W9-BUE-595

CECIL
TEXTBOOK
of MEDICINE

THE CONSULTING EDITORS

Respiratory Diseases
Critical Care Medicine

JEFFREY M. DRAZEN, M.D.
Parker B. Francis Professor of Medicine
Harvard Medical School
Chief, Pulmonary and Critical Care Division
Department of Medicine
Brigham and Women's Hospital
Boston, Massachusetts

Endocrine Diseases
Metabolic Diseases
Women's Health

GORDON N. GILL, M.D.
Professor of Medicine
University of California, San Diego
La Jolla, California
Attending Staff
UCSD Medical Center and Thornton Hospital
San Diego and La Jolla, California

Neurology

ROBERT C. GRIGGS, M.D.
Chair, Department of Neurology
Professor of Neurology, Medicine, Pathology and
   Laboratory Medicine, and Pediatrics
University of Rochester School of Medicine and
   Dentistry
Rochester, New York

Renal and Genitourinary Diseases

JUHA P. KOKKO, M.D., Ph.D.
Asa G. Candler Professor and Chairman of Medicine
Emory University School of Medicine
Atlanta, Georgia

Infectious Diseases
HIV and the Acquired Immunodeficiency Syndrome

GERALD L. MANDELL, M.D.
Professor of Medicine
Owen R. Cheatham Professor of the Sciences
Chief, Division of Infectious Diseases
University of Virginia Health Sciences Center
Charlottesville, Virginia

Gastrointestinal Diseases
Diseases of the Liver, Gallbladder, and Bile Ducts

DON W. POWELL, M.D.
Edward Randall and Edward Randall, Jr., Distinguished
   Chairman
Professor, Department of Internal Medicine
Professor, Physiology and Biophysics
University of Texas Medical Branch
Galveston, Texas

Hematologic Diseases
Oncology

ANDREW I. SCHAFER, M.D.
The Bob and Vivian Smith Professor and Chair
Department of Medicine
Baylor College of Medicine
Chief, Internal Medicine Service
The Methodist Hospital
Houston, Texas

CECIL

*T*EXTBOOK
of *M*EDICINE

21st
Edition

EDITED BY:

Lee Goldman, M.D.

Julius Krevans Distinguished Professor and Chairman
Department of Medicine
Associate Dean for Clinical Affairs
University of California, San Francisco
School of Medicine
San Francisco, California

J. Claude Bennett, M.D.

Distinguished University Professor Emeritus
University of Alabama at Birmingham
Formerly President, Spencer Professor of Medicine, and
    Chairman, Department of Medicine
University of Alabama at Birmingham
Birmingham, Alabama

W.B. SAUNDERS COMPANY
A Division of Harcourt Brace & Company
Philadelphia ▪ London ▪ Toronto ▪ Sydney

W.B. SAUNDERS COMPANY
A Division of Harcourt Brace & Company

The Curtis Center
Independence Square West
Philadelphia, Pennsylvania 19106

Library of Congress Cataloging-in-Publication Data

Cecil textbook of medicine/edited by Lee Goldman, J. Claude Bennett.—21st ed.
    p.   cm.

Includes bibliographical references and index.

ISBN 0–7216–7995–1

1. Internal medicine. I. Cecil, Russell L. (Russell La Fayette), 1881–1965.
II. Goldman, Lee, MD. III. Title: Textbook of medicine.
[DNLM: 1.   Medicine. WB 100 C3888 2000]

RC46.C423   2000   616—dc21

DNLM/DLC   98–52751

Material in the chapters listed below is in the public domain.

Chapter 15	"Immunization," by Walter A. Orenstein.
Chapter 20	"Electrical Injury," by Cleon W. Goodwin.
Chapter 47	"Pathophysiology of Heart Failure," by Barry M. Massie.
Chapter 160	"Aplastic Anemia and Related Bone Marrow Failure Syndromes," by Neal S. Young.
Chapter 220	"Wilson Disease," by William A. Gahl.
Chapter 261	"Mineral and Bone Homeostasis," by Stephen J. Marx.
Chapter 280	"Mastocytosis," by Dean D. Metcalfe.
Chapter 333	"Diphtheria," by Roland W. Sutter.
Chapter 390	"Viral Gastroenteritis," by Albert Z. Kapikian.

CECIL TEXTBOOK OF MEDICINE

ISBN 0–7216–7995–1 Set (Vols. 1 & 2)
ISBN 0–7216–7996–X Single volume

Copyright © 2000, 1996, 1991, 1988, 1985, 1982, 1979, 1975, 1971, 1963, 1959, 1955 by W.B. Saunders Company.

Copyright © 1951, 1947, 1943, 1940, 1937, 1933, 1930, 1927 by W.B. Saunders Company.

Copyright renewed 1991 by Paul Beeson.

Copyright renewed 1979 by Russell L. Cecil and Robert F. Loeb.

Copyright renewed 1987, 1975, 1971, 1965, 1961, 1958, 1955 by W.B. Saunders Company.

All rights reserved. No part of this publication may be reproduced or transmitted in any form or by any means, electronic or mechanical, including photocopy, recording, or any information storage and retrieval system, without permission in writing from the publisher.

Printed in the United States of America.

Last digit is the print number: 9   8   7   6   5   4   3   2   1

The 21st Edition of the *Cecil Textbook of Medicine*
is dedicated to our families:
Jill
and
Jeff, Daniel, Robyn
and
Nancy
and
Katya & Dave, Miller & Phil, Clark & Margie
and
Jessica, Polly, Helen

CONTRIBUTORS

RODNEY D. ADAM, M.D.
Associate Professor of Medicine and Microbiology/Immunology, University of Arizona College of Medicine, Tucson, Arizona
Venomous Snake Bites

JUDITH C. AHRONHEIM, M.D.
Professor of Medicine, New York Medical College, Valhalla; Chief, Eileen E. Anderson Section of Geriatrics, Department of Medicine, Saint Vincent's Hospital and Medical Center, New York, New York
Special Problems in the Geriatric Patient

MASOOD AKHTAR, M.D.
Clinical Professor of Medicine, University of Wisconsin Medical School—Milwaukee Clinical Campus; Director, Institute for Cardiac Rhythms, St. Luke's Medical Center, and Director, Arrhythmia Services, Milwaukee Heart Institute; St. Luke's Medical Center/Sinai Samaritan Medical Center, Milwaukee, Wisconsin
Cardiac Arrhythmias with Supraventricular Origin

ALLEN C. ALFREY, M.D.
Professor of Medicine, University of Colorado; Consultant, Veterans Administration Medical Center, Denver, Colorado
Disorders of Magnesium Metabolism

NANCY BATES ALLEN, M.D.
Associate Professor of Medicine, Duke University Medical Center, Durham, North Carolina
Wegener's Granulomatosis

ROBERT H. ALLEN, M.D.
Cleo Meador and George Ryland Scott Professor of Hematology Research and Professor of Medicine and Biochemistry, Department of Medicine, University of Colorado Health Sciences Center, Denver, Colorado
Macrocytic and Megaloblastic Anemias

JOSEPH S. ALPERT, M.D.
Robert S. and Irene P. Flinn Professor of Medicine and Head, Department of Medicine, University of Arizona Health Sciences Center, Tucson, Arizona
Pulmonary Hypertension

MICHAEL J. AMINOFF, M.D., FRCP
Professor of Neurology, University of California School of Medicine, San Francisco, California
Major Sensory Symptoms; Spinal Anatomy; Neck and Back Pain; Intervertebral Disk Disease; Inflammatory Disorders Involving the Spinal Cord; Vascular Disorders Involving the Spinal Cord

KARL E. ANDERSON, M.D.
Professor, The University of Texas Medical Branch, Galveston, Texas
The Porphyrias

HANS C. ANDERSSON, M.D.
Assistant Professor, Human Genetics Program, Tulane University Medical School, New Orleans, Louisiana
The Mucopolysaccharidoses

MICHAEL A. APICELLA, M.D.
Professor and Head, Department of Microbiology, The University of Iowa College of Medicine, Iowa City, Iowa
Meningococcal Infections

GERALD B. APPEL, M.D.
Professor of Clinical Medicine, Columbia University College of Physicians and Surgeons; Director, Clinical Nephrology, The New York–Presbyterian Hospital, New York, New York
Glomerular Disorders

FREDERICK R. APPELBAUM, M.D.
Professor and Head, Division of Medical Oncology, University of Washington School of Medicine; Member and Director, Clinical Research Division, Fred Hutchinson Cancer Research Center, Seattle, Washington
The Acute Leukemias

GORDON L. ARCHER, M.D.
Professor of Medicine and Microbiology/Immunology and Chairman, Division of Infectious Diseases, Department of Internal Medicine, Medical College of Virginia Campus of Virginia Commonwealth University, Richmond, Virginia
Staphylococcal Infections

JAMES O. ARMITAGE, M.D.
Professor and Chair, Department of Internal Medicine, University of Nebraska Medical Center, Omaha, Nebraska
Approach to the Patient with Lymphadenopathy and Splenomegaly

FRANK C. ARNETT, M.D.
Elizabeth Bidgood Chair and Professor of Internal Medicine and Pathology, University of Texas—Houston Medical School; Chief of Rheumatology, Hermann Hospital and Lyndon B. Johnson Hospital, Houston, Texas
Rheumatoid Arthritis

WILLIAM J. ARNOLD, M.D.
Executive Vice President and Medical Director, Advanced Bio-Surfaces, Inc.,
Minnetonka, Minnesota
Specialized Procedures in the Management of Patients with Rheumatic Diseases

GROVER C. BAGBY, JR., M.D.
Professor of Medicine and of Molecular and Medical Genetics, and Director, Oregon Cancer Center, Oregon Health Sciences University; Head, Hematology/Oncology Section, Portland Veterans Affairs Medical Center, Portland, Oregon
Leukopenia and Leukocytosis

DONALD S. BAIM, M.D.
Professor of Medicine, Harvard Medical School; Chief, Interventional Cardiology Section, Beth Israel Deaconess Medical Center, Boston, Massachusetts
Coronary Angioplasty

EUGENE V. BALL, M.D.

Jane Knight Lowe Professor of Medicine Emeritus, University of Alabama at Birmingham, Birmingham, Alabama

Behçet's Disease; Systemic Diseases in Which Arthritis Is a Feature; Miscellaneous Forms of Arthritis; Non-articular Rheumatism; Articular Tumors; Erythromelalgia

ROBERT W. BALOH, M.D.

Professor of Neurology and Surgery (Head and Neck), University of California, Los Angeles, Medical School, Los Angeles, California

Neuro-Ophthalmology; Smell and Taste; Hearing and Equilibrium

ALAN F. BARKER, M.D.

Professor, Internal Medicine, Pulmonary and Critical Care, Oregon Health Sciences University, Portland, Oregon

Bronchiectasis and Localized Airway/Parenchymal Disorders

A. JAMES BARKOVICH, M.D.

Professor of Radiology, Neurology, Pediatrics, and Neurosurgery, University of California, San Francisco, San Francisco, California

Neurocutaneous Syndromes; Malformations of Cortical Development; Congenital Anomalies of the Craniovertebral Junction, Spine, and Spinal Cord (Including Syringomyelia)

RICHARD J. BAROHN, M.D.

Professor and Acting Chairman of Neurology, Lois C.A. and Darwin E. Smith Distinguished Chair in Neurological Mobility Research, University of Texas Southwestern Medical Center at Dallas, Dallas, Texas

General Approach to Muscle Diseases; Muscular Dystrophies; Morphologically Distinct Congenital Myopathies; Metabolic Myopathies; Channelopathies (Non-dystrophic Myotonias and Periodic Paralyses); Inflammatory and Other Myopathies

MURRAY G. BARON, M.D.

Professor of Radiology and Chief, Division of Thoracic Radiology, Emory University, School of Medicine, Atlanta, Georgia

Radiology of the Heart

BRUCE A. BARSHOP, M.D., Ph.D.

Associate Professor of Pediatrics, Division of Biochemical Genetics, University of California, San Diego, School of Medicine, La Jolla, California

Homocystinuria

JOHN A. BARTLETT, M.D.

Associate Professor of Medicine, Duke University Medical Center, Durham, North Carolina

Management and Counseling for Persons with HIV Infection

JOHN G. BARTLETT, M.D.

Professor of Medicine and Chief, Division of Infectious Diseases and the AIDS Care Program, Johns Hopkins University School of Medicine, Baltimore, Maryland

Botulism; Tetanus; Gastrointestinal Manifestations of AIDS

NATHAN M. BASS, M.D., Ph.D.

Professor of Medicine and Medical Director, Liver Transplant Program, University of California, San Francisco, School of Medicine, San Francisco, California

Toxic and Drug-Induced Liver Disease

GEORGE A. BELLER, M.D.

Ruth C. Heede Professor of Cardiology and Professor of Internal Medicine, University of Virginia School of Medicine; Chief, Cardiovascular Division, Department of Internal Medicine, University of Virginia Health Sciences Center, Charlottesville, Virginia

Nuclear Cardiology and Computed Tomography

J. CLAUDE BENNETT, M.D.

Distinguished University Professor Emeritus, University of Alabama at Birmingham; Formerly President, Spencer Professor of Medicine, and Chairman, Department of Medicine, University of Alabama at Birmingham, Birmingham, Alabama

Medicine as a Learned and Humane Profession; Approach to the Patient with Immune Disease

NEAL L. BENOWITZ, M.D.

Professor of Medicine, Psychiatry and Biopharmaceutical Sciences and Chief, Division of Clinical Pharmacology and Experimental Therapeutics, University of California, San Francisco; Staff Physician, San Francisco General Hospital, San Francisco, California

Tobacco

JOSEPH R. BERGER, M.D.

Professor and Chairman, Department of Neurology; Professor, Department of Internal Medicine, University of Kentucky College of Medicine, Lexington, Kentucky

Introduction; Acute Viral Meningitis and Encephalitis; Poliomyelitis; The Herpesviruses; Rabies; Slow Virus Infections

JAY BERNSTEIN, M.D.

Clinical Professor of Pathology, Wayne State University School of Medicine, Detroit; Attending Pathologist and Director Emeritus, Beaumont Research Institute, William Beaumont Hospital, Royal Oak, Michigan

Anomalies of the Urinary Tract

JOSEPH R. BERTINO, M.D.

Professor of Pharmacology and Medicine, Cornell Medical College; Chairman, Molecular Pharmacology and Therapeutics, and Attending, Department of Medicine, Memorial Sloan-Kettering Cancer Center, New York, New York

Principles of Cancer Therapy

BRUCE BEUTLER, M.D.

Professor, Department of Internal Medicine, University of Texas Southwestern Medical Center at Dallas; Associate Investigator, Howard Hughes Medical Institute, Dallas, Texas

The Pathogenesis of Fever

STEVEN M. BEUTLER, M.D.

Assistant Clinical Professor, Department of Medicine, College of Medicine, University of California at Irvine, Irvine, California; Associate Director, Section of Infectious Diseases, Department of Medicine, Arrowhead Regional Medical Center, Colton, California

The Pathogenesis of Fever

GUADALUPE BILBAO, M.D.

Postdoctoral Fellow, University of Alabama at Birmingham, Birmingham, Alabama

Gene Therapy

ALAN L. BISNO, M.D.

Professor and Vice-Chairman, Department of Medicine, University of Miami School of Medicine; Chief, Medical Service, Miami Veterans Affairs Medical Center, Miami, Florida

Rheumatic Fever

BRUCE R. BISTRIAN, M.D., Ph.D., M.P.H.

Professor of Medicine, Harvard Medical School; Chief, Clinical Nutrition, Beth Israel Deaconess Medical Center, Boston, Massachusetts

Nutritional Assessment

WILLIAM A. BLATTNER, M.D.

Professor, University of Maryland, Baltimore, Institute of Human Virology; Attending Physician, Veterans Affairs Medical Center, Baltimore, Maryland

Retroviruses Other Than HIV

WILLIAM J. BLOT, Ph.D.

Adjunct Professor, Johns Hopkins University School of Hygiene and Public Health, Baltimore; Chief Executive Officer, International Epidemiology Institute, Rockville, Maryland

The Epidemiology of Cancer

JAMES R. BONNER, M.D.

Professor of Medicine and Surgery, University of Alabama School of Medicine, Birmingham, Alabama

Drug Allergy

DENNIS W. BOULWARE, M.D.

Professor of Medicine, University of Alabama at Birmingham, Birmingham, Alabama

The Painful Shoulder

ROBERT C. BOURGE, M.D.

Professor of Medicine, Radiology and Surgery and Director, Division of Cardiovascular Disease, University of Alabama at Birmingham School of Medicine, Birmingham, Alabama

Cardiac Transplantation

LAURENCE A. BOXER, M.D.

Professor of Pediatrics, University of Michigan; Director of Pediatric Hematology/Oncology, C.S. Mott Children's Hospital, Ann Arbor, Michigan

Disorders of Phagocyte Function

DAVID J. BRANDHAGEN, M.D.

Instructor of Medicine, Mayo Medical School; Consultant, Gastroenterology/Hepatology, Mayo Clinic, Rochester, Minnesota

Iron Overload (Hemochromatosis)

LAWRENCE J. BRANDT, M.D.

Professor of Medicine, Albert Einstein College of Medicine; Director, Division of Gastroenterology, Moses Campus of Montefiore Medical Center, Bronx, New York

Vascular Disorders of the Intestine

BARRY D. BRAUSE, M.D.

Clinical Professor of Medicine, Cornell University Medical College; Attending Physician, The New York Hospital and The Hospital for Special Surgery, New York, New York

Osteomyelitis

MALCOLM K. BRENNER, M.B., Ph.D.

Professor, Departments of Medicine and of Pediatrics, Baylor College of Medicine; Director, Stem Cell Transplantation, Texas Children's Hospital and The Methodist Hospital, Houston, Texas

Stem Cell Transplantation

WILLIAM J. BRITT, M.D.

Professor of Pediatrics and Microbiology, University of Alabama at Birmingham, Birmingham, Alabama

Infections Associated with Human Cytomegalovirus

SAMUEL BRODER, M.D.

Executive Vice President and Chief Medical Officer, Celera Genomics Corporation, Rockville, Maryland

Treatment of HIV Infection and AIDS

PHILIP A. BRUNELL, M.S., M.D.

Senior Consulting Physician, Laboratory of Clinical Investigation, National Institute of Allergy and Infectious Diseases, National Institutes of Health, Bethesda, Maryland

Measles; Rubella (German Measles); Varicella (Chickenpox, Shingles)

ROBERT C. BRUNHAM, M.D.

Professor and Head, Department of Medical Microbiology, University of Manitoba; Head, Section of Infectious Diseases, University of Manitoba Health Sciences Centre, Winnipeg, Manitoba, Canada

Diseases Caused by Chlamydiae

JOHN C.M. BRUST, M.D.

Professor of Clinical Neurology, Columbia University College of Physicians and Surgeons; Director, Department of Neurology, Harlem Hospital Center, New York, New York

Nutritional Disorders of the Nervous System

REBECCA H. BUCKLEY, M.D.

J. Buren Sidbury Professor of Pediatrics and Professor of Immunology, Duke University School of Medicine; Chief, Division of Allergy and Immunology, Duke University Medical Center, Durham, North Carolina

Primary Immunodeficiency Diseases

WARD E. BULLOCK, M.D.

Professor of Medicine, University of Connecticut Health Center; Attending Physician, John Dempsey Hospital, Farmington; Consultant in Infectious Diseases, Veterans Administration Hospital, Newington, Connecticut

Actinomycosis; Nocardiosis

DANIEL BURKHOFF, M.D., Ph.D.

Assistant Professor of Medicine, Attending and Director of Cardiac Research Laboratory, Columbia University College of Physicians and Surgeons, New York, New York

Cardiac Function and Circulatory Control

THOMAS BUTLER, M.D.

Professor of Internal Medicine and of Microbiology and Immunology, Texas Tech University Health Sciences Center; Chief of Infectious Diseases, University Medical Center, Lubbock, Texas

Typhoid Fever; Shigellosis

BLASE A. CARABELLO, M.D.

Professor of Medicine, Cardiology Division, Department of Medicine, Medical University of South Carolina, Charleston, South Carolina

Valvular Heart Disease

EDGAR M. CARVALHO, M.D., Ph.D.

Professor of Medicine and Clinical Immunology, Faculdade de Medecina e Escola Bahiana de Medicina; Chief of the Immunology Service, Hospital Universitário Prof. Edgard Santos—Federal University of Bahia, Salvador, Bahia, Brazil

Schistosomiasis (Bilharziasis)

STEPHEN D. CEDERBAUM, M.D.

Professor of Psychiatry and Pediatrics, University of California, Los Angeles; Attending Physician, UCLA Medical Center; Consultant in Metabolic Disorders, Kaiser Permanente of Southern California, Los Angeles, California

Diseases of the Urea Cycle

BARTOLOME R. CELLI, M.D.

Professor of Medicine, Tufts University; Chief, Division of Pulmonary and Critical Care Medicine, St. Elizabeth's Medical Center, Boston, Massachusetts

Diseases of the Diaphragm, Chest Wall, Pleura, and Mediastinum

JOHN P. CELLO, M.D.

Professor of Medicine and Surgery, University of California, San Francisco, School of Medicine, San Francisco, California

Gastrointestinal Hemorrhage and Occult Gastrointestinal Bleeding

EUGENE BING CHANG, M.D.

Martin Boyer Professor of Medicine, University of Chicago; Attending Physician, University of Chicago Hospital, Chicago, Illinois

Malabsorption Syndromes

RUSSELL W. CHESNEY, M.D.

Le Bonheur Professor and Chair of Pediatrics, University of Tennessee, Memphis; Vice President of Academic Affairs and Chief of Pediatrics, Le Bonheur Children's Medical Center, Memphis, Tennessee

Specific Renal Tubular Disorders

SANDY F.S. CHUN, M.D.

Staff Physician, Kaiser Mountain View Clinic, Mountain View, California

Mucormycosis

C. GLENN COBBS, M.D.

Professor and Vice Chairman for VA Affairs, University of Alabama at Birmingham; Chief, Medical Service, Birmingham Veterans Administration Medical Center, Birmingham, Alabama

Disease Caused by Bartonella *Species*

SIDNEY COHEN, M.D.

Professor and Chairman, Department of Medicine, Temple University School of Medicine, Philadelphia, Pennsylvania

Diseases of the Esophagus

LAWRENCE H. COHN, M.A., M.D.

Professor of Surgery, Harvard Medical School; Chief, Cardiac Surgery, Brigham and Women's Hospital, Boston, Massachusetts

Surgical Treatment of Coronary Artery Disease

ADRIANE P. CONCUS, M.D.

Lecturer, Department of Otolaryngology, Head and Neck Surgery, The University of Michigan Health System, Ann Arbor, Michigan

Head and Neck Cancer

DENNIS L. COOPER, M.D.

Associate Professor of Medical Oncology, Yale University School of Medicine, Yale–New Haven Hospital, New Haven, Connecticut

Tumor Markers

MAX D. COOPER, M.D.

Professor of Medicine, Pediatrics and Pathology, University of Alabama at Birmingham; Investigator, Howard Hughes Medical Institute, Birmingham, Alabama

Diseases of the Thymus

JAMES D. CRAPO, M.D.

Executive Vice President, Academic Affairs, and Chairman, Department of Medicine, National Jewish Medical and Research Center, Denver, Colorado

Respiratory Structure and Function

MICHAEL H. CRIQUI, M.D., M.P.H.

Professor and Vice-Chair, Department of Family and Preventive Medicine, University of California, San Diego, School of Medicine, San Diego, California

Epidemiology of Cardiovascular Disease

JEFFREY L. CUMMINGS, M.D.

The Augustus S. Rose Professor of Neurology, Director of the Alzheimer's Disease Center, Professor of Psychiatry and Biobehavioral Sciences, UCLA School of Medicine, Los Angeles, California

Disorders of Cognition

DAVID T. CURIEL, M.D.

Professor of Medicine, University of Alabama at Birmingham; Director, Gene Therapy Center, Jeanne and Ann Griffin Chair for Women's Cancer Research, University of Alabama at Birmingham, Birmingham, Alabama

Gene Therapy

JAMES W. CURRAN, M.D., M.P.H.

Dean, and Professor of Epidemiology, Rollins School of Public Health of Emory University, Atlanta, Georgia

Epidemiology of HIV Infection and AIDS

JOHN J. CURTIS, M.D.

Professor of Medicine, University of Alabama at Birmingham School of Medicine and Medical Center, Birmingham, Alabama

Treatment of Irreversible Renal Failure

JOHN J. CUSH, M.D.

Clinical Associate Professor of Internal Medicine, The University of Texas Southwestern Medical School; Chief, Division of Rheumatology, Presbyterian Hospital of Dallas, Dallas, Texas

The Spondyloarthropathies

F. MICHAEL CUTRER, M.D.

Assistant Professor of Neurology, Harvard Medical School; Director, Partners Headache Center, Massachusetts General Hospital, Brigham and Women's Hospital, Boston, Massachusetts

Headaches and Other Head Pain

DAVID C. DALE, M.D.

Professor of Medicine, University of Washington School of Medicine; Attending Physician, University of Washington Medical Center, Seattle, Washington

The Febrile Patient

TROY E. DANIELS, D.D.S, M.S.

Professor of Oral Pathology, Schools of Dentistry and Medicine, University of California, San Francisco, San Francisco, California

Diseases of the Mouth and Salivary Glands

BESS DAWSON-HUGHES, M.D.

Professor of Medicine, Tufts University School of Medicine; Chief, Calcium and Bone Metabolism Laboratory, Jean Mayer U.S.D.A. Human Nutrition Research Center on Aging at Tufts University, Boston, Massachusetts

Vitamin D

HAILE T. DEBAS, M.D.

Maurice Galante Distinguished Professor of Surgery, Department of Surgery; Dean, School of Medicine, and Vice Chancellor, Medical Affairs, University of California, San Francisco, San Francisco, California

Peptic Ulcer Disease: Surgical Therapy

LEONARD J. DEFTOS, M.D., J.D.

Professor of Medicine, University of California, San Diego; San Diego VA Medical Center, San Diego, California

Calcitonin and Medullary Thyroid Carcinoma

CARLOS DEL RIO, M.D.

Associate Professor of Medicine (Infectious Diseases) and Adjunct Associate Professor of International Health, Emory University School of Medicine and Rollins School of Public Health of Emory University, Atlanta, Georgia

Epidemiology of HIV Infection and AIDS

ANTHONY N. DEMARIA, M.D.

Professor of Medicine and Chief of Cardiovascular Medicine, University of California, San Diego, San Diego, California

Echocardiography

RICHARD D. DeSHAZO, M.D.

Professor of Medicine and Pediatrics and Chair, Department of Internal Medicine, University of Mississippi Medical Center, Jackson, Mississippi

Allergic Rhinitis; Immune Complex Diseases

ROBERT J. DESNICK, Ph.D., M.D.

Professor and Chairman, Department of Human Genetics, Mount Sinai School of Medicine, New York, New York

Lysosomal Storage Diseases

IVAN DIAMOND, M.D., Ph.D.

Professor and Vice-Chairman, Department of Neurology, Professor of Molecular and Cellular Pharmacology, and Professor of Pediatrics, University of California, San Francisco; Director, Ernest Gallo Clinic and Research Center, Department of Neurology, San Francisco, California

Alcoholism and Alcohol Abuse

ROBERT B. DIASIO, M.D.

Newman H. Waters Professor and Director, Division of Clinical Pharmacology, and Chairman, Department of Pharmacology and Toxicology, University of Alabama School of Medicine, Birmingham, Alabama

Principles of Drug Therapy

ANNA MAE DIEHL, M.D.

Professor of Medicine, Johns Hopkins University School of Medicine; Faculty, Division of Digestive Diseases, Johns Hopkins Medical Center, Baltimore, Maryland

Acute and Chronic Liver Failure and Hepatic Encephalopathy

WOLFGANG H. DILLMANN, M.D.

Professor of Medicine, University of California, San Diego, La Jolla, California

The Thyroid

EUGENE P. DIMAGNO, M.D.

Professor of Medicine, Mayo Medical School; Director, Gastroenterology Research Unit, and Consultant, Division of Gastroenterology and Hepatology, Mayo Clinic and Mayo Foundation, Rochester, Minnesota

Carcinoma of the Pancreas

CHARLES A. DINARELLO, M.D.

Professor of Medicine, University of Colorado School of Medicine; Staff Physician, University Hospital, Denver, Colorado

The Acute-Phase Response

WILLIAM E. DISMUKES, M.D.

Professor and Vice-Chairman, Department of Medicine, and Director, Division of Infectious Diseases, University of Alabama at Birmingham School of Medicine; Director, Internal Medicine Residency Training Program, University of Alabama Medical Center, Birmingham, Alabama

Introduction to the Mycoses; Histoplasmosis; Blastomycosis; Paracoccidioidomycosis; Cryptococcosis; Sporotrichosis; Candidiasis

R. GORDON DOUGLAS, JR., M.D.

Adjunct Professor of Medicine, Cornell University Medical College, New York, New York; President, Vaccine Division, Merck and Company, Inc., Whitehouse Station, New Jersey

Introduction to Viral Diseases; Other Arthropod-borne Viruses

JEFFREY M. DRAZEN, M.D.

Parker B. Francis Professor of Medicine, Harvard Medical School; Chief, Pulmonary and Critical Care Division, Department of Medicine, Brigham and Women's Hospital, Boston, Massachusetts

Asthma

MARC K. DREZNER, M.D.

Professor of Medicine, Duke University, Durham, North Carolina

Osteomalacia and Rickets

THOMAS D. DUBOSE, JR., M.D.

Professor of Internal Medicine and Integrative Biology, Pharmacology and Physiology, University of Texas, Houston, Medical School; Chief of Nephrology, Memorial Hermann Hospital; Section Chief of Nephrology, M.D. Anderson Cancer Center, Houston, Texas

Vascular Disorders of the Kidney

THOMAS P. DUFFY, M.D.

Professor of Medicine, Yale University School of Medicine; Attending Physician, Yale–New Haven Hospital, New Haven, Connecticut

Normochromic, Normocytic Anemias; Microcytic and Hypochromic Anemias

RICHARD J. DUMA, M.D., Ph.D.

Clinical Professor of Medicine, Medical College of Virginia, Virginia Commonwealth University, Richmond, Virginia; Director, Infectious Diseases, Halifax Medical Center, Daytona Beach, Florida

Pneumococcal Pneumonia

HERBERT L. DUPONT, M.D.

H. Irving Schweppe, Jr., M.D. Chair of Internal Medicine, Baylor College of Medicine; Mary W. Kelsey Professor, University of Texas, Houston; Chief, Internal Medicine, St. Luke's Episcopal Hospital, Houston, Texas

Introduction to Enteric Infections

PAUL H. EDELSTEIN, M.D.

Professor, Department of Pathology and Laboratory Medicine, University of Pennsylvania Medical Center, Philadelphia, Pennsylvania

Legionellosis

GARABED EKNOYAN, M.D.

Professor of Medicine, Baylor College of Medicine; Chief, Renal Service, Ben Taub General Hospital, Houston, Texas

Tubulointerstitial Diseases and Toxic Nephropathies

RONALD J. ELIN, M.D., Ph.D.

Professor of Pathology and Laboratory Medicine, University of Louisville, School of Medicine; Medical Director, Laboratory Medicine, University of Louisville Hospital, Louisville, Kentucky

Reference Intervals and Laboratory Values

DIANE L. ELLIOT, M.D.

Professor of Medicine, Oregon Health Sciences University, Portland, Oregon

Pregnancy: Hypertension and Other Common Medical Problems

LOUIS J. ELSAS II, M.D.

Professor of Pediatrics and Biochemistry and Director, Division of Medical Genetics, Emory University; Chief, Section of Medical Genetics, Emory Clinic and Egleston Hospital of Emory University, Atlanta, Georgia

Inborn Errors of Metabolism; Approach to the Patient with Metabolic Disease; Branched-Chain Aminoacidurias

STEPHEN H. EMBURY, M.D.

Professor of Medicine, University of California, San Francisco, School of Medicine; Physician, Division of Hematology, San Francisco General Hospital, San Francisco, California

Sickle Cell Anemia and Associated Hemoglobinopathies

ANDREW G. ENGEL, M.D.

William L. McKnight-3M Professor of Neuroscience, Mayo Medical School and Mayo Clinic, Rochester, Minnesota

Disorders of Neuromuscular Transmission

GREGORY F. ERICKSON, Ph.D.

Professor, Department of Reproductive Medicine, University of California, San Diego, School of Medicine, La Jolla, California

Ovaries and Development; Menstrual Cycle and Fertility

MARC S. ERNSTOFF, M.D.

Professor of Medicine, Dartmouth Medical School, Hanover; Professor and Chief, Hematology/Oncology, Dartmouth-Hitchcock Medical Center; Deputy Director, Norris Cotton Cancer Center, Lebanon, New Hampshire

Non-metastatic Effects of Cancer: Other Systems

LUIS R. ESPINOZA, M.D.

Professor of Medicine and Chief, Section of Rheumatology, Louisiana State University School of Medicine, New Orleans, Louisiana

Infectious Arthritis

VIRGIL F. FAIRBANKS, M.D.

Professor, Mayo Medical School; Consultant (Hematology and Hematopathology), Mayo Clinic, Rochester, Minnesota

Iron Overload (Hemochromatosis)

MICHAEL B. FALLON, M.D.

Associate Professor of Medicine, University of Alabama at Birmingham School of Medicine; Chief, Gastroenterology and Hepatology, Birmingham Veterans Administration Medical Center, Birmingham, Alabama

Hepatic Tumors

DAVID P. FAXON, M.D.

Professor of Medicine, University of Southern California, School of Medicine; Chief, Division of Cardiology, WAC and USC Medical Center and USC University Hospital, Los Angeles, California

Catheterization and Angiography

AARON FAY, M.D.

Ophthalmologist, Massachusetts Eye and Ear Infirmary, Boston, Massachusetts

Diseases of the Visual System

JUDITH ELLEN FEINBERG, M.D.

Professor of Medicine, University of Cincinnati College of Medicine; Attending Physician, University Hospital, Cincinnati, Ohio

Pneumocystis carinii Pneumonia

ROBERT FEKETY, M.D.

Professor Emeritus of Internal Medicine, Division of Infectious Diseases, Department of Internal Medicine, University of Michigan Health System, Ann Arbor, Michigan

Pseudomembranous Colitis

EVA L. FELDMAN, M.D., Ph.D.

Associate Professor of Neurology, University of Michigan, Department of Neurology, Ann Arbor, Michigan

Introduction; Hereditary Cerebellar Ataxias and Related Disorders; Hereditary Spastic Paraplegias; Motor Neuron Diseases

CALEB E. FINCH, Ph.D.

ARCO and William F. Kieschnick Professor in the Neurobiology of Aging, Andrus Gerontology Center, Department of Biological Sciences, University of Southern California, Los Angeles, California

Biology of Aging

SYDNEY M. FINEGOLD, M.D.

Professor of Medicine and Professor of Microbiology and Immunology, University of California, Los Angeles, School of Medicine; Staff Physician, Infectious Diseases Section, Veterans Administration Medical Center, West Los Angeles, Los Angeles, California

Lung Abscess

JOEL S. FINKELSTEIN, M.D.

Assistant Professor of Medicine, Harvard Medical School; Assistant Physician, Massachusetts General Hospital, Boston, Massachusetts

Osteoporosis

SUZANNE W. FLETCHER, M.D., M.Sc.

Professor, Department of Ambulatory Care and Prevention, Harvard Medical School; Physician, Harvard Pilgrim Health Care, and Senior Physician, Brigham and Women's Hospital, Boston, Massachusetts

Clinical Decision Making: Approach to the Patient

KATHLEEN M. FOLEY, M.D.

Professor of Neurology, Neuroscience and Clinical Pharmacology, Cornell University Medical College; Attending Neurologist, Department of Neurology, Memorial Sloan-Kettering Cancer Center, New York, New York

Pain

JAY W. FOX, Ph.D.

Professor of Microbiology and Director, Biomolecular Research Facility, University of Virginia School of Medicine, Charlottesville, Virginia

Venoms and Poisons from Marine Organisms

MICHAEL M. FRANK, M.D.

Samuel L. Katz Professor and Chairman, Department of Pediatrics, and Professor of Immunology and Medicine, Duke University Medical Center, Durham, North Carolina

Urticaria and Angioedema

DAVID O. FREEDMAN, M.D.

Associate Professor of Medicine and Epidemiology and International Health, University of Alabama at Birmingham; Director, UAB Travelers Health Clinic, The Kirklin Clinic, Birmingham, Alabama

Filariasis

SCOTT L. FRIEDMAN, M.D.

Irene and Dr. Arthur Fishberg Professor of Medicine and Director of Liver Research, Mount Sinai School of Medicine, New York, New York

Alcoholic Liver Diseases, Cirrhosis and Its Sequelae

VALENTIN FUSTER, M.D., Ph.D.

Professor of Cardiology; Dean for Academic Affairs; Director, The Zena and Michael A. Wiener Cardiovascular Institute; Richard Gorlin, M.D./ Heart Research Foundation; Mount Sinai Medical Center, New York, New York

Atherosclerosis-Thrombosis and Vascular Biology

ROBERT F. GAGEL, M.D.

Professor and Chairman, Department of Internal Medicine Specialties, University of Texas M.D. Anderson Cancer Center, Houston, Texas

Nonmetastatic Effects of Cancer: The Endocrine System; Calcitonin and Medullary Thyroid Carcinoma

WILLIAM A. GAHL, M.D., Ph.D.

Head, Section on Human Biochemical Genetics, Heritable Disorders Branch, National Institute of Child Health and Human Development, National Institutes of Health, Bethesda, Maryland

Wilson Disease

JOHN N. GALGIANI, M.D.

Professor of Medicine, University of Arizona; Director, Valley Fever Center for Excellence, Veterans Affairs Medical Center, Tucson, Arizona

Coccidioidomycosis

MARC B. GARNICK, M.D.

Executive Vice President, Chief Medical Regulatory Officer, Praecis Pharmaceutical INC, Cambridge, Massachusetts; Clinical Professor of Medicine, Harvard Medical School; Beth Israel-Deaconess Medical Center, Boston, Massachusetts

Tumors of the Kidney, Ureter, and Bladder

RENATE E. GAY, M.D.

Professor, University Hospital, Department of Rheumatology, Zurich, Switzerland

Connective Tissue Structure and Function

STEFFEN GAY, M.D.

Professor of Experimental Rheumatology, University Hospital, Department of Rheumatology, Zurich, Switzerland

Connective Tissue Structure and Function

LEONARD S. GETTES, M.D.

Distinguished Professor of Cardiology, Department of Medicine, University of North Carolina at Chapel Hill, Chapel Hill, North Carolina

Principles of Electrophysiology

GORDON N. GILL, M.D.

Professor of Medicine, University of California, San Diego, La Jolla; Attending Staff, UCSD Medical Center and Thornton Hospital, San Diego and La Jolla, California

Principles of Endocrinology

D. GARY GILLILAND, Ph.D., M.D.

Associate Professor of Medicine, Harvard Medical School; Associate Investigator, Howard Hughes Medical Institute; Physician, Brigham and Women's Hospital and the Dana-Farber Cancer Institute, Boston, Massachusetts

Myelodysplastic Syndrome

JOHN W. GNANN, JR., M.D.

Associate Professor of Medicine, Division of Infectious Diseases, University of Alabama at Birmingham, Birmingham, Alabama

Mumps

DAVID E. GOLAN, M.D., Ph.D.

Associate Professor of Medicine and Associate Professor of Biological Chemistry and Molecular Pharmacology, Harvard Medical School; Physician, Brigham and Women's Hospital and Dana-Farber Cancer Institute, Boston, Massachusetts

Hemolytic Anemias: Red Cell Membrane and Metabolic Defects

LEE GOLDMAN, M.D.

Julius Krevans Distinguished Professor and Chairman, Department of Medicine, Associate Dean for Clinical Affairs, University of California, San Francisco, School of Medicine, San Francisco, California

Medicine as a Learned and Humane Profession; Approach to the Patient with Possible Cardiovascular Disease

NORA GOLDSCHLAGER, M.D.

Professor of Clinical Medicine, University of California, San Francisco, School of Medicine; Director, Coronary Care Unit, San Francisco General Hospital, San Francisco, California

Electrocardiography

ELLIE J.C. GOLDSTEIN, M.D.

Clinical Professor of Medicine, University of California, Los Angeles, School of Medicine, Los Angeles; Director, R.M. Alden Research Laboratory, Santa Monica–UCLA Medical Center, Santa Monica, California

Diseases Caused by Non–spore-forming Anaerobic Bacteria

JESÚS GÓMEZ-NAVARRO, M.D.

Research Assistant Professor, Department of Hematology/Oncology, University of Alabama at Birmingham, Birmingham, Alabama

Gene Therapy

CLEON W. GOODWIN, M.D.

Johnson and Johnson Distinguished Associate Professor of Surgery, Weill Medical College of Cornell University; Director, The New York Hospital Burn Center, New York, New York

Electrical Injury

DUNCAN A. GORDON, M.D.

Professor of Medicine, University of Toronto, Faculty of Medicine; Senior Rheumatologist, Toronto Western Hospital, University Hospital Group, Toronto, Ontario, Canada

Approach to the Patient with Musculoskeletal Disease

DAVID Y. GRAHAM, M.D.

Professor of Medicine and Molecular Virology, Baylor College of Medicine; Chief, Gastroenterology, Veterans Affairs Medical Center, Houston, Texas

Peptic Ulcer Disease: Medical Therapy; Peptic Ulcer Disease: Complications

JARED J. GRANTHAM, M.D.

University Distinguished Professor, Kansas University School of Medicine and Medical Center, Kansas City, Kansas

Cystic Diseases of the Kidney

HARRY L. GREENE, M.D.

Clinical Professor, Pediatrics, Vanderbilt Medical Center, Nashville, Tennessee

Glycogen Storage Diseases; Fructose Intolerance

WILLIAM B. GREENOUGH III, M.D.

Professor of Medicine and Professor of International Health, The Johns Hopkins University School of Medicine and School of Hygiene and Public Health; Active Staff, Johns Hopkins Bayview Medical Center and Johns Hopkins Geriatric Center, Baltimore, Maryland

Cholera

EDWARD C. GRENDYS, JR., M.D.

Assistant Professor, Gynecologic Oncology, University of South Florida School of Medicine; Physician, H. Lee Moffitt Cancer and Research Institute, Tampa, Florida

Pregnancy: Neoplastic Diseases

JOHN W. GRIFFIN, M.D.

Professor, Neurology, Neuroscience and Pathology; Director, Department of Neurology, Johns Hopkins University School of Medicine; Neurologist-in-Chief, Johns Hopkins Hospital, Baltimore, Maryland

General Approach to Nerve Disease; Pathophysiology of Peripheral Neuropathies; Immune-Mediated Neuropathies; Hereditary Neuropathies; Metabolic Neuropathies; Toxic Neuropathies; Neuropathies Associated with Infectious Diseases; Entrapment and Compressive Neuropathies

ROBERT C. GRIGGS

Neurologist-in-Chief, Department of Neurology, University of Rochester Medical Center, Rochester, New York

Approach to the Patient; The Neurologic Examination; Neurogenetics; Disorders of Motor Function

JEROME E. GROOPMAN, M.D.

Professor of Medicine, Harvard Medical School; Chief, Division of Experimental Medicine, Beth Israel Deaconess Medical Center, Boston, Massachusetts

Hematology/Oncology in AIDS

ROBERT I. GROSSMAN, M.D.

Professor of Radiology, Neurosurgery, and Neurology, Chief of Neuroradiology, Department of Radiology, University of Pennsylvania Medical Center, Philadelphia, Pennsylvania

Radiologic Imaging Procedures

RICHARD L. GUERRANT, M.D.

Thomas H. Hunter Professor of International Medicine; Chief, Division of Geographic Medicine; Director, Office of International Health, University of Virginia School of Medicine, Charlottesville, Virginia

Campylobacter Enteritis; Enteric Escherichia coli Infections

LESTER M. HADDAD, M.D.

Clinical Professor of Emergency Medicine, Medical College of Georgia, Augusta; Clinical Professor of Family Medicine, Medical University of South Carolina, Charleston, South Carolina; Medical Staff, Memorial Medical Center and St. Joseph's Hospital, Savannah, Georgia

Acute Poisoning

STEPHEN M. HAHN, M.D.

Assistant Professor, University of Pennsylvania School of Medicine, Philadelphia, Pennsylvania

Oncologic Emergencies

JUDITH G. HALL, M.D., M.Sc.

Professor of Pediatrics, University of British Columbia; Head, Department of Pediatrics, British Columbia's Children's Hospital, Vancouver, British Columbia, Canada

Congenital Anomalies

PERRY V. HALUSHKA, Ph.D., M.D.

Professor of Pharmacology and Medicine, Medical University of South Carolina, Charleston, South Carolina

Prostaglandins and Related Compounds

LAURENCE A. HARKER, M.D.

Blomeyer Professor of Medicine and Director, Division of Hematology and Oncology, Emory University School of Medicine, Atlanta, Georgia

Antithrombotic Therapy

NANCY L. HARRIS, M.D.

Professor of Pathology, Harvard Medical School and Massachusetts General Hospital, Boston, Massachusetts

Non-Hodgkin's Lymphomas

GARNER T. HAUPERT, JR., M.D.

Assistant Professor of Medicine, Harvard Medical School; Associate Physician, Massachusetts General Hospital, Boston, Massachusetts

Natriuretic Hormones

FREDERICK G. HAYDEN, M.D.

Professor of Internal Medicine and Pathology, University of Virginia School of Medicine; Associate Director, Clinical Microbiology Laboratory, University of Virginia Health Sciences Center, Charlottesville, Virginia

Influenza

BARTON F. HAYNES, M.D.

Professor and Chairman, Department of Medicine, Duke University Medical Center, Durham, North Carolina

Diseases of the Thymus

LOUIS W. HECK, M.D.

Associate Professor of Medicine, Division of Clinical Immunology and Rheumatology, University of Alabama at Birmingham, Birmingham, Alabama

The Amyloid Diseases

DOUGLAS C. HEIMBURGER, M.D., M.S.

Professor of Nutrition Sciences and Medicine and Director, Cancer Prevention and Control Training Program, University of Alabama at Birmingham, Birmingham, Alabama

Nutrition's Interface with Health and Disease

J. OWEN HENDLEY, M.D.

Professor of Pediatrics, Pediatric Infectious Diseases, University of Virginia Health Sciences Center, Charlottesville, Virginia

The Common Cold

JANET B. HENRICH, M.D.

Yale School of Medicine, Women's Health Center, New Haven, Connecticut

Approach to Women's Health

MICHAEL S. HERSHFIELD, M.D.

Professor of Medicine, Duke University School of Medicine and Medical Center, Durham, North Carolina

Disorders of Purine and Pyrimidine Metabolism; Gout and Uric Acid Metabolism

HOBY P. HETHERINGTON, Ph.D.

Scientist, Medical Department, Brookhaven National Laboratory, Upton, New York; Visiting Scientist, Department of Neurosurgery, Yale University School of Medicine, New Haven, Connecticut

Newer Imaging Techniques

DOUGLAS M. HEUMAN, M.D.

Professor of Medicine, Medical College of Virginia of Virginia Commonwealth University; Director of Hepatology, McGuire Department of Veterans Affairs Medical Center, Richmond, Virginia

Diseases of the Gallbladder and Bile Ducts

WILLIAM R. HIATT, M.D.

Professor of Medicine, University of Colorado Health Sciences Center, Section of Vascular Medicine and Geriatrics; Executive Director, Colorado Prevention Center, Denver, Colorado

Atherosclerotic Peripheral Arterial Disease

RICHARD E. HILLMAN, M.D.

Professor, Department of Child Health; Professor, Department of Biochemistry; University of Missouri–Columbia School of Medicine; Director, Metabolic Genetics, University of Missouri Hospital and Clinics, Columbia, Missouri

Primary Hyperoxaluria

MARC C. HOCHBERG, M.D., M.P.H.

Professor of Medicine and Epidemiology and Head, Division of Rheumatology and Clinical Immunology, University of Maryland School of Medicine, Baltimore, Maryland

Sjögren's Syndrome

CRAIG J. HOESLEY, M.D.

Assistant Professor, Department of Medicine, University of Alabama at Birmingham, Birmingham, Alabama

Disease Caused by Bartonella *Species*

DAVID R. HOLMES, JR., M.D.

Professor of Medicine, Mayo Medical School; Consultant in Cardiovascular Diseases and Director, Cardiac Catheterization Laboratory, Mayo Clinic, Rochester, Minnesota

Cardiogenic Shock

JAY H. HOOFNAGLE, M.D.

Director, Division of Digestive Diseases and Nutrition, and Investigator, Liver Diseases Section, National Institute of Diabetes and Digestive and Kidney Diseases, National Institutes of Health, Bethesda, Maryland

Acute Viral Hepatitis; Chronic Hepatitis

EDWARD W. HOOK III, M.D.

Professor of Medicine, Division of Infectious Diseases, University of Alabama at Birmingham; Medical Director, STD Control Program, Jefferson County Department of Public Health, Birmingham, Alabama

Granuloma Inguinale (Donovanosis); Chancroid; Syphilis; Nonsyphilitic Treponematoses

PHILIP C. HOPEWELL, M.D.

Professor of Medicine, University of California, San Francisco; Associate Dean, San Francisco General Hospital, San Francisco, California

Pulmonary Manifestations of HIV Infection

RICHARD B. HORNICK, M.D.

Adjunct Clinical Professor of Medicine, University of Florida School of Medicine, Gainesville; Vice President, Medical Education, Orlando Regional Healthcare System, Orlando, Florida

Tularemia; Rickettsial Diseases

THOMAS H. HOSTETTER, M.D.

Professor of Medicine, Director of Division of Renal Diseases, University of Minnesota, Minneapolis, Minnesota

Diabetes and the Kidney

KEITH HRUSKA, M.D.

Ira M. Lang Professor of Medicine, Washington University; Director, Renal Stone Center, Barnes-Jewish Hospital, St. Louis, Missouri

Renal Calculi (Nephrolithiasis)

RUSSELL D. HULL, M.B.B.S., M.Sc.

Professor of Medicine, University of Calgary; Director, Thrombosis Research Unit, Foothills Hospital, Calgary, Alberta, Canada

Peripheral Venous Disease

GENE G. HUNDER, M.D.

Professor of Medicine, Mayo Medical School; Consultant in Rheumatology and Internal Medicine, Mayo Clinic, Rochester, Minnesota

Polymyalgia Rheumatica and Giant Cell Arteritis

DANIEL C. IHDE, M.D.

Professor of Medicine, University of South Florida; Professor of Medicine, H. Lee Moffitt Cancer Center, Tampa, Florida

Approach to the Patient with Metastatic Cancer, Primary Site Unknown

ROBERT W. IKE, M.D.

Associate Professor, Department of Internal Medicine, Division of Rheumatology, University of Michigan Medical Center, Ann Arbor, Michigan

Specialized Procedures in the Management of Patients with Rheumatic Diseases

SHARON K. INOUYE, M.D., M.P.H.

Associate Professor of Medicine, Yale University School of Medicine; Director, Elder Life Program, Yale–New Haven Hospital, and Co-director, Claude D. Pepper Older Americans Independence Center and Program on Aging, New Haven, Connecticut

Neuropsychiatric Aspects of Aging; Delirium and Other Mental Status Problems in the Older Patient

MICHAEL D. ISEMAN, M.D.

Professor of Medicine, Divisions of Pulmonary Sciences and Infectious Diseases, University of Colorado School of Medicine; Senior Staff Physician, National Jewish Medical and Research Center, Denver, Colorado

Tuberculosis

JON I. ISENBERG

Professor of Medicine, University of California, San Diego; Attending Physician, UCSD Medical Center, San Diego, California

Peptic Ulcer Disease: Epidemiology, Pathophysiology, Clinical Manifestations and Diagnosis

ERIC M. ISSELBACHER, M.D.

Instructor in Medicine, Harvard Medical School; Assistant in Medicine, Massachusetts General Hospital, Boston, Massachusetts

Diseases of the Aorta

MARK A. JACOBSON, M.D.

Associate Professor of Medicine, University of California, San Francisco; Attending Physician, San Francisco General Hospital, San Francisco, California

Ophthalmologic Manifestations of AIDS

FREDERICK A. JAKOBIEC, M.D.

Chairman, Department of Ophthalmology, Harvard Medical School; Chief of Ophthalmology, Massachusetts Eye and Ear Infirmary, Boston, Massachusetts

Diseases of the Visual System

JOSEPH JANKOVIC, M.D.

Professor of Neurology, Baylor College of Medicine; Director, Parkinson's Disease Center and Movement Disorders Clinic, Baylor College of Medicine, Houston, Texas

Introduction; Parkinsonism; Tremors; Dystonias; Choreas, Athetosis, and Ballism; Tics, Myoclonus, and Stereotypies

CHERYL A. JAY, M.D.

Assistant Clinical Professor of Neurology, University of California, San Francisco; Attending Neurologist, San Francisco General Hospital, San Francisco, California

Alcoholism and Alcohol Abuse

MARY M. JENKINS, Ph.D.

Research Associate, University of Alabama at Birmingham, Birmingham, Alabama

Hemoglobinopathies: Methemoglobinemias, Polycythemias, and Unstable Hemoglobins

ROBERT T. JENSEN, M.D.

Chief, Digestive Diseases Branch, National Institute of Diabetes and Digestive and Kidney Diseases, National Institutes of Health, Bethesda, Maryland

Pancreatic Endocrine Tumors

JOHN A. JERNIGAN, M.D.

Assistant Professor of Medicine, Emory University School of Medicine; Hospital Epidemiologist, Emory University Hospital, Atlanta, Georgia

Nosocomial Infections

WALDEMAR G. JOHANSON, JR., M.D., M.P.H.

Professor and Chairman, Department of Medicine, University of Medicine and Dentistry of New Jersey—New Jersey Medical School, Newark, New Jersey

Overview of Pneumonia; Pneumonia Caused by Aerobic Gram-Negative Bacilli; Aspiration Pneumonia

RICHARD B. JOHNSTON, JR., M.D.

Professor of Pediatrics, University of Colorado School of Medicine, National Jewish Medical and Research Center, Denver, Colorado

Whooping Cough (Pertussis)

KEITH A. JOINER, M.D.

Professor of Medicine, Cell Biology and Epidemiology; Chief, Section of Infectious Diseases; Associate Chairman, Department of Internal Medicine; Director, Investigative Medicine Program, Yale University School of Medicine, New Haven, Connecticut

Introduction to Protozoan and Helminthic Diseases

HOWARD W. JONES III, M.D.

Professor, Department of Obstetrics/Gynecology, Vanderbilt University School of Medicine and Medical Center; Director, Division of Gynecologic Oncology, Vanderbilt University Hospital, Nashville, Tennessee

Ovarian Carcinoma

KENNETH LYONS JONES, M.D.

Professor of Pediatrics, University of California, San Diego, School of Medicine, La Jolla; Staff Physician, University of California, San Diego, Medical Center, San Diego, California

Syndromes Involving Multiple Organ Systems

NATHALIE JOSSO, M.D.

Ecole Normale Supérieure; Attaché, Hôpital St. Vincent de Paul, Paris, France

Disorders of Sexual Differentiation

RALPH F. JÓZEFOWICZ, M.D.

Professor of Neurology and Medicine, University of Rochester School of Medicine and Dentistry; Attending Neurologist, Strong Memorial Hospital, Rochester, New York

The Neurologic History; Neurologic Diagnostic Procedures

JOHN A. KANIS, M.D., FRCP, FRCPath

Professor in Human Metabolism, University of Sheffield Medical School, Sheffield, United Kingdom

Paget's Disease of Bone (Osteitis Deformans)

PHILIP W. KANTOFF, M.D.

Director of the Lamb Center for Genitourinary Oncology, Dana-Farber Cancer Institute; Associate Professor of Medicine, Harvard Medical School, Boston, Massachusetts

Tumors of the Kidney, Ureter, and Bladder

ALBERT Z. KAPIKIAN, M.D., D.Sc.(Hon)

Head, Epidemiology Section, Laboratory of Infectious Diseases, National Institute of Allergy and Infectious Diseases, National Institutes of Health, Bethesda, Maryland

Viral Gastroenteritis

ALLEN P. KAPLAN, M.D.

Professor of Medicine, Medical University of South Carolina, Charleston, South Carolina

Anaphylaxis

GILLA KAPLAN, Ph.D.

Associate Professor, The Rockefeller University, New York, New York

Leprosy (Hansen's Disease)

ADOLF W. KARCHMER, M.D.

Professor of Medicine, Harvard Medical School; Chief, Division of Infectious Diseases, Beth Israel Deaconess Medical Center, Boston, Massachusetts

Antibacterial Therapy

PAUL KATZ, M.D.

Anton and Margaret Friesz Professor and Chairman, Department of Medicine; Chief Operating Officer, Georgetown University Medical Center, Washington, D.C.

Glucocorticosteroids in Relation to Inflammatory Disease

DONALD KAYE, M.D.

Professor of Medicine, MCP Hahnemann School of Medicine, Philadelphia, Pennsylvania

Salmonella Infections Other Than Typhoid Fever

JAMES W. KAZURA, M.D.

Professor of Medicine and International Health, Case Western Reserve University School of Medicine; Chief, Division of Geographic Medicine, Department of Medicine, University Hospitals of Cleveland, Cleveland, Ohio

Nematode Infections

MICHAEL J. KEATING, M.D., M.B., B.S.

Professor of Medicine; Associate Head for Clinical Research, University of Texas M.D. Anderson Cancer Center, Houston, Texas

The Chronic Leukemias

CRAIG M. KESSLER, M.D.

Professor of Medicine and Pathology; Head, Section of Hematology; Director, Division of Coagulation Laboratories; Director, Hemophilia and Thrombosis Treatment Center, Vincent T. Lombardi Cancer Center, Georgetown University Hospital and School of Medicine, Washington, D.C.

Coagulation Factor Deficiencies

CATARINA I. KIEFE, Ph.D., M.D.

Professor of Medicine and Associate Professor of Biostatistics, University of Alabama at Birmingham; Quality Management Physician Consultant to the Chief of Staff, Birmingham Veterans Affairs Medical Center, Birmingham, Alabama

Application of Statistics

ELLIOTT D. KIEFF, M.D., Ph.D.

Harriet Ryan Albee Professor, Departments of Medicine and Microbiology and Molecular Genetics, Channing Laboratory, Brigham and Women's Hospital and Harvard Medical School, Boston, Massachusetts

Infectious Mononucleosis: Epstein-Barr Virus Infection

CHARLES H. KING, M.D.

Associate Professor of Medicine, Division of Geographic Medicine, Case Western Reserve University School of Medicine; Attending Physician, University Hospitals of Cleveland, Cleveland, Ohio

Cestode Infections

BETH D. KIRKPATRICK, M.D.

Fellow, Division of Infectious Diseases, Johns Hopkins University School of Medicine, Baltimore, Maryland

Cryptosporidiosis

SAULO KLAHR, M.D.

John E. and Adaline Simon Professor of Medicine, Washington University School of Medicine; Director of Research and Scientific Affairs, Barnes–Jewish Hospital, St. Louis, Missouri

Obstructive Uropathy

SAMUEL KLEIN, M.D.

Professor of Medicine and Director, Center for Human Nutrition, Washington University School of Medicine, St. Louis, Missouri

Protein-Energy Malnutrition

JUHA P. KOKKO, M.D., Ph.D.

Asa G. Candler Professor and Chairman of Medicine, Emory University School of Medicine, Atlanta, Georgia

Rhabdomyolysis; Approach to the Patient with Renal Disease; Fluids and Electrolytes

DONALD J. KROGSTAD, M.D., A.B.

Henderson Professor and Chair, Department of Tropical Medicine, School of Public Health and Tropical Medicine; Professor and Chair, Department of Parasitology, School of Graduate Studies; Professor of Medicine, School of Medicine; Director, Tulane Center for Infectious Diseases, Tulane University, New Orleans, Louisiana

Malaria

HENRY M. KRONENBERG, M.D.

Professor of Medicine, Harvard Medical School; Chief, Endocrine Unit, Department of Medicine, Massachusetts General Hospital, Boston, Massachusetts

Multiple-Organ Syndromes: Polyglandular Disorders

CALVIN M. KUNIN, M.D.

Pomerene Professor of Internal Medicine, Ohio State University College of Medicine and Public Health; Attending Physician, Ohio State University Medical Center, Columbus, Ohio

Urinary Tract Infections and Pyelonephritis

RUBEN I. KUZNIECKY, M.D.

Professor of Neurology and Neurosurgery, University of Alabama at Birmingham; Director, UAB Epilepsy Center, University of Alabama at Birmingham, Birmingham, Alabama

Neurocutaneous Syndromes; Malformations of Cortical Development; Congenital Anomalies of the Craniovertebral Junction, Spine, and Spinal Cord (Including Syringomyelia)

ROBERT A. KYLE, M.D.

Professor of Medicine and of Laboratory Medicine, Mayo Medical School; Consultant, Division of Hematology and Internal Medicine, Mayo Clinic and Mayo Foundation, Rochester, Minnesota

Plasma Cell Disorders

PHILIP J. LANDRIGAN, M.D., M.Sc.

Ethel H. Wise Professor and Chair, Department of Community and Preventive Medicine, Mount Sinai School of Medicine, New York, New York

Principles of Occupational and Environmental Medicine

THOMAS H. LEE, M.D., M.Sc.

Associate Professor of Medicine, Harvard Medical School; Medical Director, Partners Community Health Care, Inc., Boston, Massachusetts

Interpretation of Data for Clinical Decisions

BRUCE B. LERMAN, M.D.

H. Altschul Master Professor of Medicine, Weill Medical College of Cornell University; Chief, Division of Cardiology, and Director, Cardiac Electrophysiology Laboratory, New York Hospital–Cornell Medical Center, New York, New York

Ventricular Arrhythmias and Sudden Death

BERNARD LEVIN, M.D., B.Ch.

Professor of Medicine and Vice-President for Cancer Prevention, University of Texas M.D. Anderson Cancer Center, Houston, Texas

Neoplasms of the Large and Small Intestines

STUART LEVIN, M.D., MACP

Professor of Medicine, Rush Medical School; Ralph C. Brown, M.D., Professor and Chairman, Department of Internal Medicine, Rush-Presbyterian–St. Luke's Medical Center, Chicago, Illinois

Zoonoses

WENDY LEVINSON, M.D.

Professor of Medicine and Chief, Section of General Internal Medicine, University of Chicago, Chicago, Illinois

Approach to Women's Health

MATTHEW E. LEVISON, M.D.

Professor of Medicine and Public Health and Chief, Division of Infectious Diseases, MCP Hahnemann University School of Medicine, Philadelphia, Pennsylvania

Infective Endocarditis

ALFRED J. LEWY, M.D., Ph.D.

Professor of Psychiatry, Ophthalmology, and Physiology and Pharmacology, School of Medicine, Oregon Health Sciences University, Portland, Oregon

The Pineal Gland

LAWRENCE M. LICHTENSTEIN, M.D., Ph.D.

Professor of Medicine, Johns Hopkins University School of Medicine, Baltimore, Maryland

Insect Sting Allergy

OLIVER LIESENFELD, M.D.

Senior Researcher, Institute for Infection Medicine, Free University of Berlin, Germany

Toxoplasmosis

ALDO Ā.M. LIMA, M.D., Ph.D.

Full Professor, Faculty of Medicine, Federal University of Ceará, Fortaleza, Ceará, Brazil

Schistosomiasis (Bilharziasis)

KAREN L. LINDSAY, M.D.

Associate Professor of Clinical Medicine, University of Southern California School of Medicine, Los Angeles, California

Acute Viral Hepatitis; Chronic Hepatitis

PETER E. LIPSKY, M.D.

Professor of Internal Medicine and Microbiology, University of Texas Southwestern Medical Center at Dallas, Dallas, Texas

The Spondyloarthropathies

EDISON T. LIU, M.D.

Director, Division of Clinical Sciences, National Cancer Institute, Bethesda, Maryland; Adjunct Professor of Biochemistry and Biophysics, University of North Carolina at Chapel Hill, Chapel Hill, North Carolina

Oncogenes and Suppressor Genes: Genetic Control of Cancer

ROGERIO A. LOBO, M.D.

Rappleye Professor of Obstetrics/Gynecology and Chairman of the Department, Columbia University College of Physicians and Surgeons; Director, Sloane Hospital for Women, New York Presbyterian Hospital, New York, New York

Menopause

D. LYNN LORIAUX, M.D., Ph.D.

Professor and Chairman, Department of Medicine, Oregon Health Sciences University, Portland, Oregon

The Adrenal Cortex

JOHN M. LUCE, M.D.

Professor of Medicine and Anesthesia, University of California, San Francisco; Associate Director, Medical-Surgical Intensive Care Unit, San Francisco General Hospital, San Francisco, California

Approach to the Patient in a Critical Care Setting; Respiratory Monitoring in Critical Care; Ventilator Management in the Intensive Care Unit

MICHAEL R. LUCEY, M.D.

Associate Professor of Medicine, University of Pennsylvania School of Medicine; Associate Chief, Division of Gastroenterology; Director of Hepatology; Medical Director, Liver Transplant Program, Hospital of the University of Pennsylvania, Philadelphia, Pennsylvania

Diseases of the Peritoneum, Mesentery, and Omentum

ROBERT G. LUKE, M.D.

Taylor Professor of Medicine and Chairman, Department of Medicine, University of Cincinnati College of Medicine, Cincinnati, Ohio

Chronic Renal Failure

WILLIS C. MADDREY, M.D.

Professor of Internal Medicine and Executive Vice President for Clinical Affairs, University of Texas Southwestern Medical Center at Dallas, Dallas, Texas

Parasitic, Bacterial, Fungal, and Granulomatous Liver Diseases

R. ELLEN MAGENIS, M.D.

Professor of Pediatrics and Molecular and Medical Genetics at Child Development Rehabilitation Center; Director of Clinical Cytogenetics Laboratory; Consultant to University Hospital, Oregon Health Sciences University, Portland, Oregon

Chromosomes and Their Disorders

JACQUELYN J. MAHER, M.D.

Associate Professor of Medicine, University of California, San Francisco; Attending Physician, San Francisco General Hospital, San Francisco, California

Inherited, Infiltrative, and Metabolic Disorders Involving the Liver

ADEL A.F. MAHMOUD, M.D., Ph.D.

President, Merck Vaccines, Merck Company, Inc., Whitehouse Station, New Jersey

Liver, Intestinal, and Lung Fluke Infections

STEPHEN E. MALAWISTA, M.D.

Professor of Medicine, Department of Internal Medicine, Yale University School of Medicine; Attending Physician, Yale–New Haven Medical Center, New Haven, and West Haven Veterans Affairs Medical Center, West Haven, Connecticut

Lyme Disease

HARTMUT H. MALLUCHE, M.D.

Professor and Chief, University of Kentucky, Lexington, Kentucky

Renal Osteodystrophy

GERALD L. MANDELL, M.D.

Professor of Medicine and Owen R. Cheatham Professor of the Sciences; Chief, Division of Infectious Diseases, University of Virginia Health Sciences Center, Charlottesville, Virginia

Introduction to Microbial Disease; Introduction to Bacterial Disease; Introduction to HIV and Associated Disorders

WARREN J. MANNING, M.D.

Associate Professor of Medicine and Radiology, Harvard Medical School; Associate Director, Non-invasive Cardiac Imaging, and Co-Director, Cardiac MR Center, Beth Israel Deaconess Medical Center, Boston, Massachusetts

Cardiac Magnetic Resonance Imaging; Pericardial Disease

ARIANE J. MARELLI, M.D.

Assistant Professor of Medicine, McGill University; Assistant Physician, Division of Cardiology, Department of Medicine, McGill University Health Center, Montreal, Quebec, Canada

Congenital Heart Disease in Adults

LAWRENCE F. MARSHALL, M.D.

Professor and Chair, Neurosurgery, University of California, San Diego, Medical Center, San Diego, California

Head Injury; Spine and Spinal Cord Injury

MANUEL MARTINEZ-MALDONADO, M.D.

Vice Provost for Research and Professor of Medicine, Oregon Health Sciences University, Portland, Oregon

Hereditary Chronic Nephropathies

STEPHEN J. MARX, M.D.

Chief, Genetics and Endocrinology Section, National Institute of Diabetes and Digestive and Kidney Diseases, National Institutes of Health, Bethesda, Maryland

Mineral and Bone Homeostasis

JAY W. MASON, M.D.

Professor and Chair, Department of Internal Medicine, College of Medicine, University of Kentucky, Lexington, Kentucky

Electrophysiologic Diagnostic Procedures

JOEL B. MASON, M.D.

Associate Professor of Medicine and Nutrition, Tufts University; Director, Vitamins and Carcinogenesis Program, USDA Human Nutrition Research Center on Aging at Tufts University; Staff Gastroenterologist and Acting Chief, Division of Clinical Nutrition, New England Medical Center, Boston, Massachusetts

Consequences of Altered Micronutrient Status

BARRY M. MASSIE, M.D.

Professor of Medicine, University of California, San Francisco; Director, Coronary Care Unit and Heart Failure Program, Department of Veterans Affairs Medical Center, San Francisco, California

Pathophysiology of Heart Failure

MARGARET M. McGOVERN, M.D., Ph.D.

Associate Professor, Mount Sinai School of Medicine; Associate Attending, Mount Sinai Hospital, New York, New York

Lysosomal Storage Diseases

ELIZABETH McLOUGHLIN, Sc.D.

Assistant Adjunct Professor, Department of Surgery, University of California, San Francisco; Director of Programs, Trauma Foundation, San Francisco, California

Violence and Injury

M. MOLLY McMAHON, M.D.

Associate Professor of Medicine, Endocrinology, Metabolism, and Nutrition and Internal Medicine; Director of Adult Clinical Nutrition, Mayo Clinic and Mayo Foundation, Rochester, Minnesota

Parenteral Nutrition

KENNETH R. MEEHAN, M.D.

Assistant Professor of Medicine, Georgetown University and Georgetown University Medical Center, Washington, D.C.

Non-metastatic Effects of Cancer: Other Systems

MARIO F. MENDEZ, M.D., Ph.D.

Associate Professor, Neurology and Psychiatry, UCLA School of Medicine, Los Angeles, California

Disorders of Cognition

JAY E. MENITOVE, M.D.

Clinical Professor of Medicine, Kansas University School of Medicine, Kansas City, Kansas, and University of Missouri–Kansas City School of Medicine; Executive Director and Medical Director, Community Blood Center of Greater Kansas City, Kansas City, Missouri

Blood Transfusion

STEVEN J. MENTZER, M.D.

Associate Professor of Surgery, Harvard Medical School; Division of Thoracic Surgery, Brigham and Women's Hospital and the Dana-Farber Cancer Institute, Boston, Massachusetts

Surgical Approach to Lung Disease

DEAN D. METCALFE, M.D.

Chief, Laboratory of Allergic Diseases, National Institute of Allergy and Infectious Diseases, National Institutes of Health, Bethesda, Maryland

Mastocytosis

YORK E. MILLER, M.D.

Professor of Medicine, Division of Pulmonary Sciences and Critical Care Medicine, University of Colorado School of Medicine; Staff Physician, Denver Veterans Affairs Medical Center; Program Leader, Lung Cancer Program, University of Colorado Comprehensive Cancer Center, Denver, Colorado

Pulmonary Neoplasms

DANIEL R. MISHELL, JR., M.D.

Lyle G. McNeile Professor and Chairman, Department of Obstetrics/Gynecology, University of Southern California School of Medicine; Chief of Professional Services, Women's and Children's Hospital, Los Angeles County and University of Southern California Medical Center, Los Angeles, California

Contraception

WILLIAM E. MITCH, M.D.

Garland Herndon Professor of Medicine, Emory University School of Medicine; Director, Renal Division, Emory University Hospital, Grady Hospital, Atlanta Veterans Affairs Hospital, and Crawford Long Hospital, Atlanta, Georgia

Acute Renal Failure

BEVERLY S. MITCHELL, M.D.

Professor, Departments of Medicine and Pharmacology, Lineberger Comprehensive Cancer Center, University of North Carolina at Chapel Hill, Chapel Hill, North Carolina

Disorders of Purine and Pyrimidine Metabolism

MARK E. MOLITCH, M.D.

Professor of Medicine, Center for Endocrinology, Metabolism and Molecular Medicine, Northwestern University Medical School; Attending Physician, Northwestern Memorial Hospital, Chicago, Illinois

Neuroendocrinology and the Neuroendocrine System; The Pituitary: Anterior Pituitary

MARIE-CLAUDE MONIER-FAUGERE, M.D.

Research Professor, University of Kentucky, Lexington, Kentucky

Renal Osteodystrophy

FRED MORADY, M.D.

Professor of Medicine, University of Michigan, School of Medicine; Director, Clinical Electrophysiology Laboratory, University of Michigan Medical Center, Ann Arbor, Michigan

Electrophysiologic Interventional Procedures and Surgery

GABRIELLE F. MORRIS, M.D.

Chief Resident, University of California, San Diego, Medical Center, San Diego, California

Head Injury; Spine and Spinal Cord Injury

J. GLENN MORRIS, JR., M.D., M.P.H.

Professor of Medicine and Head, Division of Hospital Epidemiology, Professor of Epidemiology and Preventive Medicine, Professor of Microbiology, University of Maryland School of Medicine, Baltimore, Maryland

Yersinia Infections

MICHAEL A. MOSKOWITZ, M.D.

Professor of Neurology, Harvard Medical School; Director, Stroke and Neurovascular Regulation Laboratory, Massachusetts General Hospital, Boston, Massachusetts

Headaches and Other Head Pain

BALFOUR M. MOUNT, M.D.

Eric M. Flanders Professor of Palliative Medicine, McGill University; Attending Physician, McGill University Health Centre, Montreal, Quebec, Canada

Care of Dying Patients and Their Families

JAMES M. MOUNTZ, M.D., Ph.D.

Professor of Radiology, Division of Nuclear Medicine, University of Alabama at Birmingham; Director of Neuronuclear Medicine, University of Alabama at Birmingham Medical Center, Birmingham, Alabama

Newer Imaging Techniques

MAURICE A. MUFSON, M.D.

Professor and Chairman, Department of Medicine, and Professor, Department of Microbiology, Marshall University School of Medicine; Active Staff, Cabell Huntington Hospital and St. Mary's Hospital, Huntington, West Virginia

Viral Pharyngitis, Laryngitis, Croup, and Bronchitis

HYMAN B. MUSS, M.D.

Professor of Medicine, University of Vermont; Director, Hematology/Oncology, Fletcher Allen Health Care, Burlington, Vermont

Breast Cancer and Differential Diagnosis of Benign Nodules

TOMOKO V. NAKAWATASE, M.D.

Assistant Clinical Professor, UCLA School of Medicine; Associate Physician, UCLA Medical Center, Los Angeles, California

Disorders of Cognition

AVINDRA NATH, M.D.

Associate Professor, Department of Neurology; Associate Professor, Department of Microbiology and Immunology, University of Kentucky College of Medicine, Lexington, Kentucky

Introduction; Acute Viral Meningitis and Encephalitis; Poliomyelitis; The Herpesviruses; Rabies; Slow Virus Infections

ROBERT K. NAVIAUX, M.D., Ph.D.

Assistant Professor, Department of Medicine, University of California, San Diego, School of Medicine, La Jolla, California

Galactosemia

FRANKLIN A. NEVA, M.D.

Head, Section on Opportunistic Parasitic Diseases, Laboratory of Parasitic Diseases, National Institutes of Health, Bethesda, Maryland

American Trypanosomiasis (Chagas' Disease)

MARIA I. NEW, M.D.

Professor and Chairman, Department of Pediatrics, Harold and Percy Uris Professor of Pediatric Endocrinology and Metabolism, Weill Medical College of Cornell University; Pediatrician-in-Chief, Department of Pediatrics, and Chief, Division of Pediatric Endocrinology, New York Hospital–Cornell Medical Center, New York, New York

Disorders of Sexual Differentiation

WILLIAM L. NYHAN, M.D., Ph.D.

Professor of Pediatrics, University of California, San Diego, School of Medicine, La Jolla; Attending Physician, UCSD Medical Center, San Diego, California

Galactosemia

JOHN A. OATES, M.D.

The Thomas F. Frist Sr. Professor of Medicine and Professor of Pharmacology, Vanderbilt University School of Medicine; Attending Physician, The Vanderbilt University Hospital, Nashville, Tennessee

Multiple-Organ Syndromes: Carcinoid Syndrome

ALBERT OBERMAN, M.D., M.P.H.

Professor and Director, Division of Preventive Medicine, Department of Medicine, University of Alabama at Birmingham School of Medicine, Birmingham, Alabama

Principles of Preventive Health Care

DANIEL T. O'CONNOR, M.D.

Professor, Department of Medicine, University of California, San Diego, School of Medicine, La Jolla; Chief, Hypertension, Veterans Affairs San Diego Healthcare System, San Diego, California

The Adrenal Medulla, Catecholamines, and Pheochromocytoma

JEFFREY W. OLIN, D.O.

Chairman, Department of Vascular Medicine, Cleveland Clinic Foundation, Cleveland, Ohio

Other Peripheral Arterial Diseases

GILBERT S. OMENN, M.D., Ph.D.

Professor, Internal Medicine, Human Genetics, Cancer Center, and Public Health, University of Michigan School of Medicine; Chief Executive Officer, University of Michigan Health System, and Executive Vice President for Medical Affairs, University of Michigan, Ann Arbor, Michigan

Cancer Prevention

SUZANNE OPARIL, M.D.

Professor of Medicine, Physiology and Biophysics, and Director, Vascular Biology and Hypertension Program, University of Alabama at Birmingham, Birmingham, Alabama

Arterial Hypertension

WALTER A. ORENSTEIN, M.D.

Director, National Immunization Program, Centers for Disease Control and Prevention, Atlanta, Georgia

Immunization

SUSAN L. ORLOFF, M.D.

Assistant Professor of Surgery, Department of Surgery, Section of Liver and Pancreas Transplantation, Hepatobiliary Surgery, Oregon Health Sciences University and Hospital; Staff Surgeon, Portland Veterans Affairs Medical Center, Portland, Oregon

Peptic Ulcer Disease: Surgical Therapy

JOSEPH G. OUSLANDER, M.D.

Professor of Medicine, Emory University School of Medicine; Director, Division of Geriatric Medicine and Gerontology, and Vice President for Professional Affairs, Wesley Woods Center of Emory University; Director, Rehabilitation Research and Development Center, Atlanta Veterans Affairs Medical Center, Atlanta, Georgia

Urinary Incontinence

MICHAEL N. OXMAN, M.D.

Professor of Medicine and Pathology, University of California, San Diego, La Jolla, California; Staff Physician, Veterans Affairs San Diego Healthcare System, San Diego, California

Enteroviruses

MILTON PACKER, M.D.

Dickinson W. Richards Professor of Medicine and of Pharmacology; Chief, Division of Circulatory Physiology; Director, Center for Heart Failure Research, Columbia University College of Physicians and Surgeons; Head, Heart Failure Center, Columbia-Presbyterian Medical Center, New York, New York

Management of Congestive Heart Failure

FRANK PARKER, M.D.

Professor of Dermatology, Department of Dermatology, Oregon Health Sciences University, Portland, Oregon

Non-metastatic Effects of Cancer: The Skin; Structure and Function of Skin; Examination of the Skin and an Approach to Diagnosing Skin Diseases; Principles of Therapy; Skin Diseases of General Importance

HENRY P. PARKMAN, M.D.

Associate Professor of Medicine; Director, GI Motility Laboratory, Temple University Hospital, Philadelphia, Pennsylvania

Diseases of the Esophagus

JOSEPH E. PARRILLO, M.D.

James B. Herrick Professor of Medicine, Rush Medical College; Chief, Division of Cardiovascular Disease and Critical Care Medicine; Director, Section of Cardiology; Medical Director, Rush Heart Institute; Rush-Presbyterian–St. Luke's Medical Center, Chicago, Illinois

Approach to the Patient with Shock; Shock Syndromes Related to Sepsis

ALAN W. PARTIN, M.D., Ph.D.

Professor of Urology, The Johns Hopkins Medical Institutions, Baltimore, Maryland

Diseases of the Prostate

PANKAJ JAY PASRICHA, M.D.

Associate Professor of Medicine; Chief, Division of Gastroenterology and Hepatology, University of Texas Medical Branch, Galveston, Texas

Gastrointestinal Endoscopy

RICHARD D. PEARSON, M.D.

Professor of Medicine and Pathology, Division of Geographic and International Medicine, Departments of Medicine and Pathology, University of Virginia School of Medicine, Charlottesville, Virginia

Advice to Travelers; Leishmaniasis; Other Protozoan Diseases

TIMOTHY A. PEDLEY, M.D.

Henry and Lucy Moses Professor of Neurology, Chairman, Department of Neurology, College of Physicians and Surgeons of Columbia University; Neurologist-in-Chief, The Neurological Institute of New York, The New York Presbyterian Hospital at Columbia-Presbyterian Center, New York, New York

The Epilepsies

NEAL S. PENNEYS, M.D., Ph.D., M.B.A.

Professor of Dermatology, St. Louis University; Associate Dean and Chief Operating Officer, University Medical Group of St. Louis University, St. Louis, Missouri

Cutaneous Signs of AIDS

WILLIAM A. PETRI, JR., M.D., Ph.D.

Professor of Medicine, Microbiology and Pathology, University of Virginia School of Medicine; Attending Physician and Associate Director of Clinical Microbiology, University of Virginia Hospitals, Charlottesville, Virginia

Relapsing Fever; Leptospirosis

JAMES M. PHANG, M.D.

Chief, Metabolism and Cancer Susceptibility Section, Basic Research Laboratory, Division of Basic Sciences, National Cancer Institute, Frederick, Maryland

The Hyperprolinemias and Hydroxyprolinemia

CLAUDE A. PIANTADOSI, M.D.

Duke University Medical Center and Durham Veterans Affairs Medical Center, Durham, North Carolina

Physical, Chemical, and Aspiration Injuries of the Lung

EDYTA C. PIROG, M.D.

Instructor of Pathology, Weill Medical College of Cornell University; Assistant Attending Pathologist, New York–Presbyterian Hospital, New York, New York

Cervical and Uterine Cancer Screening

F. XAVIER PI-SUNYER, M.D.

Professor of Medicine, College of Physicians and Surgeons, Columbia University; Chief, Division of Endocrinology, Diabetes and Nutrition, St. Luke's–Roosevelt Hospital Center, New York, New York

Obesity

PHILIP A. PIZZO, M.D.

Thomas Morgan Professor and Chair, Department of Pediatrics, Harvard Medical School; Physician-in-Chief and Chair, Department of Medicine, Children's Hospital, Boston, Massachusetts

The Compromised Host

FRED PLUM, M.D.

Professor of Neurology and Neuroscience, Department of Neurology and Neuroscience, Weill Medical College of Cornell University, New York, New York

Medicine as a Learned and Humane Profession

CAROL S. PORTLOCK, M.D.

Professor of Clinical Medicine, Cornell University Medical College; Attending Physician, Lymphoma Service, Memorial Sloan-Kettering Cancer Center, New York, New York

Hodgkin's Disease

JEROME B. POSNER, M.D.

Professor of Neurology and Neuroscience, Weill Medical College of Cornell University; Attending Neurologist, Memorial Sloan-Kettering Cancer Center, New York, New York

Non-metastatic Effects of Cancer: The Nervous System

DON W. POWELL, M.D.

Edward Randall and Edward Randall, Jr., Distinguished Chairman and Professor, Department of Internal Medicine, and Professor, Physiology and Biophysics, University of Texas Medical Branch, Galveston, Texas

Approach to the Patient with Gastrointestinal Disease; Approach to the Patient with Diarrhea; Approach to the Patient with Liver Diseases

MICHAEL PRATT, M.D., M.S., M.P.H.

Medical Epidemiologist, Centers for Disease Control and Prevention, Division of Nutrition and Physical Activity, Atlanta, Georgia

Physical Activity

JOSEF T. PRCHAL, M.D.

Professor of Medicine and Director, Comprehensive Sickle Cell Center, University of Alabama at Birmingham, Division of Hematology/Oncology, Birmingham, Alabama

Hemoglobinopathies: Methemoglobinemias, Polycythemias, and Unstable Hemoglobins

LAUREL C. PREHEIM, M.D.

Professor of Medicine, Medical Microbiology and Immunology, Creighton University School of Medicine, University of Nebraska College of Medicine; Chief, Infectious Diseases Section, Department of Veterans Affairs Medical Center, Omaha, Nebraska

Other Mycobacterioses

RICHARD W. PRICE, M.D.

Professor and Vice Chair, Department of Neurology, University of California, San Francisco; Chief, Neurology Service, San Francisco General Hospital, San Francisco, California

Neurologic Complications of HIV-1 Infection

WILLIAM A. PULSINELLI, M.D., Ph.D.

Semmes-Murphey Professor and Chairman, Department of Neurology, University of Tennessee College of Medicine, Memphis, Tennessee

Cerebrovascular Diseases—Principles; Ischemic Cerebrovascular Disease; Hemorrhagic Cerebrovascular Disease

REED EDWIN PYERITZ, M.D., Ph.D.

Professor of Human Genetics, Medicine and Pediatrics, MCP Hahnemann School of Medicine; Director, Center for Medical Genetics, Allegheny General Hospital, Pittsburgh, Pennsylvania

Marfan Syndrome; Ehlers-Danlos Syndromes; Osteogenesis Imperfecta Syndromes; Pseudoxanthoma Elasticum

ANASTACIO DE QUEIROZ SOUSA, M.D.

Professor of Medicine, Universidade Federal do Ceará, Fortaleza; Secretary of Health, State of Ceará, Ceará, Brazil

Leishmaniasis

PETER J. QUESENBERRY, M.D.

Professor of Medicine and Director, Cancer Center, University of Massachusetts Medical School, Worcester, Massachusetts

Hematopoiesis and Hematopoietic Growth Factors

THOMAS C. QUINN, M.D.

Professor of Medicine, International Health, Immunology and Molecular Microbiology, Johns Hopkins Medical Institutions; Attending Physician, Johns Hopkins Hospital and National Institutes of Health Clinical Center, Baltimore, Maryland

African Trypanosomiasis (Sleeping Sickness)

JONATHAN I. RAVDIN, M.D.

Nesbitt Professor and Chairman, Department of Medicine, University of Minnesota Medical School; Chief of Medicine, Fairview University Medical Center, Minneapolis, Minnesota

Amebiasis

ROBERT W. REBAR, M.D.

Professor, Department of Obstetrics and Gynecology, University of Cincinnati College of Medicine, Cincinnati, Ohio

Ovaries and Development; Menstrual Cycle and Fertility

ANNETTE C. REBOLI, M.D.

Associate Professor of Medicine, University of Medicine and Dentistry of New Jersey, Robert Wood Johnson Medical School of Camden; Attending Physician, Cooper Hospital/University Medical Center, Camden, New Jersey

Erysipeloid

JOHN J. REILLY, JR., M.D.

Associate Professor of Medicine, Harvard Medical School; Medical Director of Lung Transplantation, Brigham and Women's Hospital, Boston, Massachusetts

Surgical Approach to Lung Disease

DAVID A. RELMAN, M.D.

Assistant Professor of Medicine, and of Microbiology and Immunology, Stanford University, Stanford, California; Staff Physician, VA Palo Alto Health Care System, Palo Alto, California

Disease Caused by Bartonella *Species*

JACK S. REMINGTON, M.D.

Professor of Medicine, Division of Infectious Diseases and Geographic Medicine, Stanford University School of Medicine; Marcus A. Krupp Research Chair and Chairman, Department of Immunology and Infectious Diseases, Research Institute, Palo Alto Medical Foundation, Palo Alto, California

Toxoplasmosis

ROBERT R. RICH, M.D.

Executive Associate Dean and Professor of Medicine, Emory University School of Medicine, Atlanta, Georgia

The Major Histocompatibility Complex and Disease Susceptibility

RALPH M. RICHART, M.D.

Professor of Pathology in Obstetrics and Gynecology, Columbia University; Attending Pathologist, Presbyterian Hospital, New York, New York

Cervical and Uterine Cancer Screening

RICHARD K. RIEGELMAN, M.D., Ph.D.

Dean, The George Washington University School of Public Health and Health Services, Washington, D.C.

The Preventive Health Examination

JOHN M. RINGMAN, M.D.

Assistant Professor, Department of Neurology, University of California Irvine Medical Center, Orange, California

Disorders of Cognition

ROGER S. RITTMASTER, M.D.

Adjunct Professor of Physiology and Biophysics, Dalhousie University, Halifax, Nova Scotia, Canada; Principal Clinical Research Physician, Glaxo Wellcome Inc., Research Triangle Park, North Carolina

Hirsutism

ROBERT A. RIZZA, M.D.

Professor of Internal Medicine and Chair, Division of Endocrinology, Metabolism and Nutrition, Mayo School of Medicine, Rochester, Minnesota

Hypoglycemia/Pancreatic Islet Cell Disorders

JOHN P. ROBERTS, M.D.

Professor of Surgery, University of California, San Francisco; Chief of Transplant Services, University of California, San Francisco, Medical Center, San Francisco, California

Liver Transplantation

WILLIAM O. ROBERTSON, M.D.

Professor of Pediatrics—Medical Toxicology, University of Washington School of Medicine; Medical Director, Washington Poison Center, Seattle, Washington

Chronic Poisoning: Trace Metals and Others

ALAN G. ROBINSON, M.D.

Vice Provost, Medical Sciences, Executive Associate Dean, School of Medicine, UCLA School of Medicine, Los Angeles, California

The Pituitary: Posterior Pituitary

JOSEPH R. RODARTE, M.D.

Professor of Medicine and Chief, Pulmonary/Critical Care Section, Baylor College of Medicine, Houston, Texas

Chronic Bronchitis and Emphysema

GRIFFIN P. RODGERS, M.M.Sc., M.D.

Chief, Molecular and Clinical Hematology Branch, National Institute of Diabetes and Digestive and Kidney Diseases, National Institutes of Health, Bethesda, Maryland

Hemoglobinopathies: Thalassemias

JOHN L. ROMBEAU, M.D.

Professor of Surgery, University of Pennsylvania School of Medicine, Philadelphia, Pennsylvania

Enteral Nutrition

DANIEL I. ROSENTHAL, M.D.

Professor of Radiology, Harvard University; Associate Radiologist in Chief, Massachusetts General Hospital, Boston, Massachusetts

Bone Tumors

LANNY J. ROSENWASSER, M.D.

Professor of Medicine, University of Colorado Health Sciences Center; Marjorie and Stephen Raphael Chair in Asthma Research and Head, Division of Allergy and Clinical Immunology, National Jewish Medical and Research Center, Denver, Colorado

The Vasculitic Syndromes; Polyarteritis Nodosa Group

MICHAEL C. ROWBOTHAM, M.D.

Associate Professor of Clinical Neurology and Anesthesia; Director, UCSF Pain Clinical Research Center; Associate Director, UCSF–Mount Zion Pain Management Center, University of California, San Francisco, School of Medicine, San Francisco, California

Other Specific Pain Syndromes

RICHARD A. RUDICK, M.D.

Professor of Neurology, Ohio State University College of Medicine, Hazel Prior Hostetler Professor of Neurology and Director, The Mellen Center, The Cleveland Clinic Foundation, Cleveland, Ohio

Neurologic Complications in the Immunologically Compromised Host; Reye Syndrome; Multiple Sclerosis and Related Conditions; Central Nervous System Complications of Viral Infections and Vaccines

ANIL K. RUSTGI, M.D.

T. Grier Miller Associate Professor of Medicine and Genetics, University of Pennsylvania School of Medicine; Chief of Gastroenterology, Hospital of the University of Pennsylvania, Philadelphia, Pennsylvania

Neoplasms of the Stomach

MICHAEL S. SAAG, M.D.

Professor of Medicine; Director, AIDS Outpatient Clinic, University of Alabama at Birmingham, Birmingham, Alabama

Mycetoma; Dematiaceous Fungal Infections; Prevention of HIV Infection; Renal, Cardiac, Endocrine, and Rheumatologic Manifestations of AIDS

R. BRADLEY SACK, M.D., Sc.D.

Professor of International Health and Medicine, Johns Hopkins University School of Hygiene and Public Health, Baltimore, Maryland

The Diarrhea of Travelers

ROBERT A. SALATA, M.D.

Professor of Medicine, International Health, Epidemiology and Biostatistics, Case Western Reserve University; Chief, Division of Infectious Diseases, and Medical Director, University Hospitals of Cleveland, Cleveland, Ohio

Brucellosis

SYDNEY E. SALMON, M.D.

Professor of Medicine, University of Arizona School of Medicine, Tucson, Arizona

Principles of Cancer Therapy

JEFFREY H. SAMET, M.D., M.A., M.P.H.

Associate Professor of Medicine and Social and Behavioral Sciences, Boston University Schools of Medicine and Public Health; Medical Director, Addiction Services, Boston Public Health Commission, Boston, Massachusetts

Drug Abuse and Dependence

JONATHAN M. SAMET, M.D., M.S.

Professor and Chairman, Department of Epidemiology, The Johns Hopkins University School of Hygiene and Public Health, Baltimore, Maryland

Occupational Pulmonary Disorders

CLIFFORD B. SAPER, M.D., Ph.D.

James Jackson Putnam Professor of Neurology and Neuroscience, Harvard Medical School; Chairman, Department of Neurology, Beth Israel Deaconess Medical Center, Boston, Massachusetts

Autonomic Disorders and Their Management

FRED RICHARD SATTLER, M.D.

Professor of Medicine, Division of Infectious Diseases, University of Southern California School of Medicine, Los Angeles, California

Pneumocystis carinii Pneumonia

DAVID T. SCADDEN, M.D.

Associate Professor of Medicine, Harvard Medical School; Director, Immunodeficiency Disease Center, Massachusetts General Hospital, Dana-Farber/Partners Cancer Care, Boston, Massachusetts

Hematology/Oncology in AIDS

ANDREW I. SCHAFER, M.D.

The Bob and Vivian Smith Professor and Chair, Department of Medicine, Baylor College of Medicine; Chief, Internal Medicine Service, The Methodist Hospital, Houston, Texas

Approach to the Patient with Bleeding and Thrombosis; Hemorrhagic Disorders: Mixed Abnormalities; Thrombotic Disorders: Hypercoagulable States

BRUCE F. SCHARSCHMIDT, M.D.

Adjunct Professor of Medicine, University of California, San Francisco, San Francisco, California; Vice President, Chiron Corporation, Emeryville, California

Bilirubin Metabolism, Hyperbilirubinemia, and Approach to the Jaundiced Patient

RANDOLPH B. SCHIFFER, M.D.

Chair, Department of Neuropsychiatry and Behavioral Science, Texas Tech University Health Sciences Center; Chief of Service, Neuropsychiatry, University Medical Center, Lubbock, Texas

Psychiatric Disorders in Medical Practice

STEPHEN C. SCHIMPFF, M.D.

Professor of Medicine, Oncology and Pharmacology, University of Maryland School of Medicine; Chief Executive Officer, University of Maryland Medical Center; Executive Vice President, University of Maryland Medical System, Baltimore, Maryland

Diseases Caused by Pseudomonads

DAVID SCHLOSSBERG, M.D.

Professor of Medicine, Jefferson Medical College, Thomas Jefferson University; Director, Department of Medicine, Episcopal Hospital, Philadelphia, Pennsylvania

Mycoplasmal Infection; Arthropods and Leeches

EDWARD L. SCHNEIDER, M.D.

Dean, Leonard Davis School of Gerontology, Andrus Gerontology Center, University of Southern California, Los Angeles, California

Biology of Aging

THOMAS J. SCHNITZER, M.D., Ph.D.

Professor of Medicine and Director, Office of Clinical Research and Training, Northwestern University Medical School, Chicago, Illinois

Osteoarthritis (Degenerative Joint Disease)

ALAN D. SCHREIBER, M.D.

Professor of Medicine and Assistant Dean for Research, University of Pennsylvania School of Medicine, Philadelphia, Pennsylvania

Autoimmune Hemolytic Anemias

THEODORE R. SCHROCK, M.D.

Professor and J. Englebert Dunphy Chair, Department of Surgery, University of California, San Francisco, School of Medicine, San Francisco, California

Diseases of the Rectum and Anus

HARRY W. SCHROEDER, JR., M.D., Ph.D., FACMG

Professor of Medicine and Microbiology, Division of Developmental and Clinical Immunology, Departments of Medicine and Microbiology, University of Alabama at Birmingham, Birmingham, Alabama

Human Heredity

H. RALPH SCHUMACHER, JR., M.D.

Professor of Medicine, University of Pennsylvania School of Medicine; Director, Arthritis-Immunology Center, Veterans Affairs Medical Center, Philadelphia, Pennsylvania

Crystal Deposition Arthropathies; Relapsing Polychondritis; Multifocal Fibrosclerosis

PETER H. SCHUR, M.D.

Professor of Medicine, Harvard Medical School; Senior Physician, Brigham and Women's Hospital, Boston, Massachusetts

Systemic Lupus Erythematosus

CHARLES R. SCRIVER, M.D., C.M.

Alva Professor of Human Genetics and Professor of Pediatrics and Biology, McGill University; Physician and Director (Retired), DeBeve Laboratory of Biochemical Genetics, Montreal Children's Hospital Research Institute, Montreal, Quebec, Canada

The Hyperphenylalaninemias and Alkaptonuria

CYNTHIA L. SEARS, M.D.

Associate Professor, Divisions of Infectious Diseases and Gastroenterology, Department of Medicine, Johns Hopkins University School of Medicine, Baltimore, Maryland

Cryptosporidiosis; Giardiasis

MARGRETTA R. SEASHORE, M.D.

Professor of Genetics and Pediatrics, Yale University School of Medicine; Attending Physician, Yale–New Haven Hospital, New Haven, Connecticut

Genetic Counseling

CAROL E. SEMRAD, M.D.

Assistant Professor of Clinical Medicine, Columbia University College of Physicians and Surgeons; Assistant Attending Physician, New York Presbyterian Hospital, New York, New York

Malabsorption Syndromes

F. JOHN SERVICE, M.D.

Professor of Medicine, Mayo Medical School; Consultant, Division of Endocrinology, Metabolism and Nutrition, Mayo Clinic, Rochester, Minnesota

Hypoglycemia/Pancreatic Islet Cell Disorders

EMMANUEL SHAPIRA, Ph.D., M.D.

Late Director, Human Genetics Program, Karen Gore Chair in Human Genetics, Tulane University Medical School, New Orleans, Louisiana

The Mucopolysaccharidoses

CHARLES L. SHAPIRO, M.D.

Associate Professor of Medicine, Director of Breast Medical Oncology, Ohio State University, Columbus, Ohio

Tumors of the Kidney, Ureter, and Bladder

GEORGE M. SHAW, M.D., Ph.D.

Investigator, Howard Hughes Medical Institute; Director, Division of Hematology/Oncology, University of Alabama at Birmingham, Birmingham, Alabama

Biology of Human Immunodeficiency Viruses

STEVEN A. SHEA, Ph.D.

Assistant Professor of Medicine, Harvard Medical School; Associate Director, Sleep Disorders Program, Brigham and Women's Hospital, Boston, Massachusetts

Disorders of Ventilatory Control

ROBERT S. SHERWIN, M.D.

CNH Long Professor of Medicine, Director, Diabetes Endocrinology Research Center, Yale University School of Medicine; Attending Physician, Yale–New Haven Hospital, New Haven, Connecticut

Diabetes Mellitus

MARGARET A. SHIPP, M.D.

Associate Professor of Medicine, Dana-Farber Cancer Institute, Harvard Medical School, Boston, Massachusetts

Non-Hodgkin's Lymphomas

ROBERT E. SHOPE, M.D.

Professor of Pathology, University of Texas Medical Branch, Galveston, Texas

Introduction to Hemorrhagic Fever Viruses

JONAS A. SHULMAN, M.D.

Executive Associate Dean for Medical Education and Student Affairs, Professor of Medicine (Infectious Diseases), Emory University School of Medicine, Atlanta, Georgia

Anthrax

MARC SHUMAN, M.D.

Professor of Medicine, University of California, San Francisco; Chief of Hematology-Oncology, University of California Medical Center and Moffitt and Long Hospitals, San Francisco, California

Hemorrhagic Disorders: Abnormalities of Platelet and Vascular Function

MARK SIEGLER, M.D.

Lindy Bergman Professor of Medicine and Director, MacLean Center for Clinical Medical Ethics, University of Chicago, Chicago, Illinois

Clinical Ethics in the Practice of Medicine

MURRAY N. SILVERSTEIN, M.D.

Professor of Medicine, Mayo Medical School; Consultant, Division of Hematology and Internal Medicine, Mayo Clinic and Mayo Foundation, Rochester, Minnesota

Myeloproliferative Diseases

MICHAEL S. SIMBERKOFF, M.D.

Associate Professor of Medicine, New York University School of Medicine; Chief of Staff, Department of Veterans Affairs, New York Harbor Health Care System, New York Campus, New York, New York

Infections Caused by Haemophilus *Species*

ROGER P. SIMON, M.D.

Professor of Neurology, University of Pittsburgh, Pittsburgh, Pennsylvania

Disturbances of Consciousness and Arousal; Sustained Impairments of Consciousness; Brain Death; Brief Loss of Consciousness; Disorders of Sleep and Arousal; Parameningeal Infections; Neurosyphilis

JOSEPH V. SIMONE, M.D.

Professor of Pediatrics and Medicine, University of Utah; Medical Director, Huntsman Cancer Foundation and Institute, Salt Lake City, Utah

Introduction to Oncology

MARK I. SINGER, M.D.

Professor and Vice-Chairman, Department of Otolaryngology–Head and Neck Surgery, University of California, San Francisco, San Francisco, California

Head and Neck Cancer

PETER A. SINGER, M.D., M.P.H., FRCPC

Sun Life Chair and Director, University of Toronto Joint Centre for Bioethics; Staff Physician, The Toronto Hospital, Toronto, Ontario, Canada

Clinical Ethics in the Practice of Medicine

DELIA SMITH, Ph.D.

Associate Professor, University of Alabama at Birmingham School of Medicine, Birmingham, Alabama

The Eating Disorders

WILLIAM J. SNAPE, JR., M.D.

Clinical Professor of Medicine, University of California, Irvine, Irvine; Director, Motility Center, Long Beach Memorial Medical Center, Long Beach, California

Disorders of Gastrointestinal Motility

BURTON E. SOBEL, M.D.

E.L. Amidon Professor and Chair, Department of Medicine, College of Medicine; Professor of Biochemistry, University of Vermont; Physician-in-Chief, Medicine Health Care Service, Fletcher Allan Health Care, Burlington, Vermont

Acute Myocardial Infarction

KONRAD H. SOERGEL, M.D.

Professor of Medicine and Physiology, Department of Medicine, Division of Gastroenterology and Hepatology, Medical College of Wisconsin; Physician, Froedtert Memorial Lutheran Hospital, Milwaukee, Wisconsin

Pancreatitis

ANDREW H. SOLL, M.D.

Professor of Medicine, University of California, Los Angeles, School of Medicine; Staff Physician, Veterans Affairs of Greater Los Angeles Health Care System, West Los Angeles, California

Gastritis and Helicobacter pylori; Peptic Ulcer Disease: Epidemiology, Pathophysiology, Clinical Manifestations, and Diagnosis

P. FREDERICK SPARLING, M.D.

Professor of Medicine and Microbiology and Immunology, University of North Carolina School of Medicine, Chapel Hill, North Carolina

Introduction to Sexually Transmitted Diseases and Common Syndromes; Gonococcal Infections

STEPHEN A. SPECTOR, M.D.

Professor of Pediatrics and Chief, Division of Infectious Diseases; Member, Center of Molecular Genetics and Center for AIDS Research, University of California, San Diego, La Jolla, California

HIV in Pregnancy

ALLEN M. SPIEGEL, M.D.

Chief, Metabolic Diseases Branch, National Institute of Diabetes and Digestive and Kidney Diseases, National Institutes of Health, Bethesda, Maryland

The Parathyroid Glands, Hypercalcemia, and Hypocalcemia

ALAN M. STAMM, M.D.

Associate Professor of Medicine, University of Alabama at Birmingham; Attending Physician, University of Alabama at Birmingham Health System, Birmingham, Alabama

Listeriosis

DANIEL STEINBERG, M.D., Ph.D.

Professor of Medicine, University of California, San Diego, School of Medicine, La Jolla, California

The Hyperlipoproteinemias

WILLIAM F. STENSON, M.D.

Professor of Medicine, Washington University School of Medicine; Attending Physician, Barnes-Jewish Hospital, St. Louis, Missouri

Inflammatory Bowel Disease

DAVID A. STEVENS, M.D.

Professor of Medicine and Associate Chief of the Division of Infectious Diseases and Geographic Medicine, Stanford University Medical School, Stanford; Chief, Division of Infectious Diseases, Department of Medicine, Santa Clara Valley Medical Center, San Jose, California

Aspergillosis; Mucormycosis

DENNIS L. STEVENS, M.D., Ph.D.

Professor of Medicine, University of Washington School of Medicine, Seattle, Washington; Chief, Infectious Diseases, Veterans Affairs Medical Center, Infectious Disease Section, Boise, Idaho

Streptococcal Infections; Clostridial Myonecrosis and Other Clostridial Diseases

LYNNE WARNER STEVENSON, M.D.

Associate Professor of Medicine, Harvard Medical School; Director, Cardiomyopathy and Heart Failure Program, Brigham and Women's Hospital, Boston, Massachusetts

Diseases of the Myocardium

KINGMAN P. STROHL, M.D.

Professor of Medicine and Anatomy, Case Western Reserve University; Director, Center for Sleep Disorders Research, Veterans Affairs Medical Center, Cleveland, Ohio

Obstructive Sleep Apnea-Hypopnea Syndrome; Upper Airway Diseases

WADI N. SUKI, M.D.

Professor of Medicine, and of Molecular Physiology and Biophysics, and Chief, Renal Section, Baylor College of Medicine; Chief, Renal Service, The Methodist Hospital, Houston, Texas

Phosphorus Deficiency and Hypophosphatemia

JOHN B. SULLIVAN, JR., M.D.

Associate Professor and Associate Dean, University of Arizona Health Sciences Center, Tucson, Arizona

Venomous Snake Bites

WARREN R. SUMMER, M.D.

Howard A. Buechner Professor of Medicine, Louisiana State University; Chief of Pulmonary and Critical Care Medicine, Oechsner Medical Institutions, New Orleans, Louisiana

Respiratory Failure

MARIA J. SUNSERI, M.D.

Sleep Disorders Center, Pittsburgh, Pennsylvania

Disorders of Sleep and Arousal

ROLAND W. SUTTER, M.D., M.P.H. & T.M.

Acting Chief, Technical Services Branch, Vaccine Preventable Disease Eradication Division, National Immunization Program, Centers for Disease Control and Prevention, Atlanta, Georgia

Diphtheria

MORTON N. SWARTZ, M.D.

Professor of Medicine, Harvard Medical School; Chief, Jackson Firm of Medical Services, and Chief, Emeritus, Infectious Disease Unit, Massachusetts General Hospital, Boston, Massachusetts

Bacterial Meningitis

RONALD S. SWERDLOFF, M.D.

Professor of Medicine, Associate Chair of Department of Medicine, and Chief of Division of Endocrinology, University of California, Los Angeles, School of Medicine and Harbor-UCLA Medical Center; Director, Mellon Foundation Reproductive Biology Center, and Director, WHO Collaborating Center in Reproductive Biology, Harbor-UCLA Research and Education Institute, Torrance, California

The Testis and Male Sexual Function

NICHOLAS J. TALLEY, M.D., Ph.D.

Department of Medicine, University of Sydney, Sydney; Head, Division of Medicine, Nepean Hospital, Penrith, Australia

Functional Gastrointestinal Disorders: Irritable Bowel Syndrome, Non-Ulcer Dyspepsia, and Non-cardiac Chest Pain

VICTOR F. TAPSON, M.D.

Associate Professor of Medicine, Duke University School of Medicine; Medical Director, Duke University Lung Transplant Program, and Director, Pulmonary Outpatient Clinic, Duke University Medical Center, Durham, North Carolina

Pulmonary Embolism

WILLIAM R. TAYLOR, M.D.

Assistant Professor, University of California, San Diego, California

Spine and Spinal Cord Injury

AYALEW TEFFERI, M.D.

Associate Professor of Medicine, Mayo Medical School; Consultant, Division of Hematology and Internal Medicine, Mayo Clinic and Mayo Foundation, Rochester, Minnesota

Myeloproliferative Diseases

PIERRE THÉROUX, M.D.

Professor of Medicine, University of Montreal, Montreal Heart Institute Research Department, Montreal, Quebec, Canada

Angina Pectoris

C. CRAIG TISHER, M.D.

Professor of Medicine and Pathology, Folke H. Peterson Dean's Distinguished Professorship, and Senior Associate Dean, University of Florida College of Medicine; Attending Physician, Shands Hospital, Gainesville, Florida

Structure and Function of the Kidneys

GALEN B. TOEWS, M.D.

Professor of Internal Medicine, University of Michigan Medical School; Chief, Division of Pulmonary and Critical Care Medicine, University of Michigan Health System, Ann Arbor, Michigan

Interstitial Lung Disease

JOHN J. TREANOR, M.D.

Associate Professor of Medicine, Infectious Diseases Unit, University of Rochester, School of Medicine and Dentistry, Rochester, New York

Adenovirus Diseases

GERARD M. TURINO, M.D.

John H. Keating, Sr., Professor of Medicine, Columbia University College of Physicians and Surgeons; Director, James P. Mara Center for Lung Disease, St. Luke's–Roosevelt Hospital, New York, New York

Approach to the Patient with Respiratory Disease

MARK M. UDDEN, M.D.

Associate Professor of Medicine, Baylor College of Medicine; Attending Physician, Ben Taub General Hospital, Houston, Texas

Intravascular Hemolytic Anemias

ARTHUR C. UPTON, M.D.

Clinical Professor of Environmental and Community Medicine, University of Medicine and Dentistry of New Jersey, Robert Wood Johnson Medical School, Piscataway, New Jersey; Professor Emeritus, Department of Environmental Medicine, New York University School of Medicine, New York, New York

Radiation Injury

MARGOT I. VAN ALLEN, M.D., M.Sc.

Clinical Professor, Department of Medical Genetics, University of British Columbia; Senior Staff Geneticist, Provincial Medical Genetic Program, British Columbia's Children's Hospital, Vancouver, British Columbia, Canada

Congenital Anomalies

NICHOLAS A. VICK, M.D.

Professor of Neurology, Northwestern University; Head, Division of Neurology, Evanston Northwestern Healthcare, Evanston, Illinois

Intracranial Tumors; Specific Types of Brain Tumors and Their Management; Neoplasms of the Spinal Canal; Disorders of Intracranial Pressure

Z. RENO VLAHCEVIC, M.D.

Charles Caravati Professor of Medicine and Chairman, Division of Gastroenterology, Medical College of Virginia of Virginia Commonwealth University; Chief, Section of Gastroenterology, Medical College of Virginia and McGuire Department of Veterans Affairs Medical Center, Richmond, Virginia

Diseases of the Gallbladder and Bile Ducts

JOHN E. VOLANAKIS, M.D.

Professor, Department of Medicine, University of Alabama at Birmingham Medical School, Birmingham, Alabama; Scientific Director, Biomedical Sciences Research Center "A. Fleming," Athens, Greece

Complement

BRUCE D. WALKER, M.D.

Associate Professor, Harvard Medical School, Boston; Director, AIDS Research Center, Massachusetts General Hospital, Charlestown, Massachusetts

Immunology Related to AIDS

EDWARD E. WALSH, M.D.

Professor of Medicine, University of Rochester School of Medicine and Dentistry; Physician, Department of Medicine, Rochester General Hospital, Rochester, New York

Respiratory Syncytial Virus; Parainfluenza Viral Diseases

CHRISTINA WANG, M.D.

Professor of Medicine, University of California, Los Angeles, School of Medicine; Director, General Clinical Research Center, Harbor-UCLA Medical Center and Research and Education Institute, Torrance, California

The Testis and Male Sexual Function

STEVEN E. WEINBERGER, M.D.

Professor of Medicine, Harvard Medical School; Vice Chairman, Department of Medicine, Beth Israel Deaconess Medical Center, Boston, Massachusetts

Sarcoidosis

ROLAND L. WEINSIER, M.D., Dr.P.H.

C.E. Butterworth, Jr., Professor and Chair, Department of Nutrition Sciences, University of Alabama at Birmingham, Birmingham, Alabama

Diet

MYRON L. WEISFELDT, M.D.

Professor of Medicine and Chairman, Department of Medicine, Columbia University College of Physicians and Surgeons, New York, New York

Cardiac Function and Circulatory Control

RICHARD A. WEISIGER, M.D., Ph.D.

Professor of Medicine and Chief, Gastroenterology Faculty Practice, University of California, San Francisco, San Francisco, California

Hepatic Metabolism in Liver Disease; Laboratory Tests in Liver Disease and Approach to the Patient with Abnormal Tests

GERALD WEISSMAN, M.D.

Professor of Medicine and Director, Division of Rheumatology, New York University School of Medicine, New York, New York

NSAIDs: Aspirin and Aspirin-like Drugs; Tissue Injury in Rheumatic Diseases

PETER F. WELLER, M.D.

Professor of Medicine, Department of Medicine, Harvard Medical School; Chief, Division of Allergy and Inflammation; Co-Chief, Division of Infectious Diseases, Department of Medicine, Beth Israel Deaconess Medical Center, Boston, Massachusetts

Eosinophilic Syndromes

MICHAEL J. WELSH, M.D.

Professor of Medicine and of Physiology and Biophysics, University of Iowa College of Medicine; Investigator, Howard Hughes Medical Institute, Iowa City, Iowa

Cystic Fibrosis

JOHN E. WENNBERG, M.D., M.P.H.

Peggy Y. Thomson Professor for the Evaluative Clinical Sciences, Professor of Medicine, and Professor of Community and Family Medicine (Epidemiology), Dartmouth Medical School, Hanover, New Hampshire

Social and Economic Issues in Medicine

DAVID P. WHITE, M.D.

Associate Professor of Medicine, Harvard Medical School; Director, Sleep Disorders Program, Brigham and Women's Hospital, Boston, Massachusetts

Disorders of Ventilatory Control

RICHARD J. WHITLEY, M.D.

Professor of Pediatrics, Microbiology, and Medicine and Loeb Eminent Scholar Chair in Pediatrics, University of Alabama at Birmingham, Birmingham, Alabama

Antiviral Therapy (Non-AIDS); Herpes Simplex Virus Infections

MICHAEL P. WHYTE, M.D.

Professor of Medicine, Pediatrics, and Genetics, Washington University School of Medicine; Director, Metabolic Research Unit, Shriners Hospital for Children, St. Louis, Missouri

Osteonecrosis, Osteosclerosis/Hyperostosis and Other Disorders of Bone

FREDRICK M. WIGLEY, M.D.

Professor of Medicine and Director, Division of Rheumatology, Johns Hopkins University, Baltimore, Maryland

Scleroderma (Systemic Sclerosis)

C. MEL WILCOX, M.D.

Associate Professor of Medicine and Director of Clinical Research, Division of Gastroenterology and Hepatology; Chief of Endoscopy, University of Alabama at Birmingham, Birmingham, Alabama

Miscellaneous Inflammatory Diseases of the Intestine

GERHARD R. WITTICH, M.D.

Professor of Radiology, University of Texas Medical Branch, Galveston, Texas

Diagnostic Imaging Procedures in Gastroenterology

JOSEPH L. WITZTUM, M.D.

Professor of Medicine, University of California, San Diego, School of Medicine, La Jolla, California

The Hyperlipoproteinemias

RAYMOND L. WOOSLEY, M.D., Ph.D.

Professor of Pharmacology and Medicine and Chairman, Department of Pharmacology, Georgetown University Medical Center, Washington, D.C.

Antiarrhythmic Drugs

ROBERT L. WORTMANN, M.D.

Professor and Chairman, Department of Internal Medicine, The University of Oklahoma College of Medicine—Tulsa, Tulsa, Oklahoma

Idiopathic Inflammatory Myopathies

ALBERT W. WU, M.D., M.P.H.

Associate Professor, Department of Health Policy and Management; Joint Appointment: Medicine; Epidemiology, School of Hygiene and Public Health and School of Medicine, Johns Hopkins University; Attending Physician, Johns Hopkins Hospital, Baltimore, Maryland

Principles of Outcome Assessment

JOSHUA WYNNE, M.D., M.B.A.

Professor of Medicine, Wayne State University, Detroit, Michigan

Miscellaneous Conditions of the Heart: Tumor, Trauma, and Systemic Disease

JOACHIM YAHALOM, M.D.

Professor of Radiation Oncology in Medicine, Weill Medical College of Cornell University; Member and Attending, Memorial Sloan-Kettering Cancer Center, New York, New York

Hodgkin's Disease

ROBERT YARCHOAN, M.D.

Chief, HIV and AIDS Malignancy Branch, Division of Clinical Sciences, National Cancer Institute, National Institutes of Health, Bethesda, Maryland

Treatment of HIV Infection and AIDS

ERNEST L. YODER, M.D., Ph.D.

Associate Chair, Education, Department of Internal Medicine, Wayne State University School of Medicine, Detroit, Michigan

Disorders Due to Heat and Cold

NEAL S. YOUNG, M.D.

Chief, Hematology Branch, National Heart, Lung, and Blood Institute, National Institutes of Health, Bethesda, Maryland

Aplastic Anemia and Related Bone Marrow Failure Syndromes

ELIZABETH J. ZIEGLER, M.D.

Professor of Medicine, Division of Infectious Diseases, University of California, San Diego, School of Medicine, La Jolla; Attending Physician and Chief, Infectious Disease Clinic, University of California, San Diego, Medical Center, San Diego, California

Extraintestinal Infections Caused by Enteric Bacteria

KENNETH S. ZUCKERMAN, M.D.

Harold H. Davis Professor of Cancer Research, Professor of Internal Medicine and of Biochemistry and Molecular Biology, and Director, Division of Medical Oncology and Hematology, University of South Florida College of Medicine; Chief, Medicine Service, H. Lee Moffitt Cancer Center and Research Institute, Tampa, Florida

Approach to the Anemias

PREFACE

As the 21st edition of *Cecil Textbook of Medicine* ushers in the 21st century, medicine has never been more exciting and challenging. Extraordinary advances in diagnostic and therapeutic modalities, triggered by advances in molecular and cellular biology, are revolutionizing the scientific basis of medicine. One of the highest priorities of this edition is the incorporation of these molecular and cellular advances into a comprehensive yet easily understandable description of the modern pathophysiologic basis of disease. Simultaneously, medicine has seen equally revolutionary advances in the application of methodologies such as the randomized control trial, the measurement of quality-of-life, and an understanding of cost effectiveness as they apply to clinical medicine. This new edition also emphasizes the application of this new information via the concept of evidence-based medicine to clinical decision-making. This dual emphasis—molecular biology and evidence-based medicine—permeates the entire fabric of this work. Increased use of flow diagrams to guide diagnostic and therapeutic decision making is a natural outgrowth of these advances.

Just as each edition brings new authors, it also reminds us of our gratitude to past editors and authors. Previous editors of *Cecil Textbook of Medicine* include Russell Cecil, Paul Beeson, Walsh McDermott, James Wyngaarden, H. Lloyd Smith, and Fred Plum. As we welcome three new associate editors—Jeffrey M. Drazen, Don W. Powell, and Andrew I. Schafer—we also express our appreciation to editors from the previous edition on whose foundation we have built. Special appreciation is due to Fred Plum, who served as consulting editor for the neurology section for eight editions and as co-editor for the 20th edition. We also thank Robert Ockner, who served as consulting editor for gastrointestinal diseases and diseases of the liver, gallbladder, and bile ducts. We also wish to express our deepest personal gratitude to the late Thomas W. Smith, who was consulting editor for cardiovascular diseases, respiratory diseases, and critical care medicine. Our returning consulting editors for this edition, Gerald L. Mandell, Gordon N. Gill, and Juha P. Kokko, continue to make critical contributions to the selection of authors and the review of selected manuscripts. The editors, however, are fully responsible for the book as well as the integration among chapters.

This edition includes a new part on women's health, a new part on eye, ear, nose, and throat diseases, and a substantially expanded part on critical care medicine. Thirty-five chapters are totally new and address important aspects of medicine. The new chapters of this edition include "Antiarrhythmic Drugs," "Coronary Angioplasty," "Obstructive Sleep Apnea-Hypopnea Syndrome," "Ventilator Management in the Intensive Care Unit," "Rhabdomyolysis," "Urinary Incontinence," "Approach to the Patient with Gastrointestinal Disease," "Hematopoiesis and Hematopoietic Growth Factors," "Approach to the Patient with Lymphadenopathy and Splenomegaly," "Approach to Women's Health," "HIV in Pregnancy," "Menopause," "Cervical and Uterine Cancer Screening," and "Neurogenetics." Overall, this edition has 124 new authors, as well as 335 returning authors.

The tradition of *Cecil Textbook of Medicine* is that all chapters are written by distinguished experts in each field. We would also like to take this opportunity to thank several junior physicians who assisted these individuals on specific chapters: Graham Pineo ("Peripheral Venous Disease"), Eric van Sonnenberg and Brian W. Goodacre ("Diagnostic Imaging Procedures in Gastroenterology"), Sergei Kantsevoy ("Acute and Chronic Liver Failure and Hepatic Encephalopathy"), Miguel Arguedas ("Hepatic Tumors"), William Delgado ("Examination of the Skin and an Approach to Diagnosing Skin Disease" and "Skin Diseases of General Importance"), and Robert Sidbury ("Principles of Therapy" and "Skin Diseases of General Importance"). We are also most grateful for the editorial assistance in San Francisco of Stephanie Webb and in Birmingham of Cheryl Dunlap; these individuals have shown extraordinary dedication and equanimity in managing the unending flow of manuscripts, disks, figures, and permissions. At W.B. Saunders Company, Les Hoeltzel, Lynne Gery, Frank Polizzano, Tom Stringer, Jonel Sofian, and Peg Shaw have been critical to the planning and production process under the direction of Lisette Bralow, to whom we are also most indebted. Finally, we would like to thank our families—Jill, Nancy, Jeff, Daniel, Robyn, and Katya, Miller, and Clark and their respective spouses David, Philip, and Margie—for their understanding of the time and focus required to edit a book that attempts to sustain the tradition of our predecessors and to meet the needs of today's physician.

LEE GOLDMAN, M.D.
J. CLAUDE BENNETT, M.D.

NOTICE

Medicine is an ever-changing field. Standard safety precautions must be followed, but as new research and clinical experience broaden our knowledge, changes in treatment and drug therapy become necessary or appropriate. Readers are advised to check the product information currently provided by the manufacturer of each drug to be administered to verify the recommended dose, the method and duration of administration, and the contra-indications. It is the responsibility of the treating physician relying on experience and knowledge of the patient to determine dosages and the best treatment for the patient. Neither the Publisher nor the editor assumes any responsibility for any injury and/or damage to persons or property.

THE PUBLISHER

CONTENTS

PART XIII: HEMATOLOGIC DISEASES

PART XIV: ONCOLOGY

PART XV: METABOLIC DISEASES

PART XVI: NUTRITIONAL DISEASES

PART XVII: ENDOCRINE DISEASES

PART XXIII: HIV AND THE ACQUIRED
IMMUNODEFICIENCY SYNDROME

COLOR PLATES

PART I

MEDICINE AS A LEARNED AND HUMANE PROFESSION

1 MEDICINE AS A LEARNED AND HUMANE PROFESSION

Lee Goldman ▪ *Fred Plum*
▪ *J. Claude Bennett*

Becoming a physician has meaning far beyond completing medical school and residency. It is the entry to a way of life, the one characteristic common to every true profession. It may sound old-fashioned, but the learned professions are really "callings" from which the members cannot separate their lives. There are no part-time professionals; having accepted such a calling, one is bound to live it or leave it. A physician can also be a good spouse, a good parent, and a good citizen of the community; however, the role of spouse, parent, and citizen is inextricably intertwined with the calling of being a physician.

THE SCIENTIFIC INFRASTRUCTURE OF MEDICINE

Medicine is not a science, but a profession that encompasses medical science as well as personal, humanistic, and professional attributes. Nonetheless, the delivery of Western medicine depends totally on science and the scientific method. Since Flexner issued his famous report on the subject in 1910, American medical education has striven to develop a strong scientific base as an integral part of medical education at every level: pre-medical, medical, residency, and continuing medical education. Biomedical science is fundamental to understanding disease, making diagnoses, applying new therapies, and appreciating the complexities and opportunities of new technologies. The process of becoming a physician and being committed to lifelong learning requires that an individual possess the scientific base not only to acquire and appreciate new knowledge but also to see new ways for applying it to patient care. The physician must be able to understand reports of current research in the medical literature to grasp and evaluate the newest and latest approaches, no matter how complicated the field may become.

This textbook of medicine strongly emphasizes how things work, how they go awry when pathologic processes ensue, and what effect a given therapy can be expected to have in correcting abnormalities. We seek to create in our readers a yearning for a greater depth of understanding and a continuing commitment to stay at the frontier of scientific knowledge throughout their professional lives.

Medicine has advanced to an outstanding degree in the past half century. (The 100 years from 1850 to 1950 were characterized—with the important exceptions of the discovery of penicillin, sulfonamides, and insulin—by the application of chemistry and physics to biologic materials, e.g., blood and urine, or to the body, e.g., roentgenography and sphygmomanometry, and by the empiric use of medicinal chemicals.) The advances of the last 50 years have come at the most fundamental levels of science and have reflected the general explosion in scientific knowledge world-wide.

True understanding of disease processes depends on levels of scientific knowledge that are just being discovered. For example, an understanding of how proteins are synthesized, fold into their native conformation, and express their various physical properties leads to an understanding of why erythrocytes sickle, the complexities of amyloid formation and how it influences organ function, the nature of protein aggregation as a fundamental process of Alzheimer's disease, and the importance of protein-protein interaction in transmitting messages across cell membranes, within the cytoplasm, and to the nucleus of cells. An appreciation for the way G proteins function explains membrane transport, how messages transfer from the outside to the inside of cells, how microbial toxins operate, how hormones influence cell action, and how cells respond to external stimuli and are regulated in their response. Knowledge of the basic processes of DNA synthesis, mutation, and somatic alteration of gene expression explains inherited diseases and diseases that have their fundamental processes expressed in a continuous pattern of somatic alteration within a given individual. Fundamental science is crucial as a knowledge base for any member of our profession. Fortunately, for a physician studying and learning in this complex environment, medical science has become so fundamental that an understanding of a few basic and critical processes can provide insight into a wide variety of diseases.

A list of major clinical achievements in any particular branch of medicine reveals that more than 60% of the enabling discoveries arise from the category of very basic science and that these discoveries were initially made without any particular notion of how they might be applied to human disease. Breakthroughs in infectious diseases, the regulation of blood pressure, fundamental immunology, fundamental genetics, and metabolic regulation by hormones represent milestones in the course of medical history that now provide the tools to help unravel the intricacies of human disease. Despite unbelievable successes, many diseases continue to elude absolute answers: Cancer, Alzheimer's disease, many autoimmune diseases, and most psychiatric diseases are just some examples. Nonetheless, the clues now being ferreted out at the molecular level anticipate solutions of even these disorders, realistically filling future expectations with excitement and anticipation.

The scientific infrastructure that we appreciate today is the springboard for the future in which most of the readers of *Cecil Textbook of Medicine,* 21st edition, will practice. Throughout most of the recorded history of medicine, diagnoses and therapies have not been based on scientific fact, and the degree of certainty with which physicians worked was inexact, if not totally flawed. However, this situation has entirely changed: By 150 years ago things were beginning to change, and by the 20 years spanning the turn of the century, the first fundamental lights began to illuminate the "golden age of microbiology." During this period, Pasteur, working in Paris, and Robert Koch, working in Berlin, began to unravel the intricacies of infectious diseases. To define microorganisms, to understand how they cause infection and transmit diseases, and to understand the host response represented a turning point and forever established the scientific method as the basis for understanding and treating disease. It is an amazing experience to read the scientific papers from Paris and Berlin at that time because in a relatively short period those two schools of thought set us on a pathway from which medicine can never depart—that of demanding precision, of requiring experimental proof, and of building confidence by accumulating irrefutable data.

Today's medicine is more than intuition and common sense. It is precision based on a century or more of refining definitions of disease in highly specific terms. We now experience these "golden ages" in more rapid order: the discovery of antibiotics less than 60 years ago; an understanding of immunology in molecular terms within the last 30 years; and now in genetics, not just knowledge at the molecular level, but understanding how to manipulate genes for the immediate benefit of mankind.

We are indeed in the age of molecular-biophysical medicine, an influence that permeates and unifies all the traditional disciplines of medicine. Whether one is talking about inborn errors of metabolism, neurotransmitters, cytokines, oncogenes, or hormone regulation, all are being defined with exquisite detail at the molecular level. Programs aimed toward the goal of the human genome project—to sequence all the DNA within the entire genome—are moving forward with accelerating speed. The ability to define every gene, its product, and its role and explicit function has become a shared international goal.

Concurrent with these advances in fundamental human biology has been a dramatic shift in the methods for evaluating the application of scientific advances to the patient and to populations. The randomized control trial, sometimes with thousands of patients at multiple institutions, has replaced anecdote as the preferred method for measuring the benefits and uses of diagnostic or therapeutic interventions. As studies progress from those that demonstrate biologic effect, to those that elucidate dosing schedules and toxicity, and finally to those that assess true clinical benefit, the metrics of measuring outcome have also improved from subjective impressions of physicians or patients to reliable and valid measures of morbidity, quality of life, functional status, and other patient-oriented outcomes. These marked improvements in the scientific methodology of clinical investigation have expedited extraordinary changes in clinical practice, such as reperfusion therapy for acute myocardial infarction, and have demonstrated that reliance on intermediate outcomes, such as a reduction in asymptomatic ventricular arrhythmias with certain drugs, may unexpectedly increase rather than decrease mortality. Just as the physician for the twenty-first century must understand advances in fundamental biology, a similar understanding is needed of the fundamentals of clinical study design as it applies to diagnostic and therapeutic interventions.

This pattern of attaining scientific knowledge, beginning with a sick patient and moving first in a reductionist process to individual molecules and fundamental biochemical processes and then back toward an evaluation of scientifically based diagnostic and therapeutic advances, should not reduce our appreciation for the other contributors to the human condition. Advances in molecular and structural biology and the wonders of immunology and genetics must not allow us to neglect the many aspects of human psychology, anthropology, and sociology that influence the world in which we live and that play such a major role in morbidity and eventual mortality. According to the National Center for Health Statistics, behavioral causes—including alcohol, drugs, violence, suicide, smoking, and excessive aggression—generate more than half the cost to the nation for health care. We are only just beginning to grasp the impact of these factors on our nation and the world. In our joy—and sometimes arrogant pride—over achievements in molecular medicine and randomized controlled trials, we must also humbly realize that the sciences that analyze human or population behavior and attempt to improve it, as well as the way that society is structured, are indispensable to the future of medicine and must be incorporated into the discipline of our profession.

THE PHYSICIAN AS A SCIENTIST

To use scientific medicine correctly, physicians must be trained as scientists to understand and apply the thinking patterns of the scientific method, to develop an inquiring mind, to know how to design experiments and obtain data, to learn how to analyze the validity and generalizability of those data, and to use this knowledge to ask questions and provide truthful answers within defined limits of precision. Biomedical science becomes the working instrument for the physician who, by definition, practices an analytic profession. Most of these learned skills extend to the management of individual cases at the bedside, i.e., how to gather information, how to synthesize it, how to interpret it to make a full diagnostic story, and how to bring collective wisdom together in the design and execution of appropriate therapy. A central tenet of all sciences is to constantly ask, "Could my conclusion be wrong?" The rigors

of the scientific method also provide the physician with learning skills and a process of analysis that are indispensable for dealing with individual patients, as well as provide the opportunity to contribute to medical progress and the improvement of care.

The explosion in medical knowledge has led to increasing specialization and subspecialization, defined initially by organ system and more recently by locus of principal activity (inpatient as compared with outpatient), reliance on manual skills (proceduralist as compared with nonproceduralist), or participation in research. More recently, however, it is becoming increasingly clear that the same fundamental molecular and genetic mechanisms are broadly applicable across all organ systems and that the scientific methodologies of randomized trials and careful clinical observation span all aspects of medicine. Every physician must delight in learning the new, correcting the old, and perfecting the future. Much of what medicine now accomplishes depends on large-scale testing of procedures, interventions, vaccines, and new drugs. The fact that many such studies must be conducted in large populations through a multicenter approach provides an opportunity for all physicians to participate in clinical investigation in some way at some time in their professional careers. Indeed, this step is essential for the future of medicine and for physicians to move forward together as a profession.

The patient-physician interaction proceeds through a number of phases of clinical reasoning and decision making. The interaction begins with an elucidation of complaints or concerns, followed by inquiries or evaluation to address these concerns in increasingly precise ways. The process commonly requires a careful history or physical examination, ordering of diagnostic tests, integration of clinical findings with the test results, understanding of the risks and benefits of the possible courses of action, and careful consultation with the patient and family to develop future plans. Physicians can increasingly call on a growing literature of evidence-based medicine to guide the process so that benefit is maximized while respecting individual variations among different patients. When this process is approached in a rigorous scientific manner, which does not mean coldly or impersonally, the results become reproducible and generalizable over time. New information, new techniques, and new technology can be brought into the process and their contribution evaluated in a conceptualization of the scientific method often termed *continuous quality improvement*. Through such constant commitment to advancing the frontiers of medicine, physicians improve health, discover true cures, devise new ways of delivering care, and reduce ultimate health costs.

THE PHYSICIAN AS CAREGIVER

Being both professional and caring is an acquired skill. A physician can diagnose and prescribe in a technically correct and scientific, but insensitive way. The patient may be made better, even cured, but still feel unsatisfied with the interaction. In these cases, patients are likely to ask the questions: Does my physician really care? Does what happens to me matter to the physician? Does my doctor show sensitivity and compassion beyond mere technical ability? Patients want and deserve compassion and understanding. They want their physicians to be interested in them as individuals who seek advice, as well as relief from pain, disease, and suffering. They want to sense that they can safely share their deepest thoughts and their most heartfelt confidences with their physicians. In short, they want to value their physician as a trusted friend. Patients also expect to be kept informed while they are receiving competent professional service. As a caregiver, it is this sharing of oneself that is so very important.

To some it may seem odd to talk about caring as a learned skill, but it is just that. In studying to be a physician, one must learn both compassion and caring. Easy, supportive interaction with patients and others less fortunate is a skill that comes readily for some and with great difficulty for others. In learning how to demonstrate compassion, Kahlil Gibran taught us: "You give but little when you give of your possessions—it is when you give of yourself that you truly give" (*The Prophet*). The giving of oneself with ease, with grace, and with meaning is, for most persons, an acquired skill. Sometimes a deep sense of awakening within is required to release the innate sensitivity and compassion that perhaps have not been expressed since childhood. Nevertheless, these traits remain imperatives if the aim is to become a "complete physician."

When patients seek medical attention, they entrust their doctors with their very lives. The physician must earn such complete trust. Technical abilities and skilled treatment of disease alone do not suffice. Patients must believe that their physicians care about them as people, not just as patients. Physicians, in turn, must understand that they do far better as professionals if they err on the side of being human with their patients. Dag Hammarskjöld told us of "the humility that comes from others having faith in you." Without that touch of humility, physicians may be unable to understand and accept the trust that patients place in us. The physician must be willing to answer the patient's needs and also willing to undertake a long-term commitment to the patient's care. This commitment continues beyond a single insightful diagnosis or the completion of a procedure. The patient still needs care when the data come back from the clinical laboratory, the radiology department, the cardiac catheterization laboratory, or the surgical pathology laboratory. Patients continue to need help in understanding their disease, in dealing with family interactions, and in finding a caring ear when they suffer most. They often need assistance in obtaining necessary additional medical help from specialists or consultants and personal help in dealing with processes involving families and personal situations. Many patients need a link to community or social support systems. A particularly difficult time comes as physicians deal with patients who become old, frail, dependent, crippled, or cognitively impaired. These are the circumstances from which the most sensitive among us truly learn what it means to give of ourselves. Sometimes we may find once again that our patients are the best teachers.

THE PHYSICIAN AS A PROFESSIONAL

To help orient our professional compass, the American Board of Internal Medicine has promulgated a definition of "professionalism":

Definition: Professionalism in internal medicine comprises those attributes and behaviors that serve to maintain the interest of the patient above one's own self-interest.
- A commitment to the highest standards of excellence in the practice of medicine and in the generation and dissemination of knowledge.
- A commitment to the attitudes and behaviors that sustain the interests and welfare of patients.
- A commitment to be responsive to the health needs of society. Professionalism aspires to altruism, accountability, excellence, duty, service, honor, integrity, and respect for others.

The interest of the patient lies above self-interest—an indispensable attribute not only of medicine but of all professions. It has to do with our personal behavior transcending our technical abilities, our scientific knowledge, and even our attitudes of compassion and caring. What it means is that we offer to others a special sensitivity—whether they be physician colleagues, students, residents, nonphysician caregivers, patients, or their families. To remain professionals, dignity and understanding must permeate all our interactions—all our thinking, teaching, learning, and listening.

SYSTEMS OF PATIENT CARE FOR THE MILLENNIUM AND BEYOND

Students of medicine learn by didactics, observation, and directed participation. As they pass into residency, the avenues of participation become an increasingly independent course of training. In this intellectual experience of growing independence, young physicians learn how to analyze information, organize it, render compassionate and considered care, and deal with their professional colleagues, as well as with patients and their families. This historical independence of thought and action can make it difficult for many physicians who will be entering practice in the future to understand that the evolving changes in the health care delivery system will unavoidably affect that perceived level of independence.

The virtually anonymous third-party payers of the past have now emerged as aggressive, prudent purchasers who are highly competitive with other payers. Patient care in the mass is becoming a big business, at least as it relates to insurers, managed care organizations, and groups of employers. Each of these entities has virtual control of large blocks of "covered lives" (patients) and has enormous influence over whether, when, and which physicians and hospitals deliver services. The system has been evolving over the past several years because of the perceived complexity of health care delivery, the increasing costs ascribed to technology and professional subspecialization, and the sheer size of the fraction of gross national product dedicated to health care. American businesses, large and small, realize the need to exert some sort of cost brake on the health care delivery system. The federal Medicare program of health insurance for persons older than 65 years and the federal and state government Medicaid programs of health insurance for defined categories of low-income people have grown as entitlement programs, further adding to the federal deficit and the limitations of budgetary flexibility. Additionally, because this country contains large numbers of uninsured and relatively poor, underinsured people, the government should respond by developing a mechanism for universal coverage and easier access to health care.

The changing medical care environment places increasing emphasis on standards, outcomes, and accountability. As purchasers of insurance become more cognizant of value rather than just cost, outcomes ranging from rates of screening mammography to mortality rates with coronary artery bypass graft surgery become metrics by which rational choices can be made. Clinical guidelines and critical pathways derived from randomized control trials and evidence-based medicine can potentially lead to more cost-effective care, as well as better outcomes.

However, these major changes in the American health care system bring with them a number of major risks and concerns. If the concept of limited choice among physicians and health care providers is based on objective measures of quality and outcome, the channeling of patients to better providers is one reasonable definition of better selection and enlightened competition. If, however, the limiting of options is based overwhelmingly on cost rather than on measures of quality, outcomes, and patient satisfaction, the historic relationship between the patient and the truly professional physician is fundamentally compromised.

In this new environment the physician oftentimes has a dual responsibility: to the health care system as an expert who helps create standards, measures of outcome, clinical guidelines, and mechanisms to ensure high-quality, cost-effective care, as well as to individual patients who entrust their well-being to that physician to promote their best interests within the reasonable limits of the system. A health insurance system that emphasizes cost-effective care, that gives physicians and health care providers responsibility for the health of a population and the resources required to achieve these goals, that must exist in a competitive environment in which patients can choose alternatives if they are not satisfied with their care, and that places increasing emphasis on health education and prevention can have a number of positive effects. In this environment, however, physicians must beware of overt and subtle pressures that could entice them to underserve patients and thereby abrogate their professional responsibilities by putting personal financial reward ahead of their patients' welfare. The physician's responsibility to represent the patient's best interests and avoid financial conflicts by doing too little in the newer systems of capitated care provides different specific challenges but an analogous moral dilemma to the historic American system in which the physician could be rewarded financially for doing too much.

In the current health care environment, all physicians and trainees must redouble their commitment to professionalism. At the same time, the challenge to the individual physician to retain and expand the scientific knowledge base and process the vast array of new information is daunting. If, however, physicians can address these various challenges, all citizens should have easier access to outstanding health care.

Advances in medical science and increased individual responsibility for health-promoting behavior are both necessary for a fair, equitable, and cost-effective health care system that provides a level of quality acceptable to the American public. Advances in medical science are central to achieving high quality at acceptable cost. It follows that health care delivery systems must seek out proven technology to maintain their competitive position. Physicians in those organizations will have to be educated continually to provide the best professional advice regarding the adoption of new technologic advances, including information not only on their safety and efficacy but also on their effect on medical outcomes, patient satisfaction, and cost-effectiveness. From the standpoint of the physician as a professional, the future is, in a sense, a return to the past when the physician and the patient were not insulated from economic realities and psychosocial contexts. High technology and high caring are not antithetic; they go together.

Even though these economic and social changes are coming about in a rather turbulent fashion, the future stands out clearly. The practice of medicine will continue to be an exciting career pursuit and an honored profession that provides physicians a rewarding opportunity to help others. The great diagnosticians will be the ones who also have the greatest access to the newest and most comprehensive therapies. It is comprehensive medicine toward which we must strive rather than generalist medicine or subspecial-

ist medicine; it is doing whatever is necessary to treat all aspects of the patient's disease. Whether it be in the intricacies of gene therapy or in behavior modification to treat substance abuse, "comprehensive" means being able to care for individuals in the best way with the greatest depth of knowledge. For physicians of the new century, this pursuit will be professionally and personally satisfying and will be welcomed by them as well as by society as a whole.

American Board of Internal Medicine Committee on Evaluation of Clinical Competence: Project Professionalism. Philadelphia, American Board of Internal Medicine, 1994.

Smith R, Hiatt H, Berwick D: A shared statement of ethical principles for those who shape and give health care: A working draft from the Tavistock Group. Ann Intern Med 130:143, 1999.
Two careful discussions of professionalism in medicine and how it is a critical part of the health care system.

PART II

SOCIAL AND ETHICAL ISSUES IN MEDICINE

2 CLINICAL ETHICS IN THE PRACTICE OF MEDICINE

Peter A. Singer ▪ *Mark Siegler*

Clinical ethics is a practical discipline that contributes to improvement in patient care. It focuses on the central importance of patient preferences and choices in the patient-physician relationship and on the moral obligations of physicians, such as the need for honesty, competence, compassion, and respect for the patient. Clinical ethics teaches physicians about a wide range of specifically ethical issues—informed consent, truth telling, end-of-life decisions, advance directives, and increasing third-party constraints on the autonomy of both patients and physicians. Although in theory these issues have been resolved, in practice they continue to vex conscientious physicians. The most clinically important ethical issues that arise frequently in the practice of internal medicine include decision making by competent patients, substitute decision making (including advance directives) for incompetent patients, end-of-life decisions, futility, and clinical-ethical concerns in an era of cost containment and health care reform.

DECISION MAKING BY COMPETENT PATIENTS

During the past generation, the relationship between patients and physicians has become more equal. Most clinical decisions are now reached by a process of shared decision making in which physicians provide information and guidance that allow competent adult patients to base decisions on their own personal preferences, values, and goals. Competent adult patients have an ethical and legal right to accept or refuse medical care recommended by physicians, including life-sustaining treatments. Patients are in control of their own health care. In general, patients accept their physicians' recommendations because physicians and patients share the same goal—improving the patient's health status—and because patients usually trust and have confidence in both physicians' technical abilities and their commitment to the patient's welfare.

INFORMED CONSENT. The clinical-ethical process of shared decision making is mirrored by the legal doctrine of informed consent. Informed consent is defined as voluntary acceptance by a competent patient of a plan for medical care after the physician adequately discloses the proposed plan, its risks and benefits, and alternative approaches. The informed consent process applies not only to invasive surgical procedures but to every clinical decision as well. Moreover, the legal and ethical standards of informed consent are not satisfied merely by obtaining the patient's signature on a consent form but require a process of effective communication and education between the physician and patient. If the patient has decision-making capacity (see later), the physician should seek consent from the patient; if the patient lacks decision-making capacity, the physician should seek consent from the appropriate substitute decision maker. The best way for young physicians to learn how to obtain informed consent from patients is by observing a clinician who is recognized for skill in negotiating the consent process.

The patient's right to participate in treatment decisions is well recognized in law, philosophy, public policy, and clinical practice.

Perhaps the clearest *legal* statement of this right was enunciated in 1914 by Justice Cardozo: "Every human being of adult years and sound mind has the right to determine what shall be done with his body." The *philosophical* right of patients to control their own medical care is based on the principle of individual autonomy. In the 1980s, a presidential commission clearly stated that respect for patient preferences should be the basis of *public policy* in medical ethics. Moreover, evidence from *clinical* research indicates that patients who participate in their own health care decisions are more likely to implement the shared decision, express greater satisfaction with their physician, and most importantly, have improved functional outcomes in several chronic diseases.

DISCLOSURE AND TRUTH TELLING. For the purposes of informed consent, disclosure must include proposed diagnostic tests and treatments, their risks and benefits, and possible alternative approaches. Although standards for disclosure may vary from one jurisdiction to another, the physician should disclose all the information that a reasonable person in the patient's situation would want or need to know before making a decision. For example, physicians would be expected to inform patients about risks that are either highly likely to occur or less likely but very serious when they do occur, e.g., death or permanent disability. Although a subjective standard of disclosure based on an individual patient's personal view is a difficult clinical standard to achieve, physicians should try to know their patients well enough to tailor disclosure to a patient's particular situation.

Another aspect of disclosure separate from the need to obtain informed consent involves telling patients the truth about unfavorable diagnoses, such as metastatic cancer, and their prognoses. In the United States, the current medical standard is to be honest with patients and not to conceal bad news. The patient's right to know an unfavorable diagnosis, even if no further tests or treatment is proposed, is grounded in the ethical principle of respect for persons and in the implied promise by physicians to be truthful in their relationships with a patient. The real clinical skill in "telling the truth" or delivering bad news to a patient involves determining exactly what the "truth" is in a particular case and then deciding how and when it should be imparted in a culturally sensitive way that does not destroy the patient's hope.

DECISION-MAKING CAPACITY AND COMPETENCY. Decision-making capacity, a clinical concept, is the ability to understand relevant information and appreciate the consequences of a decision. Competency is the parallel legal concept. Patients who have been determined to have decision-making capacity should make their own health care decisions, based on the principle of autonomy, whereas patients determined to lack it should be protected from making bad and sometimes irreversible decisions, based on the principle of beneficence. Decision-making capacity is a dynamic state and may change quickly, as when a patient is admitted stuporous, hypotensive, and with sepsis and lacks this capacity but, 12 hours later, after appropriate treatment, is sitting in bed, conversing normally, and has regained it. Moreover, decision-making capacity is decision specific. For example, patients with substantial cognitive impairment may retain decision-making capacity to decide whether they wish to accept a recommended elective cholecystectomy.

Unfortunately, no valid and widely accepted clinical measures are available to assess decision-making capacity. Physicians should assess this capacity by asking patients whether they understand and appreciate their medical problem and the risks and benefits of the proposed treatment and why they have chosen to accept or reject it.

The physician or health care team responsible for the patient should determine whether a patient retains or has lost decision-making capacity. When doubt exists, consultation with a psychiatrist or neurologist may be helpful. Disagreements about decision-making capacity are often brought to the attention of hospital attorneys, ethics committees, or ethics consultants. In cases of irremediable conflict and if clinical circumstances permit, the ultimate judge of a patient's competency is a court. Often, however, the tempo of clinical circumstances may require physicians to make decisions by relying on clinical judgment and assistance from consultants to reach the best and most ethical determination.

SUBSTITUTE DECISION MAKING

American legal theory accords incompetent patients the same rights as competent patients to consent to or refuse diagnostic tests and treatment. In practice, however, patients who lack decision-making capacity cannot exercise this right. To address this paradox, substitute decision makers, sometimes called surrogates or proxies, are permitted to make health care decisions for a patient who lacks decision-making capacity. The overall goal of substitute decision making is to approximate the decisions that the patient would make if the patient were still capable of making a decision. Substitute decision-making policies raise two questions: Who should make decisions for a patient who lacks decision-making capacity, and by what standards should the decision be made?

The most appropriate person to make substitute decisions is someone designated by the patient while still competent, either orally or through a written proxy advance directive (see later). Other substitute decision makers, in their usual order of priority, include a spouse, adult child, parent, brother or sister, and any other relative or concerned friend. In some jurisdictions, a public official may serve as substitute decision maker for a patient who has no other decision maker available. Many states have now passed health surrogate laws that permit a substitute decision maker to be appointed without going to court when a patient lacks decision-making capacity and has no formal advance directive.

The standards for making substitute decisions for patients without decision-making capacity are, in decreasing order of priority, the patient's explicit wishes, values and beliefs, and best interests. A patient's wishes are prior expressions, while competent, that apply to the actual decision that needs to be made, such as whether the patient wants mechanical ventilation in the late stages of amyotrophic lateral sclerosis. Sometimes patients record their specific wishes in an instruction advance directive (see the next section). Values and beliefs are less specific than explicit wishes, but they allow the substitute decision maker to guess what the patient might have decided based on other past choices and the patient's general approach to life. Best interests, which are "objective" estimates of the benefits and burdens of treatment to the patient, are invoked only when the patient's wishes, values, and beliefs are unknown.

ADVANCE DIRECTIVES. The two types of advance directives are proxy directives, sometimes called durable powers of attorney for health care, which state *whom* a person wants to make treatment decisions on that patient's behalf, and instruction directives, sometimes called living wills, which state *what* treatment the person would or would not want in various situations. The person completes the advance directive when competent, and the directive generally takes effect if the person becomes incompetent. At present, advance directives are recognized legally in every state, and the federal Patient Self-Determination Act requires health care facilities to inquire whether patients have an advance directive and to inform patients of their rights under state law to complete an advance directive. Although public opinion polls indicate strong support for advance directives and although many different advance directive forms are available, relatively few Americans have filled out such directives. Recent evidence has highlighted the limited effect of advance directives on clinical outcomes, such as "do not resuscitate" orders, and on administrative outcomes, such as length of stay. Nevertheless, advance care planning has important psychosocial benefits for patients and families.

END-OF-LIFE DECISIONS

With the possible exception of informed consent, no issue in clinical ethics has been as thoroughly analyzed as end-of-life deci-

sions. Nevertheless, the spectrum of end-of-life decisions remains confusing for clinicians and the public. Three distinct practices can be delineated: decisions to forego life-sustaining treatment, euthanasia and physician-assisted suicide, and comprehensive care for dying patients that emphasizes palliation.

The right of patients to refuse medical interventions also applies to life-sustaining treatment such as cardiopulmonary resuscitation, mechanical ventilation, dialysis, and artificial nutrition and hydration, even if such a decision results in the patient's death. "Do not resuscitate" orders, in which decisions are reached to forego resuscitation if the patient has a witnessed cardiopulmonary arrest, are by far the most widely used and best-studied examples of withholding potentially life-sustaining interventions. A patient's decision to discontinue (withdraw) or not to initiate (withhold) life-sustaining treatment is not considered the moral or legal equivalent of suicide, and physician participation in such an action is not the equivalent of physician-assisted suicide. These decisions may be made by the patient or substitute decision maker and are legally and ethically permissible when clinicians follow appropriate procedures, as outlined in the previous discussions of decision making by competent patients and substitute decision making. Clinicians must understand that such actions do not place them at legal risk and often reflect the best standards of clinical practice.

In contrast to foregoing life-sustaining treatment, euthanasia and physician-assisted suicide are, at the time of this writing, prohibited in almost every legal system in the world, with one notable exception being the state of Oregon, which has legalized physician-assisted suicide. Euthanasia can be defined as an action that leads directly to the death of a patient, e.g., an injection of potassium chloride. Physician-assisted suicide can be defined as providing patients with medical means that the patient uses to commit suicide, e.g., the prescription of a large amount of barbiturates to a patient who then uses the drugs to commit suicide. The main arguments supporting physician-assisted suicide and euthanasia are based on respect for patients' freedom of choice and the claimed right of individuals to enlist a physician's assistance to end their pain and suffering. The main arguments opposing these practices include respect for human life, protection of vulnerable patients, and fear of abuse. Both proponents and opponents of physician-assisted suicide and euthanasia appeal to the role-related responsibility of being a physician to support their arguments. In 1997, the U.S. Supreme Court ruled that physician-assisted suicide is not a constitutional right and therefore state laws prohibiting or permitting the practice are not unconstitutional. Even if assisted suicide and euthanasia receive legal sanction in selected jurisdictions, physicians will still be confronted with the fundamental issue of whether such practices are ethical in a medical context.

A third practice in the spectrum of end-of-life decisions is the provision of comprehensive clinical care, including palliative care, for dying patients. Such care should include the skilled use of pain-relieving drugs, as well as attention to the patient's other physical, psychological, social, and spiritual needs. Palliative care is ethically and legally permissible, even mandatory, and is an essential component of quality clinical care of the dying. A practical problem for physicians, however, is to distinguish appropriate palliative care from euthanasia. According to guidelines developed by the Chief Coroner of Ontario, an act is considered palliative care, and not euthanasia, if (1) it is intended solely to relieve the person's suffering, (2) it is administered in response to symptoms or signs of the patient's suffering and is commensurate with that suffering, and (3) it is not the deliberate infliction of death.

FUTILITY

In contrast to a patient who refuses treatment is the situation in which patients or families wish to have certain treatments that physicians believe are futile. No ethical or legal framework has been established to address such cases. Despite numerous attempts to define futility, application of these definitions in practice has proved controversial. Physicians should distinguish among patients who are imminently dying (e.g., refractory cardiogenic shock), terminally ill (e.g., metastatic pancreatic cancer), and severely and irreversibly impaired (e.g., persistent vegetative state).

When confronted with a futility case, physicians should strive to establish consensus, based on published data where available, among the various members of the health care team regarding the appropriateness of various proposed treatment plans. The physician should communicate with the patient and family to understand their views, including their cultural, religious, and psychological perspectives. Based on this information, the physician may need to negotiate to reach consensus on a treatment plan that is acceptable to the patient and family, as well as the health care team. If consensus is not achievable, an impartial mediator may help resolve the disagreement. As a last resort, arbitration, sometimes via a formal legal approach, may be required. This process will be more effective if formalized as an institutional policy.

CLINICAL-ETHICAL CONCERNS IN MANAGED CARE

Profound changes in the financing and organization of health care in recent years have intensified old ethical challenges and posed new ones for physicians. These challenges include but are not limited to access to health care for the uninsured, conflicts of interest, organizational ethics, resource allocation, managed care gag rules, and physician compensation incentives. To maintain ethical integrity, medical practice in a managed care environment should emphasize the ability to provide quality care, the ability of physicians to serve as their patients' advocates, the right of patients to select their own physicians and to make their own health care decisions, the requirement of physicians to disclose financial incentives that could influence their clinical recommendations, and the availability of reasonable appeal mechanisms for patients or families who believe that their rights have not been honored.

CONCLUSIONS

Scientific and technologic developments in medicine have created unprecedented ethical dilemmas for physicians, and the revolution in molecular medicine will generate additional ethical problems. Clinical ethics has emerged as a new and useful component of medical practice by emphasizing that technical and ethical concerns are inseparable in the practice of medicine. Clinical ethics focuses on the continuing centrality of the patient-doctor relationship and on how patients and physicians work within existing administrative and political structures to reach mutual agreement on clinical decisions affecting the patient. In addition, clinical ethics offers a language of discourse that broadens the medical model from one that is narrowly technical to one that takes serious account of individual patient preferences. The language and content of clinical ethics have been adopted not only by patients, physicians, nurses, other health care providers, and medical educators, but also by health economists, hospital administrators, policy developers, and judges. In this regard, ethical considerations in medicine are likely to remain an important component of medical education, clinical practice, biomedical research, and the political evolution of our health care system.

Almost 2500 years ago, Plato recognized that good clinical medicine is a marriage of scientific knowledge and human care. In Book IV of *The Laws,* he described an excellent physician as one who ". . . treats disease by going into things thoroughly from the beginning in a scientific way and takes the patient and family into confidence. Thus he learns something from the sufferer. . . . He does not give prescriptions until he has won the patient's support, and when he has done so, he steadfastly aims at providing complete restoration to health by persuading the sufferer into compliance. . . ." The best clinical medicine and patient outcomes are achieved when the patient and physician have established a relationship in which technical and personal aspects of care are integrated. The practice of ethical medicine in the twenty-first century will require nothing more but demand nothing less.

www.bioethics.gov/nbac.html *Website of the U.S. National Bioethics Advisory Commission.*

www.acp-asim.org/ethics/index.html *Website of the American College of Physicians–American Society of Internal Medicine Center for Ethics and Professionalism. Includes College Ethics Manual.*

www.ama-assn.org/ethic/ethics.htm *Website containing American Medical Association's ethics activities including Council on Ethical and Judicial Affairs, Institute for Ethics, and the Education for Physicians on End-of-life Care Project.*

www.med.upenn.edu/~bioethic *Online information on bioethics from the University of Pennsylvania Center for Bioethics.*

www.utoronto.ca/jcb *Online information on bioethics from the University of Toronto Joint Centre for Bioethics.*

Jonsen AR, Siegler M, Winslade WJ: Clinical Ethics: A Practical Approach to Ethical Decisions in Clinical Medicine, 4th ed. New York, McGraw-Hill, 1998. *A practical guide to help clinicians deal with ethical problems that occur frequently in practice.*

Provides a clinical decision-making approach along with discussions of informed consent, decision-making capacity, end-of-life decisions, futility, and managed care.

Singer PA (ed): Bioethics at the Bedside. Ottawa, Canadian Medical Association, 1999. *Covers topics that will be important for clinicians in practice, including the topics in this chapter.*

3 CARE OF DYING PATIENTS AND THEIR FAMILIES

Balfour M. Mount

Too many people suffer needlessly at the end of life, both from errors of omission—when caregivers fail to provide palliative and supportive care known to be effective—and from errors of commission—when caregivers do what is known to be ineffective and even harmful.

Committee on Care at the End of Life

Death calls into question our competence as caregivers, our unconscious premises regarding the omniscience of modern medical science, and the nature of our role in end-of-life care. It raises questions concerning meaning, life, death, and immortality. It may undermine communication with our patients and their family members and result in increased isolation and despair. It is the time when it is erroneously said that "nothing more can be done," yet it is a time to relieve suffering and develop individually tailored support programs. The physician has an unparalleled opportunity to act as a catalyst to enable comfort, communication, integration, and healing.

DEFINITION AND GOALS OF PALLIATIVE CARE

Palliative care aims to improve the quality of life when treatment to cure disease and prolong life is no longer a realistic objective. It offers services designed to address the physical, psychological, social, and spiritual needs of dying patients and their families. Its goals are to relieve suffering, attain patient comfort without iatrogenic somnolence or change in affect, assist the patient and family in making the most of decreasing resources, and support those involved in a search for meaning. "Palliative care," in the broad sense of relieving suffering, is not restricted to those who are dying. The term "hospice," or an approach to care that includes medical, psychosocial, and spiritual issues, may also be used in this sense. In addition, hospice may also refer to the site of care or the organization or program that provides end-of-life care.

Although this chapter deals with care of the dying in general, a spectrum of dying trajectories may be seen, including those experiencing a sudden unexpected death; those with an anticipated death after a relatively predictable, perhaps rapid, decline; and those facing a chronic illness of uncertain duration that may either be punctuated by acute crises or be relatively stable, only later to face an eventual decline or sudden death. Although the disease trajectory will shape the window of opportunity afforded the caregiver to support the patient, in all these situations the bereavement risk associated with those left behind should be assessed.

The variety of possible dying trajectories is also a reminder of the importance of establishing a pattern of open, supportive communication with the patient and family concerning what the future may hold, their goals and aspirations, treatment options with their benefits and burdens, and their preferences for treatment intervention in relevant end-of-life settings. These discussions may lead to the completion of advance directives. They also tend to enhance coping as a result of both lessening the anxiety associated with uncertainty and promoting an enhanced sense of community in the face of adversity.

Optimal care demands full-spectrum support—physical, psychosocial, and spiritual. Such comprehensive care must involve the patient, family, and an experienced multidisciplinary team, usually composed of both health care professionals and volunteers. The great majority of terminally ill patients can be appropriately managed by their primary care physician. The primary care physician should have ready access to advice and consultation from local palliative care experts. A minority of patients may require temporary or permanent transfer to the care of a regional palliative care expert for the control of refractory distress.

Quality of life—subjective well-being—is the central concern in end-of-life care. It is suggested by the response to "How are you today?" or "How are you in yourself?" or "How is it going these days?" Quality of life does not vary with physical status alone, but is modified by all domains of personal experience—physical, psychological, social, financial, and spiritual. It is what the patient says it is, not what objective observers see.

SYMPTOM CONTROL

Attentive control of pain and other symptoms and detailed consideration of psychosocial and spiritual issues should characterize care from the time of diagnosis. When neglected until the late stages of disease, problems in these domains tend to become entrenched, interactive, and increasingly difficult to control. Vigilant prophylaxis of symptoms and attention to the nonphysical factors contributing to suffering lead to enhanced quality of life and diminished drug requirements.

The main symptoms associated with terminal illness include pain, the anorexia-cachexia syndrome, weakness and fatigue, dyspnea and cough, nausea and vomiting, mouth problems, skin problems, lymphedema, ascites, confusion, dementia, and anxiety. These symptoms can be easily monitored by physical examination or by using 0 to 10 numerical, verbal, or visual analog scales. This information should be obtained during each visit and graphed in the patient record in a manner similar to the recording of vital signs earlier in the disease process. Physical status and cognitive function should also be regularly monitored with validated instruments because of their potential for rapid change and impact on defining care needs. Chapter 27 provides a detailed review of pain and its management.

Because symptoms may change rapidly, frequent re-evaluation is an essential component of effective care of the dying (Table 3–1). Norms of care are redefined in this setting. Only investigations that may lead to a treatment that will improve quality of life are considered. Blood pressure, pulse, and temperature are not routinely monitored, whereas the frequency of bowel movements is!

Attention to detail is required for planning both assessment and care. For one very weak patient, use of a bedside commode or a bedpan and simply accepting occasional incontinence of urine and stool enabled conservation of scant energy reserves for eagerly

anticipated daily visits with his family. Bowel care for the equally weak, fiercely independent man in the next bed involved planned nonintervention while he laboriously struggled unaided to the toilet some 15 ft from his bed. A gentle offer of assistance was given ("When you wish, just let us know"), and a discussion of his need for autonomy was held with family members. Thus, radically different approaches to the details of bowel care were used for two dying men with divergent needs.

Competent care of the dying involves meticulous care of skin, mouth, and eyes; adapting activities of daily living, furniture, and utensils to accommodate progressive weakness (a favorite chair raised on blocks, a padded and raised toilet seat, a spoon with a padded handle to accommodate a weak grip); clean smooth sheets; quiet music, flowers, and a few cherished belongings; the reassuring glow of soft lighting at night; and the reliable availability of both skilled nursing and an interested physician.

Fears and misunderstandings about existing or anticipated symptoms and the effects of medication are common. The patient and family should participate in both planning and providing care. Clear explanations of symptoms and treatment options give reassurance that "the doctor understands what's going on" and "there is a plan."

COMMUNICATION ISSUES

Giving bad news is always difficult. The physician should bring to discussions of prognosis not a set of fixed rules concerning whether "to tell" or "not to tell," but an openness to examining with the patient the reality at hand. Communication that is insensitive in the interest of "telling all" or evasive, falsely optimistic, or otherwise misleading in the interest of "protecting" the patient generally risks seriously undermining the long-range credibility of the physician. Studies suggest that the majority of patients with a serious illness sense the possibility of death, whether or not they have been told. Fears are usually diminished if they can be named.

Integrating "bad news" is usually a process, not an event. Grave tidings are often repressed and simply "not heard" at the first airing. The physician should follow the pace of disclosure set by the patient and be sensitive to all forms of communication: plain language ("I fear I may be dying"), symbolic language ("I keep dreaming of a long tunnel with a candle at the end and I am afraid someone is going to blow the candle out"), and nonverbal communication (depressed facial expression, excessive muscle tension). It has been estimated that 80% of communication is nonverbal. The absence of questions does not mean that questions do not exist for the patient. The physician who says "I never tell patients they have cancer unless they ask me" risks leaving the responsibility of broaching the most sensitive and awesome questions to the one who is most vulnerable, the patient.

Discussions should be positive, yet reality oriented. "Am I dying? How long do I have?" may be responded to by "I don't know how long any of us have to live. If you are asking if it is serious enough to warrant getting your affairs in order, I would say yes, get your house in order. While you're doing that, you and I will deal with the medical problems you're experiencing."

Discussions focused on the goals of treatment minimize uncertainty and foster confidence. Involving the family in these discussions facilitates their subsequent mutual support. Sitting together, the patient, family, and doctor examine what is still possible rather than what has been lost.

"There are only three aims we can have in treating any illness, Bill—to cure, to prolong life, and to improve the quality of life. We are not going to be able to cure your tumor in the sense of making it go away permanently. But, you know, there are many medical problems we can't cure—including diabetes, arthritis, and most types of heart disease—yet many people with these conditions live meaningful lives, sometimes for longer periods than we expect.

"So 'cure' isn't an option. What about the next goal, 'to prolong life'? You could undergo surgery, but there is no sense putting you through something that wouldn't be helpful." (Surgery is often used as the first example since it presents a concrete, easily grasped image of futility.) "With treatments as they now stand, the same would be said for chemotherapy, radiotherapy, and immunotherapy." (The phrasing focuses on the limitations of current therapy, not the hopelessness of the illness.)

Table 3–1 ■ GUIDELINES FOR SYMPTOM CONTROL

1. "Nothing matters more than the bowels" (Saunders). Daily assessment needed.
2. Control of one symptom improves control of all symptoms.
3. Most symptoms are caused by multiple factors. Psychological distress may augment all symptoms.
4. "Assessment must precede treatment" (Twycross).
5. Rule out correctable factors underlying each symptom.
6. Clarify who is bothered by the symptoms: patient, family, or staff.
7. Give a simple explanation for each symptom to the patient and family. Diagrams helpful.
8. Consider the anticipated prognosis, functional status, and the patient's goals in determining appropriate treatment.
9. Discuss treatment options with patient and family and involve them in treatment planning when practical.
10. Determine what was helpful in the past.
11. Use a total-care approach employing nondrug, environmental, and other supportive measures.
12. If needed, use combinations of pharmacologic agents when differing mechanisms of action and toxicity permit.
13. Prescribe drugs prophylactically in individually optimized, regular doses for persistent symptoms.
14. Never say "Nothing more can be done." Consult or refer if comfort is not achieved.

"Does this mean nothing more can be done?" (thus naming the worst fear). "Not at all! It simply means we are at the third goal—that of focusing on the quality of life. How can we make the best of this? Let's examine that. If I understand you, the three complaints you have right now are your backache, that cough, and your loss of appetite. Let's see what we can do about each of these. . . ."

The patient and family are left with a clear understanding that the issue is not "to treat or not to treat," but an appropriate shifting in therapeutic goals by a physician who is interested, involved, and undaunted by the specter of this illness. Hope is contagious. Hope is a way through, not a way out.

Information about the expected prognosis may aid physicians in making recommendations and help the patient and family make plans, but specific estimates of an individual's survival should generally be avoided because of their inherent uncertainty. No matter how carefully phrased, such pronouncements always unsheathe a sword of Damocles that heightens anxiety and drains the ability to live fully in the moment: "I have only two more months."

Accepting the present reality, including the increasing weakness, dependence, uncertain future, and impending loss, frees the patient to choose from available options. Acceptance of that kind is not born out of despair and resignation. It is the transcendent alternative to denial. It is a path to meaning that is possible even in the face of physical deterioration and advancing disease.

FAMILY AS THE UNIT OF CARE

Terminal illness is a pressure cooker of family stress. Grief, fear, anger, and guilt abound. Long-standing interpersonal tensions tend to be accentuated. Family meetings to discuss treatment plans and identify problems and fears are a time-efficient tool highly effective in preventing impending crises, clarifying misunderstandings, and building bridges of mutual support.

A checklist of areas of inquiry is useful in family assessment (Table 3–2). Ensure that children and the elderly are informed and involved. Their exclusion often leaves them ill prepared for loss.

The bereaved are a high-risk population with an increased incidence of impaired function, medical illness, psychological distress, and even death, especially when other risk factors for bereavement morbidity are present (Table 3–3). Referral to programs offering bereavement support may be beneficial.

LOCATION OF DYING

Death has been moved from the home to the institution in industrial nations, and family members often feel ill prepared to care for dying loved ones. With careful planning, family education, mobilization of community resources, and continuing support, however, both the family and patient may benefit from experiencing this last time together in the home.

Even though more than two thirds of patients would prefer to die at home, not all of those expressing this wish will be able to live in comfort at home until death. A home-based death should not become an implied yardstick of success. The goal of care should be to support the patient and family as a unit in adapting to the realities of their needs and resources. Around-the-clock, 7-days-per-week availability of community-based services linked to backup inpatient beds enables the desired balance of maximum quality of life and efficiency in utilization of health care resources.

Home care of the dying begins with careful home assessment

Table 3–2 ■ FAMILY ASSESSMENT ISSUES

1. Identity of nuclear family, extended family, and social network
2. Characteristics of family system: roles, relationships, communication patterns
3. Presence of concurrent life crises
4. History of coping with past crises
5. Values and beliefs about death
6. Response to current illness: changes in roles and relationships
7. Family resources: physical, emotional, financial, social, spiritual
8. Immediate family needs
9. Long-range family needs

Table 3–3 ■ SELECTED BEREAVEMENT RISK INDICATORS

1. Parental grief
2. Social isolation
3. Timid, dependent personality; poorly developed coping skills
4. Short preparation time (duration of illness)
5. Ambivalent or charged relationship with deceased
6. Concurrent life crisis
7. Pining and clinging in final illness
8. Grief expression repressed by cultural or family norms
9. Disenfranchised grief: mistress, lover, divorcée, loss of a secret relationship

performed by an experienced home care team able to direct the family to needed community resources and to recommend modifications in living arrangements and furnishings to simplify care. "You will find it much easier if you rent a hospital bed. They are inexpensive. Try placing it in the living room where she can be quiet, close to the family, and able to see the children passing in the street."

"She is weaker now. You will need a handrail and small bench for the bath tub and a walker. I think you would find a commode for the bedside helpful as well."

An effective palliative home care program implies the involvement of a team. Regularly scheduled nursing visits are supplemented by emergency visits as required. A trusted physician is essential to consult in the home and collaborate with community-based nurses when the need arises. A social worker, occupational therapist, chaplain, and volunteers may all play a role. Simple, clear routines for medications and treatments are established. A sense of order and safety is fostered by around-the-clock availability of telephone consultation with experienced staff who are aware of recent changes in the patient's condition and medications. Brief respite admissions before family exhaustion sets in may help prolong the capability of home care.

A sensitive discussion with the family about what to do when their loved one dies may promote a sense of confidence and preparedness. Acknowledgment of a job well done ("You certainly have done well to keep her at home this long") helps allay feelings of inadequacy and guilt should admission to the hospital become necessary.

AS DEATH APPROACHES

During the final weeks or days of a terminal illness, frequent changes in clinical status may occur. Common crises include progressive weakness, inability to swallow, aspiration of oral intake, inability or refusal to take medications, changing levels of consciousness and orientation, restlessness, and urinary or fecal incontinence. Careful planning and prompt response to the request for emergency assistance can avoid unnecessary hospital admission.

Individualized reductions in medication doses as death approaches can prolong an alert, interactive, comfortable state, often to the moment of death. Noisy upper airway secretions ("death rattle") are troubling to the family, who will need reassurance, but they are generally not troubling to the patient. They may be reduced by early intervention with hyoscine hydrobromide, 0.4 mg given subcutaneously at intervals of 2 to 4 hours as needed.

Questions and fears that the patient and family have about death should be gently explored. The will, funeral arrangements, and a "life review" may be discussed as a means of completing unfinished business and facilitating closure.

Encourage family members, including the young, the elderly, and those from out of town, to visit earlier rather than later. Assess bereavement risks and arrange follow-up support if indicated.

Decathexis, a protective "separating off" or "turning in" by the patient, is sometimes seen as death approaches. A simple explanation may reassure the concerned family that this is not depression or rejection but a normal protective mechanism. "He doesn't need you to say much now, but your presence will help."

Take premonitions of death seriously, and watch for the need for family members to give their lingering loved one permission to die.

"It's all right, John. You can let go. You've taken care of everything. We'll miss you, but thanks to you we'll be O.K."

AT THE TIME OF DEATH

The hours that surround the death of a family member are charged with meaning for the bereaved and are usually remembered for years to come. Caregivers may use this experience to therapeutic advantage by establishing guidelines for patient and family care that facilitate subsequent grief work.

Endeavor to have someone sitting at the bedside of the imminently dying person. If the bedside companion is a family member, be sensitive to the patient's need either for support or for time to be alone with the loved one. Encourage available family members to view the body before it has been moved to the funeral home. Seeing the body facilitates acceptance of the fact of death.

When family members arrive, they need support and quiet hospitality, including a handkerchief, a cup of tea, a listening ear. Acknowledge the support given by the bereaved to the deceased during the illness.

Allow sufficient time with the body for active grieving. It may be helpful for a caregiver to unobtrusively touch the body and thus indicate that there is nothing frightening about physical contact with the body—an experience that may be highly effective in promoting closure.

Discuss whether the family wishes to have an autopsy. Many find the documentation of reality that an autopsy provides to be helpful in the months and years to come.

When death occurs in a hospital, ask the family whether they would prefer to collect and pack their loved one's personal effects, particularly if a child has died. A memento of the event such as a lock of hair or a picture may be an aid to bereavement, especially in parental grief.

Respect cultural differences in the expression of acute grief. Certain cultural groups may be extremely vocal and demonstrative in their grieving. Wails, screams, fainting attacks, and other dramatic gestures have therapeutic value for many and may be followed in a remarkably short period of time by a sense of composure and evident relief.

Acknowledge the mystery of death without offering "answers" concerning the unknowable. Honor religious rites and prayers meaningful to the bereaved.

Attendance at the death or funeral service by the physician who was involved during the illness assists review of the illness, emphasizes the value of the deceased, underscores respect for the family, and assists the physician's own grief.

THE PHYSICIAN AND DEATH

In caring for the dying, physicians are challenged in each dimension of their being. What do we do with our accumulated losses as caregivers? How do we establish a new balance in our emotional economy when an important investment has been lost? At what cost? To whom? Do our professional encounters with death leave a need for thicker defensive shells, emotional distancing, intellectualization, and acting out? The risk is minimized if we accept relief of suffering as our mandate rather than the narrower goal of fighting disease and if we attend to our own physical, psychosocial, and spiritual needs.

Chochinov HM, Breitbart W: Psychiatric Dimensions of Palliative Medicine. New York, Oxford University Press, 1999. *A detailed examination of psychiatric issues relevant to end-of-life care.*

Doyle D, Hanks GWC, MacDonald N: Oxford Textbook of Palliative Medicine, 2nd ed. New York, Oxford Medical Publications, 1998. *The gold standard reference textbook on palliative medicine.*

Field MJ, Cassel CK: Approaching Death: Improving Care at the End of Life. Washington, National Academy Press, 1997. *The Institute of Medicine and Committee on Care at the End of Life offer a detailed report concerning the experience of dying and the conditions that help people attain dignity, meaning, and comfort at the end of life.*

MacDonald N: Palliative Medicine, a Case-Based Manual. New York, Oxford University Press, 1998. *Common clinical issues in palliative care addressed in a case-based format. An ideal resource for group teaching or self-directed learning.*

Portenoy RK, Bruera E: Topics in Palliative Care. New York, Oxford University Press, 1997. *Informative reviews of topics related to delirium in cancer patients, gastrointestinal disorders in patients with advanced cancer, advances in the pharmacotherapy of pain and psychosocial adaptation to cancer.*

4 SOCIAL AND ECONOMIC ISSUES IN MEDICINE

John E. Wennberg

A great deal about medical practice that a physician would like to know is not available in this edition of the *Cecil Textbook of Medicine* or in other medical texts. Examples of desired but missing information include data on exactly whether and when to hospitalize patients with a broad variety of medical conditions, conclusive evidence on the efficacy of many common surgical procedures, or details about how patients value the outcomes of interventions that physicians are likely to recommend. In the absence of this information and relying on a traditional model of decision making that assumes that the physician is able to act as the rational agent for the patient in choosing among treatment options, the medical system has developed as an economy in which the availability of hospital beds, physicians, and other local resources determines the pattern of care.

Experts in economics have long held that the market for medical care differs from that for most goods and services because a competitive market assumes that the consumer is informed about availability, price, and market competition. Patients, by contrast, simply do not have enough information to choose their own care—and patients' widespread use of insurance means that the price of care does not closely modulate the decision to use it. In this market, the traditional remedy is to rely on professionals to control demand and for patients to delegate decision making to their physicians. The tacit agreement between patient and physician is that professionals, in fulfilling their ethical roles, prescribe only needed care. Physicians are also assumed to serve conscientiously as agents for society by ensuring that the supply of resources is adequate—but only adequate—to meet a rational level of demand. Although the physician's understood role as decision-making agent for both patient and society can be compromised by unethically inducing use for self-serving reasons, it has also been assumed that such activity is controlled by agencies, such as the Medicare program's Professional Review Organization, that patrol the market to discipline those who depart from the central consensus about what works and what patients need.

It is increasingly apparent, however, that the foundation of much of medical care is not an evidence-based professional consensus about effectiveness and value. The decision to use care, such as hospitalization for a patient with pneumonia, is often driven by availability, not explicit theory. Even when theories of care are explicit—as in treating conditions such as angina pectoris or benign prostatic hypertrophy (BPH) (for which treatment options can range from surgery to drugs or watchful waiting)—the outcomes are often not well understood. Furthermore, physicians are imperfect agents; their own preferences for treatments or outcomes often become entangled with and overpower those of the patient.

FLAWS IN THE SCIENTIFIC AND ETHICAL BASIS OF CLINICAL DECISION MAKING

For a number of conditions such as BPH, early-stage prostate cancer, or stable angina, medical theories of efficacy and professional discourse are well organized; opinions are strongly held concerning appropriate treatment, even when experts disagree. Often, disagreements cannot be resolved by appeal to evidence because adequate outcome studies have not been performed. In a market where patients rely on the profession to prescribe treatments, the existence of diverse professional opinions about the value of options invites suppliers to influence demand. In fee-for-service markets, where provider income and the financial stability of institutions depend on the level of utilization, such influence becomes inevitable.

The marked variation in the rates of surgery for BPH found in studies conducted in the state of Maine in the early 1980s exposed the lack of consensus about how patients with BPH should be treated. Rates of surgery for BPH ranged between 15% undergoing surgery by age 85 in one town and 50% in another, quite similar community. The rates were physician specific and attributable to at least two widely held and opposing theories about the benefits associated with surgery for BPH among Maine's urologists. The physicians differed in their assumptions about the nature of the underlying illness, as well as the benefits to be derived from surgery. Some believed in a preventive theory: Operate early to avoid later complications, including premature death. Others were more optimistic about untreated BPH. They argued for the quality-of-life theory: Surgery benefits most men by reducing symptoms and improving the quality of life.

The unresolved competition between the prevention and the quality-of-life theories reflected indeterminacy rooted in poor clinical science. Subsequent research showed that the preventive theory was incorrect; early surgery appears to lead to a slight decrease in life expectancy because for most men, BPH does not progress to life-threatening obstruction and the small operative mortality risk reduces life expectancy slightly. Moreover, the studies showed that urine flow, the standard used to determine the urologists' estimate of the need for (and the success of) surgery, was an extremely poor indicator of how patients themselves valued their preoperative conditions and their surgical outcomes. What did matter to patients was the degree to which their symptoms bothered them (which was not necessarily related to symptom severity) and the possible negative outcomes of surgery such as impotence and incontinence.

When patients are offered an active role in choosing treatment through shared decision making, the link between supply and utilization can be broken. When patients enrolled in two separate prepaid group practices were informed about their options for treatment of BPH through an interactive videodisk program and were provided with information specific to their own clinical situations, most elected conservative treatment. Among those with severe symptoms, only one in five chose surgery, and the per capita rates of surgery declined about 50%.

THE THRESHOLD EFFECT FOR INTERVENTION

Medical practice occurs within a context of available supply that is only rarely known to the participants—physicians generally have no idea how many beds per capita are available in their communities. The exception is the traditional health maintenance organization (HMO)—the closed-staff, pre-paid group practice model exemplified by Kaiser-Permanente and the Group Health Cooperative of Puget Sound. Such organizations know the number of people enrolled in their health plans and use population-based health planning to determine the per capita numbers of beds they provide and health workers they hire. They typically use about 150 hospital beds per 100,000 enrollees and employ physicians according to specialty-specific population-based ratios. Population-based planning is essential because the system receives a fixed amount of money for each enrollee for whom they agree to provide all "necessary" care. A fixed budget requires controlling resources, which is accomplished by setting limits on supply.

In fee-for-service markets, by contrast, neither administrators nor health care providers know the size of the population that their organizations serve. Private-sector, population-based health planning that relates supply to consumption is virtually nonexistent. Populations do not "enroll," there are no fixed budgets, and revenue is generated by providing services.

The lack of information on the quantity of local resources and the actuarial costs of local consumption supports a dynamic of market growth that is not closely constrained by the size or the health care needs of the population. An institution's growth is determined by its own perceived needs and its assumed roles in the community and the region. Size is influenced by such nonmedical factors as competition, prestige, or the expansion of professional staff to meet the critical mass required to ensure night and weekend coverage. The decision about how many specialists to train is less a function of how many are needed in a community than of the needs (and desires) of the directors of the training programs.

Increasingly, the tools of epidemiology, applied to the study of supply and utilization in local health care markets, make it possible to compare resource allocation and utilization rates among communities (and in some cases between individual hospitals) as though they were the closed and countable populations of enrollees in closed-staff HMOs. These studies reveal remarkable differences in the per capita supply of resources, even among demographically similar markets. The studies also show that variations in supply affect the threshold for clinical decision making. The effect of supply of beds on the decision for hospitalization provides a cogent example. For example, although some of Boston's beds (and some of New Haven's) are used to care for people who live outside the city, Boston has nearly 50% more beds per person in the local population than New Haven does.

The differential in population-based availability of hospital resources produces a diffuse effect on the admission threshold for most conditions. A few "demand-driven" conditions, such as myocardial infarction and hip fracture, are unaffected by the available supply of resources (because virtually all physicians, regardless of the context of supply, agree on the need to hospitalize the patient). The increments of beds and other resources in high-resource communities are used for patients with "supply-sensitive" conditions such as pneumonia, congestive heart failure, and bronchitis, which in low-rate markets are more often treated on an outpatient basis. For such conditions, hospitalization rates for people living in Boston are typically 60% higher than for residents of New Haven. Furthermore, capacity and utilization vary substantially from hospital to hospital even within these cities.

The threshold effect is not scaled simply on the severity of illness. As capacity increases, populations who are very sick as well as those who are not so sick receive more hospital care. A strong linear relationship exists between capacity and level of investment in terminal care. Yet more is not better in the dimension of life expectancy: Residents of Boston and New Haven experience the same population-based mortality rates. The effects of supply on decision making are subliminal inasmuch as neither administrators, clinicians, nor patients are directly aware of the supply context of local practice. The impact is primarily on the problem-solving tasks of medicine—the care of sick people with conditions about which medical theory is weak and evidence that one course of action is better than another is unproven.

The rise of capitation, whereby physicians and hospitals assume total responsibility for patient care for a pre-negotiated price in a variety of practice settings other than traditional HMOs, has provided additional incentives to titrate the provision of medical services to match need rather than to match the historical supply of beds or capacity. While these incentives clearly reduce overutilization, care must be taken to ensure that professionalism, combined with guidelines and perhaps regulation, does not lead to underutilization.

REMEDIES

FIND OUT WHAT WORKS. Biomedical science creates the fundamental understanding of the mechanisms of disease at the cellular and molecular levels and is a fruitful source of clinical theory and practice technologies for intervening in the lives of patients. However, its mission as a branch of applied biology does not emphasize evaluation of medical theories or communication about options. It is the job of the evaluative sciences to conduct technology assessments and outcomes research to estimate the probabilities for outcomes that matter to patients and to elucidate the importance of patient preferences in choosing treatment. Although some progress has been made, explicit policies to ensure the orderly evaluation of relevant treatment theories and the education of health professionals in evaluative sciences are not yet in place.

FIND OUT WHAT PATIENTS WANT. The success of the biomedical revolution greatly increases medical options and, by doing so, exacerbates the problem of choice in medicine. Although the assumption that physicians can make vicarious decisions that reflect the patient's true preferences may seem naive, throughout most of the history of Western medicine it did not make much difference because there were few choices. Biomedicine and technology have changed the medical landscape; many conditions can now be treated by a number of options that carry different sets of risks and benefits. Rational choice among them depends on learning how to communicate medical options in ways that enable patients to choose among effective treatments according to their own preferences. Although emphasis on the ethical and legal requirements for physicians to share decision making with patients is now greater, the striking variations in rates of surgery among communities and the association between capacity and the intensity of investment in terminal care are reminders that supply-inducing utilization remains a powerful force in medical markets. Successfully implementing shared decision making requires practice environments in which the choices patients make are not in conflict with the financial interests of health care organizations, employers, or individual providers. Creating such an environment is one of the great challenges of health care reform because breaking the link between supply and utilization creates a market in which demand emanates from patients and thus results in different per capita rates of consumption and different demands for resources.

LIMIT CAPACITY. Stability in health care markets also requires that capacity be limited in some reasonable way. Many believe that practice guidelines will discipline the decisions of physicians to bring utilization and supply into equilibrium on the basis of medical efficacy. However, the evidence from Boston and New Haven indicates otherwise. The extraordinary variations in hospitalization rates among some of the nation's most prestigious teaching hospitals suggest that the rules have no firm scientific basis; some form of population-based planning is likely to be required.

Arrow K: Uncertainty and the welfare economics of medical care. Am Econ Rev 53: 941, 1963. *A classic presentation of rational agency theory by a Nobel laureate in economics.*

Fuchs VR: Health care for the elderly: How much? Who will pay for it? Health Aff (Millwood) 18:11, 1999. *A review emphasizing the cost implications of our increasing elderly population and increasing technologic capabilities.*

Katz J: The Silent World of Doctor and Patient. London, Collier Macmillan, 1984. *An excellent review of the history of the doctor-patient relationship and the difficulty of establishing shared decision making.*

Wennberg JE, Cooper MM (eds): The Dartmouth Atlas of Health Care 1998. Chicago, American Hospital Publishing, 1998. *Recent national study of small area variations.*

PART III

AGING AND GERIATRIC MEDICINE

5 BIOLOGY OF AGING

Caleb E. Finch ▪ *Edward L. Schneider*

THE LONGEVITY REVOLUTION

As part of a remarkable revolution in human biology, the average lifespan has increased beyond 65 years in most human populations, and the fastest-growing age group is the oldest. In the United States since 1950, the age group 65 years and older has grown from 8% to 13% of the general population. The record lifespan is held by a recently deceased French woman, Jeanne Calment, who reached 122 years and 4 months. Despite impairments of vision and hearing, she appeared to be cognitively intact. It is predicted that by 2020 a total of 50 million will live to be at least 65 years of age, i.e., an increase by another 50% (Fig. 5–1). Thus aging has become a world-wide issue affecting all nations, irrespective of their economic development.

The key to maximum lifespan concerns how mortality rates change at later ages. During most of the adult lifespan, the mortality rate accelerates according to the Gompertz equation such that graphs of the log of the mortality rate for each year give a straight line when plotted against age. As a rule, the mortality rate doubles every 8 years throughout the world after puberty. However, new evidence shows that at advanced ages of 100 years or more, the acceleration of mortality rates slows considerably. It is possible that those already at advanced ages will achieve new record lifespans.

ARE DISEASE AND DISABILITY INEVITABLE WITH AGING?

We do not fully understand the powerful historical trend for increasing survival to later ages. It seems unlikely that all the improvements can be attributed to the success of medical interventions and improved public health. Obviously, the decline in infant and maternal mortality played a major role in the observed increase in life expectancy at birth during this century. However, the increases in life expectancy at *middle age* preceded the introduction of antibiotics and other major life-saving interventions. At least some groups in the United States also seem to be aging with greater health, as judged by the declining rates of death from cardiovascular and cerebrovascular disease in the last decades. Lifestyle choices such as smoking, diet, and exercise certainly have a role, but other factors may be found.

Major differences exist among populations in age-related diseases and changes that implicate environmental factors. Breast cancer, for example, has approximately a 10-fold higher incidence in Japanese women who live in California versus Japan; this difference continues throughout the adult lifespan. Within the same country, many differences can be seen. Even brain functions are subject to environmental influences, as suggested by the progressive improvement in scores on intelligence tests in different birth cohorts when tested at later ages. These examples imply that the outcomes of aging are subject to a great many environmental influences. Biologists refer to these environmentally influenced differences as *plasticity in the aging processes.*

Alzheimer's disease shows both hereditary and environmental influences. Overall, the risk increases steadily with age and afflicts about 35% of those older than 85 years (see Chapter 449). Alzheimer's disease is not a new disease, but it is becoming increasingly

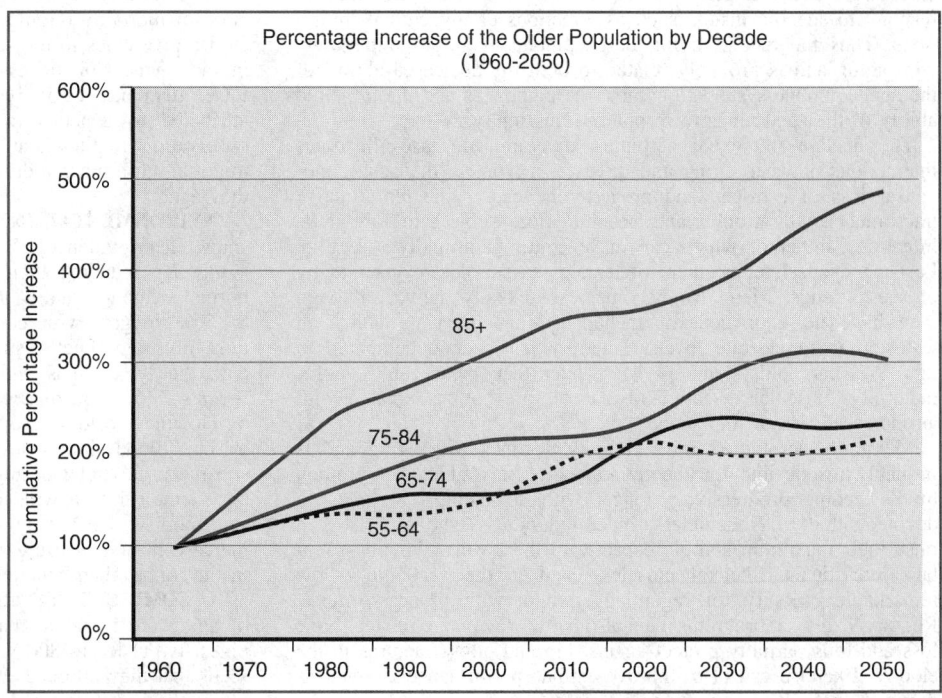

FIGURE 5–1 ▪ Past and projected increases in the elderly by decade. (From U.S. Bureau of the Census, Current Population Reports, P25-1092. Population Projections of the U.S. by Age, Sex, Race, and Hispanic Origin. U.S. Government Printing Office, Washington DC, 1992.)

prominent because of the increased numbers of individuals who are surviving to the eighth, ninth, and tenth decades. Genetic risk factors of different strengths have been mapped precisely. Familial Alzheimer's disease with early onset is strongly associated with rare mutations in the presenilin (*PS*) genes on chromosomes 1 (*PS-2*) and 14 (*PS-1*) and in the amyloid precursor protein on chromosome 21. A more common susceptibility factor is found in the apolipoprotein E gene on chromosome 19. The apoE $\epsilon4$ isoform confers a several-fold higher risk of Alzheimer's disease. Even so, some $\epsilon4/\epsilon4$ homozygotes retain mental health at ages beyond 100. Other gene associations (α_1-antichymotrypsin, α_2-macroglobulin, VLDL receptor, *FE65*) may differ in effect among populations. Higher education is associated with a lower risk of Alzheimer's disease, perhaps because persons with better cognitive function have more of a functional reserve before declining below an absolute level defined as cognitive impairment. Although education could also be a proxy for environmental effects, the mental demands of higher education may increase the synaptic density that could slow the loss of function.

AGING AND FUNCTIONAL DECLINE

Many fears about aging are related to the myth that everything declines with aging. Even genetically identical mice experience heterogeneity in their physiologic responses to aging. In aging humans, the interplay of environment and genetic diversity similarly results in increasing heterogeneity in physiologic responses. Whether drug metabolism or exercise capacity is measured, the heterogeneity of aging is manifested by the substantial increase in differences among individuals. Thus whereas pharmacologic response to specific drugs may be relatively similar among 20-year-olds, predicting the response in 80-year-olds is considerably more difficult. The normal heterogeneity of aging is further compounded in a clinical setting by the diseases acquired during a lifetime and the increased number of medications taken by older patients.

Many parameters such as resting cardiac output are relatively stable with normal aging. For other measures such as renal function as assayed by creatinine clearance, the response to aging varies widely—some individuals have a rapid decline with aging, others have moderate declines, and still others have no change at all.

Nevertheless, a number of important physiologic variables decline substantially with aging and compromise the individual's ability to respond to pathologic insults. Some of these age-dependent factors include a decrease in vital capacity, immune function, and bronchiolar ciliary movement, as well as an increase in arterial wall stiffness. These changes decrease the ability of an older body to respond to specific insults such as infections or myocardial infarctions. Thus the risk of dying of pneumonia increases remarkably with aging and is probably related to both the decreased ability of the aged immune system to combat the pathogens and the impaired ability of the aged lungs to respond to this injury.

The decline in sexual activities after mid-life also illustrates interactions between aging and disease. In women, the post-menopausal loss of estrogen and progesterone causes the reproductive tract mucosa to atrophy and become more subject to low-grade infections, either of which can make coitus painful (dyspareunia). Post-menopausal replacement of female sex steroids reverses many of these trends. Men also become less sexually active, although men have no equivalent of menopause or universal decline in testosterone to castrate levels. Paternity has been documented in men 94 years old, some 34 years later than the record age for maternity. Vascular disease and diabetes are both associated with an increased risk of impotence.

Maximum aerobic exercise capacity declines with aging and is probably responsible for the retirement of star athletes. Marathon times become progressively longer with advancing age, even in devoted athletes. Nonetheless, older individuals who exercise can raise their maximum aerobic capacity to the level of young sedentary individuals. Skeletal muscles, even in the very old, show remarkable capacity for regaining strength with proper exercise. Regular exercise programs can also slow down age-related bone loss and thus partially protect against hip and other fractures in the elderly. Exercise can also improve cardiac performance, as well as diminish the risk of hypertensive disease.

These associations suggest that with the decline of so many physiologic functions, one could die of "old age." Some death certificates have even listed "old age" as the cause of death. Careful investigation, however, usually reveals that the patient died of a recognizable disease, such as pneumonia, that might not have killed a 20-year-old but did produce the final blow to an older individual whose physiologic responses had been severely diminished with aging.

Another important relationship between aging and disease is the concept that age-dependent loss of specific cell populations may result in specific age-dependent diseases and disorders. For example, with aging comes a loss of cerebral cholinergic neurons that cannot be attributed to vascular disease or Alzheimer's disease alone. The extent of neuron loss during normal aging is controversial and hard to establish, in part because large neurons tend to shrink. Vascular changes, which are common in cerebral arteries, may impair the availability of nutrients, even without clinically recognized strokes, and over time result in damage to neurons. The brains of Alzheimer's disease victims younger than 70 years show a clear distinction from the brains of nondemented patients of the same age in the number of plaques and tangles. At very advanced ages, however, it becomes more difficult for the neuropathologist to distinguish between "normal" aging and Alzheimer's disease.

LESSONS FROM OTHER SPECIES

GENETICS OF LIFESPANS. The trends for increased survival to later ages lead to fundamental questions about the biology of aging, particularly about genetic control over the lifespan. Many species of animals have short natural lifespans that are dictated in unknown ways by their particular genes. Laboratory rodents possess the shortest lifespans among mammals, about 5 years at the maximum; domestic cats and dogs and cattle survive in the middle range to 20 years at the most; humans enjoy the upper end. The best-recognized effects of genes on the lifespan are the mutations that cause early-onset diseases.

In contrast to mammals, research on invertebrates has identified specific genes that can increase the lifespan, as well as others that decrease it. The fruitfly *Drosophila* normally lives for about 2 months, but the artificial evolution of short- and long-lived lines of flies was accomplished by choosing individuals that reproduce at younger versus later ages. The resulting selection for lifespan depended on existing genetic variation in the wild-caught flies rather than on new mutations, but the particular survival-influencing genes are still being sought. The nematode *Caenorhabditis* also possesses "survival" genes that increase the organism's lifespan, which normally takes only 3 weeks from egg to senescence. Mutants have been found that have double the lifespan because of slower acceleration of mortality (Gompertz rate). These studies on flies and nematodes give clues in the search for genes that favor longer lifespans in mammals. Nonetheless, it is sobering to the genetic view that fewer than half of individual variations in adult lifespan can be attributed to genetics in humans, mice, flies, and worms. This observation implies that lifestyle and the environment are more important for most individuals than their inherited genes in how they age.

ENVIRONMENTAL INFLUENCES ON THE LIFESPAN. Rodents show clear evidence of environmental influence in outcomes of aging. By reducing their dietary intake to about half *ad libitum* normal without vitamin or mineral deficiencies, the animals live up to 50% longer, with correspondingly slower acceleration of the mortality rate. Diet restriction also reduces age-related diseases, e.g., the lymphomas and kidney lesions, that usually kill aging rodents. Moreover, diet restriction can delay infertility during aging by slowing the loss of ovarian oocytes. Metabolic changes include a lower blood glucose level and increased insulin efficiency, opposite the usual trend during aging. These examples from other species demonstrate a wide range of environmental interventions that can modify the outcomes of aging. By implication, the recent increase in human life expectancy could be due largely to environmental rather than genetic changes.

DO SOME SPECIES ESCAPE AGING? Extremely slow patterns of aging are found in many species, especially plants. Bristlecone pines live at least 4800 years without change in the viability of the seeds that they produce each year, and 1000 years is not unusual in other conifers. Geoducks and quahogs, both bivalve mollusks, live at least 200 years. In the northern Pacific, several species of rock-fish can live at least 100 years and show no loss of fertility. Turtles may also exceed 100 years. Although no general signs of age-related dysfunction are known in these long-lived examples, detailed studies remain to be done.

To experience a complete absence of aging, an organism would be required to repair all types of injuries and rid itself of abnormal growths. Theoretically, the retention of a complete set of genes by cells throughout the body ("somatic cell genomic totipotency") could lead to replacement of any damaged tissue. Achieving this goal through the control of gene activity, however, would not confer immortality because death still overtakes individuals, even in the absence of age-related disorders.

In humans, the safest of all ages occurs at about the time of puberty, when the mortality risk through accidents and disease is about 1:2000 per year. If this risk were maintained indefinitely without the usual acceleration, the life expectancy at birth would be about 1200 years, and the last survivor in a population of 4 billion would be 25,000 years old. Although fantastic improvements over the present human lifespan may be accomplished through disease reduction, humans would still be subject to unavoidable dangers that statistically limit the ultimate lifespan.

EVOLUTIONARY THEORY OF AGING

The evolutionary view recognizes that young adults produce the most offspring; even if reproductive capacity were not subject to age-related declines, natural hazards would reduce the older population. Natural selection acts mostly on children and young adults, who are the most responsible for propagation of the species. Correspondingly, the force of natural selection against harmful or disadvantageous genes becomes progressively weaker with advancing age. As a consequence, theory predicts that mutations in the population gene pool are tolerated if any adverse effects are delayed to older ages. Among examples of genes with delayed adverse effects are hereditary Alzheimer's disease and hereditary risks of breast cancer. Many different genes may cause particular diseases of aging.

CELL BIOLOGY OF AGING

Numerous theories address specific aging changes in processes ranging from the molecular to the organ system level of function. One of the oldest is the *somatic mutation theory,* which originally focused on chromosomal genes. There is little doubt that somatic cells accumulate oncogenic mutations on a sporadic and scattered basis during the individual lifespan and that these mutations are of great importance to the age-related increase in cancer. However, relatively few nuclear genes in any cell show evidence of accumulated damage through mutations. The somatic mutation theory has been expanded to include mitochondrial DNA mutations. In certain brain regions with high concentrations of the neurotransmitter dopamine, 1 to 5% of the mitochondria may have DNA deletions that impair adenosine triphosphate production.

Free radical theories postulate that endogenously generated and highly reactive free radicals cause the somatic mutations just described. Free radicals can also damage proteins. Slowly replaced proteins such as collagen and elastin tend to show the accumulation of oxidized amino acids and the addition of glucose derivatives (glycosylation), both of which involve free radical chemistry. Some features of diabetes such as diabetic lens opacity are associated with glycosylated proteins. Antioxidants and compounds that trap free radicals may slow or reverse the oxidation of proteins during aging.

Oxidative damage from free radicals is increasingly implicated in degenerative diseases of aging. Epidemiologic studies indicate that specific antioxidants may protect individuals who are at risk for coronary artery disease, cataracts, and certain cancers. Neurodegeneration during Alzheimer's disease is also suspected to be driven by free radical mechanisms that are stimulated by β-amyloid peptide. The gene for familial amyotrophic lateral sclerosis has been mapped to the chromosomal locus for superoxide dismutase, which converts the free radical of oxygen to hydrogen peroxide, which in turn is converted to harmless water and oxygen.

Cell-aging theories are based on the finite number of possible divisions made in culture by skin fibroblasts and by most other cells obtained from humans (the Hayflick limit phenomenon). The causes of clonal aging appear to involve the activities of genes that control cell proliferation, some of which are also crucial to malignancy, such as the *p21, p53,* and *Rb* genes, which may normally serve as tumor suppressors but are commonly mutated in human cancers. Most investigators agree that the nondividing status that follows repetitive proliferation does not lead to cell death. If kept carefully, nondividing cells can live for many months in culture dishes. This observation is consistent with the fact that hearts and brains are full of cells that ceased dividing decades ago.

Cell senescence may also involve loss of DNA at the ends of chromosomes (telomeres); immortal cancer cells, as well as the germ-like cells in the gonads, are protected against telomere shortening by an enzyme called *telomerase.* When telomerase is genetically introduced, fibroblasts can bypass the Hayflick limit. It is not yet known whether these cell lines would be malignant in the body.

Programmed cell death also relates to aging. During development, excess numbers of neurons, lymphocytes, and other cells die through a genetically programmed sequence of changes called *apoptosis.* Cell death, however, can arise from other causes such as ischemia or toxins, a process referred to as *necrotic cell death.* In the aging prostate, apoptosis can be observed among benign proliferating cells. Such natural mechanisms of cell death may protect against the progression of abnormal growths during aging.

Immune theories of aging are based on the observation that with aging the primary immune response weakens as reflected by the increasing vulnerability to influenza and other infections. One factor is an increase in memory T cells at the expense of virgin T cells, with a net effect of reducing the response to novel antigens. On the other hand, a general increase is seen in low-grade autoimmune and inflammatory processes such as arthritis. The net result indicates that hyperactivity in some immune functions coexists with hypoactivity in others. Ultimately, this complex situation may be understood in terms of the regulation of genes that control the proliferation of immune cell populations.

Endocrine theories account for a wide range of physiologic changes. Certain post-menopausal dysfunctions, as noted earlier, are clearly related to the exhaustion of ovarian follicles that produce estrogen and progesterone. The loss of estrogen accelerates osteoporosis. Moreover, the beneficial effects of estrogen, which also reduces the risk of heart attacks, strokes, and possibly Alzheimer's disease, are lost at menopause. Melatonin and dehydroepiandrosterone are sometimes advertised as "miracle" hormones for aging, but there is little evidence that they benefit the outcomes of normal aging.

Neuroendocrine theories address subtle changes in the output of the pituitary that accompany aging. The decreased secretion of growth hormone, for example, is modest in most older adults. Some individuals may suffer growth hormone deficits that cause skeletal muscle atrophy, which can be corrected by growth hormone replacement therapy. Nothing, however, suggests the presence of general deficits of growth hormone that would warrant therapeutic replacement on the scale practiced for estrogen replacement after menopause. Many other age changes could be linked to altered functions of brain centers that influence the autonomic nervous system and metabolism. Such associations are largely speculative in humans.

Wear-and-tear theories include mechanical and biochemical features of aging. Insects can wear out their irreplaceable wings. Tooth and joint erosion is common during human aging. At the molecular level, endogenously produced free radicals may damage certain irreplaceable molecules.

SUMMARY

Aging changes appear to be very diverse and subject to numerous environmental and genetic influences. Aging processes thus show a great deal of plasticity and potential for modification. With the exception of the ovary, no other organ appears to have a programmed senescence in adult life that leads to predictable complete loss of function during aging in all human populations. Although some individuals carry genes that predispose them to early onset of specific degenerative diseases, there is much reason to anticipate that interventions will be possible. The reduced rates of death from ischemic heart disease in recent decades show the importance of lifestyle in the outcomes of aging. Many biologists and geriatricians are convinced that the potential for successful aging by maintaining health and independence at advanced ages is far greater than recognized by the general public.

General

Austad SN: Why We Age. What Science Is Discovering About the Body's Journey Through Life. Wiley, New York, 1997. *Excellent overview on aging of different organs and processes.*

Bodnar AG, Ouellette M, Frolkis M, et al: Extension of life-span by introduction of telomerase into normal human cells. Science 279:349, 1998. *Breakthrough on clonal senescence.*

Hazzard WR, et al: Principles of Geriatric Medicine and Gerontology, 4th ed. Health-care Management Group, 1998. *Broad coverage and many special topics.*

Schneider EL, Rowe JW: Handbook on the Biology of Aging, 4th ed. San Diego, Academic Press, 1996. *A regularly updated and authoritative source of reviews by mainstream researchers.*

Wachter K, Finch CE: From Zeus to the Salmon. The Biodemography of Aging. Washington, DC, National Academy of Sciences, 1997. *Current data on the increased human lifespan and biological interpretations of advanced age.*

Genetics of Aging

Finch CE, Tanzi RE: The genetics of aging. Science 278:407, 1997. *Summary of recent findings on the genetics of lifespans and mechanisms of aging.*

6 NEUROPSYCHIATRIC ASPECTS OF AGING

Sharon K. Inouye

OVERVIEW

The process of aging produces important physiologic changes in the central nervous system (Table 6–1), including neuroanatomic, neurotransmitter, and neurophysiologic changes. These processes in turn result in age-related symptoms and manifestations (Table 6–2) for many older persons. However, these physiologic changes develop at dramatically variable rates in different older persons, the decline being modified by factors such as diet, environment, lifestyle, genetic predisposition, disability, disease, and side effects of drugs. These changes can result in the common age-related symptoms of benign senescence, slowed reaction time, postural hypotension, vertigo or giddiness, presbyopia, presbycusis, stiffened gait, and sleep difficulties. In the absence of disease, these physiologic changes usually result in relatively modest symptoms and little restriction in activities of daily living. However, these changes decrease physiologic reserve and hence increase the susceptibility to challenges posed by disease-related, pharmacologic, and environmental stressors.

Neuropsychiatric disorders, the leading cause of disability in older persons, account for nearly 50% of functional incapacity. Severe neuropsychiatric conditions have been estimated to occur in 15 to 25% of older adults world-wide. Importantly, these condi-

Table 6-1 ■ AGE-RELATED PHYSIOLOGIC CHANGES IN THE CENTRAL NERVOUS SYSTEM

Neuroanatomic changes
  Brain atrophy
  Decreased neuron counts
  Increased neuritic plaques
  Increased lipofuscin and melanin
Neurotransmitter changes
  Decline in cholinergic transmission
  Decreased dopaminergic synthesis
  Decreased catecholamine synthesis
Neurophysiologic changes
  Decreased cerebral blood flow
  Electrophysiologic changes (slowing of alpha rhythm, increased latencies in evoked responses)

Table 6-2 ■ NEUROPSYCHIATRIC MANIFESTATIONS OF AGE-RELATED PHYSIOLOGIC CHANGES

SYSTEM	MANIFESTATION
Cognition	Forgetfulness
	Processing speed declines through adult life
	Neuropsychological declines: selective attention, verbal fluency, retrieval, complex visual perception, logical analysis
Reflexes	Stretch reflexes lose sensitivity
	Decreased or absent ankle reflexes
	Decreased autonomic and righting reflexes, postural instability
Sensory	Presbycusis (high-frequency hearing loss), tinnitus
	Deterioration of vestibular system, vertigo
	Presbyopia (decreased lens elasticity)
	Slowed pupil reactivity, decreased upgaze
	Olfactory system deterioration
	Decreased vibratory sensation
Gait/balance	Gait stiffer, slowed, forward flexed
	Increased body sway and mild unsteadiness
Sleep	Decreased sleep efficiency, fatigue
	Increased awakenings, insomnia
	Decrease in sleep stages 3 and 4
	Sleep duration more variable, more naps

tions are due to diseases that increase with age but are not part of the normal aging process. Alzheimer's disease and related dementias occur in approximately 10% of those aged 65 and older and up to 40% of those older than 85 years. Delirium occurs in 5 to 10% of all persons 65 years and older, usually in the setting of acute illness and hospitalization. Severe depression occurs in approximately 5% of older adults, with as many as 15% having significant depressive symptoms. Anxiety disorders occur in 10% of older adults. Common geriatric neuropsychiatric conditions include delirium (Chapter 444), dementia (Chapter 449.3), and depression (Chapter 450). Older individuals are also subject to substantial morbidity and functional disability from cerebrovascular disease (Chapter 470), Parkinson's disease (Chapter 460), peripheral neuropathies (Chapter 498), degenerative myelopathies such as spinal stenosis (Chapter 493) and disk disease (Chapter 494), giant cell arteritis (Chapter 295), subdural hematoma (Chapter 471), seizure disorders (Chapter 484), sleep apnea (Chapter 87), falls (Chapter 8), incontinence (Chapter 119), and impotence (Chapter 247). To diagnose these conditions, physicians must understand and perform a mental status examination and an assessment of functional capacity and know the uses and side effects of psychoactive drugs in geriatric patients.

MENTAL STATUS EXAMINATION

In addition to a detailed neurologic examination, evaluation of neuropsychiatric disturbances in older persons requires a careful mental status examination, including an assessment of mood, affect, and cognition. Brief screening tests are available to evaluate these domains and to assist in the detection of potential problems requiring further evaluation and treatment. For depression screening, scores of 6 or more on the 15-item short-form Geriatric Depression Scale (Table 6–3) indicate substantial depressive symptoms requiring further evaluation. Alternative depression screening instruments include the Center for Epidemiologic Studies—Depression Scale and the General Health Questionnaire; for cognitively impaired patients, observer-rated depression scales such as the Hamilton Depression Scale are recommended.

Early cognitive deficits can easily be missed during conversation because intellectual impairment can be readily masked with intact social skills. Given the high frequency of cognitive impairment, formal cognitive screening is recommended for all older persons. Ideally, cognitive testing should evaluate at least the general domains of attention, orientation, language, memory, visuospatial ability, and conceptualization. To exclude delirium, attention should be assessed first by asking the patient to perform a task such as repeating five digits or reciting the months backwards; the remainder of cognitive testing will not be useful in an inattentive patient. For further cognitive testing, many brief, practical screening instruments are available. The most widely used instrument is the Mini-

Table 6–3 ■ GERIATRIC DEPRESSION SCALE—SHORT FORM

1. Are you basically satisfied with your life?	yes/**NO**
2. Have you dropped many of your activities and interests?	**YES**/no
3. Do you feel that your life is empty?	**YES**/no
4. Do you often get bored?	**YES**/no
5. Are you in good spirits most of the time?	yes/**NO**
6. Are you afraid that something bad is going to happen to you?	**YES**/no
7. Do you feel happy most of the time?	yes/**NO**
8. Do you feel helpless?	**YES**/no
9. Do you prefer to stay home rather than going out and doing new things?	**YES**/no
10. Do you feel you have more problems with memory than most?	**YES**/no
11. Do you think it is wonderful to be alive now?	yes/**NO**
12. Do you feel pretty worthless the way you are now?	**YES**/no
13. Do you feel full of energy?	yes/**NO**
14. Do you feel that your situation is hopeless?	**YES**/no
15. Do you think that most people are better off than you are?	**YES**/no

Scoring: Answers indicating depression are **highlighted;** six or more highlighted answers indicate depressive symptoms.

Adapted from Yesavage J, Brink T, Rowe T, et al: Development and validation of a geriatric depression screening scale: A preliminary report. J Psychiatr Res 17:37, 1983.

Mental State Examination, a 19-item, 30-point scale that can be completed in 10 minutes (Table 6–4). A score of 25 or more generally indicates intact cognitive function, whereas a score of 24 or less requires further evaluation for potential dementia. Further bedside testing can include asking the patient to draw a clock with the hands at a set time to assess visuospatial ability and higher cortical functions. Questions to evaluate judgment and problem-solving ability in hypothetic situations, such as in a fire or when driving, can provide critical insight into the patient's ability to function safely and independently.

FUNCTIONAL ASSESSMENT

Functional impairment, defined as difficulty in performing daily activities, is common among elderly persons. Although not routinely evaluated in the standard medical assessment, determination

Table 6–4 ■ MINI-MENTAL STATE EXAMINATION

COGNITIVE DOMAIN	MAXIMUM SCORE
Orientation	
What is the (year) (season) (date) (day) (month)?	5
Where are we (city) (state) (county) (hospital) (floor)?	5
Registration	
Name 3 objects: 1 sec to say each. Ask the patient for all 3 after you have said them. Give 1 point for each correct answer. Repeat them until all 3 are learned. Count the trials and record the number.	3
Attention and calculation	
Serial 7s backward from 100 (stop after 5 answers). Alternatively, spell WORLD backward.	5
Recall	
Ask for the 3 objects repeated above. Give 1 point for each correct answer.	3
Language and praxis	
Show a pencil and watch, and ask the patient to name them.	2
Ask the patient to repeat the following: "No ifs, ands, or buts."	1
Three-stage command: "Take this paper in your right hand, fold it in half, and put it on the floor."	3
"Read and obey the following: Close your eyes."	1
"Write a sentence."	1
"Copy this design" (interlocking pentagons).	1

A score of 25 or greater signifies intact cognitive function.

Adapted from Folstein MF, Folstein SE, McHugh PR: "The Mini-Mental State": A practical method for grading the cognitive state of patients for the clinician. Journal of Psychiatric Research 12:189, 1975.

of the patient's degree of functional incapacity based on medical and neuropsychiatric conditions is critical to understanding the burden of disease and its impact on the individual's daily life. The important relationship of functional status with health in older persons is reflected in the finding that functional measures are stronger predictors of mortality after hospitalization than are admitting diagnoses. Moreover, functional measures strongly predict other important hospital outcomes in the elderly such as length of stay, functional status at discharge, future care needs, caregiver burden, risk for institutionalization, and long-term prognosis.

The functional assessment should include an assessment of the patient's ability to carry out basic self-care activities of daily living, as well as higher-level activities needed for independent living, the instrumental activities of daily living. Performance of activities of daily living reflects the ability of the patient to perform basic self-care activities, including feeding, grooming, bathing, dressing, toileting, transferring, and walking. Performance of instrumental activities of daily living reflects the ability of the patient to perform more complex tasks, including shopping, meal preparation, managing finances, housekeeping, using the telephone, taking medications, driving, and using transportation. The functional assessment is carried out with the patient or the family, and the questions ascertain whether the patient can perform these activities independently. Other related domains that should be assessed include vision, hearing, continence, nutritional status, safety, falls, living situation, social supports, and socioeconomic status.

The onset of acute functional decline is often the first and sometimes the only sign of serious acute illness in older persons and warrants immediate medical attention. Similarly, the onset or worsening of related conditions such as delirium, falls, incontinence, depression, or "failure to thrive" heralds the need for prompt medical evaluation.

PSYCHOACTIVE EFFECTS OF DRUGS IN OLDER PATIENTS

ADVERSE DRUG EVENTS IN THE ELDERLY. Iatrogenic complications occur in 29 to 38% of older hospitalized patients, with a three- to five-fold increased risk in older as compared with younger patients. Adverse drug events, the most common type of iatrogenic complication, account for 20 to 40% of all complications. The elderly are particularly vulnerable to adverse drug reactions because of multiple-drug regimens, multiple chronic diseases, relative renal and hepatic insufficiency, decreased physiologic reserve, and altered drug metabolism with aging. Moreover, inappropriate drug use has been reported in about 40% of hospitalized older patients, with more than one quarter of these patients having absolute contraindications to the drug and the others being given a drug that was unnecessary. Because 50% of adverse drug events occur in patients receiving inappropriate drugs, the potential for reducing these adverse events is substantial.

DRUGS WITH PSYCHOACTIVE EFFECTS. Nearly every class of drugs has the potential to cause delirium in a vulnerable patient, but specific drugs have been most commonly implicated (Table 6–5) and should be used with caution in older patients. Many cases of delirium or cognitive decline in older patients may be preventable through avoidance, substitution, or dose reduction of these psychoactive drugs. Long-acting benzodiazepines (e.g., flurazepam and diazepam) are particularly problematic medications for the elderly and should be avoided whenever possible. If non-pharmacologic approaches to the management of insomnia are unsuccessful, short-term use of an intermediate-acting benzodiazepine without active metabolites (e.g., lorazepam, 0.5 mg, half-life of 10 to 15 hours) is recommended. Drugs with anticholinergic effects (e.g., antihistamines, antidepressants, neuroleptics, antispasmodics) produce a panoply of poorly tolerated side effects in older patients, including delirium, postural hypotension, urinary retention, constipation, and dry mouth. Of the narcotics, meperidine causes delirium more frequently than other agents do because of an active metabolite, normeperidine. Cardiac drugs such as digitalis and antiarrhythmic agents have prolonged half-lives, narrowed therapeutic windows, and decreased protein binding in older patients. The clinician should be aware that toxicity with these agents, e.g., digoxin, can occur even at therapeutic drug levels. The H_2-receptor

Table 6–5 ■ DRUGS WITH PSYCHOACTIVE EFFECTS

Sedative/hypnotics
   Benzodiazepines (especially flurazepam, diazepam)
   Barbiturates
   Sleeping medications (chloral hydrate)
Narcotics (especially meperidine)
Anticholinergics
   Antihistamines (diphenhydramine, hydroxyzine)
   Antispasmodics (belladonna, Lomotil)
   Heterocyclic antidepressants (amitriptyline, imipramine, doxepin)
   Neuroleptics (chlorpromazine, haloperidol, thioridazine)
   Antiparkinsonian (benztropine, trihexyphenidyl)
   Atropine/scopolamine
Cardiac
   Digitalis glycosides
   Antiarrhythmics (quinidine, procainamide, lidocaine)
   Antihypertensives (β-blockers, methyldopa)
Gastrointestinal
   H_2-antagonists (cimetidine, ranitidine, famotidine, nizatidine)
   Metoclopramide (Reglan)
Miscellaneous
   Nonsteroidal anti-inflammatory drugs
   Corticosteroids
   Anticonvulsants
   Levodopa
   Lithium
Over-the-counter drugs
   Cold/sinus preparations (antihistamines, pseudoephedrine)
   Sleep aids (diphenhydramine, alcohol-containing elixirs)
   Stay Awake (caffeine)
   Nausea/gastrointestinal (Donnagel, meclizine, H_2-antagonists, loperamide)

antagonists (e.g., cimetidine, ranitidine, famotidine, nizatidine) are among the most common causes of drug-induced delirium in the elderly because of their frequent use; clinicians should strongly consider the use of less toxic alternatives (e.g., sucralfate or antacids) or dosage reduction for older patients, especially when the medication is being used for prophylaxis rather than treatment of active disease.

Psychoactive drugs account for nearly 50% of preventable adverse drug events, often in patients in whom three or more psychoactive drugs are prescribed, frequently at inappropriately high doses. Delirium and cognitive impairment are the most frequent adverse outcomes of psychoactive drugs. The use of any psychoactive drug is associated with a 4-fold increased risk of delirium or cognitive decline, but the outcomes of delirium and cognitive decline depend on the type or class of drug administered, as well as the total number of drugs received. Sedative-hypnotic drugs are associated with a 3- to 12-fold increased risk for delirium or cognitive decline, narcotics with a 2- to 3-fold increased risk, and anticholinergic drugs with a 5- to 12-fold increased risk. Moreover, when more drugs are used, not only does each carry its own individual risk for adverse outcomes, but the overall risk is also compounded by the heightened potential for drug-drug interactions. For example, if more than three drugs are added in a 24-hour period, the risk of delirium increases 4-fold. Similarly, the risk of cognitive decline increases directly with the number of drugs prescribed, from a 3-fold increased risk with two or three drugs to a 14-fold increased risk with six or more drugs.

PRINCIPLES OF DRUG THERAPY IN THE ELDERLY. Physicians should always consider whether non-pharmacologic approaches are appropriate alternatives to medications in older persons. For example, relaxation techniques, massage, and music are highly effective for the treatment of insomnia and anxiety; localized pain can often be effectively managed with local measures such as injection, heat, ultrasound, and transcutaneous electrical stimulation.

When drug therapy is required in the elderly, physicians should choose the drug with the least toxic potential and emphasize drugs that have been well tested in elderly populations (Table 6–6). Once the drug is chosen, it is often wise to start at 25 to 50% of the standard adult dosage for psychoactive drugs and increase the dose slowly. Drug regimens should be kept as simple as possible, with the fewest drugs and the fewest number of pills possible. Most importantly, the medication list should be reassessed frequently.

Table 6–6 ■ GUIDELINES FOR DRUG THERAPY IN THE ELDERLY

General principles:
   Remember that the elderly are highly sensitive to the psychoactive effects of all drugs.
   Know the pharmacology of the drugs you prescribe. Know a few drugs well.
Recommended approach:
  1. Use non-pharmacologic approaches whenever possible.
  2. Avoid *routine* use of "as needed" drugs for sleep, anxiety, pain.
  3. Choose the drug with the least toxic potential.
  4. Substitute less toxic alternatives whenever possible (antacid or sucralfate for an H_2-blocker, Metamucil/Kaopectate for Lomotil, scheduled acetaminophen/choline magnesium salicylate regimen for pain management).
  5. Reduce the dosage.
  6. "Start low and go slow."
    Start with 25–50% of the standard dose of psychoactive drugs in the elderly.
    Titrate the drug slowly.
    Set realistic end points: titrate to improvement, not elimination of symptoms.
  7. Keep the regimen simple.
  8. Regularly reassess the medication list. Have the patient bring in all bottles and review what is being taken.
  9. Re-evaluate chronic drug use since the patient is changing.
 10. Review over-the-counter medication use.

Even long-standing medications should be re-evaluated since the host is changing with age and illness. Chronic usage does not necessarily justify continued usage. The physician should review with the patient all prescribed and over-the-counter medications on a regular basis, preferably by having the patient bring in all medication bottles and indicate how each is being taken. Patients frequently underestimate the toxic potential of over-the-counter medications and may be using a variety of over-the-counter medications that could potentiate the side effects or even directly counteract the desired effects of prescription medications.

Leape LL, Brennan TA, Laird N, et al: The nature of adverse events in hospitalized patients: Results of the Harvard Medical Practice Study II. N Engl J Med 324:377, 1991. *Landmark study documenting the rate and type of adverse events in over 30,000 hospital admissions. This study revealed that drug complications were the most common type of adverse event and that the rate of adverse events rose with age.*

Some drugs that cause psychiatric symptoms. Med Lett 40:21, 1998. *This article provides a comprehensive listing of drugs with potential psychoactive effects.*

Tombaugh TN, McIntyre NJ: The Mini-Mental State Examination: A comprehensive review. J Am Geriatr Soc 40:922, 1992. *This study provides a detailed review of 26 years of information on the Mini-Mental State Examination, the most widely used cognitive screening test, including its psychometric properties, strengths, and limitations.*

7 ■ DELIRIUM AND OTHER MENTAL STATUS PROBLEMS IN THE OLDER PATIENT

Sharon K. Inouye

EVALUATION OF MENTAL STATUS CHANGE IN THE OLDER PATIENT

Mental status change, one of the most common presenting symptoms in acutely ill elders, is estimated to account for up to 30% of emergency evaluations for older patients. Importantly, mental status often serves as a barometer of the overall underlying health of an elderly patient and is commonly the only symptom of serious underlying disease. A broad range of medical, neurologic, and psychiatric conditions can lead to mental status changes (see Chapters 444, 449, and 450), and a systematic approach aids in the evaluation of suspected mental status change in an older patient (Fig. 7–1).

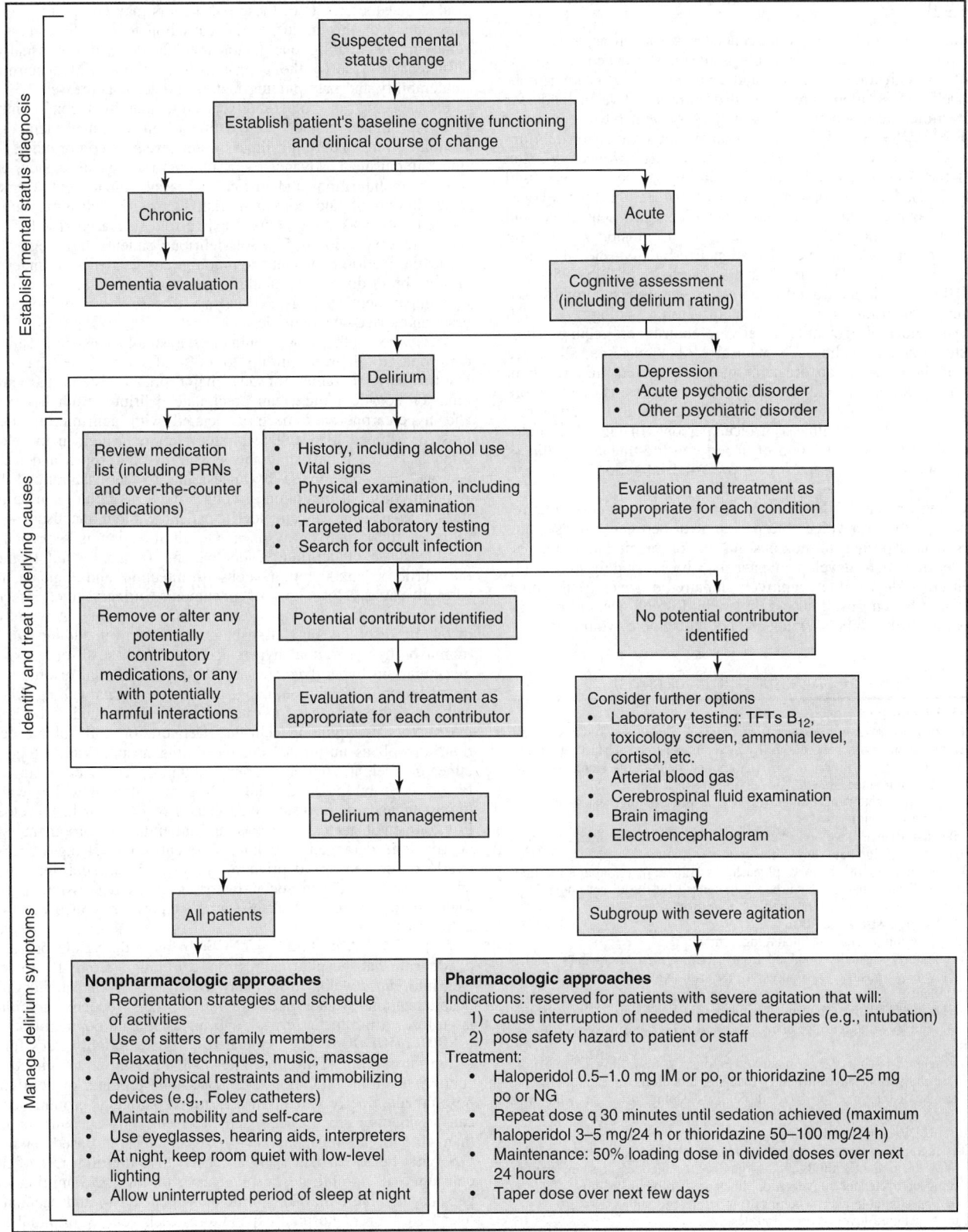

FIGURE 7–1 ■ Algorithm for evaluation of suspected mental status change in an older patient.

The first step in evaluating suspected altered mental status in an older patient is to obtain a detailed history from a reliable informant to establish the patient's baseline level of cognitive function and the clinical course of any cognitive changes. Chronic changes, i.e., changes occurring over months to years, most likely represent an underlying dementing illness, which should be evaluated accordingly (see Chapter 449). Acute changes, i.e., changes occurring over days to weeks—even if superimposed on an underlying dementia—should be further evaluated by detailed cognitive assessment to determine whether delirium is present. If features of delirium (e.g., inattention, disorganized thinking, altered level of consciousness, fluctuating symptoms) are not present, further evaluation for depression, acute nonorganic psychotic disorders, or other psychiatric conditions is indicated.

DELIRIUM

Delirium, a clinical syndrome characterized as an acute disorder of attention and cognitive function, is the most frequent complication of hospitalization for elders and a potentially devastating problem. Delirium is often unrecognized despite sensitive methods for its detection, and its complications may be preventable.

DEFINITIONS. The definition and diagnostic criteria for delirium continue to evolve. The *Diagnostic and Statistical Manual,* Version IV, of the American Psychiatric Association has been widely used (Table 7–1), but development of the criteria in this manual was based on expert consensus, and their diagnostic sensitivity and specificity have not been determined. The Confusion Assessment Method provides a simple, operationalized diagnostic algorithm with a sensitivity of 94 to 100% and a specificity of 90 to 95%.

ETIOLOGY. Similar to other common geriatric syndromes (see Chapter 8), delirium is usually of multifactorial etiology. A search for the innumerable potential underlying contributors requires clinical astuteness and a thorough medical evaluation, especially since many of these factors are treatable but, if untreated, may result in substantial morbidity and mortality. The process is made more challenging by the frequently nonspecific, atypical, or muted features of the underlying illness in older persons. In fact, delirium is commonly the only initial sign of underlying life-threatening illness such as pneumonia, urosepsis, or myocardial infarction in the geriatric population.

The development of delirium usually involves a complex interrelationship between a vulnerable patient with pertinent predisposing factors and exposure to noxious insults or precipitating factors. Thus delirium may develop in patients who are highly vulnerable to delirium—such as the cognitively impaired or severely ill—after a relatively benign insult such as a single dose of sleeping medication. Conversely, patients who are not vulnerable would be rela-

Table 7–1 ■ DIAGNOSTIC CRITERIA FOR DELIRIUM

DSM-IV Diagnostic Criteria
  A. Disturbance of consciousness (i.e., reduced clarity of awareness of the environment) with reduced ability to focus, sustain, or shift attention.
  B. A change in cognition (such as memory deficit, disorientation, language disturbance) or the development of a perceptual disturbance that is not better accounted for by a pre-existing, established, or evolving dementia.
  C. The disturbance develops over a short period (usually hours to days) and tends to fluctuate during the course of the day.
  D. Evidence from the history, physical examination, or laboratory findings indicates that the disturbance is caused by the direct physiologic consequences of a general medical condition.

The CAM Diagnostic Algorithm*
Feature 1. Acute onset and fluctuating course
  This feature is usually obtained from a family member or nurse and is shown by positive responses to the following questions: Is there evidence of an acute change in mental status from the patient's baseline? Did the (abnormal) behavior fluctuate during the day, that is, tend to come and go, or increase and decrease in severity?
Feature 2. Inattention
  This feature is shown by a positive response to the following question: Did the patient have difficulty focusing attention, for example, being easily distractible, or have difficulty keeping track of what was being said?
Feature 3. Disorganized thinking
  This feature is shown by a positive response to the following question: Was the patient's thinking disorganized or incoherent such as rambling or irrelevant conversation, unclear or illogical in flow of ideas, or unpredictable and switching from subject to subject?
Feature 4. Altered level of consciousness
  This feature is shown by any answer other than "alert" to the following question: Overall, how would you rate this patient's level of consciousness (alert [normal], vigilant [hyperalert], lethargic [drowsy, easily aroused], stupor [difficult to arouse], or coma [unarousable])?

DSM-IV = *Diagnostic and Statistical Manual of Mental Disorders,* Version IV; CAM = Confusion Assessment Method.
  *The diagnosis of delirium by CAM requires the presence of features 1 and 2 and either 3 or 4.
  From Inouye SK, van Dyck CH, Alessi CA, et al: Clarifying confusion: The Confusion Assessment Method. A new method for detection of delirium. Ann Intern Med 113:941, 1990.

tively resistant, and delirium would develop only after exposure to multiple noxious insults. Moreover, previous studies have demonstrated that the effects of these risk factors may be cumulative. The importance of this multifactorial causation to the clinician is that removing or treating one factor in isolation will not usually be sufficient to resolve the delirium. Instead, the full spectrum of vulnerability and precipitating factors should be addressed.

Predisposing, or vulnerability, factors identified consistently in previous studies include pre-existing cognitive impairment or dementia, severe underlying illness, high levels of comorbidity, functional impairment, advanced age, chronic renal insufficiency, dehydration, malnutrition, and vision or hearing impairment. Dementia is an important and consistent risk factor for delirium, with demented patients having a two- to five-fold increased risk for delirium. Moreover, 30 to 50% of delirious patients have underlying dementia. Delirious patients commonly have evidence of underlying chronic brain disease, particularly conditions associated with cognitive impairment such as Parkinson's disease, cerebrovascular disease, and space-occupying lesions.

Medications, the most common remediable cause of delirium, contribute to delirium in up to 40% of cases (see Chapter 6). Insufficiency or failure of any major organ system, particularly renal or hepatic failure, can precipitate delirium. Both hypoxemia and hypercarbia have been associated with delirium. Clinicians must be attuned to occult respiratory failure, which in the elderly often lacks the usual signs and symptoms of dyspnea and tachypnea and can be missed by measuring oxygen saturation alone. Acute myocardial infarction or congestive heart failure can be manifested as delirium in an elderly patient without the usual symptoms of chest pain or dyspnea. Occult infection is a particularly notable cause of delirium. Older patients frequently fail to mount the febrile or leukocytotic response to infection, and clinicians must carefully assess for signs of pneumonia, urinary tract infection, endocarditis, abdominal abscess, or infected joints. A variety of metabolic disorders may contribute to delirium, including hypernatremia or hyponatremia, hypercalcemia, acid-base disorders, hypoglycemia and hyperglycemia, and thyroid or adrenal disorders. Immobilization and immobilizing devices (e.g., indwelling bladder catheters, physical restraints) have been demonstrated to be important factors precipitating delirium. Dehydration and volume depletion, as well as nutritional decline during hospitalization (e.g., decline in weight, fall in serum albumin), are well-documented factors contributing to delirium. Drug and alcohol withdrawal are important and often unsuspected causes of delirium in the elderly. Environmental factors such as an unfamiliar environment, sleep deprivation, deranged schedule, frequent room changes, sensory overload, or sensory deprivation may aggravate delirium in the hospital setting. Psychosocial factors such as depression, psychological stress, pain, or lack of social supports may also precipitate delirium.

INCIDENCE AND PREVALENCE. In the elderly, the prevalence of delirium at hospital admission can range from 10 to 40%. Delirium can develop in as many as 25 to 56% of patients during hospitalization. Higher rates are found when frequent surveillance is performed in older, surgical, and intensive care populations.

EPIDEMIOLOGY. The associated hospital mortality rates for delirium range from 25 to 33%, rates as high as those associated with acute myocardial infarction and sepsis. The problem of delirium in hospitalized elderly patients has assumed particular prominence because patients aged 65 years and older currently account for more than 40% of all inpatient days of hospital care. Based on recent U.S. vital health statistics and a conservative delirium rate of 20%, delirium will complicate hospital stays for over 2.3 million older persons, involve over 17.5 million inpatient days, and account for over $4 billion of hospital expenditures each year. Substantial additional costs are incurred after hospital discharge because of the increased need for rehabilitation services, nursing home placement, and home care. These extrapolations highlight the extensive economic and health policy implications of delirium.

PATHOGENESIS. The basic pathogenesis of delirium remains unclear. Most investigators agree that delirium appears to be a functional rather than structural lesion. Electroencephalographic studies demonstrate global functional derangements in patients with delirium, characterized by generalized slowing of cortical background (alpha) activity. The leading current hypotheses view delirium as the final common pathway of many different pathogenic mechanisms culminating in a widespread reduction in cerebral oxidative metabolism with resultant impairment of cholinergic transmission. Proposed mediators examined in previous studies have included β-endorphin, somatostatin, lymphokines, tryptophan, phenylalanine metabolites, and cortisol. Although delirium has long been considered a transient syndrome, several of these basic mechanisms may not be completely reversible, particularly those resulting in hypoxic damage. Moreover, the dose and duration of the noxious insults, along with the degree of vulnerability of the patient, may also exert great influence on the ultimate reversibility of the delirium.

CLINICAL MANIFESTATIONS. The cardinal features of delirium include acute onset and inattention. Establishing the acuity of onset requires accurate knowledge of the patient's baseline cognitive function. Patients are inattentive, that is, they have difficulty focusing, maintaining, and shifting attention. They appear easily distracted and have difficulty maintaining conversation and following commands. Objectively, patients may have difficulty with simple repetitive tasks, digit spans, and recitation of months backward. Other key features include disorganization of thought processes, which is usually a manifestation of underlying cognitive or perceptual disturbances, and an altered level of consciousness, typically lethargy with reduced clarity of awareness of the environment. Although not cardinal elements, other features frequently occurring during delirium include disorientation, cognitive deficits, psychomotor agitation or retardation, perceptual disturbances such as hallucinations and illusions, paranoid delusions, and sleep-wake cycle reversal.

DIAGNOSIS AND EVALUATION. The cornerstone of evaluation of delirium is a comprehensive history and physical examination. The first step in evaluation (Table 7–2) should be to establish the diagnosis of delirium through cognitive assessment and determine whether the present condition represents an acute change from the patient's baseline cognitive function. Because cognitive impairment may not be apparent during conversation, brief cognitive screening tests such as the Mini-Mental Status Examination should be used. Attention should be further assessed with simple tests such as a forward digit span (inattention indicated by an inability to repeat five digits forward) or recitation of the months backward. The history, which should be obtained from a reliable informant, is targeted to establish the patient's baseline cognitive function and the time course of any mental status change, as well as to obtain clues about potential precipitating factors such as recent medication changes, intercurrent infections, or medical illnesses. Physical examination should include a detailed neurologic examination for focal deficits and a careful search for signs of occult infection or an acute abdominal process.

A crucial difficulty in the differential diagnosis of delirium is distinguishing a long-standing confusional state (dementia) from delirium alone or delirium superimposed on dementia. These two conditions are differentiated by the acute onset of symptoms in delirium (dementia is much more insidious) and the impaired attention and altered level of consciousness associated with delirium. The differential diagnosis also includes depression and nonorganic psychotic disorders. Although paranoia, hallucinations, and affective changes can occur with delirium, the key features of acute onset, inattention, altered level of consciousness, and global cognitive impairment will assist in the recognition of delirium. At times, the differential diagnosis can be quite difficult—particularly with an uncooperative patient or when an accurate history is unavailable. Because of the potentially life-threatening nature of delirium, it is prudent to manage the patient as having delirium and search for underlying precipitants (e.g., intercurrent illness, metabolic derangements, drug toxicity) until further information can be obtained.

Review of the medication list, including over-the-counter medications, is critical, and use of medications with psychoactive effects should be discontinued or minimized whenever possible. In the elderly, these medications may cause psychoactive effects even at dosages and measured drug levels that are within the "therapeutic range." Consideration should be given to the possibility that withdrawal from alcohol or other medications is a contributor to delirium.

Laboratory evaluation must be tailored to the individual situation (see Table 7–2). In patients with pre-existing cardiac or respiratory diseases or related symptoms, an electrocardiogram or arterial blood gas determination may be indicated. The need for cerebrospinal fluid examination remains controversial except when clearly indicated, such as in a febrile delirious patient. Brain imaging should be reserved for patients with new focal neurologic signs, for those with a history or signs of head trauma, or for patients without another identifiable cause of the delirium. The electroencephalogram, with its false-negative rate of 17% and false-positive rate of 22% in distinguishing delirious and nondelirious patients, has a limited role and is most useful for detecting an occult seizure disorder and differentiating delirium from nonorganic psychiatric disorders.

TREATMENT. In general, nonpharmacologic approaches should be used in all delirious patients and will usually be successful for symptom management. Pharmacologic approaches should be reserved for the occasional patient in whom the delirium symptoms may result in interruption of needed medical therapies (e.g., intubation, intravenous lines) or may endanger the safety of the patient or other persons. However, no drug is ideal for the treatment of delirium symptoms; any choice may further cloud the patient's mental status and obscure efforts to monitor the course of the mental status change. Thus any drug chosen should be given in the lowest dose for the shortest time possible. Neuroleptics are the preferred agents of treatment, with haloperidol and thioridazine being the most widely used agents. Haloperidol causes less orthostatic hypotension and fewer anticholinergic side effects than thioridazine does and is available in parenteral form; however, it has a higher rate of extrapyramidal side effects and acute dystonias. If parenteral administration is required, intravenous use results in rapid onset of action with a short duration of effect, whereas intramuscular use will have a more optimal duration of action. Thioridazine, which is more sedating, may be beneficial in agitated patients; its elixir form can be given by the oral or nasogastric route. The recommended starting dose is 0.5 to 1.0 mg haloperidol orally or parenterally or thioridazine, 10 to 25 mg orally, and then repeating the dose every 30 minutes after the vital signs have been rechecked until sedation has been achieved. The end point should be an awake but manageable patient. The average elderly patient who has not previously been treated with neuroleptics should require a total loading dose of no more than 3 to 5 mg of haloperidol or 50 to 100 mg of thioridazine. Subsequently, a maintenance dose consisting of half of the loading dose should be administered in divided doses over the next 24 hours, with doses tapered over the next few days as the agitation resolves.

Benzodiazepines are not recommended for the first-line treatment

---

Table 7–2 ■ EVALUATION OF DELIRIUM IN ELDERLY PATIENTS

1. Cognitive testing and determination of baseline cognitive functioning. Establish the diagnosis of delirium
2. Comprehensive history and physical examination, including careful neurologic examination for focal deficits and search for occult infection
3. Review the medication list: discontinue or minimize all psychoactive medications. Check the side effects of all medications
4. Laboratory evaluation (tailored to the individual): complete blood count, electrolytes, blood urea nitrogen, creatinine, glucose, calcium, phosphate, liver enzymes, oxygen saturation
5. Search for occult infection: physical examination, urinalysis, chest radiography, selected cultures (as indicated)
6. When no obvious cause is revealed from the above steps, further targeted evaluation is considered in selected patients:
   Laboratory tests:
     Magnesium, thyroid function tests, B_{12} level, drug levels, toxicology screen, ammonia level
   Arterial blood gas:
     Indicated in patients with dyspnea, tachypnea, any acute pulmonary process, or history of significant respiratory disease
   Electrocardiogram:
     Indicated in patients with chest or abdominal discomfort, shortness of breath, or cardiac history
   Cerebrospinal fluid examination:
     Indicated when meningitis or encephalitis is suspected
   Brain imaging:
     Indicated in patients with new focal neurologic signs or with a history or signs of head trauma
   Electroencephalogram:
     Useful in diagnosing occult seizure disorder and differentiating delirium from nonorganic psychiatric disorders

of delirium because of their tendency to cause oversedation and exacerbate the confusional state. However, they remain the drugs of choice for treatment of withdrawal syndromes from alcohol and sedative drugs (see Chapters 16 and 17).

Non-pharmacologic management techniques recommended for every delirious patient include encouraging the presence of family members, using "sitters" to be orienting influences, or transferring a disruptive patient to a private room or closer to the nurse's station for increased supervision. Interpersonal contact and communication, including verbal reorientation strategies, simple instructions and explanations, and frequent eye contact, are vital. Patients should be involved in their own care and allowed to participate in decision making as much as possible. Eyeglasses and hearing aids may reduce sensory deficits. Mobility, self-care, and independence should be encouraged, and physical restraints should be avoided, if possible, because of their tendency to increase agitation, their questionable efficacy, and their potential to cause injury. Attention must be focused on minimizing the disruptive influences of the hospital environment. Clocks and calendars should be provided to assist with orientation. Room and staff changes should be kept to a minimum. A quiet environment with low-level lighting is optimal for delirious patients. Perhaps the most important intervention is to allow an uninterrupted period for sleep at night. Nonpharmacologic approaches to relaxation, including music, relaxation tapes, and massage, can be highly effective.

PROGNOSIS. Delirium is an important independent determinant of prolonged length of hospital stay, increased mortality, increased rates of institutional placement, and functional and cognitive decline—even after controlling for age, gender, dementia, illness severity, and baseline functional status.

Delirium had previously been considered to be a reversible, transient condition, but recent studies on the duration and persistence of delirium symptoms document that delirium may be much more persistent than previously believed. In fact, delirium duration of 30 days or more is typical, and as few as 20% of patients may have complete resolution of all delirium symptoms at 6-month follow-up. Moreover, a prolonged transitional phase characterized by abnormalities in cognition, affect, or behavior appears to be quite common. In addition, delirium appears to have greater deleterious effects in patients with underlying cognitive impairment. The long-term detrimental effects are most probably related to the duration, severity, and underlying cause(s) of the delirium, as well as the vulnerability of the host (i.e., baseline cognitive impairment).

PREVENTION. The most effective intervention strategy to reduce delirium and its associated complications is primary prevention of delirium before it occurs. Ideally, preventive strategies should address important delirium risk factors and target patients at moderate to high risk for delirium at baseline (Table 7–3). On a larger scale, preventive efforts for delirium will require system-wide changes to educate physicians and nurses to improve recognition and heighten awareness of the clinical implications, provide incentives to change practice patterns that lead to delirium (e.g., immobilization, use of sleep medications, bladder catheters, and physical restraints), and create systems that enhance high-quality geriatric care (e.g., geriatric expertise, case management, clinical pathways, and quality monitoring).

Cole MG, Primeau FJ: Prognosis of delirium in elderly hospital patients. Can Med Assoc J 149:41, 1993. *Systematic review with a meta-analysis of eight studies involving 573 delirious patients on outcomes associated with delirium.*

Elie M, Cole MG, Primeau FJ, Bellavence F: Delirium risk factors in elderly hospitalized patients. J Gen Intern Med 13:204, 1998. *Review emphasizing that advanced age, underlying dementia, and serious medical illness are the principal risk factors for delirium in the hospital.*

Francis J: Delirium in older patients. J Am Geriatr Soc 40:829, 1992. *An outstanding review of the recent literature on delirium with an extensive reference list.*

Inouye SK, Bogardus ST, Charpentier PA, et al: A multicomponent intervention to prevent delirium in hospitalized older patients. N Engl J Med 340:669, 1999. *Clinical trial of a multiple risk factor reduction approach for prevention of delirium in hospitalized older medical patients.*

Rummans TA, Evans JM, Krahn LE, Fleming KC: Delirium in elderly patients: Evaluation and management. Mayo Clin Proc 70:989, 1995. *Recent review of aspects of clinical findings and management approaches.*

8 SPECIAL PROBLEMS IN THE GERIATRIC PATIENT

Judith C. Ahronheim

Biologic and chronologic ages are not well matched. Nevertheless, physiologic changes and the higher prevalence of overt and subclinical disease in late life create specific vulnerabilities and special problems.

DRUGS AND RISKS

CLINICAL PHARMACOLOGY. The elderly experience more adverse drug events than any other age group does because their exposure to larger numbers of medications provides more opportunities for medication errors and drug-drug interactions and because their altered pharmacokinetics results in enhanced sensitivity to many agents.

PHARMACOKINETIC CHANGES. Age-related physiologic changes, especially in renal function, that occur in late life reduce drug elimination, prolong drug half-life, and increase the risk of drug toxicity. Although the average glomerular filtration rate (GFR) declines approximately 50% between the third and ninth decades of life primarily as a result of hypertension and diabetes, many individuals maintain normal or nearly normal GFR in late life. Serum creatinine does not reflect the age-related decline in GFR or predict individual renal function because muscle mass, the source of serum creatinine, also declines with age.

In general, the loading dose of medications should not be altered in the presence of renal dysfunction, but subsequent doses, especially for medications that have narrow therapeutic-to-toxic ratios and are eliminated by the kidney, such as digoxin and aminoglycosides, must be adjusted according to actual renal function for any medication. Formulas such as

Creatinine clearance

$$= \frac{\text{weight (kg)} \times (140 - \text{age})}{72 \times \text{serum creatine (mg/dL)}} \quad \text{(for women, multiply result by 0.85)}$$

for rapid estimation of GFR have been validated in subgroups of elderly patients and should be used when dosing decisions are rapidly needed. However, these estimates may be inaccurate in debilitated patients with muscle wasting and in the dynamic setting of acute illness. Serum drug levels should be obtained to guide dosing of drugs with a narrow therapeutic-to-toxic ratio.

Table 7–3 ■ DELIRIUM RISK FACTORS AND POTENTIAL INTERVENTIONS

RISK FACTOR	INTERVENTIONS
Cognitive impairment	Therapeutic activities program
	Reality orientation program (reorienting techniques, communication)
Sleep deprivation	Noise reduction strategies
	Scheduling of nighttime medications, procedures, and nursing activities to allow uninterrupted period of sleep
Immobilization	Early mobilization (e.g., ambulation or bedside exercises)
	Minimizing immobilizing equipment (e.g., bladder catheters)
Psychoactive medications	Restricted use of "as needed" sleep and psychoactive medications (e.g., sedative-hypnotics, narcotics, anticholinergic medications)
	Nonpharmacologic protocols for management of sleep and anxiety
Vision impairment	Provision of vision aids (e.g., magnifiers, special lighting)
	Provision of adaptive equipment (e.g., illuminated phone dials, large-print books)
Hearing impairment	Provision of amplifying devices
	Repair of hearing aids
Dehydration	Early recognition and volume repletion

Hepatic blood flow may decrease with advancing age, but controversy exists over the extent to which age-related hepatic changes affect drug metabolism. Some but not all studies have demonstrated a decline in hepatic oxidative processes ("phase I" metabolism) in the elderly. Likewise, unanimity is lacking over whether the inducibility or inhibition of the cytochrome P-450 system, which is responsible for most oxidative drug metabolism, changes with age. In contrast, it is generally agreed that hepatic conjugation ("phase II" metabolism) is unaltered with age. Unlike oxidized metabolites, which are often active, metabolites produced by conjugation are usually inactive. Diazepam undergoes oxidation to long-acting, renally excreted metabolites, and repeated dosing may lead to delayed toxicity. In contrast, lorazepam undergoes conjugation and inactive metabolites are produced. It should not be assumed that normal conjugation of medications such as lorazepam guarantees safety because the effects of certain drugs may be enhanced in the elderly regardless of the metabolic pathway.

With advancing age, lean body mass declines and body fat increases. Thus the volume of distribution tends to be lower for water-soluble drugs and higher for fat-soluble drugs. The onset of action of a water-soluble drug such as alcohol may be earlier than expected, and the steady-state concentrations of a lipid-soluble drug such as diazepam may not be reached until later than expected. In the latter situation, toxicity may occur in a delayed and unexpected fashion, especially in the presence of active metabolites.

Serum albumin remains normal in the healthy elderly but may decline swiftly during illness owing to inflammation, impaired protein synthesis, and diminished reserves in late life. When serum albumin levels are low, standard clinical laboratory assays of drugs highly bound to albumin (such as phenytoin) may be misleading because they reflect total (bound plus free) drug and hence might prompt the clinician to raise the dose and create the potential for toxicity.

PHARMACODYNAMICS. Although the effects of some agents at the tissue level may decrease in late life, most alterations involve enhanced effects on the target or non-target organ, probably related to physiologic changes as well as the presence of overt or silent disease. Whether caused by reduced elimination (altered pharmacokinetics) or alterations in the receptor or tissue itself (pharmacodynamics), the known side effects of essentially all medications may be potentiated in the elderly.

BOWEL AND BLADDER PROBLEMS

CONSTIPATION AND FECAL IMPACTION. Contrary to popular belief, there is little evidence to indicate an increased prevalence of constipation among the community-dwelling elderly, although the use of laxatives is increased, perhaps because of traditional beliefs about what constitutes normal bowel function. Constipation may be increased among the institutionalized elderly, however, because of immobility, decreased intake of fluid and fiber, prolonged intestinal transit time, impaired anorectal sensation, neurologic disease, bowel lesions, and the use of constipating medicines. Constipating medications include but are not limited to tricyclic antidepressants, anticholinergics, some antihypertensive agents, calcium channel antagonists, opioid analgesics, aluminum-containing antacids, and bile acid resins.

An important consequence of constipation is fecal impaction, which may be manifested as fever, altered mental status, agitation, urinary retention, or paradoxical diarrhea caused by leakage around the impaction. Because of these features, fecal impaction can be mistaken for other problems and hence be treated inappropriately. Fecal impaction can usually be treated with suppositories, enemas, or manual disimpaction, but in extreme cases mechanical bowel obstruction may require surgical intervention. Prevention consists of strict attention to the patient's bowel habits, adequate hydration, adequate but not excessive dietary fiber, avoidance of constipating medications when possible, and judicious use of laxatives.

PROBLEMS WITH MICTURITION. URINARY INCONTINENCE. Urinary incontinence affects 10 to 30% of the community-residing elderly (Table 8–1). The prevalence rises among the oldest elderly and reaches at least 60 to 70% among elderly persons residing in nursing homes. The most common cause of urinary incontinence in elderly men and women is overactivity of the bladder detrusor. In this condition (called "detrusor instability"), the detrusor muscle

Table 8–1 ■ COMMON FORMS OF URINARY INCONTINENCE IN THE ELDERLY

TYPE	CAUSE OR ASSOCIATION
Urge (detrusor instability)	Post-menopause, old age, CNS disease
Stress	Increased intra-abdominal pressure superimposed on
"True"	Incompetent urethral sphincter
Reflex	Overdistended bladder
Mixed urge and stress	See above
Overflow	Incomplete bladder outlet obstruction (e.g., BPH), bladder atony (e.g., long-standing diabetes)
Pseudoincontinence	Inability to toilet, confusional states

CNS = central nervous system; BPH = benign prostatic hypertrophy.

contracts in response to inappropriately small volumes of urine, often preceded by a sense of urgency. Incontinence results if the patient is unable to get to the toilet on time or when other problems coexist such as urethral incompetence or bladder inflammation. Detrusor instability is believed to be caused by lack of inhibition of the brain stem detrusor reflex by higher cerebrocortical centers. However, most affected elderly have no clinically apparent neurologic disease.

The symptoms of detrusor instability—frequency and urge incontinence—may be ameliorated by "bladder training," which consists of prolonging the interval between voidings by using behavioral techniques. Patients who are physically disabled or cognitively impaired should be toileted frequently or on a schedule, and incontinence garments (adult diapers) may be used. Antispasmodic agents such as oxybutynin, which relaxes the bladder wall and promotes the storage of urine, presumably by inhibiting cholinergically mediated detrusor contractions, may be useful. Other medications with anticholinergic activity, such as imipramine, have been suggested for this purpose but, owing to central nervous system effects and other actions, are less well tolerated in geriatric patients.

In elderly women, post-menopausal changes in pelvic musculature contribute to urinary incontinence by leading to loss of the extrinsic support of pelvic organs and the bladder neck. Pelvic and distal urethral tissue contain estrogen and progesterone receptors, and the urethra may become patulous after menopause. In this setting, intra-abdominal pressure may easily surpass intraurethral pressure and lead to leakage of urine. This "true stress incontinence" (i.e., occurring in the absence of a detrusor contraction) typically occurs immediately after a cough or sneeze or, in severe cases, merely upon arising from a sitting position. Stress incontinence may respond to treatment with exogenous estrogens, but data in patients 75 years and older are limited. Other treatment approaches include pelvic muscle exercises and α-adrenergic agents such as phenylpropanolamine, which act on urethral α-adrenergic receptors to increase urethral tone.

Urodynamic studies are not routinely required to evaluate incontinence, but testing ranging from simple bedside observation to a series of complex tests should be considered when the history and clinical evaluation fail to explain the cause. Asymptomatic patients may exhibit involuntary detrusor contractions on cystometric testing, whereas patients with detrusor instability may have a falsely negative test if they are psychologically inhibited from emptying their bladders under testing conditions. Likewise, urodynamic testing may not be predictive of who will benefit from a specific treatment, especially in patients with multiple abnormalities.

Chronic indwelling catheters should not be used in the management of incontinence, even in patients with decubitus ulcers, because urinary tract infection develops in virtually 100% of chronically catheterized patients and chronic antibiotic suppression merely leads to the production of resistant strains of organisms. When indwelling catheters are the only alternative (as in urinary retention that cannot be managed with intermittent catheterization), antibiotic treatment should be reserved for symptomatic illness or unexplained lethargy.

URINARY RETENTION. Urinary retention is far more common in men, in whom it is most often related, at least in part, to prostatic outlet obstruction caused by benign prostatic hyperplasia. Acute urinary retention may occur in elderly men and less often in women as a result of fecal impaction, the bedridden state, immobility, or anticholinergic drugs such as tricyclic antidepressants, disopyramide, first-generation antihistamines, and drugs used to treat urinary incontinence. Diuretics can also lead to urinary retention when they produce a volume of urine that overwhelms the compromised bladder. Urinary retention may be precipitated following surgery by the prolonged effects of anesthetic agents and opioid analgesics. Urinary retention that first begins in the hospital can persist for some time but generally resolves when the the patient does not have an antecedent history of retention.

Long-standing diabetes mellitus may be associated with a "cystopathy" caused by peripheral neuropathy of the afferent limb of the spinal detrusor reflex and the resulting detrusor areflexia. However, most elderly diabetics with bladder dysfunction do not suffer from diabetic cystopathy, perhaps because of shorter disease duration in adult-onset diabetes.

It is important to distinguish frank urinary retention (the inability to void) from increased residual urine, defined as a post-void residual urine volume greater than *approximately* 50 mL. For example, in elderly women, anatomic problems such as cystocele may increase residual urine. Other patients may have incomplete bladder emptying because of modest detrusor hyporeflexia. Frank urinary retention, which may be manifested as "overflow incontinence," requires immediate attention, whereas increased post-void residual urine, which is often asymptomatic, does not in and of itself require treatment.

FALLS AND FRACTURES

Approximately one third of people 75 years and older fall at least once annually, and a key aspect of management in elderly patients is the prevention of falls. When fall-related injury occurs, it is just as important to assess the reason for the fall as to address the injury. Falls among the elderly are most commonly caused by acute or chronic neurologic disease, arthritis, musculoskeletal impairments, poor balance, postural instability, cardiac arrhythmias, generalized weakness from acute or chronic medical illness (including acute myocardial infarction), orthostatic hypotension, or impaired coordination hampering the ability to fall "well." Additional factors are visual impairments, dementia, medications with sedating properties, and antihypertensive medications, especially when they lead to overcorrection of hypertension.

The probable cause of the fall can be ascertained in 95% of cases with a careful history and physical examination alone. Further diagnostic work-up should be guided by this initial evaluation.

Although most falls in the elderly result in trivial or minor injury, approximately 5% result in injury serious enough to require hospitalization. Falls are by far the most important accidental cause of death in the geriatric population; the death rate from falls is approximately 10 per 100,000 population between the ages of 65 and 74 years, but it rises to approximately 150 per 100,000 after age 85.

Wrist and hip fractures are almost always related to a fall, whereas vertebral wedging and fractures may occur without obvious trauma. The incidence of wrist (Colles') fracture increases in mid-life among women but reaches a plateau by age 60. In contrast, the incidence of hip fracture rises steadily after age 60, and approximately 17% of men and 30% of women sustain a hip fracture by age 90. These fracture patterns may be partly related to the mechanism of falling in that an older person may lack the coordination to break a fall by quickly throwing out the arm. In addition, reduced muscle mass and subcutaneous fat may contribute to diminished absorption of energy on impact.

Hip fractures in the elderly are a surgical emergency. Initial radiographs sometimes fail to reveal a fracture. When an elderly patient has fallen and cannot stand or bear weight or has severe pain on weight bearing, the hip must be deemed fractured until proved otherwise. If repeat radiography fails to reveal a fracture on frontal and lateral views, a bone scan or magnetic resonance imaging should be done. Surgery should be performed as soon as the patient is medically stabilized because morbidity and mortality rise exponentially if surgery is delayed beyond approximately 48 hours.

Assiduous medical management of these frail patients is essential and should be directed at prevention or treatment of pneumonia, deep vein thrombosis, pulmonary embolus, pressure sores, urinary tract infection, and fecal impaction. Post-operative delirium (see Chapter 7) is common and may be due to one or more medical problems, to medications, or to prolonged effects of anesthesia.

The increased risk of fracture with aging is due not only to the tendency to fall but also to bone loss, which begins to occur after the fourth decade of life in both sexes. At the time of menopause, the rate of bone loss in women accelerates for approximately 7 years. The accelerated phase is manifested first in trabecular bone of the vertebrae and the extreme ends of long bones. In the absence of trauma, the rate of spinal compression fractures is about eight times higher, and the rate of wrist and hip fracture from all causes is about twice as high in women as in men. Recent evidence indicates that bone loss further accelerates in the last decades of life in both men and women.

Age-related bone loss is due largely to osteoporosis (see Chapter 257), but many geriatric patients also have osteomalacia (Chapter 263). Osteomalacia in the elderly is most often due to vitamin D deficiency, usually coexists with osteoporosis, and resembles the latter clinically. Vitamin D deficiency may be due to inadequate sunlight exposure, impairment in intestinal vitamin D absorption, and a reduced capacity to manufacture vitamin D in the skin.

Osteomalacia is preventable and treatable. Only about 15 minutes of sunlight exposure twice per week is needed to optimize the vitamin D status in light-skinned adults. The elderly may require somewhat more, and still more time is required in deeply pigmented persons, in whom ultraviolet light does not penetrate the melanin layer as quickly. Elderly people, regardless of race, should ingest a minimum of 800 IU/day of vitamin D and higher doses if vitamin D deficiency is documented. Much higher doses should be continued only until the deficiency is corrected because of the danger of toxicity. Excessive sunlight exposure does not produce hypervitaminosis D but should be avoided to minimize skin damage.

Substantial advances have been made in the prevention and treatment of osteoporosis in the elderly, with special emphasis on estrogen in women and biphosphonates in both women and men (see Chapter 257). Weight bearing and resistive exercise also retard bone loss. A sensible exercise program tailored to the needs and limitations of the individual patient also helps maintain mobility, muscle tone, and cardiovascular function.

It is always important to identify and address preventable causes of bone loss such as primary hyperparathyroidism, vitamin D deficiency, phosphate depletion, use of corticosteroids or heparin, cigarette smoking, excessive alcohol intake, and marginal calcium intake. Correction of negative calcium balance in elderly men and women generally requires a daily total intake of 1500 mg elemental calcium from dietary sources and supplements.

FLUID BALANCE AND ELECTROLYTE DISORDERS

Geriatric patients may become easily dehydrated after a variety of insults such as excessive environmental heat, diarrhea, or febrile illness. Underlying factors are an impaired renal concentrating ability and impaired urinary sodium conservation in response to salt deprivation as a result of progressive loss of nephrons, especially in the renal cortex, an increase in basal and stimulated levels of atrial natriuretic hormone, and a decrease in the responsiveness of the renin-angiotensin-aldosterone system. In addition, the thirst response to dehydration is diminished even among healthy elderly. All these problems are accentuated in neurologically impaired patients, who are even less likely to seek water when dehydrated. A variety of medical illnesses may therefore be complicated by or be manifested as hypernatremia, hyperosmolarity, and obtundation.

Even more common is hyponatremia caused by an exaggerated release of arginine vasopressin after an osmotic stimulus and a decreased ability to excrete a water load, in part related to the reduced GFR. Elderly patients also have a higher rate of disorders that predispose to hyponatremia, such as congestive heart failure, central neurologic impairments, and the syndrome of inappropriate antidiuretic hormone secretion (SIADH). The disproportionate occurrence of SIADH among the elderly is probably related to enhanced physiologic release of arginine vasopressin, as well as exposure to the many pharmacologic agents known to produce this syndrome.

Enteral tube feeding is also frequently associated with hyponatremia. Although hypotonic feeds may be partly to blame, hyponatremia in tube-fed patients may also be a marker for underlying central nervous system disease, which has been associated with SIADH. In neurologically impaired, tube-fed patients, attention must be paid to the amount of free water added to the feed or used to flush the feeding tube, and serum sodium must be monitored. When saline solutions are given to correct dehydration, salt deficits, or fluid-electrolyte imbalance, they must be infused cautiously and with careful monitoring to avoid heart failure.

PRESSURE SORES

Most pressure sores (decubitus ulcers) occur within the first 2 weeks of hospitalization or institutionalization. The prevalence among nursing home patients is approximately 11%, but as many as 20% of these patients have hospital-acquired pressure sores when they are admitted to the nursing home.

Pressure sores develop when extrinsic pressure on the skin exceeds the mean capillary pressure (32 mm Hg), thereby reducing blood flow and tissue oxygenation. In recumbent patients, pressures over the sacrum or greater trochanter reach as high as 100 to 150 mm Hg. Moisture, friction, and shear contribute to skin breakdown under these circumstances. Advanced age may increase the risk because of changes in the skin, including decreased thickness and vascularity of the dermal layer, delayed wound healing, and redistribution of fat from the subcutaneous to deeper layers. Conditions that increase risk include immobility, arterial insufficiency, poor nutrition, and zinc, iron, or vitamin C deficiency. Neurologic impairments reduce the spontaneous movements that normally occur during sleep. Associated urinary and fecal incontinence exacerbate the problem by creating moisture and irritation.

Pressure sores can occur anywhere on the body. Typical sites include dependent areas possessing minimal subcutaneous fat and bony prominences such as the sacrum, greater trochanter, scapula, lateral malleolus, thoracic spine, and heels.

The hallmark of prevention is avoidance of pressure, and patients at risk should be identified early. Bedridden patients should be lifted, not dragged, across the sheet. Normal skin should be kept clean and dry without the use of indwelling catheters because they do not avoid the problem of fecal soilage and may reduce nursing vigilance. An effort should be made to restore nutritional deficiencies, but nutritional repletion is not a substitute for removal of pressure and meticulous skin care.

Shallow ulcer craters should be kept clean and covered with a dressing if indicated. Uncomplicated blisters should be managed without débridement or dressing because blister fluid may enhance wound healing. Ulcers involving subcutaneous tissue may generate substantial necrotic tissue, which should be débrided. Débridement can be accomplished mechanically with dressings or enzymatically with débriding agents. Ulcers extending through fascia or involving bone, muscle, or supporting tissue require surgical débridement and often skin grafting.

A variety of appliances, dressings, and débriding methods may supplement meticulous nursing care, although clinical trials to prove their efficacy or cost-effectiveness are often lacking. Foam "egg crate" pads and mattresses redistribute pressure, and sheepskin padding absorbs moisture. Air-fluidized beds (warm air flowing through silicon beads) and alternating air pressure mattresses redistribute and reduce extrinsic pressure. Although the air-fluidized bed may help speed ulcer healing, it is expensive and difficult to clean. Wet-to-dry dressings enhance débridement of necrotic tissue, but if the dressing is not exposed to air, it macerates healthy skin and enlarges the ulcer. Inappropriate use of wet-to-dry dressings desiccates underlying tissue. Occlusive hydrocolloid dressings may enhance healing, avoid the problem of desiccation, and protect a pressure sore from external soilage. A covered wound cannot be inspected, however, and sophisticated dressings should not create a false sense of security or reduce nursing vigilance when the key to treatment lies in removal of pressure.

Ulcer craters should not be treated with topical antibiotics, which promote antimicrobial resistance without enhancing wound healing. Systemic antibiotics should be used only if obvious cellulitis or evidence of systemic infection related to the skin lesion is present.

MEDICAL DECISION MAKING FOR COGNITIVELY IMPAIRED ELDERLY

Patients have a fundamental right to accept or refuse any medical treatment. The physician must inform patients of the risks, benefits, and alternatives of proposed treatments and determine whether they have the capacity to decide. Many geriatric patients lack decisional capacity because of dementia or other neurologic impairments. Nevertheless, they have the right to refuse treatment either through an advance directive (written or oral) or through an authorized surrogate decision maker (see Chapter 2).

All efforts should be made to involve the patient in the decision-making process. Patients with limited capacity, such as those with early dementia, may still have the ability to make their own medical decisions. Decisional capacity is patient specific and decision specific and is a clinical judgment that can usually be made by a primary care physician. Family members and others often try to "protect" elderly patients out of concern that bad news will be harmful. In extreme situations, the delivery of bad news can be harmful to certain patients (such as a severely depressed patient at risk for suicide). However, in most situations, patients wish to be fully informed and participate in their own care, so it is important for the physician to assess the patient's desire for information and deliver news sensitively.

Despite the general consensus that patients may refuse any form of medical treatment, controversy surrounds the refusal of long-term enteral tube feeding, a treatment often given to patients with advanced neurologic impairment. Although the 1990 U.S. Supreme Court *Cruzan* decision affirmed the right of patients with decisional capacity to refuse tube feeding and other medical treatments, the Court left it up to individual states to set specific legal standards for refusal by patients *lacking* decisional capacity. Some states require a high level of evidence of a patient's previously expressed wishes to refuse life-sustaining treatment, whereas other states have separate legal standards for refusal of tube feeding. Physicians should familiarize themselves with state regulations.

As of this writing, lower courts have twice upheld family requests for treatment deemed medically futile by physicians. The arguments supporting such "futile" treatment have hinged on the need to maintain patient autonomy and affirm the family as the rightful decision makers for incompetent patients; they have not addressed the authority of physicians to make futility determinations. Demands for treatment in such extreme cases are rare and in the courts have been vastly outnumbered by "right-to-die" disputes, in which patients or their surrogates have refused life-prolonging treatments imposed by physicians or institutions. It is uncertain whether recent changes in the health care system and cost-cutting maneuvers will increase the number of conflicts in which patients or families demand care that the health care system is unwilling to provide.

When conflict exists, health professionals who morally object to the withdrawal of life-sustaining treatments have the right to transfer care of the patient to another physician or facility that will uphold the patient's or family's decision. They do not, however, have the right to decide unilaterally what treatments patients should have.

Ahronheim JC: Artificial nutrition and hydration in the terminally ill patient. Clin Geriatr Med 12:379, 1996. *Critical review of medical aspects with an emphasis on enteral feeding of patients with advanced neurologic impairments.*

Arnaud MJ, Baumgartner R, Morley JE, et al: Hydration and Aging. New York, Springer, 1998. *Monograph reviewing the clinical aspects and physiology of sodium and water metabolism in late life and treatment approaches in various disease states.*

Close J, Ellis M, Hooper R, et al: Prevention of falls in the elderly trial (PROFET): A randomised controlled trial. Lancet 353:93, 1999. *An interdisciplinary approach reduced recurrent falls in the elderly.*

Schwartz JB: Clinical pharmacology. *In* Hazzard WR, Blass JP, Ettinger WH, et al: Principles of Geriatric Medicine and Gerontology, 4th ed. New York, McGraw-Hill, 1999, pp 303–331. *Critical review of age-related pharmacologic principles with specific attention given to medications frequently prescribed in geriatric practice.*

Thomas DR, Allman RM (eds): Pressure ulcers. Clin Geriatr Med 13:421, 1997. *Volume devoted to the epidemiology, assessment, and management of pressure ulcers with extensive references.*

Urinary Incontinence Guideline Panel: Urinary Incontinence in Adults: Clinical Practice Guidelines. Rockville, MD, Agency for Health Care Policy and Research, 1996, AHCPR Publication No. 96-0682. *Consensus panel guidelines with extensive references.*

PART IV

PREVENTIVE HEALTH CARE

9 PRINCIPLES OF PREVENTIVE HEALTH CARE

Albert Oberman

A growing body of evidence links personal health behavior and preventive services to the reductions in mortality from the leading causes of death and disability in the United States. Advances in understanding the determinants of risk, the demand for preventive measures in health reform, and the remarkable overall downward mortality trend (Table 9–1) provide the momentum for further primary preventive efforts. Reductions in cardiovascular mortality accounted for much of the decline in total mortality. Yet life expectancy at birth in the United States (78.9 years for women and 72.5 years for men) remains considerably below that of many developed countries. Other causes of preventable morbidity and mortality such as cancer, chronic obstructive pulmonary disease, human immunodeficiency virus (HIV) infection, and homicide have escalated. Men have higher age-adjusted death rates for every cause, especially for HIV infection. Death rates strongly correlate with socioeconomic status and are higher for blacks than for whites for 8 of the 10 leading causes of death. Furthermore, there is a broad spectrum of health care delivery and prevention within the country. Use of clinical preventive services is less among those without a usual source of health care, those in lower income and education groups, and older adults.

PREVENTION STRATEGIES

The two complementary strategies for prevention are a population approach and a clinical, high-risk approach. A strong rationale exists for the population approach, in which interventions are offered on a broad scale to all segments of the population, because much of the current burden of ill health comes from the large numbers of those at moderate individual risk rather than from the few who demonstrate marked abnormalities. Since the risk for chronic diseases is generally continuous and often curvilinear, this approach shifts the entire population's risk to a lower level.

Chronic diseases commonly arise from the interaction of multiple risk factors at moderate levels rather than from single aberrant risk factors. For example, most hypertensive complications and preventable deaths come from the many persons with mild to moderate hypertension (see Chapter 55) rather than the relatively few with severe hypertension. Estimates indicate that a 3-mm Hg downward shift in the average systolic blood pressure in the United States might reduce the annual mortality from all causes by 4%, from coronary heart disease by 5%, and from stroke by 8%.

The high-risk strategy targets individuals in whom disease is judged most likely to develop and who would therefore benefit from intervention. This strategy, which is more compatible with usual medical practice, avoids the inefficiency of the population approach with its need to intervene in many who neither desire such help nor are likely to benefit. Preventive policies that focus on high-risk individuals offer substantial benefits for these individuals, but the potential impact on the total burden of disease is often disappointing.

Despite the rationale for emphasizing prevention, studies indicate that major gaps exist in the delivery of preventive health services. The main barriers include the time required, the lack of reimbursement, skepticism toward attempting behavioral change, and a health system geared to illness.

CLINICAL PREVENTIVE SERVICES

Clinical preventive services include counseling, immunization, screening tests, and reduction of the susceptibility to disease by interventions such as chemoprevention. Preventive services are often classified as primary, secondary, or tertiary. Primary prevention is directed toward preventing disease or injury before it develops; secondary prevention deals with early detection and treatment to impede the progress of pre-clinical disease. In contrast, tertiary prevention refers to rehabilitative activities after the onset of disease to minimize complications and disability. Distinguishing among these phases of prevention may be confusing. Detecting and treating hypertension could be considered secondary prevention of hypertensive disease but primary prevention of congestive heart failure and stroke. In any event, prevention can be perceived along a continuum from modification of predisposing factors, to preventing disease, to avoiding premature death and disability. The sooner the prevention, the more likely unnecessary illness, disability, and

Table 9–1 ■ DEATH RATES* FOR 1995, MALE-FEMALE AND BLACK-WHITE RATIOS FOR 1995, AND PER CENT CHANGE IN DEATH RATES 1950 TO 1995 FOR 10 LEADING CAUSES OF DEATH†— UNITED STATES

RANK/CAUSE	AGE-ADJUSTED 1995 DEATH RATE	MALE-FEMALE RATIO	BLACK-WHITE RATIO	% CHANGE 1950–1995
All causes	503.9	1.7	1.6	−40.1
1. Diseases of heart	138.3	1.8	1.5	−55.0
2. Malignant neoplasms	129.9	1.4	1.4	+3.6
3. Accidents	30.5	2.5	1.3	−47.0
4. Cerebrovascular diseases	26.7	1.2	1.8	−69.9
5. Chronic obstructive pulmonary disease	20.8	1.5	0.8	+372.7
6. HIV infection	15.6	5.0	4.7	+59.2‡
7. Diabetes mellitus	13.3	1.2	2.4	−7.0
8. Pneumonia and influenza	12.9	1.6	1.4	−50.8
9. Suicide	11.2	4.5	0.6	+1.8
10. Homicide and legal intervention	9.4	3.7	6.1	+74.1

*Per 100,000 population, age adjusted to the 1940 U.S. population.
†Based on death rates.
‡Per cent change for 1990 to 1995. Categories for coding were introduced in 1987.
From National Center for Health Statistics: Health, United States, 1996–97 and Injury Chartbook. Hyattsville, MD, Public Health Service, 1997.

Table 9–2 ■ ESTIMATION OF NON-GENETIC CONTRIBUTIONS TO DEATH IN THE UNITED STATES

	POTENTIAL CONTRIBUTING FACTORS								
DISEASES AND INJURIES	Tobacco	Diet and Exercise	Alcohol	Microbes	Toxins	Firearms	Sexual Behavior	Motor Vehicles	Illicit Drugs
Cancer	X	X	X		X		X		
Cardiovascular disease	X	X	X		X				X
Diabetes mellitus		X							
Digestive diseases/cirrhosis	X		X						
Accidents			X			X		X	X
HIV infection				X			X		X
Hepatitis			X	X			X		X
Infectious/parasitic diseases				X					
Respiratory diseases	X			X	X				X
Renal diseases					X				
Neurologic diseases				X	X				
Pneumoconioses				X	X				
Homicide/suicide			X			X		X	X
Sexually transmitted diseases				X			X		
Infant mortality							X	X	X

Modified from McGinnis MJ, Foege WH: Actual causes of death in the United States. JAMA 270:2207–2212, 1993.

premature death can be avoided. Therefore, increasing emphasis has been placed on preventing risk factors themselves. The term "primordial" prevention has been introduced for this concept.

Indiscriminate screening without adequate advice and follow-up serves no useful purpose. The periodic health examination (see Chapter 10) has evolved from a broad-based, uniform protocol to an approach that targets the prevention, detection, and treatment of specific diseases or risk factors for pre-determined age, gender, and racial groups.

Changes in the health care system and the development of national guidelines will probably draw greater attention to health promotion, disease prevention, and the interface of physician-based medical care with the public health system. Physicians should consider each disorder in terms of the potential for prevention as compared with the possibility of adverse effects from the preventive intervention.

Ample evidence connects identifiable and oftentimes preventable factors to the morbidity and mortality associated with major health problems (Table 9–2). About half of all deaths, morbidity, and disability can be attributed to such non-genetic factors, and many lifestyle changes benefit multiple systems and disorders. For example, cigarette smoking has been estimated to contribute to one in five deaths in the United States (see Chapter 13); dietary changes (see Chapter 39) may lower the occurrence of atherosclerosis, diabetes, osteoporosis, and cancer. Other important personal behavior factors affecting health include physical activity, alcohol, illicit drug use, sexual practices, and exposure to environmental toxins.

Several common misconceptions impede preventive health care. Many believe that diseases with a strong heritable component cannot be altered, but susceptibility to disease often requires the interaction of multiple genes and environmental factors for expression (see Chapter 31). In addition, chronic diseases are multifactorial, so other factors can be changed to compensate for an elevated genetic risk. The notion that prevention is less useful in older persons excludes many who would benefit most from prevention. The elderly have a greater absolute risk of disease and have been shown to adhere and respond favorably to preventive measures. In addition, life expectancy is frequently underestimated in the elderly—those who reach 65 years can now expect to live into their 80s.

With a larger aging population, decreasing fatality rates, and improved treatment of many disorders, it is essential that the focus be on primary prevention. Otherwise, the prevalence and associated morbidity of major diseases will increase and further consume available medical resources. It should be clearly understood that the purpose of prevention is not only to postpone illness to a later age but also often to prevent the diseases themselves and the resultant disability.

On average, U.S. citizens spend 85% of their 75+ years of life expectancy in a healthy state unimpaired by disabilities, disease, or injuries. The leading causes of disability-adjusted loss of years of life in developed countries over the next 25 years will probably continue to be atherosclerotic diseases, but the impact of depression, smoking-related disease, accidents, alcohol, and degenerative neurologic and rheumatologic diseases will also be substantial (Ta-

Table 9–3 ■ TEN PROJECTED LEADING CAUSES OF DISABILITY-ADJUSTED LIFE YEARS IN 2020 ACCORDING TO BASELINE PROJECTION BY REGION

DEVELOPED REGIONS		DEVELOPING REGIONS	
Rank/Disease or Injury	DALYs* (×10⁶)	Rank/Disease or Injury	DALYs (×10⁶)
All causes	160.5	All causes	1228.3
1. Ischemic heart disease	18.0	1. Unipolar major depression	68.8
2. Cerebrovascular disease	9.9	2. Traffic accidents	64.4
3. Unipolar major depression	9.8	3. Ischemic heart disease	64.3
4. Trachea, bronchus, and lung cancers	7.3	4. Chronic obstructive pulmonary disease	52.7
5. Traffic accidents	6.9	5. Cerebrovascular disease	51.5
6. Alcohol use	6.1	6. Tuberculosis	42.4
7. Osteoarthritis	5.6	7. Lower respiratory infections	41.1
8. Dementia and other degenerative and hereditary CNS disorders	5.5	8. War injuries	40.2
9. Chronic obstructive pulmonary disease	4.9	9. Diarrheal diseases	37.0
10. Self-inflicted injuries	3.9	10. HIV	34.0

DALYs = disability-adjusted life years; CNS = central nervous system; HIV = human immunodeficiency virus.
*Sum of the years of life lost to death and reduction in the value of years of life lived because of disability.
From Murray CJL, Lopez AD: Alternative projections of mortality and disability by cause 1990–2020: Global Burden of Disease Study. Lancet 349:1498–1504, 1997.

ble 9–3). All U.S. citizens should be able to reach the objective for Healthy People 2000—to attain at least 65 years of healthy life.

Murray CJL, Lopez AD: Alternative projections of mortality and disability by cause 1990–2020: Global Burden of Disease Study. Lancet 349:1498, 1997. *One of a four-part series by the authors on the Global Burden of Disease Study, which predicts worldwide trends in mortality and morbidity.*

National Center for Health Statistics: Health, United States, 1998, with Socioeconomic and Health Status Chartbook. Hyattsville, MD, Public Health Service, 1998. *A report on the health status and trends of the nation.*

National Center for Health Statistics: Healthy People 2000 Review, 1997. Hyattsville, MD, Public Health Service, 1997. *Most recent data and modifications to the objectives for Healthy People 2000: National Health Promotion and Disease Prevention Objectives.*

Report of the US Preventive Services Task Force: Guide to Clinical Preventive Services: An Assessment of the Effectiveness of 169 Interventions, 2nd ed. Baltimore, Williams & Wilkins, 1996. *The most recent authoritative recommendations for clinical preventive services.*

10 THE PREVENTIVE HEALTH EXAMINATION

Richard K. Riegelman

Integrating prevention into the practice of adult medicine is an intellectual and administrative challenge. The annual physical examination has been replaced by the periodic health examination, with intervals adjusted by age group. The complete physical examination and multiphasic screening laboratory work-up have been replaced by a focused screening history and physical examination designed to detect risk factors for disease. Laboratory testing is now guided by principles designed to select tests that are likely to produce substantial benefit to groups of individuals at affordable cost. In addition, the preventive health examination should include active therapeutic interventions, including counseling, vaccination, and chemoprophylaxis.

To help accomplish these multiple goals, groups such as the American College of Physicians, the Canadian Task Force, and the U.S. Preventive Services Task Force (USPSTF) have developed guidelines for the preventive health examination. The widely used USPSTF recommendations have been intentionally limited to procedures with adequate supportive evidence. A recommendation to screen for a disease, for instance, generally requires evidence that the disease causes substantial morbidity or mortality, that detection at the asymptomatic stage is feasible, and that early detection can alter outcome.

Thus it is important to view the USPSTF recommendations as a minimum set of guidelines that are likely to increase in number over time as further evidence accumulates and new approaches are introduced. Other organizations, especially those with a specific disease or professional focus, generally recommend more intensive or aggressive examinations.

INDIVIDUALIZING THE PREVENTIVE HEALTH EXAMINATION

In the USPSTF screening guidelines, the recommended history, physical examination, and laboratory tests for any individual are derived by considering that person's age, gender, and risk factors (Table 10–1). Of note is that efforts to base preventive approaches on evidence have led to the absence of recommendations for many tests that were previously recommended by many, such as chest radiography to detect lung cancer even among smokers, because any early detection that may occur does not generally alter a patient's prognosis. Other tests that are explicitly *not* recommended for asymptomatic, normal-risk individuals include the electrocardiogram, exercise stress testing, multiple chemistry screens, and sputum cytology testing.

CHANGES IN THE PREVENTIVE HEALTH EXAMINATION. The guidelines of the USPSTF, which is now affiliated with the Agency for Healthy Care Policy and Research, are currently undergoing a new cycle of review. Their review of colon cancer screening implies new recommendations, including annual fecal occult blood testing and periodic flexible sigmoidoscopy to reduce colorectal cancer mortality in individuals 50 years and older. The use of mammography between the ages of 40 and 50 years has been very controversial despite efforts to obtain consensus. In the absence of consensus, decisions should be left to individual patients

Table 10–1 ■ U.S. PREVENTIVE SERVICES TASK FORCE PERIODIC EXAMINATION RECOMMENDATIONS: SCREENING HISTORY, PHYSICAL EXAMINATION, AND LABORATORY WORK—AGES 19 AND OLDER

Schedule every 1 to 3 yrs of age 19–64 and every year if 65 or older

The recommended schedule applies only to the periodic visit itself. The frequency of the individual preventive services is left to clinical discretion except as indicated. The table indicates recommended ages and high-risk (HR) groups for whom the recommendations are made. Recommendations are applicable to age groups indicated in parentheses

HISTORY	PHYSICAL EXAMINATION
Dietary intake (≥19)	**Height and weight** (≥19) **Blood pressure** (≥19) **Visual acuity** (≥65) **Hearing** (≥65)
Physical activity (≥19)	**Clinical breast exam** (≥50) and **HR 19–49** —Annually over 50, women aged 35 and older with a family history of
Tobacco/alcohol/drug use (≥19)	premenopausally diagnosed breast cancer in a first-degree relative
Sexual practices (19–64)	**Testicular exam** (**HR 19–39**)—Men with a history of cryptorchidism, orchiopexy, or testicular atrophy
Functional status (≥65)	**Symptoms of TIA** (≥65)
	Complete skin exam (**HR** ≥**19**)—Persons with a family or personal history of skin cancer, increased occupational or recreational exposure to sunlight, or clinical evidence of precursor lesions (e.g., dysplastic nevi, certain congenital nevi)
	Thyroid for nodules (**HR** ≥**19**)—Persons with a history of upper body irradiation
	Auscultation for carotid bruits (**HR** ≥**40**)—Persons with risk factors for cerebrovascular or cardiovascular disease (e.g., hypertension, smoking, coronary disease, atrial fibrillation, diabetes) or those with neurologic symptoms (e.g., TIAs or a history of cerebrovascular disease)
	Complete oral cavity exam (**HR** ≥**19**)—Persons with exposure to tobacco or excessive amounts of alcohol or those with suspicious symptoms or lesions detected through self-examination

LABORATORY WORK

Nonfasting total cholesterol (≥19)

Papanicolaou smear (19–64, **HR** ≥**65**)—Pap smear every 1–3 yr. At 65 and older, only women who have not had previous documented screening in which smears have been consistently negative

Fasting glucose (**HR**≥**19**)—The markedly obese, persons with family history of diabetes, or women with a history of gestational diabetes

Rubella antibodies (**HR 19–39**)—Women lacking evidence of immunity

VDRL (**HR 19–64**)—Prostitutes, persons who engage in sex with multiple partners in areas in which syphilis is prevalent, or contacts of persons with active syphilis

Urinalysis for bacteremia (**HR 19–64**)—Persons with diabetes

Dipstick urinalysis (≥65)

Mammography (**HR 35–49;** ≥**50**)—Women aged 35 and older with a family history of premenopausally diagnosed breast cancer in a first-degree relative; otherwise every 1–2 yr beginning at age 50. See text

Table 10–1 ■ U.S. PREVENTIVE SERVICES TASK FORCE PERIODIC EXAMINATION RECOMMENDATIONS:
SCREENING HISTORY, PHYSICAL EXAMINATION, AND LABORATORY WORK—AGES 19 AND OLDER *Continued*

LABORATORY WORK

Chlamydial testing (HR 19–64)—Persons who attend clinics for sexually transmitted diseases, attend other high-risk health care facilities (e.g., adolescent and family planning clinics), or have other risk factors for chlamydial infection (e.g., multiple sexual contacts or a sexual partner with multiple sexual contacts, age younger than 20).

Gonorrhea culture (HR 19–64)—Prostitutes, persons with multiple sexual partners or a sexual partner with multiple contacts, sexual contacts of persons with culture-proven gonorrhea, or persons with a history of repeated episodes of gonorrhea

Counseling and testing for HIV infection (HR 19–64)—Persons seeking treatment for sexually transmitted disease; homosexual and bisexual men; past or present IV drug users; persons with a history of prostitution or multiple sexual partners; women whose past or present sexual partners were HIV infected, bisexual, or IV drug users; persons with long-term residence or birth in an area with high prevalence of HIV infection; or persons with a history of transfusion between 1978 and 1985

Hearing (HR 19–64)—Persons exposed regularly to excessive noise

PPD (HR ≥19)—Household members of persons with tuberculosis or others at risk for close contact with the disease (e.g., staff of tuberculosis clinics, shelters for the homeless, nursing homes, substance abuse treatment facilities, dialysis units, correctional institutions); recent immigrants or refugees from countries in which tuberculosis is common, migrant workers; residents of nursing homes, correctional institutions, or homeless shelters; or persons with certain underlying medical disorders (e.g., HIV infection)

Fecal occult blood/sigmoidoscopy (HR)—Persons 50 and older who have first-degree relatives with colorectal cancer; a personal history of endometrial, ovarian, or breast cancer; or a previous diagnosis of inflammatory bowel disease, adenomatous polyps, or colorectal cancer

Colonoscopy (HR 19–39)—Persons with a family history of familial polyposis coli or cancer family syndrome

Fecal occult blood/colonoscopy (HR ≥40)—Persons with a family history of familial polyposis coli or cancer family syndrome

Fecal occult blood/sigmoidoscopy (≥50)—See text

Bone mineral content (HR 40–64)—Premenopausal women at increased risk for osteoporosis (e.g., white race, bilateral oophorectomy before menopause, slender build) and for whom estrogen replacement therapy would otherwise not be recommended

Electrocardiogram (≥19)—Men who would endanger public safety were they to experience sudden cardiac events, e.g., commercial airline pilots. Men >40 with 2 or more cardiac risk factors (high blood cholesterol, hypertension, cigarette smoking, diabetes mellitus, family history of coronary artery disease) or sedentary or high-risk men planning to begin a vigorous exercise program

Thyroid function tests (women ≥65)

Glaucoma testing by eye specialist (≥65)

TIA = transient ischemic attack; HIV = human immunodeficiency virus; PPD = purified protein derivative.
From U.S. Preventive Services Task Force: Guide to Clinical Preventive Services, 2nd ed. Alexandria, VA, International Medical Publishing, 1996.

40 to 50 years old and their physicians. The use of screening tests for prostate cancer has not been endorsed by the USPSTF or the National Cancer Institute.

COUNSELING AS PART OF THE PREVENTIVE HEALTH EXAMINATION. The periodic preventive examination is an opportunity to provide counseling as well as screen for risk factors and disease. However, prevention and counseling should not be confined to the periodic preventive examination, and all encounters should be viewed as opportunities to identify or monitor risk factors and provide counseling. The USPSTF has identified a series of high-priority areas of counseling, which are summarized in Table 10–2.

IMPLEMENTING THE PREVENTIVE HEALTH EXAMINATION

Successful implementation of the periodic health examination requires that physicians endorse, participate in, and share responsibility for the process with the patient. The preventive health examination should not be viewed as a one-shot effort. For some patients it may be best integrated into visits for specific problems. For example, patients may be most receptive to smoking cessation recommendations when they are recovering from bronchitis.

The physician may be aided by flowsheets or checklists to organize the preventive recommendations and serve as a reminder. Many interventions can be implemented by non-physicians as a routine part of the physician's practice.

Active involvement by patients is essential to successful prevention. The recent introduction of Personal Health Guides allows patients to share in the responsibility for putting prevention into practice.

US Preventive Services Task Force: Guide to Clinical Preventive Services, 2nd ed. Baltimore, Williams & Wilkins, 1995. *A review of the methods, evidence, and recommendations of the USPSTF.*
US Public Health Service: The Clinician's Handbook of Preventive Services. Washington, DC, International Medical Publishing, 1994. *A guide to accompany the Office of Disease Prevention and Health Promotion's Put Prevention into Practice program, which also includes Personal Health Guides and patient educational materials.*
Websites increasingly provide the most up-to-date information on changes in recommendations. The following websites are useful sources of information on the USPSTF and National Institutes of Health consensus reports, respectively:
http://www.ahcpr.gov
http://www.odp.od.nih.gov/consensus/statements

Table 10–2 ■ PREVENTIVE SERVICES TASK FORCE—MAJOR ROUTINE COUNSELING RECOMMENDATIONS FOR INDIVIDUALS 19 AND OLDER

Ask to describe the use of alcohol and other drugs and counsel regarding the danger of alcohol and tobacco use in any form.

Patients with increased exposure to sunlight should be advised to protect their lips and skin.

Counsel about car safety belt use and avoidance of driving while using or after the use of alcohol or other drugs. Regular injury prevention counseling is suggested for all older adults or their caretakers.

Obtain a history of sexual practices and provide counseling on prevention of unintended pregnancy and contraceptive options to all sexually active women who do not want to become pregnant and men who do not want to have a child, as well as counseling regarding high-risk behavior and prevention of sexually transmitted diseases and HIV infection.

Routinely provide nutrition assessment and counseling.

Routinely assess patients' physical activity practices and advise a program of regular physical activity that is tailored to their health status and lifestyle.

Counsel regarding regular dental visits, brushing and flossing, use of fluoride, and avoiding foods high in sugar.

Encourage patients to keep an up-to-date list of medications with dosage and usage schedules.

11 DIET

Roland L. Weinsier

By 1996, annual health care expenditures in the United States surpassed $1 trillion and were more than 13.5% of the gross national product. Only a tiny fraction is invested in preventing disease and promoting health despite the fact that better control of fewer than 10 risk factors, including increasing exercise, decreasing smoking, wearing seat belts, and improving diet, could prevent 40 to 70% of all premature deaths, one third of all cases of acute disability, and two thirds of all cases of chronic disability. In support of this notion is the fact that age-adjusted mortality rates from coronary heart disease in the United States have decreased by more than 40% over the past 25 years; up to one third of this decline is probably attributable to diet-induced reductions in serum cholesterol levels.

NUTRITION IN DISEASE PREVENTION

Dietary recommendations aimed at reducing disease risk of the entire population can be of major benefit for the nation's health because even a relatively small reduction in risk in a large number of moderate-risk people could lead to greater benefit for the total population than a large reduction in risk for a small number of high-risk people. For example, population-wide dietary changes are especially worthwhile because most coronary disease occurs in people who have only moderate elevations in serum cholesterol (i.e., <240 mg/day), not, however, those at high risk because of very high serum cholesterol levels. Similarly, decreasing fat intake may substantially reduce the overall risk of certain cancers, even though the cancer-reducing effects for many individuals may be small or absent.

Although genetic factors certainly affect individual susceptibility, emigrating populations fairly quickly tend to acquire the disease rates of their new compatriots rather than retain the patterns of their relatives residing in their country of origin. With future advances in understanding genetic variability and its interaction with the environment, recommendations for the general population may soon be supplemented with more sophisticated, individually based dietary interventions.

DIET-DISEASE RELATIONSHIPS

Heart disease, cancer, and stroke account for two thirds of all deaths in the United States, and eating patterns parallel these vital statistics. In lieu of the high-fiber, low-fat foods of our ancestors, refined starches, sweets, saturated fats, and salt make up a major portion of today's typical American diet. In addition, diet contributes greatly to hypertension, hypercholesterolemia, and obesity, which are associated with significant morbidity.

DIETARY GUIDELINES

CURRENT PRACTICES. Fewer than one third of adults meet the goal of eating five or more vegetable servings per day, more than half consume less than one serving of fruit per day, and total dietary fiber is consistently below the minimum recommended intake of 20 g/day. Relative to the goal of at least 80% of people not salting their food at the table, only about 60 to 70% of adults report that they avoid using table salt. By contrast, based on data obtained between the late 1970s and the early 1990s, a larger proportion of adults were selecting diets lower in fat. The decline in fat intake was related to and perhaps partly a result of the four-fold increase in the percentage of adults consuming low-fat/low-calorie products. Despite the reduction in fat intake, a dramatic increase was noted in the prevalence of overweight among U.S. adults—from 25% to 33%. Whether this weight gain is due to an increase in non-fat calorie intake or a decrease in physical activity is still unresolved.

GUIDELINES. At least five reports of dietary guidelines for Americans and at least 19 reports of national dietary guidelines from outside the United States have been published. The general recommendations made in these reports are remarkably concordant, thus lending credence to the recommendations. The guidelines discussed in the following paragraphs (Table 11–1) are distilled from various recent reports, although total agreement has not been reached on every aspect.

1. Adjust energy intake for weight control.

AIM. Body mass index (BMI) should be less than 25, where BMI = weight (kilograms) ÷ height^2 (meters). Although great emphasis has been placed on reducing energy intake to control body weight, a major factor in the increasing prevalence of obesity in the United States is likely to be a decrease in total daily physical activity in the home and workplace. Data indicate that both fat

Table 11–1 ■ DIETARY GUIDELINES

Weight control	Keep body mass index (weight in kg ÷ ht^2 in meters) below 25
Fat	<25% of calories as total fat, <7% of calories as saturated fat, <300 mg/d of dietary cholesterol
Carbohydrate	>55% of calories as carbohydrates
Salt	<6 g/d
Protein	<2–3 servings/d of high-protein foods
Dairy	Up to 2–3 servings/d of low-fat dairy products
Alcohol	≤1 oz/d (2 drinks)

and total energy intake in adults have declined, whereas body weight has risen, and suggest that the average level of activity-related energy expenditure may have fallen dramatically.

2. Eat less fat, particularly saturated fat.

AIM. Total fat should be less than 25% of the calories consumed; saturated fat, less than 7% of calories; and dietary cholesterol, less than 300 mg/day. Eat less than three 3-oz servings of red meat per week (a 3-oz serving of meat is roughly the size of a deck of playing cards). Because there is no risk and great potential benefit, some experts suggest reducing total fat intake to as low as 10% of calories and totally excluding red meat.

COMMENT. Fats, whether as oil, margarine, or butter, provide over twice the calories (9 kcal/g) as carbohydrates (4 kcal/g) and protein (4 kcal/g); hence reducing all fats is the most important way to reduce energy intake and therefore reduce the risk of obesity and diabetes. Reducing saturated fat specifically lowers the risk of coronary heart disease, and decreasing total fat intake may also reduce the risk of cancers such as colon, prostate, and breast cancer.

Saturated fats are solid at room temperature and are found primarily in meat and dairy products (butter, cream, cheese, red meat) and some vegetable products (coconut, palm oil, cocoa butter, and vegetable oils that have been hydrogenated to make solid margarine). Dietary cholesterol comes only from animal products. Saturated fat and cholesterol can be reduced by substituting fish, skinned poultry, lean meats, and low- or non-fat dairy products for fatty meats and whole-milk dairy products. Recent evidence suggests that monounsaturated fats (olive oil and canola oil) are preferable to polyunsaturated fats for preventing heart disease. When polyunsaturated fats are transformed from the *cis* to the *trans* form, as when margarine is hardened into stick as opposed to tub form, the fats appear to become more atherogenic. As a replacement for saturated fats, complex carbohydrates (i.e., fruits, vegetables, whole-grain products) have some advantages over monounsaturated and polyunsaturated fats (i.e., addition of oils and margarines) in that complex carbohydrates are lower in energy density and higher in many essential nutrients and fiber.

3. Eat more foods containing complex carbohydrates and fiber.

AIM. More than 55% of the calories consumed should be carbohydrates. Eat at least seven servings of a combination of vegetables and fruits and at least six servings of a combination of unrefined starches and legumes (beans, peas).

COMMENT. Preferred carbohydrates include fresh fruit, green and yellow vegetables, whole-grain breads and cereals, beans, baked potatoes, and other unrefined starches. These foods, which are good sources of fiber and antioxidants such as β-carotene and vitamin C, substances that may protect against certain cancers, should be substituted for foods with higher energy density such as fats and simple sugars, which are conducive to obesity. The evidence for an inverse association of vegetable and fruit intake with certain cancers (especially lung cancer) is strong and consistent. High vegetable and fruit intake, which has been associated with reduced urinary calcium excretion, may also be beneficial for the prevention of bone loss. Sufficient quantities of complex carbohydrates, with their naturally high nutrient and fiber content, may obviate the need for vitamin and fiber supplements.

4. Reduce salt intake.

AIM. Salt intake should be less than 6 g/day.

COMMENT. Taste for salt is acquired and can be modified. On average, Americans consume about 10 to 12 g of salt per day, about 20 times their requirement of less than 0.5 g/day (equivalent to <200 mg of sodium). Because susceptibility to salt-induced hypertension (i.e., salt-sensitive individuals) cannot be identified easily, this recommendation is reasonable for the entire population and of specific benefit for the hypertension prone. Evidence that high sodium intake is associated with greater calcium and bone loss adds further impetus to achieve this goal, especially for women at risk for osteoporosis. Reducing sodium intake entails avoiding table salt. However, since 80% of dietary sodium generally comes from manufactured and restaurant-prepared foods, patients should be encouraged to read labels and avoid packaged and canned foods that have high sodium contents (i.e., >150 mg per serving), as well as reduce their intake of steak and soy sauce, bouillon cubes, prepared soups, chips, and crackers.

5. Use protein-rich foods in moderation.

AIM. Less than two to three servings per day of high-protein foods (i.e., poultry, fish, nuts) should be consumed. Eat less than three 3-oz servings of red meat and eggs per week.

COMMENT. At about 100 to 140 g/day, the average intake of protein in this country is well in excess of need, which is closer to 40 to 60 g/day for the average adult. Most adults can achieve an adequate intake with a diet that contains a variety of vegetables and starches, even without the use of animal products. Animal protein (such as from meat, poultry, and fish) causes increased loss of calcium in the urine and, when taken in excessive amounts, could contribute to osteoporosis. Red meat has also been associated with an increased risk of colon and other cancers, as well as with coronary artery disease.

6. Use dairy products in moderation.

AIM. Two to three servings per day of low-fat dairy products such as milk, yogurt, and cheese should be consumed.

COMMENT. The optimal intake of calcium remains uncertain, and recommendations have varied from 800 to 1500 mg/day. To achieve these levels by diet would necessitate liberal use of dairy products (e.g., 8 oz of milk provides 250 to 300 mg calcium). However, recommendations regarding the liberal use of dairy products must be tempered by several caveats: (1) Adult populations in countries with low bone fracture rates generally consume *few* dairy products and actually have low calcium intake by our standards. (2) Use of dairy products to achieve these high levels of calcium intake may not be equivalent to taking calcium supplements, which have been shown to reduce fracture rates. (3) Dairy products contain substantial amounts of protein (which increase calcium loss); dairy foods may also increase the intake of saturated fat, and their lactose content is not tolerated by a large segment of the population. (4) Milk intake can decrease iron absorption by as much as 50%, which may induce iron deficiency in persons with marginal iron status. (5) Dairy foods are not the only sources of calcium—for example, greens, spinach, broccoli, and beans contain substantial amounts. Thus it is possible that a reduction in the incidence of bone fractures may be more appropriately approached with dietary modifications other than the use of liberal amounts of dairy products; modifications might include a reduction in animal protein and salt intake, liberal use of vegetables and fruits, and if deemed appropriate, calcium supplementation.

7. Drink alcohol in moderation, if at all.

AIM. One ounce or less of pure alcohol should be consumed per day (equivalent to two cans of beer, two small glasses of wine, or two average cocktails). Pregnant women should avoid alcoholic beverages.

COMMENT. Although moderate alcohol intake is associated with a lower risk of coronary artery disease, drinking poses other risks that may offset any potential advantages. Because alcohol is high in energy density (7 kcal/g or 200 kcal/oz of ethanol), alcoholic beverages may contribute significantly to total calorie intake.

DIETARY SUPPLEMENTS

Approximately half of the adults in the United States report using nutritional supplements. In many cases they are self-prescribed. Evidence is accumulating that for some persons, supplementation with certain vitamins may be beneficial. For example, folic acid will reduce certain congenital abnormalities, and both folic acid and vitamin B_6 reduce homocysteine levels and hence may reduce the risk of coronary disease. However, the most desirable approach for the general public is to obtain the recommended levels of nutrients by eating a variety of whole foods, as described previously. When the diet is optimal, routine use of nutritional supplements may be of little benefit to most people, and unprescribed daily use of selenium and fat-soluble vitamin supplements such as β-carotene and vitamin E in amounts exceeding the recommended dietary allowances should be avoided.

SUMMARY

Experimental and epidemiologic data point strongly toward several common dietary factors that should form the foundation for daily eating patterns. These data indicate that our meals should be based mainly on whole grains, legumes (beans, peas), other vegetables, and fruit. Fats and oils should be used sparingly. If consumed, poultry and fish should be taken in moderation; red meat and eggs should be used no more than several times per week. It is less clear but likely that a healthful diet may also include low-fat dairy products in moderation and, if desired, small amounts of alcohol.

Health is increasingly dependent on lifestyle, and associations between diet and many specific diseases are becoming more clear. In this context, physicians should routinely provide nutrition counseling and/or referral to qualified nutritionists as part of routine health evaluations or whenever possible as part of a medical encounter.

Fuchs CS, Giovannucci EL, Colclitz GA, et al: Dietary fiber and the risk of colorectal cancer and adenoma in women. N Engl J Med 340:169, 1999. *Recent study showing no relation between dietary fiber and colorectal cancer or adenoma.*

National Center for Health Statistics: Healthy People 2000 Review, 1997. Hyattsville, MD, Public Health Service, 1997. *Health promotion priorities and goals for the nation in areas such as nutrition, fitness, drugs, and sexual behavior are reviewed in the context of progress made since 1990.*

National Research Council: Recommendations on diet, chronic diseases, and health. *In* Diet and Health: Implications for Reducing Chronic Disease Risk. Washington, DC, National Academy Press, 1989, pp 665–710. *Extensive review of the criteria used for formulating dietary recommendations, their implications, potential adverse consequences, and positive public health impact.*

Willett WC: Diet and health: What should we eat? Science 264:532, 1994. *An overview of specific relationships between foods and common diseases, with commentaries about the potential for disease prevention through improved nutrition.*

12 PHYSICAL ACTIVITY
Michael Pratt

Regular physical activity is an important component of a healthy lifestyle. Over the past two decades a large body of epidemiologic and clinical evidence has linked regular physical activity with a variety of health benefits. Although the strength of the data supporting these associations varies greatly from condition to condition, physical inactivity is clearly a major contributor to premature mortality and morbidity from chronic disease. To reduce the burden of disease resulting from physical inactivity, physicians should routinely assess the activity levels of their patients and provide appropriate counseling.

DEFINITIONS

Physical activity of moderate (brisk walking at 3 to 4 miles per hour) or vigorous intensity (jogging, singles tennis, moving heavy furniture) has health benefits (Table 12–1). Exercise refers to physical activity that is planned or structured and may be done to improve or maintain one or more components of physical fitness. Both physical activity and exercise are behaviors, whereas physical fitness refers to an individual's capacity to perform physical activity. Physical fitness is generally considered to consist of five components: aerobic or endurance capacity, muscular strength, muscular endurance, flexibility, and body composition.

Table 12–1 ■ DEFINING THE INTENSITY OF PHYSICAL ACTIVITY

ACTIVITY TYPE	METS*	HEART RATE†	AEROBIC CAPACITY‡
Moderate	3–6	50–70%	40–60%
Vigorous	>6	>70%	>60%

*Ratio of the metabolic rate during activity to the resting metabolic rate. One MET is defined as the energy expended while sitting quietly.
†Percentage of maximum heart rate.
‡Percentage of maximum aerobic capacity.

EPIDEMIOLOGY

National and state-based surveys indicate that approximately 30% of American adults are completely sedentary during their leisure time and another 30% to 40% are minimally active. Fewer than 40% of adults report being physically active at the recommended levels (20 minutes or more of vigorous activity at least three times per week or 30 minutes or more of moderate-intensity activity five or more times per week). Participation in leisure time physical activity appears to have increased from the 1960s through the 1980s but has reached a plateau over the past decade. Participation in physical activity declines with age and tends to be slightly higher among men than women and among whites than among members of other racial or ethnic groups. Higher levels of education and income are associated with greater participation in physical activity and account for most of the racial and ethnic differences observed for leisure time physical activity.

HEALTH BENEFITS OF PHYSICAL ACTIVITY

The physiologic and metabolic responses to exercise are at the root of the multiple health benefits associated with physical activity. Physical activity requires increased energy expenditure and imposes demands and stresses on multiple organ and enzyme systems. These demands lead to acute responses and to long-term adaptations of the circulatory, respiratory, nervous, endocrine, and skeletal systems. The most direct benefits of physical activity are cardiovascular and musculoskeletal adaptations, which increase functional capacity in these organ systems. Increased aerobic capacity and muscular strength and endurance have been well documented following training programs in individuals of all ages. Maintenance of functional capacity and strength may be especially important for preventing disability and maintaining independence among older adults. Many disease- and risk factor–specific benefits of physical activity have also been postulated. Convincing data link regular physical activity to lower rates of coronary heart disease (CHD) and colon cancer and to improvements in mental health, glucose metabolism, and bone density, but much research is needed to evaluate other possible health consequences of physical activity.

CORONARY HEART DISEASE. Classic epidemiologic studies demonstrated that heart disease was less likely to develop in conductors on double-decker buses in London than in less active drivers and that among longshoremen, the most active men had the least risk of CHD. Longitudinal studies of college alumni have shown a reduced incidence of CHD and lower CHD and all-cause mortality among regularly active men as compared with their sedentary counterparts. Previously sedentary men who initiated regular physical activity in middle age also reduced their risk of death from CHD and all causes when compared with men who remained sedentary. Increased physical fitness has been linked with lower all-cause and CHD mortality for both men and women. Overall, the risk of CHD in sedentary men is about twice that of men who are habitually active. To date, no randomized clinical trial of physical activity for the primary prevention of CHD has been conducted. However, the association of regular physical activity with reductions in CHD meets strict epidemiologic criteria for causality—the association is strong, consistent, graded, temporally appropriate, and biologically plausible (Table 12–2).

The evidence for a causal role of regular physical activity in the secondary prevention of CHD is at least as strong as that for primary prevention. Patients with CHD who engage in regular physical activity as part of a cardiac rehabilitation program have lower all-cause and CHD mortality than do non-participants 1 to 3

Table 12–2 ■ MECHANISMS BY WHICH PHYSICAL ACTIVITY PREVENTS CORONARY HEART DISEASE

Reduces elevated systolic blood pressure
Reduces elevated diastolic blood pressure
Raises HDL cholesterol
Reduces triglycerides
Reduces weight gain and enhances weight maintenance and fat distribution
Increases glucose uptake and insulin sensitivity
Reduces platelet adhesion
Enhances fibrinolysis
May reduce thrombosis
Decreases sympathetic and increases parasympathetic drive, which reduces myocardial oxygen demand
May reduce ventricular arrhythmias
May increase myocardial oxygen supply

HDL = high-density lipoprotein.

years after initial hospitalization. Exercise-based cardiac rehabilitation programs have also been shown to increase functional capacity and reduce CHD symptoms and may improve quality of life. Appropriate physical activity should be a part of the management and rehabilitation of most patients with CHD (see Chapter 60).

WEIGHT CONTROL. Individuals who are regularly active tend to weigh less and have a lower percentage of body fat than do sedentary individuals despite the fact that physically active persons are consistently observed to consume more calories than sedentary individuals. Regular physical activity increases caloric expenditure indirectly by raising the resting metabolic rate after activity, as well as directly by the activity itself. A combined program of diet and regular physical activity appears to be the most effective means of maintaining ideal body weight. Regular physical activity appears to alter body fat distribution beneficially, independent of its effects on body weight and total adiposity.

DIABETES. Physical activity increases muscle glucose uptake directly and also increases insulin sensitivity. Physical activity is commonly prescribed for managing non–insulin-dependent diabetes mellitus (NIDDM). Physical activity may also prevent NIDDM through its effects on insulin and glucose metabolism and maintenance of body weight (see Chapter 242). In well-conducted longitudinal studies, the incidence of NIDDM has been observed to be lower in regularly active male college alumni, physicians, and female nurses than their sedentary counterparts.

OSTEOPOROSIS. Physical activity may play an important role in maintaining bone mineral density, preventing osteoporosis, and reducing fractures (see Chapter 257). Bone density is reduced by bed rest and can be increased by weight-bearing activity. Regular physical activity has been demonstrated to increase bone mass in young women and reduce the decline in bone mass seen in postmenopausal women and may increase bone density in patients with osteoporosis. Postmenopausal women who walk approximately 1 mile per day have higher bone mineral density and slower rates of bone loss than do sedentary women. Regular physical activity also increases muscle mass and strength, perhaps reducing the risk of falls and protecting against fractures when falls do occur.

CANCER. Both regular physical activity and physical fitness have been associated with lower mortality from cancer in longitudinal studies. Although data for most specific cancers are limited, studies of occupational and leisure time activity indicate that physical activity is protective against colon cancer. Several studies suggest a reduced risk of breast cancer in regularly active women, but a nearly equal number of studies have failed to demonstrate this relationship. The protective effects may be mediated by reduced intestinal transit time (colon cancer) and altered endocrine function.

MENTAL HEALTH. Regular physical activity and physical fitness are positively associated with mental health and well-being. Persons who are regularly active report less anxiety and depression and lower levels of stress than do sedentary persons. Exercise programs may be useful as an adjunctive therapy for treating mild to moderate depression.

HEALTH RISKS

Physical activity is associated with risks as well as benefits. Musculoskeletal overuse injuries of the lower extremity are the most common negative consequences of physical activity. Three factors are strongly associated with a risk of musculoskeletal injury: previous injuries, increased duration of activity, and exercise intensity. The risk of injury is considerably higher with vigorous activity than with moderate activity. The clinician can reduce patients' risk of injury by making them aware of these associations and by advocating moderate physical activity and gradual increases in duration of activity.

Major cardiac events, although rare, have been associated with vigorous physical activity. The risk of cardiac arrest is transiently elevated during exercise both for those who are regularly active and to a greater extent for individuals who are irregularly active. However, the overall risk of cardiac arrest is reduced in men who are regularly active. The incidence of sudden death associated with jogging has been estimated at 1 per 360,000 hours of jogging. The majority of these deaths are due to underlying CHD. Physical activity may also exacerbate medical conditions such as asthma, and irregular exercise may make insulin dosing more challenging in diabetic patients. Nevertheless, most individuals with underlying disease or disability may still safely exercise if appropriate precautions are taken.

MEDICAL EVALUATION

Appropriate medical evaluation depends on the individual's age and health status and the type of activity undertaken. Individuals who are free of disease and who are initiating moderate-intensity physical activity such as regular walking do not require medical evaluation. Men older than 40 years and women older than 50 who wish to become vigorously active should undergo a medical examination. Persons of any age with symptomatic cardiovascular disease or multiple risk factors for cardiovascular disease require medical evaluation. Evaluation of patients with known cardiovascular disease should include a physician-supervised, symptom-limited exercise test with blood pressure and electrocardiographic monitoring; such testing is not generally thought to be mandatory in asymptomatic adults without known cardiovascular disease.

ASSESSMENT AND COUNSELING

Health professionals should routinely counsel patients to adopt and maintain an active lifestyle. The exercise prescription should consider an individual's age, health, current activity level, and readiness to initiate behavior change. Research on both quitting smoking and initiating physical activity has shown that patients move along a behavioral continuum from pre-contemplation, to contemplating change, to making a change, and finally to maintaining the new behavior. Physicians have greater success in changing their patient's physical activity practices if they can target their counseling to the patient's current activity level and behavioral stage. Brief, specific physical activity counseling reinforced by other providers, follow-up appointments, or educational materials can increase physical activity.

How much and what type of physical activity should be prescribed? The traditional exercise prescription calls for 20 or more minutes of continuous aerobic activity three to five times per week at moderate to vigorous intensity (60% of maximum heart rate or 50% of aerobic capacity). This prescription is appropriate for increasing fitness and improving health status. Reassessment of epidemiologic and clinical data on the health aspects of physical activity reveals that many of the health benefits attributable to physical activity are associated with the total quantity of activity performed even if the activity is discontinuous and of only moderate intensity. Moderate activities such as brisk walking, gardening, and stair climbing on a daily basis can have major health impacts. The Centers for Disease Control and Prevention, National Institutes of Health, Surgeon General, and the American College of Sports Medicine currently recommend that American adults participate in 30 minutes or more of moderate-intensity physical activity on most and preferably all days of the week.

The physical activity prescription can take the traditional vigorous exercise approach or follow the recommendation for daily moderate physical activity (Table 12–3). Both provide significant health benefits. Tailoring recommendations for physical activity to the patient's individual goals, interests, skills, available time, and barriers to activity increases the chance for success.

Most persons are aware that they should be more active. The physician can encourage patients to become regularly active by

Table 12–3 ■ THE EXERCISE PRESCRIPTION

Type of physical activity
  Continuous or intermittent
  Primarily aerobic
  Stretching for flexibility
  Resistance exercise for strength
Intensity
  Moderate (40–60% relative to capacity, "brisk walk")
                    OR
  Vigorous (>60% relative to capacity)
Duration
  20–60 min/d
  150–300 kcal/d
Frequency
  Daily for intermittent moderate activity
  Three or more times per week for continuous, vigorous activity
Session
  For planned exercise:
    Warm-up, 3–5 min
    Conditioning, 15–40 min
    Cool-down, 2–5 min
  For lifestyle activity: Incorporate activity into the daily routine. "Pulses" of activity should be at least 10 min long and at an intensity equal to brisk walking
Progression
  Increase duration, intensity, and frequency gradually
  Evaluate progress each visit
Warning signs
  Severe musculoskeletal pain
  Claudication
  Chest pressure, pain, or discomfort
  Unusual shortness of breath
  Dizziness, nausea, vomiting

reinforcing the importance of physical activity to health, working with the patient to help build the skills and self-confidence needed to be active, and designing a program of physical activity that fits into the individual's lifestyle.

Dunn AL, Marcus BH, Kampert JB, et al: Comparison of lifestyle and structured interventions to increase physical activity and cardiorespiratory fitness: A randomized trial. JAMA 281:327, 1999. *Lifestyle changes are as effective as a structured exercise program.*

Simons-Morton DG, Calfas KJ, Oldenburg B, Burton NW: Effects of interventions in health-care settings or physical activity on cardiorespiratory fitness. Am J Prev Med 15:413, 1998. *A review and discussion of all the controlled trials of physical activity counseling for primary and secondary prevention. This issue of the* American Journal of Preventive Medicine *also includes up-to-date reviews of physical activity interventions in a variety of settings (schools, workplace, communities) and for special populations.*

US Department of Health and Human Services: Physical Activity and Health: A Report of the Surgeon General. Atlanta, US Department of Health and Human Services, Centers for Disease Control and Prevention, National Center for Chronic Disease Prevention and Health Promotion, 1996. *An authoritative review of the health effects of physical activity and current patterns and trends of participation in physical activity in the United States.*

13 TOBACCO

Neal L. Benowitz

EPIDEMIOLOGY

Currently, about 45 million individuals in the United States are cigarette smokers, including 28% of men and 23% of women. People who are less well educated and/or have unskilled occupations are more likely to smoke. Smoking is responsible for about 430,000 preventable U.S. deaths annually. A lifelong smoker has about a one in three chance of dying prematurely from a complication of smoking. Smoking is the major preventable cause of death in developed countries.

Other forms of tobacco use include pipes and cigars (used by 8.7% of men and 0.3% of women) and smokeless tobacco (5.5% of men and 1% of women). Smokeless tobacco use in the United

States is primarily oral snuff and chewing tobacco, whereas nasal snuff is used to a greater extent in the United Kingdom.

HARMFUL CONSTITUENTS OF TOBACCO

Tobacco smoke is an aerosol of droplets (particulates) containing water, nicotine and other alkaloids, and tar. Tobacco smoke contains several thousand different chemicals, many of which may contribute to human disease. Major toxic chemicals in the particulate phase of tobacco include nicotine, benzo(a)pyrene and other polycyclic hydrocarbons, N'-nitrosonornicotine, β-naphylamine, polonium-210, nickel, cadmium, arsenic, and lead. The gaseous phase contains carbon monoxide, acetaldehyde, acetone, methanol, nitrogen oxides, hydrogen cyanide, acrolein, ammonia, benzene, formaldehyde, nitrosamines, and vinyl chloride. Tobacco smoke may produce illness via systemic absorption of toxins and/or cause local pulmonary injury by oxidant gases.

TOBACCO ADDICTION

Tobacco use is motivated primarily by the desire for nicotine. Drug addiction is defined as compulsive use of a psychoactive substance, the consequences of which are detrimental to the individual or society. Understanding addiction is useful in providing effective smoking cessation therapy. Nicotine is absorbed rapidly from tobacco smoke into the pulmonary circulation; it then moves quickly to the brain, where it acts on nicotinic cholinergic receptors to produce its gratifying effects, which occur within 10 to 15 seconds after a puff. Smokeless tobacco is absorbed more slowly and results in less intense pharmacologic effects. With long-term use of tobacco, physical dependence develops as a result of an increased number of nicotinic cholinergic receptors in the brain. When tobacco is unavailable, even for only a few hours, withdrawal symptoms often occur, including anxiety, irritability, difficulty concentrating, restlessness, hunger, craving for tobacco, disturbed sleep, and in some people, depression.

Addiction to tobacco is multifactorial, including a desire for the direct pharmacologic actions of nicotine, relief of withdrawal symptoms, and learned associations. Smokers report a variety of reasons for smoking, including pleasure, arousal, enhanced vigilance, improved performance, relief of anxiety or depression, reduced hunger, and control of body weight. Environmental cues—such as a meal, a cup of coffee, talking on the phone, an alcoholic beverage, or friends who smoke—often trigger an urge to smoke. Smoking and depression are strongly linked. Smokers are more likely to have a history of major depression than non-smokers are. Smokers with a history of depression are also likely to be more highly dependent on nicotine and have a lower likelihood of quitting. When they do quit, depression is more apt to be a prominent withdrawal symptom.

Most tobacco use begins in childhood or adolescence. Risk factors for youth smoking include peer and parental influences, behavioral problems (e.g., poor school performance), and personality characteristics such as rebelliousness or risk taking, depression, and/or anxiety, as well as genetic influences. Adolescent desire to appear older and more sophisticated, such as emulating more mature role models, is another strong motivator. Environmental influences such as advertising are also thought to contribute. Whereas smoking rates among adults have been declining over the past 30 years, initiation rates for youth have remained constant for the past 15 years. Approaches to preventing tobacco addiction in youth include educational activities in schools or in the media, reducing accessibility of tobacco to youth (such as taxation, enforcing restrictions against youth purchasing tobacco), changing the social and environmental norms, and deglamourizing smoking (restricting indoor smoking, educating parents not to smoke around children).

TOBACCO-RELATED DISEASES

Tobacco use is a major cause of death from cancer, cardiovascular disease, and pulmonary disease (Table 13–1). Smoking is also a major risk factor for peptic disease, osteoporosis, reproductive disorders, and fire-related injuries.

Table 13–1 ■ HEALTH HAZARDS OF TOBACCO USE (RISKS INCREASED BY SMOKING)

Cancer	*Reproductive Disturbances*
See Table 13–2	Reduced fertility
Cardiovascular Disease	Premature birth
Sudden death	Lower birth weight
Acute myocardial infarction	Spontaneous abortion
Unstable angina	Abruptio placentae
Stroke	Premature rupture of membranes
Peripheral arterial occlusive disease	Increased perinatal mortality
Aortic aneurysm	*Oral Disease (Smokeless Tobacco)*
Pulmonary Disease	Oral cancer
Lung cancer	Leukoplakia
Chronic bronchitis	Gingivitis
Emphysema	Gingival recession
Asthma	Tooth staining
Increased susceptibility to pneumonia	*Other*
Increased morbidity from viral respiratory infection	Earlier menopause
	Osteoporosis
	Cataract
Gastrointestinal Disease	Premature skin wrinkling
Peptic ulcer	Aggravation of hypothyroidism
Esophageal reflux	Altered drug metabolism or effects

CANCER. Smoking is the single largest preventable cause of cancer (Table 13–2). It is responsible for about 30% of cancer deaths. A number of chemicals in tobacco smoke may contribute to carcinogenesis as tumor initiators, co-carcinogens, tumor promoters, or complete carcinogens. Lung cancer is the leading cause of cancer deaths in the United States and is predominantly attributable to cigarette smoking. The risk of lung and other cancers is proportional to how many cigarettes are smoked per day and the duration of smoking. Workplace exposure to asbestos or α-radiation (see Chapter 18) (the latter in uranium miners) synergistically increases the risk of lung cancer in cigarette smokers. Alcohol use (see Chapter 16) interacts synergistically with tobacco in causing oral, laryngeal, and esophageal cancer. The mechanism of interaction may involve alcohol-solubilizing tobacco carcinogens and/or alcohol-related induction of liver or gastrointestinal enzymes that metabolize and activate tobacco carcinogens. The tobacco-related risks of bladder and kidney cancer are enhanced by occupational exposure to aromatic amines, such as found in the dye industry. Cervical cancer is more common in women who smoke, presumably the result of exposure to carcinogens in cervical secretions. Smoking appears to be involved in 20 to 30% of leukemia cases in adults, including both lymphoid and myeloid leukemia.

Table 13–2 ■ SMOKING AND CANCER MORTALITY

TYPE OF CANCER		RELATIVE RISK AMONG SMOKERS		MORTALITY ATTRIBUTABLE TO SMOKING	
		Current	Former	Percentage	Number
Lung	Male	22.4	9.4	90	82,800
	Female	11.9	4.7	79	40,300
Larynx	Male	10.5	5.2	81	2,400
	Female	17.8	11.9	87	700
Oral cavity	Male	27.5	8.8	92	4,900
	Female	5.6	2.9	61	1,800
Esophagus	Male	7.6	5.8	78	5,700
	Female	10.3	3.2	75	1,900
Pancreas	Male	2.1	1.1	29	3,500
	Female	2.3	1.8	34	4,500
Bladder	Male	2.9	1.9	47	3,000
	Female	2.6	1.9	37	1,200
Kidney	Male	3.0	2.0	48	3,000
	Female	1.4	1.2	12	500
Stomach	Male	1.5	?	17	1,400
	Female	1.5	?	25	1,300
Leukemia	Male	2.0	?	20	2,000
	Female	2.0	?	20	1,600
Cervix	Female	2.1	1.9	31	1,400

Adapted from Newcomb PA, Carbone PP: The health consequences of smoking: Cancer. Med Clin North Am 76:305, 1992.

CARDIOVASCULAR DISEASE. Cigarette smoking accounts for about 20% of cardiovascular deaths in the United States. Risks are increased for coronary heart disease, sudden death, cerebrovascular disease, and peripheral vascular disease, including aortic aneurysm. Cigarette smoking accelerates atherosclerosis and promotes acute ischemic events. The mechanisms of the effects of smoking are not fully elucidated but are believed to include (1) hemodynamic stress (nicotine increases the heart rate and transiently increases blood pressure), (2) endothelial injury and dysfunction (nitric oxide release and resultant vasodilation are impaired), (3) development of an atherogenic lipid profile (smokers have on average higher low-density lipoprotein, more oxidized low-density lipoprotein, and lower high-density lipoprotein cholesterol than non-smokers do), (4) enhanced coagulability, (5) arrhythmogenesis, and (6) relative hypoxemia because of the effects of carbon monoxide. Carbon monoxide reduces the capacity of hemoglobin to carry oxygen and impairs the release of oxygen from hemoglobin to body tissues, both of which combine to result in a state of relative hypoxemia. To compensate for this hypoxemic state, polycythemia develops in smokers, with hematocrits often 50% or more. The polycythemia also increases blood viscosity, which adds to the risk of thrombotic events.

Cigarette smoking acts synergistically with other cardiac risk factors to increase the risk of ischemic heart disease. Although the risk of cardiovascular disease is roughly proportional to cigarette consumption, the risk persists even at low levels of smoking, that is, one to two cigarettes per day. Cigarette smoking reduces exercise tolerance in patients with angina pectoris and intermittent claudication. Vasospastic angina is more common and the response to vasodilator medication is impaired in patients who smoke. The number of episodes and total duration of ischemic episodes as assessed by ambulatory electrocardiographic monitoring in patients with coronary heart disease are substantially increased by cigarette smoking. The increase in relative risk of coronary heart disease because of cigarette smoking is greatest in young adults, who in the absence of cigarette smoking would have a relatively low risk. Women who use oral contraceptives and smoke have a synergistically increased risk of both myocardial infarction and stroke.

After acute myocardial infarction, the risk of recurrent myocardial infarction is higher and survival is half over the next 12 years in persistent smokers as compared with quitters. Smoking interferes with revascularization therapy for acute myocardial infarction. After thrombolysis, the reocclusion rate is four-fold higher in smokers who continue than in those who quit. The risk of reocclusion of a coronary artery after angioplasty or occlusion of a bypass graft is increased in smokers. Cigarette smoking is not a risk factor for hypertension per se but does increase the risk of complications, including the development of nephrosclerosis and progression to malignant hypertension.

PULMONARY DISEASE. More than 80% of chronic obstructive lung disease in the United States is attributable to cigarette smoking. Cigarette smoking also increases the risk of respiratory infection, including pneumonia, and results in greater disability from viral respiratory tract infections. Pulmonary disease from smoking includes the overlapping syndromes of chronic bronchitis (cough and mucus hypersecretion), emphysema, and airway obstruction. The lung pathology produced by cigarette smoking includes loss of cilia, mucous gland hyperplasia, increased number of goblet cells in the central airways, inflammation, goblet cell metaplasia, squamous metaplasia, mucus plugging of small airways and destruction of alveoli, and a reduced number of small arteries. The mechanism of injury is complex and appears to include direct injury by oxidant gases, increased elastase activity (a protein that breaks down elastin and other connective tissue), and decreased antiprotease activity. A genetic deficiency of α_1-antiprotease activity produces a similar imbalance between pulmonary protease and antiprotease activity and is a risk factor for early and severe smoking-induced pulmonary disease.

OTHER COMPLICATIONS. Cigarette smoking increases the risk of duodenal and gastric ulcers, delays the rate of ulcer healing, and increases the risk of relapse after ulcer treatment. Smoking is also associated with esophageal reflux symptoms. Smoking produces ulcer disease by increasing acid secretion, reducing pancreatic bicarbonate secretion, impairing the gastric mucosal barrier (related to decreased gastric mucosal blood flow and/or inhibition of prostaglandin synthesis), and/or reducing pyloric sphincter tone.

Cigarette smoking is a risk factor for osteoporosis in that it reduces the peak bone mass attained in early adulthood and increases the rate of bone loss in later adulthood. Smoking antagonizes the protective effect of estrogen replacement therapy on the risk of osteoporosis in postmenopausal women.

Cigarette smoking is a major cause of reproductive problems and results in approximately 4600 U.S. infant deaths annually. Growth retardation from cigarette smoking has been termed the "fetal tobacco syndrome." Cigarette smoking causes reproductive complications by causing placental ischemia mediated by the vasoconstricting effects of nicotine, the hypoxic effects of chronic carbon monoxide exposure, and/or the general increase in coagulability produced by smoking.

Other adverse effects of cigarette smoking include premature facial wrinkling, an increased risk of cataracts, olfactory dysfunction, and fire-related injuries, the latter of which contribute significantly to the economic costs of tobacco use. Smoking reduces the secretion of thyroid hormone in women with subclinical hypothyroidism and increases the severity of clinical symptoms of hypothyroidism in women with subclinical or overt hypothyroidism, the latter effect reflecting antagonism of thyroid hormone action. Cigarette smoking also potentially interacts with a variety of drugs by accelerating drug metabolism or by the antagonistic pharmacologic actions that nicotine and/or other constituents of tobacco have with other drugs (Table 13–3).

HEALTH HAZARDS OF SMOKELESS TOBACCO

Smokeless tobacco refers to snuff and chewing tobacco. Oral snuff is placed (as a "pinch") between the lip and gum or under the tongue; chewing tobacco is actively chewed and generates saliva that is spit out (hence the term "spit tobacco"). Smokeless tobacco products are usually flavored, many with licorice, and also contain sodium bicarbonate to keep the local pH alkaline to facilitate buccal absorption of nicotine. Nicotine absorption from smokeless tobacco is similar in magnitude to that absorbed from cigarette smoking. In addition, other chemicals, including sodium, glycyrrhizinic acid (from licorice), and potentially carcinogenic chemicals such as nitrosamines are absorbed systemically.

Smokeless tobacco is addictive and is associated with an increased risk of oral cancer at the site where the tobacco is usually placed (inside the lip, under the cheek or tongue) or nasal cancer in nasal snuff users. Other oral diseases also associated with smokeless tobacco include leukoplakia, gingivitis, gingival recession, and staining of the teeth. Cardiovascular effects of smokeless tobacco include acute aggravation of hypertension or angina pectoris as a result of the sympathomimetic effects of nicotine, hypokalemia, hypertension secondary to the effects of glycyrrhizinic acid (a potent mineralocorticoid), and excessive sodium absorption resulting in aggravated hypertension or sodium-retaining disorders.

ENVIRONMENTAL TOBACCO SMOKE

Considerable evidence indicates that exposure to environmental tobacco smoke (ETS) (i.e., passive smoking) is harmful to the health of non-smokers (Table 13–4). Recently, the U.S. Environmental Protection Agency classified ETS as a class A carcinogen, which means that it has been shown to cause cancer in humans.

ETS consists of smoke that is generated while the cigarette is smoldering, as well as mainstream smoke that has been exhaled by the smoker. Seventy-five per cent or more of the total combustion product from a cigarette enters the air. The constituents of ETS are qualitatively similar to those of mainstream smoke. However, some toxins such as ammonia, formaldehyde, and nitrosamines are present in much higher concentrations in ETS than in mainstream smoke. The Environmental Protection Agency has estimated that ETS is responsible for approximately 3000 lung cancer deaths annually in non-smokers in the United States, is causally associated with 150,000 to 300,000 cases of lower respiratory tract infection in infants and young children up to 18 months of age, and is causally associated with the aggravation of asthma in 200,000 to 1 million children. An appreciation of the hazards of ETS is important to the physician because it provides a basis for advising par-

Table 13–3 ■ INTERACTION BETWEEN CIGARETTE SMOKING AND DRUGS

DRUG(S)		INTERACTION (EFFECTS COMPARED WITH NON-SMOKERS)	SIGNIFICANCE
Antipyrine	Lidocaine	Accelerated metabolism	May require high doses in smokers, reduced doses after quitting
Caffeine	Oxazepam		
Desmethyldiazepam	Pentazocine		
Estradiol	Phenacetin		
Estrone	Phenylbutazone		
Flecainide	Propranolol		
Heparin	Theophylline		
Imipramine			
Oral contraceptives		Enhanced thrombosis, increased risk of stroke and myocardial infarction	Do not prescribe to smokers, especially if older than 35
Cimetidine and other H$_2$ blockers		Lower rate of ulcer healing, higher ulcer recurrence rates	Consider using mucosal protective agents
Propranolol		Less antihypertensive effect, less antianginal efficacy; more effective in reducing mortality following myocardial infarction	Consider the use of cardioselective β-blockers
Nifedipine (and probably other calcium blockers)		Less antianginal effect	May require higher doses and/or multiple-drug antianginal therapy
Diazepam, chlordiazepoxide (and possibly other sedative-hypnotics)		Less sedation	Smokers may need higher doses
Chlorpromazine (and possibly other neuroleptics)		Less sedation, possibly reduced efficacy	Smokers may need higher doses
Propoxyphene		Reduced analgesia	Smokers may need higher doses

ents not to smoke when children are in the home, for insisting that child care facilities be smoke-free, and for recommending smoking restrictions in work sites and other public places.

BENEFITS OF QUITTING

The benefits of quitting smoking are substantial for smokers of any age. A person who quits smoking before age 50 has half the risk of dying in the next 15 years than a continuing smoker has. Smoking cessation reduces the risks of development of lung cancer, with the risk falling to half that of a continuing smoker by 10 years and one sixth that of a smoker after 15 years' cessation. The risk of acute myocardial infarction falls rapidly after quitting smoking and approaches non-smoker levels within a year of abstinence. Cigarette smoking produces a progressive loss of airway function over time that is characterized by an accelerated loss of forced expiratory volume in 1 second (FEV$_1$) with increasing age. FEV$_1$ loss to cigarette smoking cannot be regained by cessation, but the rate of decline slows after smoking cessation and returns to that of non-smokers. Women who stop smoking during the first 3 to 4 months of pregnancy reduce the risk of having a low–birthweight baby to that of a woman who has never smoked.

After quitting, smokers gain an average of 5 to 7 lb, which is perceived as undesirable and a reason not to quit by some smokers. Smokers tend to be thinner because of the effects of nicotine to increase energy expenditure and reduce compensatory increases in food consumption. After they quit smoking, ex-smokers tend to reach the weight expected had they never smoked. On balance, the benefits of quitting far outweigh the risks associated with weight gain, and patients should be counseled accordingly.

TREATMENT OF NICOTINE ADDICTION

Seventy per cent of cigarette smokers would like to quit. Spontaneous quit rates are about 1% per year. Simple physician advice to

Table 13–4 ■ HEALTH HAZARDS OF ENVIRONMENTAL TOBACCO SMOKE IN NON-SMOKERS

CHILDREN	ADULTS
Hospitalization for respiratory tract infection in first year of life	Lung cancer
Wheezing	Myocardial infarction
	Reduced pulmonary function
Middle ear effusion	Irritation of eyes, nasal congestion, headache
Asthma	
Sudden infant death syndrome	Cough

quit increases the quit rate to 3%. Minimal-intervention programs increase quit rates to 5 to 10%, whereas more intensive treatments, including smoking cessation clinics, can yield quit rates of 25 to 30%. A practical office smoking cessation program developed by the National Cancer Institute consists of "4 A's": (1) *ask* about smoking at every opportunity; (2) *advise* all smokers to stop; (3) *assist* the patient in stopping and maintaining abstinence; and (4) *arrange* follow-up to reinforce non-smoking. Assistance in quitting should include providing self-help material or quit kits, which are widely available from governmental health agencies, professional societies, and local organizations such as cancer, heart, and lung associations. The physician may offer additional education and counseling through the office (most efficiently provided by office staff and through teaching aids such as videotapes) or through referral to community smoking cessation programs. Smokers who are interested may be offered nicotine replacement or other pharmacologic therapy.

Currently, two medications have been approved for smoking cessation: nicotine and bupropion. All types of smoking cessation medications, if used properly, double smoking cessation rates when compared with placebo treatments. Nicotine replacement medications include 2- and 4-mg nicotine polacrilex gum, transdermal nicotine patches, nicotine nasal spray, and nicotine inhalers. A smoker should be instructed to quit smoking entirely before beginning nicotine replacement therapies. Optimal use of nicotine gum includes instructions not to chew too rapidly, to chew 8 to 10 pieces per day for 20 to 30 minutes each, and to use it for an adequate period for the smoker to learn a lifestyle without cigarettes, usually 3 months or longer. Side effects of nicotine gum are primarily local and include jaw fatigue, sore mouth and throat, upset stomach, and hiccups.

Several different transdermal nicotine preparations are marketed—three deliver 21 or 22 mg over a 24-hour period, and one delivers 15 mg over a period of 16 hours. All have lower-dose patches for tapering. Patches are applied in the morning and removed either the next morning or at bedtime, depending on the patch. Full-dose patches are recommended for most smokers for the first 1 to 3 months, followed by one to two tapering doses for 2 to 4 weeks each. Nicotine nasal spray, one spray into each nostril, delivers about 0.5 mg nicotine systemically and can be used every 30 to 60 minutes. Local irritation of the nose commonly produces burning, sneezing, and watery eyes during initial treatment, but tolerance develops to these effects in 1 to 2 days. The nicotine inhaler actually delivers nicotine to the throat and upper airway, from where it is absorbed similarly to nicotine from gum. It is marketed as a cigarette-like plastic device and can be used ad libitum.

Bupropion, also marketed as an antidepressant drug, is dosed at 150 to 300 mg/day for 7 days prior to stopping smoking and then at 300 mg/day for the next 6 to 12 weeks. Bupropion can also be used in combination with a nicotine patch. Bupropion in excessive doses can cause seizures and should not be used in individuals with a history of seizures or with eating disorders (bulimia or anorexia). On average, nicotine medications or bupropion treatment doubles the cessation rates found with placebo treatment, and absolute rates of smoking cessation have increased from 12% (placebo) to 24% (active medication) in clinical trials.

Follow-up office visits and/or telephone calls during and after active treatment increase long-term smoking cessation rates. Even in the best treatment circumstances, 70% or more of smokers relapse. Most smokers go through a quitting process three or four times before they finally succeed. When a quit attempt fails, the health care provider should encourage patients to try again as soon as they are ready. Cost-effectiveness studies find average costs per year of life saved of $1000 to $2000 for brief physician counseling alone and $2000 to $4000 for counseling plus medication to aid cessation. Smoking cessation treatment is much less costly per year of life saved than other widely accepted preventive therapies, including treatment of mild to moderate hypertension or hypercholesterolemia.

Benowitz NL: Pharmacology of nicotine: Addiction and therapeutics. Annu Rev Pharmacol Toxicol 36:597, 1996. *A review of the human pharmacology of nicotine, its role in producing tobacco addiction, and the basis for pharmacotherapy for nicotine addiction.*

Hughes JR, Goldstein MG, Hurt RD, Shiffman S: Recent advances in the pharmacotherapy of smoking. JAMA 281:72, 1999. *Recommends that pharmacotherapy should be made available to all smokers who wish to quit.*

Hurt RD, Sachs DPL, Glover ED, et al: A comparison of sustained-release bupropion and placebo for smoking cessation. N Engl J Med 337:1195, 1997. *Clinical trial demonstrating the benefit of bupropion in smoking cessation therapy.*

Law MR, Morris JK, Walk NJ: Environmental tobacco smoke exposure and ischemic heart disease: An evaluation of the evidence. BMJ 315:973, 1997. *Reviews environmental tobacco smoke as a cause of cardiovascular disease.*

The Smoking Cessation Clinical Practice Guideline Panel and Staff: The Agency for Health Care Policy and Research Smoking Cessation Clinical Practice Guideline. JAMA 275:1270, 1996. *Consensus recommendations on implementing smoking cessation for primary care clinicians, smoking cessation specialists, and health care administrators.*

14 VIOLENCE AND INJURY

Elizabeth McLoughlin

DEFINITIONS

Violence in the United States is a public health emergency and can be caused by institutional and personal actions. The root causes of violence include inequitable social and economic conditions. *Personal violence* is the intentional use of physical or psychological force against another person or against oneself that may result in injury or death. An *injury* is damage to tissue usually caused by excessive energy transfer. That energy can be kinetic (causing fractures, lacerations, and contusions), thermal (burns and scalds), electrical (electrocutions), or chemical (poisonings). The mechanism is somewhat different for drowning and suffocation, which result when tissue is deprived of oxygen. Injuries may be classified in many ways, primarily by type, by cause, and by intent. *Type* of injury includes, for example, a fracture, laceration, or burn. *Cause* groupings distinguish among, for example, injuries caused by a car crash, a bullet, poisons, or a fall. *Intent* categories address whether the injury was unintentional, intentionally self-inflicted (the most severe outcome being suicide), or intentionally inflicted by another (the most severe outcome being homicide). Violent injuries such as homicide and suicide are positioned at the intersection of violence in general and all injuries.

EPIDEMIOLOGY

In 1995, 6% of all deaths in the United States were caused by an injury; 8% of all hospital discharges had a first listed diagnosis of injury and 37% of all emergency department visits were for injuries. Figure 14–1 presents the burden of injury at four levels of severity. Suicide and homicide account for about 35% of deaths from injury (Table 14–1).

The leading external causes of injury death, regardless of intent, are motor vehicle traffic crashes, firearms, poisoning (primarily by drug overdose), suffocation (which includes suicide by hanging), falls, drownings, and fire. Although firearms slightly exceed motor vehicles as the primary mechanism for injury death for males, the age-related profiles are remarkably alike across the age range (Fig. 14–2). Among firearm deaths, the peak in young men is primarily homicide, whereas the peak in older men is primarily suicide. Motor vehicle deaths exceed firearm deaths in the young and the very elderly, age groups that are vulnerable to pedestrian as well as vehicle occupant deaths.

The external causes of fatal and non-fatal injury differ dramatically. In states with databases where one can compare the causes of fatal and non-fatal injury, for example, in California in 1995, falls accounted for fewer than 10% of the deaths but over one third of the hospitalizations for injury. In comparison, motor vehicles and firearms together accounted for more than half of the deaths but fewer than 20% of the hospitalizations.

Violence in families is an increasingly recognized and complex problem. Children's Protective Services determined that over 1 million children were victims of abuse or neglect in 1995. The National Family Violence Surveys estimate that 116 per 1000 women experience a violent act and 34 per 1000 experience severe violence at the hands of an intimate partner. No estimates of the prevalence of elder abuse have been made, but the problem is serious and may be increasing as the population ages.

Alcohol consumption is a major risk factor for all types of injury. In 1987, the estimated percentage of unintentional injury deaths associated with alcohol were 42% for motor vehicles, 20% for other road vehicles, 20% for water transport, 16% for air transport, 35% for falls, 45% for fires, and 38% for drowning. For suicide and homicide, the percentages of deaths associated with alcohol are estimated to be 28% and 46%, respectively.

SECULAR TRENDS IN INJURIES

Injuries are preventable. Data on injury deaths from 1910 to 1995 show a significant decrease in other (i.e., non–motor vehicle) unintentional injury death rates (Fig. 14–3). This decrease was due in part to improved safety design of occupational machinery and other protective measures, the mechanization of agriculture and

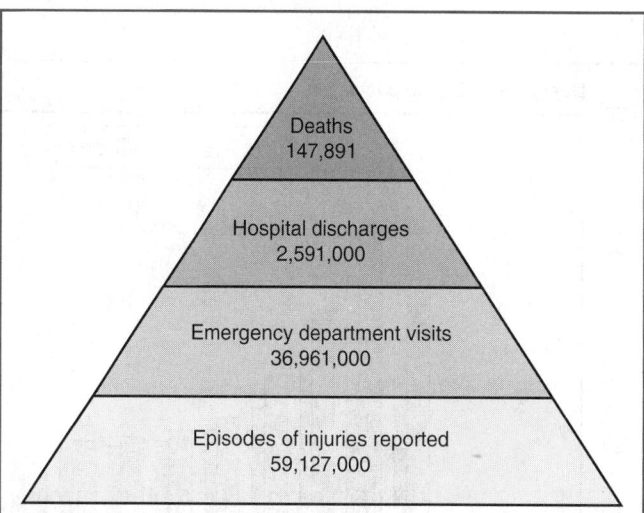

FIGURE 14–1 ■ Burden of injury: United States, 1995. (Data from National Vital Statistics System, National Hospital Discharge Survey, National Hospital Ambulatory Medical Care Survey, National Health Interview Survey. Reprinted from Fingerhut LA, Warner M: Injury Chartbook. *Health, United States 1996–97.* Hyattsville, MD, National Center for Health Statistics, 1997.)

Table 14–1 ■ NUMBERS* AND RATES† OF INJURY DEATHS IN THE UNITED STATES (1995) BY
INTENTIONALITY AND MECHANISM BY GENDER

DEATHS	TOTAL		MALES		FEMALES		
	No.	Rate†	No.	Rate†	No.	Rate†	%
All deaths	147,891	56.3	105,645	78.4	42,246	25.4	100.0
Distribution by Intentionality							
Unintentional	90,402	34.4	60,066	43.3	30,336	16.8	61.1
Suicide	31,284	11.9	25,369	18.6	5,915	4.1	21.2
Homicide	22,552	8.6	17,408	14.5	5,144	4.0	15.2
Other	3,653	1.3	2,802	2.0	851	0.5	2.5
Distribution by Mechanism							
Motor vehicle traffic	42,452	16.2	28,490	22.2	13,962	9.9	28.7
Firearms	35,957	13.7	30,724	24.1	5,233	4.0	24.3
Poisoning	16,307	6.2	11,568	8.4	4,739	3.2	11.0
Falls	11,275	4.3	6,387	3.6	4,888	1.4	7.6
Suffocation	10,376	4.0	7,106	5.1	3,270	1.7	7.0
Drowning	5,071	1.9	4,015	3.1	1,056	0.8	3.4
Fire	4,235	1.6	2,528	1.8	1,707	1.1	2.9
Other	22,218	6.7	14,827	10.2	7,391	3.4	15.0

*Excludes adverse event–related deaths (International Classification of Diseases, Injuries, and Causes of Death codes E870–E879 and E930–E949)
†Per 100,000 population. Crude rates are used for "total rate"; age-adjusted rates are used for "gender rate."
From National Vital Statistics System, 1995. Atlanta, National Center for Health Statistics, Centers for Disease Control and Prevention, 1998.

industry, labeling and packaging of drugs and toxic products, and improved medical care.

Between 1912 and 1995, unintentional work deaths per 100,000 population were reduced 90%, from 21 to 2. In 1912, an estimated 18,000 to 21,000 workers' lives were lost. In 1996, in a work force more than triple in size and producing 13 times the goods and services, there were only 4800 work-related deaths.

The death rate from motor vehicle crashes increased 10-fold from 1910 to 1930 as cars became the primary form of transportation. However, this death rate has decreased 30% in the last two decades owing in part to improved safety features in vehicles and roads, temporary lowering of speed limits, increased legal drinking age, and public intolerance of drinking and driving.

The homicide rate increased from 6 per 100,000 population in 1910 to 9 in 1930, decreased during World War II and the postwar period (1940s to 1960s) to approximately 5, and then increased to 10 in the 1980s and 1990s. Recent increases are attributed to the enormous number of guns in circulation, currently estimated to be from 150 to 200 million, one third of which are handguns. The suicide rate has shown less variability but has been consistently higher than the homicide rate throughout this century.

WAYS TO REDUCE INJURY

An example of the effectiveness of a public policy to prevent injury is the reduction in deaths and non-fatal head injuries in motorcyclists after enactment of the mandatory helmet laws. Hospital charges for injuries to California motorcyclists declined markedly in the 2 years (1992 to 1993) following enactment of the law, with charges related to head injuries falling by 58%. Certain personal and family actions can prevent injury from known hazards (Table 14–2), and enactment of certain public policies has the potential to reduce injury:

MOTOR VEHICLE CRASHES. Wear seat belts to maximize the protection offered by air bags, keep children properly restrained in the back seat, wear helmets while riding motorcycles and bicycles, and drive sober.

POLICIES. Enact or maintain motorcycle helmet laws; improve public transportation to reduce dependence on cars.

FIREARMS. Remove guns from the home (or at least store unloaded, locked, and out of reach of children).

POLICIES. Restrict the purchase and possession of handguns in the home, up to and including bans (official policy of the American

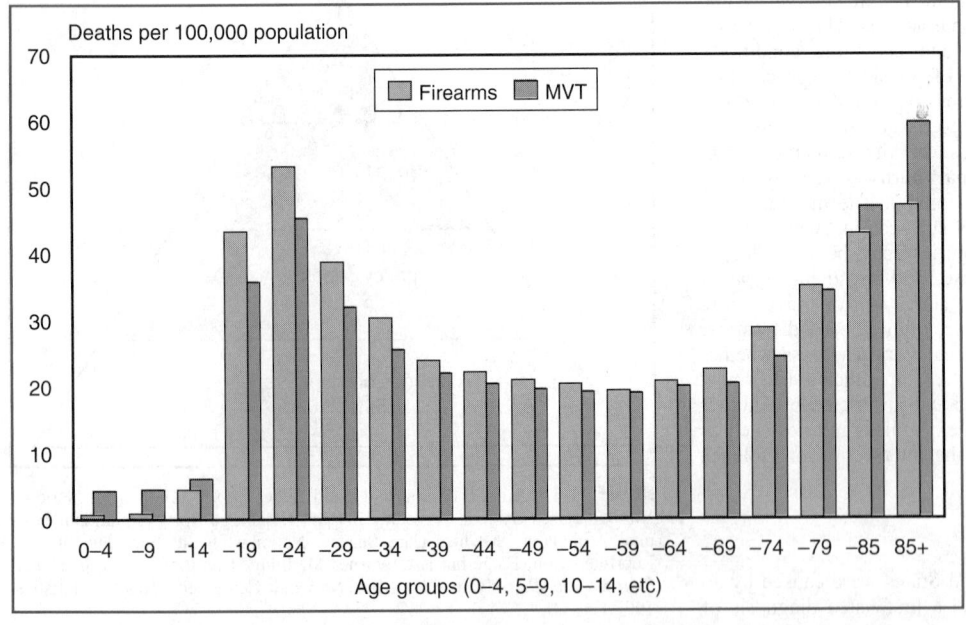

FIGURE 14–2 ■ Firearms and motor vehicle traffic crashes: male death rates by age groups, United States, 1995. (Data drawn from 1995 Injury Mortality Data, National Center for Health Statistics, Centers for Disease Control and Prevention, 1998.)

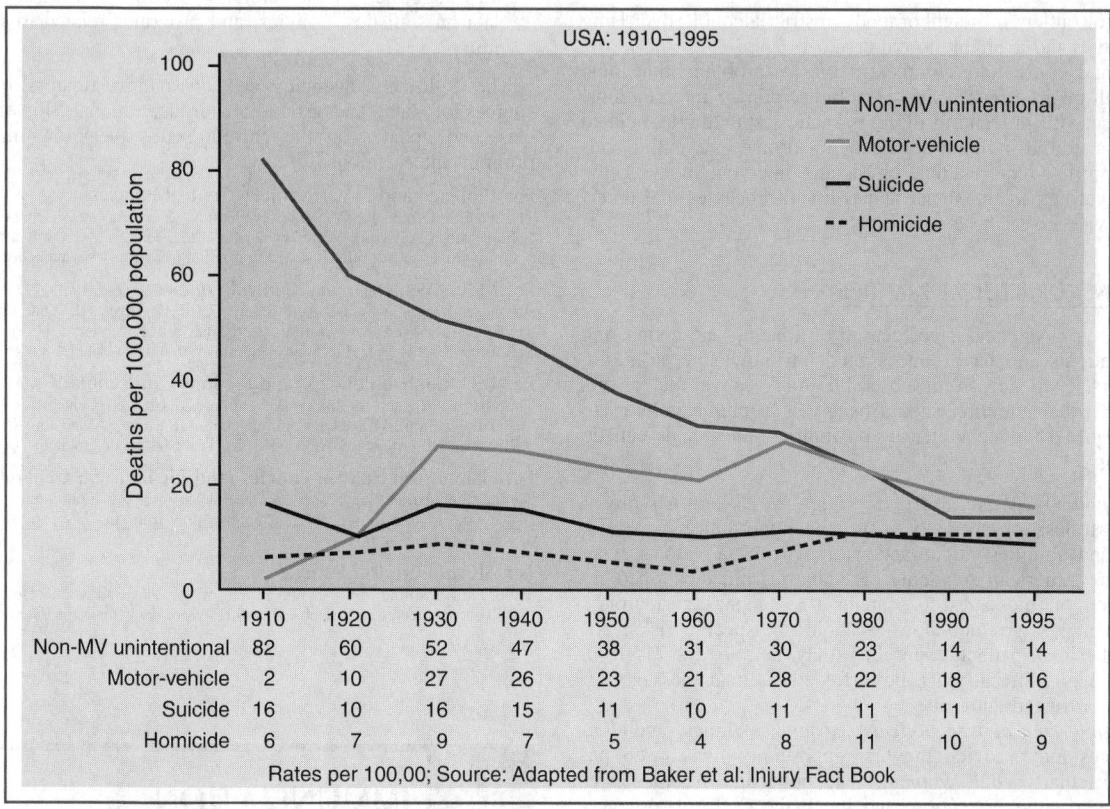

FIGURE 14-3 ■ Trends in injury death rates, United States, 1910 to 1995. (Updated from Baker SP, O'Neill B, Ginsburg MJ, et al: The Injury Fact Book. 2nd ed. New York, Oxford University Press, 1992.)

Academy of Pediatrics and the American Public Health Association).

FIRE AND BURN INJURIES. Install and maintain smoke detectors or residential sprinklers; reduce the temperature settings in residential hot water heaters to 125° F.

POLICIES. Establish mandatory flammability performance standards for cigarettes to prevent furniture ignition.

DROWNING. Wear flotation devices while boating.

POLICIES. Require four-sided isolation fences with self-latching gates on all residential pools.

FALLS. Install guards on balconies and windows in high-rise buildings; improve lighting and install handgrip devices in the home.

ALCOHOL-RELATED INJURY. Avoid binge drinking, promote alcohol moderation, and drive sober.

POLICIES. Permit community control over the number and loca-

Table 14-2 ■ SOME KEY MEASURES TO PREVENT INJURY

INJURY	FOR PUBLIC POLICY	FOR PATIENTS
Motor vehicle	Enact and enforce seat belt, child restraint, and motorcycle helmet laws.	Use seat belts, child restraints Use helmets when riding bicycles and motorcycles
Firearms	Ban assault weapons Enforce waiting period for firearm purchase	Remove firearms from home If gun in home, store locked and unloaded
Fire and burns	Mandate fire-safe cigarettes	Maintain smoke detectors; install sprinklers
Drowning	Mandate 4-sided fencing of pools	Wear flotation devices when boating
Falls		Install guards on balconies, windows; install handrails in elders' homes
Alcohol	Advocate for local control of alcohol outlets Restrict alcohol advertising that appeals to children	Drive sober Avoid binge drinking
Actions for physicians	Counsel patients about injury and prevention (see above). Identify and refer abused patients to social/legal services. Insist on adequate physical/occupational rehabilitation. Improve injury databases and use them to design preventive strategies. Become knowledgeable about and advocate sound public policies.	

tion of alcohol outlets in neighborhoods; restrict alcohol advertising that is attractive and available to children.

Violence and injuries are complex, pervasive problems that must be reduced through comprehensive, multidisciplinary interventions. As is the case with preventing diseases such as smoking-associated cancers and acquired immune deficiency syndrome, preventing violence and injuries requires that physicians intervene both at the individual level and in the social and political processes that determine the prevalence of these conditions.

IMPLICATIONS FOR MEDICAL PRACTICE

Traditionally, physicians have focused on treating and counseling individual patients and have concentrated on knowledge, attitudes, and behaviors. Evidence from successful injury prevention efforts suggests that equal attention should be given to public policies to prevent injury. To reduce violence and injuries, physicians can do the following:

1. *Counsel patients about injury risk and prevention.* All physicians, regardless of specialty, have the opportunity to advise patients and families about actions they can take to prevent injury. The American Academy of Pediatrics has developed injury prevention messages for parents that emphasize a child's developmental stages and how to avoid age-specific risks. Although physician-patient counseling may not always result in behavior change, it can be a powerful educational message delivered by a trusted authority.

2. *Identify and refer abused patients.* Hospitals, clinics, and doctors' offices may provide the first opportunity for abused patients, particularly adult women, to acknowledge the abuse, receive support, find protection, and break the cycle of violence. Medical and nursing professional organizations have prepared guidelines for institutionalizing the health care response to family violence through the development of model protocols, staff training materials, and proposed modification of intake forms for hospitals and clinics (e.g., American Medical Association guidelines). Policies and procedures should be adapted to individual hospital needs and address state-specific regulations about reporting abuse to authorities. Health care providers can best assist abused patients by working collaboratively with local social and legal services and by referring patients to these resources.

3. *Emphasize rehabilitation and community follow-up.* Tertiary prevention involves minimizing functional disability, a consequence of serious injury. Physicians can help their patients return to productive lives by ensuring that patients receive appropriate physical and occupational therapy and that they have access to community services after discharge. The independent living movement and local centers for independent living, as well as state departments of rehabilitation, can provide role models and resources for people with disabilities. Because community social and mental health services are essential for prevention and rehabilitation, physicians can serve their patients by publicly speaking out in support of these services.

4. *Improve the injury database for research and prevention.* Information about the mechanisms and intentionality of injury must be gathered by coroners, medical examiners, and health care providers through history taking and documentation in official records. The usefulness of non-fatal injury data would be increased if all states established centralized hospital and emergency department databases that included external cause of injury codes.

5. *Advocate for public policy solutions to the violence and injury problem.* Physicians have played a leadership role in injury control in such diverse areas as traffic safety, burns from tap water and clothing ignition, and firearms policy. Today's injury problems call for augmented medical leadership in policy areas. Legislators and journalists turn to physicians for information about disease and injury because physicians have daily contact with sick and injured people and can thus speak from personal experience about the problem. Informed physicians can advocate for solutions by testifying at legislative hearings, by granting media interviews, by making presentations at professional meetings, and by teaching medical students and residents about in-

jury prevention principles and strategies. The World Wide Web sites suggested in the reference section provide the most recent data on statistics, policies, and programs related to violence and injury.

The following agencies can direct investigators to additional sources of data, background materials, rationale for specific policies, and updates on the current status of policy initiatives and program interventions.

For Violence and Firearm Injury Control Policies
The Pacific Center for Violence Prevention, San Francisco General Hospital, San Francisco, CA 94100; Web: www.pcvp.org. Federal government information about criminal justice from the Justice Information Center at www.ncjrs.org.

For Motor Vehicle Injury Control Policies
Advocates for Highway and Auto Safety, 750 First Street, NE, Suite 901, Washington, DC 20002; Web: www.saferoads.org. Federal government information from the National Highway Traffic Safety Administration at www.nhtsa.dot.gov.

For Falls Control Policies (and for Injury in General)
The National Center for Injury Prevention and Control (Centers for Disease Control and Prevention), Office of Communications Resources, Mailstop K65, 4770 Buford Highway NE, Atlanta, GA 30341-3724; Web: www.cdc.gov/ncipc.

For Flame/Burn Control Policies (and for Injury in General)
Trauma Foundation, San Francisco General Hospital, San Francisco, CA 94100; Web: www.tf.org. Federal government information from the US Fire Administration at www.usfa.fema.gov.

For Alcohol Control Policies
The Marin Institute for the Prevention of Alcohol and Other Drug Problems, 24 Belvedere Street, San Rafael, CA 94901; Web: www.marininstitute.org.

15 IMMUNIZATION
Walter A. Orenstein

Immunization is one of the most cost-effective means of preventing morbidity and mortality from infectious diseases. Routine immunization, particularly of children, has resulted in decreases of 90% or more in reported cases of measles, mumps, rubella, congenital rubella syndrome, polio, tetanus, diphtheria, and pertussis. In many circumstances, immunization not only prevents morbidity and mortality but also, in the long run, reduces health care costs.

GENERAL CHARACTERISTICS OF IMMUNIZATIONS

Immunization protects against disease or the sequelae of disease through the administration of an immunobiologic: vaccines, toxoids, immune globulin preparations, and antitoxins. Protection induced by immunization can be active or passive.

ACTIVE IMMUNIZATION. Administering a vaccine or toxoid causes the body to produce an immune response against the infectious agent or its toxins. Vaccines consist of suspensions of live (usually attenuated) or inactivated microorganisms or fractions thereof. Toxoids are modified bacterial toxins that retain immunogenic properties but lack toxicity. Active immunization generally results in long-term immunity, although the onset of protection may be delayed because it takes time for the body to respond. With live attenuated vaccines, small quantities of living organisms multiply within the recipient until an immune response cuts off replication. In contrast, inactivated vaccines and toxoids contain large quantities of antigen. In the majority of recipients, a single dose of a live vaccine generally induces an immune response that closely parallels natural infection and induces long-term immunity. Killed vaccines, in contrast, often require multiple doses.

PASSIVE IMMUNIZATION. Passive immunization using immune globulins or antitoxins delivers pre-formed antibodies to provide temporary immunity. Immune globulins obtained from human blood may contain antibodies to a variety of agents, depending on the pool of human plasma from which they are prepared. Specific immune globulins are made from the plasma of donors with high levels of antibodies to specific antigens, such as tetanus immune globulin. Most immune globulins must be injected intramuscularly. Antitoxins are solutions of antibodies derived from animals immunized with specific antigens (e.g., diphtheria antitoxin). Passive immunization is usually indicated to protect individuals immediately before anticipated exposure or shortly after known or suspected exposure to an infectious agent (Table 15–1), when active immunization either is not possible or has not been adequate.

ROUTE AND TIMING OF VACCINATION. Each immunobiologic has a preferred site and route of administration. In adults, vaccines containing adjuvants should be injected intramuscularly, preferably in the deltoid muscle. For men, a 1-inch needle is adequate, whereas for women, recommended needle lengths vary from 5/8 inch for women weighing less than 60 kg to 1 inch for those weighing 60 to 90 kg and 1.5 inches for women heavier than 90 kg. Use of the buttocks is discouraged except when large volumes are required both because of the potential for damage to the sciatic nerve and because of diminished immune response to some vaccines, such as hepatitis B. Subcutaneous vaccines are also usually administered in the deltoid area, and intradermal vaccines are usually given on the volar surface of the forearm. In general, inactivated vaccines and toxoids can be given simultaneously at different sites. With vaccines that frequently cause side effects, such as cholera and inactivated typhoid vaccines, it may be best to separate administration by at least a week. With the exception of cholera and yellow fever vaccines, which should ideally be administered at least 3 weeks apart, live and inactivated vaccines can be administered at the same time. For example, measles, mumps, and rubella (MMR) vaccine can be administered with oral polio vaccine (OPV). However, with the exception of MMR and OPV, which can be administered at any interval, live vaccines not delivered on the same day should be separated by at least 1 month because immune globulin may also interfere with the take of live vaccines other than OPV; ideally, such vaccines should be administered at least 2 weeks prior or 3 to 11 months after immune globulin.

ADVERSE REACTIONS. Hypersensitivity to vaccine components such as animal proteins, antibiotics, preservatives, and stabilizers can lead to local and systemic reactions ranging from mild to severe. The egg protein contained in vaccines grown in chicken eggs (influenza and yellow fever vaccines) may cause reactions in persons allergic to eggs. In general, persons without anaphylactic-type allergies to eggs can be given these vaccines safely, but persons with anaphylactic reactions to eggs should not generally receive these vaccines except when absolutely necessary and then only under established protocols by physicians who are expert in such situations. Even though measles and mumps vaccines are grown in chick embryo tissue culture, the risk of anaphylaxis even in those with severe hypersensitivity to eggs is very low, so such persons can be vaccinated without prior testing but should be observed for at least 20 minutes and preferably 90 minutes after immunization.

No vaccine is completely safe or completely effective. Two major groups make comprehensive, detailed recommendations regarding immunization of adults: (1) the Task Force on Adult Immunization of the American College of Physicians (ACP) and The Infectious Diseases Society of America (IDSA), which publishes the *Guide for Adult Immunization*, and (2) the Advisory Committee on Immunization Practices of the U.S. Public Health Service. The latter group publishes its information in *Morbidity and Mortality Weekly Report*. Suspected adverse events temporally related to vaccinations should be reported to the Vaccine Adverse Events Reporting System (1-800-822-7967).

GENERAL CONSIDERATIONS. Immunizations for adults depend on age, lifestyle, occupation, and medical conditions (Table 15–2). All adults should have a primary series of tetanus and diphtheria toxoids with boosters of combined toxoids (Td) every 10 years. Persons born in or after 1957 should have evidence of immunity to measles, mumps, and rubella. Vaccination of susceptible adolescents and adults against varicella is desirable. Pneumococcal vac-

Table 15–1 ■ **PASSIVE IMMUNIZATIONS FOR ADULTS**

DISEASE	NAME OF MATERIAL	COMMENTS AND USE
Tetanus	Tetanus immune globulin, human	Management of tetanus-prone wounds in persons without adequate prior active immunization and treatment of tetanus
Cytomegalovirus	Cytomegalovirus immune globulin, intravenous	Prophylaxis for bone marrow and kidney transplant recipients
Diphtheria	Diphtheria antitoxin, equine	Treatment of established disease, high frequency of reactions to serum of non-human origin
Rabies	Rabies immunoglobulin, human	Post-exposure prophylaxis of animal bites
Measles	Immune globulin, human	Prevention or modification of disease in contacts of cases, not for control of epidemics
Hepatitis A	Immune globulin, human	Protection of household contacts, pre-exposure prophylaxis for travelers who need protection before immunity can be achieved with hepatitis A vaccine
Hepatitis B	Hepatitis B immune globulin, human	Prophylaxis for needlestick or mucous membrane contact with HBsAg-positive persons, for sexual partners with acute hepatitis B or hepatitis B carriers, for infants born to mothers who are carriers of HBsAg, for infants whose mother or primary caregiver has acute hepatitis B
Varicella	Varicella-zoster immune globulin	Persons with underlying disease and at risk of complications from chickenpox who have not had varicella or varicella vaccine and who are exposed to varicella. May be given post-exposure to known susceptible adults, particularly if antibody-negative
Vaccinia	Vaccinia immune globulin	Treatment of eczema vaccinatum, vaccinia necrosum, and ocular vaccinia following vaccinia (smallpox) vaccination
Erythroblastosis fetalis	Rh immune globulin	Rh-negative women who give birth to Rh-positive infants or who abort
Hypogammaglobulinemia	Immune globulin, intravenous	Maintenance therapy
Idiopathic thrombocytopenic purpura	Immune globulin, intravenous	Therapy for acute episodes
Botulism	Trivalent A, B, and E antitoxin, equine	Treatment of botulism
Snakebite	Antivenin, equine (North American coral snake antivenin)	Specific for North American coral snake, *Micrurus fulvius*
	Crotalidae, polyvalent	Effective for viper and pit viper bites, including rattlesnakes, copperheads, moccasins
Spider bite	Antivenin, equine	Specific for black widow spider, *Latrodectus mactans*, and other members of the genus

HBsAg = hepatitis B surface antigen.

Table 15–2 ■ SELECTED IMMUNIZING AGENTS INDICATED FOR ADULTS*

DISEASE	IMMUNIZING AGENT	INDICATIONS	SCHEDULE	MAJOR CONTRAINDICATIONS AND PRECAUTIONS	COMMENTS
Cholera	Inactivated vaccine	Meeting international travel requirements	Two 0.5-mL doses SC or IM or two 0.2-mL doses ID 1 wk to 1 mo apart; booster dose every 6 mo		Of limited effectiveness; cholera and yellow fever vaccine should be administered at least 3 wk apart
Diphtheria	Tetanus and diphtheria toxoids combined	All adults	Two doses IM 4 wk apart, 3rd dose 6–12 mo after 2nd dose for primary series, booster every 10 yr; no need to repeat if schedule is interrupted	History of neurologic or severe hypersensitivity reaction following a previous dose	
Hepatitis A	Inactivated hepatitis A vaccine	Travelers to highly or intermediately endemic countries, men who have sex with men; illegal drug users (injectors and non-injectors), persons who work with virus-infected primates or do research with the virus, persons with chronic liver disease, recipients of clotting factors	2 doses at least 6 mo apart for persons ≥2 years of age	Hypersensitivity to vaccine components	Should be considered for outbreak control for children and adolescents in communities with intermediate to high underlying transmission
Hepatitis B	Inactivated virus vaccine	Adolescents, health care and public safety workers potentially exposed to blood, clients and staff of institutions for the developmentally disabled, hemodialysis patients, sexually active homosexual men; users of illicit injectable drugs, recipients of clotting factors, household and sexual contacts of HBV carriers, inmates of long-term correctional facilities, heterosexuals treated for sexually transmitted diseases or with multiple sexual partners, travelers with close contact for ≥6 mo with populations with high prevalence of HBV carriage	IM; three doses at 0, 1, and 6 mo		Pregnancy should not be considered a contraindication if the woman is otherwise eligible. Health care workers who have contact with patients or blood should be tested 1–2 mo after vaccination to determine serologic response
Influenza	Inactivated influenza virus vaccine	All adults ≥65 yr; other adults with high-risk conditions; adults caring for persons with high-risk conditions, including medical personnel (see text); women who will be in 2nd or 3rd trimester of pregnancy during influenza season	Annual vaccination; see annual ACIP recommendation	Anaphylactic hypersensitivity to eggs	
Japanese encephalitis	Inactivated virus vaccine	Travelers to Asia spending at least 1 mo in endemic areas during transmission season	Three 1-mL doses SC on days 0, 7, 30; shortened schedule of 0, 7, 14 days may be used when necessary. Booster doses may be given after 2 yr	Persons with histories of urticaria at greater risk of adverse reactions to vaccine; pregnancy	No data exist on concurrent administration with vaccines other than DTP, drugs (e.g., chloroquine, mefloquine), or other biologics

Table 15–2 ■ **SELECTED IMMUNIZING AGENTS INDICATED FOR ADULTS*** *Continued*

DISEASE	IMMUNIZING AGENT	INDICATIONS	SCHEDULE	MAJOR CONTRAINDICATIONS AND PRECAUTIONS	COMMENTS
Lyme disease	Inactivated outer surface protein A (OspA)	Primarily persons who live, work, or visit areas at high or moderate risk for Lyme disease and who will have frequent or prolonged exposure to a tick-infested habitat during transmission season.	Three doses IM at 0, 1 month, and 12 months		Duration of immunity and need for boosters are unknown.
Measles	Live-virus vaccine	All adults born after 1956 without history of live vaccine on or after 1st birthday, physician-diagnosed measles, or detectable measles antibody; persons born before 1957 can generally be considered immune	One dose sufficient for most adults; 2 doses at least 1 mo apart indicated for persons entering college or medical facility employment, traveling abroad, or at risk of measles during outbreaks	Altered immunity (e.g., leukemia, lymphoma, generalized malignancy, congenital immunodeficiency, immunosuppressive therapy), immune globulin or other blood products within prior 3–11 mo depending upon dose of immune globulin or blood product received, untreated tuberculosis, anaphylactic hypersensitivity to neomycin or gelatin, pregnancy, thrombocytopenia	Persons with anaphylactic allergies to eggs may be vaccinated (see text). Vaccine should be administered to persons with asymptomatic HIV infection and should be considered for symptomatic HIV patients, except those with severe immunocompromise
Meningococcal disease	Polysaccharide vaccine containing tetravalent A, C, W135, and Y	Terminal complement component deficiencies, anatomic or functional asplenia, travelers who will live in areas with hyperendemic or epidemic diseases; may be useful during localized outbreaks	One dose		Consider revaccination after 3–5 yr for adults at increased risk of disease
Mumps	Live-virus vaccine	All adults born after 1956 without history of live vaccine on or after 1st birthday, physician-diagnosed mumps, or detectable mumps antibody; persons born before 1957 can generally be considered immune	One dose	Altered immunity (e.g., leukemia, lymphoma, generalized malignancy, congenital immunodeficiency, immunosuppressive therapy), immune globulin or other blood products within prior 3–11 mo, anaphylactic hypersensitivity to neomycin or gelatin, pregnancy, thrombocytopenia if administered with measles vaccine	Although persons born before 1957 are generally immune, vaccine can be given to adults of all ages and may be particularly indicated for post-pubertal males who are thought to be susceptible. Persons with anaphylactic allergies to eggs may be vaccinated.
Pneumococcal disease	23-valent polysaccharide vaccine	Adults with cardiovascular disease, pulmonary disease, diabetes mellitus, alcoholism, cirrhosis, cerebrospinal fluid leaks, splenic dysfunction or anatomic asplenia, Hodgkin's disease, lymphoma, multiple myeloma, chronic renal failure, nephrotic syndrome, immunosuppression, HIV infection; high-risk populations such as certain Native Americans and *all* adults ≥65 yr	One dose IM or SC. A 2nd dose should be considered 5 or more yr later for adults at high risk of disease (e.g., asplenic patients), as well as those who lose antibody rapidly (e.g., nephrotic syndrome, renal failure, transplant recipients). Revaccinate adults who received a first dose when <65 yr who are now ≥65 years and who received their vaccine at least 5 years earlier.		

Table continued on following page

Table 15–2 ■ SELECTED IMMUNIZING AGENTS INDICATED FOR ADULTS* Continued

DISEASE	IMMUNIZING AGENT	INDICATIONS	SCHEDULE	MAJOR CONTRAINDICATIONS AND PRECAUTIONS	COMMENTS
Poliomyelitis	IPV (inactivated), OPV (live attenuated)	Certain adults who are at greater risk of exposure to wild poliovirus than the general population, including travelers to countries where polio is epidemic or endemic, members of community or specific populations groups with disease caused by wild poliovirus, laboratory workers handling specimens that may contain poliovirus, health care workers in close contact with patients who may be excreting wild poliovirus, unvaccinated adults whose children will receive OPV	For unvaccinated adults, IPV is preferred: two doses SC 4 wk apart and a 3rd dose 6–12 mo after the 2nd; if less than 4 wk available before protection is needed, a single dose of OPV or IPV. For incompletely immunized adults, complete primary series with either vaccine; primary series consists of three doses of IPV or OPV; no need to restart interrupted series. A single dose of OPV or IPV can be given to adults who previously completed a primary series	OPV: immune deficiency diseases, patients with altered immune status (e.g., leukemia), household contacts of immunodeficient patients, household contacts with a family history of immunodeficiency until the immune status of individuals is established. On theoretic grounds, pregnant women should not receive IPV or OPV. However, if immediate protection is needed, IPV or OPV can be used	Adults who have not been adequately immunized against polio are at a very small risk of polio when their children are vaccinated with OPV. The child can be vaccinated with OPV regardless of the immune status of the parents. An acceptable alternative, provided that the full immunization of the child is not compromised, is to vaccinate the parents first with IPV or use an all-IPV schedule for the child
Rabies	Inactivated vaccine, HDCV, PCEC, or RVA	High-risk persons, including animal handlers, selected laboratory and field workers, and persons traveling for ≥1 mo to areas with high risk of rabies	Pre-exposure *prophylaxis:* three doses of 1.0 mL IM for HDCV, PCEC, or RVA on days 0, 7, and 21 or 28. For HDCV only, three doses of 0.1 mL ID on days 0, 7, and 21 or 28	History of severe hypersensitivity reaction	Further doses needed following exposure. If to be given concurrently with chloroquine, only IM route should be used
Rubella	Live-virus vaccine	Adults, particularly women of childbearing age, who lack history of rubella vaccine and detectable rubella-specific antibodies in serum; both males and females in institutions where rubella outbreaks may occur, such as hospitals, the military, and colleges. Persons born prior to 1957, except women who can become pregnant, can generally be considered immune	1 dose SC	Pregnancy, altered immunity (e.g., leukemia, lymphoma, generalized malignancy, congenital immunodeficiency, immunosuppressive therapy), immune globulin or other blood products within the 3–11 mo prior to vaccination, anaphylactic hypersensitivity to neomycin. Administration of blood products should not contraindicate post-partum vaccination; thrombocytopenia if administered with measles vaccine	Women should be counseled to avoid pregnancy for 3 mo
Tetanus	Tetanus and diphtheria toxoids combined	All adults	Three doses IM needed for primary series: two doses 4 wk apart, 3rd dose 6–12 mo after 2nd dose, booster every 10 yr; no need to repeat if schedule is interrupted	History of neurologic or severe hypersensitivity reaction following a previous dose	Special recommendations for wound treatment (see text). Persons with GBS within the 6 wk after immunization, particularly adults who received a prior primary series, should probably not be revaccinated in most circumstances
Typhoid fever	Heat-phenol–inactivated vaccine, Vi capsular polysaccharide vaccine, live attenuated Ty21a oral vaccine	Travelers to areas where the risk of prolonged exposure to contaminated food and water is high; may be considered for family and intimate contacts of carriers and laboratory workers who work with *Salmonella typhi*	*Inactivated vaccine:* two 0.5-mL doses SC 4 or more wk apart, boosters of 0.5 mL SC or 0.1 mL ID every 3 yr; *Vi polysaccharide vaccine:* one dose IM 0.5 mL, boosters every 2 yr; *Oral vaccine:* 4 doses on alternate days, boosters every 5 yr	Severe local or systemic reaction to a prior dose. Ty21A vaccine should not be administered to persons with altered immunity or those receiving antimicrobial agents	Efficacy only 50–77%. Food and water precautions essential. Ty21a and Vi polysaccharide vaccines preferred over heat-phenol–inactivated vaccine

Table 15–2 ■ **SELECTED IMMUNIZING AGENTS INDICATED FOR ADULTS*** *Continued*

DISEASE	IMMUNIZING AGENT	INDICATIONS	SCHEDULE	MAJOR CONTRAINDICATIONS AND PRECAUTIONS	COMMENTS
Varicella	Attenuated varicella vaccine, OKA strain	Persons, including health care workers, who have contact with patients, at high risk of complications from varicella; persons who work with children (e.g., teachers), persons in institutions that may have outbreaks (e.g., colleges), non-pregnant women of childbearing age, international travelers; desirable for other susceptible adolescents and adults	2 0.5-mL SC doses 4–8 wk apart for persons ≥13 yr of age	Immunocompromise, pregnancy, allergy to vaccine components; avoid salicylate use for 6 wk after vaccination	Adults with a history of prior varicella should be considered immune. Vaccine virus has rarely been transmitted to contacts from healthy vaccinees in whom rash developed. Women who receive vaccine should not become pregnant for 1 mo
Yellow fever	Live attenuated virus (17D strain)	Persons living or traveling in areas where yellow fever exists	One dose; booster every 10 yr	Immunocompromised persons; history of anaphylactic allergies to eggs; pregnancy on theoretic grounds, although may be given if risk is high	

*See the text and package inserts for further details, particularly regarding indications, dosage, mode of administration, side effects, and adverse reactions and contraindications.
SC = subcutaneously;   IM = intramuscularly;   ID = intradermally;   HBV = hepatitis B virus;   ACIP = Advisory Committee on Immunization Practices;   DTP = diphtheria-tetanus-pertussis;   HIV = human immunodeficiency virus;   IPV = inactivated polio vaccine;   OPV = live-virus trivalent oral polio vaccine;   HDCV = human diploid cell vaccine for rabies;   RVA = rabies vaccine absorbed;   PCEC = purified chick embryo cell culture rabies vaccine;   GBS = Guillain-Barré syndrome.

cine and annual vaccination against influenza are indicated for all adults 65 years and older and younger adults with certain medical conditions that place them at high risk of complications. Health care workers exposed to blood or blood products should receive hepatitis B vaccine. Those caring for patients at high risk of complications from influenza should receive annual vaccination. Health care workers likely to come in contact with persons transmitting measles, mumps, rubella, or varicella should be immune to those diseases.

IMMUNOCOMPROMISE. Patients with conditions that compromise their immune systems should not receive live attenuated vaccines. Such patients include those with immunodeficiency diseases, leukemia, lymphoma, and generalized malignancy and those who are immunosuppressed from therapy with corticosteroids, alkylating agents, antimetabolites, and radiation. An exception is infection with human immunodeficiency virus (HIV). Asymptomatic patients should receive MMR vaccine. MMR should be considered for symptomatic patients with HIV; however, severely immunocompromised persons should not be vaccinated. Because of the availability of enhanced-potency inactivated polio vaccine (IPV), all patients known to be infected with HIV should receive IPV instead of OPV. Patients with leukemia in remission who have not been receiving any chemotherapy for at least 3 months may receive live-virus vaccines. Short-course therapy (<2 weeks) with corticosteroids, alternate-day regimens with low to moderate doses of short-acting corticosteroids, and topical applications or tendon injections are not ordinarily contraindications to the administration of live vaccines.

Immunocompromised patients can receive inactivated vaccines and toxoids, although the efficacy of such preparations may be diminished. Patients with known HIV infection should receive pneumococcal vaccine and annual influenza vaccination.

PREGNANCY. In general, live vaccines should not be given to pregnant women because of the theoretic concern that such vaccines could adversely affect the fetus. No significant adverse events attributable to vaccination of pregnant women with MMR or varicella have been documented; nevertheless, pregnant women should not receive MMR, and women who do receive MMR or varicella

should wait 3 months or 1 month, respectively, before becoming pregnant. Polio and yellow fever vaccines should not usually be given to pregnant women unless the risk of disease is substantial. Td vaccination is especially indicated for pregnant females who are not appropriately vaccinated to prevent neonatal tetanus in their infants. Vaccination is best performed after the first trimester. All pregnant women should be screened for hepatitis B surface antigen (HBsAg). Offspring of HBsAg carrier mothers should receive hepatitis B vaccine and hepatitis B immune globulin. Women who will be in the second or third trimester of pregnancy during the influenza season should receive influenza vaccine.

INDIVIDUAL IMMUNOBIOLOGICS

Tetanus and Diphtheria

Tetanus (see Chapter 337) toxoid is one of the most effective immunizations, with over 95% protection after a primary series. The adsorbed is preferred over the fluid preparation because it induces protective levels of antitoxin that persist longer after fewer doses. A primary series consists of three doses. In persons aged 7 years or older, it should always be used in combination with diphtheria (see Chapter 333) toxoid (Td), which is more than 85% effective in preventing disease. Doses need not be repeated if the schedule is interrupted. Boosters are recommended every 10 years. An easy way to remember is to schedule immunization at the middle of each decade (e.g., 25 years, 35 years, etc.). The ACP/IDSA Task Force on Adult Immunization has recently suggested that a single Td booster at age 50 may be sufficient to maintain protective antibody levels in older adults who have received a primary series with boosters as a teenager and young adult.

After a wound, persons of unknown immunization status or those who have received fewer than three doses of tetanus toxoid should receive a dose of Td regardless of the severity of the wound. Td is also indicated for those who have previously received three or more doses if more than 10 years has elapsed since the last dose, in the case of clean, minor wounds, and if more than 5 years has elapsed for all other wounds. Tetanus immune globulin should be administered simultaneously at a separate site to persons who have not received at least three doses of toxoid and who have wounds that are not clean and minor. Most reactions to Td consist of local inflammation and low-grade fever. However, Guillain-Barré syndrome and brachial neuritis have very rarely been associated with tetanus toxoid.

Measles

Measles (see Chapter 381) immunization is recommended for all persons born in or after 1957 who lack evidence of prior physician-diagnosed measles or laboratory evidence of immunity or appropriate vaccination. Prior to 1989, appropriate vaccination consisted of a single dose of live vaccine administered on or after the first birthday. Now, a routine two-dose schedule is recommended: the first dose, which is 93 to 98% effective, at 12 to 15 months of age and the second dose at entry to primary school. By 2001, all children from kindergarten through the 12th grade should have a second dose. Most adults are considered to have been appropriately vaccinated if they received one dose of vaccine administered on or after their first birthday. Some adults, however, who are at increased risk of measles (health care workers with direct patient contact, students in college, international travelers) should receive a second dose of vaccine unless they have documentation of prior physician-diagnosed measles or serologic evidence of immunity. Persons embarking on foreign travel should ideally have received two doses or have other evidence of measles immunity. Persons born before 1957 are usually immune as a result of natural infection and do not require vaccination, although vaccination is not contraindicated if they are believed to be susceptible.

During outbreaks of measles in institutions, all persons at risk who have not received two doses or who lack other evidence of measles immunity should be vaccinated. Measles vaccine is usually administered along with mumps and rubella vaccine (MMR) to ensure immunity against all three diseases. Individuals already immune to one or more of the components, however, may receive MMR without harm.

Measles vaccine is contraindicated for pregnant women on theoretic grounds, for persons with moderate to severe acute febrile illnesses, and for persons with altered immunocompetence, except those with HIV infection who are not severely immunocompromised. Patients with anaphylactic reactions to eggs can be vaccinated without prior skin testing.

In approximately 5 to 15% of susceptible recipients of measles vaccine, temperatures of 39.4° C or higher develop between 5 and 12 days after vaccination and last 1 to 2 days. Transient rashes develop in about 5%. Thrombocytopenic purpura has been reported rarely after MMR. The overall rate of reactions after the second dose of a measles-containing vaccine is substantially lower than after the first dose. Encephalopathy or encephalitis following measles vaccination has been reported at a rate lower than the background or expected rate.

Rubella

Rubella (see Chapter 382) vaccine is indicated for susceptible adults born in 1957 or later and for susceptible women of any age who are considering becoming pregnant. Persons without a prior history of vaccination on or after the first birthday or laboratory evidence of immunity should be considered susceptible. A single dose of vaccine is 95% or more effective. Many persons receive two doses of rubella vaccine via the two-dose schedule of MMR.

Follow-up of 305 susceptible women who received rubella vaccines within 3 months of the estimated date of conception has failed to reveal any evidence of defects compatible with congenital rubella syndrome in their offspring. Nevertheless, vaccine is contraindicated in pregnant women on theoretic grounds, and conception should be delayed for 3 months after rubella vaccination.

Reactions occur only in susceptible persons. Arthralgia, usually of the small peripheral joints, develops in up to 40% of susceptible adults, and frank arthritis develops in 10 to 20%. Joint symptoms usually begin 1 to 3 weeks following vaccination and persist for 1 day to 3 weeks. Very rarely have chronic recurrent or persistent joint symptoms developed following vaccination, but controlled

studies have shown that the incidence of these events in vaccinees is similar to that of non-vaccinees. Other infrequent adverse events include transient peripheral neuritis and pain in the arms and legs. Thrombocytopenic purpura has been reported rarely when rubella vaccine is administered as MMR. Rubella vaccine is contraindicated for persons with moderate to severe acute febrile illnesses and for persons with reduced immunocompetence. When given with measles vaccine, it may be administered to those with asymptomatic HIV infection and considered for those with symptomatic infection without severe immunocompromise. Rubella vaccine is grown in human diploid cells and can be administered without problems to persons with allergy to eggs.

Mumps

Mumps (see Chapter 384) vaccine is indicated for all persons, especially susceptible males, without a prior history of vaccination on or after the first birthday, physician-diagnosed mumps, or laboratory evidence of immunity. Most persons born prior to 1957 can be considered immune as a result of natural infection, although vaccination is not contraindicated if such persons are thought to be susceptible. In clinical trials, a single dose of vaccine has induced seroconversion in more than 90% of recipients.

Adverse events following mumps vaccine are uncommon—fever, parotitis, and allergic manifestations. Thrombocytopenic purpura has been reported rarely in those administered MMR. Mumps vaccine is contraindicated for pregnant women on theoretic grounds, for persons with moderate to severe acute febrile illnesses, and for persons with altered immunocompetence. When combined with measles vaccine, it may be given to those with asymptomatic HIV infection and considered for those with symptomatic infection if they are not severely immunocompromised. Patients with anaphylactic reactions to eggs can be vaccinated without skin testing (see Measles earlier).

Varicella

A live attenuated varicella vaccine (Oka strain) was licensed in March 1995. The vaccine protects 70 to 90% of recipients against any disease and more than 95% of recipients against severe disease. Breakthrough infections in persons who have previously seroconverted have been reported in 2 to 4% per year following vaccination with the licensed product. Such breakthroughs are typically mild and average fewer than 50 lesions as compared with several hundred lesions in unvaccinated persons with varicella. Breakthrough illnesses do not appear to increase in incidence or severity with increasing time since vaccination, a finding compatible with long-term protection following initial vaccination. Persons 13 years or older require two doses at least 4 weeks apart to achieve seroconversion rates of approximately 99%, a rate comparable to that in younger children after one dose.

The most common side effect is soreness at the injection site, which is reported in 25 to 35% of recipients 13 years or older. Varicella-like rashes at the injection site (median of two lesions) have been reported in 3% of recipients in this age group after the first dose and in 1% after the second dose. Non-localized rashes with a median of five lesions have been reported in 5.5% of recipients after the first dose and in 0.9% after the second dose. The incidence of herpes zoster (shingles) is substantially lower than would be expected after natural varicella (see Chapter 383). Although more severe events occurring in temporal relation to the vaccine have been reported very rarely, a causal relationship has not been established. Transmission of vaccine virus to a contact is extremely rare and appears to take place only with vaccinees in whom a varicella-like rash has developed.

Varicella vaccine is indicated routinely for all children. Persons with a prior history of varicella disease can be considered immune and do not need vaccination. Whereas a negative or unknown history of disease is predictive of susceptibility in children, many adults with such histories are immune. Serologic screening of adults in some situations may be cost-effective, provided that identified susceptible adults are vaccinated. The vaccine is contraindicated in the immunocompromised, those with anaphylactic allergies to vaccine components, and pregnant women. Varicella vaccine is more temperature sensitive than other vaccines used in the United States. It must be stored frozen at −15° C or colder to retain potency. It should be discarded if not used within 30 minutes of reconstitution.

Hepatitis B

Hepatitis B (see Chapter 149) vaccine is the first vaccine that can prevent cancer (an estimated 800 persons per year in the United States die of hepatitis B–related liver cancer; many times more do so in the developing world). It can also prevent acute and chronic complications of hepatitis B, including an estimated 4000 deaths annually from cirrhosis and 250 deaths annually from fulminant hepatic disease in the United States. The original hepatitis vaccine in the United States consisted of purified, inactivated, alum-adsorbed, 22-nm HBsAg particles obtained from human plasma. Currently produced vaccines are derived from inserting the gene for HBsAg into *Saccharomyces cerevisiae*. Hepatitis B vaccine, the first licensed vaccine made by using recombinant techniques, produces adequate antibody responses in more than 90% of normal adults and more than 95% of normal infants, children, and adolescents when administered in a three-dose series. The dosage depends on the product, the age group, and the underlying clinical condition and can be determined by consulting the package insert. The duration of vaccine-conferred immunity is not known, although follow-up of vaccinees for 11 years indicates persistence of protection against clinically significant infections (i.e., detectable viremia and clinical disease). Booster doses are not currently recommended. Vaccine must be injected intramuscularly, preferably in the deltoid.

Because strategies targeting hepatitis B vaccine use only to high-risk populations have not had a significant impact on hepatitis B incidence, universal vaccination is now recommended. Universal infant vaccination is presently recommended for all populations. All adolescents who have not been previously vaccinated should be immunized. Universal screening for HBsAg is recommended for all pregnant women, with administration of three doses of vaccine and one dose of hepatitis B immune globulin recommended for infants of carrier mothers.

The major side effect is soreness at the injection site. Alopecia, which is usually reversible, has been reported very rarely. Among adults receiving plasma-derived vaccine, the risk of Guillain-Barré syndrome is increased after the first dose, but the overall increase, if real, is very small and is outweighed by the substantial benefits of vaccination. Recombinant vaccine, which is now the standard, does not appear to increase the risk of Guillain-Barré syndrome. There is no risk of acquiring HIV infection from either vaccine.

Influenza

Annual influenza (see Chapter 379) vaccination is indicated for adults at high risk of complications from the disease: persons with chronic cardiopulmonary disorders, residents of nursing homes or other chronic care facilities, persons aged 65 or older, patients with other chronic diseases (such as diabetes mellitus, kidney dysfunction, hemoglobinopathies, and immunosuppression) who have required regular medical follow-up or hospitalization in the prior year, and children receiving long-term aspirin therapy. Women who will be in the second or third trimester of pregnancy during the influenza season (usually late December through mid-March) should also be vaccinated. In addition, transmission of influenza to high-risk patients can be reduced by annually vaccinating health care workers and household contacts of high-risk patients.

The efficacy of influenza vaccine varies with the host's condition and the degree to which antigens in the vaccine match viruses in circulation the following season. Current vaccines contain whole or split inactivated viruses of three major antigenic types—A (H3N2), A (H1N1), and B. Provided that the match is good, vaccine efficacy is usually 70 to 90% in normal healthy young adults. Efficacy is substantially lower, often between 20 and 40%, in the institutionalized elderly; nevertheless, it appears to be 60 to 80% protective against pneumonia and death. Ideally, vaccines should be administered between October and mid-November of each year, although earlier in the autumn suffices if circumstances require.

Persons with anaphylactic allergies to eggs should not be immunized. The most common side effect is soreness at the injection site. Fever, malaise, and myalgia may begin 6 to 12 hours after vaccination and persist for 1 to 2 days, although such reactions are most common in children exposed to vaccine for the first time.

Severe allergic reactions are rare. If current influenza vaccines cause Guillain-Barré syndrome, it is likely to be very rare, on the order of 1 case per million doses. A live attenuated trivalent influenza vaccine for intranasal administration may soon become available.

Pneumococcal Vaccine

Pneumococcal vaccine consists of purified polysaccharide capsular antigens from the 23 types of *Streptococcus pneumoniae* that are responsible for 85 to 90% of the bacteremic disease in the United States (see Chapter 319). Most adults, including the elderly and patients with alcoholic cirrhosis and diabetes mellitus, have a two-fold or greater rise in type-specific antibodies within 2 to 3 weeks of vaccination. Although the serologic response is generally acceptable, estimates of vaccine efficacy in preventing disease vary widely. Efficacy may be lower in some patients, such as those with alcoholic cirrhosis or Hodgkin's disease. There is good evidence that vaccination is approximately 60% effective against bacteremic pneumococcal disease, which accounts for an estimated 50,000 cases annually. However, evidence regarding efficacy against pneumonia in high-risk populations is not clear. Regardless, the preponderance of information supports the use of pneumococcal vaccine in high-risk populations, including all persons older than 65 years.

Immunity may decrease 5 or more years after initial vaccination; boosters should therefore be considered at that time for adults at highest risk of disease, such as asplenic patients, as well as for those who lose antibody rapidly, such as patients with nephrotic syndrome or renal failure. Persons older than 65 years who received a dose more than 5 years earlier when they were younger than 65 years should be revaccinated.

Local reactions are frequent. Fewer than 1% of vaccinees experience severe local reactions or systemic illness such as fever and malaise. Severe events such as anaphylaxis are rare. Because of the rarity of severe reactions in revaccinated patients, persons with indications for vaccination but with unknown histories of prior vaccination should be vaccinated.

Special efforts should target hospitalized patients. Approximately two thirds of patients later admitted with pneumococcal disease had been hospitalized for other reasons within the preceding 5 years.

Poliomyelitis

The last documented cases of indigenously acquired poliomyelitis (see Chapters 389 and 476) caused by wild polioviruses in the United States were reported in 1979. All indigenous cases since 1981, approximately 8 per year, have been linked epidemiologically and/or via laboratory tests to OPV exposure. Between 1980 and 1994, the overall risk of acquiring vaccine-associated polio was 1 case for every 2.4 million doses distributed. The risk is more than 3000 times higher for immunodeficient persons than normal recipients. Vaccine polioviruses may spread from recipients to contacts, and cases among the latter account for more than one third of the total vaccine-associated cases. A goal has been established to eradicate wild poliovirus from the world by the end of 2000. Between 1988, when the goal was announced, and 1997, cases of polio reported world-wide have decreased by 85% and indigenous wild poliovirus transmission has been eliminated from the Americas since late 1991. Because of the lower risk of wild virus exposure and the continued occurrence of vaccine-associated polio with an all-OPV schedule, all major immunization advisory groups have changed recommendations for routine immunization. A primary series of four doses of IPV, or two doses of IPV followed by two doses of OPV, is an acceptable alternative for vaccinating children. OPV, even for just the first two doses, should be restricted to special situations such as refusal of IPV, imminent international travel, and a child who is behind in immunizations and for whom an all-IPV regimen would be a barrier to catching up.

The Advisory Committee on Immunization Practices prefers the sequential IPV/OPV schedule for public health reasons to take advantage of the individual protection of IPV as well as the gut immunity induced by OPV, which can immunize contacts and enhance community protection; this schedule should reduce vaccine-associated polio by 50 to 75%. With further progress in polio eradication, an all-IPV schedule is envisioned prior to stopping vaccination, probably by 2001.

Adults are at increased risk of paralytic disease from receiving OPV; routine vaccination of adults is therefore not warranted given the small risk of exposure to wild virus in the United States. The major indication for adult vaccination is travel to areas where wild poliovirus is endemic or epidemic. For previously unvaccinated adults, IPV is indicated. Adult travelers who have histories of partial vaccination should complete a primary series of three doses of either IPV or OPV. Adults who formerly received three doses should receive a booster of OPV or IPV. Health care personnel who come in contact with wild viruses should be immune to polio. IPV is the vaccine of choice in such persons to protect both the recipient and any immunocompromised persons with whom the health care worker has contact from exposure to OPV. Parents of children to be vaccinated with OPV may elect to receive IPV before vaccinating their child or alternatively elect to give their children all IPV.

A primary series of both OPV and IPV consists of three doses. A fourth dose is administered to children at school entry. The sequential schedule requires four doses to obtain the full benefits of both vaccines. No serious side effects of IPV have been reported. OPV should never be given to immunocompromised individuals or to a child living in a household with immunocompromised persons.

Hepatitis A

Two inactivated hepatitis A (see Chapter 149) vaccines are available in the United States. Seroconversion rates after a single dose of either vaccine in persons older than 2 years exceed 95%. Antibody levels shown to be protective in animals develop in almost all persons. The most common side effect has been tenderness and soreness at the injection site. Although rare and more serious adverse events have been reported in temporal association with vaccination, a causal relationship has not been established.

The vaccine is indicated primarily for persons traveling to countries, primarily the developing world, with high or intermediate endemicity for hepatitis A. In addition, children living in communities with high rates of endemic hepatitis A (anti–hepatitis A prevalence of 30 to 40% by 5 years of age) should be vaccinated. Health care workers have not been shown to be at higher risk than the general population for hepatitis A and do not need routine immunization. Although food handlers are not at increased risk of hepatitis A when compared with the general population, the consequences of infection or suspected infection in this group, which can lead to extensive public health investigations, may make vaccination cost-effective in some settings. Hepatitis A vaccine should be given to children 2 years of age or older to control outbreaks in communities with high rates of prior infection and be considered for communities with intermediate levels of prior infection (anti-hepatitis A seroprevalence of 10 to 25% by 5 years of age). In 1999, the Advisory Committee on Immunization Practices voted to recommend universal vaccination of children who reside in states or counties with an average annual incidence rate of hepatitis A between 1987 and 1997 of ≥20/100,000 population. Universal vaccination may also be considered for areas with average annual incidence rates between 10 and 20/100,000. Doses vary by age and product. All schedules call for a second dose at least 6 months after the first dose with a permissible range for one of the products as long as 18 months after the initial dose. Vaccines are not indicated for children younger than 2 years because of the absence of adequate data on safety and efficacy.

Lyme Disease

On December 21, 1998, the Food and Drug Administration licensed LYMErix (Smith Kline Beecham Biologicals). The vaccine contains lipidated recombinant outer-surface protein A (OspA) of *Borrelia burgdorferi*, the cause of Lyme disease in the United States. The vaccine works by inducing antibodies against OspA, an antigen expressed on the surface of the spirochete in the tick vector. Expression of OspA is either very limited or absent when spirochetes infect humans. When an infected tick feeds on blood with antibodies to OspA, the blood kills the spirochetes in the tick gut prior to the time transmission can take place. The vaccine was found to be 49% effective after two doses at 0 and 1 month and 76% effective after

three doses at 0, 1, and 12 months in persons 15 to 70 years of age. Efficacy was higher against asymptomatic infection, 83% and 100%, after two or three doses, respectively. Another unlicensed product as of February 1999 containing purified OspA produced by Pasteur, Merrieux, Loynaught reported efficacies of 68% and 92% after two or three doses, respectively, in persons 18 to 92 years of age.

The major side effect of LYMErix is local reactions (24.1% vs. 7.6% in placebo recipients). Myalgias, influenza-like illness, fever, and chills were all significantly higher in vaccinees than placebo recipients, but their attributable risk was 1.4% or less. The vaccine is indicated primarily for persons living or working in endemic tick-infested areas or visitors who will have substantial exposure during transmission season. The duration of immunity and hence the need for boosters is unknown.

Meningococcal Polysaccharide Vaccine

A quadrivalent meningococcal polysaccharide vaccine containing serogroups A, C, Y, and W135 is now available. These groups account for approximately 50% of meningococcal disease in the United States (see Chapter 329). Serogroup A and C vaccines have had 85 to 100% efficacy in epidemic settings, whereas vaccines for the other groups have documented good immunogenicity in adults. The duration of immunity is unknown, although protection in older children and adults probably persists for at least 3 years. Protection in pre-school children may be shorter. Routine vaccination is not recommended in the United States because of the low risk of infection. A single dose is indicated for high-risk persons. Vaccination may also be useful during localized epidemics of serogroups in the vaccine. Meningococcal vaccine may be offered to travelers and persons who will live in areas with hyperendemic or epidemic disease, e.g., the "meningitis belt" of sub-Saharan Africa stretching from Mauritania to Ethiopia.

Revaccination should be considered 2 to 3 years after primary immunization for children younger than 4 years at the initial vaccination. Revaccination 3 to 5 years after the initial dose may also be considered for older adolescents and adults at continued risk. The major side effects are local reactions lasting 1 to 2 days.

Rabies

Rabies (see Chapter 478) vaccine is indicated for pre-exposure prophylaxis of high-risk persons, including animal handlers, selected laboratory and field workers, and persons traveling for more than 1 month to areas where rabies is a constant threat. The pre-exposure regimen consists of either three 1.0-mL intramuscular injections on days 0, 7, and 21 or 28 for all rabies vaccines or, for the human diploid cell vaccine only, three 0.1-mL intradermal injections on days 0, 7, and 21 or 28. Testing for serum antibody or a booster every 2 years is indicated for persons with continuing risk. Post-exposure treatment depends on prior exposure to vaccine (see Chapter 478). Human rabies immune globulin is indicated for previously unvaccinated persons who are exposed.

VACCINES INTENDED PRIMARILY FOR INTERNATIONAL TRAVELERS

Yellow Fever

Yellow fever (see Chapter 391) now occurs only in areas of South America and Africa. Vaccination with a single dose of the live attenuated 17D strain of virus confers protection to almost all recipients for at least 10 years. Boosters are recommended every 10 years for those at risk. Side effects are uncommon. Yellow fever vaccine should not be given to immunocompromised persons or those with anaphylactic allergies to eggs. The vaccine is contraindicated in pregnant women on theoretic grounds, although if such women must travel to a high-risk area, they may be vaccinated.

Typhoid Vaccine

Three types of vaccines, a live attenuated Ty21a oral vaccine, a parenteral heat-phenol–inactivated vaccine, and a capsular polysaccharide vaccine (ViCPS), appear to be of comparable efficacy (50 to 77%). Typhoid (see Chapter 340) vaccine is indicated primarily for travelers to areas where the risk of prolonged exposure to contaminated food and water is high. The vaccine is not optimally effective; food and water precautions are still essential. The vaccine may also be considered for family or other intimate contacts of typhoid carriers and laboratory workers who work with *Salmonella typhi*. For adults and children 6 years and older, any of the vaccines may be used. For Ty21a, one enteric-coated capsule is taken every other day for four doses. Alternatively, a single dose of the ViCPS vaccine or two doses of heat-phenol–inactivated vaccine separated by 4 or more weeks may be given. The duration of protection with Ty21a is not known; repetition of the primary series is recommended every 5 years for persons at risk. Boosters are recommended every 2 years for the ViCPS vaccine and every 3 years for recipients of the heat-phenol–inactivated vaccine if they continue to be at risk. The ViCPS vaccine can be given to children as young as 2 years. The heat-phenol–inactivated vaccine can be used in children 6 months or older.

Adverse reactions are much less common after the Ty21a and the ViCPS vaccines than after the inactivated vaccine. Thus, whenever feasible, the Ty21a and ViCPS vaccines are preferred.

Cholera

Cholera (see Chapter 344) vaccines offer only about 50% protection after completion of a primary series of two doses 1 week to 1 month apart. Peak protection appears about 2 months after the last dose, and protection wanes by 3 to 6 months. Vaccination often results in significant local reactions accompanied by fever. Neurologic reactions are rare. The major indication is to meet requirements imposed by some countries for entry.

Japanese Encephalitis Vaccine

Japanese encephalitis (see Chapter 392) vaccine is primarily indicated for travelers to Asia who will spend a month or longer in endemic areas during the transmission season, especially if travel will include rural areas. In all instances, travelers should be advised to take personal precautions to reduce exposure to mosquito bites. The vaccine appears to be 80 to 91% effective in preventing clinical disease. The primary series consists of three subcutaneous 1-mL doses given on days 0, 7, and 30 (see Table 10–2). A shortened schedule given on days 0, 7, and 14 may be used when necessary. Booster doses may be given after 2 years. Local reactions are common and occur in about 20% of vaccinated persons, and systemic symptoms of fever, headache, chills, nausea, and abdominal pain have been noted in about 10%. A delayed urticaria-angioedema syndrome may occur a median of 12 hours after the first dose of vaccine and up to 2 weeks after the second dose. Vaccinees should be observed for at least 30 minutes after inoculation and, during the subsequent 10 days, should remain in areas with ready access to medical care. The vaccine is contraindicated for pregnant women on theoretic grounds, but if such women travel to an endemic, high-risk area, they may be vaccinated.

OTHER VACCINES

A number of other vaccines used in selected circumstances include smallpox (vaccinia) vaccine, which is used by the military and laboratory workers who handle orthopoxviruses; BCG (bacille Calmette-Guérin) vaccine to prevent tuberculosis, which has very limited use in the United States; anthrax vaccine, which is indicated in selected high-risk populations; and plague vaccine, which may be considered for workers at risk and for some travelers. In addition, trivalent botulism antitoxin is available for the treatment of suspected cases of botulism.

Although not available today, a number of vaccines are under development and may be licensed in the future. For example, extensive field trials have occurred or are planned with pneumococcal and meningococcal conjugate vaccines, acellular pertussis vaccines in adults, and human immunodeficiency virus. Because of the biotechnology revolution, it is likely that many more vaccines will become available in the future.

ACP Task Force on Adult Immunization and Infectious Diseases Society of America: Guide for Adult Immunization, 3rd ed. Philadelphia, American College of Physicians, 1994, pp 1–218. *An excellent comprehensive guide covering all aspects of adult immunization. A must for the physician who cares for adults, whether in primary, secondary, or tertiary care.*

Centers for Disease Control: Update on Adult Immunization. Recommendations of The Advisory Committee on Immunization Practices (ACIP). MMWR 40(RR-12):1, 1991. *A compendium of ACIP statements on immunizations for adults, as well as valuable information on other aspects of immunization. Somewhat dated at this point. More current ACIP statements on individual vaccines are published as available in the* Morbidity and Mortality Weekly Report, *Recommendations and Reports Supplement.*

Centers for Disease Control and Prevention: General recommendations on immunization: Recommendations of The Advisory Committee on Immunization Practices (ACIP). MMWR 43(RR-1):1, 1994. *A comprehensive review of vaccination schedules, precautions, contraindications, and adverse events, as well as information about federal laws on injury compensation and record keeping.*

Centers for Disease Control and Prevention: Health Information for International Travel. Washington, DC, US Government Printing Office, 1996–1997. *A complete guide for the international traveler, including required and recommended vaccinations. Revised every 1 to 2 years.*

Centers for Disease Control and Prevention: Update: Vaccine side effects, adverse reactions, contraindications, and precautions—Recommendations of the Advisory Committee on Immunization Practices (ACIP). MMWR 45(RR-12):1, 1996. *A comprehensive evaluation of the Institute of Medicine reports on adverse events with modifications, where appropriate, in precautions and contraindications.*

Committee on Infectious Diseases, American Academy of Pediatrics: Report of the Committee on Infectious Diseases, 23rd ed. Elk Grove Village, IL, American Academy of Pediatrics, 1997, pp 1–764. *The "Red Book" is published every 2 to 3 years and addresses in a comprehensive manner vaccination of children and adolescents, as well as other issues relating to prevention, control, and treatment of infectious diseases.*

National Immunization Program (NIP), Centers for Disease Control and Prevention. *The NIP has established toll-free numbers for answering questions from both the general public and physicians: 1-800-232-2522 (English), 1-800-232-0233 (Spanish). Inquiries can be made to the NIP by e-mail: nipinfo@cdc.gov or the NIP web site at www.cdc.gov/NIP.*

Plotkin SA, Orenstein WA: Vaccines, 3rd ed. Philadelphia, WB Saunders, 1999, pp 1–1230. *A thorough review of each of the available vaccines, vaccine-preventable diseases, and etiologic agents. Covers such topics as vaccine production, handling, indications, adverse events, and public health impact.*

16 ALCOHOLISM AND ALCOHOL ABUSE

Ivan Diamond ■ *Cheryl A. Jay*

DEFINITIONS

Alcoholism is characterized by addiction to ethanol. In contrast to behavioral and socioeconomic definitions of alcoholism, in a medical setting alcoholism is a chronic disease in which the alcoholic craves and consumes ethanol uncontrollably, becomes *tolerant* to its intoxicating effects with repetitive drinking, and has symptoms and signs of alcohol withdrawal (*physical dependence*) when drinking is stopped. Individuals who drink excessively without evidence of dependence have an *alcohol abuse* disorder. *Binge drinking* refers to bouts of excessive drinking for several days at a time. The distinction between alcoholism and alcohol abuse has practical implications since alcoholics require more intensive medical intervention.

ETIOLOGY

Genetic susceptibility and environmental factors interact to produce alcoholism, often in families. Twin studies show that a monozygotic twin of an alcoholic is more likely to be alcoholic than is a dizygotic twin. Such studies yield broad heritability estimates of 50%, which suggests that about half the variance for the development of alcoholism may be attributed to genetic factors. Even stronger support for genetic vulnerability to alcoholism comes from adoption studies. Children of alcoholic parents who were adopted early in life by non-alcoholic parents are over three times more likely to become alcoholics than are control adoptees. This pattern is particularly evident for "male-limited" alcoholism in fathers and sons with antisocial, impulsive, novelty-seeking behavior, who often begin drinking as children or early adolescents. Adoption studies suggest that this type of alcoholism in the biologic father is a much greater predictor for alcoholism in the son than is the environment in which the boy is raised.

PREVALENCE

A recent U.S. survey found the 12-month prevalence of alcohol abuse and alcoholism to be 2.5% and 7.2%, respectively; the lifetime prevalence was 9.4% and 14.1%. At least twice as many men are alcoholic as women. Coexisting psychiatric abnormalities include antisocial personality disorder, schizophrenia, depression, anxiety disorders, and drug abuse. Alcoholism and alcohol abuse affect 20% or more of ambulatory and hospitalized patients. Physicians should be aware that steady employment and social stability do not exclude the diagnosis. Alcoholism develops in individuals of all races and socioeconomic classes; only 5% of alcoholics fit the "skid row" stereotype.

EPIDEMIOLOGY

Nearly two thirds of Americans older than 14 years drink alcoholic beverages. Their per capita consumption is the equivalent of 9.7 gallons of whiskey, 89 gallons of beer, or 31 gallons of wine per year. Heavy drinkers account for half of the alcohol consumed and nearly all of the socioeconomic and medical complications of alcoholism and alcohol abuse. The annual cost of these problems to American society is about $100 billion, a figure that includes costs to treat alcoholism and related medical complications and lost productivity. Excessive alcohol consumption ranks as the third leading preventable cause of death, behind cigarette smoking and obesity, and accounts for 5% of the total U.S. mortality, or about 100,000 deaths annually.

PATHOGENESIS

ETHANOL ABSORPTION, DISTRIBUTION, AND ELIMINATION. Ethanol is absorbed completely from the gastrointestinal tract and is detected in the blood within minutes of ingestion. About 25% enters the bloodstream from the stomach and 75% from the intestine, but gastrointestinal absorption is also affected by food; the rate of drinking; the concentration, amount, and type of alcoholic beverage; variations in gastrointestinal motility; and gender. Most foods in the stomach delay gastric absorption, and high concentrations of alcohol in the stomach can cause pylorospasm, which slows gastric emptying and retards intestinal absorption. Rapid gastric emptying or gastrectomy increases rates of alcohol absorption from the small intestine. Alcohol vapor can also be absorbed through the lungs. Women have lower gastric alcohol dehydrogenase activity and hence have higher blood alcohol concentrations than men do after consuming similar amounts of ethanol per kilogram of body weight.

Ethanol readily crosses biologic membranes, particularly in the brain, and equilibrates rapidly into total body water. Ninety to 98% is removed in the liver, and the remainder is excreted by the kidneys, lungs, and skin. Elimination proceeds at a constant rate, independent of the blood alcohol concentration (zero-order kinetics); a 70-kg man can metabolize 5 to 10 g ethanol per hour. Since the average drink contains 12 to 15 g ethanol, blood alcohol levels continue to rise when an individual drinks at a rate greater than metabolism; however, when drinking is discontinued, blood levels fall by about 10 to 25 mg/dL/hour.

ETHANOL METABOLISM. Ethanol oxidation to acetaldehyde by alcohol dehydrogenase in the liver is the rate-limiting step and accounts for more than 90% of ethanol metabolism in vivo. Alcohol dehydrogenase has a high affinity for ethanol and accounts for essentially all ethanol oxidation at low to moderate doses. When the blood alcohol concentration is high, however, a microsomal ethanol-oxidizing system with a lower affinity for ethanol can also generate acetaldehyde (Fig. 16–1). This oxidizing system can be induced by ethanol to accelerate drug metabolism in the liver (see Chapter 148). Barbiturates have a similar effect, which accounts for the metabolic cross-tolerance between these agents.

Acetaldehyde is converted to acetate by aldehyde dehydrogenase, a metabolic event with important clinical ramifications. For example, in 50% of Japanese and other Asian people, a genetic variation in an aldehyde dehydrogenase isoenzyme results in reduced enzyme activity in vivo. Shortly after drinking alcohol, affected individuals have increased blood acetaldehyde levels and experience an alcohol-flush reaction characterized by vasodilatation with facial flushing, hot sensations, tachycardia, and hypotension. These unpleasant experiences appear to deter drinking; Japanese and Chinese people with this isoenzyme have a lower rate of alcoholism. Pharmacologic inhibition of aldehyde dehydrogenase can cause severe aversive symptoms after drinking alcohol and is the reason why disulfiram (Antabuse) has been used to discourage drinking. Disulfiram inhibits aldehyde dehydrogenase (and other sulfhydryl-containing enzymes), but it is not ordinarily toxic when taken therapeutically without ethanol. After drinking alcohol, however, patients on prophylactic disulfiram therapy have significant increases in blood acetaldehyde levels, and a more severe *acetaldehyde syndrome* develops. They can experience dysphoria, intense palpitations, sweating, thirst, throbbing headache, dyspnea, nausea and vomiting, weakness, vertigo, and syncope. Moreover, other drugs that likewise inhibit aldehyde dehydrogenase, such as metronidazole (Flagyl), may also make patients ill if they drink ethanol. Disulfiram does not cure alcoholism and is not widely used.

In peripheral tissues, acetate derived from acetaldehyde is converted to acetyl coenzyme A and subsequently to CO_2 and water. Complete oxidation of ethanol yields 7.1 kcal/g, and ethanol may account for 5 to 10% of the total caloric intake in the United States. Alcoholics often obtain 50% of their calories from ethanol, and serious nutritional deficiencies, particularly protein, thiamine, folate, and pyridoxine deficiency, develop in many (Table 16–1) (see Chapter 231). Moreover, as a consequence of ethanol metabolism, alcoholics are prone to hypoglycemia (Chapter 243), lactic acidosis (Chapter 102), hyperuricemia (Chapter 299), and hypertriglyceridemia (Chapter 206). Binge drinking, inadequate diet, and severe vomiting on a background of chronic alcohol consumption can lead to alcoholic ketoacidosis (see Chapter 102).

CLINICAL MANIFESTATIONS

ALCOHOL INTOXICATION. The blood-brain barrier to ethanol is virtually non-existent, and shortly after drinking, the concentra-

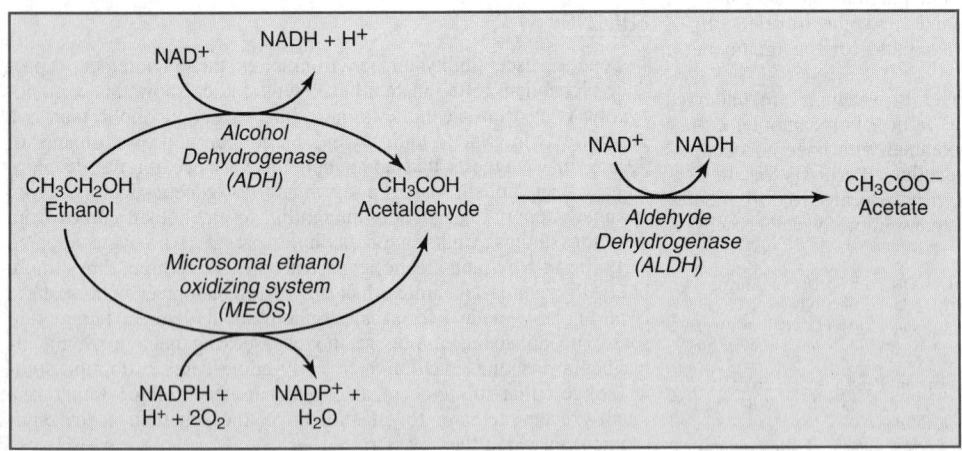

FIGURE 16–1 ■ Ethanol metabolism. Alcohol dehydrogenase (ADH) predominates at low to moderate ethanol doses. The microsomal ethanol-oxidizing system (MEOS) is induced at high ethanol levels or chronic exposure and by certain drugs. Aldehyde dehydrogenase (ALDH) inhibition (genetic or drug induced) leads to acetaldehyde accumulation.

Table 16–1 ■ ALCOHOL-RELATED MEDICAL DISORDERS

AFFECTED ORGAN OR SYSTEM	DISORDERS

Nutrition	Deficiencies of
	  Vitamins: Folate, thiamine, pyridoxine, niacin, riboflavin
	  Minerals: Magnesium, zinc, calcium
	  Protein

Metabolites and electrolytes	Hypoglycemia, ketoacidosis, hyperlipidemia, hyperuricemia, hypomagnesemia, hypophosphatemia
GI tract	Liver: Fatty liver, hepatitis, cirrhosis Gut: Esophagitis, gastritis Pancreatitis
Nervous system	Brain: Hepatic encephalopathy, Wernicke-Korsakoff syndrome, cerebellar degeneration, central pontine myelinolysis, Marchiafava-Bignami disease, dementia Neuromuscular: Neuropathy, myopathy Amblyopia
Cardiovascular	Heart: Arrhythmia, cardiomyopathy Hypertension
Bone marrow	Macrocytosis, anemia, thrombocytopenia, leukopenia
Endocrine	Pseudo–Cushing's syndrome, testicular atrophy, amenorrhea
Other	Traumatic injury Aerodigestive neoplasms Osteopenia Fetal alcohol syndrome

tion of alcohol in the brain is nearly the same as in the blood. In a non-alcoholic, intoxication occurs at blood alcohol levels of 50 to 150 mg/dL (Table 16–2), and legal intoxication ranges from 80 to 100 mg/dL in most states. After two to three average drinks (12 oz beer, 5 oz wine, or 1.5 oz 80-proof spirits), the blood alcohol concentration approaches the legal limit, depending on body weight and gender; women may achieve higher blood alcohol concentrations with fewer drinks. A general "rule of thumb" is that ethanol metabolism removes one drink per hour. Symptoms vary directly with the rate of drinking and are more severe when blood alcohol concentrations are rising than falling. Most individuals feel euphoric, lose social inhibitions, and manifest expansive, sometimes garrulous behavior; others may become gloomy, belligerent, or even explosively combative. Some people do not experience euphoria but become sleepy after moderate drinking; they rarely abuse alcohol. Neurologic signs of intoxication include impaired cognition, slurred speech, incoordination, mild truncal ataxia, and slow or irregular eye movements. Signs of increased sympathetic activity include mydriasis, tachycardia, and skin flushing. Cerebellar and vestibular function deteriorates at higher blood alcohol levels, and drunkenness is characterized by dysarthria, more severe ataxia, nystagmus, and diplopia. Patients may become lethargic with bradycardia, reduced blood pressure, and diminished respirations, sometimes complicated by vomiting and pulmonary aspiration. In non-tolerant individuals, stupor and coma may supervene at 400 mg/dL, and fatalities occur above this level, usually because of respiratory

depression with respiratory acidosis and hypotension. The median lethal dose for ethanol is approximately 450 mg/dL. Other central nervous system depressants such as narcotics and sedative-hypnotics act synergistically with alcohol.

Alcoholic blackouts sometimes complicate acute alcohol intoxication during the consumption of large amounts of ethanol. These episodes, which can occur in alcoholics or sporadic drinkers, are characterized by amnesia for several hours without impaired consciousness. The patient reports an inability to remember new events but has no difficulty with long-term memory or immediate recall. These symptoms resemble the syndrome of transient global amnesia (see Chapters 449 and 470). Ethanol can depress myocardial function at moderate doses, and binge drinking can cause arrhythmias, or the *holiday heart syndrome* (see Chapter 64). Relaxation of vascular smooth muscle causes vasodilation, which can lead to hypothermia, particularly in cold environments.

TOLERANCE TO ALCOHOL. A reduced response to ethanol, or tolerance, develops both acutely and chronically during drinking and is due to adaptive changes in the central nervous system, not ethanol metabolism. *Acute tolerance* occurs during a single episode of drinking and is characterized by greater intoxication at a given blood alcohol concentration when the level is rising than when falling (Mellanby effect). *Chronic tolerance* occurs in alcoholics and is characterized by greater resistance to the intoxicating effects of ethanol; they may appear to be sober at levels of 400 to 500 mg/dL, concentrations known to produce stupor, coma, or death in naive individuals. The highest blood alcohol level reported is 1510 mg/dL in an ambulatory chronic alcoholic who had stopped drinking 3 days earlier. Tolerance appears to be due to ethanol-induced changes in gene expression and intracellular signaling cascades involving neurotransmitter receptors, ion channels, and protein kinases.

NATURAL HISTORY OF ALCOHOLISM. Most people who consume alcohol begin drinking in adolescence or early adulthood. Up to half of male drinkers have alcohol-related problems such as blackouts, fighting, or a single alcohol-related arrest during their late teens or early twenties. Most learn to moderate their alcohol consumption by their late twenties. Those who continue to accumulate alcohol-related problems often become alcoholic. Craving and uncontrolled drinking accompanied by tolerance and symptoms of withdrawal signal the development of alcoholism. Episodes of abstention and failed efforts to control drinking are common and highlight the relapsing and remitting course of the disease. Some alcoholics achieve long-term sobriety on their own; those who do not face increased mortality from trauma and medical complications.

ALCOHOL WITHDRAWAL SYNDROME. Ethanol is a central nervous system depressant. In alcoholics, the nervous system appears to adapt to chronic exposure to ethanol by increasing the activity of neural mechanisms that counteract alcohol's depressant effects. When drinking is abruptly reduced or discontinued, these adaptive neural mechanisms are left unrestrained by ethanol, and physical dependence is manifested by a hyperexcitable *alcohol withdrawal syndrome*. The alcohol withdrawal syndrome typically evolves in a recognizable temporal sequence (Fig. 16–2) and consists of tremulousness, disordered perceptions, seizures, and delirium tremens of varying severity.

TREMULOUSNESS. Tremor, the earliest, most common, and most apparent symptom, begins about 6 to 8 hours after the last drink, usually the morning after an overnight abstinence ("morning shakes"). Tremor is generalized, coarse, and rapid and often accompanied by irritability, nausea, and vomiting. The patient usually senses an inner tremulousness even when the tremor is not severe. Self-treatment is usually a morning drink to "quiet the nerves," followed by drinking for the rest of the day. If the alcoholic does not resume drinking, tremor intensifies by 24 to 36 hours and is exacerbated by motor activity or stress. The tremor can be so severe that it interferes with walking, eating, or speech. Accompanying symptoms and signs of sympathetic hyperactivity are also apparent. The patient is increasingly anxious and easily startled by minor stimuli and complains of insomnia and anorexia. Increased sweating, facial flushing, mydriasis, tachycardia, and mild hypertension are noted. Most abnormalities subside in a few days, but increased arousal and anxiety may persist for 2 weeks.

Table 16–2 ■ BLOOD ETHANOL LEVELS AND SYMPTOMS

BLOOD ETHANOL LEVELS (mg/dL)	SYMPTOMS	
	Sporadic Drinkers	Chronic Drinkers
50–100	Euphoria, gregariousness, incoordination	Minimal or no effect
100–200	Slurred speech, ataxia, labile mood, drowsiness, nausea	Sobriety or incoordination Euphoria
200–300	Lethargy, combativeness Stupor, incoherent speech Vomiting	Mild emotional and motor changes
300–400	Coma	Drowsiness
>500	Respiratory depression, death	Lethargy, stupor, coma

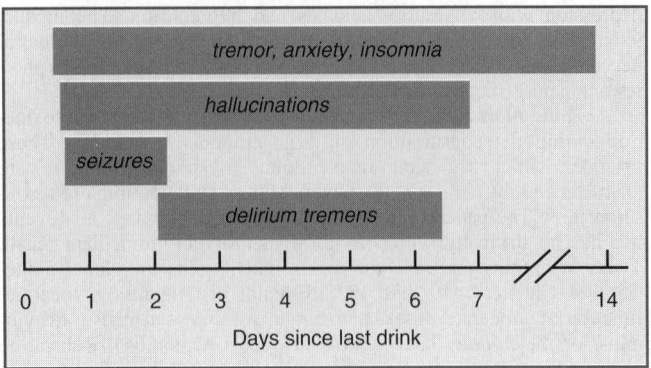

FIGURE 16–2 ■ Time course of alcohol withdrawal.

DISORDERED PERCEPTIONS. Disordered perceptions accompany tremor and sympathetic hyperactivity in approximately 25% of patients, become most pronounced at 24 to 36 hours, and clear in a few days. Often, vivid nightmares interfere with sleep; while awake, ordinary visual, auditory, and tactile experiences become distorted and misinterpreted. Isolated and prolonged auditory hallucinations may develop in alcoholics undergoing withdrawal (*alcoholic hallucinosis*) despite being alert, oriented, and without memory loss. Hallucinations may persist for weeks even though other signs of ethanol withdrawal have improved and the patient is less agitated and tremulous. In the absence of sympathetic hyperactivity, persistent auditory hallucinations may be confused with acute schizophrenia (see Chapter 450). However, alcoholic hallucinosis is closely associated with ethanol withdrawal and usually subsides in weeks to months.

ALCOHOL WITHDRAWAL CONVULSIONS. Generalized tonic-clonic seizures develop in about one third of alcoholics, most often within 12 to 24 hours after reducing or stopping drinking. Some propose that the first seizure in alcoholics may be a consequence of ethanol toxicity. However, ethanol dependence is followed by withdrawal seizures in animals, particularly in mice bred to have convulsions during withdrawal, thus suggesting a role for genetic vulnerability in humans. Ethanol withdrawal seizures usually follow chronic daily drinking but can also occur after 5 to 7 days of binge drinking. Alcoholics who have seizures during one episode of withdrawal are likely to have them again when alcohol withdrawal is repeated. One isolated convulsion or several seizures may occur, usually within a 6-hour period. Focal seizures are less common and indicate a cerebral lesion, either old or new. Status epilepticus occurs in about 3% of cases, and ethanol withdrawal accounts for about 15% of all patients evaluated for status epilepticus. Status epilepticus is a medical emergency and requires immediate treatment with anticonvulsants (see Chapter 484).

DELIRIUM TREMENS. Delirium tremens, the most alarming manifestation of the ethanol withdrawal syndrome, occurs in about 5% of alcoholics. It consists of agitated arousal, global confusion and disorientation, insomnia, and vivid, often threatening hallucinations and delusions. Signs of sympathetic hyperactivity include tremor, mydriasis, tachycardia, fever, and intense diaphoresis. In contrast to tremulousness, disordered perceptions, and seizures, which appear earlier after withdrawal, delirium tremens begins abruptly within 2 to 4 days of abstinence, sometimes as a surprising development in an unrecognized alcoholic admitted to the hospital for other reasons. Patients are terrified by their hallucinations and can be combative, destructive, and very dangerous. Episodes of delirium tremens last from 1 to 3 days and end as abruptly as they begin. However, relapses occur, and the disorder may continue for days to weeks with intervening periods of lucidity. When signs of sympathetic hyperactivity are absent, it may be difficult to distinguish delirium tremens from an acute psychosis. However, the diagnosis is usually suggested by the evolution of symptoms in a chronic alcoholic undergoing withdrawal. The differential diagnosis includes alcoholic hypoglycemia, overdose with anticholinergic agents, intoxication with amphetamines, cocaine, and phencyclidine, and withdrawal from other sedating drugs. Metabolic disturbances,

cerebral infection, encephalitis, meningitis, sepsis, or thyrotoxicosis should also be considered.

DIAGNOSIS

Alcohol-related problems are common in medical practice, and physicians should be alert to their diverse clinical manifestations. End-organ complications such as ulcers, hepatitis, cirrhosis, pancreatitis, cardiomyopathy, or peripheral neuropathy should prompt consideration of alcoholism as an underlying cause. Recurrent trauma, particularly skeletal fractures, sleep disorders, fatigue, depression, sexual dysfunction, and labile hypertension, should also arouse suspicion of alcoholism. Hospitalization may precipitate the unexpected appearance of an alcohol withdrawal syndrome within several days of admission.

Physicians should identify individuals who do not meet the criteria for alcohol dependence but who drink alcohol at levels that pose potential health risks. Laboratory-based screening such as elevated mean corpuscular volume (MCV) or γ-glutamyl transpeptidase (GGTP) may help the physician in confronting patient denial, but elevated MCV or GGTP values are neither specific for alcoholism nor sufficiently sensitive to serve as effective screens. Simple screening questionnaires such as the CAGE (Fig. 16–3) outperform laboratory measures in detecting excessive alcohol consumption in a variety of clinical settings. Because advice and discussion by a concerned physician are simple, cost-effective ways to reduce heavy drinking, routine screening for alcohol disorders is recommended, particularly in primary care.

Complex ethanol-drug interactions must also be considered when prescribing medications to patients who use alcohol. Ethanol potentiates the central nervous system depressant effects of narcotic, sedative, and psychoactive drugs (see Chapter 26), and patients for whom these agents are prescribed should be counseled explicitly about this interaction. In contrast, the induction of microsomal enzymes in the liver by ethanol accelerates the elimination of drugs metabolized by these enzymes (see Chapter 26). As a result, ethanol can decrease drug efficacy by lowering the amount of active drug available or increase toxicity and promote unusual side effects caused by drug metabolites.

TREATMENT

ACUTE ALCOHOL INTOXICATION. Mild to moderate ethanol intoxication requires no specific therapy. Severe acute alcohol intoxication, defined by a depressed level of consciousness, can be fatal and is a medical emergency. Administration of sedatives to intoxicated patients who are agitated and combative can lead to stupor, coma, and respiratory arrest from synergistic depressant effects and should be avoided. The immediate history should include information about the quantity of alcohol consumed, the rate of drinking, use of other drugs including methanol and ethylene glycol, complicating medical and psychiatric disorders, and prior alcohol abuse or alcoholism. If the patient is stuporous and unable to walk, the airway must be evaluated immediately. Indications for endotracheal intubation and assisted ventilation include marked hypoventilation, accumulating secretions, or coma. Complications such as hypoglycemia, meningitis, subdural hematoma, and hepatic encephalopathy must be considered. Evidence of head trauma or focal cerebral signs suggests urgent intracranial pathology, and a computed tomography scan should be performed immediately. Otherwise, routine scans for alcohol intoxication are not indicated. Gastric lavage may be performed if the obtundation is due to recent and massive alcohol consumption, but it must be preceded by endotracheal intubation. Hemodialysis should be considered if the blood alcohol concentration exceeds 500 mg/dL or when methanol or ethylene glycol has been ingested concurrently.

After a history and physical examination, patients with adequate vital signs and acceptable mental status but without evidence of other disorders can be kept calm under observation until sobriety returns. However, medical information is usually incomplete, and it is often necessary to anticipate complications commonly associated with severe alcohol intoxication or alcoholism. Routine blood counts and laboratory studies may uncover anemia (see Chapter 159), hypokalemia, hypophosphatemia, and hypomagnesemia.

STEP I: ASK about alcohol use

Consumption
per week
per occasion

CAGE questions (1 point for each yes answer):
Have you ever felt that you should **C**ut down on your drinking?
Have people **A**nnoyed you by criticizing your drinking?
Have you ever felt bad or **G**uilty about your drinking?
Have you ever had a drink first thing in the morning to steady your nerves or to get rid of a hangover (**E**ye opener)?

Men: >14 drinks/week or >4 per occasion
Women: >7 drinks/week or >3 per occasion
or
CAGE score ≥1

STEP II: ASSESS for alcohol-related problems

At risk:
Drinking above recommended levels or in high-risk situations
Personal or family history of alcohol-related problems
Current alcohol-related problems:
CAGE score 1–2 (in past year)
Evidence of alcohol-related medical or behavioral problems

May be alcohol-dependent:
CAGE score ≥3 or ≥1 of the following:
preoccupied with drinking
unable to stop once started
drinking to avoid withdrawal symptoms
tolerance

STEP III: ADVISE appropriate action

State medical concerns about drinking
Agree on plan of action:

At risk or current problems:
Advise to cut down
Set specific drinking goal

Alcohol dependent:
Advise to abstain
Refer to specialist

STEP IV: MONITOR patient progress

All patients:
Consider scheduling separate follow-up visit or phone call
Review progress and reinforce efforts at each follow-up visit

Patients referred for alcohol treatment:
Review updates from treatment specialist
Monitor for depression and anxiety

FIGURE 16–3 ■ Screening and brief intervention for alcohol problems in clinical practice.

Alcoholic hypoglycemia (see Chapter 243) can be evaluated rapidly by a bedside blood glucose determination. If laboratory results are delayed, 12.5 to 25 g glucose should be given intravenously but must be preceded by or accompanied by 100 mg intravenous thiamine to avoid precipitating Wernicke's encephalopathy (see Chapter 489). Alcoholic ketoacidosis (see Chapter 102) will be improved by infusion of 5% dextrose in half-normal saline, also with thiamine. If the blood alcohol level is too low to account for obtundation or if improvement does not occur as expected, it is necessary to search for other causes of stupor and coma (see Chapter 444), including other sedating agents.

ALCOHOL WITHDRAWAL SYNDROME. Alcoholics stop drinking for many reasons, including serious alcohol-related medical, surgical, or psychiatric conditions. Hence symptoms or signs of trauma, infection, liver disease, gastritis, pancreatitis, arrhythmia, or electrolyte disturbance should be sought. One hundred milligrams of thiamine should be given intravenously to all patients undergoing ethanol withdrawal to prevent or treat Wernicke's encephalopathy (see Chapter 489) and should be followed by daily multivitamins.

The alarming symptoms of ethanol withdrawal are best managed by substituting another central nervous system depressant. However, alcoholics undergoing withdrawal are very resistant to sedatives (cross-tolerance), so large doses are often required to calm their agitation. Benzodiazepines are widely used to manage tremulousness and disordered perceptions during ethanol withdrawal. The goal is to suppress symptoms and produce mild sedation, and the drug dosage is adjusted to the severity of the withdrawal reaction. Treatment includes managing delirium and autonomic stability and preventing seizures. A sedative-hypnotic agent, typically a benzodiazepine, is prescribed as a substitute for alcohol, and the dose is tapered over several days. Patients with mild tremulousness and few associated symptoms usually respond to oral diazepam, 5 to 10 mg every 4 to 6 hours. The dosage is then reduced by 20 to 25% on successive days or increased if symptoms of ethanol withdrawal return. β-Blockers are useful ancillary therapy; they attenuate the symptoms of autonomic hypersensitivity but are not anticonvulsants and do not appear to reduce delirium. Detoxification can be carried out with close monitoring in an outpatient setting in socially stable patients with mild withdrawal. If withdrawal is more severe or accompanied by significant medical, surgical, or psychiatric illness or the patient is in an unstable social setting, inpatient detoxification may be needed. In such instances, benzodiazepines such as diazepam (Valium), chlordiazepoxide (Librium), oxazepam (Serax), or lorazepam (Ativan) are administered orally or parenterally in doses sufficient to keep the patient calm. Benzodiazepines should not be given intramuscularly because of inconsistent absorption. Patients may require hourly medication at doses that would be fatal in non-tolerant individuals. The first several days of severe alcohol withdrawal may require intravenous administration of total daily diazepam doses exceeding 400 mg (or the equivalent of other benzodiazepines) to achieve mild sedation. Multivitamin and thiamine supplementation should be continued, as should meticulous attention to electrolyte status. The benzodiazepine dosage can then be tapered by approximately 20 to 25% on successive days, with an increase in dosage if withdrawal symptoms recur. Once the symptoms of ethanol withdrawal are suppressed, it is necessary to avoid oversedation and the danger of respiratory depression by carefully titrating the dose of diazepam to just keep the patient calm.

Alcohol withdrawal seizures can often be managed with intravenous benzodiazepines such as diazepam or lorazepam. Phenytoin does not prevent seizures during withdrawal. Management of status epilepticus is the same as in other situations (see Chapter 484). Alcoholics are at increased risk for head trauma and central nervous system infection; studies to exclude these more serious diagnostic possibilities should be performed when seizures occurring in the setting of withdrawal display focal features or are accompanied by a prolonged post-ictal state or when status epilepticus intervenes. Long-term anticonvulsant therapy is not indicated for typical alcohol withdrawal seizures.

Delirium tremens requires hospitalization and vigorous management in an intensive care setting. Mortality has reached 15% in the past, primarily because of injuries or associated medical disorders complicated by hyperthermia and dehydration. Volume depletion accompanying delirium tremens may cause circulatory collapse, and fluid losses can require replacement of 4 to 10 L in the first day. The goal of treatment is to control behavior and suppress symptoms without danger to the patient. Five to 10 mg or more of diazepam is given intravenously every 5 to 15 minutes until the patient is calm, and maintenance therapy is continued every 1 to 4 hours, as needed. Initially, as much as 200 mg of diazepam may be required before the agitation subsides. Seizures are unusual in patients with delirium tremens and should be evaluated promptly because of the possibility of meningitis or other disorders. Coexisting hepatic and cardiac disease may complicate fluid management, and the possibility that sedative agents may precipitate hepatic encephalopathy should be kept in mind.

ALCOHOLISM AND ALCOHOL ABUSE. Alcoholics and alcohol abusers come to medical attention because of alcohol-related medical or psychiatric conditions, by referral from social service or criminal justice agencies, or through screening in clinical practice. Family members provide valuable collateral history. Physicians should confront alcoholics in a firm but non-judgmental fashion, educate them about health risks, and assess their motivation to stop drinking (see Fig. 16–3). Heavy drinkers should be counseled to reduce consumption. It is valuable to establish a contract with the patient to decrease drinking and return for follow-up assessments. Alcoholics should be referred to a rehabilitation program but may first require inpatient detoxification. Diverse psychosocial interventions have been tested; all are equally effective, and a successful outcome is related more to interested personal intervention than to psychotherapy matched to the patient's condition. Medication may be a useful adjunct in some instances. Disulfiram can be helpful in highly selected patients. The opiate antagonist naltrexone (ReVia), the only other agent currently approved by the Food and Drug Administration (FDA) for the treatment of alcoholism, appears to decrease the relapse rate in abstinent alcoholics. Acamprosate, a drug not yet approved by the FDA, has also shown promising results in clinical trials.

Intervention is more effective earlier in the course of the illness, before the onset of associated medical disorders. Alcoholics who continue to drink shorten their lifespans by at least 15 years. Many alcohol-related medical complications such as ulcer disease, acute pancreatitis, hepatitis, myopathy, and neuropathy stabilize or regress with continued abstinence. Others such as cirrhosis with portal hypertension, Wernicke-Korsakoff syndrome, or dilated cardiomyopathy frequently cause permanent disability or death. About half of socially stable, middle-class alcoholics remain sober for at least a year after rehabilitation. Alcoholics Anonymous and Al-Anon provide low-cost support for alcoholics and their families in virtually all communities in the United States.

Litten RZ, Allen JP: Medications for alcohol, illicit drug, and tobacco dependence: An update of research findings. J Subst Abuse Treat 16:105, 1999. *New approaches to alcohol dependence.*

O'Connor PG, Schottenfeld RS: Patients with alcohol problems. N Engl J Med 338: 592–602, 1998. *A useful review of the diagnosis and treatment of alcohol-related problems.*

Saitz R, O'Malley SS: Pharmacotherapies for alcohol abuse: Withdrawal and treatment. Med Clin North Am 81:881, 1997. *A helpful review of the pathophysiology, treatment goals, and medication options for alcohol withdrawal and dependence.*

Schorling JB, Buchsbaum DG: Screening for alcohol and drug abuse. Med Clin North Am 81:845, 1997. *An excellent summary of the rationale for alcohol screening in primary care, use of screening questionnaires such as the CAGE, and practical guidelines for brief physician intervention.*

US Department of Health and Human Services: Ninth Special Report to the US Congress on Alcohol and Health. Rockville, MD, National Institute on Alcohol Abuse and Alcoholism, 1996. *A comprehensive discussion of the major biomedical and socioeconomic problems of alcoholism and alcohol abuse.*

17 DRUG ABUSE AND DEPENDENCE

Jeffrey H. Samet

Drug abuse as a health problem has grown in prominence as a consequence of several developments: Over a million drug arrests occur in the United States each year, injection drug use has become a major transmission risk for human immunodeficiency virus (HIV) infection, and costs are enormous, $177 billion in the United States in 1991. Medical complications of drug abuse are predominantly infectious but span organ systems and range from cocaine-related cardiac arrhythmia to the neuropsychiatric effects of hallucinogens.

DEFINITIONS. The terms drug (or substance) "dependence" and drug "abuse" have specific clinical meanings (Table 17–1). Dependence is the more severe disorder and is frequently associated with physiologic in addition to psychological manifestations. *Tolerance* and *withdrawal* are the major physiologic manifestations of drug dependence. Tolerance is defined as either a need for increased

Table 17–1 ■ DIAGNOSTIC CRITERIA FOR DEPENDENCE AND DRUG ABUSE

DEPENDENCE (≥3 NEEDED)	ABUSE (≥1 FOR 12 MO)
1. Tolerance	1. Recurrent substance use resulting in failure to fulfill major role obligations at work, school, or home
2. Withdrawal	2. Recurrent substance use in situations in which it is physically hazardous
3. The substance is often taken in larger amounts over a longer period than intended	3. Recurrent substance-related legal problems
4. Any unsuccessful effort or a persistent desire to cut down or control substance use	4. Continued substance use despite having persistent or recurrent social or interpersonal problems caused or exacerbated by the effects of the substance
5. A great deal of time is spent in activities necessary to obtain the substance or recover from its effects	Never met criteria for dependence
6. Important social, occupational, or recreational activities given up or reduced because of substance use	
7. Continued substance use despite knowledge of having had persistent or recurrent physical or psychological problems that are likely to be caused or exacerbated by the substance.	

amounts of the substance to achieve intoxication or the desired effect or a diminished effect with continued use of the same amount of the substance. Withdrawal is manifested by a characteristic syndrome with sudden abstinence, but it may be relieved or avoided if the same or a closely related substance is taken. The other criteria for dependence relate to the pattern of drug use (i.e., taken in a larger amount or longer period than intended); effects on life activities (i.e., great deal of time spent on activities to obtain, use, or recover from the substance; reduction in social, occupational, or recreational activities as a result of substance use); and the psychological need to use the substance (i.e., use despite awareness of adverse consequences, persistent desire for the substance, or inability to control its use).

A diagnosis of substance abuse requires the recurrent use of a substance over a 12-month period with subsequent adverse consequences (e.g., failure to fulfill a major role at work, school, or home; legal problems; persistent interpersonal problems) or placement of an individual in high-risk, physically hazardous situations. Addiction is a chronic, relapsing illness characterized by compulsive drug seeking and use.

The degree of harm associated with occasional drug use or "experimentation" is difficult to quantify, and no definition has been formally assigned to the use of illicit drugs with consequences less than those associated with the abuse definition. However, fear of progression to abuse or dependence, the potential morbidity of any use of drugs such as cocaine, the criminality associated with drug use, and the high-risk behavior while under the influence of a drug are the basis of recommendations to proscribe use of these substances.

ETIOLOGY. A minority of people who ever experiment with an illicit drug progress to a clinical drug abuse diagnosis. The cofactors responsible for progression to dependence and abuse are only partially defined. Genetic susceptibility, social context of the drug use, and co-morbid psychiatric conditions are each considered important factors affecting an individual's potential for subsequent problems. Twin studies suggest that genetics plays a role in a person's positive or negative perception of a drug's effect. The social context in which drug abuse develops and is expressed is very important. For example, returning Vietnam War veterans addicted to heroin were relatively easy to treat in comparison to addicts on the streets of the United States, in part because the veterans had become addicted in a setting different from the one they found on return home and were exposed to few enduring environmental cues. Psychiatric co-morbidity, particularly depression and panic disorders, appears to be a high-risk condition for the development of drug abuse, as well as possible consequences of this abuse.

Use of appropriate narcotic analgesic medication to care for acute painful conditions is not an etiology of drug abuse. Similarly, narcotic medication for cancer patients with chronic pain does not lead to opioid abuse. Unfortunately, inappropriate fear of drug abuse is one reason for the undertreatment of pain with opioid medications.

DRUG OF ABUSE: HEROIN AND OTHER OPIOIDS

CLASSIFICATION. Opioids, including naturally occurring alkaloids (opiates derived from the poppy plant *Papaver somniferum*), semisynthetic compounds (chemically altered alkaloids), and synthetic agents, are potent analgesics and produce an intense euphoria associated with nausea, drowsiness, miosis, and a decrease in respiration, pulse, and blood pressure. Opioids are also valued for their calming, antitussive, and antidiarrheal effects. Depending on their effect on opioid cell membrane receptors, they may be classified as agonists (morphine, heroin, methadone), partial agonists-antagonists (buprenorphine), or antagonists (naloxone, naltrexone). These drugs have led to a vast array of medical complications because of both their abuse potential and their parenteral route of administration.

HISTORY. Opioids were commonly used in many settings in 19th century America. The drug was supplied freely by physicians to treat symptoms of pain, anxiety, cough, and diarrhea. Opiates were also available without restriction in commercial medicinal remedies.

In 1806, a pure substance was isolated from opium and named "morphine" after the Greek god of dreams "Morpheus." By the middle of the century, the advent of the hypodermic needle allowed this inexpensive, standard-strength agent to become a highly effective pain-killing and calming therapy. Smoking opium, which has no medicinal value, also rose in the latter half of the century. In 1898, heroin was commercially introduced by the Bayer Company as an antitussive and was used as therapy for morphine addiction. The increasing recognition of the perils of opiate addiction, its identification with foreign groups and internal minorities, and concern over the estimated prevalence of 250,000 opiate users in 1900 led to a series of state and federal measures culminating in the Harrison Narcotic Act in 1914, which legislated controls over the importation and distribution of opiates.

Opiate use remained a problem in the early 20th century despite both interdiction efforts and the development and dismantling of narcotic clinics that maintained narcotic addicts with prescription drugs. In the 1920s, narcotic abuse became a predominantly underground activity. Efforts to treat narcotic addiction as a medical problem were limited until the advent of methadone maintenance therapy in the 1960s. Heroin use increased during the Vietnam War, when almost half of the enlisted men experimented with opioids. Heroin use decreased in the 1980s but has been on the rise since the 1990s.

EPIDEMIOLOGY. In the United States, an estimated 2.5 million people have reported prior use of heroin, and more than 100,000 addicts are enrolled in over 700 methadone maintenance programs. These programs are generally located in large cities, with the highest concentration in the northeastern United States.

In 1995, an estimated 141,000 individuals became new heroin users, an upward trend over the previous 5 years comparable to the increases seen in the epidemic of the late 1960s. New initiates in 1995–1996 were likely to be young (90% younger than 26 years) and non-injecting (77% have never injected but rather smoke, sniff, or snort heroin). Opiates were reported to have been used at least once by 1.3% of 18- to 25-year-olds in 1996. Polysubstance abuse is increasingly common, with as many as 50% of male and 25% of female narcotic addicts meeting the criteria for alcohol dependence within the first 5 years of active drug treatment. Concurrent use of alcohol, stimulants, sedatives, and/or marijuana occurs in three quarters of narcotic addicts. Nicotine is the most common substance used together with opiates.

BIOMOLECULAR MECHANISMS OF ACTION. Opioids exert their effects on specific receptors for three distinct families of endogenous opioid peptides: enkephalins, endorphins, and dynorphins. In the central nervous system, three major classes of opioid receptors with unique selectivity and pharmacologic profiles have been identified: μ, κ, and δ. Subtypes of these major classes ($\mu 1$, $\mu 2$, $\kappa 1$, $\kappa 2$, $\kappa 3$, $\delta 1$, $\delta 2$) have been elucidated primarily by the use of selective receptor antagonists. μ-Receptor activity is associated with the most prominent manifestations of morphine and heroin:

respiratory depression, analgesia, euphoria, and the development of dependence. It is thought that opioid peptides acting as neurotransmitters or neuromodulators exert their actions at neuronal synapses.

CLINICAL PHARMACOLOGY. Heroin may be injected intravenously or subcutaneously, snorted, smoked, or ingested. The parenteral and inhaled routes of administration result in the most rapid delivery of drug to the brain and are hence the most potentially addicting. As the purity of street heroin has increased from less than 5% in the 1960s to 1980s to varying levels up to 80% in the 1990s, its non-parenteral administration has risen. Heroin may be used intermittently or regularly. Intermittent users either quit or become regular users within 1 to 3 years. Given the drug's half-life, regular users require two to four daily doses to avoid withdrawal symptoms.

Heroin's initial effect is an intense euphoria described as a "rush" or "kick," compared in intensity and pleasure to an orgasm, that lasts 45 seconds to several minutes. The initial effects may be perceived as a turning in the stomach with tingling and warmth. A user's first experience may be unpleasant because of nausea, vomiting, and anxiety, but these effects decrease or become less of a concern to the user over time. The intense euphoria is followed by an intoxicated pleasant feeling referred to as "nodding," with decreased respiration and peristalsis. The depressant effect of heroin on the central nervous system is marked, particularly after parenteral administration. Sedation, mental clouding, decreased visual acuity, heavy feeling in the extremities, light sleep with vivid dreams, and reduction in anxiety are typical, at least until tolerance develops. Physical signs include miosis, decreased heart rate, and lowered blood pressure. In addition to these effects on opioid receptors, heroin causes the release of histamine, which may result in itching, scleral injection, and hypotension.

High levels of tolerance develop rapidly with regard to respiratory depression, analgesia, sedation, vomiting, and euphoric properties. Little tolerance develops for miosis or constipation, so a heroin addict with an acutely painful medical condition may complain of insufficient analgesia despite pinpoint pupils. Cross-tolerance is common among opioids.

From the patient's perspective, withdrawal from heroin is a dreaded clinical condition, a mix of emotional, behavioral, and physical signs and symptoms (Table 17–2). Although very unpleasant, it is not life-threatening. The timing of withdrawal symptoms, which are directly related to clearance of the drug, begins 4 to 8 hours after the last dose of heroin. The acute withdrawal syndrome will peak in intensity after 36 to 72 hours and resolve over a period of 5 to 7 days.

In addition to the acute abstinence syndrome, a protracted abstinence syndrome occurs and lasts 6 months or more. In contrast to the hyperadrenergic characteristics of the primary withdrawal syndrome (tachycardia, hypertension, elevated temperature, miosis, and diaphoresis), the period afterward can consist of sluggishness, sleep disturbance, and malaise. Craving can recur for years after cessation of drug use. An understanding of the nature of recovery from heroin use is important for setting appropriate expectations for both the patient and the health care provider.

CLINICAL COMPLICATIONS. Most opioid-related medical complications occur as a result of the spread of infectious agents by injection drug use among heroin addicts. The manifestations of these medical complications are protean but frequently non-specific, such as fever, malaise, weight loss, pain, or dyspnea. The underly-

Table 17–2 ■ SIGNS AND SYMPTOMS OF WITHDRAWAL FROM OPIOIDS AND COCAINE

Opioid Withdrawal	
Vital signs	Tachycardia, hypertension, fever
Central nervous system	Craving, restlessness, insomnia, muscle cramps, yawning, miosis
Eyes, nose	Lacrimation, rhinorrhea
Skin	Perspiration, piloerection
Gastrointestinal	Nausea, vomiting, diarrhea
Cocaine Withdrawal	
Crash	Depression, fatigue
Withdrawal	Anxiety, high craving
Extinction	Normalization of mood, episodic craving

ing etiologies include endocarditis, cellulitis, HIV disease, hepatitis, pneumonia, and a variety of abscesses. Additionally, specific syndromes have been attributed to direct toxic effects of the opioid itself.

Reports of infectious complications of intravenous drug use before 1970 included falciparum malaria, tetanus, endocarditis, and acute hepatitis. Although the former two are now rare, hepatitis B and C are exceedingly common and serologically detectable in a large majority of heroin addicts both in the United States and abroad.

The major cardiac complication of opiate abuse is bacterial endocarditis (see Chapter 326) caused by injection drug use. *Staphylococcus aureus* is the most frequently reported bacterial isolate, and the tricuspid valve is the most common valve involved. Uncommon organisms such as *Serratia* and *Pseudomonas* have been described in specific geographic regions, so knowledge of local epidemiologic trends regarding endocarditis in injection drug users is important. Left-sided valvular infection is associated with a worse prognosis, as are the uncommon gram-negative and fungal infections.

Opiate abusers normally have acute rather than subacute endocarditis. The initial clinical finding can be fever alone in half the cases, or fever may be associated with pulmonary infiltrates from right-sided emboli or systemic embolic phenomena such as arthritis, abscess, and osteomyelitis. The diagnosis of endocarditis in a febrile injection drug user is difficult because of the poor sensitivity and specificity of readily available clinical and laboratory data. Thus, blood cultures are essential for these patients. If adequate outpatient follow-up is not possible, hospitalization is generally recommended until initial blood culture results are known. The sensitivity and specificity of echocardiography vary greatly among various studies but are not adequate to exclude endocarditis. Initial presumptive therapy for methicillin-resistant species may be considered, depending on the local epidemiology. Other cardiac complications associated with opioid abuse include toxic cardiomyopathy, abnormalities of the conduction system such as QT prolongation, ST-T wave changes, and cor pulmonale.

The most common pulmonary complication is bacterial pneumonia, which is present in one third of injection drug users evaluated for fever. The risk for this infection probably results from a combination of factors: cough suppression, hypoventilation, immune dysfunction, and aspiration during periods of clouded sensorium. Pulmonary hypertension can result from "talc granulomatosis," the development of diffuse pulmonary granulomas caused by the intravenous injection of foreign substances, most notably talc. Other pulmonary complications associated with opiate abuse include acute pulmonary edema, bronchospasm, septic pulmonary emboli, and infectious or chemical mediastinitis.

Renal complications of opiate abuse include acute diseases (myoglobinuria, necrotizing angiitis, glomerulonephritis associated with endocarditis or hepatitis) and chronic diseases (nephrotic syndrome, renal failure, renal amyloidosis). The pathology most commonly found in heroin-associated nephrotic syndrome is focal and diffuse glomerulosclerosis (see Chapter 106). In HIV-infected patients, HIV-associated nephropathy is also found (see Chapter 417).

Between 50 and 90% of patients in methadone maintenance clinics have positive serologic studies for hepatitis B and C. Hepatitis A and delta are also common. Complications of these infections (see Chapter 150) range from chronic asymptomatic antigenemia to chronic active hepatitis, cirrhosis, and hepatocellular carcinoma.

Neurologic complications of opioid abuse are both infectious and non-infectious. Seizures, most often generalized, are the most common non-infectious complication. The etiology of seizures includes overdose, with centrally mediated respiratory depression and hypoxia, and cerebral infarction. Other neurologic complications include transverse myelitis, brachial and lumbosacral plexitis, peripheral neuropathies, and myopathies. Meningitis, mycotic aneurysm, and abscesses (epidural, subdural, and brain) are well-described infectious conditions resulting from injection drug use. In HIV-infected patients, HIV-associated neurologic infectious and non-infectious diseases are common (see Chapter 411).

Psychiatric conditions among opioid abusers are very common and include alcohol abuse/dependence, major depression, phobic disorders, and antisocial personality, all of which have a greater

than 15% lifetime prevalence. Men are four to seven times more likely to have an antisocial personality than women are; women more commonly have depression. Women abusers are at high risk of being victims of violence.

Immunologic abnormalities among heroin addicts were described before the acquired immune deficiency syndrome epidemic. In vitro, morphine decreases the number of T lymphocytes, and naloxone, an opiate antagonist, can reverse this decrease. The hypergammaglobulinemia of addicts, presumably resulting from repeated antigenic stimulation, is the explanation given for a high rate of false-positive indirect syphilis serologic test results. The long-term consequences of opioid-related immunologic effects are not clear. The most prominent clinical endocrine effect is amenorrhea.

The associated medical complications of HIV infection in drug users mirror that of non-injection drug users with HIV infection with a few of caveats. HIV-infected drug users have an increased frequency of bacterial pneumonia and a decreased frequency of Kaposi's sarcoma. HIV infection among family members is strikingly common in these HIV-infected patients. HIV testing with appropriate counseling should be strongly recommended for all opioid abusers. Behavioral changes to promote the use of condoms, bleach to clean injection equipment, and the avoidance of sharing of needles can reduce HIV transmission. Needle exchange programs are efficacious in reducing the harm of heroin addiction.

DRUG OF ABUSE: COCAINE AND OTHER PSYCHOSTIMULANTS

CLASSIFICATION. Cocaine, an alkaloid extracted from coca leaves, and other psychostimulants (e.g., amphetamine, methamphetamine) rapidly increase the concentration of several neurotransmitters in synaptic junctions and stimulate the sympathetic and central nervous system. This stimulation may be manifested as increased alertness, energy, talkativeness, diminished appetite, and altered sexual function; sympathetic signs include tachycardia, mydriasis, and hyperthermia. Topical cocaine is used in otolaryngologic procedures, and psychostimulants are used either for their stimulant effects or for their paradoxical calming effect in some patients with attention deficit disorder.

HISTORY. The earliest recorded use of cocaine in the form of ingested coca leaf occurred as far back as 3000 B.C. In 1860, cocaine was isolated and incorporated into tonics, teas, and wines. In the 1880s, an Atlanta druggist patented a product that contained two naturally occurring stimulants, cocaine and caffeine, and eventually became known as Coca-Cola; until 1903 it contained approximately 60 mg of cocaine per 8-oz serving. In the late 19th century, reports of cocaine addiction surfaced, and its use was restricted after passage of the Harrison Narcotic Act of 1914. The abuse potential of amphetamines led to their being listed as schedule II drugs, which are defined as having a high potential for abuse with severe liability to cause psychic or physical dependence.

EPIDEMIOLOGY. In 1996 an estimated 1.7 million Americans, 0.8% of the population aged 12 and older, had used cocaine in the prior month. Approximately 652,000 Americans used cocaine for the first time in 1995, and about 30 million have used cocaine at least once. Use is higher in the 18- to 34-year-old age groups (1.5 to 2.0%), in men than in women (1.1% versus 0.5%), in urban areas, and among those with less education. Although current cocaine use was highest in the unemployed (2.4%), 73% of adult users were employed full or part time. Current cocaine use was similar for whites (0.8%), blacks (1.0%), and Hispanics (1.1%).

BIOMOLECULAR MECHANISMS OF ACTION. Cocaine increases neurotransmitter concentrations at the synaptic terminal by blocking the reuptake of norepinephrine, dopamine, and serotonin and potentiating the release of these monoamines. In the heart, both α- and β-adrenergic receptors are stimulated.

Dopamine activates the ventral tegmental–nucleus accumbens pathway, a major component of the brain reward system. The system is complex, with at least five dopamine receptor subtypes with distinct molecular and pharmacologic properties. D_1, D_2, and D_3 receptors have been implicated in the reinforcing actions of cocaine. Cocaine's ability to block sodium channels in neuronal cells accounts for its local anesthetic actions. Chronic use of cocaine leads to dysregulation of the brain's dopaminergic systems. Possible degeneration of dopaminergic terminals in the brains of cocaine addicts is suggested by positron emission tomographic studies in which cocaine binding to dopamine transporters in the basal ganglia and thalamus is decreased.

CLINICAL PHARMACOLOGY. Cocaine can be smoked, orally ingested, applied to mucous membranes, or injected intravenously. Cocaine hydrochloride, a water-soluble powder often mixed with adulterants, can be used by all routes except that it cannot be smoked because it decomposes when burned. Freebase or crack cocaine vaporizes before decomposition and can thus be smoked.

The route of administration determines the amount of cocaine absorbed and the rapidity of its uptake in the brain. Swallowed or snorted (intranasal) cocaine penetrates biologic membranes poorly and undergoes 70 to 80% hepatic transformation. Cocaine administered intravenously or smoked is absorbed rapidly and directly into the systemic circulation to the brain. The onset of action varies according to the route of administration: oral, peak effect in 1 hour; intranasal, 3 to 5 minutes for onset with a peak effect in 30 to 60 minutes; intravenous, onset in 12 to 16 seconds, with 10 to 20 minutes' duration of effect; and smoked, onset in 6 to 8 seconds with 5 to 10 minutes' duration of effect. Cocaine has an elimination half-life of 30 to 60 minutes. Less than 5% of cocaine appears unchanged in urine. Cocaine's two major metabolites are benzoylecgonine and ecgonine methyl ester. Both are inactive, and the former is the main target in urine testing (Table 17–3). Casual users can progress to high-dose users with compulsive and uncontrollable bingeing. During a binge, cocaine is administered every 10 to 30 minutes, generally over a period of 4 to 24 hours or more. Cocaine-dependent individuals typically binge several times a week, each followed by days of abstinence.

The acute effects of cocaine include intense euphoria, increased energy and self-confidence, enhanced mental acuity and sensory awareness (including sexual), decreased appetite, and sympathomimetic symptoms. Withdrawal symptoms are the inverse of the acute effects: depressed mood, lack of energy, limited interest in the environment, hyperphagia, hypersomnia, anxiety, and craving. The withdrawal syndromes of cocaine-dependent individuals are not as consistent or well depicted as those of alcohol or opioid withdrawal. Chronic users become tolerant to its acute effects; symptoms of anxiety, agitation, inability to concentrate, and loss of sexual drive predominate. Even beyond the initial withdrawal period, craving leading to relapse can be precipitated by conditioned cues in which the pleasurable effects of cocaine use are associated with particular settings.

CLINICAL MANIFESTATIONS. The most common medical complications of cocaine use involve the brain and the heart: altered mental status, seizures, chest pain, palpitations, and syncope. Sudden death can occur by a variety of mechanisms: arrhythmias, status epilepticus, intracerebral hemorrhage, and centrally mediated respiratory arrest.

Cocaine use leads to ischemia and myocardial infarction as a result of increased myocardial demand because of tachycardia and hypertension, to diffuse and local coronary spasm in normal or atherosclerotic arteries, and to a propensity to thrombus formation secondary to blood stasis in narrowed arteries and increased platelet aggregability. Myocardial infarction is unrelated to the dose of cocaine ingested, the frequency of use, or the route of administration; first-time, recreational, and habitual users are all at risk. Almost 90% of cocaine-associated myocardial infarctions occur in men. Most chest pain develops within minutes, but pain can be delayed up to 15 hours after use.

Other cardiac complications include supraventricular and ventricular arrhythmias, cardiomyopathy, and myocarditis. Arrhythmias are attributed to direct toxic effects and a cocaine-induced hyperadrenergic state. Myocardial damage may be similar to that seen in pheochromocytoma, in which norepinephrine excess results in a non-specific pathologic finding, contraction band necrosis.

Cocaine addiction is frequently associated with psychiatric diseases such as depression, anxiety, phobia, attention deficit, and antisocial personality disorders. High doses can result in transient psychosis, delirium, paranoid ideation, bizarre behavior, and suicide attempts.

Other complications of cocaine use include vascular headaches, rhabdomyolysis with acute renal failure, placental abruption, erosion of dental enamel, gingival ulceration, chronic rhinitis, perforated nasal septum, pulmonary edema, and sexual dysfunction. Sexually transmitted diseases, including HIV, have been strongly associated with cocaine use; HIV testing should be considered in any patient with a cocaine abuse diagnosis. Ingested packets of cocaine can rupture and cause acute toxic reactions and cardiovascular collapse.

Other Specific Drug: Methamphetamine

The synthetic psychostimulant methamphetamine, which is a particularly potent form of amphetamine, is highly addictive, cheaper, and longer lasting than cocaine. Nicknames include "speed," "crank," and "zip"; the smokable form is called "ice" or "crystal." Chronic use has been associated with violent behavior.

DRUG OF ABUSE: MARIJUANA AND OTHER CANNABINOIDS

Marijuana is the common name applied to the leaves, stems, and tops of the plant *Cannabis sativa*, which contains cannabinoids, the most active of which is Δ^9-*trans*-tetrahydrocannabinol (THC). It is generally smoked but can be eaten, mixed in food or tea. Tolerance and physical dependence are not major clinical problems. The changes in the brain, cardiovascular system, and lungs are acute and reversible. Marijuana or purified oral THC may be effective therapy for nausea in some patients.

Cannabinoids are the most commonly used illicit drugs in the world, with approximately 250 million users. An estimated 10.1 million Americans, 4.7% of the population aged 12 and older, are current marijuana or hashish users, and nearly 70 million Americans have used marijuana in their lifetime. From 1992 to 1995, the use of marijuana among youth aged 12 to 17 more than doubled and was similar among both boys and girls; whites, blacks, and Hispanics; metropolitan and non-metropolitan areas; and geographic regions.

Cannabinoids bind to specific receptors for the endogenous ligand anandamide: CB1 in the brain and CB2 in the periphery. G-protein activation occurs as a result of the receptor binding and has three effects: inhibition of adenylate cyclase, increased potassium ion conductance, and decreased calcium ion conductance. CB1 receptors are concentrated in the globus pallidus, hippocampus, cerebral cortex, cerebellum, and striatum.

Smoked marijuana results in a variety of acute changes within 3 minutes that peak within 20 to 30 minutes; when ingested, onset takes 30 to 60 minutes and the peak effect occurs after 2 to 3 hours. An average cigarette contains 2.5 to 5.0 mg of THC, and 50 to 60% is absorbed. THC is lipophilic and distributed rapidly throughout the body. Because of slow release from adipose tissue, THC or its metabolites can be found in urine 2 to 10 days after use in non-chronic users and 36 days after use in chronic users (see Table 17–3).

Most effects last 2 to 3 hours after inhalation; psychomotor effects can last 11 hours. Effects include conjunctival injection, mild euphoria, impaired memory, dry mouth, motor incoordination,

Table 17–3 ■ URINE TESTING FOR ABUSED DRUGS

DRUG	COMPOUND DETECTED	URINE DETECTION TIME
Heroin	Morphine 6-Acetylmorphine	1–3 d
Codeine	Codeine Morphine	1–3 d
Methadone	Methadone	2–4 d
Cocaine	Benzoylecgonine	1–3 d
Amphetamine	Amphetamine	2–4 d
Methamphetamine	Methamphetamine, amphetamine	2–4 d
Marijuana	Tetrahydrocannabinol	1–3 d for casual use, up to 30 d for chronic use
Phencyclidine	Phencyclidine	2–7 d for casual use, up to 30 d for chronic use
Benzodiazepines	Oxazepam, diazepam, other benzodiazepines	Up to 30 d
Barbiturates	Amobarbital, secobarbital, other barbiturates	2–4 d for short acting, up to 30 d for long acting

time-space distortion, increased visual and auditory awareness, increased hunger, sleepiness, and spontaneous laughter; some may experience nausea, headaches, tremors, decreased muscle strength, and increased anxiety. Few chronic effects have been attributed to marijuana use, but an amotivational syndrome has been described in which young people lose goal-directed behavior with regard to school or work.

DRUGS OF ABUSE: LSD AND OTHER HALLUCINOGENS

Hallucinogen use results predominantly in changes in thought, perception, and mood. Minimal impairment occurs in memory or intellect. This class of drugs is not generally associated with stupor, narcosis, or excessive stimulation. Users do not exhibit craving. The two major categories of hallucinogens are indolamines (e.g., lysergic acid diethylamide [LSD], dimethyltryptamide, psilocybin) and phenylethylamines (e.g., 2,5-dimethoxy-4-methylamphetamine, methylene dioxyamphetamine, methylene dioxymethamphetamine, mescaline). Related drugs include phencyclidine (PCP), nutmeg, morning glory seeds, catnip, nitrous oxide, and amyl or butyl nitrite. These drugs have no appropriate clinical role.

In the United States the lifetime prevalence of hallucinogen use was 9.7% in 1996; over 20 million individuals have used hallucinogens at least once. Lifetime prevalence varied by race: higher in whites than Hispanics and blacks. The male-to-female ratio of use was constant across races at 2 to 3:1. LSD was widely used on college campuses in the 1960s. The 1970s and early 1980s saw a decline in the use of most hallucinogens. In the 1990s, hallucinogen use has increased among high school students, college students, and young adults aged 19 to 28.

The classic hallucinogens are structurally similar to many major neurotransmitters, but serotonin (5-hydroxytryptamine [5-HT]) agonist or partial agonist properties have most consistently been associated with its actions. These drugs bind at 5-HT2A and 5-HT2C receptors with high affinity. These receptors are found in greatest density in brain cortical regions (cerebral cortex, claustrum, caudate putamen, globus pallidus, ventral pallidum, islands of Calleja, mamillary nuclei, and inferior olive) and may have a role in depression and suicide.

Hallucinogen use results in an altered perception of one's environment marked by a subjective feeling of enhanced mental activity, perceptual distortions, visual hallucinations, sharpened sense of hearing, and a reduced ability to tell the difference between one's self and one's surrounding. These drugs can produce sympathomimetic effects, including mydriasis, flushed face, fine tremor, piloerection, high blood pressure, hyperthermia, and hyperglycemia. Adverse effects of a specific hallucinogen are highly variable among individuals and even in the same individual at different times. Panic attacks and psychosis are the two major adverse effects. Clinically "desired" effects and adverse effects will also vary by specific hallucinogen. These altered perceptions can be associated with paranoid delusions, manic or depressed behavior, and confusion. Aggressive behavior has been described with psychosis; in particular, PCP has been implicated in violent crimes. The psychotic episodes can last hours or days, and flashbacks can occur. The event may be simple visual images or a complex emotional experience resembling prior drug experiences. It can occur days or weeks after the last dose and is more common in heavy users. Precipitants for flashbacks are anxiety, stress, fatigue, emergence into a dark environment, and marijuana. It is not known whether prolonged psychotic episodes occur only in individuals predisposed to psychosis (i.e., underlying psychiatric disease) or whether the use of hallucinogens, particularly chronic use or high doses, can lead to such complications.

Panic reactions may or may not be associated with hallucinations. Individuals can be highly stimulated, frightened, and fearful of losing their mind. This drug effect is more likely to occur in individuals with limited experience with hallucinogens. Physiologic and psychological manifestations are those of classic panic attacks: palpitations, high blood pressure, hyperthermia, perspiration, exaggerated anxiety, loss of contact with reality, depersonalization, paranoia, and confusion. Although tolerance can develop with hallucinogens, the clinical syndrome is unusual inasmuch as chronic use is uncommon. No clinically significant withdrawal symptoms are known. Concerns about chronic use include decreased intellect, organic brain syndrome, and possibly "chromosomal damage," although definitive correlations have not been established.

The use of hallucinogens may be detected in the acute setting while examining a patient with toxic manifestations or may be noted when obtaining a history of drug use. After diagnosis, it is important to obtain a history of other substance abuse and psychiatric illness, as well as a neurologic evaluation. No specific laboratory tests are required; a urine toxicologic screen for other drugs of abuse is recommended (see Table 17–3).

LSD is often sold as postage stamp–size papers impregnated with varying doses of LSD, from 50 to more than 300 μg. Doses of 20 μg can lead to psychological effects, with doses of 100 μg causing hallucinogenic psychoactive manifestations within 1 to 2 hours. Clearing of symptoms begins in 10 to 12 hours, although symptoms of fatigue and tension can persist for an additional 24 hours.

PCP, also known as phencyclidine or angel dust, was originally developed as an anesthetic in the 1950s but was abandoned because of frequent postoperative delirium and hallucinations. It can be obtained in various forms (powder, liquid, tablet, capsule, or sprayed on other drugs such as marijuana) and administered by several routes (smoked, ingested, snorted, or injected intravenously). The drug is water soluble and lipophilic, so it penetrates fat stores and has a long half-life, up to 3 days. Casual use by smoking on a weekly basis is most common, although some have reported continuous intake lasting 2 days or longer. A pronounced pharmacologic characteristic of PCP is its analgesia and amphetamine-like stimulation in addition to hallucination. Ataxia, slurred speech, nystagmus, and numbness are commonly observed at doses of 1 to 10 mg. Emotional withdrawal, catatonic posturing resembling schizophrenia, and physical violence can result from its use.

DRUG OF ABUSE: BENZODIAZEPINES AND OTHER SEDATIVES

Benzodiazepines and the less commonly used barbiturates are legitimate therapeutic drugs with abuse potential. These drugs are designated as schedule IV substances by the Drug Enforcement Agency and the Food and Drug Administration. Schedule IV drugs have a low potential for abuse and lead to limited physical or psychological dependence.

Non-medical use of tranquilizers and sedatives occurred in fewer than 2% of U.S. adults in 1996. Thus the magnitude of the problem is substantially less than that of opioids, psychostimulants, and marijuana and occurs largely in individuals who also abuse other substances. This finding is consistent with the experience in laboratory animals, who do not exhibit repeated self-administration, a standard measure of addictive potential, when exposed to benzodiazepines.

All benzodiazepines studied are capable of producing physiologic dependence even when used in low doses over prolonged periods as may be seen in clinical practice. The key to the diagnosis of benzodiazepine or other sedative abuse is evidence of inappropriate drug-taking behavior, including escalation in dose, obtaining prescriptions from multiple physicians, or taking the drug for reasons other than those for which it was prescribed. Physiologic dependence should not imply that inappropriate drug-taking behavior exists. Before initiating clinical use of benzodiazepines and other sedatives, a careful medical history must be obtained regarding current and prior substance abuse. Although not absolutely contraindicated, particular caution and extra monitoring are appropriate in patients with such a history.

DRUG ABUSE TREATMENT AND PREVENTION OF RELAPSE

Patients with illicit drug use will benefit from treatment only if they recognize that their substance use is a problem. The transtheoretical model considers a patient on a continuum from pre-contemplation (denial) toward maintenance (abstinence/recovery) (Fig. 17–1). The clinical approach should be tailored to the patient's readiness to change behavior and enter treatment.

The major goals of drug abuse treatment are detoxification, abstinence initiation, and relapse prevention. Treatment can be both pharmacologic and non-pharmacologic. Commonly, pharmacologic approaches are offered by physicians specializing in addiction.

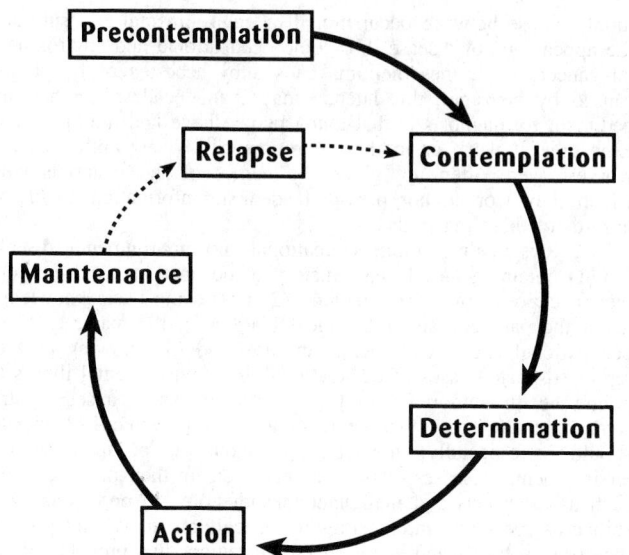

FIGURE 17–1 ■ Graphic depiction of the Prochaska and DiClemente model for readiness for behavioral change.

Some form of psychosocial treatment is the backbone of substance abuse treatment, be it psychotherapy, behavioral therapy, or counseling. Issues addressed in these encounters include teaching coping skills, changing reinforcement contingencies, fostering management of painful affects, addressing motivation, improving interpersonal functioning, enhancing social supports, and fostering compliance with and retention in pharmacotherapy. Much of this work is done by substance abuse providers. However, physicians are in an excellent position to detect drug abuse by exploring this history when confronted by a possible drug abuse–related clinical manifestation.

The active ingredients of brief intervention have been summarized by the acronym *FRAMES:* (1) *feedback* of personal risk or impairment (e.g., sharing abnormal test results, discussing medical complications), (2) emphasis on personal *responsibility* to change, (3) clear *advice* to change, (4) a *menu* of different change options, (5) provider *empathy,* and (6) enhancement of patient *self-efficacy* or optimism. Physicians can refer to substance abuse treatment specialists; self-help groups or Narcotics Anonymous is often part of a successful abstinence maintenance program.

Pharmacologic treatment of *opioid* abuse can be approached in three ways: agonist substitution, antagonist treatment, or symptomatic treatment. With detoxification, the goal is amelioration of the symptoms of heroin or other opioid withdrawal by methadone (agonist substitution) with a slow taper over a period of 1 to 6 months, by clonidine (symptomatic treatment) for 5 to 7 days, or by a combination of clonidine and naltrexone (antagonist treatment) for 3 to 5 days. The latter regimen appears to shorten the course of withdrawal, but long-term outcomes such as relapse prevention remain unclear. A promising but at present investigational treatment involves the use of buprenorphine (agonist/antagonist), which has the advantage of a better safety profile than pure agonists and, unlike methadone, does not produce significant physical dependence. Hospitalized opioid-dependent patients may be treated with methadone for withdrawal symptoms by any physician. However, methadone is not available for the treatment of opioid addiction after discharge, except in specially licensed treatment facilities.

Short-term detoxification with methadone is not effective in leading to long-term abstinence.

Prevention of relapse to active heroin abuse has been most commonly attempted by substitution of a safer drug (e.g., methadone, *l*-acetyl-α-methadol) with similar pharmacologic properties to relieve the craving and withdrawal and to partially block the euphoric effects of heroin (Table 17–4). In an already-detoxified patient, a less common alternative is to use an opioid antagonist (e.g., naltrexone) that effectively blocks agonist stimulation. Methadone is not adequate treatment for acute pain syndromes.

Physicians can promote harm reduction measures, such as those for injection drug users, while emphasizing the importance of drug abuse treatment: participation in needle exchange programs, avoidance of "shooting galleries" to obtain or administer drugs, and instructions to never share "works" (injection equipment). Such interventions, which can be delivered by physicians to drug abusers, have played a crucial role in international efforts to limit the spread of HIV infection.

Cocaine abuse is treated by psychotherapy, behavioral therapy, and 12-step programs. Acupuncture has been used for detoxification and relapse prevention. As yet, no pharmacologic agent has consistently been effective in reducing cocaine use or craving. Dopamine agonists, antidepressants, and other drugs have been studied, but none are currently recommended. No antidote is known for acute cocaine overdose.

Marijuana use rarely requires acute treatment in the medical setting. Reassurance is generally sufficient to manage the occasional dysphoric manifestations. Occasionally, anxiety reactions require specific therapy with benzodiazepines; rarely, psychotic reactions are treated with haloperidol.

Specific therapy for the complications of *hallucinogen* use is non-pharmacologic and involves emotional reassurance and a calm supportive environment. No specific antagonists for any of the hallucinogens are clinically available. Clinical outcomes are not improved by enhancing excretion of these compounds. Medications are required only if the patient cannot be adequately controlled, in which case anxiolytic drugs are recommended. Neuroleptics are not recommended because they may exacerbate the anticholinergic effects of adulterants in the ingested drug.

Discontinuation of *benzodiazepines* can be accomplished in dependent patients by prescribing a regimen of very gradual dose reduction. Alternatively, another long-acting sedative-hypnotic can be substituted for the drug of abuse and gradually withdrawn. In each case, it is important to attempt to verify that the patient has no alternative sources for these medications. In the case of treatment for each drug described, medical follow-up after the acute toxic manifestations is essential to address substance abuse issues and possible coexisting medical and psychiatric problems.

Leshner AI: Addiction is a brain disease, and it matters. Science 278:45, 1997. *A concise overview of drug addiction by the Director of the National Institute on Drug Abuse. Addiction is portrayed as a chronic, relapsing disease of the brain that can have a profound impact on both personal and public health.*
National Consensus Development Panel on Effective Medical Treatment of Opiate Addiction: Effective medical treatment of opiate addiction. JAMA 280:1936, 1998. *A comprehensive review.*
O'Connor PG, Samet JH, Stein MD: Management of hospitalized intravenous drug users: Role of the internist. Am J Med 96:551, 1994. *Reviews common clinical dilemmas faced by internists when managing the care of injection drug users in the inpatient hospital setting.*
Samet JH, O'Connor PG, Stein MD (eds): Alcohol and drug abuse. Med Clin North Am, July 1997. *This in-depth review of a spectrum of drug abuse and alcohol issues addresses detection, treatment, and special populations of substance abusers from a broad physician perspective.*

Table 17–4 ■ RELAPSE PREVENTION FOR OPIOID ABUSE

MEDICATION	DOSE	DOSING INTERVAL	MECHANISM	PRESCRIBING REGULATIONS	WITHDRAWAL*
Methadone	60–100 mg orally	Daily	Agonist	Yes	++
LAAM	30–100 mg orally	q2–3d	Agonist	Yes	++
Buprenorphine	8–16 mg sublingually	q1–2d	Agonist/antagonist	Not yet FDA approved	+
Naltrexone	50 mg oral	Daily	Antagonist	No	–

LAAM = *l*-acetyl-α-methadol; FDA = Food and Drug Administration.
*++ = moderate; + = mild; – = none.

18 PRINCIPLES OF OCCUPATIONAL AND ENVIRONMENTAL MEDICINE

Philip J. Landrigan

In their jobs, people can be exposed to dangerous chemicals, hazardous physical agents, and emotional stress, and they can suffer trauma. Any of these occupational exposures can cause disease—sometimes immediately and sometimes after an interval of years or decades.

In addition, tens of millions of people are regularly exposed to environmental toxins. Some are exposed to high levels in well-publicized disasters such as radiation at Chernobyl, but many more are chronically exposed to lower levels. Air pollution, lead, radon, and pesticides are examples of environmental agents that can cause illness and death.

Occupational and environmental toxins cause a broad range of illnesses, and these diseases can involve virtually every organ system. They include classic, well-described diseases such as lung cancer and malignant mesothelioma in workers exposed to asbestos, cancer of the bladder in dye workers, pneumoconiosis in coal miners, leukemia and lymphoma in people exposed to benzene, skin cancer in farmers and sailors chronically exposed to the sun, and chronic bronchitis in workers exposed to dust particles. Occupational illnesses also include newer entities recognized only in recent years such as dementia in persons exposed to solvents, sterility in men and women exposed to certain pesticides, asthma and bronchitis in children and adults chronically exposed to particulate air pollution, and carpal tunnel syndrome in workers engaged in repetitive, stressful wrist motion. Some of these diseases are acute; others are chronic. Some are manifested through obvious symptoms, whereas others involve more subtle degrees of dysfunction.

In the United States, occupational exposure accounts each year for approximately 6500 traumatic deaths from injury, 13.2 million non-fatal injuries, 60,000 deaths from disease, and 860,000 cases of work-related illness. The total costs, direct medical expenses plus indirect economic losses, are estimated to be $171 billion annually, nearly 3% of the gross domestic product of the United States. In the environment, the Centers for Disease Control and Prevention estimate that nearly 1 million children suffer from lead poisoning and that tens of thousands have asthma induced by indoor and outdoor air pollution.

Occupational and environmental exposures always need to be considered in the differential diagnosis. Because of the enormous numbers exposed and the wide range of illnesses, the possibility of occupational or environmental exposure to toxins needs to be considered in the evaluation of every patient.

CLINICAL DIAGNOSIS OF OCCUPATIONAL AND ENVIRONMENTAL DISEASE

Occupational and environmental diseases are underdiagnosed. Many are incorrectly attributed to other causes because frequently these diseases are not distinct in their clinical features and can closely resemble chronic diseases caused by other factors. Examples include (1) lung cancer caused by asbestos, radon, or beryllium that is incorrectly attributed to cigarette smoking; (2) severe abdominal pain caused by lead poisoning that is erroneously diagnosed as acute appendicitis (some such cases have resulted in unnecessary laparotomy); (3) dementia caused by organic solvents that is attributed to "old age" or to ethanol ingestion; (4) renal failure caused by chronic exposure to lead or cadmium that is ascribed to "idiopathic factors"; and (5) hearing loss caused by noise that is incorrectly attributed to presbycusis.

Only if a careful history of toxic occupational and environmental exposure is taken in these cases can a correct diagnosis be made. A barrier to accurate diagnosis is the long latency that must commonly elapse between occupational or environmental exposure and the appearance of disease. For some occupational and environmental cancers (e.g., mesothelioma caused by asbestos or lymphoma caused by benzene), this latency may span decades. Another impediment to diagnosis is that many people have had multiple toxic exposures at work or in the environment. At least until recently, workers were often not given the names of the materials with which they worked nor provided adequate information about the hazards of these materials.

The keys to diagnosing occupational and environmental disease are (1) obtaining an adequate history of occupational and environmental exposure for every patient, (2) possessing basic knowledge about the pathogenesis and clinical features of the major types of occupational and environmental disease, and (3) knowing how to report suspected cases of occupational and environmental illness to public health authorities so that additional cases caused by the same exposure can either be recognized or prevented. Physicians should be especially knowledgeable about the occupational and environmental diseases that commonly occur in their practice areas, such as asbestosis and malignant mesothelioma in port cities with shipyards, pesticide intoxication in agricultural areas, and poisonings from solvents and exotic metals in regions that produce microelectronics.

OCCUPATIONAL AND ENVIRONMENTAL HISTORY

The history is the single most important instrument for obtaining information on the role of occupational and environmental factors in causing disease. Information about current and past exposure should routinely be sought in every patient at several logical points when taking a history. At each juncture, a few brief screening questions should be asked systematically. Then if suspicious information is elicited, more detailed follow-up questions are needed. A routine screen for occupational and environmental disease consists of the following items:

1. In the *history of the present illness,* pay attention to any temporal relationship between the onset of illness and toxic exposure in the workplace or the environment. For example, did symptoms begin shortly after the patient started a new job? Did they abate during vacation and then recrudesce after the patient resumed work? Were they related to the introduction of a new chemical or process? Did they correlate with episodes of pollution? Were there similar illnesses among coworkers or neighbors? Were the individuals who were more heavily exposed the more severely affected? A possible occupational cause should be sought in every case of acute trauma (in children and adolescents as well as adults) and in every case of repetitive trauma, e.g., carpal tunnel syndrome.
2. In the *medical history,* obtain a list of current and principal past occupations and industries of employment. Each patient should be asked whether illness ever developed as a consequence of the work.
3. In the *review of systems,* routinely ask every patient: "Do you now or have you previously had occupational or environmental exposure to asbestos, lead, fumes, chemicals, dust particles, loud noise, radiation, or other toxic factors?" Also ask all patients whether they believe that any of these factors may have caused or contributed to their illness. Even if a postulated connection between exposure and disease initially appears tenuous, such suspicions always need to be considered carefully.

DETAILED EXPOSURE HISTORY. If information from the routine interview suggests an occupational or environmental cause, the physician should obtain a more detailed history of toxic exposure. Data on the duration and intensity of exposure are particularly important. It is necessary to learn how the patient worked with the suspected toxin and to consider how the material may have been absorbed. Information should be obtained on all jobs ever held, places of employment, products manufactured, and materials with which the patient worked.

If toxic exposure is identified or strongly suspected and an occupational or environmental cause seems likely, further follow-up inquiries may need to be made through the patient's labor union, companies where the patient has been employed, company physicians, or state or local health departments. Information on toxic

Table 18–1 ■ SELECTED LIST OF SENTINEL HEALTH EVENTS (OCCUPATIONAL)—
OCCUPATIONALLY RELATED UNNECESSARY DISEASE, DISABILITY, AND UNTIMELY DEATH

CONDITION	INDUSTRY/OCCUPATION	AGENT
Pulmonary tuberculosis	Physicians, medical personnel	*Mycobacterium tuberculosis*
Plague, tularemia, anthrax, rabies, and other infections	Farmers, ranchers, hunters, veterinarians, laboratory workers	Various infectious agents
Rubella	Medical personnel, intensive care personnel	Rubella virus
Hepatitis	Daycare center staff, orphanage staff, medical personnel	Hepatitis A, B, and C viruses
Acquired immune deficiency syndrome (AIDS)	Health care personnel	HIV
Ornithosis	Bird breeders, pet shop staff, poultry producers, veterinarians, zoo staff	*Chlamydia psittaci*
Malignant neoplasm of nasal cavities	Woodworkers, cabinet and furniture makers	Hardwood dust, formaldehyde
	Radium chemists and processors	Radium
	Nickel smelting and refining workers	Nickel
Malignant neoplasm of larynx	Asbestos industries and users	Asbestos
Malignant neoplasm of trachea, bronchus, and lung	Asbestos industries and users	Asbestos
	Topside coke oven workers	Coke oven emissions
	Uranium and fluorspar miners	Radon daughters
	Smelters, processors, users	Chromates, nickel, arsenic
	Mustard gas formulators	Mustard gas
	Ion exchange resin makers, chemists	Bis(chloromethyl) ether
Mesothelioma	Asbestos industries and users	Asbestos
Malignant neoplasm of bone	Radium chemists and processors	Radium
Malignant neoplasm of scrotum	Automatic lathe operators, metalworkers	Mineral/cutting oils
	Coke oven workers, petroleum refiners	Soot and tar
Malignant neoplasm of bladder	Rubber and dye workers	Benzidine, naphthylamine, auramine, 4-nitrophenyl
Malignant neoplasm of kidney	Coke oven workers	Coke oven emissions
Lymphoid leukemia	Radiologists	Ionizing radiation
	Rubber industry, chemical industry	Benzene, 1,3-butadiene, ethylene oxide
Myeloid leukemia	Rubber industry, chemical industry	Benzene, 1,3-butadiene, ethylene oxide
	Radiologists	Ionizing radiation
Erythroleukemia	Rubber industry, chemical industry	Benzene, 1,3-butadiene, ethylene oxide
Non-autoimmune hemolytic anemia	Whitewashing and leather industry	Copper sulfate
	Electrolytic processes, smelting	Arsine
	Plastics industry	Trimellitic anhydride
Aplastic anemia	Chemical manufacture	TNT, benzene
	Radiologists, radium chemists	Ionizing radiation
Agranulocytosis or neutropenia	Explosives and pesticide industries	Phosphorus
	Pesticides, pigments, pharmaceuticals	Inorganic arsenic, benzene, 1,3-butadiene
Toxic encephalitis	Battery, smelter, and foundry workers	Lead
Parkinson's disease (secondary)	Manganese processing, battery makers, welders	Manganese
Peripheral neuropathy	Pesticides, pigments, pharmaceuticals	Arsenic and arsenic compounds
	Furniture refinishers, degreasing operations	Hexane
	Plastics, rayon industries	Methyl butyl ketone, copper disulfide, other solvents
	Explosives industry	TNT
	Battery, smelter, and foundry workers	Lead
	Dentists, chloralkali plants, battery makers	Mercury
	Plastics industry, paper manufacturing	Acrylamide
	Microwave and radar technicians	Microwaves
	Radiologists	Ionizing radiation
	Blacksmiths, glass blowers, bakers	Infrared radiation
	Moth repellent formulators, fumigators	Naphthalene
Hearing loss	Many industries	Excessive noise
Raynaud's phenomenon (secondary)	Lumberjacks, chain sawyers, grinders	Vibration
	Vinyl chloride polymerization industry	Vinyl chloride monomer
Extrinsic asthma	Jewelry alloy and catalyst makers	Platinum
	Polyurethane, adhesive, paint workers	Isocyanates
	Plastics, dye, insecticide makers	Phthalic anhydride
	Foam workers, latex makers, biologists	Formaldehyde
	Bakers	Flour
	Woodworkers, furniture makers	Red cedar and other wood dust
Pneumoconiosis of coal workers	Coal miners	Coal dust
Asbestosis	Power plant workers	Asbestos
	Asbestos industries	
	Construction workers	
	Demolition workers	
	Building maintenance workers	
	Firefighters	
Silicosis	Quarrymen, sandblasters, miners, silica processors; ceramic industries and foundries	Silica
Talcosis	Talc processors	Talc
Chronic beryllium disease of the lung	Beryllium alloy workers, ceramic and cathode ray tube makers, nuclear reactor workers	Beryllium
Byssinosis	Cotton industry workers	Cotton, flax, hemp, and cotton-synthetic dust
Acute bronchitis, pneumonitis, and pulmonary edema from fumes and vapors	Alkali and bleach industries	Chlorine
	Silo fillers, arc welders	Nitrogen oxides
	Paper, refrigeration, oil industries	Sulfur dioxide
	Plastics industry	Trimellitic anhydride

Table continued on following page

Table 18–1 ■ SELECTED LIST OF SENTINEL HEALTH EVENTS (OCCUPATIONAL)—
OCCUPATIONALLY RELATED UNNECESSARY DISEASE, DISABILITY, AND UNTIMELY DEATH *Continued*

CONDITION	INDUSTRY/OCCUPATION	AGENT
Toxic hepatitis	Solvent users, dry cleaners, plastics industry	Carbon tetrachloride, chloroform, trichloroethylene
	Explosives and dye industries	Phosphorus, TNT
	Fumigators, fire extinguisher formulators	Ethylene dibromide
Acute or chronic renal failure	Battery makers, plumbers, solderers	Inorganic lead
	Electrolytic processes, smelting	Arsine
	Battery makers, jewelers, dentists	Inorganic mercury
	Fire extinguisher makers	Carbon tetrachloride
	Antifreeze manufacturers	Ethylene glycol
Male infertility	Pesticide formulators and applicators	Dibromochloropropane
Contact and allergic dermatitis	Leather tanning, poultry dressing plants, packing, adhesives and sealant industry, boat building and repair	Irritants (e.g., cutting fish oils, solvents, acids, alkalis, allergens)

From Rutstein DD, Mullan RJ, Frazier TM, et al: Sentinel health events (occupational): A basis for physician recognition and public health surveillance. Am J Public Health 73: 1054, 1983. © APHA.

substances used in a workplace may be legally available to patients under the Records Access Standard and Hazard Communication Standard of the Occupational Safety and Health Administration and under state and local "right-to-know" laws.

REPORTING AND REFERRAL. If the diagnostic interview indicates or strongly raises suspicion that disease is due to toxic occupational or environmental exposure, the physician is required in most jurisdictions to report the case to state or local public health authorities. Many episodes of these diseases are in essence common-source outbreaks of highly preventable illness. Prompt reporting can lead to identification of additional cases earlier and to prevention by abating a common exposure source.

The physician may require access to specialized referral sources in occupational and environmental medicine. Two national organizations that maintain listings of occupational and environmental specialist physicians are the American College of Occupational and Environmental Medicine (Arlington Heights, IL) and the Association of Occupational and Environmental Clinics (Washington, DC). Other valuable resources are the U.S. Public Health Service's National Institute for Occupational Safety and Health (Cincinnati, OH), and the Centers for Disease Control and Prevention (Atlanta).

ESTABLISHING THE DIAGNOSIS OF OCCUPATIONAL OR ENVIRONMENTAL ILLNESS

If the history suggests an occupational or environmental cause, the following fundamental principles help make a diagnosis of occupational or environmental disease:

1. *Biologic Plausibility.* The likelihood that a disease is of occupational or environmental origin increases if the disease has previously been seen in other patients with the same or similar exposure, if a biologic mechanism is known, or if the disease has been seen in laboratory animals experimentally exposed to the chemical (or to a similar chemical). However, many thousands of chemicals to which workers are regularly exposed in industry and that have been dispersed into the environment have never been laboratory-tested for their toxicity. Therefore, the possibility always exists of diagnosing a disease entity that has never previously been recognized, e.g., malignant mesothelioma in workers exposed to asbestos, hepatic angiosarcoma in workers exposed to vinyl chloride, and cancer of the bladder in aniline dye workers.
2. *Dose Response.* The likelihood of occupational or environmental causation increases if the disease occurs more commonly and more seriously in more heavily exposed members of a population. However, in the case of occupational and environmental carcinogens, there are no threshold levels of exposure below which safety is ensured; any exposure to these agents is potentially carcinogenic, although heavier exposure carries greater risk. In addition, agents that are allergens or chemical sensitizers can cause symptoms at very low exposure levels.

SENTINEL HEALTH EVENTS. To help physicians establish link-

ages between occupational exposure and disease, a sentinel health event is defined as "an unnecessary disease, disability or untimely death which is occupationally related." By scanning the list in Table 18–1, physicians can identify work-related illnesses or exposures that may occur in their patients. Additionally, they can identify occupations and industries that may be pertinent to their local practice areas. This selected list also represents an accessible starting point for developing competence in the differential diagnosis of occupational and environmental disease.

Goldman RH, Peters JM: The occupational and environmental health history. JAMA 246:2831, 1991. *A concise, systematic approach to history taking.*
Leigh JP, Markowitz SB, Fahs M, et al: Occupational illness and injury in the United States: Estimates of costs, morbidity, and mortality. Arch Intern Med 157:1557, 1997.
Rom WN: Environmental and Occupational Medicine, 3rd ed. Boston, Little, Brown, 1998. *The classic reference in the field.*
Rosenstock L, Cullen M: Clinical Occupational Medicine, 2nd ed. Philadelphia, WB Saunders, 1994. *A useful guide to common occupational and environmental health problems.*

19 RADIATION INJURY

Arthur C. Upton

The term *radiation injury* denotes any abnormality of form or function caused by electromagnetic waves or accelerated atomic particles. The term is often also applied to the harmful effects of high-intensity ultrasound and electromagnetic fields. Because the different types of radiation differ markedly in their biologic effects, each must be dealt with separately in terms of the injuries that they can cause.

IONIZING RADIATION

Ionizing radiation occurs as electromagnetic waves of extremely short wavelength (Fig. 19–1) and also as accelerated atomic particles (e.g., electrons, protons, neutrons, α-particles). The injuries caused by ionizing radiation include mutagenic, carcinogenic, and teratogenic effects, as well as various acute and chronic tissue reactions such as erythema, cataract of the lens, sterility, and depression of hematopoiesis.

ETIOLOGY. The biologic effects of ionizing radiation result from damage to DNA and other vital molecules by locally deposited energy. Doses of ionizing radiation are therefore measured in terms of energy deposition (Table 19–1).

All humans are continuously exposed to natural background ionizing radiation from (1) cosmic rays; (2) radium and other radioactive elements in the earth's crust; (3) potassium-40, carbon-14, and other radionuclides normally present in human tissues; and (4)

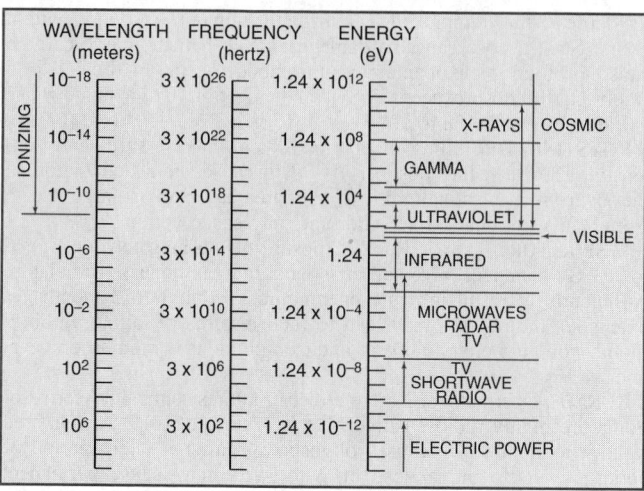

FIGURE 19–1 ■ The electromagnetic spectrum. (From Mettler FA, Upton AC: Effects of Ionizing Radiation, 2nd ed. Philadelphia, WB Saunders, 1995.)

inhaled radon and its daughter elements (Table 19–2). In people residing at mile-high elevations such as in Denver, the contribution from cosmic rays may be increased two-fold, and at jet aircraft altitudes it may exceed 0.005 mSv (1 Sv = 100 rem) per hour. Likewise, in regions where the earth's crust is rich in radium, the contribution from this radionuclide may be similarly increased. However, exposure of the bronchial epithelium to inhaled radon and its daughters accounts for two thirds of ionizing radiation.

Among man-made sources of radiation, the largest source is from x-rays used in medical diagnosis. Smaller amounts of radiation are also received from radioactive minerals in building materials, phosphate fertilizers, and crushed rock; radiation-emitting components of TV sets, smoke detectors, and other consumer products; radioactive fallout from atomic weapons; and nuclear power.

Workers in various occupations are exposed to additional doses of ionizing radiation, depending on their job assignments and working conditions. The average annual effective dose received by monitored radiation workers in the United States is less than 1 mSv, and fewer than 1% approach the maximum permissible dose limit (50 mSv) in any given year.

INCIDENCE, PREVALENCE, AND EPIDEMIOLOGY. Precise data on the frequency of injuries caused by ionizing radiation are not available. Injuries attributable to excessive occupational exposure, although prevalent among radiation workers in the era preceding modern safety standards, are seldom encountered in the United States today. However, tens of thousands of inhabitants had to be evacuated from the surrounding area as a result of the 1986 Chernobyl accident, which caused radiation sickness in more than 200 emergency workers, including 31 fatalities, and released enough radioactivity to result in a collective dose equivalent commitment of 600,000 person-Sv for the population of the northern hemisphere. Less catastrophic but more numerous than reactor accidents have been accidents with medical and industrial γ-ray sources, which are occasionally serious enough to be fatal.

Another public health concern is the larger population risk of cancer from exposure to background ionizing radiation. To date,

however, no definite evidence of such effects has been observed in populations residing in areas of high natural background radiation, and no more than 3% of all cancers in the general population are thought to be attributable to natural background ionizing irradiation, although a larger percentage of lung cancers may be attributable to indoor radon. Also of concern are heritable abnormalities resulting from the mutagenic and clastogenic effects of radiation, which have yet to be observed in humans although they are well documented in other organisms. From the available evidence it is inferred that such effects probably account for less than 1% of all genetically determined disease in the human population.

Prenatal irradiation has been observed in the past to cause death, malformations, cataracts, mental retardation, impairment of growth, and behavioral disorders, depending on the dose and the developmental stage of the embryo at the time of its exposure. Special precautions to avoid exposing the embryo now largely prevent such complications.

PATHOGENESIS. Ionizing radiation colliding randomly with atoms and molecules in its path gives rise to ions and free radicals that break chemical bonds and cause other molecular alterations, ultimately injuring the affected cells. Any molecule may be thus altered, but DNA is the critical biologic target because of the limited redundancy of its genetic information. A dose of radiation large enough to kill the average dividing cell (2 Sv) causes hundreds of lesions in its DNA molecules. Most such lesions are reparable, but those produced by a densely ionizing radiation (e.g., proton or α-particle) are generally less reparable than those produced by a sparsely ionizing radiation (e.g., x-ray or γ-ray).

Unrepaired or misrepaired damage to DNA may be expressed in the form of mutations, the frequency of which approximates 10^{-5} to 10^{-6} per locus per sievert. Because the mutation rate tends to increase in proportion to the dose, it is inferred that a single ionizing particle traversing a genetic target may suffice to cause a mutation. Radiation damage can also cause changes in chromosome number and structure, the yields of which are well enough characterized that their frequency in lymphocytes can serve as a biologic dosimeter.

Radiation damage to genes, chromosomes, and other vital organelles may kill cells, especially dividing cells, which are radiosensitive as a class. Measured in terms of proliferative capacity, the survival of dividing cells tends to decrease exponentially with increasing dose; rapid exposure to 1 to 2 Sv generally reduces the surviving population of such cells by about 50%. Except for lymphocytes and oocytes, which tend to die in interphase, most cells killed by irradiation die in mitosis.

Although the killing of cells is a stochastic process, too few cells are killed by a dose below 0.5 Sv to cause clinically detectable injury in most organs other than the testis and those of the embryo. The killing of dividing progenitor cells, if sufficiently extensive, can interfere with the orderly replacement of senescent cells, especially in tissues such as the epidermis, bone marrow, and intestinal epithelium, which are characterized by a high rate of normal cell turnover. The timing of the resulting atrophy (Fig. 19–2) varies, depending on the cell population dynamics within the tissue in question; in organs such as the liver and vascular endothelium, which are characterized by slow cell turnover, expression of the injury is delayed. If the volume of tissue exposed is small or if the dose is accumulated slowly, the effects of irradiation may be coun-

Table 19–1 ■ RADIATION QUANTITIES AND DOSE UNITS

QUANTITY	DOSE UNIT	DEFINITION
Radioactivity	Becquerel (Bq)	One disintegration per second
Absorbed dose	Gray (Gy)	Energy deposited in tissue (1 J/kg)
Equivalent dose	Sievert (Sv)	Absorbed dose weighted for quality (potency) of the radiation
Effective dose	Sievert (Sv)	Equivalent dose weighted for sensitivity of the exposed organs
Collective effective dose	Person-Sv	Effective dose applied to a population
Committed effective dose	Sievert (Sv)	Effective dose from a given intake of radioactivity to be received over a period extending into the future

Modified from Phillips TL: Radiation injury. In Wyngaarden JB, Smith LH Jr, Bennett JC (eds): Cecil Textbook of Medicine, 19th ed. Philadelphia, WB Saunders, 1992, p 2351.

Table 19–2 ■ AVERAGE AMOUNTS OF IONIZING RADIATION RECEIVED ANNUALLY FROM DIFFERENT SOURCES BY A RESIDENT OF THE UNITED STATES

SOURCE	DOSE*	
	mSv	%
Natural		
Radon†	2.0	55
Cosmic	0.27	8
Terrestrial	0.28	8
Internal	0.39	11
Total natural	2.94	82
Artificial		
X-ray diagnosis	0.39	11
Nuclear medicine	0.14	4
Consumer products	0.10	<0.3
Occupational	<0.01	<0.03
Nuclear fuel cycle	<0.01	<0.03
Nuclear fallout	<0.01	<0.03
Miscellaneous‡	<0.01	<0.03
Total artificial	0.63	18
Total Natural and Artificial	~3.6	100

*Average effective dose.
†Average effective dose to bronchial epithelium.
‡Department of Energy facilities, smelters, transportation, etc.
Modified from Health Effects of Exposure to Low Levels of Ionizing Radiation: BEIR V. Washington, DC, National Academy of Sciences, National Academy Press, 1990.

teracted in part by compensatory regenerative hyperplasia of surviving cells.

CLINICAL MANIFESTATIONS. Ionizing radiation injuries encompass a diversity of tissue reactions that vary markedly in dose-response relationships, manifestations, timing, and prognosis (Table 19–3). Except for mutagenic and carcinogenic effects, the reactions generally result from the killing of sizable numbers of cells in the exposed tissues and are not detectable unless the dose of radiation exceeds a substantial threshold. For this reason, the reactions are called *non-stochastic* (or *deterministic*) effects, in contrast to mutagenic and carcinogenic effects, which are presumed to have no thresholds and are considered to be *stochastic* in nature. The existing data, however, do not exclude the possibility that these effects may have thresholds in the millisievert dose range, and the existence of adaptive responses to radiation (e.g., DNA repair processes) has been interpreted by some observers to support the hypothesis that the net effects of small doses may actually be beneficial ("radiation hormesis").

Tissues in which cells proliferate rapidly are generally the first to exhibit radiation injury. In such tissues, mitotic inhibition and cytologic abnormalities may be detectable immediately after irradiation, whereas ulceration, fibrosis, and other degenerative changes may not appear until months or years later (see Fig. 19–2).

SKIN. After rapid exposure to a dose of 6 Sv or more, erythema typically appears within a day, lasts a few hours, and is followed 2 to 4 weeks later by one or more waves of deeper and more prolonged erythema, as well as epilation. Brief exposure to a dose in excess of 10 to 20 Sv may cause transepithelial injury, with moist desquamation, necrosis, and ulceration within 2 to 4 weeks. The ensuing fibrosis of the underlying dermis and vasculature may lead to atrophy and a second wave of ulceration months or years later.

BONE MARROW AND LYMPHOID TISSUE. A dose of 2 to 3 Sv delivered rapidly to the whole body sufficiently destroys lymphocytes

to depress the lymphocyte count and immune response within hours. Such a dose can also damage enough hematopoietic cells to cause profound leukopenia and thrombocytopenia within 3 to 5 weeks. If the dose exceeds 5 Sv, fatal infection and/or hemorrhage is likely to result (Table 19–4).

INTESTINE. The killing of epithelial stem cells is sufficiently extensive after an acute dose of 10 Sv to cause rapid denudation of the overlying intestinal villi. If the area affected is large, death from a fatal dysentery-like syndrome may ensue within days.

RESPIRATORY TRACT. Rapid exposure of the lung to a dose of 6 to 10 Sv damages alveolar cells and the pulmonary vasculature sufficiently to result in acute pneumonitis within 1 to 3 months. If extensive, the process may lead to fatal respiratory failure within 6 months or pulmonary fibrosis and cor pulmonale months or years later.

GONADS. Spermatozoa are relatively radioresistant, but spermatogonia are highly radiosensitive; that is, a dose of 0.15 Sv delivered rapidly to both testes causes oligospermia after a latent period of about 6 weeks, and a dose of 2 to 4 Sv may cause permanent sterility. Oocytes are also radiosensitive; a dose of 1.5 to 2.0 Sv delivered to both ovaries causes temporary sterility, and a larger dose causes permanent sterility, depending on the woman's age at the time of exposure.

LENS OF THE EYE. Acute exposure of the lens to more than 1 Sv may lead within months to a microscopic posterior polar opacity, and 2 to 3 Sv received in a single brief exposure or 5.5 to 14 Sv accumulated over a period of months may result in a vision-impairing cataract.

OTHER TISSUES AND ORGANS. Other tissues and organs, except for those of the embryo, are relatively less radiosensitive. All tissues, however, are relatively more radiosensitive when rapidly growing.

WHOLE-BODY RADIATION INJURY. Brief exposure of a major part of the body to more than 1 Sv may cause the acute radiation syndrome, which is characterized by (1) an initial prodromal stage of malaise, anorexia, nausea, and vomiting; (2) an ensuing latent period; (3) a second (main) phase of illness; and (4) either recovery or death (see Table 19–4). The main phase of the illness usually takes one of four primary forms: (1) hematologic, (2) gastrointestinal, (3) neurovascular, or (4) pulmonary, depending on the size and anatomic distribution of the dose.

LOCALIZED OR REGIONAL RADIATION INJURY. In contrast to the acute radiation syndrome, manifestations of which are dramatic and relatively prompt, reactions to localized irradiation in most tissues tend to evolve more slowly and to not produce symptoms or signs unless the volume of tissue irradiated and the dose are large. When the injury is produced by a radionuclide, it follows the anatomic distribution of the radionuclide and the resulting radiation, which may be influenced by the physicochemical state in which the radionuclide is encountered as well as its portal of entry into the body.

HERITABLE (GENETIC) EFFECTS OF RADIATION. Radiation-induced heritable mutations and chromosomal abnormalities, although well documented in other organisms, have yet to be observed in humans despite over four decades of intensive study of more than 76,000 children of Japanese atomic bomb survivors, in whom no definite evidence of heritable radiation effects has been detectable in terms of untoward pregnancy outcomes, neonatal deaths, malignancies, balanced chromosomal rearrangements, sex chromosome aneuploidy, alterations in serum or erythrocyte protein phenotypes, changes in gender ratio, or disturbances in growth and development. On the basis of the existing evidence it is inferred that a dose of at least 1.0 Sv is required to double the rate of heritable mutations in human germ cells and that, consequently, less than 1% of all genetically determined disease is attributable to natural background irradiation.

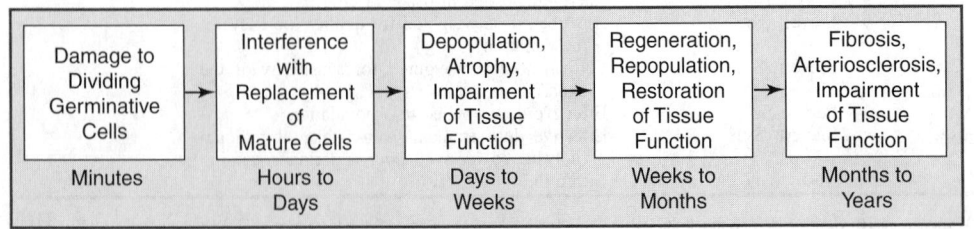

FIGURE 19–2 ■ Characteristic sequence of events in the pathogenesis of the non-stochastic effects of ionizing radiation. (From Upton AC: Radiological science. *In* Detels R, Holland W, McEwen J, Omenn GS [eds]: Oxford Textbook of Public Health, 3rd ed. New York, 1997, by permission of Oxford University Press.)

Table 19–3 ■ ESTIMATED APPROXIMATE THRESHOLD DOSES OF CONVENTIONALLY FRACTIONATED X-RADIATION FOR CLINICALLY DETRIMENTAL EFFECTS IN VARIOUS TISSUES

ORGAN	INJURY AT 5 YEARS	THRESHOLD DOSE (Gy)*	IRRADIATION FIELD (AREA)
Skin	Ulcer, severe fibrosis	55	100 cm²
Oral mucosa	Ulcer, severe fibrosis	60	50 cm²
Esophagus	Ulcer, stricture	60	75 cm²
Stomach	Ulcer, perforation	45	100 cm²
Small intestine	Ulcer, stricture	45	100 cm²
Colon	Ulcer, stricture	45	100 cm²
Rectum	Ulcer, stricture	55	100 cm²
Salivary glands	Xerostomia	50	50 cm²
Liver	Liver failure, ascites	35	Whole
Kidney	Nephrosclerosis	23	Whole
Urinary bladder	Ulcer, contracture	60	Whole
Testis	Permanent sterility	5–15	Whole
Ovary	Permanent sterility	2–3	Whole
Uterus	Necrosis, perforation	>100	Whole
Vagina	Ulcer, fistula	90	5 cm²
Breast, child	Hypoplasia	10	5 cm²
Breast, adult	Atrophy, necrosis	>50	Whole
Lung	Pneumonitis, fibrosis	40	Lobe
Capillaries	Telangiectasia, fibrosis	50–60	—
Heart	Pericarditis, pancarditis	40	Whole
Bone, child	Arrested growth	20	10 cm²
Bone, adult	Necrosis, fracture	60	10 cm²
Cartilage, child	Arrested growth	10	Whole
Cartilage, adult	Necrosis	60	Whole
CNS (brain)	Necrosis	50	5 cm²
Spinal cord	Necrosis, transection	50	Whole
Eye	Panophthalmitis, hemorrhage	55	Whole
Cornea	Keratitis	50	Whole
Lens	Cataract	5	Whole
Ear (inner)	Deafness	>60	Whole
Thyroid	Hypothyroidism	45	Whole
Adrenal	Hypoadrenalism	>60	Whole
Pituitary	Hypopituitarism	45	Whole
Muscle, child	Hypoplasia	20–30	Whole
Muscle, adult	Atrophy	>100	Whole
Bone marrow	Hypoplasia	2	Whole
Bone marrow	Hypoplasia, fibrosis	20	Localized
Lymph nodes	Atrophy	33–45	—
Lymphatics	Sclerosis	50	—
Fetus	Death	2	Whole

*Dose causing effect in 1 to 5% of exposed persons.
From Rubin P, Casarett GW: A direction for clinical radiation pathology: The tolerance dose. *In* Vaeth JM (ed): Frontiers of Radiation Therapy and Oncology. Basel, Karger, 1972; and Nonstochastic effects of ionizing radiation. ICRP Publication 41. Ann ICRP 14:1, 1984, with kind permission from Elsevier Science Ltd, The Boulevard Langford Land, Kidlington OX5 1GB, UK.

CARCINOGENIC EFFECTS OF RADIATION. Many but not all types of benign and malignant growths have been observed as inducible by irradiation. The induced growths characteristically take years or decades to appear and possess no features distinguishable from those arising through other causes. With few exceptions, moreover, they have been detectable only after relatively large doses (>0.5 Sv) and have varied with the type of neoplasm as well as the age and gender of the exposed population. Because the existing data do not suffice to describe the dose-incidence relationship precisely or define how long after irradiation the risk of cancer may remain

Table 19–4 ■ SYMPTOMS, THERAPY, AND PROGNOSIS OF WHOLE-BODY IONIZING RADIATION INJURY

	0–1 Sv	1–2 Sv	2–6 Sv	6–10 Sv	10–20 Sv	>50 Sv
Therapeutic needs	None	Observation	Specific treatment	Possible treatment	Palliative	Palliative
Vomiting	None	5–50%	>3 Gy, 100%	100%	100%	100%
Time to nausea, vomiting	—	3 hr	2 hr	1 hr	30 min	<30 min
Main locus of injury	None	Lymphocytes	Bone marrow	Bone marrow	Small bowel	Brain
Symptoms and signs	—	Moderate leukopenia	Leukopenia, hemorrhage, epilation	Leukopenia, hemorrhage, epilation	Diarrhea, fever, electrolyte imbalance	Ataxia, coma, convulsions
Critical period	—	—	4–6 wk	4–6 wk	5–14 d	1–4 hr
Therapy	Reassurance	Observation	Transfusion of granulocytes, platelets; antibiotics	Transfusion; antibiotics; bone marrow transplant	Fluids and salts; possible bone marrow transplant	Palliative
Prognosis	Excellent	Excellent	Guarded	Guarded	Poor	Hopeless
Lethality	None	None	0–80%	80–100%	100%	100%
Time of death	—	—	2 mo	1–2 mo	2 wk	1–2 d
Cause of death	—	—	Infection, hemorrhage	Hemorrhage, infection; pneumonitis	Enteritis, infection	Cerebral edema

Modified from Phillips TL: Radiation injury. *In* Wyngaarden JB, Smith LH Jr, Bennett JC (eds): Cecil Textbook of Medicine, 19th ed. Philadelphia, WB Saunders, 1992, p 2354.

elevated in an exposed population, assessment of the risks of low-level irradiation must be based on assumptions about these parameters. Such assessments (Table 19–5) have depended heavily on findings in atomic bomb survivors, whose overall incidence of cancer appears to have increased as a linear non-threshold function of their radiation dose. Such estimates cannot be assumed to predict the risk of cancer attributable to a dose accumulated over a period of weeks, months, or years, however, because experiments with laboratory animals have shown the carcinogenic potency of x-rays or γ-rays to decrease by a factor of 2 to 10 if the exposure is sufficiently prolonged.

EFFECTS OF PRENATAL IRRADIATION. The embryo is especially vulnerable to death if exposed before implantation, and it is susceptible to malformations and other developmental disturbances if exposed during subsequent stages in organogenesis. Evidence also suggests that the embryo and fetus are sensitive to the carcinogenic effects of radiation. Among various disturbances in growth and development, the dose-dependent increase in frequency of severe mental retardation and the dose-dependent decrease in IQ test scores in atomic bomb survivors who were irradiated between the 8th and the 15th week and, to a lesser extent, the 16th and the 25th week after conception are particularly noteworthy.

DIAGNOSIS. Any facility likely to deal with radiation injuries should be able to cope with such injuries and should have personnel on call who are appropriately trained and equipped for the purpose. At the outset, to evaluate the dose and to determine whether the patient has been contaminated with radionuclides, the nature of the exposure and any measurements by film badges or other detectors should be reviewed in detail. If exposure to radionuclides is known or suspected, radioactivity measurements of the whole body, skin, other tissue, blood, urine, and/or body fluid may be indicated to identify the isotope(s) and evaluate the dose. Malaise, anorexia, nausea, and vomiting suggest a total-body dose larger than 1 Sv, as do signs of erythema, hemorrhage, or infection in the skin, conjunctivae, or mucous membranes. The depth of lymphopenia within the first 24 hours also varies with the size of the total-body dose. Although the granulocyte count may be temporarily elevated during the first 24 to 48 hours, the rapidity with which it and the platelet count fall in the ensuing 2 to 4 weeks also varies with the total-body dose. Cytogenetic analysis of cultured lymphocytes for chromosomal aberrations can provide another useful index of exposure.

TREATMENT. In managing radiation injury, good medical judgment and first aid come first. Hence even if the patient has been heavily irradiated, the patient should be evaluated for other forms of injury such as burns, mechanical trauma, and smoke inhalation.

Table 19–5 ■ ESTIMATED LIFETIME RISK OF CANCER OF VARIOUS ORGANS ATTRIBUTABLE TO 0.1-Sv RAPID IRRADIATION

TYPE OR SITE OF CANCER	EXCESS CANCER DEATHS PER 100,000	
	No.	%*
Stomach	110	17
Lung	85	2
Colon	85	7
Leukemia (excluding CLL)	50	14
Urinary bladder	30	12
Esophagus	30	8
Breast	20	2
Liver	15	8
Gonads	10	3
Thyroid	8	40
Bone	5	12
Skin	2	30
Remainder	50	1
Total	500	3

CLL = chronic lymphocytic leukemia.
*Per cent increase in the expected risk of death from cancer of the same organ in a non-irradiated population.
Modified from 1990 Recommendations of the International Commission on Radiological Protection. ICRP Publication 60. Ann ICRP 21:3, 1991, with kind permission from Elsevier Science Ltd, The Boulevard Langford Land, Kidlington OX5 1GB, UK.

If radioactive contamination is known or suspected, those handling the patient should wear gloves and other protective clothing and take precautions to isolate all contaminated objects.

Apart from symptomatic treatment, management of the hematologic form of acute radiation syndrome is similar to that used for pancytopenic leukemia, including reverse isolation, antibiotics to combat infection, granulocyte and platelet transfusions as needed, and intravenous fluids as required to combat dehydration and electrolyte loss (see Chapter 177). Colony-stimulating factors and interleukin may be beneficial in patients exposed to 6 to 10 Sv. Bone marrow transplantation (see Chapter 182) may be life saving after a dose of 7 to 10 Sv if a suitably matched donor is available; hence specimens of marrow and peripheral blood for tissue typing should be obtained as early as possible.

For localized injuries, treatment depends on the anatomic location and severity. Dry and moist desquamation of the skin, which are the most common injuries requiring treatment, are usually managed adequately by simple cleansing. Large or ulcerated lesions, on the other hand, should be covered with lanolin and closed dressings that are changed regularly; severe injuries may require resection of necrotic tissue and skin grafting.

In the event of radioactive contamination, steps should be taken to minimize the uptake and retention of isotope. For example, contaminated areas should be rinsed; the mouth, nose, and bronchial tree lavaged; and the gastrointestinal tract purged, if necessary. Additional measures to inhibit the uptake and retention of specific radionuclides may also be indicated.

PROGNOSIS. After a total-body dose of 2 Sv or less, survival is probable with little or no treatment; in the 2- to 10-Sv range, appropriate treatment can afford a high rate of survival. If the injury is localized, the prognosis depends on the nature and severity of the reaction. Although recovery is the rule after minor, acute reactions, delayed reactions tend to be irreversible and progressive.

PREVENTION. Because the mutagenic and carcinogenic effects of ionizing radiation have no thresholds, unnecessary exposure should be avoided and any doses to radiation workers and patients should be kept as low as reasonably achievable, with particular care that they not exceed the relevant maximum permissible doses, such as 50 mSv/year occupational whole-body radiation. Facilities using radiation or radiation sources should be appropriately designed and equipped and should provide specialized training and supervision for all workers who may be occupationally exposed. Because indoor radon accounts for the bulk of the public's exposure to ionizing radiation, measures to limit excessive doses from this source are also warranted.

NON-IONIZING RADIATION

ULTRAVIOLET RADIATION. The ultraviolet (UV) radiation spectrum (see Fig. 19–1) is subdivided, for convenience, into three bands: UVA, or "black light," 400 to 320 nm; UVB, 320 to 280 nm; and UVC, which is germicidal, 280 to 100 nm. UV radiation does not penetrate deeply into human tissues, so the injuries it causes are confined chiefly to the skin and eyes.

ETIOLOGY. The largest source of UV radiation for the public is sunlight, which varies in intensity with latitude, elevation, and season. Important man-made sources include sun and tanning lamps, welding arcs, plasma torches, germicidal and black-light lamps, electric arc furnaces, hot-metal operations, mercury-vapor lamps, and some lasers. Low-intensity sources include fluorescent lamps and certain laboratory equipment.

INCIDENCE AND PREVALENCE. Reactions of the skin to UV radiation, common among fair-skinned people, include sunburn, skin cancers (basal cell and squamous cell carcinomas and to a lesser extent melanomas), aging of the skin, solar elastosis, and solar keratosis. Injuries of the eye include photokeratitis, which may result from brief exposure to a high-intensity UV radiation source ("welder's flash") or more prolonged exposure to intense sunlight ("snow blindness"); cortical cataract; and pterygium.

PATHOGENESIS. The effects of UV radiation are primarily attributable to its absorption in DNA; pyrimidine dimers are produced and cause mutational changes in exposed cells. Sensitivity to UV radiation may be increased by DNA repair defects (as in xeroderma pigmentosum), by agents (e.g., caffeine) that inhibit repair enzymes, and by photosensitizing agents (e.g., psoralens, sulfonamides, tetracyclines, nalidixic acid, sulfonylureas, thiazides, pheno-thiazines, furocoumarins, and coal tar) that produce UV radiation–absorbing DNA photoproducts. The carcinogenic action of UV radiation is mediated through direct effects on the exposed cells and depression of local immunity. UVB in sunlight, although far less intense than UVA, plays a more important role in sunburn and skin carcinogenesis, but UVA also contributes to skin carcinogenesis, tanning, some photosensitivity reactions, and aging of the skin.

CLINICAL ASPECTS. See Parts XXVII (Skin Diseases) and XXVI (Eye Diseases).

PREVENTION. Excessive exposure to sunlight or other sources of UV radiation should be avoided, especially in fair-skinned individuals. Protective clothing, UV radiation–screening lotions or creams, and UV radiation–blocking sunglasses should be used. To protect occupationally exposed workers, the National Institute of Occupational Safety and Health has recommended a limit of 1.0 mW/cm² for periods longer than 1000 seconds and 1000 mW/cm² (1.0 J/cm²) for periods of 1000 seconds or less. Globally, the protective layer of ozone in the stratosphere is being depleted by chlorofluorocarbons and other air pollutants, and every 1% decrease in ozone is expected to increase the UV radiation reaching the earth by 1 to 2% and thereby increase the rates of non-melanotic skin cancer by 2 to 6%.

VISIBLE LIGHT. Visible light consists of electromagnetic waves varying in wavelength from 380 nm (violet) to 760 nm (red) (see Fig. 19–1). Too little illumination can cause eyestrain or seasonal affective disorder, whereas too bright a light can injure the retina.

ETIOLOGY. Bright, continuously visible light normally elicits an aversion response to protect the eye against injury, so few sources of light other than the sun in a solar eclipse are large and bright enough to cause a retinal burn under normal viewing conditions.

PATHOGENESIS. Photochemical reactions in the retina from sustained exposure to intensities exceeding 0.1 mW/cm², such as can result from fixing on a bright source of light, may suffice to produce photochemical blue-light injury, and brief exposure of the retina to intensities exceeding 10 W/cm², depending on image size, may cause a retinal burn.

CLINICAL ASPECTS. See Part XXVI (Eye Diseases).

PREVENTION. Common sense usually suffices to prevent excessive exposure of the retina to light; however, in situations involving potential exposure to high-intensity sources such as carbon arcs or lasers, appropriate training, proper design of equipment, and protective eye shields are important.

INFRARED RADIATION. Infrared radiation consists of electromagnetic waves ranging in wavelength from 7×10^{-5} m to 3×10^{-2} m. The injuries caused by infrared radiation are chiefly burns of the skin and cataracts of the lens of the eye.

ETIOLOGY. Potentially hazardous sources include furnaces, ovens, welding arcs, molten glass, molten metal, and heating lamps.

INCIDENCE AND PREVALENCE. The warning sensation of heat usually prompts aversion in time to prevent burning of the skin by infrared radiation; however, the lens of the eye is vulnerable because it lacks the ability to sense or dissipate heat. As a result, glass blowers, blacksmiths, oven operators, and those working around heating and drying lamps are at increased risk of infrared radiation–induced cataracts.

CLINICAL ASPECTS. See Parts XXVI and XXVII.

PREVENTION. Control of infrared radiation hazards requires appropriate shielding of its sources, training of potentially exposed persons, and use of protective clothing and goggles.

MICROWAVE RADIATION. Microwave and radiofrequency radiation consists of electromagnetic waves ranging in frequency from about 3 kHz to 300 GHz. The injuries caused by microwave and radiofrequency radiation consist primarily of burns of the skin and other tissues. Microwave and radiofrequency radiation can also interfere with cardiac pacemakers and other medical devices.

ETIOLOGY. Sources of microwave and radiofrequency radiation are used widely in radar, television, radio, other telecommunications systems, various industrial operations (e.g., heating, welding, and melting of metals; processing of wood and plastic; high-temperature plasma), household appliances (e.g., microwave ovens), and medical applications (e.g., diathermy and hyperthermia).

INCIDENCE AND PREVALENCE. Isolated cases of skin burns, thermal injury to deeper tissues, and even death from hyperthermia have been caused by industrial microwave and radiofrequency radiation sources. Burns have also resulted from faulty or improperly

used household microwave ovens and from the overexposure of patients with impaired cutaneous pain and temperature senses that usually warn of impending injury. Other effects reported in the literature but as yet inconclusively documented include cataract of the lens, impairment of fertility, developmental disturbances, neurobehavioral abnormalities, depression of immunity, and increased risk of cancer.

PATHOGENESIS. The biologic effects of microwave and radiofrequency radiation are primarily thermal in nature. Because of the deep penetration of these types of radiation, the cutaneous burns they cause tend to involve dermal and subcutaneous tissues and heal slowly.

CLINICAL ASPECTS. See Part XXVII (Skin Diseases).

PREVENTION. Microwave and radiofrequency radiation sources must be properly designed and shielded, and potentially exposed persons, especially those with cardiac pacemakers or other sensitive devices, must be properly trained and supervised. In general, detectable heating of tissue requires microwave and radiofrequency radiation power densities greater than 10 W/cm²; avoidance of such exposure, as prescribed by existing federal standards, suffices to prevent injury.

EXTREMELY LOW-FREQUENCY ELECTROMAGNETIC FIELDS. Extremely low-frequency electromagnetic fields range in frequency from 1 to 3000 Hz, including the 50- to 60-Hz fields associated with alternating currents in electric power distribution systems and appliances. Exposure to such fields is not known to be hazardous, but data suggesting that it may cause reproductive abnormalities and carcinogenic effects have aroused public health concern.

ETIOLOGY. The earth is surrounded by a naturally occurring electromagnetic field ranging in frequency from the low end of the extremely low-frequency region to radiofrequencies that exist briefly as a result of lightning discharges. Localized electromagnetic fields are also generated by electric power lines, transformers, motors, household appliances, video display tubes, and various medical devices, notably nuclear magnetic resonance (NMR) imaging systems. These localized fields are generally stronger than naturally existing ones; for example, electromagnetic field flux densities near common household appliances may range up to 270 mG, as compared with the average value of 0.6 mG for the earth's magnetic field.

INCIDENCE AND PREVALENCE. Exceptionally strong fields may affect electrically active tissues (nerves, neuromusculature, heart) and cardiac pacemakers and may raise body temperature. In addition, conflicting epidemiologic studies have evaluated the possibility that (1) residential exposure of children to weaker electromagnetic fields may increase their risk of leukemia, (2) occupational exposure of male utility workers may increase their risk of brain cancer and leukemia, and (3) chronic exposure of pregnant women through video display tubes may increase their risk of miscarriage and of bearing children with birth defects; none of these links have been established.

PATHOGENESIS. Evaluation of epidemiologic data is complicated by the lack of any known biologic basis for the effects of extremely low-frequency electromagnetic fields on tissue, especially because the 60-Hz currents emanating from normal nerve and muscle activity are far stronger than those attributable to 1- to 10-mG external 60-Hz fields. Such fields have nevertheless been reported to influence ion transport, melatonin secretion, and tumor promotion in some model systems.

PREVENTION. Persons with pacemakers should avoid electromagnetic fields stronger than 0.5 mT, such as exist around transformers, accelerators, NMR systems, and other electric devices; areas containing such fields should be posted with warning signs. Exposure of workers should also be limited, in accordance with natural guidelines.

ULTRASOUND. Although frequently classified with non-ionizing radiation, ultrasound actually consists of mechanical vibrations at inaudibly high frequencies (i.e., >16 kHz) and is not a component of the electromagnetic spectrum. Deleterious effects from prolonged exposure to high-power ultrasound include headache, malaise, tinnitus, vertigo, hypersensitivity to light and sound, and peripheral neuritis. Low-level exposure to ultrasound has not been conclusively shown to cause injury, but the possibility of adverse effects on embryos has been speculated but not documented.

ETIOLOGY. High-power, low-frequency ultrasound is used widely in science and industry for cleaning, degreasing, plastic welding, liquid-extracting, atomizing, homogenizing, and emulsifying operations, as well as in medicine for such applications as lithotripsy. Low-power, high-frequency ultrasound is used widely in analytic work and in medical diagnosis (e.g., ultrasonography).

INCIDENCE AND PREVALENCE. Low-frequency ultrasound, transmitted through the air or through bodily contact with the generating source, has been observed to cause a variety of problems in occupationally exposed workers, including headache, earache, tinnitus, vertigo, malaise, photophobia, hyperacusis, peripheral neuritis, and autonomic polyneuritis. Similar complaints may result from excessive exposure to high-frequency ultrasound through bodily contact with the source; however, adverse effects have not been demonstrated to result from exposure to high-frequency ultrasound at the low power levels used in medical ultrasonography.

PATHOGENESIS. The biologic effects of ultrasound are similar in mechanism to those of mechanical vibration.

PREVENTION. Protection against ultrasound injury requires appropriate isolation and insulation of generating sources, as well as proper training and ear protective devices for those working around such sources. Yearly audiometric and neurologic examinations of such workers are also advisable.

American Conference of Governmental Industrial Hygienists: 1997 Threshold Limit Values and Biological Exposure Indices. Cincinnati, American Conference of Governmental Industrial Hygienists, 1997. *An authoritative listing of recommended maximum permissible occupational exposure limits of radiation of all types.*

Mettler FA, Kelsey CA, Ricks RC: Medical Management of Radiation Accidents. Boca Raton, FL, CRC Press, 1990. *An excellent and comprehensive review of the management of people accidentally exposed to ionizing radiation.*

Mettler FA, Upton AC: Medical Effects of Ionizing Radiation, 2nd ed. Philadelphia, WB Saunders, 1994. *A comprehensive review of the effects of ionizing radiation on human beings.*

National Academy of Sciences/National Research Council: Possible Health Effects of Exposure to Residential Electric and Magnetic Fields. Washington, DC, National Academy Press, 1997. *An authoritative review of the possible health hazards of residential electric and magnetic fields.*

1990 Recommendations of the International Commission on Radiological Protection. ICRP Publication 60. Ann ICRP 21:3, 1991. *An authoritative statement of the principles and procedures for protection against ionizing radiation.*

20 ELECTRICAL INJURY

Cleon W. Goodwin

DEFINITION AND PREVALENCE

Electrical injury is manifested in a variety of forms ranging from cardiopulmonary arrest and minimal tissue damage to devastating electrocution and vaporization of major body parts. Tissue damage is a direct consequence of the flow of electrical current, which causes both thermal tissue damage and electrical breakdown of cell membranes. The extent of injury is proportional to current, voltage, duration of exposure, cellular architecture, and whether the electricity is alternating or direct current. Alternating current, the more common cause of electrical injury, is more dangerous than direct current because it can produce tonic muscle contractions and the victim may be unable to release the source of electricity. Furthermore, cardiac arrest and coma frequently accompany electrocution with alternating current, and these events are most likely to occur at current frequencies of 50 to 60 cycles per second. As frequency increases above 60 cycles per second, tissue damage and the risk of cardiac arrest decrease. Tissue damage caused by line voltages less than 1000 V is arbitrarily designated low-voltage injury. High-tension electrical injury is caused by line voltages greater than 1000 V.

Electricity causes injury by four mechanisms: direct contact, conduction, arc, and secondary ignition. Low-voltage electrical sources

produce direct injury at the point of contact. Skin and subcutaneous tissue are involved most commonly, although occasionally muscle and bone beneath the cutaneous burn may be damaged. High-voltage current not only causes direct injury at the point of contact but also damages tissues that conduct the electricity through the body. Arc burns occur without the source of electricity actually contacting the body surface. Very high voltages are required to produce charge transfer, and when arcing occurs, extremely high temperatures (3000° C) are produced. The duration of the arc is brief, and the "flash" injury produced is usually limited to the body surface. A variant of arc injury occurs when electrical current being conducted along a body part surfaces and flashes over into the axilla and other flexion creases. Finally, burns occur when the electrical source ignites clothing and other flammable materials. Very deep flame burns may occur, especially if the patient is unconscious. The victim may not be able to verify the actual circumstances, so evaluation and management must assume that diverse multisystem effects of electrical injury may be present.

In an adult, electrical burns are occupational hazards. However, in recent years the increasing number of electrical injuries reflects the technologic sophistication of society. Sport parachuting, hot air ballooning, and installation of home radio and television antennas have become common causes of electrical injuries. In urban environments, electric-powered mass transit conduits are one of the most common sources of such injuries. Household appliances cause most electrical injuries in children. Lightning injury affects all age groups, especially in rural areas. Electrical injuries represent 1 to 5% of burn center admissions and up to 15% of deaths.

PATHOGENESIS

Meticulous laboratory investigations have verified that tissue damage associated with electrical injury occurs when electrical energy is converted to thermal energy and causes joule heating of tissue. The resulting injury is a thermal burn that produces physiologic responses similar to those caused by other mechanisms of thermal injury. Skin represents the initial barrier to current flow and is an effective insulator for deeper tissues. After electrical contact and the onset of current flow, the skin undergoes coagulation necrosis and desiccates. With low-voltage injuries, the charred skin at the point of contact terminates current flow and limits the extent of injury. The skin surrounding the contact point may sustain an arc burn as the increase in skin resistance terminates current flow (Fig. 20–1). At high voltages (>1000 V), skin resistance is initially overcome and current flow through deep tissue in the body is relatively unimpeded. Except for bone, these internal tissues act as a volume conductor offering little resistance to flow. Current flow is terminated when the tissue at the point of electrical contact desiccates and resistance increases markedly. At this point, electrical arcing frequently occurs. The charred tissue then acts as an electrical insulator. Deep tissue damage is related to the density of

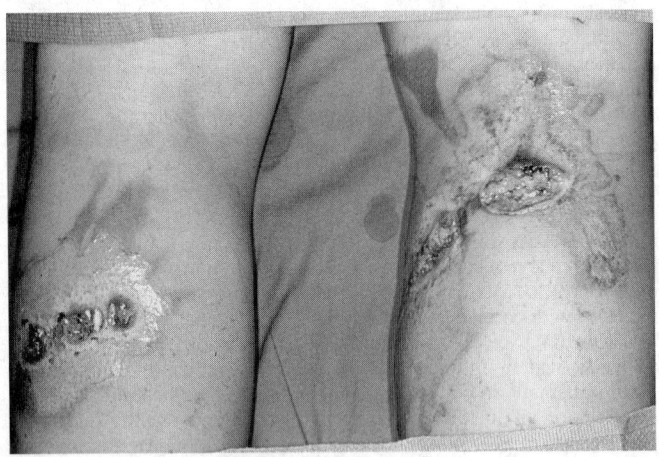

FIGURE 20–1 ■ Charring of the skin of both calves indicates points of contact with a high-voltage electrical current. These contact points are surrounded by full-thickness cutaneous burns caused by arcing of current. The extent of deep tissue destruction is often not related to the size of the cutaneous manifestations of the injury.

current flow through these tissues. Heat production and hence thermal injury depend on the density of current flow. In body parts with small cross-sectional areas such as an extremity, current density is high and tissue destruction is severe. In large cross-sectional areas such as the trunk, current density is reduced and deep injuries are unusual. Superficial tissues cool faster than deep tissues. Because bone has high resistance to current flow, it heats to higher temperatures than the surrounding soft tissue does. As a result, the most severely damaged soft tissues are usually muscle and nerves directly adjacent to bone, a position almost impervious to clinical detection. The most severe cutaneous and deep injuries are adjacent to contact sites, and damage decreases with increasing distance from contact points.

Recent investigations strongly suggest that in addition to joule heating of tissue, direct effects of electricity on the electrical and architectural properties of cell membranes are responsible for much of the resulting tissue damage, especially during the early phase of current flow. Experimental studies have shown that rhabdomyolysis and neurolysis may occur after electrical contact associated with only small increases in tissue temperature.

The extent of tissue injury appears to be determined at the time of electrical contact. Progressive soft tissue injury probably does not occur despite the clinical observation that muscle that seems to be viable immediately after electrical injury appears necrotic several days later. In addition, electrical energy may cause lesser degrees of damage without producing coagulation necrosis. This phenomenon may explain the transient abnormalities of visceral organ function that follow electrical injury. In the heart, this minor damage may have disastrous consequences. Electrically injured patients who experience fatal cardiac arrest demonstrate focal necrosis of the myocardium and the specialized tissue of the sinus and atrioventricular nodes, as well as contraction band necrosis of the smooth muscle cells of the coronary arteries.

CLINICAL MANIFESTATIONS

High-voltage electrical injuries commonly involve multiple organ systems and dictate treatment in specialized burn centers with broad multidisciplinary capabilities. Many of the abnormalities produced by electrocution may not be reflected by the surface appearance of the electrical burn but may become clinically apparent at any time during hospitalization. Consequently, meticulous serial examination and documentation of electrically injured patients are necessary both for medical and legal assessment and for planning.

CARDIOPULMONARY ARREST. Cardiopulmonary arrest is common in patients with high-voltage electrical injuries, particularly lightning injury. Arrhythmias, conduction disturbances, and infarct patterns may be present on the admission electrocardiogram. Most arrhythmias are transitory, whereas conduction delays and infarct patterns are likely to be permanent. In the few patients who have undergone long-term cardiac function studies and angiography, these permanent electrocardiographic findings do not appear to represent physiologic abnormalities.

BURN WOUND. In patients who survive to be admitted to the hospital, the electrical burn itself becomes a major focus of treatment. Most high-voltage electrical injuries are characterized by

contact burns at locations where the electrical current has entered or left the body. These contact burns are typically charred and excavated, and deeper anatomic structures may be visible in the depths of the wound (Fig. 20–2). Contrary to popular notions, these contact wounds have no unique characteristics that identify them as so-called entrance or exit sites. These contact areas are usually surrounded by less severe burns of variable depth. If ignition of clothing has occurred, the patient may have extensive cutaneous burns unrelated to the site of electrical contact.

Underlying injury to major muscle compartments is accompanied by edema formation, which may be accentuated by concomitant fluid resuscitation. When the tissue pressure beneath this muscle fascia increases, signs of vessel and nerve compression appear. Loss of sensation, pain, and decreased pulses indicate the presence of a compartment syndrome. Palpation often demonstrates tense muscle compartments, especially when the affected extremity is compared with an opposite unburned extremity. Even with good blood flow, the burned extremity may be cool to touch and have no palpable pulse. Therefore, circulatory integrity is best judged by Doppler ultrasonography of distal pulses. Compartment pressure can be measured directly, and pressures greater than 30 to 40 mm Hg are associated with tissue damage.

ACUTE RENAL FAILURE. Acute renal failure manifested as early oliguria or anuria is not uncommon after electrical injury and is caused by two mechanisms. First, gross underestimation of the extent of injury and fluid resuscitation requirements rapidly leads to hypovolemia and oliguria. In many patients the majority of severely damaged tissue is muscle that is hidden from view, and the need for fluid replacement may not be appreciated immediately. Second, necrotic muscle releases myoglobin, which is directly toxic to renal tubular cells. Hypovolemia potentiates the toxicity of myoglobin in the tubules unless high urine flow is maintained (see Chapter 99). Visible myoglobinuria indicates massive acute muscle necrosis and impending renal failure. Life-threatening electrolyte abnormalities often accompany massive muscle injury and myoglobinuria.

NERVOUS SYSTEM. The electrical injury may involve both the central and the peripheral nervous system. A thorough neurologic examination on admission is essential; because of the delayed appearance of many neurologic complications, serial examination should continue throughout the hospitalization. Both normal and abnormal function should be documented. Because extremities sustain the majority of direct electrical injuries, associated peripheral nerves are most often damaged at the time of contact. Such injuries are usually permanent and may determine the ultimate salvageability of the extremity. Some patients may also have signs of peripheral neuropathy in locations anatomically distant from the sites of electrical injury. The mechanism responsible is not known, but fortunately these deficits are usually reversible. Motor involvement is more common than sensory abnormalities. Several days to weeks after an electrical injury, a polyneuritis syndrome may affect nerves away from the sites of surface injury. Associated deficits may only partially resolve. Immediate signs of spinal cord symptoms tend to be temporary and readily reversible. Spinal cord injuries of delayed

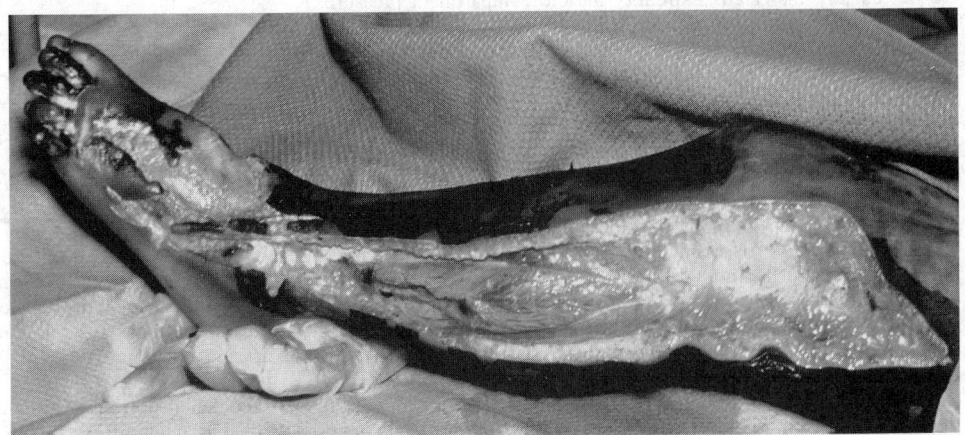

FIGURE 20–2 ■ This severely burned lower extremity had no evidence of arterial circulation. Fasciotomy incisions were placed along the mid-medial and mid-lateral planes to decompress all muscle compartments. The incisional margins have separated because of massive edema in the proximal region of the incision. Necrotic muscle with overlying vessel thrombosis is seen distally. After the patient was stabilized, exploration and débridement were carried out in the operating room.

onset are more often permanent or only partially reversible and are manifested as transverse myelitis, ascending paralysis, hemiplegia, or related syndromes.

FRACTURES. Early evaluation should include assessment for skeletal trauma. Long-bone fractures frequently accompany falls, and fractures of the vertebral column may be produced by tetanic contraction of the paraspinous muscle at the time of electrocution. Both types of fractures can be identified on appropriate radiographs.

INTERNAL ORGANS. Electrical injuries to the major viscera most commonly occur when the body wall overlying an organ is in direct contact with the electrical current. Otherwise, the volume of the torso is large by comparison with the extremities and allows the electrical current to be distributed over a large cross-sectional area at relatively low resistance. As a result, direct injury to internal organs rarely occurs. Dysfunction of the liver, pancreas, and gut may occur during hospitalization but usually reflects the patient's underlying condition rather than the unique effects of electrical injury.

TREATMENT

CARDIOPULMONARY RESUSCITATION. Cardiopulmonary arrest is common after electrical injury, and resuscitative efforts should be instituted immediately. Patients in whom cardiac arrest has occurred frequently respond to cardiopulmonary resuscitation (see Chapters 53 and 93), particularly after lightning injury. Cardiac monitoring or telemetry is advisable for 48 hours in all patients, and continued monitoring is needed only if arrhythmias persist. The choice of antiarrhythmic agent is dictated by the nature of the rhythm disturbance. All persistent electrocardiographic alterations should receive thorough cardiologic investigation once the acute electrical injury has healed.

FLUID THERAPY. As with any other tissue injury, fluid loss into damaged tissue is one of the major physiologic derangements after electrical burns. Intravascular volume is replenished with lactated Ringer's solution sufficient to maintain a urinary output of 50 to 75 mL/hour. If the patient has grossly visible myoglobinuria, urinary output should be increased to 100 to 150 mL/hour by raising the fluid infusion rate. The increased urine production facilitates dilution of myoglobin and its washout from renal tubules. If myoglobinuria is severe or urinary output remains low despite an increased rate of fluid administration, mannitol (12.5 g) should be added to each liter of lactated Ringer's solution. Adding sodium bicarbonate to the resuscitation solution alkalinizes the urine and also increases the solubility and hence excretion of myoglobin.

WOUND MANAGEMENT. Wound care involves treating both the cutaneous and deep soft tissue injuries. Immediately after electrical injury, second- and third-degree cutaneous wounds should be débrided, cleansed, and treated with topical antimicrobial burn creams. Mafenide acetate (Sulfamylon) is preferred for electrical injuries because of its superior ability to penetrate deeply injured tissue and its anticlostridial properties. Tetanus immunization should be updated as needed (see Chapter 15). Prophylactic antibiotics have not been shown to decrease episodes of infection and are not usually indicated. Extremity muscle compartment pressures should be monitored by physical palpation and by Doppler ultrasonography of major arterial pulses. Tissue manometry using needle-tipped transducers appears to reflect compartmental pressures, and measurements greater than 30 to 40 mm Hg are indications for surgical decompression. If the extremity has been injured by a circumferential third-degree burn, escharotomy should be performed. If the compartment symptoms persist, fasciotomy involving all major compartments is indicated, usually in an operating room. Although fasciotomy may allow preservation of nutrient blood flow to potentially viable tissue, it is likely that the ultimate extent of the tissue damage has already been determined at the time of the electrical injury and progressive tissue loss seldom occurs.

Dead tissue promotes infection, which may be life-threatening, and definitive treatment of electrical burns is directed toward the timely removal of necrotic tissue; however, amputation of electrically injured extremities is not always required. Technetium-99m pyrophosphate scintigraphy is the most common diagnostic technique used within the first 24 hours to define viable as compared with non-viable tissue in wounds whose surface appearance may not reflect deeper injuries. Normal isotopic uptake reflects normal perfusion, whereas totally non-viable tissue exhibits no uptake. Areas of potentially reversible injury demonstrate increased isotope uptake, and serial scanning may be useful in determining the need for débridement. In extremities with intact flow of the major arteries, arteriography may be helpful. Truncation of flow to nutrient muscle branches indicates irreversible injury. Finally, the viability of deep tissue is determined most accurately by serial surgical exploration of the injured extremity.

The timing of surgical intervention and the extent of débridement are determined by the stability of the patient and the nature of the burn wound. Generally, initial exploration and débridement may commence at the end of the resuscitation phase, within 24 to 48 hours of injury. Distal portions of electrocuted extremities that are desiccated and mummified should be amputated. More proximally, it may be impossible to determine grossly the extent of deep tissue injury. These areas should be thoroughly explored via fasciotomy incisions if previously placed. All muscle groups should be inspected, especially those against bone. Only obviously necrotic tissue is removed, and every attempt should be made to salvage viable tissue. This approach requires daily wound examination and sequential operative débridement until all necrotic tissue is removed. Intervening complications such as intractable hyperkalemia, severe myoglobinuria, or infection may force abandonment of this sequential approach and necessitate urgent amputation at a relatively high level. It is rarely advisable to proceed to early closure after amputation, and definitive closure of the débrided wound is performed only when all necrotic tissue has been removed. Similarly, excising or grafting full-thickness cutaneous burns may be delayed until this time. Long-term care requires multidisciplinary rehabilitation and prosthetic services.

LATE COMPLICATIONS

A number of apparently related late complications that occur a few months to several years after injury may develop in patients sustaining electrical injuries. As with cutaneous burns, post-traumatic stress disorders develop in more than half of electrically injured patients, especially if a body part has been lost. Associated psychiatric symptoms respond well to psychotherapy and medication. Contractures require extensive rehabilitative care and reconstructive surgery. Cholelithiasis occurs with increased frequency in patients who have sustained electrical burns. Cataracts are particularly troublesome and occur in up to 6% of electrically injured patients. The physical examination performed on admission of such patients should include a careful ophthalmologic evaluation to identify pre-existing cataracts. Although vision loss may be extensive, surgical correction is highly effective.

Centers for Disease Control and Prevention: Lightning-associated deaths—United States, 1980–1995. MMWR 47:391, 1998.
Lee RC: Injury by electrical forces: Pathophysiology, manifestations, and therapy. Curr Probl Surg 34:677, 1997.
Leikin JB, Aks SE, Andrews S, et al: Environmental injuries. Dis Mon 43:809, 1997.

21 CHRONIC POISONING: TRACE METALS AND OTHERS

William O. Robertson

DEFINITION. Our chemical environment was recognized as a threat to health early in history. Well-documented outbreaks of occupational mercury and lead "poisonings" had been recorded and preventive measures implemented by 200 BC. In the Middle Ages, arsenic poisoning was used as a political weapon. In more recent times, we have seen increasing recognition of industrial toxins, "accidental poisoning" in childhood, purposeful overdoses in adults, adverse reactions to drugs, medication mixups in hospitals, and environmental hazards for us all. The common theme is that the patient's metabolic and genetic variability determine the impact of a given molecule in such hereditary disorders as phenylketonuria, glucose-6-phosphate dehydrogenase deficiency, and others. As our understanding of life has expanded, the connotation of poisoning has undergone substantial evolution.

ETIOLOGY. New analytical techniques can promptly and completely identify poisonings and have uncovered the causes of such diverse entities as Minamata disease (teratogenesis consequent to methyl mercury), an outbreak of ascending paralysis affecting more than 4000 with more than 400 deaths in Iraq (also caused by methyl mercury), the "gray syndrome" in premature infants (caused by chloramphenicol), mesotheliomas induced by asbestos, and an epidemic of angiosarcoma of the liver among industrial workers (caused by vinyl chloride). Nevertheless, many unknowns remain and justify careful prospective monitoring of industry, of the home, and of the environment. Unfortunately, the combination of more "synthetic chemicals," vastly more precise testing techniques, a press far more devoted to Rachel Carson's *Silent Spring* than to DuPont's "better living through chemistry," and an increasingly litigious society has created an era of "toxic torts" and its consequences, plus a very anxious and concerned public and profession.

Many metals and non-metals in trace amounts are capable of causing human disease, especially after chronic or repetitive exposure. In some cases, poisoning is a consequence of workplace exposure. In others, the disease results from using prescription or non-prescription medicines or as an adverse effect of medical procedures such as hemodialysis. Occasionally, such poisoning results from attempts at suicide or homicide.

Over the past few decades, increased awareness of the health consequences of industrial substances, more stringent federal and state regulations, and fear of lawsuits have resulted in a healthier workplace. However, the majority of the potentially exposed work force is employed by small industries that may not have implemented protective measures.

Knowledge of the subtle consequences of chronic, low-level trace element exposure is still grossly inadequate. For example, acute lead poisoning in children or adults is readily diagnosed, but the consequences of increased body lead burdens in the absence of the anemia, colic, or clinically apparent encephalopathy and its clinical significance, if any, is not well understood.

The interrelationships among trace elements are also poorly understood. For example, copper smelter workers are exposed not only to copper but also to lead, zinc, arsenic, gold, silver, cadmium, and mercury; in these workers, pneumonitis or other acute illnesses may result from two or more metals acting in concert. In other instances, excesses or deficits of a trace element may act indirectly by inducing deficiency or toxicity of another trace element.

LEAD

ETIOLOGY. In the past, lead poisoning was ascribed to pica (abnormal ingestion) among children living in dilapidated houses with peeling layers of lead-based paints. In the past two decades lead intoxication has occurred with decreasing frequency, in part related to less use of lead in paint and leaded gasoline. Several studies relate environmental lead contamination to traffic density patterns, with leaded gasoline the major culprit.

It is estimated that more than 800,000 American workers have potentially significant lead exposure. Lead and other metal smelter workers or miners, welders, storage battery workers, and pottery makers are particularly heavily exposed. Workers in auto manufacturing, ship building, paint manufacture, and printing industries are also at substantial risk, as are house painters and those who repair old houses.

Lead-soldered kettles and cans and lead-glazed pottery can release lead when acidic fluids are stored or cooked in them. Demolition workers and those employed in firing ranges have become poisoned from intensive aerosol exposure. In the southern United States, moonshine whiskey is an important cause of poisoning. The stills are connected with lead solder, and old radiators containing lead are used as condensers; 20 to 90% of moonshine samples contain lead in the potentially toxic range.

In past centuries, lead acetate was added to wine to sweeten it, a deception that was eventually made punishable by death. Recently, adding lead to various herbal and folk medicines has resulted in poisoning. Retained bullets can result in lead poisoning, especially if a joint is involved, because synovial fluid appears to be a good solvent for lead. The interval between lodging of the bullet and clinical evidence of lead poisoning has ranged from 2 days to 40 years. Lead poisoning has also occurred in adults who have eaten fowl and inadvertently ingested lead pellets. Children have been poisoned by swallowing lead household objects, such as lead curtain weights, that are then retained in the gastrointestinal tract for a prolonged time. Gasoline sniffing can produce lead poisoning; the organic tetraethyl lead appears to have a proclivity for the nervous system.

In a sense we are all lead poisoned; before the Industrial Revolution, the total body burden of lead was about 2 mg, whereas currently in industrialized societies, the whole-body content is about 200 mg. Each day, an average of 150 to 250 μg is ingested, 5 to 10% of which is absorbed. In children, the percentage is even higher.

CLINICAL MANIFESTATIONS. The major toxic effects of lead are referable to the abdomen, the blood, and the nervous system.

GASTROINTESTINAL TRACT. The exact pathogenesis of lead colic remains uncertain. The crampy, diffuse, often intractable abdominal pain may be accompanied by nausea, vomiting, anorexia, constipation, or occasionally diarrhea. The pain may be confined to the epigastric, periumbilical, or other areas of the abdomen and may simulate a variety of surgical and non-surgical diseases.

BLOOD. Lead interferes with a variety of red cell enzyme systems, including δ-aminolevulinic acid dehydratase and ferrochelatase. The former is needed to conjugate levulinic acid to form porphobilinogen; the latter facilitates the incorporation of iron into protoporphyrin IX. The red cell abnormalities include punctate basophilic stippling. Anemia is frequent in severe acute lead poisoning and may be normocytic normochromic but usually is microcytic hypochromic. Moreover, an inherited deficiency in δ-aminolevulinic acid dehydratase can cause lead intoxication at modest blood lead levels.

NERVOUS SYSTEM. The central nervous system (CNS) symptoms at first are vague and are often mistakenly disregarded. These manifestations include irritability, incoordination, memory lapses, labile affect, sleep disturbances, restlessness, listlessness, paranoia, headache, lethargy, and dizziness. In more serious cases, manifestations include syncope-like attacks, disorientation, flaccidity, severe mental impairment, ataxia, vomiting, cranial nerve palsies, localized neurologic signs, psychosis, somnolence, seizures, blindness, and coma. Severe lead encephalopathy is not restricted to children. Occasionally, the brain manifestations mimic a space-occupying lesion. The cerebrospinal fluid may be under increased pressure and may show an increased protein content. Papilledema has been reported, as have grayish deposits surrounding the optic disc and optic atrophy. Frank encephalopathy is an ominous prognostic sign for both mortality and persistent brain damage. Most children who experience two or more bouts of clinically evident encephalopathy have neurologic residua. Tetraethyl lead (organic lead) poisoning causes euphoria, nervousness, insomnia, hallucinations, convulsions, and frank psychosis.

Peripheral nerve involvement is seen more often in adults than in children. Wristdrop and footdrop occur most often; the former, depending on type of occupation, may be asymmetric, and there may be paresthesias. The spinal cord may also be involved, with manifestations having some similarity to those of amyotrophic lateral sclerosis.

Over the past generation, increasing evidence has arisen of subtle brain damage in the absence of clinical evidence of encephalopathy. Inordinate body burdens of lead may result in mentation difficulties, emotional lability, deficits in intelligence and memory, impaired psychomotor and visual motor function, slowed nerve conduction, and behavioral aberrations in both children and adults, even in the absence of overt evidence of poisoning. These changes are postulated to occur at blood levels of 40 μg/dL (or even less in young children). However, the scientific community is sharply divided about the clinical significance of these observations.

OTHER CLINICAL MANIFESTATIONS. In adults, the kidneys are often involved (see Chapter 107), the characteristic lesion being interstitial nephritis; as the disease progresses, glomerular filtration rate falls. Polyarthralgias, mild hepatic dysfunction, and dysuria may also occur. Occasionally, arrhythmias and cardiomegaly have been reported, as have abnormalities of liver function. Lead readily crosses the placenta and is thought to be responsible for an increased incidence of spontaneous abortion and miscarriage and possibly for impairing the fetal CNS.

DIAGNOSIS. In the adult, a high index of suspicion and a careful examination of the peripheral blood for basophilic stippling are mandatory; for occupational workers, lead screening is warranted. Blood lead levels are readily determined by atomic absorption spectrophotometry or anodic stripping voltometry. Urinary coproporphyrin levels are increased because lead interferes with incorporation of iron into heme. Erythrocyte protoporphyrin (EP) can be measured rapidly fluorometrically; both EP and zinc protoporphyrin (ZPP) are reliable indicators of lead poisoning but are also elevated in iron-deficiency anemia. Table 21–1 lists some indications of undue lead absorption.

Additional industrial exposure should not be permitted if blood levels exceed 25 to 40 $\mu g/dL$. Currently, 26 states have lead registries to monitor all lead analytic determinations in the state in an attempt to curtail problems.

TREATMENT. Three agents have been used to form tight complexes with lead and thus promote its biologic inactivation and elimination from tissues (Table 21–2). Dimercaprol (British antilewisite, BAL) is given in oil intramuscularly; calcium disodium edetate (calcium versenate) can be given either intramuscularly or intravenously; and D-pencillamine is administered by mouth. Chelation should be undertaken only after careful consideration for those with milder evidence of poisoning, because each of the agents may be associated with significant adverse effects. Because most of the body lead is stored in the bones, clinical improvement and reduction in blood lead levels (or reduction in EP or ZPP) may be temporary, to be followed by increases in blood lead concentrations and clinical evidence of repoisoning owing to mobilization of lead from bone. In such cases, chelating agents may need to be readministered. Newer, less toxic oral dimercaprol analogues dimercaptosuccinic acid and dimercaptopropanesulfonate have been introduced with the hope of enhancing efficacy and reducing complications.

Treatment is ordinarily successful in extra-CNS disease but may not be so in patients with encephalopathy. Various degrees of mentation deficits may remain in both children and adults.

Although the Centers for Disease Control and Prevention (CDC) has said the acceptable blood concentration of lead for children is 10 $\mu g/dL$, debate continues to rage about that specific number. Blood lead levels have fallen dramatically in the United States (and some other countries) in the past 25 years, but no measurable increase in IQ has followed; if anything, hyperactivity, aggressiveness, and antisocial behavior have all increased.

MERCURY

ETIOLOGY. Mercury has been used for at least 2000 years. More than 60 occupations involve mercury exposure, including chloralkali work; manufacture of pesticides, insecticides, and fungicides; manufacture of mercury-containing instruments, lamps, neon lights, batteries, paper, paint, dye, electrical equipment, and jewelry; and dentistry. Exposure in dental offices has diminished substantially in recent years, however.

In addition to occupational or industrial exposure, poisoning has resulted from inadvertent contamination of grains by mercury-containing pesticides as well as from accidental or intentional ingestion

Table 21–1 ■ POSITIVE SCREENING TESTS INDICATING UNDUE LEAD ABSORPTION

Whole-blood lead	Children	>10 $\mu g/dL$
	Adults	>30 $\mu g/dL$
Whole-blood erythrocyte protoporphyrin or zinc protoporphyrin	Children	>35 $\mu g/dL$*
	Adults	>50 $\mu g/dL$

*This value is unsettled.

Table 21–2 ■ CHELATION REGIMENS

	CHILDREN*	ADULTS*	DURATION
CaNa$_2$ EDTA	50 mg/kg/d IM† or IV, or 1500 mg/m²/24 hr (severe disease); 1000 mg/m²/d (mild-moderate intoxication)	1.0 g IV in 5% dextrose twice daily, or 2.0 g/d IM in divided doses; longer term, 1 g IM 3 × per week† until lead burden reduced to satisfactory levels	3 to 5 days
BAL	3 mg/kg/dose IM, or 300–450 mg/m²/24 hr IM (Given in divided doses every 4 hr)	2.5 mg/kg/dose IM	3 to 5 days
Penicillamine	30 mg/kg/d PO	1.0–1.5 g/d PO	Until blood lead and FEP‡ levels approach normal§
2,3-Dimercaptosuccinic acid (DMSA)‖	10 mg/kg tid for 5 days 10 mg/kg then bid for 14 days		

*CaNa$_2$ EDTA and BAL are ordinarily used together for symptomatic illness.
†Procaine must be used for IM injections of CaNa$_2$ EDTA.
‡FEP = free erythrocyte protoporphyrin.
§Must be monitored carefully because toxicity occurs in up to 20% of cases.
‖Orphan drug approved only for children.

or injection of elemental mercury or mercury-containing compounds. In the past, mercury was administered medicinally as a component of cathartics, teething powders, and antihelminthics. Today, mercury compounds have no bonafide place in therapeutic medicine.

CLINICAL MANIFESTATIONS AND TREATMENT. The biologic effects, tissue distribution, and toxicity of mercury depend on the form in which it is introduced into the body.

METALLIC MERCURY. Elemental mercury is a liquid at environmental temperatures but vaporizes with agitation as well as gentle heating. Bulk mercury is used in dental amalgams; up to 10% of dental offices have excessive mercury vapor levels; and accidental spillage can lead to mercury poisoning. The greatest exposure to metallic mercury is in industry. Heavy aerosol exposure to mercury produces chills, fever, cough, chest pain, and hemoptysis; roentgenograms show diffuse pulmonary infiltrates. Oxidized elemental mercury is readily absorbed from the alveoli; subsequently it can enter the brain. With mild exposure, the manifestations are likely to be subtle and diagnosis is difficult. Insomnia, nervousness, mild tremor, impaired judgment and coordination, decreased mental efficiency, emotional lability, headache, fatigue, loss of sexual drive, and depression are early manifestations and are often mistakenly ascribed to psychogenic causes. Abdominal cramps, dermatitis, and diarrhea may also occur, and the victim may complain of a metallic taste. As the poisoning becomes more severe, persistent involuntary tremors of the extremities are noted. Thereafter, other signs of mercury poisoning may appear, including amblyopia, polyneuropathy, erythroderma, acrodynia, joint pains, swollen gums with a blue line around the teeth, sialorrhea, and paresthesias. The major manifestation of chronic mercury vapor exposure may be renal damage, including the nephrotic syndrome. The wide range of clinical findings after elemental mercury exposure appears to relate in part to the rate of oxidation of mercury to its salts and the rapidity of their subsequent excretion through the kidneys, saliva, and urine.

Because the body's metabolism of mercury, blood and urine levels may be unreliable and clear evidence of poisoning may be documented only after administering drugs that augment mercury excretion in the urine. In most cases, improvement occurs after removal from exposure or treatment with appropriate chelating agents.

In contrast, ingesting even large amounts of metallic mercury usually produces no clinical disturbance. Aspiration of liquid mercury into the lungs is also usually benign, although roentgenologic visualization of mercury globules may be evident for many years. Even after intravenous injection of mercury, there may be no abnormalities other than roentgenologic densities in the lungs or subcutaneous tissue or mild respiratory distress.

INORGANIC MERCURY. Exposure to the salts of mercury (i.e., $HgCl_2$ and Hg_2Cl_2) occurs primarily in industry and results from ingestion. $HgCl_2$ is far more toxic than Hg_2Cl_2. The major manifestations are gastrointestinal and renal, with proteinuria, granular casts in the urinary sediment, the nephrotic syndrome, and pyuria from tubular damage. In some cases, severe oliguria and even anuria may occur. Additionally, diarrhea, abdominal pain, hepatic dysfunction, and lesser evidence of CNS disease may be found. Rhabdomyolysis with striking muscle enzyme elevation and acrodynia have also been reported.

ORGANOMERCURIALS. Methyl mercury—a devastating teratogen found in fungicides—is well absorbed from the intestinal tract, is widely distributed in the body, and readily passes through the placenta into the fetus and also into breast milk. About 10% localizes in the brain, and the ensuing damage is largely irreversible. Major epidemics have resulted from industrial contamination of water, with subsequent biotransformation of elemental and inorganic mercury into methyl mercury that was ingested by fish who were subsequently consumed by humans. Other epidemics have resulted from using grains contaminated by organic mercurial pesticides or animal ingestion of seeds treated with mercury. The epidemics in the Minamata and Niigata regions of Japan and in Iraq, Guatemala, Pakistan, and the United States have resulted in a high death rate and an appalling amount of permanent brain damage. In addition to the milder symptoms listed under elemental mercury poisoning, CNS manifestations include severe paresthesias, dysarthria, ataxia, visual field constriction, hearing loss, blindness, microcephaly, spasticity, paralysis, and coma.

ARSENIC

ETIOLOGY. Arsenic is ubiquitous in nature; it is present in the earth's crust in concentrations of 2 to 5 parts per billion. It is found in inordinately high concentrations in some well water. It is used in the glass, pigment, textile, tanning, and bronze-plating industries; in wood preservation; in a variety of metal alloys; in veterinary medicines; in some herbicides, insecticides, and rodenticides; in fire salts to produce multicolored flames; and by farmers and vintners. American industry uses about one half of the world's production of arsenic trioxide. Arsenic poisoning has also resulted from using certain herbal preparations, from ingesting illegal (moonshine) whiskey, from burning arsenate-treated wood, and from administering arsenic-containing folk and prescription medicines.

Elemental arsenic is not toxic even if ingested in substantial amounts. There are three toxic forms of arsenic: pentavalent salts, trivalent salts, and arsine gas. The arsenic in the earth's crust and in most foods is in the pentavalent form, the least toxic form. Trivalent arsenic, which is more toxic, accumulates in the body more readily than the pentavalent form. Arsenic gas (arsine) is extraordinarily toxic; it is formed by the hydrolysis of metallic arsenide or by the action of acids or nascent hydrogen on arsenical compounds, especially in the refining of certain metals. Arsine is used in the electronics industry and can be liberated in sewage plants.

CLINICAL MANIFESTATIONS. *Arsine gas* poisoning is usually overwhelming and frequently fatal. The onset of symptoms after exposure is usually between 1 and 6 hours. Fever, headache, muscle pains, nausea, vomiting, epigastric pain, dysuria, and explosive diarrhea characterize the acute episode. Because arsenic preferentially binds to red blood cells, hemolytic anemia and hemoglobinuria occur early, and red cell ghosts may be seen in the peripheral blood. There may also be profound hypoxia and cyanosis. Renal failure due to acute tubular necrosis (occasionally due to cortical necrosis) occurs in the first few days after onset of symptoms. This may be accompanied by shock and encephalopathy, characterized by agitation and disorientation. Both bone marrow depression and myocardial damage may occur. Those who do not die of intractable vascular collapse often develop subacute manifestations of arsenic poisoning (see later). Those who recover may develop chronic renal failure.

ARSENIC INGESTION. Depending on dose and form, arsenic ingestion can be insidious or overwhelming with cramping abdominal pain and diarrhea. Other acute manifestations include nausea, vomiting, dysphagia, cyanosis, headache, hematuria, and weakness. Hyperesthesia, muscle cramps, conjunctivitis, syncope, excessive thirst, periorbital swelling, epistaxis, and tinnitus may also occur. The patient may complain of a metallic taste, and there may be a garlic odor to the breath, which can also occur with selenium, tellurium, phosphorus, and dimethyl sulfoxide (DMSO) poisoning.

Other manifestations that may occur in the first week include jaundice, hematuria, and hepatomegaly with hepatic enzyme abnormalities; electrocardiographic abnormalities; a cardiomyopathy that can be lethal; pericarditis; rhabdomyolysis; pulmonary edema; evidence of encephalopathy; seizures; renal dysfunction; kidney failure with acute tubular necrosis; and respiratory muscle paralysis.

The most prominent manifestation after the first week of illness is symmetric polyneuropathy. At first, sensory manifestations predominate, the patient complaining of a burning sensation in a stocking-glove distribution. Motor involvement follows almost immediately with diminished or absent reflexes and severe weakness. Occasionally the neuropathy is unilateral. Prolonged encephalopathy and/or psychosis has been reported in a few instances. In cases of subacute poisoning, Aldrich-Mees lines (transverse white bands) may be seen in the nails; like the garlic odor, these may be seen in other trace element intoxications.

Chronic exposure is associated with cutaneous lesions, particularly hyperpigmentation (arsenic melanosis) and hyperkeratoses located primarily on the palms and soles. Alopecia and so-called raindrop depigmentation may also occur. In 5 to 10% of those chronically exposed, skin cancers appear after latent periods of 5 to more than 25 years; these tend to be multiple and are situated mainly on the trunk and upper extremities. An epidemic of skin cancers is underway in India after arsenic-contaminated deep well waters replaced bacteriologically contaminated surface water. In the United States, the most frequent cause of such skin lesions in past years was the medicinal use of Fowler's solution, an inorganic trivalent arsenical. Currently, most cases arise after occupational exposure, but a small number have been ascribed to chronic exposure to well water with high arsenic content. Epidemiologic studies on gold ore and tin miners, vineyard workers, laborers in sheep-dip factories, and smelter workers show a clear increase in the incidence of squamous cell carcinoma of the lung, the risk of bronchogenic cancer correlating with the intensity and duration of arsenic trioxide exposure, and all are potentiated by smoking.

DIAGNOSIS. Skin, nails, and hair do not usually contain arsenic until 2 to 4 weeks after exposure, but occasionally hair accumulation can occur more rapidly. If the diagnosis is suspected, arsenic concentrations can be measured in blood, urine, hair, or nails by atomic absorption spectrophotometry or neutron activation techniques, but, as with mercury, accurate interpretation can be difficult.

TREATMENT. The treatment of choice is dimercaprol (BAL). It should be given within the first 24 hours after exposure. If BAL is given later, it is less likely that improvement will be observed, and in many cases the peripheral neuropathy is refractory to treatment. Exchange transfusion or dialysis shortly after the onset of acute illness has also been reported to be beneficial. Penicillamine may also be useful, as may orally administered 2,3-dimercaptosuccinic acid (DMSA).

TRACE ELEMENTS WHOSE TOXICITY IS IN LARGE PART ASSOCIATED WITH HEMODIALYSIS

ZINC. The normal adult body zinc content is 1.5 to 3.0 g. Usually, daily intake ranges from 5 to 35 mg. Zinc is bound to metallothioneins synthesized in the liver and is excreted by both the urine and the gastrointestinal tract. It has a strong affinity for red cells and plasma proteins. Consequently, there is no loss across dialysis membranes; instead, depending on the dialysate, blood zinc concentrations may increase markedly during hemodialysis. There appear to be two well-documented zinc sources: adhesive plaster (containing zinc oxide) used to prevent dialysis coils from unwinding and the water of the dialysis fluid.

The manifestations of zinc toxicity do not necessarily correlate well with plasma or whole-blood zinc levels. Nausea, vomiting, anorexia, lethargy, irritability, weakness, abdominal pain, and anemia are the most frequent manifestations. Other manifestations may include diarrhea, muscle pain, lymphadenopathy, hyperamylasemia with or without pancreatitis, intestinal bleeding, thrombocytopenia, oliguria, hypotension, and renal failure with tubular necrosis. Injecting large amounts of zinc has resulted in death. Intestinal manifestations may supervene after either orally or parenterally induced zinc intoxication.

Welders, smelter workers, and solderers are exposed to aerosolized zinc and may experience zinc fume fever, characterized by chills, fever, myalgias, a metallic taste, cough, nausea, lethargy, and occasionally hemoptysis. There may be diffuse roentgenologic infiltrates and pulmonary dysfunction. Ordinarily, all manifestations disappear rapidly after cessation of exposure. If more prolonged pulmonary dysfunction occurs, it is thought to result from the effects of other metals to which the workers are simultaneously exposed.

ALUMINUM. Aluminum-induced dialysis dementia can be a fatal disease. The tap water used during dialysis is often to blame. Some waters naturally contain high concentrations of aluminum. In other cases, aluminum sulfate had been added to the community water supply to remove organic materials. In still other cases, the dialysis fluid appeared to be less responsible than aluminum-containing gels administered by mouth to reduce phosphate levels. If oral aluminum hydroxide is administered to non-dialyzed patients suffering from renal failure, the encephalopathy syndrome rarely occurs in adults; young children appear to be particularly at risk. Dialysis encephalopathy occurs only after repeated dialyses, usually spanning months or years. Peritoneal dialysis can also be complicated by encephalopathy.

Early manifestations include malaise, memory loss, and a characteristic speech disturbance. As the disease progresses, dysarthria, asterixis, myoclonic twitches, dementia, somnolence, and seizures occur. The electroencephalogram shows slowing, together with bursts of delta activity and high-voltage, symmetric spikes. Using reverse osmosis or deionization treatment has markedly reduced the incidence of severe dialysis dementia, but there is increasing evidence of a mild form of encephalopathy in chronic dialysis patients, characterized by psychomotor dysfunction, memory defects, weakness, and mild myoclonus.

Unusual manifestations of aluminum intoxication include myalgias, proximal myopathy, and severe skeletal pain caused by profound osteodystrophy that is unresponsive to vitamin D and is followed by fractures. Aluminum is deposited at the calcified bone-osteoid junction, and bone formation is impaired (see Chapters 261, 263, and 266). Aluminum also interferes with parathyroid function, and it may be associated with cardiomyopathy. Aluminum toxicity is also characterized by a poorly understood microcytic anemia that may be related in part to aluminum binding to transferrin and interfering with iron incorporation into heme.

Those involved in aluminum processing or manufacturing, pottery or explosive making, or welding may be exposed to aluminum aerosols. Pulmonary granulomas, fibrosis, and, in some cases, postfibrosis emphysema may supervene. In bauxite smelters this is known as Shaver's disease. Those involved in aluminum smelting may develop wheezing, chest tightness, and evidence of airway obstruction (potroom asthma).

Serum aluminum levels often do not reflect body loads. Intoxication may be documented by a deferoxamine mobilization test, but it can temporarily exacerbate the encephalopathy.

Although frequently lethal, in some cases the encephalopathy has regressed after intake of oral aluminum is curtailed. Treatment with deferoxamine, which complexes with aluminum, may be beneficial. Those with uremia should also be wary of community water supplies with inordinately high concentrations of aluminum.

COPPER. Copper levels may be inordinately high in the dialysis water if the water is supplied through copper plumbing. Copper is a potent red cell toxin, damaging cell membranes and inhibiting a variety of red cell enzymes. Major manifestations of toxicity include hemolysis and gastrointestinal disturbances. Nausea, vomiting, diarrhea, abdominal pain, fever, chills, hemolytic anemia, jaundice, hemoglobinuria, and severe myalgias all occur frequently. Myoglobinemia, necrotizing pancreatitis, hepatic necrosis, and profound leukocytosis may also occur.

Copper poisoning may also occur after intentional or accidental ingestion. Hematemesis, melena, hepatic necrosis, and shock may supervene.

Those exposed to metallic copper industrially may develop transient pulmonary manifestations (metal fume fever) and, rarely, green hair. These disappear rapidly when exposure is stopped.

COBALT. Patients with renal failure may have elevated tissue cobalt levels, often as a result of oral intake to combat anemia. Toxicity includes nausea, vomiting, anorexia, tinnitus, peripheral neuropathy, goiter resulting from blockage of iodine uptake, neurogenic deafness, hyperlipidemia, optic atrophy, and renal tubular damage.

Persons exposed to cobalt industrially may occasionally develop cardiomyopathy. Workers exposed to finely powdered cobalt may develop pulmonary interstitial fibrosis and cor pulmonale. Cobalt is often a component of alloys that are used in joint prostheses. Cases have been reported of joint pains, spontaneous dislocation of the prosthesis, and bone necrosis starting 9 months to 4 years postoperatively, apparently caused by a reaction to the cobalt in the alloy.

OTHER METALS. Tissue *tin* concentrations, especially in the liver, are also increased in patients undergoing hemodialysis. However, tin levels are even higher in uremic patients who have not been dialyzed. As of yet, no definite clinical disease has been associated with these increased body tin burdens.

Patients undergoing maintenance hemodialysis are often treated with *iron* for anemia. In such patients, parenteral and occasionally oral iron administration may be followed by hemosiderosis and occasionally by hemochromatosis. Serum ferritin concentrations may exceed 500 ng/mL. A proximal myopathy has also been described. Treatment with deferoxamine may reduce the body iron burden in impending or actual hemosiderosis.

CADMIUM

ETIOLOGY. Over 10 million pounds of cadmium are used industrially every year in the United States. The metal is a component of alloys; it is used to manufacture electrical conductors and in electroplating; and it is present in ceramics, pigments, dental prosthetics, plastic stabilizers, and storage batteries. It is also a by-product of zinc smelting and is used in the photographic, rubber, motor, and aircraft industries. Smelters, metal-processing furnaces, and the burning of coal and oil are responsible for much of the cadmium in air.

CLINICAL MANIFESTATIONS. *Acute intoxication* by cadmium fumes produces a characteristic clinical picture. Four to 10 hours after exposure, dyspnea, cough, and substernal discomfort supervene, often accompanied by prominent myalgias, fatigue, headache, and vomiting. In more severe cases, wheezing, hemoptysis, and progressive dyspnea caused by pulmonary edema may occur and may be accompanied by hypotension and renal failure.

In most cases, the pulmonary manifestations resolve rapidly, but pulmonary function abnormalities may not disappear for months; in these cases, vital capacity is reduced, and there is a restrictive defect. Occasionally, pulmonary edema is lethal.

Ingesting large amounts of cadmium results in nausea, vomiting, and abdominal pain, often accompanied by weakness, prostration, and myalgias. The onset of the gastroenteritis occurs shortly after ingestion and usually lasts for less than 24 hours.

Chronic cadmium exposure by aerosol for at least 10 years has resulted in emphysema in a small number of cases. The emphysema is not accompanied by bronchitis and may appear many years after industrial exposure has stopped. Workers exposed for at least 10 years also may suffer olfactory nerve damage; in some cases, this progresses to total anosmia.

The most frequent long-term consequence of aerosol or oral exposure is proteinuria. After prolonged and heavy contact, cadmium urinary excretion continues for years and is associated with damage to the proximal tubule. On occasion, the proteinuria may be accompanied by glycosuria and aminoaciduria. Only infrequently are the proteinuria and tubular damage followed by progressive renal failure.

NICKEL

ETIOLOGY. Nickel is used in various alloys, iron shell casings, ball bearings, and heart and joint prostheses. It is also used in nickel plating; as a catalyst; in magnetic tapes, dyes, and paints; and in acrylic plastics. It is found in petroleum and coal, in diesel fuels, and in soil and air. Municipal incinerators may contribute to the ambient air nickel concentrations.

Nickel is a potent contact allergen; the most frequent adverse effect for humans is nickel dermatitis, which may be both persistent and severe. Serious systemic reactions have occurred in allergic persons from nickel-containing dental prostheses, jewelry, pacemakers, or even fluids given intravenously through a nickel-containing needle. Prosthetic joints and heart valves have failed because of a reaction to the nickel in the prosthesis. In cases of recalcitrant nickel dermatitis, restriction in dietary nickel may be helpful.

CLINICAL MANIFESTATIONS AND TREATMENT. By far, the most toxic of the nickel compounds is nickel carbonyl, created by a reaction between nickel and carbon monoxide. Industrial aerosol exposure is followed immediately by headache, drowsiness, substernal pain, nausea, and vomiting. After a latent period of 1 to 5 days, the victim experiences fever, chills, dyspnea, a feeling of chest tightness, cough that is sometimes productive of blood-tinged sputum, muscle pains, weakness, and fatigue. Hepatic enzyme concentrations may be considerably elevated. In severe cases, cyanosis, progressive respiratory difficulties, and convulsions ensue, and death may follow. The treatment of choice is diethyl dithiocarbamate (Dithiocarb); dimercaprol (BAL) is an alternative but less effective therapeutic agent. Although overwhelming pneumonitis caused by nickel carbonyl is now rare, milder pulmonary toxicity in occupations such as welding probably goes unrecognized under the general rubric of metal fume fever.

CARCINOGENESIS. Nickel is considered a potent respiratory tract carcinogen. Studies of nickel refinery workers have shown a fivefold increase in risk of lung cancer, a 150-fold increase in the risk of nasal cancer, and a substantially increased risk of laryngeal cancer. Occupations most at risk among nickel workers are roasting, smelting, and electrolysis. Workers developing lung, laryngeal, and nasal cancers have usually been exposed for at least 10 years. Biopsies of nasal mucosa show potentially precancerous epithelial dysplasia in a substantial percentage of nickel workers. The cancer risk is so great that workers heavily exposed for over 10 years should probably have annual nasal mucosa biopsies as well as sputum cytologic studies and roentgenologic examinations every 4 to 6 months in an attempt at secondary prevention. The incidence of respiratory tract cancer in nickel workers depends on both the extent of nickel exposure and the effects of co-carcinogens, in particular, cigarette tobacco. Except for nickel miners and refinery workers, industrial nickel exposure has not been convincingly associated with increased risk of cancer.

OTHER TOXIC METALS

Thallium

ETIOLOGY AND PATHOGENESIS. Thallium is used in optical lenses, jewelry, low-temperature thermometers, semiconductors, luminescent tubes, dyes and pigments, scintillation counters, and fireworks. It forms a stainless alloy with silver and a corrosion-resistant alloy with lead and may be a byproduct of lead and zinc production. In some areas, it is still a component of rodenticides, pesticides, and insecticides. Thallium can enter the body through the respiratory tract, gastrointestinal tract, or skin. Like many other trace metals, thallium has a strong affinity for sulfhydryl groups and thus interferes with many enzyme systems. Additionally, it enters the cell, exchanging for intracellular potassium.

CLINICAL MANIFESTATIONS. Poisoning can be acute and overwhelming after suicidal ingestion, or it can be chronic and subtle. In acute poisoning, manifestations include nausea, vomiting, hematemesis, headache, lethargy, abdominal pain, diarrhea that may be bloody, insomnia, myalgias, muscle weakness, fever, hyperhidrosis, excessive thirst, confusion, delirium, seizures, coma, and respiratory failure. At least 10% of acutely poisoned persons die.

Among those who survive at least a week or who are exposed to smaller amounts of thallium, the most predictable manifestations are a combined sensory and motor, often painful, peripheral neuropathy and alopecia. Although the head alopecia is total, the facial, axillary, and pubic hair is spared, as is the inner one third of the eyebrows. Motor manifestations may predominate, and the ascending, predominantly motor paralysis may mimic Guillain-Barré

syndrome. Abdominal colic, nausea, and vomiting occur frequently in both the acute and the subacute forms of thallium toxicity and may so dominate the clinical picture that a diagnosis of acute appendicitis is made. Other manifestations of subacute intoxication include dementia, headache, fatigue, sleep disorders, intractable thirst, hallucinations, blindness caused by optic neuritis, impotence, amenorrhea, a blue discoloration of the gingivae, centrilobular hepatic necrosis, renal tubular necrosis, orthostatic hypotension, paralytic ileus, and myoclonic twitches. Multiple cranial nerves may be involved, but the eighth nerve is almost always spared. The electrocardiogram may show arrhythmias and changes similar to those associated with hypokalemia.

DIAGNOSIS. Thallium can be measured in blood and urine, but blood levels are often deceptively low even during clinically apparent poisoning. Because thallium is excreted in the urine, thallium determinations on 24-hour specimens are more reliable.

In some cases there is no history of occupational, environmental, or intentional exposure. Unexplained abdominal pain, neurologic abnormalities, and alopecia suggest the diagnosis.

TREATMENT. Treatment consists of hemodialysis, which can remove up to half the thallium body burden, and probably administration of Prussian blue. Prussian blue, or activated charcoal given by mouth, adsorbs thallium, so that fecal thallium concentrations increase. The half-life of thallium in the body is about 1 month, and repeated dialyses are usually needed.

PROGNOSIS. As many as 30% of those poisoned suffer some residual effects. The neuropathy may persist for many months before resolving, and some are left with variable amounts of dementia, neuropathy, ataxia, visual impairment, alopecia, and myoclonus.

Selenium

ETIOLOGY. Selenium is well absorbed from both the gastrointestinal tract and the lungs. The amount normally ingested varies markedly, depending on the local soil selenium content and on the geographic origins of foods consumed. The element is widely used in pigment, glass, electronics, ceramics, and steel industries, and it has gained popularity with both traditional and alternative medicine for its antioxidant properties.

CLINICAL MANIFESTATIONS. In humans a selenium deficiency syndrome has been clearly defined in human toddlers. Moreover, in the Republic of China, diffuse cardiomyopathy (Keshan disease) has been associated with low soil and blood selenium levels, and the incidence of the disease apparently has been strikingly reduced by selenium supplementation.

Selenium toxicity syndromes in humans can be divided into acute and chronic poisoning. Subjects with inordinate exposure to selenium fumes experience one or more of the following: intestinal disturbances, giddiness, apathy, lassitude, pallor, nervousness, depression, hair and nail loss, a garlic odor to the breath, and a metallic taste. Sore throat, dyspnea, and cough may also be noted. Symptoms usually disappear after removal from the occupational exposure. In those ingesting excessive selenium, symptoms and signs include nausea, vomiting, abdominal pain, diarrhea, anorexia, fatigue, sore throat, arthralgias, emotional lability, a metallic taste, a garlic odor to the breath, brittle nails, brittle hair, hair loss, a bronze color to the skin, hepatic dysfunction, and diffuse dermatitis. Increased selenium burdens may be associated with an increased prevalence of dental caries.

EPIDEMIOLOGY. A most impressive epidemic of chronic selenium intoxication was observed in China in the 1960s. Subacute and chronic selenium toxicity may be seen with an increasing frequency because selenium is being promoted as a non-prescription supplement.

Manganese

Manganese toxicity occurs primarily in miners who have been exposed to manganese dioxide aerosols for prolonged periods. The manifestations, known as manganic madness, are limited to the CNS. The manganese is concentrated primarily in the basal ganglia and cerebellum, accounting for the extrapyramidal Parkinson-like facies, the rigidity, and the difficulty in walking. Other manifestations include compulsive behavior (including singing, dancing, fighting, and running), explosive and involuntary laughter, headache, muscular weakness, tremors, somnolence, dystonia, hypotonia, retropulsion and propulsion, dementia, speech disturbances, irritability, sialorrhea, impotence, hypersomnia, and memory defects. In some cases, psychosis may be the dominant feature. Manganese contamination of dialysates or ingestion has been associated with abdominal pain, liver dysfunction, and evidence of pancreatitis. The molecular mechanism remains unclear, and no effective therapy exists.

Barium

Barium compounds are used in printing; in the production of paints, glass, paper, leather, soap, and rubber; in ceramics, plastic, steel, oil, textile, and dye industries; as fuel additives; and in insecticides, rodenticides, and depilatories. After accidental or intentional ingestion of large amounts, abdominal pain, vomiting, and increased peristalsis occur. If enough is absorbed, potassium is displaced intracellularly, resulting in profound hypokalemia, which in turn may produce flaccid paralysis, potentially dangerous cardiac arrhythmias, renal failure, and respiratory paralysis. Poisoning has also been described after barium chloride skin burn. Treatment consists of potassium administration and efforts to promote barium excretion. Severe allergic reaction has followed barium enema; whether this is due to the barium or preservatives is not clear.

Contact with barium also causes a benign pneumoconiosis that may occur after 1 or more years of aerosol exposure. Chest roentgenograms show extensive, very dense bilateral nodules up to 4 to 5 mm in diameter. There is no prominent fibrosis and no clinically significant disease; the nodules often regress after occupational exposure is stopped.

Boron

There are few reports of actual boron toxicity despite significant acute exposures. Ingesting boric acid can result in nausea; vomiting; diarrhea; anemia; seizures; a variety of skin eruptions characterized by intense erythema, desquamation, and exfoliation; and striking alopecia. Additionally, occupational aerosol exposure to diborane (B_2H_6) in high-energy fuels can produce acute pulmonary edema that resolves after the exposure is discontinued. Exposure to liquid boron hydride (B_5H_9) can produce dementia, cortical blindness, deafness, seizures, acidosis, and cardiac arrest. A subacute mild organic brain syndrome has also been observed.

Antimony

Industrial antimony toxicity is very rare, as is intentional ingestion or inadvertent poisoning from antimony released from inexpensive enamelware. Manifestations of acute poisoning include nausea, abdominal pain, weakness, headache, vomiting, diarrhea, hematemesis, myalgias, liver function abnormalities, acute renal tubular dysfunction, electrolyte abnormalities, and circulatory collapse. Gaseous SbH_3 (stibine) is as toxic as arsine, producing CNS toxicity and hemolysis. After antimonial injection for medicinal purposes, adverse effects include nausea, vomiting, cough, and muscle and joint pain. Hepatic dysfunction can occur, as can cardiac arrhythmias, including Adams-Stokes syndrome. Antimony is also considered one of the metals capable of causing metal fume fever. Treatment of oral ingestion consists of lavage, administration of activated charcoal, and administration of dimercaprol or the less toxic analogues dimercaptosuccinic acid or dimercaptopropanesulfonic acid.

Chromium

Chromium is used extensively in metal and galvanizing industries and in the manufacture of dyes, enamel, and paints. Chromate exposure is associated with an increased incidence of lung and certain upper respiratory tract cancers. Additionally, chromium-exposed workers may show evidence of proximal renal tubule dysfunction and commonly suffer nasal septum perforations.

Molybdenum

In animals, molybdenum produces diarrhea, anemia, alopecia, diminished growth, and bone and joint abnormalities. No clearly defined molybdenum toxicity syndrome has been reported in humans.

Platinum

The major adverse effects observed in platinum workers are allergic pulmonary reactions, including bronchial asthma.

Plutonium

In experimental models, plutonium, because of its radioactivity, is a potent carcinogen. Workers have been generally well protected, but recent data suggest that occupational exposure may be a significant problem. Some still-controversial epidemiologic studies have suggested that accidental community exposure has resulted in an increase in frequency of certain cancers and fetal malformations.

Tellurium

Used particularly in rubber, metallurgic, and electronics industries, tellurium can cause giddiness, headache, nausea, a metallic taste, and a garlic smell to the breath. In animals, tellurium causes neuropathy, but this has not been convincingly demonstrated in humans.

Tin

Tin can be released into beverages or foods from tin cans; ingestion can produce nausea, vomiting, abdominal pain, and diarrhea. Such toxicity occurs infrequently. Additionally, there have been occasional reports of neurologic abnormalities after exposure to organic tin, including the triethyl, trimethyl, and triphenyl tins, which are used primarily in agriculture for their bactericidal, fungicidal, antiparasitic, and molluscacidal properties. Manifestations include ataxic dysmetria, disorientation, seizures, nystagmus, impaired vision, hearing loss, headache, vertigo, paresthesias, intracranial hypertension, paresis, and polyneuropathy. Aerosol exposure to tin may result in stannosis, which is a mild pneumoconiosis with dense bilateral infiltrates but usually no pulmonary dysfunction.

Vanadium

Vanadium is used in alloys and in the steel and chemical industries. Its inhalation can result in neurasthenia, anorexia, vertigo, throat pain, nasal irritation (even nasal hemorrhage), and acute bronchitis characterized by a cough that is sometimes accompanied by a whoop. The nasal mucosa of vanadium-exposed workers shows vascular hyperemia and round cell infiltration.

Greenburg MI, Hamilton RJ, Phillips SD: Occupational, Industrial and Environmental Toxicology, St. Louis: Mosby, 1997.
Haddad LM, Shannon MW, Winchester JF: Clinical Management of Poisoning and Drug Overdose, Philadelphia: WB Saunders, 1998.
Comprehensive textbooks covering chronic poisonings with trace metals and other elements.

PART V

PRINCIPLES OF EVALUATION AND MANAGEMENT

22 CLINICAL DECISION MAKING: APPROACH TO THE PATIENT

Suzanne W. Fletcher

When a patient sees a doctor, the patient is seeking help—to regain or retain health. The physician's task is to work for the patient's health. The doctor does so by trying to attenuate disease, by relieving discomfort, by assisting the patient with any disability, by preventing premature death, and by maximizing contentment. Some have summarized these activities as tackling "the five Ds" of health—disease, discomfort, disability, death, and dissatisfaction. In the best of circumstances, the doctor is able to prevent disease and help the patient remain healthy. In some cases, none of the goals is achieved, but even then the physician must select from the full range of potential options in an attempt to improve the patient's course.

In most clinical encounters the patient presents basic questions to the doctor: Am I sick? What is causing my illness? Will it go away? Will it kill me? Can you make me well? Better? Can you help me stay well?

These questions set the stage for making a diagnosis, determining prognosis, carrying out treatment, promoting health, and preventing disease. This is the bulk of daily clinical work. Although young physicians learn these skills one at a time, the master clinician blends them so skillfully that often it is difficult to discern which is occurring at any given moment. For example, when obtaining a history or performing a physical examination to arrive at a diagnosis, the master clinician all the while is considering prognosis and is treating the patient with appropriate attention, empathy, consolation, and therapeutic information, thus ensuring that the patient feels better just for having been with the doctor.

DIAGNOSIS

Diagnosis is accomplished with history taking, physical examination, and laboratory testing. Although modern medicine has shifted attention toward the laboratory, even today most of the diagnosis is accomplished through history taking and physical examination, which narrow the diagnostic possibilities before laboratory testing is used. And it is through history taking and physical examination that the doctor humanizes the medical encounter for the patient and sets the stage for successful treatment.

MEDICAL HISTORY. There are standard sections to a complete medical history (Table 22–1). It is usual, but not necessary, to obtain the complete history when a physician and patient meet for the first time. During follow-up visits, active medical problems are the focus. If the patient's presenting complaint is urgent, it may not be feasible to obtain a complete medical history—for example, when a patient is admitted to the intensive care unit or seen in the emergency department, the presenting problem prevails. In every case, the doctor should start with what is most important in the history and, according to circumstances, adjust the rest of the history taking. The patient's medical history will unfold over time and should be augmented at each subsequent doctor-patient encounter.

HISTORY OF THE PRESENT ILLNESS. For each major symptom, the doctor must determine *what* (e.g., pain, nausea, weakness), *where* (part of body), *when* (e.g., continuous, intermittent, time of day), *how much* (severity), *chronologic course* (beginning of symptom, end, improvement, worsening), and what makes the symptom *better* or *worse*. It is important to determine what medical care the patient has already received for the problem, including laboratory tests previously performed, their results, the diagnosis reached, the treatment given, whether the patient adhered to the treatment, and results of the treatment. Finally, the physician must seek answers to questions that narrow the diagnostic possibilities. This step, the most difficult part of obtaining an understanding of the present illness, requires a great deal of diagnostic skill and knowledge. Skilled clinicians form diagnostic hypotheses early in the patient's story and are able to ask specific questions, the answers to which confirm or exclude a given diagnostic possibility. Parts of the history of the present illness, such as the description of symptoms and treatment compliance, are best obtained from the patient, whereas others, such as details about previously performed laboratory tests and treatment, are best acquired from medical sources.

CLINICAL INTERVIEW TECHNIQUE. The interaction of a doctor and patient during the medical interview is a marvelous mixture of art and science. The art is the interaction of two unique human beings; the science is the interaction of the biologic and behavioral bases of medicine.

Each physician must develop an interviewing technique that is comfortable and true to his or her own personality. Interview style also necessarily varies according to the particular patient. Some patients are loquacious, others come right to the point, and still others are mute. Some patients want to control the encounter, some are passive, a few are hostile. The doctor needs to adjust the interview accordingly. But at every encounter, the patient must be treated with both courtesy and dignity.

Table 22–1 ■ THE PATIENT'S MEDICAL HISTORY

Description of patient
  Age, gender, race, occupation, and, for women, parity
Chief complaint
  Four or five words, preferably quoting the patient, stating the purpose of the visit and the duration of the complaint. Occasionally the patient states a request (e.g., "I need a flu shot") instead of a complaint.
Other physicians involved in the patient's care
  Name, address, telephone number, and relationship to the patient
History of the present illness
  For each major symptom, what, where, when, how much, chronologic course, what makes the symptom better or worse, past medical care, questions to narrow diagnostic possibilities
Past medical history
  Previous illnesses and hospitalizations, immunizations, medications the patient takes, allergies, and alcohol, tobacco, and drug habits
Social and occupational history
  Description of a typical day in the patient's life and how the present illness affects it, social supports (family, friends, and colleagues) available to the patient, and occupational history
Family history
  History of genetically related diseases in the patient's family and longevity and cause of death of family members
Review of systems
  Systematic review of major organ systems: skin, hematopoietic system (including lymph nodes), head, eyes, ears, nose, mouth, throat, neck, breasts, and respiratory, cardiovascular, gastrointestinal, genitourinary, musculoskeletal, nervous, endocrine, and psychiatric systems

It is the physician's task to manage the pace and direction of the interview. At the outset, the doctor should introduce himself or herself and address the patient by name. It is helpful to indicate how long the encounter is likely to last. The physician should focus total attention on the patient. A few minutes of complete attention is better than 30 minutes of distracted interaction.

In relating a history, most patients do not follow the precise order just outlined. The patient may include bits and pieces of social and family history while describing the current complaint. It is the physician's job to fashion order out of the story while still allowing the patient a chance to tell the story in his or her own way. Giving the patient this chance increases the likelihood of patient satisfaction with the clinical encounter as well as increases the patient's willingness to follow the doctor's advice about treatment. In addition, many doctors enjoy listening to their patients. Over a lifetime, a physician meets patients from almost every class, race, educational level, profession, moral persuasion, and personality type. Listening to patients' stories told in their own way reveals the rich variety of humanity.

After introductions, the physician asks why the patient has come. Then the doctor should listen. If questions are needed to help the patient along, they should be open ended and non-specific. After a few minutes, the doctor should begin to direct the interview more actively, by facilitating the patient's story with more directed questions. Often, it helps to summarize the history during the interview. Finally, the doctor must narrow the diagnostic possibilities with appropriate questions.

If time is short, the doctor must take charge of the interview more quickly; but in almost all circumstances, the patient should be given a chance to tell his or her story. If the physician takes charge too quickly, not only do patient satisfaction and cooperation decrease, but the chances for a missed diagnosis increase. This risk of a missed diagnosis is especially relevant when the patient is uncomfortable or afraid to speak openly, as with teenage pregnancies or cases of sexual abuse.

PAST MEDICAL HISTORY, SOCIAL HISTORY, FAMILY HISTORY, AND REVIEW OF SYSTEMS. These sections are far more routine than the history of the present illness, and the questions in each section are best memorized. The doctor should explain briefly each new section so that the patient understands the shift in topic. ("Now I would like to ask you about other illnesses you may have had in the past.") Start with general questions. ("Have you ever been sick before?")

Usually, the social history seems least relevant for diagnosis and therefore physicians most frequently shorten or omit it. However, learning about a patient's daily life, how the current illness is affecting it, and what social supports the patient can call on for assistance are particularly important when trying to fashion an effective treatment for the patient.

Because most questions in the latter sections of the medical history are standard, answers can be obtained by giving the patient a printed questionnaire or by using a computerized questionnaire. Both are organized in a branching manner, so that affirmative answers can be explored further.

PHYSICAL EXAMINATION. The physical examination is done with the five senses, and probably a sixth as well. Physicians in training should practice the complete examination on as many patients as possible to master all parts thoroughly. A complete examination, with a thorough neurologic and pelvic examination, takes even skillful examiners a good deal of time. Sometimes, because of time, the doctor may have to conduct a complete examination over several visits.

Several principles are important every time a physician performs a physical examination. The physician must demonstrate respect for the patient, making sure to expose private parts of the body only for as long as necessary for a careful examination. The physical examination should follow a standard order and be performed in a systematic manner. It should be as comfortable as possible for the patient and require a minimum amount of shifting and changing of position. The more uncomfortable parts of the examination, such as the rectal and pelvic examinations, generally should be performed last.

The physical examination begins with inspection, which starts on entering the room. Next come the vital signs. The physician always should examine carefully those parts of the body related to the reason for the patient's visit. Whenever necessary, objective measurements—such as number and size of the nodes, breadth of the liver, circumference of the calf—should be taken, not only for accurate assessment of the clinical course but also for more precise communication with other clinicians who may next see the patient.

Physicians should strive to improve their physical examination skills throughout their careers. One approach is to choose one part of the examination and practice it on every patient seen during a given period. For example, a few weeks of extra attention to the thyroid improve those examination skills even if none of the patients so examined has thyroid disease.

Questioning and examining the patient are types of diagnostic tests and should be evaluated scientifically just as laboratory tests are. Some questions and examination techniques produce more accurate results than others. For example, the many different ways of examining the breast are not equally good for detecting lumps. Clinicians should master examination techniques that research has shown to be most accurate.

LABORATORY TESTS. Laboratory tests have become a standard part of the doctor-patient encounter; their correct use is complex and subject to a number of scientific principles (see Chapter 23). The physician must also explain clearly to the patient the purpose and use of tests. Although generally used for diagnosis or screening, occasionally a laboratory test may have a therapeutic impact. For example, a patient with chest pain may be reassured after having a normal exercise stress test.

PROGNOSIS

It is important to tell the patient the diagnosis (writing it down often helps) and discuss what to expect from the clinical course of the condition. For many patients, the prognosis of the illness is their greatest concern. If the illness is likely to resolve without sequelae, reassurance is often all that is needed.

The most difficult prognoses to discuss are those for fatal illnesses, especially many cancers. Most patients want to know even bad prognoses, but how much a physician tells a given patient should be determined primarily by the patient, not the physician. The physician has the duty to make the patient aware of his or her willingness to discuss the prognosis. Often detailed discussions are best conducted at follow-up visits, after the two have had a chance to get to know each other. The best physicians blend honest fact and hope together, helping the patient through the complicated steps of shock, denial, depression, and acceptance of a fatal illness. Most importantly, they make it clear that they will not abandon the patient.

Doctors should educate themselves about the clinical course of the medical illnesses they encounter. No matter the import of the disease, they should learn how long, on average, for example, the pain of herpes zoster continues, the headache of sinusitis persists, and the patient with class IV congestive heart failure lives.

TREATMENT AND PREVENTION

Increasingly, patients visit doctors not for diagnosis but for treatment of ongoing medical problems. Even when a doctor must make the diagnosis, it is important to remember that making a diagnosis alone cannot improve the health of a patient; only treatment and prevention can.

Two general principles should be kept in mind about treatment. First, the physician should treat the patient as well as the disease. With every clinical encounter, the physician should strive to ensure that the patient feels better just for having been with the doctor. When prescribing specific treatment, alleviation of symptoms, especially pain and nausea, is often as important to the patient as, for example, prescribing antibiotics for an infection. Second, successful treatment of an illness, especially outside the hospital, usually requires the patient's active participation.

THERAPEUTIC PROCEDURES. Therapeutic procedures, such as surgery, irradiation, angioplasty, and chemotherapy, as well as invasive diagnostic tests and screening procedures, such as genetic testing, must be explained thoroughly to the patient; often, signed consent must be obtained. The physician must help the patient understand what will happen during the procedure, the hoped-for outcome and its probability, and the adverse effects of the procedure and their probabilities. Informed consent is a medicolegal requirement, but, just as important, it is a cornerstone of excellent clinical care. Technologic advances in medicine are complex, often costly, and rarely without the potential for adverse complications. Substantial clinical skill is required to obtain true informed consent. The physician should act as the patient's advocate. The patient should be given the necessary facts but not overwhelmed with incomprehensible technical details or a long list of terrifying and improbable adverse effects. The physician should freely give professional advice but clearly communicate that the final decision is the patient's. If the patient remains undecided about a procedure after a thorough discussion, in most cases it is best to delay the decision. A patient who feels pressured by the doctor to undergo a risky procedure may be particularly upset if complications arise.

MEDICATIONS. Compliance with physicians' medication orders is a given when the patient is in a hospital, but this is certainly not true in the ambulatory setting. With ambulatory patients it is especially important to explain to the patient, in simple terms, the medication, its purpose, its dosage schedule, and how long it should be continued.

It is useful to ask the patient to bring all medicines to each follow-up visit. Many patients do not know the names of their medicines; discussing pills in bottles is easier than reviewing medication names. Often the doctor can make a rough estimate of medication compliance by the level of pills in the bottle—although for ongoing prescriptions patients may combine bottles or refill prescriptions before beginning to take the medication in a particular bottle, thus making accurate compliance measurement impossible. Sometimes the physician discovers that the patient does not have one of the prescribed medicines or is taking medication prescribed by another physician. For each medicine discussed, the doctor should ask how often the patient is taking it and if there are any problems. If the patient is taking the medicine incorrectly, the physician can determine whether the problem is misunderstanding of the dosage schedule, forgetfulness, an adverse side effect, the cost of the drug, or some other reason.

To help the patient take prescribed medication, the physician should follow a few commonsense rules. The most important determinant of medication compliance is the number of medicines prescribed. Parsimony is key. In general, and especially for a patient on multiple medications, the doctor should strive for simple once- or twice-daily dosage schedules of the least expensive effective medication. At follow-up visits, the fewer the medication changes, the better. For patients who have trouble remembering to take their medicines, written instructions or pill containers with alarms can help. Sometimes the physician can refer the patient to special pharmacy or nursing programs for help with medicine compliance.

PREVENTION AND HEALTH MAINTENANCE. Preventive and health maintenance activities, such as routine mammograms, smoking cessation, and influenza vaccines, are indicated periodically according to guidelines based on age, gender, and clinical status. Prompting systems, such as a prevention checklist, help incorporate appropriate prevention activities into the doctor-patient encounter. If there is no checklist or other system in place, the doctor should briefly consider what preventive activities are indicated in a patient of the given age and gender (see Chapter 10) and perform them.

Doctors perform four types of preventive and health maintenance activities: (1) screening examinations to identify asymptomatic disease or risk factors, (2) immunizations to prevent subsequent disease, (3) lifestyle counseling to stop harmful habits and promote healthful ones, and (4) prescribing chemoprophylaxis, such as hormone replacement therapy. The most difficult of these activities is counseling lifestyle changes. Before beginning counseling, the patient's motivation for change should be determined. If the patient is motivated, and most patients are, counseling should concentrate on the actual steps the patient should take. Follow-up is especially important. Most patients fail the first few times they attempt to make a lifestyle change. If that happens, the doctor should encourage the patient to keep trying and avoid being judgmental. Success with even a small percentage of patients can lead to substantial health benefits. If doctors succeed in helping only 10% of their patients who smoke to break the habit, it has been estimated that more than 1 million American lives would be saved.

WRAP-UP

After taking the medical history, performing the physical examination, reviewing what laboratory tests are being ordered and why,

and discussing recommended treatment and preventive activities, the doctor and patient should discuss follow-up plans and what to do if a problem occurs before the scheduled follow-up visit. The patient should be given the physician's name, *in writing,* and should know how to contact the doctor if the need arises. These steps are particularly important in the practice of internal medicine, in which most patient care involves chronic medical problems rather than episodic illness. The patient should be given a chance to ask any questions he or she may have. Arrangements should be made for the doctor to contact the patient with appropriate laboratory test results. At the end of the visit, the doctor should indicate that it was good to see the patient.

SUMMARY

A successful doctor-patient encounter requires a great deal of synthesis and judgment on the doctor's part. The physician must be thinking of many different elements at once, not only the diagnostic possibilities but also the prognostic implications, how and what to communicate to the patient, how to help the patient feel as comfortable as possible, which laboratory tests and therapy to choose, and how to explain them clearly to the patient. These elements must be addressed and updated constantly throughout the interview, often simultaneously. The doctor must translate all thought processes into effective interactions with the patient and must work to develop a partnership with the patient so that medically indicated diagnostic tests and treatments that are acceptable to the patient are identified and used. Overriding all of these activities, the doctor must keep asking how to improve and enhance the health of the patient, how to change those five Ds.

Paradoxically, modern medicine, with its powerful technologies for diagnosis and treatment, requires more than ever that the physician emphasize one of medicine's most ancient activities, that of being a teacher. Fittingly, society requires that the doctor work with—not on—the patient. Although physicians may come to have a good deal of influence with some of their patients, the best carefully avoid trying to have power over their patients. Like great physicians of old, they know the truth of the classic maxim that the secret of the care of the patient is caring for the patient.

Lipkin M, Putnam SA, Lazare A (eds): The Medical Interview. Clinical Care, Education, and Research. New York, Springer, 1995. *A textbook on the medical interview and related skills.*

Ramsey PG, Curtis R, Paauw DS, et al: History-taking and preventive medicine skills among primary care physicians: An assessment using standardized patients. Am J Med 104:152, 1998. *Primary care physicians may miss important information on the initial patient visit; structured questionnaires may help avoid this problem.*

Schneiderman H, Peixoto AJ: Bedside Diagnosis: An Annotated Bibliography of Literature on Physical Examination and Interviewing, 3rd ed. Philadelphia, American College of Physicians, 1997. *Lists references collected from a computerized search of the medical literature from 1974 through 1996 and other materials collected by the authors.*

Simel DL, Rennie D: The clinical examination: An agenda to make it more rational. JAMA 277:572, 1997. *An editorial updating the JAMA series of review articles on The Rational Clinical Examination.*

U.S. Preventive Services Task Force: Guide to Clinical Preventive Services, 2nd ed. Baltimore, Williams & Wilkins, 1996. *A complete guide and rationale for clinical preventive services.*

23 INTERPRETATION OF DATA FOR CLINICAL DECISIONS

Thomas H. Lee

Key functions in the professional lives of all physicians are the collection and analysis of clinical data. Decisions must be made on the basis of these data, including which therapeutic strategy is most appropriate for the patient or whether further information should be gathered before the best strategy can be chosen. This decision-making process is a blend of science and art, in which the physician must synthesize a variety of concerns, including what is the patient's most likely outcome with various management strategies, what is the patient's worst possible outcome, and what are the patient's preferences among these strategies?

Only rarely does the physician enjoy true certainty regarding any of these issues, so a natural inclination for physicians is to seek as much information as possible before making a decision. That approach ignores the dangers inherent in the collection of information. Some of these dangers are direct, such as the risk of cerebrovascular accident associated with coronary angiography. Other dangers are indirect, such as the possibility that performance of a blood culture might lead to a contaminant result that might, in turn, lead to further blood cultures, unnecessary antibiotic therapy, and prolongation of hospitalization.

An additional concern is the cost of information-gathering, including the direct costs of the tests themselves and the indirect costs that flow from decisions made on the basis of the test results. In health care today, and for the foreseeable future, complete physicians must be able to consider costs and include management of care among their core competencies. The available pool of resources for health care is not expanding as quickly as the demands posed by medical advances and the aging of the population. If resources are to be available to care for the sick patients who are most likely to benefit from them, physicians must be skillful at identifying low-risk patients and then exercise discretion on the use of resources for them.

For the physician, there are three key questions in this sequence. Should I get a test to improve my assessment of diagnosis or prognosis? Which test is the best test? Which therapeutic strategy is most appropriate for this patient?

SHOULD I ORDER A TEST?

The decision of whether to order a test depends on the physician's and the patient's willingness to pursue a management strategy with the current degree of uncertainty. This decision is influenced by several factors, including the patient's attitudes toward diagnostic and therapeutic interventions (e.g., a patient with claustrophobia might prefer an angiogram to magnetic resonance imaging), as well as the information provided by the test itself. A decision *not* to obtain a specific test should also be considered an information-gathering strategy, because the data collected while a patient is observed often reduce uncertainty about diagnosis and outcome.

The impact of information from tests is often expressed as *probabilities* (Table 23–1). A probability of 1.0 implies that an event is certain to occur, whereas a probability of 0 implies that the event is impossible. When all the possible events for a patient are assigned probabilities, these estimates should sum to 1.0.

It is often useful to use *odds* to quantify uncertainty instead of

Table 23–1 ■ KEY DEFINITIONS*

Probability = A number between 0 and 1 that expresses an estimate of the likelihood of an event.
Odds = The ratio of [the probability of an event] to [the probability of the event not occurring].

Test Performance Characteristics
Sensitivity = Percentage of patients with disease who have an abnormal test result.
Specificity = Percentage of patients without disease who have a normal test result.
Positive predictive value (PV+) = Percentage of patients with an abnormal test result who actually have disease.
Negative predictive value (PV−) = Percentage of patients with a normal test result who do not have disease.

Bayesian Analysis
Pre-test (or prior) probability = the probability of a disease before the information is acquired.
Post-test (or posterior) probability = the probability of an event after new information is acquired.

$$\text{Pre-test (or prior) odds} = \frac{\text{Pre-test probability of disease}}{(1 - \text{pre-test probability of disease})}$$

$$\text{Likelihood ratio} = \frac{\text{Probability of result in diseased persons}}{\text{Probability of result in non-diseased persons}}$$

*Note that *disease* can mean a condition, such as coronary artery disease, or an outcome, such as postoperative cardiac complications.

probability. Odds of 1:2 suggest that the likelihood of an event is only half the likelihood that the event will not occur. The relationship between odds and probability is expressed in the formula

$$\text{Odds} = p/(1-p)$$

where p is the probability of an event.

Performance Characteristics

Key terms for the description of test performance include *sensitivity* and *specificity*. It is critical to note that these parameters describe the test and are in theory true regardless of the patient population to which the test is applied. However, research studies that describe test performance are often based on highly selected patient populations; hence, test performance may deteriorate when tests are applied in clinical practice. For example, the result of a test for prostatic cancer such as a prostate-specific antigen test may rarely be abnormal if evaluated in a low-risk population such as high school students. On the other hand, false-positive abnormal prostate-specific antigen test results are common when the test is performed in men with benign prostatic hypertrophy.

Although researchers are interested in the performance of tests, the true focus of medical decision making is the patient. Therefore, physicians are more interested in the probability that a patient has a specific disease or outcome if a test result is normal or abnormal— that is, the predictive values of positive or negative test results. These predictive values are extremely sensitive to the population from which they are derived. For example, an abnormal exercise test result in an asymptomatic patient has a much lower positive predictive value than that same test result in a patient with a history of exertional substernal chest pressure. Bayes' theorem (see later) provides a framework for analyzing the interaction between test results and a patient's pre-test probability of a disease.

As useful as the performance characteristics may be, they are limited by the fact that few tests truly provide dichotomous (i.e., "positive" or "negative") test results. Tests such as exercise tests have several parameters (e.g., ST-segment deviation, exercise duration, hemodynamic response) that provide insight into the patient's condition, and the "normal range" for many blood tests (e.g., prostate-specific antigen) varies markedly depending on the age of the tested population and one's willingness to "miss" patients with disease. In addition, tests that require human interpretation (e.g., radiologic studies) are particularly subject to variability in the reported results.

Bayes' Theorem

The impact of a test result on a patient's probability of disease was first quantified by Thomas Bayes, an eighteenth century English clergyman who developed a formula for the probability of disease in the presence of a positive test result. The classic presentation of Bayes' theorem is complex and difficult to use. A more simple form of this theorem is known as the *odds ratio* form, which describes the impact of a test result on the pre-test odds (see Table 23–1) of a diagnosis or outcome for a specific patient.

To calculate the post-test odds of disease, pre-test odds are multiplied by the *likelihood ratio* (LR) for a specific test result. The mathematical presentation of this form of Bayes' theorem is as follows:

$$\text{Post-test odds} = (\text{Pre-test odds}) \times (\text{LR})$$

The likelihood ratio is the probability of a particular test result in patients with the disease divided by the probability of that same test result in patients without disease. In other words, the likelihood ratio is the test result's sensitivity divided by the false-positive rate. A test of no value (e.g., flipping a coin and calling "heads" an abnormal result) would have a likelihood ratio of 1.0, because half of patients with disease would have "positive" test results, as would half of patients without disease. Therefore, this test would have no impact on a patient's odds of disease. The farther a likelihood ratio is above 1.0, the more that test result raises a patient's probability of disease. For likelihood ratios less than 1.0, the closer the ratio is to 0, the more it lowers a patient's probability of disease.

When displayed graphically (Fig. 23–1), a test of no value (dot-

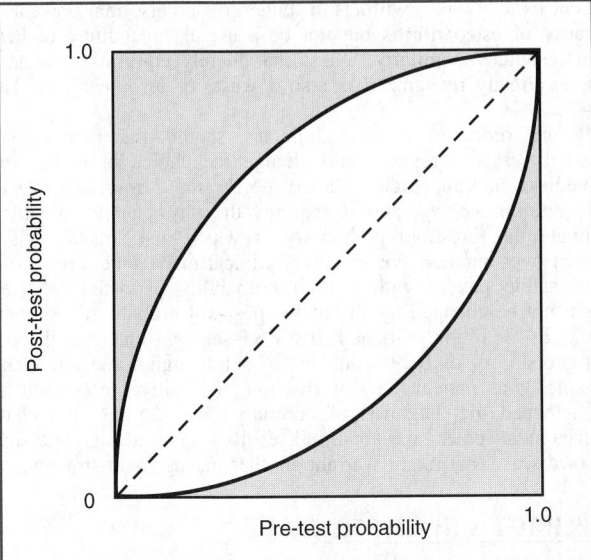

FIGURE 23–1 ▪ Impact of various test results on the patient's probability of disease. The *x* axis depicts a patient's probability of disease before a test. If the test is of no value, the post-test probability (dotted line) is no different from the pre-test probability. An abnormal test result raises the post-test probability of disease, as depicted by the concave-downward arc, whereas a normal test result lowers the probability.

ted line) does not change the pre-test probability, whereas an abnormal or normal result from a useful test moves the probability up or down, respectively. Note that, for a patient with a high pre-test probability of disease, an abnormal test result changes the patient's probability only slightly, but a negative test result leads to a marked reduction in the probability of disease. Similarly, for a patient with a low pre-test probability of disease, a normal test has little impact but an abnormal test result markedly raises the probability of disease.

For example, consider how various exercise test results influence a patient's probability of coronary disease (Table 23–2). For a patient whose clinical history, physical examination, and electrocardiographic findings suggest a 50% probability of disease, the pre-test odds of disease are 1.0. Likelihood ratios for various test results are developed by pooling data from published literature. Note that the "sensitivity" of an exercise test with no ST-segment changes is the rate of such test results in patients with coronary disease and the specificity is the percentage of patients without coronary disease who do *not* have this test result.

When the likelihood ratios for various test results are multiplied times the pre-test odds to calculate post-test odds, the odds decrease for patients without ST-segment changes but increase for

patients with 1 or 2 mm of ST-segment change. Post-test odds can be converted to post-test probabilities according to the following formula:

$$Probability = Odds/(1 + odds)$$

The calculations quantify how the absence of ST-segment changes reduces a patient's probability of disease, whereas ST-segment depression raises the probability of disease.

This form of Bayes' theorem is also useful for showing how the post-test probability of disease is influenced by the patient's pre-test probability of disease. For example, if a patient's clinical data suggest a *probability* of coronary disease of only 0.1, the *pre-test odds* of disease would be only 0.11. For such a low-risk patient, an exercise test with no ST-segment changes would lead to post-test probability of coronary disease of 4%, whereas 1-mm or 2-mm ST-segment changes would lead to a post-test probability of disease of 33% or 55%, respectively.

Even if clinicians rarely perform the calculations that are described in Bayes' theorem, there are important lessons from this theorem that are relevant to principles of test ordering (Table 23–3). The most critical of these lessons is that the interpretation of test results must incorporate information about the patient. Thus, an abnormal test result in a low-risk patient may not be a true indicator of disease. Similarly, a normal test result in a high-risk patient should not be taken as evidence that disease is not present.

Figure 23–2 provides an example of the post-test probabilities for positive and negative results for a test with a sensitivity of 85% and a specificity of 90% (e.g., thallium scintigraphy for diagnosis of coronary artery disease). In a high-risk population with a 90% prevalence of disease, the positive predictive value of an abnormal result is 0.99, compared with just 0.31 for the same test result obtained in a low-risk population with a 5% prevalence of disease. Similarly, the negative predictive value of a normal test result is greater in the low-risk population than the high-risk population.

Multiple Testing

Clinicians frequently obtain more than one test aimed at addressing the same issue and at times are confronted with conflicting results. If these tests are truly "independent"—that is, the tests do not have the same basis in pathophysiology—then it may be appropriate to use the post-test probability obtained through performance of one test as the pre-test probability for the analysis of the impact of the second test result.

However, if the tests are not independent, then this strategy for interpretation of serial test results can be misleading. For example, suppose a low-risk patient has an abnormal lung ventilation-perfusion scan. Obtaining that same test result over and over will not truly raise that patient's probability of coronary disease further and further. In this extreme case, the tests are identical; therefore, serial

Table 23–2 ▪ **EXAMPLE OF ODDS RATIO FORM OF BAYES' THEOREM**

Question: What is the probability of coronary disease for a patient with a 50% pre-test probability of coronary disease who undergoes an exercise test if that patient develops (a) no ST-segment changes, (b) 1 mm of ST-segment depression, or (c) 2 mm of ST-segment depression?
Step 1. Calculate the pre-test odds of disease:

$$p/(1 - p) = 0.5/(1 - 0.5)$$
$$= 0.5/0.5$$
$$= 1.0$$

Step 2. Calculate the likelihood ratios for the various test results, using the formula LR = Sensitivity/(1 − specificity). (Data from pooled literature.)

TEST RESULT	SENSITIVITY	SPECIFICITY	LIKELIHOOD RATIO
No ST-segment changes	0.34	0.15	0.4
1 mm ST-segment depression	0.66	0.85	4.4
2 mm ST-segment depression	0.33	0.97	11

Step 3. Calculate the post-test odds of disease, and convert those odds to post-test probabilities:

TEST RESULT	PRE-TEST ODDS	LIKELIHOOD RATIO	POST-TEST ODDS	POST-TEST PROBABILITY
No ST-segment changes	1	0.4	0.4	0.29
1 mm ST-segment depression	1	4.4	4.4	0.81
2 mm ST-segment depression	1	11	11	0.92

Table 23-3 ■ **PRINCIPLES OF TEST ORDERING AND INTERPRETATION**

1. The interpretation of test results depends on what is already known about the patient.
2. No test is perfect; clinicians should be familiar with their diagnostic performance (see Table 23-1) and never believe that a test "forces" them to pursue a specific management strategy.
3. Tests should be ordered if they may provide *additional* information beyond that already available.
4. Tests should be ordered if there is a reasonable chance that the data will influence patient care.
5. Two tests that provide similar information should not both be ordered.
6. When choosing between two tests that provide similar data, use the test that has lower costs and/or causes less discomfort and inconvenience to the patient.
7. Clinicians should seek all of the information provided by a test, not just a positive or negative result.
8. The cost-effectiveness of strategies using non-invasive tests should be considered in a manner similar to that of therapeutic strategies.

testing adds no information. More commonly, clinicians are faced with results from tests with related but not identical bases in pathophysiology, such as ventilation-perfusion scintigraphy and pulmonary angiography.

Regardless of whether tests are independent, the performance of multiple tests increases the likelihood that an abnormal test result will be obtained in a patient without disease. For example, if a chemistry battery includes 20 tests and the normal range for each test has been developed to include 95% of healthy individuals, the chance that a healthy patient will have a normal result for any specific test is 0.95. However, the probability that all 20 tests will be normal is $(0.95)^{20}$, or 0.36. Thus, most healthy people can be expected to have at least one abnormal result. Hence, unless screening test profiles are used thoughtfully, false-positive results can subject patients to unnecessary tests and procedures.

Threshold Approach to Decision Making

Even if a test provides information, that information may not actually change care. For example, a radiograph of a knee in a patient who is not willing to undergo surgery may reveal the severity of osteoarthritis but not be a useful expenditure of health care resources. Similarly, a test that merely confirms a diagnosis that is already recognized is also a waste of resources (see Table 23-3).

Before ordering a test, clinicians should therefore consider whether that test result could change the choice of management strategies. This approach is called the *threshold approach to medical decision making*, and it requires the physician to be able to estimate the threshold probability at which one strategy will be chosen over another. For example, clinical management for a clinically stable patient with a high probability of coronary disease might not be changed by any of the post-test probabilities shown in Table 23-2. If that patient had no ST-segment changes, the post-test probability of 0.29 would still be too high for a clinician to consider that patient free of disease. A positive test result that strengthened the diagnosis of coronary disease might not change management, unless the abnormal results suggested a greater severity of disease that might warrant another management strategy.

WHICH TEST IS THE BEST TEST?

If the clinician decided that more information is needed to reduce uncertainty, and if it appears possible that tests might lead to a change in management strategies, the question arises of which test is most appropriate. Several factors influence this decision, including patient preferences, the risk associated with the tests, and the diagnostic performance of the alternative tests.

Diagnostic performance of a test is often summarized in terms of sensitivity and specificity, but, as demonstrated in the example in Table 23-2, these parameters depend on which threshold (e.g., 1 mm vs. 2 mm of ST-segment change) is used. A low threshold for calling a test abnormal might lead to excellent sensitivity for detecting disease, but at the expense of a false-positive rate. Conversely, a threshold that led to few false-positive results might cause a clinician to miss many cases of true disease.

The receiver operating characteristic (ROC) curve is a graphic form of describing this trade-off and providing a method for comparing test performance (Fig. 23-3). Each point on the curve describes the sensitivity and the false-positive rate for a different

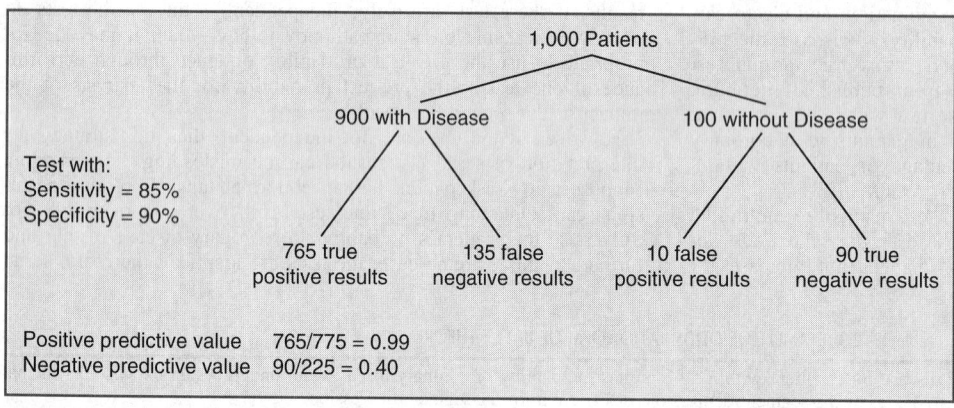

A

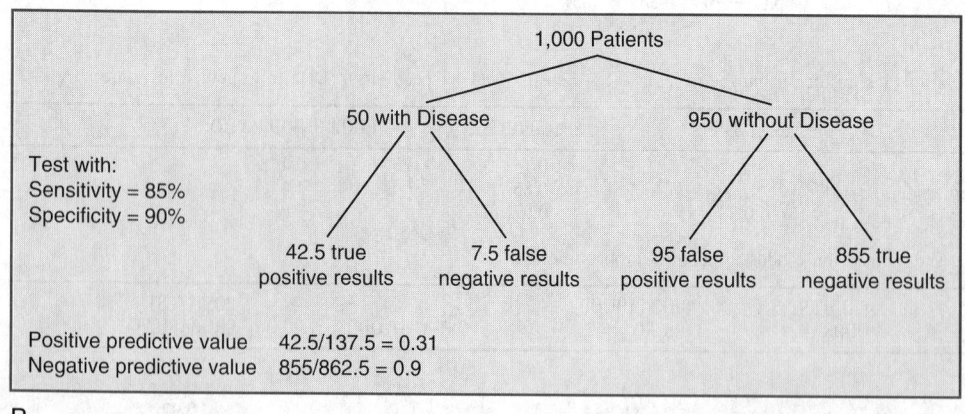

B

FIGURE 23-2 ■ Interpretation of test results in high- and low-risk patients. *A*, High-risk population (90% prevalence of disease). *B*, Low-risk population (5% prevalence of disease).

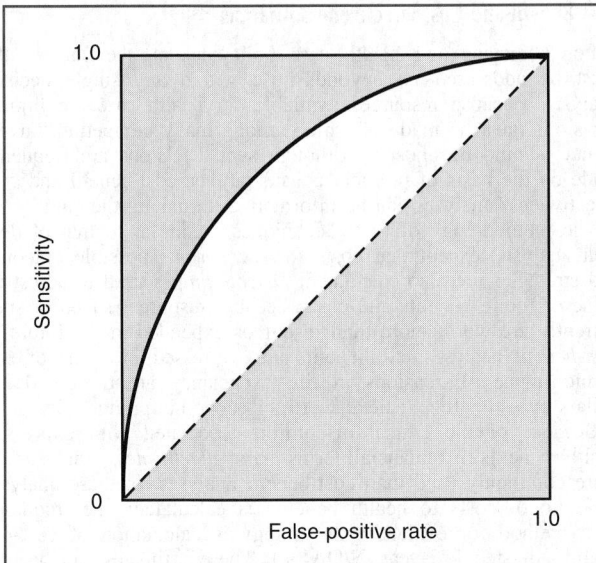

FIGURE 23–3 ■ Receiver operating characteristic curve. The points on the curve reflect the sensitivity and false-positive (1 − specificity) rates of a test at various thresholds. As the threshold is changed to yield greater sensitivity for detecting the outcome of interest, the false-positive rate rises. The better the test, the closer the curve comes to the upper left hand corner. A test of no value (e.g., flipping a coin) would lead to a curve with the course of the dotted line. The area under the curve is often used to compare alternative testing strategies.

threshold for abnormality for a test. A test of no value would lead to a curve with the course of the dotted line, whereas a misleading test would be described by a curve that was concave upward (not shown).

The more accurate the test, the closer its ROC curve comes to the upper left corner of the graph—which would indicate a test threshold that had both excellent sensitivity and a low false-positive rate. The closer an ROC curve comes to the upper left corner, the greater the area under the curve. The area under their respective ROC curves can thus be used to compare the information provided by two tests.

Even if one test is superior to another as demonstrated by a greater area under its ROC curve, the question still remains as to what value of that test should be considered abnormal. The choice of threshold depends on the purpose of testing and on the consequences of a false-positive or false-negative diagnosis. For example, if the goal is to screen the population for a disease that is both potentially fatal and potentially curable, a threshold with excellent sensitivity is appropriate even if it leads to frequent false-positive results. In contrast, if a test is used to confirm a diagnosis that is likely to be treated with an invasive procedure, a threshold with high specificity will be preferred. For example, only 1 mm of ST-segment depression might be the appropriate threshold when exercise electrocardiography was used to evaluate the possibility of coronary disease in a patient with chest pain. However, if the question was whether to perform coronary angiography in search of severe coronary disease that might benefit from revascularization, a threshold of 2 mm or more would be more appropriate.

CHOOSING A STRATEGY

Physicians and patients ultimately must use clinical information to make decisions. These choices are usually made after consideration of a variety of factors, including information from the clinical evaluation, patient preferences, and expected outcomes with various management strategies. Insight into the impact of these considerations can be improved through the performance of decision analysis (Table 23–4).

The first step in a decision analysis is to define the problem clearly; this step often requires writing out a statement of the issue so it can be scrutinized for any ambiguity. After the problem is defined, the next step is to define the alternative strategies.

For example, consider the question of what management strategy is most appropriate for patients who present with a first episode of

Table 23–4 ■ STEPS IN PERFORMANCE OF DECISION ANALYSIS

1. Frame the question.
2. Create the decision tree.
   a. Identify the alternative strategies.
   b. List the possible outcomes for each of the alternative strategies.
   c. Describe the sequence of events as a series of decision nodes and chance nodes.
3. Choose a time horizon for the analysis.
4. Determine the probability for each chance outcome.
5. Assign a value to each outcome.
6. Calculate the expected utility for each strategy.
7. Perform sensitivity analysis.

postmenopausal bleeding. The four basic alternatives for the initial evaluation are (1) office endometrial biopsy; (2) dilatation and curettage (D&C); (3) hysterectomy; and (4) observation unless bleeding recurred.

The expected outcomes for these strategies depend in part on the sensitivity and specificity of the diagnostic procedures (D&C, endometrial biopsy). Assumptions must be made about the next step if the first test was non-diagnostic. Thus, the four basic management strategies actually include at least eight different "game plans" (Table 23–5). A wide range of other factors influence the findings of the analysis: the effectiveness and likely compliance with medical therapy for complex hyperplasia, the risk that complex hyperplasia would progress to endometrial cancer, and the expected outcomes with surgery or radiation therapy for endometrial cancer.

These estimates are needed to make estimates for each strategy's predicted life expectancy and direct medical costs. These outcomes usually differ for patients of different ages and with different underlying risks for the outcomes of interest—in this case, cancer and complex hyperplasia. Optimal strategies are unlikely to be the same for an elderly patient with a short life expectancy and low risk of cancer as for a younger patient with a long life expectancy and a high risk of cancer.

The credibility of the decision analysis depends on the credibility of these estimates. Unfortunately, published reports often do not provide information on the outcomes of interest for specific patient subsets (e.g., women aged 50 to 59 years or women over age 80 years), or there may not have been sufficient statistical power within patient subsets for the findings to be statistically significant. Furthermore, randomized trial data are relevant to the populations included in the trial; hence, the extension of the findings to other genders, races, and age groups requires assumptions by those performing the analysis. For many issues, expert opinion must be used to derive a reasonable estimate of the outcome.

For many diseases, the potential outcomes are more complex than perfect health or death. With chronic diseases, patients may live many years in a condition somewhere between these two, and the goal of medical interventions may be to improve quality of life rather than extend survival. Thus, the value of life in imperfect health must be reflected in decision analyses. These values are, by convention, expressed on a scale of 0 to 100, where 0 indicates the worst outcome and 100 is the best outcome.

Life expectancy and quality of life estimates are combined in many decision analyses to calculate *quality-adjusted life years*. For

Table 23–5 ■ EVALUATION STRATEGIES FOR POSTMENOPAUSAL BLEEDING

INITIAL TEST	SECOND TEST IF FIRST WAS NON-DIAGNOSTIC	THIRD TEST IF SECOND WAS NON-DIAGNOSTIC
1. No work-up*	No further work-up*	
2. Office biopsy	No further work-up	
3. Office biopsy	D&C	No further work-up
4. Office biopsy	D&C	Hysterectomy
5. Office biopsy	Hysterectomy	
6. D&C	No further work-up	
7. D&C	Hysterectomy	
8. Hysterectomy		

*Assumes that, if bleeding recurred, patients would undergo work-up at a future date.

Adapted from Feldman S, Berkowitz RS, Tosteson ANA: Cost effectiveness of strategies to evaluate postmenopausal bleeding. Obstet Gynecol 81:968–975, 1993.

Table 23-6 ■ ESTIMATED COST-EFFECTIVENESS OF SOME LIFE-PROLONGING OR LIFE-SAVING INTERVENTIONS

CATEGORY	INTERVENTION	COST/LIFE-YEAR
Transportation	Grooved pavement on highways	$29,000
	Collapsible steering columns in cars	$67,000
	Airbags	$120,000
Toxins	Chlorination of drinking water	$3,100
	Radon remediation in homes with levels	
	• ≥8.11 pCi/L	$35,000
	• ≥4 pCi/L	$140,000
	Asbestos exposure standard of 0.2 (vs. 2.0) fibers/cc in construction industry	$29,000,000
Medicine	β-Blocker treatment after myocardial infarction for:	
	• High-risk survivors	$3,000
	• Low-risk survivors	$17,000
	Cervical cancer screening:	
	• Every 3 years for women age 65+	≤$0
	• Annually for women beginning at age 20	$82,000
	Immunization for all infants and pre-school children	≤$0
	Lovastatin for:	
	• Men age 35–54 years with heart disease and total cholesterol ≥ 250 mg/dL	≤$0
	• Women age 35–44 with no heart disease and total cholesterol ≥ 300 mg/dL	$1,200,000
	Annual stool guaiac colon cancer screening for:	
	• People age 55+	≤$0
	• People age 40+	1,300
	Sclerotherapy for esophageal bleeding in alcoholics	≤$0
	Heart transplantation for patients < age 55 and favorable prognosis	$3,600
	Universal (vs. category-specific) precautions to prevent human immunodeficiency virus transmission	$890,000
	Influenza vaccination for all citizens	$140

Adapted from Tengs TO, Adams ME, Pliskin JS, et al: Five-hundred life-saving interventions and their cost effectiveness. Risk Analysis 15:369–390, 1995.

example, a strategy that leads to a 10-year life expectancy with such severe disability that utility of the state of health is only half that of perfect health would have a quality-adjusted life expectancy of 5 years. With such adjustments to life-expectancy data, the impact of interventions that improve quality of life but do not extend it can be compared with those that extend life but do not improve its quality.

After the value and the probability of the various outcomes have been estimated, the expected utility of each strategy can be calculated. In comparing the different strategies available at a decision node, the analysis generally selects the option with the highest expected utility. At chance nodes, the expected utility is the weighted average of the utility of the various possible branches.

After the analysis has been performed with the baseline assumptions, *sensitivity analyses* should be performed in which these assumptions are varied over a reasonable range. These analyses can reveal which assumptions have the most influence over the conclusions and identify threshold probabilities at which the conclusions would change. For example, the decision analysis comparing various strategies for evaluation of postmenopausal bleeding found that initial office biopsy resulted in slightly better or comparable life expectancy compared with D&C or initial hysterectomy, but this finding would be reversed if different assumptions for the procedural complication rates were used or if the clinical consequences of an initial misdiagnosis were considered more severe.

Cost-Benefit and Cost-Effectiveness Analysis

For clinicians and health care policymakers, the choices that must be addressed go beyond those within any single decision analysis. Because resources available for health care are limited, decisions must be made of which among many competing "investments" should be chosen. Although such decisions are frequently made on the basis of political considerations, cost-benefit and cost-effectiveness analyses can be informative in making the choices.

The methodology of these techniques is similar to that of decision analysis, except that costs for the various possible outcomes and strategies are also calculated. *Discounting* is used to adjust the value of future benefits and costs, because resources saved or spent currently are worth more than resources expended in the future. In *cost-benefit* analyses, all benefits are expressed in terms of economic impact. Extensions in life expectancy are translated into dollars by estimating societal worth or economic productivity.

Because of the ethical discomfort associated with expressing health benefits in financial terms, *cost-effectiveness* analyses are more commonly used than cost-benefit analyses. In these analyses, the ratio of costs to health benefits is calculated; one frequently used method for evaluating a strategy is calculation of cost-per-quality-adjusted life year ($/QALY). These estimates can be used to compare strategies and identify settings in which strategies that may be more expensive (e.g., coronary angiography) may "purchase" quality-adjusted life years at a lower cost than less-aggressive strategies (e.g., observation).

Cost-effectiveness analyses can provide important insights into the relative attractiveness of different management strategies and can also help guide policymakers in decisions about which technologies to make available on a routine basis. It is important to emphasize that no medical intervention can have an attractive cost-effectiveness if its effectiveness has not been proven. Furthermore, the cost-effectiveness of an intervention depends heavily on the patient population in which it is applied. Thus, a very inexpensive intervention will have a poor cost-effectiveness ratio if it is used in a low-risk population that is unlikely to benefit from it. In contrast, an expensive technology can have an attractive cost-effectiveness ratio if used in patients with a high probability of benefiting from it. Table 23–6 shows cost-effectiveness estimates from published literature for some common medical and non-medical interventions. Such estimates should only be used with understanding of the population for which they are relevant.

Balas EA, Kretschmer RAC, Gnann W, et al: Interpreting cost analyses of clinical interventions. JAMA 279:54–57, 1998. *This article reviews basic principles for capturing cost information and assesses the extent to which published studies adhere to these principles.*

Richardson WS, Detsky AS: Users' guides to the medical literature: VII. How to use a clinical decision analysis: A. Are the results of the study valid? Evidence-based Medicine Working Group. JAMA 273:1292–1295, 1995. *Part of an excellent series on critical assessment of literature on tests and other procedures. This installment addresses issues related to clinical decision analysis.*

Tengs TO, Adams ME, Pliskin JS, et al: Five-hundred life-saving interventions and their cost effectiveness. Risk Analysis 15:369–390, 1995. *This article includes cost-effectiveness estimates on a wide range of life-saving interventions including health care and public health strategies.*

24 APPLICATION OF STATISTICS

Catarina I. Kiefe

The knowledge on which clinicians base medical decisions is growing explosively. Epidemiologic concepts of study design, data quality, and validity of inferences are key to the understanding and use of the medical literature (see Chapter 25). The appropriate use of statistical tools is a necessary but not sufficient component of a good study.

In the medical literature, investigators publish their findings using *descriptive statistics* to summarize data and *inferential statistics* to test hypotheses. Judgment is required in the choice of statistical tools as well as in the interpretation of statistical analyses. Physicians need a basic understanding of statistics to be informed users of the medical literature and to know whether and when to apply data in the literature to benefit their patients.

DESCRIPTIVE STATISTICS

Many clinical variables, such as systolic blood pressure, are measured on a continuous numeric scale. For these continuous variables, appropriate measures of "central location" include a *mean* (average), *median* (50th percentile or middle value), and *mode* (most common value). Measures of dispersion quantify the amount of variability exhibited by variables. For those continuous variables distributed in a bell-shaped fashion (*Gaussian or normal distribution*), the mean ± 1.96 *standard deviations (SD)* defines an interval *containing 95% of the observed values*. The *standard error of the mean (SEM)* measures the precision of the estimate of the mean itself. The SEM is always smaller than the SD, and it is not appropriate to use the SEM directly as a measure of dispersion. When a variable has a bell-shaped distribution, the sample mean ±1.96 × SEM represents the *95% confidence interval* for the mean. The length of this confidence interval describes the precision of the mean estimate. For example, if a study reports that mean systolic blood pressure is 123 mm Hg, SD = 10 mm Hg, and SEM = 2 mm Hg, then 95% of the population represented by this study should have a systolic blood pressure between 103 and 143 mm Hg, and if 100 similar studies were performed, 95 of them would be expected to yield a mean systolic blood pressure within the confidence interval from 119 to 125 mm Hg. Asserting that the mean is within its 95% confidence interval is true 95% of the time.

Many variables of clinical interest are not continuous. Vital status after a myocardial infarction is a *dichotomous (nominal)* variable taking on only the two values "alive" or "dead." Major blood group (A, B, AB, or O) is also a nominal variable, with individuals classified into one of four categories, without intrinsic order to the categories. On the other hand, stage of breast cancer is an *ordinal variable*. The values are "ordered" in a meaningful manner, for example, stage IV breast cancer is more advanced than stage II. However, the progression from stage I to stage II is quite different from the progression from stage III to stage IV. Therefore, one-unit increments have very different implications from what they would have for a continuous variable. Nominal and ordinal variables are usually described using the absolute numbers and proportions of individuals in each category; means and SDs are not appropriate for such variables.

HYPOTHESIS TESTING

Much clinical research is concerned with detecting associations between an exposure (e.g., tobacco smoking) and a disease (e.g., lung cancer) or between an intervention and a clinical response or outcome (see Chapter 25). For a typical study, investigators first develop a hypothesis: for example, that the mean systolic blood pressure in a group given an antihypertensive agent is lower than the mean pressure in a group given a placebo. Next, the investigators sample the populations of interest (e.g., the treatment and control groups) and measure the variable of interest (e.g., systolic blood pressure). A *null hypothesis* of no effect, or no difference between groups, is formulated. In this example, the null hypothesis would be that the two groups, treatment and control, were drawn from the same underlying population. If the null hypothesis is true and the study is well designed, any observed difference in mean systolic blood pressure between the two groups would be due to random sampling and differences between the two groups should be no greater than the magnitude that would be expected by chance.

With a well-designed study, inferences based on population samples apply to the entire population. The underlying assumption is that the samples, which are the treatment and control groups, are selected at random. Any systematic violation of this assumption, such as preferentially including individuals on a low-salt diet in the treatment group, would introduce bias and jeopardize the validity of inferences to be drawn from the study. However, statistics would not speak to this study flaw. If a difference between two population samples is observed (e.g., systolic blood pressures are lower in the treatment than in the control group), then the key statistical ques-

tion is whether this difference could have been due to random sampling (i.e., chance).

The likelihood that an observed difference or an even more extreme difference is due to chance alone is called the *P value*. If a certain difference between mean systolic blood pressures in treatment and control groups were observed, $P < .05$ would mean that given that the null hypothesis is true, there is a less than 5% likelihood that this or a larger difference is due to chance. Thus, if the P value is small, it is unlikely that an observed difference is due to chance, the null hypothesis is rejected, and it is inferred that there are real population differences (i.e., a real association between treatment and systolic blood pressure). The conventional level for "small" has been traditionally accepted, arbitrarily, as .05.

Although an association may be demonstrated with statistical tools, association does not necessarily establish causality. For example, a statistical association between pancreatic cancer and coffee drinking has been observed and published. However, after lengthy debates in the scientific community, coffee is not generally accepted as a cause of pancreatic cancer. The decision of whether an association is due to cause and effect involves much more than statistics. Factors contributing to this decision include biologic plausibility, strength of association, consistency of association across well-designed studies performed in different settings, and dose-response effect.

A small P value safeguards against the risk that a chance finding in a particular sample will mistakenly lead to rejection of a null hypothesis that is actually true. Progressively lower P values strongly suggest that the observed data are inconsistent with the null hypothesis. The error of rejecting a true null hypothesis, commonly called type I error, occurs when chance leads to the conclusion that differences or associations exist when in reality they do not (e.g., believing that systolic blood pressure was lowered by a particular treatment when the observed differences were no more than random variation). For type I error, which is also called alpha error or significance level, the traditional acceptable upper limit is .05.

In contrast, type II error occurs when a large P value leads to the incorrect conclusion that a difference does not exist, and hence the null hypothesis is incorrectly accepted. An example would be to conclude mistakenly that systolic blood pressure was not lowered by treatment, when in reality treatment is effective even though it did not work to a degree greater than potentially explainable by chance in the study at hand. Type II error, also called the beta error, may occur because the study lacks the statistical power to demonstrate a true association or difference. The power of the study (i.e., the probability of detecting a difference or an association that really exists) is 1−beta. The power of the study increases as the sample size increases, as the acceptable alpha error increases, and if the magnitude of the difference that is considered clinically significant is increased. Power decreases with increasing variability in the data. A common mistake is to conclude that an effect does not exist because a study with low power failed to demonstrate a statistically significant result. The critical reader should beware of type I errors when a study demonstrates a "positive" effect and should consider the possibility of type II errors when a study is negative.

Impressively small P values may correspond to effects of small magnitude when a study has a very large sample size. For example, if a study reported a mean drop of 1 mm Hg ($P < .001$) in systolic blood pressure for a certain medication, this result would possess a high degree of statistical significance but no clinical significance, especially given alternative methods to lower blood pressure.

Tests of statistical significance help safeguard against the possibility that chance could threaten a study's internal validity. Other threats such as bias, other variables that may confound the findings, or faulty data are not addressed by statistical significance testing. Both investigators and readers may overestimate a study's external validity; that is, they may generalize the results demonstrated by the data to a population inadequately represented in their study sample. For example, the benefits of cholesterol-lowering medications were initially demonstrated only in middle-aged, mostly white, men. Because these initial studies were well designed and conducted, their internal validity was not questioned. However, the extent to which these results could be extrapolated to older individuals, women, or minorities could not be determined from the original studies and continues to engender debate and to guide additional research.

TESTS OF STATISTICAL SIGNIFICANCE

Once a hypothesis is clearly formulated and data have been collected to test that hypothesis, standard statistical procedures, commonly called tests of statistical significance, interpret the data and assign P values. The choice of statistical tests depends on the nature of the data. In the example of the antihypertensive trial, in which the goal is to compare the mean systolic blood pressure for subjects given placebo with that of subjects given active drug, the appropriate test of statistical significance if the blood pressure distributions are bell shaped is the unpaired Student t test. If the antihypertensive trial included three (or more) randomization groups, such as diet, drugs, and placebo, analysis of variance, often called ANOVA, is the most appropriate test of statistical significance. Both the Student t test and ANOVA assign P values to the differences between randomization groups.

ANOVA and t test are parametric tests, which assume that data follow certain distributions described by parameters, such as the traditional bell-shaped curves. Conversely, non-parametric tests (Table 24–1) do not assume that data follow any pre-specified distributions and are preferable when the actual data are not consistent with the underlying parametric assumptions of a bell-shaped distribution.

In some studies, it is more appropriate to have each subject serve as his or her own control rather than having a placebo group composed of patients who received inactive medication. Observations in the same patient with and without an intervention, which may be given in active and control periods of time that are assigned randomly and in a blinded fashion, call for the use of the *paired Student t test.*

A different situation arises when a dichotomous variable is the outcome of interest. For example, investigators studying the effect of β-blockers on mortality after myocardial infarction might randomize subjects into two groups: one receiving a β-blocker and the other receiving a placebo. The null hypothesis would be that the proportion of deaths is the same in both groups. The appropriate test of statistical significance in this case is the *chi-square*; if the study has very small numbers, an alternative is the Fisher exact test.

Certain situations call for evaluating the association between two continuous variables. For example, one might hypothesize that systolic blood pressure increases linearly with age. Mathematically, this relationship may be represented by the model

$$\text{Systolic blood pressure} = a + b(age)$$

with blood pressure and age varying with the individual and with fixed values a (regression constant) and b (regression slope or regression coefficient) to be determined. *Linear regression* provides a P value for the null hypothesis that $b = 0$ (i.e., blood pressure and age are not correlated with each other) and supplies values for the coefficients a and b. Furthermore, linear regression determines whether this model fits a given data set reasonably well. Assuming

normally distributed data, the *Pearson correlation coefficient*, usually denoted by r, is a measure of the strength of linear association between age and systolic blood pressure; r is always between -1 and 1, and r^2 (always between 0 and 1) measures how much of the variability in systolic blood pressure is explained by age. For example, a Pearson correlation coefficient of 0.6 would mean that approximately 36% (0.6^2) of the variability in systolic blood pressure is explained by age.

MULTIVARIABLE METHODS

Frequently, the complexity of clinical phenomena defies reduction to a simple equation with only one independent variable. For example, factors such as weight may be associated with other factors, such as age, but also affect blood pressure independent of age. A simple linear regression model neglects this *confounding variable* (weight) and may distort the association between blood pressure and age. More sophisticated methods, such as the multiple regression method, can adjust for confounding variables and better model the relationship of systolic blood pressure, the dependent or outcome variable, with independent variables, which are age and weight (Table 24–2):

$$\text{Systolic blood pressure} = a + b(age) + c(weight)$$

Multiple linear regression determines the coefficients a, b, and c, assesses the goodness of fit of the model with the data, and calculates a P value for each coefficient. The method can consider multiple potential independent variables.

When the dependent variable is dichotomous rather than continuous and several continuous and/or nominal independent variables are being considered, multiple *logistic* regression is preferable to multiple *linear* regression. When the independent variable is nominal with more than two categories, discriminant analysis or newer types of multiple regression analysis are appropriate. An alternative non-parametric multivariate technique constructs classification and regression trees that sequentially determine which independent variables add significant information in subgroups defined by previously selected, significant, independent variables.

Cox proportional hazards regression is used when the outcome variable is the time to occurrence of a certain event. For example, a randomized controlled trial evaluating two different treatments for lung cancer might use survival time as its outcome variable. Cox regression models the effect of the treatment on survival time while adjusting for variables such as age, gender, and stage at diagnosis. The difference between Cox regression and multiple logistic regression is that the outcome variable in Cox regression is continuous, such as survival time, and the outcome in multiple logistic regression is dichotomous, such as survival at 5 years.

Multivariable modeling, which has become deceptively easy to perform with powerful statistical software, is subject to misuse, especially when the approach violates the underlying assumptions of the multivariate method. Another problem is commonly called *overfitting*. For example, suppose that a multivariate model is used to study the effect of β-blockers on mortality after myocardial infarction in 200 subjects, of whom 20 die. In addition to the use of β-blockers, other independent variables in the model could be age, gender, co-morbidity, left ventricular ejection fraction, and many others. Inclusion of so many independent variables may lead

Table 24–1 ■ RECOMMENDED STATISTICAL APPROACHES TO VARIOUS TYPES OF DATA AND SITUATIONS

WHO OR WHAT IS BEING STUDIED?	CHARACTERISTICS OF THE DATA		
	Continuous*	Ordinal	Nominal
Two groups of different people	Unpaired t test	Mann-Whitney rank-sum test	Chi-square test or Fisher exact test
Three or more groups of different people	Analysis of variance	Kruskal-Wallis statistic	Chi-square test
Before and after in the same matched people	Paired t test	Wilcoxon signed-rank test	McNemar's test
Association of two variables with each other†	Linear regression and Pearson correlation coefficient	Spearman correlation coefficient	Contingency coefficients

*And with a distribution that at least approximates a bell-shaped curve.
†If *both* do not meet the criteria for the type of data, choose the column farther to the right that is consistent with both variables.

MULTIVARIABLE METHODS	DEPENDENT VARIABLE
Multiple linear regression	Continuous
Multiple logistic regression	Dichotomous
Cox proportional hazards	Time to outcome event
Discriminant analysis	Nominal
Classification and regression trees	Dichotomous (but can be nominal or time to outcome event)

to *overfitting,* because the number of outcome events (i.e., deaths) is so low that the model is unreliable. In general, analysis should consider no more than one potential independent variable for every 5 to 10 outcome events in the study.

Statistics are safeguards against random sampling error that can cause erroneous inferences. Statistics cannot compensate for other threats to the validity of clinical research, such as bias or faulty data, and have the potential to be both misunderstood and misused.

Bailar JC III, Mosteller F (eds): Medical Uses of Statistics, 2nd ed. Boston, NEJM Books, 1992. *Essays on using statistics in medicine geared toward statistical ideas and their current use, not computational details. Addresses "why" rather than "how" questions.*

Concato J, Feinstein AR, Holford TR: The risk of determining risk with multivariable models. Ann Intern Med 118:201, 1993. *Useful review article that reports on how multivariable models are being used in medical journals, while establishing a framework to critique their use.*

Daniel WW: Biostatistics: A Foundation for Analysis in the Health Sciences, 7th ed. New York, John Wiley & Sons, 1999. *Introductory statistical textbook with few mathematical prerequisites. Exercises use data sets available from a website.*

Last JM: A Dictionary of Epidemiology, 3rd ed. New York, Oxford University Press, 1995. *A practical reference book, small in dimension (180 pages) but invaluable to the physician who wants to quickly look up epidemiological or statistical terms.*

Sackett DL, Haynes RB, Guyatt GH, et al: Clinical Epidemiology: A Basic Science for Clinical Medicine, 2nd ed. Boston, Little, Brown, 1991. *Practical, insightful, and entertaining, this expanded, updated version of a classic series on how to read the medical literature clarifies statistical concepts, emphasizing their use in clinical practice and clinical research.*

25 PRINCIPLES OF OUTCOME ASSESSMENT

Albert W. Wu

Physicians treat patients to improve or maintain their health. For some complaints such as an isolated symptom, it is evident when the patient's health has improved. In other cases, the effects of treatment may not be immediately apparent. For a given patient, it is often difficult to know what treatment or course of action is likely to lead to the best outcome. Furthermore, several kinds of outcomes may be important in evaluating a treatment.

Traditionally, data obtained from a medical history, physical examination, and laboratory tests form the basis of treatment evaluation and include parameters such as clinical events, physical findings, laboratory abnormalities, symptoms, and mortality. However, these conventional measures are less representative of the effects of treatment on the patient's overall health because much of the emphasis in medicine has shifted from delivering acute care to treating chronic diseases. New approaches use standardized questions to assess quality of life and patient satisfaction and use insurance claims data to examine costs. As issues of cost-effectiveness and quality improvement become increasingly important, so does outcome assessment.

DEFINITIONS

Outcomes research, which is a comprehensive approach to determining the effects of medical care, entails the use of a variety of data sources and measurement methods. Outcomes research includes the rigorous determination of what does and does not work in medical care and how different providers compare with regard to their effects on patient outcome.

In outcomes research, *efficacy* refers to how a treatment works in ideal circumstances when delivered to selected patients by providers most skilled at providing it. *Effectiveness* refers to how a treatment works under ordinary conditions by the average practitioner for the typical patient. Efficacy is often measured in clinical trials, whereas effectiveness is better measured in observational studies.

Outcome assessment plays an important role in studies of quality of care. Excellent quality care maximizes the benefits and minimizes the risks to the patient, adheres to professional standards, is consistent with patient expectations and preferences, and achieves efficiency in the use of resources. According to Donabedian's widely accepted model of quality of care, it is necessary to assess the "structure, process, and outcomes" of care when monitoring quality. Structure refers to stable elements that form the basis of the health system, such as the type of facility, administrative organization, and provider qualifications. Process refers to what happens in the medical interaction and includes the technical and interpersonal skills of the physician and other providers. Process measures compare care with relevant standards. In this framework, outcomes are the measurable events and observations that are presumed to occur in part as a result of the structure and process of medical care.

THE IMPORTANCE OF OUTCOME ASSESSMENT

Factors that have led to the current interest in patient outcomes include the rising cost of health care, changes in the organization and financing of care, findings of unexplained variation in physicians' practice patterns, recognition of the limitations of available information about the effects of many treatments, and increased adoption of a model of shared patient and physician decision making. The cost of medical care in the United States has grown from $250.1 billion and 9.2% of the gross domestic product in 1980 to $1.035 trillion and 14% of the gross domestic product by 2000. Desire to control the growth rate in medical expenditure, coupled with evidence that some medical procedures may be performed inappropriately, has created incentives to assess the relative effectiveness of different treatments. Elimination of treatments deemed less effective could result in reductions or reallocation of resources to treatments that produce greater benefits.

The growth of pre-paid care and prospective payment for hospital care has promoted increased competition among health care providers. Managed care organizations and insurers now compete for corporate buyers, and individual physicians compete for inclusion on preferred provider lists. Most of the competition currently involves price and services offered, but "report cards" detailing the performance of health plans, institutions, and individual physicians on a variety of outcomes can demonstrate value and improve consumers' choices. The emergence of managed care as the predominant model of practice in the United States has also led to concern about erosion in the quality of care to achieve cost savings.

Researchers have documented substantial geographic differences in the use of medical procedures for apparently similar patients. For example, in 1992–1993, among women on Medicare who had breast cancer surgery, the proportion who had breast-sparing surgery (as opposed to total mastectomy) varied by a factor of 33, from 1.4% to 48.0% (Fig. 25–1). Related studies have shown that the per capita costs of hospitalization for residents of Boston are about twice those for residents of New Haven. Whether these differences reflect overuse in high-use areas or underuse in low-use areas requires additional information. Striking differences may also be seen in outcomes depending on whom the patient sees for care. For example, as many as 5 additional deaths per 100 are related to which cardiac surgeon performs coronary bypass surgery. Although some patients receive unneeded procedures, it is estimated that 25% of people with serious coronary artery disease are not offered indicated revascularization.

Recognition of the considerable uncertainty facing practicing physicians has led to calls for the practice of "evidence-based medicine." Such an approach combines pathophysiologic rationale,

Percentage of Inpatient Breast Cancer Surgery in Medicare Women That Was Breast Sparing

By Hospital Referral Region (1992-93)

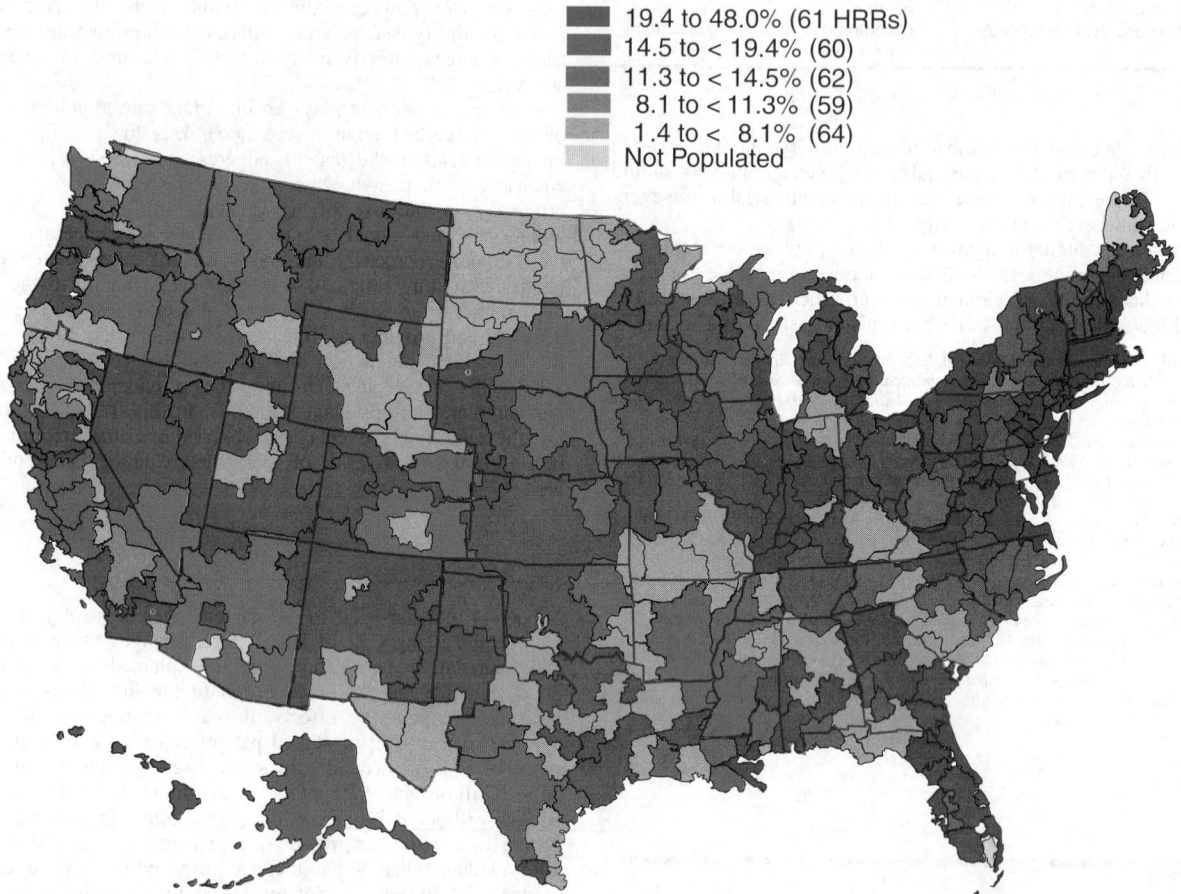

■ 19.4 to 48.0% (61 HRRs)
■ 14.5 to < 19.4% (60)
■ 11.3 to < 14.5% (62)
■ 8.1 to < 11.3% (59)
■ 1.4 to < 8.1% (64)
  Not Populated

FIGURE 25–1 ■ Breast-sparing surgery was more widely and commonly used in the Northeast than elsewhere in the United States; regionally, its use was lowest in the South, Midwest, and Northwest. (From Wennberg JE, Cooper MM [eds]: Dartmouth Atlas of Health Care. © Trustees of Dartmouth College.)

caregiver experience, and patient preferences with valid and current evidence from clinical research.

The traditional model of clinical decision making, in which patients delegate choice to the physician, is being replaced by a model of shared decision making, in which patients actively participate in the choice of treatment. In choosing among treatment options, this model requires increased emphasis on patient preferences for risks and outcomes, as well as increased patient understanding (see Chapter 2).

For all of the reasons stated above, activity directed at outcome assessment has grown rapidly. Since 1986, the Health Care Financing Administration has reported hospital mortality rates for specific conditions. Since 1987, the Joint Commission on Accreditation of Health Care Organizations has shifted from traditional structural measures of quality assurance to quality assessment based on outcomes adjusted for the severity of patients' disease. The National Committee on Quality Assurance, an independent accrediting body for managed care organizations, has worked since 1989 to develop measures of plan performance.

TYPES OF HEALTH OUTCOMES

Outcomes research considers a broad range of indicators, including conventional clinical measures such as mortality, disease or treatment complications, persistence of pathology, physiologic or laboratory abnormalities, deformity, signs and symptoms, and adverse clinical events. In addition, outcomes research considers the patient's perspective of quality of life and satisfaction with care.

Other relevant outcomes include the use of health care resources and the costs and economic losses caused by disability or death (Table 25–1).

MEASUREMENT STANDARDS

To be useful, a test must meet standards for reliability, validity, responsiveness, and interpretability (Table 25–2). *Reliability* concerns the extent to which a measuring procedure yields consistent results on repeated trials. *Validity* is the degree to which a test measures what it is intended to measure, e.g., whether a pain questionnaire actually measures pain rather than the patient's mood. *Responsiveness* is the ability of a test to detect clinically meaningful changes. For example, if a treatment results in an important improvement in health-related quality of life, a measure should be able to detect that difference. For results to be useful, measurements must also be expressed in terms that clinicians can understand.

PATIENT-ASSESSED OUTCOMES

QUALITY OF LIFE. Several terms are used almost interchangeably to refer to the concept of "health," including health status, functional status, quality of life, and health-related quality of life. In 1948 the World Health Organization defined health as "a state of complete physical, mental, and social well-being, and not merely

Table 25-1 ■ HEALTH OUTCOMES

OUTCOME	EXAMPLE FOR A PATIENT WITH MYOCARDIAL INFARCTION
Clinical	
Mortality	Death in hospital
Pathology	Coronary artery narrowing
Non-fatal clinical event	Stroke
Hospital re-admission	Re-admission within 30 d of hospital discharge
Complication of disease or treatment	Sternal wound infection after coronary artery bypass grafting
Physiologic test	Ejection fraction
Laboratory test	Troponin level
Symptom	Angina pectoris
Patient-Reported	
Health-related quality of life	Ability to perform usual physical activities
Satisfaction with care	Patient ratings of overall quality of care
Cost	
Utilization of health services	Number of physician visits
Direct cost	Cost of physician visits and prescription medications
Indirect cost	Loss of income from missed days of work

Table 25-3 ■ DIMENSIONS OF HEALTH-RELATED QUALITY OF LIFE

DIMENSION	DESCRIPTION
Physical functioning	Activities of daily living, strenuous activities
Mental health	Anxiety, depression, well-being, behavioral and emotional control
Social functioning	Quantity and quality of social contacts
Role functioning	Ability to perform work or usual activities
Cognitive functioning	Attention, memory, concentration
Energy	Energy and fatigue
General health perceptions	Global self-assessment of health
Pain	Severity and frequency of pain
Symptoms	Nausea, headache, dizziness, etc.
Sexual functioning	Performance and satisfaction
Sleep	Quantity and quality of sleep

the absence of disease and infirmity." Bergner identified five dimensions of *health status*: (1) genetic and inherited characteristics; (2) biochemical, physiologic, and anatomic condition, including impairment of systems, disease, signs, and symptoms; (3) *functional status*, which includes performance of the usual activities of life such as self-care, physical activities, and work; (4) mental condition, which includes positive and negative feelings; and (5) health potential, including longevity and prognosis.

Quality of life is a broad concept that encompasses a person's assessment of all aspects of that person's experience. Because quality of life includes important dimensions of life that are distant from conventional medical concern (e.g., achievement and spiritual fulfillment), it is useful to focus on aspects of quality of life that may be affected by therapeutic measures. *Health-related quality of life* encompasses several dimensions of health status that are directly experienced by the person, e.g., physical functioning, mental health, cognitive functioning, social and role functioning, energy, general health perceptions, symptoms, sexual functioning, and sleep (Table 25-3).

STRUCTURE OF MEASURES AND MODES OF ADMINISTRATION. Measurements of health-related quality of life require indicators of different dimensions. Some measures consist of a single global health item such as the question "Would you say your health is excellent, very good, good, fair, or poor?" However, most instruments consist of a series of questions or "items" that are summed to yield a score for each specific dimension.

Questionnaires can be self-administered or given by trained interviewers. Interviews are labor intensive but ensure compliance and minimize misinterpretation. Interviews may be conducted in person,

Table 25-2 ■ MEASUREMENT STANDARDS

STANDARD	DEFINITION	EXAMPLE
Reliability	Does the instrument produce the same results if reapplied to the same situation?	CD4 lymphocyte counts repeated for the same individual yield the same results.
Validity	Does the instrument really measure what it purports to?	Scores on a pain questionnaire are highly correlated with scores on established pain measures.
Responsiveness	Is the instrument capable of identifying small but clinically significant changes?	The mean score on a functional status questionnaire increases significantly with the use of inhaled corticosteroids for asthma.

by telephone, or with computer assistance. Sometimes a surrogate respondent is used to estimate the responses that would be obtained from an unreliable or inarticulate patient.

TYPES OF QUALITY-OF-LIFE MEASURES. Two basic approaches are used to assess quality of life: generic and disease-specific. The format of measures may be single indices, health profiles, or utility measures.

Generic instruments are designed for use across different diseases, treatments, settings, and patient groups. The major advantage is that they can be used in any population and allow comparisons of the relative impact of various health interventions. However, they may be unresponsive to changes in specific conditions and may be too general to guide clinical decision making. *Disease-specific* measures focus on dimensions of health related to a particular disease, population, symptom, or problem and may be more responsive to a change in the patient's condition than a generic instrument. For example, the Health Assessment Questionnaire (Fries, 1982), widely used in studies of arthritis, includes questions about handgrip strength and pain. Disease-specific measures are more easily understood by clinicians but are frequently less well tested than generic instruments.

Single indices attempt to reduce several concepts to a unidimensional scale. For example, the Karnofsky Performance Status score (Karnofsky, 1948), which is commonly used in cancer trials, combines information about the ability to work, to perform normal activities without assistance, and to care for personal needs. Single indices are brief but are less reliable than multi-item scales and generally yield limited information.

Health profiles attempt to measure all important dimensions of health-related quality of life. For example, the *Sickness Impact Profile* (Bergner, 1981) assesses a physical dimension (including ambulation, mobility, body care, and movement), a psychosocial dimension (including social interaction, alertness behavior, communication, and emotional behavior), and additional domains including eating, work, home management, sleep and rest, and recreation and pastimes. The *SF-36 Health Survey* (Ware, 1992) is a relatively brief (36-item), widely used questionnaire that assesses several dimensions of health, including general health perceptions, physical functioning, role limitations because of physical health, role limitations because of mental health, social functioning, pain, mental health, and energy (Fig. 25-2).

Utility measures are derived from economic and decision theory. The term *utility* refers to the value placed by the individual on a particular health state. Utility is summarized as a score ranging from 0.0, representing death, to 1.0, representing perfect health. In economic analyses, utilities are used to justify devoting resources to a treatment. Because utility measures weight the duration of life according to its quality, they can be used to generate quality-adjusted life-years. However, because they are expressed as a single score, they do not provide detail about how specific aspects of patients' lives are affected. The *Quality of Well-being Scale* (Kaplan, 1988) is a widely used instrument that combines questions about various dimensions of functional status with community-derived preferences for these states.

PATIENT SATISFACTION. *Patient satisfaction* refers to patients' subjective evaluations of their health care. Patient ratings of care reflect what patients think is important about the quality of care, including the doctor-patient relationship and their perception of the

ACTIVITIES	Yes, Limited A Lot	Yes, Limited A Little	No, Not Limited At All
	(circle one number on each line)		
a. Vigorous activities, such as running, lifting heavy objects, participating in strenuous sports	1	2	3
b. Moderate activities, such as moving a table, pushing a vacuum cleaner, bowling, or playing golf	1	2	3
c. Lifting or carrying groceries	1	2	3
d. Climbing several flights of stairs	1	2	3
e. Climbing one flight of stairs	1	2	3
f. Bending, kneeling, or stooping	1	2	3
g. Walking more than a mile	1	2	3
h. Walking several blocks	1	2	3
i. Walking one block	1	2	3
j. Bathing or dressing yourself	1	2	3

FIGURE 25–2 ■ Sample questions assessing physical functioning from the SF-36 Health Survey. (From Ware JE, Snow KK, Kosinski M, et al: SF-36 Health Survey: Manual and Interpretation Guide. Boston, The Health Institute, 1993.)

adequacy of diagnosis and therapy. They also predict patients' subsequent behavior, including how well they comply with the medications prescribed, whether they return to the same physician or go elsewhere, and whether they recommend a physician to others. The method used to elicit a patient's judgments about care can affect the results dramatically. For example, when the response choices use the word *satisfied*, most patients choose the best possible answer. Rating scales (e.g., excellent to poor) result in a better distribution of responses. The Patient Satisfaction Questionnaire (Ware, 1988) and the Medical Outcomes Study 9-item Visit Rating Form (Rubin, 1993) are examples of carefully constructed instruments to assess general medical care and specific physician visits.

COST STUDIES

The basic formula of a cost study is a cost-benefit ratio. Studies most often examine direct costs (the costs of treatment itself) but may also include estimates of indirect costs (the costs of disability or loss of livelihood, both actual and potential) (Table 25–4). *Cost-identification* studies enumerate the cost of applying a treatment to a specified population under a particular set of conditions. These studies describe the natural history of costs without comparing the benefits of one intervention with those of alternatives. *Cost-benefit* studies compare the monetary costs of a treatment with the cost

Table 25–4 ■ TYPES OF COST STUDIES

KIND OF COST STUDY	DESCRIPTION
Cost-identification	Enumerates cost of applying a treatment to a specified population under a particular set of conditions
Cost-benefit	Compares the costs of treatment and cost savings resulting from benefits of the treatment in dollar terms
Cost-effectiveness	Compares the costs and benefits of a treatment in terms of reduced mortality or morbidity such as years of life saved or quality-adjusted life-years saved
Cost-utility	Compares the cost and benefits of a treatment in terms of utility scores

savings that result from the benefits of that treatment. A limitation is that all benefits, including decreased mortality, are expressed in dollar terms. Moreover, techniques for assigning value to a human life are controversial. *Cost-effectiveness* analysis compares the costs and benefits of a treatment in terms of reduced mortality or morbidity, such as years of life saved. *Cost-utility* analysis expresses the costs and benefits of treatment in terms of utility scores, such as cost per quality-adjusted life-year gained.

STUDY DESIGN

Outcome assessments use a variety of research designs, including experiments (e.g., randomized controlled trials) and observational studies (e.g., cross-sectional, cohort, and case-control studies) (see Chapter 23). Meta-analysis is used to pool data from many studies. Appropriateness studies examine whether treatments are used on patients who are likely to benefit from them and are not used on those unlikely to benefit. Each of these study designs has strengths and limitations (Table 25–5).

RANDOMIZED CONTROLLED TRIALS. The randomized controlled trial involves selecting representative subjects, randomly assigning them to treatment and control groups, and monitoring them for the outcomes of interest. The randomized double-blind placebo-controlled trial is considered the gold standard for evaluating a treatment's efficacy. The experimental design allows the greatest control over the influence of confounding variables and permits causal inferences. However, randomized controlled trials also have shortcomings. Data collection is time consuming and costly. Many research questions are not suitable for experimental designs, such as when ethical concerns prohibit placebo controls or when outcomes are rare. Although blinding study subjects and physicians to treatment assignment is possible in studies of medications, it is more difficult when studying medical and surgical procedures. Even though randomized controlled trials provide data on treatment efficacy, their inclusion and exclusion criteria and the selected nature of study volunteers often limit their generalizability.

OBSERVATIONAL STUDIES. Rather than assigning patients to a treatment of interest, observational studies examine the outcomes of medicine as it is practiced. In *cross-sectional studies*, all variables are measured at a single point in time. Although cross-sectional studies are relatively inexpensive and can provide useful descriptions of the prevalence of diseases, treatments, and outcomes, they provide weak evidence for causal associations because they do not account for temporal relationships.

In *cohort studies*, patients are monitored over a certain period.

Table 25–5 ■ STUDY DESIGNS

DESIGN	STRENGTHS	WEAKNESSES
Experiment	Strongest evidence for cause and effect	Expensive Long duration Unsuitable for many questions Not useful for rare outcomes Limited generalizability
Cross-sectional	Short duration May study several outcomes Controls subject selection Controls measurements Yields prevalence	Does not establish causal relationships Unmeasured differences between groups
Cohort	Establishes sequence of events Avoids bias in measuring predictors Yields incidence, relative risk, excess risk	Relatively expensive Long duration Requires large sample size Not useful for rare outcomes
Case-control	Useful for rare conditions Relatively inexpensive Short duration Yields odds ratio	Potential sampling bias Limited to one outcome variable Does not yield prevalence, incidence, or relative risk
Meta-analysis	Increases statistical power for outcomes Helpful when studies disagree	Quality of secondary data varies Requires combining data from different studies

Prospective cohort studies can provide evidence for cause-and-effect relationships between predictors and outcomes because the predictors are measured before the outcomes occur. If some patients receive a treatment and some do not, evidence for effectiveness can also be estimated. In some cases, observational studies may use a *quasi-experimental design* to take advantage of "natural experiments," such as introducing a new treatment or changing insurance coverage. As in clinical trials, prospective data collection is expensive and time consuming, and cohort studies are not useful when outcomes are rare.

In *case-control studies*, the prevalence of risk factors in a sample of subjects who have a disease or outcome (the cases) is compared with that in a sample who do not (the controls). Case-control studies are inexpensive and uniquely efficient for studying rare conditions. However, a case-control study can examine only one outcome because cases are selected on this basis. In addition, because cases and controls are selected separately and data on predictors are collected retrospectively, these studies are susceptible to bias.

All observational studies are subject to significant confounding effects because groups may differ with regard to measured or unmeasured characteristics. Risk-adjustment methods are used to control for factors that are unequally distributed between groups and that may be related to patient outcomes, such as patient demographics and severity of illness. However, inferences must be made cautiously because unmeasured variations in patients, practitioners, and processes may be the real explanation for differences in outcomes.

META-ANALYSIS LITERATURE SYNTHESIS. Literature synthesis can be used to characterize the extent and quality of medical evidence and to summarize findings of existing studies. *Meta-analysis* is a systematic synthesis of the literature that uses standardized statistical methods (see Chapter 24) to obtain a quantitative estimate of the effect of a particular intervention by aggregating the effects reported in many studies. Its main purposes are to identify gaps in knowledge, increase statistical power for primary outcomes by combining studies that are too small to be conclusive, and resolve controversy when studies disagree. Its primary disadvantage is that it relies on secondary data. If those data are inadequate, little additional information can be generated. In addition, it may be difficult to combine data from studies conducted at different times and using different methods on different patient populations.

APPROPRIATENESS STUDIES. Appropriateness studies establish standard indications against which the use of a particular medical intervention is judged. Methods to develop "indications" involve careful analysis of what is known and the use of expert physicians to fill in gaps in knowledge and come to consensus about indications. Appropriateness studies can be incorporated into guidelines to help practicing physicians decide under what circumstances a procedure should or should not be performed.

DATA SOURCES

Outcomes research uses a variety of sources of data, including patient questionnaires, medical records, and claims and administrative data files (Table 25–6).

PATIENT QUESTIONNAIRES. Outcomes research frequently uses a questionnaire-based approach to assess patient outcomes. Patients are commonly asked about their ability to function, how they feel, and their satisfaction with the care received. Sometimes, subjective data from patients can provide valuable information that may not be evident from physiologic measurements. Surprisingly, studies have shown that patient-reported measures can be at least as reliable as conventional biochemical or physiologic indices. However, although patient reports provide a unique perspective, measures must be chosen with care. Data collection requires the cooperation of patients and providers, and selective non-participation can threaten generalizability. Study designs must recognize the limitations of patient recall and the fact that patients' evaluations of outcome may be affected by their expectations.

MEDICAL RECORD REVIEW. Detailed clinical information can be collected unobtrusively by retrospective review of medical records. To maximize reliability, abstraction must be performed by trained reviewers with a clinical background. Data obtained by this method are limited by the level and accuracy of documentation and the completeness of the medical record.

CLAIMS AND ADMINISTRATIVE DATA. Claims data analysis uses data files, such as those maintained by the Medicare program, to explore patterns of care and clinical outcomes. The database on all Medicare beneficiaries and providers includes demographics, characteristics of hospitals and other providers, expenditures, diagnoses, procedures, dates of service, and complications. Available data include a longitudinal record of health care utilization and medical costs for all claims submitted since 1991.

Medicare data have revealed striking variations in clinical practice, particularly in the performance of diagnostic and therapeutic procedures. They also provide population-based descriptions of the frequency of death and complications associated with various diagnoses and procedures and are used to monitor trends over time. However, several problems limit the value of claims data for assessing medical effectiveness or evaluating the quality of care. Claims data may not contain enough detail about clinical features thought to affect prognosis, such as the stage of colon cancer. Thus it may be difficult to identify clinically relevant patient groups and control adequately for clinical factors likely to affect outcome.

CHALLENGES

Many challenges remain before outcome assessment can be applied to full advantage. In particular, there are large gaps in our understanding of how the structure and process of care influence patient outcomes.

Clinical trials are needed to examine the effectiveness as well as the efficacy of existing and newly developed treatments and procedures. Studies that measure the effectiveness of treatments must examine short- and long-term outcomes. To examine the effectiveness of services, to disseminate information, and to evaluate the quality of medical care, data systems must be able to characterize variation in treatments and outcomes. Better research tools and measurement techniques are needed, including more reliable, valid,

Table 25–6 ■ DATA SOURCES FOR OUTCOME ASSESSMENTS

DATA SOURCE	ADVANTAGES	DISADVANTAGES
Patient surveys	Provide the patient's perspective Provide reliable data	Labor intensive Requires cooperation of patient ± providers Selective non-participation Patient may have trouble with recall Evaluations of outcome affected by expectation
Chart abstraction	Unobtrusive Detailed clinical information Can be performed retrospectively	Costly Labor intensive May be unreliable Variables may not be recorded consistently
Claims data	Unobtrusive Low cost Large number Broad cross-section of patients	Data lack clinical detail for identifying patient groups or risk adjustment May be inaccurate

and understandable measures of patient-reported outcomes tested in more diverse populations. Better risk-adjustment models are needed to facilitate valid reports and comparisons of patient outcomes. Finally, to improve decision making in the care of individual patients, students and clinicians must learn to understand and integrate evidence for effective practices with clinical expertise, pathophysiologic knowledge, and patient preferences.

Brook RH, Kamberg CJ, McGlynn EA: Health system reform and quality. JAMA 276: 476, 1996. *Review of eight important questions about trade-offs between cost and quality to be considered in the changing health care system.*

Dartmouth Medical School Center for the Evaluative Clinical Sciences: The Dartmouth Atlas of Health Care in the United States 1998. Chicago, American Hospital Publishing, 1998. *Easy-to-read tables and graphs demonstrate that in health care, geography is destiny. Striking regional variations and idiosyncratic patterns are shown for services such as hospitalization, terminal care, and elective surgery.*

Guyatt GH, Naylor CD, Juniper E, et al: Users' guides to the medical literature. XII How to use articles about health-related quality of life. JAMA 277:1232, 1997. *Guidelines to help clinicians judge the appropriateness and usefulness of data on health-related quality of life for a given situation.*

Hulley SB, Cummings SR: Designing Clinical Research. An Epidemiologic Approach. Baltimore, Williams & Wilkins, 1988. *Highly accessible primer that walks the reader step by step from conceiving a research question, through designing a study, to writing a grant proposal.*

Spilker B: Quality of Life and Pharmacoeconomics in Clinical Trials, 2nd ed. Philadelphia, Lippincott-Raven, 1996. *A 127-chapter compendium of review articles and descriptions of the majority of leading health measurement methods; most chapters are written by the developers themselves.*

26 PRINCIPLES OF DRUG THERAPY

Robert B. Diasio

It is generally appreciated that under different conditions a drug may produce diverse effects, ranging from none to a desirable effect or, in other cases, an undesirable, toxic effect. The physician caring for the patient must learn how to individualize the drug dosage under different conditions to ensure effective and safe therapy. This requires knowing both pharmacokinetics—examining the movement of a drug over time through the body—and pharmacodynamics—relating drug concentration to drug effect (Fig. 26–1). In this chapter, a review of the basic concepts of pharmacokinetics and pharmacodynamics is presented, followed by guidelines on

how to use this information to optimize therapeutic applications. Finally, drug interactions and adverse drug responses are discussed with advice on how both can be recognized and minimized in clinical practice.

PHARMACOKINETIC PRINCIPLES

ADMINISTERING DRUGS. The most straightforward means of administering a drug into the systemic circulation is by intravenously injecting it as a bolus. With this route, the full amount of a drug is delivered to the systemic circulation almost immediately. The same dose may also be administered as an intravenous infusion over a longer time, resulting in a decrease in the peak plasma concentration as well as an increase in the time the drug is present in the circulation. Many other routes of administration can be used, including sublingual, oral, transdermal, rectal, inhalation, subcutaneous, and intramuscular; each of these routes carries not only a potential delay in the time it takes the drug to enter the circulation but also the possibility that a large fraction of it will never reach the circulation.

ABSORPTION. Absorption refers to the transfer of a drug from the site where it was administered to the systemic circulation. Most drugs use passive diffusion to cross a membrane barrier and enter the systemic circulation. Because passive diffusion in this setting depends on the concentration of the solute at the membrane surface, the rate of drug absorption is affected by the concentration of free drug at the absorbing surface. Factors that influence the availability of free drug affect drug absorption from the administration site; this effect can be exploited to design medications that provide a slow release of drug into the circulation by prolonging drug absorption. With certain sustained-released oral preparations, the rate of dissolution of the drug in the gastrointestinal tract determines the rate at which the drug is absorbed (e.g., time-released antihistamines). Similarly, a prolonged drug effect can be obtained by using transdermal medications (e.g., nitroglycerin) or intramuscular depot preparations (e.g., benzathine penicillin G).

FIRST-PASS EFFECT. Some drugs that are administered orally are absorbed relatively well into the portal circulation but are metabolized by the liver before reaching the systemic circulation. Because of this "first-pass" or "presystemic" effect, for some drugs, the oral route may therefore be less suitable than other routes of administration. A good example is nitroglycerin, which is well absorbed but efficiently metabolized during the first pass through the liver. The same drug can achieve adequate systemic levels when given sublingually or transdermally.

BIOAVAILABILITY. The extent of absorption of drug into the sys-

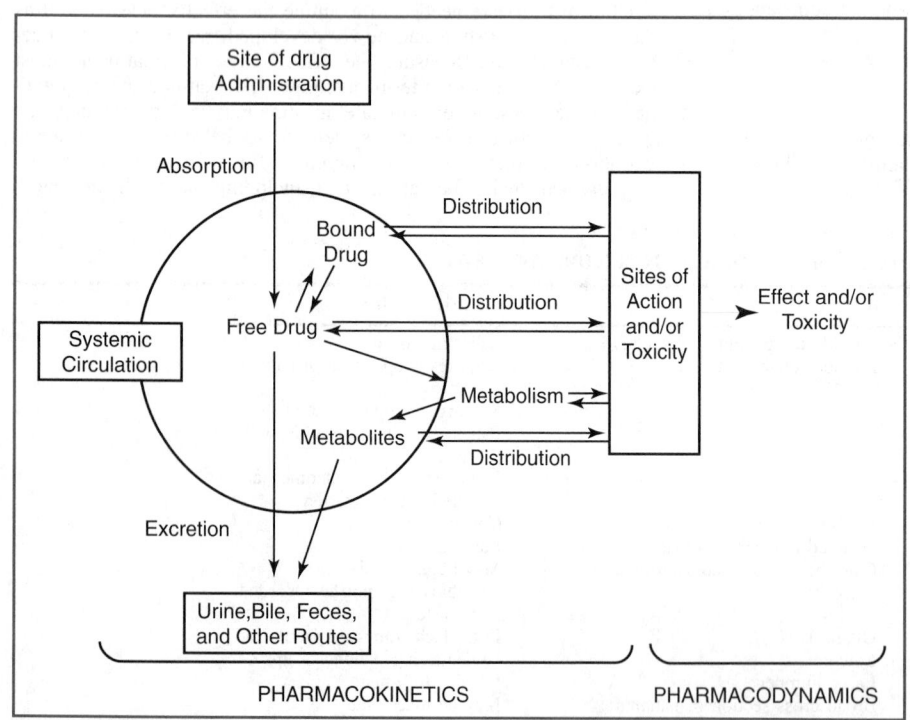

PHARMACOKINETICS   PHARMACODYNAMICS

FIGURE 26–1 ■ Schematic of drug movement through the body, from site of administration to production of drug effect. The relationship between pharmacokinetics and pharmacodynamics is shown.

temic circulation may be incomplete. The bioavailability of a particular drug is the fraction (F) of the total drug dose that ultimately reaches the systemic circulation from the site of administration. This fraction is calculated by dividing the amount of the drug dose that reaches the circulation from the administration site by the amount of the drug dose that would enter the systemic circulation following direct intravenous injection into the circulation (essentially the total dose). Bioavailability, or F, can therefore range from 0, in which no drug reaches the systemic circulation, to 1.0, in which essentially all of the drug is absorbed. The bioavailability of a drug in different formulations may change because the overall absorption may differ. This variability has become a recent concern with the increasing use of generic preparations.

DISTRIBUTION. After delivery of a drug into the systemic circulation either directly by intravenous injection or after absorption, the drug is transported throughout the body, initially to the well-perfused tissues and later to areas that are less perfused. The distribution phase can best be assessed by plotting the drug's plasma concentration on a log scale versus time on a linear scale (Fig. 26–2). The initial phase, from immediately after administration through the rapid fall in concentration, represents the distribution phase, during which a drug rapidly disappears from the circulation and enters the tissues. This is followed by the elimination phase (see later), when drug in the plasma is in equilibrium with drug in the tissues. It is during this latter phase that the drug's plasma concentration is thought to be related to drug effect.

VOLUME OF DISTRIBUTION. The volume of distribution (VD) is a term used to relate the amount of drug in the body to the concentration of drug in the plasma. It is calculated by dividing the dose that ultimately gets into the systemic circulation by the plasma concentration at time zero (C_{p0}).

$$VD = \frac{dose}{C_{p0}} \quad (1)$$

The C_{p0} can be calculated by extrapolating the elimination phase back to time zero (see Fig. 26–2). The volume of distribution is best considered the "apparent VD" because it represents the apparent volume needed to contain the entire amount of the drug, assuming that the drug is distributed throughout the body at the same concentration as in the plasma. Table 26–1 lists pharmacokinetic data for 20 commonly used drugs from several drug classes, demonstrating the wide variation in VD. Thus, digoxin can be seen to have a large VD (>5 L), whereas valproic acid has a relatively small VD (0.15 L). As discussed later, the VD is a useful pharmacokinetic term for calculating the loading dose and in appreciating how various changes can affect a drug's half-life.

ELIMINATION. Drugs are removed from the body by two major mechanisms: hepatic elimination, in which drugs are metabolized in the liver and excreted through the biliary tract, and renal elimina-tion, in which drugs are removed from the circulation by either glomerular filtration or tubular secretion. For the vast majority of drugs, the rates of hepatic and renal elimination are proportional to the plasma concentration of the drug. This relationship is often described as a "first-order" process. Two measurements are used to evaluate elimination: clearance and half-life.

CLEARANCE. The efficiency of elimination can be described by assessing how the drug clears from the circulation. Drug clearance is a measure of the volume of plasma cleared of drug per unit of time. It is similar to the measurement used clinically to assess renal function—the creatinine clearance—which is the volume of plasma from which creatinine is removed per minute. Total drug clearance (Cl_{tot}) is the rate of elimination by all processes (El_{tot}) divided by the plasma concentration of the drug (C_p):

$$Cl_{tot} = \frac{El_{tot}}{C_p} \quad (2)$$

Drugs may be cleared by several organs, with renal and hepatic clearance being the two major mechanisms. Total drug clearance (Cl_{tot}) can therefore be best described as the sum of clearances by each organ. For must drugs this is essentially the sum of the renal and hepatic clearance:

$$Cl_{tot} = Cl_{Ren} + Cl_{Hep} \quad (3)$$

Table 26–1 demonstrates the wide variation in clearance values among commonly used medications, with some drugs (e.g., ethosuximide and phenobarbital) having relatively low clearances (<5 mL/min) and other drugs (e.g., aspirin and mexiletine) having relatively high clearances (>500 mL/min). Amikacin, gentamicin, and tobramycin are almost entirely cleared by the kidneys, whereas drugs such as aspirin, carbamazepine, and phenytoin are cleared less than 5% by the kidneys.

Drug clearance is affected by several factors, including (1) blood flow through the organ of clearance; (2) protein binding to the drug; and (3) the activity of the clearance processes in the organs of elimination (e.g., glomerular filtration rate [GFR] and tubular secretion in the kidney or enzyme activity in the liver). Drug clearance is not affected by distribution of drug throughout the body (VD) because clearance mechanisms act only on drug in the circulation.

HALF-LIFE. The amount of time needed to eliminate a drug from the body depends on both the clearance and the volume of distribution. The first-order elimination constant (k_e) represents the proportion of the apparent volume of distribution that is cleared of drug per unit of time during the exponential disappearance of drug from the plasma over time (elimination phase).

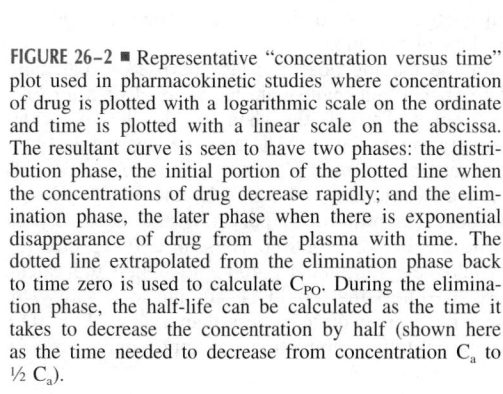

FIGURE 26–2 ▪ Representative "concentration versus time" plot used in pharmacokinetic studies where concentration of drug is plotted with a logarithmic scale on the ordinate and time is plotted with a linear scale on the abscissa. The resultant curve is seen to have two phases: the distribution phase, the initial portion of the plotted line when the concentrations of drug decrease rapidly; and the elimination phase, the later phase when there is exponential disappearance of drug from the plasma with time. The dotted line extrapolated from the elimination phase back to time zero is used to calculate C_{PO}. During the elimination phase, the half-life can be calculated as the time it takes to decrease the concentration by half (shown here as the time needed to decrease from concentration C_a to ½ C_a).

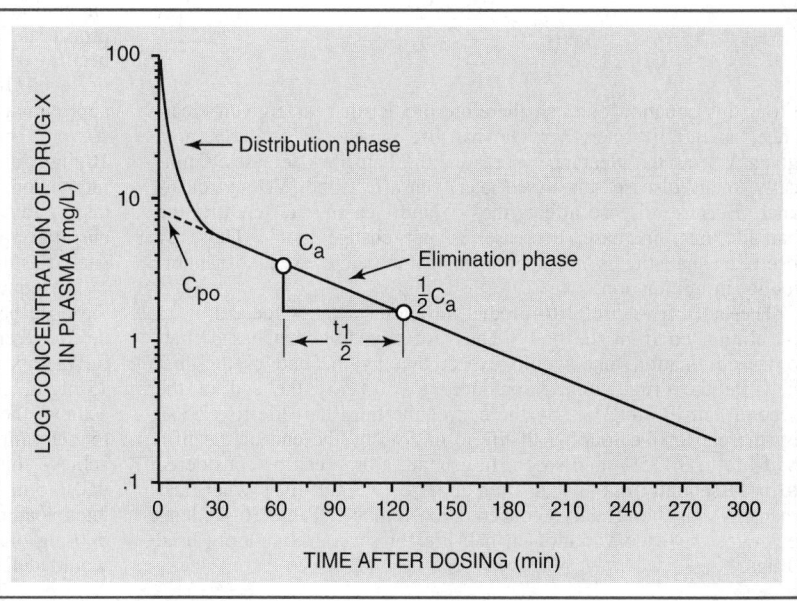

Table 26–1 ■ PHARMACOKINETIC PARAMETERS FOR SOME COMMONLY USED DRUGS

	V_D (liters/kg)	PROTEIN BINDING (%)	TOTAL Cl (ml/min)	% OF Cl_{tot} AS RENAL Cl	HALF-LIFE (hr)	THERAPEUTIC RANGE (mg/L)
Amikacin	0.25	<10	100	94–98	2–3	5–20 (TR) 20–30 (PK)
Aspirin (acetylsalicylic acid)	0.14–0.18	80–90	575–725	<2	0.2–0.3	20–250
Carbamazepine	1.2	75–90	50–125	1–3	12–17	4–12
Digoxin	5–7.3	20–30	75	50–70	34–44	0.5–2.0
Disopyramide	0.6–1.4	50–65	1.3–1.4	40–60	4–10	2–4
Ethosuximide	0.7	<10	3	20	60	40–100
Gentamicin sulfate	0.22–0.3	<10	60	>95	1.5–4 4–8 (PK)	0.5–2.0 (TR)
Lidocaine	3	60–80	700	<10	1.5–2.0	1–5
Lithium carbonate	0.7–1	0	20–40	95–99	20–270	4–1.4*
Mexiletine	5.4	75	500–850	15	8–10	0.7–2.0
Penicillin G	0.5–0.7	45–68	—	20	0.4–0.9	Variable
Phenobarbital	0.6–0.7	20–45	4	25	2–6 days	<10–40*
Phenytoin	0.4–0.8	88–93	—	<5	7–26	10–20
Primidone	0.6	<20	45–100	15–25	10–12	5–12
Procainamide	2.2	14–23	470–600	40–70	2.5–4.7	4–8
Quinidine sulfate	2	80	180–300	10–20	6–8	0.3–6.0
Theophylline	0.3–0.7	60	36–50	<10	4–16	5–20
Tobramycin	0.25–0.30	<10	70	>95	2–4 4–8 (PK)	0.5–2.0 (TR)
Valproic acid	0.15	80–95	7	<10	5–20	50–100
Vancomycin	0.4–1.0	52–60	65	85	4–6	5–10 (TR) 25–35 (PK)

TR = trough value; PK = peak value.

*Therapeutic range varies depending on indication for drugs (e.g., *lithium carbonate*–range 0.4–1.3 mg/L, appropriate for affective schizophrenia disorder; whole range 1.0–1.4 mg/L appropriate for mania; *phenobarbital*—concentration <10 mg/L appropriate for anticonvulsant, 40 mg/L appropriate as hypnotic.

$$k_e = \frac{Cl}{V_D} \qquad (4)$$

The value of this constant for a particular drug can be determined by plotting drug concentration versus time on a log-linear plot (see Fig. 26–2) and measuring the slope of the straight line obtained during the exponential (elimination) phase.

The time needed to eliminate the drug is best described by the drug half-life ($t_{1/2}$), which is the time required during the elimination phase (see Fig. 26–2) to decrease the plasma concentration of the drug by half. Mathematically, the half-life is equal to the natural logarithm of 2 (representing a reduction of drug concentration to half) divided by k_e. Substituting for k_e from equation 4 and calculating the natural logarithm of 2, the half-life can therefore be represented by the following equation:

$$t_{1/2} = \frac{0.693\ V_D}{Cl} \qquad (5)$$

From this equation one can therefore predict that, at a given clearance, as the V_D increases, the half-life increases. Similarly, at a given V_D, as the clearance increases, the half-life decreases. Clinically, many disease states (see later) can affect both V_D and clearance. Because disease affects the V_D and clearance differently, the half-life may increase, decrease, or not change much. Thus, by itself, the half-life is not a good indicator of the extent of abnormality in elimination.

The half-life is useful to predict how long it takes for a drug to be eliminated from the body. Thus, for any drug that has a first-order elimination, one would expect that by the end of the first half-life the drug would be reduced to 50%, by the end of the second half-life to 25%, by the end of the third half-life to 12.5%, by the end of the fourth half-life to 6.25%, by the end of the fifth half-life to 3.125%, and so on. In general, a drug can be considered to be essentially eliminated after three to five half-lives when less than 10% of the effective concentration remains. Table 26–1 demonstrates the wide variation in half-life for several commonly used drugs.

APPLYING PHARMACOKINETIC PRINCIPLES

USING A LOADING DOSE. To attain a desired therapeutic concentration rapidly, a loading dose is often used. In determining the amount of drug to be given, the physician must consider the "volume" within the body into which the drug may distribute. This volume is best described by the apparent V_D. The loading dose can be calculated by multiplying the desired concentration by the V_D.

$$\text{Loading dose} = \text{desired concentration} \times V_D \qquad (6)$$

Administering the entire loading dose rapidly may produce an initially high peak concentration that results in toxicity. This problem can be avoided either by administering the loading dose as a divided dose or by varying the rate of access to the circulation—for example, by administering the drug as an infusion (with intravenous drug) or by taking advantage of the slower access to the circulation from various other routes (e.g., oral dose). This approach is illustrated by phenytoin (see Table 26–1), which may need to be administered with a loading dose to achieve a therapeutic level (10 to 20 mg/L) rapidly. Because the V_D for phenytoin is approximately 0.6 L/kg, the loading dose calculated from equation 6 would be 420 mg/L to attain a minimally therapeutic level of 10 mg/L in a 70-kg adult. Administering 420 mg of phenytoin by intravenous bolus carries the risk of cardiac arrest and death. By taking advantage of the reduced bioavailability (F = 0.8) and slow absorption of oral phenytoin, the loading dose can be safely administered as an oral dose of 500 mg.

The equation for the loading dose can also be used to calculate the dose needed to "boost" an inadequate blood level of drug to a desired therapeutic range. Thus, if the phenytoin level is observed on therapeutic monitoring to be 5 mg/L and the desired level is 15 mg/L, it is necessary to multiply the difference needed to achieve the desired concentration (10 mg/L) by the V_D (0.6 L/kg) to determine the dose (in milligrams per kilogram) necessary to achieve this drug level after distribution. Thus, in a 70-kg individual, 0.6 mg/kg would be multiplied by 70 kg to obtain the calculated loading dose (420 mg) that could be administered safely. A 500-mg oral dose with a bioavailability less than 1 (e.g., F = 0.8) would deliver to the systemic circulation the approximate amount

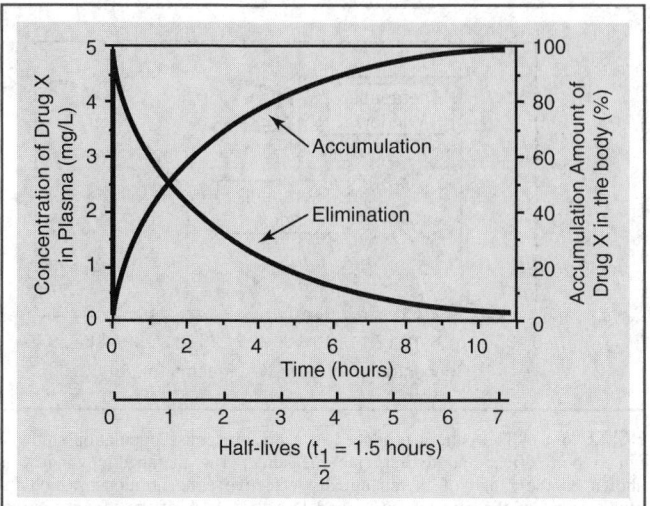

FIGURE 26-3 ▪ Representative plot of the "mirror image" relationship between elimination of drug (after drug is discontinued) and accumulation of drug (during infusion). The plot shows the concentration on the left y-axis and time on the upper x-axis. The lower x-axis shows the time in half-lives, and the y-axis on the right shows the percentage of drug in the body. After three to five half-lives, elimination is essentially complete and accumulation is essentially at a steady state.

needed and avoid the risks associated with rapid intravenous administration.

DETERMINING DRUG ACCUMULATION. Continuing to administer a drug, either as a prolonged infusion or as repeated doses, results in accumulation until a "steady state" occurs. Steady state is the point when the amount of drug being administered equals the amount being eliminated so that the plasma and tissue levels remain constant. The elimination half-life determines not only the time of drug elimination but also the time course of drug accumulation. This "mirror image" pattern of drug accumulation and elimination is shown graphically in Figure 26–3. As with drug elimination, three to five half-lives determine the time it takes to reach steady state during drug accumulation. Whereas drugs with short half-lives accumulate rapidly, drugs with long half-lives require a longer time to accumulate, with a potential delay in achieving therapeutic drug levels. For drugs with long half-lives, a loading dose may be needed to rapidly achieve drug accumulation and a more rapid therapeutic effect.

With each change in drug dose or rate of infusion, a change in steady state occurs. Although not obvious for drugs with short half-lives, the effects of dose adjustments for drugs with longer half-lives are delayed, with the time varying directly with the drug's half-life.

USING A MAINTENANCE DOSE. After steady state is reached in three to five half-lives with either a continuous infusion or intermittent doses, the rate of drug administered equals the rate of drug eliminated. For an intravenous drug, the administration rate is the infusion rate (I), whereas for a drug administered by another route (e.g., oral dose) the administration rate is the dose per unit time (D/t). From equation 3 the rate of elimination (total) can be seen to equal the $Cl_{tot} \times C_p$ Therefore, it follows with an intravenously administered drug, because the infusion rate equals the elimination rate at steady state, that:

$$I \times Cl_{tot} \times C_p \tag{7}$$

Similarly, with an orally administered drug, the dose administered per unit time equals the elimination rate at steady state, with the result that

$$D/t = Cl_{tot} \times C_p \tag{8}$$

These equations demonstrate the direct relationship between the dose and the resultant plasma concentration at steady state. This relationship is independent of the distribution of the drug. By using these equations, it is possible to determine the infusion rate or the interval and dose needed to achieve and maintain a specified drug concentration in the plasma.

When administered intermittently, a drug approaches steady-state concentration over time with a pattern similar to that observed with continuous infusion (Fig. 26–4). With intermittent drug administration, such as with an oral dose, the drug concentration fluctuates; the magnitude of fluctuation between the "peak" and "trough" concentrations depends on the interval of administration, drug half-life, absorption characteristics, and site of administration. The effect of a change in the interval of administration for an oral drug is shown in Figure 26–4. As the intervals decrease below the half-life, the fluctuation decreases and approaches the curve produced by an intravenous infusion. Orally administered drugs may reach the blood stream more rapidly, attaining a higher peak concentration with one formulation, whereas the same drug administered as a time-released formulation is absorbed more slowly, with a lower peak concentration but lasting longer in the plasma. Finally, the

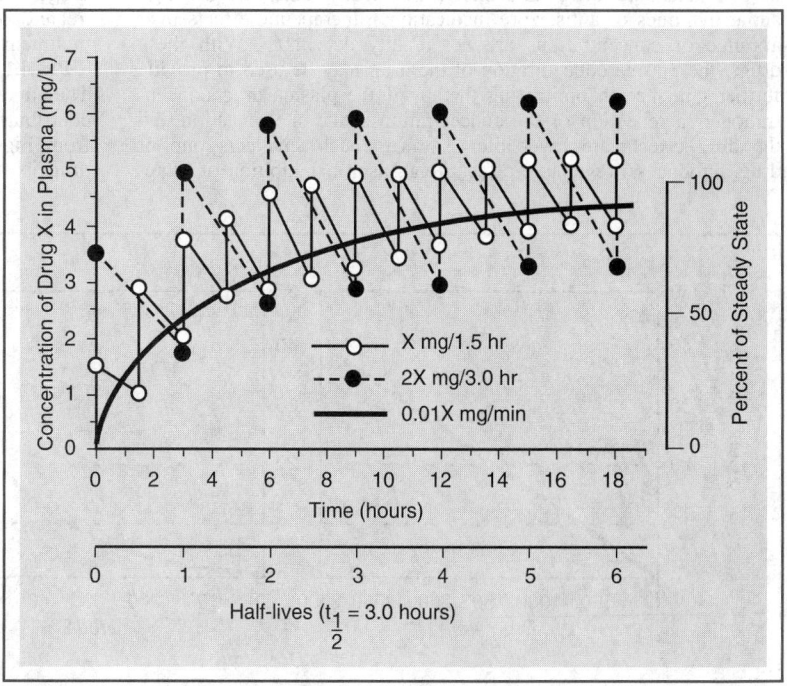

FIGURE 26–4 ▪ The accumulation of drug over time approaching a steady state is shown. Time is depicted in both hours (upper x-axis) and half-lives (lower x-axis, demonstrating that in three to five half-lives steady state is reached). The solid line depicts the pattern produced by an infusion of a hypothetical drug at a dose of 0.01X. The solid circles with the hatched line show the pattern resulting from orally administering a 2X dose every 3 hours, and the open circles with the solid line represent the pattern produced by orally administering a dose X every 1.5 hours.

same drug administered via different routes may have very different plasma profiles not only because of differing absorption characteristics but also because of other effects such as first-pass metabolism.

DECREASING THE DRUG LEVEL. At times it may be necessary to decrease the plasma drug level while maintaining therapy, e.g., when signs of toxicity become apparent or a potentially dangerously high concentration of drug is noted when monitoring drug levels (see later). The most effective and rapid response is to discontinue the drug, with the length of time off the drug determined by the estimated drug half-life in the specific patient. After discontinuing the drug for a time based on the drug's half-life, the value for total clearance (Cl_{tot}) of the drug can be used to determine what infusion rate (I) (equation 7) or dose and interval (D/t) (equation 8) must be used to achieve the new desired concentration (C_p).

DOSE-DEPENDENT PHARMACOKINETICS

Although the above pharmacokinetic principles can be a guide to the dose of most drugs, not all drugs behave the same when the dose is increased. Most drugs are eliminated following first-order or linear kinetics, with the amount of drug eliminated directly proportional to the concentration of drug in the plasma (Fig. 26–5A). A few drugs have a different pattern when eliminated. Three of the most commonly used drugs that exhibit this different pharmacokinetic pattern are ethanol, phenytoin, and salicylate. These drugs have dose-dependent, non-linear, saturation kinetics. As the dose of drug increases and the concentration of drug in the plasma in turn rises, the relative amount of drug being eliminated falls (i.e., the clearance decreases) until the rate of drug metabolism is at its maximum. At this point drug elimination is said to be "zero-order," and the drug concentration in plasma starts to increase much more (no longer a linear relationship) with each subsequent increase in dose (see Fig. 26–5B).

MONITORING DRUG CONCENTRATION AS A GUIDE TO THERAPY

Although published pharmacokinetic data (usually population averages) such as are listed in Table 26–1 are useful to determine initial drug dosing, dose modification may still be needed in the individual patient. For some drugs (e.g., antihypertensives or anticoagulants), the therapeutic effects (e.g., blood pressure or coagulation) can be easily quantified over a range of concentrations, permitting adequate drug adjustment. For many other drugs (e.g., antiarrhythmics or antiseizure medications), therapeutic effects over a range of concentrations are not readily detectable. With these drugs, the plasma concentration of the drug may be used to provide further guidance in optimizing therapy if the plasma drug concentration is a reflection of the concentration at the site of action and the drug effects are reversible. A third, much smaller group of drugs produces irreversible effects (e.g., aspirin inhibition of plate-

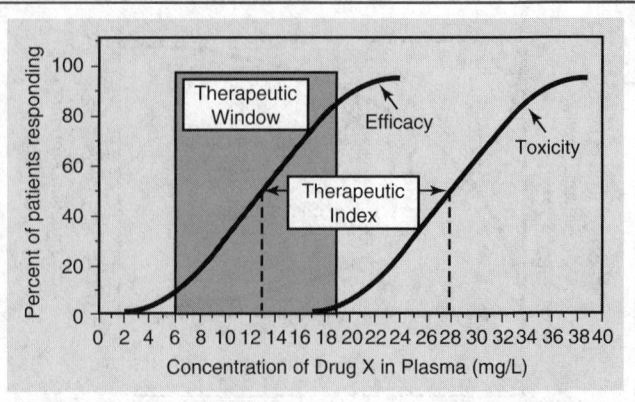

FIGURE 26–6 ■ The pattern produced in a dose-response population study in which both effect and toxicity are measured. The therapeutic window is shown as the range of therapeutically effective concentrations, which includes most of the efficacy curve and less than 10% of the toxicity curve. The therapeutic index is calculated by dividing the 50% value on the toxicity curve by the 50% value on the efficacy curve.

let aggregation). With these drugs, plasma drug concentration does not correlate with drug effect, and drug monitoring is therefore not useful.

To use drug concentrations as a guide to therapy, it is necessary to establish a range of concentrations from minimally to maximally efficacious with tolerable toxicity. This range of concentrations, or "therapeutic window," is usually determined from a dose-response curve generated from a population of patients who have been closely examined for therapeutic and toxic effects (Fig. 26–6). This graph may also be used to determine the "therapeutic index." This useful measure of drug toxicity is calculated by dividing the 50% value from the toxicity curve by the 50% value of the efficacy curve. Because these curves are generated from population data, the values may not be applicable for all individuals.

Table 26–1, in addition to providing useful pharmacokinetic data, also lists therapeutic ranges for several commonly used drugs for which measuring the drug concentration and knowing the therapeutic range may be useful in clinical management. Many of these drugs are typically used to treat serious or life-threatening diseases. It is essential to avoid inadequate doses because therapeutic effect is needed. At the same time, excessive doses must be avoided because of the risk of toxicity with many of these drugs that have a small therapeutic index. It is not necessary to assay drug levels for drugs used in non-critical diseases (no problem if inadequately treated) or for which the therapeutic index is large (therefore overtreatment is not likely to produce toxicity).

PROBLEMS WITH INTERPRETING DRUG CONCENTRATION. The time of blood collection, perhaps more than any other factor, contributes to the misinterpretation of drug levels. As can be seen from Figure 26–2, if sampling is performed too early, while the drug is still in the distribution phase, the drug level may be high

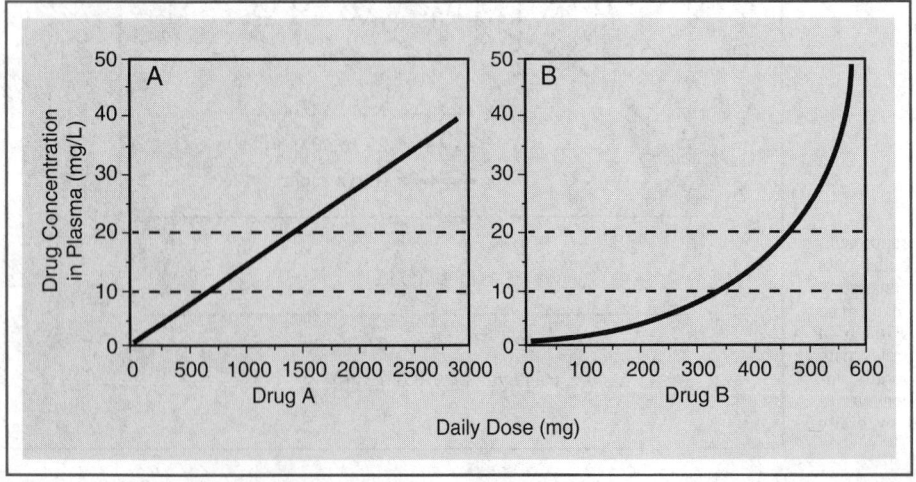

FIGURE 26–5 ■ The effect of increasing dose on serum concentration for drug A, which follows first-order or linear kinetics, and drug B, which follows zero-order or nonlinear (or saturable) kinetics.

and not reflect drug concentration at the site of action. Therefore, it is important to sample after the distribution phase.

For many drugs administered intermittently, a trough level, obtained immediately before administering the next dose, is most useful for making decisions regarding dose adjustments (see Table 26–1). For drugs that are administered by infusion or intermittently at short intervals (see Fig. 26–4), the best time to draw blood is during steady state.

Protein binding is another major factor that contributes to the misinterpretation of drug levels. Free drug (not bound to protein and thus able to equilibrate with tissues and interact with the site of action) is the critically important drug concentration when making therapeutic decisions. However, many drugs are tightly bound to plasma protein. Table 26–1 shows that many commonly used drugs, such as aspirin, carbamazepine, phenytoin, and valproic acid, have protein binding greater than 75%. Because many of the commonly used drug assays determine total drug concentration (which includes both protein-bound drug and free drug), assessment of the "true" free drug concentration may be inaccurate, particularly if the fraction of drug bound to protein varies. Second, the drug's binding may be decreased by disease or other drugs, leading to increased unbound drug levels that alter the interpretation of the measured drug concentrations. Both kidney and liver disease can change the binding of certain drugs (e.g., phenytoin) to protein because of a decrease in protein (e.g., decreased albumin as in nephrotic syndrome or liver disease) or as a result of competition for protein binding by endogenously produced substances (e.g., uremia in kidney disease or hyperbilirubinemia in liver disease). Similarly, other drugs may compete for binding to protein. A major problem that occurs secondary to the just-discussed changes in protein binding is that free drug is not typically measured in many of the common drug assays used by most clinical laboratories. Last, it should be noted that changes in drug binding to protein can also affect the pharmacokinetics of the drug, the main effect being on the V_D, which increases as protein binding decreases.

The usefulness of a drug assay is also limited by physiologic changes that may alter the response at a particular drug concentration. An example of this pharmacodynamic change is the response produced at a certain digoxin level in the presence of altered electrolyte concentration (e.g., potassium, calcium, or magnesium). Tolerance, a reduced response to a given concentration of drug with continued use, is another pharmacodynamic change that may alter how a drug concentration is interpreted. Tolerance is commonly observed with the continued use of narcotics (e.g., in terminal cancer patients); initially adequate pain control is noted at a given drug concentration, but after chronic administration the same drug concentration is no longer associated with pain relief.

ADJUSTING DRUG DOSE WITH DISEASE

KIDNEY DISEASE. The major questions to be answered in determining whether drug dosage needs to be adjusted in the setting of kidney disease include (1) Is the drug primarily excreted through the kidneys? and (2) Are increased drug levels likely to be associated with toxicity? If both are true, it is likely that with decreased renal clearance a drug will accumulate and become toxic. With renal failure it is therefore necessary to adjust the dosing regimen of such drugs, particularly for a drug with a long half-life and small therapeutic index (e.g., digoxin).

To obtain the desired concentration over time in the presence of decreased clearance, adjustments can be made by (1) decreasing the dose while maintaining the dose interval (DD); (2) maintaining the dose but increasing the interval between doses (II); or (3) a combination of both (DD and II). Table 26–2 shows how these three different methods are used for several commonly used drugs (previously characterized in Table 26–1 as to their pharmacokinetic properties with normal renal function) that require dosage adjustment with renal dysfunction. Although it may be possible with these adjustments to achieve an average concentration similar to that with normal renal function, there may be concomitant marked changes in the magnitude of peak and trough values. In choosing the type of drug adjustment the physician should consider not only the therapeutic index of the drug but also (1) whether an effective concentration needs to be achieved quickly and maintained within a narrow range (i.e., there is a need to maintain an average drug

Table 26–2 ∎ ADJUSTMENT OF DRUG DOSAGE IN RENAL FAILURE

DRUG	TYPE OF ELIMINATION	HALF LIFE (hrs) Normal	HALF LIFE (hrs) End-Stage Renal	Method*	GFR (mL/min) >50	GFR (mL/min) 10–50	GFR (mL/min) <10	Removed by Dialysis†
Amikacin	Renal	2–3	30	DD	60–90%	30–70%	20–30%	Yes
				II	12 hr	12–18 hr	24 hr	
Aspirin	Hepatic (renal)	2–19	Unchanged	II	4 hr	4–6 hr	Avoid	Yes
Carbamazepine	Hepatic (renal)	35	?	DD	Unchanged	Unchanged	75%	No
Digoxin	Renal (non-renal 15–40%)	36–44	80–120	DD	Unchanged	25–75%	10–25%	No
				II	24 hr	36 hr	48 hr	
Disopyramide	Renal + hepatic	5–8	10–18	II	Unchanged	12–24 hr	24–40 hr	No
Ethosuximide	Hepatic, renal	55	60	DD	Unchanged	Unchanged	75%	Yes
Gentamicin sulfate	Renal	2	24–48	DD	60–90%	30–70%	20–30%	Yes
				II	8–12 hr	12 hr	24 hr	
Lidocaine	Hepatic (renal < 20%)	1.2–2.2	1.3–3.0	DD	Unchanged	Unchanged	Unchanged	No
Lithium carbonate	Renal	14–28	Prolonged	DD	Unchanged	50–75%	25–50%	Yes
Mexiletine	Hepatic (renal)	8–13	16	DD	Unchanged	Unchanged	50–75%	Yes
Penicillin G	Renal (hepatic)	0.5	6–20	DD	Unchanged	75%	25–50%	Yes
				II	6–8 hr	8–12 hr	12–16 hr	
Phenobarbital	Hepatic (renal 30%)	60–150	117–160	II	Unchanged	Unchanged	12–16 hr	Yes
Phenytoin	Hepatic (renal)	24	8	DD	Unchanged	Unchanged	Unchanged	No
Primidone	Hepatic (renal <20%)	8	12	II	8 hr	8–12 hr	12–24 hr	Yes
Procainamide	Renal (hepatic 7–24%)	2.5–4.9	5.3–5.9	II	4 hr	6–12 hr	8–24 hr	Yes
Quinidine sulfate	Hepatic (renal 10–50%)	5.0–7.2	4–14	II	Unchanged	Unchanged	Unchanged	Yes
Theophylline	Hepatic	3–12	?	DD	Unchanged	Unchanged	Unchanged	Yes
Tobramycin	Renal	2.5	56	DD	60–90%	30–70%	20–30%	Yes
				II	8–12 hr	12 hr	24 hr	
Valproic acid	Hepatic	Biphasic 1 and 12	10	DD	Unchanged	Unchanged	Unchanged	No
Vancomycin	Renal	6–8	200–250	II	24–72 hr	72–240 hr	240 hr	No

GFR = glomerular filtration rate.
*Method: DD (alone)—decrease dose (maintain same interval).
II (alone)—increase interval between doses (maintain dose).
DD and II (together)—combination of both approaches.
†Dialysis refers to hemodialysis.

concentration and avoid trough levels when the drug is ineffective); and (2) whether toxicity is associated with elevated drug concentrations (i.e., toxicity with peak drug concentration).

Renal drug clearance has been shown to correlate with creatinine clearance (whether the drug uses glomerular filtration or tubular secretion); therefore, any adjustment of drug dose in kidney disease can use the creatinine clearance to calculate the dose needed because the renal drug clearance is proportional to the creatinine clearance. The creatinine clearance, which is used as an estimate of GFR, may be directly calculated from the serum creatinine using the following equation:

$$Cl_{Cr} = \frac{(140 - age) \times weight\ (kg)}{72 \times serum\ creatinine\ (mg/dL)} \qquad (9)$$

(The value should be multiplied by 0.85 for females) (*Note:* This calculation applies only when the serum creatinine is less than 5 mg/dL and the renal function is not rapidly changing.)

USING CLEARANCE FOR DOSE ADJUSTMENT. The dose of a drug used in renal insufficiency ($Dose_{D-RI}$) can be shown to be proportional to the dose used with normal renal function ($Dose_D$) in the same ratio as the clearance of the drug in renal insufficiency (Cl_{D-RI}) to the clearance with normal renal function (Cl_D). Thus, by rearranging, the $Dose_{D-RI}$ is defined as

$$Dose_{D-RI} = Dose_D \times \frac{Cl_{D-RI}}{Cl_D} \qquad (10)$$

One can estimate the Cl_{D-RI} by multiplying the Cl_D by the ratio of the creatinine clearance in renal insufficiency (Cl_{Cr-RI}) over the Cl_{Cr} with normal renal function.

$$Cl_{D-RI} = Cl_D \times \frac{Cl_{Cr-RI}}{Cl_{Cr}} \qquad (11)$$

It must be remembered, as shown in equation 3, that total clearance is the sum of clearance by renal and non-renal (typically hepatic) mechanisms. Thus, any non-renal clearance is assumed to remain normal, and only the renal clearance is adjusted, with total clearance being reduced only to the extent that renal clearance is reduced. The dose may then be calculated from the total (adjusted) clearance and the desired plasma concentration using either equation 7 or 8. However, the calculated dose is only an initial guide to the dose needed. By monitoring the drug response and/or the plasma drug concentration at various times after initial dosing, further dose adjustments can be made as necessary. From a practical perspective, most clinical dose adjustment of drugs in the presence of renal dysfunction can be guided by published tables that recommend reductions based on changes in GFR (see Table 26–2) and the effectiveness of dialysis in removing the drug.

LOADING DOSE IN RENAL INSUFFICIENCY. For those drugs that are typically administered with a loading dose with normal renal function, the same regimen may be used with renal insufficiency to ensure that the desired concentration is rapidly achieved. For other drugs that typically are administered without a loading dose with normal renal function, the presence of a prolonged half-life with renal insufficiency may delay drug accumulation to steady state. In this setting, a loading dose (equal to the amount needed to reach steady state with normal renal function) would be required.

ADDITIONAL CONSIDERATIONS IN RENAL INSUFFICIENCY. Because of individual differences among patients, the approaches outlined earlier should be considered only initial approximations to prevent ineffective (too low) or toxic (too high) doses. In planning further maintenance therapy, it is desirable to monitor blood levels to guide further dosing.

If a metabolite of the drug is responsible for effect or toxicity and accumulates in renal failure, the drug level alone may not provide sufficient guidance for planning therapy in the setting of renal insufficiency. Thus, the major metabolite of procainamide is *N*-acetylprocainamide, which has similar toxicity to the parent drug but only modest antiarrhythmic activity. In the setting of renal failure, *N*-acetylprocainamide may accumulate dramatically because it is more dependent on renal elimination. Thus, measuring procain-

amide levels alone does not accurately assess either the levels needed for antiarrhythmic effect or the risk of toxicity.

LIVER DISEASE. Although many drugs are biotransformed in the liver, it is not possible to make any general recommendations for drug dose adjustments in liver disease. Unlike renal disease, no useful laboratory test is available on which to base dose adjustments. It has been suggested that if the liver's capacity to produce protein (reflected by albumin concentration and the prothrombin time) is significantly reduced, the clearance of drugs metabolized by the P-450 enzymes is probably also reduced.

One special situation that can develop with chronic liver disease and may require dose adjustment is the presence of portacaval shunts. This condition produces not only a potential hemodynamic alteration, leading to decreased hepatic blood flow with accompanying decreased clearance, but also possible bypassing of a first-pass effect, resulting in higher concentrations of drug reaching the systemic circulation. Drugs with a large hepatic extraction that are typically administered orally (e.g., propranolol) may then appear in the systemic circulation with higher, potentially toxic concentrations.

HEMODYNAMIC DISEASES. Decreased cardiac output or hypotensive conditions lead to decreased perfusion of the organs, including those responsible for eliminating drugs. As noted earlier with primary kidney disease, the dose can be adjusted for decreased renal perfusion by using the creatinine clearance. The effect of decreased hepatic blood flow on pharmacokinetics is more difficult to assess. For drugs that have a high hepatic extraction (e.g., lidocaine), decreased hepatic blood flow suggests a need to reduce doses.

Altered hemodynamics may also affect the distribution of selected drugs. Drugs that have a relatively large VD (e.g., lidocaine, procainamide, and quinidine) may be affected by conditions leading to hypotension, such as shock resulting in a decrease in the apparent VD. With a reduced VD the loading dose of a drug should be reduced to avoid potentially toxic drug levels.

In general, in the setting of severely compromised hemodynamics, it is advisable to be conservative, avoiding potentially toxic loading and maintenance doses of drugs. Drug levels and the clinical status should be monitored closely and drug doses should be adjusted as necessary.

APPROACH TO DRUG OVERDOSE

The pharmacokinetic principles discussed earlier can be useful to determine the best approach to drug removal in the setting of a drug overdose, particularly if hemodialysis or hemoperfusion is contemplated. The major goal is to increase the overall clearance of drug, removing a substantial fraction of the total body load of drug. Examining the VD and Cl values can provide some guidance. For drugs with a very large VD (e.g., digoxin in Table 26–1), only a small amount of drug can be removed because clearance affects only the amount of drug present in the plasma, and a large portion of the drug in the body is outside the plasma compartment. Similarly, for drugs with very high clearance values, hemoperfusion may only minimally increase the overall clearance and therefore is not indicated. Table 26–2 provides data for determining whether hemodialysis is likely to be useful to remove several commonly used drugs.

USING DRUGS IN THE ELDERLY

Administering drugs to the elderly is perhaps the most challenging area in adult therapeutics (see Chapter 8) because of several factors, including (1) the increasing likelihood of multiple illnesses, often with multisystemic involvement; (2) the need for these patients to be on multiple drugs (often prescribed by different physicians); and (3) the increasing probability of altered pharmacokinetics and pharmacodynamics. These factors together contribute to significantly increased frequency of drug interactions and adverse drug responses in this group of patients.

PHARMACOKINETIC CHANGES WITH AGE. These changes can be secondary to the effects of general physiologic changes of aging, such as the change in body composition, or to specific changes in pharmacokinetically important organs (e.g., kidneys or liver). The distribution of drugs tends to change dramatically with age, mainly because of changes in body composition. Most typical is the increase in total body fat with the accompanying decrease in lean body mass and total body water. Changes may also occur in the concentration of plasma proteins, particularly albumin, which decreases as the liver ages. The changes in distribution are manifest as a change in the apparent volume of distribution. For water-soluble drugs that are not bound to plasma proteins, the apparent V_D is reduced, in contrast to lipid-soluble drugs, for which the V_D is increased. Minimal changes in metabolism accompany aging, but these alone cannot typically account for altered pharmacokinetics.

Excretion can be altered in the elderly. The clearance of a number of drugs is decreased. Both cardiac output and blood flow to the kidneys and liver may also be decreased. GFR may be reduced by as much as 50%. Hepatic elimination of drugs is less affected except for drugs with a high hepatic clearance (e.g., lidocaine). The elimination half-life of many drugs is increased with aging as a consequence of a larger apparent V_D and a decreased hepatic or renal clearance (see equation 5).

PHARMACODYNAMIC CHANGES WITH AGE. These changes are a result of changes in the responsiveness of the target organ. They require using smaller drug doses in the elderly, even if the pharmacokinetics are unchanged. Many examples exist of such changes with drugs commonly used in the elderly; for example, antianxiety drugs and drugs from the sedative-hypnotic class may produce increased central nervous system depression in the elderly at concentrations that are well tolerated in younger adults. Similarly, anticoagulants (e.g., warfarin) may produce hemorrhage in the elderly at concentrations that are well tolerated in younger individuals.

GENERAL RECOMMENDATIONS. Several general principles apply to drug use in the elderly: (1) The clearance of drugs eliminated by the kidneys may be reduced by 50%; (2) drugs that are eliminated primarily by the liver typically do not require adjustment for age except for those with high hepatic clearances, which may be affected by age-related decrease in hepatic blood flow; (3) because of potential for increased target-organ sensitivity in the elderly, only the lowest effective dose should be used; and (4) frequent reviews of the patient's drug history should be conducted, including not only prescription but also over-the-counter medications, keeping in mind the increased potential risk for drug interactions and adverse drug responses.

INTERACTIONS BETWEEN DRUGS

Because patients are typically treated today with multiple agents even for a single disease, the possibilities for drug interactions are great. In general, most clinically important drug interactions typically involve a drug with a low therapeutic index (e.g., warfarin) and an easily detectable pharmacologic effect (e.g., bleeding), such that a small increase in the amount of drug produces a significant effect (toxicity).

EPIDEMIOLOGY. It is difficult to accurately assess the prevalence of drug interactions in either the inpatient or ambulatory settings, particularly because no formal surveillance mechanism is currently available. The risk for drug interactions appears to be increasing, particularly for critically ill, hospitalized patients who frequently are taking more than 10 medications.

ETIOLOGY. There are basically two types of drug interaction: (1) pharmacokinetic drug interactions, caused by a change in the amount of drug or active metabolite at the site of action, and (2) pharmacodynamic drug interactions (without a change in pharmacokinetics), due to a change in drug effect.

Pharmacokinetic Drug Interactions

Less Drug at the Site of Action

DECREASED ABSORPTION. The gastrointestinal lumen is perhaps the best example of an area where two or more drugs have the opportunity to interact, resulting in decreased drug absorption. Several examples, including commonly used drugs, illustrate this type of interaction. For many of these drugs, a physicochemical interaction prevents the drug(s) from being absorbed. Drugs such as colestipol and cholestyramine (resins used to lower cholesterol and bind bile acids) can also bind other drugs simultaneously present in the gastrointestinal lumen. Among the drugs that can be bound are digoxin and warfarin. Because many other drugs can also be bound, it is generally recommended that other drugs not be administered within 2 hours of colestipol or cholestyramine. Metal ions

(e.g., aluminum, calcium, and magnesium that are present in antacids and iron in supplements to treat iron deficiency) may form insoluble complexes with tetracyclines, which can act as chelating agents. Other commonly used medications that decrease absorption include kaolin-pectin suspensions used to treat diarrhea. These medications can significantly inhibit the absorption of co-administered drugs (e.g., digoxin).

Drugs that are particularly susceptible to pH changes may have decreased absorption when co-administered with drugs that either affect gastric acidity or alter the extent of exposure to low pH. Thus, H_2-receptor antagonists such as cimetidine, ranitidine, and famotidine may elevate gastric pH, which can in turn inhibit the dissolution and subsequent absorption of drugs that are weak bases (e.g., ketoconazole). Medications that delay gastric emptying (e.g., belladonna alkaloids) can increase the degradation of a co-administered acid-labile drug (e.g., levodopa), resulting in decreased absorption.

ALTERED DISTRIBUTION. Drugs that use the same active transport process to reach their site of action can compete at the level of transport, resulting in lower levels of drug reaching the site of action. The classic example of this type of interaction is guanidinium-type antihypertensives co-administered with tricyclic antidepressants, phenothiazines, and certain sympathomimetic amines (e.g., ephedrine), which block the antihypertensive effects of the former.

INCREASED METABOLISM. A number of drugs (e.g., barbiturates such as phenobarbital, phenytoin, ethanol, glutethimide, griseofulvin, rifampin, and toxic compounds such as cigarette smoke and certain chlorinated hydrocarbons) can increase hepatic metabolism of other drugs (e.g., corticosteroids, cyclophosphamide, cyclosporine, certain β-adrenergic blockers, theophylline, and warfarin) by inducing the activity of the cytochrome P-450 mixed-function oxidase (CYP) system.

More Drug at the Site of Action

INCREASED ABSORPTION. Any drug that increases the rate of gastric emptying (e.g., metoclopramide) can potentially increase the absorption of acid-unstable drugs. Also, drugs that decrease intestinal motility (e.g., anticholinergics) may increase the absorption of drugs that are relatively poorly absorbed (e.g., digoxin tablets) by increasing the contact time of the drug with the absorbing surface.

ALTERED DISTRIBUTION. Drugs bound to protein are limited in their distribution (particularly to the site of action) and are not available for metabolism or excretion. Drugs can compete with each other for binding to plasma proteins, resulting in drug interactions. For example, sulfonamides can displace barbiturates bound to serum albumin, leading to increased levels of free barbiturates with possible toxicity.

DECREASED METABOLISM. One of the most impressive drug interactions is produced when one drug inhibits the metabolism of another drug, leading to the second drug accumulating and thus significantly risking toxicity. For example, this type of interaction results from using 6-mercaptopurine, an antileukemic drug with a low therapeutic index, with allopurinol, often used in this setting to control hyperuricemia. The interaction may result in potentially life-threatening toxicity.

Some drugs can inhibit the metabolism of many other drugs. For example, cimetidine can inhibit the metabolism of diazepam, imipramine, lidocaine, propranolol, quinidine, theophylline, and warfarin. Amiodarone inhibits the metabolism of calcium channel blockers, flecainide, phenytoin, quinidine, and warfarin. Of particular importance with amiodarone is its half-life of 1 to 2 months, so that it continues to inhibit drug metabolism for several months after being discontinued.

Other drugs are notable in that their metabolism is inhibited by a variety of different drugs. The metabolism of the commonly used anticoagulant warfarin is inhibited not only by cimetidine and amiodarone but also by many other drugs, including alcohol, allopurinol, disopyramide, disulfiram, metronidazole, phenylbutazone, sulfinpyrazone, and trimethoprim-sulfamethoxazole. Similarly, the metabolism of phenytoin is also inhibited by additional drugs, including chloramphenicol, clofibrate, dicumarol, disulfiram, isoniazid (slow acetylators), phenylbutazone, and valproic acid.

Although most of the examples just noted involved enzymes metabolizing the drug in the liver, it should be noted that drug-metabolizing enzymes located outside the liver may also be affected by certain drugs. The best known example is monoamine oxidase, which can be affected by non-specific monoamine oxidase inhibitors, resulting in the accumulation of catecholamines at multiple sites after their release in response to eating tyramine-containing foods.

DECREASED EXCRETION. Drugs can compete for the active transporters present in the kidney. Most of these interactions involve the acid transporters. The best-known interaction is the probenecid inhibition of penicillin transport, leading to decreased penicillin clearance with resultant increased plasma levels—an interaction that was used in the past to maximize penicillin therapy. A similar inhibitory effect on renal excretion of methotrexate can be produced by salicylates, phenylbutazone, and probenicid. The active transport of basic drugs (e.g., procainamide) can also be inhibited by other drugs (e.g., cimetidine or amiodarone).

Pharmacodynamic Drug Interactions

With pharmacodynamic interactions, drugs interact at the level of the receptor or may produce additive effects by acting at separate sites on cells. An example of the first is the interaction of propranolol and epinephrine, which blocks β-adrenergic receptors with the result that the α-adrenergic effects of epinephrine are unopposed. This undesirable interaction can result in severe hypertension.

Many examples exist of additive effects between drugs. Aspirin, which can produce increased bleeding time by acting on platelets, can interact with warfarin, which affects clotting. The result is an increased risk of hemorrhage. Similarly, cardiac drugs such as β-adrenergic blockers and calcium channel blockers, when co-administered, have additive negative inotropic effects, resulting in an increased risk of cardiac failure.

DIAGNOSING AND PREVENTING DRUG INTERACTIONS. To recognize the presence of a drug interaction, the index of suspicion must be high whenever multiple drugs are used together. Because of the ever-increasing list of known and suspected drug interactions, it is impossible for a clinician to remember all or even a significant number of the possible interactions.

Several clinical settings should raise concern about the possibility of drug interactions: (1) The use of any drug with a low therapeutic index (Table 26–3) should be suspect. (2) As the number of drugs being used concurrently increases, there is a disproportionately greater risk of drug interactions, particularly with more than 10 drugs. (3) Critically ill patients who have multisystemic disease with compromised renal, hepatic, cardiac, or pulmonary function have an increased risk of drug interactions. This risk may be even higher for patients with the acquired immunodeficiency syndrome, who have an immunocompromised state as well as being on a great number of drugs. (4) Patients with various behavioral and psychiatric disorders (e.g., drug abusers taking a large number of prescription drugs, illicit drugs, and alcohol) are at risk to develop drug interactions.

Several steps can be taken to prevent drug interactions: (1) In taking the medical history, it is important to document all the drugs the patient is taking, including prescription, over-the-counter, and other addictive drugs. (2) It is desirable to minimize the number of drugs the patient is taking by frequently reviewing the patient's drug list to ensure that each drug continues to be needed. (3) There should be a high degree of suspicion when medications with a low therapeutic index known to have a high risk of drug interactions (see Table 26–3) are used. (4) High-risk clinical settings, such as

Table 26–3 ▪ DRUGS WITH LOW THERAPEUTIC INDICES AT HIGH RISK FOR ADVERSE DRUG RESPONSE AND DRUG INTERACTIONS

Anticoagulants
Antiarrhythmics
Anticonvulsants
Digoxin
Lithium carbonate
Oral hypoglycemics
Theophylline

occur with critically ill patients, should raise suspicion of adverse drug interactions. (5) Adverse drug interactions should be considered in the differential diagnosis whenever any change occurs in a patient's course.

ADVERSE REACTIONS TO DRUGS

An adverse drug response is an undesired effect produced by a drug at standard doses, which typically necessitates reducing or stopping the suspected agent and may require treatment for the noxious effect produced. Further harm may occur with continued or future therapy with the drug.

EPIDEMIOLOGY. The actual incidence of adverse drug responses is somewhat difficult to quantify, because many cases are not recognized. Several large studies have demonstrated that the incidence may approach 20% for outpatients (even higher for patients on more than 15 drugs) and 2 to 7% for inpatients. Recent meta-analyses of several prospective studies indicate that adverse drug reactions may be the fourth to sixth leading cause of death in hospitalized patients. It is clear from recent surveys that a relatively small group of drugs (see Table 26–3) continues to be implicated in most of the reported adverse drug responses. Current trends suggest that the incidence of adverse drug responses is likely to increase as a result of an increase in the number of both prescribed and over-the-counter medications.

ETIOLOGY. Most adverse drug responses are caused by either (1) exaggerated (but predictable) pharmacologic effect of the drug or (2) toxic or immunologic effect of drug or metabolite (not typically expected).

EXAGGERATED (PREDICTABLE) RESPONSE TO A DRUG. Exaggerated drug responses that cause adverse drug effects may be due to any condition that causes either altered pharmacokinetics or pharmacodynamics (discussed earlier).

Recently there has been interest in the role of genetic factors as a cause of increased susceptibility to adverse drug responses, primarily through an effect on drug metabolism. Genetic polymorphism of drug metabolizing enzymes can account for variability in pharmacokinetics and drug effect observed in population studies. Three of the best-studied polymorphisms are the debrisoquine/sparteine, N-acetylation, and mephenytoin polymorphisms. These are each associated with an autosomal recessive inheritance and together are responsible for the metabolism of approximately 40 drugs (Table 26–4). Individuals with autosomal recessive genes are "poor metabolizers" with potentially altered pharmacokinetics that result in elevated plasma drug concentrations and can lead to toxicity. These defects are not noted until the patient is given the drug. They are often described as being "pharmacogenetic" syndromes.

Other genetic defects do not specifically affect metabolism and hence do not produce a range of quantitative changes. These defects can produce "qualitative" defects and are often associated with structural defects. The classic example is glucose-6-phosphate dehydrogenase (G6PD). Individuals who are deficient in this enzyme cannot tolerate oxidative stress that is produced by some drugs, leading to hemolysis (see Chapter 164). Drugs that can produce this clinical picture include aspirin, nitrofurantoin, primaquine, probenecid, quinidine, quinine, sulfonamides, sulfones, and vitamin K. Another similar defect is deficiency of methemoglobin reductase, which results in an inability to maintain iron in hemoglobin in the ferrous state, causing methemoglobinemia after exposure to oxidizing drugs such as nitrites, sulfonamide, or sulfones.

TOXIC OR IMMUNOLOGIC (UNPREDICTABLE) RESPONSE TO DRUG. This type of adverse drug response is not predictable and is not obviously due to either an increase in drug concentration (pharmacokinetic) or drug effect (pharmacodynamic). Toxic responses include direct reactions between drug and a specific organ (e.g., platinum-containing drugs such as cisplatin can produce direct toxicity in the kidney and the eighth cranial nerve). With other drugs, metabolism of the drug to an active intermediate must first occur. With a standard dose of acetaminophen, no untoward effects occur because the relatively small amount of reactive metabolite formed by oxidative metabolism is rapidly detoxified by reduced glutathione. In the presence of an overdose, the glutathione is depleted and the remaining reactive metabolite can then damage the liver. Understanding the mechanism of this toxicity has provided a rationale for treating acetaminophen overdose. Thus, sulfhydryl-containing

Table 26-4 ■ GENETIC POLYMORPHISMS OF DRUG-METABOLIZING ENZYMES

TYPE	PRIMARY DRUG EXAMPLES	OTHER DRUGS THAT ARE SUBSTRATES	INCIDENCE OF "POOR METABOLIZERS" IN WHITES (%)	ENZYME INVOLVED
Debrisoquine-sparteine polymorphism	Debrisoquine, sparteine, bufuralol	Antidepressants, antiarrhythmics, β-adrenergic-receptor blocking drugs, codeine, dextromethorphan, neuroleptics	5–10	Cytochrome P-450 IID6 (CYP2D6)
Mephenytoin polymorphism	Mephenytoin	Mephobarbital, hexobarbital, diazepam, omeprazole	4 (Japanese, Chinese, 15–20)	Cytochrome P-450 IIC (CYP2C)
Acetylation polymorphism	Isoniazid, sulfadiazine	Isoniazid, hydralazine, phenelzine, procainamide, dapsone, sulfamethazine, sulfapyridine, aminoglutethimide, aminosalicylic acid, sulfadiazine, sulfasalazine	40–70 (Japanese, 10–20)	N-Acetyltransferase (NAT₂)
Methyl-conjugation polymorphism	Catecholamines	L-Dopa, methyldopa	25–30	Catechol-O-methyltransferase (COMT)

compounds (e.g., N-acetylcysteine), which can complex with the reactive metabolite, can be administered to reduce the amount of "free" toxic metabolite present, thereby protecting the liver.

Immunologic reactions to drugs (Table 26–5) in general are not produced by the drug alone. Like other small molecular weight compounds (<1000 daltons), they are typically not antigenic themselves. When a drug or reactive metabolite combines with a protein to form a drug-protein complex, it can become antigenic, capable of eliciting an immune response.

Perhaps the most impressive form of drug allergy is anaphylaxis, which is due to an IgE-mediated hypersensitivity. Many drugs from different classes have been shown to produce this type of drug allergy (see Table 26–5). The best-known example is the anaphylactic response produced by penicillin, which can occur after administering penicillin by any route. Skin testing with penicillin G, penicilloic acid, or penicilloyl-polylysine can identify patients at risk and should be used in patients with suspected penicillin allergy who need to be treated with penicillin. If the skin test is positive,

Table 26-5 ■ SOME NOTABLE ADVERSE DRUG REACTIONS

I. Multisystemic Manifestations
  A. Anaphylaxis
    1. Macromolecules
      Allergenic extracts
      Dextrans (including iron dextran)
      Enzymes
        Asparaginase
        Chymopapain
        Trypsin
      Heparin
      Hormones (e.g., ACTH, insulin)
      Human gamma globulin
      Monoclonal antibodies
      Protamine
      Vaccines
      Antisera
    2. Diagnostic agents
      Fluorescein
      Iodinated contrast media
    3. Antimicrobials
      Aminosalicylic acid
      Amphotericin B
      Cephalosporins
      Cinoxacin
      Clindamycin
      Demeclocycline
      Ethambutol
      Kanamycin
      Lincomycin
      Nalidixic acid
      Penicillins
      Streptomycin
      Sulfonamides
      Tetracyclines
      Vancomycin
    4. Other drugs, including nonsteroidal anti-inflammatory drugs (NSAIDs)
      Aspirin
      Benzyl alcohol
      Bleomycin
      Cisplatin
      Colchicine

      Cromolyn
      Cytarabine
      Dantrolene
      Ethylenediamine
      Etoposide
      Flucytosine
      Glucocorticoids
      Indomethacin
      Lidocaine
      Local anesthetics
      Mephyton
      Meprobamate
      Niacin
      Opiates
      Pentamidine
      Probenecid
      Procainamide
      Sulfite
      Thiopental
      Tolmetin
      Triamterene
      Tubocurarine and other muscle-relaxing agents
      Vitamin B₁₂
  B. Serum sickness
    1. Macromolecules
      Dextrans
      Heparin
      Hormones (e.g., insulin, ACTH)
      Vaccines
      Antisera
    2. Antimicrobials
      Cephalosporins
      Griseofulvin
      Lincomycin
      Minocycline
      Penicillins
      Streptomycin
      Sulfonamides
    3. Other drugs
      Barbiturates
      Hydralazine
      Phenylbutazone
      Phenytoin
      Procarbazine

      Propylthiouracil
  C. Drug fever
    1. Antimicrobials
      5-Aminosalicylic acid
      Amphotericin B
      Cephalosporins
      Erythromycin
      Isoniazid
      Kanamycin
      Nitrofurantoin
      Norfloxacin
      Penicillins
      Pyrazinamide
      Quinine
      Streptomycin
      Sulfonamides
      Tetracyclines
    2. Other drugs
      Allopurinol
      Captopril
      Heparin
      Hydantoins
      Hydralazine
      Hydrochlorothiazide
      Methyldopa
      Penicillamine
      Phenobarbital
      Pneumococcal vaccine
      Procainamide
      Propylthiouracil
      Quinine
  D. Vasculitis
      Allopurinol
      Atenolol
      Busulfan
      Carbamazepine
      Colchicine
      Diphenhydramine
      Ethionamide
      Furosemide
      Hydantoins
      Hydroxyurea
      Ibuprofen
      Indomethacin
      Isoniazid
      Meprobamate
      Methamphetamine

      Naproxen
      Penicillins
      Phenothiazines
      Phenylbutazone
      Propranolol
      Propylthiouracil
      Streptokinase
      Sulfonamides
      Tetracyclines
      Thiazide diuretics
      Vaccines
  E. Systemic lupus erythematosus syndrome
      5-Aminosalicylic acid
      Chloroquine
      Chlorpromazine
      Ethosuximide
      Griseofulvin
      Hydralazine
      Isoniazid
      Methyldopa
      Nitrofurantoin
      Penicillamine
      Penicillins
      Phenytoin
      Procainamide
      Propylthiouracil
      Quinidine
      Tetracycline
      Tocainide
      Trimethadione
II. Skin
  A. Urticaria and angioedema
    1. Antimicrobials
      5-Aminosalicylic acid
      Aminoglycosides
      Cephalosporins
      Isoniazid
      Metronidazole
      Miconazole
      Nalidixic acid
      Penicillins
      Quinine
      Rifampin
      Spectinomycin
      Sulfonamides

Table continued on following page

Table 26–5 ■ SOME NOTABLE ADVERSE DRUG REACTIONS *Continued*

2. Other drugs
   Asparaginase
   Aspirin and other NSAIDs
   Calcitonin
   Chloral hydrate
   Chorambucil
   Cimetidine
   Cyclophosphamide
   Daunorubicin
   Doxorubicin
   Ergotamine
   Ethchlorvynol
   Ethosuximide
   Ethylenediamine
   Glucocorticoids
   Melphalan
   Penicillamine
   Phenothiazines
   Procainamide
   Procarbazine
   Quinidine
   Tartrazine
   Thiazide diuretics
   Thiotepa
B. Morbilliform-maculopapular rash
   1. Antimicrobials
      5-Aminosalicylic acid
      Cephalosporins
      Erythromycin
      Gentamicin
      Penicillins
      Streptomycin
      Sulfonamides
   2. Other drugs
      Allopurinol
      Barbiturates
      Captopril
      Coumarin
      Gold salts
      Hydantoins
      Thiazide diuretics
C. Toxic epidermal necrolysis, erythroderma, and exfoliative dermatitis
   Allopurinol
   Amikacin
   Captopril
   Carbamazepine
   Chloral hydrate
   Chlorambucil
   Chloroquine
   Chlorpromazine
   Cyclosporine
   Diltiazem
   Ethambutol
   Ethylenediamine
   Glutethimide
   Gold salts
   Griseofulvin
   Hydantoins
   Hydroxychloroquine
   Minoxidil
   Nifedipine
   NSAIDs
   Penicillin
   Phenobarbital
   Rifampin
   Spironolactone
   Streptomycin
   Sulfonamides
   Trimethadione
   Trimethoprim
   Tocainide
   Vancomycin
   Verapamil
D. Erythema multiforme
   Acetaminophen
   Barbiturates
   Carbamazepine
   Chloroquine

Chlorpropamide
Clindamycin
Ethambutol
Ethosuximide
Gold salts
Hydantoins
Hydralazine
Hydroxyurea
Mechlorethamine
Meclofenamate
Penicillins
Phenolphthalein
Phenylbutazone
Rifampin
Streptomycin
Sulfonylureas
Sulindac
Vaccines
E. Photosensitive
   1. Topical
      Fluorouracil
      Hexachlorophene
      Para-aminobenzoic acid esters
      Promethazine
      Sulfanilamide
   2. Systemic
      Carbamazepine
      Chlorpromazine
      Griseofulvin
      Imipramine
      Lincomycin
      Nalidixic acid
      Naproxen
      Norfloxacin
      Phenothiazines
      Piroxicam
      Quinethazone
      Sulfonamides
      Sulfonylureas
      Thiazide diuretics
      Triamterene
F. Fixed drug eruptions
   Acetaminophen
   5-Aminosalicylic acid
   Aspirin
   Barbiturates
   Benzodiazepines
   Chloroquine
   Dapsone
   Dimenhydrinate
   Diphenhydramine
   Gold salts
   Hydralazine
   Hyoscine
   Ibuprofen
   Iodides
   Meprobamate
   Methenamine
   Metronidazole
   Penicillins
   Phenobarbital
   Phenolphthalein
   Phenothiazines
   Phenylbutazone
   Procarbazine
   Pseudoephedrine
   Quinine
   Saccharin
   Streptomycin
   Sulfonamides
   Tetracyclines
G. Erythema nodosum
   Bromides
   Oral contraceptives
   Penicillin
   Sulfonamides
H. Contact dermatitis
   Ambroxol
   Amikacin
   Antihistamines
   Bacitracin

Benzalkonium chloride
Benzocaine
Benzyl alcohol
Cetyl alcohol
Chloramphenicol
Chlorpromazine
Clioquinol
Colophony
Ethylenediamine
Fluorouracil
Formaldehyde
Gentamicin
Glucocorticoids
Glutaraldehyde
Heparin
Hexachlorophene
Iodochlorhydroxyquin
Lanolin
Local anesthetics
Minoxidil
Naftin
Neomycin
Nitrofurazone
Opiates
Para-aminobenzoic acid
Parabens
Penicillins
Phenothiazines
Proflavine
Propylene glycol
Streptomycin
Sulfonamides
Thimerosal
Timolol
III. Lungs
   A. Asthma
      Aspirin and other NSAIDs
      Cromolyn
      Sulfite
      Tartrazine
      Occupational exposures to:
         Cephalosporins
         Glutaraldehyde
         Pancreatic enzymes
         Papain
         Penicillins
         Psyllium
         Thimerosal
   B. Eosinophilic pneumonitis
      5-Aminosalicylic acid
      Azathioprine
      Captopril
      Carbamazepine
      Chlorpropamide
      Chlorpromazine
      Cromolyn
      Desipramine
      Gold salts
      Imipramine
      Nitrofurantoin
      Penicillins
      Phenytoin
      Sulfonamides
      L-Tryptophan
   C. Fibrotic and pleural reactions
      Bleomycin
      Busulfan
      Cyclophosphamide
      Gold salts
      Hydralazine
      Hydrochlorothiazide
      Melphalan
      Methotrexate
      Methysergide
      Mitomycin
      Nitrofurantoin
      Procarbazine
IV. Liver
   A. Cholestatic
      Chlorzoxazone

Erythromycin estolate
Ethchlorvynol
Imipramine
Nalidixic acid
Nitrofurantoin
Phenothiazines
Sulfamethoxazole
Sulfonylureas
Troleandomycin
B. Hepatocellular
   5-Aminosalicylic acid
   Amphotericin B
   Azapropazone
   Ethacrynic acid
   Furosemide
   Gold salts
   Griseofulvin
   Halothane
   Hydantoins
   Isoniazid
   Methyldopa
   Monoamine oxidase inhibitors
   Nitrofurantoin
   Propylthiouracil
   Pyrazinamide
   Quinidine
   Rifampin
   Sulfonamides
   Trimethadione
C. Chronic active hepatitis
   Methyldopa
   Nitrofurantoin
V. Kidney
   A. Glomerulitis
      Allopurinol
      Captopril
      Gold salts
      NSAIDs
      Penicillamine
      Penicillins
      Phenytoin
      Probenecid
      Sulfonamides
      Thiazide diuretics
   B. Interstitial nephritis
      Allopurinol
      Aztreonam
      Captopril
      Carbamazepine
      Cephalosporins
      Chloramphenicol
      Cimetidine
      Ciprofloxacin
      Colistin
      Furosemide
      Minocycline
      NSAIDs
      Penicillins, especially methicillin
      Phenytoin
      Polymyxin B
      Rifampin
      Sulfonamides
      Tetracycline
      Thiazide diuretics
VI. Bone marrow and blood cells
   A. Bone marrow aplasia
      Chloramphenicol
      Gold salts
      Mephenytoin
      Penicillamine
      Phenylbutazone
      Trimethadione
   B. Anemia
      Acetaminophen
      5-Aminosalicylic acid
      Captopril
      Cephalosporins
      Chlorpromazine
      Cisplatin

Table 26–5 ■ SOME NOTABLE ADVERSE DRUG REACTIONS *Continued*

Hydantoins	C. Thrombocytopenia	Isoniazid	D. Granulocytopenia
Ibuprofen	Acetaminophen	Levodopa	Captopril
Insulin	Acetazolamide	Meprobamate	Cephalosporins
Isoniazid	Acetylsalicylic acid	Methyldopa	Chloral hydrate
Levodopa	5-Aminosalicylic acid	Penicillamine	Chlorpropamide
Mefenamic acid	Carbamazepine	Phenylbutazone	Penicillins (semisynthetic)
Melphalan	Chloramphenicol	Procainamide	Phenothiazines
Methyldopa	Chlorpheniramine	Quinidine	Phenylbutazone
Methylsergide	Cimetidine	Quinine	Phenytoin
Penicillins	Digitoxin	Ranitidine	Procainamide
Quinidine	Diltiazem	*Rauwolfia* alkaloids	Propranolol
Quinine	Ethchlorvynol	Rifampin	Tolbutamide
Rifampin	Gold salts	Sulfonamides	E. Lymphoid hyperplasia
Sulfonamides	Heparin	Sulfonylureas	Phenytoin
Sulfonylureas	Hydantoins	Thiazide diuretics	Mephenytoin

Adapted from Reed CE: Drug allergy. *In* Wyngaarden JB, Smith LH Jr, Bennett JC (eds): Cecil Textbook of Medicine, 19th ed. Philadelphia, WB Saunders, 1992, pp 1480–1481.

the patient must undergo desensitization before receiving penicillin. If the skin test is negative, penicillin can be administered but with caution.

DIAGNOSIS. Although it should be clear from the previous discussion that many of the well-known adverse drug effects are due to a relatively small group of drugs, it should be emphasized that every drug can potentially cause an adverse drug response. Therefore, the physician should always consider the possibility of an adverse drug response in the differential diagnosis even if none has been reported previously for the particular drug. Table 26–5 lists a number of diverse clinical presentations associated with adverse drug responses. In many instances it is readily apparent that a specific drug has produced an adverse drug response, such as the appearance of a rash in an otherwise healthy patient who recently has been started on a single drug (e.g., penicillin). In other cases, the effect produced by the drug may be difficult to discern from other disease states. In still other cases, the adverse effect may mimic the illness being treated (e.g., an arrhythmia developing in a patient being treated with an antiarrhythmic drug).

From a public health perspective, it is highly desirable to have a mechanism available for detecting, cataloging, and tracking the incidence and severity of adverse drug responses not only for drugs at various stages of development but also for drugs that were approved earlier. The Food and Drug Administration (FDA) tries to track adverse drug events through a voluntary reporting program, MedWatch. Health care professionals are encouraged to report any adverse events or product problems on a one-page form that can then be sent by mail, fax, or modem to the FDA. Although various methods for surveying adverse drug responses have been proposed, it is ultimately the cooperation of alert clinicians and health care professionals that must be encouraged.

Bennett WM: Drug Prescribing in Renal Failure: Dosing Guidelines for Adults, 3rd ed. Philadelphia, American College of Physicians, 1994. *This manual provides useful data for adjusting doses in patients with renal dysfunction, including those on dialysis.*

Doucet J, Chassagne P, Trivalle C, et al: Drug-drug interactions related to hospital admissions in older adults: A prospective study of 1000 patients. J A Geriatr Soc 44:944, 1996. *Study of the frequency, nature, and side effects of drug-drug interactions in geriatric patients consecutively admitted to an inpatient facility.*

Guengerich FP: Role of cytochrome P450 enzymes in drug-drug interactions. Adv Pharmacol 43:7, 1997. *Many adverse drug-drug interactions are secondary to pharmacokinetic changes that can be explained by alterations of P-450 catalyzed reactions.*

Harder S, Thurmann P: Clinically important drug interactions with anticoagulants. Clin Pharmacokinet 30:416, 1996. *Review of clinically important drug interactions that occur with commonly used anticoagulant drugs.*

Lam YW, Banerji S, Hatfield C, Talbert RL: Principles of drug administration in renal insufficiency. Clin Pharmacokinet 32:30, 1997. *Current review of principles that should be used in managing drug use in the presence of renal insufficiency (118 references).*

Lazarou J, Pomeranz BH, Corey PN: Incidence of adverse drug reactions in hospitalized patients: A meta-analysis of prospective studies. JAMA 279:1200, 1998. *Determination of the proportion of US hospitalized patients who are affected by serious or fatal drug reactions.*

Rizack MA: The Medical Letter Handbook of Adverse Drug Interactions. New Rochelle, The Medical Letter, 1998. *This paperback handbook provides a relatively comprehensive listing of drugs thought to produce interactions, with a description of adverse effects, their probable mechanisms, clinical recommendations, and original references.*

Westphal JF, Brogard JM: Drug administration in chronic liver disease. Drug Safety 17:47, 1997. *Guidelines for drug administration in the presence of liver disease (225 references).*

■ PROBLEMS OF OVERARCHING IMPORTANCE AND TRANSCENDING ORGAN SYSTEMS

27 PAIN

Kathleen M. Foley

Pain is the most common symptom for which patients seek medical evaluation. Several national patient surveys have emphasized the magnitude of pain as a public health issue, citing its negative impact on patients' functional status and quality of life.

Improved medical and diagnostic methods, coupled with recent advances in our understanding of central nervous system (CNS) pain modulatory systems and their neuroanatomic and neuropharmacologic correlates, have led to specialized and innovative applications of pain management strategies. The consensus in pain therapy is that pain patients are managed most effectively by a multidisciplinary approach, using the expertise of a wide range of health care professionals. To facilitate clinical research and patient care, the International Association for the Study of Pain has proposed a taxonomy of pain syndromes to serve as a universal classification, with a working definition of pain as "an unpleasant sensory and emotional experience associated with either actual or potential tissue damage, or described in terms of such damage."

The physician's therapeutic task is twofold: to discover and treat the cause of the pain or to treat the pain itself, whether or not the underlying cause is treatable. In the majority of clinical pain syndromes, pain therapy serves to palliate the symptom. For such patients, the goal of pain treatment should be to improve the patient's quality of life by facilitating his or her functional status and social interactions.

TYPES OF PAIN

Clinically, pain can be classified *temporally* as acute or chronic; *quantitatively* as mild, moderate, or severe; *physiologically* as somatic, visceral, or neuropathic, and *etiologically* as medical or psychogenic.

TEMPORAL CHARACTERISTICS. Patients with *acute pain* usually give a clear description of its location, character, and timing, leading to an etiologic diagnosis. Objective signs and associated autonomic nervous system hyperactivity with tachycardia, hypertension, and diaphoresis are present. The setting of the pain, its meaning, and its duration influence the patient's ability to tolerate it. Acute pain (e.g., postoperative pain, acute traumatic pain) is usually self-limited. *Subacute pain* develops over several days, and *episodic pain* occurs for set periods of time on a recurring basis. *Chronic pain* is the persistence of pain for 3 months or longer. The acute signs of autonomic nervous system hyperactivity disappear with adaption to the pain. Chronic pain leads to significant changes in personality, lifestyle, and functional ability, compromising the patient's quality of life. Multidisciplinary approaches to treatment play a critical role in addressing the multidimensional aspects of the pain. Other commonly used terms to describe pain include *baseline pain,* which refers to the average pain intensity expressed for 12 or more hours in a 24-hour period, and *breakthrough pain,* which is a transient increase in pain resulting from volitional factors (e.g., incident pain on movement) and non-volitional factors (e.g., flatulence).

QUANTITATIVE CHARACTERISTICS. The intensity of pain is used to describe its severity. Pain intensity is the major factor in choosing drug therapy, and the use of a reliable pain intensity scale can enormously affect appropriate patient treatment. Numerous studies have shown that health care professionals underestimate patients' pain intensity, particularly if patients report pain as moderate or severe. This observation is one of the common causes of the undertreatment of pain. The repeated use of validated pain intensity scales, such as categorical scales, numerical scales, and visual analogue scales, can facilitate appropriate pain assessment and treatment. Categorical scales use verbal reports and ask patients to describe their pain as mild, moderate, severe, or excruciating. Numerical scales ask patients to rate their pain as a number from 0 to 10 with 0 at "no pain" and 10 being the "worst possible pain." Visual analogue scales consist of a 10-cm line anchored on either end by the two points, "no pain" and "worst possible pain," and the patient is asked to mark on the line the intensity of his or her pain.

PHYSIOLOGIC CHARACTERISTICS. Somatic pain results from activation of peripheral receptors and somatic sensory efferent nerves without injury to the peripheral nerve or CNS. The pain can be either sharp or dull, but it is typically well-localized and describable. Visceral pain results from visceral nociceptive receptors and visceral efferent nerves being activated and is characterized by a deep, aching, cramping sensation often referred to cutaneous sites. Neuropathic pain results from direct injury to peripheral receptors, nerves, or the CNS. It is typically described as burning or dysesthetic and often occurs in an area of sensory loss (e.g., postherpetic neuralgia). Recent experimental pain models in animals and humans have provided the opportunity to study neuropathic pain and its phenomena of "windup," whereby spinal neurons become abnormally active after repetitive C-fiber stimulation, and "central sensitization," whereby neurons decrease activation thresholds, enlarge their receptive fields, and fire spontaneously. These phenomena account for the clinical signs of allodynia (pain associated with non-nociceptive stimuli) and hyperalgesia (increased pain with nociceptive stimuli) that occur with nerve injury. N-methyl-D-aspartate (NMDA)-receptor antagonists such as ketamine, amantadine, and dextromethorphan block these phenomena and prevent neuropathic pain in animals and humans. Clinical trials are in progress to define the safety and efficacy of these agents.

ETIOLOGIC CHARACTERISTICS. Patients with chronic pain can generally be classified into one of three major etiologic groups, allowing for some overlap. The first group includes patients with chronic pain associated with structural disease. Such pain (e.g., metastatic cancer, sickle-cell disease, rheumatoid arthritis) is usually characterized by prolonged episodes of pain alternating with pain-free intervals or by unremitting pain waxing and waning in severity. Successful treatment of the pain is closely allied with disease treatment, but in certain instances, treating the pain is the only therapeutic goal (e.g., the dying patient with pain). Psychological factors may play an important role in exacerbating or relieving the pain, but analgesic drugs are often the mainstay of therapy.

The second group comprises patients who suffer from *psychophysiologic disorders* causing pain. In these patients, structural disease, such as a herniated disc or torn ligament, may once have been present, but psychological factors have caused chronic physiologic alterations, such as muscle spasms, which produce pain long after the underlying defect has healed. Typically, such patients are physically inactive and spend much of their time thinking and talking about their pain, often leading to social and emotional isolation. Patients are more impaired by the "chronic illness behavior" than by a defined pathologic condition. They usually respond poorly to analgesic drugs and often suffer from iatrogenic complications such as adverse drug reactions and ineffective surgical procedures. Successful treatment can be expected only through a structured rehabilitation program designed to modify pain behaviors and not through medical intervention that corrects pathologic conditions. Multidisciplinary pain clinics that diagnose and treat these intractable chronic pain syndromes exist in many centers and should be used to evaluate and treat such patients.

Patients in the third group complain of pain that appears to have neither a structural nor a physiologic basis. These patients probably suffer from somatic delusions. Such patients usually have serious psychiatric disorders, and the history of their pain is so vague and bizarre and its distribution so unanatomic as to suggest the diagnosis. These patients are rare, respond poorly to pain treatment strategies alone, and require psychiatric treatment with a variable response rate.

ASSESSMENT OF PAIN

The approach to assessing the patient with pain begins with the premise that to manage pain, the physician must understand its multidimensional nature and must establish a relationship of mutual trust with the patient (Table 27–1). The diagnosis of the specific pain syndrome and a complete understanding of the psychological state of the patient are not often achieved at the initial evaluation. A comprehensive assessment involves taking a careful history, performing a detailed medical, neurologic, and psychological evaluation, developing a series of diagnosis-related hypotheses, and ordering the appropriate diagnostic studies. The history of the pain complaint should include the patient's description of the site of the pain, its quality, its exacerbating and relieving factors, its temporal pattern, its associated symptoms and signs, its interference with activities of daily living, and its response to previous and current analgesic therapies.

Multiple pain complaints are common in patients with chronic medical illness and need to be prioritized and classified. In evaluating the patient with pain, it is imperative to clarify his or her current level of anxiety and depression and to obtain a history of previous psychiatric illness to define the psychological risk. Does

Table 27–1 ■ CLINICAL ASSESSMENT OF PAIN

1. Believe the patient's complaint of pain.
2. Take a careful history of the pain complaint to place it temporally in the patient's history.
3. Assess the characteristics of each pain, including site, referral pattern, and aggravating and relieving factors.
4. Clarify the temporal aspects of the pain: acute, subacute, chronic, episodic, intermittent, breakthrough, or incident.
5. List and prioritize each pain complaint.
6. Evaluate the response to previous and current analgesic therapies.
7. Evaluate the psychological state of the patient.
8. Ask if the patient has a past history of alcohol or drug dependence.
9. Perform a careful medical and neurologic examination.
10. Develop a series of diagnosis-related hypotheses.
11. Order and personally review the appropriate diagnostic procedures.
12. Design the diagnostic and therapeutic approach to suit the individual.
13. Provide continuity of care from evaluation to treatment to ensure patient compliance and to reduce patient anxiety.
14. Reassess the patient's response to pain therapy.
15. Discuss advance directives for managing pain of dying patients.

the patient have a past history or family history of acute or chronic pain? Information on how the patient has handled previous painful events may provide insight into whether the patient has demonstrated chronic illness behavior. A personal or family history of alcohol or drug dependence may explain why the patient may be fearful or refuse to take opioid drugs. Because each patient has his or her own understanding of the meaning of pain, it is useful to have the patient elaborate this meaning. Does he or she think it represents recurrent tumor, in the case of a patient with cancer? Or is he or she convinced that it is simply arthritis? The more serious the nature of the pain diagnosis, the more likely the patient's understanding of its meaning may produce psychological distress. Data suggest that psychological factors play a significant role in accounting for the differences in pain experiences among patients with the same pain diagnosis or illness. Awareness of the common psychiatric syndromes—anxiety and depression—that occur in patients with pain can facilitate the diagnosis during pain complaint assessment.

Although it is crucial to know as much as possible about the individual patient with pain, such information may not be readily available in the first interview and, in some instances, may never be available because the patient lacks the intellectual competence to define clearly those various components. It is also necessary to verify the history from a family member who may provide information that the patient is unable or unwilling to provide: the family member may be more objective in assessing the disability of the patient who underreports his or her symptoms. Similarly, if a patient is a poor historian, a family member may provide essential information that may alter the diagnostic approach. In short, all attempts should be made to compile a careful history and to define the medical, neurologic, and psychological profile of the pain complaint.

In cases of advanced disease, it is crucial to request that the patient define what he or she would do if the pain is intractable or intolerable. Has the patient seen someone die a painful death? Does he or she have suicidal thoughts or a pact with a family member because of the pain? Does the patient have a family history of suicide? Does he or she have drugs in reserve for such an event or a gun in the house that might be used if the patient feels desperate? Such questions may allow the patient openly to discuss his or her fears of pain, and such open discussions can allow the treating physician to define the options for care and reassure the patient of his or her commitment to appropriate and adequate pain control. Patients rarely offer this information unless requested, so it is crucial that a repertoire of specific questions be developed that can be integrated into the initial history taking.

No patient should be evaluated inadequately because of a significant pain problem. Early management of the pain while investigating the source markedly improves the patient's ability to participate in the necessary diagnostic procedures. During the initial evaluation of the pain complaint, alternative methods of pain control including anesthetic and neurosurgical approaches should be considered, (e.g., the temporary use of local anesthetics via an epidural catheter to manage pain from a vertebral body collapse or intravenous opioids to control acute severe abdominal pain). These approaches should be considered not just when all else fails but rather be an integral part of the assessment. Continual reassessment of the response provides the best method to validate the initial diagnosis. However, in those patients in whom the effect of therapy is less than predicted or in whom the pain is exacerbated, reassessment of the treatment approach or a search for a new cause of the pain should be considered. In developing the diagnostic and therapeutic approach to suit the individual, careful judgment should be used in choosing diagnostic approaches that directly affect the choice of the therapeutic strategy or answer a specific question. The random use of diagnostic procedures in patients with pain is inappropriate and may have an adverse effect on their quality of life. This principle applies most commonly to patients with advanced cancer, in whom painful diagnostic procedures are inappropriate because they simply confirm the existence of disease for which treatment is unavailable or inappropriate. Lastly, in developing a strategy for managing pain in patients with advanced cancer or incurable medical diseases, it is important for the physician to know the patient's decisions about resuscitation, living wills, and symptom management if he or she becomes incompetent (see Chapter 3). These discussions improve the physician's ability to care for the pain patient with advanced disease appropriately and humanely.

MANAGEMENT OF PAIN

Recent advances in pain research provide the scientific rationale for using new, improved methods of treatment, including better and more effective use of standard drug therapy (non-opioid, opioid, and adjuvant analgesic drugs), the development of new drugs, the use of novel methods and routes of drug administration, and the use of selective anesthetic and neurosurgical approaches to control pain. The Agency for Health Care Policy and Research guidelines for management of acute postoperative pain and cancer pain establish standards of care for using analgesic, anesthetic, and neurosurgical approaches.

DRUG THERAPY. Analgesic drugs can be divided into three groups. In group I, the non-opioid analgesics, such as aspirin and acetaminophen and the non-steroidal, anti-inflammatory drugs (NSAIDs), act both peripherally and, in some instances, centrally, through inhibition of various enzyme systems (e.g., cyclooxygenase (see Chapter 29). In group II, the opioid agonist and antagonist drugs activate opioid receptors in the central and peripheral nervous systems. In group III, the adjuvant analgesic drugs produce analgesia in certain pain states (e.g., amitriptyline paroxetine, galapentin in neuropathic pain) or potentiate the opioid analgesics.

These three groups represent the mainstay of drug therapy for patients with acute and chronic pain. Their effective use requires an understanding of their pharmacologic characteristics and appropriate selection of a particular drug individualized to the needs of the patient and the specific pain syndrome.

NON-OPIOID ANALGESICS. Aspirin, acetaminophen, and the NSAIDs are the first-line agents for management of mild to moderate pain; in patients with severe pain, these drugs potentiate the effects of opioid analgesics. Non-opioid analgesics have a ceiling effect, and their long-term use is compromised by gastrointestinal and hematologic side effects. The choice and use of these drugs must be individualized, with the patient receiving maximal levels of one drug before another is tried. If pain control is ineffective or the non-opioid agents are poorly tolerated, opioid analgesics are indicated.

OPIOID ANALGESICS. Drugs in this class vary in potency, efficacy, and adverse effects. They are classified as agonist or antagonist drugs depending on their ability to bind to the opiate receptor and produce analgesia. The opioid agonist drugs, such as morphine, bind to specific opiate receptors, resulting in analgesia. These agents are commonly used for moderate to severe pain. The opioid antagonist drugs block the effect of morphine at its receptor. Included in this category is a group of drugs with analgesic properties referred to as the mixed agonist-antagonist drugs. These drugs are often used in acute postoperative pain but are of limited use in chronic pain management because they produce psychotomimetic effects with increasing doses. Only pentazocine is available in oral form and only in combination with naloxone, aspirin, and acetaminophen; this preparation precipitates withdrawal in opioid-dependent patients.

Effective use of opioid analgesics requires balancing the desirable effects of pain relief with the undesirable side effects of nausea, vomiting, mental clouding, sedation, tolerance, and physical dependence. These undesirable effects may impose a practical limit on the dose one can give a particular patient. Studies suggest that aggressive treatment of opioid-induced side effects can facilitate dose titration, maximize analgesia, and minimize these effects. Much of the difficulty encountered with the clinical use of opioids arises from individual variation, consisting of differences in response of specific patients to the same drug or dose.

Within general guidelines for the rational use of analgesics in patients with acute and chronic pain (Table 27–2), individualization of drug treatment is the cardinal rule of management. Both the type of pain and its intensity should dictate the drug selection, allowing the physician to start with a specific drug for a specific type of pain. To ensure adequate dosing schedules, one must know the clinical pharmacology of the opioid analgesics, including the relative potency of the drug, the duration of analgesic effect, its half-life, and the equianalgesic dose for both oral and parenteral routes

Table 27–2 ■ GUIDELINES FOR THE USE OF ANALGESICS IN THE MANAGEMENT OF PAIN

1. Start with a specific drug for a specific type of pain.
2. Individualize the choice of drug, dose, timing, and route of administration.
3. Know the pharmacology of the drug prescribed.
   a. Relative potency of the drug
   b. Duration of the analgesic effect
   c. Pharmacokinetics of the drug
   d. Equianalgesic doses of the drug and its route of administration
4. Administer analgesics on a regular basis.
5. Use a combination of drugs to provide additive analgesia.
   a. Opioid plus non-opioid (e.g., aspirin, acetaminophen, and NSAIDs)
   b. Opioids plus adjuvants (e.g., hydroxyzine and dextroamphetamine)
6. Gear the route of administration to the patient's needs:

Oral	Transdermal
Buccal	Subcutaneous
Sublingual	Intravenous
Transmucosal	Intrathecal
Intranasal	Intraventricular
Rectal	

7. Anticipate and treat side effects:

Sedation	Constipation
Respiratory depression	Multifocal myoclonus
Nausea and vomiting	Seizures

8. Know the differences among tolerance, physical dependence, and psychological dependence.
9. Prevent and treat acute withdrawal.
10. Know how to manage the tolerant patient:
    Use combinations of non-opioid and opioid drugs.
    Use combinations of drug therapy, anesthetic, and neurosurgical procedures.
    Switch to an alternative opioid analgesic starting with one fourth to one half the equianalgesic dose and titrate to analgesia.
    Use epidural local anesthetics alone or in combination with opioids.
11. Reassess the nature of the pain.
12. Do not use placebos to assess pain.

of administration (Tables 27–3 and 27–4). For example, the plasma half-lives of the opioids vary widely and do not correlate with their analgesic time course. Both methadone, with a half-life of 15 to 30 hours and levorphanol with a half-life of 12 to 16 hours produce analgesia for 4 to 6 hours. With repeated doses, these drugs accumulate in plasma and can result in excessive sedation and respiratory depression. It is often necessary to adjust the dosing schedule considering both the patient's degree of pain relief and the plasma half-life of the drug. Knowledge of the equianalgesic doses when a switch is made from one route of administration to another prevents undermedication. Medication should be administered on a regular basis with the interval between doses based on the duration of analgesic effect. The pharmacologic objective is to maintain the plasma level of the drug above the "minimal effective concentration" for pain relief. The time required to reach steady-state after repeated administration depends on the half-life of the drug; full assessment of the analgesic efficacy of a drug regimen may take 24 hours for a drug such as morphine, or up to 5 to 7 days for methadone.

Combining drugs enables the physician to improve pain relief without escalating the opioid dose. Several combinations have proven effective, including an opioid plus a non-opioid (aspirin, acetaminophen, or ibuprofen), an opioid plus an amphetamine (dextroamphetamine, 10 mg), and an opioid plus an antihistamine (100 mg of IM hydroxyzine). Drugs such as diazepam and chlorpromazine do not provide additive analgesia and may produce additive sedation. Oral administration of drugs is the most practical route, but the choice must be made according to the patient. Several routes or methods of drug administration have been developed to maximize analgesic effects and minimize the undesirable side effects associated with the standard methods. The approaches that are the most commonly used for managing acute or chronic pain with chronic medical illness include slow-release morphine preparations effective for 8 to 24 hours; rectal, intranasal, sublingual, and transdermal and continuous subcutaneous and intravenous infusions for patients who are unable to tolerate oral analgesics because of gastrointestinal obstruction or malabsorption and in whom repeated parenteral dosing is difficult because of limited muscle mass or a bleeding diathesis; and epidural and intrathecal opioid administration via temporary catheters or implanted pumps. This last approach minimizes the distribution of drug to receptors in the brain stem and cerebral hemispheres, reduces the side effects of systemic administration, and is effective in selected patients with chronic cancer and non-malignant pain who are unable to tolerate the excessive sedation or mental clouding associated with an oral or parenteral route.

Patient-controlled analgesia (PCA) is a useful approach to treat both acute pain associated with medical illness (postoperative pain, sickle cell pain) and chronic cancer-related pain. Parenteral infusions (intravenous or subcutaneous) of opioids can be self-administered by the patient using specially designed computerized pumps that can be set to deliver specific amounts of drug on demand or by continuous infusion. These devices allow patients to control their own pain management. Studies demonstrate that patients using PCA use less medication than patients who receive PRN medications for postoperative or chronic pain.

Side effects of the opioid analgesics should be anticipated and treated. Sedation and drowsiness vary with the drug, the dosage, and the route of administration. Useful approaches to counteract the sedative effects include reducing the individual dose and prescribing it more frequently; using dextroamphetamine (2.5 to 10 mg) or methylphenidate (5 to 15 mg) in combination with the morning opioid dose; switching to a different opioid—from morphine to hydromorphone or methadone; and discontinuing all other sedative drugs.

Respiratory depression is the most serious adverse effect, but tolerance develops rapidly, allowing for prolonged use and dose escalation for chronic pain. If respiratory depression occurs, it can be reversed by administering the specific opioid antagonist, nalox-

Table 27–3 ■ ORAL NON-OPIOID ANALGESIC DRUGS

DRUG	INDICATIONS	EQUIANALGESIC DOSE	STARTING DOSE (mg/24 HR)	COMMENTS
Aspirin	Often used in combination with opioids	650	650	Contraindicated in hepatic and renal dysfunction; avoid during pregnancy, in hemolytic disorders, and, if possible, in combination with steroids
Choline magnesium trisalicylate	Like aspirin	ND	750–1500	Minimal impact on platelet function
Acetaminophen	Like aspirin	650	650	
Ibuprofen	Higher analgesic potential than aspirin	ND	200–400	Like aspirin
Fenoprofen	Like ibuprofen	ND	200–400	Like aspirin
Diflunisal	Longer duration of action than ibuprofen; higher analgesic potential than aspirin	ND	500–1000	Like aspirin
Naproxen	Like diflunisal	ND	250–1500	Like aspirin

ND = Analgesic relative potency studies are not available to determine equianalgesic dose to aspirin.

Table 27–4 ■ OPIOID ANALGESIC DRUGS

CLASS	DRUG	INDICATIONS	EQUIANALGESIC DOSE	STARTING DOSE (mg/24 HR)	COMMENTS
Morphine-like agonist, mild to moderate pain	Codeine	Often used in combination with non-opioid analgesics	32–65*	32–65	Commonly used as first drug
	Oxycodone	Shorter acting; combination with non-opioid analgesics limits dose escalation	5*	5–10	Fewer side effects than codeine, available alone or in combination with aspirin and acetaminophen
	Meperidine	Shorter acting; biotransformed to normeperidine, a toxic metabolite	50*	50–100	Normeperidine accumulates with repetitive dosing, causing CNS excitation; not for use in patients with renal dysfunction or receiving monoamine oxidase inhibitors
	Propoxyphene hydrochloride (Darvon)	Used in combination with non-opioid analgesics; long half-life; biotransformed to potentially toxic metabolite (norpropoxyphene)	65–130*	65–130	Propoxyphene and metabolite accumulate with repetitive dosing; overdose complicated by convulsions
Mixed agonist/antagonist	Pentazocine	Used in combination with non-opioids	50*	50–100	May cause psychotomimetic effects; may precipitate withdrawal in opioid-dependent patients. Oral combination with naloxone to discourage parenteral abuse
	Butorphanol (Stadol)	Used in combination with non-opioids	2*	2–4	May cause psychotomimetic effects; may precipitate withdrawal in opioid-dependent patients; only available in intranasal and intramuscular preparations
Morphine-like agonists, moderate to severe pain	Morphine MSIR MS Contin Roxanol Kadian	Used for chronic pain, available in oral liquid, tablets, slow-release preparations, and rectal and parenteral routes	10–60†	30–60	Standard of comparison for opioid-type analgesics; morphine-6-glucuronide, active metabolite, accumulates in renal failure
	Hydromorphone (Dilaudid)	Like morphine	1.5–8.0†	4–8	Slightly shorter acting, high-potency IM dosage form available for tolerant patients
	Methadone (Dolophine)	Like morphine; may accumulate with repetitive dosing, causing excessive sedation	10–20†	10–20	Good oral potency; long plasma half-life (15–30 hr)
	Levorphanol (Levo-Dromoran)	Like methadone	2–4†	2–4	Long plasma half-life (12–16 hr)
	Fentanyl (Duragesic)	Like morphine, but available in a transdermal preparation applied every 3 days	NA	25–100 µg TD	Useful in patients who are unable to take drugs orally and require continuous opioid dosing
	Oxycodone (OxyContin)	Like morphine	15/30†	5–10	Available in immediate-release and slow-release tablets
	Oxymorphone	Like morphine, less histamine effect	1/10 PR	10 PR	Rectal and parenteral preparations only

*Equianalgesic doses for mild to moderate pain compared with 650-mg aspirin.
†Equianalgesic doses by IM/oral routes for severe pain compared with 10 mg IM morphine standard.
IM = Intramuscular; CNS = central nervous system; PR = per rectum; TD = transdermal.

one in a dose of 0.4 mg/ml. In patients who are receiving chronic opioids for pain and who develop respiratory depression, diluted doses of naloxone (0.4 mg in 10 mL of saline) should be infused slowly to reverse the respiratory depression and to prevent severe withdrawal symptoms and recurrence of pain.

Opioids have emetic properties. The occurrence of nausea and vomiting with one drug does not mean that all produce similar symptoms. Changing to a different opioid or using an antiemetic in combination can obviate this effect. Tolerance rapidly develops to the emetic effects of opioids so that after several days antiemetics often can be discontinued. Constipation should be prevented by providing a regular bowel regimen including cathartics, stool softeners, and careful attention to diet. Opioids can produce multifocal myoclonus. The most common offender is meperidine because its active metabolic, normeperidine, accumulates and can cause seizures. Because the half-life of the normeperidine is 16 hours, it may take several days for toxic side effects to clear. Multifocal myoclonus occurs more commonly in patients with renal dysfunc-

tion receiving the meperidine. Such patients should be switched to alternative drugs such as fentanyl or methadone, which are not predominantly cleared by the kidney. Morphine has an active metabolite that accumulates in renal dysfunction and has been reported to play a role in its side effects. To prevent withdrawal, patients should be slowly tapered off their opioids; 25% of the total daily opioid dose prevents the development of abstinence symptoms. Tolerance is common in patients receiving opioid analgesics chronically for pain. The earliest sign is the decrease in the duration of effective analgesia. For reasons not well understood, the rate of tolerance development varies greatly among patients with pain. Increased opioid requirements are most commonly associated with disease progression rather than tolerance alone. With the development of tolerance, increases in the frequency or the dose of the opioid are required to provide continued pain relief. Because the analgesic effect is a logarithmic function of the dose of the opioid, doubling of the dose may be needed to restore full analgesia. There appears to be no limit to the development of tolerance; and with appropriate dose adjustments, patients can continue to obtain pain relief. Cross-tolerance among the opioid analgesics is not complete, therefore, changing to an alternative opioid at a starting dose of one fourth to one half of the predicted equianalgesic dose may be advantageous.

Tolerance is distinct from physical dependence, which is characterized by the appearance of withdrawal signs after drugs are abruptly discontinued, and from psychological dependence, which is epitomized by a concomitant behavioral pattern of drug abuse characterized by craving a drug for other than pain relief and overwhelming involvement in its procurement and use. The profound fear of causing psychological dependence plays a major role in physicians' reluctance to prescribe opioid analgesics, particularly in patients with non-malignant pain and in patients with cancer in the early phases of their disease. From the available data based on studies on the chronic use of opioids in patients with cancer, few patients develop psychological dependence on the drug. This issue is controversial in management of patients with chronic non-malignant pain, but data indicate that such patients can be treated effectively with chronic opioid therapy. Guidelines for the use of chronic opioid therapy in non-malignant pain have been developed (Table 27–5).

ADJUVANT ANALGESICS. Some drugs increase the analgesic effects of the opioids, counteract their side effects, or act as analgesics themselves. Clear evidence suggests the analgesic efficacy of carbamazepine, baclofen, and pimozide in trigeminal neuralgia and of the tricyclic antidepressants in neuropathic pain. Similarly, several psychostimulants are effective in counteracting opioid-induced sedation (dextroamphetamine and methylphenidate) and in improving analgesia (dextroamphetamine and caffeine). For the other drugs in this group, anecdotal or survey data suggest their usefulness in various types of neuropathic pain (Table 27–6), and the physician must consider the risks and benefits of polypharmacy when trying to provide analgesia for patients with difficult and complex pain syndromes. Certain phenothiazines also have potent analgesic effects. Methotrimeprazine (Levoprome) has an analgesic potential close to that of morphine (15 mg IM is equivalent to 10 mg IM morphine). This drug also has sedative and antiemetic properties again useful for severe pain in patients tolerant to opioid analgesics. In treating neuropathic pain, the tricyclic antidepressants are efficacious. For lancinating neuropathic pains, not only carbamazepine and phenytoin but valproate and gabapentin have been reported to be effective. Mexiletine, an oral local anesthetic, demonstrates analgesic properties in patients with painful diabetic neuropathy. Corticosteroids have been reported to be useful as general purpose adjuvant analgesics. They ameliorate pain in patients with bone metastases and produce beneficial effects on appetite, nausea, mood, and fatigue. They have most commonly been used in patients with breast or prostate cancer to improve quality of life.

Specific adjuvants used in managing cancer pain have specialized effects (e.g., bisphosphonates) in malignant bone pain. The physician should become familiar with this class of compounds and consider their use in sequential trials to improve patients' quality of life and functional status.

ALTERNATE METHODS OF PAIN CONTROL. A variety of non-pharmacologic therapeutic approaches can be used alone or in combination with analgesic drugs. These include physical therapy, trigger point injections, transcutaneous nerve stimulation, and a variety of behavioral approaches—all of which should be familiar to general physicians. Pain experts should be consulted before using anesthetic and neurosurgical approaches.

PHYSICAL THERAPY. Chronic pain is commonly associated with reduced physical activity and splinting or immobilization of the injured body part. A graded exercise program with appropriate use of splints and braces and reactivation of the injured part plays a pivotal role in re-establishing the functional status of the patient. Local rubbing and transcutaneous electrical stimulation for "counterirritation" may help to mobilize the patient with localized pain. Trigger point injections with either saline or a local anesthetic provide dramatic relief of painful muscle spasm.

COGNITIVE BEHAVIORAL THERAPY. Cognitive behavioral interventions including coping skills and modification of thoughts, feelings, and behaviors can help reduce the perception of distress caused by pain. Some patients may be able to use relaxation tech-

Table 27–5 ■ GUIDELINES FOR MANAGING CHRONIC OPIOID THERAPY FOR NON-MALIGNANT PAIN

1. Opioid therapy should be considered only after all other reasonable attempts at analgesia have failed.
2. A history of substance abuse, severe character pathology, and chaotic home environment should be viewed as relative contraindications.
3. A single practitioner should take primary responsibility for treatment.
4. Patients should give informed consent before the start of therapy; points to be covered include recognition of the low risk of true addiction as an outcome, potential for cognitive impairment with the drug alone and in combination with sedative/hypnotics, likelihood that physical dependence will occur (abstinence syndrome possible with acute discontinuation), and understanding by female patients that children born when the mother is on opioid maintenance therapy will likely be physically dependent at birth.
5. After drug selection, doses should be given around the clock; several weeks should be agreed on as the period of initial dose titration; and although improvement in function should be continually stressed, all should agree to at least partial analgesia as the appropriate goal of therapy.
6. Failure to achieve at least partial analgesia at relatively low initial doses in the non-tolerant patient raises questions about the potential treatability of the pain syndrome with opioids.
7. Emphasis should be given to attempts to capitalize on improved analgesia by gains in physical and social function; opioid therapy should be considered complementary to other analgesic and rehabilitative approaches.
8. In addition to the daily dose determined initially, patients should be permitted to escalate dose transiently on days of increased pain; two methods are acceptable: (a) prescription of an additional 4 to 6 "rescue doses" to be taken as needed during the month; (b) instruction that one or two extra doses may be taken on any day but must be followed by an equal reduction of dose on subsequent days.
9. Initially, patients must be seen and drugs prescribed at least monthly. When stable, less frequent visits may be acceptable.
10. Exacerbations of pain not effectively treated by transient, small increases in dose are best managed in the hospital, where dose escalation, if appropriate, can be observed closely and a return to baseline doses can be accomplished in a controlled environment.
11. Evidence of drug hoarding, acquisition of drugs from other physicians, uncontrolled dose escalation, or other aberrant behaviors must be carefully assessed. In some cases, tapering and discontinuing opioid therapy are necessary. Other patients may appropriately continue therapy within rigid guidelines. Consideration should be given to consulting with an addiction specialist.
12. At each visit, assessment should specifically address:
    a. Comfort (degree of analgesia)
    b. Opioid-related side effects
    c. Functional status (physical and psychosocial)
    d. Existence of aberrant drug-related behaviors
13. Use of self-report instruments may be helpful but should not be required.
14. Documentation is essential and the medical record should specifically address comfort, function, side effects, and the occurrence of aberrant behaviors repeatedly during the course of therapy.

From Portenoy RK: Opioid therapy for chronic nonmalignant pain: Current status. *In* Fields HL, Liebeskind JC (eds): Progress in Pain Research and Management, vol 1. Seattle, IASP Press, 1994, p 247.

niques to reduce muscular tension and emotional arousal or to enhance pain tolerance. Other approaches, including meditation, imagery, music therapy, and biofeedback can reduce participatory anxiety that may lead to avoidance behaviors. Successful use of these therapies requires a cognitively intact patient and a health care professional skilled in their application.

ANESTHETIC AND NEUROSURGICAL APPROACHES. These approaches are most effective in treating patients with well-defined pain. Several factors are important in selecting an appropriate procedure for each patient. The role of these approaches is limited because diffuse pain problems rather than focal ones are the most common. Their use is limited by the number of professionals who have expertise in the performance of these procedures. Many of these procedures are most useful in patients with a limited lifespan; yet such patients often consider their pain to be an important marker for their disease and are frightened by the potential, although unlikely complications of these procedures. As a result, these procedures are often performed late in the course of the illness, and full evaluation of their effectiveness and duration of action is limited by the patient's overriding medical problems. These procedures are often not very effective in managing neuro-

Table 27–6 ■ ADJUVANT ANALGESIC DRUGS

CLASS	DRUG	INDICATIONS	STARTING DOSE (mg) RANGE/24 HR	COMMENTS
Anticonvulsants	Phenytoin	Neuropathic pain, acute lancinating type	100, 100–300	Use in paroxysmal nerve pain
	Carbamazepine	Acute lancinating type	100, 200–800	Use in paroxysmal nerve pain; start with low doses; titrate slowly
	Valproate	Neuropathic pain; acute lancinating type	125, 1000–3000	Anecdotal reports of efficacy in neuropathic pain
	Gabapentin	Neuropathic pain	300, 300–1200	Controlled studies report efficacy in neuropathic pain
Antidepressants	Amitriptyline, nortriptyline, desipramine, paroxetine*	Neuropathic pain (e.g., postherpetic neuralgia)	10, 25–>150 10–>40*	Start at low dose and titrate slowly; have analgesic properties
Stimulants	Dextroamphetamine	Somatic and visceral postoperative pain and chronic pain	2.5, 5–10	Additive analgesia in combination with opioids; reduces sedative effects
	Methylphenidate		5, 5–15	
	Caffeine	Counteracts opioid-induced sedation	200, 200–400	
Antihistamines	Hydroxyzine	Somatic and visceral pain	25, 25–100	Additive analgesia in combination with opioids; antiemetic, antianxiety properties
Phenothiazine	Methotrimeprazine	Somatic and visceral pain; useful in opioid-tolerant patients with gastrointestinal obstruction and pain	5 IM 5–20 IM	Has antianxiety and antiemetic effects; available only in IM preparation
Steroids	Prednisone	Somatic and neuropathic pain (e.g., inflammatory pain, reflex sympathetic dystrophy)	5, 5–60	Anti-inflammatory, antiemetic, analgesic effects
	Dexamethasone	Somatic and neuropathic pain (e.g., inflammatory pain, reflex sympathetic dystrophy)	0.5, 0.5–16	
Miscellaneous	Baclofen	Paroxysmal pain of trigeminal neuralgia and central pain states	10, 10–80	May be used with carbamazepine in trigeminal neuralgia
	Pimozide	Refractory trigeminal neuralgia	2, 4–12	Adverse effects include acute dystonia and akathesias
	Mexiletine	Neuropathic pain; useful in diabetic neuropathy	150, 150–600	Dose-response studies have not been done
	Clonidine	Neuropathic pain; intrathecal and transdermal use	0.1–1	Additive analgesia to opioid by intrathecal route

*Refers to dose range for paroxetine.

pathic pain except for the use of local anesthetics. They are most helpful in managing somatic and visceral pain. One approach uses nitrous oxide for patients with far-advanced disease to provide additive analgesia. Nitrous oxide, administered with oxygen through a non-rebreathing facemask in concentrations from 25 to 75% has been demonstrated to be useful when combined with systemic opioid analgesics to control pain and anxiety in patients with advanced disease and pain. Similarly, intravenous barbiturates to manage dying patients who have inadequate analgesia or uncontrollable symptoms and who request that they be maintained in a sedated state represents another type of anesthetic approach.

A series of anecdotal reports and controlled studies support the use of intravenous, subcutaneous, transdermal, intrapleural, and epidural local anesthetics in managing patients with somatic, visceral, and neuropathic pain. Intravenous lidocaine represents both a diagnostic and a therapeutic treatment in patients with neuropathic pain. If such patients obtain an analgesic response, a trial of oral mexiletine or the use of continuous subcutaneous lidocaine may be considered. Transdermal lidocaine in a 2%, 5%, and 10% ointment has been reported to be useful in patients with superficial hyperesthesia, dysesthesias, and significant allodynia. Spreading the ointment on the painful site can often provide transient pain relief. This effect has been best demonstrated in patients with postherpetic neuralgia. Intrapleural local anesthetics are useful for acute pain in the chest wall and have been adapted for managing chronic cancer pain. Intermittent and continuous epidural infusions of local anesthetics are useful to manage difficult chronic pain associated with metastatic disease below the waist, often involving the sacrum and lumbosacral plexus. The use of continuous low-dose infusions of local anesthetics is associated with minimal systemic side effects.

Peripheral nerve blocks are used both diagnostically to localize the nerve distribution and therapeutically to interrupt pain transmission within a determined nerve distribution. This technique is limited to areas of the body in which interruption of both motor and sensory function does not interfere with the patient's functional status. This approach, therefore, is most commonly used in patients who have pain in the head, chest, or abdomen. These techniques are most useful in patients with somatic pain; neuropathic pain is rarely controlled by peripheral nerve blocks alone. Examples of successful blocks include gasserian ganglionic blocks for craniofacial pain, intercostal blocks for chest wall pain, and paravertebral blocks for radicular pain. In patients with somatic pain who respond to a local anesthetic block, neurolytic blockade with either alcohol or phenol may provide more prolonged relief. A block produced by phenol tends to be less profound and of shorter duration than one produced by alcohol. Epidural and intrathecal neurolytic blocks are used primarily to manage patients with far-advanced disease whose pain is either unilateral in the chest or abdomen or midline in the perineum. These blocks are less useful in managing upper and lower limb pain associated with brachial and lumbosacral plexopathy because of the high risk of motor weakness associated with effective neurolytic blockade by this route. Patients should be selected for management with epidural or intrathecal agents on the basis of the following criteria: exhaustion of appropriate antitumor approaches; clear clinical and radiologic definition of the pain; poor candidacy for percutaneous cordotomy; failure of opioid, non-opioid, and adjuvants to produce adequate analgesia without significant side effects: and at least 75% pain relief in response to diagnostic epidural or intrathecal blocks.

The neurosurgical approaches include neuroablative, neurostimulatory, and neuropharmacologic approaches. Neuroablative procedures involve producing a surgical or radiofrequency lesion along the nociceptive neural pathway. Sectioning the posterior roots (rhizotomy), producing a lesion in the lateral dorsal horn (dorsal root entry zone lesion), and interrupting the ascending spinothalamic pathway (cordotomy) are examples of neuroablative procedures performed for pain relief. Cordotomy, either percutaneous or open, is the most common neuroablative procedure used to manage chronic pain, most commonly associated with cancer. It is the procedure of choice for patients with unilateral pain below the waist who have a relatively short life expectancy. Cordotomy is usually effective for 1 to 3 years with dysesthesias substituting for analgesia in patients living longer than 3 years. Pain in the chest wall or upper extremity may be successfully treated initially with cordotomy, but extensive data demonstrate that with time, the level of analgesia drops, limiting the effectiveness of this approach. Somatic pain appears to be most responsive to cordotomy; visceral and neuropathic pain are less responsive for reasons that are not fully understood. Percutaneous cordotomy can be performed in a supine, awake patient through a lateral C1-C2 approach. Such a lesion interrupts pain and temperature on the contralateral side of the lesioned site. Patients typically report spontaneous relief of pain in this lesioned area. Pain relief can be obtained in 60 to 80% of patients immediately after cordotomy; results at 6 to 12 months are 40 to 50%. Dorsal rhizotomy is the next most common neuroablative procedure used; it is performed by sectioning the posterior sensory rootlets, and a specific localized dermatomal pain level can be identified. It can be performed by an operative section of the nerve or by a neurolytic block. This procedure is commonly used in patients with chest wall pain from tumor invasion and results in improved analgesia in 50 to 80% of patients treated.

Other neuroablative procedures rarely used to manage patients with chronic pain include dorsal root entry zone lesions, myelotomy, and cingulotomy. Neurostimulatory procedures involving the peripheral nerve and spinal cord are generally based on the gate therapy of pain. Various percutaneous electrical nerve stimulators are available to treat chronic neuropathic pain. These devices deliver various patterns of electrical stimulation and take the form of either transcutaneous electrical nerve stimulation or implanted devices producing nerve stimulation. Controversy exists about the usefulness of these techniques. The dorsal column–stimulating technique involves introducing an electrode into the epidural or intrathecal space and advancing it to the appropriate level overlying the dorsal columns. Once in place, the electrode is implanted subcutaneously, and an external transmitting electrode is placed over the receiving electrode and connected to a transmitter. The main indications for placing a dorsal column stimulator are intractable dysesthetic or deafferentation pain of the limbs or trunk. This procedure is effective in 43 to 75% of patients and carries a low morbidity rate. Its most common complication is failure of the device itself, which occurs in up to 10% of patients. Placing stimulating electrodes in the medial thalamus has also been reported to be useful for managing neuropathic pain from injury to the central and peripheral nervous systems. These anesthetic and neurosurgical approaches are most commonly performed by a pain expert in referral centers. They should be reserved for patients who have failed other pain management approaches and to whom the risks and benefits have been carefully explained.

MANAGEMENT OF CANCER PAIN

The management of cancer pain attempts to integrate assessment techniques, drug therapy, and anesthetic, neurosurgical, and behavioral approaches as well as to stress continuity of care (Fig. 27–1). Treatment of cancer pain must begin with a careful diagnostic assessment that addresses not only the medical nature of pain, but also its psychological and social components. At the time of assessment, a plan is developed to treat both the cancer, if possible, and the pain itself. If the anticancer treatment is effective, pain relief usually occurs, and the drugs used for analgesia can be discontinued without difficulty. Pain relief begins with analgesic drugs moving from non-opioid drugs alone or in combination with adjuvant drugs, through weak opioids to strong opioids. If pain relief is achieved with this program, no further therapy is necessary. In patients with severe, persistent pain unresponsive to analgesic drugs or in whom the side effects of the drugs are not tolerated, physicians should first try switching to an alternate analgesic. If the pain is unresponsive to analgesic drugs and is localized (e.g., intercostal pain from tumor infiltration of the chest wall), neurolytic blocks are indicated. If the pain is unilateral and below the waist, cordotomy should be considered. For more diffuse pain unresponsive to analgesics, neuropharmacologic procedures, including nitrous oxide inhalation, may be considered. Behavioral approaches, which include relaxation techniques, breathing exercises, and cognitive control of pain, serve as adjuvants and should be integrated into the management of patients with chronic pain. Whatever techniques of pain management are used in patients with cancer, the physician is

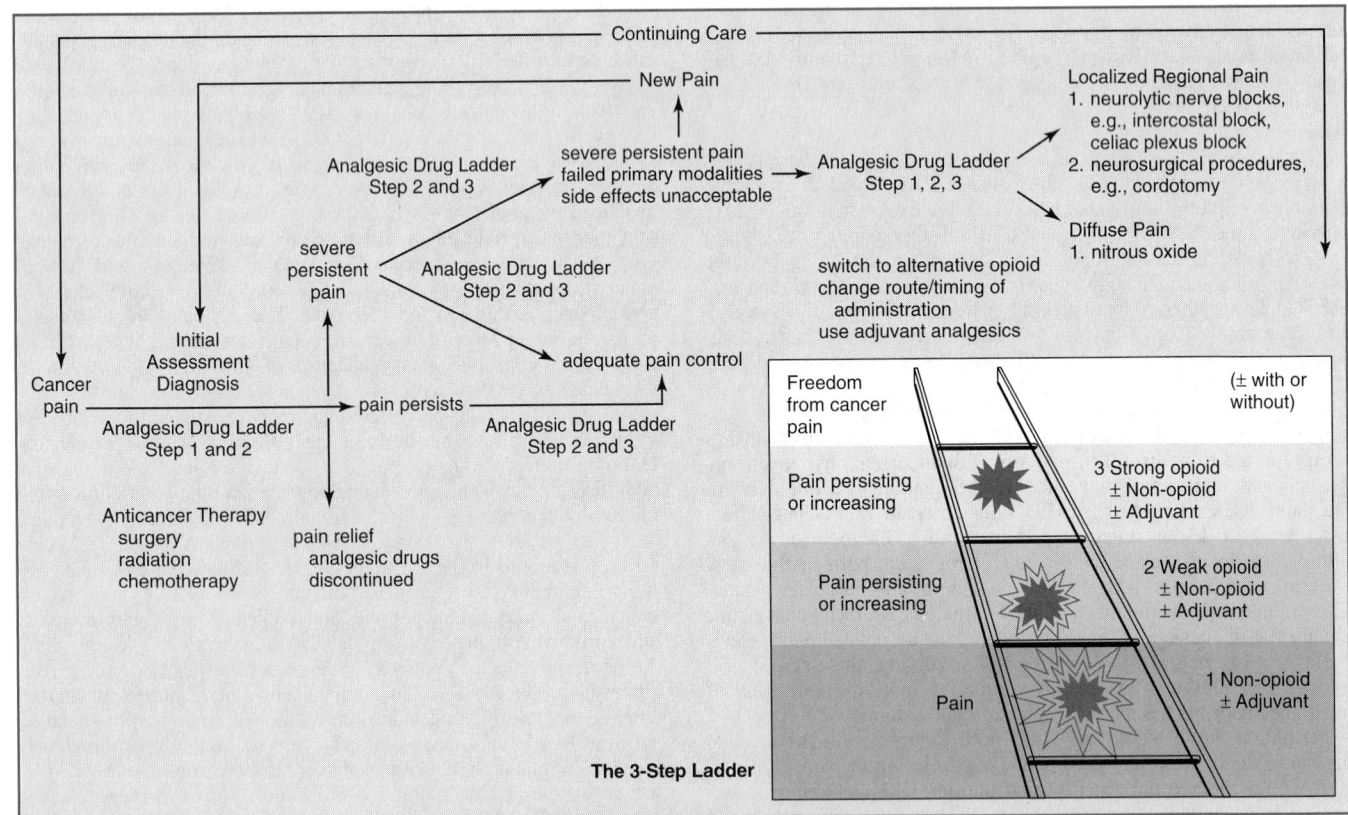

FIGURE 27–1 ■ Algorithm for the management of cancer pain.

responsible for delivering continuing care, constantly reassessing both the diagnosis and the treatment to achieve optimal relief of pain and suffering for both the patient and the family.

Doyle D, Hanks GWC, MacDonald N: Oxford Textbook of Palliative Medicine, 2nd ed. London, Oxford University Press, 1998. *An excellent compendium of pain assessment and analgesic pharmacotherapy of pain.*

Foley KM, Cherny NI: Guidelines for the care of the dying. Hematol Oncol Clin North Am 10(1):261–286, 1996. *This monograph addresses pain assessment and treatment of cancer pain.*

Jacox A, Carr DB, Payne R, et al: Management of Cancer Pain. Clinical Practice Guideline No. 9. AHCPR Publication No. 94-0592. Rockville, MD, Agency for Health Care Policy and Research, US Department of Health and Human Services, Public Health Service, March 1994. *A concise summary of the appropriate treatment of cancer pain.*

Portenoy RK, Kanner RM: Pain Management Theory and Practice. Philadelphia, FA Davis, 1996. *A comprehensive review of common neurologic pain syndromes and their therapy.*

28   GLUCOCORTICOSTEROIDS IN RELATION TO INFLAMMATORY DISEASE

Paul Katz

For more than 50 years, glucocorticosteroids have been extremely important agents in treating diseases characterized by inflammation and exaggerated immune responses. The pioneering work of Hench and colleagues in rheumatoid arthritis demonstrated the possible potency of these agents in such pathologic states. Although substantial advances have been made in our understanding of the mechanisms by which glucocorticosteroids exert beneficial effects, considerable gaps in our knowledge remain. Despite extensive data regarding the *in vitro* and *in vivo* activities of these drugs, it is probable that glucocorticosteroids have different beneficial activities in different diseases.

The challenge of glucocorticosteroid therapy continues to be the counterbalancing of desirable anti-inflammatory and immunosuppressive actions versus undesirable pharmacologic activities. Regrettably, more precise understanding of the mechanisms of action of glucocorticosteroids has not resulted in the development of regimens with minimal toxicity.

PHARMACOLOGY

The variety of glucocorticosteroid preparations available for systemic use (Table 28–1) differ in their relative anti-inflammatory potency, potential for sodium retention, and plasma and biologic half-lives. In general, shorter-acting preparations such as prednisone and prednisolone are preferable to longer-acting agents such as dexamethasone because tapering to an alternate-day schedule cannot be accomplished with drugs with prolonged (i.e., >24 hours) biologic half-lives. Additionally, hydrocortisone and cortisone are rarely used to treat inflammatory and immunologically mediated diseases because of the considerable mineralocorticoid activity that accompanies their use.

MECHANISMS OF ACTION

Glucocorticosteroids exert anti-inflammatory and immunosuppressive actions through several pathways. Nonetheless, all effects are mediated by changes in the circulatory kinetics of leukocytes, alterations in the function of inflammatory cells, and modification of soluble mediators (Table 28–2).

Regardless of which of the these mechanisms is examined, the initial subcellular events are initiated by glucocorticosteroid binding to cytoplasmic receptors that are reasonably comparable though heterogeneous among different leukocytes. The 800-amino acid receptor consists of three domains that differ in function: a hormone or ligand-binding carboxyl terminal region, a DNA-binding domain, and an amino terminal immunogenic area. After glucocorticosteroid-receptor interaction, the complex traverses nuclear pores, binds to DNA at specific sites, leads to changes in the transcription rates of glucocorticosteroid-sensitive genes, and results in regulation of the synthesis of those proteins participating in the inflammatory response.

EFFECTS ON LEUKOCYTE CIRCULATORY KINETICS. The profound but transient effects of glucocorticosteroids on leukocyte trafficking differ depending on cell type. Irrespective of white blood cell type and regardless of duration of therapy or dosing interval, these effects are maximal at 4 to 6 hours after administration. In part, these effects derive from glucocorticosteroid action on vascular endothelial cells, including alterations in the expression of adhesion molecules, changes in cytokine secretion, and decreased expression of major histocompatibility complex (MHC) class II antigens (see Chapter 278).

A significant neutrophilia is observed 4 to 6 hours after glucocorticosteroids because neutrophils have an increased intravascular half-life, increased bone marrow release, and decreased egress from the circulation to extravascular sites of inflammation. By 24 hours, the neutrophilia resolves unless further doses are given. Although glucocorticosteroids induce a transient increase in circulating neutrophils, these cells have a decreased ability to migrate to extravascular sites.

Neutrophilia (see Chapter 172) is accompanied by lymphopenia because of the temporary migration of selected lymphocytes to bone marrow and spleen. A significant T lymphocytopenia occurs with a selective egress from the circulation of CD4+ "helper-inducer" T cells, whereas CD8+ "cytotoxic-suppressor" T cells are relatively resistant to these effects (see Chapter 270). B lymphocytes are less susceptible to glucocorticosteroid-induced effects than T cells, with little alteration in intravascular number or composition. Natural killer cells, identified by CD16 expression, are similarly resistant. Monocytes, however, migrate to extravascular locales within the time frame of other glucocorticosteroid-associated changes. Eosinophils and basophils transiently exit the circulation, although the exact sites of migration are unknown; eosinophils are, however, reduced at areas characterized by immediate hypersensitivity reactions.

These glucocorticosteroid-induced transient changes in the intravascular leukocyte pool occur regardless of dosing intervals or duration of therapy. These effects mitigate the ability of inflammatory cells to participate in inflammatory and immunologically mediated reactions, thereby inducing a favorable effect, but also diminish leukocyte participation in eliminating microbial invaders.

Table 28–1 ■ GLUCOCORTICOSTEROID PREPARATIONS

	ANTI-INFLAMMATORY POTENCY	EQUIVALENT DOSE (mg)	SODIUM-RETAINING POTENCY	PLASMA HALF-LIFE (min)	BIOLOGIC HALF-LIFE (h)
Hydrocortisone	1	20	2+	90	8–12
Cortisone	0.8	25	2+	30	8–12
Prednisone	4	5	1+	60	12–36
Prednisolone	4	5	1+	200	12–36
Methylprednisolone	5	4	0	180	12–36
Triamcinolone	5	4	0	300	12–36
Betamethasone	20–30	0.6	0	100–300	36–54
Dexamethasone	20–30	0.75	0	100–300	36–54

From Garber EK, Targoff C, Paulus HE: *In* Paulus HE, Furst DE, Droomgoole SH (eds): Drugs for Rheumatic Diseases. New York, Churchill Livingstone, 1987, p 446.

Table 28–2 ■ EFFECT OF GLUCOCORTICOSTEROIDS ON INFLAMMATORY AND IMMUNE RESPONSES

Effects on Leukocyte Circulatory Kinetics (transient and maximal 4 to 6 hours after administration)
1. Neutrophilia
2. Monocytopenia
3. Lymphocytopenia—selective depletion of CD4+ T cells
4. Eosinopenia
5. Basophilopenia

Effects on Leukocyte Function
1. Neutrophils: Little effect on chemotaxis, phagocytosis, and killing
2. Monocytes: Suppression of chemotaxis, cidal activity, and surface receptor expression
3. Eosinophils: Decreased chemotaxis and killing
4. T lymphocytes: Cutaneous anergy; suppression of activation, proliferation, and differentiation; reduced cytotoxic (CD8) responses
5. B lymphocytes: Reduction in serum immunoglobulins; no effect on response to injected antigens; decreased activation and proliferation
6. Natural killer cells: No effect on cytotoxic activity

Effects on Soluble Mediators
1. Decreased production of prostaglandins, histamine, and leukotrienes
2. Decreased production of IL-1, IL-2, interferon-γ, and tumor necrosis factor-α
3. Little effect on complement
4. Decreased clearance of antigen-antibody complexes from circulation

CHANGES IN LEUKOCYTE FUNCTION. Just as leukocytes vary in responsiveness to glucocorticosteroid-induced circulatory changes, similar variability is observed in their intrinsic functional capabilities. Although neutrophils are quite sensitive to changes in trafficking after glucocorticosteroid administration, these cells are relatively refractory to glucocorticosteroid-associated changes in function. Thus, chemotaxis, lysosomal enzyme release, and killing are either resistant to glucocorticosteroid effects or affected only with high doses. Conversely, cells of the monocyte-macrophage series are functionally sensitive to glucocorticosteroid effects with reduced chemotaxis, killing activity, and surface receptor expression of class II antigens, Fc receptors, and receptors for the third component of complement (C3). Eosinophil chemotactic and cytotoxic functions are also reduced by glucocorticosteroids.

A variety of lymphocyte functions, including activation, proliferation, and differentiation, are sensitive to glucocorticosteroids. Although glucocorticosteroids do not affect T-cell activation, down-regulation of RNA synthesis decreases proliferation, which can be reversed *in vitro* with exogenous interleukin (IL)-2. Mitogen- and antigen-induced proliferative responses are reduced *in vitro*; the *in vivo* counterpart of these responses, cutaneous delayed-type hypersensitivity, is similarly impaired within 2 weeks of starting drug therapy. Similar effects on the mixed lymphocyte reaction occur and may in part explain the utility of glucocorticosteroids in reversing allograft rejection. Cytotoxic T-cell (CD8+) responses are depressed by in vivo glucocorticosteroids.

Unlike T cells, B-lymphocyte function is only modestly affected by glucocorticosteroid therapy. Within 1 month of glucocorticosteroid therapy, reduction in serum immunoglobulins is noted because of increased catabolism. Antibody responses to injected antigens are not impaired. In vitro, glucocorticosteroids suppress B-cell activation with abrogation of cell enlargement, expression of activation antigens, and responses to B-cell activators. Once *in vitro* activation and proliferation have occurred, immunoglobulin and antibody production are unaffected by glucocorticosteroids. The cytotoxic activities of natural killer cells are resistant to *in vitro* and *in vivo* glucocorticosteroids.

EFFECTS ON SOLUBLE MEDIATORS. Glucocorticosteroids may mediate some of the aforementioned activities by affecting soluble mediators. Prostaglandins arise from arachidonic acid after the action of phospholipase A₂ (PLA_2) on phospholipids. Glucocorticosteroids block prostaglandin production through effects on the inhibitors of PLA_2, called lipocortins, or directly on enzyme production. Additionally, transcription of the enzyme cyclooxygenase, which catalyzes the metabolism of arachidonic acid to prostaglandins, may also be blocked by glucocorticosteroids (see Chapter 29). IL-1, interferon-gamma, IL-6, and tumor necrosis factor-α pro-

duction and/or release are suppressed by glucocorticosteroids. However, other monocyte-derived cytokines, such as migration inhibitory factor, are unaffected by glucocorticosteroids. Substantial effects on the T cell–derived cytokine IL-2 are observed. Glucocorticosteroids inhibit IL-2 synthesis, likely through effects on gene expression by suppressing RNA transcription, translation, and degradation, resulting in decreased production of this cytokine. Additionally, glucocorticosteroids block IL-2–directed protein phosphorylation as well as the release of other T cell–derived mediators.

Basophil-derived histamine and leukotriene secretion are abrogated by glucocorticosteroids. In general, complement metabolism is clinically unaffected, although these drugs may have some effects on release of C3 and factor B. Glucocorticosteroids inhibit the production of a variety of fibroblast-derived mediators, including prostaglandins, glycosoaminoglycans, and IL-1. These effects may be clinically relevant in the inflammatory arthritides. The clearance of antigen-antibody (i.e., immune) complexes from the circulation is decreased by glucocorticosteroids; this effect, which may be important in the therapy for autoimmune diseases, appears to be mediated by down-regulation of reticuloendothelial Fc receptor activity.

CLINICAL USE OF GLUCOCORTICOSTEROIDS

GENERAL PRINCIPLES OF THERAPY. The decision to implement therapy with glucocorticosteroids must be derived from a precise understanding of these agents and the often formidable adverse reactions that accompany their use. These drugs have important roles in treating entities such as hypoadrenalism (see Chapter 240) and malignancy (see Chapter 198), in which the replacement is physiologic or aimed at a life-threatening disease. For inflammatory and immunologically related disorders, however, it is incumbent on the treating physician to determine that glucocorticosteroids are the appropriate form of treatment and that other nonglucocorticosteroid approaches are unlikely to be equally beneficial. When glucocorticosteroid treatment becomes desirable, if not mandatory, efforts must focus on minimizing glucocorticosteroid side effects while maintaining therapeutic efficacy. Generally, these goals can be at least partially attained by using short-acting glucocorticosteroid medications at the lowest possible dose and the greatest dosing interval for the shortest period of time.

SYSTEMIC GLUCOCORTICOSTEROID THERAPY. INITIATING AND TAPERING THERAPY. For most inflammatory and immunologically mediated diseases, short-acting glucocorticosteroid preparations are desirable (see Table 28–1). In general, plasma half-life correlates with biologic half-life; use of preparations with longer half-lives, such as dexamethasone, is associated with a greater likelihood of adverse effects. Therefore, shorter-acting glucocorticosteroids such as prednisone or prednisolone are preferable to longer-acting preparations. These agents are also more amenable to being tapered to alternate-day regimes to reduce side effects.

Therapy is usually initiated as a single oral morning dose of prednisone (0.5 to 1.0 mg/kg). A morning dose is preferable to dosing later in the day because morning administration mimics the natural diurnal variation in cortisol levels. When more potent anti-inflammatory and immunosuppressive effects are desired, the total daily dose can be divided into three to four doses, given the short half-life of this drug. Unfortunately, this regimen is associated with a greater likelihood of adverse effects and hypothalamic-pituitary-adrenal axis suppression; therefore, as quickly as possible, efforts should be undertaken to consolidate the split-dose schedule to a single morning dose. For example, 15 mg of prednisone given four times per day is reduced to 20 mg three times daily, then to 30 mg twice daily, and, finally, to a single dose of 60 mg. The duration of each of these steps is dictated by the patient's tolerance and by control of the underlying disease; in general, this consolidation of dose should be accomplished within 3 weeks.

The once-daily regimen is maintained until the disease is stable and clinical improvement is recognized or deemed unlikely or side effects develop. Tapering should not be undertaken until the disease process is clinically quiescent, at which time reduction to an alternate-day regimen should be initiated with the goal of administering enough prednisone on the high-dose, or "on," day to suppress disease activity on the low-dose, or "off," day. This approach permits a return to normal hypothalamic-pituitary-adrenal axis function while reducing the risk of glucocorticosteroid side effects, especially opportunistic infection.

The possibility of hypothalamic-pituitary-adrenal suppression in patients receiving chronic glucocorticosteroid therapy is particularly problematic, particularly around times of stress, such as surgery. Although hypothalamic-pituitary-adrenal suppression is generally dependent on daily and cumulative doses as well as duration of treatment, it may be impossible to anticipate which patients will require supplemental glucocorticosteroids. A variety of tests have been proposed to determine the integrity of the hypothalamic-pituitary-adrenal axis, but the impact of exogenous corticotropin on serum cortisol may be the most valuable. Recent work has suggested that the amount of supplemental glucocorticosteroids required during surgery can be estimated by ascertaining the "amount" of stress (minor, moderate, or severe) anticipated in the perioperative period, with an upward adjustment of daily hydrocortisone (25 mg for minor stress; 50–75 mg for moderate stress, 100–150 mg for major stress) for up to 3 days.

Several protocols for tapering to an alternate-day regimen have been used. For example, the single daily dose may be reduced in 5- to 10-mg decrements to one half of the initial dose. The dose on the "on" day can be doubled while the dose on the "off" day is gradually decreased. Therefore, once a daily dose of 30 mg of prednisone is achieved, the patient is changed to a regimen of 60 mg/day alternated with 30 mg/day, with subsequent 5-mg reductions on the low-dose day weekly until a 15-mg daily level is reached. This dose is then reduced in 2.5-mg amounts until discontinuation, at which point a 60-mg alternate-day regimen has been attained. Once alternate-day therapy has been realized, gradual reductions in glucocorticosteroids should be attempted. An alternate approach is to reach a total daily dose of 30 mg/day and then reduce the drug on the low-dose day. These tapering schemes are feasible only when relatively short-acting glucocorticosteroids are used; longer-acting drugs have biologic half-lives of more than 24 hours, thereby negating the beneficial effects of an alternate-day regimen.

Clearly, this protocol is not uniformly effective. Failures may occur if the attempt to begin tapering is premature because the disease is still active, if the dose is reduced too rapidly, if the decrements in dose are too large, if not enough prednisone is administered on the "on" day, or if glucocorticosteroid "withdrawal" symptoms (e.g., myalgias, arthralgias, fever) are confused with a recrudescence of the disease. In some instances, tapering can be facilitated by using glucocorticosteroid-sparing drugs that help control the primary disease as glucocorticosteroids are reduced. For example, non-steroidal anti-inflammatory agents, cytotoxic drugs (e.g., methotrexate, azathioprine, and cyclophosphamide), and other agents may permit tapering to alternate-day glucocorticosteroid regimens. Clearly, however, these agents may also have associated toxicities that limit utility.

ALTERNATIVES TO ORAL THERAPY. In many circumstances it may be appropriate to administer glucocorticosteroids locally or to use systemic regimens that may reduce the likelihood of adverse effects. Topical and ophthalmic preparations can often control cutaneous (see Chapters 521 and 522) and ocular (see Chapter 512) disease, respectively, without appreciable systemic absorption of the preparation. Similarly, glucocorticosteroids administered nasally for allergic rhinitis (see Chapter 274), by inhalation for asthma or lower airway disease (see Chapter 74), and intra-articularly or by soft tissue injection for musculoskeletal inflammatory conditions may control the underlying disease without the adverse effects of systemic therapy. However, these methods of delivering drugs can also cause local toxicity and must be used with caution. Deflazacort, an oral glucocorticosteroid preparation not currently available in the United States, has been reported to have fewer adverse reactions, particularly osteoporosis, than conventional glucocorticosteroids.

When local glucocorticosteroid therapy and even systemic daily oral treatment are inadequate to control the underlying disease, intermittent, short-term, high-dose intravenous methylprednisolone can be used in inflammatory and immunologically mediated diseases, using 3- to 5-day regimens at 20 mg/kg/day or 1 g/m²/day. Pulse regimens have been successfully used in systemic lupus erythematosus with renal disease, some forms of vasculitis, rheumatoid arthritis, ankylosing spondylitis, and Goodpasture's syndrome. The precise mechanism(s) of the beneficial actions of such "pulse" ther-

apy is unclear, particularly because these protocols are often efficacious even when superimposed on daily glucocorticosteroid usage.

Pulse therapy has been associated with arrhythmias and sudden death, probably because of shifts in electrolytes in patients with underlying electrolyte abnormalities, conduction system disturbances, or diuretic therapy. In these settings, electrocardiographic monitoring is advisable while the drug is slowly administered over 1 to several hours. Other reported adverse reactions with pulse therapy include seizures and systemic infections, but the precise relationship of the reactions to pulse glucocorticosteroids is unclear because the therapy is commonly given to critically ill patients. Current indications for pulse regimens have included recrudescence of disease despite chronic glucocorticosteroid therapy, a flare of disease activity in the setting of glucocorticosteroid side effects, the need to control disease until another modality (e.g., cytotoxic drug) becomes effective, and the onset of a rapidly progressive glucocorticosteroid-responsive syndrome.

COMPLICATIONS OF GLUCOCORTICOSTEROID THERAPY

Prolonged systemic glucocorticosteroid therapy is invariably associated with toxicity (Table 28–3). In general, side effects depend on daily dose, dosing frequency, and duration of treatment, and emphasize the need to treat with alternate-day regimens or the lowest daily dose possible for as briefly as feasible. Hypothalamic-pituitary-adrenal axis suppression may occur with less than 2 weeks of systemic therapy and may be persistent despite cessation of the drug. The integrity of the hypothalamic-pituitary-adrenal axis in the setting of glucocorticosteroid therapy can be determined by measuring the change in serum cortisol level after cosyntropin infusion (see Chapter 240).

In general, the most effective way of preventing or minimizing the adverse effects of glucocorticosteroids is to reduce their dosage; unfortunately, this may not always be feasible. It is particularly important to monitor patients closely for the development of infection; typical signs of infection may be masked by glucocorticosteroid treatment. Glucocorticosteroid-induced osteoporosis (see Chapter 257) is especially problematic in older individuals, particularly those who are estrogen deficient. Calcium supplementation and postmenopausal estrogen repletion are also helpful. Cyclical, oral

Table 28–3 ▪ SIDE EFFECTS OF GLUCOCORTICOSTEROID THERAPY

Characteristic early in therapy: essentially unavoidable
  Insomnia
  Emotional lability
  Enhanced appetite or weight gain or both
Common in patients with underlying risk factors or other drug toxicities
  Hypertension
  Diabetes mellitus
  Peptic ulcer disease
  Acne vulgaris
Anticipated with use of sustained and intense treatment: minimize risk by conservative dosing regimens and steroid-sparing agents when possible
  Cushingoid habitus
  Hypothalamic-pituitary-adrenal suppression
  Infection diathesis
  Osteonecrosis
  Myopathy
  Impaired wound healing
Insidious and delayed: likely dependent on cumulative dose
  Osteoporosis
  Skin atrophy
  Cataracts
  Atherosclerosis
  Growth retardation
  Fatty liver
Rare and unpredictable
  Psychosis
  Pseudotumor cerebri
  Glaucoma
  Epidural lipomatosis
  Pancreatitis

From Boumpas DT, Chrousos GP, Wilder RL, et al: Glucocorticoid therapy for immune-mediated diseases: Basic and clinical correlates. Ann Intern Med 119:1198, 1993.

bisphosphonates prevent glucocorticosteroid-induced loss of bone mineral density in the spine and hip and may be the preferred therapy.

Boumpas DT, Chrousos GP, Wilder RL, et al: Glucocorticoid therapy for immune-mediated diseases: Basic and clinical correlates. Ann Intern Med 119:1198, 1993. *Clinically relevant information about how glucocorticosteroids work. Update on usage and side effects.*

Lamberts SWJ, Bruining HA, De Jong FH: Corticosteroid therapy in severe illness. N Engl J Med 337:1285, 1997. *Complete summary of the literature on the use of supplemental, "stress" glucocorticoids in patients receiving chronic therapy.*

29 NSAIDS: ASPIRIN AND ASPIRIN-LIKE DRUGS

Gerald Weissmann

HISTORY

SALICYLATES. On June 2, 1763, the Royal Society received a communication from Reverend Edward Stone of Chipping Norton in Oxfordshire. Its opening lines are probably unmatched in clinical pharmacology: "Among the many useful discoveries which this age has made, there are very few which better deserve the attention of the public than what I am going to lay before your Lordship. There is a bark of an English tree, which I have found by experience to be a powerful astringent and very efficacious in curing aguish and intermittent disorders."

The tree was the willow (*Salix alba*), the astringent bark of which contains salicin, the glycoside of salicylic acid. Stone had discovered that salicylates reduced the fever and aches produced by a variety of acute, shiver-provoking illnesses, or agues.

The salicylate most commonly used is acetylsalicylic acid, aspirin. At its low doses (80 to 325 mg/day), acetylsalicylic acid is used to prevent coronary and cerebral thrombosis by virtue of its antiplatelet effect. Intermediate, over-the-counter doses (650 mg to 3 g/day) are used as analgesics and antipyretics. Finally, for 100 years very high doses (> 3 g/day) have been used to reduce the redness and swelling of joints in rheumatic fever, gout, and rheumatoid arthritis.

Aspirin and other salicylates have a variety of other biologic effects, only some of which are related to their use in medicine today. Salicylates can dissolve corns on the toes—a keratolytic effect; provoke loss of uric acid from the kidneys—their uricosuric property; and kill bacteria in vitro—their antiseptic action. But cell biologists also use aspirin and salicylates to inhibit anion transport across cell membranes, to interfere with the activation of white blood cells, and to uncouple oxidative phosphorylation by isolated mitochondria. Finally, molecular biologists use salicylates to activate genes that code for heat-shock proteins in the lampbrush chromosomes of *Drosophila*, to influence mitogen-activated protein kinases, and to induce ceramide-mediated apoptosis in cancer cells.

Hippocrates (fourth century BC) had advocated the chewing of willow leaves to relieve the pains of childbirth, and there are references by Pliny (first century) and Galen (second century) to the analgesic property of willow, but it was Stone who put extract of willow bark into our pharmacopoeia as an effective antipyretic agent.

By 1828, at the Pharmacologic Institute of Munich, Büchner isolated a tiny amount of the active glycoside, salicin, in the form of bitter-tasting yellow, needle-like crystals. Two years later, Leroux, in Paris, improved on the extraction procedure and obtained 1 ounce of salicin from 3 pounds of the bark. By 1838, Raffaele Pira of Pisa described how he obtained a pure substance from salicin by hydrolyzing the glycoside in a CrO_3-mediated oxidation via an aldehyde intermediate.

Willow bark was not alone in providing a rich natural source of salicylates. Meadowsweet (*Spiraea ulmaria*) yielded ample quanti-

ties of an ether-soluble oil from which *Spirsäure*, the same *acide salicylique* of Pira, was crystallized. Oil of wintergreen, a traditional remedy for aguish disorders, also was shown to contain the methyl ester of salicylic acid from which *acide salicylique* could be prepared.

Forced to compete with the French and British dye industries, which supplied their textile mills with pigments imported from overseas colonies, the Germans responded by inventing cheap aniline dyes, creating in their train such giant enterprises as I. G. Farben. By 1833, the pharmacist E. Merck of Darmstadt had obtained a clean preparation of salicin that was less expensive by half than the impure willow extracts used as antipyretics, but an inexpensive, pure, acceptable remedy was not available until 1860, when Kolbe and his students at Marburg succeeded in the first synthesis of salicylic acid and its sodium salt from phenol, CO_2, and sodium. The availability of cheap salicylic acid spread its clinical use far and wide.

SALICYLATES AS ANTI-INFLAMMATORY DRUGS. In 1876, Stricker and Ries reported the first successful treatment of acute rheumatism by sodium salicylate at doses of 5 to 6 g/day. Almost simultaneously, Maclagan reported his results with salicylic acid and salicin at similar dosage levels.

Stricker and Ries and Maclagan found that salicylates reduce not only fever and pain but also redness and swelling. That anti-inflammatory property was next used to advantage by the Parisian Germain See, who, in 1877, introduced high-dose salicylates, both acid salicylique and salicin, as effective treatments for gout and "chronic poly-arthritis."

ASPIRIN AND ACETAMINOPHEN. In 1898, Felix Hofmann, an aniline dye chemist at the Friedrich Bayer-Eberfeld division of I. G. Farben, searched for less acidic derivatives to avoid gastric irritation and focused on acetyl derivatives of sodium salicylate. Acetylsalicylic acid proved more palatable and less irritating to the stomach. Hofmann took the material to his supervisor, Heinrich Dreser, head of Bayer's laboratory of pharmacology, who called the new drug aspirin, the *a* from acetyl and the *spirin* from the German *Spirsäure*.

Competitors entered the field as markets expanded for other drugs that could reduce fever and pain. Based on anecdotal accounts from Alsace that a product formed from aniline treated with vinegar made a useful febrifuge, Karl Morner, in 1889, synthesized the material—acetanilide—and isolated its metabolites. Acetanilide itself, unfortunately, caused bone marrow depression and anemias in a distinct number of patients, so other derivatives were sought. Acetanilide and the widely used phenacetin are metabolized to N-acetyl-*p*-aminophenol, which by various anagramatic combinations yields the generic names acetaminophen in the United States and paracetamol in the United Kingdom. In 1955, acetaminophen acquired a trade name in the United States that was to make it famous: Tylenol—also from acetyl-*p*-aminophenol.

Neither acetanilide nor phenacetin proved as useful as aspirin for treating rheumatic fever or rheumatoid arthritis because they were not anti-inflammatory. By comparison, trials of steroids versus aspirin and sodium salicylate showed that salicylates at doses high enough to yield plasma levels of 25 to 35 mg/dL (6 to 9 g/day) were as effective anti-inflammatory agents as cortisone or prednisone in rheumatic fever.

NSAIDs INHIBIT PROSTAGLANDIN SYNTHESIS

The most important recent contribution to the story of aspirin-like drugs was made by John Vane and colleagues, who found that aspirin-like drugs inhibited the biosynthesis of prostaglandin (PG) E_2 and PGF_{2a} from radiolabeled arachidonic acid in studies in vitro. Moreover, they found that platelets taken from volunteers given aspirin and indomethacin 1 hour before venipuncture failed to make prostaglandins in response to thrombin and that catecholamine-induced release of prostaglandins from canine spleens could be inhibited by indomethacin, albeit less consistently than by aspirin.

Aspirin-like drugs inhibit the enzyme that transforms arachidonic acid to the stable PGE_1 and PGE_2. The constitutive enzyme, cyclooxygenase 1, is a 70-kd homodimer localized to microsomal membranes. First called "prostaglandin synthase," then "cyclooxygenase," today it is known as "prostaglandin H synthase," or COX-1 (Fig. 29–1). This enzyme catalyzes two reactions: the *bis*-dioxy-

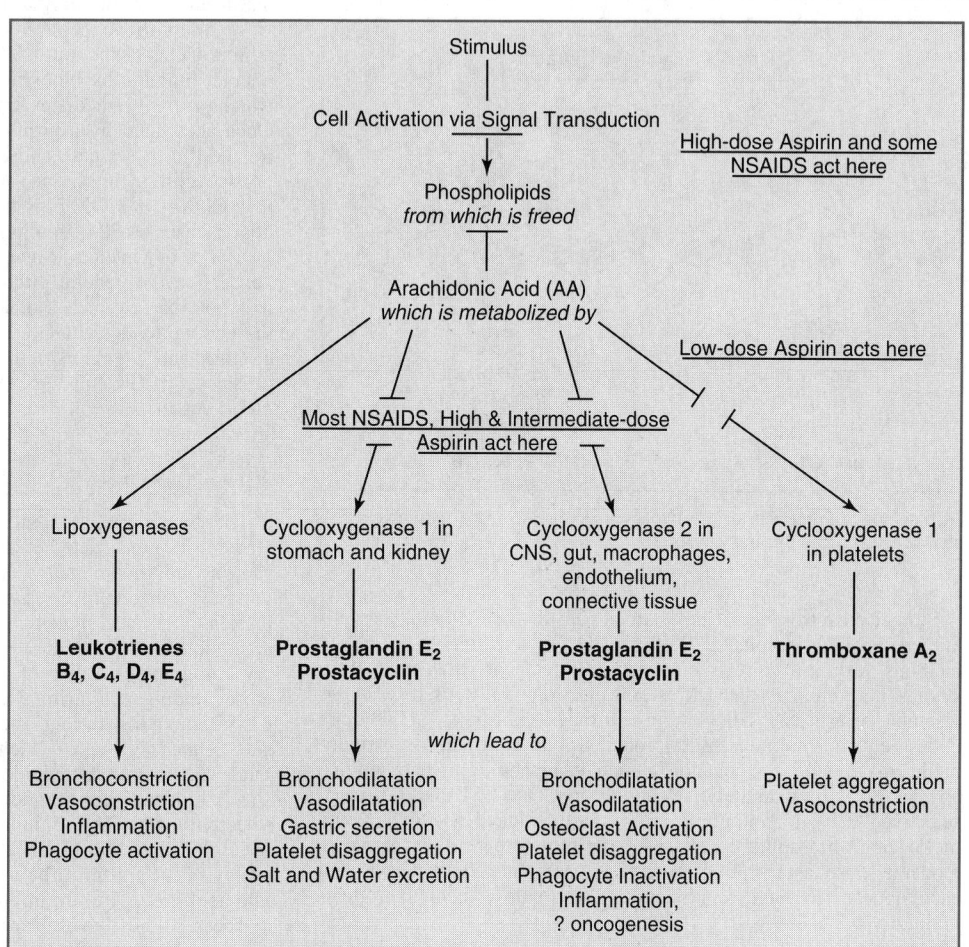

FIGURE 29–1 ■ The inflammatory cascade.

genation of arachidonic acid to form PGH$_2$ (cyclooxygenase activity) and the reduction of hydroperoxides to the corresponding alcohols (peroxidase activity). PGH synthase—and its inducible analogue COX-2—form stable prostaglandins of the E and F series via the unstable endoperoxide intermediates PGG$_2$ and PGH$_2$. The endoperoxides, critical for platelet function, are transformed by platelets to a most potent vasoconstricting and platelet-aggregating substance, thromboxane A$_2$ (TxA$_2$). Vane had also isolated a potent vasodilator, prostacyclin (PGI$_2$), which was again made from arachidonate by the cyclooxygenase of endothelial cells. Because platelets make TxA$_2$, which constricts the smooth muscle of blood vessels, and because blood vessel walls make prostacyclin I$_2$, which powerfully relaxes blood vessels and inhibits platelet aggregation, the hunt was on for ways to inhibit the synthesis of thromboxane but not prostacyclin.

Vane and his associates, in the 1970s, had amassed convincing evidence that the prostaglandin hypothesis of aspirin action was largely correct. Almost all aspirin-like drugs (by then generally called "nonsteroidal anti-inflammatory drugs," or NSAIDs) inhibit prostaglandin synthetase, and the potency of these drugs (ID$_{50}$) parallels their clinical potency or their effect in experimental animals (e.g., aspirin was anywhere from 1/40 to 1/200 as active as indomethacin and from 1/5 to 1/50 as active as ibuprofen). NSAIDs inhibit PG synthetase, but central analgesics such as morphine or codeine, antihistamines, antiserotonin drugs, and cortisone and its analogues do not.

Vane argued that stable prostaglandins not only were produced at sites of inflammation but also, alone or in concert with other mediators, could provoke all the cardinal signs of inflammation. Indeed, PGE$_1$ and PGE$_2$ *do* induce vasodilation; they promote edema when dilated blood vessels have been made leaky by histamine; they produce fever when injected either into the cerebral ventricles or directly into the anterior hypothalamus; and they sensitize pain receptors of the skin to such other pain-provoking hu-

mors as bradykinin or histamine. By comparison, acetaminophen ineffectively inhibits prostaglandin synthesis by enzyme preparations from a variety of tissues but is effective against the synthetase from brain. And although non-acetylated salicylates are roughly 1/10 as potent as aspirin in vitro, studies of urinary prostaglandin metabolites showed that sodium salicylate effectively diminishes excretion of these metabolites in humans. Sodium salicylate also effectively reduces prostaglandin release in models of experimental inflammation in animals.

CYCLOOXYGENASES 1 AND 2

Many cyclooxygenase products (e.g., PGE$_2$, PGI$_2$) are clearly associated with inflammation in vivo. Within the past decade, however, thanks to the work of Needleman, Hershman, and others, it is now known that there are two PGH$_2$ synthase isozymes (COX-1 and COX-2), which share 62% homology at the message and protein level. Despite the close relationship of the complement DNAs for COX-1 and COX-2, the messenger RNAs for these two isozymes differ greatly with respect to size—2.8:3.0 kb and 4.1 kb for COX-1 and COX-2, respectively. The major difference between these two isozymes is that COX-1 is present in many cells constitutively but COX-2 is expressed only after it is induced by tumor necrosis factor-α (TNFα), interleukin 1 (IL-1), interleukin 8 (IL-8), or lipopolysaccharide (see Fig. 29–2). By unknown means, aspirin inhibition of COX-2 leads to the generation of 15-hydroxyeicosatetraenoic acid (15-HETE) and its probable metabolite, 14,15-diHETE, which is a potent inhibitor of neutrophil O$_2$ generation. Engagement of two lipoxygenases (5- and 15-) leads to the synthesis of lipoxins A$_4$ and B$_4$. Neutrophils treated with aspirin release both LXA$_4$ and its 15-epi metabolite 15-epi-LTXA$_4$; these compounds are as potent as glucocorticoids in animal models of inflammation.

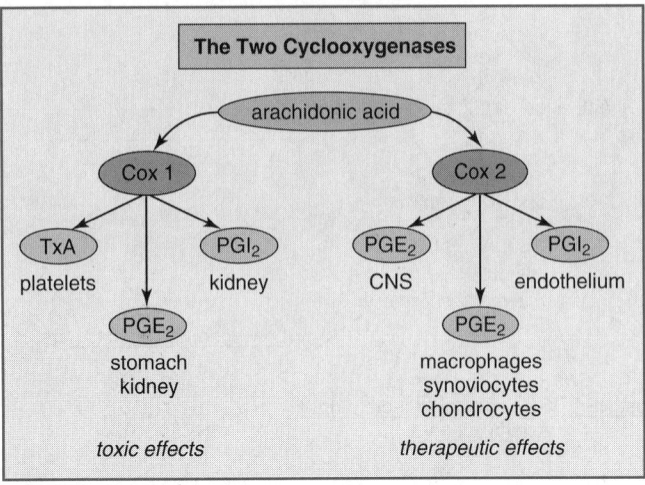

FIGURE 29–2 ■ Properties of the two cyclooxygenases. Cox 1 = cyclooxygenase 1; Cox 2 = cyclooxygenase 2.

Studied in retrospect, it now is claimed that one or another well-known NSAID inhibits COX-1 or COX-2 selectively; but assay methods vary and there is only partial agreement between in vitro studies and clinical data. Most of the commonly used NSAIDs resemble aspirin and salicylate in that they inhibit both COXs more or less equally (sulindac, flurbiprofen, S-ibuprofen, naproxen, indomethacin). On the other hand, the active metabolite of nabumetone appears to be moderately selective for COX-2. Three far more selective "COX-2 inhibitors" are in early clinical use (celecoxib, meloxicam, nimesulide); each has been shown to be as effective as moderate-dose aspirin in short-term studies of inflammation, and each appears to have significantly fewer side effects than dual-inhibitory NSAIDs.

INHIBITION OF COX-1 EXPLAINS NSAID SIDE EFFECTS

Perhaps the most persuasive aspect of the prostaglandin hypothesis, as modified after the discovery of COX-2, was its explanation of the clinical side effects of NSAIDs. A major problem with NSAIDs at anti-inflammatory doses is that they provoke stomach irritation and peptic ulceration. Aspirin is the worst offender in this regard. The irritation derives from the need for endogenous prostaglandins by the gastric mucosa to regulate its overproduction of acid and to synthesize the mucous barrier that prevents its self-digestion. It is clear that the constitutive synthase is the enzyme affected by NSAIDs and that addition of an exogenous PGE_1 analogue (misoprostol) can prevent and/or treat NSAID-induced peptic ulcers.

Moreover, most NSAIDs promote salt and water retention, especially when heart or liver disease compromises renal blood flow. NSAIDs block the formation of the vasodilator PGI_2 by kidney cells, and renal blood supply is reduced even further. It is no surprise, therefore, to learn that kidney and stomach are rich in COX-1 and that selective COX-2 inhibitors are less toxic to these organs.

Another side effect of NSAIDs—but not sodium salicylate—is aspirin-sensitivity syndrome in those genetically susceptible, which results in wheezing, sneezing, and polyp formation. These consequences are due to the diversion of arachidonate from blocked COXs to the 5-lipoxygenase pathway, which is not inhibited by NSAIDs. It is by means of the lipoxygenase pathways that leukotrienes (LT) C, D, and E are formed, and these have been implicated in aspirin hypersensitivity. Tinnitus, a common side effect that high-dose aspirin shares with sodium salicylate, has been attributed by some to COX-1–dependent synthesis of PGEs by cells of the inner ear.

Finally, the most common side effect of NSAIDs, and especially of aspirin, is their interference with platelet function. Patients on these drugs sometimes suffer untoward bleeding after tooth extraction, minor surgery, or trauma. Weiss and Aledort, in 1967, showed that aspirin inhibits normal platelet aggregation both in vitro and in vivo. With the exception of sodium salicylate, all NSAIDs that inhibit COX-1, the only COX expressed in thrombocytes, inhibit platelet function by blocking formation of endoperoxides and TxA_2, which are intermediates in platelet stimulus-response coupling. Once acetylated by aspirin, COX-1 of platelets remains inactivated for the life of the cell, and thromboxane cannot be made. However, prostacyclin synthesis in endothelial cells, which can synthesize new COX-1 or COX-2, is inhibited no more than a few days. Low-dose aspirin (<325 mg/day) can irreversibly block COX-1 activity of a pool of platelets in the portal circulation even before salicylate appears in the general circulation. These observations explain why it is possible, by means of low-dose aspirin, to inhibit formation of the endoperoxides (PGG_2, PGH_2) and TxA_2—all of which promote clotting and vasoconstriction—without blocking the synthesis of prostacyclin (PGI_2), which inhibits platelet function and dilates blood vessels.

THE MODES OF ACTION OF ASPIRIN-LIKE DRUGS

The interaction of NSAIDs with COX-1 and COX-2 has been studied in great detail. Lands and Kulmacz showed earlier that aspirin and indomethacin interact in a complex, biphasic fashion with the enzyme, whereas other NSAIDs such as ibuprofen, naproxen, and meclofenamate simply interfere with the binding of arachidonate to its oxidation site. Recent biochemical and x-ray crystallographic studies of both COX-1 and COX-2 have extended these findings: aspirin irreversibly acetylates Ser 530 of both COXs, blocking further access of arachidonic acid to their active site. Other NSAIDs—including salicylic acid itself—sterically hinder access of arachidonic acid to the channel in which the active site is hidden. This channel is somewhat larger in COX-2, and the selectivity of COX-2 inhibitors depends on the presence of a valine-isoleucine substitution at 523. The gatekeeper of the channel in both COXs appears to be arginine 123, which bonds to the carboxylic acid group present in clinically useful NSAIDs.

These studies have clearly defined the mechanism whereby aspirin-like drugs inhibit the biosynthesis of stable prostaglandins. However, the hypothesis that locally produced prostaglandins are the major mediators of inflammation has been only partly substantiated. Although Vane's proposal that all NSAIDs inhibit the transformation of arachidonic acid to stable prostaglandins (i.e., PGE_2 and PGI_2) has turned out to be largely correct, this proposition cannot be generalized to all products of the arachidonic acid cascade and to all NSAIDs at all dosages. The three major antipyretic, analgesic drugs exert diverse effects on prostaglandin biosynthesis (Table 29–1). When used to treat rheumatic diseases in dosages of more than 3 g/day, high-dose aspirin has antipyretic, anti-inflammatory, and analgesic effects and can inhibit the synthesis of prostaglandins in disrupted cell preparations. However, at the intermediate dosage indicated for analgesia (650 mg every 3 to 4 hours), aspirin has antipyretic and analgesic but not anti-inflammatory activity. Finally, at its lowest clinically effective dosage (80 to 325 mg/day), aspirin exerts only an antiplatelet effect (COX-1 inhibition). Plasma levels of salicylate in individuals given intermediate doses of aspirin are sufficient to inhibit prostaglandin biosynthesis in vivo by kidneys, platelets, and vascular endothelium, whereas low doses of aspirin, which treat or prevent coronary or cerebral thrombosis, yield barely detectable plasma levels of salicylate. To achieve an anti-inflammatory effect, high-dose aspirin must provide a plasma concentration of 18 to 30 mg/dL. Those observations suggest two possibilities: either the COX-2 of inflammation is relatively insensitive to aspirin—a notion without experimental support—or high-dose aspirin differs in mode of action from more modest aspirin regimens.

NONPROSTAGLANDIN EFFECTS OF NSAIDs

Further evidence that aspirin-like drugs exert clinical effects that do not depend on inhibiting prostaglandin biosynthesis can be drawn from the properties of sodium salicylate and acetaminophen. Although sodium salicylate shares many of the properties of aspirin, it fails to inhibit prostaglandin biosynthesis in disrupted cell

Table 29–1 ■ EFFECTS OF COMMONLY USED ANALGESIC AND ANTIPYRETIC AGENTS

	ACETYLSALICYLIC ACID			SODIUM SALICYLATE	TRADITIONAL NSAIDs	SELECTIVE COX-2 INHIBITORS	ACETAMINOPHEN
	Low Dose*	Intermediate Dose*	High Dose*				
Antipyretic	0	+	+	+	+	+	+
Analgesic	0	+	+	+	+	+	+
Anti-inflammatory	0	0	+	+	+	+	0
Inhibit prostaglandin synthesis of platelets	+	+	+	0	+	0	0
Inhibit prostaglandin synthesis systemically	0	+	+	±	+	+	0
Inhibit colon cancer	?	+	?	?	+	?	0
Retard Alzheimer's disease	?	+	?	?	+	?	0
Prevent coronary, cerebral thrombosis	+	+	?	?	?	0	0

*Low dose, 80 to 325 mg/d; intermediate dose, 650 mg to 3 g/d; high dose > 3 g/d.

preparations at concentrations that may be achieved in plasma. Moreover, clinical studies show that because non-acetylated salicylates do not inhibit platelet function in vitro or ex vivo, they do not cause bleeding. Indeed, acetaminophen, which also fails to inhibit prostaglandin biosynthesis, does not affect platelet aggregation, nor is it anti-inflammatory. It must therefore be concluded that pain and fever can effectively be reduced without inhibiting the synthesis of prostaglandins at all.

Moreover, stable prostaglandins (PGE_1, PGE_2, PGI_2) possess not only proinflammatory but also anti-inflammatory properties. For example, these compounds produce vasodilation, act in synergy with complement component C5a or LTB_4 to produce edema, mediate fever and myalgia in response to IL-1, act in synergy with bradykinin to provoke pain, and also inhibit the function of T-suppressor cells.

On the other hand, high doses of these stable prostaglandins inhibit inflammation in animal models of arthritis, and much lower doses inhibit inflammation induced by local skin irritants. Since the early 1970s, it has been known that PGI_2 and stable prostaglandins of the E type inhibit the activation in vitro of neutrophils, platelets, and mononuclear phagocytes by interfering with their stimulus-response/coupling. In these cells, NSAIDs increase cellular cyclic adenosine monophosphate levels, which are regulated by means of prostaglandin receptors. The relevance in vivo of these data obtained in vitro is supported by the observation that experimental arthritis or glomerulonephritis in rats can be reduced with systemic PGE_1.

As a class, NSAIDs are planar organic anions that partition across the lipid bilayers of plasma membranes in accordance with the Nernst equation. The more acidic the pH, as at inflammatory sites, the greater the lipophilicity of NSAIDs, which subsequently interfere with cell function, including assembly of a superoxide anion-generating system by a cell-free, membrane-rich preparation from neutrophils, the activity of phospholipase C in mononuclear cells, the 12-hydroperoxyeicosatetraenoic acid peroxidase in platelets, and signal transduction in neutrophils and lymphocytes.

The first effect of aspirin-like drugs on cell metabolism was found to be the uncoupling of oxidative phosphorylation by isolated mitochondria. More recent studies have shown that aspirin, but not acetaminophen, alters the uptake of precursor arachidonate and its insertion into the membranes of cultured human monocytes and macrophages. Salicylates also inhibit anion transport across a variety of cell membranes. Again, the capacity of salicylates to inhibit anion movements is not shared by acetaminophen. Finally, NSAIDs inhibit synthesis of cartilage proteoglycan and bone metabolism, both in vitro and in vivo, by mechanisms that do not depend on inhibiting COX-1 or COX-2. It is a matter of clinical concern that some classes of NSAIDs (e.g., salicylates), but not all (e.g., piroxicam), inhibit proteoglycan synthesis, thereby promoting loss of cartilage matrix.

Aspirin-like drugs affect stimulus-response coupling in the most abundant cells of acute inflammation: neutrophils. Neutrophils injure tissues by releasing proteases, inflammatory peptides, reactive oxygen species such as O_2^- and H_2O_2, and lipid irritants such as platelet-activating factor and LTB_4. Activation of the neutrophil in response to soluble stimuli (chemoattractants) or to immune complexes follows general pathways of stimulus-response coupling secretory cells and is inhibited by all NSAIDs studied so far. NSAIDs—indomethacin, piroxicam, diclofenac, and ibuprofen (at micromolar concentrations) and salicylates (at millimolar concentrations)—inhibit the cell-cell aggregation of human neutrophils induced by chemoattractants and mediated by the cell surface adhesion molecule CD11b/CD18. Although all NSAIDs inhibit aggregation, only some inhibit enzyme release and/or O_2^- generation. Millimolar concentrations of sodium salicylate and aspirin, which are achieved in the high-dose treatment of rheumatoid arthritis or rheumatic fever, are required to inhibit the aggregation of neutrophils. However, at these concentrations sodium salicylate does not interfere with the activation of platelets or synthesis of TxA_2. In contrast, aspirin at 1/10 to 1/100 of these concentrations inhibits platelet aggregation and completely inhibits thromboxane biosynthesis through its effect on PGH synthase. It is therefore likely that the shared anti-inflammatory effects of aspirin and sodium salicylate are related to their common inhibition of neutrophil activation rather than to their divergent actions on prostaglandin biosynthesis. In contrast to aspirin and sodium salicylate, acetaminophen does not affect neutrophil aggregation.

Inhibitory effects of NSAIDs on neutrophil activation in vitro can also be demonstrated in patients. Indeed, neutrophils derived from the synovial fluid of patients with rheumatoid arthritis produce less superoxide anion after 10 days of therapy with piroxicam, whereas cells from normal volunteers given ibuprofen or piroxicam for 3 days fail to aggregate normally in response to chemoattractants. Sodium salicylate, an ineffective inhibitor of PGH synthase in vitro, is as effective as aspirin at inhibiting neutrophil activation. At anti-inflammatory concentrations, NSAIDs appear to uncouple transmembrane receptors with their effector molecules in the plasmalemma, including those regulated by guanine nucleotide-binding (G) proteins.

Recent work on the mechanism of action of high-dose aspirin and salicylate in vitro (i.e., 1–5 mM) has shown that salicylates (1) induce apoptosis in colonic cancer cells—which overexpress COX-2—via a ceramide-dependent pathway, (2) inhibit the disposition and traffic to the nucleus of such cytoplasmic transcription factors as the glucocorticoid receptor and its attendant heat-shock proteins, (3) interfere with the translocation of NF_kB in response to $TNF\alpha$, other cytokines, or tissue factor; and (4) interfere with the activation of the AP-1 promoter site, which is critical to metalloprotease synthesis. Salicylates also disrupt several cascades of protein kinase activation, including the p38 and the ras $\rightarrow$ raf-1 $\rightarrow$ MEK $\rightarrow$ p44$^{erk\ 1}$, p42$^{erk\ 2}$ signaling pathways. Finally, high-dose aspirin has variable transcriptional and translational effects on nitric oxide synthases (e.g., iNOS, cNOS). None of these in vitro actions of salicylates is duplicated by acetaminophen. Consequently, these molecular targets, as well as COX, have been implicated in newly documented effects of prolonged NSAID use and intermediate-dose aspirin on prevention of (1) colon cancer in animals and humans, (2) retardation of the progression of Alzheimer's disease in adults, and (3) eliciting Reye's syndrome in children. These effects on Alzheimer's disease and colon cancer are *not* limited to aspirin in intermediate doses; indeed, other NSAIDs such as sulindac or piroxicam may be even superior. Acetaminophen, however, is ineffective.

Another argument against a unitary mode of action of aspirin-like drugs comes from the cell biology of marine sponges, which are both the most primitive and most ancient of animal creatures. The activation of sponge cells in the course of cell-cell aggregation is not influenced by stable prostaglandins, nor do sponge cells contain COX activity. Nevertheless, aggregation of marine sponge cells is inhibited by NSAIDs—either by high-dose aspirin or sodium salicylate and by 12 other NSAIDs tested, but not by acetaminophen. Because the concentrations of NSAIDs that inhibit aggregation of marine sponges are the same as those that inhibit neutrophil aggregation and because marine sponges cannot make prostaglandins, these effects, like those on human neutrophils, are unlikely to result from their inhibition of prostaglandin synthesis.

Hawkey CJ: COX-2 inhibitors. Lancet 353:307–314, 1999. *A comprehensive review of this new class of drugs.*

Luong C, Miller A, Barnett J, et al: Flexibility of the NSAID binding site in the structure of human cyclooxygenase-2. Nat Struct Biol 3:927, 1996. *A readable account of how NSAIDs fit into the groove of the enzyme. A tour de force of structural biology.*

Pierpoint WS: The natural history of salicylic acid: Plant product and mammalian medicine. Interdisc Sci Rev 22:45, 1997. *A literate review, from a botanical perspective, of what salicylates do in plants and humans. There are as many similarities as differences.*

Pillinger MH, Capodici C, Han G, et al: Inflammation and anti-inflammation: Gating of cell/cell adhesion at the level of mitogen-activated protein kinases. Ann NY Acad Sci 832:1, 1997. *Evidence that aspirin blocks integrin-mediated neutrophil aggregation in which the MAP-kinases play a critical role.*

Pillinger MH, Capodici C, Rosenthal R, et al: Modes of action of aspirin-like drugs: Salicylates inhibit Erk activation and integrin-dependent homotypic neutrophil adhesion. Proc Natl Acad Sci U S A, 95:14540–14545, 1998.

Riendeau D, Charleson S, Cromlish W, et al: Comparison of the COX-1 inhibitory properties of nonsteroidal anti-inflammatory drugs (NSAIDs) and selective COX-2 inhibitors, using sensitive microsomal and platelet assays. Can J Physiol Pharmacol 74:1088, 1997. *A comprehensive study that discusses the difficulties of deciding whether one or another NSAID is selective for COX-1 or COX-2.*

Stewart WF, Kawas C, Corrada M, et al: Risk of Alzheimer's disease and duration of NSAID use. Neurology 48:626, 1997. *Aspirin and NSAID use clearly reduce the risk; patients taking NSAIDs other than aspirin fare better. A pioneer study.*

Vane JR, Bonting RM: Mechanism of action of aspirin-like drugs. Semin Arthritis Rheum 26(Suppl 1):2, 1997. *A fine discussion of how COX-1 and COX-2 explain the toxicities and therapeutic effects, respectively, of aspirin-like drugs.*

Weiss HA, Forman D: Aspirin, non-steroidal anti-inflammatory drugs and protection from colorectal cancer: A review of the epidemiological evidence. Scand J Gastroenterol 220(Suppl 1):137, 1996. *A critical look at the doses required and the probity of the evidence. It looks good for NSAIDs now, but the last word is not in.*

30 NEWER IMAGING TECHNIQUES

James M. Mountz ■ Hoby Hetherington

Imaging technology continues to advance the accuracy of diagnosis. Computers have become vital tools for radiologic clinical practice and have advanced the cost-effectiveness of imaging. Picture archiving and communications systems (PACS) have emerged as an important part of digital imaging technology. They enable image and multimedia data distribution, archiving, and transmission. The workstation is becoming the contact between a PACS and the radiologist or referring physician.

ADVANCES IN CONVENTIONAL IMAGING MODALITIES

ULTRASONIC TECHNIQUES. Endoluminal ultrasonography has allowed the imaging of anatomy by inserting small ultrasonic probes into the major vessels or other body lumina to visualize nearly all organ systems of the body. Ultrasound probes are designed to pass through the instrument channel of ordinary fiberoptic or video endoscopes.

Intravascular ultrasonography (IVUS) is composed fundamentally of a miniature ultrasound (US) transducer mounted at the end of a catheter. This catheter-based system, when introduced into an adequately sized blood vessel, produces real-time, two-dimensional (2D), cross-sectional images of the vascular structure. High-resolution images of vascular lumen, vessel wall, and vascular plaque are achievable (Fig. 30–1).

Applications for IVUS include guiding and evaluating endovascular interventional procedures, correlating IVUS results with histology in diseased vessels, early detection and sonographic tissue characterization of atherosclerosis, and three-dimensional (3D) voxel modeling of vascular structures by computerized reformation of 2D cross-sectional images.

With new techniques in transvaginal US, higher resolution allows earlier diagnosis of fetal developmental anomalies. Transvaginal echography is used to examine asymptomatic patients at risk for repeated abortion in the first trimester of pregnancy. It has been established that a reliable echographic finding—the normal sequential appearance of the yolk sac of the embryo and the presence of normal fetal heart activity—can be used prognostically for the future course of pregnancy. Transvaginal US is playing an increasingly important role in detecting congenital heart defects among patients with high risk for fetal anomalies (see Chapter 57); they are usually performed at 12 to 16 weeks' gestation. When a prenatal diagnosis of a structural abnormality is made, the health care team can outline a management strategy to optimize the care and support given to the fetus, mother, and family. Transvaginal US in the early second trimester is a useful tool both for detecting fetal cardiac structural defects and for providing anatomic evaluation of multiple organ systems in fetal development.

Other endoluminal US modalities (e.g., transrectal or transesophageal US) may also be used to assess extraluminal anatomy and pathology, within the limits of the depth of penetration of the transducer. For example, a 20-MHz mechanical linear probe can be used within the upper gastrointestinal tract, pancreatic duct, biliary tree, and colon. US probes are best used for high-resolution imaging of focal endoscopically visible lesions. Endoscopic visualization enables direction of the probe to the lesion of interest.

ANGIOGRAPHIC TECHNIQUES. Digital subtraction angiography

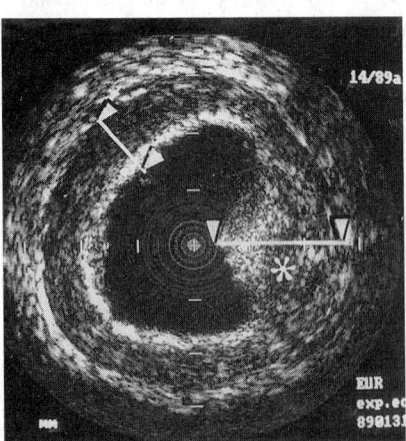
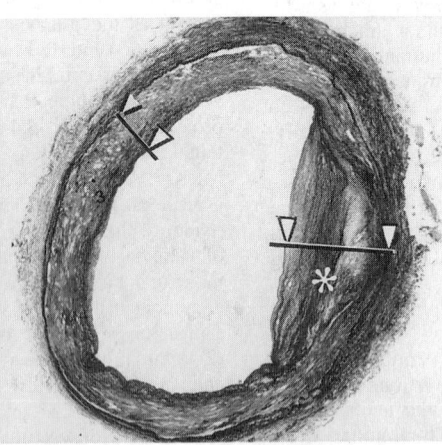

FIGURE 30–1 ■ Ultrasonic cross-sectional image (left) obtained in vitro (at 40 MHz) with the corresponding photomicrograph of the histologic cross section (right) obtained from a superior mesenteric artery. Bright echoes of the internal elastic lamina and adventitia circumscribe the hypoechoic media. A distinct media was observed echographically in the absence of a lesion (at 10 o'clock). In the presence of an extensive lesion (asterk) the media becomes invisible echographically. The corresponding histologic section reveals absence of the media in this region. (Verhoeff–van Gieson stain [calibration 1 mm], magnification ×6.) (From Gussenhoven EJ, Frietman PAV, The SHK, et al: Assessment of medial thinning in atherosclerosis by intravascular ultrasound. Am J Cardiol 68:1625, 1991.)

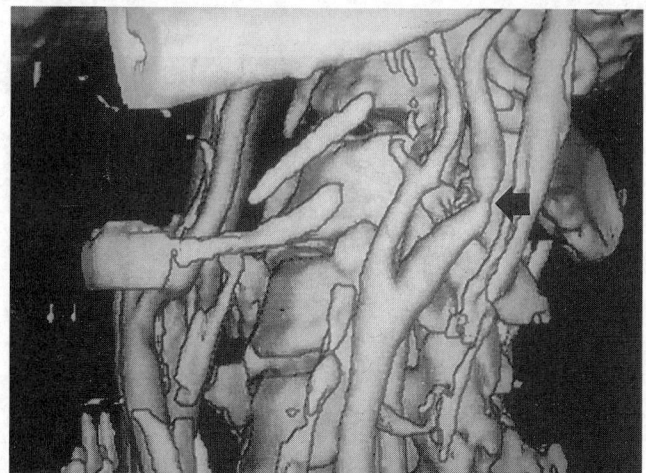

FIGURE 30-2 ■ Three-dimensional–rendered image from spiral CT of the neck. The bones and opacified vessels are clearly seen. A stenotic lesion of the left internal carotid artery distal to the bifurcation is identified (arrow). (Courtesy of Jerry Arenson, Elscint, Inc., Hackensack, NJ.)

(DSA) is a valuable and frequently used diagnostic technique that allows the physician to evaluate vascular anatomy and pathology. More recently, 3D time-of-flight magnetic resonance angiography (MRA) and intra-arterial DSA have been used to compare pre- and postoperative evaluation of the carotid bifurcation. Although MRA is emerging as an accurate modality for imaging carotid bifurcations, significant limitations still exist in its ability to demonstrate the intracranial circulation.

Color-flow duplex surveillance of graft patency is a valuable tool to evaluate peripheral bypass procedures. For example, color-aided duplex Doppler sonography can exclude transplant renal artery stenosis and determine the feasibility and safety of intra-arterial DSA in hypertensive renal allograft recipients on an outpatient basis. This imaging modality allows renal angiography to be reserved for those patients with an inconclusive US study.

Spiral CT couples continuous tube rotation with continuous scan table movement to compile continuous anatomic information without establishing arbitrary boundaries at section interfaces as in conventional CT. The unique method of data collection of the spiral CT scanner has been combined with dynamic intravenous (IV) contrast material bolus protocols to image the abdominal vasculature, including the aorta, renal arteries, and splanchnic circulation. Through various techniques of image processing, including surface renderings and maximum intensity projection (MIP) image display, it is possible to obtain excellent anatomic detail of the aorta and its major branches. Vessel contrast on spiral CT scans is

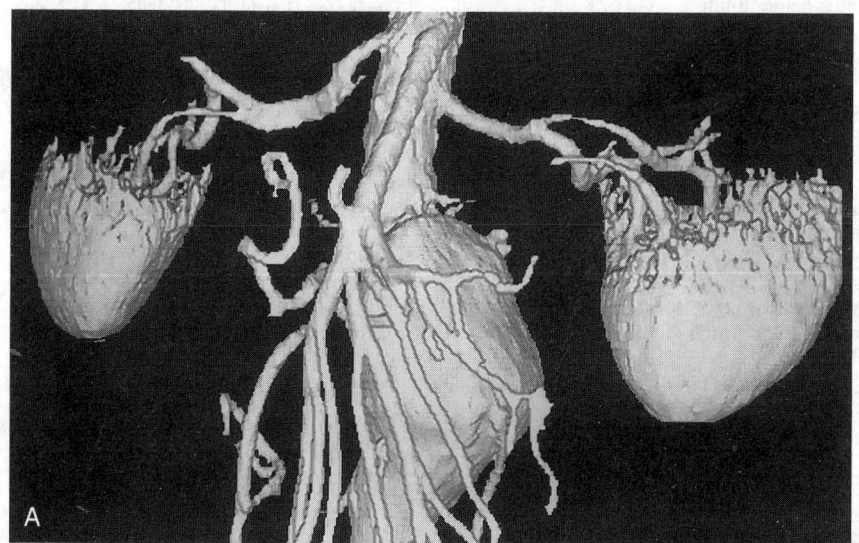

FIGURE 30-3 ■ Abdominal aortic aneurysm. Three-dimensional (3D) image (A), maximum intensity projection (MIP) image (B), and cross-sectional images (C) of a 5-cm aneurysm. Mural thrombus within the aneurysm is best seen on the transverse slice. The relationship to the renal arteries is seen on the 3D and MIP images. The upper portions of the kidneys are not visualized on the 3D image because scanning begins before the contrast material reaches the capillary beds. The lower portions of the kidneys are visualized because the capillaries fill during the 30 seconds required for scanning from top to bottom. (From Mogavero GT, Wass JL, Kopecky KK: Angiography among top applications for spiral CT. Diagn Imaging [Spiral CT suppl] November:10–14, 1993.)

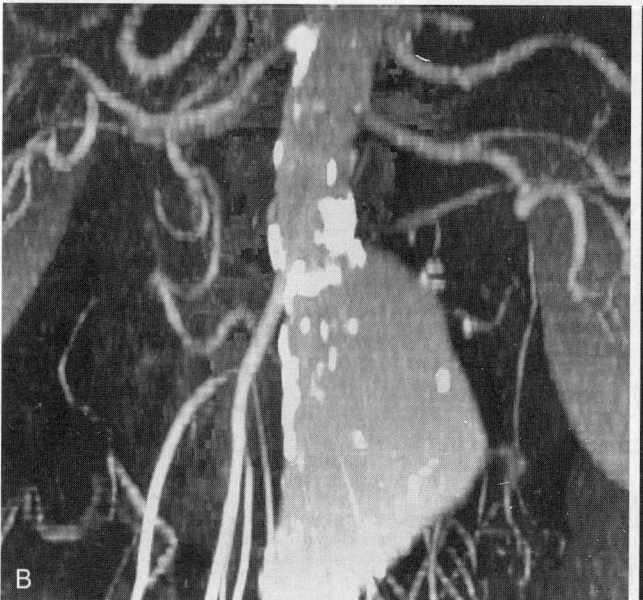

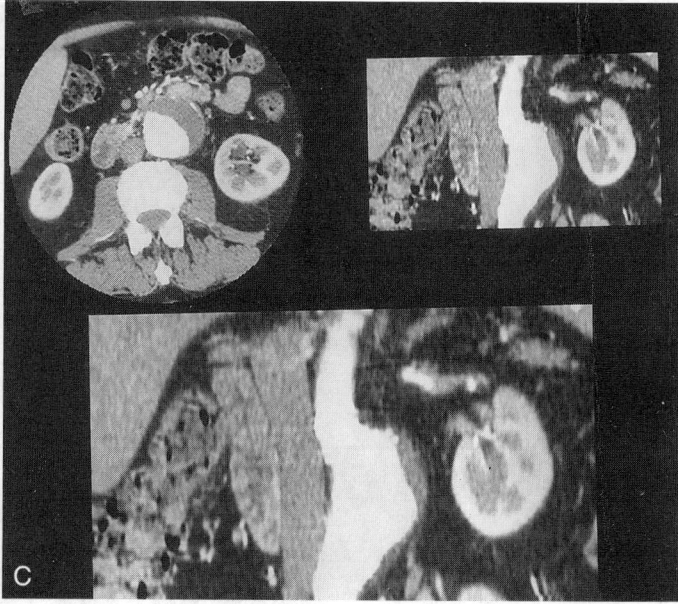

excellent and can be used in evaluating pulmonary embolism, renal artery stenosis, the degree of carotid artery stenosis (Fig. 30–2), and other pathologic conditions including celiac bypass graft occlusion, abdominal aortic dissection, and abdominal aortic aneurysm (Fig. 30–3).

MAGNETIC RESONANCE IMAGING (MRI) (see Chapters 45 and 443)

MRI has become a powerful tool for clinical diagnosis. Four areas that should experience rapid growth during the next several years are (1) cardiac imaging of function and coronary angiography, (2) brain functional imaging, (3) spectroscopic imaging of metabolite content, including the neurotransmitter GABA (gamma amino butyric acid) in the human brain, and (4) high field high-resolution imaging (Table 30–1). Just as much of the progress over the last 10 years was made possible by the availability of higher field superconducting magnets (0.5T to 1.5T), similar improvements should be expected from the increasing use of the next generation of high field magnets—4T, and most recently 7 and 8T systems.

BRAIN FUNCTIONAL IMAGING. Images collected using a gradient echo sequence are sensitive to the oxygenation state of the cerebral venous system. Specifically, regions that increase their oxyhemoglobin:deoxyhemoglobin ratio show increases in image signal intensity. When performing a mental or physical task, blood flow to the affected area of the brain increases, typically outstripping the requirement for oxygen utilization. This in turn causes the venous system to have a higher oxyhemoglobin:deoxyhemoglobin content, thereby enhancing its signal intensity. By subtracting images acquired before and during the activating task, the region of the brain associated with the task is highlighted. This method has been used to localize the effects of visual stimulation, various motor functions, and word association. In the past several years this method has also been used clinically to localize various brain functions to plan surgery. The activation (those regions of the brain that show a significant increase in signal) is thresholded and then overlaid on a high-resolution anatomic image for reference (Fig. 30–4).

SPECTROSCOPIC IMAGING. In epilepsy, measurements of N-acetyl aspartate (NAA), a specific marker of neurons, has allowed a noninvasive determination of neuronal loss and damage, permitting lateralization of the affected areas. Similar measurements in Alzhei-

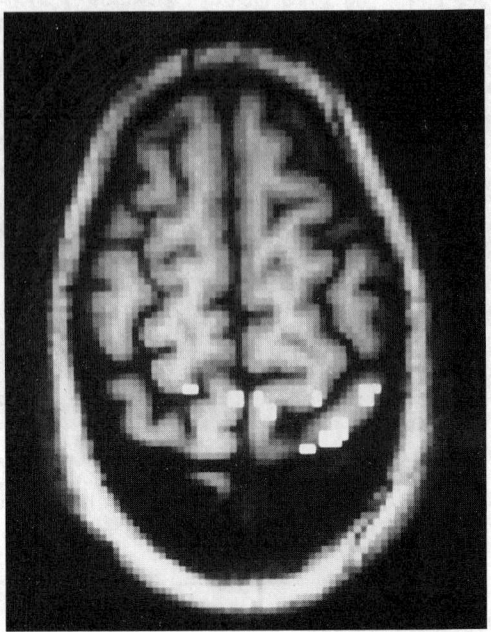

FIGURE 30–4 ■ Functional brain activation image. The regions of the brain showing activation during finger tapping are highlighted and overlaid on an MRI of the same section. (Courtesy of Donald Tweig, PhD, and Graeme Mason, PhD, University of Alabama at Birmingham.)

mer's disease may also prove useful in localizing affected brain regions. In multiple sclerosis, measurements of choline—a compound that becomes elevated during membrane breakdown—permits an assessment of the degree of active demyelination. Recent methods have permitted the planar and multislice imaging of these compounds at spatial resolutions of less than 0.2cc. In a multiple sclerosis patient, affected regions display significant deviations in the ratios of creatine/NAA and choline/NAA from control levels. Recent efforts have focused on extending these measurements to enable the visualization of neurologically active compounds such as

Table 30–1 ■ MAJOR CLINICAL APPLICATIONS OF IMAGING PROCEDURES*

MODALITY	COMPUTED TOMOGRAPHY	GENERAL NUCLEAR MEDICINE	MRI	SPECT	^{18}F-FDG PET	PET	MRSI	fMRI
Cancer								
Primary	+++	+	++	+	+			
Metastatic	+	+++ *Bone scan*	+	++^{111}In-MoAb	++Whole-body PET			
Nodal metastasis	+	+	+	+	+++ *FDG*			
Brain								
Epilepsy	+		++	+++ *Ictal rCBF*	+++ *Interictal FDG*		+	
Dementia	+	+	+	+++ *rCBF*	++FDG	+		
Psychiatry	+			++	++FDG	++^{11}C *Neurotransmitters*		
Brain function				++^{133}Xe rCBF	++FDG	+++^{15}OH$_2$O	+	++
Heart								
Cardiac perfusion		+++^{201}Tl-201		++^{201}Tl- and ^{99m}Tc-MIBI SPECT		+^{13}N ammonia		
Cardiac viability		+^{99m}Tc-RBCs RNV		+^{201}Tl- and gated ^{99m}Tc-MIBI SPECT	+++ *FDG*			

*Image modalities providing the best diagnostic value for major disease categories: 3+ is the best, 2+ provides near equivalent information, 1+ is useful but as a secondary choice, and blanks have little clinical utility. General nuclear medicine includes routine technetium-99m ^{99m}(Tc)–labeled tracers for planar imaging. RNV is radionuclide ventriculography performed by obtaining equilibrium gated blood pool cardiac images of ^{99m}Tc-labeled red blood cells (RBCs). Single photon emission computed tomography (SPECT) includes imaging of brain regional cerebral blood flow (rCBF) tracers such as ^{99m}Tc-HMPAO, cardiac perfusion tracers such as thallium-201 (^{201}Tl) and ^{99m}Tc-sestamibi (^{99m}Tc-MIBI), and indium-111–labeled monoclonal antibodies (^{111}MoAb) used for tumor imaging. The most widely used PET tracer, fluorine-18–labeled fluorodeoxyglucose (^{18}F-FDG), is used for metabolic imaging in many diseases. The positron-emitting isotopes (^{11}C, ^{15}O, and ^{13}N) are more limited in their clinical utilization. Magnetic resonance spectroscopic imaging (MRSI) and functional magnetic resonance imaging (fMRI) can be performed on conventional 1.5T magnets but are best on high field scanners.

glutamate and GABA. Using this methodology, the effects of various anti-epileptics and mood altering substances on GABA levels can be determined. As these methods become more routine, spectroscopic studies will no longer be limited to the diagnosis of pathological changes in cell types, but will serve as sensitive probes of brain function and metabolism.

HIGH-RESOLUTION IMAGING. The improved signal-to-noise ratio at 4.1T permits images of the human brain with 250 to 500 μM in plane resolution (a factor of 2 to 4 higher than that commonly obtained at 1.5T) from tomographic slices 3 mm thick. The higher resolution improves visualization of the basal ganglia and thalamus, frequently the site of small strokes (Fig. 30–5A). The images display excellent definition of a number of anatomic features of the brain (caudate head, globus pallidus, and putamen). The greater spatial resolution and gray/white matter contrast combine to improve the definition of the hippocampus, critical to diagnose temporal lobe epilepsy (see Fig. 30–5B). The enhanced T_2^* contrast and high spatial resolution enable visualization of small

cerebral vessels, which may aid in the diagnosis of idiopathic Parkinson's disease (see Fig. 30–5C). Finally, the T_2^* contrast and high spatial resolution enable visualization of small cerebral vessels, which are not detectable in conventional clinical imaging studies (see Fig. 30–5D).

ADVANCES IN NUCLEAR MEDICINE IMAGING

BRAIN SPECT APPLICATIONS. Single photon emission computed tomography (SPECT) can be performed using a standard Anger camera to acquire multiple views of the radiotracer distribution over 360 degrees and reconstruct the radioactivity distribution of 3D space. The data are stored in a pixel matrix that can be displayed in the transverse, coronal, and sagittal planes.

The radionuclide technetium-99m hexamethylpropyleneamine ox-

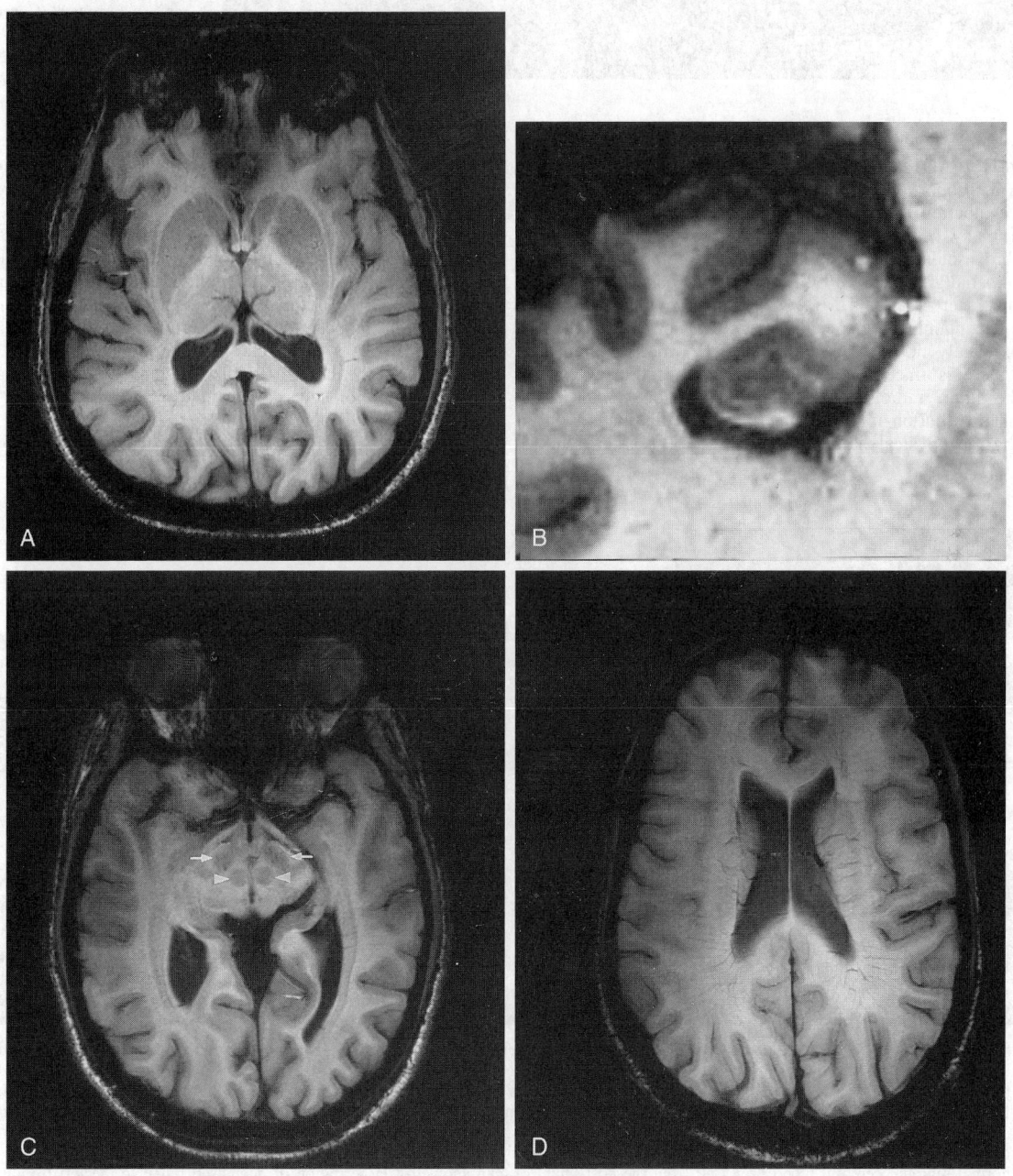

FIGURE 30–5 ■ *A,* High-resolution MRI (460 m in plane resolution from a 3-mm section) of a healthy human brain acquired at 4.1T at the level of the thalamus. *B,* Magnified portion of a coronal MRI of a healthy human brain displaying the internal structure of the hippocampus. *C,* Axial image at the level of the red muclei (arrowheads) and substantia nigra (arrows). *D,* Axial image displaying the multitude of small venous vessels.

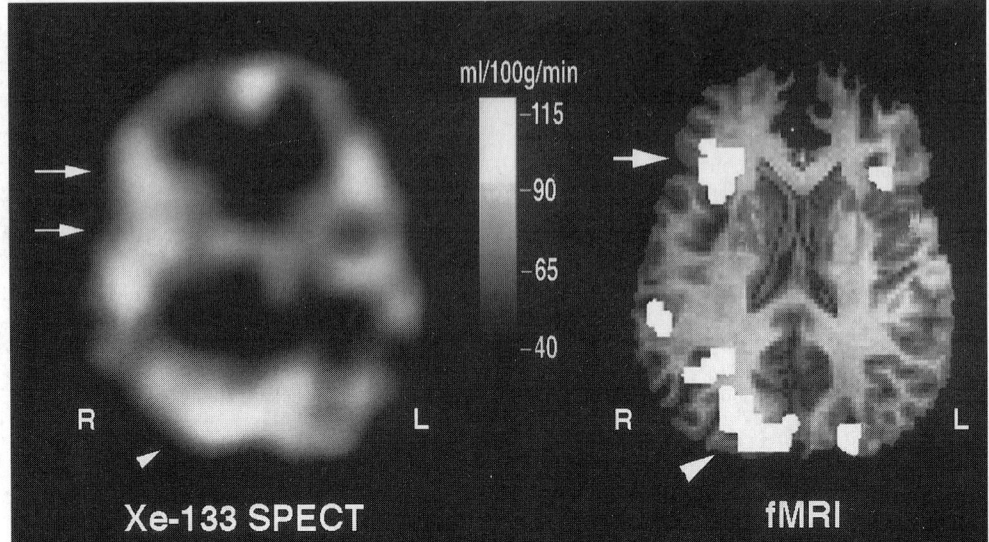

FIGURE 30–6 ■ Images from a normal subject performing a mental rotation task. The xenon-133 SPECT image (left) shows increases in blood flow to the right parieto-occipital (arrowhead) and right frontal cerebral hemisphere (arrows). The fMR BOLD image (right) shows areas of activation (white squares) in the same brain regions (arrows). (Courtesy of Georg Deutsch, PhD, and Donald Tweig, PhD, University of Alabama at Birmingham.)

ime (Tc-99m HMPAO) is a brain blood flow tracer that is extracted by the brain in proportion to regional cerebral blood flow (rCBF). Brain rCBF evaluation is extremely useful clinically to evaluate the diagnosis of many central nervous system diseases including dementia, cerebrovascular disease, epilepsy, and psychiatric disorders.

Activation paradigm brain SPECT is possible because of rapid uptake of the tracer Tc-99m HMPAO (essentially within the time that the blood containing the tracer makes a first pass through the brain, approximately 30 to 45 seconds after IV injection), during which time there is tracer uptake, incorporation, and irreversible trapping. The brain radioisotopic tracer distribution retains this fixed cerebral distribution in essence permanently, dissipating only as dictated by the physical half-life of the tracer ($t_{1/2}$ = 6 hours).

Owing to the irreversible binding and nonredistribution, this isotopic distribution is the end result of the actual brain SPECT image, which may commence many minutes after tracer injection and requires approximately 30 minutes acquisition time.

The rCBF uptake pattern over a short time interval (e.g., days) within the same subject is highly reproducible because the anatomy, location of brain functional regions, and brain metabolic activity do not appear to change significantly. As a result, the tracer Tc-99m HMPAO is especially well suited for brain activation studies because the change in distribution between mental states can yield information regarding which brain regions are responsible for the specific functional state under study.

The recent development of Xe-133 dynamic brain SPECT imag-

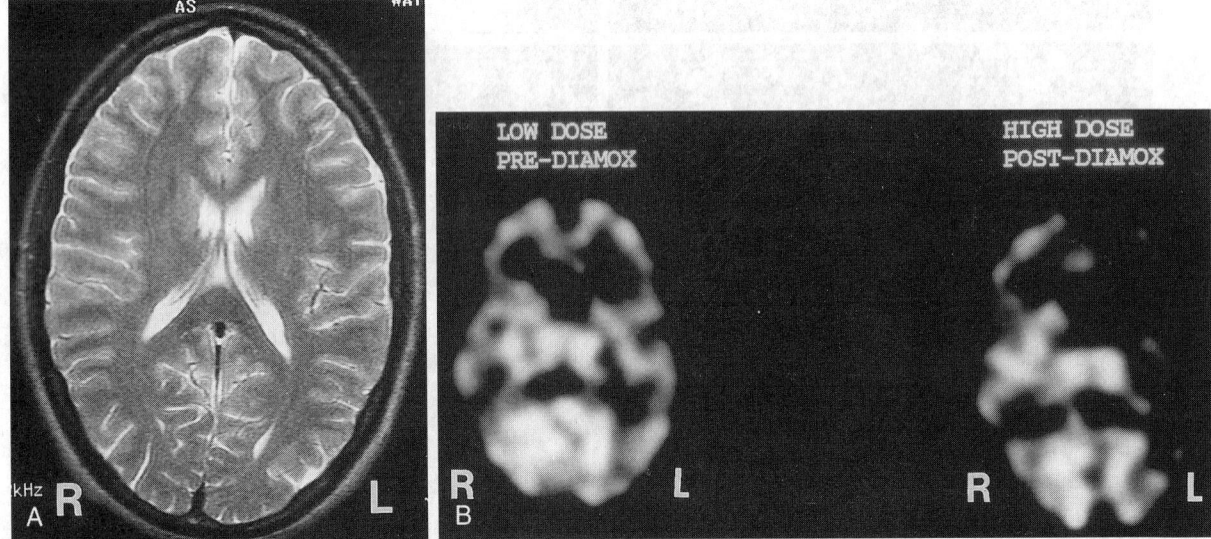

FIGURE 30–7 ■ *A*, A 58-year-old man complained of transient neurologic deficits of motor function involving the right upper and lower extremities. Angiography showed 100% blockage of the left internal carotid artery. Owing to compromised cerebral blood flow, evaluation for a surgical revascularization procedure was performed. The illustrated MRI is normal. (From Mountz JM, Deutsch G, Khan SH: Regional cerebral blood flow changes in stroke image by Tc-99m HMPAO SPECT with corresponding anatomic image comparison. Clin Nucl Med 18:1067, 1993). *B*, An acetazolamide (Diamox) vascular stress test was performed to determine if the viability of the left internal carotid vascular territory was in jeopardy. The pre-Diamox SPECT scan demonstrates normal regional cerebral blood flow (left), but the post-Diamox scan showed a large region of decreased rCBF to the left frontal, temporal, and parietal lobes, representing severe rCBF compromise to the entire distribution of the left internal carotid artery (right). This case exemplifies the ability of the brain to provide effective vascular collateral supplies to the territory of a major arterial blockade. The cerebrovascular stress test clearly revealed the limitations of this collateral circulation. (From Mountz JM, Deutsch G, Kuzniecky R, et al: Brain SPECT: 1994 update. In Freeman LM [ed]: Nuclear Medicine Annual 1994. New York, Raven Press, 1994.)

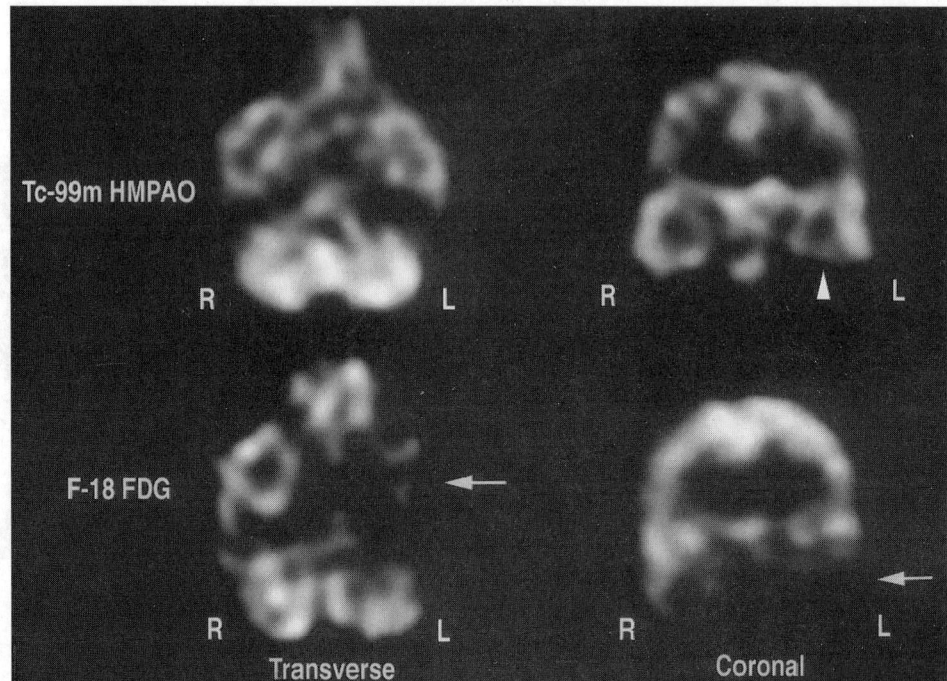

FIGURE 30-8 ■ Interictal transverse and coronal rCBF SPECT images from a 19-year-old man with temporal lobe epilepsy (top). Only slightly decreased perfusion is seen in the medial left temporal lobe (arrowhead). Hypometabolism in the left temporal lobe (characteristic of temporal lobe epilepsy) is clearly visualized (arrows) on the ^{18}F-FDG coincidence camera images (bottom).

ing provides several advancements for measuring brain activation states. Following the inhalation of Xenon/air mixture, this technique measures Xe-133 clearance for each pixel from a rapidly acquired series of tomographic scans and provides absolute quantification of rCBF in units of ml/100g/min. This technique also has greater sensitivity in detection of blood flow changes in the brain as compared to conventional rCBF brain SPECT. The major current limitation is that these scans have relatively low resolution due to the low counts per pixel acquired in the rapid scanning procedure and the low energy photon emission of Xe-133.

Functional brain imaging can now be extended to measure the subtle changes in brain activity associated with thinking. For example, the mental rotation task produces prominent right parietal and right frontal lobe activation, which is evident on both the Xe-133

and BOLD MRI images (Fig. 30–6). These procedures have the potential to detect congnition and thought as well as abnormal brain activation patterns attributable to psychiatric disease and may eventually lead to a more accurate anatomically-based categorization of psychiatric illness.

Regional CBF brain SPECT can identify patients at risk for stroke who may benefit from neurosurgical revascularization procedures. Pharmacologic manipulation to detect cerebrovascular insufficiency is also possible using the cerebral vasodilator acetazolamide (Diamox). Diamox stress tests use a protocol employing two sequential brain SPECT scans. The first SPECT scan (rest scan) is obtained after injecting Tc-99m HMPAO (5 mCi) at rest. Then Diamox (1 gram) is administered intravenously and, after a 20 minute waiting period for vasoreactive change, a second higher

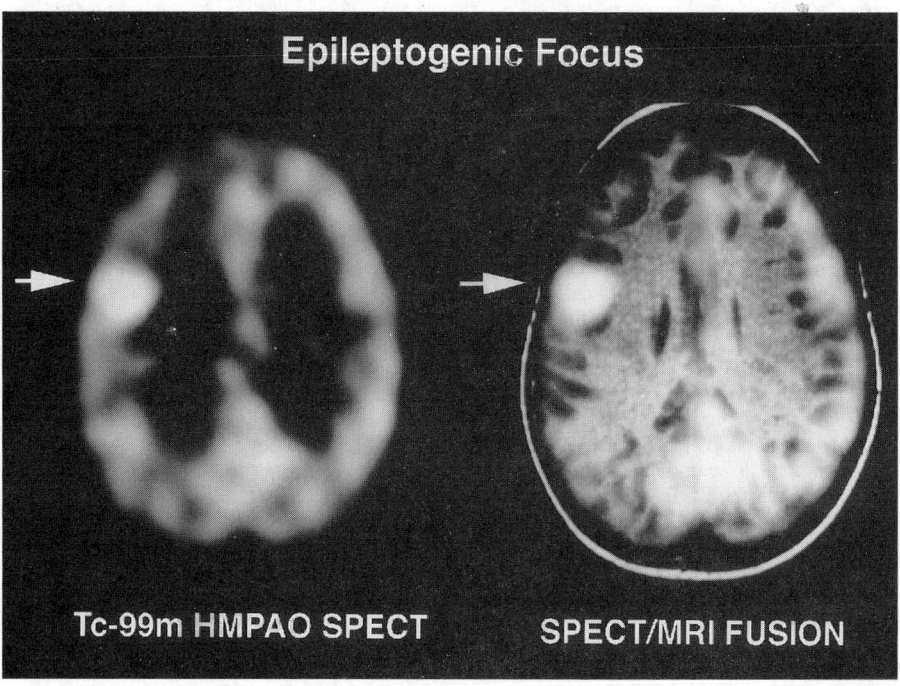

FIGURE 30–9 ■ An ictal ^{99m}Tc-HMPAO SPECT scan section from a 9-year-old boy with intractable non-localizable seizures (left) shows a region of marked hyperperfusion in the right dorsolateral frontal lobe (arrow). The patient's SPECT scan was registered and overlaid to its corresponding location on the patient's MRI to produce a "fusion" image (right).

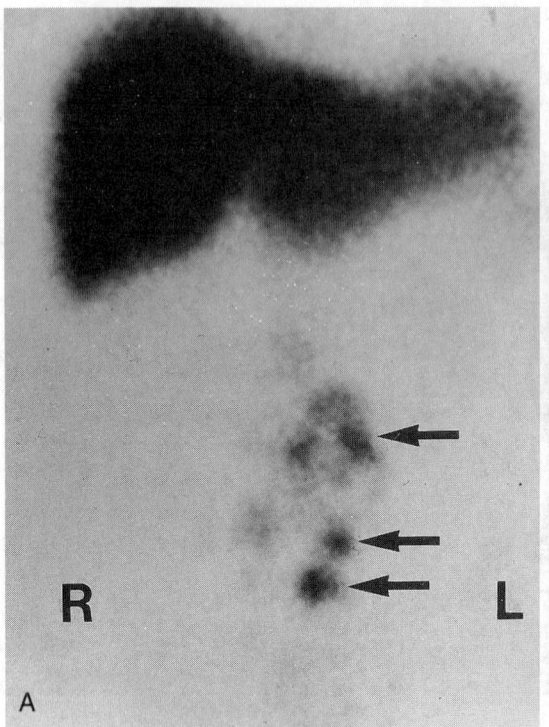
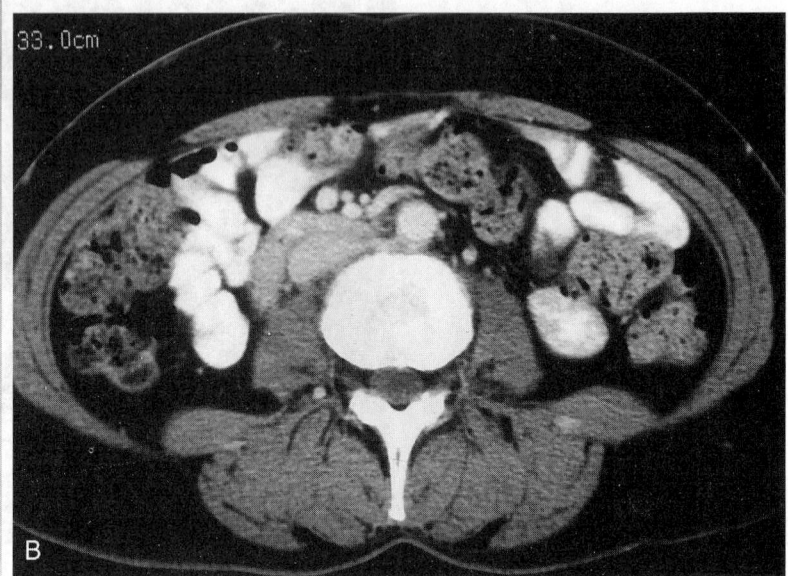

FIGURE 30–10 ■ *A*, A 47-year-old woman was evaluated for metastatic ovarian carcinoma. After the injection of 6 mCi of indium-111–labeled CYT-103, numerous regions of increased tracer uptake representing metastatic carcinoma were found. Even in retrospect, the metastatic disease could not be identified on contrast medium–enhanced CT. *B*, A CT scan section through the level of the lower abdomen of the same patient shows no definite abnormalities. This illustrates the high sensitivity for detecting metastases that can be obtained using indium-111–labeled monoclonal antibody tracers.

dose of Tc-99m HMPAO (20 mCi) is injected and the patient undergoes a second brain SPECT scan (stress scan) (Fig. 30–7). During the stress scan the vascularly comprised territories of brain blood flow show a relative decrease in tracer uptake compared with the rest scan.

Functional metabolic abnormalities and rCBF changes have been known to occur in partial seizures for many years. The development of coincidence SPECT cameras capable of imaging the two 511 KeV photons from positron emitting tracers will greatly increase the clinical application of F-18 Fluorodeoxyglucose (F-18 FDG) for evaluation of diseases of the brain and heart and in the detection of primary and metastatic neoplastic disease. These cameras can perform both conventional nuclear medicine imaging and "PET" imaging. Fluorine-18 has sufficient half life (109 minutes) to be distributed regionally, further permitting its widespread routine use in diagnostic nuclear medicine (Fig. 30–8).

The rationale for injecting Tc-99m HMPAO during the ictal phase of a seizure is based on the observation that rCBF is temporally and focally increased during the ictal phase of a seizure in patients with extra-temporal lobe epilepsy. The precise region of this neuronal hyperexcitability can be localized because Tc-99m HMPAO has rapid uptake without redistribution. When the patient is stabilized after the seizure, the subsequent brain SPECT scan several hours later reflects the dramatic increase in rCBF that occurred during the first few seconds of the seizure (not the actual rCBF at the time of the scan). This injection and scan procedure is most revealing in extra-temporal lobe epilepsy patients without clear localization by any other laboratory or imaging criteria. In extra-temporal lobe epilepsy (particularly frontal lobe epilepsy), ictal rCBF brain SPECT studies are extremely useful in localizing the seizure focus. In patients undergoing limited brain resection guided by the abnormal rCBF brain SPECT scan, the ictal SPECT findings accurately localize the brain region responsible for seizures, as confirmed by the pathology of the resected tissue as well as the seizure-free postsurgery course (Fig. 30–9).

Cerebral necrosis following brain tumor therapy is a significant problem. Distinction between necrosis and residual or recurrent viable tumor cannot be accurately evaluated by either CT or MRI because conventional anatomic neuroimaging modalities depend on alterations in blood-brain barrier permeability in order to evaluate tumor size. Functional imaging of metabolic activity allows clear distinction between new, recurrent, or residual, viable, high-grade glioblastoma and brain necrosis. Functional imaging not only can determine tumor grade and viability status but also can measure tumor size. SPECT imaging using the radioisotopes thallium-201 (Tl-201) and Tc-99m 2-methoxy-isobutyl-isonitrile (Tc-99m MIBI) have been shown to be both sensitive and specific for detecting viable portions of high-grade brain tumor. Tl-201 acts as a potassium analog and is taken up into the metabolically active tumor cell based on the increased Na$^+$ K$^+$-ATPase enzyme activity.

Brain SPECT has also made significant advances in using neuronal receptor-binding tracers to evaluate brain disease. The iodine-123–labeled tracer ((S)-(−)-3-iodo-2-hydroxy-6-methoxy-N-[(1-ethyl-2-pyrrolidinyl)-methyl]benzamide [iodine-123 IBZM]) is an example of a tracer that can map the dopamine D-2 receptor and has been used to investigate dopamine receptor distributions in movement disorders and schizophrenia. Muscarinic acetylcholine receptor distribution has been evaluated in Alzheimer's disease using the iodine-123-labeled tracer ((R)-3-quinuclidinyl-4-iodobenzilate [iodine-123 QNB]). The central benzodiazepine receptor distribution in epilepsy patients has been evaluated with iodine-123–labeled iomazenil. These tracer studies have elucidated the role of neurochemical receptors in the pathogenesis of neurologic and psychiatric disorders; this understanding is important for the development of pharmacologic therapies specifically targeted for these receptors.

MOLECULAR NUCLEAR MEDICINE IMAGING. Monoclonal antibodies have played an important role in the development of this target-specific imaging method. For example, a radiolabeled monoclonal antibody, indium-III CYT-103 (OncoScint CR/OV), is used for clinical imaging of colorectal and ovarian carcinoma (Fig. 30–10).

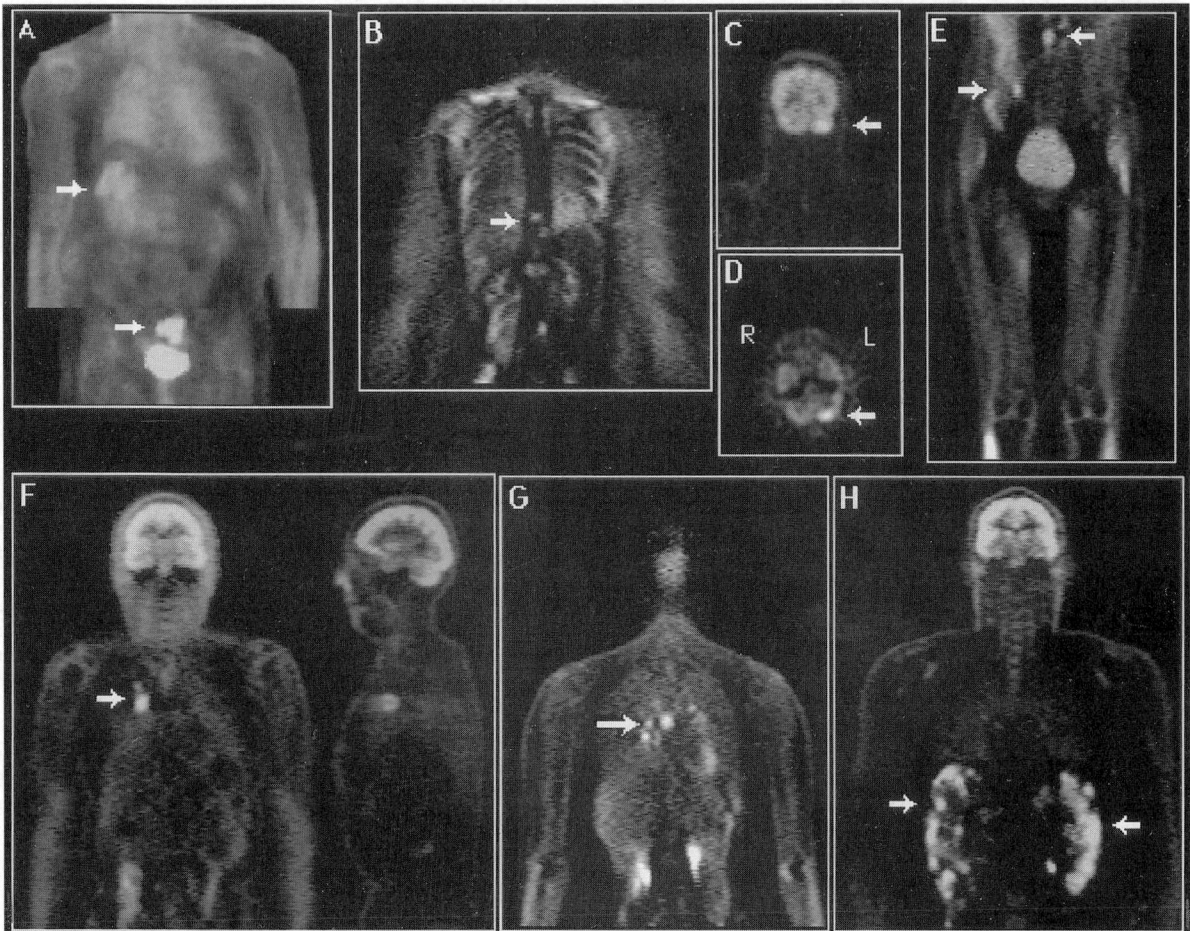

FIGURE 30–11 ▪ Whole-body ¹⁸F-FDG PET scans. All scans were obtained on the Siemens 931 tomograph after injection of 10 mCi of ¹⁸F-FDG (after a 40-minute uptake period) using the whole-body acquisition and processing technique. The images were not corrected for attenuation. *A,* Projection image (2D) of the torso of a patient with primary colorectal carcinoma (lower arrow) with metastases to the liver (upper arrow). The patient was fasting; therefore, very little myocardial uptake is evident. Selected coronal tomographic sections (*B* and *C*) and transaxial (*D*) images are from a breast cancer patient with metastases to the spine (*B,* multiple lesions at level of arrow and below) and the cerebellum (*C* and *D*). *E,* Coronal tomographic image illustrating abdominal metastases (arrows) in a patient with ovarian carcinoma. *F,* Coronal and sagittal tomographic image through the torso and head of a patient with a primary bronchogenic carcinoma (arrow). *G,* Coronal tomographic image of a patient with Hodgkin's disease with involvement of multiple thoracic nodes (arrow). *H,* Coronal tomographic image of a patient with metastatic melanoma to the liver and spleen (arrows). (From Hawkins RA, Hoh C, Dahlbom M, et al: PET cancer evaluation with FDG. J Nucl Med 32:1555, 1991.)

POSITRON EMISSION TOMOGRAPHY (PET). Methods for whole-body PET imaging have been used in a variety of cancers, including colorectal carcinoma, lung cancer, head and neck cancer, primary and metastatic brain tumor, breast carcinoma, lymphoma, melanoma, bone cancer, and other soft tissue cancers (Fig. 30–11). A variety of radiopharmaceuticals are currently included in clinical tumor-imaging protocols, including metabolic substrates such as fluorine-18 fluorodeoxyglucose (fluorine-18 FDG).

Deyn PP, Dierckx RA, Alavi A, Pickut BA (eds): Brain SPECT in Neurology and Psychiatry. London, John Libbey & Co, 1997. *Extensive description of many clinical applications of brain SPECT imaging.*

Hoh CK, Schiepers C, Seltzer MA, et al. PET in oncology: Will it replace the other modalities? Seminars in Nuclear Medicine, 27:94–106, 1997. *Review of the current clinical applications of positron emission tomography in oncology.*

Kremkau FW, Merritt CR, Carson PL, et al. The American Institute of Ultrasound in Medicine and the Society of Radiologists in Ultrasound: Future directions in diagnostic US. Radiology, 209:305–11, 1998. *Description of contemporary applications of ultrasound in medicine.*

Springer SP, Deutsch G (eds): Left Brain Right Brain: Perspectives from Cognitive Neuroscience, 5th ed. New York, WH Freeman & Co, 1998. *Relationship between brain anatomy and brain function.*

PART VI

PRINCIPLES OF HUMAN GENETICS

31 HUMAN HEREDITY

Harry W. Schroeder, Jr.

Genetics as an experimental science owes its origins to Gregor Mendel and his cross-breeding of garden peas in 1865. He identified specific physical characteristics *(phenotypes),* such as seed color and plant height, that could be transmitted from one generation to the next. Each phenotype was ascribed to hereditary factors, later designated *genes,* that were inherited in pairs, one each from the male and female parent. True-breeding plants *(homozygotes)* inherited identical factors from the parental plants, whereas non–true-breeding plants *(hybrids* or *heterozygotes)* inherited alternative factors *(alleles)* from each parent. Some alleles were shown to have a greater effect on the phenotype of hybrids than others. In the case of a *dominant* allele, a single copy of the gene was sufficient to produce the same phenotype seen in homozygous organisms. Latent or *recessive* genes could not be detected by studying the phenotype of the hybrid parent. Detecting these genes in the hybrid required breeding the plants and demonstrating the presence of offspring that bore the recessive phenotype. Mendel's experiments led to the formulation of the laws of *unit inheritance* (that factors retain their identity from generation to generation and do not blend in the hybrid), of *segregation* (that two members [alleles] of a single pair of factors [genes] are never found in the same gamete but always segregate), and of *independent assortment* (that members of different pairs of genes [non-alleles] assort to gametes independently of one another). These laws were first applied to human disease by Sir Archibald Garrod in his studies of "inborn errors of metabolism" in 1908 (see Chapter 32).

Genetic information is encoded in the sequence of a linear polymer of purine and pyrimidine bases termed *deoxyribonucleic acid* (DNA). Each purine or pyrimidine pairs with a complementary base (A:T and G:C) (Table 31–1) to form two antiparallel polynucleotide strands that are twisted into a double helix. Each strand is thus complementary to the other. DNA strands are covered with histone and non-histone proteins that allow them to be supercoiled and twisted into compact structures termed *chromosomes.* There are 23 pairs of chromosomes per somatic nucleus, 22 pairs of autosomes numbered by descending size, and 1 pair of sex chromosomes (X + X, female; X + Y, male). These chromosomes are located in the nucleus of the cell. During *mitosis,* the chromosomes are unwound and the DNA is split apart and copied. Each replicated strand creates a complete copy of the original DNA double helix, allowing the transmission of a complete set of genetic information into each daughter cell. In *meiosis,* a reduction division of genetic information occurs. Allelic chromosomes are paired, duplicated, and separated. Only one of the allelic pair of chromosomes is allowed to segregate into the gamete. Thus, a *diploid* germ cell gives rise to a *haploid* sperm or egg that contains an assortment of one of each of the 23 pairs of allelic chromosomes in the parental cell. During fertilization, sperm and egg unite to create a zygote with a complete set of 46 chromosomes. These fundamental properties of DNA and cell division are the basis of Mendel's laws of unit inheritance, segregation, and independent assortment.

The central dogma of molecular genetics holds that each gene encodes one polypeptide (Fig. 31–1). Each human cell contains approximately 3.9×10^9 base pairs of DNA per haploid genome, or enough to encode about 1 million polypeptides of average length. Estimates of the number of structural genes in humans range from 50,000 to 100,000; thus, more than 90% of DNA does not encode peptide sequences. Non-coding DNA often plays a major role in the regulation of gene expression (see Fig. 31–1).

Table 31–1 ■ THE GENETIC CODE

1ST	2ND								3RD
	U		C		A		G		
U	UUU	Phe	UCU	Ser	UAU	Tyr	UGU	Cys	U
	UUC	Phe	UCC	Ser	UAC	Tyr	UGC	Cys	C
	UUA	Leu	UCA	Ser	UAA	Stop	UGA	Stop	A
	UUG	Leu	UCG	Ser	UAG	Stop	UGG	Trp	G
C	CUU	Leu	CCU	Pro	CAU	His	CGU	Arg	U
	CUC	Leu	CCC	Pro	CAC	His	CGC	Arg	C
	CUA	Leu	CCA	Pro	CAA	Gln	CGA	Arg	A
	CUG	Leu	CCG	Pro	CAG	Gln	CGG	Arg	G
A	AUU	Ile	ACU	Thr	AAU	Asn	AGU	Ser	U
	AUC	Ile	ACC	Thr	AAC	Asn	AGC	Ser	C
	AUA	Ile	ACA	Thr	AAA	Lys	AGA	Arg	A
	AUG	Met	ACG	Thr	AAG	Lys	AGG	Arg	G
G	GUU	Val	GCU	Ala	GAU	Asp	GGU	Gly	U
	GUC	Val	GCC	Ala	GAC	Asp	GGC	Gly	C
	GUA	Val	GCA	Ala	GAA	Glu	GGA	Gly	A
	GUG	Val	GCG	Ala	GAG	Glu	GGG	Gly	G

Three adjacent bases of RNA form a codon that specifies 1 of 20 different amino acids or 1 of 3 termination codons. A = adenine; C = cytosine; G = guanine; U = uridine. (In DNA, thymine [T] replaces uridine). The first base in the codon is identified on the left, the second base is identified at the top of the chart, and the third base is identified on the right. Each codon is followed by the amino acid it encodes. The amino acids are identified by their standard three-letter code. Ala = alanine; Arg = arginine; Asn = asparagine; Asp = aspartic acid; Cys = cysteine; Gln = glutamine; Glu = glutamic acid; Gly = glycine; His = histidine; Ile = isoleucine; Leu = leucine; Lys = lysine; Met = methionine; Phe = phenylalanine; Pro = proline; Ser = serine; Thr = threonine; Trp = tryptophan; Tyr = tyrosine; and Val = valine. Stop = termination codon.

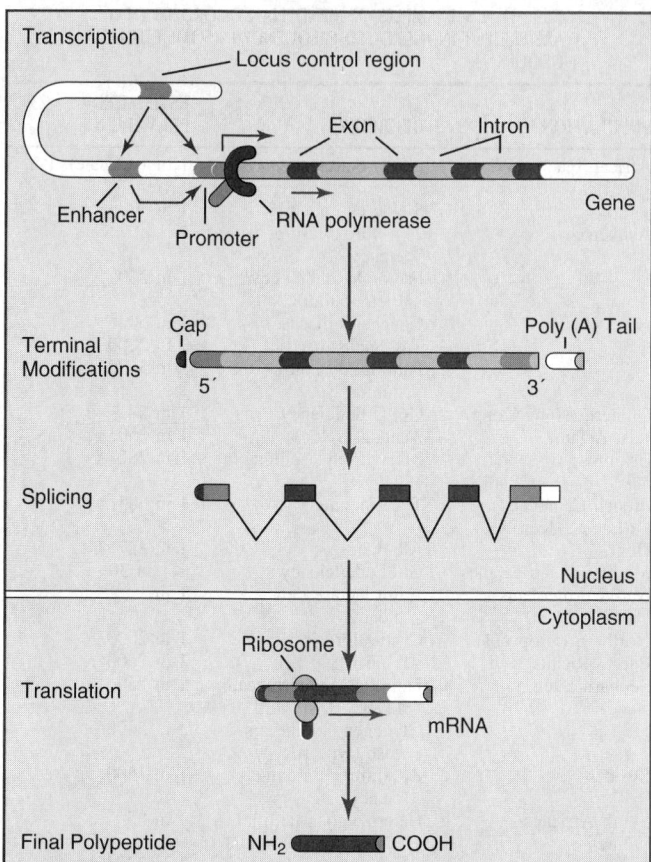

FIGURE 31-1 ■ The flow of genetic information from gene to polypeptide proceeds in a stepwise fashion. Located near the gene are DNA control regions that specify the transcription start site *(promoters)*, define the tissue specificity of the gene *(enhancers)*, and control the use of linked genes during ontogeny *(locus control regions)*. The regions of DNA that specify the sequence of a polypeptide chain, or structural genes, are organized into discrete units *(exons)* that are separated by noncoding sequences *(introns)*. The sequence of the DNA is *transcribed* in the nucleus into RNA, a less stable nucleic acid that can be turned over rapidly. The termini of the RNA are modified to partially stabilize the final product, and the intervening introns are spliced out, generating messenger ribonucleic acid *(mRNA)*. The mRNA is transported from the nucleus to the cytoplasm, where it is *translated* by ribosomes into polypeptide strands.

Non-coding DNA can also play a structural role in the function of the cell such as forming regions important for the structural stability of the chromosome (e.g., *matrix-associated regions*) or specialized sequences that define the ends of the chromosome *(telomeres)* and the site of attachment at the time of meiosis and mitosis *(centromeres)*. However, approximately 10% of cellular DNA consists of a repetitive sequence that has been randomly inserted throughout the genome. Although the function of this repetitive DNA is unknown, its presence has proven useful for gene mapping studies.

RECOMBINATION

Genes linked and transmitted by chromosomes seem to violate Mendel's laws of independent assortment and segregation because effectively there would be only 23 sets of genes. During the process of meiosis, allelic chromosomes are brought into close juxtaposition (Fig. 31-2). Single-strand breaks occur in the chromosomes and allow bridges, or *chiasmata*, to form between homologous portions of the chromosomes. This *crossing-over* of DNA strands allows allelic chromosomes to *recombine*, forming patchwork or *chimeric* chromosomes that contain portions of each of the parental chromosomes. Although recombination can occur anywhere in the chromosome, only a limited number of chiasmata form during each meiosis. Two genes that are on opposite ends of the chromosome may thus behave as if they were on different chromosomes, whereas recombination is less likely between genes

that are very close in their primary sequence to each other. The increased frequency of the joint inheritance of two genes that are closely linked on a chromosome is termed *linkage disequilibrium*.

Distances between genes on a chromosome can be quantified by their physical distance from each other in millions of base pairs *(megabases)* or by their genetic distance, as measured by the frequency of recombination between the two genes per generation. One per cent of genetic recombination is known as a *centimorgan*. On average, 1 centimorgan covers approximately 1 megabase of DNA. However, the relationship between linear and genetic distance is not absolute. The frequency of recombination, and thus the genetic distance between genes in specific regions of the genome, may differ depending on the sequence or the ancillary proteins that cover the DNA. Recombination frequencies in selected regions of the genome differ in male and female gametes, implying that segments of chromosomes can be handled differently by testicular and ovarian cells. This disparity can lead to differences in the function of alleles, depending on whether they have been inherited from the mother or the father, a process termed *imprinting*.

MUTATION

Broadly defined, a *mutation* is a stable, heritable alteration in the DNA sequence that can be passed from a cell to its progeny. From the standpoint of evolution, mutations are essential to generate sufficient genetic diversity to permit species to adapt to their environment through the mechanism of "natural selection." The normal rate of mutation is approximately 10^{-7} base pair changes per generation; thus, on average, individuals pass on 390 base pair changes to their offspring. Alterations of DNA sequence in cells of the body that do not give rise to germ cells are termed *somatic mutations*. Although by definition these alterations are not transmitted to the gametes, the mutations are passed on to the progeny of the

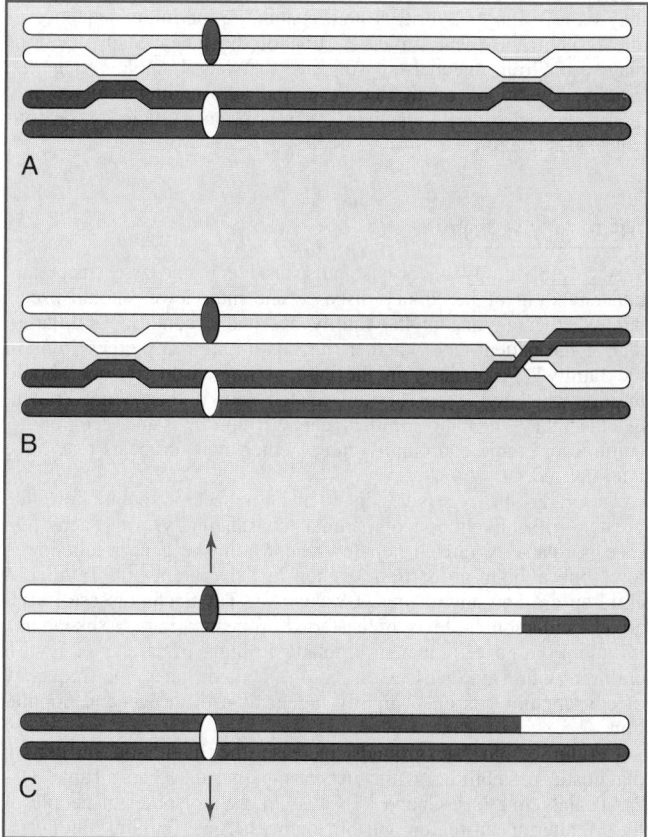

FIGURE 31-2 ■ Crossing-over and chiasmata formation. *A,* During meiosis, homologous chromatids are attached to each other at sites of sequence identity. *B,* Single-stranded breaks allow bridges or chiasmata to form. *C,* Crossing-over of the DNA strands allows the allelic chromatids to recombine, generating a chimeric chromatid.

mutated cells. Somatic mutations in *oncogenes,* for example, underlie the development of many cancers (see Chapter 191).

Mutations may involve millions of base pairs in the structure of a chromosome, as in duplications, deletions, and translocations of a portion of one chromosome to another (see Chapter 34). Mutations can involve an entire human genome of 3.9 billion base pairs, as in triploidy, in which a third copy of the entire chromosomal complement occurs. At the other extreme, a mutation can be minute and involve a small deletion or insertion or it can be a replacement of only a single base pair *(point mutation).* Point mutations in coding regions may be of three types: (1) a *synonymous* or *silent* mutation (about 23% of random base substitutions in coding regions), in which the base replacement does not lead to a change in the amino acid but only to a different codon for the same amino acid; (2) a *missense* or *replacement* mutation (about 73% of base substitutions in coding regions), in which the base change results in substitution of one amino acid for another; and (3) a *nonsense* mutation (about 4% of base substitutions in coding regions), in which the base change generates one of the termination codons. Deletions or insertions that occur in a coding region can alter the reading frame distal to the mutation *(frameshift* mutations). Frameshift mutations frequently alter the protein sequence and can lead to premature peptide termination by generating a stop codon.

The functional consequences of mutations may vary depending on the location of the mutation. Enzymes, for example, exhibit a hierarchy of resistance to mutation. The catalytic site is exquisitely sensitive, and a single mutation may abrogate function. The hydrophobic core provides structural stability for the molecule, and amino acid changes may result in an unstable protein product that is temperature sensitive, falling apart at high temperature. Finally, portions of the hydrophilic exterior may serve primarily to promote solubility, and changes in amino acid sequence that preserve polarity may have minimal consequences.

Large deletions may interrupt a coding region and cause an absence of one or more closely linked protein products. If the deletion removes a bridge between two coding regions, the result may be a fusion or hybrid protein containing the initial sequence of one protein and the terminal portion of the other. Such deletions may result from unequal crossing over between homologous genes. Finally, alterations of the DNA in the surrounding regions may lead to changes in RNA splicing, transcriptional efficiency, or control of tissue expression.

THE FAMILY HISTORY

A careful family history is indispensable in the assessment and understanding of hereditary disease. The interviewer should ascertain whether anyone in the family has had a condition similar to that of the patient, and whether this condition or any other "runs in the family." Particularly in the case of rare disorders, one should inquire whether the parents are related and, if this is not known, whether they or their families came from the same geographic, cultural, or ethnic community and whether their forebears may have intermarried.

The rarer the recessive disorder in a specific population, the greater is the likelihood of parental consanguinity. Tay-Sachs disease is relatively rare in non-Jews, in whom the gene frequency is low, but a high proportion of non-Jewish parents of Tay-Sachs children are consanguineous. By contrast, Tay-Sachs disease is relatively common in Jews of eastern European origin (Ashkenazis), in whom the gene frequency is relatively high. In parents of Jewish children with Tay-Sachs disease in the United States, the frequency of consanguinity is only slightly higher than in the general population.

Certain ethnic backgrounds increase the likelihood of certain diagnostic possibilities while decreasing that of others (Table 31–2). Thalassemia (see Chapter 167) is chiefly a disorder of people of the Mediterranean region and of Southeast Asia, familial Mediterranean fever (see Chapters 171 and 297) is a disorder of Armenians and Sephardic Jews, acatalasia is a disease of Japanese and Koreans, and gout (see Chapter 299) is very common among the Maori. By contrast, cystic fibrosis (see Chapter 76) is rare in African blacks, phenylketonuria (see Chapter 209) is uncommon in Jews,

Table 31–2 ■ EXAMPLES OF MENDELIAN DISORDERS THAT ARE PRESENT IN INCREASED FREQUENCY IN SOME ETHNIC GROUPS

POPULATION	DISORDER	ESTIMATED PREVALENCE
African blacks (West Africa)	G6PD deficiency	1 in 10 (male), 1 in 5 (female)
	Sickle cell anemia	1 in 500
Ashkenazi Jews	21-Hydroxylase deficiency	1 in 30
	Factor XI deficiency (hemophilia C)	1 in 200
	Gaucher's disease	1 in 600
	Tay-Sachs disease	1 in 2000
	Familial dysautonomia	1 in 3600
Chinese (Hong Kong)	G6PD deficiency	1 in 28
East Asians	Acatalasia	1 in 250
Eskimos	21-Hydroxylase deficiency	1 in 282
French Canadians (Lac St. Jean)	Tyrosinemia	1 in 685
Hopi	Albinism	1 in 227
Mediterranean peoples	G6PD deficiency	<1 in 30
Native Americans	Adult lactase deficiency	1 in 1
Northern Europeans	Cystic fibrosis	1 in 2000
Puerto Ricans	Albinism	1 in 2000
Sephardic Jews	Familial Mediterranean fever	1 in 250
	Glycogen storage disease (type III)	1 in 5400
Swedes	α_1-Antitrypsin deficiency	1 in 1500
South Africans (whites)	Heterozygous familial hypercholesterolemia	1 in 85
	Porphyria variegata	1 in 330
Thais	Hemoglobin E	1 in 200

and sickle cell anemia (see Chapter 169) does not occur in Northern Europeans.

PEDIGREE ANALYSIS

The chief method to study an inherited disease in humans is to observe its pattern of distribution in families or *kindreds,* that is, its pattern in a *pedigree* (Fig. 31–3). The construction of a pedigree begins with the individual first detected, who is referred to as the *proband* or *index case.* The pedigree pattern allows one to judge whether the distribution conforms to mendelian principles of segregation and assortment and thus represents single-factor inheritance. Patterns that do not conform to mendelian principles may represent

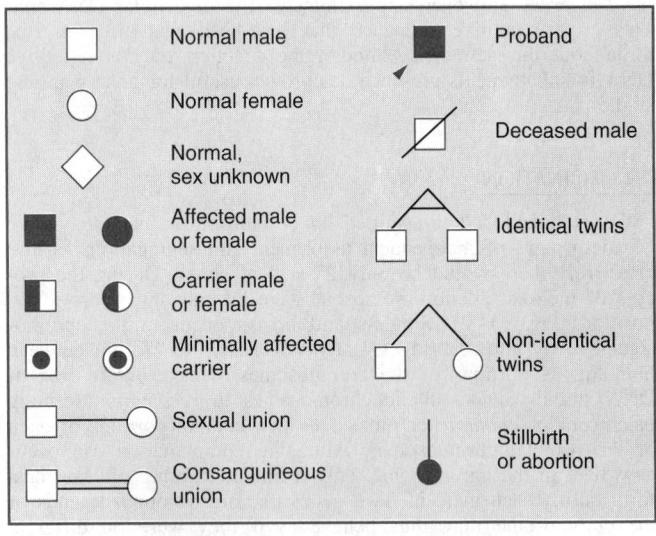

FIGURE 31–3 ■ Standard pedigree symbols.

polygenic traits in which a number of genes each contributes a minor effect. Valid pedigrees depend on accurate and extensive information about the kindred. This information is likely to be more reliable when based on detection by the physician than when based on memory.

MAPPING THE HUMAN GENOME

The International Human Genome Project began in 1990 with the stated goals of developing genetic and physical maps and determining the complete DNA sequence of the human genome. Elucidation of the genetic maps has been aided by the development of several novel molecular techniques. One very useful technique takes advantage of repetitive sequences found in the genome, such as runs of di-, tri-, or tetranucleotide repeats (e.g., CA_n, CAG_n, or $CAGA_n$). The repeat regions are subject to considerable evolutionary slippage, resulting in duplications and deletion. By means of the polymerase chain reaction (PCR), DNA oligonucleotide probes that bind uniquely to either side of a repeat region can be used to rapidly amplify and visualize the size of the repeat. These size variations create a number of different alleles, or PCR *markers,* for each repeat region. A series of markers on each chromosome can be used to create a genetic linkage map of the genome. The more closely a marker is linked to the gene or trait of interest, the more likely it is that the marker will be transmitted to the offspring along with that gene. By analyzing the inheritance of a series of markers in families with genetic disease, it becomes possible to find the rough location of the disease gene. The second type of genome map, the physical map, is an actual assemblage of DNA clones lined up in the same order as they appear on the chromosome. Determination of the actual sequence of the genome has been aided by the rapid development of automated sequence analyzers. As this chapter is written, 5% of the genome has been sequenced and the goal is to complete the sequence by the year 2005.

The ultimate goal is to use this mapping and sequence information to isolate and study the structure and function of genes that can contribute to the development of disease. A number of disease genes that function in a simple mendelian fashion, most notably the genes for cystic fibrosis, neurofibromatosis (see Chapter 522), Huntington's disease (see Chapter 463), familial breast cancer (see Chapter 258) and others, have already been isolated.

MONOGENIC DISORDERS

Disorders caused by single mutant genes show one of four simple (mendelian) patterns of inheritance: (1) autosomal dominant, (2) autosomal recessive, (3) X-linked dominant, or (4) X-linked recessive. Dominant traits are those expressed in the heterozygote (as well as in the homozygote or hemizygote). Recessive traits are those expressed in the homozygotes (or hemizygotes) but silent in the heterozygote. The terms *dominant* and *recessive* refer to the phenotypic expression of the trait, not to the expression of the gene. Thus, it is incorrect to speak of a dominant or recessive gene. A gene is either expressed or not expressed. Whether the trait is considered dominant or recessive often depends on the level of observation. Sickle cell anemia is a recessive trait; that is, it requires a double dose of the abnormal gene for expression at the clinical level. Nevertheless, the sickle gene is expressed in single dose as well, giving rise to carriers with SA hemoglobin. In a state of reduced oxygen tension, red blood cells in SA carriers may sickle. Recessive traits may thus be *codominant* when viewed biochemically at the level of the gene product or dominant in an altered environment.

With few exceptions, each of the more than 3000 mendelian diseases is rare. The overall population frequency of monogenic disorders is about 10 per 1000 live births, comprising about 7 per 1000 dominants, about 2.5 per 1000 recessives, and about 0.4 per 1000 X-linked conditions (Table 31–3).

If a particular disease shows a mendelian pattern of inheritance, its pathogenesis, no matter how complex, is likely due to a single abnormal gene. For example, in homozygous patients with sickle cell (SS) disease, such seemingly unrelated disturbances as hemolytic anemia, painful crises, nephropathy, vascular occlusions, and *Salmonella* osteomyelitis are all physiologic consequences of a sin-

Table 31–3 ■ ESTIMATED PREVALENCE OF SELECTED MONOGENIC DISORDERS IN THE UNITED STATES

DISORDER	ESTIMATED PREVALENCE
Autosomal Dominant	
von Willebrand's disease	1 in 125
Familial hypercholesterolemia	1 in 500
Acute intermittent porphyria	1 in 500 (psychiatric admissions)
Polycystic kidney disease	1 in 1,250
Hypertrophic obstructive cardio- myopathy	1 in 1,500
Huntington's disease	1 in 2,500
Hereditary spherocytosis	1 in 5,000
Acute intermittent porphyria	1 in 10,000
Osteogenesis imperfecta tarda	1 in 15,000
Marfan syndrome	1 in 20,000
Autosomal Recessive	
Hemochromatosis	1 in 400
Sickle cell anemia	1 in 625 (US/blacks)
Cystic fibrosis	1 in 2,500 (US/whites)
α_1-Antitrypsin deficiency	1 in 4,000
Tay-Sachs disease	1 in 3,000 (US/Jews)
Cystinuria	1 in 7,000
Phenylketonuria	1 in 10,000
Albinism	1 in 10,000 (US/blacks)
21-Hydroxylase deficiency	1 in 14,000
Albinism	1 in 18,000 (US/whites)
Mucopolysaccharidoses (all types)	1 in 25,000
Glycogen storage disease (all types)	1 in 50,000
Galactosemia	1 in 57,000
Wilson's disease	1 in 100,000
Homocystinuria	1 in 200,000
X-Linked	
G6PD deficiency	1 in 10 (US/blacks)
Fragile X syndrome	1 in 1,500 (males)
Duchenne muscular dystrophy	1 in 7,000 (males)
Hemophilia (A + B)	1 in 10,000 (males)

gle missense mutation, resulting in a single amino acid substitution in both β-globin chains of hemoglobin ($\alpha_2\beta_2$). When two or more phenotypic characters are controlled by a single gene, that gene is said to have *pleiotropic* effects.

AUTOSOMAL DOMINANT TRAITS. Autosomal genes are those genes situated on chromosomes other than the X or Y. When there are two alleles—A and a—at a locus, three possible genotypes exist: *AA, Aa,* and *aa.* Genotypes *AA* and *aa* are *homozygotes; Aa* is a *heterozygote.*

Dominant traits are fully manifest in the presence of a gene in the heterozygous state, that is, when only one abnormal gene *(mutant allele)* is present and the corresponding partner allele on the homologous chromosome is normal. Figure 31–4 shows a typical pedigree of transmission of an autosomal dominant trait. The following features are characteristic: (1) each affected individual has an affected parent (unless the condition arose by a new mutation in a germ cell that formed the individual); (2) an affected individual usually bears an equal number of affected and unaffected offspring; (3) males and females are affected in equal numbers; (4) each gender can transmit the trait to male and female; (5) normal children of an affected individual have only normal offspring; and (6) when the trait does not impair viability or reproductive capacity, *vertical* transmission of the trait occurs through successive generations. Three or more generations of male-to-male transmission argue against X-linkage of a rare gene.

Many autosomal dominant disorders show two additional characteristics that are not seen in recessive disorders: (1) marked variability in severity, or *expressivity,* and (2) delayed age at onset. Dominant traits in humans often exert only mild effects and are thus not completely dominant in a mendelian sense. Occasionally, the expression of the abnormal gene is so weak that a generation appears to be skipped because the carrier of the abnormal gene is clinically normal. When this is the case, the trait is said to be *nonpenetrant.* When a gene of a dominant trait exists in the homozygous state, the effect may be very severe, perhaps lethal. Examples are common in animals, in which experimental matings can be constructed, but are rare in humans, because matings of two affected heterozygotes are exceptional. One example is homozygous

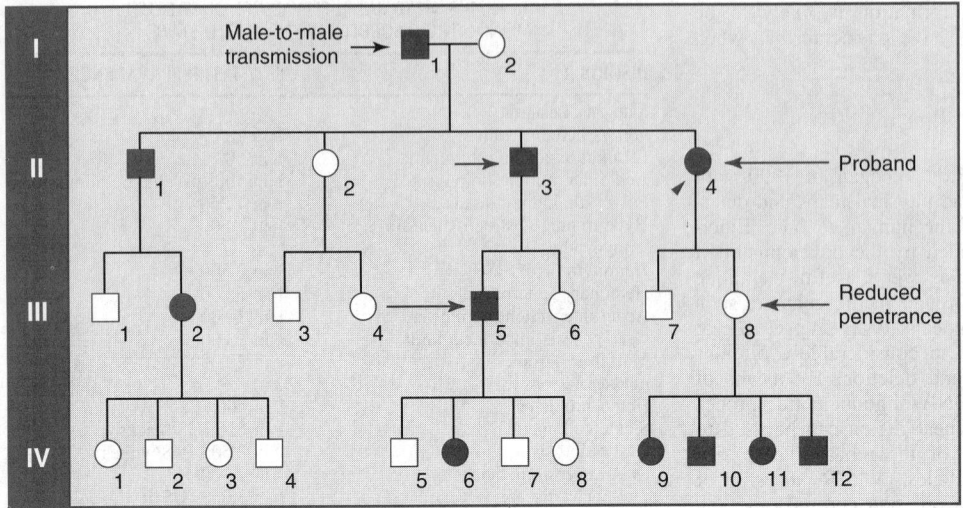

FIGURE 31–4 ■ Pedigree of an autosomal dominant trait. Solid symbols indicate those affected. The generation is indicated by roman numerals, and individuals in each generation are sequentially assigned roman numerals. Three generations of male-to-male transmission provide strong evidence of the autosomal dominant transmission of the trait. Although the likelihood of inheriting the disease gene is 50% for each offspring, by chance alone all or none of the children in individual families may be affected. By phenotype, individual III.8 does not express the trait. (See text for further details.)

familial hypercholesterolemia. Others possibly include achondroplasia and Osler-Weber-Rendu syndrome. Delayed age at onset is seen in Huntington's disease and adult polycystic kidney disease. These disorders do not become manifest clinically until adult life, even though the mutant gene has been present since conception.

In every autosomal dominant disease some affected persons owe their disorder to a new mutation rather than to an inherited allele. Because a reasonable estimate of the frequency of mutation is on the order of 5×10^{-6} mutation per allele per generation (or $\sim 1 \times 10^{-8}$ mutation per codon) and because a dominant trait requires a mutation in only one of the parental gametes, one would expect that about 1 in 100,000 newborns would possess a new mutation in any given gene. Many mutations are silent or recessive and are not manifest in a single gene dose. However, others cause a defective gene product that gives rise to a dominant trait.

Regions of trinucleotide repeats, such as $(CAG)_n$, appear to be at increased risk for slippage during DNA replication. The longer the repeat, the higher the risk of slippage. In genes that contain such repeats, this process appears to be the basis of *anticipation,* wherein the manifestations of a mutation are apparent at a younger age in each succeeding generation. Examples include myotonic dystrophy and the children of fathers with Huntington's disease.

The percentage of patients with dominant disorders that represent new mutations is inversely proportional to the effect of the disease on biologic fitness (i.e., survival to adult life) and reproductive capacity. If a dominant mutation produces early death or absolute infertility, genetic transmission is impossible, and all cases represent new mutations. In tuberous sclerosis, the severe mental retardation reduces biologic fitness to about 20% of normal and the proportion of cases due to new mutations is about 80%. In dominant conditions such as familial hypercholesterolemia, in which there is no reduction in biologic fitness, virtually all cases have a family pedigree showing classic vertical transmission.

For some genes, new mutations appear to be more frequent in the germ cells of fathers of relatively advanced age. Both Marfan syndrome (see Chapter 215) and achondroplastic dwarfism display a "paternal age effect." Fathers of sporadic cases of both conditions are an average of 5 to 7 years older than the general population of fathers or than fathers who transmit these syndromes because of an inherited mutation. Diagnosis of a new mutation must exclude low expressivity of the trait in the carrier parent and also mistaken paternity.

Study of the molecular basis of autosomal dominant disorders has yielded a number of novel insights. Because in a dominant disorder the mutation expressed in only 50% of the gene product may be sufficient to cause disease, mutations can involve proteins that regulate complex metabolic pathways (e.g., membrane receptors as in familial hypercholesterolemia), and structural or non-enzymic proteins (e.g., hemoglobin or collagen) or a membrane protein (e.g., in hereditary spherocytosis). However, in hereditary retinoblastoma, the autosomal dominant trait reflects an absence of the *rb* gene on one allele and is non-penetrant until a somatic mutation occurs on the second allele, creating a homozygous state. In this case, the autosomal dominant trait reflects increased susceptibility to the consequences of a second mutation. Conditions such as these emphasize that the distinction between recessive and dominant inheritance is one of perception and detection.

AUTOSOMAL RECESSIVE DISORDERS. Autosomal recessive conditions are clinically apparent only in the homozygous state, that is, when both alleles at a particular genetic locus are mutant alleles. In most autosomal recessive disorders the clinical presentation tends to be more uniform than in dominant diseases, and the onset is often early in life. Figure 31–5 shows a typical pedigree of an autosomal recessive trait. The following features are characteristic: (1) the parents are clinically normal; (2) only siblings are affected; (3) males and females are affected in equal proportions; (4) if an affected individual marries a homozygous normal person, none of the children is affected but all are heterozygous carriers; (5) if an affected individual marries a heterozygous carrier, one half of the children are affected, and the pedigree pattern superficially suggests a dominant trait; (6) if two individuals who are homozygous for the same mutant gene marry, all of their children are affected; (7) if both parents are heterozygous at the same genetic locus, one fourth of their children are homozygous affected, on average one fourth are homozygous normal, and one half are heterozygous carriers of the same mutant gene; and (8) the less frequent the mutant gene is in the population, the greater the likelihood that the affected individual is the product of consanguineous parents.

In actual practice, unless the kinship is very large, the ratio of affected to unaffected sibs is frequently greater than 1:4. Including probands in the enumeration loads the results in favor of the trait. In a sibship of 10 or more children, the loading factor is not pronounced. However, in all ascertainable one-child sibships the involvement is 100%, in two-child sibships it is 67% (when the fundamental probability is 50%), in three-child sibships it is 57%, and so on. In small sibships a correction must be made for *bias of ascertainment.* The simplest method is to exclude the proband from the calculation and to determine the proportion of affected children among the remaining siblings.

A *completely recessive* disease is one in which the heterozygote is clinically normal. When some features of the disease are detectable in the heterozygote, the disease is sometimes said to show *intermediate inheritance,* or to be *incompletely recessive* or *incompletely dominant.* The ambiguity of these terms from classic genetic studies of phenotypes is further emphasized by results of different methods of detecting gene effects. In many instances of completely recessive inheritance, refined laboratory observations enable the recognition of the trait in the clinically normal heterozygote. In Tay-Sachs disease, for example, clinically normal parents and some siblings can be shown to be heterozygotes by assay of hexosaminidase A in leukocytes. With the advent of molecular techniques,

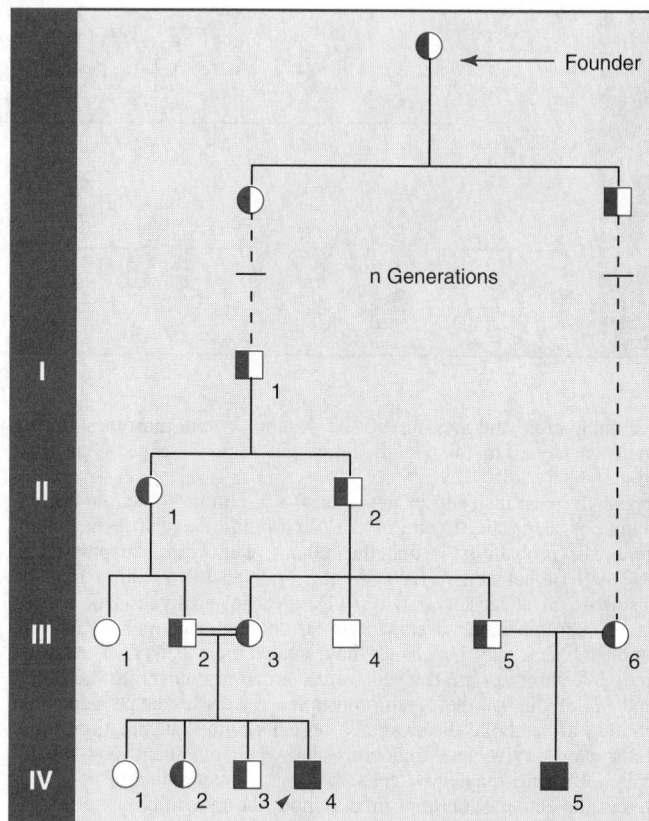

FIGURE 31–5 ■ Pedigree of an autosomal recessive trait. Note that both parents (III.2 and III.3) of the affected proband (IV.4) are heterozygous for the trait. Two siblings of the proband are carriers, and one is normal (IV.1). The double line (═══) indicates that the parents of the proband are related by descent (first cousins). In isolated populations, individuals are more likely to share a common ancestor (the founder). Although technically not consanguineous, marriage in an inbred society often leads to a higher risk for having affected offspring. (See text for further details.)

detection of heterozygotes by direct mutation analysis is becoming increasingly feasible. Because of its importance in genetic counseling, detecting healthy heterozygous carriers of genes that, in the homozygous state, cause overt disease is one of the most significant aspects of medical genetics.

In pure form a recessive disease requires the inheritance of identical mutant genes from both parents. When the mutant genes are rare, the likelihood that any two unrelated parents are carriers for the same defect is small. Inheriting two different mutant genes derived from the same locus gives rise to *heteroallelic compounds.* The classic example is Hb SC disease, in which different abnormal β-globin genes have been inherited from each parent. As we identify and sequence a broad array of disease genes, many more such examples are being found. Alternative mutations contribute to varied manifestations of disorders of the same gene. Within a family, affected individuals are likely to have the same mutations. Therefore, ascertaining the effects of a mutation in a proband can have predictive value for other members of the family.

If the parents of a child with a recessive disorder have a common ancestor who carried a mutant gene, the likelihood that two of the descendants would each have inherited the gene increases. The less frequent the gene, the stronger is the likelihood that an affected individual has resulted from a consanguineous mating. First cousins share, on the average, one eighth of their genes. When two first cousins marry, an offspring has, on the average, one sixteenth of the loci homozygous for a gene derived from a common ancestor. In general, offspring of a first-cousin mating are slightly more likely to have congenital malformations, as well as mental defects and metabolic diseases, than are children born to unrelated parents.

Increased frequency of consanguinity is not observed if the recessive disease is common. Sickle cell anemia, phenylketonuria, cystic fibrosis, and Tay-Sachs disease are examples in which the carrier (heterozygote) state is frequent in certain populations and in which consanguinity is usually not present in the parents. Consanguinity would also not be expected in dominant or X-linked traits or genetic compounds. When the disease allele is identical, it is likely that the gene was in fact inherited from a distant common ancestor, or *founder.*

A high percentage of recessive disorders involves abnormalities

of enzyme proteins. In most reactions the normal maximal enzyme activity is greatly in excess of catalytic requirements; that is, the concentration of a substrate is usually maintained at a point well below saturation for the enzyme that metabolizes it. Hence a reduction to 50% of normal activity in a heterozygote does not impair the health of the carrier, whereas a total or nearly total deficiency may result in a serious inborn error of metabolism (see Chapter 32).

X-LINKED INHERITANCE. Diseases or traits that result from genes located on the X chromosome are termed X-linked. Because the female has two X chromosomes, she may be either heterozygous or homozygous for the mutant gene, and the trait may exhibit recessive or dominant expression. The terms *X-linked dominant* and *X-linked recessive* refer only to expression of the trait in females. The male has only one X chromosome and therefore is *hemizygous* for X-linked traits. Males can be expected to express X-linked traits regardless of their recessive or dominant behavior in the female. This accounts for the large numbers of X-linked diseases. Males transmit their X chromosome to all of their daughters, making them all obligate carriers of an X-linked disease trait. Affected males do not transmit an X chromosome to their sons; thus, an important feature of X-linked inheritance is the absence of male-to-male transmission.

Because the female carries two X chromosomes in each cell, it might be expected that the concentrations of proteins determined by genes on the X chromosome would be twice that of males. This is not the case, and the explanation is provided by the process of X-inactivation first proposed by Mary Lyon, termed *lyonization* in her honor. Although both X chromosomes are active early in ontogeny, with differentiation one of the X chromosomes becomes inactive, condensing to form a *Barr body.* Inactivation is random, so each cell has an equal probability that the paternally or maternally derived X chromosome will be inactivated. Once one of the two X chromosomes is inactivated, the same X chromosome remains inactive throughout all subsequent cell divisions. Thus, on the average one half of the cells of a female express the X chromosome of her father and one half that of her mother. The single exception to this rule is a 2.5-megabase region at the tip of the X chromosome that shares homology with the tip of the Y chromosome, allowing

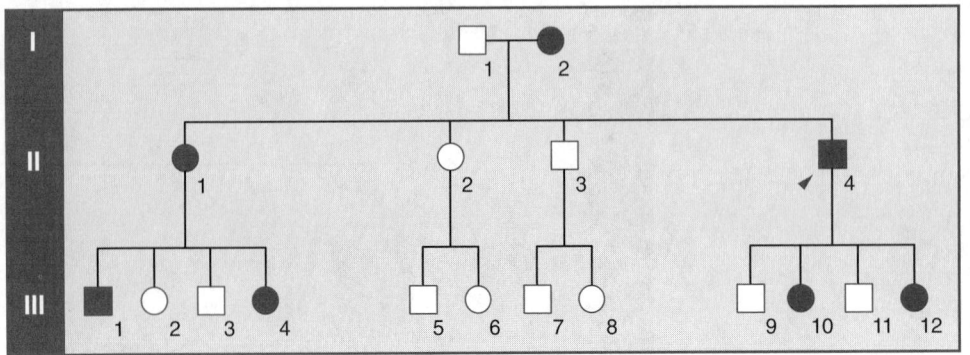

FIGURE 31–6 ■ Pedigree of a dominant X-linked trait. Unlike autosomal dominant inheritance, dominant X-linked traits cannot be passed from a father to a son. (See text for further details.)

recombination and pairing of the X and Y chromosomes during meiosis. Genes in this pseudoautosomal region escape X-inactivation.

For the vast majority of genes on the X chromosome, the normal female is a mosaic. If one of the X chromosomes carries a mutant gene, the probability is that the mutant phenotype is expressed in one half of her cells. However, this statistical probability may be disturbed in at least two ways: (1) Because inactivation of one of the X chromosomes occurs early in development and is random, some females may by chance have many more cells that carry an active X chromosome derived from one parent than from the other; and (2) if one of the X chromosomes carries a mutant gene that confers a metabolic disadvantage on cells with that mutation, these cells may survive less frequently during development, and the female offspring may have cells that carry predominantly or exclusively the active X chromosome without the mutation.

X-LINKED DOMINANT TRAITS. This mode of inheritance (Fig. 31–6) is uncommon. Its characteristic features are as follows: (1) females are affected about twice as often as males; (2) heterozygous females transmit the trait to both genders with a frequency of 50%; (3) hemizygous affected males transmit the trait to all of their daughters and none of their sons; and (4) the expression is more variable and generally less severe in heterozygous females than in hemizygous affected males. Examples of X-linked dominant inheritance include the Xg(a+) blood group, vitamin D–resistant (hypophosphatemic) rickets (see Chapter 263), and pseudohypoparathyroidism (see Chapter 264).

Some rare X-linked dominant disorders occur only in the heterozygous female, because the condition is lethal in the hemizygous affected male. Additional characteristics of this form of inheritance are as follows: (1) an affected mother transmits the trait to one half of her daughters (heterozygotes) and (2) an increased frequency of abortions occurs in affected women, the abortions representing affected male fetuses. Examples of disorders that appear to fit this mode of inheritance include incontinentia pigmenti, focal dermal hypoplasia, orofaciodigital syndrome, and hyperammonemia caused by ornithine transcarbamylase deficiency.

X-LINKED RECESSIVE TRAITS. This mode of inheritance (Fig. 31–7) is relatively common. Its characteristic features are as follows: (1) The disorder is fully expressed only in the hemizygous affected male. (2) Heterozygous females are usually normal; occasionally, they may exhibit mild features of the disorder; rarely they may be almost as severely affected as the hemizygous affected male (this variability is attributed to the probability that a disproportionate percentage of *normal* X chromosomes of the heterozygous female may have been inactivated early in development. (3) On average, a heterozygous female transmits the trait to one half of her sons (hemizygous affected), but the other half are normal. (4) On average, one half of daughters of a heterozygous female are carriers and one half are normal. (5) All daughters of an affected male married to a normal female are carriers, and no sons of such a union are affected (no father-to-son transmission). (6) In the rare event of the union of an affected male and a heterozygous female, one half of the daughters are homozygous affected and one half are

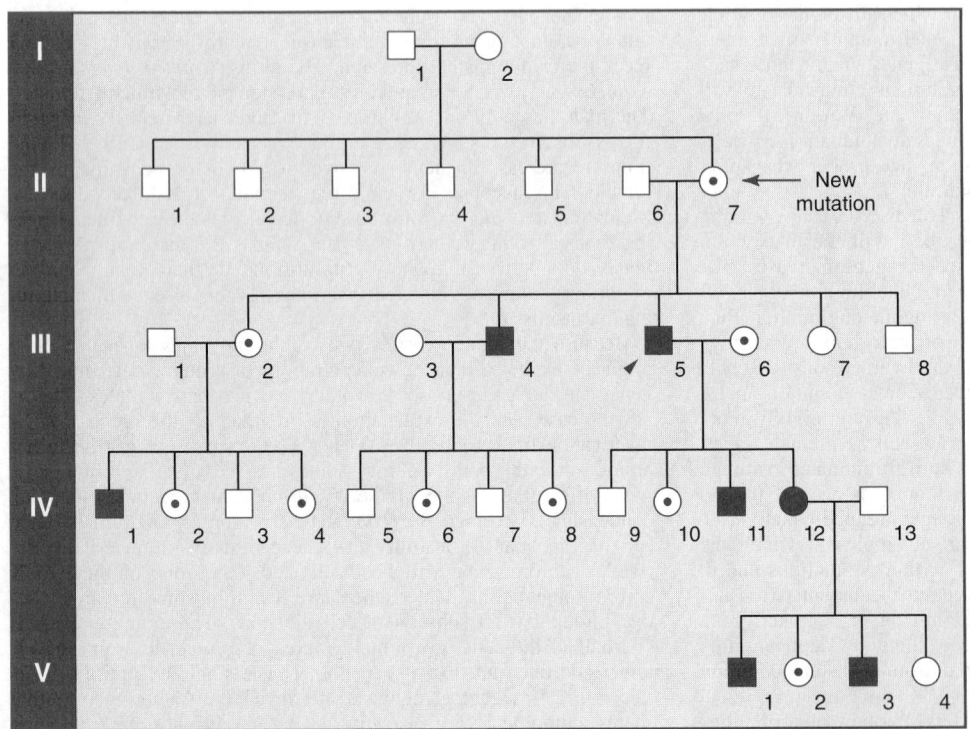

FIGURE 31–7 ■ Pedigree of an X-linked recessive trait. Individual II.7 is the youngest daughter of a family of six siblings. She has two affected sons and five normal brothers. Most likely, the mutation took place in the aged father during spermatogenesis (I.1). The proband (III.5) unfortunately married a female carrier and thus had an affected daughter (IV.12). All of her sons will be affected (e.g., V.1 and V.3). (See text for further details.)

heterozygous carriers; one half of sons are hemizygous affected (maternal inheritance), and one half are normal. Thus, in this situation, one half of all offspring are affected. (7) If the trait is rare, parents and relatives are normal except for male relatives in the female line; for example, on average, one half of maternal uncles are affected. This "uncle and nephew" pattern gives rise to an *oblique* pedigree pattern, in contrast to the vertical pattern of autosomal dominant conditions and the horizontal pattern of autosomal recessive conditions.

Examples of X-linked recessive conditions include hemophilia A, Duchenne's muscular dystrophy, the Lesch-Nyhan syndrome, glucose-6-phosphate dehydrogenase deficiency, and Fabry's disease. In several of these (e.g., Duchenne's muscular dystrophy and Fabry's disease), heterozygous females may exhibit mild or even moderately severe forms of the disease. Colorblindness is also an X-linked inherited trait, but it is sufficiently frequent (occurring in about 8% of white males) that the occurrence of homozygous colorblind females is not rare.

It is important to distinguish between X-linked inheritance and *sex-influenced autosomal dominant inheritance*. Baldness and hemochromatosis are examples of autosomal dominant and recessive traits that are sex influenced. Heterozygous females express the gene for baldness only when a source of testosterone becomes available (e.g., a masculinizing tumor of the ovary). Homozygous females rarely develop clinical hemochromatosis because menstruation and pregnancy mitigate the accumulation of iron.

Y-LINKED INHERITANCE. A gene on the Y chromosome is transmitted through the father to all of his sons and none of his daughters. Only a small number of genes are located on the Y chromosome. Among them is the dominant gene for maleness, *SRY*.

POLYGENIC INHERITANCE

Most phenotypic traits are determined by many genes collaborating at different loci rather than by single gene effects. Polygenic inheritance is suggested for traits that show continuous variation in the form of a normal distribution curve. Height and intelligence are examples of polygenic traits in which the extremes of the distribution are not necessarily considered abnormal. Parents and offspring, and usually siblings also, have 50% of their genes in common. Second-degree relatives share on average one fourth of all genes ($\frac{1}{2}^2$), and third-degree relatives (cousins) share one eighth ($\frac{1}{2}^3$). As the degree of relation becomes more distant, the probability of inheriting the same combination of genes is reduced and the degree of resemblance is likely to be less.

Many of the common chronic diseases of adults (e.g., essential hypertension, diabetes mellitus, hyperuricemia, hypercholesterolemia, coronary artery disease, and schizophrenia) and the common birth defects of children (e.g., cleft palate and lip and congenital heart disease) that tend to run in families fit best into the category of *multifactorial genetic disease*. This category should be suspected

when the pedigree of a disease does not support inheritance in a simple dominant or recessive manner. Multifactorial genetic diseases have both a polygenic component and an environmental component of causative factors. In the population at large, *risk* genes are present in low frequency. If any one individual has a particularly large number of risk genes, the latent disorder becomes overt. When an individual inherits just the right combination of risk genes, he or she passes beyond a "risk threshold" at which environmental factors may determine the expression and severity of disease (Fig. 31–8). For another family member to develop the same disease, that individual would have to inherit the same or a very similar combination of genes. The likelihood of such an occurrence is clearly greater in first-degree than in more distant relatives. The chances of another relative inheriting the right combination of risk genes also decrease as the number of genes required to express a given trait increases. Elegant and complex mathematical models have been advanced for polygenic-multifactorial disease, but these should not obscure the fact that each of the risk genes must express itself, like any other gene, by way of a specific biochemical product. Eventually, the vague concept of genetic susceptibility of polygenic inheritance must yield to the basic premise that genes control the synthesis of specific proteins with specific functions. The major histocompatibility locus or human leukocyte antigen system was one of the first genetic loci to be prominently associated with disease susceptibility (see Chapter 278). Currently, the techniques and tools of the Human Genome Project are being used to identify risk genes for common diseases, such as type I diabetes mellitus (see Chapter 242).

Multifactorial or polygenic inheritance must not be confused with *genetic heterogeneity*. Hypercholesterolemia and hyperuricemia behave as multifactorial traits when viewed at the population level. At the family level, however, it is sometimes possible to identify a single mutation that is mainly responsible for the disease in that family. Examples include (1) familial hypercholesterolemia, an autosomal dominant trait present in about 5% of subjects with premature myocardial infarctions, which in single-gene dosage produces atherosclerosis in the absence of any extraordinary environmental factor, and (2) hypoxanthine-guanine phosphoribosyltransferase deficiency, an X-linked recessive trait present in about 0.5% of subjects with gout, which in the hemizygous state produces marked purine overproduction without any relationship to obesity or alcohol consumption.

MITOCHONDRIAL INHERITANCE

Each mitochondrion contains several circular chromosomes that code for certain ribosomal and transfer RNAs and for 13 polypeptides involved in oxidative phosphorylation, the chief function of the mitochondrion. The mitochondrial code differs from that of nuclear DNA and that of any contemporary prokaryote; it is similar

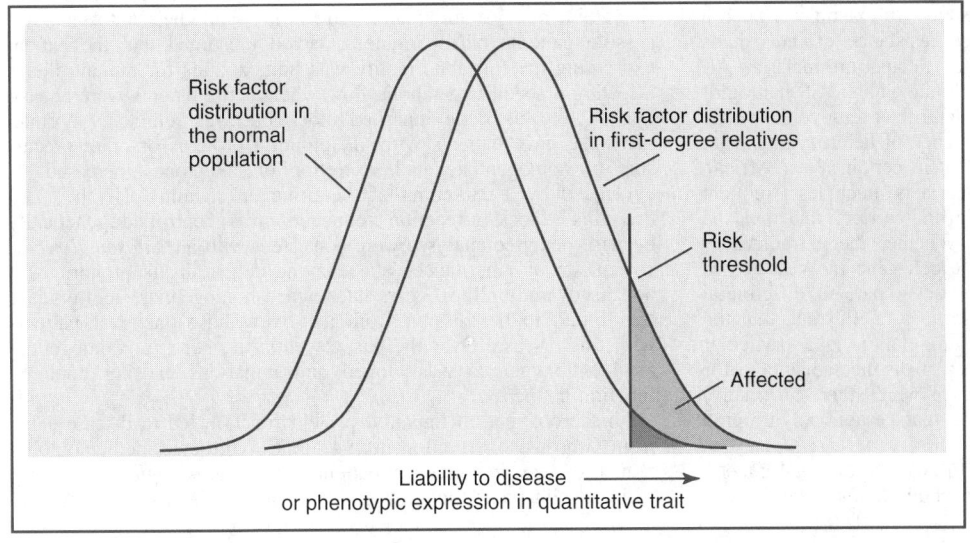

FIGURE 31–8 ■ The darkly shaded area represents the proportion of the population at risk for expression of a disease that conforms to a polygenic multifactorial model of inheritance. The shared inheritance of genes leads to an increased prevalence of disease among the relatives of affected individuals. This increased prevalence is most evident among first-degree relatives (hatched area).

to that of bacteria. Mitochondrial inheritance is exclusively matrilineal. Diseases that are thought to involve mitochondrial mutations include Leber's hereditary optic atrophy, infantile bilateral striatal necrosis, and myoclonic epilepsy with "ragged red fibers."

GENE FREQUENCY

The distribution of a mutant gene in the general population may be calculated on the basis of the Hardy-Weinberg equation. If the frequency of a particular gene A is p, then that of its alternative allele is $(1 - p) = q$. Three genotypes are found in the population: those who are homozygous *AA,* those who are heterozygous *Aa,* and those who are homozygous *aa.* In a randomly mating population, the frequencies of these genotypes are in the proportion p^2 *(AA),* 2 pq *(Aa),* and q^2 *(aa).* An important consequence of this distribution is that irrespective of the initial frequency of the genes A and *a* in the population, the proportion of the three genotypes tends to remain constant in succeeding generations, provided that there is no difference in biologic fitness of any of the genotypes. If viability or fertility among the three genotypes is unequal, if individuals migrate into or out of the population, or if mating is not random, the frequency calculations require considerable correction. In small populations major changes in gene frequency can occur on the basis of chance alone.

If the frequency of a recessive disease in a particular population is known, the frequency of heterozygous carriers and of the abnormal gene can be calculated. Thus, for a recessively inherited disease aa (q2) with a frequency of 1 per 10,000 (e.g., albinism), the frequency of the gene *a* (q) is 1 per 100, and that of heterozygous carriers is $2 \times p \times q = 2 \times 99/100 \times 1/100 =$ approximately 1 in 50. Thus, in this particular example there are 200 clinically unaffected carriers of the abnormal gene for every affected individual. Table 31–3 lists the frequency of several inherited diseases. Cystic fibrosis, a recessively inherited disease, has a prevalence in the white population of about 1 per 2500 (q^2); thus, the frequency of the gene (q) is 1 in 50 and of heterozygous carriers is approximately 1 in 25, or 4% of the white population. A similar calculation with respect to sickle cell anemia among African-Americans in the United States ($q^2 = 1/625$) yields a frequency of heterozygous carriers of 1 in 12.5, or 8% of this population.

The frequency of most genes in the population is relatively stable. When a gene is rare and severely disadvantageous, the rate of its introduction into a population by spontaneous mutation is balanced by the rate of elimination of the disadvantageous gene by natural selection. The frequency of the disadvantageous gene, however, can be stabilized at a high level if the heterozygotes are slightly favored (increased biologic fitness) and leave a greater number of progeny than does either homozygote. When a rare form of a species is present at a frequency that cannot be maintained by recurrent mutation alone, a *balanced polymorphism* is said to exist. Usually, this means that the rarer of two allelic forms occurs with a frequency of at least 1% of the population. When this is found, *heterozygote advantage* should be suspected. An example of such a balanced polymorphism is the increased resistance of individuals heterozygous for the sickle cell trait to falciparum malaria. Although persons with sickle cell disease (homozygotes, SS hemoglobin) often die before they can reproduce and thus remove the sickle cell gene from the population, the prevalence of heterozygotes (SA hemoglobin) may nevertheless reach 40% in certain West African populations. Death from falciparum malaria is much less frequent in carriers of the sickle cell trait than in non-carriers, and thus the heterozygote does have an advantage. Whether the extraordinary frequency of heterozygotes for the sickle cell gene in West Africa is due entirely to differential mortality or in part to differential fertility is uncertain, but this example suffices to illustrate that the effects of genes can be assessed only in relation to a particular environment. In most instances, however, a distinct advantage for the heterozygote of a polymorphic trait (of which there are many) cannot be demonstrated, and it is likely that certain polymorphic traits are genetically neutral.

The term *genetic load* has been used to describe the total genetic disability of a population. It comprises both a *mutational load,* based on recurrent mutation of a normal gene to a lethal or sublethal gene, and a *segregational load,* resulting from segregation of the harmful gene from advantaged heterozygotes, as in the example of sickle cell heterozygotes discussed earlier. Each individual has been estimated to have three to eight genes, which, if homozygous instead of heterozygous, would be lethal. The relative contribution of the segregational and mutational loads to the total genetic load is uncertain.

Knowledge of the genetic basis of susceptibility for specific diseases is likely to aid in disease prevention as well as therapy. Associated with these benefits, however, is the risk of discrimination against healthy at-risk individuals who may never develop a disorder. Thus, in addition to learning how to use this new knowledge for patient care, internists must gain the wisdom to use genetic information appropriately and confidentially.

Beaudet AL, Scriver CR, Sly WS, et al: Introduction to Human Biochemical and Molecular Genetics. New York, McGraw-Hill, 1990. *A historical perspective and summation of what we know about basic principles of human genetics, which emphasizes causes (mutations), pathogenesis, and therapy.*

King RA, Rotter JI, Motulsky AG: The Genetic Basis of Common Diseases. New York, Oxford University Press, 1992. *A review of the hereditary basis of diseases with a prevalence of 1% or greater in the population.*

Online Mendelian Inheritance in Man. Center for Medical Genetics, Johns Hopkins University (Baltimore, MD) and National Center for Biotechnology Information, National Library of Medicine, (Bethesda, MD), 1997. World Wide Web URL: http://www.ncbi.nlm.nih.gov/omim/ *A catalogue of autosomal dominant, autosomal recessive, and X-linked phenotypes, with brief descriptions and literature references for each.*

Rimoin DL, Connor JM, Pyeritz RE: Emery and Rimoin's Principles and Practice of Medical Genetics, 3rd ed. New York, Churchill Livingstone, 1997. *An authoritative textbook of medical genetics.*

Scriver CR, Beaudet AL, Sly WS, et al: The Metabolic Basis of Inherited Disease, 7th ed. New York, McGraw-Hill, 1995. *Authoritative discussions of all inborn errors of metabolism for which there is a substantial body of metabolic or biochemical information.*

Vogel F, Motulsky AG: Human Genetics: Problems and Approaches, 3rd ed. Berlin, Springer-Verlag, 1997. *A superb treatment of the principles of human genetics.*

32 INBORN ERRORS OF METABOLISM

Louis J. Elsas II

Metabolism is a collective term for integrated biochemical processes of the intact organism, differentiated organ, cell, and subcellular organelle. Normal metabolism enables economical homeostasis for the organism by maintaining anabolic and catabolic flow of substrates to products. In the early twentieth century, Sir Archibald Garrod recognized heritable blocks in normal human metabolic flow that conformed to mendelian mechanisms of inheritance. He first coined the term *inborn error of metabolism* in his Croonian Lectures of 1908, in which he described four diseases—alkaptonuria, albinism, cystinuria, and pentosuria—and their autosomal recessive patterns of inheritance. Garrod presumed that the patient expressing the full abnormality was homozygous for mutant alleles affecting a specific metabolic flow whereas the parents were heterozygous for this same inherited block but were clinically normal. When he gave patients with alkaptonuria proteins or other precursors of homogentisic acid, excretion of alkaptones increased, as evidenced by a darkening of the urine on standing. He theorized that this "block-in-reaction sequence" was controlled genetically because pedigree analyses were consistent with an *autosomal recessive* mode of inheritance. The enzyme defect in alkaptonuria was not discovered until 50 years later, when homogentisic acid oxidase was found to be missing from the liver and kidneys of patients with this disease. Over the past 2 years, the gene for homogentisate-1,2-dioxygenase was cloned and mutations causing impaired function defined.

First proof that an impaired protein function led to disease came from Gibson's observation in 1948 that erythrocyte methemoglobin reductase was impaired in patients with *methemoglobinemia.* By 1952, Pauling and Ingram had identified an abnormal hemoglobin

Proteins act as follows:
1. Catalyze plasma membrane functions
   a. Substrate transport
   b. Cellular signaling (receptors)
2. Catalyze major cellular metabolic pathways in the cytosol, lysosome, peroxisome, mitochondria, and nucleus
3. Circulate in blood and provide and maintain various functions (clotting; metal, lipid, or vitamin transport; immunity; oxygen transport; regulation of proteases, hormones, adhesion proteins)
4. Maintain structural integrity of organs and organelles (collagen, elastin, actin, dystrophin, fibrillins)

structure in *sickle cell anemia*. During this same period, Cori and Cori identified a deficiency of hepatic glucose-6-phosphatase in *von Gierke's disease* or *type I glycogen storage disease* and thus confirmed Garrod's theory by defining a block in the flow of hepatic glucose production from its stored glycogen.

It is important to understand that variations in human proteins do not usually produce disease. Heritable diversity in hemoglobins, phosphoglucomutase, lactate dehydrogenase, red blood cell acid phosphatase, haptoglobins, immunoglobins, and so forth were discovered and defined for normal populations. In some cases, diversity is required for optimal health, as with the immunoglobulin proteins and the switch from fetal to adult hemoglobins. Several mechanisms produce a normal diversity of proteins. For example, the β-globin gene has many nucleotide sequence variations that produce different amino acid changes in the primary protein structure without producing a functional change. When no functional change occurs, the alteration is considered a *polymorphism*. Normal protein variation can occur through normal gene rearrangements, as exemplified by the formation of immunoglobins, giving rise to required variations in response to foreign antigens (see Chapter 270). Here, gene rearrangements occur in response to antigens to produce protein diversity. Alternative splicing of RNA is another mechanism for protein variation. Examples are the insulin receptor, elastin, thyroid peroxidase, and tyrosine hydroxylase. Organ specificity and subcellular localization for evolutionarily conserved genes also occur through post-translational modification of their encoded proteins. Glycosylation of proteins directed to the plasma membrane receptors or for secretion is an example of this post-translational mechanism for normal protein diversity in the human organism.

The relatively rare circumstance in which a change in a protein impairs function is called a *mutation* and may produce an inborn error of metabolism. True mutations provide insight into the functional role of the normal protein in human metabolism. Inborn errors of metabolism are classified here in accordance with the organ, cell, and subcellular location of normal protein function (Table 32–1) and the abnormal mechanisms that interfere with the normal metabolic flow resulting from impaired proteins (Table 32–2). By understanding the pathophysiologic mechanisms producing disease, the normal function and cellular location were defined for these proteins. As science progresses in protein and gene replacement therapy, this approach to disease classification provides a practical working model for clinical intervention.

One important clinical aspect in defining the genetic component

1. Accumulation to toxic concentrations of substrates in a blocked catabolic reaction. *Examples:* maple syrup urine disease, glucose-galactose malabsorption, galactosemia
2. Production of toxic byproducts through a normally minor pathway. *Examples:* tyrosinemia type I and adenosine deaminase deficiency
3. Deficiency of an end-product in an anabolic pathway. *Examples:* albinism, orotic aciduria, and Zellweger's syndrome
4. Loss of regulation resulting in overproduced intermediates to toxic levels. *Examples:* congenital adrenal hyperplasia, intermittent porphyria, familial hypercholesterolemia

of a metabolic disease, as well as the environmental causes, is that one can predict, intervene in, and prevent the disease by a variety of stratagems. In general, the severity of an inborn error of metabolism depends on the degree of protein impairment rendered by the genetic mutation. Thus, a "leaky" mutation may not be expressed until adulthood, whereas a complete block in the same metabolic pathway is lethal in infancy. The pathophysiologic mechanisms outlined in Table 32–2 may occur individually or combine to produce loss in homeostasis and a disease state. The extent of disease and the clinical outcome in the complex human organism involve not only a specific genetic block but also alternate metabolic pathways (*epigenetic* phenomena) and the environment. Clinical outcome depends on (1) the ability to engineer the environment and to accommodate for impaired protein function through alternate pathways and (2) the timeliness of environmental and medical intervention in preventing irreversible organ damage.

Many disorders are produced by mutant proteins that impair the transport of nutrients into cells (Table 32–3). *Familial glucose-galactose malabsorption syndrome* exemplifies defective transporter protein, resulting in specific accumulation of non-transported glucose to toxic concentrations in the intestinal lumen. Direct evidence for the genetic control of intestinal glucose transport in humans was obtained by in vitro studies of jejunal biopsy material from families in which the affected members express refractory diarrhea on ingesting D-galactose or D-glucose. Biopsy material from asymptomatic first-degree relatives demonstrated partial impairment of this transport function and defined autosomal recessive inheritance. These physiologic data suggested that a single mutant gene affected sodium-dependent, active glucose transport by human jejunal (and proximal renal tubular) microvilli. Expression cloning of active glucose transport has now confirmed the presence of energy- and sodium-dependent glucose transporter genes, their deduced amino acid sequences, and specific codon changes producing syndromes of familial glucose-galactose malabsorption and renal glycosuria.

Now a family of active and facilitative glucose transporter genes is known to be differentially expressed by specific organs and there are a large number of inherited defects involving the plasma membrane transport of glucose. Glucose transporters represent a family of proteins whose definitions of function evolved after their cloning and molecular genetic analyses (Table 32–4). Comparing the data from families with renal glycosuria and glucose-galactose malabsorption, it became evident that different Na^+-dependent active glucose transporters were present in kidney and gut epithelium. The SGLT1 is shared by kidney and gut, whereas SGLT2 functions predominantly in kidney alone and causes renal glycosuria without glucose-galactose malabsorption (see Table 32–4). An insulin-responsive, facilitative glucose transporter (GLUT4) is not Na^+-dependent and is expressed primarily in insulin-responsive tissues (fat cells, skeletal muscle). More than one glucose transporter is expressed by most cells. For example, the jejunal epithelial cell uses SGLT1 to concentrate glucose from its luminal surface into the cytosol, then effluxes glucose at its basal-lateral surfaces through GLUT2. GLUT2 is also involved in regulating the amount of glucose transporter into β cells of the pancreas, a process that regulates glucose stimulation of insulin release. Indirect evidence indicates that mutations in the GLUT2 gene are "sensitivity genes" involved in regulating insulin secretion.

Many diseases characterized by "hormone resistance" are caused by another family of proteins that function in the plasma membrane. The concept of failure to respond to hormone stimulation originated in the early 1940s with a description of *pseudohypoparathyroidism* (see Chapter 264). Heritability of resistance to parathormone was suggested before the existence of parathormone receptors, hormone-sensitive adenylate cyclases, or guanine nucleotide-binding proteins was known.

Diseases caused by defective transmembrane binding and signaling include *Laron's dwarfism*, which results from growth hormone receptor (GHR) defects. Deletions in the *GHR* gene of Asian Jews are defined. Phenotypic characteristics are *proportionate dwarfism*, hypoglycemia, craniofacial disproportion with a doll-like face, balding, frontal bossing, truncal obesity, and wrinkled skin. In this disorder, growth hormone concentration is elevated in blood, pe-

Table 32–3 ■ DISEASES CAUSED BY PLASMA MEMBRANE TRANSPORTER PROTEIN MUTATIONS

DISEASE	TISSUE AFFECTED	SUBSTRATE	MODE OF INHERITANCE	CLINICAL EXPRESSION
B_{12} malabsorption	Ileum	Vitamin B_{12}	Autosomal recessive	Juvenile
Blue diaper syndrome	Gut	Tryptophan	Autosomal recessive	Hypercalcemia
Congenital chloridorrhea	Gut	Chloride	Autosomal recessive	Diarrhea, alkalosis
Cystic fibrosis	Apical epithelia	Chloride	Autosomal recessive	Lung, intestinal obstruction
Cystinuria	Kidney + gut	Cystine + lysine, arginine, ornithine	Autosomal recessive	Renal lithiasis (cystine)
Familial hypophosphatemic rickets	Kidney + gut	Phosphate	X-linked dominant	Rickets
Folate deficiency	Lymphocyte, erythrocyte	Methyl tetrahydrofolate	Autosomal recessive	Aplastic anemia
Glucose-galactose malabsorption	Gut + kidney	Glucose and galactose	Autosomal recessive	Refractory diarrhea
Hartnup's syndrome	Gut + kidney	Neutral amino acids	Autosomal recessive	Nicotinic acid deficiency (pellagra)
Hereditary hypophosphatemic rickets	Kidney	Phosphate	Autosomal dominant	Growth restriction, rickets, hypercalciuria
Hereditary renal hypouricemia	Kidney	Uric acid	Autosomal recessive	Urolithiasis (uric acid)
Hereditary spherocytosis	Erythrocyte	Sodium	Autosomal recessive	Hemolytic anemia
Hyperdibasic aminoaciduria (type I)	Kidney	Lysine Arginine Ornithine	Autosomal dominant	? Symptoms
Iminoglycinuria	Kidney + gut	Glycine Proline Hydroxyproline	Autosomal recessive	Benign ?
Isolated lysinuria	Kidney + gut	Lysine	Autosomal recessive	Growth failure, seizures
Lysinuric protein intolerance (type II)	Kidney, fibroblasts, hepatocytes, gut	Lysine	Autosomal recessive	Growth restriction, hyperammonemia, mental retardation
Methionine malabsorption (oasthouse disease)	Gut	Methionine	Autosomal recessive ?	Mental retardation, white hair, failure to thrive
Renal glycosuria	Kidney	Glucose	Autosomal recessive	Benign glycosuria
Renal tubular acidosis (type I)	Distal renal tubule	H^+ secretion, citrate, calcium	Autosomal dominant	Hypokalemia, growth restriction, nephrocalcinosis
Renal tubular acidosis (type II)	Proximal renal tubule	Bicarbonate	"Familial"	Hyperchloremic metabolic acidosis

ripheral tissue responses are decreased, and insulin-like growth factor-1 concentrations in blood are low. An autosomal recessive mode of inheritance is defined. Causes for dominant or polygenic symmetrical growth restriction may result from mutations in the hypothalamic pituitary trophic proteins, in growth hormone, in GHR, and in post-receptor signaling. The *GHR* gene is found on chromosome 5p13-p12, and many different mutations account for disorders of stature in this gene. *Familial hypercholesterolemia* defines a phenotype of autosomal dominant hypercholesterolemia, early-onset heart disease, and decreased low-density lipoprotein (LDL)-cholesterol binding and uptake by plasma membrane. This disorder affects a significant number of individuals in the general population, an estimated 1 in 500. An autosomal dominant mode of inheritance for early-onset adult heart disease is caused by many different mutations in the LDL-cholesterol receptors. The dysfunction of LDL receptors results in a loss in the cell's ability to down-regulate endogenous cholesterol synthesis and accumulation of LDL cholesterol in the vascular space. Increased intracellular and intravascular accumulation of LDL-cholesterol results in atherosclerosis and heart disease in the third and fourth decades of life (see Table 32–2). The gene for the LDL-cholesterol receptor is found on chromosome 19p13.1–13.2. The rare disorder, *leprechaunism*, has become a prototypic inborn error of severe insulin resistance and loss of cellular signal transduction through the insulin receptor.

Affected infants have low birth weight, acanthosis nigricans, cystic changes in organs, and loss of glucose homeostasis. Affected patients have remarkably elevated plasma insulin concentrations above 500 mIU/mL. Specific impairment in iodine-125–labeled insulin binding is evident in cells cultured from patients, and a spectrum of mutations produces a spectrum of severe insulin-resistant syndromes (leprechaunism, Rabson-Mendenhall, and type A diabetes with acanthosis nigricans). Obligate heterozygotes (parents) of patients with leprechaunism have partially impaired insulin binding and glucose tolerance curves suggesting type II diabetes mellitus.

Sequencing of the complementary DNA (cDNA) for the insulin receptor indicated that both its α and β subunits are encoded by a single cDNA of 5 kb length. A large 120-kb gene is located on chromosome 19p13.2. In families with leprechaunism and other variations of severe insulin resistance, several different mutations are known (Table 32–5). These mutations impair synthesis, receptor transfer to the plasma membrane, binding of insulin, autophosphorylation, and receptor signaling (see Table 32–5). Thus, mutations in the insulin receptor gene exemplify clinical *heterogeneity* in inborn errors of metabolism produced by intra-allelic variations. This term signifies that different mutations produce different severity and variation of diseases even though they result from mutations in the same gene. Membrane receptors transduce signals to

Table 32–4 ■ HUMAN GLUCOSE TRANSPORTERS

	PROTEIN kd (AA)	mRNA SIZE (kb)	CHROMOSOMAL LOCALIZATION	EXPRESSION IN TISSUE AND CELLS	FUNCTION	DISORDER
GLUT1	55 (492)	2.8	lp35 → p31.3	Blood-brain barrier, erythrocyte fibroblast	Basal glucose transport across most cells, including blood-brain barrier	Seizures with low cerebrospinal fluid and normal blood glucose
GLUT2	58 (524)	2.8 3.4 5.4	3q26.1 → q26.3	Liver, kidney, intestine, beta cell of the pancreas	Low-affinity glucose transport	Defective insulin secretion in diabetes
GLUT3	54 (496)	2.7 4.1	12p13.3	Neurons, fibroblast, placenta, testes	Basal glucose transport High affinity	?
GLUT4	55 (509)	2.8 3.5	17p13	Fat, skeletal muscle, heart	Insulin-stimulated glucose transport	Defective insulin-stimulated transport ?NIDDM
GLUT5	50 (501)	2.0	1p32 → p22	Small intestine	Fructose transport	?
GLUT7 (rat)	52 (528)	?	?	Liver microsome	Glucose release from endoplasmic reticulum	Type 1d glycogen storage disease
Concentrative Glucose Transporters						
SLGT1	75 (664)	2.2 2.6 4.8	22q11 → qter	Intestine, kidney (medulla)	Intestinal absorption, renal reabsorption, high affinity (2Na:1 glucose)	Glucose-galactose malabsorption
SLGT2	76 (672)	2.4 3.0 3.5 4.5	16p11.2	Kidney (cortex)	Low affinity, high capacity (1Na:1 glucose)	Renal glycosuria

NIDDM = non–insulin-dependent diabetes mellitus.

Table 32–5 ■ MUTATIONS IN THE INSULIN RECEPTOR (IR) GENE CAUSING INHERITED INSULIN RESISTANCE

SYNDROME	DISEASE MECHANISM	SYNDROME	DISEASE MECHANISM
Recessive Inheritance		Type A Insulin Resistance	
Leprechaunism		1363 T → G Phe362 → Val	Defective processing by IR
1597 A → G Lys460 → Glu	Defective insulin binding	Homozygous	
2233 C → T Gln672 → STOP	Reduced number of IR	1604 A → G Asn462 → Ser	Defective insulin binding
476 G → C Arg86 → Pro	Defective binding	617 G → A Trp133 → STOP	Reduced mRNA
Homozygous	Activation of glucose transport and phosphotransfer	2424 G → T Arg735 → Ser	Defective cleavage IR
		Homozygous	
917 T → C Leu233 → Pro	Defective processing by IR	3197 G → A Arg993 → Gln	Defective kinase
Homozygous		3217 G → T Arg1000 → STOP	Decreased mRNA
310 G → A Gly31 → Arg	Defective processing by IR	Delta exon 14	Receptor truncation
Not determined		Not determined	
2908 C → T Arg897 → STOP	Reduced mRNA	Lipodystrophy	
Noncoding region IR gene	Reduced mRNA	Ile485 → Thr	(?)
1333 C → T Arg372 → STOP	Reduced mRNA	**Dominant Inheritance**	
Noncoding region IR gene	Reduced mRNA	Type 1 insulin resistance	Defective phosphorylation
Del 1159-1161 Del Asn281	Defective binding (?)	3176 C → T Pro986 → Leu	Defective phosphorylation
Splice error intron 13		3242 G → T Gly1008 → Val	Defective phosphorylation
302 T → C Val28 → Ala	(?)	Del 3300 → Ter Del 1013	Truncated receptor
1315 G → C Gly366 → Arg			Defective phosphorylation
850 A → G His209 → Arg	Defective processing by IR	3619 G → A Ala1134 → Thr	Defective phosphorylation
Homozygous		3623 C → A Ala1135 → Glu	Defective phosphorylation
Rabson-Mendenhall Syndrome		3678 G → A Met 1153 → Ile	Defective phosphorylation
264 C → A Asn15 → Lsy	Defective processing by IR	3818 G → C Trp1200 → Ser	
3217 → C → T Arg1000 → STOP	Reduced mRNA	Type II (non–insulin-dependent diabetes mellitus	
Splice error intron 4	Reduced mRNA	3421 A → G Lys1068 → Glu	Defective phosphorylation
nt 2617 (del 5) 801x		3710 G → A Arg1164 → Gln	Defective kinase

proteins bound on the inner cytoplasmic surface (second messengers). Thus, the insulin receptor transfers its signal by phosphotransfer to the insulin receptor signal protein 1 (IRS-1), a protein of 180 kd. The *IRS-1* gene is located on chromosome 2q, is rich in tyrosine residues, and acts as the phosphotransfer second messenger. Although no mutations in humans are as yet defined in IRS-1, some membrane receptors that signal through cyclic nucleotides have mutations in their signaling (G) proteins. An example is *Albright's hereditary osteodystrophy* or *pseudohypoparathyroidism* (see Chapter 264). A heterogeneous group of mutations has now been found in the gene for the parathormone receptor's guanine nucleotide-binding protein (G_sa), which links the receptor to adenylate cyclase and stimulates cyclic adenosine monophosphate when the receptor is occupied by parathormone. This gene for G_sa is located on chromosome 20q13, and both deletions and missense mutations are defined that produce Albright's hereditary osteodystrophy. Interestingly, somatic mutations in arginine 201 of the same gene turn the G_sa protein constitutively "on" and produce another disease, the McCune-Albright-Sternberg syndrome, which includes non-ossifying bone tumors and premature puberty.

Inborn errors affecting proteins of the cytosolic compartment within a cell are the more "traditional" inborn errors of metabolism (Table 32–6). They impair the catalytic reactions of anabolic or catabolic pathways and are usually classified by the type of micromolecules altered. Thus, we consider here the disorders of sugar, amino acid, purine, and organic acid metabolism.

Galactose metabolism is important in infancy because the primary carbohydrate source of human milk is lactose, a disaccharide composed of glucose and galactose. Classic *galactosemia* results from mutations in the gene for galactose 1-phosphate uridyltransferase [GALT]. The gene is found on chromosome 9p13, and its cDNA codes for a protein of 379 amino acids. A common mutation is a substitution of arginine for glutamine at codon 188 (Q188R). This mutation eliminates GALT activity and produces classic neonatal disease. If not treated, the infant suffers liver, central nervous system, and renal damage and may succumb to bacterial sepsis. Variant forms of galactosemia with other mutations in the GALT gene are known to produce GALT activity, ranging from 3% to 25% of normal. If excess lactose is ingested, cataracts, premature ovarian failure, and growth and mental restriction may not be recognized until adulthood. When individuals with these disorders are detected early, as with population-based newborn screening programs (see Chapters 37 and 201), disease is prevented by replacing lactose with sucrose in the infant's formula and by the patient's adhering to a diet restricted in galactose throughout life.

Phenylalanine is an essential amino acid for growth whose anabolic products include tyrosine, thyroid hormone, adrenergic neurotransmitters, and melanin. *Phenylketonuria* (PKU) (see Chapter 209) is caused by mutations in the gene encoding the phenylalanine hydroxylase protein, the first enzyme in this anabolic flow that catalyzes tyrosine production.

Albinism is an example of an inborn error in an anabolic pathway in which the pathophysiologic mechanism is directly related to the lack of an end product (see Mechanism 3, Table 32–2). Tyrosine is converted by the action of a cytosolic tyrosinase first to dopa and then to dopamine. Dopamine can then be converted either to the red-yellow pigment pheomelanin or to the black-brown pigment eumelanin. These reactions occur in the melanosomes produced in the melanocytes and exported to the keratinocytes. Color of skin is an inherited factor that depends on several genes and is a function of the intensity of the pigment in the skin and not the number of melanocytes, which is constant for all humans. Although skin color is a polygenic trait, single genes can have a profound effect on this color, as evidenced by the albino phenotype. In humans, *oculocutaneous albinism* (OCA) is inherited as an autosomal recessive trait. X-linked forms of *ocular albinism* also exist. Individuals with OCA are classified as either tyrosinase negative or positive for tyrosine activity in hair bulbs. Tyrosinase-negative individuals form no pigment, and the gene for tyrosinase has been localized to chromosome 11q14 and many mutations are defined. A tyrosine-positive OCA has been associated with an autosomal recessive gene located on chromosome 15q11-13 (the P gene) and X-linked ocular albinism caused by *OCA-1* gene mutations. A wide variation in phenotypic expression of albinism is reported from very severe neurologic deficiency with ocular and sarcomatous skin cancers to mild cosmetic problems.

Inborn errors of the urea cycle (see Chapter 211) are represented by defects in the integration of both anabolic and catabolic pathways and the distribution of catalytic proteins between mitochondria and cytosol. The role of the urea cycle is to convert ammonia, a byproduct of protein breakdown, to urea and to synthesize arginine and ornithine. Reactions to complete this anabolic cycle require three mitochondrial enzymes, three cytosolic enzymes, and two mitochondrial transporter proteins. Inherited disorders affecting the function of each of five enzymes are known. Individuals with defects in any of the enzymes present with varying degrees of hyperammonemia caused by protein ingestion or a catabolic state. With the exception of the gene for ornithine transcarbamylase found on the short arm of chromosome X, the other four proteins are encoded on autosomes and defects are inherited as autosomal recessive traits. Many principles involved in the pathophysiology of inborn errors of metabolism are exemplified by disorders of the urea cycle.

A group of inborn errors of metabolism is caused by mutations in nuclear genes that encode mitochondrial proteins. Collectively, they are considered disorders of organic acid metabolism (Table 32–7). For example, branched-chain α-ketoacid dehydrogenase is a multienzyme complex located on the matrix side of the mitochondrial inner membrane in all tissues. When any of these proteins is impaired, the autosomal recessive disorder *maple syrup urine disease* may result (see Chapter 212). In addition to nuclear-encoded genes, 13 proteins of mitochondrial complexes involved in oxidative phosphorylation are encoded in the mitochondrial DNA genome. Only complex II is encoded entirely by the nuclear genome. A wide range of disorders affecting the eye, brain, and muscle are caused by mutations in mitochondrial DNA. The heritability of these disorders is distinguished from those caused by mutations in

Table 32–6 ■ DISEASES CAUSED BY IMPAIRED CYTOSOLIC ENZYMES

DISORDER	ENZYME DEFECT	PHENOTYPE	INHERITANCE
Carbohydrates			
Fructosuria	Fructokinase	Benign	Autosomal recessive
Hereditary fructose intolerance	Fructose 1-phosphate aldolase	Liver dysfunction, early death	Autosomal recessive
Galactosemia	Galactose-1-P-uridyl transferase	Liver dysfunction, cataracts, sepsis, mental retardation, death	Autosomal recessive
Hereditary fructose 1,6-*bis*-phosphate deficiency	Fructose 1,6 *bis*-phosphatase	Apnea, ketosis, lactic acidosis	Autosomal recessive
Amino Acids			
Phenylketonuria	*p*-Hydroxyphenylalanine hydroxylase	Mental retardation (teratogenic)	Autosomal recessive
Tyrosinemia			
Type II	Tyrosine aminotransferase	Palmar bullae, corneal lesions	Autosomal recessive
Type I	Fumarylacetoacetate hydrolase	Succinyl acetone accumulation	Autosomal recessive
Homocystinuria	Cystathionine B synthase	Marfanoid habitus, arterial thrombosis, lens dislocation, mental retardation	Autosomal recessive
Hyperornithinemia	Ornithine aminotransferase	Gyrate atrophy of the retina	Autosomal recessive
Lesch-Nyhan syndrome	Hypoxanthine phosphoribosyltransferase	Neurologic dysfunction with self-destructive tendency	X-linked

Table 32–7 ■ ORGANIC ACIDEMIAS: DISORDERS OF METABOLISM BY MITOCHONDRIAL PROTEINS

DISORDER	ENZYME DEFECT	INHERITANCE
Isovaleric acidemia	Isovaleryl CoA dehydrogenase	Autosomal recessive
Methylcrotonic aciduria	3-Methylcrotonyl CoA carboxylase	
Glutoconic aciduria	3-Methylglutaconyl CoA hydralatase	
Glutaric aciduria (1)	3-Hydroxy-3-methylglutaryl CoA lyase	
Mevalonic aciduria	Mevalonate kinase	
Thiolase deficiency	2-Methylacetoacetyl CoA thiolase	
Isobutyric aciduria	3-Hydroxyisobutyryl CoA deacylase	
Propionic aciduria	Propionyl CoA carboxylase	Autosomal recessive
Methylmalonic aciduria	Methylmalonyl CoA mutase	Autosomal recessive
Lactic acidosis	Pyruvate dehydrogenase	Autosomal recessive
	Pyruvate decarboxylase	
Acyl-CoA dehydrogenase deficiencies	Short-, medium-, and long-chain fatty acyl CoA dehydrogenase	Autosomal recessive
Branched-chain α-ketoacidemia	Branched-chain α-ketoacid dehydrogenase	Autosomal recessive
Respiratory chain defects	Electron transfer factor (ETF) deficiency	Autosomal recessive
Glutaric acidemia type II	Multiple acyl CoA dehydrogenases	Autosomal recessive
Leber's optic atrophy	Mitochondrial oxidative phosphorylation complexes	Maternal
Myoclonic epilepsy and ragged red fibers	Mitochondrial oxidative phosphorylation complexes	Maternal
Leigh's disease	Mitochondrial oxidative phosphorylation complexes	Maternal

nuclear DNA by being transmitted through affected mothers to all of her offspring. Males do not transmit mitochondrial mutations to their offspring, thus the term *maternal inheritance* (see Table 32–7).

Another group of inborn errors of metabolism is collectively categorized as *lysosomal disorders* (see Chapter 208) to indicate the subcellular localization of these impaired proteins. Most of these enzymes are involved in breakdown of endocytosed membrane components and when defective result in accumulation of their nondegraded substrates in the lysosomes and macrophages of affected organs.

I-cell disease is an inborn error of post-translational processing of proteins directed to the lysosome. Clarification of this pathophysiology led to an understanding of the mechanisms by which lysosomal enzymes are polarized to remain in lysosomes. Patients with I-cell disease have inherited defects in the recognition markers required to direct enzymes to the endocytic receptor of plasma membrane and to its capture in the acidic milieu of the lysosome. Patients lack all cellular lysosomal enzymes. Instead, empty lysosomes look like inclusion bodies (hence, "I cell"). The misdirected lysosomal enzymes are secreted and are present in excess in plasma but are missing from cells. These extracellular enzymes were found to lack mannose 6-phosphate residues, and this observation led to an understanding of the post-translational mechanisms by which enzymes are both directed to the lysosome and recaptured into endosomes by adding phosphorylated mannose to their protein structure. Individuals with I-cell disease lack this phosphotransferase activity.

Inborn errors affecting single enzymes in the degradative pathway for mucopolysaccharides and gangliosides helped define the steps required for the breakdown of these complex macromolecules. Disorders of mucopolysaccharide metabolism (see Chapter 214) include Hurler's syndrome; Scheie's syndrome; Hunter's syndrome; Sanfilippo's syndrome types A, B, C, and D; Morquio's syndrome types A and B; and Sly's syndrome. Disorders of ganglioside metabolism include Fabry's disease, Gaucher's disease, Niemann-

Pick disease, Tay-Sachs disease, I-cell disease, fucosidosis, mannosidosis, sialidosis, and aspartylglycosaminuria.

Another group of inborn errors of metabolism defined by altered organelle function are *peroxisomal diseases* (Table 32–8). Peroxisomes are radiodense organelles of 0.5 to 1 nm diameter bounded by a single trilaminar membrane. Both anabolic and catabolic reactions occur in this organelle. Primary pathways synthesize plasmalogens (unique fatty acids containing vinyl ethers), cholesterol, and bile acids. Other biosynthetic reactions include gluconeogenesis from amino acids and the formation of oxalic acid by the action of alanine-glyoxylate aminotransferase (see Chapter 205). Catabolic reactions include breakdown of hydrogen peroxide by peroxisomal catalase, a traditional protein of the peroxisome; polyamine oxidation; purine breakdown; ethanol oxidation; phytanic acid hydroxylation; and pipecolic acid degradation. A major function of the peroxisome is β-oxidation of very long chain fatty acids, those longer than 24 carbons.

An understanding of the importance of a number of reactions that occur in the peroxisome has come from identifying patients with either defects in individual biochemical pathways or lack of peroxisomes. The targeting signal for peroxisomal proteins may lie in their carboxyl terminal end, and mutations in the alanine-glyoxylate aminotransferase have resulted in mistargeting of this enzyme to mitochondria with consequent *familial hyperoxaluria* (see Chapter 205).

Disorders affecting the peroxisome are of two types: type 1, the absence of the peroxisome itself caused by defects in its assembly processes; and type 2, the absence of specific enzymes from the peroxisomal milieu caused by mutations in phosphotransfer or specific enzyme structure. These disorders are listed in Table 32–8.

Several inborn errors are caused by abnormalities in proteins that function in the nucleus and are involved in DNA repair (see class 2, Table 32–1). Patients expressing these inherited disorders carry a high risk for developing cancers. Among these inborn errors of DNA metabolism are both rare disorders, such as xeroderma pigmentosum, Bloom syndrome, ataxia-telangiectasia, Fanconi's anemia, and diseases associated with early aging such as progeria and Werner syndrome, as well as more common adult-onset nonpolyposis colon cancer. Collectively, the disorders show an increased sensitivity and delayed repair of damaged DNA due to ultraviolet, x-ray, alkylating cross links, or "normal" variation.

A large number of inborn errors involve proteins that circulate in blood (see class 3 of Table 32–1). Stable circulating proteins in blood perform a variety of functions, including immunologic, hemostatic, regulatory, hormonal, and interorgan transport of trace metals, lipids, and other nutrients. Some inherited disorders affecting circulating proteins are tabulated in Table 32–9. Proteins involved in oxygen transport, coagulation, and immunity are detailed in other chapters, but the pathophysiologic mechanisms and genetic approaches of screening, diagnosis, and intervention to prevent an expected outcome make them appropriate to consider here as inborn errors of metabolism.

Table 32–8 ■ INBORN ERRORS OF PEROXISOMES

Disorders of peroxisomal biogenesis
  Zellweger's syndrome (cerebrohepatorenal syndrome)
  Neonatal adrenoleukodystrophy
  Infantile Refsum's disease
  Hyperpipecolic acidemia
  Leber's amaurosis
  Rhizomelic chondrodysplasia punctata (Conradi's syndrome)
Peroxisomal 3-oxoacyl CoA thiolase deficiency
Peroxisomal acyl CoA oxidase deficiency
X-linked adrenoleukodystrophy (impaired lignoceroyl CoA and hexacosanoyl CoA ligase)
Adult Refsum's disease (phytanic acid α-hydroxylase deficiency)
Acatalasemia (H_2O_2 oxidoreductase deficiency)

Table 32–9 ▪ SOME INBORN ERRORS OF PROTEINS THAT CIRCULATE IN BLOOD

FUNCTIONAL CLASS	PROTEIN	PHENOTYPE
Transport	Ceruloplasmin	Wilson's disease
	Albumin	Analbuminemia
	Hemoglobin	Hemoglobinopathies
	α-Lipoprotein	Analphalipoproteinemia
	β-Lipoprotein	Abetalipoproteinemia
	Transcobalamin II	Megaloblastic anemia
Hormones	Growth hormone	Pituitary dwarfism
	Insulin	Diabetes mellitus (insulin-dependent)
	Somatomedin	Pituitary dwarfism
Coagulation	Factors I–XIII	Coagulopathies
	Kininogen	Kininogen deficiency
	Prekallikrein	Prekallikrein deficiency
Immune system	Complement components	Hypocomplementemias
	Immunoglobulins	Hypogammaglobulinemias
Inhibitors	α1-Antitrypsin	Pulmonary emphysema and/or cirrhosis
	C′1 esterase inhibitor	Angioneurotic edema

Abnormal structural proteins produce inborn errors such as Marfan syndrome (fibrillin), osteogenesis imperfecta (collagen type I), spondyloepiphyseal dysplasia (collagen type II), and Sack's syndrome (collagen type III) (see Chapters 215 to 218). These disorders exemplify class 4 of inborn errors of metabolism (see Table 32–1). The enzymes involved in post-translational processing of these proteins may also cause these syndromes. An example is Ehlers-Danlos syndrome type VI in which collagen lysylhydroxylase deficiency produces excess poorly hydroxylated collagen. Inborn errors of matrix proteins are exemplified by disorders of collagen metabolism. More than 20 different genes dispersed on 9 chromosomes are currently known to code for more than 11 different types of collagen. These disorders are detailed in Chapters 215 to 218, and 283.

Elsas L, Priest J: Medical genetics. *In* Sodeman W, Sodeman T (eds): Pathologic Physiology Mechanisms of Disease, 7th ed. Philadelphia, WB Saunders, 1985. *A traditional compilation of pathophysiologic mechanisms producing inherited diseases.*

Longo N, Elsas L: Human glucose transporters. *In* Advances in Pediatrics, vol 45, 1998. *A review of glucose transporters and insulin responsivity.*

Online Mendelian Inheritance in Man. National Center for Biotechnology Information: http://www3.ncbi.nlm.nih.gov./Omim/. *An up-to-date electronic review of inherited disorders of man.*

Scriver CR, Beaudet AL, Sly WS, et al: The Metabolic Basis of Inherited Disease, 7th ed. New York, McGraw-Hill, 1995. *A three-volume resource for inherited metabolic diseases.*

33 GENE THERAPY

Jesús Gómez-Navarro ▪ *Guadalupe Bilbao* ▪ *David T. Curiel*

Gene therapy is a relatively new method of therapeutic intervention targeted at the level of cellular gene expression. In this approach, altering a pathophysiologic state is achieved by delivering nucleic acids into a cell. These nucleic acids may be genes, portions of genes, oligonucleotides, or ribonucleic acid. In conventional therapeutics, as in pharmacotherapy, altering a cell or tissue phenotype is accomplished by altering cell physiology or metabolism at the level of protein expression. For gene therapy, this is accomplished by changing the pattern of expression of the genes whose products may thus achieve the desired effect on the cellular phenotype. From a conceptual standpoint, gene therapy strategies may offer the potential to achieve a much higher level of specificity of action by virtue of the highly specific control and regulatory mechanisms of gene expression that may be targeted in this technique. Additionally, interceding at an earlier stage in disease pathogenesis may offer greater potential to achieve fundamental changes in phenotypic parameters of disease with a more favorable outcome. Lastly, using the body to produce therapeutic proteins, potentially in only certain tissues, has practical advantages of its own.

Gene therapy was initially conceptualized as a method to treat acquired genetic diseases. In this regard, more than 5000 monogenetic disorders exist in which the entirety of the disease state may be attributed to a single lesion at a specific genetic locus. Replacing or augmenting a defective gene by delivering its wild-type counterpart thus offers a potential means to rectify definitively the pathogenic basis of the disease state. Inherited genetic diseases, however, are not the only logical targets for gene therapy. The underlying basis for a variety of acquired disorders may be shown to be accumulated lesions in specific genetic loci, as in malignancies associated with mutations in dominant and recessive oncogenes. In these instances also, if the pathogenic basis is established to be lesions in cellular genes, a logical strategy is replacing or adding the mutated genes with the wild-type counterpart to perform the deficient function.

The indications for this form of therapy must be established. The first and foremost criterion for any gene therapy is that the aberrant gene being targeted must be well characterized. In addition, it must be shown that the defined genetic abnormalities are the basis of the observed pathogenesis of the disease state. If the logic of genetic intervention thus exists, clearly defined endpoints of the therapy intervention must exist and an alternate, effective therapy for the targeted disease must not exist. This reflects the fact that, at this juncture, gene therapy is still a radical, experimental therapy that may be justified only in this context.

Certain minimum criteria of potential efficacy also must be met. As a first step, it must be possible to deliver the therapeutic gene to the target cells of interest. After delivery, the introduced gene must be expressed at an appropriate level for the desired effect and for sufficient time for this effect to be achieved. Additionally, the delivery and expression of the therapeutic gene must be safe for the target cell and, by extension, for the individual being treated. From a conceptual standpoint, it must be recognized that these goals are all interrelated and, furthermore, that all of them must be addressed to rationally implement any gene therapy strategy. Clinical experience with gene therapy during the past decade shows that serious toxicity is not a problem. Most importantly, it is now evident that a variety of gene transfer maneuvers can alter favorably the cellular phenotype in vitro, although a fundamental limitation exists owing to an insufficient gene delivery and expression into target cells in vivo.

In practice, gene therapy implementation in human clinical trials has used two distinct strategies to meet the aforementioned criteria. In selected instances, target cells may be removed from the body, genetically modified extracorporeally, and then reintroduced into the patient. This ex vivo strategy has been applied in those contexts in which the technical capacity exists to readily harvest and manipulate the relevant target cell. As an alternative strategy, the in vivo approach involves directly delivering the therapeutic gene to the relevant target cells in situ in an intact individual. Whereas both approaches have been used in human clinical trials, the preponderance of strategies to date have employed the ex vivo approach. Although this method may offer certain advantages in selected contexts, it must be recognized that using this route presents the technical difficulty associated with accomplishing direct in vivo delivery.

The advantages of the ex vivo approach are that it allows gene transfer to the target cells in a defined, in vitro setting, in which delivery efficiencies may be optimized. This approach also allows the modified cells to be characterized from the standpoint of safety before they are reintroduced to the patient. Despite these advantages, this method may be limited to very select settings in which target cells can be propagated ex vivo; at present, this is viable for a very limited set of tissue types. The in vivo approach in theory overcomes this limitation of target tissue accessibility. Delivery in vivo, however, is fraught with considerably greater complexities than the ex vivo approach. Thus, the gene transfer vector in the direct-delivery approach must achieve delivery in the context of significant host barriers, including humoral, reticuloendothelial, and immunologic factors. This dichotomy highlights the reason why the

Table 33–1 ■ CLINICAL USE OF GENE TRANSFER SYSTEMS

TYPE	VECTOR SYSTEM	CLINICAL TRIALS*	DISTINGUISHING FEATURES
Nonviral	Liposomes	30	Repetitive administration feasible, inefficient gene delivery, transient expression
	Naked DNA or RNA (injection, gene gun, electroporation)	6	Easy preparation, inefficient gene delivery, transient expression
	Molecular conjugates	—	Flexible design, inefficient gene delivery, transient expression, unstable in vivo
Viral	Retrovirus	63	Integrates into the chromosome of dividing cells, unstable in vivo
	Adenovirus	34	Highly efficient in vivo; production in large numbers makes infection of tissues more efficient; tropism can be modified; induces potent inflammation and immunity
	Poxvirus (vaccinia)	15	Extensive clinical experience with parent virus; large insert capacity; induces potent inflammation and immunity
	Adeno-associated virus	1	Nonpathogenic; integrates into the chromosome; low insert capacity; difficult to scale-up
	Herpes simplex virus	1	Highly efficient in vivo; very large insert capacity; cytotoxic
	Chimeric vectors (e.g., Ad/Retro)	—	Combine features of component genetic vectors
	Lentivirus	—	Integrates into the chromosome of *both* dividing and nondividing cells; not yet available as a well-characterized production system

*Registered in the NIH Office of Recombinant DNA Activities at the end of 1998.

ability to accomplish in vivo gene delivery currently represents the greatest challenge to implementing gene therapy strategies. Earlier protocols were principally of the ex vivo type and relied on recombinant retroviruses as gene transfer vehicles.

The technology to derive recombinant retroviruses that can efficiently transfer genes has been sufficiently developed that these vectors have been used for a majority of human protocols (Table 33–1) They can accomplish effective gene transfer to a variety of target cells despite being rendered replication incompetent by genomic deletions. In addition, because these viruses are integrative, they can produce permanent genetic modifications of target cells with the consequence of long-term heterologous gene expression. Whereas the vectors are suited for ex vivo modification of target cells, a variety of limitations have restricted their use in strategies to accomplish direct, in vivo gene transfer. The retrovirus requires proliferative target cells to mediate effective gene transfer. One exception are lentiviruses, the class of retrovirus that includes hu-

man immunodeficiency virus, which can integrate also in nondividing cells. An additional obstacle for retroviruses is the high susceptibility of the virus particle to humoral factors that ablate its gene-transfer capacity. Thus, the basic biology of recombinant retroviruses has been an additional factor restricting initially implemented gene therapy protocols to strategies using ex vivo methodologies.

To circumvent the limitations associated with recombinant retroviruses, alternative vector systems have been developed (see Table 33–1). These systems include both non-viral and viral approaches to accomplish gene transfer. In both of these approaches, the goal is to develop a system that can deliver genes in vivo after systemic administration. This development is a step toward deriving a "targetable-injectable" vector—a vector that can deliver therapeutic genes selectively to target cells after direct, in vivo administration. The development of such a vector system would have two very important consequences for potential gene therapy strategies: (1) it

FIGURE 33–1 ■ Methods to modify the adenoviral cellular tropism. Viral tropism is determined by the fiber and its recognition region in the terminus, or "knob" (dotted circle). Binding of the virus to target cells can be modified via either immunologic or genetic methods. Immunologic targeting involves the attachment of molecular conjugates incorporating antibodies against the fiber knob and ligands specific for cognate receptors in target cells. Genetic targeting involves the genetic modification of the fiber gene to generate fiber chimeras with novel ligand specificity. Note that in both cases, binding capacity to a non-native target cellular receptor is accompanied by ablation of the endogenous binding to the adenovirus primary receptor (coxsackievirus and adenovirus receptor [CAR]).

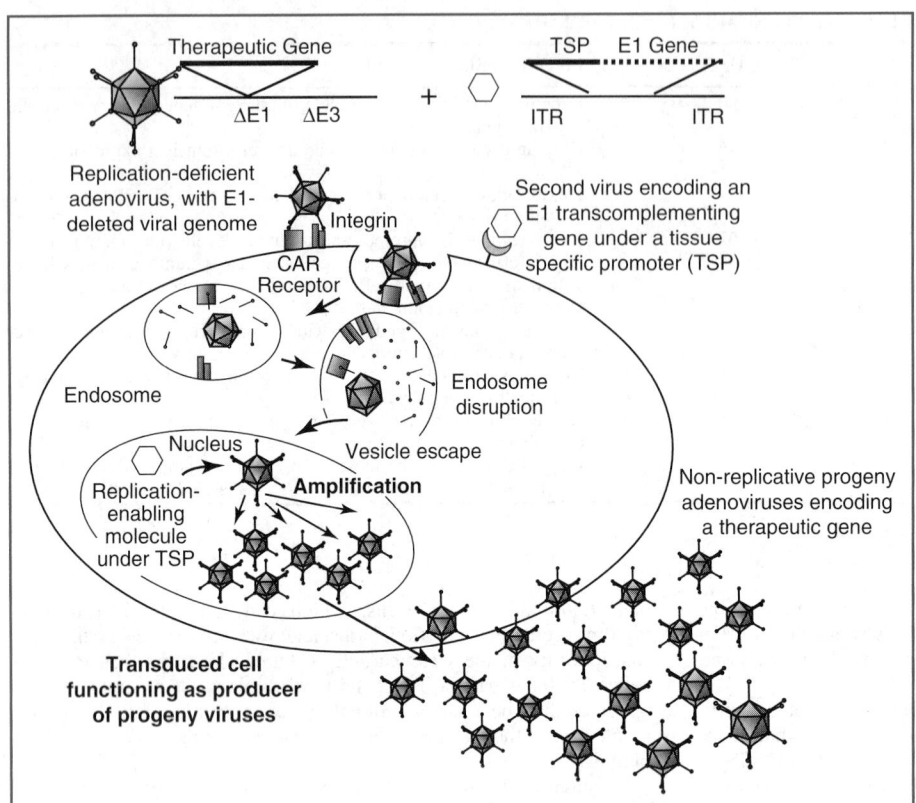

FIGURE 33–2 ■ Amplification of gene transfer by replicative viral vector systems. Replication-deficient adenoviruses can be genetically complemented in vivo in cells co-infected with a second vector that encodes the deleted replication-enabling molecules. Tissue- or tumor-specific promoters can regulate the expression of these proteins, thus limiting the occurrence of viral replication to the target tissue. Progeny virus leads to infection of neighboring cells, increased local viral inoculum, and augmentation of therapeutic gene expression.

would allow the implementation of a variety of gene therapy strategies targeted to cell or tissue types that cannot currently be modified ex vivo, and (2) it would allow gene therapy to be carried out in a context other than its present restriction to highly specialized tertiary care medical centers possessing the support facilities involved in ex vivo approaches.

A variety of nonviral systems have been developed and used in strategies to directly deliver genes in vivo. Liposomes are artificial lipid bilayer vesicles containing the foreign deoxyribonucleic acid (DNA). Their design overcomes the potential safety hazards associated with viral gene sequences contained in the viral vectors. Whereas initial formulations were associated with significant target cell toxicity, newer agents appear more promising in this regard. These vectors, delivered to select target organs after direct in vivo delivery, have been used in human clinical trials targeting pulmonary disorders and a wide variety of malignancies. Despite this systemic stability, delivery is at present non-specific, because the liposomes lack any mechanism to achieve targeting. This goal is the principal logic behind the design of molecular conjugate vectors. These synthetic molecules exploit the endogenous cellular receptor–mediated pathway to transfer genes. Their design characteristics allow a degree of targeting not available in other systems,

although a limited systemic stability may undermine the realization of that ability.

Non-retroviral viral vectors being actively developed include recombinant adenoviruses, the parvovirus adeno-associated virus (AAV), and vectors based on the herpes simplex virus. Adenoviruses have been evaluated for their ability to be directly delivered in vivo to a variety of organ systems, including the lung, liver, brain, and vasculature. Extensive characterization of the virus has made possible the introduction of numerous modifications in its genome and biochemical composition that overcome some of its limitations. Principal among them are the genetic and antibody-based modifications of the viral tropism (Fig. 33–1), the design of replicative vectors (Fig. 33–2), and the incorporation of immuno-modulatory genes. The AAV vector is less highly developed but has also been associated with practical problems, including a very limited heterologous DNA-carrying capacity as well as very low viral titers. Herpes simplex vectors were developed for highly efficient gene transfer into neuronal tissues, but replication-deficient vectors with high capacity and low cytotoxicity have recently found utility in other contexts, such as bone marrow–derived cells and malignant tissues.

The rapid appearance of alternative systems, including targeted

Table 33–2 ■ GENE THERAPY APPROACHES FOR THE TREATMENT OF CANCER

STRATEGY	CLINICAL TRIALS*	MOLECULAR MECHANISM OF ANTICANCER EFFECT
Mutation compensation	6	Inhibition of expression of dominant oncogene
	18	Augmentation of deficient tumor-suppressor genes
	2	Abrogation of autocrine growth factor loops (single chain antibodies)
Molecular chemotherapy	36	Selective delivery of toxin or toxin gene to cancer cells
Genetic immunopotentiation	54	In vitro transduction—augmentation of tropism or cell killing capacity of tumor-infiltrating lymphocytes; genetic modification of irradiated tumor cells
	47	In vivo transduction—administration of costimulatory molecules or cytokines; immunization with virus encoding tumor-associated antigens
Viral-mediated oncolysis	2	Tumor cell lysis by viral vector replication.

*Registered in the NIH Office of Recombinant DNA Activities at the end of 1998.

vectors built on available viral-based systems (see Fig. 33–1), predicts that additional strategies can achieve the central goal of targeted gene delivery after the targeted vector is administered directly in vivo. Furthermore, chimeras have been designed that adopt favorable features of parental vectors.

Initial strategies to accomplish gene therapy were designed for inherited genetic disorders. Since the first human clinical trial of gene therapy in 1990, a variety of genetic diseases—ADA deficiency, cystic fibrosis, Gaucher's disease, Canavan's disease, hyperlipidemia—have been treated using gene therapy. Specific strategies to treat a variety of other disorders are being developed, but the central problem of delivering genes to target cells has limited more general use of these methods for inherited genetic disorders.

Gene therapy is also rational in the context of acquired genetic disorders and thus has been used to target cancer; the overwhelming number of human gene therapy protocols in trial have been for cancer therapy. A variety of approaches have been developed based on the molecular pathogenesis of cancer. Specific strategies include the following: (1) a wild-type tumor suppressor gene for recessive oncogene mutations, (2) inhibitory gene constructs for dysregulated or overexpressed dominant oncogenes, (3) toxin genes selectively delivered to cancer cells to eradicate them, and (4) immunomodulatory genes to increase the immunogenicity of tumors (Table 33–2). Each of these specific strategies has a counterpart in human protocols that have been approved for clinical trials. Interestingly, these strategies have begun to be applied to inhibit or destroy the tumor vasculature.

Gene transfer may represent a therapeutic strategy applicable to contexts outside of genetic diseases. The ability to modulate specific patterns of gene expression may represent a viable option in certain inflammatory, vascular, and immune-mediated disorders. In this regard, specific genetic methods of abrogating selected patterns of gene expression have been shown to alter disease pathogenesis in models of inflammatory and fibrotic lung disease, rheumatoid arthritis, postischemic hepatic injury, postcatheterization arterial stenosis, peripheral artery disease, and organ graft rejection. Gene therapy thus offers a means for highly selected ablation of specific gene expression patterns. Using techniques of "anti-sense" inhibition or "single-chain antibodies," the informational flow from genes through the level of protein is interrupted based on sequence-specific hybridization or by antibody-antigen binding specificity. This strategy offers the potential to intervene with a level of specificity at multiple sites in the gene expression pathway not achievable using classic pharmacological therapies.

Thus, gene therapy may ultimately represent another form of pharmacotherapy, albeit a form with mostly improved potentials based on exploitation of the exquisite specificity offered by the cellular apparatus of gene expression. As vector technology achieves the basic ability to deliver therapeutic genes quantitatively, and specifically, into target cells, it is anticipated that promising results already observed in preclinical studies will translate quickly into the clinic for amelioration of a variety of diseases.

Andezion WF: Human gene therapy. Nature 392:25–30, 1998. *In-depth analysis of vector technology for gene transfer.*

Bilbao G, Feng M, Rancourt C, et al: Adenoviral/retroviral vector chimeras: A novel strategy to achieve high-efficiency stable transduction in vivo. FASEB J 11:624–634, 1997. *Novel, chimeric vector systems may be engineered to capitalize on favorable aspects of available gene therapy vectors.*

Roth JA, Cristiano RJ: Gene therapy for cancer: What have we done and where are we going? J Natl Cancer Inst 89:21–39, 1997. *First comprehensive account of results obtained in clinical trials of gene therapy for patients with cancer.*

URL: http://www.nih.gov/od/orda/protocol.pdj. *Updated list of human gene therapy clinical trials registered by the NIH Office of Recombinant DNA Activities.*

Verma I, Somia N: Gene therapy—promises, problems and prospects. Nature 389: 239–242, 1997. *State-of-the-art summary of gene therapy.*

34 CHROMOSOMES AND THEIR DISORDERS

R. Ellen Magenis

Cytogenetics is the study of chromosomes and their behavior as they relate to transmission of the genetic material from parent to offspring. Errors in chromosome behavior and structure are the cause of a wide range of clinical syndromes.

Every nucleated somatic cell in the human has a complete genome of about 6×10^9 base pairs of DNA, with an uncoiled total length of approximately 2 meters. The genome is packaged by supercoiling into 46 chromosomes, consisting of 22 pairs of homologous chromosomes (identical in regard to morphology and constituent gene loci) and 1 pair of sex chromosomes (X and Y), one partner of each pair being derived from the mother and one from the father. The 46 chromosomes in metaphase vary in length from 2 to 12 μm. The genes are arranged along the chromosomes in linear order, with each gene having a precise position or locus. Genes that have their loci on the same chromosome are said to be *syntenic;* genes that are close together on the same chromosome and tend to travel together during meiosis (little crossing-over) are said to be *linked.* Alternate forms of a gene that occupy the same locus are called *alleles.* Any one chromosome bears only a single allele at a given locus, although in the population as a whole there may be multiple alleles, any one of which can occupy that specific locus.

CELL DIVISION. The number of chromosomes found in somatic cells is constant and is termed the *diploid* (2n) number. Each gamete, however, has only half the diploid number and is said to be *haploid* (n). To maintain this regularity, two types of cell division occur: *mitosis,* which is the cell division occurring in somatic tissues during growth and repair, and *meiosis,* which is the specialized form of cell division occurring when gametes form.

MITOSIS. The function of mitosis is to distribute and maintain the continuity of the genetic material in every cell of the body. This process consists of a number of different phases, which results in an equal distribution of the chromosomes to the two daughter cells. The cell cycle has four stages: mitosis (M), gap$_1$ (G$_1$), synthesis (S), and gap$_2$ (G$_2$). The G$_1$ phase follows mitosis, during which RNA and protein synthesis occurs. S is the period during which DNA replication takes place and the DNA content of the cell doubles, and G$_2$ is the period during which energy requirements for cell division are built up and any repair of errors in DNA synthesis takes place. Mitosis has four phases: (1) prophase, during which the duplicated chromosomes condense into microscopically visible bodies; (2) metaphase, during which the chromosomes continue to contract and line up on the metaphase plate; (3) anaphase, when the chromatids of the chromosomes separate at the centromeres; and (4) telophase, when the separated chromatids gather and the cell divides.

MEIOSIS. This process occurs only during the formation of the gametes and results in four daughter cells, each with the haploid number of chromosomes. In males, each primary spermatocyte forms four functional spermatids that develop into sperm, whereas in females, each oocyte forms only one ovum, the remaining products of meiosis being nonfunctional polar bodies.

Processes fundamental to meiosis include chromosome pairing, chromosome crossing-over, and chromosome segregation. These processes result in halving the chromosome number, regular distribution of chromosomes to daughter cells, and independent assortment of the genetic material from both the cross-over events and maternal-paternal homologue distribution in meiosis I. The ultimate result ensures genetic variability.

METHODS FOR THE PREPARATION OF CHROMOSOMES. Because non-dividing chromosomes cannot be analyzed, live dividing cells are required for chromosome analysis. The cell type most commonly used is the mitogenically stimulated peripheral blood lymphocyte. Skin fibroblasts, bone marrow cells, amniotic fluid cells, chorionic villus cells, and tumor cells are also used for special tests. Dividing cells are accumulated at metaphase. To accomplish this, a drug (Colcemide) that destroys the mitotic spindle is added to the culture medium toward the end of the culture period. The cells are subjected to hypotonic treatment followed by fixation and spreading on microscope slides. The slides are then stained.

Staining techniques may result in either a non-banded or a banded appearance of the chromosomes. Laboratories today use at least one of several banding techniques; this results in a great deal of additional information. These methods provide a means to precisely identify each chromosome and extra or missing chromosomes as well as the exact localization of breakpoints in chromosome rearrangements.

HIGH-RESOLUTION CHROMOSOMES. Cells are synchronized with the use of a methotrexate (or other) block; the block is released and the cells harvested at the times predicted to "catch" the chromosomes in late prophase or early metaphase, revealing more bands. With this approach, a band level of over 800 per haploid set can be achieved, which allows detection of a number of microdeletion syndromes (Fig. 34–1).

MOLECULAR CYTOGENETICS. Fluorescence in situ hybridization (FISH) is a recent advance in clinical cytogenetic technology that bridges the gap between molecular genetics and cytogenetics. Selected DNA sequences at least 2 to 3 kilobases long are used as probes. Probes are labeled by nick translation, usually with biotin or digoxigenin and then denatured by heat. Chromosomes are prepared by routine methods and are denatured using formamide and heat. The probe(s) is applied to these metaphase preparations and allowed to reanneal. The hybridization site(s) is detected by using fluorochrome-conjugated reagents and fluorescence microscopy.

FISH allows the detection of submicroscopic deletions, subtle rearrangements, and small duplications; and it can identify marker chromosomes and the content of multiple rearranged chromosomes. FISH is also useful for detecting aneuploidy (extra or missing chromosomes) in interphase cells in cancers.

HUMAN CHROMOSOME NOMENCLATURE. The 46 human chromosomes consist of three types, designated by the position of the centromere or primary constriction. These are metacentric, sub-

metacentric, and acrocentric, depending on whether the position of the centromere is median, submedian, or near terminal. Each individual chromosome pair can be recognized when banding techniques are used, and the chromosomes are numbered from 1 to 22 in descending order of length. In the female, the two sex chromosomes—designated X chromosomes—are identical, whereas in the male the two sex chromosomes—designated X and Y—are morphologically different.

The nomenclature used to describe the chromosomes and their bands, variants, and rearrangements is described in detail by the International System of Human Cytogenetic Nomenclature (ISCN). A shorthand notation is used to describe the chromosome complement of an individual. In this notation the number of chromosomes is specified first, followed by the listing of the sex chromosomes. Thus, a normal female karyotype is designated 46,XX and a normal male karyotype is designated 46,XY. Any deviations of the autosomes are written after the sex chromosomes. An individual autosome is referred to by its number, its short arm by the letter p, and its long arm by the letter q. A + or − sign written before a designated chromosome indicates that the chromosome is extra (+) or missing (−); for example, 47,XX + 21 describes a female with 47 chromosomes, including an extra chromosome 21 in addition to the 46 chromosomes of the normal karyotype.

To describe a translocation between two autosomes the small letter t is used outside parentheses and the chromosome numbers are inside: for example, 46,XY,t(9;21)(q34;p11). This indicates a male with a normal number of chromosomes and a reciprocal translocation between the long arm of chromosome 9 and short arm of chromosome 21 with designated breakpoints.

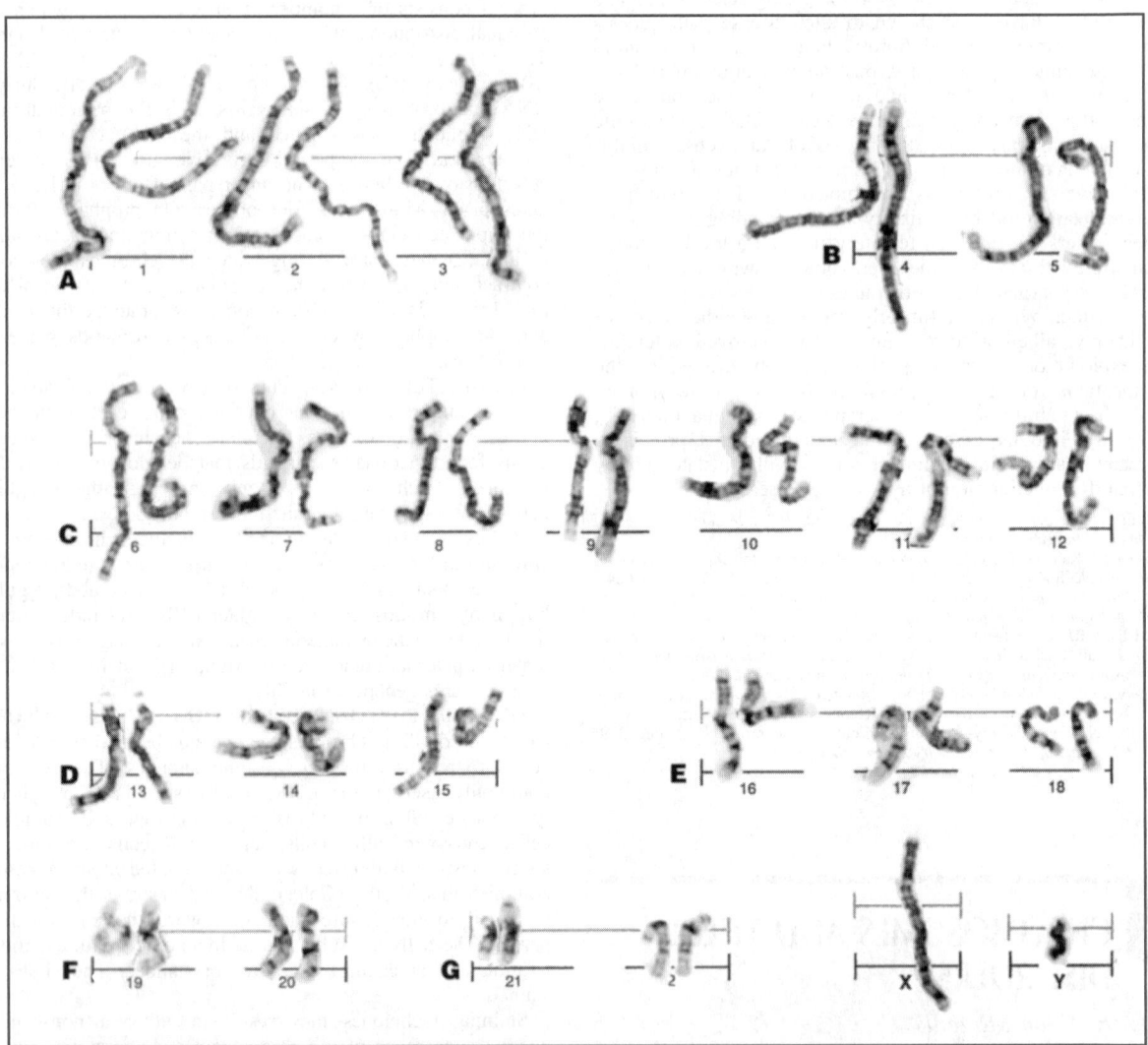

FIGURE 34–1 ■ Normal Giemsa-banded (G-band) male karyotype at the 850-band stage. This band level is the best to look for microdeletions, although the long chromosomes tend to curve and overlapping of chromosomes is frequent.

Chromosome abnormalities can be divided into two classes: abnormalities of number and structure.

ABNORMALITIES OF CHROMOSOME NUMBER. These arise from non-disjunction, that is, from the failure of two homologous chromosomes in the first division of meiosis or of two sister chromatids in either mitosis or the second division of meiosis to pass to opposite poles of the cell. Non-disjunction results in cells with abnormal chromosome numbers. If these cells are gametes, fertilization results in a zygote with an abnormal chromosome number. If non-disjunction occurs during an early cleavage division of a zygote, then chromosomal mosaicism (two or more cell lines differing in chromosome complement) may result.

ABNORMALITIES OF CHROMOSOME STRUCTURE. These result from chromosome breakage and reunion. When a chromosome breaks it can rejoin in its old form (restitution) or it can rejoin with another broken chromosome (reunion). Reunion leads to a structural rearrangement that can be balanced or unbalanced. If it is balanced, the amount of genetic material is presumed to be identical to that found in a normal cell; and there is a simple rearrangement of the distribution of this material. Types of balanced rearrangements include balanced reciprocal translocations, Robertsonian translocations, and inversions. Balanced chromosome rearrangements do not usually lead to any clinical change. If the rearrangement is unbalanced, this indicates loss or gain of chromosome material. Such unbalanced rearrangements in meiotic cells usually result in changes in the clinical phenotype.

CHROMOSOME DELETION. Deletion is the loss of a chromosome segment after chromosome breakage (Fig. 34–2A and B). Deletions may be terminal or interstitial or result in ring chromosomes.

CHROMOSOME DUPLICATION. Duplication is the addition of a chromosome segment and may be the result of breakage reunion or of replication error (see Fig. 34–2C). The isochromosome shown in Figure 34–2D has both a deleted short arm and a duplicated long arm, or deletion and duplication.

INVERSIONS. These result from two chromosome breaks with inversion of the intervening segment and can be detected only by altered position of the centromere or by chromosome banding studies that show a changed banding sequence (see Fig. 34–2E). Inversions result in disturbances in chromosome pairing and in the formation of unbalanced as well as balanced gametes.

BALANCED RECIPROCAL TRANSLOCATION. This results from exchange of chromosome segments between non-homologous chromosomes (see Fig. 34–2F). An individual carrying such a rearrangement has a higher frequency of abnormal gametes as the result of a disturbance in chromosome pairing at meiosis. Such individuals themselves have a balanced chromosome complement and are clinically normal, but they may have a high risk of having congenitally malformed children and/or spontaneous abortions. Normal children may also be born. Such persons require careful genetic counseling (see Chapter 37).

ROBERTSONIAN TRANSLOCATION. This is a specific type of unequal reciprocal translocation that occurs between acrocentric chromosomes, resulting in a new metacentric chromosome formed from two acrocentric chromosomes. Such rearrangements may be important in the transmission of Down syndrome when one of the chromosomes involved is chromosome 21. If the structural change occurs in the early embryo, mosaicism with some cells normal and some with the structural abnormality may result.

CONSEQUENCES OF CHROMOSOME IMBALANCE

FETAL LOSS. Through the processes of meiosis and mitosis, regular distribution of the chromosomes to daughter cells generally occurs. However, errors in these processes are frequent and account for a large portion of fetal loss. It is estimated that at least 50% of all conceptuses are lost in the first 2 to 3 weeks after conception, most due to major chromosome abnormalities. Chromosome studies of spontaneously aborted first-trimester fetuses show a chromosome abnormality rate of close to 50%. The most common abnormalities, each occurring in about 25% of the chromosomally abnormal cases, are 45,X, missing a sex chromosome, and triploidy with three sets of chromosomes (3n). The remainder include trisomy for any of the autosomes with the exception of chromosome 1, which has been

seen only in studies of the early zygote. Among the trisomies, trisomy 16 is the most frequent. No autosomal monosomies have been detected; it is postulated that they do occur at the same rate as the trisomies, as would be predicted from segregation events, but are so severely impaired that implantation does not occur.

TRIPLOIDY. Triploidy is characterized by cystic degeneration of the placenta, sometimes appearing as a hydatidiform mole, with an accompanying fetus. The fetus is small for gestational age and has low-set ears and syndactyly. There is a markedly increased incidence of toxemia of pregnancy, and eclampsia may ensue. By using chromosome heteromorphisms as a tool and molecular techniques for confirmation, it has been shown that most triploidy is due to double fertilization of a single egg.

The true mole may be confused with triploidy because it also has cystic degeneration of the placenta, the cysts appearing in grapelike clusters. However, there is no accompanying fetus and the chromosomes are always apparently normal 46,XX. Both sets of chromosomes are paternal in origin, with no maternal contribution, likely the result of fertilization of an empty egg. The malignant potential of the true mole is high, whereas triploidy is rarely associated with malignancy.

45,X FETUSES. The 45,X fetuses are markedly edematous and have large cystic masses encircling the neck. They are small for gestational age and generally have characteristic facial features.

AUTOSOMAL TRISOMY. Only three autosomal trisomies survive to term: trisomies of chromosomes 13, 18, and 21. Most trisomies 13 and 18 are lost before term, and those that survive to term usually live no more than 1 year. About 70% of trisomy 21 conceptions die before term; with modern treatment, many of those individuals doing well after birth may survive to old age. Mosaicism for autosomal trisomy along with a normal cell population may modify the phenotype and allow survival.

BIRTH DEFECTS/PATTERNS OF MALFORMATION. Seven to 10 per cent of stillbirths and neonatal deaths are due to chromosome imbalance; trisomy 18 and trisomy 13 are frequent in this group. At least 0.5 to 1% of all liveborns have chromosome abnormalities. These chromosome abnormalities result in multiple major and/or minor malformations that occur in recognizable patterns essentially specific to the particular chromosome or chromosome segment.

DYSMORPHOLOGY. Dysmorphology is the study of malformations secondary to abnormal embryonic or fetal development. Malformations may be the result of inborn errors in morphogenesis or the result of exposure to teratogenic agents; the latter may mimic malformations due to altered genetic control.

Dysmorphology is still primarily a descriptive discipline. To diagnose the abnormal, an appreciation of normal biologic variation is important. Diversity of facial features and body habitus in individuals, families, and ethnic groups must be considered. Minor malformations having no medical significance such as epicanthal folds or low-set ears should be looked for in the physical examination because they may serve as clues to more serious defects and/or help in defining specific syndromes. Major malformations affecting a part of an organ, an entire organ, or a larger region of the body that are of medical consequence may be the result of imbalance of large or small chromosome segments, but small chromosome abnormalities such as some microdeletions may not result in any major malformations.

CHROMOSOMAL SYNDROMES

A syndrome is a characteristic overall pattern of anomalies presumed to be causally related.

NUMERICAL ABNORMALITIES. Abnormalities of the sex chromosomes (e.g., 45,X; 47,XXX; 47,XXY; 47,XYY) are the most frequently found chromosome aberrations among live newborns and individuals studied later because of suspect clinical features.

Sex chromosome abnormalities in general have less severe phenotypic consequences than do those caused by autosomal imbalance. This is due to lyonization (x-inactivation) of all X chromosomes except one; e.g., the XXX female will have two X chromosomes inactivated, the XX normal female, one.

LYONIZATION. In females, the sex chromosomes are identical in

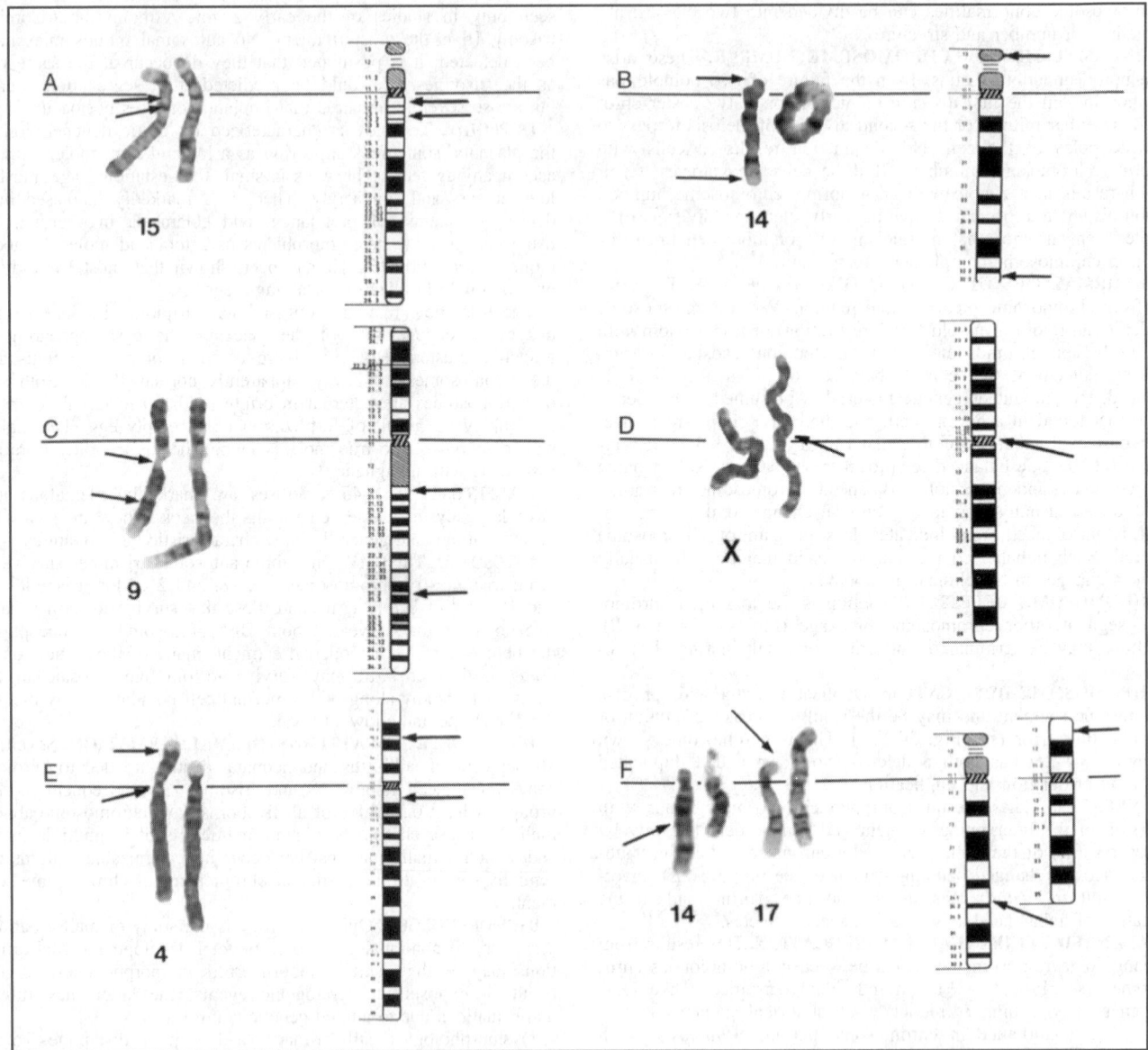

FIGURE 34–2 ■ Partial karyotypes illustrating several types of structural chromosome aberrations. The abnormal chromosomes are placed on the right of each pair. *A,* Interstitial deletion: Chromosomes 15 from a patient with Angelman syndrome. Ideogram and chromosomes are at the 850-band stage. Arrows on the ideogram and normal 15 indicate the small segment deleted. This same deletion is seen in 75 to 80% of patients with Prader-Willi syndrome. *B,* Ring chromosome: Chromosomes 14 from a patient with nonspecific mental retardation. Both ends of the abnormal chromosome have very small deletions; the broken ends are joined in the form of a ring. Chromosomes are at the 550 band stage. *C,* Duplication: Chromosomes 9 at about the 850-band level. In the right-hand chromosome 9 there is an interstitial duplication of a large segment on the long arm, delineated by the arrows on the normal chromosome. The patient had multiple minor anomalies and mental retardation. *D,* Isochromosomes with duplication-deficiency: X-chromosomes from a patient with Turner syndrome. Chromosomes at the 550-band stage show a deletion duplication, in this case due to isochromosome formation. Both arms of the abnormal chromosome are long arms; the short arm is missing. One explanation for this recurring characteristic abnormality is centromere misdivision. The arrow points to the centromere of the abnormal chromosome. *E,* Inversion: balanced chromosome 4 pericentric inversion delineated by arrows, from a normal woman. This inversion chromosome segregated throughout her family. Chromosomes are at the 550-band stage. *F,* Translocation: balanced reciprocal translocation between chromosomes 14 and 17 from a normal individual. Arrows indicate breakpoints. Ideogram is at the 550-band level as are the chromosomes 14; the chromosomes 17 are between the 550- and 850-band length. This likely is due to position in the metaphase spread; chromosomes at the periphery are often longer than those at the center.

size and are genetically homologous chromosomes (as in the case of autosomes); however, in the normal diploid interphase cell, one of the X chromosomes forms a condensed heterochromatic body called the *Barr body.* This condensation, together with evidence from coat color pattern in mice, led Lyon to hypothesize *X inactivation.* She stated (1) in each somatic cell there is inactivation of all but one of the X chromosomes; (2) this process occurs early in development and is random with respect to maternally or paternally derived X chromosomes in different cells; and (3) once a particular X chromosome is inactive, it is inactive in all daughter cells.

This hypothesis is important with regard to several aspects of X chromosome gene expression: (1) It reveals the mechanism for dosage compensation, a process that equalizes the amount of X chromosome gene expression between females with two X chromosomes and males having only one X chromosome; (2) it explains some of the phenotypic effects associated with additional or missing sex chromosomes, or the occasional manifesting XX carrier of an X-linked recessive disorder; and (3) it indicates the complexity of testing for carrier status of X-linked diseases.

Evidence that dosage compensation has taken place in males

SYNDROME	DESCRIPTION
Velocardiofacial/(Sprintzen) DiGeorge	*Common:* cleft palate; conotruncal heart defects (interrupted aortic arch, tetralogy of Fallot, right side aortic arch, ventriculoseptal defect) *Also present:* pharyngeal hypotonia, retrognathia, malar flatness, small anomalous ears, tortuous retinal vessels, slender tapered digits, scoliosis, short stature *Face:* long with narrow palpebral fissures, thickening of helical rims; nose is prominent with squared nasal root, philtrum is long, mouth is often held open; velopharyngeal incompetence with or without cleft palate
Prader-Willi	*Face:* narrow bifrontal diameter, almond-shaped eyes, thin upper lip, down-turned mouth *Genitalia:* particularly male, are hypoplastic; hypogonadism; delayed puberty *Other:* truncal obesity after age 1 to 4 years
Angelman	Small head; occiput is flat, often with a pronounced occipital groove. Eyes may be mildly wide spaced and deep set, nose is mildly prominent, mouth is large, teeth widely spaced. Ataxic gait. Happy demeanor.

chromosome abnormalities differs greatly for males and females. Large duplications and deletions in the female with an accompanying normal X almost always result in Turner syndrome, whereas they are lethal in the male. A specific structural abnormality, isochromosome Xq (two copies of the X long arm joined with the missing short arm) is common among girls with Turner syndrome, comprising 20% of the total abnormal karyotypes.

Microdeletions and duplications may show little effect in the carrier female but have syndromic consequences for the male. For example, microdeletion Xp22.32 in the male results in ichthyosis, chondrodysplasia punctata, short stature, and mental retardation. When the deletion is somewhat larger and includes the Kallman gene, inability to smell and hypogonadotropic hypogonadism occur in addition to the other features. In all instances of X microdeletion

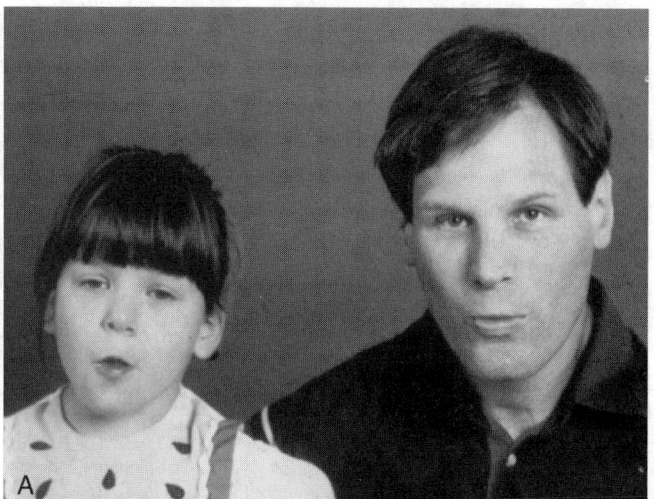

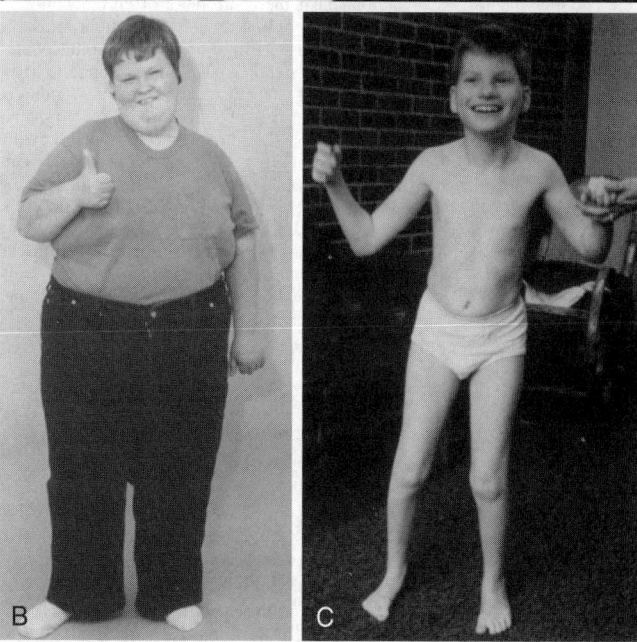

FIGURE 34–3 ■ *A,* Father and daughter with velocardiofacial syndrome. Note masklike facial features and lack of ability to purse the lips for whistling. The father had had repair of a congenital heart defect (tetralogy of Fallot); the child had a normal heart. A small deletion of chromosome 22 long arm is found in most cases, sometimes detected only with molecular-cytogenetic techniques. *B,* Twenty-year-old man with Prader-Willi syndrome. He has a de novo deletion of the proximal long arm of chromosome 15, which occurred on the chromosome 15 homolog inherited from his father. *C,* Twelve-year-old boy with Angelman syndrome. He is ataxic and unable to walk without help, is happy and alert, but is severely mentally retarded and has no speech. He has the same de novo deletion as the patient in Figure 34–3B, but the deletion occurred on the chromosome 15 inherited from his mother.

with XXY or females with XXX is the fact that interphase cells in these cases have one or two condensed heterochromatic (Barr) bodies.

THE 45,X LIVEBORN (TURNER SYNDROME). The most consistent features found in girls with a missing sex chromosome are short stature, usually beginning before birth, and gonadal dysgenesis. Although eggs may be present in the newborn gonad, early attrition takes place and eggs have disappeared by puberty. There is puffiness of the hands and feet usually disappearing in childhood, low posterior hairline and short and/or webbed neck, excessive pigmented nevi, deep-set nails, short fourth metacarpal, narrow maxilla, prominent ears, horseshoe kidney, and heart defect (usually coarctation of the aorta). Pubertal development usually does not occur in the absence of hormonal treatment.

47,XXY (KLINEFELTER SYNDROME). This condition occurs in about 1 in 500 males and is the most common cause of male infertility. These males are tall with long limbs, have testes that remain small after puberty, have gynecomastia, are dull mentally (about 20% with IQ < 80), and are immature in behavior.

47,XXX. There are no characteristic major or minor malformations found in 47,XXX females; almost all appear normal at birth. Height, weight, and head circumference are generally normal, although the head may be at a lower centile than height and weight. Language is usually delayed, and IQ is lower than normal, particularly lower than the IQ of siblings. Behavioral and social problems and emotional immaturity are the rule. Normal sexual development generally occurs; although apparently not frequent, both 47,XXX and 47,XXY individuals have been reported in offspring of females with this condition.

47,XYY. The 47,XYY karyotype has elicited much public interest because of the reports of association with criminality. Occurrence of the karyotype is common, occurring in about 1 in 1000 male births. These males are tall and may have mild fine motor problems, impulsive behavior, and temper outbursts. Although most affected males blend into the general population, it is now recognized, after correction for earlier ascertainment bias, that there is an excess of aberrant or criminal behavior as compared with 46,XY males. Such behaviors may occur even with IQ scores as high as 146. However, the average IQ of 47,XYY males is somewhat lower than that of normal males.

48,XXXX; 48,XXXY; 49,XXXXX; 49,XXXXY. In general, as additional X chromosomes are added, the phenotypic consequences become more severe. Mental retardation is constant, dysmorphia is evident, stature tends to be small, and skeletal anomalies may occur. Facial features may suggest Down syndrome.

STRUCTURAL ABNORMALITIES. The outcome of structural X

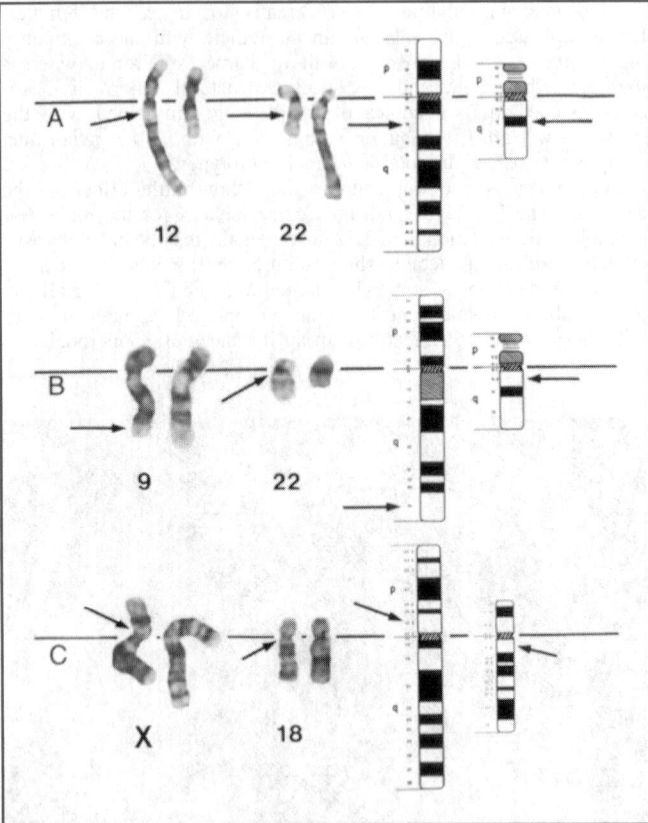

FIGURE 34-4 ■ Partial karyotypes from three specific cancers illustrating recurring rearrangements in specific cancer types. The ideograms on the right are at the 400-band stage. *A,* Chromosomes 12 and 22 from a clear cell sarcoma. There is a breakpoint near the centromere of chromosome 12 long arm; arrow indicates the break site on the far left normal chromosome 12 and on the ideogram. The material distal to the break site is translocated to chromosome 22 as part of an apparently balanced exchange. Arrow points to breakpoint site on the normal chromosome 22 and ideogram. *B,* Chromosomes 9 *(far left)* and 22 from a patient with chronic myelogenous leukemia. Arrows point to break sites on the normal chromosomes beyond which the material on the abnormal chromosomes has been exchanged. This rearrangement results in a new fusion gene (BCR on chromosome 22 and *ABL* oncogene on 9) that alters the function of certain hematopoietic cells. *C,* Translocation between the proximal short arm of the X chromosome and the proximal long arm of chromosome 18 is the hallmark of synovial sarcoma. Arrows point to the breakpoint region on the normal chromosomes (left chromosome of each pair) while the rearranged chromosomes are on the right. The fusion product has not yet been characterized.

syndromes in the male, mothers should have chromosome analysis performed because the carrier rate is high.

FRAGILE X. Clinical features in this syndrome vary even in the male, and carrier females often have minimal expression. This chromosome aberration also is not expressed in all who carry the defect, particularly females, making diagnosis of the condition difficult. The fragile X chromosome appears as a recurrent break at the same site in Xq27 in 4 to 50% of cells. The syndrome is frequent, occurring in 2 to 6% of retarded males. Birth weight is usually high and the head relatively large. The face is long and narrow with prominent chin and ears. There is usually macroorchidism. Mental retardation is moderately severe. About 15% exhibit autistic features.

With the finding of CGG trinucleotide repeat sequences in excess in the fragile X mental retardation 1 gene (*FMR-1*) in affected males, a molecular test has become available that can reliably diagnose carriers.

X/Y TRANSLOCATIONS. The XX male with short stature, infantile testes, and mild intellectual difficulties is almost always the result of a cryptic translocation between the distal X short arm and distal Y short arm with transfer of the *SRY* gene (sex reversal Y) from the Y to the X.

Y-CHROMOSOME SYNDROMES. Mosaicism for loss of the Y chromosome (45,X/46,XY) has varying results, probably depending on the percentage of cells missing a Y chromosome in the developing gonad. Peripheral blood cell mosaicism is compatible with normal male phenotype, with genital ambiguity, and with mixed gonadal dysgenesis or full Turner syndrome. In the latter case, surgical extirpation and pathologic examination of the dysgenetic gonads are recommended because of the danger of gonadoblastoma.

Deletion of the distal short arm of the Y when it includes the *SRY* gene results in a female with gonadal dysgenesis and usually also lymphedema, as in Turner syndrome. However, these individuals are usually not short and may have excellent muscle strength.

AUTOSOMAL ANEUPLOIDY

Of the three autosomal trisomies that may survive to a term birth, only one allows long-term survival—trisomy 21 (Down syndrome). Trisomy 21 syndrome is both common and well known, the features described by Down almost 130 years ago. It was the first syndrome known to have a chromosomal cause, the extra chromosome discovered by Lejeune in 1959. Increased incidence of the condition with increased maternal age was suspected by Mitchell in 1876 and shown statistically by Penrose in 1933. This increased incidence has led to the use of amniocentesis for prenatal diagnosis of Down syndrome in older mothers.

About 95% of individuals with Down syndrome have trisomy 21; the other 5% have translocation, predominantly Robertsonian translocation between 14 and 21.

Clinical features do not differ between trisomy and translocation cases unless the translocation involves more distal breakpoints on chromosome 21. Clinical features in the newborn include hypotonia, hyperextensible joints, excess skin on back of neck, flat facial profile, slanted palpebral fissures, overfolded helices, protruding tongue, short fifth fingers with single creases, single palmar creases, and plantar furrow. In the older individual, Brushfield spots may be more evident, strabismus and nystagmus may occur, fissured lips and furrowed tongue are common, pectus carinatum or excavatum may appear, and small genitalia may be noted. Moderate mental retardation is a constant feature. Congenital heart defects are present in about 50% of cases. There is an increased susceptibility to infection and an immunoglobulin imbalance. Antithyroid antibodies are found frequently as is an increased rate of hypothyroidism.

AUTOSOMAL STRUCTURAL ABNORMALITIES

There is an almost unlimited number of different ways in which the 22 pairs of autosomes can be broken with pieces lost (deletions) or reattached (translocations, duplications). Therefore, numerous described syndromes occur owing to imbalance of such chromosome segments. Four such syndromes are summarized to illustrate certain points; all are microdeletion syndromes recognized by their recurring patterns of anomalies before recognition of their chromosomal origin. Other well-known syndromes that have been shown to be due to microdeletions are Williams syndrome (del 7q), Rubinstein-Taybi syndrome (del 16p), and Miller-Dieker lissencephaly syndrome (del 17p).

DEL(22)(q11q11) VCF (SPRINTZEN) AND DIGEORGE MICRO-DELETION SYNDROMES. Velocardiofacial (VCF or Sprintzen) syndrome and DiGeorge syndrome are now recognized to be the result of deletion of a small portion of the long arm of chromosome 22 near the centromere. The *syndrome appears to be extremes along a clinical continuum* not specifically related to the size of the deletion. The condition in some individuals is so mild that the individual blends into the normal population. The true incidence of this syndrome is unknown, but it may be as common as Down syndrome.

Although the deletion of chromosome 22(q11) may be so small that it cannot be detected at the microscope without FISH, major malformations may be present (Table 34-1 and Fig. 34-3A). Mild to moderate mental retardation may be present, and speech is hypernasal even without clefting. Absent thymus, tonsils, and adenoids and hypocalcemia in infancy have been noted. Affect is often very bland, including facial expression; phobias and psychosis may appear in adolescents and adults.

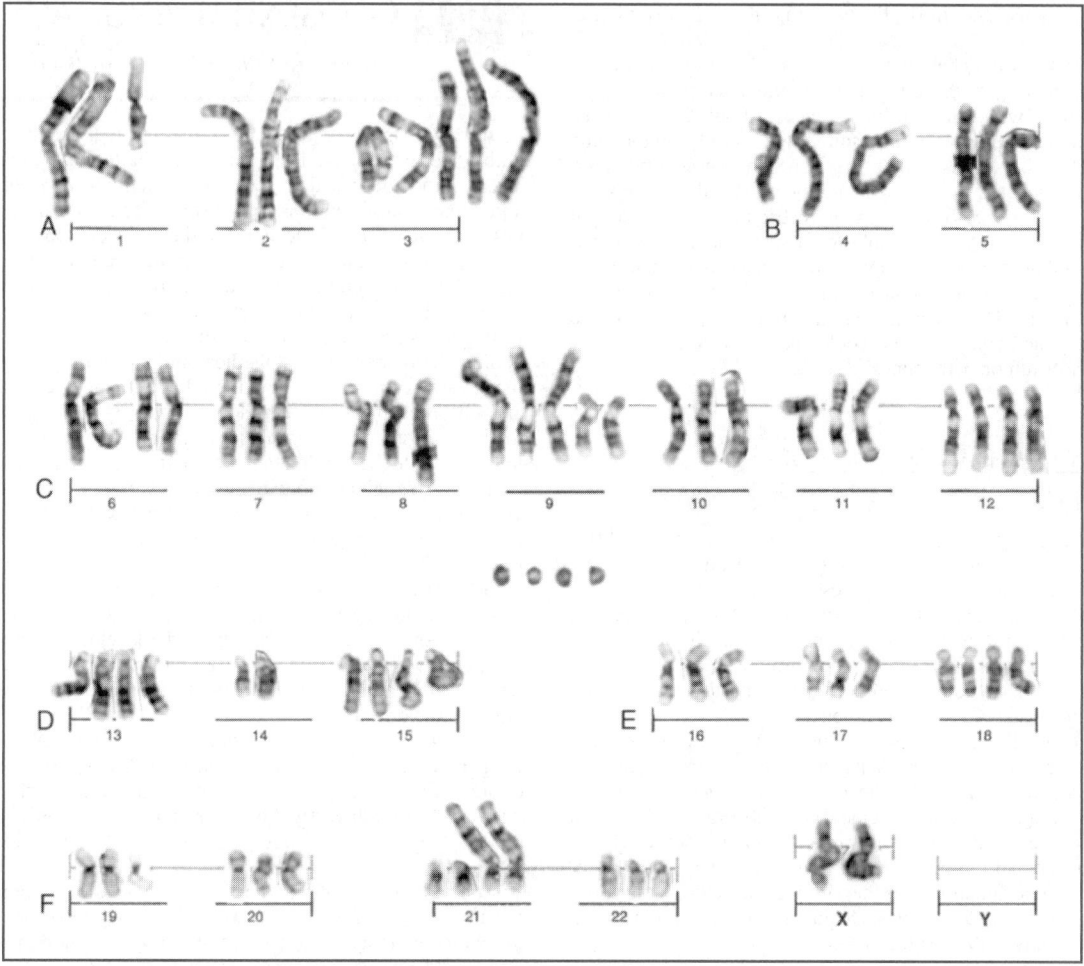

FIGURE 34–5. ■ Karyotype from a metastatic malignant melanoma illustrating the complex numerical and structural abnormalities usually seen. The structural abnormalities involve chromosomes 1, 3, 4, 6, 8, 9, 14, and 21; and there are four small unidentifiable ring chromosomes. Note that all five chromosomes 9 are abnormal, with missing short arms, replaced in three with material from another chromosome.

PRADER-WILLI AND ANGELMAN SYNDROMES. Prader-Willi syndrome was first described in 1956; that it is a chromosomal microdeletion syndrome was not known until 1981, when a small deletion of the proximal long arm of chromosome 15 was recognized. Clinical findings uniquely change with age. In the newborn period and infancy the infant may be so hypotonic that a primary muscle disorder is suspected; however, muscle biopsy and other neuromuscular studies show no abnormality. The infant is difficult to feed and weight gain is slow, as is motor development. The infant improves over time; and at some time after age 12 months and before 6 years, rapid increase in weight occurs and the child becomes progressively morbidly obese in the absence of intervention. Physical features are described in Table 34–1 and Figure 34–3B. Behavior problems are frequent in older children; stubbornness and obsessive-compulsive behavior are common, and temper tantrums may be sudden and severe.

In 1987 it was first reported that individuals with Angelman syndrome, a condition that clinically is very different from Prader-Willi syndrome, have a chromosome 15 proximal long arm deletion indistinguishable from that seen in Prader-Willi syndrome. Angelman syndrome is characterized by normal size at birth and normal appearance; incoordinated suck and swallow, resulting in feeding difficulties; developmental delay noted at about age 6 months; limited babbling; absent speech; ataxic gait; happy disposition with frequent smiles and laughter; excessive drooling; and seizures. Table 34–1 and Figure 34–3C list physical features. After these individuals learn to walk around age 3 to 5, activity becomes almost ceaseless.

PARENTAL ORIGIN. As early as 1983, chromosome heteromor-

phism studies of individuals with Prader-Willi syndrome and their parents showed that in all cases the deletion of chromosome 15 had occurred on a paternally derived chromosome. Similar parental origin studies, using molecular techniques in addition to chromosome heteromorphisms of individuals with Angelman syndrome, have shown that the chromosome 15 deletion in all instances occurred on the maternally transmitted chromosome. These data forced the recognition that there must be gender-specific differences in the expression of certain genes in some regions of the human genome.

UNIPARENTAL DISOMY. Some cases of Angelman syndrome and of Prader-Willi syndrome do not involve a cytogenetically visible deletion. In almost all the non-deletion Prader-Willi syndrome cases, parental origin studies have identified characteristics that heretofore were thought *not* to occur in the human—findings of uniparental disomy, a situation in which both chromosomes 15 are maternal in origin and no paternal chromosome 15 is present. About 5% of the cases of non-deletion Angelman syndrome have shown uniparental disomy with two copies of chromosome 15 of paternal origin and no maternal copy. These findings further suggest that a gene or genes in the region 15q11 have differential expression, depending on the gender of the parent, now termed *imprinting*.

IMPRINTING. Imprinting is the differential epigenetic modification of certain maternal and paternal genes in the zygote that results in the differential expression of the parental alleles during development and in the adult. This phenomenon affects only certain regions of the human genome, one region being that involved in Prader-Willi syndrome and Angelman syndrome on the proximal long arm of chromosome 15. Several hypotheses have been formulated to explain this, the most likely being that of methylation differences.

RETINOBLASTOMA. The malignant tumor retinoblastoma is hereditary, originating in the eye. It is inherited as an autosomal dominant disorder with reduced penetrance. About 5% of these patients have a constitutional chromosomal deletion of chromosome 13, band q14. This suggests that the gene for susceptibility to retinoblastoma is located in the segment deleted and that it must be a tumor-suppressor gene. Studies using restriction fraction length polymorphism linked to the retinoblastoma locus have shown that loss of the homologous normal retinoblastoma gene is necessary for the tumor to develop. This would constitute the second event, the primary event being the constitutional mutation or deletion of the retinoblastoma gene. These events would then fit Knudsen's "two-hit" hypothesis in tumor pathogenesis.

ACQUIRED CHROMOSOMAL ABNORMALITIES

Cancer Cytogenetics

Current thinking regarding the role of chromosome abnormalities in the pathogenesis of cancer is that the chromosomal change affects cancer-promoting or cancer-suppressor genes, altering the stable normal behavioral characteristics of the cell to the unstable behavior typical of malignancy. These changes may occur through either loss or gain of a chromosome or chromosomal segment or rearrangement of chromosomal material that might alter function by virtue of an altered gene or fusion of genes.

With loss of material due to terminal deletion it is suspected that there is concurrent loss of suppressor gene(s), but, if interstitial, the rejoined new segments may alter function of the splice point genes so that control is altered or a combined gene is formed. Gain of a chromosome or segment conceivably results in a dose effect of contained genes resulting in altered dynamics. Translocations recombine genes; gene function may be eliminated, new fusion genes created, and regulation damaged such that inactivation, activation, or up-regulation may occur (Fig. 34–4).

Over time, further chromosomal changes (evolution) usually occur in cancers as they progress, causing complex numerical and structural alterations. Although typical evolution is known for some malignancies as in chronic myelogenous leukemia, it is not known for most types of cancer (Fig. 34–5).

Cancer Categories

Cancers are classified in three major categories: (1) hematologic malignancies, (2) lymphomas, and (3) solid tumors. Although tremendous advances have been made in the study of solid tumors, much more information is known in diagnosis, prognosis, and treatment of the leukemias (see Chapters 176 and 177). This is so despite the far greater numbers of solid tumors, because of difficulties in obtaining the appropriate solid tumor tissue, and culturing and obtaining good-quality chromosomes. Nevertheless, because there have been many improvements, many laboratories can perform solid tumor cytogenetics.

The number of recognized recurrent chromosome abnormalities in all categories is now large. For many cancers, malignancy behavior, prognosis, and treatment modalities may be determined by the specific chromosomal change(s).

Gorlin RJ, Cohen MM, Levin LS: Syndromes of the Head and Neck. New York, Oxford University Press, 1990. *Almost encyclopedic in scope; the one you take to the clinic with you.*

Heim S, Mitelman F: Cancer Cytogenetics. New York, Wiley-Liss, 1995. *The overall most useful cancer cytogenetics text.*

Jones KL: Smith's Recognizable Patterns of Human Malformation. Philadelphia, WB Saunders, 1997. *The favorite text on syndromes, now updated.*

Mitelman F (ed): An International System for Human Cytogenetic Nomenclature. Basel, S. Karger, 1995. *This volume presents internationally accepted guidelines for naming and numbering human chromosomes, normal and abnormal.*

Rimoin DL, Connor JM, Pyritz RE: Emery and Rimoin's Principles and Practice of Medical Genetics. New York, Churchill Livingstone, 1997. *An excellent practical text of medical genetics containing outstanding chapters on basic and clinical cytogenetics.*

Schinzel A: Catalog of Unbalanced Chromosome Aberrations in Man. Berlin, Walter de Gruyter & Co, 1984. *For its age useful but needs to be brought up-to-date.*

35 CONGENITAL ANOMALIES

Margot I. Van Allen ▪ *Judith G. Hall*

DEFINITION. Structural abnormalities that result from errors in embryogenesis or the fetal period are called *congenital anomalies*. These anomalies, which are also sometimes referred to as major and minor malformations and birth defects, can occur in all organ systems and parts of the body, either in isolation or in association with other anomalies. *Severe anomalies* are defined as structural anomalies that require medical and/or surgical treatment and are cosmetically significant. *Mild anomalies* are structural alterations posing no significant health or social burdens. When multiple congenital anomalies occur together and are etiologically related they may result from *syndromes*, including monogenic (see Chapter 31) and chromosome disorders (see Chapter 34). An *association* refers to the non-random statistical association of two or more anomalies not known to be etiologically related. A *sequence* refers to a pattern of congenital anomalies that results from a single primary abnormal event in embryogenesis (malformation), from a single mechanical factor (deformation), or from a disruptive event (disruption).

PREVALENCE. Severe congenital anomalies are identified in 2 to 3% of all newborns born in North America. Higher rates of congenital anomalies are reported in underdeveloped countries and during periods of famine and war. This rate doubles in the first year of life as congenital anomalies not diagnosed in the neonate become clinically apparent. By 5 years of age, 7 to 10% of all children have been diagnosed with at least one severe congenital anomaly. Some congenital anomalies do not present until adulthood, either causing clinical disease (e.g., Berry aneurysm), identified coincidentally with diagnostic investigations for unrelated disorders (e.g., horseshoe kidney), or discovered at postmortem examination (e.g., bicornuate uterus).

Approximately 15% of newborns have one or more mild structural anomalies. Those with two mild anomalies have a 10% risk of a severe anomaly, and those with three or more mild anomalies have a 20% risk for a severe anomaly.

Congenital anomalies and genetic disorders pose a significant burden on health care services and are important contributors to pediatric morbidity and mortality. In North America, over half of all North American children evaluated in subspecialty medical clinics or admitted to hospitals are seen for treatment of disorders resulting from congenital abnormalities. Two thirds of the deaths of infants and children in pediatric hospitals in developed countries are caused by an underlying congenital anomaly. The effect of congenital anomalies on health care in adults is not known. Genetic disorders and genetic predisposition to certain diseases are major contributors to health care costs at all ages.

The rate of congenital anomalies and chromosomal abnormalities is higher in miscarried fetuses and stillborn infants, compared with liveborn infants (Table 35–1). Prenatal screening of pregnancies with maternal serum triple screen markers and ultrasound studies done at 16 to 19 weeks of pregnancy can identify approximately half of all congenital anomalies. Positive screening tests warrant urgent referral to a medical center with expertise in fetal diagnosis and treatment.

PATHOGENESIS AND ETIOLOGY. Congenital anomalies result

Table 35–1 ▪ RATE OF CONGENITAL ANOMALIES AND CHROMOSOMAL ANOMALIES

PATIENT GROUP	CONGENITAL ANOMALIES	CHROMOSOMALLY ABNORMAL
Miscarried embryos	30%	60%
Miscarried fetuses (<20 weeks' gestation)	12.2%	29.2%
Stillborn fetuses (>20 weeks' gestation)	7.2%	6.0%
Liveborns	2–3% at birth 7–10% at 5 years old	0.57%

from abnormal embryogenesis and histogenesis during the embryonic (up to 8 weeks post fertilization) and fetal (9–40 weeks) periods, respectively. By the end of 8 weeks post fertilization, the embryo has taken human form and most organs are fully formed and located in their final position in the body. Exceptions include external genitalia (12 weeks), abdominal wall closure (10 weeks), heart (postnatal closure of patent ductus arteriosus and defect of the atrial septum secundum), brain, and dental structures (Table 35–2). The pathogenesis of congenital anomalies is divided into malformations, deformations, disruptions, and dysplasias (Table 35–3).

There are many different causes of congenital anomalies (*etiologic heterogeneity*), and there can be variation in the clinical presentation of individuals with the same disorder (*phenotypic heterogeneity*). A specific congenital anomaly is rarely pathognomonic for a specific syndrome or genetic disorder (Table 35–4).

A number of human teratogens have been identified to cause congenital anomalies. Specific information on potential teratogenic effects of an exposure can be obtained through teratogen information services, computerized databases, and reference books. The most common teratogen used during pregnancy is alcohol, followed by cocaine, and related drugs. Commonly used medications frequently encountered in practice that are teratogenic include anticonvulsants, angiotensin-converting enzyme inhibitors, antineoplastic agents, isotretinoin, warfarin (Coumadin), tetracycline, and thalidomide. Common in utero infections that affect the embryo and fetus include rubella, syphilis, toxoplasmosis, human immunodeficiency virus, herpes virus, cytomegalovirus, parvovirus, coxsackie virus, hepatitis, Venezuelan equine encephalitis, and varicella-zoster. Maternal conditions resulting in metabolic teratogens and other effects on the fetus include poor nutrition and starvation, diabetes mellitus, untreated hypothyroidism (including iodine deficiency), hyperthyroidism, hyperparathyroidism, systemic lupus erythematosus, myasthenia gravis, alcoholism, phenylketonuria, Rh isoimmunization, homocystinuria, adrenal hyperactivity, and myotonic dystrophy.

CLINICAL MANIFESTATIONS. Congenital anomalies most commonly present in infants younger than 2 months of age or are detected prenatally with fetal sonograms.

Evaluation of the congenital anomaly includes an accurate anatomic description with respect to appearance, size, shape, location, consistency and density, continuity with surrounding structures, patency, color, and whether contiguous structures are distorted, lost, or malformed. Associated structural anomalies should be documented and described, including mild anomalies and birth marks. Accurate anthropometric measures of body length, weight, occipital-frontal head circumference, and facial and other body structures need to be recorded and compared to standardized tables. A complete physical examination of all organ systems including the central nervous system may identify occult anomalies not apparent on examination of external features.

Pertinent historical information includes age at presentation, appearance at the time of presentation and change with time, previous treatment and investigations, functional expectations, and current and future plans for treatment. A review of systems should be done, with emphasis on identification of symptoms related to associated structural anomalies that commonly occur in association with the presenting anomaly. Examples of common associations are

VACTERL (*v*ertebral, *a*nal, *c*ardiac, *t*racheoesophageal, *r*enal, and *l*imb anomalies) and CHARGE (*c*oloboma, *h*eart defect, *a*tresia choanae, *r*etarded growth, *g*enital anomalies, and *e*ar anomalies). The patient is assessed for sensory deficits, particularly those affecting hearing and vision.

The presence of associated structural anomalies, increased minor anomalies, abnormal growth parameters, and dysmorphic facial features indicates an underlying syndrome, genetic disorder, or chromosomal abnormality. Gestalt diagnosis is frequently possible for common syndromes, such as Down syndrome. The majority of associations require further diagnostic investigations and assistance with computerized databases before a final diagnosis is possible.

In fetuses and newborns, emphasis is placed on pregnancy history (length of gestation; complications such as bleeding, infections, fevers, high blood pressure, and those relating to delivery; gestational diabetes; maternal age and medical problems; medications and other exposures; onset of fetal movement); placenta and umbilical cord pathology; diagnostic investigations during the pregnancy; previous pregnancy history; and special concerns that the pregnant mother had that she believes may have caused the problem.

Aborted embryos and fetuses need a complete autopsy, histologic examination, radiography, photographic documentation, cultures for infections, and other investigations as indicated. Pathologic examination of the placenta, membranes, and umbilical cord is indicated in every birth with a structural anomaly or pregnancy complication.

Table 35–3 ■ SCHEMATIC REPRESENTATION OF THE DIFFERENT TYPES OF ERRORS OF MORPHOGENESIS RESULTING IN CONGENITAL ANOMALIES AND THEIR DEFINITION

ERROR OF MORPHOGENESIS	DEFINITION
Normal development	Normal development
Malformation	Morphologic defect of an organ, part of an organ, or a larger part of the body resulting from an intrinsically abnormal developmental process
Disruption	Morphologic defect of an organ, part of an organ, or a larger region of the body resulting from the extrinsic breakdown of, or an interference with, an originally normal developmental process
Deformation	Morphologic defect resulting in an abnormal form, shape, or position of a part of the body caused by mechanical forces
Dysplasia	Morphologic defect resulting from the abnormal organization of cells into tissues

Table 35–2 ■ EMBRYONIC TIMING OF COMMON CONGENITAL ANOMALIES

STRUCTURAL ANOMALIES	EMBRYONIC ERROR IN MORPHOGENESIS	LATEST TIME POSTCONCEPTION
Anencephaly	Failure of closure of the anterior neural tube	26 days
Cleft lip	Failure of closure of embryonic component parts of the lip (42% associated with cleft palate)	36 days
Branchial sinus and/or cyst	Remnant of fusion of primary or secondary palate	10 weeks
Cardiac anomalies	Variable	Variable
Transposition of the great vessels	Errors in directional development of the bulbus cordis septum	34 days
Ventricular septal defect	Failure of closure of ventricular septum	6 weeks
Limb anomalies	Variable	Variable
Radial aplasia	Failure of formation of the radius	38 days
	Failure of separation of the digits	
Syndactyly		6 weeks
Omphalocele	Failure of anterior closure of the abdominal wall in the midline	10 weeks
Diaphragmatic hernia	Failure of closure of the retroperitoneal canal	6 weeks

Table 35-4 ■ ETIOLOGY OF CONGENITAL ANOMALIES

ETIOLOGY	%
Monogenic	7.5
Chromosomal	6
Multifactorial	20
Congenital infection	2-3
Maternal diabetes	1.5
Other maternal illnesses	<1.5
Maternal medication	1-2
Unknown	>50

When evaluating a teratogen exposure, the clinician should determine the name of the agent, dosage, route, blood levels when appropriate, any symptoms of toxicity, and gestation of exposure with reference to the last menstrual period or dating fetal sonogram. Other pertinent information includes the woman's age and medical conditions, whether there was an overdose or suicide attempt, pregnancy complications, and pertinent family history.

In infants and children, as well as in individuals with intellectual disabilities, a history of developmental milestones should be determined. Informal developmental screening and/or formal developmental or intelligence testing is important for overall management, and at times diagnosis. In school-aged children, school performance, IQ, special abilities and weaknesses, interests, and goals should be evaluated. In adults, assessment of level of education, special education programs, vocational training, current occupation, career choice, and social situation can help determine a patient's abilities. In general, individuals with congenital anomalies are more likely to be underestimated rather than overestimated in their abilities. In particular, certain minor anomalies of the face can give an appearance that is interpreted by educators and others as indicative of "retardation" (e.g., blepharophimosis).

Many adults with congenital anomalies have received treatment as infants or young children and have no or poor recollection of their prior medical condition. Medical records may be the only source of information about the anomaly. Alternatively, history from parents or older siblings can sometimes be helpful. Many individuals with congenital anomalies of one organ system have associated structural anomalies that may present after childhood with clinical signs and symptoms specific for the involved organ system. Other signs of undiagnosed congenital anomalies include the presence of increased minor structural anomalies, certain skin lesions, abnormal growth, developmental delay, and mental retardation.

Family history is as important in assisting in the diagnosis of a disorder as other investigations. A three-generation pedigree should be obtained, with specific reference to other family members having a similar, associated, or other congenital anomaly; medical illnesses; early death; stillbirths and miscarriages; prolonged hospitalizations; institutionalization; mental retardation; learning disabilities; growth disorders; relatedness (e.g., first cousins); ethnic origins; and concerns previously identified by the family such as non-paternity and incest. Medical records and examination of other family members may be indicated.

Diagnosis of the cause of a congenital anomaly is important because it facilitates the prediction of an overall prognosis and natural history of the disorder. A differential diagnosis is helpful in directing investigations for potential complications and the presence of anomalies as well as the exclusion of disorders that may have a more severe outcome. Preventative health care by early detection and treatment of potential complications of a specific disorder improves the quality of life of the patient.

DIAGNOSTIC INVESTIGATIONS. Diagnostic investigations should be directed toward determining whether the congenital anomaly is isolated or if there are associated anomalies of the same or other organ systems. Indications for chromosome studies are summarized in Table 35-5.

RECURRENCE RISKS. Recurrence risks for common isolated structural anomalies are given in Table 35-6. These tables are only applicable after exclusion of monogenic, syndromic, chromosomal, and other possible causes for the congenital anomaly. A specific family may have an unrecognized monogenic disorder, and the

Table 35-5 ■ INDICATION FOR CHROMOSOME STUDIES

Stillbirths or neonatal deaths (7%)
Multiple congenital anomalies (23%)
Small for gestational age (10%)
Facial dysmorphia with a single major congenital anomaly
Significant mental retardation (12%)
Postnatal growth retardation
Microcephaly
Couple with more than two miscarriages

recurrence risk may actually be higher (i.e., 25 to 50%) (see section on genetic disorders).

TREATMENT. Some structural anomalies are surgically correctable. More commonly, the congenital anomaly is not amenable to surgical treatment or requires multiple staged surgeries or operative palliation. Individuals with disabling or multiple congenital anomalies usually require expertise of many medical and surgical specialists knowledgeable in the natural history of the disorder and are best managed by multidisciplinary teams. Treatment plans include management of the medical and surgical problems related to the congenital anomaly, including physiotherapy, occupational therapy, prostheses, treatment of sensory deficits, interviews with social workers, and addressing of issues of education for optimal intellectual outcome, as well as employment opportunities and psychosocial development.

PROGNOSIS. The prognosis for a disorder depends on the specific structural anomaly or anomalies. When a diagnosis of a syndrome or a chromosomal or genetic disorder is made, review of previous medical history can provide information on long-term prognosis and the natural history of the disorder.

PREVENTION AND PRENATAL DIAGNOSIS. The use of folic acid supplementation, preferably with other multivitamins preconceptually and during the first 3 months of pregnancy, is recommended to reduce the risk of congenital anomalies. Prospective cohort and case-control studies have demonstrated a reduced rate of occurrence and recurrence of neural tube defects. The occurrence/recurrence of other congenital anomalies, particularly those due to multifactorial inheritance, may also be reduced. These include nonsyndromic cleft lip/palate and some types of limb reduction, heart, and urinary tract anomalies. Current recommendations from the Centers for Disease Control and Prevention are that all women of reproductive age receive at least 0.4 mg of folic acid supplementation a day. For couples at increased risk for recurrence of neural tube defects, women should take 4.0 mg of folic acid supplementation a day while planning pregnancy and for the first 3 months of pregnancy. A healthy, well-balanced diet abundant in fresh fruits and vegetables is also recommended. In many cases there are other micronutrient deficiencies, making it beneficial to take a multivitamin supplement including folic acid. At least half of all pregnancies are unplanned, so ideally vitamin supplementation is taken irrespective of deliberate pregnancy planning. Women eating selected diets (e.g., vegetarians and those with gluten enteropathy) are at risk for vitamin B_{12} deficiency and would benefit by taking

Table 35-6 ■ RECURRENCE RISKS FOR COMMON CONGENITAL ANOMALIES

CONGENITAL ANOMALY	NORMAL PARENTS, ONE AFFECTED CHILD: RISK FOR SUBSEQUENT CHILD	ONE AFFECTED PARENT: RISK FOR OFFSPRING
Cleft lip and palate	4% unilateral lip 5.6% bilateral lip	3.2%
Cleft palate	2%	6%
Clubfoot	3%	3%
Ventricular septal defect	4-5%	3-4%
Auricular septal defect	3%	3.5%
Neural tube defect	5%	3%
Congenital dislocation of the hip	3.5%	3.5%
Pyloric stenosis	3.2% (if brother affected) 6.5% (if sister affected)	25.4% (if mother affected) 4.2% (if father affected)
Renal abnormalities	9%	

multivitamins in addition to folic acid. High doses of folic acid are contraindicated in the presence of vitamin B_{12} deficiency and may interfere with seizure control for women on anticonvulsants.

Prenatal diagnosis of recurrence of a number of congenital anomalies is possible, depending on the disorder, using diagnostic fetal ultrasound and fetal echocardiograms at 16 to 19 weeks of pregnancy. Prenatal testing with chorionic villi sampling, amniocentesis, and/or fetal blood sampling can diagnose almost all chromosomal disorders, some genetic disorders, and some structural anomalies (see section on prenatal diagnosis).

COUNSELING ABOUT A CONGENITAL ANOMALY. Talking to a family once a congenital anomaly has been identified is rarely easy, in particular when the affected individual is a fetus or a newborn. It is the responsibility of the health care professional to provide affected adults or parents and guardians of affected fetuses and children with sufficient and accurate information about the disorder so that they can make an informed decision regarding the medical and surgical management, obtain resource information in the community, and establish an appropriate social support network.

Families and individuals will usually go through an acute grief reaction when congenital anomalies are identified. Individuals vary in their personal response to the news, which is usually bad. Stages of the grief reaction include denial manifested as refusal to accept the diagnosis, anger, and seeking someone to blame; a sense of loss and grieving for the expected normal child is acutely present and may continue for many years. These feelings are followed by resignation, acceptance, and the search for meaningful and useful action. Depending on the stage of grief reaction, information provided by the health care professional will be received in a variety of ways. Careful documentation of the content of the counseling is important, because selective memory is common. Health care professionals need to communicate directly with each other rather than relying on the patient or family members as intermediaries for information.

Gilbert-Barness E: Potter's Pathology of the Fetus and Infant. St. Louis, Mosby–Year Book, 1997. *A definitive text on the pathology of congenital anomalies, particularly those that are lethal.*
Hall GH, Froster-Iskenius UG, Allanson JE: Handbook of Normal Physical Measurements. New York, Oxford University Press, 1989. *A concise handbook containing normative data on all the anthropometric and growth measurements needed by physicians.*
Harper PS: Practical Genetic Counselling, 4th ed. London, Butterworth, 1993. *A practical manual for information on congenital anomalies and genetic disorders for the practicing physician. It is particularly good for information on recurrence risks for isolated structural anomalies and a brief summary of the differential diagnosis of the most common causes of common structural anomalies.*
Jones KL: Smith's Recognizable Patterns of Human Malformation, 5th ed. Philadelphia, WB Saunders, 1997. *A practical approach to diagnosis of common syndromes, genetic disorders, and chromosomal abnormalities. Each disorder has clinical photographs and a summary of the pertinent features.*
Rimoin DL, Connor JM, Pyeritz RE: Emery and Rimoin's Principles and Practice of Medical Genetics, 3rd ed. New York, Churchill Livingstone, 1996. *A detailed text which provides specific clinical information and up-to-date research knowledge on genetic disorders.*
Stevenson RE, Hall JG, Goodman RM: Human Malformations and Related Anomalies. New York, Oxford University Press, 1993. *The most definitive book available on congenital anomalies.*

36 SYNDROMES INVOLVING MULTIPLE ORGAN SYSTEMS

Kenneth Lyons Jones

The emergence of dysmorphology/clinical genetics as a specialty has led, over the past 20 years, to the recognition of a large number of multiple malformation syndromes. Although many of these disorders are due to the effect of a single altered gene, others are the result of a chromosome abnormality or of a teratogen such as alcohol. The majority of these conditions become apparent in early infancy or childhood, but adolescent and adult patients with such conditions may initially present to internists and primary care physicians. The reader is referred to the textbooks listed at the end of this chapter for general background information and diagnostic approaches to these disorders.

The purpose of this chapter is to present information regarding the natural history of some of the more commonly recognized patterns of human malformation to provide a framework for managing adults with these disorders. In addition, data regarding etiology emanating from some of the newer molecular techniques are presented when available. Characteristics of these disorders are summarized in Table 36–1.

WILLIAMS SYNDROME

Ocular problems involve both esotropia and hyperopia. The mean IQ of adults is in the mid-50s (range, 17 to 87). A specific cognitive profile including relative strengths in language and auditory rote memory and weakness in the ability to visualize an object as a set of parts and construct a replica of it from those parts has been documented. The vast majority of individuals with Williams syndrome live with their parents, in group homes, or in supervised apartments. Although the most common cardiovascular defect is supravalvular aortic stenosis (occurring in about 70% of patients), pulmonary artery stenosis, aortic hypoplasia, and other vascular stenoses have been documented. Progression of the vascular stenosis, including hypoplasia of the aorta and renal artery stenosis, has been documented. The extent to which peripheral vascular lesions contribute to the hypertension is unknown. The presence of ectopic calcium deposits and hypercalcinuria indicates that the error in calcium metabolism assumed to be limited to early childhood does not disappear with age in all cases. Hyperparathyroidism secondary to the hypercalcinuria is often present. Gastrointestinal problems include obesity with subsequent diabetes mellitus, chronic constipation, peptic ulcer disease, cholelithiasis, and diverticulitis; and genitourinary problems include ureteral reflux and bladder diverticula associated with recurrent infection. Nephrocalcinosis and renal insufficiency have been documented. Musculoskeletal defects including lordosis and limitation of joint movements are progressive.

Although most individuals with Williams syndrome represent sporadic cases within otherwise normal families, parent-to-child transmission has been documented, implicating autosomal dominant inheritance. Studies using fluorescent in situ hybridization and quantitative Southern analysis indicate that both inherited and sporadic cases of Williams syndrome are associated with a deletion of one elastin allele located within chromosome subunit 7q11.23. However, studies suggest that haploinsufficiency for the LIM-kinase gene, which is contiguous with elastin, may account for the cognitive abnormalities in this disorder.

NOONAN SYNDROME

Although rarely severe, mental deficiency occurs in approximately 25% of cases of Noonan's syndrome. Congenital heart defects occur frequently and include pulmonary valve stenosis due to a dysplastic or thickened valve, atrial septal defect, asymmetrical septal hypertrophy, cardiomyopathy, and ventricular septal defect. Other problems that might affect long-term follow-up are uncommon. Rare cases of autoimmune thyroiditis have been documented. A small penis and cryptorchidism associated with delayed sexual development and infertility have been noted in some males. Most females are fertile. Malignant hyperthermia has been documented frequently. Hematologic abnormalities including Factor XI deficiency, von Willebrand's disease, and thrombocytopenia occur.

Although most cases of this disorder are sporadic, parent-to-child transmission has been documented, implicating autosomal dominant inheritance as the cause. A gene for this disorder has been mapped to 12q22-qter. However, non-linkage has been documented in at least one family, indicating genetic heterogeneity. Because of the marked variability in expression of this disorder, in many cases a mildly affected parent is initially diagnosed after the birth of a severely affected child.

BECKWITH-WIEDEMANN SYNDROME

Beckwith-Wiedemann syndrome (BWS) is the best known and most frequently recognized overgrowth syndrome. With increasing

Table 36–1 ■ COMMON ABNORMAL SIGNS AND SYMPTOMS OF SYNDROMES BY SYSTEM

SYNDROME	PRINCIPAL FEATURES	OCULAR	IQ	NEURO	CARDIOVASCULAR Hypertension	Anomaly	ENDO	GI	GU	MS	TUMOR	OTHER
Williams	Prominent lips, hoarse voice, cardiovascular defect	+	+	+	+	+	+	+	+	+	−	−
Noonan	Neck webbing, pectus excavatum, pulmonic stenosis	−	+	−	−	+	+	−	+	+	−	Hematologic
Beckwith-Wiedemann	Overgrowth, macrocrania, poor coordination	−	−	−	−	+	+	−	−	+	+	−
Sotos	Overgrowth, macrocrania, poor coordination	−	+	−	−	+	+	−	−	−	+	−
Prader-Willi	Obesity, hypogenitalism, behavioral abnormalities	+	+	−	+		+	−	+	+	−	−
Stickler	Flat facies, myopia, spondyloepiphyseal dysplasia	+	−	−	−	+	−	−	−	+	−	Cleft palate Hearing loss
Fetal alcohol	Microcephaly, short palpebral fissures, long smooth philtrum	+	+	+	−	+	−	−	−	+	−	−
Velocardiofacial	Cleft palate, cardiac defect, characteristic facies	−	+	−	−	+	+	−	−	−	−	Psychosis Immune deficiency
Bardet-Biedl	Pigmentary retinopathy, obesity, renal abnormalities	+	+	−	+	+	+	−	+	+	−	−
Werner	Cataract, gray sparse hair, skin changes	+	−	+	+	+	+	−	+	+	+	Short stature Metastatic calcifications

age, the typical facial features become less obvious. In the newborn period, the face is round to oval. Prominent cheeks give the impression of a narrow forehead. The tongue is extremely prominent through mid-childhood. By adolescence, the tongue no longer protrudes and the glabellar nevus, so prominent in early infancy, has faded. Creases on the ear lobes and indentations or pits on the posterior rim of the helix are typical at all ages. Regarding the overgrowth, height remains at or above the 95th percentile throughout adolescence whereas weight remains between the 75th and 95th percentiles. Spontaneous pubertal development occurs at an appropriate time for chronologic age. Cardiovascular anomalies including both structural defects and cardiomegaly occur in approximately one third of patients. Malignant tumors, the majority of which include Wilms' tumor, adrenal carcinoma, and hepatoblastoma, occur in approximately 7% of cases. Although no consensus has been forthcoming regarding screening, most clinicians recommend abdominal and renal ultrasound scans at least every 6 months up to elementary school age and then at yearly intervals until adolescence.

The gene for BWS is located at 11p15.5. In a normal situation, the maternal copy of this gene is inactivated such that a normal individual has only one active copy of the gene functioning at any one time (i.e., the paternal copy). BWS is one of a number of genetic disorders in which the presence of the phenotype depends on whether the gene has been inherited from the father or the mother, a mechanism known as genomic imprinting (see Chapter 31). In the case of BWS, the phenotype occurs as a result of a variety of different situations that produce a dosage imbalance or two rather than one active copy of the gene. For example, chromosomal abnormalities that cause duplication of the BWS locus at 11p15.5 result in the BWS phenotype if they are paternally derived and thus associated with two active copies of the gene. Chromosomal inversions and translocations involving the BWS locus produce the phenotype if they are inherited from the mother. Presumably, disrupting the locus activates a gene that is normally inactive. Also, the BWS phenotype has been seen in conjunction with paternal disomy, a situation in which both BWS loci are inherited from the father, giving two copies of the gene.

SOTOS SYNDROME

Although marked overgrowth in Sotos syndrome is a consistent feature during infancy and childhood, adult height is usually within the normal range. The head, which is large at birth, remains so throughout life. In adulthood, mandibular growth is striking, and the chin becomes long and narrow. Mild mental deficiency with an average IQ of 72 has been reported in 85% of cases. Abnormal results of glucose tolerance testing have been observed in 14% of

cases, and tumors including Wilms' tumor, hepatocellular carcinoma, mixed parotid tumor, vaginal epidermoid carcinoma, osteochondroma, cavernous hemangioma, hairy pigmented nevus, and intestinal polyposis occur in less than 5% of the cases. Regarding cause, the majority of cases represent sporadic events in otherwise normal families. However, at least five families have been reported in which both parent and offspring are affected, suggesting autosomal dominant inheritance.

PRADER-WILLI SYNDROME

Although severe hypotonia, failure to thrive, and hypogenitalism characterize Prader-Willi syndrome in early life, hyperphagia, obesity, and the appearance of bizarre behavior that intensifies with advancing age usually become manifest by age 6 years. The insatiable appetite—leading in many cases to morbid obesity, limited sexual function, and severe behavioral abnormalities—results in significant problems that can have a devastating effect on the ability of adults with this disorder to successfully adapt to their families and society. Mental retardation, which occurs in the vast majority of affected individuals, is mild in 63%, moderate in 31%, and severe in the remainder. Almost three fourths of affected individuals receive special education and function at a sixth grade level or below in reading and at a third grade level or below in mathematics. Secondary sexual characteristics are delayed and remain immature in the vast majority of cases. Sixty percent of females have amenorrhea, and the remaining 40% begin to menstruate between ages 10 and 28 years (average, 17 years). Obesity (see Chapter 228), sometimes severe enough to require gastric bypass surgery, contributes significantly to the health problems associated with this disorder, including elevated blood pressure, stroke, respiratory difficulties, and diabetes mellitus. Although sleep apnea has not been documented, rapid eye movement–related oxygen desaturation is common and the severity is significantly correlated with the severity of the obesity.

Typical maladaptive behaviors include temper tantrums, arguing, irritability, stubbornness, lying, skin picking, obsessions, and defiance. Aging may be associated with confusion, withdrawal, and fatigue.

More than 50% of affected individuals have a chromosome deletion involving band q11-12 of the long arm of chromosome 15. In all individuals with Prader-Willi syndrome, the origin of the deletion is the paternal parent. Individuals in whom the parental origin of the same deletion (15q11-12) is maternal have Angelman's syndrome—a disorder associated with severe mental retardation, a "puppet-like" gait, and paroxysms of laughter. Evidence that the expression of the clinical phenotype in these two conditions depends on the genetic material from the parent of origin gives

further credence to the concept of genomic imprinting. Additional support for the concept of imprinting in these disorders comes from the observation that some individuals with Prader-Willi syndrome, who have no evidence of a chromosome deletion, have inherited both chromosomes 15 from their mother, whereas some individuals with Angelman's syndrome who have no evidence of a chromosome deletion have inherited both chromosomes 15 from their father. The inheritance of both members of a chromosome pair from one parent is referred to as uniparental disomy. Recognizing that uniparental disomy occurs in some cases of Prader-Willi syndrome and Angelman's syndrome indicates that these parents have genetic information in 15q11-12 that derives from only their mothers or their fathers, respectively. From a practical standpoint, recurrence risk for Prader-Willi syndrome is most likely less than 1 in 1000, and it is unlikely to occur in individuals with deletion of 15q.

STICKLER SYNDROME

Marked variability of expression exists for this autosomal dominant disorder. Ophthalmologic abnormalities require the greatest follow-up. Although 75% of patients develop myopia by age 20, it does not occur in some patients until after age 50. Retinal detachment, leading to blindness, usually does not occur until after age 20. Mitral valve prolapse occurs in 50% of cases. Progressive degenerative arthropathy predominantly involving weight-bearing joints most commonly becomes a problem after age 30, leading in some cases to total hip replacement. Hearing loss, both sensorineural and conductive, frequently occurs.

FETAL ALCOHOL SYNDROME

Prenatal exposure to alcohol is the most common recognizable cause of mental retardation. Most characteristic are short palpebral fissures and a long smooth philtrum that lacks lateral vertical ridges. Growth deficiency, both prenatal and postnatal, is typical. Head circumference is most severely affected. Although patients remain short and microcephalic after the onset of puberty, the facies becomes less distinctive and weight frequently is increased for height. Myopia can become a significant problem. Although the range of IQ scores varies widely, average IQ is approximately 65. For a group of adolescents and adults (mean age, 18 years), academic performance ranged from second to fourth grade levels, with deficiency in arithmetic most severe. Maladaptive behaviors including poor concentration and attention, impulsivity, and periods of high anxiety frequently occur; and secondary disabilities including mental illness, disrupted school experiences, trouble with the law, and alcohol abuse and drug problems are common. Although the majority of affected individuals are born to alcoholic women, problems with intellectual performance have been associated with prenatal exposure to as little as 1 ounce of absolute alcohol per day.

VELOCARDIOFACIAL SYNDROME

One of the most common multiple malformation syndromes associated with oral clefting, the velocardiofacial syndrome is usually associated with submucous cleft palate or, even more likely, velopharyngeal incompetence with hypernasal speech. Ventricular septal defect with or without a right aortic arch is the most common cardiac defect. The characteristic facies includes vertical maxillary excess with a long face, a prominent nose with a squared nasal root and narrow alar base, a retruded mandible, and minor ear anomalies. Learning disabilities and mild intellectual impairment occur frequently, with IQ ranging from 70 to 90. Hypocalcemia secondary to hypoparathyroidism (see Chapter 264) occurs infrequently in infancy but is virtually never a management problem after childhood. An excessive number of infections have been reported in a number of individuals with this condition. The extent to which this may relate to an immunologic deficiency is unclear. However, abnormal T-cell function and absent thymic tissue have been documented in a few instances, and adenoid hypoplasia has been noted frequently. Of perhaps the greatest concern relative to natural history, a number of affected individuals have developed psychiatric disorders, primarily chronic schizophrenia with paranoid delusions with onset varying between ages 10 and 21. Regarding etiology,

velocardiofacial syndrome is an autosomal dominant condition. Affected patients have been shown to have an interstitial deletion of chromosome 22q11. Of significance, this is the same region that is deleted in some cases of the DiGeorge sequence, a disorder that involves developmental defects of the third and fourth pharyngeal pouches, leading to thymic and parathyroid hypoplasia and cardiac defects. Based on a number of clinical studies in which a child with the DiGeorge sequence was born to a parent with velocardiofacial syndrome, it is now believed that the two disorders represent different manifestations of the same genetic defect.

BARDET-BIEDL SYNDROME

Visual acuity deteriorates rapidly with age such that by age 30 more than 90% of patients are legally blind, the result of severe retinal dystrophy. Markedly constricted visual fields, severe abnormalities of color vision, raised dark-adaptive thresholds, and extinguished or minimal rod-and-cone responses on electroretinography occur in the majority of cases. Mental deficiency is usually mild to moderate. Although structural and/or functional abnormalities of the kidneys associated in 50% of cases with hypertension occur in the vast majority of adults with this disorder, symptomatic renal impairment occurs in only a small minority. Genital hypoplasia manifested by small testes and a very small penis occurs in most males. Although no male with this disorder has reproduced, a few women have given birth. The hypogonadism has been described as primary germinal hypoplasia and also as hypogonadotrophic. Postaxial polydactyly, syndactyly, and brachydactyly are common. This is an autosomal recessive genetically determined condition with marked variability of expression even between affected siblings. Three different loci, one on chromosome 16q21, a second on chromosome 11q, and a third on chromosome 3, have been identified.

WERNER SYNDROME

Usually, Werner syndrome is not diagnosed until young adulthood, with graying of the hair occurring at an average age of 20 the earliest sign. This is followed by skin changes, primarily atrophy involving the face and distal extremities; loss of hair; development of an abnormally thin, high-pitched, or hoarse voice; visual symptoms or detection of cataracts; skin ulcers; and, lastly, diabetes at a mean age of 34. Vascular calcifications, most commonly involving vessels of the legs, have been noted in all major vessels, including the aorta. Hypertension occurs in about 50% of cases. Coronary artery disease is common. Hypogonadism, reduced fertility, and diabetes mellitus occur frequently. Testicular atrophy is the most striking pathologic feature of this disorder. Approximately 10% of patients develop malignant tumors, especially sarcomas and meningiomas. The mean stature of affected males is 61 inches and that of affected females is 57.5 inches. Death occurs at an average age of 47, with a range from ages 31 to 63. The two most common causes of death are malignancies and vascular accidents. Werner syndrome is caused by a recessive mutation that has been mapped to chromosome 8p. Fibroblasts from skin biopsy specimens grow more slowly, assume a senescent morphology more rapidly, and assume a markedly reduced lifespan in vitro. DNA repair is normal. Karyotype preparations show a normal number of chromosomes but multiple stable chromosome rearrangements, including deletion of a portion of a single chromosome and translocations involving several chromosomes, as well as an increase in chromosome breakage.

General References

Borgaonkar DS: Chromosomal Variation in Man, 7th ed. New York, Wiley-Liss, 1994. *A catalog of chromosomal variants and anomalies.*
Briggs GC, Freeman RK, Yaffe SJ: Drugs in Pregnancy and Lactation, 4th ed. Baltimore, Williams & Wilkins, 1994. *A reference guide to fetal and neonatal risk that provides practical information regarding the effects of a large number of drugs on the fetus.*
Buyse ML (ed): Birth Defects Encyclopedia. New York, CV Mosby, 1990. *A massive multiauthored reference book listing all known birth defects regardless of cause, with descriptions, illustrations, and references. For on-line search and retrieval, contact Maxwell Online, Inc., 8000 Westpark Drive, McLean, VA 22102 (telephone, 800-055-0906).*
Jones KL: Smith's Recognizable Patterns of Human Malformation, 5th ed. Philadelphia, WB Saunders, 1997. *This short "bible" for description of malformation syn-*

dromes has many useful photographs and accounts of many different types of defects.

McKusick V: Mendelian Inheritance in Man, 11th ed. Baltimore, Johns Hopkins University Press, 1994. *Standard reference source listing definite and possible monogenic diseases, traits, and syndromes with short descriptions and literature citations. Continuously updated and also available with computer access. Contact OMIM User Support, Welch Medical Library, 1830 E. Monument Street, Baltimore, MD 21205 (telephone, 301-955-7058).*

Schinzel A: Catalogue of Unbalanced Chromosome Aberrations in Man. New York, W de Gruyter, 1984. *The definitive detailed reference for unbalanced chromosomal aberrations.*

Shepard TH: Catalog of Teratogenic Agents, 8th ed. Baltimore, Johns Hopkins University Press, 1995. *The most comprehensive reference for teratogens in humans and animals.*

Williams Syndrome

Ewart AK, Morris CA, Atkinson D, et al: Hemizygosity at the elastin locus in a developmental disorder, Williams syndrome. Nat Genet 5:11, 1993. *Hemizygosity at the elastin locus is identified in four familial and five sporadic cases of Williams syndrome.*

Frangiskakis JM, Ewart AK, Morris CA, et al: *LIM-kinase 1 hemizygosity implicated in impaired visuospatial constructive cognition.* Cell 86:59, 1996.

Morris CA, Leonard CO, Dilts C, et al: Adults with Williams syndrome. Am J Med Genet (Suppl) 6:102, 1990. *A detailed clinical summary of 29 adults with Williams syndrome.*

Noonan Syndrome

Allanson JE, Hall JG, Hughes HE, et al: Noonan syndrome: The changing phenotype. Am J Med Genet 21:507, 1985. *A review documenting the changing phenotype from the newborn period to adulthood.*

Jamieson CR, Van der Burgt, Brady AF et al: Mapping a gene for Noonan syndrome to the long arm of chromosome 12. Nat Genet 8:357, 1994. *Results of a genome-wide linkage analysis in a large family with Noonan syndrome.*

Mendez HMM, Opitz JM: Noonan syndrome: A review. Am J Med Genet 21:493, 1985. *An excellent review of the complete spectrum of defects.*

Beckwith-Wiedemann Syndrome

Hall JG: Nontraditional inheritance. Growth Genet Horm 6:1, 1990. *An overview of genetic phenomena, including imprinting, which are not explained by traditional mendelian concepts.*

Normal AM, Read AP, Clayton-Smith J, et al: Recurrent Wiedemann-Beckwith syndrome with inversion of chromosome 11p11.2p15.5. Am J Med Genet 42:638, 1992. *Possible mechanisms giving rise to this disorder are discussed.*

Sotos Syndrome

Wit JM, Beemer FA, Barth PG, et al: Cerebral gigantism (Sotos syndrome), compiled data of 22 cases. Eur J Pediatr 144:131, 1985. *An in-depth study of the clinical features, growth, bone age, cranial CT scans, and plasma somatomedin activity of 22 children with Sotos' syndrome.*

Prader-Willi Syndrome

Butler MG: Prader-Willi syndrome: Current understanding of cause and diagnosis. Am J Med Genet 35:319, 1990. *Review of all aspects (including detailed cytogenetics) of the syndrome.*

Dykens EM, Hodapp RM, Walsh K, et al: Adaptive and maladaptive behavior in Prader-Willi syndrome. J Am Acad Child Adolesc Psychiatry 31:1131, 1992. *Examination of the development and profiles of adaptive and maladaptive behavior of 21 adults and adolescents.*

Greenswag LR: Adults with Prader-Willi syndrome, a survey of 232 cases. Dev Med Child Neurol 29:145, 1987. *Review with special attention to adults.*

Stickler Syndrome

Lieberfarb RM, Hirose T, Holmes LB: The Wagner-Stickler syndrome, a study of 22 families. J Pediatr 99:394, 1981. *Review of spectrum of defects documenting the variable expression.*

Fetal Alcohol Syndrome

Streissguth AP, Clarren SK, Jones KL: Natural history of the fetal alcohol syndrome: A ten-year follow-up of eleven patients. Lancet 2:85, 1985. *Long-term follow-up of the original children described with this disorder.*

Streissguth AP, Aase JM, Clarren SK et al: Fetal alcohol syndrome in adolescents and adults. JAMA 265:1961, 1991. *Manifestations in 61 adolescents and adults.*

Velocardiofacial Syndrome

Driscoll DA, Spinner NB, Budarf ML, et al: Deletions and microdeletions of 22q11.2 in VCFS. Am J Med Genet 44:261, 1992. *A review of the karyotypic abnormalities in velocardiofacial syndrome.*

Scrambler PJ, Kelly D, Williamson R, et al: The velo-cardio-facial syndrome is associated with chromosome deletions which encompasses the DiGeorge syndrome locus. Lancet 339:1138, 1992. *Deletions of the DiGeorge syndrome critical region are described in a group of patients with velocardiofacial syndrome.*

Bardet-Biedl Syndrome

Green JS, Parfrey PS, Harnett JD, et al: The cardinal manifestations of Bardet-Biedl syndrome, a form of Laurence-Moon-Biedl syndrome. N Engl J Med 321:1002, 1989. *Spectrum of clinical features in 32 patients ascertained through the Canadian National Institute of the Blind.*

Harnett JD, Green JS, Cramer BC, et al: The spectrum of renal disease in Laurence-Moon-Biedl syndrome. N Engl J Med 319:615, 1988. *Review of abnormalities of renal structure and function.*

Leppert M, Baird L, Anderson KL et al: Bardet-Biedl syndrome is linked to DNA markers on chromosome 11q and is genetically heterogeneous. Nat Genet 7:108, 1994. *Results of linkage analysis in 31 families with Bardet-Biedl syndrome.*

Werner Syndrome

Epstein CJ, Martin GM, Schultz AL, et al: Werner's syndrome: A review of its symptomatology, natural history, pathologic features, genetics. and relationship to the natural aging process. Medicine 45:177, 1966. *A detailed summary of clinical and laboratory characteristics of 125 cases of Werner's syndrome.*

Thomas W, Rubenstein M, Goto M, et al: A genetic analysis of the Werner syndrome region on human chromosome 8p. Genomics 16:685, 1993.

37 GENETIC COUNSELING

Margretta R. Seashore

Genetic counseling can be defined as a process in which individuals or family members obtain information about a genetic condition that may affect them. The purpose of genetic counseling is to enable individuals and families to make important decisions about marriage, reproduction, and health management based on the facts of the genetic situation for which a risk is perceived. This process is part of a thorough genetic evaluation in which the diagnosis is made or confirmed, the genetic model is developed, the information is communicated, the options are discussed, and psychosocial support is offered. Any breakdown in this progression may lead to information being misunderstood, misinterpreted, or misused.

DIAGNOSIS

The first step in genetic counseling is to confirm the diagnosis. The worst error that can be made is to provide an elegant and sophisticated analysis for the wrong disorder. The importance of this step cannot be overemphasized. Many persons have been given a general diagnosis, such as mental retardation, for which there can be a multitude of genetic as well as non-genetic explanations. The increasing definition of the molecular pathology of many disorders has heightened the importance of recognizing genetic heterogeneity. For example, at least 20 different forms of muscular dystrophy have been identified that are clinically similar. Both X-linked and autosomal recessive forms are known. At least two, Becker's and Duchenne's dystrophy, are X-linked conditions that are allelic but clinically quite distinct. Differentiations of this kind must be made with as much accuracy as possible if the patient and family are to be given the most precise answers.

The confirmation of the diagnosis uses five medical tools, four of which are very familiar to all clinicians. They are medical records, medical history, physical examination, laboratory tests, and molecular genetic analysis. The importance of reviewing medical records seems obvious; yet it can be a difficult task to accomplish completely. Validation of the rate of progression of symptoms and signs, the development of the present physical findings, and the results of prior laboratory tests is best done from the medical records. In addition, the status of family members can sometimes be assessed from examination of their medical records. Often the medical geneticist has been told of a relative who "had the same problem" only to learn from that individual's medical records that the relative's problem was entirely different.

The medical history provides clues to the beginnings and progression of symptoms and signs that may provide valuable hints to diagnosis. The pattern of progression in the degenerative neurologic disorders provides important diagnostic information. A history of more than two spontaneous miscarriages may suggest a chromosomal translocation in one parent. Early death of infants in the pedigree may suggest an inborn error of intermediary metabolism.

The physical examination again provides the opportunity to consider genetic heterogeneity. For example, there are many genetic causes of short stature. The details of the physical examination may provide the information to determine the correct genetic diagnosis. Precise measurement of anthropometric features can be compared with values in the literature and the diagnostic considerations narrowed. Careful examination of other family members may be needed before the presence of the condition can be excluded in them.

Laboratory tests often provide helpful diagnostic information to complete the genetic diagnosis. Radiographic appearance of bones is often the critical information in diagnosing the chondrodystro-

Adult polycystic kidney disease	Neurofibromatosis type 1
Alport's syndrome	Neurofibromatosis type 2
Duchenne's muscular dystrophy	Ornithine transcarbamylase deficiency
Cystic fibrosis	Phenylketonuria
Fragile-X syndrome	Sickle cell anemia
Gaucher's disease	Spinocerebellar ataxias
Hemophilia A	Tay-Sachs disease
Huntington's disease	Thalassemias
Multiple endocrine neoplasia	Wiskott-Aldrich syndrome
Myotonic dystrophy	

phies, for example. Measurement of enzyme activity, analysis of proteins, and karyotype of chromosomes can aid in the specific diagnosis of a condition.

The development of molecular diagnostic tools that can provide precise definition of the mutation or utilize linkage to a specific genetic marker has revolutionized genetic counseling. In the past, the chromosomal location of specific genes was inferred from pedigree information for the X chromosome and linkage to specific protein markers for autosomes. Now the chromosomal location of many more genes is known, linkage to specific DNA markers has been established, and many genes of clinical importance have been cloned and sequenced. It is likely that within the next two decades, the entire human genome will be mapped and entirely sequenced. More than 4000 genes have now been mapped to specific locations in the human genome. Many of these comprise specific genes or linkage markers for some of the more than 6000 established single gene conditions that appear in the McKusick catalog of mendelian phenotypes. The number of conditions that show linkage to known genetic markers or to anonymous DNA probes grows daily. These new tools can be used to enhance the precision of genetic diagnosis and counseling. Table 37–1 lists examples of many of the genetic conditions that can be diagnosed using these molecular tools. This list is being expanded at a rapid rate and should not be considered complete. At least one disease has been mapped to each chromosome (Table 37–2). Any condition mapped to a specific chromosomal location can theoretically be diagnosed using molecular methods, given the appropriate molecular probes and informative family members.

THE GENETIC MODEL

The next essential step—development of the genetic model—should be taken before the genetic counseling visit with the patient and family takes place. The patient has come with the question "what is it and is it inherited?" Arrival at a diagnosis leads to the

answer to the first part of the question. The second part is crucial to the process of genetic counseling. Development of the genetic model requires the family history, the precise diagnosis, and knowledge of the possible genetic mechanisms. The diagramming of the pedigree from the family history may fit such an obvious genetic model that further analysis is simple. When the physical examination and laboratory studies are typical of a recognized genetic condition such as Duchenne's muscular dystrophy and the pedigree demonstrates a clear pattern of X-linked inheritance, developing the genetic model is straightforward. More often, however, the pedigree is less clear. Where there is familial aggregation without an obvious mendelian pattern or the individual is the only affected member of the family at present, all possible genetic mechanisms must be considered and excluded or confirmed. The genetic model must then be used to identify those at risk for the condition.

Three general genetic mechanisms must be considered: chromosomal, mendelian, and multifactorial. The chromosomal disorders should be considered as a possible explanation for multiple anomalies, mental retardation, recurrent miscarriages, and unexplained stillbirths (see Chapter 34). Empirical figures must be used to predict the recurrence of chromosomal abnormalities in a family. These range between 1% and 10%, and the literature must be consulted with reference to the specific situation.

When a clear mendelian pattern is seen and the disorder is a recognized mendelian condition, counseling is based on that pattern. When the family history fails to demonstrate a mendelian pattern, the diagnosis is reviewed and the medical literature consulted to determine the inheritance pattern for the specific disorder. In autosomal recessive conditions the birth of an affected child may be the first signal that a set of parents is heterozygous for a rare recessive condition. Here the genetic model depends on the correct diagnosis and the known inheritance pattern for that disorder. For X-linked conditions, the decision must be made whether the affected individual represents a new mutation or inheritance from a heterozygous mother who by chance has no affected relatives. In the past, Bayesian calculations based on the pedigree have been the mainstay of this kind of analysis. Today, however, molecular diagnostic tools have refined the ability to determine heterozygosity in this situation. For dominantly inherited conditions, the literature must be consulted to determine the proportion of patients who represent new mutations, a figure that can approach 50%. When a new mutation appears to be the explanation, others in the family are not at risk, but each offspring of the affected individual has a 50% risk of inheriting the gene. Variable expression can confound the analysis of a family demonstrating an autosomal dominant condition. Gonadal mosaicism for the mutation accounts for rare recurrences in families in which neither parent is affected with the dominant condition and no test can exclude it. In general, however, the absence of the condition in any other family member makes the likelihood high that the patient represents a new mutation. Frequently, no mendelian hypothesis can be sustained yet there is familial aggregation of the disorder. Many conditions, such as neural tube defects and cleft lip and palate, appear to be multifactorial in origin with both genetic and environmental components. Genetic counseling for these conditions must rely on empirical figures for the specific condition.

Table 37-2 ■ EXAMPLES OF ONE CONDITION MAPPED TO EACH CHROMOSOME

GENETIC CONDITION	MAP LOCATION
Charcot-Marie-Tooth neuropathy 1	1q22
Neurosensory, non-syndromic recessive deafness	2p23-p22
von Hippel-Lindau syndrome	3p26-p25
Huntington's disease	4p16.3
Familial polyposis of the colon	5q21-p22
Congenital adrenal hyperplasia	6p21.3
Cystic fibrosis	7q31.2
Langer-Gideon syndrome	8q24.11-q24.13
Friedreich's ataxia	9q13-q21
Multiple endocrine neoplasia IIB	10q11.2
Wilms' tumor-aniridia syndrome	11p13
Stickler's syndrome	12q14
Wilson's disease	13q14-q21
Familial hypertrophic cardiomyopathy 1	14q12
Familial spastic paraplegia	15q11.1
Adult-type polycystic kidney disease	16p13
Neurofibromatosis	17q11.2
Kidd blood group	18q11-q12
Myotonic dystrophy	19q13.2-q13.3
Alagille syndrome	20p12
Alzheimer's disease	21q21.3-q22.05
NF2 (bilateral acoustic neuroma)	22q12.2
Duchenne's muscular dystrophy	Xp21.2

THE COUNSELING PROCESS

Once the genetic model has been established, this information can be communicated to the patient and family. The process of genetic counseling itself has the following components: transferring information about the genetic risks, putting the risks in perspective, providing a summary of the disorder, and discussing the options. It must begin with the individual who brought the original question. An explanation of the genetic risks requires imparting factual information using scientific concepts that are not familiar to everyone. It is important that the facts on which the genetic model is based be clearly explained. However, it is neither possible nor desirable to present an entire course in medical genetics to the anxious patient and family. Therefore, the relevant facts must be carefully culled from the counselor's knowledge and communicated clearly. It is important to remember that persons may be very anxious and find

Table 37-3 ■ SOME CONDITIONS THAT HAVE BEEN
DIAGNOSED PRENATALLY

DISORDER	DIAGNOSTIC METHOD
All defined chromosomal disorders	Cytogenetic analysis
Adrenoleukodystrophy	DNA and long-chain fatty acids
Cystinosis	Cystine transport
Cystic fibrosis	DNA analysis
Duchenne's muscular dystrophy	DNA analysis
Ectodermal dysplasia	Fetoscopy, skin biopsy
Fabry's disease	α-Galactosidase A
Fragile-X syndrome	DNA analysis
Gaucher's disease	β-Glucosidase; DNA analysis
GM$_2$-gangliosidosis I (Tay-Sachs)	Hexosaminidase A
Hemoglobinopathies	DNA analysis
Hemophilia A	DNA analysis
Metachromatic leukodystrophy	Aryl sulfatase A
Mucopolysaccharidosis I (Hurler's)	α-L-iduronidase
Neural tube defects: spina bifida, anencephaly	α-Fetoprotein, ultrasound, amniotic fluid acetylcholinesterase
Omphalocele	α-Fetoprotein, ultrasound
Congenital malformations: hydrocephalus, limb, cardiac, renal anomalies	Ultrasound
Skeletal dysplasias	Ultrasound/DNA analysis
Phenylketonuria	DNA analysis

See Milunsky (1998) for more information.

it difficult to absorb complex material, especially if they are fearful about the implications of the information. The strategy of first presenting a brief summary of the conclusions and their implications, stating that the evidence for this conclusion will presently be discussed, can allay some fears and relieve some of the distraction that prevents families from hearing this kind of information.

If the condition is a chromosome disorder, the structure and ways of identifying chromosomes must be mentioned and the specific disorder illustrated. Using teaching aids such as diagrams and photographs of chromosomes is helpful, with the normal situation providing a frame of reference. When the condition is a mendelian disorder, the basic concepts of single gene inheritance must be discussed briefly, but the discussion should center on the mode of inheritance involved in the particular family and not be clouded with a great deal of extraneous material about other modes of inheritance. Families without a prior family history of the disorder may have difficulty with the fact that the disorder has never been seen in their family. An explanation of heterozygosity may help clarify autosomal recessive inheritance. Autosomal dominant inheritance is easy to understand when there are other affected individuals and the pedigree demonstrates a clear vertical pattern. More difficult for the family to understand is the new mutation. As in the chromosome disorders, the use of such teaching aids as gene diagrams, sample pedigrees, and other models may be extremely valuable.

A second important component of genetic counseling is putting the risk in perspective. Many workers in the field have noted that

Table 37-4 ■ INDICATIONS FOR GENETIC COUNSELING

Advanced parental age
    Maternal age over 35
    Paternal age over 50
Family history of inherited disease
Risk of chromosome disorder
    Previous child with chromosomal abnormality
    Parent with known chromosomal translocation
Heterozygote screening based on ethnicity
    Tay-Sachs, Canavan (Ashkenazi-Jewish; French Canadian)
    Thalassemias (Mediterranean, Arab, Indo-Pakistani)
    Sickle cell anemia (West African, Mediterranean, Arab, Indo-Pakistani, Turkish, Southeast Asian)
Pregnancy screening abnormality
    Maternal serum α-fetoprotein
    Maternal serum triple screen
    Ultrasound examination

Table 37-5 ■ REPRODUCTIVE OPTIONS FOR FAMILIES WITH
GENETIC RISKS

Adoption
Reproductive assistance
    In vitro fertilization with a donor egg
    Artificial insemination by donor
Prenatal diagnosis

perception of risk may be of more importance in family decision making than the actual numerical value of the risk. This perception depends on at least two factors: (1) risk compared to background risk and (2) overall burden, a combination of risk and severity. A risk of 1 in 4 of recurrence in a second child, in the case of phenylketonuria, for example, is very much greater than a risk of 1 in 10,000 in the general population. Conversely, a risk of 1 in 10,000 may sound high to a couple who believe that the chances of something being wrong with an unborn child are 1 in a million. The presentation of such risk figures can change the perception of that risk. For example, a 1 in 4 chance of recurrence of phenylketonuria is also a 3 to 1 chance against recurrence. The burden of judgment is a very personal one. Physical handicap may be a severe burden for one family, whereas another may find that tolerable but mental handicap unacceptable. Helping families to think about risks in these ways is an important component of genetic counseling.

Modern molecular tools have allowed some families to take advantage of presymptomatic diagnosis for inherited disorders such as antitrypsin deficiency, Huntington's disease, and breast cancer. The issues these families face depend on how they will be able to use that information. If treatment or prevention of disease is possible, the information may be welcomed. If, as in Huntington's disease, the affected person faces catastrophic outcome without any possible intervention, the choice to take the test may be a very difficult one. The physician must help the patient weigh the risks and benefits and discuss the impact of the results before the patient chooses testing.

Genetic counseling also includes a description of the disorder. Many persons go to their local library in an attempt to find literature about the disorder or ask medical friends to do so. Often this results in misinformation or information that is out of date. Providing written material about the disorder is often helpful. Many genetic counseling clinics have pamphlets, booklets, and other literature to provide. The family should also be furnished with a written report of the counseling summarizing the important points.

REPRODUCTIVE OPTIONS AND PRENATAL DIAGNOSIS

If risk to future unborn children is at issue, the family at risk for a genetic disorder must be told about the reproductive options available. Prenatal diagnosis is an important reproductive option that must be discussed. Appropriate referral to experts in areas of alternative reproductive options must be made. Aside from refraining from having children at all, the options can enhance the chances of having healthy children for the family at risk.

The methods in prenatal diagnosis depend on imaging the fetus, examining DNA in cells of fetal origin, analyzing chromosomes in fetal cells, examining analytes, and measuring proteins and enzymes in cells of fetal origin. The major autosomal and sex chromosomal aneuploidies can be diagnosed in this way, along with chromosomal rearrangements, deletions, insertions, and the like. Any DNA-based diagnosis that can be performed on cells can be performed on fetal cells.

Measurement of α-fetoprotein, human chorionic gonadotropin, and unconjugated estrogen in maternal serum (triple screen) allows detection of an estimated 60 to 70% of fetuses with Down syndrome or trisomy 18 regardless of maternal age and is recommended regardless of prior risk. Indications, diagnostic uses, and risks of mid-trimester amniocentesis, chorionic villus sampling, and fetal blood sampling by cordocentesis are shown in the Tables 37-1 to 37-6. Recent studies of chorionic villus sampling suggest a small (1/3000–1/1000) risk of limb hypoplasia in infants born after that procedure. Fetoscopy is done only when other diagnostic avenues have failed and is used to visualize fetal anatomy and to perform biopsy of fetal tissues, such as liver or skin.

Table 37-6 ■ PRENATAL DIAGNOSIS METHODS

METHOD	USE	RISK
Ultrasonography	Estimated fetal age Assess growth Evaluate anatomy and organ function	None recognized
Amniocentesis or chorionic villus sampling (CVS)	Fetal cells: analyze DNA, chromosomes proteins Amniotic fluid: analyze proteins, measure analytes of fetal origin	Amniocentesis (15–20 weeks) ≤0.5% risk miscarriage CVS (9–11 weeks) ≤2% risk miscarriage
Periumbilical blood sampling	Fetal blood: analyze cells, measure serum analytes	≤2% risk miscarriage

It is crucial that the pregnant woman undergoing prenatal diagnosis be given extremely clear counseling. Spelling out clearly the expectations and limitations of the testing before any procedures is critical. The diagnoses that are being sought must be explained. It is very easy for the woman to conclude that a normal test result shows that the infant will be "normal," when in fact a short list of pathologic conditions for which her risk was increased has been excluded. Normalcy is never completely assured. After these conditions have been excluded, the pregnancy stands at the same risk for other potential problems as others in the general population.

Much more difficult is the situation in which the result of the test is not normal. Although this possibility is best discussed beforehand and the options considered, it is no longer considered necessary that the woman make a decision before she learns the test results. The implications of the diagnosis must be reviewed with care, sensitivity, and accuracy. The options for the woman are to terminate the pregnancy or to carry it to term. Rarely, surgical or medical treatment of the identified fetus can be offered, but this may be experimental, uncertain, and risky. The decision to termi-

nate a pregnancy must be made in collaboration with the obstetrician who will perform the procedure so that the process can be described and possible complications reviewed. The choice of procedure depends on the stage of pregnancy; the complications are specific to the particular procedure. Psychosocial support after the procedure is crucial. Most families who elect to terminate a pregnancy go through a period of grieving for the loss of the hoped-for normal child. Many such pregnancies were planned and wanted. The family should be offered the chance to visit with the genetic counselor to discuss their normal feelings of sadness and loss and to join a support group if one is available. There is no evidence for long-term psychological sequelae of genetic pregnancy termination.

Thoughtful genetic counseling challenges the skills of the physician in diagnosis, analysis, communication, and support. Rarely is it the province of only one person, but rather it requires the collaborative efforts of an experienced team. From the initial evaluation through development of the genetic model and identification of those at risk to completion of the transfer of information, the use of these skills enables patients and their families to make intelligent, informed, and reasoned decisions for their futures.

Geller GBJ, Green MJ, Press N, et al: Genetic testing for susceptibility to adult-onset cancer: The process and content of informed consent: Consensus Development Conference. JAMA 277:1467–1474, 1997. *Informative about the psychological aspects of genetic counseling, the impact of genetic information, and the challenge of information transfer.*
Frets P, Duivenvoorden H, et al: Factors influencing the reproductive decision after genetic counseling. Am J Med Genet 35:496–502, 503–509, 1990. *Another in the series of articles on the psychodynamics of genetic counseling.*
Kessler S: Psychological aspects of genetic counseling: XI. Nondirectiveness revisited. Am J Med Genet 72:164–171, 1997. *Thoughtful review of genetic counseling techniques.*
Kevles D, Hood L: The Code of Codes: Scientific and Social Issue in the Human Genome Project. Cambridge, MA, Harvard University Press, 1992. *Scholarly treatment of the social impact of the new molecular genetics.*
McKusick V: Mendelian Inheritance in Man, 10th ed. Baltimore, Johns Hopkins University Press, 1992. *Exhaustive catalog of mendelian phenotypes.*
Milunsky A: Genetic Disorders and the Fetus, Diagnosis, Prevention and Treatment, 3rd ed. New York, Plenum Press, 1998. *Extensive textbook on prenatal diagnosis.*

PART VII

CARDIOVASCULAR DISEASES

38 APPROACH TO THE PATIENT WITH POSSIBLE CARDIOVASCULAR DISEASE

Lee Goldman

Patients with cardiovascular disease may present with a wide range of symptoms and/or signs, each of which may be caused by non-cardiovascular conditions. Conversely, patients with substantial cardiovascular disease may be asymptomatic. Because cardiovascular disease is by far the leading cause of death in the United States and other developed countries, it is critical that patients be carefully evaluated to detect early cardiovascular disease, that symptoms or signs of cardiovascular disease be evaluated in detail, and that appropriate therapy be instituted. A wide array of improvements in diagnosis, therapy, and prevention have contributed to an impressive decline in age-adjusted cardiovascular death rates in the United States since the late 1960s. However, because of the increase in the number of persons older than 40 years, the absolute number of deaths from cardiovascular disease in the United States has not declined.

In evaluating the patient with known or suspected heart disease, the physician must quickly determine whether a potentially life-threatening condition exists. In such situations, the evaluation must focus on the specific issue at hand and be accompanied by the rapid performance of appropriately directed additional tests. Examples of potentially life-threatening conditions include acute myocardial infarction (see Chapter 60), unstable angina (see Chapter 59), suspected aortic dissection (see Chapter 66), pulmonary edema (see Chapter 48), and pulmonary embolism (see Chapter 84).

HISTORY FOR DETECTION OF CARDIOVASCULAR SYMPTOMS
(Table 38-1)

Patients may spontaneously complain of a variety of cardiovascular symptoms, but sometimes these symptoms are elicited only by obtaining a careful and complete medical history. In patients with known or suspected cardiovascular disease, questions about cardiovascular symptoms are key components of the history of present illness; in other patients, these issues remain a fundamental part of the review of systems.

Chest Pain

Chest discomfort or pain is the cardinal manifestation of myocardial ischemia due to coronary artery disease or any condition that causes myocardial ischemia via an imbalance of myocardial oxygen demand as compared with myocardial oxygen supply (see Chapter 59). New, acute, often ongoing pain may indicate an acute myocardial infarction, unstable angina, or aortic dissection; a pulmonary

Table 38-1 ■ CARDINAL SYMPTOMS OF CARDIOVASCULAR DISEASE

Chest pain or discomfort
Dyspnea, orthopnea, paroxysmal nocturnal dyspnea, wheezing
Palpitations, dizziness, syncope
Cough, hemoptysis
Fatigue, weakness
Pain in extremities with exertion (claudication)

cause such as acute pulmonary embolism or pleural irritation; a musculoskeletal condition of the chest wall, thorax, or shoulder; or a gastrointestinal abnormality such as esophageal reflux or spasm, peptic ulcer disease, or cholecystitis (Table 38-2). The chest discomfort of myocardial infarction commonly occurs without an immediate or obvious precipitating clinical cause and builds in intensity over at least several minutes; the sensation can range from annoying discomfort to severe pain (see Chapter 60). Although a variety of adjectives may be used by patients to describe the sensation, physicians must be suspicious of any discomfort, especially if it radiates to the neck, shoulder, or arms. The chest discomfort of unstable angina is clinically indistinguishable from that of myocardial infarction except that the former may be more clearly precipitated by activity and be more rapidly responsive to antianginal therapy (see Chapter 59). Aortic dissection (see Chapter 66) classically presents with the sudden onset of severe pain in the chest that radiates to the back; the location of the pain often provides clues to the location of the dissection: ascending aortic dissections commonly present with chest discomfort radiating to the back, whereas dissections of the descending aorta commonly present with back pain radiating to the abdomen. The presence of back pain or a history of hypertension or other predisposing factors, such as Marfan's syndrome, should prompt a careful assessment of peripheral pulses, to see if the great vessels are affected by the dissection, and of the chest radiograph, to evaluate the size of the aorta. If this initial evaluation proves at all suspicious, further testing with transesophageal echocardiography, computed tomography, or magnetic resonance imaging is indicated. The pain of pericarditis (see Chapter 65) may simulate that of an acute myocardial infarction: it may be primarily pleuritic or it may be continuous. Key physical findings include a pericardial rub. The pain of pulmonary embolism (see Chapter 84) is commonly pleuritic in nature and is associated with dyspnea; hemoptysis may also be present. Pulmonary hypertension (see Chapter 56) of any cause may be associated with chest discomfort with exertion, and it is commonly associated with severe dyspnea and often with cyanosis.

Recurrent, episodic chest discomfort may be noted with angina pectoris as well as with a large number of cardiac and non-cardiac causes (see Chapter 59). A variety of stress tests can be used to provoke reversible myocardial ischemia in susceptible individuals and to help determine whether such ischemia is the pathophysiologic explanation for the chest discomfort (see Chapter 59).

Dyspnea

Dyspnea, which is an uncomfortable awareness of breathing, is commonly due to cardiovascular or pulmonary disease. In cardiovascular conditions, dyspnea is usually caused by increases in pulmonary venous pressure due to left ventricular failure (see Chapters 47 and 48) or valvular heart disease (see Chapter 63). Orthopnea, which is an exacerbation of dyspnea when the patient is recumbent, is due to increased work of breathing because of either increased venous return to the pulmonary vasculature or loss of gravitational assistance in diaphragmatic effort. Paroxysmal nocturnal dyspnea is severe dyspnea that awakens a patient at night and forces the assumption of a sitting or standing position to achieve gravitational redistribution of fluid.

In heart failure, dyspnea is typically noted as a hunger for air and a need or an urge to breathe. The feeling that breathing requires increased work or effort is more typical of airway obstruction or neuromuscular disease. A feeling of chest tightness or constriction during breathing is typical of bronchoconstriction, which is commonly caused by obstructive airway disease but may also be seen in pulmonary edema. A feeling of heavy breathing, rapid

Table 38–2 ■ CAUSES OF CHEST PAIN

CONDITION	LOCATION	QUALITY	DURATION	AGGRAVATING OR RELIEVING FACTORS	ASSOCIATED SYMPTOMS OR SIGNS
Cardiovascular Causes					
Angina	Retrosternal region; radiates to or occasionally isolated to neck, jaw, epigastrium, shoulder, or arms—left common	Pressure, burning, squeezing, heaviness, indigestion	<2–10 min	Precipitated by exercise, cold weather, or emotional stress; relieved by rest or nitroglycerin; atypical (Prinzmetal's) angina may be unrelated to activity, often early morning	S_2, or murmur of papillary muscle dysfunction during pain
Rest or unstable angina	Same as angina	Same as angina but may be more severe	Usually <20 min	Same as angina, with decreasing tolerance for exertion or at rest	Similar to stable angina, but may be pronounced; transient cardiac failure can occur
Myocardial infarction	Substernal and may radiate like angina	Heaviness, pressure, burning, constriction	Sudden onset, 30 min or longer but variable	Unrelieved by rest or nitroglycerin	Shortness of breath, sweating, weakness, nausea, vomiting
Pericarditis	Usually begins over sternum or toward cardiac apex and may radiate to neck or left shoulder; often more localized than the pain of myocardial ischemia	Sharp, stabbing, knifelike	Lasts many hours to days; may wax and wane	Aggravated by deep breathing, rotating chest, or supine position; relieved by sitting up and leaning forward	Pericardial friction rub
Aortic dissection	Anterior chest; may radiate to back	Excruciating, tearing, knifelike	Sudden onset, unrelenting	Usually occurs in setting of hypertension or predisposition such as Marfan's syndrome	Murmur of aortic insufficiency, pulse or blood pressure asymmetry; neurologic deficit
Pulmonary embolism (chest pain often not present)	Substernal or over region of pulmonary infarction	Pleuritic (with pulmonary infarction) or angina-like	Sudden onset; minutes to <1 hr	May be aggravated by breathing	Dyspnea, tachypnea, tachycardia; hypotension, signs of acute right ventricular failure, and pulmonary hypertension with large emboli; rales, pleural rub, hemoptysis with pulmonary infarction
Pulmonary hypertension	Substernal	Pressure; oppressive	Similar to angina	Aggravated by effort	Pain usually associated with dyspnea; signs of pulmonary hypertension
NONCARDIAC CAUSES					
Pneumonia with pleurisy	Localized over involved area	Pleuritic localized	Brief or prolonged	Painful breathing	Dyspnea, cough, fever, dull to percussion, bronchial breath sounds, rales, occasional pleural rub
Spontaneous pneumothorax	Unilateral	Sharp, well localized	Sudden onset, lasts many hours	Painful breathing	Dyspnea; hyperresonance and decreased breath and voice sounds over involved lung
Musculoskeletal disorders	Variable	Aching	Short or long duration	Aggravated by movement; history of muscle exertion or injury	Tender to pressure or movement
Herpes zoster	Dermatomal in distribution	Burning, itching	Prolonged	None	Vesicular rash appears in area of discomfort
Esophageal reflux	Substernal, epigastric	Burning, visceral discomfort	10–60 min	Aggravated by large meal, postprandial recumbency; relief with antacid	Water brash
Peptic ulcer	Epigastric, substernal	Visceral burning, aching	Prolonged	Relief with food, antacid	
Gallbladder disease	Epigastric, right upper quadrant	Visceral	Prolonged	May be unprovoked or follow meals	Right upper quadrant tenderness may be present
Anxiety states	Often localized over precordium	Variable; location often moves from place to place	Varies; often fleeting	Situational	Sighing respirations, often chest wall tenderness

From Andreoli TE, Bennett JC, Carpenter CCJ, Plum F: Evaluation of the patient with cardiovascular disease. *In* Cecil Essentials of Medicine. 4th ed. Philadelphia, WB Saunders, 1997, pp 11–12.
S_4 = fourth heart sound.

breathing, or a need to breathe more is classically associated with deconditioning.

Palpitations

Palpitations describe a subjective sensation of an irregular or abnormal heartbeat. Palpitations may be caused by any arrhythmia (see Chapters 51 and 52) with or without important underlying structural heart disease. Palpitations should be defined in terms of the duration and frequency of the episodes, the precipitating and related factors, and any associated symptoms of chest pain, dyspnea, lightheadedness, or syncope. It is critical to use the history to determine whether the palpitations are caused by an irregular or a regular heartbeat. The feeling associated with a premature atrial or ventricular contraction, often described as a "skipped beat" or a "flip-flopping of the heart," must be distinguished from the irregularly irregular rhythm of atrial fibrillation and the rapid but regular rhythm of supraventricular tachycardia. Associated symptoms of chest pain, dyspnea, lightheadedness, dizziness, or sweating suggest an important effect on cardiac output and mandate further evaluation. In general, evaluation begins with ambulatory electrocardiography (ECG) (Table 38–3), which is indicated in patients who have palpitations in the presence of structural heart disease or substantial accompanying symptoms.

Lightheadedness or *syncope* (see Chapters 50 and 447) can be caused by any condition that decreases cardiac output (e.g., bradyarrhythmia, tachyarrhythmia, obstruction of the left ventricular or right ventricular inflow or outflow, cardiac tamponade, aortic dissection, or severe pump failure), by reflex-mediated vasomotor instability (e.g., vasovagal, situational, or carotid sinus syncope), or orthostatic hypotension. Neurologic diseases (e.g., migraine headaches, transient ischemic attacks, or seizures) also can cause transient loss of consciousness. The history, physical examination, and ECG are often diagnostic of the cause of syncope. Syncope caused by a cardiac arrhythmia usually occurs with little warning. Syncope with exertion or just after concluding exertion is typical of aortic stenosis and hypertrophic obstructive cardiomyopathy. In many patients, additional testing will be required to document central ner-

vous system disease, the cause of reduced cardiac output, or carotid sinus syncope. When the history, physical examination, and ECG do not provide helpful diagnostic information that points toward a specific cause of syncope, it is imperative that patients with heart disease or an abnormal ECG be tested with continuous ambulatory ECG monitoring to diagnose a possible arrhythmia; in selected patients, formal electrophysiologic testing may be indicated (see Chapter 50). In patients with no evident heart disease, tilt testing (Chapter 50) can help detect reflex-mediated vasomotor instability.

Other Symptoms

Non-productive *cough* is often an early manifestation of elevated pulmonary venous pressure and otherwise unsuspected heart failure. *Fatigue* and *weakness* are common accompaniments of advanced cardiac disease and reflect an inability to perform normal activities. A variety of approaches have been used to classify the severity of cardiac limitations ranging from Class I (little or no limitation) to Class IV (severe limitation) (Table 38–4). *Hemoptysis* is a classic presenting finding in patients with pulmonary embolism, but it is also common in patients with mitral stenosis, pulmonary edema, bronchiectasis, and bronchitis. *Claudication,* which is pain in the extremities with exertion, should alert the physician to possible peripheral arterial disease (see Chapters 67 and 68).

The Complete Medical History

The complete medical history should include a thorough review of systems, family history, social history, and past medical history. The review of systems may reveal other symptoms that suggest a systemic disease as the cause of any cardiovascular problems. The family history should focus on premature atherosclerosis or evidence of familial abnormalities, such as may be found with various causes of the long QT syndrome (see Chapter 49) or hypertrophic cardiomyopathy (see Chapter 64).

The social history should include specific questioning about cigarette smoking, alcohol intake, and use of illicit drugs. The past medical history may reveal prior conditions or medications that suggest systemic diseases, ranging from chronic obstructive pulmonary disease, which may explain a complaint of dyspnea, to hemochromatosis, which may be a cause of restrictive cardiomyopathy. A careful history to inquire about recent dental work or other procedures is critical if bacterial endocarditis is part of the differential diagnosis.

PHYSICAL EXAMINATION FOR DETECTION OF SIGNS OF CARDIOVASCULAR DISEASE

The cardiovascular physical examination, which is a subset of the complete physical examination, provides important clues to the diagnosis of asymptomatic and symptomatic cardiac disease and may reveal cardiovascular manifestations of non-cardiovascular diseases. The cardiovascular physical examination begins with careful measurement of the pulse and blood pressure. If aortic dissection (see Chapter 66) is a consideration, blood pressure should be measured in both arms and, preferably, in at least one leg. When coarctation of the aorta is suspected (see Chapter 57), blood pressure must be measured in the leg as well as in the arms. Discrepancies in blood pressure between the two arms can also be caused by atherosclerotic disease of the great vessels. Pulsus paradoxus, which is a decrease in the systolic blood pressure of more than the usual 10 mm Hg drop in inspiration, is typical of pericardial tamponade (see Chapter 65).

General Appearance

The respiratory rate may be increased in patients with heart failure. Patients with pulmonary edema are usually markedly tachypneic and may have labored breathing. Patients with advanced heart failure may have Cheyne-Stokes respirations.

Systemic diseases such as hyperthyroidism (see Chapter 239), hypothyroidism (see Chapter 239), rheumatoid arthritis (see Chapter 286), scleroderma (see Chapter 290), and hemochromatosis (see Chapter 221) may be suspected from the patient's general appearance. Marfan's syndrome (see Chapter 215), Turner's syndrome (see Chapter 249), Down syndrome (see Chapter 34), and a variety of congenital anomalies may also be readily apparent.

Table 38–3 ■ AHA/ACC GUIDELINES FOR USE OF DIAGNOSTIC TESTS IN PATIENTS WITH PALPITATIONS*

AMBULATORY ELECTROCARDIOGRAPHY

Class I	Palpitations, syncope, dizziness
Class II	Shortness of breath, chest pain, or fatigue (not otherwise explained, episodic and strongly suggestive of an arrhythmia as the cause because of a relation of the symptom with palpitation)
Class III	Symptoms not reasonably expected to be due to arrhythmia

ELECTROPHYSIOLOGIC STUDY

Class I	1. Patients with palpitations who have a pulse rate documented by medical personnel as inappropriately rapid and in whom electrocardiographic recordings fail to document the cause of the palpitations
	2. Patients with palpitations preceding a syncopal episode
Class II	Patients with clinically significant palpitations, suspected to be of cardiac origin, in whom symptoms are sporadic and cannot be documented; studies are performed to determine the mechanisms of arrhythmias, to direct or provide therapy, or to assess prognosis
Class III	Patients with palpitations documented to be due to extracardiac causes (e.g., hyperthyroidism)

ECHOCARDIOGRAPHY

Class I	Arrhythmias with evidence of heart disease
	Family history of genetic disorder associated with arrhythmias
Class II	Arrhythmias commonly associated with, but without evidence of, heart disease
	Atrial fibrillation or flutter
Class III	Palpitation without evidence of arrhythmias
	Minor arrhythmias without evidence of heart disease

*Class I, general agreement the test is useful and indicated; class II, frequently used, but there is a divergence of opinion with respect to its utility; class III, general agreement the test is not useful.

AHA/ACC = American Heart Association/American College of Cardiology.

From Goldman L, Braunwald E, eds. *Primary Cardiology.* Philadelphia: WB Saunders, 1998, p 126.

Table 38–4 ■ A COMPARISON OF THREE METHODS OF ASSESSING CARDIOVASCULAR DISABILITY

CLASS	NEW YORK HEART ASSOCIATION FUNCTIONAL CLASSIFICATION	CANADIAN CARDIOVASCULAR SOCIETY FUNCTIONAL CLASSIFICATION	SPECIFIC ACTIVITY SCALE
I	Patients with cardiac disease but without resulting limitations of physical activity. Ordinary physical activity does not cause undue fatigue, palpitation, dyspnea, or anginal pain.	Ordinary physical activity, such as walking and climbing stairs, does not cause angina. Angina with strenuous or rapid or prolonged exertion at work or recreation.	Patients can perform to completion any activity requiring ≥7 metabolic equivalents, e.g., can carry 24 lb up 8 steps; carry objects that weigh 80 lb; do outdoor work (shovel snow, spade soil); do recreational activities (skiing, basketball, squash, handball, jog/walk 5 mph).
II	Patients with cardiac disease resulting in slight limitation of physical activity. They are comfortable at rest. Ordinary physical activity results in fatigue, palpitations, dyspnea, or anginal pain.	Slight limitation of ordinary activity. Walking or climbing stairs rapidly, walking uphill, walking or stair climbing after meals, in cold, in wind, or when under emotional stress, or only during the few hours after awakening. Walking more than 2 blocks on the level and climbing more than one flight of ordinary stairs at a normal pace and in normal conditions.	Patient can perform to completion any activity requiring ≥5 metabolic equivalents but cannot and does not perform to completion activities requiring ≥7 metabolic equivalents, e.g., have sexual intercourse without stopping, garden, rake, weed, roller skate, dance fox trot, walk at 4 mph on level ground.
III	Patients with cardiac disease resulting in marked limitation of physical activity. They are comfortable at rest. Less than ordinary physical activity causes fatigue, palpitations, dyspnea, or anginal pain.	Marked limitation of ordinary physical activity. Walking 1 to 2 blocks on the level and climbing more than one flight in normal conditions.	Patient can perform to completion any activity requiring ≥2 metabolic equivalents but cannot and does not perform to completion any activities requiring ≥5 metabolic equivalents, e.g., shower without stopping, strip and make bed, clean windows, walk 2.5 mph, bowl, play golf, dress without stopping.
IV	Patient with cardiac disease resulting in inability to carry on any physical activity without discomfort. Symptoms of cardiac insufficiency or of the anginal syndrome may be present even at rest. If any physical activity is undertaken, discomfort is increased.	Inability to carry on any physical activity without discomfort—anginal syndrome *may be* present at rest.	Patient cannot or does not perform to completion activities requiring ≥2 metabolic equivalents. *Cannot* carry out activities listed above (Specific Activity Scale, Class III).

From Goldman L, et al: Comparative reproducibility and validity of systems for assessing cardiovascular functional class: Advantages of a new specific activity scale. Circulation 64:1227, 1981. Reproduced by permission of the American Heart Association.

Ophthalmologic Examination

Examination of the fundi may show diabetic or hypertensive retinopathy or the Roth's spots typical of infectious endocarditis. Beading of the retinal arteries is typical of severe hypercholesterolemia. Osteogenesis imperfecta, which is associated with blue sclerae, is also associated with aortic dilatation and mitral valve prolapse. Retinal artery occlusion may be caused by an embolus from clot in the left atrium or left ventricle, a left atrial myxoma, or atherosclerotic debris from the great vessels. Hyperthyroidism may present with exophthalmos and typical stare, whereas myotonic dystrophy, which is associated with atrioventricular block and arrhythmia, is often associated with ptosis and an expressionless face.

Jugular Veins

The external jugular veins help in assessment of mean right atrial pressure, which normally varies between 5 and 10 cm H_2O; the height (in centimeters) of the central venous pressure is measured by adding 5 cm to the height of the observed jugular venous distension above the sternal angle of Louis. The normal jugular venous pulse, best seen in the internal jugular vein (and not seen in the external jugular vein unless insufficiency of the jugular venous valves is present), includes an a wave, caused by right atrial contraction; a c wave, reflecting carotid artery pulsation; an x-descent; a v wave, which corresponds to isovolumetric right ventricular contraction and is more marked in the presence of tricuspid insufficiency; and a y descent, which occurs as the tricuspid valve opens and ventricular filling begins (Fig. 38–1). Abnormalities of the jugular venous pressure and pulse are useful in detecting conditions such as heart failure, pericardial disease, tricuspid valve disease, and pulmonary hypertension (Table 38–5).

Carotid Pulse

The carotid pulse should be examined in terms of its volume and contour. The carotid pulse (Fig. 38–2) may be increased in frequency and may be more intense than normal in patients with a higher stroke volume due to aortic regurgitation, arteriovenous fistula, hyperthyroidism, fever, or anemia. In aortic regurgitation or arteriovenous fistula, the pulse may have a bisferious quality. The carotid upstroke is delayed in patients with valvular aortic stenosis

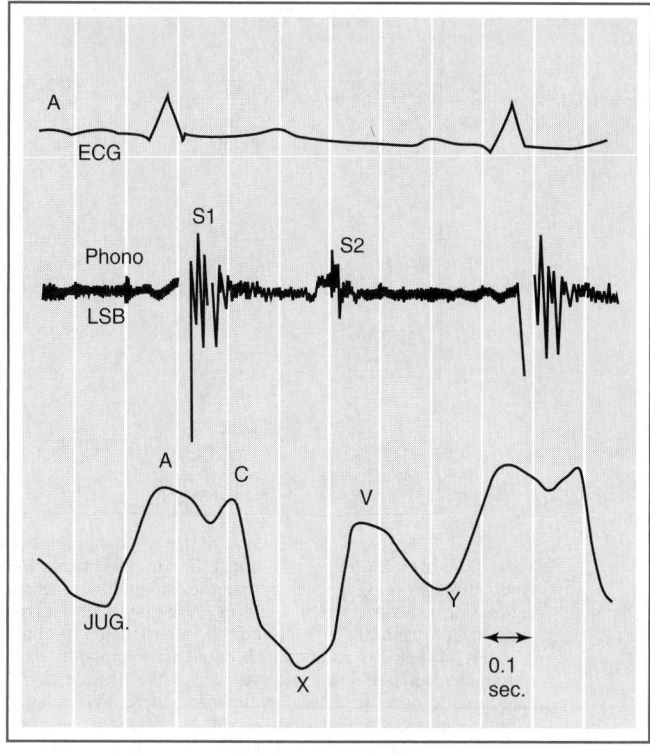

FIGURE 38–1. ■ Normal jugular venous pulse.

Table 38–5 ■ **ABNORMALITIES OF THE VENOUS PRESSURE AND PULSE AND THEIR CLINICAL SIGNIFICANCE**

1. Positive hepatojugular reflux—suspect congestive heart failure, particularly left ventricular systolic dysfunction (echocardiography recommended).
2. Elevated systemic venous pressure without obvious 'x' or 'y' descent and quiet precordium and pulsus paradoxus—suspect cardiac tamponade (echocardiography recommended).
3. Elevated systemic venous pressure with sharp 'y' descent, Kussmaul's sign and quiet precordium—suspect constrictive pericarditis (cardiac catheterization and MRI or CT recommended).
4. Elevated systemic venous pressure with a sharp brief 'y' descent, Kussmaul's sign, and evidence of pulmonary hypertension and tricuspid regurgitation—suspect restrictive cardiomyopathy (cardiac catheterization and MRI or CT recommended).
5. A prominent 'a' wave with or without elevation of mean systemic venous pressure—exclude tricuspid stenosis, right ventricular hypertrophy due to pulmonary stenosis, and pulmonary hypertension (echo-Doppler study recommended).
6. A prominent 'v' wave with a sharp 'y' descent—suspect tricuspid regurgitation (echo-Doppler or cardiac catheterization to determine etiology).

From Heart Disease: A Textbook of Cardiovascular Medicine. Edited by Eugene Braunwald. 5th ed. Philadelphia: WB Saunders, 1997.

(see Chapter 63) and has a normal contour but diminished amplitude in any cause of reduced stroke volume.

Cardiac Inspection and Palpation

Inspection of the precordium may reveal the hyperinflation of obstructive lung disease or unilateral asymmetry of the left side of the chest because of right ventricular hypertrophy before puberty. Palpation may be performed with the patient either supine or in the left lateral decubitus position; the latter moves the left ventricular apex closer to the chest wall and increases the ability to palpate the point of maximal impulse and other phenomena. Low-frequency phenomena such as systolic heaves or lifts from the left ventricle (at the cardiac apex) or right ventricle (parasternal in the third or fourth intercostal space) are best felt with the heel of the palm. With the patient in the left lateral decubitus position, this technique may also allow palpation of an S_3 gallop in cases of advanced heart failure and/or an S_4 gallop in cases of poor left ventricular

distensibility during diastole. The left ventricular apex is more diffuse and may sometimes be frankly dyskinetic in patients with advanced heart disease. The distal palm is best for feeling thrills, which are the tactile equivalent of cardiac murmurs. By definition, a thrill denotes a murmur of grade 4/6 or louder. Higher-frequency events may be best felt with the fingertips; examples include the opening snap of mitral stenosis or the loud pulmonic second sound of pulmonary hypertension.

Auscultation

The first heart sound (Fig. 38–3), which is largely produced by closure of the mitral and—to a lesser extent—the tricuspid valves, may be louder in patients with mitral valve stenosis and intact valve leaflet movement and less audible in patients with poor closure due to mitral regurgitation (see Chapter 63). The second heart sound is caused primarily by closure of the aortic valve, but closure of the pulmonic valve is also commonly audible. In normal individuals, the louder aortic closure sound occurs first, followed by pulmonic closure. With expiration the two sounds are virtually superimposed, whereas with inspiration the increased stroke volume of the right ventricle commonly leads to a discernible splitting of the second sound. This splitting may be fixed in patients with an atrial septal defect (see Chapter 57) or a right bundle branch block. The split may be paradoxical in patients with left bundle branch block or other causes of delayed left ventricular emptying. The aortic component of the second sound is increased in intensity in the presence of systemic hypertension and decreased in intensity in patients with aortic stenosis. The pulmonic second sound is increased in the presence of pulmonary hypertension.

Early systolic ejection sounds are related to forceful opening of the aortic or pulmonic valve; such sounds are common in congenital aortic stenosis, with a mobile valve; in hypertension, with forceful opening of the aortic valve; and in healthy young individuals, especially when cardiac output is increased. Midsystolic or late systolic clicks are most commonly caused by mitral valve prolapse (see Chapter 63). Clicks are relatively high-frequency sounds that are best heard with the diaphragm of the stethoscope.

The third heart sound corresponds to rapid ventricular filling during early diastole. It may occur in normal children and young adults, especially if stroke volume is increased. However, after about age 40 years, a third heart sound should be considered abnormal; it is caused by conditions that increase the volume of

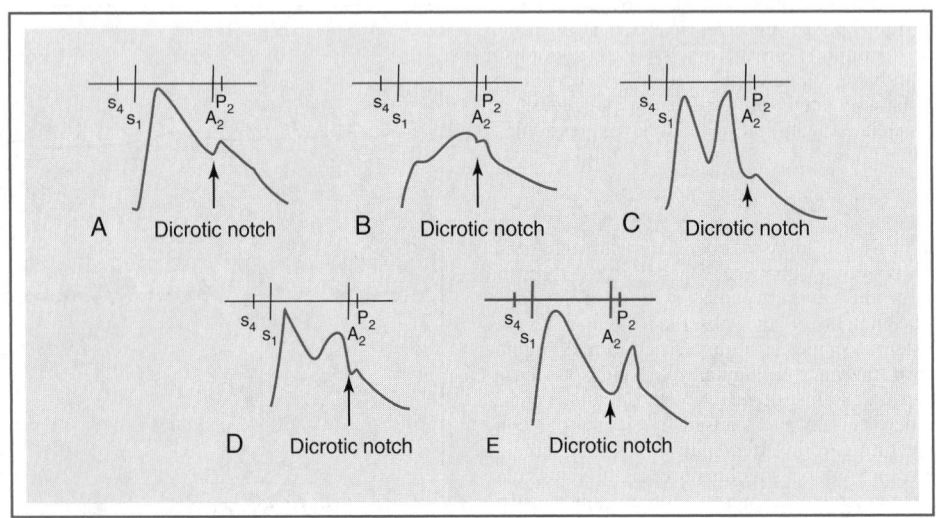

FIGURE 38–2. ■ Schematic diagrams of the configurational changes in the carotid pulse and their differential diagnosis. Heart sounds are also illustrated. *A*, Normal. *B*, Anacrotic pulse with slow initial upstroke. The peak is close to the second heart sound. These features suggest fixed left ventricular outflow obstruction such as valvular aortic stenosis. *C*, Pulsus bisferiens, with both percussion and tidal waves occurring during systole. This type of carotid pulse contour is most frequently observed in patients with hemodynamically significant aortic regurgitation or combined aortic stenosis and regurgitation with dominant regurgitation. It is rarely observed in patients with mitral valve prolapse or in normal individuals. *D*, Pulsus bisferiens in hypertrophic obstructive cardiomyopathy. It is rarely appreciated at the bedside by palpation. *E*, Dicrotic pulse results from an accentuated dicrotic wave and tends to occur in sepsis, severe heart failure, hypovolemic shock, cardiac tamponade, and after aortic valve replacement. S_4 = atrial sounds; S_1 = first heart sound; A_2 = aortic component of the second heart sound; P_2 = pulmonary component of the second heart sound). (From Chatterjee, K: Bedside evaluation of the heart: The physical examination. *In* Chatterjee, K et al [eds]: Cardiology: An Illustrated Text/Reference. Philadelphia, JB Lippincott, 1991 pp 3.11–3.51.)

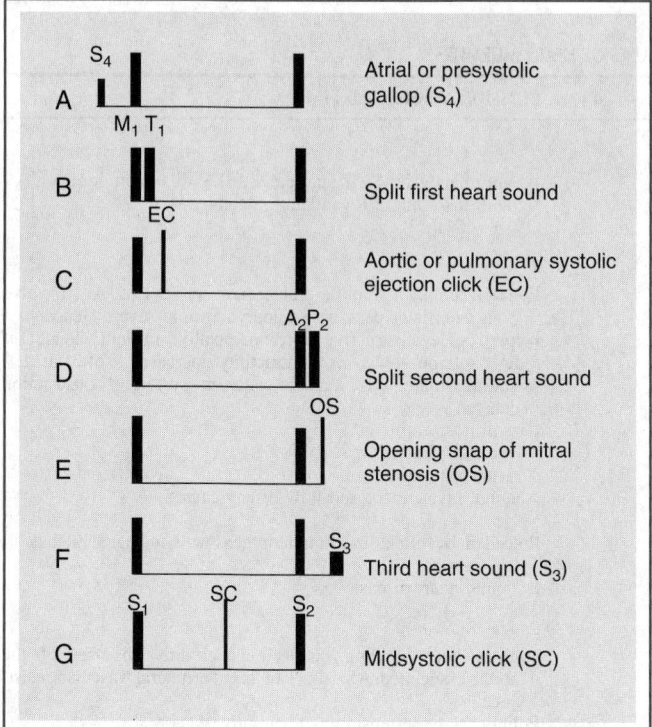

A S_4 Atrial or presystolic gallop (S_4)
    $M_1 T_1$

B Split first heart sound
    EC

C Aortic or pulmonary systolic ejection click (EC)

D $A_2 P_2$ Split second heart sound

E OS Opening snap of mitral stenosis (OS)

F S_3 Third heart sound (S_3)

G S_1 SC S_2 Midsystolic click (SC)

FIGURE 38–3. ■ Timing of the different heart sounds and added sounds. (Modified and reproduced, with permission, from Wood P: Diseases of the Heart and Circulation, 3rd ed. Lippincott, 1968.)

ventricular filling during early diastole (such as mitral regurgitation) or that increase pressure in early diastole (such as advanced heart failure). A left ventricular S_3 gallop is best heard at the apex, whereas the right ventricular S_3 gallop is best heard at the fourth intercostal space at the left parasternal border; both are best heard with the bell of the stethoscope. A fourth heart sound is rarely heard in young individuals but is common in adults older than 40 or 50 years because of reduced ventricular compliance during atrial contraction; it is a nearly ubiquitous finding in patients with hypertension, heart failure, or ischemic heart disease.

The opening snap of mitral and, less commonly, tricuspid stenosis occurs at the beginning of mechanical diastole, prior to the onset of the rapid phase of ventricular filling. An opening snap is high-pitched and is best heard with the diaphragm; this differential frequency should help distinguish an opening snap from a third heart sound on physical examination. An opening snap can commonly be distinguished from a loud pulmonic component of the second heart sound by the differential location (mitral opening snap at the apex, tricuspid opening snap at the left third or fourth intercostal space, pulmonic second sound at the left second intercostal space) as well as by the longer interval between the second heart sound and the opening snap.

Heart murmurs may be classified as systolic, diastolic, or continuous (Table 38–6). Murmurs are graded by intensity on a scale of 1 to 6. Grade 1 is faint and appreciated only by careful auscultation; 2, readily audible; 3, moderately loud; 4, loud and associated with a palpable thrill; 5, loud and audible with the stethoscope only partially placed on the chest; 6, loud enough to be heard without the stethoscope on the chest. Systolic ejection murmurs usually peak in early to midsystole when left ventricular ejection is maximal; examples include fixed valvular, supravalvular, or infravalvular aortic or pulmonic stenosis. The murmur of hypertrophic obstructive cardiomyopathy has a similar ejection quality, although its peak may be later in systole when dynamic obstruction is maximal (see Chapter 64). Pansystolic murmurs are characteristic of mitral or tricuspid regurgitation or with a left-to-right shunt from conditions such as a ventricular septal defect (left ventricle to right ventricle). A late systolic murmur is characteristic of mitral valve prolapse (see Chapter 63) or ischemic papillary muscle dysfunction. Ejection quality murmurs may also be heard in patients with normal valves but increased flow, such as occurs with marked anemia,

fever, or bradycardia due to congenital complete heart block; they may also be heard across a valve that is downstream from increased flow due to an intracardiac shunt. Maneuvers such as inspiration, expiration, standing, squatting, and handgripping can be especially useful in the differential diagnosis of a murmur; however, echocardiography will commonly be required to make a definitive diagnosis of both cause and severity (Table 38–7).

High-frequency, early-diastolic murmurs are typical of aortic regurgitation and pulmonic regurgitation from a variety of causes. The murmurs of mitral and tricuspid stenosis begin in early to middiastole and tend to diminish in intensity later in diastole in the absence of effective atrial contraction, but they tend to increase in intensity in later diastole if effective atrial contraction is present.

Continuous murmurs may be caused by any abnormality that is associated with a pressure gradient in both systole and diastole: examples include a patent ductus arteriosis, ruptured sinus of Valsalva aneurysm, arteriovenous fistula (of the coronary artery, pulmonary artery, or thoracic artery), or a mammary soufflé. In some situations, murmurs of two coexistent conditions (e.g., aortic stenosis and regurgitation; atrial septal defect with a large shunt and resulting flow murmurs of relative mitral and pulmonic stenosis) may mimic a continuous murmur.

Abdomen

The most common cause of hepatomegaly in patients with heart disease is hepatic engorgement from elevated right-sided pressures associated with right ventricular failure of any cause. Hepatojugular reflux is elicited by pressing on the liver and showing an increase in the jugular venous pressure; it indicates advanced right ventricular failure or obstruction to right ventricular filling. Evaluation of the abdomen may also reveal an enlarged liver caused by a systemic disease such as hemochromatosis or sarcoidosis, which may also affect the heart. In more severe cases, splenomegaly and ascites may also be noted. Large, palpable, polycystic kidneys are commonly associated with hypertension. A systolic bruit suggestive of renal artery stenosis or an enlarged abdominal aorta is a clue of atherosclerosis.

Extremities

Extremities should be evaluated for peripheral pulses, edema, cyanosis, and clubbing. Diminished peripheral pulses suggest peripheral arterial disease (see Chapters 67 and 68). Delayed pulses in the legs are consistent with coarctation of the aorta and are also seen after aortic dissection.

Edema is a cardinal manifestation of right-sided heart failure. When due to heart failure, pericardial disease, or pulmonary hypertension, the edema is usually symmetrical and progresses upward from the ankles; each of these causes of cardiac edema is commonly associated with jugular venous distention and often with hepatic congestion. Unilateral edema suggests thrombophlebitis or proximal venous or lymphatic obstruction. Edema in the absence of evidence of right- or left-sided heart failure suggests renal disease, hypoalbuminemia, myxedema, or other noncardiac causes.

Cyanosis is a bluish discoloration caused by reduced hemoglobin exceeding about 5 g/dL in the capillary bed. Central cyanosis is seen in patients with poor oxygen saturation due to a reduced inspired oxygen concentration or inability to oxygenate the blood in the lungs (e.g., as a result of advanced pulmonary disease, pulmonary edema, pulmonary arteriovenous fistula, or right-to-left shunting); it may also be seen in patients with marked erythrocytosis. Methemoglobinemia (see Chapter 168) can also present with cyanosis. Peripheral cyanosis may be caused by reduced blood flow to the extremities due to vasoconstriction, heart failure, or shock. *Clubbing,* which is loss of the normal concave configuration of the nail as it emerges from the distal phalynx, is seen in patients with chronic central cyanosis and in patients with pulmonary abnormalities such as lung cancer.

Examination of the Skin

Examination of the skin may reveal bronze pigmentation typical of hemochromatosis, jaundice characteristic of severe right-sided heart failure or hemochromatosis, or capillary hemangiomas typical of Osler-Weber-Rendu disease, which is also associated with pul-

Table 38-6 ■ SOME COMMON CAUSES OF HEART MURMURS*

	USUAL LOCATION	COMMON ASSOCIATED FINDINGS
Systolic		
Holosystolic		
Mitral regurgitation (MR)	apex → axilla	↑ with handgrip; S₃ if marked MR; LV dilatation common
Tricuspid regurgitation (TR)	LLSB	↑ with inspiration; RV dilatation common
Ventricular septal defect (VSD)	LLSB → RLSB	Often with thrill
Early-midsystolic		
Aortic valvular stenosis (AS)	RUSB	
Fixed supravalvular or subvalvular	RUSB	Ejection click if mobile valve; soft or absent A₂ if valve immobile; later peak associated with more severe stenosis
Dynamic infravalvular	LLSB → apex + axilla	Hypertrophic obstructive cardiomyopathy; murmur louder if LV volume lower or contractility increased, softer if LV volume increased†; can be later in systole if obstruction delayed
Pulmonic valvular stenosis (PS)	LUSB	↑ with inspiration
Infravalvular (infundibular)	LUSB	↑ with inspiration
Supravalvular	LUSB	↑ with inspiration
"Flow murmurs"	LUSB	Anemia, fever, increased flow of any cause‡
Mid-late Systolic		
Mitral valve prolapse (MVP)	LLSB or apex → axilla	Preceded by click; murmur lengthens with maneuvers that ↓ LV volume*
Papillary muscle dysfunction	Apex → axilla	Ischemic heart disease
Diastolic		
Early Diastolic		
Aortic regurgitation (AR)	RUSB, LUSB	High-pitched, blowing quality; endocarditis, diseases of the aorta, associated AS; signs of low peripheral vascular resistance
Pulmonic valve regurgitation (PR)	LUSB	Pulmonary hypertension as a causative factor
Mid-late Diastolic		
Mitral stenosis (MS), tricuspid stenosis (TS)	Apex, LLSB	Low-pitched; in rheumatic heart disease, opening snap commonly precedes murmur; can be due to increased flow across normal valve‡
Atrial myxomas	Apex (L), LLSB (R)	"Tumor plop"
Continuous		
Venous hum	Over jugular or hepatic vein or breast	Disappears with compression of vein or pressure of stethoscope
Patent ductus arteriosis (PDA)	LUSB	
Arteriovenous (AV) fistula		
Coronary	LUSB	
Pulmonary, bronchial, chest wall	Over fistula	
Ruptured sinus of Valsalva aneurysm	RUSB	Sudden onset

*See also Chapters 57 and 63.

†LV (left ventricular) volume is decreased by standing or during prolonged, forced expiration against a closed glottis (Valsalva maneuver); it is increased by squatting or by elevation of the legs; contractility is increased by adrenergic stimulation or in the beat after a post-extrasystolic beat

‡Including a left-to-right shunt through an atrial septal defect for tricuspid or pulmonic flow murmurs and a ventricular septal defect for pulmonic or mitral flow murmurs.

LUSB = left upper sternal border (2nd–3rd intercostal spaces); RUSB = right upper sternal border (2nd–3rd intercostal spaces); LLSB = left lower sternal border (4th intercostal space); RLSB = right lower sternal border (4th intercostal space).

monary arteriovenous fistulas and cyanosis. Infectious endocarditis may be associated with Osler's nodes, Janeway's lesions, or splinter hemorrhages (see Chapter 326). Xanthomata are subcutaneous deposits of cholesterol seen on the extensor surfaces of the extremi-

Table 38-7 ■ SENSITIVITY AND SPECIFICITY OF BEDSIDE MANEUVERS IN THE IDENTIFICATION OF SYSTOLIC MURMURS

MANEUVER	RESPONSE	MURMUR	SENSITIVITY (%)	SPECIFICITY (%)
Inspiration	↑	RS	100	88
Expiration	↓	RS	100	88
Valsalva maneuver	↑	HC	65	96
Squat to stand	↑	HC	95	84
Stand to squat	↓	HC	95	85
Leg elevation	↓	HC	85	91
Handgrip	↓	HC	85	75
Handgrip	↑	MR & VSD	68	92
Transient arterial occlusion	↑	MR & VSD	78	100

Modified with permission from Lembo NJ, Dell'Italia LJ, Crawford MH, et al.: Beside diagnosis of systolic murmurs. N Engl J Med 318:1572–1578, 1988. Copyright 1988 Massachusetts Medical Society. All rights reserved.

RS = right-sided; HC = hypertrophic cardiomyopathy; MR = mitral regurgitation; VSD = ventricular septal defect.

ties or on the palms and digital creases; they are found in patients with severe hypercholesterolemia.

Laboratory Studies

All patients with known or suspected cardiac disease should have an ECG and chest radiograph. The ECG (see Chapter 42) will help identify rate, rhythm, conduction abnormalities, and possible myocardial ischemia. The chest radiograph (see Chapter 41) will yield important information on chamber enlargement, pulmonary vasculature, and the great vessels.

Blood testing in patients with known or suspected cardiac disease should be targeted to the conditions in question. In general, a complete blood cell count, thyroid indices, and lipid levels are part of the standard evaluation.

Echocardiography (see Chapter 43) is the most useful test to analyze valvular and ventricular function. Using Doppler flow methods, both stenotic and regurgitant lesions can be quantified. Transesophageal echocardiography is the preferable method for evaluating possible aortic dissection and for identifying clot in the cardiac chambers. Radionuclide studies (see Chapter 44) can measure left ventricular function, assess myocardial ischemia, and determine whether ischemic myocardium is viable.

Stress testing using exercise or pharmacologic stress is useful to precipitate myocardial ischemia that may be detected by ECG abnormalities, perfusion abnormalities on radionuclide studies, or transient wall motion abnormalities on echocardiography. These tests are often critical in diagnosis of possible myocardial ischemia (see Chapter 59) and in establishment of prognosis in patients with known ischemic heart disease.

Cardiac catheterization (see Chapter 46) can precisely measure gradients across stenotic cardiac valves, judge the severity of intracardiac shunts, and determine intracardiac pressures. Coronary angiography provides a definitive diagnosis of coronary disease and is a necessary prelude to coronary revascularization with percutaneous transluminal coronary angioplasty (see Chapter 61) or coronary bypass graft surgery (see Chapter 62).

Continuous ambulatory ECG monitoring can help diagnose arrhythmias. A variety of newer technologies allow for longer-term monitoring in patients with important but infrequently occurring symptoms (see Chapter 50). Formal invasive electrophysiologic testing can be useful in the diagnosis of ventricular or supraventricular wide-complex tachycardia, and it is critical for guiding a wide array of new invasive electrophysiologic therapies (see Chapter 53).

SUMMARY

The history, physical examination, and laboratory evaluation should help the physician to establish the etiology of any cardiovascular problem; identify and quantify any anatomic abnormalities; determine the physiologic status of the valves, myocardium, and conduction system; determine functional capacity; estimate prognosis; and provide primary and/or secondary prevention. Key preventive strategies, including diet modification, recognition and treatment of hyperlipidemia, cessation of cigarette smoking, and adequate physical exercise, should be part of the approach to every patient, with or without heart disease.

Braunwald E: The clinical examination. In Goldman L, Braunwald E (eds): Primary Cardiology. Philadelphia, WB Saunders, 1998, pp 27–43.
Braunwald E: Examination of the patient. In Braunwald E (ed): Heart Disease, 5th ed. Philadelphia, WB Saunders, 1997, pp 1–14.
Chatterjeee K: Physical examination. In Topol EJ (ed): Textbook of Cardiovascular Medicine. Philadelphia, Lippincott-Raven, 1998, pp 293–332.
Topol EJ: The history. In Topol EJ (ed): Textbook of Cardiovascular Medicine. Philadelphia, Lippincott-Raven, 1998, pp 285–292.
More detailed descriptions of the cardiac history and physical examination.

39 EPIDEMIOLOGY OF CARDIOVASCULAR DISEASE
Michael H. Criqui

TYPES OF CARDIOVASCULAR DISEASE

The three major clinical manifestations of atherosclerotic cardiovascular disease (CVD) include coronary heart disease (CHD) (see Chapters 58, 59, and 60), stroke (see Chapter 470), and peripheral arterial vascular disease (PVD) (see Chapter 67). Atherosclerosis can also be found in other arterial beds, especially the renal arteries, where it causes about two thirds of cases of renal artery stenosis (see Chapters 55 and 112).

IMPORTANCE OF CARDIOVASCULAR DISEASE

DISEASE IMPACT. In 1997, more than 57 million Americans were estimated to have some form of CVD: 50 million had hypertension, 14 million had CHD, and 4 million had suffered a stroke. More than 1 in 5 Americans currently have some form of CVD.

Each year, about 1 million deaths in the United States, or about 42% of all deaths, are due to CVD. One sixth of CVD deaths occur in persons younger than age 65 years. On an annual basis, about 1.5 million Americans suffer myocardial infarction (MI), about 500,000 die of CHD, about 500,000 have strokes, and about 150,000 die of stroke.

SECULAR TRENDS. The death rate from CHD has fallen over

40% since 1968 (Fig. 39–1). Stroke mortality has continued to decline throughout the twentieth century. These observations have raised the question of whether this decline in mortality is due to a true reduction in incidence at the population level, which could logically be attributed to improved prevention, or simply to a decline in case-fatality rates, which would presumably be attributable mostly to better treatment. Several studies have evaluated this question, and the consensus is that both prevention and therapy have contributed, so that both population incidence rates and case-fatality rates have declined.

Despite this decline, CVD is still the leading cause of death in developed countries by a considerable margin. In addition, by 1990, CHD and stroke already ranked as the second and third leading causes of mortality even in developing regions.

ECONOMIC IMPACT. Despite the age-adjusted decline in mortality from CVD in the United States and many Western countries, CVD paradoxically poses an increasing economic burden, due largely to two factors: (1) an aging population, which keeps the actual numbers of CVD cases relatively stable, and (2) technologic improvements, which allow more aggressive and extensive therapy. For example, both hospital discharges and deaths from congestive heart failure, which is a frequent consequence of chronic CHD, have increased substantially in the past decade, as have the number of CVD operations and procedures.

NATURAL HISTORY OF CARDIOVASCULAR DISEASE

Arterial lesions begin as fatty streaks, often early in life (see Chapter 58). Studies of teenagers and young adults who were victims of accidental and other non-CVD causes of mortality show early fatty streaks, and these changes have correlated with traditional CVD risk factors. These fatty streaks can progress to raised lesions, which can progressively occlude the lumen of the artery.

Symptoms that typically occur in vascular beds well before the lesions completely occlude the lumen include angina pectoris from lesions in the coronary arteries (see Chapter 59), transient ischemic attacks from lesions in the cerebrovascular arteries (see Chapter 470), and intermittent claudication from lesions in the arteries in the lower extremities (see Chapter 67). Although each of these pain syndromes has a classic prototype, patients can present with quite atypical symptoms despite significant disease. Unfortunately, many patients either do not experience symptoms or ignore warning symptoms, and their first presentation may be a severe or fatal MI or stroke.

RISK FACTORS FOR CVD

TYPES OF STUDIES. The epidemiology of CVD has been evaluated in a number of study designs including ecologic, case-control, cross-sectional survey, prospective cohort, and clinical trial designs. In general, the strength of the causal inference one can draw from a study increases along this continuum, with policy changes typically appropriate only when supported by solid clinical trial evidence.

UNMODIFIABLE CVD RISK FACTORS. Several CVD risk factors are essentially immutable. These are older age, male gender, and a family history of CVD. Nonetheless, these risk factors are important to consider in evaluating an individual patient at risk.

CIGARETTE SMOKING. Cigarette smoking, along with dyslipidemia and hypertension, is considered one of the three major risk factors for CHD, thromboembolic stroke, and PVD. Event rates are three to four times higher in regular smokers, with a dose-response relationship. Unlike most other CVD risk factors, cigarette smoking can be eliminated entirely, but not easily (see Chapter 13). For CHD, the benefits of quitting smoking are dramatic—CHD incidence in ex-smokers falls to near non-smoking levels in 2 years.

DYSLIPIDEMIA. Dyslipidemia is probably a better term than hyperlipidemia because it includes all lipid and lipoprotein abnormalities, such as low levels of high-density lipoprotein (HDL)-cholesterol (hypoalphalipoproteinemia), which can be a potent risk factor. Early epidemiologic studies confirmed that elevated serum cholesterol level was an independent risk factor for CVD, with a strong dose-response relationship that is exponential at higher levels of

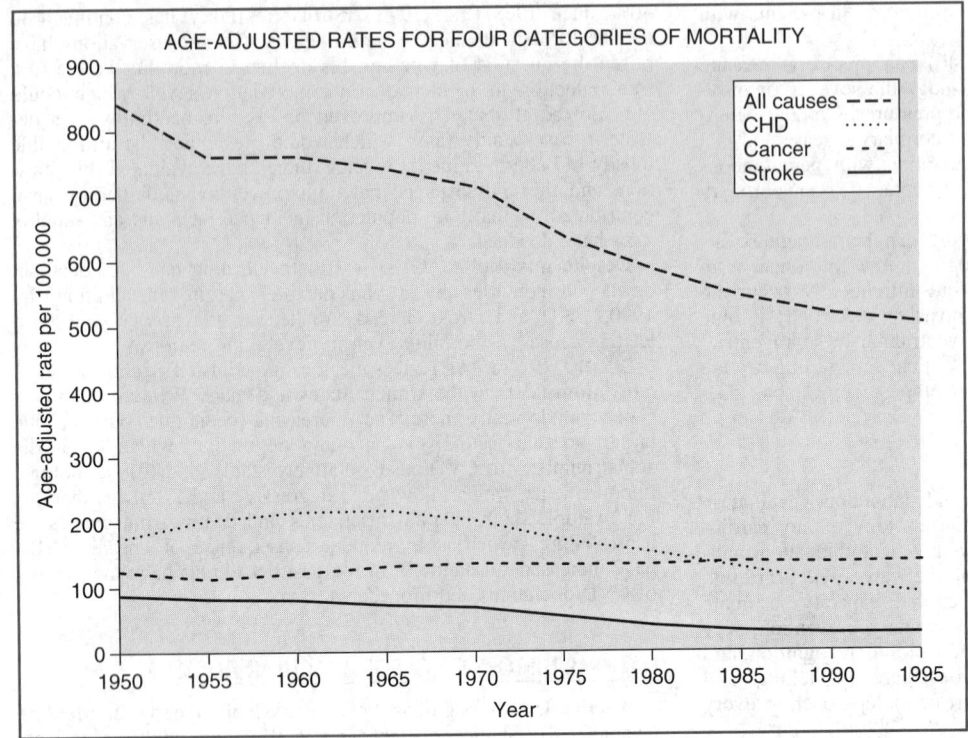

FIGURE 39–1 ■ Age-adjusted rates per 100,000 for four categories of mortality.

cholesterol. Although much of the interindividual variability in cholesterol is genetic, dietary consumption of cholesterol, saturated fat, and *trans*-fatty acids (typically formed by partial hydrogenation [saturation] of unsaturated vegetable fat) increases serum cholesterol.

Total cholesterol is carried on three lipoproteins in the blood, resulting in three separate cholesterol fractions with differing prognostic significance—very-low-density lipoprotein (VLDL)-cholesterol, low-density lipoprotein (LDL)-cholesterol, and HDL-cholesterol. LDL-cholesterol is positively related and HDL-cholesterol is inversely related to CVD incidence. VLDL-cholesterol is a close surrogate for serum triglycerides when the triglyceride level is less than 400 mg/dL. Triglycerides may be independently related to CVD in some subgroups in the population, such as persons with diabetes or low HDL-cholesterol.

Lp(a) is a lipoprotein identical to LDL except for the addition of a highly glycosylated protein, apolipoprotein (a). The similarity of the amino acid sequences of Lp(a) and plasminogen suggests the possibility of a connection between atherogenesis and thrombosis. Lp(a) has been associated with elevated CHD risk in several, but not all, epidemiologic studies. Intervention, however, is somewhat problematic, with only niacin and estrogen showing some effect in lowering Lp(a).

The best single lipid measure in predicting risk is the total cholesterol/HDL-cholesterol ratio (Fig. 39–2). Total cholesterol includes LDL-cholesterol, VLDL-cholesterol (a triglyceride surrogate), and HDL-cholesterol, while the denominator is the protective HDL-cholesterol. Ratios below 3 are ideal, 3 to 5 are average, and those above 5 represent elevated risk, but risk continues to rise throughout the range of total cholesterol/HDL-cholesterol values. In addition to being the best predictor of CVD outcomes in epidemiologic studies, a decrease in the total cholesterol/HDL-cholesterol ratio is also a better predictor of treatment benefit than changes in any other lipid or lipoprotein parameter in clinical trials.

HYPERTENSION. Elevated blood pressure is a potent risk factor for all forms of atherosclerotic CVD and is the dominant risk factor for stroke (see Chapter 469). In epidemiologic studies, there is a graded relation between the level of blood pressure, even at the lowest levels, and CVD outcomes. Early trials in severe hypertension unequivocally demonstrated the benefits of reducing very high blood pressure levels, with a sharp reduction in both morbidity and mortality from CVD. Meta-analyses of pharmacologic treatment of mild hypertension have also shown benefit. Multiple classes of antihypertensive drugs are now available, and extensive research is needed to determine the optimal drug regimen for a given patient, because some evidence suggests different drugs affect CVD outcomes differently despite similar reductions in blood pressure. For example, the short-acting dihydropyridine calcium channel blockers may increase CHD risk. In most patients, blood pressure, and often other CVD risk factors as well, can be improved to a greater or

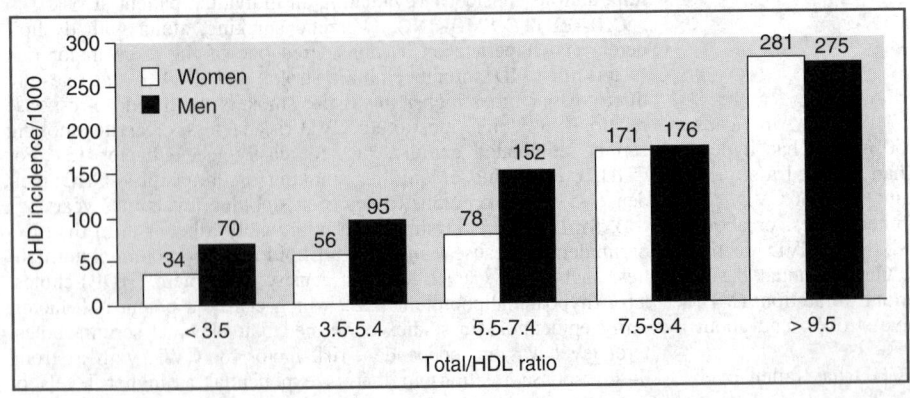

FIGURE 39–2 ■ Age-adjusted 7-year total CHD incidence per 1000 by total cholesterol/HDL-cholesterol ratio. (From Kannel WB: Am Heart J 114:413–419, 1987.)

lesser degree by lifestyle changes, including weight loss, exercise, and a diet that is rich in fruits and vegetables and avoids excess sodium and alcohol.

Systolic pressure rises with age throughout life in Western populations, whereas diastolic pressure plateaus in late mid-life and decreases somewhat thereafter. However, recent trials of blood pressure lowering in isolated systolic hypertension in the elderly have shown dramatic benefits for both stroke and CHD, with the absolute benefit of treatment remaining stable or even rising with increasing age.

PHYSICAL INACTIVITY. Persons who exercise more or are better conditioned are at lower CVD risk. Recent evidence shows significant changes in multiple risk factors with exercise, including improved insulin resistance, blood pressure, HDL-cholesterol, fibrinolysis, and triglycerides. Randomized trials of cardiac rehabilitation for secondary prevention also suggest benefit. Physical inactivity is now commonly considered one of the four major risk factors for CVD. Prior concerns about the possible acute risk of exercise for cardiac ischemia in susceptible persons are clearly outweighed by the benefits for most individuals; nevertheless, it is appropriate to evaluate high-risk individuals before beginning an exercise program.

DIABETES MELLITUS. Patients with either type I or II diabetes mellitus, also called insulin-dependent and non–insulin-dependent diabetes mellitus, respectively, are at increased risk of CVD (see Chapter 242). In type II diabetes, the risk is approximately doubled in men and increased fourfold in women, sharply attenuating the typical relative protection in women. In type I diabetes the risks are even higher, particularly in patients with proteinuria.

Patients with type II diabetes mellitus commonly exhibit evidence of insulin resistance well before the onset of chemical diabetes. Insulin resistance and type II diabetes are typically accompanied by one or more of a number of metabolic abnormalities: elevated insulin, glucose, blood pressure, and triglyceride levels, as well as lower HDL-cholesterol levels. Although LDL-cholesterol levels are typically normal, the LDL particles tend to be smaller and denser and may be more atherogenic, although it is not yet known if this effect is independent of accompanying hypertriglyceridemia. Evidence suggests correction of the lipid abnormalities in type II diabetes substantially decreases CHD risk. However, controversy persists as to whether reduction of glucose levels will improve macrovascular risk. New oral agents that lower glucose and insulin and improve insulin resistance may help resolve this issue. With weight loss and exercise, insulin resistance improves, triglyceride levels decrease, LDL particles become larger and less dense, HDL-cholesterol increases, and hypertension tends to improve.

OBESITY. Obesity (see Chapter 11) contributes to increased CVD risk by aggravating known CVD risk factors, including hypertension, insulin resistance, low HDL-cholesterol, and hypertriglyceridemia. However, even adjusting for these risk factors, obesity appears to contribute independently to CVD risk. Although the body mass index, defined as weight/height^2, has been the traditional measure of obesity in epidemiologic studies, measures of central obesity or abdominal fat, such as the waist/hip ratio, may be better predictors of CVD risk.

ALCOHOL. Alcohol (see Chapter 16) at less than 1 drink up to 3 drinks per day is protective against CHD. Thrombotic stroke and PVD show similar associations. This protective effect appears to be mediated by increases in HDL-cholesterol, as well as by possible effects on coagulation and fibrinolytic factors. For non-atherosclerotic CVD, such as hemorrhagic stroke and cardiomyopathy, risk is increased by alcohol consumption. At higher levels of alcohol consumption (3+ drinks per day), blood pressure increases, arrhythmias may be induced, rebound hypercoagulability may develop, direct myocardial damage can occur, and total CVD risk is increased. Maximum overall benefit for alcohol is reached at a single drink per day, and consumption of more than 2 drinks per day is associated with increases in morbidity and mortality from total cardiovascular causes, cirrhosis, accidents and violence, and certain cancers. Of particular concern is the consistent increase in breast cancer in women observed in epidemiologic studies even with only modest levels of drinking. In addition, the benefit of alcohol for CHD is essentially limited to older persons at relatively high risk of CHD, whereas younger persons and persons at lower risk of CHD have minimal benefit but could easily suffer alcohol-related harm. For the just mentioned reasons, and given the high

abuse potential of alcohol, it seems unwise to recommend alcohol for cardioprotection.

THROMBOTIC AND FIBRINOLYTIC FACTORS. In recent years, increasing attention has been paid to factors influencing the "second" CVD epidemiology, that is, thrombosis and fibrinolysis, as opposed to atherogenesis. The most consistent and reproducible risk factor in this group is fibrinogen, and epidemiologic studies have reported consistent and independent associations of fibrinogen with CHD, stroke, and PVD. Several other coagulation factors have showed associations in some studies, including Factor VII, Factor VIII, and various measures of platelet aggregability. Low-dose aspirin therapy inhibits platelet aggregation, which reduces CVD risk, but can increase the risk of bleeding.

Plasminogen activator inhibitor 1 (PAI-1) has also been correlated with both MI and carotid disease. Tissue-type plasminogen activator (t-PA) has shown both positive and inverse associations with CVD, with the counterintuitive positive associations possibly explained by ongoing fibrinolysis, which similarly may explain the findings of an elevated D-dimer level in CVD patients.

HOMOCYSTEINE. Numerous studies have shown homocysteine to be a strong, independent risk factor for CVD, including CHD, stroke, and PVD. The potential for intervention is theoretically quite good, since folic acid supplementation alone or in combination with other B vitamins is known to lower total plasma homocysteine levels. Many individuals with normal homocysteine levels may show hyperhomocysteinemia after methionine loading. Clinical trials are in progress to determine whether reduction in homocysteine with folic acid reduces the associated CVD risk. Positive trial results would indicate an inexpensive, relatively safe intervention for patients with, or at risk for, CVD.

INFECTION AND INFLAMMATION. Recent research has given support to an old theory that infectious agents may be involved in the pathogenesis of atherosclerosis. The evidence is perhaps strongest for *Chlamydia pneumoniae,* which has been isolated from atherosclerotic plaques, and patients with CVD have been shown to have elevated titers. In addition, after MI, *Chlamydia pneumoniae* titer levels may predict CVD events, and treatment with macrolide antibiotics may reduce recurrent CVD events. In animals, herpesviruses can stimulate atherosclerosis, and cytomegalovirus titers have been reported to be increased in some studies of CVD patients. Evidence for other infectious agents, such as *Helicobacter pylori,* is weaker than for cytomegalovirus and *Chlamydia pneumoniae.*

The link of infection to atherogenesis and thrombosis is unclear, but inflammation is likely involved. For example, inflammatory markers such as C-reactive protein may predict future fatal and non-fatal CHD events in men.

GONADAL HORMONES. There have been numerous reports of the association of both endogenous and exogenously administered estrogens and androgens with CVD risk factors and CVD events in men and women. The most convincing and clinically relevant data show a sharp reduction in CVD events in postmenopausal women using hormone replacement therapy with either unopposed estrogen or estrogen/progestin combinations. Estrogen raises HDL-cholesterol, lowers LDL-cholesterol, and appears to have a direct, immediate beneficial effect on arterial tone and flow. Definitive proof of any beneficial effects of hormone replacement therapy in women is being examined in trials of both primary and secondary prevention, but the one randomized secondary prevention trial surprisingly showed no benefits. New "designer estrogens" such as raloxifene are now available, with apparently fewer overall risks, but perhaps lesser benefits for CVD.

PSYCHOSOCIAL FACTORS. Psychosocial factors such as anger, anxiety, depression, hostility, type A behavior, and various measures of social support have been associated with occurrence or recurrence of CVD. In addition, measures of cardiovascular physiologic reactivity have been correlated with CVD outcomes. Currently, inadequate data are available to prove whether or not psychosocial interventions can reduce CVD risk.

SYNERGY OF RISK FACTORS. CVD risk factors appear to interact synergistically in producing risk (Table 39–1). The observed rate of CHD death in men who smoke, have serum cholesterol levels greater than or equal to 250 mg/dL, and have diastolic blood pressures greater than or equal to 90 mm Hg is nearly twice as great as would be predicted by adding the risk attributable to each

Table 39–1 ■ 10-YEAR AGE-ADJUSTED CHD MORTALITY RATES NATIONAL COOPERATIVE POOLING PROJECT

NUMBER OF RISK FACTORS*	ACTUAL RATE/1000	PREDICTED ADDITIVE RATE/1000†
0	13	—
1	23	—
2	44	33
3	82	43

*Risk factors: cigarette smoking, cholesterol ≥ 250 mg/dL, diastolic blood pressure ≥ 90 mm Hg.

†Because any one risk factor has an attributable rate of 10/1000, the predictive additive rate for two risk factors = 13 + 10 + 10 = 33; for three risk factors, 13 + 10 + 10 + 10 = 43.

From Criqui MH, et al: Prev Med 9:525–533, 1980.

of these three risk factors to the baseline risk. Multivariate statistical models have confirmed the multiplicative effect of CVD risk factors acting in concert. These data also imply that control of one risk factor will provide a substantial preventive benefit in persons with multiple risk factors.

RISK FACTORS IN PRIMARY AND SECONDARY PREVENTION. Primary prevention refers to preventing CVD in healthy persons. Secondary prevention refers to preventing recurrent CVD and death in patients with extant CVD. The major difference between primary and secondary prevention is that event rates are much greater in secondary prevention, approximately 10-fold higher, and the proportion of morbidity and mortality due to CVD is much higher. These simple facts have major clinical implications. First, the short-term benefit of intervention for a given patient is much greater in absolute terms in secondary prevention. Second, if a given intervention has any hazard, such as bleeding from antiplatelet therapy or cancer from hormone replacement therapy in women, such a hazard is likely to be relatively greater in primary prevention, where CVD event rates in the near term are relatively low.

In general, CVD risk factors and preventive interventions have similar effects on outcomes in primary and secondary prevention. For example, smoking cessation after MI cuts recurrent CHD risk in half and cholesterol lowering after MI can reduce new CHD events by about 35% (see Chapter 60).

GENDER ISSUES. The epidemiology of CVD in women and men is quite similar. Except for gonadal hormones, risk factors produce quite similar relative risks in men and women. The major gender difference is the greater age-specific CVD risk of men, particularly at younger ages. Because absolute CVD risk is lower overall in women, the incremental risk produced by a given risk factor tends to be less, except for diabetes, in which both the relative and incremental risks for heart disease are greater in women.

ETHNIC ISSUES. Minority ethnic groups are increasing as a proportion of the total U.S. population, with Hispanics being the fastest growing group. Considerable evidence exists for differences in CVD epidemiology between whites and both African-Americans and Native Americans. For example, African-Americans have higher blood pressures and worse hypertensive outcomes than whites, and some Native American groups have a sharp excess of diabetes. Data also suggest excess obesity and diabetes in Hispanics and a high risk of insulin resistance and CHD among emigrants from the Indian subcontinent to Western countries.

SUBCLINICAL CVD

Tests for subclinical CVD in the cerebral circulation include cerebral magnetic resonance imaging, retinal photography, and carotid duplex imaging; in the coronary circulation, cardiac magnetic resonance imaging, echocardiography, ambulatory electrocardiography, and ultrafast electron beam computed tomography (EBCT); and in the peripheral arteries, pulse wave velocity, reactive hyperemia, duplex imaging of the lower extremity arteries, and systolic blood pressures at the ankle (ankle-brachial index [ABI]) and toe (TBI) relative to the arm systolic pressure. Current evidence for prognostic significance is strongest for carotid duplex and the ABI, where significant carotid stenosis or an ABI less than 0.9 independently predicts a fourfold or greater increase in future CVD events.

Coronary calcification on EBCT correlates reasonably well with anatomic coronary stenosis and predicts CVD events short term. However, long-term studies of EBCT are not yet available (see Chapter 44).

THE CONTINUUM FROM RISK FACTORS TO SUBCLINICAL DISEASE TO CLINICAL DISEASE. It is unclear why some persons can tolerate higher levels of CVD risk factors whereas others develop clinical CVD despite "normal" risk factor levels. Now that numerous traditional and newer CVD risk factors have been identified, research needs to be focused on the transition from risk factors to subclinical disease to clinical disease and on the key factors in this transition. It is likely that atherosclerotic, thrombotic, fibrinolytic, and vascular reactive influences are all important at various transition points, and a better understanding of this natural history of CVD will allow more appropriate and targeted therapy.

Criqui MH, Golomb BA: Epidemiologic aspects of lipid abnormalities. Am J Med 105; 485–575, 1998. *Updated review of the epidemiology of dyslipidemias, with a discussion of the relative importance of various lipid and lipoprotein measurements.*

Joint National Committee: The Sixth Report of the Joint National Committee on Prevention, Detection, Evaluation, and Treatment of High Blood Pressure. National Institutes of Health, National Heart, Lung and Blood Institute. NIH publication No. 98-4080. Bethesda, MD, National Institutes of Health, 1997. *Background and current recommendations for blood pressure measurement, evaluation, prevention, and treatment, including a chapter on special populations and situations.*

McGovern PG, Pankow JS, Shahar E, et al: Recent trends in acute coronary heart disease: Mortality, morbidity, medical care, and risk factors. N Engl J Med 334: 884–890, 1996. *A solid analysis of CHD trends in a major U.S. metropolitan area (Minneapolis-St. Paul), indicating the decline in CHD can be explained by both the declining incidence of MI in the population and the improved survival of MI patients.*

O'Leary DH, Polak JF, Kronmal RA, et al: Carotid-artery intima and media thickness as a risk factor for myocardial infarction and stroke in older adults. N Engl J Med 340:14–22, 1999. *A clear demonstration of the independent prognostic significance of a measure of subclinical CVD for subsequent myocardial infarction and stroke.*

40 CARDIAC FUNCTION AND CIRCULATORY CONTROL

Daniel Burkhoff ■ *Myron L. Weisfeldt*

The heart is a muscular pump connected to the systemic and pulmonary vascular systems. Working together, the job of the heart and vasculature is to maintain adequate circulation of blood to the organs at rest and during periods of exercise. To understand perturbations that cause symptoms and disease, it is first necessary to understand the normal anatomy and physiology of the heart, its interaction with the vascular system, and its regulation by the autonomic nervous system.

ANATOMY OF THE HEART

The left ventricle, which is an axisymmetrical, truncated ellipsoid with walls approximately 1 cm thick, is constructed from billions of cardiac muscle cells (myocytes) connected end to end at their *gap junctions* to form a network of branching muscle fibers that wrap around the chamber in a highly organized manner. The right ventricle is a roughly crescent-shaped structure formed by a 3- to 5-mm-thick sheet of myocardial fibers (the *right ventricular free wall*) that interdigitate at the anterior and posterior insertion points with the muscle fibers of the outer layer of the left ventricle. The right and left ventricular chambers share a common wall, the *interventricular septum*, that divides the chambers. Both the right and left atria are thin-walled muscular structures that receive blood from a low-pressure venous system. The *tricuspid valve* in the right heart and the *mitral valve* in the left heart separate each atrium from its associated ventricle, prohibit backward flow during forceful contraction of the ventricles, and are attached to fibrous rings that encircle each valve annulus. The central regions of these valves attach via *chordae tendineae* to *papillary muscles* that emerge from the ventricular walls. The predominant factor that determines valve opening and closure is the pressure gradient that exists between the ventricle and the atrium. However, the papillary muscles contract synchronously with the other heart muscles and aid in maintaining proper valve leaflet position, thus helping to prevent regurgitant flow during contraction. A second set of tissue valves, the *aortic valve* and the *pulmonary valve*, separate each ventricle from its accompanying arterial connection and ensure unidirectional flow by preventing blood from flowing from the artery back into the ventricle. Pressure gradients across these valves are the major determinants of whether they are open or closed.

CARDIAC MUSCLE PHYSIOLOGY

The ability of the ventricles to generate blood flow and pressure derives from the ability of individual myocytes to shorten and generate force. Myocytes are tubular structures. During contraction, the muscles shorten and generate force along their long axis. Force production and shortening of cardiac muscle are created by regulated interactions among contractile proteins, which are assembled in an ordered and repeating structure called the *sarcomere* (Fig. 40–1). The lateral boundaries of each sarcomere are defined on both sides by a band of structural proteins to which the so-called *thin filaments* attach. The *thick filaments* are centered between the Z lines and are held in register by a strand of proteins at the central M line. Alternating light and dark bands, as seen in cardiac muscle under light microscopy, result from the alignment of thick and thin filaments and give cardiac muscle its typical striated appearance.

The thin filaments are composed of linearly arranged globular actin molecules. The thick filaments are composed of bundles of myosin strands, with each strand having a tail, a hinge, and a head region. The tail regions bind to each other in the central portion of the filament, and the strands are aligned along a single axis. The head regions extend out from the center of the thick filament in both directions to create a central bare zone and head-rich zones on both ends of the thick filament. Each actin globule has a binding site for the myosin head. The hinge region allows the myosin head to protrude from the thick filament and make contact with the actin filament. In addition to the actin binding site, the myosin head contains an enzymatic site that cleaves the terminal phosphate molecule of adenosine triphosphate (ATP, myosin ATPase) to provide the energy used for repeatedly generating force. Force is produced when myosin binds to actin and, with the hydrolysis of ATP, the head rotates and extends the hinge region. The force generated by a single sarcomere is proportional to the number of actin-myosin bonds. The state of actin-myosin binding following ATP hydrolysis is referred to as the *rigor state* because in the absence of additional ATP the actin-myosin bond will persist and maintain high muscle tension. Relaxation, which requires uncoupling of the actin-myosin bond, occurs when a new ATP molecule binds to the ATPase site on the myosin head.

Actin-myosin interactions are regulated by troponin and tropomyosin. Tropomyosin is a thin protein strand that sits on the actin strand and, under normal resting conditions, covers the actin-myosin binding site, inhibits the interaction of actin and myosin, and prevents force production. Troponin, which is associated with tropomyosin, has calcium binding sites. When calcium binds to troponin, a conformational change causes the tropomyosin molecule to be pulled away from the actin-myosin binding site; as a result, inhibition of the actin-myosin interaction is eliminated, thus allowing force to be produced. This arrangement of proteins provides a means by which variations in intracellular calcium can readily modify instantaneous force production. The rise and fall of calcium levels during each beat is the basis for the cyclic rise and fall of muscle force. The greater the peak calcium, the greater the number of potential actin-myosin bonds and the greater the amount of force production.

EXCITATION-CONTRACTION COUPLING. The sequence of events that lead to myocardial contraction is triggered by electrical depolarization of the cell; electrical depolarization increases the probability of sarcolemmal calcium channel opening, which in turn results in calcium influx into the cell (Fig. 40–2). A rise in calcium concentration then occurs in the subsarcolemmal space near the *lateral cisternae* of the sarcoplasmic reticulum. This rise in local calcium concentration causes the release of a larger pool of calcium stored in the sarcoplasmic reticulum through calcium release channels called *ryanodine receptors*, which are found in high concentration near the lateral cisternae. The mechanisms by which the subsarcolemmal rise in calcium concentration results in calcium release from the sarcoplasmic reticulum, a process referred to as *calcium-induced calcium release*, are not fully elucidated; the recently discovered tight anatomic coupling between the sarcolemmal calcium channels and ryanodine receptors has suggested that conformational changes of calcium channel proteins can directly influence the properties of the ryanodine receptor. The calcium released from the sarcoplasmic reticulum diffuses through the myofilament lattice and is available for binding to troponin, which disinhibits actin and myosin interactions and results in force production.

Calcium release is rapid and does not require energy because of the large calcium concentration gradient between the sarcoplasmic reticulum and the cytosol during diastole. In contrast, removal of calcium from the cytosol and from troponin occurs up a concentration gradient and is an energy-requiring process. Calcium sequestration is primarily accomplished by pumps on the sarcoplasmic reticulum membrane that consume ATP (sarcoplasmic reticulum Ca^{2+}-ATPase pumps); these pumps are located in the central portions of the sarcoplasmic reticulum and are in close proximity to the myofilaments. Sarcoplasmic reticulum Ca^{2+}-ATPase activity is regulated by the phosphorylation status of another sarcoplasmic reticulum protein, phospholamban. To maintain calcium homeostasis, an amount of calcium equal to what entered the cell through the sarcolemmal calcium channels must also exit with each beat. This equilibrium is accomplished primarily by the sarcolemmal

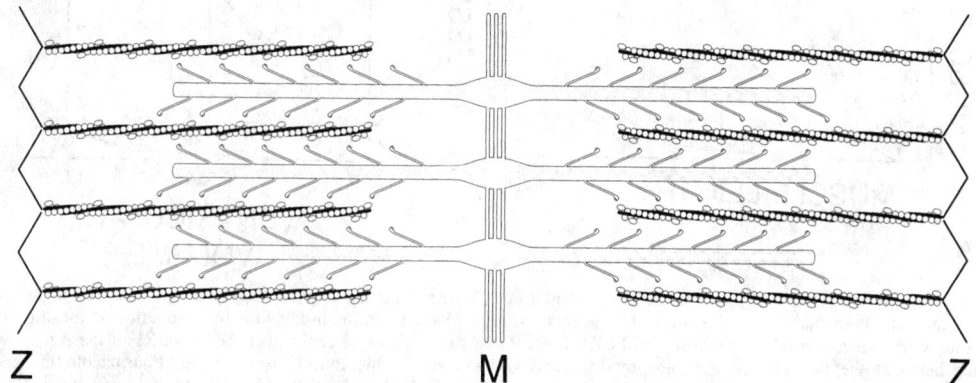

FIGURE 40–1 ■ Basic structure of the sarcomere. Thin filaments composed of actin with the associated regulatory proteins tropomyosin and troponin insert into structural proteins at the Z line, which define the boundaries of the sarcomere. Thick filaments composed of myosin sit between the thin filaments and send their heads out in proximity to the actin molecules. During diastole (state of low intracellular calcium), tropomyosin strands block the interactions between actin and myosin. The thick filaments are kept in register at their centers by structural proteins at the M line. During systole (state of high calcium), calcium binds to troponin, which causes tropomyosin to shift away from the myosin binding site on actin, thus allowing the actin-myosin interactions that underlie force generation.

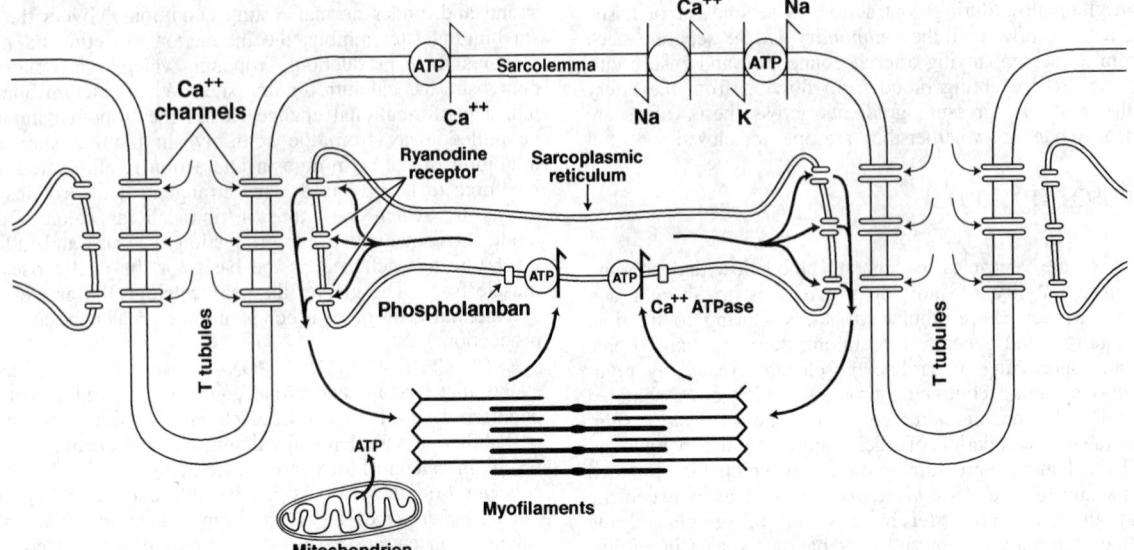

FIGURE 40–2 ■ Important features of the cardiac cell with an emphasis on aspects related to calcium metabolism. Arrows indicate calcium fluxes. The contraction cycle begins with calcium entering the cell via calcium channels and inducing the release of calcium from the lateral cisternae of the sarcoplasmic reticulum. This calcium binds to myofilaments and allows cross-bridge interactions that lead to force generation. A majority of the cytosolic systolic calcium is sequestered at the middle portion of the sarcoplasmic reticulum by the adenosine triphosphate (ATP)-dependent calcium pump; the activity of these pumps is modified by the phosphorylation status of phospholamban. The sodium-calcium exchanger removes an amount of calcium during diastole equal to what entered through calcium channels to maintain calcium homeostasis. The sodium-potassium pump (an ATP-dependent pump) influences intracellular sodium concentrations, which in turn can influence the activity of the sodium-calcium exchanger and thus influence intracellular calcium and contractility.

sodium-calcium exchanger, a transmembrane protein that translocates calcium across the membrane down its concentration gradient in exchange for sodium ions moved in the opposite direction. Sodium homeostasis is in turn regulated largely by the ATP-requiring sodium-potassium pump on the sarcolemma.

FORCE-LENGTH RELATIONS. In addition to calcium, cardiac muscle length exerts a major influence on force production (Fig. 40–3). Because each muscle is composed of a linear array of sarcomere bundles from one end of the muscle to the other, muscle length is directly proportional to the average sarcomere length.

Changes in sarcomere length alter the geometric relationship between thick and thin filaments. For myofilaments in general, optimal force is achieved when sarcomere length is about 2.2 to 2.3 μm, the length that provides optimal overlap of thick and thin filaments. As sarcomere length is decreased below about 2.0 μm, the tips of apposing thin filaments hit each other, the thick filaments approach the Z lines, and the distance between thick and thin filaments increases. Each of these factors contributes to a reduction in force with decreasing sarcomere length. In skeletal muscle, when sarcomeres are stretched beyond 2.3 μm, force de-

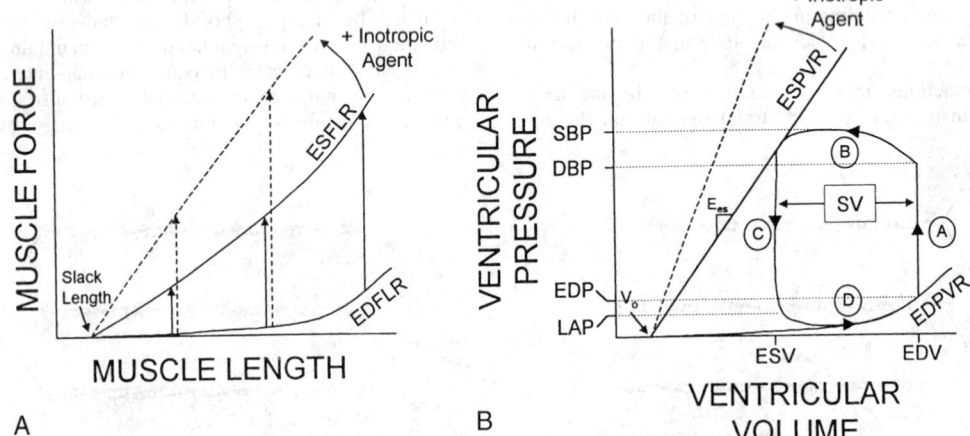

FIGURE 40–3 ■ *A*, Relationship between muscle length and force. When stretched from the slack length (the length at which no force is generated), both diastolic and systolic forces increase and result in the end-diastolic force-length relationship (EDFLR) and the end-systolic force-length relationship (ESFLR). ESFLR rises much more steeply than the EDFLR, so the force developed (difference between the two curves, indicated by the arrows) increases as the muscle is stretched. Pharmacologic agents that increase contractile strength (contractility) have little effect on the EDFLR, but the ESFLR increases and consequently the force developed at any given length increases. *B*, An analogous situation exists for the intact ventricle: Contractile properties are characterized by end-diastolic and end-systolic pressure-volume relations (EDPVR and ESPVR, respectively). The slack length in muscle corresponds with V_0, the volume at which no pressure is generated. The ESPVR is nearly linear and characterized by a slope, E_{es}, that varies in relation to contractility. The pressure-volume loop sits within the boundaries defined by the EDPVR and ESPVR. The four phases of the cardiac cycle are indicated by isovolumic contraction (A), ejection (B), isovolumic relaxation (C), and filling (D). EDV = end-diastolic volume; ESV = end-systolic volume; DBP = diastolic aortic blood pressure; SBP = peak systolic blood pressure; EDP = end-diastolic pressure; LAP = left atrial pressure; SV = stroke volume.

creases because fewer myosin heads can reach and bind with actin; skeletal muscle can typically operate in this so-called *descending limb* of the sarcomere force-length relationship. In cardiac muscle, however, constraints imposed by the sarcolemma prevent myocardial sarcomeres from being stretched beyond 2.3 μm, even under conditions of severe heart failure when very high stretching pressures are imposed on the heart.

Force-length relationships are conveniently used to characterize systolic and diastolic contractile properties of cardiac muscle. These relationships are measured by holding the ends of an isolated muscle strip and measuring the force developed at different muscle lengths while preventing the muscle from shortening (*isometric contractions*). As the muscle is stretched from its slack length (the length at which no force is generated), both the resting (end-diastolic) tension and the peak (end-systolic) tension increase. The end-diastolic force-length relationship is non-linear and exhibits a shallow slope at small lengths and a steeper slope at larger lengths, which is a reflection of the non-linear mechanical restraints imposed by the sarcolemma and extracellular matrix to prevent overstretch of the sarcomeres. End-systolic force increases with increasing muscle length to a much greater degree than does end-diastolic force. The difference in force at end-diastole as compared with end-systole increases as muscle length increases and indicates a greater amount of developed force as the muscle is stretched. This fundamental property of cardiac muscle is called the *Frank-Starling law of the heart* in recognition of its two discoverers. If a drug increases the amount of calcium released to the myofilaments (for example, epinephrine, which belongs to a class of drugs referred to as *inotropic* agents), the end-systolic force-length relationship will be shifted upward and at any given length the muscle can generate more force. Inotropic agents typically do not affect the end-diastolic force-length relationship. In view of the prominent effect of muscle length on force generation, the intrinsic strength of cardiac muscle, commonly referred to as muscle *contractility*, should be indexed by the end-systolic force-length relationship and not simply by peak force generation.

FROM MUSCLE TO CHAMBER. Muscle length and the force generated by muscles in the walls of the ventricles are interrelated with the volume and pressure within the chambers. It is intuitively clear that as ventricular chamber volume varies, so too do muscle and sarcomere lengths. Ventricular pressure is related to the force within the walls and the geometry of the chamber. For the left ventricle, which has a roughly circular cross-section, Laplace's law for thick-walled structures provides an approximation of this relationship: $P \approx 2 \cdot T \cdot h/R$, where P is the pressure within the chamber, T is the tension developed by the muscle (force/unit cross-sectional area), h is the wall thickness, and R is the internal radius of the chamber. From this equation it is clear that chamber pressure depends on both tension and muscle length (because muscle length is related to chamber volume, which is related to chamber radius). Because of the complex structure and geometry of the right ventricle, no simple analytic equation can describe this interrelationship; however, the underlying principle is the same.

Just as end-systolic and end-diastolic force-length relationships can be used to characterize the systolic and diastolic properties of cardiac muscle fibers, so too can end-systolic and end-diastolic *pressure-volume relationships* be used to characterize the peak systolic and end-diastolic properties of the ventricular chambers. Analogous to muscle, the end-diastolic pressure-volume relationship is non-linear, with a shallow incline at low pressures and a steep rise at pressures in excess of 20 mm Hg. However, the end-systolic pressure-volume relationship is typically linear, and as for muscle, ventricular pressure-generating capability is increased as ventricular volume is increased. Also analogous to muscle, the end-systolic pressure-volume relationship is used to index ventricular chamber *contractility*. Because the end-systolic pressure-volume relationship is roughly linear, it can be characterized by a slope and volume axis intercept. The slope of the line, which has units of myocardial stiffness or volume elastance (mm Hg/mL) is called E_{es} (*end-systolic elastance*), and the volume axis intercept (analogous to slack length of the muscle) is referred to as V_0. When muscle *contractility* is increased (for example, by administration of an *inotropic* agent), the slope of the end-systolic pressure-volume relationship (E_{es}) increases, whereas little change occurs in V_0 (discussed further below).

THE CARDIAC CYCLE. The heart beats roughly once every second and repeatedly cycles through a sequence of hemodynamic events that can be divided into four phases. This cycle can be summarized by tracking the time course of change in ventricular pressure and volume along with atrial and aortic pressures in relation to events noted on the electrocardiogram (Fig. 40–4). At end-diastole, ventricular pressure is at its resting level (*end-diastolic pressure*) and ventricular volume is at its maximal value (*end-diastolic volume*). Aortic pressure declines gradually during this period as the blood ejected into the aorta during the prior ventricular contraction discharges to the peripheral circulation. Just before the onset of ventricular systole, atrial contraction provides a final boost to ventricular volume. As ventricular contraction begins about 120 milliseconds later, pressure rises inside the ventricular chamber and exceeds the pressure in the atrium; this pressure differential causes the mitral valve to close. Ventricular pressure is still less than that of the aorta, so the aortic valve remains closed. Because both valves are closed, no blood enters or leaves the ventricle during this time; this first phase is called *isovolumic contraction*. As systole progresses, ventricular pressure eventually exceeds that of the aorta, so the aortic valve opens. As muscular contraction continues, blood is ejected from the ventricle into the aorta, and ventricular volume decreases during the *ejection* phase of the cycle. As contraction of the cardiac muscle reaches its maximal effort (end of systole), ejection ends as ventricular volume reaches its lowest point (*end-systolic volume*). The amount of blood ejected is called the stroke volume (SV) and equals the difference between end-diastolic and end-systolic volume. The *ejection fraction* (EF), defined as the percentage of end-diastolic volume (EDV) ejected during a contraction (EF = 100 · SV/EDV), provides a practical means of indexing heart strength in the clinical setting. As the muscles relax, ventricular pressure falls below that in the aorta, and the aortic valve closes. Muscular relaxation proceeds, and pressure continues to fall. Ventricular volume is constant during this phase of *isovolumic relaxation* because both the mitral and aortic valves are closed. Eventually, ventricular pressure falls below the pressure in the left atrium; the mitral valve opens and blood can flow from the atrium into the ventricle during the *filling* phase.

The four phases of the cardiac cycle are also illustrated by a *pressure-volume diagram* (see Fig. 40–3). The plot of instantaneous ventricular pressure versus volume for one cardiac cycle forms a loop called the *pressure-volume loop*, which sits within the boundaries defined by the end-diastolic and end-systolic pressure-volume relationships. The right ventricle, coupled with the right atrium and the pulmonary artery, undergoes a sequence of events nearly identical to that of the left ventricle except that the magni-

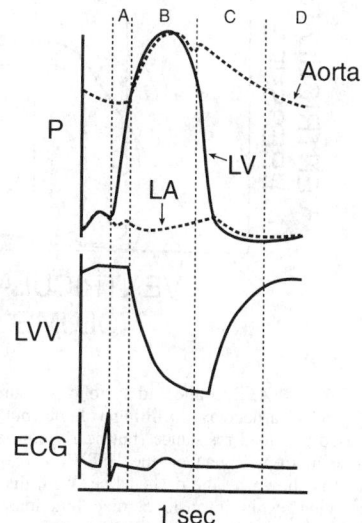

FIGURE 40–4 ■ Time sequence of events during a single cardiac cycle. Pressures (P) in the aorta, left ventricle (LV), and left atrium (LA) are shown. The four phases of the cardiac cycle are also illustrated: isovolumic contraction (A), ejection (B), isovolumic relaxation (C), and filling (D).

Table 40–1 ■ RANGE OF NORMAL RESTING VALUES

Pressure
  Central venous (mean): 0–5 mm Hg
  Right atrial (mean): 0–5 mm Hg
  Right ventricular (systolic/diastolic): 20–30/0–5 mm Hg
  Pulmonary artery (systolic/diastolic): 20–30/8–12 mm Hg
  Left atrial (mean): 8–12 mm Hg
  Left ventricular (systolic/diastolic): 100–150/8–12 mm Hg
  Aortic (systolic/diastolic): 100–150/70–90 mm Hg
Volume-related measures
  Right ventricular end-diastolic volume: 70–100 mL
  Left ventricular end-diastolic volume: 70–100 mL
  Stroke volume: 40–70 mL
  Cardiac index: 2.5–4.0 L/min/m²
  Ejection fraction: 55–70%
Arterial resistance
  Systemic vascular resistance: 10–20 mm Hg·min/L
  Pulmonary vascular resistance: 0.5–1.5 mm Hg·min/L

tudes of the peak pressures are approximately one sixth that of the left ventricle (Table 40–1).

DETERMINANTS OF CARDIAC PERFORMANCE. Two primary measurements of overall cardiovascular performance are arterial blood pressure and cardiac output (mean arterial blood flow) because both adequate blood pressure and adequate cardiac output are necessary to maintain life. In general terms, these aspects of cardiac performance depend on four fundamental factors: *preload, afterload, ventricular contractility,* and *heart rate.*

Preload, which refers to the degree to which sarcomeres are stretched just before the onset of systole, is generally defined for the ventricle as either end-diastolic pressure or end-diastolic volume—two parameters that are interrelated by the nonlinear end-diastolic pressure-volume relationship. As for myocytes, ventricular pressure and flow-generating capacity vary with the *preload* (Frank-Starling law of the heart); a decrease in preload corresponds to a decrease in both end-diastolic volume and pressure, which are associated with decreases in peak pressure and stroke volume (Fig. 40–5). An increase in preload leads to an increase in ventricular pressure and flow generation, but there are limits to how high preload pressures can be increased; left ventricular end-diastolic pressures in excess of about 20 to 25 mm Hg typically cause exudation of fluid into the alveoli, and the resulting pulmonary edema limits blind oxygenation.

Afterload refers to the physical forces that must be overcome for myocytes to shorten and for the ventricle to eject blood. From the point of view of myocardium, peak arterial pressure provides a measure of the peak stress experienced by myocytes because stress is related to pressure according to Laplace's law. In the absence of left ventricular outflow obstruction, arterial pressure is an appropriate index for quantifying myocyte afterload in vivo. Another parameter to characterize the ventricular afterloading properties of the arterial system is *total peripheral resistance,* which predominantly relates to the vasomotor tone of the resistance vessels. Total peripheral resistance (TPR) is calculated as the ratio between the mean pressure drop across the arterial system (mean arterial pressure [MAP] minus mean venous pressure [VP]) and cardiac output (CO): TPR = (MAP − VP)/CO. When compared with the baseline pressure-volume loop, the loop obtained with increased total peripheral resistance (but a similar preload volume) exhibits a higher peak pressure and a decrease in stroke volume and ejection fraction (see Fig. 40–5).

Contractility refers to the intrinsic strength of the cardiac muscle (*myocardial contractility*) or the ventricle (*ventricular contractility*), independent of external conditions imposed by either preload or afterload. Inotropic agents such as epinephrine change muscle contractility and therefore induce shifts of the end-systolic pressure-volume relationship and changes in cardiac performance. When compared with the baseline pressure-volume loop, the loop obtained at increased contractility exhibits a greater pressure, stroke volume, and ejection fraction despite a constant preload volume and arterial resistance. Although the end-systolic pressure-volume relationship fundamentally provides a load-independent index of ventricular contractility, it is difficult to measure in patients and is usually limited to the research setting. Although ejection fraction is influenced by afterload resistance as well as by changes in contractility, the ejection fraction can help assess response to therapy and is a strong correlate of survival in cardiac disease. Thus despite theoretic limitations, the ejection fraction provides a simple and useful clinical indicator of overall left ventricular contractile strength.

The importance of *heart rate* in determining cardiac performance is readily appreciated by noting that cardiac output measured in liters per minute is equal to the amount of blood ejected at each heart beat (stroke volume in liters per beat) multiplied by the number of beats per minute. Because blood pressure is related to cardiac output and total peripheral resistance, heart rate variations also provide a means of influencing mean arterial pressure. Thus the ability to vary the heart rate provides an effective means of influencing cardiovascular performance.

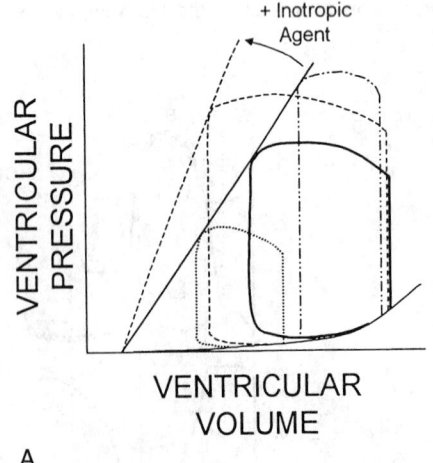

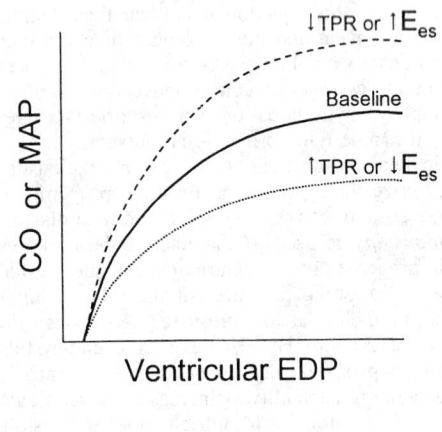

A   B

FIGURE 40–5 ■ *A,* Baseline end-systolic pressure-volume relationship (ESPVR) and pressure-volume loop shown by the solid lines. The effect of a decrease in filling volume (but constant vascular resistance) on the loop is shown by the dotted line. The effect of increased afterload resistance (but nearly constant preload volume) on the loop is shown by the dotted-dashed line. The effect of a positive inotropic agent on the ESPVR and on the pressure-volume loop with constant afterload resistance and nearly constant preload is shown by the dashed line. With the exception of the inotropic agent, the changes in pressure and stroke volume do not reflect changes in intrinsic cardiac function. *B,* The interdependence between indices of ventricular pump performance (e.g., cardiac output [CO] and mean arterial pressure [MAP]) are summarized by Frank-Starling curves that plot these indices as a function of filling pressure and vary with changes in heart contractile strength (E$_{es}$) and with total systemic peripheral resistance (TPR). The nature of this interdependence is summarized according to modern theories of ventricular vascular coupling according to the following equations: CO ≈ HR·[EDV − V$_0$]/[1 + TPR/(T·E$_{es}$)], and MAP ≈ [EDV − V$_0$]/[T/TPR + 1/E$_{es}$], where T is the duration of the cardiac cycle (i.e., T = 60/HR) HR is heart rate, and EDV is end-diastolic volume.

Cardiac output and mean arterial pressure can be related to the measures of preload, afterload, contractility, and heart rate (see Fig. 40–5B) by Frank-Starling curves. These curves plot end-diastolic pressure versus either cardiac output or mean arterial pressure to provide an overall characterization of left ventricular pump function in practical terms and to demonstrate the dependence of pump function on afterload resistance and contractility.

DETERMINATION OF MYOCARDIAL OXYGEN CONSUMPTION AND ENERGY METABOLISM. The heart relies almost exclusively on oxidation of fatty acids and glucose as an immediate source of energy. The heart normally extracts free fatty acids preferentially from the coronary perfusion for oxidative energy production. Under conditions of limited oxygen supply, this preference is changed to glucose. Greater energy is consumed in metabolizing free fatty acids than in metabolizing glucose. Under most conditions, anaerobic metabolism provides very limited energy. Severe hypoxia with high coronary flow produces lactate and anaerobic ATP. The much more common condition of ischemia with acidosis results in little anaerobic energy. Under most steady-state circumstances, the heart is dependent on the availability of molecular oxygen to continue its function.

The oxygen and energy consumption of the heart is determined principally through its contractile activity. Three major independent hemodynamic or mechanical factors contribute to myocardial oxygen consumption by the heart: heart rate, the tension developed by the heart during contraction or systole, and the contractile state or contractility of the heart. Only 10% or less of the total oxygen consumption of the heart is used to maintain functions other than contraction; if the heart ceases to beat but is kept alive, it will consume approximately 10% of the normal amount of oxygen. A very modest reserve exists for "storing" oxygen, oxidative capacity, or anaerobic substrate. Thus, without the availability of oxygen (e.g., hypoxia, ischemia, carbon monoxide poisoning), heart function deteriorates remarkably rapidly, essentially on a beat-to-beat basis.

Because oxygen consumption is determined principally by the contractile activity of cardiac muscle, a more rapid heart rate requires greater oxygen consumption. If the heart rate rises from 60 to 180 beats per minute during exercise or stress, oxygen consumption will increase three-fold over the basal value.

Myocardial oxygen consumption is also related to contractile tension and the contractile state as indexed by the total *pressure-volume area* (Fig. 40–6). Oxygen consumption is linearly correlated with the total pressure-volume area, so if the heart were to contract under isovolumic conditions because of infinitely high afterload resistance to ejection, all the energy produced by the heart would be internal, potential energy because no external work would be performed despite the oxygen consumed. As tension decreases to within the physiologic afterload range, external stroke work is performed and potential energy is also produced; oxygen consumption is proportional to the total of the two.

A simpler index of myocardial oxygen consumption for an intact heart is the *rate-pressure product*. With this index, the heart rate is multiplied by the peak systolic pressure and used as an index of oxygen demand or consumption. Although this index ignores the contribution of the contractile state, the rate-pressure product provides a reasonable index of oxygen consumption when the contractile state is unchanged or relatively stable.

With an increase in the contractile state, an additional obligatory increase in oxygen consumption is produced above what is related to heart rate and tension. Evidence suggests that the increased oxygen consumption with an increase in the contractile state is due to the increased sarcoplasmic reticular ATPase activity required to sequester the increased amount of cycling calcium that underlies the increase in contractility.

CORONARY BLOOD FLOW: METABOLIC AND NEUROHORMONAL REGULATION. The volume of coronary or myocardial blood flow under normal conditions is largely regulated by myocardial oxygen demands. Because the heart extracts 90% or more of the oxygen needed from the coronary blood, the striking increases in oxygen consumption that occur with high tension development, higher heart rates, and/or high contractility are met almost entirely by increases in coronary blood flow. High myocardial oxygen consumption and high coronary flow are characteristic of exercise.

The predominant mechanisms involved in this augmentation of coronary blood flow from normal values of 60 to 100 mL/100 g/

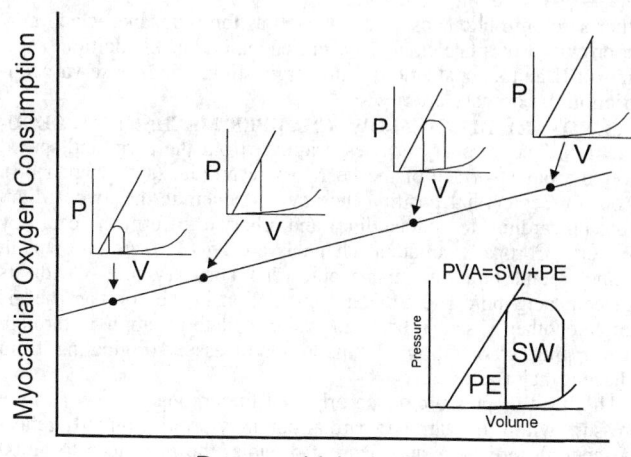

Pressure-Volume Area

FIGURE 40–6 ■ The total pressure-volume area (PVA), which equals the sum of the stroke work (SW, area contained within the pressure-volume loop, PVL) and the potential energy (PE, area contained between the end-systolic and end-diastolic pressure-volume relationships and the isovolumic relaxation portion of the PVL), is linearly related to oxygen consumption. The insets show various PVLs and their corresponding PVA–oxygen consumption point on the curves. An ejecting beat at low filling volume (left) has a lower oxygen consumption than an isovolumic beat at the same filling volume (second from the left). For isovolumic contractions, there is no external SW; all generated energy is PE. When filling is increased, the PVA increases for both ejecting and isovolumic contractions in proportion to the increase in PVA. The non-zero y-axis intercept indicates the substantial energy requirements for basal metabolism and for calcium cycling, which are not directly related to energy for force generation. At increased contractility, the PVA–oxygen consumption curve shifts upward in a parallel manner, which is related largely to the fuel required for cycling the increased amount of calcium present at the increased contractility.

minute to values that are six-fold higher are metabolic factors, especially adenosine released from mildly ischemic myocardial and other cells. Adenosine is the byproduct of the breakdown of ATP to adenosine monophosphate and then to adenosine. A second control of the magnitude of coronary blood flow under increased workload or demand conditions is nitric oxide, which is produced by coronary vascular endothelial cells and has a direct local vasodilating effect on coronary arteries and the more distal bed. Nitric oxide is a byproduct in a number of reactions that lead to an increase in the activity of nitric oxide synthase, an enzyme that produces nitric oxide from the amino acid L-arginine. In addition to adenosine and nitric oxide, other longer-acting coronary vasodilators such as bradykinin, prostaglandins, and CO_2 may have a direct effect in maintaining coronary artery blood flow.

Coronary artery mechanical changes also contribute to regulation of coronary flow. As coronary arteries are stretched by higher luminal pressure, they constrict; as pressure within the coronary artery is reduced, the artery dilates. These very potent changes, which help maintain coronary blood flow under circumstances of altered coronary flow hemodynamics but maintained oxygen demands, are termed autoregulatory mechanisms for coronary blood flow.

In addition to the metabolic and other factors that lead to coronary vasodilatation, a series of factors can lead to coronary arterial vasoconstriction. The exact roles of these vasoconstricting factors in health and disease are unclear, but in disease these factors may have a profoundly important effect. A local regulating factor is the endothelin system, which consists of peptides synthesized and controlled locally within small arteries or arterioles that have a profound vasoconstricting effect on the resistance arteries within the coronary circulation. Constricting endothelins may be produced at the site of coronary artery atherosclerotic lesions and lead to vasoconstriction at those sites. In addition, at sites of coronary artery atherosclerosis where the endothelium is disrupted or abnormal, circulating vasoconstrictor substances gain access to smooth muscle receptors that are ordinarily covered by coronary arterial endothelium. These substances include circulating serotonin, 5-hydroxytryptamine, and other serotonin-like substances, as well as thromboxane, which may be produced by platelets or adjacent endothelium. In addition, angiotensin II and sympathetic α_1-adrenergic stimulation cause vasoconstriction in coronary arteries.

CORONARY BLOOD FLOW: CHAMBER MECHANICAL REGULATION. The coronary arteries originate from the aorta and spread over the outer surface of the heart or epicardium (see Chapter 46). From this epicardial position the arteries penetrate the myocardium from epicardium to endocardium and arborize to form the capillary network. Coronary collateral channels are 25 to 50 or 100 μm in diameter and link one major epicardial coronary artery with its adjacent neighbor. The collateral circulation in the coronary bed is not like other vascular beds, in which collateralization is through overlapping arborization of small blood vessels originating from adjacent major arteries.

The head of pressure at the origin of the coronary artery and the pressure within the large epicardial coronary arteries directly reflect the central aortic pressure. During diastole, the resistance to blood flow from the coronary arteries is largely from the tone of resistance vessels. During systole, coronary perfusion pressure (which equals aortic pressure) is determined by the left ventricular intracavitary pressure. In turn, cavitary pressure equals the pressure within the inner myocardial wall. It is not surprising, then, that the endocardial coronary arteries are remarkably compressed during systole. The systolic pressure within the thick left ventricular wall toward the epicardial surface is not nearly as high as the endocardial portion of the wall. Therefore, coronary blood flow occurs both during systole and diastole toward the epicardium but is essentially exclusively limited to diastole in the subendocardium.

In addition, if left ventricular workload is increased or myocardial contractility or function is decreased, left ventricular diastolic pressure will increase. This increase in diastolic pressure will act as a compressor force on the subendocardial vessels and limit myocardial blood flow during this critical period of diastole. Finally, the influence of heart rate on coronary blood flow, particularly to the subendocardium, is important and dramatic. As the heart rate increases, the period of diastole between beats becomes shorter and shorter. This limitation of coronary flow to the subendocardium during tachycardia can have profound effects in the setting of coronary artery disease and heart failure such that drugs that block tachycardia during exercise may be very useful therapeutically.

NEUROHORMONAL REGULATION OF THE CARDIOVASCULAR SYSTEM. The major components of the neurohormonal systems that regulate cardiovascular function are the sympathetic and parasympathetic components of the autonomic nervous system and the renin-angiotensin system. The major attributes of the sympathetic nervous system in responding rapidly to stress are the ability to increase the heart rate, increase myocardial contractility, and regulate vascular tone in the various organs. Most of these functions are performed by the sympathetic nervous system through release of norepinephrine at the nerve endings throughout the circulation. Under more profound stress, the sympathetic nervous system elaborates epinephrine from the adrenal gland. Norepinephrine and epinephrine act through the α-adrenergic vasoconstricting mechanisms in the periphery, but both increase contractility by stimulating α- and β-adrenergic receptors in the heart. Epinephrine has a more striking β-adrenergic effect than norepinephrine does, especially at low circulating levels. Through these β-adrenergic actions, epinephrine profoundly increases the heart rate and, at the same time, induces vasodilatation of the central arterial bed, thereby reducing impedance to left ventricular ejection. The coronary circulation operates in a mixed fashion, with evidence of coronary artery vasoconstriction occurring in response to α-adrenergic stimulation and vasodilation in response to lower doses of epinephrine.

The most important parasympathetic innervation is that of the sinoatrial and atrioventricular nodes, where these nerves slow the firing rate of pacemaker tissue and slow conduction in the atrioventricular node. The neurotransmitter for the parasympathetic nervous system is acetylcholine. Ventricular muscle is poorly innervated by the parasympathetic nervous system and vagal tone has very little effect on contractility under normal resting conditions; however, increased vagal tone will depress myocardial contractility when sympathetic tone is high. At rest, the heart rate is under control of the parasympathetic nervous system rather than the sympathetic

system. Thus β-adrenergic blocking drugs have little effect on the heart rate at rest and markedly reduce augmentation of the heart rate, particularly at high levels of exercise.

The sympathetic nervous system also has a profound vasoconstrictive effect on the venous system, particularly the capacitance bed within the splanchnic or abdominal circulation. Thus in forms of stress with rapid loss of blood or fluids, the venous constriction effects of sympathetic stimulation can be life saving.

The renin-angiotensin system is a second coordinated system that regulates blood pressure, peripheral vasoconstriction, and contractility in a fashion complementary to the sympathetic nervous system. Generally, action of the renin-angiotensin system is not nearly as immediate or profound as that of the sympathetic nervous system, but it operates principally as an intermediate- and long-term regulator. Under pathologic conditions such as heart failure, the system can remain chronically activated. Renin is a hormone released by macula densa cells within the juxtaglomerular apparatus of the kidney under conditions of decreased perfusion to the kidney, decreased delivery of sodium to the macula densa, or increasing sympathetic activity. Once renin is released, it acts exclusively through production of angiotensin II, a very potent peripheral vasoconstrictor and coronary arterial constrictor, within the circulation and at individual organ sites. Angiotensin II induces release of the sodium-retaining hormone aldosterone from the adrenal gland. All these actions tend to retain sodium in the circulation and increase arterial blood pressure. Angiotensin, which is also a very potent stimulus to both myocardial and peripheral vessel hypertrophy, promotes the release of norepinephrine from peripheral sympathetic nervous system sites.

CARDIOVASCULAR RESPONSE TO EXERCISE. High levels of exercise require truly remarkable augmentation of heart function and performance, as well as adaptation of the peripheral circulation. Enhanced blood flow is needed to the exercising muscles and restriction of blood flow away from those parts of the body that are not essential during the period of exercise. Blood flow is also augmented to the skin and oral mucosa for dissipation of the heat produced by exercising muscles.

Oxygen consumption for the entire body during strenuous exercise increases approximately 18-fold. Two thirds of this increase in oxygen consumption results from greater cardiac output and the remaining third from an increase in oxygen extraction from arterial blood. Arterial oxygen saturation usually remains near 100%, whereas venous oxygen saturation decreases from approximately 75% to 25%. This increase in oxygen extraction is mostly related to the increase in blood flow to the exercising muscle, which essentially extracts most of the oxygen within the blood. The increase in blood flow to the exercising muscle occurs as a result of an increase in arterial pressure and perfusion of the exercising limbs and profound vasodilation of the arteries of the exercising muscle. Arterial dilation is a consequence of the release of potassium and other vasodilating substances from the exercising muscle. Whereas overall cardiac output may increase 6-fold, blood flow to the exercising muscle may increase 40- or 50-fold from rest to exercise.

This increase in blood flow to the exercising muscle and the increase in skin blood flow increase venous return to the heart. The heart accommodates this increase in venous return by augmenting cardiac function remarkably. The major element in this increase in cardiac function in normal young individuals is an augmentation in sympathetic drive to the heart and a withdrawal of vagal tone. The heart rate is increased, contractility is increased (resulting in increased ventricular ejection and an increase in the ventricular ejection fraction), ejection and filling rates are increased, aortic impedance is decreased, and systolic blood pressure is increased.

In a young individual, withdrawal of vagal tone and greater sympathetic drive during maximal exercise increase the heart rate from 60 to 70 beats per minute at rest to 170 to 200 beats per minute. At this rapid heart rate, not only must ejection of blood be more rapid, but it is also essential to use mechanisms to augment the rate of filling the heart. These increases in contractility with associated increases in the velocity of ejection and filling occur as a result of augmented sympathetic drive to the heart, which increases the amount of calcium cycling within the cell and also increases the rate of sarcoplasmic reticulum ATPase activity to hasten calcium sequestration.

Another sympathetic adaptation during exercise is arterial vasodilation of the aorta and central arteries. This β-sympathetic central arterial vasodilation decreases the impedance to left ventricular ejection, but the augmentation in cardiac output is so great that even though impedance is lowered, systolic arterial blood pressure rises. The final mechanism available to the heart to augment cardiac function beyond that created by the withdrawal of vagal tone and the increase in sympathetic tone is an enhancement of preload (the Frank-Starling mechanism). A young individual at maximum exercise uses this mechanism very little, but when the sympathetic nervous system is blocked or when the sympathetic response is limited by aging or chronic heart failure, then preload recruitment operates as a reserve mechanism to augment cardiac output during exercise. With increased preload, the left ventricle (and presumably the right ventricle) dilate acutely to a larger diastolic volume. This increase in diastolic volume results in stretching of myocardial fibers and augmentation of pump function.

PHYSIOLOGIC PRINCIPLES UNDERLYING HEART FAILURE. Heart failure is an inability of the heart to provide sufficient blood flow to meet the metabolic demands of the body (see Chapter 47). Heart failure can occur by three primary physiologic mechanisms: increased work, decreased function of the heart, and altered filling of the heart. For many types of chronic increase in workload, the heart adapts very significantly by increasing its size or volume and by increasing its muscle mass through hypertrophy. The ventricles dilate in response to volume overload from endurance exercise or aortic and mitral regurgitation, anemia, and hyperthyroidism. With long-term pressure overload such as in hypertension or aortic or pulmonary valve obstruction, pressure overload hypertrophy occurs. The ventricle can generate greater pressure at the same volumes. This same type of hypertrophy also occurs in athletes who perform exercises that increase blood pressure but do not increase volume, such as weight lifting.

AGE CHANGES IN THE CARDIOVASCULAR SYSTEM. In the cardiovascular system, intrinsic cardiac muscle function, the inotropic response to non-sympathetic mediators, and coronary perfusion are well maintained with age. With age, however, cellular hypertrophy occurs because of both cell dropout and increased stiffening of the vascular tree; the result is increased afterload on the left ventricle. As a result of the hypertrophy, systole is prolonged.

Large arteries stiffen with age. Thus even without hypertension, an age-related increase in impedance to ejection, a greater systolic load, and an increased pulse wave velocity occur. In addition, the *chronotropic* (i.e., heart rate response) and inotropic response to sympathetic mediation is diminished, so states that put sudden loads on the left ventricle, such as acute hypertension or myocardial infarction, have more severe consequences in the elderly. Also, disease and stress may produce less compensatory hypertrophy in the elderly and therefore place more stress on the left ventricle with age.

With exercise or other forms of stress, the effects of a decreased β-sympathetic response in the elderly are dominant. Older individuals have less of an increase in heart rate and contractility and a larger increase in impedance. Fortunately, the intrinsic cardiac muscle reserve is adequate to compensate for these limitations in exercise response if no cardiac disease is present. In the presence of disease, however, cardiac reserve is diminished. Therefore, older individuals or victims of acute myocardial infarction or heart failure have much greater difficulty during exercise because the heart rate rises less, load or impedance is greater, and preload recruitment may already be near the maximally tolerated level.

Katz AM: Physiology of the Heart, 2nd ed. New York, Raven Press, 1992. *Comprehensive text of the current understanding of cellular and biochemical cardiac control.*

Lakatta EG, Gerstenblith G, Weisfeldt ML: The aging heart: Structure, function and disease. *In* Braunwald E (ed): Heart Disease, 5th ed. Philadelphia, WB Saunders, 1997, p 1687. *Review of aging of the circulatory system.*

Sagawa K, Maughan L, Suga H, Sunagawa K: Cardiac Contraction and the Pressure-Volume Relationship. New York, Oxford University Press, 1988. *Comprehensive text of the current basis of understanding of pump function of the heart.*

■ SPECIALIZED DIAGNOSTIC PROCEDURES

41 RADIOLOGY OF THE HEART

Murray G. Baron

The heart casts a homogeneous shadow on the chest film. No internal detail can be seen within its contours because the radiodensities of blood, myocardium, and other cardiac tissues are so similar that one cannot be distinguished from the others. Only two borders of the heart, where it contacts the radiolucent, air-containing lung, can be discerned in any one projection. Changes in the size and/or shape of the chambers of the heart and the great vessels usually alter the shape of the cardiac silhouette. However, because the heart is a three-dimensional structure and all of the cardiac chambers are not border forming in any projection, multiple views are required for complete evaluation. With the advent of echocardiography, the need for this "cardiac series" has disappeared. However, a remarkable amount of information regarding the heart is presented on standard frontal and lateral films of the chest. Because these films are a part of most routine medical examinations, they are a useful tool for detecting disease, as well as evaluating the severity of known disease, documenting the progress of the disease, and assessing the efficacy of treatment.

RADIOLOGIC ANATOMY

On a frontal chest film, the right cardiac border has two components: a straight vertical upper half formed by the superior vena cava and a gently convex lower half representing the lateral wall of the right atrium (Fig. 41–1). The break in the contour of this border of the heart indicates the caval-atrial junction. Some patients are able to lower their diaphragms sufficiently during inspiration to uncover a small, straight segment of the inferior vena cava between the diaphragm and the right atrium.

The left cardiac border is composed of four distinct segments. The uppermost bulge represents the aortic knob, the most distal portion of the aortic arch where it turns downward to become the descending aorta. The prominence below the knob is formed by the main pulmonary artery and the subvalvular portion of the outflow tract of the right ventricle. The lowermost third of this border represents the anterolateral wall of the left ventricle. Between this bulge and that of the pulmonary artery is a short, flat, or slightly concave segment where the left atrial appendage reaches the border of the heart.

In the lateral view (see Fig. 41–1C), the anterior border of the cardiac silhouette is formed by the body and the outflow tract of the right ventricle. The heart lies in the anterior portion of the chest, and the right ventricle abuts the lower third of the sternum. Both the outflow tract and pulmonary artery slope posteriorly. Air-containing lung interposed between this portion of the heart and the anterior chest wall forms the "retrosternal clear space." The posterior border of the heart extends from the carina to the diaphragm. Its upper half is formed by the back of the left atrium, whereas the lower half represents the posterior wall of the left ventricle. The shadow of the inferior vena cava is usually seen in the lateral projection to extend obliquely upward and anteriorly from the diaphragm to enter the posterior aspect of the right atrium. The lowermost posterior contour of the left ventricle curves anteriorly and

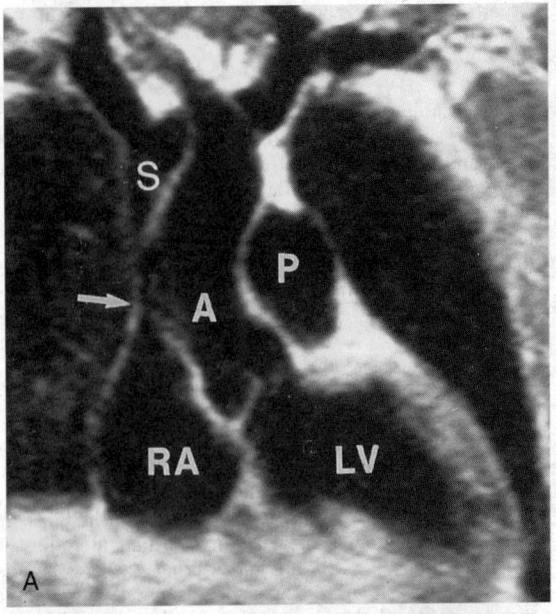

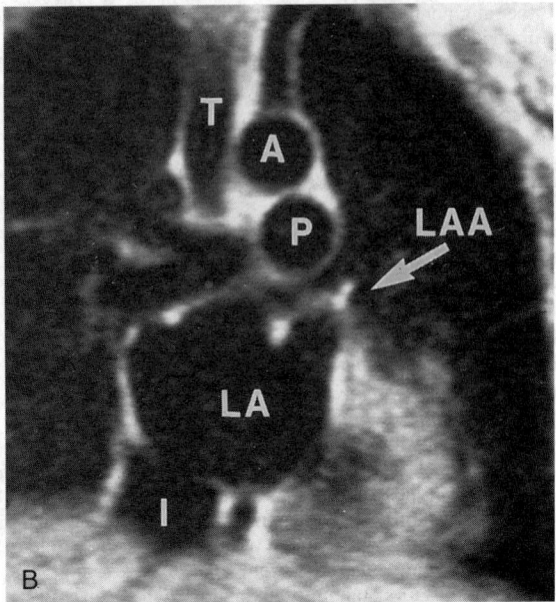

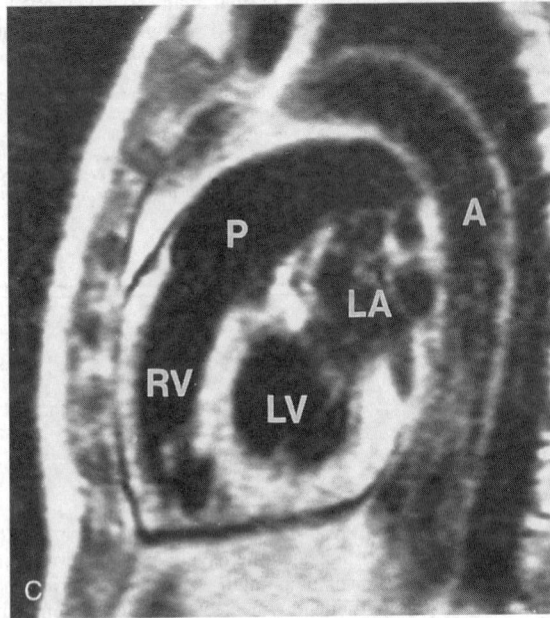

FIGURE 41–1 ■ Normal radiographic anatomy, magnetic resonance images. *A,* Coronal section at the level of the aortic valve. The right border of the cardiac silhouette is formed by the superior vena cava (S) and the right atrium (RA). The arrow indicates the caval-atrial junction. The lower portion of the left cardiac border is formed by the left ventricle (LV). A = ascending aorta; *P* = main pulmonary artery. *B,* Coronal section at the level of the left atrium. The upper portion of the left cardiac border is formed by the aorta (A), main pulmonary artery (P), and left atrial appendage (LAA). LA = left atrium; I = inferior vena cava; T = trachea. *C,* Sagittal section near the midline. The right ventricle (RV) forms the anterior surface of the heart, which abuts the sternum. The pulmonary artery (P) extends upward and posteriorly from the ventricle. The posterior border of the heart is formed by the left atrium (LA) and left ventricle (LV).

crosses the inferior vena cava about 2 cm above the left side of the diaphragm.

Alterations in the contour of the heart usually reflect dilation and/or hypertrophy of the chambers. Many times the pattern of these changes, together with the appearance of the pulmonary vasculature, points to a specific underlying cardiac abnormality. Chest films are most sensitive for detecting chamber dilation. Cardiac hypertrophy is more difficult to recognize inasmuch as the thickened myocardium tends to encroach on the ventricular lumen more than extending outward and enlarging the cardiac silhouette. With severe hypertrophy, as in hypertrophic cardiomyopathy, the heart enlarges to the left and the apex becomes blunted and rounder than usual. This appearance is not pathognomonic.

HEART SIZE

A normal-sized heart does not guarantee the absence of cardiac disease. Angina, for example, no matter how severe, does not

affect heart size until the left ventricle decompensates. Similarly, patients with restrictive cardiomyopathy may be in severe congestive failure with a normal-appearing heart. On the other hand, an enlarged heart always indicates the presence of cardiac or pericardial disease. Therefore, accurate evaluation of heart size is important.

The cardiothoracic ratio is measured by dropping a vertical line through the heart and measuring the greatest distance to the right and left cardiac borders (Fig. 41–2). The sum of the two is the transverse cardiac diameter. The transverse thoracic diameter is the greatest width of the chest, measured from the inner surfaces of the ribs. Dividing the cardiac diameter by the chest diameter gives the cardiothoracic ratio. A value of less than 0.6 can be considered within the limits of normal. Setting this value at 0.5, as is often done, produces too many false-positive results.

In most cases, exact measurement of the cardiac silhouette is not necessary, and a reasonably experienced observer can achieve an acceptable degree of accuracy by visual estimation. The single greatest effect on apparent cardiac size is the degree of inspiration. The volume of the heart is essentially constant throughout the

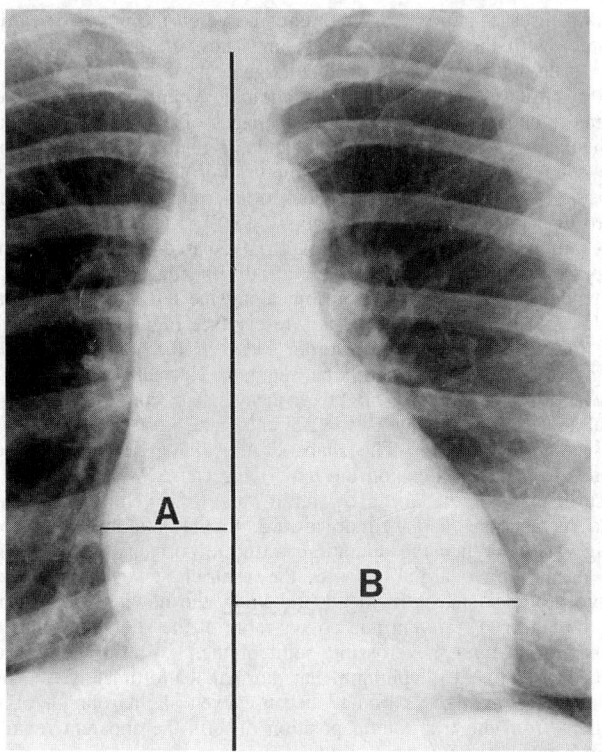

FIGURE 41–2 ■ Measurement of the transverse cardiac diameter. Severe aortic stenosis with a 95-mm systolic gradient across the valve is present. The heart, although considerably hypertrophied, is normal in size and configuration. A vertical line is drawn through the heart. The greatest distances to the right cardiac border (A) and to the left cardiac border (B) are then measured. Transverse cardiac diameter = A + B.

cardiac cycle. With expiration, as the diaphragm moves up, the vertical diameter of the heart is shortened and its transverse diameter increases. Because heart size is estimated primarily from its width, the heart appears larger on expiratory films. The degree of

inspiration can be determined from the relationship of the diaphragm to the ribs. On a properly positioned frontal chest film, a reasonable degree of inspiration is indicated if the diaphragm is lowered to at least the level of the posterior portion of the 9th rib.

When the anteroposterior diameter of the chest is small, the heart may be compressed between the sternum and the spine so that it splays to one or both sides. For this reason, the heart often appears enlarged in patients with the straight back syndrome or with a pectus excavatum deformity of the sternum. An epicardial fat pad (actually it is truly extrapleural fat outside the pericardium) can occur in one or both cardiophrenic angles and makes the heart appear larger than it actually is. The cardiophrenic angle often appears obtuse or the cardiac apex is indistinct. In addition, the slightly more radiolucent image of the fat can usually be distinguished from the greater density of the heart.

A change in size of the cardiac silhouette can also occur between systole and diastole. This point is important because chest films are exposed at random with reference to the cardiac cycle, and the apparent size of the heart may be different on two films of the same patient made at different times. In the majority of cases, the difference in the transverse cardiac diameter between systole and diastole is small, no more than several millimeters. However, in younger patients, especially the more athletic with a slow heart rate and a large stroke volume, phasic change in the normal cardiac diameter can be as much as 2 cm.

CHAMBER ENLARGEMENT

LEFT ATRIUM. Dilation of the left atrium alone, in the absence of a left-to-right shunt, is most often due to disease of the mitral valve, although it can also result simply from atrial fibrillation. The two "popular" radiologic signs of left atrial enlargement—a double contour within the right cardiac border and elevation of the left main bronchus—are both accurate when present, but are insensitive. They are not seen in about half the cases of mitral valve disease. To produce a discernible margin within the cardiac silhouette in the frontal projection, the thickness of the heart must increase sharply at some point. This increase in thickness occurs in mitral disease when the left atrium enlarges and protrudes posteri-

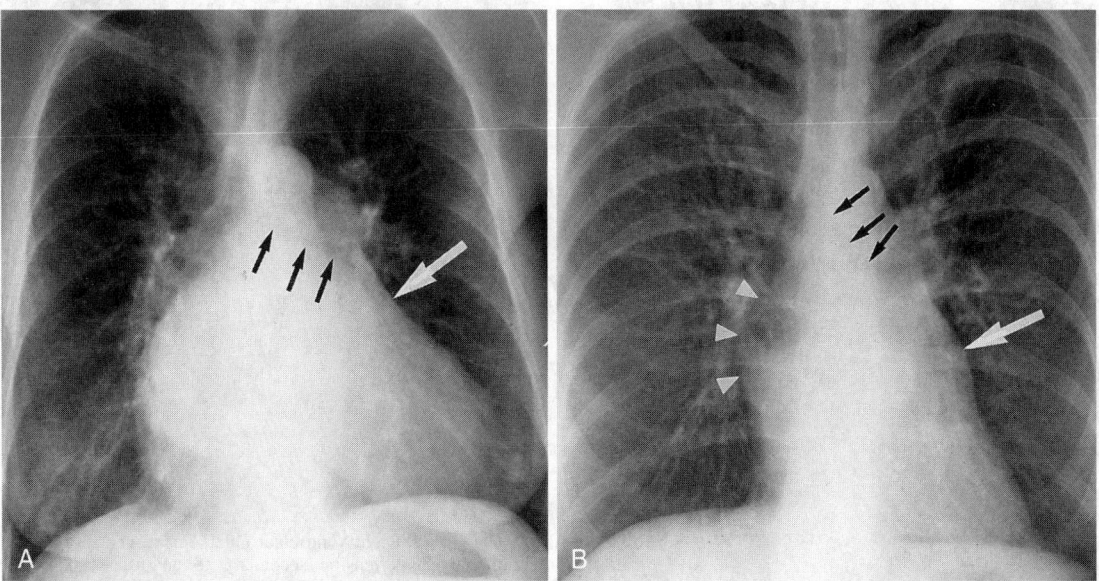

FIGURE 41–3 ■ Left atrial enlargement in mitral valve disease. *A,* Patient 1: The enlarged left atrium causes the central portion of the cardiac silhouette to be abnormally dense. The right border of the atrium is seen within the right side of the cardiac silhouette. The left main bronchus *(small arrows)* is elevated. The region of the left atrial appendage *(white arrow)* is slightly concave because this structure was resected at a previous mitral commissurotomy. *B,* Patient 2: The enlarged left atrial appendage bulges from the left side of the heart *(white arrow),* whereas the body of the atrium *(arrowheads)* extends beyond the right atrium to form a part of the right heart border. No double density is seen within the heart, and the left main bronchus *(small arrows)* is not elevated.

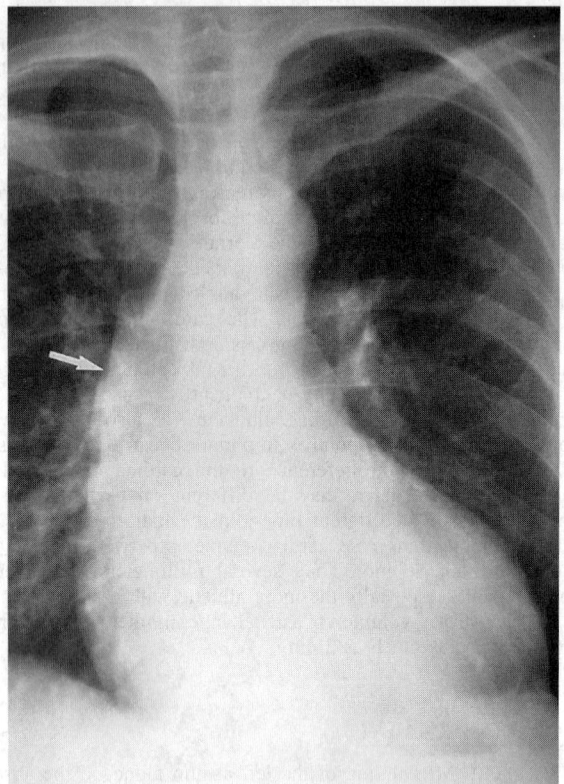

FIGURE 41–4 ▪ Left ventricular dilatation, aortic insufficiency. The apex of the heart is displaced downward and to the left. The ascending aorta *(arrow)* is diffusely dilated. The pulmonary vasculature is normal.

mitral disease, it forms a continuous curve on the posterior cardiac border with the enlarged left atrium. Thus, the double contour is not seen with mild left atrial enlargement or in severe cases of mitral disease. Furthermore, the radiologic technique used for chest films is chosen to provide optimal images of the lungs. The heart, when enlarged, is underexposed, and the double contour may not be seen within its opaque silhouette. For the same reason, the position of the left main bronchus often cannot be clearly visualized through the mediastinal shadow.

A more sensitive sign of left atrial enlargement in the frontal projection is dilation of the left atrial appendage. The appendage extends anteriorly from the atrium along the left side of the heart, below the level of the pulmonary artery (see Fig. 41–1B). It forms the part of the left heart border between the pulmonary artery segment and the left ventricular segment. Normally, the border of the appendage is flat or slightly concave. Any convexity is abnormal and usually indicates left atrial enlargement.

LEFT VENTRICLE. The shape of the dilated left ventricle depends to a large extent on the underlying cause. When it is due to insufficiency of the aortic or mitral valve, the ventricle elongates and its apex is displaced downward, to the left, and posteriorly (Fig. 41–4). When the dilatation is due to coronary artery disease or primary myocardial disease, the ventricle tends to assume a more globular shape. In the lateral view, the downward extension of the enlarged left ventricle covers more of the vena caval shadow than normal, and the crossing point of their posterior borders occurs nearer to the diaphragm than normal. Unfortunately, the usefulness of this sign is limited because even slight rotation of the patient from the true lateral position distorts the apparent relationship between the two structures.

Enlargement of the left ventricle produces a smoothly curved dilatation of the lower portion of the cardiac silhouette. A localized bulge in this contour most often represents a ventricular aneurysm (Fig. 41–5). Dilatation of the left ventricle is usually associated with elevation of left ventricular end-diastolic pressure. The latter increases the resistance to left atrial emptying and can result in dilation of the atrium. Therefore, left atrial enlargement in the

orly from the back of the heart. The right border of the left atrium is then silhouetted where it abuts the right lung and its contour is seen within the cardiac silhouette (Fig. 41–3A). This pattern is not apparent with lesser degrees of left atrial enlargement. Conversely, when the right atrium also enlarges, as is common in long-standing

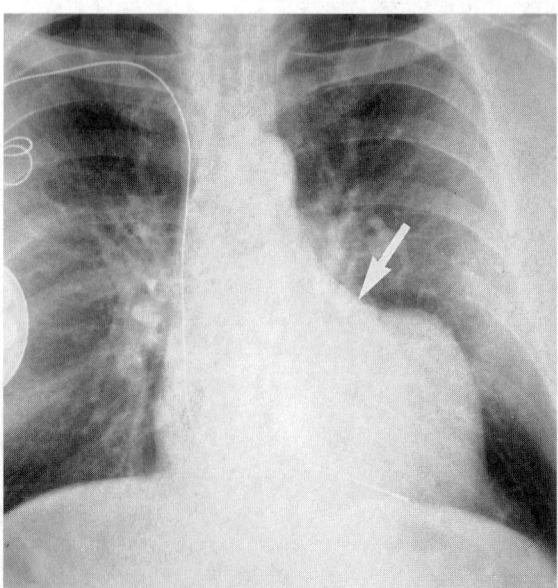

FIGURE 41–5 ▪ Left ventricular aneurysm. A bulge on the lower portion of the left cardiac border, formed by the anterolateral wall of the left ventricle, represents a ventricular aneurysm. The patient had suffered a myocardial infarct 1 year previously. The left atrial appendage segment *(arrow)* is normal. A transvenous pacemaker has been inserted through the right subclavian vein. The electrode tip is situated in the apex of the right ventricle.

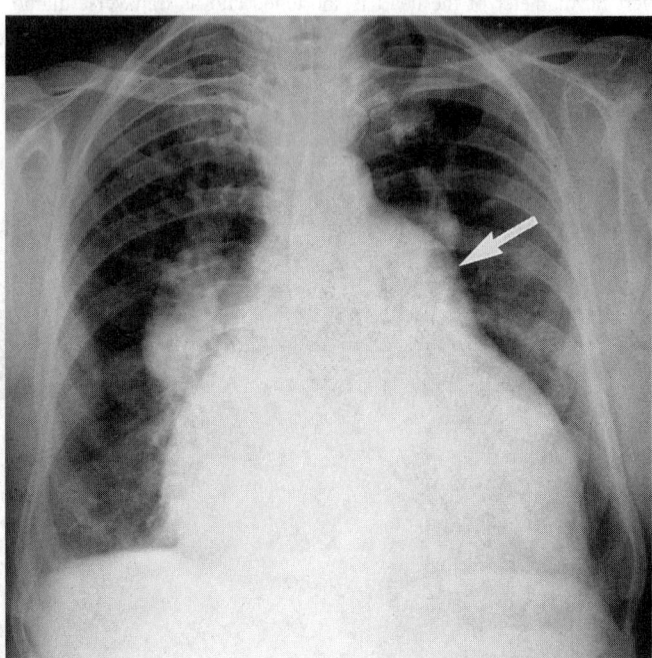

FIGURE 41–6 ▪ Right ventricular enlargement seen in a patient with resistive pulmonary hypertension secondary to an atrial septal defect. The main pulmonary artery *(arrow)* and the right pulmonary artery are markedly dilated. The left pulmonary artery was also dilated but is hidden by the heart in this view. The sudden "cutoff" of the vascular shadows just beyond the hila is characteristic of resistive pulmonary hypertension. Enlargement of the right ventricle is elevating the cardiac apex and displacing it to the left. Accentuation of the curvature of the lower right cardiac border and enlargement of the cardiac silhouette to the right are caused by dilatation of the right atrium.

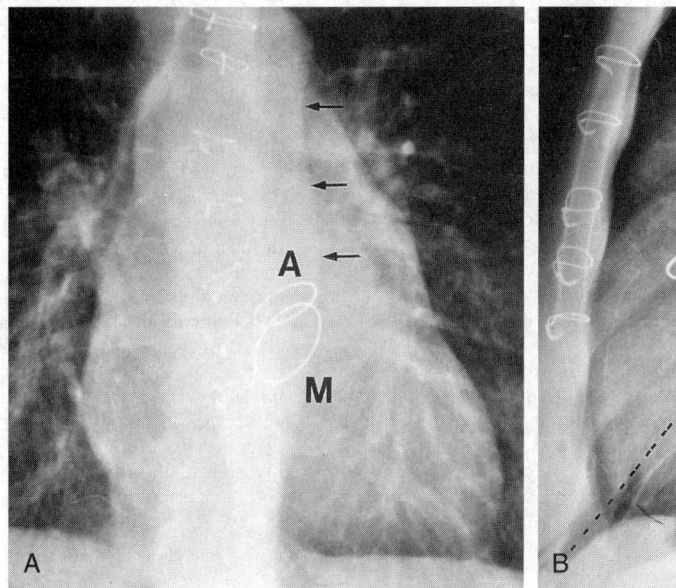

FIGURE 41-7 ■ Location of the mitral and aortic valves. Both the mitral and aortic valves have been replaced by porcine heterografts. The circular stents indicate the location and tilt of each valve. M = mitral valve; A = aortic valve. *A,* Frontal projection. The two valves are normally in contact with each other, and it is difficult to separate them in the frontal projection. Furthermore, on a routinely exposed film, calcific deposits are not easily seen because of the overlapping shadows of the descending aorta *(arrows)* and the spine. *B,* Lateral projection. The valves can be differentiated on the lateral view by drawing a line from the left main bronchus *(arrow)* to the anterior costophrenic sulcus. The aortic valve lies above this line and the mitral valve below it.

presence of a large left ventricle does not necessarily indicate the presence of mitral valve disease.

RIGHT ATRIUM. Enlargement of only the right chambers of the heart is seen in severe pulmonary hypertension without coexisting left heart failure, in bacterial endocarditis of the tricuspid and/or pulmonic valve, and in the carcinoid syndrome. Dilatation of the right atrium causes an accentuation and outward bowing of the curvature on the lower half of the right cardiac contour in the frontal view. With greater degrees of dilatation, the cardiac silhouette enlarges to the right (Fig. 41–6).

RIGHT VENTRICLE. The right ventricle is the most difficult of the four cardiac chambers to evaluate on chest films. Except for a small area in the subpulmonic region, the chamber is not border forming in the frontal projection. Even moderate right ventricular enlargement may produce no abnormality in this view other than some elevation of the main pulmonary artery. As right ventricular size increases, the transverse diameter of the heart enlarges to the left, and the cardiac apex becomes blunted and elevated (see Fig. 41–6). Enlargement of either or both ventricles displaces the apex

of the heart to the left. It is not often possible to distinguish between biventricular enlargement or dilatation of one or the other of the ventricles.

As the right ventricle enlarges, its area of contact with the sternum increases and tends to obliterate the retrosternal clear space in the lateral view. This sign is non-specific inasmuch as it also depends on the shape of the chest and the size of the left ventricle, as well as the size of the right ventricle.

CALCIFICATION

Calcific deposits, because they have a greater radiodensity than the cardiac soft tissues, can be seen within the cardiac silhouette. Valvular calcification most often involves the mitral and aortic valves and usually indicates significant stenosis. The calcium is deposited in irregular clumps near the valve commissures. Because the two valves are in contact—inserting on a common fibrous tendon—determining which valve is calcified may be difficult.

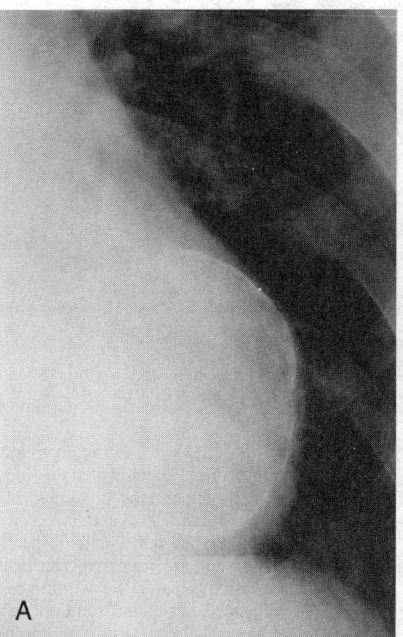
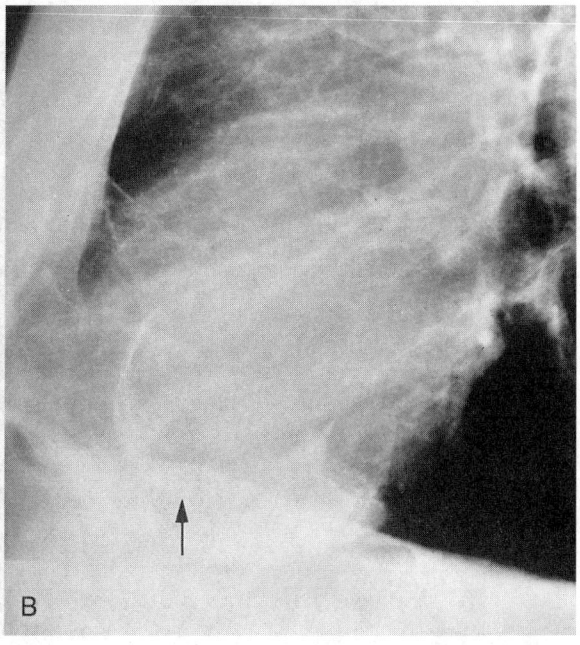

FIGURE 41-8 ■ Calcified myocardial infarcts. *A,* Patient 1: Frontal projection of an anterolateral left ventricular aneurysm. The fine calcific line outlines an anterolateral aneurysm of the left ventricle. The calcific deposit is much finer than that seen with pericardial calcification. The patient had suffered a myocardial infarction several years earlier. *B,* Patient 2: Lateral projection of a septal infarction. The curvilinear calcific deposit is within the scarred lower portion of the ventricular septum. The infarct extended posteriorly along the base of the heart to involve the diaphragmatic wall of the left ventricle *(arrow).*

Both lie within the midportion of the cardiac silhouette in the frontal projection, just to the left of the spine (Fig. 41–7A). They can be separated by fluoroscopy: the axis of motion of the aortic valve approaches the vertical, whereas the orbit of motion of the mitral valve is oriented nearer the horizontal. The distinction can also be made on lateral chest films. If a line is drawn from the left main bronchus, seen as a dark, circular shadow superimposed on the lowermost part of the trachea, to the anterior costophrenic angle, the mitral valve lies below the line and the aortic valve above it (see Fig. 41–7B). Calcification of the mitral annulus, most common in elderly women, can be distinguished from valvular calcification in that mitral calcification forms a heavy, relatively smooth curvilinear shadow in the form of an O or a C.

Calcification of the myocardium in coronary artery disease indicates a previous transmural infarct and frequently a ventricular aneurysm. The calcified scar is visualized as a fine, curvilinear density, most commonly on the anterolateral aspect of the heart, where it is seen best in the frontal view (Fig. 41–8A), or in the lower portion of the interventricular septum, where it is seen best in the lateral projection (see Fig. 41–8B). Calcification of the pericardium is usually coarser and tends to occur in clumps. Often, pericardial calcium is distributed primarily over the interventricular sulcus and the atrioventricular grooves, but when extensive, the deposits may coalesce and completely surround the heart (Fig. 41–9).

Calcification of the coronary arteries is a specific sign of complicated atheromatous plaque in which previous hemorrhage has occurred. Not uncommonly, this type of plaque, which may not produce significant narrowing of the vessel, is the site of thrombosis and vascular occlusion leading to myocardial infarction. Although the calcium is often not deposited in the areas of high-grade stenosis, a very strong correlation exists between the extent of coronary artery calcification and the extent of coronary arterial sclerosis.

Calcification of the coronary arteries is difficult to visualize on chest films because the deposits are thin and their shadows are blurred by the motion of the heart. Fluoroscopy is more sensitive but not as accurate as fast computed tomographic scanning for detecting or quantifying coronary artery calcification. Radiologic detection of coronary artery calcification is the only current noninvasive method for directly visualizing atheromatous disease in the coronary arterial walls.

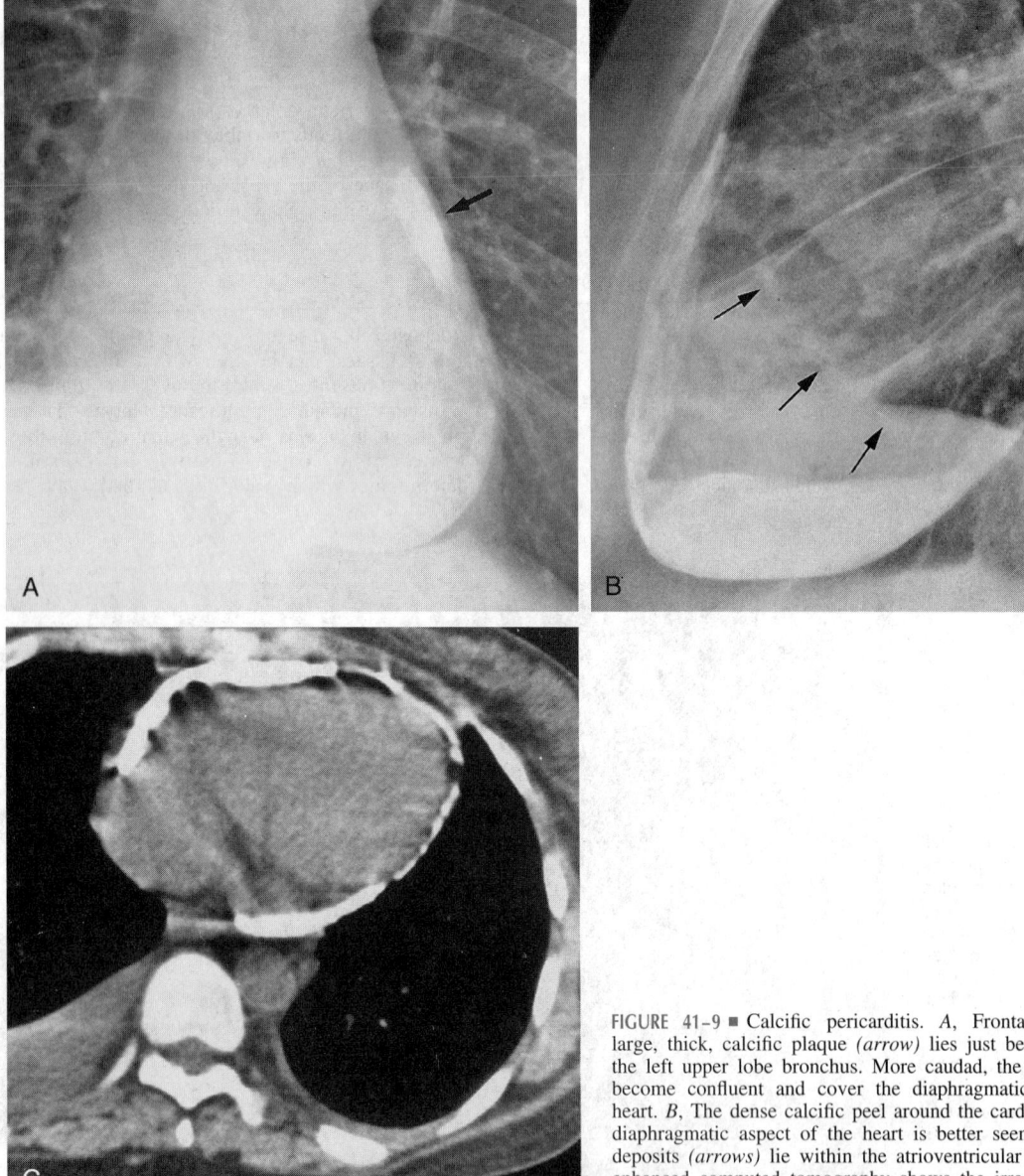

FIGURE 41–9 ■ Calcific pericarditis. *A,* Frontal projection. A large, thick, calcific plaque *(arrow)* lies just below the level of the left upper lobe bronchus. More caudad, the calcific deposits become confluent and cover the diaphragmatic surface of the heart. *B,* The dense calcific peel around the cardiac apex and the diaphragmatic aspect of the heart is better seen. Linear calcific deposits *(arrows)* lie within the atrioventricular sulcus. *C,* Nonenhanced computed tomography shows the irregular, thick, calcific peel almost encircling the heart.

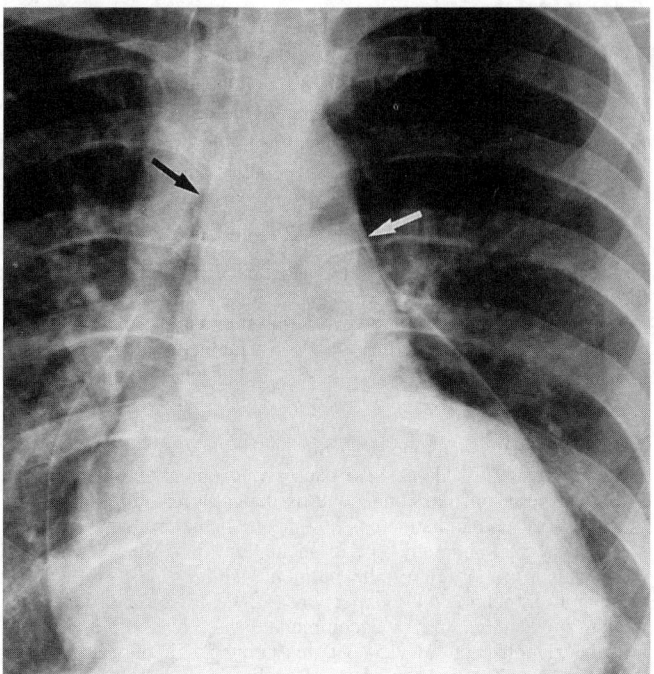

FIGURE 41–10 ▪ The superior pericardial reflection with effusion following a tap. During pericardiocentesis, some of the withdrawn fluid was replaced with air. The normal pericardium is now outlined between the intrapericardial air and the air in the lungs and is seen as a thin linear shadow along the outer border of the cardiac silhouette. The film is made in the erect position and the air has risen to the highest point of the pericardial cavity *(arrows)*, above the level of the pulmonary hila and almost reaching the aortic arch.

PERICARDIAL EFFUSION

The pericardium completely invests the heart, except for a small area on its posterior surface between the entrances of the pulmonary veins and the superior and inferior venae cavae. When fluid accumulates in the pericardium, the sac distends smoothly to enlarge the cardiac silhouette and give it a flask-shaped appearance. A similar shape can occur with a dilated, failing heart.

Differentiation of the two conditions is readily made from the appearance of the pulmonary hila on a frontal chest film. The pericardial sac extends onto the great vessels and up to or slightly above the level of the bifurcation of the main pulmonary artery

(Fig. 41–10). As the sac distends with fluid, it tends to overlap and obscure the hilar vessels. On the other hand, when the heart fails, the vessels become congested and appear more prominent than normal (Fig. 41–11).

Posterior displacement of the epicardial fat line is a second reliable sign of pericardial effusion. In adults, fat is often insinuated between the myocardium and the visceral pericardium (the epicardium) and is sometimes seen in the lateral projection as a curvilinear, radiolucent shadow paralleling the anterior aspect of the heart. The anterior surface of the parietal pericardium borders the retrosternal mediastinal fat. The soft tissue density between these two fat lines therefore represents the pericardium, the epicardium, and the fluid between them. When normal, this stripe is no more than 1 to 2 mm thick. As fluid accumulates in the pericardial sac, the epicardial fat line is displaced posteriorly and the pericardial stripe widens (Fig. 41–12).

PULMONARY VASCULATURE

Almost all of the linear shadows in the lung represent large and medium-sized pulmonary arteries and veins. The terminal branches of the vessels are too small to be visualized as individual structures. The same is true of the interstitial tissues that support the alveoli and form the primary and secondary interlobular septa. However, summation of the minimal densities cast by these structures gives the pulmonary fields an overall grayish cast. The large vessels are seen because their soft tissue density is set off against the surrounding air-containing alveoli.

The caliber of the pulmonary vessels reflects the volume of blood flowing through the lungs. When this volume is diminished because of a right-to-left shunt, venous blood bypasses the pulmonary vessels and consequently these vessels are smaller in caliber and the lungs appear abnormally radiolucent. Increased size and prominence of the pulmonary vessels, both central and peripheral, usually indicate an increase in pulmonary blood flow secondary to a left-to-right shunt (Fig. 41–13A). The vessels in the lower as well as the upper lung fields are dilated. Although pulmonary arteries and veins also become abnormally prominent in heart failure, the vessels are not usually sharply outlined, and additional signs of pulmonary venous hypertension or interstitial edema are present.

The vessels to the lower lobes carry about 60 to 70% of the pulmonary blood flow and are normally of greater caliber than the vessels to the upper lobes. As pulmonary venous pressure increases, the lower lobe vessels become constricted, so more blood is distributed to the upper lobes, which makes their vessels more prominent. This redistribution of the pulmonary vasculature is a

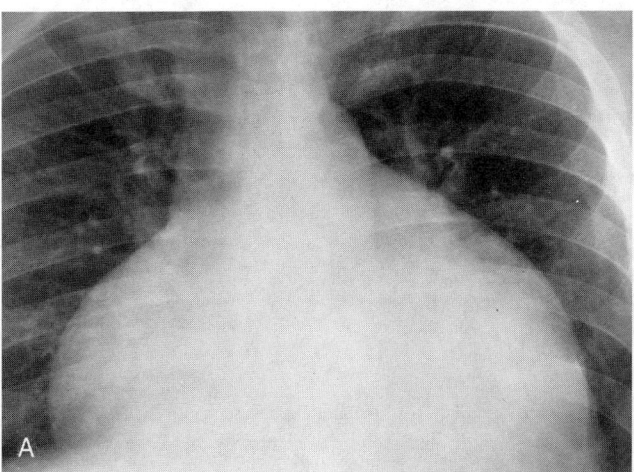
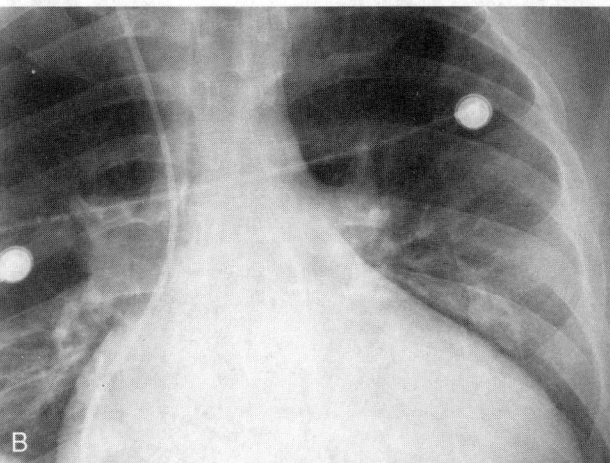

FIGURE 41–11 ▪ Hilum overlay sign. *A*, Pericardial effusion. The heart is diffusely enlarged. Its silhouette extends outward and obscures the hilar shadows in each lung. *B*, Dilated cardiomyopathy. The heart is diffusely enlarged. The failing left ventricle has caused congestion of the hilar vessels and they are more prominent than normal.

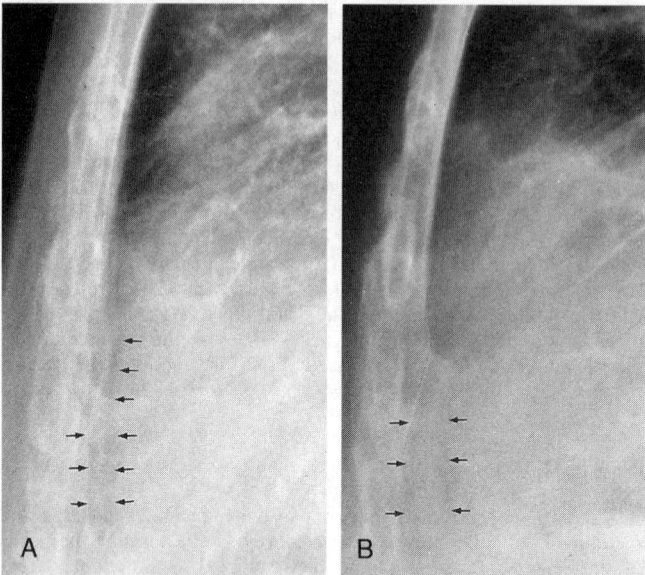

FIGURE 41–12 ■ Pericardial effusion with posterior displacement of the epicardial fat line. The two lines of arrows point to the substernal fat and the subepicardial fat layers. *A*, Normal. The fine line of soft tissue density between the fat layers represents the epicardium, the pericardium, and the fluid between them. *B*, Same patient with a pericardial effusion. The epicardial fat line is displaced posteriorly, and the pericardial stripe is abnormally wide.

reliable sign of pulmonary venous hypertension (see Fig. 41–13*B*), although it is often difficult to recognize unless quite marked. With a sufficient further increase in venous pressure, pulmonary edema develops.

PULMONARY EDEMA. Normally, extravascular circulation of fluid in the lungs from the capillaries through the interstitium and back to the blood stream by way of the lymphatics is constant. When pulmonary venous pressure increases, more and more fluid leaks from the capillary bed, the capacity of the lymphatics to remove the fluid is exceeded, and the interstitium becomes waterlogged. Because the interlobular septa in the outer portions of the lung bases are oriented parallel to the x-ray beam on an erect film, when thickened, they are seen as parallel, short horizontal lines extending to the pleural surfaces (Kerley B lines). Kerley A lines also represent thickened interlobular septa, but they are longer and are seen in the upper lung fields. These lines are within the depth of the lung and usually do not reach the pleural surface. Most of the other septa, even when thickened, are too fine to be identified as individual structures. However, the summation pattern creates random "noise" on the film that obscures the shadows of the pulmonary vessels (Fig. 41–14). A "ground-glass" appearance of the lung fields without identifiable vascular markings within them is characteristic of interstitial pulmonary edema. The patient is usually severely tachypneic at this stage, but rales may not be present. Interstitial edema also causes thickening of the bronchial walls and peribronchial connective tissue and a resulting increase in the thickness and indistinctness of the bronchial walls where they are projected on end. This "peribronchial cuffing" is best visualized in the superior portion of the pulmonary hila, where the anterior segmental bronchus of the upper lobes is viewed on end. When the interstitium can no longer accommodate the excess fluid, it spills into the alveoli (Fig. 41–15). At this point, as air bubbles through the fluid, the typical auscultatory findings of pulmonary edema appear.

PULMONARY ARTERIAL HYPERTENSION. Resistive pulmonary hypertension can result from a left-to-right intracardiac shunt, mitral valve disease, or extracardiac disease such as repeated episodes of pulmonary embolization. The central pulmonary arteries become grossly dilated. Instead of gradually tapering as they bifurcate, a sudden, sharp change in the caliber of the vessels is noted. The size and number of the smaller arterial branches decrease, which makes them look like a "pruned tree" (see Fig. 41–6). With severe pulmonary hypertension, the right heart chambers may dilate. The radiographic appearance of pulmonary hypertension is relatively specific but not sensitive. Clinically significant hypertension can be present with a normal-appearing pulmonary vascular bed.

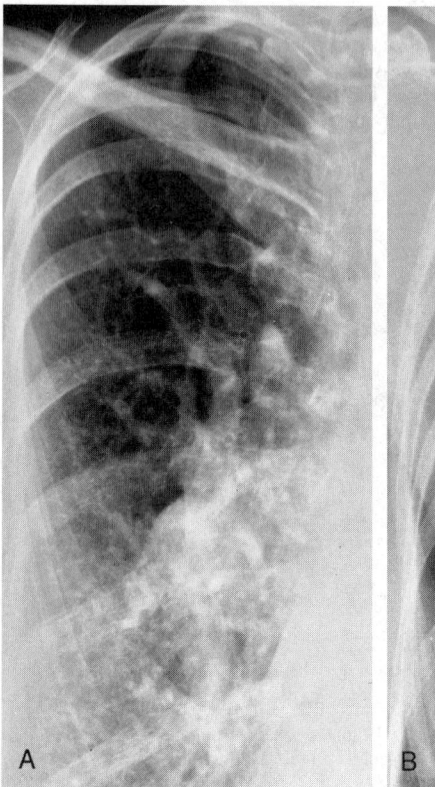

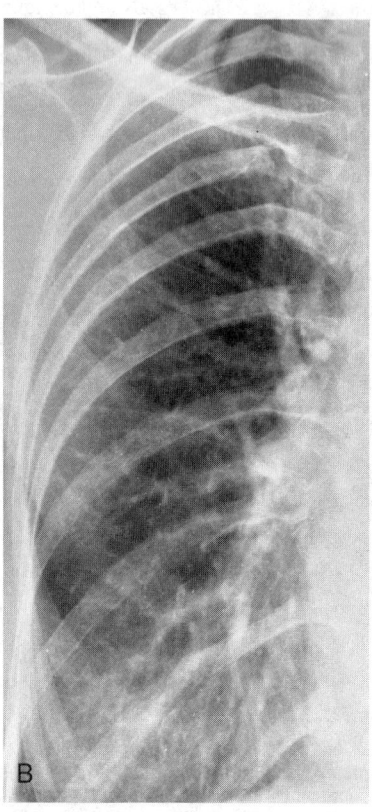

FIGURE 41–13 ■ Pulmonary vasculature. *A*, Atrial septal defect, left-to-right shunt. All pulmonary vessels, to the lower lobes as well as the upper lobes, are dilated, which is indicative of increased blood flow. *B*, Mitral stenosis, pulmonary venous hypertension with redistribution of the pulmonary vasculature. The lower lobe vessels are constricted and the upper vessels, which now carry more blood, are of greater caliber.

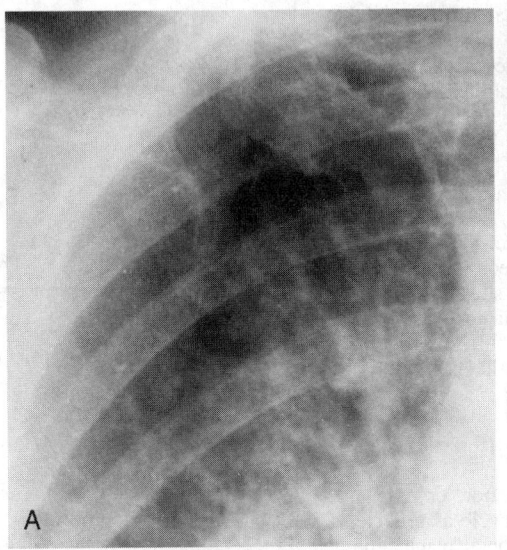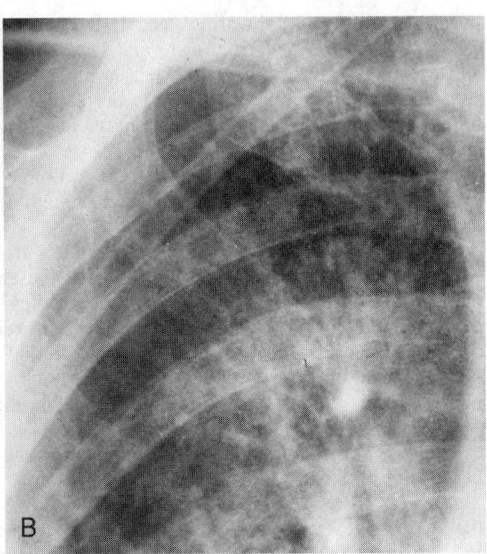

FIGURE 41–14 ■ Interstitial pulmonary edema. *A,* Close-up of the right upper lobe; portable film of a patient with an acute myocardial infarct. The pulmonary vessels are well outlined. *B,* Two days later, the patient became tachypneic. No abnormal auscultatory findings were present in the lungs. Radiographically, the lung fields are noisy, with numerous random shadows obscuring the outline of the pulmonary vessels. The appearance and the time sequence of the changes are characteristic of interstitial pulmonary edema.

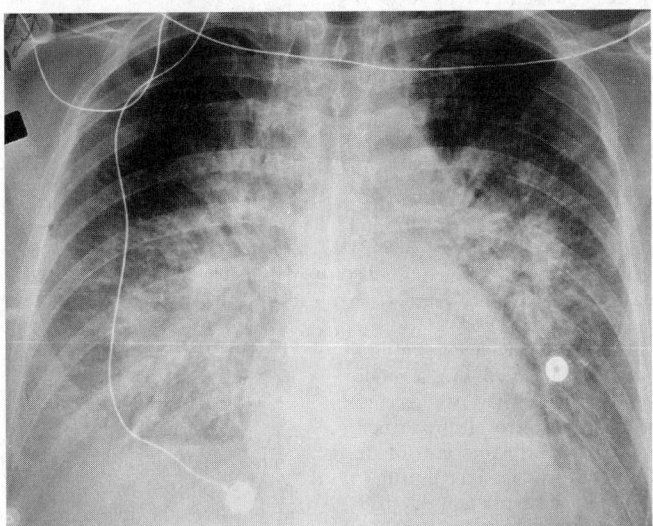

FIGURE 41–15 ■ Alveolar pulmonary edema, acute myocardial infarction. Patchy areas of consolidation can be seen in the perihilar regions of both lungs. Dilatation of the heart after a massive myocardial infarction may not be seen for the 1st 24 to 48 hours.

Baron MG: Radiology of the pericardium. *In* Gooding CA (ed): Diagnostic Radiology, 1991. Berkeley, University of California, 1991.

Budoff MJ, Georgiou D, Brody A, et al: Ultrafast computed tomography as a diagnostic modality in the detection of coronary disease. A multi-center study. Circulation 93:898, 1996.

Milne ENC: The radiologic distinction of cardiogenic and non-cardiogenic edema. AJR Am J Roentgenol 144:879, 1985.

Nakamori N, Doik K, MacMahon H, et al: Effect of heart-size parameters computed from digital chest radiographs on detection of cardiomegaly. Invest Radiol 6:546, 1991.

Reed JC: Chest radiology: Plain film patterns and differential diagnosis, 4th ed. St. Louis, CV Mosby, 1997. *A useful text.*

pulses occurs within the conduction system of the heart. When excited, or depolarized, atrial and ventricular myocardial muscle fibers contract. The electrical currents produced by these electrical impulses spread through the body and are recorded from the body surface by applying electrodes at various body surface points and connecting them to a recording apparatus.

The ECG is a valuable diagnostic tool to evaluate conduction delay of atrial and ventricular electrical impulses, origin of arrhythmias, myocardial ischemia and infarction, atrial and ventricular hypertrophy, pericarditis, the effect of cardiac drugs (especially digitalis and certain antiarrhythmic agents), disturbances in electrolyte balance (especially potassium), the function of electronic cardiac pacemakers, and systemic diseases that affect the heart. A patient with heart disease may have a normal ECG, and a normal individual may have an abnormal ECG.

42 ELECTROCARDIOGRAPHY

Nora Goldschlager

The electrocardiogram (ECG) is a recording of the electrical potentials produced by cardiac tissue. Formation of electrical im-

LEAD SYSTEMS

12-LEAD ECG (I, II, III, aVR, aVL, aVF, V1–6). *Bipolar* standard leads (I, II, and III) record electrical potentials in the frontal plane. Electrodes are applied to the arms and legs; the right leg electrode serves as the ground. Lead I reflects the potential difference between the left and right arms, lead II the potential difference between the left leg and right arm, and lead III the potential difference between the left leg and left arm. The electrical potential recorded from any one extremity is the same regardless of where the electrode is placed on the extremity. In a patient with tremor, an ECG relatively free of muscle "noise" can be obtained by applying the electrodes to the upper portions of the limbs. In exercise testing and in ambulatory ECG recordings, the electrodes are applied near or on the torso.

A *unipolar* lead records electrical potentials from the small area of tissue underlying the lead, as well as all the electrical events of the cardiac cycle as viewed from that recording site. The frontal plane unipolar leads (aVR, aVL, and aVF) are related to the standard bipolar leads (I, II, and III). The precordial (V) leads record potentials in the horizontal plane without being influenced by potentials from an "indifferent" electrode (Table 42–1). Esophageal leads record atrial and ventricular potentials as seen from the esophagus, and intracardiac leads record potentials from the chamber or site in which they are positioned.

THE CARDIAC VECTOR. The frontal plane vector, or axis, is the sum of the electrical potentials of the cardiac cycle as reflected in the frontal plane of the body. By combining frontal plane bipolar leads I, II, and III with frontal plane unipolar leads aVR, aVL, and aVF, a hexaxial reference system that illustrates all six leads of the frontal plane can be constructed (Fig. 42–1); and the mean QRS, P, and T wave vectors in the frontal plane can be approximated by determining their net magnitudes and direction in any two of the three standard leads. The normal QRS axis lies between 0 and +110 degrees; superior axis deviation (between −45 and −90 degrees) and right axis deviation (between +110 and ±180 degrees) are considered abnormal. Leftward deviation of the mean frontal plane QRS axis can occur with advancing age in the absence of clinically overt heart disease. Both the normal frontal plane P wave and T wave axes usually correspond to the normal QRS axis and point in the same general direction. The unipolar precordial leads approximate the electrical potentials (vectors) in the horizontal plane.

MONITOR LEADS. Although any ECG lead or leads can be used in a specialized clinical area such as a coronary care unit, a modified bipolar chest lead (MCL) is most common. The positive electrode is placed in the V_1 position and the negative electrode near the left shoulder; a third electrode is placed at a remote area of the chest and serves as the ground. This "MCL$_1$" lead is useful to evaluate cardiac rhythm. Bipolar lead II is also often used. It is important that the monitoring lead be documented on any recorded rhythm strips so as to avoid erroneous diagnoses based on improper interpretation of P-QRS morphologies depicted in that lead. To monitor the patient for ST and T wave abnormalities due to ischemia, the positive electrode can be placed in any position that has been previously noted to show the abnormality.

THE ECG GRID. ECG paper is graph paper with horizontal and vertical lines at 1-mm intervals (Fig. 42–2) with a heavier line

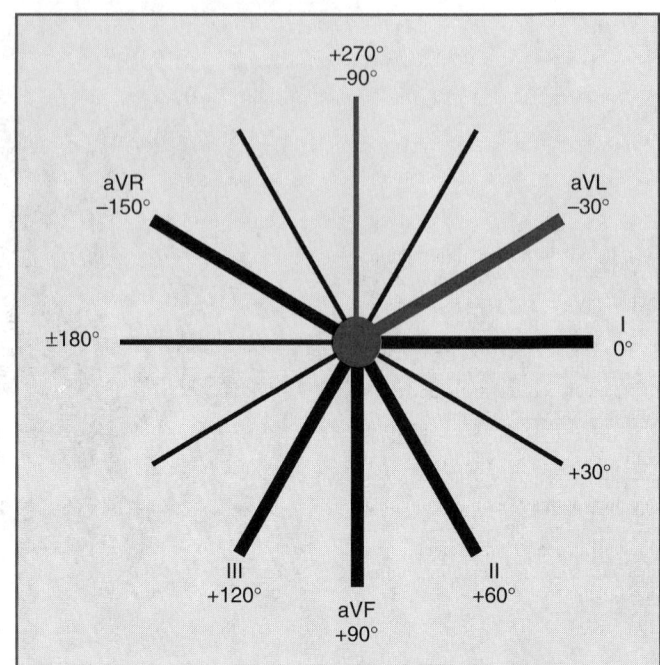

FIGURE 42–1 ■ Hexaxial reference system depicting frontal plane ECG leads. By convention, the positive pole of lead I is designated as 0 degrees and the negative pole as ± 180 degrees; the positive pole of aVF as +90 degrees and the negative pole as +270 degrees or −90 degrees; the positive pole of aVR as +210 degrees or −150 degrees; and the positive pole of aVL as +330 degrees or −30 degrees. If a perpendicular line is drawn through the center of a given lead axis, any electrical force (vector) oriented in the positive half of the electrical field records an upright deflection in that lead; any force oriented in the negative half of the electrical field records a downward deflection. (Adapted from Goldschlager N, Goldman MJ: Principles of Clinical Electrocardiography, 13th ed. Norwalk, CT, Appleton & Lange, 1989. The McGraw-Hill Cos., Inc.)

every 5 mm. Time is measured along the horizontal lines with 1 mm = 0.04 second. Voltage is measured along the vertical lines and is expressed as millimeters (10 mm = 1 mV). In routine clinical practice, the recording speed is 25 mm per second. The usual calibration is a 1-mV signal that produces a 10-mm deflection. "Double standard," sometimes useful for identifying the atrial rhythm in patients with tachycardia, produces a 20-mm deflection; "half standard," useful when a markedly increased voltage precludes optimal visualization of QRS morphology, produces a 5-mm deflection; and "quarter standard," useful when recording intracardiac electrograms, produces a 2.5-mm deflection. Every ECG should be accompanied by a standard in order to interpret the tracing properly; currently available page-writing ECG machines, which can record multiple leads simultaneously, automatically inscribe the selected standard. The recording speed is also automatically inscribed in currently available page-writing machines, and should also be noted: 50 mm/second recordings can be misinterpreted as bradycardia or as abnormally long PQRST intervals, whereas 12.5 mm/second recordings can be misinterpreted as tachycardia or as abnormally short PQRST intervals.

CELLULAR ELECTROPHYSIOLOGY OF THE HEART (Chapter 49)

CELL DEPOLARIZATION AND REPOLARIZATION. Four electrophysiologic events are involved in generating the ECG: (1) impulse formation in the primary pacemaker of the heart (usually the sinoatrial [SA] node); (2) impulse transmission through specialized conduction fibers; (3) activation (depolarization) of myocardial tissue; and (4) repolarization (recovery) of the myocardium. The potential difference between the inside and outside of the cell is known as the resting membrane potential, which is determined mainly by the 30:1 intracellular to extracellular potassium gradient

Table 42–1 ■ POSITION OF UNIPOLAR PRECORDIAL LEADS ON THE BODY SURFACE

LEAD	PRECORDIAL POSITION
V_1	Fourth intercostal space, right sternal border
V_2	Fourth intercostal space, left sternal border
V_3	Equidistant between V_2 and V_4
V_4	Fifth intercostal space, left midclavicular line; all subsequent leads (V_{5-9}) are taken in the same horizontal plane as V_4
V_5	Anterior axillary line
V_6	Midaxillary line
V_7	Posterior axillary line
V_8	Posterior scapular line
V_9	Left border of the spine
$V_{3R–9R}$	Right side of the chest in the same location as the left-sided leads V_{3-9}; V_{2R} is therefore the same as V_1

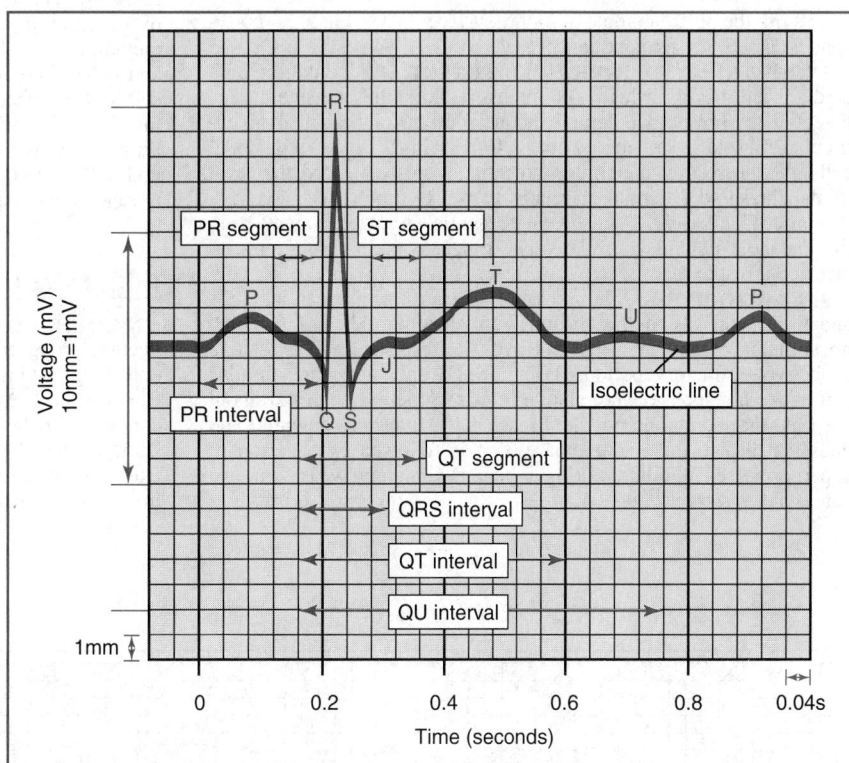

FIGURE 42–2 ■ Schematic illustration of the ECG grid and normal complexes, intervals, and segments. (Adapted from Goldschlager N, Goldman MJ: Principles of Clinical Electrocardiography, 13th ed. Norwalk, CT, Appleton & Lange, 1989. The McGraw-Hill Cos., Inc.)

across the membrane. The resting potential in most cardiac cells, with the exception of those of the SA and atrioventricular (AV) nodal areas, is − 80 to − 90 mV.

When cell depolarization begins, an abrupt change occurs in membrane permeability to sodium. Sodium and, to a lesser extent, calcium ions enter the cell through their respective channels, resulting in a sharp rise of intracellular potential to about ± 20 mV. This phase of depolarization is designated *phase 0* and reflects the sodium-dependent fast inward current typical of working myocardial cells and Purkinje fibers. The maximum rate of depolarization of ventricular cells is 200 volts/second, and that of atrial cells is 100 to 200 volts/second. Pacemaker cells in the SA and AV nodes are depolarized by a calcium-dependent slow inward current. Under some abnormal conditions, such as ischemia, cells whose fast inward sodium current is inhibited are depolarized by slow inward calcium currents.

Following cell depolarization, the potential gradually returns to resting potential. This repolarization process is characterized by *phase 1*—an initial rapid return of intracellular potential to 0 mV, largely the result of sodium channels closing; *phase 2*—a plateau

resulting from calcium entering slowly into the cell; and *phase 3*—return of the intracellular potential to resting level, resulting from potassium extruding out of the cell. At the end of phase 3, the normal resting potential is re-established, and the excess of sodium and a deficit of potassium ions are rectified by a sodium pump. In calcium-dependent cells (SA and AV nodal cells) the phases of repolarization are less well demarcated.

The summation of all phase 0 potentials of atrial myocardial cells results in the P wave inscribed in the surface ECG. Phase 2 corresponds to the PR segment, which follows the P wave, and phase 3 corresponds to the T_a wave of atrial repolarization. The summation of phase 0 potentials of ventricular myocardial cells

Table 42–2 ■ COMMON CAUSES OF AV CONDUCTION DELAYS

Hypervagotonia (often associated with sinus bradycardia or sinus arrhythmia)
Digitalis
β-Blocking drugs
Some calcium channel–blocking drugs (verapamil, diltiazem)
Class III antiarrhythmic agents (sotalol, amiodarone)
Coronary artery disease
Lenegre's disease (diffuse fibrosis of the conduction system)
Infiltrative heart disease
Aortic root disease (syphilis, spondylitis)
Calcification of the mitral and/or aortic anulus
Acute infectious disease
Myocarditis

Table 42–3 ■ SOME CAUSES OF BUNDLE BRANCH BLOCK PATTERN

Clinically normal individual
Lenegre's disease (idiopathic fibrosis of the conduction tissue)
Lev's disease (calcification of the cardiac skeleton)
Cardiomyopathy
  Dilated
  Hypertrophic (concentric or asymmetric)
  Infiltrative
    Tumor
    Chagas' disease
    Myxedema
    Amyloidosis
Ischemic heart disease
  Acute myocardial infarction
  Remote myocardial infarction
  Coronary artery disease without myocardial infarction
Aortic stenosis
Infective endocarditis with abscesses in the conduction system
Cardiac trauma
Hyperkalemia
Ventricular hypertrophy
Rapid heart rates
Massive pulmonary embolism

results in the QRS complex in the surface ECG. Phase 2 corresponds to the ST segment and phase 3 to the T wave.

EXCITATION AND THRESHOLD POTENTIAL. Excitation of a cardiac cell occurs when a stimulus reduces the transmembrane potential to threshold potential (about -60 mV in atrial and ventricular muscle cells and about -40 mV in SA and AV nodal cells). If the resting membrane potential is raised toward the level of the threshold potential, a relatively weak stimulus can evoke a response. Conversely, if the resting potential is lowered away from the threshold potential, a relatively stronger stimulus is required to produce a response.

REFRACTORINESS. The refractory period of myocardial cells and tissue consists of the absolute refractory period, during which no stimulus of any intensity can evoke a response, and a relative (effective) refractory period, during which only a strong stimulus can evoke a response. The relative refractory period begins at about the time the membrane potential reaches the threshold potential and ends just before the end of phase 3; it is followed by a period of supernormal excitability, during which a relatively weak stimulus can evoke a response.

CONDUCTION VELOCITY. The velocity at which electrical impulses spread through the heart depends on the intrinsic properties of different portions of the conduction system and myocardium, including size, shape, and orientation of muscle cells, and presence and type of connective tissue. Conduction of action potentials from cell to cell occurs over specialized intercellular channels or gap junctions. Conduction velocity is most rapid in the His bundle and Purkinje system (about 2 m/second) and slowest in the SA and AV nodes (0.01 to 0.02 m/second); conduction in atrial and ventricular muscle is about 1 m/second.

THE NORMAL ELECTROCARDIOGRAM

NORMAL COMPLEXES (see Fig. 42–2). The *P wave* is the deflection produced by atrial depolarization; it is normally 0.12 second long or less and is directed leftward and inferiorly in the frontal plane. An abnormally long P wave signifies an interatrial conduction delay. The QRS complex represents ventricular depolarization. The *Q (q) wave* is the initial negative deflection resulting from the onset of ventricular depolarization; the *R (r) wave* is the first positive deflection resulting from ventricular depolarization;

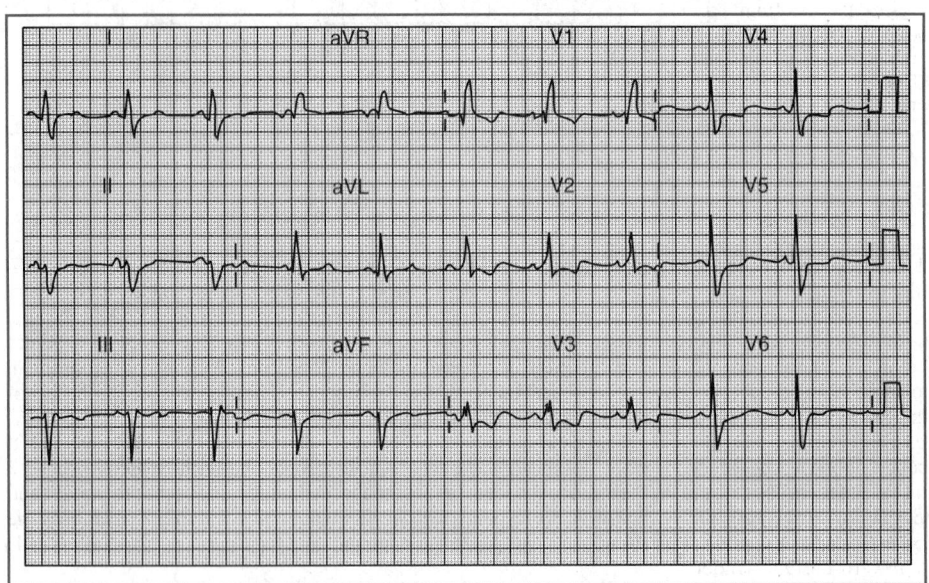

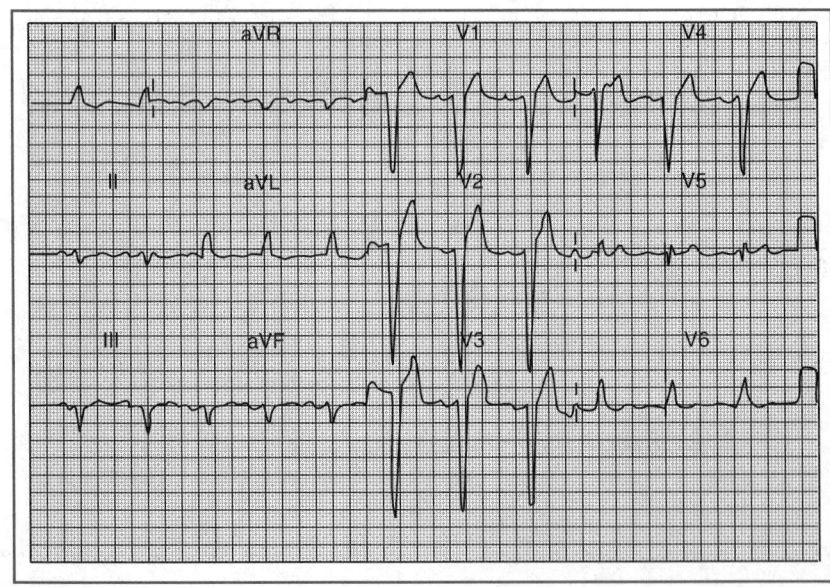

FIGURE 42–3 ■ *A*, 12-lead ECG illustrating a markedly superior mean frontal plane QRS axis and right bundle branch block (deep, wide S wave in leads I, aVL, and V_{5-6} and rsR' in V_1). The ST segments are downsloping and depressed in leads overlying the region of conduction delay and thus may represent secondary abnormalities. The QU interval is also abnormally prolonged. *B*, 12-lead ECG illustrating left bundle branch block, indicated by the notched broad QRS complex in leads overlying the left ventricle (I, aVL, V_{5-6}).

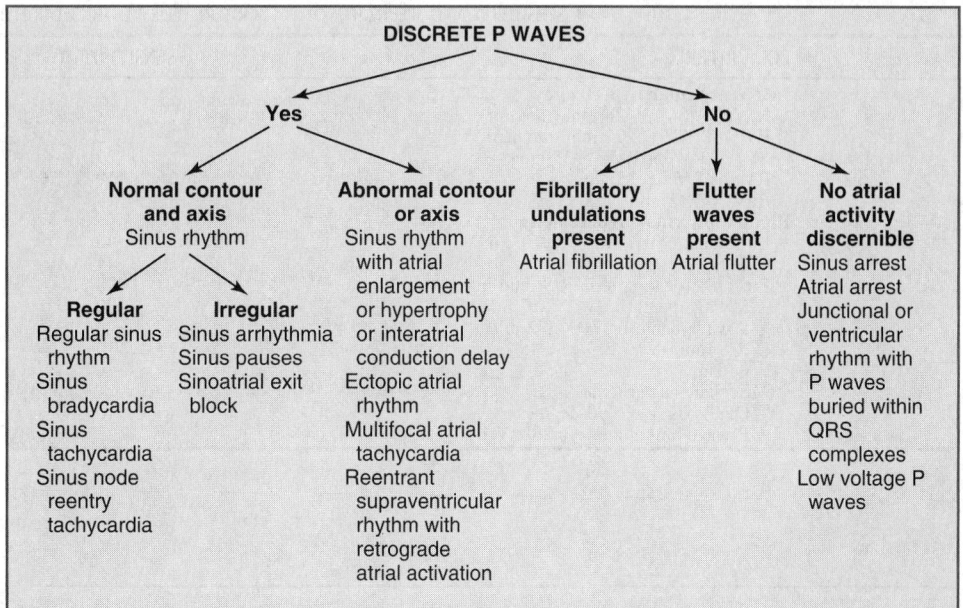

FIGURE 42-4 ■ An approach to the interpretation of the ECG.

and the *S (s) wave* is the negative deflection of ventricular depolarization that follows the first positive (R) wave. A *QS wave* signifies a negative deflection that does not rise above the baseline. An *R′ (r′) wave* is a second positive deflection and follows an S wave; a negative deflection that follows the r′ is termed the s′ wave; if an s wave does not follow the initial R wave, the second positive deflection is still termed an R′ (r′) wave, and the QRS complex is described as an Rr′ (rR′) complex. Capital letters (Q, R, S) refer to waves over 5 mm; lowercase letters (q, r, s) refer to waves under 5 mm. The morphology (and axis) of the QRS complex provides information regarding ventricular hypertrophy, myocardial infarction, and conduction delays in the bundle branches and myocardium. The *T wave* is the deflection produced by ventricular repolarization. The *U wave* is the (usually positive) deflection following

the T wave and preceding the subsequent P wave; it is thought to be due to repolarization of the intraventricular (Purkinje) conduction system and is often accentuated in left ventricular hypertrophy. In some circumstances, such as hypokalemia and hypomagnesemia, the U wave is thought to represent an oscillatory membrane potential, called an *afterdepolarization*. Negative U waves, best seen in leads V_{4-6}, can be seen in acute myocardial ischemia (where they are insensitive but relatively specific markers of left anterior descending coronary artery disease), and left ventricular hypertrophy from any cause.

NORMAL INTERVALS. The *RR interval* is the interval between two consecutive R waves. If the ventricular rhythm is regular, this interval in seconds (or fractions of a second) divided into 60 (seconds) equals the heart rate per minute. If the ventricular rhythm

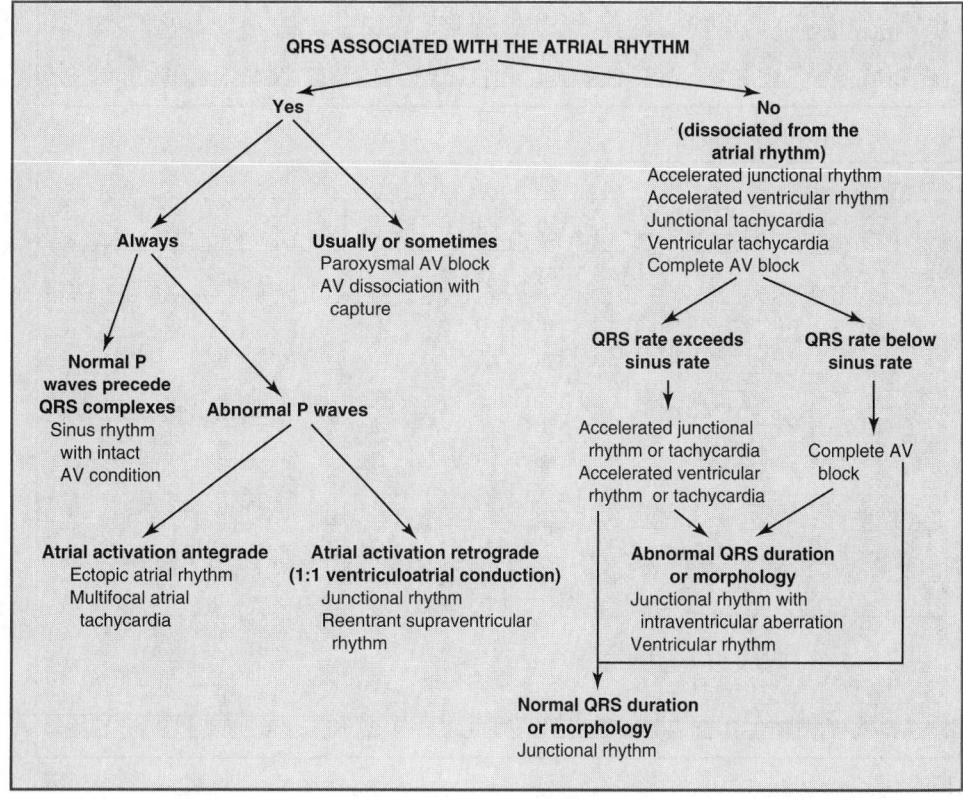

FIGURE 42-5 ■ The QRS rhythm.

Table 42–4 ■ SENSITIVITY AND SPECIFICITY OF ECG CRITERIA FOR VENTRICULAR HYPERTROPHY

ECG CRITERIA	SENSITIVITY (%)	SPECIFICITY (%)
Left ventricular hypertrophy		
RaVL + SV$_3$ > 28 mm (men) or		
RaVL + SV$_3$ > 20 mm (women)	42	95
SV$_1$ + RV$_5$ or RV$_6$ > 35 mm	29	93
RV$_5$ or RV$_6$ ≥ 25 mm	19	97
RaVL > 11 mm	18	97
Right ventricular hypertrophy		
Limb lead criteria R in I ≤ 0.2 mV	40	98
S$_2$ S$_2$ S$_3$	44	75
Precordial lead criteria R/S ratio in V$_1$ > 1	28	99
R wave height in V$_1$ > 0.7 mV	30	97
S wave depth in V$_1$ < 0.2 mV	22	100
R/S ratio in V$_5$ or V$_6$ < 1.0	10	100
QR in V$_1$	—	100
Miscellaneous criteria		
QRS axis > + 90 degrees	16	100
P wave amplitude > 0.25 mV in II, III, aVF, V$_1$, or V$_2$	22	99

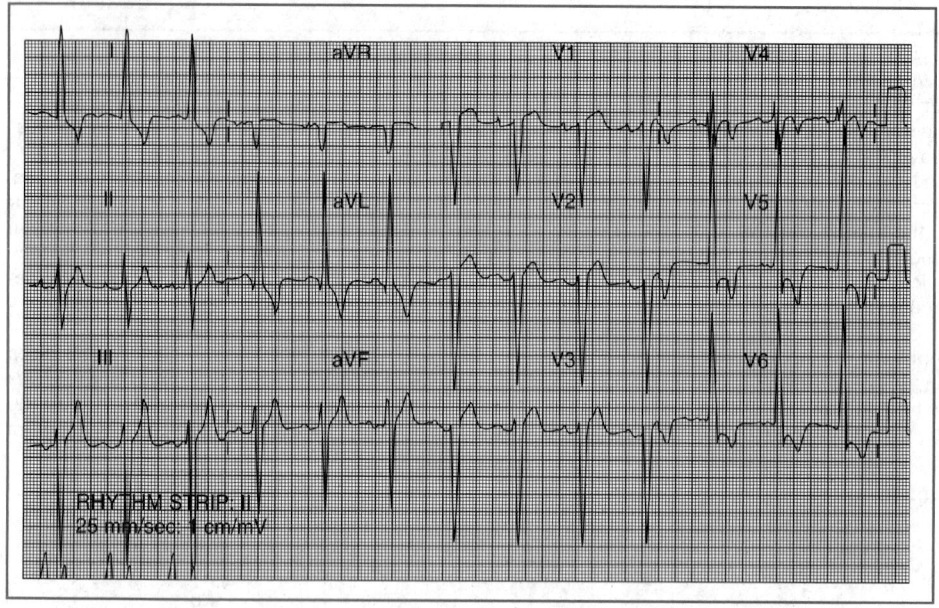

A

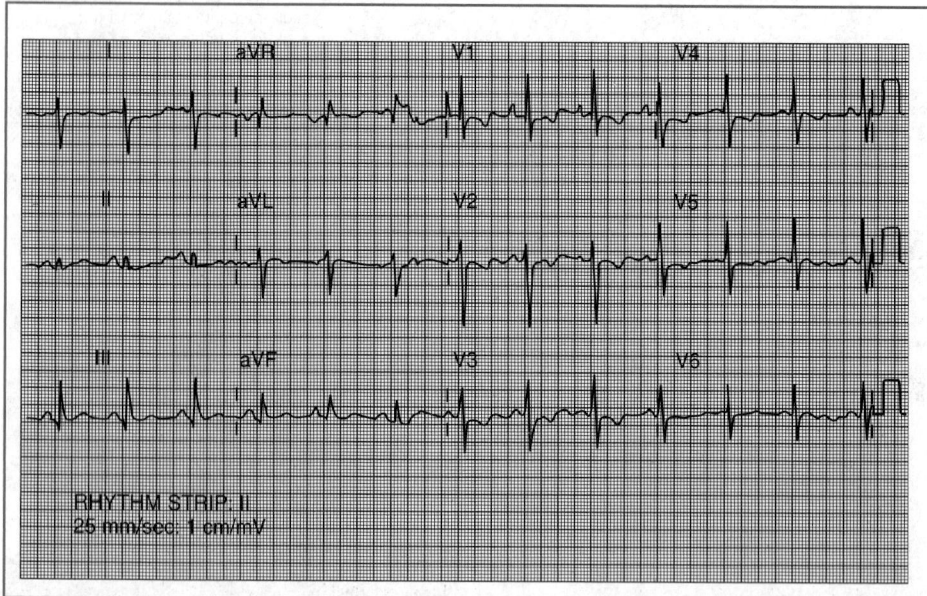

B

FIGURE 42–6 ■ *A,* 12-lead ECG showing left ventricular hypertrophy with accompanying leftward deviation of the mean frontal plane QRS axis to about −40 degrees and depressed downsloping ST-T waves in leads overlying the left ventricle. The P waves are broad and notched, consistent with left atrial enlargement, a common accompaniment of left ventricular hypertrophy. *B,* 12-lead ECG showing right ventricular hypertrophy with accompanying rightward deviation of the mean frontal plane QRS axis to > 120 degrees and depressed downsloping ST-T waves in leads overlying the right ventricle. The P waves are tall in lead II (exceeding 2.5 mm) and V$_1$, consistent with right atrial enlargement.

is irregular, the number of R waves in a specific number of seconds is counted and converted into number per minute. The *PP interval* is the interval between two consecutive P waves. In regular sinus rhythm, the PP interval is the same as the RR interval. When the ventricular rhythm is irregular or when atrial and ventricular rhythms are regular but their rates are different from each other, the PP interval, measured from the same point on two successive P waves, is computed in the same manner as the ventricular rate. The *PR interval* measures the AV conduction time and includes the time required for atrial depolarization, normal conduction delay in the AV node (approximately 0.07 second), and impulse propagation through the His bundle and bundle branches, to the onset of ventricular depolarization. The normal PR interval is 0.12 to 0.20 second and is related both to heart rate and to prevailing autonomic tone (Table 42–2).

The *QRS interval* represents ventricular depolarization time. The upper limit of normal is 0.11 second. Conduction delay in the bundle branches or in myocardial tissue results in a prolonged QRS interval. If the conduction delay is in one of the bundle branches, a specific ECG pattern of right or left bundle branch "block" is recorded (Table 42–3; Fig. 42–3).

The *QT interval* represents the duration of electrical systole and varies with heart rate and autonomic nervous system input. It includes the *QT segment*, which reflects calcium balance: A prolonged QT segment suggests hypocalcemia, whereas a short QT segment indicates hypercalcemia. The *QU interval* represents total ventricular repolarization time, including that of the Purkinje fibers. When the end of the T wave is not distinguished owing to superimposition of a U wave, the *QU interval* is measured in place of the QT interval. An abnormally prolonged QU interval is potentially clinically significant in patients with ischemia, syncope, or ventricular arrhythmias and potassium and magnesium imbalance.

NORMAL SEGMENTS AND JUNCTIONS. The *PR segment* is measured from the end of the P wave to the onset of the QRS complex; it is normally isoelectric but is often depressed in patients with ventricular hypertrophy or chronic pulmonary disease. PR segment depression can carry over into the subsequent ST segment, mimicking true ST segment depression. The *J junction* defines the point at which the QRS complex ends and the ST segment begins; it may not be easily discernible during rapid heart rates and in patients with hyperkalemia.

The *ST segment* begins at the J point and ends at the onset of the T wave. This segment is usually isoelectric but may vary from − 0.5 to + 2 mm in the precordial leads; it is considered elevated or depressed compared with that portion of the baseline between the end of the T wave and the beginning of the P wave (TP segment). ST segment abnormalities are very important diagnostically in acute myocardial ischemia and infarction and in pericarditis. The *TP segment* defines the portion of the tracing between the end of the T wave and the beginning of the next P wave; at normal heart rates, it is usually isoelectric. At rapid heart rates the P wave encroaches on the T wave, eliminating the TP segment.

In addition to the standard 12-lead ECG, recordings are used during exercise or pharmacologic stress testing to document myocardial ischemia, for ambulatory monitoring to detect arrhythmias or ischemic ST segment abnormalities, and for transtelephonic monitoring in patients with cardiac pacemakers or frequent rhythm disturbances. Newer ECG techniques such as body surface mapping (in which instantaneous depolarization and repolarization are plotted) and signal-averaged electrocardiography (in which the QRS complex is filtered to assess the presence of abnormal low-amplitude terminal potentials to predict the risk of an arrhythmic event) are now available (see Chapter 50).

The availability of computerized ECG interpretation allows for rapid initial screening, which may be useful in some clinical circumstances; however, physician overread is mandatory for accurate interpretation.

STEPS IN ANALYZING AN ECG

Identify the atrial rhythm and measure its rate (Fig. 42–4). Establishing the rate allows the atrial rhythm to be characterized as bradycardia (rate <60 per minute), normal (rate between 60 and 100 per minute), and tachycardia (rate >100 per minute). If atrial and ventricular rates are different from each other, their rates must be determined separately. Determine the regularity or irregularity of the rate. Irregular rhythms should be further described as totally irregular ("irregularly" irregular as, for example, in atrial fibrillation) or regular with periods of irregularity ("regularly" irregular as, for example, in atrial bigeminy).

Determine the P wave axis, duration, and morphology to provide information about the focus or origin of the atrial rhythm and whether the atria are being depolarized antegradely or retrogradely. If the atrial rhythm is sinus, the P wave morphology and duration can suggest the presence of atrial enlargement or hypertrophy (Fig. 42–5).

Identify the ventricular rate and whether it is regular or irregular. Ascertain whether it is associated with the atrial rhythm and what their relationships are: Is there one P wave for each QRS complex? Do the P waves precede or follow the QRS complexes? What is the PR interval? Is it constant or does it change?

Determine the QRS axis and duration, and describe the QRS morphology. The duration, morphology, and axis of the QRS complexes can help define the origin of the ventricular rhythm. Rhythms originating above the ventricles usually use the normal His-Purkinje system to active ventricular muscle, and the QRS complexes are narrow and normal-appearing unless bundle branch block is present. QRS complexes originating from ventricular tissue, however, are broad and bizarre. If the ventricles are depolarized using the normal His-Purkinje pathways, the QRS morphology (including voltage), duration, and axis can suggest the presence of left and/or right ventricular hypertrophy (Table 42–4; Fig. 42–6).

Finally, *compare the present ECG with previous records.*

Goldberger AL: Clinical Electrocardiography, A Simplified Approach, 6th ed. St. Louis, CV Mosby, 1998.

43 ECHOCARDIOGRAPHY

Anthony N. DeMaria

Echocardiography is a non-invasive technique that evaluates cardiac anatomy and function with images and recordings produced by sound energy. Although introduced as a one-dimensional technique in the early 1970s, echocardiography has evolved into a two- and even three-dimensional imaging modality that is also capable of deriving hemodynamic data from measures of blood flow velocity using the Doppler principle. Cardiac ultrasonography is currently the primary modality employed to assess valvular, pericardial, and congenital heart diseases, as well as cardiac masses. It also has an established role in the assessment of left ventricular (LV) structure and performance, the evaluation of myocardial infarction, and the detection of coronary artery disease.

PHYSICAL PRINCIPLES

Sound energy produces a series of sinusoidal cycles of alternating compression and rarefaction as it travels through a medium. Sound of a frequency above the audible range of 20,000 cycles/sec is termed *ultrasound;* it travels as a beam that obeys the laws of reflection and refraction. When directed into the thorax and aimed at the heart, a sound beam travels in a straight line until it encounters a boundary between structures with different acoustical impedance, such as between blood and tissue. At such surfaces, a portion of the energy is reflected or refracted, and the remaining attenuated signal is transmitted distally. A cardiac image is then constructed from the reflected energy, or echoes.

In practice, the ultrasound signal is both produced and received by a single hand-held transducer that converts electrical to mechanical (sound) energy and vice versa. The central component of the transducer is a piezoelectric crystal whose ionic structure changes shape to produce sound waves when exposed to an electric current. This same crystal is deformed by the reflected sound wave to produce an electrical signal. Echocardiographic images and recordings are constructed in the form of a display of the distance between individual cardiac structures and the transducer. Specifically, electronic circuitry within the instrument measures the transit time for the beam to travel from the transducer to a given structure and back again, and then it calculates distance from transit time using the velocity of sound in soft tissue of 1540 m/sec. The structure is then displayed on the image at the calculated distance. Because interrogating beams can be repetitively transmitted at rates of up to 1000 per second, the movement of structures can be tracked as they change their positions relative to the transducer over time.

The earliest echographs used a single beam to record the structure and motion of a small region of the heart over time, so-called M-mode echocardiography. Subsequently, multiple ultrasound beams were combined to produce a wedge-shaped tomographic image of cardiac anatomy, referred to as two-dimensional echocardiography. The spatial orientation provided by two-dimensional echocardiography was a marked advance, but the typical frame rates of 20 to 30/min provide less temporal resolution than M-mode. Miniaturization of ultrasonic transducers enabled incorporation into standard gastroscopes to perform transesophageal echocardiography or into cardiac catheters to yield intravascular ultrasound images. Transesophageal echocardiography has been of particular value in studying posteriorly located cardiac structures such as the left atrial appendage or in supplying high-resolution images in patients who are difficult to examine by the transthoracic approach. Echocardiography has been performed in conjunction with exercise or pharmacologic stress to evaluate coronary artery disease or, most recently, with the administration of contrast agents to facilitate endocardial definition and evaluate myocardial perfusion.

The sound energy reflected by blood cells is not of sufficient amplitude to be detected by conventional methods. Therefore, blood flow recordings are performed using the Doppler principle. Specifically, when a sound signal is reflected by moving blood cells, the frequency of the signal is changed (the Doppler shift). The resultant frequency shift depends on the direction and velocity of blood flow relative to the transducer. Frequency shift signals can be recorded for a single range-gated point along the beam (pulsed Doppler) or all composite points along the beam (continuous-wave Doppler) and can be displayed as a graphic record of velocity plotted against time (spectral Doppler). Pulsed Doppler enables localized assessment of flow velocity and turbulence but cannot record high velocities due to an artifact termed *aliasing*. Continuous-wave Doppler cannot localize flow but can accurately measure the high velocities produced by disturbed flow. The velocity and direction of flow can also be estimated for multiple points along multiple beams and be displayed as color signals superimposed on standard black and white tissue images (color Doppler flow imaging). Flow velocity, which is related to the pressure gradient across any orifice, provides a mechanism to calculate pressures from velocities within the central circulation using a simplification of the Bernoulli equation.

Several technical factors are important to understand the limitations of echocardiography in clinical practice. Air and bone present an impediment to ultrasound transmission, and good image quality requires that the ultrasound beam have clear access to cardiac structures. Thus, echocardiographic imaging may be limited or impossible in some patients, such as those with severe lung disease or marked obesity. In addition, structures that are not perpendicular to the beam may not reflect adequate energy to be recorded, a phenomenon referred to as *dropout*. Artifacts may also be produced by high levels of background noise or by the increasing width of the imaging beam as it propagates away from the transducer. In regard to Doppler recordings, velocity is a vectorial entity that has magnitude and direction; the beam must be parallel to or within 20 degrees of the direction of flow to record velocity accurately.

ECHOCARDIOGRAM IMAGES AND MEASUREMENTS

The conventional two-dimensional echocardiographic examination consists of wedge-shaped sector images acquired from a number of standard views obtained with different transducer orientations. Doppler recordings can be obtained in any view but are of greatest value when the beam is parallel to flow direction (e.g., transmitral and transaortic flow is best evaluated from the apical view).

A variety of measurements can be derived from echocardiographic recordings. Because the images are tomographic, any individual view may not be representative of the whole. Moreover, areas of dropout may limit measurements based on the entire perimeter of the chamber. Therefore, simple one-dimensional measurements (e.g., LV dimension, LV wall thickness, left atrial dimension) are usually relied on most heavily. However, calculation of LV volumes and ejection fraction is usually possible using a variety of algorithms based on assumed LV geometry and correlate well with those obtained by other techniques such as angiography.

Echocardiography enables the derivation of a number of hemodynamic parameters. Flow volume through an orifice can be calculated as the product of the orifice cross-sectional area derived from echocardiographic images multiplied by velocity measurements provided by pulsed Doppler. Such measurements can be made for flow through any valve or in the ascending aorta or pulmonary artery. Volumetric flow calculations are applied in estimating stroke volume and cardiac output. In normal persons, the volume of blood entering the LV through the mitral valve (LV inflow) equals that exiting the LV through the aortic valve (LV outflow). In the presence of isolated mitral or aortic regurgitation, a greater volume of blood will inflow or outflow the ventricle, respectively; the difference between inflow and outflow measures represents regurgitant volume. A similar approach underlies the calculation of valve area by the continuity equation. The continuity equation is based on the fact that the volume of flow proximal to a stenotic valve is equal to that through the orifice. Since the area and velocity can be measured proximal to the orifice and the velocity can be measured through the orifice, the continuity equation yields the orifice area. Transmitral LV filling patterns by pulsed Doppler can be analyzed for evidence of diastolic dysfunction, manifested by a marked increase in either early or atrial flow velocities or a change in early deceleration rate. Diminished velocities with a slow early diastolic deceleration indicate impaired relaxation, whereas increased velocities and rapid deceleration in early diastole indicate augmented stiffness and a restrictive pattern of filling. A simplification of the Bernoulli equation as $4 \times$ (peak velocity)^2 can be used to measure the pressure gradient across any orifice. Gradient measurement is useful not only in quantifying valve stenosis but also in evaluating pulmonary artery, left atrial, and LV pressures from tricuspid, mitral, and aortic regurgitant jets, respectively.

CLINICAL APPLICATIONS

Echocardiography is useful to evaluate patients with a murmur that might be indicative of an important cardiac condition, for evaluation of unexplained dyspnea or edema, to detect a potential source of systemic emboli, to evaluate an abnormal electrocardiogram that may be suggestive of an old myocardial infarction or pericardial disease, to evaluate unexplained syncope of potential cardiac etiology, and sometimes to evaluate patients with chest pain (Table 43–1). It is also useful for the evaluation of a variety of suspected specific disorders of cardiac valves, cardiac muscle, the pericardium, and the great vessels (Table 43–2).

Valvular Heart Disease

STENOSIS. Echocardiography is unsurpassed in its ability to detect and quantify valvular heart disease (see Chapter 63). Normal valve leaflets are well visualized by echocardiography and appear as thin, rapidly moving structures with an excursion extending to the borders of the chamber or great vessel into which they open. Doppler examination of normal valves depicts forward blood flow of maximal velocities below 1.7 m/sec, without evidence of regur-

Table 43–1 ■ INDICATIONS FOR ECHOCARDIOGRAPHY BY SIGNS AND SYMPTOMS

Murmur (not functional)
Dyspnea
Edema
Systemic embolus
Evaluation of abnormal electrocardiogram (question of old myocardial infarction or pericarditis)
Unexplained syncope of potential cardiac etiology
Abnormal heart size on chest radiograph
Chest pain

Table 43–2 ■ INDICATIONS FOR ECHOCARDIOGRAPHY BY DISORDERS

Valvular stenosis Valvular regurgitation Infectious endocarditis Mitral prolapse Prosthetic valves	For diagnosis or to assess hemodynamic severity or ventricular function
Myocardial ischemia Myocardial infarction	To assess presence, area, and complications
Chronic coronary artery disease	To assess left ventricular dysfunction
Heart failure	To determine etiology and ventricular function
Pericardial disease Cardiac masses Great vessel abnormalities Pulmonary disease	To identify and for follow-up
Hypertension	If left ventricular function will influence decision
Arrhythmias	If heart disease is suggested

gitation. Flow through the semilunar valves exhibits a progressive rise and fall in systole, whereas that through the atrioventricular valves is characterized by a bimodal pattern, with high flow velocities on valve opening in early diastole and after atrial contraction just before the next systole.

Stenotic valves are invariably apparent on an echocardiogram (Fig. 43–1) and are characterized by marked thickening and an obvious decrease in the extent of opening excursion. High-intensity echocardiographic signals indicative of calcification are usually observed. Two-dimensional echocardiographic images of the mitral orifice are readily obtainable, and planimetry of these structures yields estimates of valve area in mitral stenosis that correlate well with values obtained by cardiac catheterization and surgery. However, the orifice of the aortic valve leaflets is often difficult to identify with certainty by transthoracic echocardiography, and aortic stenosis severity cannot be accurately assessed by ultrasound imaging. The quantitation of aortic stenosis typically relies on Doppler measurements. Measurements of peak and mean transvalvular aortic gradient can be readily derived from the maximal transvalve Doppler velocity when subjected to the simplified Bernoulli equation. Similar Doppler approaches can be taken to measure mitral stenosis severity, although peak gradient is a less physiologic measure of the severity of mitral obstruction than aortic obstruction. An alternate approach to assessing the severity of mitral stenosis utilizes the rate of transmitral flow deceleration in early diastole by Doppler, calculated as the time for the Doppler velocity to fall to one half of the pressure equivalent (pressure half-time). Although encountered less frequently, tricuspid and pulmonic stenosis can be quantitatively assessed using the same techniques.

The accuracy of echocardiography in the assessment of valvular stenosis is so high that cardiac catheterization currently is believed to be indicated only in those patients with technically poor ultrasound examination, in those whom the echocardiographic data are not consistent with signs and symptoms of disease, or to define coronary artery anatomy.

REGURGITATION. With valvular regurgitation, there often is a divergence between anatomy and function. Thus, anatomically abnormal valves may not be regurgitant, whereas normal-appearing valves may be accompanied by severe regurgitation. Accordingly, two-dimensional ultrasonic imaging is of greatest value in establishing the specific etiology of valvular regurgitation, whereas Doppler techniques provide the primary method for the detection and quantitation of these abnormalities. Echocardiographic images are also of value in providing evidence of LV or left atrial volume overload. Of the etiologies of mitral regurgitation identifiable by echocardiography, mitral prolapse and torn chordae tendineae are of particular significance. Mitral prolapse, or superior/posterior displacement of the mitral leaflets behind the annulus into the left atrium in systole, is usually midsystolic and best diagnosed by echocardiography. Associated abnormalities include valvular thickening and redundancy, annular dilatation, and perhaps aortic enlargement. Although initially believed quite common, application of

strict diagnostic criteria to the parasternal long-axis view has revised estimates of prevalence downward. In torn chordae, the flail portion of the mitral apparatus can usually be visualized and typically signifies a large regurgitant volume.

The presence of regurgitation is readily identifiable by the retrograde flow of blood emanating from the affected valve into the receiving chamber by color flow Doppler (Figs. 43–2 and 63–2). Regurgitant jets may be observed in normal subjects, most commonly for the tricuspid and pulmonic valves, but are rarely observed with normal aortic or mitral valves. Quantitation of valvular regurgitation is based on four basic approaches: (1) the documentation of differences between LV inflow and LV outflow as determined by volumetric calculations; (2) detection of retrograde flow in the descending aorta for aortic regurgitation and into the pulmonary veins with mitral regurgitation; (3) assessment of the size of the regurgitant jet by color Doppler imaging; and (4) derivation of regurgitant flow rate, volume, and effective orifice area from volume calculations or analysis of the convergence signal proximal to the regurgitant leaflets. The rate of jet deceleration may also be of value in quantifying regurgitation, particularly for the aortic valve. Each of these approaches is limited by imprecision of measurement and the influence of confounding variables. Therefore, the quantitation of valvular regurgitation by echocardiography is less accurate than that of valvular stenosis and is best achieved as the cumulative result of analyzing all possible criteria.

The non-invasive evaluation of prosthetic heart valves has long been fraught with difficulty. The foreign materials with which prosthetic valves are made characteristically result in reverberation artifacts and in severe attenuation and shadowing of ultrasound signals, rendering ultrasound images difficult to interpret. Two-dimensional echocardiographic imaging is of greatest value in determining that artificial valves are properly seated, exhibit free movement of the occluder device, and are free from external masses such as thrombi or vegetations. Doppler, the predominant modality for the assessment of prosthetic valves by ultrasound, provides data regarding abnormalities of transvalvular velocity, gradient, and the presence or absence of valvular regurgitation. Due to artifacts, transesophageal echocardiography may be required for adequate examination of prosthetic valves, particularly those in the mitral position.

Infective Endocarditis

Echocardiography has assumed an important role in diagnosing and assessing the hemodynamic consequences, complications, prognosis, and need for surgery in patients with infective endocarditis (see Chapter 326). The hallmark of infective endocarditis on echocardiography is a vegetation (see Fig. 63–4), which can be detected in more than 80% of cases as a focal valvular thickening without restrictive leaflet motion. The presence of vegetation is associated with an increase in heart failure, emboli, and need for surgical intervention. Echocardiography is also extremely valuable in detecting complications of infective endocarditis such as periannular abscess and valve perforation or tear. Transesophageal echocardiography is more accurate than transthoracic echocardiography in assessing endocarditis, particularly in regard to complications and prosthetic valves.

Ischemic Heart Disease

Disease of the coronary arteries is by far the most common cause of heart disease, and echocardiography is assuming an emerging role in assessing this disorder. Although echocardiography cannot regularly visualize the coronary arteries, it provides important information regarding coronary artery disease through the evaluation of LV performance. Detection of regional dyssynergy is of value in identifying and sizing acute myocardial infarction (see Chapter 60). Furthermore, cardiac ultrasound is the modality of choice for assessing the complications of acute myocardial infarction such as ventricular septal defect, ruptured papillary muscle, pseudoaneurysm, and thrombi.

The provocation of regional contractile abnormalities by treadmill or bicycle exercise or by pharmacologic stress imposed by inotropic or vasodilator drugs can be applied to diagnose and assess the physiologic significance of coronary artery disease (CAD). Stress echocardiography has been shown to be superior to stress

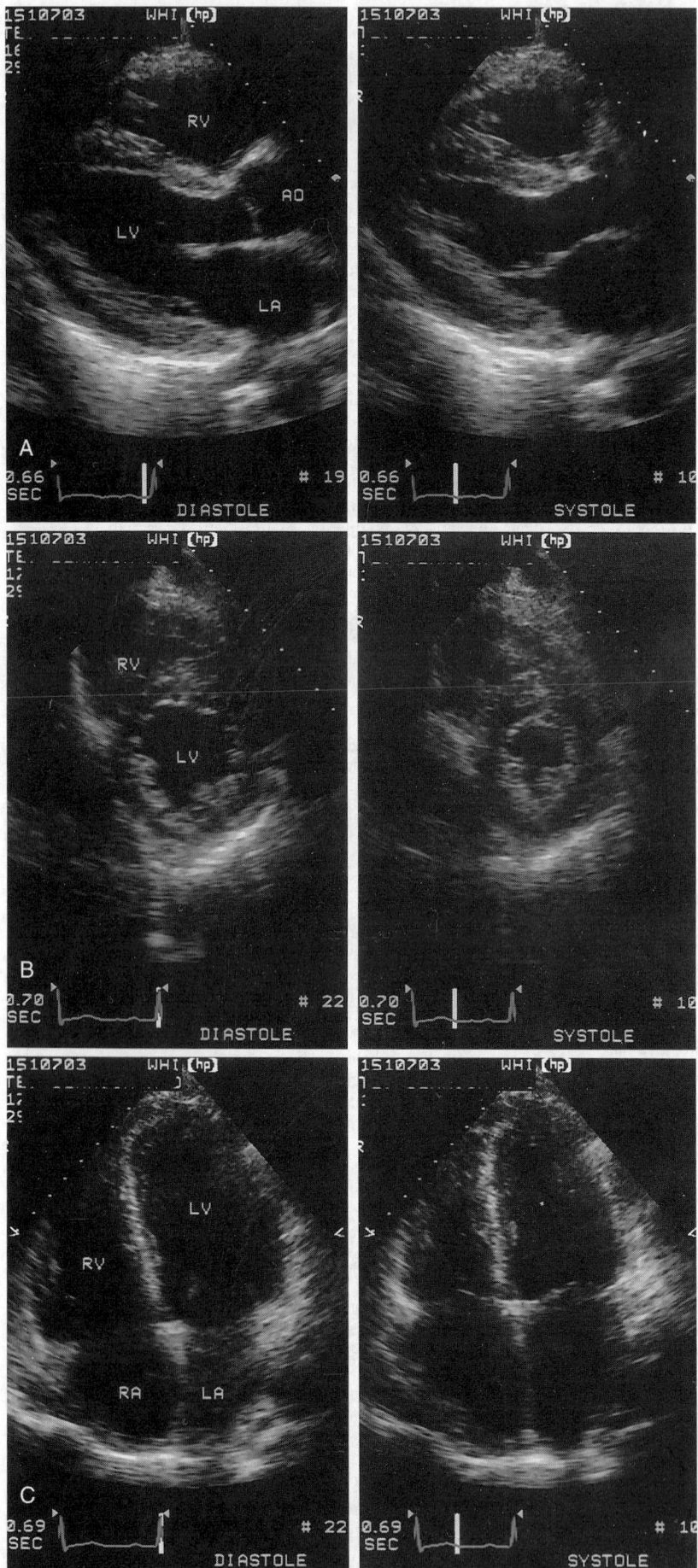

FIGURE 43–1 ■ Normal two-dimensional transthoracic echocardiogram in systole and diastole. A, With the transducer in the left parasternal location, images can be obtained parallel to the longitudinal axis of the left ventricle. This long-axis view depicts an elliptical left ventricle as visualized from the left shoulder, with the apex to the left and the base to the right. B, With the transducer in the left parasternal location, a perpendicular (short-axis) view of the left ventricle is obtained. The left ventricle appears as a circular cross-section in the short-access view. C, Positioning the transducer at the apical impulse provides images of the perimeter of all four cardiac chambers and both the mitral and tricuspid valves (four-chamber view).

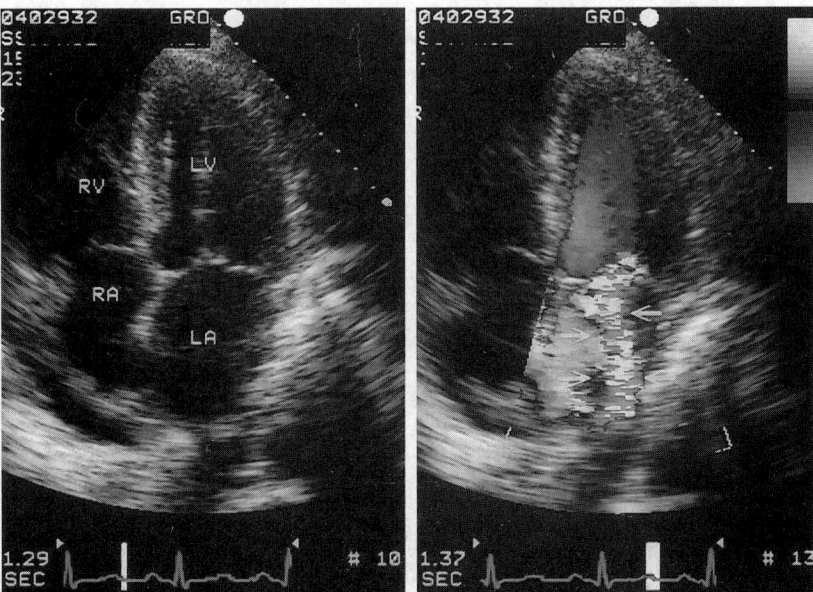

FIGURE 43–2 ■ Mitral regurgitation. The four-chamber apical view in systole is demonstrated with (left panel) and without (right panel) superimposed color Doppler flow imaging. A clear-cut mitral regurgitant jet can be seen emanating from a pre-acceleration area in the mitral orifice and penetrating backward into the left atrium (arrows). LV = left ventricle; LA = left atrium; RA = right atrium.

electrocardiography in the identification of CAD, yields similar results to radionuclide techniques, and provides prognostic information (see Chapter 44).

Documentation of enhanced contraction of hypokinetic or akinetic segments by cardiac ultrasound in response to low-dose inotropic stimulation with dobutamine is a good marker of viable myocardium, especially when high-dose stimulation induces recurrent contractile dysfunction.

Cardiomyopathy

Primary disease of the myocardium independent of other cardiovascular structures such as coronary arteries or valves (cardiomyopathy) has multiple causes, is often idiopathic, and is generally a diagnosis of exclusion. Echocardiography forms the cornerstone of the diagnostic strategy for cardiomyopathy (see Chapter 64). The approach aims first to classify the pathophysiology of the disorder as dilated (myocyte necrosis, profound dilation, and systolic dysfunction), hypertrophic (disproportionate septal thickening, obstructive or non-obstructive), or restrictive (generalized wall thickening with both systolic and diastolic impairment). Classification is based on LV cavity size, wall thickness, and systolic contraction. Dilated

cardiomyopathy (Fig. 43–3) is characterized by dilation, near-normal wall thickness, and severe global hypokinesis. Hypertrophic cardiomyopathy may be concentric hypertrophy (Fig. 43–4) or asymmetrical septal hypertrophy (Fig. 43–5) with normal contraction and often LV outflow tract obstruction due to systolic anterior movement of the mitral valve. Restrictive cardiomyopathy is characterized by generalized wall thickening, modest generalized hypokinesis, and evidence of impaired diastolic function. Causes associated with dilated myopathy include infection, inflammation, toxins, collagen vascular disease, and musculoskeletal disease. Hypertrophic cardiomyopathy is familial, whereas restrictive cardiomyopathy is associated with infiltrative processes such as amyloidosis and hemochromatosis. Echocardiography can establish and assess the severity of cardiomyopathy in nearly all cases, although cardiac catheterization or biopsy is occasionally necessary.

Echocardiography plays a particularly important role in hypertrophic obstructive cardiomyopathy. Because asymmetrical septal hypertrophy and systolic anterior motion are fundamental manifestations of the disorder and are best detected by tomographic techniques, echocardiography is the modality of choice for diagnosis. The presence of mitral regurgitation and extent of hypertrophy can

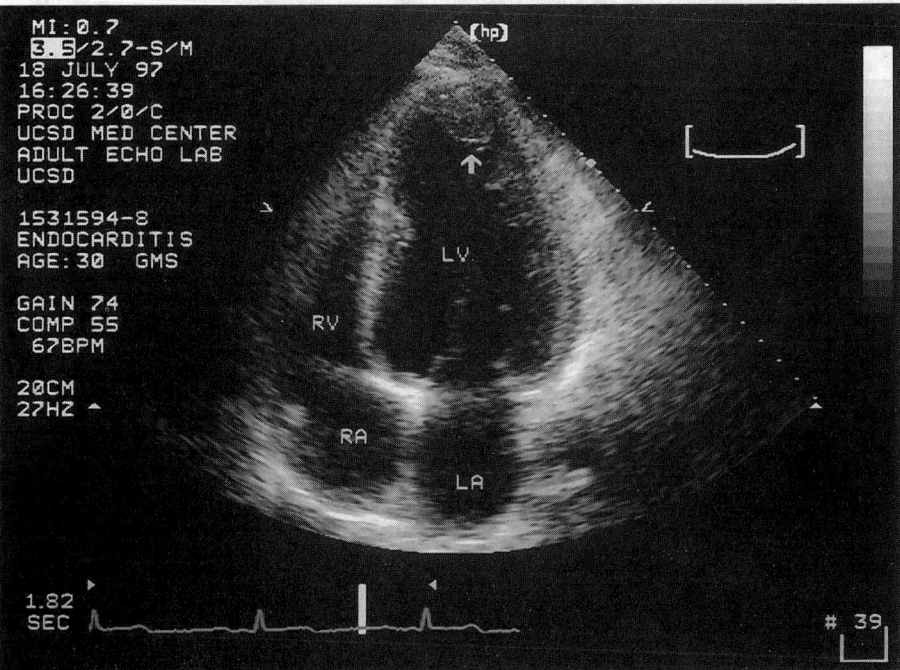

FIGURE 43–3 ■ Dilated left ventricle with clot. An apical view of a four-chamber echocardiogram in a patient with dilated cardiomyopathy. The left ventricle is enlarged and spherical; a thrombus is seen at the cardiac apex (arrow). LV = left ventricle; LA = left atrium; RA = right atrium.

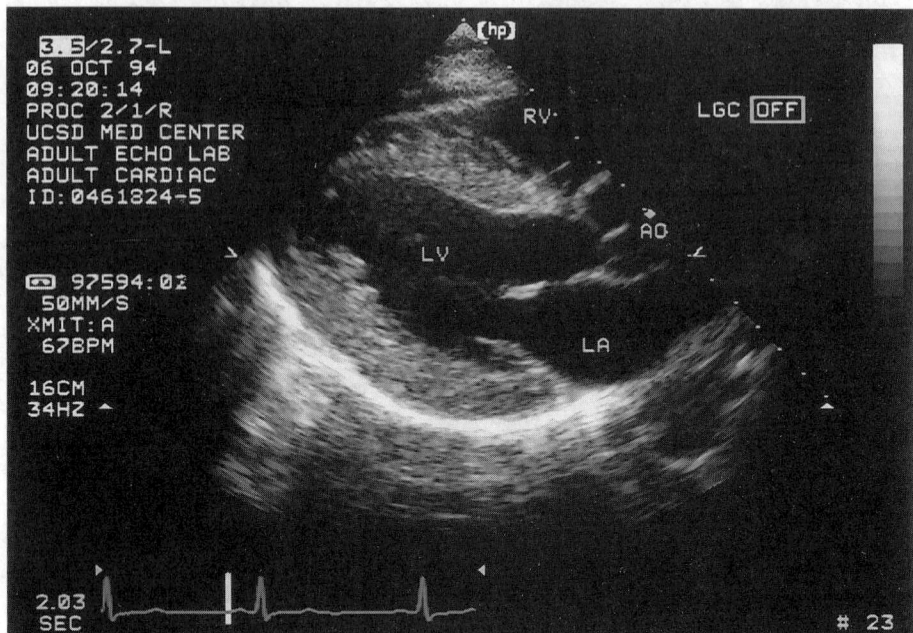

FIGURE 43-4 ■ Concentric hypertrophy. The parasternal long-axis view obtained in a patient with concentric hypertrophy due to systemic hypertension. The distance between calibration dots on the right is 10 mm so the wall thickness is 13 mm for both the septum and the posterior wall. Ao = aorta.

also be defined. In addition, echocardiography can detect dynamic subvalvular obstruction and quantify the gradient by virtue of the Bernoulli approach.

Congenital Heart Diseases

Congenital heart diseases represent fundamental distortions of cardiac anatomy (see Chapter 57). Echocardiography is a particularly valuable technique to assess these disorders and has largely eliminated the need for cardiac catheterization. Echocardiography can distinguish the anatomic right ventricle from the left ventricle by the presence of a moderator band, coarser trabeculae, an infundibulum, and an atrioventricular valve positioned closer to the cardiac apex. An oval orifice is readily identified by echocardiography in patients with bicuspid aortic valves. Atrial septal defects are characterized by right ventricular enlargement and paradoxical anterior motion of the septum in systole; in the absence of pulmonary

hypertension, both the orifice and shunt of an atrial septal defect may be visualized by two-dimensional echocardiography and color Doppler imaging. In ventricular septal defects, the primary presentation often consists of shunt flow depicted by color Doppler imaging. Measurement of cardiac chamber size and pulmonary artery pressure enables a comprehensive evaluation of these disorders.

Cardiac Masses

Echocardiography is the modality of choice for the diagnosis and evaluation of cardiac mass lesions such as tumors and clots (see Fig. 43-3). Cardiac masses must be distinguished from ultrasonic artifacts, which manifest inappropriate motion, lack border definition, and are often unattached to a cardiac surface.

Cardiac thrombi may be located in the left atrium or left ventricle. Most left atrial clots are due to atrial fibrillation or mitral valve disease and are found in the left atrial appendage, which is not well

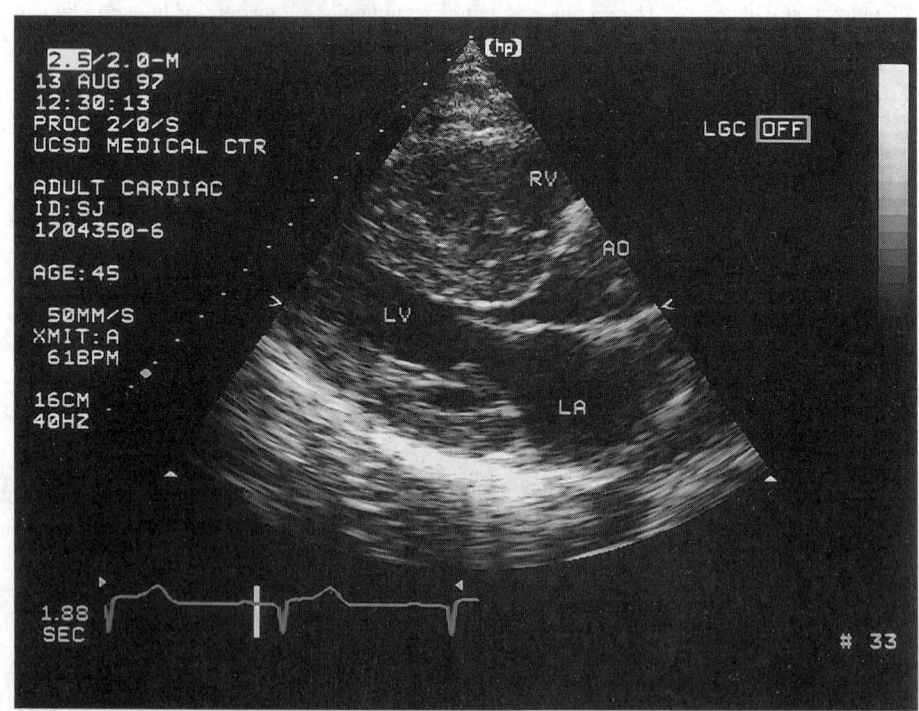

FIGURE 43-5 ■ Hypertrophic cardiomyopathy. The parasternal long-axis view obtained in a patient with hypertrophic cardiomyopathy in diastole. As can be seen, the thickness of the interventricular septum exceeds that of the posterior basal left ventricular wall by a factor of 2.

FIGURE 43–6 ■ Echocardiographic approach to cardiomegaly. The initial step in the evaluation of a patient with evidence of cardiomegaly involves examining the echocardiogram to determine whether the enlargement is due to pericardial effusion or whether it involves the right ventricle or left ventricle alone or in combination. If isolated right ventricular enlargement is present, the potential causes are enumerated. If left ventricular enlargement is found, the physician must next determine whether there are associated structural abnormalities such as valvular or congenital heart disease. If no associated anatomic abnormalities are present, the observation of segmental dyssynergy points strongly toward underlying coronary artery disease. If generalized global dyssynergy is present, the echocardiogram should distinguish the presence or absence of increased wall thickening. Conditions associated with increased wall thickening include infiltrative processes associated with restrictive cardiomyopathy and hypertrophy associated with hypertension or hypertrophic cardiomyopathy. A dilated left ventricle with global dyssynergy in the absence of hypertrophy may represent dilated cardiomyopathy or generalized left ventricular dysfunction due to widespread coronary artery disease (sometimes referred to as ischemic cardiomyopathy).

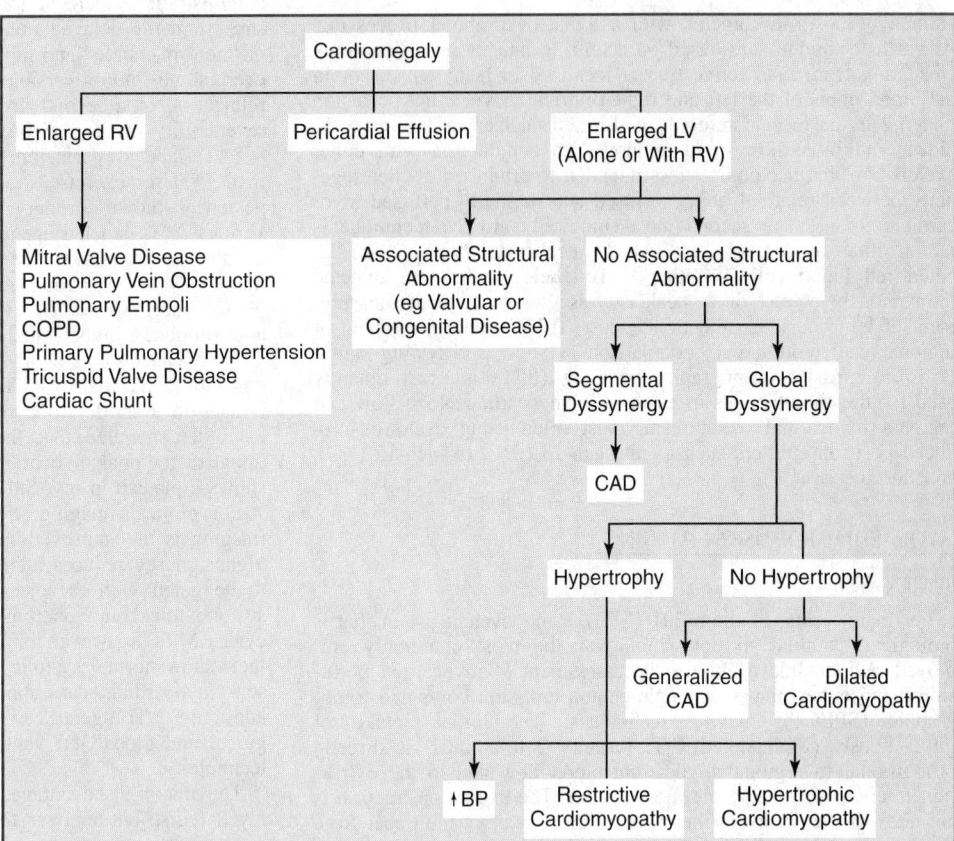

visualized by transthoracic echocardiography. Therefore, left atrial clots are best evaluated by transesophageal echocardiography, which may also detect spontaneous contrast due to extreme stasis of blood flow. Conversely, LV thrombi are characteristically caused by coronary artery disease or cardiomyopathy, are located in the LV apex, and are easily identified by transthoracic echocardiography. The presence of wall motion abnormalities helps distinguish these lesions from artifacts. An increase in the size and mobility of thrombi on an echocardiogram appears to increase the risk of embolization.

Cardiac tumors (see Chapter 70) occur uncommonly and may be intracavitary or intramural. Myxoma, the most common form of cardiac tumor, is located in the atrium in over 75% of cases. Left atrial myxoma is usually manifested by the presence of a pedicle and broad movement into and out of the mitral valve orifice during diastole and systole, respectively. Intramyocardial tumors typically present as asymmetrical localized thickening of one area of the ventricular wall.

Pericardial Disease

Pericarditis often occurs in the absence of any detectable abnormalities on an echocardiogram and is usually recognized only when accompanied by effusion, which is readily identified as a clear space surrounding the heart between epicardium and pericardium (see Chapter 65). The severity of pericardial effusion may be generally assessed by the size of the space and the presence of right ventricular and right atrial compression. However, optimal evaluation of the physiologic significance of pericardial effusion is obtained by demonstrating a greater than 25% decrease in transmitral flow velocity during inspiration by Doppler. On occasion, fibrin strands, clots, or tumors may be visualized in the fluid. Echocardiography also provides an excellent guide for performing pericardiocentesis by identifying the site of the greatest fluid accumulation.

Pericardial constriction is both less common and less well detected by echocardiography than is effusion. Although cardiac ultrasound may occasionally provide evidence of pericardial thickening or calcification, it is not as accurate for this purpose as is computed tomography. The predominant abnormality observed with constric-

tive pericarditis is inappropriate septal motion (perhaps due to restrained cardiac movement) and a greater than 20% variation of peak transmitral velocity with respiration. As with other manifestations of constrictive pericarditis, these findings may also be seen in severe chronic obstructive pulmonary disease.

Unexplained Cardiomegaly

Echocardiography is the procedure of choice to evaluate unexplained cardiomegaly detected by chest radiography (Fig. 43–6). It can readily discriminate a large left ventricle, with or without right ventricular enlargement, and detect pericardial effusions. Echocardiography is also very helpful in determining the causes of enlargement of the left and right ventricles.

ACC/AHA Practice Guidelines. ACC/AHA Guidelines for the Clinical Application of Echocardiography: Executive Summary: A report of the American College of Cardiology/American Heart Association Task Force on Practice Guidelines (Committee on Clinical Application of Echocardiography). J Am Coll Cardiol 29:862–879, 1997. *Consensus guidelines for appropriate ordering of echocardiograms.*

Otto C (ed): The Practice of Clinical Echocardiography. Philadelphia: WB Saunders, 1997. *A comprehensive textbook.*

44 NUCLEAR CARDIOLOGY AND COMPUTED TOMOGRAPHY

George A. Beller

NUCLEAR CARDIOLOGY

The techniques of nuclear cardiology permit the non-invasive imaging of the myocardium and cardiac blood pools under stress and resting conditions using radionuclide imaging agents and gamma or positron cameras with associated computer processing. All such techniques are based on acquiring images of radioactivity emanating from radioactive tracers localized in heart muscle or in the blood pools of the left and right ventricle. Myocardial perfusion imaging is the most commonly performed nuclear cardiology technique, and it is most often employed in conjunction with either exercise or pharmacologic stress intended to produce flow heterogeneity between relatively hypoperfused and normally perfused myocardial regions. The second most commonly utilized technique is radionuclide angiography, in which technetium-99m (^{99m}Tc)–labeled red blood cells or other ^{99m}Tc-labeled agents are injected intravenously at rest or at peak exercise for subsequent measurement of left ventricular ejection fraction (LVEF) and assessment of regional wall motion with comparison of stress and resting states. Positron emission tomographic imaging (PET) is predominantly used for the simultaneous assessment of myocardial blood flow and regional myocardial metabolism, most often using cyclotron-produced positron emitters such as nitrogen-13 (^{13}N), oxygen-15 (^{15}O), and fluorine-18 (^{18}F).

MYOCARDIAL PERFUSION IMAGING

Imaging Agents

For many years, thallium-201 (^{201}Tl), a monovalent cation that is biologically similar to potassium, was the most commonly employed radionuclide agent for the assessment of myocardial perfusion using either planar or single-photon emission computed tomographic (SPECT) imaging techniques. The initial uptake of intravenously administered ^{201}Tl (usually 2 to 3 mCi) is directly proportional to regional myocardial blood flow and to the extraction fraction of ^{201}Tl by the myocardium. The extraction fraction is an index of the ability of the myocardium to extract the tracer from the blood pool in the first pass through the coronary circulation. The extraction fraction for ^{201}Tl under normal conditions is approximately 85%. After the initial phase of myocardial uptake, there is continuous exchange of myocardial ^{201}Tl and ^{201}Tl in the blood pool that recirculates from the systemic compartment. ^{201}Tl is continually washed out of normally perfused myocardium and replaced by circulating ^{201}Tl from residual activity in the blood compartment. This process of continuous exchange forms the basis of the phenomenon of ^{201}Tl "redistribution," which is defined as total or partial reversibility (i.e., resolution) of initial post-stress defects by

the time of repeat imaging at 3 to 4 hours after initial tracer administration. Defects that show no redistribution between the stress and the delayed images are designated as being "persistent" or "non-reversible" and most often represent myocardial scar. However, some "non-reversible" defects at 4 hours will resolve with reinjection of a second dose of ^{201}Tl in the resting state. Delayed reversibility suggests viable but underperfused myocardium.

^{99m}Tc-labeled perfusion agents now are more commonly used than ^{201}Tl for exercise stress testing to evaluate patients with suspected or known coronary heart disease (CHD) (Fig. 44–1). Of the various ^{99m}Tc-labeled agents, ^{99m}Tc-sestamibi and ^{99m}Tc-tetrofosmin are the most common. ^{99m}Tc-sestamibi, an isonitrile, is superior in many ways to ^{201}Tl for myocardial perfusion imaging. The 140-keV photon energy peak of ^{99m}Tc is optimal for gamma camera imaging and produces higher quality images than those generated using ^{201}Tl. Because of its short half-life (6 hours), 10 to 15 times larger doses of ^{99m}Tc than of ^{201}Tl can be administered, yielding superior images in a shorter time period. Experimental and clinical studies have demonstrated that the uptake of ^{99m}Tc-sestamibi is proportional to regional myocardial blood flow, and, like ^{201}Tl, this agent shows a plateau in myocardial uptake at hyperemic flows.

For clinical imaging, the major advantage of ^{99m}Tc perfusion imaging is the improved specificity for detecting CHD because its higher energy reduces attenuation artifacts and permits the images to be gated with the electrocardiogram (ECG) to assess regional systolic thickening on tomographic images throughout the cardiac cycle. Mild non-reversible defects that represent attenuation artifacts show normal systolic thickening, whereas if such areas represent myocardial scar, abnormal thickening will be observed. In addition, ^{99m}Tc agents can provide simultaneous assessment of regional and global left ventricular function using the gated SPECT technology.

The major disadvantage of ^{99m}Tc-sestamibi is its negligible delayed redistribution over time after a single intravenous injection; as a result, separate stress and rest injections must be administered to identify regions of reversible myocardial ischemia. Some laboratories employ dual-isotope rest ^{201}Tl/stress ^{99m}Tc-sestamibi imaging in which patients undergo ^{201}Tl imaging at rest and then immediately afterward undergo ^{99m}Tc-sestamibi imaging during stress. Reversibility is identified by comparing the perfusion pattern on the stress ^{99m}Tc-sestamibi images with the pattern on the baseline resting ^{201}Tl images. The major advantage of this technique is the marked decrease in imaging time.

Quantitation of SPECT perfusion images also enhances accuracy

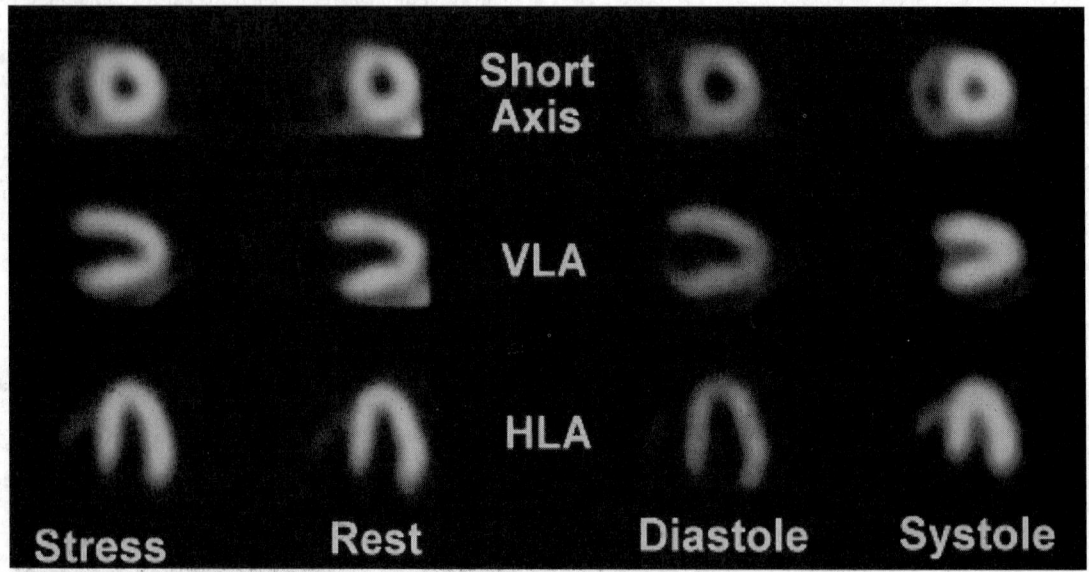

FIGURE 44–1 ■ Stress and rest SPECT studies (left two columns) in a normal patient, showing representative short-axis, vertical long-axis (VLA), and horizontal long-axis (HLA) images. Note the uniform uptake of ^{99m}Tc-sestamibi on both the stress and the rest tomograms consistent with homogeneous regional myocardial blood flow. The right two columns show the end-diastolic and end-systolic images acquired during stress and demonstrate uniform systolic thickening in all myocardial segments. The left ventricular cavity size is greater on images acquired during diastole compared with systole, consistent with a normal left ventricular ejection fraction. The "brightness" of the images at end-systole correlates directly with the degree of systolic thickening.

for differentiating artifacts due to attenuation or variants of normal from defects due to regional myocardial underperfusion. One quantitative approach utilizes polar maps or "bull's-eye plots" in which circumferential maximal count profiles of short-axis slices of the left ventricle are converted into polar coordinate profiles. The apex is in the center of the map, and the base of the left ventricle is depicted at the outer edge, yielding a two-dimensional representation of three-dimensional image information. Alternatively, regional tracer activity can be expressed as a percent of peak activity, which is normalized to 100%. Images from an individual patient are compared with a normal database for detection of significant perfusion abnormalities.

Detection of Coronary Heart Disease (Table 44-1)

Exercise or pharmacologic stress ^{201}Tl or ^{99m}Tc-sestamibi SPECT imaging in patients with chest pain yields a sensitivity for detecting CHD in the 85% to 90% range. The specificity for excluding CHD is in the 85% range for ^{99m}Tc-sestamibi SPECT imaging and increases to 90% using gated images. Both exercise or pharmacologic SPECT ^{201}Tl and exercise or pharmacologic SPECT ^{99m}Tc perfusion imaging have sensitivities and specificities that are superior to exercise ECG testing alone. Radionuclide stress perfusion imaging is of particular value compared with exercise ECG testing alone in (1) patients with resting ECG abnormalities such as those seen with left ventricular hypertrophy, digitalis effect, Wolff-Parkinson-White syndrome, and intraventricular conduction abnormalities; and (2) patients who fail to achieve more than 85% of maximum predicted heart rate. Approximately 40% of patients with a low-to-intermediate pretest likelihood of CHD who manifest ST-segment depression have no evidence for CHD (false-positive findings). The addition of stress perfusion imaging can assist in differentiating true-positive from false-positive exercise-induced ST-segment depression.

Pharmacologic Stress Imaging

Certain patients are unable to exercise to adequate heart rates and workloads on exercise stress testing protocols. In these patients, pharmacologic stress testing using vasodilators such as dipyridamole or adenosine, or inotropic agents such as dobutamine or arbutamine, is an alternative to exercise for detecting physiologically significant coronary artery stenoses. The basis for vasodilator perfusion imaging relates to the concept of coronary flow reserve. When blood flow is maximally increased with an intravenously administered vasodilator, an impairment in the flow reserve capacity in a stenotic artery compared with the large flow increase in a normal non-stenotic vascular bed results in a "relative" inhomogeneity of myocardial perfusion between normal and stenotic beds. If ^{201}Tl or ^{99m}Tc-sestamibi is injected during peak vasodilation in the

presence of a hemodynamically significant coronary stenosis with reduced flow reserve, a heterogeneity of tracer uptake will be observed as defects on post-stress images acquired soon after tracer injection. Sensitivity and specificity for CHD detection are comparable for dipyridamole and adenosine. Dobutamine stress is preferred in patients who have bronchospasm or a history of asthma or who have consumed caffeine, which is an adenosine receptor antagonist, within 12 hours before testing. Patients who experience side effects such as hypotension and chest pain during dipyridamole or adenosine infusion should be treated with intravenous aminophylline, an adenosine antagonist that immediately reverses these side effects.

Assessment of Prognosis

One of the chief applications of stress myocardial perfusion imaging is the identification of patients at either high or low risk for future ischemic cardiac events. Numerous studies have shown that the extent of hypoperfusion on post-stress SPECT perfusion images provides important incremental prognostic information when added to clinical variables, the resting LVEF, exercise ECG stress test variables, and even coronary artery anatomy. Patients with chest pain and a normal myocardial perfusion scan at peak exercise or under vasodilator stress have a subsequent cardiac event rate of less than 1% per year and are generally appropriate candidates for medical therapy. Conversely, patients with high-risk imaging results (Table 44-2), such as depicted in Figure 44-2, may benefit from

Table 44-2 ■ HIGH-RISK RESULTS IN EXERCISE MYOCARDIAL PERFUSION SCANNING

Abnormal regional perfusion in regions supplied by two or more coronary arteries (e.g., defects in the left anterior descending artery and left circumflex artery territories)

Extensive reversible defects, even if only in the region of one major coronary artery (e.g., defects in the anterior wall, septum, and apex corresponding to the left anterior descending coronary artery territory)

Large defect size (>20% of the left ventricular myocardium) on quantitative single-photon emission computed tomography

Increased lung thallium-201 uptake best assessed by quantitating the lung:heart thallium-201 ratio

Transient ischemic left ventricular cavity dilation in the stress as compared with the resting state

Adapted with permission from Beller GA: Radionuclide perfusion imaging techniques for evaluation of patients with known or suspected coronary artery disease. Adv Intern Med 42:139, 1997.

Table 44-1 ■ RADIONUCLIDE TESTING TO DIAGNOSE ISCHEMIC HEART DISEASE

INDICATION	TEST	CLASS
1. Diagnosis of symptomatic and selected patients at high risk for asymptomatic myocardial ischemia	Exercise or pharmacologic myocardial perfusion imaging, including PET*	I
	Exercise RNA	IIa
2. Assessment of ventricular performance (rest or exercise)	RNA†	I
	Gated sestamibi imaging	IIb
3. Assessment of myocardial viability in patients with left ventricular dysfunction in planning revascularization	Rest-distribution Tl-201 imaging	I
	Stress-redistribution-reinjection Tl-201 imaging	I
	PET imaging with FDG	I
	Dobutamine RNA	IIb
	Post-exercise RNA	IIb
	Post-NTG RNA	IIb
4. Planning PTCA—identifying lesions causing myocardial ischemia, if not otherwise known	Exercise or pharmacologic myocardial perfusion imaging	I
	Exercise RNA	IIa
5. Risk stratification before noncardiac surgery	Pharmacologic or exercise perfusion imaging	I
6. Screening of asymptomatic patients with low likelihood of disease	All tests	III

Class I = usually appropriate and considered useful; class II = acceptable but usefulness less well established; class IIa = weight of evidence in favor of usefulness; class IIb = can be helpful but not well established by evidence; class III = generally not appropriate.

*The relative cost of positron emission computed tomography (PET), thallium (Tl)-201 or technetium (Tc)-99m agents and lesser availability of PET must be considered when selecting this technique.

†RNA can be accomplished by first-pass imaging of a technetium-based myocardial perfusion agent.

FDG = ^{18}F-2-deoxyglucose; RNA = radionuclide angiography; NTG = nitroglycerine; PTCA = percutaneous transluminal coronary angioplasty.

Adapted with permission from Ritchie JL, Bateman TM, Bonow RO, et al: Guidelines for clinical use of cardiac radionuclide imaging. Report of the American College of Cardiology/American Heart Association Task Force on Assessment of Diagnostic and Therapeutic Cardiovascular Procedures (Committee on Radionuclide Imaging), developed in collaboration with the American Society of Nuclear Cardiology. J Am Coll Cardiol 25:521–547, 1995.

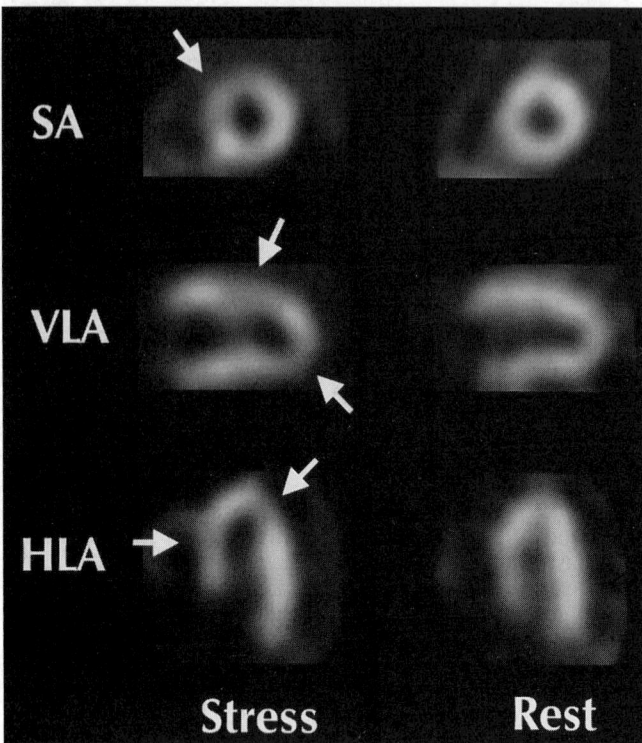

FIGURE 44–2 ■ Stress and rest single-photon emission computed tomographic ^{99m}Tc-sestamibi images obtained in a patient with chest pain. There is a significant decrease in ^{99m}Tc-sestamibi uptake in the anterior wall, septum, inferior wall, and apex consistent with extensive stress-induced ischemia. The resting study shows the reversibility of defects in all these regions. This patient also demonstrated more than 2.0 mm of horizontal ST-segment depression at 4 minutes of exercise on the Bruce protocol. Abbreviations are the same as in Figure 44–1.

early referral for invasive strategies, including revascularization, even if symptoms are mild.

Exercise or pharmacologic stress perfusion imaging also provides useful prognostic information for predischarge risk stratification in patients who have experienced an uncomplicated myocardial infarction. Demonstration of defects remote from the zone of infarction, which indicate underlying multivessel disease, evidence for residual ischemia within the infarct zone, or both, identify patients with an increased risk of reinfarction and subsequent cardiac death. Patients with only a non-reversible defect within the zone of infarction have a better long-term outcome unless the total defect size exceeds 15% of the left ventricular myocardium.

Patients with peripheral vascular disease may be limited by claudication and not manifest exertional angina despite substantial CHD. Preoperative pharmacologic stress perfusion imaging offers a non-invasive strategy for the detection of physiologically important coronary stenoses that may be associated with an increased risk of early and late cardiac events after peripheral vascular or aortic surgery. Patients who benefit most from preoperative risk assessment utilizing pharmacologic stress perfusion imaging are those at an intermediate risk of having underlying CHD based on clinical and resting ECG variables. Patients with evidence for inducible ischemia on preoperative perfusion imaging likely will benefit from improved preoperative medical therapy and may also benefit from coronary angiography and coronary revascularization performed before the planned elective vascular surgical operation.

Determination of Myocardial Viability with SPECT or PET imaging

SPECT perfusion imaging, particularly with ^{201}Tl, is performed only in the resting state to identify residual myocardial viability in zones corresponding to severe regional wall motion abnormalities in patients with CHD and depressed left ventricular function. When severe left ventricular dysfunction is caused by "hibernation,"

which is a state of chronic reduced contractility because of substantial ischemia, and not by irreversible myocardial necrosis, ^{201}Tl uptake is preserved at rest. ^{201}Tl is injected at rest, and images are acquired 10 minutes and 4 hours later. Areas of resting hypoperfusion that are viable and contributing to hibernation will show initial defects on early images and delayed redistribution or mild non-reversible defects on delayed images. If ^{201}Tl uptake ultimately exceeds 50% of peak uptake in these regions, there is a 70% to 75% probability that regional myocardial function will improve after successful revascularization. Controversy still exists with respect to the value of resting ^{99m}Tc-sestamibi or ^{99m}Tc-tetrofosmin imaging for determination of viability.

Regional myocardial metabolism can be non-invasively assessed utilizing PET tracers such as ^{18}F-2-deoxyglucose (FDG) or carbon-11 (^{11}C)-acetate. FDG is a glucose analogue that is initially taken up in myocardial cells and is trapped by conversion to FDG-6 phosphate. FDG is impermeable to the cell membrane and remains within viable cells at high concentrations for more than 40 to 60 minutes. The magnitude of FDG activity on PET images is indicative of the rate of myocardial glucose consumption. Under conditions of hibernation, increased FDG uptake reflects substrate utilization in the glycolytic pathway. Increased FDG activity on clinical PET images in areas of diminished regional blood flow as determined by ^{13}N ammonia imaging is characteristic of myocardial viability. Such areas of blood flow/FDG mismatch usually demonstrate improved regional function after coronary revascularization. Regions of the heart that show both diminished ^{13}N uptake and FDG uptake (a "match" pattern) represent predominantly non-viable myocardium, and such segments have only a 10% to 15% probability of demonstrating improved systolic function after revascularization. The clearance of ^{11}C acetate after intravenous injection is reflective of oxidative metabolism. Under conditions of ischemia and diminished oxidative metabolism, ^{11}C acetate clearance is prolonged.

Patients with CHD with predominantly viable myocardium as the cause of left ventricular dysfunction have better survival and more improvement of heart failure symptoms after revascularization compared with patients whose left ventricular dysfunction is caused by extensive regions of scar, who do not benefit from revascularization and should be treated medically and, if necessary, with cardiac transplantation. The non-invasive determination of myocardial viability in patients with CHD and very low LVEF, with or without signs and symptoms of heart failure, is often helpful in choosing therapeutic options (Fig. 44–3).

IMAGING OF VENTRICULAR FUNCTION

Global and segmental ventricular function can be accurately evaluated using gated cardiac blood pool imaging with either the *first-pass* method or the *equilibrium* method to provide a radionuclide angiogram or ventriculogram. Ventricular volumes both at rest and during exercise, as well as right and left ventricular ejection fractions, can be measured. A uniform diminution of left ventricular systolic function without segmental wall motion abnormalities suggests non-ischemic dilated cardiomyopathy, whereas depressed global left ventricular function associated with segmental wall motion abnormalities suggests ischemic heart disease.

For these radionuclide angiographic techniques, the optimum blood pool label is one that is specific for the patient's own red blood cells. Red blood cells can be labeled—in vivo or in vitro—with ^{99m}Tc. For the in vivo technique of labeling red blood cells, unlabeled stannous pyrophosphate that is reconstituted in normal saline is injected intravenously 15 to 10 minutes before injection of 15 to 30 mCi of ^{99m}Tc pertechnetate. This process results in the appropriate labeling of the blood pools of the left and right ventricle to be imaged with a gamma camera.

First-pass radionuclide angiography analyzes rapidly acquired image frames to observe the fate of a bolus of ^{99m}Tc as it traverses the venous system to the right side of the heart, pulmonary artery, lungs, left atrium, and left ventricle. Several cardiac cycles can be sampled continuously as the bolus of ^{99m}Tc passes through the right and then the left ventricles. Time-activity curves are generated by measuring radioactive counts in the blood pools over time. Ejection fraction values are obtained by dividing the stroke counts (end-

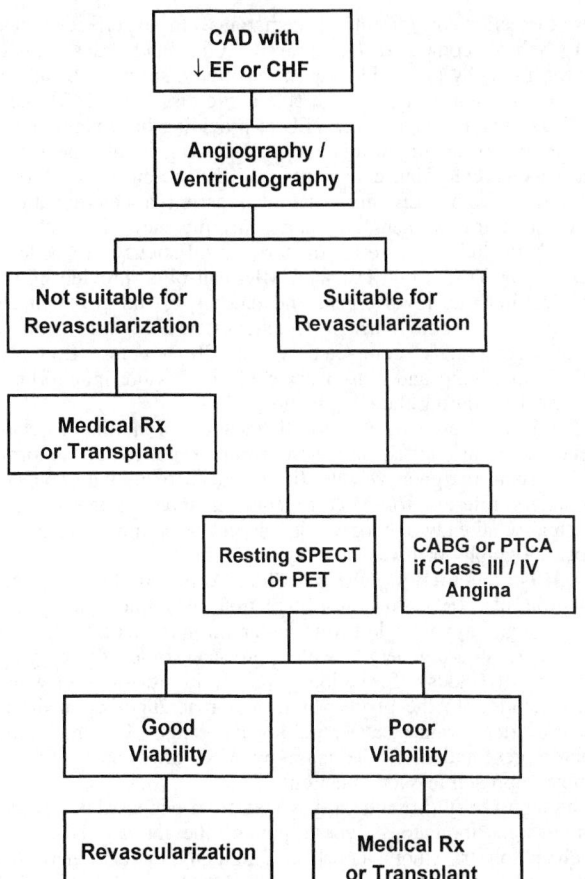

FIGURE 44–3 ■ Decision-making algorithm for the assessment of patients with ischemic cardiomyopathy. All such patients should undergo coronary angiography and ventriculography, and those patients not suitable for revascularization should undergo vigorous medical treatment and subsequent transplantation if criteria for such an intervention are met. In patients whose coronary vessels are suitable for revascularization, a resting single-photon emission computed tomographic (SPECT) study, positron emission tomographic (PET) study, or low-dose dobutamine echocardiogram can help identify hibernating but viable myocardium that may benefit from coronary revascularization. In contrast, patients with poor viability in areas of abnormal myocardial function would best be treated medically or considered for cardiac transplantation. An exception to this strategy is in patients who have severe angina and who usually should undergo revascularization to alleviate symptoms and improve quality of life without a prior assessment of myocardial viability. EF = ejection fraction; CHF = congestive heart failure; CABG = coronary artery bypass graft surgery; PTCA = percutaneous transluminal coronary angioplasty; Rx = prescription/treatment.

diastolic counts minus end-systolic counts) by the end-diastolic counts. It is also possible to estimate end-systolic and end-diastolic volumes. The *first-pass* radionuclide angiography approach is well suited for detection of left-to-right intracardiac shunts (see Chapter 57). First-pass radionuclide angiography can also be determined immediately after the injection of ^{99m}Tc-sestamibi or ^{99m}Tc-tetrofosmin, thereby permitting the immediate assessment of left ventricular function as well as assessment of myocardial perfusion.

The *equilibrium* radionuclide angiographic approach is performed after thorough mixing of ^{99m}Tc-labeled blood cells within the intravascular compartment. Because the ^{99m}Tc remains within the blood pool, serial imaging studies can be acquired over several hours. Acquisition of the images is synchronized with the QRS complex on the ECG through a multigated approach by which each cardiac cycle is divided into multiple frames. From the frame images accumulated during multiple cardiac cycles, both regional wall motion and global left ventricular function can be evaluated in a cine mode.

A non-imaging nuclear probe or "nuclear stethoscope" can be used for the continuous monitoring of left ventricular function. This miniaturized device is placed over the region of the left ventricle on the chest wall and yields time-activity curves for each cardiac cycle from which ejection fractions can be calculated. No images are generated. Recently, an ambulatory variant of this nuclear probe has been introduced to permit continuous ambulatory monitoring of left ventricular function during activity.

ULTRAFAST COMPUTED TOMOGRAPHY

Ultrafast computed tomography (CT), also referred to as electron-beam CT (EBCT), images calcification associated with atherosclerotic plaques in coronary arteries. Autopsy studies have shown a significant relationship between the amount of calcium deposited in coronary arteries and the severity of underlying coronary atherosclerotic disease. Ultrafast CT can accurately measure coronary calcification with a high degree of reproducibility (Fig. 44–4). Ultrafast CT scanning can identify obstructive coronary disease with an approximate 75% sensitivity and 80% specificity in *symptomatic* patients. However, the extent of calcification does not correlate with stenosis severity, although it does predict an increased risk of future cardiac events. Furthermore, about 50% of soft plaques without calcification on intracoronary ultrasound will be missed by ultrafast CT. The most likely future clinical application of ultrafast CT may be to diminish greatly the likelihood of significant CHD in asymptomatic patients younger than 60 years of age with multiple risk factors for CHD; in this setting, however, it is not clear whether ultrafast CT will be preferable to exercise electrocardiography or exercise or stress perfusion scintigraphy. Ultrafast CT may also be useful for detecting myocardial fat infiltration and diagnosing arrhythmogenic right ventricular dysplasia.

CONVENTIONAL COMPUTED TOMOGRAPHIC SCANNING

Perhaps the most frequently used clinical application of conventional CT imaging in patients with cardiovascular disease is the assessment of disorders of the aorta, such as suspected dissecting aortic aneurysm (see Chapter 66). Conventional CT with contrast medium enhancement has a high sensitivity for diagnosing an aneurysm, can accurately measure its diameter, and can determine the

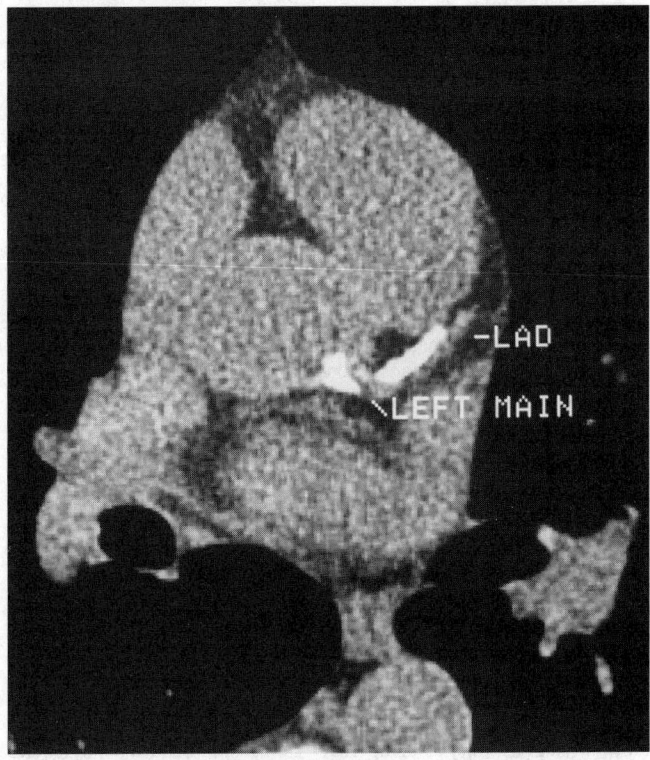

FIGURE 44–4 ■ Example of an electron beam CT scan (ultrafast CT) showing heavy calcium deposits in the left main and left anterior descending (LAD) coronary arteries. (Courtesy of Alan D. Guerci, M.D., The Heart Center, St. Francis Hospital, Roslyn, NY.)

presence or absence of intraluminal thrombus. CT is also highly accurate for identifying the intimal flap and differentiating the true from the false lumen. Conventional CT can accurately detect pericardial cysts, neoplastic pericardial infiltration, pericardial effusion, and pericardial thickening as seen in chronic constrictive pericarditis.

Achenbach S, Moshage W, Ropers D, et al: Value of electron-beam computed tomography for the noninvasive detection of high-grade coronary-artery stenoses and occlusions. N Engl J Med 339:1964–71, 1998. *Electron-beam CT may be useful to detect or rule out high-grade coronary-artery stenoses and occlusions.*

Arad Y, Spadaro LA, Goodman K, et al: Predictive value of electron beam computed tomography of the coronary arteries: 19-month follow-up of 1173 asymptomatic subjects. Circulation 93:1951, 1996.

Beller GA: Radionuclide perfusion imaging techniques for evaluation of patients with known or suspected coronary artery disease. Adv Intern Med 42:139, 1997.

Hachamovitch R, Berman DS, Kiat H, et al: Exercise myocardial perfusion SPECT in patients without known coronary artery disease: Incremental prognostic value and use in risk stratification. Circulation 93:905, 1996.

Hendel RC, Chaudhry FA, Bonow RO: Myocardial viability. Curr Probl Cardiol 21:145, 1996.

Ritchie JL, Bateman TM, Bonow RO, et al: Guidelines for clinical use of cardiac radionuclide imaging. Report of the American College of Cardiology/American Heart Association Task Force on Assessment of Diagnostic and Therapeutic Cardiovascular Procedures (Committee on Radionuclide Imaging), developed in collaboration with the American Society of Nuclear Cardiology. J Am Coll Cardiol 25:521–547, 1995.

Taillefer R, DePuey EG, Udelson JE, et al: Comparative diagnostic accuracy of Tl-201 and Tc-99m sestamibi SPECT imaging (perfusion and ECG-gated SPECT) in detecting coronary artery disease in women. J Am Coll Cardiol 29:69, 1997.

45 CARDIAC MAGNETIC RESONANCE IMAGING

Warren J. Manning

More than any other imaging technique, cardiac magnetic resonance imaging (MRI) offers the promise of dramatically changing our choice of technologies to evaluate patients with known or suspected cardiac disease. The combined attributes of superior image quality and flexibility for assessment of cardiac anatomy, ventricular function, great vessel and coronary blood flow, and myocardial perfusion give MRI tremendous potential for evaluation of the cardiovascular system. Although current clinical applications of MRI are limited to relatively specific conditions (Table 45–1), rapid evolution of the technology over the past decade will probably continue and thereby further define the expanding clinical role of cardiac MRI. Given the relative cost disadvantage of MRI in comparison to other non-invasive technologies such as ultrasound and nuclear cardiology, MRI's clinical role will probably depend on strategies that eliminate the need for other imaging tests such as echocardiography or diagnostic coronary angiography.

The most common imaging approaches are the spin-echo (black blood) and gradient-echo (bright blood with areas of turbulence depicted as regions of low signal intensity) techniques. For cardiac MRI applications, electrocardiographic (ECG) gating is almost always essential. Spin-echo imaging is commonly used to assess cardiac anatomy, whereas gradient-echo imaging is more commonly used for cine-imaging (e.g., ventricular and valvular function). Exogenous intravenous contrast (gadolinium-diethylenetriamine pentaacetic acid) may be helpful in some situations but is generally not needed for most current cardiac applications.

THORACIC AORTA AND GREAT VESSELS. Over the past decade, cardiac MRI has had its greatest clinical impact on assessment of the thoracic aorta in patients with known or suspected thoracic aortic aneurysm or aortic dissection (Fig. 45–1). Transverse, coronal, and sagittal images using ECG gating spin-echo techniques are typically acquired. The "sine qua non" of aortic dissection (see Chapter 66) is the identification of an intimal "flap" separating the true and false lumens. Cine gradient-echo imaging is often obtained to define flap mobility and blood flow in both lumens. Eccentric aortic wall thickening may also be seen and possibly represents an

early dissection or intramural hematoma. In experienced hands, MRI, helical computed tomography (CT), and transesophageal echocardiography (TEE) have high sensitivity, specificity, and accuracy for the identification of thoracic aortic dissection. MRI and CT have specific advantages over TEE in providing information regarding the full extent of the dissection, including involvement of the great vessels, entry and exit points, and the presence of a thrombosed lumen. Both TEE and MRI also permit a determination of aortic valve involvement and aortic insufficiency, although valve morphology and the severity of aortic insufficiency are better appreciated by TEE. Both TEE and MRI can often provide information regarding the involvement and patency of the proximal coronary arteries. With current techniques, MRI assessment can generally be safely completed within 30 minutes. Both ECG rhythm monitoring and non-invasive blood pressure monitoring are recommended during the examination.

MRI is also quite useful for delineation of aortic coarctation, patent ductus arteriosus, and more complex congenital abnormalities involving the great vessels. In general, patients with congenital lesions are referred for MRI to confirm and/or better define an abnormality already identified or suspected on prior imaging by echocardiography or invasive x-ray angiography.

CARDIAC TUMORS AND MASSES. Although the high spatial resolution of MRI allows for depiction of intracavitary tumors/masses (e.g., myxoma, left ventricular thrombi) (see Chapter 70), these "masses" are generally well appreciated by echocardiographic methods. MRI adds information primarily in situations in which a mass extends into the myocardium and/or neighboring mediastinal structures (e.g., venae cavae, pulmonary veins). The three-dimensional representation of the mass by MRI often helps guide the surgical approach in such situations.

Although rarely difficult to diagnose from echocardiographic images, benign lipomatous hypertrophy of the interatrial septum as visualized on transthoracic echocardiography or TEE may sometimes lead to the misdiagnosis of an atrial septal "tumor." The characteristic, very intense signal from fatty tissue readily allows for the MRI diagnosis of this benign disorder.

PERICARDIUM AND PERICARDIAL EFFUSIONS. The normal pericardium is seen as a thin black line between visceral and parietal pericardial fat on spin-echo MRI. Normal pericardial thickness is 0.8 to 2.6 mm. In patients with constrictive cardiomyopathy, the thickened pericardium is readily appreciated by MRI. CT is also valuable in this situation and is better for specific assessment of pericardial *calcifications* (see Chapters 64 and 65). It should be remembered, however, that although both MRI and CT will accurately quantify focal pericardial thickening, the presence of thickened pericardium is not diagnostic of constrictive physiology.

CONGENITAL HEART DISEASE. MRI is quite useful for the as-

Table 45–1 ■ CURRENT CLINICAL APPLICATIONS FOR CARDIAC MRI

1. Diagnosis and serial evaluation of thoracic aorta
   Aneurysm
   Dissection
   Hematoma
   Coarctation
2. Assessment of simple and complex congenital heart disease
   Spatial relationships of aorta, pulmonary arteries, cardiac chambers, venous system
   Identification of anomalous coronary arteries
   Quantitation of intracardiac shunt
3. Quantitation of ventricular volumes, ejection fraction, mass
   Quantitative left and right ventricle volumes, ejection fraction, mass
   Regional and global systolic function
4. Primary or secondary cardiac tumors
   Especially tumors that involve extracardiac structures
5. Pericardial disease
   Constriction
   Pericardial effusions—especially loculated effusions
6. Assessment of specific cardiomyopathies
   Hypertrophic cardiomyopathy—distribution of hypertrophy
   Sarcoidosis
   Hemochromatosis
   Right ventricular dysplasia
7. Future
   Coronary artery integrity
   Atherosclerotic plaque
   Myocardial perfusion

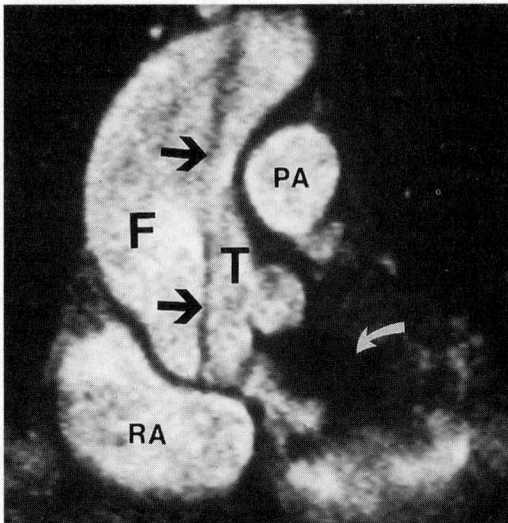

FIGURE 45-1 ■ Ascending aortic dissection: coronal orientation, gradient-echo sequence. Note that the dissection flap (black arrows) begins immediately superior to the aortic valve leaflet. Flow (white signal) is seen in both the true (T) and false (F) lumen. Signal void (turbulence) is seen in the left ventricular cavity immediately below the aortic valve and is caused by associated aortic insufficiency (curved white arrow). PA = pulmonary artery. RA = right atrium.

sessment of both simple and complex congenital heart disease (see Chapter 57). Although atrial septal defects and ventricular septal defects in adults are generally well appreciated by transthoracic echocardiography and/or TEE, phase-contrast MRI can be quite valuable in quantifying the ratio of pulmonary to systemic flow. MRI is particularly valuable for assessing congenital heart disease outside the cardiac chambers, such as aortic coarctation or anomalous pulmonary venous drainage, and in patients with complex congenital heart disease who have undergone corrective or palliative surgery.

Although MRI assessment of the native coronary arteries for obstructive disease remains to be defined, the newer breath-hold segmented gradient-echo methods readily identify anomalous coronary arteries (Fig. 45–2) (see Chapter 57). While uncommon, with a prevalence of only 1 to 2%, an anomalous vessel that courses between the aorta and pulmonary artery is associated with an in-

creased risk of sudden death and myocardial infarction in young adults. Even among patients with anomalous coronary arteries identified by invasive x-ray angiography, the course of the anomalous vessel may be misinterpreted because of the projection method, thus making MRI a preferred technique.

QUANTITATIVE ASSESSMENT OF VENTRICULAR VOLUMES AND MASS. Although rarely used clinically because of its relative cost disadvantage in comparison with echocardiography or radionuclide angiography, MRI is considered the "gold standard" for the *quantitative* assessment of left and right ventricular volumes and ejection fraction, as well as regional systolic function. When compared with echocardiography, which has suboptimal results in a substantial number of patients, breath-hold cine-MRI can be readily performed in nearly all patients in less than 10 minutes. Semiautomated methods allow for delineation of the endocardial and epicardial borders with very high accuracy/reproducibility and for determination of ventricular volumes, stroke volume, and ejection fraction. MRI may be especially valuable for eliciting quantitative information regarding left ventricular mass and regression of hypertrophy in response to antihypertensive therapy or aortic valve replacement. The accurate evaluation of *right* ventricular volumes and ejection fraction is also relatively unique to MRI.

CARDIOMYOPATHIES. The ability of MRI to acquire images of the entire heart in true tomographic planes makes it ideal for the evaluation of patients with hypertrophic cardiomyopathies, especially patients with focal hypertrophy. Investigative MRI "tagging" methods may also be helpful in the further assessment of patients with hypertrophic cardiomyopathy, but this application remains to be more fully elucidated.

In specific conditions, cardiac MRI is also useful in the assessment of patients with dilated cardiomyopathy. In addition to biventricular volumetric and mass data, MRI may confirm excess iron deposition as the cause of depressed systolic function in a patient with suspected hemochromatosis. With spin-echo imaging, depressed myocardial signal intensity correlates with systolic function, as well as the severity of iron deposition. In contrast, focal signal enhancement may be found with other diseases such as sarcoidosis or myocarditis. In the absence of clinical suspicion, however, routine MRI in dilated cardiomyopathy is currently not suggested.

Spin-echo MRI can be used to identify transmural or focal fatty infiltration in the right ventricular free wall (Fig. 45–3) of patients with suspected right ventricular dysplasia, a condition associated with ventricular arrhythmias and sudden death and in which the right ventricular free wall myocardium is diffusely or focally replaced with fatty or fibrous tissue (see Chapters 52 and 57). Asso-

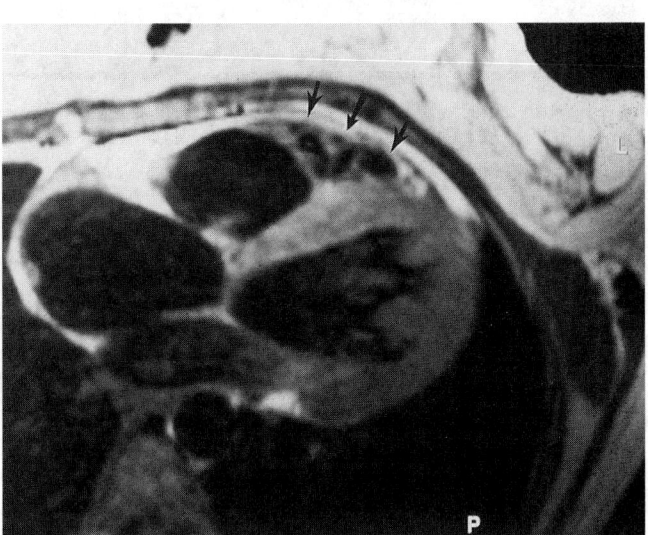

FIGURE 45-2 ■ Anomalous left coronary artery: transverse image, gradient-echo sequence. The normal right coronary artery (white arrow) may be seen with the anomalous left coronary artery (black arrow) traversing between the aorta (Ao) and right ventricular outflow tract (RVOT).

FIGURE 45-3 ■ Transverse spin-echo magnetic resonance image acquired during ventricular systole in a patient with right ventricular dysplasia (RVD). Note the mildly dilated right ventricular cavity. The right ventricular free wall (arrows) is thin with enhanced/bright signal within the wall consistent with fatty replacement. (Courtesy of J.P. Ridgway and U.M. Sivananthan, Leeds General Infirmary, Leeds, England.)

ciated focal wall thinning and systolic dysfunction are also often present.

SPECIAL CONSIDERATIONS FOR MRI IN CARDIAC PATIENTS. In addition to general restrictions regarding MRI (intracranial clips, transcutaneous electrical nerve stimulation units, intra-auricular implants, etc.), special considerations are also needed when performing MRI in cardiac patients. Nearly all current clinical cardiac MRI uses ECG gating to minimize artifacts (blurring) related to bulk cardiac motion. Although the presence of an irregular rhythm (atrial fibrillation, frequent ventricular or atrial ectopic activity) is not a contraindication to MRI, image quality is often suboptimal in these settings and alternative imaging methods should be considered.

MRI is considered safe for both bioprosthetic and mechanical heart valves (except for pre–series 6000 Starr-Edwards prostheses), but signal loss and image distortion will occur in the region immediately surrounding the prosthesis. Similarly, sternotomy wires and thoracic vascular clips are not a contraindication to imaging, but localized artifacts are common.

Patients with cardiac pacemakers and automatic implantable cardiodefibrillators should *not* undergo MRI because of concern regarding pacemaker reprogramming, direct stimulation of the heart during gradient switching, and/or localized heating in the lead system. Similarly, patients with pulmonary artery catheters that include pacing or thermistor wires should not undergo MRI.

Hundley WG, Li HF, Lange RA, et al: Assessment of left-to-right intracardiac shunting by velocity-encoded, phase-difference magnetic resonance imaging. A comparison with oximetric and indicator dilution techniques. Circulation 91:2955, 1995. *Demonstration of MR quantitation of pulmonary:systemic flow in 21 patients with intracardiac shunts.*

Magnetic resonance imaging. *In* Marcus: Cardiac Imaging, 2nd ed. Philadelphia, WB Saunders, 1996, pp 629–792. *Excellent overview of basic MR principles, contrast agents, and clinical applications of MRI to the cardiovascular system.*

McConnell MV, Ganz P, Selwyn AP, et al: Identification of anomalous coronary arteries and their anatomic course by magnetic resonance coronary angiography. Circulation 92:3158, 1995. *Report demonstrating the clinical utility of MR coronary angiography in patients with suspected anomalous coronary anatomy.*

Nagel E, Lehmkuhl HB, Bocksh W, et al: Noninvasive diagnosis of ischemia-induced wall motion abnormalities with the use of high-dose dobutamine stress MRI: comparison with dobutamine stress echocardiography. Circulation 99:763–770, 1999. *Identifies role for MRI.*

Shellock FG, Kanal E: Bioeffects and safety of MR procedures. *In* Edelman RR, Hesselink JR, Zlatkin MB (eds): Clinical Magnetic Resonance Imaging, 2nd ed. Philadelphia, WB Saunders, 1996, pp 391–434. *Excellent review of contraindications to MR scanning, including tables and references for many prostheses, implanted clips, etc.*

Weisskoff RM, Edelman RR: Basic principles of MRI. *In* Edelman RR, Hesselink JR, Zlatkin MB (eds): Clinical Magnetic Resonance Imaging, 2nd ed. Philadelphia, WB Saunders, 1996, pp 3–51. *Very good review of MR physics.*

46 CATHETERIZATION AND ANGIOGRAPHY

David P. Faxon

Cardiac catheterization and angiography provide the detailed assessment of both anatomy and physiology of the heart and vasculature and are the gold standard for assessment of cardiac disease. The technique was first applied to humans by Werner Forssmann in 1929, but it was expanded into a diagnostic tool by Andre Cournard and Dickinson Richards; in 1956, all three shared the Nobel Prize for their discovery. Selective coronary angiography was introduced by Mason Sones in 1963 and further modified by Melvin Judkins. Cardiac catheterization is now the second most common operative procedure in the United States, with nearly 2 million procedures performed per year.

INDICATIONS. Cardiac catheterization is most commonly performed to determine the nature and extent of a suspected cardiac problem in a symptomatic patient in whom surgical or interventional therapy is anticipated (Table 46–1). It is also used to exclude the presence of significant disease when findings from other modalities, such as stress testing or echocardiography, are equivo-

Table 46–1 ▪ INDICATIONS FOR CARDIAC CATHETERIZATION AND ANGIOGRAPHY

I. Coronary Artery Disease
  A. Asymptomatic or symptomatic
    1. High risk for adverse outcome based on non-invasive testing
    2. After resuscitation from cardiac arrest or sustained ventricular tachycardia
  B. Symptomatic
    1. Severe angina on medical therapy
    2. Unstable angina (high or intermediate risk)
    3. Acute myocardial infarction
      a. Primary reperfusion with angioplasty
      b. Recurrent ischemic episodes during hospitalization
      c. Shock or hemodynamic instability
      d. Mechanical complications such as mitral regurgitation or ventricular septal defect
    4. Chest pain of uncertain origin and non-invasive testing is equivocal
    5. High-risk patients undergoing non-cardiac surgery

II. Valvular Heart Disease
  A. Aortic stenosis
    1. Symptomatic patients (angina, heart failure, syncope) with suspected severe aortic stenosis
    2. Hypertrophic cardiomyopathy with angina
  B. Aortic regurgitation
    1. Symptomatic patients (angina, heart failure, syncope) with suspected severe aortic regurgitation
    2. Asymptomatic patients with progressive cardiac enlargement or reduction of ejection fraction
  C. Mitral stenosis
    1. Symptomatic patients (dyspnea, heart failure, emboli) with suspected severe mitral stenosis
  D. Mitral regurgitation
    1. Symptomatic patients (dyspnea, heart failure, emboli) with suspected severe mitral regurgitation

III. Other
  A. Congenital heart disease
    1. Before cardiac surgery or percutaneous correction
  B. Pericardial disease
    1. Symptomatic patients with suspected constrictive pericarditis or tamponade
  C. Vascular disease
    1. Aortic dissection or aneurysm with suspected concomitant coronary disease
  D. Congestive heart failure
    1. New onset
    2. Suspected to be secondary to coronary artery disease
  E. Cardiac transplantation
    1. Presurgical and postsurgical evaluation

Adapted from American College of Cardiology/American Heart Association Ad Hoc Task Force on Practice Guidelines: ACC/AHA Guidelines for Coronary Angiography. Circulation 99:2345–2357, © 1999. Reproduced with permission.

cal or when the patient continues to be severely symptomatic and a definitive diagnosis is important in the patient's management.

Because coronary angiography is the only technique capable of accurately defining the severity and extent of coronary disease, it is essential in the assessment of patients being considered for revascularization. If coronary disease is unlikely and non-invasive testing can accurately define the cardiac abnormality, then cardiac catheterization may not be necessary in young adults or children with simple congenital anomalies, such as atrial septal defect, or young adults with valvular heart disease, such as aortic stenosis or mitral stenosis. Even then, valuable prognostic information often can be gathered from the hemodynamic measurements at the time of cardiac catheterization.

CONTRAINDICATIONS AND RISKS. The risks of cardiac catheterization and coronary angiography are low, with a 0.05% risk of myocardial infarction, 0.07% risk of stroke, and a reported mortality of 0.1%. These risks, however, are increased substantially in certain subsets of patients, such as those patients undergoing an emergency procedure, patients having an acute myocardial infarction, and patients who are hemodynamically unstable. In patients who require catheterization as a prelude to a potentially lifesaving intervention, there are no absolute contraindications, but relative contraindications include acute renal failure, pulmonary edema, bacteremia, acute stroke, active gastrointestinal bleeding, and documented anaphylactic reaction to contrast dye.

Of all the potential complications, contrast medium–induced allergic reactions and contrast medium–induced renal failure are particularly important because they are common, even in relatively healthy patients, and precautions can reduce these risks. For example, the frequency of allergic reactions is 5% and life-threatening anaphylactic reactions occur in 0.1% of angiographies. Pretreatment of patients with prior allergic reactions with corticosteroids, antihistamines, and H_2 antagonists can substantially reduce the risk of a subsequent reaction. Contrast medium–induced renal failure occurs in 3 to 7% of all patients but is most common in patients with diabetes and/or pre-existing renal failure, in whom the incidence is 12 to 30%. Preprocedural and postprocedural hydration for 12 hours with 0.5 normal saline at 50 mL/hour reduces the risk of subsequent renal failure. Diabetics on metformin should have the drug withdrawn 48 hours before the procedure to reduce the risk of contrast medium–induced lactic acidosis.

TECHNIQUE. Patients should be fasting and sedated, but awake, for the procedure. Antibiotics are not necessary. Oral anticoagulation should be stopped before the procedure, but emergent cardiac catheterization can be performed on full anticoagulation or even after the recent administration of thrombolytic agents.

VASCULAR ACCESS. The vast majority of procedures are performed percutaneously through the femoral artery and vein. A brachial (or radial or, rarely, axillary) approach is used when peripheral vascular disease precludes access from the lower extremity or when early ambulation after the procedure is critical. After the femoral approach, 4 to 6 hours of local compression and bed rest is desirable before the patient ambulates and is discharged.

RIGHT-SIDED HEART CATHETERIZATION. The most commonly used catheter is a balloon flotation catheter that is introduced into the femoral, brachial, subclavian, or internal jugular vein and then passed with or without fluoroscopic guidance into the right atrium, right ventricle, and pulmonary artery. If necessary, hemodynamic measurement of oxygen saturations can be obtained as the catheter is passed into the pulmonary artery. Once in the pulmonary artery, inflation of the balloon at the tip of the catheter occludes the smaller pulmonary arteries and allows for measurement of the pulmonary capillary wedge pressure, which is nearly always an accurate reflection of left atrial pressure. With a thermistor-tipped balloon, thermal dilution cardiac output can also be obtained.

LEFT-SIDED HEART CATHETERIZATION. The left-sided cardiac structures can be accessed from the femoral, brachial, radial, or axillary artery. The catheters are passed retrograde under fluoroscopic guidance into the ascending aorta. Because embolization of a clot from a catheter in the arterial circulation could lead to a stroke, heparin is frequently used. Hemodynamic measurements and oxygen saturations are also obtained.

Occasionally, left-sided heart catheterization can be accomplished by a needle-tipped catheter that punctures the atrial septum from the right atrial side to enter the left atrium; the needle is withdrawn, and the catheter is advanced to the left ventricle. This technique is reserved for situations in which the left ventricle cannot be accessed by the retrograde approach, such as in patients who have aortic valve prostheses, or when mitral valvuloplasty or invasive electrophysiology studies are being done.

HEMODYNAMIC ASSESSMENT. PRESSURE MEASUREMENTS. The measurement of intracardiac pressure is an essential component of cardiac catheterization and is performed through fluid-filled catheters that are attached to an external pressure transducer (Table 46–2). The shape and magnitude of the waveforms provide important diagnostic information. For example, an elevated mean right atrial pressure associated with a rapid y descent and an early rise (square root sign), with equalization of right atrial, right ventricular diastolic, left atrial, and left ventricular diastolic pressures is characteristic of *constrictive pericarditis. Cardiac tamponade* (see Chapter 65), on the other hand, results in equalization of diastolic chamber pressures but without a prominent y descent. A large v wave (two times greater than the mean pressure) in the right atrium or left atrium suggests severe *tricuspid* or *mitral regurgitation,* respectively. Simultaneous recording of pressures in the proximal and distal cardiac chambers can allow for assessment of valvular stenosis. For instance, a pressure gradient in diastole between the pulmonary capillary wedge or left atrial pressure and the left ventricle is found in patients with *mitral stenosis.* A gradient between the aorta and left ventricular systolic pressure is present when *aortic stenosis* (see Chapter 63) occurs (Fig. 46–1). Simultaneous measurement of blood flow is important in assessment of valvular disease. In the presence of regurgitation, an increasing gradient is

Table 46–2 ■ NORMAL HEMODYNAMIC MEASUREMENTS

	RANGE
Pressures (mmHg)	
Right heart	
Right atrium (mean, a wave, v wave)	0–5, 1–7, 1–7
Right ventricle (peak systole, end-diastole)	17–32, 1–7
Pulmonary artery (peak systole, diastole, mean)	17–32, 4–13, 9–19
Pulmonary capillary wedge (mean)	4–12
Left heart	
Left atrium (mean, a wave, v wave)	4–12, 4–15, 4–15
Left ventricle (peak systole, end-diastole)	90–140, 5–12
Aorta (peak systole, diastole, mean)	90–140, 60–90, 70–105
Cardiac Output and Resistances	
Cardiac index (L/min/m²)	2.8–4.2
Arteriovenous oxygen difference (vol%)	3.5–4.8
Systemic vascular resistance (dyne-sec-cm⁻⁵)	900–1400
Pulmonary vascular resistance (dyne-sec-cm⁻⁵)	40–120
Oxygen consumption (mL/min)	115–140

evident because of an increase in blood flow across the valve. When a premature ventricular contraction induces a large pressure gradient between the aorta and left ventricle as well as a reduction in pulse pressure in the aorta (Brockenbrough effect), *hypertrophic obstructive cardiomyopathy* (see Chapter 64) is suggested. *Severe aortic regurgitation* (see Chapter 63) causes an elevation in aortic systolic pressure, a fall in aortic diastolic pressure, and equalization of the end-diastolic pressures in the ventricle and aorta.

CARDIAC OUTPUT Cardiac output can be measured by the direct Fick method, by indicator dilution methods, or by angiographic techniques. The Fick method is the most accurate in low cardiac output states, whereas the indicator dilution method is most accurate in high output conditions. When an accurate assessment of cardiac output is essential (e.g., when assessing the degree of valvular stenosis), both Fick and indicator dilution techniques are frequently used. The Fick principle states that the amount of a substance taken up or released by an organ is the product of its blood flow and the arterial-venous difference in the concentration of the substance. Because oxygen can be reliably measured, the Fick method determines oxygen consumption by measuring inhaled and exhaled oxygen content and the arterial and venous blood oxygen content. The formula for calculating Fick cardiac output is:

$$\text{Cardiac output (L/min)} = \frac{\text{Oxygen consumption (mL } O_2/\text{min)}}{\text{Arterial-venous oxygen difference (vol \% } \times 10)}$$

where the arterial-venous oxygen difference = 1.39 (O_2 carrying capacity of blood) × hemoglobin (g/dL) × (arterial-oxygen saturation difference).

The indicator dilution method is based on the Stewart-Hamilton equation, in which cardiac output is determined by the following formula:

$$\text{Cardiac output} = \frac{I \times 60}{cm \times t}$$

where I = amount of indicator injected, 60 = sec/min, cm = mean indicator concentration (mg/L), and t = total indicator circulatory time in seconds. The indicator dilution method involves injection of a substance that can be measured in blood. The indicator is injected at one site and sampled at another. Because the completeness of the mixing of the indicator is critical, injection and sampling are optimally done in cardiac chambers that are not adjacent to each other, for example, injection into the right atrium and sampling in the pulmonary artery. Thermodilution techniques are most common: temperature is the indicator, and the mean change in temperature is the indicator concentration that is sampled distally. Because cardiac output varies with body size, it is customary to calculate the cardiac index (L/min/m²) by dividing cardiac output by body surface area.

VALVE AREAS AND RESISTANCES. The resistance to blood flow can be calculated in a manner similar to Ohm's law of electrical resistance, as the ratio of the mean pressure gradient to the flow.

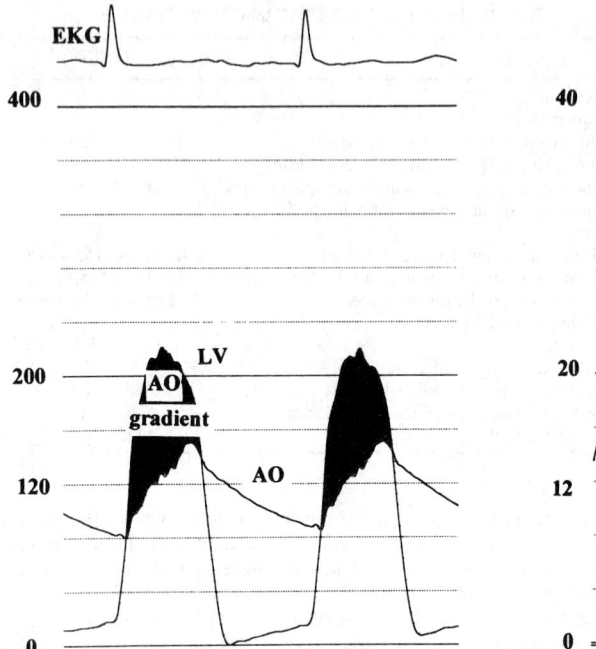

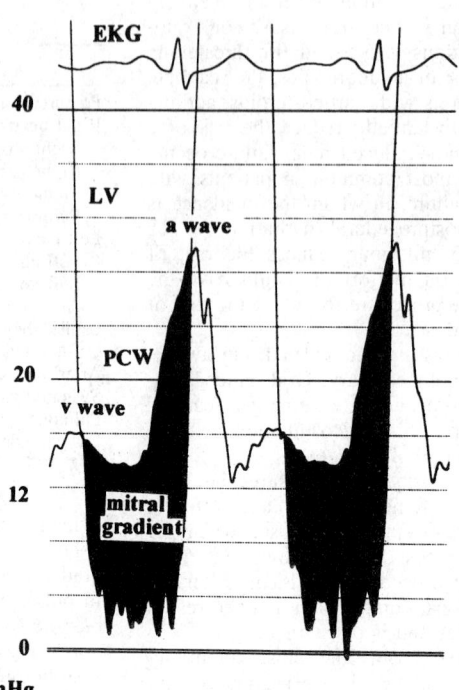

FIGURE 46–1 ■ Examples of the hemodynamic findings in aortic and mitral stenosis. In the left panel, simultaneous recording of aortic (AO) and left ventricular (LV) pressure shows a 50-mm Hg systolic pressure gradient. In the right panel, there is a 15-mm Hg diastolic gradient between the pulmonary capillary wedge pressure (PCW) and left ventricular pressure (LV). The a wave in the PCW tracing is larger than the v wave, indicating increased resistance to left ventricular filling in this patient.

$$\text{Resistance} = \frac{\text{Mean pressure gradient}}{\text{Mean flow}}$$

The resistance through the systemic circulation is calculated as the mean aortic pressure minus the mean right atrial pressure, divided by cardiac output, multiplied by 80 to convert to dynes-seconds-cm^{-5}. Likewise, pulmonary vascular resistance is calculated as mean pulmonary artery pressure minus mean pulmonary capillary wedge pressure multiplied by 80 divided by cardiac output. The valve area in stenotic valves is the inverse of resistance. The most commonly used formula for calculation of valve stenosis is the Gorlin formula, where K is the constant (44.3 for aortic valve and 37.7 for mitral valve).

$$\text{Valve area} = \frac{\text{Flow across the valve}}{K \times \sqrt{\text{valvular gradient}}}$$

Severe aortic stenosis is considered to be present when the mean valvular gradient is greater than 50 mm Hg and the aortic valve area is less than or equal to 0.8 cm^2. For the mitral valve, a valve area of less than 1.0 cm^2 is considered severe.

SHUNTS. Patients with known or suspected congenital heart disease (see Chapter 57) should have hemodynamic assessment and estimation of the location and degree of cardiac shunting if present. Estimation of the shunt can be made by changes in oxygen saturation, as well as by angiography. Measurement of oxygen saturation in each of the cardiac chambers and vessels can detect a "step up"

in oxygen content in the right side of the heart when a left-to-right shunt is present or a "step down" in the oxygen content in the left side of the heart when a right-to-left shunt is present. Systemic blood flow can be calculated by the Fick principle by obtaining oxygen saturations from the aorta and both venae cavae. Pulmonary blood flow is calculated using oxygen saturations from the pulmonary artery and left atrium. The shunt ratio (pulmonary blood flow: systemic blood flow) measures the severity of a shunt; for an atrial or ventricular septal defect, a shunt ratio of greater than 1.5 to 1 is considered significant.

CARDIAC ANGIOGRAPHY. Angiography is almost always performed during cardiac catheterization by injecting an iodine-containing radiopaque contrast agent. These agents are highly viscous and can cause cardiac arrhythmias and adverse hemodynamic changes due to ionic changes, volume expansion, and negative inotropic effects. Use of more expensive, low osmolar, non-ionic agents reduces these adverse effects.

AORTOGRAPHY. Aortography allows for the assessment of the aortic size and the extent of aortic regurgitation. It also determines the location of coronary bypass grafts, if present.

LEFT VENTRICULOGRAPHY. Left ventriculography is frequently performed with coronary angiography, because it allows for assessment of left ventricular size and function as well as the presence and extent of mitral regurgitation (Fig. 46–2). Left ventricular volume in end-diastole and end-systole can be calculated by the area-length method (normal = 70 ± 20 mL and 25 ± 10 mL, respectively). The difference between end-diastole and end-systole is the stroke volume. Cardiac output is calculated by multiplying the stroke volume times the heart rate. The ratio of angiographic stroke

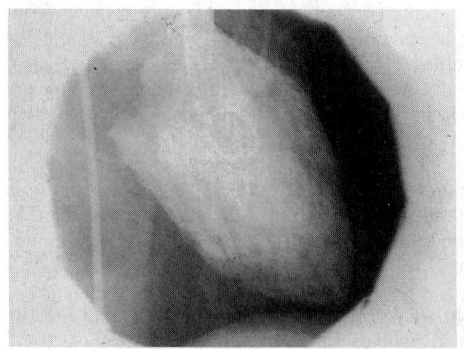

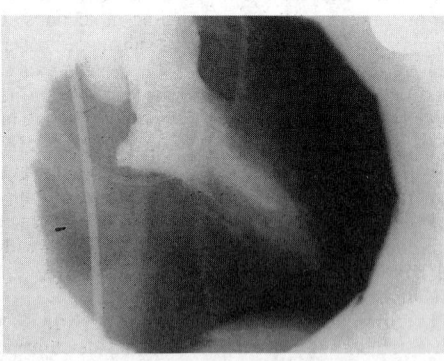

FIGURE 46–2 ■ An example of left ventriculography. The ventricular contour is seen in diastole in the left panel and in systole in the right panel.

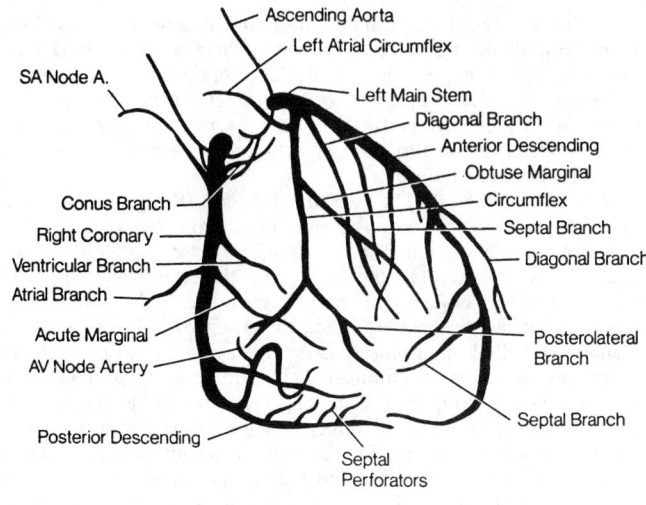

RAO

LAO

FIGURE 46–3 ■ The coronary vessels in the right and left anterior oblique view are shown. The major arteries are the left main, left anterior descending, circumflex, and right coronary arteries. (From Yang SS, Bentivoglio LG, Maranhao V, Goldberg H [eds]: From Cardiac Catheterization Data to Hemodynamic Parameters. © 1988. Used by permission of Oxford University Press, Inc.)

volume to end-diastolic volume is the ejection fraction, which is an estimate of contractile function. Normal ejection fraction ranges from 0.5 to 0.7. Wall motion abnormalities, which are usually indicative of coronary artery disease, can also be assessed during angiography and classified as hypokinetic (reduced motion), akinetic (no motion), or dyskinetic (paradoxical motion). Estimation of

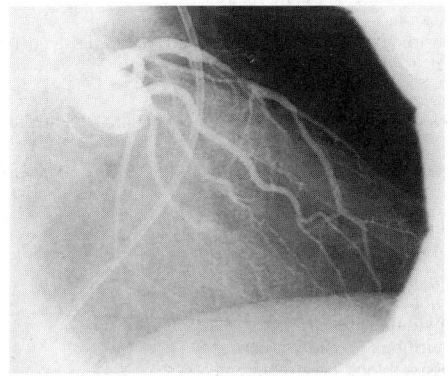

FIGURE 46–4 ■ An example of a significant stenosis in the left anterior descending coronary artery.

mitral regurgitation by angiography uses a semi-quantitative technique by which 1+ is minimal regurgitation into the left atrium in systole, 2+ is mild to moderate regurgitation of contrast to outline the left atrium, 3+ is moderate to severe regurgitation from which the left atrium becomes as dense as the left ventricle, and 4+ is severe regurgitation by which the left atrium becomes more dense than the left ventricle. Usually 3 to 4+ mitral regurgitation is considered to be of hemodynamic significance and a relative indication for mitral valve surgery.

CORONARY ANGIOGRAPHY. Coronary angiography defines the coronary anatomy, the degree of obstruction of the coronary arteries, and the states of any coronary artery bypass grafts by means of injection of a contrast agent selectively in the ostium of the right or left coronary artery or bypass conduit (Figs. 46–3 and 46–4). The degree of obstruction is expressed as the percent stenosis, which is the ratio of the most severely narrowed segment in any view compared with the "normal" proximal and/or distal segment. A narrowing of greater than 50% of the diameter is considered significant. Visual assessments can overestimate the severity of the stenosis, but quantitative techniques reduce the variability of the measurement. The normal coronary vasculature can be highly variable but generally includes three major vessels: left anterior descending, left circumflex, and right coronary artery, with the first two emanating from the left main artery. A *right dominant* circulation occurs when the posterior wall of the left ventricle is served by the right coronary artery, and a *left dominant* circulation when it is served by the left circumflex artery; it is *co-dominant* when served by both.

ADJUNCTIVE METHODS TO ASSESS CORONARY STENOSIS. Coronary angiography is limited to assessment of changes in the lumen diameter. Because atherosclerosis is a diffuse process, angiography can underestimate the severity of the disease and does not provide direct assessment of the physiologic significance of a stenosis. Intravascular ultrasound uses a small, flexible catheter with a 20- to 30-mHz transducer at its tip that can be passed over an angioplasty guidewire into the coronary artery. Accurate assessment of the degree of atherosclerosis and the percent stenosis can be obtained by this technique. Intracoronary Doppler flow measurements use a Doppler probe mounted on a small angioplasty-type guidewire. Measurement of the change in flow velocity before and after coronary vasodilation with agents such as adenosine can provide an estimate of coronary flow reserve and help assess the severity of the stenosis. A significant reduction in coronary flow reserve is present when the ratio of flow at rest to flow after vasodilation is less than 2:1. Measurement of blood flow velocity and coronary artery diameter before and after administration of acetylcholine can assess the possibility that coronary vasospasm or abnormalities in coronary endothelial function are present. Both intravascular ultrasound and Doppler flow studies are most commonly used in conjunction with interventional procedures.

American College of Cardiology/American Heart Association Ad Hoc Task Force on Practice Guidelines: ACC/AHA Guidelines for Coronary Angiography. Circulation 99:2345, 1999. *The most up-to-date review of coronary angiography and indications for the procedure.*

Baim DS, Grossman W (eds): Cardiac Catheterization, Angioplasty, and Intervention, 5th ed. Philadelphia, Williams & Wilkins, 1996. *A comprehensive text.*

Topol EJ (ed): Textbook of Cardiovascular Medicine. Philadelphia, Lippincott–Raven, 1998. *A comprehensive text.*

47 PATHOPHYSIOLOGY OF HEART FAILURE

Barry M. Massie

HEART FAILURE

DEFINITION. Heart failure is a heterogeneous syndrome in which an abnormality of cardiac function is responsible for the inability of the heart to pump blood at an output sufficient to meet the requirements of metabolizing tissues and/or to do so only at abnormally elevated diastolic pressures or volumes. The heart failure syndrome is characterized by (1) signs and symptoms of intravascular and interstitial volume overload, including shortness of breath, rales, and edema; and/or (2) manifestations of inadequate tissue perfusion, such as impaired exercise tolerance, fatigue, and renal dysfunction. Heart failure may occur as a result of impaired myocardial contractility (systolic dysfunction, characterized as reduced left ventricular ejection fraction), increased ventricular stiffness or impaired myocardial relaxation (diastolic dysfunction, which is often associated with a preserved left ventricular ejection fraction), a variety of other cardiac abnormalities (including obstructive or regurgitant valvular disease, intracardiac shunting, or disorders of heart rate or rhythm), or states in which the heart is unable to compensate for increased peripheral blood flow or metabolic requirements. In adults, left ventricular involvement is almost always present even if the manifestations are primarily those of right ventricular dysfunction (fluid retention without dyspnea or rales). Heart failure may result from an acute insult to cardiac function, such as a large myocardial infarction (MI), or more commonly, as a result of a chronic process. The focus in this chapter is on the syndrome of *chronic* heart failure, because the common causes, such as myocardial infarction (see Chapter 60), valvular disease (see Chapter 63), and myocarditis (see Chapter 64) as well as cardiogenic shock (see Chapter 95) are discussed elsewhere.

EPIDEMIOLOGY. Heart failure is growing in incidence and prevalence and is associated with rising mortality rates. Although these trends primarily reflect the strong association between heart failure and advancing age, they also are influenced by the rising prevalence of precursors such as hypertension, dyslipidemia, and diabetes in industrialized societies and the improved long-term survival of patients with ischemic and other forms of heart disease. The annual incidence of new cases of heart failure rises from less than 1/1000 patient-years below age 45, to 10/1000 above age 65, and as high as 30/1000 (3%) in individuals older than 85 years. Prevalence figures follow a similar exponential pattern, increasing from 0.1% below age 50 to 55 to nearly 10% above age 80. In the United States, there are an estimated 4.8 million heart failure patients, of whom approximately 75% are age 65 or older. Although the relative incidence and prevalence of heart failure are somewhat lower in women than men, women constitute at least half of the cases because of their longer life expectancy.

The prognosis of patients with heart failure remains poor despite advances in therapy. Of patients who survive the acute onset of heart failure, only 35% of men and 50% of women are alive after 5 years. Although it is difficult to predict prognosis in individual patients, patients with symptoms at rest (Class IV) have a 30 to 70% annual mortality rate, those symptomatic with mild activity (Class III) have mortality rates of 10 to 20% annually, and those with symptoms only with moderate activity (Class II) still have a 5 to 10% annual mortality rate. Mortality rates are higher in older patients, men, and those with reduced ejection fractions and underlying coronary heart disease. In the United States, nearly 1 million hospitalizations each year with a primary diagnosis of heart failure account for 6 million hospital days. The estimated cost of heart failure management ranges from $15 to 40 billion annually, depending on the formula used.

ETIOLOGY AND PREVENTION. Any condition that causes myocardial necrosis or produces chronic pressure or volume overload can induce myocardial dysfunction and heart failure. In developed countries, the causes of heart failure have changed greatly over the past several decades. Valvular heart disease, with the exception of calcific aortic stenosis, has declined markedly, whereas coronary heart disease has become the predominant cause in both men and women, being responsible for 60 to 75% of cases. Hypertension, although less frequently the primary cause of heart failure than in the past, continues to be a factor in 75%, including the majority of those with coronary disease.

Treatment of hypertension, with a focus on the systolic pressure, reduces the incidence of heart failure by 50%. Importantly, this intervention remains effective even in patients older than 75 years of age (see Chapter 55). Any intervention that reduces the risk of a first or recurrent MI will also reduce the incidence of heart failure

(see Chapter 39). For example, in post-MI patients, β-blockers, antihyperlipidemic agents, antithrombotic therapy, and coronary revascularization can prevent the development of heart failure. In patients with reduced ejection fractions, angiotensin-converting enzyme (ACE) inhibitors and β-blockers prevent or delay progressive left ventricular dysfunction and dilatation and, thereby, the onset or worsening of heart failure.

PATHOGENESIS. DIFFERING MECHANISMS OF HEART FAILURE. Heart failure is a syndrome that may result from many cardiac and systemic disorders (Table 47–1). Some of these disorders do not, at least initially, involve the heart, and therefore the term *heart failure* may be confusing. However, even the high output states may present as the classic findings of exertional dyspnea and edema—so-called *high-output heart failure*—that resolve if the underlying disorder is eliminated. If persistent, these conditions may secondarily impair myocardial performance as a result of chronic volume overload or direct deleterious effects on the myocardium. Other conditions, including the mechanical abnormalities, disorders of rate and rhythm, and pulmonary abnormalities, do not primarily affect myocardial function but are not infrequent causes of heart failure.

ABNORMALITIES OF CARDIAC FUNCTION. (Table 47–2) **Systolic**

Table 47–1 ▪ PATHOGENESIS OF HEART FAILURE

I. Impaired Systolic (Contractile) Function
  A. Ischemic damage or dysfunction
    1. Myocardial infarction
    2. Persistent or intermittent myocardial ischemia
    3. Hypoperfusion (shock)
  B. Chronic pressure overloading
    1. Hypertension
    2. Obstructive valvular disease
  C. Chronic volume overload
    1. Regurgitant valvular disease
    2. Intracardiac left-to-right shunting
    3. Extracardiac shunting
  D. Non-ischemic dilated cardiomyopathy
    1. Familial/genetic disorders
    2. Toxic/drug-induced damage
    3. Immunologically mediated necrosis
    4. Infectious agents
    5. Metabolic disorders
    6. Infiltrative processes
    7. Idiopathic conditions

II. Diastolic Function (Restricted Filling, Increased Stiffness)
  A. Pathologic myocardial hypertrophy
    1. Primary (hypertrophic cardiomyopathies)
    2. Secondary (hypertension)
  B. Aging
  C. Ischemic fibrosis
  D. Restrictive cardiomyopathy
    1. Infiltrative disorders (amyloidosis, sarcoidosis)
    2. Storage diseases (hemochromatosis, genetic abnormalities)
  E. Endomyocardial disorders

III. Mechanical Abnormalities
  A. Intracardiac
    1. Obstructive valvular disease
    2. Regurgitant valvular disease
    3. Intracardiac shunts
    4. Other congenital abnormalities
  B. Extracardiac
    1. Obstructive (coarctation, supravalvular aortic stenosis)
    2. Left-to-right shunting (patent ductus)

IV. Disorders of Rate and Rhythm
  A. Bradyarrhythmias (sinus node dysfunction, conduction abnormalities)
  B. Tachyarrhythmias (ineffective rhythms, chronic tachycardia)

V. Pulmonary Heart Disease
  A. Cor pulmonale
  B. Pulmonary vascular disorders

VI. High Output States
  A. Metabolic disorders
    1. Thyrotoxicosis
    2. Nutritional disorders (beri-beri)
  B. Excessive blood flow requirements
    1. Chronic anemia
    2. Systemic arteriovenous shunting

Table 47–2 ■ MAJOR DETERMINANTS OF CARDIAC PERFORMANCE

Ventricular systolic function (contractility)
Ventricular diastolic function
   Relaxation
   Stiffness
Ventricular preload
Ventricular afterload
Cardiac rate and conduction
Myocardial blood flow

Function. In the normal ventricle, stroke volume increases over a wide range of end-diastolic volumes (the Frank-Starling effect). If contractility (or the inotropic state of the myocardium) is enhanced, such as during exercise or catecholamine stimulation, this increase is correspondingly greater. In the failing heart with depressed contractility, there is relatively little increment in systolic function with further increases in left ventricular volume, and the ventricular function curve is shifted downward and flattened (see also Chapter 40). In the clinical setting, systolic dysfunction is characterized by depressed stroke volume despite elevated ventricular filling pressures. The resulting symptoms are those of pulmonary or systemic congestion, activity intolerance, and organ dysfunction.

Assessment of systolic function clinically is more problematic. The most useful measure is the left ventricular ejection fraction (stroke volume/end-diastolic volume, usually expressed as a percent), which reflects a single point on the ventricular function curve. However, the ejection fraction is "load dependent," meaning that alterations in afterload (see later) can affect it independent of contractility. In addition, mitral regurgitation, which facilitates ejection into the low pressure left atrium, may lead to an overestimation of systolic function by the ejection fraction. Nonetheless, with the exceptions indicated earlier, when the ejection fraction is normal (above 55% in most laboratories), systolic function is usually adequate. Mild (40–50%), moderate (30–40%), and severe (<30%) reductions in ejection fraction are associated with reduced survival and, in the severe range, with reduced functional reserve if not overt symptoms of heart failure. Cardiac output, in contrast, is a poor measure of systolic function, because it can be markedly affected by heart rate, systemic vascular resistance, and the degree of left ventricular dilatation.

Diastolic Function. Diastole is the part of the cardiac cycle between aortic valve closure and mitral valve closure. Diastole consists of three phases: (1) active relaxation, (2) the conduit phase, and (3) atrial contraction. If relaxation is delayed or if the myocardium is abnormally stiff (e.g., a steeper relationship between change in pressure to change in volume; $\Delta P/\Delta V$ is excessively steep), passive filling may be impaired and atrial pressures are abnormally elevated. In this setting of a non-compliant ventricle (compliance is the inverse of stiffness, e.g., the change in volume for a given change in pressure), atrial contraction is responsible for a disproportionately large amount of diastolic filling.

The importance of abnormalities of diastolic function in the pathogenesis of heart failure is being increasingly appreciated. Because relaxation is energy dependent, it is frequently impaired in the presence of ischemia or hypoxemia. Recurring myocardial ischemia, pathologic myocardial hypertrophy, chronic volume overload, and aging are all associated with increased interstitial fibrosis and poor relaxation.

In the left ventricle with diastolic dysfunction, left ventricular filling pressures rise because of the compliance changes, with resulting left atrial hypertension and pulmonary congestion. Cardiac output may be reduced if ventricular filling is sufficiently impaired. With activity, these abnormalities are exaggerated, with resulting exertional dyspnea and exercise intolerance.

Ventricular Preload. In the intact heart, preload is best characterized by the end-diastolic volume or pressure, which are indirect indicators of end-diastolic fiber length (see Chapter 40). The performance of the normal ventricle is highly preload dependent, but the failing heart operates at high preloads and on the flat part of the ventricular function curve (see Fig. 40–3). Thus, unlike the normal ventricle, a modest decrease in preload will have little effect on left ventricular filling pressures, whereas an increase in preload will not improve systolic function but will further worsen pulmonary congestion. Thus, preload reduction by diuresis or by reducing venous return with venodilating agents will generally have a beneficial clinical effect in heart failure.

Ventricular Afterload. Left ventricular afterload is frequently equated with arterial pressure or systemic vascular resistance, but a more accurate measurement of afterload is systolic wall stress, defined as [(pressure × the radius of the left ventricle)] divided by [(2 × the thickness of the left ventricle)] (see Chapter 40). Thus, at any given arterial pressure, afterload is increased in a dilated thin ventricle and lower with a smaller or thicker ventricle. Increased afterload has an effect quite similar to that of depressed contractility, so afterload reduction can improve cardiac performance.

Heart Rate and Rhythm. Heart rate affects cardiac performance by two mechanisms. Increasing heart rate enhances the inotropic state by upregulating cytosolic calcium concentrations. Second, heart rate is an important determinant of cardiac output and is the primary mechanism by which cardiac output is matched to demand in situations such as exercise. Because stroke volume is relatively fixed in the failing heart, heart rate becomes the major determinant of cardiac output. However, chronic tachycardia impairs ventricular performance, and cardiac function often improves with control of tachyarrhythmias such as atrial fibrillation.

Optimal cardiac performance depends on a well-coordinated sequence of contraction. Normal atrioventricular conduction times (0.16–0.20 sec) enhance the contribution of atrial contraction to left ventricular filling, which is particularly important in the noncompliant ventricle. Patients with heart failure frequently have intraventricular conduction abnormalities, which result in dysynchronous contractions, such that the septum and parts of the anterior wall begin contracting only after systole has ended in other regions.

Myocardial Blood Flow and Oxygen Requirements. In the normal heart, myocardial blood flow is closely coupled to oxygen requirements and it is not ordinarily considered a determinant of cardiac performance. However, myocardial ischemia is associated with a rapid decline in contractile function that may persist long beyond the episode (myocardial stunning). Chronically inadequate blood flow may lead to a reduction in contractility, which serves to reestablish the balance between oxygen delivery and demands (hibernation). Low arterial diastolic pressures may interfere with the autoregulatory reserve of the coronary circulation, which is limited at diastolic pressures below 60 mm Hg. Endothelial dysfunction, which is common in heart failure patients, may also limit blood flow. At the same time, tachycardia, increased afterload, and substantial left ventricular hypertrophy increase myocardial oxygen requirements. Thus, inadequate myocardial blood flow plays an important role in the pathogenesis of cardiac dysfunction, sometimes even in patients without obstructive coronary disease.

THE HEART FAILURE SYNDROME

Chronic heart failure is a multifaceted syndrome with diverse presentations (Fig. 47–1). The initial manifestations of hemodynamic dysfunction are a reduction in stroke volume and a rise in ventricular filling pressures, perhaps in the basal state but more consistently under conditions of increased systemic demand for blood flow. These changes have downstream effects on cardiovascular reflexes and systemic organ perfusion and function, which in turn stimulate a variety of interdependent compensatory responses involving the cardiovascular system, neurohormonal systems, and alterations in renal physiology. It is this constellation of responses that lead to the characteristic pathophysiology of the heart failure syndrome. Recognition of the role of neurohormonal activation in heart failure has grown with the increasing understanding of its pathophysiology and with evidence that blockade of some of these responses can have a profound effect on the natural history of the disease (Table 47–3). The number of hormonal systems known to be activated in heart failure continues to grow.

NEUROHUMORAL RESPONSES. THE SYMPATHETIC NERVOUS SYSTEM. Initial activation of the sympathetic nervous system probably results from reduced pulse pressures, which stimulate arterial baroreceptors, and renal hypoperfusion. Evidence for its activation comes from elevated levels of circulating norepinephrine, direct sympathetic nerve recordings showing increased activity, and increased norepinephrine release by several organs, including the

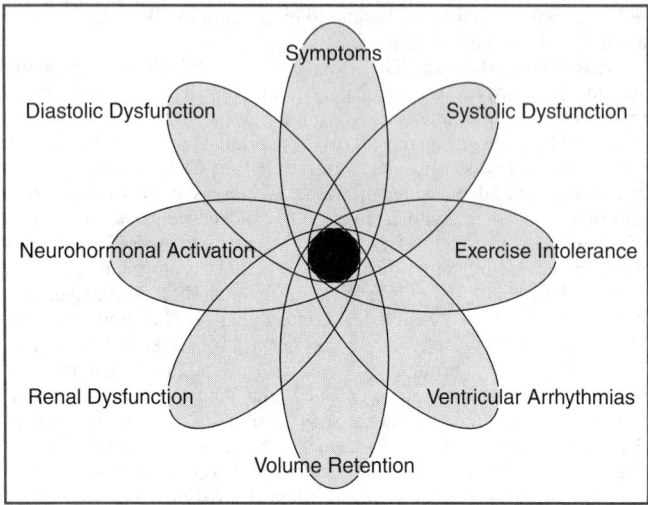

FIGURE 47–1 ■ Pathophysiology of heart failure, illustrated by Venn diagram.

heart. As cardiac function deteriorates, responsivity to norepinephrine diminishes, as evidenced by baroreceptor desensitization and down-regulation of cardiac adrenergic receptors and signal transduction. This densensitization, in turn, may further stimulate sympathetic responses.

The adaptive role of norepinephrine is to stimulate heart rate and myocardial contractility and to produce vasoconstriction. All of these actions serve to reverse the depression of cardiac output and blood pressure. However, elevated levels of plasma norepinephrine are associated with worse prognosis, although it is unclear whether this is a cause-and-effect relationship. There is also convincing, albeit circumstantial, evidence that norepinephrine has adverse effects on the myocardium. In this regard, β-adrenoceptor blockade, which for many years has been considered dangerous in heart failure because it deprives the heart of important compensatory stimulation, consistently improves left ventricular function and prognosis as well. The role of other catecholamines in heart failure remains undefined.

THE RENIN-ANGIOTENSIN-ALDOSTERONE SYSTEM. Elements of the renin-angiotensin-aldosterone system are activated relatively early in heart failure. The presumptive mechanisms of induction include renal hypoperfusion, β-adrenergic system stimulation, and hyponatremia. All may be further activated by diuretic therapy. Angiotensin II increases blood pressure by vasoconstriction and enhances glomerular filtration both by increasing renal pressure and maintaining glomerular flow by its intrarenal hemodynamic effects. Aldosterone causes sodium retention, which serves to restore normal cardiac output by enhancing intravascular volume. However,

Table 47–3 ■ **NEUROHORMONES THAT MAY BE INCREASED IN CHRONIC HEART FAILURE**

Norepinephrine
Epinephrine
Plasma and tissue renin activity
Angiotensin II
Aldosterone
Prostaglandins
Vasopressin
Neuropeptide Y
Vasoactive intestinal peptides
Natriuretic peptides
Endothelin
Endorphins
Calcitonin gene-related peptide
Growth hormone
Cortisol
Proinflammatory cytokines
Neurokinin A
Substance P

these adaptations have deleterious consequences. Excessive vasoconstriction can depress left ventricular function, and sodium retention worsens the already elevated ventricular filling pressures. There is also experimental evidence indicating that angiotensin II may have pathologic effects on the myocardium and induce vascular hypertrophy, while aldosterone induces myocardial fibrosis. The striking success of ACE inhibitors and, more recently, spironolactone in improving the natural history of heart failure suggests that the adverse effects of renin-angiotensin-aldosterone activation may outweigh their benefit.

OTHER NEUROHORMONAL SYSTEMS. Levels of several natriuretic peptides are consistently elevated in heart failure, and they may counterbalance the vasoconstricting and sodium retaining actions of the renin-angiotensin-aldosterone and sympathetic nervous systems. It does, however, appear that responses to these natriuretic hormones are down-regulated, so that they do not have the same diuretic effects in chronic heart failure that they manifest in normal individuals. Elevated circulating and tissue levels of vasodilating prostaglandins may improve glomerular hemodynamics, and inhibitors of prostaglandin synthesis (including aspirin and other nonsteroidal anti-inflammatory agents) interfere with the hemodynamic and renal actions of ACE inibitors.

Endothelin and arginine vasopressin are elevated in many heart failure patients, and interference with their actions may promote vasodilation and diuresis. Arginine vasopressin induces vasoconstriction through a vascular (V-1) receptor and reduces free water clearance through a renal tubular (V-2) receptor. The endothelins cause prolonged vasoconstriction, reductions in glomerular filtration, mesangial hypertrophy, bronchoconstriction, and pulmonary arteriolar constriction. The endothelins are particularly attractive targets for therapy.

CYTOKINE ACTIVATION. Circulating levels of a number of proinflammatory cytokines, including tumor necrosis factor-α, interleukin-1β, and interleukin-6, are elevated in patients with relatively severe heart failure and may be involved in the syndrome of cardiac cachexia. These cytokines may also induce contractile dysfunction, myocardial fibrosis, and myocyte necrosis, perhaps by mediating some of the deleterious responses to catecholamines and angiotensin-II.

ALTERED RENAL PHYSIOLOGY. In most patients with chronic heart failure, the kidneys are anatomically and structurally normal. Reduced blood pressure, diminished stroke volume, and reduced renal perfusion pressure and flow are sensed as reduced blood volume by the high-pressure baroreceptors and the juxtaglomerular apparatus that maintain cardiovascular homeostasis. In chronic heart failure, these receptors become desensitized, generating reduced afferent responses. The low-pressure intracardiac pressure and volume receptors also desensitized. Thirst and fluid intake may be increased as a result of activation of the cerebral thirst center. Thus, although heart failure is usually associated with a normal or even increased blood volume, it is paradoxically characterized by activation of the same homeostatic responses as those to hemorrhage and shock; the result is abnormal retention of sodium and water. In advanced heart failure, usually characterized by low cardiac output and/or hypotension (or with co-existing renal vascular disease), the glomerular filtration rate may become so severely reduced that sodium and fluid retention becomes refractory to diuretic therapy.

LEFT VENTRICULAR REMODELING AND PROGRESSION OF HEART FAILURE. After an initial insult precipitates heart failure, progressive alterations occur in myocardial structure and function owing to continuing damage by the underlying process as well as responses to hemodynamic stresses and neurohormonal activation. The left ventricle progressively dilates and changes from the normal ellipsoid shape to a more spherical geometry. This "remodeling" is accompanied by changes in the cardiac interstitium, leading to altered orientation of the myofibrils and progressive fibrosis. The result is more discoordinate and less effective contraction. Both ACE inhibitors and β-blockers slow, halt, or even reverse this remodeling process, thus preventing left ventricular dilatation, geometric distortion, and deterioration in contractile function.

CLINICAL PRESENTATION OF HEART FAILURE

Heart failure may present acutely in a de novo manner, chronically, or as an acute exacerbation of chronic heart failure.

Acute Heart Failure

Acute heart failure usually presents as shortness of breath, culminating, sometimes in a matter of minutes, with pulmonary edema. A more subacute presentation is of progressive dyspnea associated with systemic fluid retention over a period of days to a few weeks. The precipitous form usually suggests extensive acute damage, most commonly as an ongoing or recent MI. Other such insults include the acute development of valvular regurgitation from ruptured chordae tendineae, bacterial endocarditis, or aortic dissection or of rapidly progressive myocarditis or toxic damage. The syndrome may progress to cardiogenic shock (see Chapter 95).

Rapid diagnosis by non-invasive testing, early cardiac catheterization, and, in some cases, endomyocardial biopsy is critical. Treatment is cause specific and may include early coronary revascularization, valve repair or replacement, or supportive care (inotropic support, intra-aortic balloon pumping, ventricular assist devices). If not reversed, cardiac transplantation (see Chapter 71) may be the best option for appropriate candidates.

Chronic Heart Failure

LEFT- AND RIGHT-SIDED HEART FAILURE. In adults, the great majority of patients with heart failure have abnormalities of the left ventricle as the underlying cause. Nonetheless, the clinical presentation may be variable, sometimes suggesting predominantly or even exclusively right ventricular dysfunction. The manifestations of left ventricular dysfunction are related to elevated filling (diastolic) pressures, which are transmitted backward to the left atrium and pulmonary veins, or inadequate cardiac output. The former results in dyspnea, sometimes at rest but usually with activity, and, when severe, pulmonary edema, classically associated with rales and possibly pleural effusions. The cardiac output may be insufficient to support peripheral organ function, causing exertional muscle fatigue, impaired renal function and salt excretion, or even depressed mentation.

Right-sided heart failure results from either chronic right ventricular pressure overload (e.g., pulmonary hypertension due to cor pulmonale or pulmonary vascular disease) or to intrinsic dysfunction of the right ventricle or its valves. However, it is important to emphasize that the most common cause of right ventricular pressure overload is left-sided heart dysfunction resulting in pulmonary hypertension. When the symptoms and signs of left-sided heart failure are absent or difficult to elicit, the physician may inappropriately seek a primarily right-sided pathology. The primary manifestations of right-sided failure are related to chronically elevated right atrial and systemic venous pressures: jugular venous distention, peripheral edema, ascites, hepatic and bowel edema, and varied gastrointestinal complaints.

HEART FAILURE WITH PRESERVED SYSTOLIC FUNCTION. Myocardial mechanisms that lead to the syndrome of heart failure can be differentiated into conditions that depress left ventricular systolic function and those that occur despite preserved contractility. Although arbitrary, a left ventricular ejection fraction threshold of 45 to 50% is often employed for this distinction.

Until the recent widespread use of non-invasive assessments of left ventricular function, heart failure with preserved systolic function was considered unusual in the absence of valvular abnormalities or other specific and uncommon causes. However, it is now recognized that 20 to 40% of heart failure patients have normal ejection fractions. In the ongoing Cardiovascular Health Study, a population-based study of more than 5000 patients age 65 and older, more than 70% of patients developing heart failure had normal or only mildly impaired systolic function. Indeed, it is likely that the large majority of elderly heart failure patients have primarily diastolic dysfunction as the cause.

Although there are many potential causes of heart failure with preserved systolic function, most patients have current hypertension or a history of treated hypertension; the resulting left ventricular hypertrophy and increased fibrosis are probably responsible for increased chamber stiffness. Ischemic heart disease may also contribute to heart failure with preserved systolic function, probably by virtue of subendocardial fibrosis or as a result of acute, intermittent ischemic dysfunction. Diabetes mellitus is often present, especially in women. Age itself is a critical predisposing factor because it causes loss of myocytes (apoptosis), increased fibrosis with shifts to more rigid forms of collagen, and loss of vascular compliance.

The mortality rates of patients with preserved systolic function are lower than those with low ejection fractions but remain higher than the general population, even in comparison with similarly older aged individuals. However, hospitalization and rehospitalization rates for these patients are comparable to those with reduced ejection fractions, and there are few data on treatment to guide physicians in the management of these patients.

Although heart failure patients with preserved systolic function are often considered to have *diastolic dysfunction,* there are many other explanations for this presentation, some of which are reversible or warrant specific therapy (Table 47–4). The first two questions are whether the patient's symptoms are due to heart failure of any type and whether important valvular abnormalities were missed. Ejection fraction measurements may be inaccurate, particularly when their technical quality is suboptimal. Regurgitant valve diseases may lead to a dissociation between the ejection fraction and underlying myocardial dysfunction, because in this setting the afterload may be very low. There are also a number of conditions in which left ventricular function is transiently impaired but subsequently measured ejection fractions may be normal; intermittent ischemia, presenting as episodic heart failure ("flash pulmonary edema") is the most important, because revascularization may be indicated. Severe hypertension with subsequent treatment and transient arrhythmias may also have temporary effects on ejection fraction. Some patients with alcoholic cardiomyopathy may exhibit very rapid recovery in ejection fraction when they cease drinking.

The remaining patients most likely have diastolic dysfunction as the underlying disorder. Unfortunately, the non-invasive measurement of diastolic function remains problematic. The most common test used, Doppler echocardiography, is neither sensitive nor specific for diastolic dysfunction. Particularly in the elderly, Doppler mitral valve filling patterns show impaired early diastolic filling in the majority of subjects, whether or not they have evidence of heart failure. Thus, diastolic dysfunction is basically a diagnosis of exclusion based on accompanying conditions and circumstantial evidence.

FACTORS PRECIPITATING ACUTE DECOMPENSATION OF CHRONIC HEART FAILURE. Many patients with chronic heart failure maintain a stable course and then abruptly present with acutely or subacutely worsening symptoms. Although this decompensation may reflect unrecognized gradual progression of the underlying disorder, a number of precipitating events must be considered and, if present, addressed (Table 47–5). An important focus is on changes in medications (by patient or physician), diet, or activity. Superimposed new or altered cardiovascular conditions, such as arrhythmias, ischemic events, hypertension, or valvular abnormalities, should be considered. Systemic processes such as fever, infection, or anemia may also cause cardiac decompensation.

Table 47–4 ■ CAUSES OF (AND ALTERNATIVE EXPLANATIONS FOR) HEART FAILURE WITH PRESERVED SYSTOLIC FUNCTION (LEFT VENTRICULAR EJECTION FRACTION >45–50%)

Inaccurate diagnosis of heart failure (e.g., pulmonary diseases, obesity)
Inaccurate measurements of ejection fraction
Systolic function overestimated by ejection fraction (e.g., mitral regurgitation)
Episodic, unrecognized systolic dysfunction
  Intermittent ischemia
  Arrhythmia
  Severe hypertension
  Alcohol
Diastolic dysfunction
  Abnormalities of myocardial relaxation
    Ischemia
    Hypertrophy
  Abnormalities of myocardial compliance
    Hypertrophy
    Aging
    Fibrosis
    Diabetes
    Infiltrative diseases (amyloidosis, sarcoidosis)
    Storage diseases (hemachromatosis)
    Endomyocardial diseases (endomyocardial fibrosis, radiation, anthracyclines)
Pericardial diseases (constriction, tamponade)

Table 47–5 ■ FACTORS THAT MAY PRECIPITATE ACUTE DECOMPENSATION OF CHRONIC HEART FAILURE

Discontinuation of therapy (patient non-compliance or physician initiated)
Initiation of medications that worsen heart failure (calcium antagonists, β-blockers, non-steroidal, anti-inflammatory drugs, antiarrhythmic agents)
Iatrogenic volume overload (transfusion, fluid administration)
Dietary indiscretion
Alcohol consumption
Increased activity
Pregnancy
Exposure to high altitude
Arrhythmias
Myocardial ischemia or infarction
Worsening hypertension
Worsening mitral or tricuspid regurgitation
Fever or infection
Anemia

EVALUATION OF THE PATIENT WITH POSSIBLE HEART FAILURE

Symptoms of Heart Failure

The common symptoms of heart failure are well known but are frequently absent and variably specific for this condition. The symptoms generally reflect, but may be dissociated from, the hemodynamic derangements of elevated left- and right-sided pressures and impaired cardiac output or cardiac output reserve.

DYSPNEA. Dyspnea, or perceived shortness of breath, is the most common symptom of patients with heart failure. In the majority of patients, dyspnea is present only with activity or exertion. The underlying mechanisms are multifactorial. The most important is pulmonary congestion with increased interstitial or intra-alveolar fluid, which activates juxtacapillary J receptors, which in turn stimulate a rapid and shallow pattern of breathing. Increased lung stiffness may enhance the work of breathing, leading to a perception of dyspnea. Central regulation of respiration may be disturbed in more severe heart failure, resulting in disordered sleep patterns and sleep apnea. Cheyne-Stokes respiration, or periodic breathing, is not uncommon in advanced heart failure, is usually associated with low output states, and may be perceived by the patient (and the patient's family) as either severe dyspnea or transient cessation of breathing. Hypoxia, which is uncommon in heart failure patients unless there is accompanying pulmonary disease, suggests the presence of pulmonary edema. Dyspnea is a relatively sensitive symptom of heart failure, provided a careful history is taken of the patient's level of activity, but dyspnea may become less prominent with the onset of right ventricular failure and tricuspid regurgitation, which may lead to lower pulmonary venous pressures. It should also be noted that dyspnea is a common symptom of patients with pulmonary disease, obesity, and anemia and in sedentary individuals.

ORTHOPNEA AND PAROXYSMAL NOCTURNAL DYSPNEA. Orthopnea is dyspnea that is positional, occurring in the recumbent or semirecumbent position. It occurs due to the increase in venous return from the extremities and splanchnic circulation to central circulation with changes in posture, with resultant increases in pulmonary venous pressures and pulmonary capillary hydrostatic pressure. Nocturnal cough may be a manifestation of this process and is an underrecognized symptom of heart failure. Orthopnea is a relatively specific symptom of heart failure, although it may occur in patients with pulmonary disease who breathe more effectively in an upright posture and in individuals with significant abdominal obesity or ascites. However, most patients with mild or moderate heart failure do not experience orthopnea when they are adequately treated.

Paroxysmal nocturnal dyspnea (PND) is an attack of acute, severe shortness of breath awakening the patient from sleep, usually 1 to 3 hours after the patient retires. Symptoms usually resolve over a period of 10 to 30 minutes after the patient arises, often gasping for fresh air from an open window. PND results from increased venous return and mobilization of interstitial fluid from the extremities and elsewhere, with accumulation of alveolar edema. PND almost always represents heart failure, but it is a relatively uncommon finding.

ACUTE PULMONARY EDEMA. Pulmonary edema results from transudation of fluid into the alveolar spaces as a result of acute rises in capillary hydrostatic pressures due to an acute depression of cardiac function or to an acute rise in intravascular volume. The initial symptoms may be cough or progressive dyspnea. Because alveolar edema may precipitate bronchospasm, wheezing is not uncommon. If the edema is not treated, the patient may begin coughing up pink (or blood tinged), frothy fluid and become cyanotic and acidotic.

EXERCISE INTOLERANCE. Activity or exercise intolerance is, together with dyspnea, the most characteristic symptom of chronic heart failure. Intuitively, it might be assumed that exercise would be limited by shortness of breath due to rising pulmonary venous pressures and pulmonary congestion. Although this mechanism may contribute, it is only one of many operating. Blood flow to exercising muscles is impaired, both as a result of reduced cardiac output reserve and impaired peripheral vasodilation; oxygen delivery is limited and early fatigue ensues. Heart failure is also associated with additional abnormalities of skeletal muscle itself, including biochemical changes and alterations in fiber types, which increase muscle fatigue and impair muscle function. Finally, heart failure may adversely affect respiratory muscle function and ventilatory control.

FATIGUE. Fatigue is a very common, if non-specific, complaint of patients with heart failure. Perhaps the most common origin of this complaint is muscle fatigue. Fatigue may also be a non-specific response to the systemic manifestations of heart failure, such as chronic increases in catecholamines and circulating levels of cytokines, sleep disorders, and anxiety.

EDEMA AND FLUID RETENTION (ASCITES, PLEURAL EFFUSION, PERICARDIAL EFFUSION). Elevated right atrial pressures increase the capillary hydrostatic pressures in the systemic circulation, with resultant transudation. The location of edema fluid is determined by position (e.g., dependent) and accompanying pathology. Most commonly, edema accumulates in the extremities and resolves at night when the legs are not dependent. Edema may occur only in the feet and ankles; but if it is more severe, it may accumulate in the thighs, scrotum, and abdominal wall. Edema is more likely and more severe in patients with accompanying venous disease (or who have had veins harvested for coronary bypass surgery) and those on calcium channel blockers, which themselves cause edema.

Fluid may also accumulate in the peritoneal cavity and in the pleural or pericardial space. Ascites occurs as a result of elevated pressures in the hepatic, portal, and systemic veins draining the peritoneum. Ascites is unusual in heart failure and almost always is associated with peripheral edema. Most commonly, there is severe tricuspid regurgitation, with potential damage to the liver. Otherwise, significant primary liver disease should be suspected as an exacerbating factor or cause of ascites. Pleural effusions are fairly common in chronic heart failure, especially when it is accompanied by both left- and right-sided manifestations. The effusions result from an increase in transudation of fluid into the pleural space and impaired lymphatic drainage due to elevated systemic venous pressures. Pericardial effusions are far less frequent but may occur.

ABDOMINAL AND GASTROINTESTINAL SYMPTOMS. Passive congestion of the liver may lead to right upper quadrant pain and tenderness and even mild jaundice. Usually only mild elevations of transaminase levels and modest increases in bilirubin levels are observed. With severe, acute rises in central venous pressures, especially when associated with systemic hypotension, a severe congestive and ischemic hepatopathy may occur with striking elevations in liver function tests and hypoglycemia. Recovery is usually rapid and complete if the hemodynamic abnormalities are corrected.

Bowel wall edema may lead to early satiety (a common symptom in heart failure), nausea, diffuse abdominal discomfort, malabsorption, and a rare form of protein-losing enteropathy. The potential role of heart failure in producing these non-specific gastrointestinal symptoms is often overlooked, leading to extensive diagnostic testing or unnecessary discontinuation of medications.

SLEEP DISORDERS AND CENTRAL NERVOUS SYSTEM (CNS) MANIFESTATIONS. Periods of nocturnal oxygen desaturation to below 80 to 85% are relatively common in patients with heart failure, coincide with episodes of apnea, and often are preceded or followed by episodes of hyperventilation. These are similar to, and may represent truncated forms of, Cheyne-Stokes respiration. These episodes reflect altered CNS ventilatory control and have been associated with diminished heart rate variability. Supplemental oxygen appears to reverse some of the ventilatory disorders, and the apneic spells respond to nasal positive-pressure ventilation. In some patients, these interventions may have a striking beneficial effect on fatigue and other symptoms of heart failure.

Aside from the common complaint of fatigue, which may in part be CNS in origin, brain function is not affected in most patients with heart failure. However, in advanced heart failure, cerebral hypoperfusion may cause impairment of memory, irritability, limited attention span, and altered mentation.

CARDIAC CACHEXIA. In chronic, severe heart failure, unintentional chronic weight loss may occur, leading to a syndrome of cardiac cachexia. The etiology of this syndrome is unclear, but it may result from a number of factors, including elevated levels of proinflammatory cytokines (e.g., tumor necrosis factor), elevated metabolic rates, loss of appetite, and malabsorption. Cardiac cachexia carries a poor prognosis.

Physical Findings

The physical findings associated with heart failure generally reflect elevated ventricular filling pressures and, to a lesser extent, reduced cardiac output. Importantly, in chronic heart failure many of these findings are absent, often obscuring the correct diagnosis.

APPEARANCE AND VITAL SIGNS. Compensated patients may be quite comfortable, but patients with more severe symptoms are often restless, dyspneic, and pale or diaphoretic. Although the heart rate is usually at the high end of the normal range or above (>80 beats per minute), it may be lower in chronic, stable patients. Premature beats or arrhythmias are common. Pulsus alternans (alternating amplitude of successive beats) is a sign of advanced heart failure (or a large pericardial effusion). The blood pressure may be normal or high, but in advanced heart failure it is usually on the low end of normal or below.

JUGULAR VEINS AND NECK EXAMINATION. Examination of the jugular veins is one of the most useful aspects of the evaluation of heart failure patients. The jugular venous pressure should be quantified in centimeters of water (normal 8 cm or less) by estimating the level of pulsations above the sternal angle (and arbitrarily adding 5 cm in any posture). The presence of abdominal-jugular reflux should be assessed by putting pressure on the right upper quadrant of the abdomen for 30 seconds and avoiding an induced Valvsalva maneuver; a positive finding is a rise in the jugular pressure of at least 1 cm. Either an elevated jugular venous pressure or abnormal abdominal-jugular reflux has been reported in 80% of patients with advanced heart failure. No other simple sign provides nearly as high a sensitivity.

An additional important finding in the neck is evidence of tricuspid regurgitation—a large cv wave, usually associated with a high jugular venous pressure. This finding is confirmed by hepatic pulsations, which can be detected during the abdominal-jugular reflux determination. The carotid pulses should be evaluated for evidence of aortic stenosis, and thyroid abnormalities should be sought.

PULMONARY EXAMINATION. Although dyspnea is the most common symptom of patients with heart failure, the pulmonary examination is usually unremarkable. Rales, representing alveolar fluid, are a hallmark of heart failure; when present in patients without accompanying pulmonary disease, they are highly specific for the diagnosis. However, in chronic heart failure, they are usually absent, even in patients known to have pulmonary capillary wedge pressures above 20 mm Hg (normal <12 mm Hg). Thus, left ventricular failure cannot be excluded by the absence of rales. Pleural effusions, which are indicative of bilateral heart failure in patients with appropriate symptoms, are relatively rare.

CARDIAC EXAMINATION. The cardiac examination is a critical part of the evaluation of the patient with heart failure, but more for identification of associated cardiac abnormalities than the assessment of its severity. Assessment of the point of maximal impulse may provide information concerning the size of the heart (enlarged if displaced below the fifth intercostal space or lateral to the midclavicular line) and its function (if sustained beyond one third of systole or palpable over two interspaces). Additional precordial pulsations may indicate a left ventricular aneurysm. A parasternal lift is valuable evidence of pulmonary hypertension.

The first heart sound (S_1) may be diminished in amplitude when left ventricular function is poor, and the pulmonic component of the second heart sound (P_2) may be accentuated when pulmonary hypertension is present. An apical third heart sound (S_3) is a strong indicator of significant left ventricular dysfunction but is present only in a minority of patients with low ejection fractions and elevated left ventricular filling pressures. A fourth heart sound (S_4) is not a specific indicator of heart failure, but it is usually present in patients with diastolic dysfunction. An S_3 at the lower left or right sternal border or below the xiphoid indicates right ventricular dysfunction. Murmurs may indicate the presence of significant valvular disease as the cause of heart failure, but mitral and tricuspid regurgitation are also common secondary manifestations of severe ventricular dilatation and dysfunction.

EXAMINATION OF THE ABDOMEN AND EXTREMITIES. The size, pulsatility, and tenderness of the liver should be evaluated as evidence of passive congestion and tricuspid regurgitation. Ascites and edema should be sought and quantified.

Radiographic Findings

Although the standard posteroanterior and lateral chest radiograph provides limited information about chamber size, the presence of overall cardiomegaly (a cardiothoracic ratio above 0.50) is a strong indicator of heart failure or another cause of cardiomegaly (especially valvular insufficiency). However, nearly 50% of heart failure patients do not have this high a cardiothoracic ratio.

Most patients with acute heart failure, but only a minority of those with chronic heart failure, will have evidence of pulmonary venous hypertension (upper lobe redistribution, enlarged pulmonary veins) or interstitial (haziness of the central vascular shadows or increased central interstitial lung markings) or pulmonary (perihilar or patchy peripheral infiltrates) edema. The absence of these findings reflects both the subjectivity of interpretation and the increased capacity of the lymphatics to remove interstitial and alveolar fluid in chronic heart failure. This absence of radiographic findings is consistent with the absence of rales in most patients with chronic heart failure despite markedly elevated pulmonary venous pressures. Pleural effusions are important adjunctive evidence of heart failure. Characteristically, these are more common and larger on the right than left side, reflecting the greater pleural surface area of the right lung.

THE ELECTROCARDIOGRAM. The major importance of the electrocardiogram is to evaluate cardiac rhythm, identify prior MI, and detect evidence of left ventricular hypertrophy. Prior MIs suggest that the cause is ischemic cardiomyopathy with systolic dysfunction. Left ventricular hypertrophy is a non-specific finding but may point toward left ventricular diastolic dysfunction if the ejection fraction is not depressed.

ECHOCARDIOGRAPHY. Newer modalities for non-invasive diagnostic testing have revolutionized the diagnosis of heart failure. The most useful procedure is the transthoracic echocardiogram (see Chapter 43), which provides a quantitative assessment of left ventricular function, which can, in the presence of appropriate symptoms and signs, confirm the presence of heart failure due to systolic dysfunction or indicate whether the patient has heart failure with preserved systolic function. The echocardiogram also provides a wealth of additional valuable information, including assessment of left and right ventricular size, regional wall motion (as an indicator of prior MI), evaluation of the heart valves, and diagnosis of left ventricular hypertrophy. The echocardiogram has generally replaced the chest radiograph in the diagnostic assessment of heart failure.

Making the Diagnosis of Heart Failure

The diagnosis of heart failure is straightforward when a patient presents with classic symptoms and accompanying physical findings. However, in patients with chronic heart failure, the diagnosis is often delayed or missed entirely because no single sign or symptom is diagnostic (Table 47–6).

The most frequent symptoms, dyspnea and fatigue, are not specific for heart failure, especially in the older population, although their presence should always lead to a more complete evaluation. The more specific symptoms of orthopnea, PND, and edema are much less common. Although the physical examination may be helpful, characteristic physical findings may be absent. Unfortu-

Table 47–6 ▪ SENSITIVITY, SPECIFICITY, AND PREDICTIVE VALUE OF SYMPTOMS AND PHYSICAL FINDINGS FOR DIAGNOSING HEART FAILURE

SYMPTOM OR SIGN	SENSITIVITY* (%)	SPECIFICITY* (%)	PREDICTIVE ACCURACY* (%)
Exertional dyspnea	66	52	23
Orthopnea	21	81	2
Paroxysmal nocturnal dyspnea	33	76	26
History of edema	23	80	22
Resting heart rate >100 beats per minute	7	99	6
Rales	13	91	21
Third heart sound	31	95	61
Jugular venous distention†	10	97	2
Edema (on examination)	10	93	3

*See Chapter 23 for definitions.

†Reported to have much higher sensitivity (57%) and predictive accuracy (67%) at rest and even better sensitivity (81%) and predictive accuracy (81%) with abdominal jugular reflux in another series (Butman SM, et al: J Am Coll Cardiol 22:968–974, 1993).

Adapted from Harlan WR, et al: Ann Intern Med 86:133–138, 1977.

nately, the chest radiograph, on which many physicians rely, adds relatively little to the clinical evaluation.

Thus, the key to making the timely diagnosis of chronic heart failure is to maintain a high degree of suspicion, particularly in high-risk patients (those with coronary artery disease, chronic hypertension, diabetes, histories of heavy alcohol use, and advanced age). When these patients present with any of the symptoms or physical findings suggestive of heart failure, additional testing (see later) should be undertaken, generally beginning with echocardiography.

Differential Diagnosis

Although it is not difficult to make the definitive diagnosis of heart failure in a patient presenting with the classic symptoms and signs, several alternative diagnoses need to be considered in less clear-cut situations, such as in the patient with normal left ventricular function and less definitive clinical evidence. The most important differentiation is between heart failure and pulmonary disease. In this setting, pulmonary function testing or additional tests to characterize lung pathology may be helpful. When left ventricular systolic function is normal, it sometimes may be difficult to make a conclusive determination of the relative role of heart failure as compared with other concomitant conditions, such as severe obesity, chronic anemia, or other systemic illnesses; in some patients, a therapeutic trial (see Chapter 48) may be diagnostic.

EVALUATION AND FOLLOW-UP OF THE HEART FAILURE PATIENT

Once the diagnosis of heart failure is made, the goal of additional testing is to identify potentially correctable or specifically treatable cases and to obtain further information necessary for future management.

Routine Diagnostic Assessment

LABORATORY TESTING. An extensive battery of laboratory tests is not required for most patients with heart failure. Routine testing should include a complete blood cell count (to detect anemia and systemic diseases with hematologic manifestations), measurement of renal function and electrolytes including magnesium (to exclude renal failure and to provide a baseline for subsequent therapy), liver function tests (to exclude accompanying liver pathology and provide a baseline), and blood sugar and lipid testing (to diagnose diabetes and dyslipidemia, both of which should be managed aggressively in heart failure patients).

A few additional tests may be indicated. Thyrotoxicosis, and to a lesser extent hypothyroidism, may cause heart failure and may be difficult to diagnose clinically, especially in older patients. Many guidelines recommend thyroid function tests in all patients, or at least in the elderly and in those with atrial fibrillation. Hemochro-

matosis (see Chapter 221) is a potentially treatable cause of heart failure; particularly if there is accompanying diabetes or hepatic disease, serum ferritin levels are indicated. Sarcoidosis (see Chapter 81) is another potentially treatable cause, although it would be unusual not to have evidence of accompanying lung disease. Amyloidosis (see Chapter 297) should be considered in patients with other manifestations, but treatment of the cardiac manifestations is rarely successful, except with heart transplantation.

ASSESSMENT OF LEFT VENTRICULAR FUNCTION. Although heart failure is a syndrome with many pathogenic mechanisms, the most common are left ventricular systolic dysfunction and left ventricular diastolic dysfunction. In some patients it may be nearly impossible to distinguish between these two forms of heart failure by clinical evaluation, because both may present with the same symptoms and with only subtle differences on physical examination. However, it is essential to distinguish between these two entities, because they may require different diagnostic evaluations and different therapeutic approaches (see Chapter 48). The most useful and practical test is the echocardiogram (see Chapter 43); alternative approaches include radionuclide measurements of ejection fraction (see Chapter 44) and left ventriculography if cardiac catheterization (see Chapter 46) is being performed. All these tests allow the detection of significant systolic dysfunction; diastolic dysfunction can sometimes be documented (see Chapter 43) but is often identified primarily as a process of exclusion in those with preserved systolic function.

Additional Diagnostic Evaluation

ASSESSMENT FOR CORONARY ARTERY DISEASE. Coronary artery disease is the most common cause of heart failure in industrialized societies. Although it is often known whether a patient has coronary disease based on a prior history of MI or positive results in an angiogram or non-invasive test, in some patients it may be silent. There are two reasons to identify the coexistence of heart failure and coronary disease: first, to treat symptoms that may be due to ischemia; and, second, to improve prognosis (see Chapter 62). A prudent approach is to subdivide heart failure patients into three groups: (1) those with clinical evidence of ongoing ischemia (active angina or a possible ischemic equivalent), (2) those who have had a prior MI but do not currently have angina, and (3) those who may or may not have underlying coronary disease. The first group of patients may be most expeditiously evaluated by coronary angiography, because they stand to benefit in terms of symptoms and also probably have more extensive ischemia. In the second group are patients with heart failure and prior MI who by other criteria (age, absence of other major co-morbid conditions) are otherwise good candidates for coronary revascularization; they should generally undergo non-invasive stress testing in conjunction with nuclear myocardial perfusion imaging or echocardiography. These procedures identify individuals with extensive ischemic, but viable myocardium, whose prognosis and symptoms may also be improved with revascularization. The third group, patients without either angina or prior MI, are much less likely to benefit from an evaluation for asymptomatic coronary disease.

MYOCARDIAL BIOPSY. There is no rationale for routine myocardial biopsy in patients with heart failure, even in the subgroup without apparent coronary disease. Few entities that might be detected are amenable to specific therapy, and those that are (hemochromatosis, sarcoidosis) can usually be detected by their other manifestations or other procedures. A possible exception is acute fulminant myocarditis (see Chapter 64), particularly the entities of eosinophilic and giant cell myocarditis, which may respond to immunosuppressive therapy. A potential exception is the patient being evaluated for cardiac transplantation (see Chapter 71), because the presence of some entities may preclude this procedure.

ASSESSMENT OF EXERCISE CAPACITY. Quantitative assessment of exercise capacity provides additional insight into prognosis over the clinical evaluation and measurements of cardiac function, particularly when a detailed history of activity tolerance cannot be obtained. Exercise testing with measurements of peak oxygen uptake by respiratory gas exchange has become a routine part of the transplant evaluation (see Chapter 71), because it provides an indication of need for early intervention and an additional method for follow-up. However, in most patients, such testing is not necessary. Emphasis should be placed on eliciting each patient's maximum tolerated activity and the minimum activity associated with symptoms; both can be followed from visit to visit, as a guide to management.

ASSESSMENT OF ARRHYTHMIAS. Ventricular arrhythmias are extremely common in patients with chronic heart failure, with 50 to 80% of patients exhibiting non-sustained ventricular tachycardia during 24-hour monitoring. Because approximately 50% of cardiac deaths in these patients are sudden, these arrhythmias have been viewed with concern. However, in multivariate analyses, asymptomatic ventricular arrhythmias carry little independent prognostic significance when the severity of symptoms, ejection fraction, and presence of concurrent coronary disease are taken into account. Furthermore, arrhythmias are no more predictive of sudden death than of total mortality. Thus, further evaluation of asymptomatic arrhythmias is not warranted. In contrast, ventricular arrhythmias associated with syncope or hemodynamic compromise must be taken seriously and require further evaluation and treatment (see Chapter 52).

Follow-Up Evaluation

After the diagnosis of heart failure is confirmed and the initial evaluation is complete, there is little need for further testing beyond the laboratory tests (primarily renal function and electrolytes) necessary to monitor therapy. Once the status of ventricular function is known, there are few indications for retesting. Exceptions are monitoring for transplantation and important changes in clinical status (e.g., marked deterioration in a patient previously known to have preserved left ventricular function, occurrence of new murmurs in conjunction with declining status).

Instead, the key to successful follow-up is the careful tracking of clinical symptoms and patient weights, which often involves interviewing not only the patient but also family members, who may be more aware of changes in status than the patient. Continuity of care and seamless transitions from the inpatient to outpatient setting are critical aspects of optimal management. Patients with advanced heart failure and those requiring frequent hospitalization require special handling. Programs that provide telephone-based tracking of daily weights and symptoms can detect deterioration in time to intervene before the need for hospitalization. Although these programs may be costly, several evaluations have found them to be cost effective. Because the management of these patients requires considerable experience and expertise, specialized heart failure programs and clinics have been developed and may provide additional benefit compared with traditional care.

Dauterman KW, Massie BM, Gheorghiade M: Heart failure associated with preserved systolic function: A common and costly clinical entity. Am Heart J 135:S310–S319, 1998. *Review of the epidemiology, mechanisms, and therapy of this common form of heart failure.*

Eichhorn EJ. New insights into dilated cardiomyopathy. Cardiol Clin 16:603, 1998. *Monograph with chapters on the etiology, pathophysiology, and treatment of heart failure.*

Massie BM, Shah NB: Evolving trends in the epidemiologic factors of heart failure: Rationale for preventive strategies. Am Heart J 133:703–712, 1997. *Review of statistics on incidence, prevalence, mortality, hospitalizations for heart failure, and discussion of preventative approaches to reduce its impact.*

Poole-Wilson PA, Colucci WS, Massie BM, et al (eds): *Heart Failure: Scientific Principles and Clinical Practice.* New York, Churchill Livingstone, 1997. *Comprehensive text, with coverage of basic mechanisms, pathophysiology, diagnosis, and treatment of heart failure.*

Schrier RW, Fassett RG. Pathogenesis of sodium and water retention in cardiac failure. Renal Failure 20:773, 1998. *Excellent review of the mechanisms underlying the primary manifestation of heart failure.*

48 MANAGEMENT OF HEART FAILURE

Milton Packer

The cardinal manifestations of heart failure (see Chapter 47) are (1) dyspnea and fatigue, which may limit exercise tolerance, and (2) fluid retention, which may lead to pulmonary and peripheral edema. Both abnormalities can impair the functional capacity and

quality-of-life of affected individuals. In addition, by its very nature, heart failure is a progressive disorder. With time, the functional limitations imposed by the disease become increasingly apparent, and eventually patients experience symptoms at rest or on minimal exertion. This progression is directly related to the inexorable deterioration of cardiac structure and function, which can occur without any recurrence of the initial injury to the heart. Once initiated, heart failure advances (often silently) and leads inevitably to a recurrent need for medical care and hospitalization and, finally, to the death of the patient.

APPROACH TO THE PATIENT WITH HEART FAILURE

Defining the Cause of Heart Failure

The primary step in the management of heart failure is to identify and characterize the nature of the underlying cardiac disorder. A careful history may reveal the past occurrence of a myocardial infarction (MI) (see Chapter 60), valvular disease (see Chapter 63), hypertension (see Chapter 55), myocarditis (see Chapter 64), thyroid disease (see Chapter 239), or ingestion of cardiotoxic substances. Direct inquiry may also identify any associated disorders (e.g., anemia, arrhythmias, ischemia, or renal dysfunction) or concomitant medications (e.g., calcium channel blockers, antiarrhythmic drugs, and non-steroidal anti-inflammatory drugs) that can exacerbate the syndrome of heart failure or complicate its management. The physical examination may indicate the presence of cardiac enlargement, valvular disorders, or congenital heart disease (see Chapter 57) or evidence of a systemic disease that may lead to or contribute to heart failure.

Although the history and physical examination may provide important clues about the nature of the underlying cardiac abnormality, such information may occasionally be misleading, because patients with risk factors for one disease may have an unrelated cardiac disorder. Hence, regardless of the clinical impressions formed during the initial evaluation, the physician should define the precise nature of the underlying disorder by performing an invasive or non-invasive imaging test of the cardiac chambers. The single most useful diagnostic test is the two-dimensional Doppler flow echocardiogram. This test allows the physician to determine if the primary abnormality is pericardial, myocardial, valvular, or vascular and, if it is myocardial, whether the dysfunction is primarily systolic or diastolic (see Chapter 47). This distinction is critical, because surgery is the primary approach to the management of most pericardial, valvular, or vascular disorders whereas pharmacologic strategies are the primary approach to the management of myocardial disorders.

The focus in this chapter is on the management of patients with left ventricular systolic dysfunction, which is the cause of heart failure in 70% of patients presenting with the syndrome. The management of patients with a hypertrophic cardiomyopathy (see Chapter 64) or with disorders of the pericardium (see Chapter 65), valves (see Chapter 63) or great vessels (see Chapter 66) is discussed in the chapters specifically devoted to these topics.

Mechanisms Leading to Heart Failure

There are four distinct phases in the evolution of heart failure (Fig. 48–1): (1) the initial cardiac injury, (2) neurohormonal activation and cardiac remodeling, (3) fluid retention and peripheral vasoconstriction, and (4) contractile failure.

Causes of Cardiac Injury

A variety of disorders can injure the myocardium and lead to systolic dysfunction. About two thirds of patients with systolic dysfunction have coronary artery disease; and in these patients, the occurrence of an acute MI is usually the injurious event that triggers the decline in ejection fraction. These patients characteristically show regional abnormalities of wall motion in the myocardial segments that are perfused by the obstructed coronary arteries, and the left ventricle is typically more severely affected than the right. In the remaining one third of patients, the coronary vessels appear normal; the ventricle is globally (rather than regionally) hypokinetic; and the right and left ventricles are generally affected to a similar degree. The source of myocardial injury in patients with a

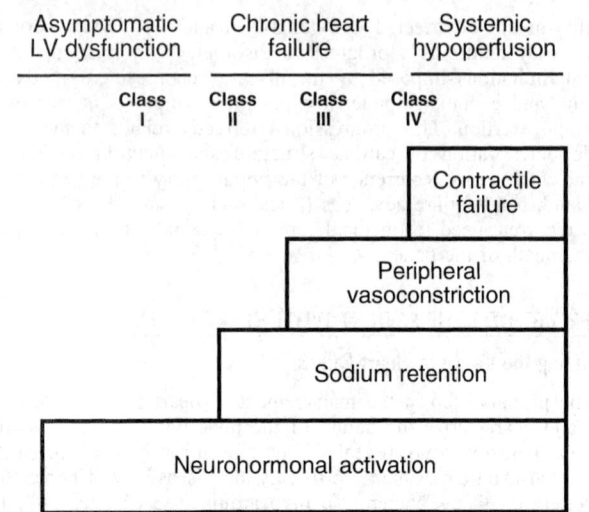

FIGURE 48–1 ■ Mechanisms contributing to the development of heart failure at each stage of the disease. This diagram should be used in conjunction with Figure 48–2; see text for details. The classes designated at the top of the page refer to the functional classification developed by the New York Heart Association. According to this classification system, patients may have symptoms at rest (Class IV), on less than ordinary exertion (Class III), on ordinary exertion (Class II), or only at levels that would cause symptoms in normal individuals (Class I).

non-ischemic cardiomyopathy may be a prior infection (e.g., myocarditis), exposure to a cardiac toxin (e.g., alcohol, cocaine, or cancer chemotherapeutic agent), or a systemic disorder (e.g., hypothyroidism or hyperthyroidism). However, no cause of myocardial injury may be found; such patients are considered to have an idiopathic dilated cardiomyopathy.

Is it important to identify the cause of myocardial injury in a patient with systolic dysfunction due to a cardiomyopathy? Coronary arteriography and non-invasive imaging studies can indicate the presence and functional consequences of coronary artery disease, and myocardial biopsy may identify the presence of inflammatory or infiltrative disorders of the heart. Yet, it remains unclear how the information generated by these tests should be used, because there is little evidence that anti-ischemic interventions can improve clinical outcomes in patients with heart failure due to advanced systolic dysfunction who do not have angina, and most infiltrative or inflammatory disorders are not reversible. Indeed, most treatable sources of myocardial injury can be identified by history or by simple blood tests (e.g., thyroid function tests).

Neurohormonal Activation and Cardiac Remodeling

Regardless of the source of myocardial injury, once a critical mass of the left ventricle is injured, heart failure becomes a progressive, self-reinforcing process, whether or not the initial insult recurs or is adequately treated. The principal manifestation of such progression is a change in the geometry of the left ventricle such that the chamber enlarges and becomes more spherical; this process is referred to as cardiac remodeling. This change in chamber size not only increases the hemodynamic stresses on the walls of the failing heart and depresses its performance but also increases the magnitude of regurgitant flow through the mitral and tricuspid valves. These effects, in turn, serve to sustain and exacerbate the remodeling process, leading to a progressive decline in left ventricular ejection fraction. Remodeling is an essential step in the transition from the initial cardiac injury to asymptomatic ventricular dysfunction to symptomatic heart failure.

What factors are responsible for, or accelerate, the process of left ventricular remodeling? Although many mechanisms may be involved, there is substantial evidence that the activation of endogenous neurohormonal systems (see Chapter 47) plays a critical role in cardiac remodeling and thereby in the progression of heart failure. These systems are activated early after an acute myocardial injury, and their activity is progressively enhanced as the disorder advances. Elevated circulating or tissue levels of norepinephrine, angiotensin II, and endothelin can act (alone or in concert) to

affect adversely the structure and function of the failing heart. These neurohormonal factors not only increase the hemodynamic stresses on the heart by causing peripheral vasoconstriction, but they may also exert a direct toxic effect on the heart by causing myocytes to undergo a process of programmed cell death (apoptosis). Neurohormonal factors can also stimulate the process of myocardial fibrosis, which can further alter the architecture and impair the performance of the failing heart. Interestingly, the initial activation of neurohormonal systems and cardiac remodeling that follows a myocardial injury is commonly asymptomatic. Although the ejection fraction is depressed and may deteriorate further, the patient commonly shows no evidence of symptoms or fluid retention for long periods of time. This is the phase referred to as asymptomatic left ventricular dysfunction.

Fluid Retention and Peripheral Vasoconstriction

As the process of physiologic deterioration continues, the activation of neurohormonal systems not only adversely affects the heart but begins to exert a deleterious effect on the kidneys and peripheral blood vessels. The sympathetic nervous system and renin-angiotensin system act on the kidneys to retain sodium and water and act on peripheral blood vessels to cause vasoconstriction. Both of these mechanisms increase the loading conditions in the failing heart, which can in turn lead to symptoms of pulmonary congestion and exercise intolerance. This is the phase referred to as chronic heart failure. As cardiac function deteriorates, hemodynamic factors emerge and can exacerbate the functional derangements of the kidneys and peripheral vessels produced by neurohormonal systems. A decline in renal blood flow impairs the ability of the kidneys to excrete salt and water, and an increase in sodium content of peripheral vessels can impair their dilatory capacity. Similarly, a decline in regional blood flow can attenuate the physiologic actions of endogenous natriuretic peptides that normally counteract vasoconstrictor mechanisms. Over time, the interplay of hemodynamic and neurohormonal factors leads to worsening of symptoms and a deterioration of clinical status, often with little additional decrease in the left ventricular ejection fraction.

Contractile Failure

As the disease advances, the myocardium eventually loses a critical mass of functioning myocytes and can no longer sustain forward flow and peripheral perfusion. Despite the decline in cardiac performance, the patient survives because the inotropic and vasoconstrictor effects of the sympathetic nervous system and the renin-angiotensin system act to support cardiac contractility and systemic pressures, at least in the short term. The renal retention of salt and water is intense, but the resulting expansion of intravascular volume fails to support the circulation and acts only to exacerbate pulmonary and peripheral congestion. This precarious state cannot be sustained; the threat to the circulation is so immediate that the patient can be stabilized only by intensive medical care in a hospital. The phase of contractile failure frequently characterizes the terminal stages of the disorder.

The evolution through these four stages of heart failure may occur slowly or rapidly, the rate of progression being determined by the severity of the initial cardiac injury and the intensity of neurohormonal activation. Death may occur during any of the four phases, although it is commonly sudden in patients with minimal or mild symptoms and is usually related to pump failure in patients with advanced symptoms.

Defining an Appropriate Therapeutic Strategy

Each of the four phases of heart failure requires a specific therapeutic approach (Fig. 48–2). For patients who have not yet suffered an initial cardiac insult, every effort should be made to minimize the occurrence and impact of diseases that can injure the heart. For patients who have developed left ventricular dysfunction but remain asymptomatic, physicians should interfere with the neurohormonal systems that can cause cardiac remodeling and lead to the development of clinical heart failure. For patients who have developed symptoms, the primary goals are to alleviate fluid retention, lessen disability, and reduce the risk of further progression and death. These goals generally require a strategy that combines diuretics (to control salt and water retention), with neurohormonal interventions (to minimize the deleterious effects of the sympathetic nervous system and renin-angiotensin systems) and that frequently

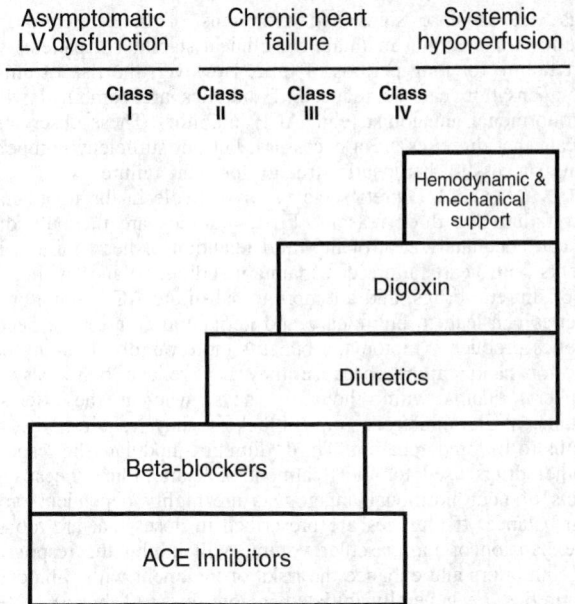

FIGURE 48-2 ■ Treatment strategies appropriate to each stage of heart failure. This diagram should be used in conjunction with Figure 48-1; see text for details. The classes designated at the top of the page refer to the functional classification developed by the New York Heart Association (see legend to Figure 48-1).

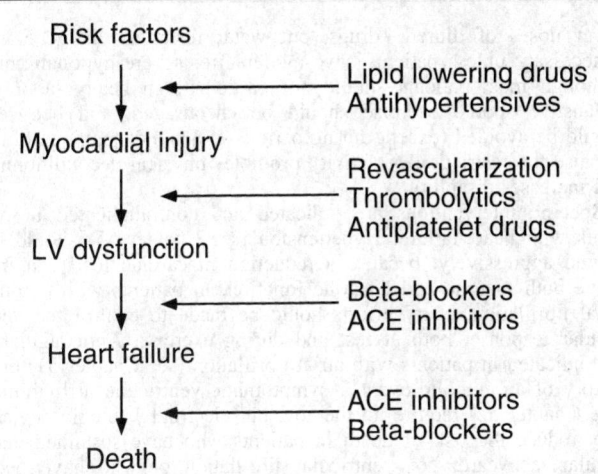

FIGURE 48-3 ■ Sequence of steps in the evolution and progression of heart failure. Also identified are interventions that have been shown to inhibit each step in the process and thus can favorably affect the natural history of the disease.

adds hemodynamic interventions (to enhance cardiac performance and reduce peripheral vasoconstriction). Finally, for patients hospitalized with immediately life-threatening heart failure, the principal objectives are to stabilize the precarious state of the circulation and to maintain end-organ function until precipitating factors have resolved or until a definitive solution can be formulated to treat the underlying disease. Such patients generally require intensive hemodynamic or mechanical support (see Chapter 95). These observations suggest that neurohormonal mechanisms are dominant in the early phases of heart failure, whereas hemodynamic mechanisms play an increasingly critical role as the disease advances to its terminal phase.

Both neurohormonal and hemodynamic interventions can improve the performance of the failing heart, but they do so in distinct ways. On the one hand, drugs can increase ejection fraction by directly stimulating the contractility of individual myocyte cells. This approach (used by positive inotropic agents) can produce immediate hemodynamic benefits but may exacerbate the deleterious actions of neurohormonal systems and thereby the process of cardiac remodeling. As a result, positive inotropic agents may be useful in the short-term management of patients hospitalized with immediately life-threatening disease, but long-term treatment with these agents may increase morbidity and mortality. On the other hand, drugs can increase ejection fraction by antagonizing the neurohormonal activation that can impair the function and viability of cardiac cells. This approach (used by angiotensin-converting enzyme [ACE] inhibitors and β-adrenergic receptor blockers) can slow the progression of heart failure and reduce the risk of major cardiac events in patients with asymptomatic left ventricular dysfunction or established symptoms of heart failure. However, in patients with end-stage disease, neurohormonal antagonists can undermine the homeostatic mechanisms that are critical for the support of cardiac contractility and systemic pressures. These observations indicate that the treatment of heart failure should be targeted to the mechanisms that drive the disease process during each phase of the disorder.

PREVENTION OF HEART FAILURE

Heart failure can be prevented by decreasing the risk of the initial cardiac injury or, if the injury has already occurred, by decreasing the early and continuing loss of myocardium. Specific interventions can alter the development and progression of heart failure during each phase of the disease (Fig. 48–3).

DECREASE THE RISK OF THE INITIAL CARDIAC INJURY.

The treatment of hyperlipidemia and hypertension in high-risk patients can reduce the risk of MI and, as a result, the likelihood of developing heart failure. In patients with hypercholesterolemia and a history of angina or MI, treatment with a lipid-lowering agent has been shown to decrease the risk of death and of heart failure. In patients with systolic or diastolic hypertension without a history of heart disease, antihypertensive therapy decreases the risk of stroke and of heart failure; these benefits are particularly marked in patients with a previous MI.

DECREASE THE LIKELIHOOD OF DEVELOPING HEART FAILURE AFTER CARDIAC INJURY. The aggressive treatment of patients *during* an acute MI can reduce the *extent* of the initial myocardial injury. In patients who are in the middle of an acute MI, reperfusion with percutaneous transluminal coronary angioplasty and thrombolytic agents can minimize the loss of myocardium and can thereby reduce the risk of developing subsequent heart failure in patients with an uncomplicated MI and decrease the risk of death in patients whose MI is complicated by heart failure.

Furthermore, the aggressive treatment of patients after an acute MI can reduce the extension of the initial injury to other segments of the myocardium. In patients with a recent MI, treatment with a β-blocker reduces the risk of reinfarction and of death, especially in those with heart failure at the start of treatment (see Chapter 60). Similarly, use of an ACE inhibitor in patients with a recent MI reduces the risk of reinfarction, heart failure, and death, especially in those with left ventricular dysfunction at the start of treatment. Combined neurohormonal blockade (ACE inhibitors and β-blockers) may produce complementary benefits.

Finally, in patients with established ischemic or non-ischemic left ventricular systolic dysfunction (ejection fraction < 35–40%) with no or minimal symptoms of heart failure, treatment with an ACE inhibitor can reduce the risk of developing heart failure. Similarly, in patients with a history of heart failure after an acute MI, treatment with an ACE inhibitor or a β-blocker may reduce the risk of death.

OUTPATIENT TREATMENT OF HEART FAILURE

The goals of outpatient management of patients with symptoms of heart failure due to systolic dysfunction of the left ventricle are (1) the control of fluid retention; (2) the control of neurohormonal activation (to reduce morbidity and mortality); and (3) the control of symptoms and disability.

General Measures

Several general measures are advisable for most patients with chronic heart failure. Obese patients should lose weight, smokers should stop using cigarettes, and concomitant cardiac conditions and risk factors (e.g., hyperlipidemia) should be actively managed. Moderate sodium restriction is usually indicated to permit use of lower doses of diuretic drugs, but water restriction is generally unnecessary unless patients have moderate or severe hyponatremia. Although most patients should not participate in heavy labor or exhaustive sports, exercise should be encouraged, and bed rest should be avoided (except during periods of acute decompensation), because the restriction of activity promotes physical deconditioning and increases disability.

Specific interventions are indicated and contraindicated in patients with heart failure. Hypertension (see Chapter 55) should be treated aggressively, because a reduction in cardiac load can improve both systolic and diastolic function. In patients with chronic atrial fibrillation, every effort should be made to control the ventricular response, both at rest and during exercise. Anticoagulants are indicated in patients with atrial fibrillation (see Chapter 51) or a history of an embolic event. Asymptomatic ventricular arrhythmias (see Chapter 52) require no therapy, but electrophysiologic devices may reduce the risk of death in patients who have sustained ventricular tachycardia or ventricular fibrillation or who have been resuscitated from sudden death. Patients with heart failure are predisposed to the proarrhythmic effects of antiarrhythmic drugs and the cardiodepressant effects of calcium channel blockers, and such agents should be avoided. Non-steroidal anti-inflammatory drugs can inhibit the effects of diuretics and ACE inhibitors and can worsen both cardiac and renal function.

Drugs for the Control of Fluid Retention

The first step in the treatment of patients with chronic heart failure is the control of fluid retention. This step is generally not necessary in patients with asymptomatic left ventricular systolic dysfunction.

Diuretics

Diuretics interfere with the sodium retention of heart failure by inhibiting the reabsorption of sodium and chloride at specific sites in the renal tubules. Of the commonly used agents, furosemide, torsemide, and bumetanide act at the loop of Henle (i.e., loop diuretics); thiazides and metolazone act in the distal tubule; and potassium-sparing diuretics act at the level of the collecting duct.

All diuretics increase urine volume and sodium excretion, but these agents differ in their pharmacologic properties. The loop diuretics increase the fractional excretion of sodium up to 20 to 25% of the filtered load, enhance the clearance of free water, and maintain efficacy even when renal perfusion and function are impaired. In contrast, the thiazide diuretics increase the fractional excretion of sodium to only 5 to 10% of the filtered load, tend to decrease free water clearance, and lose their effectiveness in patients with only moderately impaired renal perfusion and function. Consequently, the loop diuretics have emerged as the preferred diuretic agents for patients with heart failure.

CLINICAL EFFECTS. Controlled trials have shown that diuretic

drugs can decrease signs and symptoms of fluid retention, but diuretics alone cannot maintain the clinical stability of patients with heart failure for long periods of time. However, the risk of clinical decompensation can be reduced if diuretics are combined with a neurohormonal antagonist (e.g., ACE inhibitor). These observations indicate that diuretics are a necessary, but not sufficient, component of any successful therapeutic strategy for heart failure.

CLINICAL USE. Diuretics play a pivotal role in the treatment of heart failure for three reasons. First, diuretics are the only drugs that can adequately control the fluid retention of heart failure. Few patients with heart failure can maintain sodium balance without the use of diuretic drugs, and attempts to substitute ACE inhibitors for diuretics can lead to pulmonary and peripheral congestion. Second, diuretics produce symptomatic benefits more rapidly than any other drug for heart failure, because they can relieve pulmonary and peripheral edema within hours or days, whereas the effects of digitalis, ACE inhibitors, or β-blockers may require weeks or months to become apparent. Third, diuretics modulate the responses to other drugs used for the treatment of heart failure, because the effects of neurohormonal antagonists are highly dependent on sodium balance. If diuretics are prescribed in doses that are too low, the expansion of intravascular volume will inhibit the response to ACE inhibitors and enhance the risks of treatment with β-blockers.

Diuretics are generally initiated in low doses (Table 48–1), and the dose is increased until signs and symptoms of fluid retention are alleviated. Once this goal has been achieved, treatment with the diuretic is continued long term to prevent the recurrence of salt and water retention. Although diuretics are commonly prescribed at a constant daily dose, the doses of these drugs should ideally be adjusted based on changes in the patient's body weight. As heart failure advances and renal function declines, patients will become resistant to the effects of low doses of these drugs and will respond only when high doses are used or when diuretics with different renal tubular sites of action are used in combination. Non-steroidal anti-inflammatory drugs can decrease the efficacy and increase the risk of diuretics and should be avoided.

CLINICAL PRECAUTIONS. The principal adverse effects of diuretics include (1) electrolyte depletion, (2) neurohormonal activation, and (3) hypotension and azotemia. Other types of side effects may occur (e.g., rash, hearing difficulties), but these are generally idiosyncratic or occur with the use of very large doses.

ELECTROLYTE DEPLETION. Diuretics can cause the depletion of potassium and magnesium, which can predispose patients to serious cardiac arrhythmias, particularly in the presence of digitalis therapy. The loss of electrolytes is related to enhanced delivery of sodium to distal sites in the renal tubules and the exchange of sodium for other cations, a process that is potentiated by activation of the renin-angiotensin-aldosterone system. Concomitant administration of ACE inhibitors, angiotensin II receptor blockers, or aldosterone antagonists can prevent the loss of electrolytes caused by diuretics.

NEUROHORMONAL ACTIVATION. Diuretic drugs may increase the activation of endogenous neurohormonal systems in patients with

Table 48–1 ■ DRUGS RECOMMENDED FOR GENERAL USE IN CHRONIC HEART FAILURE

	STARTING DOSE	SUBSEQUENT DOSES
Diuretics		
Furosemide	20–40 mg once or twice daily	Titrate to achieve dry weight (up to 400 mg/d)
Torsemide	10–20 mg once or twice daily	Titrate to achieve dry weight (up to 200 mg/d)
Bumetinide	0.5–1.0 mg once or twice daily	Titrate to achieve dry weight (up to 10 mg/d)
Metolazone	2.5–5.0 once daily	Titrate to achieve dry weight (up to 20 mg/d)
Angiotensin-Converting Enzyme Inhibitors		
Captopril	6.25 mg twice daily	Titrate to target dose (50 mg three times daily)
Enalapril	2.5 mg twice daily	Titrate to target dose (10–20 mg twice daily)
Lisinopril	2.5–5.0 mg once daily	Titrate to target dose (20–35 mg once daily)
Ramipril*	1.25–2.5 mg twice daily	Titrate to target dose (5 mg twice daily)
Quinapril	10 mg twice daily	Target dose not established (not >40 mg twice daily)
Fosinopril	5–10 mg once daily	Target dose not established (not >40 mg once daily)
β-Receptor Blockers		
Carvedilol	3.125 mg twice daily	Titrate to target dose (6.25–25 mg twice daily)
Bisoprolol*	1.25 mg once daily	Titrate to target dose (10 mg once daily)
Metoprolol* (sustained-release)	12.5–25 mg daily	Titrate to target dose (200 mg once daily)
Aldosterone Antagonists		
Spironolactone	12.5–25 mg once daily	Titrate to target dose (25 mg once daily)
Digitalis Glycosides		
Digoxin	0.125–0.25 mg once daily	Target dose not established (not >0.5 mg/day)

*Drugs not approved by the U.S. Food and Drug Administration for use in the management of chronic heart failure, April, 1999.

heart failure. Such activation may increase the risk of disease progression, unless patients are receiving concomitant treatment with a neurohormonal antagonist (ACE inhibitor or sympathetic antagonist).

HYPOTENSION AND AZOTEMIA. Although the use of diuretics can lower blood pressure or cause azotemia, these changes are generally asymptomatic and require no specific treatment. The dose of diuretic should not be reduced for asymptomatic changes in blood pressure or renal function if the patient has signs of fluid overload.

Drugs That Antagonize Neurohormonal Mechanisms

Drugs that interfere with the actions of endogenous neurohormonal systems (e.g., the renin-angiotensin system and the sympathetic nervous system) can relieve the symptoms of heart failure by antagonizing the vasoconstriction caused by an increase in neurohormonal activity. Yet, their major advantage over traditional treatments is their ability to inhibit the cardiotoxic effects of the neurohormonal system and thereby retard the progression of heart failure. As a result, neurohormonal interventions have emerged as essential agents in the management of heart failure. Two types of neurohormonal antagonists have been approved for the treatment of heart failure by the U.S. Food and Drug Administration (FDA): (1) ACE inhibitors, which interfere with the actions of the renin-angiotensin system; and (2) β-adrenergic receptor blockers, which interfere with the actions of the sympathetic nervous system.

Angiotensin-Converting Enzyme Inhibitors

ACE inhibitors interfere with the renin-angiotensin system by inhibiting the enzyme responsible for the conversion of angiotensin I to angiotensin II. However, the benefits of these drugs may not be entirely explained by their actions on the renin-angiotensin system. Because the ACE is identical to kininase II, ACE inhibition not only interferes with the formation of angiotensin II but also enhances the action of kinins (Fig. 48–4); kinin potentiation may be more important than angiotensin suppression in mediating the effects of ACE inhibitors. The favorable effects of ACE inhibitors on cardiac remodeling may not be seen with angiotensin II receptor antagonists, and this advantage of ACE inhibitors is abolished by the co-administration of kinin antagonists. Moreover, the hemodynamic and prognostic benefits of ACE inhibitors may be attenuated by the co-administration of aspirin, which blocks kinin-mediated prostaglandin synthesis.

Five ACE inhibitors have been approved for the treatment of chronic heart failure by the FDA: captopril, enalapril, lisinopril, quinapril, and fosinopril (see Table 48–1). Ramipril is approved for the treatment of heart failure after an acute MI.

CLINICAL EFFECTS. All ACE inhibitors approved for the treatment of heart failure have been shown in double-blind, placebo-controlled trials to produce hemodynamic and clinical benefits. Treatment with these drugs improves left ventricular ejection fraction and decreases left ventricular chamber size; both actions suggest a favorable effect on the process of cardiac remodeling. ACE inhibitors relieve dyspnea, prolong exercise tolerance, and reduce the need for emergency care for worsening heart failure. These benefits are seen in patients with mild, moderate, and severe symptoms, whether or not they are treated with digitalis. However, ACE inhibitors should not be used before (or instead of) diuretics in patients with a history of fluid retention, because diuretics are needed to maintain sodium balance and prevent the development of peripheral and pulmonary edema. Nevertheless, ACE inhibitors may reduce the need for large doses of diuretics and potassium supplements and may attenuate many of the adverse metabolic effects of aggressive diuretic therapy (e.g., hypokalemia and hyponatremia).

In addition, several long-term trials have shown that ACE inhibitors can reduce the risk of death and retard the progression of heart failure in patients with an ischemic or non-ischemic cardiomyopathy who are already receiving digitalis and diuretics. In the Studies of Left Ventricular Dysfunction (SOLVD) Treatment Trial, the use of enalapril in patients with mild-to-moderate symptoms was associated with a 16% reduction in all-cause mortality ($P = .004$) and a 26% decrease in the risk of death or hospitalization for heart failure ($P < .001$) (Fig. 48–5). In the Co-operative North Scandinavian Enalapril Survival Study (CONSENSUS), the use of enalapril in patients with severe symptoms was associated with a 27% reduction in the risk of death ($P = .003$). When the results of all studies are combined, ACE inhibitors appear to reduce both the risk of

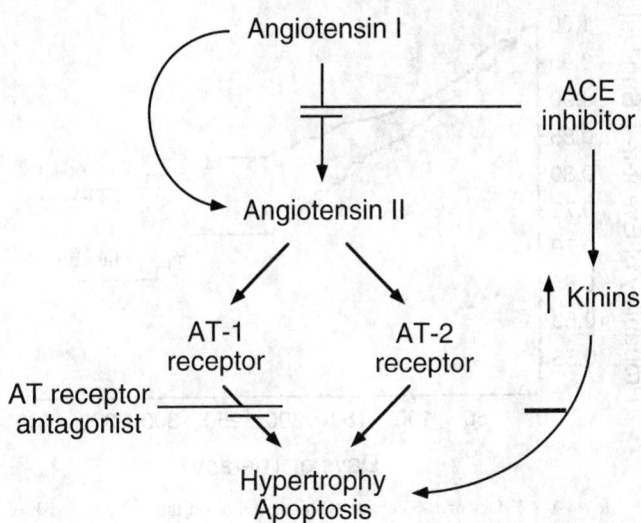

FIGURE 48–4 ■ Effects of angiotensin-converting enzyme (ACE) inhibitors and angiotensin (AT) receptor antagonists on the renin-angiotensin pathway. ACE inhibitors interfere with the formation of angiotensin II and inhibit the degradation of kinins; both effects can inhibit hypertrophy and programmed cell death (apoptosis). In contrast, AT receptor antagonists inhibit the interaction of angiotensin with the AT-1 receptor but have little effect on kinins.

death and the risk of hospitalization for heart failure by 20 to 30%. Furthermore, ACE inhibitors produce greater effects on survival than a combination of direct-acting vasodilators (e.g., hydralazine and isosorbide dinitrate). ACE inhibitors have also been shown to reduce mortality rates in patients with impaired left ventricular function or heart failure after an acute MI (see Chapter 60).

CLINICAL USE. Because of their ability to improve the natural history of heart failure, all patients with heart failure due to left ventricular systolic dysfunction should receive an ACE inhibitor unless they are unable to tolerate the drug or have a contraindication to it. Physicians should not withhold treatment with an ACE inhibitor until the patient becomes resistant to treatment with other drugs, because such patients might die during the period of delay and such deaths might have been prevented if treatment with the ACE inhibitor had been initiated earlier. The available data do not justify withholding ACE inhibitors from any specific subset of patients, even patients with low blood pressures or impaired renal function. Treatment is generally maintained even in patients who do not experience symptomatic benefits.

Treatment with an ACE inhibitor is generally initiated in low

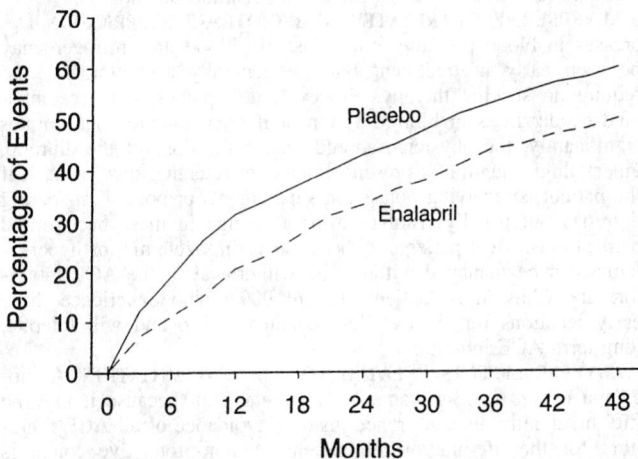

FIGURE 48–5 ■ Effect of ACE inhibition with enalapril on the combined risk of death and hospitalizations for heart failure. The SOLVD treatment trial enrolled 2569 patients with primarily Class II and III symptoms treated with digitalis and diuretics. Use of enalapril was associated with a 26% reduction in risk ($P < 0.001$).

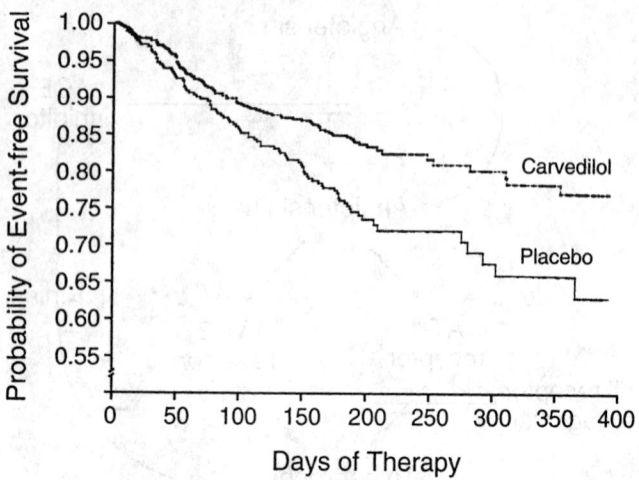

FIGURE 48–6 ■ Effect of β-blockade with carvedilol on the combined risk of death and hospitalizations for cardiovascular reasons. The U.S. Carvedilol Program enrolled 1094 patients with primarily Class II and III symptoms treated with digitalis, diuretics, and an ACE inhibitor. Use of carvedilol was associated with a 38% reduction in risk ($P < 0.001$).

doses followed by gradual increments in dose if lower doses have been well tolerated. In general, the dose of ACE inhibitor is increased until the doses are similar to those used in the clinical trials that established the ability of these drugs to reduce morbidity and mortality. Examples of starting doses of ACE inhibitors include captopril, 6.25 mg three times a day; enalapril, 2.5 mg twice daily; or lisinopril, 2.5 to 5.0 mg once daily (see Table 48–1). Examples of target doses of ACE inhibitors include captopril, 50 mg three times a day; enalapril, 10 to 20 mg twice daily; and lisinopril, 20 to 35 mg once daily. High doses are more effective than low doses in reducing the risk of hospitalization. The clinical effects of therapy may take weeks or months to become apparent.

Because fluid retention can attenuate the effects of ACE inhibitors, physicians should ensure that the dose of diuretics is optimized before initiating treatment. Close monitoring of diuretic therapy is also needed after initiation of treatment, because the dose of diuretic may need to be reduced if the patient experiences symptomatic decreases in blood pressure or clinically important declines in renal function. Non-steroidal anti-inflammatory drugs can decrease the efficacy and increase the risks of ACE inhibitors and should be avoided.

CLINICAL PRECAUTIONS. The adverse effects of ACE inhibitors can be attributed to the two principal pharmacologic actions of these drugs: (1) those related to the effects of angiotensin suppression and (2) those related to the effects of kinin potentiation.

ADVERSE EFFECTS RELATED TO ANGIOTENSIN SUPPRESSION. Decreases in blood pressure or increases in blood urea nitrogen may be seen early in treatment but are generally asymptomatic and require no specific therapy. However, if hypotension is accompanied by dizziness or blurred vision or if renal function deteriorates significantly, the physician should reduce the dose of the diuretic, unless fluid retention is present. Potassium retention may be seen if the patient is receiving potassium supplements or potassium-sparing diuretics but usually resolves after a change in these background medications. Most patients with hypotension, azotemia, or hyperkalemia can be managed without the withdrawal of the ACE inhibitor; and, thus, most patients (about 90%) who experience these early reactions remain excellent candidates for, and will tolerate, long-term ACE inhibition.

ADVERSE EFFECTS RELATED TO KININ POTENTIATION. Angioedema occurs in less than 1% of patients, but because it may be life threatening, its occurrence justifies avoidance of all ACE inhibitors for the lifetime of the patient. A non-productive cough is observed in 5 to 15% of patients receiving ACE inhibitors; it usually appears within the first several months of therapy, disappears within 1 to 2 weeks of discontinuing treatment, and recurs within days of rechallenge. When a patient receiving an ACE inhibitor complains of cough, other causes should be considered

(especially pulmonary congestion), and the ACE inhibitor should be implicated only after the physician confirms that the cough disappears after withdrawal of the drug and recurs after rechallenge. Because the cough is related to a common action of all ACE inhibitors, its occurrence frequently requires the withdrawal of the ACE inhibitor and the use of alternative approaches to interfering with the renin-angiotensin system (e.g., angiotensin II receptor antagonists).

β-Adrenergic Receptor Blockers

Although most physicians have been taught to avoid the use of β-blockers in patients with heart failure, recent evidence indicates that these drugs can produce important clinical benefits in this disorder. Like ACE inhibitors, β-blockers interfere with the deleterious actions of an endogenous neurohormonal system, which can adversely affect the failing heart by promoting cell death, hypertrophy, ischemia, arrhythmias, vasoconstriction, and fluid retention. Insofar as these deleterious effects are mediated through three distinct adrenergic receptors (α_1, β_1, and β_2), agents that block multiple receptors may provide greater protection against catecholamine-induced cardiomyopathy than drugs that block only one receptor. This hypothesis is being prospectively evaluated in a large-scale clinical trial.

Of available β-blockers, only carvedilol has been approved by the FDA for the treatment of heart failure. Other β-blockers (metoprolol and bisoprolol) have also been effective in large-scale trials and may be approved in the future.

CLINICAL EFFECTS. Several β-blockers have been shown in double-blind, placebo-controlled trials to produce hemodynamic and clinical benefits. Treatment with these drugs improves left ventricular ejection fraction and decreases left ventricular chamber size; both actions suggest a favorable effect on the process of cardiac remodeling. β-Blockers relieve symptoms and improve clinical status; these benefits have been seen in patients with mild-to-moderate and moderate-to-severe symptoms, whether or not they are treated with digitalis. β-Blockers are generally used together with ACE inhibitors in clinical practice; combined use of both neurohormonal antagonists can be expected to produce additive benefits.

In addition, several long-term trials have shown that β-blockers can reduce the risk of death and retard the progression of heart failure in patients with an ischemic or non-ischemic cardiomyopathy who are already receiving digitalis, diuretics, and ACE inhibitors. In the U.S. Carvedilol Program, the use of carvedilol in patients was associated with a 65% reduction in all-cause mortality ($P = .0001$) and a 36% decrease in the risk of death or hospitalization for a cardiovascular reason ($P < .001$) (Fig. 48–6). In the Second Cardiac Insufficiency Bisoprolol Study (CIBIS), the use of bisoprolol was associated with a 32% reduction in the risk of death ($P < .001$) and a 32% decrease in the frequency of being hospitalized for heart failure ($P < .0001$). In the Metoprolol CR/XL Randomized Trial in Heart Failure (MERIT-HF) study, the use of metoprolol was associated with an approximately 35% reduction in the risk of death ($P < .001$). When the results of all studies are combined, β-blockers appear to reduce both the risk of death and the risk of hospitalization for heart failure by 30 to 40% in patients already receiving ACE inhibitors. The magnitude of the effects are similar regardless of the cause or severity of heart failure, but there is little experience with the use of these drugs in patients with symptoms at rest. β-Blockers have also been shown to reduce mortality rates in patients with impaired left ventricular function or heart failure after an acute MI.

CLINICAL USE. Because β-blockers can favorably modify the natural history of heart failure, all patients with heart failure due to left ventricular systolic dysfunction should receive a β-blocker unless they have a contraindication to its use or are unable to tolerate treatment with the drug. β-Blockers should not be withheld until the patient is shown to be resistant to treatment with other drugs, because such patients might die or experience worsening of their disease during the period of delay and such progression might have been prevented if treatment with the β-blocker had been initiated earlier. Treatment is generally maintained even in patients who do not experience symptomatic benefits. However, there are insufficient data on the efficacy and safety of β-blocker use in patients with Class IV symptoms or those receiving intravenous drugs for heart failure to justify the use of these drugs in those with end-stage disease. In addition, patients with bronchospastic disease or advanced heart block should not receive treatment with these drugs.

Treatment with a β-blocker is generally initiated in very low doses followed by gradual increments in dose if lower doses have been well tolerated (see Table 48–1). In general, the dose of these drugs is increased until doses are achieved similar to those used in the clinical trials that established the ability of these drugs to reduce morbidity and mortality. Examples of starting doses of β-blockers include carvedilol, 3.125 mg twice daily; bisoprolol, 1.25 mg/day; and metoprolol (sustained-release), 12.5 mg/day. Examples of long-term doses of β-blockers include carvedilol, 6.25–25 mg twice daily; bisoprolol, 10 mg/day; and metoprolol (sustained-release), 200 mg/day. As in the case of ACE inhibitors, the clinical effects of therapy may take weeks or months to become apparent.

Because fluid retention can increase the risks of β-blockade, physicians should ensure that the dose of diuretics is optimized before initiating treatment. Close monitoring of diuretic therapy is also needed after initiation of treatment, because an increase in the dose of diuretic may be required if the patient experiences a significant increase in body weight or worsening symptoms of heart failure.

CLINICAL PRECAUTIONS. Like ACE inhibitors, β-blockers can produce unwanted side effects that result directly from changes in neurohormonal activity. These adverse reactions occur during initiation of therapy but are generally mild in severity, can be managed by changes in concomitant therapy, usually subside after several days or weeks of treatment, and, thus, infrequently lead to the withdrawal of treatment. In clinical trials, most patients (> 85%) with heart failure were able to tolerate short- and long-term therapy with these drugs.

HYPOTENSION. Vasodilatory side effects may be seen within 24 to 48 hours of initiation of therapy or after increments in dose but usually subside with repeated dosing without any change in the dose of the β-blocker or background medications. Physicians can minimize the risk of hypotension by administering the β-blocker and the ACE inhibitor at different times of the day.

FLUID RETENTION. Initiation of therapy with a β-blocker can produce fluid retention, which is usually manifest as an asymptomatic increase in body weight but may be severe enough to cause worsening symptoms of heart failure. Increases in body weight are generally seen within 3 to 5 days of initiation of therapy or after increments in dose. Physicians should ask patients to weigh themselves daily, and asymptomatic increases in weight should be treated promptly by increasing the dose of concomitantly administered diuretics until the patient's weight is restored to pretreatment levels.

BRADYCARDIA AND HEART BLOCK. Therapy with a β-blocker can produce decreases in heart rate and alterations in cardiac conduction that may lead to bradycardia or heart block. These changes are usually asymptomatic but may be severe enough to cause symptomatic hypotension. If the heart rate declines to less than 50 beats per minute or second or third heart block is observed, the dose of β-blocker should be decreased. Cardiac pacing might be considered to allow the use of β-blockade in selected patients.

Aldosterone Antagonists

Although generally classified in the category of potassium-sparing diuretics, drugs that block the actions of aldosterone (e.g., spironolactone) act to antagonize an endogenous neurohormonal mechanism that may adversely affect the heart independent of its effects on sodium balance. In the Randomized Aldactone Evaluation Study (RALES) trial, the addition of low doses of spironolactone (12.5–25 mg/day) to patients with current or recent Class IV symptoms receiving ACE inhibitors decreased the risk of death by 25 to 30% and the risk of hospitalization for heart failure by approximately 35% ($P < .001$). Although this result has not yet been replicated, the use of low doses of spironolactone merits consideration in patients with advanced heart failure. Such use, however, is not currently approved by the FDA.

Drugs Used to Relieve Symptoms and Lessen Disability

Digitalis

The digitalis glycosides exert their effects in patients with heart failure by virtue of their ability to inhibit sodium-potassium adenosine triphosphatase (Na^+, K^+-ATPase). Inhibition of this enzyme in

the heart results in an increase in cardiac contractility; and for many decades, the benefits of digitalis in heart failure were ascribed to this positive inotropic action. However, by inhibiting Na^+, K^+-ATPase in vagal afferents, digitalis acts to sensitize cardiac baroreceptors, which, in turn, reduce the outflow of sympathetic impulses from the central nervous system. In addition, by inhibiting Na^+, K^+-ATPase in the kidney, digitalis reduces the renal tubular reabsorption of sodium; the resulting increase in the delivery of sodium to the distal tubules leads to the suppression of renin secretion. These observations have led to the hypothesis that, in addition to increasing contractile force, digitalis may produce important vasodilatory effects by attenuating the activation of neurohormonal systems.

Although a variety of digitalis glycosides have been used in the treatment of heart failure for the past 200 years, the most commonly used preparation in the United States is digoxin. Digoxin is the principal glycoside that has been evaluated in placebo-controlled trials.

CLINICAL EFFECTS. Controlled studies have shown that digoxin can improve symptoms, quality of life, and exercise tolerance in patients with mild-to-moderate heart failure. These benefits are seen regardless of the underlying rhythm (sinus rhythm or atrial fibrillation), cause of heart failure (ischemic or non-ischemic cardiomyopathy), or concomitant therapy (with or without ACE inhibitors). The addition of digoxin produces favorable effects on clinical status and ejection fraction, and the withdrawal of digoxin is followed by hemodynamic and clinical deterioration. However, in a long-term controlled clinical trial, digoxin did not reduce the risk of death and was associated with only a modest reduction in the combined risk of death and hospitalization. These results indicate that the primary benefit of digoxin in heart failure is to alleviate symptoms and improve clinical status.

CLINICAL USE. Digoxin provides a convenient, inexpensive, and well-tolerated means of improving the clinical status of patients with heart failure. However, the finding that the drug has little effect on the progression of heart failure has minimized any mandate for its early use; and, thus, it can be prescribed at any time if symptoms persist after the use of other drugs. Digoxin is a preferred agent in patients with heart failure who have atrial fibrillation and a rapid ventricular response (see Chapter 51). The drug is not recommended for use in patients who have no symptoms or for the stabilization of patients with acutely decompensated heart failure.

Digoxin is usually initiated and maintained at a dose of 0.25 mg/day (see Table 48–1). Lower doses are indicated in patients who are elderly (> 70 years) or in those with impaired renal function (serum creatinine > 1.5 mg/dL). Higher doses may be needed to control the ventricular response in patients with atrial fibrillation. Although serum digoxin levels are commonly used to guide the administration of digoxin, there is little evidence to support this approach. There is no relation between drug levels and efficacy in patients in sinus rhythm, and patients with atrial fibrillation are better monitored by their heart rate response than by drug levels.

CLINICAL PRECAUTIONS. The principal adverse effects of digoxin include (1) cardiac arrhythmias (e.g., ectopic and re-entrant cardiac rhythms and heart block); (2) gastrointestinal symptoms (e.g., anorexia, nausea and vomiting); and (3) neurologic complaints (e.g., visual disturbances, disorientation, and confusion). These side effects are commonly associated with serum digoxin levels greater than 2 ng/mL, but digitalis toxicity may occur with lower digoxin levels, particularly if hypokalemia or hypomagnesemia coexist. The concomitant use of quinidine, verapamil, spironolactone, flecainide, propafenone, and amiodarone can increase serum digoxin levels and may increase the risk of adverse reactions. Patients with advanced heart block should not receive the drug unless a pacemaker is in place.

Low doses of digoxin are well tolerated by most patients with heart failure. Adverse effects occur primarily when the drug is administered in large doses, but large doses are generally not needed to produce clinical benefits. Nevertheless, there is persistent concern that digitalis may exert deleterious cardiovascular effects in the long term at doses that appear to be well tolerated in the short term. In a large-scale trial, the use of digoxin in doses that produced serum levels below the toxic range appeared to increase the frequency of hospitalizations and deaths related to cardiovascular events other than heart failure. These observations raise the possibility that even low doses of digoxin can adversely affect the heart.

Algorithm for the Management of Chronic Heart Failure

The evidence summarized in this section can be synthesized into an algorithm that can guide the management of patients with symptoms of heart failure (Fig. 48–7).

Step 1: Establish the Diagnosis of Heart Failure

Patients who are limited in their ability to exercise or perform activities of daily living because of dyspnea or fatigue should be evaluated for the presence of heart failure. During the initial evaluation, the clinician should obtain a two-dimensional echocardiogram, which can identify disorders of the valves, pericardium, or great vessels that may be corrected surgically and can quantify the type and magnitude of ventricular dysfunction. Patients with systolic dysfunction (ejection fraction ≤ 40%) should be distinguished from patients with preserved left ventricular function (> 40%).

Every effort should be made to identify and treat concomitant conditions (e.g., anemia, thyroid disorders) or withdraw concomitant medications (e.g., calcium channel blockers, antiarrhythmic drugs, and non-steroidal anti-inflammatory drugs) that may exacerbate the syndrome of heart failure. Patients who are in respiratory distress, have evidence for poor end-organ perfusion or fluid overload, or have a serious complicating illness should be hospitalized for treatment with intravenous agents (e.g., diuretics, vasodilators and/or positive inotropic agents) to achieve rapid stabilization of their clinical condition.

Step 2: Initiate Therapy With a Diuretic to Stabilize the Symptoms

Because of the critical importance of fluid retention, the use of diuretics is warranted in most patients with symptoms of heart failure, together with a moderate degree of sodium restriction. The dose of diuretic should be adjusted until there is no evidence of fluid retention, as reflected either by resolution of peripheral edema

or normalization of jugular venous pressure. After these early goals are achieved, treatment with the diuretic should be continued long term to prevent the recurrence of fluid retention, and the doses of diuretics should be continually re-evaluated to maintain patients free of edema and at dry weight. If this approach is not followed, the resulting underutilization of diuretics will not only undermine the ability of these drugs to relieve symptoms but will also adversely affect the patient's ability to respond favorably and safely to ACE inhibitors and β-blockers. As heart failure advances and renal function declines, patients may become resistant to the effects of low doses and will respond only when high doses are used or a second diuretic (e.g., metolazone) is added.

Step 3: Use ACE Inhibitors and β-Blockers to Stabilize the Disease

Because diuretics do not prevent disease progression, patients with heart failure due to systolic dysfunction should not be treated with a diuretic alone, even if their symptoms are alleviated with the use of diuretic drugs. Patients who respond favorably to diuretics should receive additional therapy with agents that block the actions of neurohormonal systems (ACE inhibitors and β-blockers). The use of neurohormonal inhibitors should not be reserved for patients who are refractory to diuretics, because patients might die during the period of delay and patients with end-stage heart failure and persistent fluid retention often respond poorly to ACE inhibitors and β-blockers. In patients with mild, moderate, or severe heart failure, treatment with the ACE inhibitor should be started first, initially in low doses, and every effort should be made to maintain treatment if patients experience early intolerance. Changes in diuretics may be needed to minimize the risk of adverse reactions. In patients with Class II or III heart failure, treatment with a β-blocker should be added to the ACE inhibitor, regardless of the degree of clinical improvement with the ACE inhibitor. Therapy should be initiated in low doses followed by appropriate increments in dose, and every effort should be made to maintain treatment if patients experience early intolerance. As with ACE inhibitors, changes in diuretics may be needed to minimize the risk of adverse reactions. In patients with recent or current Class IV symptoms, the addition of spironolactone to the ACE inhibitor merits consideration.

Optimal effects on disease progression can be achieved only by using both an ACE inhibitor and a β-blocker in combination. ACE inhibition appears to reduce the risk of death and of hospitalization by 20 to 30%, and the addition of a β-blocker to the ACE inhibitor produces a further 30 to 40% reduction in the risk of a major clinical event. However, treatment with ACE inhibitors and a β-blocker should not be initiated at the same time. Therapy with a β-blocker should be started after the patient has been stabilized on appropriate doses of the ACE inhibitor.

Step 4: Add Therapy With Digoxin in Patients With Persistent Symptoms

Because the benefits of digoxin are largely related to its ability to improve symptoms and clinical status, the drug may be used at any time to alleviate symptoms. Some physicians prescribe digoxin to all symptomatic patients with systolic dysfunction receiving a diuretic, whereas others reserve digoxin for patients who remain symptomatic despite the use of diuretics, ACE inhibitors, and β-blockers. Digoxin should be a preferred agent in patients whose heart failure is associated with atrial arrhythmias (e.g., atrial fibrillation).

Other Therapeutic Strategies in Patients With Heart Failure

Drugs Used in Patients Intolerant of ACE Inhibitors

Two types of drugs are available for patients who cannot tolerate treatment with an ACE inhibitor. Neither approach is recommended in patients who can tolerate an ACE inhibitor without difficulty.

ANGIOTENSIN RECEPTOR BLOCKERS. Angiotensin II receptor antagonists (e.g., losartan, valsartan, irbesartan, eprosartan, candesartan) interfere with the actions of the renin-angiotensin system by blocking the interaction of angiotensin II with its receptor (see Fig. 48–4). This mechanism, distinct from that of ACE inhibitors, is not associated with the accumulation of kinins; thus, the effects of

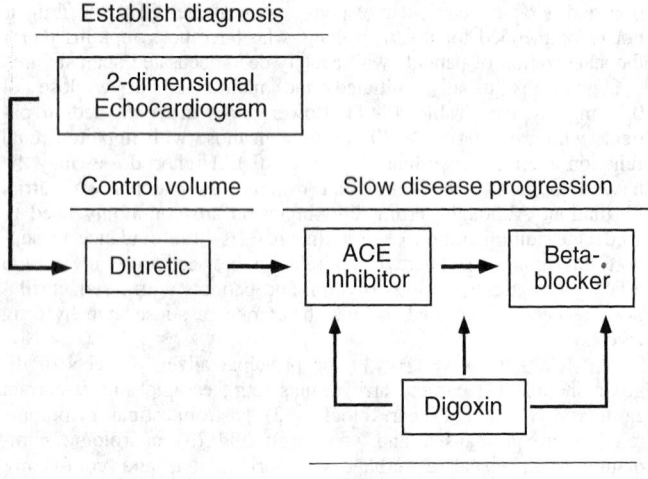

Establish diagnosis

FIGURE 48–7 ■ Algorithm for the management of chronic heart failure. *Step 1: Establish the diagnosis.* A two-dimensional echocardiogram can quantify the type and magnitude of ventricular dysfunction and can identify disorders of the valves, pericardium, or great vessels that may be corrected surgically. *Step 2: Control volume with the use of diuretics.* The dose of diuretic should be adjusted until there is no evidence of fluid retention, as reflected either by resolution of peripheral edema or normalization of jugular venous pressure. *Step 3: Slow disease progression with the use of ACE inhibitors and β-blockers.* Even if symptoms are controlled with a diuretic, ACE inhibitors and β-blockers should be used together to reduce the risk of death and hospitalization. (There is little information about the use of β-blockers in patients with Class IV symptoms.) *Step 4: Treat any residual symptoms with digoxin.* Some physicians prescribe digoxin to all symptomatic patients with systolic dysfunction receiving a diuretic, whereas others reserve digoxin for patients who remain symptomatic despite the use of a diuretic, ACE inhibitor, and β-blocker.

these drugs in heart failure may differ from those reported for ACE inhibitors. In controlled trials, angiotensin II antagonists have not been shown consistently to improve the symptoms of heart failure or to enhance exercise tolerance, and their effects on the risk of death and hospitalization have not been defined. Hence, although several angiotensin II receptor antagonists have been approved for use in hypertension by the FDA, none has yet been approved for the treatment of heart failure. Accordingly, angiotensin II receptor antagonists should not be used for the treatment of heart failure in patients who have no prior exposure to an ACE inhibitor, and these drugs should not be substituted for ACE inhibitors in patients who are tolerating ACE inhibitors without difficulty. Angiotensin II antagonists may be used in patients who cannot tolerate an ACE inhibitor because of cough or angioedema.

HYDRALAZINE AND ISOSORBIDE DINITRATE. Although direct-acting vasodilators can produce favorable short-term hemodynamic effects in patients with heart failure, their long-term use has not improved symptoms and has increased the risk of heart failure and death in controlled clinical trials. Of the agents evaluated, only a combination of isosorbide dinitrate and hydralazine has produced some encouraging results. The combination of these two direct-acting vasodilators has been reported to reduce the risk of death in patients with heart failure receiving digitalis and diuretics. However, this vasodilator combination has no effect on the frequency of hospitalizations, and many patients fail to tolerate long-term treatment with these drugs. Furthermore, when compared with ACE inhibitors, the nitrate-hydralazine combination is associated with a higher risk of death, despite greater benefits on exercise fraction and exercise tolerance. Finally, there is little experience with the use of hydralazine and isosorbide dinitrate in patients receiving an ACE inhibitor or a β-blocker. For all of these reasons, neither hydralazine nor isosorbide dinitrate (alone or in combination) is approved by the FDA for the treatment of heart failure.

Therefore, the combination of hydralazine and isosorbide dinitrate is not used for the treatment of heart failure in patients who have no prior exposure to an ACE inhibitor, and these drugs should not be substituted for ACE inhibitors in patients who are tolerating ACE inhibitors. The combined use of hydralazine and isosorbide dinitrate may be used in patients who cannot tolerate an ACE inhibitor because of hypotension or renal insufficiency. There is little evidence to support the use of nitrates alone or hydralazine alone in the management of chronic heart failure.

Drugs Used for the Treatment of Coexistent Cardiac Disorders

Many patients with heart failure have coexistent cardiac disorders that require active management. Revascularization should be strongly considered in patients with heart failure who have angina, because it may reduce the risk of major cardiac events. Nitrates and β-blockers and amlodipine may be used if revascularization cannot be performed or is unsuccessful. Diuretics, ACE inhibitors, and β-blockers are excellent choices for the treatment of patients who have heart failure and hypertension.

Atrial arrhythmias are common in patients with heart failure; and if accompanied by a rapid ventricular response, they can exacerbate the severity of symptoms and possibly accelerate progression of the underlying disease. Although the prevention of atrial arrhythmias would be highly desirable, this goal cannot be effectively or safely achieved with most antiarrhythmic drugs. The agent most likely to suppress atrial arrhythmias in patients with heart failure is amiodarone, but the substantial toxicity of the drug has justifiably discouraged its widespread use. As a result, many physicians do not attempt to restore sinus rhythm in patients with an established atrial arrhythmia but instead focus on controlling the rate of the ventricular response with digitalis and β-blockers and reducing the risk of embolic events with anticoagulants. If a slow ventricular response cannot be achieved in this manner, amiodarone or radiofrequency ablative procedures (see Chapter 51) should be considered.

Most patients with heart failure have frequent and complex ventricular arrhythmias; but when asymptomatic, these do not presage or contribute to the occurrence of sudden death and thus do not require therapy. The appearance of ventricular arrhythmias in these patients is likely to reflect the severity of the underlying cardiac disease and thus may respond to interventions that reduce the risk of disease progression. In addition, every effort should be made to correct electrolyte imbalances if these are found. In patients who

have an immediate life-threatening ventricular arrhythmia (sustained ventricular tachycardia or ventricular fibrillation) or who have been resuscitated from sudden death, use of an implantable cardioverter-defibrillator may reduce the risk of a lethal recurrence (see Chapter 52).

Because of stasis of blood in dilated hypokinetic cardiac chambers, patients with a dilated cardiomyopathy are at increased risk of cardiac thrombi and embolic events. Yet, it is unclear whether all patients with a depressed ejection fraction should receive treatment with anticoagulant drugs, even if they are known to harbor a cardiac thrombus. Most cardiac thrombi detected by echocardiography do not embolize, and most embolic events are related to thrombi that were not visualized. Anticoagulation is recommended primarily for patients with a previous embolic event or atrial fibrillation.

Drugs To Be Avoided in Patients with Heart Failure

Patients with heart failure can improve dramatically after the withdrawal of drugs that are known to affect cardiac function adversely or that interact unfavorably with drugs of established benefit.

ASPIRIN AND NON-STEROIDAL ANTI-INFLAMMATORY DRUGS. Prostaglandins play an important role in circulatory homeostasis and in the action of many drugs used to treat heart failure. These substances are endogenous vasodilators that act to unload the heart when peripheral vessels are constricted and can support glomerular filtration when renal perfusion is compromised. The natriuretic actions of diuretics and the vasodilatory effects of ACE inhibitors are mediated in part by the release of endogenous prostaglandins. For all of these reasons, the administration of agents that block prostaglandin synthesis can produce worsening cardiac and renal function and can lead to clinical deterioration, particularly in patients with compromised renal perfusion who are receiving diuretics and ACE inhibitors. As a result, most patients with heart failure should not receive non-steroidal anti-inflammatory agents.

Whether the recommendation to avoid inhibitors of prostaglandin synthesis applies to aspirin remains controversial. Aspirin is widely prescribed to patients with heart failure, either to reduce the risk of recurrent myocardial ischemic events in patients with coronary artery disease or to decrease the frequency of systemic embolic events in patients with normal coronary arteries. However, by interfering with kinin-mediated prostaglandin synthesis, aspirin can attenuate the hemodynamic actions of ACE inhibitors in patients with heart failure. In large multicenter trials, the use of aspirin was associated with a loss of the effects of ACE inhibitors on survival and an attenuation of the effects of these drugs on cardiovascular morbidity. As a result, some physicians prefer to use a non-aspirin platelet inhibitor (e.g., clopidogrel; see Chapter 188) in patients with heart failure who are receiving ACE inhibitors.

CALCIUM CHANNEL BLOCKERS. Although calcium channel blockers are peripheral vasodilators, these agents have not improved the symptoms of heart failure or enhanced exercise tolerance. Instead, the short- and long-term administration of these drugs has caused serious adverse cardiovascular reactions, including profound hypotension, worsening heart failure, pulmonary edema, and cardiogenic shock. These deleterious responses have been observed with short- or long-acting formulations of the same drug (e.g., nifedipine) as well as with the older and newer members of this class (e.g., felodipine and mibefradil). As a result, clinicians should not use calcium channel blockers for the treatment of heart failure, and most calcium channel blockers should be avoided for the treatment of angina, atrial fibrillation, or hypertension in patients with heart failure. Of the available agents, only amlodipine has strong evidence supporting its safety in patients with advanced disease.

ANTIARRHYTHMIC AGENTS. Antiarrhythmic agents can suppress ventricular arrhythmias in patients with heart failure, but these agents have not been shown to reduce the risk of sudden death. Instead, the short- and long-term administration of these drugs has caused serious adverse cardiovascular reactions, including worsening heart failure, life-threatening proarrhythmia, and death. These deleterious responses have been observed with most types of antiarrhythmic agents, including Class I (encainide, flecainide, and mexiletine) and Class III (D-sotalol) drugs (see Chapter 54). Mixed results have been reported with amiodarone. As a result, antiarrhythmic therapy should not be used to treat patients with heart failure who have asymptomatic ventricular arrhythmias, regardless of their frequency or complexity. Antiarrhythmic drugs may be useful for patients with rapid atrial fibrillation or for those with hemodynamically destabilizing ventricular tachycardia or ventricular fibrillation.

OUTPATIENT INTRAVENOUS POSITIVE INOTROPIC THERAPY. Although positive inotropic agents (e.g., dobutamine and milrinone) can produce striking hemodynamic benefits when given intravenously for short periods of time, long-term use of these drugs has not been shown to produce symptomatic benefits and has been associated with an increase in the risk of death. Such toxicity has been reported with all types of agents of this class (except for digitalis), whether these have been prescribed orally or intravenously or administered continuously or intermittently. Because of the lack of data demonstrating efficacy and important concerns about toxicity, the use of intermittent intravenous positive inotropic therapy cannot be recommended as a long-term treatment strategy, even in patients with end-stage heart failure.

TREATMENT OF PATIENTS HOSPITALIZED FOR HEART FAILURE

Most patients with heart failure can be managed as outpatients, but nearly one third of patients with heart failure require hospitalization each year. The major syndromes requiring hospitalization include (1) fluid overload resistant to orally administered diuretics (e.g., refractory peripheral edema); (2) severe respiratory distress with or without hypoxemia (e.g., acute pulmonary edema); and (3) refractory symptoms with poor end-organ perfusion requiring intravenous therapy. Each syndrome represents an exaggerated expression of each of the pathophysiologic mechanisms that play a role in the evolution of heart failure; that is, refractory edema reflects excessive sodium and water retention; acute pulmonary edema is the result of extreme vasoconstriction; and refractory symptoms associated with systemic hypoperfusion are the ultimate consequence of contractile failure. Aspects of these syndromes frequently coexist in the same patient.

These syndromes share a common therapeutic approach: that is, because of their immediate life-threatening nature, physicians must rely on short-term hemodynamic interventions to achieve clinical stability as rapidly as possible. If the syndromes are the result of changes in diet or medications or the advent of a treatable complicating illness (e.g., arrhythmia, pneumonia or renal failure), the hemodynamic support can be gradually withdrawn, and a long-term outpatient stretegy can be implemented. However, if these syndromes represent the end-stage of a terminal disease that is refractory to medical therapy, hemodynamic support must be continued until a definitive mechanical solution can be devised (e.g., cardiac transplantation; see Chapter 71). In either case, neurohormonal activation is not a therapeutic target in patients who are hospitalized for the treatment of decompensated heart failure. Indeed, by supporting cardiac contractility and systemic blood pressure, the activation of the sympathetic nervous system and renin-angiotensin system may help to maintain circulatory homeostasis in acutely ill patients. The administration of neurohormonal antagonists (ACE inhibitors and β-blockers) in this setting is frequently ineffective and may be deleterious.

Fluid Overload Refractory to Oral Diuretics (Refractory Peripheral Edema)

Patients with heart failure are frequently hospitalized for the treatment of edema that persists despite the use of diuretics. These patients typically present with a marked increase in body weight, associated with pleural effusions, ascites, and massive peripheral edema. The degree of fluid retention can become so severe that the edema itself becomes incapacitating and may require mechanical removal of fluid for relief of symptoms. A frequent cause of this syndrome is non-compliance with diet or medications; and when such is the case, clinical stability can usually be achieved rapidly by restoring the patient's earlier therapeutic regimen. However, in some patients, the occurrence of refractory edema is indicative of advancing right and left ventricular failure. By causing mesenteric congestion, right ventricular failure can impair the rate of absorp-

tion of diuretics; by causing renal hypoperfusion, left ventricular failure can impede the delivery of diuretics to active sites in the renal tubules. As a result, as heart failure advances, patients become increasingly resistant to the effects of diuretic drugs and require larger and larger doses to achieve a therapeutic response.

Management of Refractory Peripheral Edema

Several strategies should be considered in the management of patients with refractory edema. Non-steroidal anti-inflammatory drugs, which can decrease the efficacy and increase the risk of diuretics, should be withdrawn. Vasodilators (especially ACE inhibitors) may reduce renal perfusion pressure and attenuate the effects of furosemide; they should be used cautiously. Diuretics acting on the loop of Henle (e.g., furosemide) should be selected and administered intravenously to ensure their rapid entry into the blood stream in high concentrations. If the patient fails to respond to the intravenous administration of large doses of furosemide, the physician may add a second diuretic with a different renal tubular site of action (e.g., metolazone). A combination of two diuretics can produce a dramatic increase in urine output, but such a regimen is commonly accompanied by striking (and occasionally life-threatening) degrees of hypokalemia. If a combination of intravenous furosemide and oral metolazone proves ineffective, these diuretics should be co-administered with drugs that increase renal blood flow (e.g., dopamine alone or combined with dobutamine). Finally, if the edema becomes refractory to all pharmacologic interventions, hemofiltration or peritoneal dialysis may be useful in restoring fluid balance in selected patients.

Regardless of the severity of fluid retention, every effort should be made to achieve dry weight, even if achievement of this goal requires a prolonged hospitalization. Patients discharged prematurely with residual edema due to an inadequate diuresis are commonly readmitted to the hospital for refractory edema within several weeks. In contrast, patients who achieve dry weight frequently become responsive to conventional treatments for heart failure and have a lower risk of recurrent hospitalization.

Pulmonary Congestion (Acute Pulmonary Edema)

One of the most common clinical presentations of advanced left ventricular failure is the syndrome of pulmonary congestion. These patients complain of dyspnea at rest and have pulmonary rales on physical examination. Pulmonary congestion may be the first evidence of heart failure in patients without a history of cardiac disease; it may appear in patients who are already hospitalized for an acute cardiac disorder (e.g., MI); or it may complicate the course of a patient with long-standing heart failure. If severe, abrupt, and accompanied by clinical evidence of sympathetic overactivity (tachycardia, diaphoresis and vasoconstriction), the syndrome is designated as acute pulmonary edema. Acute pulmonary edema may also be triggered by non-cardiac disorders, including direct injury to the alveolar-capillary membrane, high-altitude stress, catastrophes of the central nervous system, narcotic overdose, or pulmonary embolism.

Regardless of its cause, pulmonary edema reflects the transudation of fluid into the alveolar space and arises from an imbalance in the factors that regulate the transport of fluid from the pulmonary microcirculation to the interstitial space of the lung. When the cause of the syndrome is cardiac, pulmonary edema results from the rapid onset of intense peripheral vasoconstriction that leads to a marked increase in pulmonary venous pressures. The profound constriction of systemic arteries and veins causes a sudden and dramatic redistribution of blood from peripheral reservoirs to the pulmonary circuit, causing the pulmonary capillary hydrostatic pressure in the lung to exceed the capillary colloid osmotic pressure. However, the transudation of fluid into the alveoli cannot occur if pulmonary blood flow is impaired; thus, patients with an elevated pulmonary vascular resistance or depressed right ventricular function rarely develop acute pulmonary edema.

Management of Pulmonary Edema

Several general measures are advisable for most patients with pulmonary congestion. Every effort should be made to identify an underlying precipitating factor, because its correction is often critical to the success of treatment. Patients usually feel most comfortable resting in bed in the upright position with the legs dependent. Special attention should be devoted to maintaining adequate oxygenation, which can be achieved by increasing the concentration of inspired oxygen or (if necessary) by endotracheal intubation and mechanical ventilation.

Given the importance of peripheral vasoconstriction in the pathogenesis of pulmonary edema, pharmacologic dilation of peripheral vessels represents the critical element in any successful approach to management. This goal can be achieved with the use of (1) morphine; (2) loop diuretic drugs (e.g., furosemide); and (3) direct-acting vasodilators (e.g., nitroglycerin and nitroprusside). Because of the need for rapid and reliable treatment, these interventions are generally administered intravenously.

MORPHINE. Morphine remains the most effective single agent for the treatment of acute cardiogenic pulmonary edema. The drug acts specifically to antagonize the peripheral vasoconstrictor effects of the sympathetic nervous system; the resultant vasodilatation leads to an immediate and dramatic decline in pulmonary arterial and venous pressures, leading directly to symptomatic improvement. The precise site of the vasodilation produced by morphine is uncertain. The magnitude of venodilation produced by the drug in the limbs is insufficient to explain its effects on pulmonary flow and pressures; instead, morphine appears to act primarily to increase the pooling of blood in the splanchnic circulation. In addition, morphine blunts the chemoreceptor-mediated ventilatory reflexes that trigger the severe tachypnea that accompanies pulmonary edema; by doing so, the drug reduces the work of breathing and thereby oxygen demand.

Morphine is administered in intermittent doses of 2 to 4 mg intravenously (up to 10–15 mg), until dyspnea is relieved and diaphoresis subsides. The former reflects the acute decline in pulmonary blood flow and pulmonary venous pressures; the latter indicates a decline in the activity of the sympathetic nervous system. Patients should be monitored for respiratory depression, which can be reversed by narcotic antagonists.

LOOP DIURETICS. All diuretics increase urine output in patients with pulmonary edema, but loop diuretics can produce dramatic clinical benefits even before a diuresis has materialized. These immediate benefits are related to the peripheral arterial and venous dilatation produced by these drugs, which results from their ability to enhance the release of prostaglandins from the kidney. Non-loop diuretics do not exert this direct vasodilator action. Although loop diuretics act quickly to increase sodium excretion, the rapidity of diuresis does not determine the clinical response to treatment, because vasodilation (not diuresis) is the principal mechanism of symptom relief. Indeed, an increase in urine output is generally not seen until peripheral signs of vasoconstriction have resolved.

Furosemide is the loop diuretic most commonly used in the treatment of pulmonary edema. The dose of the drug is determined by the prior exposure of the patient to diuretic therapy. In patients who have not received loop diuretics, treatment is usually begun with low doses (40–80 mg intravenously), whereas patients who have received long-term therapy may require large doses of the drug (120–200 mg intravenously). Furosemide is usually well tolerated, but hypotension may occur when the drug is administered to patients with acute heart failure after an acute MI. In such patients, pulmonary congestion may be primarily related to diastolic dysfunction.

NITROPRUSSIDE AND NITROGLYCERIN. By stimulating guanylate cyclase within the vascular smooth muscle cell, both nitroprusside and nitroglycerin exert dilating effects on arterial resistance and venous capacitance vessels and thereby lower pulmonary blood flow and pulmonary venous pressures. Nitroprusside differs from nitroglycerin in several ways: (1) nitroprusside has greater effects on arterial resistance vessels and thus is more likely to produce hypotension; (2) nitroprusside causes greater activation of neurohormonal mechanisms and thus is more likely to produce rebound phenomena after abrupt withdrawal; and (3) the prolonged infusion of nitroglycerin (but not nitroprusside) is accompanied by a loss of the drug's hemodynamic effects (pharmacologic tolerance).

Therapy with both nitroprusside and nitroglycerin is usually initiated as a continuous low-dose intravenous infusion, the rate of which is increased to achieve specific hemodynamic or clinical goals. Nitroglycerin (1–50 μg/kg/min) is considered the agent of choice in patients with underlying ischemic heart disease; nitroprusside (0.2–5.0 μg/kg/min) is preferred for patients who have severe hypertension or valvular regurgitation. Hypotension is the most common side effect of both nitroprusside and nitroglycerin; thus, infusions of the drugs require close continuous monitoring of vital signs. Symptomatic hypotension is frequently associated with

bradycardia (not tachycardia), particularly when nitroglycerin is used. Both drugs can cause pulmonary vasodilatation, which can aggravate arterial hypoxemia in patients with ventilation-perfusion abnormalities. Long-term (> 48 hour) infusions of both drugs is fraught with difficulties (i.e., the development of hemodynamic tolerance with nitroglycerin and the risk of cyanide and thiocyanate toxicity with nitroprusside). Hence, these drugs should generally be used only for brief periods.

MECHANICAL VENTILATION AND PHLEBOTOMY. If dyspnea, diaphoresis, and peripheral vasoconstriction persist or if the syndrome becomes immediately life threatening, mechanical ventilation can improve oxygenation and reduce the redistribution of blood into the pulmonary circuit. If this fails to stabilize the course of the patient, the removal of 250 to 500 mL of blood by phlebotomy can produce a rapid reduction in pulmonary blood volume and dramatic clinical improvement.

Refractory Symptoms Associated With Systemic Hypoperfusion

The most serious presentation of heart failure in the hospitalized patient is the syndrome of refractory heart failure, which is characterized by hemodynamic instability and systemic hypotension. Patients complain of dyspnea and fatigue at rest and have objective evidence of poor peripheral perfusion, as reflected by low systemic blood pressure, diminished mental alertness, cool extremities, and decreased urine output. Laboratory evaluation frequently reveals hyponatremia and azotemia. Refractory heart failure may represent the first evidence of heart disease; it may appear in patients who are already hospitalized for an acute cardiac disorder (e.g., MI); or it may complicate the course of a patient with long-standing heart failure. If severe, abrupt, and accompanied by clinical evidence of sympathetic overactivity, the syndrome is designated as cardiogenic shock (see Chapter 95).

The central feature of refractory heart failure is a deterioration of cardiac performance to a level incompatible with adequate perfusion of peripheral organs. Although patients characteristically present with very low blood pressures, the level of systemic pressure may not accurately reflect the adequacy of perfusion. Some patients have very low blood pressures but maintain excellent end-organ perfusion and function (e.g., patients with heart failure receiving ACE inhibitors). In others, blood pressure is preserved by intense peripheral vasoconstriction even though cerebral and renal function is severely compromised. In either case, the degree of circulatory compromise is so profound and the state of the circulation is so precarious that small changes in physiologic variables can readily provoke end-organ failure or death. The primary goal of treatment is the restoration of clinical stability and adequate perfusion to all organs of the body.

Management of Refractory Heart Failure

Several general measures are indicated in all patients with refractory heart failure. Immediate hospitalization (usually in a critical care unit) is essential. Non-invasive assessment of ventricular function may be useful to quantify the magnitude of ventricular dysfunction and to allow the diagnosis of surgically correctable lesions (e.g., papillary muscle rupture, ventricular septal defect, prosthetic valve thrombosis). Invasive hemodynamic monitoring may be helpful in characterizing the hemodynamic derangement and guiding the use of pharmacologic agents. Daily measurements of urine output and body weight are useful in monitoring fluid balance.

The most important therapeutic measures in the treatment of refractory heart failure are (1) fluid management; (2) the use of intravenous positive inotropic agents; (3) the use of intravenous vasoconstrictor agents; and (4) mechanical and surgical interventions.

FLUID MANAGEMENT. In general, patients should be maintained at dry weight as long as this goal can be achieved without compromising peripheral perfusion. Although fluids are commonly administered with the goal of maintaining the pulmonary capillary wedge pressure at a specific level, there is little evidence that this approach improves the outcome of patients. Similarly, although pulmonary-artery balloon-flotation catheters are frequently used to perform hemodynamic measurements, physicians should recognize that the level of cardiac output does not assess the adequacy of peripheral perfusion and that the level of pulmonary capillary wedge pressure is influenced not only by intravascular volume but also by changes in cardiac contractility, diastolic function, mitral valve function, and the peripheral circulation. Hence, the clinical response to fluid administration may provide more useful information than isolated measurements of cardiac output or ventricular filling pressures.

INTRAVENOUS POSITIVE INOTROPIC AGENTS. Positive inotropic drugs can produce hemodynamic and clinical benefits not only by stimulating cardiac contractility but also by exerting dilatory effects on peripheral blood vessels. Cardiac output is increased and pulmonary wedge pressures are decreased, usually with little change in systemic blood pressure. All positive inotropic agents used in the treatment of refractory heart failure act by increasing myocardial levels of cyclic adenosine monophosphate, either by increasing its synthesis (e.g., dobutamine) or by decreasing its degradation (e.g., milrinone). However, milrinone differs from dobutamine in several ways: (1) because it is a more effective vasodilator, milrinone produces greater decreases in pulmonary wedge pressure and greater decreases in blood pressure than dobutamine; (2) because it is a long-acting agent, adverse effects persist for longer periods with milrinone than dobutamine; and (3) pharmacologic tolerance commonly occurs with dobutamine, but not with milrinone. A combination of dobutamine and milrinone may be particularly useful in selected patients, but such a regimen should be used cautiously because both drugs can produce tachycardia, myocardial ischemia, and serious arrhythmias.

Dobutamine is administered as a continuous intravenous infusion, initially at a rate of 3 to 6 μg/kg/min (without a bolus), and the rate may be increased up to 10 to 15 μg/kg/min. Milrinone is generally initiated with a bolus dose of 0.5 μg/kg, followed by a continuous infusion at a rate of 0.375 to 0.75 μg/kg/min. Short-term infusions of both drugs (alone or in combination) can be effective in the treatment of refractory heart failure, especially when systemic blood pressures are relatively preserved. However, long-term continuous or intermittent infusions can increase the risk of cardiac events (including death) and should be avoided.

INTRAVENOUS VASOCONSTRICTOR AGENTS. Two vasoconstrictor agents are commonly used to support systemic blood pressure in patients with refractory heart failure: dopamine and levarterenol. Dopamine is an endogenous catecholamine that interacts with dopamine receptors (both DA_1 and DA_2 subtypes), β_1 (but not β_2) adrenergic receptors, and α-adrenergic receptors in the heart and peripheral circulation. As a result of these interactions, the drug causes vasodilation (owing to its agonist effects on DA_1 receptors), stimulates cardiac contractility (owing to its agonist effects on β_1 receptors), and causes constriction of peripheral arterial and venous vessels (owing to its agonist effects on α_1-receptors). The hemodynamic effects of dopamine depend largely on the dose of the drug administered. Low doses (< 2 μg/kg/min), which stimulate DA_1 and DA_2 receptors, act to dilate the renal and splanchnic circulations. Moderate doses (2–5 μg/kg/min), which activate β_1-receptors, increase cardiac output but produce little change in pulmonary wedge pressure, heart rate, or systemic vascular resistance. High doses (> 5 μg/kg/min), which stimulate α_1-receptors, increase pulmonary wedge pressure, blood pressure, and heart rate and may reduce renal blood flow. Dopamine may be useful in the treatment of both pulmonary congestion and peripheral hypoperfusion. In normotensive patients with pulmonary congestion, low doses of dopamine increase renal blood flow and are used alone (or in combination with dobutamine) to potentiate the diuretic actions of furosemide. In hypotensive patients with peripheral hypoperfusion, large doses of dopamine are used to support systemic blood pressure (see Chapter 95).

Levarterenol is the commercial preparation of the endogenous catecholamine, norepinephrine, which stimulates both α_1- and β_1-receptors when administered in therapeutic doses. Because of its lack of DA_1-receptor effects, levarterenol increases systemic vascular resistance and blood pressure more than dopamine, and the degree of systemic vasoconstriction may be sufficient to reduce renal blood flow even though cardiac output is increased as a result of β_1-receptor stimulation. Consequently, levarterenol is used only in patients with shock whose blood pressure cannot be supported adequately with dopamine (see Chapter 95). Levarterenol is generally infused in doses ranging from 0.03 to 0.12 μg/kg/min.

Both dopamine and levarterenol can cause serious adverse effects. Stimulation of α-receptors can cause intense peripheral vaso-

constriction, which may reduce peripheral perfusion and (if extravasated during infusion) can cause local tissue necrosis. Stimulation of β-receptors can lead to serious atrial and ventricular arrhythmias and myocardial ischemia. Stimulation of DA_1-receptors may cause nausea and vomiting.

MECHANICAL AND SURGICAL INTERVENTIONS. If pharmacologic interventions fail to stabilize the patient with refractory heart failure, mechanical and surgical interventions may provide effective circulatory support (see Chapter 62). These include intra-aortic balloon counterpulsation; left ventricular assist device; and cardiac transplantation (see Chapter 71). A number of experimental surgical procedures have also been developed to support the failing heart (cardiomyoplasty and partial resection of the left ventricle); but despite a high level of initial enthusiasm, the results to date have been variable, unpredictable, and largely disappointing.

Intra-aortic balloon counterpulsation has been useful in the management of cardiogenic shock that is caused by acute myocardial ischemia or infarction (see Chapter 95), particularly when there is a coexisting mechanical defect (e.g., ventricular septal defect or papillary muscle rupture). Short-term use of ventricular assist devices has produced dramatic hemodynamic and clinical benefits, but long-term use of these devices has been associated with a high risk of infection and thromboembolic events. Ventricular assist devices have been primarily used to provide temporary circulatory support for patients awaiting transplantation, but there is interest in the permanent implantation of these devices as a long-term treatment strategy. A controlled clinical trial to evaluate this possibility is now in progress. Cardiac transplantation (see Chapter 71) is an effective treatment for refractory heart failure, with a survival rate of 80 to 90% at 1 year and 60 to 70% at 5 years, usually with a markedly improved quality of life, despite the risks of organ rejection, immunosuppression, and allograft vasculopathy. These outcomes exceed the results with any medical or surgical intervention available for the management of patients with advanced heart failure, but such outcomes are comparable (and perhaps somewhat inferior) to the results with medical therapy in patients with mild or moderate heart failure. Hence, cardiac transplantation should be considered only for patients with refractory symptoms. The utility of transplantation is limited by the small number of donor hearts.

ACC/AHA Task Force on Practice Guidelines: Guidelines for the evaluation and management of heart failure. Circulation 92:2764–2784, 1995.

CIBIS Investigators and Committees: The Cardiac Insufficiency Bisoprolol Study (CIBIS-II), a randomized trial. Lancet 353:9–13, 1999. *Beta-blocker therapy improved survival in patients with stable class III or IV heart failure.*

The Digitalis Investigation Group: The effect of digoxin on mortality and morbidity in patients with heart failure. N Engl J Med 336:525–533, 1997. *Digitalis reduced hospitalization rates but did not reduce mortality rates.*

Heart Failure Guideline Panel: Heart Failure: Evaluation and Care of Patients with Left Ventricular Systolic Dysfunction. Rockville, MD: US Department of Health and Human Services, Agency for Health Care Policy and Research, 1994. Clinical Practice Guideline Number 11. AHCPR publication No. 94-0612.

Lechat P, Packer M, Chalon S, et al: Clinical effects of β-adrenergic blockade in chronic heart failure: A meta-analysis of double-blind, placebo-controlled, randomized trials. Circulation 98:1184–1191, 1998.

Packer M, Bristow MR, Cohn JN, et al, for the U.S. Carvedilol Heart Failure Study Group: The effect of carvedilol on morbidity and mortality in patients with chronic heart failure. N Engl J Med 334:1349–1355, 1996.

Packer M, Cohn JN: Consensus recommendations for the management of chronic heart failure. Am J Cardiol 83(2A):1A–38A, 1999. *A comprehensive review.*

49 PRINCIPLES OF ELECTROPHYSIOLOGY

Leonard S. Gettes

BASIC PRINCIPLES

The heart is able to initiate an impulse, conduct this impulse to atrial and ventricular myocytes, and integrate the activation of individual myocytes to produce the most efficient contractile sequence.

The ability of myocytes to respond to an impulse by depolarizing and then repolarizing reflects the movement of ions across hexameric protein channels that span the phospholipid sarcolemmal membrane. Opening and closing of these channels, resulting from changes in the configuration of protein subunits, regulates ionic flow into and out of the cell. These conformational changes in protein subunits occur in response to changes in transmembrane voltage, in which case the channel is termed voltage gated, or in response to various neurotransmitters, enzymes, metabolic products, or ions, in which case the channel is termed ligand gated.

The transmembrane movement of ions generates the transmembrane action potential, which has five phases (Fig. 49–1A). Phase 0, the upstroke, is caused by the movement of sodium and/or calcium ions into the cell and reaches a level of close to +30 mV (the inside of the cell is positive with respect to the extracellular space). The currents thus generated are the rapid sodium inward current (I_{Na}) and the slow calcium inward current (I_{Ca}). Phase 1, the spike of the action potential, is attributed to rapid inactivation of the sodium current and activation of a short-lived, transient outward current referred to as I_{to}. Phase 2, the plateau phase of the action potential, is caused by the balance created by the calcium inward current as it slowly deactivates and a potassium outward current, I_K, which is slowly activated. The magnitude of this potassium outward current increases with time, and its increase, coupled with eventual deactivation of the calcium inward current, leads to the end of the plateau and the onset of phase 3, the phase of rapid repolarization. The terminal portion of rapid repolarization is caused by the activation of yet another potassium outward current termed I_{K1}, which helps restore the action potential to its resting level. Phase 4, the phase between action potentials, represents electrical diastole, during which most cells have no change in transmembrane voltage, which remains close to −85 mV (the inside of the cell is negative with respect to the extracellular space). However, some cells may depolarize spontaneously during diastole and consequently reach the threshold for activation of the inward current and produce a spontaneous action potential (see Fig. 49–1B). These cells are the pacemaker cells and are responsible for spontaneous impulse formation. The ionic currents responsible for spontaneous diastolic depolarization include a decaying outward current and an inward current activated by hyperpolarization, which is carried by sodium ions and is referred to as I_f. A background inward current carried by sodium ions (I_{Na-B}) is also present and contributes to spontaneous depolarization. The cells in the sinoatrial or sinus node, which is the primary pacemaker region, lack the rapid sodium inward current system; their upstroke is generated by the slow inward calcium current. Thus the rate of rise of their action potentials is slower than that of cells having the rapid sodium inward current.

The action potential configuration of cardiac cells varies with the location, size, and function of the various cell types (Fig. 49–2). The sinus node is a spindle-like structure located near the junction of the superior vena cava and the right atrium. Modulation of the rate of spontaneous diastolic depolarization in the sinus node by sympathetic and parasympathetic stimulation results in either speeding or slowing. However, the sinus node spontaneously depolarizes even when denervated, a capability that permits transplanted hearts to beat spontaneously.

Impulses formed in the sinus node spread radially first to depolarize the right and then the left atrium, which is the source of the P wave on the body surface electrocardiogram (ECG). These impulses are then funneled into the atrioventricular (AV) node, a process facilitated by the three internodal tracts of specialized atrial fibers that extend from the sinus to the AV node. The AV node is located on the right side of the interatrial septum, just anterior to the ostium of the coronary sinus and superior to the septal leaflet of the tricuspid valve. The cells in the upper portion of the AV node, like the cells in the sinus node, lack the rapid sodium inward current; the upstroke of their action potentials is due to activation of the slow inward calcium current, and the speed of conduction in this region is very slow. The PR interval on the ECG is due in large part to this slow conduction.

The AV node is the only way for the impulse to travel across the fibrous valve rings that constitute the skeleton of the heart and separate the atria from the ventricles, unless tracts of myocardial cells bridge the AV junction and thereby bypass either all or part of the AV node. These bypass tracts, referred to as Kent bundles, offer alternative pathways from the atria to the ventricles. These cells do possess the rapid sodium inward current and thus conduction in these tracts is more rapid than in the AV node. Impulses traversing these tracts reach the ventricle before those crossing the AV node and cause ventricular pre-excitation. Pre-excitation is associated with a unique ECG pattern referred to as Wolff-Parkinson-White (see Chapter 51). These pathways also permit the development of re-entry circuits between the atria and the ventricles and are an important cause of tachyarrhythmias in patients with otherwise normal hearts.

On exiting the AV node, the impulse is conducted very rapidly to ventricular myocytes via a specialized connecting system consisting of the anatomically distinct common His bundle and the right and left bundle branches. The bundle branches give rise to the terminal Purkinje fiber network, which lines the endocardial surface of both ventricles and carries the impulse to the ventricular myocardial cells. The cells of the His-Purkinje system are larger in diameter, depolarize and conduct more rapidly, and have a longer action potential duration than do the working cells in either the atria or the ventricles. Their activation occurs during the latter portion of the PR segment of the body surface ECG.

Depolarization of the ventricles is initiated by depolarization of the interventricular septum from the left ventricular to the right ventricular side. The right and left ventricles then depolarize simultaneously and sequentially from apex to base and from endocardium to epicardium. This sequential depolarization of the ventricu-

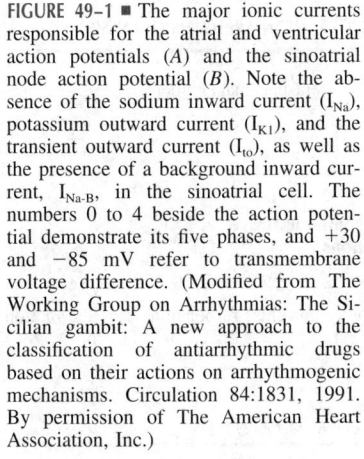

FIGURE 49–1 ■ The major ionic currents responsible for the atrial and ventricular action potentials (A) and the sinoatrial node action potential (B). Note the absence of the sodium inward current (I_{Na}), potassium outward current (I_{K1}), and the transient outward current (I_{to}), as well as the presence of a background inward current, I_{Na-B}, in the sinoatrial cell. The numbers 0 to 4 beside the action potential demonstrate its five phases, and +30 and −85 mV refer to transmembrane voltage difference. (Modified from The Working Group on Arrhythmias: The Sicilian gambit: A new approach to the classification of antiarrhythmic drugs based on their actions on arrhythmogenic mechanisms. Circulation 84:1831, 1991. By permission of The American Heart Association, Inc.)

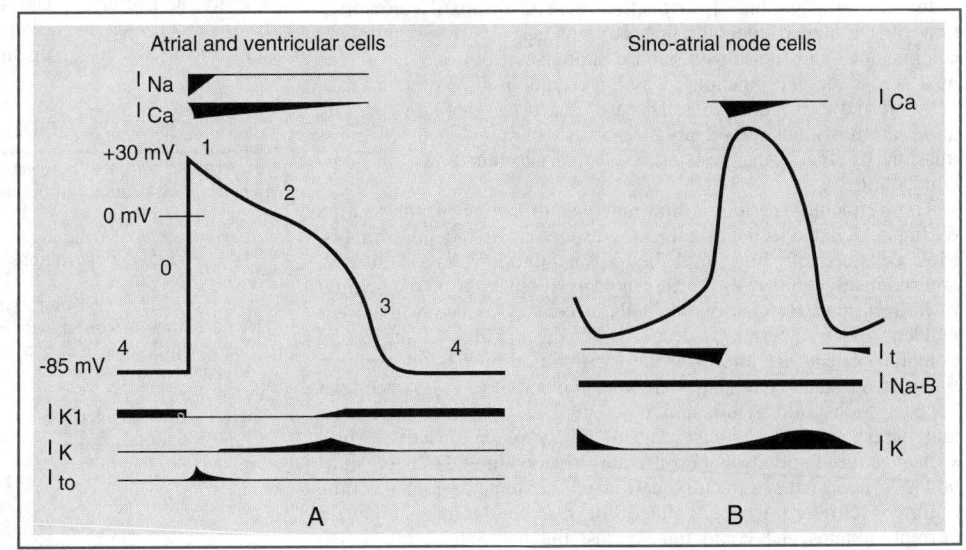

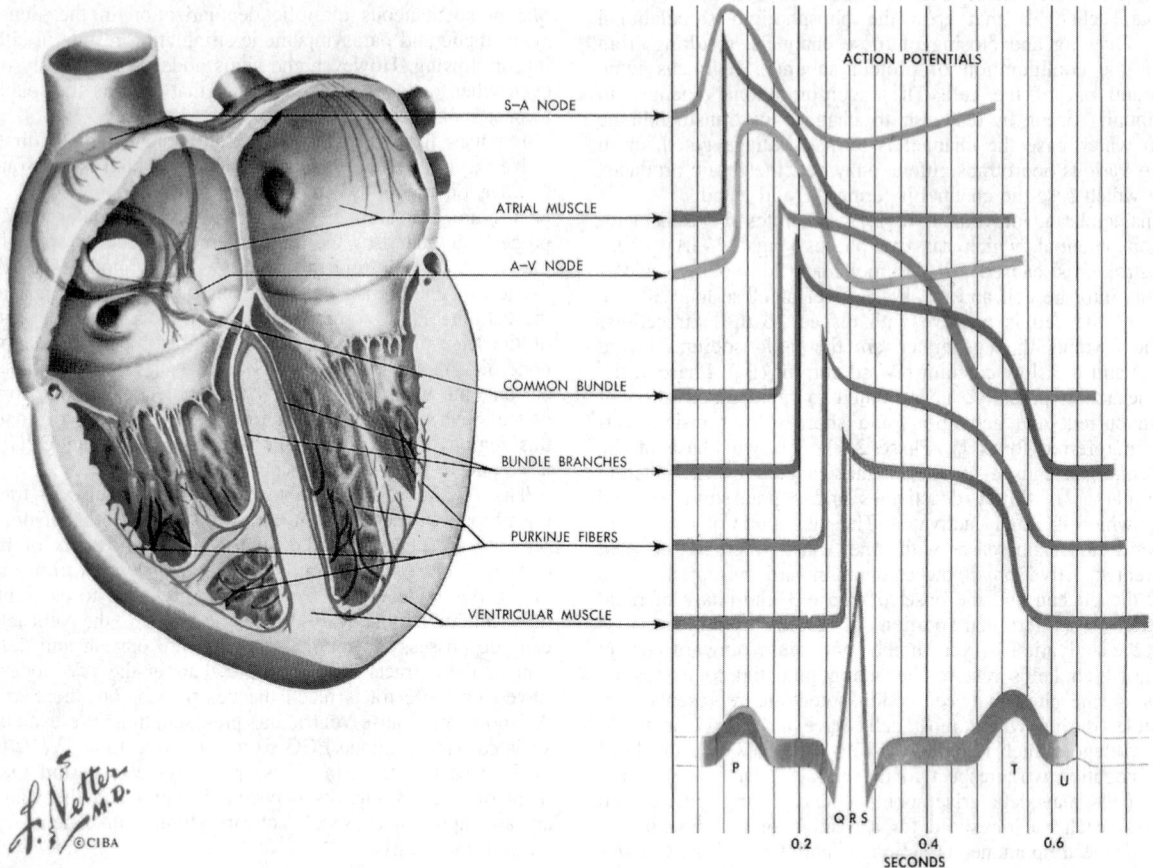

FIGURE 49–2 ■ The relationship of action potentials recorded from various portions of the specialized conducting system and from the atrial and ventricular muscle to each other and to the simultaneously recorded body surface electrocardiogram. (From The Ciba Collection of Medical Illustrations, vol 5, Heart.)

lar fibers, followed by their sequential repolarization, is responsible for the QRS complex, the ST segment, and the T wave of the body surface ECG.

The clusters of spontaneously depolarizing cells within the sinus node are the dominant pacemakers of the heart. However, other cells are able to assume pacemaker capabilities if the sinus node is depressed by disease or drugs or if impulse transmission from the atria to the ventricle across the AV node is blocked. These subsidiary pacemakers reside in the atria, AV node, and the His-Purkinje system. Their intrinsic rate is slower than that of the sinus node and decreases progressively from the sinus node to the distal His-Purkinje system.

Impulse propagation, or conduction, depends primarily on activation of the inward depolarizing currents carried by sodium and calcium ions and the transmission of impulses from one cell to the next across the gap junctions, which are composed of protein channels referred to as connexons. Diseases and drugs that slow the rate at which individual cells depolarize or that inhibit cell-to-cell transmission by increasing resistance of the gap junction will slow conduction.

The refractory period is the interval following depolarization during which the cell is unable to respond to a second stimulus. Most cells are refractory until the transmembrane voltage returns to approximately −60 mV, the threshold for activation of the sodium inward current. Refractoriness in these cells is termed voltage dependent and is determined primarily by the duration of the action potential plateau. Factors that alter the duration of the action potential plateau, such as changes in rate, temperature, or extracellular concentrations of calcium and potassium, as well as sympathetic and parasympathetic agonists and a variety of cardioactive drugs, will alter the duration of the refractory period. In cells of the sinus and AV nodes, the refractory period may extend beyond the time required to return to the voltage for reactivation of the inward current systems and could thus outlast the duration of the action

potential. This period is termed time-dependent, or post-repolarization, refractoriness and can be induced by some antiarrhythmic drugs, acute ischemia, and hyperkalemia.

PATHOPHYSIOLOGY OF CARDIAC ARRHYTHMIAS

Bradyarrhythmias and tachyarrhythmias may occur as a result of abnormalities in impulse formation, in impulse propagation, or in repolarization (Table 49–1).

ABNORMALITIES IN IMPULSE FORMATION. Abnormalities in impulse formation may result from enhanced automaticity, triggered activity, and re-entry. The normal and latent pacemaker fibers may, for reasons such as inflammation or ischemia, become unusually sensitive to events or agents that increase the rate of spontaneous

Table 49–1 ■ **FACTORS IMPORTANT IN ARRHYTHMOGENESIS**

Abnormalities in Impulse Formation
Enhanced automaticity in normal or latent pacemaker fibers
Triggered activity
  Early afterdepolarizations
  Delayed afterdepolarizations
Re-entry
Abnormalities in Impulse Propagation
Decreased rate of rise in action potential upstroke
  Increased resistance at gap junctions
  Myocardial fibrosis
Abnormalities in Repolarization
Changes in characteristics of ionic currents responsible for the action
  potential plateau:
  K outward currents
  Na inward current
  Ca inward current
Inhomogeneous Changes in Conduction and Refractoriness

depolarization. Such events and agents include a decrease in extracellular potassium, β-adrenergic agonists, myocardial fiber stretch, and depolarizing currents during acute ischemia.

Abnormalities in impulse formation may also result from abnormal depolarization occurring during or after repolarization. Those occurring during repolarization are termed early afterdepolarizations, whereas those occurring during the early portion of phase 4 after repolarization has been completed are termed delayed afterdepolarizations. When these afterdepolarizations reach the threshold potential for activation of either the sodium or the calcium inward current, they may "trigger" a propagated response; when runs of such "triggered" responses occur in sequence, they may be responsible for ventricular tachycardia.

Early afterdepolarizations can be induced by a variety of interventions that have in common the ability to lengthen the action potential duration either by delaying activation of the potassium outward currents or by delaying inactivation of the sodium inward current. These changes prolong the QT interval on the body surface ECG. Abnormalities in one of several genes that determine the protein structure of the potassium channels or the sodium channels are responsible for a congenital syndrome characterized by prolongation of the QT interval on the ECG (see Chapter 52). Directacting antiarrhythmic drugs such as those with class Ia characteristics and those with class III characteristics (see Chapter 54) block the plateau potassium currents, prolong the duration of the action potential and the QT interval on the ECG, and may be associated with early afterdepolarizations and ventricular tachycardia of the torsades de pointes variety (see Chapter 52).

Delayed afterdepolarizations are attributed to an inward current that results from the oscillation of intracellular calcium following its release from the sarcoplasmic reticulum. Such afterdepolarizations can be induced by digitalis glycosides and are believed to be an important cause of the atrial and ventricular tachycardias caused by these drugs. Delayed afterdepolarizations and triggered rhythms have also been associated with β-adrenergic agonists, a decrease in extracellular potassium, acute ischemia and reperfusion, and caffeine. Each of these interventions is also capable of enhancing phase 4 diastolic depolarization (Table 49–2). Thus distinction between arrhythmias caused by triggered activity and those caused by enhanced automaticity is often difficult.

ABNORMALITIES IN IMPULSE PROPAGATION. Abnormalities in impulse propagation may be physiologic, pharmacologic, or pathologic. They may be asymptomatic or a cause of symptomatic bradyarrhythmias. In addition, such abnormalities are an important component of the substrate permitting the development of re-entry.

Interruption of conduction in either bundle branch by fibrosis or calcification may cause right or left bundle branch block. Such blocks cause characteristic ECG changes (see Fig. 42–3) but, by themselves, are asymptomatic. Complete block in both bundle branches, in the common His bundle, or in the AV node may inhibit the transmission of impulses from the atria to the ventricles and cause high-grade or complete AV block and the emergence of slow escape pacemakers (see Chapter 51). Block in the AV node may be physiologic secondary to an increase in vagal tone and can be seen in well-trained young athletes. It may also be caused by drugs that act on the AV node either by enhancing the effects of acetylcholine, such as the digitalis glycosides and the β-adrenergic blocking agents, or by directly affecting the AV nodal fibers, such as the calcium channel blocking agents. These drugs may also cause incomplete AV block, in which some but not all of the supraventricular impulses are conducted to the ventricles. Conduc-

tion block in the His bundle is rarely if ever physiologic and is most often caused by disease; it too may result in incomplete as well as complete AV block.

Conduction in the atrial and ventricular myocardium may be diffusely slowed by drugs that act directly on the myocardium and by an increase in extracellular potassium and may eventually lead to asystole or cardiac arrest. Conduction may also be slowed or blocked regionally, i.e., in only a portion of the ventricular myocardium. For example, acute ischemia or infarction induces regional conduction slowing via an increase in extracellular potassium, a decrease in extracellular pH, the accumulation of lysophosphoglycerides, a fall in intracellular pH, and an increase in intracellular calcium. These extracellular and intracellular events slow the rate at which the individual cells depolarize and cause cell-to-cell uncoupling. As the infarction heals, the presence of fibrosis in the infarcted region leads to anatomic barriers that interfere with the spread of excitation and cause conduction abnormalities.

Regional conduction abnormalities may form part of the substrate for re-entry, an important cause of atrial and ventricular premature beats and rhythms. Re-entry is the mechanism responsible for atrial flutter and fibrillation (see Chapter 51), for most cases of ventricular tachycardia (see Chapter 52), and for ventricular fibrillation (see Chapter 52). It is also responsible for paroxysmal AV reciprocating or re-entrant tachycardias, such as those occurring in patients with ventricular pre-excitation or Wolff-Parkinson-White syndrome (see Chapter 51). Re-entry reflects the ability of an impulse to re-enter a portion of the myocardium that has previously been excited to establish a self-sustaining, re-entry circuit. Re-entry requires a unidirectional block, which is defined as the inability of an impulse to conduct in one direction while still being able to conduct in the opposite or retrograde direction. A unidirectional block is usually caused by inhomogeneities in conduction and refractoriness in the fibers that make up the re-entry circuit. The other requirement for re-entry is that the relationship between the speed of conduction and the recovery of excitability, termed the refractory period of the cells within the re-entry circuit, be such that the impulse is able to excite the tissue at the site of the block and then to re-enter the previously excited tissues. In Wolff-Parkinson-White syndrome, for example, the non-premature beat travels to the ventricle via both the AV node and the bypass tract and extinguishes itself when the wave fronts collide (see Fig. 51–4). However, because of differences in the refractory periods of the AV node and the bypass tract, a properly timed atrial premature beat may be able to enter the AV nodal pathway but then be blocked in the bypass tract. When this impulse travels through the ventricular myocardium to reach the distal portion of the blocked pathway, the blocked pathway will now have recovered its excitability and will be capable of conducting the impulse in a retrograde direction. This impulse re-excites the atrium and the antegrade nodal pathway and establishes the re-entry circuit. A later premature beat will travel down both pathways, whereas an earlier premature beat will not conduct in either pathway because both will be refractory. Re-entry can also occur in or close to the AV node itself because of the existence of fiber tracts with differing electrophysiologic characteristics. In some types of atrial flutter, a re-entrant pathway has been identified within the right atrium.

Re-entry may also occur if the circuit is determined by functional rather than anatomic characteristics. In patients with acute myocardial infarction, for example, the inhomogeneous slowing of conduction in the ischemic region, coupled with inhomogeneities in

Table 49–2 ▪ ELECTROPHYSIOLOGIC EFFECTS OF FACTORS ASSOCIATED WITH ARRHYTHMIAS

FACTOR	ABNORMAL IMPULSE FORMATION	ABNORMAL IMPULSE PROPAGATION	ABNORMAL REFRACTORINESS
Catecholamines	++	+	+
Acetylcholine	++	++	+
Increased K^+_e	—	+++	++
Decreased K^+_e	+++	—	++
Cardioactive drugs	+++	+++	+++
Acute ischemia	++	+++	+++
Infarction/fibrosis	+	+++	++
Cardiac dilation	++	+	+

K^+_e = extracellular potassium.

refractoriness, may create a functional obstacle that permits the establishment of one or more re-entry circuits.

Inhomogeneities in conduction and refractoriness are responsible for creating the substrate for re-entrant arrhythmia in the setting of both the anatomically and functionally defined re-entry circuits. However, re-entry also requires a trigger to initiate the arrhythmia. In AV re-entrant tachyarrhythmias and in atrial fibrillation and flutter, the trigger is usually an atrial premature beat, whereas in ventricular tachycardias and ventricular fibrillation, the trigger is usually a ventricular premature beat. These premature beats may occur as a result of abnormalities in impulse formation secondary to enhanced automaticity, triggered activity, or spontaneous re-entry.

Cascio WE, Johnson TA, Gettes LS: Electrophysiologic changes in ischemic ventricular myocardium: I. Influence of ionic, metabolic, and energetic changes. J Cardiovasc Electrophysiol 6:1039, 1995. *An in-depth discussion of the causes of the electrophysiologic abnormalities associated with acute ischemia. It includes an extensive and up-to-date bibliography.*

Priori SG, Barhanin J, Hauer RN, et al: Genetic and molecular basis of cardiac arrhythmias: Impact on clinical management. Circulation 99:518, 1999. *Practical advice on diagnosis and management.*

Zipes DP, Jalife J: Cardiac Electrophysiology from Cell to Bedside, 2nd ed. Philadelphia, WB Saunders, 1995. *A large and extensive multiauthored text that explores in varying degrees of detail all of the issues discussed in this chapter.*

50 ELECTROPHYSIOLOGIC DIAGNOSTIC PROCEDURES

Jay W. Mason

Clinical cardiac electrophysiology relies on a large and growing array of tests for diagnosis of cardiac arrhythmias and for estimation of risk for sudden death (Table 50–1).

ELECTROCARDIOGRAPHY (See Chapter 42)

The 12-lead electrocardiogram (ECG) provides powerful predictions of the site of atrioventricular block (see Chapter 51), the location of accessory fibers in the Wolff-Parkinson-White syndrome (see Chapter 51), the reentry mechanism in certain supraventricular tachyarrhythmias (see Chapter 51), and the site of origin and drug responsiveness of certain ventricular tachycardias (see Chapter 52). The ECG is often used as a means of detecting incipient antiarrhythmic drug toxicity, as in the case of excessive QRS widening by class IC drugs or QT prolongation by class IA and III drugs (see Chapter 54). The importance of recording a 12-lead ECG during symptoms of potential arrhythmic etiology cannot be over-emphasized, as uncertainty regarding the true cause of symptoms persists when ECG documentation is lacking. Treadmill and other forms of exercise stress testing with ECG monitoring are useful to induce exercise-related arrhythmias for diagnosis, to evaluate the efficacy of drugs in suppressing arrhythmias, and to evaluate the propensity of class IC antiarrhythmic drugs, such as flecainide and propafenone (see Chapter 54), to promote exercise-induced ventricular tachycardia.

QT dispersion correlates more powerfully with disease states than does the QT interval, an indirect ECG measurement of total cardiac repolarization time that has prognostic and therapeutic significance. Dispersion of the QT interval is measured in various ways, all of which estimate the difference between the longest and shortest QT intervals on a single 12-lead tracing. QT dispersion is generally less than 60 ms in normal persons, 60 to 80 ms in patients with previous myocardial infarction, 80 to 100 ms in patients with left ventricular hypertrophy, and 100 to 120 ms in patients with the long QT syndrome. QT dispersion, which likely reflects local disparities in repolarization, predisposes to ventricular fibrillation. T-wave alternans, or fluctuations in the amplitude of the T wave, is a related measure that also has been correlated with arrhythmia risk.

SIGNAL-AVERAGED ECG. Typically a standard 12-lead ECG is recorded with amplifier filter settings that accept frequencies between 0.1 and 150 Hz. Most of the frequencies of the QRS complex are between 25 and 150 Hz, but muscle artifact and other noncardiac signals also reside in that range. Thus, small, high-frequency myocardial signals that might contain useful information cannot be detected within the background noise by the standard ECG. Signal averaging can detect meaningful low-amplitude signals because they occur during each QRS complex, whereas the background noise occurs either randomly or independent of the cardiac rhythm. The signal-averaged ECG (SAECG) averages 100 or more QRS complexes to identify reproducible, low-amplitude cardiac signals, most importantly, low-amplitude potentials that are in the terminal portion of the QRS complex and are predictive of ventricular tachycardia in patients with previous myocardial infarction, independent of left ventricular function and other risk predictors. SAECG has also been proven helpful in identifying patients whose unexplained syncope may be caused by tachycardia. However, SAECG does not identify patients with coronary disease and a low left ventricular ejection who will survive longer with an implanted cardioverter-defibrillator after coronary artery bypass surgery. For this and other reasons, SAECG is not routinely used, even by cardiac electrophysiologists.

HOLTER MONITORING. The Holter monitor, developed in the early 1960s by Holter and colleagues as a long-term tape recording of the cardiac rhythm, has become an indispensable and highly refined tool for cardiac rhythm analysis and risk prediction. Present day systems record 24 hours of rhythm data using three distinctly different technologies for data storage and analysis: tape recording for subsequent analysis, digital recording with real-time analysis, and digital storage for subsequent analysis. Recording to print 24 hours of cardiac rhythm is still the dominant technology because real-time analysis systems are subject to errors owing to the lack of human interaction to eliminate artifact and correct misclassification of beats.

The original sole objective of Holter monitoring was to record the cardiac rhythm continuously so as to capture episodes of arrhythmia; but multifaceted analysis, including classification and quantification of normal and abnormal beats, characterization of tachyarrhythmias, identification and quantification of bradyarrhythmias and pauses, detection of ST-segment changes, and correlation of these events with symptoms, is now possible. These analyses are enormously useful in determining the need for antiarrhythmic drug therapy, estimating antiarrhythmic drug effects, and identifying the need for cardiac pacing.

When cardiac rhythm data are digitized for analysis, every recorded R-R interval can be calculated. A variety of conditions, including heart failure and previous myocardial infarction, modify either the autonomic input to the heart or its ability to respond to the input and thereby decrease the variability of the heart rate. Loss of heart rate variability in patients with diseases such as heart failure and prior myocardial infarction is probably the combined result of reduced vagal influence and increased sympathetic activity, which is known to promote ventricular fibrillation. Decreased heart rate variability predicts mortality in patients with ventricular ectopy after myocardial infarction independent of other factors, and it may help select patients who will benefit from interventions. Heart rate variability is largely a result of vagal activity, which is known to be protective against ventricular fibrillation.

The QT interval varies directly with heart rate and can be affected by cardiac disease. For example, some forms of the long QT syndrome result in enhanced prolongation of QT interval at slower heart rates. The QT interval may also be altered independent of heart rate, such as in patients after myocardial infarction, in whom the QT interval is abnormally long. Computer programs have been developed to automate measurement of the QT interval from Holter-monitor recordings. Lengthening of QT interval may be predictive of an adverse outcome, and altered variability of the QT interval may be a more specific indicator of risk.

Episodes of ST segment depression not associated with symptoms on Holter monitor are predictive of the presence and severity of coronary artery disease and are presumed to be the result of silent ischemic episodes. Although both false-positive and false-negative ST-segment shifts occur, and there is controversy over the interpretation and appropriate therapeutic response to Holter-

Table 50–1 ■ ARRHYTHMIA DIAGNOSTIC TESTS

TEST	INDICATION OR USE	ADVANTAGES AND LIMITATIONS
12-lead electrocardiogram (ECG)	Documentation of arrhythmia, prediction of arrhythmia mechanism and of antiarrhythmic drug toxicity	ECG is readily available, but other tests may be required for definitive arrhythmia diagnosis
QT dispersion	Estimation of the risk of sudden death	Though an independent predictor, accuracy is insufficient as a basis for therapy
Signal-averaged ECG	Estimation of risk of ventricular tachyarrhythmia	A positive test tips the scale toward therapy or invasive procedures when available data are equivocal, but decisions cannot be based on this test alone
T-waves alternans recording	Estimation of sudden death risk	There is not yet much experience with this technique
Holter monitor		
Rhythm recording	Detection and quantitation of frequent arrhythmias	Provides rich data for diagnosis and assessment of antiarrhythmic therapy, but not useful for detection of infrequent events
Heart rate variability	Estimation of sudden death risk	Possibly the most accurate predictor of the risk of sudden death
QT variability	Estimation of sudden death risk	Utility not yet adequately studied
ST segment monitoring	Detection of coronary ischemia	Although proven to predict coronary events, efficacy of intervention unclear
Event monitor	Detection of infrequent arrhythmias	
Body surface potential map	Measurement of regional cardiac electrical activity	Superior to 12-lead ECG for localizing abnormalities, but not in general clinical use
Electrophysiologic study		
Automaticity measurement	Evaluation of sinus node and subsidiary pacemaker function	Relatively insensitive but specific marker of sinus node disease
Conduction and refractoriness measurement	Detection of conduction system disease and risk of AV block	Accurately describes existing refractoriness and conduction, but a relatively insensitive predictor of AV block
Tachycardia induction	Identification of the mechanism of tachyarrhythmia and of possible cause of syncope and other symptoms	Invaluable in management of tachyarrhythmias, but weakened by excessive false-positive responses
Pharmacologic study	Prediction of the efficacy of antiarrhythmic drugs	Useful but less important with advent of implanted cardioverter defibrillators
Device assessment	Evaluation of pacemaker and implanted cardioverter defibrillator function	Irreplaceable
Activation mapping	Identification of arrhythmia mechanisms and of targets for ablation	Critically important for invasive treatment of tachyarrhythmias, but much less useful for ventricular tachycardia associated with coronary artery disease
Tilt test	Detection of cardioinhibitory and vasodepressor mechanisms of syncope	The most important new diagnostic tool for syncope; false-positive rate not adequately defined.

monitor–detected silent ischemia, it is clear that these episodes are independently predictive of ischemia-related adverse events.

EVENT MONITORING. Holter monitoring is limited to relatively short periods of continuous ECG recording. When the objective is to record the cardiac rhythm during symptomatic episodes that occur infrequently (less often than daily), event monitoring is the diagnostic procedure of choice, unless the symptoms are even less frequent than monthly.

Event monitors are designed for intermittent capture of the cardiac rhythm over long periods of time. The system is typically provided to the patient for a month, during which time he or she can make heart rhythm recordings as often as symptoms occur. One variety of event monitor depends on semichronic lead placement. The patient is instructed in electrode removal and replacement and usually reattaches the leads one or more times each day. The system records the ECG into a loop buffer that continuously refreshes previous data. The duration of memory, varying from seconds to several minutes, is usually programmable. The patient records symptomatic events by pressing an event button. The recorder freezes a period of previously recorded data and continues to record the rhythm in real time according to previously programmed instructions. Other recorders are applied by the patient, often with wrist bands or hand-held chest electrodes, during symptomatic episodes. These instruments are less complex and do not require continuous attachment of electrodes; but because they have no memory of the preceding cardiac rhythm and require time to be applied, they are useful only for patients whose spells last for a few minutes and who can always have the recorder nearby. Both varieties of recorders can transmit rhythm strips over the telephone to centralized receivers, where they can be analyzed and promptly brought to the physician's attention. A more recent implantable device can monitor the rhythm continuously without interruption for months or years, retain arrhythmia episodes in memory, and telemetrically relay the stored information to a receiver without the need for external lead attachments.

BODY SURFACE POTENTIAL MAPPING. Body surface potential mapping (BSPM) places 200 or more electrodes circumferentially around the entire surface of the thorax. BSPM is better than the 12-lead ECG to estimate regional heterogeneity of repolarization and to locate accessory pathways. However, the specialized equipment and data interpretation required with BSPM have limited its clinical utility.

ELECTROPHYSIOLOGIC STUDY

Electrophysiologic (EP) study involves use of temporary or permanent cardiac electrodes for direct recording and pacing of the heart, for both diagnostic and therapeutic purposes. The most common indications for EP study are supraventricular tachycardia (see Chapter 51), ventricular tachycardia (see Chapter 52), and sudden death (see Chapter 52). Other important indications include atrioventricular block, sinus node dysfunction, and syncope of unknown cause (see Chapter 51).

PACING AND RECORDING TECHNIQUES. Catheters with one to a dozen or more electrodes are inserted through veins and arteries and placed under fluoroscopic guidance into a variety of locations in the heart for recording and pacing. The primary measurement is the timing of each recorded signal to detect locally abnormal conduction times and sequences of activation. Other important measurements include local repolarization times, local tissue refractoriness, and spontaneous pacemaker activity.

During most EP studies, a catheter is placed just across the tricuspid valve in the region of the bundle of His, where a sharp, high-frequency deflection is identified between the atrial and ventricular depolarizations during sinus rhythm. The presence and timing of this deflection determine sites of atrioventricular block and mechanisms of tachyarrhythmia.

Programmed electrical stimulation, or precisely timed pacing, is used to evaluate conduction over normal and abnormal pathways and to initiate tachyarrhythmias for detailed analysis. When supraventricular tachycardia is being studied, multiple atrial sites, including the coronary sinus, are paced and recorded to determine the mechanism of the tachycardia (see Chapter 51), including potential sites for catheter ablation (see Chapter 53). When ventricular tachycardia or sudden death are the indications for study, ventricular pacing and recording are emphasized. When syncope of uncertain cause is being evaluated, the study should assess the ability of the sinus node and atrioventricular conduction system to withstand pacing stress as well as the vulnerability of the heart to initiation of both ventricular and supraventricular tachyarrhythmias.

PHARMACOLOGIC TESTING. The majority of both supraventricular and ventricular tachyarrhythmias can be initiated by programmed stimulation during EP study. Prevention of their initiation by an antiarrhythmic drug predicts long-term drug efficacy, so pharmacologic testing is a common indication for EP study. However, Holter monitoring also predicts the efficacy of antiarrhythmic therapy, and a large, randomized trial found no difference in the accuracy of predictions made by EP study and Holter monitoring. Because of recent demonstrations of superior efficacy of implanted cardioverter-defibrillator devices in comparison to antiarrhythmic drugs in patients with ventricular tachyarrhythmias (see Chapters 52 and 53), pharmacologic EP testing has been partially supplanted by device implantation.

DEVICE ASSESSMENT. With increased use of implanted devices for control of supraventricular and ventricular tachyarrhythmias, assessment of these devices has become a major component of EP testing (see Chapter 53). In patients with recurrent ventricular tachycardia, arrhythmia initiation and termination is performed to define effective sensing and pacing algorithms to be programmed in the implanted device's memory. In patients with ventricular fibrillation, the effectiveness of lead placement and of the delivery of the defibrillating shock is tested. Effective pacemaker settings are determined by EP study. In patients with recurrent, persistent atrial fibrillation, atrial defibrillator devices are tested in much the same way as ventricular devices to ascertain the accuracy of arrhythmia detection and termination.

ACTIVATION SEQUENCE MAPPING

In patients with reentrant supraventricular tachyarrhythmias unresponsive to medical therapy, ablation is usually performed via catheter delivery of an ablative agent, usually radiofrequency energy, to a specific myocardial site involved in arrhythmogenesis (see Chapter 53). Most patients undergo a complex intracardiac electrophysiologic mapping procedure prior to the ablation to locate the appropriate target tissue.

Mapping of the sequence of electrical activation of the heart is a procedure of major importance in diagnosis and management of resistant cardiac arrhythmias. The objective of mapping is to determine the mechanism of the arrhythmia, such as delineation of a large reentrant pathway and segments within it that might be responsive to therapy. In other cases, a small focus of origin of a tachycardia may be identified for subsequent ablation. Mapping compares the time of electrical activation of the tissue in contact with an electrode to a fiducial time point, such as the onset of the QRS complex. The process is repeated until enough sites have been recorded to permit construction of an activation map showing the relative time of activation at each site, thereby demonstrating the direction and velocity of the activation wave front. Most mapping catheters bear multiple electrodes so that several sites can be recorded simultaneously. Newer mapping arrays deployed by intravascular catheters include noncontact probes with numerous closely spaced electrodes on their surfaces for recording endocardial signals from a distance, and "basket" arrays that spring out to contact the chamber walls when advanced beyond the catheter lumen. Pathologic rhythms need be sustained for only a few beats if many mapping sites are recorded simultaneously. Powerful data acquisition systems allow the clinician to see an immediate display of activation data. Useful mapping data can be obtained from all four cardiac chambers, as well as from the pulmonary artery, the aortic root, the coronary sinus, the coronary veins, and the coronary arteries. Activation mapping is also performed during open-chest cardiac surgical procedures. Body surface potential mapping can estimate the activation sequence on the cardiac surface. This technique can approximately localize accessory pathways in the Wolff-Parkinson-White syndrome but has not yet reached the level of accuracy needed to guide therapy.

TILT TESTING

When no cause for syncope is apparent, head-up tilt testing may reveal a neurocardiogenic origin. Most tilt protocols involve a 30-minute baseline measurement period followed by elevation of the table to 60 degrees for up to 45 minutes. Heart rate and the blood pressure are always monitored. In some laboratories, multiple ECG leads, intra-arterial pressure, an electroencephalogram, respirations, thoracic impedance (to estimate stroke volume), and cerebral blood flow velocity by transcranial Doppler ultrasound are also measured. The classic response in a patient with neurocardiogenic syncope is a sudden and precipitous fall in both heart rate and blood pressure (Fig. 50–1). In some patients, the blood pressure drops without a fall in heart rate.

Neurocardiogenic syncope includes the well-known vasovagal faint. In all forms of neurocardiogenic syncope, autonomic reflexes inappropriately dilate arterial resistance vessels and may inhibit the activity of the sinus node and lower pacemakers. In some cases, initiation of the reflex results from excessive stimulation of cardiac

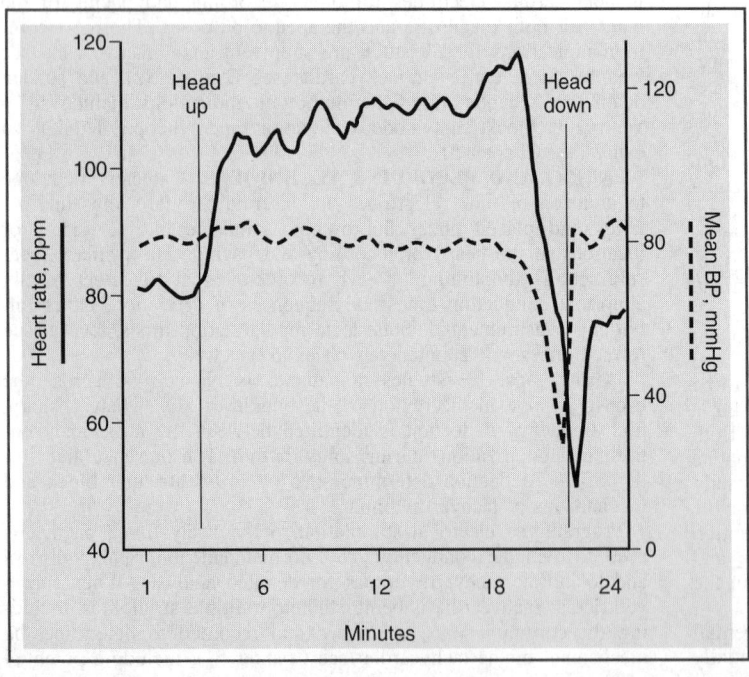

FIGURE 50–1 ■ Head-up tilt test performed on an 18-year-old woman with a history of syncope associated with pain, preceded by a prodrome of dizziness, graying vision, and diaphoresis. A similar prodrome preceded syncope during the test. Note the precipitous, nearly simultaneous, decline of heart rate and blood pressure after an initial rise in heart rate. Vital signs returned to normal rapidly after the head was lowered. (Courtesy of Robert F. Sprung, University of Utah.)

Table 50–2 ■ DIAGNOSTIC APPROACH TO PALPITATIONS, DIZZINESS, AND SYNCOPE

CONDITION	MOST COMMON CAUSES	ORDER OF DIAGNOSTIC TESTING
Palpitations	PACs, PVCs, SVT including AF, VT, AVB, psychiatric disorder	History and examination → Holter or event monitor, depending on frequency of symptoms → Exercise stress test if exercise related → EPS if symptoms suggest sustained arrhythmia
Dizziness	Cardiac arrhythmia, medications, vestibular disorder, cerebellar disease, psychiatric disorder	History and examination → Holter or event monitor, depending on frequency of symptoms → ENT or neurologic consultation → Tilt test → EPS if symptoms are severe and arrhythmia has not been excluded
Syncope	Cardiac arrhythmia, neurocardiogenic reflex, medications, psychiatric disorder	History and examination → Event monitor → Tilt test → SAECG → EPS if arrhythmia still suspected → Glucose tolerance test → Neurologic or psychiatric consultation

PACs = premature atrial contractions; PVCs = premature ventricular contractions, SVT = supraventricular tachycardia; AF = atrial fibrillation; VT = ventricular tachycardia; AVB = atrioventricular block; SAECG = signal-averaged ECG; EPS = electrophysiologic study.

mechanoreceptors caused, for example, by dehydration or venous blood pooling, and leading to a compensatory increase in cardiac contractile force and then to mechanoreceptor activation. Many other triggers of the inhibitory reflexes also are likely involved.

Treatment is directed at inhibiting the potential triggers of the reflex. Support stockings prevent venous blood pooling, fludrocortisone expands blood volume, β-blockers and disopyramide reduce the force of cardiac contraction, scopolamine and other anticholinergic agents block vagal inhibition, and anxiolytics mitigate fright and panic responses.

DIAGNOSTIC APPROACH TO PALPITATIONS, DIZZINESS, AND SYNCOPE (Table 50–2)

Palpitations, dizziness, and syncope are among the most common complaints. In many cases, a specialist is not needed to diagnose and treat these symptoms.

PALPITATIONS. Palpitations are often described as a fluttering sensation or a "flip-flop" in the chest. They are usually due to atrial or ventricular extrasystoles and usually do not require further evaluation, especially if cardiac auscultation or palpation of the pulse are consistent with single premature beats. When presyncope accompanies the palpitations, evaluation is necessary. Most patients with benign palpitations do not require therapy. In fact, antiarrhythmic drug therapy is inappropriate except for very frequent and highly symptomatic ectopy or more advanced forms of arrhythmia (see Chapters 51 and 52).

DIZZINESS. The term "dizziness" includes lightheadedness, disequilibrium, vertigo, and presyncope, and thus has numerous potential etiologies. The history is paramount in determining the appropriate work-up for dizziness. Many patients, especially elderly individuals, experience postural hypotension associated with standing, especially after stooping or bending over. If the physical examination is normal, further evaluation of these patients is usually unnecessary. If the problem is loss of balance or vertigo (see Chapters 447 and 517), a noncardiac etiology should be sought. When presyncope, defined as near loss of consciousness, is not postural in origin, it deserves further evaluation similar to what is recommended for frank syncope.

SYNCOPE. The medical history is by far the most important tool in the evaluation of syncope. A carefully documented history will divulge the likely cause in many patients and should always be the principal determinant of further evaluation. If the syncopal spell was witnessed, it is essential to speak directly to the witness as part of a complete history.

Most syncopal spells have a cardiovascular etiology. The most common cardiovascular causes are arrhythmia and neurocardiogenic syncope (in essence, an exaggerated vasovagal response). Bradyarrhythmic syncope is usually caused by sinoatrial nodal disease or atrioventricular conduction disease (see Chapter 51). Patients with sinus node disease usually experience presyncope rather than syncope. When they experience true syncope, they usually have several seconds of warning symptoms before fainting. Drop attacks associated with His-Purkinje disease, or Morgagni-Stokes-Adams attacks, are usually more abrupt. Tachyarrhythmic syncope may occur with or without warning, depending on the rhythm. SVT and VT are usually accompanied by a warning and usually abate spontaneously. The patient often is aware of rapid heart action before losing consciousness. VF causes abrupt syncope and rarely abates

without cardioversion. Neurocardiogenic syncope is usually heralded by dizziness and other symptoms but may be very abrupt. Often the event is preceded by a change in posture to sitting or standing, a prolonged period of standing with little movement, or an inciting incident such as venipuncture.

Psychogenic syncope is probably the second most common cause of fainting. The spells are usually recurrent, usually witnessed, and rarely associated with injury due to the fall. Though a psychogenic cause may be suspected at the initial interview, the diagnosis can be made only if cardiovascular and neurologic causes are excluded.

Neurologic causes of syncope are much less common (see Chapter 447) and include epileptic seizures and transient ischemia involving the vertebrobasilar arterial bed. Epilepsy is suspected when seizure activity is noted or a typical postictal state follows the event. A seizure does not guarantee a neurologic cause, because cardiovascular collapse can rarely cause a typical seizure complex. However, seizure activity induced by hypotension is usually very brief and may not be associated with incontinence or a postictal state.

Holter monitoring has only a secondary role in evaluation of syncope and is likely to be helpful only in patients with daily episodes. Event monitoring is more useful. In difficult cases, especially patients who experience severe spells less frequently than monthly, an EP study or an implantable loop recorder may be the only means for diagnosis.

Cain ME, Anderson JL, Arnsdorf MF, et al: Signal-averaged electrocardiography. J Am Coll Cardiol 27:238–249, 1996. *This is an authoritative article that covers all the relevant literature regarding methods and use of signal-averaged electrocardiography.*

Linzer M, Yang EH, Estes NA, et al: Diagnosing syncope: 1. Value of history, physical examination, and electrocardiography: Clinical Efficacy Assessment Project of the American College of Physicians; 2. Unexplained syncope. Ann Intern Med 126:989–996; 127:76–86, 1997. *These two articles contain most of the relevant information and references on diagnostic evaluation of syncope with helpful interpretation by the authors.*

Pepine CJ, Sharaf B, Andrews TC, et al: Relation between clinical, angiographic and ischemic findings at baseline and ischemia-related adverse outcomes at 1 year in the Asymptomatic Cardiac Ischemia Pilot study: ACIP Study Group. J Am Coll Cardiol 297:1483–1489, 1997. *A prospective study providing the most complete delineation to date of the clinical significance of silent ischemia in patients with known coronary artery disease.*

Task Force of the European Society of Cardiology and the North American Society of Pacing and Electrophysiology: Heart rate variability: Standards of measurement, physiologic interpretation, and clinical use. Circulation 93:1043–1065, 1996. *This lengthy article provides one-stop shopping for information on heart rate variability.*

Zinetbaum P, Josephson ME: Evaluation of patients with palpitations. N Engl J Med 338:1369–1373, 1998. *A review article with a practical approach to this common problem.*

51 CARDIAC ARRHYTHMIAS WITH SUPRAVENTRICULAR ORIGIN

Masood Akhtar

The atria and ventricles are electrically insulated from each other by fibrous tissue that is the anatomic atrioventricular (AV) junction.

The fibrous structures in the AV junction are the annuli of the mitral and tricuspid valves and the fibrous portion of the interventricular septum. In the absence of an electrical bridge, the atrial impulses cannot cross this fibrous gap. Normally, the AV node and the His-Purkinje system (HPS) provide the only electrical conduit. In some individuals, additional electrical bridges connect the atria with ventricles directly, bypassing these normal pathways and forming the basis for pre-excitation syndromes such as Wolff-Parkinson-White (WPW) syndrome.

Any arrhythmia arising above the bifurcation of the His bundle into the right and left bundle branches is classified as supraventricular. The resultant QRS complex morphology can either be normal or may be wide due to bundle branch or fascicular block (aberrant conduction) or conduction over an accessory pathway (anomalous conduction or pre-excitation). Supraventricular cardiac arrhythmias can be broadly categorized into tachyarrhythmias or bradyarrhythmias.

TACHYARRHYTHMIAS

Supraventricular tachyarrhythmias can occur either as isolated premature complexes or in the form of non-sustained or sustained tachycardias. The most frequent definition of non-sustained tachycardias is an arrhythmia with a rate of more than 100 beats per minute lasting three beats or more but less than 30 seconds. Sustained tachycardia is a prolonged episode of tachycardia lasting 30 seconds or more or terminated earlier with an intervention such as intravenous medication, overdrive pacing, or direct current electrical cardioversion.

Premature Atrial Complexes

ELECTROCARDIOGRAPHIC AND ELECTROPHYSIOLOGIC FEATURES. Premature atrial complexes (PACs) can arise from any part of the left or right atrium. The P wave morphology depends on the origin but differs from sinus rhythm unless PACs arise near the upper right atrial junction with the superior vena cava, that is, close to the location of sinus node. The P wave always precedes the QRS complex (Fig. 51–1A); and if it encounters the absolute refractory period of the AV node or the His-Purkinje system, the P wave will be blocked and not be followed by a QRS complex. A blocked PAC may be confused with second-degree AV block, unless its prematurity is recognized by the PP interval shortening or with sinus node dysfunction (SND) if it is inconspicuous. Distortion of the ST-T segment is often a clue to the presence of a P wave. When a premature QRS complex has the morphology of the underlying sinus rhythm but is not preceded by a P wave, it is labeled as AV junctional (see Fig. 51–1B). When two or more morphologically distinct P waves result in a rate less than 100 beats per minute, the rhythm is termed *wandering atrial pacemaker*.

Premature complexes from the atria or AV junction usually

Table 51–1 ■ SUPRAVENTRICULAR TACHYCARDIAS

Atrial Tachycardias
  Sinus tachycardia
  Sinus node re-entry
  Atrial tachycardia
    Unifocal
    Multifocal
  Atrial flutter
  Atrial fibrillation
AV Junctional Tachycardia
  AV re-entry (Wolff-Parkinson-White syndrome)
    Orthodromic
    Antidromic
  AV nodal re-entry
    Common
    Uncommon
Non-paroxysmal Junctional
Automatic Junctional Tachycardia

AV = atrioventricular.

maintain the same intraventricular conduction pattern seen during sinus complexes; that is, if the sinus rhythm shows a normal QRS complex or bundle branch block pattern, the same configuration will be expected during the premature complexes (Fig. 51–2B). However, if the premature complexes are relatively early (i.e., closely coupled), they can encroach on the refractory period of the right or left bundle branches, resulting in aberrant conduction and producing a right or left bundle branch or fascicular block pattern (see Fig. 51–1A) despite normal intraventricular conduction during sinus rhythm. Closely coupled PACs also frequently initiate sustained or non-sustained supraventricular tachycardias.

Sustained Supraventricular Tachycardias

Supraventricular tachycardias can be broadly categorized into atrial and AV junctional (Table 51–1). Atrial tachycardias are independent of AV nodal conduction such that with effective vagal maneuvers (e.g., carotid sinus massage, Valsalva) AV block occurs but the atrial process continues. Conversely, most AV junctional tachycardias require propagation through the AV node to continue, so AV junctional tachycardias generally terminate if vagal maneuvers induce AV nodal block.

Atrial Tachycardias

SINUS TACHYCARDIA. Sinus tachycardia is usually due to an enhancement of normal automaticity seen in settings of increased adrenergic drive. Because sympathetic stimulation or vagal withdrawal also enhance AV nodal conduction, the PR interval does not prolong despite sinus rate acceleration. The P wave configuration is the same as with sinus rhythm—upright in leads II, III, and aV$_F$ (see Fig. 51–2B) and biphasic in V$_1$—because of the normal sequence with which the sinus node depolarizes the two atria. The

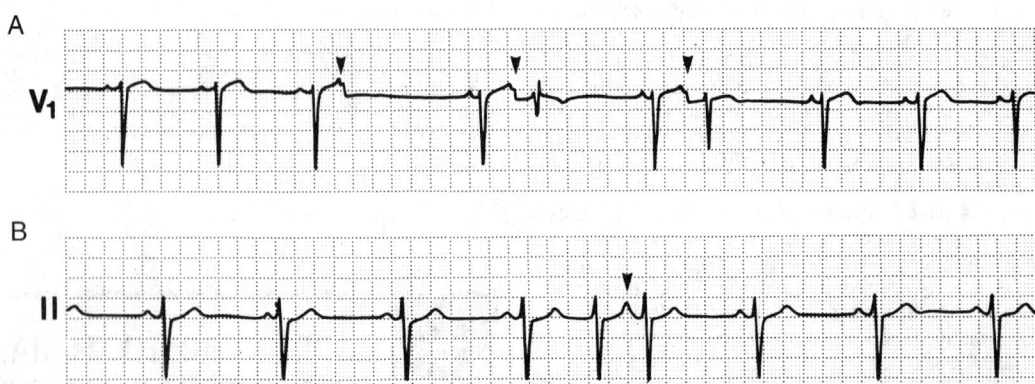

FIGURE 51–1 ■ Isolated premature complexes. *A,* Three premature atrial complexes (PACs) (arrows). The first one blocks and the remaining two conduct to the ventricles with different QRS morphology than sinus complexes owing to encroachment of premature impulses on the refractory period of the His-Purkinje system (aberrant conduction). *B,* Premature junctional complex (5th complex). Note the similarity of QRS complex between the sinus and premature beat that is not preceded by a P wave. The next sinus P wave (arrow) occurs on time and conducts to the ventricles. ECG leads are labeled. (Modified from Akhtar M: Examination of the heart: V. The electrogram. With permission from the American Heart Association.)

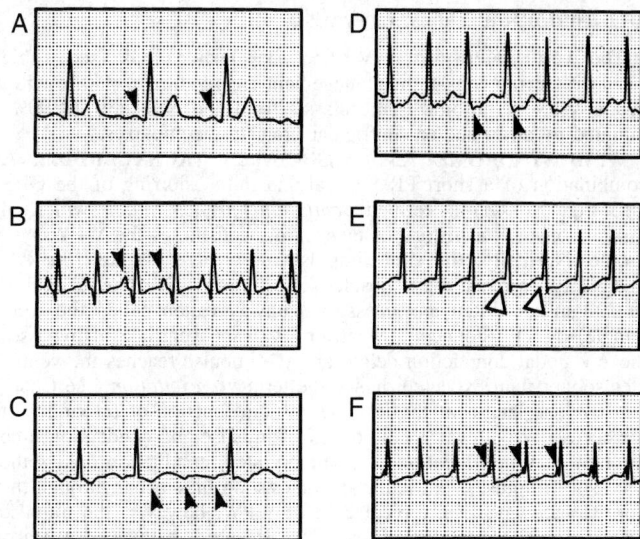

FIGURE 51-2 ■ P-QRS relationship in supraventricular tachycardia. Sinus rhythm (A), usual type of sinus tachycardia (B), and unifocal atrial tachycardia (C) are shown. Note the positive P wave and normal PR interval during sinus tachycardia. Atrial tachycardia (C) originates in the low atrium (negative P wave) and is accompanied by variable degree of AV block. The P wave during AV junctional re-entry follows the QRS and is in the ST segment during AV re-entry (D) and buried in the QRS complex during common AV nodal re-entry (E). Non-paroxysmal junctional tachycardia where the atria and ventricles are independently stimulated is shown (F). Resultant AV dissociation occurs because the junctional rate accelerates and competes with the sinus mechanism. Note the gradual march of P waves in and out of the QRS. ECG lead II in all panels.

atrial rate during sinus tachycardia seldom exceeds 200 beats per minute and is generally less than 150 beats per minute.

SINUS NODE RE-ENTRY. The P wave morphology is similar to sinus rhythm, but the underlying mechanism is re-entry in the

region of the sinus node. Unlike the physiologic form of sinus tachycardia, which has a gradual onset and termination, sinus node re-entry starts and ends abruptly. As with many other atrial re-entrant tachycardias, sinus node re-entry is generally triggered by a PAC. Sudden acceleration of the atrial rate prolongs the PR interval or even leads to AV nodal block due to the expected physiologic delay in AV nodal conduction unless concomitant sympathetic stimulation facilitates AV nodal conduction. The atrial rates range between 150 and 250 beats per minute. Depending on the state of AV conduction, 1:1 AV conduction or a variable degree of AV block may be noted.

ATRIAL TACHYCARDIA. Any tachycardia arising above the AV junction that has a P wave configuration different than sinus rhythm is called atrial tachycardia (see Fig. 51–2C). In general, impulses arising in the superior portion of the right or left atrium produce a positive P wave in the inferior leads (i.e., leads II, III, and aV$_F$), whereas those arising in the lower or inferior portions result in negative P waves in the same leads. Atrial tachycardias can result from enhanced normal automaticity, abnormal automaticity, triggered activity, and re-entry (see Chapter 49). The re-entrant forms can be easily reproduced in the electrophysiology laboratory with electrical stimulation of the atria (see Chapter 50). When the P wave configuration is uniform from beat to beat, the tachycardia is unifocal, whereas the term *multifocal atrial tachycardia* implies several different P wave morphologies. Atrial rates range between 100 and 250 beats per minute, and the ventricular response depends on the status of AV conduction; a 1:1 P wave/QRS complex ratio is common with rates less than 200 beats per minute, whereas at higher rates various degrees of block (e.g., 3:2, 2:1, 3:1) are common (see Fig. 51–2C). Both atrial rates and AV conduction can be markedly altered by cardioactive drugs, particularly antiarrhythmic agents (see Chapter 49).

ATRIAL FLUTTER. Atrial flutter causes regular atrial rates ranging from 250 to 350 beats per minute (300 being the most common) (Fig. 51–3A, B). Common atrial flutter, with "sawtooth" appearance in leads II, III, and aV$_F$, has a fairly uniform route of

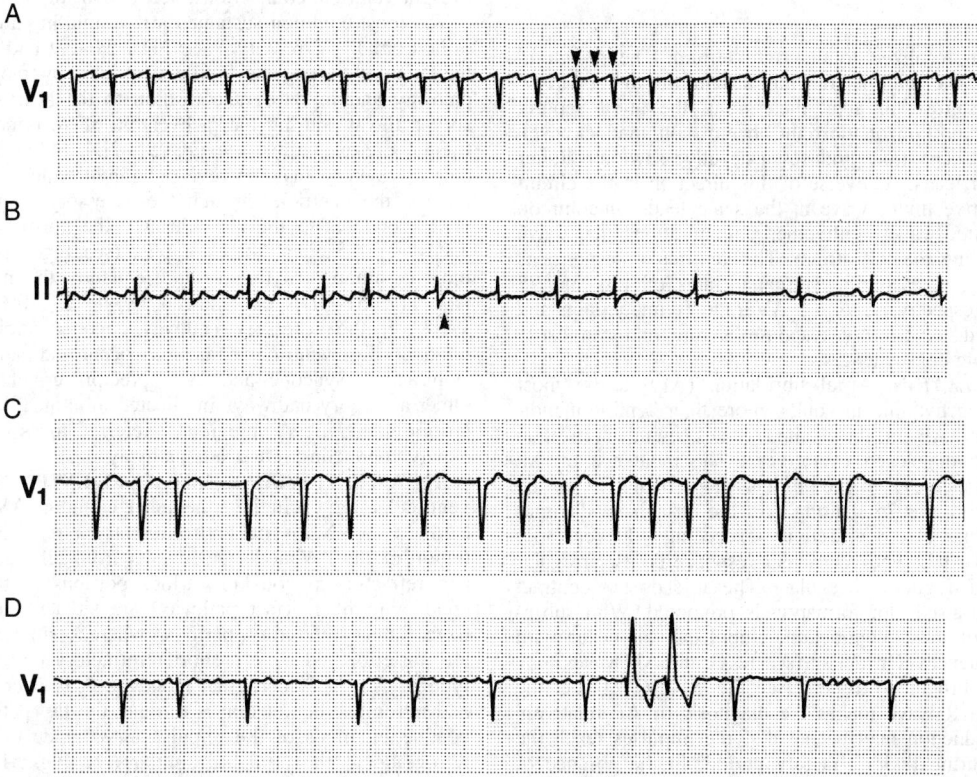

FIGURE 51-3 ■ Atrial flutter and atrial fibrillation. A, Regular narrow QRS tachycardia with ventricular rate of 150 beats per minute, most commonly seen in atrial flutter with 2:1 AV block. B, With a higher degree of AV block, the flutter waves can be more clearly seen, and in this case, the atrial flutter converted briefly to atrial fibrillation (at the arrow) and then to sinus rhythm. C and D, Atrial fibrillation. In C the atrial activity is difficult to identify, but it is quite clear in D; in both tracings the RR intervals are irregularly irregular. Two consecutive QRS complexes due to aberrant conduction (right bundle branch block) are noted in D. (Modified from Akhtar M: Examination of the heart: V. The electrogram. With permission from the American Heart Association.)

VENTRICULAR PREEXCITATION

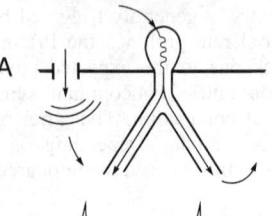

A

ORTHODROMIC TACHYCARDIA

B

ECG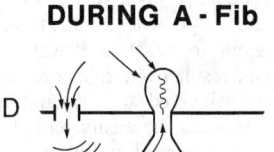

ANTIDROMIC TACHYCARDIA

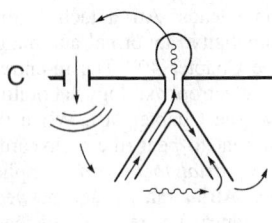

C

PREEXCITATION DURING A - Fib

D

FIGURE 51–4 ■ Wolff-Parkinson-White syndrome. *A,* Ventricular pre-excitation (short PR and delta wave) due to earlier ventricular activation via the accessory pathway. *B,* Narrow QRS tachycardia with anterograde conduction over the AV node–His-Purkinje syndrome and retrograde propagation via the accessory pathway (orthodromic tachycardia). *C,* The reversal of this re-entrant circuit produces antidromic tachycardia with regular and pre-excited complexes. *D,* During atrial fibrillation, preferential conduction over the accessory pathway produces rapid irregular pre-excited complexes. (Modified from Akhtar M: Examination of the heart: V. The electrogram. With permission from the American Heart Association.)

impulse propagation localized to the right atrium. The re-entrant impulse travels over the anterolateral right atrium, through a narrow isthmus in the posteroseptal area, then along the atrial septum toward the superior portion of the right atrium (counterclockwise). Incidental left atrial activation produces a negative sawtooth flutter wave in the inferior leads. A reverse of this direction in the circuit could cause a positive flutter wave in the same leads (uncommon or clockwise). Flutter waves with other configurations may have other origins including the left atrium. The ventricular response is usually 2:1 or 4:1, representing ventricular rates of 150 and 75 beats per minute, respectively. A 3:1 AV ratio is uncommon and fairly well tolerated. A 1:1 AV response is rare and can cause serious hemodynamic consequences.

ATRIAL FIBRILLATION. Atrial fibrillation (AF) is the most common sustained arrhythmia in adults: more than 2 million individuals suffer from AF in the United States, with more than 160,000 new cases diagnosed every year. The incidence of AF increases with advancing age and afflicts more than 6% of the population older than age 75. During AF, the atria have disorganized, rapid, irregular electrical activity exceeding 400 beats per minute (see Fig. 51–3C). The ventricular response is also irregular and quite variable (irregularly irregular). The atria do not contract effectively, so intra-atrial clot formation is promoted. With subsequent resumption of atrial contraction, embolism can occur with devastating consequences. On the surface ECG, the AF waves may be coarse, fine, or difficult to discern (see Fig. 51–3C, D), but the irregularity of the RR wave makes the diagnosis of AF relatively easy. Aberrant conduction may be noted if the impulses reach the bundle branches during their refractory period. In the absence of accessory pathways, the average ventricular response via the AV node–HPS is seldom more than 200 and is generally less than 150 beats per minute. However, with a rapidly conducting accessory pathway, ventricular rates can exceed 300 beats per minute and precipitate ventricular fibrillation.

Atrioventricular Junctional Tachycardia

The vast majority of AV junctional tachycardias (see Table 51–1) requiring long-term management are re-entrant. AV re-entry in the WPW syndrome is the classic form and is usually (>90%) initiated by atrial and/or ventricular premature complexes.

WPW SYNDROME AND ASSOCIATED TACHYCARDIAS. A combination of a short PR interval and initial slurring of the QRS (see Fig. 51–4A) is termed *ventricular pre-excitation,* which in association with a history of tachycardia constitutes the WPW syndrome. Normally, the sinus impulse must travel through the AV node–HPS to reach the ventricles, resulting in a PR interval of 120 to 200 msec. When an accessory pathway (often called the Kent bundle) directly connects the atrium with the ventricle, it bypasses the AV nodal conduction delay; and the impulse reaches the ventricles sooner than expected, hence the term *pre-excitation* (see Chapter 49). The length of the PR interval is a function of proximity of the accessory pathway to the origin of impulse and conduction time through it. When location or relatively slow conduction delays the accessory impulse, ventricular depolarization may occur through the normal pathway. In a typical case of WPW, however, the impulse reaches the ventricle first through the accessory pathway and starts the QRS earlier, resulting in a shorter PR interval (see Fig. 51–3A). Because the initial QRS activation is due to muscle to muscle conduction, as opposed to Purkinje to muscle activation during normal QRS, the beginning of the QRS is slurred and produces a so-called delta wave. Soon after, ventricular activation also starts through the normal pathway and is more rapidly spread through the ventricular myocardium, resulting in a fusion QRS activation with a rapid inscription after the delta wave. If the atrial or sinus impulse never reaches the ventricle through the accessory pathway due either to delayed arrival at or lack of antegrade conduction over the accessory pathway, the abnormality is termed the *concealed WPW syndrome,* because retrograde conduction through the accessory pathway may be intact and able to cause orthodromic tachycardia. The most common accessory pathway (>50%) is in the left ventricle free wall, that is, left atrial to left ventricle connection. Posteroseptal pathways (connecting the right atrial with left ventricle) are the next most common (30%). Right free wall and anteroseptal accessory pathways, both of which are right atrium to right ventricle connections, account for the remaining.

The most common sustained arrhythmia in patients with WPW is orthodromic AV re-entry (see Figs. 51–2D and 51–4B), in which the impulse propagates to the ventricles by means of the normal pathway and in retrograde fashion to the atria through the accessory pathway; during the tachycardia, there is no evidence of ventricular pre-excitation (see Fig. 51–2D). In rare instances, the circuit of re-entry may be reversed (antidromic) so that the impulse reaches the ventricle through the accessory pathway and in retrograde conducts to the atria through the normal pathway and produces a pre-excited QRS complex (see Fig. 51–4C). The second most common arrhythmia and frequently the most serious is AF (see Fig. 51–4D), experienced by up to 40% of patients with WPW. If the accessory pathway conducts rapidly during AF, a relatively fast ventricular rate may occur and cause severe hypotension and/or syncope and even precipitate ventricular fibrillation. Other accessory pathways implicated in clinical tachycardias are the atriofascicular fibers (previously referred to as Mahaim fibers) and slowly conducting retrograde pathways.

ATRIOVENTRICULAR NODAL RE-ENTRY. In the absence of ventricular pre-excitation, the most common AV junctional tachycardia is AVNR. The entire re-entry circuit is localized to the region of the AV node and results from differences of conduction and refractory periods in various portions of the AV node. Fast conducting fibers (fast pathway) are situated more anteriorly and have longer refractory periods, whereas slower-conducting fibers are posterior and have a shorter refractory period. In the common type of AVNR, anterograde conduction is over the slow pathway and retrograde conduction is through the fast pathway such that the conduction times of the impulse anterograde to the ventricles and retrograde to the atria are similar (see Fig. 51–2E), resulting in near simultaneous P and QRS complexes. The retrograde P wave therefore is either obscured by the QRS complex (see Fig. 51–2E) or alters the appearance of the terminal portion of the QRS and may be recognized in the early part of the ST segment. Less frequently, the direction of conduction through the re-entry circuit is reversed, with anterograde conduction to the ventricle over the fast pathway and retrograde conduction to the atria via the slow pathway; the result is a shorter PR interval. If the P wave follows the T wave, its retrograde morphology (i.e., negative in leads II, III, and aV_F) is clearly recognizable. Sustained AVNR and AV re-entry together account for more than 75% of cases frequently labeled as paroxysmal atrial tachycardia (PAT).

NON-PAROXYSMAL JUNCTIONAL TACHYCARDIA. Non-paroxysmal junctional tachycardia arises within the region of the His bundle and activates the ventricles with a QRS morphology similar to sinus beats (see Fig. 51–2*F*). Retrograde conduction through the AV node may or may not take place. If there is retrograde block, sinus rhythm remains uninterrupted, and the sinus P wave also blocks when the AV node is refractory because of retrograde AV nodal penetration of the junctional impulse; AV dissociation may result (see Fig. 51–2*F*). A 1:1 P wave/QRS complex relationship may occur, and if the P wave is negative, junctional origin is suggested. Ventricular rates seldom exceed 150 beats per minute, and when the rate is less than 100 beats per minute the term *accelerated junctional rhythm* is applied. The underlying mechanism is enhanced normal automaticity.

AUTOMATIC JUNCTIONAL TACHYCARDIA. The main difference between automatic junctional tachycardia and non-paroxysmal junctional tachycardia on the surface electrocardiogram is the rate. In the automatic variety, rates are faster (range, 130–200 beats per minute). This arrhythmia can be episodic or persistent. Because the rates are fairly comparable to paroxysmal AV junctional re-entrant tachycardia and the QRS complex morphology is similar to sinus beats, the presence of AV dissociation is the main electrocardiographic distinction from re-entrant arrhythmias. The underlying etiology is abnormal automaticity in the AV junction.

Clinical Features of Supraventricular Tachycardia

The usual type of sinus tachycardia is caused by increased metabolic demands from high adrenergic states such as fever, physical exertion, hypovolemia, heart failure, sympathomimetic or parasympatholytic medications, thyrotoxicosis, and pheochromocytoma. All other supraventricular tachycardias represent abnormalities of rhythm and commonly produce tachycardia-related symptoms, including palpitation, racing of the heart, dizziness, shortness of breath, chest discomfort, presyncope, and sometimes frank syncope. Incessant supraventricular tachycardia and uncontrolled ventricular rates in AF can cause tachycardia-related cardiomyopathy, which is reversible with control of these arrhythmias.

Atrial dilation, fibrosis, and acute or chronic inflammatory states involving atrial myocardium or pericardium may cause atrial tachycardias. Multifocal atrial tachycardia is relatively frequent in the presence of chronic pulmonary disease. AF is often associated with aging, hypertension, valvular and pulmonary diseases, acute and chronic coronary disease, hyperadrenergic states, and metabolic abnormalities such as thyrotoxicosis. AF may also be noted in the absence of any detectable cardiac pathology—lone AF. The risk of thromboembolism in AF increases with age, diabetes mellitus, hypertension, previous embolic episodes, valvular disease, and heart failure. The lowest incidence, less than 1% annually, is in patients younger than 65 years of age with lone AF.

Re-entrant tachycardias have an abrupt onset and an abrupt ending, particularly when terminated with vagal maneuvers or intravenous medications. Even though a functioning accessory pathway is a congenital abnormality, its clinical manifestation can occur at any age. If no electrocardiogram is done, asymptomatic ventricular pre-excitation can go undetected for many years. When discovered, ventricular pre-excitation can mimic inferior or anteroseptal myocardial infarction, right ventricular hypertrophy, and right and left bundle branch block. WPW is not clearly associated with mitral valve prolapse or hypertrophic cardiomyopathy, but single and multiple right-sided accessory pathways are more common with Ebstein's anomaly.

Non-paroxysmal AV junctional tachycardia is frequently seen with high adrenergic drive, that is, after myocardial infarction or cardiac surgery, with sympathomimetic and parasympatholytic agents, or with digitalis toxicity. Automatic junctional tachycardia is not known to be associated with any particular cardiovascular pathology.

Therapy for Supraventricular Tachyarrhythmias (Table 51–2; see also Chapters 48 and 49)

ACUTE THERAPY. Isolated premature beats seldom pose any significant risk, do not cause severe arrhythmic symptoms, and hence do not warrant aggressive therapy. Conversely, sustained or prolonged repeated episodes of non-sustained supraventricular tachycardias generally require effective therapy. An acute episode of junctional tachycardia from either AV nodal re-entry or AV re-entry can be terminated with vagal maneuvers such as carotid massage, which produce a marked sinus slowing and AV nodal block. In most atrial tachycardias, adenosine and/or vagal stimulation produce enough AV block to unmask the atrial origin of the tachycardia. However, some atrial tachycardias, particularly those arising near the sinus node, may also terminate after adenosine administration. Intravenous β-blockers and calcium channel blockers can also be used for the same purpose. For sustained control of ventricular rate during atrial tachycardia, AF, or atrial flutter-fibrillation, intravenous esmolol and diltiazem are quite effective. If ventricular response during AF is through a rapidly conducting accessory pathway, intravenous digitalis and calcium channel blockers are contraindicated and procainamide is a better choice. Atrial tachycardias, including atrial flutter or AF, may convert spontaneously or convert after treatment of an underlying cause such as hypoxia or heart failure or after cessation of precipitating medications; when these rhythms persist, direct-current cardiover-

Table 51–2 ▪ DRUGS AND DOSES USED TO TREAT SUPRAVENTRICULAR TACHYCARDIAS

DRUG	IV BOLUS	IV INFUSION	ORAL DOSE
Digoxin	0.5–1.0 mg		0.125–0.5 mg/d
Adenosine	6–12 mg		
β-Blockers			
Esmolol	5 μg/kg/min	3 μg/kg/min	
Propranolol	1–3 mg		10–40 mg tid
Calcium channel blockers			
Verapamil	5–15 mg		80–120 mg tid/qid
Diltiazem	15–25 mg	15 mg/hr	120 mg bid/tid
Class IA			
Procainamide	10–15 mg/kg	5 mg/kg	750–1500 mg qid
Quinidine			300–600 mg qid
Disopyramide			100–200 mg tid
Class IC			
Flecainide			50–200 mg bid
Propafenone			150–300 mg tid
Class III			
Ibutilide	1–2 mg		
Sotalol			80–160 mg bid
Amiodarone	2–3 mg/kg	0.5–1 mg/min	800–160 mg/d for 7 to 10-day loading dose then 100–400 mg/d

sion is usually required (see Chapter 53). Whenever more rapid control of supraventricular tachycardia is desired, for example, in patients with myocardial ischemia or hypotension, direct-current cardioversion is the best solution (see Chapter 53).

LONG-TERM MANAGEMENT. For symptomatic patients with sustained AV junctional re-entry, control can sometimes be achieved with digitalis, β-blockers, and calcium channel blockers or with Class I and Class III drugs (see Chapter 54); however, radiofrequency ablation is now the preferred choice for most symptomatic sustained regular re-entrant supraventricular tachycardias described earlier (see Chapter 53). Digitalis is contraindicated in patients with overt pre-excitation during sinus rhythm.

In patients with atrial tachycardia, atrial flutter, or AF, ventricular rate control is possible through relative AV nodal block with digitalis, β-blockers, and calcium channel blockers (see Table 51–2). For termination or prevention of atrial tachyarrhythmias, Class Ia, Ic, or III drugs are usually needed (see Chapter 54). If the nature and origin of a specific supraventricular tachycardia is known, the potential benefit of antiarrhythmic drugs can be deduced (see Chapter 54). Sotalol and amiodarone are currently the most effective drugs for long-term control of AF and flutter (see Table 51–2).

Anticoagulation therapy with warfarin is recommended in all patients with AF older than 65 years of age or who have risk factors for thromboembolism and have no contraindication to anticoagulation. The international normalized ratio (INR) goal is 2.0 to 3.0, unless mitral stenosis is present, in which case the target is an INR of 2.5 to 3.5. Aspirin may be better than no treatment for patients who cannot tolerate warfarin.

BRADYARRHYTHMIAS

Bradyarrhythmias (Table 51–3) can be broadly classified into SND and AV blocks.

Sinus Node Dysfunction

Among the various pacemaker cells distributed throughout the cardiac conduction system, the sinus node has the highest rate of automaticity and therefore it functions as the dominant pacemaker (see Chapter 49). The usual sinus rate varies between 60 and 100 beats per minute, determined by physiologic need and modulated through the autonomic nervous system. SND has several different manifestations, including sinus bradycardia, sinoatrial (SA) exit block, sinus arrest, and bradycardia-tachycardia syndrome.

SINUS BRADYCARDIA. Rates less than 60 beats per minute are usually described as bradycardia (Fig. 51–5A). In healthy persons, however, rates of 50 beats per minute are not unusual, and rates as low as 30 beats per minute may be recorded during sleep. Sinus bradycardia of clinical significance is usually defined as persistent rates less than 45 beats per minute while awake. SND may also be manifested by the failure to accelerate the sinus rate (lack of chronotropic response) in response to situations such as exercise, heart failure, fever, sympathomimetic drugs, or parasympatholytic drugs. It is important to determine that SND including sinus bradycardia

---

Table 51–3 ■ **BRADYCARDIAS**

Sinus Node Dysfunction
　Sinus bradycardia <45/min
　Sinoatrial exit block
　　First degree
　　Second degree
　　Third degree
　Sinus arrest
　Bradycardia-tachycardia syndrome
Atrioventricular Block
　First degree
　Second degree
　　Mobitz type I (Wenckebach phenomenon)
　　Mobitz type II
　　Higher degree (e.g., 2:1, 3:1)
　Third degree
　　Atrioventricular node
　　His-Purkinje system

---

in a given individual is not secondary to cardioactive drugs such as β-blockers and calcium channel blockers.

SINOATRIAL EXIT BLOCK. The sinus node may fire, but the impulse to the atrium can be delayed or periodically interrupted with loss of P wave (see Fig. 51–5B); this abnormality, termed *SA exit block,* has been confirmed by intracardiac recordings. However, because sinus node activity is not recorded on the surface ECG, the diagnosis of SA exit block is made from analysis of PP intervals. First-degree SA exit block is difficult to determine from the surface ECG. Diagnosis of second-degree SA block (type I, II, and higher degrees) can be more easily established. In type I SA block (SA Wenckebach or Mobitz type I), the PP interval progressively shortens after a pause (reflecting the dropped P wave), and then the cycle repeats. In Mobitz II or type II second-degree SA block, a sudden absence of an expected P wave is noted, and the pause is a multiple of the dominant PP cycle. With a higher degree of block, two or more P waves may be missing. A subsidiary pacemaker from the AV nodal junction usually emerges during these circumstances. Third-degree SA block means complete absence of sinus P waves (see Fig. 51–5C). Atrial response to other stimuli, such as retrograde activation from AV junctional or atrial pacing, suggests third-degree SA block rather than sinus arrest; in the absence of sinus node recording, however, such a diagnosis is difficult to make.

SINUS ARREST. Sudden disappearance of P waves could be due to either SA exit block or cessation of sinus node pacemaker function. The two are difficult to distinguish unless the resultant PP interval has a predictable periodicity or is a multiple of sinus PP cycle (see Fig. 51–5B). SA exit block and sinus arrest must be distinguished from blocked PACs (see Fig. 51–5D) and sinus arrhythmia. Blocked PACs are likely to distort the ST-T segment and reset the sinus node so that the PP cycle with a blocked APC is less than two PP intervals. Sinus arrhythmia, which is a physiologic variation of PP change, usually follows the respiratory cycle (phasic sinus arrhythmia). The non-phasic variety may result in an abrupt sinus pause and may be confused with SND.

BRADYCARDIA-TACHYCARDIA SYNDROME. Because SND often represents atrial disease processes (e.g., fibrosis, degeneration, inflammation), coexistence of atrial tachyarrhythmias with bradycardia is not surprising. When an atrial tachycardia such as AF is terminated, the underlying rhythm may reveal sinus bradycardia, SA exit block, or even complete atrial standstill with an escape rhythm from a lower pacemaker in the AV node, the HPS, or the ventricles.

Atrioventricular Blocks

When atrial activity can be clearly identified and fails to produce a ventricular response, AV block exists. In a resting state, the normal AV node is capable of conducting up to 200 impulses per minute. With facilitation of AV nodal conduction due to adrenergic stimulation or vagal withdrawal, this rate can reach 250 impulses per minute and even 300 impulses per minute in exceptional cases. Therefore, with rapid atrial tachycardia, atrial flutter, and AF, some degree of AV block (in the AV node) is expected. AV block is defined when some impulses do not reach the ventricle during normal sinus rhythm or sinus tachycardia.

Electrophysiologic and Electrocardiographic Features

FIRST-DEGREE AV BLOCK (prolonged AV conduction or PR interval with 1:1 P-QRS relationship). The normal PR interval is 120 to 200 msec. Because the PR interval incorporates intra-atrial, AV nodal, and HPS conduction, it could be prolonged because of conduction delay in any of these areas. The intra-atrial conduction time can be estimated from the onset of the P wave on surface ECG to the onset of atrial deflection on the His bundle electrogram. The AH interval represents conduction through the AV node and is normally 60 to 140 msec; the HPS time estimated by HV interval is 35 to 55 msec. When the PR interval is prolonged, delay is usually in the AV node (Fig. 51–6A); intra-atrial conduction delays and abnormal HPS conduction time seldom prolong the PR interval more than 200 msec and are highly unlikely to prolong it to more than 300 msec. Block in the AV node or within the His bundle does not alter the QRS complex morphology compared with sinus rhythm; if a fascicular or bundle branch block occurs, infra-His block is likely.

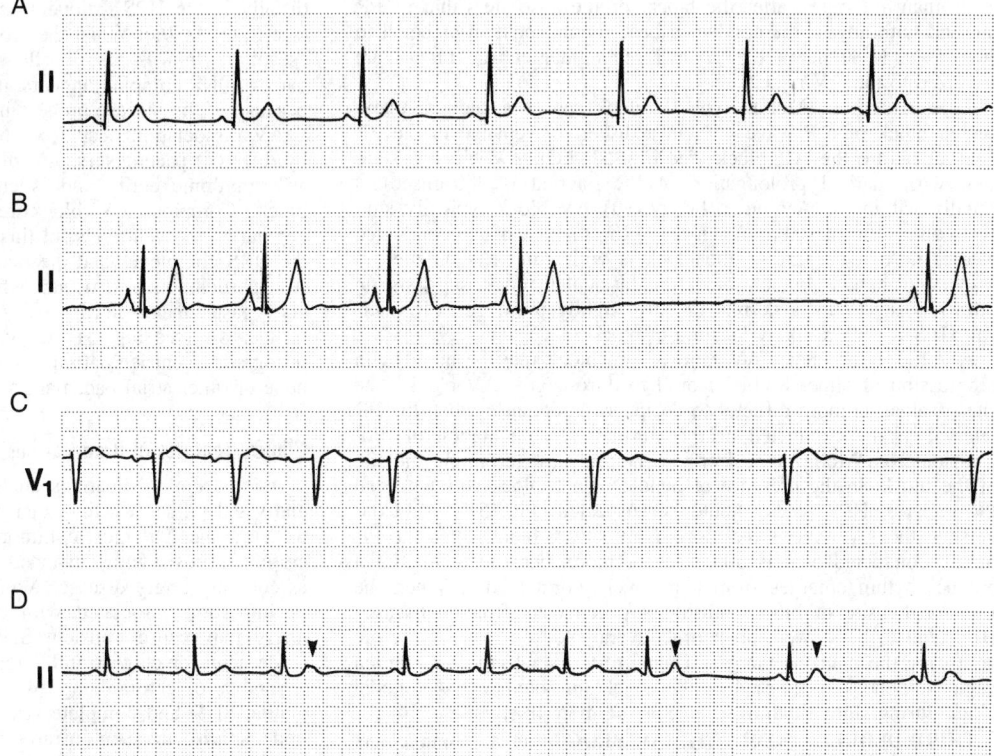

FIGURE 51–5 ■ Sinus node dysfunction. *A*, Sinus bradycardia, with sudden loss of sinus activity (no P waves) in *B* and *C*. Sinus rhythm resumes after a 4.5-second pause (*B*), whereas junctional rhythm emerges as a subsidiary mechanism in *C*. The exact cause (i.e., sinoatrial exit block vs. sinus arrest) cannot be determined from the surface ECG in these examples. In *D*, blocked PACs (note distortion of the T wave at arrows compared with sinus cycles) mimic sinus node dysfunction.

SECOND-DEGREE AV BLOCK (intermittent AV conduction). With second-degree AV block, some P waves fail to produce a QRS complex. In type I, also called Mobitz type I or Wenckebach phenomenon, there is a progressive increase in the PR interval, despite a constant PP rate, until a P wave blocks and the cycle is repeated (see Fig. 51–6*B*). Any P-QRS ratio can be seen (e.g., a 3:2, 4:3, 5:4). In a typical Wenckebach phenomenon, the PR interval after the block is the shortest. The largest increase in PR interval occurs after the second conducted beat; therefore, the RR interval after the pause, which contains the blocked P wave, progressively shortens until the next pause (see Fig. 51–6*B*). The Wenckebach phenomenon can be found in all cardiac conducting tissues, but the magnitude of PR prolongation or shortening from beat to beat is maximum in the AV node and therefore most noticeable. The AV node is the likely site of block when the PR interval increment with any subsequent PP cycle exceeds 100 msec, PR shortening is

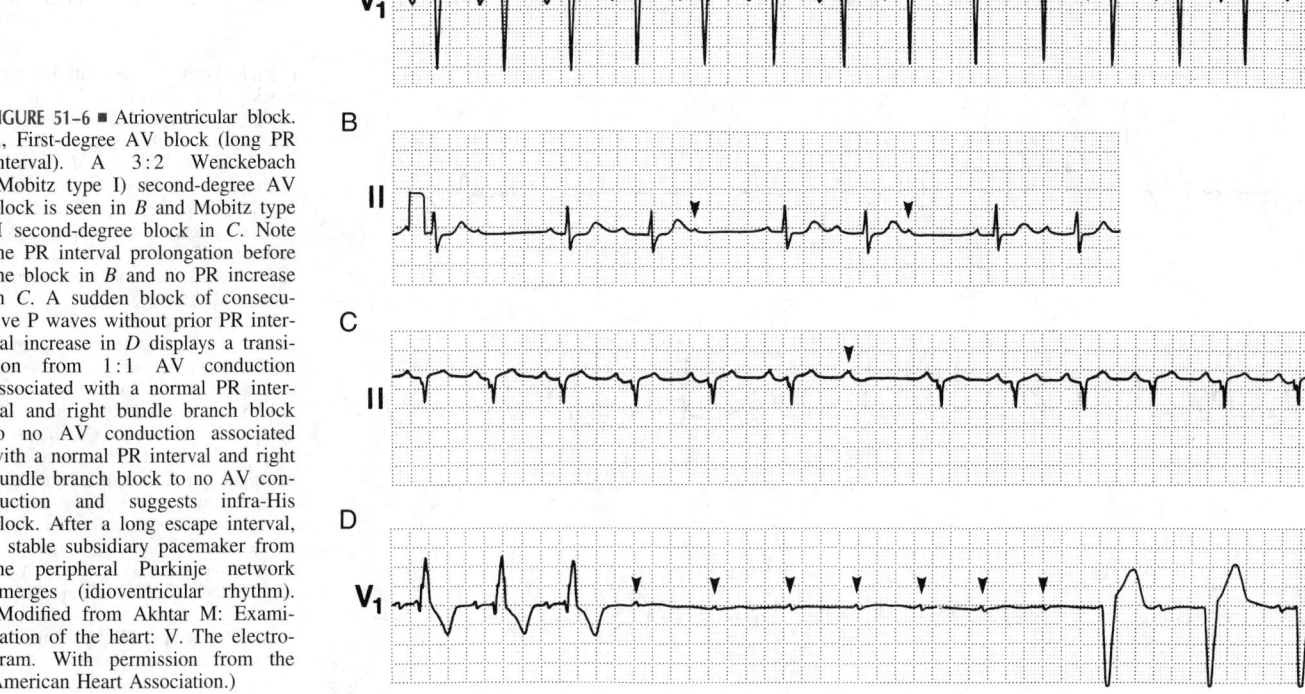

FIGURE 51–6 ■ Atrioventricular block. *A*, First-degree AV block (long PR interval). A 3:2 Wenckebach (Mobitz type I) second-degree AV block is seen in *B* and Mobitz type II second-degree block in *C*. Note the PR interval prolongation before the block in *B* and no PR increase in *C*. A sudden block of consecutive P waves without prior PR interval increase in *D* displays a transition from 1:1 AV conduction associated with a normal PR interval and right bundle branch block to no AV conduction associated with a normal PR interval and right bundle branch block to no AV conduction and suggests infra-His block. After a long escape interval, a stable subsidiary pacemaker from the peripheral Purkinje network emerges (idioventricular rhythm). (Modified from Akhtar M: Examination of the heart: V. The electrogram. With permission from the American Heart Association.)

more than 100 msec after the block, or the absolute value of PR interval with any of the conducted beats is greater than or equal to 300 msec. Most but not all type I second-degree AV blocks are localized to the AV node.

Type II AV, or Mobitz type II, block causes a sudden, unexpected block of a P wave without a discernible change in the PR interval before the AV block (see Fig. 51–6C). AV block associated with marked prolongation of PR interval (≥300 msec) is usually within the AV node, but type II AV block typically suggests disease in the HPS. When the QRS complex of the conducted beat is normal or narrow, the block is within the His bundle; an associated bundle branch block or fascicular block suggests an infra-His site. With a normal or only slightly prolonged PR interval, HPS is a more likely location of block.

A 2:1, 3:1, or higher AV ratio of AV block may be noted with progression of either Mobitz I or II to third-degree AV block. The site of block is more difficult to decipher, particularly when the PR interval of the conducted beat is normal. Documentation of progression from Mobitz type I or II is helpful in determining the site of the block. In the presence of bundle branch block and a normal PR interval, HPS block should be suspected (Fig. 51–7A). Conversely, the AV node is the more likely site of block when the PR of the conducted beat is 300 msec or more, because a junctional escape rhythm emerges from a relatively normal HPS. When the HPS is the site of block, subsidiary pacemakers from a diseased HPS tend to be slower and permit several blocked P waves before an escape mechanism emerges. Therefore, in the absence of marked vagal influences, a 3:1 or 4:1 ratio is seldom noted with AV nodal block during sinus rhythm, so HPS is the more likely site of block.

THIRD-DEGREE (COMPLETE) AV BLOCK (no AV conduction). Complete failure of impulse propagation along the AV conduction system necessitates emergence of subsidiary pacemaker distal to the site of block. Normally, the rate of resting pacemaker activity is highest in the sinus node (60–100 beats per minute), followed by the AV junction (40–60 beats per minute) and the bundle branch–Purkinje system (20–40 beats per minute). When the tissues expected to function as subsidiary pacemakers are abnormal, the rates may be even slower. During intact AV conduction, all of the subsidiary pacemakers remain suppressed (overdrive suppression). With abrupt cessation of AV conduction, the first subsidiary pacemaker response (often referred to as escape beat) is almost always slower than the subsequent rate from the same subsidiary foci; the rate of the emergent pacemaker below the site of block gradually accelerates (warm-up phenomenon) to its usual anticipated rate.

When the AV node is the site of third-degree AV block, the AV junctional pacemakers drive the ventricular rates (see Fig. 51–7B). The QRS complex morphology is similar to sinus beats and nor-mally warms up to 40 to 60 beats per minute. With infra-His block, the escape rhythm shows a wide QRS complex, originates distally in the HPS (idioventricular), and has a relatively slow rate (see Fig. 51–7C). When the block is within the His bundle and the escape rhythm is also in the His bundle distal to the block, a narrow QRS complex appears at a slower than expected escape rate because of the disease process involving the junctional pacemakers.

AV dissociation occurs when the atria and ventricles are driven by different pacemakers. AV dissociation per se does not represent an arrhythmic entity and is either due to AV or ventriculoatrial block. Complete AV block requires a subsidiary pacemaker to depolarize the ventricles; in this situation, the P wave is faster than the QRS complexes and the two are unrelated (see Fig. 51–7B, C). AV dissociation also occurs when the rate of subsidiary pacemakers is faster than a normal sinus, such as non-paroxysmal junctional tachycardia (see Fig. 51–2F) or ventricular tachycardia; if there is retrograde (ventriculoatrial) block, the atria are driven by the SA node or other atrial pacemakers.

Clinical Features of Bradycardias

Aside from medications such as digitalis, antiarrhythmic drugs, and vagal influences, the exact cause for SND is frequently difficult to determine. The most common causes for SND are muscle degeneration, fibrosis with advanced age, and/or cardiac pathology such as coronary artery disease. Acute inferior wall myocardial ischemia or infarction associated with disease of proximal right coronary artery may cause transient SND. Other, less common causes include acute or chronic inflammation from myocarditis or pericarditis and prior cardiac surgery with trauma to the sinus node. Congenital SND and complete atrial standstill with no detectable sinus node activity are seen on rare occasions.

AV nodal blocks can be caused by digitalis, antiarrhythmic drugs, and vagal influences. Involvement of the AV junctional area with any inflammatory or other disease process can result in AV nodal block of varying degrees. The most common cause of chronic AV block in the HPS is progressive fibrosis and/or calcification in the HPS with aging or myocardial fibrosis from any cause. Because of the proximity of aortic and mitral valves to the distal His bundle and proximal bundle branches, annular calcification or valve surgery can cause acute or chronic intra-His and infra-His block. Myocardial infiltration by an infectious agent (i.e., Chagas' disease) is an important cause of chronic heart block in Latin American countries. Acute inferior wall ischemia and/or infarction can cause various degrees of AV nodal block because of ischemia in the nodal artery distributions. Involvement of HPS during acute anterior MI can lead to bundle branch block and/or AV block.

Sinus bradycardia and various degrees of AV nodal blocks are

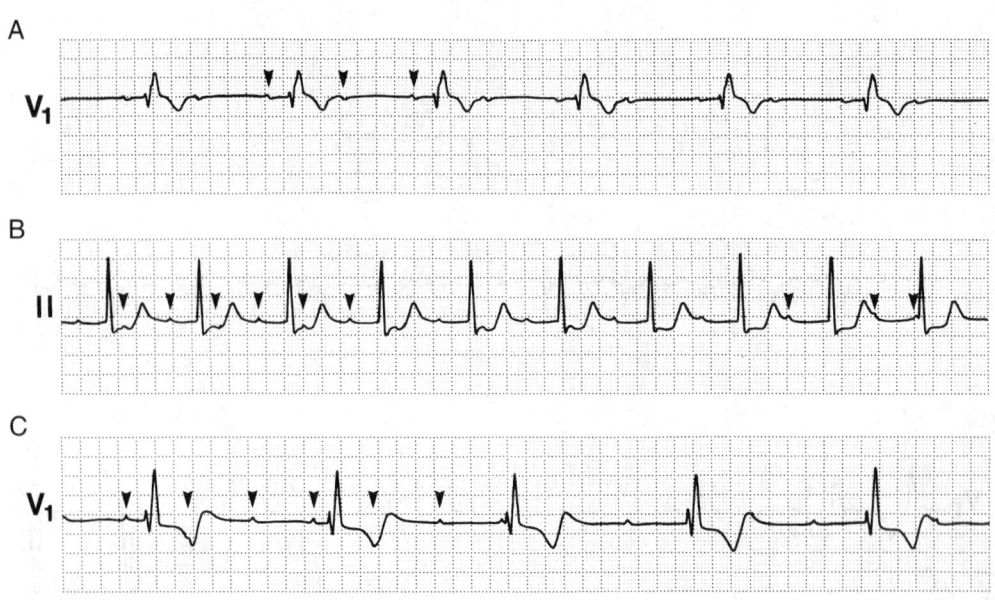

FIGURE 51–7 ■ 2:1 and third-degree block. *A*, A 2:1 AV ratio, a slightly prolonged PR interval of conducted beats, right bundle branch block. The site of block is difficult to determine from the surface ECG. *B* and *C*, Third-degree block. The escape mechanism has a narrow QRS complex in *B* at a rate of 50 beats per minute and suggests intranodal block and a junctional subsidiary pacemaker. The escape mechanism in *C* is from the peripheral Purkinje network (idioventricular), as indicated by its slow rate (33 beats per minute) and wide complexes. In both panels, the atrial rates are constant and unrelated to ventricular rates, which are also constant but driven by a slower subsidiary pacemaker located distal to the sites of block (AV dissociation). The appropriate ECG leads are labeled. (Modified from Akhtar M: Examination of the heart: V. The electrogram. With permission from the American Heart Association.)

also noted during sleep even in otherwise healthy people. Asymptomatic first- and second-degree AV block, particularly when partially or completely reversed by exercise, points toward a benign condition. Persistent second- and third-degree AV nodal block during the waking hours and during activity is abnormal and is often associated with symptoms of bradycardia, including dizziness, fatigue, exertional dyspnea, aggravation of heart failure, near-syncope, or syncope. Third-degree AV block with a good junctional escape mechanism that accelerates during exercise, as often noted in patients with congenital AV block, may remain asymptomatic. Patients with congenital heart block may not appreciate their potential for more active lifestyle because of the lack of a reference point but feel much better when an appropriate heart rate acceleration can be achieved after pacemaker therapy.

Bradycardias of all types may also be secondary to profound vagal influences, as seen with neurally mediated syndromes such as vasovagal episodes, vomiting, abdominal surgery, and upper and lower gastrointestinal invasive procedures. Periods of prolonged sinus arrest and AV nodal block with marked suppression of subsidiary pacemaker can occur and lead to symptomatic asystole. Vasovagal (neurocardiogenic) syndromes are a rather common cause of syncope in relatively healthy populations (see Chapter 50); in the vast majority of these cases, vasodepression (hypotension) is the primary cause of syncope, and rate control alone does not relieve symptoms.

Therapy for Bradycardias

Asymptomatic SND or AV nodal block require no therapy. Acute management of symptomatic SND and second- and third-degree AV block includes administration of intravenous atropine (1.0 mg) or isoproterenol (usually 1–2 μg/min infusion) to increase the heart rate. Temporary cardiac pacing may be needed. When SND or AV block is due to transient abnormalities, such as drug-induced or acute ischemic syndromes, temporary pacing is usually sufficient; however, when infra-His or intra-His block is suspected (e.g., exercise-induced AV block or asymptomatic Mobitz type II block) and the site can be documented with His bundle recording, permanent pacing is indicated. For all forms of persistent symptomatic SND or second- or third-degree AV block, permanent pacing is the therapy of choice (see Chapter 53). Nevertheless, even prolonged paroxysmal asystole due to neurocardiogenic mechanism is not an indication for permanent pacing; instead, pharmacologic therapy that relieves hypotension will control bradycardiac symptoms as well. As a general rule, bradycardia in individuals younger than 55 years of age is vagal in origin and does not require permanent pacing unless proven otherwise.

Akhtar M: Techniques of electrophysiologic testing. *In* Alexander RW, Schlant R, Fuster V (eds): Hurst's The Heart, 9th ed. New York, McGraw-Hill, 1998, pp 955–967.

Myerburg R, Kessler K, Castellanos A: Recognition, clinical assessment and management of arrhythmias and conduction disturbances. *In* Alexander RW, Schlant R, Fuster V (eds): Hurst's The Heart, 9th ed. New York, McGraw-Hill, 1998, pp 873–941. *Well referenced chapters pertinent to supraventricular arrhythmias.*

52 VENTRICULAR ARRHYTHMIAS AND SUDDEN DEATH

Bruce B. Lerman

PREMATURE VENTRICULAR COMPLEXES

ELECTROCARDIOGRAPHIC FEATURES. Premature ventricular complexes (PVCs) are ubiquitous arrhythmias that are recognized on the surface electrocardiogram (ECG) by their wide (generally > 120 msec) and bizarre QRS morphology, occurring independently of atrial activation (P waves). Very late cycle PVCs may follow a P wave that occurs on time and are identified by a shorter than

normal PR interval. PVCs may be due to enhanced automaticity, triggered activity, or re-entry.

Most PVCs are followed by a "compensatory pause" because the PVC fails to conduct retrogradely to the atria and therefore cannot affect or reset the electrical activity of the sinus node. The interval between the first sinus beat and the PVC plus the interval between the PVC and the next sinus beat equals two normal sinus intervals (Fig. 52–1). Occasionally, PVCs may be interpolated between two sinus beats (i.e., produce no pause) and, rarely, PVCs may penetrate and reset the sinus node.

PVCs may be isolated or occur in groups. Two consecutive PVCs are termed a *couplet*. Three or more consecutive PVCs at a rate of 100 beats per minute or more are termed *ventricular tachycardia* (VT). Single PVCs may occur sporadically or as bigeminy (every other beat is a PVC), trigeminy (every third beat is a PVC), or higher-order periodicities. A given patient may manifest PVCs with two or more different morphologies, in which case the ectopy is termed *multiform*. Single PVCs, regardless of whether or not they occur sporadically or in a periodic pattern, are sometimes referred to as "simple" ventricular ectopy, whereas multiform PVCs, very closely coupled PVCs (so-called R-on-T), ventricular couplets, and non-sustained VT are referred to as "complex" ventricular ectopy. Fusion beats result from simultaneous activation of the ventricle by a normally conducted supraventricular beat and a concurrent PVC and have a morphology with some similarities to both the supraventricular and ventricular beats.

EPIDEMIOLOGY. Ventricular ectopy is exceedingly rare in infants but increases in frequency with age. PVCs occur in patients with and without structural heart disease. Holter monitoring (see Chapter 50) reveals at least one PVC in 40 to 75% of normal adults and complex ventricular ectopy in 5 to 10% of normal adults. PVCs occur with greater frequency and complexity in patients with structural heart disease, especially ischemic and valvular heart disease and idiopathic cardiomyopathy. PVCs may also occur in the setting of drug toxicity (e.g., digitalis intoxication) or electrolyte disturbances (e.g., hypokalemia).

PROGNOSIS. PVC frequency and complexity have no prognostic significance for patients without structural heart disease. Among patients with prior myocardial infarction, both frequent (>10 PVCs/hr) and complex ventricular ectopy are associated with an increased risk of death. However, this risk is strongly concentrated in patients with depressed left ventricular function. Likewise, among patients with valvular heart disease, sudden death is rare when ventricular function is normal (e.g., uncomplicated mitral valve prolapse), but risk increases when complex ventricular ectopy is observed in the setting of depressed left ventricular function. R-on-T PVCs may be somewhat more likely to result in ventricular fibrillation (VF) or polymorphic VT than later coupled PVCs. However, this relationship is weak and has limited prognostic utility.

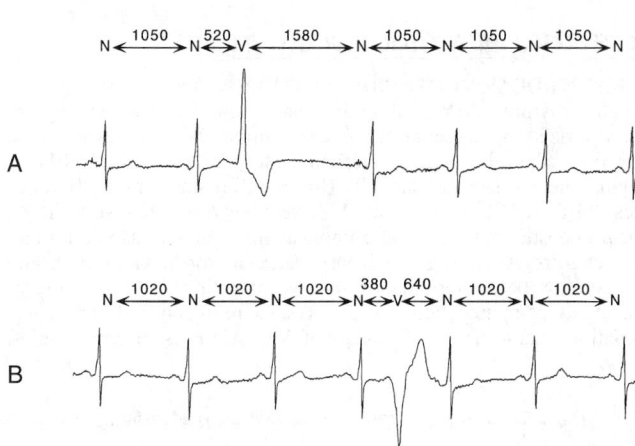

FIGURE 52–1 ■ Multiform premature ventricular contractions (PVCs). *A,* PVC followed by a compensatory pause. *B,* Recording from the same individual demonstrates an interpolated PVC of a different morphology. Tracings are from lead I. N = normal sinus beat; V = ventricular premature beat; intervals given in milliseconds.

Sustained re-entrant ventricular arrhythmias likely result from the interaction of a critically timed triggering event (PVC) with an appropriate substrate (myocardial scarring resulting in mechanical as well as electrical ventricular dysfunction). However, owing to the high prevalence of ventricular ectopy in patients with structural heart disease, the predictive value for future events is low. Even among patients for whom PVCs indicate a poor prognosis, antiarrhythmic drug therapy aimed specifically at suppressing PVCs does not necessarily provide benefit. Suppression of PVCs with encainide, flecainide, or moricizine actually results in a significant increase in mortality in patients with frequent PVCs after myocardial infarction.

TREATMENT. Because there is no evidence that treatment directed at suppressing PVCs improves overall mortality, the primary indication for treatment is to relieve symptoms. Although most PVCs are asymptomatic, in some patients they may result in troubling palpitations. Frequent PVCs may also cause a pounding sensation in the neck due to cannon a waves from atrioventricular dissociation. Because PVCs result in a reduced stroke volume, patients with very frequent PVCs may occasionally have fatigue, exertional intolerance, dyspnea, and lightheadedness.

Most patients with symptomatic PVCs in the absence of structural heart disease can be managed with a β-blocker. Class I or Class III antiarrhythmic drugs may be considered, but the potential for proarrhythmia and organ toxicity must be weighed (see Chapter 54). An alternative to antiarrhythmic drug therapy for highly symptomatic patients, particularly for those without structural heart disease whose PVCs originate from the right ventricular outflow tract, is radiofrequency catheter ablation of the arrhythmogenic focus (see Chapter 53).

PARASYSTOLE

Ventricular parasystole results when an automatic focus arises from the ventricles and fires independently of supraventricular impulses conducted through the AV node. Classically, a surrounding region of depressed conductivity protects the focus by creating complete entrance block that prevents supraventricular beats from resetting the focus. Independence of the parasystolic focus from the underlying rhythm is demonstrated by variable coupling intervals between the ectopic beats and the preceding sinus beats as well as a fixed minimum time interval between PVCs, with any longer interectopic intervals being integer multiples of this minimum interval (reflecting exit block from the parasystolic focus) (Fig. 52–2).

The entrance block surrounding the parasystolic focus can be partial rather than complete, so conducted supraventricular beats may influence depolarization of the parasystolic focus and either delay or accelerate its next discharge. Clinically, parasystole may manifest as sporadic PVCs or as bigeminy or trigeminy. Although generally benign, parasystolic rhythms may result in PVCs at a critical point during repolarization (R on T) and precipitate VF.

ACCELERATED IDIOVENTRICULAR RHYTHM

ELECTROCARDIOGRAPHIC FEATURES. Accelerated idioventricular rhythm (AIVR) describes an ectopic ventricular rhythm characterized by three or more consecutive PVCs occurring at a rate faster than the normal ventricular escape rate of 30 to 40 beats per minute but slower than VT. However, no single rate differentiates "fast" AIVR from "slow" VT. Because AIVR has very different prognostic and therapeutic implications than VT, it is important to recognize AIVR's gradual onset, acceleration ("warm-up"), and deceleration before termination (consistent with an automatic mechanism) as compared with the paroxysmal initiation and abrupt termination characteristic of re-entrant VT. AIVR is generally brief, lasting less than 1 minute, and is suppressed when the sinus rate exceeds its rate.

CLINICAL MANIFESTATIONS. AIVR occurs most often in the setting of acute myocardial infarction (MI), particularly after reperfusion, and usually resolves spontaneously. AIVR is also observed in patients with rheumatic heart disease, dilated cardiomyopathy, acute myocarditis, hypertensive heart disease, digitalis intoxication, and cocaine intoxication, as well as in patients without structural heart disease. It is generally benign and, because most runs of AIVR are brief and asymptomatic, requires no specific treatment. If patients with left ventricular dysfunction do not tolerate AIVR owing to the loss of AV synchrony, increasing the atrial rate with atropine or by pacing suppresses AIVR.

VENTRICULAR TACHYCARDIA (VT)

DEFINITIONS. VT, which originates below the bundle of His at a rate greater than 100 beats per minute, is a wide complex rhythm that may be monomorphic (uniform) or polymorphic with beat to beat changes in the QRS configuration (Fig. 52–3). Sustained VT persists for 30 seconds or more or requires termination because of hemodynamic instability. Sustained polymorphic VT is usually unstable and often degenerates into VF. Sustained monomorphic VT may be stable for long periods of time or, in the setting of faster rates or myocardial ischemia, may degenerate into polymorphic VT or VF. Torsades de pointes (TdP), a particular form of polymorphic VT, has a characteristic morphology ("twisting around a point") and is associated with prolongation of the QT interval on the surface ECG.

ELECTROCARDIOGRAPHIC FEATURES. It is important to distinguish monomorphic VT from supraventricular tachycardia with aberrant conduction, because both present as wide complex tachycardias (Table 52–1). Features on the surface ECG permit differentiation of VT from supraventricular tachycardia with an overall accuracy that approaches 90%. Atrioventricular dissociation, which can be identified on the surface ECG in 25% of VTs, strongly suggests a ventricular origin. However, the presence of a one-to-one atrioventricular relationship does not necessarily imply a supraventricular origin, because a substantial minority of patients with VT have one-to-one retrograde conduction from the ventricles to the atria during tachycardia. Capture and fusion beats are also suggestive of VT but are usually seen only during slow VT. A capture beat represents activation of the ventricles by a supraventricular impulse that conducts via the His-Purkinje system. This beat prematurely "captures" both ventricles during VT and therefore results in a single narrow QRS interposed between wide tachycardia complexes. Other features on the surface ECG that permit differentiation of VT from supraventricular tachycardia include QRS width, axis, and morphology. Although helpful in most situations, these morphologic criteria are not 100% specific. An irregular wide complex rhythm with essentially a single QRS morphology raises the possibility of atrial fibrillation with ventricular pre-excitation (see Chapter 51), particularly in patients without structural heart disease.

Other diagnostic measures include the response of the tachycardia to vagal maneuvers and adenosine. Most VT is insensitive to vagal maneuvers such as carotid sinus massage and Valsalva, as well as to adenosine, whereas most forms of supraventricular tachycardia terminate or persist with transient high-grade atrioventricular block in response to these maneuvers. However, idiopathic right ventricular outflow tract VT in patients with normal hearts may also terminate with vagal maneuvers and adenosine.

CLINICAL MANIFESTATIONS AND ACUTE TREATMENT. Patients with monomorphic VT may present with sudden cardiac death or symptoms of impaired consciousness, such as syncope or near-syncope. Associated symptoms may include chest pain, dyspnea, and palpitations. Occasionally, patients with VT and slow rates

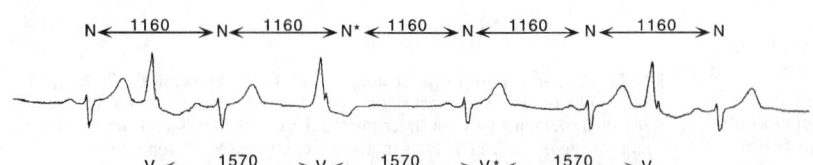

FIGURE 52–2 ■ Parasystole: Sinus rhythm with a competing ventricular parasystolic focus. N = normal sinus beat; V = ventricular parasystolic beat; N* = timing of normal sinus discharge (occurring during the ventricular refractory period); V* = timing of ventricular parasystolic discharge (occurring during the ventricular refractory period); intervals in milliseconds.

Figure 52–3 ■ Ventricular tachyarrhythmias. *A,* Rhythm strip demonstrating monomorphic ventricular tachycardia. *B,* An example of polymorphic ventricular tachycardia. *C,* An example of ventricular fibrillation. All tracings are from lead V1.

may be asymptomatic, and hemodynamic stability is unreliable in distinguishing VT from supraventricular tachycardia.

Physical examination during VT may reveal signs of cardiogenic shock, including pulselessness, apnea, cool extremities, and cyanosis. Physical examination may reveal hypotension or signs of heart failure, such as pulmonary rales or jugular venous distention. Characteristic features during VT include cannon a waves and variable intensity of the first heart sound, both of which result from atrioventricular dissociation.

Acute therapy for VT depends on the degree of hemodynamic instability that accompanies the arrhythmia. For minimally symptomatic patients without hypotension (systolic blood pressure > 90 mm Hg), pharmacologic therapy should be initiated. Intravenous lidocaine is often chosen as a first-line agent because it can be administered rapidly (bolus dose of 1–1.5 mg/kg, followed by additional boluses of 0.5–0.75 mg/kg at 5–10 minute intervals, up to a maximal dose of 3 mg/kg) and maintained with an infusion (1–4 mg/min). If lidocaine is ineffective, alternatives include intravenous procainamide (maximal dose 17 mg/kg), at an infusion rate up to 20–30 mg/min, or intravenous amiodarone (15 mg/min over 10 min, followed by 1 mg/min over the next 6 hours and then 0.5 mg/min over 18 hours) (see Chapter 54). If pharmacologic therapy is unsuccessful for hemodynamically stable VT, synchronized cardioversion with a direct-current shock may be required, beginning with 50–100 J and increasing to 360 J if necessary.

For patients with severe signs or symptoms during VT, such as

Table 52–1 ■ ELECTROCARDIOGRAPHIC CHARACTERISTICS OF VENTRICULAR TACHYCARDIA

Atrioventricular Relationship
Atrioventricular dissociation
Sinus capture beats
Fusion beats
QRS Width
Left bundle branch block: >160 msec
Right bundle branch block: >140 msec
QRS Axis
Extreme left axis (−90 to −180°)
Right-axis deviation in the presence of left bundle branch block (+90 to +180°)
QRS Morphology
Right bundle branch block
  Morphology in V1
    Monophasic R wave
    Biphasic (qR or RS)
    Triphasic with R > R′
  Morphology in V6
    R/S ratio < 1
Left bundle branch block
  Morphology in V1
    Broad R wave (>30 msec)
    Onset of R wave to nadir of S wave > 60 msec
    Notched downstroke in lead V1
  Morphology in V6
    QR or QS complex
Onset of R wave to nadir of S wave > 100 msec in any precordial lead
Absence of RS wave in any precordial lead
Positive or negative precordial concordance

chest pain or myocardial ischemia, heart failure or shortness of breath, decreased level of consciousness, or hypotension (systolic blood pressure <90 mm Hg), immediate synchronous cardioversion is indicated, with subsequent intravenous antiarrhythmic therapy to maintain sinus rhythm. After resuscitation from VT, the patient must be evaluated for a possible primary cause, such as electrolyte imbalance, acid-base disturbance, hypoxemia, drug toxicity, and myocardial ischemia.

DIAGNOSIS AND TREATMENT. Invasive electrophysiologic testing (see Chapter 50) can guide pharmacologic (see Chapter 54) or device-based therapy (see Chapter 53) in patients with sustained monomorphic VT and previous MI. In these patients, a sustained ventricular tachyarrhythmia can be induced with programmed stimulation in approximately 90%.

ISCHEMIC HEART DISEASE. VT during acute MI may be monomorphic or polymorphic. Sustained ventricular arrhythmias within the first 48 hours of an acute MI do not convey an increased risk of future spontaneous arrhythmias. Coronary revascularization or antianginal medical therapy may be sufficient to control arrhythmias due to acute ischemia. Antiarrhythmic medications, such as lidocaine, are also useful to control recurrent arrhythmias in this setting. Polymorphic VT and VF can also result from coronary vasospasm, which may occur in diseased or normal coronary arteries.

Sustained monomorphic VT occurs most frequently in patients with prior MI and depressed left ventricular function. VT arises from the border zone of the myocardial infarction, where viable myocytes scattered within areas of fibrosis form a chronic substrate for re-entry. VT may occur days to decades after the myocardial infarction, with an incidence that declines with time. The strongest risk factors for sustained ventricular arrhythmias late after myocardial infarction are depressed left ventricular function and increased frequency and complexity of ventricular ectopy. Patients with a left ventricular ejection fraction less than 30% after MI have a nearly threefold increased risk of mortality or arrhythmic events.

Patients with VT beyond the first 48 hours after MI have a high recurrence rate, with an annual risk that approaches 30% in the absence of treatment. In general, coronary revascularization does not reduce the risk of recurrent VT arising from a chronic substrate after a remote MI, and definitive antiarrhythmic therapy is required. Randomized trials have demonstrated the superiority of automatic cardioverter-defibrillators over antiarrhythmic medications in patients with sustained monomorphic VT. Catheter ablation may have an adjunctive role for controlling frequent ventricular arrhythmias.

CARDIOMYOPATHY (see Chapter 64). Both monomorphic and polymorphic VT occur in patients with non-ischemic dilated cardiomyopathy, likely because of re-entry in regions of fibrosis. The signal-averaged electrocardiogram and invasive programmed stimulation (see Chapter 50) have limited sensitivity and specificity for predicting future risk. Polymorphic VT, and to a lesser extent monomorphic VT, occur in hypertrophic cardiomyopathy owing to myocyte disarray, fibrosis, and/or ischemia, which provide a substrate for re-entry.

ARRHYTHMOGENIC RIGHT VENTRICULAR DYSPLASIA. Arrhythmogenic right ventricular dysplasia is a cardiomyopathy characterized by myocyte loss with fibroadipose replacement of the right ventricle. The condition is usually sporadic, but familial forms have been identified. Arrhythmogenic right ventricular dysplasia causes sudden cardiac death in adolescents and young adults. Patients develop re-entry involving diseased portions of the right ventricle but rarely develop right ventricular failure.

The surface ECG during sinus rhythm characteristically demonstrates an R′ (epsilon wave) in lead V_1 and T-wave inversions in the anterior precordial leads. Echocardiography (see Chapter 43) and right ventriculography demonstrate abnormalities of the right ventricle, including wall motion abnormalities and aneurysmal dilatation. Magnetic resonance imaging and electron-beam computed tomography (see Chapters 44 and 45) can demonstrate fatty replacement of the right ventricle, thinning of the right ventricular wall, and wall motion abnormalities. Endomyocardial biopsy may demonstrate characteristic fatty replacement and fibrosis but has limited sensitivity owing to the patchy nature of the cardiomyopathy. During invasive electrophysiologic testing, multiple morphologies of monomorphic VT may be inducible, usually with a left bundle branch block configuration.

Therapeutic modalities for treating arrhythmogenic right ventricular dysplasia include antiarrhythmic medication and implantation of a cardioverter-defibrillator. Catheter ablation, while rarely curative, may ameliorate frequent ventricular arrhythmias.

POSTOPERATIVE TETRALOGY OF FALLOT. Patients who have undergone surgical repair of tetralogy of Fallot via right ventriculotomy are at an increased risk of sudden death and VT. Tachycardia is due to re-entry around the right ventriculotomy scar in the infundibulum. Catheter or surgical ablation or resection is effective in preventing recurrent VT.

BUNDLE BRANCH REENTRY. Patients with dilated cardiomyopathy and disease in the His-Purkinje system are prone to develop a specific form of VT known as bundle branch re-entry, in which the right and left bundle branches participate in a macro re-entrant tachycardia circuit. The tachycardia typically demonstrates a left bundle branch block morphology and is often associated with presyncope or syncope. The diagnosis is made with invasive electrophysiologic testing, and the tachycardia may be cured by catheter ablation of one of the bundle branches.

IDIOPATHIC VENTRICULAR TACHYCARDIA. Idiopathic VT in patients without structural heart disease commonly arises from the right ventricular outflow tract and has a left bundle branch block morphology and inferior axis. It may present as a sustained arrhythmia facilitated by exercise or as repetitive non-sustained VT and, unlike other forms of VT, terminates in response to vagal maneuvers, adenosine, β-blockers, and verapamil. Like more common forms of VT, it also responds to Class I antiarrhythmic medication (see Chapter 54). Arrhythmogenesis is triggered by increased levels of cyclic adenosine monophosphate and intracellular calcium overload. Right ventricular outflow tract tachycardia can be cured by catheter ablation (see Chapter 53).

A less common form of idiopathic VT, known as fascicular tachycardia, arises from re-entry in the region of the left posterior fascicle, is characterized by a right bundle branch block morphology and superior axis, and characteristically terminates in response to verapamil. As with right ventricular outflow tract VT, fascicular VT can be cured by catheter ablation.

LONG QT SYNDROME. The *congenital* long QT syndromes include the Jervell and Lange-Nielsen syndromes (autosomal recessive and associated with congenital sensorineural deafness), the Romano-Ward syndrome (autosomal dominant and associated with normal hearing), and other congenital long QT syndromes. Genetic abnormalities responsible for the Romano-Ward syndrome include heterozygous mutations of the *KVLQT1, HERG,* and *SCN5A* genes on chromosomes 11, 7, and 3, respectively; a locus on chromosome 4 has also been identified. Both the *KVLQT1* and *HERG* genes code for potassium channels. Failure of these channels to activate normally prolongs the action potential duration and provokes early afterdepolarizations. The *SCN5A* gene codes for sodium channel subunits; failure of this channel to inactivate also prolongs the action potential duration. Heterozygous mutations in the *KVLQT1* gene result in the Romano-Ward syndrome, whereas homozygous mutations result in the Jervell and Lange-Nielsen syndrome. This suggests that QT prolongation is a dominantly inherited phenotype whereas congenital deafness is recessively inherited.

The corrected QT interval (QT_c) is usually greater than 0.46 in

men and 0.47 in women, although affected individuals may have QT intervals that fall within the normal range. The QT interval fails to shorten normally or may prolong with exercise. Other features on the surface ECG include bifid or notched T waves, T-wave alternans, and sinus bradycardia.

Patients with the long QT syndrome are at risk for TdP, which may result in syncope or sudden cardiac death. Slow ventricular rates or ventricular pauses can precipitate TdP due to bradycardia-dependent prolongation of the QT interval; alternatively, in some forms of the long QT syndrome, catecholamine stimulation, such as fright or exertion, may facilitate TdP.

Long-term therapies for patients with the congenital long QT syndrome include β-blockade, permanent pacing, left-sided cervicothoracic sympathetic ganglionectomy, and implantation of a cardioverter-defibrillator. Patients with the *SCN5A* mutation may potentially respond to the sodium channel blocker mexiletine.

The *acquired* long QT syndrome predisposes to TdP and is usually related to electrolyte abnormalities such as hypokalemia and hypomagnesemia, tricyclic antidepressants, phenothiazines, non-sedating antihistamines such as terfenadine and astemizole (whose levels may be elevated by drugs that inhibit hepatic metabolism such as ketoconazole), macrolide antibiotics such as erythromycin, pentamidine, probucol, cisapride, and Class IA and Class III antiarrhythmic medications. A liquid protein diet, starvation, central nervous system disease, and bradyarrhythmias may also predispose to TdP. Therapy for the acquired long QT syndrome is directed at reversing the metabolic abnormalities or withholding the offending medication. Infusion of magnesium and temporary pacing decrease the QT interval and prevent pause-dependent arrhythmias, whereas isoproterenol is a temporizing measure to increase the sinus rate. Class IB antiarrhythmic medications (see Chapter 54), which tend to shorten the action potential duration and decrease the QT interval, may also be used.

DIGITALIS TOXICITY. Ventricular arrhythmias seen in digitalis toxicity include single PVCs, non-sustained VT, and sustained polymorphic or monomorphic VT. Some digitalis-toxic rhythms are due to triggered activity from intracellular calcium overload that results from inhibition of the Na^+/K^+ ATPase. A characteristic digitalis-toxic rhythm is bidirectional tachycardia, characterized by a right bundle branch block configuration and alternating right- and left-axis deviations. Therapy for severe digitalis-toxic arrhythmias includes infusion of digoxin immune Fab fragments, which may be life saving. Alternatives are Class IB antiarrhythmic medications such as lidocaine and phenytoin (see Chapter 54).

VENTRICULAR FLUTTER AND FIBRILLATION

DEFINITIONS. Ventricular fibrillation (VF) is a malignant arrhythmia characterized by disorganized electrical activity resulting in a failure of sequential cardiac contraction and the inability to maintain cardiac output (see Fig. 52–3). If not promptly terminated, VF results in hypoxemia and eventually sudden cardiac death. Ventricular flutter is an extremely rapid, hemodynamically unstable VT that typically progresses to VF. The evaluation and management of ventricular flutter should parallel that for VF.

ETIOLOGY. With rare exceptions, VF occurs in patients with underlying structural heart disease, especially ischemic heart disease with left ventricular systolic dysfunction. In patients resuscitated from an episode of VF, it is imperative to identify the cause of the arrhythmia (see Sudden Cardiac Death) and to search for evidence of an acute ischemic event. Patients who survive an episode of VF within 48 hours of an acute MI generally have a good prognosis, with a 2% recurrence rate at 1 year.

De novo VF can be caused by myocardial ischemia, which results in complex changes in the electrophysiologic properties of the ventricle, including delays in conduction and changes in refractoriness, that potentiate the multiple re-entrant wavefronts that characterize VF. Alternatively, PVCs during the vulnerable period of ventricular repolarization (R-on-T phenomenon) may initiate VF. Prolonged VT may result in hypotension and myocardial ischemia, causing degeneration of VT to VF.

ELECTROCARDIOGRAPHIC FEATURES. The ECG during ventricular flutter is characterized by a sinusoidal QRS complex, without a distinct ST segment or T wave, at a rate of 240 to 280 beats per minute. In contrast, VF is an irregular rhythm with an undulating low-amplitude baseline without organized QRS complexes or T waves.

SUDDEN CARDIAC DEATH

DEFINITIONS AND INCIDENCE AND PREVALENCE. Half of all cardiac deaths are sudden, accounting for approximately 300,000 deaths per year in the United States. Sudden cardiac death (SCD) is death due to instantaneous, unanticipated circulatory collapse within 1 hour of initial symptoms and is often, but not always, due to a cardiac arrhythmia. Nearly 90% of all sudden natural deaths have a cardiac etiology, and 80% of these are attributable to coronary artery disease (Table 52–2). In recent years, the incidence of SCD has declined in parallel with the decrease in coronary artery disease, likely due to a reduction in cardiac risk factors, more effective secondary preventive measures, improved resuscitative efforts, and expansion of emergency medical services. Similar to acute MI, SCD has a circadian pattern with a primary peak in the morning hours after awakening. Prodromal symptoms in the 2 weeks preceding collapse may include fatigue, dyspnea, and chest pain. Risk factors for SCD are identical to those for coronary artery disease and include age, male gender, hypertension, tobacco use, hypercholesterolemia, and left ventricular hypertrophy.

Holter monitor data indicate that approximately 85% of the rhythms leading to SCD are ventricular tachyarrhythmias, with the remaining 15% due to bradyarrhythmias. Among tachyarrhythmias, 75% are due to VT, either monomorphic (two thirds) or polymorphic (one third), and 25% are due to TdP and primary VF. When VT precedes VF, it usually persists for 30 seconds to 3 minutes before degenerating into VF. Therefore, by 4 minutes after collapse, VF is identified in nearly 90% of SCD cases, whereas asystole is identified in 10%. As more time elapses, asystole and electromechanical dissociation are identified in approximately 60% of victims, suggesting that these rhythms reflect prolonged hypoxemia and likely explain the lower long-term survival in SCD patients presenting with asystole.

ETIOLOGY. Most survivors of cardiac arrest have structural heart disease, especially coronary artery disease. VF may be the first manifestation of coronary artery disease in as many as 25% of patients with ischemic heart disease. Only 20% of patients have evidence for a new Q wave MI at the time of cardiac arrest, whereas a remote MI is present in 40 to 80% of victims.

Dilated cardiomyopathy, which may be idiopathic or due to viral myocarditis, sarcoidosis, hemachromatosis, or amyloidosis (see Chapter 64), accounts for 10 to 15% of survivors of SCD. In patients with dilated cardiomyopathy, the risk of SCD is related to symptomatic status. For example, the annual mortality in patients who are NYHA functional Class II is estimated to be 5 to 15%, of which 50 to 80% is due to SCD. In patients who are functional Class IV, the annual mortality is 30 to 70%, of which 5 to 30% are arrhythmogenic. Another cause of SCD is valvular heart disease, which is frequently associated with ventricular hypertrophy and/or dilated atria. In younger patients, particularly those who arrest during physical activity, causes such as hypertrophic cardiomyopathy (with or without outflow obstruction), arrhythmogenic right ventricular dysplasia, the long QT syndrome, anomalous origin of the coronary arteries, and the Wolff-Parkinson-White syndrome (for those patients who can conduct rapidly over the accessory pathway during atrial fibrillation) should be considered. Other causes include repair of congenital anomalies such as transposition of the great arteries and tetralogy of Fallot (see Chapter 57). In a small subset of patients, no structural heart disease is detected.

PATHOGENESIS. Although SCD is not usually associated with an acute Q-wave MI, transient ischemia often precedes SCD. In patients with stable high-grade atherosclerotic plaques (> 75% occlusion) but no previous MI or unstable ischemia, VF may be due to coronary vasospasm. The true prevalence and significance of ischemia in precipitating VF is unknown, especially because ischemic ST segments changes are rarely present at the time of SCD. The electrophysiologic consequences of acute ischemia that ultimately result in VF are mediated through acidosis, potassium efflux from the cell with membrane depolarization, increased intracellular calcium, and an increase in adrenergic tone.

RISK STRATIFICATION. Because the incidence of SCD is 0.1 to 0.2% in the general population, preventive measures will only be

meaningful and cost-effective for those patients who are identified as high risk. However, the relatively poor sensitivity, specificity, and predictive value of risk factors often diminish the utility of specific recommendations. Most data regarding risk stratification have been derived from post-MI patients, in whom the left ventricular dysfunction, particularly an ejection fraction less than 30%, is the strongest independent predictor of SCD. Frequent or complex ventricular ectopy, commonly defined as 10 or more PVCs per hour, is a usual co-morbidity of myocardial dysfunction and also an independent predictor of SCD. The risks of left ventricular dysfunction and ventricular ectopy are additive. For example, the combination of an ejection fraction less than 30% and 10 or more PVCs per hour carries a far greater risk of SCD than either risk factor alone. However, as the Cardiac Arrhythmia Suppression Trial showed (Table 52–3), suppression of a ventricular ectopy does not necessarily improve prognosis. Late potentials on the signal-averaged ECG (see Chapter 50) also identify post-MI patients at risk of VT/VF, particularly in patients with an ejection fraction less than 40%.

In general, reduced baroreceptor sensitivity and decreased heart rate variability, both reflections of diminished parasympathetic tone, are associated with increased arrhythmic events after MI. The predictive role of electrophysiologic testing in post-MI patients without sustained ventricular arrhythmias is unclear. Some data have shown no prognostic value, whereas other data show an association between inducible sustained VT and future arrhythmic events (see Table 52–3).

DIAGNOSIS. In assessing prognosis and planning a treatment strategy, it is useful to classify SCD as either primary (without a clear trigger) or secondary. A primary episode has a 10 to 30% one-year recurrence rate, whereas most secondary episodes are associated with recurrence rates less than 2%. Identifiable reversible precipitants of secondary VF include transient ischemia possibly related to vasospasm; hypokalemia due to diuretics; hyperkalemia secondary to renal failure, angiotensin-converting enzyme inhibitors, prostaglandin inhibitors, or potassium-sparing diuretics; proarrhythmia secondary to antiarrhythmics, tricyclics, and antihistamines; or substance abuse with drugs such as cocaine and amphetamines. Therapy is directed toward removing or treating the acute precipitant. SCD related to acute ischemia in the absence of prior MI is often associated with severe proximal occlusive disease, normal left ventricular function, normal signal-averaged ECG, and non-inducibility (absence of VT) during electrophysiological study.

Most patients should undergo comprehensive evaluation of myocardial function and coronary anatomy. Echocardiography is useful for excluding hypertrophic cardiomyopathy and valvular heart disease (see Chapter 43), magnetic resonance imaging for diagnosing arrhythmogenic right ventricular dysplasia (see Chapter 45), and myocardial biopsy for identifying infiltrative diseases such as myocarditis, amyloidosis, hemochromatosis, and sarcoidosis (see Chapter 64). Coronary angiography should be performed to assess coronary occlusive disease and to exclude coronary artery anomalies (see Chapters 46 and 59). Myocardial perfusion scintigraphy provides complementary data for assessing ischemic burden (see Chapter 44). Left ventricular function can be assessed by contrast ventriculography, radionuclide ventriculography, or echocardiography.

Evaluation of SCD survivors also includes Holter monitoring and/or electrophysiologic testing (see Chapter 50). However, the Electrophysiological Study Versus Electrocardiographic Monitoring (ESVEM) trial showed a 50% two-year recurrence of ventricular tachyarrhythmias in patients in whom antiarrhythmic drugs successfully suppressed PVCs. These data suggest a dissociation between PVC suppression and recurrence of VT; PVCs may represent a marker of left ventricular dysfunction rather than a trigger of SCD, or the arrhythmogenic substrate may change over time.

In SCD survivors, sustained monomorphic VT is inducible by electrophysiologic testing (see Chapter 50) in 40 to 50% and polymorphic VT in 10 to 20%; in 30 to 50%, no sustained arrhythmia is induced. In patients with ischemic heart disease and left ventricular dysfunction, inducibility of sustained VT carries a poor prognosis. However, a low ejection fraction is associated with a poor prognosis, regardless of whether sustained VT is inducible; for example, patients with an ejection fraction of 30% or less and who are non-inducible have a 25% arrhythmia recurrence rate at 1 year,

Table 52–2 ▪ CAUSES AND CONTRIBUTING FACTORS IN SUDDEN CARDIAC DEATH

I. Coronary Artery Abnormalities
 A. Coronary atherosclerosis
  1. Chronic ischemic heart disease with transient supply/demand imbalance—thrombosis, spasm, physical stress
  2. Acute myocardial infarction
  3. Chronic atherosclerosis with change in myocardial substrate
 B. Congenital abnormalities of coronary arteries
  1. Anomalous origin from pulmonary artery
  2. Other coronary atrioventricular fistula
  3. Origin of left coronary artery from right sinus of Valsalva
  4. Origin of right coronary artery from left sinus of Valsalva
  5. Hypoplastic or aplastic coronary arteries
  6. Coronary-intracardiac shunt
 C. Coronary artery embolism
  1. Aortic or mitral endocarditis
  2. Prosthetic aortic or mitral valves
  3. Abnormal native valves or left ventricular mural thrombus
  4. Platelet embolism
 D. Coronary arteritis
  1. Polyarteritis nodosa, progressive systemic sclerosis, giant cell arteritis
  2. Mucocutaneous lymph node syndrome (Kawasaki's disease)
  3. Syphilitic coronary ostial stenosis
 E. Miscellaneous mechanical obstruction of coronary arteries
  1. Coronary artery dissection in Marfan's syndrome
  2. Coronary artery dissection in pregnancy
  3. Prolapse of aortic valve myxomatous polyps into coronary ostia
  4. Dissection or rupture of sinus of Valsalva
 F. Functional obstruction of coronary arteries
  1. Coronary artery spasm with or without atherosclerosis
  2. Myocardial bridges
II. Hypertrophy of Ventricular Myocardium
 A. Left ventricular hypertrophy associated with coronary atherosclerosis
 B. Hypertensive heart disease without significant coronary atherosclerosis
 C. Hypertrophic myocardium secondary to valvular heart disease
 D. Hypertrophic cardiomyopathy
  1. Obstructive
  2. Non-obstructive
 E. Primary or secondary pulmonary hypertension
  1. Advanced chronic right ventricular overload
  2. Pulmonary hypertension in pregnancy
III. Myocardial Diseases and Heart Failure
 A. Chronic congestive heart failure
  1. Ischemic cardiomyopathy
  2. Idiopathic congestive cardiomyopathy
  3. Alcoholic cardiomyopathy
  4. Hypertensive cardiomyopathy
  5. Post-myocarditis cardiomyopathy
  6. Postpartum cardiomyopathy
 B. Acute cardiac failure
  1. Massive acute myocardial infarction
  2. Acute myocarditis
  3. Acute alcoholic cardiac dysfunction
  4. Ball-valve embolism in aortic stenosis or prosthesis
  5. Mechanical disruptions of cardiac structures
   a. Rupture of ventricular free wall
   b. Disruption of mitral apparatus
    (1) Papillary muscle
    (2) Chordae tendineae
    (3) Leaflet
   c. Rupture of interventricular septum
  6. Acute pulmonary edema in noncompliant ventricles
IV. Inflammatory, Infiltrative, Neoplastic, and Degenerative Processes
 A. Acute viral myocarditis with or without ventricular dysfunction
 B. Myocarditis associated with the vasculitides
 C. Sarcoidosis
 D. Progressive systemic sclerosis
 E. Amyloidosis
 F. Hemochromatosis
 G. Idiopathic giant cell myocarditis
 H. Chagas' disease
 I. Cardiac ganglionitis
 J. Arrhythmogenic right ventricular dysplasia
 K. Neuromuscular diseases (e.g., muscular dystrophy, Friedreich's ataxia, myotonic dystrophy)
 L. Intramural tumors
  1. Primary
  2. Metastatic

 M. Obstructive intracavitary tumors
  1. Neoplastic
  2. Thrombotic
V. Diseases of the Cardiac Valves
 A. Valvular aortic stenosis/insufficiency
 B. Mitral valve disruption
 C. Mitral valve prolapse
 D. Endocarditis
 E. Prosthetic valve dysfunction
VI. Congenital Heart Disease
 A. Congenital aortic or pulmonic valve stenosis
 B. Right-to-left shunts with Eisenmenger's physiology
  1. Advanced disease
  2. During labor and delivery
 C. After surgical repair of congenital lesions (e.g., tetralogy of Fallot)
VII. Electrophysiologic Abnormalities
 A. Abnormalities of the conducting system
  1. Fibrosis of the His-Purkinje system
   a. Primary degeneration (Lenègre's disease)
   b. Secondary to fibrosis and calcification of the "cardiac skeleton" (Lev's disease)
   c. Postviral conducting system fibrosis
   d. Hereditary conducting system disease
  2. Anomalous pathways of conduction
 B. Prolonged QT interval syndrome
  1. Congenital
   a. With deafness
   b. Without deafness
  2. Acquired
   a. Drug effect
   b. Electrolyte abnormality
   c. Toxic substances
   d. Hypothermia
   e. Central nervous system injury
 C. Idiopathic ventricular fibrillation
  1. Absence of identifiable structural or functional causes
  2. Sleep-death in Southeast Asians
   a. Bangungut
   b. Pokkuri
   c. Nonlaitai
VIII. Electrical Instability Related to Neurohumoral and Central Nervous System Influences
 A. Catecholamine-dependent lethal arrhythmias
 B. Central nervous system related
  1. Psychic stress, emotional extremes
  2. Auditory-related
  3. "Voodoo" death in primitive cultures
  4. Diseases of the cardiac nerves
  5. Congenital QT interval prolongation
IX. Sudden Infant Death Syndrome and Sudden Death in Children
 A. Sudden infant death syndrome
  1. Immature respiratory control functions
  2. Susceptibility to lethal arrhythmias
  3. Congenital heart disease
  4. Myocarditis
 B. Sudden death in children
  1. Eisenmenger's syndrome, aortic stenosis, hypertrophic cardiomyopathy, pulmonary atresia
  2. After corrective surgery for congenital heart disease
  3. Myocarditis
  4. Unexplained
X. Miscellaneous
 A. Sudden death during extreme physical activity
 B. Mechanical interference with venous return
  1. Acute cardiac tamponade
  2. Massive pulmonary embolism
  3. Acute intracardiac thrombosis
 C. Dissecting aneurysm of the aorta
 D. Toxic/metabolic disturbances
  1. Electrolyte disturbances
  2. Metabolic disturbances
  3. Proarrhythmic effects of antiarrhythmic drugs
  4. Proarrhythmic effects of noncardiac drugs
 E. Mimics of sudden cardiac death
  1. "Cafe coronary"
  2. Acute alcoholic states ("holiday heart")
  3. Acute asthmatic attacks
  4. Air or amniotic fluid embolism

From Meyerburg RJ, Castellanos A: Cardiac arrest and sudden cardiac death. In Braunwald E (ed): Heart Disease: A Textbook of Cardiovascular Medicine, 5th ed. Philadelphia. WB Saunders, 1997, pp 748–749.

Table 52–3 ■ CLINICAL TRIALS FOR PREVENTION OF SUDDEN CARDIAC DEATH

STUDY	BACKGROUND/ PREMISE	PURPOSE	ENTRY CRITERIA	DESIGN	OUTCOME
CAST	PVCs in survivors of MI are a risk factor for SCD	Assess whether suppression of PVCs with antiarrhythmic drugs reduces risk of SCD	Asymptomatic/mildly symptomatic PVCs (≥6/hr) post MI	1. Primary prevention 2. Drug titration with encainide, flecainide, or morizicine to assess PVC suppression 3. Randomized: suppressive drug vs. placebo 4. Endpoint: arrhythmic death	Antiarrhythmic drugs; 1. Increase overall mortality 2. Increase risk of SCD
CAMIAT	Frequent or repetitive PVCs post MI increase mortality 1–2 years after event	Assess effect of amiodarone on risk of VF	1. Post MI 2. ≥10 PVCs/hr or ≥(1) 3 beat run	1. Primary prevention 2. Randomized: amiodarone vs. placebo 3. Endpoint: resuscitated VF or arrhythmic death	1. Amiodarone reduces VF and arrhythmic death (relative risk reduction: 38%) 2. No difference between groups in overall mortality
EMIAT	Patients post MI with ↓ EF are at increased risk for SCD	Assess whether amiodarone reduces mortality in patients post MI with ↓ EF	1. Post MI 2. EF ≤ 40%	1. Primary prevention 2. Randomized: amiodarone vs. placebo 3. Primary endpoint: mortality	1. No difference in mortality between amiodarone and placebo 2. 35% risk reduction in arrhythmic deaths with amiodarone
SWORD	Patients post MI and ↓ EF have increased mortality	Assess whether d-sotalol compared with placebo reduces mortality	1. Recent MI 2. EF ≤ 40%	1. Primary prevention 2. Randomized: d-sotalol vs. placebo 3. Endpoint: mortality	1. d-sotalol associated with increased mortality 2. Increased mortality presumed secondary to proarrhythmia
GESICA	Patients with severe CHF are at increased risk for SCD	Assess effect of amiodarone on mortality in patients with CHF	1. CHF 2. EF ≤ 35%	1. Primary prevention 2. Randomized: amiodarone vs. standard treatment 3. Primary endpoint: mortality	1. 28% risk reduction in mortality with amiodarone 2. 27% risk reduction in SCD
CHF-STAT	Patients with CHF and asymptomatic PVCs are at increased risk of SCD	Assess effect of amiodarone vs. placebo on mortality in patients with CHF	1. CHF 2. EF ≤ 40% 3. ≥10 PVCs hr	1. Primary prevention 2. Randomized: amiodarone vs. placebo 3. Primary endpoint: mortality	1. No difference in mortality between amiodarone and placebo 2. Amiodarone more effective in suppressing PVCs and improving EF
CASH	Survivors of SCD are at high risk for recurrent event	Assess relative efficacy of class I, II, and III drugs and ICD	1. Survivor of SCD due to VF/VT	1. Secondary prevention 2. Randomized: propafenone vs. metoprolol vs. amiodarone vs. ICD 3. Endpoint: mortality	1. Propafenone arm aborted because of increased mortality vs. ICD
CASCADE	Survivors of SCD are at high risk for recurrent event	Assess efficacy of amiodarone vs. other antiarrhythmic drugs	1. Out-of-hospital VF 2. VF not associated with Q wave MI	1. Secondary prevention 2. Randomized: amiodarone vs. other antiarrhythmics; antiarrhythmics guided by EPS and/or Holter 3. Endpoints: cardiac mortality, SCD	1. Amiodarone more effective than conventional Rx in preventing SCD recurrence 2. Absence of recurrence at 2 years: amiodarone 82% vs. conventional Rx 69%
MADIT	Patients with NSVT, post MI, and ↓ EF have 30% 2-year mortality	Assess whether prophylactic ICD vs. conventional medical therapy improves survival	1. Prior MI 2. EF ≤ 35% 3. NSVT (≥3–30 beats; 120/min) 4. Inducible but non-suppressible VT with antiarrhythmic drug during EPS	1. Primary prevention 2. Randomized: ICD vs. conventional medical therapy 3. Endpoint: mortality	1. Prophylactic ICD improves survival (Hazard ratio: 0.46)
AVID	Patients who survive VF or hypotensive VT are at increased risk for recurrence	Assess relative efficacy of ICD vs. antiarrhythmic drugs on mortality	1. VF (or) 2. Sustained VT + EF ≤ 40%	1. Secondary prevention 2. Randomized: ICD vs. antiarrhythmic drugs 3. Endpoint: mortality	1. ICD reduces mortality compared with antiarrhythmic drugs 2. Relative risk reduction (1 & 3 yrs): 39% & 31%
CABG Patch	Patients with CAD, ↓ EF, and (+) SAECG are at increased risk of SCD	Assess effect of prophylactic ICD at time of elective CABG surgery on survival	1. CAD 2. EF ≤ 35% 3. (+) SAECG	1. Primary prevention 2. Randomized: ICD vs. control 3. Endpoint: mortality	1. No difference in mortality between ICD and control patients

AVID = Antiarrhythmics versus implantable defibrillators; CAD = coronary artery disease; CAMIAT = Canadian Amiodarone Myocardial Infarction Arrhythmia Trial; CASCADE = Cardiac Arrest in Seattle: Conventional Versus Amiodarone Drug Evaluation; CASH = Cardiac Arrest Study Hamburg; CAST = Cardiac Arrhythmia Suppression Trial; CHF = congestive heart failure; EF = ejection fraction; EMIAT = European Myocardial Infarct Amiodarone Trial; EPS = electrophysiologic study; GESICA = Grupo de Estudio de la Sobrevida en la Insuficiencia Cardiaca en Argentina; ICD = implantable cardioverter defibrillator; MADIT = Multicenter Automatic Defibrillator Implantation Trial; MI = myocardial infarction; NSVT = nonsustained ventricular tachycardia; PVCs = premature ventricular contractions; SCD = sudden cardiac death; SAECG = signal averaged electrocardiogram; SWORD = Survival With Oral d-Sotalol; VF = ventricular fibrillation; VT = ventricular tachycardia; CABG = coronary artery bypass grafting.

whereas non-inducible patients with an ejection fraction greater than 30% have a 10 to 15% recurrence rate. In patients with SCD and idiopathic dilated cardiomyopathy, sustained monomorphic VT is rarely induced. Furthermore, neither the inability to induce VT nor the ability of drugs to suppress inducible polymorphic VT or VF is a predictor of a favorable outcome.

THERAPY. ACUTE MANAGEMENT. The most important factor that determines the outcome of cardiac arrest is the time to defibrillation. Another significant factor is the initial rhythm identified. VT is associated with the best prognosis, followed by VF; patients with asystole or electromechanical dissociation rarely survive. Optimal chances for survival occur when cardiopulmonary resuscitation (CPR) is initiated within 4 minutes of the arrest and advanced cardiac life support, including intubation, intravenous medications, and defibrillation, is implemented within 8 minutes. A key element for success is bystander initiation of CPR. The automatic external defibrillator, which recognizes VF and delivers high-energy shocks, allows lay persons and non-medical personnel to function as first responders.

Despite public education in bystander CPR and efforts to train emergency medical technicians, early in-hospital mortality is 50 to 60%, and less than 25% of patients with out-of-hospital SCD survive to discharge from the hospital, underscoring the importance of primary and secondary prevention. As many as one third of deaths are attributable to heart failure or cardiogenic shock; 90% who will recover from coma with meaningful function do so by the third hospital day.

PRIMARY AND SECONDARY INTERVENTION. Primary preventive approaches to SCD prophylactically treat patients identified as being at high risk and generally include reduction or elimination of myocardial ischemia with antianginal agents and/or coronary revascularization. Regardless of whether or not residual ischemia is present, initial therapy in all patients without contraindications should include a β-blocker, which consistently reduces SCD (30–45%) as well as total mortality (25–60%) in survivors of MI. Results are similarly persuasive in patients with heart failure who can tolerate β-blockers. The beneficial effects of β-blockers in prevention of SCD occur independently of their limited effect on PVC suppression. Angiotensin-converting enzyme inhibitors also reduce SCD and overall mortality in survivors of MI with left ventricular ejection fraction less than or equal to 35% (see Chapter 60).

In general, with the exception of amiodarone, antiarrhythmic drugs have proven proarrhythmic and have not improved survival (see Table 52–3), demonstrating that suppression of PVCs is not an appropriate surrogate for prevention of SCD. In contrast, amiodarone reduces arrhythmic deaths in MI survivors who have an ejection fraction of 40% or less with either frequent PVCs or nonsustained VT, and amiodarone and β-blockers may be synergistic in their benefits. However, amiodarone does not appear to improve overall mortality, and approximately 5% of patients discontinue the drug because of pulmonary toxicity.

Implantable cardioverter-defibrillators (ICDs) have reduced mortality in MI survivors who have a low ejection fraction, with either non-sustained VT or inducible sustained VT that is not suppressed with procainamide. ICDs have not, however, been shown to decrease mortality in patients undergoing elective coronary revascularization who have reduced left ventricular function and a positive signal-averaged ECG.

In patients with heart failure due to non-ischemic cardiomyopathy, amiodarone appears to reduce total mortality, SCD, and deaths due to heart failure. It does not, however, confer benefit in patients with congestive heart failure due to ischemic cardiomyopathy.

Long-term outcome is poor in survivors of SCD, with a 50% mortality rate within 3 years. Coronary revascularization is the principal mode of secondary prevention in patients with significant coronary disease, with normal ventricular function, and in whom VT cannot be induced during electrophysiologic study. Revascularization is not effective, however, in preventing VT in patients with sustained monomorphic VT due to scar from a previous MI; treatment with catheter ablation or map-guided subendocardial resection may be effective. Because the likelihood of antiarrhythmic suppressibility is low and its long-term effectiveness poor (50% recurrence at 2 years), antiarrhythmic therapy is seldom considered a reliable

means of secondary prevention. Amiodarone is currently the most effective antiarrhythmic medication, but randomized trials show that an ICD is considerably more effective in reducing total mortality.

Antiarrhythmics Versus Implantable Defibrillators (AVID) Investigators: A comparison of antiarrhythmic-drug therapy with implantable defibrillators in patients resuscitated from near fatal arrhythmias. N Engl J Med 337:1576, 1997. *Multicenter secondary prevention trial.*

Domonski MJ, Zipes DP, Schron E: Treatment of sudden cardiac death: Current understanding from randomized trials and future directions. Circulation 95:2694, 1997. *Review of primary and secondary preventive trials.*

Moss AJ, Hall WJ, Cannon DS, et al: Improved survival with an implantable defibrillator in patients with coronary artery disease at high risk for ventricular arrhythmia. N Engl J Med 35:1993, 1996. *Multicenter primary prevention trial.*

Priori SG, Burhanin J, Hauer RN, et al: Genetic and molecular basis of cardiac arrhythmias: Impact on clinical management. Circulation 99:518, 1999. *Review of the molecular and genetic aspects of inherited arrhythmias.*

53 ELECTROPHYSIOLOGIC INTERVENTIONAL PROCEDURES AND SURGERY

Fred Morady

PACEMAKERS

PACEMAKER GENERATORS AND LEADS. Pacemaker batteries, which are lithium iodide cells that typically have a life span of 7 to 8 years, now often weigh less than 30 g. They usually are implanted subcutaneously in the infraclavicular area. Programmability of many different variables has become standard, as has the ability of the pacemaker to provide diagnostic and telemetric data.

Pacemaker leads usually are bipolar, with the distal electrode serving as the cathode. Unipolar leads are less commonly used because of the potential for pacing chest wall muscles and for inhibition of pacing by skeletal muscle myopotentials. The leads are inserted into the heart either percutaneously through a subclavian vein or by cutdown into a cephalic vein. Atrial leads usually are positioned in the right atrial appendage, and ventricular leads are placed in the right ventricular apex. Fixation to the myocardium is achieved either passively with tines or actively with a screw mechanism. Newer electrode designs, such as porous carbon or steroid-eluting electrodes, have resulted in lower acute and chronic pacing thresholds.

PACING MODES. The mode of pacing is described in shorthand fashion by a three- to five-letter code. The first letter designates the chamber being paced (A for atrium, V for ventricle, D for dual-chamber); the second letter designates the chamber being sensed (A, V, D, or O for no sensing); the third letter designates whether the pacemaker functions in an inhibited (I) or tracking mode (T), in both modes (D), or asynchronously (O); and the fourth letter indicates whether the pacemaker is capable of rate-modulation independent of atrial activity. An additional fifth letter may be used to designate the capability for antitachycardia pacing (P), delivery of shocks (S), or both (D). The most commonly employed pacing modes are VVI (pacing and sensing within the ventricle in inhibited fashion), VVIR (VVI plus rate-responsiveness), and DDD (pacing and sensing of atrium and ventricle, both in inhibited and tracking fashion).

The most appropriate pacing mode must always be determined on an individualized basis, the goal being to meet the patient's physiologic needs with the simplest system possible. For example, in a patient with chronic atrial fibrillation who has symptomatic pauses but not chronotropic incompetence, a VVI pacemaker is sufficient. However, if the patient also has chronotropic incompetence, a VVIR pacemaker is necessary to restore a normal rate-response to exercise. In a patient with high-degree atrioventricular (AV) block and normal sinus node function, DDD pacing is optimal. However, if a patient with high-degree AV block also has sinus node dysfunction, the ideal pacing mode is DDDR.

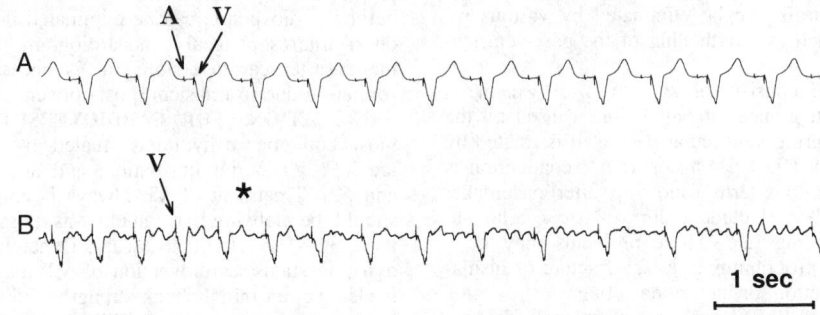

FIGURE 53–1 ■ Rhythm strips from a Holter monitor in a patient with complete atrioventricular block, sinus bradycardia, paroxysmal atrial fibrillation, and a rate-responsive dual-chamber pacemaker with mode-switching capability. *A*, When the patient is in sinus rhythm, the pacemaker functions in a DDDR mode, with synchronized atrial and ventricular pacing at 105 beats per minute while the patient is walking. *B*, At the onset of an episode of atrial fibrillation, there is tracking of the atrium that results in ventricular pacing at 140 beats per minute, which is the upper rate limit of the pacemaker. Within 2 seconds (asterisk), the mode-switch feature results in VVIR pacing, and the ventricular pacing rate gradually falls to 70 beats per minute, which is the lower rate limit of the pacemaker. A = atrial stimulus; V = ventricular stimulus.

In patients who have paroxysmal atrial fibrillation and high-degree AV block, no single pacing mode is optimal. DDD pacing is ideal when the patient is in sinus rhythm, but during atrial fibrillation DDD pacing may result in tracking of the atrium at the upper rate limit of the pacemaker. Conversely, VVIR pacing, which is ideal during atrial fibrillation, will not provide AV synchrony during periods of sinus rhythm. The development of mode-switching pacemakers has solved this dilemma. Mode-switching pacemakers are capable of pacing in the DDD mode during sinus rhythm and automatically switching to rate-responsive ventricular pacing during atrial fibrillation or other supraventricular arrhythmias (Fig. 53–1).

INDICATIONS FOR A PERMANENT PACEMAKER (Tables 53–1 and 53–2). In general, pacemakers are implanted either to alleviate symptoms caused by bradycardia or to prevent severe symptoms in patients who are likely to develop symptomatic bradycardia. The most common bradycardia-induced symptoms are dizziness or lightheadedness, syncope or near-syncope, exercise intolerance, or symptoms of heart failure. Because these symptoms are non-specific, documentation of an association between symptoms and bradycardia should be obtained before pacemaker implantation. If the bradycardia is persistent, such as in a patient who presents with complete AV block, a simple electrocardiogram may be sufficient to document the need for a pacemaker. If the bradycardia is intermittent, other diagnostic testing, such as 24-hour ambulatory monitoring, a continuous loop recorder, or an electrophysiology test (see Chapter 50) may be needed to document a relationship between symptoms and bradycardia.

After a symptomatic bradycardia has been documented, a correctable cause for the bradycardia should be excluded before a pacemaker is implanted. Correctable causes for symptomatic bradycardias include hypothyroidism, an overdose with drugs such as digitalis, electrolyte disturbances, and several categories of medications, most commonly β-adrenergic blocking agents (administered either orally or in the form of eyedrops for glaucoma), calcium channel blocking agents, and antiarrhythmic medications (see Chapter 51). At times, a pacemaker is necessary to allow continued treatment with a medication that is responsible for the bradycardia, such as in a patient who develops symptomatic sinus bradycardia after initiation of therapy with a β-adrenergic blocking agent for paroxysmal atrial fibrillation associated with a rapid ventricular response.

COMPLICATIONS OF PACEMAKERS. Complications related to the implantation procedure occur in less than 2% of patients and include pneumothorax, perforation of the atrium or ventricle, lead dislodgement, infection, and erosion of the pacemaker pocket. Thrombosis of the subclavian vein occurs in 10 to 20% of patients and is more likely in the presence of multiple leads; it rarely causes symptoms.

Pacemaker-mediated tachycardia is a possible complication of DDD pacing when the atrial lead senses retrograde depolarizations because of ventriculoatrial conduction. The resulting tachycardia often has a rate equal to the upper rate limit of the pacemaker.

Table 53–1 ■ CLASS I INDICATIONS* FOR IMPLANTATION OF A PERMANENT PACEMAKER

I. Atrioventricular Block
  A. Third-degree atrioventricular block associated with symptoms
  B. Third-degree atrioventricular block with pauses ≥3 seconds or with an escape rate <40 beats per minute in awake patients
  C. Postoperative atrioventricular block that is not expected to resolve
  D. Second-degree atrioventricular block associated with symptoms
  E. Chronic bifascicular or trifascicular block with intermittent third-degree atrioventricular block or type II second-degree atrioventricular block
II. Atrioventricular Block Associated with Myocardial Infarction
  A. Second- or third-degree atrioventricular block in the His-Purkinje system
  B. Transient second- or third-degree infranodal atrioventricular block and associated bundle branch block
  C. Persistent, symptomatic second- or third-degree atrioventricular block
III. Sinus Node Dysfunction
  A. Symptomatic sinus bradycardia or sinus pauses
  B. Symptomatic chronotropic incompetence
IV. Carotid Sinus Syndrome: Recurrent Syncope or Near-Syncope due to Carotid Sinus Syndrome

Table 53–2 ■ CLASS II INDICATIONS* FOR IMPLANTATION OF A PERMANENT PACEMAKER

I. Atrioventricular Block
  A. Asymptomatic third-degree atrioventricular block with an escape rate ≥40 beats per minute
  B. Asymptomatic Mobitz II second-degree atrioventricular block
  C. Asymptomatic Mobitz I second-degree atrioventricular block in the His-Purkinje system
  D. Bifascicular or trifascicular block and syncope without identifiable cause
  E. His-ventricular interval >100 msec
  F. Pacing-induced block in the His-Purkinje system
II. Atrioventricular Block Associated with Myocardial Infarction: persistent second- or third-degree atrioventricular block at the level of the atrioventricular node
III. Sinus Node Dysfunction: heart rate ≤40 beats per minute, without clear association between symptoms and bradycardia
IV. Neurocardiogenic Syncope: recurrent neurocardiogenic syncope associated with significant bradycardia reproduced by tilt-table testing.

*Class I indications are conditions for which there is general agreement that a pacemaker is indicated.
Please see the Cheitlin et al reference on page 252 (J Am Coll Cardiol 31:1175–1209, 1998).

*Class II indications are conditions for which pacemakers are often used, without unanimous agreement among experts that a pacemaker is necessary.
Please see the Cheitlin et al reference on page 252 (J Am Coll Cardiol 31:1175–1209, 1998).

Pacemaker-mediated tachycardia can be eliminated by various re-programming maneuvers, such as lengthening of the post-ventriculoatrial refractory period.

The pacemaker syndrome consists of symptoms of weakness, lightheadedness, exercise intolerance, or palpitations caused by the absence of AV synchrony during ventricular pacing. It is treated by restoring AV synchrony with DDD pacing or, if AV conduction is intact, AAI pacing. During long-term follow-up after pacemaker implantation, potential problems include failure to pace, failure to capture, and changes in pacing rate. These problems may be a manifestation of suboptimal programming, a lead fracture or insulation break, generator malfunction, or battery depletion.

TEMPORARY PACEMAKERS. Temporary pacemaker leads generally are inserted percutaneously into an internal jugular or subclavian vein, or by cutdown into a brachial vein, then positioned under fluoroscopic guidance in the right ventricular apex and attached to an external generator. Temporary pacing is used to stabilize patients awaiting permanent pacemaker implantation, to correct a transient symptomatic bradycardia due to drug toxicity or a metabolic defect, or to suppress torsades de pointes by maintaining a rate of 85 to 100 beats per minute until the causative factor has been eliminated. Temporary pacing may also be used in a prophylactic fashion in patients at risk of symptomatic bradycardia during a surgical procedure or high-degree AV block in the setting of an acute myocardial infarction. The most common complication of temporary pacemakers is infection; this risk is minimized by limiting the use of a pacemaker lead to 48 hours. In emergent situations, ventricular pacing can be instituted immediately by transcutaneous pacing using electrode pads applied to the chest wall.

TRANSTHORACIC CARDIOVERSION AND DEFIBRILLATION

MECHANISM OF ACTION. Direct-current defibrillators store an electrical charge and discharge it across two paddle electrodes in a damped, sinusoidal waveform. The shock terminates arrhythmias caused by re-entry by simultaneously depolarizing large portions of the atria or ventricles, thereby causing re-entry circuits to extinguish (see Chapters 51 and 52).

A non-synchronized shock that is delivered coincident with the T wave during supraventricular tachycardia or ventricular tachycardia (VT) may precipitate ventricular fibrillation (VF). *Cardioversion* refers to the termination of supraventricular tachycardia or VT by delivery of a shock in synchrony with the QRS complex. When shocks are delivered to terminate VF, synchronization to the QRS complex is not necessary, and this process is referred to as *defibrillation*.

TECHNIQUE. Whenever cardioversion or defibrillation is performed on an elective basis, the patient should be in a fasting state. Intravenous access to a peripheral vein should be established, and oxygen, suction, and equipment needed for airway management should be readily available. Transthoracic shocks are painful, and drugs commonly used for anesthesia or amnesia include short-acting barbiturates such as methohexital or a short-acting amnestic agent such as midazolam. In the anteroapical configuration, one electrode is positioned to the right of the sternum at the level of the second intercostal space, and the second electrode is positioned at the midaxillary line, lateral to the apical impulse. In the anteroposterior configuration, an electrode is placed to the left of the sternum at the fourth intercostal space, and the second electrode is positioned posteriorly, to the left of the spine, at the same level as the anterior electrode. These two electrode configurations result in similar success rates of cardioversion and defibrillation.

An important variable affecting the success of cardioversion/defibrillation is the shock strength. Other technique-dependent variables that maximize energy delivery to the heart include firm paddle pressure, delivery of the shock during expiration, and repetitive shocks. Patient-related variables that may decrease the probability of successful cardioversion/defibrillation include metabolic disturbances, a long arrhythmia duration, some antiarrhythmic drugs such as amiodarone, and a body weight more than 80 kg.

Because cardioversion of atrial fibrillation (see Chapter 51) may be complicated by thromboembolism, anticoagulation with warfarin is generally necessary for 3 weeks before cardioversion and for 1 month after cardioversion whenever atrial fibrillation has been present for 48 hours or more. The 3-week period of anticoagulation before cardioversion can be eliminated if no atrial thrombi are seen on a transesophageal echocardiogram, but anticoagulation for 1 month after cardioversion still is necessary to prevent thrombus formation due to transient, post-conversion atrial stunning.

INDICATIONS FOR CARDIOVERSION/DEFIBRILLATION. The most common arrhythmias treated by cardioversion/defibrillation are VF, VT, atrial fibrillation, and atrial flutter (see Chapters 51 and 52). Treatment of VF always is emergent, and a 200-J shock should be delivered as quickly as possible, followed by one or more 360-J shocks if necessary. Depending on the patient's hemodynamic status, cardioversion of VT may be elective or emergent; if elective, an initial shock strength of 50 J is appropriate, followed by higher energy levels if additional shocks are needed. An initial energy level of 50 J is appropriate for cardioversion of atrial flutter. In atrial fibrillation, in which cardioversion usually is performed on an elective basis, an initial shock of 100 to 200 J is appropriate, depending on the patient's body weight. Shocks of 300 to 360 J then are used if necessary. If atrial fibrillation must be treated on an urgent basis, for example, in a patient with the Wolff-Parkinson-White syndrome who has a very rapid ventricular rate and hemodynamic compromise, an initial shock of 200 J should be followed by 360-J shocks, as needed. Because the defibrillation energy requirement is a probability function and not a discrete value, subsequent shocks may be effective for cardioversion/defibrillation even when the first 360-J shock is ineffective.

COMPLICATIONS OF CARDIOVERSION/DEFIBRILLATION. Asynchronous shocks may precipitate VF. Rarely, VF may occur even when shocks are synchronized to the QRS complex. The risk of post-shock ventricular arrhythmias is increased in the presence of a supratherapeutic plasma concentration of digitalis, so cardioversion in the presence of digitalis toxicity should be avoided.

Transient ST-segment elevation may occur after cardioversion and usually is of no clinical consequence. Mild myocardial necrosis occasionally may occur if a total energy exceeding 425 J is delivered in a short period of time. Another rare complication of cardioversion is pulmonary edema, which may be due to transient left ventricular dysfunction.

Post-shock bradycardia or asystole may occur because of vagal discharge or an underlying sick sinus syndrome. At times, atropine or emergent transcutaneous pacing may be necessary. In patients who have a pacemaker or implantable cardioverter-defibrillator (ICD), the shocking electrodes should be positioned as far away from the generator as possible and the generator and pacing threshold should be checked afterward.

IMPLANTABLE CARDIOVERTER-DEFIBRILLATORS

IMPLANTABLE CARDIOVERTER-DEFIBRILLATOR PULSE GENERATORS AND LEADS. ICDs now weigh as little as 116 g, are multiprogrammable, have improved detection algorithms, are capable of antitachycardia and antibradycardia (including dual-chamber) pacing, can deliver biphasic shocks at strengths of less than 1 to 42 J, and provide a record of the electrograms recorded during arrhythmia episodes. With the development of pulse generators small enough to implant in the infraclavicular area and endocardial leads that are inserted transvenously, the implantation procedure has been greatly simplified and now is very similar to that of permanent pacemakers.

A single lead that contains a pacing-sensing electrode and two defibrillating coils can be used. If adequate defibrillation is not achieved with a single lead configuration, a subcutaneous patch electrode or subcutaneous array can be added. In another commonly used configuration, the pulse generator itself functions as an electrode, and a lead that has a pacing-sensing electrode at its tip and a distal defibrillating coil electrode is positioned at the right ventricular apex. Multiple other combinations of a chest wall patch electrode with defibrillating electrodes in the right ventricular apex, superior vena cava, or coronary sinus also can be used.

INDICATIONS. ICDs have become first-line therapy in patients who have survived an episode of VF not associated with acute myocardial infarction or who have had an episode of hemodynamically significant, sustained VT (see Chapter 52). ICDs also are implanted in patients at high risk of cardiac arrest, including patients with idiopathic, dilated cardiomyopathy and unexplained syncope or patients with coronary artery disease, ejection fraction less than 35%, spontaneous episodes of non-sustained VT, and inducible sustained VT not suppressed by procainamide in the electrophysiology laboratory (see Chapter 52). The results of several ongoing clinical trials may expand the indications for prophylactic use of ICDs.

PROGRAMMING OF IMPLANTABLE CARDIOVERTER-DEFIBRILLATORS. Testing is performed at the time of implantation to determine the energy requirement for defibrillation. A safety margin of at least 10 J should be present; for example, if the maximum output of the pulse generator is 32 J, successful defibrillation should be achieved with shocks of 22 J or less in strength. If the patient has had episodes of VT, antitachycardia pacing can be evaluated and programmed as needed to terminate the VT. Appropriate programming of the device is performed during pre-discharge testing.

With ICDs that are tiered-therapy devices, as many as two VT zones and one VF zone are available to provide individualized therapy for ventricular arrhythmias that have different rates. The rate threshold and various sequences of antitachycardia pacing and low- and/or high-energy shocks can be programmed for each of the two VT zones. The VF zone is a high-rate zone in which high-energy shocks are delivered. Optimal programming is important for many reasons, including minimizing patient discomfort, reducing the chance of syncope with an arrhythmia episode, maximizing the battery life of the pulse generator, and preventing inappropriate shocks.

COMPLICATIONS. Complications related to the implantation procedure include pneumothorax, myocardial perforation, and infection, all of which should have an incidence less than 1%. Complications associated with the subcutaneous or submuscular pocket into which the device is placed include hematoma formation and erosion of the pocket. The endocardial leads that are used in the ICD system occasionally become dislodged shortly after implanta-

tion, necessitating a second procedure to reposition the leads. Other lead complications include a fracture or insulation breakdown, either of which may result in a failure to defibrillate. A lead fracture also may result in artifact that mimics VF and triggers inappropriate shocks.

Patients who have an ICD do not require evaluation every time they experience a device discharge. However, urgent evaluation is necessary if the patient experiences flurries of discharges. Analysis of stored electrograms often reveals the underlying problem (Fig. 53–2). The frequent shocks may be appropriate shocks triggered by flurries of VT or VF; if a correctable cause such as a metabolic defect or proarrhythmic drug cannot be identified, antiarrhythmic drug therapy and/or catheter ablation should be used to eliminate these arrhythmia flurries. Flurries of shocks may be triggered by atrial fibrillation with a rapid ventricular response, in which case aggressive management of the atrial fibrillation is indicated. In addition, flurries of shocks may be a manifestation of a lead fracture, in which case lead replacement is necessary.

In patients who require both a pacemaker and an ICD, precautions must be taken to avoid device interactions. Pacemaker stimuli that occur during an episode of VF may result in failure of the ICD to detect the VF. In addition, sensing of pacemaker stimuli by an ICD may result in inappropriate shocks.

RADIOFREQUENCY CATHETER ABLATION

TISSUE EFFECTS OF RADIOFREQUENCY ENERGY. Radiofrequency ablation is a percutaneous catheter technique that can permanently eliminate a variety of supraventricular and VTs that previously required either chronic pharmacologic treatment for suppression or surgery for cure. Radiofrequency energy is delivered through an electrode catheter whose tip is in contact with tissue that is critical to maintenance of the tachycardia. The radiofrequency energy results in resistive heating of the tissue and irreversible tissue destruction when the tissue temperature exceeds 50° C. The lesions that are created are 5 to 6 mm in diameter and 2 to 3 mm deep. Chronic lesions demonstrate coagulation necrosis and are well demarcated.

PROCEDURAL ASPECTS. Diagnostic electrophysiologic testing (see Chapter 50) and radiofrequency ablation often are performed during the same procedure, commonly on an outpatient basis. Various pacing techniques and/or an infusion of isoproterenol are used to induce the patient's arrhythmia, allowing the specific mechanism of the tachycardia to be determined. Depending on the type of tachycardia, sites in the heart are targeted for ablation based on the results of mapping (see Chapter 50) or as guided by specific anatomic landmarks. Radiofrequency energy is delivered, typically in applications of 1 minute, at a power setting sufficient to result in adequate tissue heating of 60 to 70° C.

RADIOFREQUENCY ABLATION OF SUPRAVENTRICULAR ARRHYTHMIAS. AV nodal re-entrant tachycardia (see Chapter 51), the most common type of paroxysmal supraventricular tachycardia, is eliminated by radiofrequency ablation of either the "fast" or "slow" limb of the re-entry circuit. For slow pathway ablation, which is the preferred technique, target sites for ablation are located in the posteroseptal right atrium, near the ostium of the coronary sinus. Slow pathway ablation has a success rate of 98 to 100% and is associated with a 0 to 1.3% risk of high-degree AV block.

Left-sided accessory pathways are ablated using either a retrograde aortic or transseptal approach, and those that are right-sided or septal are ablated using a venous approach. Detailed mapping of the accessory pathway is essential for identification of an appropriate ablation site, and the ablation catheter is positioned either on the atrial or ventricular aspect of the mitral or tricuspid annulus. The success rate of accessory pathway ablation is 90 to 98%, and the complication rate is 2 to 3%. A fatal complication occurs in less than 0.1% of patients. The most common non-fatal but serious complications are cardiac tamponade due to mechanical perforation of the heart by an electrode catheter and high-degree AV block in patients with a septal accessory pathway.

Detailed mapping also is needed to identify sites for ablation of atrial tachycardias (see Chapter 51). Most atrial tachycardias arise

A

B

C

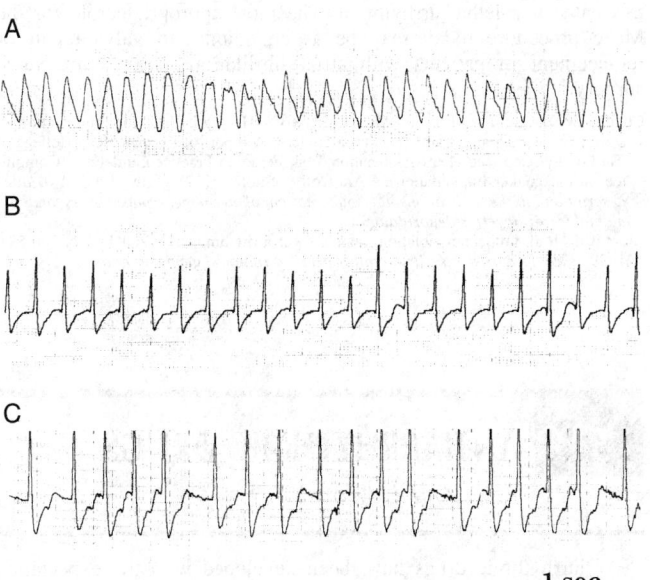

1 sec

FIGURE 53–2 ■ Exmples of stored electrograms obtained several hours after three different patients had experienced a flurry of shocks from an implantable cardioverter-defibrillator and showing the rhythm recorded by the device immediately before a shock was delivered. *A,* In this patient, the stored electrogram demonstrates ventricular tachycardia, rate 300 beats per minute, indicating tht the shock was appropriate. He was treated with amiodarone to reduce the frequency of episodes of ventricular tachycardia. *B,* This patient received shocks because of paroxysmal supraventricular tachycardia at a rate of 206 beats per minute, which exceeded the programmed rate cut-off of 170 beats per minute. He underwent radiofrequency ablation of the paroxysmal supraventricular tachycardia and received no further inappropriate shocks. *C,* The stored electrograms in this patient indicate that the patient received inappropriate shocks that were triggered by atrial fibrillation, rate 180 beats per minute. The rate cut-off of the device in this patient was 150 beats per minute. This patient was trated with a β-blocker to keep the ventricular rate less than 150 beats per minute during atrial fibrillation.

in the right atrium and are mapped using a venous approach, but left atrial tachycardias are mapped using a transseptal approach. Assuming that the atrial tachycardia is arising only at one site, the success rate of ablation is approximately 90%, and complications are rare.

Type I atrial flutter (see Chapter 51) arises in the right atrium and can be eliminated by radiofrequency ablation directed at a critical isthmus in the low right atrium, between the tricuspid annulus and the inferior vena cava. The success rate of this type of ablation is approximately 90%, and the risk of a serious complication is less than 1%.

In patients with drug-refractory atrial fibrillation (see Chapter 51) associated with an uncontrolled ventricular rate, either radiofrequency ablation or modification of the AV node can improve symptoms, functional capacity, and left ventricular function. In AV node ablation, third-degree AV block is intentionally induced; the success rate is 100%, and all patients require a permanent pacemaker. In the AV node modification procedure, the intent is to slow the ventricular rate without creating the need for a pacemaker. The success rate of the modification procedure is 75%, and the remaining 25% of patients require a pacemaker because of intentional or unintentional ablation of the AV node. Both types of procedures may be associated with a late, 1 to 2% risk of sudden death.

Two other ablation procedures that may prove to be helpful in patients with atrial fibrillation are the creation of linear lesions in the right and/or left atrium to eliminate atrial fibrillation and ablation of a focal source of paroxysmal atrial fibrillation, usually within one of the pulmonary veins. At present, these types of ablation procedures are investigational, and their efficacy and safety remain to be determined.

Inappropriate sinus tachycardia also can be managed with radiofrequency ablation. The sinus node, located in the high lateral right atrium, is targeted for ablation. The success rate is 90%, and 10% of patients require a pacemaker because of an inadequate atrial escape rate.

Because of a very favorable risk-benefit ratio, radiofrequency ablation is appropriate first-line therapy for any patient with paroxysmal supraventricular tachycardia, the Wolff-Parkinson-White syndrome, or type I atrial flutter who is symptomatic enough to warrant therapy (see Chapter 51). In the case of atrial flutter other than type I, atrial fibrillation, and inappropriate sinus tachycardia, an ablation procedure is appropriate only in patients with severe symptoms who are refractory to medication.

RADIOFREQUENCY ABLATION OF VENTRICULAR TACHYCARDIA. Radiofrequency ablation has been used as first-line treatment for idiopathic VT. The most common type of idiopathic VT arises in the outflow tract of the right ventricle and has a left bundle branch block configuration and superior axis. Another type of idiopathic VT has a right bundle branch block configuration and a superior axis and arises in the inferoapical left ventricle (see Chapter 52). The success rate of radiofrequency ablation of these types of VT has been 85 to 100%, and complications have been rare.

In patients with coronary artery disease, VT usually arises in diseased tissue adjacent to an area of prior infarction in the left ventricle. Because the disease process is diffuse instead of focal and because VT may originate at multiple sites, radiofrequency ablation of VT usually is not curative in patients with coronary artery disease. More often, radiofrequency ablation is used as adjunctive therapy with an ICD or with antiarrhythmic drug therapy. In the setting of coronary artery disease, the success rate of radiofrequency ablation of VT has been 65 to 95%, with a serious complication occurring in less than 2% of patients.

ARRHYTHMIA SURGERY

WOLFF-PARKINSON-WHITE SYNDROME. At present, surgical accessory pathway ablation may be indicated for the occasional patient with the Wolff-Parkinson-White syndrome who has potentially dangerous arrhythmias and in whom radiofrequency catheter ablation is unsuccessful. When performed by an experienced surgeon, the success rate of surgical accessory pathway ablation approaches 100% and the risk of a serious complication is low.

Intraoperative mapping is necessary to establish the location of the accessory pathway, which then can be ablated either cryosurgically using an epicardial approach or by direct dissection using an endocardial approach.

VENTRICULAR TACHYCARDIA IN PATIENTS WITH CORONARY ARTERY DISEASE. Subendocardial resection may be appropriate at the time of another surgical cardiac procedure in patients with coronary artery disease and recurrent, sustained, monomorphic VT. The substrate for monomorphic VT in patients with coronary artery disease usually lies within visually apparent scar tissue surrounding an area of prior myocardial infarction (see Chapter 52). Subendocardial resection has been successful in eliminating VT when performed either on a visual basis, with resection or cryoablation of all visually apparent scar tissue, or on a map-guided basis, with resection or cryoablation limited to the areas found to be participating in the generation of the VT. At centers experienced in this type of operation, the success rate of subendocardial resection has been 85 to 90%, and the operative mortality rate has been in the range of 5 to 10%. Although subendocardial resection has the potential advantage of preventing recurrences of VT, the relatively high operative mortality rate has discouraged its widespread use.

ATRIAL FIBRILLATION. In the past few years, the Maze procedure has been developed in an attempt to cure atrial fibrillation. A series of incisions are made in specific regions of the left and right atria to subdivide the atria into parts too small to sustain atrial fibrillation, and an isthmus of tissue is left between the subdivisions to allow both for normal atrial activation by the sinus node and for restoration of atrial transport function. Because the incisions are anatomically determined, intraoperative mapping is not necessary. With the most recent refinements in the Maze procedure, the operative mortality rate has been 2%, more than 90% of patients have had no recurrences of atrial fibrillation during long-term follow-up, and approximately 25% of patients have required a permanent pacemaker because of pre-existing or surgically induced chronotropic incompetence.

Although these results are impressive, many patients are reluctant to undergo an open-heart procedure associated with a risk of death to treat a non-lethal arrhythmia. The most appropriate role for the Maze procedure today may be as an adjunct to valve repair or replacement in patients with atrial fibrillation who require valve surgery.

Cheitlin MD, Conill A, Epstein AE, et al: ACC/AHA guidelines for implantation of cardiac pacemakers and antiarrhythmia devices: A report of the American College of Cardiology/American Heart Association Task Force on Practice Guidelines (Committee on Pacemaker Implantation). J Am Coll Cardiol 31:1175–1209, 1998. *A detailed description of the indications for implantation of permanent pacemakers and implantable cardioverter-defibrillators.*

Morady F: Radiofrequency ablation treatment for arrhythmias. N Engl J Med, 340:534, 1999. *A comprehensive review of all aspects of radiofrequency ablation.*

54 ANTIARRHYTHMIC DRUGS

Raymond L. Woosley

Antiarrhythmic drugs have been developed with the expectation that they would extend and/or improve life for many patients with cardiovascular disease, and especially those with a history of life-threatening arrhythmias. However, their usefulness has been limited by ineffectiveness and/or toxicity. In mortality trials, benefit has not been seen, and worsened mortality has been observed with several drugs. Therefore, care must be taken in deciding the mode of treatment, or in fact whether to treat with drugs at all.

Many antiarrhythmic agents are available today, but no agent is completely effective for all patients, and every agent has the potential for causing serious toxicity. Drug selection is often empirical, and known side effects may prohibit the use of certain classes of drugs for a specific patient.

Because of discouraging results with Class I sodium channel blocking drugs (e.g., quinidine, encainide, flecainide, moricizine) in the Cardiac Arrhythmic Suppression Trial (CAST), Class III drugs that prolong the action potential duration have been developed. Amiodarone may improve mortality in some patients, but the d-isomer of sotalol increases mortality after myocardial infarction. More recently, a trial of dofetilide failed to improve mortality but provided reassuring results that mortality was not increased.

CLASSIFICATION OF ANTIARRHYTHMIC DRUGS

Antiarrhythmic drugs are often classified according to their electrophysiologic effects with approaches such as the Vaughan Williams classification (Fig. 54–1). However, most antiarrhythmic drugs have multiple actions; hence their pharmacology is complex and may differ in different cardiac tissues. Furthermore, many antiarrhythmic agents have pharmacologically active metabolites whose production varies extensively within the population and whose activity may be quite different than the parent compound.

CLASS I DRUGS. Drugs having Class I action possess "local anesthetic" or "membrane-stabilizing" activity by blocking of the fast inward sodium channel to produce a decrease in the maximum depolarization rate, Vmax, of the action potential (phase 0) and slow intracardiac conduction (see Fig. 49–1). Class IA drugs, including quinidine, procainamide, and disopyramide, increase ventricular refractoriness and prolong the QT interval. Class IB drugs, including lidocaine, mexiletine, and tocainide, are modest sodium channel blockers that shorten the action potential duration (APD) and refractoriness with little effect on PR, QRS, or QT intervals. Class IC drugs, including flecainide and propafenone, are potent sodium channel blockers that slow conduction velocity, have little effect on repolarization, and increase PR and QRS intervals but cause little change in the QT interval.

CLASS II DRUGS. Class II drugs are β-adrenergic antagonists, which are effective for supraventricular arrhythmias and tachyarrhythmias caused by excessive sympathetic activity but are of limited efficacy for severe, life-threatening ventricular arrhythmias. Although their exact mechanism is unknown, they are the only drugs found effective in preventing sudden cardiac death in survivors of prior myocardial infarction.

CLASS III DRUGS. Class III drugs' predominant effect is to prolong the duration of the cardiac action potential and refractoriness. Examples include amiodarone, sotalol, bretylium, ibutilide, and N-acetylprocainamide (NAPA), which is the major metabolite of procainamide.

CLASS IV DRUGS. Class IV drugs are calcium channel antagonists. Currently, only verapamil and diltiazem are used as antiarrhythmics.

Because of the many limitations of the Vaughan Williams classification, "The Sicilian Gambit" classification system has been developed based on the differential effects of antiarrhythmic drugs on channels, receptors, and transmembrane pumps (see Fig. 54–1). For example, quinidine, a Class IA drug, is a sodium channel antagonist with the ability to block potassium channels and antagonize acetylcholine and catecholamines at cholinergic and α-adrenergic receptors, respectively. One would expect conduction slowing, increased APD (and refractoriness), and vasodilation to result from these three actions of quinidine.

POLYMORPHIC METABOLISM. Because antiarrhythmic drugs have a narrow therapeutic index, variable metabolism and clearance often cause clinical effects. For example, many antiarrhythmic agents, especially in Class I, are substrates or inhibitors for a cytochrome P-450 (CYP) that is genetically absent in 7% of whites and 1 to 2% of blacks and Asians. These individuals have markedly decreased clearance of mexiletine, flecainide, and propafenone. Because other drugs may compete for or inhibit this enzyme, there is a risk of serious interactions between these drugs and timolol, metoprolol, quinidine, fluoxetine, and perhaps others.

DRUGS

Lidocaine (Xylocaine)

CLINICAL APPLICATIONS. Lidocaine is very often the drug of first choice for the acute suppression of ventricular arrhythmias.

Antiarrhythmic Drug Actions

Vaughn-Williams Class	Drug	Channels			Receptors				Clinical effects				ECG changes
		Na	Ca	K	α	β	ACh	Ado	Pro-Arrhy	LV Fx	Heart rate	Extra cardiac	
I A	Quinidine	Mod		High	Low		Mod		High			High	A
	Procainamide	Mod		Mod					Mod			High	
	Disopyramide (Norpace)	Mod		Mod			Mod		Low	↓↓		Mod	
I B	Lidocaine (Xylocaine)	Low							Low			Mod	B
	Mexiletine (Mexitil)	Low							Low			Mod	
I C	Propafenone (Rythmol)	High				Mod			Mod	↓↓	↓	Low	C
	Flecainide (Tambocor)	High							Mod	↓↓		Low	
II	β adrenergic antagonists					Mod			Low	↓	↓↓		
III	Bretylium (Bretylol)			High	Ag/An	Ag/An			Low		↓		
	Sotalol (Betapace)			High		Mod			Low	↓	↓↓		
	Amiodarone (Cordarone)	Low	Low	High	Mod	Mod			Low		↓↓	High	
	Ibutilide (Corvert)	Ag		Mod					High			Low	
IV	Verapamil (Calan, Isoptin)		High						Low	↓↓	↓		
	Diltiazem (Cardizem)		Mod						Low	↓	↓		
Misc	Adenosine (Adenocard)							Ag	Low		↓		

Antagonist
Relative Potency
○ Low ◐ Moderate ● High
△ = Agonist
▲ = Agonist/Antagonist

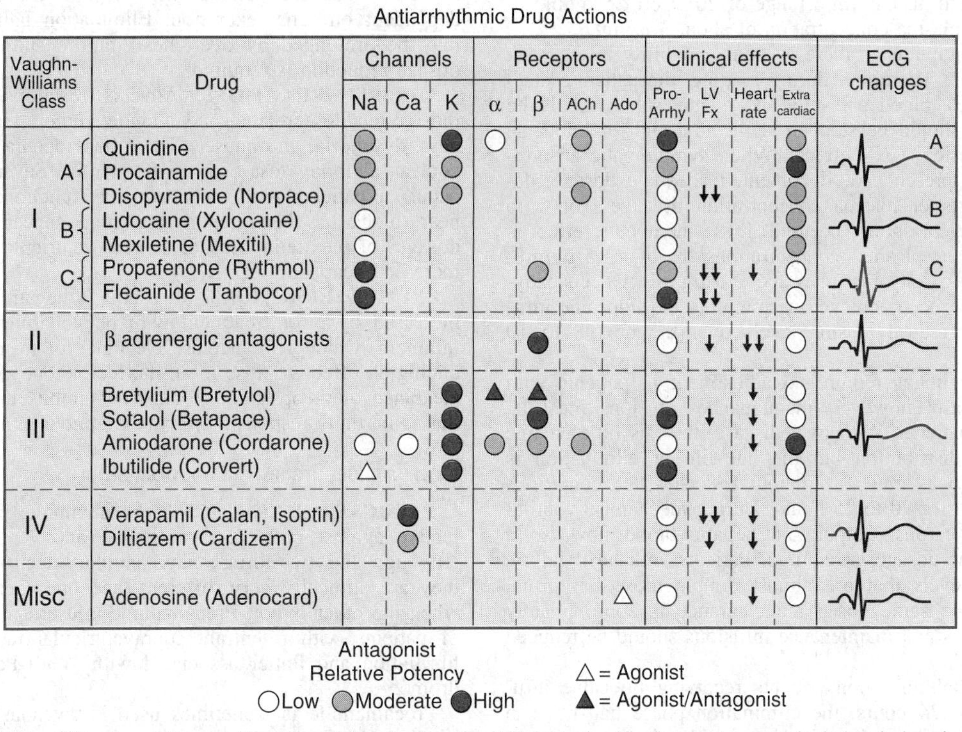

FIGURE 54–1. ■ This figure is a modification of the Sicilian Gambit drug classification system and includes designation by the Vaughan Williams system. The sodium channel blockers are subdivided into the A, B, and C subgroups based on their relative potency. The targets of antiarrhythmic drugs, listed across the columns, are the ion channels (sodium, calcium, and potassium) and the receptors (α-adrenergic, β-adrenergic, cholinergic [ACH], and adenosinergic [ADO]). The next columns compare the drugs' clinical actions. These include proarrhythmic potential (Proarrhy), effect on left ventricular function (LV Fx), effects on heart rate (Heart Rate), and potential for extra cardiac side effects (Extra Cardiac). The ECG tracings indicate the changes (in color) that are caused by usual dosages of the drug (i.e., PR interval, QRS interval, and QT interval). The drugs are listed in rows with their brand names shown in parentheses. The symbols in the table indicate the drugs' relative potency as agonists or antagonists. The solid triangle indicates the biphasic effects of bretylium initially to release norepinephrine and act as an agonist and subsequently to block further release and act as an antagonist of adrenergic tone. The number of arrows and their direction indicate the magnitude and direction of effect of the drugs on heart rate and left ventricular function (i.e., inotropy).

Although such therapy does not reduce total mortality, it decreases the incidence of primary ventricular fibrillation in patients with documented acute myocardial infarction. Because of lidocaine's complex pharmacokinetics, a monitored environment is desirable to permit evaluation of patient response and detection of toxicity.

MECHANISM OF ACTION. Lidocaine reduces Vmax and produces shortening or no change in APD and effective refractory period (ERP) of normal Purkinje fibers, unlike quinidine and procainamide, which additionally block potassium channels and lengthen APD. Lidocaine has little effect on the electrophysiology of the normal conduction system; in patients with conduction system abnormalities, it has variable effects.

CLINICAL PHARMACOLOGY. The two desethyl metabolites of lidocaine that are excreted by the kidneys have less antiarrhythmic potency than the parent drug and may contribute to the production of central nervous system (CNS) side effects. Antiarrhythmic activity is correlated with lidocaine's concentration in the central compartment, and the half-life of distribution out of this compartment is rapid (8 min). The time required to reach steady-state conditions is 8 to 10 hours in normal individuals and up to 20 to 24 hours in some patients with heart failure and/or liver disease, whose elimination half-life is much longer than the 1.5 to 2 hours in normal subjects.

DOSAGE AND ADMINISTRATION. Lidocaine's primary use is for acute rapid suppression of ventricular arrhythmias. Single intravenous boluses will achieve only transient therapeutic effects because the drug is rapidly distributed out of the plasma and myocardium. For a stable patient, a total loading dose of lidocaine should be 3 to 4 mg/kg administered as a series of doses over 20 to 30 minutes. For example, after injection of an initial dose of 1 mg/kg over 2 minutes, a series of three loading "boluses" can be administered slowly (50 mg each over 2 minutes) 8 to 10 minutes apart, while the patient is continuously observed for the development of side effects.

At the time of initiation of the loading regimen, a maintenance infusion, designed to replace ongoing losses due to drug elimination, should be started, usually in a range of 20 to 60 μg/kg/min to achieve the desired plasma concentration of about 3 μg/mL.

Even in normal individuals, there is great variability in the peak plasma concentration. Therefore, during loading, the patient's electrocardiogram (ECG), blood pressure, and mental status should be monitored; loading should be stopped at the first sign of lidocaine excess, usually transient CNS effects. When symptomatic arrhythmias persist in the presence of documented adequate dosage, defined by side effects or plasma concentration in excess of 5 to 7 μg/mL, another agent should be used. Little therapeutic effect is evident at lidocaine plasma concentrations below 1.5 μg/mL, whereas the risk of toxicity increases above 5 μg/mL. Once steady-state conditions have been achieved, terminating the lidocaine infusion will gradually reduce plasma levels over the next 8 to 10 hours.

Initial loading regimens require no adjustment in patients with renal or liver disease; however, maintenance infusions must be decreased in such patients. With liver disease, there is little change in the volume of distribution but the half-life of elimination is prolonged greatly to as much as 5 hours; steady-state conditions will not be achieved for 20 to 25 hours. During mechanical ventilation, there is low cardiac output and hepatic blood flow, so a decrease in lidocaine dosage is required. Patients with heart failure achieve lidocaine levels that are almost double those in normal individuals given the same dose, and clearance is approximately halved; loading doses and maintenance infusions should be reduced by 50%.

In post–myocardial infarction patients receiving lidocaine infusions for more than 24 hours, the elimination phase half-life can increase up to 50%. An increase in plasma lidocaine occurring at this time often reflects an elevation in plasma levels of α-1-acid glycoprotein (AAG), to which lidocaine binds, rather than an increase in active drug. In this situation, the lidocaine dosage should not be reduced, provided the patient is monitored closely for toxicity and has no adverse side effects.

ADVERSE REACTIONS. CNS symptoms are the most frequent side effects of lidocaine administration. A rapid bolus can induce seizures. With more gradual attainment of excessive levels, drowsiness, dysarthria, dysesthesia, and even coma may occur. Lidocaine

can depress cardiac function, leading to decreased lidocaine clearance, and produce an even greater increase in lidocaine concentrations. Sinus node dysfunction can also occur.

DRUG INTERACTIONS. An additive or synergistic depression of myocardial function or conduction may occur during combined therapy with other antiarrhythmic agents, especially during conversion from lidocaine to another agent. A pharmacokinetic drug interaction between propranolol and lidocaine produces higher than expected plasma concentrations of lidocaine. Cimetidine decreases splanchnic, and hence liver, blood flow, decreases lidocaine's volume of distribution, and inhibits the enzymes responsible for lidocaine metabolism.

Mexiletine (Mexitil)

CLINICAL APPLICATIONS. Mexiletine is used in the treatment of ventricular arrhythmias and has, on occasion, been effective in treating refractory arrhythmias. Success rates vary between 6% and 60% but are usually less than 20%. Mexiletine does not prolong the QT interval, and therefore it can be useful in patients with a history of torsades de pointes or long QT syndrome when quinidine, sotalol, procainamide, and disopyramide are contraindicated.

CLINICAL PHARMACOLOGY. Mexiletine has little first-pass metabolism but is eliminated primarily by hepatic metabolism with only 10 to 15% being excreted unchanged in the urine. Its half-life of elimination is between 8 and 20 hours (9 to 12 hours for healthy subjects), with the time needed to reach steady state ranging between 1 and 3 days.

DOSAGE AND ADMINISTRATION. Mexiletine therapy should be initiated with a low dosage and increased at 2- to 3-day intervals until efficacy or intolerable side effects such as tremor or other CNS symptoms develop. With normal renal function, the recommended initial oral mexiletine dosage is 200 mg every 8 hours. As with most drugs having extensive liver metabolism, clearance will be widely variable within the population. This is especially true for mexiletine because CYP2D6, responsible for its metabolism, is missing in 7% of the white population.

All patients with renal failure should be given low initial doses, especially because patients with hepatic CYP2D6 deficiency are dependent on renal excretion. Elimination half-life and clearance may be prolonged by overt heart failure and hepatic failure, and dosage reduction is required.

ADVERSE REACTIONS. Adverse reactions to mexiletine are most often dose related and include tremor, visual blurring, dizziness, dysphoria, and nausea. Thrombocytopenia and a positive antinuclear antibody test occur infrequently. Severe bradycardia may occur in patients with sinus node dysfunction, and worsening of heart block has been reported at high concentrations. Usual oral dosages of mexiletine do not depress ventricular function or induce increased heart failure.

DRUG INTERACTIONS. Mexiletine's hepatic metabolism can be increased by prior treatment with phenobarbital, phenytoin, or rifampicin, which will increase clearance of mexiletine, possibly reducing an effective dose to an ineffective one. Mexiletine decreases clearance of theophylline. Quinidine inhibits the CYP2D6 enzyme that is partially responsible for mexiletine clearance.

Procainamide (Pronestyl-SR, Procan-SR)

CLINICAL APPLICATIONS. Procainamide, like quinidine, is effective against both supraventricular and ventricular arrhythmias. Although the two drugs have similar electrophysiologic effects, they are clinically very different, and one agent may be effective when the other is not. Procainamide is useful in acute management of patients with re-entrant supraventricular tachycardia and atrial fibrillation and flutter associated with Wolff-Parkinson-White syndrome.

Procainamide is sometimes used intravenously to suppress ventricular arrhythmias occurring immediately after myocardial infarction or to convert sustained ventricular tachycardia when lidocaine is ineffective. Because it takes approximately 20 minutes to administer a loading dose of procainamide safely, its use is limited to those clinical situations in which adequate time is available.

MECHANISM OF ACTION. Procainamide slows conduction and decreases automaticity and excitability of atrial and ventricular myocardium and Purkinje fibers. Because of its effect on potassium channels, it also prolongs APD and refractoriness. Compared with quinidine, procainamide has very little vagolytic activity and causes less prolongation of the QT interval. Its major metabolite, *N*-acetyl-procainamide (acecainide, NAPA), has predominantly Class III antiarrhythmic activity; it prolongs APD and refractoriness in both atrial and ventricular myocardium and prolongs the QT interval.

CLINICAL PHARMACOLOGY. Procainamide is rapidly absorbed and 100% orally bioavailable. About 15% of procainamide is bound to serum proteins. Procainamide's short half-life of elimination of 2 to 4 hours in patients with normal renal function has led to the use of sustained-release preparations, which can be given every 3 to 6 hours.

Slightly more than half of the general population are phenotypic rapid acetylators of procainamide and quickly convert it to NAPA. The usually effective plasma concentrations are 4 to 8 μg/mL for procainamide and 7 to 15 μg/mL for NAPA. Plasma concentrations should be monitored to determine compliance and prevent toxicity.

DOSAGE AND ADMINISTRATION. When administered intravenously, procainamide can be given as a constant 25-minute loading infusion of 275 μg/min/kg or by a series of doses (100 mg delivered over 3 minutes) given every 5 minutes up to a total dose of 1 g. If the loading infusion is well tolerated with no hypotension and less than 25% QRS or QT widening, the maintenance intravenous infusion is 20 to 60 μg/kg/min.

With normal renal and cardiac function, the initial recommended oral maintenance dose is 50 mg/kg/day in the sustained-release form every, 6 to 8 hours. Because the electrophysiologic effects of procainamide and NAPA are quite different, monitoring of patients receiving procainamide should include measurement of plasma concentrations of both agents to determine their relative concentrations. Patients with the rapid acetylator phenotype or impaired renal function may develop high plasma concentrations of NAPA and should be monitored to maintain NAPA levels well below 20 μg/mL. With renal dysfunction or a low cardiac output, procainamide and especially NAPA in usual doses may accumulate to potentially toxic levels.

ADVERSE REACTIONS. Up to 40% of patients discontinue procainamide in the first 6 months due to adverse reaction. Arrhythmia may be aggravated, including the development of torsades de pointes most often due to NAPA; therefore, procainamide should not be used in patients with a long QT syndrome, a history of torsades de pointes, or hypokalemia. Fifteen to 20% of patients develop a a lupus-like syndrome that regresses with discontinuation of the drug. Procainamide can cause agranulocytosis, so a white blood cell count should be obtained every 2 weeks for the first 3 months.

DRUG INTERACTIONS. Unlike quinidine, procainamide does not cause an increase in digoxin levels. Procainamide's clearance is reduced by 10 to 50% by cimetidine or ranitidine, which block its renal tubular secretion.

Disopyramide (Norpace)

CLINICAL APPLICATIONS. Disopyramide (Class IA) is effective against a broad range of supraventricular and ventricular arrhythmias, with an antiarrhythmic profile similar to that of quinidine and procainamide. Its negative inotropic and anticholinergic actions frequently limit its usefulness.

DOSAGE AND ADMINISTRATION. A loading dose is not recommended with disopyramide because of the risk of heart failure or anticholinergic side effects. The usually effective dosage for disopyramide is 100 to 400 mg two to four times daily, to a maximal dose of 800 mg/day. Therapy should begin with low doses to allow ample time for steady-state equilibrium.

Rapid fluctuations in plasma concentration are difficult to avoid because of disopyramide's saturable protein binding. The generally accepted therapeutic range for total (free and bound) disopyramide is 2 to 5 μg/mL but should not be strictly relied upon.

DRUG INTERACTIONS. Phenytoin, rifampicin, and phenobarbital induce hepatic metabolism of disopyramide, increase its elimination, and potentially reduce its antiarrhythmic effect. Significant depression of myocardial contractility may result from the combined administration of disopyramide with β-adrenergic or calcium channel antagonists; these combinations should be avoided in patients with impaired ventricular function.

Quinidine

CLINICAL APPLICATIONS. Quinidine (Class IA) is used for a variety of supraventricular and ventricular arrhythmias, including conversion of atrial fibrillation, atrial flutter or supraventricular

tachycardia, and suppression of ventricular extrasystoles and ventricular tachycardia. However, meta-analysis of six placebo-controlled trials in patients with atrial fibrillation showed a small but statistically significant increase in mortality in the patients treated with quinidine. Because of the similarity to the results in CAST, these results should be assumed to be valid until a definitive prospective study is available.

CLINICAL PHARMACOLOGY. Although quinidine sulfate is usually administered every 6 hours, its elimination half-life varies from 3 to 19 hours. Oral bioavailability is approximately 70%. Quinidine is inactivated or eliminated by both hepatic metabolism (50 to 90%) and renal elimination (10 to 30%). Several active metabolites vary among individuals.

DOSAGE AND ADMINISTRATION. Quinidine is available as sulfate, gluconate, and polygalacturonate, and the quinidine content varies among these at 83%, 62%, and 60%, respectively. The usually effective dosage of quinidine sulfate ranges from 800 to 2400 mg/day, with the maximum recommended single dose being 600 mg. Doses of other forms should be adjusted based on quinidine content. Elderly patients often require lower dosages of quinidine because of both reduced clearance and volume of distribution. Because the half-life varies from 3 to 19 hours, doses should be adjusted only every 2 to 4 days to prevent unexpected drug accumulation. The range of therapeutic plasma concentrations measured using assays that differentiate quinidine from its metabolites is 0.7 to 5.5 μg/mL. Intravenous therapy with quinidine is potentially hazardous and rarely indicated.

No adjustment in initial dosage is needed for patients with renal or hepatic disease, but lower than usual total plasma concentrations can produce toxicity in patients with decreased protein binding due to hepatic failure. Patients with rapid quinidine elimination, often due to induction of hepatic metabolism caused by other drugs, may require doses of up to 600 mg every 6 hours.

Patients with congenital long QT syndrome, hypokalemia, or a history of torsades de pointes should not be given quinidine because of their increased risk for torsades de pointes. For patients with heart failure, quinidine can cause proarrhythmia and precipitate digitalis toxicity; quinidine titration should begin at a lower dose. The dose of any concomitant cardiac glycoside should be reduced and monitored, and the potassium level should be maintained above 4 mEq/L.

The direct negative inotropic effects of quinidine are usually offset by its vasodilatory effect, so oral quinidine is usually well tolerated hemodynamically in patients with reduced ventricular function or heart failure; however, the risk of quinidine-induced torsades de pointes is potentiated in patients with heart failure in the setting of bradycardia and low serum magnesium or potassium levels.

ADVERSE REACTIONS. Marked prolongation of the QT interval can occur with usual or even low doses, and the risk of torsades de pointes is markedly increased. This arrhythmia may be responsible for quinidine syncope, which occurs in as many as 5 to 10% of patients within the first days of quinidine treatment, and for quinidine-induced sudden death. For patients who develop torsades de pointes, treatment with pacing or isoproterenol is usually very effective. Magnesium sulfate injection has also been recommended as initial therapy, but controlled trials are not currently available.

Because quinidine acts via α-adrenergic blockade to produce vasodilatation, hypotension may occur, especially in patients concomitantly receiving nitrates or other vasodilators. Other adverse effects include diarrhea, vomiting, tinnitus, and rarely thrombocytopenia; conduction block can occur in patients with pre-existing conduction system disease. In patients treated with quinidine for atrial flutter without prior atrioventricular nodal blockade by digitalis, sudden increases in antrioventricular conduction and rapid ventricular rates may develop due to quinidine's anticholinergic effects.

DRUG INTERACTIONS. Quinidine metabolism is inhibited by cimetidine and induced by phenytoin, phenobarbital, and rifampicin. Clinical digoxin toxicity has been described in 20 to 40% of patients receiving concurrent quinidine and digoxin. Quinidine is a potent inhibitor of the hepatic cytochrome P-450 specific for debrisoquine metabolism (CYP2D6), although it is not metabolized by this specific P-450 isozyme.

Propafenone (Rythmol)

CLINICAL APPLICATIONS. Propafenone (Class IC) is similar to other antiarrhythmic agents in overall efficacy and patient tolerance for many types of arrhythmias, including supraventricular arrhythmias.

CLINICAL PHARMACOLOGY. Propafenone has a marked structural similarity to propranolol and can produce clinically significant β-adrenergic inhibition. As with mexiletine and flecainide, patients deficient in CYP2D6 have very slow elimination of propafenone and develop significant β-receptor antagonism at low doses.

DOSAGE AND ADMINISTRATION. Effective dosages range from 300 to 900 mg/day in two to four divided doses. Propafenone dosage should not be changed more frequently than every 3 days because of slow elimination of the parent drug in poor metabolizers and slow accumulation of metabolites in extensive metabolizers. Drug interactions occur with many antidepressants and neuroleptics. Quinidine results in higher propafenone concentrations. Combination with β-blockers should be avoided.

Flecainide (Tambocor)

CLINICAL APPLICATIONS. Flecainide (Class IC) is very effective in suppressing a variety of ventricular and supraventricular tachycardias. The finding of increased mortality in patients with ischemic heart disease has generally restricted its use to treat supraventricular arrhythmias in patients without known coronary artery disease. Its negative inotropic actions restrict its use to patients having moderately well-preserved ventricular function.

CLINICAL PHARMACOLOGY. Most of flecainide is metabolized by CYP2D6 in the liver to compounds that are not pharmacologically active. Because flecainide is also eliminated by the kidneys to a considerable extent, the enzyme deficiency usually has little effect on its pharmacokinetics except in patients with renal insufficiency.

DOSAGE AND ADMINISTRATION. Patients with supraventricular tachycardia should receive 50 mg every 12 hours as a starting dose; after 3 to 4 days, the dose can be adjusted up to 100 to 150 mg every 12 hours based on clinical response. Because 7% of white patients with renal failure do not have the CYP2D6 enzyme and because flecainide is usually eliminated by both metabolism and renal excretion, all patients with renal failure should be given very low dosages and have the doses titrated very carefully.

ADVERSE REACTIONS. Flecainide can induce proarrhythmic events even when prescribed as recommended, especially in patients with severe heart disease. Flecainide produces a measurable decrease in left ventricular function in most patients and can depress sinus node activity in patients with pre-existing sinus node dysfunction; it also prolongs the QRS and PR intervals on the surface ECG. Flecainide increases pacing thresholds by as much as 200% and must be used with caution in pacemaker-dependent patients. It also increases the threshold for electrical defibrillation in patients with defibrillators.

DRUG INTERACTIONS. Cimetidine reduces flecainide clearance and prolongs its half-life. Digoxin, propranolol, and amiodarone increase flecainide levels.

β-RECEPTOR ANTAGONISTS

β-Receptor antagonists (β-blockers) are usually considered as relatively equivalent members of a class of agents that block adrenergic agonists at the β-receptor. Unfortunately, there are few comparative trials to evaluate their equivalence as antiarrhythmic agents and to determine the dosages at which they might have equivalence. They are generally considered to be effective for arrhythmias associated with excessive sympathetic stimulation (e.g., pheochromocytoma) or arrhythmias associated with exercise or acute myocardial infarction. The antiarrhythmic efficacy of β-blockers are thought to be due to two actions: blockade of the post-synaptic cardiac receptor and "membrane stabilizing activity." The direct membrane effect produces shortening of the action potential in vitro but requires concentrations far higher than can be achieved clinically. However, for some drugs in this class, it is important to consider other ancillary actions that might augment or impede their efficacy. For example, the Class III action (potassium channel blockade) of sotalol augments its antiarrhythmic potency, whereas

the intrinsic sympathomimetic activity of pindolol is thought to impede antiarrhythmic efficacy. β-Blockers such as propranolol, atenolol, and metoprolol are generally considered to be effective in supraventricular arrhythmias such as atrioventricular nodal re-entry, atrial fibrillation, or atrial flutter. Esmolol, an ultra–short-acting β-blocker with a half-life of 9 minutes, is useful for slowing ventricular response to atrial fibrillation or flutter for short periods of time, such as after surgery. Chronic therapy with β-blockers is also effective in preventing life-threatening arrhythmias in many patients with the congenital long QT syndrome, especially those whose symptoms are associated with adrenergic stimulation.

Although β-blockers are generally considered to be ineffective or even contraindicated in patients with sustained ventricular tachycardia, they are often useful, especially when combined with other antiarrhythmic agents, for prevention of recurrent episodes of ventricular tachycardia. Although they are not usually very effective in suppressing premature ventricular contractions, they are often able to reduce the troublesome symptoms of palpitations and, more importantly, in patients with prior myocardial infarction, reduce the associated risk of sudden death.

The dosages of β-blockers required for treatment of arrhythmias are generally similar to those required for treatment of hypertension or angina. In some patients, higher dosages (equivalent to >320 mg/day of propranolol) are required to suppress ventricular arrhythmias, but these dosages are also associated with a higher incidence of fatigue and potentially serious depression.

Bretylium (Bretylol)

CLINICAL APPLICATIONS AND PHARMACOLOGY. Bretylium (Class III) is effective acute therapy of ventricular tachycardia and/or ventricular fibrillation. Because it produces complex indirect effects through the autonomic nervous system, it should be reserved for patients who have failed to respond to lidocaine. Bretylium is eliminated almost entirely unchanged in the urine, and clearance correlates well with creatinine clearance.

DOSAGE AND ADMINISTRATION. The usual intravenous dosage for bretylium is 5 mg/kg given by rapid injection into a central intravenous line during cardiac emergencies and by a loading infusion of the same dose over 10 to 20 minutes in less acute situations to reduce nausea and vomiting. The loading dose should be repeated after 20 minutes if the arrhythmia is still present. Maintenance infusions of 1 to 4 mg/min should be given depending on body size and renal function. Heart rhythm and blood pressure should be monitored carefully, especially during the first few hours of bretylium therapy. In patients with renal insufficiency, bretylium clearance is reduced and half-life is prolonged; therefore, the maintenance infusion for bretylium should be reduced to the lowest effective dosage.

ADVERSE REACTIONS. When bretylium is given by rapid intravenous injection, many patients experience nausea and vomiting. Increased ventricular arrhythmias can occur and lead to more frequent cardioversion. The reduction in peripheral vascular resistance can cause symptomatic hypotension in patients who are volume depleted or have fixed valvular obstruction.

Sotalol (Betapace)

CLINICAL APPLICATIONS AND PHARMACOLOGY. Sotalol blocks β-receptors and increases the QT interval and cardiac refractoriness. This unique combination of properties makes sotalol effective in suppressing a variety of supraventricular and ventricular arrhythmias; however, sotalol increases instability in patients with ventricular arrhythmias after a myocardial infarction.

Peak plasma concentrations are seen 2.5 to 4 hours after a dose. It is eliminated by the kidneys unchanged with a half-life of approximately 12 hours.

DOSAGES AND ADMINISTRATION. The recommended initial dose of sotalol is 80 mg every 12 hours. In patients with relatively normal renal function, steady state will occur in 2 to 3 days. In patients who do not respond and have QT intervals less than 500 ms, the dosage may be increased to 160 mg twice daily and, if necessary, to 240 mg twice daily.

Because sotalol is mainly eliminated unchanged in the urine, the dosing interval should be 24 hours if the creatinine clearance is between 30 and 60 mL/min and every 36 to 48 hours if it is between 10 and 30 mL/min. Because of the increased risk of torsades de pointes and heart failure, patients with reduced cardiac output should be given lower doses and monitored carefully.

ADVERSE REACTIONS. A major concern with sotalol treatment is the occurrence of torsades de pointes, which occurs with an overall incidence of approximately 2%. It is more common in females, in patients with heart failure, and in those with a history of sustained ventricular tachycardia (7%). The incidence of torsades de pointes should be minimized by careful screening for predisposing factors such as bradycardia, baseline prolongation of the QT interval, and hypokalemia; by careful dose escalation beginning at 160 mg/day; and by limiting the maximum QT interval prolongation to less than 550 msec. The incidence of new or worsened heart failure is only about 3%. Other side effects typical of β-blockers are to be expected.

DRUG INTERACTIONS. Concomitant use of sotalol with agents that prolong repolarization has the potential to increase the likelihood of torsades de pointes. No pharmacokinetic interactions have been seen with sotalol.

Amiodarone (Cordarone)

CLINICAL APPLICATIONS. Amiodarone is approved by the Food and Drug Administration only for life-threatening ventricular arrhythmias refractory to other available forms of therapy. Nevertheless, numerous trials describe its efficacy in the conversion and slowing of atrial fibrillation, AV nodal re-entrant tachycardia, and tachycardias associated with the Wolff-Parkinson-White syndrome. The reasons for amiodarone's restrictive labeling include its documented potentially lethal complications, the difficulties associated with its variable time for onset of action, and multiple dangerous drug interactions. Large clinical trials of oral amiodarone in patients with prior myocardial infarction or heart failure have either been negative or demonstrated a reduction in sudden death but not total mortality. Unlike the Class IC drugs, amiodarone does not increase mortality and may have a small benefit in some patient populations. Intravenous amiodarone can be used for recurrent life-threatening ventricular tachycardia or fibrillation; hypotension is the major side effect.

CLINICAL PHARMACOLOGY. Amiodarone is slowly absorbed from the gastrointestinal tract, and bioavailability varies over a fourfold range. It is extensively metabolized to its desethyl metabolite (DEA); and little; if any, is excreted unchanged in the urine. Concentrations of DEA, which has antiarrhythmic potency equal to or greater than amiodarone, vary from 0.4 to 2.0 times that of amiodarone during chronic therapy. After intravenous administration, the measured half-life in plasma is from 4.8 to 68.2 hours. Slow redistribution of drug out of adipose and muscle tissues leads to slow and extremely variable elimination from plasma, with half-lives ranging from 13 to 103 days in the steady state.

DOSAGE AND ADMINISTRATION. Without a loading dose, amiodarone requires several weeks to months before producing its antiarrhythmic action. Large intravenous dosages or oral loading dosages can hasten the onset of therapeutic effects. Large clinical trials have utilized a loading dose of 600 to 800 mg daily for 14 days. The usual maintenance dose varies from 200 to 600 mg/day, and, because of the severity of adverse reactions, the lowest effective dosage should be prescribed. Patients with supraventricular arrhythmias may respond to lower dosages than those with ventricular arrhythmias.

For intravenous administration, the manufacturer recommends a three-phase infusion over the first 24 hours: 150 mg over 10 minutes, followed by 360 mg over the next 6 hours, followed by 0.5 mg/min. The drug can be continued at this rate, but monitoring of plasma concentrations is recommended. An additional 150 mg can be infused over 10 minutes for those patients who continue to have recurrent ventricular tachycardia or fibrillation or whose arrhythmia recurs during downward titration of the infusion.

Amiodarone concentrations are usually between 1 and 2 μg/mL during effective oral therapy. Similar concentrations of DEA accumulate during therapy and, although unproven, are likely to contribute to antiarrhythmic efficacy. Monitoring of plasma concentrations is of limited value, but levels of amiodarone above 3 to 4 μg/mL for prolonged periods of time are associated with a higher incidence of adverse effects.

ADVERSE REACTIONS. Intravenous amiodarone at dosages greater than 5 mg/kg decreases contractility and peripheral vascular resistance, producing severe hypotension in some instances. This effect may be due to the effects of the diluent polysorbate 80, because oral administration at usual dosages improves myocardial contractility.

The safety of amiodarone is controversial. The early reports and some recently completed trials found it to be very well tolerated, but experience in the United States has revealed a very high incidence of intolerable and sometimes lethal reactions.

The most serious adverse reaction is lethal interstitial pneumonitis, which may be more common in patients with pre-existing lung disease. Monitoring is essential because the pneumonitis is reversible if detected early. A chest radiograph every 3 months may be useful, but serial pulmonary function tests are of little value. Hyperthyroidism or hypothyroidism is seen in about 4% of patients. Accumulation of corneal microdeposits is almost uniform during long-term therapy and can progress to interfere with vision. Some white patients notice a slate-gray or bluish discoloration of sun-exposed areas of the skin. Thirty percent or more of patients have abnormally elevated serum hepatic enzyme levels, and progression to jaundice and cirrhosis has been reported.

DRUG INTERACTIONS. Amiodarone interferes with the clearance of many drugs such as digoxin, warfarin, quinidine, procainamide, disopyramide, mexiletine, and propafenone. The elimination of many other drugs may be impaired by amiodarone, and the lowest effective dosage should be sought.

Ibutilide (Convert)

CLINICAL APPLICATIONS. Ibutilide is a Class III drug for rapid conversion of recent onset atrial fibrillation or flutter. It has not yet been tested in other arrhythmias or in patients with atrial fibrillation or flutter of long duration (>90 days). It should not be given to patients who have hypokalemia, hypomagnesemia, or a QTc more than 440 msec at baseline. In controlled studies, ibutilide has terminated the arrhythmia in 5 to 88 minutes in approximately 44% of patients treated with 1 mg followed by either 0.5 or 1 mg; approximately 20% of patients responded to the first infusion and approximately 25% of those not responding to the first infusion responded to the second infusion.

CLINICAL PHARMACOLOGY. Ibutilide is available at this time only for intravenous administration. When given over 10 minutes, it distributes rapidly in a multi-exponential fashion with the clinically relevant component having a half-life from 2 to 12 hours (mean = 6 hours). The drug is mainly eliminated by oxidative hepatic metabolism and systemic clearance is rapid. Because formal drug interaction studies have not been performed, it is not possible to anticipate which enzymes are likely responsible for its elimination.

DOSAGE AND ADMINISTRATION. The recommended dose for a patient over 60 kg is 1 mg; if the patient weighs less than 60 kg, 0.01 mg/kg should be given over 10 minutes. For patients whose arrhythmias have not converted by 10 minutes after completion of the first dose, a second dose of equal size can be administered.

ADVERSE REACTIONS. The most serious adverse reaction is torsades de pointes, which was seen in 1.7% of patients in premarketing experience. The risk of torsades de pointes is higher in patients who are female and/or who have reduced ventricular function or electrolyte disorders.

CALCIUM CHANNEL BLOCKERS

Verapamil and diltiazem are useful in the management of supraventricular tachycardia, when they are administered to slow the ventricular rate in patients with atrial fibrillation or flutter and to treat and prevent atrioventricular nodal re-entrant tachycardia. Intravenous diltiazem is useful for the temporary control of rapid ventricular rate during atrial fibrillation and flutter. In controlled clinical trials, conversion to sinus rhythm is no more likely with diltiazem than with placebo. The usual dosages for calcium channel blockers for acute treatment are verapamil, 2.5 to 5 mg intravenously over 2 to 4 minutes, with another 5 to 10 mg if necessary 15 to 30 minutes later to a maximum total dose of 20 mg, or diltiazem either as an intravenous bolus of 0.25 mg/kg (about

20 mg) over 2 minutes, with a second dose of 0.35 mg/kg if necessary, or as a continuous infusion at 5 to 10 mg/hr with maximum dose of 15 mg/hr and maximum duration of 24 hours.

Adenosine (Adenocard)

CLINICAL APPLICATIONS AND PHARMACOLOGY. By directly slowing atrioventricular nodal conduction, adenosine is very effective for the acute conversion of paroxysmal supraventricular tachycardia caused by re-entry involving the atrioventricular node. Because of the fleeting and relatively selective action of adenosine on the atrioventricular node, it may be used as a diagnostic tool in patients with narrow or wide complex tachycardia. However, it is preferable to make the correct diagnosis before giving any drugs because of the risk of adverse effects.

After rapid intravenous injection, the half-life of elimination has been estimated as 1.5 to 10 seconds. The drug is rapidly metabolized in the plasma and in cells to form inosine and adenosine monophosphate. Maximal pharmacologic effects are seen within 10 to 20 seconds when given into a central line.

DOSAGE AND ADMINISTRATION. Adenosine should be injected intravenously into a proximal tubing site and flushed quickly with saline. For adults the initial dose is 6 mg injected over 1 to 2 seconds. If the arrhythmia persists, a 12-mg dose can be injected 1 to 2 minutes later. An alternative regimen is an initial dose of 50 μg/kg incremented by 50 μg/kg until the paroxysmal supraventricular tachycardia is terminated or side effects become intolerable.

ADVERSE REACTIONS. Adenosine is contraindicated in patients with sick-sinus syndrome or second- or third-degree heart block unless the patient has a functioning artificial pacemaker. Because of the rapid clearance of adenosine, side effects such as facial flushing, dyspnea, or chest pressure persist less than 60 seconds. Other less frequent side effects include nausea, lightheadedness, headache, sweating, palpitations, hypotension, and blurred vision.

DRUG INTERACTIONS. Dipyridamole pretreatment increases the potency of adenosine, probably because it blocks its cellular uptake; carbamazepine may potentiate the actions of adenosine. Caffeine and theophylline antagonize the actions of adenosine.

Kuhlkamp V, Mewis C, Mermi J, et al: Suppression of sustained ventricular tachyarrhythmias: A comparison of d,l-sotalol with no antiarrhythmic drug treatment. J Am Coll Cardiol 33:46–52, 1999. *In a randomized trial of 93 patients with an implantable defibrillator for ventricular fibrillation, d,l-sotalol significantly reduced recurrent ventricular tachycardia; there was no difference in mortality in the two groups.*

Myerburg RJ, Mitrani R, Interian A, Castellanos A: Interpretation of outcomes of antiarrhythmic clinical trials: Design features and population impact. Circulation 97:1514–1521, 1998.

Roden DM: Risks and benefits of antiarrhythmic therapy. N Engl J Med 331:785–791, 1994.

Woosley RL, Roden DM: The Sicilian Gambit approach to antiarrhythmic drug actions. *In* Members of the Sicilian Gambit (eds): Antiarrhythmic Therapy: A Pathophysiologic Approach. Armonk, NY, Futura Publishing, 1994, pp 85–101.

55 ARTERIAL HYPERTENSION

Suzanne Oparil

High blood pressure (BP) is a major health problem throughout the industrialized world because of its high prevalence (approximately 25% of all adults and over 60% of persons older than 60 years in the United States) and its association with increased risk of cardiovascular disease. Advances in diagnosing and treating hypertension have played a major role in the dramatic declines in coronary heart disease (−49%) and stroke (−58%) mortality that have occurred in the last 25 years. Major progress has been made in public awareness of the importance of high BP, in introducing antihypertensive therapies, and in controlling high BP in the population over this period. However, the most recent data from the National Health and Nutrition Examination Survey for 1991–1994 indicate that awareness, treatment, and control rates for high BP have actually declined in the current decade (Table 55–1). Of even greater concern is that the cardiovascular complications of high BP are increasing: Since 1993, age-adjusted stroke rates have risen, the

Table 55–1 ■ AWARENESS, TREATMENT, AND CONTROL OF HIGH BLOOD PRESSURE IN ADULTS*

	NHANES II 1976–80	NHANES III (PHASE 1) 1988–91	NHANES III (PHASE 2) 1991–94
Awareness	51%	73%	68.4%
Treatment	31%	55%	53.6%
Control†	10%	29%	27.4%

*NHANES = National Health and Nutrition Examination Survey. Adults aged 18 to 74 years with systolic blood pressure of 140 mm Hg or greater or diastolic of 90 mm Hg or greater or taking antihypertensive medication.

†Systolic BP, <140 mm Hg; diastolic BP, <90 mm Hg.

From Burt V, et al: Prevalence of hypertension in the US adult population: Results from the third National Health and Nutrition Examination Survey. Hypertension 23: 305, 1995; and Joint National Committee on Prevention, Detection, Evaluation, and Treatment of High Blood Pressure: Sixth Report of the Joint National Committee on Prevention, Detection, Evaluation, and Treatment of High Blood Pressure (JNC VI). Arch Intern Med 157:2413, Copyright 1997, American Medical Association.

slope of the age-adjusted rate of decline in coronary heart disease has leveled off, and the incidence of end-stage renal disease and the prevalence of heart failure have increased. These alarming trends support a need for greater emphasis on public awareness of the problem of high BP and on more aggressive approaches to antihypertensive treatment and BP control by caregivers.

DEFINITION

BP in human populations is distributed normally, and the cutoff point for high BP is arbitrary. The diagnosis of hypertension in adults is made when the average of two or more diastolic BP measurements on at least two subsequent visits is 90 mm Hg or more or when the average of multiple systolic BP readings on two or more subsequent visits is consistently greater than 140 mm Hg (Table 55–2). The patient should be clearly informed that a single elevated reading does not constitute a diagnosis of hypertension but is a sign that further observation is required. *Isolated systolic hypertension* is defined as systolic BP of 140 mm Hg or greater and diastolic BP less than 90 mm Hg. *Essential, primary,* or *idiopathic hypertension* is systemic hypertension of unknown cause. More than 95% of all cases of hypertension are in this category. *Secondary hypertension* (Table 55–3), i.e., systemic hypertension of known cause, accounts for fewer than 5% of all cases of systemic hypertension. The importance of identifying patients with secondary hypertension is that they can sometimes be cured by surgery or by specific medical treatment. Thus the morbidity and mortality of potentially ineffective empirical medical therapy can be avoided and the cumulative cost of medical treatment reduced.

Malignant hypertension is the syndrome of markedly elevated BP (diastolic BP usually greater than 120 to 140 mm Hg) associated with papilledema. *Accelerated hypertension* is the syndrome of markedly elevated BP associated with hemorrhage and exudates

Table 55–2 ■ CLASSIFICATION OF BLOOD PRESSURE FOR ADULTS

CATEGORY	SYSTOLIC (mm Hg)		DIASTOLIC (mm Hg)
Optimal	<120	and	<80
Normal	<130	and	<85
High-normal	130–139	or	85–89
Hypertension			
Stage 1	140–159	or	90–99
Stage 2	160–179	or	100–109
Stage 3	≥180	or	≥110

Subjects should not be taking antihypertensive drugs and not be acutely ill.

Isolated systolic hypertension is defined as systolic greater than 140 mm Hg and diastolic BP less than 90 mm Hg and staged appropriately (e.g., 170/82 mm Hg is defined as stage 2 isolated systolic hypertension). In addition to classifying stages of hypertension on the basis of average BP levels, clinicians should specify the presence or absence of target organ disease and additional risk factors. This specificity is important for risk classification and treatment (see Table 55–8).

Optimal BP with respect to cardiovascular risk is less than 120/80 mm Hg. However, unusually low readings should be evaluated for clinical significance.

BP is based on the average of two or more readings taken at each of two or more visits after an initial screening.

From Joint National Committee on Prevention, Detection, Evaluation, and Treatment of High Blood Pressure: The Sixth Report of the Joint National Committee on Prevention, Detection, Evaluation, and Treatment of High Blood Pressure (JNC VI). Arch Intern Med 157:2413, Copyright 1997, American Medical Association.

Table 55-3 ■ CAUSES OF SECONDARY HYPERTENSION

Systolic and Diastolic Hypertension
Renal
   Renal parenchymal disease
      Acute glomerulonephritis
      Chronic nephritis
      Collagen vascular disease
      Diabetic nephropathy
      Hydronephrosis
      Polycystic disease
   Renal vascular disease
   Renal transplantation
   Renin-secreting tumors
Endocrine
   Adrenal
      Primary aldosteronism
      Overproduction of 11-deoxycorticosterone (DOC), 18-OH-DOC, and
         other mineralocorticoids
      Congenital adrenal hyperplasia
      Cushing's syndrome
      Pheochromocytoma
   Extra-adrenal chromaffin tumors
   Hyperparathyroidism
   Acromegaly
   Pregnancy-induced hypertension
   Sleep apnea
   Coarctation of the aorta
Neurologic disorders
   Dysautonomia
   Increased intracranial pressure
   Quadriplegia
   Lead poisoning
   Guillain-Barré syndrome
   Postoperative hypertension
Drugs and chemicals
   Amphetamines
   Antidepressants
   Appetite suppressants
   Cocaine
   Cyclosporine
   Erythropoietin
   Ethanol
   Glucocorticoids
   Mineralocorticoids, including licorice and carbenoxolone
   Monoamine oxidase inhibitors
   Nasal decongestants
   Non-steroidal anti-inflammatory agents
   Oral contraceptives
   Phenothiazines
   Tyramine
Isolated Systolic Hypertension
Aging, with associated aortic rigidity
Increased cardiac output
   Thyrotoxicosis
   Anemia
   Aortic valvular insufficiency
Decreased peripheral vascular resistance
   Arteriovenous shunts
   Paget's disease of bone
   Beriberi

From Oparil S, Calhoun DA: High blood pressure. Scientific American Medicine, vol 1. Dale DC, Federman DD (eds): Scientific American, New York, 1998, Sect 1, Subsect III, p 1–14.

(grade 3 Kimmelstiel-Wilson retinopathy). If untreated, accelerated hypertension commonly progresses to a malignant phase. Both accelerated and malignant hypertension are associated with widespread degenerative changes in the walls of resistance vessels. These syndromes are characterized by extreme BP elevations, sudden onset, fulminant course, and evidence of severe, generalized vascular damage, including grade 3 or 4 Kimmelstiel-Wilson retinopathy, hypertensive encephalopathy, hematuria, and renal dysfunction. Malignant hypertension is usually fatal unless treated promptly and vigorously. If BP can be controlled, and it usually can be, the prognosis depends on the state of renal function.

People with *high-normal BP* tend to maintain pressures that are above average for the general population and are at greater risk of definite hypertension and of experiencing non-fatal and fatal cardiovascular events than the general population. As a group, these people manifest increased cardiac output, a more rapid heart rate,

and higher left ventricular ejection fractions than either the normotensive population or the population of patients with stable hypertension.

White coat hypertension refers to the situation in which a patient's BP is elevated when measured by a physician or other health care personnel but normal when measured outside the health care setting. The syndrome is best diagnosed by 24-hour ambulatory BP monitoring or home BP monitoring but may be suspected with any reliable BP measurements outside the health care setting.

INCIDENCE AND PREVALENCE

The prevalence of high BP increases with age (Fig. 55–1). High BP, an extremely common health problem in the geriatric population, afflicts approximately 65% of the population in the 65- to 74-year-old group. Blacks have a higher prevalence of hypertension than whites (38% versus 29%), and men have a higher overall prevalence of hypertension than women (33% versus 27%). Hypertension is more common in men than in women up to approximately age 50; after that age, hypertension is more common in women. Blacks tend to have more severe hypertension than whites. The prevalence of isolated systolic hypertension increases sharply with age: less than 5% in those younger than 50 years but up to 22% in those 80 years and older.

ETIOLOGY AND PATHOGENESIS OF ESSENTIAL HYPERTENSION AND ITS CARDIOVASCULAR COMPLICATIONS

Essential hypertension tends to cluster in families and represents a collection of genetically based diseases and/or syndromes with a number of underlying inherited biochemical and pathophysiologic factors (Fig. 55–2). In most cases, high BP results from a complex interaction of genetic, environmental, and demographic factors. The recent search for genes that contribute to the development of essential hypertension has found that the disorder is polygenic in origin. However, with several exceptions (such as angiotensinogen and α-adducin), the particular genes involved are still being sought.

Hypertension, in concert with other cardiovascular risk factors, leads to atherosclerosis (see Chapter 39) and other forms of vascular pathology by damaging the endothelium. If hypertension is accompanied by hyperlipidemia, as it is in more than 40% of the U.S. population, lipid-rich atherosclerotic plaques develop. In the absence of hyperlipidemia, intimal thickening occurs. Non-atherosclerotic hypertension-induced vascular damage can lead to stroke and end-stage renal disease, and increased afterload related to systemic hypertension is a leading cause of congestive heart failure. Furthermore, the neurohumoral factors that contribute to the pathogenesis of hypertension, including increased sympathetic nervous system activity and enhanced angiotensin II production, are independent causes of myocardial hypertrophy and vascular remodeling.

RISKS OF HYPERTENSION

The risk of cardiovascular disease mortality is positively related to both systolic and diastolic BP over the entire range. Follow-up data from more than 350,000 middle-aged men screened for the Multiple Risk Factor Intervention Trial show that the relative risk of cardiovascular mortality doubled when systolic BP was in the high-normal range (130 to 139 mm Hg) and diastolic BP was in the stage 1 hypertensive range (95 to 99 mm Hg) (Fig. 55–3). The risk for end-stage renal disease in participants of the Multiple Risk Factor Intervention Trial with high-normal BP (130 to 139/85 to 89 mm Hg) was double that for participants with "optimal" blood pressures. Furthermore, data from the Framingham Heart Study show two-fold and three-fold increases in the risk of congestive heart failure in hypertensive (stages 1 and 2) men and women, respectively, when compared with normotensive persons in the population.

DIAGNOSIS

INITIAL EVALUATION. The initial evaluation of a hypertensive patient should determine baseline BP, assess the degree of target

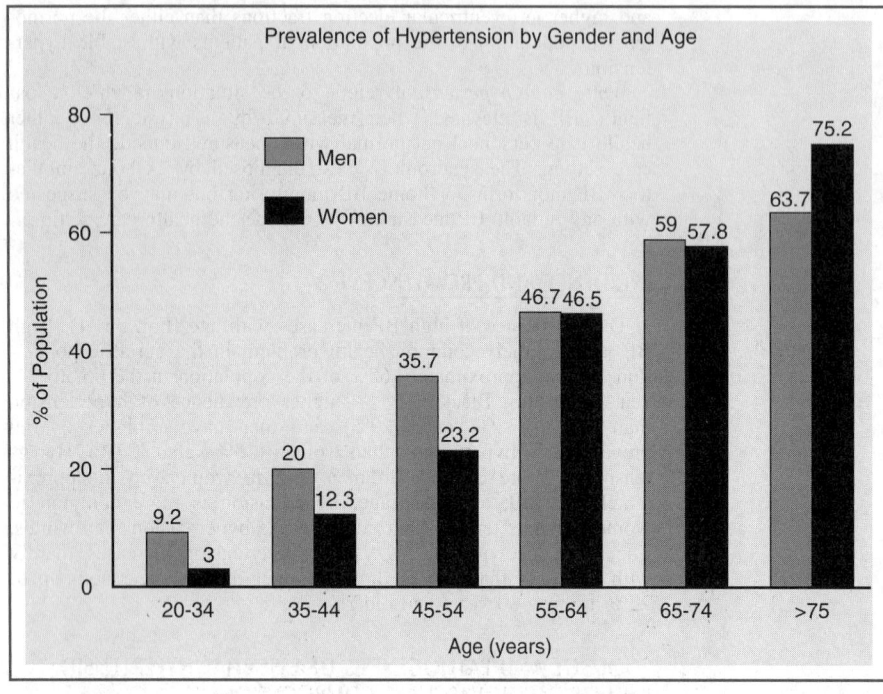

Prevalence of Hypertension by Gender and Age

FIGURE 55-1 ■ Prevalence rates of high blood pressure in the United States by gender and age from the Third National Health and Nutrition Examination Survey. Results are based on the average of three blood pressure measurements with systolic blood pressure of 140 mm Hg or less and/or diastolic blood pressure of 90 mm Hg or less. (From Burt VL, Cutler JA, Higgins M: Trends in the prevalence, awareness, treatment and control of hypertension in the adult US population: Data from the Health Examination Surveys, 1960 to 1991. Hypertension 26:60 1995.)

organ disease and the presence or absence of concomitant cardiovascular disease, screen for secondary causes of hypertension, identify other cardiovascular risk factors, and characterize the patient (gender, race, age, lifestyle, concomitant illnesses) to facilitate the choice of therapy (in particular, drug selection), and define that patient's prognosis.

BLOOD PRESSURE MEASUREMENT. Accurate and reproducible measurement of BP by the cuff technique is the most crucial part of the diagnostic evaluation and the follow-up of the patient. BP should be measured in a standardized fashion with the patient sitting after 5 or more minutes of rest and 30 or more minutes after smoking or ingestion of caffeine. A mercury sphygmomanometer is preferred; acceptable alternatives include a recently calibrated aneroid manometer or a validated electronic device attached to an arm cuff. Finger devices are unacceptable. Two or three measurements should be taken at each visit, and at least 2 minutes should be

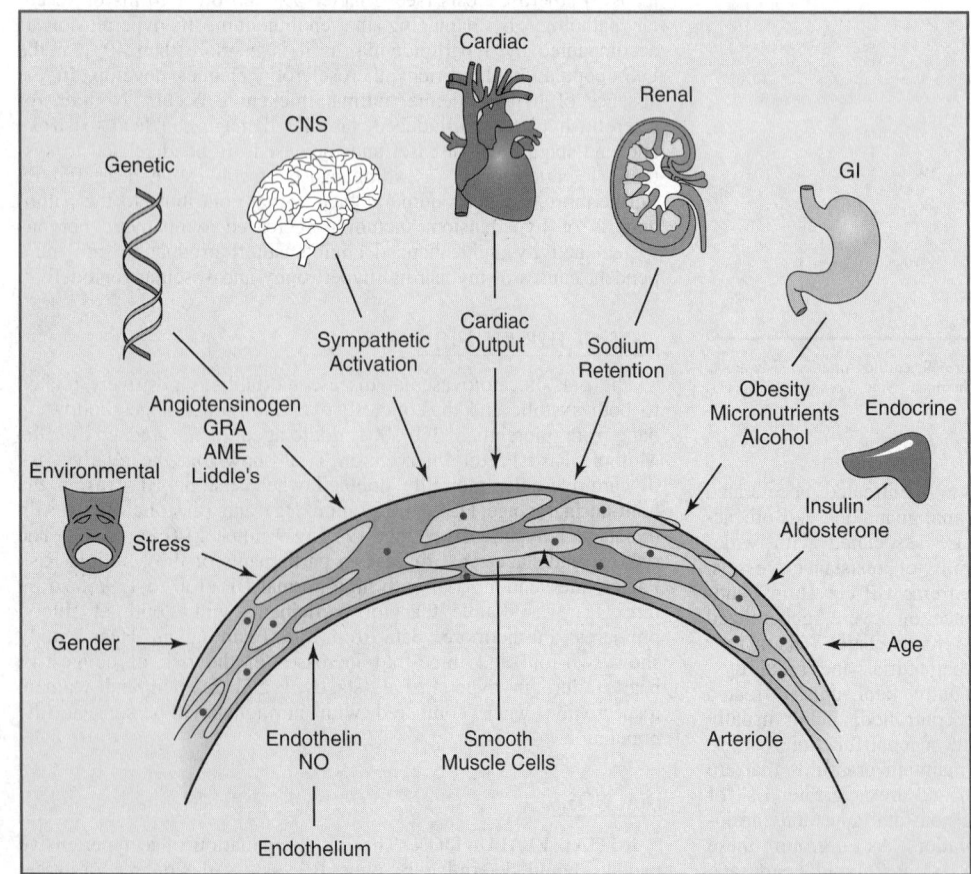

FIGURE 55-2 ■ Pathophysiologic factors most frequently implicated in the development of hypertension. These factors represent a combination of genetic and environmental influences.

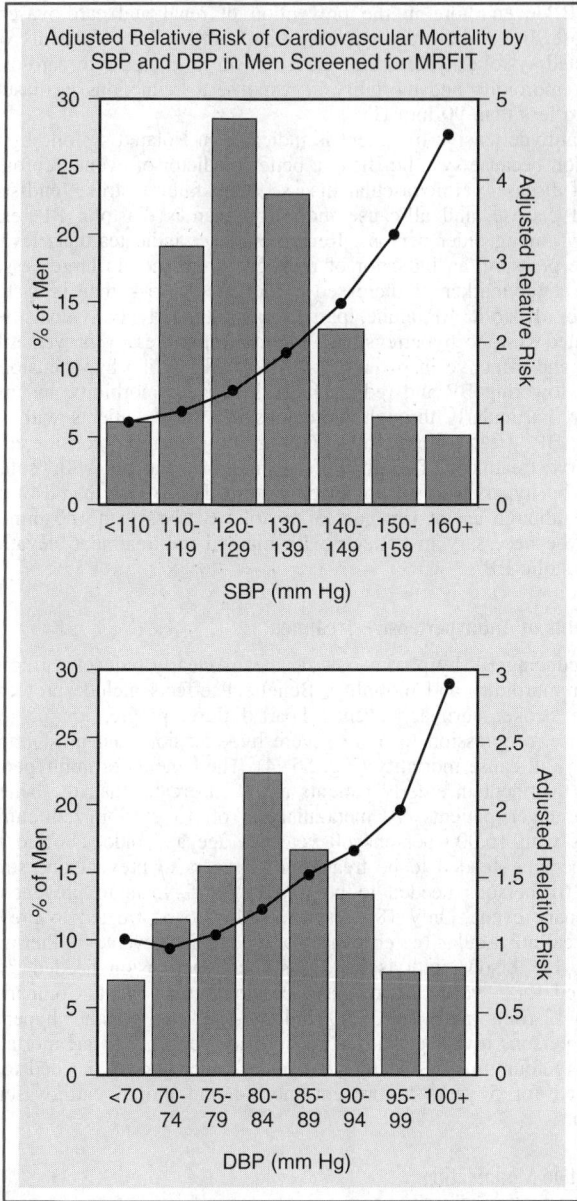

FIGURE 55–3 ■ Adjusted relative risk of cardiovascular mortality by systolic and diastolic blood pressure in men screened for the Multiple Risk Factor Intervention Trial. (From National High Blood Pressure Education Program Working Group report on primary prevention of hypertension. Arch Intern Med 153:186, Copyright 1993, American Medical Association.)

and the efficacy of treatment is augmented by considering both office and out-of-office BP measurements. Self-measurement of BP has several potential advantages, including distinguishing sustained hypertension from white coat hypertension, assessing response to antihypertensive treatment, improving adherence to treatment by making the patient a "partner" in the therapeutic plan, and decreasing costs by reducing the need for frequent office BP checks. The superiority of home or workplace BP measurements depends on the use of accurate and calibrated BP monitors, as well as careful and repeated instruction on how to measure BP.

MEDICAL HISTORY. A careful, complete history should be obtained and a physical examination performed in all patients before antihypertensive therapy is started. The medical history should focus on identifying known, remediable causes of high BP, establishing the presence or absence of target organ disease and cardiovascular disease, and identifying other cardiovascular risk factors or co-morbid conditions that might affect prognosis or treatment. Discussion of family history should include mention of familial diseases associated with secondary hypertension, including familial renal disease, polycystic kidney disease (see Chapter 115), medullary thyroid cancer (see Chapter 265), pheochromocytoma (see Chapter 241), and hyperparathyroidism (see Chapter 264). Discussion of the patient's personal habits should include physical activity, ethanol consumption, and diet. All current medications should be considered, in particular, agents that may exacerbate existing hypertension or antagonize or adversely interact with drug therapy (see Table 55–3). The physician should also begin assessing the patient's understanding of the illness and willingness to alter lifestyle if necessary.

PHYSICAL EXAMINATION. The physical examination should include height; weight; funduscopic examination; verification of hypertension in the contralateral arm; a careful examination of the neck, abdomen, and extremities for bruits; neurologic assessment; and if coarctation of the aorta is suspected (see Chapter 57), blood pressure measurement in the leg. Criteria for both treatment and prognosis are affected by the presence of target organ disease.

LABORATORY EVALUATION. Pre-treatment laboratory tests can be restricted to those generally performed as part of a routine medical checkup evaluation: complete blood count; urinalysis; serum potassium, sodium, and creatinine levels; fasting blood glucose; low- and high-density lipoprotein cholesterol levels; and a 12-lead electrocardiogram. These tests help assess the presence and severity of target organ disease and other cardiovascular risk factors and can be used as a baseline for monitoring the effects of antihypertensive treatment. Serial electrocardiograms and echocardiograms (see Chapters 42 and 43) may help assess the effects of hypertension and antihypertensive treatment on the heart, but their clinical utility in managing an individual patient is unclear.

TREATMENT

The goal of antihypertensive therapy is to reduce overall cardiovascular risk and thus cardiovascular morbidity and mortality. In any given patient, the decision to initiate therapy is governed by the risk of cardiovascular disease, which is determined by the extent of the BP elevation and the presence or absence of target organ disease and/or additional cardiovascular risk factors (Table 55–4). Consensus guidelines stratify hypertensive patients into risk groups for therapeutic decisions (Table 55–5). Risk group A includes patients with high-normal BP or stage 1, 2, or 3 hypertension who do not have clinical cardiovascular disease, target organ damage, or other risk factors. Persons with stage 1 hypertension in risk group A are candidates for a trial (up to 1 year) of vigorous lifestyle modification with BP monitoring. If the BP goal is not achieved, pharmacologic therapy should be added. For those with stage 2 or stage 3 hypertension, immediate drug therapy is warranted. Risk group B includes patients with hypertension who do not have clinical cardiovascular disease or target organ damage but who do have one or more of the major cardiovascular risk factors other than diabetes mellitus. This group contains the large majority of patients with high BP. If multiple risk factors are present, immediate drug therapy should be considered. Lifestyle modification and management of reversible risk factors should accompany drug treat-

allowed between readings. The width of the BP cuff should be about two thirds the width of the arm (15 cm in most adults), and more important, the bladder within the cuff should encircle at least 80% of the arm. Falsely elevated readings can be obtained when the bladder is too short, and the error is magnified if the cuff is also too narrow. Many patients will require a large adult cuff.

To obtain an accurate systolic BP, the cuff should be inflated rapidly to at least 30 mm Hg above systolic BP, as determined by palpating the radial artery. This approach is necessary to avoid underestimating the BP because of the auscultatory gap, which is an unexplained disappearance of Korotkoff sounds for some interval between systole and diastole. The systolic reading is taken as the level of BP at which clear Korotkoff sounds are heard with each heartbeat (Korotkoff phase I). The diastolic reading is taken at the level when sounds disappear (Korotkoff phase V).

Measurement of BP by patients or family members and/or automated ambulatory BP monitoring often helps verify the diagnosis and assess the severity of hypertension. BP values obtained outside the office setting have consistently been shown to be lower and to better correlate with target organ disease than BP measurements by health care personnel. Therefore, assessment of the need to treat

Table 55-4 ■ MAJOR CARDIOVASCULAR RISK FACTORS

Smoking
Dyslipidemia
Diabetes mellitus
Age older than 60 yr
Sex (men or postmenopausal women)
Family history of cardiovascular disease: women younger than 65 or men
  younger than 55 yr
Target Organ Damage/Clinical Cardiovascular Disease
Heart diseases
  Left ventricular hypertrophy
  Angina/prior myocardial infarction
  Prior coronary revascularization
  Heart failure
Stroke or transient ischemic attack
Nephropathy
Peripheral arterial disease
Retinopathy

From Joint National Committee on Prevention, Detection, Evaluation, and Treatment of High Blood Pressure: The Sixth Report of the Joint National Committee on Prevention, Detection, Evaluation, and Treatment of High Blood Pressure (JNC VI). Arch Intern Med 157:2413, Copyright 1997, American Medical Association.

ment. Risk group C includes patients with hypertension or high-normal BP who have clinically manifested cardiovascular disease or target organ damage. Patients who have high-normal BP accompanied by renal insufficiency (see Chapter 104), heart failure, or diabetes mellitus (see Chapter 242) should be considered for immediate pharmacologic therapy. Appropriate lifestyle modifications should be used as adjunctive treatment.

The initial goal of antihypertensive therapy for most patients is to lower diastolic BP to levels less than 90 mm Hg and systolic BP to less than 140 mm Hg with minimal adverse effects. More aggressive BP goals (130/85 mm Hg or lower) are recommended for patients with concomitant diabetes mellitus or renal insufficiency. Furthermore, when self-measurement of BP or automated ambulatory BP measurements are used to guide therapy, a reasonable BP goal is less than 135/85 mm Hg. For patients with renal insufficiency and proteinuria greater than 1 g/24 hours, a BP goal of 125/75 mm Hg or less is recommended. The ultimate theoretic goal is to achieve optimal BP levels with respect to cardiovascular risk, i.e., less than 120/80 mm Hg. However, such aggressive BP lowering is poorly tolerated by many patients and therefore impractical for the general population of hypertensive patients. Furthermore, concerns have been raised that reducing diastolic BP to levels less than 85 mm Hg may increase the risk of ischemic heart disease, presumably secondary to coronary hypoperfusion, the so-called J-curve hypothesis. This concern appears to be most relevant to hypertensive patients with pre-existing coronary artery disease and to those with a pulse pressure greater than 60 mm Hg. Data that support this hypothesis are predominantly retrospective and inconclusive, and large prospective clinical trials have failed to substantiate the J-curve hypothesis. Recent data support the value of lower-

ing BP even more in the prevention of renal and cardiovascular disease. In addition, clinical trial data from studies of patients with isolated systolic hypertension have shown no increase in cardiovascular morbidity and mortality in response to reductions in diastolic BP to less than 90 mm Hg.

Antihypertensive treatment is indicated in isolated systolic hypertension because systolic BP is a better predictor of events (coronary heart disease, cardiovascular disease, heart failure, stroke, end-stage renal disease, and all-cause mortality) than is diastolic BP, especially among older persons. Recent evidence indicates that elevated pulse pressure, an indicator of reduced compliance in large vessels, is a better marker of increased cardiovascular risk than is systolic BP or diastolic BP alone, particularly in elderly individuals with isolated systolic hypertension. Pharmacologic therapy is well tolerated and effective in patients with isolated systolic hypertension in both lowering BP and reducing cardiovascular morbidity and mortality, particularly through reductions in stroke. Patients with systolic BP greater than 160 mm Hg are generally considered to deserve treatment. The goal of treatment in patients with isolated systolic hypertension is to lower systolic BP to less than 140 mm Hg, although an interim goal of systolic BP less than 160 mm Hg may be necessary in patients with marked pre-treatment elevations in systolic BP.

Benefits of Antihypertensive Treatment

Reducing BP by pharmacologic means clearly reduces cardiovascular morbidity and mortality. Beneficial effects include protection from stroke, coronary events, heart failure, progression of renal disease, progression to more severe hypertension, and most importantly, all-cause mortality (Fig. 55-4). The benefits of antihypertensive treatment in elderly patients are even greater than the benefits in younger patients. A meta-analysis of 13 randomized clinical trials with 16,000 persons 60 years of age and older showed that 43 persons needed to be treated for 5 years to prevent one stroke and 61 persons needed to be treated for 5 years to prevent one coronary event. Only 18 persons needed to be treated to prevent one cardiovascular (cerebrovascular or cardiac) event. Furthermore, only 15 persons with isolated systolic hypertension needed to be treated for 5 years to prevent a cardiovascular event. Comparison with 12 trials involving 33,000 middle-aged and younger hypertensive persons revealed that for all outcomes except cardiac mortality, two to four times as many younger as older persons needed to be treated for 5 years to prevent morbid and mortal cardiovascular events.

Lifestyle Modification

OVERALL RECOMMENDATIONS. Non-pharmacologic interventions (lifestyle modifications) are generally beneficial in reducing a variety of cardiovascular risk factors, including high BP, and in promoting good health and should therefore be used in all hypertensive patients, either as definitive treatment or as an adjunct to drug therapy (Fig. 55-5). Although permanent modifications in diet and lifestyle are difficult to achieve and have never been shown in

Table 55-5 ■ TREATMENT STRATEGIES AND RISK STRATIFICATION

BP STAGE (mm Hg)	RISK GROUP A (NO RISK FACTORS, NO TOD/CCD)	RISK GROUP B (AT LEAST 1 RISK FACTOR, NOT INCLUDING DIABETES; NO TOD/CCD)	RISK GROUP C (TOD/CCD AND/OR DIABETES, WITH OR WITHOUT OTHER RISK FACTORS)
High-normal (130–139/85–89)	Lifestyle modification	Lifestyle modification	Drug therapy Lifestyle modification
Stage 1 (140–159/90–99)	Lifestyle modification (up to 12 mo)	Lifestyle modification (up to 6 mo)	Drug therapy Lifestyle modification
Stages 2 and 3 (≥160/≥100)	Drug therapy Lifestyle modification	Drug therapy Lifestyle modification	Drug therapy Lifestyle modification

For example, a patient with diabetes and a blood pressure of 142/94 mm Hg plus left ventricular hypertrophy should be classified as having stage 1 hypertension with target organ disease (left ventricular hypertrophy) and with another major risk factor (diabetes). This patient would be categorized as *stage 1, risk group C* and be recommended for immediate initiation of pharmacologic treatment.

For patients with multiple risk factors, clinicians should consider drugs as initial therapy plus lifestyle modifications.

Drug therapy is indicated for those with heart failure, renal insufficiency, diabetes, and high-normal BP.

TOD/CCD = target organ disease/clinical cardiovascular disease.

From Joint National Committee on Prevention, Detection, Evaluation, and Treatment of High Blood Pressure: The Sixth Report of the Joint National Committee on Prevention, Detection, Evaluation, and Treatment of High Blood Pressure (JNC VI). Arch Intern Med 157:2413, Copyright 1997, American Medical Association.

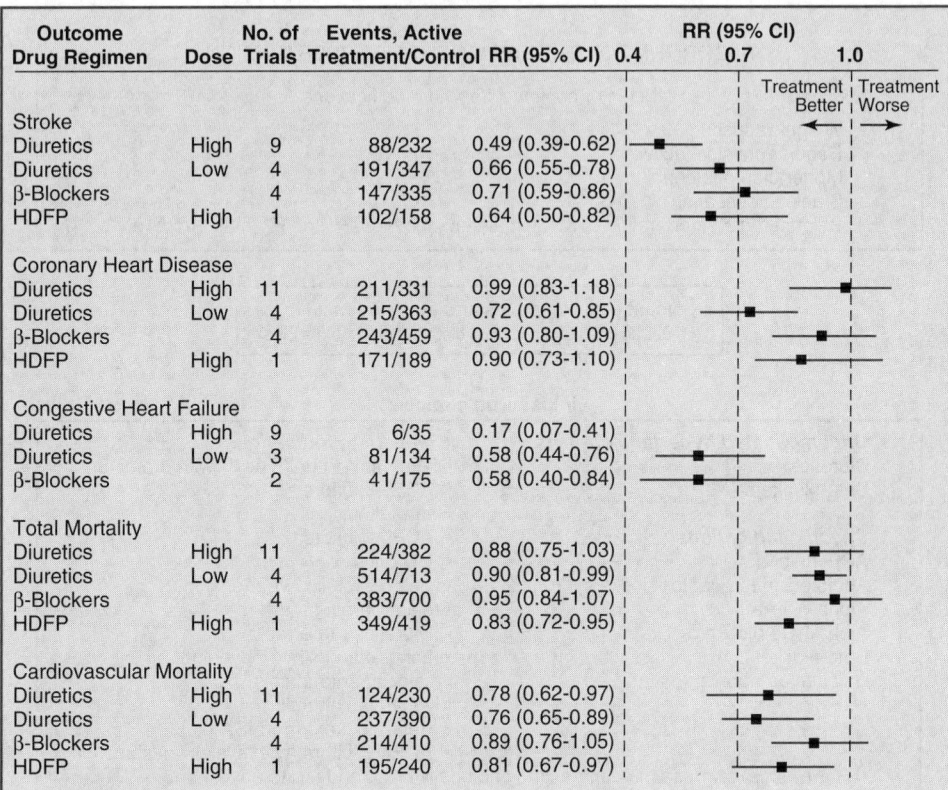

Outcome Drug Regimen	Dose	No. of Trials	Events, Active Treatment/Control	RR (95% CI)
Stroke				
Diuretics	High	9	88/232	0.49 (0.39-0.62)
Diuretics	Low	4	191/347	0.66 (0.55-0.78)
β-Blockers		4	147/335	0.71 (0.59-0.86)
HDFP	High	1	102/158	0.64 (0.50-0.82)
Coronary Heart Disease				
Diuretics	High	11	211/331	0.99 (0.83-1.18)
Diuretics	Low	4	215/363	0.72 (0.61-0.85)
β-Blockers		4	243/459	0.93 (0.80-1.09)
HDFP	High	1	171/189	0.90 (0.73-1.10)
Congestive Heart Failure				
Diuretics	High	9	6/35	0.17 (0.07-0.41)
Diuretics	Low	3	81/134	0.58 (0.44-0.76)
β-Blockers		2	41/175	0.58 (0.40-0.84)
Total Mortality				
Diuretics	High	11	224/382	0.88 (0.75-1.03)
Diuretics	Low	4	514/713	0.90 (0.81-0.99)
β-Blockers		4	383/700	0.95 (0.84-1.07)
HDFP	High	1	349/419	0.83 (0.72-0.95)
Cardiovascular Mortality				
Diuretics	High	11	124/230	0.78 (0.62-0.97)
Diuretics	Low	4	237/390	0.76 (0.65-0.89)
β-Blockers		4	214/410	0.89 (0.76-1.05)
HDFP	High	1	195/240	0.81 (0.67-0.97)

FIGURE 55-4 ■ Meta-analysis of controlled clinical trials of the effects of antihypertensive treatment with diuretics and/or β-blockers on cardiovascular outcomes and total mortality. (From Psaty BM, Smith NL, Siscovick, DS, et al: Health outcomes associated with antihypertensive therapies used as first-line agents. JAMA 277:739, Copyright 1997, American Medical Association.)

controlled trials to reduce cardiovascular disease morbidity or mortality, they may lower BP and obviate the need for drug treatment or reduce the dosage requirements of antihypertensive drugs to control BP.

Therapy should be tailored to the individual characteristics of each patient, such as weight reduction and exercise for an overweight patient and moderation in alcohol consumption for a heavy drinker. A reasonable generalized approach for all patients includes (1) reduced dietary sodium and increased calcium and potassium from food sources, (2) weight loss for overweight patients, (3) regular physical activity, (4) moderation of alcohol consumption, and (5) smoking cessation. Such an approach has been shown to produce significant sustained reductions in BP while reducing overall cardiovascular risk.

Two clinical trials, one with a comprehensive food plan that supplied the recommended dietary allowances of all the major nutrients and the other with a diet rich in fruits, vegetables, and low-fat dairy products and reduced in saturated and total fat, produced reductions in BP comparable with or greater than those usually seen with monotherapy for stage 1 hypertension. The Dietary Approaches to Stop Hypertension (DASH) trial showed BP reductions of 11.4/5.5 mm Hg in hypertensive persons receiving the diet rich in fruits, vegetables, and low-fat dairy products when compared with control subjects ingesting a so-called usual American diet, with dietary sodium intake and weight held constant. Furthermore, the DASH "combination diet" produced reductions in BP of 3.5/2.1 mm Hg in subjects without hypertension. Thus in well-motivated patients with stage 1 or 2 hypertension, modifying lifestyle effectively lowers BP and may be more important than the initial choice of antihypertensive drug. The same lifestyle modification strategies that are effective in treating hypertensive patients may also be useful in the primary prevention of essential hypertension.

WEIGHT REDUCTION. A clear, direct relationship is seen between body weight and BP (see Chapter 11). Overweight individuals (body mass index, >27.8 for men and >27.3 for women) have an increased incidence of hypertension and increased cardiovascular risk. Weight loss is closely correlated with reduction in BP and is potentially the most efficacious of all non-pharmacologic measures to treat hypertension. Weight loss also enhances the efficacy of antihypertensive drugs. This effect is independent of dietary

sodium restriction and is seen in both obese and non-obese hypertensive individuals. Weight loss also reduces overall cardiovascular risk and tends to improve the patient's self-image and sense of well-being. Patients should avoid appetite suppressants, which contain sympathomimetics such as phenylpropanolamine that can elevate BP. Moreover, the appetite suppressant drugs fenfluramine and phentermine have been withdrawn from the market because of cardiovascular toxicity, including serious mitral, aortic, and tricuspid regurgitant lesions and, rarely, pulmonary hypertension. Weight reduction through a combination of dietary caloric restriction and increased physical activity is recommended for all overweight hypertensive individuals. Because sustained weight reduction is so difficult to achieve, more emphasis should be placed on prevention of weight gain, particularly in younger individuals with high-normal BP and in families with a high prevalence of hypertension.

INCREASED PHYSICAL ACTIVITY. At least 30 minutes of moderate-intensity physical activity such as brisk walking, bicycling, or yard work three times a week (preferably once a day) can lower BP in both normotensive and hypertensive individuals (see Chapter 12). Additional benefits of regular physical activity include weight loss, enhanced sense of well-being, improved functional health status, and reduced risk of cardiovascular disease and all-cause mortality. Accordingly, regular aerobic physical activity is recommended for all hypertensive individuals, including those with target organ damage. Patients with advanced or unstable cardiovascular disease may require medical evaluation before initiation of exercise or a medically supervised exercise program.

MODERATION OF ALCOHOL INTAKE. Alcohol consumption elevates BP, both acutely and chronically, and cross-sectional studies have demonstrated an association between increased BP and increased levels of alcohol consumption (see Chapter 16). Furthermore, excessive alcohol intake appears to cause resistance to antihypertensive therapy. Moderate alcohol consumption may reduce overall cardiovascular risk in the general population, but whether any risk reduction also occurs in the hypertensive population is uncertain. Alcohol consumption is not recommended for hypertensive non-drinkers; for drinkers, intake should be limited to 1 oz of alcohol (2 oz of 100-proof whiskey, 8 oz of wine, or 24 oz of beer) a day in most men and half that amount in women and small men.

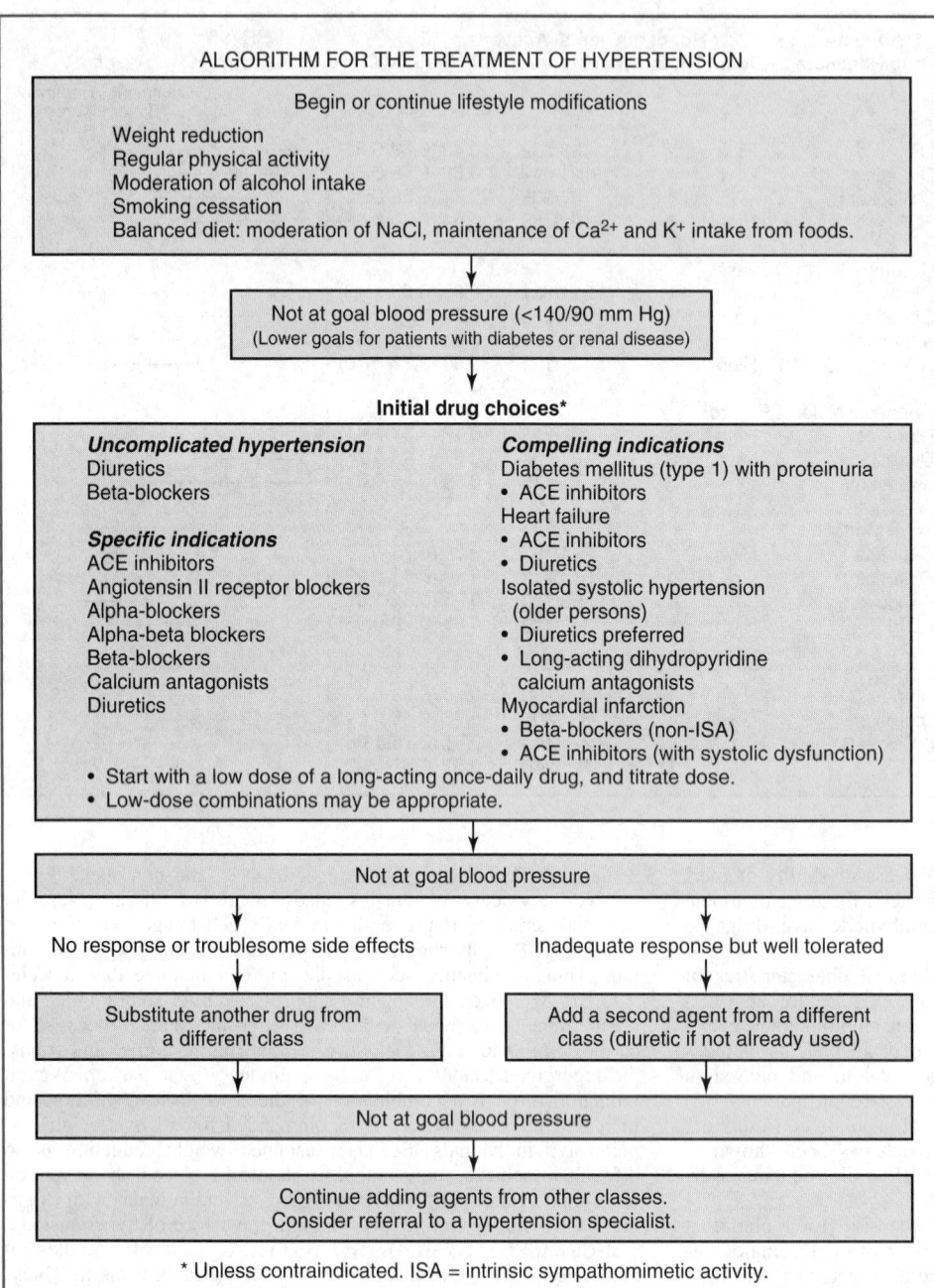

ALGORITHM FOR THE TREATMENT OF HYPERTENSION

Begin or continue lifestyle modifications

Weight reduction
Regular physical activity
Moderation of alcohol intake
Smoking cessation
Balanced diet: moderation of NaCl, maintenance of Ca^{2+} and K^+ intake from foods.

Not at goal blood pressure (<140/90 mm Hg)
(Lower goals for patients with diabetes or renal disease)

Initial drug choices*

Uncomplicated hypertension
Diuretics
Beta-blockers

Specific indications
ACE inhibitors
Angiotensin II receptor blockers
Alpha-blockers
Alpha-beta blockers
Beta-blockers
Calcium antagonists
Diuretics

Compelling indications
Diabetes mellitus (type 1) with proteinuria
• ACE inhibitors
Heart failure
• ACE inhibitors
• Diuretics
Isolated systolic hypertension
 (older persons)
• Diuretics preferred
• Long-acting dihydropyridine
 calcium antagonists
Myocardial infarction
• Beta-blockers (non-ISA)
• ACE inhibitors (with systolic dysfunction)

• Start with a low dose of a long-acting once-daily drug, and titrate dose.
• Low-dose combinations may be appropriate.

Not at goal blood pressure

No response or troublesome side effects

Inadequate response but well tolerated

Substitute another drug from a different class

Add a second agent from a different class (diuretic if not already used)

Not at goal blood pressure

**Continue adding agents from other classes.
Consider referral to a hypertension specialist.**

* Unless contraindicated. ISA = intrinsic sympathomimetic activity.

FIGURE 55–5 ■ Treatment algorithm for patients with essential hypertension. If the goal blood pressure is not achieved in response to a given intervention, the additional interventions indicated in the lower boxes are added. ACE = angiotensin-converting enzyme. (Adapted from Joint National Committee on Prevention, Detection, Evaluation, and Treatment of High Blood Pressure: The Sixth Report of the Joint National Committee on Prevention, Detection, Evaluation, and Treatment of High Blood Pressure [JNC VI]. Arch Intern Med 157:2413, Copyright 1997, American Medical Association.)

RESTRICTING DIETARY SODIUM. High sodium intake has generally been related to BP elevation, particularly in hypertensive individuals, but studies evaluating the antihypertensive efficacy of moderate dietary sodium restriction in unselected patients with essential hypertension have not demonstrated a large benefit. Recent meta-analyses of published studies have shown small but consistent reductions in BP in hypertensive individuals who participated in clinical trials of salt restriction. Furthermore, the magnitude of the decrease in BP in any individual did not correlate with the reduction in salt intake.

Recent evidence suggests that dietary salt restriction may have adverse effects. An observational study of a large cohort of hypertensive persons, all of whom were advised to restrict their sodium intake, showed that men in the lowest quartile of sodium excretion had a four-fold greater risk of heart attack than did those in the highest quartile. This observation, as yet unconfirmed in prospective, controlled trials, raises the possibility that sodium restriction may be harmful for some hypertensive persons. In addition, increased BP levels have been observed in some hypertensive pa-

tients when dietary sodium intake is reduced. The observed heterogeneity in BP response to restricted dietary sodium has given rise to attempts to classify hypertensive patients as "salt sensitive" or "salt resistant" and to develop biochemical indices of salt sensitivity. Patients with low renin activity, such as the elderly and black patients, are more likely to respond to sodium restriction with a decrease in BP.

Sodium restriction can minimize diuretic-induced hypokalemia, facilitates BP control with diuretics, and should be encouraged in patients who are receiving diuretics. Moderate sodium restriction (4 to 6 g of salt per day) can generally be recommended to hypertensive patients, with the realization that only a subset will benefit. Such sodium restriction can be accomplished by not adding salt to food during preparation or at the table and avoiding processed foods containing salt as the preservative. Salt substitutes, in which sodium is replaced with potassium, are useful in hypertensive patients who do not have renal dysfunction.

MAINTENANCE OF DIETARY CALCIUM INTAKE. An inverse relationship has been observed between dietary calcium intake and

Table 55–6 ■ ANTIHYPERTENSIVE DRUG THERAPY FOR PATIENTS WITH CO-MORBID CONDITIONS

INDICATION	DRUG THERAPY
Compelling Indications unless Contraindicated	
Diabetes mellitus (type 1) with proteinuria	ACE inhibitors
Heart failure	ACE inhibitors, diuretics
Isolated systolic hypertension (older patients)	Diuretics (preferred), calcium channel blockers (long-acting dihydropyridine)
Myocardial infarction	β-Blockers (non-intrinsic sympathomimetic activity), ACE inhibitors (with systolic dysfunction)
Favorable Effects on Co-morbid Conditions	
Angina	β-Blockers, calcium channel blockers (long acting)
Atrial tachycardia and fibrillation	β-Blockers, calcium channel blockers (non-dihydropyridine)
Cyclosporine-induced hypertension	Calcium channel blockers
Diabetes mellitus (type I and II) with proteinuria	ACE inhibitors (preferred), calcium channel blockers
Dyslipidemia	α-Blockers
Essential tremor	β-Blockers (non-cardioselective)
Heart failure	Carvedilol, angiotensin II receptor blockers, low-dose β-blockers
Hyperthyroidism	β-Blockers
Migraine	β-Blockers (non-cardioselective), calcium channel blockers (non-dihydropyridine)
Osteoporosis	Thiazides
Benign prostatic hyperplasia	α-Blockers
Renal insufficiency (except in renovascular hypertension and creatinine ≥265.2 mmol/L [3 mg/dL])	ACE inhibitors
Potential Unfavorable Effects on Co-morbid Conditions	
Bronchospastic disease	β-Blockers
Depression	β-Blockers, central α-antagonists, reserpine
Diabetes mellitus (types I and II)	β-Blockers, high-dose diuretics
Dyslipidemia	β-Blockers (non-intrinsic sympathomimetic activity), diuretics (high dose)
Gout	Diuretics
2nd- and 3rd-degree heart block	β-Blockers, diltiazem, verapamil
Heart failure	Calcium channel blockers (except amlodopine, felodipine)
Liver disease	Labetalol, methyldopa
Peripheral vascular disease	β-Blockers
Pregnancy	ACE inhibitors, angiotensin II receptor blockers
Renal insufficiency	Potassium-sparing agents
Renovascular disease	ACE inhibitors, angiotensin II receptor blockers

Note: Angiotensin II receptor blockers may be useful in the same clinical settings as ACE inhibitors, but this has not yet been demonstrated in controlled clinical trials.
ACE = angiotensin-converting enzyme.
From Joint National Committee on Prevention, Detection, Evaluation, and Treatment of High Blood Pressure: The Sixth Report of the Joint National Committee on Prevention, Detection, Evaluation, and Treatment of High Blood Pressure (JNC VI). Arch Intern Med 157:2413, Copyright 1997, American Medical Association.

BP in the general population. Furthermore, 75 to 90% of adults in the United States fail to consume the recommended daily allowance of calcium (1000 mg for adults younger than 65 years; 1500 mg for adults older than 65 years). Clinical studies of the BP-lowering effects of calcium supplements have produced mixed results, but the recent DASH trial showed that a diet rich in low-fat dairy foods is associated with major reductions in BP in both normotensive and hypertensive persons. Although the DASH trial was not designed to identify the specific components of the diet that are effective in reducing BP, it is likely that calcium and vitamin D derived from food sources contributed to the effects of the diet on BP. Maintaining the recommended calcium intake, preferably from food sources, is also beneficial for preventing osteoporosis and perhaps gastrointestinal malignancy.

MAINTENANCE OF DIETARY POTASSIUM INTAKE. An inverse relationship between dietary potassium intake and BP has been demonstrated, and high dietary potassium intake may lower BP in hypertensive patients. Inadequate potassium intake may increase BP. Hypertensive patients should maintain adequate potassium intake (50 to 90 mmol/day) by eating fresh fruits and vegetables. Potassium supplementation should be avoided or used only with extreme caution in patients with renal insufficiency, in diabetics, and in patients receiving potassium-sparing diuretics. Hypokalemia (see Chapter 102.3), whether caused by diuretic use or poor dietary intake, should be treated. Hypokalemia should be particularly avoided in patients receiving digoxin and in patients with known coronary artery disease inasmuch as it predisposes to arrhythmia. Potassium-sparing diuretics should be considered in patients who are hypokalemic before initiation of diuretic therapy or in whom hypokalemia develops while receiving a non–potassium-sparing diuretic.

OTHER INTERVENTIONS. Other lifestyle modifications, including relaxation and stress reduction, caffeine restriction, magnesium supplementation, changing the fat content of the diet, and garlic and onion consumption, have not been shown to produce sustained benefits in BP control.

Pharmacologic Therapy

GENERAL CONSIDERATIONS. Monotherapy with most antihypertensive drugs effectively controls BP in fewer than 50% of patients. Furthermore, changes in or discontinuance of treatment is frequent: several large studies of hypertensive patients have shown that 50 to 70% of new treatments were changed or discontinued within the first 6 months. Whether these high discontinuance rates reflect adverse effects of the drugs, poor efficacy, or other factors is uncertain, but this inconsistency in treatment probably contributes to poor BP control rates and the progression of target organ damage in the hypertensive population.

Non-adherence to prescribed therapy is a major problem in the management of hypertensive patients, and maximizing adherence is more important than choosing a specific drug regimen. A variety of factors, including cost of the medication and related care, inadequate patient education, complexity of the regimen, the patient's level of literacy and education, and the adverse effects of the medication, contribute to non-adherence to antihypertensive regimens. Clues to non-compliance include frequently missed appointments, failure to manifest the expected biologic effects of prescribed drugs such as heart rate slowing with β-adrenergic blockers, and alcohol and substance abuse.

The establishment of a good relationship with the patient and free and open communication about hypertension, its complications, and the goals and pitfalls of treatment are critical in enhancing compliance. Educational messages can also be delivered by office personnel. A positive and supportive approach to treatment—with the message that a drug regimen that is effective can be found for most patients—yields the best results.

GENERAL TREATMENT STRATEGIES. The initial choice of antihypertensive drug treatment is a topic of great interest and controversy for a variety of reasons, including the development of new drugs with real or perceived advantages over existing agents, cost issues, the lack of morbidity and mortality data for the newer agents, and a paucity of data comparing the efficacy and tolerability of agents from different classes. In the Captopril Prevention Project, captopril and conventional antihypertensive therapy with diuretics or β-blockers had similar efficacies in preventing cardiovascular morbidity and mortality in nearly 11,000 randomized patients. The Treatment of Mild Hypertension Study found that representatives of five of the major classes of antihypertensive agents (diuretics, α-adrenergic blockers, β-adrenergic blockers, angiotensin-converting enzyme [ACE] inhibitors, and calcium channel blockers) were equally effective in lowering BP and improving various outcome measures. The Veterans Affairs study found that a sustained-release preparation of the calcium channel blocker diltiazem had a small but statistically significant advantage in controlling BP. Neither study had the power to compare the effects of the treatments on cardiovascular outcomes.

Long-term, controlled clinical trials are needed to clarify the benefits and risks of cardiovascular outcomes associated with BP reduction with different classes of antihypertensive agents, particularly in patients with multiple cardiovascular risk factors. Clinical trials in progress around the world, with a projected patient enrollment of 200,000, are addressing this issue. Current data indicate that short-acting dihydropyridine calcium channel blockers are associated with an increased risk of adverse cardiovascular outcomes when compared with other medications and should be avoided.

For the minority of hypertensive patients without co-morbid conditions, target organ damage, or concomitant cardiovascular risk factors, drug therapy should begin with a diuretic or a β-blocker (see Fig. 55–5) because these are the only antihypertensive drugs that have been shown in randomized controlled trials to reduce cardiovascular morbidity and mortality and they are less costly and hence more cost-effective than the newer classes of drugs. For most patients, however, co-morbid conditions may dictate the choice of another class of drug and/or avoidance of diuretics and β-blockers for initial therapy (see Fig. 55–5, Table 55–6). For patients with coexistent diabetes mellitus or cardiovascular disease, randomized controlled trials have provided compelling indications for initial drug choices from specific drug classes. It is reasonable to individualize treatment on the basis of each patient's personal needs with respect to convenience, cost, and quality of life and, specifically, to initiate treatment with the agent that is expected to be best tolerated and is most likely to be effective in lowering BP over time. Long-acting agents are preferable because adherence to therapy and consistency of BP control are superior with once-a-day dosing.

When monotherapy is unsuccessful, a second agent, usually of a different class, should be added. Alternatively, low-dose, fixed-dose combination drugs can be used (Table 55–7). Low doses of drugs with different mechanisms of action may have additive or synergistic effects on BP with minimal dose-dependent adverse effects and the convenience of single-tablet dosing. In contrast, traditional fixed-dose combinations, which contain full conventional doses of each component, should be reserved for patients who do not respond adequately to monotherapy.

After therapy has been initiated, patients should be seen every 1 to 4 weeks (depending on the severity of hypertension) to titrate the antihypertensive drug dosage and every 3 to 4 months once BP control is achieved. They should be encouraged to measure and record their own BP levels at home or in the workplace as an aid to adherence and improved BP control. Recommended dose ranges for individual drugs are listed in Table 55–8 (see Table 55–7 for dose ranges for combination agents); common adverse effects are summarized in Table 55–9.

Patients whose BP cannot be controlled with an appropriate and optimal three-drug regimen that includes a diuretic and who are

Table 55–7 ■ COMMON COMBINATION AGENTS FOR TREATMENT OF HYPERTENSION

GENERIC NAME	TRADE NAME (MANUFACTURER)	DAILY DOSE (PILLS/d)	PILL CONTENT (mg/mg)
Centrally Acting Agents and Diuretics			
Clonidine/chlorthalidone	Combipres (Boehringer-Ingelheim)	1–2	0.1/15, 0.2/15, 0.3/15
Reserpine/HCTZ	Hydropres (Merck)	1–2	0.125/25, 0.125/50
Combination Diuretics			
HCTZ/amiloride	Moduretic (Merck)	1–2	50/5
HCTZ/spironolactone	Aldactazide (Searle)	1–2	25/25, 50/50
HCTZ/triamterene	Maxzide (Bertek)	1–2	25/37.5, 50/75
	Dyazide (SmithKline Beecham)	1–2	25/37.5
ACE Inhibitors and Diuretics			
Benazepril/HCTZ	Lotensin HCT (Novartis)	1	5/6.25, 10/12.5, 20/12.5, 20/25
Captopril/HCTZ	Generic (Mylan)	2–3	25/15, 25/25, 50/15, 50/25
Enalapril/HCTZ	Vaseretic (Merck)	1–2	5/12.5, 10/25
Lisinopril/HCTZ	Zestoretic (Zeneca)	1–2	10/12.5, 20/12.5, 20/25
	Prinzide (Merck)	1–2	10/12.5, 20/12.5, 20/25
Moexipril/HCTZ	Uniretic (Schwarz)	1–2	7.5/12.5, 15/25
Calcium Channel Antagonists and ACE Inhibitors			
Amlodipine/benazepril	Lotrel (Novartis)	1–2	2.5/10, 5/10, 5/20
Diltiazem/enalapril	Teczem (Hoechst Marion Roussel)	1–2	180/5
Felodipine/enalapril	Lexxel (Astra)	1–2	5/5
Verapamil/trandolapril	Tarka (Knoll)	1	180/2, 240/1, 240/2, 240/4
Angiotensin II Antagonists and Diuretics			
Losartan/HCTZ	Hyzaar (Merck)	1	50/12.5
Valsartan/HCTZ	Diovan HCT (Novartis)	1	80/12.5, 160/12.5
β-Blockers and Diuretics			
Atenolol/chlorthalidone	Tenoretic (Zeneca)	1	50/25, 100/25
Bisoprolol/HCTZ	Ziac (Lederle)	1–2	2.5/6.25, 5/6.25, 10.6.25
Metoprolol/HCTZ	Lopressor HCTZ (Novartis)	1–2	50/25, 100/25, 100/50
Propranolol/HCTZ	Inderide (Wyeth-Ayerst)	1–2	40/25, 80/25
Propranolol LA/HCTZ	Inderide LA (Wyeth-Ayerst)	1	80/50, 120/50, 160/50
Timolol/HCTZ	Timolide (Merck)	1–2	10/25
Vasodilators and Diuretics			
Prazosin/polythiazide	Minizide (Pfizer)	2–4	1/0.5, 2/0.5, 5/0.5

HCTZ = hydrochlorothiazide; ACE = angiotensin-converting enzyme; LA = long acting.

Table 55–8 ■ COMMON ANTIHYPERTENSIVE DRUGS IN AMBULATORY TREATMENT OF HYPERTENSION

GENERIC NAME	TRADE NAME (MANUFACTURER)	ADULT MAINTENANCE DOSE (mg/d)	FREQUENCY OF ADMINISTRATION (TIMES/d)	DURATION OF ACTION (hr)
Adrenergic Inhibitors				
Central α_2 agonists				
Clonidine	Catapres (Boehringer-Ingelheim)	0.2–0.6	2	6–12
Clonidine patch	Catapres-TTS (Boehringer-Ingelheim)	1 patch (0.1, 0.2, 0.3 mg)	Weekly	7 d
Guanabenz	Wytensin (Wyeth-Ayerst)	8–64	2	8–12
Guanfacine	Tenex (Robins)	1–3	1	12–24
Methyldopa	Aldomet (Merck)	500–2000	2	6–12
β-Adrenergic blockers				
Acebutolol	Sectral (Wyeth-Ayerst)	400–1200	1 or 2	12–24
Atenolol	Tenormin (Zeneca)	50–100	1	24
Carteolol	Cartrol (Abbott)	2.5–10	1	24
Betaxolol	Kerlone (Searle)	10–20	1	24
Bisoprolol	Zebeta (Lederle)	2.5–20	1	24
Metoprolol	Lopressor (Novartis)	100–450	1 or 2	12
Metoprolol sustained release	Toprol XL (Astra)	50–400	1	24
Nadolol	Generic (Mylan)	40–320	1	24
Penbutolol	Levatol (Schwarz Pharma)	20	1	24
Pindolol	Generic	10–60	2	6–12
Propranolol	Inderal (Wyeth-Ayerst)	40–640	2	6–12
Propranolol sustained release	Inderal LA (Wyeth-Ayerst)	80–640	1	24
Timolol	Blocadren (Merck)	20–60	2	6–12
α_1-Adrenergic blockers				
Doxazosin	Cardura (Pfizer)	2–16	1	24
Prazosin	Minipress (Pfizer)	2.5–20	2 or 3	3–6
Terazosin	Hytrin (Abbott)	1–20	1	24
Mixed α- and β-adrenergic blockers				
Carvedilol	Coreg (SmithKline Beecham)	12.5–50	2	7–10
Labetalol	Normodyne (Schering) Trandate (Glaxo Wellcome)	200–2400	2	3–6
Diuretics				
Thiazides and related sulfonamides				
Chlorthalidone	Hygroton (Rhone-Poulenc Rorer)	12.5–100	1	24–72
	Thalitone (Monarch)	15–50	1	24–72
Hydrochlorothiazide	HydroDIURIL (Merck)	12.5–50	1–2	12–18
Indapamide	Lozol (Rhone-Poulenc Rorer)	1.25–5.0	1	18–24
Metolazone	Mykrox (Medeva)	0.5–1.0	1–2	12
	Zaroxolyn (Medeva)	2.5–5.0	1–2	12–24
Loop diuretics				
Bumetanide	Generic (Mylan)	0.5–2.0	2	1–4
Ethacrynic acid	Edecrin (Merck)	50–400	2	3–6
Furosemide	Lasix (Hoechst Marion Roussel)	80–600	2	3–6
Torsemide	Demadex (Boehringer Mannheim)	5–10	1	8–12
Potassium-sparing diuretics				
Amiloride	Midamor (Merck)	5–20	1	24
Spironolactone	Aldactone (Searle)	50–400	1–2	3–6
Triamterene	Dyrenium (SmithKline Beecham)	50–300	1–2	3–6
Angiotensin-Converting Enzyme Inhibitors				
Benazepril	Lotensin (Novartis)	10–80	1 or 2	12–24
Captopril	Generic (Mylan)	75–450	2–3	4–8
Enalapril	Vasotec (Merck)	5–40	1 or 2	12–24
Fosinopril	Monopril (Bristol-Myers Squibb)	10–80	1 or 2	12–24
Lisinopril	Prinivil (Merck) Zestril (Zeneca)	10–40	1	24
Moexipril	Univasc (Schwarz-Pharma)	7.5–30	1 or 2	12–24
Quinapril	Accupril (Parke-Davis)	10–80	1 or 2	12–24
Ramipril	Altace (Hoechst Marion Roussel)	2.5–20	1 or 2	12–24
Trandolapril	Mavik (Knoll)	1–4	1	24
Angiotensin II Antagonists				
Candesartan cilexetil	Atacand (Astra)	8–32	1 or 2	24
Irbesartan	Avapro (Sanobil)	75–300	1	24

Table continued on following page

Table 55–8 ■ COMMON ANTIHYPERTENSIVE DRUGS IN AMBULATORY TREATMENT OF HYPERTENSION *Continued*

GENERIC NAME	TRADE NAME MANUFACTURER)	ADULT MAINTENANCE DOSE (mg/d)	FREQUENCY OF ADMIN- ISTRATION (TIMES/d)	DURATION OF ACTION (hr)
Losartan	Cozaar (Merck)	25–100	1 or 2	12–24
Telmisartan	Micardis (Boehringer In- gelheim)	40–80	1	24
Valsartan	Diovan (Novartis)	80–320	1	24
Calcium Channel Antagonists				
Dihydropyridines				
Amlodipine	Norvasc (Pfizer)	2.5–10	1	24
Felodipine	Plendil (Astra)	2.5–10	1	24
Isradipine	DynaCirc (Novartis)	5–20	2	3–6
	DynaCirc CR (Novartis)	5–20	1	24
Nifedipine	Procardia XL (Pfizer) Adalat CC (Bayer)	30–90	1	24
Nicardipine	Generic	60–120	2	12
Nisoldipine	Sular (Zeneca)	20–60	1	12–24
Non-dihydropyridines				
Diltiazem	Cardizem SR (Hoechst Marion Roussel)	120–360	2	12
	Cardizem CD (Hoechst Marion Roussel)	120–360	1	24
	Dilacor XR (Watson)	120–540	1	24
	Tiazac (Forest)	120–540	1	24
Verapamil	Calan SR (Searle)	120–480	1	24
	Covera-HS (Searle)	180–480	1 (at bedtime)	24
	Isoptin SR (Knoll)	120–480	1 or 2	12–24
	Verelan (Lederle)	120–480	1	24

LA = long acting; SR = sustained release.

adherent to the regimen have *resistant hypertension*. The most common treatable cause of resistant hypertension is volume overload, and these patients frequently benefit from the addition of a diuretic—a loop diuretic if they have concomitant renal dysfunction. Re-evaluation for secondary causes of hypertension and possible referral to a hypertension specialist are indicated.

Step-down therapy, i.e., withdrawing antihypertensive medication under close monitoring, should be attempted in patients with stage 1 or stage 2 hypertension whose BP has been adequately controlled for a year or more. Doses should be titrated slowly downward and medications discontinued one at a time, if possible. Step-down therapy is generally most effective for patients who are also making lifestyle modifications.

SPECIAL PATIENT GROUPS. SECONDARY HYPERTENSION. Clues from the medical history, physical examination, initial laboratory evaluation and clinical course help identify the 5% of hypertensive patients with specific causes for the disorder (see Table 55–3, Fig. 55–6). Patients with the more common and treatable forms of secondary hypertension share the characteristics outlined in Figure 55–6. The signs, symptoms, and physical and laboratory findings that point to a specific secondary etiology for hypertension may appear as part of the initial evaluation or may emerge in the course of follow-up, especially in conjunction with a disappointing response to usual medical therapy. Because some of these conditions can be superimposed on underlying chronic essential hypertension, it is particularly important to remain alert for these diagnoses in patients who have been treated for prolonged periods but whose hypertension is progressively more difficult to control.

RENOVASCULAR HYPERTENSION. Renovascular disease is the most common (1 to 2%) cause of curable/treatable secondary hypertension. Any lesion that obstructs either large or small renal arteries can cause renovascular hypertension. The most common and clinically important of these are intrinsic lesions of the large vessels (see Chapter 112) because they can be physically treated and the hypertension either cured or ameliorated. Of patients with renovascular hypertension, atherosclerotic disease is found in 75% overall and in nearly all elderly patients, whereas fibrous or fibromuscular disease is found in 25%, including the vast majority of younger patients.

The usefulness of screening tests for renovascular hypertension is highly variable, so patients should be referred to high-volume centers for testing. Patients most likely to have renovascular hypertension include those with hypertension of abrupt onset, especially in the young or in late middle-aged or elderly patients; those with

malignant hypertension or sudden acceleration of benign hypertension; and those who fail to respond to medical therapy. An upper abdominal bruit, particularly one that is systolic-diastolic or continuous in timing, is high pitched, and radiates laterally from the midepigastrium, occurs in one half to two thirds of patients with surgically proven renovascular hypertension. A precipitous drop in BP and/or acute deterioration in renal function in response to ACE inhibitor therapy suggests possible bilateral renal artery stenosis and warrants evaluation. A definitive diagnosis of renal artery stenosis is made by *selective renal angiography,* which defines the anatomy of the stenotic renal artery and hence provides information needed to plan the approach to revascularization. With the advent of safe and highly effective percutaneous techniques for renal revascularization, most angiographers now proceed immediately to angioplasty and use the BP response as a test of the functional significance of the lesion.

The natural history of renal artery stenosis is progressive arterial occlusion with loss of renal function. The treatment of choice is revascularization via angioplasty or surgery. For patients with obstruction of renal blood flow caused by an ostial stenosis at the origin of the renal artery and those who have unsuccessfully undergone balloon angioplasty, renal artery stents are useful in maintaining renal artery patency. Renal revascularization is seldom successful in curing hypertension in middle-aged or elderly patients with atherosclerotic disease but is useful in improving the ease of BP control with medical therapy and in preserving renal function. For patients in whom revascularization is not possible, strict BP control with medication should be attempted. Use of an ACE inhibitor or an angiotensin II receptor antagonist, alone or in combination with a diuretic, is preferred, except in those with bilateral renal artery stenosis, renal artery stenosis in a solitary kidney, or unilateral renal artery stenosis with severe parenchymal disease in the contralateral kidney. Renal function and serum potassium levels must be monitored closely, particularly when therapy is initiated. ACE inhibitors and angiotensin II receptor antagonists induce acute, reversible renal failure in this subset of patients as a result of impaired autoregulation of glomerular filtration secondary to blockade of the intrarenal renin-angiotensin system when renal artery perfusion pressure is reduced. Normal autoregulation of the glomerular filtration rate, which depends on an intact intrarenal renin-angiotensin system, is lost when the renin-angiotensin system is interrupted with these drugs.

Renal size and function must be carefully monitored in patients being treated medically for renovascular hypertension, even if BP is

Table 55-9 ■ COMMON ADVERSE EFFECTS OF ANTIHYPERTENSIVE DRUGS

DRUGS	ADVERSE EFFECTS	PRECAUTIONS AND SPECIAL CONSIDERATIONS
Diuretics		
Thiazides and related sulfonamides	Hypokalemia, hyperuricemia, glucose intolerance, hypercholesterolemia, hypertriglyceridemia, sexual dysfunction	May be ineffective in renal failure; hypokalemia increases digitalis toxicity; hyperuricemia may precipitate acute gout
Loop diuretics	Same as for thiazides	Effective in chronic renal failure; cautions regarding hypokalemia and hyperuricemia same as above; hyponatremia may occur, especially in the elderly
Potassium-sparing agents	Hyperkalemia	Danger of hyperkalemia in patients with renal failure or diabetes or those receiving ACE inhibitors
Amiloride	Sexual dysfunction	—
Spironolactone	Gynecomastia, mastodynia, sexual dysfunction	—
Adrenergic Antagonists		
β-Adrenergic blockers	Bradycardia, fatigue, insomnia, bizarre dreams, sexual dysfunction, hypertriglyceridemia, decreased HDL cholesterol	Should not be used in patients with asthma, chronic obstructive pulmonary disease, 2nd- or 3rd-degree heart block, and sick sinus syndrome; use in congestive heart failure requires careful titration, special precautions; use with caution in patients with diabetes and peripheral vascular disease; sudden withdrawal of these drugs may be hazardous
Central α-agonists	Drowsiness, dry mouth, fatigue	Rebound hypertension may occur with abrupt discontinuance
Methyldopa	—	May cause liver damage and positive direct Coombs' test (rare hemolytic anemia)
Reserpine	Sexual dysfunction, nasal congestion, lethargy	Contraindicated in patients with a history of depression; use with caution in patients with a history of peptic ulcer
α₁-Adrenergic blockers	"1st-dose" syncope, orthostatic hypotension, weakness, palpitations, dizziness, headache, fluid retention	Use cautiously in elderly patients
Combined α- and β-adrenergic blockers	Nausea, fatigue, dizziness, headache, orthostatic hypotension	Use with caution in patients with cardiac failure, chronic obstructive pulmonary disease, sick sinus syndrome, 2nd- or 3rd-degree heart block, diabetes
Vasodilators		
Vasodilators	Headache, tachycardia, fluid retention	May precipitate angina in patients with coronary heart disease
Hydralazine	Positive antinuclear antibody (without other changes)	Lupus syndrome may occur (rare at recommended doses)
Minoxidil	Hypertrichosis, ascites (rare)	May cause or aggravate pleural and pericardial effusions
Angiotensin-Converting Enzyme Inhibitors		
ACE inhibitors	Cough, taste disturbances, rash, hyperkalemia, angioedema (rare)	Can cause reversible acute renal failure in patients with bilateral renal artery stenosis; contraindicated in pregnancy because of possible teratogenic effects; neutropenia may occur in patients with autoimmune collagen disorders
Angiotensin II Antagonists		
Angiotensin II antagonists	Hyperkalemia, angioedema (very rare)	May cause reversible acute renal failure in patients with bilateral renal artery stenosis; contraindicated in pregnancy because of possible teratogenic effects
Calcium Channel Antagonists		
Calcium channel antagonists	Headache, hypotension, dizziness	Use with caution in patients with congestive heart failure, heart block, sick sinus syndrome, bradycardia
Dihydropyridines	Ankle edema, flushing, increase in heart rate, gingival hypertrophy	
Diltiazem	1st-degree heart block, bradycardia, worsening of systolic dysfunction	
Verapamil	Constipation, 1st-degree heart block, bradycardia	

ACE = angiotensin-converting enzyme; HDL = high-density lipoprotein; HMG CoA = hepatic hydroxymethylglutaryl coenzyme A.

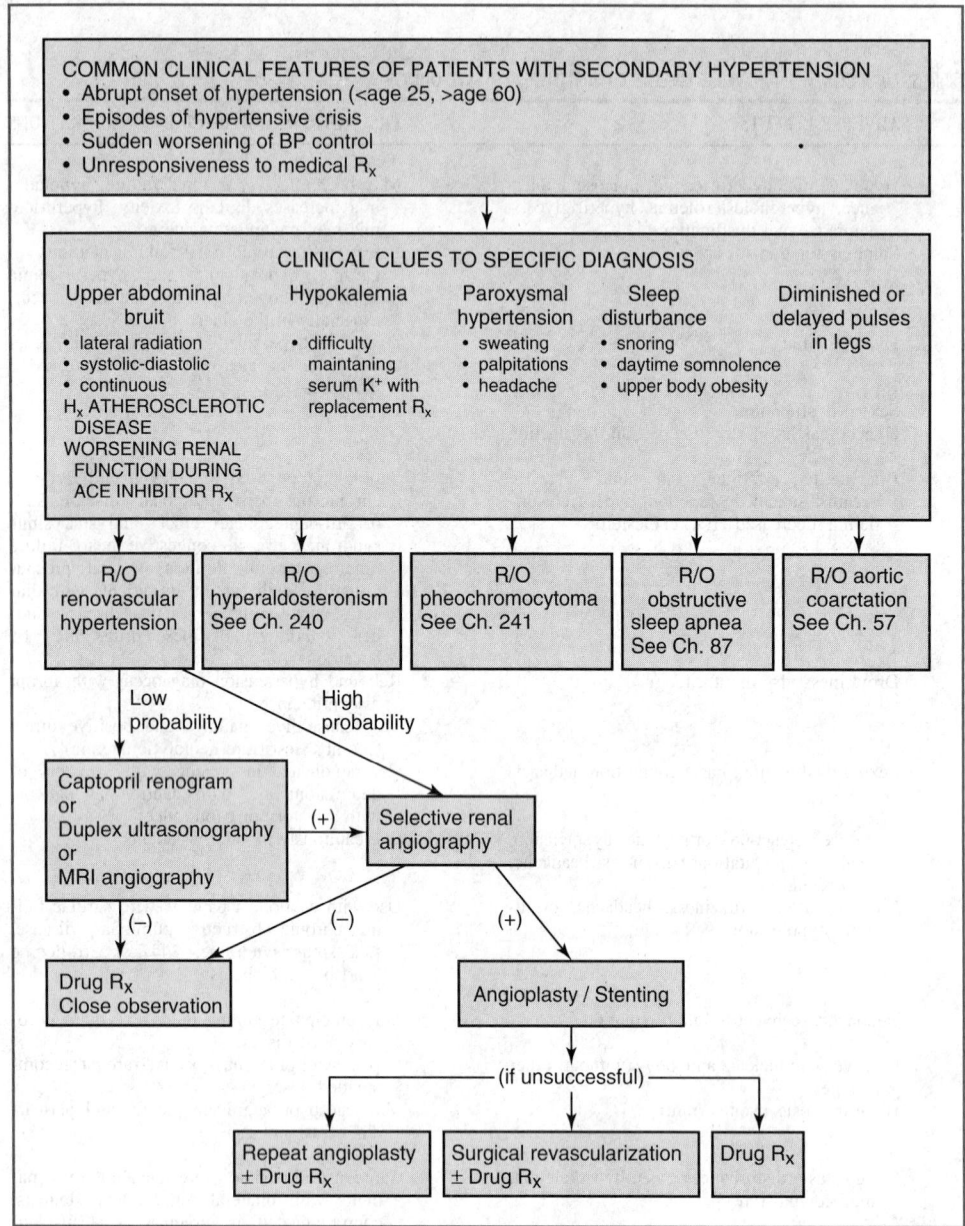

FIGURE 55–6 ■ Algorithm for identifying patients for evaluation of secondary causes of hypertension.

satisfactorily controlled. Renal function can deteriorate and renal mass can be lost very rapidly in patients with atherosclerotic disease who are treated medically. Significant reduction in renal size is the most sensitive index of loss of renal mass. Serial (every 3 to 6 months) estimates of renal size are important for monitoring patients who are receiving medical treatment for renovascular hypertension.

ADRENAL DISEASE. Primary aldosteronism (see Chapter 240) and pheochromocytoma (see Chapter 241) are relatively rare causes of hypertension that are clinically important because the associated hypertension can usually be cured with appropriate surgical or targeted drug therapy.

OBSTRUCTIVE SLEEP APNEA. Approximately 50% of patients with obstructive sleep apnea (see Chapter 87) are hypertensive, whereas up to 30% of hypertensive patients have sleep apnea. Recurrent hypoxia induced by sleep apnea may trigger sustained increases in peripheral resistance and cardiac output, in part secondary to chronic sympathetic activation, and thereby elevate BP. Alternatively, hypertension and sleep apnea may simply share risk factors, such as age and obesity, and occur independently. Effective treatment of sleep apnea benefits BP control, so all patients being

evaluated for hypertension should be questioned for the possibility of sleep apnea.

ORAL CONTRACEPTIVE–INDUCED HYPERTENSION. A small percentage of women who use oral contraceptives experience the onset of hypertension, which resolves by stopping oral contraceptive therapy. The diagnosis of oral contraceptive–induced hypertension can be made by documenting the onset of hypertension de novo during contraceptive therapy and resolution of the hypertension upon drug withdrawal. This form of hypertension usually begins during the first year of taking oral contraceptives.

CO-MORBID CONDITIONS. Co-morbid conditions, principally target organ damage and major cardiovascular risk factors, that influence the choice of antihypertensive therapy have been demonstrated in 50 to 70% of patients with essential hypertension, particularly in the elderly. Other common conditions that may influence drug selection include benign prostatic hypertrophy and osteoporosis (see Table 55–6). Agents that have added benefit for patients with these conditions should be considered as part of the treatment program, although additional drugs may be needed to bring the BP under control. Agents that have adverse effects on these co-morbid conditions should generally not be selected as first- or second-line

EMERGENCY	RECOMMENDED TREATMENT	DRUGS TO AVOID
Hypertensive encephalopathy	Nitroprusside, labetalol, fenoldopam, nicardipine	β-Blockers, clonidine, methyldopa
Subarachnoid hemorrhage	Nimodipine, nitroprusside, fenoldopam, labetalol	β-Blockers, clonidine, methyldopa, diazoxide
Ischemic stroke	Nitroprusside, fenoldopam, labetalol	β-Blockers, clonidine, methyldopa, diazoxide
Intracerebral hemorrhage	No treatment, nitroprusside, fenoldopam, labetalol	β-Blockers, clonidine, methyldopa, diazoxide
Myocardial ischemia or infarction	IV nitroglycerin, labetalol, calcium antagonists, nitroprusside	Hydralazine, diazoxide
Left ventricular failure	Nitroprusside, IV nitroglycerin	β-Blockers, labetalol
Aortic dissection	β-Blocker with nitroprusside or trimethaphan, labetalol	Hydralazine, diazoxide
Hyperadrenergic states (cocaine overdose, clonidine withdrawal, pheochromocytoma, diet pills, amphetamines)	Phetolamine, labetalol, nitroprusside, clonidine (for clonidine withdrawal only)	β-Blockers without α-antagonism
Acute renal insufficiency	Fenoldopam, nitroprusside, nicardipine, labetalol	β-Blockers, trimethaphan
Eclampsia	Magnesium sulfate, hydralazine, labetalol, calcium antagonists	ACE inhibitors, diuretics, trimethaphan
Postoperative crisis	Labetalol, fenoldopam, nitroglycerin, nicardipine, nitroprusside	Trimethaphan

ACE = Angiotensin-converting enzyme.

therapy but may be needed to control BP in patients with resistant hypertension who also have one of these co-morbid conditions.

DIABETES MELLITUS. Hypertension is twice as common in diabetics as in the general population, and diabetics with hypertension have a greatly increased risk of cardiovascular disease when compared with either normotensive diabetics or hypertensives without diabetes. Non-pharmacologic approaches, including weight loss, exercise, and decreased alcohol consumption, benefit both glucose and BP control. ACE inhibitors are recommended first-line agents for treating hypertension in diabetic patients, particularly patients with type I diabetes and/or diabetic nephropathy, because they reduce proteinuria and slow the rate of deterioration in renal function. Angiotensin II receptor blockers may have similar beneficial effects, but the clinical trials needed to test their benefits are not yet completed. Calcium channel blockers, α-blockers, and low-dose diuretics are also preferred agents because of their favorable or neutral effects on glucose and lipid metabolism and on renal function. Potassium supplements and potassium-sparing diuretics should be used with caution in diabetics because of the frequent occurrence of hyporeninemic hypoaldosteronism and consequent hyperkalemia in patients with diabetic nephropathy. Because of the aggressive nature of target organ disease development in diabetics, a lower BP goal (<130/85 mm Hg) is recommended.

OLDER PERSONS. Older persons benefit more from antihypertensive treatment than younger people do, at least in the short term. Therefore, aggressive treatment of high BP is strongly indicated in this group. However, older persons tend to be more sensitive to pharmacologic intervention, so antihypertensive medication should be prescribed cautiously at roughly half the usual recommended starting dose, and doses should be titrated upward slowly (6- to 8-week intervals). Elderly persons are more prone to orthostatic hypotension because of decreased sensitivity of their baroreceptors, so supine and standing BP should be checked regularly to avoid orthostatic hypotension. Low-dose diuretics and long-acting dihydropyridine calcium channel blockers are recommended as preferred agents because they have been shown in randomized clinical trials to prevent cardiovascular events and mortality in this group.

CORONARY ARTERY DISEASE. Antihypertensive therapy is strongly indicated in this high-risk group, but treatment should be initiated cautiously and patients monitored carefully to avoid rapid reductions in BP, which may precipitate myocardial ischemia. Accordingly, short-acting calcium channel blockers and oral clonidine should be particularly avoided in this group. β-Blockers have antianginal properties and are useful in the secondary prevention of acute myocardial infarction and sudden cardiac death. ACE inhibitors are indicated after myocardial infarction with left ventricular systolic dysfunction inasmuch as they have been shown in randomized controlled clinical trials to prevent heart failure and mortality in such patients. The utility of angiotensin II receptor antagonists in this context remains to be established in clinical trials.

HEART FAILURE. Hypertension is a major cause of left ventricular failure, and control of high BP improves left ventricular function, slows the progression of heart failure, and prevents death in heart failure patients. ACE inhibitors, used alone or in combination with diuretics and digoxin, have been shown in many clinical trials to both prevent heart failure and reduce morbid and mortal events in heart failure patients. A recent clinical trial has shown superiority of the angiotensin II receptor antagonist losartan over the ACE inhibitor captopril in reducing mortality in older patients with heart failure; further study is needed to establish the general utility of angiotensin II receptor antagonists in this condition. Alternative therapies include the combination of hydralazine with isosorbide dinitrate, the α, β-blocker carvedilol, and low-dose β-blockers. The long-acting dihydropyridine calcium channel blockers amlodipine and felodipine are safe in patients with heart failure; other calcium channel blockers should be avoided.

RENAL DISEASE. High BP is both a cause and a result of progressive renal dysfunction, often leading to end-stage renal disease, particularly in black individuals. Hypertensive patients with even slight elevations in serum creatinine levels have already suffered significant renal damage and should be evaluated thoroughly to rule out reversible causes of renal failure and treated aggressively (goal BP, <130/85 mm Hg or ≤125/75 mm Hg in the presence of >1-g proteinuria in 24 hours) to prevent progression of the disease. Multidrug therapy is usually needed to accomplish this goal, and an ACE inhibitor should be included in the regimen unless contraindicated. An initial small transient increase in serum creatinine (<1 mg/dL) is to be expected when BP is first lowered with antihypertensive treatment in these patients; greater increases or persistent increases are clues to the presence of renal vascular disease. Loop diuretics are generally needed for volume and BP control in patients with serum creatinine levels of 2.5 mg/dL or greater; potassium-sparing diuretics should be avoided in this group.

HYPERTENSIVE CRISIS. Hypertensive crises are subclassified as *hypertensive urgencies* or *emergencies*, depending on evidence of ongoing target organ damage. In the absence of neurologic, cardiovascular, or renal deterioration and funduscopic abnormalities, patients with severely elevated BPs (>200/120 mm Hg) do not require immediate BP reduction. However, with evidence of ongoing target organ damage, patients with severely elevated BPs should be immediately treated with parenteral medications, usually in an intensive care unit. A BP of 190/130 mm Hg may be well tolerated in a patient with chronic hypertension, whereas that BP reading in another patient may precipitate acute renal insufficiency, left ventricular failure, cerebral edema, or another vascular crisis, thereby creating a medical emergency. The triggering mechanism for the arteriolar lesion responsible for the development of accelerated or malignant hypertension is unknown but has been related to the absolute level or rate of rise of arterial pressure, the presence of disseminated intravascular clotting, or activation of the renin-angiotensin system. The syndrome is perpetuated by the deposition of fibrin in arteriolar walls, which leads to retinopathy, renal damage, and increased renin release.

Usually the cause of any particular hypertensive crisis is not known, and therapy must be empirical. Patients with *hypertensive emergencies* require parenteral antihypertensive therapy administered in an intensive care setting (Table 55–10). When the cause is

Table 55–11 ■ ANTIHYPERTENSIVE DRUGS FOR MANAGEMENT OF HYPERTENSIVE EMERGENCY

DRUGS	INTRAMUSCULAR (mg*)	SINGLE DOSE (mg*)	CONTINUOUS INFUSION (μg/kg/min)	ONSET OF ACTION	ADVERSE EFFECTS
Parenteral Agents **Direct vasodilators**					
Sodium nitroprusside (Nipride)	—	—	0.5–10	Instantaneous	Nausea, vomiting, muscle twitching, apprehension, sweating, thiocyanate intoxication
Fenoldopam (Corlopam)	—	—	0.1–0.8	5 min	Hypotension, nausea, vomiting, headache, flushing
Nicardipine (Cardene)	—	5/hr initially, titrated upward by 1–2.5/hr every 15 min as needed up to 15/hr	—	1–5 min	Hypotension, flushing, headache, diaphoresis, dizziness, nausea, tachycardia
Diazoxide (Hyperstat)	—	50–100 at 5- to 10-min intervals until satisfactory BP response is achieved	Rarely used	3–5 min	Tachycardia, palpitations, flushing, headache, nausea, vomiting, aggravation of angina or congestive heart failure or both, hyperglycemia, hyperuricemia, hypotension
Hydralazine (Apresoline)	10–40 min at 30-min intervals until satisfactory BP response is achieved	10–20 at 30-min intervals until satisfactory BP response is achieved	Rarely used	30 min intramuscularly, 5–10 min intravenously	Tachycardia, palpitations, flushing, headache, vomiting, aggravation of angina or congestive heart failure or both
Sympathetic Blocking Drugs **Ganglion blocking agents**					
Trimethaphan camsylate (Arfonad)	—	—	4–90	5–10 min	Urinary retention, paralytic ileus, paralysis of pupillary reflex and eye accommodation, dry mouth, orthostatic hypotension
CNS-active agents					
Methyldopa hydrochloride (Aldomet ester)	—	250–500; may be repeated at 6-hr intervals	—	2–3 hr	Drowsiness
α-Adrenergic receptor blocking agents					
Phentolamine (Regitine)	5–15	5–15 (rapid injection essential)	—	Instantaneous	Tachycardia, flushing
Labetalol	—	20 mg initially over 2 min, then 40–80 mg at 10-min intervals as needed up to 300 mg total	2 mg/min to a total dose of 300 mg	Instantaneous	Postural dizziness with or without postural hypotension; paradoxical pressor responses have been reported; nausea, vomiting, scalp tingling, burning in throat and groin

*Start with the lowest dose shown. Subsequent doses and intervals of administration should be adjusted according to blood pressure response. Constant surveillance is mandatory.

known, specific treatment should be instituted whenever possible (Table 55–11).

Symptoms of hypertensive crisis include headache, malaise, dizziness, blurred vision, chest pain, palpitations, and shortness of breath. Clinical and laboratory signs of hypertensive crisis include funduscopic changes (arteriolar narrowing, arteriovenous nicking, hemorrhage, exudates, papilledema); changes related to renal insufficiency; microangiopathic hemolytic anemia; signs of left ventricular dysfunction (S_4 and S_3 gallops, jugular venous distention, cardiomegaly, tachycardia, pulmonary edema); and evidence of increased intracranial pressure (confusion, somnolence, stupor, neurologic deficits, seizures). Patients with hypertensive emergencies may have stroke, subarachnoid hemorrhage, intracranial hemorrhage, aortic dissection, left ventricular failure, or myocardial ischemia. Importantly, however, severely elevated BP is often discovered coincidentally without any related signs or symptoms.

Evaluation of a patient with a hypertensive crisis includes a pertinent history, with a special attempt to elicit symptoms related to the cause or consequences of the severely elevated BP. Physical examination includes a determination of supine, sitting, and standing BP; neurologic evaluation; funduscopic examination; cardiac auscultation with evaluation of left ventricular size and function; and palpation of distal pulses. Chest radiography, electrocardiography, complete blood cell count with blood smear, and renal profiles and urinalysis should be performed. If by history, physical examination, or laboratory data the patient has evidence of ongoing (new or worsening) target organ damage, the patient should be considered to be having a medical emergency.

The goal in treating *hypertensive emergencies* is a prompt but gradual reduction in BP to just above normotensive levels. Precipitous or excessive reductions in BP may impair the body's ability to autoregulate blood flow and could cause target organ hypoperfusion. Ideally, BP should be reduced to 150 to 160/100 to 110 mm Hg and maintained at that level for a few days. Then, with initiation or reinitiation of long-term therapy, BP can slowly be returned to the normotensive range.

Hypertensive urgencies do not require immediate BP reduction, but rather initiation of maintenance therapy without acute oral loading for effective and sustained BP reduction. The prior practice of immediately reducing BP with oral loading of clonidine, nifedipine, or other rapid-acting antihypertensive agents exposes the patient to the unnecessary risk of acute end-organ hypoperfusion secondary to abrupt, uncontrolled decreases in BP and should be discouraged. However, after initiating maintenance therapy or adjusting existing therapeutic regimens, early follow-up is essential to ensure the efficacy of and compliance with prescribed therapy.

Appel LJ, Moore TJ, Obarzanek E, et al: A clinical trial of the effects of dietary patterns on blood pressure. N Engl J Med 336:1117, 1997. *This randomized, controlled feeding study compared the BP effects of a diet rich in fruits and vegetables and a "combination" diet rich in fruits, vegetables, and low-fat dairy products and with reduced saturated and total fat with a control diet that was low in fruits, vegetables, and dairy products with a fat content typical of the average American diet. Sodium intake and body weight were maintained constant. The "combination" diet reduced BP by 11.4/5.5 mm Hg in hypertensives and 3.5/2.1 mm Hg in normotensives, thus offering a novel nutritional approach to preventing and treating hypertension.*

Hansson L, Lindholm LH, Niskanen L, et al: Effect of angiotensin-converting-enzyme inhibition compared with conventional therapy on cardiovascular morbidity and mortality in hypertension: The Captopril Prevention Project (CAPPP) randomised trial. Lancet 353:611–16, 1999. *Captopril and conventional treatment did not differ in efficacy in preventing cardiovascular morbidity and mortality.*

Joint National Committee on Prevention, Detection, Evaluation, and Treatment of High Blood Pressure: The Sixth Report of the Joint National Committee on Prevention, Detection, Evaluation, and Treatment of High Blood Pressure (JNC VI). Arch Intern Med 157:2143, 1997. *Detailed recommendations for diagnosis and pharmacologic and non-pharmacologic treatment of systemic hypertension.*

Mulrow CD, Cornell JA, Herrera CR, et al: Hypertension in the elderly: Implications and generalizability of randomized trials. JAMA 272:1932, 1994. *A meta-analysis of randomized trials of antihypertensive therapy showing greater short-term benefit in elderly than younger patients. The limitations of randomized clinical trials are discussed.*

Psaty BM, Smith NL, Siscovick DS, et al: Health outcomes associated with antihypertensive therapies used as first-line agents. JAMA 277:739, 1997. *A meta-analysis of 18 long-term randomized trials of antihypertensive drugs including 48,220 individuals treated for an average of 5 years showed significant treatment-related reductions in stroke, coronary heart disease, congestive heart failure, and total and cardiovascular mortality.*

Staessen JA, Fagard R, Thijs L, et al: Randomized double-blind comparison of placebo and active treatment for older patients with isolated systolic hypertension. Lancet 350:757, 1997. *Placebo-controlled trial demonstrating that treating isolated systolic hypertension with the intermediate-acting calcium channel blocker nitrendipine as the beginning drug reduced total and non-fatal stroke by 42% and 44%, respec-*

tively, after only 2 years of follow-up. The study was stopped early because of this large benefit; other cardiovascular end points showed improvement, which in many cases did not attain statistical significance, perhaps because of the abbreviated follow-up period.

56 PULMONARY HYPERTENSION

Joseph S. Alpert

Pulmonary hypertension is defined as pressure within the pulmonary arterial system elevated above the normal range. Pulmonary hypertension may be acute or chronic; right ventricular (RV) failure may develop in either setting as a result of the increase in RV pressure work. Severe pulmonary hypertension even affects left ventricular (LV) function: RV dilatation secondary to severe pulmonary hypertension causes the interventricular septum to shift to the left, thereby decreasing LV volume and compliance.

A variety of pathologic disorders can cause pulmonary hypertension. These entities lead to changes in pulmonary circulatory function that elevate pulmonary pressure. Certain normal physiologic events can also elevate pulmonary pressures. For example, exercise-induced increases in cardiac output result in moderate elevations in pulmonary arterial pressure. Increased blood viscosity secondary to increased red cell mass (e.g., polycythemia vera) can also cause pulmonary hypertension. Moreover, increased resistance in any of the various vascular zones of the pulmonary circulation can lead to pulmonary hypertension. For example, increased pulmonary arteriolar resistance in a patient with congenital heart disease causes severe, chronic pulmonary hypertension. Finally, elevated pulmonary venous pressure in the setting of LV failure or mitral stenosis is associated with an immediate increase in pulmonary arterial pressure to maintain forward blood flow through the lungs despite the increase in pulmonary venous pressure.

Chronic pulmonary hypertension is an important cause of RV failure in the United States. Many of the 30,000 individuals who die each year of chronic obstructive pulmonary disease (COPD) succumb to RV failure resulting from pulmonary hypertension. In addition, approximately 200,000 deaths occur yearly from acute pulmonary embolism, a common cause of sudden-onset pulmonary hypertension and acute RV failure.

HEMODYNAMICS OF THE PULMONARY CIRCULATION

In normal individuals at sea level, pulmonary arterial blood pressure is quite low because pulmonary arteriolar resistance is low—one-twelfth of the value found in the systemic circulation. Therefore, normal mean pulmonary arterial pressure is only 12 to 15 mm Hg (Table 56–1). Normal left atrial pressure is also low at 6 to 10 mm Hg. Consequently, the driving pressure or pressure gradient across the pulmonary vascular bed is only 6 to 12 mm Hg; that is, a normal cardiac output of 5 to 6 L/min flows across the pulmonary vascular bed to the left atrium with a pressure drop of 6 to 12

Table 56–1 ■ NORMAL VALUES AT SEA LEVEL AND AT ALTITUDE FOR RESTING PULMONARY PRESSURES

VARIABLE	SEA LEVEL	14,900 FEET
Pulmonary arterial pressure (mm Hg, systolic/diastolic, mean)	20/12, 15	38/14, 25
Left atrial pressure (mm Hg)	5	5
Gradient (difference) between pulmonary arterial mean pressure and left atrial pressure (mm Hg)	10–12	20
Pulmonary vascular resistance (dynes-sec-cm⁵)	120	266

Modified from Fishman AP: Pulmonary hypertension. *In* Wyngaarden JB, Smith LH Jr, Bennett JC (eds): Cecil Textbook of Medicine, 19th ed. Philadelphia, WB Saunders, 1992, p 270.

mm Hg. This compares with a pressure drop of approximately 90 mm Hg across the systemic circulation.

The distensibility and low vascular resistance of the pulmonary circulation are the result of the thin muscular medial layer of the pulmonary arterioles. Systemic arterioles have a medial muscle layer that is considerably thicker. The lower resistance and hence pressure within the pulmonary circuit, compared with its systemic counterpart, are reflected in the right ventricle, which is less than half as thick as the left ventricle.

Pressure within the pulmonary arteries (Ppa) is directly proportional to three factors: the pressure within the pulmonary veins (Ppv), the cardiac output (CO), and the pulmonary vascular resistance (PVR). This relationship is expressed in the following formula:

$$Ppa = CO \times PVR + Ppv$$

Pulmonary hypertension develops when flow or resistance to flow across the pulmonary vascular bed increases. As already noted, a variety of physiologic and pathophysiologic mechanisms can lead to such increases in pulmonary pressures (e.g., exercise). In normal individuals, marked increases in RV cardiac output during severe exertion are associated with small increments in pulmonary arterial pressure; pulmonary pressure increases minimally during exercise in normal persons because pulmonary vascular resistance falls with increasing cardiac output. This fall in vascular resistance is due in part to arteriolar vasodilation and in part to opening or recruitment of previously closed microvessels.

Another "physiologic" cause of pulmonary hypertension is hypoxia, which is associated with ascent from sea level. The pulmonary hypertension of altitude results from hypoxic arteriolar vasoconstriction.

Other factors that may affect pulmonary pressures are blood viscosity, intrathoracic pressure, and endogenous vasoactive substances. Poiseuille's law predicts that pressure change along a tube containing a moving fluid is directly proportional to the viscosity of the contained fluid. Therefore, marked increases in the number of red blood cells per cubic milliliter of blood produce elevations in blood viscosity that can cause pulmonary hypertension. Another factor that can increase pulmonary arterial pressure is elevation in intrathoracic pressure, which is directly transmitted to the pulmonary vasculature. Increased intrathoracic pressure contributes to the pulmonary hypertension observed in patients who are being mechanically ventilated, especially if positive end-expiratory pressure (PEEP) ventilation is used.

Dysfunctional pulmonary vascular endothelium plays an important role in the pathophysiology of pulmonary hypertension. Normal endothelium releases growth factors and cytokines that regulate vascular smooth muscle tone, proliferation, and migration. Dysfunctional endothelium leads to vasoconstriction and intravascular thrombus formation. A variety of pulmonary vascular endothelial abnormalities have been demonstrated in patients with pulmonary hypertension, including impaired endothelium-dependent vasodilatation, decreased elaboration of vasodilating nitric oxide and prostacyclin, elevated circulating levels of the potent vasoconstrictor endothelin, and increased levels of various clotting factors such as fibrinopeptide A, Factor VIIIc, von Willebrand factor, and plasminogen activator inhibitor.

PATHOPHYSIOLOGY OF PULMONARY HYPERTENSION

A number of different pathophysiologic scenarios can produce pulmonary hypertension: increases in pulmonary flow, vascular resistance, blood viscosity, intrathoracic pressure, and vasoactive substances. "Hyperkinetic" pulmonary hypertension can be seen in patients with congenital heart disease (see Chapter 57) who have extensive left-to-right cardiac shunts that produce a large pulmonary blood flow (Table 56–2).

Pulmonary hypertension can be divided into three classes based on the location of the abnormal increase in pulmonary vascular resistance: precapillary, passive, and reactive. Patients with increased pulmonary arteriolar and/or arterial resistance are classified as having *precapillary* pulmonary hypertension. The pathologic

Table 56–2 ■ PATHOPHYSIOLOGY OF PULMONARY HYPERTENSION

MECHANISM	DISEASE ENTITIES
Increased pulmonary blood flow	Congenital heart disease with left-to-right shunts; marked increase in cardiac output (e.g., severe anemia); severe bronchiectasis with systemic-to-pulmonary artery shunts
Abnormalities in the pulmonary arteries: Increased resistance to flow or loss of cross-sectional area	Pulmonary embolism; pulmonary fibrosis; sarcoidosis; scleroderma; extensive pulmonary resection; severe COPD; thoracic deformities (e.g., kyphoscoliosis, severe pectus excavatum); schistosomiasis; extensive neoplastic or inflammatory infiltration
Abnormalities in the pulmonary arterioles: vasoconstriction and/or obliteration	Hypoxia (e.g., altitude); COPD, hypoventilation syndromes, (e.g., sleep apnea); acidosis; toxic substances; primary pulmonary hypertension
Abnormalities in pulmonary veins or venules: elevated pulmonary venous pressure and vascular resistance	Left atrial hypertension (e.g., mitral stenosis, left ventricular failure); pulmonary venous thrombosis; pulmonary veno-occlusive disease; mediastinitis (e.g., methysergide-induced sclerosing mediastinitis)
Increased blood viscosity	Polycythemia vera; leukemia with very high leukocyte counts
Increased intrathoracic pressure	COPD; mechanical ventilation, especially with positive end-expiratory pressure

COPD = Chronic obstructive pulmonary disease.

changes involve the pulmonary circulation proximal to the pulmonary capillaries (i.e., in the pulmonary arterioles and/or arteries). Pulmonary arterial pressure is increased, but pulmonary capillary wedge and pulmonary venous pressures are normal. The gradient between the mean pulmonary arterial pressure and the pulmonary capillary or pulmonary venous pressures is greater than 12 mm Hg. Examples include hypoxic pulmonary hypertension (increased arteriolar resistance) and pulmonary embolism (increased arterial resistance) (see Chapter 84).

Individuals with increased pulmonary venous pressure secondarily causing pulmonary arterial hypertension are said to exhibit *passive* pulmonary hypertension because the increase in pulmonary arterial pressure occurs passively—without active pulmonary arterial vasoconstriction. Pulmonary arterial, capillary, and venous pressures are all elevated. The gradient between the mean pulmonary arterial pressure and the pulmonary capillary or pulmonary venous pressures is less than or equal to 12 mm Hg. Examples of passive pulmonary arterial hypertension include mitral stenosis (see Chapter 63) and LV failure (see Chapter 47).

The third form of pulmonary arterial hypertension is termed *reactive* and contains elements of both precapillary and passive pulmonary hypertension. Reactive pulmonary hypertensive patients have elevated pulmonary venous pressure as well as pulmonary arteriolar vasoconstriction. The gradient between the mean pulmonary arterial pressure and the pulmonary capillary or pulmonary venous pressures is greater than 12 mm Hg. Patients with reactive pulmonary arterial hypertension usually have long-standing mitral stenosis.

Increased resistance to blood flow through the pulmonary arterial circulation can be the result of large pulmonary emboli or loss of pulmonary arterial cross-sectional area from various disease entities (e.g., pulmonary fibrosis, extensive pulmonary resection, vasculitis, or infiltration of the lung with tumor). Increased pulmonary arteriolar resistance is commonly the result of hypoxia and/or acidosis, which cause pulmonary arteriolar vasoconstriction. Certain specific vasoactive chemical compounds (e.g., pyrrolizidine alkaloids and anorectic drugs) can also increase pulmonary arteriolar tone. Patients with congenital heart disease with left-to-right shunts can develop markedly increased pulmonary arteriolar vascular resistance through a pathophysiologic process that begins as vasoconstriction and ends with obliteration and loss of pulmonary microvessels.

Primary pulmonary hypertension is the result of abnormal increases in pulmonary arteriolar tone. The resultant pulmonary hypertension in these patients leads to thickening of the intimal and medial layers of the pulmonary arterioles, which, in turn, further exacerbates the degree of pulmonary hypertension. A vicious spiral is thereby engendered in which ever-increasing levels of pulmonary arterial hypertension lead to further arteriolar thickening, which leads to worsening pulmonary hypertension. This pathophysiologic sequence is also seen in patients with congenital heart disease who develop pulmonary vascular disease and pulmonary hypertension.

Increased pulmonary venous pressure and vascular resistance are other causes of pulmonary hypertension: increased pulmonary venous pressure leads to augmented pulmonary capillary and pulmonary arterial diastolic pressure. Pulmonary arterial systolic and mean pressure must increase in this setting to maintain forward cardiac output. Disease entities that increase pulmonary venous pressure and resistance to blood flow include pulmonary venous thrombosis (e.g., sickle cell anemia, pulmonary venous occlusive disease, mitral stenosis, and LV failure).

DIAGNOSIS OF PULMONARY HYPERTENSION

Accurate non-invasive measurement of pulmonary arterial blood pressure can be obtained with the Doppler echocardiogram, but the physician must rely on clinical information obtained from the history and physical examination to select individuals for Doppler echocardiographic examination.

HISTORY AND PHYSICAL EXAMINATION. Patients with mild to moderate pulmonary hypertension are often asymptomatic. Individuals with more severe pulmonary hypertension usually complain of dyspnea on exertion secondary to exercise-induced decreases in cardiac output and increases in pulmonary arterial pressure. Other symptoms can include easy fatigability, exertional chest discomfort and/or syncope, cough, hemoptysis, and, rarely, hoarseness secondary to compression of the left recurrent laryngeal nerve by a dilated left pulmonary artery.

Physical examination (Table 56–3) in the patient with pulmonary arterial hypertension usually reveals one or more of the following signs: increased intensity of the pulmonic component of S_2, a diastolic murmur of pulmonic regurgitation in patients with severe pulmonary hypertension, evidence of RV dilatation (left parasternal lift or heave), or signs of RV failure (jugular venous distention, RV S_3 gallop that increases in intensity with inspiration), hepatomegaly, ascites, and/or peripheral edema. Patients with severe emphysema

Table 56–3 ■ COMMONLY USED CLINICAL CLUES SUGGESTING THE DIAGNOSIS OF PULMONARY HYPERTENSION

Increased loudness of the pulmonic component of the second heart sound
Right ventricular enlargement on physical examination: left parasternal impulse or lift
Signs of right ventricular failure present on physical examination: jugular venous distention, right ventricular S_3, hepatomegaly, ascites, hepatojugular reflux, peripheral edema
Right ventricular hypertrophy on the ECG
Enlargement of the right ventricle and/or pulmonary arteries on the chest radiograph, echocardiogram, radionuclide ventriculogram, or CT/MRI
Pulmonary arterial systolic blood pressure >30 mm Hg by Doppler echocardiography or catheterization

and increased thoracic anteroposterior diameter may not display the findings usually associated with advanced pulmonary hypertension because chest expansion makes palpation and auscultation more difficult.

THE ELECTROCARDIOGRAM. Electrocardiographic (ECG) diagnosis of RV hypertrophy (RVH) is often the first suggestion that pulmonary hypertension is present (Table 56–4). However, the finding of RVH by ECG is often a late finding in patients with pulmonary hypertension. Acute RV strain (an S wave in lead I and a Q wave and inverted T wave in lead III) develops in patients with major pulmonary embolism. Chronic RV pressure overload leads to right-axis deviation and an R/S ratio greater than 1.0 in lead V_s (see Fig. 42–6*B*). A new incomplete or complete right bundle branch block may also be observed.

ECHOCARDIOGRAPHY AND DOPPLER ECHOCARDIOGRAPHY. Echocardiographic findings usually present in patients with pulmonary hypertension include RV dilatation and/or hypertrophy, right atrial dilatation, and the paradoxical septal wall motion associated with RV volume overload (see Table 56–4). Doppler studies predict with considerable accuracy the level of pulmonary arterial systolic and mean pressures. Associated pathologic entities (e.g., mitral stenosis) can also be identified and their severity quantitated.

Table 56–4 ■ LABORATORY FINDINGS IN PATIENTS WITH PULMONARY HYPERTENSION

DISEASE ENTITY	ECG	CHEST X-RAY	OTHER USEFUL TESTS	CATHETERIZATION
Precapillary Pulmonary Hypertension				
PPHT	RVH	↑↑ RA, ↑ RV, clear lungs with tapered periph. arteries	PFTs nl; lung scan nl or min. abn	PAP ↑↑, nl PCW, ↑ RAP, PAgram nl
Pulmonary embolism	nl or acute cor pulmonale ($S_1Q_3T_3$ or new IRBBB or RBBB)	nl or infiltrate, unilateral pulm. effusion	abnl ABGs; ↓ Po₂, ↑ pH, ↓ Pco₂; lung scan: seg. perf. defects, nl ventil. scan	PAP ↑, nl PCW, RAP nl or ↑; + PAgram
Disorders of ventilation	nl or RVH	Specific abnl in various entities	ABGs, PFTs: abnl	PAP ↑, PCW nl, RAP nl or ↑
Congenital heart disease	RVH	Clear lungs, ↑↑ PA, ↑ RV, tapered distal arteries, specific abnl in various entities	Cardiac echo: specific abnl in various entities	↑↑ PAP, nl PCW, RA ↑ or nl, ↓ arterial Po₂
Passive Pulmonary Hypertension				
Mitral stenosis	AF or NSR, LAE, RVH, or no VH	Pulm. congestion, ↑ LA, ↑ RV	Echo: LAE, abnl MV, nl LV	Gradient across MV, PAP ↑ PCW ↑, RAP nl or ↑
Left ventricular failure	Abnl depends on specific entity: LVH, MI, BBB	↑↑ or ↑ LV, ↑ LA, ↑ or nl RV, pulm. congestion	Echo: abnl LV function, LAE	Abnl LV function, ↑ LVEDP, ↑ PCW, ↑ PAP
Reactive Pulmonary Hypertension				
Long-standing mitral stenosis	AF, RVH	↑↑ PA, ↑↑ RV, ↑↑ LA, pulm. congestion	Echo: very abnl MV, ↑↑ RV, ↑↑ LA	MV gradient, PCW ↑↑, ↑↑ PAP, ↑ RAP
Pulmonary veno-occlusive disease	RVH	↑↑ PA, ↑↑ RV	Lung scan: nl or minor defects	Absent MV gradient, PCW ↑ or nl, LAP nl, LVP nl

Abbreviations: PPHT = primary pulmonary hypertension; PA = pulmonary artery; RV = right ventricle; RA = right atrium; LV = left ventricle; LA = left atrium; PAP = pulmonary artery pressure; RAP = right atrial pressure; LVP = left ventricular pressure; PCW = pulmonary capillary pressure; LAP = left atrial pressure; nl = normal; abnl = abnormal or abnormality; pulm. = pulmonary; ABGs = arterial blood gases; PFTs = pulmonary function tests; seg. = segmental; PAgram = pulmonary angiogram; RVH = right ventricular hypertrophy; LVH = left ventricular hypertrophy; NSR = normal sinus rhythm; VH = ventricular hypertrophy; LAE = left atrial enlargement; AF = atrial fibrillation; MI = myocardial infarction; BBB = bundle branch block; LVEDP = left ventricular end-diastolic pressure; min. = minimal; MV = mitral valve; periph. = peripheral; perf. = perfusion; ventil. = ventilation; + = positive; ↑↑ = markedly increased; ↑ = increased; ↓ = decreased.

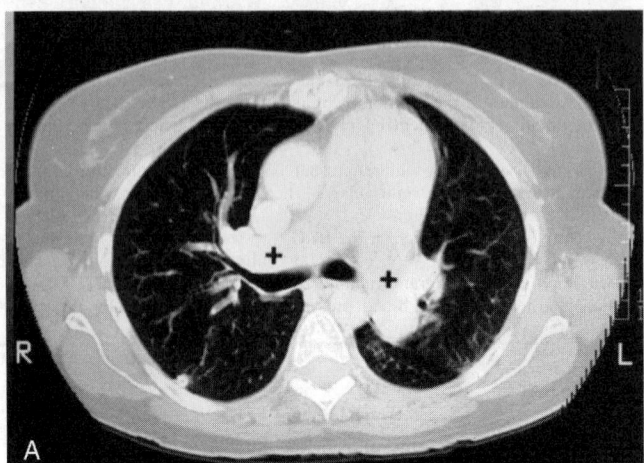

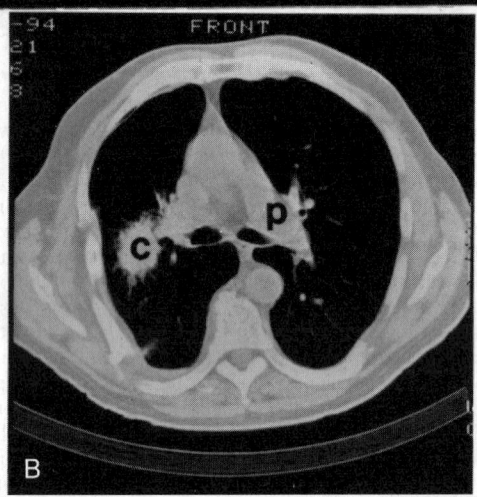

FIGURE 56–1 ■ A, MRI from a 47-year-old woman with an atrial septal defect and pulmonary vascular disease producing severe pulmonary hypertension. Note the marked enlargement of the main pulmonary arteries (+) and the dearth of peripheral pulmonary arteries ("pruning"). (Courtesy of Dr. Howard I. Molitch, Radiology Department, University of Arizona Health Science Center.) B, MRI from a 62-year-old man with severe, chronic asthmatic bronchitis leading to pulmonary hypertension. Note the markedly enlarged left main pulmonary artery (p). There is a bronchogenic carcinoma in the right lung (c). (Courtesy of Dr. Theron W. Ovitt, Radiology Department, University of Arizona Health Science Center.)

RADIONUCLEAR DIAGNOSTIC TECHNIQUES. A number of radionuclide diagnostic studies are useful in patients with known or suspected pulmonary hypertension. Pulmonary scintigraphy is the most sensitive non-invasive diagnostic test for pulmonary embolism, but it is not very specific (see Table 56–4). RV and LV size and function can be measured using radionuclear ventriculography in patients in whom adequate echocardiographic studies are unobtainable. Certain pulmonary conditions that may cause pulmonary hypertension (e.g., sarcoidosis; see Chapter 81) are associated with abnormal gallium lung scans.

COMPUTED TOMOGRAPHY (CT) SCANNING/MAGNETIC RESONANCE IMAGING (MRI). Tomographic studies of the chest with CT or MRI (see Chapters 44 and 45) often yield important information about cardiac and/or pulmonary pathologic changes in patients with pulmonary hypertension. RV and LV size and shape are clearly visualized, as are the major pulmonary arteries. Pulmonary parenchymal alterations are also disclosed (Fig. 56–1). Spiral CT scans can also visualize pulmonary emboli in major pulmonary arteries.

CARDIAC CATHETERIZATION AND ANGIOGRAPHY. Precise measurement of pulmonary arterial, capillary, and venous pressures are obtained by right-sided, and at times left-sided, heart catheterization. Pressures may be unexpectedly low if the patient has undergone vigorous diuresis before the hemodynamic study. Precapillary pulmonary hypertension can be distinguished from venous (also termed *passive*) pulmonary hypertension by hemodynamic observations (see Table 56–4). Cardiac catheterization also identifies patients with congenital or acquired intracardiac shunts and pulmonary hypertension. The severity of RV failure can be quantitated.

Pulmonary angiography is the most accurate technique for identifying pulmonary embolism (Fig. 56–2). Angiographic studies are usually combined with hemodynamic measurements of right-sided heart function.

SPECIFIC ENTITIES ASSOCIATED WITH PULMONARY HYPERTENSION

Myriad disease entities are associated with pulmonary hypertension (see Table 56–2). For many of these conditions, pulmonary hypertension is an epiphenomenon (i.e., the major pathophysiologic abnormality is not the increased pressure in the pulmonary vascular bed). On the other hand, there are diseases for which pulmonary hypertension is the central theme.

PRECAPILLARY PULMONARY HYPERTENSION. PRIMARY PULMONARY HYPERTENSION. Although primary pulmonary hypertension (PPHT) is an uncommon disease, it represents the purest form of pulmonary hypertension without other disease entities present. Because the increase in vascular resistance is present in the

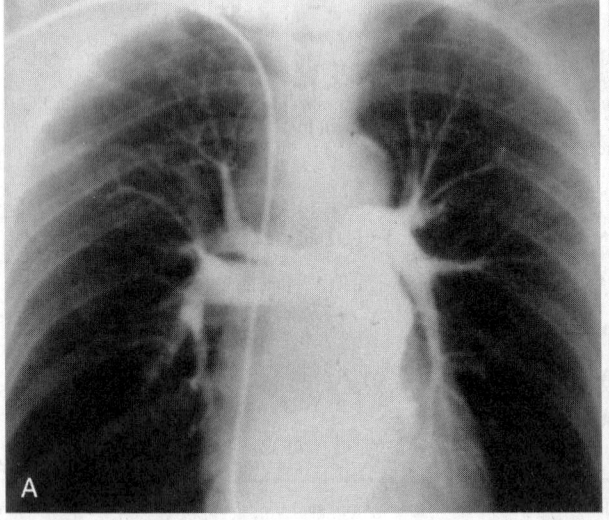

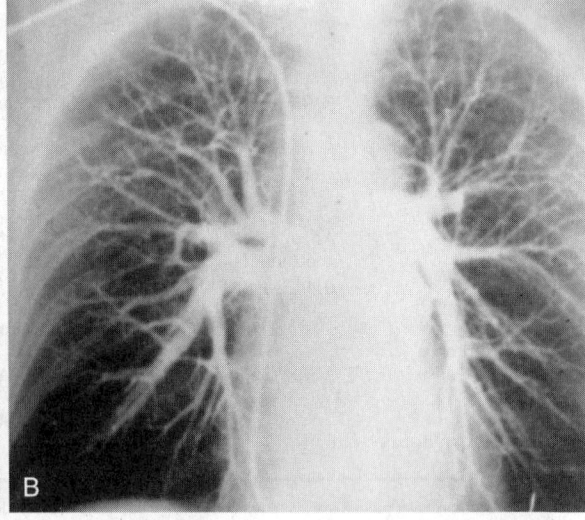

FIGURE 56–2 ■ Pulmonary angiography in a 67-year-old man with massive pulmonary embolism. A, Angiogram was obtained hours after the patient presented with dyspnea at rest, hypotension, and right ventricular failure. B, Angiogram was obtained 2 weeks later, after 2 weeks of anticoagulation. Note the filling defects and vessel cut-offs in the initial angiogram, with marked improvement in the follow-up study.

pulmonary arterioles, PPHT is one of the forms of precapillary pulmonary hypertension.

PPHT is a disease of unknown cause, although abnormal pulmonary vascular reactivity seems to underlie this condition in many individuals. For example, pulmonary vascular endothelial function is abnormal in PPHT: circulating endothelin and thromboxane levels are elevated, whereas nitric oxide and prostacyclin levels are diminished.

Some authorities argue that recurrent episodes of asymptomatic pulmonary embolism lead to PPHT. In support of this theory is the common autopsy finding of clinically silent organizing or recanalized pulmonary thrombi in the pulmonary arterial bed. However, these thrombi may be the result of *in situ* thromboses. Abnormalities of coagulation such as increased platelet reactivity and defective fibrinolysis have been described in patients with PPHT.

A number of pathologic findings are common to all patients with PPHT: intimal thickening and fibrosis in small pulmonary arteries and arterioles; increased medial thickening of small muscular pulmonary arteries and arterioles; necrotizing arteritis and fibrinoid necrosis in small muscular pulmonary arteries; and dilated, thin-walled side branches to muscular pulmonary arteries called plexiform lesions.

The majority of patients with PPHT come to medical attention late in the course of the illness. Women with PPHT outnumber men with PPHT 3 to 4:1. Familial or autosomal dominant inheritance is occasionally observed. This genetic defect appears to be localized to chromosome 2 (2q31-q32). Patients usually complain of exertional dyspnea without orthopnea and fatigue. Other complaints include exertional syncope, angina-like chest discomfort, palpitations, cough, and hemoptysis. Physical examination discloses findings consistent with pulmonary hypertension with or without RV failure (see Table 56–3). Routine laboratory tests are usually unremarkable. The aforementioned abnormalities in platelet function and fibrinolysis may be observed. The ECG reveals signs of RVH and, at times, right atrial enlargement. Chest radiographs disclose clear lung fields, enlarged central pulmonary arteries, and marked tapering of peripheral pulmonary arteries. Pulmonary function test results are usually normal except for arterial blood gases, which disclose evidence of hyperventilation: low $Paco_2$ and normal or modestly reduced Po_2.

Pulmonary scintigraphy is usually normal or demonstrates minor subsegmental defects. Patients with advanced PPHT may develop hypotension during pulmonary scintigraphy secondary to obstruction of a portion of the remaining pulmonary microvessels. Pulmonary angiography is a diagnostically important but clinically dangerous procedure in patients with PPHT. Angiography demonstrates small tapering pulmonary arteries in a "pruned tree" pattern and absence of pulmonary emboli. Hypotension or frank shock may develop during angiography in patients with PPHT. Consequently, small selective injections of angiographic dye are preferred.

The differential diagnosis of PPHT includes mitral stenosis, recurrent pulmonary embolism, congenital cardiac defects with severe pulmonary vascular disease, sickle cell anemia, collagen vascular disease, and rare entities such as cor triatriatum.

PULMONARY EMBOLISM. Acute pulmonary embolism (see Chapter 84) is one of the most common causes of pulmonary hypertension in the United States. The cause of the increase in pulmonary arterial pressure is obstruction of the pulmonary arterial bed by embolized thrombus and the resulting release of vasoactive substances. Therefore, pulmonary embolism represents another example of precapillary pulmonary hypertension.

Massive embolism, defined as thrombus obstructing 50% or more of the pulmonary arterial circulation, is associated with pulmonary arterial systolic pressures in the range of 50 to 60 mm Hg in individuals without prior heart or lung disease. Patients with heart and/or lung disease and pre-existing pulmonary hypertension may demonstrate pulmonary arterial systolic pressures that are considerably higher. Pulmonary hypertension is relieved in patients with acute pulmonary embolism as the degree of embolic obstruction declines. Chronic pulmonary hypertension secondary to unresolved embolism is rare. It is usually the result of multiple episodes of symptomatic but unrecognized pulmonary embolism.

Patients may present with dyspnea and tachypnea at rest, pleuritic chest discomfort, or hypotension. Physical examination discloses clear lungs or localized rales and/or wheezes. Signs of RV dilatation and/or failure are usually restricted to patients with mas-

sive embolism. Abnormal arterial blood gases (decreased Po_2 and Pco_2 and increased pH) are common in acute pulmonary embolism. The ECG is abnormal only in patients with massive embolism, disclosing the pattern of acute RV strain (S_1, Q_3, T_3). The chest radiograph is often normal, or it may reveal unilateral platelike atelectasis and/or a small pleural effusion. Pulmonary ventilation/perfusion scintigraphy is the most useful non-invasive test in patients with acute pulmonary embolism, demonstrating segmental perfusion defects that fail to ventilate. Pulmonary angiography represents the diagnostic gold standard for the diagnosis of pulmonary embolism: intraluminal filling defects are identified in patients with acute embolism (see Fig. 56–2). The differential diagnosis includes congestive heart failure and a variety of pulmonary or pleural infectious processes (e.g., bacterial pneumonia or viral pleuritis).

DISORDERS OF VENTILATION. A number of ventilatory disorders (see Chapter 90) cause pulmonary hypertension by three different pathophysiologic sequences: hypoxic vasoconstriction, anatomic restriction of the pulmonary vascular bed, and a combination of both vasoconstriction and restriction of the vasculature. Patients with high-altitude pulmonary hypertension or COPD develop pulmonary vasoconstriction and hypertension secondary to alveolar hypoxia. Patients with COPD exacerbate existing hypoxic pulmonary vasoconstriction by means of acidemia secondary to CO_2 retention.

Anatomic restriction of the pulmonary vascular bed as a cause of pulmonary hypertension is seen in patients with sarcoidosis and idiopathic pulmonary fibrosis. The combination of vasoconstriction and anatomic restriction of the vascular bed is observed in patients with kyphoscoliotic pulmonary disease.

In patients with ventilatory disorders and pulmonary hypertension, the symptoms and signs of pulmonary hypertension (see Table 56–3) are mixed with the clinical manifestations of the underlying pulmonary disorder. Similarly, laboratory abnormalities depend on the underlying pulmonary disease. For example, ECG evidence of RVH may be obscured in patients who have COPD with marked hyperinflation. In general, the ECG is a reasonably reliable marker for RVH in patients with pulmonary hypertension secondary to restriction of the pulmonary vascular bed. However, the ECG is much less reliable in patients with vasoconstrictive pulmonary hypertension. The differential diagnosis of pulmonary hypertension is extensive in patients with ventilatory disorders (see Table 56–2).

CONGENITAL HEART DISEASE WITH SEVERE PULMONARY VASCULAR DISEASE. Patients with congenital cardiac lesions (see Chapter 57) and left-to-right shunts may develop progressive pulmonary vascular disease with associated pulmonary hypertension. As pulmonary vascular disease progresses, pulmonary hypertension worsens and the magnitude of the left-to-right shunt declines. Eventually, there is minimal shunting of blood or even a net right-to-left shunt that results in arterial desaturation, so-called Eisenmenger's reaction. The pathologic changes associated with severe pulmonary vascular disease resemble those observed in patients with PPHT. A number of different congenital cardiac defects can be associated with Eisenmenger's reaction, including atrial septal defect, ventricular septal defect, patent ductus arteriosus, and more complex lesions such as transposition of the great arteries (see Fig. 56–1A). As in PPHT, the long-term prognosis is guarded for these patients, although it is better than once thought.

Patients with Eisenmenger's reaction usually complain of dyspnea on exertion. They may also experience angina-like chest discomfort, hemoptysis, and exertional syncope. The ECG discloses RVH, and the chest radiograph demonstrates clear lung fields, central pulmonary arterial enlargement, and marked tapering of distal pulmonary arteries. Echocardiography and/or catheterization with angiography usually reveals the correct diagnosis. The differential diagnosis includes PPHT, severe mitral stenosis, and a variety of end-stage pulmonary diseases.

PASSIVE PULMONARY HYPERTENSION. MITRAL STENOSIS. Increased left atrial pressure in patients with mitral stenosis is accompanied by pulmonary arterial hypertension. Pulmonary hypertension is largely reversible in these patients after successful valvuloplasty or valve replacement. Rarely, pulmonary hypertension fails to regress in patients with severe and long-standing mitral stenosis.

Patients complain of dyspnea on exertion, fatigue, and occasionally hemoptysis. Physical examination discloses the typical murmur of mitral stenosis and evidence of RV enlargement. The patient is often in atrial fibrillation. The ECG may reveal RVH; left atrial enlargement is commonly present. The chest radiograph demonstrates pulmonary congestion and RV and left atrial enlargement. Echocardiography and/or cardiac catheterization with angiography confirms the diagnosis. The differential diagnosis includes PPHT, a variety of entities leading to LV failure, and the rare condition cor triatriatum.

LEFT VENTRICULAR FAILURE. Any disease that causes LV failure with resultant left atrial hypertension is accompanied by pulmonary hypertension. The most common causes of LV failure include coronary artery disease, systemic hypertension, and cardiomyopathy. Patient complaints are similar to those expressed by individuals with mitral stenosis. The physical examination often reveals the underlying cause of LV failure (e.g., the murmur of aortic stenosis combined with abnormal carotid upstroke and LV enlargement). An LV S_3 is commonly present in patients with overt LV failure regardless of cause. The ECG findings depend on the underlying cause of LV failure (e.g., myocardial infarction in a patient with coronary artery disease). The chest radiograph usually reveals pulmonary congestion as well as LV enlargement. The differential diagnosis of LV failure includes mitral stenosis, aortic stenosis, coronary artery disease with myocardial infarction, hypertensive heart disease, cardiomyopathy, and other less common entities affecting the left ventricle (e.g., myocarditis).

REACTIVE PULMONARY HYPERTENSION. A small number of patients with many years of passive pulmonary hypertension develop pulmonary arteriolar vasoconstriction (i.e., precapillary pulmonary hypertension), on top of pre-existing passively elevated pulmonary arterial pressure. In these individuals, pulmonary arterial pressure is elevated disproportionately to the level of pulmonary venous pressure. The gradient between mean pulmonary arterial pressure and pulmonary capillary or venous pressure is more than 12 mm Hg. Medial hypertrophy and possibly intimal hyperplasia are found in pulmonary arterioles of patients with reactive pulmonary hypertension. The most common disease entity resulting in reactive pulmonary hypertension is long-standing mitral stenosis. Other pathologic conditions that cause pulmonary venous hypertension (e.g., aortic stenosis or LV failure secondary to myocardial infarction) commonly result in the patient's death before reactive pulmonary hypertension becomes severe.

Patients with reactive pulmonary hypertension are usually very symptomatic. Dyspnea and fatigue are the dominant complaints. The physical examination usually reveals RV enlargement and other findings associated with severe pulmonary hypertension. The ECG demonstrates RVH; the chest radiograph shows RV enlargement and very large central pulmonary arteries. Marked cardiomegaly secondary to RV dilation is often present. Successful mitral valvuloplasty or valve replacement often results in marked amelioration of reactive pulmonary hypertension. However, some elevation in pulmonary arterial pressure may persist secondary to permanent loss of pulmonary microvessels.

Pulmonary veno-occlusive disease is a poorly understood condition characterized by diffuse involvement of pulmonary veins and venules. Affected veins demonstrate fibrous narrowing or obliteration of the lumen. The result is severe, chronic pulmonary venous and capillary hypertension that eventually results in irreversible reactive pulmonary arterial hypertension. Patients complain of dyspnea and fatigue; the clinical picture may resemble advanced mitral stenosis or PPHT.

TREATMENT OF PULMONARY HYPERTENSION

Because a variety of disease entities with varying pathophysiologic abnormalities lead to pulmonary hypertension, it is impossible to recommend one specific remedy for all forms of increased pulmonary vascular pressure (Fig. 56–3). In general, however, effective therapy should reduce pulmonary vascular resistance directly. If pulmonary pressures are reduced proportionately to a decrease in cardiac output, little therapeutic gain is achieved. General therapeutic measures include supplementing inspiratory oxygen, correcting acid-base abnormalities, and ensuring that inspired air is cool, dry, and free of inhaled irritants.

Patients with PPHT represent a difficult therapeutic challenge because increased pulmonary vascular abnormalities may be so far advanced that they cannot be ameliorated when these individuals come to medical attention. Therefore, survival statistics are often poor for these patients. When first seen, many patients with PPHT have lost microvasculature, rendering pulmonary hypertension irreversible; cardiopulmonary or pulmonary transplantation is the only effective means of therapy. Earlier in the course of the illness, however, pulmonary vasoconstriction may still be present. Intravenous prostacyclins (epoprostenol) and calcium channel blockers

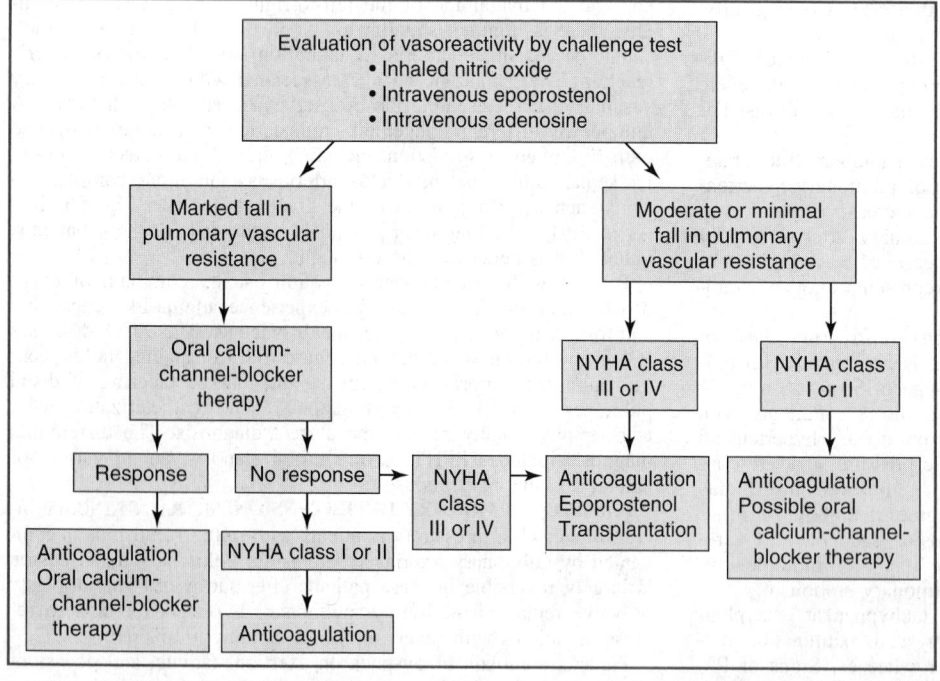

FIGURE 56–3 ■ Algorithm for the management of primary pulmonary hypertension. NYHA = New York Heart Association. (From Rubin LJ: Primary pulmonary hypertension. N Engl J Med 336:116, 1997. Copyright © 1997, Massachusetts Medical Society. All rights reserved.)

given in high doses (e.g., diltiazem, 120 mg three times a day) can lower pulmonary vascular resistance by dilating pulmonary resistance vessels if vasoconstriction is still present. In patients with PPHT and residual pulmonary vasoconstriction, therapy with epoprostenol and calcium channel blockers has been shown to reduce pulmonary arterial pressure and vascular resistance, leading to regression of RVH and probably to prolonged survival. Unfortunately, only 25 to 30% of patients with PPHT respond to oral calcium channel blocker therapy. A substantially larger proportion of patients respond to intravenous epoprostenol. Early studies with aerosolized and oral prostacyclin analogues appear promising. Lifelong anticoagulation is advised for these individuals, who are at high risk for pulmonary embolism.

Patients with acute pulmonary embolism can usually be successfully managed with intravenous heparin followed by oral warfarin therapy. Thrombolytic therapy, surgical thrombectomy, and venous interruption are helpful in selected patients (see Chapter 84).

Therapy for patients with disorders of ventilation varies, depending on the particular pulmonary disorder. Thus, patients with COPD may experience a lowering of pulmonary arterial pressure when given supplemental inspiratory oxygen, bronchodilators, and appropriate antibiotics for bronchial or pulmonary infection. Patients with high-altitude pulmonary hypertension improve with supplemental inspiratory oxygen or return to sea level. Kyphoscoliotic pulmonary disease may improve after appropriate corrective orthopedic surgery. Individuals with severe pulmonary sarcoidosis may experience amelioration when given corticosteroids.

Patients with congenital heart disease complicated by pulmonary vascular disease may require cardiopulmonary or pulmonary transplantation if pulmonary vascular changes are advanced. If there is a reversible component to the increased pulmonary vascular resistance in these individuals, it can often be identified by measuring pulmonary arterial resistance during inspiration of 100% oxygen. In patients with reversibly increased pulmonary vascular resistance, successful obliteration of the left-to-right shunt may result in subsequently lower vascular resistance. However, in some patients, pulmonary vascular resistance continues to increase despite closing the congenital cardiac defect.

In patients with passive pulmonary hypertension, pulmonary arterial pressure and resistance usually fall after successful therapy for the condition that produced the elevated pulmonary venous pressure. Thus, relieving mitral valvular obstruction in patients with mitral stenosis results in decreased pulmonary venous and arterial pressures and pulmonary vascular resistance. Similarly, successful therapy for LV failure leads to lower pulmonary pressures and resistance. Even patients with long-standing mitral stenosis and reactive pulmonary hypertension usually demonstrate a marked improvement in pulmonary pressures and resistance after relieving mitral valvular obstruction. Patients with pulmonary veno-occlusive disease usually require cardiopulmonary or pulmonary transplantation because the diagnosis is made late in the course of the illness. In many instances, the diagnosis of pulmonary veno-occlusive disease is first made when the involved lungs are examined pathologically after removal for cardiopulmonary or pulmonary transplantation.

Abenhaim L, Moride Y, Brenot F, et al: Appetite-suppressant drugs and the risk of primary pulmonary hypertension. N Engl J Med 335:609, 1996. *Administration of the appetite suppressant drug, fenfluramine, and its derivatives is associated with the development of primary pulmonary hypertension.*

Barst RJ, Rubin LJ, Long WA, et al: A comparison of continuous intravenous epoprostenol (prostacyclin) with conventional therapy for primary pulmonary hypertension. N Engl J Med 334:296, 1996. *Continuous intravenous infusion of epoprostenol produced symptomatic and hemodynamic improvement as well as prolonged survival in patients with severe primary pulmonary hypertension.*

Fishman AP: Aminorex to Fen/Phen: An epidemic foretold. Circulation 99:556, 1999. *Anorexigenic drugs cause pulmonary hypertension.*

Frank H, Mlczoch J, Huber K, et al: The effect of anticoagulant therapy in primary and anorectic drug-induced pulmonary hypertension. Chest 112:714, 1997. *Anticoagulant therapy is associated with improved survival and quality of life in patients with primary pulmonary hypertension.*

Hinderliter AL, Willis PW, Barst RJ, et al: Effects of long-term infusion of prostacyclin (epoprostenol) on echocardiographic measures of right ventricular structure and function in primary pulmonary hypertension. Circulation 95:1479, 1997. *Prostacyclin therapy has beneficial effects on RV structure and function in patients with primary pulmonary hypertension.*

Moraes D, Loscalzo J: Pulmonary hypertension: Newer concepts in diagnosis and management. Clin Cardiol 20:676, 1997. *A review of various forms of pulmonary hypertension including discussion of pathophysiology, diagnosis, and therapy.*

Rubin LJ: Primary pulmonary hypertension. N Engl J Med 336:111, 1997. *Excellent review of pathophysiology, pathogenesis, diagnosis, and therapy of primary pulmonary hypertension.*

57 CONGENITAL HEART DISEASE IN ADULTS

Ariane J. Marelli

GENERAL PRINCIPLES

Over the past four decades, the convergence of major progress in medicine, pediatrics, and cardiovascular surgery has resulted in the survival to adulthood of an increasingly large number of patients with complex structural heart lesions. Adult physicians are becoming increasingly responsible for these patients, commonly in concert with a cardiologist and a tertiary care facility.

DEFINITIONS

Patients can be subdivided into three categories according to their surgical status. Patients may be unoperated or surgically palliated or may have undergone physiologic repair. Congenital heart lesions can be classified as *acyanotic* or *cyanotic*. Cyanosis refers to a blue discoloration of the mucous membranes resulting from an increased amount of reduced hemoglobin. Central cyanosis occurs when the circulation is mixed because of a right-to-left shunt.

A *native lesion* refers to an anatomic lesion present at birth. Acquired lesions, naturally occurring or as a result of surgery, are superimposed on the native anatomy. *Palliative* interventions are performed in patients with cyanotic lesions and are defined as operations that serve either to increase or decrease pulmonary blood flow while allowing a mixed circulation and cyanosis to persist (Table 57–1). *Physiologic* repair applies to procedures that provide total or nearly total anatomic and physiologic separation of the pulmonary and systemic circulations in complex cyanotic lesions and result in patients who are acyanotic.

Eisenmenger's complex refers to flow reversal across a ventricular septal defect (VSD) when pulmonary vascular resistance exceeds systemic levels. *Eisenmenger's physiology* is used to designate the physiologic response in a broader category of shunt lesions in which a right-to-left shunt occurs in response to an elevation in pulmonary vascular resistance. *Eisenmenger's syndrome* is a term applied to common clinical features shared by patients with Eisenmenger's physiology.

Each congenital lesion can influence the course of another. For example, the physiologic consequences of a VSD will be different if it occurs in isolation or in combination with pulmonary stenosis. A *simple lesion* is defined as either a shunt lesion or an obstructive lesion of the right or left heart occurring in isolation. A *complex lesion* is a combination of two or more abnormalities.

ETIOLOGY

In 90% of patients, congenital heart disease is attributable to multifactorial inheritance; only 5 to 10% of malformations are due

Table 57–1 ■ PALLIATIVE SURGICAL SHUNTS FOR CONGENITAL HEART LESIONS

PALLIATIVE SHUNT	ANASTOMOSIS
Systemic Arterial–to–Pulmonary Artery Shunts	
Classic Blalock-Taussig	Subclavian artery to PA
Modified Blalock-Taussig	Subcalvian artery to PA (prosthetic graft)
Potts anastomosis	Descending aorta to left PA
Waterston's shunt	Ascending aorta to right PA
Systemic Venous–to–Pulmonary Artery Shunts	
Classic Glenn	SVC to right PA
Bidirectional Glenn	SVC to right and left PA
Bilateral Glenn	Right and left SVC to right and left PA

PA = pulmonary artery; SVC = superior vena cava.
From Marelli A, Mullen M. Clin Paediatr 4:189, 1996.

to primary genetic factors, either chromosomal or related to a single mutant gene. The most common defect observed in patients with *chromosomal aberrations* is a VSD, which is observed in 90% of patients with trisomy 13 and 18. Defects of the endocardial cushions and the ventricular septum are observed in 50% of patients with Down's syndrome (trisomy 21). The most frequently observed defects in patients with Turner's syndrome (45,X) are aortic coarctation, aortic stenosis, and atrial septal defect (ASD). Abnormalities involving the chromosomal band 22q11 can result in a group of syndromes, the most common of which is the DiGeorge syndrome. The shared phenotypic features are designated CATCH-22 syndromes, i.e., a combination of cardiac defects, abnormal facies, thymic hypoplasia, cleft palate, and hypocalcemia. The recurrence risk for families with a child who carries a congenital cardiac malformation due to a chromosomal anomaly is related to the recurrence risk of the chromosomal anomaly itself.

Typically, *single mutant genes* are also associated with syndromes of cardiovascular malformations, although not every patient with the syndrome will have the characteristic cardiac anomaly. Examples include osteogenesis imperfecta (autosomal recessive) associated with aortic valve disease, the Jervell and Lange-Nielsen (autosomal recessive) and the Romano-Ward (autosomal dominant) syndromes associated with a prolonged QT interval and sudden death, and the Holt-Oram (autosomal dominant) syndrome, in which an ASD occurs with a range of other skeletal anomalies. Noonan's syndrome is associated with pulmonary stenosis, ASD, and hypertrophic cardiomyopathy. Osler-Weber-Rendu telangiectasias are associated with pulmonary arteriovenous fistulas.

The *risk of recurrence* when the mother carries a sporadically occurring congenital lesion varies from 2.5 to 18% depending on the lesion. Obstructive lesions of the left ventricular outflow tract have the highest recurrence rates in offspring. When the father carries the lesion, 1.5 to 3% of the offspring are affected. When a sibling has a congenital cardiac anomaly, the risk of recurrence in another sibling varies from 1 to 3%.

INCIDENCE AND PREVALENCE

Congenital cardiac malformations occur at a rate of 8 per 1000 live births, which corresponds to approximately 32,000 infants with newly diagnosed congenital heart disease each year in the United States. An estimated 20% die within the first year of life—a substantial decrease from the reported 40% in the late 1960s. Each year an estimated 20,000 surgical procedures are performed to correct circulatory defects in patients with congenital malformations. Approximately 80% of the first-year survivors live to reach adulthood. The estimated prevalence of adults with congenital heart disease in the United States is now about 900,000.

Bicuspid aortic valve occurs in about 2% of the general population, is the most common congenital cardiac anomaly encountered in adult populations, and accounts for up to half of operated cases of aortic stenosis in adults (see Chapter 63). ASDs constitute 30 to 40% of cases of congenital heart disease seen in adults, with ostium secundum ASD accounting for 7% of all congenital lesions. A solitary VSD accounts for 15 to 20% of all congenital lesions and is the most common congenital cardiac lesion observed in the pediatric population; its high spontaneous closure rates explain the lesser prevalence in adults. Patent ductus arteriosus (PDA) accounts for 5 to 10% of all congenital cardiac lesions in infants with a normal birthweight. Pulmonary stenosis and coarctation of the aorta account for 3 to 10% of all congenital lesions.

Tetralogy of Fallot is the most common cyanotic congenital anomaly observed in adults. Together with complete transposition of the great arteries (TGA), these lesions account for 5 to 12% of congenital heart disease in infants. More complex lesions such as tricuspid atresia, univentricular heart, congenitally corrected TGA, Ebstein's anomaly, and double-outlet right ventricle account for 2.5% or less of all congenital heart disease.

APPROACH TO THE PATIENT

Congenital heart disease is a lifelong condition during which the patient and the lesion evolve concurrently. A patient may have

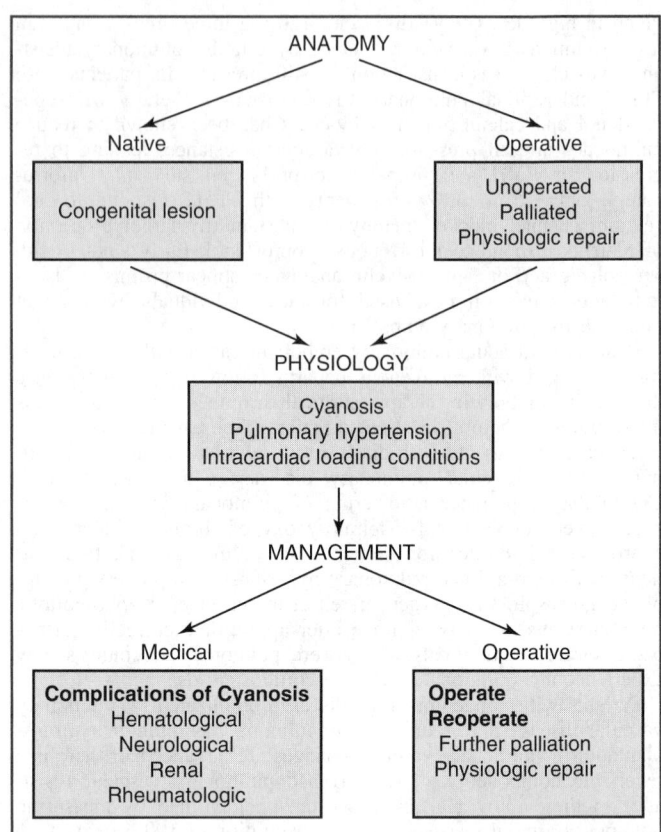

FIGURE 57–1 ■ The goals of complete clinical assessment are to define anatomy and physiology to determine appropriate management.

been monitored for many years because of an erroneous diagnosis made in infancy or childhood when diagnostic techniques were more limited. The approach to adults with congenital heart disease (Fig. 57–1) should answer the following questions: What is the native anatomy? Has this patient undergone surgery for the condition? What is the physiology? What can and should be done for this patient both medically and surgically? And importantly, who should do it?

If the patient has not undergone surgery, the question is why? If the patient is palliated, has the degree of cyanosis progressed as evidenced by a drop in systemic saturation or a rise in hemoglobin? If the patient has undergone a physiologic repair, what procedure was performed? Are residual lesions present and have new lesions developed as a consequence of surgery? The patient's *physiology* is determined by the presence or absence of cyanosis, pulmonary hypertension, adequate filling of the cardiac chambers, and any resulting medical complications.

A clinical assessment, 12-lead electrocardiogram, chest radiograph, and baseline oxygen saturation should be part of every initial assessment. Two-dimensional transthoracic echocardiography (see Chapter 43), Doppler, and color flow imaging are used to establish the diagnosis and monitor the evolution of documented hemodynamic complications. *Transesophageal echocardiographic* (TEE) examination is particularly useful in adults and is increasingly important during interventional catheter-guided therapy and surgery. *Magnetic resonance imaging* (MRI) (see Chapter 45) and computed tomography (see Chapter 44) are useful adjuncts. *Cardiac catheterization* for congenital heart disease has shifted from pure diagnosis to include intervention. Coronary arteriography is recommended for adults older than 40 years in whom surgical intervention is contemplated.

Pulmonary Hypertension

Pulmonary hypertension secondary to structural disease of the heart or circulation can occur with or without an increase in pulmonary vascular resistance. Pulmonary vascular obstructive disease occurs when pulmonary vascular resistance rises and becomes fixed and irreversible. In the most common congenital anomalies, pulmonary hypertension occurs as a result of increased pulmonary blood flow because of a native left-to-right shunt. Examples include ASD, a moderate size VSD, PDA, and a variety of complex lesions. The rate at which pulmonary hypertension progresses to become pulmonary vascular obstructive disease varies from one lesion to another and depends at least in part on the source of pulmonary blood flow. Pulmonary hypertension typically develops in patients with an ASD after the fourth decade, with Eisenmenger's syndrome being a late complication seen in only 5 to 10% of cases. In contrast, in patients with a large VSD or persistent PDA, progressive elevation in pulmonary vascular resistance occurs rapidly because the pulmonary vascular bed is exposed not only to the excess volume of the left-to-right shunt, but also to systemic arterial pressures. As a result, Eisenmenger's complex develops in approximately 10% of patients with a large VSD during the first decade. Surgical pulmonary artery banding is a palliative measure aimed at decreasing pulmonary blood flow and protecting the pulmonary vascular bed against the development of early pulmonary vascular obstructive disease.

If forward flow from the right heart is insufficient, native collaterals and/or surgical shunts provide an alternative source of pulmonary blood flow (see Table 57–1). With large surgical shunts, however, direct exposure of the pulmonary vascular bed to the high pressures of the systemic circulation causes pulmonary vascular obstructive disease. As a result, systemic-to-pulmonary arterial shunts are currently less favored in neonates and infants, in whom systemic venous–to–pulmonary arterial shunts are now preferred.

Eisenmenger's Syndrome

The term *Eisenmenger's syndrome* should be reserved for patients in whom pulmonary vascular obstructive disease is present and pulmonary vascular resistance is fixed and irreversible. These findings in combination with the *absence of left-to-right shunting* render the patient inoperable.

The clinical manifestations of Eisenmenger's syndrome include dyspnea on exertion, syncope, chest pain, congestive heart failure, and symptoms related to erythrocytosis and hyperviscosity. On physical examination, central cyanosis and digital clubbing are hallmark findings. Systemic oxygen saturations typically vary between 75 and 85%. The pulse pressure will narrow as the cardiac output falls. Examination of jugular venous pressure can reveal a dominant *a wave* reflecting a non-compliant right ventricle until tricuspid insufficiency is severe enough to generate a large *v wave*. A prominent right ventricular impulse is felt in the left parasternal border in end-expiration or in the subcostal area in end-inspiration. A palpable pulmonary artery is commonly felt. The pulmonary component of the second heart sound is increased and can be felt in the majority of cases. Pulmonary ejection sounds are common when the pulmonary artery is dilated with a structurally normal valve. Right atrial gallop is heard more frequently when the *a wave* is dominant. A murmur of tricuspid insufficiency is common, but the inspiratory increase in the murmur (Carvallo's sign) disappears when right ventricular failure occurs. In diastole, a pulmonary insufficiency murmur is often heard. The 12-lead electrocardiogram shows evidence of right atrial enlargement, right ventricular hypertrophy, and right axis deviation. Chest radiographic findings include a dilated pulmonary artery segment, cardiac enlargement, and diminished pulmonary vascular markings (see Fig. 41-6). Echocardiography will confirm the right-sided pressure overload and pulmonary artery enlargement, as well as the tricuspid and pulmonary insufficiency. Cardiac catheterization is indicated if doubt exists about the potential reversibility of the elevated pulmonary vascular resistance in a patient who might otherwise benefit from surgery.

Systemic Complications of Cyanosis

Cyanosis occurs when persistent venous-to-arterial mixing results in hypoxemia. Adaptive mechanisms to increase oxygen delivery include an increase in oxygen content, a rightward shift in the oxyhemoglobin dissociation curve, a higher hematocrit, and an increase in cardiac output. When cyanosis is not relieved, chronic hypoxemia and erythrocytosis result in hematologic, neurologic, renal, and rheumatic complications.

Hematologic complications of chronic hypoxemia include erythrocytosis, iron deficiency, and bleeding diathesis. Hemoglobin and hematocrit levels, as well as red cell indices, should be checked

regularly and correlated with systemic oxygen saturation levels. Symptoms of hyperviscosity include headaches, faintness, dizziness, fatigue, altered mentation, visual disturbances, paresthesias, tinnitus, and myalgia. Symptoms are classified as mild to moderate when they interfere with only some activities, or they can be marked to severe and interfere with most or all activities. Patients with *compensated erythrocytosis* establish an equilibrium hematocrit at higher levels in an iron-replete state with minimal symptoms. Patients with *decompensated erythrocytosis* manifest unstable, rising hematocrit levels and experience severe hyperviscosity symptoms.

In the iron-replete state, moderate to severe hyperviscosity symptoms typically occur when hematocrit levels exceed 65%. If no evidence of dehydration is present, removal of 500 mL of blood over a 30- to 45-minute period should be followed by quantitative volume replacement with normal saline or dextran (Fig. 57–2). The procedure may be repeated every 24 hours until symptomatic improvement occurs.

Hemostatic abnormalities can occur in up to 20% of cyanotic patients with erythrocytosis. Bleeding is usually mild and superficial and leads to easy bruising, skin petechiae, or mucosal bleeding, but epistaxis, hemoptysis, or even life-threatening postoperative bleeding can occur. A variety of clotting factor deficiencies and qualitative and quantitative platelet disorders have been described.

Treatment for spontaneous bleeding is dictated by its severity and the abnormal hemostatic parameters (Fig. 57–3). For severe bleeding, platelet transfusions, fresh-frozen plasma, vitamin K, cryoprecipitate, and desmopressin have been used. Reduction in erythrocyte mass also improves hemostasis, so cyanotic patients undergoing surgery should have prophylactic phlebotomy if the hematocrit is greater than 65%.

Iron deficiency is common in cyanotic adult patients because of excessive bleeding or phlebotomy. In contrast to normocytic erythrocytosis, which is rarely symptomatic at hematocrit levels less than 65%, iron deficiency may be manifested by hyperviscosity symptoms at hematocrit levels well below 65%. The treatment of choice is not phlebotomy but oral iron repletion until a rise in hematocrit is detected, typically within 1 week.

Neurologic complications, including cerebral hemorrhage, can be caused by hemostatic defects and are most often seen after inappropriate use of anticoagulant therapy. Patients with right-to-left shunts may be at risk for paradoxical cerebral emboli. Focal brain injury may provide a nidus for brain abscess if bacteremia supervenes. Attention should be paid to the use of air filters in peripheral intravenous lines to avoid paradoxical emboli through a right-to-left shunt.

Prophylactic phlebotomy has no place in the prevention of cerebral arterial thrombosis. Indications for phlebotomy are the occurrence of symptomatic hyperviscosity in an iron-repleted patient and prevention of excessive bleeding perioperatively.

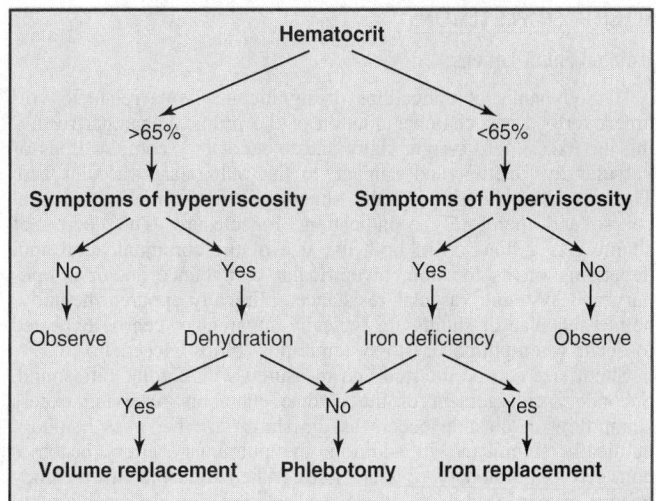

FIGURE 57–2 ■ Treatment algorithm for erythrocytosis of cyanotic congenital heart disease.

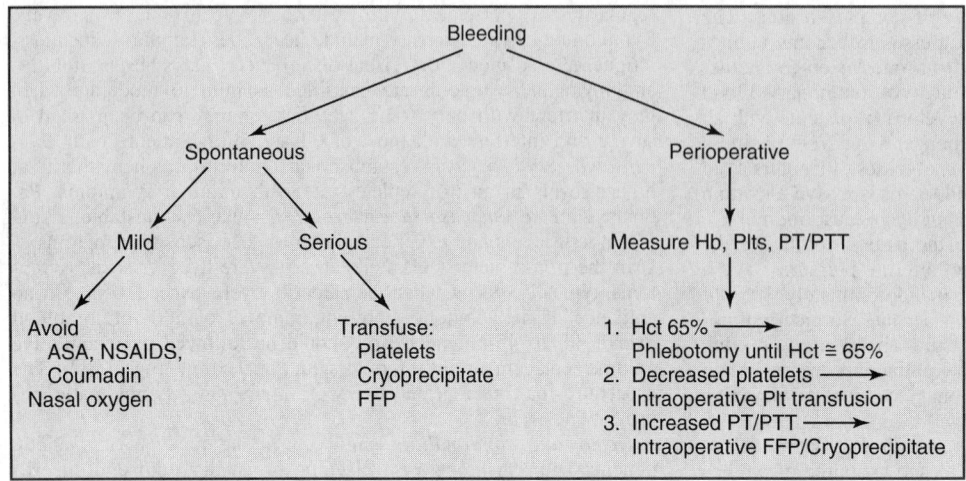

FIGURE 57–3 ■ Treatment algorithm for bleeding diathesis of cyanotic congenital heart disease. FFP = fresh-frozen plasma; Hb = hemoglobin; Hct = hematocrit; Plts = platelets; PT = prothrombin time; PTT = partial thromboplastin time.

Chronic oxygen therapy is unlikely to benefit hypoxemia secondary to right-to-left shunting in the setting of a fixed pulmonary vascular resistance. Chronic oxygen therapy results in mucosal dehydration with an increased incidence of epistaxis and is therefore not recommended.

Renal dysfunction can be manifested as proteinuria, hyperuricemia, or renal failure. Focal interstitial fibrosis, tubular atrophy, and hyalinization of afferent and efferent arterioles can be seen on renal biopsy. Increased blood viscosity and arteriolar vasoconstriction can lead to renal hypoperfusion with progressive glomerulosclerosis. Hyperuricemia is commonly seen in patients with cyanotic congenital heart disease and is thought to be due mainly to the decreased reabsorption of uric acid rather than overproduction from erythrocytosis. Asymptomatic hyperuricemia need not be treated because lowering uric acid levels has not been shown to prevent renal disease or gout.

Rheumatologic complications include gout and hypertrophic osteoarthropathy, which is thought to be responsible for the arthralgias affecting up to a third of patients with cyanotic congenital heart disease. In patients with right-to-left shunting, megakaryocytes released from the bone marrow bypass the lung and are entrapped in systemic arterioles and capillaries where they release platelet-derived growth factor, which promotes local cell proliferation. Digital clubbing and new osseous formation with periostitis occur and cause the symptoms of arthralgia. Symptomatic hyperuricemia and gouty arthritis can be treated as necessary with colchicine, probenecid, or allopurinol; non-steroidal anti-inflammatory drugs are best avoided given the baseline hemostatic anomalies in these patients.

SPECIFIC SIMPLE LESIONS

Isolated Shunt Lesions

Hemodynamic complications of significant shunts relate to volume overload and chamber dilation of the primary chamber receiving the excess left-to-right shunt and to secondary complications of valvular dysfunction and damage to the pulmonary vascular bed. The size and duration of the shunt will determine the clinical course and therefore the indications for closure. The degree of shunting is a function of both the size of the communication and, depending on its location, biventricular compliance and/or pulmonary and systemic vascular resistance. Clinically apparent hemodynamic sequelae of shunts are typically apparent or can be expected to occur when pulmonary-to-systemic flow ratios exceed 1.5 to 1.

Shunt size can be inferred and measured with cardiac ultrasound. Secondary enlargement of the cardiac chambers receiving excess shunt flow in diastole occurs as the shunt size becomes hemodynamically significant; in addition, the pulmonary artery becomes enlarged as pulmonary pressure rises. When tricuspid insufficiency occurs primarily from right ventricular dilatation or secondary to pulmonary hypertension, the regurgitant jet can be used to estimate the pulmonary pressure as another indicator of shunt significance. When the pulmonary-to-systemic flow (Qp:Qs) exceeds 2:1, the

volume of blood in both circulations can be estimated by comparing the stroke volume at the pulmonary and aortic valves. Shunt detection and quantification can also be obtained by using a first-pass radionuclide study. As a bolus of radioactive substance is injected into the systemic circulation, the rise and fall of radionuclide activity can be measured in the lungs. When a shunt is significant, the rate of persistent activity in the lungs over time can be used to calculate the shunt fraction. For both echocardiographic and radionuclide quantification of shunt size, sources of error are multiple. The most predictable results are obtained only in experienced laboratories. Uncertainty about the physiologic significance of a borderline shunt can be minimized by integrating serial determinations from multiple clinical and relevant diagnostic sources rather than basing management decisions on a single calculated shunt value.

Atrial Septal Defect

Classification of ASDs is based on anatomic location. Most commonly, an *ostium secundum* ASD occurs in the central portion of the interatrial septum as a result of an enlarged foramen ovale or excessive resorption of the septum primum. The combination of a secundum ASD and acquired mitral stenosis is known as *Lutembacher's syndrome*, the pathophysiology of which will be determined by the relative severity of each. Abnormal development of the embryologic endocardial cushions result in a variety of atrioventricular canal defects, the most common of which consists of a defect in the lower part of the atrial septum in the *ostium primum* location, typically accompanied by a cleft mitral valve and mitral regurgitation. The *sinus venosus* defect, which accounts for 2 to 3% of all interatrial communications, is located superiorly at the junction of the superior vena cava and right atrium and is generally associated with anomalous drainage of the right-sided pulmonary veins into the superior vena cava or right atrium. Less commonly, interatrial communications can be seen at the site of the coronary sinus, typically associated with an anomalous left superior vena cava.

The *pathophysiology* is determined by the effects of the shunt on the heart and pulmonary circulation. Right atrial and right ventricular dilatation occurs as shunt size increases with pulmonary-to-systemic flow ratios greater than 1.5:1.0. Superimposed systemic hypertension and coronary artery disease modify left ventricular compliance and favor left-to-right shunting. Mitral valve disease can occur in up to 15% of patients older than 50 years. Right heart failure, atrial fibrillation, or atrial flutter can occur as a result of chronic right-sided volume overload and progressive ventricular and atrial dilatation. Stroke can result from paradoxical emboli, atrial arrhythmias, or both. A rise in pulmonary pressure occurs because of the increased pulmonary blood flow. Pulmonary hypertension is unusual before 20 years of age but is seen in 50% of patients older than 40 years. The overall incidence of pulmonary vascular obstructive disease is 15 to 20% in patients with ASD. Eisenmenger's disease with reverse shunting, a late and rare complication of isolated secundum ASD, is reported in 5 to 10% of patients.

DIAGNOSIS. Although most patients are minimally symptomatic in the first three decades, more than 70% become impaired by the fifth decade. Initial *symptoms* include exercise intolerance, dyspnea on exertion, and fatigue caused most commonly by right heart failure and pulmonary hypertension. Palpitations, syncope, and stroke can occur with the development of atrial arrhythmias.

On *physical examination* most adults have a normal general physical appearance. When Holt-Oram syndrome is present, the thumb may have a third phalanx or it may be rudimentary or absent. With an uncomplicated non-restrictive communication between both atria, the a and v waves are equal in amplitude. Precordial palpation typically discloses a normal left ventricular impulse unless mitral valve disease occurs. Characteristically, if the shunt is significant, a right ventricular impulse can be felt in the left parasternal area in end-expiration or in the subxiphoid area in end-inspiration. A dilated pulmonary artery can sometimes be felt in the second left intercostal space. On auscultation, the hallmark of an ASD is the wide and fixed splitting of the second heart sound. Pulmonary valve closure, as reflected by P_2, is delayed because of right ventricular overload and the increased capacitance of the pulmonary vascular bed. The A_2-P_2 interval is fixed because the increase in venous return elevates the right atrial pressure during inspiration, thereby decreasing the degree of left-to-right shunting and offsetting the usual phasic respiratory changes. In addition, compliance of the pulmonary circulation is reduced from the high flow, thus making the vascular compartment less susceptible to any further increase in blood flow. A soft mid-systolic murmur generated by the increased flow across the pulmonary valve is usually heard in the second left interspace. In the presence of a high left-to-right shunt volume, increased flow across the tricuspid valve is heard as a mid-diastolic murmur at the lower left sternal border. With advanced right heart failure, evidence of systemic venous congestion is present.

The *electrocardiogram* characteristically shows an incomplete right bundle branch pattern (Fig. 57–4). Right axis deviation and atrial abnormalities, including a prolonged PR interval, atrial fibrillation, and flutter, are also seen. Typically, the chest radiograph shows pulmonary vascular plethora with increased markings in both lung fields consistent with increased pulmonary blood flow (see Fig. 41–13). The main pulmonary artery and both its branches are dilated. Right atrial and right ventricular dilatation can be seen. *Cardiac ultrasound* is diagnostic and provides important prognostic information. Ostium primum and secundum ASDs are easily identifiable with transthoracic imaging, but a sinus venosus ASD can be

missed unless specifically sought. For more accurate visualization of the superior interatrial septum and localization of the pulmonary veins, TEE is very useful. With Doppler, pulmonary artery pressures can be quantified, and the Qp:Qs can be measured.

MANAGEMENT. The decision to close an ASD is based on the size of the shunt and the presence or absence of symptoms. In the presence of a significant shunt, closure of an ASD before 25 years of age without evidence of pulmonary hypertension results in a long-term outcome that is similar to that of age- and sex-matched controls. Closure of a significant asymptomatic shunt is generally indicated up to age 40; after age 40, closure is indicated in symptomatic patients with significant shunts because it results in improved survival, prevention of deterioration in functional capacity, and improvement in exercise capacity as compared with patients treated medically. Advanced age greater than 60 years is not a contraindication to ASD closure in the presence of a significant shunt because a significant number of patients will show evidence of symptomatic improvement.

Uncomplicated secundum ASDs may be closed surgically in children and adults with minimal operative mortality, in the range of 1 to 3% or less. Preoperative pulmonary artery pressure and the presence or absence of pulmonary vascular disease are important predictors of successful surgical outcome.

Small, centrally located defects can be occluded by using a transcatheter technique in a cardiac catheterization laboratory. Advantages of this approach include the avoidance of sternotomy and cardiopulmonary bypass. Complications, including device fracture with embolization and residual shunts, should decrease as newer devices are used.

Ventricular Septal Defect

For anatomic classification of VSDs, the interventricular septum can be divided into four regions. Defects of the membranous septum, or infracristal VSDs, are located in a small translucent area beneath the aortic valve and account for up to 80% of VSDs. These VSDs typically show a variable degree of extension into the inlet or outlet septum, hence their designation as "perimembranous." Infundibular defects or supracristal outlet VSDs occur in the conal septum above the crista supraventricularis and below the pulmonary valve. Inlet defects are identified at the crux of the heart between the tricuspid and mitral valves and are usually associated with other anomalies of the atrioventricular canal. Defects of the trabecular or muscular septum can be multiple and occur distal to the septal attachment of the tricuspid valve and toward the apex.

The pathophysiology and clinical course of VSDs depend on the size of the defect, the status of the pulmonary vascular bed, and the effects of shunt size on intracardiac hemodynamics. Unlike ASDs, the size of a VSD may decrease with time. Approximately half of all native VSDs are small, and more than half of them will close spontaneously; moderate or even large VSDs may also close in 10% or fewer of cases. The highest closure rates are observed in the first decade of life; spontaneous closure in adult life is unusual.

Patients who have a small defect with trivial or mild shunts are defined as those with a Qp:Qs of less than 1.5 and normal pulmonary artery pressure and vascular resistance. Patients with moderate defects have a Qp:Qs ratio of greater than 1.2 and elevated pulmonary artery pressure but not elevated pulmonary vascular resistance. Patients with a large and severe defect have an elevated Qp:Qs ratio with high pulmonary pressure and elevated pulmonary vascular resistance. Eisenmenger's complex develops in about 10% of patients with VSDs, usually when there is no resistance to flow at the level of the defect, which can be as large as the aorta. When a systolic pressure gradient is present between the ventricles, the physiologic severity may be trivial or mild but can also be moderate or severe.

Minimal or mild defects usually cause no significant hemodynamic or physiologic abnormality. A moderate or severe defect will cause left atrial and ventricular dilatation consistent with the degree of left-to-right shunting. Shunting across the ventricular septum occurs predominantly during systole when left ventricular pressure exceeds that on the right; diastolic filling abnormalities occur in the left atrium. With moderate or severe defects, the right heart becomes affected as a function of the rise in pulmonary pressure and pulmonary blood flow.

DIAGNOSIS. An adult with a VSD will most commonly have a

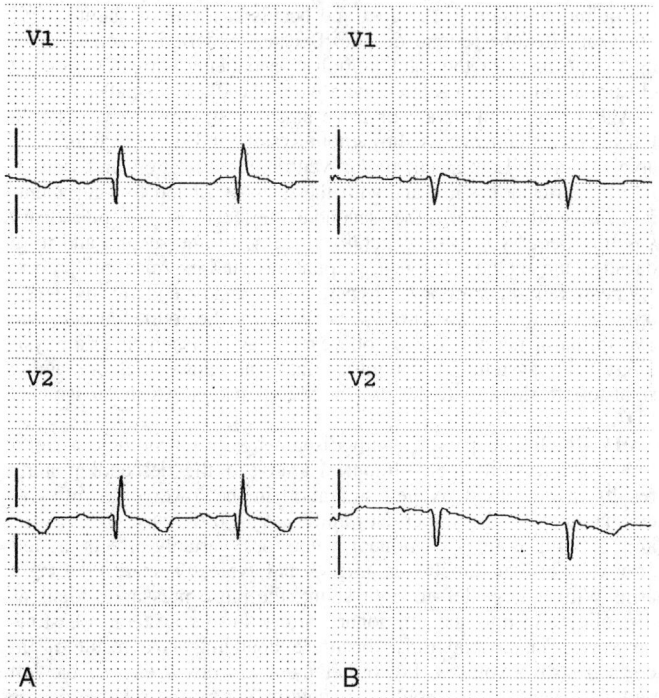

FIGURE 57–4 ■ Electrocardiographic hallmark in atrial septal defect. Right precordial leads V$_1$ and V$_2$ illustrate two variants of an incomplete right bundle branch block pattern: *A,* shows the rSr′ pattern; *B,* shows the ′rsR′ pattern.

small restrictive lesion that either was small at birth or may have undergone some degree of spontaneous closure. A second group of patients consists of those with unoperated large non-restrictive VSDs who have had Eisenmenger's complex for most of their lives. Patients with a moderately sized defect are typically symptomatic as children and are therefore more likely to have repair at a young age.

Patients with a trivial or mild shunt across a small restrictive VSD are usually asymptomatic. Physical examination discloses no evidence of systemic or pulmonary venous congestion, and jugular venous pressure is normal. A thrill may be palpable at the left sternal border. Auscultation reveals a normal S_1 and S_2 without gallops. A grade 4 or louder, widely radiating, high-frequency, pansystolic murmur is heard maximally in the third or fourth intercostal space and reflects the high pressure gradient between the left and right ventricles throughout systole. The striking contrast between a loud murmur and an otherwise normal cardiac examination is an important diagnostic clue. The electrocardiogram and chest radiograph are also normal in small VSDs.

At the other end of the spectrum are patients with Eisenmenger's complex (see above). Between these two extremes are patients with a moderate defect, whose pathology reflects a combination of pulmonary hypertension and left-sided volume overload resulting from a significant left-to-right shunt. In adults, shortness of breath on exertion can be the result of both pulmonary venous congestion and elevated pulmonary pressure. On physical examination, a diffuse palpable left ventricular impulse will occur with a variable degree of right ventricular hypertrophy and an accentuated second heart sound. A systolic murmur persists as long as pulmonary vascular resistance is below systemic resistance. The electrocardiogram commonly shows left atrial enlargement and left ventricular hypertrophy. The chest radiograph will show shunt vascularity with an enlarged left atrium and ventricle. The degree of pulmonary hypertension will determine the size of the pulmonary artery trunk.

Echocardiography can identify the defect and determine the significance of the shunt by assessing left atrial and ventricular size, pulmonary artery pressure, and the presence or absence of right ventricular hypertrophy. Cardiac catheterization is reserved for those in whom surgery is considered. Adults with a small defect of no physiologic significance need not be studied invasively. Those with Eisenmenger's complex have severe pulmonary vascular disease and are not surgical candidates. Patients who have a moderate size shunt that appears hemodynamically significant and in whom pulmonary pressures are elevated are most likely to benefit from direct measurements of pulmonary vascular resistance and reactivity.

MANAGEMENT. All patients with a VSD of any size require endocarditis prophylaxis (see Chapter 326). Patients with Eisenmenger's complex have pulmonary vascular resistance that is prohibitive to surgery. For this group of patients, management will center on the medical complications of cyanosis (see above). In a minority of patients with small defects, complications can relate to progressive tricuspid insufficiency caused by septal aneurysm formation or to acquired aortic insufficiency when an aortic cusp becomes engaged in the high-velocity jet flow generated by the defect. The intermediate group of patients with a defect of moderate physiologic significance should have surgical closure unless contraindicated by high pulmonary vascular resistance.

Late results following operative closure of isolated VSDs include residual patency in up to 20% of patients, only about 5% of whom need a reoperation. Rhythm disturbances after surgical closure of VSDs include tachyarrhythmias and conduction disturbances. Right bundle branch block occurs in one to two thirds of patients, whereas first-degree atrioventricular block and complete heart block occur in fewer than 10%. Sudden cardiac death following surgical repair of VSD occurs in 2% of patients.

Patent Ductus Arteriosus

The ductus arteriosus connects the descending aorta to the main pulmonary trunk near the origin of the left subclavian artery (Fig. 57–5). Normal postnatal closure results in fibrosis and degenerative changes in the ductal lumen, leaving in its place the residual ligamentum arteriosum, which rarely can become part of an abnormal vascular ring. When the duct persists, significant calcification of the aortic ductal end is observed.

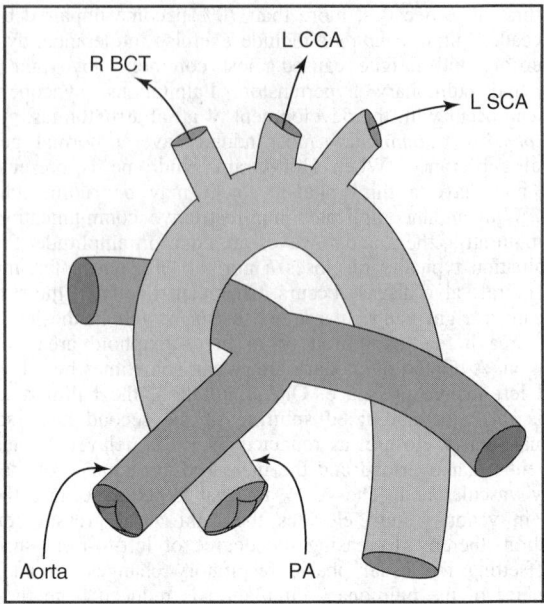

FIGURE 57–5 ■ The anatomy of a patent ductus arteriosus is shown. Note the relation between the position of the ductus and the right and left brachiocephalic vessels. BCT = brachiocephalic; CCA = common carotid artery; L = left; PA = pulmonary artery; PDA = patent ductus arteriosus; R = right; SCA = subclavian artery.

The physiologic consequences of a PDA are determined by its size and length, as well as by the ratio of pressure and resistance of the pulmonary and aortic circulations on either end of the duct. If systolic and diastolic pressure in the aorta exceeds that in the pulmonary artery, aortic blood flows continuously down a pressure gradient into the pulmonary artery and then returns to the left atrium. The left atrium and subsequently the left ventricle dilate, whereas the right heart becomes progressively affected as pulmonary hypertension develops.

A small PDA has continuous flow throughout the entire cardiac cycle without left heart dilatation, pulmonary hypertension, or symptoms. Patients with a small PDA, although protected from hemodynamic complications of a significant left-to-right shunt, remain at risk for infectious endarteritis, which usually develops on the pulmonary side of the duct and occurs at a rate of about 0.45% per year after the second decade. Because endarteritis accounts for up to one third of the total mortality in patients with PDA, ductal closure should be considered even when the PDA is small.

A PDA is of moderate or large size but still restrictive when a left-to-right shunt occurs throughout systole and diastole is of variable duration. Left atrial and/or ventricular dilatation and pulmonary hypertension will vary with the quantity of left-to-right shunting, as well as with the secondary effects on the pulmonary vascular bed. Symptoms generally increase by the second and third decades and include dyspnea, palpitations, and exercise intolerance. As heart failure, pulmonary hypertension, and/or endarteritis develops, mortality rises to 3 to 4% per year by the fourth decade, and two thirds of patients die by 60 years of age. Eisenmenger's physiology with systemic or suprasystemic pulmonary pressure and a right-to-left shunt will develop in 5% of patients with an isolated PDA.

DIAGNOSIS. In patients with Eisenmenger's physiology, a right-to-left shunt from the pulmonary artery to the descending aorta results in decreased oxygen saturation in the lower extremities as compared with the upper extremities; this difference in cyanosis and clubbing is most prominent in the toes, variably affects the left arm via the left subclavian artery, and typically spares the right arm. With a large left-to-right shunt, the pulse pressure widens as diastolic flow into the pulmonary artery lowers systemic diastolic pressure. The arterial pulse becomes bounding as a result of increased stroke volume. Precordial palpation discloses variable left and right ventricular impulses as determined by the relative degree of left-sided volume overload and pulmonary hypertension. In the presence of a continuous aortopulmonary gradient, the classic "machinery" murmur of a PDA can be heard at the first or second left intercostal space below the left clavicle. As the pulmonary pressure rises, the diastolic component of the murmur becomes progressively shorter. With the development of Eisenmenger's physiology and equalization of aortic and pulmonary pressure, the entire murmur may disappear and the clinical findings are dominated by pulmonary hypertension.

In adult patients with a significant left-to-right shunt, the *electrocardiogram* shows a bifid P wave in at least one limb lead consistent with left atrial enlargement and a variable degree of left ventricular hypertrophy. The PR interval is prolonged in about 20% of patients. In older patients, the *chest radiograph* shows calcification at the location of the PDA. Characteristically, the ascending aorta and pulmonary artery are dilated, and the left-sided chambers are enlarged. *Echocardiography* may not directly visualize the PDA but can accurately identify it by a Doppler signal that often parallels the length of the murmur. Left heart dilatation and pulmonary hypertension can be quantified and monitored. Cardiac catheterization to assess pulmonary vascular resistance is commonly indicated before closure.

MANAGEMENT. After ligation of a PDA in infancy or early childhood, bacterial endocarditis prophylaxis is not required, cardiac function is commonly normal, and no special follow-up is required. In patients with an audible PDA by auscultation but without Eisenmenger's disease, the combined risk of endarteritis, heart failure, and late mortality provides the rationale for shunt closure. If pulmonary artery pressure and/or pulmonary vascular resistance are substantially elevated, preoperative evaluation should assess the degree of reversibility. With Eisenmenger's disease, closure is contraindicated.

The PDA can be closed surgically or via transcatheter methods. Reported operative mortality rates vary from less than 1% in uncomplicated PDA to as high as 8% in the presence of substantial pulmonary hypertension. Transcatheter or coil occlusion is an accepted procedure in adults. The widely used Rashkind prosthesis has a residual shunt rate of less than 10% at 3-year follow-up. Small residual defects that are detected by echocardiography but are not associated with an audible murmur or hemodynamic findings do not appear to carry a significant risk for endarteritis.

Aortopulmonary Window

An aortopulmonary window is typically a large defect across the adjacent segments of both great vessels above their respective valves and below the pulmonary artery bifurcation. The pathophysiology is similar to that of a PDA. The shunt is usually large, so pulmonary vascular resistance rises rapidly and abolishes the aortopulmonary gradient in diastole. The murmur is usually best heard at the third left intercostal space. With a right-to-left shunt, differential cyanosis never occurs because the shunt is proximal to the brachiocephalic vessels. Differentiation of an aortopulmonary window from a PDA can usually be confirmed with echocardiography; the left-to-right shunt is seen in the main pulmonary artery in the former as compared with the left pulmonary artery bifurcation in the latter. Cardiac catheterization confirms the diagnosis and hemodynamics. Surgical repair is necessary unless pulmonary vascular obstructive disease precludes closure.

Pulmonary Arteriovenous Fistulas

Pulmonary arteriovenous fistulas can occur as isolated congenital disorders or as part of generalized hereditary hemorrhagic telangiectasia, or the Osler-Weber-Rendu syndrome. These fistulas typically occur in the lower lobes or the right middle lobe and can be small or large, single or multiple. The arterial supply usually comes from a dilated, tortuous branch of the pulmonary artery.

The most common finding is that of abnormal opacity on a chest radiograph in a patient with buccal ruby patches or in an otherwise healthy adult who has mild cyanosis. Shunting between deoxygenated pulmonary arterial blood and the oxygenated pulmonary venous blood results in a physiologic right-to-left shunt. The degree of shunting is typically small and not significant enough to result in dilatation of the left atrium and ventricle. Heart failure is unusual. Hemoptysis can result if a fistula ruptures into a bronchus. In patients with hereditary hemorrhagic telangiectasia, angiomas occur on the lips and mouth, as well as the gastrointestinal tract, and on pleural, liver, and vaginal surfaces. Epistaxis is most common, but cerebrovascular accidents can also occur. Patients with hereditary hemorrhagic telangiectasia can have symptoms that resemble those of a transient ischemic attack even in the absence of right-to-left shunting. On physical examination, cyanosis and club-

bing can be notable or barely detectable. Auscultation can disclose soft systolic or continuous non-cardiac murmurs on the chest wall adjacent to the fistula. The murmur typically increases with inspiration. The electrocardiogram is usually normal. The chest radiograph will show one or more densities, typically in the lower lobes or in the right middle lobe. An echocardiogram can confirm the presence of the fistula by showing early opacification of the left atrium in the absence of any other intracardiac communication when saline is injected into a peripheral vein. The absence of a hemodynamically significant shunt can be confirmed by documenting normal cardiac chamber size.

If the hypoxemia is progressive or if a neurologic complication is documented to have occurred because of paradoxical emboli, fistula closure should be considered. Options include percutaneous catheter techniques if the fistula is small and accessible or a pulmonary wedge resection or lobectomy if the fistula is large. Multiple or recurrent fistulas create a major therapeutic challenge.

Isolated Obstructive Lesions of the Right and Left Ventricular Outflow Tract

Complications of obstructive lesions of the outflow tract relate to the secondary effects of exposure to pressure overload in the chamber proximal to the obstruction. The inability to increase systemic or pulmonary blood flow in the face of a fixed obstruction can cause exercise intolerance, inadequate myocardial perfusion, ventricular arrhythmias, and sudden death.

Right Ventricular Outflow Tract Obstruction

Obstruction of the right ventricular outflow tract can occur at the level of the pulmonary valve (see below), above it in the main pulmonary artery or its branches, or below it in the right ventricle itself. *Supravalvar and branch pulmonary artery stenoses* are important and common complications of patients with the tetralogy of Fallot (see below). Residual supravalvar pulmonary stenosis is sometimes seen after palliative pulmonary artery banding to decrease pulmonary blood flow in patients with large left-to-right shunts. Congenital branch pulmonary artery stenosis can occur in isolation or with valvar pulmonary stenosis, shunt lesions, or a variety of syndromes. Patients with Noonan's syndrome have a characteristic phenotypic facial appearance, short stature, and webbed neck; cardiac lesions may include a dysplastic pulmonary valve, left ventricular hypertrophic cardiomyopathy, and peripheral pulmonary artery stenosis. Supravalvar pulmonary stenosis can be seen with supravalvar aortic stenosis in the Williams elfin facies syndrome.

Pulmonary atresia refers to an absent, imperforate, or closed pulmonary valve, which typically occurs in conjunction with other malformations. Pulmonary atresia with a non-restrictive VSD is a complex cyanotic malformation discussed later.

Primary *infundibular stenosis* with an intact ventricular septum can result from a fibrous band just below the infundibulum. In a *double-chambered right ventricle*, obstruction is caused by anomalous muscle bundles that divide the right ventricle into a high-pressure chamber below the hypertrophied muscle bundles and a low-pressure chamber above the bundles and below the valve. The clinical features will vary depending on the presence or absence of other lesions such as pulmonary valvar stenosis or VSD.

Valvar Pulmonary Stenosis

Isolated congenital *valvar pulmonary stenosis* is a common lesion caused by a bicuspid valve in 20% of cases, a dysplastic valve caused by myxomatous changes and severe thickening in 10% of cases, and an abnormal trileaflet valve in most of the remaining cases. Fusion of the leaflets results in a variable degree of thickening and calcification in older patients.

Twenty-five year survival of patients with valvar pulmonary stenosis is greater than 95% but is worse in those with severe stenosis and peak systolic gradients greater than 80 mm Hg. For patients with mild (<50–mm Hg gradients) and moderate (50– to 80–mm Hg gradients) pulmonary stenosis, bacterial endocarditis, complex ventricular arrhythmias, and progression of the stenosis are uncommon.

DIAGNOSIS. A patient with moderate or even severe pulmonary stenosis may be asymptomatic. With severe stenosis, exercise intolerance can be associated with pre-syncope and ventricular arrhythmias. Progressive right heart failure is the most common cause of death. On *physical examination* of patients with significant pulmonary stenosis, jugular venous pressure has a dominant a wave reflecting a non-compliant right ventricle. Palpation discloses a sustained parasternal lift of right ventricular hypertrophy. An expiratory systolic ejection click is characteristic if the leaflets are still mobile. In moderate or severe stenosis, a grade 3 or louder systolic murmur can be heard and felt in the second left interspace. The length of the murmur increases as it peaks progressively later in systole with an increasing degree of obstruction. If right heart failure occurs, tricuspid insufficiency and systemic venous congestion develop. The *electrocardiogram* can show right axis deviation and tall, peaked right atrial P waves in lead II. With more than mild stenosis, the R wave exceeds the S wave in lead V_1. On chest radiography, the main pulmonary artery can be dilated even if the stenosis is mild. Characteristically, the left pulmonary artery is more dilated than the right because of the leftward direction of the high-velocity jet. A variable degree of right ventricular hypertrophy will be manifested as right-sided chamber enlargement. Echocardiography can establish the diagnosis and determine the severity by Doppler ultrasound.

MANAGEMENT. For gradients less than 50 mm Hg, conservative management is indicated and exercise should not be limited. Because progression is uncommon, repeat echocardiography can be performed at about 5-year intervals in the absence of symptoms. For gradients greater than 80 mm Hg, balloon valvuloplasty or surgical valvulotomy should be performed. For gradients of 50 to 80 mm Hg, intervention is generally recommended particularly in symptomatic patients.

Left Ventricular Outflow Tract Obstruction

Stenosis of the left ventricular outflow tract can occur at, below, or above the aortic valve. Discrete *subaortic stenosis*, most commonly caused by a fibromuscular ring located just below the valve, accounts for 15 to 20% of all cases of congenital obstruction of the left ventricular outflow tract. Concomitant aortic insufficiency occurs in 50% of cases. Supravalvar aortic stenosis occurs as a result of thickened media and intima above the aortic sinuses; early coronary atherosclerosis or even ostial coronary obstruction can occur.

Congenital Valvar Aortic Stenosis

The normal aortic valve has three cusps and commissures. A unicuspid aortic valve accounts for the majority of cases of severe aortic stenosis in infants (see also Chapter 63). A *bicuspid aortic valve*, which is the most common congenital cardiac malformation, functions normally at birth but often becomes gradually obstructed as calcific and fibrous changes occur; prolapse of one or both cusps can cause aortic insufficiency.

The pathophysiology of aortic stenosis depends not only on its severity but also on the age at diagnosis. When a functionally normal bicuspid aortic valve becomes stenotic in adulthood because of degenerative changes, criteria for diagnosis and intervention parallel those for other forms of acquired aortic stenosis (see Chapter 63). When the valve is congenitally stenotic, myocardium with a lifelong exposure to pressure overload behaves differently than if the hemodynamic burden occurred later in life.

The estimated overall 25-year survival rate for patients with congenital valvar aortic stenosis diagnosed in childhood is 85%. Children with initial peak cardiac catheterization gradients less than 50 mm Hg have long-term survival rates of over 90%, as opposed to survival rates of 80% in those with gradients of 50 mm Hg or greater.

DIAGNOSIS. Symptoms include angina, exertional dyspnea, presyncope, and syncope and may progress to heart failure. The auscultatory hallmark of a bicuspid aortic valve is an audible systolic ejection click that is typically of a higher pitch than the first heart sound and is best heard not at the cardiac base but at the apex. The sound is caused by sudden movement of the stenotic valve as it moves superiorly in systole and is followed by the typical aortic stenosis murmur (see Chapter 63). When significant calcification of the valve results in reduced mobility, the ejection sound is no longer heard. The diagnosis is easily confirmed by two-dimensional echocardiography, with which the number and orientation of aortic cusps can readily be identified.

MANAGEMENT. Conservative management is generally indicated for mild stenosis with a peak gradient of less than 25 mm Hg, but close supervision is required because 20% of these patients will require an intervention during long-term follow-up. Unlimited athletic participation is allowed only for asymptomatic patients with peak gradients of less than 20 to 25 mm Hg, a normal electrocardiogram, and a normal exercise test. For children who are symptomatic or have gradients greater than 30 mm Hg but do not have significant aortic insufficiency, transcatheter aortic valvotomy is preferred. Aortic valvuloplasty can be considered in young adults, but calcification limits its success and valve replacement is usually required (see Chapter 63). For adults, treatment decisions are similar to those for aortic stenosis from other causes.

Coarctation of the Aorta

Aortic coarctation typically occurs just distal to the left subclavian artery at the site of the aortic ductal attachment or its residual ligamentum arteriosum. Less commonly the coarctation ridge lies proximal to the left subclavian. A bicuspid aortic valve is the most common coexisting anomaly, but VSDs and PDAs are also seen. "Pseudocoarctation" refers to buckling or kinking of the aortic arch without the presence of a significant gradient.

The most common complications of aortic coarctation are systemic hypertension and secondary left ventricular hypertrophy with heart failure. Systemic hypertension is caused by decreased vascular compliance in the proximal aorta and activation of the renin-angiotensin system in response to renal artery hypoperfusion below the obstruction. Left ventricular hypertrophy occurs in response to chronic pressure overload. Congestive heart failure occurs most commonly in infants and then after 40 years of age. The high pressure proximal to the obstruction stimulates the growth of collateral vessels from the internal mammary, scapular, and superior intercostal arteries to the intercostals of the descending aorta. Collateral circulation increases with age and contributes to perfusion of the lower extremities and the spinal cord. This mechanism, although adaptive in a patient who has not undergone surgery, accounts for significant morbidity during surgery when the motor impairment results from inadequate protection of spinal perfusion. Aneurysms occur most notably in the ascending aorta and in the circle of Willis. Premature coronary disease is thought to be related to the resulting hypertension. Complications, including bacterial endarteritis at the coarctation site or more commonly endocarditis at the site of a bicuspid aortic valve, cerebrovascular complications, myocardial infarction, heart failure, and aortic dissection, occur in 2 to 6% of patients, more frequently in those with advancing age who have not undergone surgery.

DIAGNOSIS. Young adults may be asymptomatic with incidental systemic hypertension and decreased lower extremity pulses. Coarctation should always be considered in adolescents and young adult males with unexplained upper extremity hypertension. The pressure differential can cause epistaxis, headaches, leg fatigue, or claudication. Older patients have angina, symptoms of heart failure, and vascular complications.

On *physical examination*, the lower half of the body is typically slightly less developed than the upper half. The hips are narrow and the legs are short, in contrast to broad shoulders and long arms. Blood pressure measurements should be obtained in each arm and one leg; an abnormal measurement is a less than 10 mm Hg increase in popliteal systolic blood pressure as compared with arm systolic blood pressure. The diastolic pressure should be the same in the upper and lower extremities. A pressure differential of more than 30 mm Hg between the right and the left arms is consistent with compromised flow in the left subclavian artery. Right brachial palpation characteristically reveals a strong or even bounding pulse as compared with a slowly rising or absent femoral, popliteal, or pedal pulse. Examination of the eyegrounds can reveal tortuous or corkscrew retinal arteries. Precordial palpation is consistent with left ventricular pressure overload. On auscultation, a systolic ejection sound reflecting the presence of a bicuspid aortic valve should be sought. The coarctation itself generates a systolic murmur heard posteriorly, in the mid-thoracic region, the length of which correlates with the severity of the coarctation. Over the anterior of the chest, systolic murmurs reflecting increased collateral flow can be heard in the infraclavicular areas and the sternal edge or in the axillae.

In adult coarctation, the most common finding on the *electrocardiogram* is left ventricular hypertrophy. *Chest radiographic* findings are diagnostic. Location of the coarctation segment between

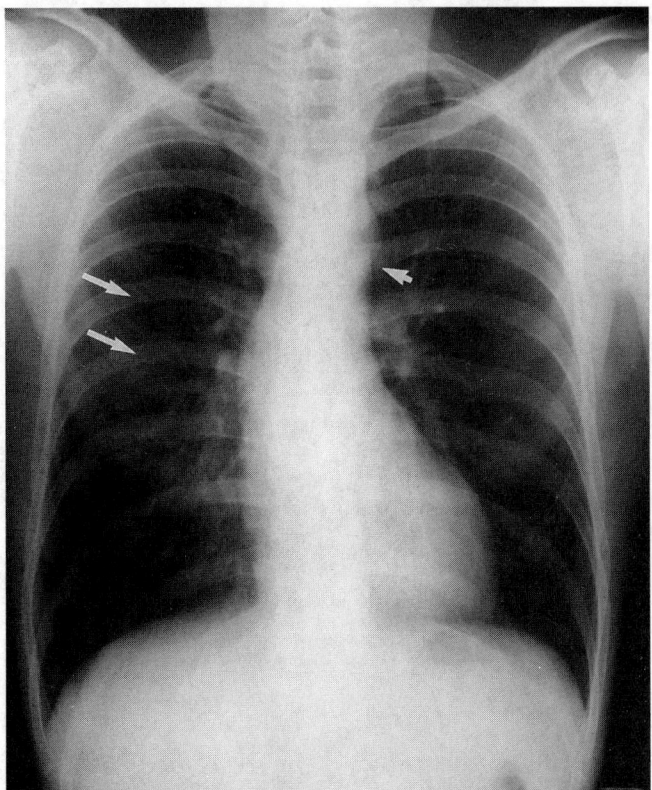

FIGURE 57-6 ■ Chest radiograph of a patient with coarctation of the aorta showing the radiographic "3" formed by the dilated subclavian artery above and the dilated aorta below (short arrow). Note the notching best seen at the level of the 7th and 8th ribs (long arrows). The dilated ascending aortic segment can also be seen.

the dilated left subclavian artery above and the leftward convexity of the descending aorta below results in the "3 sign" (Fig. 57-6). Bilateral rib notching as a result of dilation of the posterior intercostal arteries is seen on the posterior of the third to eighth ribs when the coarctation is located below the left subclavian. Unilateral rib notching sparing the left ribs is observed when the coarctation occurs proximal to the left subclavian artery. Transthoracic *echocardiography* documents the gradient in the descending aorta and determines the presence of left ventricular hypertrophy. MRI (see Chapter 45) is the best modality for visualizing the anatomy of the descending aorta. *Cardiac catheterization* should measure pressures and assess collaterals when surgery is contemplated.

MANAGEMENT. Repair is considered in patients with gradients greater than 30 mm Hg on cardiac catheterization. Fifty per cent of patients repaired when older than 40 years have residual hypertension, whereas those who have undergone surgery between the ages of 1 and 5 years have a less than 10% prevalence of hypertension on long-term follow-up. Balloon angioplasty is the treatment of choice for focal recoarctation in previously operated patients.

Anomalies of the Sinuses of Valsalva and Coronary Arteries

Sinus of Valsalva Aneurysms

At the base of the aortic root, the aortic valve cusps are attached to the aortic wall, above which three small pouches, or sinuses, are seated. The right coronary artery originates from one sinus and the left main coronary artery from a second; the third is called the noncoronary sinus. A weakness in the wall of the sinus can result in aneurysm formation with or without rupture. In over 90% of cases the aneurysm involves the right or non-coronary cusp. Rupture typically occurs into the right heart at the right atrial or ventricular level with a resulting large left-to-right shunt driven by the high aortic pressure.

A previously asymptomatic young man typically has chest pain and rapidly progressing shortness of breath sometimes after physical strain. The physical examination is consistent with significant

heart failure. Even if the communication is between the aorta and the right heart, biventricular failure is not unusual. The classic murmur is loud and continuous, often with a thrill. A murmur of aortic insufficiency secondary to damage to the adjacent aortic valve may be superimposed. The chest radiograph shows volume overload of both ventricles with evidence of shunt vascularity and pulmonary venous congestion. The echocardiogram is diagnostic. Cardiac catheterization can verify the integrity of the coronary artery adjacent to the ruptured aneurysm.

Even though symptoms may abate as the heart dilates, progressive cardiac decompensation typically results in death within 1 year of the rupture. A ruptured sinus of Valsalva aneurysm therefore requires urgent surgical repair.

Coronary Artery Fistulas

Fistulas arise from the right or left coronary arteries and in 90% of cases drain into the right ventricle, the right atrium, or the pulmonary artery in order of decreasing frequency. Typically, young patients are asymptomatic, but supraventricular arrhythmias are seen with progressive dilatation of the intracardiac chambers. Angina can occur as the fistula creates a coronary steal by diverting blood away from the myocardium. Congestive heart failure is seen with large fistulas. A continuous murmur heard in a young, otherwise normal acyanotic, asymptomatic patient should raise suspicion of the diagnosis. Most fistulas are associated with a small shunt and hence the murmur is often less than grade 3 and is heard in the precordial area. Unless the shunt is large, the electrocardiogram is normal, as is the chest radiograph. The echocardiogram, especially the TEE, is diagnostic. Percutaneous transcatheter closure with coil embolization is preferred, but surgical ligation is also an alternative.

Anomalous Origin of the Coronary Arteries

The left main coronary artery normally arises from the left sinus of Valsalva and courses leftward, posterior to the right ventricular outflow tract. The right coronary artery arises from the right sinus of Valsalva and courses rightward to the right ventricle. Isolated ectopic or anomalous origins of the coronary arteries (see Fig. 45-2) are seen in 0.6 to 1.5% of patients undergoing coronary angiography.

The most common anomaly is ectopic origin of the left circumflex artery from the right sinus of Valsalva, followed by anomalous origin of the right coronary artery from the left sinus and anomalous origin of the left main coronary artery from the right sinus. If the anomalous coronary artery does not course between the pulmonary artery and aorta, the prognosis is favorable. Risks of ischemia, myocardial infarction, and death are greatest when the left main coronary artery courses between both great vessels.

Coronary arteries can also originate from the pulmonary trunk. If both the right and left arteries originate from the pulmonary trunk, death usually occurs in the neonatal period. If only the left anterior descending coronary artery originates from the pulmonary trunk, the rate of survival to adulthood is approximately 10%, depending on the development of collateral retrograde flow to the anomalous artery from a normal coronary artery. This collateral flow may cause a continuous murmur along the left sternal border, congestive heart failure from the large shunt, and a coronary steal syndrome as blood is diverted away from the normal artery.

A single coronary ostium can provide a single coronary artery that branches into right and left coronary arteries, the left then giving rise to the circumflex and the anterior descending arteries. The ostium can originate from the right or left aortic sinus. The coronary circulation is functionally normal unless one of the branches passes between the aorta and the pulmonary artery.

Diagnostic procedures include angiography, MRI, and TEE. For an anomalous coronary artery that originates from the pulmonary artery, surgical reimplantation into the aorta is preferred. For an anomalous artery that courses between the pulmonary artery and aorta, a bypass graft to the distal vessel is preferred.

SPECIFIC COMPLEX LESIONS

Tetralogy of Fallot

Tetralogy of Fallot, the most common cyanotic malformation, is characterized by superior and anterior displacement of the subpulmonary infundibular septum, which causes the tetrad of pulmonary stenosis, VSD, aortic override, and right ventricular hypertrophy. The VSD is perimembranous in 80% of cases. Additional cardiac anomalies include a right-sided aortic arch in up to 25% of patients. An anomalous left anterior descending artery originating from the right coronary cusp and crossing over the right ventricular outflow tract is seen in 10% of cases. Other associated anomalies include ASD, left superior vena cava, defects of the atrioventricular canal, and aortic insufficiency. With pulmonary atresia, pulmonary blood flow occurs via aortic-to-pulmonary collaterals. Life expectancy is limited unless staged reconstructive surgery is performed.

The physiology in unrepaired tetralogy of Fallot is determined by the severity and location of the pulmonic outflow obstruction and by the interaction of pulmonary and systemic vascular resistance across a non-restrictive VSD. Because the pulmonary stenosis results in a relatively fixed pulmonary resistance, a drop in systemic vascular resistance as occurs with exercise is associated with increased right-to-left shunting and increasing cyanosis. A child who squats after running is attempting to reverse the process by increasing systemic vascular resistance by crouching with bent knees. Native pulmonary blood flow is typically insufficient. Unless a PDA has remained open, a cyanotic adult will typically have undergone a palliative procedure to increase pulmonary blood flow.

Examination of unrepaired patients reveals central cyanosis and clubbing. The right ventricular impulse is prominent. The second heart sound is single and represents the aortic closure sound with an absent or inconspicuous P_2. Typically, little or no systolic murmur is heard across the pulmonary valve because the more severe the obstruction, the more right-to-left shunting occurs and the less blood flows across a diminutive right ventricular outflow tract. A diastolic murmur of aortic insufficiency is often heard in adults. In the presence of a palliative systemic arterial–to–pulmonary artery shunt, the high-pressure gradient generates a loud continuous murmur. In a patient who has not undergone surgery, progressive infundibular stenosis and cyanosis occur. Before the advent of palliative surgery, mortality rates were 50% in the first few years of life and survival past the third decade was unusual.

Complete surgical repair consists of patch closure of the VSD and relief of the right ventricular outflow tract obstruction. Adequate pulmonary blood flow is ensured by reconstructing the distal pulmonary artery bed. Previous palliative shunts are usually taken down. Complete repair in childhood yields a 90 to 95% 10-year survival rate with good functional results, and 30-year survival rates may be as high as 85%. Total correction with low mortality and a favorable long-term follow-up is possible even in adulthood.

After repair, residual pulmonary stenosis, proximal or distal, with a right ventricular pressure greater than 50% of systemic occurs in up to 25% of patients. Some degree of pulmonary insufficiency is common, particularly if a patch has been inserted at the level of the pulmonary valve or if a pulmonary valvotomy has been performed. Residual VSDs can be found in up to 20% of patients. Patients may be asymptomatic or may have symptoms related to long-term complications following surgical repair. Symptoms can reflect residual right ventricular pressure or volume overload or arrhythmias at rest or with exercise. Angina can occur in a young patient if surgical repair has damaged an anomalous left anterior descending artery as it courses across the right ventricular outflow tract. In acyanotic adults, clubbing commonly regresses. A right ventricular impulse is often felt as a result of residual pulmonary insufficiency or stenosis. Typically, no functioning pulmonary valve is present and hence the second heart sound is still single. A systolic murmur can represent residual pulmonary stenosis, residual VSD, or tricuspid insufficiency. A diastolic murmur can reflect aortic or pulmonary insufficiency. Ventricular arrhythmias are common following repair, with an incidence of sudden death as high as 5%.

The electrocardiogram in unrepaired tetralogy of Fallot will show right axis deviation, right atrial enlargement, and dominant right ventricular forces over the precordial leads. The most common finding following repair is complete right bundle branch block, which is seen in 80 to 90% of patients. The chest radiograph typically shows an upturned apex with a concave pulmonary artery segment giving the classic appearance of a "boot-shaped" heart. Figure 57–7 demonstrates the findings in an adult following repair. The apex is persistently upturned although the pulmonary artery

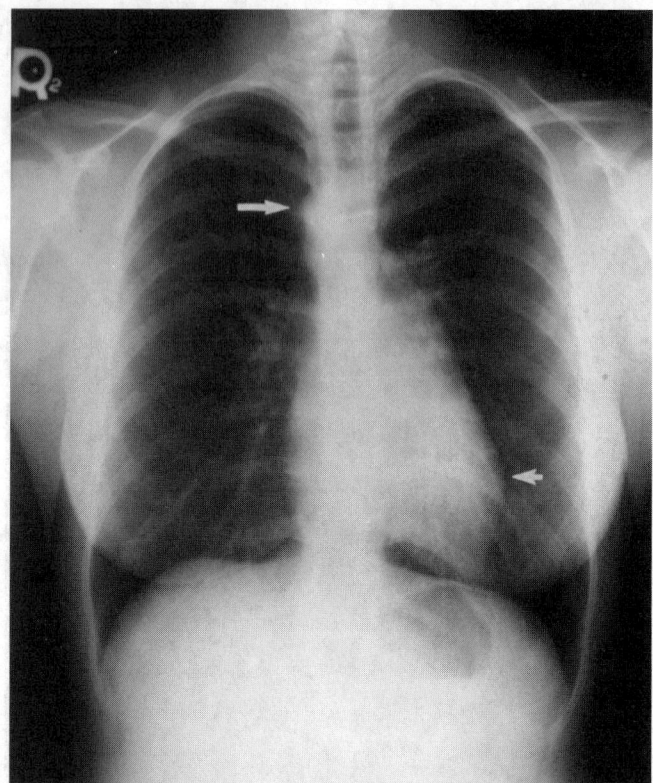

FIGURE 57–7 ■ Chest radiograph of an adult after tetralogy of Fallot repair. A right aortic arch with rightward indentation of the trachea (long arrow) can be seen. The right ventricular apex remains upturned (short arrow). Note the sternal wires consistent with intracardiac repair, thus clarifying the fullness of the pulmonary artery segment often seen after extensive enlargement of the right ventricular outflow tract.

segment is no longer concave. Echocardiography can confirm the diagnosis and document intracardiac complications in repaired and unrepaired patients. Shunt patency can be determined by Doppler. MRI can accurately document stenosis in the distal pulmonary artery bed. Cardiac catheterization is reserved for patients in whom operative or reoperative treatment is contemplated or in whom the integrity of the coronary circulation needs to be verified.

Patients with a change in exercise tolerance, angina, or evidence of heart failure, as well as those with symptomatic arrhythmias and/or syncope, should be referred for complete evaluation. Surgical *reintervention* is generally considered when right ventricular pressure is more than two thirds systemic because of residual right ventricular outflow tract obstruction.

Complete Transposition of the Great Arteries

Complete TGA is the second most common cyanotic lesion, and surgically corrected adults are increasingly common. In simple TGA, the atria and ventricles are in their normal positions but the aorta arises from the right ventricle and the pulmonary artery arises from the left ventricle. When the aorta is anterior and rightward with respect to the pulmonary artery, as is most common, D-transposition is present. The native anatomy has the pulmonary and systemic circulations in parallel, with deoxygenated blood recirculating between the right side of the heart and the systemic circulation whereas oxygenated blood recirculates from the left side of the heart to the lungs. The condition is incompatible with life unless a VSD, PDA, or ASD is present or an ASD is created; a hemodynamically significant VSD is present in 15% of cases. Subpulmonary obstruction of the *left* ventricular outflow tract occurs in 10 to 25% of cases.

The *Senning* or *Mustard atrial baffle repairs*, which were the first corrective procedures, redirect oxygenated blood from the left atrium to the right ventricle so that it may be ejected into the aorta while deoxygenated blood detours the right atrium and heads for the left ventricle and into the pulmonary artery. Although this operation results in acyanotic physiology, the right ventricle assumes a permanent position under the aorta and pumps against systemic pressures, a lifelong task for which it was not designed. When the subpulmonary obstruction is significant, the *Rastelli* procedure reroutes blood at the ventricular level by tunneling the left ventricle to the *aorta* inside the heart through a VSD. A conduit is then inserted outside the heart between the left ventricle and aorta. More recently, the *arterial switch operation* transects the aorta and pulmonary artery above their respective valves and switches them to become realigned with their physiologic outflow tracts and appropriate ventricles. The proximal coronary arteries are translocated from the sinuses of the native aorta to the neo-aorta (native pulmonary artery). In this operation, each ventricle reassumes the role that it was embryologically destined to fulfill.

If an adult patient is cyanotic and has a native intracardiac shunt or a palliative shunt, referral to an appropriate facility should be undertaken to explore the possibility of intracardiac repair. At the current time, adults with TGA most commonly have undergone an *atrial baffle repair*, with an expected 15-year survival rate of 75% and a 20-year survival rate of 70%. For patients with an atrial baffle procedure, symptoms include exercise intolerance, palpitations caused by bradyarrhythmias or atrial flutter, and right ventricular failure. Typically the patient is acyanotic unless a baffle leak exists. The clinical findings are determined by the presence or absence of systemic right ventricular failure. On auscultation, the second heart sound is classically single. The electrocardiogram reveals sinus bradycardia, but nodal rhythms and heart block occur as the patient ages. The chest radiograph shows a variable degree of right ventricular enlargement. Echocardiography can be used to confirm the diagnosis and explore related abnormalities. Cardiac catheterization is performed when an operation or reoperation is contemplated. Reoperation is performed in approximately 20% of patients for baffle-related complications, progressive left ventricular outflow tract stenosis, or severe tricuspid regurgitation.

Congenitally Corrected Transposition of the Great Arteries

In congenitally corrected TGA, the great arteries are transposed, the ventricles are inverted, but the atria remain in their normal position. The systemic circulation (left atrium, morphologic right ventricle, and aorta) and pulmonary circulation (right atrium, morphologic left ventricle, and pulmonary artery) are in series. The patient is therefore acyanotic unless an intracardiac shunt is also present. The right ventricle is aligned with the aorta and performs lifelong systemic work, which accounts in part for its eventual failure. Associated lesions include a VSD, pulmonary stenosis, and Ebstein's malformation of the left-sided tricuspid valve. Complete heart block develops at a rate of 2% per year. Patients with congenitally corrected TGA and no other associated defects can remain free of symptoms until the sixth decade, at which time significant atrioventricular valve regurgitation, failure of the right (systemic) ventricle, supraventricular arrhythmias, and heart block occur.

Right-Sided Ebstein's Anomaly

The septal and posterior cusps of the tricuspid valve are largely derived from the right ventricle as it liberates a layer of muscle that skirts away from the cavity to become valve tissue. When this process occurs abnormally, the posterior and septal cusps of the tricuspid valve remain tethered to the muscle and adhere to the right ventricular surface—hence the diagnostic hallmark of Ebstein's anomaly, apical displacement of the septal tricuspid leaflet.

In right-sided Ebstein's anomaly of the tricuspid valve, the right heart consists of three anatomic components: right atrium proper, true right ventricle, and the atrialized portion of the right ventricle between the two. The displaced septal and posterior tricuspid leaflets lie between the atrialized right ventricle and the true right ventricle. In mild Ebstein's anomaly, the degree of tricuspid leaflet tethering is only mild, the anterior leaflet retains mobility, and the size of the true right ventricle is only mildly reduced. Severe Ebstein's anomaly is associated with severe tethering of the tricuspid leaflet tissue and a diminutive, hypocontractile true right ventricle. Functionally the valve is regurgitant because it is unable to appose its three leaflets during ventricular contraction. Valvular regurgitation and asynchronous, abnormal right ventricular function cause the dilatation and right heart failure observed in the more severe forms of the lesion. The wide spectrum of severity of the anomaly is based on the degree of tricuspid leaflet tethering and

the relative proportion of atrialized and true right ventricle. The most common associated cardiac defect, a secundum ASD or patent foramen ovale, is reported in over 50% of patients. On physical examination, a clicking "sail sound" is heard as the second component of S_1 when tricuspid valve closure becomes loud and delayed.

The 12-lead electrocardiogram typically shows highly peaked P waves with a wide, often bizarre-looking QRS complex. Pre-excitation occurs in 20% of patients; supraventricular tachyarrhythmias, atrial fibrillation, and atrial flutter occur in 30 to 40% of patients and constitute the most common findings in adolescents and adults with right-sided Ebstein's anomaly.

When patients of all ages are taken together, the predicted mortality is approximately 50% by the fourth or fifth decade. Surgical options include replacement or repair of the tricuspid valve and closure of the ASD. The feasibility of tricuspid valvuloplasty depends on the size and mobility of the anterior tricuspid leaflet, which is used to construct a unicuspid right-sided valve.

Atrioventricular Canal Defect

Embryologic septation of the atrioventricular canal results in closure of the inferior portion of the interatrial septum and the superior portion of the interventricular septum. Septation is achieved with the growth of endocardial cushions, which also contribute to development of the mitral and tricuspid valves. Hence the nomenclature "atrioventricular canal defect" or "endocardial cushion defect" is used to designate this group of anomalies.

A *partial atrioventricular canal defect* refers to an ostium primum ASD with a cleft mitral valve. The anomaly is manifested as a hemodynamic combination of an ASD with a variable degree of mitral regurgitation. The 12-lead electrocardiogram shows the typical findings of left axis deviation with a Q wave in leads I and aVL and a prolonged PR interval. The echocardiogram shows a defect in the inferior portion of the interatrial septum and a cleft mitral valve.

A *complete atrioventricular canal defect* is an uncommon defect consisting of a primum ASD, an inlet VSD that usually extends to the membranous interventricular septum, and a common atrioventricular valve. Unoperated adults usually have Eisenmenger's syndrome unless concomitant pulmonary stenosis has protected the pulmonary vascular bed or the VSD has undergone spontaneous closure, in which case the physiologic consequences are similar to those of a partial atrioventricular canal.

Surgical repair of an atrioventricular defect consists of closing the interatrial and/or interventricular communication with reconstruction of the common atrioventricular valve or closure of the cleft in the mitral valve. An adult who has undergone repair may have significant residual regurgitation of the mitral or tricuspid valve. Even after surgery, acquired subaortic obstruction can occur in the long left ventricular outflow tract, which has a classic "gooseneck deformity" on cardiac angiography.

Univentricular Heart and Tricuspid Atresia

The terms single ventricle, common ventricle, and univentricular heart have been used interchangeably to describe the "double-inlet ventricle," in which one ventricular chamber receives flow from both the tricuspid and mitral valves. In 75 to 90% of cases, the single ventricle is a morphologic left ventricle. Obstruction of one of the great arteries is common, and life expectancy is short without an operation. The patients most likely to survive to adulthood palliated or, rarely, unoperated have a single ventricle of the left morphologic type with pulmonary stenosis protecting the pulmonary vascular bed.

In tricuspid atresia, no orifice is found between the right atrium and right ventricle, and an underdeveloped or hypoplastic right ventricle is present. The morphologic left ventricle is consistently normally developed and therefore becomes the single functional ventricle. Typically, blood flows into the right atrium then through an obligatory ASD and to the left atrium, where it then proceeds to the left ventricle. Variable features include a VSD, abnormal position of the great arteries, and a variable relative degree of pulmonary stenosis, all of which are used to classify tricuspid atresia. Unoperated, 50% of patients die in the first 6 months and 90% in the first decade.

Adult patients will rarely be unoperated. They may be acyanotic after the Fontan operation; if cyanotic and palliated, the patient may benefit from further palliation or may be eligible for the Fontan operation. With the Glenn shunt or the Fontan operation, a direct anastomosis is created between the systemic venous and pulmonary circulations. Venous blood flows passively from the systemic veins to the pulmonary circulation and returns oxygenated to a left-sided atrium and into the single functional ventricle, which then pumps oxygenated blood into the systemic circulation. The Glenn anastomosis diverts part of the systemic venous return to the lungs, whereas the Fontan procedure makes the patient acyanotic by diverting the entire systemic venous circulation to the pulmonary vascular bed. For optimum results, a successful Fontan operation requires low pulmonary vascular resistance, preserved single ventricular function, and an unobstructed anastomosis between the systemic veins and the pulmonary arteries. At 5-year follow-up, 80% or more of Fontan survivors are in New York Heart Association Functional Class I or II, with successful pregnancy reported in a small number of patients. When patients of all ages are considered together, 10-year survival rates vary from 60 to 70%. Late deaths are due to reoperation, arrhythmia, ventricular failure, and protein-losing enteropathy.

VASCULAR MALFORMATIONS

Aortic Arch Anomalies

VASCULAR RINGS AND OTHER ARCH ANOMALIES. One of the most frequent developmental errors of the aortic arch is an aberrant right subclavian artery originating distal to the left subclavian and coursing rightward behind the esophagus at the level of the third thoracic vertebrae. Although the finding is frequent, symptoms are uncommon. When symptoms occur, the term *dysphagia lusoria* has been used in reference to swallowing difficulties that result from esophageal compression. Abnormal development of the brachial arches and dorsal aorta can result in a variety of anomalies that lead to the formation of *vascular rings* around the trachea and esophagus. The outcome is often benign, but symptoms of respiratory compromise or dysphagia warrant surgery. When the left pulmonary artery arises from the right and passes leftward between the trachea and esophagus, a *pulmonary artery sling* occurs. Symptoms of tracheal compression warrant correction.

A *right aortic arch* occurs when the aortic arch courses toward the right instead of the left. Mirror-image branching is the most common anatomic variant. In the vast majority of cases, this anomaly coexists with other congenital lesions, notably the tetralogy of Fallot.

Anomalous Venous Connections

ANOMALIES OF SYSTEMIC VENOUS RETURN. A *persistent left superior vena cava* can be fortuitously diagnosed on a chest radiograph or on echocardiography. Its clinical relevance depends on development of the coronary sinus. If the coronary sinus is normally formed, typically the left superior vena cava drains into the right atrium through the coronary sinus. If the coronary sinus is not normally developed, the persistent left superior vena cava drains into the left atrium and cyanosis results from the obligatory right-to-left shunt. The latter commonly occurs with an ASD or a complex cardiac anomaly. Venous return above the renal veins can be abnormal with *inferior vena cava interruption* and azygos or hemiazygos continuation. In the former, inferior vena cava flow above the renal veins continues into the azygos vein, which courses normally up the right of the spine to empty into the junction between the superior vena cava and right atrium. In a less common anatomic arrangement, the caval flow empties into a hemiazygos vein, which empties into a persistent left superior vena cava. The finding rarely occurs in isolation but can be seen in patients with associated simple or complex malformations.

ANOMALIES OF PULMONARY VENOUS RETURN. In *partial anomalous pulmonary venous return,* one or more but not all four pulmonary veins are not connected to the left atrium. The most common pattern has the right pulmonary veins connected to the superior vena cava, usually with a *sinus venosus* ASD. Anomalous connection of the right pulmonary veins to the inferior vena cava

results in a chest radiographic shadow that resembles a Turkish sword, hence the designation "*scimitar syndrome.*" Associated anomalies include hypoplasia of the right lung, anomalies of the bronchial system, hypoplasia of the right pulmonary artery, and dextroposition of the heart. Partial anomalous pulmonary venous return results in a left-to-right shunt physiology similar to that of an ASD.

In *total anomalous pulmonary venous return,* all the pulmonary veins connect abnormally to either the right atrium or one of the systemic veins above or below the diaphragm. Concurrent obstruction of the pulmonary veins is present when drainage occurs below the diaphragm and variable when drainage occurs above it. An ASD is essential to sustain life. One third of cases occur with major complex cardiac malformations.

In *cor triatriatum,* the pulmonary veins drain into an accessory chamber that is usually connected to the left atrium through an opening of variable size. The hemodynamic consequences are determined by the size of this opening and are similar to those of mitral stenosis. If symptoms of pulmonary venous hypertension occur, surgical treatment is indicated.

CARDIAC MALPOSITIONS

The normal heart is left sided and hence the designation levocardia. Cardiac malpositions are defined in terms of the intrathoracic position of the heart in relation to the position of the viscera (visceral situs), which are usually concordant with the position of the atria. That is, when the liver is on the right and the stomach is on the left, the atrium receiving systemic venous blood (right atrium) is right sided and the atrium receiving pulmonary venous blood (left atrium) is left sided. Asplenia and polysplenia syndromes are associated with a variety of complex cardiovascular malformations.

DEXTROCARDIA AND MESOCARDIA. In *dextrocardia* the heart is on the right side of the thorax with or without situs inversus. When the heart is right sided with inverted atria, a right-sided stomach, and a left-sided liver, the combination is *dextrocardia with situs inversus.* In this arrangement, also called *mirror-image dextrocardia,* the ventricles are inverted, but so are the viscera and therefore the atria. The heart usually functions normally, and the diagnosis is often fortuitous. The heart sounds are louder on the right side of the chest and the liver is palpable on the left. The chest radiograph shows a right-sided cardiac apex with a lower left hemidiaphragm and a right-sided stomach bubble. The electrocardiogram shows an inverted P and T wave in lead I with a negative QRS deflection and a reverse pattern between aVR and aVL. A mirror-image progression is seen from V_1 to a right-sided V_6 lead. An echocardiogram should be performed to ensure that intracardiac anatomy is normal. When *dextrocardia with situs solitus* occurs, the ventricles are inverted but not the viscera and therefore not the atria. Associated severe cardiac malformations are typical. In mesocardia, the heart is centrally located in the chest with normal atrial and visceral anatomy. The apex is central or rightwardly displaced on the chest radiograph. Typically, no associated cardiac malformations are present.

SPECIALIZED ISSUES

ENDOCARDITIS PROPHYLAXIS. Prolonged survival of patients with complex congenital heart disease has resulted in a population at increased risk for infective endocarditis (see Chapter 326). Infection most commonly affects sites of turbulent blood flow on the low-pressure side of gradients. Such sites include restrictive VSDs, PDAs, a cleft mitral valve, aortic coarctation (most often at the site of an associated bicuspid aortic valve), and prosthetic shunts, valves, and conduits in a postoperative patient. The risk of endocarditis associated with isolated low-pressure lesions in the right heart is low.

Endocarditis should be suspected early and cultures obtained before antibiotic therapy is begun. Current recommendations for the prevention of bacterial endocarditis apply to most congenital heart lesions, with the exception of an isolated ASD and surgically repaired ASD, VSD, or PDA without residual shunting beyond 6 months after repair.

EXERCISE. The goal of exercise evaluation is to assess the func-

Table 57-2 ■ EXERCISE RECOMMENDATIONS IN ADULTS WITH CONGENITAL HEART DISEASE

CONDITION	UNRESTRICTED	LOW/MODERATE INTENSITY*	PROHIBITED
ASD†	No PHT. No arrhythmia. Normal ventricular function	PA pressure >40 mm Hg *with* normal ETT; no arrhythmia	Eisenmenger's
VSD†	Small. No PHT. No arrhythmia; normal ventricular function	Moderate VSD	Eisenmenger's
PDA†	Small. No PHT. No arrhythmia; normal ventricular function	PA pressure > 40 mm Hg *with* normal ETT; no arrhythmia	Eisenmenger's
Coarctation‡	Gradient ≤20 mm Hg arm to leg; normal BP at rest and exercise	Gradient ≥20 mm Hg arm to leg *with* normal BP and normal ETT	Gradient ≥ 50 mm Hg arm to leg *or* aortic aneurysm
PS	Gradient <50 mm Hg. No arrhythmia; normal ventricular function	Gradient ≥50 mm Hg	Gradient ≥ 70 mm Hg *or* ventricular arrhythmia
AS	Gradient ≤ 20 mm Hg, normal ECG, normal ETT; asymptomatic	Gradient > 20 mm Hg *with* normal ECG, normal ETT; asymptomatic	Gradient ≥ 50 mm Hg *or* ventricular arrhythmia
TOF after repair	Normal RV pressure. No shunt. No arrhythmia	Increased RV pressure *or* moderate PR *or* SVT	RV pressure ≥ 65% systemic *or* ventricular; arrhythmia on ETT *or* severe PR
Mustard or Senning		No cardiomegaly, arrhythmia, or syncope. Normal ETT	Cardiomegaly *or* arrhythmia at rest or exercise
c-TGA unoperated	No cardiomegaly. Mild TR. No arrhythmia; normal ETT	Moderate RV dysfunction, moderate TR. No arrhythmia	Severe TR *or* uncontrolled arrhythmia
Ebstein's	Mild Ebstein's. No arrhythmia. Operated with mild TR	Moderate TR *with* no arrhythmia	Severe Ebstein's *or* uncontrolled arrhythmia
Fontan		Normal O₂ saturation *with* near-normal ETT and ventricular function	Moderate/severe MR/TR *or* uncontrolled arrhythmia

*Based on peak dynamic and static components of exercise during competition for individual sports (see credit line).
†Unoperated or 6 months after surgery.
‡Unoperated or 1 year after surgery.
AS = aortic stenosis; ASD = atrial septal defect; BP = blood pressure; c-TGA = corrected transposition of the great arteries; ECG = electrocardiogram; ETT = exercise tolerance test; MR = mitral regurgitation; PA = pulmonary artery; PDA = patent ductus arteriosus; PHT = pulmonary hypertension; PR = pulmonary regurgitation; PS = pulmonary stenosis; RV = right ventricle; SVT = supraventricular tachyarrhythmia; TOF = tetralogy of Fallot; TR = tricuspid regurgitation; VSD = ventricular septal defect.
Based on guidelines recommended in Graham TP, Bricker TJ, James FW, et al: Task Force 1: Congenital Heart Disease, 26th Bethesda Conference. Eligibility for competition in athletes with cardiovascular abnormalities. Reprinted with permission from the American College of Cardiology; *J Am Coll Cardiol* 24:867, 1994.

tional results of therapeutic interventions and provide guidelines for exercise prescriptions. Patients with residual hemodynamic lesions or unrepaired congenital cardiac anomalies should be evaluated on an annual basis with physical examination, an electrocardiogram, and a cardiac ultrasound if indicated. Pertinent additional tests may include Holter monitoring and exercise testing. Attention should be directed to the detection of pulmonary hypertension, arrhythmias, myocardial dysfunction, and symptoms such as exercise-induced dizziness, syncope, dyspnea, or chest pain.

A series of exercise guidelines have been proposed for major groups of congenital heart defects (Table 57–2). Patients beyond 6 months after repair of a single shunt lesion without pulmonary hypertension, arrhythmias, or evidence of myocardial dysfunction can participate in all sports. In patients with residual shunts, if the peak pulmonary artery pressure is less than 40 mm Hg in the absence of ventricular dysfunction or significant arrhythmias, patients can enjoy a free range of activity. Patients with elevated pulmonary vascular resistance are at risk of sudden death during intense exercise; although most self-limit their activity, participation in competitive sports is contraindicated. Patients with aortic and pulmonary stenosis should be counseled as recommended earlier, according to gradient severity. For patients with uncomplicated aortic coarctation, athletic participation is permitted if the arm-leg blood pressure gradient is 20 mm Hg or less at rest and the peak systolic blood pressure during exercise is normal. For patients after tetralogy of Fallot repair, repair of TGA, and the Fontan operation, exercise recommendations will vary according to residual ventricular function and the presence or absence of arrhythmias.

Connelly MS, Webb GD, Somerville J, et al: Canadian Consensus Conference on Adult Congenital Heart Disease 1996. Can J Cardiol 14:395, 1998. *An international panel of experts gathered to offer a unique, practical, and up-to-date series of guidelines for the management of all the major congenital lesions seen in adults.*
Marelli AJ, Moodie DS: Adult congenital heart disease. In Topol EJ (ed): Textbook of Cardiovascular Medicine. Philadelphia, Lippincott-Raven, 1998, pp 769–796. *Provides more specific information on management issues related to specific lesions.*
Perloff JK: The Clinical Recognition of Congenital Heart Disease, 4th ed. Philadelphia, WB Saunders, 1994. *Classic and unique textbook. Detailed description of diagnostic features of all congenital lesions.*
Perloff JK, Child JS: Congenital Heart Disease in Adults, 2nd ed. Philadelphia, WB Saunders, 1998. *Problem oriented rather than lesion oriented. Comprehensive coverage of all medical complications of congenital cardiac disease.*
Perloff JK, Marelli AJ, Miner PD: Risk of stroke in adults with cyanotic congenital heart disease. Circulation 87:1954, 1994. *Study that puts to rest the inappropriate practice of prophylactic phlebotomy to prevent stroke in adults with cyanotic heart disease.*

58 ATHEROSCLEROSIS-THROMBOSIS AND VASCULAR BIOLOGY

Valentin Fuster

Atherothrombotic cardiovascular disease is a diffuse condition involving the heart (coronary arteries), brain (carotid, vertebral, and cerebral arteries), and peripheral arteries. Indeed, most of the risk factors that apply to one arterial bed also apply to the others. It is, therefore, not surprising that the presence of one atherosclerotic cardiovascular disease increases the risk of developing others.

MORPHOLOGY OF CORONARY ATHEROSCLEROSIS-THROMBOSIS

The Normal Artery

The normal artery (Fig. 58–1) consists essentially of a tube with an *intima* covered by a continuous layer of endothelial cells that maintains the circulating blood flow (antithrombotic), acts as a barrier to entry of circulating materials into the vessel wall, and regulates smooth muscle cell function; the *media* of pure smooth muscle cells, which contract and maintain the tone of the artery wall, and of extracellular matrix or fibrils (elastin, collagen, and proteoglycans), which provide supportive structure; and the *adventitia* of loose connective tissue (fibroblasts, extracellular matrix, and vasa vasorum).

Atherosclerosis-Thrombosis

Atherosclerosis is the descriptive term for thickened and hardened lesions of the medium and large muscular and elastic arteries. This lesion is lipid rich, in contrast to *arteriosclerosis*, which is the

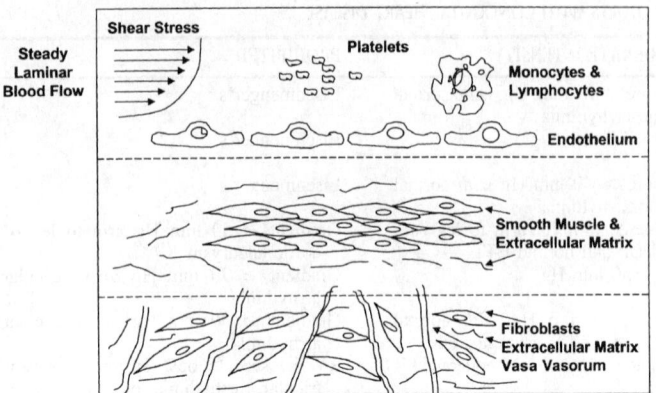

FIGURE 58–1 ■ Normal artery.

generic term for thickened and stiffened arteries of all sizes. In atherosclerosis, lesions occur within the innermost layer of the artery (the intima) and are largely confined to this region of the vessel. They are generally eccentric and, if they become complicated by thrombosis, can occlude the artery and cause ischemia or necrosis, with the characteristic clinical sequelae of myocardial infarction (MI), cerebral infarction, or gangrene of the extremities.

Classification and Phases of the Lesions of Atherosclerosis-Thrombosis

Progression of the atherosclerotic plaque in any arterial bed can be subdivided into five phases (Fig. 58–2). Phase 1 consists of a small lesion that is commonly found in persons younger than age 30 and that may progress over several years. Type I lesions consist of macrophage-derived foam cells that contain lipid droplets; type II lesions contain both macrophages and smooth muscle cells with extracellular lipid deposits; and type III lesions contain smooth muscle cells surrounded by extracellular connective tissue, fibrils, and lipid deposits.

Phase 2 vulnerable lipid-rich plaques are prone to disruption because of their high lipid content. The lesion is categorized morphologically as one of two variants. Type IV plaques consist of confluent cellular lesions with a great deal of extracellular lipid intermixed with fibrous tissue, whereas type Va plaques possess an extracellular lipid core covered by a thin fibrous cap. Phase 2 can evolve into acute phase 3 or 4, and either of these can evolve into a fibrotic phase 5.

Phases 3 and 4 consist of the acute complicated type VI lesions. Disruption of a type IV or Va lesion leads to the formation of a mural thrombus that does not completely occlude the artery (phase 3) or of an occlusive thrombus (phase 4) that may result in an acute coronary syndrome.

Changes in the geometry of the disrupted plaque and in the organization of the thrombus by connective tissue can lead to the more occlusive and fibrotic type Vb or Vc lesions of phase 5. These lesions may cause angina or MI or, if the preceding stenosis and ischemia produce a protective collateral circulation, may occlude without symptoms.

VASCULAR BIOLOGY OF CORONARY ATHEROSCLEROSIS-THROMBOSIS

The Early Dynamic Process of Lipoprotein Transport in Plaque Formation

Chronic minimal injury to the arterial endothelium is physiologic and is often the result of a disturbance in the pattern of blood flow at bending points and near bifurcations of the arterial tree. Local shear forces are probably enhanced in hypertension. In addition, chronic minimal endothelial injury or dysfunction, leading to accumulation of lipids and monocytes (macrophages), is produced by hypercholesterolemia, advanced glycation end-products in diabetes, chemical irritants in tobacco smoke, circulating vasoactive amines, immune complexes, and infections (see Figs. 58–2 and 58–3).

Most lipids deposited in the atherosclerotic lesions are derived from plasma low-density lipoproteins (LDLs) that enter the vessel wall through the injured or dysfunctional endothelium. All major cell types within the vessel wall and atherosclerotic lesions can oxidize LDLs, but the endothelial cell is probably critical in these very early stages by mildly oxidizing LDLs. Mildly oxidized LDLs (or minimally modified LDLs) and regional low shear and turbulent flow may play an initial role in monocyte recruitment by inducing the endothelial expression of two adhesive cell surface glycoproteins, intercellular adhesion molecule-1 and vascular cell adhesion molecule-1. After monocytes adhere to the surface of the vessel wall, other specific molecules, such as a specific chemotactic protein or monocyte chemotactic protein-1 and monocyte colony-stimulating factor, may attract and modify monocytes within the subendothelial space. After entering the vessel wall, monocytes differentiate into macrophages. They may be responsible for converting mildly oxidized LDLs into highly oxidized LDLs, which

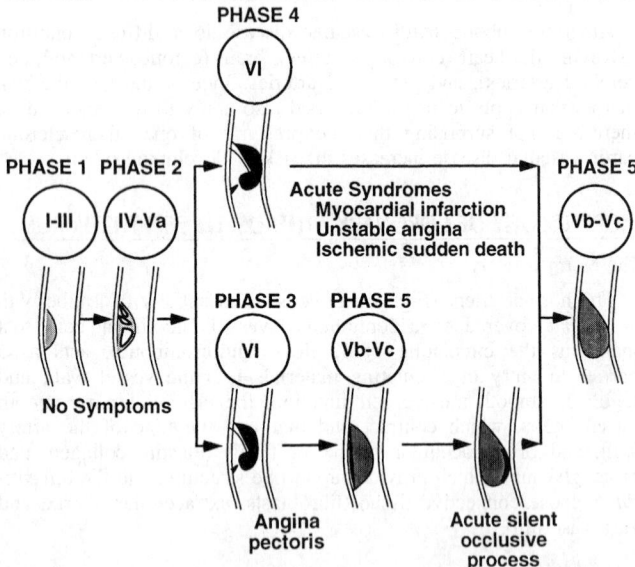

FIGURE 58–2 ■ Phases and lesion morphology of the progression of coronary atherosclerosis according to gross pathologic and clinical findings. (Modified with permission from Fuster V, et al: Circulation 90:2126–2146, 1994.)

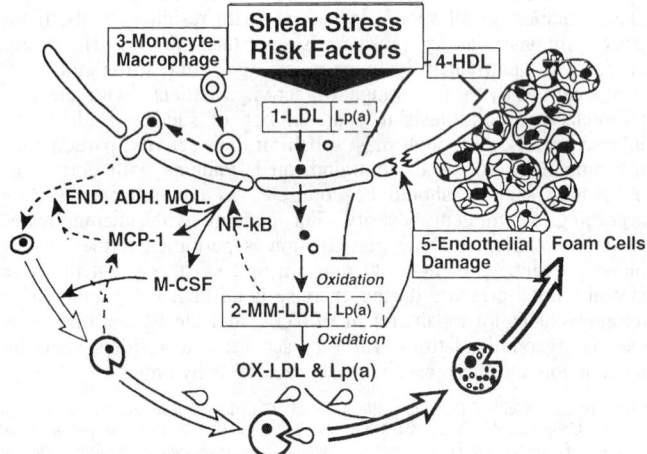

FIGURE 58–3 ■ Schematic of pathogenesis of phase I of progression: chronic endothelial injury and risk factors—influx, accumulation, and fate of lipids and monocyte-macrophages. ENDOT. = endothelial; END. ADH. MOL. = endothelial adhesion molecule; HDL = high-density lipoprotein; LDL = low-density lipoprotein; Lp(a) = lipoprotein (a); MCP-1 = monocyte chemotactic protein-1; M-CSF = monocyte colony-stimulating factor; MM = minimally modified; NF-κB = necrosis factor κB; OX = oxidized. (Modified with permission from Steinberg D: Circulation 84:1420–1425, 1991; and Steinberg D: Oxidative modification of LDL and atherogenesis. Circulation 95:1062–1072, 1997.)

bind to the scavenger receptors of macrophages and enter the cells, converting them into foam cells.

High-density lipoproteins (HDLs) may protect against excess lipid accumulation in the vessel wall by inhibiting the oxidation of LDLs or its subsequent effects. HDLs may also contribute to reverse cholesterol transport, which is active LDL removal from the vessel wall and from the macrophages or foam cells.

Macrophages or foam cells, after saturation with lipid and before or after their death, can liberate a large number of products, including oxidized LDLs and free radicals, which cause further endothelial damage. Such early alteration of the endothelium from the lumen (shear forces and risk factors) and from the vessel wall (macrophages) may lead to local vasoconstriction. Thus, the endothelium can profoundly affect vascular tone by releasing relaxing factors, such as prostacyclin and nitric oxide, and contracting factors, such as endothelin-1. Under physiologic conditions, nitric oxide appears to predominate, but in early atherogenesis the endothelial damage may cause these cells to generate more mediators that enhance constriction and fewer mediators that enhance dilation. When the endothelium disappears as a result of the damage, the de-endothelialized surface is exposed to circulating platelets, the platelet-derived growth factors (released from platelets as well as from macrophages, injured endothelial cells, and smooth muscle cells) cause intimal smooth muscle cell proliferation and synthesis of extracellular matrix. Cardiovascular risk factors known to affect the epicardial coronary arteries also affect coronary microcirculatory function, with a tendency for vasoconstriction that may contribute to anginal pain.

The earliest atherosclerotic lesion, the so-called fatty streak or type III lesion, represents a dynamic balance of the entry and exit of lipoproteins as well as the development of the extracellular matrix. A decrease in lipoprotein entry (such as by modifying risk factors and thus endothelial injury) will likely result in a predominance of lipoprotein exit and final scarring. However, an increase of lipoprotein entry can predominate over the efflux and scarring, resulting in the vulnerable, lipid-rich type IV and Va plaques that are prone to disruption.

The Vulnerable Lipid-Rich Plaque and Its Disruption

Type IV and Va plaques are commonly composed of an abundant crescentic mass of lipids, separated from the vessel lumen by a discrete component of extracellular matrix (see Figs. 58–2 and 58–4). The relatively small coronary lesions by angiography may be associated with acute progression to severe stenosis or total occlusion and may eventually account for as many as two thirds of the patients in whom unstable angina or other acute coronary syndromes develop. This unpredictable and episodic progression is most likely caused by disruption of type IV and V plaques with subsequent thrombus formation, which changes the plaque geometry and leads to acute or intermittent plaque growth and acute occlusive coronary syndromes.

Plaques that undergo disruption tend to be relatively small and soft; they have a high concentration of cholesterol esters, rather than of free cholesterol monohydrate crystals. This rather passive phenomenon of plaque disruption is related to physical forces and occurs most frequently between the lipid core and the lumen where the fibrous cap is thinnest, most heavily infiltrated by foam cells, and, therefore, weakest. This physical vulnerability to disruption depends on three factors:

1. Circumferential wall stress or cap "fatigue," which in part relates to a combination of the thickness and collagen content of the fibrous cap covering the core, the blood pressure, and the radius of the lumen; long-term repetitive cyclic stresses may weaken the plaque and increase its vulnerability to fracture, ultimately leading to sudden and unprovoked (i.e., untriggered) mechanical failure.
2. Location, size, and consistency of the atheromatous core.
3. Blood flow characteristics, particularly the impact of flow on the proximal aspect of the plaque (i.e., configuration and angulation of the plaque).

In addition, there is also an active phenomenon of plaque disruption related to macrophage activity. Macrophages can degrade extracellular matrix by phagocytosis or by secreting proteolytic en-

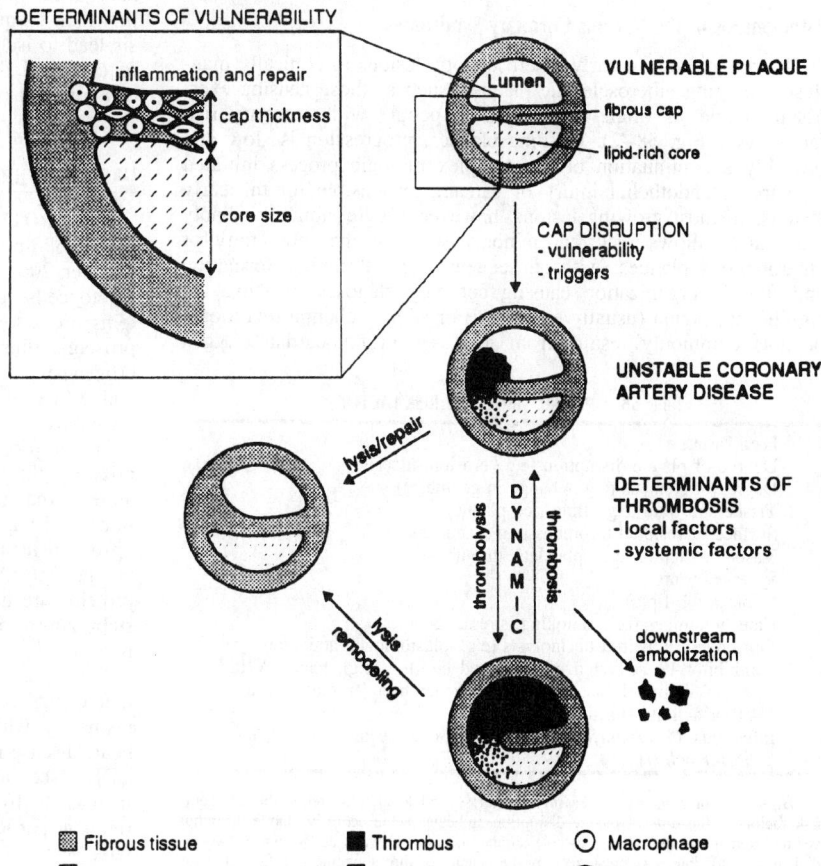

FIGURE 58–4 ■ Pathogenesis of a frequent type of unstable angina: anatomic changes (plaque disruption and thrombosis) leading to acute coronary syndromes and subsequent plaque remodeling. An element of vasoconstriction is usually present (see text for detailed description). (Modified with permission from Theroux P, Fuster V: Circulation 97:1195–1206, 1998.)

zymes such as plasminogen activators and a family of matrix metalloproteinases (collagenases, gelatinases, and stromelysins) that may weaken the fibrous cap, predisposing it to disruption. Moreover, foam cells may induce programmed cell death (apoptosis) of the surrounding smooth muscle cells and so predispose to the active phenomenon of plaque disruption.

Acute Thrombosis, Occlusive or Mural

Disruption of a vulnerable or unstable plaque with a subsequent change in plaque geometry and thrombosis results in a type VI or complicated lesion (see Fig. 58–2 and Table 58–1). Occasionally, the thrombus will be occlusive and manifest clinically as an MI, unstable angina, or sudden coronary death. However, it seems that such a thrombus more often is non-occlusive or mural, causes no symptoms, and, by self-organization, contributes to the progression of atherosclerosis. Multiple risk factors predispose to acute occlusive thrombosis, whereas the patient with fewer risk factors is more likely to have simple mural thrombosis and progressive atherogenesis.

SUBSTRATE-DEPENDENT THROMBOSIS. There is striking heterogeneity in the composition of human atherosclerotic plaques, even in the same individual, and the disruption of plaques exposes different vessel wall components to blood. The lipid core, characteristic of vulnerable plaques and abundant in cholesterol ester, is the most thrombogenic.

TISSUE FACTOR–DEPENDENT THROMBOSIS. Tissue factor (TF), a small-molecular-weight glycoprotein, initiates the extrinsic clotting cascade and is believed to be a major regulator of coagulation, hemostasis, and thrombosis. TF forms a high-affinity complex with coagulation Factors VII/VIIa; and TF/VIIa complex activates Factors IX and X, which in turn lead to thrombin generation. In a normal artery, TF antigen is present only in the adventitia. In atherosclerotic plaques, TF antigen is present in the various cells and extracellularly in the lipid-rich core, particularly in areas with dense macrophage or foam cell content. The lipid-rich core exhibits the most intense TF staining, and there is a strong relationship of TF antigen with macrophages. TF in the lipid core is probably what confers the thrombogenicity of the disrupted vulnerable plaque.

Pathogenesis of the Various Coronary Syndromes

The progression of early atherosclerotic lesions to clinically manifest, enlarging atherosclerotic plaques, such as those causing exertional angina, is often more rapid in people with coronary risk factors (see Fig. 58–2). In some plaques, progression is slow and probably a continuation of the complex biologic process initiated by chronic endothelial injury or damage responsible for the early lesions. In most growing lesions, however, progression is probably rapid and follows recurrent minor fissures of the most fatty or atheromatous plaques, with subsequent mural thrombus formation and fibrotic organization causing coronary stenoses. If these are significant, angina (usually exertional) or silent ischemia (exertional or not) commonly results from increases in myocardial oxygen

demand that outstrip the ability of stenosed coronary arteries to increase oxygen delivery.

In contrast, unstable angina or ischemia, non–Q-wave MI, and Q-wave MI (on occasion these acute syndromes may also be silent), which represent a continuum of the disease process, are usually characterized by an abrupt reduction in coronary flow. The predisposing coronary lesion is frequently only mildly to moderately stenotic, which suggests that plaque disruption with superimposed thrombus rather than the severity of the underlying lesion is the primary determinant of acute occlusion. The presence of local and systemic thrombogenic risk factors at the time of plaque disruption may modify the extent and duration of thrombus deposition and account for the variety of pathologic and acute clinical manifestations (see Table 58–1).

In unstable angina, a relatively small erosion or fissuring of an atherosclerotic plaque may lead to an acute change in plaque structure and a reduction in coronary blood flow, resulting in exacerbation of angina. Transient episodes of thrombotic vessel occlusion at the site of plaque damage may occur, leading to angina at rest. This thrombus is usually labile and results in temporary vascular occlusion, perhaps lasting only 10 to 20 minutes. In addition, release of vasoactive substances by platelets (serotonin and thromboxane A_2), the vasoconstrictive effect of thrombin, and vasoconstriction secondary to endothelial vasodilator dysfunction may contribute to a reduction in coronary flow. Overall, alterations in perfusion and myocardial oxygen supply probably account for two thirds of episodes of unstable angina; the remainder may be caused by transient increases in myocardial oxygen demand.

In non–Q-wave MI, more severe plaque damage results in more persistent thrombotic occlusion, perhaps lasting up to 1 hour. Only about one fourth of patients with non–Q-wave MI have an infarct-related vessel occluded for more than 1 hour, but the distal myocardial territory is usually supplied by collaterals. Therefore, spontaneous thrombolysis, resolution of vasoconstriction, and presence of collateral circulation are important in preventing the formation of Q-wave MI by limiting the duration of myocardial ischemia. In Q-wave MI, larger plaque fissures result in the formation of a fixed and persistent thrombus, which leads to an abrupt cessation of myocardial perfusion for more than 1 hour, resulting in transmural necrosis of the involved myocardium. Some cases of sudden coronary death probably involve a rapidly progressive coronary lesion in which plaque disruption (mild or severe) and resultant thrombosis lead to ischemic and fatal ventricular arrhythmias in the absence of collateral flow. Platelet microemboli may also contribute to the development of sudden ischemic death.

VASCULAR BIOLOGY OF RISK FACTORS

LIPOPROTEINS. Lipoproteins are high-molecular-weight complexes of lipid and protein that circulate in the blood plasma (see Chapter 206). Their physiologic functions include transport of lipids to cells for energy, growth requirements, or storage. Lipoproteins are also metabolic precursors of biologic regulators such as prostaglandins, thromboxanes, and leukotrienes. LDLs promote atherogenesis by affecting one or several of the processes of influx and efflux of the vessel wall. Elevated LDL levels also promote thrombosis formation.

HDLs promote cholesterol efflux from atherosclerotic lesions, possibly through a receptor-mediated mechanism. In addition, it appears that HDLs inhibit the oxidation and subsequent accumulation of LDL-cholesterol. Observational data and experiments in vitro and in transgenic mice suggest that HDLs containing apo A-I but not apo A-II are protective, whereas HDLs with both apolipoproteins are neutral. Apo A-I has been identified as a prostacyclin-stabilizing factor, suggesting another possible mechanism of benefit.

Evidence is growing that triglyceride-rich lipoproteins are important contributors to the development of coronary disease. Mechanisms by which hypertriglyceridemia may contribute to coronary heart disease risk include increased thrombogenicity; "small, dense" LDLs (see later section on diabetes), postprandial lipidemia with increased chylomicron and very low density lipoprotein (VLDL) remnant particles, decreased HDL levels, and insulin resistance (see later section on diabetes). An elevated lipoprotein(a) [Lp(a)] level in plasma may be a significant risk factor for coronary disease,

---

Table 58–1 ■ THROMBOGENIC RISK FACTORS*

Local Factors
Degree of plaque disruption (e.g., erosion, ulcer)
Degree of stenosis (e.g., change in geometry)
Tissue substrate (e.g., lipid-rich plaque)
Surface of residual thrombus (e.g., recurrence)
Vasoconstriction (e.g., platelets, thrombin)
Systemic Factors
Cholesterol, Lp(a)
Catecholamines (e.g., smoking, stress, cocaine)
Fibrinogen, impaired fibrinolysis (e.g., plasminogen activator-inhibitor-1), activated platelets and clotting (e.g., Factor VIIa, von Willebrand factor, thrombin generation [fragment 1 and 2], or activity [fibrinopeptide A])
Infections (? *Chlamydia pneumoniae*, cytomegalovirus, *Helicobacter pylori*)

*High risk: presumably by the presence of several local or systemic thrombogenic risk factors at the time of plaque disruption, indicates acute occlusive labile thrombus versus fixed mural thrombus (unstable angina and non–Q wave and Q wave myocardial infarction); low risk: presumably by the paucity of thrombogenic risk factors at the time of plaque disruption, indicates only mural thrombus (progressive atherogenesis).

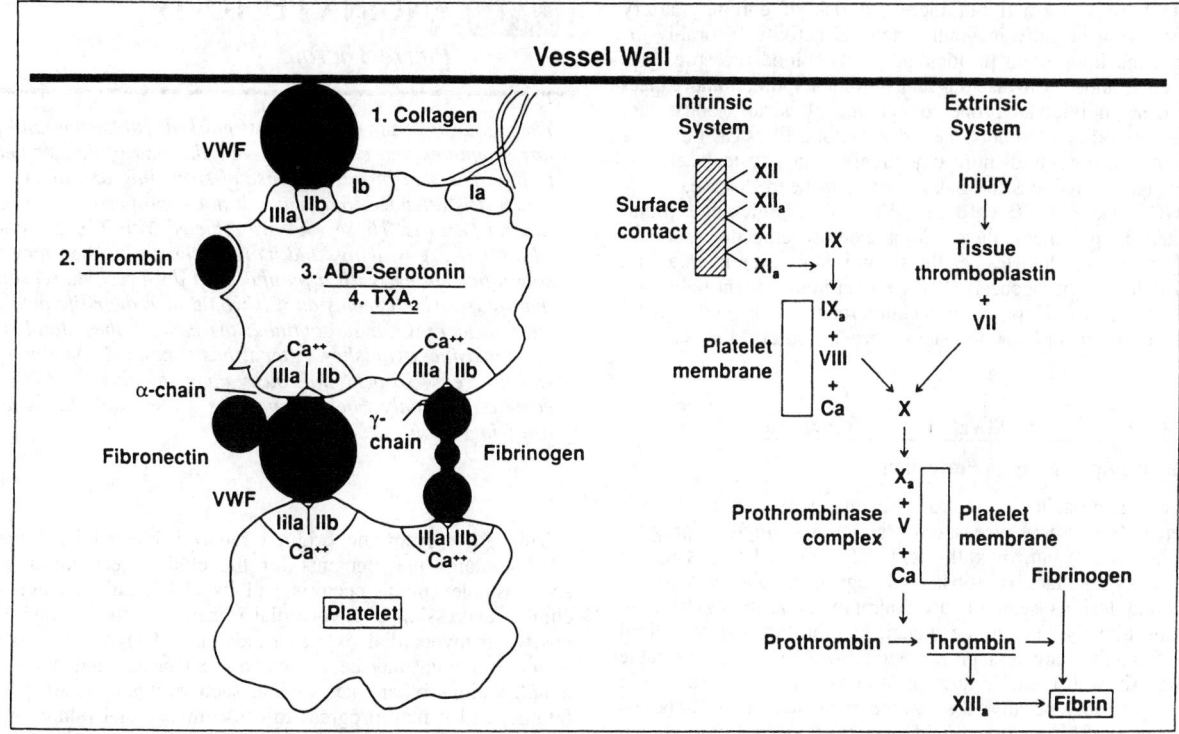

FIGURE 58–5 ■ Interactions among platelet membrane receptors (glycoproteins Ia, Ib, and IIa/IIIa). Adhesive macromolecules, the disrupted vessel wall **(left panel),** and a flow chart of the intrinsic and extrinsic systems of the coagulation cascade **(right panel).** In the left panel, Arabic numerals indicate the pathways of platelet activation that are dependent on collagen (1), thrombin (2), adenosine phosphate and serotonin (3), and thromboxane A_2 (4); there are also some reports that suggest the binding of von Willebrand factor (polymeric protein) to collagen or heparin. Note the interaction in the right panel between clotting factors (XII, XIIa, XI, XIa, IX, IXa, VII, VIII, X, Xa, and V) and the platelet membrane. (Reproduced with permission from Fuster V, et al: N Engl J Med 326:310–318, 1992. Copyright © 1992, Massachusetts Medical Society. All rights reserved.)

particularly in the presence of elevated LDL-cholesterol, although this risk has not been well characterized, and the distribution of Lp(a) levels in some ethnic populations is highly skewed.

DIET. Serum cholesterol and LDL-cholesterol concentrations are strongly associated with dietary intakes of total fat, saturated fatty acids, and cholesterol. Saturated fat intake is associated with increased thrombogenicity. Salt intake is associated with elevated blood pressure in susceptible persons. Importantly, a number of other effects of dietary components such as *trans*-fatty acids, marine oils, fiber, and others have been suggested as beneficial.

HYPERTENSION. In the setting of elevated blood pressure, endothelial dysfunction promotes atherogenesis by attenuating responses to endothelium-dependent vasodilators, increasing vascular permeability to macromolecules (including lipoproteins), and increasing endothelin production and leukocyte adherence. In addition, hypertension may also be associated with phenotypic changes in vascular smooth muscle cells that increase their proliferative potential and their response to growth factors.

SMOKING. A variety of observational data suggest that smoking exerts its atherogenic effects by inducing an elevation in blood fibrinogen concentration, enhancing platelet reactivity (possibly as a result of increased catecholamine levels), and increasing whole-blood viscosity by inducing secondary polycythemia. In addition, altered vascular reactivity induced by endothelial dysfunction or nicotine, or both, promotes increases in vascular tone. Smoking also lowers HDL-cholesterol and promotes oxidation of LDL-cholesterol, presumably owing to the exposure of the latter to free radicals present in cigarette smoke.

DIABETES. Insulin resistance in patients with type II diabetes or in patients with poorly controlled type I diabetes is accompanied by hyperinsulinemia, which may, in turn, elevate circulating insulin-related growth factors such as insulin growth factor-1. In chronic hyperglycemia, glycated proteins and various local growth factors can stimulate the proliferation of the fibromuscular component of the mature atherosclerotic plaque. Levels of lipoproteins such as LDL-cholesterol may not be abnormal in patients with

diabetes mellitus; however, lipoproteins may be glycated, resulting in abnormal function. Hypertriglyceridemia with HDL depletion is the characteristic lipid profile of insulin resistance and poorly controlled diabetes. As an important consequence of hypertriglyceridemia, abnormalities in the metabolism of triglyceride-rich lipoproteins result in modifications of LDL structure, so as to produce a smaller, denser, so-called subclass B form of LDL, which has markedly enhanced atherogenicity. Abnormalities of Lp(a) levels also are widespread in patients with poorly controlled diabetes.

SYSTEMIC THROMBOGENIC RISK FACTORS. Thrombotic mechanisms contribute not only to acute events after plaque activation but also to atheroma growth (see Table 58–1 and Fig. 58–5). Aside from the thrombogenic effect of high levels of cholesterol (circulating platelet and/or monocyte-TF activator), a high catecholamine drive such as in cigarette smoking, emotional stress, or cocaine use may enhance thrombogenicity, perhaps by inducing vasoconstriction, and directly trigger plaque disruption.

Several hemostatic determinants, including fibrinogen, von Willebrand factor, and Factor VIIa, have been associated with an increased risk of cardiovascular disease; however, the association with fibrinogen is the most powerful and most consistent. Increased plasminogen activator inhibitor-1 and tissue-type plasminogen activator antigen (most likely a marker for endothelial dysfunction) are associated with an increased risk of cardiovascular events; elevated tissue-type plasminogen activator activity, by contrast, is associated with a decreased risk of events.

Systemic infections (e.g., with *Chlamydia pneumoniae,* cytomegalovirus, and *Helicobacter pylori*) may be linked to atherosclerotic disease and its thrombotic complications; increased antibody titers have, in some studies, been associated with future adverse events in post-MI patients. Infectious agents may activate circulating monocytes and lymphocytes and create a hypercoagulable state (through synthesis and activation of TF and platelet interaction, raising fibrinogen levels, and so on).

OBESITY AND PHYSICAL INACTIVITY. Obesity predisposes to hyperlipidemia, diabetes, and hypertension, but obesity itself is associated with only a small but increased risk of coronary artery atherosclerosis, principally in youth. Physical activity favorably influences plasma lipoprotein profiles, adiposity, blood pressure, glucose tolerance, and cardiovascular and pulmonary functional capacity; moreover, individuals prone to become physically active are also prone to modify favorably their risk factors. Physical fitness, a condition that is measured more objectively than physical activity, also independently reduces the risk of coronary heart disease.

GENETIC FACTORS (FAMILY HISTORY). Single-gene mutations influence lipid metabolism. Complex polygenic disorders include hypertension, diabetes mellitus, and homocysteinemia and also contribute to atherogenesis. However, currently identifiable genetic abnormalities only partially account for the risk predicted by a positive family history for premature coronary artery disease.

VASCULAR BIOLOGY OF PREVENTIVE APPROACHES

Lipid-Modifying Approaches to Prevention

Aggressive approaches to retard or even reverse atherosclerosis can significantly decrease disease progression and improve prognosis (see Chapter 39) but, overall, yield only minimal regression of atherosclerosis. The lack of substantial regression observed in the atherosclerotic lesions seen on arteriography is probably because such lesions already tend to be advanced, fibrotic, and less lipid rich; therefore, they are less prone to reabsorption or to favorable remodeling. The substantial reduction in coronary events from lipid lowering is probably because the marked reduction in LDL-cholesterol stimulates efflux of the liquid or esterified cholesterol from the plaques; also, deposition of cholesterol crystals in the vessel wall predominates over the influx of LDL-cholesterol. Consequently, there is a decrease in the softness of the plaque and presumably in the physical or passive phenomenon of plaque disruption. There is also evidence of a decrease in the number and activity of the macrophages and, therefore, in the active phenomenon of plaque disruption and vessel wall–dependent thrombogenicity.

Antithrombotic Approaches to Prevention and Treatment

If atherosclerotic plaque disruption cannot be prevented, antiplatelet and anticoagulant agents still can be beneficial (see Chapter 188 and Fig. 58–5). Aspirin, which is effective in unstable angina and acute MI as well as in primary and secondary prevention, interferes with only one of the four pathways of platelet activation, the one dependent on thromboxane A_2. The other three pathways—one dependent on adenosine diphosphate and serotonin, a second on collagen, and a third on thrombin—remain unaffected, as does the coagulation system. Combination therapy with a platelet inhibitor (aspirin or a ticlopidine type of drug to inhibit the adenosine diphosphate pathway) and an anticoagulant agent (intravenous heparin, subcutaneous low-molecular-weight heparin, or oral warfarin) may have an additive effect. Newer antithrombotic approaches act by either blocking the early stage of thrombin-related platelet activation, such as the specific antithrombins hirudin and hirulog, or by blocking the late stage of receptor glycoprotein IIb/IIIa-related platelet activation.

Fuster V, Fallon JT, Nemerson Y: Coronary thrombosis. Lancet 348(Suppl):S7–S10, 1996.

Fuster V, Gotto AM, Libby P, et al: Pathogenesis of coronary disease: The biologic role of risk factors. J Am Coll Cardiol 27:964–1047, 1996. *These two papers by Fuster and colleagues present an overview of the pathogenesis of coronary artery disease (atherosclerosis and thrombosis) and the biological pathogenetic role of risk factors.*

Libby P, Egan D, Skarlatos S: Roles of infectious agents in atherosclerosis and restenosis: An assessment of the evidence and need for future research. Circulation 96:4095–4103, 1997.

Ross R: Atherosclerosis—an inflammatory disease. N Engl J Med 1998, 340:115–126, 1999. *The papers by Libby and colleagues and by Ross review the role of inflammation (accumulation and activity of monocytes and lymphocytes) and the possible role of infectious agents in coronary artery disease.*

Steinberg D: Oxidative modification of LDL and atherogenesis. Circulation 95:1062–1072, 1997. *This paper outlines the role by which lipid oxidation and metabolism play a role in coronary artery disease.*

Theroux P, Fuster V: Acute coronary syndromes. Circulation 97:1195–1206, 1998. *This paper links the pathogenetic mechanisms of coronary artery disease with the clinical presentation of acute coronary syndromes.*

59 ANGINA PECTORIS

Pierre Theroux

There is a disorder of the breast marked with strong and peculiar symptoms and considerable for the kind of danger belonging to it. . .The seat of it, and sense of strangling and anxiety with which it is attended, may make it not improperly be called Angina pectoris. Those who are afflicted with it, are seized, while they are walking, and more particularly when they walk soon after eating, with a painful most disagreeable sensation in the breast, which seems as if it would take their life away, if it were to increase or to continue: the moment they stand still, all this uneasiness vanishes. After it has continued some months, it will not cease so instantaneously upon standing still; and it will come on, not only when the persons are walking, but when they are lying down. . .

Heberden

This quote from the original report published by Heberden in 1772 contains the elements for the clinical recognition of stable and unstable angina pectoris and its classification. Angina is one clinical expression of myocardial ischemia. Ischemia rapidly develops when myocardial oxygen needs exceed myocardial oxygen delivery. Ischemia may be clinically silent or associated with clinical manifestations other than angina, such as dyspnea, arrhythmias, or fatigue; and it may progress to cause myocardial infarction (MI) or sudden death (see Chapter 60). Atherosclerosis, which is the most frequent cause of myocardial ischemia, may evolve for years without symptoms. Conversely, chest pain can result from a variety of causes of myocardial ischemia other than atherosclerosis or from non-ischemic causes of cardiac or non-cardiac origin.

DEFINITION. Angina may be defined by the stability or nonstability of its manifestation, its provocation factors, or its pathophysiology. The clinical diagnosis of *stable angina* is first based on symptom recognition. Stable angina is usually reproducible in an individual patient and is consistent over time. In most patients, it is precipitated by effort, relieved by rest, and related to fixed stenoses of one or more epicardial coronary arteries. *Unstable angina* is diagnosed clinically when a patient has new-onset angina (by definition, any patient with new-onset angina has a brief interval of instability), increasing angina (angina that is more frequent, more prolonged, or precipitated by less effort than before), or angina occurring at rest. Most commonly, unstable angina is caused by a clot superimposed on a fixed coronary obstruction (see Chapters 58 and 60), although the definition of unstable angina remains clinical and is not based on specific pathophysiology.

Angina is most commonly precipitated by increasing effort; in stable angina, this degree of effort is reasonably predictable from day to day in an individual patient. Some patients have angina during exercise but then the discomfort disappears with continued exercise (*walk-through angina*). *Nocturnal angina* may occur in two forms: one type develops soon after a patient lies down because of an increase in venous return that increases myocardial oxygen demand beyond the capacity of supply; a second type may occur several hours later and is related to increases in myocardial oxygen demand or vasospasm. *Postprandial angina* develops during or soon after meals because of an increased oxygen demand in the splanchnic vascular bed.

The underlying pathophysiologic basis of angina may be due to fixed coronary obstruction, clot superimposed on a fixed coronary obstruction, or vasospasm on a coronary artery lesion of variable severity. In addition, angina can be caused by situations associated with excess myocardial oxygen demand, with a lower threshold for angina when high left ventricular diastolic pressures impede myocardial blood flow during diastole.

ETIOLOGY. Angina is most commonly caused by atherosclerotic narrowing of one or more epicardial coronary arteries. It can also occur when myocardial ischemia develops despite normal epicardial coronary arteries. For example, patients with aortic stenosis (see Chapter 63) or hypertrophic cardiomyopathy (see Chapter 64) have marked increases in myocardial oxygen demand because of myocardial hypertrophy. In syndrome X, patients with normal epicardial coronary arteries may develop true myocardial ischemia and angina because of the failure to have normal vasodilation of the resistance vessels with exercise or other stimuli.

The diagnosis of angina requires documentation of the presence of myocardial ischemia. Conversely, some patients can have substantial coronary artery disease and even demonstrable myocardial ischemia by diagnostic testing yet not experience angina.

PATHOPHYSIOLOGY. Proper evaluation and treatment of patients with angina require an understanding of basic pathophysiologic mechanisms of coronary circulation and myocardial ischemia. Ischemia is the consequence of an imbalance between myocardial oxygen supply and oxygen demand. Myocardial oxygen demand is enhanced by increases of heart rate, blood pressure, myocardial contractility, and left ventricular size. Myocardial oxygen supply is critically dependent on coronary blood flow, intraluminal coronary patency, coronary perfusion pressure, the hemoglobin oxygen content of the blood, and the duration of diastole.

MYOCARDIAL ENERGETICS. Myocardial metabolism is essentially aerobic. Free fatty acids and protons accumulate within a few seconds after oxygen deprivation as contractile function ceases; ST segment changes ensue within minutes, followed by appearance of chest pain. The major determinants of myocardial oxygen consumption associated with heart contraction are, in decreasing order of importance, heart rate, wall tension generated during systole (afterload), the inotropic state of the myocardial cell (contractility), and end-diastolic volume (preload) (see Chapter 40).

CORONARY CIRCULATION. Myocardial oxygen extraction is high in the basal state (75% at rest, 90% during ischemia), and adaptation of the heart to increased demand is achieved mainly through vasodilatation of coronary resistance vessels. Coronary blood flow can increase fivefold to sixfold during exercise from resting values of 0.8 mL/g/min because of the ability of the coronary circulation to autoregulate in response to changes in perfusion pressure and oxygen demand. The autoregulation is modulated by sympathetic and parasympathetic neural influences, metabolic factors (primarily adenosine, a potent vasodilator produced by oxidative phosphorylation of adenosine nucleotides that are produced when adenosine triphosphate utilization exceeds production), and many important vasoactive substances, such as nitric oxide, produced by or acting through the endothelium. Coronary perfusion of the left ventricle occurs mainly during diastole when wall tension, and hence coronary resistance, is lowest. The gradient in intramyocardial tension, highest in the subendocardium and lowest in the subepicardium, makes the subendocardial areas more sensitive to ischemia; more severe ischemia progresses transmurally from the subendocardial to the subepicardial areas.

A gradient of pressure across the coronary obstruction builds up as the severity of luminal obstruction increases. The pressure drop through a stenosis is influenced mainly by the cross-sectional area of the stenosis (Δ pressure = 1/area^2 × length of stenosis × flow rate). A reduced distal pressure is associated with vasodilatation, which limits the coronary reserve (i.e., the potential for any further increase in flow).

Stenoses of more than 75% of the cross-sectional area (corresponding to more than 50% of the luminal diameter by coronary angiography) can result in ischemia when the energy requirements are high, as in physical exercise in stable effort angina. The threshold to ischemia decreases as the severity of the obstruction increases. The extreme is chest pain at rest because of severe stenosis with inadequate collateral circulation or because of thrombus formation or dynamic occlusion by inappropriate vasoconstriction: thrombus formation is the common cause of acute coronary syndromes, whereas coronary spasm is the cause of Prinzmetal's variant angina.

THE ENDOTHELIUM. The endothelium is a very active surface that produces potent vasoactive, anticoagulant, procoagulant, and fibrinolytic substances. Prostacyclin derived from the metabolism of arachidonic acid relaxes smooth muscle cells and inhibits platelet aggregation through an increase in the intracellular concentration of cyclic adenosine monophosphate. Nitric oxide, also produced by the endothelium, increases the intracellular content of cyclic guanine monophosphate and mediates the vasodilator response to shear rate and a variety of vasoactive products, such as acetylcholine, adenosine diphosphate, bradykinin, and serotonin. This nitric oxide system, although important, is very fragile and becomes ineffective

in atherosclerotic vessels and when the endothelium is rendered dysfunctional by the presence of risk factors such as smoking, hypercholesterolemia, hypertension, and diabetes mellitus. Endothelin produced by the endothelium is a potent vasoconstrictor with prolonged effect.

THE ACTIVE PLAQUE. Atherosclerosis is a highly dynamic process involving a build-up of cellular events: oxidative stress, endothelial dysfunction, monocytic infiltration, foam cell formation, production of cytokines, expression of adhesion molecules, and proliferation and migration of smooth mucosal cells (see Chapter 58). The culprit lesion in unstable angina is characterized by an exaggeration of the inflammatory reaction with dense neutrophils, lymphocytes, and mast cell infiltration and secretion of metalloproteinases that are matrix degradation molecules; of cytokines that mediate the inflammatory process; and of growth factors. Degeneration of the plaque and thinning of its cap are eventually associated with rupture at regions of high shear stress. The plaque rupture exposes procoagulant and proaggregant substances to flowing blood, triggering thrombus formation. Tissue factor abundant in macrophages within the plaque forms a complex with circulating Factor VIIa. The complex triggers the intrinsic and extrinsic pathways of the coagulation system to form the tenase complex; Factor Xa converts prothrombin into thrombin. Circulating platelets adhere through surface glycoprotein receptors to von Willebrand factor and to collagen. Platelet activation is associated with shape change and secretion of potent proaggregant, procoagulant, and vasoactive substances from their granules and, importantly, with a configuration change of the platelet membrane receptor glycoprotein IIb/IIIa. The receptor then becomes competent to recognize and bind the arginine/glycine/aspartic acid (RGD) sequence of fibrinogen and other ligands, resulting in platelet bridging and platelet clot formation. Thrombus formation typically occurs on plaques that are of moderate severity (40 to 60% lumen diameter reduction), rich in cholesterol and cholesterol esters, and with a thin cap. The ischemia that results from the more severe obstruction can be more or less severe to cause transmural or subendocardial ischemia and more or less sustained to cause myocardial necrosis or transient ischemia.

DIAGNOSIS AND CLASSIFICATION. The various classifications of angina have been inspired by considerations of etiology, assessment of severity and/or prognosis, and treatment.

STABLE (EFFORT) ANGINA. The cardinal manifestation of effort angina is chest pain triggered by exercise and promptly relieved by rest. The pain usually builds up rapidly within 30 seconds and disappears in decrescendo within 5 to 15 minutes, and more promptly when nitroglycerin is used. Chest pain is variably described but is typically a tightness, squeezing, or constriction; however, some patients describe an ache, a feeling of dull discomfort, indigestion, or burning pain. The discomfort is most commonly midsternal and radiates to the neck, left shoulder, and left arm. It can also be precordial or radiate to the jaw, teeth, right arm, back, and, more rarely, to the epigastrium. Episodes of discomfort that are less than 1 minute or more than 30 minutes in duration are unlikely to be stable angina, but prolonged episodes can be consistent with unstable angina, especially if associated with ischemic electrocardiographic changes. When discomfort is considered clinically typical for angina, about 80% of individuals will have demonstrable coronary artery disease and evidence of myocardial ischemia; however, 20% of patients, including a higher percentage of younger patients without risk factors, will have no evidence of myocardial ischemia despite the typical complaints. The probability of coronary artery disease varies by age range, gender, and characteristics of symptoms (Table 59–1).

Although angina of any severity (see Table 38–4) can be stable by this definition, Class IV angina as well as worsening or new-onset angina are usually termed *unstable angina*. The intensity of pain ranges from mild to very severe discomfort. Some patients do not note any pain or discomfort but rather an "anginal equivalent" of shortness of breath, dizziness, or fatigue. The characteristics as well as triggers are variable among patients but usually reproducible in a given patient.

Atypical angina describes symptoms that are suggestive of angina but unusual with regard to location, characteristics, triggers, or duration. In patients with atypical angina symptoms, the prevalence of underlying coronary artery disease and myocardial ischemia

Table 59–1 ■ PROBABILITY OF CORONARY ARTERY DISEASE BY AGE, GENDER, AND SYMPTOMS

AGE (YR)	GENDER	TYPICAL/DEFINITE ANGINA PECTORIS†	ATYPICAL/PROBABLE ANGINA PECTORIS†	NONANGINAL CHEST PAIN†	ASYMPTOMATIC†
30–39	Men	Intermediate	Intermediate	Low	Very low
	Women	Intermediate	Very low	Very low	Very low
40–49	Men	High	Intermediate	Intermediate	Low
	Women	Intermediate	Low	Very low	Very low
50–59	Men	High	Intermediate	Intermediate	Low
	Women	Intermediate	Intermediate	Low	Very low
60–69	Men	High	Intermediate	Intermediate	Low
	Women	High	Intermediate	Intermediate	Low

From Gibbons RJ, Balady GJ, Beasley JW, et al: ACC/AHA guidelines for exercise testing: Executive summary. A report of the American College of Cardiology/American Heart Association Task Force on Practice Guidelines (Committee on Exercise Testing). Circulation 96:345–354, 1997.

No data exist for patients <30 or >69 years, but it can be assumed that prevalence of coronary artery disease increases with age. In a few cases, patients with ages at the extremes of the decades listed may have probabilities slightly outside the high or low range.

†High indicates >90%; intermediate 10%–90%; low, <10%; and very low, <5%.

ranges from 20 to 50%; the presence of risk factors increases the likelihood of the disease. In women and the elderly, the clinical features of angina may be more atypical, the initial manifestations more subtle, and the various non-invasive tests less reliable indicators of the absence or presence of coronary artery disease. Although coronary disease occurs on average 10 years later in women than in men, the prognosis may be worse.

Effort or stress angina is typically associated with a greater than or equal to 75% reduction in the cross-sectional diameter of one or more of the large epicardial coronary arteries, resulting in inadequate myocardial oxygen supply when demands are increased. The severity of angina should be graded by a careful history using a standardized classification system (see Table 38–4).

UNSTABLE ANGINA. The key clinical feature of unstable angina is rapid aggravation of symptoms, as manifested by more severe, more frequent, or more prolonged pain; pain less promptly relieved with nitroglycerin; or pain occurring at rest or at a decreasing threshold of exercise. Unstable angina covers a wide spectrum of clinical severity and is considered an intermediary syndrome between stable angina and MI. It implies a pathophysiologic process related to an abrupt decrease in myocardial oxygen delivery. Unstable angina has been classified as *new-onset angina* if symptoms were manifested in the previous 2 months with a component of progression in the pattern of angina; *crescendo angina*, when previously present symptoms exacerbate; *acute coronary insufficiency* when the chest pain is prolonged for 20 minutes or more; and *post-infarction angina* when chest pain recurs in the 4 weeks that follow an MI. Unstable angina occurring within 6 months after a percutaneous intervention procedure (see Chapter 61) is considered a different entity because it is most often related to a restenosis at the site of the previous dilatation. One way to categorize unstable angina is to use the Braunwald classification system, which is based on severity, clinical circumstances, associated electrocardiographic changes, and intensity of treatment (Table 59–2).

ACUTE CORONARY SYNDROMES. Unstable angina is part of the broader diagnosis of *acute coronary syndromes* that include sudden cardiac death, MI with ST segment elevation, non–Q-wave MI, and the complications associated with percutaneous coronary interventions. These syndromes mark rapid progression in the severity of coronary artery obstruction generally caused by an obstructing intravascular thrombus.

The clinical presentation of a *non–Q-wave MI* (see Chapter 60) is often indistinguishable from unstable angina because each may be characterized by prolonged ischemic chest pain. Treatment of the two conditions is also generally similar. The diagnosis of non–Q-wave MI is clinically suspected when the pain is prolonged and associated with persistent ST-T changes. The diagnosis is made, however, only after documentation of myocardial necrosis by elevated plasma levels of creatine kinase (CK) and of its MB isoenzyme (CK-MB); troponin I and troponin T levels are also elevated. A small elevation of troponin I or T can be present with normal CK and CK-MB values; this leakage is thought to indicate minor cell necrosis or severe ischemia and identifies a high-risk subset of patients with unstable angina. It may be a marker of distal embolization with shedding of thrombogenic material from a complex plaque.

VARIANT ANGINA. Prinzmetal's Variant Angina. Prinzmetal's variant angina is associated with transient ST-segment elevation, occurring most often at rest and in the early morning hours. The episodes of chest pain may be repetitive or intermittent with periods of exacerbation; episodes are promptly relieved by nitroglycerin. Syncope during an episode of chest pain is infrequent but strongly suggestive of the syndrome. Prinzmetal's variant angina is caused by an occlusive spasm typically in a normal or minimally diseased coronary artery. Raynaud's phenomenon and migraine have been described in some patients, suggesting that the syndrome may be part of a more generalized vasospastic disorder.

Angina With Normal Coronary Angiography (Syndrome X, Microvascular Angina). Angina may be caused by microvascular dysfunction without detectable lesions or spasm in the large coronary vessels. The diagnosis requires objective documentation of ischemic pain, with ST-segment changes or a transient regional perfusion defect, or of endothelial dysfunction with limited flow reserve with pharmacologic provocation. The chest pain episodes are often triggered by emotional stress and commonly occur in clusters. The prognosis is favorable.

DIFFERENTIAL DIAGNOSIS. Non-cardiac precipitants of myocar-

Table 59–2 ■ CLASSIFICATION OF UNSTABLE ANGINA

Severity

Class I — New-onset, severe, or accelerated angina

Patients with angina of less than 2 months' duration, severe or occurring three or more times per day, or angina that is distinctly more frequent and precipitated by distinctly less exertion; no rest pain in the last 2 months

Class II — Angina at rest; subacute

Patients with one or more episodes of angina at rest during the preceding month but not within the preceding 48 hours

Class III — Angina at rest; acute

Patients with one or more episodes at rest within the preceding 48 hours

Clinical Circumstances

Class A — Secondary unstable angina

A clearly identified condition extrinsic to the coronary vascular bed that has intensified myocardial ischemia (e.g., anemia, infection, fever, hypotension, tachyarrhythmia, thyrotoxicosis, hypoxemia secondary to respiratory failure)

Class B — Primary unstable angina

Class C — Postinfarction unstable angina (within 2 weeks of documented myocardial infarction)

Electrocardiogram

Without/with transient ST-segment deviations or T-wave changes

Intensity of Treatment

1. Absence of treatment or minimal treatment
2. Occurring in presence of standard therapy for chronic stable angina (conventional doses of oral β-blockers, nitrates, and calcium antagonists)
3. Occurring despite maximally tolerated doses of all three categories of oral therapy, including intravenous nitroglycerin.

Adapted from Braunwald E: Unstable angina: A classification. Circulation 80:410, 1989.

Cardiac, Ischemic Pain
Coronary atherosclerosis
Coronary, non-atherosclerotic causes
  Coronary spasm
  Coronary thrombosis
  Cocaine-induced chest pain
  Disorders of the microcirculation
  Congenital abnormality of the coronary circulation (e.g., anomalous origin of the left anterior descending coronary artery from the pulmonary artery)
Non-coronary causes
  Tachycardia
  Increased afterload (e.g., aortic valve stenosis, hypertrophic cardiomyopathy, left ventricular hypertrophy, and hypertension)
  Increased preload (e.g., aortic regurgitation)
  High inotropic state (e.g., adrenergic stimulation)
Cardiac, Non-ischemic
  Pericarditis
  Aortic dissection
Non-cardiac
  Gastrointestinal (e.g., esophageal spasm, reflux, rupture; ulcer)
  Psychogenic (e.g., anxiety, depression, cardiac psychosis)
  Pulmonary (e.g., pulmonary embolism, pneumothorax, pleuritic pain, pulmonary hypertension)
  Neuromuscular (e.g., costochondritis, Tietze's syndrome, herpes zoster, thoracic outlet syndrome)

dial ischemia include anemia, thyrotoxicosis, hypoxemia, and severe pulmonary disease (see Tables 38–2 and 59–3). Myocardial ischemia of a cardiac cause other than atherosclerosis develops in aortic valve stenosis, hypertension with left ventricular hypertrophy, hypertrophic cardiomyopathy, paroxysmal tachycardia, cocaine-induced chest pain, and congenital abnormalities of the coronary circulation. Non-ischemic cardiac causes of chest pain include pericarditis and aortic dissection. Non-cardiac, non-ischemic chest pain includes esophageal reflux and spasm, neuromuscular disorders, bronchopulmonary disease, and psychogenic factors.

No historical points, physical examination findings, or tests are faultless in the diagnosis of angina. Rather, the probability of angina is evaluated. The likelihood of coronary artery disease is influenced by age, gender, and other coronary risk factors (hyperlipidemia, smoking, hypertension), as well as by the clinical history of chest pain (see Table 59–1).

PHYSICAL EXAMINATION. The cardiopulmonary physical examination may be totally normal in patients with stable angina, even during an anginal attack. During ischemia, however, pulmonary rales, a transient S_4 or S_3 gallop, a sustained or dyskinetic left ventricular impulse, a transient mitral regurgitation murmur caused by papillary muscle dysfunction, or paradoxical splitting of S_2 (from transient left ventricular dysfunction or left bundle branch block) may be appreciated. The presence of hypertension, xanthomata, xanthelasma, corneal arcus, diminished pulses, or vascular bruits (see Chapter 67) raises the likelihood that the patient has coronary atherosclerosis. The physical examination may also help diagnose other causes of chest discomfort, including costochondritis and pulmonary disorders, as well as non-ischemic causes of cardiac chest pain, including aortic dissection or pericarditis (see Table 38–2).

DIAGNOSTIC WORK-UP. Laboratory Evaluation. Routine blood work cannot establish or exclude the diagnosis of angina but is important to assess abnormalities that may precipitate or worsen angina and to distinguish unstable angina from a non–Q-wave MI. The laboratory evaluation should therefore include a complete blood cell count to exclude anemia, which may precipitate or worsen angina; thyroid function tests to exclude hyperthyroidism, which may also precipitate or worsen angina; and assessment of renal function to exclude renal insufficiency as a precipitating or aggravating cause. Enzyme markers (troponin T, troponin I, CK-MB) help distinguish unstable angina from a non–Q-wave MI (see Chapter 60). Patients should be routinely evaluated for coronary risk factors, including an evaluation for hyperlipidemia (see Chapter 206), diabetes mellitus (see Chapter 242), and possibly, homocystine levels.

Elevated levels of C-reactive protein and of fibrinogen may identify patients with angina at higher risk for developing unstable

angina or MI. However, these tests are not presently recommended for the routine care of individual patients.

Resting Electrocardiogram. The resting electrocardiogram (ECG) obtained at times other than during episodes of chest pain has limited value. Some patients may have ST-segment or T-wave abnormalities suggestive of ischemia; others may have Q waves as markers of prior MI. By comparison, a 12-lead ECG may be extremely valuable in patients with unstable angina when it shows ST-T changes consistent with ischemia. Similar changes can be found on the ECG obtained *during* ischemia in patients with stable angina.

Provocative Testing. Provocative testing uses exercise or pharmacologic stress to precipitate myocardial ischemia. Ischemia is diagnosed by ST-T changes on the ECG, a perfusion defect on perfusion scintigraphy, or a regional wall motion abnormality on two-dimensional echocardiography. However, some patients with angina pectoris and significant underlying coronary artery disease may have negative results on these various provocative tests. Conversely, a positive test can be a false positive. Furthermore, patients with *silent ischemia* may have positive results in the absence of angina pectoris.

Exercise electrocardiography significantly enhances the value of the ECG for detecting myocardial ischemia and making the presumptive diagnosis of ischemic heart disease. The exercise ECG is most likely to indicate ischemia when the ST changes are horizontal or downsloping, are more than 1 mV (Fig. 59–1), occur during the early stages of exercise or at a low workload, persist for several minutes after exercise, and are accompanied by symptoms consistent with angina. The appearance of a new mitral regurgitation murmur, a 10-mm Hg or greater drop in blood pressure, or typical anginal pain during exercise add to the diagnostic value. False-positive results are most common in patients with underlying left ventricular hypertrophy or interventricular conduction abnormalities on the resting ECG, a pre-excitation syndrome such as the Wolff-Parkinson-White syndrome, electrolyte abnormalities, or digitalis use. ST-segment changes in patients with a lower clinical probability of angina pectoris are more likely to be a false-positive result than are the same changes in patients with higher clinical probability of the disease. The risk associated with exercise testing is low (1 per 10,000 tests) if the test is avoided in patients with significant aortic stenosis, severe hypertension, or severe heart failure.

A variety of exercise test protocols (Table 59–4) are used to measure exercise performance and, in patients with positive test results, the functional class (see Table 38–4). The sensitivity of exercise electrocardiography for detecting coronary artery disease is about 70%, and its specificity for excluding coronary artery disease

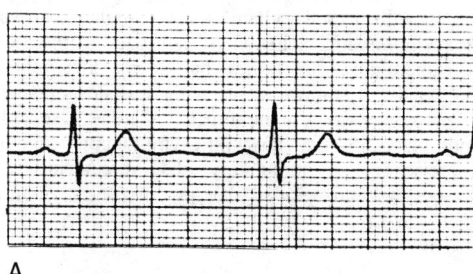

A

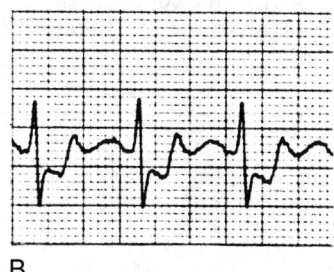

B

FIGURE 59–1 ■ Classic electrocardiographic ST-segment depression of myocardial ischemia. *A,* Normal lead V_5 at rest. *B,* Lead V_5 with 2- to 3-mm ST-segment depression during exercise.

Table 59-4 ▪ COMMON EXERCISE TEST PROTOCOLS

PROTOCOL	STAGE	DURATION (MIN)	GRADE (%)	RATE (MPH)	METABOLIC EQUIVALENTS AT COMPLETION	FUNCTIONAL CLASS
Modified	1	3	0	1.7	2.5	III
Bruce protocol*	2	3	10	1.7	5	II
	3	3	12	2.5	7	I
	4	3	14	3.4	10	I
	5	3	16	4.2	13	I
Naughton protocol†	0	2	0	2	2	III
	1	2	3.5	2	3	III
	2	2	7	2	4	III
	3	2	10.5	2	5	II
	4	2	14	2	6	II
	5	2	17.5	2	7	I

*Commonly used in ambulatory patients.
†Commonly used in patients with recent myocardial infarction, unstable angina, or other conditions that are expected to limit exercise.
From Goldman L, Braunwald E: Primary Cardiology. Philadelphia, WB Saunders, 1998, p 237.

is about 75% (Table 59–5). The predictive value is influenced by the prior probability of ischemic heart disease (see Table 59–1).

Perfusion scintigraphy using thallium-201 or technetium-99 sestamibi (see Chapter 44) is commonly performed in conjunction with exercise or dipyridamole injection. Myocardial scintigraphy can also localize the site of active ischemia in patients with more than one-vessel disease and hence help plan an interventional procedure (see Chapters 61 and 62). The sensitivity and specificity of perfusion scintigraphy using either the planar or the single-photon emission computed tomographic imaging techniques are generally somewhat better than for exercise electrocardiography. A false-negative result can be encountered in patients with three-vessel disease and global left ventricular ischemia.

Echocardiography (see Chapter 43) with exercise has a sensitivity and specificity at least equivalent to those of exercise electrocardiography. When performed after the infusion of dobutamine, stress echocardiography has been associated with a sensitivity of 86 to 96% for diagnosing coronary disease and a specificity of 66 to 95% for excluding it.

Positron emission tomography can assess myocardial perfusion and metabolism and diagnose coronary disease with sensitivities and specificities that may approach 95%. However, this more expensive test is not widely available and generally is not needed for the diagnosis (see Chapter 44).

Continuous electrocardiographic monitoring allows detection of otherwise clinically silent ischemia. Many patients with symptomatic angina also have multiple additional episodes of asymptomatic ischemia with a total ischemic burden higher than suspected. Control of asymptomatic ischemia by approaches that rely on reduction of ischemic burden rather than focus on symptoms may improve prognosis in some patients with episodes of silent ischemia. For example, the Asymptomatic Cardiac Ischemia Pilot (ACIP) randomized 558 patients with asymptomatic ischemia and a positive exercise test or ambulatory ECG monitoring to angina-guided therapy, ischemia-guided therapy, or routine revasculariza-

tion. Rates of death or MI after 2 years of follow-up were 12.1%, 8.8%, and 4.7%, respectively.

In patients with angina and a previous MI or symptoms of heart failure, left ventricular function should be assessed quantitatively by echocardiography (see Chapter 43) or nuclear techniques (see Chapter 44). The combination of multivessel disease and poor left ventricular function is associated with a poor enough prognosis to consider a mechanical revascularization procedure (see later). Quite often, segmental dysfunction can be caused by stunned myocardium (transient dysfunction due to acute ischemia) or hibernating myocardium (poorly functioning myocardium due to chronic hypoperfusion). These conditions should be recognized because they can be reversible with appropriate treatment.

When selecting a diagnostic test (Table 59–6), it is important to realize that the predictive value of the test is dependent on the prevalence of the disease as determined by the Bayes theorem; thus, the post-test likelihood of coronary artery disease is influenced by the pretest prevalence of the disease. Therefore, in populations with low or high prevalence of coronary artery disease, the probability of disease is little influenced by the test's results; the

Table 59-5 ▪ APPROXIMATE SENSITIVITIES AND SPECIFICITIES OF COMMON TESTS TO DIAGNOSE CORONARY ARTERY DISEASE

	SENSITIVITY	SPECIFICITY
Exercise electrocardiography		
>1 mv ST depression	0.70	0.75
>2 mv ST depression	0.33	0.97
>3 mv ST depression	0.20	0.99
Perfusion scintigraphy		
Planar	0.83	0.88
SPECT	0.86–0.88	0.60–0.68
Echocardiography		
Exercise	0.83–0.87	0.74–0.80
Pharmacologic stress	0.86–0.96	0.66–0.95

SPECT = single-photon emission computed tomography.

Table 59-6 ▪ SUGGESTED NON-INVASIVE TESTS IN DIFFERENT TYPES OF PATIENTS WITH STABLE ANGINA

Exertional angina, mixed angina, walk-through angina, postprandial angina with or without prior myocardial infarction
  A. Normal resting ECG: treadmill exercise ECG test
  B. Abnormal uninterpretable resting ECG: exercise myocardial perfusion scintigraphy (thallium-201-sestamibi)
  C. Unsuitable for exercise, unable to exercise adequately: dipyridamole or adenosine myocardial perfusion scintigraphy, dobutamine stress echocardiography
Atypical chest pain with normal or borderline abnormal resting ECG or with nondiagnostic stress ECG, particularly in women: exercise myocardial perfusion scintigraphy
Vasospastic angina: ECG during chest pain, ST segment depressed during ambulatory ECG
Dilated ischemic cardiomyopathy with typical angina or for assessment of the extent of hibernating myocardium: assessment of regional and global ejection fraction by radionuclide ventriculography or two-dimensional echocardiography, radionuclide myocardial perfusion scintigraphy; in selected patients, flow and metabolic studies with positron emission tomography
Syndrome X: initially treadmill exercise stress ECG (after demonstration of presence of normal coronaries; coronary blood flow reserve can be assessed non-invasively by positron emission tomography)
Known severe aortic stenosis or severe hypertrophic cardiomyopathy with stable angina: exercise stress tests are contraindicated; dipyridamole or adenosine myocardial perfusion scintigraphy in selected patients. Coronary angiography is preferred and should be done if surgery is planned.
Mild aortic valvular disease or hypertrophic cardiomyopathy with typical exertional angina: treadmill myocardial perfusion scintigraphy under strict supervision or dipyridamole or adenosine myocardial perfusion scintigraphy

ECG = elecrocardiogram.
From Goldman L, Braunwald E: Primary Cardiology. Philadelphia, WB Saunders, 1998, p 242.

Table 59-7 ■ RISK STRATIFICATION IN UNSTABLE ANGINA

	GRADIENT IN RISK		
	High	Intermediate*	Low*
Early Risk Evaluation (Hospital Admission)			
Clinical presentation	Prolonged chest pain Hemodynamic compromise during pain Transient S_3	Chest pain at rest	New-onset exertional angina More severe exertional angina
ECG: T wave	Deep T waves in anterior leads ST-segment elevation Pseudonormalization ST-segment depression $\geq$1 mV	T-wave changes ST-segment depression <1 mV	No ST-segment/T-wave changes
Troponin T, troponin I tests	Elevated	Elevated	Normal
In-Hospital Risk Stratification			
Evolution	Recurrent ischemia	Inducible ischemia Silent ischemia	No recurrent pain No silent or inducible ischemia

*Mainly determined by the absence of high-risk features. Other determinants of risk are older age, previous bypass surgery, previous myocardial infarction, and co-morbid conditions such as diabetes mellitus, renal failure, and obstructive coronary disease.

diagnostic yield is maximal in patients with less typical presentations and hence intermediate probabilities.

An additional indication to perform provocative testing is to gain insight into the severity of the disease for prognostic stratification. Poor prognostic indicators are more than 2 mV ST-segment depression within the first 3 minutes of exercise, a downsloping shape and depth of ST-segment depression of 2 mV, and persistence of the changes during the recovery phase for more than 5 minutes. Exercise-induced hypotension suggests multivessel disease.

Coronary arteriography is not usually indicated for diagnostic purposes except in some individuals to exclude with certainty the diagnosis of coronary disease and in some patients with otherwise unexplained symptoms. Arteriography can also be useful to diagnose vasospastic angina by performing coronary angiography after injection of ergonovine or acetylcholine, which causes a focal vasospasm in patients with Prinzmetal's variant angina. The usual indication for coronary arteriography is to explore the possibility of percutaneous coronary transluminal angioplasty (PTCA) or coro-

Table 59-8 ■ THERAPEUTIC APPROACH FOR STABLE ANGINA

General medical therapy—cessation of smoking: control of hypertension, diabetes, and hyperlipidemia: regular exercise and reduction of weight; aspirin if not contraindicated

Medical therapy in patients with stable angina in the absence of specific indications for revascularization to improve prognosis and prevent symptoms (β-blockers); pre-exercise prophylaxis (nitroglycerin); add long-acting nitrates and then calcium channel blockers as needed; goal is acceptable exercise capacity and quality of life and prevention of frequent or severe ischemia; revascularization therapy (catheter-based revascularization or surgical revascularization procedure depending on anatomic considerations) unless contraindications of refractory angina, frequent or severe symptomatic ischemia, unacceptable quality of life, or intolerable side effects of medications

Indications for revascularization therapy to improve prognosis in the absence of other major life-limiting diseases

Significant left main coronary artery stenosis → coronary artery bypass surgery

Significant three-vessel coronary artery disease with or without associated left main coronary artery stenosis and with or without normal left ventricular ejection fraction → coronary artery bypass surgery, including internal mammary arteries as conduits

Double-vessel coronary artery stenosis, including proximal left anterior descending coronary artery stenosis → coronary artery bypass surgery or catheter-based revascularization

Other single- or double-vessel coronary artery stenosis → catheter-based revascularization or coronary artery bypass surgery

In elderly (older than age 75 years) patients, patients with other life-limiting diseases, or patients needing urgent noncardiac surgery, catheter-based revascularization may be preferable when either type of revascularization is reasonable from a coronary perspective

In patients with moderately to severely depressed left ventricular ejection fraction with angina or angina equivalent with or without signs of heart failure → surgical revascularization if feasible

From Goldman L, Braunwald E: Primary Cardiology. Philadelphia, WB Saunders, 1998, p 255.

nary artery bypass graft (CABG) surgery to correct limiting symptoms, improve the quality of life, and improve prognosis.

Considering the different yield of various tests and the costs involved, it is important to select the tests that will be most appropriate in different types of patients (Table 59–6).

UNSTABLE ANGINA. Unstable angina is a heterogeneous syndrome with regard to causes, clinical manifestations, severity, and prognosis. The severity of the underlying coronary artery disease is also variable: 5 to 10% may have left main vessel disease; 40%, three-vessel disease; 25%, two-vessel disease; 20%, one-vessel disease; and 10%, no significant coronary artery stenoses. Most of the latter do not truly have unstable angina but rather another cause of pain mimicking its clinical presentation. The diagnosis requires careful clinical recognition followed by stratification of patients into groups at high, intermediate, or low risk of subsequent complications (Table 59–7). More aggressive therapeutic strategies are generally recommended in higher-risk patients.

TREATMENT. STABLE ANGINA. Management of angina targets control of symptoms, prevention of the complications of MI and death, as well as corrective measures to control the underlying atherosclerotic process, halt its progression, and promote its regression (Table 59–8). Counseling is important for teaching the nature and causes of the disease and its manifestations, risks, therapeutic approaches, and medical follow-up. It should focus on the individual patient's risk factors, taking socioeconomic status into account.

Prevention of Death and Myocardial Infarction. *Medical Management.* Antiplatelet therapy is indicated in all patients with coronary artery disease. The therapy is effective in all risk categories, including MI, unstable angina, stable angina, silent ischemia, and after CABG or PTCA. In the Antiplatelet Trialists Group meta-analysis of more than 100,000 patients from 145 randomized controlled trials, the odds of MI, stroke, or vascular death were reduced overall by more than 25% by antiplatelet therapy. Aspirin is the most common first choice, but clopidogrel, a thienopyridine derivative closely related to ticlopidine, is an alternative. In the Clopidogrel versus Aspirin in Patients at Risk of Ischemic Events (CAPRIE) randomized trial, patients receiving a 75-mg daily dose of clopidogrel had an 8.7% lower rate of the combined endpoint of stroke, MI, and vascular death compared with patients on 325 mg/day of aspirin ($P = 0.04$). Clopidogrel was significantly better in patients enrolled because of peripheral vascular disease and nonsignificantly better in patients with a previous stroke; aspirin was non-significantly better in patients enrolled because of a previous MI. Clopidogrel was associated with fewer gastrointestinal side effects, slightly more cutaneous reactions, no excess total bleeding, and no excess in leukopenia or thrombocytopenia compared with aspirin. Because of this favorable side effect profile, clopidogrel may be preferred over ticlopidine, which has also been shown useful in secondary prevention of vascular events. Clopidogrel and ticlopidine are antagonists of the adenosine diphosphate receptors in platelets. Aspirin irreversibly inhibits platelet cyclooxygenase and prevents formation of thromboxane A_2.

Warfarin (Coumadin) at a therapeutic international normalized ratio is also effective after MI, particularly in patients with atrial

Table 59–9 ■ CLINICAL USE OF NITROGLYCERIN AND NITRATES

COMPOUND	DOSE	CLINICAL EFFECTS	USE
Nitroglycerin			
Sublingual or buccal spray	0.15 to 1.5 mg	Relief of angina within 2 min	Before or at onset of pain
Ointment	7.5 to 15 mg	Antianginal benefit for 8–12 hr	Prophylaxis of pain
Transdermal	>50 mg/24 hr applied for 12 hr	Effective 8–16 hr	Patch on for 12 hr, then off
Intravenous	5 to 1000 mg/min for 24–48 hr	Ongoing; increasing dose may be required	Unstable angina
Isosorbide dinitrate			
Sublingual	2.5 to 15 mg	Same as nitroglycerin sublingual but slower	Before onset of pain
Oral	5–80 mg/d	Antianginal effect for 10–12 hr	Prophylaxis
Isosorbide-5-mononitrate			
Oral	20 mg twice daily	Antianginal effect for 8–12 hr	Prophylaxis
Slow release	60 to 240 mg/d	Antianginal effect for 12–18 hr	Prophylaxis

fibrillation or when left ventricular dysfunction is present. The combination of low-dose warfarin with aspirin is probably no better than aspirin alone to prevent recurrent MI. Paradoxically, warfarin was shown useful when added to aspirin in a primary prevention trial in high-risk individuals.

Based on the results of many studies that have shown a protective effect of β-blockers in secondary prevention after MI, it may be extrapolated that these medications will also be protective in patients with unstable angina and stable angina. Inhibitors of the angiotensin converting enzyme and probably also of the angiotensin receptor prolong life in patients with heart failure or depressed left ventricular ejection fraction and are routinely indicated; the potential of these drugs to prevent MI is being investigated in large clinical trials.

PTCA and CABG. CABG is indicated for prolongation of life in patients with left main vessel disease or in patients with three-vessel disease and left ventricular dysfunction regardless of symptoms. CABG or PTCA is also generally indicated for three-vessel disease with normal ventricular function or for proximal left anterior coronary artery disease when ischemia is documented.

Control of Symptoms. Effective antianginal therapy relieves myocardial ischemia by improving oxygen supply and/or reducing demand.

Medical Management. Myocardial oxygen demand is reduced by β-blockers, nitrates, and calcium antagonists. Nitrates and calcium antagonists are also coronary vasodilators. Nitroglycerin (Table 59–9) produces immediate vasodilation; venous and arteriolar vasodilatation reduces preload and afterload on the heart, and coronary vasodilatation relieves inappropriate coronary vasoconstriction. Administered sublingually or by oral spray, nitroglycerin is the cornerstone of therapy to terminate an angina attack; the efficacy is immediate in Prinzmetal's angina and is rapid in rest and effort angina. Long-acting nitrates administered orally or transdermally are effective to prevent angina and improve tolerance to exercise. A period of the day free of exposure is recommended to avoid tachyphylaxis. Nitroglycerin is exogenous nitric oxide and may overcome some of the problems associated with deficient production in the dysfunctional endothelium.

β-Blocker therapy (Table 59–10) helps reduce the hemodynamic stress imposed on a fragile lesion; these medications also reduce heart rate at rest and during exercise and reduce blood pressure.

Calcium channel antagonists (Table 59–11) are potent vasodilators to relieve coronary artery spasm. They also reduce myocardial oxygen needs by a variable effect on heart rate, blood pressure, and contractility. Selection of the best agent for an individual patient is influenced by many considerations, including associated disease and tolerance to the drugs. A controversy exists on possible deleterious effects on mortality for calcium antagonists, particularly short-acting nifedipine. Diltiazem and verapamil are contraindicated in patients with left ventricular dysfunction occurring after MI. Patients with hypertension will benefit from β-blockers or calcium antagonists. β-Blockers are used only with caution in diabetic patients. Patients with heart failure will benefit from nitrates and low-dose β-blockers. Active bronchospasm is a contraindication to β-blockers; cardioselective β-blockers may, however, be tested. The dihydropyridine calcium channel blockers may be advantageous when a bradyarrhythmia is present. A β-blocker, diltiazem, or verapamil is useful in patients who have tachyarrhythmias.

Revascularization. PTCA (see Chapter 61) and CABG (see Chapter 62) result in an immediate relief of the obstruction to blood flow and are indicated to treat unacceptable symptoms in patients with stable angina (see Table 59–8). With PTCA, symptomatic and angiographic improvement is expected in more than 90% of patients, with a complication rate below 10%. The risk of complications (death <1%; MI, 8%; abrupt vessel closure requiring urgent surgery, 1%) decreases with more experience, improved technology, stent implantation, and use of intravenous glycoprotein IIb/IIIa antagonists.

Elective CABG is associated with a mortality rate as low as 0.2%. The risk of CABG is affected by many factors, including age, co-morbid diseases, left ventricular function, and the extent of coronary artery disease. Internal mammary artery grafts are clearly associated with a better short- and long-term outcome.

For single-vessel disease, both PTCA and CABG can provide substantial symptomatic relief, but neither has been documented to improve survival. In patients with multivessel disease, PTCA and CABG appear to have equivalent results in terms of death and MI, with PTCA allowing patients to return to work sooner and CABG being associated with fewer symptoms and better exercise tolerance. CABG is preferred over PTCA in patients with diabetes mellitus. The choice between CABG and PTCA is often influenced by local expertise as well as by patient and physician preference.

Table 59–10 ■ CLINICAL USE OF β-BLOCKERS

COMPOUND	INTRINSIC SYMPATHOMIMETIC ACTIVITY*	HALF-LIFE (HR)	CLEARANCE	USE
Non-cardioselective				
Propranolol	–	1–6	Liver	40–80 mg bid to qid
Propranolol long-acting	–	8–11	Liver	80–360 mg/d
Nadolol	–	20–40	Kidney	40–240 mg/d
Sotalol	–	7–18	Kidney	40–160 mg bid
Trinolol	–	4–5	Liver-kidney	10–15 mg bid
Cardioselective				
Alebutolol	++	8–13	Liver-kidney	200–600 mg bid
Atenolol	–	6–7	Kidney	50–200 mg/d
Metoprolol	–	3–7	Liver	50–200 mg bid

*Presence commonly associated with maintenance or increase in heart rate; absence associated with decrease in heart rate

Table 59–11 ■ PROPERTIES OF CALCIUM CHANNEL BLOCKING DRUGS IN CLINICAL USE

DRUGS	VASCULAR SELECTIVITY*	USUAL DOSE	PLASMA HALF-LIFE	SIDE EFFECTS
Dihydropyridines				
Nifedipine	3.1	Immediate release: 20–40 mg 3 times daily Slow release: 30–180 mg once daily	4 hr	Hypotension, dizziness, flushing, nausea, constipation, edema
Amlodipine	†	5–10 mg once daily	30–50 hr	Headache, edema
Felodipine	5.4	5–10 mg once daily	11–16 hr	Headache, dizziness
Isradipine	7.4	2.5–10 mg twice daily	8 hr	Headache, fatigue
Nicardipine	17.0	20–40 mg three times daily	2–4 hr	Headache, dizziness, flushing, edema
Nisoldipine	†	20–40 mg once daily	2–6 hr	Similar to nifedipine
Nitrendipine	14.4	20 mg once or twice daily	5–12 hr	Similar to nifedipine
Other				
Bepridil	‡	200–400 mg once daily	24–40 hr	Arrhythmias, dizziness, nausea
Diltiazem	0.3	Immediate release: 30–80 mg 4 times daily Slow release: 120–320 mg once daily	3–4 hr	Hypotension, dizziness, flushing, bradycardia
Verapamil	1.3	Immediate release: 80–160 mg three times daily Slow release: 120–480 mg once daily		Hypotenison, myocardial depression, heart failure, edema

Adapted from Katzung, B.G., and Chatterjee, K.: Vasodilators and the treatment of angina. *In* Katzung B.G. (ed.): *Clinical Pharmacology*. Norwalk, CT, Appleton & Lange, 1994, pp. 171–187. Appeared in Goldman L, Braunwald E: *Primary Cardiology*. Philadelphia, WB Saunders, 1998.
*Numerical data give the ratio of vascular potency to cardiac potency; higher numbers indicate greater vascular, less cardiac potency.
†Significant degree of vasodilatation greater than myocardial depression.
‡Myocardial depression greater than vasodilatation.

UNSTABLE ANGINA. Based on clinical characteristics, patients can also be divided into those with high, intermediate, and low risk of death or non-fatal MI in the short term (Table 59–7). The treatment of unstable angina includes interventions to control pain, interventions that reduce myocardial oxygen demand, and interventions that are designed to increase myocardial oxygen supply. Intravenous or sublingual nitroglycerin (up to three sublingual nitroglycerin tablets at 5-minute intervals) is administered for the relief of chest pain and is followed by an intravenous infusion of nitroglycerin (beginning at 5 to 10 g/min and increasing by up to 10 g/min every 5 minutes as needed and tolerated). The goal is to switch patients to oral or topical nitrates when they have been asymptomatic for 24 hours. Morphine may be given in doses of 2 to 5 mg intravenously, repeated once or twice after 15 to 30 minutes to relieve symptoms.

Aspirin should be started immediately at an initial dose of 160 to 325 mg followed by 80 to 160 mg/day. For patients who cannot tolerate aspirin, clopidogrel, 75 mg/day (or ticlopidine, 250 mg twice daily) is an appropriate alternative; because the full antiplatelet effects of these drugs may be delayed for a few days, an alternative is to use a 300-mg loading dose of clopidogrel. Intravenous heparin should be started on all patients at high or intermediate risk immediately and be continued for 2 to 5 days until the patient has been free of chest pain for at least 24 hours or a coronary intervention procedure is performed. The recommended dose is 80 units/kg as an intravenous bolus followed by 8 units/kg/min by infusion to keep the activated partial thromboplastin time at one and one-half to two times control values. Low molecular-weight heparin (see Chapter 188), which may be preferred to standard heparin, can be administered subcutaneously to produce a sustained and reproducible anticoagulation response, with no need for monitoring. Low-molecular-weight heparins have less platelet effects and only rarely cause heparin-induced thrombocytopenia. Their risk of bleeding is not, however, less than that of unfractionated heparin. Two recent trials have shown a superiority of subcutaneous enoxaparin (1 mg or 100 anti–Factor X units per kilogram) administered twice daily for 48 hours to 8 days after admission. One trial with nadroperin and one with dalteparin have not shown a superiority over unfractionated heparin. Prolonged administration after hospital discharge was not associated with additional benefit in these trials.

Intravenous glycoprotein IIb/IIIa antagonists have been extensively investigated in recent years. Significant benefit has been demonstrated in coronary angioplasty with abciximab, eptifibatide, and tirofiban, and in the management of unstable angina and non–Q-wave MI with eptifibatide and tirofiban. The drugs are continued during coronary angiography and during percutaneous coronary interventions if they are performed. The recommended dose of tirofiban is 0.4 μg/kg/min for 30 minutes followed by an infusion of 0.1

μg/kg, and that of eptifibatide is an 180-μg/kg bolus followed by an infusion of 2.0/kg/min; it is recommended to reduce the dose of eptifibatide if coronary angioplasty is performed. Optimal antithrombotic therapy of unstable angina and non–Q-wave MI and prevention of death and MI is achieved with a combination of aspirin, heparin, and a GPIb/IIIa antagonist.

β-Blockers are indicated in patients at high risk for adverse events unless contraindications such as hypotension, marked bradycardia, substantial left ventricular failure, atrioventricular block, or more than mild bronchospastic airway disease co-exist. Therapy is begun intravenously in patients with evolving pain and is followed by oral therapy to a target of 50 to 60 beats per minute: metoprolol (5 mg by slow intravenous bolus repeated every 5 minutes for a total initial dose of 15 mg followed in 1 to 2 hours by 25 to 100 mg orally every 12 hours); propranolol (0.5–1 mg intravenously followed in 1 to 2 hours by 40–80 mg orally every 6 to 8 hours); atenolol (as two 5-mg intravenous doses 5 minutes apart followed by 50–100 mg/day orally); or esmolol (in an intravenous infusion of 0.1 mg/kg/min titrated by 0.05 mg/kg/min every 10 to 15 minutes until the desired response has been achieved or a maximum dose of 0.2 mg/kg/min is given).

Calcium channel antagonists are useful primarily for patients with vasospastic angina, especially documented Prinzmetal's angina. In patients with non-vasospastic angina, short-acting nifedipine should never be used in the absence of β-blockade because it might increase the risk of MI.

Mechanical Revascularization. In patients with refractory ischemia despite medical therapy, mechanical revascularization with either PTCA or CABG should be performed whenever possible. Intra-aortic balloon counterpulsation is indicated as a bridge to revascularization in the unstable patient.

Randomized trials have shown that the rates of death or MI are not reduced by a routine aggressive management strategy as compared with a conservative strategy, provided that angiography followed by indicated intervention is performed in patients who have persistent or recurrent ischemia, heart failure, left ventricular ejection fraction below 50%, malignant ventricular arrhythmias, or a clearly high-risk, positive, non-invasive study. The early aggressive strategy is associated with less angina and lower rates of hospital readmission during follow-up.

CONTROL OF THE UNDERLYING ATHEROSCLEROTIC PROCESS. Correction of coronary risk factors improves prognosis in patients with coronary artery disease and may be associated with regression of the disease. An aggressive program for correction of risk factors is therefore mandated in patient management. Indeed, in many patients the long-term benefits may exceed those of revascularization procedures. The program should include smoking cessation; control of blood cholesterol, blood sugar, and hypertension; and physical fitness. Lipid-lowering drugs, particularly HMG CoA reductase inhibitors (see Chapter 206) are indicated for their potential to alter plaque content and prevent plaque activation.

Antiplatelet Trialists' Collaboration: Collaborative overview of randomized trials of antiplatelet therapy: I. Prevention of death, myocardial infarction, and stroke by prolonged antiplatelet therapy in various categories of patients. BMJ 308:81, 1994. *The meta-analysis of 145 randomized trials of more than 100,000 patients documented clearly the efficacy of antiplatelet therapy for the management of the acute manifestations of coronary artery disease, for its secondary prevention, and, in some instances, for primary prevention.*

Bypass Angioplasty Revascularization Investigation (BARI) Investigators: Comparison of coronary bypass surgery with angioplasty in patients with multivessel disease. N Engl J Med 335:217, 1996. *The randomized trial of PTCA versus coronary artery bypass surgery in patients with multivessel disease did not show any difference in 5-year survival, although subsequent revascularization was required more often after PTCA. For treated diabetics, however, 5-year survival was significantly better after CABG than after PTCA.*

CAPRIE Steering Committee: A randomized, blinded, trial of clopidogrel versus aspirin in patients at risk of ischaemic events. Lancet 348:1329, 1996. *The trial compared clopidogrel to aspirin for secondary prevention of cardiovascular events in patients with a previous stroke, previous myocardial infarction, or peripheral vascular disease. Clopidogrel was slightly, but significantly, better than aspirin. The side effect profile of the drug was also favorable.*

Cohen M, Demers C, Gurfinkel EP, et al, for the Efficacy and Safety of Subcutaneous Enoxaparin in Non-Q-Wave Coronary Events Study Group: Low molecular weight heparin versus unfractionated heparin for unstable angina and non–Q-wave myocardial infarction. N Engl J Med 337:447, 1997. *The randomized double-blind trial compared treatment with enoxaparin, a low-molecular-weight heparin, to unfractionated heparin in hospitalized patients with unstable angina or non–Q-wave myocardial infarction; aspirin was administered to all patients. The risk of death, myocardial infarction, or recurrent angina was reduced with the low-molecular-weight heparin.*

Coumadin Aspirin Reinfarction Study (CARS) Investigators: Randomized double-blind trial of fixed-dose warfarin with aspirin after myocardial infarction. Lancet 350:389, 1997. *In this trial of 8803 patients who had had a myocardial infarction, the addition of low, fixed-dose warfarin combined with low-dose aspirin did not provide benefit beyond that achieved with aspirin monotherapy.*

Heberden W: Some account of a disorder of the breast. Med Trans Coll Physicians Lond 2:59, 1772. *Original description of angina pectoris published in 1772 remains up-to-date; it also accounts for the progression from stable angina to unstable angina.*

Henderson RA, Pocock SJ, Sharp SJ, et al: Long-term results of RITA-1 trial: Clinical and cost comparisons of coronary angioplasty and coronary-artery bypass grafting. Lancet 352:1419, 1998. *Initial strategies of PTCA and CABG led to similar long-term results in terms of survival and avoidance of myocardial infarction and to similar long-term health-care costs.*

Theroux P, Fuster V: Acute coronary syndromes: Unstable angina and non–Q wave myocardial infarction. Circulation 97:1195, 1998. *A comprehensive review.*

60 ACUTE MYOCARDIAL INFARCTION

Burton E. Sobel

DEFINITIONS AND HISTORICAL CONSIDERATIONS

Acute myocardial infarction (MI) is a focus of necrosis resulting from inadequate tissue perfusion; it is accompanied by consequent hypoxia, accumulation of deleterious metabolites, and signs and symptoms reflective of myocardial cell death. Anoxia without decreased perfusion can cause MI but does so only rarely. MI refers also to the "typical" clinical syndrome that results from such ischemia and that is manifested by signs and symptoms such as crushing chest pain and diaphoresis, malignant ventricular arrhythmia, heart failure, or shock. However, MI can also present as sudden cardiac death, or presentations can be atypical and clinically silent or subtle, with new-onset or accelerated angina, atypical chest pain mimicking "indigestion," impaired cerebral perfusion with syncope, or signs simulating those of a cerebrovascular accident or altered mental states. Coronary thrombosis, recognized as a potential cause as early as 1910, was established unequivocally as the pathophysiologic cause by early angiographic study of afflicted patients. Early catastrophic complications of MI include ventricular fibrillation, rupture of the ventricular free wall, ventricular septal rupture (with shock and left-to-right shunting), and papillary muscle rupture (with

profound mitral or tricuspid regurgitation). Later complications include ventricular mural thrombus with peripheral embolization and cerebrovascular accident, heart failure with or without ventricular true or pseudoaneurysm, ventricular dilation and remodeling, and infarct expansion. The initial presentation is often sudden cardiac death. Progression of underlying coronary artery disease in survivors of acute MI may result in unstable angina pectoris, "silent ischemia" (with electrocardiographic [ECG] changes without symptoms), recurrent MI, or sudden death.

INCIDENCE AND ETIOLOGY

Incidence

Diagnosed coronary artery disease is present in as many as 7 million Americans and kills more than 500,000 annually. Sudden death, precluding hospitalization, occurs in more than 350,000 cases. Even among those who die after the prehospital phase, death is most often sudden. MI accounts for 750,000 hospital admissions in the United States annually. The impressive decline in age-adjusted death rates attributable to acute MI since the mid-1970s, a decrease of as much as 47% according to some estimates, probably reflects a decreased incidence of coronary atherosclerosis, better treatment of chronic coronary artery disease, and marked improvements in the care of patients who suffer an MI. Nevertheless, because of population growth, the total number of MI-related deaths in the United States has not declined. MI too often leaves survivors afflicted with or prone to heart failure, and coronary artery disease remains responsible for more years of potential life lost before age 65 years, regardless of gender or race, than any other illness.

Etiology

Although most MIs result from thrombotic occlusion superimposed on coronary atherosclerosis, severe atherosclerotic disease may exist for years with no change in severity of effort-induced angina. A seminal precipitating factor of acute coronary syndromes, including unstable angina, sudden cardiac death, and acute MI, is hemorrhagic rupture or fissuring of a fat-laden, unstable atheroma with consequent thrombosis (see Chapter 58). Q-wave MIs (previously called *transmural*) appear to result when occlusive thrombi persist, as documented angiographically in more than 90% of patients with acute MI. Non–Q-wave MIs (previously called *subendocardial*) result from incomplete or spontaneously recanalized thrombotic occlusions after ischemia that are persistent enough to elicit necrosis; reocclusion with early recurrent MI is common. The distinction between Q-wave and non-Q-wave MI is often blurred by early revascularization procedures that can interrupt development of what otherwise would have become a Q-wave MI.

Risk factors for MI parallel those for atherosclerosis in general (see Chapters 39 and 58) and include diabetes mellitus, hypertension, truncal obesity, smoking, increased levels of low-density-lipoprotein (LDL) cholesterol, decreased levels of high-density-lipoprotein (HDL) cholesterol, elevated levels of plasma homocysteine, increased levels of lipoprotein (a), a positive family history for atherosclerosis, and, in some studies, increased levels of triglycerides. Other genetic variations with a less clear link to coronary atherosclerosis include polymorphisms in the plasminogen activator inhibitor type-1, thrombomodulin, and angiotensin-converting enzyme genes.

Soon after MI, changes such as hyperglycemia or elevated triglyceride levels may be inappropriately interpreted as being indicative of diabetes or hyperlipidemia, when in fact they reflect transiently impaired insulin release because of reduced pancreatic blood flow, augmented glycogenolysis secondary to catecholamine release, increased gluconeogenesis secondary to 17 hydroxy (OH) corticosteroid release, increased concentrations of plasma free fatty acids, and augmented hepatic synthesis of triglycerides. Conversely, decreased cholesterol levels secondary to hepatic dysfunction may be misinterpreted as an absence of hypercholesterolemia that would otherwise have been evident; the fall in LDL cholesterol levels is greater than that of total cholesterol levels and may persist for 6 to 8 weeks.

Rare causes of acute MI (Table 60–1) other than atherosclerosis include coronary arterial emboli secondary to infective or marantic

Table 60–1 ■ CONDITIONS OTHER THAN CORONARY ATHEROSCLEROSIS THAT MAY CAUSE ACUTE MYOCARDIAL INFARCTION

Coronary emboli	Causes include aortic or mitral valve lesions, left atrial or ventricular thrombi, prosthetic valves, fat emboli, intracardiac neoplasms, infective endocarditis, and paradoxical emboli
Thrombotic coronary artery disease	May occur with oral contraceptive use, sickle cell anemia and other hemoglobinopathies, polycythemia vera, thrombocytosis, thrombotic thrombocytopenic purpura, disseminated intravascular coagulation, antithrombin III deficiency and other hypercoagulable states, macroglobulinemia and other hyperviscosity states, multiple myeloma, leukemia, malaria, and fibrinolytic system shutdown secondary to impaired plasminogen activation or excessive inhibition
Coronary vasculitis	Seen with Takayasu's disease, Kawasaki's disease, polyarteritis nodosa, lupus erythematosus, scleroderma, rheumatoid arthritis, and immune-mediated vascular degeneration in cardiac allografts
Coronary vasospasm	May be associated with variant angina, nitrate withdrawal, cocaine or amphetamine abuse, and angina with "normal" coronary arteries
Infiltrative and degenerative coronary vascular disease	May result from amyloidosis, connective tissue disorders (such as pseudoxanthoma elasticum), lipid storage disorders and mucopolysaccharidoses, homocystinuria, diabetes mellitus, collagen vascular disease, muscular dystrophies, and Friedreich's ataxia
Coronary ostial occlusion	Associated with aortic dissection, luetic aortitis, aortic stenosis, and ankylosing spondylitis syndromes
Congenital coronary anomalies	Including Bland-White-Garland syndrome of anomalous origin of the left coronary artery from the pulmonary artery, left coronary artery origin from the anterior sinus of Valsalva, coronary arteriovenous fistula or aneurysms, and myocardial bridging with secondary vascular degeneration
Trauma	Associated with and responsible for coronary dissection, laceration, or thrombosis (with endothelial cell injury secondary to trauma such as angioplasty); radiation; and cardiac contusion
Augmented myocardial oxygen requirements exceeding oxygen delivery	Encountered with aortic stenosis, aortic insufficiency, hypertension with severe left ventricular hypertrophy, pheochromocytoma, thyrotoxicosis, methemoglobinemia, carbon monoxide poisoning, shock, and hyperviscosity syndromes

endocarditis (often associated with drug abuse or collagen vascular disease, respectively), calcium deposits or thrombi from prosthetic or calcified valves, ventricular mural thrombi, atrial thrombi or myxomas, coronary thrombosis caused by trauma or by use of oral contraceptives in women, vasculitis, vasospasm (idiopathic or associated with cocaine or amphetamine abuse), coronary vascular degeneration (including accelerated atherosclerosis) after cardiac transplantation, and inflammatory small vessel coronary disease (0.1- to 1.0-mm diameter vessels) associated with diabetes, collagen vascular diseases, or disorders affecting extracellular matrix. Occasionally, acute MI may occur with the angiographic syndrome X (angina with "normal" coronary arteries) or variant angina (see Chapter 59), because of diminished elaboration of nitric oxide or increased release of vasoconstrictors, such as endothelin. Acute MI may also be a consequence of failed coronary revascularization. Thus, closure of the instrumented artery is seen in 1% or more of patients after percutaneous transluminal coronary angioplasty (PTCA), even when stenting is employed; early closure of coronary artery bypass grafts occurs in up to 5% of patients; and approximately 5% of patients have acute reocclusion after thrombolysis for an acute MI.

PATHOLOGY AND PATHOPHYSIOLOGY

Pathology

Coronary atherosclerosis is especially prominent at branch points of vessels (see Chapter 58). Lipid-rich soft plaques with thinned fibrous caps are particularly prone to rupture, which precipitates an acute coronary event.

The spectrum of myocardial injury depends not only on the intensity of impaired myocardial perfusion but also on its duration. Accordingly, no conventional microscopic or gross changes may be evident in hearts of patients who die suddenly as a result of an acute coronary event. Typical MI is manifest by coagulation necrosis followed ultimately by fibrosis. Contraction-band necrosis occurs when ischemia is followed by reperfusion or accompanied by massive adrenergic stimulation, often with myocytolysis.

In patients who die with a history of preceding unstable angina, morphologic manifestations of frank MI may be lacking. However, one can see platelet microemboli and vascular mural thrombosis, which are of diverse age and indicate repetitive thrombotic phenomena initiated by dynamic changes in complicated atherosclerotic plaques. In victims of MI with ECG changes, the presence of Q waves after complete resolution of the insult generally indicates a larger MI, but the previously made distinction between transmural and nontransmural MI cannot be made based on ECG

criteria, and this old terminology has been replaced by the terms Q-wave and non-Q-wave MI, respectively.

Pathophysiology

The right and left coronary arteries arise most commonly independently from individual ostia associated with right and left aortic valve cusps. The left anterior descending (LAD) and circumflex coronary arteries arise at the left main coronary artery bifurcation and supply the anterior left ventricle, the bulk of the interventricular septum, the apex, and the lateral and posterior left ventricular walls (see Chapter 46). The right coronary artery generally supplies the right ventricle, the posterior third of the interventricular septum, the inferior wall (diaphragmatic surface) of the left ventricle, and a portion of the posterior wall of the left ventricle (via the posterior descending branch). When the posterior descending coronary artery that supplies the posterior interventricular septum arises from the left circumflex artery, the circulation is called left dominant. More often, the posterior descending artery arises from the right coronary artery (right dominant circulation). The posterior left ventricular branch of the right coronary artery supplies the atrioventricular (AV) node in 90% of subjects. Another right coronary artery branch (in 55% of subjects) supplies the sinus node. The right ventricle is supplied by the right coronary artery. Although the posterior division of the left bundle branch has a dual blood supply (from both the left and right coronary arteries), the anterior fascicles of the left bundle and the right bundle are each supplied primarily by branches of the LAD artery.

In view of anatomic considerations, it is not surprising that right coronary artery occlusion is manifested frequently by sinus bradycardia, AV block, right ventricular MI, or left ventricular MI of modest extent. However, markedly impaired left ventricular function with pulmonary congestion or edema indicative of extensive injury and intraventricular conduction defects, such as hemiblock, is more typical of left coronary artery occlusion. With left ventricular inferior wall MI, hypotension is common not only because of vagotonia, but also because of activation of chemoreceptors initiating the Bezold-Jarisch reflex and accumulation of adenosine in the infarct zone secondary to local inhibition of adenosine deaminase that can be antagonized pharmacologically by administration of aminophylline.

If coronary recanalization is not induced relatively promptly (spontaneously, mechanically, surgically, or with fibrinolytic drugs), regional myocardial perfusion may not be sustained despite restoration of patency (the "no-reflow" phenomenon) because of endothelial cell swelling, presence of platelet and leukocyte plugs, or complement-mediated microvascular inflammation. In addition to hypoxia, decreased removal of noxious metabolites, including potassium, calcium, amphiphilic lipids, and oxygen-centered free radicals, impairs ventricular performance and may evoke lethal arrhythmias. Inflammation of endocardial surfaces and stasis associated with dyskinesis can lead to ventricular mural thrombi. Epicardial inflammation may initiate pericarditis, which is seen with more than 20% of Q-wave infarcts.

SYSTOLIC FUNCTION. Even transitory deprivation of oxygen and accumulation of metabolites promptly cause diminished diastolic relaxation, abnormal regional systolic contractile function and wall thickening, abnormal wall motion, diminished cardiac cycle–dependent variation of backscattered ultrasound, and, if extensive, diminished stroke volume. Restoring perfusion may promptly restore function of myocardium that exhibits decreased function because of decreased perfusion ("hibernating" myocardium). Often, however, impaired function persists for some period of time after blood flow is restored and before the myocardium recovers ("stunning"). In general, hypokinesis and akinesis reflect the locus and extent of myocardial injury. Expansion of MI and ventricular dilatation (so-called ventricular remodeling) begin within hours after the onset of MI with thinning of the infarct zone and realignment of layers of tissue within and adjacent to it. Rupture, seen in as many as 10% of fatal MIs before the thrombolytic therapy era, may result, particularly when cardiogenic shock, hemodynamically significant arrhythmia, or antecedent history of hypertension with ventricular hypertrophy is present. Rupture, often heralded by abrupt hypotension, bradycardia, and atypical T-wave changes, may occur also with small MIs because the well-preserved ventricular function can increase wall stress.

A ventricular aneurysm, which is an outward bulging of a non-contracting segment, is seen with early cardiac imaging in as many as 20% of patients with Q-wave MI. Clinically, aneurysms may be recognized only later, manifested by heart failure, recurrent ventricular arrhythmia, or recurrent emboli. They may be accompanied by persistent ST-segment elevation in ECGs obtained 6 weeks or more after MI.

As left ventricular end-diastolic volume and pressure increase because of impaired regional contractility and relaxation, intramural diastolic ventricular pressure increases and myocardial perfusion declines. Peripheral arterial vasoconstriction and systemic venous constriction can no longer offset declining stroke volume, and blood pressure falls. With decreased cardiac output and accelerated heart rate, coronary flow declines. Because coronary artery disease is usually generalized, ischemia "at a distance" may be evident as ECG changes or may result in a vicious circle in which stuttering MI ultimately leads to profound left ventricular failure and cardiogenic shock.

Normally perfused zones initially may exhibit compensatory hyperkinesis with excessive wall thickening in systole. However, as the heart dilates over a period of 24 to 48 hours, hyperkinesis regresses.

DIASTOLIC FUNCTION. Very early after the onset of MI, relaxation of ischemic myocardium decreases. Impaired relaxation leads to increased left ventricular end-diastolic volume and pressure (LVEDP). The increased LVEDP results in ventricular dilation, elevated pulmonary venous pressure, decreased pulmonary compliance, interstitial and (ultimately) alveolar pulmonary edema, hypoxemia, and exacerbation of myocardial ischemic injury. As the infarct thins and shrinks, and if infarct expansion does not predominate, ventricular dilatation may regress, and diastolic cardiac and pulmonary pressures may return toward normal.

RIGHT VENTRICULAR FUNCTION. Impaired right ventricular function was recognized initially in the extreme, when right coronary artery occlusion led to gross right ventricular MI. However, similar manifestations can occur when inferior left ventricular MI and left circumflex occlusion exist with a left dominant circulation. Acute right ventricular dysfunction diminishes cardiac output disproportionally to left ventricular injury. High-grade bradyarrhythmias are common, including those resulting from third-degree heart block. Occasionally, profound arterial oxygen desaturation can develop because of augmented right atrial pressure and right-to-left shunting through a patent foramen ovale. The hemodynamic changes resemble many of those seen with pericardial constriction or tamponade (see Chapter 65).

COMPENSATORY MECHANISMS. Adaptations reflect the locus and extent of infarction. With large anterior MIs, reflex-augmented sympathoadrenal and vagal discharge may give rise to tachycardia, ventricular arrhythmia, and bradycardia (sinus node depression or heart block), as well as pallor, cutaneous vasoconstriction, and diaphoresis. Initially, compromised cardiac output is maintained by the combination of increased heart rate and ventricular dilatation with recruitment of the Frank-Starling mechanism. Right ventricular MI most dramatically impairs hemodynamics early in its course. As healing progresses and the right ventricle becomes less compliant, its conduit function is restored, permitting maintenance of cardiac output at the expense of augmentation of right ventricular filling pressure. In addition, recovery of right ventricular contractile performance is a prominent and remarkable feature of right ventricular MI. With left ventricular inferior wall MI, with or without concomitant right ventricular involvement, bradycardia (sinus node depression, AV block) and hypotension are frequent and are often indicative of excessive vagal tone.

EFFECTS OF MI ON ORGANS OTHER THAN THE HEART. Augmentation of pulmonary venous pressure may cause diminished pulmonary compliance, dyspnea, pulmonary vascular redistribution (detectable radiographically), interstitial and alveolar pulmonary edema, respiratory decompensation, and hypoxemia. Cerebral hypoperfusion may result in restlessness or, rarely, psychosis. Coupled with dyspnea in the elderly, it may be manifested only as confusion and combativeness. Increased sympathoadrenal tone reflected by markedly elevated plasma catecholamine levels and adrenocortical stimulation may be prominent as well. Plasma concentrations of atrial natriuretic peptide decrease initially but then increase, perhaps because of heart failure and atrial stretch. Elevated plasma concentrations of vasopressin, angiotensin (with β-adrenergic stimulation of renin release), and aldosterone contribute to fluid retention and hyponatremia. Impaired pancreatic blood flow inhibits insulin secretion.

In addition to the typical increase in erythrocyte sedimentation rate and leukocytosis, modestly increased levels of plasma fibrinogen and augmented circulating plasminogen activator inhibitor type-1 (PAI)-1 occur as part of the acute phase reaction to MI. Impaired fibrinolysis and augmented platelet activation by circulating catecholamines may predispose to continuing coronary and ventricular mural thrombosis. Plasma viscosity increases because of increased fibrinogen, α_2-globulins, and hemoconcentration, several days after the onset of MI, most markedly when left ventricular failure or shock supervenes.

DETERMINANTS OF PROGNOSIS. Immediate survival depends primarily on whether ventricular fibrillation (VF) occurs, and if so, whether it can be treated instantly. Community-based emergency systems that have defibrillators and appropriately trained personnel, rapid hospitalization, and, in some instances, dedicated chest pain facilities for patients with suspected evolving MI have improved early survival. Even among hospitalized patients, death is often attributable to VF, which can, of course, often be interrupted by immediate defibrillation.

Judging from ambulatory ECGs and recordings obtained in coronary care units, lethal arrhythmias associated with acute MI are primary VF (i.e., VF in the absence of severe heart failure) in 85% or more instances. Only rarely is electrical asystole responsible. The association between primary VF and "warning arrhythmias" (high-grade ventricular ectopy and R-on-T phenomena) is not strong, although ectopy as well as VF may reflect intermittent or severe ischemia with compromised ventricular performance exacerbating ischemia, thereby predisposing to VF. Use of routine prophylactic lidocaine appears to be associated with *increased* mortality, and pharmacologic suppression of ventricular ectopy per se does not necessarily increase survival. In fact, suppression with type IA or IC agents, β-blockers, calcium channel blockers, or type III agents (see Chapter 54) may increase the incidence of asystole in patients being treated with lidocaine by suppressing ventricular escape mechanisms in the event of sinus arrest or complete heart block.

In some instances, mortality may result from VF secondary to cardiac decompensation accompanying profound heart failure, hypotension, or shock (secondary VF). Accordingly, determinants of late mortality include "infarct size," measured enzymatically or by other means at the time of the index MI. Late mortality is also related to diminished left ventricular ejection fraction and elevated left ventricular end-systolic and end-diastolic volumes.

Late mortality is also a reflection, in part, of the likelihood of recurrent MI and the frequency and severity of episodic ischemia, both of which may reflect progression of underlying atherosclerotic coronary artery disease and thrombosis. Complex ventricular ectopy after hospital discharge correlates with subsequent mortality. Most late cardiac death is sudden, arrhythmic death.

THE STATUS OF THE INFARCT-RELATED ARTERY. Coronary thrombolysis and mechanical revascularization have revolutionized primary treatment of acute MI largely because they salvage myocardium when implemented early after the onset of ischemia. In addition, however, a more modest prognostic benefit of an open infarct-related artery may be evident even when recanalization can be induced only 6 hours or more after onset of symptoms, when salvaging substantial amounts of jeopardized ischemic myocardium is no longer likely. An open infarct-related artery may improve ventricular function, improve collateral blood flow, decrease infarct expansion, decrease ventricular aneurysm formation, improve ventricular remodeling, diminish left ventricular dilatation, decrease late arrhythmia associated with ventricular aneurysms, and decrease mortality. The lowest mortality is associated with prompt induction of or spontaneous restoration of flow in the infarct-related artery to near normal (Thrombolysis in Myocardial Infarction [TIMI] grade 3).

SIGNS AND SYMPTOMS

"Typical" Q-wave MI may be manifested by prodromal symptoms of fatigue, chest discomfort, or malaise in the days preceding the event, or it may occur suddenly, without warning. Onset of MI occurs more often in the early morning hours, perhaps in part because of the increased catecholamine-induced platelet aggregation and increased concentrations in blood of PAI-1 after awakening. Onset is generally not directly associated with severe exertion, but concomitant with exertion, the immediate risk of MI increases by six-fold on average and by as much as 30-fold in very sedentary people.

Typical pain is intense, severe, unremitting for 30 to 60 minutes, and retrosternal, often radiating down the ulnar aspect of the left arm and into the neck, to the left shoulder, jaw, or teeth. Occasionally the pain is epigastric. The pain is classically described as crushing or squeezing, but it also may be described as an ache, burning pain, indigestion, or a feeling of fullness or "gas." Diaphoresis, weakness, a sense of impending doom, profound restlessness, confusion, presyncope, hiccuping (presumably reflecting irritation of the phrenic nerve or diaphragm), nausea and vomiting, and palpitations may be present. Decreased systolic ventricular performance accounts for impaired perfusion of vital organs and reflex-mediated compensatory responses to hypotension, such as restlessness and impaired mentation, pallor, cutaneous vasoconstriction and sweating, tachycardia, and prerenal failure. Impaired left ventricular diastolic function leads to pulmonary vascular congestion with shortness of breath and tachypnea and may lead to pulmonary edema with orthopnea. Impaired right ventricular diastolic function leads to systemic venous hypertension, edema, hepatomegaly, and further compromise of left ventricular filling and cardiac output.

MI may be clinically silent (in as many as 25% of elderly patients, a population in whom 50% of MIs occur), with the diagnosis established only retrospectively by ECG criteria. The patient may recall only an episode of "indigestion" or nothing. Stoicism, an unusually high pain threshold, disorders such as diabetes mellitus that impair function of the nervous system, or obtundation caused by medications or impaired cerebral perfusion may prevent recognition of typical chest pain.

PHYSICAL FINDINGS TYPICAL OF ACUTE MI

Typical clinical findings can be summarized as follows:

GENERAL APPEARANCE. Pallor, diaphoresis, restlessness.

VITAL SIGNS. Heart rate is often increased secondary to sympathoadrenal discharge, ventricular ectopy, accelerated idioventricular rhythm, ventricular tachycardia, atrial fibrillation or flutter, or other supraventricular arrhythmias, the latter being rare unless atrial MI or heart failure is present. Bradyarrhythmias may be present and attributable to impaired sinus node function. AV nodal block or infranodal block may be evident. The blood pressure is generally elevated initially with arterial vasoconstriction, in contrast to the case of acute pulmonary embolism, in which initial hypotension is frequent. However, with right ventricular MI or severe left ventricular dysfunction, hypotension occurs. The respiratory rate may be increased in response to pulmonary congestion or anxiety. Coughing, wheezing, and production of frothy sputum may occur. Fever is usually present within 24 to 48 hours, with the temperature curve generally parallel to the time course of elevations of creatine kinase (CK) levels in blood. Fever may exceed 39° C.

FUNDUSCOPIC EXAMINATION. Manifestations of atherosclerotic vascular disease include copper wiring of arterioles. Antecedent long-standing hypertension may be reflected by arterial narrowing and hemorrhages. Conditions predisposing to atherosclerosis, such as diabetes with microaneurysms, may be evident. Funduscopic examination is particularly important to detect hemorrhage and neovascular proliferation, which require monitoring if fibrinolytic agents are used.

ARTERIAL AND VENOUS PULSES. Pulsus alternans, although rare, may reflect impaired left ventricular function, as may decreased amplitude and brevity of the carotid pulse secondary to decreased stroke volume. Jugular venous distention may accompany right ventricular MI or right ventricular failure secondary to profound left ventricular dysfunction and pulmonary hypertension.

CHEST. Rales or wheezes secondary to pulmonary venous hypertension are common with extensive left ventricular MI. Pleural effusions generally occur only with biventricular failure.

HEART. Lateral displacement of the apex impulse, dyskinesis, a palpable S_4 gallop, and a soft S_1 sound may indicate diminished contractility of the compromised left ventricle. Paradoxical splitting of S_2 may reflect left bundle branch block or prolongation of the pre-ejection period with delayed aortic valve closure despite decreased stroke volume. Accentuated S_4 and S_3 gallops may reflect increased left ventricular volume. A mitral regurgitation murmur indicative of either papillary muscle dysfunction or rupture or annulus dilatation may be audible even if cardiac output is diminished markedly. A systolic murmur and thrill indicative of ventricular septal rupture may be heard, and a pericardial friction rub may be evident. Premature ventricular beats, brief runs of ventricular tachycardia, or accelerated idioventricular rhythm are common.

ABDOMEN. Hepatojugular reflux may be elicited even when hepatomegaly is not marked.

EXTREMITIES. Peripheral cyanosis, edema, and pallor may indicate vasoconstriction, and diminished cardiac output may reflect right ventricular dysfunction or failure.

NEUROLOGIC FINDINGS. Patients with acute MI are prone to frank cerebrovascular insults as a result of ventricular mural thrombi and consequent embolization (with an incidence of approximately 1%). Recrudescence of signs or symptoms of a previously sustained cerebrovascular accident may occur secondary to diminished cerebral perfusion. Conversely, the incidence of MI in patients with cerebrovascular accidents is substantial.

The incidence of MI appears to be greater, and its prognosis worse, in patients with depression. MI may precipitate reactive depression whether or not β-adrenergic blocking agents or other central nervous system (CNS)-active agents are administered.

LABORATORY DETERMINATIONS

The objectives of laboratory testing include determination of the presence or absence of MI (diagnosis and differential diagnosis); characterization of the locus, nature (Q-wave or non–Q-wave), and extent of MI (estimation of infarct size); detection of recurrent ischemia or MI (extension of MI); detection of early and late complications of MI; and estimation of prognosis. Laboratory evaluation is particularly helpful in the presence of co-morbid conditions that may affect prognosis and influence care, such as diabetes, renal or hepatic failure, anemia, bleeding disorders, and respiratory failure.

The complete blood count and platelet count (which often decreases after heparin is given) are useful not only diagnostically but also in assessing suitability for treatment with thrombolytic drugs. The leukocyte count may be normal initially, but it generally increases within 2 hours and peaks in 2 to 4 days, with predominance of polymorphonuclear leukocytes and a shift to the left.

Elevations persist generally for 1 to 2 weeks. Other components of the acute-phase reaction contribute to elevations of the erythrocyte sedimentation rate (ESR) within 48 hours with subsequent changes that parallel those in the leukocyte count. Because of increased pulmonary pressure, and sometimes systemic venous pressure, contraction of plasma volume is common after acute MI and is manifested not only by hemoconcentration but also by prerenal failure with elevation of plasma creatinine and blood urea nitrogen levels. Arterial blood gases should be assayed if necessary to evaluate hypoxemia resulting from pulmonary congestion, atelectasis, or ventilatory impairment secondary to complications of MI or excessive sedation or analgesia. Fingertip oximetry may be adequate in the absence of CO_2 retention and can obviate the need for arterial puncture and bleeding in patients treated with thrombolytic drugs. However, normal oxygen saturation does not exclude impending respiratory failure. The chest radiograph is useful in determining the presence or absence of cardiomegaly, pulmonary edema, pleural effusions, Kerley B lines, and other criteria of heart failure. A small cardiac silhouette and clear lung fields in a patient with systemic hypotension may indicate relative or absolute hypovolemia. A large cardiac silhouette with similar hemodynamics may reflect hemopericardium and tamponade or right ventricular MI compromising cardiac output. Chest radiographic findings indicative of pulmonary venous hypertension may occur later and persist longer because of delay in fluid shifts among vascular, interstitial, and alveolar spaces.

ECG FINDINGS. Sequential ECG findings remain hallmarks of diagnosis despite the occasional occurrence of MI without any acute changes and the nonspecific nature of some of the ECG changes that may be seen (Fig. 60–1). The diagnosis can be established with certainty when typical ST elevation persists for hours and is followed by inversion of T waves within the first few days and development of Q waves subsequently. However, initial ST depression or T-wave inversion is difficult to differentiate from that seen with ischemia without MI or in unrelated conditions (Table 60–2). ST-segment depression followed by T-wave inversion without evolution of Q waves can result from non–Q-wave MI or subendocardial ischemia without MI. Q-wave MI cannot be differentiated from non–Q-wave MI initially if ST elevation is lacking and Q waves have not yet developed. True posterior wall MIs may present with precordial ST depression, inverted and hyperacute T waves, or both. ST elevation and upright hyperacute T waves may be evident with right-sided chest leads. Right ventricular MI com-

Table 60–2 ■ CONDITIONS ASSOCIATED WITH ECG CHANGES THAT MAY OBSCURE OR SIMULATE THOSE INDICATIVE OF ACUTE MI

ABNORMALITY	EXAMPLE
Intraventricular conduction abnormalities	Left bundle branch block, left anterior superior fascicular block, infranodal arborization block, right ventricular transvenous or epicardial pacing
Electrolyte disturbances	Hypokalemia or hyperkalemia, hypocalcemia
Pre-excitation	
Early repolarization	
Cerebrovascular accident	
Myocarditis	Inflammatory, infiltrative, viral, collagen vascular disorders, pheochromocytoma, cardiac allograft rejection, neuromuscular disorders such as muscular dystrophy and Friedreich's ataxia
Left ventricular hypertrophy	Hypertrophic cardiomyopathy, dilated cardiomyopathy, valvular heart disease, hypertension
Right ventricular hypertrophy	Cor pulmonale, acute pulmonary embolus, pneumothorax
Cardiac tumors	
Pericarditis	

ECG = electrocardiographic; MI = myocardial infarction.

monly is manifested by ST elevation or Q waves detectable in right-sided precordial leads. The appearance of abnormalities in a large number of ECG leads often indicates extensive injury or concomitant pericarditis. Anterior and anterolateral MIs tend to involve more left ventricular myocardium than inferior or true posterior MIs. Hyperacute (symmetrical and often, but not necessarily, pointed) T waves are frequently an early sign of MI at any locus.

MACROMOLECULAR MARKERS OF MI. Detection of elevated concentrations in plasma of macromolecules released from irreversibly injured myocardium has become the definitive diagnostic criterion of MI. The MB isoenzyme of CK, cardiac troponin I, and troponin T egress from irreversibly injured ischemic myocardium within several hours after the onset of the insult, and their elevated concentrations in plasma constitute sensitive diagnostic findings. These macromolecules are abundant in myocardium and are virtually absent from most other tissues. Characteristic sequential changes of plasma CK-MB include elevations above normal within 4 hours, a two- to ten-fold peak in 16 to 24 hours, and a return to

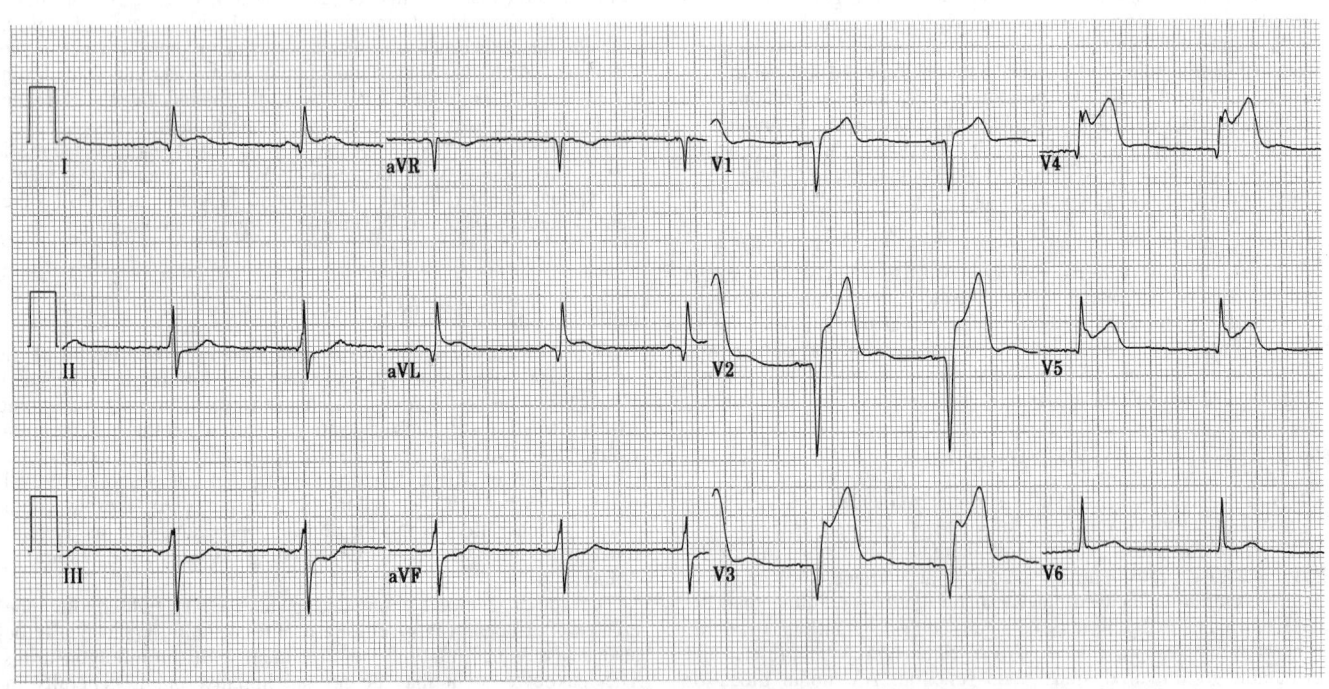

FIGURE 60–1 ■ ECG tracing showing an acute anterior-lateral MI. Note ST elevation in leads I, L, and V$_{1-6}$ with Q waves in V$_{1-4}$. (Courtesy of Dr. Thomas Evans.)

Table 60-3 ■ SERUM MARKERS OF ACUTE MYOCARDIAL INFARCTION

| | | CARDIAC TROPONINS | | | |
	MYOGLOBIN	cTnI	cTnT	CK-MB	MB-ISOFORMS
Molecular weight (kD)	17	23	33	86	86
First detectable (hr)	1–2		2–4	3–4	2–4
100% sensitivity (hr)	4–8		8–12	8–12	6–10
Peak (hr)	4–8		10–24	10–24	6–12
Duration (d)	(0.5–1.0)	5–10	5–14	2–4	0.5–1.0

cTnI = cardiac specific troponin I; cTnT = cardiac specific troponin T.

Adapted with permission from Adams J, Abendschein D, Jaffe A: Biochemical markers of myocardial injury: Is MB creatine kinase the choice for the 1990s? Circulation 88: 750–763, 1993.

baseline within 3 to 4 days (Table 60–3). The magnitude and persistence of elevations are useful in estimating the extent of MI. Analysis of subforms (isoforms) of individual isoenzymes of CK can provide accurate estimates of the time of onset of MI, the time of occurrence of recanalization, and, possibly, earlier detection of MI than can be obtained on the basis of isoenzyme or total CK analysis.

The cardiac-specific troponins T and I also rise within 4 to 6 hours after the onset of MI, and they peak within about 24 hours; however, they continue to be elevated for 10 to 14 days and hence are also useful for later diagnosis. Available data suggest that the troponins are only slightly more likely than CK-MB to be elevated at the time that the patient first presents to the emergency department. Elevated troponin levels, either assayed quantitatively in the regular laboratory or semiquantitatively with hand-held devices in the emergency department, can also help predict which patients with clinical unstable angina (see Chapter 59) will subsequently develop serious complications. False-positive CK-MB elevations are found with skeletal muscle inflammation or necrosis, with renal failure, and, rarely, with other conditions. False-positive troponin T but not troponin I elevations occur in patients with renal insufficiency. The ratio of LDH_1/LDH_2 isoenzymes remains elevated for several days after acute MI and is useful for late diagnosis, but it is now rarely assayed given the availability of troponin assays. Concentrations of other enzymes and proteins, such as total CK, aspartate serum transaminase (AST), myoglobin, and myosin light chains, rise in patients with acute MI but are rarely assessed because of their low specificities for acute MI.

IMAGING. The preferred non-invasive modality to evaluate regional wall motion and overall ventricular performance is usually color-flow Doppler transthoracic echocardiography. Both sensitivity and specificity of abnormal wall motion for acute MI exceed 90%, particularly in patients without previous MI. Assessment of segmental function and overall left ventricular performance provides prognostic information and is essential when MI is extensive, as judged by enzymatic criteria or complicated by shock or profound heart failure, in part to identify potentially surgically correctable complications and to detect ventricular true or false aneurysms or thrombi (see Fig. 43–3). In patients with ventricular thrombi, treatment entails administration of fibrinolytic drugs, anticoagulants, or both. Imaging is useful also to detect pericardial effusion, concomitant valvular or congenital heart disease, and marked depression of ventricular function that may interdict treatment in the acute phase with β-adrenergic blockers. Echocardiography is also helpful in delineating recovery of stunned or hibernating myocardium. Doppler echocardiography is particularly useful to estimate the severity of mitral or tricuspid regurgitation, detect ventricular septal defects secondary to rupture, assess diastolic function, monitor cardiac output calculated from flow velocity and aortic outflow tract area estimates, and estimate pulmonary artery systolic pressure. When right ventricular MI is suspected, or when left ventricular MI is superimposed on a previous insult or associated with ECG phenomena (such as left bundle branch block) that obscure diagnosis, assessment of right ventricular function and delineation of regional wall motion may be particularly helpful.

Positron-emission tomography with tracers of intermediary metabolism, perfusion, or oxidative metabolism permits quantitative assessment of the distribution and extent of impairment of myocardial oxidative metabolism and regional myocardial perfusion (see

Chapter 44). It can also define the efficacy of therapeutic interventions designed to salvage myocardium and has been used diagnostically to differentiate reversible from irreversible injury in hypoperfused zones.

DIFFERENTIAL DIAGNOSIS

The diagnosis is straightforward when the history of acute MI is typical, the initial ECG is abnormal and is followed by definitive sequential changes, and cardiac-specific macromolecule levels are elevated in the initial or subsequent plasma samples with typical sequential changes. A presumptive diagnosis can be made when any two of these criteria are present. Unfortunately, however, the diagnosis may be obscure in patients seen very early after the onset of MI and in those with ECG manifestations of previous ischemic or other types of heart disease, electrocardiographically silent infarcts, or atypical presentations. Without the aid of laboratory tests and cardiac imaging, differentiation from ischemia without MI (e.g., aortic stenosis in the elderly [see Chapter 63], ischemia attributable to right ventricular overload, new-onset or unstable angina, or inadequate myocardial perfusion in markedly hypertrophied left ventricles or in association with marked aortic insufficiency) and from pericarditis (see Chapter 65), accompanied by pain simulating that of MI, may be difficult (see Table 38–2). A critical differential diagnostic consideration is aortic dissection (see Chapter 66), which should be suspected whenever pain is severe yet atypical, radiates to the back, is accompanied by pulse or blood pressure inequalities in the arms or legs, or is not associated with ECG changes typical of MI.

Pleurodynia, pulmonary embolism or infarction (see Chapter 84), pneumothorax (see Chapter 86), pneumonitis, musculoskeletal pain associated with bursitis, the shoulder-hand syndrome, pectoral lymphadenopathy, herpes zoster before eruption of the typical vesicles, myalgia, and costochondritis may simulate MI superficially, but these can usually be differentiated easily on the basis of physical findings, results of laboratory tests, and chest radiography (see Table 38–2). Pain originating in the abdomen from cholecystitis or cholelithiasis, pancreatitis, hepatitis, duodenal or gastric ulcer, gastritis, esophagitis, esophageal spasm, or esophageal reflux associated with a hiatal hernia may masquerade as MI, but the correct diagnosis can be made by careful evaluation and sequential testing to exclude MI and confirm alternative causes of symptoms.

In the initial evaluation, definitive diagnosis often cannot be made immediately, and it is less important than appropriate assessment (Fig. 60–2), interim management, and rapid triage (Table 60–4). For patients with a clinical history suggestive of acute MI and an ST segment elevation of 1 mm or more in two or more leads, consistent with acute MI and not known to be long-standing, the presumptive diagnosis is acute MI; urgent coronary recanalization should be attempted with the use of thrombolytic agents, primary angioplasty, or a combination of the two (Fig. 60–3). Other patients present with strong evidence of an acute ischemic event that may prove to be a non-Q-wave MI, unstable angina, or even the beginning of a Q-wave MI; they commonly have ST-segment and T-wave changes consistent with ischemia, a clinical syndrome consistent with unstable angina (see Chapter 59), or both. Urgent treatment should be begun for non–Q-wave MI and unstable angina (Fig. 60–4), and the patient should be moved expeditiously to a coronary intensive care unit, monitored step-down or intermediate

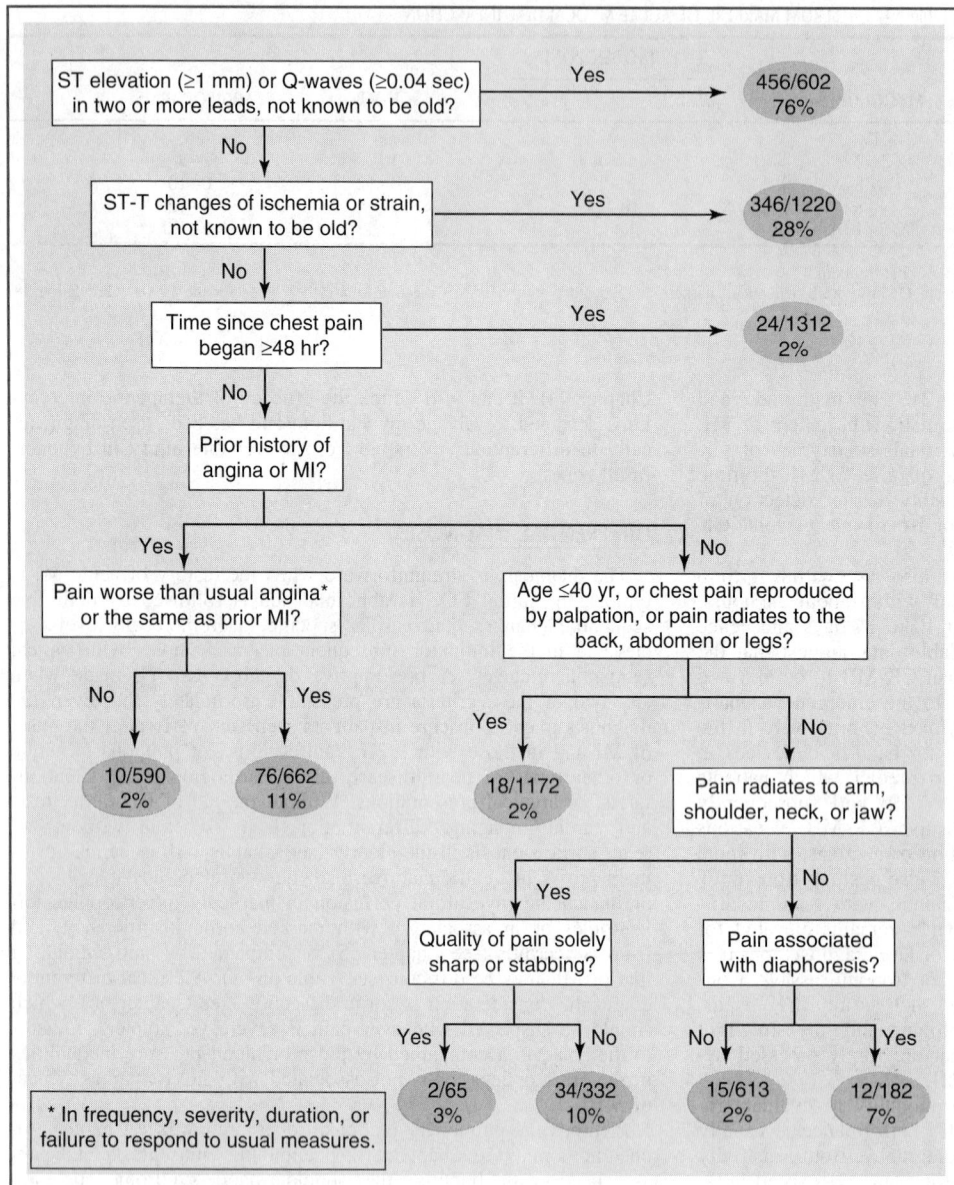

FIGURE 60–2 ■ Flow diagram for estimating the risk of acute MI in emergency settings in patients with acute chest pain. For each clinical subset, the numerator is the number of patients with the set of presenting characteristics who developed an MI, whereas the denominator represents the total number of patients presenting with that characteristic or set of characteristics. (Adapted from Pearson SD, Goldman L, Garcia TB, et al: Physician response to a prediction rule for the triage of emergency department patients with chest pain. J Gen Intern Med 9:241–247, 1994. Reprinted by permission of Blackwell Science, Inc.)

care unit, or the catheterization laboratory. Initial evaluation and management of patients with some characteristics suggestive of MI or unstable ischemic heart disease, but without a convincing clinical story or ECG findings, is more difficult. Such patients have been shown in several large studies to have a 1 to 5% probability of acute MI and a low risk of developing complications that require intensive care. They can be monitored in intermediate care or step-down units or, as is now commonly practiced, be observed for 6 to 12 hours in an emergency department or chest pain evaluation/observation unit that provides continuous ECG monitoring and resuscitative facilities, but not intensive nursing coverage. In such units, sequential testing with blood sampling for cardiac enzyme determinations (see above) and ECGs are performed every 3 to 4 hours for 6 to 12 hours. If patients do not show evidence of myocardial necrosis, recurrent ischemia, hemodynamic abnormalities, or arrhythmias, they are suitable for risk stratification with exercise stress testing or stress echocardiography or scintigraphy before being discharged (see below). Very low-risk patients can be discharged without further observation or evaluation if the clinical presentation is sufficiently atypical, the ECG is normal, and alternative explanations for the chest discomfort are obvious.

Intensive care is generally indicated for patients with ischemic ECG changes in two or more leads (ST-segment elevation, ST-segment depression, or T-wave inversion consistent with MI or ischemia) and for patients without such changes if they have two or more of the following: known coronary disease with pain that is unstable in terms of frequency, duration, intensity, or failure to respond to usual measures; hypotension (defined as systolic blood pressure below 110 mm Hg); major new atrial tachyarrhythmias, ventricular tachyarrhythmias, or heart block; or rales above the bases, which are indicative of substantial heart failure. Patients without any ischemic ECG changes but with any one of these manifestations or with new onset of chest pain consistent with unstable angina are appropriate candidates for intermediate or step-down care. An evaluation/observation unit alternative is an appropriate option for patients with known coronary disease whose presentation is not highly suggestive of unstable angina and for patients with new-onset symptoms suggestive of acute ischemic heart disease but without ischemic ECG changes, a convincing diagnosis of new-onset unstable angina, or the hemodynamic or arrhythmic criteria noted above.

CARE OF THE PATIENT

The focus of treatment differs in the prehospital, hospital (coronary care unit and step-down unit), and convalescent phases despite considerable overlap of objectives in each.

INTENSIVE CARE

1. Major ischemic electrocardiographic (ECG) changes in ≥2 leads, not known to be old:
   a. ST elevation of 1 mm or more or Q-waves of 0.04 sec or more
      or
   b. ST depression of 1 mm or more or T-wave inversion consistent with ischemia
      or
2. Any two of the following, with or without major ECG changes:
   a. Unstable known coronary disease (in terms of frequency, duration, intensity, or failure to respond to usual measures)
   b. Systolic blood pressure below 110 mm Hg
   c. Major new arrhythmias (new-onset atrial fibrillation, atrial flutter, sustained supraventricular tachycardia, second-degree or complete heart block, or sustained or recurrent ventricular arrythmias)
   d. Rales above the bases

INTERMEDIATE CARE/STEPDOWN UNIT

Patients who do not meet criteria for intensive care but who either:
1. Have one unstable characteristic:
   a. Unstable known coronary disease
   b. Systolic blood pressure below 110 mm Hg
   c. Rales above the bases
   d. Major arrhythmias (new-onset atrial fibrillation, atrial flutter, sustained supraventricular tachycardia, second-degree or complete heart block, or sustained or recurrent ventricular arrhythmias)
2. A patient with new onset of very typical ischemic heart disease that meets the clinical criteria for unstable angina and that is occurring now at rest or with minimal exertion

EVALUATION/OBSERVATION UNIT

1. Other patients with new-onset symptoms that may be consistent with ischemic heart disease but that are not associated with ECG changes or a convincing diagnosis of unstable ischemic heart disease at rest or with minimal exertion
2. Some patients with known coronary disease whose presentation does not suggest a true worsening but for whom further observation is thought to be beneficial

HOME WITH OFFICE FOLLOW-UP IN 7–10 DAYS TO DETERMINE WHETHER FURTHER TESTING IS NEEDED

Other patients

*Except in patients in whom other serious noncoronary causes of chest pain are being considered, such as possible aortic dissection or pulmonary embolism, where the triage will be dictated by the appropriate evaluation for these other possible diagnoses.

Treatment in the Prehospital Phase

Most death caused by MI occurs early and is attributable to primary ventricular fibrillation (VF). Thus, initial objectives are immediate ECG monitoring, reversal of VF should it occur, and rapid transfer to facilitate prompt coronary recanalization. Community-based systems in Belfast, Ireland; Columbus, Ohio; Los Angeles; and Seattle have documented conclusively the effectiveness of rapid response by rescuers (e.g., police and firefighters) trained in defibrillation. Approximately 65% of deaths caused by MI occur in the first hour. More than 60% (39% of those in patients who would otherwise succumb) can be prevented by defibrillation initiated by a bystander or a first-responding rescuer. Additional objectives of prehospital care by paramedical and emergency personnel include adequate analgesia (generally with morphine), reduction of excessive sympathoadrenal and vagal stimulation pharmacologically, treatment of hemodynamically significant or symptomatic ventricular arrhythmias (generally with lidocaine), and support of cardiac output, systemic blood pressure, and respiration.

Prehospital administration of tissue-type plasminogen activator (t-PA), aspirin, and heparin to patients with bona fide MI by paramedics, guided by ECG findings within 90 minutes of the onset of symptoms, improves outcome compared with thrombolysis begun after hospital arrival. It is indicated for patients in whom thrombolysis will be the preferred approach to coronary reperfusion.

Atropine (0.5 mg, IV, given at 5-minute intervals to a maximum of 2 to 4 mg) is particularly useful to counteract excessive vagal tone that often underlies bradyarrhythmias and hypotension. It is indicated when heart rate is disproportionately diminished with respect to blood pressure, when hypotension (sometimes secondary to morphine administration) is refractory despite augmentation of left ventricular filling pressure, or when impaired AV nodal conduction accompanied by Wenckebach block is evident. If bradycardia persists, transthoracic pacing may be life-saving.

Emergency Department Treatment

Emergency department treatment begins with a focused cardiovascular history and physical examination, establishment of intravenous access, performance of a 12-lead ECG, and continuous rhythm monitoring. All patients with suspected MI should be given 160 to 325 mg of aspirin to chew unless a documented aspirin allergy is present. Baseline cardiac enzyme levels should be obtained. Initial stabilization in patients with suspected MI and ongoing acute chest pain should include sublingual nitroglycerine, which may be repeated for two additional doses at 5-minute intervals if pain persists in patients who do not have contraindications such as hypotension (systolic blood pressure less than 90 mm Hg), bradycardia, tachycardia, or findings suggestive of right ventricular infarction (see above).

Refractory or severe pain should be treated symptomatically with intravenous morphine, meperidine, or pentazocine. Repeated intravenous doses of 4 to 8 mg of morphine at intervals of 5 to 15 minutes can be given with relative impunity until the pain is relieved or toxicity is manifested by hypotension, vomiting, or depressed respiration. Should toxicity occur, a morphine antagonist such as naloxone can reverse it.

Blood pressure and pulse must be monitored in an attempt to keep the systolic blood pressure above 100 mm Hg and, optimally, below 140 mm Hg. Relative hypotension may be treated with elevation of the lower extremities or administration of fluids, except in patients with concomitant pulmonary congestion, in whom treatment for cardiogenic shock may be required (see Chapter 95). Atropine, in doses similar to those given in the prehospital phase, may increase blood pressure if hypotension reflects bradycardia or excess vagal tone.

Oxygen should be given to avoid hypoxemia. High concentrations may be counterproductive because of vasoconstriction and lack of augmented myocardial oxygen delivery in normoxemic patients. Patients requiring mechanical ventilation require special measures (see Chapter 93).

Triage decisions are guided by assignment of patients to subsets. For patients with probable MI who are appropriate candidates for reperfusion because of 1 mm or more of new ST elevation in two or more leads, or presumably new bundle branch block in the setting of a typical clinical syndrome, plans should be made for prompt treatment to induce recanalization even while the patient is in the emergency department. Alternatives include intravenous thrombolysis (started immediately in the emergency department) or immediate transfer to the cardiac catheterization laboratory for primary percutaneous transluminal coronary angioplasty (PTCA) (see below). For patients whose clinical presentations and ECGs strongly suggest ischemia, especially those with ECG ST-segment depression or T-wave inversion, thrombolysis is not recommended, but transfer to either a coronary care unit (CCU) or an intermediate care/step-down unit should be preceded by institution of anti-ischemic therapy (see below) for suspected non–Q-wave infarction or unstable angina. Lower-risk patients without obvious ischemia should be observed and monitored in either a step-down/intermediate care unit or a chest pain evaluation/observation unit (see above).

Treatment in the Hospital Phase

CCUs have reduced early mortality from acute MI by approximately 50%, initially by providing immediate defibrillation and more recently by facilitating implementation of beneficial interventions. The latter include administration of intravenous medications and therapy designed to limit the extent of MI, salvage jeopardized ischemic myocardium, and recanalize infarct-related arteries, as well as diagnosis and treatment of other conditions.

CORONARY RECANALIZATION. Alternatives for coronary recanalization include intravenous thrombolytic agents or catheter-based approaches. Thrombolysis can be accomplished with a variety of intravenous medications and regimens (see Chapter 188), with or without the use of adjunctive therapies. Catheter-based recanalization with PTCA, with or without stenting, can induce

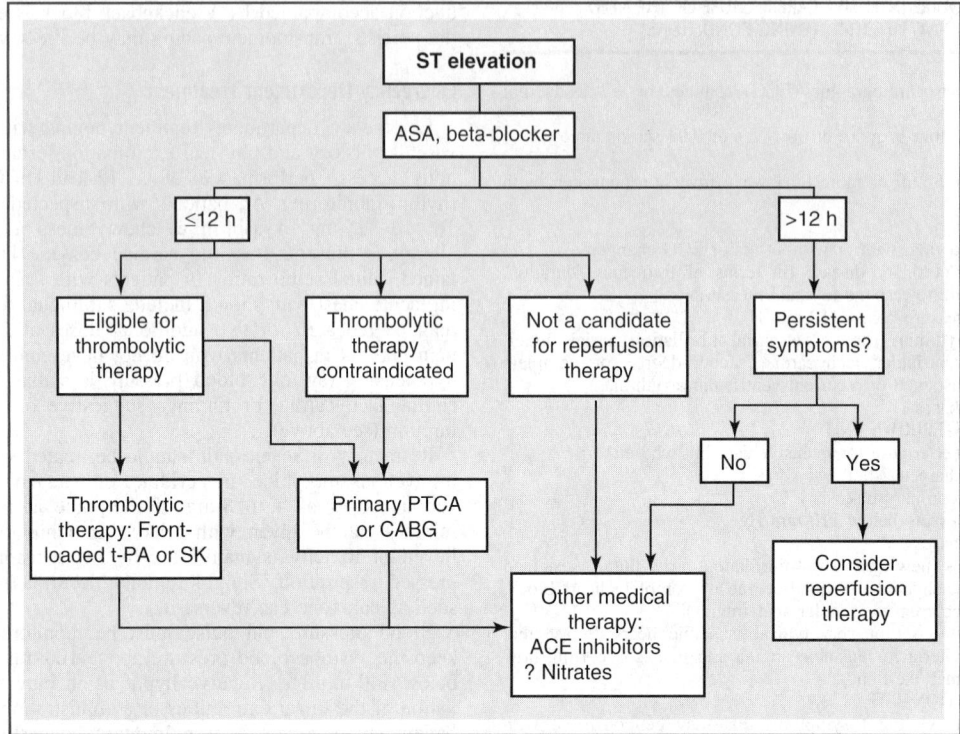

FIGURE 60–3 ▪ Recommendations for management of patients with ST elevation. All patients with ST-segment elevation on the ECG should receive aspirin (ASA), β-adrenergic blockers (in the absence of contraindications), and an antithrombin (particularly if tissue-type plasminogen activator [t-PA] is used for thrombolytic therapy). Whether heparin is required in patients receiving streptokinase (SK) remains a matter of controversy; the small additional risk for intracranial hemorrhage may not be offset by the survival benefit afforded by adding heparin to SK therapy. Patients treated within 12 hours who are eligible for thrombolytics should expeditiously receive either frontloaded t-PA or an alternative such as reteplase, Eminase, or SK or be considered for primary percutaneous transluminal coronary angioplasty (PTCA). Primary PTCA is also to be considered when thrombolytic therapy is absolutely contraindicated. Coronary artery bypass graft (CABG) may be considered if the patient is seen in less than 6 hours from the onset of symptoms. Individuals treated after 12 hours should receive the initial medical therapy noted above and, on an individual basis, may be candidates for reperfusion therapy or angiotensin-converting enzyme (ACE) inhibitors (particularly if left ventricular function is impaired). (Modified from Antman EM: Medical therapy for acute coronary syndromes: An overview. *In* Califf RM [ed]: Atlas of Heart Diseases, VIII. Philadelphia, Current Medicine, 1996.)

patency in more infarct-related arteries (about 90% compared with about 50 to 80% for pharmacologic thrombolysis) with less residual stenosis, less recurrent ischemia, lower risks of reocclusion, and less need for later mechanical revascularization (see Chapter 61). Catheter-based approaches also avoid the risk of bleeding, including intracerebral bleeding, seen with thrombolytic medications. Patients who are treated with primary PTCA generally have shorter lengths of stay and consume fewer medical resources than patients treated with IV thrombolysis. Several randomized trials have demonstrated that rapidly available primary PTCA performed by skilled operators for acute MI is associated with long-term outcomes similar to those achieved with the use of IV thrombolytic medications, although this comparison remains a topic of active investigation. Disadvantages of primary PTCA include the fact that the procedure is highly dependent on the skill of the operator and that immediate access to highly skilled operators is necessary.

Data from non-randomized studies suggest an advantage for primary PTCA in patients with acute MI complicated by cardiogenic shock. It is clearly the treatment of choice in patients with contraindications to thrombolytic agents (see below). It is currently unclear whether certain subsets of patients do better with PTCA or thrombolysis. For example, in patients with type II diabetes, elective PTCA is inferior to coronary artery bypass surgery, and it may be the case that similar or other characteristics will ultimately guide the choice among reperfusion therapies in acute MI.

The first generation of fibrinolytic drugs (see Chapter 188), typified by streptokinase, urokinase, acetylated plasminogen streptokinase activator complexes (APSAC), reteplase, and nPA, induce activation of circulating plasminogen and clot-associated plasminogen indiscriminately. First-generation drugs invariably elicit a systemic lytic state characterized by depletion of circulating fibrinogen, plasminogen, and hemostatic proteins, and by marked elevation of concentrations of fibrinogen degradation products in plasma.

Second-generation drugs, typified by t-PA and single-chain urokinase plasminogen activator and including recently developed agents such as TNK, activate plasminogen in the fibrin domain preferentially compared with free plasminogen in the circulation. Thus, they exhibit clot selectivity. In optimal regimens, they induce clot lysis without inducing a systemic lytic state, are less prone to predispose to hemorrhage that requires transfusion compared with non–clot-selective agents, and are effective in inducing recanalization in 80 to 90% of infarct-related arteries within 90 minutes. Thus, in contrast to intravenous streptokinase, which is effective in recanalizing approximately 50% of infarct-related arteries, 75 to 80% are recanalized with t-PA.

Coronary thrombolysis with intravenously administered activators of plasminogen improves ventricular function and decreases mortality, especially early after MI, particularly when initiated within a few hours after the onset of ischemia. Even when initiated later, up to 6 hours or more after the onset of MI, restoration of patency of the infarct-related artery may confer an early mortality benefit, perhaps reflecting improved collateral blood flow, improved ventricular remodeling and function, decreased infarct expansion, decreased arrhythmogenicity, decreased ventricular aneurysm formation, and decreased late arrhythmia associated with those aneurysms that do develop.

The properties of second generation agents translate into clinical benefits. For example, in the GUSTO trial, significant improvements in 24-hour mortality, 30-day mortality, 1-year mortality, and survival without a disabling stroke were evident (Table 60–5).

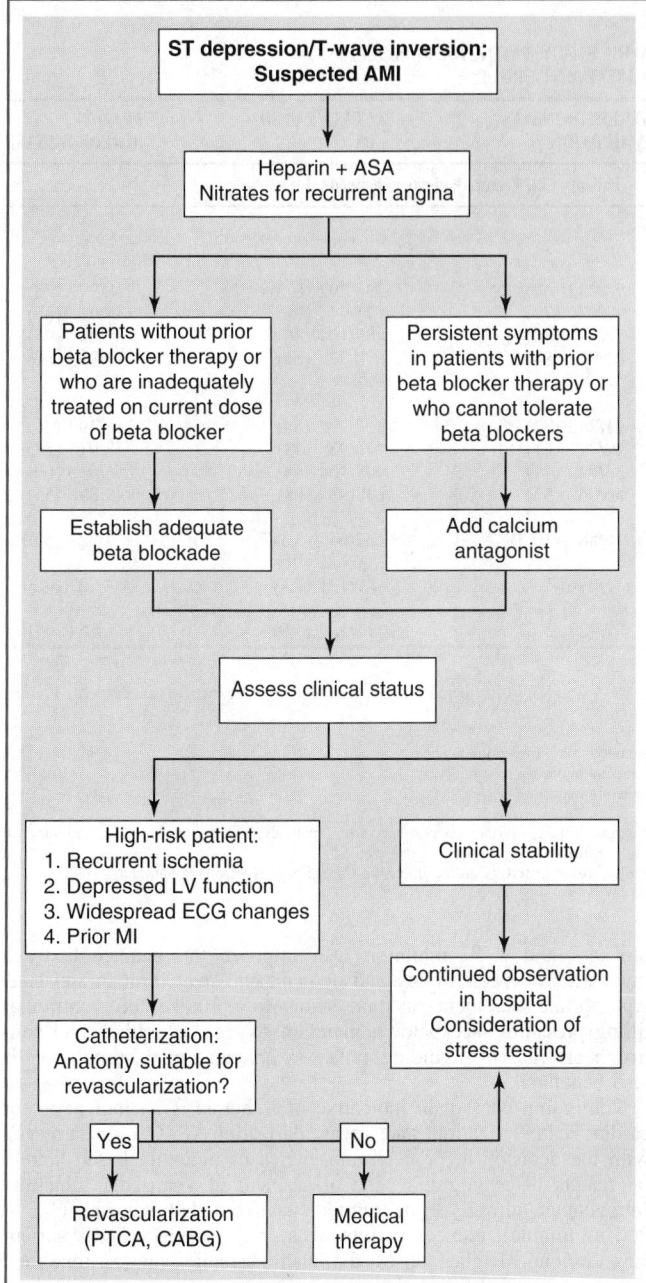

FIGURE 60-4 ■ Recommendations for management of patients with acute myocardial infarction (MI) without ST elevation. All patients without ST elevation should be treated with an antithrombin and aspirin (ASA). Nitrates should be administered for recurrent episodes of angina. Adequate β-adrenergic blockade should then be established; when this is not possible or contraindications exist, a calcium antagonist can be considered. High-risk patients should be triaged to cardiac catheterization with plans for revascularization if they are clinically suitable; patients who are clinically stable can be treated more conservatively, with continued observation in the hospital and consideration of a stress test to screen for myocardial ischemia. LV = left ventricular; ECG = electrocardiographic; PTCA = percutaneous transluminal coronary angioplasty; CABG = coronary artery bypass graft. (Modified from Antman EM: Medical therapy for acute coronary syndromes: An overview. In Califf RM [ed]: Atlas of Heart Diseases, VIII. Philadelphia, Current Medicine, 1996.

The risks of coronary thrombolysis include bleeding, much of which is confined to sites of vascular access. Marked depletion of fibrinogen or prolongation of the bleeding time may be markers of pharmacologic effects that lead to bleeding. With thrombolysis, the incidence of hemorrhagic stroke is increased, but the risk of thrombotic or embolic stroke is somewhat reduced, and overall any small increase in fatal cerebrovascular accidents is more than offset by the favorable impact on survival.

Plasminogen activators should not be given to patients with active internal bleeding or a bleeding diathesis, suspected aortic dissection, recent trauma, intracranial neoplasm, or hypertensive crisis. Relative contraindications include prolonged or traumatic cardiopulmonary resuscitation, peptic ulcer disease, remote cerebrovascular accident, and hepatic failure. Safety has not been established for pregnant women, although it has been for menstruating women. In general, use of thrombolytic agents has been well demonstrated to be effective in patients 75 years or younger who present with suspected Q-wave MI within 6 hours after the onset of symptoms, and in whom contraindications are not present. Although the absolute risk of complications is greater in the elderly, overall mortality reduction is at least as great in this group, because the prognosis with MI managed conservatively is also worse than that for younger patients. Treatment may be helpful in some patients first seen 6 to 12 hours after the onset of symptoms, particularly those with stuttering infarcts. It has not been demonstrated to be effective in patients with non–Q-wave MI or unstable angina.

Clinical efficacy of coronary thrombolysis depends on the frequency, rapidity, and persistence of recanalization, all of which depend not only on the intensity of fibrinolysis, but also on the inhibition of coagulation and platelet-induced thrombosis, which undoubtedly occur concomitantly. Presently, intravenous heparin is the agent of choice, coupled with orally administered aspirin. Alternatives include low-molecular-weight heparin, other inhibitors of coagulation (such as hirudin), and antagonists of binding of fibrinogen to the platelet surface glycoprotein IIb/IIIa receptor (such as abciximab, eptifibatide, tirofiban, and orbofiban). These and similar agents are undergoing intense evaluation for assessment of their potential utility alone or in various combinations with fibrinolytic agents. They are particularly promising because platelet activation results in profound augmentation of thrombin generation. Even optimally effective coronary thrombolysis is compromised by early thrombotic reocclusion in 6 to 20% of patients with initial recanalization unless vigorous conjunctive anticoagulation is initiated immediately.

Treatment may require use of thrombolytic medications and mechanical revascularization. For example, use of low-dose IV t-PA combined with early PTCA appears to be superior to PTCA alone. Emergency coronary artery bypass grafting (CABG) may be needed in patients who fail to respond to PTCA with stenting, and it is feasible soon after the administration of intravenous thrombolytic agents if necessary. Despite a high perioperative mortality rate for CABG within 24 hours of failed pharmacologic thrombolysis or PTCA, subsequent 1-year mortality among survivors may be as low as 2% and no different from that in those who have survived CABG implemented later after MI. Because this higher early mortality rate may reflect higher severity, CABG appears to be a worthwhile option in patients who fail other efforts to establish reperfusion and who experience ongoing major complications.

Contrary to initial expectations, not all patients treated with thrombolytic drugs should be subjected to obligatory early cardiac catheterization and angioplasty. A strategy comprising arteriography and angioplasty in only those patients who exhibit recurrent or persistent symptoms and signs of ischemia appears to be safer (Table 60–6) and as effective as obligatory angiography for all patients in preserving ventricular function and reducing mortality. Rescue PTCA (i.e., PTCA performed when occlusion has proven to be refractory to coronary recanalization with fibrinolytic drugs), is indicated for patients with left anterior descending coronary artery lesions or cardiogenic shock.

OTHER PREVENTIVE THERAPY IN THE ACUTE HOSPITAL PHASE. β-Adrenergic blockers are of benefit when begun intravenously within 4 hours of the onset of pain and continued long-term. Mortality, sudden death, and infarct size are reduced in patients with Q-wave MI. Patients with unstable angina may benefit similarly and have a reduced incidence of MI. Contraindications include hypotension, bradycardia, heart failure that is severe or worsens with the medications, second- or third-degree AV block or marked first-degree AV block, and a history of reactive airways disease. Patients with insulin-dependent diabetes mellitus and peripheral vascular disease can be treated with caution. Among the many available regimens, two commonly used approaches are IV atenolol, 5 to 10 mg followed by 50 to 100 mg/day, or metoprolol,

Table 60–5 ■ RESULTS OF THE GUSTO-1 ANGIOGRAPHIC STUDY: PATENCY AND REOCCLUSION
OF THE INFARCT-RELATED ARTERY, ACCORDING TO TREATMENT GROUP*

VARIABLE	STREPTOKINASE + SC HEPARIN	STREPTOKINASE + IV HEPARIN	ACCELERATED t-PA	t-PA + STREPTOKINASE
	Patients with Feature/Patients Examined (%)			
Patency				
Open vessels, TIMI grades 2 and 3 combined				
At 90 min	159/293 (54)	170/283 (60)	236/292 (81)†‡	218/299 (73)‡
At 180 min	77/106 (73)	72/97 (74)	71/93 (76)	77/91 (85)
At 24 hr	64/83 (77)	74/92 (80)	89/104 (86)	87/93 (94)§
At 5–7 days	67/93 (72)	81/96 (84)	70/83 (84)¶	71/89 (80)
Complete reperfusion, TIMI grade 3				
At 90 min	85/293 (29)	91/283 (32)	157/292 (54)‡ǁ	114/299 (38)
At 180 min	37/106 (35)	40/97 (41)	40/93 (43)	48/91 (53)
At 24 hr	42/83 (51)	38/92 (41)	47/104 (45)	56/93 (60)
At 5–7 days	47/93 (51)	56/96 (58)	48/83 (58)	49/89 (55)
Reocclusion				
From TIMI grade 2 at 90 min to grade 0 or 1 at follow-up	3/56 (5.4)	6/58 (10.3)	2/64 (3.1)	4/72 (5.6)
From TIMI grade 3 at 90 min to grade 0 or 1 at follow-up	4/54 (7.4)	1/69 (1.4)	9/121 (7.4)	4/92 (4.3)
Overall reocclusion	7/110 (6.4)	7/127 (5.5)	11/185 (5.9)	8/164 (4.9)

SC = subcutaneous; IV = intravenous; t-PA = tissue plasminogen activator.
*Overall patency rates (TIMI 2 and 3 flow) at 90 min and complete reperfusion rates (TIMI 3 flow only) at 90 min are superior with the regimen of accelerated t-PA and intravenous heparin with similar reocclusion rates in all four groups.
†$P = 0.032$ for the comparison of this group with the group given t-PA with streptokinase.
‡$P < 0.001$ for the comparison of this group with the groups given streptokinase with subcutaneous or intravenous heparin.
§$P < 0.001$ for the comparison of this group with the group given streptokinase with subcutaneous heparin.
¶$P = 0.032$ for the comparison of this group with the group given streptokinase with subcutaneous heparin.
ǁ$P < 0.001$ for the comparison of this group with the group given t-PA with streptokinase.
From the GUSTO Angiographic Investigators: The effects of tissue plasminogen activator, streptokinase, or both on coronary-artery patency, ventricular function, and survival after acute myocardial infarction. N Engl J Med 329:1618, 1993. Copyright 1993, Massachusetts Medical Society. All rights reserved.
From Battle RW, Sobel BE: Coronary thrombolysis for treatment of acute myocardial infarction. Brown D (ed): Cardiac Intensive Care. Philadelphia, WB Saunders, 1998.

5 mg, IV, repeated for a total of three doses followed by 50 to 100 mg/day given orally.

Angiotensin-converting enzyme (ACE) inhibitors are useful for long-term therapy (see below) and also appear to benefit patients who have no evidence of hypotension if administration is begun within the first 24 hours after onset of MI. Alternatives include captopril, 12.5 to 50 mg given orally twice a day, enalapril, 5 to 40 mg given orally daily or twice a day, or any one of newer agents, including lisinopril, quinapril, or ramipril, in pharmacologically equivalent doses. Calcium channel blockers have not been shown to be beneficial in acute MI, and because they may exert deleterious side effects alone or when given with other medications, they should generally be avoided. Treatment with both β-adrenergic

Table 60–6 ■ OUTCOME AFTER INVASIVE VERSUS CONSERVATIVE MANAGEMENT*

EVENT	MANAGEMENT STRATEGY AFTER THROMBOLYSIS		
	Invasive (%)	Conservative (%)	P Value
Death	5.2	4.7	0.49
Death or reinfarction	10.9	9.7	0.25
Coronary artery bypass grafting	11.9	10.5	0.18
Intracranial hemorrhage	0.9	0.7	0.70
Any adverse endpoint†	13.0	10.6	0.04

*The percentages of adverse clinical events during the initial 42 days of follow-up are shown in these results from a study of 3262 patients with Q-wave infarction randomized to treatment with (invasive strategy) or without (conservative strategy) obligatory angiography and angioplasty early after acute myocardial infarction treated initially with tissue-type plasminogen activator (t-PA). The invasive strategy was not superior.
†Death, nonfatal reinfarction, intracranial hemorrhage, or coronary bypass grafting after angioplasty.
Adapted from The TIMI Group; Comparison of invasive and conservative strategies after treatment with intravenous tissue plasminogen activator in acute myocardial infarction: Results of the thrombolysis in myocardial infarction (TIMI) phase II trial. N Engl J Med 320:618, 1989. Inclusion and exclusion criteria are delineated in the referenced article.

blockers and ACE inhibitors can improve the balance between myocardial oxygen supply and demand and may limit infarct size. Appropriate treatment of fluid status to optimize left ventricular filling pressures (see below), maintain oxygen saturation, and control heart rate by avoiding reflex sympathoadrenal stimulation is also beneficial.

Continuing chest pain indicative of ischemia is an indication for cardiac catheterization and revascularization (PTCA or surgery), with the decision to proceed and choice of modality based largely on results of angiography and assessment of ventricular function. Intravenous nitroglycerin, titrated to avoid hypotension (10 to 200 μg/minute), reduces peripheral arterial resistance and ventricular afterload. Higher doses diminish systemic venous tone and blood pressure, thereby potentially (paradoxically) exacerbating ischemia. Favorable effects are probably mediated by diminished afterload and preload and decreased LVEDP, facilitating myocardial perfusion. Tolerance to continuously administered intravenous nitrates occurs rapidly, often within hours.

GENERAL CARE IN THE CCU. General measures commonly include use of stool softeners to avoid constipation, straining, and consequent circulatory derangements. Prophylaxis (oral sucralfate, 1 g given twice a day), or an H_2-antagonist (famotidine, ranitidine, or cimetidine, given orally or IV at 6- to 12-hour intervals) for stress ulcers is appropriate for patients at high risk, including those with sepsis, hypotension or shock, bleeding diathesis, a requirement for prolonged mechanical intervention, or elevated intracranial pressure. Antipyretics (e.g., acetaminophen) should be used to prevent or suppress the fever that is typically seen in the first 24 to 48 hours and its consequent tachycardia. Patients with uncomplicated MI need be confined to bed for only 1 day. Physical activity should be limited (bed-chair regimen) throughout the CCU stay, with gradual and carefully monitored resumption of ambulatory activity in the late hospital phase. Educational programs targeting smoking cessation, lipid lowering, and treatment of hypertension as indicated, in addition to phased rehabilitation programs, should be initiated early during the hospital course for patients with uncomplicated MI. Sedative, anxiolytic, and hypnotic drugs at night may be helpful, but these cannot replace optimal communication by compassionate physicians and nurses and the reassurance it provides.

Prophylaxis and Treatment of Arrhythmia

Continuous ECG monitoring is essential for 48 to 72 hours after the onset of MI, and optimally throughout hospitalization by telemetry to detect VF and numerous arrhythmias that may occur. Some patients develop VF because of augmentation of myocardial oxygen requirements, impaired ventricular performance with consequent exacerbation of ischemia, or both.

Both primary and secondary (to hemodynamic decompensation, hypoxemia, electrolyte disturbances, or progressive cardiac or pulmonary failure) VF should be treated by immediate electrical countershock (see Chapter 53). Fibrillation may be confused with electrical asystole when the vector of VF is perpendicular to the axis of the recording lead used for monitoring. True asystole requires confirmation with multiple leads and differentiation from fine VF. If the distinction between VF and asystole cannot be made with certainty, VF should be assumed to be present. Other established components of cardiopulmonary resuscitation and advanced cardiac life support are invaluable, but the primacy of immediately restoring effective cardiac rhythm cannot be overemphasized. Electrical countershock should be implemented immediately, rather than deferred until after implementation of endotracheal intubation and other emergency measures. If true electrical asystole is documented, immediate external, transvenous, or transthoracic cardiac pacing is essential, although prognosis in this situation is grim.

After successful resuscitation from VF, lidocaine should be administered by continuous infusion (20 to 50 μg/kg of body weight per minute), particularly in the presence of frequent, closely coupled, multiform, or repetitive ventricular premature complexes or ventricular tachycardia. Blood levels should be maintained in the range of 2 to 5 μg/mL. Recurrent VF that is refractory to lidocaine may be suppressed after a considerable lag period by IV bretylium, given in 5- to 10-mg/kg doses, or by amiodarone, given as a 0.75 μg/kg loading dose followed by infusion of 5 to 10 μg/kg/ minute or 150 mg over 10 minutes, followed by 60 mg/hour for 6 hours and 30 mg/hour for 18 hours, to 48 to 72 hours, total duration of infusion, with concomitant initiation of treatment with oral amiodarone. Other promising antifibrillatory drugs are currently being investigated in the United States.

Prophylactic lidocaine administration is not indicated when the patient is in a setting in which defibrillation can be implemented immediately and pharmacologic treatment can be initiated promptly, because its adverse effects (CNS depression; seizures; proarrhythmic, asystolic, and cardiodepressant effects) may offset potential benefit. However, repeated bolus injections of 0.5 to 1.0 mg/kg of body weight, given every 5 minutes to a total of 4 mg/kg, followed by maintenance infusions of 1 to 2 mg/minute, are used in selected situations in which non-sustained (VT) or other high-grade ventricular arrhythmias cause hemodynamic compromise or cannot be controlled by other means in the first few hours after the onset of MI, when the risk of primary VF is greatest. Assessment and treatment should focus on electrolyte and pH derangements and their correction. β-Blockers and magnesium sulfate may be useful.

VF or VT in the first 48 hours is often secondary to ischemia or reperfusion and does not require invasive evaluation. Sustained VT occurring later does require invasive evaluation, which often includes implantation of an implantable cardioverter-defibrillator (ICD). The need for treatment of late, non-sustained VT is controversial. Flecainide, encainide, and sotalol suppress the arrhythmia, but they also appear to increase mortality. Amiodarone and moricizine have not increased survival. β-Blockers are useful when mild or modest LV dysfunction is present. If severe dysfunction is evident, treatment should be guided by results of electrophysiologic studies (see Chapter 50). Torsades de pointes may respond to overdrive pacing or IV magnesium sulfate. Accelerated idioventricular rhythm should not be treated unless hemodynamic decompensation occurs, in which case sequential or atrial overdrive pacing or atropine may be effective. Magnesium sulfate (administered as 1 g over 5 minutes, IV, followed by an 8-g infusion over 24 hours) did not reduce mortality in one large clinical trial, but the reason may have been its late implementation.

SUPRAVENTRICULAR ARRHYTHMIAS. Treatment of these arrhythmias is the same as that used when they occur under other circumstances (see Chapter 51) and is indicated when they impair hemodynamics or compromise myocardial viability by augmenting oxygen requirements. Sinus tachycardia is usually secondary to excessive sympathoadrenal tone associated with extensive MI and impaired ventricular performance, pericardial inflammation with irritation of the sinus node, relative or absolute hypovolemia, hypoxemia secondary to pulmonary venous congestion and respiratory impairment, heart failure, or other potentially remediable factors. Atrial fibrillation or flutter, though uncommon, may indicate heart failure or atrial MI. In the absence of the Wolff-Parkinson-White syndrome, these conditions should be treated with β-blockers, calcium channel blockers, or digitalis glycosides (see Chapters 51 and 54). Calcium channel blockers are, however, potentially hazardous, especially in the presence of hypotension or poor left ventricular function. A short-acting β-adrenergic blocker such as esmolol may be helpful initially to control ventricular rate. When decompensation is evident, rapid atrial pacing (to terminate atrial flutter) or electrical cardioversion (to terminate either atrial fibrillation or flutter) should be used (see Chapter 53).

BRADYARRHYTHMIAS (see CHAPTER 51). Sinus bradycardia occurs often, particularly in patients with inferior MI. If it is refractory to atropine, it may require temporary transvenous pacing. A wandering atrial pacemaker or first-degree AV block rarely requires specific treatment. Higher degrees of AV block or AV block associated with hypotension refractory to atropine (or, in refractory patients, aminophylline, given to compete for adenosine receptors) may require sequential pacing to sustain hemodynamics.

In patients with inferior wall MI, long-term pacing is needed only rarely, even when (1) high degrees of heart block persist throughout the hospital phase, (2) sinus node function is markedly impaired, (3) Mobitz type II second- or third-degree block occurs intermittently, or (4) block is associated with newly acquired bundle branch block or other criteria of conduction system impairment. Although implemented often in the setting of anterior MI with high-degree or prolonged AV block, long-term pacing may not improve survival after MI, because the mortality is so high with the extensive MI that is frequently responsible for the block. Nevertheless, temporary transvenous pacing may stabilize hemodynamics, and long-term pacing may be justified prophylactically in patients at high risk. Recently refined external transcutaneous pacers may be helpful on a short-term basis when transvenous pacing cannot be implemented expeditiously.

Hemodynamic Manifestations

Hemodynamic observations can be useful in guiding therapy (Table 60–7).

HEMODYNAMIC SUBSETS. Patients are categorized with respect to cardiac output (increased, normal, or diminished), systemic arterial blood pressure (increased, normal, or diminished, with or without increased or decreased systemic vascular resistance), and the presence or absence of pulmonary venous hypertension (elevated pulmonary arterial wedge pressure).

Patients without diminished systemic arterial blood pressure or pulmonary venous hypertension may have normal or hyperdynamic hemodynamics (the latter reflected by a high cardiac output, with or without hypertension caused by sympathoadrenal stimulation). Systemic arterial hypotension may be attributable to relative or absolute hypovolemia or to right ventricular MI (generally reflected by elevated systemic venous pressure). Rarely, it reflects decreased peripheral vascular resistance caused by vagotonia or sepsis. The noncompliant left ventricle requires augmented filling pressure to sustain cardiac output. Accordingly, relative hypovolemia may exist despite moderately elevated left ventricular filling pressure. Central venous pressure cannot be relied on for assessment of left ventricular volume.

Right ventricular failure, with or without concomitant tricuspid regurgitation, leads to increased central venous pressure without concomitantly increased pulmonary venous or pulmonary arterial occlusive pressure, which is indicative of left atrial pressure. Clinical findings often resemble those of pericardial effusion or constriction, but echocardiography can easily make the distinction. Pulmonary venous hypertension without systemic arterial hypotension is

Table 60–7 ■ HEMODYNAMIC SUBSETS AMONG PATIENTS WITH ACUTE MYOCARDIAL INFARCTION

SUBSET		SYSTEMIC ARTERIAL BLOOD PRESSURE	CARDIAC INDEX (L/m²/min)	LEFT VENTRICULAR FILLING PRESSURE (PULMONARY ARTERY OCCLUSIVE PRESSURE) (mm Hg)
I	Normal hemodynamics	Normal	2.7 ± 0.5	≤ 12
II	Hyperdynamic state	Increased	>3.0	<12
III	Hypovolemia*	Decreased	≤ 2.7	≤ 9
IV	Left ventricular failure			
	A. Mild	Normal	≤ 2.5	>18
	B. Severe	Normal or decreased	≤ 1.8	≥ 22
V	Cardiogenic shock	Decreased	≤ 1.8	≥ 18
VI	Shock attributable to right ventricular infarction†	Decreased	≤ 1.8	≤ 18

*Relative hypovolemia may result in hypertension even if pulmonary artery pressure is moderately elevated (≤ 18 mm Hg) if left ventricular compliance is decreased owing to infarction or failure.

†Central venous (systemic venous) pressure is often markedly elevated (upper limit of normal = 6 mm Hg).

Adapted from Forrester JS, et al: Medical therapy of acute myocardial infarction by application of hemodynamic subsets. N Eng! J Med 295:1404, 1976.

often indicative of left ventricular failure (differentiated as mild or severe in terms of normal or depressed cardiac output). Profound hypotension and pulmonary venous hypertension are manifestations of cardiogenic shock (see Chapter 95). The vicious circle of cardiogenic shock—progressive MI with declining cardiac output, further compromise of perfusion, and, ultimately, extensive necrosis with profound failure and shock—is generally irreversible without prompt mechanical support of the circulation and coronary revascularization with thrombolytic drugs, angioplasty, or surgery.

In general, hemodynamic status reflects the extent of left ventricular MI. However, an MI of modest extent superimposed on a previous MI can profoundly compromise hemodynamics. Initial impairment of ventricular performance may exceed that attributable to irreversible injury because of myocardial stunning. Right ventricular involvement may compromise cardiac output more than anticipated from the extent of left ventricular injury alone.

PATIENTS REQUIRING INVASIVE MONITORING. Most MI patients do not require hemodynamic monitoring with right-sided heart catheterization and/or invasive arterial pressure monitoring. Patients with peripheral hypoperfusion despite initial administration of fluids to replete or expand vascular volume and those with severe, refractory, or progressive heart failure, refractory arrhythmias, persistent pain, or hemodynamic instability should be evaluated by balloon flotation right-sided heart catheter hemodynamic monitoring. Patients with pulmonary congestion indicative of pulmonary venous hypertension, reflected by physical findings or chest roentgenographic abnormalities, usually can be managed conservatively.

Monitoring catheters should generally be introduced through compressible sites, preferably the internal jugular vein, particularly because of the high likelihood that thrombolytic agents will be used early in the treatment of MI. They should remain in place for no more than 72 hours to avoid the risk of infection, and they can often be removed much more promptly. Sometimes, ascertaining systemic and pulmonary venous pressure, cardiac output, and peripheral vascular resistance is sufficient for subsequent management without the need for continuous monitoring. In other instances, the effects of vasodilators, diuretics, agents with positive inotropic effects, and therapeutic alterations of vascular volume should be monitored over the ensuing 48 to 72 hours.

Alternatively, echocardiography can be used to assess left ventricular performance, the presence and severity of mitral regurgitation, ventricular and atrial chamber dimensions, and pulmonary arterial systolic pressure. Such observations, coupled with careful, repeated physical examinations and assessment of oxygen saturation, can often guide therapy less invasively.

TREATMENT TAILORED TO HEMODYNAMICS. Invasive hemodynamic monitoring in patients with clinically complicated acute MI permits rapid delineation of left ventricular filling pressure, effective vascular volume, the presence or absence of mitral regurgitation and its severity, ventricular septal rupture (with oximetry), right ventricular systolic and diastolic pressure and function, and cardiac output and peripheral vascular resistance. Hemodynamic measurements can also guide therapy in the following manner (Table 60–8):

1. Hypertensive patients with increased cardiac output and normal pulmonary artery wedge pressure may benefit from infusions of β-adrenergic blockers, such as esmolol, to reduce myocardial oxygen requirements.

Table 60–8 ■ THERAPEUTIC INTERVENTIONS TAILORED TO SPECIFIC HEMODYNAMIC SUBSETS

	HEMODYNAMIC SUBSET	INTERVENTION	REMARKS
I	Normal hemodynamics	None required	
II	Hyperdynamic state	β-Adrenergic blockade	Analgesics and anxiolytic drugs may be helpful.
III	Hypovolemia	Intravenous fluids to augment effective vascular volume	Marked increases in pulmonary artery occlusive pressure reflecting pulmonary venous hypertension and increased left ventricular filling pressure may occur if heart failure is unmasked or exacerbated; manifestations may include dyspnea, hypoxemia, bronchospasm and rales, and pulmonary congestion evident radiographically
IV	Left ventricular failure		
	A. Mild	Systemic arterial vasodilators	Diuretics may be useful if failure is refractory
	B. Severe	Systemic arterial vasodilators and diuretics	Cardiotonic agents may be helpful if hypotension supervenes, but their use can exacerbate the imbalance between myocardial oxygen requirements and supply; thus, sympathomimetic and dopaminergic agents may be helpful, but their beneficial effect on hemodynamics is usually only transitory, and their use may exacerbate ischemic injury
V	Cardiogenic shock	Coronary recanalization and circulatory support	
VI	Shock attributable to right ventricular infarction	Augmentation of vascular volume and cardiotonic agents	

Adapted from Forrester JS, et al: Medical therapy of acute myocardial infarction by application of hemodynamic subsets. N Engl J Med 295:1404, 1976.

2. Hypotension associated with relative or absolute hypovolemia reflected by lack of substantial elevation (>18 mm Hg) of pulmonary capillary wedge pressure (an estimate of left ventricular filling pressure) generally responds to augmentation of vascular volume with IV fluids. Pulmonary artery wedge pressure should be monitored to preclude fluid overload leading to pulmonary edema. Hypotension with markedly elevated right ventricular diastolic, right atrial, and central venous pressures may implicate right ventricular MI, which often responds to augmented vascular volume and stimulation of contractility with cardiotonic agents, such as dobutamine, dopamine, or β-adrenergic agonists. Systemic arteriolar vasodilators secondarily decrease impedance of right ventricular outflow if they ameliorate left ventricular failure and can be used when systemic arterial diastolic pressure is adequate.

3. Sudden and profound hypotension may reflect a catastrophic insult, such as pulmonary embolism (manifested by pulmonary arterial hypertension and hypoxemia) or rupture of the ventricular septum (detectable by augmented right ventricular and pulmonary artery pressure associated with an oxygen step-up in the right ventricle). Alternatively, it may reflect left ventricular papillary muscle rupture with mitral regurgitation, manifested by large V waves in the pulmonary artery wedge pressure recording. When caused by free wall rupture with hemopericardium, hemodynamic manifestations of pericardial tamponade are apparent, with a diastolic pressure plateau in all four cardiac chambers, impaired right ventricular filling, and confirmatory echocardiographic findings of pericardial fluid and diastolic right atrial and right ventricular collapse (see Chapter 65). Mechanical insults should be treated by immediate surgery if hemodynamic stability cannot be maintained without pharmacologic and circulatory support. Surgery can be delayed for 1 to 2 weeks if stability can be maintained without such measures, and if the patient can be monitored meticulously.

4. Hypotension associated with markedly elevated pulmonary capillary wedge pressure generally indicates severely impaired left ventricular performance and cardiogenic shock (see Chapter 95). Supportive measures and cardiotonic agents are generally ineffective unless the ischemia can be relieved by coronary thrombolysis, angioplasty, or surgery. Mechanical circulatory support may be necessary to obtain definitive diagnostic information pertinent to potentially remediable insults, such as septal or free wall rupture, mitral regurgitation, or coronary reocclusion. Intra-aortic balloon counterpulsation or circulatory support with a left ventricular assist device may be particularly useful as a temporizing measure or as a bridge to cardiac transplantation.

5. Pulmonary venous hypertension with normal systemic arterial pressure indicates relative or absolute excess of vascular volume and left ventricular failure, which should be treated with vasodilators to reduce both ventricular preload and afterload, diminish the commonly associated mitral regurgitation accompanying left ventricular failure, and diminish left atrial and pulmonary venous hypertension. Intravenous nitroprusside, nitroglycerin, or parenteral or oral ACE inhibitors may be effective. Caution must be exercised to avoid marked changes in concentrations of plasma electrolytes. If pulmonary congestion is severe or pulmonary edema is present, but cardiac output is reasonably well maintained and associated with adequate systemic arterial blood pressure, loop diuretics can contract vascular volume by removing fluid; they also have salutary pulmonary venodilatory effects. Rarely, peritoneal dialysis, ultrafiltration, or phlebotomy with reinfusion of cellular elements may be employed. Hemodialysis is dangerous because of the risk of precipitous changes in filling pressures and cardiac performance. Cardiotonic agents (dobutamine or dopamine, digitalis, and phosphodiesterase inhibitors, such as amrinone or milrinone) may be necessary but entail the risk of exacerbating imbalance between myocardial oxygen supply and demand.

6. Hypotension, with or without pulmonary venous hypertension indicative of left ventricular failure, is generally associated with increased peripheral vascular resistance in patients with MI. In rare instances, vascular resistance may be decreased, in which case dobutamine or, alternatively, vasoconstrictors (such as dopamine in relatively high doses; epinephrine, particularly if cardiac rate is not accelerated; and, rarely, although usually fruit-

lessly, norepinephrine) may be indicated. The decrease in resistance is often caused by other factors, such as occult sepsis (see Chapter 96). In patients with profound ventricular failure, circulatory support with intra-aortic balloon counterpulsation or left ventricular assist devices may facilitate performance of diagnostic catheterization and identification and treatment of surgically remediable lesions.

NON–Q-WAVE MI

Non–Q-wave MI, which is often suspected on the basis of ischemic ECG changes as well as other signs or symptoms consistent with myocardial ischemia, is confirmed by abnormalities of cardiac enzymes (see above). A non–Q-wave MI is relatively more common in patients with pre-existing symptomatic coronary disease, elderly individuals, and patients with the clinical syndrome of unstable angina (see Chapter 59). The incidence of acute arrhythmias and heart failure is generally less in non–Q-wave than in Q-wave MI, but when non–Q-wave MI is superimposed on substantial prior myocardial necrosis, all of the complications seen with Q-wave MI may also be seen with non–Q-wave MI. Conversely, because non–Q-wave MI may be a manifestation of incomplete or non-sustained thrombotic coronary occlusion, the late incidence of reocclusion, repeat MI, or sudden cardiac death is as high as it is after Q-wave MI. Although some have recommended more aggressive diagnostic angiography and mechanical revascularization in patients with Q-wave compared with non–Q-wave MI, recent data indicate that the criteria should be similar for both. Thus, an aggressive approach can be reserved for patients who have recurrent symptoms or who are at high risk. All of the therapies that reduce long-term complication rates after Q-wave MI appear to be beneficial after non–Q-wave MI. The principal difference in the management of non–Q-wave as compared with Q-wave MI is that thrombolytic agents have not been shown to be beneficial for patients with non–Q-wave MI. Instead, treatment focuses on the use of aspirin and intravenous heparin, analogous to their use in the syndrome of unstable angina (see Chapter 59). In fact, the syndromes of unstable angina and non–Q-wave MI may overlap. The elevations in troponin I and troponin T, seen often with unstable angina, may indicate that non–Q-wave MI is present.

OTHER COMPLICATIONS

PERICARDITIS (see Chapter 65) Pericarditis rarely occurs after non–Q-wave MI, but it occurs in up to 20% of patients after Q-wave MI, usually between 1 day and about 6 weeks after the acute event. Symptoms are similar to those seen with acute pericarditis of other etiologies. Aspirin is the treatment of choice; corticosteroids and other nonsteroidal anti-inflammatory drugs may interfere with myocardial healing. The incidence of pericarditis appears to have been reduced by effective acute recanalization.

RECURRENT ISCHEMIA, INFARCT EXTENSION, OR REINFARCTION. These complications may be the cause of recurrent pain in the hours, days, or weeks after MI. Most patients have recurrent ECG changes, which are very helpful in distinguishing true recurrent ischemia from other non-cardiac causes of pain. Patients with recurrent ischemia—spontaneously, at low exercise levels during risk stratification studies, or during physical activity—should be evaluated and managed aggressively. If the pain occurs at rest or at low levels of activity, diagnostic angiography should be performed, followed by coronary revascularization as indicated (see Chapters 46, 61, and 62).

STRUCTURAL COMPLICATIONS. Rupture of a papillary muscle, which causes acute mitral (and rarely tricuspid) regurgitation, or of the ventricular septum, which causes an acute left-to-right shunt, leads to acute hemodynamic compromise. Most affected patients will have a new systolic murmur, but the murmur may be surprisingly soft in the presence of markedly diminished cardiac output. When these complications are suspected, the diagnosis must be confirmed or excluded rapidly, usually by transthoracic echocardiography with Doppler flow imaging. Patients are usually managed with aggressive afterload reduction, sometimes including intra-aortic balloon counterpulsation. Urgent surgical consultation should be obtained for consideration of repair, commonly with simultaneous CABG surgery.

CARDIAC RUPTURE. Rupture of the free wall of the left ventricle usually presents with pericardial tamponade (see Chapter 65), cardiogenic shock (see Chapter 95), and cardiovascular collapse. Some patients develop false left ventricular aneurysms, which are localized ruptures that cause less severe hemodynamic compromise initially. In both situations, immediate pericardiocentesis should be followed by prompt surgical repair.

STEP-DOWN CARE

Patients with uncomplicated MI require CCU care generally for no more than 48 to 72 hours. Subsequent care is often facilitated by 1 to 3 days in a step-down unit equipped with telemetry for continuous ECG monitoring; however, with entirely uncomplicated MI treated with effective reperfusion, patients may be discharged directly from the CCU. In patients who have been treated with thrombolytic agents, heparin can be discontinued after 2 to 3 days, and secondary prevention of thrombosis can be continued with daily aspirin or other oral antiplatelet drugs, including IIb/IIIa antagonists that are under investigation for this purpose.

Therapeutic objectives during step-down care include (1) immediate recognition and treatment of VT, VF, and bradycardia caused by sinus node dysfunction or AV block; (2) daily clinical and appropriate laboratory monitoring for prompt detection and treatment of complications, including deep venous thrombosis, pulmonary embolism, post-MI pericarditis, left ventricular thrombi, ventricular true or false aneurysms, or catastrophic mechanical complications (including cardiac rupture); (3) treatment to minimize

the risk of recurrent MI; (4) assessment of prognosis based on evaluation of left ventricular function, exercise tolerance, and the severity of spontaneous or inducible ischemia; and (5) gradual and judicious progressive ambulation followed by a rehabilitation program after discharge. Complications detected by telemetry (e.g., episodic ischemia with ST-segment deviation, arrhythmia, heart block, new-onset bundle branch block, tachycardia with minimal exertion), physical findings suggestive of heart failure, markedly impaired ventricular performance documented echocardiographically, or manifestations of recurrent coronary occlusion, such as recurrent pain, unexplained tachycardia, exacerbation or appearance of heart failure, hypotension, or impaired ventricular performance, as well as manifestations of ischemia (e.g., recurrent chest pain), justify coronary arteriography before discharge from the hospital, with mechanical revascularization if indicated.

RISK STRATIFICATION

Before hospital discharge, it is critical to determine what interventions should be undertaken to optimize prognosis (Fig. 60–5). Prognosis is influenced by the burden of residual coronary disease, the extent of residual left ventricular function, and, to a lesser extent, the presence or severity of arrhythmia.

All post-MI patients should have a functional assessment of cardiac performance. Alternatives include a submaximal exercise test with exercise ECG, an exercise or stress myocardial perfusion scintigram with thallium or sestamibi, or an exercise or stress echocardiogram. Exercise is generally preferred to pharmacologic stress for patients who are able to exercise on a treadmill, whereas pharmacologic stress with dobutamine or dipyridamole is preferred for patients who cannot exercise. ECG criteria are usually considered adequate for patients without baseline ECG abnormalities, whereas perfusion scintigraphy or echocardiography is preferred for patients with underlying ECG changes or for those taking medica-

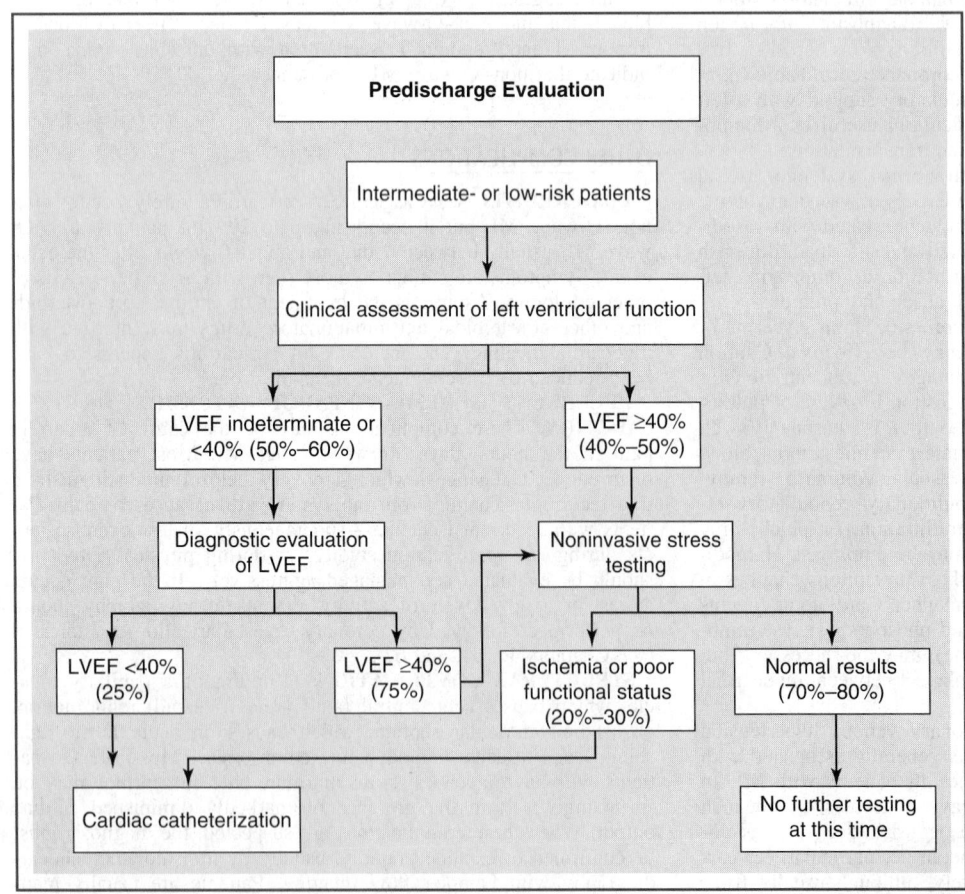

FIGURE 60–5 ■ Flow diagram for predischarge risk stratification. LVEF = left ventricular ejection fraction.

tions, such as digoxin, that might confound ECG interpretation. If the stress test is negative, further diagnostic evaluation for ischemia can entail a symptom-limited test 3 to 6 weeks later. However, if either the pre-discharge or subsequent post-discharge test evokes more than mild ischemia (such as ≥2 mm ST-segment depression on ECG or a markedly positive perfusion scintigram or stress echocardiogram, hypotension with ischemia, or a very low working capacity), coronary angiography should be performed and followed by revascularization as indicated.

Patients with left ventricular ejection fractions below 40% have a poor prognosis and are likely to benefit from aggressive therapy to prevent ventricular remodeling and subsequent heart failure and death. All patients with a recurrent MI, or an anterior MI, or with symptomatic heart failure before or concomitant with an MI should have an echocardiogram to assess left ventricular function. Because patients with three-vessel disease and left ventricular dysfunction have a better prognosis with CABG, and perhaps with PTCA, than with medical therapy, patients with ejection fractions below 40% should undergo coronary angiography unless there are contraindications to subsequent revascularization.

Patients who develop VF or sustained VT in the early hours after MI are not clearly at increased risk for late recurrences of the arrhythmia. However, if such arrhythmias occur more than 48 hours after the onset of the acute MI, patients should be evaluated with electrophysiologic testing with consideration of implantation of an ICD (see Chapter 53). Continuous ambulatory ECG (Holter) monitoring, previously used routinely in many post-MI patients, is not generally helpful.

CONVALESCENCE AND REHABILITATION

The objectives of management during convalescence include use of interventions to retard or prevent progression of atherosclerosis, prevent recurrent symptomatic ischemia and MI, and prevent late complications, such as systemic embolization or heart failure. These objectives can be accomplished in part with lifestyle changes as well as with medical interventions.

CHOLESTEROL REDUCTION. LDL cholesterol should be reduced to 100 mg/dL or less with diet and 3-hydroxy-3-methylglutaryl coenzyme A (HMG CoA) reductase inhibitors (see Chapter 206). Effective reduction of the cholesterol level decreases the incidence of recurrent events and cardiovascular mortality.

SMOKING CESSATION. Smoking cessation is imperative (see Chapter 13).

MEDICAL THERAPY TO PREVENT REINFARCTION. Use of β-blockers for at least 3 to 5 years reduces the incidence of coronary events, cardiovascular mortality, and all-cause mortality in patients who can tolerate these medications, including patients with left ventricular dysfunction. By comparison, calcium channel blockers have not been shown to reduce cardiovascular or all-cause mortality in the chronic setting or in the short term, and their use may limit the use of β-blockers or ACE inhibitors because these classes of medications share some similar side effects; therefore, calcium channel antagonists generally should not be used.

Use of aspirin leads to a 25% or greater reduction in the risk of reinfarction, cardiovascular mortality, and all-cause mortality in survivors of MI (see Chapter 188) and is appropriate in the absence of specific contraindications. In patients with contraindications, alternative antiplatelet agents (see Chapter 188) should be used. Warfarin is indicated for 3 to 6 months for patients who have been documented by echocardiography to have left ventricular mural thrombus, extensive akinesis, left ventricular aneurysm, or marked heart failure.

EXERCISE REHABILITATION AND SOCIAL SUPPORT. Physical conditioning improves exercise capacity and may reduce the incidence of recurrent ischemic events. In patients with a negative symptom-limited exercise test 3 to 6 weeks post-MI, exercise can be increased progressively, preferably initially as part of a formal rehabilitation program that often includes smoking cessation, diet modification, and weight loss. The level of exercise should be titrated with respect to the results of the symptom-limited exercise test and the patient's symptomatic status.

Because of the strong association between depression and adverse prognosis, as well as the risks of social isolation, addressing such issues as family and social support, return to work, and counseling to facilitate sexual function is essential. For some patients, formal counseling and/or antidepressant medications may be indicated.

HYPERTENSION AND LEFT VENTRICULAR FUNCTION. Indefinite use of ACE inhibitors is indicated in patients with an ejection fraction below 40%, heart failure associated with the MI or after it, a left ventricular aneurysm, or a large region of akinesis. ACE inhibitors reduce progression to heart failure, reduce cardiac and all-cause mortality, and may reduce the incidence of recurrent MI.

Because of the benefits of β-blockers and ACE inhibitors in post-MI patients, they are generally the first-line agents for treatment of hypertension. Diuretics should be added if hypertension is not well controlled by these medications or substituted if contraindications to their use exist. Calcium channel blockers should generally be avoided.

OTHER MEDICAL FACTORS. Diabetes should be controlled with oral agents and/or insulin as indicated. Estrogens improve lipid profiles in post-menopausal women and may have a direct vasodilatory effect on the coronary circulation. However, data from clinical trials on the risks and benefits of hormone replacement therapy are inconclusive in post-MI patients.

Elevated homocysteine levels appear to be an additional risk factor for progressive atherosclerosis. These levels can be reduced with administration of folic acid beginning at a dose of 400 μg to 1 mg/day. The utility of vitamin E remains conjectural.

Antiarrhythmic agents other than β-blockers, and perhaps amiodarone, can worsen prognosis in post-MI patients. Therapy of symptomatic ventricular arrhythmias and treatment of survivors of sudden cardiac death are generally accomplished with the use of an ICD, although amiodarone is appropriate in some circumstances (see Chapter 52).

DETECTION OF PROGRESSIVE DISEASE. The post-MI patient is usually seen in follow-up monthly for several months, then quarterly, and then at least twice per year, even in the absence of recurrent signs or symptoms. Risk factors, medications, lifestyle habits, and psychosocial support should be monitored and managed rigorously. Subsequent follow-up is similar to that for the patient with stable angina pectoris.

THE OUTLOOK

Early mortality associated with acute MI has declined markedly since the late 1960s. Before the advent of CCUs, hospital mortality was approximately 30%. Aggressive defibrillation reduced it by half. Protection of jeopardized ischemic myocardium and early pharmacologic coronary recanalization followed by mechanical revascularization, when indicated have lowered mortality even further; mortality is approximately 5% among patients younger than 75 years who have no contraindications to thrombolysis in whom treatment can be initiated within several hours after the onset of symptoms. Aggressive early revascularization, especially with stents and the use of platelet IIb/IIIa receptor antagonists, as well as vigorous treatment with cholesterol-lowering agents, offers considerable additional promise in secondary prevention for reducing the frequency of coronary events and enhancing survival. Consolidating these gains requires close observation and management of patients throughout convalescence to facilitate recognition and prevention of recurrent ischemia and retard progression of coronary artery disease, and implementation of vigorous medical, mechanical, and surgical intervention when required.

ACC/AHA Task Force on Practice Guidelines: ACC/AHA guidelines for the management of patients with acute chest myocardial infarction. J Am Coll Cardiol 28: 1328–1428, 1996.

Ambrosioni Z, Borghi C, Magnani B, for the Survival of Myocardial Infarction Long-Term Evaluation (SMILE) Study Investigators: The effect of the angiotensin-converting-enzyme inhibitor zofenopril on mortality and morbidity after anterior myocardial infarction. N Engl J Med 332:80–85, 1995. *An important study confirming the benefit of ACE inhibitors in improving survival, particularly in patients with left ventricular function that has been compromised by anterior MI.*

Antman EM, Tanasijevic MJ, Thompson B, et al: Cardiac-specific troponin I levels to predict the risk of mortality in patients with acute coronary syndromes. N Engl J Med 335:1342–1349, 1996. *In patients with acute coronary syndromes, cardiac troponin I levels provide useful prognostic information and permit the early identification of patients with an increased risk of death.*

Cannon CP, McCabe CH, Borzak S, et al, and the TIMI 12 Investigators: A randomized trial of an oral platelet glycoprotein IIb/IIIa inhibitor, sibrafiban, in patients post an acute coronary syndrome: Results of the TIMI 12 Trial. Circulation 97:340–349, 1998. *Demonstration of the safety of an oral antiplatelet agent in patients with acute coronary syndromes in a pilot study.*

The Cardiac Arrhythmia Suppression Trial Investigators: Preliminary report: Effect of encainide and flecainide on mortality in a randomized trial of arrhythmia suppression after MI. N Engl J Med 321:406, 1989. *A noteworthy report of the unexpected adverse influences of type 1c antiarrhythmic agents when used to treat ventricular ectopy in asymptomatic patients who have sustained an acute MI.*

Chen J, Radford MJ, Wang Y, et al: Do "America's best hospitals" perform better for acute myocardial infarction? N Engl J Med 340:286–292, 1999. *Hospitals with better reputations had better outcomes, probably due to higher rates of using aspirin and B-blockers.*

Cohen M, Demers C, Gurfinkel EP, et al: A comparison of low-molecular-weight heparin with unfractionated heparin for unstable coronary artery disease. N Engl J Med 337:7, 447–452, 1997. *Evidence that low-molecular-weight heparin is superior to standard, unfractionated heparin in preventing recurrent cardiac events in patients who have sustained an acute coronary event.*

Ellis SG, Ribiero da Sliva E, Heyndrickx G, et al, for the RESCUE Investigators: Randomized comparison of rescue angioplasty with conservative management of patients with early failure of thrombolysis for acute anterior myocardial infarction. Circulation 90:2280–2284, 1994. *The incidence of heart failure and death is decreased by rescue angioplasty in patients in whom initial pharmacologic thrombolysis fails to recanalize the critical vessel underlying an acute, anterior wall MI.*

Gersch BJ, Chesebro JH, Braunwald E, et al, and the TIMI II Investigators: Coronary artery bypass graft surgery after thrombolytic therapy in the thrombolysis in myocardial infarction trial, phase II (TIMI II). J Am Coll Cardiol 25:395–402, 1995. *A study that lays to rest the fear that surgery is associated with an unduly high risk of complications in patients treated initially with a clot-selective thrombolytic drug.*

Gruppo Italiano per lo Studio della Streptochi-nasi nell'Infarto Miocardico (GISSI): Long-term effects of intravenous thrombolysis in acute MI: Final report of the GISSI study. Lancet 2:871, 1987. *The pivotal report that demonstrated improved survival after coronary thrombolysis in patients with acute MI.*

The GUSTO Investigators: An international randomized trial comparing four thrombolytic strategies for acute MI. N Engl J Med 329:673, 1993. *A pivotal study that demonstrates that coronary thrombolysis with tissue-type plasminogen activator (t-PA) is superior to streptokinase in improving survival after acute MI under conditions in which optimal regimens for anticoagulation with heparin are used with each thrombolytic agent.*

Hall AS, Murray GD, Ball SG, on behalf of the AIREX Study Investigators: Follow-up study of patients randomly allocated ramipril or placebo for heart failure after acute myocardial infarction: AIRE Extension (AIREX) Study. Lancet 349:1493–1497, 1997. *Robust evidence that administration of ramipril to patients with clinically defined heart failure after acute MI results in a survival benefit that is not only large in magnitude, but is also sustained over many years.*

Hamm CW, Goldmann BU, Heeschen C, et al: Emergency room triage of patients with acute chest pain by means of rapid testing for cardiac troponin T or troponin I. N Engl J Med 337:1648–1653, 1997. *Bedside tests for cardiac-specific troponins are highly sensitive for the early detection of myocardial-cell injury in acute coronary syndromes. Negative test results are associated with low risk and allow rapid and safe discharge of patients with an episode of acute chest pain from the emergency room.*

Jaffe AS: New markers for myocardial infarction: Are they needed? Contemp Intern Med 9:8, 6–13, 1997. *A comparison of the diagnostic characteristics of diverse macromolecular markers of myocardial injury emphasizing the high sensitivity and specificity of cardiac troponins (I and T) and their more protracted elevations compared with concentrations of MB-CK.*

Lenderink T, Simoons ML, Van Es GA, et al: Benefit of thrombolytic therapy is sustained throughout 5 years and is related to TIMI perfusion grade 3 but not grade 2 flow at discharge. Circulation 92:1110–1116, 1995. *Demonstration of the persistence of initial benefit conferred by coronary thrombolysis on survival and the markedly lower mortality seen when recanalization is associated with more complete reperfusion.*

Peterson ED, Show LJ, Califf RM: Risk stratification after myocardial infarction. Ann Intern Med 126:561–582, 1997. *American College of Physicians' clinical practice guidlines with a useful approach to risk stratification in post-MI patients.*

Sacks FM, Pfeffer MA, Moye LA, et al: Effect of pravastatin on coronary events after myocardial infarction in patients with average cholesterol levels. Cholesterol and Recurrent Events Trial Investigators. N Engl J Med 335:1001–1009, 1996. *An important demonstration of the benefit of pharmacologic lowering of LDL cholesterol in patients with overt coronary artery disease whose cholesterol levels are within the conventionally defined normal range.*

Sobel BE: Interpretation of results of clinical trials in coronary thrombolysis. Fibrinolysis Proteolysis 11:17–21, 1997. *A review delineating pitfalls in interpreting results in which diverse thrombolytic drugs are compared, and the need to consider results in the context of time to treatment, adequacy and nature of anticoagulation, time to implementation of patency, time to and frequency of reocclusion, and nature of the study population.*

The TIMI Study Group: Comparison of invasive and conservative strategies after treatment with intravenous tissue plasminogen activator in acute MI: Results of the thrombolysis in MI (TIMI) phase II trial. N Engl J Med 320:618, 1989. *A definitive report from a large number of centers comparing survival after coronary thrombolysis with that following obligatory early angiography and demonstrating the advantages of a conservative strategy that focuses on thrombolysis alone.*

Weaver DW, Cerqueira M, Hallstrom A, et al: Prehospital-initiated vs hosptial-initiated thrombolytic therapy: The MITI trial. JAMA 270:1211–1216, 1993. *An important study showing a 99% survival if thrombolysis with t-PA, aspirin, and heparin is initiated in MI patients within 90 minutes after notification of emergency services.*

61 ■ CORONARY ANGIOPLASTY

Donald S. Baim

Catheter-based (non-surgical) techniques have become the most common form of myocardial revascularization. More than 400,000 procedures are performed annually in the United States alone, compared with some 300,000 surgical bypass operations.

HISTORICAL BACKGROUND

In 1977, after several years of refinement in the peripheral circulation, the first human percutaneous transluminal coronary angioplasty (PTCA) was performed by Greuntzig using a balloon-tipped catheter. This catheter was introduced by femoral arterial puncture, advanced across the target lesion in its smaller (collapsed) configuration, and then inflated within the stenosis to produce the desired luminal enlargement (Fig. 61–1). Fewer than 1000 procedures were performed annually through 1981.

At first, it was estimated that no more than 5% of patients who were eligible for coronary artery bypass grafting (CABG) would be candidates for PTCA. Even among carefully selected candidates with proximal, concentric, non-calcified single-vessel disease, the failure rate was about 20%, including major complications (death, myocardial infarction, emergency bypass surgery) in 8% (Table 61–1). Despite many improvements over the next decade, the experience with PTCA exposed four fundamental weaknesses of balloon dilatation: (1) failure to cross some lesions with the balloon; (2) inability to dilate certain rigid (calcified) or elastic (eccentric) lesions; (3) local plaque disruption (dissection) that interfered with antegrade coronary flow and required emergency bypass surgery to correct; and (4) renarrowing (re-stenosis) of the dilated segment in the first year in 40% of patients who had an initially successful procedure, such that another revascularization procedure was required in more than 20% of patients.

In an effort to overcome these fundamental limitations, newer devices include endoluminal metallic scaffolds (stents) and devices for the removal of plaque mass from the target lesion (atherectomy). As these devices were tested, refined, and introduced into clinical practice, their superior performance in terms of higher success rates and lower rates of complications and re-stenosis have reduced the role for "stand-alone" balloon PTCA to roughly 20% of interventions. However, balloon angioplasty is still widely used in an "adjunctive" role to pre-dilation, to help facilitate the passage of a new device, or to post-dilation, so as to maximize the degree of luminal enlargement obtained by a new device. The goal is to provide consistently wide luminal patency through strategies dictated by lesion morphology, with no major acute complications and

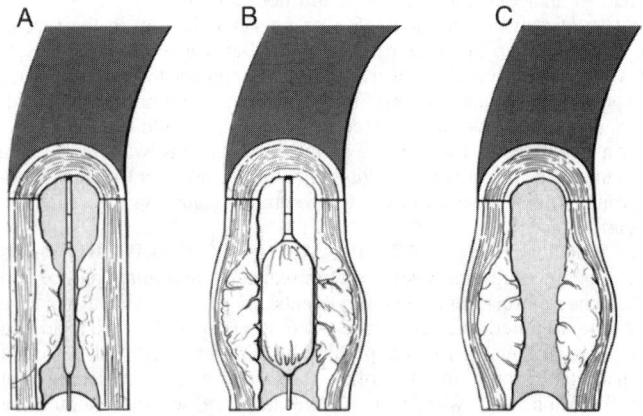

FIGURE 61–1 ■ Conventional balloon angioplasty, showing the cracking of the intimal plaque and the elastic recoil of the vessel wall following balloon deflation. (From Baim DS: New devices for catheter intervention. Hospital Pract 28:41, 1993. © 1993, The McGraw-Hill Companies. Illustration by Laura Duprey.)

Table 61-1 ■ EVOLUTION OF CORONARY ANGIOPLASTY PROCEDURES AND RESULTS*

	NHLBI (1981)	NHLBI (1985–1986)	NHLBI (1997)	BIDMC (1997)
No. of patients	1155	1802		2372
Age >65	12%	27%		48%
Prior MI	21%	37%		
Prior CABG	9%	13%	28%	30%
Vessels treated				
Left main	1.3%	0.6%	1.0%	2.3%
Left anterior descending	63.1%	48.3%	38%	34.9%
Circumflex	6.4%	15.7%	21%	21.6%
Right	25.3%	29%	34%	29.4%
Saphenous graft	3.3%	4.9%	4%	11.1%
Multiple vessels	5%	22%		25.6%
Devices used				
Balloon only	100%	100%	31%	19.5%
Stent	0%	0%	58%	68.8%
Rotational atherectomy	0%	0%	9%	13.8%
Directional atherectomy	0%	0%	1%	3.7%
Lesion success	66.8%	87.8%	93.8%	94.2%
Major adverse events†				
Death	1.2%	1.0%	1.0%	0.8%
MI	4.9%	4.3%	2.6%	2.2%
Emergency bypass	5.8%	3.4%	0%	0.2%

*Despite patients who are older, sicker, and more unstable, the results of catheter intervention (success, major complications) have improved consistently with improving technology (particularly with the introduction of newer interventional devices).
†In settings other than acute MI.
NHLBI = National Heart Lung and Blood Institute PTCA registries in 1970–1981, 1985–1986. NHLBI 1997 data are preliminary (Williams DO, personal communication); BIDMC = experience at the author's institution in 1997; MI = myocardial infarction; CABG = coronary artery bypass grafting.

a low chance (10–15%) of developing re-stenosis that would require a repeat revascularization procedure during the next year.

INDICATIONS

The fundamental indication for the performance of catheter-based coronary intervention is an anatomically approachable lesion or lesions that are responsible for clinical ischemia and for which angioplasty rather than surgery or continued medical therapy constitutes the preferred approach in a patient who understands the risks and benefits of the therapeutic alternatives. Initially, the anatomic restrictions were driven by the limited capabilities of early balloon catheters. Current equipment allows treatment of distal, diffuse, calcified lesions of multiple coronary arteries or previously constructed saphenous vein bypass grafts. Total occlusions of a coronary artery may also be treated, but with a lower success rate (65% vs. 95%) owing to the inability to cross some chronic occlusions with the guidewire. Expansion to the treatment of multivessel disease occurred progressively in the late 1980s, to the point where 30 to 40% of procedures now involve treatment of more than one lesion. A variety of randomized trials between PTCA and CABG for patients with multivessel disease conducted during that period indicated generally equivalent 5-year mortality (except for patients with diabetes, in whom surgical mortality was lower than PTCA). However, more patients treated initially by PTCA required a repeat revascularization procedure (another PTCA or CABG) to treat restenosis. Because of the recent successes of new devices, particularly stents, in improving percutaneous procedural outcome, several trials of PTCA with stenting versus CABG are underway.

The clinical indications for catheter-based intervention may include any of the manifestations of myocardial ischemia. Patients with stable but severe or life-limiting angina refractory to medical therapy are generally referred for diagnostic catheterization including coronary angiography, as may be some patients with mild or no symptoms but in whom non-invasive test results suggest coronary lesions for which the prognosis may be improved by revascularization (see Chapter 59). If a suitable lesion or lesions are found to explain the clinical manifestations, the definitive catheter-based intervention can generally be performed as an extension of the same procedure—about 25% of diagnostic catheterizations proceed to an interventional procedure during the same sitting, whereas another 35% are referred for surgery. If patients with unstable angina (particularly new-onset angina or recent progression to rest pain) can be stabilized initially with medical therapy, diagnostic cardiac catheterization with "angioplasty stand-by" can be performed 24 to 48 hours after admission. Alternatively, because about 80% of patients with unstable angina proceed to coronary angiography and about 50% proceed to revascularization within the next 6 weeks of admission, some recommend early catheterization in all patients to decrease length of stay, time to return to work, and the number of readmissions to the hospital, without increasing overall rates of death or myocardial infarction.

More recently, there has been growing interest in the use of catheter techniques for revascularization of patients with acute myocardial infarction (see Chapter 60). Although the earlier trials showed that immediate or routine 18- to 48-hour delayed PTCA offered little incremental clinical benefit to thrombolysis except in patients with ongoing spontaneous or exercise-induced ischemia, there is now substantial evidence that proceeding directly to PTCA (without the thrombolytic agent) can improve outcome and probably decrease costs if the procedure can be performed by experienced interventionalists within 90 minutes of the patient's arrival at the hospital.

PROCEDURE

After any hemodynamic measurements and baseline angiography (see Chapter 46), the diagnostic coronary catheters are removed and exchanged for an appropriate "guiding catheter" that will remain securely in the coronary ostium, serving as a conduit through which the therapeutic devices can be advanced and intermittent puffs of radiographic contrast medium can be given to define the location of devices relative to target lesions. Once the guiding catheter is in place, a small "guidewire" (0.010–0.018 inch diameter) is negotiated into the desired vessel, across the target lesion, and well into the distal circulation. This guidewire then serves as a rail over which subsequent therapeutic devices are advanced. With achievement of a satisfactory result (<30% residual stenosis, no significant dissections of plaque at or adjacent to the treatment site, and normal distal flow), other target lesions may be addressed.

At the end of the procedure, patients should be free of chest pain or new electrocardiographic abnormalities, but they should be followed closely for the next several hours for chest pain or electrocardiographic changes that might be suggestive of closure of one of the treated vessels, for dehydration due to the osmotic load of iodinated contrast, or for bleeding or loss of distal pulses at the catheter introduction site. Although mild elevations (up to three times normal) of the creatine kinase MB fraction are seen in more than 15% of interventional patients, their importance is still the subject of much debate.

Follow-up should include immediate contact for recurrent chest pain or puncture site complaints. Otherwise, a routine visit at 2 to 4 weeks (combined with a repeat stress test, if desired) can give a clear picture of the patient's symptomatic response to the intervention and serve as a useful baseline should the patient redevelop symptoms. The symptoms of re-stenosis of the dilated segment develop in about 15% of patients and usually begin as mild exertional discomfort. If the nature of the symptoms and timing of their onset (6 weeks to 6 months after intervention) are typical, plans should be made for repeat catheterization and possible repeat intervention. Vague or atypical symptoms may be evaluated further by a functional stress test before proceeding to repeat catheterization. Symptoms developing more than 6 to 9 months after the procedure are more likely due to a new or progressive lesion at another site than to re-stenosis.

COMPLICATIONS

Despite its similarity to percutaneous diagnostic catheterization (see Chapter 46), therapeutic cardiac catheterization carries significantly higher risk, including about a 1% risk each for death, Q-wave myocardial infarction, or emergent bypass surgery. Most of this risk depends on baseline conditions (age, left ventricular function, extent of coronary disease, other co-morbid conditions), coronary anatomy, and the response of the target lesions to treatment. In the period before stenting (pre-1994), balloon dilatation would frequently produce local dissections that could lead within minutes to hours to "abrupt closure" of the dilated segment and require emergent re-dilation or CABG, with the latter carrying about 6% mortality and up to a 50% risk of a Q-wave myocardial infarction. In the stent era (see later), arteries with even marginally imperfect results are generally stented, reducing current emergency CABG rates well below 1%. The widespread use of newer platelet IIb/IIIa receptor blockers (in addition to aspirin and intravenous heparin) has also helped decrease the incidence of thrombotic/occlusive complications of catheter-based intervention.

Other coronary complications include perforation (with or without tamponade) caused by mechanical or laser atherectomy devices or guidewires (<1%), "snow plow" occlusion of side branches that originate within a treated main vessel segment, and "no reflow" of the distal circulation owing to either particulate embolization or intense vasoconstriction of the distal microcirculation. There is about a 1% risk of local complications (bleeding, false aneurysm, occlusion) at the arterial entry site.

STENTS

More than 20 different designs and several broad classes of stents now exist (Fig. 61–2), including balloon expandable versus self-expanding stents and slotted tube versus wire coil construction, but not all are currently approved for use in the United States. Until recently, the most experience has been with the balloon-expandable, slotted tube (Palmaz-Schatz) stent, which was approved for use in the United States in 1994 based on two randomized trials that showed higher procedural success, less residual narrowing acutely, and less re-stenosis (to more than a 50% narrowing) at angiography 6 months after the procedure.

With complete stent expansion, post-procedure aspirin plus ticlopidine can reduce the stent thrombosis rate to about 1%. Because of the risk of neutropenia with ticlopidine, patients should have a complete blood cell count every 2 weeks for the 2 to 4 weeks while they are on the drug. Newer oral agents such as clopidogrel are now available to replace ticlopidine.

The original indication for stenting was a focal de novo lesion (i.e., not a re-stenosis after a prior intervention) in a 3-mm diameter native vessel—a subgroup that accounts for only about 10% of current interventions. A second stent (the Gianturco-Roubin balloon expandable coil) was approved for use in reversing acute or threatened abrupt closure after PTCA. By 1998, however, stent use climbed to more than 50% of all U.S. coronary interventions, based on treatment of other types of lesions, including prior re-stenosis

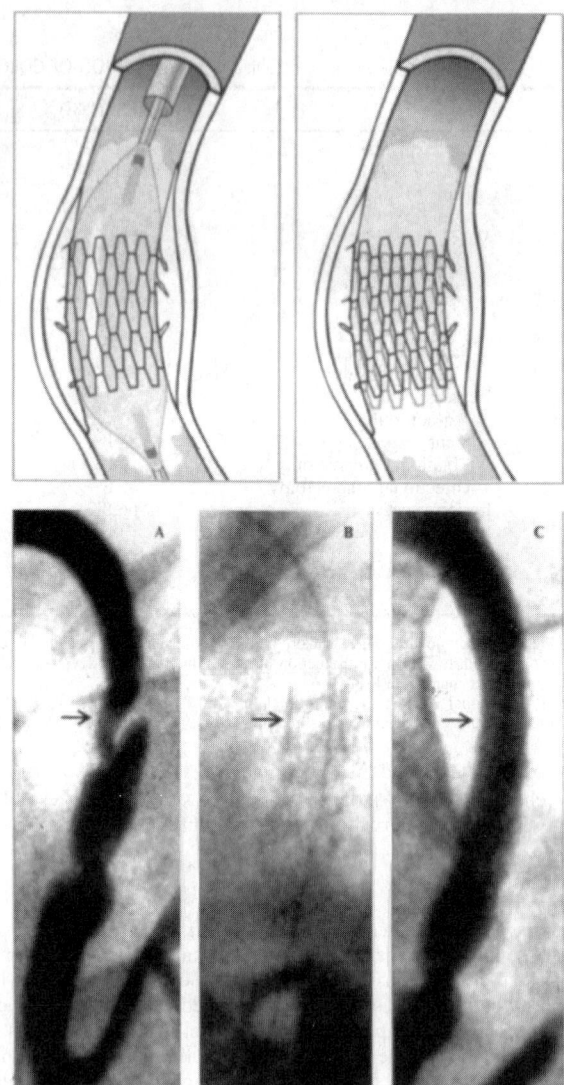

FIGURE 61–2 ■ Intracoronary stent, trapping intimal dissections and resisting elastic recoil to provide a large smooth lumen, as seen in the example of a saphenous vein graft lesion before, during, and after stent placement. (From Baim DS: New devices for catheter intervention. Hospital Pract 28:41, 1993. © 1993, The McGraw-Hill Companies. Illustration by Laura Duprey.)

after a non-stent device, stenotic saphenous vein grafts, total occlusions (after successful pre-dilatation), vessels smaller than 2.7 mm, long or diffuse disease, acute myocardial infarction, and bifurcation lesions. As the spectrum of lesions has expanded, the original two designs proved to be inadequate. As a result, second-generation stents, which were designed to enhance the performance in one or more of these categories, are now available and widely used, with data suggesting similar (<1%) thrombosis rates and, with full expansion, low angiographic re-stenosis rates of 15 to 20%.

However, the mere placement of a stent does not prevent re-stenosis: stents simply provide a larger acute lumen diameter by tacking up dissections and resisting recoil of the vessel wall. This larger acute lumen has a device-independent effect to reduce re-stenosis. It appears that the acute result determines late outcome more than the device used to achieve it. Although stents are the most effective current method to optimal acute results, neointimal hyperplasia can cause stenosis within the stent. Various catheter techniques for removing this material and re-dilating the lumen have been used to treat in-stent re-stenosis, but patients with recurrent re-stenotic episodes commonly require CABG to provide sustained relief. Various adjunctive therapies such as β or γ radiation, newer drugs, and gene therapy are being evaluated for their potential to attenuate this hyperplastic response and reduce the stent re-stenosis rate.

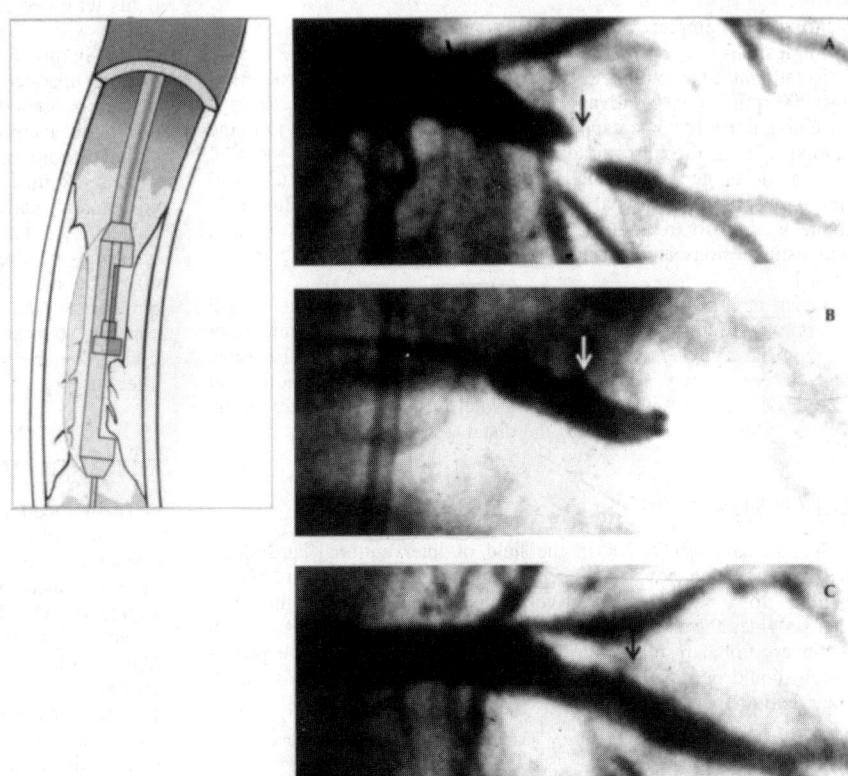

FIGURE 61-3 ▪ Directional coronary atherectomy. The windowed housing is advanced across the target lesion and oriented toward the bulk of the plaque. Low-pressure inflation of the balloon on the opposite side of the housing presses the plaque into the window of the device, where it is excised and trapped by advancement of a spinning blade. (From Baim DS: New devices for catheter intervention. Hospital Pract 28:41, 1993. © 1993, The McGraw-Hill Companies. Illustration by Laura Duprey.)

ATHERECTOMY DEVICES

Although both conventional PTCA and stents displace the obstructive plaque outward and out of the flow lumen, atherectomy devices actually remove plaque from the lesion and the body. The first such device is the directional coronary atherectomy (DCA) system (Fig. 61–3), which uses a windowed steel cylinder with a spinning cutting blade to excise, trap, and remove atheromatous material. Initial (1993–1994) studies with this device suggested little clinical benefit and more risk as compared with balloon PTCA, but recent studies with better acute results demonstrated somewhat reduced re-stenosis with comparable safety. Use of this technique, however, is currently limited to specific anatomic situations such as non-calcified ostial and bifurcation lesions because

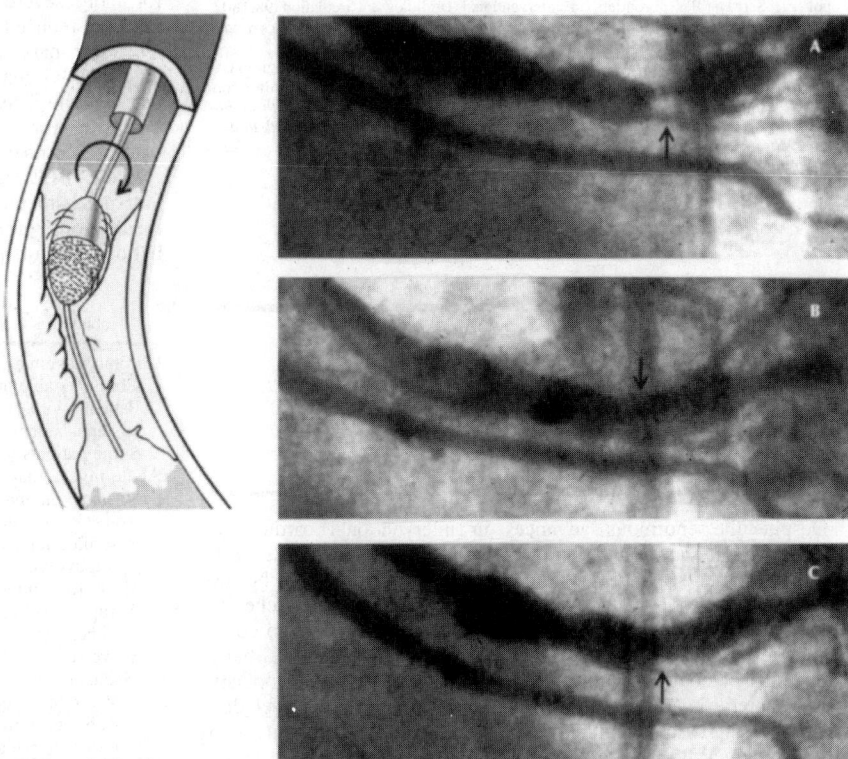

FIGURE 61-4 ▪ Rotational atherectomy (Rotablator). The diamond-chip coated burr (spinning at nearly 200,000 rpm) grinds the plaque into microscopic particles as it is slowly advanced across the lesion over a guidewire. (From Baim DS: New devices for catheter intervention. Hospital Pract 28:41, 1993. © 1993, The McGraw-Hill Companies. Illustration by Laura Duprey.)

stenting is a simpler means to the same end for most other anatomic lesions.

Rotational atherectomy uses a football-shaped burr that rotates at 180,000 rpm as it is advanced through the target lesion over a special guidewire. Microscopic diamond chips embedded into the leading half of the burr abrade even calcified plaque and convert it into particles generally smaller than a white blood cell (25 μm) that pass through the distal microcirculation (Fig. 61–4). This technique is used to treat most calcified lesions, long diffuse disease, and ostial lesions at the origin of a coronary artery or a coronary branch.

Laser atherectomy uses fiberoptic catheters to transmit pulsed lasers of different wavelengths to the plaque. In general, laser therapy has shown no incremental benefit over mechanical means. One exception may be the crossing of those total occlusions that cannot be crossed with a guidewire, where use of a small fiberoptic wire may create a channel into the distal vessel.

CONCLUSION

In 23 years (1977–2000), the field of interventional cardiology has gone from a novelty procedure applicable to less than 5% of patients to a safe and effective mainstream therapeutic modality that provides the majority of revascularization (see Table 61–1). To achieve optimal results, consensus panels suggest that these procedures should be done only by individuals performing more than 75 interventions per year.

Baim DS, Grossman W (eds): Cardiac Catheterization, Angiography and Intervention 5th ed. Baltimore, Williams & Wilkins, 1996. *Standard textbook resource for details about procedures, results, and clinical trial data.*

Kong DF, Califf RM, Miller DP, et al: Clinical outcomes of therapeutic agents that block the platelet IIb/IIIa integrin in ischemic heart disease. Circulation 98:2829, 1998. *Summary of the trials of various agents in this class, which decrease the incidence of death, MI, and emergency repeat intervention (mostly the incidence of non-Q wave infarctions) after catheter-based revascularization.*

Pocock SJ, Henderson RA, Rickards AF, et al: Meta-analysis of randomized trials comparing coronary angioplasty with bypass surgery. Lancet 346:1184, 1995. *An excellent overview of the several randomized trials comparing conventional balloon angioplasty to surgery for the treatment of patients with multivessel coronary artery disease. Acute results and 5-year mortality are equivalent (except perhaps in patients with diabetes, in whom surgery may be preferred), but patients treated initially by angioplasty more frequently require a repeat catheter intervention or bypass surgery to manage re-stenosis of the treated segment. Trials using newer devices (with lower rates of re-stenosis than conventional balloon angioplasty) are in progress.*

Topol EJ, Serruys PW: Frontiers in interventional cardiology. Circulation 98:1802, 1998. *Review of current state of the art and expected future directions in coronary angioplasty.*

Weaver WD, Simes J, Betriu A, et al: Comparison of primary coronary angioplasty and intravenous thrombolytic therapy for the therapy of acute myocardial infarction. JAMA 278:2093, 1997. *Earlier trials have demonstrated the superiority of thrombolytic drugs (e.g., rt-PA) over conventional management of acute myocardial infarction. More recent trials show further improvement by immediate (direct) angioplasty of the infarct-related vessel.*

especially left main coronary obstruction and particularly in patients with decreased left ventricular function.

The wide spectrum of patients who now undergo CABG contrasts sharply to the carefully selected patients with single-vessel disease operated on in 1967 by Favaloro and his colleagues. Patients considered for CABG today tend to be considerably older and more acutely ill, to more likely to have diabetes mellitus, and to have more advanced diffuse arterial disease and more left ventricular dysfunction than in previous decades. CABG has become an integral part of the overall strategy of treating patients with unstable angina and acute evolving myocardial infarction, either primarily or after failure of other therapies (see Chapters 59 and 60). The increasingly wide spectrum of operative indications requires considerable ingenuity, better operative techniques including coronary bypass conduits, markedly improved myocardial protection, and more sophisticated techniques for life support during and after surgery.

INDICATIONS FOR CORONARY ARTERY BYPASS SURGERY

The indications for CABG (Table 62–1) include patients who have one or more significant lesions with greater than 70% luminal diameter in the coronary arterial system and either have failed intensive medical therapy and/or angioplasty for treating chronic angina or who have specific abnormalities for which CABG improves prognosis independent of any symptomatic benefit. An anatomic indication for CABG regardless of symptoms includes a greater than or equal to 70% diameter stenosis of the left main coronary artery unless absolutely contraindicated by other co-morbid conditions. Similarly, acute failure of a percutaneous coronary intervention (see Chapter 61) of any vessel may require emergency CABG. Patients with triple-vessel disease and concomitant left ventricular dysfunction have a better prognosis with CABG even if they have few or no symptoms. Patients who undergo CABG should not have other life-threatening co-morbidities.

CHRONIC STABLE ANGINA. These patients, who represent the largest group of patients considered for CABG, have effort angina or stress-related angina that is not adequately controlled by medical therapy or for which medical therapy results in side-effects or diminished functional capacity (see Chapter 59). For patients with multivessel disease, CABG results in fewer subsequent procedures and less angina than percutaneous transluminal coronary angioplasty (Table 62–2). CABG is generally preferred over angioplasty for more severe disease, especially three-vessel disease accompanied by reduced ventricular function, and is first-choice treatment when coronary lesions are not amenable to angioplasty. Occasionally, CABG may be considered for a patient with single-vessel disease who is symptomatic despite medical treatment, who is not a candidate for or who has failed angioplasty, and whose single diseased coronary artery is unusually large and dominant.

UNSTABLE AND/OR NON–Q WAVE INFARCTION ANGINA. Patients with unstable angina should be stabilized, if possible, by medications, but in the severest cases they may require intra-aortic balloon support pump for the stabilization of hemodynamics, relief

---

Table 62–1 ■ INDICATIONS FOR CORONARY ARTERY BYPASS SURGERY

Chronic ischemia
  Chronic stable angina not adequately controlled by medical therapy
  Patients with anatomy for which CABG will prolong survival (left main stenosis or triple-vessel disease with left ventricular dysfunction)
  Some patients with "silent" ischemia
Acute myocardial ischemia
  Unstable angina
  Non–Q wave infarction
  Postinfarction angina
  Acute evolving myocardial infarction
  Myocardial infarction with shock
  Abrupt vessel closure after angioplasty
With other cardiac operations
  Valve surgery
  Mechanical sequelae of myocardial infarction:
    Ventricular septal defect
    Ruptured septal defect
    Left ventricular aneurysm

---

62 SURGICAL TREATMENT OF CORONARY ARTERY DISEASE

Lawrence H. Cohn

Despite the enormous advances in interventional cardiology, thrombolytic therapy, and pharmacologic therapy of patients with coronary heart disease (CHD), surgical therapy continues to be the most comprehensive method of direct reperfusion of the ischemic human myocardium. Approximately 300,000 patients undergo coronary artery bypass grafting (CABG) annually for one of many indications of acute and chronic myocardial ischemia. Angioplasty (see Chapter 61) is now generally indicated for single-vessel disease and some cases of multivessel disease, but CABG continues to be the treatment of choice for severe multivessel coronary disease,

Table 62–2 ■ CABG vs PTCA FOR MULTIVESSEL CORONARY DISEASE

END POINT	POCOCK ET AL.*		BARI STUDY†	
	CABG (n = 1303)	PTCA (n = 1336)	CABG (n = 914)	PTCA (n = 915)
	Percentage of Patients			
Death	2.8	3.1	10.7	13.7
Death or MI	8.5	8.1	19.6	21.3
Repeated CABG	0.8	18.3‡	0.7	20.5‡
Repeated CABG or PTCA	3.2	34.5‡	8.0	54.0‡
More than mild angina	12.1	17.8‡	—	—

Adapted from Bittl JA: Advances in coronary angioplasty. N Engl J Med 335:1290–1302, 1996. Copyright 1996 Massachusetts Medical Society. All rights reserved.

BARI = Bypass Angioplasty Revascularization Investigators; CABG = coronary artery bypass grafting; PTCA = percutaneous transluminal coronary angioplasty; MI = myocardial infarction.

* This study was a meta-analysis of the results of six trials at 1 year. Patients with multivessel disease were studied.

† Data were obtained from the BARI investigators. Patients with multivessel disease were studied. The results reported are for the 5-year follow-up.

‡ $P < .05$.

of anginal symptoms, and amelioration of electrocardiographic abnormalities. A national prospective randomized study showed that stabilizing patients before CABG is far preferable to operating on patients in a truly unstable condition; after stabilization, operative mortality is similar to elective surgery. The angiographic patterns of obstructive disease for patients with non–Q wave myocardial infarction are the same as those of unstable angina, and patients are considered for operation with the same degree of aggressiveness as are patients with unstable angina, provided that they are otherwise good candidates for surgery (see Chapter 60).

EVOLVING MYOCARDIAL INFARCTION. A number of cardiac centers with excellent logistic set-ups have performed large numbers of operations in these patients with excellent results and reduction or prevention of myocardial necrosis. However, angioplasty of the infarct-related vessel has generally become the intervention of choice in these patients.

POSTINFARCTION ANGINA. A major advance in therapy for coronary disease has been the aggressive treatment by CABG of postinfarction angina, which may occur within hours to days of the completed myocardial infarction (see Chapter 60). Results of surgery for this syndrome are similar to those for unstable angina, provided that the patient is not in shock preoperatively.

MYOCARDIAL INFARCTION WITH CARDIOGENIC SHOCK. CABG is an alternative to angioplasty for the aggressive treatment of myocardial infarction with cardiogenic shock, which is usually caused by one or cumulative infarctions of at least 40% of the left ventricle. Careful evaluation of residual left ventricular function in non-ischemic areas and of the anatomy of the distal coronary vessels is critical because patients with poor residual myocardial function or poor distal vessels do not do well after CABG. Operative mortality in the best of centers is 25 to 30%.

SILENT ISCHEMIA. Patients with "silent" ischemia (see Chapter 59) may present with an episode of "sudden death" after physical exertion (see Chapter 52) or with positive results on screening tests. Data now suggest that patients with severe hemodynamic alterations during or after exercise testing and with multivessel disease are especially good candidates for CABG.

CORONARY BYPASS WITH OTHER CARDIAC OPERATIONS. When a mechanical abnormality complicates acute myocardial infarction and requires operation, such as a ventricular septal defect, ruptured or dysfunctional papillary muscle that produces mitral regurgitation, left ventricular aneurysm, pseudoaneurysm, or left ventricular rupture, coronary bypass is often done adjunctively (see Chapter 60). These sequelae of a Q-wave myocardial infarction may occur days to weeks after the original infarction and are often associated with multiple-vessel coronary disease requiring CABG.

A high percentage of adults with valvular heart disease (see Chapter 63) have coexistent coronary artery lesions. These patients require a concomitant CABG because of the increased demand for coronary blood flow to the left ventricular myocardium imposed by the hemodynamic burden produced by the valve lesion. In the evaluation of an adult patient older than age 40 for valvular heart surgery, coronary arteriography is generally indicated. In some series of patients operated on for aortic valve disease, 30 to 40% of

the patients require concomitant CABG. The long-term outlook for patients with valve disease and coronary disease, despite the fact that the coronary disease may be grafted completely, is not as satisfactory as for those who have valve disease without coexisting coronary artery disease.

BASIS OF SURGICAL TREATMENT OF CORONARY HEART DISEASE

In the CABG operation (Fig. 62–1), a conduit is sutured distal to the obstructing lesion in the artery and then connected proximally to either the aorta or naturally by in situ connection such as the internal thoracic artery to the subclavian artery. The reversed autogenous saphenous vein graft continues to be a reliable and flexible conduit for coronary bypass, but the best readily available conduit is the internal thoracic (mammary) artery, which runs under

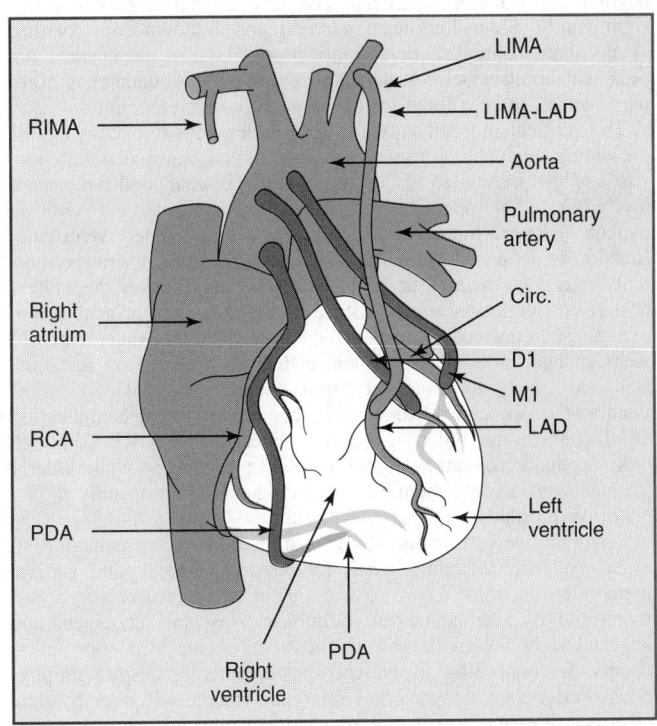

FIGURE 62–1 ■ The classic quadruple coronary bypass operation. Three autogenous saphenous vein grafts are placed from the aorta into the posterior descending coronary artery, a diagonal branch of the left coronary artery, and the circumflex marginal coronary artery. The most important graft is the left internal mammary artery directly applied in situ to the left anterior descending coronary artery. Variations of this theme include the applications of the right internal mammary artery directly to the right coronary artery or the posterior descending coronary artery and the use of other autogenous arterial grafts.

the chest wall bilaterally, supplying blood to the chest wall and breast. These arteries may be dissected off the chest wall and used as a conduit to a coronary artery beyond the blockage, particularly the left anterior descending coronary artery. The advantages of this conduit are a better size relationship to the coronary artery into which it is anastomosed, its natural in situ connection to the subclavian artery obviating a proximal anastomosis, and the major clinical advantage of significantly improved long-term patency over that of any other conduit, thus reducing the need for reoperation. It is the bypass graft of choice, particularly for the left anterior descending coronary artery. More recently, the right internal thoracic artery, the right gastroepiploic artery, and especially the radial artery have been used for autogenous arterial conduits for coronary bypass surgery. Artificial grafts, at the present time, have not been developed to the point that they are satisfactory to maintain long-term patency in 1- to 2-mm coronary arteries.

Operations are performed on cardiopulmonary bypass with moderate systemic hypothermia and using cardioplegic solutions administered both in the ascending aorta (antegrade) and in the coronary sinus (retrograde) to render the heart totally flaccid and motionless, markedly reducing myocardial energy requirements while performing these precise anastomoses. Hemodilution and other blood salvage techniques to minimize blood loss and avoid blood transfusions are extensively used.

Minimally invasive CABG is performed through small incisions, sometimes on the beating heart without concomitant cardiopulmonary bypass, but data as yet are too incomplete to evaluate this new approach. It is currently performed in no more than about 5% of CABG operations. A newer experimental alternative for patients with refractory symptoms but without bypassable vessels is direct myocardial revascularization using surgical or catheter-based lasers to create direct channels between the left ventricular cavity and the ischemic myocardium.

Over the 30 years that CABG has been performed several facts have become clear. Complete revascularization—placing a graft beyond every major significant coronary arterial stenosis—yields significantly better long-term survival and freedom from cardiac events than incomplete revascularization. Thus, in the average patient with multivessel coronary artery disease who undergoes coronary bypass, at least three to four bypass grafts are common.

The surgical mortality after CABG varies with the acuity of the presenting clinical syndromes, the state of left ventricular function, size and diffuseness of the coronary artery disease, and patient comorbidities. The operative mortality in a multivessel CABG in patients younger than 60 years of age with good left ventricular function is about 1%. In acute ischemic syndromes, operative mortality may vary from 2 to 25%, depending on whether the indication is postinfarction angina with a normal ventricle or acute myocardial infarction with cardiogenic shock. Patients older than 70 years of age, particularly women, and those operated on for acute ischemic events have an increased operative risk. The rates of ventilator dependency, stroke, and other organ system complication are higher in the older age group undergoing CABG. Although older patients tolerate elective CABG exceedingly well, elderly patients with acute ischemic syndromes have a significantly higher operative mortality.

Postoperative care of the CABG patient consists of managing all organ systems, including renal, pulmonary, cerebral, and general metabolic functions. Low cardiac output after cardiac surgery is monitored by cardiac output, pulmonary vascular resistance, and left and right ventricular filling pressures. Acute atrial fibrillation occurs in about 30% of patients postoperatively despite prophylaxis. Perioperative myocardial infarction diagnosed either by new electrocardiographic Q waves or significant enzyme elevations occurs in 2 to 5% of cases. Postoperative antiplatelet therapy is important and includes daily aspirin to prevent platelet "stickiness" in the grafts.

One of the major morbid factors associated with patients undergoing CABG is stroke. Stroke rate in the previous decade has been about 7% in the older-than-70 group undergoing CABG, but it has been reduced by the use of a single aortic cross-clamp during the anastomoses to prevent a showering of platelet emboli to the brain. With the use of these techniques, the stroke rate is now 3% or less, but cognitive dysfunction without focal motor defects occurs in another 3% of patients.

CORONARY BYPASS REOPERATIONS

Coronary bypass surgery is palliative. Unless the atheromatous coronary disease is controlled biochemically, symptoms may recur as a result of progression of native disease and/or disease in the bypass grafts, and reoperation may be required. Increased use of the internal thoracic artery bypass graft to at least the left anterior descending artery delays reoperation significantly. Indications for reoperative CABG are similar to primary operative indications, but ischemia should be well documented before undertaking reoperations because the risk is somewhat higher (5 to 8%) and the benefits to be gained are somewhat less than with primary operation. Operative risk is higher, owing to the possibility of myocardial ischemia from manipulating partially obstructed atheromatous grafts and the increased risk of bleeding from adhesions. Currently, by using a "no touch" technique with early onset of femorofemoral cardiopulmonary bypass and improved retrograde cardioplegia myocardial protection, the risk of reoperative surgery has now decreased almost to that of primary operations.

LATE RESULTS OF CORONARY BYPASS SURGERY

The current operative mortality has stabilized at 2 to 5% despite the increased number of aged patients, complexity of disease, numbers of reoperations, left ventricular dysfunction, and extension of the operation to almost all forms of acute myocardial ischemia. The probability of long-term survival and prevention of late cardiac events is also related to the function of the left ventricle, complete revascularization, type of conduits used (internal thoracic arteries vs. saphenous veins), and, to some extent, patient rehabilitation. In general, the 5-year survival rate of patients with multivessel disease completely revascularized is 90 to 95% and the 10-year survival is 85 to 90%. The long-term graft patency is clearly better with an internal thoracic artery than with a saphenous vein (95% vs. 75 to 80% at 5 years). In the long term, patients with left main coronary stenosis or with severe triple-vessel disease and perhaps some forms of two-vessel disease have improved survival and protection from cardiac events over similar patients treated medically (Fig. 62–2). Effects on ventricular function are less easy to document, but it is apparent that the ischemic or "stunned" myocardium may show significant improvements in left ventricular function after CABG, and, moreover, CABG may prevent further deterioration of function in the severely dysfunctional left ventricle.

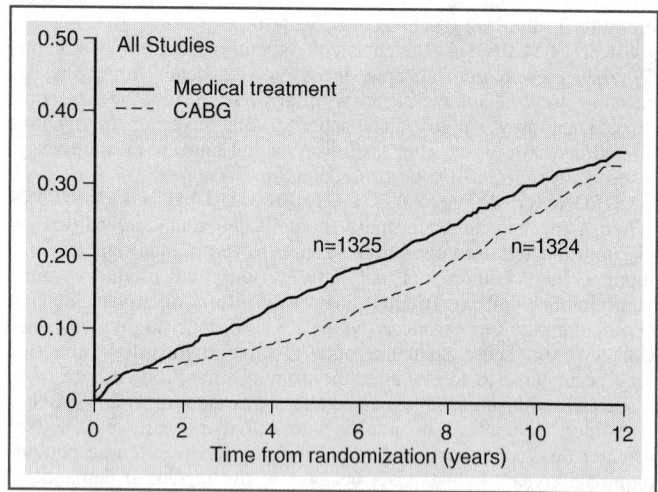

FIGURE 62–2 ■ Survival curve for overall population of patients in seven randomized studies of medical treatment versus coronary artery bypass grafting (CABG) for chronic stable angina. (From Yusuf S, Zucker D, Peduzzi P, et al: Effect of coronary artery bypass graft surgery on survival: Overview of 10-year results from randomised trials by the Coronary Artery Bypass Graft Surgery Trialists Collaboration. Lancet 344:563, 1994.)

American College of Cardiology/American Heart Association: Guidelines and Indications for Coronary Artery Bypass Graft Surgery: A report of the American College of Cardiology/American Heart Association Task Force on Assessment of Diagnostic and Therapeutic Cardiovascular Procedures (Subcommittee on Coronary Artery Bypass). J Am Coll Cardiol 17:543, 1991. *A multispecialty, multiorganizational compendium of the guidelines for performing coronary artery bypass graft surgery. Summarizes medical and surgical literature in 50 comprehensive and authoritative pages of indications for this important operation.*

Borst C, Gründeman PF: Minimally invasive coronary artery bypass grafting: An experimental perspective. Circulation 99: 400–403, 1999. *An update on the potential of this new technique.*

Hlatky MA, Bacon C, Boothroyd D, et al: Cognitive function 5 years after randomization to coronary angioplasty or coronary artery bypass graft surgery. Circulation 96: II–11, 1997.

63 VALVULAR HEART DISEASE

Blase A. Carabello

The cardiac valves permit unobstructed forward blood flow through the heart when they are open while preventing backward flow when they are closed. Most valvular heart diseases cause either valvular stenosis with obstruction to forward flow or valvular regurgitation with backward flow. Valvular stenosis imparts a pressure overload on the left or right ventricle because those chambers must generate higher than normal pressure to overcome the obstruction to pump blood forward. Valvular regurgitation imparts a volume overload on the heart, which now must pump additional volume to compensate for that which is regurgitated. When valve disease is severe, these hemodynamic burdens can lead to ventricular dysfunction, heart failure, and sudden death (Table 63–1). In almost every instance, the definitive therapy for severe valvular heart disease is mechanical restoration of valve function.

AORTIC STENOSIS

ETIOLOGY. BICUSPID AND OTHER CONGENITALLY ABNORMAL AORTIC VALVES. Approximately 1% of the population is born with a bicuspid aortic valve; there is a male predominance (see Chapter 57). Whereas this abnormality usually does not cause a hemodynamic disturbance at birth, bicuspid aortic valves tend to deteriorate with age. Approximately one third of such valves become stenotic, another third become regurgitant, and the remainder cause only minor hemodynamic abnormalities. The initial insult responsible for bicuspid aortic valve stenosis is unknown, but eventually thickening and calcification of the leaflets inhibit opening and stenosis develops, usually in the fourth, fifth, and sixth decades of life.

Sometimes congenital aortic stenosis from a unicuspid, bicuspid, or even abnormal tricuspid valve causes symptoms during childhood and requires correction by adolescence. Occasionally, these congenitally stenotic aortic valves escape detection until adulthood, and the diagnosis is then usually made in the third and fourth decades of life.

TRICUSPID AORTIC VALVE STENOSIS. Some patients born with apparently normal tricuspid aortic valves develop thickening and calcification similar to that which occurs in bicuspid valves. When aortic stenosis develops in previously normal tricuspid aortic valves, it usually does so in the sixth to eighth decades of life. Why previously normal aortic valves degenerate in some patients but not in others is unknown. However, the initial lesion has many characteristics of an atherosclerotic plaque, and there is some association between tricuspid aortic valve stenosis and risk factors for atherosclerotic coronary heart disease.

RHEUMATIC VALVULAR HEART DISEASE. Rheumatic valve disease is now a rare cause of aortic stenosis in developed countries. In virtually every case, the mitral valve is also detectably abnormal.

PATHOPHYSIOLOGY AND ITS RELATIONSHIP TO SYMPTOMS. The presence or absence of the classic symptoms of aortic stenosis—angina, syncope, and the symptoms of heart failure—is the key to the natural history of the disease. Before the onset of symptoms, survival is similar to that for the normal population and sudden death is rare. However, once the classic symptoms develop, survival declines precipitously. Approximately 35% of patients with aortic stenosis present with angina. Of these, 50% will be dead in 5 years unless aortic valve replacement is performed. Approximately

15% present with syncope; of these, 50% will be dead in only 3 years unless the aortic valve is replaced. Of the 50% who present with the symptoms of congestive heart failure, 50% will be dead in 2 years without aortic valve replacement. In all, only 25% of patients with symptomatic aortic stenosis survive 3 years in the absence of valve replacement, and the annual risk of sudden death ranges from 10% in patients with angina to 15% with syncope to 25% with heart failure. Prompt recognition of symptoms and evaluation for possible severe aortic stenosis is crucial in managing the disease.

The normal aortic valve area is 3 to 4 cm², and little hemodynamic disturbance occurs until the orifice is reduced to about one third of normal, at which time a systolic gradient develops between the left ventricle and aorta. Left ventricular and aortic pressures normally are nearly equal during systole. However, in aortic stenosis, intercavitary left ventricular pressure must increase above aortic pressure to produce forward flow across the stenotic valve and to achieve an acceptable downstream pressure (see Fig. 46–1). There is a geometric progression in the magnitude of the gradient as the valve area narrows. Given a normal cardiac output, the gradient rises rapidly from 10 to 15 mm Hg at valve areas of 1.5 to 1.3 cm² to about 25 mm Hg at 1.0 cm², 50 mm Hg at 0.8 cm², 70 mm Hg at 0.6 cm², and 100 mm Hg at 0.5 cm². The rate of progression of aortic stenosis varies widely from patient to patient; it may remain stable for many years or increase as rapidly as 15 mm Hg per year.

A major compensatory response to the increased left ventricular pressure of aortic stenosis is the development of concentric left ventricular hypertrophy. The Laplace equation, stress (s) = pressure (p) × radius (r)/2 × thickness (th), indicates that the force on any unit of left ventricular myocardium (afterload) varies directly with ventricular pressure and radius and inversely with wall thickness. Thus, as pressure increases, it can be offset by increased left ventricular wall thickness (concentric hypertrophy). The determinants of left ventricular ejection fraction are contractility, preload, and afterload. By normalizing afterload, the development of concentric hypertrophy helps preserve ejection fraction and cardiac output despite the pressure overload. However, although hypertrophy clearly serves a compensatory function, it also has a pathologic role and is in part responsible for the classic symptoms of aortic stenosis.

ANGINA. In general, angina occurs from myocardial ischemia when left ventricular oxygen (and other nutrient) demand exceeds supply, which is predicated on coronary blood flow. In normal subjects, coronary blood flow can increase 5- to 8-fold under maximum metabolic demand, but in aortic stenosis this reserve is limited. Reduced coronary blood flow reserve may be caused by a relative diminution of capillary ingrowth to serve the needs of the hypertrophied left ventricle or by a reduced transcoronary gradient for coronary blood flow because of the elevated left ventricular end-diastolic pressure. Restricted coronary blood flow reserve appears responsible for angina in many patients who have aortic stenosis despite normal epicardial coronary arteries. In other patients, angina is due to increased oxygen demand when inadequate hypertrophy allows wall stress, a key determinant of myocardial oxygen consumption, to increase.

SYNCOPE. Syncope usually occurs because of inadequate cerebral perfusion. In aortic stenosis, syncope is usually related to exertion. It may result when exertion causes a fall in total peripheral resistance that cannot be compensated by increased cardiac output because output is limited by the obstruction to left ventricular outflow; this combination reduces systemic blood pressure and cerebral perfusion. In addition, high left ventricular pressures during exercise may trigger a systemic vasodepressor response that lowers blood pressure and produces syncope. Cardiac arrhythmias, possibly caused by exertional ischemia, also cause hypotension and syncope.

HEART FAILURE. In aortic stenosis, both contractile dysfunction (systolic failure) and failure of normal relaxation (diastolic failure) occur and cause symptoms. The extent of ventricular contraction is governed by contractility and afterload. In aortic stenosis, contractility (the ability to generate force) is often reduced. The mechanisms of contractile dysfunction may include abnormal calcium handling, microtubular hyperpolymerization causing an internal viscous load on the myocyte, and myocardial ischemia. In some cases, contractile function is normal but hypertrophy is inadequate to

Table 63–1 ■ SUMMARY OF SEVERE VALVULAR HEART DISEASE

	AORTIC STENOSIS	MITRAL STENOSIS	MITRAL REGURGITATION	AORTIC REGURGITATION
Etiology	Idiopathic calcification of a bicuspid or tricuspid valve Congenital Rheumatic	Rheumatic fever Annular calcification	Mitral valve prolapse Ruptured chordae Endocarditis Ischemic papillary muscle dysfunction or rupture Collagen vascular diseases and syndromes Secondary to LV myocardial diseases	Annuloaortic ectasia Hypertension Endocarditis Marfan syndrome Ankylosing spondylitis Aortic dissection Syphilis Collagen vascular disease
Pathophysiology	Pressure overload upon the LV with compensation by LV hypertrophy. As disease advances, reduced coronary flow reserve causes angina. Hypertrophy and afterload excess lead to both systolic and diastolic LV dysfunction.	Obstruction to LV inflow increases left atrial pressure and limits cardiac output mimicking LV failure. Mitral valve obstruction increases the pressure work of the right ventricle. Right ventricular pressure overload is augmented further when pulmonary hypertension develops.	Places volume overload on the LV. Ventricle responds with eccentric hypertrophy and dilatation, which allow for increased ventricular stroke volume. Eventually, however, LV dysfunction develops if volume overload is uncorrected.	*Chronic* Total stroke volume causes hyperdynamic circulation, induces systolic hypertension and thus causes both pressure and volume overload. Compensation is by both concentric and eccentric hypertrophy. *Acute* Because cardiac dilation has not developed, hyperdynamic findings are absent. High diastolic LV pressure causes mitral valve preclosure and potentiates LV ischemia and failure.
Symptoms	Angina Syncope Heart failure	Dyspnea Orthopnea PND Hemoptysis Hoarseness Edema Ascites	Dyspnea Orthopnea PND	Dyspnea Orthopnea PND Angina Syncope
Signs	Systolic ejection murmur radiating to neck Delayed carotid upstroke S$_4$, soft or paradoxic S$_2$	Diastolic rumble following an opening snap Loud S$_1$ Right ventricular lift Loud P$_2$	Holosystolic apical murmur radiates to axilla, S$_3$ Displaced PMI	*Chronic* Diastolic blowing murmur Hyperdynamic circulation Displaced PMI Quincke pulse DeMusset's sign, etc. *Acute* Short diastolic blowing murmur Soft S$_1$
ECG	LAA LVH	LAA RVH	LAA LVH	LAA LVH
Chest Radiograph	Boot-shaped heart Aortic valve calcification on lateral view	Straightening of left heart border Double density at right heart border Kerley B lines Enlarged pulmonary arteries	Cardiac enlargement	*Chronic* Cardiac enlargement Uncoiling of the aorta *Acute* Pulmonary congestion with normal heart size
Echocardiographic Findings	Concentric LVH Reduced aortic valve cusp separation Doppler shows mean gradient ≥ 50 mm Hg in most severe cases	Restricted mitral leaflet motion Valve area ≤ 1.0 cm^2 in most severe cases Tricuspid Doppler may reveal pulmonary hypertension	LV and left atrial enlargement in chronic severe disease Doppler: large regurgitant jet	*Chronic* LV enlargement Large Doppler jet PHT < 400 msec *Acute* Small LV, mitral valve preclosure
Catheterization Findings	Increased LVEDP Transaortic gradient 50 mm Hg AVA ≤ 0.7 in most severe cases	Elevated pulmonary capillary wedge pressure Transmitral gradient usually >10 mm Hg in severe cases MVA < 1.0 cm^2	Elevated pulmonary capillary wedge pressure Ventriculography shows regurgitation of dye into left ventricle	Wide pulse pressure Aortography shows regurgitation of dye into LV Usually unnecessary
Medical Therapy	Avoid vasodilators Digitalis, diuretics, and nitroglycerin in inoperable cases	Diuretics for mild symptoms Anticoagulation in atrial fibrillation Digitalis, β-blockers, verapamil or diltiazem for rate control	Vasodilators in acute disease No proven therapy in chronic disease (but vasodilators commonly used)	*Chronic* Vasodilators in chronic asymptomatic disease with normal left ventricular function *Acute* Vasodilators
Indications for Surgery	Appearance of symptoms in patients with severe disease (see text)	Appearance of more than mild symptoms Development of pulmonary hypertension Appearance of persistent atrial fibrillation	Appearance of symptoms EF < 0.60 ESD ≥ 45 min	*Chronic* Appearance of symptoms EF < 0.55 ESD ≥ 55 min *Acute* Even mild heart failure Mitral valve preclosure

AVA = aortic valve area; EF = ejection fraction; ESD = end-systolic diameter; LAA = left atrial enlargement; LV = left ventricle; LVEDP = left ventricular end-diastolic pressure; LVH = left ventricular hypertrophy; MS = mitral stenosis; MVA = mitral valve area; PMI = point of maximal impulse; PND = paroxysmal nocturnal dyspnea; PHT = pressure half-time; RVH = right ventricular hypertrophy.

normalize wall stress and leads to excessive afterload. Excessive afterload in turn inhibits ejection, reduces forward output, and leads to heart failure.

The increased wall thickness that helps to normalize stress unfortunately increases diastolic stiffness. Even if muscle properties remain normal, higher filling pressure is required to distend a thicker ventricle. As aortic stenosis advances, collagen deposition also stiffens the myocardium and adds to the diastolic dysfunction.

DIAGNOSIS. PHYSICAL EXAMINATION. The diagnosis of aortic stenosis is usually first suspected when the classic systolic ejection murmur is heard during physical examination. The murmur is loudest in the aortic area and radiates to the neck. In some cases, the murmur may disappear over the sternum and reappear over the left ventricular apex giving the false impression that the murmur of mitral regurgitation is also present (Gallivardan's phenomenon). The intensity of the murmur increases with cycle length because longer cycles are associated with greater aortic flow. In mild disease, the murmur peaks in intensity in early or mid systole. As stenosis severity worsens, the murmur peaks progressively later in systole. Perhaps the most helpful clue to the severity of aortic stenosis by physical examination is the characteristic delay in the carotid pulse with the diminution in its volume (see Fig. 38–2); in elderly patients, however, increasing carotid stiffness may pseudo-normalize the carotid upstrokes. The left ventricular apical impulse in aortic stenosis is not displaced but is enlarged and forceful. The simultaneous palpation of a forceful left ventricular apex beat together with a delayed and weakened carotid pulse are persuasive clues that severe aortic stenosis is present. The S_1 in aortic stenosis is usually normal. In congenital aortic stenosis when the valve is not calcified, S_1 may be followed by a systolic ejection click. In calcific disease, S_2 may be single and soft when the aortic component is lost because the valve neither opens nor closes well. In some cases, delayed left ventricular emptying due to left ventricular dysfunction may create paradoxical splitting of S_2. An S_4 gallop is common. In advanced disease, pulmonary hypertension and signs of right-sided failure are surprisingly common.

Because of the dire consequences of missing the diagnosis of symptomatic aortic stenosis, the physician must have a low threshold for obtaining an echocardiogram whenever the possibility of aortic stenosis cannot be excluded by physical examination. Asymptomatic patients with suspicious murmurs benefit from early diagnosis to allow both the patient and the physician to be more vigilant regarding possible early signs and symptoms and to guide the use of prophylactic regimens to prevent bacterial endocarditis (see Chapter 326).

NON-INVASIVE EVALUATION. The electrocardiogram in aortic stenosis usually demonstrates left ventricular hypertrophy. However, in some cases of even severe aortic stenosis, electrocardiographic left ventricular hypertrophy is absent, possibly owing to the lack of left ventricular dilatation. Left atrial abnormality is common because the stiff left ventricle increases left atrial afterload and causes the left atrium to dilate.

The chest radiograph in aortic stenosis is usually non-diagnostic. The cardiac silhouette is usually not enlarged but may assume a boot-shaped configuration. In advanced cases there may be signs of cardiomegaly and pulmonary congestion; aortic valve calcification may be seen in the lateral view.

Echocardiography. Echocardiography is indispensable to assess the extent of left ventricular hypertrophy, systolic ejection performance, and aortic valve anatomy (Fig. 63–1). Doppler interrogation of the aortic valve makes use of the modified Bernoulli equation (gradient = 4 × velocity^2) to assess the severity of the stenosis. As blood flows from the body of the left ventricle across the stenotic valve, the flow rate must accelerate for the volume to remain constant. Doppler interrogation of the valve detects this increase in velocity to estimate the valve gradient.

CARDIAC CATHETERIZATION. When echocardiography demonstrates severe aortic stenosis and the patient has one or more of the classic symptoms of the disease, aortic valve replacement should be performed. Because most patients with aortic stenosis are of the age in which coronary disease is common, cardiac catheterization to perform coronary arteriography is usually accomplished before surgery. When the hemodynamic diagnosis is unclear, right- and left-sided heart catheterization should be performed to obtain a transaortic valvular pressure gradient and cardiac output, which are used to calculate the aortic valve area by the Gorlin formula:

$$A = \frac{CO/SEP \times HR}{44.3 \sqrt{h}}$$

where CO = cardiac output (mL/min), SEP = systolic ejection period (sec), HR = heart rate, and h = mean gradient.

THERAPY. SURGERY. The only effective therapy for aortic stenosis is aortic valve replacement. As noted earlier, once the symptoms of aortic stenosis develop, the 3-year mortality is 75% without aortic valve replacement. However, once the valve is replaced, survivorship returns nearly to normal. Even octogenarians benefit

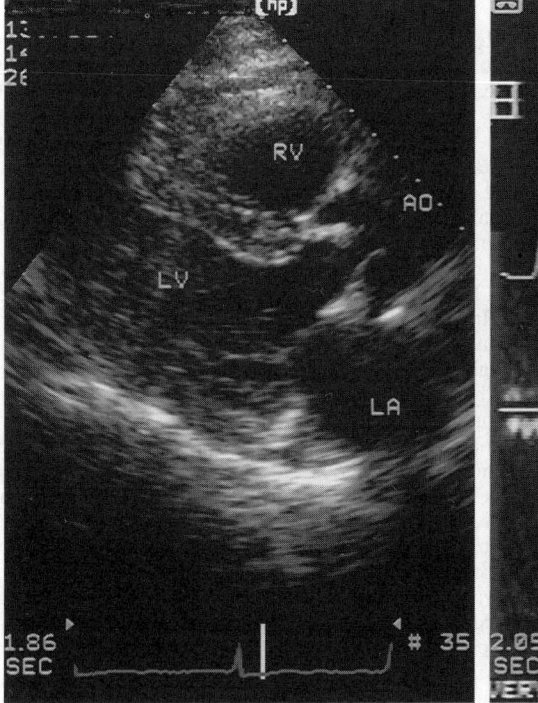
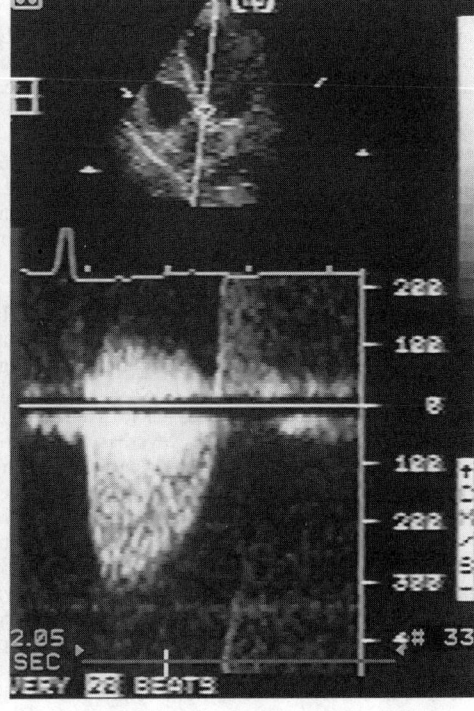

FIGURE 63–1 ■ Doppler echocardiogram obtained in a patient with aortic stenosis. The left panel shows thickened aortic valve leaflets that dome into the aorta with restricted opening in systole. The right panel shows a miniaturized apical four-chamber view at top with Doppler cursor through the aorta, while the bottom panel shows a continuous-wave spectral Doppler signal with a peak velocity of 3 m/sec. The peak valve gradient can be calculated as 4 × 3^2 or 36 mm Hg. (Courtesy of Dr. Anthony DeMaria.)

from valve replacement unless other co-morbid factors preclude surgery, so aortic valve replacement should not be denied simply on the basis of age, nor should valve replacement be denied because ejection fraction is reduced; the excess afterload imposed by the stenotic valve is relieved with valve replacement, and depressed ejection performance usually improves dramatically after surgery. The exception to this rule is severely reduced ejection fraction in the face of only a small aortic valve gradient where the severity of the aortic stenosis may be overestimated because of the failing left ventricle has difficulty opening a mildly to moderately stenotic valve. In such cases, left ventricular muscle dysfunction either has another cause or is often so severe that it does not recover after valve replacement.

BALLOON AORTIC VALVOTOMY. In acquired calcific aortic stenosis, leaflet restriction results from heavy calcium deposition in the leaflets themselves and is not due to commissural fusion. Thus, balloon aortic valvotomy is relatively ineffective in improving aortic stenosis, usually resulting in a residual gradient of 30 to 50 mm Hg and a valve area of 1.0 cm². Mortality after this procedure is similar to that of untreated patients. Thus, balloon aortic valvotomy is only used palliatively in cases in which aortic valve replacement is impossible because of co-morbidity or impractical when immediate temporary relief is required because of the demands of other non-cardiac conditions.

MEDICAL THERAPY. The only medical therapy indicated in aortic stenosis is antibiotic prophylaxis to prevent bacterial endocarditis (see Chapter 326). Otherwise, the patient either is asymptomatic and requires no therapy or is symptomatic and requires surgery. In patients with heart failure awaiting surgery, diuretics can be used cautiously to relieve pulmonary congestion. Nitrates may also be used carefully to treat angina pectoris. Although vasodilators, especially angiotensin-converting enzyme inhibitors, have become a cornerstone of the therapy for heart failure, they are not recommended in aortic stenosis. With fixed valvular obstruction to outflow, vasodilation reduces pressure distal to the obstruction without increasing cardiac output and may cause syncope. When surgery and valvoplasty are unsuccessful or impossible, digitalis and diuretics can be used to improve symptoms with the understanding that they will not improve life expectancy.

MITRAL STENOSIS

ETIOLOGY. In almost all cases of acquired mitral stenosis, the cause is rheumatic heart disease. Occasionally, severe calcification of the mitral annulus can lead to mitral stenosis in the absence of rheumatic involvement. Mitral stenosis is three times more common in women and usually develops in the fourth and fifth decades of life. Although the disease has become rare in developed countries because of the waning incidence of rheumatic fever, mitral stenosis is still prevalent in developing nations where rheumatic fever is common.

PATHOPHYSIOLOGY. At the beginning of diastole, a transient gradient between the left atrium and left ventricle normally initiates left ventricular filling. After early filling, left atrial and left ventricular pressures equilibrate. In mitral stenosis, obstruction to left ventricular filling increases left atrial pressure and produces a persistent gradient between the left atrium and the left ventricle (see Fig. 46–1). The combination of elevated left atrial pressure (and therefore pulmonary venous pressure) and restriction of inflow into the left ventricle limits cardiac output. Although myocardial involvement from the rheumatic process occasionally affects left ventricular muscle function, the muscle itself is normal in most patients with mitral stenosis. However, in approximately one third of patients with mitral stenosis, left ventricular ejection performance is reduced despite normal muscle function, owing to reduced preload (from inflow obstruction) and increased afterload due to reflex vasoconstriction caused by reduced cardiac output.

Because the right ventricle generates most of the force that propels blood across the mitral valve, the right ventricle incurs the pressure overload of the transmitral gradient. In addition, secondary but reversible pulmonary vasoconstriction develops, further increasing pulmonary artery pressure and the burden on the right ventricle. As mitral stenosis worsens, right ventricular failure develops.

DIAGNOSIS. HISTORY. Patients with mitral stenosis usually remain asymptomatic until the valve area is reduced to about one third its normal size of 4 to 5 cm². Then the symptoms typical of left-sided failure—dyspnea on exertion, orthopnea, and paroxysmal nocturnal dyspnea—develop. As the disease progresses and right ventricular failure occurs, ascites and edema are common. Hemoptysis, which is common in mitral stenosis but uncommon in other causes of left atrial hypertension, develops when high left atrial pressure ruptures anastomoses of small bronchial veins. In some cases, a very large left atrium may impinge on the left recurrent laryngeal nerve, causing hoarseness (Ortner's syndrome), or may impinge on the esophagus, causing dysphagia.

PHYSICAL EXAMINATION. Although mitral stenosis produces a typical and diagnostic physical examination, the diagnosis is frequently missed because the auscultatory findings may be subtle. Palpation of the precordium finds a quiet apical impulse. If pulmonary hypertension and right ventricular hypertrophy have developed, the examiner will note a parasternal lift. S_1 is typically loud and may be the most prominent physical finding of the disease. A loud S_1 is present because the transmitral gradient holds the mitral valve open throughout diastole until ventricular systole closes the fully opened valve with a loud closing sound. In far-advanced disease, however, the mitral valve may be so damaged that it neither opens nor closes well, so S_1 may become soft. S_2 is normally split; the pulmonic component is increased in intensity if pulmonary hypertension has developed. Left-sided S_3 and S_4 gallop sounds, which represent the ventricular and atrial components of rapid left ventricular filling, are exceedingly rare in mitral stenosis because obstruction at the mitral valve prevents rapid filling. S_2 is usually followed by an opening snap. The distance between S_2 and the opening snap provides a reasonable estimation of left atrial pressure and therefore an estimate of the severity of the mitral stenosis. The higher the left atrial pressure, the sooner the left atrial pressure and the falling left ventricular pressure of early ventricular relaxation equilibrate. It is at this equilibration point that the mitral valve opens and the opening snap occurs. Thus, when left atrial pressure is high, the opening snap closely (0.06 sec) follows S_2. Conversely, when left atrial pressure is relatively normal, the snap occurs later (0.12 sec) and may mimic the cadence of an S_3 gallop. The opening snap is followed by the classic low-pitched early-diastolic mitral stenosis rumble, which increases in length as the mitral stenosis worsens. This murmur can be inaudible if the patient has a relatively low resting cardiac output. However, modest exercise, such as isometric handgrip, may accentuate the murmur's intensity. If the patient is in sinus rhythm, atrial systole may produce a presystolic accentuation of the murmur. If pulmonary hypertension has developed, the pulmonic component of S_2 will increase in intensity to become as loud or louder than the aortic component. With pulmonary hypertension, a diastolic blowing murmur of pulmonary insufficiency (Graham Steell) is often heard, although in many cases a coexistent murmur of mild aortic insufficiency is mistaken for this murmur. Neck vein elevation, ascites, and edema will be present if right ventricular failure has developed.

NON-INVASIVE EVALUATION. If the patient is in sinus rhythm, left atrial abnormality is usually present on the electrocardiogram. However, atrial fibrillation is common. If pulmonary hypertension has developed, there is often evidence of right ventricular hypertrophy.

On the chest radiograph, left atrial enlargement produces straightening of the left heart border and a double density at the right heart border owing to the combined silhouettes of the right atrium and left atrium. Pulmonary venous hypertension produces increased vascularity. Kerley B lines, which represent thickening of the pulmonary septa due to chronic venous engorgement, may also be seen.

The echocardiogram produces excellent images of the mitral valve and is the most important diagnostic tool in confirming the diagnosis (Fig. 63–2). Transthoracic echocardiography or, if necessary, transesophageal echocardiography will make the diagnosis in nearly 100% of cases and accurately assess its severity. Mitral stenosis, like aortic stenosis, can be quantified by assessing the transvalvular gradient using the modified Bernoulli principle. The stenosis is considered mild when the calculated or planimetered valve area is more than 1.75 cm², moderate at 1.25 to 1.75 cm², moderately severe at 1.0 to 1.25 cm², and severe at less than 1.0 cm².

FIGURE 63-2 ■ An en fosse view of a stenotic mitral valve in the short-axis view of the left ventricle is shown on the left. Planimetry for the mitral valve orifice yielded an area of 1.09 cm². The M-mode echocardiogram on the right has been aligned with the appropriate structures on the left. It demonstrates the restricted opening of the mitral valve in diastole associated with the classic diastolic rumbling murmur. (From Assey ME, Usher BW, Carabello BA: The patient with valvular heart disease. In Pepine CJ, Hill JA, Lambert CR [eds]: Diagnostic and Therapeutic Cardiac Catheterization, 2nd ed, p 709. Baltimore, Williams & Wilkins, 1994.)

During echocardiography, the suitability of the valve for balloon valvotomy can also be assessed (see later). If even mild tricuspid regurgitation is present, the systolic gradient across the tricuspid valve can be used to gauge the pulmonary artery pressure, which is an important prognostic factor in mitral stenosis because prognosis worsens as pulmonary pressure increases.

CARDIAC CATHETERIZATION. Cardiac catheterization is usually unnecessary to assess the severity of mitral stenosis. However, because many patients with mitral stenosis are of an age when coronary disease might be present, coronary arteriography is usually performed if cardiac surgery is anticipated or if the patient has coexistent angina. In such cases, it is not uncommon to perform left- and right-sided heart catheterizations to confirm the transmitral gradient and to calculate the valve area from the Gorlin formula (see earlier).

THERAPY. MEDICAL THERAPY. Asymptomatic patients with mitral stenosis and sinus rhythm require no therapy. Symptoms of mild dyspnea and orthopnea can be treated with diuretics alone. Once symptoms worsen to more than mild, or if pulmonary hypertension develops, mechanical correction of the stenosis rather than medical therapy is preferable because mechanical intervention improves longevity in severely symptomatic patients.

Patients with mitral stenosis who develop atrial fibrillation usually decompensate because the rapid heart rate reduces diastolic filling time and in turn increases left atrial pressure and decreases cardiac output. Therefore, the heart rate must be controlled promptly, preferably with an infusion of diltiazem or esmolol for acute atrial fibrillation or with oral digoxin, a β-blocker, or a calcium channel blocker in chronic atrial fibrillation. Once rate is controlled, anticoagulation and conversion to sinus rhythm should be undertaken either pharmacologically or with direct-current countershock (see Chapter 51). If sinus rhythm cannot be maintained, mechanical intervention is usually done with the hope that sinus rhythm can be restored after the obstruction to atrial outflow is corrected.

Because patients with concomitant mitral stenosis and atrial fibrillation have an extraordinarily high risk of systemic embolism, they are anticoagulated with warfarin, targeting an international normalized ratio (INR) of 2.5 to 3.5. Anticoagulation is warranted in all such patients unless there is a serious contraindication to its use.

MECHANICAL THERAPY. Once symptoms progress past early New York Heart Association Class II, that is, symptoms with more than ordinary activity, or if pulmonary hypertension develops, prognosis is reduced unless the mitral stenosis is relieved. In most instances, an excellent result can be obtained from percutaneous balloon val-

votomy. Unlike aortic stenosis, in mitral stenosis there is fusion of the valve leaflets at the commissures. Balloon dilatation produces a commissurotomy and a substantial increase in valve area that appears to persist for at least a decade. Suitability for balloon valvotomy is partially determined during echocardiography. Patients with pliable valves, little valvular calcification, little involvement of the subvalvular apparatus, and less than moderate mitral regurgitation are ideal candidates. However, even when valve anatomy is not ideal, valvotomy may be attempted in cases of advanced age or in situations in which co-morbid risk factors increase surgical risk. In otherwise healthy patients with unfavorable valve anatomy, surgery to perform an open commissurotomy or valve replacement is undertaken.

MITRAL REGURGITATION

ETIOLOGY. The mitral valve is composed of the mitral annulus, the leaflets, the chordae tendineae, and the papillary muscles. Abnormalities of any of these structures may lead to mitral regurgitation. The most common cause of mitral regurgitation in the United States is mitral valve prolapse, which is responsible for approximately two thirds of all cases and comprises a number of diseases including myxomatous degeneration of the valve. Myocardial ischemia leading to papillary muscle dysfunction or infarction is the next most common cause, accounting for approximately a fourth of all cases. Annular calcification, endocarditis, collagen vascular disease, and rheumatic heart disease are less common causes. Recently, use of the weight loss agents dexfenfluramine, fenfluramine, and possibly phentermine has been implicated in causing valve damage.

Mitral regurgitation can be subdivided on the basis of chronicity. Common causes of severe acute mitral regurgitation include ruptured chordae tendineae, ischemic papillary muscle dysfunction or rupture, and infective endocarditis. Chronic severe mitral regurgitation is more likely to be due to myxomatous degeneration of the valve, rheumatic heart disease, or annular calcification.

PATHOPHYSIOLOGY. The pathophysiology of mitral regurgitation can be divided into three phases, as shown in Figure 63-3. In acute mitral regurgitation of any cause, the sudden option for ejection of blood into the left atrium "wastes" a portion of the left ventricular stroke volume as backward rather than forward flow. The combined regurgitant and forward flows cause a volume overload of the left ventricle, stretching existing sarcomeres toward their maximum length. Thus, use of the Frank-Starling mechanism is maximized, and end-diastolic volume increases concomitantly.

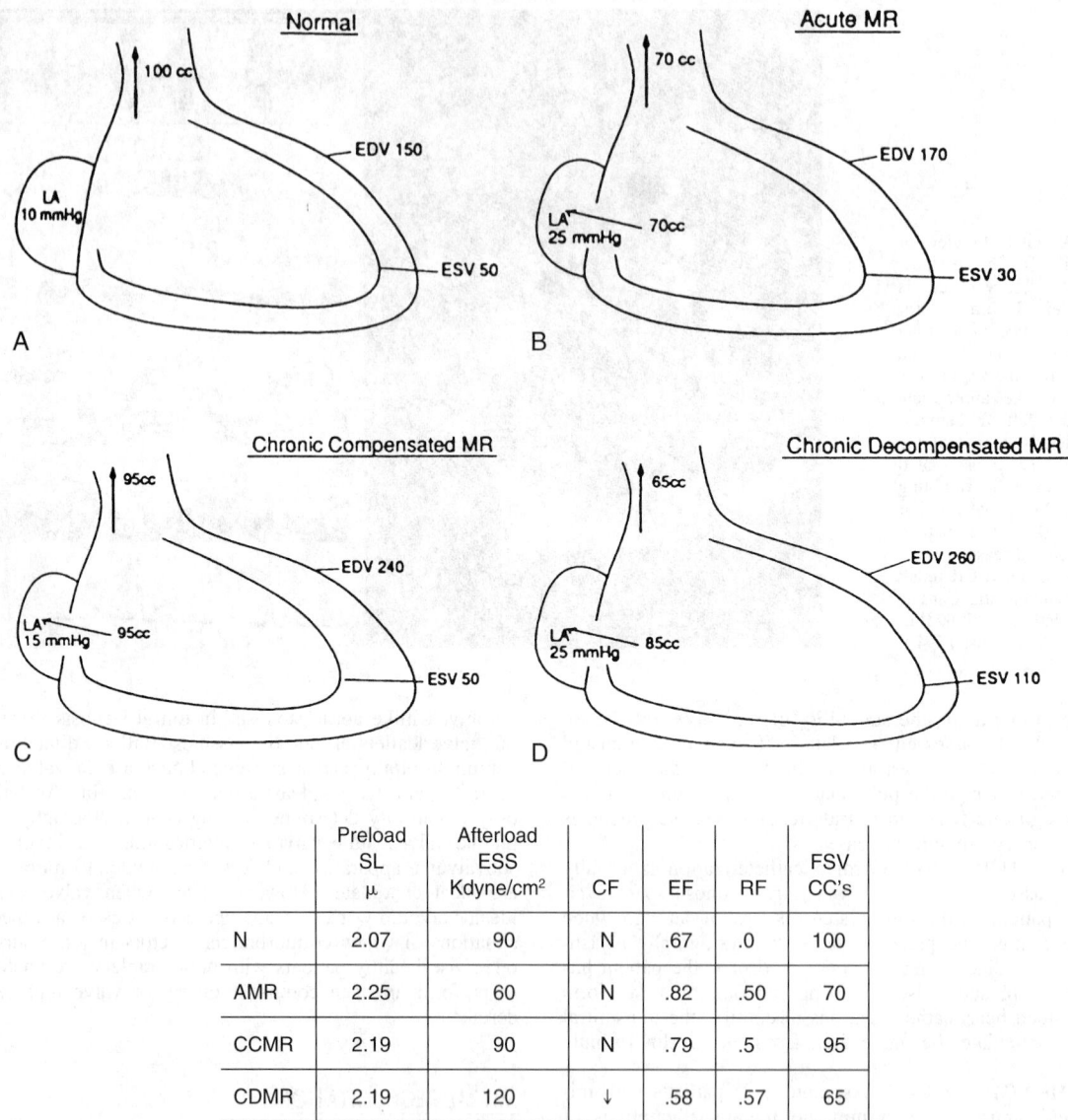

	Preload SL μ	Afterload ESS Kdyne/cm²	CF	EF	RF	FSV CC's
N	2.07	90	N	.67	.0	100
AMR	2.25	60	N	.82	.50	70
CCMR	2.19	90	N	.79	.5	95
CDMR	2.19	120	↓	.58	.57	65

FIGURE 63-3 ■ *Panel A:* Normal physiology (N) is compared with *panel B:* physiology of acute mitral regurgitation (AMR). Acutely the volume overload increases preload (sarcomere length, SL) and end-diastolic volume (EDV) increases from 150 to 170 mL. Unloading of the left ventricle by the presence of the regurgitant pathway decreases afterload (end-systolic stress [ESS]) and end-systolic volume (ESV) falls from 50 to 30 mL. These changes result in an increase in ejection fraction (EF). However, because 50% of the total left ventricular stroke volume (regurgitant fraction [RF]) is ejected into the left atrium (LA), forward stroke volume (FSV) falls from 100 to 70 mL. At this stage, contractile function (CF) remains normal. *Panel C:* Chronic compensated mitral regurgitation (CCMR). In this phase of mitral regurgitation, eccentric cardiac hypertrophy has developed and end-diastolic volume has increased substantially. Increased end-diastolic volume combined with normal contractile function permits ejection of a larger total stroke volume and therefore a larger forward stroke volume than in the acute phase. Left atrial enlargement permits lower left atrial pressure. Because the radius term in the Laplace equation has increased with increasing left ventricular volume, afterload and end-systolic volume return to normal. *Panel D:* Chronic decompensated mitral regurgitation (CDMR). In this stage, contractile dysfunction causes a large increase in end-systolic volume with a fall in both total and forward stroke volume. Additional left ventricular enlargement leads to worsening mitral regurgitation. However, the relatively favorable loading conditions in this phase still permit a normal ejection fraction despite contractile dysfunction. (From Carabello BA: Mitral regurgitation: I. Basic pathophysiologic principles. Mod Concepts Cardiovasc Dis 57[10]:57, 1988.)

The regurgitant pathway unloads the left ventricle in systole because it allows ejection into the relatively low impedance left atrium, in turn reducing end-systolic volume. Although increased end-diastolic volume and decreased end-systolic volume both act in concert to increase total stroke volume, forward stroke volume is subnormal because a large portion of the total stroke volume is regurgitated into the left atrium. This regurgitant volume increases left atrial pressure, so the patient experiences heart failure with low cardiac output and pulmonary congestion despite normal left ventricular contractile function.

In many cases, severe acute mitral regurgitation necessitates emergent surgical correction. However, patients who can be managed through the acute phase may then enter the phase of compen-

sation. In this phase, eccentric left ventricular hypertrophy and increased end-diastolic volume, combined with normal contractile function, allow for ejection of a sufficiently large total stroke volume to allow forward stroke volume to return toward normal. Left atrial enlargement allows for accommodation of the regurgitant volume at a lower filling pressure. In this phase, the patient may be relatively asymptomatic even during rather strenuous exercise.

While severe mitral regurgitation may be tolerated for many years, the lesion eventually causes left ventricular dysfunction. The now damaged ventricle has impaired ejection performance and end-systolic volume increases. In turn, greater left ventricular residual volume at end-systole increases end-diastolic volume and end-diastolic pressure, and the symptoms of pulmonary congestion may reappear. Additional left ventricular dilatation may worsen the amount of regurgitation by causing further enlargement of the mitral annulus and malalignment of the papillary muscles. Although there is substantial contractile dysfunction, the increased preload and the presence of the regurgitant pathway, which tends to normalize afterload despite ventricular enlargement, augment ejection fraction and may maintain it in a relatively normal range.

The causes of left ventricular contractile dysfunction in mitral regurgitation may relate to loss of contractile proteins and abnormalities in calcium handling. In at least some cases, contractile dysfunction is reversible by timely mitral valve replacement.

DIAGNOSIS. The standard symptoms of left-sided congestive heart failure should be sought. An attempt to discover potential causes should be made by questioning for a prior history of a heart murmur or abnormal cardiac examination, rheumatic heart disease, endocarditis, myocardial infarction, or the use of anorexigenic drugs.

PHYSICAL EXAMINATION. Volume overload of the left ventricle displaces the apical impulse downward and to the left. S_1 may be reduced in intensity, whereas S_2 is usually physiologically split. In severe mitral regurgitation, S_2 is followed by S_3, which does not necessarily indicate heart failure but reflects rapid filling of the left ventricle by the large volume of blood stored in the left atrium during systole. The typical murmur of mitral regurgitation is a holosystolic apical murmur that often radiates toward the axilla. There is a rough correlation between the intensity of the murmur and the severity of the disease, but this correlation is too weak to use in clinical decision making because the murmur may be soft when cardiac output is low. Unlike aortic stenosis, the murmur intensity usually does not vary with the RR interval. In acute mitral regurgitation, the presence of a large V wave may produce rapid equilibration of left atrial and left ventricular pressure, reducing the driving gradient and shortening the murmur. Pulmonary hypertension may develop and produce right-sided signs including a right ventricular lift, increased P_2, and, if right ventricular dysfunction has developed, signs of right-sided heart failure.

NON-INVASIVE EVALUATION. The electrocardiogram usually shows left ventricular hypertrophy and left atrial abnormality. The chest radiograph usually demonstrates cardiomegaly; the absence of cardiomegaly indicates either that the mitral regurgitation is mild or that it has not been chronic enough to allow cardiac dilatation to occur.

Echocardiography demonstrates the extent of left atrial and left ventricular enlargement. Ultrasonic imaging of the mitral valve is excellent and therefore offers clues to the mitral valve abnormalities responsible for the regurgitation. Color flow Doppler interrogation of the valve helps assess the severity of regurgitation, but since this technique images flow velocity rather than actual flow, it is subject to errors in interpretation. The Doppler technique is excellent for excluding the presence of mitral regurgitation and for distinguishing between mild and severe degrees; however, color flow Doppler examination may not be sufficient for more exact quantification of mitral regurgitation or to determine if the severity of the lesion is sufficient to cause eventual left ventricular dysfunction. When the severity of mitral regurgitation is in doubt or if mitral valve surgery is contemplated, cardiac catheterization is helpful in resolving the severity of the lesion; it should include coronary arteriography in patients older than age 40 or with symptoms suggesting coronary disease (see Chapter 46).

MEDICAL THERAPY. Severe Acute Mitral Regurgitation. In severe acute mitral regurgitation, the patient is usually symptomatic with heart failure or even shock. The goal of medical therapy is to increase forward cardiac output while concomitantly reducing regurgitant volume (see Chapter 48). Arterial vasodilators reduce systemic resistance to flow and thereby preferentially increase aortic outflow and simultaneously decrease the amount of mitral regurgitation and left atrial hypertension. If hypotension already exists, vasodilators such as nitroprusside will lower blood pressure further and cannot be used. In such cases, intra-aortic balloon counterpulsation is preferred if the aortic valve is competent. Counterpulsation increases forward cardiac output by lowering ventricular afterload while augmenting systemic diastolic pressure.

Chronic Asymptomatic Mitral Regurgitation. Vasodilator therapy is clearly effective in the treatment of acute mitral regurgitation and in chronic aortic regurgitation (see later). However, perhaps because afterload is usually not increased in chronic asymptomatic

mitral regurgitation, vasodilators have had little effect in reducing left ventricular volume or in improving normal exercise tolerance in mitral regurgitation.

In patients with *symptomatic* mitral regurgitation, angiotensin-converting enzyme inhibitors have been demonstrated to reduce left ventricular volumes and to improve symptoms. However, mitral valve surgery rather than medical therapy usually is preferred in most symptomatic patients with mitral regurgitation. When atrial fibrillation is present, chronic anticoagulation should achieve the same INR goal as for mitral stenosis.

SURGICAL THERAPY. The timing of mitral valve surgery must weigh the risks of the operation and of a prosthesis, if one is inserted, versus the risk of irreversible left ventricular dysfunction if surgery is delayed unwisely. For most other types of valve disease, surgical correction usually requires the placement of a prosthetic valve, but in mitral regurgitation the native valve can often be repaired. Because conservation of the native valve obviates the risks of a prosthesis, the option of mitral valve repair should influence the patient and physician toward earlier operation.

TYPES OF MITRAL VALVE SURGERY. "Standard" Mitral Valve Replacement. In the standard mitral valve replacement, the mitral valve leaflets and its apparatus are removed and a prosthetic valve is inserted. Although this operation almost guarantees mitral valve competence, destruction of the mitral valve apparatus is problematic. It is clear that the mitral valve apparatus has a much wider physiologic function than simply to prevent mitral regurgitation. The apparatus is responsible for coordinating left ventricular contraction and for helping to maintain the efficient prolate ellipsoid shape of the left ventricle. Destruction of the apparatus leads to a sudden fall in left ventricular function and an often permanent decline in postoperative ejection fraction. Thus, this operation is used only in circumstances in which the native valve cannot be repaired, such as in severe rheumatic deformity or in ischemic mitral regurgitation.

Mitral Valve Replacement With Apparatus Preservation. In this procedure, a prosthetic valve is inserted but the continuity between the native leaflets and the papillary muscles is maintained. This procedure has the advantage of ensuring mitral valve competence while preserving the left ventricular functional aspects of the mitral apparatus. Even if only the posterior leaflets and chordae are preserved, the patient benefits both from improved postoperative ventricular function and better survival. In many cases, it is possible to preserve both anterior and posterior chordal attachments, although anterior continuity can be associated with left ventricular outflow tract obstruction. Although the patient benefits from both restored mitral valve competence and maintenance of left ventricular function, insertion of a prosthesis still carries all prosthesis-associated risks.

Mitral Valve Repair. When feasible, mitral valve repair is the preferred operation. Repair restores valve competence, maintains the functional aspects of the apparatus, and avoids insertion of a prosthesis. Repair is most applicable in cases of posterior chordal rupture; anterior involvement and rheumatic involvement make repair more difficult. In all cases, the feasibility of repair depends on the pathoanatomy that is causing the mitral regurgitation and on the skill and experience of the operating surgeon.

TIMING OF SURGERY. Symptomatic Patients. Most patients with the symptoms of dyspnea, orthopnea, or fatigue should undergo surgery irrespective of which operation is performed because they already have lifestyle limitations from their disease. Furthermore, the mere presence of symptoms may worsen prognosis despite relatively well-preserved left ventricular function. The onset or worsening of symptoms is a summary of the patient's pathophysiology and may give a broader view of cardiovascular integrity than any single measurement of pressure or function.

Asymptomatic Patients With Left Ventricular Dysfunction. The onset of left ventricular dysfunction in mitral regurgitation may occur without causing symptoms. Early surgery is warranted to prevent muscle dysfunction from becoming severe or irreversible. Whether valve repair or replacement is eventually performed, survival is prolonged to or toward normal if surgery is performed before ejection fraction declines to less than 0.60 or before the left ventricle is unable to contract to an end-systolic dimension of 45 mm. Thus, patients with severe mitral regurgitation should be followed yearly with a history, a physical examination, and an echocardiographic evaluation of left ventricular function. Once the patient reports symptoms or echocardiography demonstrates the onset of left ventricular dysfunction, surgery should be undertaken.

Asymptomatic Elderly Patients. Patients older than 75 years of age may have poor surgical results, especially if coronary disease is present or if mitral valve replacement rather than repair must be performed. Thus, while elderly patients with symptoms refractory to medical therapy may benefit from surgery, there is little compelling reason to commit elderly *asymptomatic* patients to a mitral valve operation.

MITRAL VALVE PROLAPSE

Mitral valve prolapse occurs when one or both of the mitral valve leaflets prolapses into the left atrium superior to the mitral valve annular plane during systole. The importance of mitral valve prolapse varies from patient to patient. In some cases, prolapse is simply a consequence of normal left ventricular physiology without significant medical impact, while in other cases there is severe valvular deformity associated with an increased risk of stroke, arrhythmia, endocarditis, and progression to severe mitral regurgitation. Examples of the former situation are those that produce a small left ventricle (i.e., the Valsalva maneuver or atrial septal defect), in which reduction of ventricular volume causes relative lengthening of the chordae tendineae and subsequent mitral valve prolapse. At the other end of the spectrum, severe redundancy and deformity of the valve, which occurs in myxomatous valve degeneration, clearly increases the risk of the complications noted earlier.

DIAGNOSIS. HISTORY. Most patients with mitral valve prolapse are asymptomatic. However, in some cases, mitral valve prolapse is associated with a symptom complex including palpitation, syncope, and chest pain. The exact cause-and-effect relationship between the presence of mitral valve prolapse and these symptoms has been difficult to draw. In some cases, chest pain is associated with a positive thallium scintigram indicating the presence of true ischemia despite normal epicardial coronary arteries, perhaps because excessive tension on the papillary muscles increases oxygen consumption and causes ischemia. Palpitation, syncope, and presyncope, when present, are linked to autonomic dysfunction, which seems to be more prevalent in mitral valve prolapse.

PHYSICAL EXAMINATION. On physical examination, the mitral valve prolapse syndrome produces characteristic findings of a midsystolic click and a late systolic murmur. The click occurs when the chordae tendineae are stretched taut by the prolapsing mitral valve in mid-systole. As this occurs, the mitral leaflets move past their coaptation point, permit mitral regurgitation, and cause the late systolic murmur. Maneuvers that make the left ventricle smaller, such as the Valsalva maneuver, cause the click to come earlier and the murmur to be more holosystolic and often louder. In some cases of echocardiographically proven mitral valve prolapse, neither the click nor the murmur is present; in other cases, only one of these findings is present.

NON-INVASIVE EVALUATION. Echocardiography is useful to prove that prolapse is present, to image the amount of regurgitation and its physiologic effects, and to discern the pathoanatomy of the mitral valve. Although an echocardiogram is not necessary to diagnose prolapse in patients with the classic physical findings, the echocardiogram adds significant prognostic information because it can detect those patients who have specifically abnormal valve morphology and in whom most of the complications of the disease occur.

About a decade ago it became clear that the mitral annulus did not exist in a single plane but had a saddle-back shape. Thus, prolapse demonstrated in the four-chamber echocardiographic view should be confirmed in the parasternal long-axis view. Echocardiographic diagnoses made before the understanding that the mitral valve plane was multidimensional (circa 1987) may have been made in error.

CLINICAL COURSE. Most patients with mitral valve prolapse have a benign clinical course; even for complication-prone patients with redundant and misshapen mitral leaflets, complications are relatively rare. Approximately 10% of patients with thickened leaflets suffer either infective endocarditis, stroke, progression to severe mitral regurgitation, or sudden death. The progression to severe mitral regurgitation varies with gender and age, and men are approximately twice as likely to progress as women. By the age of 50 years, only approximately 1 in 200 men requires surgery to correct mitral regurgitation. However, by age 70, the risk increases to approximately 3%.

THERAPY. Because most patients with mitral valve prolapse are asymptomatic, therapy is unnecessary. Patients with mitral valve prolapse and its characteristic murmur should observe standard endocarditis prophylaxis (see Chapter 326). On the other hand, patients with otherwise normal valve leaflets shown to prolapse during echocardiography with no heart murmur do not require endocarditis precautions. Patients with clearly abnormal valves but no murmur fall into a middle category of endocarditis risk where a firm recommendation about prophylaxis cannot be made. In patients with palpitation and autonomic dysfunction, β-blockers are often effective in relieving symptoms. Low-dose aspirin therapy has been recommended for patients with redundant leaflets because these patients have a slightly increased risk of stroke. However, no data from large studies are available to support this contention. In patients developing severe mitral regurgitation, the therapy is the same as for other causes of mitral regurgitation.

AORTIC REGURGITATION

ETIOLOGY. Aortic regurgitation is caused either by abnormalities of the aortic leaflets or by abnormalities of the proximal aortic root. Leaflet abnormalities causing aortic regurgitation include bicuspid aortic valve, infective endocarditis, rheumatic heart disease and anorexigenic drugs. Common aortic root abnormalities that cause aortic regurgitation include Marfan syndrome (see Chapter 215), hypertension-induced annuloaortic ectasia, aortic dissection (see Chapter 36), syphilis (see Chapter 365), ankylosing spondylitis (see Chapter 287), and psoriatic arthritis (see Chapter 287). Acute aortic regurgitation is usually caused by infectious endocarditis or aortic dissection.

PATHOPHYSIOLOGY. As with mitral regurgitation, aortic regurgitation imparts a volume overload on the left ventricle because the left ventricle must pump the forward flow entering from the left atrium as well as the regurgitant volume returning through the incompetent aortic valve. As with mitral regurgitation, compensation for the volume overload occurs from the development of eccentric cardiac hypertrophy, which increases chamber size and allows the ventricle to pump a greater total stroke volume and therefore a greater forward stroke volume. Ventricular enlargement also allows the left ventricle to accommodate the volume overload at a lower filling pressure. However, unlike mitral regurgitation, in aortic regurgitation the entire stroke volume is ejected into the aorta. Because pulse pressure is proportional to the stroke volume and the elastance of the aorta, the increased stroke volume increases systolic pressure. Systolic hypertension leads to afterload excess, which does not occur in mitral regurgitation unless the cardiac output is low enough to cause systemic arterial constriction. Not surprisingly, ventricular geometry also differs between mitral and aortic regurgitation because the afterload excess in aortic regurgitation causes a modest element of concentric as well as eccentric hypertrophy.

In acute aortic insufficiency, such as might occur in infective endocarditis, severe volume overload of the previously unprepared left ventricle results in a sudden fall in forward output while precipitously increasing left ventricular filling pressure. It is probably this combination of pathophysiologic factors that leads to rapid decompensation, presumably because the gradient for coronary blood flow is severely diminished, in turn causing ischemia and a progressive deterioration in left ventricular function. In acute aortic insufficiency, reflex vasoconstriction increases peripheral vascular resistance. In compensated chronic aortic insufficiency, vasoconstriction is absent, and vascular resistance may actually be reduced and contribute to the hyperdynamic circulation observed in such patients.

CLINICAL PRESENTATION. SYMPTOMS. The most common symptoms from chronic aortic regurgitation are those of left-sided heart failure, that is, dyspnea on exertion, orthopnea, and fatigue. In acute aortic regurgitation, cardiac output and shock may develop rapidly. The onset of symptoms in chronic aortic regurgitation usually heralds the onset of left ventricular systolic dysfunction. However, some patients with symptoms have apparently normal systolic function, and symptoms may be attributed to diastolic dysfunction. Other patients may have ventricular dysfunction yet remain asymptomatic.

Angina may also occur in patients with aortic insufficiency, but less commonly than in aortic stenosis. The cause of angina in aortic regurgitation is probably multifactorial. Coronary blood flow reserve is reduced in some patients because diastolic runoff into the left ventricle lowers aortic diastolic pressure while increasing left ventricular diastolic pressure—these two influences lower the driving pressure gradient for flow across the coronary bed. When angina occurs in aortic regurgitation, it may be accompanied by flushing. Other symptoms include carotid artery pain and an unpleasant awareness of the heartbeat.

DIAGNOSIS. PHYSICAL EXAMINATION. Aortic regurgitation produces a myriad of signs because a hyperdynamic, enlarged left ventricle ejects a large stroke volume at high pressure into the systemic circulation. Palpation of the precordium finds a hyperactive apical impulse displaced downward and to the left. S_1 and S_2 are usually normal. S_2 is followed by a diastolic blowing murmur heard best along the left sternal border with the patient sitting upright. In mild disease the murmur may be short, heard only in the beginning of diastole when the gradient between the aorta and left ventricle is highest. As the disease worsens, the murmur may persist throughout diastole. A second murmur, a mitral valve rumble, is heard at the left ventricular apex in severe aortic insufficiency. Although the cause is still debated, this Austin Flint murmur is probably produced as the regurgitant jet impinges on the mitral valve and causes it to vibrate.

In chronic aortic regurgitation, the high stroke volume and reduced systemic arterial resistance result in a wide pulse pressure, which generates a plethora of signs. These include Corrigan's pulse (sharp upstroke and rapid decline of the carotid pulse), de Musset's sign (head bobbing), Duroziez's sign (combined systolic and diastolic bruits created by compression of the femoral artery with the stethoscope), and Quincke's pulse (systolic plethora and diastolic blanching in the nail bed when gentle traction is placed on the nail). Perhaps the most reliable of physical signs indicating severe aortic regurgitation is Hill's sign, an increase in the femoral systolic pressure of 40 mm Hg or more compared with systolic pressure in the brachial artery.

Unlike chronic aortic insufficiency with its myriad of clinical signs, acute aortic insufficiency may have a very subtle presentation. The eccentric hypertrophy, which compensates chronic aortic insufficiency, has not yet had time to develop and thus the large total stroke volume responsible for most of the signs of chronic aortic insufficiency is absent. The only clues to the presence of acute aortic insufficiency may be a short diastolic blowing murmur and reduced intensity of S_1. This latter sign occurs because high diastolic left ventricular pressure closes the mitral valve early in diastole (mitral valve preclosure), so that when ventricular systole occurs, only the tricuspid component of S_1 is heard.

NON-INVASIVE EVALUATION. The electrocardiogram in aortic insufficiency is non-specific but almost always demonstrates left ventricular hypertrophy. The chest radiograph shows an enlarged heart, often with uncoiling and enlargement of the aortic root.

Echocardiography is the most important non-invasive tool for assessing both the severity of aortic insufficiency and its impact on left ventricular geometry and function (Color Plate 1A). During echocardiography, left ventricular end-diastolic dimension, end-systolic dimension, and fractional shortening are determined. Aortic valve anatomy and aortic root anatomy can be assessed and the cause of the aortic regurgitation often determined. Color flow Doppler examination of the aortic valve helps quantify the severity of aortic regurgitation by assessing the depth and width to which the diastolic jet penetrates the left ventricle. Another way to assess the severity of aortic regurgitation is the pressure half-time method: continuous-wave Doppler interrogation of the aortic valve displays the decay of the velocity of retrograde flow across the valve. In mild aortic insufficiency, the gradient across the valve is high throughout diastole and its rate of decay is slow, producing a long Doppler half-time (the time it takes the velocity to decay from its peak to that value divided by the square root of 2). In severe aortic regurgitation there is rapid equilibration between pressure in the aorta and the pressure in the left ventricle, and the Doppler half-time is short. If mitral valve preclosure is detected in acute aortic insufficiency, urgent surgery is necessary. In cases in which the severity of aortic insufficiency is in doubt, catheterization to perform aortography is useful in resolving the issue.

THERAPY. MEDICAL THERAPY. Asymptomatic Patients With Normal Left Ventricular Function. Because aortic regurgitation increases left ventricular afterload, which in turn worsens the aortic regurgitation, afterload-reducing drugs are efficacious in the treatment of the disease. Patients who are symptomatic or manifest left ventricular dysfunction should undergo aortic valve surgery. For *asymptomatic* patients with normal left ventricular function, afterload reduction is recommended because it delays or reduces the need for aortic valve surgery without any adverse effects once surgery finally was carried out. Currently, the best prognostic data are for nifedipine, but other vasodilators including angiotensin-converting enzyme inhibitors and hydralazine have also demonstrated hemodynamic improvement for aortic regurgitation and may prove to be at least equally beneficial.

Acute Aortic Regurgitation. Once any of the symptoms or signs of heart failure develop, even if mild, medical mortality is high, approaching 75%. Therapy with vasodilators, such as nitroprusside, may help improve the patient's condition before surgery but is not a substitute for surgery. In patients with acute aortic regurgitation caused by bacterial endocarditis (see Chapter 326), surgery may be delayed to permit a full or partial course of antibiotics, but persistent, severe aortic regurgitation requires emergency valve replacement. Even when blood cultures have recently been positive and antibiotic therapy has been of brief duration, valve reinfection rate is low, zero to 10%. Thus, emergent surgery should not be withheld simply because the duration of antibiotic therapy has been brief.

SURGICAL THERAPY. The Timing of Aortic Valve Surgery. Although some patients may be able to undergo successful aortic valve repair to restore aortic valve competence, most patients will require insertion of an aortic valve prosthesis. Patients with advanced symptoms are at increased risk for a suboptimal surgical outcome whether or not they have evidence of left ventricular dysfunction. Thus, patients should undergo aortic valve replacement before symptoms impair lifestyle. It also is clear that asymptomatic patients who manifest evidence of left ventricular dysfunction benefit from surgery. Because loading conditions differ between aortic and mitral regurgitation, the objective markers for the presence of left ventricular dysfunction also differ. In aortic regurgitation, once ejection fraction falls below 0.55 or end-systolic dimension exceeds 55 mm, postoperative outcome is impaired, presumably because these markers indicate that left ventricular dysfunction has developed. Thus, surgery should occur before these benchmarks are reached.

TRICUSPID REGURGITATION

ETIOLOGY. Tricuspid regurgitation is usually secondary to a hemodynamic load on the right ventricle rather than to a structural valve deformity. Diseases that cause pulmonary hypertension, such as chronic obstructive airway disease or intracardiac shunts, lead to right ventricular dilatation and subsequent tricuspid regurgitation. Because most of the force that is needed to fill the left ventricle is provided by the right ventricle, left ventricular dysfunction leading to elevated left ventricular filling pressure also places the right ventricle under a hemodynamic load and can eventually lead to right ventricular failure and tricuspid regurgitation. In some instances, tricuspid regurgitation may be caused by pathology of the valve itself. The most common cause of primary tricuspid regurgitation is infective endocarditis, usually stemming from drug abuse and unsterile injections. Other causes include carcinoid syndrome, rheumatic involvement of the tricuspid valve, myxomatous degeneration, right ventricular infarction, and mishaps during endomyocardial biopsy.

DIAGNOSIS. The symptoms of tricuspid regurgitation are those of right-sided heart failure, including ascites, edema, and occasionally right upper quadrant pain. On physical examination, tricuspid regurgitation produces jugular venous distention accentuated by a large v wave as blood is regurgitated into the right atrium during systole. Regurgitation into the hepatic veins causes hepatic enlargement and liver pulsation. Right ventricular enlargement is detected as a parasternal lift. Ascites and edema are common.

The definitive diagnosis of tricuspid regurgitation is made during echocardiography. Doppler interrogation of the tricuspid valve demonstrates systolic disturbance of the right atrial blood pool. Echocardiography can also be used to determine the severity of pulmonary hypertension, to measure right ventricular dilatation, and to assess whether the valve itself is intrinsically normal or abnormal.

THERAPY. The therapy for secondary tricuspid regurgitation is usually aimed at the cause of the lesion. Thus, if left ventricular failure has been responsible for right ventricular failure and tricuspid regurgitation, the standard therapy for improving left ventricular failure (see Chapter 48) will lower left ventricular filling pressure, reduce secondary pulmonary hypertension, relieve some of the hemodynamic burden of the right ventricle, and partially restore tricuspid valve competence. If pulmonary disease is the primary cause, therapy is directed toward improving lung function (see Chapter 75). Vasodilators, so useful in the treatment of left-sided heart failure, are often ineffective in treating pulmonary hypertension itself. Thus, medical therapy directed at tricuspid regurgitation itself is usually limited to diuretic use.

Surgical intervention for the tricuspid valve is rarely entertained in isolation. However, if other cardiac surgery is planned in a patient with severe tricuspid regurgitation, ring annuloplasty or tricuspid valve repair is often attempted to ensure postoperative tricuspid competence. Tricuspid valve replacement is often not well tolerated and is now rarely performed except when severe deformity, as often seen in endocarditis or carcinoid disease, precludes valve repair.

PULMONIC STENOSIS

Pulmonic stenosis is a congenital disease resulting from fusion of the pulmonic valve cusps (see Chapter 57). It is usually detected and corrected during childhood, but occasionally cases are diagnosed for the first time in adulthood. Symptoms of pulmonic stenosis include angina and syncope. Occasionally, patients develop symptoms of right-sided heart failure. During physical examination, the uncalcified valve in pulmonic stenosis produces an early systolic ejection click on opening. During inspiration, the click diminishes or even disappears because increased flow into the right side of the heart during inspiration partially opens the pulmonic valve in diastole so systole causes less of an opening sound. The click is followed by a systolic ejection murmur, which radiates to the base of the heart. If the transvalvular gradient is severe, right ventricular hypertrophy develops and produces a parasternal lift.

The diagnosis of pulmonic stenosis is confirmed during echocardiography, which quantifies the transvalvular gradient as well as the degree of right ventricular hypertrophy and dysfunction.

THERAPY. In asymptomatic patients with a gradient of less than 25 mm Hg, no therapy is required. If symptoms develop or the gradient exceeds 50 mm Hg, balloon commissurotomy is effective in reducing the gradient and relieving symptoms.

POSTOPERATIVE CARE OF PATIENTS WITH SUBSTITUTE HEART VALVES

Different types of prosthetic valves have different advantages and disadvantages (Table 63–2). After a prosthetic valve has been inserted, a baseline echocardiogram should be obtained to provide a reference point should valve dysfunction be suspected at a later date. Echocardiography then need not be repeated unless there is a change in clinical status or in physical findings. The major causes of valve dysfunction are infectious endocarditis, clot, and valve degeneration. Dysfunction is most commonly manifested by valvular regurgitation, but valvular stenosis can also occur with clot, vegetations, or degeneration, especially degeneration of a bioprosthesis.

Whenever a patient with a prosthetic heart valve develops a temperature greater than 100°F, endocarditis must be excluded by blood culture; for fever with signs of sepsis, broad-spectrum antibiotics must be begun while awaiting culture results. For patients

Table 63–2 ■ ADVANTAGES AND DISADVANTAGES OF SUBSTITUTE CARDIAC VALVES

TYPE OF VALVE	ADVANTAGES	DISADVANTAGES
Bioprosthesis (Carpentier-Edwards; Hancock)	Avoid anticoagulation in patients with sinus rhythm	Durability limited to 10–15 years Relatively stenotic
Mechanical valves (St. Jude; Medtronic-Hall; Starr-Edwards)	Good flow characteristics in small sizes Durable	Require anticoagulation
Homografts and autografts	Anticoagulation not required Durability increased over that of bioprostheses	Surgical implantation technically demanding

with bioprosthetic valves, mechanical prostheses, and homografts, endocarditis prophylaxis should be used at the time of procedures that have a high risk for bacteremia (see Chapter 326). Whether prophylaxis is necessary for pulmonary autografts is currently unclear, but physicians usually prescribe prophylaxis for such patients.

All patients with a mechanical heart valve require anticoagulation. Recommended INR values range from 2.0 for the young normotensive patient in sinus rhythm with an aortic valve prosthesis to 3.5 for the patient with atrial fibrillation and a mitral valve prosthesis. Aspirin, at doses of 325 mg, is recommended in addition to warfarin to reduce the risk of valve thrombosis in patients with mechanical prosthetic valves at higher risk for thromboembolic complications.

Bonow RO, Carabello B, de Leon AC Jr, et al: ACC/AHA guidelines for the management of patients with valvular heart disease: Executive summary. A report of the American College of Cardiology/American Heart Association Task Force on Practice Guidelines (Committee on Management of Patients with Valvular Heart Disease). Circulation 98:1949, 1998. *Consensus guidelines that provide a useful approach to common valvular abnormalities.*

Carabello BA, Crawford FA Jr: Valvular heart disease. N Engl J Med 337:32, 1997.

Enriquez-Sarano M, Schaff HV, Orszulak TA, et al: Valve repair improves the outcome of surgery for mitral regurgitation: A multivariate analysis. Circulation 91:1022, 1995.

Gaasch WH, Sundaram M, Meyer TE: Managing asymptomatic patients with chronic aortic regurgitation. Chest 111:1702, 1997.

Otto CM, Burwash IG, Legget ME, et al: Prospective study of asymptomatic valvular aortic stenosis: Clinical, echocardiographic, and exercise predictors of outcome. Circulation 95:2262, 1997.

64 DISEASES OF THE MYOCARDIUM

Lynne Warner Stevenson

Cardiomyopathy means heart muscle disease and distinguishes disorders originating in the myocardium from those in which myocardial dysfunction results from other cardiovascular disease. General usage, however, frequently also includes the diffuse dilation and hypocontractility that can result from severe coronary artery disease and is termed *ischemic cardiomyopathy*. Among the estimated 4.0 to 4.7 million patients in the United States with heart failure, 5 to 10% are generally considered to have primary cardiomyopathy.

GENERAL PRESENTATION

Patients presenting with cardiac dysfunction of any cause often describe progressive exertional intolerance, reflecting inadequate cardiac output reserve or excessive elevation in ventricular filling pressures. Elevated filling pressures at rest can cause orthopnea, supine cough, and paroxysmal nocturnal dyspnea (see Chapter 47). Right-sided congestion can cause discomfort during bending, abdominal discomfort, anorexia, and peripheral edema, although edema is often absent, particularly in younger patients. These symptoms are common in all types of cardiomyopathy and in fact are common to all cardiac diseases when filling pressures become elevated. The term *congestive heart failure* describes this syndrome of elevated filling pressures but not the cause of heart failure nor the type of cardiomyopathy.

In some patients, tachyarrhythmias or bradyarrhythmias may be the presenting symptom of cardiomyopathy. Chest pain occurs in almost one third of patients with cardiomyopathy despite normal epicardial coronary arteries and may result from pulmonary hypertension, pericardial involvement, microvascular ischemia, or unknown factors. Systemic emboli arising from dilated ventricles or atria and frequently associated with atrial fibrillation are occasionally the first sign of cardiomyopathy.

Once a patient has been recognized to have symptoms or signs consistent with heart failure, the diagnosis can often be established on the basis of physical examination, but it is generally confirmed by echocardiography (Fig. 64–1). Although the classification of cardiomyopathies implies rigid distinctions, there is a blurring of the spectrum that extends from restrictive disease through disease with normal ejection fraction and impaired ventricular filling to borderline hypertrophy and classic hypertrophic cardiomyopathy. Although the myocardial pathology differs markedly, the clinical manifestations of elevated filling pressures and fluid retention feature prominently throughout this spectrum.

Specific cardiac conditions such as coronary artery disease or valvular heart failure are often suggested by the history, physical examination, and echocardiogram but may require cardiac catheterization for confirmation and quantification. Evaluation should determine whether heart failure results from excessive peripheral cardiac demand, such as in chronic severe anemia (generally requiring a hemoglobin level less than 8 mg/dL), or peripheral arteriovenous shunt, such as in Paget's bone disease or occasionally in patients with a large fistula for dialysis. Tachycardia-induced cardiomyopathy, most commonly observed in children and young adults, can result in adults from supraventricular or slow ventricular tachycardias when rates are chronically or frequently above 120 to 140 beats per minute and is completely reversible. If these other conditions are absent or inadequate to explain the cardiac dysfunction,

the next task is to distinguish among dilated, restrictive, and hypertrophic cardiomyopathy by echocardiography.

DILATED CARDIOMYOPATHY

Dilated cardiomyopathy is characterized by increased left ventricular or biventricular dimensions with decreased ventricular ejection fraction (Table 64–1). Myocardial contractility is severely impaired and labeled "systolic failure." Abnormalities in diastolic function often reflect excessive volume overload and are generally less marked than in restrictive or hypertrophic cardiomyopathy. At the time of diagnosis, half of the patients are younger than 55 and one third have New York Heart Association Class III or IV symptoms. Evidence from population screening suggests a higher frequency of asymptomatic disease than previously recognized.

Etiology

Dilated cardiomyopathy has many causes (Table 64–2) that lead to the syndrome. A brief primary injury such as toxic exposure may be fatal to some myocytes, after which the increased burden of pressure and volume stimulates hypertrophy in the surviving myocytes. This hypertrophy initially preserves global function but can eventually lead to progressive functional impairment. One mechanism leading to progressive deterioration late after an initial injury may be the triggering of programmed cell death, known as "apoptosis." Some chronic exposures, such as to ethanol, may reversibly impair global contractility without directly causing cell injury but cause irreversible dysfunction if continued chronically. Inflammatory myocarditis may combine irreversible cell death with reversible depression from inflammatory mediators such as cytokines. Many injuries may also affect the collagen scaffolding of the myocardium, influencing stiffness and the potential for ventricular dilation. Most cardiomyopathies reflect the sum of irrevocable my-

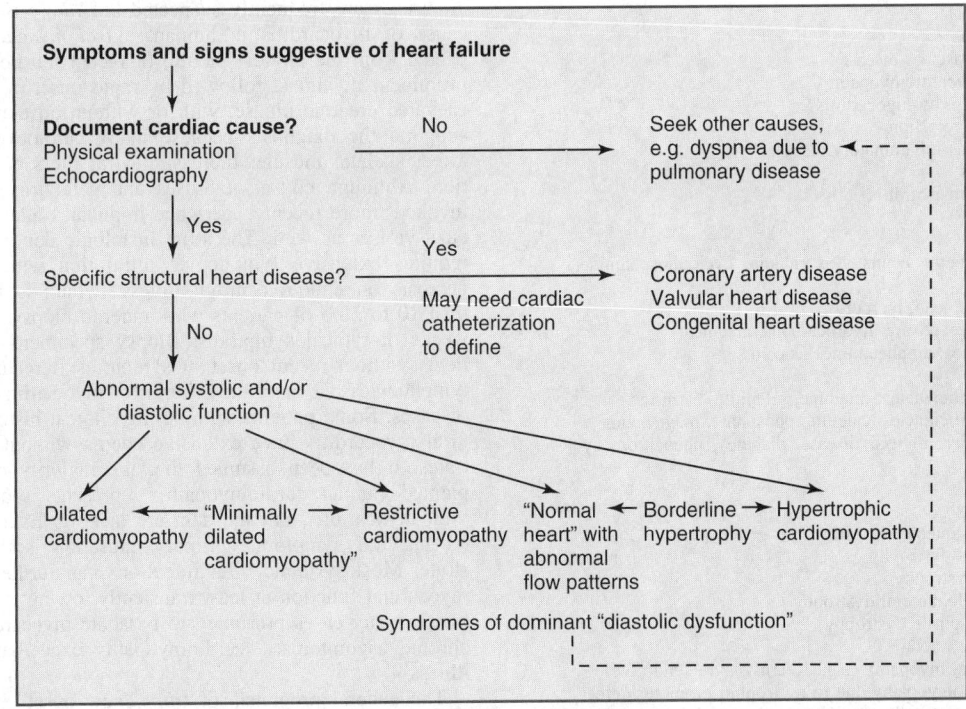

FIGURE 64–1 ■ Initial approach to classification of cardiomyopathy. The evaluation of symptoms or signs consistent with heart failure first includes confirmation that they can be attributed to a cardiac cause. Although this is often apparent from routine physical examination, echocardiography serves to confirm cardiac disease and provides clues to the presence of other cardiac disease, such as focal abnormalities, suggesting primary valve disease or congenital heart disease. Having excluded these conditions, cardiomyopathy is generally considered to be dilated, restrictive, or hypertrophic, as shown in Figure 64–2. Patients with apparently normal cardiac structure and contraction are occasionally found to demonstrate abnormal intracardiac flow patterns consistent with diastolic dysfunction but should also be evaluated carefully for other causes of their symptoms. Most patients with so-called diastolic dysfunction will also demonstrate at least borderline criteria for left ventricular hypertrophy, frequently in the setting of chronic hypertension and diabetes. A moderately decreased ejection fraction without marked dilation or a pattern of restrictive cardiomyopathy is sometimes referred to as "minimally dilated cardiomyopathy," which may either represent a distinct entity or a transition between acute and chronic disease.

Table 64–1 ■ PROFILES OF SYMPTOMATIC CARDIOMYOPATHY

	DILATED	RESTRICTIVE	HYPERTROPHIC
Ejection fraction (normal ≥55%)	<30%	25–50%	>60%
Left ventricular diastolic dimension (normal <55 mm)	≥60 mm	<60 mm	Often decreased
Left ventricular wall thickness	Decreased	Normal or increased	Markedly increased
Atrial size	Increased	Increased; may be massive	Increased
Valvular regurgitation	Mitral first during decompensation; tricuspid regurgitation in late stages	Frequent mitral and tricuspid regurgitation	Mitral regurgitation
Common first symptoms*	Exertional intolerance	Exertional intolerance	Exertional intolerance; may have chest pain
Congestive symptoms*	Left before right, except right prominent in young adults	Right often exceeds left	Primary exertional dyspnea
Risk for arrhythmia	Ventricular tachyarrhythmia; conduction block in Chagas' disease, giant cell myocarditis, and some families. Atrial fibrillation.	Ventricular uncommon except in sarcoidosis; conduction block in sarcoidosis and amyloidosis; atrial fibrillation.	Ventricular tachyarrhythmias Atrial fibrillation

*Left-sided symptoms of pulmonary congestion; dyspnea on exertion, orthopnea, paroxysmal nocturnal dyspnea. Right-sided symptoms of systemic venous congestion: discomfort on bending, hepatic and abdominal distention, peripheral edema.

Table 64–2 ■ MAJOR CAUSES OF DILATED CARDIOMYOPATHY

Inflammatory
  Infectious myocarditis
    Viral
    Rickettsial
    Bacterial
    Mycobacterial
    Spirochetal
    Parasitic
    Fungal
  Non-infectious
    Collagen vascular disease
    Peripartum cardiomyopathy
    Hypersensitivity myocarditis
    Transplant rejection
  Granulomatous inflammatory disease
    Sarcoidosis
    Giant cell myocarditis
Toxic
  Alcohol
  Chemotherapeutic agents: doxorubicin, cyclophosphamide, interferon
  Heavy metals: lead, mercury
  Occupational exposure: hydrocarbons, arsenicals
  Catecholamines: amphetamines, cocaine
Metabolic
  Nutritional deficiencies: thiamine, selenium, carnitine
  Electrolyte deficiencies: calcium, phosphate, magnesium
  Endocrinopathy: thyroid disease, diabetes, pheochromocytoma
  Obesity
Familial
  Cardiac and skeletal myopathy
    Duchenne's dystrophy
    Becker's dystrophy
    Facioscapulohumeral dystrophy
    Erb's limb-girdle dystrophy
    Friedreich's ataxia
  Mitochondrial myopathy (e.g., Kearns-Sayre syndrome)
  Isolated cardiomyopathy due to dystrophin promoter defect
  Some cases of arrhythmogenic right ventricular dysplasia
  Associated with other systemic diseases
  Susceptibility to immune-mediated myocarditis
Overlap with Restrictive Cardiomyopathy
  Hemochromatosis
  Amyloidosis
  Sarcoidosis
Idiopathic
  Primary left ventricular or biventricular cardiomyopathy
  Arrhythmogenic right ventricular dysplasia

ocyte loss plus secondary abnormalities, some of which may be reversible, in the remaining myocardium that continues to function under stress.

Myocarditis

Viral Myocarditis

Most of our conception of viral myocarditis derives from murine animal models in which initial viral replication can be exacerbated by exercise and immunosuppression. Subsequently, active replication ceases, although some viral DNA may still be detectable, and thymus-derived lymphocytes appear to cross react with myocardial cells. Infected animals may die, recover, or develop dilated hearts with areas of fibrosis.

Viruses are frequently suspected but rarely isolated as the direct cause of myocarditis in humans. *Viral myocarditis* may be suspected from the clinical picture of recent febrile illness, often with prominent myalgias, followed by rapid onset of cardiac symptoms. Elevated creatine kinase, with or without an elevated MB fraction, supports the diagnosis because many cardiotropic infections also affect skeletal muscle. Increasing viral titers confirm recent infection. Although coxsackieviruses and echoviruses have often been invoked, more recent experience implicates adenoviruses and influenza viruses as well. The strict histologic definition of myocarditis requires extensive lymphocyte infiltration with adjacent myocyte necrosis on endomyocardial biopsy, which is identified in fewer than 10 to 20% of patients who undergo biopsy within the first few weeks of typical symptoms. Biopsy specimens obtained from patients without recent onset of symptoms frequently show scattered lymphocytes but meet the criteria for myocarditis in fewer than 5% of cases. Some patients with strong clinical history for recent postviral myocarditis have extensive edema without lymphocytic infiltrates. It has been assumed that the majority of otherwise unexplained human cardiomyopathy represents sequelae of previous viral myocarditis, but the data are lacking. Even with a history of recent viral symptoms, primary causation is difficult to demonstrate. Most systemic viral infections can further depress impaired myocardial function at least transiently, owing to induction of cytokines. Many cases presumed to be acute myocarditis may represent chronic asymptomatic cardiomyopathy exacerbated by acute viral illness.

The general prognosis of truly "new onset" heart failure attributed to recent viral infection is major improvement in left ventricular function in up to half of patients, which can occur whether or not an initial biopsy met criteria for myocarditis. Treatment of biopsy-proven acute myocarditis, presumed to be postviral, has included azathioprine, prednisone, and more recently cyclosporine, but there has been no proven benefit in controlled trials. The rationale for immunosuppressive therapy is based in part on the dramatic response of transplant rejection, which has equivalent histology. The hope remains that some patients who show a progressive downhill course and persistent inflammation may benefit from immunosuppression. A common current approach to the patient with recent symptom onset is to defer biopsy and observe the patient closely during treatment of heart failure. (An exception would be the patient in whom tachyarrhythmias or conduction disturbances complicate new-onset heart failure, raising the possibility of giant cell myocarditis or sarcoidosis, which might be diagnosed on biopsy, as described later.) If deterioration continues during the months after referral, the prognosis for recovery becomes very poor and biopsy may then be considered, with the intent to treat a patient with positive findings with a brief trial of immunosuppression in the hopes of averting the need for cardiac transplantation.

Occasionally, acute viral myocarditis may present over a few days with a "fulminant" picture, characterized by fevers and often by compromise of hepatic and renal as well as cardiac function. Such patients are assumed to be undergoing active viral infection during which immunosuppression would be deleterious. On rare occasions, it has been necessary to support the patient with mechanical ventricular assist devices until the equally likely outcomes of dramatic improvement or cardiac demise (possibly transplantation) declare themselves within the next week. Biopsy, which could be complicated by the coagulopathy that frequently accompanies the acute syndrome, may show severe edema with or without dramatic lymphocyte infiltration but is generally deferred in "fulminant myocarditis."

Cardiomyopathy defined by echocardiographic abnormalities occurs in 10 to 40% of patients clinically infected with the human immunodeficiency virus (HIV). Lymphocytic myocarditis has been found in up to 50% of autopsied hearts. The causative role of the HIV virus is difficult to isolate from the contribution of other co-infecting organisms such as cytomegalovirus and their related cytokine secretion. The role of secondary factors is supported by the frequent improvement observed in impaired ventricular function. Detecting viral particles in myocytes, however, supports a direct causation. Pericardial effusions as well as myocarditis may occur.

Other Infections Causing Myocarditis

Numerous infectious agents have been associated with myocarditis (see Table 64–2). *Chagas' disease* (see Chapter 423), due to infection with *Trypanosoma cruzi,* carried by the reduviid bug, affects up to 15% of the rural population in South America and is also common in Central America. The acute tissue-invasive phase can present as myocarditis but is usually silent. Subsequent progression of myocardial disease occurs over years, with a predilection to develop apical aneurysms and right bundle branch block. Destruction of parasympathetic ganglia may contribute to cardiac dysfunction as well as impaired gastrointestinal motility. The chronic process has been attributed to a triggered autoimmune reaction, but frequent eruption of generalized trypanosomal infection during immunosuppression after transplantation for chronic Chagas' disease suggests continued infection. Once patients have developed symptomatic heart failure, 5-year survival is 20%. There is no specific therapy for the chronic stage of the disease, although pacemaker implantation may decrease deaths from heart block.

Toxoplasmosis (see Chapter 425) can cause myocarditis, with intermittent rupture of cysts in the myocardium leading to atypical chest pain, arrhythmias, pericarditis, and symptomatic heart failure. The endomyocardial biopsy may show focal lymphocytic infiltration and, rarely, a fortuitous cyst. Diagnosis is made from antibody titers. Therapy is with pyrimethamine and sulfadiazine, on which relapses are common.

Lyme carditis classically refers to presentation with conduction system abnormalities due to infection with *Borrelia burgdorferi,* diagnosed serologically. There have, however, been isolated cases of heart failure attributed to this infection.

Non-infectious Myocarditis

Myocardial inflammation may occur without preceding infection. It can be associated with systemic inflammatory disorders such as polymyositis or systemic lupus erythematosus, although pericarditis and coronary artery vasculitis are more common. Hypersensitivity reactions, particularly to drugs, can cause myocarditis characterized by infiltration of eosinophils in addition to lymphocytes. Such hypersensitivity is frequently unsuspected and may complicate cardiomyopathy of other causes; it may be suspected from peripheral eosinophilia and confirmed by endomyocardial biopsy. Response to

withdrawal of the offending agent and to corticosteroid therapy is often seen.

Rejection after cardiac transplantation is the paradigm for lymphocyte-mediated myocarditis (see Chapter 71). Lessons derived from this "model" include (1) the frequent and rapid reversibility of myocardial depression during immunosuppression, (2) the potential importance of non-cellular mediators such as antibodies and cytokines even when cellular infiltration is mild or absent, and (3) the association between chronic immune stimulation and coronary vascular disease. The average transplant recipient experiences one to two episodes of rejection requiring enhanced immunosuppression. Only 10% of rejection episodes cause clinical compromise, and 95% of all episodes resolve.

Heart failure developing during the last month of pregnancy and first 3 months post partum is termed *peripartum cardiomyopathy.* The frequency is between 1 in 3,000 and 1 in 15,000 deliveries, with increased risk for mothers with older age, increased parity, twins, malnutrition, toxemia, or hypertension. Lymphocytic myocarditis has been found in 30 to 50% of biopsy specimens, suggesting an immune component postulated to be cross-reactivity between uterine and cardiac myocyte proteins or an enhanced susceptibility to viral myocarditis. Presentation is usually with orthopnea and excessive dyspnea on minimal exertion, most often within the first weeks after delivery when excess volume of pregnancy would normally be mobilized. The major differential diagnosis is of pre-existing cardiac disease aggravated by pregnancy. The prognosis of peripartum cardiomyopathy is for improvement to normal or near-normal ejection fraction during the next 6 months in over half of patients. Diuretics should be used as needed to facilitate post-partum diuresis. It has been recommended that breast feeding, which requires vigorous hydration, be discontinued. It is not known whether therapy with angiotensin-converting enzyme inhibitors improves the likelihood of recovery.

Granulomatous Disease

Although considered to be distinct diseases, cardiac sarcoidosis and giant cell myocarditis are both characterized by granulomatous infiltration, ventricular arrhythmias, and conduction block. In addition, both infectious and non-infectious immune causes have been suggested for each.

Sarcoidosis is a multisystem granulomatous disease that often presents in young adults and is more common in blacks (see Chapter 81). Although cardiac involvement is found in up to half of autopsies, clinical cardiac involvement occurs in fewer than 10% of patients, who can present with ventricular tachyarrhythmias, or less often with heart failure and reduced left ventricular ejection fraction. There is often less initial ventricular dilation with sarcoidosis than with other dilated cardiomyopathy, so it may be present as either a dilated or restrictive cardiomyopathy. Biopsy diagnosis of sarcoidosis from extracardiac sites is often adequate for the diagnosis in a patient with typical cardiac abnormalities. Gallium scan may be useful to demonstrate cardiac inflammation. Cardiac biopsy may show granulomas (Fig. 64–2); however, because of the focal distribution of the lesions, the specimens obtained are frequently non-diagnostic.

Immunosuppression with corticosteroids has been associated with improvement of arrhythmias, although in general an implantable defibrillator would be considered after demonstration of significant ventricular arrhythmias. Additional immunosuppressive agents have occasionally been added. Moderate left ventricular dysfunction may also improve with immunosuppressive therapy, although severe heart failure due to sarcoidosis may worsen rapidly regardless of therapy. It should be recognized that therapy leads granulomas to "resolve" into fibrosis, sometimes forming ventricular aneurysms that may be more common after corticosteroid therapy.

Giant cell myocarditis accounts for 10 to 20% of biopsy-positive cases of myocarditis. Onset is usually rapid with chest pain, fever, and hemodynamic compromise. There is a higher incidence of ventricular tachycardia and atrioventricular block than in lymphocytic myocarditis. Giant cell myocarditis has been associated with thymomas, thyroiditis, pernicious anemia, and systemic lupus erythematosus. The rapid time course and diffuse histology of the disease suggest that it is distinct from sarcoidosis, although some believe that it may be related. Immunosuppression is frequently

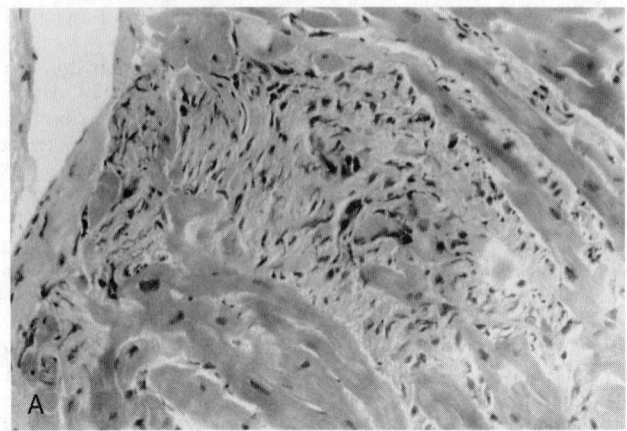

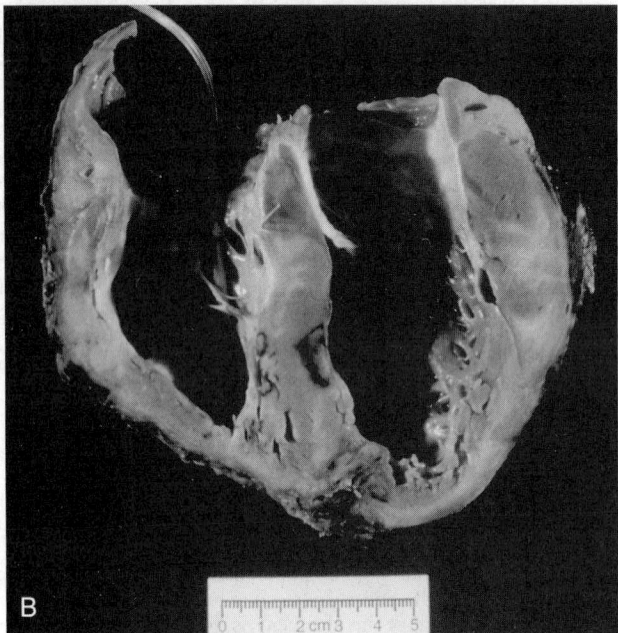

FIGURE 64–2 ■ *A,* Endomyocardial biopsy specimen from a patient with asymptomatic pulmonary sarcoidosis who presented with syncope and new heart failure. Shown is a large granuloma with slightly more active inflammation than the usual non-caseating sarcoid granuloma. *B,* Gross specimen from the same patient who had been treated with corticosteroid therapy for sarcoidosis, showing the heart removed 4 months later at the time of cardiac transplantation. Histologic examination revealed no further evidence of active inflammation, which was replaced by numerous areas of fibrosis (white areas on the gross specimen). The dark area on the septum is a site where radiofrequency ablation had been performed at one of the multiple foci of ventricular tachycardia. (Courtesy of Dr. Gayle Winters, Department of Pathology, Brigham and Women's Hospital, Boston, MA.)

employed but is not predicted to improve the clinical course, which is usually one of rapid deterioration and death from failure and refractory ventricular tachyarrhythmias. For eligible candidates, heart transplantation is generally performed as soon as possible.

When ventricular tachyarrrhythmias are a major feature of new-onset heart failure, particularly in a young person, endomyocardial biopsy is generally indicated to determine whether granulomatous inflammation is present, even though the more likely diagnosis will be a negative biopsy or lymphocytic myocarditis. If granulomatous inflammation is severe and accompanied by clinical decompensation and a left ventricular ejection fraction less than 20 to 25%, transplantation should be considered early in patients with otherwise good organ function, whether the diagnosis appears to be sarcoidosis or giant cell myocarditis.

Toxic Causes

Many substances have been reported to cause acute cardiac injury or chronic cardiomyopathy. In the United States, ethanol contributes to more than 10% of cases of heart failure. Alcohol and its direct metabolite acetaldehyde are direct cardiotoxins acutely and chronically. It is important to recognize that ethanol can contribute to heart failure with another primary cause, such as coronary artery disease. This myocardial depression is initially reversible but if sustained can lead to irreversible injury characterized histologically by vacuolization, mitochondrial abnormalities, and fibrosis. Even in chronic stages, however, the heart failure represents a sum of reversible and irreversible depression. The amount of alcohol necessary to produce symptomatic cardiomyopathy in susceptible individuals is not known but has been estimated to be six drinks (about 4 ounces of pure ethanol) a day for 5 to 10 years. Frequent binging without heavy daily consumption may also be sufficient. Alcoholic cardiomyopathy can develop in patients without social evidence of an alcohol problem. It is crucial to convince them of the value of abstention, which leads to improvement in at least half of patients with severe symptoms, some of whom normalize left ventricular ejection fraction. Patients with other causes of heart failure should also avoid alcohol.

Doxorubicin (Adriamycin) cardiotoxicity causes characteristic histologic changes on endomyocardial biopsy, with vacuolar degeneration and myofibrillar loss. Potential mechanisms of cardiotoxicity include free radical formation, release of histamines and catecholamines, and effects on mitochondrial function and nucleic acid synthesis. Between 5 and 10% of patients receiving at least 450 mg/m² of body surface area develop overt heart failure, but more than half of patients receiving multiple courses have 10% decline in resting ejection fraction. Patients with higher doses and lower baseline ejection fractions have higher risk for clinical heart failure. The dysfunction may continue to progress, with 63% of pediatric patients who have received at least 500 mg/m² having some cardiac dysfunction detected after 10 years. Patients with a history of doxorubicin therapy may be particularly susceptible to a superimposed insult, such as cardiac ischemia, alcohol, or viral infection, and may improve if the new insult is relieved. Clinical status may also improve with supportive hemodynamic therapy to reduce filling pressures and systemic vascular resistance, even though the heart is often relatively non-dilated.

Cyclophosphamide has been associated with more acute cardiac dysfunction during therapy or the first few weeks, frequently with decreased electrocardiographic voltage. Pericarditis with effusion has been seen, and increased left ventricular mass has been attributed to hemorrhagic necrosis. Ifosfamide is a newer, similar compound that can cause acute severe heart failure and malignant ventricular arrhythmias. Death from cardiogenic shock and recovery of normal left ventricular function have both been reported.

Metabolic Causes

Cardiomyopathy has been associated with *catecholamine excess,* which may injure the heart by compromising the coronary microcirculation but also through direct toxic effects on myocytes exposed to excessive stimulation and calcium loading. Pheochromocytoma can cause a reversible cardiomyopathy, as can heavy use of cocaine, which inhibits the reuptake of catecholamines.

Nutritional deficiencies are not commonly implicated in cardiomyopathy in developed Western countries. Thiamine deficiency can lead to beri-beri heart disease, which is initially a vasodilated state with high cardiac output, later deteriorating to low output. Thiamine deficiency can result from poor nutrition in some Asian areas and to alcoholism but has also been reported in teenagers with diets dominated by processed foods. Abnormal regulation of carnitine can cause dilated or restrictive forms of cardiomyopathy, particularly in children. Calcium deficiency due to hypoparathyroidism, gastrointestinal abnormalities, or chelation directly compromises myocardial contractility, as does deficiency of phosphate, which is needed for high-energy compounds. Hypophosphatemia may occur in alcoholism, in diabetes, during recovery from malnutrition, and in hyperalimentation. Magnesium, a cofactor for thiamine-dependent reactions and for sodium-potassium adenosine triphosphatase, may be depleted by impaired absorption or increased renal excretion.

Endocrinopathies have multiple systemic effects that may affect the heart. Hyperthyroidism may impair cardiac reserve, in part due to tachycardia and to enhanced adrenergic sensitivity in addition to direct affects of triiodothyronine. Hypothyroidism depresses contractility and conduction and may cause pericardial effusions. Diabetes has been associated with cardiomyopathy independently of the epicardial coronary atherosclerosis for which it is a risk factor. Particularly in combination with hypertension, cardiomyopathy with diabetes may present a picture in which diastolic function is more impaired than systolic function. In addition to aggravating heart failure by increasing demand, massive obesity is implicated as a cause of cardiomyopathy with increased ventricular mass and decreased contractility, which improve after weight loss.

Familial Cardiomyopathy

Inherited genetic factors have been implicated in familial dilated cardiomyopathy, although with less frequency and more varied inheritance patterns than in hypertrophic cardiomyopathy. Many of the early examples described varying degrees of cardiomyopathy associated with specific conduction system abnormalities. The most distinct examples of familial cardiomyopathies are the *neuromyopathic disorders* (see Chapter 506) such as Duchenne muscular dystrophy and Becker's X-linked slowly progressive muscular dystrophy, both caused by mutations in the gene for dystrophin, a cytoskeletal protein. More recently, a deletion in a cardiac promoter region associated with this gene was demonstrated in a family with X-linked cardiomyopathy without skeletal myopathy.

Mitochondrial myopathies are maternally transmitted, such as the Kearns-Sayre syndrome of cardiomyopathy, ophthalmoplegia, retinopathy, and cerebellar ataxia. The mitochondrial abnormalities frequently cause skeletal as well as cardiac myopathic changes that can be rapidly progressive in young adulthood.

In addition to abnormalities of muscle proteins and metabolism, heritable factors may influence susceptibility to external triggers for anticardiac immune responses. Kindreds have been described with heart failure presenting after viral infection or during pregnancy. Although previously thought to be rare, familial involvement has now been described in up to 20% of cases of dilated cardiomyopathy.

Arrhythmic right ventricular dysplasia (ARVD) is characterized by focal fibrous-fatty replacement of the right ventricle. The right ventricular free wall and the atria are primarily involved, giving rise to ventricular and supraventricular arrhythmias, which are often the presenting symptom. Proposed causes include congenital hypoplasia of myocardial tissue and focal injury with fibrous replacement. Some patients present with left ventricular dysfunction, without initial recognition of the right ventricular abnormalities, which are often unappreciated on routine echocardiography. Although many cases are spontaneous, there are kindreds with varied expression, the best known of which is the Naxos syndrome originating from the Mediterranean area, in which the affected family members share strikingly curly hair and palmar hyperkeratosis.

Overlap with Restrictive Cardiomyopathy

Diseases causing primarily restrictive cardiomyopathies (see later) can occasionally overlap to cause a picture consistent with dilated cardiomyopathy, particularly when the ventricle is not severely dilated. *Hemochromatosis* and *sarcoidosis* should be considered when evaluating all cardiomyopathy, although they are more often considered with the restrictive diseases. *Amyloidosis* is less commonly confused with dilated than with hypertrophic cardiomyopathy but should be considered for a thick-walled ventricle with moderately depressed contractile function.

Increasing understanding of processes leading to heart failure and particularly of the genetic contribution have reduced the number of cases with no known etiology. Even after careful evaluation, however, the majority of cases of dilated cardiomyopathy are still considered to be *idiopathic*, of unknown cause.

Evaluation of Dilated Cardiomyopathy

History

The history for a patient with dilated cardiomyopathy is gradual exertional intolerance and onset of congestive symptoms, occasionally including chest pain, syncope, or clinical embolic events. An acute presentation may reflect a new problem, such as hyperthyroidism, superimposed on an unrecognized chronic cardiomyopathy of other origin. Rapid development over days to weeks, however, suggests postviral or giant cell myocarditis. Chest pain, typical of pericarditis or mimicking acute myocardial infarction, may result from acute myocarditis, as can ventricular arrhythmias in the ab-

sence of detectable left ventricular dysfunction. Regardless of cause, however, many patients describe an upper respiratory syndrome during the preceding 6 months, as do most people without cardiomyopathy. Adequate history regarding alcohol and cocaine use requires tactful diligence. Family history of possible cardiomyopathy may be helpful, with careful questioning about sudden deaths attributed to "massive heart attacks." Other specific clues such as toxic occupational exposure, residence in rural South America, or frequent exposure to raw meat products can suggest specific causes.

The history should also include careful questioning to elucidate symptoms indicative of the level of hemodynamic compensation, because the majority of heart failure symptoms result from hemodynamic abnormalities of intracardiac filling pressures or systemic perfusion. The presence of orthopnea, which may be indicated by supine cough as well as by dyspnea, indicates elevated left ventricular filling pressures (congestion) at rest. Dyspnea on minimal exertion such as dressing or walking to the bathroom usually is also indicative of elevated resting filling pressures, whereas dyspnea on moderate exertion such as two flights of stairs or two blocks generally indicates low cardiac output reserve. Anorexia, early satiety, and abdominal discomfort usually indicate elevated right-sided heart filling pressures, often with secondary tricuspid regurgitation.

The history for patients without evidence of resting congestion should quantitate their activity as precisely as possible (see Chapter 38). The history should also include specific elucidation of recent pre-syncope or syncope that could indicate dysrhythmic events and the need for specific electrophysiologic evaluation. In addition, patients should be asked specifically about symptoms that may indicate cerebral or peripheral embolic events.

General Cardiac Examination

Common components of the examination for all patients with suspected cardiac disease should address systemic circulatory compensation, evidence of intracardiac abnormalities, and any extracardiac clues to etiology. Elevated filling pressures at rest are diagnosed from elevated jugular venous pressures, abnormal hepatojugular reflux, hepatic distention and ascites, peripheral edema, and the presence of rales, the last three being perhaps the best-known but least sensitive signs of congestion in chronic heart failure. Adequacy of perfusion is best assessed in patients with regular rhythm by blood pressure, specifically the difference between systolic and diastolic, which generally exceeds 25% of systolic if the cardiac index is over 2.2 L/min/m². Cool legs and arms often reflect severe hypoperfusion, but hands and feet can be cool in anyone who is anxious. Vague mental status, inattention, or lapses into sleep during conversation may indicate cerebral hypoperfusion. Pulsus alternans or periodic breathing may be detected in some patients with marked decompensation. If resting hemodynamics appear to be normal, functional cardiac reserve may be assessed initially by a 6-minute walk around the corridor and more objectively by exercise testing analyzing oxygen uptake and anaerobic threshold.

In dilated cardiomyopathy, the left ventricular impulse is often displaced far laterally, although considerable posterior dilation can occur without detectable lateral displacement. The impulse is generally diffuse but not sustained. For restrictive cardiomyopathy, the impulse is less displaced and is often accompanied by a very prominent S_4. Any process leading to secondary right-sided heart failure may cause a separate right ventricular impulse to be felt along the left sternal border beneath the xiphoid process during inspiration. S_3 sounds are often heard, with or without accompanying S_4 sounds, in any cardiomyopathy, with increasing prominence of the S_3 for a given patient frequently reflecting more ventricular volume overload. Absence of gallop rhythms does not mean that heart failure is absent, because many patients never manifest them. Mitral regurgitation is usually significant once hemodynamic decompensation has developed but is not always audible. This murmur, heard best in the axilla, may overlap with a sternal area murmur of tricuspid regurgitation, which generally develops later during decompensation. A short medium-pitched murmur of pulmonic regurgitation may occur early in diastole in patients with marked pulmonary hypertension.

Laboratory Assessment (Table 64–3)

In dilated cardiomyopathy, the electrocardiogram usually shows left ventricular dilation, with poor R wave progression and higher voltage in V_6 than in V_5. Marked decrease in voltage suggests amyloidosis or pericardial effusion. Left atrial abnormality is generally present. Atrial fibrillation may be present. Left bundle branch block occurs in approximately 20%, and many other patients have non-specific QRS prolongation. Right bundle branch block is less common, except in Chagas' disease. Prolongation of the PR interval is common and has been associated with worse survival in some series. More profound conduction block may suggest giant cell myocarditis, sarcoidosis, or amyloidosis. Non-specific T-wave abnormalities are usually present.

The chest radiograph usually shows cardiomegaly, although in some patients marked left ventricular dilation occurs posteriorly before the silhouette enlarges on the anteroposterior view. The degree of cardiomegaly on radiography often reflects more the degree of right than left ventricular dilation, which may explain its prognostic significance, because right ventricular failure carries a more ominous prognosis.

Low sodium and chemistries indicating compromise of renal and hepatic function usually reflect the degree of hemodynamic compromise rather than any specific cause. Creatine kinase levels may be elevated in acute myocarditis, reflecting both cardiac and skeletal myositis, and they may also be elevated in the chronic dystrophies. Serial viral titers may support a diagnosis of myocarditis, and titers for toxoplasmosis, Chagas' disease, or antistreptolysin may also be considered. Peripheral blood eosinophilia should stimulate search for a systemic allergic reaction that could be causing a hypersensitivity myocarditis or for a parasitic disease, and consideration of endocardial restrictive disease (see later). Serologic evidence of active collagen vascular disease should raise the question of cardiac involvement. A sensitive assay for thyroid-stimulating hormone is usually an adequate screen for thyroid disease. Other endocrinologic diagnoses, particularly pheochromocytoma, should be entertained but do not all need to be excluded by extensive laboratory testing. Studies of iron and transferrin should exclude hemochromatosis (see Chapter 221).

As discussed earlier, echocardiography is the initial cardiac laboratory examination in most patients, identifying left ventricular and often right ventricular dilation and hypocontractility and allowing distinction of dilated cardiomyopathy from other forms of cardiomyopathy (see Fig. 64–1). In addition, primary valve disease and septal defects can be detected if present. Primary mitral regurgitation may be difficult to distinguish from mitral regurgitation secondary to dilated heart failure but is more likely if the leaflets or chordae tendineae are abnormal. In general, congestive symptoms with severe mitral regurgitation and ejection fraction greater than 30% are due to primary valve disease or restrictive cardiomyopathy, whereas mitral regurgitation secondary to ventricular dilation develops at lower ejection fractions. Focal wall motion abnormalities often result from coronary artery disease but are common in Chagas' disease and in sarcoidosis and may be seen in any cardiomyopathy. Disproportionate left ventricular hypertrophy may implicate previous hypertension or "burned out" hypertrophic cardiomyopathy as primary causes.

Nuclear imaging may occasionally be useful to diagnose inflammatory conditions but has limited sensitivity and specificity. Focal thallium defects make coronary disease more likely but are also found in non-ischemic cardiomyopathy.

Coronary arteriography should be seriously considered in most patients presenting with dilated heart failure to exclude coronary artery anomalies or atherosclerotic disease. Cardiac catheterization may be needed to confirm a diagnosis of primary valve disease suspected from echocardiography. Determining cardiac output and filling pressures with right-sided heart catheterization may be useful to confirm information from the clinical assessment and to guide subsequent therapy when hemodynamic decompensation is present.

The only definite indications for endomyocardial biopsy are monitoring of cardiac transplant rejection and anthracycline cardiotoxicity. Biopsy is often considered in patients presenting with less than 3 to 6 months of symptoms, among whom lymphocytic myocarditis is detected in 5 to 20%, without clear therapeutic implications. Patients with prominent ventricular arrhythmias and rapid deterioration may undergo biopsy to look for giant cell myocarditis, which carries a high likelihood of requiring imminent transplantation, or sarcoidosis, which may improve with corticosteroid therapy. Endomyocardial biopsy is often performed in patients in whom the clinical suspicion of amyloidosis is high but cannot otherwise be confirmed (see later).

On biopsy, the majority of patients with chronic cardiomyopathy show abnormalities of varying myocyte size, nuclear hypertrophy ("box-car" nuclei), and fibrosis; although considered "diagnostic," these findings do not have unique therapeutic implications. Diagnoses commonly made on endomyocardial biopsy that may affect therapy are transplant rejection, anthracycline cardiotoxicity, giant cell myocarditis, amyloidosis, sarcoidosis, hypereosinophilic syndrome, hemochromatosis, and, occasionally, other metabolic storage diseases. Sampling error limits recognition of toxoplasmosis or Chagas' disease and can lead to false-negative biopsies for sarcoidosis as well. In the individual patient, decisions regarding biopsy must reflect the likelihood that a diagnosis will be made, with its therapeutic and prognostic implications. The utility of biopsy will expand as new biochemical analyses supersede the current techniques of staining and microscopy.

General Therapy and Prognosis

Patients with recent-onset cardiomyopathy have almost a 50% chance of substantial recovery, which is lower in patients with the most severe compromise at presentation. For patients with chronic cardiomyopathy of unknown cause, the prognosis is determined by the stability or deterioration of their left ventricular function and hemodynamic compensation. In general, prognosis parallels the functional class at which they can be maintained, with a 1-year mortality of less than 10% for Class I patients with dilated cardiomyopathy, 10 to 15% for Class II patients, 20 to 25% for Class III patients, and up to 50% for patients who remain Class IV despite aggressive therapy to relieve congestion. Other major prognostic factors include left ventricular ejection fraction, the exact value of which becomes less predictive once it is below 25% and symptoms are severe. Larger left ventricular diastolic dimension is a robust predictor of worse outcome at every stage of heart failure. Decrease in left ventricular ejection fraction and/or increase in dimensions over time are ominous. Preservation of right ventricular function predicts better outcome. Serum sodium and peak oxygen consumption with exercise are useful prognostic factors. Elevated serum norepinephrine and other neuroendocrine abnormalities have been used experimentally but are less often measured clinically.

Patients considered to have a recent active process with some potential for improvement, such as postviral or peripartum cardiomyopathy, are often advised to avoid vigorous exercise for the next 3 to 6 months. This proscription is derived weakly from data that

---

Table 64–3 ■ LABORATORY EVALUATION OF CARDIOMYOPATHY

Routine Initial Evaluation
Electrocardiogram*
    Chest radiograph*
    Two-dimensional and Doppler echocardiogram*
    Chemistry:
        Serum sodium,* potassium,* glucose, creatinine, blood urea nitrogen
        Albumin,* total protein,* liver function tests, serum iron, ferritin
        Creatine kinase
        Thyroid-stimulating hormone
    Hematology:
        Hemoglobin/hematocrit*
        White blood cell count with differential, including eosinophils*
        Erythrocyte sedimentation rate
Initial Evaluation in Selected Patients
    Titers for suspected infection:
        Acute viral (coxsackie virus, echovirus, influenza virus)
        Human immunodeficiency virus, Epstein-Barr virus
        Lyme disease, toxoplasmosis
        Chagas' disease
    Serologies for active rheumatologic disease
    Endomyocardial biopsy

*Included for general initial evaluation of heart failure according to guidelines from Konstam MA, et al. Heart failure: Evaluation and care of patients with left ventricular systolic dysfunction. Agency for Health Care Policy and Research, U.S. Dept. of Health and Human Services, Rockville, MD, 1994.

swimming enhanced mortality in the murine model of acute viral myocarditis and from anecdotal human experience. Patients should be advised, however, to remain mobile, continue regular walking, and avoid daytime bed rest, which leads to deconditioning and depression.

When no cause dictates specific therapy, it is important to rule out contributing factors, such as thyroid disease or rapid atrial fibrillation, which could be treated. If there are no such factors, the therapy for cardiomyopathy is as described for various stages of heart failure (see Chapter 48), with prescription of angiotensin-converting enzyme inhibitors in almost all patients, digitalis glycosides in many, and diuretics and additional vasodilators as dictated by the hemodynamic profile. β-blocking agents improve ventricular function and appear to decrease the progression of disease in stable heart failure but are not indicated in patients with recent or ongoing decompensation. When symptoms of congestion or dyspnea on minimal exertion persist despite empiric therapy with angiotensin-converting enzyme inhibitors, diuretics, and digoxin, compensation can frequently be restored and maintained on a regimen tailored to hemodynamic goals, which include near-normal filling pressures. For patients who are truly refractory to medical therapy but have no other conditions that would compromise long-term survival, cardiac transplantation may be considered (see Chapter 71). Among the investigational surgical therapies for heart failure, benefits have not yet been demonstrated in a controlled trial of cardiomyoplasty, which is contraindicated in Class IV patients. Left ventricular reduction surgery (Batista procedure) is associated with up to a 30% need for acute mechanical devices or transplantation, and the benefits for other patients remain to be defined.

RESTRICTIVE CARDIOMYOPATHIES

The restrictive cardiomyopathies are the least common of the three major categories of cardiomyopathy. Although characterized primarily by decreased distensibility ("diastolic dysfunction"), the restrictive cardiomyopathies are frequently accompanied by some degree of depressed contractility and ejection fraction ("systolic dysfunction"). Hemodynamically, end-diastolic pressures and consequently atrial pressures are elevated initially, with relative preservation of cardiac output until disease is advanced. Although classically considered to be "non-dilated" with normal ventricular dimensions, many restrictive cardiomyopathies are associated with some global or focal ventricular dilation, although less than for equivalent degrees of congestive symptoms in the primary dilated cardiomyopathies. The atria, however, frequently become very enlarged after chronic exposure to high filling pressures.

The initial challenge is to distinguish restrictive cardiomyopathy from dilated cardiomyopathy or pericardial disease (see Chapter 65). Echocardiography in restrictive disease usually shows left ventricular diastolic dimension less than 6 to 6.5 cm and ejection fraction of more than 30%. Symptomatic congestion, the major clinical feature of *restrictive* cardiomyopathy, rarely occurs in primary *dilated* cardiomyopathy until after the ejection fraction is below 30%. Echocardiographic profiles of abnormal relaxation and diastolic filling are helpful in confirming physiologic impairment in patients with near-normal ejection fraction but are less helpful in distinguishing restrictive from other cardiomyopathy, in which the degree of volume overload determines filling pattern. The difficult distinction between primary restrictive disease and extrinsic pericardial disease often requires comparison of right and left ventricular filling during invasive hemodynamic measurement and pericardial imaging by computed tomography or magnetic resonance imaging, particularly in patients with a history of mediastinal radiation, which can cause both myocardial and pericardial disease.

Most restrictive cardiomyopathies result from deposition of abnormal substances in the myocardium (Table 64–4). These are commonly divided into "infiltrative" diseases, in which the abnormal substance is largely between the myocytes, and "storage" diseases, in which abnormal substances accumulate within myocytes.

Infiltrative Disease

Amyloidosis (see Chapter 297) is the most common cause of infiltrative cardiomyopathy. Clinically evident cardiac amyloidosis usually results from primary amyloidosis or the amyloidosis associated with multiple myeloma, in which immunoglobulin light chains

Table 64–4 ■ CAUSES OF RESTRICTIVE CARDIOMYOPATHIES
Infiltrative
Amyloidosis
Sarcoidosis
Gaucher's disease—glucocerebroside-laden macrophages
Hurler's disease—mucopolysaccharide-laden macrophages
Storage
Hemochromatosis
Fabry's disease
Glycogen storage diseases
Fibrotic
Radiation
Scleroderma
Metabolic
Carnitine deficiency
Defects in fatty acid metabolism
Endocardial
Possibly related diseases
Tropical endomyocardial fibrosis
Hypereosinophilic syndrome (Löffler's endocarditis)
Carcinoid syndrome
Radiation
Doxorubicin
Dilated cardiomyopathy overlap
Early stage ("minimally dilated cardiomyopathy")
Partial recovery from dilated cardiomyopathy
Myocardial metabolic defects
Idiopathic

are the major amyloid protein. Instead of an immunoglobulin, however, amyloid deposits in familial amyloidosis contain an abnormal prealbumin (transthyretin) associated with different specific point mutations, many of which involve the kidney or liver without cardiac compromise. Secondary amyloidosis and senile amyloidosis rarely cause clinical cardiac involvement.

Amyloid infiltration of the interstitium stiffens the ventricles and also replaces some contractile elements (Fig. 64–3). Although it is also found in the atria, it is not extensive enough to prevent atrial dilation. Deposits frequently affect the conduction system, leading to bradyarrhythmias. When amyloid also surrounds the arterioles, it may compromise the microcirculation, further impairing systolic and diastolic function and leading to anginal chest pain in some patients.

Like other cardiomyopathies, the earliest symptom may be dyspnea with exertion. Congestion occurs earlier in the course than with dilated cardiomyopathy, frequently with disproportionate right-sided

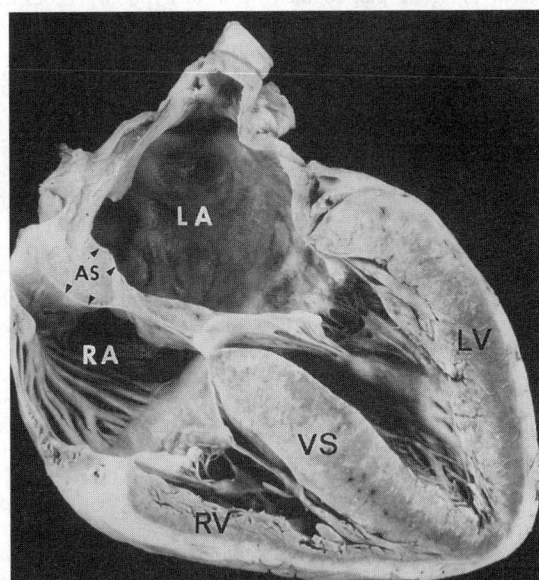

FIGURE 64–3 ■ A necropsy specimen of an amyloid heart demonstrating the thickened ventricular septum (VS), atrial septum (AS), and free walls of the left ventricle (LV) and right ventricle (RV), and the dilated left atrium (LA). (Courtesy of Dr. William Edwards, Mayo Clinic, Rochester, MN.)

congestive symptoms of abdominal discomfort and peripheral edema. Syncope may reflect sinus or atrioventricular node involvement. Occasional angina may be due to small vessel ischemia. Some patients may present with orthostatic hypotension due to amyloid autonomic neuropathy. Evidence of involvement elsewhere such as carpal tunnel syndrome, skin friability, or nephrotic syndrome may also suggest the diagnosis of amyloidosis.

Electrocardiograms characteristically show markedly decreased voltage despite increased wall thickness on echocardiography. Specific diagnosis in some cases can be made from a characteristic sparkling refractile pattern on echocardiography. Up to 80% of patients have a monoclonal protein identified from either serum or urine. Biopsy of subcutaneous fat or the rectum frequently reveals amyloidosis. Endomyocardial biopsy, which carries a higher risk of perforation in the amyloid-infiltrated heart, reveals infiltration in the interstitium and around the coronary vasculature with deposits that are pale pink on hematoxylin-eosin stain and are birefringent with the specific Congo red stain. Symptomatic patients generally have more than 25% of myocardial areas involved.

Once amyloidosis has been associated with heart failure, the median survival is less than 1 year, with less than 5% five-year survival. Most deaths occur suddenly. Patients with familial amyloidosis may have a slower course than those with a monoclonal gammopathy. Making the diagnosis is important to exclude potential candidates for cardiac transplantation, after which amyloidosis can recur rapidly. Symptomatic therapy focuses on the congestive picture. Vasodilator therapy is less effective than in dilated cardiomyopathy, owing to less pronounced systolic dysfunction, greater reliance on high filling pressures, and the frequently accompanying autonomic neuropathy, which predisposes to postural hypotension. Digoxin has not been associated with clear benefit and may carry increased toxicity, particularly through aggravating conduction block. Therapy with colchicine or the combination of melphalan and prednisone for patients with associated monoclonal gammopathy has yielded response rates of only 20 to 30%.

Sarcoidosis (see Chapter 81) of the heart can cause a picture of reduced left ventricular ejection fraction with variable degrees of ventricular dilation. It can present as either restrictive or dilated cardiomyopathy (discussed earlier under Granulomatous Disease).

Storage Diseases

Although amyloidosis and sarcoidosis are seen around myocytes, compromise from the storage diseases results primarily from intracellular accumulation. *Hemochromatosis* is the most common example in adults, frequently arising from an autosomal recessive disorder in the gene that regulates iron absorption. The estimated frequency of homozygosity for the mutant allele is 5 per 1000. In the absence of the genetic defect in iron regulation, hemochromatosis can result from iron overload due to hemolytic anemia and transfusions. Iron is deposited primarily in the perinuclear areas of myocytes. Disrupted cellular architecture and mitochondrial function lead to cell death and replacement fibrosis. The atrioventricular node may be involved. The degree of left ventricular dilation is variable, leading to both dilated and restrictive pictures, with the restrictive aspects dominating earlier in the course. Dilation is generally to left ventricular diastolic dimensions of less than 60 mm, but ejection fractions in severe cases are often less than 30%, unlike the other restrictive diseases. The diagnosis is generally made from the clinical picture, serum iron studies, and genetic testing but may be confirmed by endomyocardial biopsy tissue stained for iron. Early diagnosis is important, because phlebotomy and iron chelation therapy may improve cardiac function before cell injury has become irreversible. Deaths from hemochromatosis result more from cirrhosis and liver carcinoma than from cardiac disease.

Specific metabolic enzyme deficiencies can lead to abnormal metabolites accumulating in the myocardium, causing increased ventricular mass and restrictive cardiomyopathy. Fabry's disease (see Chapter 208) results in intracellular glycolipid accumulation in myocardium and valves, vessel walls, skin, cornea, kidneys, gastrointestinal tract, and central nervous system. Mortality from this X-linked disorder in men results from multiple organ involvement in the fourth or fifth decade. Some heterozygous women have also developed cardiomyopathy. Glycogen storage disease (see Chapter 203) results from enzyme deficiencies that lead to excessive deposition of normal glycogen in myocardium, skeletal muscle, and liver. The most common is type II, Pompe's disease, associated with dramatic thickening of ventricular septal and free walls, large QRS amplitude, short PR interval, and death usually within the first few years of life. Gaucher's disease (see Chapter 203) of glucocerebroside metabolism and Hurler's disease of mucopolysaccharide metabolism result in infiltration of the myocardium by cells filled with abnormal metabolites and may more properly be considered with the infiltrative cardiomyopathies.

Fibrotic Restrictive Cardiomyopathy

Restrictive myocardial disease can occur with diffuse fibrotic changes in the absence of abnormal substance accumulation. Radiation for thoracic malignancy (see Chapter 19) can produce restrictive cardiomyopathy, usually presenting within several years, although occasionally up to 15 years later. Patients treated with both doxorubicin and radiation may be at higher risk. This consequence of radiation is less common, however, than pericardial disease, from which it must be distinguished.

Fibrosis in the scleroderma heart (see Chapter 290) accumulates in the interstitium but may also result from small vessel ischemia with microinfarction. Left ventricular dilation is uncommon, and the congestive symptoms may be refractory to therapy.

Endocardial Restrictive Cardiomyopathy

The picture of restrictive cardiomyopathy can be caused also by specific involvement of the endocardium with relative sparing of the remaining ventricular wall thickness. In equatorial Africa, endomyocardial fibrosis accounts for 15 to 25% of cardiac deaths. It can involve either ventricle, most commonly both, with dense thickening of the ventricular inflow tracts and atrioventricular valves while sparing the underlying myocardium and systolic function. Diuretics can decrease but rarely resolve the congestive symptoms. Extensive surgical resection has been performed for otherwise refractory disease, but with high perioperative morbidity and mortality.

Endomyocardial fibrosis may represent part of the spectrum of hypereosinophilic syndrome (see Chapter 173) (Löffler's endocarditis), characterized by persistent eosinophilia of more than 1500 eosinophils/mm³ without other cause leading to dysfunction of the heart, lungs, and other organs. The eosinophilic contents are thought to injure the endocardium, which is then the site of platelet thrombi and fibrosis. The cardiac apices may be obliterated, creating a characteristic echocardiographic picture. The mitral and tricuspid valves are affected, leading to prominent atrioventricular valve regurgitation. The thrombotic surface can be the origin of multiple systemic emboli. Geographic, infectious, and metabolic factors have been implicated but not verified. Immunosuppressive therapy can reduce the burden of eosinophils and the cardiac injury caused by the eosinophilic granules.

Endocardial injury can also result from the 5-hydroxyindoleacetic acid released by carcinoid tumors. The major sites affected are the tricuspid valve and right ventricular endocardium.

Idiopathic Restrictive Cardiomyopathy

Restrictive cardiomyopathy may occasionally be diagnosed in the absence of any specific cause. Although isolated systolic function may be relatively normal, the ejection fraction is usually in the 30 to 45% range, in which cardiac output may become compromised from restricted filling and secondary valvular regurgitation. For a given patient with slightly reduced left ventricular ejection fraction and slightly elevated left ventricular volume, overt congestive symptoms and abnormal diastolic filling pattern suggest a restrictive cardiomyopathy, whereas a relative lack of symptoms is more consistent with a "minimally dilated cardiomyopathy." Some patients who demonstrate marked improvement of left ventricular function after an obvious dilated cardiomyopathy attributed to viral infection or alcohol may be left with an ejection fraction greater than 40% but significant exertional dyspnea related to reduced compliance. Restrictive disease occasionally occurs in families, in whom a genetic defect affecting myofilament relaxation has been postulated but not identified.

Therapy and Prognosis of Restrictive Cardiomyopathy

Because systolic function is relatively preserved, some patients with restrictive disease may be misdiagnosed for many years as hypochondriacal or deconditioned. Prolonged exposure to elevated filling pressures can cause irreversible pulmonary hypertension, analogous to that with mitral stenosis, and occasionally true cardiac cirrhosis before diagnosis. When congestive symptoms develop, they may be dominated by refractory pleural effusions, ascites, and sometimes dramatic cachexia. Therapy with diuretics is helpful but not curative. The theoretical rationale for calcium channel blockers to improve diastolic relaxation has not been confirmed by clinical results; a reduction in venous return without a concomitant improvement in ventricular compliance can markedly reduce cardiac output. Despite relatively preserved ejection fraction, these patients can sometimes be helped only with cardiac transplantation, which should be done before severe inanition develops. In general, survival with restrictive disease is slightly better than for patients with a similar severity of symptoms but lower ejection fraction from dilated cardiomyopathy.

HYPERTROPHIC CARDIOMYOPATHY

Classic

Etiology and Physiology

Hypertrophic cardiomyopathy is a common genetic abnormality that may occur in as many as 1 in 500 persons and results from any of more than 50 mutations in the sarcomeric proteins β-myosin heavy chain, cardiac troponin T, α-tropomyosin, and myosin-binding C genes. Generally inherited in an autosomal dominant pattern, the mutations may also occur spontaneously. The phenotypic expression of the disease varies markedly between and within families.

The cardinal features are marked left ventricular hypertrophy not due to other cardiac disease, frequently with asymmetrical involvement of the septum, accompanied by supranormal ejection fraction and decreased left ventricular systolic cavity dimension (Fig. 64–4). Pathologically, the myocytes show marked disarray in a characteristic whorled pattern and disorganization of the larger muscle bundles as well. The descriptor "obstructive" or "non-obstructive" refers to whether a pressure gradient that impedes left ventricular outflow can be detected at rest or with maneuvers that decrease left ventricular volume. Previous names for this syndrome included asymmetrical septal hypertrophy, hypertrophic obstructive cardiomyopathy, and idiopathic hypertrophic subaortic stenosis, but these have been largely replaced by the term *hypertrophic cardiomyopathy*.

The affected ventricle is hypercontractile with a supranormal ejection fraction, at times almost obliterating the left ventricular cavity. Diastolic distensibility is markedly limited, leading to elevated filling pressures that can cause shortness of breath. Filling pressures rise further and aggravate dyspnea when the heart rate accelerates during exercise or atrial fibrillation. Myocardial ischemia despite the absence of epicardial coronary artery disease can cause anginal-type chest pain owing to the increased oxygen demands and reduced oxygen delivery for the hypertrophied ventricle with high intracavitary pressures.

Outflow obstruction, present or inducible in about 25% of patients, is caused by apposition of the anterior mitral valve leaflet to the septum and can elevate filling pressures further and compromise forward output. When present, the midsystolic gradient can approach levels seen in severe aortic stenosis. The gradient may be elicited or enhanced by maneuvers that decrease left ventricular volume, such as vasodilation, the Valsalva maneuver, or standing after squatting. Enhanced contractility also aggravates the gradient, as for the beat after a premature ventricular contraction (Brockenbrough phenomenon). Handgrip increases systemic resistance and decreases the gradient. Syncope can result from an increased gradient leading to decreased cardiac output, from elevated intraventricular pressures activating vagal reflexes, or from ventricular arrhythmias arising within the areas of abnormal myocyte organization.

Most patients present between ages 20 and 40, although occasional patients present after age 50. Presenting symptoms may be dyspnea on exertion, chest pain, palpitations, or syncope. When syncope occurs, it is generally during or shortly after heavy exer-

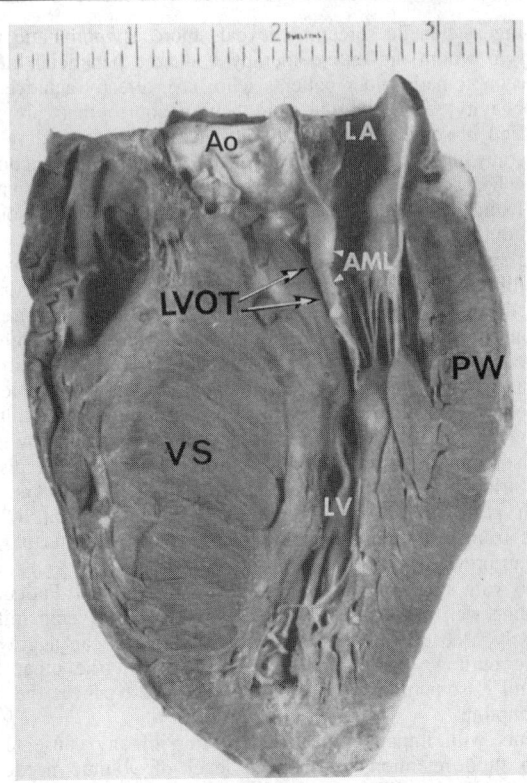

FIGURE 64–4 ■ One of the original cases of hypertrophic cardiomyopathy, demonstrating the marked hypertrophy of the ventricular septum (VS) in contact with the anterior mitral leaflet (AML), impinging on the left ventricular outflow tract (LVOT). The left ventricular (LV) cavity is severely reduced. Ao = aorta; LA = left atrium. (From Teare D: Asymmetric hypertrophy of the heart in young adults. Br Heart J 20:1, 1958. Labels superimposed.)

tion. Cardiac examination in asymptomatic patients may be unrevealing except for a slightly prominent left ventricular impulse. Decreased compliance during atrial filling may lead to a palpable and audible S_4 gallop. When present, the murmur is usually best heard at the left lower sternal border and represents a sum of the outflow murmur and mitral regurgitation. It is typically harsh and increases in intensity with the maneuvers described earlier, which decrease ventricular size. When a gradient impedes ejection, the carotid impulse may transmit both an early and late systolic pulse. An enhanced wave in the jugular venous pulse usually reflects decreased right ventricular compliance because of the abnormal septum rather than right-sided heart failure.

Echocardiography establishes the diagnosis of hypertrophy. Classic asymmetrical septal hypertrophy is defined as a septal–posterior wall thickness ratio of at least 1.5, but asymmetry is not necessary to diagnose hypertrophic cardiomyopathy. Doppler interrogation can identify resting gradients. Cardiac catheterization is often performed to quantify the gradient and in older patients to exclude coexistent coronary disease as a component of chest pain. Electrocardiographic abnormalities most commonly include left ventricular hypertrophy and increased Q waves occasionally misdiagnosed as infarction. Left atrial abnormality may be detected in the P waves, and a short PR interval with slurred QRS upstroke may be misdiagnosed as pre-excitation.

Considerable debate exists over appropriate screening for hypertrophic cardiomyopathy, which is the most common cause identified in sudden deaths occurring in athletes. It is unclear to what degree the increased recognition in athletes results from the addition of physiologic to pathologic ventricular hypertrophy, the superimposition of sudden autonomic surges predisposing to arrhythmias during competition, or their high public profile.

Therapy

Therapy for Symptoms

The controversy regarding therapy in asymptomatic patients is increasing as genetic screening reveals more asymptomatic young patients in whom preventive therapy could be beneficial but also more asymptomatic older patients who have already achieved normal longevity, suggesting a more benign course than previously recognized in some people. In the absence of data regarding benefits, therapy in asymptomatic patients is generally not encouraged except when accompanied by severe hypertrophy, such as ventricular wall thickness over the equivalent of 35 mm in adults, or by a marked outflow gradient (Fig. 64–5).

Once symptoms are present, therapy is directed to improve diastolic filling and perhaps reduce myocardial ischemia and to reduce sudden death. β-Adrenergic blocking drugs and verapamil are most commonly used to address symptoms. A major action of both is to improve diastolic filling by increasing the duration of diastole as heart rate decreases. Additional effects on reducing inotropic state may decrease myocardial oxygen consumption directly, thus decreasing any ischemia, and decrease generation of an outflow gradient. Disopyramide decreases the inotropic state but can also increase atrioventricular conduction if atrial fibrillation occurs; so, if used, it is usually combined with a β-blocking agent. Clinical benefits from disopyramide may decrease over time, and it is less used than previously.

β-Blocking agents are generally the initial treatment. Patients not responding well to this therapy may respond well to verapamil, and conversely. Because of its vasodilation, verapamil can aggravate a dynamic outflow gradient in some patients. On the other hand, verapamil is sometimes used initially when chest pain is the dominant symptom.

Patients with impaired diastolic function of any cause tend to develop fluid retention beyond the level of volume needed for optimal ventricular filling. Diuretics should be used to treat obvious fluid retention, but caution is needed to avoid excessive diuresis to a volume-depleted state that would compromise cardiac output and increase a provokable gradient.

Atrial fibrillation occurs commonly in hypertrophic cardiomyopathy, perhaps even more commonly than in other conditions associated with chronically elevated atrial pressures. Because of the deleterious effects of rapid ventricular rates and loss of the atrial kick on ventricular filling and symptoms of congestion, vigorous attempts to achieve and maintain sinus rhythm are warranted, most commonly with amiodarone. When sinus rhythm cannot be maintained, amiodarone may also be useful for maintaining slow ventricular response, facilitated also by β-blockers or verapamil, which are often not in themselves sufficient. For refractory fast ventricular rates, it may be necessary to ablate the atrioventricular node and provide permanent dual-chamber pacing. Anticoagulation is strongly indicated for patients with a history of atrial fibrillation, even if sinus rhythm has been restored, owing to the high risk of embolic events with recurrence.

Truly refractory symptoms are uncommon but should be addressed according to whether systolic performance is preserved and whether or not there is outflow obstruction (resting gradient usually ≥ 50 mm). It is estimated that fewer than 5% of hypertrophic cardiomyopathy patients have refractory severe symptoms and major outflow obstruction. For those patients, dual-chamber pacing has often been tried, with variable results. Septal reduction procedures abolish or substantially reduce the gradient in over 90% of cases, with persistent symptomatic improvement in 70%. Approaches include surgical myotomy-myectomy or alcohol injection into the septal coronary artery. Mitral valve replacement may also improve the gradient by reducing apposition of the valve leaflet to the septum and may also be considered when there are intrinsic abnormalities of the mitral valve contributing to mitral regurgitation, whether or not obstruction is present.

In perhaps 5% of patients, hypertrophic cardiomyopathy may "burn out" into a condition more typical of dilated heart failure, with thinner walls and no outflow gradient but persistence of mitral regurgitation. Residual diastolic stiffness renders such patients less likely to have marked ventricular dilation and more likely to have symptoms of congestion at left ventricular ejection fractions that are not severely reduced (often in the range of 30 to 40%, as opposed to usual dilated cardiomyopathy in which severe symptoms are rare above an ejection fraction of 25%). Such patients should discontinue verapamil and disopyramide, continue β-blocking agents only at low doses with caution, and begin therapy with angiotensin-converting enzyme inhibitors, with diuretics as needed for fluid retention. Cardiac transplantation may be considered in these patients, in whom deterioration may occur rapidly.

Therapy for Sudden Death

With hypertrophic cardiomyopathy, sudden death accounts for most of the annual mortality, which is reported as 3 to 4% in referral centers and 1% in less selected populations. There are multiple potential causes of syncope and sudden death in hypertrophic cardiomyopathy, with the most common being primary and secondary ventricular tachyarrhythmias. Patients at highest risk are those who have already had sustained ventricular tachycardia or sudden death and young patients with either a family history of two or more sudden deaths or, in some cases, a genetic mutation associated with high risk of sudden death. These patients in general receive therapy with either amiodarone or an implantable cardioverter-defibrillator. Patients with syncope should also be carefully evaluated for specific arrhythmic causes.

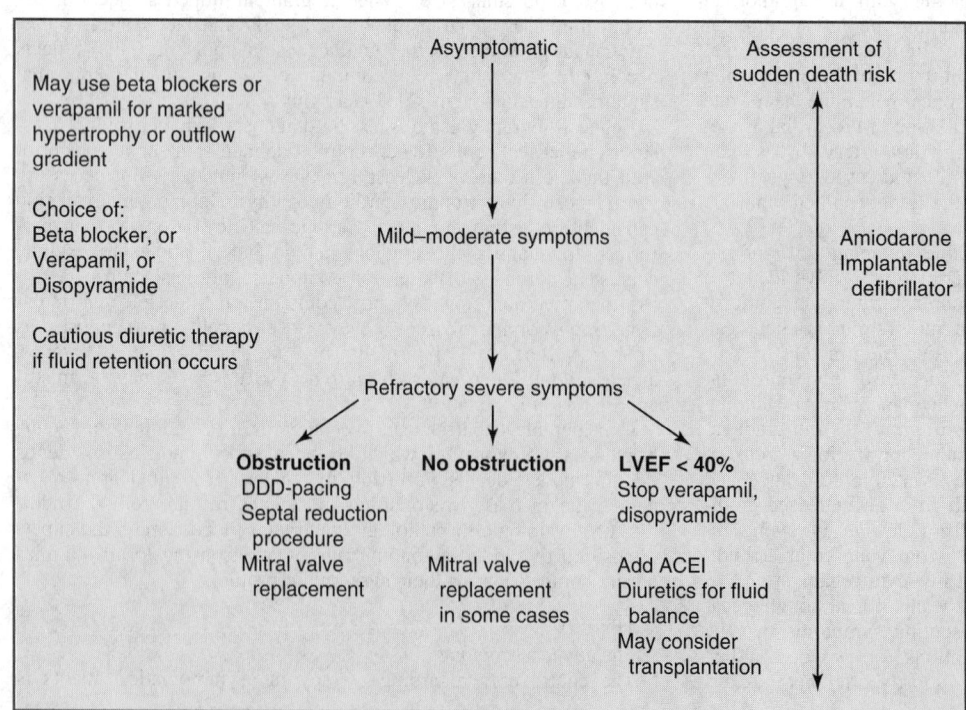

FIGURE 64–5 ■ Approach to therapy of hypertrophic cardiomyopathy according to the severity of symptoms. Risk for sudden death should be considered regardless of symptomatic status. LVEF = left ventricular ejection fraction; ACEI = angiotensin-converting enzyme inhibitor.

For patients not included in the high-risk groups just mentioned, risk stratification has been difficult. Short runs of non-sustained ventricular tachycardia are not currently considered an indication for prophylactic treatment. It does appear possible, however, to define a relatively low-risk group by the following: no family history of premature death, no sustained or non-sustained ventricular tachycardia on Holter monitoring, absence of a marked outflow gradient, absence of marked ventricular hypertrophy (> 20 mm) or left atrial enlargement, and no exercise-induced hypotension. Although these low-risk patients may not need to be restricted from vigorous activity, it has been recommended that all patients with hypertrophic cardiomyopathy avoid intense training and competition.

Apical Giant T-Wave Hypertrophy

A separate entity of apical hypertrophic cardiomyopathy has been recognized, predominantly in Japan, where it accounts for one fourth of hypertrophic cardiomyopathy. It is characterized by systolic apical obliteration that creates a "spadelike" cavity on angiography and frequently by giant negative T waves in the precordial electrocardiogram. There is no intraventricular gradient. Symptoms are usually mild. Malignant ventricular arrhythmias appear less commonly than in other forms of hypertrophic cardiomyopathy. Some patients, particularly elderly women, have marked symmetrical hypertrophy, which is disproportionate to the degree of their hypertension.

Spectrum of Dominant Diastolic Dysfunction

Many more patients have moderate concentric hypertrophy without any characteristics of classic genetic hypertrophic cardiomyopathy or the apical hypertrophic cardiomyopathy. Although the majority of these reflect chronic hypertension and do not have any symptoms of cardiac disease, there is an increasing recognition that some of these patients develop typical symptoms of congestion, with elevated filling pressures, fluid retention, and pulmonary edema. The clinical syndrome overlaps that of restrictive disease with normal or mildly reduced left ventricular ejection fraction but abnormal diastolic flow patterns. This picture is particularly common in older patients with a history of hypertension and diabetes mellitus. The major focus of symptomatic therapy is usually the reduction of filling pressures to levels as low as can be tolerated, which includes judicious use of diuretics, control of hypertension, and reduction of heart rate. Whereas angiotensin-converting enzyme inhibitor use is indicated in patients with reduced left ventricular ejection fraction and is a good choice for control of hypertension, it is reasonable but not specifically demonstrated to have cardiovascular benefits in patients with minimally reduced, preserved, or enhanced left ventricular ejection fraction. Atrial fibrillation often leads to clinical decompensation both because of increased rate and loss of the atrial contribution to ventricular filling.

Kasper EK, Agema WRP, Hutchins GM, et al: The causes of dilated cardiomyopathy: A clinicopathologic review of 673 consecutive patients. J Am Coll Cardiol 23:586, 1994. *Results of systematic endomyocardial biopsy in a large referral population. Results are representative of other series except for a slightly higher incidence of myocarditis, which included "borderline myocarditis."*

Kelly DP, Straus AW: Inherited cardiomyopathies. N Engl J Med 330:913, 1994. *A thoughtful summary of the identification of specific genetic defects causing cardiomyopathy.*

Spirito P, Seidman CE, McKenna WJ, Maron BJ: The management of hypertrophic cardiomyopathy. N Engl J Med 336:775–785, 1997. *An excellent synthesis of current and evolving therapies for hypertrophic cardiomyopathy.*

Wynne J, Braunwald E: The cardiomyopathies and myocarditides: Toxic, chemical and physical damage to the heart. In Braunwald E (ed): Heart Disease: A Textbook of Cardiovascular Medicine. Philadelphia, WB Saunders, 1997, p 1404. *A definitively detailed and referenced source of information on all of the clinical aspects of the cardiomyopathies.*

65 PERICARDIAL DISEASE

Warren J. Manning

NORMAL PERICARDIAL ANATOMY AND FUNCTION

The pericardium is composed of two distinct layers: the fibrous parietal pericardium, which provides a protective sac around the heart to prevent sudden cardiac dilation and minimize bulk cardiac motion, and the inner, visceral pericardium intimately related to the surface of the heart. These two layers are separated by 10 to 50 mL of clear fluid, an ultrafiltrate of plasma produced by the visceral pericardium. This fluid acts as a lubricant to minimize frictional forces between the heart and surrounding structures. In health, the intrapericardial pressure is slightly negative.

CONGENITAL PERICARDIAL ABNORMALITIES. Although congenital total absence of the pericardium does not appear to be associated with clinical disease, partial or localized absence of pericardium, specifically around the left atrium, may be associated with focal herniation and subsequent strangulation. This condition, usually diagnosed by thoracic computed tomography (CT) or magnetic resonance imaging (MRI), has been associated with atypical chest pain or sudden death; therefore, surgical repair is often recommended when a partial pericardial defect is confirmed. Benign pericardial cysts are quite rare and often seen as rounded or lobulated structures adjacent to the usual cardiac silhouette on the chest radiograph; both thoracic CT and MRI (Fig. 65–1) are useful for the diagnosis of these cysts.

Acquired pericardial disease may have numerous etiologies, most of which produce responses that are pathophysiologically and clini-

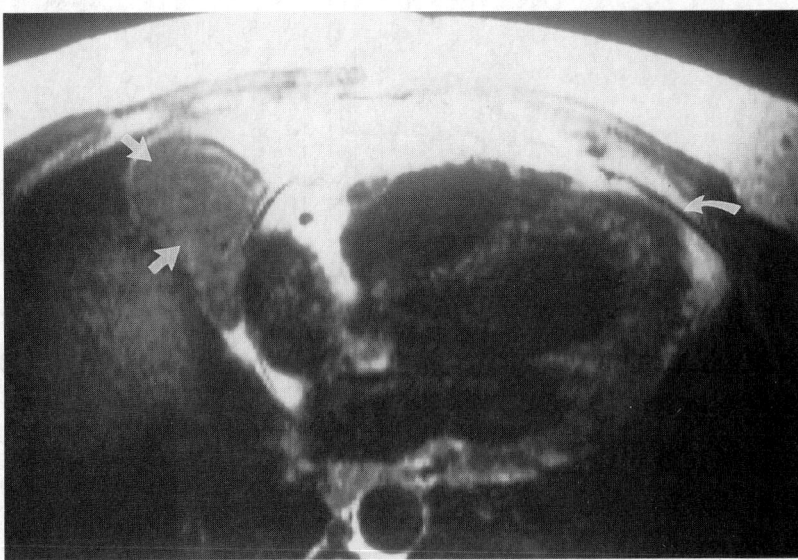

FIGURE 65–1 ■ Transverse (axial) magnetic resonance image. Note the anterior pericardial cyst (straight white arrows). Also note the normal pericardium (curved white arrow). (Courtesy of Robert R. Edelman, MD.)

Table 65–1 ■ ETIOLOGY OF PERICARDITIS

Infectious Pericarditis
    Viral (coxsackie A and B, echovirus, mumps, adenovirus, HIV)
    Mycobacterium tuberculosis
    Bacterial (*Pneumococcus, Streptococcus, Staphylococcus, Legionella*)
    Fungal (histoplasmosis, coccidioidomycosis, candidiasis, blastomycosis)
    Other (syphilis, parasites)
Non-infectious Pericarditis
    Idiopathic
    Neoplasm
        Metastatic (lung cancer, breast cancer, melanoma, lymphoma)
        Primary (mesothelioma)
    Renal failure
    Trauma
    Irradiation (especially for breast cancer, Hodgkin's disease)
    Myocardial infarction
    Hypothyroidism
    Aortic dissection
    Chylopericardium (thoracic duct injury)
    Trauma
        Post-pericardiotomy
        Chest wall injury/trauma
Hypersensitivity Pericarditis
    Collagen vascular disease (systemic lupus erythematosus, rheumatoid
        arthritis, scleroderma, acute rheumatic fever)
    Drug induced (procainamide, hydralazine, isoniazid)
    Post–myocardial infarction (Dressler's syndrome)

cally similar. These responses most frequently result in acute pericarditis, pericardial effusion, or constrictive pericarditis.

ACUTE PERICARDITIS

The most common clinical pathologic process involving the pericardium is acute pericarditis. Although multiple causes are possible (Table 65–1), the most common is viral infection. Classically, this disorder is characterized by chest pain, a pericardial friction rub, electrocardiographic (ECG) changes, and pericardial effusion. It is often brief in duration and uncomplicated, although vigilance for progression to tamponade is always prudent.

CLINICAL FEATURES. Chest pain of acute infectious (viral) pericarditis typically develops in younger adults 1 to 2 weeks after a "viral illness." The symptoms are sudden and severe in onset, characteristically with retrosternal and/or left precordial pain and referral to the back and trapezius ridge. Pain may be *preceded* by low-grade fever (in contrast to myocardial infarction, in which the

pain precedes the fever). Although radiation to the arms in a manner similar to myocardial ischemia may also occur, it is less common. The pain is often pleuritic (e.g., accentuated by inspiration or coughing) and may also be aggravated (supine or left lateral decubitus posture) or relieved (upright posture) by changes in posture.

The physical examination in patients with acute pericarditis is most notable for a pericardial friction rub. Although classically described as triphasic, with systolic and both early (passive ventricular filling) and late (atrial systole) diastolic components, more commonly a biphasic (systole and diastole) or a monophasic rub may be heard. The rub may be transient as well as positional. Also common are a resting tachycardia (rarely atrial fibrillation) and, if the etiology is infectious, a low-grade fever.

DIAGNOSTIC TESTING. ECG changes (Fig. 65–2) are common, particularly with infectious etiologies because of associated inflammation of the superficial epicardium. During the initial few days, diffuse (limb leads and precordial leads) ST segment elevations occur in the absence of reciprocal ST segment depression. PR segment depression is also common and reflects atrial involvement. After several days, the ST segments normalize and then the T waves become inverted (in contrast to the ECG changes seen with myocardial infarction, in which the temporal relationship of the T wave inversions is earlier and precedes normalization of the ST changes). In the setting of a large pericardial effusion, loss of R wave voltage (absolute R wave magnitude of 5 mm or less in limb leads and 10 mm or less in precordial leads) and electrical alternans (Fig. 65–3) may also be seen (see Pericardial Effusion below).

If the pericardial effusion is not significant, the chest radiograph is often unrevealing, although a small left pleural effusion may be seen. An elevated erythrocyte sedimentation rate and mild elevation of the white blood cell count are also common.

TREATMENT. In the absence of significant pericardial effusion (see below), treatment is primarily directed at relieving the patient's symptoms. Non-steroidal anti-inflammatory agents such as indomethacin (25 to 50 mg three times daily) are generally quite effective, although aspirin (325 to 650 mg three times daily) may also be used. Glucocorticoids (prednisone, 20 to 60 mg/day) may be useful for resistant situations. Anti-inflammatory agents should be continued at a constant dose until the patient is afebrile and asymptomatic for 1 week, followed by a gradual taper over the next several weeks. The use of warfarin and/or heparin should be avoided if possible to minimize the risk of hemopericardium, but anticoagulation may be required in the setting of atrial fibrillation. Avoidance of vigorous physical activity is also recommended during the acute and early convalescent period.

Viral and idiopathic pericarditis is usually self-limited. However,

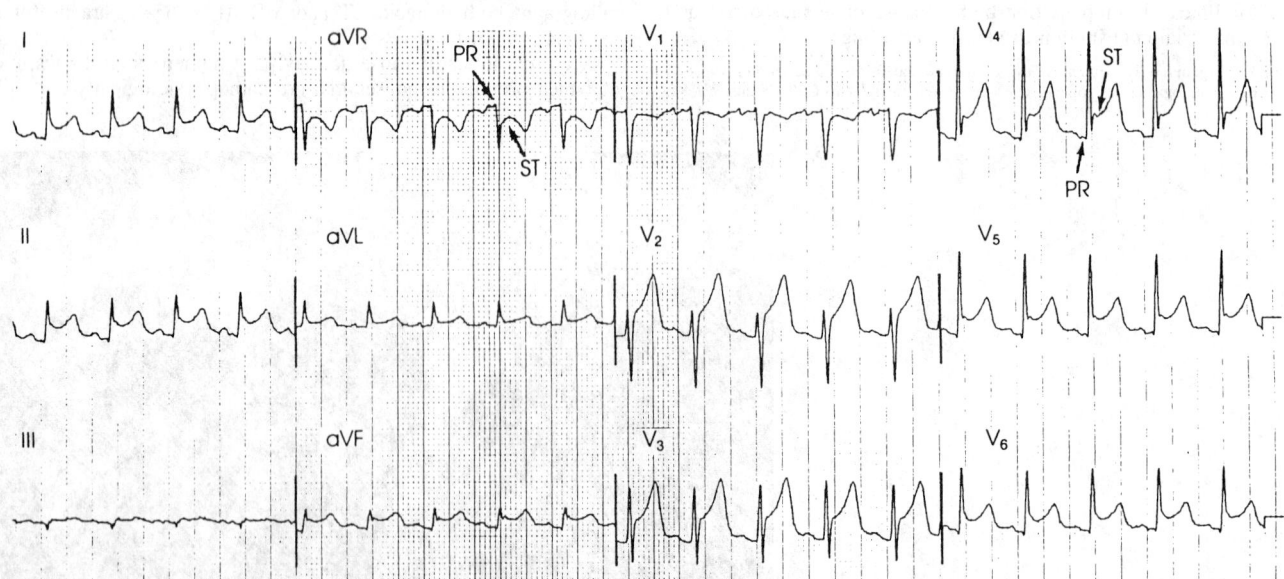

FIGURE 65–2 ■ Twelve-lead electrocardiogram from a patient with acute pericarditis. Note the diffuse ST-T wave changes along with PR elevation in lead aVR and PR segment depression in leads II and aVF and in the precordial leads. (Courtesy of Ary L. Goldberger, MD.)

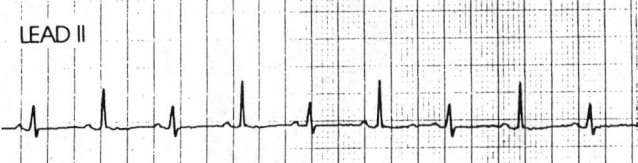

LEAD II

FIGURE 65–3 ■ Lead II rhythm strip taken from a patient with acute pericarditis complicated by a very large pericardial effusion and tamponade physiology. Note the resting sinus tachycardia with relatively low voltage and electrical alternans. (Courtesy of Ary Goldberger, MD.)

up to a quarter of patients may have recurrent symptoms. For this group, prolonged treatment with colchicine, 1 mg/day, or pericardiectomy should be considered. Patients with recurrent pericarditis are at increased risk for progression to constrictive pericarditis (see below).

PERICARDIAL EFFUSION

Excess fluid may develop in the pericardial space in all forms of pericardial disease. Most commonly, the fluid is exudative and reflects pericardial injury/inflammation. Serosanguineous effusions are typical of tuberculous and neoplastic disease but may also be seen in uremic and viral/idiopathic disease or in response to mediastinal irradiation. Hemopericardium is most commonly seen with trauma, myocardial rupture following myocardial infarction, catheter-induced myocardial or epicardial coronary artery rupture, aortic dissection with rupture into the pericardial space, or primary hemorrhage in patients receiving anticoagulant therapy (often after cardiac valve surgery). Chylopericardium is quite rare and results from leakage or injury to the thoracic duct.

Although the presence of pericardial effusion is indicative of underlying pericardial disease, the clinical relevance of pericardial effusion is most closely associated with the rate of collection, intrapericardial pressure, and subsequent development of tamponade physiology. A rapidly accumulating effusion, as in hemopericardium caused by trauma, may result in tamponade physiology with collection of only 100 to 200 mL. By comparison, a more slowly developing effusion may allow for gradual stretching of the pericardium, with effusions exceeding 1500 mL in the absence of hemodynamic embarrassment.

DIAGNOSIS OF PERICARDIAL EFFUSION. Pericardial effusion is often suspected clinically when the patient has symptoms and signs of tamponade physiology (see below), but it may also be first suggested by unsuspected cardiomegaly on the chest radiograph, especially if loss of the customary cardiac borders and a "water bottle" configuration are noted (Fig. 65–4). Fluoroscopy, which may display minimal or absent motion of cardiac borders, is commonly performed when myocardial or epicardial coronary artery perforation is suspected during a diagnostic or interventional percutaneous procedure.

In most situations, two-dimensional transthoracic echocardiography is the diagnostic imaging procedure of choice for the evaluation and semiquantitative assessment of suspected pericardial effusion (Fig. 65–5). In emergency situations, it can be performed at the bedside, with the subcostal four-chamber view being the most informative imaging plane. This imaging plane is particularly relevant because it allows the size and location of the effusion to be assessed from an orientation that determines whether the effusion can be drained percutaneously. Transudative effusions typically appear relatively "echo lucent" (Fig. 65–6A), whereas organized/exudative and hemorrhagic effusions have an "echo-filled" or a "ground-glass" appearance (see Fig. 65–6B). Stranding, which may be appreciated in the setting of organized or chronic effusions, suggests an inability to drain the effusion fully by percutaneous approaches. In patients with very large effusions, which are associated with electrical alternans, the heart may appear to swing freely within the pericardial sac.

CARDIAC TAMPONADE. Accumulation of fluid in the pericardium with a resultant increase in pericardial pressure and impairment of ventricular filling results in cardiac tamponade. This complication of pericarditis may be fatal if it is not quickly recognized and aggressively treated. The hallmarks of cardiac tamponade are

65 Pericardial Disease ■ 349

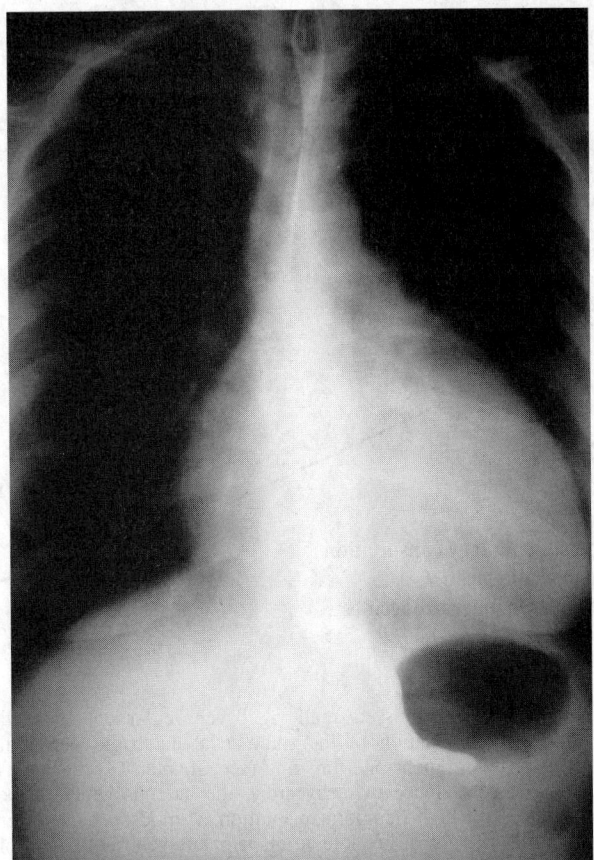

FIGURE 65–4 ■ Posteroanterior (PA) chest radiograph in a patient with a large pericardial effusion. Note the loss of customary heart borders and a "water bottle" configuration. (Courtesy of Sven Paulin, MD.)

increased intracardiac pressure and the resulting impaired ventricular filling and depressed cardiac output. In tamponade, ventricular filling is impaired throughout diastole; by comparison, early diastolic filling is relatively normal with pericardial constriction. Invasive hemodynamic assessment will reveal equalization of right and left atrial as well as right and left ventricular diastolic pressures. Tamponade may not be an "all or none" phenomenon; mild or "low-pressure" tamponade can be seen when intrapericardial pressures are only modestly elevated with resultant equalization of atrial pressures but not diastolic ventricular pressures.

CLINICAL FEATURES OF CARDIAC TAMPONADE. The clinical features of cardiac tamponade may mimic those of heart failure, with dyspnea on exertion, orthopnea, and hepatic engorgement. A number of clinical features help distinguish cardiac tamponade from constrictive pericarditis and restrictive cardiomyopathy (Table 65–2). The typical physical examination with tamponade includes jugular venous distention with a prominent x descent (Fig. 65–7), sinus tachycardia with hypotension, a narrow pulse pressure, elevated (>10 mm Hg) pulsus paradoxus, and distant heart sounds. The pulsus paradoxus may be apparent with palpation, but more commonly it is measured with a sphygmomanometer during slow respiration; direct arterial monitoring is not generally necessary for quantification. A small (<10 mm Hg) pulsus is normal and is related to the ventricles being confined within the pericardium and sharing a common septum. With inspiration, right ventricular filling is enhanced, thereby displacing the interventricular septum toward the left ventricle and exaggerating the reduction in left ventricular filling and resultant stroke volume. The exaggerated pulsus is not specific for tamponade; it may also be present with hypovolemic shock, chronic obstructive pulmonary disease, and bronchospasm.

ECHOCARDIOGRAPHY AND CARDIAC TAMPONADE. For patients in whom the history and/or physical examination is suggestive of tamponade, emergency echocardiography is imperative and generally diagnostic. Echocardiographic evidence of tamponade physiol-

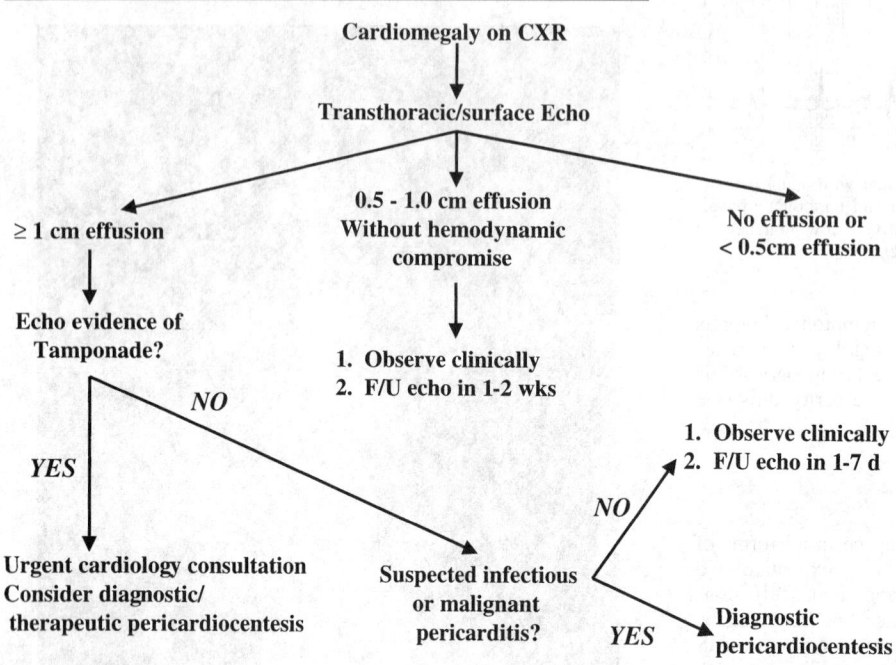

Cardiomegaly on CXR

↓

Transthoracic/surface Echo

≥ 1 cm effusion

**0.5 - 1.0 cm effusion
Without hemodynamic
compromise**

**No effusion or
< 0.5cm effusion**

**Echo evidence of
Tamponade?**

NO

YES

1. **Observe clinically**
2. **F/U echo in 1-2 wks**

1. **Observe clinically**
2. **F/U echo in 1-7 d**

NO

**Urgent cardiology consultation
Consider diagnostic/
therapeutic pericardiocentesis**

**Suspected infectious
or malignant
pericarditis?**

YES

**Diagnostic
pericardiocentesis**

FIGURE 65–5 ■ Schematic for the clinical management of patients with cardiomegaly on chest x-ray (CXR) and suspected pericardial effusion in patients with normal left ventricular systolic function and normal thyroid-stimulating hormone (TSH). (Adapted from Lorell BH: Pericardial disease. *In* Goldman L, Braunwald E [eds]: Primary Cardiology. Philadelphia, WB Saunders, 1998, p 440.)

ogy includes a compressed/small right ventricular chamber with late-diastolic invagination of the right atrial and right ventricular free wall on two-dimensional imaging (see Chapter 43). Because of the frequent coexistence of tachycardia, the latter is generally best appreciated with high–temporal resolution M-mode echocardiography. Localized right atrial, left atrial, and left ventricular diastolic collapse may also be seen and are particularly relevant for loculated effusions such as those following trauma and cardiac surgery. Pseudoprolapse of the mitral valve may be seen because of the compressed left ventricular cavity. When surface echocardiography is inadequate, as in a post-thoracotomy patient or a patient with chest wall trauma, transesophageal echocardiography may be helpful. Thoracic CT and MRI may be particularly valuable for delineation of loculated pericardial effusions. In addition to diastolic invagination, M-mode echocardiography may demonstrate exaggerated inspiratory septal motion and variation in the duration of

aortic valve opening. Finally, Doppler echocardiography may be used to assess transtricuspid and transmitral flow profiles and demonstrate the exaggerated peak E wave response seen in tamponade. It is important to note that many of these typical echocardiographic findings may be absent in patients with significant pulmonary artery hypertension.

TREATMENT OF CARDIAC TAMPONADE. When tamponade is suggested clinically and confirmed on echocardiographic examination, immediate treatment may be life-saving. When time allows, right heart catheterization should be performed to confirm elevated intrapericardial pressure and "equalization" of right atrial, left atrial, pulmonary capillary wedge, right ventricular diastolic, and left ventricular diastolic pressure. If echocardiography demonstrates at least 1 cm of fluid anterior to the mid-right ventricular free wall and apex, percutaneous pericardiocentesis can generally be safely performed. During this procedure, a small catheter is advanced over a

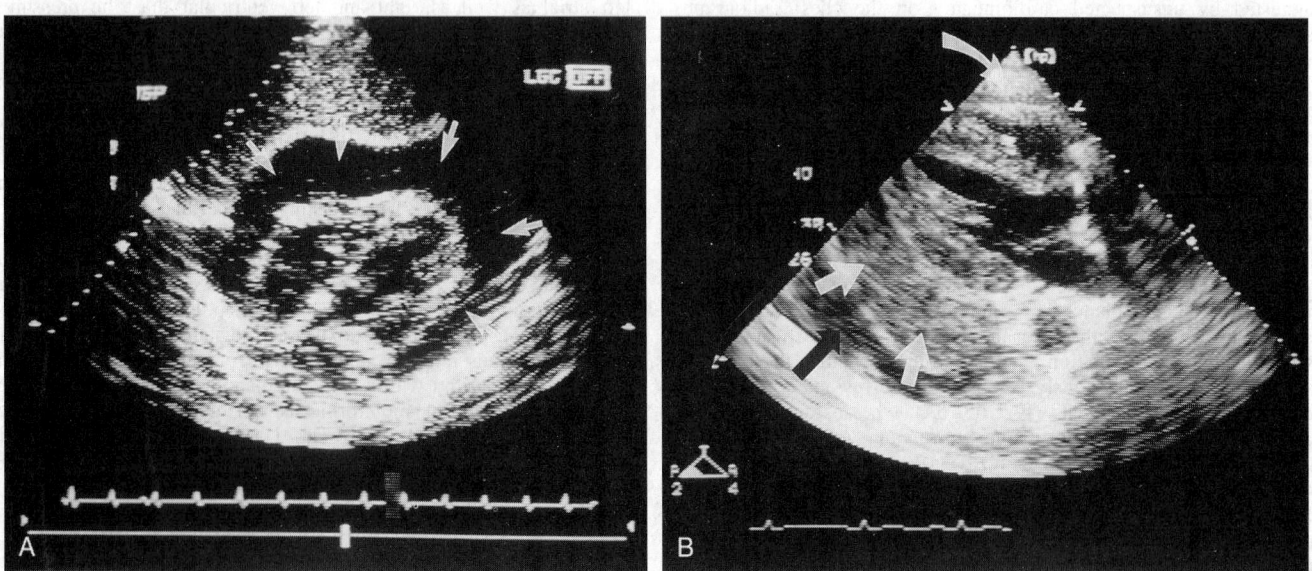

FIGURE 65–6 ■ *A*, Transthoracic echocardiogram from the subcostal approach. Note the large echo-lucent area/pericardial effusion (white arrows) surrounding the heart. The right ventricle is compressed. *B*, Transthoracic echocardiogram from the parasternal long-axis window in another patient. Note the large "echo-filled" pericardial effusion posterior (straight white arrows) to the left ventricle and anterior (curved white arrow) to the right ventricle. This patient had a hemorrhagic pericardial effusion that developed several weeks after aortic valve replacement and treatment with chronic warfarin. A pleural effusion (black arrow) is also seen. LV = left ventricle.

Table 65–2 ■ COMPARISON OF PHYSICAL EXAMINATION AND DIAGNOSTIC TESTS FOR CARDIAC TAMPONADE, CONSTRICTIVE PERICARDITIS, AND RESTRICTIVE CARDIOMYOPATHY

CHARACTERISTIC	CARDIAC TAMPONADE	CONSTRICTIVE PERICARDITIS	RESTRICTIVE CARDIOMYOPATHY
Clinical			
Pulsus paradoxus	+	+/−	−
Prominent y descent	−	+	−
Prominent x descent	+	+	−
Kussmaul's sign	−	+	−
S₃ or pericardial "knock"	−	+	+
S₄	−	−	+
ECG			
Low voltage	+	+	+
Abnormal P waves	−	+	+/−
Electrical alternans	+	−	+
Chest Radiograph			
Cardiomegaly	+	−	−
Pericardial calcification	−	+	−
Echocardiography			
Pericardial effusion	+	−	−
Pericardial thickening	−	+	−
Small right ventricle	+	−	−
Thickened myocardium	−	−	+
Enhanced respiratory variation in E wave	+	+	−
CT/MRI			
Pericardial thickening	−	+	−
Pericardial calcification	−	+	−
Cardiac Catheterization			
Equalization of pressures	+	+	−
Abnormal myocardial biopsy	−	−	+

ECG = electrocardiogram; CT = computed tomography; MRI = magnetic resonance imaging.

needle inserted into the pericardial cavity. Echocardiographic guidance is particularly useful for smaller effusions or if pericardiocentesis is performed by less experienced operators. As much fluid as possible is removed, with monitoring of filling pressures. Unless the etiology has already been identified, pericardial fluid should be sent for evaluation (including culture and cytology). A flexible catheter may be left in the pericardial space for several days to avoid early reaccumulation.

Hemodynamically significant effusions of less than 1 cm, organized or multiloculated effusions, or focal effusions confined to the posterior or lateral cardiac borders or around the atria should be approached surgically via a limited thoracotomy/mediastinoscopy and pericardial window. If the effusion is related to a malignancy and aggressive chemotherapy is not being administered, reaccumulation in the ensuing weeks or months is the norm, and elective surgery should be considered before hospital discharge. Hemorrhagic effusions related to cardiac trauma or aortic dissection are also best managed by emergency surgery (if available) or in combination with very temporizing pericardiocentesis. If the patient is in extremis, emergency pericardiocentesis should be performed at the bedside.

APPROACH TO EFFUSION WITHOUT TAMPONADE. For patients with suspected pericardial effusion, transthoracic echocardiography is the initial test of choice and in most patients will be definitive in confirming the presence or absence of a significant pericardial effusion (loculated effusions may be better identified by CT or MRI). If a small (0.5 to 1.0 cm) "echo-lucent" pericardial effusion is seen, the patient can generally be observed with a follow-up echocardiogram in 1 to 2 weeks (sooner if clinical deterioration is evident). If the follow-up study demonstrates a smaller effusion, subsequent echocardiograms are not necessary (unless the patient's clinical condition changes). Assuming a clinical history of "viral" pericarditis, assessment of renal function and thyroid-stimulating hormone is reasonable, but the results will probably be normal. A tuberculin skin test should be performed routinely. One should also exclude a drug-induced etiology (e.g., cromolyn, hydralazine, isoniazid, phenytoin, procainamide, reserpine).

In the setting of a moderate (1 to 2 cm) or large (>2 cm) pericardial effusion, treatment and follow-up are dependent on the clinical scenario and echocardiographic findings. If the patient is clinically unstable and tamponade is suggested (see above), urgent cardiology consultation and diagnostic/therapeutic pericardiocentesis should be planned. If the patient is hemodynamically stable and tamponade is not suggested, the patient can be observed and a follow-up study performed in 1 to 7 days. The initial evaluation is the same as listed earlier for a small effusion. Follow-up echocardiographic studies should be continued until the size of the effusion has decreased, but they need not be repeated until complete resolution. If bacterial or malignant pericarditis is suspected, diagnostic pericardiocentesis should be performed even in the absence of clinical instability or suggestion of tamponade; tuberculous pericarditis is best diagnosed by pericardial biopsy. A complete blood count with differential, platelet count, and coagulation parameters should also be assessed. Anticoagulation with heparin or warfarin should be discontinued unless the patient has a mechanical heart valve or atrial fibrillation. Blood cultures are indicated if an infectious etiology is suspected. Complement, antinuclear antibodies, and the sedimentation rate may be helpful if systemic lupus erythematosus is

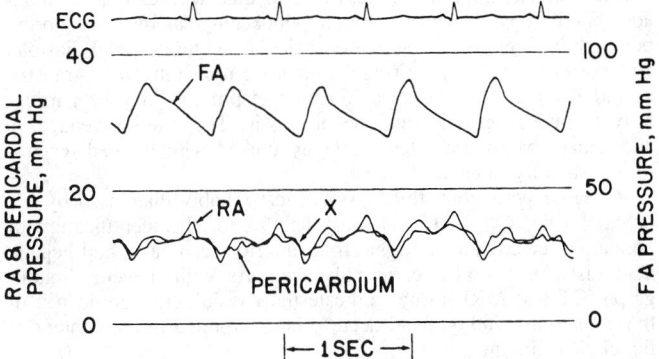

FIGURE 65–7 ■ Simultaneous right atrial (RA), intrapericardial, and femoral artery pressure recordings in a patient with cardiac tamponade. Note the elevated and equilibrated intrapericardial and RA pressures with a prominent *x* descent and blunted *y* descent suggestive of impaired right atrial emptying in early diastole. The arterial pulse pressure is narrowed. (From Lorell BH: Profiles in constriction, restriction and tamponade. *In* Baim DS, Grossman W [eds]: Cardiac Catheterization, Angiography, and Intervention, 5th ed. Philadelphia, Williams & Wilkins, 1996, p 812.)

being considered, although isolated pericardial effusion is unlikely to be the first manifestation of this disorder. Pericarditis following myocardial infarction (Dressler's syndrome) is far less common today. Given experimental laboratory evidence that some of the non-steroidal agents promote left ventricular aneurysm formation in this setting, aspirin is the preferred agent for pain relief. The presence of an "echo-filled" effusion should raise concern for hemorrhagic or organized pericarditis, which may progress to constriction.

CHRONIC PERICARDIAL EFFUSIONS. Tuberculous pericarditis is the most common cause of chronic pericardial effusion. Frequently, pericardial calcification is also present and can be appreciated by thoracic CT. Symptoms are those of a chronic systemic illness with weight loss, fatigue, and dyspnea on exertion. Chest radiographic evidence of pulmonary tuberculosis, analysis of gastric aspirates, and tuberculin skin tests should be performed. Pericardial biopsy is more commonly diagnostic of tuberculous pericarditis than is pericardial fluid staining or culture.

Hypothyroidism/myxedema is another common cause of very large pericardial effusions, especially in the elderly. The effusion is commonly first identified on a chest radiograph and is often seen in the absence of resting tachycardia. Measurement of thyroid-stimulating hormone is diagnostic. Both the effusion and coexistent cardiomyopathy will respond to hormone replacement. In the absence of hemodynamic compromise, pericardiocentesis is often not needed in this situation.

CONSTRICTIVE PERICARDITIS

Constrictive pericarditis is an uncommon condition with impairment of mid and late ventricular filling from a thickened/noncompliant pericardium. In the classic form, fibrous scarring and adhesions of both pericardial layers lead to obliteration of the pericardial cavity. Early ventricular filling is unimpeded, but diastolic filling is subsequently abruptly reduced as a result of the inability of the ventricles to fill because of physical constraints imposed by a rigid, thickened, and sometimes calcified pericardium. In less developed countries, tuberculosis remains the most common cause of chronic constrictive pericarditis, whereas in the United States, tuberculosis is infrequently the culprit. Constriction may be associated with malignancy (lung cancer, breast cancer, lymphoma), histoplasmosis, mediastinal irradiation, purulent or recurrent viral pericarditis, rheumatoid arthritis, uremia, chest trauma or hemopericardium, and cardiac surgery. Constriction may follow cardiac surgery by several weeks to months and may occur decades after chest wall irradiation. The "cause" may not be identified in many patients.

PATHOPHYSIOLOGY. The normal pericardium is 3 mm or less in thickness. With chronic constriction, especially from tuberculosis, the pericardium may thicken to 10 mm or greater, calcify, and intimately involve the epicardium. In subacute constriction, calcification is less prominent, and the pericardium may be only minimally thickened. As with cardiac tamponade, the pathophysiology of constriction includes impaired diastolic ventricular filling, which leads to elevated venous pressure. However, tamponade and constriction have many important differences (see Table 65–2). With constriction, the impairment in ventricular filling is minimal in early diastole, and a prominent y descent is present. Subsequently, diastolic pressure rises abruptly when cardiac volume reaches the anatomic limit set by the non-compliant pericardium; by comparison, in tamponade, ventricular filling is impaired throughout diastole. Diastolic pressure remains elevated until the onset of systole. This prominent y descent with an elevated plateau of ventricular pressure has been termed the "dip and plateau" or "square root" sign (Fig. 65–8); by comparison, in tamponade the y descent is absent. Stroke volume and cardiac output are reduced because of impaired filling, whereas intrinsic systolic function of the ventricles may be normal or only minimally impaired.

PHYSICAL EXAMINATION. In constriction, the most prominent physical finding is an abnormal jugular venous pulse. Central venous pressure is elevated and displays prominent x and y descents. For patients in sinus rhythm, the x descent is coincident with the carotid pulse. The y descent, which is absent or diminished in tamponade, is most prominent and abbreviated because of a rapid

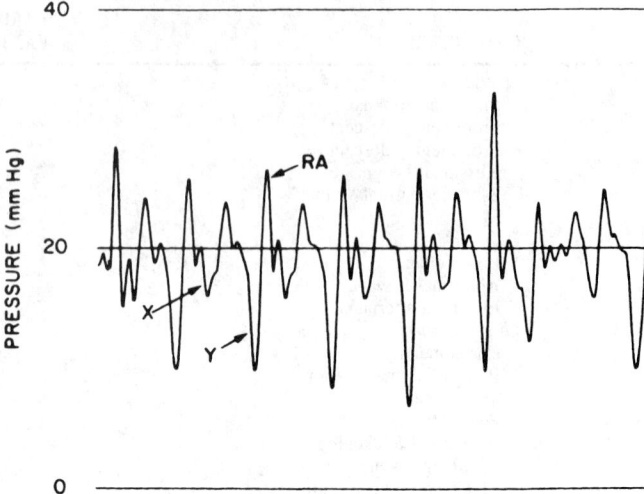

FIGURE 65–8 ■ Right atrial (RA) pressure recording from a patient with constrictive pericarditis. Note the elevation in pressure and prominent y descent corresponding to rapid early diastolic right atrial emptying. (From Lorell BH: Profiles in constriction, restriction and tamponade. *In* Baim DS, Grossman W [eds]: Cardiac Catheterization, Angiography, and Intervention, 5th ed. Philadelphia, Williams & Wilkins, 1996, p 812.)

rise in pressure in mid-diastole. A diagnosis of constriction should always be suspected in patients with a prominent y descent in the setting of dyspnea, weakness, anorexia, peripheral edema, hepatomegaly, splenomegaly, and ascites. The pulse pressure is often narrowed, but pulsus paradoxus is usually absent. Pleural effusions are common. The clinical picture may mimic hepatic cirrhosis, but with distended neck veins. Venous pressure often fails to fall with inspiration (Kussmaul's sign), and arterial pulse pressure is normal or reduced. The apical pulse is often poorly defined, and heart sounds may be distant. A loud third heart sound, the "pericardial knock," may be audible very early after aortic valve closure because of the sudden deceleration in ventricular filling.

DIAGNOSTIC TESTS. The ECG of patients with constriction is often abnormal and displays low QRS voltage, especially in the limb leads, P mitrale, and non-specific ST-T wave changes. Atrial fibrillation may be present in a third of patients. The chest radiograph may demonstrate pericardial calcification in tuberculous constriction, but the finding of pericardial calcification is not diagnostic for constriction. Cardiac size may be small, normal, or enlarged. Surface echocardiography is less helpful than with cardiac tamponade, but it may display pericardial thickening/calcification, abrupt posterior deflection of the interventricular septum at end-diastole, and posterior wall "flat tiring." Enhanced transmitral and transtricuspid Doppler E wave variation with respiration may be particularly helpful in establishing the diagnosis. The inferior vena cava and hepatic veins are often markedly dilated with blunted respiratory variability in caval diameter.

Increased pericardial thickness is most reliably diagnosed by CT or MRI (Fig. 65–9). CT is more helpful for the identification of pericardial calcification. Right atrial, inferior vena cava, and hepatic vein distention is also commonly seen. As with the chest radiograph, CT and MRI do not indicate the physiologic significance of these anatomic findings and need to be interpreted in the context of the clinical findings.

At cardiac catheterization, patients with chronic constrictive pericarditis usually have elevation (≥15 mm Hg) and equalization (within 5 mm Hg) of right atrial, right ventricular diastolic, pulmonary capillary wedge, and left ventricular diastolic pressure. Right ventricular end-diastolic pressure is often one third of systolic pressure, and pulmonary artery hypertension is mild. Cardiac output is usually depressed. Right atrial pressure is characterized by a preserved x descent with a prominent early diastolic y descent. The right atrial pressure fails to decrease appropriately or may rise

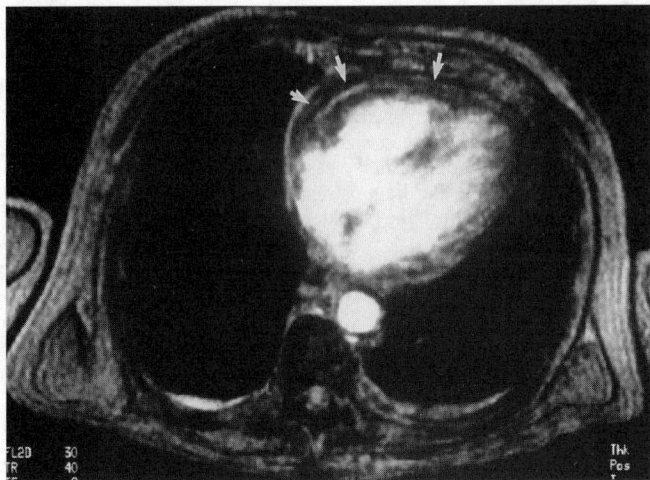

FIGURE 65-9 ■ Transverse magnetic resonance image. Note the markedly thickened pericardium (white arrows) in this 35-year-old man who had received radiation therapy for Hodgkin's disease 20 years earlier and was seeking medical attention for progressive dyspnea on exertion.

during inspiration. Both right and left ventricular diastolic pressures display an early diastolic dip followed by a plateau (Fig. 65–10)—although this finding may be difficult to appreciate if the patient is tachycardic or in atrial fibrillation.

TREATMENT. Constrictive pericarditis may occasionally reverse spontaneously when it develops in the setting of acute pericarditis. More commonly, the natural history of this disease is one of progression with declining cardiac output and progressive renal and hepatic failure. Surgical stripping/removal of both layers of the adherent pericardium is the definitive therapy. The benefits of pericardial stripping may be modest initially but will continue to be manifested over the ensuing months. Operative mortality is generally low but may exceed 5 to 15% in the most advanced cases. The

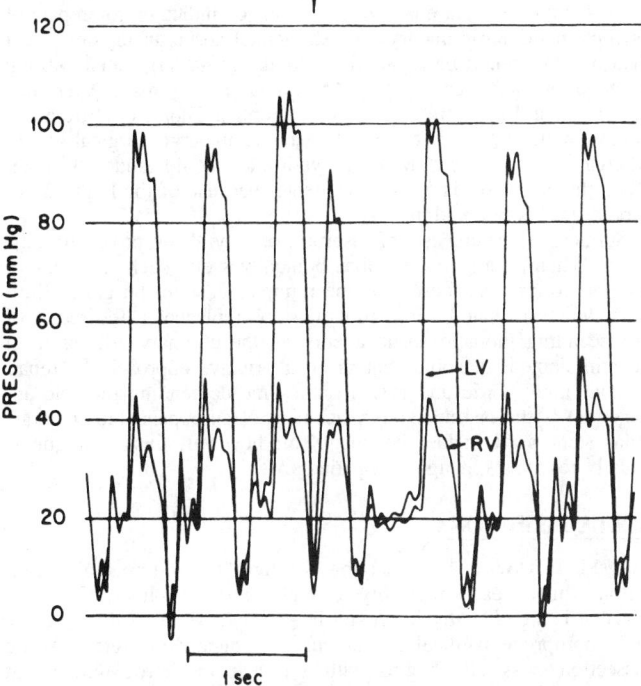

FIGURE 65-10 ■ Simultaneous left (LV) and right (RV) ventricular pressure recordings in a patient with constrictive pericarditis. Note the equilibration of LV and RV diastolic pressures and the "dip and plateau" most apparent with the prolonged diastole. (From Lorell BH: Profiles in constriction, restriction and tamponade. *In* Baim DS, Grossman W [eds]: Cardiac Catheterization, Angiography, and Intervention, 5th ed. Philadelphia, Williams & Wilkins, 1996, p 804.)

surgical risk is related to the extent of myocardial involvement and the severity of secondary hepatic and/or renal dysfunction. For patients with suspected tuberculous constriction, antituberculous therapy should be administered before and after pericardial surgery.

EFFUSIVE-CONSTRICTIVE PERICARDITIS

Effusive-constrictive pericarditis is characterized by the combination of a tense pericardial effusion in the presence of visceral pericardial constriction and may represent an intermediate stage in the development of constrictive pericarditis. Causes of effusive-constrictive pericarditis are the same as those associated with constriction, and the clinical features resemble those of both tamponade and constriction. Physical examination demonstrates pulsus paradoxus and a prominent x descent in the absence of a y descent. The cardiac silhouette is generally enlarged because of the associated pericardial effusion, whereas the ECG displays low QRS voltage and non-specific ST-T wave changes. Surface echocardiography may demonstrate an "echo-filled" pericardial effusion with thickened pericardium and fibrinous pericardial bands. Although this echocardiographic appearance should heighten suspicion, the diagnosis is generally made after successful pericardiocentesis. Rather than normalizing after pericardiocentesis, intracardiac pressures remain elevated with a "square root" sign in the ventricular tracings and development of a prominent y descent in the atrial and jugular venous pressure pulses. A Kussmaul sign may also be evident. Treatment by excision of both visceral and parietal pericardium is usually effective.

Adler Y, Finkelstein Y, Guindo J, et al: Colchicine treatment for recurrent pericarditis. A decade of experience. Circulation 97:2183, 1998. *Colchicine is often effective.*

Cujec B, Brockington GM, Schwartz SL, Pandian NG: Echocardiography in pericardial disease. *In* Skorton DJ, Schelbert HR, Wolf GL, Brundage BH (eds): Marcus Cardiac Imaging: A companion to Braunwald's Heart Disease, 2nd ed. Philadelphia, WB Saunders, 1996, pp 404–419. *Beautiful illustrations of characteristic echocardiographic findings.*

Lorell BH: Pericardial diseases. *In* Braunwald E (ed): Heart Disease: A Textbook of Cardiovascular Medicine, 5th ed. Philadelphia, WB Saunders, 1997, pp 1478–1534. *Comprehensive with an extensive list of references.*

Oh JK, Hatle LK, Seward JB, et al: Diagnostic role of Doppler echocardiography in constrictive pericarditis. J Am Coll Cardiol 23:154, 1994. *Study of the role of Doppler echocardiography in the discrimination of constrictive and restrictive cardiomyopathy.*

Shabetai R (ed): Disease of the pericardium. Cardiol Clin 8:1, 1990. *Comprehensive review, well illustrated and referenced.*

66 DISEASES OF THE AORTA

Eric M. Isselbacher

The aorta is composed of three tissue layers. The intima is a thin inner layer lined with endothelial cells. The middle layer, or media, is the thickest layer of the aortic wall and is composed of sheets of elastic tissue that give the aorta tremendous tensile strength. The outermost layer, or adventitia, is made mostly of collagen and carries the vasa vasorum, which nourish the aortic wall.

The ascending aorta is about 3 cm wide and 5 cm long and is located in the anterior mediastinum. Its most proximal portion (just above the aortic valve) is known as the aortic root and is made up of the three sinuses of Valsalva. In the superior mediastinum, the ascending aorta meets the aortic arch, which gives rise to the brachiocephalic arteries. The descending thoracic aorta courses posteriorly and is about 2.5 cm in diameter and 20 cm in length. After crossing the diaphragm, it becomes the abdominal aorta, which is normally 2.0 cm in width and about 15 cm in length before it bifurcates into the two common iliac arteries.

AORTIC ANEURYSMS

DEFINITION. An aortic aneurysm is a pathologic dilatation of the aorta. Aneurysms are described in terms of their location, size, shape, and etiology. The shape of an aneurysm is *fusiform* when there is symmetrical dilatation of the aorta and *saccular* when the dilatation involves mainly one wall. In addition, there may be a *false aneurysm* or *pseudoaneurysm* when the aorta is enlarged, owing to dilatation of only the outer layers of the vessel wall, such as occurs with a contained rupture of the aortic wall.

Aneurysms may involve any part of the aorta, but abdominal aortic aneurysms are much more common than thoracic aneurysms. Abdominal aortic aneurysms are four to five times more common in men than in women and have a prevalence of at least 3% in persons older than 50 years of age. Among thoracic aortic aneurysms, aneurysms of the descending aorta are most common, followed by those involving the ascending aorta; aneurysms of the aortic arch are quite uncommon. Descending thoracic aortic aneurysms may extend distally and involve the abdominal aorta, creating a thoracoabdominal aortic aneurysm.

ETIOLOGY. Atherosclerosis is the major underlying cause of abdominal aortic aneurysms. The infrarenal aorta tends to be most severely affected by the atherosclerotic process and is accordingly the common site for aortic aneurysm formation. The mechanism by which atherosclerosis leads to the growth of aneurysms remains uncertain. Recent evidence suggests that the atherosclerotic thickening of the aortic intima reduces diffusion of oxygen and nutrients from the aortic lumen to the media, in turn causing degeneration of the elastic elements of the media and a weakening of the aortic wall. As the wall begins to dilate, tension on the wall increases according to Laplace's law (tension is proportional to the product of the pressure and the radius), thereby promoting further expansion of the aneurysm. In addition to atherosclerotic factors, there appears to be a genetic predisposition to the development of abdominal aortic aneurysms as well: up to 28% of first-degree relatives of those with abdominal aortic aneurysms may be affected.

Although atherosclerosis is also a common cause of aneurysms of the descending thoracic aorta, the most important cause of aneurysms of the ascending thoracic aorta is degeneration of the elastin and collagen within the media of the aortic wall. When this process is severe it is known as *cystic medial necrosis*, which histologically appears as smooth muscle cell necrosis and degeneration of elastic layers within the media. Cystic medial necrosis is found in almost all patients with Marfan syndrome (see Chapter 215), placing this group at very high risk for aortic aneurysm formation. Among patients without overt evidence of connective tissue disease, it is unclear what specifically predisposes to the development of such medial degeneration. However, a history of hypertension is a common risk factor. Syphilis was once a common cause of thoracic aortic aneurysms, with degeneration of the aortic media during the secondary phase of the disease producing a weakening of aortic wall. However, syphilis has now become a rarity. Other rare causes of thoracic aortic aneurysms include infectious aortitis, great vessel arteritis, aortic trauma, and aortic dissection.

CLINICAL MANIFESTATIONS. The large majority of abdominal and thoracic aortic aneurysms are asymptomatic when they are discovered incidentally on a routine physical examination or imaging study. When patients with abdominal aortic aneurysms experience symptoms, pain in the hypogastrium or lower back is the most frequent complaint. The pain tends to have a steady gnawing quality that may last for hours or days. Aneurysm expansion or impending rupture may be heralded by new or worsening pain, often of sudden onset. With actual rupture, the pain is often associated with hypotension and the presence of a pulsatile abdominal mass.

Patients with thoracic aortic aneurysms may experience chest pain or, less often, back pain. Vascular complications include aortic insufficiency (sometimes with secondary heart failure), hemoptysis, and thromboembolism. An enlarging aneurysm may produce local mass effects due to compression of adjacent mediastinal structures, producing symptoms such as coughing, wheezing, dyspnea, hoarseness, recurrent pneumonia, or dysphagia.

DIAGNOSIS. Abdominal aortic aneurysm may be palpable on physical examination, although obesity may obscure even large aneurysms. Typically, abdominal aortic aneurysms are hard to size accurately by physical examination alone, because adjacent structures often make an aneurysm feel larger than it really is. Thoracic aortic aneurysms, on the other hand, usually cannot be palpated at all.

The definitive diagnosis of an aortic aneurysm is made by radiologic examination. Abdominal aortic aneurysms can be detected and sized by either abdominal ultrasonography or computed tomography (CT). Ultrasound is extremely sensitive and is the most practical method to use in screening for aortic aneurysms. CT is even more accurate and can size an aneurysm to within a diameter of ± 2 mm. Although CT is less practical than ultrasound as a screening tool, once the diagnosis has been made it is the preferred modality for following the serial changes in aneurysm size over time.

Thoracic aortic aneurysms are frequently recognized on chest radiographs, often producing widening of the mediastinal silhouette, enlargement of the aortic knob, or displacement of the trachea from midline. CT is an excellent modality for detecting and sizing thoracic aneurysms and, again, is particularly useful for following aneurysm size over time. Transthoracic echocardiography, which generally visualizes the aortic root and ascending aorta well, is useful for screening patients with Marfan syndrome because this group is at particular risk for aneurysms involving this portion of the aorta.

PROGNOSIS. The major concern in managing an aortic aneurysm is its tendency to rupture. The majority of aneurysms expand over time, and the risk of rupture increases with aneurysm size. Abdominal aortic aneurysms of less than 4.0 cm have only a 0 to 2% risk of rupture, whereas those larger than 5.0 cm have a 22% risk of rupture within 2 years. The overall mortality in those who rupture an abdominal aortic aneurysm is 80%, including a mortality of 50% even for those who reach the hospital. Thoracic aneurysms of less than 5.0 cm in size typically expand slowly and rarely rupture, but the rate of growth and risk of rupture increase significantly when the aneurysms are 6.0 cm or larger. Similar to what is seen with abdominal aneurysms, the rupture of thoracic aneurysms has a high early mortality of 76% at 24 hours.

TREATMENT. The goal of medical therapy for patients with aortic aneurysms is to attempt to reduce the risk of aneurysm expansion and rupture. β-blockers are the mainstay because they are effective in reducing both aortic pressure and the abrupt rise in pressure during systole so as to reduce the force of the blood striking the aortic wall. Aneurysms should be followed closely with serial imaging studies (such as CT) to detect any progressive enlargement over time that may indicate the need for surgical repair.

Aortic aneurysms that produce symptoms due to aneurysm expansion, vascular complications, or compression of adjacent structures should be repaired. Size is the major indicator for repair of asymptomatic aortic aneurysms. Abdominal aortic aneurysms larger than 6.0 cm should be repaired, as should those larger than 5.0 cm in good operative candidates. Abdominal aneurysms greater than 4.0 cm should be monitored every 6 months. Thoracic aortic aneurysms greater than 6.0 cm in size should undergo surgical repair, whereas patients with Marfan syndrome should undergo repair when the aneurysm is 5.5 cm or greater because of the high risk of rupture in this population.

Surgical repair consists of insertion of a synthetic prosthetic tube graft. When aneurysms involve branch vessels, such as renal or mesenteric arteries, these must be reimplanted into the graft. Similarly, when a dilated aortic root must be replaced in the repair of an ascending thoracic aortic aneurysm, the coronary arteries must be reimplanted. In some centers an alternative approach for repair of abdominal aortic aneurysms (and some descending thoracic aneurysms) is the percutaneous placement of an expandable endovascular stent graft inside the aneurysm; however, this technique is usually reserved for high-risk patients.

AORTIC DISSECTION

DEFINITION. Aortic dissection is a rare but life-threatening condition with an early mortality as high as 1% per hour. However, survival is significantly improved if the diagnosis is made promptly and appropriate medical and/or surgical therapy instituted. Aortic dissection classically begins with a tear in the aortic intima that exposes a diseased medial layer to the systemic pressure of intraluminal blood. The blood then penetrates into the media, cleaving it into two layers longitudinally and producing a blood-filled false lumen within the aortic wall. This false lumen then propagates distally (or sometimes retrograde) a variable distance along the aorta from the site of intimal tear.

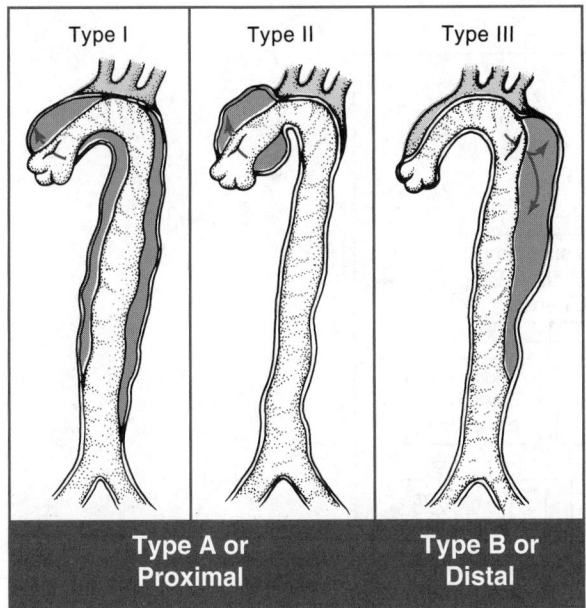

FIGURE 66-1 ■ Classification systems for aortic dissection. (From Isselbacher EM, Eagle KA, DeSanctis RW: Diseases of the aorta. *In* Braunwald E [ed]: Heart Disease: A Textbook of Cardiovascular Medicine, 5th ed, p 1555. Philadelphia, WB Saunders, 1997.)

The location of an aortic dissection may be described according to one of several classification systems (Fig. 66–1). Two thirds of aortic dissections are type A (proximal) and the other one third is type B (distal). The classification schemes all serve the same purpose, which is to distinguish those dissections that involve the ascending aorta from those that do not. Involvement of the ascending aorta carries a high risk of early rupture and death from cardiac tamponade, so prognosis and management differ according to the extent of aortic involvement. Dissections are also classified according to their duration, with those present for less than 2 weeks considered acute and those present for 2 weeks or more considered chronic.

ETIOLOGY. Disease of the aortic media, with degeneration of the medial collagen and elastin, is the most common predisposing factor for aortic dissection. Patients with Marfan syndrome have classic cystic medial degeneration and are at particularly high risk of aortic dissection at a relatively young age. The peak incidence of aortic dissection in patients without Marfan syndrome is in the sixth and seventh decades of life, and men are affected twice as often as women. A history of hypertension is present in the large majority of cases, whereas a bicuspid aortic valve or coarctation of the aorta are less common. Rarely, aortic dissection may occur in a young woman during the peripartum period. Iatrogenic trauma from intra-aortic catheterization procedures or cardiac surgery may also cause aortic dissection.

CLINICAL MANIFESTATIONS. Severe pain, occurring in 74 to 90% of cases, is the most common presenting symptom of aortic dissection. The pain may be retrosternal, in the neck or throat, interscapular, in the lower back, abdominal, or in the lower extremities depending on the location of the aortic dissection. Indeed, the pain may migrate as the dissection propagates distally. Thoracic pain is often of sudden onset and at its most severe at the start. It is sometimes described as "tearing," "ripping," or "stabbing." Patients may also present with acute aortic insufficiency, right coronary artery occlusion, hemopericardium, syncope, a cerebrovascular accident, or ischemic peripheral neuropathy.

Hypertension is a common finding on physical examination and is present in most of those with distal aortic dissection. Hypotension may also occur, particularly among those with proximal dissections, and is usually due to rupture into the pericardium or severe aortic insufficiency. Lastly, the finding of *pseudohypotension* may be present, in which there is a falsely low measure of upper extremity blood pressure due to involvement of a subclavian artery by the dissection. Similarly, pulse deficits are a common finding on physical examination, particularly among patients with proximal

aortic dissections, when there is involvement of the subclavian, carotid, or femoral arteries. Aortic insufficiency is another important physical finding that occurs in more than one half of those with a proximal dissection. However, paradoxically, when acute aortic insufficiency is severe the murmur may not be appreciable, so a widened pulse pressure and congestive heart failure should raise suspicion of its presence.

Vascular complications from aortic dissection include compromise of a coronary artery causing myocardial ischemia or infarction. Involvement of the brachiocephalic arteries may produce a stroke or coma, whereas compromise of the spinal arteries may produce paraplegia. When a dissection extends into the abdominal aorta, there may be compromise of flow to one or both renal arteries producing acute renal failure that may exacerbate hypertension. Mesenteric ischemia or frank infarction may present as abdominal pain. Finally, the dissection may extend distally to the aortic bifurcation and compromise or occlude one of the common iliac arteries producing a femoral pulse deficit and lower-extremity ischemia.

It is often an abnormality on a chest radiograph that first raises the suspicion of aortic dissection. However, the findings on chest radiography are non-specific and rarely diagnostic. An enlarged mediastinal silhouette is the most common finding, present in 81 to 90% of cases. A left pleural effusion is commonly seen in those with involvement of the descending thoracic aorta and, when small, typically represents a transudate from the inflamed aortic wall. A normal chest radiograph does not exclude the diagnosis of aortic dissection. Electrocardiographic findings in aortic dissection are non-specific.

DIAGNOSIS. Once there is clinical suspicion of aortic dissection it is essential to confirm or exclude the diagnosis promptly with an imaging study (Fig. 66–2). Several imaging modalities can accurately diagnose the presence of aortic dissection, including aortography, CT (see Chapter 44), magnetic resonance (MR) imaging (see Chapter 45), and transesophageal echocardiography (TEE) (see Chapter 43). Each institution must determine which of these modalities is most appropriate as an initial diagnostic approach based on the availability of each and the skill and experience of those who perform and interpret the diagnostic studies.

Nevertheless, when suspicion of aortic dissection is high, a TEE (Fig. 66–3) is the most rapid way to provide sufficient detail to enable the surgeon to take the patient directly to the operating room. When clinical suspicion is low (i.e., when one wants to "rule out" aortic dissection) contrast medium–enhanced CT (Fig. 66–4) is preferred because it is entirely non-invasive. If TEE is not readily available, contrast medium–enhanced CT is the test of choice in both high- and low-probability patients.

TREATMENT. The goal of initial medical therapy for acute aortic dissection is to halt any further progression of the aortic dissection and to reduce the risk of rupture. Whenever there is a suspicion of aortic dissection, such therapy should be instituted immediately while imaging studies are ordered rather than waiting until the diagnosis is confirmed. The initial goal is to reduce the force of ventricular contraction and reduce systolic blood pressure to 100 to 120 mm Hg, or to the lowest level that maintains cerebral, cardiac, and renal perfusion. Intravenous labetalol, which acts as both an α- and a β-blocker, may be particularly useful in aortic dissection for controlling both hypertension and contractile force. After labetalol or a pure β-blocker has been administered, intravenous nitroprusside should be added to titrate blood pressure minute by minute as needed. If β-blockers are contraindicated, calcium channel blockers may be useful.

When patients present with significant hypotension, pseudohypotension should first be carefully excluded. True hypotension may be due to rupture of the dissection into the pericardium, producing hemopericardium and cardiac tamponade. Such patients should be treated with volume expansion and taken to surgery as quickly as possible because their early mortality is extremely high. Pericardiocentesis should be performed only as a last resort because it may precipitate hemodynamic collapse and death.

After initial medical therapy has been instituted and the diagnosis of aortic dissection confirmed, definitive therapy must be determined. Whenever an acute dissection involves the ascending aorta, surgical repair is indicated to minimize the risk of life-threatening

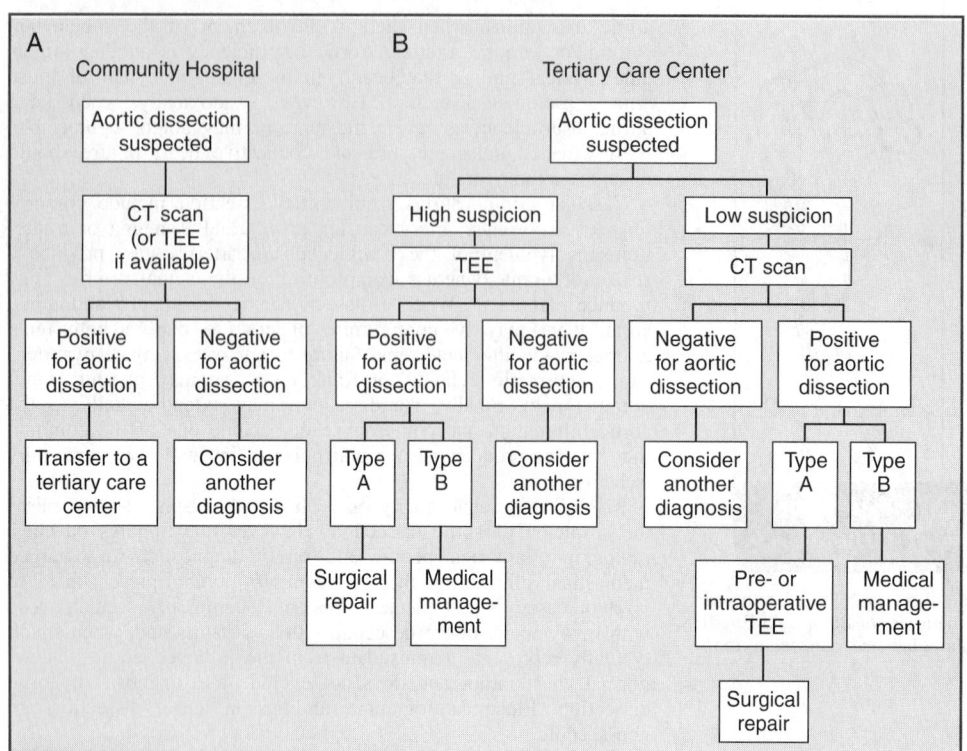

FIGURE 66-2 ■ Suggested algorithms for the evaluation of suspected acute aortic dissection. *A,* Approach used in many community hospitals where cardiac surgery is not performed. *B,* Approach used in many tertiary care centers where transesophageal echocardiography and cardiac surgery are both available. TEE = transesophageal echocardiography; CT = computed tomography.

complications such as rupture, cardiac tamponade, severe aortic insufficiency, or stroke. On the other hand, those with acute dissections confined to the descending aorta are at much lower risk of such complications and tend to fare as well with medical therapy as with surgical repair. However, when a type B dissection is associated with a serious complication, such as end-organ ischemia, surgery is indicated. Patients with chronic type A dissections can be managed medically, because they have already survived the early period of high mortality associated with acute proximal dissections.

PROGNOSIS. Patients with acute aortic dissection who survive the initial hospitalization generally do well thereafter, whether treated medically or surgically. However, late complications, such as aortic insufficiency, recurrent dissection, aneurysm formation, and aneurysm rupture can occur. Medications to control hypertension and reduce ventricular contractility can dramatically reduce the incidence of such late complications and should therefore be continued indefinitely. β-blockers are the drug of choice in this setting, but typically a second or third agent will need to be added to achieve the goal of a systolic blood pressure below 120 mm Hg.

Patients are at highest risk of complications during the first 2 years after aortic dissection. Progressive aneurysm expansion typically occurs without symptoms, so patients must be observed closely with serial aortic imaging at 6-month intervals for the first 2 years and annually thereafter provided that the anatomy is stable.

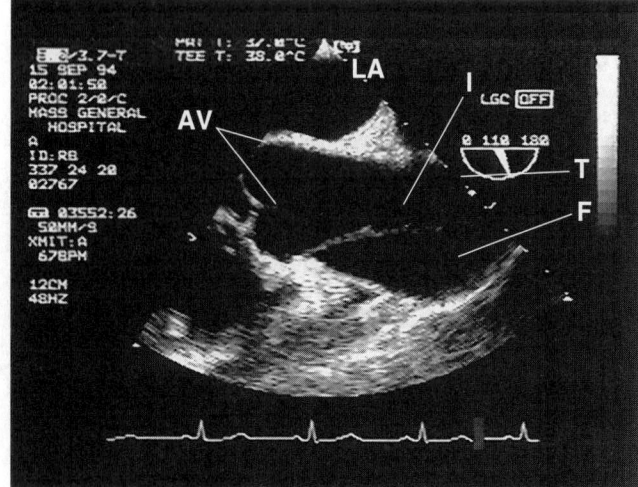

FIGURE 66-3 ■ A transesophageal echocardiogram of the ascending aorta in long axis in a patient with a type A aortic dissection. The aortic valve (AV) is on the left, and the ascending aorta extends to the right. Within the aorta is an intimal flap (I) that originates at the level of the sinotubular junction. The true (T) and the false (F) lumens are separated by the intimal flap. LA = left atrium. (From Isselbacher EM, Eagle KA, DeSanctis RW: Diseases of the aorta. *In* Braunwald E [ed]: Heart Disease: A Textbook of Cardiovascular Medicine, 5th ed, plate 11. Philadelphia, WB Saunders, 1997.)

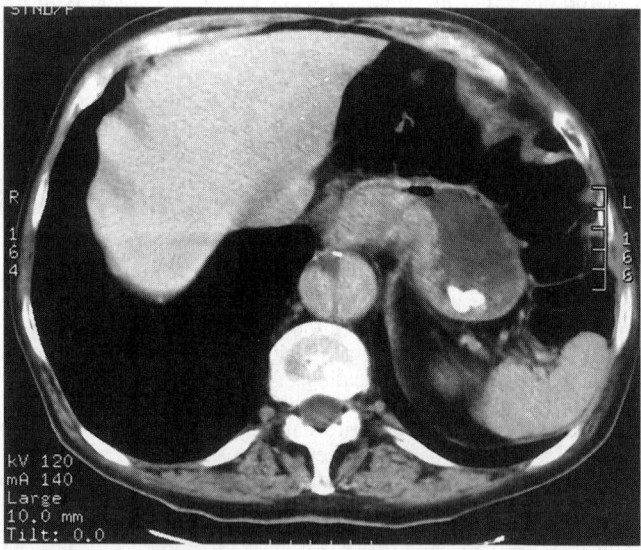

FIGURE 66-4 ■ A contrast medium–enhanced CT scan of the chest at the level of the diaphragm showing an intimal flap (I) separating the two lumens of the descending thoracic aorta in a type B aortic dissection. (From Isselbacher EM, Eagle KA, DeSanctis RW: Diseases of the aorta. *In* Braunwald E [ed]: Heart Disease: A Textbook of Cardiovascular Medicine, 5th ed, p 1561. Philadelphia, WB Saunders, 1997.)

INTRAMURAL HEMATOMA OF THE AORTA

Intramural hematoma of the aorta is an atypical form of aortic dissection. It is believed to occur when there is rupture of the vasa vasorum within the aortic media that results in a contained hemorrhage within the medial layer. This hematoma may then propagate longitudinally along a variable length of the aorta; but since the intimal layer remains intact, the hematoma does not communicate with the aortic lumen. Thus, it was initially termed *aortic dissection without intimal rupture*. Although intramural hematoma of the aorta is clinically indistinguishable from aortic dissection, on cross-sectional imaging it appears as a crescentic thickening around the aortic wall rather than as a true and false lumen separated by an intimal flap. The presence of an intramural hematoma may be missed on aortography. The prognosis and management of intramural hematoma is essentially the same as described earlier for classic aortic dissection.

TAKAYASU'S ARTERITIS

DEFINITION. Takayasu's arteritis is a chronic inflammatory disease of unknown etiology that involves the aorta and its branches. The mean age at onset is 29, with women affected eight times as often as men. It occurs more often in Asia and Africa than in Europe or North America. An early stage, characterized by active inflammation involving the aorta and its branches, progresses at a variable rate to a later sclerotic stage with intimal hyperplasia, medial degeneration, and obliterative changes. The majority of the resulting arterial lesions are stenotic, but aneurysms may occur as well. The aortic arch and brachiocephalic vessels are most often affected, and the disease tends to be most pronounced at branch points in the aorta. The abdominal aorta is also commonly involved, and the pulmonary artery is sometimes involved. The disease may be diffuse or patchy, with affected areas separated by lengths of normal aorta.

CLINICAL MANIFESTATIONS. The majority of patients initially present with symptoms of a systemic inflammatory process such as fever, night sweats, arthralgias, and weight loss. However, there is often a delay of months to years between the onset of symptoms and the time the diagnosis is made. At the time of diagnosis, 90% of patients have entered the sclerotic phase and suffer symptoms of vascular insufficiency, typically with pain in the upper (or less often lower) extremities. There will often be absent pulses and diminished blood pressures in the upper extremities, and the condition has therefore earned the name *pulseless disease*. There may be bruits over affected arteries. Significant hypertension (due to renal artery involvement) occurs in more than half of patients, but its presence may be difficult to recognize, owing to the diminished pulses. Aortic insufficiency may result from proximal aortic involvement. Heart failure may result from either the hypertension or the aortic insufficiency. Involvement of the ostia of the coronary arteries may cause angina or myocardial infarction. Carotid artery involvement may cause cerebral ischemia or stroke. Abdominal angina may result from mesenteric artery compromise.

The overall 15-year survival for those diagnosed with Takayasu's arteritis is 83%, with the majority of deaths due to stroke, myocardial infarction, or heart failure. The survival rate for those with major complications of the disease is as low as 66%, whereas it may be as high as 96% for those without a major complication.

DIAGNOSIS. Laboratory abnormalities during the acute phase include an elevated erythrocyte sedimentation rate, a mild leukocytosis, anemia, and elevated immunoglobulin levels. The diagnosis is best made by aortography, which reveals stenosis of the aorta and stenosis or occlusion of its branch vessels, often with post-stenotic dilatation or associated aneurysms.

TREATMENT. Corticosteroids are the primary therapy for the acute inflammatory stage and may be effective in improving the constitutional symptoms, lowering the erythrocyte sedimentation rate, and slowing disease progression. Cyclophosphamide or methotrexate may be used when corticosteroid therapy alone is ineffective. It is unknown whether medical therapy reduces the risk of major complications or prolongs life.

Balloon angioplasty can dilate stenotic lesions of the aorta and renal arteries. Surgery may be necessary to bypass or reconstruct key segments such as the coronary, carotid, or renal arteries or to treat aortic insufficiency. Ideally, when possible, surgery should not be performed during the inflammatory phase.

GIANT CELL ARTERITIS

Giant cell arteritis (see Chapter 295) is more common than Takayasu's arteritis. Its etiology is also unclear, but it tends to occur in an older population, with a mean age of 67. It typically affects medium-sized arteries, but in 15% of cases it will involve the aorta and branches of the aortic arch. Narrowing of the aorta is rare, but weakening of the ascending aortic wall may lead to localized thoracic aortic aneurysms and secondary aortic insufficiency. Narrowing of the branches of the aortic arch produces symptoms similar to those seen in Takayasu's arteritis. Because the temporal artery is commonly involved, the diagnosis is usually made with a temporal artery biopsy. Management involves the use of high-dose corticosteroid therapy, to which the disease is usually responsive.

Cigarroa JE, Isselbacher EM, DeSanctis RW, Eagle KA: Diagnostic imaging in the evaluation of suspected aortic dissection: Old standards and new directions. N Engl J Med 328:35, 1993. *A comprehensive summary of the four imaging modalities that are used to diagnose aortic dissection. Both the diagnostic strengths and practical utility of each technique are discussed.*

Isselbacher EM, Eagle KA, DeSanctis RW: Diseases of the aorta. *In* Braunwald E (ed): Heart Disease: A Textbook of Cardiovascular Medicine, 5th ed. Philadelphia, WB Saunders, 1997, pp 1546–1581.

Lederle FA, Simel DL: Does this patient have abdominal aortic aneurysm? JAMA 281: 77, 1999. *Emphasizes the limitation of the physical examination for diagnosing abdominal aortic aneurysm.*

Nienaber CA, von Kodolitsch Y, Petersen B, et al: Intramural hemorrhage of the thoracic aorta. Circulation 92:1465, 1995. *An important retrospective study demonstrating that both the presentation and the natural history of intramural hematoma of the aorta are essentially the same as seen in classic aortic dissection.*

Shores J, Berger KR, Murphy EA, Pyeritz RE: Progression of aortic dilatation and the benefit of long-term beta-adrenergic blockade in Marfan's syndrome. N Engl J Med 330:1335, 1994. *An important study that demonstrated the beneficial effect of β-blockers in slowing the progression of aortic aneurysms.*

The UK Small Aneurysm Trial Participants: Mortality results for a randomized controlled trial of early elective surgery or ultrasonographic surveillance for small abdominal aortic aneurysm. Lancet 352:1649, 1998. *Ultrasonographic surveillance is as good as immediate surgery for aneurysms below 5 cm.*

67 ATHEROSCLEROTIC PERIPHERAL ARTERIAL DISEASE

William R. Hiatt

DEFINITION

Peripheral arterial disease (PAD) from atherosclerotic occlusion of the arterial circulation to the lower extremities is usually part of a systemic disorder of atherosclerosis affecting other major circulations. The disease may be manifested by intermittent claudication or severe chronic leg ischemia related to the severity of the hemodynamic obstruction and reduced perfusion to skeletal muscle and skin of the lower extremity.

ETIOLOGY

PAD is caused by atherosclerosis and has an etiology and pathogenesis similar to that of atherosclerosis in other circulations (see Chapter 58). In contrast to coronary heart disease, women have the same risk of development of PAD as men. Patients with type II diabetes mellitus have a four-fold increased risk of PAD as compared with a two-fold increased risk of myocardial infarction or stroke. However, the severity of PAD is not directly correlated with glycemic control but rather with the coexistence of cardiovascular risk factors in addition to diabetes. The risk of PAD increases 10% with a 10-mg/dL increase in total cholesterol. Whereas an elevated low-density lipoprotein cholesterol level is highly associated with the development of coronary disease, reduced high-density lipoprotein cholesterol and increased triglyceride levels are more often associated with PAD. Cigarette smoking is associated with a three- to four-fold increase risk for PAD and is synergistic with other risk factors; the prevalence of cigarette smoking in the PAD population is approximately twice that of the general population. As with coronary heart disease, PAD risk is doubled in hypertensive patients. Elevated homocysteine levels promote PAD as well as coronary heart disease. Patients with hypercoagulable states more commonly have venous thrombosis and thromboembolism but may also have peripheral arterial thrombosis, particularly younger patients.

INCIDENCE AND PREVALENCE

The incidence of intermittent claudication in men ranges from 6 per 10,000 at 30 to 44 years of age to 61 per 10,000 at 65 to 74 years of age. In women, the incidence ranges from 3 per 10,000 at 30 to 44 years of age up to 54 per 10,000 at 65 to 74 years of age. The prevalence of PAD based on ankle-brachial blood pressure ratios is approximately 3% in persons younger than 60 years and increases to 20% in those older than 70 years. In these same studies, the prevalence of symptomatic claudication was less than half the prevalence of PAD. Severe chronic leg ischemia affects fewer than 1 million adults in the United States. In natural history studies, 10% of patients with claudication progress to ischemic rest pain, ulceration, gangrene, or limb loss.

When patients with PAD are assessed by history alone, the physician will recognize the presence of significant coronary disease only 20 to 40% of the time. However, when these patients are evaluated with non-invasive testing such as dipyridamole-stress thallium, the prevalence of coexistent significant coronary disease is 60%; when evaluated by angiography, the prevalence is as high as 90%. The prevalence of critical cerebrovascular disease is also markedly increased in patients with PAD.

The cardiovascular mortality in patients with PAD is six-fold higher than in age-matched control patients and is almost exclusively due to death from myocardial infarction and stroke. In one study of persons with an average age of 66 years, healthy individuals had an approximate 80% 10-year survival rate, patients with asymptomatic PAD (defined as an ankle-brachial index [ABI] less than 0.95) had an approximate 55% 10-year survival rate, patients with intermittent claudication resulting from peripheral atherosclerosis had a 40% 10-year survival rate, and those with severe chronic leg ischemia had only a 25% 10-year survival rate. These data emphasize the need to treat PAD as a systemic disorder in addition to focusing on symptoms affecting the lower extremity.

PATHOPHYSIOLOGY

HEMODYNAMICS. The hemodynamic significance of arterial stenosis is a function of not only the per cent stenosis but also flow velocity across the lesion. For example, resting blood flow velocity in the femoral artery may be as low as 20 cm/second; at this velocity a stenosis will not become hemodynamically significant until it is 90% occlusive, after which flow and pressure rapidly decrease with increasing obstruction. With exercise in a normal extremity, however, flow velocity may increase to as high as 150 cm/second; at these higher flow velocities a stenosis becomes hemodynamically significant at approximately 50%. Thus patients with claudication will have normal flow to skeletal muscle at rest but markedly impaired flow to meet metabolic demand with exercise.

The hemodynamic significance of arterial occlusive disease can easily be assessed by measuring the systolic blood pressure in the ankle and forming a ratio of that pressure to the systolic blood pressure in the arm. In a normal extremity with exercise, ankle blood pressure increases in proportion to the increase in arm blood pressure. With PAD, however, ankle blood pressure will become markedly reduced following exercise.

Patients with PAD often have numerous arterial segments involved. When blood flow in the extremity is reduced at *rest*, symptoms of severe chronic leg ischemia will develop. In contrast to claudication (in which the supply-demand mismatch involves skele-

tal muscle with exercise), severe leg ischemia affects the most distal portion of the extremity with ischemia to the skin and subcutaneous tissues of the forefoot. These patients have ischemic rest pain, distal ulceration, and gangrene.

METABOLIC AND NEUROLOGIC ABNORMALITIES. In patients *with claudication*, the ABI is not well correlated with exercise performance on a treadmill or the severity of symptoms in the community setting. The pathogenesis of PAD is initiated by atherosclerotic occlusion of the major conduit vessels in the lower extremity, but over time the disease affects skeletal muscle and neurologic and metabolic function, which leads to further impairment in muscle performance and functional status. Key factors include deconditioning and skeletal muscle injury, which is characterized as distal axonal denervation leading to loss of muscle fibers and mild atrophy of the affected muscle. Oxidative metabolism is severely impaired in patients with PAD beyond what can be explained simply by the reduction in blood flow. Patients with PAD have impaired resynthesis of phosphocreatine and abnormally high levels of adenosine diphosphate; they may also accumulate intermediates of oxidation such as acylcarnitines. Treatment should focus not only on improving the hemodynamic state of the patient but also on modifying factors such as alterations in skeletal muscle metabolism and function.

CLINICAL FEATURES

HISTORY. Chronic arterial insufficiency of the lower extremity causes two very characteristic types of pain, intermittent claudication and ischemic rest pain, often with ulceration or gangrene. Claudication is derived from the Latin word meaning to limp, which accurately describes the gait pattern of the patient at the onset of symptoms. Depending on the level and extent of the PAD, the patient may have claudication affecting the buttock and thigh (iliac occlusive disease), calf (most commonly), or foot (rarely).

Claudication is caused by reversible muscle ischemia and is characterized by cramping and aching in the affected muscle. The discomfort develops only during exercise and steadily increases with walking until the patient has to stop because of intolerable pain. The discomfort is quickly relieved by rest without change of position. Claudication may occur in one leg only (40% of the time) or affect both legs (60% of the time). The physician should ascertain severity by the distance that the patient can walk before experiencing discomfort (initial claudication distance) and before being forced to stop (absolute or maximal claudication distance). Any recent change should be determined.

Foot claudication is rare and usually seen in thromboangiitis obliterans (see Chapter 68) rather than atherosclerotic PAD. The complaint is usually of a painful ache or cramp in the forefoot associated only with walking. Patients also complain of a persistently cold foot at night.

Ischemic (or nocturnal) rest pain is a severe form of pain that diffusely involves the foot distal to the tarsal bones, although it may be localized to the vicinity of an ischemic ulcer or gangrenous toe. The progression from claudication to rest pain reflects severe arterial occlusive disease with inadequate blood flow to the distal end of the extremity at rest. The pain typical occurs at night when the patient assumes the horizontal position without gravity to help arterial flow. The pain may become so severe that it is not relieved even by substantial doses of narcotics.

RISK FACTOR EVALUATION. All patients should have a smoking history that defines current smoking status and previous pack-years. Diabetes can be evaluated by a fasting and post-prandial blood sugar and/or hemoglobin A_{1C} level. A complete lipid profile should be obtained, including measurements of low- and high-density lipoprotein cholesterol and triglycerides. Blood pressure should be routinely measured. Screening for elevated homocysteine levels should be strongly considered.

PHYSICAL EXAMINATION. A complete physical examination should be performed to evaluate the patient for systemic hypertension, cardiac murmurs or arrhythmias, carotid bruits, or an abdominal aortic aneurysm. The skin of the legs, especially the foot, should be inspected for color changes, ulceration, infection, or trauma from poorly fitting shoes.

Palpation of all arterial pulses should be performed, including the brachial, femoral, and pedal arteries. Absence of a femoral pulse indicates inflow disease of the iliac arteries. Patients with a palpable femoral pulse but absent pedal pulses have disease confined to the femoropopliteal or infrapopliteal arteries. Bruits of the aorta or femoral vessels reflect turbulent flow and are markers of systemic atherosclerosis. Any patient with a femoral bruit or absent pedal pulses should be suspected of having PAD and should have ankle blood pressure measured.

With severe claudication or ischemic rest pain, calf muscles atrophy, hair is lost over the dorsum of the toes and foot, and toenails thicken. More advanced ischemic atrophy results in a shiny, "skeletonized" appearance. Severely affected limbs will also display pallor on elevation because of inadequate arterial pressure and flow; rubor on dependency occurs with very restricted arterial inflow and chronic dilatation of the peripheral vascular bed.

Severe chronic leg ischemia can cause ulceration initially affecting the most distal aspect of the toes. These ulcers are painful, do not bleed when manipulated, and often have a dark necrotic base. The foot may be edematous from being continually kept in the dependent position in an attempt to relieve the ischemic pain. Gangrene usually begins with the toes and forefoot and may occur separately from ulceration.

LABORATORY EVALUATION. All patients with suspected PAD should have an ECG. Elevations in the hematocrit and/or platelet count can result in hyperviscosity with an associated decrease in peripheral perfusion. Significant anemia reduces the oxygen content and decreases oxygen delivery. An elevated erythrocyte sedimentation rate suggests inflammatory causes of vascular disease, including vasculitis (see Chapter 292). In patients with significant lung disease, arterial saturation should be measured to determine whether a low saturation could exacerbate peripheral oxygen delivery. Renal function should be evaluated because chronic renal failure is a significant risk factor for PAD and patients with PAD are at risk for renovascular hypertension and renal insufficiency.

An occasional patient with PAD will have acute thrombotic occlusion of a peripheral vessel from in situ thrombosis or an embolus from a more proximal site. These patients may need a coagulation screen consisting of (but not limited to) factor V Leiden, protein S, protein C, antithrombin III, and other tests of coagulation.

DIFFERENTIAL DIAGNOSIS. Pain from arthritis of the hip or knee is often present at rest and exacerbated by exercise. With cessation of exercise, the pain may not improve unless the patient rests and unloads the joint. Claudication-like symptoms may also arise from spinal stenosis, which is due to osteophytic narrowing of the lumbar neurospinal canal (see Chapter 494). These symptoms are usually lower extremity numbness and weakness produced by standing or increasing lumbar lordosis rather than just ambulation. The symptoms are relieved not simply by rest but also by sitting down or leaning forward to straighten out the lumbar spine.

Venous insufficiency (the sequela of thrombophlebitis) causes swelling and discomfort in the calf with standing and often worse swelling with prolonged walking (see Chapter 69). Patients with severe venous insufficiency may complain of venous claudication from calf swelling (not ischemic cramping) with exercise. Peripheral neuropathies are common in the elderly but are associated with a continuous burning sensation in the foot that is unaffected by exercise; a history of diabetes or alcoholism is common. Older individuals also complain of nocturnal cramps in the calf that are not vascular in origin. Tightness and discomfort in the calf precipitated by exercise may sometimes result from a chronic compartment compression syndrome; such patients are often athletes with large calf muscles. Calf claudication may also develop in athletes from popliteal entrapment caused by external muscle compression of the popliteal artery.

PERIPHERAL VASCULAR STUDIES. Measurement of systolic blood pressure in the ankle by Doppler ultrasound has become the standard for the initial evaluation of all patients with vascular disease (Fig. 67–1). Doppler detects blood flow velocity in the arms and posterior tibial and dorsalis pedis arteries of each ankle for calculation of the ABI, which is the ankle blood pressure divided by the arm blood pressure. No single cutoff value defines an abnormal ABI, but a ratio of 0.95 or less suggests the presence of PAD and a ratio of 0.90 or greater should be considered diagnostic. The vascular disease can be further localized by taking several pressure measurements in the thigh and calf (segmental limb pressures). In patients with iliac occlusive disease, the thigh-

brachial index is reduced, whereas patients with disease more distal in the leg may have a normal thigh-brachial index but reduced calf and ankle-brachial indices.

Patients with claudication but normal ABIs at rest require treadmill testing to define changes in hemodynamics. Normal individuals will increase their ankle blood pressure with exercise, whereas those with arterial disease will have a decrease in ankle blood pressure and ABI.

In patients with severe limb ischemia and non-healing ulcers, the ABI is usually less than 0.50 and the ankle systolic pressure is less than 50 mm Hg. Transcutaneous oximetry also provides information on the adequacy of the peripheral circulation for wound healing. The normal resting transcutaneous oxygen tension is greater than 60 mm Hg, but values of 40 mm Hg or greater are usually associated with good wound healing. However, when values are less than 20 mm Hg, blood flow is insufficient to heal a wound and additional measures must be taken to reperfuse the extremity.

VASCULAR IMAGING. Color-assisted duplex ultrasound can detect stenoses and measure flow at a particular arterial segment or bypass graft. Invasive arteriography, which is the most accurate means of defining arterial anatomy, is indicated only when the patient is being considered for angioplasty or vascular surgery. Magnetic resonance angiography is noninvasive and useful in selected patients to identify tibial vessels for bypass in severe PAD.

ASSESSMENT OF FUNCTIONAL STATUS. When compared with healthy individuals of the same age, patients with claudication have a 50 to 60% reduction in peak treadmill performance, a severity similar to that of patients with severe congestive heart failure. Patients are typically tested at a slow speed not to exceed 2 miles/hour, with the treadmill grade beginning at 0% and increasing 2% every 2 minutes until maximal symptoms prevent further exercise. The time or distance at which claudication pain is first noted is termed the initial claudication distance, and the maximal walking performance is termed the absolute claudication distance; therapy to improve claudication will result in an increase in both. A 25 to 50% increase in treadmill performance is considered clinically significant. Several questionnaire measures of functional status, such as the Walking Impairment Questionnaire, have been developed and validated in patients with PAD and are useful adjuncts to treadmill testing.

MEDICAL TREATMENT

Medical therapy in patients with PAD should be designed to reduce cardiovascular morbidity and mortality by treating systemic atherosclerosis and to improve functional status and limb preservation by relieving claudication and severe leg ischemia. Smoking cessation is critical to delay the progression of PAD and reduce cardiovascular morbidity and mortality. Several large clinical trials have shown the benefit of lowering cholesterol levels in patients with coronary atherosclerosis; although similar studies have not been performed in patients with PAD, the current aggressive recommendations for lipid therapy are similar to those for secondary prevention in persons with coronary artery disease (see Chapters 60 and 206). Aggressive control of blood sugar has not been shown to modify the natural history of PAD, but normalization of blood sugar is an important goal to mitigate against the complications of this disease in other circulations. Although clinical trials have not assessed the benefits of lowering blood pressure on the peripheral circulation, the goals for lowering blood pressure should be similar in patients with PAD as in other forms of cardiovascular disease (see Chapter 60). Recent well-designed studies have not found any adverse effects on claudication with β-blocker use. Aggressive blood pressure reduction with any medication will reduce perfusion pressure into the limb and may result in a slight worsening of claudication, but this side effect should not alter the blood pressure goal. Homocysteine elevation is a well-described risk factor for PAD, but the benefits of lowering homocysteine levels have not yet been demonstrated. Nevertheless, vitamin therapy with folic acid is often recommended for elevated levels (see Chapter 231).

Aspirin in patients with PAD reduces the risk of cardiovascular mortality by approximately 25%. Clopidogrel, an antagonist of adenosine diphosphate–induced platelet aggregation, provides a

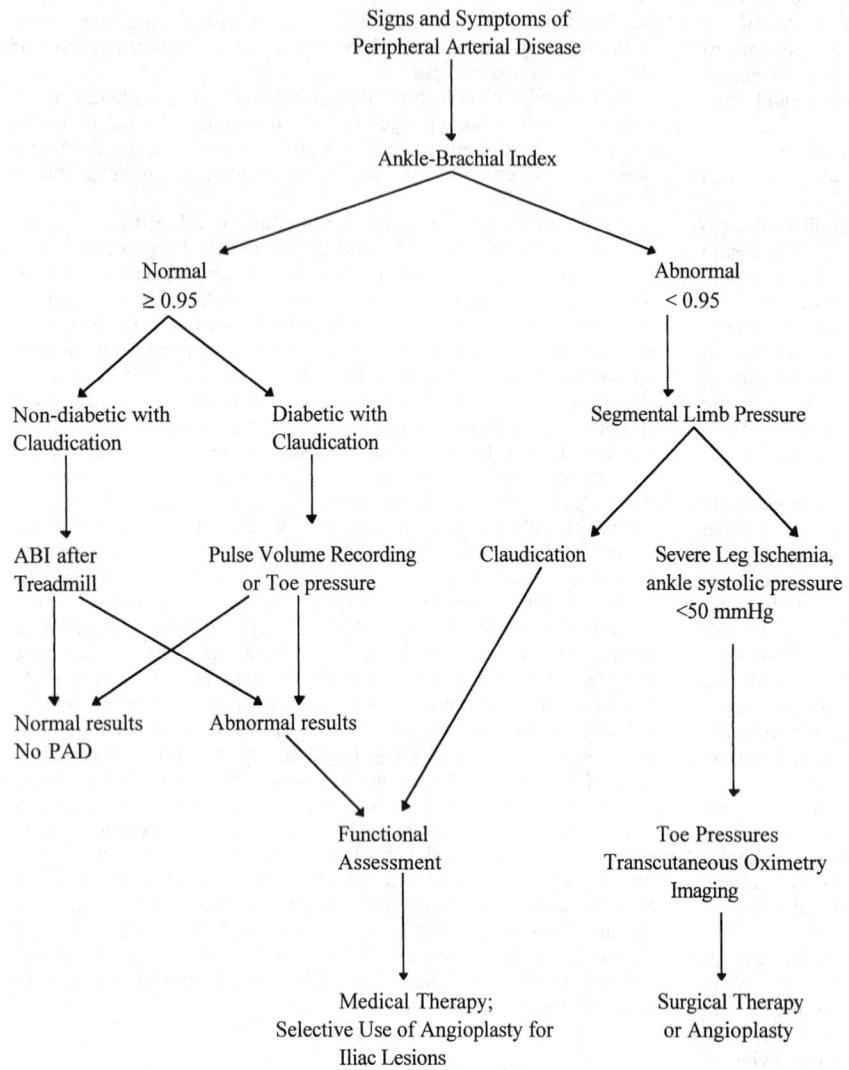

Signs and Symptoms of
Peripheral Arterial Disease

↓

Ankle-Brachial Index

Normal
≥ 0.95

Abnormal
< 0.95

Non-diabetic with
Claudication

Diabetic with
Claudication

Segmental Limb Pressure

ABI after
Treadmill

Pulse Volume Recording
or Toe pressure

Claudication

Severe Leg Ischemia,
ankle systolic pressure
<50 mmHg

Normal results
No PAD

Abnormal results

Functional
Assessment

Toe Pressures
Transcutaneous Oximetry
Imaging

Medical Therapy;
Selective Use of Angioplasty for
Iliac Lesions

Surgical Therapy
or Angioplasty

FIGURE 67–1 ■ Peripheral vascular diagnosis. ABI = ankle/brachial index; PAD = peripheral arterial disease.

23% relative risk reduction in the incidence of vascular death, myocardial infarction, and stroke when compared with aspirin in patients with PAD. In terms of symptomatic relief, a more promising agent is cilostazole, which has antiplatelet and vasodilating properties and has been shown to improve treadmill performance and functional status by questionnaire. Propionyl-L-carnitine is a naturally occurring compound that improves skeletal muscle metabolism and is also effective in treating the symptoms of claudication. Pentoxifylline lowers blood viscosity and may improve flow in the microcirculation; several clinical trials have shown a modest effect on treadmill exercise performance, but most patients perceive no benefit from it. Treatments such as vascular endothelial growth factor or fibroblast growth factor have shown promise in selected patients under experimental conditions, but randomized, blinded studies will be needed to prove efficacy.

EXERCISE THERAPY. Supervised exercise training is a well-documented treatment to relieve claudication and improve exercise performance. Typically, the initial workload on the treadmill is set at the speed and grade that precipitated claudication during the evaluation treadmill test. For training purposes, patients should be able to walk between 3 and 5 minutes at this workload until they achieve a moderately severe level of claudication pain. The patient steps off the treadmill and rests until the pain subsides and then repeats this activity for approximately 40 to 60 minutes per training session. The speed and grade of the treadmill are increased on a regular basis to induce a training effect. Results of this program are typically a 100 to 200% increase in peak exercise performance, an improvement comparable to that achieved with surgery or angioplasty without the side effects of pharmacologic therapy and without the morbidity and mortality of interventional procedures. How-

ever, the training benefit is maintained only if patients continue with their exercise program. Home-based exercise and simple recommendations to exercise are much less effective than supervised programs. Unfortunately, there are very few supervised training programs across the country, and third-party payers often do not reimburse for exercise training.

For severe leg ischemia, medical treatments are quite limited. Analgesics may also be needed, and spinal cord stimulation may reduce ischemic pain. Topical antibiotics, growth factors, and débriding agents have not been effective in treating ulcerated lesions of the lower extremity. Patients in whom cellulitis develops around an ischemic ulceration should be treated with systemic antibiotics. Chelation therapy has no benefit.

INVASIVE THERAPIES

INDICATIONS FOR SURGERY OR ANGIOPLASTY. Invasive therapies should be limited to patients who fail initial medical treatment, have severe disability as defined by validated questionnaires or treadmill testing, and have an appropriate anatomic lesion for bypass or angioplasty (Fig. 67–2).

Angioplasty guidelines emphasize that more proximal lesions have better patency rates and durability than do more distal lesions (Table 67–1). Below the inguinal ligament, the initial success and long-term patency rates have been less well studied but are not as good as for more proximal lesions.

SURGERY. Surgery is principally used to treat severe chronic leg ischemia rather than claudication because of the associated morbidity and mortality of surgery, the relatively benign natural history of

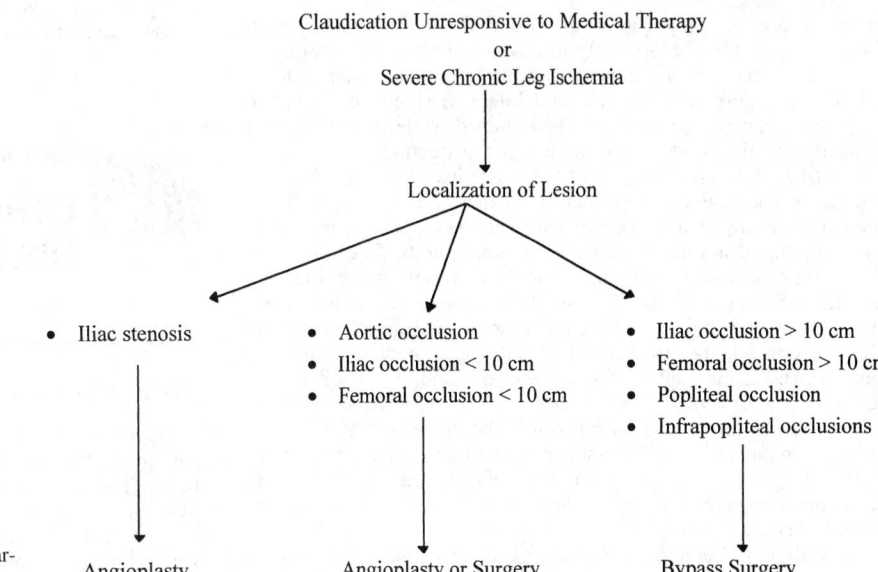

Claudication Unresponsive to Medical Therapy
or
Severe Chronic Leg Ischemia

Localization of Lesion

- Iliac stenosis

- Aortic occlusion
- Iliac occlusion < 10 cm
- Femoral occlusion < 10 cm

- Iliac occlusion > 10 cm
- Femoral occlusion > 10 cm
- Popliteal occlusion
- Infrapopliteal occlusions

Angioplasty

Angioplasty or Surgery

Bypass Surgery

FIGURE 67–2 ■ Interventional therapy for peripheral arterial disease.

claudication, and the efficacy of medical (particularly exercise) therapies. In aortoiliac disease, prosthetic materials are usually implanted. Aortoiliac surgery is associated with an average mortality of 3% and morbidity of 8%. In patients with femoropopliteal disease, the best conduit is saphenous vein. Femoropopliteal surgery with vein bypass is associated with a mortality of 2%, morbidity of 5 to 10%, and a 5-year patency rate of 70 to 80%. The use of prosthetic material (required if a vein is not available) reduces 5-year patency rates to 50%. Distal femorotibial operations for limb salvage have a similar morbidity and mortality as femoropopliteal surgery but slightly lower 5-year patency rates of 50 to 60%.

Additional cardiac evaluation should be considered in patients undergoing peripheral vascular or aortic surgery because the risk of cardiovascular morbidity and mortality can be as high as 30%. Several clinical decision rules have been proposed to separate patients into low- and high-risk groups. For example, patients with PAD and three or more of the following factors are at high risk for surgery: Q waves on the electrocardiogram (or a history of prior myocardial infarction), congestive heart failure, angina, diabetes, and age older than 70 years. Additional risk stratification can be obtained by using dipyridamole thallium scintigraphy (see Chapter 44) or stress echocardiography with dipyridamole or dobutamine (see Chapter 43). An abnormal result would presumably lead to coronary revascularization before the planned peripheral vascular intervention. However, the wisdom of this approach has not been validated. At present, patients who need vascular surgery (e.g., to prevent limb loss) but are believed to be high risk on clinical grounds should have aggressive intraoperative monitoring of central and peripheral hemodynamics and modulation of their sympathetic responses during anesthesia. Only patients with extensive, symptomatic coronary artery disease in whom the coronary disease is more severe or life-threatening than the PAD should undergo additional evaluation for cardiac revascularization. This approach will

obviously result in exposing the patient to two invasive procedures with the attendant increased risk.

ACUTE ARTERIAL ISCHEMIA

Acute arterial ischemia can be caused by occlusion of an existing bypass graft, embolism, or native vessel thrombosis. Patients may have sudden onset of claudication, rest pain, or a cool or cold extremity. The physician must assess the current circulation status and the limb's viability, as well as the nature of previous operations.

The most important initial assessment is viability. The majority of acutely ischemic limbs will be salvageable; skeletal muscle can generally tolerate 6 hours of warm ischemia before irreversible loss. Paralyzed, insensate extremities with fixed skin mottling and hard calf musculature are not salvageable and require primary amputation as soon as the patient is medically prepared for the procedure. The decision to proceed with limb salvage in marginal cases usually relies on the judgment of the vascular surgeon.

The extremity is often pale and cool to palpation; pulses are absent. It is particularly important to palpate the femoral as well as pedal pulses. The ability to palpate pedal pulses is often limited, even in the hands of experienced vascular surgeons. Therefore, unless pulses are grossly obvious, Doppler should be used to determine signals at the three major tibial arteries in the ankle. Any audible Doppler signal should prompt measurement of ankle pressure at that site to calculate an ABI.

GRAFT OCCLUSION. The most common cause of acute arterial ischemia is occlusion of an existing bypass graft. Patients have either rest pain or increasing claudication, depending on the degree of acute change in ischemia.

Initial management requires rapid therapeutic heparin anticoagu-

Table 67–1 ■ RESULTS OF ANGIOPLASTY AND SURGERY FOR PERIPHERAL ARTERIAL DISEASE

TREATMENT	MORTALITY (%)	MORBIDITY (%)	PATENCY RATES (%)		
			3 yr	5 yr	10 yr
Aortoiliac					
Angioplasty	<1	5–14	70–78	58	—
with stent	<1	8–13	81	—	—
Surgery	3	8	—	88–91	82–87
Femoropopliteal					
Angioplasty	<1	7	56	51	—
with stent	<1	2	67	—	—
Surgery (vein)	2	5–10	—	70–80	—
Surgery (prosthetic)	2	5–10	—	50	—
Femorotibial	3–5	10–20	—	50–60	

lation to prevent propagation of thrombus. A vascular surgeon should be consulted immediately to assess the timing of arteriography and surgery. Management of co-morbid diseases such as heart failure, respiratory insufficiency, and infection should be initiated, and central venous access should be obtained while preserving arm veins as potential conduits for vascular reconstruction.

EMBOLISM (CARDIAC/ARTERIAL). Cardiac embolism is most commonly encountered in patients who have pre-existing valvular heart disease, mural thrombus of the ventricle or atrium, or underlying rhythm disturbances (e.g., atrial fibrillation). The most frequent sites of lower extremity embolization are the aortic and femoral bifurcations. Patients may suffer severe ischemia because of a lack of existing collateral circulation at the time of occlusion. The decision whether to proceed directly to surgery for embolectomy versus angiography with catheter-directed thrombolysis depends on the severity of the ischemia. Thrombolysis takes more time to relieve the occlusion but offers the advantage of complete thrombus removal (often incomplete with blind catheter extraction) and avoids endothelial balloon trauma, which often leads to later fibrointimal hyperplasia and branch stenosis/occlusion of the involved arteries.

Arterial-arterial embolization (atheroembolism) may be spontaneous or iatrogenic. Patients with spontaneous atheroembolism have painful, cyanotic digit(s) of acute onset. If embolization is ipsilateral, iliac or femoral artery sources are more likely; bilateral findings indicate an aortic source. Aneurysms of the aorta and femoral and popliteal arteries are also causes. The patient will have a normal or only slightly diminished ABI because the circulation from the digital arteries to the embolic source must be relatively uninterrupted. Cases of iatrogenic atheroembolism occur after aortic catheterization procedures. The clinical picture of limb atheroembolism in this setting can vary from mild livedo reticularis to severe limb pain/cyanosis and eventual tissue loss with concurrent elevated plasma muscle enzymes and myoglobinuria (see Chapter 99). The diagnosis of cholesterol emboli can be confirmed by skin biopsy of peripheral lesions demonstrating cholesterol crystals in the capillaries. Rising creatinine, oliguria, and urine eosinophils are present in patients with renal atheroemboli. Arteries that are occluded by atheroembolic material usually cannot be reopened surgically because of the small particle/vessel size. Similarly, most patients with catheter-induced atheroembolism have diffuse aortic disease not amenable to surgical treatment. An exception occurs when catheter-induced atheroembolism calls attention to an arterial aneurysm as the suspected source of the embolic material.

NATIVE ARTERY THROMBOSIS. Native artery thrombosis occurs in two common scenarios: (1) A native artery becomes acutely occluded in a patient with a known or unknown hypercoagulable state (frequently with previous subclinical thromboses of small arteries). (2) Acute thrombosis in the iliac artery secondary to catheter trauma from coronary angiography develops in a patient with severe aortoiliac occlusive disease (as a result of either dissection of the iliac artery from the catheter or overzealous compression and occlusion of the groin post-catheterization). The primary goals in this setting are to make the diagnosis (baseline ABI before cardiac catheterization is critical), determine the level of ischemia, determine the viability of the distal end of the limb, achieve rapid therapeutic heparin anticoagulation, and make appropriate plans for diagnostic angiography (usual) or urgent surgical exploration (unusual).

Baumgartner I, Pieczek A, Manor O, et al: Constitutive expression of phVEGF165 after intramuscular gene transfer promotes collateral vessel development in patients with critical leg ischemia. Circulation 97:1114, 1998. *Early data suggesting a possible benefit.*

CAPRIE Steering Committee: A randomized, blinded trial of clopidogrel versus aspirin in patients at risk of ischaemic events (CAPRIE). Lancet 348:1329, 1996. *The benefits of antiplatelet therapy are defined in a large clinical trial.*

de Vries SO, Hunink MGM: Results of aortic bifurcation grafts for aortoiliac occlusive disease: A meta-analysis. J Vasc Surg 26:558, 1997. *The results of aortoiliac surgery are provided.*

Hiatt WR, Hirsch AT, Regensteiner JG, et al: Clinical trials for claudication. Assessment of exercise performance, functional status, and clinical end points. Circulation 92:614, 1995. *A description of the exercise testing and questionnaire methods is provided in this article.*

Hunink MGM, Wong JB, Donaldson MC, et al: Revascularization for femoropopliteal

disease: A decision and cost-effectiveness analysis. JAMA 274:165, 1995. *The expected results from angioplasty and surgery are compared.*

Nehler MR, Hiatt WR: Exercise therapy for Claudication. Ann Vasc Surg 13:109, 1999. *Guidelines to this useful intervention.*

68 OTHER PERIPHERAL ARTERIAL DISEASES

Jeffrey W. Olin

LIVEDO RETICULARIS

Livedo reticularis is characterized by a reticular, fishnet, or lacy pattern on the skin of the lower extremities and other parts of the body. This pattern is red or blue and caused by deoxygenated blood in the surrounding horizontally arranged venous plexus.

Primary or benign livedo reticularis occurs most commonly in young women between the ages of 20 and 40. Ulceration generally does not occur with this form of the disease, which may be due to vasomotor instability or hyperreactivity of the dermal blood vessels. It is intensified by cold exposure and relieved by rewarming, and it may occur in association with Raynaud's phenomenon or disease.

Secondary livedo reticularis occurs in association with atheromatous embolization (see later), polyarteritis nodosa, systemic lupus erythematosus, leukocytoclastic vasculitis, other connective tissue diseases, therapy with amantadine, and various neurologic or endocrine diseases and in patients receiving large doses of vasopressors such as epinephrine, norepinephrine, and dopamine. Livedo reticularis is also one of the many skin manifestations of the antiphospholipid antibody syndrome. In Sneddons's syndrome there is the combination of livedo racemosa (a variant of livedo reticularis) and small vessel ischemic disease of the brain, producing transient ischemic attack or stroke. Approximately 50% of patients with Sneddon's syndrome have elevated levels of anticardiolipin antibodies.

In livedoid vasculopathy or livedoid vasculitis, extensive livedo reticularis surrounds a painful, ischemic-appearing ulceration located on the anterior or posterior portion of the lower leg. Pathologically, there is thrombosis of the microvasculature with little or no active inflammatory component. Small doses of tissue plasminogen activator (10 mg intravenously daily for 14 days) may be very effective in treating the ulcerations. Atrophe blanche is a variant of livedoid vasculopathy. These ulcerations generally occur around the ankle or foot. They have a white or yellowish base with poor granulation tissue and are exquisitely painful and quite difficult to heal.

The benign variety of livedo reticularis often needs no treatment other than measures to keep the body part as warm as possible. In patients with secondary livedo reticularis, therapy should be directed at the underlying cause.

ATHEROMATOUS EMBOLIZATION

Atheromatous embolization (cholesterol embolization) refers to the embolization of cholesterol crystals or platelet fibrin aggregates to the extremities or one or more organs. Atheromatous emboli usually originate from ulcerated or stenotic atherosclerotic plaques or aneurysms that are primarily in the thoracic or abdominal aorta, iliac, or carotid artery.

Atheromatous embolization of the kidneys is a common histologic finding and may occur in 15 to 30% of patients with severe aortic atherosclerosis or aneurysm of the abdominal aorta. Increasing aortic plaque thickness, protruding aortic atheroma, and mobile aortic atheroma are associated with a high likelihood for atheromatous embolization. Atheromatous embolization may be spontaneous, but it occurs more often after cardiac catheterization, percutaneous transluminal coronary angioplasty, peripheral or cerebrovascular arteriography, or peripheral angioplasty. Pathologically, arterioles are filled with biconvex cholesterol crystals, which produce a foreign body reaction in which polymorphonuclear leukocytes, macrophages, and multinucleated giant cells appear several days to several weeks after the inciting event.

The most common clinical manifestations (Table 68–1) are skin changes, which occur in over one third of patients and are generally found in the lower extremities but may be seen in the trunk, over the buttocks, and rarely in the upper extremities. These manifestations include livedo reticularis (embolization to the dermal blood vessels), purple or blue toes, splinter hemorrhages, gangrenous digits or ulcerations, and nodules in the presence of palpable foot pulses.

Atheroembolic renal disease is a small vessel occlusive disease leading to uncontrolled hypertension and advanced or end-stage renal disease (see Chapter 112). Atheromatous embolization may also involve the gastrointestinal tract and produce ischemic bowel with generalized abdominal pain, nausea, vomiting, melena, or hematochezia. Cholesterol emboli to the gallbladder may produce acute gangrenous cholecystitis, whereas emboli to the pancreas can cause acute pancreatitis.

Cardiac manifestations of atheroemboli include angina pectoris and myocardial infarction. Patients may develop amaurosis fugax or blindness caused by retinal artery occlusion. A Hollenhorst plaque (yellow, highly refractile atheromatous material) may be present at the bifurcation of retinal blood vessels. Stroke, headache, confusion, organic brain syndrome, dizziness, and spinal cord infarction can occur. Accompanying fever, weight loss, anorexia, fatigue, myalgias, headache, nausea, vomiting, or diarrhea may suggest a necrotizing vasculitis, infective endocarditis, or malignancy.

DIAGNOSIS. Atheromatous embolization is frequently overlooked or misdiagnosed. No single laboratory test is diagnostic. Nonspecific findings such as elevation in the erythrocyte sedimentation rate, leukocytosis, or anemia may be present. Increased levels of serum amylase, hepatic transaminases, blood urea nitrogen, or serum creatinine may be noted if the pancreas, liver, or kidney is involved. The urine sediment may be abnormal but is non-specific. Eosinophilia may be present early in the course, and hypocomplementemia has been reported in a small number of series. Biopsy remains the most specific way to make the diagnosis, but it is often not required because the clinical findings may be highly suggestive of atheromatous embolization.

On arteriography, a markedly irregular and shaggy aorta may be demonstrated. Transesophageal echocardiography may detect mobile, protruding atheroma, which are associated with a very high risk for future embolization.

Atheromatous embolization may mimic a vasculitis, such as polyarteritis nodosa or leukocytoclastic vasculitis, or suggest an underlying malignancy, non-bacterial thrombotic endocarditis, subacute bacterial endocarditis, multiple myeloma, the antiphospholipid antibody syndrome, or atrial myxoma. A cardiac source of emboli should always be excluded.

TREATMENT. The treatment of atheromatous embolization should be directed toward three goals: (1) removal of the source of atheromatous material (by surgery, percutaneous transluminal angioplasty, stent implantation or stent grafts); (2) symptomatic care of the end organ where the emboli are located; and (3) risk factor modification to prevent the progression of disease.

Local care of ischemic ulcers is important, and chemical or surgical sympathectomy may be helpful. Although intravenous ilo-

prost (a prostaglandin analogue) is very useful in the healing of ischemic ulcerations secondary to atheromatous embolization, it is not available in the United States. Patients should be on antiplatelet therapy with aspirin or clopidogrel. Use of anticoagulants such as heparin or warfarin should be avoided unless there is a large mobile atheroma, which may have a significant amount of attached thrombus, in the aorta. If a vasospastic component is present, a calcium channel blocker may be effective in relieving some of the symptoms.

In the past, surgical bypass therapy was the standard for treating patients with atheromatous embolization of the thoracic and abdominal aorta, whereas patients who were poor surgical risks often underwent ligation of the common femoral arteries followed by an extra-anatomic bypass such as an axillobifemoral bypass. Now, however, covered stents (stent grafts), which can be inserted in the thoracic or abdominal aorta for aneurysms or occlusive disease, represent a new investigational technique with a relatively low morbidity and mortality.

Patients with atheromatous embolization generally have advanced atherosclerosis and poor prognosis. All patients should receive aggressive risk factor modification to slow the progression of atherosclerosis and improve overall cardiac and cerebrovascular morbidity and mortality.

THROMBOANGIITIS OBLITERANS (BUERGER'S DISEASE)

Thromboangiitis obliterans (Buerger's disease) is a non-atherosclerotic segmental, inflammatory disease that most commonly affects the small and medium-sized arteries and veins in the upper and lower extremities. The etiology of Buerger's disease is unknown, but there is an extremely strong association with heavy tobacco use, and progression of disease is closely linked to continued use.

Patients with Buerger's disease may be hypercoagulable, and some have antiendothelial cell antibodies, anticollagen antibodies, circulating immune complexes, and/or impaired endothelial-dependent vasorelaxation. There is also an increase in cellular sensitivity to type I and III collagen (normal constituents of human arteries) in patients with thromboangiitis obliterans.

INCIDENCE AND PREVALENCE. Buerger's disease has a worldwide distribution, but it is more prevalent in the Middle, Near, and Far East than in North America and Western Europe. The prevalence of Buerger's disease among patients with peripheral arterial disease varies from a low of 0.5 to 5.6% in Western Europe to a high of 60 to 89% in India, Korea, and Japan and in Ashkenazi Jews in Israel.

PATHOLOGY. In the acute phase of thromboangiitis obliterans, a highly inflammatory thrombus affects both the arteries and veins. The lesion is characterized by acute inflammation involving all coats of the vessel wall, especially of the veins in association with occlusive inflammatory cellular thrombosis. Around the periphery of the thrombus, there are often polymorphonuclear leukocytes with karyorrhexis, the so-called microabscess in which one or more multinucleated giant cells may be present. The acute phase lesion is followed by an intermediate phase in which there is progressive organization of the acute occlusive thrombus in the arteries and

Table 68–1 ■ CLINICAL MANIFESTATIONS OF ATHEROMATOUS EMBOLIZATION

Skin	Purple or blue toes	Gastrointestinal	Abdominal pain
	Gangrenous digits		GI bleeding
	Livedo reticularis		Ischemic bowel
	Nodules		Acute pancreatitis
Kidney	Uncontrolled hypertension	Constitutional	Fever
	Renal failure	symptoms	Weight loss
			Malaise
Neurologic	Transient ischemic attack		Anorexia
	Amaurosis fugax		
	Stroke		
	Hollenhorst plaque		
Cardiac	Myocardial infarction or ischemia		

From Bartholomew JR, Olin JW: Atheromatous embolization. *In* Young JR, Olin JW, Bartholomew JR (eds): Peripheral Vascular Diseases, 2nd ed. St. Louis, C.V. Mosby, 1996.

veins; there may be persistence of a prominent, inflammatory cellular infiltrate within the thrombus. The chronic phase or end-stage lesion is characterized by complete organization of the occlusive thrombus with extensive recanalization, prominent vascularization of the media and adventitia, and perivascular fibrosis.

CLINICAL MANIFESTATIONS. Classically, Buerger's disease occurs in a young male smoker with the onset of symptoms before the age of 40 to 45 years, but 20 to 25% of patients with Buerger's disease may be women. Buerger's disease usually begins with ischemia of the distal small arteries and veins. As the disease progresses, it may involve more proximal arteries, but involvement of large arteries is unusual.

Patients may present with claudication of the foot, legs, and occasionally the arms and hands. Foot or arch claudication may be the presenting manifestation and is often mistaken for an orthopedic problem. Seventy-five to 80% present with ischemic rest pain and/or ulcerations. Two or more limbs are almost always involved, and angiographic abnormalities are consistently found in limbs that are not yet clinically involved. Superficial thrombophlebitis and Raynaud's phenomenon each occur in approximately 40% of patients.

A positive Allen's test indicates the distal nature of thromboangiitis obliterans and its involvement of the lower and upper extremities to help differentiate it from atherosclerosis. In this test, the physician simultaneously occludes both the radial and ulnar arteries. When pressure is released from either artery, there should be prompt filling from that artery with the return of color to the hand. A positive test result is indicated when color does not return to the blanched hand.

DIAGNOSIS. No specific laboratory tests aid in the diagnosis of Buerger's disease, but tests should exclude vasculitis, hypercoagulable states, antiphospholipid antibodies, and a proximal source of emboli. On arteriography, the proximal arteries are normal, and the disease is most often infrapopliteal in the lower extremities and distal to the brachial artery in the upper extremities. There may be multiple vascular occlusions with collaterization around the obstruction (corkscrew collaterals), similar to what may be seen in other small vessel occlusive diseases such as CREST syndrome or scleroderma, but the arteriographic appearance of Buerger's disease may also be identical to that seen in patients with systemic lupus erythematosus, rheumatoid vasculitis, mixed connective diseases, and antiphospholipid antibody syndrome. However, these other diseases can usually be established or excluded by other tests. Patients with Takayasu's arteritis or giant cell arteritis present with proximal vascular involvement and can readily be distinguished from Buerger's disease.

TREATMENT. The cornerstone of therapy for thromboangiitis obliterans is the complete discontinuation of cigarette smoking or the use of tobacco in any form. Quitters will almost always avoid amputations, whereas 40% or more of patients who continue tobacco use will progress to one or more amputations.

All other forms of therapy (calcium channel blockers, antibiotics, anticoagulants, sympathectomy) are palliative. In a prospective, randomized trial, intravenous iloprost was superior to aspirin at 28 days in relieving rest pain and healing of all trophic change. At 6 months, 88% of patients receiving iloprost responded to therapy, compared with 21% in the aspirin group, and only 6% underwent amputation in the iloprost group, compared with 18% in the aspirin group. However, intravenous iloprost is not available for use in the United States. In a recently reported double-blind, placebo-controlled, randomized trial, oral iloprost was slightly more effective than placebo in relieving rest pain but not in healing ischemic ulcerations.

Surgical bypass is not a viable option in most patients because there may not be a distal target vessel with which to bypass. Sympathectomy and implantable spinal cord stimulators are of unproven benefit. Vascular endothelial growth factor is under active study.

VASOSPASTIC DISEASES AND VASCULAR DISEASES ASSOCIATED WITH CHANGES IN ENVIRONMENTAL TEMPERATURES

Raynaud's Phenomenon

Raynaud's phenomenon is the abrupt onset of digital pallor and/or cyanosis in response to cold exposure or stress. Classic manifestations of Raynaud's phenomenon are the triphasic color response consisting of pallor, cyanosis, and reactive hyperemia. Primary Raynaud's phenomenon (Raynaud's disease) denotes patients who have no underlying cause, whereas secondary Raynaud's phenomenon (also known as Raynaud's phenomenon) is associated with or caused by some other systemic illness or disease process (Table 68–2).

Raynaud's phenomenon is common in patients with connective tissue diseases. Approximately 90% of patients with scleroderma (see Chapter 290) experience Raynaud's phenomenon, and it is a component of the CREST (calcinosis, Raynaud's phenomenon, esophageal dismotility, sclerodactyly, telangiectasias) syndrome. These patients have small vessel occlusive disease that may lead to digital pitting or ulceration and eventual amputation.

The β-adrenergic receptor antagonists are the most common drugs to cause Raynaud's phenomenon because they block the vasodilatory β receptors and thus leave the vasoconstrictive α receptors unopposed. Ergotamine preparations and polyvinyl chloride exposure also can cause Raynaud's phenomenon.

Raynaud's phenomenon is common in individuals who use vibratory tools such as pneumatic hammers, chain saws, sanders, and

---

Table 68–2 ▪ CONDITIONS ASSOCIATED WITH SECONDARY RAYNAUD'S PHENOMENON

Connective tissue diseases	**Trauma**
Scleroderma or CREST syndrome	Vibratory tools, grinders, sanders
Systemic lupus erythematosus	Thermal injury
Rheumatoid arthritis	Electric shock injury
Mixed connective tissue disease	Percussive injury
Polymyositis, dermatomyositis	Hypothenar hammer syndrome
Sjögren's syndrome	**Hematologic abnormalities**
Arterial occlusive diseases	Cryoglobulinemia and cryofibrinogenemia
Vasculitis	Cold agglutinin disease
Thromboangiitis obliterans (Buerger's disease)	Myeloproliferative diseases
Thromboembolism	Hyperviscosity syndrome
Thoracic outlet syndrome	**Neurologic disorders**
Atherosclerosis of extremities (rare)	Carpal tunnel syndrome
Drugs and toxins	Reflex sympathetic dystrophy
Beta-adrenergic blocking agents	Stroke
Ergotamine preparations	Intervertebral disk disease
Methysergide	Poliomyelitis
Vinblastine	Syringomyelia
Bleomycin	**Other**
Cisplatin	Hypothyroidism
Polyvinyl chloride	Pulmonary hypertension
Estrogen	Arteriovenous fistula
Heavy metals	Neoplasms
	Renal failure

grinders; the syndrome has also been described in typists, pianists, meat cutters, and sewing machine operators. Continued use of vibratory tools can lead to a chronic occlusive small vessel vascular disease.

Trauma to the distal ulnar artery (several centimeters distal to the wrist) may occur with activities such as pounding with the palm of the hand, karate, or other activities that traumatize the hypothenar eminence and lead to an aneurysm or pseudoaneurysm of the distal ulnar artery. Thrombus within the aneurysm may then embolize to the fingers, or the distal ulnar artery may thrombose.

PATHOGENESIS. The initial manifestation of Raynaud's phenomenon occurs when the digits turn white due to intense vasoconstriction or spasm of the digital arteries. At this point there is total cessation of blood flow and the digits are often numb. As the arterial vasoconstriction becomes less severe, postcapillary venule constriction causes the blood in the capillaries and veins to become deoxygenated, thus producing the cyanotic appearance. When rewarming occurs, there is a markedly increased blood flow producing reactive hyperemia to the digits (red color).

CLINICAL MANIFESTATIONS. The symptoms of Raynaud's phenomenon may include pallor, cyanosis, and reactive hyperemia. The triphasic color response occurs in 4 to 65% of patients. Exposure to the cold is the typical precipitating factor, but emotional lability may also cause or exacerbate attacks in some patients. Vasospastic attacks usually occur only in the fingers, but vasospasm can occur in the toes, nose, ears, lips, and other body parts.

In primary Raynaud's disease, the physical examination is normal between attacks. However, in patients with secondary Raynaud's phenomenon, the presence of pits or ulcerations on the fingertips may be present in patients with scleroderma, CREST syndrome, or thromboangiitis obliterans. An abnormal result of the Allen test on physical examination indicates fixed arterial obstruction.

DIAGNOSIS. The diagnosis of Raynaud's phenomenon is not difficult when based on the patient's description of the attacks. Patients with persistent cyanosis or persistent hyperemia generally have some other condition other than Raynaud's phenomenon. In Raynaud's disease, vasospastic attacks are precipitated by exposure to the cold or emotional stimuli, there is bilateral involvement of the extremities without gangrene, and, after 2 years or more of symptoms, there is no evidence of underlying systemic diseases that could be responsible for the vasospastic attacks (Table 68–3).

To evaluate systemic illnesses, a serologic evaluation should include a complete blood cell count, multiphasic serologic analysis, urinalysis, Westergren sedimentation rate, C-reactive protein, antinuclear antibody, extractable nuclear antigen, anti-DNA, cryoglobulins, complement, anticentromere antibodies, and SCL70 scleroderma antibodies. In addition, nail-fold capillaroscopy can be performed to help confirm a diagnosis of CREST syndrome or scleroderma in patients in whom the symptoms are not clear.

The non-invasive vascular laboratory (pulse volume recordings) is useful in identifying the degree of digital arterial occlusive disease (fixed ischemia) and predicting whether ischemic ulcerations on the digits will heal. Arteriography is not routinely advocated.

TREATMENT. In patients with mild vasospastic attacks, reassurance about the benign nature of the disease and instructions on how to prevent attacks are often all that is needed. Patients should limit the amount of exposure to the cold and should dress warmly and protect not only their extremities but also their entire body. Smoking should be avoided because nicotine causes intense vaso-

constriction. β-blocking agents may exaggerate the symptoms of Raynaud's phenomenon. Mittens are better than gloves for keeping the hands warm. Patients need to be especially careful when handling cold objects. Hand and foot warming devices (battery operated or chemical) may be helpful. Conditioning techniques or biofeedback are sometimes helpful in controlling vasospastic episodes.

Patients who have infrequent attacks of Raynaud's phenomenon may benefit from a short-acting calcium channel blocker such as nifedipine, 10 to 20 mg, 30 minutes to 1 hour before going out into the cold. When vasospasm occurs more frequently, the extended-release preparations of nifedipine (30–90 mg daily), amlodipine (2.5–10 mg daily), or diltiazem (120-300 mg daily) are effective. The α_1-adrenergic receptor antagonists such as prasozin or terazosin can also decrease the severity, frequency, and duration of vasospastic attacks in patients.

Nitroglycerin can be used topically in patients, whereas prostacyclin can be given intravenously. The angiotensin-converting enzyme inhibitor captopril has shown some benefit in uncontrolled trials, but other vasodilators such as niacin and papavarine are not beneficial.

Although sympathectomy may be beneficial in the short term, with about a 50% improvement rate, the vasospastic attacks may recur after a period of 6 months to 2 years. Some patients with severe disease have had success with digital sympathectomy.

PROGNOSIS. The prognosis in patients with Raynaud's disease is excellent. There is no mortality associated with this condition. In a long-term study involving 307 patients with primary Raynaud's disease, 38% had stable disease, 36% improved, 16% worsened, and the syndrome disappeared in 10%. The prognosis associated with secondary Raynaud's phenomenon depends on the underlying condition that has caused it.

Pernio (Chilblains)

Pernio (a Latin word that literally means frostbite; however, its synonym chilblains is an Anglo-Saxon term that means cold sore) are localized inflammatory lesions of the skin as a result of abnormal response to the cold. Up to 50% of women developed pernio in war time conditions in northern Europe. Pernio is now less common but is still seen in the temperate, humid climates of northwestern Europe and in the northern United States.

Pernio develops in susceptible individuals who are exposed to non-freezing cold. The pathologic changes include edema of the papillodermis, vasculitis characterized by perivascular infiltration (with lymphocytes) of the arterioles and venules of the dermis, thickening and edema of the blood vessel walls, fat necrosis, and chronic inflammatory reaction with giant cell formation.

Pernio most commonly occurs in young women between the ages of 15 and 30 but may occur in older individuals or in children. Acute pernio may develop 12 to 24 hours after exposure to the cold. Single or multiple erythematous, purplish, edematous lesions appear accompanied by intense itching or burning. These lesions may have a yellowish or brownish discoloration and may be associated with some flaking. They tend to affect the toes and dorsum of the proximal phalanges. The lesions of acute pernio are usually self-limited, although they may lead to recurrent disease. The arterial circulation is normal on physical examination and in the non-invasive vascular laboratory. Chronic pernio occurs when

Table 68–3 ■ DIFFERENTIATING PRIMARY FROM SECONDARY RAYNAUD'S PHENOMENON

	PRIMARY RAYNAUD'S PHENOMENON (RAYNAUD'S DISEASE)	SECONDARY RAYNAUD'S PHENOMENON (RAYNAUD'S PHENOMENON)
Sex	Usually female	Male or female
Onset of symptoms	Usually <40 years old	Any age
Distribution of vasospasm	All digits; bilateral	One or more digits; may be unilateral
Evidence of structural abnormalities (+Allen's test, absent pulses)	Absent	Present
Digital pits or ulcerations	Absent	Present
Laboratory test (ESR, CRP, ANA, RF, nailfold capillaroscopy)	Normal	May be abnormal
Prognosis	Excellent	Depends on underlying disease

From Bacharach M, Olin JW; Heart Disease and Stroke 3:255–259, 1994.

repeated exposures to the cold results in the persistence of lesions with subsequent scarring and atrophy. Characteristically, the lesions begin in the fall or winter and disappear in the spring or early summer. In advanced cases, the seasonal variation may disappear and chronic occlusive vascular disease may develop.

In the typical form, the patient develops violet or yellow-brown blisters and shallow ulcers on the toes that burn and itch. The lesions first appear in the fall or winter and disappear each spring. The differential diagnosis of pernio includes recurrent, erythematous, nodular, and ulcerative lesions such as erythema induratum, nodular vasculitis, erythema nodosum, and cold panniculitis. The skin lesions of pernio may look similar to atheromatous embolization (see earlier), and an arteriogram may sometimes be required.

Prevention is the best of form of therapy. Cold exposure should be minimized as much as possible. In a randomized trial, nifedipine reduced the pain and facilitated the healing process. The severe itching may be treated with a local application of an antipruritic agent.

Acrocyanosis

Acrocyanosis, which is a persistent blue or cyanotic discoloration of the digits, occurs most commonly in the hands and may worsen with exposure to cold and improve with rewarming. The primary form is a benign cosmetic condition, but it may also be seen in patients with connective tissue diseases, thromboangiitis obliterans, and diseases associated with central cyanosis. The exact pathophysiologic abnormality is not clear but may be vasospasm in the cutaneous arteries and arterioles with compensatory dilatation in the postcapillary venules.

Ulceration or tissue loss is unusual, and the overall prognosis is excellent. Patients should be advised to keep their extremities warm. Drugs such as α-adrenergic blocking agents or calcium channel blockers may be helpful.

Frostbite

Frostbite is freezing of tissues resulting from exposure to cold. It may occur in above-freezing temperatures under circumstances such as wetness, strong wind, or high altitude.

A person's response to cold is aimed at conserving the core (internal body) temperature as well as the viability of the extremity. Heat loss is reduced by peripheral vasoconstriction caused by sympathetic stimulation and catecholamine release. Maintenance or augmentation of body heat is accomplished by muscular activity such as shivering. However, the heat production from shivering cannot be sustained for more than a few hours because of the depletion of glycogen, which is the source of heat during shivering. The extremities are also protected by the "hunting reaction," which consists of irregular, 5- to 10-minute cycles of alternating periods of vasoconstriction and vasodilatation that protect the extremities against excessive sustained vasoconstriction at minimal loss of internal body temperature. However, when the body is exposed to cold of a magnitude or duration so as to threaten the internal body temperature, this mechanism fails. Because the disruption of core temperature is more deleterious to the body than peripheral vasoconstriction, conservation of core temperature takes precedence over rewarming of the extremities, and the hunting response is replaced by continuous and more intense vasoconstriction that promotes frostbite by means of ice crystal formation, cellular dehydration, and thrombosis of the microvasculature.

Soon after exposure to the cold, pain develops and gradually progresses to numbness; the frozen part turns white because of intense vasoconstriction. With rewarming or thawing, the circulation is restored and the affected parts become hyperemic. Edema may first occur within hours of thawing and remains for days or weeks. Blisters appear within the first 24 hours and are reabsorbed within 1 to 2 weeks, after which a black eschar may persist. Overactivity of the sympathetic nervous system is manifested by hyperhidrosis or a burning sensation.

Seventy per cent of victims develop chronic sequelae including cold sensitivity, pain, and sensory disturbances, often resembling a reflex sympathetic dystrophy. Frostbite arthritis may occur in particularly severe cases.

It is important to establish the depth of the frostbite and determine if the tissue is viable, which may not be obvious on initial clinical examination but is usually determined weeks or months after the cold injury when the demarcation zone appears and the dead tissue is sloughed.

TREATMENT. In mild cases of frostbite, the only necessary treatment may be daily whirlpool baths with bed rest. However, treatment of deep frostbite should be considered a medical emergency because the early institution of medical therapy may reduce the amount of subsequent tissue loss. Thawing, the mainstay of therapy, should not be implemented if the patient may be re-exposed to cold because refreezing of thawed tissue promotes further tissue damage. Walking on a frozen limb produces substantially less damage than walking on a thawed limb.

After transfer to a medical facility, frozen tissue should be rapidly rewarmed in a water bath of 40 to 42° C (104–108° F) for 15 to 30 minutes until complete thawing has occurred. After thawing, reappearance of normal color signifies the re-establishment of blood flow. Thawing is often a very painful process and may require the administration of narcotics.

After thawing, the extremity should be cleansed twice daily in a whirlpool bath with an aseptic solution at 35 to 37° C (95–99° F). Care should be taken to prevent and treat secondary infections. Tetanus prophylaxis should be administered. A frostbite protocol consisting of débridement of clear blisters with a topical application of aloe vera, oral ibuprofen, and daily hydrotherapy is highly effective. An important principle is to avoid early débridement or amputation, which is indicated only when infected gangrene or generalized sepsis occurs.

Erythromelalgia

Erythromelalgia literally means red, painful extremities. It may be classified as the primary or idiopathic category, which may be non-familial or familial. The secondary category is associated with other diseases, the most common being myeloproliferative disorders such as polycythemia vera and essential thrombocythemia. Other diseases associated with secondary erythromelalgia include hypertension, diabetes, rheumatoid arthritis, gout, spinal cord disease, multiple sclerosis, systemic lupus erythematosus, cutaneous vasculitis, and viral infection; and it may also result from therapy with various drugs (e.g., nifedipine, nicardipine, verapamil, bromocriptine, and pergolide). The histology varies from normal to arterial occlusion with thrombus formation.

Erythromelalgia is characterized by the clinical triad of erythema, burning pain, and increased temperature usually of the extremities. The feet, especially the soles, are more commonly involved than the hands. The peripheral pulses are generally normal in the primary type and variable in secondary erythromelalgia. The symptoms may occur in "attacks" that last for minutes to hours and occasionally days and are precipitated by a warm environment. Exercise and dependency tend to exacerbate symptoms. Patients seek relief by exposing the affected extremity to a cooler environment, such as placing the extremity in cold water, walking on a cold floor barefoot, or running the air conditioner even in the winter.

Other causes of painful erythematous extremities include reflex sympathetic dystrophy, atherosclerotic peripheral arterial disease (see Chapter 67), and thromboangiitis obliterans (Buerger's disease). Erythromelalgia may precede the clinical appearance of a myeloproliferative disorder by several years, so patients older than age 30 should be monitored periodically with blood cell counts.

The treatment of erythromelalgia is often difficult and frustrating. In secondary erythromelalgia, treatment of the underlying disease (phlebotomy in patients with polycythemia vera and normalization of the platelet count in patients with thrombocythemia) may relieve the symptoms. Aspirin is the most effective modality available particularly for patients with erythromelalgia secondary to myeloproliferative disorders. Other therapies with variable success include methysergide, ephedrine, non-steroidal anti-inflammatory drugs, phenoxybenzamine, nitroglycerine, sodium nitroprusside, corticosteroids, and surgical sympathectomy.

Popliteal Artery Entrapment Syndrome

In the popliteal artery entrapment syndrome there is compression of the popliteal artery due to a congenital anatomic abnormality or an abnormal muscle or fibrous band. The most frequent abnormality is when the medial head of the gastrocnemius muscle compresses the popliteal artery causing medial deviation of the popliteal artery.

The clinical presentation is in a healthy, "athletic type" male complaining of typical claudication symptoms in the absence of premature atherosclerosis. Disappearance of the pulse with passive dorsiflexion of the foot or active plantar foot flexion against resistance may suggest the diagnosis. Duplex ultrasound may help, and computed tomography (CT) or magnetic resonance imaging (MRI) can confirm the diagnosis; on arteriography, the characteristic finding is a medial deviation of the popliteal artery with post-stenotic dilatation. Other diseases that can cause midpopliteal occlusion include cystic adventitial disease, thrombosed popliteal artery aneurysm, and atherosclerosis of the superficial femoral and popliteal arteries. The primary treatment of popliteal artery entrapment syndrome is surgical.

Cystic Adventitial Disease

In cystic adventitial disease, gelatinous fluid accumulates in an arterial wall cyst and then the cyst encroaches on the vessel lumen, resulting in stenosis or occlusion. The cyst arises in the outer portion of the media or subadventitial layer, most commonly in the popliteal artery. Cystic adventitial disease is an isolated lesion not associated with a systemic process, and the precise pathophysiologic mechanism is unknown.

The disease predominates in men with an approximate ratio of 5:1, and the mean age at diagnosis is about 45 years. Claudication is the most frequent symptom. The pulses may disappear on flexion of the knee (Ishikawa's sign). However, if the artery is occluded, no pulses will be palpable.

Pulse volume recordings may show the characteristic drop in blood pressure and change in waveform configuration in the affected limb. A perivascular cystic structure may be visualized on duplex ultrasound. CT or MRI can show the anatomy in the popliteal region. CT-guided needle aspiration can partially but usually not completely remove the high viscosity and gelatinous fluid. If arterial occlusion has occurred, catheter-directed thrombolytic therapy and/or surgical resection is indicated.

Fibromuscular Dysplasia of the Extremities

Although fibromuscular dysplasia (in particular, medial fibroplasia) is most common in the renal and carotid arteries (see Chapter 112), it may also occur in peripheral arteries of the extremity (iliac, superficial femoral, popliteal, tibial, subclavian, axillary, radial, and ulnar). These lesions may be asymptomatic or may produce a difference in blood pressure between the two limbs with paresthesias, claudication, or critical limb ischemia.

The typical arteriographic appearance of "a string of beads" is virtually pathognomonic of medial fibroplasia. Long, smooth areas of narrowing are characteristic of intimal fibroplasia but may also be seen with Takayasu's arteritis (see Chapter 57) and giant cell arteritis (see Chapters 57 and 295).

Therapy should be reserved for symptomatic disease. Under most circumstances, percutaneous balloon dilatation is the treatment of choice.

Creager MA, Halperin JL, Coffman JD: Raynaud's phenomenon and other vascular disorders related to temperature. *In* Loscalzo J, Creager MA, Dzau VJ (eds): Vascular Medicine. Boston, Little, Brown, 1996, pp 965–997. *The most comprehensive review of the pathophysiology, clinical features, and treatment of Raynaud's phenomenon published to date.*

di Marzo L, Cavallaro A, Mingoli A, et al: Popliteal artery entrapment syndrome: The role of early diagnosis and treatment. Surgery 122:26–31, 1997. *The authors describe the clinical outcome in 30 patients with popliteal artery entrapment syndrome and make a strong case for early diagnosis and treatment.*

Hashmi MA, Rashid M, Haleem A, et al: Frostbite: Epidemiology at high altitude in the Karakoram mountains. Ann R Coll Surg Engl 80:91–95, 1998. *A retrospective review of 1500 cases of frostbite that occurred during a 10-year period in a tertiary care center in northeastern Pakistan.*

Kalgaard OM, Seem E, Kvernebo K: Erythromelalgia: A clinical study in 87 cases. J Intern Med 242:191–197, 1997. *The largest series of patients with erythromelalgia reported in the western literature.*

Krozon I, Tunick PA: Atheromatous disease of the thoracic aorta: Pathologic and clinical implications. Ann Intern Med 126:629–637, 1997. *A comprehensive review of recent developments in the diagnosis and management of atherosclerosis of the thoracic aorta as a source of embolization.*

Olin JW, Lie JT: Thromboangiitis obliterans (Buerger's disease). *In* Loscalzo J, Creager MA, Dzau VJ (eds): Vascular Medicine. Boston, Little, Brown, 1996, pp 1033–1049. *A detailed review of Buerger's disease with all of the important references related to this entity.*

69 PERIPHERAL VENOUS DISEASE

Russell D. Hull

Deep vein thrombosis (DVT) usually begins in the deep veins of the calf muscles. When confined to the calf veins, DVT carries a low risk of clinically important pulmonary emboli, but the DVT may propagate into the proximal venous system, where it becomes a serious and potentially life-threatening disorder. Although most clinically important pulmonary emboli (see Chapter 84) arise from thrombi in the popliteal or proximal deep veins of the leg, they may also arise from the iliac or deep pelvic veins, renal veins, inferior vena cava, or the right side of the heart. Less commonly, thrombosis may involve the axillary and subclavian venous systems; upper extremity DVT can also cause pulmonary emboli.

Superficial thrombophlebitis involves the superficial veins of the lower or sometimes the upper extremity, is commonly associated with the presence of varicose veins or pregnancy, and may be precipitated by trauma. Superficial thrombophlebitis may be associated with DVT, particularly when the more proximal superficial veins in the thigh are involved. Indeed, if any doubt exists, objective tests for DVT should be performed.

With the exception of thrombolytic therapy for some pulmonary emboli, management of DVT and pulmonary embolism is basically the same. The diagnostic approach to patients with venous thromboembolism (VTE) may involve the lungs or the legs, and prevention of pulmonary embolism is essentially the prevention of DVT.

ETIOLOGY AND PATHOGENESIS

VTE often complicates the course of sick, hospitalized patients but may also affect ambulant and otherwise apparently healthy individuals. Pulmonary embolism remains the most common preventable cause of hospital death and is responsible for approximately 150,000 to 200,000 deaths per year in the United States. Most patients who die of pulmonary embolism succumb suddenly or within 2 hours of the acute event, before therapy can be initiated or can take effect. Effective prophylaxis against VTE is now available for most high-risk patients.

Venous thrombi are composed predominantly of fibrin and red cells and have a variable platelet and leukocyte component. The factors that predispose to the development of VTE are venous stasis, activation of blood coagulation, and vascular damage. Protective mechanisms that counteract these thrombogenic stimuli include (1) inactivation of activated coagulation factors by circulating inhibitors (e.g., antithrombin III [ATIII], α_2-macroglobulin, α_1-antitrypsin, and activated protein C), (2) clearance of activated coagulation factors and soluble fibrin polymer complexes by the reticuloendothelial system and by the liver, and (3) dissolution of fibrin by fibrinolytic enzymes derived from plasma and endothelial cells and digestion of fibrin by leukocytes. Various coagulation abnormalities (see Table 187–1) and other risk factors predispose to VTE (Table 69–1).

CLINICAL FEATURES

The clinical features of venous thrombosis include leg pain, tenderness, swelling, a palpable cord, discoloration, venous distention, prominence of the superficial veins, and cyanosis. In most patients who have clinically suspected DVT, the symptoms and signs are non-specific; in more than 50% of these patients, the clinical suspicion of DVT is not confirmed by objective testing. Conversely, patients with relatively minor symptoms and signs may have extensive venous thrombosis.

Upper extremity DVT involving the subclavian, axillary, and brachial veins is often caused by strenuous exercise and is more common in males than females. Other risk factors include central venous catheters and previous venous thrombosis, but limited studies have shown little relationship to the presence of hypercoagulable states. Unilateral swelling, distention of superficial veins, cyanosis, and a palpable cord in the axillary vein are common clinical

Table 69–1 ■ FACTORS PREDISPOSING TO VENOUS THROMBOEMBOLISM

Surgical and nonsurgical trauma
Previous venous thromboembolism
Immobilization
Malignant disease
Heart failure
Leg paralysis
Age (>40 yr)
Obesity
Estrogens and oral contraceptives
Inherited or acquired disorders
  Antithrombin III deficiency
  Protein C or S deficiency
  Activated protein C resistance (Factor V Leiden)
  Prothrombin mutant
  Homocysteinemia
  Heparin-induced thrombocytopenia
  Antiphospholipid syndrome

manifestations. The diagnosis is best confirmed by compression ultrasonography, color flow Doppler imaging, or ascending contrast venography.

Pulmonary emboli originate from thrombi in the proximal deep veins of the leg in 90% or more of patients (see Chapter 84). Other less common sources of pulmonary emboli include the deep pelvic veins, the renal veins, the inferior vena cava, the right ventricle, and the axillary veins. Pulmonary embolism occurs in 50% of patients with objectively documented proximal leg vein thrombosis; many of the emboli are asymptomatic. Usually, only part of the thrombus embolizes, and 50 to 70% of patients with angiographically documented pulmonary emboli have detectable deep venous thrombosis of the legs at the time of initial evaluation. The clinical significance of pulmonary embolism depends on the size of the embolus and the cardiorespiratory reserve of the patient.

DIFFERENTIAL DIAGNOSIS

A number of conditions can mimic venous thrombosis (Table 69–2), but without objective testing it is often impossible to exclude venous thrombosis. The cause of symptoms can often be determined by careful follow-up after a diagnosis of venous thrombosis has been excluded by objective testing. In some patients, however, the cause of pain, tenderness, and swelling remains uncertain.

Objective Tests for Diagnosis of Venous Thrombosis

Objective tests used in the diagnosis of venous thrombosis include B-mode ultrasonography (commonly with color flow Doppler), impedance plethysmography (IPG), and ascending venography. The only laboratory test of proven value in the diagnosis and management of DVT is the D-dimer test.

Real-time *B-mode ultrasound,* preferably with *Doppler assessment,* has become the standard technique for the evaluation of patients with clinically suspected DVT. Prospective studies have shown that the single criterion of vein compressibility is highly

Table 69–2 ■ ALTERNATIVE DIAGNOSES IN 87 CONSECUTIVE PATIENTS WITH CLINICALLY SUSPECTED VENOUS THROMBOSIS AND NEGATIVE VENOGRAMS*

DIAGNOSIS	PATIENTS (%)
Muscle strain	24
Direct twisting injury to the leg	10
Leg swelling in paralyzed limb	9
Lymphangitis, lymphatic obstruction	7
Venous reflux	7
Muscle tear	6
Baker's cyst	5
Cellulitis	3
Internal abnormality of the knee	2
Unknown	26

*The diagnosis was made once venous thrombosis had been excluded by venography.

sensitive and specific for the detection of *proximal* DVT (sensitivity and specificity, both >95%). Other ultrasound criteria are insensitive, non-specific, or both. Doppler ultrasonography is still not sufficiently sensitive for the detection of isolated calf vein thrombosis; serial testing is required to detect proximal extension. Serial ultrasound, based on the now-confirmed concept that calf vein thrombi are clinically important only when they extend into the proximal veins and are reliably detected by ultrasound, is a useful clinical approach. A positive result is highly predictive of acute proximal DVT and warrants anticoagulation, whereas anticoagulant therapy can be safely withheld in symptomatic patients who have negative results by serial ultrasound (Fig. 69–1).

IPG is sensitive and specific for proximal DVT in symptomatic patients, but it is insensitive for calf DVT; a normal result cannot exclude this diagnosis. In patients with clinically suspected DVT, positive IPG results guide therapeutic decisions in the absence of clinical conditions known to produce false-positive results.

Although IPG has high sensitivity and specificity for the detection of symptomatic DVT, it lacks sensitivity for the detection of asymptomatic DVT in patients who have had surgery, such as total hip replacement, or in trauma patients. In such circumstances, the only reliable method for detecting DVT is bilateral ascending venography.

False-positive IPG results may occur with disorders that interfere with arterial inflow or venous outflow, including severe heart failure, constrictive pericarditis, severe arterial insufficiency, hypotension, and external compression of veins. Most of these disorders are readily recognized clinically. The test cannot be performed on patients who are in plaster casts or who cannot be adequately positioned because of immobilization or pain.

Doppler ultrasound and IPG are both highly sensitive and specific in the diagnosis of proximal DVT in symptomatic patients, but Doppler ultrasonography is more sensitive for detecting symptomatic calf vein thrombosis and more accurate for detecting proximal DVT in patients with increased central venous pressure or arterial insufficiency and DVT in patients whose leg is in a removable cast, who are in traction, or who have had distal leg amputation. However, both IPG and Doppler ultrasonography lack sensitivity and specificity for the detection of asymptomatic venous thrombosis in patients who have undergone surgery. Doppler ultrasonography (or even real-time B-mode ultrasonography without Doppler) has generally replaced IPG as the most popular noninvasive test for the detection of venous thrombosis.

Venography, the gold standard objective method for the diagnosis of DVT, requires considerable experience to execute and interpret accurately. The most reliable criterion for DVT is an intraluminal filling defect that is constant in all films and is seen in numerous projections. Other abnormalities such as non-filling of a segment of the deep venous system or non-filling of the entire deep venous system above the knee may be caused by technical artifacts. Even in the best of circumstances, it may be impossible to cannulate a vein on the dorsum of the foot, thus making ascending

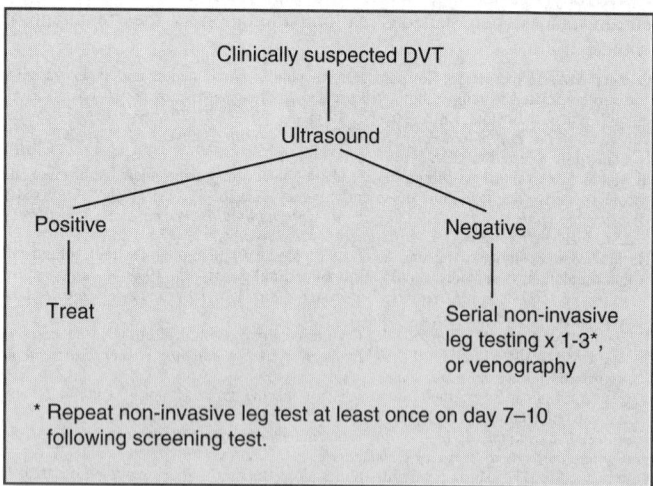

FIGURE 69–1 ■ Algorithm for the diagnosis of deep vein thrombosis (DVT) in patients with no evidence of pulmonary embolism.

venography impossible. Venography is also associated with pain in the foot while dye is being injected or 1 to 2 days after injection. The procedure may be complicated by superficial phlebitis and even DVT in 1 to 2% of patients with normal results on venography. Other less common complications include dye hypersensitivity or aggravation of renal insufficiency. The risks of venography must be carefully weighed against its benefits, and ultrasonography has largely replaced contrast venography in symptomatic patients because of its widespread availability.

D-dimer, which can be measured rapidly by a number of enzyme-linked immunosorbent assays or less reliably by latex agglutination, has a high negative predictive value for excluding suspected VTE. The combination of a negative D-dimer, a non-diagnostic lung scan, and a low clinical probability of DVT or the combination of a normal D-dimer and normal ultrasound or IPG may sufficiently exclude DVT so that further diagnostic testing can be safely limited and anticoagulation avoided.

However, the main limitation of D-dimer testing is that patients with suspected venous thrombosis frequently have significant comorbid disease or are elderly; the majority of these patients have abnormal D-dimer assays. The findings in two clinical trials that a single repeat venous ultrasound at 1 week could safely exclude the diagnosis of DVT has made the use of clinical probabilities and D-dimer testing less relevant.

For patients with suspected DVT, screening compression ultrasound should be the first test; patients who are positive should be treated. Patients with a negative screening ultrasound should undergo serial non-invasive leg testing one to three times (minimum of one test at 1 week). If a diagnosis is urgently required, venography may be used. In centers using a D-dimer assay of proven validity, patients with a negative ultrasound and low clinical probability require no further testing or treatment if the D-dimer test is negative. Because patients with a high or intermediate clinical probability still require serial non-invasive leg tests or venography despite a negative ultrasound and negative D-dimer, D-dimer assay adds little to the evaluation of such patients.

The diagnosis of upper extremity DVT can be made by compression ultrasonography, with or without color flow Doppler imaging, or by venography. Many patients with suspected upper extremity venous thrombosis have negative objective studies that exclude the diagnosis. Pulmonary embolism frequently complicates upper extremity DVT and may be the initial manifestation; objective testing for pulmonary emboli is required if the diagnosis will alter management. In patients with superficial thrombophlebitis, objective testing should be performed whenever DVT is suspected, particularly in patients with extensive phlebitis.

PREVENTION OF VENOUS THROMBOEMBOLISM

Without prophylaxis, the frequency of DVT ranges from less than 10% in low-risk patients to 40 to 80% in high-risk patients, and the frequency of fatal pulmonary embolism ranges from 0.1 to 0.8% in patients undergoing elective general surgery, 2 to 3% in patients undergoing elective hip replacement, and 4 to 7% in patients undergoing surgery for a fractured hip (Table 69–3). Factors increasing the risk of postoperative venous thrombosis include advanced age, malignancy, previous VTE, obesity, heart failure, and paralysis.

Two approaches can be taken to prevent DVT and the resulting risk of fatal pulmonary embolism: Secondary prevention involves the early detection and treatment of subclinical DVT by screening postoperative patients with sensitive, objective tests, and primary prophylaxis against DVT involves either drugs or physical methods. Primary prophylaxis is preferred in most clinical circumstances, and prevention of DVT and pulmonary embolism is more cost-effective than treatment of complications when they occur. Secondary prevention by case-finding studies should be reserved for patients in whom primary prophylaxis is either contraindicated or relatively ineffective.

The primary prophylactic measures most commonly used are low-dose or adjusted-dose unfractionated heparin, low-molecular-weight heparin (LMWH), oral anticoagulants (to an international normalized ratio [INR] of 2.0 to 3.0), and intermittent pneumatic leg compression (Table 69–4). More recently, specific antithrombin agents, e.g., hirudin and bivalirudin (Hirulog), have become available. Other less common measures include aspirin and intravenous dextran. Combined modalities such as graduated compression stockings or intermittent pneumatic leg compression along with pharmacologic agents may have an additive effect. Despite the convincing evidence for the efficacy and safety of prophylactic regimens, prophylaxis tends to be underutilized, even in high-risk patients.

TREATMENT OF VENOUS THROMBOSIS

The objectives of treatment in patients with VTE are to prevent death from pulmonary embolism, prevent recurring VTE, and prevent the post-phlebitic syndrome. Anticoagulant drugs, especially heparin, LMWH, and warfarin, constitute the cornerstone of treatment of DVT. For selected patients, thrombolysis, thrombectomy, and inferior vena cava filters are appropriate.

HEPARIN THERAPY. The anticoagulant activity of unfractionated heparin depends on a unique pentasaccharide that binds to ATIII and potentiates the inhibition of thrombin and activated Factor X (Xa) by ATIII. About one third of all heparin molecules contain the unique pentasaccharide sequence regardless of whether they are low- or high-molecular-weight fractions. It is the pentasaccharide sequence that confers the molecular high affinity for ATIII. In addition, heparin catalyzes the inactivation of thrombin by Cofactor II, which acts independently of ATIII.

Heparin also increases the release of tissue factor pathway inhibitor; binds to numerous plasma and platelet proteins, to endothelial cells, and to leukocytes; and increases vascular permeability. The anticoagulant response to a standard dose of heparin varies widely

Table 69–3 ■ RISK OF VENOUS THROMBOEMBOLISM ASSESSED BY OBJECTIVE TESTING

RISK CATEGORY	CALF VEIN THROMBOSIS	PROXIMAL VEIN THROMBOSIS	FATAL PULMONARY EMBOLISM
High risk	40–80%	10–30%	1–5%
Major orthopedic surgery on the lower limbs			
General urologic surgery in patients older than 40 yrs with a recent history of DVT or PE			
Extensive pelvic or abdominal surgery for malignant disease			
Moderate risk	10–40%	2–10%	0.1–0.8%
General surgery in patients older than 40 yrs that lasts 30 min or more, in patients younger than 40 yrs taking oral contraceptives, and in women older than 35 yrs having emergency cesarean section			
Low risk	<10%	<1%	<0.01%
Minor surgery, i.e., <30 min, in patients older than 40 yrs without additional risk factors			
Uncomplicated surgery in patients younger than 40 yrs without additional risk factors			

DVT = deep vein thrombosis; PE = pulmonary embolism.
Modified with permission from Clagett GP, Anderson FA, Heit J, et al: Prevention of venous thromboembolism. Chest 108:312S, 1995.

Table 69–4 ■ SPECIFIC RECOMMENDATIONS FOR
PROPHYLAXIS FOR VARIOUS CLINICAL RISK CATEGORIES

PATIENT CATEGORY	PROPHYLAXIS RECOMMENDATION
Moderate risk	
General abdominal, thoracic, gynecologic, or urologic surgery; medical patients	Low-dose unfractionated heparin or LMWH, IPC in patients at high risk of bleeding
Pregnancy with previous DVT	Low-dose heparin or adjusted-dose heparin
Moderate to high risk	
Neurosurgery	IPC
High risk	
Elective hip replacement	LMWH, warfarin, IPC
Elective knee replacement	LMWH, IPC
Hip fracture	LMWH, warfarin
Spinal cord injury with paralysis	LMWH, IPC

See Table 188–4 for dose recommendations for various LMWH preparations.
LMWH = low-molecular-weight heparin; IPC = intermittent pneumatic leg compression; DVT = deep vein thrombosis.

among patients, so the anticoagulant response to heparin should be monitored by using either the activated partial thromboplastin time (aPTT) or heparin levels to titrate the dose in an individual patient.

LOW-MOLECULAR-WEIGHT HEPARIN. Standard heparin is polydispersed, with a mean molecular weight ranging from 10 to 16 kd. LMWH, by comparison, has a mean molecular weight of 4 to 5 kd.

The LMWHs commercially available are made by different processes (such as nitrous acid, alkaline, or enzymatic depolymerization), and they differ chemically and pharmacokinetically. The clinical significance of these differences, however, is unclear. The doses of each of the different LMWHs have been established empirically.

When compared with unfractionated heparin, LMWHs have greater bioavailability when given by subcutaneous injection and a longer duration of anticoagulant effect (permitting once- or twice-daily administration), and because the anticoagulant response (anti-Xa activity) to LMWH is highly correlated with body weight, a fixed dose can be administered. Laboratory monitoring is not necessary with LMWH; in fact, little correlation is seen between anti-Xa activity and either bleeding or recurrent thrombosis. Three LMWHs and one heparinoid have been approved for use in the United States, and four LMWHs are approved for clinical use in Canada.

RECOMMENDED REGIMENS. In pooled data from a number of clinical trials, subcutaneous unmonitored LMWH results in a reduction in major bleeding and mortality when compared with unfractionated heparin for the treatment of proximal DVT. Furthermore, LMWH used predominantly out of hospital is as effective and safe as intravenous unfractionated heparin given in the hospital. Oral warfarin therapy can be started simultaneously. Subcutaneous LMWH treatment is continued for 5 to 6 days and discontinued subsequently when the INR is therapeutic (INR above 2.0) on 2 consecutive days.

Another approach to anticoagulant therapy for VTE is a combination of continuous intravenous heparin and oral warfarin, with both started simultaneously. The suggested length of the initial intravenous heparin therapy is 5 days. Exceptions include patients who require immediate medical or surgical intervention, such as thrombolysis or insertion of a vena cava filter, or patients at very high risk of bleeding. Heparin is continued until the INR has been within the therapeutic range (2 to 3) for 2 consecutive days.

The efficacy of heparin therapy depends on achieving a critical therapeutic level of heparin within the first 24 hours of treatment. The critical therapeutic level is an aPTT 1.5 times the mean of the control value or the upper limit of the normal aPTT range within the first 24 hours of treatment. This aPTT corresponds to a heparin blood level of 0.2 to 0.4 U/mL by the protamine sulfate titration assay and 0.35 to 0.70 U/mL by the anti–Factor Xa assay. Because of the wide variability in the aPTT and in heparin blood levels with different reagents and even with different batches of the same reagent, each laboratory must establish its own minimal therapeutic

level. Although subtherapeutic aPTT values are strongly correlated with recurrent thromboembolism, the relationship between supra-therapeutic aPTT and bleeding (aPTT ratio of 2.5 or more) is less definite. Indeed, bleeding during heparin therapy is more closely related to underlying clinical risk factors than to aPTT elevation above the therapeutic range. To avoid underdosing or overdosing with heparin, standardized nomograms based on a patient's weight are recommended (Table 69–5).

COMPLICATIONS OF HEPARIN THERAPY. The main adverse effects of heparin therapy include bleeding, thrombocytopenia, and osteoporosis. Patients at particular risk are those who have had recent surgery or trauma or those who have other clinical factors that predispose to bleeding while taking heparin, such as peptic ulcer, occult malignancy, liver disease, other hemostatic defects, age older than 65 years, and female gender.

Management of bleeding while undergoing heparin therapy will depend on the location and severity of bleeding, the risk of recurrent VTE, and the aPTT. Heparin therapy should be discontinued temporarily or permanently. Patients with recent VTE may be candidates for insertion of an inferior vena cava filter. If urgent reversal of heparin effect is required, protamine sulfate can be administered.

Heparin-induced thrombocytopenia is a well-recognized complication of heparin therapy that usually occurs within 5 to 10 days after heparin treatment has started. Approximately 1 to 2% of patients receiving unfractionated heparin will experience a fall in the platelet count to less than the normal range or a 50% fall in the platelet count within the normal range. In the majority of cases, this mild to moderate thrombocytopenia appears to be a direct effect of heparin on platelets and is of no consequence. However, an immune thrombocytopenia mediated by IgG antibody directed against a complex of PF4 and heparin develops in approximately 0.1 to 0.2% of patients receiving heparin. The development of thrombocytopenia may be accompanied by arterial or venous thrombosis, which may lead to serious consequences such as death or limb amputation. The diagnosis of heparin-induced thrombocytopenia, with or without thrombosis, must be made on clinical grounds because the assays with the highest sensitivity and specificity are not readily available. When the diagnosis of heparin-induced thrombocytopenia is made, administration of heparin in all forms must be stopped immediately. In patients requiring ongoing anticoagulation, the heparinoid danaparoid or hirudin may be used. Warfarin is another alternative, but it should probably not be started until one of the aforementioned agents has been used for 3 or 4 days to suppress thrombin generation. The defibrinogenating snake venom Arvin has been used quite extensively in the past but, like the use of plasmapheresis or intravenous gamma globulin infusion, will probably be replaced by other agents. Insertion of an inferior vena cava filter is often indicated.

Osteoporosis has been reported in patients receiving unfractionated heparin in dosages of 20,000 U/day (or more) for more than 6 months. Demineralization can progress to fracture of vertebral bodies or long bones, and the defect may not be entirely reversible.

Protamine sulfate has been shown to reduce clinical bleeding in patients experiencing bleeding while receiving heparin or LMWHs, presumably by neutralizing the high-molecular-weight fractions of heparin that are thought to be most responsible for bleeding.

THROMBOLYTIC THERAPY. Thrombolytic therapy may benefit

Table 69–5 ■ WEIGHT-BASED NOMOGRAM FOR INITIAL
INTRAVENOUS HEPARIN THERAPY

aPTT	DOSE (IU/kg)
Initial dose	80 bolus, then 18/hr
<35 sec (<1.2×)*	80 bolus, then 4/hr
35–45 sec (1.2–1.5×)	40 bolus, then 2/hr
46–70 sec (1.5–2.3×)	No change
71–90 sec (2.3–3.0×)	Decrease infusion rate by 2/hr
>90 sec (>3.0×)	Hold infusion 1 hr, then decrease infusion rate by 3/hr

*Figures in parentheses show comparison with control.
aPTT = activated partial thromboplastin time.
Adapted from Raschke RA, Reilly BM, Guidry JR, et al: The weight-based heparin dosing nomogram compared with a "standard care" nomogram. A randomized controlled trial. Ann Intern Med 119:874–881, 1993.

selected patients with acute massive venous thrombosis, such as those with phlegmasia cerulea dolens. In most patients with acute DVT, however, the indication for thrombolytic therapy remains controversial, and most patients do well with unfractionated heparin or LMWH. Currently, randomized clinical trials have yielded no definitive evidence that thrombolytic therapy is associated with improved benefit by prevention of the post-phlebitic syndrome.

THROMBECTOMY. Thrombectomy has been recommended in patients with massive iliofemoral thrombosis, particularly patients with vascular insufficiency and in whom thrombolytic therapy is contraindicated. These patients tend to have recurrent thrombosis after thrombectomy, and the procedure has fallen into disrepute in most centers. The finding of a free-floating thrombus on ultrasound has been another indication for urgent thrombectomy. However, a recent clinical trial reported no difference in outcomes for patients with free-floating thrombi and patients with proximal venous thromboses that were not free floating. Adequate anticoagulation is therefore the most important aspect of management.

INFERIOR VENA CAVA INTERRUPTION. The main indications for the insertion of an inferior vena caval filter for DVT are acute VTE and an absolute contraindication to anticoagulant therapy and the very rare instance of objectively documented recurrent VTE during adequate anticoagulant therapy. Prophylactic placement may be considered in very high-risk patients, including those with cor pulmonale or a previous history of thromboembolism who are in high-risk situations because of acetabular fracture or who have cancer. Patients who have had pulmonary embolectomy either surgically or via percutaneous catheters should have inferior vena caval filters inserted.

In a recent treatment trial of patients randomized to receive or not receive an inferior vena cava filter, the mortality and rate of major bleeding were not different at 2 years in the two groups, thus suggesting that interruption of the inferior vena cava may be unnecessary in patients who can receive adequate anticoagulant therapy. Because inferior vena cava filters were associated with an increased rate of recurrent DVT, patients receiving filters may require long-term anticoagulation.

UPPER EXTREMITY DEEP VEIN THROMBOSIS. Treatment of upper extremity DVT is the same as for proximal venous thrombosis, i.e., LMWH or heparin and then warfarin for at least 3 months. Patients with recent-onset upper extremity DVT have been treated with thrombolytic agents, but clinical trials have not demonstrated that the use of thrombolytic agents decreases long-term sequelae. The rare patient with thoracic outlet obstruction may benefit from surgery.

TREATMENT OF SUPERFICIAL THROMBOPHLEBITIS. In the absence of associated DVT, treatment of superficial thrombophlebitis is usually confined to symptomatic relief with analgesia and rest of the affected limb. The exception is patients with superficial thrombophlebitis involving a large segment of the long saphenous vein, particularly when it occurs above the knee. These patients should be treated with either LMWH or heparin, with or without oral anticoagulant therapy, or by superficial venous ligation. The presence of associated DVT requires the usual treatment with heparin and warfarin for at least 3 months.

ORAL ANTICOAGULANT THERAPY. Coumarin derivatives (primarily warfarin), the oral anticoagulants of choice, exert their anticoagulant effect by inhibition of the vitamin K–dependent γ-carboxylation of coagulation Factors II, VII, IX, and X; the result is the synthesis of immunologically detectable but biologically inactive forms of these coagulation proteins. Warfarin also inhibits the vitamin K–dependent γ-carboxylation of proteins C and S. Therefore, vitamin K antagonists such as warfarin create a biochemical paradox by producing an anticoagulant effect caused by the inhibition of procoagulants (Factors II, VII, IX and X) and a potentially thrombogenic effect by impairing the synthesis of naturally occurring inhibitors of coagulation (proteins C and S). Heparin and warfarin treatment should overlap by 4 to 5 days when warfarin treatment is initiated in patients with thrombotic disease.

The anticoagulant effect of warfarin is delayed until the normal clotting factors are cleared from the circulation, and the peak effect does not occur until 36 to 72 hours after drug administration. During the first few days of warfarin therapy, the prothrombin time mainly reflects the depression of Factor VII, which has a half-life of 5 to 7 hours. Equilibrium levels of Factors II, IX, and X are not reached until about 1 week after the initiation of therapy. The use of small initial daily doses (e.g., 5.0 to 10 mg) is the preferred approach for initiating warfarin treatment.

The dose-response relationship to warfarin therapy varies widely among individuals, and therefore the dose must be carefully monitored to prevent overdosing or underdosing. A number of drugs interact with warfarin, and patients must be warned against taking any new drugs without their physician's knowledge.

LABORATORY MONITORING AND THERAPEUTIC RANGE. The laboratory test most commonly used to measure the effects of warfarin is the one-stage prothrombin time. The prothrombin time is sensitive to reduced activity of Factors II, VII, and X, but it is insensitive to reduced activity of Factor IX. The INR is the prothrombin time ratio obtained by testing a given sample against the World Health Organization reference thromboplastin.

Warfarin is administered in an initial dosage of 5.0 to 10 mg/day for the first 2 days. The daily dose is then adjusted according to the INR. Heparin therapy is discontinued on the fourth or fifth day after initiation of warfarin therapy, provided that the INR is prolonged into the recommended therapeutic range (INR of 2.0 to 3.0). Because some individuals are either fast or slow metabolizers of the drug, selection of the correct dosage of warfarin must be individualized by making frequent INR determinations. Once the anticoagulant effect and patient's warfarin dose requirements are stable, the INR should be monitored at regular intervals (every 2 to 4 weeks) throughout the course of warfarin therapy for VTE. However, with factors that may produce an unpredictable response to warfarin (e.g., concomitant drug therapy), the INR should be monitored frequently to minimize the risk of complications caused by poor anticoagulant control.

LONG-TERM TREATMENT OF VENOUS THROMBOEMBOLISM

Patients with established DVT or pulmonary embolism require long-term anticoagulant therapy to prevent recurrent disease. Warfarin therapy is highly effective and is preferred in most patients. In patients with proximal vein thrombosis (popliteal, femoral, or iliac vein thrombosis), long-term therapy with warfarin reduces the frequency of objectively documented recurrent VTE from 47% to 2%. A warfarin regimen with an INR of 2.0 to 3.0 markedly reduces the risk of bleeding (from 20% to 4%) without loss of effectiveness in comparison with more intense doses.

All patients with a first episode of VTE should receive warfarin therapy for 3 to 6 months because shorter durations have resulted in higher rates of recurrent VTE. In patients with a continuing risk factor that is potentially reversible (e.g., prolonged bed rest), therapy should be continued for at least 3 months or until the risk factor is reversed. Warfarin treatment for more than 6 months is indicated for patients with recurrent VTE or in patients who have a continuing risk factor for VTE. The optimum duration of therapy in patients with recurrent VTE is the subject of ongoing clinical trials, but the current recommendation is to continue oral anticoagulant therapy for at least 12 months in patients with a first recurrence and indefinitely for those who have more than one recurrence.

RECURRENT VENOUS THROMBOSIS

The diagnosis of recurrent DVT is problematic, particularly if previous studies are not available for review. Abnormalities persist on ultrasound for more than 12 months in the majority of patients, and IPG remains abnormal at 3 months in approximately 30% of patients. If these tests have reverted to negative and then become positive with a symptomatic recurrence or if a new defect is detected in the same or the contralateral leg, the diagnosis is quite evident. Similarly, a new intraluminal filling defect on repeat venography is diagnostic, and a new defect on ventilation-perfusion lung scanning is helpful in making the diagnosis of pulmonary embolism. A normal D-dimer assay may exclude recurrent venous thrombosis.

Clagett GP, Anderson FA, Geerts WH, et al: Prevention of venous thromboembolism. Chest 114(Suppl.):5315, 1998. *Evidence based recommendations from the Fifth American College of Chest Physicians Consensus on Anti-Thrombotic Therapy.*

Collins R, Scrimgeour A, Yusef S, et al: Reduction in fatal pulmonary embolism and venous thrombosis by perioperative administration of subcutaneous heparin. N Engl J Med 318:1162, 1998. *A meta-analysis of a large number of clinical trials support-*

ing the use of prophylactic low-dose heparin in reducing the incidence of postoperative venous thrombosis and more importantly in reducing the incidence of fatal pulmonary embolism.

Kearon C, Gent M, Hirsh J, et al: A comparison of three months of anticoagulation with extended anticoagulation for a first episode of idiopathic venous thromboembolism. N Engl J Med 340:901, 1999. *More than 3 months of anticoagulation is preferred.*

Lensing AWA, Bueller HR: Objective tests for the diagnosis of venous thrombosis. *In* Hull RD, Pineo GF (eds): Disorders of Thrombosis. Philadelphia, WB Saunders, 1996, pp 239–257. *Comprehensive review of the currently available objective tests used for the diagnosis of venous thrombosis in patients who are either symptomatic or asymptomatic.*

Nicolaides AN, Bergqvist D, Hull R: Prevention of VTE: International consensus statement. Int Angiol 16:3, 1997. *This report summarizes recommendations for the prevention and treatment of arterial and venous thrombotic disorders.*

70 MISCELLANEOUS CONDITIONS OF THE HEART: TUMOR, TRAUMA, AND SYSTEMIC DISEASE

Joshua Wynne

CARDIAC TUMORS

Although the heart is resistant to the development of primary malignancies, it is a frequent site of secondary involvement by metastatic tumors. Most primary cardiac tumors are benign, whereas all secondary tumors are malignant (Fig. 70–1). Primary tumors of the heart are noted in 1 per 2000 to 4000 unselected autopsies, whereas metastatic involvement may be found in up to 20% of cancer patients. Recognition of cardiac involvement by tumor is often delayed because of a low index of suspicion, yet it is usually detectable by standard non-invasive techniques (echocardiography, computed tomography, and magnetic resonance imaging). The clinical features of a patient with a cardiac tumor are determined less by the histology of the tumor than by its location and size. Intracavity tumors typically involve a cardiac valve and may produce valve dysfunction (with obstruction and/or regurgitation). Intramyocardial tumors may be clinically silent or may lead to arrhythmia or heart block. Intrapericardial tumors generally become apparent when they compress the heart chambers, usually by tamponade from an effusion but occasionally by constriction. Con-

versely, the tumor type most directly determines management and prognosis.

The most common primary tumor in adults is myxoma, whereas rhabdomyomas predominate in children. Other tumors include fibromas, lipomas, and fibroelastomas. Only an occasional malignant primary tumor is encountered, usually a sarcoma. Secondary tumor involvement of the heart is much more common than a primary neoplasm and is dominated by cancers of the lung and breast, which is a reflection of their relative frequency overall. Together they account for more than half of all cases of cardiac tumors. Cardiac involvement by lymphomas, esophageal cancer, leukemia, and melanoma is also common, as is occasional involvement by other malignancies.

INTRAPERICARDIAL TUMORS. Tumor involvement of the heart most commonly occurs by contiguous spread and direct extension of neoplasms involving the chest cavity, usually with invasion of the pericardium. Lung and breast cancers typically invade the heart in this manner and, because of their relative frequency, make pericardial involvement the most common manifestation of secondary tumors, often with attendant pericardial effusion and cardiac tamponade. Because tumor invasion often extends beyond the pericardial space to involve the myocardium as well, expectations of long-term therapeutic success are often very low. Nevertheless, pericardiocentesis (often guided by echocardiography), balloon pericardiotomy, or surgical drainage and limited pericardiectomy ("pericardial window") are often life-saving short- and intermediate-term palliative procedures. Even very debilitated patients may benefit from a subxiphoid pericardiectomy, a quick and low-morbidity procedure that may provide brief palliation.

INTRACAVITY TUMORS. The most common intracavity tumor is the *myxoma*, a benign polypoid neoplasm of endocardial origin that is usually located within the left atrium and attached to the interatrial septum. Sometimes it is also seen in the right atrium and rarely in the ventricles. Myxomas are found most commonly in women between 30 and 60 years of age and are usually an isolated finding. On occasion they are familial or occur in association with other systemic abnormalities (such as pigmented skin lesions and non-cardiac tumors). Although they may not be clinically apparent when small, myxomas usually produce findings secondary to tumor embolization, mitral valve obstruction, and constitutional symptoms such as fever, malaise, and arthralgias. During diastole, a left atrial myxoma may be drawn into the mitral orifice and produce obstruction to blood flow from the left atrium to the left ventricle, thus simulating rheumatic mitral stenosis. Even the physical examination may be misleading, with a tumor "plop" simulating an opening snap and a diastolic rumble similar to the murmur found with rheumatic involvement.

If the diagnosis is suspected, echocardiography (often using the transesophageal approach) provides the definitive diagnosis; most myxomas are discovered when embolization or valve dysfunction

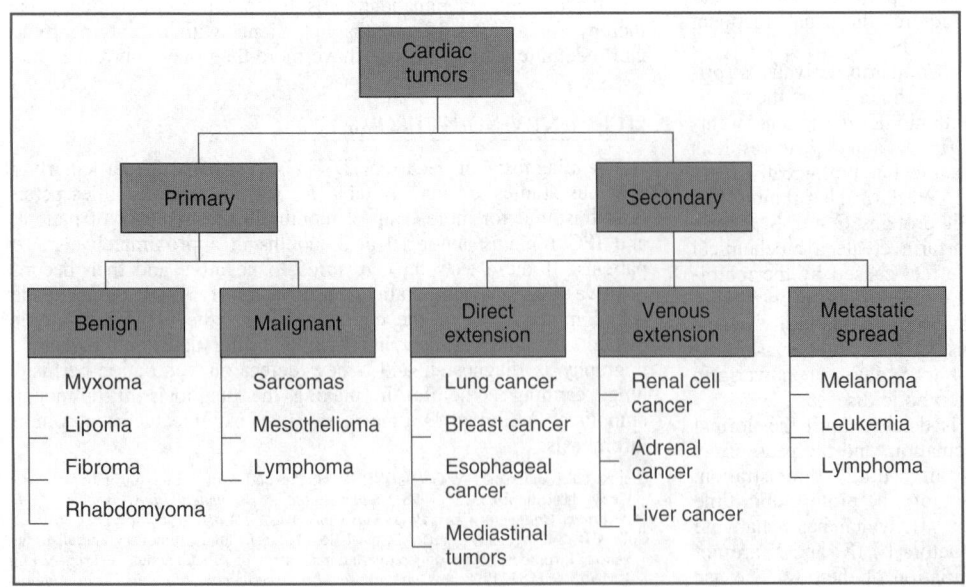

FIGURE 70–1 ■ Classification of the most common primary and secondary tumors. (Adapted from Salcedo EE, Cohen GI, White RD, Davison MG: Cardiac tumors: Diagnosis and management. Curr Probl Cardiol 17:75, 1992.)

leads to an echocardiographic study. Once diagnosed, the tumor is removed surgically, which is usually a low-risk procedure that results in cure. Myxomas can be multiple or recurrent, so even after successful removal, continued surveillance is indicated.

Other intracavity tumors are uncommon. Papillary fibroelastomas are frond-like excrescences that typically arise from a cardiac valve (often the mitral) and are usually detected incidentally during echocardiography. They may produce symptoms by virtue of systemic or coronary embolization and are usually amenable to surgical excision. Angiosarcomas occur in men more frequently than women and have a predilection for the pericardium and right atrium, where they may cause obstruction and attendant right-sided congestive heart failure. A unique type of cardiac involvement that occurs most commonly with renal cell carcinoma (and occasionally with adrenal and hepatic neoplasms) consists of extension of the tumor via the inferior vena cava, with resultant tumor involvement of the right atrial cavity.

INTRAMYOCARDIAL TUMORS. The least common location for cardiac tumors is within the myocardium, where the tumors may be clinically silent, produce arrhythmias, or protrude into a cardiac chamber with attendant obstructive features. Lipomas are encapsulated benign primary cardiac tumors that are often clinically silent. Sarcomas (angiosarcomas, rhabdomyosarcomas, fibrosarcomas) often demonstrate widespread cardiac involvement, with protrusion into the cardiac chambers and extension into the pericardial space. No good therapy is available for these tumors.

Secondary tumor involvement is usually the result of hematogenous or lymphatic spread and is frequently seen with melanoma, leukemia, and lymphoma.

CARDIAC TRAUMA

Cardiac damage may result from trauma as a consequence of either penetrating or non-penetrating injury. The usual cause of penetrating trauma is a bullet or stab wound, whereas deceleration injuries as a consequence of automobile accidents are the most common cause of non-penetrating injury. Either type often results in death before the patient comes to medical attention, usually from hemopericardium and attendant tamponade or massive hemorrhage.

NON-PENETRATING INJURY. The most common manifestation of blunt trauma is myocardial contusion, often the result of impact of the chest wall against the steering wheel. Although the diagnosis of contusion is straightforward when new electrocardiographic changes or arrhythmias are noted, the diagnosis is more difficult in the typical chest trauma patient. In such cases, demonstration of new regional left ventricular wall motion abnormalities on echocardiography or radionuclide ventriculography helps secure the diagnosis. Measurement of myocardial enzyme levels has been disappointing in assessing the diagnosis or prognosis of presumed myocardial contusion. The prognosis is generally excellent if the patient is otherwise clinically stable after myocardial contusion. Other less common manifestations of blunt trauma include traumatic ventricular septal defect, myocardial rupture and/or pseudoaneurysm formation, coronary artery trauma with myocardial infarction, valvular regurgitation, and pulmonary artery rupture.

The most feared complication of blunt trauma is traumatic transection of the descending aorta, which occurs just distal to the ligamentum arteriosum. It results from the shear forces that occur during deceleration injury as the more mobile aortic arch continues to move anteriorly while the descending aorta remains fixed because of its attachment to the posterior mediastinum. It is usually fatal if not rapidly repaired surgically. However, occasional patients may show long-term survival even without operative repair.

PENETRATING INJURY. Bullet and stab wounds, the most common form of penetrating trauma, usually result in hemopericardium with tamponade or in exsanguination, depending on the site of injury. Associated cardiac damage is not uncommon, including traumatic valvular regurgitation, intracardiac shunts, and occasionally, coronary artery injuries. Immediate thoracotomy is indicated when life-threatening hemorrhage or tamponade is present; repair of any associated cardiac defects can often wait for definitive diagnosis and management at a later time.

CARDIAC INVOLVEMENT IN SYSTEMIC DISEASE

CARCINOID. More than 50% of patients with carcinoid syndrome (see Chapter 245) metastatic to the liver have cardiac involvement, usually consisting of thickening and scarring of the endocardium and the tricuspid and/or pulmonary valves (often both) and producing both stenosis and regurgitation. Left-sided valvular involvement, myocardial metastases, and pericardial effusions occur on occasion. These endocardial changes may be produced by serotonin and other vasoactive substances released by the tumor. Morphologically similar valvular abnormalities have been seen with the anorectic agents fenfluramine and phentermine. Dyspnea is a common finding, and right heart failure may contribute to the death of one third of these patients. Systemic symptoms and survival can be improved if treatment shrinks the hepatic metastases or effectively blocks serotonin with a somatostatin analogue. In selected patients, valve replacement (often with a bioprosthesis) has resulted in significant symptomatic improvement with a one-third to nearly two-thirds perioperative mortality.

CARDIOTOXICITY OF CANCER THERAPY. Cardiotoxicity following chemotherapy (see Chapter 198) is most common with doxorubicin (Adriamycin) and consists of dose-related systolic (and diastolic) dysfunction that may produce clinical congestive heart failure months to years after treatment. Although less common with current dosing schemes that use more frequent but lower doses than prior regimens, doxorubicin cardiotoxicity continues to be associated with a poor prognosis and significant mortality. Detection of early or subclinical cardiotoxicity is difficult but best accomplished by monitoring for a fall in resting or exercise left ventricular ejection fraction with radionuclide ventriculography or echocardiography. Periodic percutaneous right ventricular endomyocardial biopsy may be more predictive but is not widely used. Concomitant use of the iron chelator dexrazoxane in selected patients appears to offer some degree of protection from the toxic cardiac effects of the anthracyclines. Cardiotoxicity appears to be potentiated in the setting of mediastinal irradiation, pre-existing cardiac disease, young or advanced age, and concomitant administration of other chemotherapeutic drugs. Girls treated for childhood cancer have a greater risk than boys for the development of late cardiotoxicity. The best treatment is discontinuation of doxorubicin treatment, after which improvement sometimes results. Once congestive heart failure appears, the use of digitalis, diuretics, and vasodilators usually results in significant symptomatic improvement.

Cardiotoxicity may also be seen with cyclophosphamide, which occasionally produces fatal hemorrhagic myocardial necrosis. Myocardial ischemia and infarction can occur during 5-fluorouracil infusions, and some but not all patients appear to respond to nitrates. Paclitaxel (Taxol) has, on rare occasion, been associated with a variety of often asymptomatic arrhythmias and abnormalities of the cardiac conduction system.

Cardiotoxicity as a consequence of radiation therapy has declined in frequency with better shielding of the heart, use of improved dosing schedules, and use of multiple radiation portals (see Chapter 19). Nevertheless, cardiac damage occurring months and years after radiation therapy continues to be seen, most commonly consisting of pericardial inflammation and effusion that may progress to chronic constrictive pericarditis. Other manifestations include accelerated coronary artery atherosclerosis (often involving the coronary ostia), myocardial fibrosis, and occasionally valvular dysfunction and abnormalities of the conducting system.

NON-BACTERIAL THROMBOTIC (MARANTIC) ENDOCARDITIS. Sterile verruciform platelet-fibrin masses are found adherent to the mitral and aortic valves in the absence of underlying inflammation in about 1% of autopsies in patients with a variety of malignant tumors and various non-neoplastic disorders. Seen most commonly in mucin-producing adenocarcinomas, they are also found in malignant melanoma and various liquid tumors. Detectable by echocardiography, they may be found in up to 20% of cancer patients during life. Systemic emboli occur in about half of these patients, with the brain a frequent site of involvement. Anecdotal reports have suggested that heparin may be efficacious, but definitive data are lacking.

ENDOCRINE DISORDERS. The heart is often involved in diabetics (see Chapter 242), although debate continues about whether diabetes is associated with a unique cardiomyopathy or whether the observed cardiac abnormalities are simply a consequence of the coronary artery disease and hypertension that so frequently accompany diabetes. Hyperthyroidism (see Chapter 239) commonly results in a hyperkinetic cardiovascular state manifested by a fall in systemic vascular resistance, an increase in cardiac output, and enhanced left ventricular emptying. Other effects include atrial fibrillation and, especially with pre-existing heart disease, congestive heart failure. Patients with coronary artery disease often experience an exacerbation of angina pectoris. Hypothyroidism may be associated with hypertension, bradycardia, and a pericardial effusion that rarely progresses to cardiac tamponade. Because myocardial ischemia is often exacerbated in myxedematous patients with pre-existing coronary artery disease as therapy is begun, thyroid hormone replacement should be started with very low doses that are increased slowly. Pheochromocytomas (see Chapter 241) are associated with histologic evidence of catecholamine-induced myocardial damage in about 50% of patients. Focal myocardial contraction band necrosis, inflammation, and fibrosis are seen histologically but only occasionally result in clinical congestive heart failure. Treatment with adrenergic receptor blockers (initially α and then β) is usually effective in treating both the hypertension and the cardiotoxicity before surgery to remove the tumor.

INFILTRATIVE DISEASES. Amyloidosis (see Chapter 297), hemochromatosis (see Chapter 221), and sarcoidosis can cause infiltrative myocardial diseases leading to cardiomyopathy (see Chapter 64). Treatment focuses on the systemic disease process.

NEUROMUSCULAR DISEASES. Cardiac involvement is common in Friedreich's ataxia, with symmetric or asymmetric left ventricular hypertrophy often grossly resembling hypertrophic cardiomyopathy. Associated ST segment and T wave abnormalities of the electrocardiogram are common. In Duchenne's muscular dystrophy (see Chapter 506), a peculiar form of myocardial necrosis principally involves the posterobasal portion of the left ventricle and the adjacent papillary muscle. The echocardiogram is often distinctive, as is the electrocardiogram, which demonstrates tall R waves in the right precordial leads and deep Q waves in the limb and lateral precordial leads. Myotonic dystrophy produces a variety of electrocardiographic abnormalities, especially abnormalities of atrioventricular conduction with the attendant risk of syncope and sudden death. Myocardial involvement is uncommon.

COLLAGEN VASCULAR DISEASES. Although demonstrable cardiac involvement is common in rheumatoid arthritis, clinical manifestations are rare. The endocardium, myocardium, or pericardium may be involved, but the most common manifestation is pericarditis, with a variable amount of pericardial effusion. Cardiac valvular involvement occurs in more than 50% of patients with systemic lupus erythematosus and in one third of patients with the antiphospholipid syndrome in the absence of lupus. The lesions consist of valvular thickening and sterile vegetations that may be evanescent but produce valve regurgitation in one quarter of patients. Although usually asymptomatic and clinically quiescent, over time the valvular abnormalities result in significant cardiovascular morbidity and mortality from embolism, infective endocarditis, and heart failure.

In progressive systemic sclerosis (see Chapter 290), focal myocardial necrosis and fibrosis may occur and culminate in a dilated cardiomyopathy. Ankylosing spondylitis and the associated seronegative arthropathies (Reiter's syndrome, psoriatic arthritis) may involve the proximal aortic root and produce clinically important aortic regurgitation.

Edoute Y, Haim N, Rinkevich D, et al: Cardiac valvular vegetations in cancer patients: Prospective echocardiographic study of 200 patients. Am J Med 102:252, 1997. *A study of the echocardiographic findings and clinical course of 200 patients with a variety of solid tumors; valvular vegetations were found in 19% of patients (a quarter of whom had systemic emboli), but only in 2% of controls.*

Pretre R, Chilcott M: Blunt trauma to the heart and great vessels. N Engl J Med 336: 626, 1997. *A summary of the clinical features of blunt trauma to the cardiovascular system. Specific suggested guidelines for the management of suspected myocardial contusion are particularly useful.*

Reynen K: Cardiac myxomas. N Engl J Med 333:1610, 1995. *An encyclopedic well-referenced review of cardiac myxomas.*

Roberts WC: Primary and secondary neoplasms of the heart. Am J Cardiol 80:671, 1997. *A descriptive review article by the noted cardiac pathologist who has contributed many of the original observations about tumor involvement of the heart.*

Roldan CA, Shively BK, Crawford MH: An echocardiographic study of valvular heart disease associated with systemic lupus erythematosus. N Engl J Med 335:1424, 1996. *The definitive echocardiographic study of the valvular abnormalities in systemic lupus erythematosus. Transesophageal echocardiography was performed in 69 patients with lupus (84% of whom had a repeat study), with comparison to a control population.*

Shan K, Lincoff AM, Young JB: Anthracycline-induced cardiotoxicity. Ann Intern Med 125:47, 1996. *A well-referenced summary of articles dealing with anthracycline cardiotoxicity.*

71 ▪ CARDIAC TRANSPLANTATION

Robert C. Bourge

Cardiac transplantation, once considered an experimental procedure, has emerged as the therapy of choice for appropriately selected patients with life-threatening, irremediable heart disease. The procedure and its postoperative medical regimen result in significant morbidity and mortality, and they are warranted only if the prognosis of the underlying cardiac disease is sufficiently grave.

The incidence of congestive heart failure increases with age and affects more than 400,000 people in the United States every year (see Chapter 47); transplantation is a therapeutic option for many of these patients. As survival after cardiac transplantation has markedly improved, the population of long-term survivors has grown. Primary care physicians, as well as cardiologists not based at cardiac transplant centers, often assist in the care of these patients, most often in consultation with cardiac transplant physicians. In addition, a physician may be called on to assist in the management and evaluation of a potential cardiac donor.

THE CARDIAC TRANSPLANT RECIPIENT

Indications for Cardiac Transplantation (Table 71–1)

Patients who are dependent on intravenous inotropic support or mechanical cardiac support or who have undergone mechanical cardiac replacement are at the highest priority for cardiac transplantation. Other indications include class IV heart failure and symptoms at rest despite optimal medication therapy (1-year survival of <50%) or class III heart failure despite maximal medical therapy (1-year survival of 30 to 70%) (see Chapters 47 and 48). Patients with class II symptoms may benefit from evaluation and subsequent transplantation if concomitant cardiac conditions, such as uncontrollable ventricular arrhythmias, adversely affect predicted survival. Patients with sustained ventricular tachycardia that is refractory to all forms of therapy, including the placement of an implantable cardioverter-defibrillator (ICD) (see Chapter 53), should also be considered for cardiac transplantation.

In the United States, the most common underlying cause of heart failure leading to cardiac transplantation is ischemic coronary heart disease (CHD). Most large studies have shown that patients with

---

Table 71–1 ▪ INDICATIONS FOR CONSIDERATION FOR CARDIAC TRANSPLANTATION (CONSIDER REFERRAL TO CARDIAC TRANSPLANT CENTER)

Irremediable cardiac disease with estimated mortality of more than 25–30% at 1 yr; survival without transplantation is estimated from heart disease etiology, disease duration, hemodynamics, functional capacity, and presence or absence of cardiac arrhythmias

Unacceptable quality of life primarily due to cardiac disease limitations

Acceptable social and financial support

Acceptable neurocognitive function

Absence of significant psychological or pathologic disorders or substance abuse

Transplantation surgical risk acceptable from a technical standpoint

Absence of co-morbid conditions that would significantly limit post-transplantation survival or significantly worsen post-transplantation quality of life, including advanced physiologic age, coexistent systemic illness with poor prognosis, irreversible pulmonary hypertension, acute pulmonary thromboembolism, severe peripheral and/or cerebrovascular disease, irreversible renal or liver disease, active peptic ulcer, active diverticulitis, diabetes mellitus with significant end-organ disease, severe obesity, severe osteoporosis, and active severe infection

Adapted from Costanzo MR, Augustine SA, Bourge R, et al: Selection and treatment of candidates for heart transplantation (Tables 1 and 2). Circulation 92:3593–3621. 1995.

heart failure secondary to CHD have a higher mortality than those with non-ischemic causes.

The second most common disease leading to cardiac transplantation is idiopathic dilated cardiomyopathy (see Chapter 64). Factors that correlate with a high mortality, and hence suggest potential benefit from cardiac transplantation, include (1) a peak oxygen consumption on an exercise gas exchange stress test of less than 11 to 14 mL/kg per minute; (2) a low plasma sodium level, especially after intensive medical management; (3) high right ventricular and/or left ventricular filling pressures (a very high right atrial or jugular venous pressure and/or pulmonary capillary wedge pressure), especially after medical management; (4) a very low ejection fraction (<15 to 20%; not predictive alone, however); (5) complex ventricular arrhythmias; (6) a very large left ventricular cavity (end-diastolic maximal dimension >70 to 75 mm); and (7) the need for recurrent hospitalization to treat worsening symptoms despite maximum medical therapy. Other less common cardiac diseases that may be treated with cardiac transplantation include sarcoidosis (especially if limited to the heart), restrictive cardiomyopathy, hypertrophic cardiomyopathy, congenital heart disease (not amenable to surgical palliation or correction), and valvular heart disease (when the risk of cardiac surgery is prohibitively high).

Evaluation for Cardiac Transplantation

EVALUATION OF UNDERLYING DISEASE AND ESTIMATION OF RISK OF MORTALITY. The evaluation for cardiac transplantation, which should generally be performed at an experienced cardiac transplantation center, typically involves identifying the underlying cardiac disease (if not already established), considering other acceptable (or preferable) treatment options, evaluating the patient for co-morbid conditions that may limit survival or increase morbidity after transplantation, and educating the patient (and family) regarding the rigors of the post-transplant medical regimen. The complete history and physical examination help to direct further tests.

The transplantation evaluation includes an assessment of the immunologic state of the potential recipient. Typically, a panel (or percentage) reactive antibody (PRA) study by cytotoxic methods or flow cytometry is performed to assess for the presence or absence of pre-existing antibodies to other (non-"self") human leukocyte antigens. A high PRA predicts a higher likelihood of post-transplant rejection and death. Patients with a high PRA require a negative crossmatch between their sera and a potential donor's lymphocytes before transplantation; a very high PRA may preclude transplantation.

EVALUATION FOR CO-MORBID CONDITIONS AND OTHER ISSUES. Any major coexisting medical condition that would not be reversible with better cardiac function is a relative contraindication to transplantation, but active severe infection and neoplasm are the two near-absolute contraindications. Because post-transplant compliance is so critical, psychological instability and substance abuse are strong relative contraindications. When in doubt, a transplant physician should be consulted to determine potential eligibility.

An evaluation of social and financial resources is very important during the transplantation evaluation. The charges for the initial cardiac transplantation hospitalization and for follow-up procedures are formidable, even if no post-transplant complications occur; medications alone can cost $6000 to $20,000 for the first year after transplantation. Most insurance carriers and Medicare help defray some of the costs, but the patient's portion may be significant. An assessment of an individual patient's need for financial support after transplantation should be performed before transplantation, especially because noncompliance due to inability to pay for medications is life-threatening.

PATIENT AND FAMILY EDUCATION. The decision by an institution to offer cardiac transplantation includes a responsibility to assist in the ongoing medical care of the patient. The prospective organ recipient should understand the individualized risks involved with the decision to proceed with transplantation, including the possible complications that may occur.

Recipient Medical Care: "The Waiting List"

Occasionally, a patient is deemed too well to be listed for transplantation (i.e., when the estimated risk of transplantation is higher than the risk of continued medical care or a surgical intervention). Most patients should be re-evaluated at intervals of 3 to 6 months until either (1) the underlying cardiac problem improves or resolves, which occasionally occurs; or (2) worsening symptoms or risk factors for death develop and prompt the decision to proceed with transplantation.

In the United States, the responsibility for cadaveric donor organ procurement and distribution is contracted to the United Network for Organ Sharing (UNOS) and its regional organ procurement organizations (OPOs). Patients are "listed" for transplantation by being placed on a national computerized list maintained by UNOS. Donor organs are distributed by location of the donor (within an OPO), ABO blood type, body size, and, occasionally, the need for specialized immunologic testing. Organ distribution is also based on the amount of time that a patient has been listed and a status system that varies slightly within different regions. Patients are typically listed as follows:

UNOS Status 1a: Inpatient on mechanical ventricular assist for ≤30 days, total artificial heart, intra-aortic balloon, extracorporeal membrane oxygenator, mechanical ventilation, high dose inotropic agents and continuous hemodynamic monitoring, or expected to live <7 days (these patients have highest priority).

UNOS Status 1b: Patient with mechanical assist implanted for >30 days, non–high dose continuous inotropic agent infusion (inpatient or outpatient).

UNOS Status 2: All others active on transplant list.

UNOS Status 7: Temporarily inactive.

About 2,500 patients receive transplants annually, but of about 4000 to 4500 patients newly listed annually for heart transplantation, almost 85% will still be awaiting cardiac transplantation at the end of the year. As a result, 10 to 30% of listed patients die before an appropriate donor is located. Once the decision is made to list the patient, the goal of ongoing medical care is to improve and maintain the patient's functional class and quality of life and to avoid medical complications that could delay or prevent transplantation.

THE CARDIAC DONOR

Identifying and Evaluating a Cardiac Donor

In general, any brain-dead patient younger than 45 to 55 years who has adequate heart function is a potential cardiac donor. Even with the Uniform Anatomical Gift Act, it is estimated that only 10 to 20% of potential cardiac donors are procured in the United States. This is in part owing to the failure of medical professionals optimally to pursue organ donation with a brain-dead patient's family. Physicians should consult the local or regional organ procurement organization regarding potential donors so that appropriate measures can be instituted to optimize the likelihood of successful donations. Physicians should also encourage their patients to become donors—donor status is stated on the driver's license in many states.

THE TRANSPLANT PROCEDURE

The cardiac transplantation admission begins with an urgent evaluation for occult infection or other medical problems not previously recognized. The patient is placed on cardiopulmonary bypass, which is timed to minimize the period of bypass for the recipient and the period of ischemia (during which the allograft is not perfused) for the donor heart. The recipient's heart is then replaced with the donor heart, with suture lines placed (and "connections" therefore made) in the ascending aorta, pulmonary artery, and either the right atrium or, more recently favored by many centers, the superior and inferior vena cavae. Allograft electrical activity and contraction usually begin spontaneously as oxygenated blood is supplied, or they do so after direct current is applied. In the modern era, in the absence of significant pre-operative debilitation or co-morbid problems, postoperative care is usually routine, with discharge to local housing possible at about 5 to 7 days after surgery. Prior to discharge, the recipient is instructed about post-transplant medical care and precautions.

MEDICAL CARE AFTER TRANSPLANTATION

Routine Post-Transplant Follow-up

The maximum mortality from two of the most common causes of death following transplant—allograft rejection and infection—occurs during the first days to 6 to 8 weeks after transplantation. Endomyocardial biopsies are typically performed once per week for the first 4 to 8 weeks, and then at gradually longer intervals.

ROUTINE IMMUNOSUPPRESSION. Immunosuppression begins with the preoperative administration of azathioprine and often cyclosporine. Intraoperative corticosteroids are often given and continued intravenously in the immediate postoperative period. Cyclosporine and azathioprine are started soon after surgery and may be given intravenously until oral medications are tolerated.

Routine chronic immunosuppression for most patients consists of triple-drug therapy, which usually includes prednisone, azathioprine, and cyclosporine. Because higher dosages of cyclosporine may induce renal insufficiency, doses are subsequently tapered over 1 to 3 months to target cyclosporine levels. Tacrolimus (Prograf) is occasionally substituted for cyclosporine in patients with persistent or recurrent rejection and is also occasionally used in women and children to avoid the hirsutism associated with cyclosporine.

Prednisone doses are tapered and, in some centers, discontinued if no significant rejection occurs during tapering. In general, the azathioprine dose is lowered if the white blood cell count consistently falls below 4000 to 5000 cells/mL. Mycophenolate mofetil (CellCept) may be superior to azathioprine and is preferred in some centers.

PROPHYLACTIC DRUG ADMINISTRATION/IMMUNIZATIONS. Immunosuppressed patients should not receive certain live viral vaccines (see Chapter 15), and Sabin oral polio vaccine should not be given to close contacts of transplant patients because viral shedding occurs. Routine use of influenza vaccine, although controversial, is of little risk and may offer some protection.

The 3-hydroxy-3-methylglutaryl co-enzyme A (HMG CoA) reductase inhibitors (usually pravastatin or simvastatin, based on available data) reduce the allograft vasculopathy, lower the incidence of cardiac rejection, and may improve post-transplant survival. Diltiazem is also routinely used at many transplant centers, as it may also lower the risk of cardiac allograft rejection; diltiazem also increases cyclosporine levels, resulting in reduced cyclosporine dosing and an overall savings in drug costs.

Post-Transplant Medical Problems

ALLOGRAFT REJECTION. INCIDENCE. Cardiac rejection may be cell mediated (cellular rejection), the most common form, and/or antibody mediated (humoral rejection). Hyperacute humoral rejection in the immediate postoperative period is due to preformed antibodies to the HLA type of the donor heart and results in sudden severe allograft dysfunction and often death. Cellular rejection, which leads to substantive or chronic rejection, is characterized initially by a mononuclear infiltrate. Higher grades of rejection are classified according to the presence and extent of myocyte infiltration, myocyte necrosis, hemorrhage, and/or vasculitis. The incidence of cardiac rejection is highest early after transplantation and subsequently decreases to a low but constant rate (Fig. 71–1).

DETECTION. Symptoms and signs associated with rejection may be nonspecific and include malaise, lethargy, fatigue, low-grade fever, and mood changes, or they may be cardiac-specific, such as dyspnea, lower blood pressure, jugular venous distention, a new S_3 or S_4 gallop, or a new supraventricular arrhythmia.

Depressed cardiac function after cardiac transplantation, with or without hemodynamic changes, is usually caused by acute rejection. Surveillance endomyocardial biopsies, especially within the first 6 months after transplantation, remain the standard for detecting early signs of rejection.

THERAPY. The therapy of cardiac rejection, which may include bolus oral or intravenous administration of steroids, OKT3, Atgam, plasmapheresis, and augmentation of the patient's existing immunosuppressive drug regimen, should be administered under the supervision of an experienced transplant physician, preferably at the patient's transplant center.

INFECTION. About one third of patients develop a serious infection post-transplant (defined as requiring intravenous antibiotics and/or considered to be life-threatening) during the first year after transplant, and infection remains the most common cause of death in the first year. Lung and bloodborne infections are most common, accounting for 50% of serious infections. The risk of a bacterial infection is highest in the early postoperative period. The risk of a viral infection is highest at 1 to 1.5 months, fungal infection within the first month, and protozoal infection from 2 to 5 months following transplant.

MALIGNANCY. Immunosuppressed transplant recipients of any

Table 71–2 ■ **MEDICAL CARE AFTER TRANSPLANTATION**

DURING FIRST 6 TO 8 WK AFTER OPERATION
Recipient resides within a reasonable distance from the center, usually with a family member or friend for support and observation
Discharge goal is 5 to 7 days after operation
Patient seen twice weekly as an outpatient with directed history and physical to assess for signs or symptoms of infection, rejection, or allograft dysfunction
Routine studies (weekly during first 6 to 8 wk)
    Chest radiograph to screen for infection
    ECG to evaluate allograft conduction system
    Echocardiogram with Doppler to assess left and right ventricular function and valve function
    Blood work to evaluate liver or kidney dysfunction
    Serum or whole blood cyclosporine (or tacrolimus) levels to guide dosing
    White blood cell and platelet counts and hematocrit to assess response to azathioprine (or mycophenolate) and screen for excessive effect
Encourage establishment of long-term exercise program and proper nutrition (low fat)
Counsel regarding expected lifestyle changes and stress
2 TO 24 MO AFTER OPERATION
Visit every 3 mo with examination and routine studies noted above
AFTER 24 MO AFTER OPERATION
Twice yearly as above, plus coronary angiography, with or without intracoronary ultrasound study, or stress echocardiography
PROPHYLACTIC DRUG ADMINISTRATION/IMMUNIZATIONS

Prophylaxis Against	Drug
Oropharyngeal *Candida* infections (thrush)	Oral daily clotrimazole or nystatin until steroid dose is minimized
Herpes zoster (shingles)	Varicella-zoster immunization if negative serology prior to transplant; oral acyclovir for 1 yr post-transplantation for all patients
Cytomegalovirus (primarily in seronegative recipient of heart from seropositive donor)	Ganciclovir (Cytovene), IV for 2–4 wk, then orally for 8–10 wk
Pneumocystis carinii (especially in endemic areas)	Oral trimethoprim-sulfamethoxazole (Bactrim), 3 times per week for 1 yr
Toxoplasma gondii (therapy in seronegative recipients of heart from seropositive donor)	Pyrimethamine and sulfadiazine (or clindamycin in sulfa-allergic patients) for 6 mo
Cardiac allograft vasculopathy (allograft coronary artery disease)	Pravastatin, 10–40 mg q.h.s., indefinitely, as tolerated; use with caution initially due to increased risk of rhabdomyolysis

FIGURE 71-1 ■ Rejection incidence over time following initial cardiac transplantation for 4766 patients with follow-up of at least 12 months. The incidence of rejection episodes, calculated as the number per 100 patients occurring each month after transplant, is highest in the first month following transplantation (34 rejections per 100 patient-months) and then rapidly declines over time. The average rejection rate after the first year following transplantation is 1.07 rejections per 100 patient-months. (Data from the Cardiac Transplant Research Database and includes information about the population who received cardiac transplants from January 1990 throught December 1997 at 42 major U.S. transplant centers.) (The author would like to thank David C. Naftel, Ph.D., University of Alabama at Birmingham, Birmingham, AL, for his assistance with data analysis and preparation of the figures.)

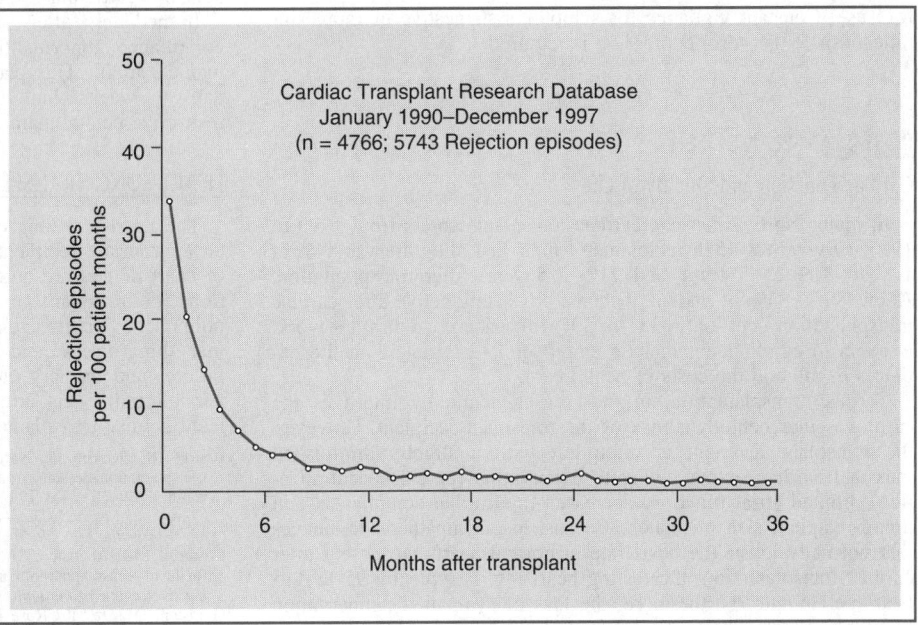

organ have an estimated risk of developing a malignancy of 1 to 2% per year. The overall risk is 6%, approximately 100 times that of the non-transplant age-controlled population, and is most notable for squamous cell carcinoma of the skin, lymphoma (including so-called lymphoproliferative disease), Kaposi's sarcoma, other sarcomas, and carcinomas of the vulva, perineum, kidney, and hepatobiliary system.

MEDICATION-RELATED PROBLEMS. Cyclosporine-induced hypertension occurs in more than 90% of heart transplant recipients within the first year. Antihypertensive drug dosing should allow for diurnal blood pressure changes, with dosing timed to have a peak effect in the morning. To control blood pressure, vasodilators (direct and calcium channel blocking drugs) and angiotensin-converting enzyme inhibitors are equally effective. If possible, β-adrenergic blocking drugs should be avoided, because the denervated heart relies on circulating catecholamines to increase heart rate and systolic function with exercise.

Cyclosporine commonly decreases glomerular filtration rate and raises the serum creatinine. Acute nephrotoxicity may occur with the first perioperative dose of cyclosporine (see Chapter 105.2) because of drug-induced renal afferent arteriolar vasoconstriction superimposed on chronic renal hypoperfusion from a low cardiac output. Cyclosporine also appears to have dose-dependent toxic effects on the renal tubules and can cause renal tubular acidosis.

Hepatic dysfunction, which occurs in up to 10% of patients following transplantation, may be the result of many causes, including intraoperative or perioperative hepatic hypoperfusion, a response to cyclosporine or azathioprine, or viral hepatitis. Cyclosporine-induced hepatotoxicity is dose-dependent and usually occurs when serum levels are extremely high.

Cyclosporine decreases urate clearance by the kidney; hyperuricemia and gout commonly occur. Allopurinol is associated with a decrease in azathioprine metabolism, and azathioprine dosing must therefore be adjusted accordingly. Non-steroidal anti-inflammatory drugs should be avoided, if possible, because of their nephrotoxic effects. Short-term colchicine may be very useful, but long-term use can increase immunosuppression and cause bone marrow toxicity.

Cyclosporine is metabolized by the cytochrome P-450 enzyme pathway and therefore interacts with numerous medications and substances that are metabolized by or that influence that enzyme system (including alcoholic beverages). Many drugs, including certain antibiotics, may directly worsen the renal toxicity of cyclosporine. Physicians should not prescribe any medication without first determining its compatibility with cyclosporine. Corticosteroid use after transplantation may result in or worsen glucose intolerance

and hyperlipidemia and may precipitate osteoporosis and its complications (see Chapter 28). The most common adverse effect associated with azathioprine is bone marrow toxicity, most commonly leukopenia and less commonly thrombocytopenia, megaloblastic anemia, red cell aplasia, and reticulocytopenia, which usually appears 7 to 14 days after initial dosing or elevations in dosing.

DRUG EFFECTS ON THE CARDIAC ALLOGRAFT. Although postganglionic parasympathetic neurons remain in the donor heart, transplanted hearts are effectively denervated because conduction does not traverse the atrial anastomotic suture lines. Any drug that affects the heart via either a change in vagal tone or a direct increase in sympathetic nerve activity has little effect on the transplanted heart. However, systemic effects still occur. Thus, for example, atropine, which increases heart rate primarily by a vagolytic effect, does not increase the heart rate in cardiac allograft recipients. However, it still has non-cardiac effects such as dry mouth, mydriasis, cycloplegia, constipation, and urinary retention.

The denervated heart is, however, more sensitive to both β-adrenergic agonists (e.g., isoproterenol) and β-adrenergic antagonists. Ocular β-blockers can occasionally cause profound bradycardia. Isoproterenol, by virtue of its chronotropic effect, is used routinely to stimulate heart rate in cases of sinus node dysfunction early after transplantation. The denervated heart is hypersensitive to adenosine; if adenosine is administered to convert supraventricular tachycardia, it should be given at 25% of the usual dose.

CARDIAC ALLOGRAFT VASCULOPATHY. Cardiac allograft vasculopathy affects all vessels in the transplanted heart (including veins) and leads to vessel lumen obliteration. It is the leading cause of death after the first year of transplantation. Depending on the means used to detect it, the incidence of the disease ranges from 10 to 50% at 1 year to 50 to 90% at 5 years after transplantation. Histologically, the disease manifests as hyperplasia of smooth muscle cells, intimal proliferation, mononuclear cell infiltration of the intima, and the presence of lipid-laden macrophages in all areas of the vessel wall. The process is thought to be multifactorial in origin, but it probably stems from an initial and/or ongoing immunologically mediated or infection-induced (e.g., cytomegalovirus) injury to the vascular endothelium. The therapy of the disease involves coronary angioplasty, the placement of intracoronary stents, and consideration of retransplantation.

SOCIAL AND PSYCHOLOGICAL PROBLEMS. Adapting to life after cardiac transplant involves an interplay of many variables, including the patient's pretransplant condition; the duration of illness; and the patient's personality, intelligence, social support, and financial support. End-stage cardiac patients often become depressed; after transplantation, early exhilaration followed by mild to moderate depression is common, possibly as a result of corticosteroid use. Constant vigilance for symptoms suggestive of more significant or longer-term depression is required.

POST-TRANSPLANT LIFE

Cardiac Function and Quality of Life

In major North American cardiac transplant centers from 1990 to 1995, survival for 4515 recipients of their first allograft was 84% at 1 year, 81% at 2 years, and 71% a 5 years after transplantation. About 80 to 85% of patients become physically active after cardiac transplantation, but only 33 to 50% of patients return to work. Barriers to employment include employers' fears regarding the patient's health and the costs of health care.

Cardiac transplantation, in most cases, markedly improves the cardiovascular hemodynamics of the transplant recipient. However, the transplant recipient is often left with a slightly diminished maximal cardiac output owing to denervation (neural decentralization), limited atrial function, decreased myocardial compliance, and donor-recipient size mismatch. Because parasympathetic influences that normally lower the heart rate in normal hearts are absent after cardiac transplantation, the resting heart rate is typically 95 to 115 beats per minute. Furthermore, the loss of sympathetic innervation blunts the normal increases in heart rate and contractility that occur with exercise, with low cardiac filling pressures, and after vasodilation. The cardiac allograft increases cardiac output primarily by an increase in filling pressure and secondarily in response to circulating catecholamines. In transplant recipients, the native and donor

atria do not contract in unison, further decreasing the atrial component of ventricular filling.

Immediately after transplantation, the cardiac allograft exhibits compliance abnormalities as evidenced by a restrictive hemodynamic pattern. This pattern usually gradually improves over a few days to weeks, but 10 to 15% of recipients develop a chronic restrictive hemodynamic pattern (see Chapter 64).

HEART-LUNG TRANSPLANTATION (see Chapter 89)

The heart and lung can be transplanted en bloc from a donor to an appropriate recipient in a single operation, but fewer than 20% of heart donors are potential heart-lung donors. The primary indications for transplant are congenital cardiac abnormalities and severe pulmonary hypertension (Eisenmenger's complex); irremediable primary lung disease and associated severe secondary right ventricular failure; and primary end-stage cardiac disease and secondary irreversible pulmonary arterial hypertension, which would preclude isolated cardiac transplantation.

Bourge RC, Kirklin JK, Naftel DC, McGiffin DC: Predicting outcome after cardiac transplantation, lessons from the Cardiac Transplant Research Database. Curr Opin Cardiol 12:136–145, 1997. *A review of the early publications of the Cardiac Transplant Research Database, which outlines methods of outcomes analysis in the heart transplant population.*

Costanzo MR, Augustine SA, Bourge R, et al: Selection and treatment of candidates for heart transplantation. Circulation 92:3593–3621, 1995. *An excellent and comprehensive review of the topic with excellent references.*

Goldstein DJ, Oz MC, Rose EA: Implantable left ventricular assist devices. N Engl J Med 339:1522–1533, 1998. *A review of use of currently available devices as a bridge to cardiac transplantation. Offers an excellent scheme for patient selection for device implantation.*

Hunt SA: Current status of cardiac transplantation. JAMA 280:1692–1698, 1998. *A relatively short overview of the history, physiology, and current status of heart transplantation directed to the non-transplant physician. Well-referenced.*

PART VIII

RESPIRATORY DISEASES

72 APPROACH TO THE PATIENT WITH RESPIRATORY DISEASE

Gerard M. Turino

The process of respiration includes many structural and functional components (see Chapter 73) in addition to the lungs, such as the nose, pharynx, sinuses, chest cage and musculature, pleura, diaphragm, extrathoracic airways, cerebral regulatory respiratory centers, and cardiovascular system. In addressing the patient with pulmonary disease, the physician must maintain a circumspect approach to possible pathogenic factors. Pulmonary infiltrates on chest film may be a manifestation of a pulmonary infection or primary lung tumor, but they may also be the result of metastatic cancer from extrapulmonary sites. Pulmonary densities of various types on chest film may be caused by generalized systemic diseases such as lupus erythematosus (see Chapter 289), scleroderma (see Chapter 290), rheumatoid arthritis (see Chapter 286), or embolic disease (see Chapter 84). Abnormal blood gas analysis findings may result from defective regulation of ventilation rather than intrinsic lung disease.

The lungs contribute to the vital processes of all other organ systems. Pulmonary oxygen and carbon dioxide exchange is necessary for metabolism and acid-base homeostasis. The pulmonary circulation is subject to hemodynamic disturbances originating in the cardiac chambers, but it may be affected by primary pulmonary hypertension (see Chapter 56). The lungs are the gaseous and particulate interface between the external atmosphere and the body, so lung function must be considered in terms of exposure to atmospheric toxins. Also, lung cells are not only responsible for normal respiratory and circulatory functions of the lung but also contribute to extrapulmonary processes, such as blood pressure control by the action of angiotensin-converting enzyme, which resides on pulmonary endothelium.

HISTORY

A detailed account of the patient's primary symptoms is essential, but other critical information includes the amount of exposure to (1) tobacco smoke (including passive exposure); (2) atmospheric pollutants, such as nitrogen dioxide, beryllium, asbestos, coal, and silica dust (see Chapter 21); (3) fumes from industrial processes; and (4) animal danders. If the patient is exposed to a potentially toxic industrial process, precise historical details on the place and duration of occupational exposure are necessary. The family history of lung disease with respect to asthma, allergies, cystic fibrosis (CF), lung cancer, and emphysema is also important. A family history of emphysema may be present in cases of serum α_1-antitrypsin deficiency. Living in certain regions of the country may predispose to histoplasmosis (see Chapter 394) or coccidioidomycosis (see Chapter 395). Infections such as *Pneumocystis carinii* pneumonia, chronic sinusitis, pneumococcal pneumonia, and tuberculosis are recognized common complications of human immunodeficiency virus (HIV) infection, so the history should explore the possibility of exposure to HIV infection (see Chapter 412).

A history of the medications taken previously and currently is necessary to evaluate certain pulmonary infiltrative lesions, such as interstitial pulmonary fibrosis as a complication of therapy with bleomycin, cyclophosphamide, methotrexate, or nitrofurantoin. Bronchospasm may be initiated or exacerbated by β-adrenergic blocking drugs. Cough and angioneurotic edema are occasional complications of angiotensin-converting enzyme inhibitor drugs.

PHYSICAL EXAMINATION (Table 72–1)

Obesity can affect the mechanics of breathing and can predispose a patient to sleep apnea. An increased thoracic anteroposterior (AP) diameter may be evidence of obstructive lung disease and pulmonary hyperinflation, whereas shortening and deformation of the thorax, as occurs in kyphoscoliosis of the spine, may cause a restrictive breathing pattern. Lagging of one side of the chest may be evidence of unilateral fibrothorax or atelectasis. Accessory muscles of ventilation are frequently used in severe airway obstruction.

If there is audible wheezing on ventilation, airway obstruction in the tracheobronchial tree must be distinguished from obstruction in the larynx and pharynx. Extrathoracic airway obstruction in the upper airway is frequently more marked during the inspiratory phase, whereas lower airway obstruction is more marked in the expiratory phase. The presence of nasal voice and/or tenderness over sinus regions of the face may be a manifestation of acute or chronic sinus disease. Full inspection of the nose and pharynx is essential to detect polyps or septal deviations, which can cause obstruction or postnasal secretions.

Table 72–1 ■ PHYSICAL SIGNS OF PULMONARY DISEASE

PATHOGENIC PROCESS	CHEST WALL MOTION AND CONFIGURATION	BREATH SOUNDS	PERCUSSION	FREMITUS
Asthmatic and bronchitic airway obstruction	Increased AP diameter, use of accessory muscles of ventilation	May be decreased; prolonged expiration; inspiratory and expiratory wheezes and rhonchi	Hyperresonant	Decreased
Airway obstruction of emphysema	Increased AP diameter, reduced chest wall musculature with general weight loss, use of accessory muscles of ventilation	Markedly diminished; prolonged expiratory phase; may be rhonchi	Hyperresonant	Decreased
Atelectasis	Inspiratory lag on affected side	Absent over affected area	Dullness	Decreased
Consolidation of acute pneumonia	Splinting of chest wall on affected side	Bronchial breath sounds, whispered pectoriloquy, rales and/or rhonchi	Dullness	Increased
Pleural effusion	Lag on affected side	Absent or decreased	Flatness	Absent
Pneumothorax	Lag on affected side, tracheal deviation away from affected side	Absent	Hyperresonant	Absent
Diffuse alveolitis or fibrosis	Restricted inspiratory and expiratory excursion	May be increased with diffuse fine rales	Decreased resonance or normal	Increased or normal

A loud pulmonary second sound, a right ventricular heave, jugular venous distention, and peripheral edema may be manifestations of primary or secondary pulmonary hypertension, whereas systemic hypertension, left ventricular enlargement, or gallop sounds may be manifestations of poor left ventricular function and may suggest heart failure as a cause of pulmonary symptoms. Clubbing of the fingers may be a manifestation of carcinoma of the lung, but it is frequently present in cystic fibrosis with hypoxemia and in severe bronchiectasis as well as in hypoxemia associated with congenital heart disease (see Chapters 57, 76, and 77).

EVALUATING BLOOD GAS COMPOSITION AND PULMONARY FUNCTION TESTING

In many patients, an arterial blood gas measurement is essential to establish or exclude significant hypoxemia and/or hypercapnia. Unless the patient is severely hypoxemic with polycythemia and visible cyanosis, significant degrees of hypoxemia can be undetected clinically unless blood gas composition is measured. Similarly, significant degrees of hypercapnia may be present without symptoms of somnolence or headache.

Pulmonary function testing, sometimes including blood gas measurements during rest and exercise, can characterize and quantify pulmonary dysfunction. Simple spirometry can quantify airway obstruction and determine the response to bronchodilator therapy. Lung volume measurements can establish whether the air-containing volume of the lung is reduced and a restrictive pattern of lung disease (as occurs in interstitial alveolitis, sarcoidosis, or fibrosis) is present. The pulmonary diffusing capacity is a sensitive measurement of interstitial reactions of the lung, such as interstitial alveolitis and fibrosis (see Chapter 78), in which the surface area of the pulmonary capillary membrane is reduced and the thickness of the alveolar capillary membrane is increased. In airway obstructive disease, diffusing capacity can determine the presence of pulmonary emphysema. A low diffusing capacity indicates alveolar destruction and the presence of emphysema as a primary process or in association with chronic bronchitis or asthma.

Detection of pulmonary hypertension and estimates of pulmonary artery pressure can be provided by echocardiography. For more thorough evaluation of the hemodynamics of the pulmonary circulation, measurements of pulmonary artery pressure and pulmonary vascular resistance should be obtained by right heart catheterization. When indicated, a pulmonary angiogram can be obtained if pulmonary embolism is suspected clinically and a ventilation-perfusion scan is not definitive.

RADIOLOGIC TECHNIQUES FOR THE DIAGNOSIS OF PULMONARY LESIONS

CHEST FILMS. The standard PA and lateral chest roentgenograms can indicate diaphragmatic and rib cage abnormalities as well as the air-containing volumes of each lung. They also define the presence of opacities, cavitary lesions, pneumothoraces, atelectasis, pleural fluid or pleural thickening, cardiac size and chamber contours, pulmonary congestion, pulmonary edema, and enlargement of the pulmonary arteries.

COMPUTED TOMOGRAPHY. Computed tomographic (CT) scans can easily measure relative tissue density, homogeneity, the relationship of parenchymal opacities to bronchi and adjacent vascular structures, and the location and extent of lymphadenopathy. Unlike conventional CT, which requires the patient to take discrete breathholds for each slice acquired, helical (spiral) CT allows volumetric data acquisition with a single breathhold and hence provides better detection of small lung lesions and pulmonary nodules, faster imaging for dynamic vascular studies, and the ability to perform three-dimensional reconstruction.

The rapidity of helical CT saves time and reduces risk in critically ill patients and permits use of a smaller bolus of contrast for detailed studies of vascular anomalies, aneurysms, or pulmonary emboli. Sections as precise as 1 mm apart can be obtained for a pulmonary nodule without respiratory motion artifacts. Helical CT also provides a more accurate assessment of mediastinal and hilar lymph nodes as well as direct extension of lung neoplasms to the mediastinum, pleura, or chest wall. Helical CT is essential for the assessment of focal lung disease and often can distinguish between a granuloma and primary bronchogenic carcinoma.

POSITRON EMISSION TOMOGRAPHIC (PET) SCANNING. By PET scan, a high uptake of labeled glucose characterizes most lung cancers. In single pulmonary nodules for which no previous radiographic examinations are available to assess a change in size, the normal uptake of glucose by PET scan may allow for continued observation, whereas increased uptake of labeled glucose would mandate resection.

MAGNETIC RESONANCE IMAGING (MRI). MRI has limited value in the chest and is best used in studying the heart, vascular anatomy, and masses or lymph nodes of the mediastinum (see Chapter 45). It can be helpful when the use of iodinated contrast agents is contraindicated.

INTERVENTIONAL RADIOGRAPHIC TECHNIQUES. Radiographic CT or ultrasound guidance has greatly added to the accuracy and reliability of needle biopsies of intraparenchymal and mediastinal masses. Similarly, pleural collections and lung abscesses can be drained using guided catheter techniques.

INVASIVE TECHNIQUES IN PULMONARY DIAGNOSIS

To evaluate suspected pulmonary neoplasm or to investigate hemoptysis, fiberoptic bronchoscopy is essential and may include sampling of bronchial cells by brushing or bronchial biopsy or, when indicated, bronchoalveolar lavage to determine the cell composition in alveoli.

If pleural disease is detected, pleural fluid analysis and pleural biopsy are helpful diagnostically. Thoracoscopy is an effective technique to evaluate lesions on the pleura or periphery of the lung by biopsy or local resection.

MAJOR SYMPTOMATIC MANIFESTATIONS OF PULMONARY DISEASE

Although a wide array of pathologic factors can produce respiratory symptoms and signs, the five common manifestations of pulmonary disease that require evaluation are (1) cough, (2) shortness of breath or dyspnea, (3) chest pain, (4) hemoptysis, and (5) a solitary pulmonary nodule.

COUGH WITH AND WITHOUT SPUTUM. Cough results from transmission of nervous impulses to the integrative cough centers in the brain from sensory stimuli in the tracheobronchial tree. Cough may be a transient or persistent symptom. Common causes of transient cough are inflammatory reactions on the surface of the trachea or bronchial branches, usually from bacterial or viral infections. Occasionally, noxious vapors in the atmosphere can induce cough (e.g., tobacco smoke, volatile chemical compounds, and vehicular exhaust). For persistent cough, one of the most prominent causes is an allergic inflammatory reaction of the bronchi associated with asthma; cough may be the earliest presenting manifestation, preceding complaints of shortness of breath or wheezing.

Another common cause of tracheobronchial irritation is regurgitation of acidic gastric contents into the tracheobronchial tree during sleep. Such regurgitation and aspiration result from failure of gastric emptying due to gastric outlet obstruction or an incompetent gastroesophageal junction (see Chapter 124). Many individuals regurgitate gastric and esophageal contents during sleep and are totally unaware of this phenomenon.

An important cause of persistent cough is a tumor in the tracheobronchial tree that leads to distortions of the bronchial wall and increases stimuli to the cough center. In any patient with persistent cough, and particularly in smokers, the possibility of a bronchial carcinoma or adenoma must be considered. Extrabronchial lesions that cause cough include a mediastinal or esophageal tumor, an aortic aneurysm that compresses a bronchus, or an enlarged left atrium compressing the left main bronchus. Sinusitis with persistent nasal secretions into the pharynx and upper airway is a frequent cause of therapy-resistant chronic cough.

Diagnostic investigations of cough include chest radiography and, if necessary, sinus radiography and CT of the thorax. When indicated, bronchoscopy and laryngoscopy should be performed. The presence, type, and amount of sputum can be useful in differential diagnosis. Acute onset of sputum with cough suggests acute

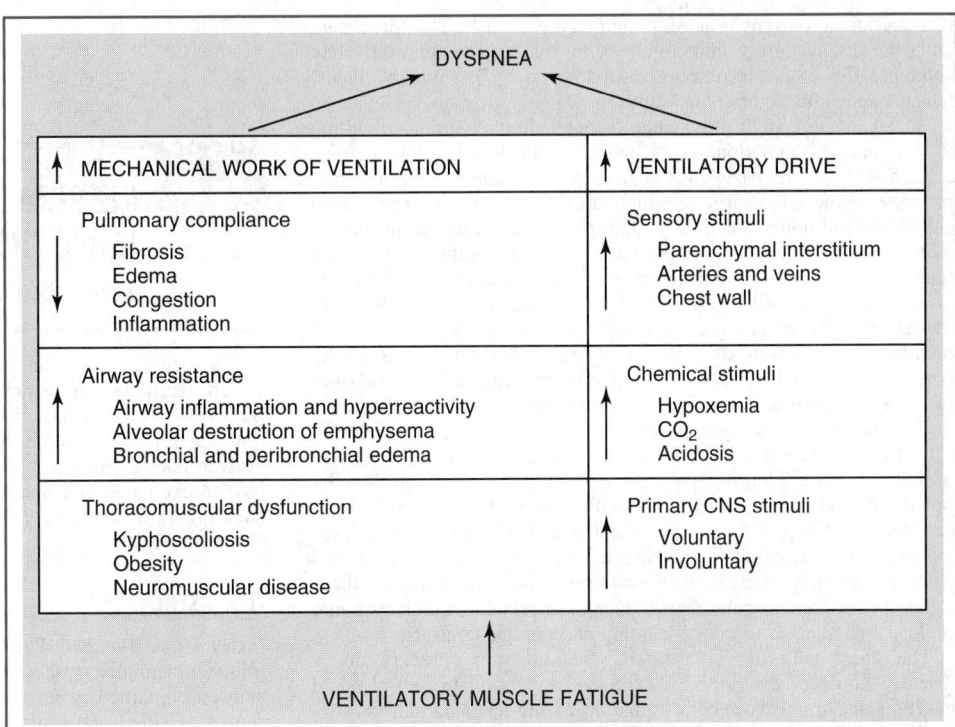

FIGURE 72–1 ■ The symptom of dyspnea can best be related to increases in the mechanical work of breathing and/or increases in ventilatory drive as a result of the effect of different pathogenic factors on ventilatory mechanics and increased ventilatory stimuli. Ventilatory muscle fatigue is an added factor (see text).

pulmonary infection or sinusitis. Long-standing sputum production, usually in the morning, is characteristic of chronic bronchitis from smoking. Large volumes of sputum throughout the day are characteristic of bronchiectasis or lung abscess. Foul-smelling sputum suggests anaerobic infection associated with lung abscess. In asthma, sputum production may vary throughout the day. Yellow or green sputum, due to the release of myeloperoxidase by leukocytes, is usually a sign of infection.

SHORTNESS OF BREATH. "Shortness of breath," "a feeling of not being able to get enough air," and "labored breathing" are all terms used by patients to describe the symptom of dyspnea. The cause of dyspnea may be pulmonary disease, circulatory disease, or both. It is the physician's responsibility to define the causative mechanisms of shortness of breath so that diagnostic techniques and therapies can be directed appropriately. The most consistent correlate of the symptom of dyspnea is increased mechanical work of breathing, usually brought on by increased airway resistance as occurs in asthma, chronic bronchitis, and emphysema, or decreased

distensibility of the lungs as occurs in interstitial fibrotic reactions (Fig. 72–1). In the latter diseases, increased effort is required to produce a higher negative pressure in the pleural space to inflate the lungs. The increased mechanical work done on the lungs to overcome obstruction to air flow or decreased distensibility is perceived as an increased effort to breathe and produces the symptom of dyspnea.

An increased drive to ventilate may also cause dyspnea. Such stimuli include hypoxia, usually when arterial oxygen tensions are less than 60 mm Hg, and stimuli from inflamed lung parenchyma, as occur in bacterial pneumonia or alveolitis and that drive the respiratory centers of the brain. These stimuli often lower the resting carbon dioxide pressure (PCO_2) to less than the normal level of 40 mm Hg and cause dyspnea, especially on mild exertion.

Patients with pulmonary emboli may present with shortness of breath and a normal chest roentgenogram. However, the inefficiency of the embolized lung for gas exchange requires abnormally high ventilatory rates to maintain a normal arterial PCO_2. Unless

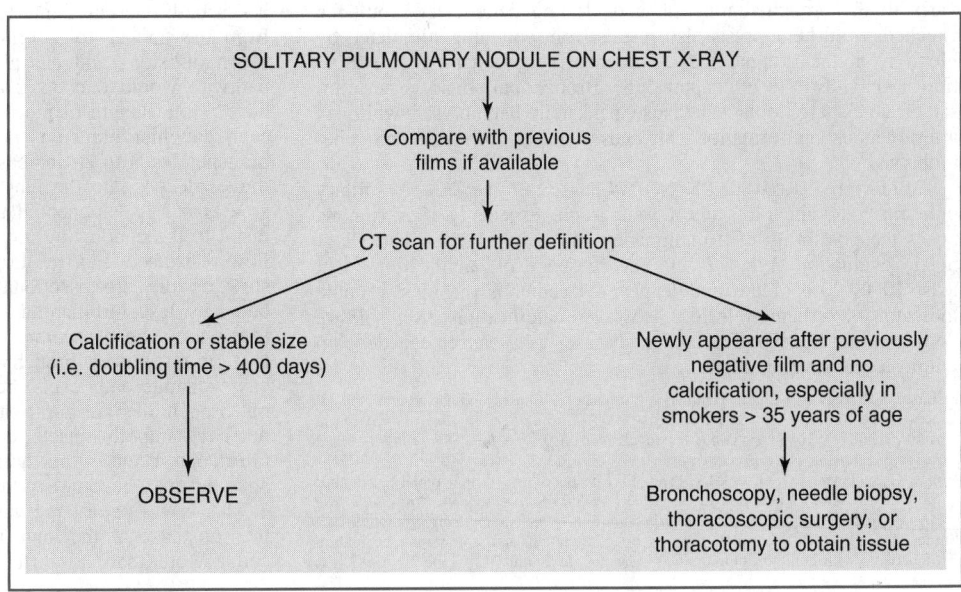

FIGURE 72–2 ■ Steps in the evaluation of the solitary pulmonary nodule.

Karlinsky JB (eds): Textbook of Pulmonary Diseases. Philadelphia, Lippincott-Raven, 1998, pp 283–310. *A thorough discussion of the use of history, physical examination, and radiologic findings for differential diagnosis of lung diseases.*

this particular presentation of pulmonary embolism is appreciated, embolic disease goes unrecognized in many patients until they suddenly die or are extremely incapacitated by pulmonary hypertension and right ventricular failure.

Because of the high prevalence of heart disease and heart failure in the general population, many patients with dyspnea have cardiac abnormalities. The basis of the dyspnea is usually a high filling pressure of the left ventricle, which causes high left atrial pressures and high pulmonary capillary and pulmonary arterial pressures, which in turn increase the pulmonary blood volume and reduce lung compliance. If the pulmonary capillary pressure is in the range of 25 mm Hg, capillary fluid will transudate into the pulmonary matrix, thereby reducing lung compliance, increasing the work of breathing, and causing dyspnea (see Chapter 47). Echocardiography (see Chapter 43) is diagnostic of abnormal ventricular or valvular function and should be performed in any patient in whom the cause of dyspnea is not readily apparent.

CHEST PAIN. Chest pain is also a common presenting symptom of lung disease. Pleuritic pain is sharp and severe, magnified by breathing, and may be associated with a pleural friction rub. Pericarditis (see Chapter 65) causes chest pain that may not be related to breathing and often is relieved by leaning forward; pericardial friction rubs may be audible in synchrony with the heartbeat. Pleuropericardial friction rubs may induce pain related to breathing and be heard in relation to both breathing and cardiac contraction.

The chest pain of myocardial ischemia from coronary artery disease should be discernible on the basis of its relation to physical exertion and its characteristic radiation to the left shoulder or arm, neck, and jaw (see Chapter 38). The chest pain of pulmonary embolism may also be characterized by a feeling of anterior chest pressure, which may persist for hours and be related to pulmonary hypertension (see Chapter 84).

HEMOPTYSIS. The most common cause of hemoptysis is pneumonia or pulmonary infection, including bronchiectasis (see Chapter 77). Bloody streaking of purulent sputum occurs during pneumonia or severe bronchitis and subsides as the infection is treated. The sudden appearance of hemoptysis without other cause must be considered a possible manifestation of lung tumor, either benign or malignant. Such hemoptysis necessitates full investigation with a chest radiograph, CT scan, and bronchoscopy (see Chapter 72). A pulmonary embolism that leads to pulmonary infarction almost always results in hemoptysis (see Chapter 84); it is usually associated with a pulmonary infiltration as a manifestation of infarction, which occasionally leads to a cavity in the lung parenchyma. Pulmonary tuberculosis, especially with cavity formation, is a prominent cause of hemoptysis, especially in patients with HIV infection. Hemoptysis is not uncommon in cystic fibrosis of the lung and can be severe and even life-threatening. A certain proportion of patients have sudden and usually mild hemoptysis for which no cause can be found; such episodes may result from a ruptured blood vessel or varix in the bronchial mucosa, and clotting parameters should be checked. Mild hemoptysis also results from coughing stimulated by blood from the oropharynx; comprehensive oropharyngeal evaluation is diagnostic (see Chapter 515). Bronchopulmonary aspergillosis or an aspergilloma can cause persistent hemoptysis, while an arteriovenous malformation can cause sudden, life-threatening hemoptysis.

SOLITARY PULMONARY NODULE (see Chapter 72). A solitary pulmonary nodule on a chest radiograph, especially if it is new, poses the possibility of a malignancy and requires immediate diagnostic evaluation (Fig. 72–2). The presence of calcification in at least 10 to 20% of the nodule near its center is the most reliable indicator of a benign lesion. However calcification of a solitary nodule is not specific for benign disease, as a cancer can develop within a scar or granuloma.

Fishman AP, Editor-in-Chief: Fishman's Pulmonary Diseases and Disorders, 3rd ed. New York, McGraw-Hill, 1998, pp 361–393. *A thorough review and analysis of the relationship of pulmonary symptoms to clinical and physiologic abnormalities in a range of pulmonary disorders.*

Hoh CK, Schiepers C, Seltzer MA, et al: PET in oncology: Will it replace the other modalities? Semin Nucl Med 27:94, 1997. *An informative review of the diagnostic role of positron emission tomography in relation to other tumor imaging modalities.*

Snider GL, Gale ME: Section III. Approach to the clinical and radiographic evaluation of patients with common pulmonary syndromes. *In* Baum GL, Crapo JD, Celli BR,

73 | RESPIRATORY STRUCTURE AND FUNCTION

James D. Crapo

The primary function of the lung is to enable gas exchange, which facilitates movement of oxygen into the bloodstream and removal of carbon dioxide (CO_2). In addition, the respiratory system carries out a large number of other ventilatory-related and nonventilatory functions. The complex effects of lung structure on its gas exchange and nonventilatory functions are critical to understanding how the lung responds to both intrapulmonary and systemic diseases.

LUNG STRUCTURE

UPPER AIRWAYS. The nasopharynx plays a critical role in humidifying inhaled gases and in clearing particles and reactive substances contained in those gases. In addition to contributing to the senses of smell and taste, the nasopharynx removes a large fraction of inhaled particles and reactive gases. Turbulent gas flow past the nasal turbinates and the right-angle turn at the posterior pharynx cause impaction of most large particles before inhaled gas enters the trachea. In addition, very highly soluble or reactive gases may be almost completely removed by the nasopharynx. Lymphoid tissue at the posterior pharynx plays a role in immune processing at this critical junction of the body with its external environment.

AIRWAYS. The primary airways consist of the trachea, the bronchi, and smaller bronchioles. The adult human trachea is approximately 25 cm in length and 2.5 cm in diameter and is given a somewhat rigid shape by 15 to 20 horseshoe-shaped cartilaginous rings. The posterior portion of the trachea, representing the membranous portion or open part of the cartilaginous rings, contains the trachealis muscle. The trachea divides into two main-stem bronchi, which then rapidly divide in an irregular dichotomous pattern into progressively smaller bronchi. Cartilaginous support surrounding or partly surrounding bronchi continues for a number of generations, at which point the airways are termed *bronchioles.* As the size of the cartilage decreases in smaller bronchi, the relative mass of smooth muscle becomes more prominent, and these medium-sized bronchi can be a significant site of bronchoconstriction. Smooth muscle becomes more scarce, as it extends into the bronchioles and is virtually absent from terminal bronchioles. The shortest path from the trachea to a terminal bronchiole involves approximately seven divisions and has a total length of 7 to 8 cm. The longest pathway would encounter approximately 25 branch divisions and have a total length of more than 22 cm. The cross-sectional area of each daughter branch is decreased, but the increasing number of branches leads to an increase in the total cross-sectional area as air moves deeper into the lung. The increase in airway cross-sectional area is nearly exponential and leads to a fall in airway resistance distal to the conducting airways. As a result, the primary site of air flow resistance is in the large, central airways. Gas flow rates also slow as the cross-sectional area increases and the flow pattern becomes less turbulent and more laminar. The final airway segments are termed *terminal bronchioles,* which then branch into two to four respiratory bronchioles (airway segments with alveolar or gas exchange outpockets) before entering alveolar ducts. The terminal bronchioles are approximately 250 μm in internal diameter, do not have smooth muscle, and are covered only with a thin, serous fluid coat. They are not normally a site of significant airway resistance but may become so during a number of disease processes.

The airways and large vessels in the lung make up about 10% of the substance of the lung and account for about 25% of the lung cells. More than 40 different cell types are found in the lungs, representing virtually every major class of tissue. The most common type of cell in the lung is the capillary endothelial cell, which represents almost 40% of the cells in the alveolar gas-exchange region. The epithelial cells lining the airways include ciliated cells, secretory cells, basal cells, and mucous cells, as well as mucus-secreting glands. Under normal conditions the airway epithelium has a low rate of cell turnover, but these cells can potentially be exposed to a variety of inhaled carcinogens and are the site of origin of the most common cancer in humans. The upper airways in the human lung are covered by a thick mucous coat, which can be more than 10 μm thick. The mucous covering of the airways thins in more distal lung and becomes a thin serous coat over the terminal airways, leaving this region of the lung most vulnerable to inhaled reactive substances. The small airways, in conjunction with the most proximal portions of the alveolar gas-exchange region, are the primary sites at which lung injury is caused by most inhaled substances.

The lungs are divided into three lobes on the right and two on the left and have a normal total of ten segments on the right and eight segments on the left side. A lung lobule, which is the smallest unit separated by fibrous septa, is approximately 2 cm in size and contains about four to eight terminal bronchioles.

ALVEOLAR REGION. The alveolar region is a branching system of alveolar ducts whose walls are made up of alveoli. The number of alveolar duct branches ranges from 3 to 13, ending in alveolar sacs whose walls are composed of alveolar outpockets. The human lung contains about 500 million alveoli that are each roughly spherical and about 225 μm in diameter. The mouths of the alveoli, which form the walls of alveolar ducts and alveolar sacs, contain large collagen and elastin bundles, whereas adjacent alveoli are interconnected by collagen fibers laced through the alveolar walls. The connective tissue bundles lining alveolar duct walls are arranged in a spiral or helical fashion and are critical in determining the overall structure and compliance of the gas-exchange region (Fig. 73–1).

Gas exchange occurs across alveolar walls that have a high vascular content, with the surface area of subadjacent capillaries virtually matching that of the alveolar surface (Fig. 73–2). Capillary blood is separated from air by a fine tissue sheet whose thickness can be as little as 0.5 μm. This tissue sheet, in the thin portions of the alveolar septa, consists of a highly attenuated epithelial cell, basement membrane, and a highly attenuated endothelial cell. The efficient function of the lung as a gas-exchange surface depends on there being a low tissue resistance to diffusion of O_2 and CO_2 molecules, a large alveolar surface for gas exchange, and a relatively large capillary blood volume uniformly distributed below the alveolar surface. In a normal human, the total surface area of the alveolar region of the lung is about 100 m², or approximately the size of a tennis court. The human lung contains

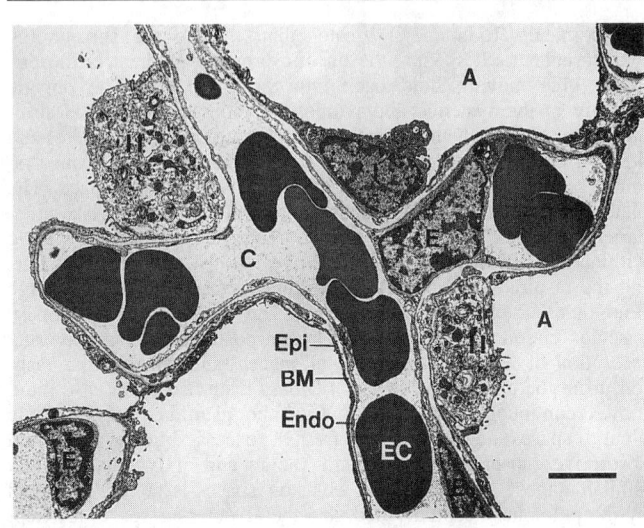

FIGURE 73–2 ■ Transmission electron micrograph of a normal human lung illustrating relationships of the alveolar air spaces (A) to pulmonary capillaries (C). Alveolar septal tissues include epithelial type I cells (I), epithelial type II cells (II), and capillary endothelial cells (E). Note the thin alveolar septal tissue barrier over much of the surface. The barrier for O_2 diffusion across the thin portions of the septa into erythrocytes (EC) consists of the epithelium (Epi), a common basement membrane (BM), and the endothelium (Endo) (bar = 4μm). (Modified from Crapo JD, Bevry BE, Gehr P, et al: Cell number and cell characteristics of the normal human lung. Am Rev Respir Dis 125:740, 1982.)

approximately 200 mL of blood in the pulmonary capillaries, which have a microvascular surface area approximately equal to the alveolar surface.

Surface tension at the air-liquid interface over the alveolar surface is reduced dramatically by the presence of a phospholipid monolayer distributed uniformly over an aqueous subphase lining the alveolar surface. This alveolar lining layer is known as *surfactant* and, by lowering the surface tension, it both enables alveoli to be stable at low lung volumes and allows alveolar volume to change with a relatively small expenditure of energy. The alveolar epithelial surface is covered by two types of specialized epithelial cells. Ninety-eight per cent of the alveolar surface is covered by type I alveolar epithelial cells, which are large cells, each covering an enormous surface area (approximately 5000 μm² per cell) with a thin, highly attenuated cytoplasm that minimizes the thickness of the air-blood barrier. About 2% of the alveolar surface is covered by the highly metabolic, cuboidal-alveolar type II epithelial cells. These cells secrete surfactant and carry out a number of other biologic functions, including regeneration of the alveolar epithelium, transport of electrolytes and fluids across the epithelium to maintain "dry" alveolar air spaces, and secretion of substances that help regulate immune and inflammatory functions in the lung.

LYMPHATICS. The lung has an extensive lymphatic system that clears fluid from both the pleural space and the lung. The pleural network lies in the visceral pleura lining the outer lung surface and connects to the deep or parenchymal plexus, which follows the bronchovascular bundles and the lobular septa. The two systems connect at the boundaries between lobes or lobules and the pleura, and both systems drain toward hilar lymph nodes through larger lymphatic channels equipped with valves. The parenchymal lymphatic channels begin at the level of respiratory bronchioles. Alveolar walls do not contain lymphatic channels. The pleural space is also lined by a parietal pleura, which is the pleural membrane on the chest wall side. The balance of oncotic and hydrostatic pressures in the capillaries lining the parietal and visceral pleuras is different owing to the fact that parietal pleura capillaries are supplied by the systemic vasculature. Mean capillary hydrostatic pressure in the parietal pleura is about 25 cm H_2O. The visceral pleura capillaries, which derive primarily from the low-pressure pulmonary vascular circuit, have a mean capillary pressure of 5 to 10 cm H_2O. Under normal conditions, the oncotic pressure in blood is

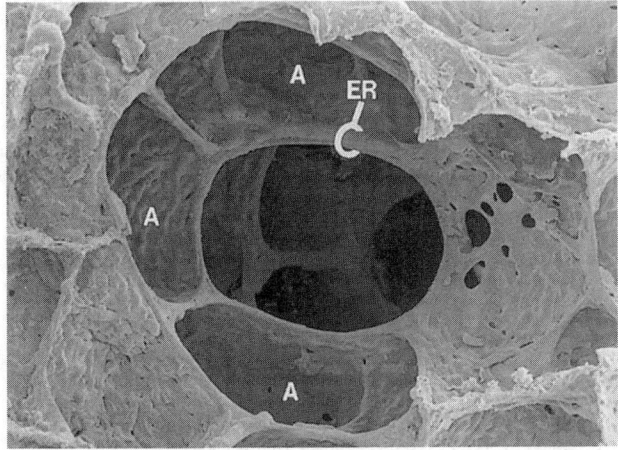

FIGURE 73–1 ■ Scanning electron micrograph of human lung showing an alveolar duct with concentrically arranged alveoli (A). The free edge of an alveolar septum is reinforced with thick bundles of connective tissue that form the entrance rings (ER) (×380). (From Gehr P, Bachofen M, Weibel ER: The normal human lung: Ultrastructure and morphometric estimation of diffusing capacity. Respir Physiol 178:112, 1978.)

approximately 15 cm H_2O greater than that in the surrounding extravascular tissues; thus, the oncotic pressure gradient is the primary force moving fluid back into the capillaries. The oncotic pressure in the systemic and pulmonary capillary systems is similar. The effects of the normal hydrostatic and oncotic pressure differences in pleural capillaries lead to fluid movement from systemic capillaries in the parietal pleura into the pleural space. The pleural fluid can be absorbed either into low-pressure visceral or parietal pleural lymphatics or into pulmonary capillaries lying within the visceral pleura. The negative intrathoracic pressures during the respiratory cycle also contribute to the presence of a large fluid flux out of the parietal pleura. The low-pressure pulmonary vascular circuit creates an even larger positive gradient favoring resorption of fluid from the pleural spaces (and, in a similar fashion, from the alveolar air spaces). Unless disturbed by disease, fluid moves continuously into and out of the pleural spaces, but the pleural spaces are maintained free of excess fluid by the high absorptive capacity of the visceral pleura and of lymphatics. In a similar manner, any fluid in alveolar air spaces is rapidly absorbed by the pulmonary capillary bed, and the alveolar air spaces are kept "dry" and thereby available for gas exchange. Diseases that affect the permeability barrier created by pulmonary capillary walls, disturb pulmonary lymphatic drainage, or increase pulmonary hydrostatic pressure can alter these forces, leading to rapid accumulation of pleural effusions and/or intraalveolar flooding.

CLEARANCE. The lung has a large surface area exposed to the external environment. More than 99% of the mass of particles inhaled under normal conditions are cleared by the nasopharynx and larger airways in the lung. Particles impacting the upper airways are primarily cleared by the epithelial mucociliary escalator. Airway epithelial cells are covered by a mucous coat that increases in thickness as it moves upward. This mucous coat is continually moved proximally by the ciliated cells lining all levels of the airways. Under normal conditions, once airway mucus reaches the posterior pharynx, it is swallowed; up to 1 L of fluid moves by this pathway from the lungs to the gastrointestinal tract each day.

Small particles ($<10\ \mu m$ in aerodynamic diameter) have a finite probability of reaching alveolar gas exchange surfaces. Once particles deposit in the alveolar region, clearance is primarily via alveolar macrophages. In the normal lung, each alveolus contains about 12 macrophages, and this number may be 2 to 10 times greater in the proximal alveoli of a smoker or an individual exposed to high levels of environmental air pollutants. These free-moving cells on the alveolar surface process inhaled particles, antigens, bacteria, and viruses by phagocytosis. A critical function of the lung is to clear and/or process inhaled antigens and infectious agents or other toxic material without stimulating an amplified immune response. Although the alveolar surface is constantly bombarded with inhaled materials, the thin, delicate alveolar septa are generally maintained in a noninflamed state, and gas exchange is undisturbed. A variety of chemical and structural elements contribute to regulation of immune processes in the lung, creating a milieu in which widely dispersed inhaled particulate material or infectious agents can be processed without creating an exaggerated or unnecessary immune response. Disorders in these immune regulatory pathways, which are at the present time poorly understood, are likely to be important elements of hyperimmune or inflammatory lung diseases.

METABOLISM. Although gas exchange is the obvious primary function of the lung, the lung also has several critical metabolic functions. The lung contains the only capillary bed in the body through which 100% of the blood passes on each circulation. Thus, the lung is in a critical position to act as a mechanical filter of the blood and to regulate vascular levels or responses to a variety of small peptides. Angiotensin-converting enzyme on the lung endothelial surfaces plays a critical role in regulating systemic blood pressure, both by metabolizing bradykinin and by activating angiotensin I to angiotensin II. The lung has an active uptake pathway for a variety of vasoactive amines or peptides. The lung vascular bed is also a primary site where circulating polymorphonuclear leukocytes are sequestered. Under normal conditions, approximately half of the circulating polymorphonuclear leukocytes are sequestered in the pulmonary capillary bed. These neutrophils are available both for rapid response to invading inhaled pathogens in the lung and for distribution through the systemic circulation, although

the regulation, function, and control of these lung-sequestered neutrophils are not yet well defined.

PHYSIOLOGIC FUNCTION

PULMONARY FUNCTION TESTS. Pulmonary function tests provide an objective measurement of lung function. They can be used to assess both heart and lung function, identify basic functional categories of lung disorders, assess responses to a variety of inhalation injuries, and assess lung injury occurring via the pulmonary circulation. Although an enormous array of pulmonary function parameters can be measured, the primary parameters of value to the practicing physician (Table 73–1) include basic measurements of lung volumes. Spirometric examination is the most commonly used test and consists of measurement of the pattern of air movement into and out of the lungs during controlled ventilatory maneuvers. The primary spirometric parameters of interest are forced expiratory volume in 1 second (FEV_1), forced vital capacity (FVC), and the ratio of FEV_1 to vital capacity (VC) (FEV_1/FVC). Carbon monoxide (CO) diffusing capacity (DL_{CO}) and arterial blood gases are the other most commonly helpful pulmonary function parameters.

LUNG VOLUMES. The lungs and the chest wall are elastic structures that function in parallel to determine the gas volume in the lungs at rest and the work involved in various breathing maneuvers. Functional residual capacity (FRC) is defined as the volume of gas in the lung at rest when the elastic inward pull of the lung is balanced by the outward pull of the chest wall and diaphragm (Fig. 73–3). FRC is the most reproducible of the pulmonary function tests because it is independent of patient effort. The gas remaining in the lung at the end of a maximal exhalation maneuver is termed *residual volume*. Total lung capacity (TLC) is the volume of gas contained in the lungs at the end of a maximal inspiration maneuver.

In healthy persons, lung volumes vary according to gender, age, height, and ethnic group. In determining predicted normal values, it is essential to have standardized data that closely approximate the subject's characteristics. Using 95% confidence intervals for the predicted normal values is recommended as the best index for determining whether a given subject is within or outside the predicted normal range. A simple and commonly used substitute for 95% confidence intervals is to define as abnormal a measured lung functional parameter that falls below 80% of its predicted normal. Thus, $\pm 20\%$ of predicted normal is a crude estimator of the range of values of pulmonary function found in a normal population.

Total gas in the lungs is commonly measured by one of three methods: (1) washout of an inert gas (N_2), (2) equilibration with an inert test gas, or (3) whole-body plethysmography. Lung volume measurements initially determine FRC because that lung volume is most easily reproduced by the patient and is independent of patient compliance. Exhalation from FRC gives the expiratory reserve volume (ERV). Residual volume (RV) can then be calculated by subtracting ERV from FRC. TLC can be calculated by adding the VC to the residual volume. Accurate measurements of lung volume done by washing out nitrogen (N_2) or by equilibrating with an inert test gas (helium) require that the test gas communicate to or from all compartments of the lung. All gas-containing compartments must be freely washed out or exchanged. Poorly communicating blebs or bullae can cause lung volumes to be significantly underes-

Table 73–1 ■ PULMONARY FUNCTION TESTS

Lung volume	
TLC	Total lung capacity
FRC	Functional residual capacity
ERV	Expiratory reserve volume
RV	Residual volume
Expiratory flow	
FEV_1	Forced expiratory volume (in 1 second)
FVC	Forced vital capacity
FEV_1 %	FEV_1/FVC ratio (expressed as %)
Diffusing capacity	
DL_{CO}	Diffusing capacity for carbon monoxide
Arterial blood gases	
PaO_2	Arterial O_2 pressure
$PaCO_2$	Arterial CO_2 pressure
pH	

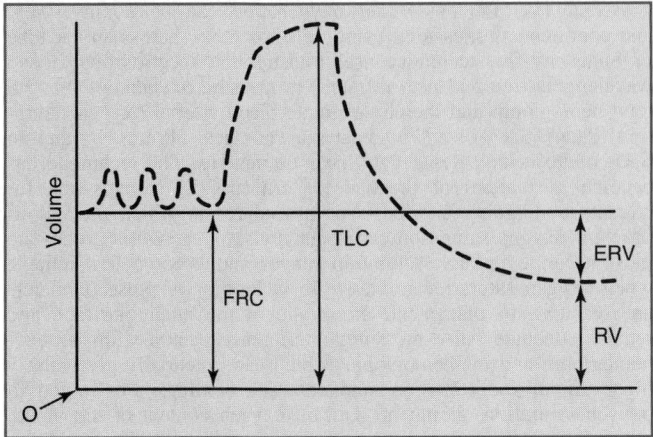

FIGURE 73-3 ■ Ventilatory tracing showing normal resting ventilation followed by a forced inhalation to total lung capacity (TLC) and then a forced exhalation to residual volume (RV). Functional residual capacity (FRC) is the resting lung volume at the end of a normal exhalation. Expiratory reserve volume (ERV) is the volume of air that can be exhaled from FRC down to RV.

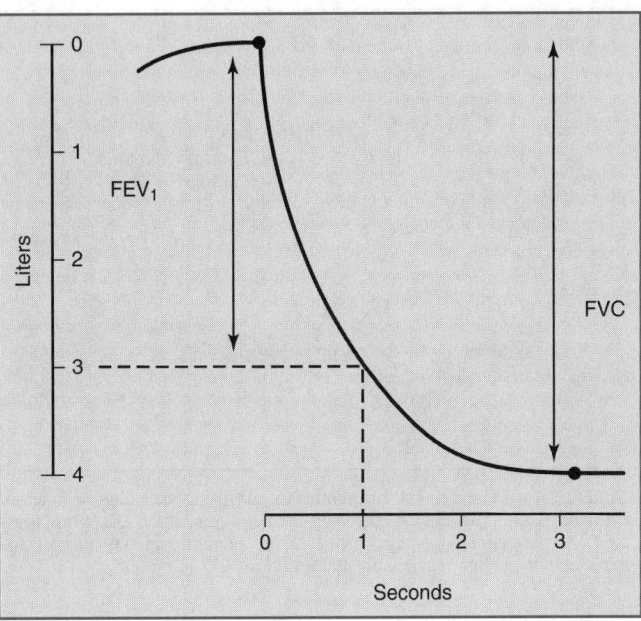

FIGURE 73-4 ■ A portion of a normal spirogram showing the forced exhalation from total lung capacity. FEV_1 is the volume exhaled in 1 second, and forced vital capacity (FVC) is the total volume that can be forcibly exhaled from total lung capacity.

timated when using N_2 washout or helium dilution techniques. Lung volumes can also be measured by body plethysmography, which involves placing the subject in a large air-tight box and having him or her breathe through a mouthpiece connected to the outside. A shutter occludes the mouthpiece, and as the subject pants against the closed shutter, the volume of gas in the chest is compressed and expanded, creating a similar change in gas volume in the box. By measuring either changes in pressure in the box or flow through a calibrated orifice in the box, the total volume of gas in the thorax can be calculated. This calculation uses Boyle's law, which states that the pressure times the volume of a gas is a constant at a constant temperature. Body plethysmography measures all gas contained in the thorax and does not require that bullae or blebs be communicating for their volume to be measured.

Finally, posteroanterior and lateral chest radiographs can be used to estimate lung volumes using planimetry. This technique estimates thoracic gas volume from the projected area of the lungs on two perpendicular views of the chest.

SPIROMETRIC MEASUREMENTS OF EXPIRATORY FLOW. With common computerized equipment, more than 20 spirometric variables are often reported. The use of large numbers of variables can lead to false-positive findings, and it is recommended that only a few basic variables from the lung spirogram be used. Among the most useful variables are FEV_1, FVC, and the ratio of FEV_1 to FVC (Fig. 73-4). FVC is the maximal volume of air that can be exhaled during a forced exhalation beginning at TLC. FEV_1 is the volume of gas that can be exhaled during the first 1 second of a forced exhalation maneuver beginning at TLC. Spirometric measurements of lung function are most useful when the patient has physical findings, symptoms, or risk factors suggesting pulmonary disease. Lung functional studies can be used to define the basic class of a lung disorder, evaluate the severity of the abnormality being quantitated, or follow the progression of the disease process. It has been shown that physicians cannot consistently and reliably identify obstructive and restrictive ventilatory defects from history taking or physical examination. Age-related declines in lung function must be considered in evaluating test results. Nonsmokers lose FEV_1 at a rate of 20 to 30 mL/year. In some smokers, this rate of decline can increase by two- to three-fold. In smokers younger than 35 years, quitting smoking can result in an increase in lung function. In smokers older than 35 years who quit smoking, the rate of decline of lung function generally slows to the normal rate associated with aging.

The magnitude of functional impairment in obstructive lung disease can be assessed using pulmonary function testing (Table 73-2). When the predicted FEV_1 is close to 4 L, the subject should not have a history of a significant exercise impairment until the FEV_1 falls below 3 L/second. In that individual, an FEV_1 between 2 to 3 L/second would be consistent with a history of mild exercise limitation. Mild exercise limitation means that the subject is able to

walk significant distances but cannot do so at high rates of speed. An FEV_1 of between 1 to 2 L/second is consistent with a moderate degree of exercise impairment, meaning that intermittent rest periods are required to walk significant distances or to climb stairs. An FEV_1 less than 1 L/second predicts a severe exercise impairment, limiting the person to very short walking distances, perhaps restricting him or her to home. These guidelines for assessing severity of an exercise impairment in obstructive lung disease must be adjusted for age and body size in the same manner that predicted FEV_1 varies. It is important to correlate predicted functional capacity by pulmonary function testing with the history of exercise limitation described by the patient. A significant difference in the functional capacity predicted by pulmonary function testing with that described by the patient can be an important indicator of the presence of nonpulmonary disease processes.

DIFFUSING CAPACITY. The diffusing capacity of the lung is defined as the lung's ability to take up an inhaled nonreactive test gas, such as CO, which binds to hemoglobin (Fig. 73-5). CO binds to hemoglobin with a high affinity so that virtually all the CO that reaches an alveolar space, crosses the alveolar air-blood barrier, and reaches a red cell will bind to hemoglobin and thus be removed from the exhaled gas. Measurement of lung-diffusing capacity is critically influenced by three parameters: (1) the ability of the test gas to reach the alveolar gas-exchanging surfaces, (2) the ability of the test gas to cross the alveolar septa, and (3) the mass of red cells in the pulmonary capillary bed available to bind the test gas. A defect in any one of the above three components influences measured lung-diffusing capacity. Airways obstruction and ventilation-perfusion mismatching prevent the test gas from reaching the alveolar gas-exchange surfaces and lower the diffusing

Table 73-2 ■ ASSESSMENT OF EXERCISE LIMITATION IN OBSTRUCTIVE LUNG DISEASE

FEV_1 (L/sec)	IMPAIRMENT*
>3	None
2–3	Mild
1–2	Moderate
<1	Severe

*This assumes a middle-aged person of normal body size having a predicted FEV_1 of close to 4 L. Applying this simple formula commonly requires some adjustment for age and body size.

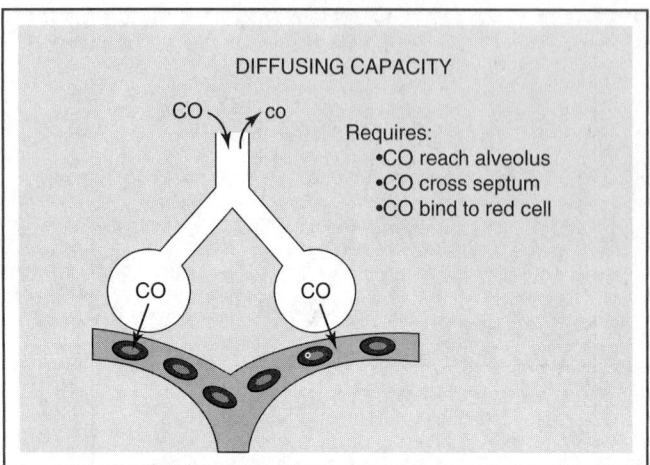

DIFFUSING CAPACITY

CO → co

Requires:
- CO reach alveolus
- CO cross septum
- CO bind to red cell

CO   CO

FIGURE 73–5 ▪ Measurement of pulmonary diffusing capacity for carbon monoxide (CO). The critical elements in measurement of DL_{CO} are illustrated. An altered DL_{CO} may be due to an alteration in any one of the fundamental elements required for the uptake of CO in the lung.

capacity in proportion to the maldistribution of ventilation. Thickening of the air-blood barrier can increase the resistance of gas movement across the tissue barrier, increasing diffusing capacity. Alveolar filling, as in pulmonary edema, reduces the alveolar surface area available for test gas exchange. Finally, the volume of red cells in the alveolar capillary bed is crucial in determining how much CO is retained in the capillary bed. Of the parameters that influence CO uptake in the lung during a diffusing capacity measurement, the uniformity of ventilation and the volume of red cells in the pulmonary capillary bed dominate the overall reaction kinetics. Diffusing capacity measurements are less sensitive to changes in thickness of the air-blood barrier because CO has a high capacity for diffusion across pulmonary tissues.

The normal values for CO diffusing capacity vary widely between laboratories, and both the absolute values and their reproducibility are strongly influenced by the measurement techniques. Diffusing-capacity measurements are most commonly useful in following changes in a patient's lung function when measured by consistent techniques applied by the same laboratory.

ABNORMALITIES OF CO-DIFFUSING CAPACITY. Based on the above discussion, it should be apparent that DL_{CO} can be altered in patients with a variety of cardiopulmonary disorders. Disorders of distribution of ventilation such as chronic obstructive pulmonary disease (COPD) and asthma are perhaps the most common causes of disordered diffusing capacity. Because of the high sensitivity of DL_{CO} to changes in pulmonary capillary blood volume, any disorder that alters pulmonary capillary blood volume significantly changes DL_{CO}. Thus, mitral stenosis or heart failure, by increasing pulmonary vascular volumes, can increase DL_{CO}. When heart failure is sufficiently severe to produce pulmonary edema, the alveolar filling decreases the surface area available for interaction with the test gas and may decrease measured DL_{CO}. Anemia or polycythemia can alter measured DL_{CO}, although the reported value is commonly corrected for changes in blood red cell content by measuring hemoglobin in venous blood near the time the test is carried out. Pulmonary vascular disorders such as pulmonary emboli and vasculitis can decrease the volume of blood in the pulmonary capillary bed and thereby decrease DL_{CO}. It is also decreased in patients with a loss of lung tissue, either by surgical resection or by destruction of the lung by a disease process such as emphysema. Finally, DL_{CO} may be decreased by interstitial lung diseases, which are characterized by interstitial fibrosis and thickening of the air-blood barrier. These processes were originally thought to be alveolar capillary block syndromes in which the block was thought to be an enhanced tissue thickness that the CO molecules had to cross to reach the pulmonary vascular bed. It is now recognized that these diseases also destroy the pulmonary capillary bed and that the primary cause for a low DL_{CO} in these conditions is a decrease in capillary blood volume rather than an alveolar capillary block associated with thickening of the blood-gas barrier.

PULSE OXIMETRY. Blood oxygenation can be noninvasively and continuously measured using pulse oximetry across an ear lobe or fingertip. This technique uses transmission spectroscopy at two wavelengths (red and near-infrared) to measure oxyhemoglobin and total hemoglobin and thereby estimate blood arterial oxygen saturation (SaO_2). SaO_2 of 80% indicates a PaO_2 near 50 mm Hg, and an SaO_2 of 90% indicates a PaO_2 near 60 mm Hg. The technique has become a standard of practice for critically ill patients and for patients undergoing anesthesia or procedures in which precipitous drops in oxygen saturation can occur. Pulse oxygenation probes are most accurate in high saturation ranges and become less reliable when oxygen saturation is below 75%. Probes for pulse oximeters are sensitive to placement, are prone to movement artifact, and require adequate pulse pressure; interference occurs with carboxyhemoglobin and methemoglobin, which can potentially give falsely high estimates of SaO_2 in smokers. The readings are limited to oxygen saturation, giving no data on oxygen content of the blood, which cannot be determined without measurement of hemoglobin content. Rapid changes in hemoglobin content or in distribution of perfusion may not be reflected in SaO_2. Thus, although the pulse oximeter is a valuable monitoring tool and is reasonably accurate under most conditions, its reliability will diminish as the clinical situation deteriorates; at this time, other methods of assessing the adequacy of tissue oxygen delivery should be used.

DISORDERS OF VENTILATION

Lung diseases are commonly divided into two broad categories—obstructive lung disease and restrictive lung disease—based on fundamental differences in the pulmonary function assessment.

OBSTRUCTIVE VENTILATORY DISORDERS. This term is used for the constellation of diseases characterized by limitation of expiratory air flow. The primary criterion for air flow obstruction is a reduced FEV_1/FVC%. In the presence of a normal or elevated TLC, the absolute value of the FEV_1 can be used to estimate severity of the obstructive lung disease. The obstruction may be caused by a variety of airway diseases including chronic bronchitis, bronchiectasis, and mucous gland hyperplasia, leading to physical obstruction or plugging of airways. In emphysema, extensive destruction of alveolar and/or airway walls occurs, leading to loss of elasticity and collapse of airway walls during exhalation, thus trapping gas in the distal lung. Emphysema is also associated with abnormalities of diffusing capacity due to extensive destruction of the alveolar capillary bed. Reversible forms of airway obstruction, such as asthma, are classified as obstructive lung diseases in which the abnormality is primarily due to restriction of size of the airway walls by inflammation, enhanced muscular tone, and/or enhanced mucus secretion. If underlying tissue destruction does not occur, this form of obstructive lung disease can be reversible.

RESTRICTIVE VENTILATORY DISORDERS. This class of lung dysfunction is characterized by fibrotic reactions of the alveolar septa and commonly includes the walls of small airways. The increased fibrotic tissue increases the elastic recoil in parenchymal lung tissue, and because these walls are interconnected to airway walls, the airways can be held open. The hallmarks of restrictive lung diseases are a low TLC and a fall in FVC. When caused by a fibrotic process, it is associated with smaller alveoli having thickened walls, increased amounts of elastic and connective tissue, and destruction of portions of the pulmonary capillary bed. Airways are generally held open by enhanced elastic recoil. The enhanced elastic recoil increases the resistance against inspiration, making it difficult for the patient to inhale and lowering the FVC. The enhanced elastic recoil facilitates rapid exhalation; thus FEV_1/FVC% is generally increased in patients with restrictive lung diseases. Other forms of restrictive ventilatory impairment can include (1) diseases of the chest wall with altered chest wall compliance (obesity, kyphoscoliosis); (2) neuromuscular diseases in which the patient has difficulty carrying out ventilatory maneuvers (Guillain-Barré syndrome, myasthenia gravis); (3) diseases of the pleura, which may entrap the lung (extensive pleural thickening); (4) space occupying lesions in the lung (tumors, cardiac enlargement, pleural effusions); and (5) removal of portions of the lungs via surgical resection.

Table 73–3 gives the common changes in lung volumes in various classes of restrictive lung diseases. Note that fibrotic lung diseases cause significant decreases in all lung volumes as the

Table 73–3 ■ LUNG VOLUMES IN RESTRICTIVE LUNG DISEASES

	PULMONARY FIBROSIS	OBESITY (CHEST WALL RESTRICTION)	NEUROMUSCULAR DISORDERS
TLC	↓	↓	↓
FRC	↓	↓	Normal
ERV	↓	↓ ↓	↓
RV	↓	Normal	↑
Collapse point	Zero	RV	FRC

fibrosis creates a smaller, less compliant lung. In contrast, massive obesity tends to preserve the RV because the underlying lung is normal and the primary problem is inspiring against the excess weight of the chest wall. The ERV is often markedly reduced out of proportion to the other lung volumes in obesity, and the FRC approaches RV as the heavy chest wall pushes the "zero energy point" downward. Neuromuscular diseases create a restrictive lung disorder in which all lung volumes move closer to FRC. These patients lack the respiratory strength to fully inhale or exhale from FRC and thus have a low TLC with an elevated RV. The simplified analysis shown in Figure 73–4 assumes that other processes such as atelectasis are not complicating the classic presentation of these forms of restrictive lung disease.

EXERCISE. Most pulmonary function measurements are taken while the subject is at rest. Defects in pulmonary function can be brought out by assessing pulmonary function under conditions of exercise. In addition, complaints of fatigue or exercise limitation can be more rigorously assessed by complete cardiopulmonary exercise testing in which cardiac and pulmonary function are simultaneously quantified under conditions of gradually increasing exercise. Measurements of heart rate, electrocardiogram, arterial blood gases, and exhaled gases can allow simultaneous assessment of cardiac and pulmonary function and can both separate disorders of heart and lung function and distinguish these from exercise limitation due to poor cooperation or deconditioning. These tests can also facilitate the diagnosis of pulmonary vascular and parenchymal infiltrative diseases.

Crapo RO: Pulmonary function testing. N Engl J Med 331:25, 1994. *Review of methods of performing pulmonary function tests as well as the standards and limitations in their interpretation.*

European Respiratory Society: Clinical exercise testing with reference to lung diseases: Indications, standardization and interpretation strategies: ERS Task Force on Standardization of Clinical Exercise Testing (review). Eur Respir J 10:2662–2689, 1997. *This consensus report gives the internationally accepted approach to the proper use of exercise testing to evaluate lung disease.*

Mercer RR, Crapo JD: Normal anatomy and defense mechanisms of the lung. *In* GL Baum, JD Crapo, BR Celli, JB Karlinsky JB (eds): Textbook of Pulmonary Disease, 6th ed. Philadelphia, Lippincott-Raven, 1998, pp 23–45. *Review of how lung structure and design influence function and the ability of lung clearance mechanisms to handle inhaled pollutants.*

74 ASTHMA

Jeffrey M. Drazen

DEFINITION

Asthma is a clinical syndrome of unknown etiology characterized by three distinct components: (1) recurrent episodes of airway obstruction that resolve spontaneously or as a result of treatment; (2) an exaggerated bronchoconstrictor response to stimuli that have little or no effect in nonasthmatic subjects, a phenomenon known as *airway hyperresponsiveness;* and (3) inflammation of the airways as defined by a variety of criteria.

EPIDEMIOLOGY AND STATISTICS

Asthma is an extremely common disorder affecting men and women equally; approximately 5% of the adult population of the United States has signs and symptoms consistent with a diagnosis

of asthma. Although most cases begin before the age of 25 years, asthma may develop at any time throughout life.

The worldwide prevalence of asthma has increased more than 30% since the late 1970s. The greatest increases in asthma prevalence have occurred in countries that have recently adopted an "industrialized" lifestyle. In addition, the burden of severe asthma has fallen disproportionately on socioeconomically disadvantaged dwellers in the inner city. The reasons for the overall increase in asthma prevalence or the disproportionate fraction of cases in the inner city are not known.

Asthma is among the most common reasons to seek medical treatment; in the United States, asthma is responsible for about 15 million annual outpatient visits to physicians and for nearly 2 million annual inpatient hospital days of treatment. The yearly direct and indirect costs of asthma care are more than $6 billion dollars, with more than 80% of these costs attributable to direct expenditures on medical care encounters or asthma medications.

PATHOLOGY AND PATHOGENESIS

Pathology of Asthma

The pathology of mild asthma, as delineated by bronchoscopic and biopsy studies, is characterized by edema and hyperemia of the mucosa and by infiltration of the mucosa with lymphocytes bearing the T_H2 phenotype, mast cells, and eosinophils. These cells produce interleukin (IL)-3, IL-4, and IL-5, and thereby create a microenvironment that promotes the synthesis of immunoglobulin E (IgE), an important allergic effector molecule. Chemokines, such as eotaxin, RANTES, MIP1α, and IL-8, produced by epithelial and inflammatory cells, serve to amplify and perpetuate the inflammatory events within the airway. As a result of these inflammatory insults, the airway wall is thickened by the deposition of type III and type V collagen below the true basement membrane (Fig. 74–1). In more severe chronic asthma, the airway walls thicken as a result of hypertrophy and hyperplasia of airway glands and secretory cells, hyperplasia of airway smooth muscle, and further deposition of submucosal collagen. The shedding of airway epithelium may lead to a denuded airway. These changes occur in a patchy fashion in mild intermittent asthma and become more widespread as the disease becomes more chronic and severe. Morphometric studies of airways from asthmatic subjects have demonstrated airway wall thickening of sufficient magnitude to increase airflow resistance and enhance airway responsiveness. In severe asthma, the airway wall is thickened markedly; in addition, patchy airway occlusion occurs by a mixture of hyperviscous mucus and clusters of shed airway epithelial cells.

The episodic airway narrowing that constitutes an asthma attack results from obstruction of the airway lumen to airflow. Although it is now well established that infiltration of the airway with inflammatory cells—especially eosinophils—and mast cells occurs in asthma, the links between these cells and the pathobiologic processes that account for asthmatic airway obstruction have not been clearly delineated. Three possible, but not mutually exclusive, links have been postulated: (1) constriction of airway smooth muscle, (2) thickening of the airway epithelium, and (3) the presence of liquids within the confines of the airway lumen. Among these mechanisms, the constriction of airway smooth muscle due to the local release of bioactive mediators or neurotransmitters is the most widely accepted explanation for the acute reversible airway obstruction in asthma attacks. Several bronchoactive mediators are thought to be the agents causing airway obstruction in the asthmatic.

Mediators of the Acute Asthmatic Response

ACETYLCHOLINE. Acetylcholine released from intrapulmonary motor nerves causes constriction of airway smooth muscle through direct stimulation of muscarinic receptors of the M_3 subtype. The potential role for acetylcholine in the bronchoconstriction of asthma primarily derives from the observation that atropine and its congeners have proven therapeutic efficacy in asthma.

HISTAMINE. Histamine, or β-imidazolylethylamine, was identified as a potent endogenous bronchoactive agent more than 90 years ago. Mast cells, which are prominent in airway tissues obtained from patients with asthma, constitute the major pulmonary source of histamine. Clinical trials with novel potent antihistamines

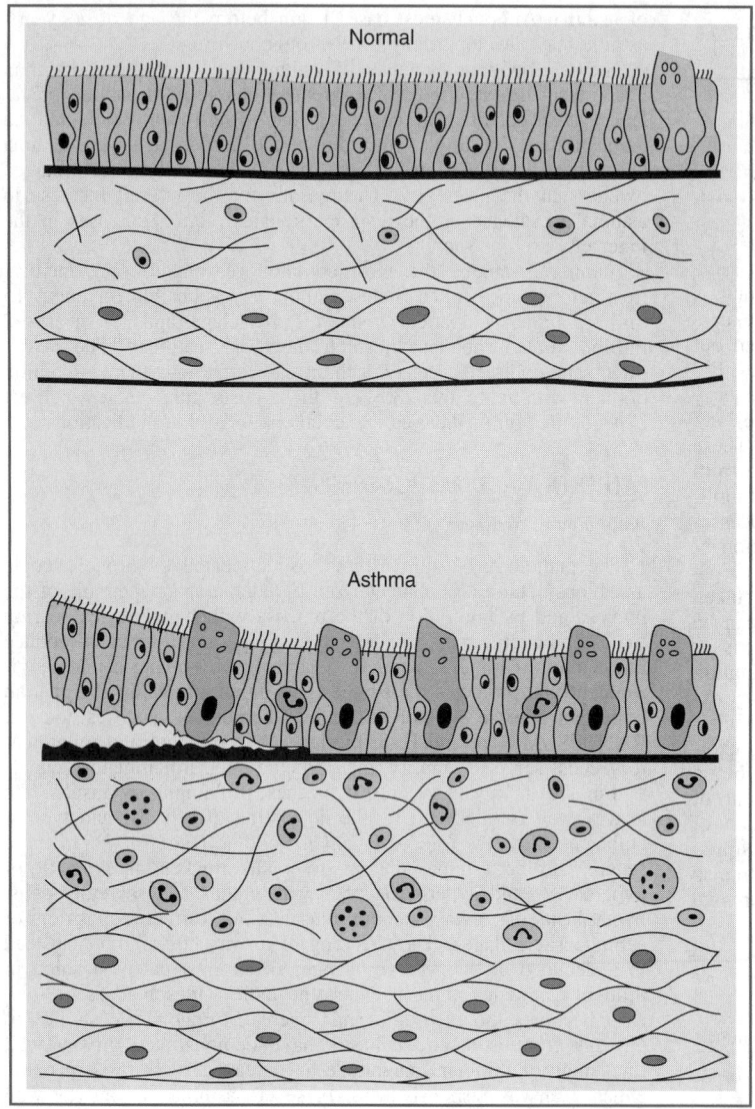

Normal

Asthma

FIGURE 74–1 ■ Schematic renderings of airway anatomy from a normal subject (*top*) and a mildly allergic asthmatic subject (*bottom*). The airway in the asthmatic patient exhibits subepithelial fibrosis, edema, and inflammatory cell infiltration.

indicate a minor role for histamine as a mediator of airway obstruction in asthma.

KININS. Bradykinin and related molecules are cleaved from plasma precursors by the actions of enzymes known as *kallikreins;* at least one type of kallikrein is released from activated mast cells. Bradykinin is a potent bronchoconstrictor mediator when administered exogenously. It is also unique among asthmatic mediators in that the sensation of dyspnea evoked by exogenous administration of bradykinin has been shown to mimic the subjective sensations reported by patients during spontaneously occurring asthmatic episodes.

LEUKOTRIENES. The cysteinyl leukotrienes—namely LTC_4, LTD_4, and LTE_4, as well as the dihydroxy leukotriene, LTB_4—are derived by the lipoxygenation of arachidonic acid released from target cell membrane phospholipids during cellular activation. 5-Lipoxygenase, the 5-lipoxygenase-activating protein, and LTC_4 synthase make up the cellular protein/enzyme content needed to produce the cysteinyl leukotrienes. The production of LTB_4 requires 5-lipoxygenase, the 5-lipoxygenase-activating protein, and LTA_4 epoxide hydrolase. Mast cells, eosinophils, and alveolar macrophages have the enzymatic capability to produce cysteinyl leukotrienes from their membrane phospholipids, whereas polymorphonuclear leukocytes produce exclusively LTB_4, which is predominantly a chemoattractant molecule; LTC_4 and LTD_4 are potent contractile agonists on airway smooth muscle. Clinical trials with leukotriene receptor antagonists or synthesis inhibitors have shown significant clinical efficacy in the treatment of chronic persistent asthma, lead-

ing to the conclusion that the leukotrienes are important mediators of the asthmatic response.

NEUROPEPTIDES. Neuropeptides are small peptides found in pulmonary nerves. Two prophlogistic peptides, substance P and neurokinin A (substance K), are found in the terminal axon dendrites of certain sensory nerves. When these nerves are stimulated by appropriate sensory stimuli, their peptides are released into the airway microenvironment. The released peptides transduce signals through binding at NK_1 and NK_2 receptors, thereby causing constriction of airway smooth muscle and bronchovascular leak. In contrast to these contractile peptides, vasoactive intestinal peptide, a bronchodilator peptide also found in pulmonary nerves, is believed to play a homeostatic role in the airways. The contractile/inhibitory action of substance P, neurokinin A, and vasoactive intestinal peptide is regulated by specific peptidases located at or near the site of their action or release. As a consequence, inhibition of the function of these peptidases enhances the biologic effects of these peptides. The availability, as experimental tools, of nonpeptide antagonists at neuropeptide receptors may lead to elucidation of the role of these peptides in the asthmatic response; for the present, their role in asthma is speculative.

NITRIC OXIDE. Nitric oxide (NO·) is produced enzymatically by airway epithelial cells and by inflammatory cells found in the asthmatic lung. Free NO· has a half-life on the order of seconds in the airway and is stabilized by conjugation to thiols to form RS-NO. Both NO· and RS-NO have bronchodilator actions and may play a homeostatic role in the airway. Paradoxically, high levels of

NO·, when co-available with superoxide anion, may form toxic oxidation products, such as peroxynitrite (OONO⁻), which could damage the airway. Patients with asthma have higher than normal levels of NO· in their expired air, and these levels decrease after treatment with glucocorticoids. Thus, the primary role of NO· in asthma may be as a proinflammatory molecule, and levels of exhaled NO· may serve as a marker of asthmatic airway inflammation.

PLATELET-ACTIVATING FACTOR. Platelet-activating factor (PAF), a phospholipid with an ether-linked fatty acid (C_{16}-C_{20}) in the sn-1 position, an acetyl moiety in the sn-2 position, and phosphatidylcholine in the sn-3 position, is derived from lyso-PAF by the action of specific acetyltransferases and is produced by a variety of inflammatory cells, including mast cells and eosinophils. PAF transduces its effects through action at a well-characterized receptor and has a potential role in asthma as an inducer of airway hyperresponsiveness and inflammation. Although this role has not been established via pharmacologic intervention, population-based observations show the importance of PAF in asthma. In Japan a disproportionate number of asthmatics with severe, as compared with mild, asthma are known to harbor a functionally important mutation in the gene encoding the enzyme that degrades PAF. Because individuals with the dysfunctional gene probably have higher levels of PAF in the airway microenvironment and have more severe asthma, it has been inferred that the presence of PAF contributes to asthma severity.

Physiologic Changes in Asthma

The consequence of the airway obstruction induced by smooth muscle constriction, thickening of the airway epithelium, or free liquid within the airway lumen is an increased resistance to airflow, which is manifested by increased airway resistance (Raw) and decreased flow rates throughout the vital capacity. At the onset of an asthma attack, obstruction occurs at all airway levels; as the attack resolves, these changes reverse—first in the large airways (i.e., mainstem, lobar, segmental, and subsegmental bronchi) and then in the more peripheral airways. This anatomic sequence of onset and reversal is reflected in the physiologic changes observed during resolution of an asthmatic episode (Fig. 74–2). Specifically, as an asthma attack resolves, flow rates first normalize at a high point in the vital capacity, and only later at a low point in the vital capacity. Because asthma is an airway disease, no primary changes occur in the static pressure-volume curve of the lungs. However, during an acute attack of asthma, airway narrowing may be so severe as to result in airway closure, with individual lung units closing at a volume that is near their maximal volume. This closure results in a change of the pressure-volume curve such that, for a given contained gas volume within the thorax, elastic recoil is decreased, which in turn further depresses expiratory flow rates.

Additional factors influence the mechanical behavior of the lungs during an acute attack of asthma. During inspiration in an asthma attack, the pleural pressure drops far below the 4 to 6 cm H_2O subatmospheric pressure usually required for tidal airflow. The expiratory phase of respiration also becomes active as the patient tries to force air from the lungs. As a consequence, peak pleural pressures during expiration, which normally are only a few centimeters of water above atmospheric pressure, may be as high as 20 to 30 cm H_2O above atmospheric pressure. The low pleural pressures during inspiration tend to dilate airways, whereas the high pleural pressures during expiration tend to narrow airways. During an asthma attack, the wide pressure swings coupled with alterations in the mechanical properties of the airway wall lead to an expiratory airflow resistance that is much higher than the inspiratory airflow resistance.

The respiratory rate is usually rapid during an acute asthmatic attack. This tachypnea is driven not by abnormalities in arterial blood gas composition, but rather by stimulation of intrapulmonary receptors with subsequent effects on central respiratory centers. One consequence of the combination of airway narrowing and rapid airflow rates is a heightened mechanical load on the ventilatory pump. During a severe attack, the load can increase the work of breathing by a factor of 10 or more and can predispose to fatigue of the ventilatory muscles. The patchy nature of asthmatic airway narrowing results in a maldistribution of ventilation ($\dot{V}$) relative to pulmonary perfusion ($\dot{Q}$). A shift occurs from the normal preponderance of $\dot{V}$/$\dot{Q}$ units, with a ratio of near unity, to a

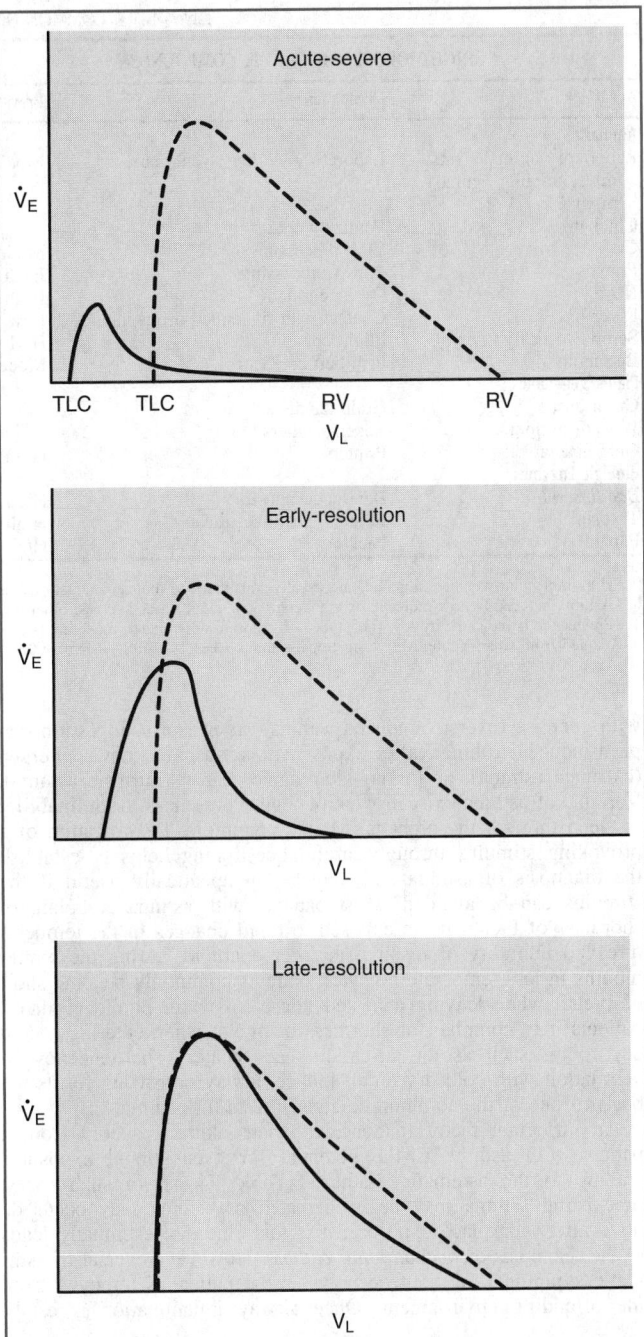

FIGURE 74–2 ■ Schematic flow-volume curves in various stages of asthma; in each figure the dashed line depicts the normal flow-volume curve. Predicted and observed total lung capacity (TLC) and residual volume (RV) are shown in the top panel. E = expiratory flow rate; V_L = lung volume.

distribution with a large number of alveolar-capillary units, with a $\dot{V}$/$\dot{Q}$ ratio of less than unity. The net effect is to induce arterial hypoxemia. In addition, the hyperpnea of asthma is reflected as hyperventilation with a low arterial P_{CO_2}.

CLINICAL PRESENTATION

History

During an asthma attack patients seek medical attention for shortness of breath accompanied by cough, wheezing, and anxiety. The degree of breathlessness experienced by the patient is not closely related to the degree of airflow obstruction but is often influenced by the acuteness of the attack. Dyspnea may occur only

Table 74–1 ■ COMMON OCCUPATIONAL CAUSES OF ASTHMA

HIGH-MOLECULAR-WEIGHT COMPOUNDS*			LOW-MOLECULAR-WEIGHT COMPOUNDS†		
Agent	Occupation	Prevalence‡	Agent	Occupation	Prevalence‡
Animals			Metals		
Laboratory animals (rats, mice, rabbits, guinea pigs)	Laboratory workers, veterinarians	Moderate	Platinum	Platinum refining	High
			Vanadium	Hard metal industry	High
Chicken	Poultry workers		Other		
Crab	Crab processing	Moderate	Trimetallic anhydride	Epoxy resin, plastics	High
Prawns	Prawn processing	High	Toluene diisocyanate	Polyurethane industries, varnishing, plastics	Moderate
Hoya	Oyster farmers	High			
River fly	Contact with riverside power plants	Low	Western red cedar	Carpenters, cabinet makers, sawmill workers	Low-moderate
Screw worm fly	Flight crews	High			
Bee moth	Fish bait breeders	Moderate	Azidocarbonamide	Plastic and rubber workers	Moderate
Plants/Vegetables			Formalin	Hospital workers	
Grain dust	Grain handlers		Urea formaldehyde	Insulation workers, affected homeowners	
Wheat/rye flour	Bakers, millers				
Gum acacia	Printers	High			
Biologic Enzymes					
Bacillus subtilis	Detergent industry	High			
Trypsin	Plastics, pharmaceutical	High			
Papain	Packing	High			

*High-molecular-weight compounds are usually considered to induce occupational asthma via an allergic mechanism.
†Asthma induced by low-molecular-weight compounds that act as haptens; other mechanisms also exist but are not clearly elucidated.
‡Prevalence is indicated by low (i.e., ≤3% of exposed individuals); moderate (i.e., 3 to 20% of exposed individuals); or high (i.e., >20% of exposed individuals).
Adapted from Chan-Yeung M: Occupational asthma. Chest 98:148S–161S, 1990.

with exercise (exercise-induced asthma), after aspirin ingestion (aspirin-induced asthma), after exposure to a specific known allergen (extrinsic asthma), or for no identifiable reason (intrinsic asthma). Variants of asthma exist in which cough, hoarseness, or an inability to sleep through the night is the only symptom. Identification of a provoking stimulus through careful questioning helps to establish the diagnosis of asthma and may be therapeutically useful if the stimulus can be avoided. Most patients with asthma complain of shortness of breath when exposed to rapid changes in the temperature and humidity of inspired air. For example, during the winter months in less temperate climates, patients commonly become short of breath when leaving a heated house; in warm humid climates, patients may complain of shortness of breath when entering a cold dry room, such as an air-conditioned theater. The tendency of ventilation with cold dry air to induce airway narrowing forms the basis of one of the common diagnostic tests for asthma.

An important factor to consider when taking a history from a patient with asthma is the potential for occupational exposures leading to the asthmatic diathesis (Table 74–1). In such cases, preexisting asthma may be exacerbated or asthma may occur de novo after workplace exposure; it is this clue that eventually leads to the diagnosis of *occupational asthma*. However, reversal of asthmatic symptoms may not occur when the patient is removed from the offending environment. Once airway inflammation is estab-

Table 74–2 ■ DIFFERENTIAL DIAGNOSIS OF WHEEZING OTHER THAN ASTHMA

Common
Acute bronchiolitis (infectious, chemical)
Aspiration (foreign body)
Bronchial stenosis
Cardiac failure
Chronic bronchitis
Cystic fibrosis
Eosinophilic pneumonia
Uncommon
Airway obstruction due to masses
  External compression
    Central thoracic tumors, superior vena cava (SVC) syndrome, substernal thyroid
  Intrinsic airway
    Primary lung cancer, metastatic breast cancer
Carcinoid syndrome
Endobronchial sarcoid
Pulmonary emboli
Systemic mastocytosis
Systemic vasculitis (polyarteritis nodosa)

lished, it can resolve quickly; in some cases, however, it may take years for the clinical manifestations of occupational exposure to resolve.

Physical Examination

VITAL SIGNS. Common features of acute asthma attacks include a rapid respiratory rate (often 25 to 40 breaths per minute), tachycardia, and pulsus paradoxus (an exaggerated inspiratory fall in the systolic pressure). The magnitude of the pulsus is related to the severity of the attack.

THORACIC EXAMINATION. Inspection may reveal that patients experiencing acute attacks of asthma are using their accessory muscles of ventilation; if so, the skin over the thorax may be retracted into the intercostal spaces during inspiration. The chest is usually hyperinflated, and the expiratory phase is prolonged relative to the inspiratory phase. Percussion of the thorax demonstrates hyperresonance, with loss of the normal variation in dullness due to diaphragmatic movement. Auscultation reveals wheezing, which is the cardinal physical finding in asthma but does not establish the diagnosis (Table 74–2). Wheezing, commonly louder during expiration but heard during inspiration as well, is characterized as polyphonic in that more than one pitch may be heard simultaneously. Accompanying adventitious sounds may include rhonchi, which are suggestive of free secretions in the airway lumen, or rales, which are indicative of localized infection or heart failure. The loss of intensity or the absence of breath sounds in a patient with asthma is an indication of severe airflow obstruction.

Laboratory Findings

PULMONARY FUNCTION FINDINGS. A decrease in airflow rates throughout the vital capacity is the cardinal pulmonary function abnormality during an asthmatic episode. The peak expiratory flow rate (PEFR), the forced expiratory volume in the first second (FEV_1), and the maximal midexpiratory flow rate (MMEFR) are all decreased in asthma. In very severe asthma, dyspnea may be so severe as to prevent the patient from performing a complete spirogram. In this case, if 2 seconds of forced expiration can be recorded, useful values for PEFR and FEV_1 can be obtained. It cannot be overemphasized that gradation of attack severity (Table 74–3) *must* be assessed by objective measures of airflow; no other methods yield accurate and reproducible results. As the attack resolves, the PEFR and the FEV_1 increase toward normal in concert while the MMEFR remains substantially depressed; as the attack resolves further, the FEV_1 and the PEFR may normalize while the MMEFR remains depressed (see Fig. 74–2). Even when the attack has resolved clinically, residual depression of the MMEFR is not

TEST	% OF PREDICTED VALUE	ASTHMA SEVERITY
PEFR	≥80%	
FEV₁	≥80%	No spirometric abnormalities
MMEFR	≥80%	
PEFR	≥80%	
FEV₁	≥70%	Mild asthma
MMEFR	55–75%	
PEFR	≥60%	
FEV₁	45–70%	Moderate asthma
MMEFR	30–50%	
PEFR	<50%	
FEV₁	<50%	Severe asthma
MMEFR	10–30%	

PEFR = peak expiratory flow rate; MMEFR = maximal midexpiratory flow rate; FEV_1 = forced expiratory volume in the first second.

uncommon; this depression may resolve over a prolonged course of treatment. If the patient is able to cooperate such that more complete measurements of lung function can be made, lung volume measurements will demonstrate an increase in both total lung capacity (TLC) and residual volume (RV); the changes in TLC and RV resolve with treatment.

ARTERIAL BLOOD GASES. Blood gas analysis need not be undertaken in individuals with mild asthma. If the asthma is of sufficient severity to merit prolonged observation, however, blood gas analysis is indicated; in such cases, hypoxemia and hypocarbia are the rule. With the subject breathing room air, the PaO_2 is usually between 55 and 70 mm Hg and the $PaCO_2$ between 25 and 35 mm Hg. At the onset of the attack, an appropriate pure respiratory alkalemia is usually evident; with attacks of prolonged duration, the pH normalizes as a result of a compensatory metabolic acidemia. A normal $PaCO_2$ in a patient with moderate to severe airflow obstruction is reason for concern, as it may indicate that the mechanical load on the respiratory system is greater than can be sustained by the ventilatory muscles and that respiratory failure is imminent. When the $PaCO_2$ rises in such settings, the pH falls quickly, because the bicarbonate stores have become depleted as a result of renal compensation for the prolonged preceding respiratory alkalemia. Because this chain of events can take place rapidly, close observation is indicated for asthmatics with "normal" $PaCO_2$ levels and moderate to severe airflow obstruction.

OTHER BLOOD FINDINGS. Asthmatic subjects are frequently atopic; thus, blood eosinophilia is common. In addition, elevated serum levels of IgE are often documented; epidemiologic studies indicate that asthma is unusual in subjects with low IgE levels. If indicated by the patient's history, specific radioallergosorbent tests (RASTs), which measure IgE directed against specific offending antigens, can be conducted. In rare instances during severe asthma attacks, serum concentrations of aminotransferases, lactate dehydrogenases, muscle creatine kinase, ornithine transcarbamylase, and antidiuretic hormone may be elevated.

RADIOGRAPHIC FINDINGS. The chest radiograph of a subject with asthma is often normal. Severe asthma is associated with hyperinflation, as indicated by depression of the diaphragm and abnormally lucent lung fields. Complications of severe asthma, including pneumomediastinum or pneumothorax, may be detected radiographically. In mild to moderate asthma without adventitious sounds other than wheezing, a chest radiograph need not be obtained; if the asthma is of sufficient severity to merit hospital admission, a chest radiograph is advised.

ELECTROCARDIOGRAPHIC FINDINGS. The electrocardiogram, save for sinus tachycardia, is usually normal in acute asthma. However, right axis deviation, right bundle branch block, "P pulmonale" or even ST-T wave abnormalities may arise during severe asthma and resolve as the attack resolves.

SPUTUM FINDINGS. The sputum of the asthmatic patient may be either clear or opaque with a green or yellow tinge. The presence of color does not invariably indicate infection, and examination of a Gram-stained and Wright-stained sputum smear is indicated. Often the sputum contains eosinophils, Charcot-Leyden crystals (crystallized eosinophil lysophospholipase), Curschmann's spirals (bronchiolar casts composed of mucus and cells), or Creola

bodies (clusters of airway epithelial cells with identifiable cilia), which can affect color without the presence of infection.

Differential Diagnosis

Asthma is easy to recognize in a young patient without comorbid medical conditions who has exacerbating and remitting airway obstruction accompanied by blood eosinophilia. A rapid response to bronchodilator treatment is usually all that is needed to establish the diagnosis. However, in the patient with cryptic episodic shortness of breath, airway challenge testing by a laboratory familiar with this procedure is indicated. Challenge testing, performed during minimal airway obstruction, determines the presence and magnitude of airway hyperresponsiveness. In such tests, subjects are exposed to increasing amounts of inhaled bronchoconstrictor agonists or breathe graded levels of cold dry air. Subjects with asthma usually require smaller amounts of a stimulus to reach a given endpoint in airway response than do nonasthmatic subjects. Airway hyperresponsiveness strongly suggests asthma, whereas its absence does not exclude asthma as a possibility. However, in the absence of airway hyperresponsiveness, other causes of wheezing (see Table 74–2) should be investigated.

TREATMENT

The treatment of asthma is directed at airway obstruction and inflammation; resolution of obstruction should be documented by objective measures such as FEV_1 or PEFR. Inexpensive and easy-to-use peak flowmeters make the latter measurement feasible in virtually all cases. Asthma treatment has two components. The first is the use of acute reliever (rescue) agents (i.e., bronchodilators) for acute asthmatic airway obstruction. The second is the use of controller treatments, which modify the asthmatic airway environment such that acute airway narrowing, requiring rescue treatments, occurs much less frequently.

In a given individual, the intensity of asthma treatment depends on the severity of disease. It is now well established that asthma is a chronic disease that should, in all but its mildest forms, be treated chronically. The treatment scheme outlined below is based on, but is not a precise copy of, the 1997 revision of the U.S. National Asthma Education and Prevention Program Guidelines for Asthma Treatment.

Classification of Asthma Severity

Asthma is classified by the severity of its presentation into one of four categories. *Mild intermittent asthma* is the term used to describe the condition in the largest group of patients with asthma. Patients in this diagnostic classification have normal or near normal lung function, infrequent asthma symptoms, usually sleep through the night without difficulty, and need to use asthma rescue medications infrequently. The only treatment needed for such patients is an inhaled medium-acting bronchodilator (see below). Indeed, if a patient is able to maintain a normal functional status and airway function using no more than a single 200-actuation metered-dose inhaler a month, no further treatment is required. Patients with *mild persistent asthma* have normal or near normal lung function on most occasions but have asthma symptoms daily, have difficulty sleeping one or two nights a week, and use their asthma rescue medications so frequently that a single 200-actuation canister is inadequate to provide a month's treatment. Such patients require a controller agent, such as an inhaled corticosteroid, an antileukotriene agent, or cromolyn sodium, in addition to their rescue treatment. Despite therapy with a single controller agent, patients with *moderate or severe persistent asthma* have persistently abnormal lung function, have asthma symptoms more than once daily, and have difficulty sleeping many nights a week. These patients require multiple asthma medications to achieve adequate disease control, and their care is best directed by an asthma care specialist.

Reliever Treatments

β-**ADRENERGIC AGENTS.** β-Adrenergic agents given by inhalation are the mainstay of bronchodilator treatment for asthma. Constricted airway smooth muscle relaxes in response to stimulation of β_2-adrenergic receptors. β-Adrenergic agonists with varying degrees of β_2-selectivity are available for use in inhaled (by nebulizer or metered-dose inhaler), oral, or parenteral preparations. Patients with mild intermittent asthma should be treated with a moderate-duration β_2-selective inhaler on an as-needed basis. This treatment should consist of two "puffs" from the inhaler, with the first and second puffs separated by a 3- to 5-minute interval, which is thought to allow enough time for the first "puff" to dilate narrowed airways, thus giving the agent better access to affected areas of the lung. Patients should be instructed to exhale to a comfortable volume, to breathe in very slowly (such as they would when sipping hot soup), and to actuate the inhaler as they inspire. Inspiration to near TLC is followed by holding the breath for 5 seconds to allow the deposition of smaller aerosol particles in more peripheral airways. Patients should receive specific instructions for correct inhaler use. Aerosol "spacers" are available from many manufacturers for patients who have difficulty coordinating inspiration and inhaler actuation. In addition, novel devices improve inhaler coordination by actuating the inhaler only when the inspiratory flow pattern is within certain well-defined limitations.

ANTICHOLINERGICS. For more than a century, atropine has been known to be useful in the treatment of asthma. Its mechanism of action is thought to be inhibition of the effects of acetylcholine released from the intrapulmonary motor nerves that run in the vagus and innervate airway smooth muscle. The adverse central nervous system effects of atropine, which limited its utility in the past, have been overcome with the development of ipratropium bromide, available for use in a metered-dose inhaler. Although ipratropium bromide has a salutary effect on cough in asthma and is useful as an adjunct to inhaled β_2-agonists in chronic stable asthma, it has not been shown to be as effective for the treatment of acute asthmatic bronchospasm as inhaled β_2-agonists.

Controller Treatments

INHALED CORTICOSTEROIDS. Inhaled corticosteroids, which have less systemic impact for a given level of therapeutic effect than systemic steroids, are effective controller treatments for patients with persistent asthma. A wide variety of inhaled corticosteroid products are on the market in the United States (Table 74–4), with little solid data to guide the physician in choosing among them. All available products have been shown to be effective treatments for persistent asthma; the major unresolved controversy is the potential for systemic effects, including growth retardation in children, loss of bone mineralization, cataracts, and glaucoma. An adverse effect common to all inhaled corticosteroids, at recommended doses, is oral thrush; the risk and severity of this complication can be reduced by means of aerosol spacers and good oropharyngeal hygiene (i.e., rinsing out the mouth by gargling after dosing).

ANTILEUKOTRIENES. Agents with the capacity to inhibit the synthesis (zileuton [Zyflo]) or action (montelukast [Singulair], pranlukast [Onon or Ultair], zafirlukast [Accolate]) of the leukotrienes are effective controller medications for the patient with mild or moderate persistent asthma. These treatments can be used on their own for mild persistent asthma or in combination with inhaled steroids for more severe asthma. Because these products are relatively new to the marketplace, the reader is advised to seek recent information concerning the details of their prescription.

LONG-ACTING β-AGONISTS. In contrast to medium-acting β-agonists, the only long-acting β-agonist currently available in the United States (salmeterol [Serevent]) has a slow onset of action and a duration of action of nearly 12 hours; it is considered a controller rather than a bronchodilator agent. Salmeterol has been shown to provide effective asthma control in patients with mild intermittent asthma when given as either the sole controller agent or in concert with inhaled corticosteroids. The major unresolved question with respect to the use of long-acting β_2-agonists is the long-term effect of an agent that is thought not to modify the biology of the asthmatic airway.

THEOPHYLLINE. Theophylline and aminophylline are bronchodilators of moderate potency that are useful in both inpatient and outpatient management of asthma. Theophylline is sold in a large number of formulations that allow therapy to proceed with daily or twice-daily dosing. The mechanism by which theophylline exerts its effects has not been established with certainty but is probably related to the inhibition of certain forms of phosphodiesterase. The utility of theophylline is limited by its toxicity and by wide variations in the rate of its metabolism, both in a single individual over time and among individuals in a population. As a result of this variability, monitoring of plasma theophylline levels is indicated to ensure that patients are treated appropriately. Acceptable plasma levels for therapeutic effects are between 10 and 20 $\mu g/mL$; higher levels are associated with gastrointestinal, cardiac, and central nervous system toxicity, including anxiety, headache, nausea, vomiting, diarrhea, cardiac arrhythmias, and seizures. These last catastrophic complications may occur without antecedent mild side effects when plasma levels exceed 20 $\mu g/mL$. Because of these potentially life-threatening complications of treatment, plasma levels need to be measured with great frequency in hospitalized patients receiving intravenous aminophylline and less frequently in stable outpatients receiving one of the long-acting theophylline preparations. Most asthma care providers use dosing amounts and intervals to achieve steady-state theophylline levels of 10 to 14 $\mu g/mL$, thereby avoiding the toxicity associated with decrements in metabolism. Treatment with theophylline is recommended only for patients with moderate or severe persistent asthma who are receiving controller medications, such as inhaled steroids or antileukotrienes, but whose asthma is not adequately controlled.

SYSTEMIC CORTICOSTEROIDS. Systemic corticosteroids are effective for the treatment of moderate to severe persistent asthma as well as occasional severe exacerbations of asthma that occur in a patient with otherwise mild asthma. The mechanism of their therapeutic effect in asthma has not been established.

No consensus has been reached on the specific type, dose, or duration of corticosteroid to be used in the treatment of asthma. In nonhospitalized patients with asthma refractory to standard therapy, a steroid "pulse" with initial doses of prednisone on the order of 40 to 60 mg/day, tapered to zero over 7 to 14 days, is recommended. For patients who cannot stop taking steroids without having recurrent uncontrolled bronchospasm despite the addition of multiple other controller treatments, alternate-day administration of oral steroids is preferable to daily treatment. For patients whose asthma requires in-hospital treatment but is not considered life-threatening, an initial intravenous bolus of 2 mg/kg of hydrocortisone, followed by continuous infusion of 0.5 mg/kg/hour, has been shown to be beneficial within 12 hours. In attacks of asthma that are considered life-threatening, the use of intravenous methylprednisolone (125 mg every 6 hours) has been advocated. In each case, as the patient improves, oral steroids are substituted for intravenous steroids, and the oral dose is tapered over 1 to 3 weeks; addition of inhaled steroids to the regimen when oral steroids are started is strongly recommended.

Table 74–4 ■ DOSES OF INHALED CORTICOSTEROIDS AVAILABLE FOR ASTHMA TREATMENT IN THE UNITED STATES*

STEROID NAME		DOSAGE		
Generic	Trade	μg/Actuation	Starting Dose	COMMENTS
Beclomethasone	Beclovent	42	2 puffs b.i.d.	Available in 2 strengths; prescription must indicate strength
	Vanceril	84		
Budesonide	Pulmicort	200	2 puffs b.i.d.	Available only in the dry powder Turbuhaler
Flunisolide	AeroBid	250	2 puffs b.i.d.	
Fluticasone	Flovent	44, 110, or 220	2 puffs b.i.d. (44 μg/puff)	Available in 3 strengths; prescription must indicate dose level; Available in pressurized MDI or as dry powder
Triamcinolone	Azmacort	100	2 puffs b.i.d.	

*Products marketed as of March 1999. Agents are listed in alphabetical order by generic name.

OTHER CONTROLLER DRUGS. Cromolyn sodium and nedocromil sodium are nonsteroid inhaled treatments that have proven beneficial in the management of mild to moderate persistent asthma. They appear to be most useful in pediatric populations or when an identifiable stimulus (such as exercise or allergen exposure) elicits an asthmatic response.

The use of systemic gold (as in rheumatoid arthritis), methotrexate, or cyclosporine has been suggested as adjunctive treatment for patients with severe chronic asthma who cannot otherwise discontinue high-dose corticosteroid treatment. However, these agents are experimental, and their routine use is not advocated.

Specific Treatment Scenarios

CONCURRENT PULMONARY INFECTION. In some patients, acute exacerbations of asthma may be due to concurrent infection, which will require targeted therapy (see Chapters 75, 77, and 82).

ASPIRIN-INDUCED ASTHMA. Approximately 5% of patients with moderate to severe persistent asthma develop asthma when they ingest agents that inhibit cyclooxygenase, such as aspirin and other nonsteroidal anti-inflammatory drugs. Such patients quite often have difficult-to-manage asthma, with nasal polyposis and chronic sinusitis even in the absence of exposure to agents that inhibit cyclooxygenase. It has been established that all the physiologic manifestations of aspirin sensitivity can be attributed to leukotriene excess; thus, the treatment of choice for such individuals is a leukotriene pathway inhibitor.

ASTHMA IN THE EMERGENCY DEPARTMENT. When a patient with asthma presents for acute emergency care, objective measures of the severity of the attack, including quantification of pulsus paradoxus and measurement of airflow rates (PEFR or FEV_1), should be evaluated in addition to the usual vital signs. If the attack has been prolonged and failed to respond to treatment with bronchodilators and high-dose inhaled steroids before arrival at the emergency department, intravenous steroids (40 to 60 mg of methylprednisolone) should be administered. Treatment with inhaled β-agonists should be repeated at 20- to 30-minute intervals until the PEFR or FEV_1 rises to greater than 40% of the predicted values. If this point is not reached within 2 hours, admission to the hospital for further treatment is strongly advocated.

When patients have PEFR and FEV_1 values that are greater than 60% of their predicted value on arrival in the emergency department, treatment with inhaled β_2-agonists alone is likely to result in an objective improvement in airflow rates. If significant improvement takes place in the emergency department, such patients can usually be treated as outpatients with inhaled β_2-agonists and an additional controller agent.

For patients whose PEFR and FEV_1 values are between 40% and 60% of the values predicted at the time of initial evaluation in the emergency care setting, a plan of treatment varying in intensity between the two cited above is indicated. Failure to respond to treatment by objective criteria (PEFR or FEV_1) within 2 hours of arriving at the emergency department is an indication for more intense therapy.

STATUS ASTHMATICUS. The asthmatic subject whose PEFR or FEV_1 does not increase to greater than 40% of the predicted value with treatment, whose $PaCO_2$ increases without improvement of indices of airflow obstruction, or who develops major complications such as pneumothorax or pneumomediastinum should be admitted to the hospital for close monitoring. Frequent treatments with inhaled β-agonists, intravenous aminophylline (at doses yielding maximal plasma levels), and high-dose intravenous steroids are indicated. Oxygen should be administered by face mask or nasal cannula in amounts sufficient to achieve SaO_2 values between 92% and 94%; a higher FiO_2 promotes absorption atelectasis and provides no therapeutic benefit. If objective evidence of an infection is present, appropriate treatment for that infection should be given. If no improvement is seen with treatment, and respiratory failure appears imminent, bronchodilator treatment should be intensified to the maximum tolerated by the patient. If indicated, intubation of the trachea and mechanical ventilation can be instituted; in this case the goal should be to provide a level of ventilation just adequate to sustain life but *not sufficient to normalize arterial blood gases.* For example, a $PaCO_2$ of 55 to 65 mm Hg, or even higher, is acceptable for a patient in status asthmaticus.

THE PREGNANT ASTHMATIC. Asthma may be exacerbated, remain unchanged, or remit during pregnancy. There need not be substantial departures from the ordinary management of asthma during pregnancy. However, no unnecessary medications should be administered; systemic steroids should be used sparingly to avert fetal complications, and certain drugs should be avoided, including tetracycline (as a treatment for intercurrent infection), atropine and atropine-like drugs (which may cause fetal tachycardia), terbutaline (which is contraindicated during active labor because of its tocolytic effects), and iodine-containing mucolytics (such as saturated solution of potassium iodide). Moreover, use of prostaglandin F_2 as an abortifacient should be avoided in asthmatics.

Barnes PJ: Drug therapy: Inhaled glucocorticoids for asthma. N Engl J Med 332:868–875, 1995. *Concise description of the role of inhaled steroids in asthma.*

Barnes PJ, Pedersen S, Busse WW: Efficacy and safety of inhaled corticosteroids: New developments. Am J Respir Crit Care Med 157:S1–S53, 1998. *Recent update on steroid efficacy and toxicity.*

Drazen JM, Israel E, Boushey HA, et al: Comparison of regularly scheduled with as-needed use of albuterol in mild asthma. N Engl J Med 335:841–847, 1996. *Demonstrates the safety of regular use of inhaled albuterol.*

Drazen JM, Israel E, O'Byrne PM: Treatment of asthma with drugs modifying the leukotriene pathway. N Engl J Med 340:197–206, 1999. *Review of anti-leukotriene treatment.*

Israel E, Cohn J, Dube L, Drazen JM: Effect of treatment with zileuton, a 5-lipoxygenase inhibitor, in patients with asthma: A randomized controlled trial. JAMA 275:931–936, 1996. *Controlled trial demonstrating the efficacy of 5-lipoxygenase inhibitors in asthma.*

National Heart Lung and Blood Institute, NHLBI/WHO Workshop Report: Global Strategy for Asthma Management and Prevention: Global Initiative for Asthma. Bethesda, MD, National Heart Lung and Blood Institute, publication 95-3659, 1995. *World guidelines for asthma treatment.*

75 CHRONIC BRONCHITIS AND EMPHYSEMA

Joseph R. Rodarte

DEFINITIONS

Chronic bronchitis and emphysema, which are two distinct pathologic conditions, share similar symptoms and frequently coexist. Patients with either or, more commonly, both conditions are usually classified as having chronic obstructive lung disease or chronic obstructive pulmonary disease (COPD). COPD is a chronic, slowly progressive disease and is the fourth most common cause of death in the United States. Death due to COPD increased 47% between 1979 and 1993. COPD is often underdiagnosed and makes unrecognized or unrecorded contributions to the mortality of other conditions affecting the elderly. For example, even mild COPD increases the risk of serious respiratory complications from anesthesia and surgery.

Within the spectrum of chronic bronchitis and emphysema are patients who have many of the features of asthma (see Chapter 74); also, patients with asthma may develop irreversible airway obstruction. Although there are no generally accepted diagnostic criteria, these patients are commonly referred to as having asthmatic bronchitis.

EPIDEMIOLOGY

Both chronic bronchitis and emphysema are strongly associated with cigarette smoking. The prevalence of COPD increased dramatically with the increased incidence of cigarette smoking by men in the 1930s and 1940s. The lower prevalence in women is believed to be due to their lower smoking rates rather than to a protective hormonal effect. The prevalence of COPD in women has been increasing with increased smoking rates; if current trends continue, COPD will soon be as common in women as in men.

Recent national data indicate that 5.4% of adults have clinically significant airway obstruction from bronchitis and 0.8% from emphysema; overall about 16 million persons in the United States have COPD. Because the disease is seriously underdiagnosed, as many as 30 million persons may be affected. In 1993, direct health care costs were estimated at $14.7 million. In addition, when patients with COPD are hospitalized for unrelated diagnoses, they have longer stays and greater costs. Indirect costs, such as from disability and days lost from work, are much greater.

PATHOGENESIS

All mammalian lungs share the property that expiratory airflow increases monotonically with expiratory effort until some critical threshold pressure difference between the pleural surface and the airway opening is reached. Beyond that threshold, flow becomes fixed and does not increase further with further increases of expiratory effort. The hallmark of chronic obstructive lung disease is a reduction of maximal expiratory flow rate. This reduction of flow rate independent of the underlying pathologic process produces much of the pathophysiologic features and disability of these diseases. In the absence of effective treatment for either chronic bronchitis or emphysema, and because of their almost universal coexistence and the difficulty in assessing the contribution of each to a reduced maximal airflow, little effort to separate them has been made until recently. Most epidemiologic studies of the natural history and treatment of COPD have not attempted to determine the relative contribution of emphysema to the airway obstruction. Other diseases associated with chronic airway obstruction include bronchiolitis obliterans associated with chronic lung transplant rejection (see Chapter 89), bronchiectasis (see Chapter 77), cystic fibrosis (see Chapter 76), lymphangiomyomatosis, sarcoidosis (see Chapter 81), and histiocytosis. Because COPD is such a common disease, it coexists with many lung diseases (e.g., pneumoconiosis) that do not of themselves cause airway obstruction.

Chronic Bronchitis

Chronic bronchitis is a clinical diagnosis requiring patients to have a chronic cough productive of sputum for at least 3 months a year for at least 2 consecutive years in the absence of other diseases, such as asthma, bronchial tumors, bronchiectasis, or chronic lung infections. However, only a minority of patients with chronic bronchitis develop clinically significant airway obstruction.

Rare patients develop chronic bronchitis with minimal or no history of cigarette smoking or other exposures associated with the condition. Smoking exposure is usually quantified by the product of packs of cigarettes per day times the number of years smoked. It is not uncommon to find individuals with a 60 pack-year smoking history who have normal lung function, but it is virtually impossible to find someone with 90 pack-year exposure and normal lung function. Only about one of six chronic cigarette smokers develops clinically significant disease. Why do some smokers develop COPD is not known. There is a strong familial association of COPD due to chronic bronchitis, but the underlying genetics are unknown. Abnormalities of cytokines and pro-inflammatory mediators are believed to play an important etiologic role. Viral infections may trigger chronic bronchitis; futhermore, in patients with established chronic bronchitis, viral or bacterial infections are a common cause of acute exacerbations and may be a significant explanation for progression in patients who have stopped smoking.

COPD is generally an insidious and slowly progressive disease. In our sedentary society, patients may lose 50% of their lung function before symptoms develop. Many patients report no complaints except for a tendency to have prolonged cough after an upper respiratory infection, until a particular "bad chest cold," after which they have had progressive dyspnea. In the past, physicians believed such patients had a slowly progressive decrease in function but belittled or denied symptoms until some particular incident. However, epidemiologic studies confirm that patients with mild subclinical disease can develop respiratory infections that do not cause patients to seek medical attention but nevertheless are associated with substantial and irreversible decreases in lung function.

The pathology of chronic bronchitis is bronchial inflammation, which differs from the eosinophilic inflammation of asthma (see Chapter 74). In the large airways, increases in the size and number of mucous glands and goblet cells are noted. Smooth muscle increases, and partial destruction of bronchial cartilage and adventitial fibrosis occurs. A neutrophilic infiltrate is present, which is much less dramatic than the inflammatory infiltrates seen in asthma. In the small airways, the lumen may be completely occluded by mucus and inflammatory cell infiltrates, and fibrosis is present in the bronchiolar walls.

Emphysema

Emphysema, which is a pathologic diagnosis, consists of enlargement of the terminal air spaces due to destruction of alveolar walls. In pure emphysema, the conducting airways are normal. The two important forms of emphysema are centrilobular and panlobular. In centrilobular emphysema, which is usually associated with cigarette smoking, alveolar destruction occurs initially around the respiratory bronchioles; within each affected acinus, more normal alveoli surround a central core of emphysema. As the lesion progresses, the entire lobule is involved; as a result, panlobular emphysema develops. However, in some cases of relatively mild emphysema, panlobular alveolar destruction occurs throughout each affected lobule while adjacent areas remain virtually normal. Centrilobular emphysema is often worse in the apices of the upper lobes and superior segments of the lower lobes, but the reason for this distribution is unknown. Panlobular emphysema is either uniform or may predominate in the lower lobes.

Emphysema, particularly the panlobular variety, has been known to have a strong familial component since the late 1960s, when it was noted that some patients from families with a high incidence of early-onset, severe emphysema had decreased α_1-globulin levels on protein electrophoreses. They were discovered to be deficient in an acute-phase protein that is secreted by the liver into the bloodstream and is now called α_1-antitrypsin because it inhibits pancreatic trypsin as well as neutrophilic leukocyte elastase. This discovery was responsible for the current paradigm for the etiology of emphysema. Noxious substances in cigarette smoke injure the alveolar epithelium and cause a release of inflammatory mediators, which attract activated neutrophils to the alveolar region. These activated neutrophils release leukocyte elastase, which is an important component of their antimicrobial action. Damage to host tissues is minimized by antiprotease activity: diffusion of α_1-antitrypsin from the plasma in areas of increased vascular permeability, as a result of inflammation, is the major factor that neutralizes leukocyte elastase. In the absence of α_1-antitrypsin, neutrophil elastase remains active, destroys alveolar walls, and produces panlobular emphysema. Of a number of abnormal alleles of α_1-antitrypsin, the most common and significant allele is termed "Z"; heterozygotes for the Z allele have lower α_1-antitrypsin blood levels than do normal subjects, but they do not have clinical disease. In contrast, homozygous ZZ individuals who smoke usually develop severe emphysema in their 30s and 40s. Individuals who do not smoke and who live in areas with good air quality may not develop clinically significant abnormal lung function until their 60s. It is believed all ZZ genotype individuals will develop emphysema and abnormal lung function during a normal life span, but in some individuals the disease may not be severe enough to become debilitating.

The gene frequency for α_1-antitrypsin deficiency is 2 to 3% in Northern European populations, so one in 1600 to 4000 births are homozygous ZZ. Even though α_1-antitrypsin deficiency represents a small fraction of patients with emphysema, it is believed that an imbalance between proteases and antiproteases in the lung is responsible for most emphysema. Endotracheal instillation of trypsin or elastase in experimental animals produces panlobular emphysema similar to that observed in humans.

Decline in Maximal Expiratory Flow

To understand how maximal expiratory flow is reduced in bronchitis and emphysema, it is necessary to understand what determines maximal expiratory flow in the normal lung. The lung develops when the bronchial tree buds into primordial mesenchymal tissue. The conducting airways can be thought of as tubes that lie in tunnels, whose lengths and diameters increase with increases in lung volume. Thus, to the first approximation, the pressure surrounding the intraparenchymal airways is pleural pressure. The lung is inflated by the difference between alveolar and pleural pressure, which stresses the lung tissue. The airways are also distended by the difference between intraluminal pressure and pleural pressure. During expiration, pleural pressure is increased above the subatmospheric pressure required to maintain static inflation of the lung at that volume. Alveolar pressure is increased by the same amount, and expiratory flow occurs down this pressure gradient. Expiratory flow is associated with a decrease of pressure in the airways because of frictional losses in the gas and conversion of pressure into kinetic energy when gas velocity increases as the total cross-sectional area of the tree decreases several hundredfold from the most peripheral airways to the central airways. With sufficient expiratory effort to produce positive pleural pressure, intraluminal airway pressure falls below pleural pressure. When this occurs, flow reaches a critical velocity, called *wave speed* in the airway, analogous to the speed of sound. Inspiratory flow increases monotonically with increases in inspiratory effort. However, during expiration, flow increases only until a critical threshold is reached, after which flow becomes fixed. Therefore, maximal flow at any given lung volume is determined by the elastic recoil of the lung at that volume (which determines not only the diameter of the elastic airways but also the amount of pressure that can be dissipated during expiration before intraluminal airway pressure falls below pleural pressure) and by the geometry of the airway (which determines how much flow can occur before the elastic recoil pressure is dissipated). Maximal flow decreases with volume because of a reduction in elastic recoil, which is the driving pressure, and because airway diameter decreases with the decreasing transmural pressure. With age, the lung loses elasticity; maximal expiratory flow decreases with age because of this reduction in the lung's elastic recoil. At the lung volume at which elastic recoil falls to zero, air cannot be forced from the lung by increasing pleural pressure because the airways collapse. The air remaining in the lung at this time, termed the *residual volume,* increases with age from approximately 20% of maximal volume to more than 50% in older subjects. The maximum volume of the lungs, termed *total lung capacity,* is determined by the balance of forces between the maximally activated inspiratory muscles and the inward elastic recoil of the lung and chest wall. Total lung capacity does not change with age in normal individuals, presumably because the decreased lung elasticity is balanced by stiffening of the chest wall and decreased inspiratory muscle force.

Any narrowing of the airway lumen due to the changes in chronic bronchitis, increased mucus in the lumen, or fibrosis of the wall will decrease the amount of flow that can occur before the elastic recoil pressure is dissipated. Decreased lung recoil also reduces maximal flow because of reduced driving pressure and decreased distending pressure on the airways. Patients with severe emphysema can have residual volumes near their predicted normal total lung capacity so that both their maximal flow and static elastic recoil are markedly reduced at all lung volumes, but the relationship between flow and recoil is the same as that in a normal individual at very low lung volumes.

Because of the phenomenon of flow limitation, maximal expiratory flow is a measure of the integrity of the lung independent of patient effort once the threshold effort is achieved. Lung elastic recoil is difficult to measure and is rarely used clinically. Because the functional effects of reduced maximal flows are not dependent on the cause of the reduction, flow-volume curves (Figs. 75–1 and 75–2) display the pertinent physiology.

CLINICAL MANIFESTATIONS

Effects of Reduced Maximal Airway Flow

During quiet breathing, respiratory muscles are relaxed at end expiration. At this volume, also called the *functional residual capacity* (FRC), the inward recoil of the lung is balanced by the outward recoil of the chest wall. Normal breathing occurs by activation of the inspiratory muscles to increase volume and gradual relaxation, allowing exhalation back to FRC. In young normal individuals, maximal flow at FRC is 5 to 6 times higher than that required for normal breathing, and ventilation can be increased more than tenfold by an increase in both tidal volume and flow rates during maximal exercise. In the elderly, maximal flow in the tidal volume range is reduced so that it approaches tidal flow. Elderly subjects can still increase their ventilation substantially (when needed for exercise) by inspiring to very high lung volumes.

In normal individuals, maximal exercise capacity is determined

by the cardiovascular system rather than by the lungs, although in the exceptionally fit geriatric athletes, ventilation may be limiting. However, with COPD, maximal flow at the volume at which lung inward recoil matches chest wall outward recoil is less than required for tidal breathing, so FRC becomes dynamically determined. With severe COPD, patients may utilize maximal flow over most of expired tidal volume, and the expiratory flows are so low that patients interrupt expiration by inspiring before reaching the relaxation volume (Fig. 75–3). The relaxed chest wall may increase pleural pressure sufficiently to achieve maximal flow without expiratory effort and produce a positive pleural pressure during expiration. Because airway resistance is high, pleural pressure is quite negative during inspiration. The increased pleural pressure swings affect venous return and may cause neck vein distention during expiration; these swings also affect cardiac output and increase the normal amplitude of blood pressure oscillations with respiration. With severe COPD, expiratory flow is so limited that tidal respiration can be achieved only near total lung capacity; subjects cannot increase ventilation to any significant extent and are unable to accomplish any sustained exercise. Although the FEV_1 is the most commonly used measure of lung function in COPD, it is not a comprehensive measure of lung physiology. Exercise capacity is correlated with FEV_1 but with considerable variability. As a general rule, patients' activity is significantly limited when the FEV_1 falls to about 50% of predicted normal. Patients with FEV_1 less than one-third of predicted are often completely incapacitated, so that even tying the shoes causes severe dyspnea.

In patients with emphysema, the decreased lung recoil allows inhalation to higher volumes and an increase in TLC, which is an adaptive mechanism for producing higher flows than possible at normal volumes. The diaphragm, which is chronically operating at a shorter length, adapts like other skeletal muscles by dropping out sarcomeres. However, the capacity for remodeling the chest is not unlimited, and TLC can increase only by 40 to 50%. Patients with bronchitis and not emphysema also increase their TLC, presumably because continuous breathing at high lung volumes causes the lung to remodel. Patients with primarily bronchitis tend to have a lower TLC than patients with predominantly emphysema.

Because COPD does not affect the lung uniformly, ventilation and perfusion distribution is impaired. Areas with low ventilation-perfusion ratios cause arterial hypoxia, which cannot be rectified by increasing ventilation to restore arterial CO_2 to normal. Therefore, patients' ventilatory requirements for any given oxygen uptake are increased, which further exacerbates the mechanical impairment. Ultimately, the work of breathing becomes so great that patients hypoventilate, retain CO_2, and develop further arterial hypoxemia. Destruction of the pulmonary capillary bed and arterial hypoxia ultimately produce pulmonary hypertension and right ventricular failure (cor pulmonale). The hypoxia associated with severe COPD exacerbates diseases associated with tissue ischemia, such as coronary artery disease.

Patients with pure emphysema tend to be extremely dyspneic and have limited exercise capacity because of their ventilatory mechanics, but they may maintain reasonably normal blood gas values and pulmonary artery pressure until very late in the course of disease. In contrast, subjects with predominantly bronchitis of the same severity tend to have more ventilation-perfusion abnormalities, worse hypoxia, and cor pulmonale earlier in the course of the disease. However, exceptions to these general patterns are frequent, especially because most patients have combinations of bronchitis and emphysema.

DIAGNOSIS

Mild to Moderate Disease

HISTORY. Chronic bronchitis and emphysema are insidious diseases. Many smokers have coughed for so long that they consider it normal and will not acknowledge chronic cough on review of symptoms, even though they cough during the examination. Most patients with chronic cough do not have airway obstruction. Many patients with up to 50% reduction in lung function do not complain of shortness of breath, and many individuals with no cardiopulmo-

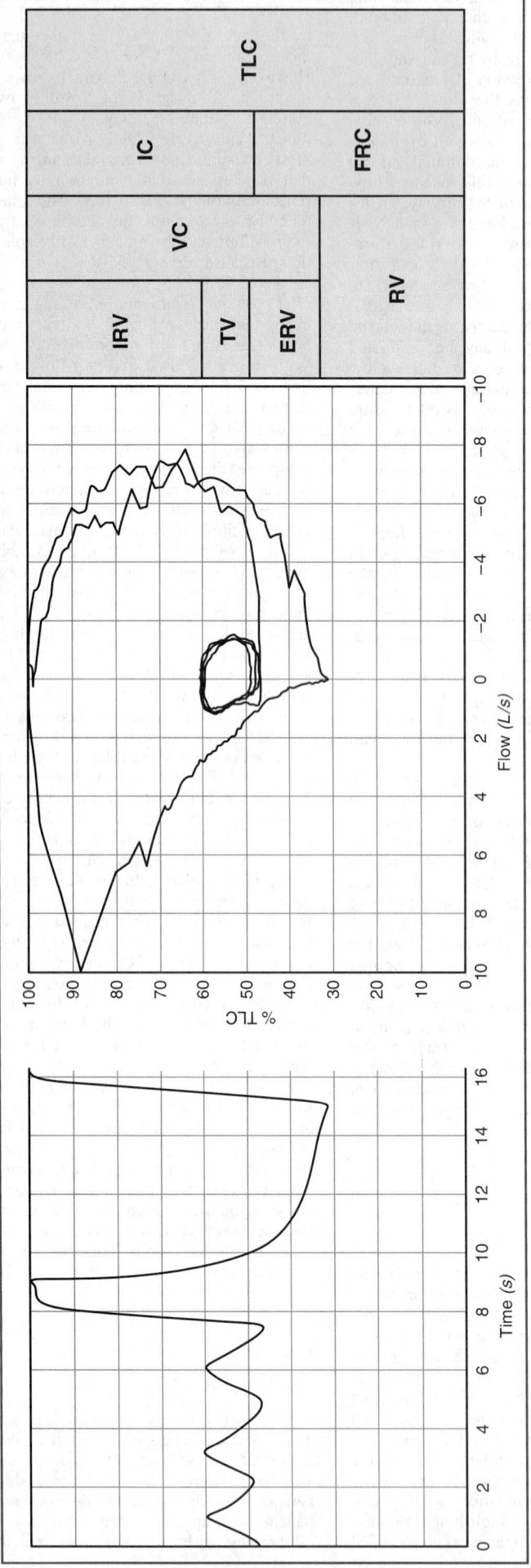

FIGURE 75–1 ■ On the left is a spirogram tracing of inspired and expired volume as a function of time. In the middle is a plot of inspiratory and expiratory flow as a function of volume. On the right are the static lung volumes defined by spirometry and an independent measure of absolute lung volume, which is defined as the gas contained in the respiratory system from the upper airway to the alveolar region. The data on the spirogram are for a normal 65-year-old subject breathing quietly, then making a maximal inspiration and an expiration using maximal expiratory effort. The flow-volume curve for the maximal expiratory effort shows that flow initially rises quickly to a maximum and then decreases monotonically and almost linearly with expired volume. Maximal flow is much greater than the flow utilized during quiet breathing. The nomenclature for the lung volumes in the block diaphragm on the right is presented in Chapter 73.

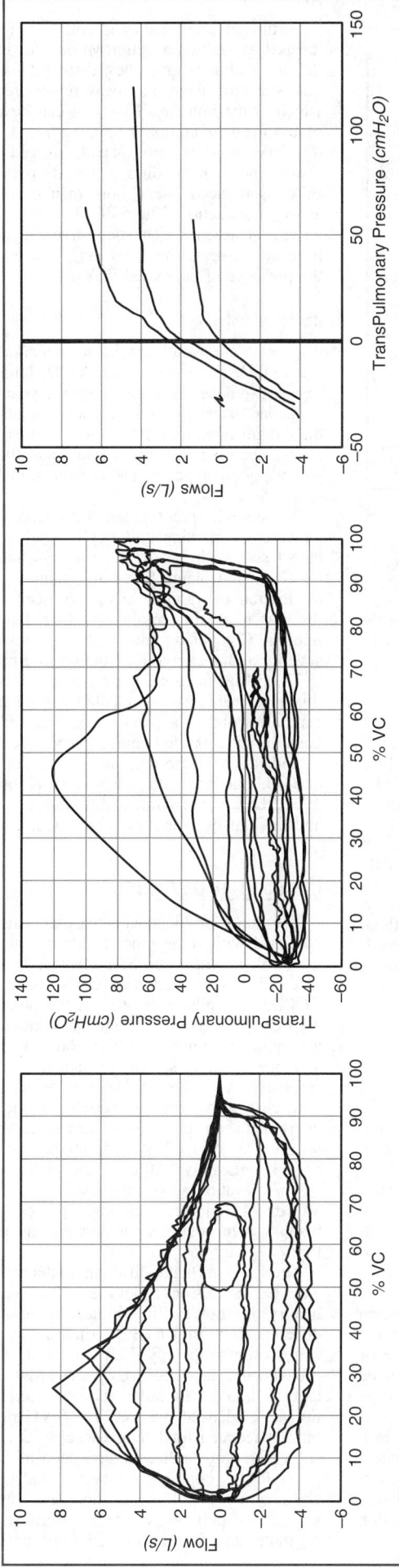

FIGURE 75–2 ■ This figure shows data obtained from a normal 65-year-old man. The left panel shows flow as a function of lung volume during successive vital capacities of increasing effort. The middle panel shows pleural pressure estimated from measurements of intraesophageal pressure measured simultaneously, also plotted against volume. Inspiratory flow increases monotonically with effort at all volumes, but expiratory flow over the lower two-thirds of the vital capacity (VC) increases over the first few efforts and then becomes constant during subsequent efforts. The pressure-volume relationships on the right confirm variable expiratory effort at volumes at which flow is constant. This phenomenon is more clearly displayed in the right panel in which simultaneously measured pressure and flow are plotted at 25%, 50%, and 75% of expired VC. This figure delineates the physiologic parameters important for the understanding of COPD. At zero flow, the pleural pressure decreases with increasing lung volume, reflecting the static elastic recoil pressure-volume relationship of the lung. At higher lung volumes, the initial slope of the pressure-flow relationship is steeper, because airway diameter is larger when the difference between pleural airway pressure is larger. Inspiratory flow increases monotonically but monotonically, with increasingly negative pleural pressures. In contrast, during expiration, flow increases with increasing pleural pressure only until a threshold value is reached, and then it becomes fixed. For efforts exceeding this threshold value, maximal flow is determined by intrinsic properties of the lung and not by effort; therefore, maximal flow is a measure of lung properties. The properties that determine maximal flow are the elastic recoil of the lung (the zero flow intercept on this figure) and the size of the airways at each recoil, which determines the slope of the pressure-flow curve. Thus, maximal flow can be reduced because of a reduced airway size and a decreased pressure-flow slope (chronic bronchitis) or from a reduced lung recoil (emphysema). In this normal person, the recoil for the curve with the lowest flow occurred when 75% of VC was expired, which is about 50% of normal TLC. In a patient with severe emphysema, this same lung recoil and maximal flow may occur at a volume above 100% of predicted total lung capacity (TLC).

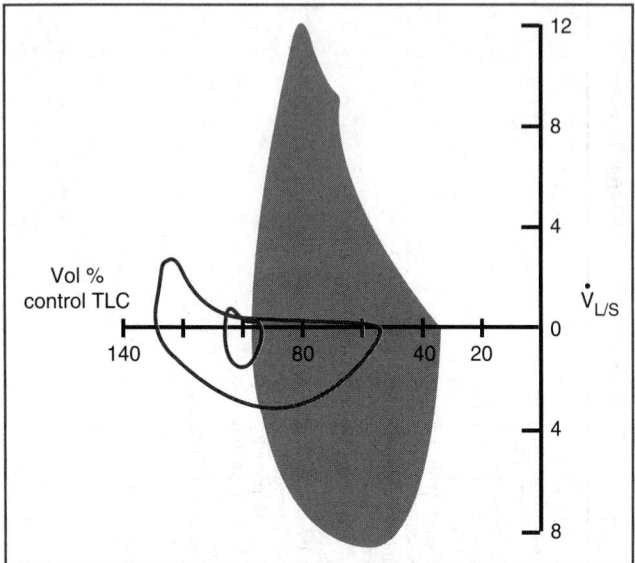

FIGURE 75–3 ■ Flow-volume relationships during quiet breathing and maximal effort in a normal individual and an individual with moderately severe emphysema. The shaded area reflects normal relationships. The lines show tidal and maximal flow-volume relationships in moderately severe COPD. Total lung capacity (TLC) and residual volume (RV) are increased, and vital capacity (VC) is decreased. The patient is using maximal expiratory flow during quiet breathing. Expiratory flow can be increased to meet the ventilatory demands of exercise only by breathing at even higher lung volumes.

nary disease will complain of mild shortness of breath on a questionnaire because they cannot comfortably do as much as they previously did because of age, obesity, or deconditioning. Therefore, the specificity and sensitivity of chronic cough, mild dyspnea, and even sputum production are low.

PHYSICAL EXAMINATION. Physical signs can be minimal or nonexistent. Patients with excessive secretions may have rhonchi (predominantly expiratory) due to secretions in large airways, but they do not necessarily have reduced maximal flow. Conversely, breath sounds can be normal to reduced in intensity without wheezes or rhonchi. Even the most experienced pulmonary physicians specializing in care of patients with airway obstruction cannot accurately assess mild to moderate reductions in maximal expiratory flow on clinical examination.

Moderate to Severe Disease

HISTORY. Experienced clinicians often miss moderate to severe disease in patients who seek medical attention for unrelated conditions and do not complain of chronic cough or dyspnea. However, by the time FEV_1 falls below 50% of predicted, most patients experience significant symptoms. Nevertheless, patients may not complain of dyspnea because they avoid activities that produce it.

PHYSICAL EXAMINATION. Because patients are breathing at very high lung volumes, they may appear to have a barrel chest at rest similar to a normal person at maximal inflation. Patients commonly have an increased respiratory rate, and close inspection reveals use of the strap muscles in their neck during inspiration. They may show jugular venous distention during expiration when semirecumbent. The left ventricular border may be medial to the left midclavicular line, and heart sounds are often faint because of hyperinflation. The pulmonic second sound may be accentuated relative to the aortic second sound. The level of a diaphragm, as judged by percussion in the posterior chest wall, may move less than 2 cm between maximal inspiration and expiration. Breath sounds may be barely audible, or there may be high-pitched wheezing during expiration. With end-stage emphysema, patients generally lose weight. With extreme increases in lung volume, the lower rib cage may move inward during inspiration because contraction of the diaphragm may pull the rib cage inward.

Spirometry

Fortunately, spirometry is both a simple and inexpensive screening test as well as a definitive diagnostic test for COPD. Although the flow-volume curves best display the physiologic parameters, the gold standard diagnostic measurement remains the traditional FEV_1, which is the volume of air that can be exhaled in the first second of a forced expiration beginning at TLC (see Chapter 73). Since the FEV_1 must be less than the forced vital capacity (FVC), it is also reduced in conditions that decrease all lung volumes. If the FEV_1 is reduced much more than the FVC, then the diagnosis is airway obstruction. The FVC is also reduced as RV increases with airway obstruction. The definitive diagnosis of airway obstruction is to demonstrate that total lung capacity is normal or increased in the presence of decreased FEV_1.

Radiologic Studies

Routine chest radiographs are remarkably insensitive for diagnosing COPD. In far-advanced COPD, lung peripheral vascular markings are reduced, the diaphragm appears flattened, the rib cage is expanded laterally, and the heart appears small because the low diaphragm makes the heart more vertical than normal. Increased air is also seen between the sternum and the heart on lateral views. In patients with hypoxia, the central pulmonary arteries are enlarged (Fig. 75–4).

Patients with predominantly bronchitis may show increased bronchovascular markings, although less than those observed with bronchiectasis. With panlobular emphysema, bullae can often be detected on the plain chest radiograph. In less severe cases, a slight diminution of vascular markings occurs in the outer one-third of the lung relative to midlung regions, but this is an extremely subtle finding. Computed tomography is the best method to assess the severity and anatomic distribution of emphysema (Fig. 75–5).

The diffusion capacity for carbon monoxide (DL_{CO}) measures the flux of tracer doses of inhaled carbon monoxide into the alveolar capillaries and is a measure of perfused alveolar capillary surface area. In patients with mild to moderate obstruction, DL_{CO} provides an indication of the contribution of emphysema to airway obstruction. In patients with severe airway obstruction (FEV_1 less than 40%), however, technical difficulties arise in performing the test, and low values cannot be interpreted.

DIFFERENTIAL DIAGNOSIS

The major problem with the diagnosis of COPD is not that it is confused with some other condition, but, like hypertension, that it is not diagnosed at all. Some have extended this analogy to suggest that FEV_1 should be "the fifth vital sign." Due to the seriousness of COPD, its insidious onset, and the potential to halt its progression with early diagnosis, the emphasis should be on case finding in the asymptomatic phase. With the advent of microprocessors, accurate and inexpensive spirometry should be generally available. All smokers, ex-smokers without a recent measurement, and persons with chronic or recurrent cough, dyspnea on exertion, or wheezing or rhonchi on physical examination should undergo spirometric testing. A normal FEV_1 for all practical purposes excludes clinically significant COPD. If the FEV_1 is associated with a reduced FEV_1/VC ratio and is not caused by a concomitant reduction in the VC due to another pathologic process involving the lungs, chest wall, or neuromuscular apparatus, the patient has airway obstruction.

The most difficult differential diagnosis is asthma (see Chapter 74). No confusion should exist in the young individual with a history of atopy and intermittent symptoms. Elderly-onset asthma is differentiated from COPD primarily by the degree of reversibility in response to therapy. Left ventricular failure (see Chapter 47) can produce dyspnea and even acute onset of wheezing, so-called cardiac asthma. Heart failure patients frequently have airway obstruction as evidenced by low FEV_1/FVC ratio, but they typically also have a reduced total lung capacity. On physical examination, they show signs of cardiac failure, such as cardiomegaly, an S_3 gallop, and rales, as opposed to wheezes and rhonchi on auscultation. The chest radiograph shows cardiomegaly and pulmonary vascular congestion or pulmonary edema. Because of the dominant role of cigarette smoking in the etiology of both COPD and ischemic

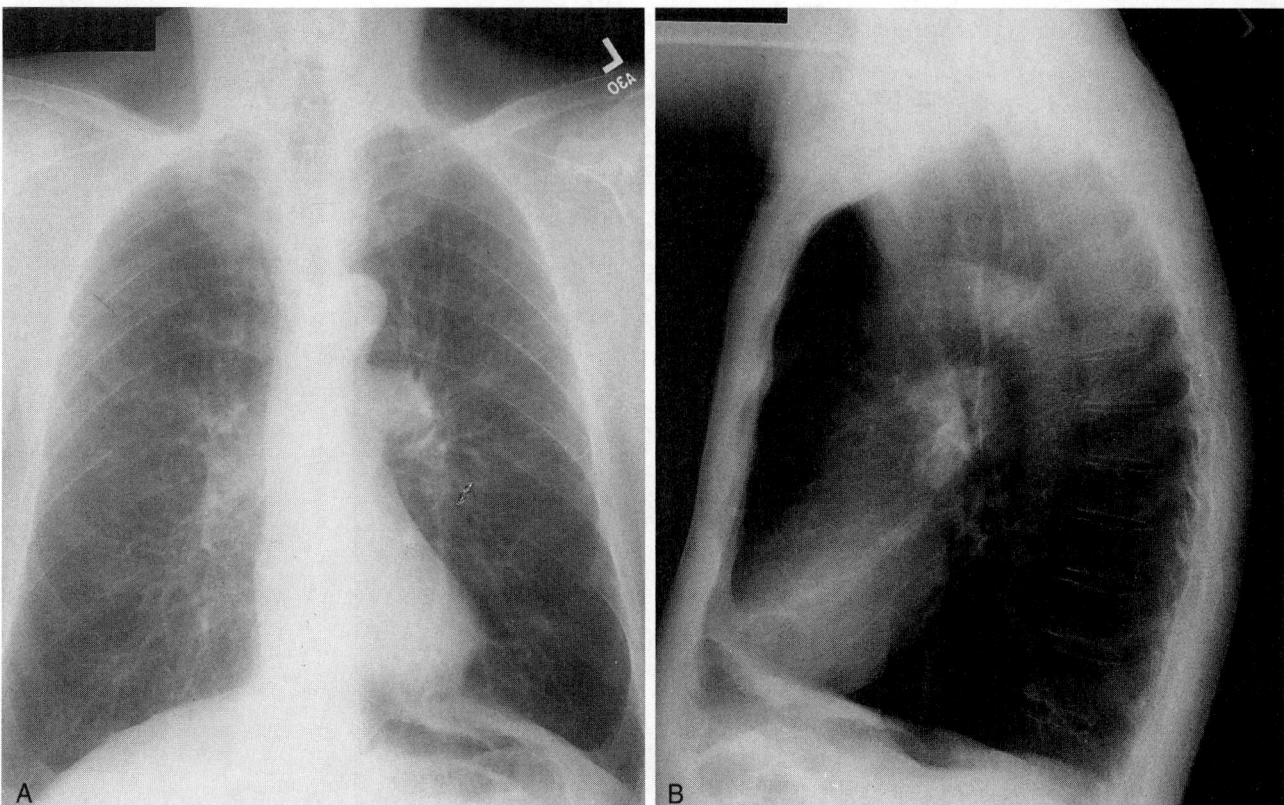

FIGURE 75–4 ■ Posteroanterior (PA) and lateral roentgenograms of the thorax in a patient with emphysema. The most obvious abnormalities are those associated with increased lung volume. The lungs appear dark because of increase air relative to tissue. The diaphragms are caudal to their normal position and appear flatter than normal. The heart is oriented more vertically than normal because of caudal displacement of the diaphragm, and the transverse diameter of the rib cage is increased; as a result, the width of the heart relative to the rib cage on the PA view is decreased. The space between the sternum and the heart and great vessels is increased on the lateral view.

cardiomyopathy, they frequently coexist. Other conditions that produce chronic airway obstruction, such as cystic fibrosis (see Chapter 76), bronchiectasis (see Chapter 77), immotile cilia syndrome, and chondromalacia, are identified by their additional features. Intrinsic or extrinsic lesions that obstruct the major airways, trachea, and larynx are rare but are commonly mistaken for asthma in younger individuals and COPD in older individuals. Extrathoracic conditions (see Chapter 515) are commonly characterized by inspiratory stridor; with spirometry, inspiratory flow is reduced much more than expiratory flow. Intrathoracic tracheal lesions cause characteristic alteration of the flow-volume curve in which the normal dependence of expiratory flow on lung volume is not present (see Chapter 73).

TREATMENT

Current recommendations of the American Thoracic Society (Fig. 75–6) include commonly used but controversial treatments for which no good efficacy data exist. For subjects who are still smoking, cessation is the most important intervention to alter the clinical course.

COPD is incurable. Lung function declines with age in normal persons; in smokers who develop COPD, the decline is greatly accelerated. Patients who are identified and quit smoking in the presymptomatic stage experience only modest improvement in lung function, but thereafter, the rate of decline in quitters parallels that in normal individuals. In non-smokers, FEV_1 declines 30 to 40 mL/year. In smokers, the annual decline may be threefold to fourfold greater. Early detection through screening of at-risk individuals will delay or even prevent the onset of symptoms and disability if smoking is discontinued as a result; cigarette smoking is a difficult addiction to treat (see Chapter 13), but some patients will be given incentive to quit after being informed by a physician that they have lung disease caused by their smoking.

Most patients with COPD have at least some increase in FEV_1 with bronchodilators, and many others can be shown to have a therapeutic effect with more sensitive physiologic tests. Virtually all patients with symptomatic COPD are prescribed chronic inhaled bronchodilator therapy. Drug administration by the inhalation route

FIGURE 75–5 ■ High-resolution computed axial tomographic 1-mm thick cross-section of the thorax of a patient with emphysema. Rather than bronchi and blood vessels surrounded by homogeneous gray parenchyma, multiple dark holes alternate with less involved parenchyma. The superior segments of the lower lobes are located posteriorly in both hemithoraces. The right lung (on the left in the figure) is more diseased than the left lung.

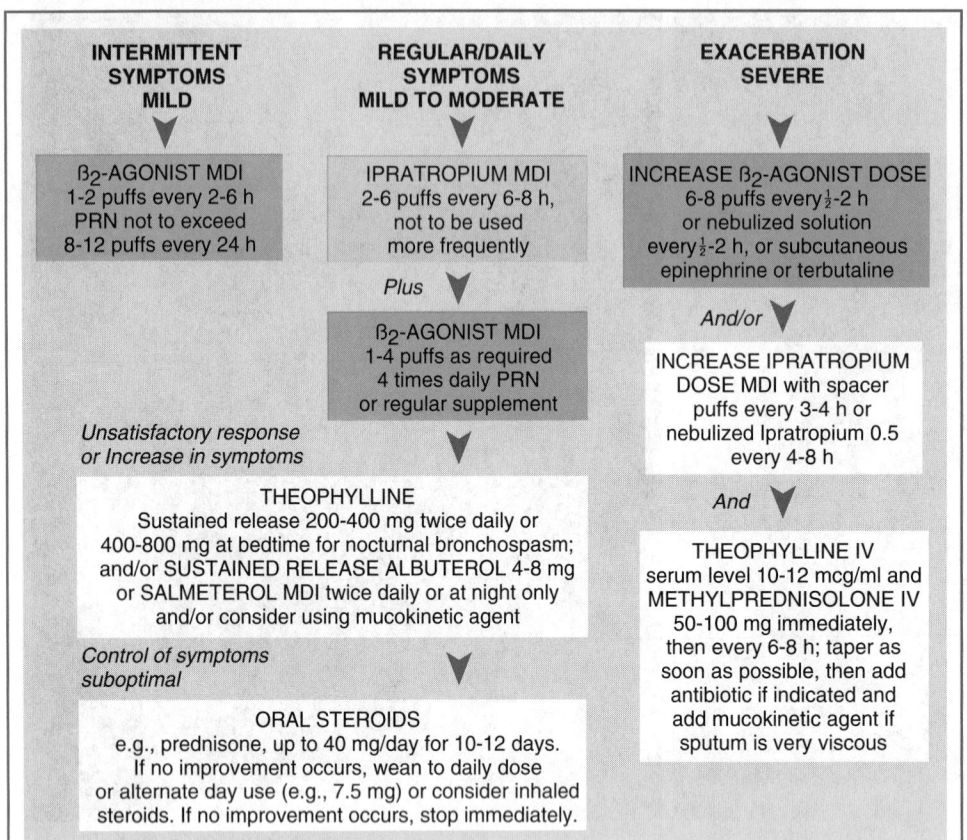

FIGURE 75–6 ■ Approach to the treatment of COPD.

minimizes systemic side effects. In contrast with asthma, patients with COPD are usually more responsive to anticholinergic medications than to β_2-agonists. Systemic anticholinergic agents are problematic in elderly men because of the risk of urinary retention and glaucoma. However, nonabsorbable anticholinergics, such as ipratropium, administered by metered-dose inhaler (MDI) 3 to 4 times a day, have local effects with minimal systemic absorption. Highly specific β_2-agonists, such as albuterol, have minimal cardiac effects. In moderate to severe disease, both drugs are recommended, and combination therapy in a single MDI has recently become available.

Because many patients with COPD have features of asthma, patients with severe exacerbations are frequently given therapeutic trials of systemic steroids (20 to 30 mg/day of prednisone); some patients whose disease has a reversible component have a beneficial response in terms of improved pulmonary function, and at 10 to 20 mg/day can be continued if needed. Many physicians prescribe inhaled nonabsorbable steroids, the newest of which is fluticasone, taken by MDI twice daily, chronically for COPD patients, although efficacy has not been demonstrated by well-designed clinical trials. In the past, oral theophylline, 300 mg twice daily in a long-acting formulation, was used in COPD because the long-acting oral formulation provided bronchodilatation throughout the night. However, theophylline is a relatively weak bronchodilator with a narrow margin between therapeutic and toxic ranges, and its use is decreasing now that long-acting β-agonists, such as salmeterol, given by MDI, have become available. Various expectorants and cough suppressants have been employed for symptomatic relief, but none is of proven efficacy; they are rarely routinely prescribed by pulmonologists.

The clinical course of COPD is marked by exacerbations that appear to be infectious, with increased dyspnea and sputum production. The sputum changes from clear or white to purulent, and increased neutrophils are present on the sputum smear. Bacterial sputum cultures are often positive for potential pathogens, such as *Haemophilus influenzae*, but these findings are difficult to interpret because the patients' lower airways are frequently colonized by

bacteria. The patients do not commonly have significant fever or an increase in chronic low-grade neutrophilic leukocytosis. Sometimes these exacerbations may lead to frank bacterial pneumonia, which is frequently a terminal event. Most pulmonary physicians believe it is important to intervene early in the course of an exacerbation with antibiotics (e.g., azithromycin [Zithromax], 250 mg twice daily on the first day and every day thereafter for 5 days) and short courses of oral steroids.

Patients with COPD are susceptible to bacterial and viral pneumonia, which, because of already-reduced lung function, carry a high risk of mortality in these patients. Therefore, all COPD patients should have pneumococcal vaccinations and annual influenza vaccinations. COPD patients with arterial PO_2 less than 50 mm Hg at rest are subject to development of pulmonary hypertension and right ventricular failure (cor pulmonale). Continuous oxygen therapy has been demonstrated to prolong life in these patients.

Patients who experience oxygen (O_2) desaturation with exercise should use O_2 during exercise. In most patients, O_2 saturations decrease during sleep. Patients with PO_2 not justifying continuous O_2 therapy should have overnight O_2 saturation monitored by percutaneous oximetry; O_2 should be used during sleep if necessary to maintain saturation at 90% or more. In most COPD patients, O_2 saturation can be restored to near normal by low-flow (1 to 2 L/minute) O_2 delivered by nasal cannula. Portable liquid O_2 systems are compact and lightweight, so that even debilitated patients can carry them using a shoulder strap or can drag them on wheels without much difficulty.

Optimal medical care for advanced COPD includes pulmonary rehabilitation. Pulmonary rehabilitation does not improve lung function, but it does increase sustainable exercise capacity and improve quality of life. Many patients with COPD are debilitated and depressed. They become anxious and are frightened by their dyspnea. Pulmonary rehabilitation improves their physical fitness, teaches them to accomplish activities of daily living with less dyspnea, educates them about their disease, increases their sense of power and control, and reduces anxiety. Group sessions provide effective therapy for situational depression and identify individuals with major depression who will benefit from referral to a psychiatrist.

Potential surgical options for patients with COPD include focal tissue lung resections or lung transplantation (see Chapter 89). Lung reduction surgery is currently the subject of a multi-center trial.

PROGNOSIS

Many patients with end-stage disease ($FEV_1 < 35\%$) seem to stabilize and maintain that level of function for a number of years. This clinical observation is probably largely a survivor effect in that patients with function at this level whose FEV_1 decreases by more than 100 mL/year do not survive. Patients may survive several exacerbations, even requiring mechanical ventilation, before succumbing to the disease. Many deaths from COPD are from respiratory complications associated with other conditions that would have much lower mortality if not complicated by concurrent COPD.

ACCP/AACVPR Pulmonary Rehabilitation Guidelines Panel: Pulmonary rehabilitation: Joint ACCP/AACVPR evidence-based guidelines. Chest 112:1363–1396, 1997. *Includes review of the evidence base for the efficacy of the various components of pulmonary rehabilitation.*

American Thoracic Society: Standards for the diagnosis and care of patients with chronic obstructive pulmonary disease. Am J Respir Crit Care Med 152 (5 suppl): S77–S120, 1995. *Official statement on terminology, diagnostic criteria, and treatment guidelines.*

Niederman MS: Introduction: Mechanisms and management of COPD: We can do better—it's time for a re-evaluation. Chest 113(suppl 4):233S–283S, 1998. *State-of-the-art review of COPD.*

Utz JP, Hubmayr RD, Deschamps C: Lung volume reduction surgery for emphysema: Out on a limb without a NETT. Mayo Clin Proc 73:552–566, 1998. *Review of the history, rationale, and results of surgery for emphysema up to the time of publication.*

76 CYSTIC FIBROSIS

Michael J. Welsh

DEFINITION

Cystic fibrosis (CF) is an autosomal recessive genetic disease caused by mutations in the gene encoding the cystic fibrosis transmembrane conductance regulator (CFTR). It is relatively common, with an incidence of 1 in 2000 to 3000 whites; and approximately 30,000 persons in the United States are affected. It is estimated that about 1 in 20 to 25 whites carry mutations in the CFTR gene; carriers are completely asymptomatic. The disease affects several different organs, but most of current morbidity and 90 to 95% of mortality result from chronic pulmonary infections. Pancreatic insufficiency is also a common cause of morbidity.

HISTORICAL PERSPECTIVE

The first known reference to CF is an adage from northern European folklore: "Woe to that child which when kissed on the forehead tastes salty. He is bewitched and soon must die." That saying describes the salty sweat that is the basis of an important diagnostic test and early mortality. The first pathologic and clinical description came in 1938, when the disease was called cystic fibrosis of the pancreas. The severity and frequency of lung disease was soon appreciated. Since then, marked improvements have occurred in diagnosis, clinical management, understanding, and treatment of the disease. As a result, the current median survival is approximately 30 years.

In addition to its importance as a clinical disease, the study of CF is important because it provides an instructive example of the pathway of discovery in the investigation of a genetic disease. Because it was one of the earliest diseases identified by positional cloning, a review of the advances, problems, and opportunities that physicians and scientists have encountered since discovery of the

CFTR gene may presage events that will be repeated and varied as an increasing number of disease-associated genes are discovered.

PATHOGENESIS AND PATHOLOGY

The gene for CFTR was positionally cloned in 1989. The gene encodes a 1480 amino acid protein that belongs to a family of proteins called *a*denosine triphosphate (ATP) *b*inding *c*assette (ABC) transporters. Several members of this family are clinically important including the multidrug resistance protein (MDR), the sulfonylurea receptor (SUR), the transporter associated with antigen processing (TAP-1/TAP-2), and the Stargardt macular dystrophy protein (ABCR). Although most ABC transporters form membrane pumps, CFTR forms a Cl^- permeable ion channel that is regulated by phosphorylation. It contains five domains: two membrane-spanning domains, each composed of six membrane spanning sequences, that contribute to the formation of the Cl^- conducting pore; two nucleotide-binding domains that bind and hydrolyze ATP to gate the channel; and a regulatory (R) domain that stimulates channel opening when it is phosphorylated by cyclic adenosine monophosphate (cAMP) dependent kinase. CFTR is located in the apical (lumen-facing) membrane of epithelium in the pulmonary airways, pancreatic duct, intestine, and biliary ducts, and in the apical and basolateral membranes of the sweat gland duct (Fig. 76–1).

The most common CF mutation is a 3 base pair deletion that causes the loss of a phenylalanine at position 508 (ΔF508). The ΔF508 mutation occurs on about 70% of CF chromosomes; the percentage is somewhat higher in persons of northern European descent. More than 700 other mutations and variations have been discovered in the gene, with only a handful accounting for more than 1% of mutations. CFTR protein with the ΔF508 mutation is made in the endoplasmic reticulum, but it is misfolded. As a result, it is recognized by the cellular quality control system, which prevents its traffic to the Golgi complex and then the apical membrane, instead targeting it for degradation by the proteosome. Although it is not normally delivered to the cell membrane, the ΔF508 protein retains significant Cl^- channel activity. Thus, correction of the defective processing could provide a novel approach to treatment. It is now appreciated that there are four general classes of mutation. Class I mutations in the CFTR gene cause the loss of CFTR Cl^- channel activity by generating an incomplete messenger RNA (mRNA) due to premature stop signals, frame shifts, and abnormal splice sites. Class II mutations, such as ΔF508, cause misfolding. Class III and IV mutations generate correctly localized proteins, which either do not open appropriately or which form pores that do not allow the normal passage of Cl^-, respectively. At least some of the variability in the clinical disease can be explained by variations in the severity of the specific mutation. However, other genes and environmental factors may modify the clinical course. Thus at the present time it is not possible to counsel patients accurately about prognosis based on their genotype.

Knowledge that CFTR is an epithelial Cl^- channel, combined with an appreciation of the epithelial physiology of organs affected by the disease has allowed some insight into the pathogenesis and manifestations of the disease (Fig. 76–2). The water impermeable sweat gland duct absorbs NaCl through Na^+ channels and CFTR Cl^- channels as sweat flows from the secretory coil to the surface of the skin. In CF, loss of CFTR prevents absorption of Cl^- and, because of the requirements for electroneutrality, absorption of Na^+. As a result, sweat emerges onto the skin with high Cl^- and Na^+ concentrations. In pancreatic ducts, CFTR Cl^- channels are important for alkalinization and hydration of the pancreatic secretions as they flow from the pancreatic acinar cells to the intestine. In CF, loss of CFTR prevents this process and causes obstruction of the small pancreatic ducts, thereby blocking the output of pancreatic enzymes. Ultimately the organ atrophies. A similar scenario appears to apply in the liver; loss of CFTR Cl^- channels disrupts normal salt and water balance in the small biliary ducts, causing their obstruction. It seems likely that obstruction of the small ducts in the male genital tract also leads to the atrophy, fibrosis, or absence of the vas deferens, tail and body of the epididymis, and seminal vesicles. In the ileum, CFTR Cl^- channels play a central

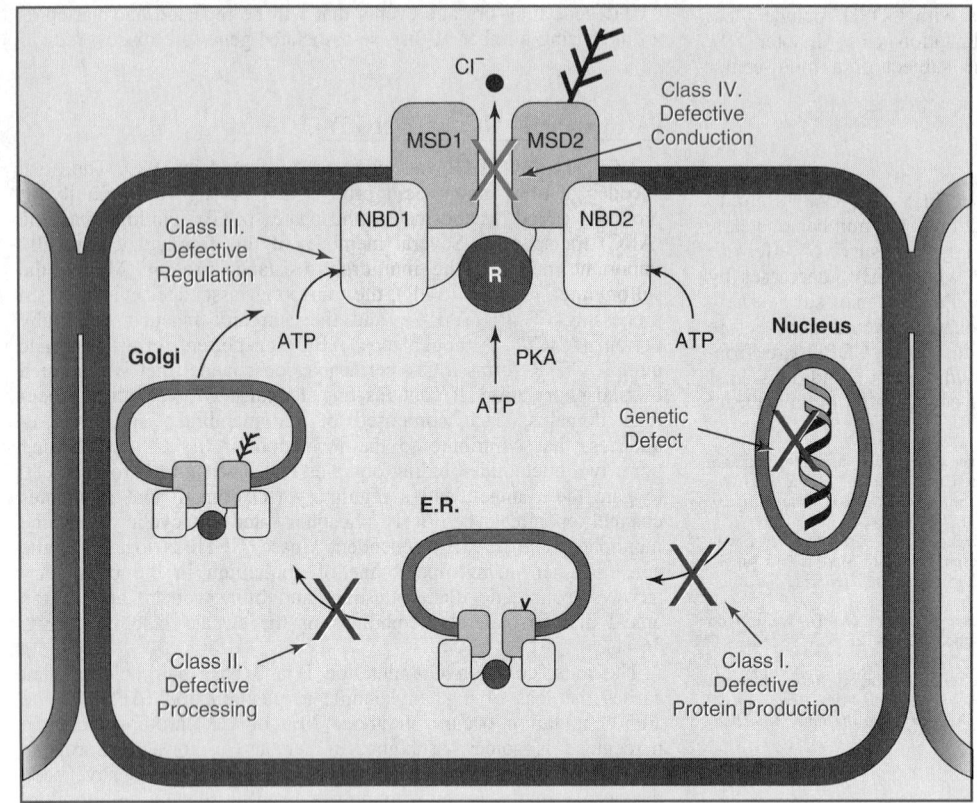

FIGURE 76–1 ▪ Biosynthesis and function of CFTR in an epithelial cell. Glycosylation is indicated by the orange branched structure. Domains of CFTR are labeled as MSD (membrane-spanning domains), NBD (nucleotide-binding domains), and R (regulatory domain). Loss of CFTR function can result from four different classes of mutation. The ΔF505 mutation is a class II defect. (From Welsh MJ, Smith AE: Molecular mechanisms of CFTR chloride channel dysfunction in cystic fibrosis. Cell 73:1251–1254, 1993.)

role in salt and water secretion. Disruption of this process is thought to produce thick, dehydrated intestinal contents that obstruct the ileum in the newborn, causing meconium ileus and producing meconium ileus-equivalent later in life.

Repeated bacterial infections of the airways, the hallmark of CF lung disease, are due to a host defense defect localized to the lung; normal lungs transplanted into a CF patient do not become infected, patients are not predisposed to infections elsewhere, and antibiotics are the most effective treatment. Normal lungs are protected from inhaled and aspirated bacteria by several defense systems, including mucociliary clearance, phagocytic cells (such as macrophages and neutrophils), and the innate immune system, consisting of several antimicrobial factors. These factors include lysozyme, lactoferrin, and small peptides, such as β-defensins. In CF, the activity of antimicrobial factors may be inhibited by an increased NaCl concentration in the thin layer of liquid covering the airway surface. Inhibition of the antimicrobial activity of the innate immune system might give inhaled bacteria an advantage in colonizing the airway surface. Other hypotheses to explain the patho-

genesis of CF airway disease include increased binding of bacteria to CF airway epithelial cells, reduced mucociliary clearance in CF, increased Na$^+$ absorption with dehydration of airway surface liquid, and defective phagocytosis of bacteria in CF.

Chronic infection is associated with an intense inflammatory response with an abundance of neutrophils. A profusion of cytokines and proinflammatory stimuli also lead to submucosal gland hypertrophy and increased mucus output. The combination of increased mucus, abundant neutrophils, and inflammatory debris that includes DNA, actin, and other macromolecules produces a thick, viscous, purulent sputum that obstructs airways. The progressive inflammation and infection damage the airways, leading to bronchitis, progressive bronchiectasis, and respiratory failure.

CLINICAL MANIFESTATIONS

Patients with CF can present at several ages with a variety of clinical manifestations. For example, they may present as newborns with meconium ileus, as infants or children with failure to thrive, or from childhood to adulthood with recurrent respiratory tract infections. These and other symptoms can mimic those found in a variety of other diseases.

Lung Disease

Clinical Presentation

Cough is usually the earliest manifestation. At first it is intermittent, occurring with what appear to be acute respiratory illnesses. Coughing is worse at night and on awakening. The cough is sometimes accompanied by wheezing, particularly in infants and young children. Episodes of cough tend to persist longer than expected for an acute respiratory illness and, with time, occur more and more frequently. As the disease progresses, the cough becomes productive of thick, purulent, often green sputum. Patients may have symptoms of bronchitis for several years or even a decade or two. Eventually, however, exacerbations of cough and sputum production are accompanied by dyspnea, reduced appetite, and weight loss. Exercise tolerance decreases as the disease progresses. Acute exacerbations improve with intensive therapy but tend to increase in frequency and severity until the patient develops symptoms of

FIGURE 76–2 ▪ Model of electrolyte transport by normal and CF airway epithelium. The apical membrane of normal epithelium contains CFTR Cl$^-$ channels and ENaC Na$^+$ channels. The paracellular pathway between the cells through the tight junctions also shows some permeability to ions.

bronchiectasis (see Chapter 77). Physical findings depend on the stage of the disease. At first crackles are intermittent, occurring with exacerbations. Lung sounds may be decreased due to hyperinflation. As the disease progresses, rales and rhonchi are common and continuous.

Laboratory Evaluation

SPUTUM CULTURE. Early in the disease, CF airways become colonized with bacteria, which are virtually impossible to eliminate. *Staphylococcus aureus* and *Haemophilus influenzae* are often found initially. However, with time *Pseudomonas aeruginosa* becomes very common, often as a mucoid species. Although mucoid *P. aeruginosa* is occasionally cultured from patients with other lung diseases, its presence in sputum should immediately alert the physician to the possibility of CF. *Burkholderia cepacia* is also common in CF, especially later in the course of the disease. Quantitative sputum cultures are sometimes of value in evaluating the response to antibiotic therapy.

RADIOLOGIC EVALUATION. With standard chest radiographs, hyperinflation may be the first finding, followed by peribronchial cuffing, which creates linear opacities. Impaction of mucus and changes consistent with bronchiectasis are observed as the disease progresses. For reasons that remain unknown, the right upper lobe is often the first and most severely involved. High-resolution chest computed tomography (CT) reveals early changes of bronchiectasis that may be widespread before conventional radiographs show any change. Hilar adenopathy is uncommon. Changes of pulmonary hypertension become obvious late in the disease.

PULMONARY FUNCTION. The first changes are of airways obstruction, particularly of the small airways. Spirometry shows reduced air flow rates, including a decreased forced expiratory volume in one second (FEV_1), FEV_1/forced vital capacity (FVC) ratio, and maximal midexpiratory flow (MMEF). The ratio of residual volume to total lung capacity is often increased. Changes consistent with airway obstruction may even be present in infants. Evidence of airway hyperreactivity is common. The arterial PO_2 tends to decrease with time due to ventilation-perfusion mismatching. Only in the late-stage disease is the PCO_2 increased and chronic respiratory acidosis apparent. The course of the disease and the response to therapy are often followed by serial measurement of spirometry, lung volumes, and oxygenation.

Complications

PNEUMOTHORAX. Pneumothorax (see Chapter 86) is a well-recognized complication, and the incidence increases with age. Although it is occasionally an incidental finding on the chest radiograph, it is often associated with chest pain, dyspnea, and hemoptysis. Indications for chest tube placement are the same as for pneumothorax from other causes. The rate of recurrence is high; pleural sclerosis may be required to prevent recurrences.

HEMOPTYSIS. Hemoptysis becomes common as patients develop bronchiectasis. Blood-streaked sputum is the most frequent finding. Massive hemoptysis occurs in approximately 1% of patients and is usually associated with an exacerbation of the chronic respiratory infection. Treatment is usually directed at the underlying pulmonary disease; but when hemoptysis is life-threatening, surgery or bronchial artery embolization may be required.

DIGITAL CLUBBING. Digital clubbing, which occurs in nearly all patients with CF, is often discovered at the time the lung disease becomes symptomatic. Hypertrophic pulmonary osteoarthropathy may occur in up to 15% of patients, especially adolescents and adults; its symptoms may correlate with exacerbations of the pulmonary disease.

UPPER AIRWAY DISEASE. Loss of CFTR function in airway epithelium causes disease not only of the intrapulmonary airways but also of the upper airways. Chronic rhinitis is very common. The sinuses are almost universally involved, as evidenced by opacification on plain radiography or magnetic resonance imaging (MRI), but acute or chronic sinusitis is not common. Nasal polyps occur in 15 to 20% of patients and occasionally require resection to prevent nasal obstruction. Of note, epithelial cells isolated from resected nasal polyps are critical in producing model systems used in research on pathogenesis and novel therapies. When surgery is scheduled to resect nasal polyps, a CF research center should be contacted, as the polyps are a valuable research resource.

ALLERGIC BRONCHOPULMONARY ASPERGILLOSIS (see

Chapter 401). Although more than 50% of patients have antibodies to *Aspergillus fumigatus,* only a small number develop allergic aspergillosis. Expectoration of rusty brown sputum plugs is suggestive of this condition.

COR PULMONALE. Late in the disease, untreated hypoxemia and progressive loss of functional lung may produce pulmonary artery hypertension and right ventricular failure (see Chapter 56).

RESPIRATORY FAILURE. Respiratory failure becomes increasingly difficult to manage as the disease worsens. Because patients with CF rely on cough to clear their airways, they often respond poorly to mechanical ventilation, which is generally instituted only if there is an acute or reversible precipitating event.

Pancreatic Disease

Failure of the exocrine pancreas (see Chapter 141) occurs in approximately 85% of patients. It is almost universal in patients homozygous for the ΔF508 mutation. Some mutations appear to produce CFTR with sufficient residual function to prevent complete pancreatic failure, although the pancreas is usually not normal. Obstruction of ducts, loss of acinar cells, and pancreatic enzyme deficiency lead to malabsorption of protein, fat, and fat-soluble vitamins. Bulky, foul-smelling stools are often difficult to flush. If left untreated, patients with pancreatic insufficiency may show a failure to thrive, weight loss, and growth inhibition. Weight loss can also be associated with severe respiratory disease and an increased work of breathing.

Symptoms of pancreatitis (see Chapter 141) occur in a small percentage of adolescents and adults, particularly patients who have retained some pancreatic function. Although the islets of Langerhans are relatively spared, destruction of the pancreas can cause endocrine pancreatic dysfunction in approximately 7% of all patients and is more common in adults. The presentation of symptomatic hyperglycemia is similar for patients with CF and type 1 diabetes. If diabetes occurs, insulin therapy should be initiated because oral agents are ineffective. Interestingly, the frequency of pancreatic disease in CF led to the discovery that patients with idiopathic and chronic pancreatitis have a higher than expected frequency of mutations in the CFTR gene, despite the absence of other findings of CF.

Gastrointestinal Disease

Symptoms of gastrointestinal disease are common in CF, although they are rarely life-threatening if properly managed. Meconium ileus, which occurs in approximately 18% of CF newborns, is virtually diagnostic. Small bowel obstruction, "distal intestinal obstruction syndrome," occurs in approximately 3% of patients, and intermittent abdominal pain, perhaps from partial obstruction, is much more common. Another cause of abdominal pain is intussusception, which usually requires surgical intervention. Rectal prolapse occurs occasionally in children but infrequently in adults.

Genitourinary Disease

More than 95% of males are sterile because of atrophy of wolffian duct structures. Spermatogenesis is intact, and retrieval of sperm has been used for in vitro fertilization. Interestingly, males with infertility due to congenital bilateral absence of the vas deferens, but no other symptoms of CF, also have an increased prevalence of mild mutations in the CFTR gene and/or sequence variations that decrease the number of functional transcripts. It may be that the vas deferens is the tissue most sensitive to a decrease in functional CFTR, followed by the lung and then the pancreas. Females with CF also have a reduced fertility due to poor nutrition, chronic lung infections, and/or the presence of a thick plug of mucus at the cervical os. Women with severely compromised pulmonary and nutritional status may show an accelerated deterioration during pregnancy.

Hepatobiliary Disease

Focal biliary cirrhosis appears to be increasing as patients live longer. The severity varies widely, with evidence in many patients limited to an elevated alkaline phosphatase level. Obstructive biliary tract disease occurs in approximately 4% of patients. In severe cases, patients develop hepatosplenomegaly, jaundice, ascites, and edema. Hematemesis from esophageal varices is a severe complication that may require endoscopy and sclerosis of affected vessels. Hepatic insufficiency may require liver transplantation.

Other Abnormalities

The increased salt loss in CF sweat can lead to salt depletion, especially with heat stress. Volume depletion and metabolic alkalosis are uncommon but serious complications. Enlarged submandibular, sublingual, and submucosal glands are commonly observed on physical examination. The parotid glands are not enlarged. Adult patients may develop osteoporosis due to poor nutrition or vitamin deficiency. Psychosocial issues in dealing with a lethal disease need to be recognized and treated appropriately.

DIAGNOSIS

Meconium ileus, pancreatic insufficiency, typical pulmonary manifestations, and/or a history of CF in the immediate family should prompt the consideration of a CF diagnosis. One or two of these, when combined with a positive sweat Cl⁻ test, make the diagnosis almost certain. Occasionally, DNA testing or measurement of the voltage across the nasal epithelium is helpful in establishing the diagnosis.

THE SWEAT Cl⁻ TEST. An increased concentration of Na^+ and Cl^- in sweat is one of the most consistent findings in CF. The sweat Cl^- should be measured by an experienced laboratory using pilocarpine iontophoresis, and it should always be repeated. A sweat Cl^- level greater than 60 mEq/L, when accompanied by the major clinical manifestations, is sufficient to make the diagnosis. Only 2% of CF patients will have a normal sweat Cl^- level.

GENETIC TESTING. If the diagnosis is strongly suspected, DNA testing may provide definitive evidence of CF. DNA testing, which is readily available from a few commercial and university laboratories, is also of value for detection of carriers, genetic counseling, and prenatal screening. Some tests that can be performed from buccal swab specimens report on 70 of the most common mutations, which yields a detection rate of approximately 90% for northern European whites.

In the absence of a positive sweat test or the detection of CF mutations on both chromosomes, evidence for the diagnosis has been established in some research laboratories by measurement of the voltage across the nasal epithelium. This test evaluates the function of CFTR Cl⁻ channels in airway epithelium.

COURSE OF THE DISEASE

The course is punctuated by exacerbations of lung disease followed by improvement with intensive therapy. Exacerbations are characterized by an increased frequency and severity of cough, increased sputum production, a change in the color or appearance of the sputum, increased dyspnea (especially with exertion), reduced appetite, and a feeling of chest congestion. These findings are accompanied by an increased respiratory rate, use of accessory muscles of respiration, and increased rales, rhonchi, and wheezes. Laboratory evaluation may show worsening pulmonary function, new infiltrates on chest radiograph, and leukocytosis.

The lung disease is progressive. Patients with an FEV_1 less than 30% predicted, an arterial Po_2 less than 55 mm Hg, or an arterial Pco_2 greater than 50 mm Hg have 2-year mortality rates above 50%. Among patients with the same FEV_1, there is a greater relative risk for females and younger patients.

TREATMENT

Antibiotics

Exacerbations of lung disease usually require an intensive course of parenteral antibiotics for 2 to 3 weeks. The choice of antibiotics is based on sputum cultures to identify and test the susceptibility of organisms. *P. aeruginosa* is a particularly common pathogen, and therefore the combination of an aminoglycoside and a β-lactam antibiotic are commonly used. Emergence of antibiotic-resistant organisms is a serious problem, especially with *P. aeruginosa* and *B. cepacia*.

Although *P. aeruginosa* is rarely eradicated, an important benefit is gained by decreasing the net bacterial load with intensive intravenous antibiotics. As the number of organisms decreases, airway inflammation is reduced, thereby decreasing airway destruction and the accompanying systemic symptoms. The response to therapy is assessed by improvement of symptoms, of pulmonary function, and, in some cases, of quantitative bacterial counts in sputum. During therapy, serum concentrations of aminoglycosides must be measured frequently, because CF patients usually require higher-than-normal antibiotic doses due to increased clearance rates and increased volumes of distribution.

Use of quinolone antibiotics has been appealing because they can be administered orally. Unfortunately, resistant strains of *P. aeruginosa* and *S. aureus* have become common. Delivery of long-term maintenance antibiotics or quarterly administration of antibiotics in an attempt to suppress chronic infection and the development of bronchiectasis is being studied. A potential risk of such strategies is more rapid development of highly resistant strains of bacteria.

Administration of antibiotics by inhalation is attractive because the concentration at the airway surface can be increased into the range required for bacterial killing, and systemic toxicity can be minimized. Using optimal nebulizers, aerosolized high-dose tobramycin can reduce the density of *P. aeruginosa* and improve FEV_1.

Chest Physiotherapy

Chest percussion and postural drainage are mainstays of treatment designed to clear purulent secretions. Other recent approaches to physiotherapy, as well as high-frequency chest compression with an inflatable vest and airway oscillation with a flutter valve, are of benefit for some patients.

Bronchodilators

Beneficial effects of β-adrenergic agonists and anticholinergic agents (see Chapters 74 and 75) have been demonstrated in short-term studies. Bronchodilator therapy should be considered during exacerbations and in hospitalized patients. However, the benefit of long-term bronchodilator therapy remains controversial.

Deoxyribonuclease

DNA released from neutrophils forms long fibrils that contribute to the viscosity of CF sputum. By cleaving the DNA, inhaled, recombinant human deoxyribonuclease I can increase the cough clearance of sputum and decrease the frequency of respiratory exacerbations that require intravenous antibiotics. It is often prescribed for patients with purulent sputum and airway obstruction.

Anti-Inflammatory Agents

Glucocorticoids have improved lung function in some studies, but adverse effects have tempered enthusiasm for their use. Very high doses of ibuprofen have been reported to slow the rate of decline in FEV_1, but frequent monitoring of serum concentrations is required, and long-term safety data are not available.

Pancreatic Enzymes and Nutrition

The frequency of pancreatic dysfunction means that pancreatic enzymes are critical for nutrition. Enzymes are administered at mealtimes as enteric-coated capsules. The number of capsules is adjusted based on weight gain or loss, abdominal cramping, and the character of stools. High doses of delayed-release pancreatic enzymes have been associated with colonic strictures. The fat-soluble vitamins A, D, and E are administered routinely, and vitamin K may be given sporadically for bleeding or to correct a prolonged prothrombin time. Patients are encouraged to eat a balanced diet, and an increase in total calories is encouraged. For some children and for patients with anorexia, supplemental feedings through percutaneous gastrostomy or duodenostomy is recommended. In general, the better the nutritional state, the slower the decline in pulmonary function.

Other Considerations

Attention should be paid to adequate salt intake during hot weather. Exercise is encouraged for its effects on the cardiovascular system, physical conditioning, and the promotion of cough. Adequate immunizations, including influenza, are mandatory. Supplemental oxygen should be given to patients with hypoxemia. Cigarette smoke, including passive smoke, should be avoided. Other air pollutants can have adverse effects, although their role in pulmonary deterioration is not certain. Lung transplantation (see Chapter 89) should be considered for patients with an FEV_1 less than 30% predicted.

Novel Treatments

Conceptually, the simplest approach to treating this disease would be to transfer a normal CFTR gene or cDNA into the affected cells. Correction of approximately 5 to 10% of airway epithelial cells could correct the electrolyte transport defect, and the airway epithelium is accessible to local inhalant delivery. Studies using recombinant viral and nonviral vectors in animals and humans indicate that gene transfer is possible, but at present it is not efficient enough. Additional problems include limited persistence of expression and development of an immune response to some vectors. Progress in this area of research has been substantial and it is hoped that successful gene therapy will become a reality. Other experimental approaches include attempts to modulate ion transport of the airway epithelium by compensating for the loss of CFTR Cl^- channels. Although amiloride has been evaluated to inhibit Na^+ transport, in multicenter trials the rate of decline in pulmonary function was not different in control and amiloride groups. Attempts to retarget CFTR containing the $\Delta F508$ mutation to the cell surface (class II mutations), to suppress stop mutations (class I), and to increase the opening of channels present at the cell surface (class III) are under investigation.

PROGNOSIS

Therapeutic regimens for CF have continued to improve. By the year 2000, nearly half of patients with CF will be adults. The dramatic improvement in the length and quality of life have been the result of aggressive treatment, attention to the details of treating a complex disease that affects numerous organs, and vigilant monitoring and treatment of early lung disease.

Crystal RG: Transfer of genes to humans: Early lessons and obstacles to success. Science 270:404–410, 1995. *Discussion of the prospects for and barriers to gene therapy of CF and other diseases.*

Davis PB, Drumm M, Konstan MW: Cystic fibrosis. Am J Respir Crit Care Med 154:1229–1256, 1996. *Description of the relationship between the genetic defect and the pathogenesis, including a focus on inflammation.*

Quinton PM: Physiological basis of cystic fibrosis: A historical perspective. Physiolog Rev 79:53–522, 1999. *Review of the physiologic basis for the pathogenesis of the disease with extensive references.*

Ramsey BW: Management of pulmonary disease in patients with cystic fibrosis. N Engl J Med 335:179–188, 1996. *Well-referenced recent discussion of current and experimental approaches to treating CF lung disease. Includes general and specific recommendations.*

Welsh MJ, Smith AE: Molecular mechanisms of CFTR chloride channel dysfunction in cystic fibrosis. Cell 73:1251–1254, 1993. *Discussion of how mutations disrupt CFTR function, examples of mutations in each class, and consideration of implications.*

77 BRONCHIECTASIS AND LOCALIZED AIRWAY/ PARENCHYMAL DISORDERS

Alan F. Barker

BRONCHIECTASIS

Pathophysiology and Etiology

Bronchiectasis, which is an acquired disorder of the major bronchi and bronchioles, is characterized by permanent abnormal dilation and destruction of bronchial walls. The affected areas show a

variety of changes including transmural inflammation, mucosal edema (cylindrical bronchiectasis), cratering and ulceration (cystic bronchiectasis) with bronchial neovascularization, and distortion due to scarring or obstruction from repeated infection (varicose bronchiectasis). The obstruction often leads to postobstructive pneumonitis that may temporarily or permanently damage the lung parenchyma. The induction of bronchiectasis requires two factors: (1) an infectious insult; and (2) impairment of drainage, airway obstruction, and/or a defect in host defense.

AIRWAY OBSTRUCTION DUE TO FOREIGN BODY ASPIRATION. Clinical examples of airway obstruction causing bronchiectasis include previous foreign body aspiration or encroaching lymph nodes (middle lobe syndrome). Bronchiectasis as a sequela of foreign body aspiration generally occurs in the right lung and in the lower lobes or the posterior segments of the upper lobes. Although less common than repeated or severe infection, it is important to identify the presence of airway obstruction (as with foreign body aspiration) because surgical resection often produces a cure. Although witnessed or recognized aspiration is uncommon, an episode of choking and coughing or unexplained wheezing or hemoptysis should raise the suspicion of a foreign body.

Particulate aspiration is typically associated with an altered state of consciousness due to stroke, seizures, inebriation, or emergent general anesthesia. The foreign body is often unchewed food or part of a tooth or crown. Delayed or ineffective therapy and poor nutrition may contribute to prolonged pneumonitis with resultant focal bronchiectasis.

HUMORAL IMMUNODEFICIENCY. Patients with hypogammaglobulinemia usually present in childhood with repeated sinopulmonary infections. In adults, the history may include frequent episodes of "sinusitis" and "bronchitis." Establishing the diagnosis of humoral immunodeficiency is important, because γ-globulin replacement can diminish or even prevent further respiratory tract infections and lung damage. Intravenous immunoglobulin augmentation should be administered when levels of immunoglobulin (Ig) G, A, and M are less than 5 to 10% of normal values. In patients with isolated IgG subclass deficiency, tests of humoral competency, such as serologic response to *Haemophilus influenzae* or pneumococcal vaccine, may be required for diagnosis.

CYSTIC FIBROSIS (See Chapter 76). The major respiratory diseases in cystic fibrosis (CF) are sinusitis and bronchiectasis; the latter may be the sole feature of CF in adults. Clues suggesting the presence of this disorder are upper lobe radiographic involvement and sputum cultures showing mucoid *Pseudomonas aeruginosa*.

YOUNG SYNDROME. Patients with Young syndrome exhibit clinical features similar to CF including bronchiectasis, sinusitis, and obstructive azoospermia. They are often middle-aged males identified during evaluation for infertility. They do not have increased sweat chloride values, pancreatic insufficiency, or genetic abnormalities. No cause has been identified.

RHEUMATIC DISEASES. Rheumatoid arthritis and Sjögren syndrome can be complicated by bronchiectasis (see Chapter 286). The arthropathy and sicca features are usually advanced when the bronchiectasis becomes apparent. In some cases, however, bronchiectasis occurs before the rheumatic disease. These patients generally have mild arthritis, and other causes for the bronchiectasis (such as tuberculosis) may be present.

DYSKINETIC CILIA. Although immotile cilia were originally described in the respiratory tract and sperm of patients with Kartagener syndrome (dextrocardia, sinusitis, bronchiectasis), many other patients have dyskinetic cilia leading to poor mucociliary clearance, repeated respiratory infections, and subsequent bronchiectasis.

PULMONARY INFECTIONS. A number of pulmonary infections have been associated with the development of bronchiectasis. Some individuals with presumed viral or *Mycoplasma* infection develop repeated respiratory infections and bronchiectasis. In addition to direct tissue injury, a sequela of virulent infections (tuberculosis) may include enlarged and caseous lymph nodes around bronchi or damaged airways that predispose to bacterial colonization (see Chapter 358). The recent recognition of bronchiectasis in acquired immunodeficiency syndrome (AIDS) illustrates the accelerated destructive interaction between repeated infections and impaired host defense. Childhood whooping cough (pertussis) is now of historical interest in the pathogenesis of bronchiectasis. It is unclear whether many of these children had secondary bacterial pneumonia. *Mycobacterium avium-intracellulare* (MAI) has traditionally been considered a secondary pathogen in an abnormal host (AIDS) or in already damaged lung (bullous emphysema). However, presumed normal hosts have developed bronchiectasis with primary MAI infections.

ALLERGIC BRONCHOPULMONARY ASPERGILLOSIS. *Aspergillus* may also be associated with bronchiectasis (see Chapters 75 and 401). This disorder should be suspected in patients with a long history of asthma that is resistant to bronchodilator therapy and is associated with a cough productive of sputum plugs or mucopurulence. Allergic bronchopulmonary aspergillosis probably represents a hyperimmune reaction to the presence of the *Aspergillus* organism rather than true infection.

CIGARETTE SMOKING. A causal role for cigarette smoking in bronchiectasis has not been shown. However, smoking and repeated infections may worsen pulmonary function and accelerate the progression of already present disease.

Clinical Findings

Patients often report frequent bouts of "bronchitis" requiring therapy with repeated courses of antibiotics (see Chapter 376). Symptoms in most patients include daily cough productive of mucopurulent phlegm, intermittent hemoptysis, pleurisy, and shortness of breath. In bronchiectasis, bleeding can be brisk; it is often associated with acute infective episodes and is produced by injury to superficial mucosal neovascular bronchial arterioles. Physical findings on chest examination include crackles, rhonchi, and/or wheezing. Digital clubbing is rare.

Diagnostic Evaluation

The diagnostic evaluation is designed to confirm the diagnosis of bronchiectasis, to identify potentially *treatable* underlying causes, and to provide functional assessment (Table 77–1). Imaging of the chest is always necessary to confirm the diagnosis. However, a defined etiology is found in fewer than 50% of patients with suspected bronchiectasis.

CHEST RADIOGRAPHY. The chest radiograph is abnormal in most patients with bronchiectasis, and this, in combination with the clinical findings, may be sufficient to establish the diagnosis. Suspicious but not diagnostic radiographic findings include plate-like atelectasis, dilated and thickened airways (tram or parallel lines; ring shadows on cross-section), and irregular peripheral opacities that may represent mucopurulent plugs. The distribution of changes also may be helpful. A central (perihilar) distribution of the abnormal shadowing is suggestive of allergic bronchopulmonary aspergillosis, whereas predominant upper lobe distribution is suggestive of cystic fibrosis.

HIGH-RESOLUTION COMPUTED TOMOGRAPHIC SCANNING. High-resolution computed tomography (HRCT) of the chest has become the defining modality for diagnosis of bronchiectasis. The major features of bronchiectasis on HRCT include airway dilatation and bronchial wall thickening (Fig. 77–1). HRCT is indicated in the following settings: a patient with suspicious clinical findings but a relatively normal chest radiograph; a patient whose chest radiograph is abnormal (e.g., pneumonic infiltrate) and underlying bronchiectasis is strongly suspected; a patient for whom management decisions, such as surgical resection of the abnormal areas of

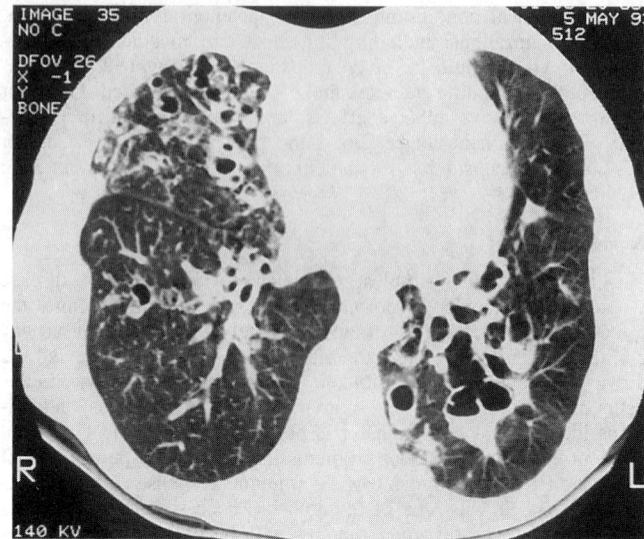

FIGURE 77–1 ■ Chest HRCT of a patient with bronchiectasis shows dilated and thickened airways in both lungs. Airways on the left have grape-like clusters of varicose bronchiectasis.

lung, depend on the extent of bronchiectasis; and patients in whom the presence or absence of other confounding diseases, such as chronic obstructive lung disease or interstitial lung disease, needs to be defined.

In addition to dilated airways and thickened bronchial walls, the CT scan may also demonstrate other findings, such as consolidation of a segment or lobe (from pneumonia), which can be seen in bronchiectasis but is not diagnostic as an isolated finding; enlarged lymph nodes, which may be indicative of reaction to infection; or areas of low attenuation and vascular disruption, probably due to the distorting effect of inflammatory small airways and suggestive of emphysema.

BRONCHOSCOPY. Bronchoscopy is an important diagnostic tool in focal (segmental or lobar) bronchiectasis to examine for obstruction by a foreign body, tumor, structural deformity, or extrinsic compression from lymph nodes. Bronchoscopy plays a key role in patients with hemoptysis to help localize the bleeding to a lobe so that appropriate intervention can be performed.

PULMONARY FUNCTION TESTS. Pulmonary function testing allows a functional assessment of the impairment induced by bronchiectasis. Spirometry before and after the administration of a bronchodilator is adequate in most patients. Obstructive impairment (reduced or normal forced vital capacity [FVC], low forced expiratory volume in 1 second [FEV_1], and/or FEV_1-FVC ratio) is the most frequent finding, but a very low FVC is also seen in advanced disease in which much of the lung has been destroyed.

Treatment of Bronchiectasis

Because infection plays a major role in causing and perpetuating bronchiectasis, a cornerstone of therapy is to reduce the microbial load and attendant inflammatory mediators. Antibiotics are used to treat an acute exacerbation and to prevent recurrent infection by suppression or eradication of pathogens.

ACUTE EXACERBATION. The diagnosis of an acute exacerba-

Table 77–1 ■ BRONCHIECTASIS: DIAGNOSTIC FEATURES OF ASSOCIATED CONDITIONS

CONDITION	DIAGNOSTIC TEST	ABNORMAL RESULT
Immunodeficiency	Quantitative Ig G, A, M	All low; rarely, isolated subclass G is low
Ciliary dyskinesia	Respiratory mucosa biopsy (examine by electron microscopy)	Ciliary struts or spokes broken or missing
Bronchopulmonary aspergillosis	IgE	High, often >1000
	Types I and III skin tests; precipitins	Positive
	Fungal sputum cultures	Positive about 50% of time
Mycobacterium avium-intracellulare	Mycobacterial sputum culture/DNA probe	Positive in about two-thirds of patients
Cystic fibrosis	Sweat chloride	>55–60 mEq/L
	Sputum culture	*Pseudomonas aeruginosa*
	Genetic testing	ΔF508 most frequent
Foreign body aspiration	Bronchoscopy	Lobar or segmental obstruction

tion depends on symptomatic changes rather than any specific laboratory feature. Acute bacterial infections are usually heralded by increased sputum production with enhanced viscosity, often accompanied by lassitude, shortness of breath, and pleuritic chest pain. Systemic complaints such as fever and chills are generally absent, and the chest radiograph rarely shows new infiltrates. The colonizing bacterial flora is usually similar to that in patients with chronic bronchitis. As a result, antimicrobial agents that are effective against *Streptococcus pneumoniae* and *H. influenzae* should generally be chosen. Recommended regimens that are well tolerated and inexpensive include trimethoprim-sulfamethoxazole, one double-strength tablet given twice daily, or amoxicillin, 500 mg every 8 hours.

The duration of therapy is not well defined, but a minimum of seven to 10 days has become frequent practice. Sputum culture and sensitivity to help define antibiotic selection and resistance patterns are indicated in patients who fail to respond to the initial antibiotic or who have repeated symptomatic attacks in a short interval.

PREVENTION. Less clear is the role of suppressive antibiotic regimens (Table 77–2). Three colonizing organisms that contribute to symptomatic episodes and are particularly problematic and difficult to eradicate include *Pseudomonas aeruginosa*, MAI, and *Aspergillus* species. *P. aeruginosa* is almost impossible to eradicate in patients with bronchiectasis; ciprofloxacin is currently the only effective oral agent against this organism, but resistance often develops after one to two treatment cycles. Aerosolized tobramycin or intravenous antibiotics are often needed when *Pseudomonas* causes repeated symptomatic episodes. MAI and *Aspergillus* species are often harbored in damaged lung tissue and bronchiectatic airways. Guidelines to help decide infectivity with MAI or *Aspergillus* include: symptomatic episodes not responding to antibacterial agents; two or more independent positive sputum cultures; new infiltrates on chest radiograph with sputum culture growing either organism; and HRCT showing diffuse nodular opacities with MAI infection. For the treatment of MAI infection, a four-drug regimen of clarithromycin, 500 mg twice daily, or azithromycin, 250 mg/day, rifampin, 600 mg/day, ethambutol, 15 mg/kg/day, and streptomycin, 15 mg/kg two to three times a week for the first 8 weeks as tolerated, has been recommended by the American Thoracic Society; therapy is continued until the patient is culture-negative for 12 months. For patients with *Aspergillus* infection or allergic bronchopulmonary aspergillosis, a prolonged course of itraconazole (400 mg/day) reduces the sputum load and improves clinical outcome in some patients.

BRONCHIAL HYGIENE. Bronchiectasis is the prototypical disease for which secretion loosening or thinning, combined with enhanced removal techniques, should be salutary. This approach is particularly important in patients in whom tenacious secretions are not reduced with appropriate antibiotic administration. Potential therapies include hydration, nebulization with saline solutions and mucolytic agents, mechanical techniques, bronchodilators, and corticosteroids.

HYDRATION AND NEBULIZATION. General hydration with oral liquids and nebulization with saline solutions or mucolytic agents are important considerations in the management of bronchiectasis. The mucolytic agent acetylcysteine is beneficial in some patients when delivered by nebulization.

PHYSIOTHERAPY. Mechanical techniques to loosen viscid secretions followed by gravitational positioning should be effective if followed assiduously. Chest percussion techniques include hand clapping of the chest by an assistant or application of a mechanical vibrator to the chest wall. Bronchiectasis most often follows a middle or lower lobe distribution. As a result, head-down positioning is needed for postural drainage but may be difficult or uncomfortable for many patients. When physiotherapy is performed regu-

larly, three to four times daily, enhanced sputum mobilization occurs in many patients. However, patients often do not take the time (15 to 30 minutes per session), do not have assistance to do vibratory techniques, or cannot tolerate proper positioning to get maximal benefit. Alternatives for patients who cannot perform chest physiotherapy include hand-held postexpiratory pressure devices or flutter valves, which facilitate secretion drainage by maintaining airway patency.

BRONCHODILATORS. Airway reactivity, presumably due to transmural inflammation, is often present in patients with bronchiectasis. Aerosol bronchodilator therapy, as used in chronic bronchitis (see Chapter 75), may be appropriate but has not been studied in patients with bronchiectasis.

ANTI-INFLAMMATORY MEDICATION. Because inflammation plays a major role in bronchiectasis, corticosteroid therapy might theoretically be beneficial. However, systemic steroids can further depress host immunity and promote increased bacterial and fungal colonization and even perpetuation of infection. One practical approach involves oral systemic prednisone therapy (20 to 30 mg/day for 2 days, tapering completely over 10 to 14 days) along with antibacterial therapy at the time of acute exacerbations. Regular inhaled steroids could be considered at other times.

HEMOPTYSIS. Bleeding in bronchiectasis can be brisk and life-threatening. It is often associated with acute infective episodes and is produced by injury to superficial mucosal neovascular bronchial arterioles. Bronchoscopy may help localize the bleeding to a lobe or segment. If an interventional radiology service is available, selective bronchial arterial embolization becomes the treatment of choice, because it will preserve lung tissue. Thoractomy and resection may still be necessary if bleeding persists.

SURGERY. The combination of impaired defense mechanisms and recurrent infection often results in bronchiectasis becoming a diffuse lung disease with little opportunity for surgical cure. Nevertheless, surgery may help some patients, even if it does not cure or eliminate all areas of bronchiectasis.

The major indications and goals for surgery in bronchiectasis include: removal of destroyed lung partially obstructed by a tumor or the residue of a foreign body; reduction in acute infective episodes occurring in the same pulmonary segment; reduction in overwhelming purulent and viscid sputum production from a specific lung segment; elimination of bronchiectatic airways causing poorly controlled hemorrhage; or removal of an area suspected of harboring resistant organisms, such as MAI or *Aspergillus*. Surgical intervention is often combined with an aggressive antibiotic and bronchodilator regimen to reduce bacterial infection and allow better drainage.

The immediate goal of surgical extirpation includes removal of the most involved segments or lobes with preservation of nonsuppurative or nonbleeding areas. Middle and lower lobe resections are most often performed. Surgical mortality varies from 2 to 12%, depending on patient selection. Complications include empyema, hemorrhage, prolonged air leak, and poorly expanding remaining lung due to persistent atelectasis or suppuration.

LUNG TRANSPLANT. Patients with suppurative lung disease were initially considered poor candidates for lung transplantation due to the potential persistence of infection that might worsen during prolonged immunosuppression. More than 1000 patients with CF have received bilateral lung or heart-lung transplantation with a survival at 1 year of 70%. Almost 200 patients with non-CF bronchiectasis have undergone bilateral lung or heart-lung transplantation; no survival data are available. Timing and selection for lung transplantation in patients with bronchiectasis are similar to the guidelines for individuals with cystic fibrosis (see Chapter 76).

Table 77–2 ■ ANTIBIOTIC STRATEGIES TO SUPPRESS BACTERIAL INFECTIONS IN PATIENTS WITH BRONCHIECTASIS

STRATEGY	EFFECTIVENESS	ISSUES/PROBLEMS
Daily antibiotic	Moderately effective	Resistance will develop; orovaginal yeast
7–14 days of antibiotic alternating with 7–14 days of no antibiotic	Well tolerated and effective	Resistance after several cycles
Aerosol antibiotic (tobramycin)	Effective for virulent Gram-negative organisms	Requires nebulizer and bronchodilator
Intermittent intravenous antibiotics	Effective; reserve for severe bronchitis and/or resistant organism(s)	Maybe only rescue therapy; most expensive

CONGENITAL CYSTIC DISEASES OF THE LUNG

Lung cysts involve abnormal foregut branching or development. The cyst lining contains airway or alveolar epithelium. Cysts communicate poorly with normal airway or lung tissue. Cysts are usually clinically apparent in childhood but occasionally remain unrecognized until later in life. Presentations include an abnormal chest radiograph with a localized cyst, irregular focal infiltrate, pneumonia that resolves slowly or recurs in the same location, compression of normal lung or mediastinal structure, or hemoptysis. Although the chest radiograph may show a focal abnormality or even a well-developed cyst, CT of the chest with contrast or MRI is needed to define the location (lung, mediastinum, or abdomen), vascular supply, and degree of compression of other structures.

Of these rare disorders, the two that may present in adults are bronchogenic cysts and pulmonary sequestration. Bronchogenic cysts rarely produce symptoms. Commonly, an asymptomatic mass is noted at the cardiophrenic angle or along the heart border on a chest radiograph. CT of the chest usually distinguishes a bronchogenic cyst from a pericardial or esophageal cyst, diaphragmatic hernia, or tumor. Unless the cyst is infected or compresses other structures, no intervention is required.

Pulmonary sequestration is characterized by nonfunctioning pulmonary parenchyma that has no connection to the tracheobronchial airways. The blood supply is from a systemic artery, usually the aorta. Pulmonary sequestrations may be intralobar (75% of all sequestrations), in which the abnormal lung is within a normal lobe and does not have a separate visceral pleura, or extralobar (25% of all sequestrations), in which the abnormal lung is separate from a normal lobe and surrounded by its own visceral pleura. Extralobar sequestrations may be seen at or below the diaphragm. Repeated pneumonia in the same lobe or segment is a feature. The lower lobes (left and posterior segments more often than right) are the most affected areas. The chest radiograph shows an infiltrate, atelectasis, and sometimes a cystic mass accompanied by a tubular extension to the mediastinum suspicious for a feeding vessel. Aortography, CT with contrast, or magnetic resonance imaging (MRI) will confirm the diagnosis (aberrant blood supply) and define the anatomy. Surgical resection with attention to the systemic feeding vessel is the treatment of choice and is usually curative.

HYPERLUCENT LUNG. Areas of lung with reduced markings on a chest radiograph are considered hyperlucent. At one extreme is a pneumothorax (see Chapter 86), with complete absence of markings due to air in the pleural space that causes collapse of lung tissue; patients with pneumothorax are almost always symptomatic and have chest pain and shortness of breath. At the other extreme are lung parenchymal collections of air, and sometimes fluid; patients are commonly asymptomatic and the disorder is usually noted on a routine chest radiograph. These collections, which may compress surrounding lung or airways and lead to infection, respiratory impairment, rupture, and pneumothorax may be due to a variety of causes. *Developmental cysts* are lined by respiratory epithelium and contain air and fluid; *congenital lobar hyperinflation* or *emphysema* is a localized anomaly that almost always presents in infancy with respiratory distress due to compression of an airway or normal lung. Occasionally an older individual presents with a chest radiograph showing focal hyperlucency. Lobar emphysema usually has areas of vasculature, whereas a pneumothorax has complete absence of markings. Surgical resection of the lobe is indicated in individuals with respiratory impairment from compressed lung or mediastinal shift. *Blebs* develop after barotrauma during mechanical ventilation; *pneumatoceles* are noted after staphylococcal or *Pneumocystis* pneumonia, and are similar to blebs; and *bullae* are due to alveolar destruction in severe emphysema and are sometimes amenable to surgical decompression (see Chapter 89).

Hyperlucency of an entire lung (Swyer-James or Macleod's syndrome) is unilateral bronchiolitis obliterans. Histopathologic specimens show fibrosis in and around small airways. The genesis is presumed to be remote virulent respiratory viral or atypical bacterial infection or toxic fume inhalation. Exertional dyspnea and cough are occasional symptoms. Inspiratory and expiratory chest CT imaging studies demonstrate complete unilateral hyperlucency and air trapping of the affected lung with normal appearance of the contralateral lung. No specific intervention is required.

ATELECTASIS. Atelectasis, or collapse, is hypoventilation of the lung (Fig. 77–2). Atelectasis may include the whole lung due to an intrinsic main-stem mass or extrinsic compression from lymph node enlargement. Lobar, segmental, or subsegmental regions may be involved. The decreased ventilation and sustained blood flow leads to ventilation-perfusion mismatch and hypoxemia.

Platelike or discoid atelectasis refers to the appearance on chest radiograph of horizontal or curvilinear lines. This type of atelectasis is seen after surgery or lengthy recumbency with conditions such as

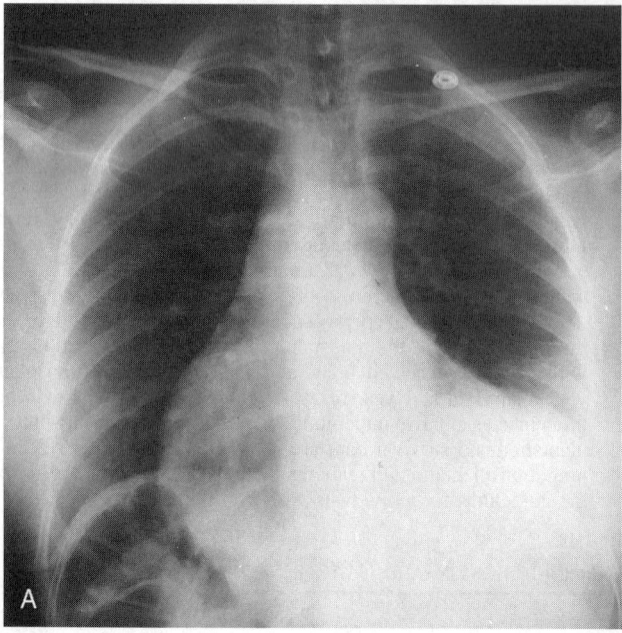

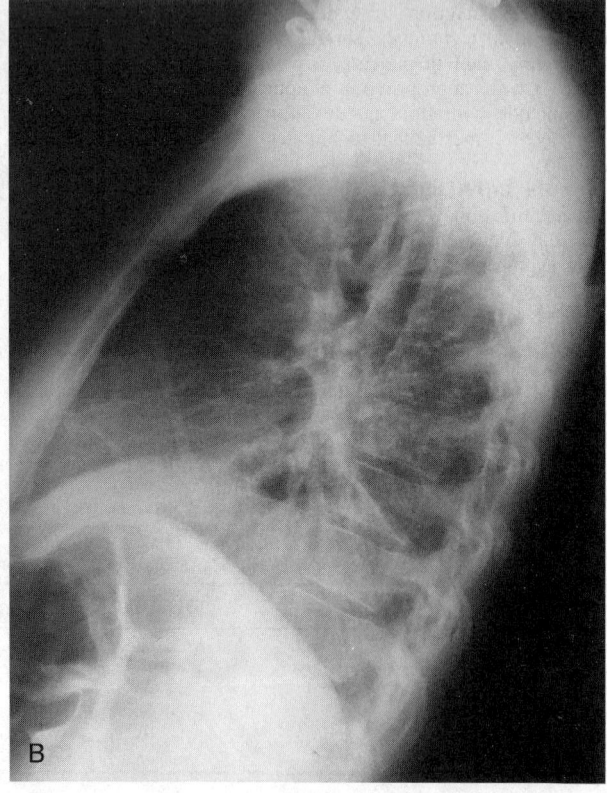

FIGURE 77–2 ■ Chest films of a patient with left lower lobe atelectasis. *A*, The PA film shows on the left opacity over the heart, loss of the diaphragmatic contour, and diagonal line of the major fissure. *B*, The lateral projection shows an elevated left diaphragm.

stroke or head or spinal injuries. Sustained chest pain of any etiology may also lead to splinting and platelike atelectasis.

Patchy atelectasis occurs in any air-space filling disease such as pulmonary hemorrhage, pulmonary edema, or respiratory distress syndrome. Fluid-filled alveoli and loss of surfactant contribute to patchy areas of infiltrate.

Passive, relaxation, or compression atelectasis occurs when the lung recoils to a smaller volume due to a process in the adjacent pleural space such as pneumothorax or pleural effusion. Obstructive atelectasis can be caused by an obstructed bronchus due to an intrinsic process, such as a tumor or mucus plug, or an extrinsic process, such as lymph nodes (middle lobe syndrome).

Rounded atelectasis is a round mass-like density abutting the pleura. It is caused by pleural scar that invaginates and contracts lung tissue. Rounded atelectasis is almost always seen in the setting of asbestos pleural disease.

Diagnosis and Treatment

The chest radiograph is a key diagnostic tool. Volume loss is almost always present and involves displacement of a lobar fissure, the mediastinum, or diaphragm to the affected area or side. Diagnosis and management of segmental or lobar obstructive atelectasis includes bronchoscopy. An intrinsic mass can be visualized and biopsied for cytologic analysis. Mucus plugs can be removed by lavage and suctioning. Rounded atelectasis must be distinguished from a tumor mass; CT scan may confirm the pleural thickening and the invaginating lung tissue. For patients at bedrest or with other risks for developing platelike atelectasis, attention to deep breathing, mobilization, analgesic medication for chest pain, and bronchial hygiene will improve gas exchange and prevent pneumonia. For patchy atelectasis, treatment is directed at the underlying disease and to the types of measures that also enhance lung volume in platelike atelectasis. Passive atelectasis requires attention to the pleural space process, such as evacuation of a pneumothorax or drainage of a pleural effusion.

Delen FM, Barker AF: New concepts in diagnosis and management of bronchiectasis. Semin Respir Crit Care Med, in press, 1999. *An updated review.*

Louie HW: Pulmonary sequestration: 17 year experience at UCLA. Am Surg 59:801, 1993. *Relatively large surgical series; good discussion of use of imaging.*

Patel SR, Meeker DP, Biscotti CV, et al: Presentation and management of bronchogenic cysts in the adult. Chest 106:79, 1994. *Seventeen-year review at one institution of 18 patients; 65 references.*

Stockley RA: Bronchiectasis, a management problem. Br J Dis Chest 82:209, 1988. *Emphasizes medical management. Some of antibiotic strategies not available in the United States.*

78 INTERSTITIAL LUNG DISEASE

Galen B. Toews

GENERAL DESCRIPTION

The interstitial lung diseases (ILDs) represent a large and heterogeneous group of lower respiratory tract disorders that are considered together because of several consistent themes among their clinical, radiographic, and physiologic presentations (Table 78–1). They also share certain pathogenic mechanisms and histopathologic features. The target structure in ILDs is the alveolar interstitium, which encompasses the space between the alveolar epithelium and the capillary endothelium, including the connective tissues surrounding blood vessels, lymphatic vessels, and airways. Although distinctive pathologic changes may be present, the common denominator among ILDs is that they are all characterized by widespread disruption of alveolar walls with loss of functional alveolar capillary units and accumulation of collagenous scar tissue. In the majority of cases, disrupted alveolar architecture is the consequence of inflammatory injury, followed by a dysfunctional process of wound repair.

The array of conditions that lead to ILDs is so broad and includes so many diverse, rare disorders that a comprehensive con-

Table 78–1 ■ CLINICAL CLASSIFICATION OF INTERSTITIAL LUNG DISEASE (ILD)

PRIMARY LUNG DISEASES
Idiopathic pulmonary fibrosis*
Sarcoidosis*
Bronchiolitis obliterans with organizing pneumonia*
Lymphocytic interstitial pneumonia
Histiocytosis X
Lymphangioleiomyomatosis

ILD ASSOCIATED WITH SYSTEMIC RHEUMATIC DISORDER
Rheumatoid arthritis*
Systemic lupus erythematosus*
Scleroderma*
Polymyositis-dermatomyositis*
Sjögren's syndrome
Mixed connective tissue disease*
Ankylosing spondylitis

ILD ASSOCIATED WITH DRUGS OR TREATMENTS
Antibiotics*
Anti-inflammatory agents
Cardiovascular drugs*
Antineoplastic agents*
Illicit drugs
Dietary supplements
Oxygen
Radiation
Paraquat

ENVIRONMENT/OCCUPATION–ASSOCIATED ILD
Organic dusts/hypersensitivity pneumonitis (>40 known agents)
    Farmer's lung*
    Air conditioner-humidifier lung*
    Bird breeder's lung*
    Bagassosis
Inorganic dusts
    Silicosis*
    Asbestosis*
    Coal workers' pneumoconiosis*
    Berylliosis
Gases/fumes/vapors
    Oxides of nitrogen
    Sulfur dioxide
    Toluene diisocyanate
    Oxides of metals
    Hydrocarbons
    Thermosetting resins

ALVEOLAR FILLING DISORDERS
Diffuse alveolar hemorrhage
Goodpasture's syndrome
Idiopathic pulmonary hemosiderosis
Pulmonary alveolar proteinosis
Chronic eosinophilic pneumonia*

ILD ASSOCIATED WITH PULMONARY VASCULITIS
Wegener's granulomatosis
Churg-Strauss syndrome
Hypersensitivity vasculitis
Necrotizing sarcoid granulomatosis

INHERITED DISORDERS
Familial idiopathic pulmonary fibrosis
Neurofibromatosis
Tuberous sclerosis
Gaucher's disease
Niemann-Pick disease
Hermansky-Pudlak syndrome

*Disorders that are the most common causes of ILD or less common conditions in which ILD is a prominent manifestation of disease.

sideration of all diagnostic possibilities is impossible. Faced with this daunting task, a clinician must appreciate the value and limitations inherent in each step of a diagnostic evaluation. Virtually all ILDs may involve breathlessness, exercise intolerance, progressive respiratory insufficiency, and diffuse parenchymal abnormalities on chest roentgenogram. Therefore, the key element of the history is carefully to identify the exposures to exogenous agents and symptoms of associated systemic illnesses that point to specific conditions. The physical examination may suggest the presence of ILDs, but occasionally, ancillary findings (such as evidence of a pleural effusion or a systemic rheumatic disease) also suggest or discount specific diagnoses. The radiographic features of ILDs may be entirely nonspecific or may be tremendously valuable in narrowing the diagnostic possibilities. Pulmonary function testing is most useful for demonstrating physiologic abnormalities consistent with ILDs and for managing patients and assessing responses to therapy. Only occasionally does physiologic testing help narrow the differential diagnosis. Having sifted through this initial evaluation, the clinician is often left with only a presumptive diagnosis. The accompanying dilemma is to decide when to obtain tissue for histopathologic examination, knowing that even lung biopsy findings may be nonspecific; this difficult and complex decision is highly individualized, based not only on the differential diagnosis at hand but also on the realization that the implications for therapy and outcome may vary dramatically among individuals.

EPIDEMIOLOGY

The prevalence of ILDs is estimated to be 20 to 40 per 100,000 of the population. ILD accounts for 100,000 hospital admissions yearly. The increased use of pneumotoxic drugs to treat malignant and cardiovascular disease and given for organ transplantation, and the increased identification of occupationally induced ILDs are likely to contribute to an increased incidence.

PATHOGENESIS

ILDs are the result of the superimposed processes of inflammation and tissue injury and attempted repair (Fig. 78–1). If the events associated with a self-limited inflammatory response are altered, the result may be a persistent inflammatory response with ongoing injury and structural derangement rather than normal repair.

The causes of most ILDs are not known. Bacteria, viruses, fungi, toxic agents, and environmental agents have all been implicated. Causative agents may activate resident pulmonary inflammatory or immune cells, which in turn generate inflammatory or immune responses. Alternatively, the causative agents may directly injure epithelial or endothelial cells. In this instance, the inflammatory response might be initiated by the injured tissue.

INTRA-ALVEOLAR INFLAMMATION. The earliest detectable lesion in ILDs is a lower respiratory tract inflammatory exudate. Macrophages, neutrophils, and lymphocytes are all present in increased numbers in the alveolar walls and the alveolar air spaces. Cellular recruitment can be divided into four steps: (1) sequestration of inflammatory cells in pulmonary vessels, (2) transmigration of the vascular wall, (3) migration through extracellular matrix, and (4) selective tissue retention. A number of cytokines are released and adhesion receptors are upregulated on endothelial cells at sites of inflammation (see Chapter 277). Selectins are critical for leukocytes to attach to endothelial cells. Leukocyte deformability also is important in the sequestration of cells in the lung. Directed migration of inflammatory cells in ILDs depends on cytokines and chemokines. Chemoattractants involved include leukotriene B4 (LTB4), interleukin-8 (IL-8), and C5a for neutrophils; C5a, fibronectin fragments containing the RGD cell-binding domain and monocyte chemoattractant protein-1 (MCP-1) for monocytes; and IL-1 and RANTES in the case of lymphocytes. Alveolar macrophages, endothelial cells, fibroblasts, and epithelial cells are all important sources of these cytokines.

Specific immune responses are also generated. T lymphocytes are activated following the recognition of major histocompatibility complex (MHC)–associated antigens on the surface of antigen-presenting cells such as dendritic cells and recruited monocytes. An immune response results in an increase in immunocompetent cells in involved pulmonary tissues.

INJURY. Epithelial cell injury is a hallmark of ILDs. Oxidants, proteases, immune and inflammatory cells, and viral infections have all been proposed as mechanisms of injury. Loss of the epithelial barrier results in transudation of plasma and the formation of a fibrin-rich exudate. Epithelial cells are lost and the alveolar basal lamina may be destroyed. The persistence and activation states of inflammatory cells (macrophages, lymphocytes, polymorphonuclear leukocytes) likely determine the type and amount of alveolar wall injury.

INTRA-ALVEOLAR FIBROSIS/ALVEOLAR COLLAPSE. Whether the repair process results in fibrosis or in a return to normal lung anatomy depends, in part, on the success of clearing the intra-alveolar exudate and debris. The forming alveolar exudate contains a new group of cytokines and mediators, including growth factors (platelet-derived growth factor [PDGF], transforming growth factor-β [TGF-β], insulin-like growth factor-1 [IGF-1]), arachidonic acid metabolites (5-lipoxygenase [5-LO] products, and prostaglandin E_2 [PGE$_2$]), fibronectin, thrombin, and fibrinopeptides. Alveolar epithelial cells and macrophages regulate both the formation and clearance of intra-alveolar fibrin. Urinary plasminogen activator (u-PA) generates plasmin, which dismantles intra-alveolar fibrin. If the intra-alveolar exudate is not cleared, the exudate is invaded by fibroblasts and new blood vessels. Formation of new blood vessels in the organizing exudate is regulated by angiogenic (interleukin-8 [IL-8]), and angiostatic factors, (interferon-gamma inducible protein-10 [IP-10]). Under the influence of growth factors, epithelial cells proliferate and produce new matrix proteins, converting the fibrin-rich exudate into scar. Proliferating type II epithelial cells eventually resurface the organized exudate. Alveolar surface area is lost as a result of intraluminal fibrosis and also as a result of alveolar collapse. Connective tissue deposition in these collapsed airspaces results in irreversible loss of gas exchange units.

CLINICAL PRESENTATION

HISTORY. Breathlessness is the most prevalent complaint. Initially, dyspnea develops only on exertion. This symptom is often denied or attributed to other causes (out of shape, overweight, viral infection). As the disease progresses, dyspnea occurs even at rest. Nonproductive cough and fatigue are also prominent complaints. Cough is a frequent complaint in patients with bronchiolitis obliterans organizing pneumonia (BOOP), eosinophilic pneumonia, and idiopathic pulmonary fibrosis. Pleuritic chest pain may occur with ILDs associated with systemic rheumatic disease and some drug-induced disorders. Pleuritic chest pain and sudden worsening of dyspnea should suggest spontaneous pneumothorax, a characteristic finding in lymphangioleiomyomatosis, neurofibromatosis, tuberous sclerosis, and pulmonary histiocytosis X. Hemoptysis may be the presenting complaint of patients who have diffuse alveolar hemorrhage syndromes or in lymphangioleiomyomatosis, but it is infrequent in other ILDs. Hemoptysis should prompt a search for complications such as pulmonary embolus, superimposed infection, or malignancy. Substernal chest discomfort may be noted late in the disease due to pulmonary hypertension.

If a specific diagnosis is made, it is most often because of information gathered during history. Many patients will have an obvious underlying disease. In others, a careful history will reveal an environmental or occupational cause. A detailed, lifelong occupational history must be obtained, because ILDs have long latency periods between occupational exposure and onset of symptoms and radiographic abnormalities (see Chapter 80). Exposure to agents that cause ILDs may also occur as a result of hobbies or recreational activities (bird breeder's lung, wood dust worker's lung, farmer's lung, sauna taker's disease). Accordingly, exposures outside the occupational setting should also be explored. Specific questions relating to medications that induce ILDs must be asked. The agents to which the patient has been exposed and the circumstances, intensity, and duration of exposure must be determined. Fever and chills are common symptoms in hypersensitivity pneumonitis and are often temporally related to the workplace or to hobbies. Symptoms may diminish or disappear after a weekend, vacation, or an absence from the workplace for several days, only to reappear on return. Patients with idiopathic pulmonary fibrosis or BOOP may date the onset of their symptoms to a preceding upper respiratory tract infection.

A smoking history should be obtained. Ninety per cent of patients with histiocytosis X are active smokers. The pulmonary component of Goodpasture's syndrome occurs in only 20% of affected individuals who are nonsmokers, but it occurs in 100% of affected individuals who are smokers. Hypersensitivity pneumonitis is very

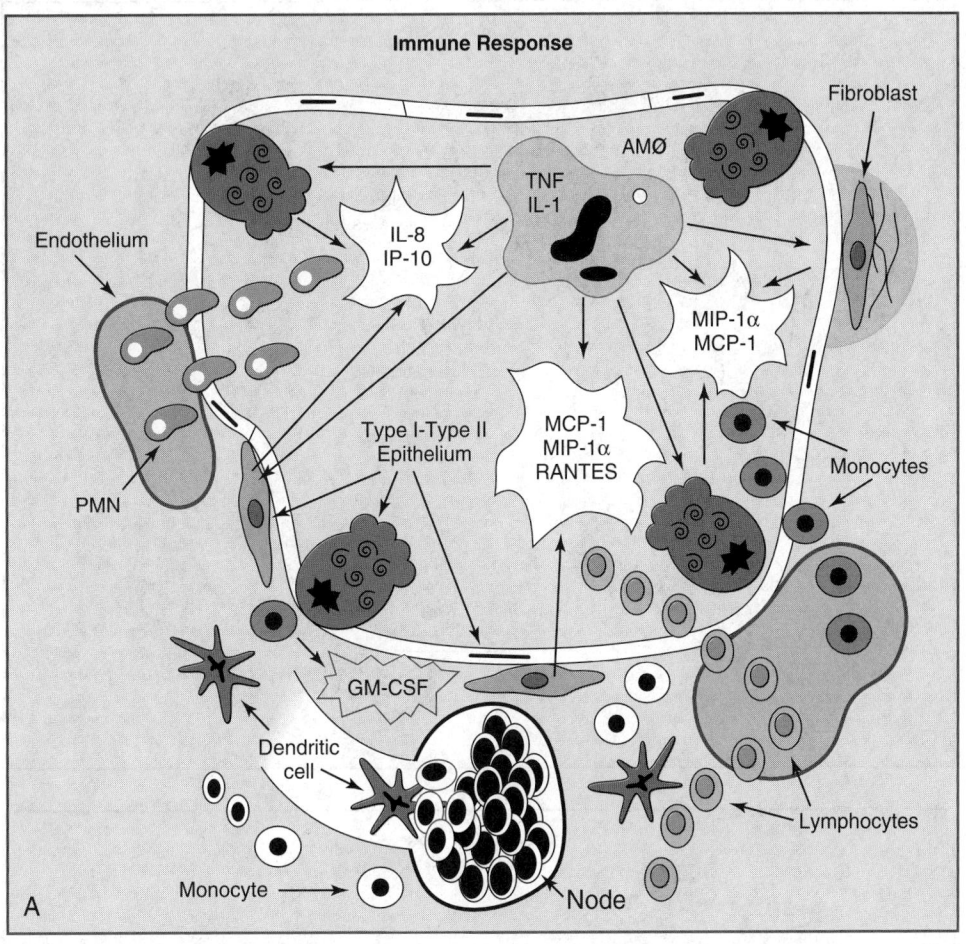

Immune Response

Fibroblast

Endothelium

PMN

AMØ

TNF
IL-1

IL-8
IP-10

MIP-1α
MCP-1

Type I-Type II
Epithelium

MCP-1
MIP-1α
RANTES

Monocytes

GM-CSF

Dendritic
cell

Lymphocytes

Monocyte

Node

A

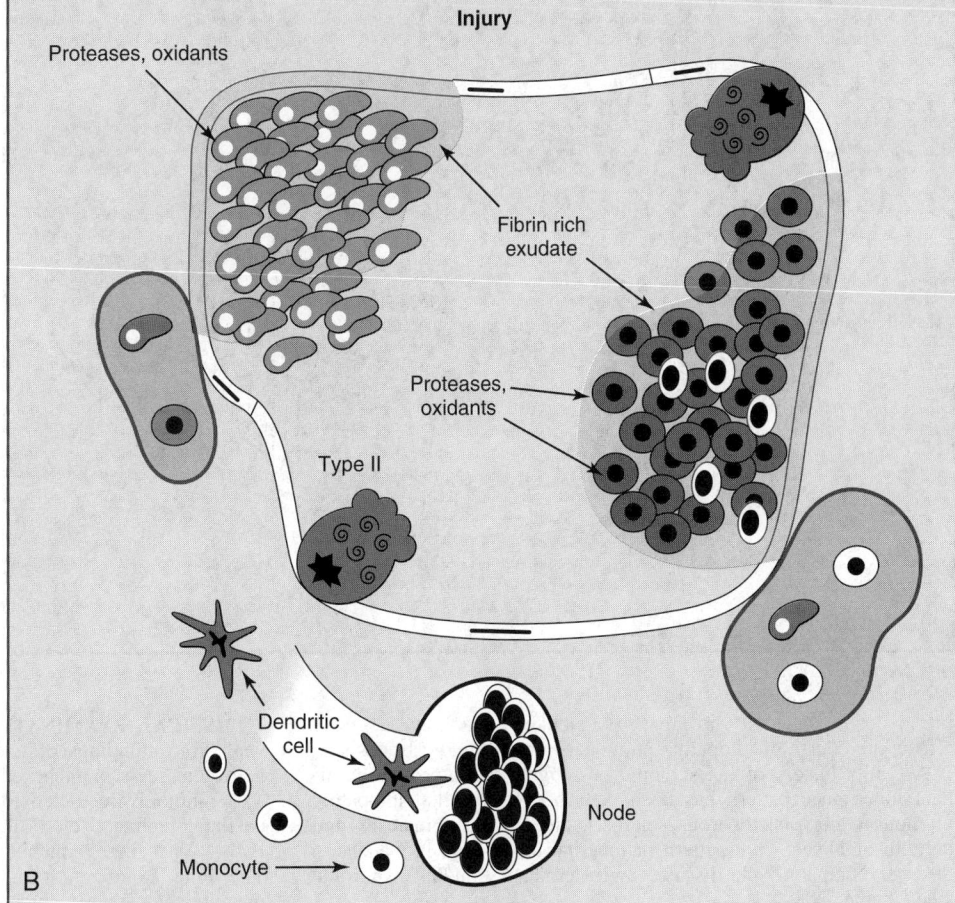

Injury

Proteases, oxidants

Fibrin rich
exudate

Proteases,
oxidants

Type II

Dendritic
cell

Node

Monocyte

B

FIGURE 78–1 ■ Pathogenesis of interstitial lung disease. *A,* Immune response: The development of an intra-alveolar exudate of polymorphonuclear leukocytes or mononuclear cells depends on inflammatory cell sequestration in pulmonary vessels. Chemokines cause leukocytes to emigrate into the parenchymal and alveolar spaces. Specific cellular immunity depends on migration of antigen-presenting cells to local nodes, clonal expansion of specific lymphocytes, and recirculation of these lymphocytes to the lung. *B,* Injury: Inflammatory cell products (oxidants, proteases) cause epithelial cell injury, epithelial cell loss, and basal lamina destruction. A fibrin-rich exudate forms.

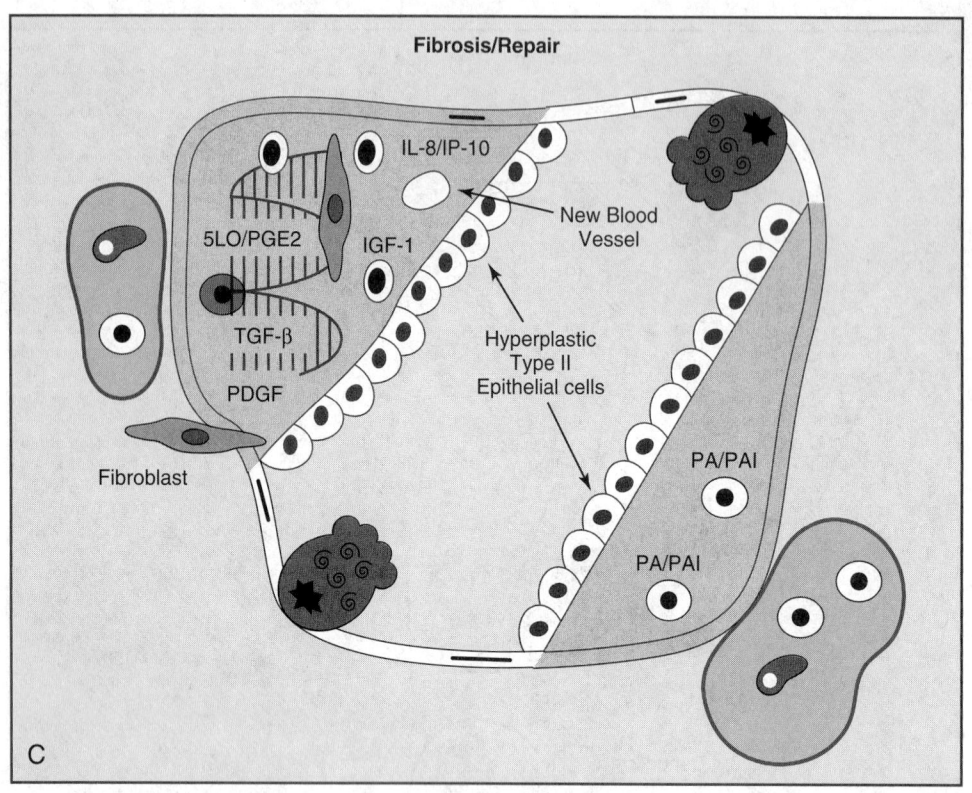

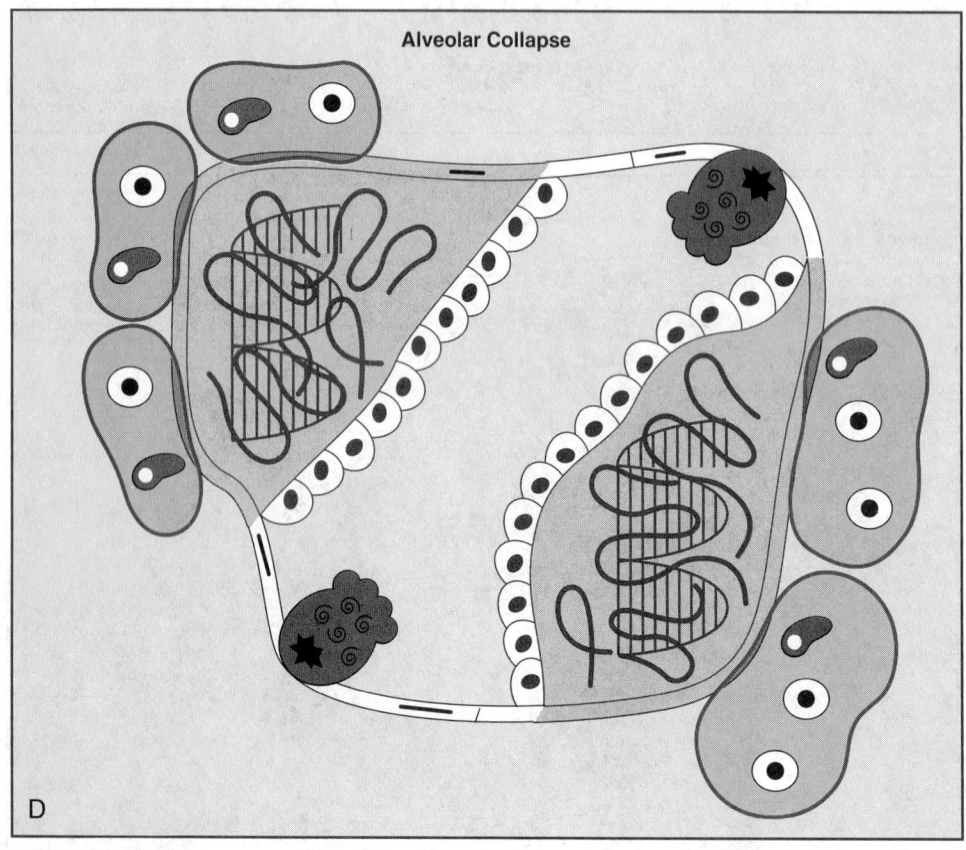

FIGURE 78–1 *Continued* ■ *C,* Fibrosis/repair: Repair of damaged alveoli requires clearance of plasma proteins and fibrin-rich matrix components, restoration of damaged extracellular matrix, regulated angiogenesis, and replacement of epithelial cells. Plasminogen activator (uPA) generates plasmin, which removes the fibrin-rich matrix on which fibroblasts migrate. If matrix proteins are not cleared, fibroblasts migrate into injured alveolar spaces, multiply, and produce additional matrix proteins. The fibrotic process is regulated by cytokines, growth factors, and arachidonic acid metabolites. The balance of angiogenic (IL-8) and angiostatic factors (e.g., IP-10) regulates the formation of new blood vessels in the organizing exudate. Re-epithelialization involves epithelial cell migration and proliferation. *D,* Alveolar collapse: Collapse results from loss of basal lamina. Folded basal lamina is found in areas of new matrix formation. Multiple alveoli may collapse to form a conglomerate scar.

infrequent in patients who are active smokers. Smoking adversely affects the course of idiopathic pulmonary fibrosis and asbestosis.

A family history of ILDs should be sought. An autosomal dominant inheritance pattern has been described for familial idiopathic pulmonary fibrosis, tuberous sclerosis, and neurofibromatosis, and an autosomal recessive pattern of inheritance is found in Gaucher's disease, Niemann-Pick disease, and Hermansky-Pudlak syndrome (see Chapter 208).

PHYSICAL EXAMINATION. The physical examination may reveal typical findings of underlying causes, such as systemic rheumatic disorders or inherited diseases. In other patients, the findings are commonly restricted to the cardiopulmonary system. Bilateral, basilar, crepitant Velcro-like rales are found in most patients with ILDs. Wheezing, rhonchi, and coarse rales are occasionally heard. The lung examination may be normal. With advanced disease, patients may have tachypnea and tachycardia, even at rest. Clubbing of the fingers and toes is a common but nonspecific finding in many fibrotic lung disorders; it is most often seen in patients with idiopathic pulmonary fibrosis and is unusual in sarcoidosis. The syndrome of hypertrophic pulmonary osteoarthropathy is rare. The new appearance of digital clubbing in a patient with known ILD should prompt a search for a complicating lung malignancy. The heart examination is normal early in the course of the disease. Later, with the onset of pulmonary hypertension and cor pulmonale, an accentuated P_2, tricuspid insufficiency, a right ventricular heave, and peripheral edema may be noted. Physical findings characteristic of associated diseases (e.g., rash of systemic lupus erythematosus [SLE], skin changes of scleroderma) may be noted.

LABORATORY STUDIES. Laboratory tests can either confirm or suggest a diagnosis in ILD, but these studies are seldom diagnostic. Rheumatoid factor and antinuclear antibodies are occasionally present in patients with ILD, but their presence does not necessarily indicate an underlying collagen vascular disorder. Plasma immunoglobulin may be elevated, but this finding is nonspecific. If hypersensitivity pneumonitis is suspected, serum-precipitating antibodies to a limited number of inhaled organic antigens may be measured. Tests for antineutrophil cytoplasmic antibodies (ANCA) should be obtained if Wegener's granulomatosis is suspected. Tests for anti-basement membrane antibodies should be obtained when Goodpasture's syndrome (see Chapter 106) is suspected. The electrocardiogram (ECG) is usually normal in ILDs. With progressive loss of alveolar capillary units, the ECG may demonstrate a pattern of right atrial and ventricular strain.

CHEST RADIOGRAPHY. The chest radiograph plays a major role in establishing the presence of ILDs and may suggest a specific diagnosis (Table 78–2). The majority of ILDs cause infiltrates in the lower lung zones. A diffuse ground glass pattern is seen early in the disease. More typically, a chest radiograph demonstrates nodules, linear (reticular) infiltrates, or a combination of the two (reticulonodular infiltrates). On chest radiography, alveolar filling disorders produce a diffuse abnormality, characterized by ill-defined alveolar nodules (acinar rosettes); air bronchograms may be noted in these patients. As the disease progresses, the infiltrates become coarser and lung volume is lost. Cystic areas (honeycomb

Table 78–2 ■ RADIOGRAPHIC FEATURES THAT SUGGEST SPECIFIC CAUSES OF INTERSTITIAL LUNG DISEASE

HILAR OR MEDIASTINAL LYMPHADENOPATHY
Sarcoidosis
Berylliosis
Silicosis (eggshell calcification)
Lymphocytic interstitial pneumonia
Amyloidosis
Gaucher's disease

PLEURAL DISEASE
Asbestosis (pleural effusion, thickening, plaques, mesothelioma)
Systemic rheumatic disorders
Lymphangioleiomyomatosis (chylous effusion)
Nitrofurantoin
Radiation pneumonitis

PNEUMOTHORAX
Histiocytosis X
Lymphangioleiomyomatosis
Neurofibromatosis
Tuberous sclerosis

PRESERVED LUNG VOLUMES OR HYPERINFLATION
Bronchiolitis obliterans organizing pneumonia
Chronic hypersensitivity pneumonitis
Histiocytosis X
Lymphangioleiomyomatosis
Neurofibromatosis
Sarcoidosis
Tuberous sclerosis

UPPER LOBE DISTRIBUTION
Ankylosing spondylitis
Berylliosis
Histiocytosis X
Silicosis
Chronic hypersensitivity pneumonitis
Necrobiotic nodules of rheumatoid arthritis

pattern) appear late in the course of ILDs. Five to 10% of patients with biopsy-proven disease have a normal chest radiograph.

HIGH-RESOLUTION COMPUTED TOMOGRAPHY. High-resolution thin-section computed tomography (HRCT), using thin (1- to 2-mm) sections without the use of contrast, offers advantages over standard chest radiography in detecting early ILD, diagnosing the specific ILD, and quantifying extent of ILD. HRCT can detect ILD in subjects with normal chest radiographs in asbestosis, silicosis, sarcoidosis, and scleroderma. HRCT abnormalities may be present before pulmonary function tests are abnormal, but, conversely, HRCT may be normal in biopsy-proven ILD. Normal findings on HRCT should not be used to exclude ILD. HRCT is valuable for identifying a suitable site for transbronchial or open lung biopsy.

PULMONARY FUNCTION TESTS. Physiologic testing can document the physiologic abnormalities associated with ILD, determine the severity, and determine the course and response to treating ILD. The classic physiologic alterations in ILD include reduced lung volumes (vital capacity, total lung capacity [TLC]), reduced diffusing capacity (DL_{CO}), and a normal or supernormal ratio of forced expiratory volume in 1 second (FEV_1) to forced vital capacity (FVC). Static lung compliance is decreased (decreased lung volume for any given transpulmonary pressure), and maximal transpulmonary pressure is increased (a very high negative pressure must be generated to open the fibrotic alveoli). Exceptions to this classic presentation are histiocytosis X, lymphangioleiomyomatosis, neurofibromatosis, sarcoidosis, and tuberous sclerosis, in which primary airway disease results in an increase in TLC and airflow limitation. A mixed restrictive and obstructive pattern is also seen in BOOP.

Arterial blood gas analysis typically shows mild hypoxemia. Carbon dioxide retention is rare, even late in the course of the disease. Most patients with ILD have marked increases in minute ventilation both at rest and at exercise, resulting in reduced partial pressure of carbon dioxide (PcO_2) and compensated respiratory alkalosis. The increased minute ventilation is accomplished by increases in respiratory rate rather than in tidal volume. Hyperventilation is not due to abnormalities in acid-base status or to hypoxemia, but rather to an increased stimulation of the respiratory center from neural signals arising from altered mechanoreceptors in the deranged lung parenchyma. The exercise tolerance of ILD patients is markedly limited. With exercise, arterial partial pressure of oxygen (PO_2) falls and the PcO_2 remains constant. Hypoxemia in patients with ILDs results from abnormal ventilation-perfusion relationships and from diffusion abnormalities. The abnormalities in diffusion, which were originally believed to be the result of thickened alveolar walls, are now recognized to be due to loss of capillary cross-sectional area and the passage of red blood cells through functioning pulmonary capillaries at a rate that is too rapid to permit full saturation of hemoglobin. Arterial pH is usually normal in ILDs but can fall with exercise as a result of anaerobic metabolism in oxygen-deprived muscles.

BRONCHOSCOPIC STUDIES. Bronchoscopy should be performed when tissue abnormalities are distributed in the bronchovascular bundle, an alveolar filling disorder is present, or an infectious disease is suspected. The distinctive histologic abnormalities of sarcoidosis, lymphangitic carcinomatosis, and lymphangioleiomyomatosis are usually found in the bronchovascular bundle; transbronchial biopsy may demonstrate their characteristic lesions. Bronchoalveolar lavage (BAL) is diagnostic if an infectious agent or neoplastic cell is noted in the lavage specimen. BAL is also used to analyze the cellular constituents, cellular products, and proteins of the distal air spaces of the lung. A predominance of eosinophils in conjunction with an appropriate clinical/radiographic picture can diagnose eosinophilic pneumonia. An asbestos body count of more than 1 per milliliter of BAL fluid documents significant asbestos exposure. In histiocytosis X, ultrastructural studies of BAL mononuclear cells reveal the typical Birbeck granule of the Langerhans cell. Special stains for surfactant may reveal a sufficient abnormality to enable a diagnosis of alveolar proteinosis. However, BAL usually is nonspecific and it is not routinely indicated because of its limited ability to predict the underlying pathology (fibrosis versus inflammation), to stage disease, or to predict response to therapy.

LUNG BIOPSY. The diagnosis of most ILDs depends on histologic studies of lung parenchyma. Transbronchial biopsy should be

RECIPIENT SELECTION GUIDELINES
Untreatable, end-stage interstitial lung disease
Substantial limitation of daily activities
Limited life expectancy (<12 to 18 mo)
No other significant medical disease
Ambulatory, good rehabilitation potential
Acceptable nutritional status
Acceptable psychosocial profile and support system

RELATIVE CONTRAINDICATIONS
Presence of active systemic disease
Significant disease of other organ systems
Significant psychosocial problems, substance abuse, or history of noncompliance
Poor nutritional status
Poor rehabilitation potential

performed if sarcoidosis or alveolar filling diseases are likely. An open-lung or thoracoscopic biopsy is required to secure a specific diagnosis and accurately stage most cases of ILD in patients who do not have systemic rheumatic disease or drug-induced injury. Open or thoracoscopic biopsy is performed if the diagnosis remains questionable after reviewing the clinical, radiographic, bronchoalveolar lavage, and transbronchial biopsy data, and if the patient is not at high risk for this procedure because of age or other serious medical disease. The mortality rate for open lung biopsy is less than 1%, and the morbidity is less than 3%. A specific diagnosis is established in 90% of cases.

GENERAL APPROACH TO THERAPY. The principal aims of therapy are (1) to remove exposure to injurious agents, (2) to suppress inflammation to prevent further destruction of the pulmonary parenchyma, and (3) to palliate the manifestations of these diseases. Corticosteroids are the mainstay of therapy. The initial treatment of choice is prednisone, 1 mg/kg of ideal body weight per day (maximum, 60 mg/day) given in one dose for 1 month, followed by 40 mg/day given for 2 months. The dose is gradually tapered (5 mg/week) over several months to a maintenance dose of 15 to 20 mg/day. The rate of taper should be individualized using clinical and physiologic parameters. Corticosteroids are continued until pulmonary function is stable for 1 year. Relapses require returning to high-dose steroids, but their efficacy in this circumstance is usually limited. Cytotoxic agents or immunosuppressive agents may be used in patients who do not improve on steroid therapy or who cannot tolerate corticosteroids. Cyclophosphamide, 1 to 2 mg/kg of ideal body weight, may be useful. Azathioprine has been suggested as an alternative agent.

Supplemental oxygen is recommended for patients who have an arterial oxygen tension of less than 55 mm Hg at rest or with exercise. Patients with cor pulmonale and right ventricular failure or those with significant erythrocytosis should also receive oxygen therapy. Respiratory tract infections should be treated promptly. Influenza and pneumococcal vaccines should be given.

Lung transplantation is now an accepted therapy for patients with end-stage ILD that is refractory to medical therapy (Table 78–3; see Chapter 89). Single-lung transplantation is the preferred therapy for most patients. Two-year survival ranges from 60 to 80%, with most deaths being due to infections that complicate immunosuppressive therapy or to chronic allograft rejection.

PRIMARY LUNG DISEASE

IDIOPATHIC PULMONARY FIBROSIS. Idiopathic pulmonary fibrosis is the classic fibrotic lung disease, but it also remains the most enigmatic ILD. The exact prevalence of idiopathic pulmonary fibrosis is unknown, but it is estimated to occur in 5 per 100,000 population. Typically, idiopathic pulmonary fibrosis is diagnosed in patients between ages 40 and 60 years. No geographic, gender, racial, or seasonal predilections have been noted. Most patients present with the insidious onset of breathlessness with exercise and a dry, nonproductive cough. Constitutional symptoms including fever, fatigue, weight loss, myalgia, and arthralgia are present in some patients. Chest examination reveals late inspiratory fine (Vel-

cro) rales at the lung bases. A right-sided heave, an augmented P_2, and an S_3 gallop are present in late stages of disease. Chest radiographs typically show a reticular or reticulonodular infiltrate that is most prominent in the lower lung zones. Multiple cystic or honeycombed areas with translucencies measuring 0.5 to 1 cm in diameter are seen late in the course of the disease and indicate a poor prognosis. Spontaneous pneumothorax may occur secondary to rupture of honeycomb cysts. Early in the course of the disease, HRCT findings include a patchy air-space opacification or ground-glass lung density that disproportionately involves peripheral (subpleural) and basilar regions but does not obscure the underlying lung parenchyma. The interlobular septa are thickened. These findings are thought to correlate with alveolar septal inflammation and the filling of air spaces by mononuclear cells (Fig. 78–2). Later, a predominantly lower lung zone reticular infiltrate is present, which consists largely of thickened interlobular septa. Honeycombing and subpleural fibrosis are also present (Fig. 78–3). Physiologic testing reveals a restrictive impairment with normal airflow parameters. The DL_{CO} frequently is reduced; this reduction may precede the restrictive abnormalities. Arterial blood gases may be normal or reveal hypoxemia (secondary to ventilation-perfusion mismatch) and respiratory alkalosis. The resting PO_2 usually falls with exercise equivalent to walking up a single flight of stairs.

Lung tissue obtained by thoracoscopic or open lung biopsy is required to establish the diagnosis of idiopathic pulmonary fibrosis. Alveolar walls are thickened by an inflammatory cell response. Alveolar epithelial cells and their basement membranes are abnormal. Alveolar cell hyperplasia and metaplasia are noted. Later in the course of the disease, capillaries are lost, and increased numbers of mesenchymal cells and deranged collagen fibers are noted. The disease is patchy (nonhomogeneous) in its distribution until late in the course of disease. Extensive ground-glass opacities with minimal honeycombing on HRCT identifies individuals likely to respond to corticosteroids. By contrast, honeycomb cysts are predictive of minimal or no response to therapy. Lung biopsy findings that are predictive of responsiveness to therapy include active inflammation and minimal fibrosis.

The mean survival after diagnosis of idiopathic pulmonary fibrosis is 5 to 7 years. Few patients experience spontaneous regression or stabilization; accordingly, the great majority of patients require treatment. Corticosteroids (see above) are the mainstay of therapy, although favorable clinical response occurs in only 10 to 20% of patients. Lung transplantation (see Chapter 89) is a beneficial therapy for selected patients who are unresponsive to medical therapy and have end-stage disease.

SARCOIDOSIS. Sarcoidosis (see Chapter 81) is a multisystem granulomatous disease characterized by noncaseating granulomas and derangement of normal tissue architecture. It often presents as ILD.

BRONCHIOLITIS OBLITERANS ORGANIZING PNEUMONIA (BOOP). BOOP is a clinical entity that shares certain features of

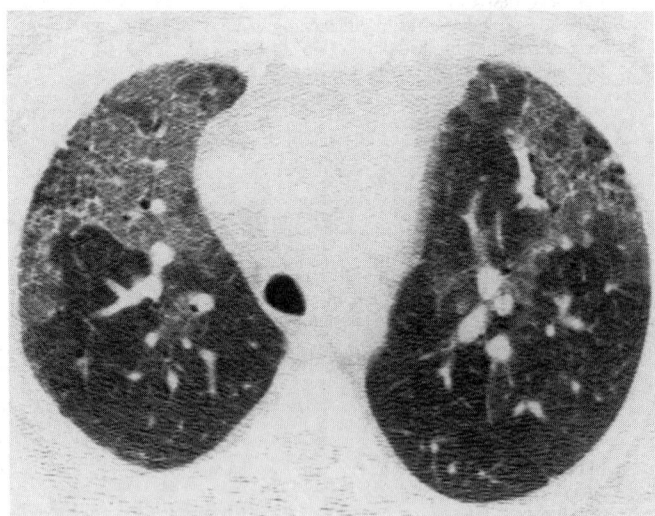

FIGURE 78–2 ■ Idiopathic pulmonary fibrosis. High-resolution computed tomographic scan from patient with biopsy-proven idiopathic pulmonary fibrosis shows patchy, peripheral ground-glass opacification, and small honeycomb cysts.

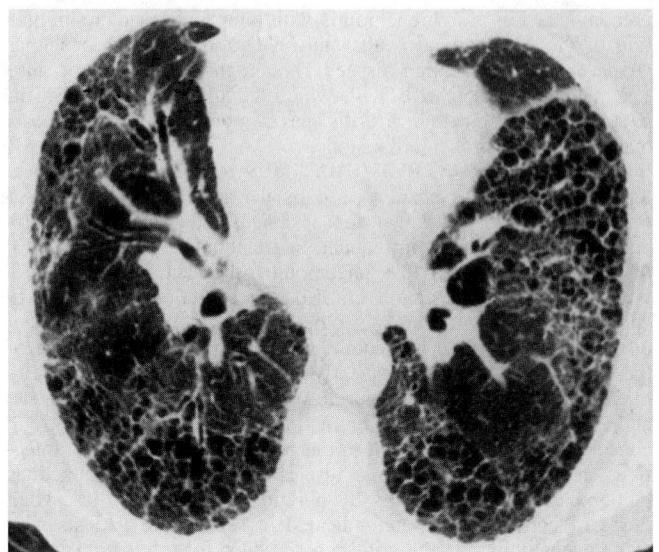

FIGURE 78-3 ■ Idiopathic pulmonary fibrosis. High-resolution computed tomographic scan from a patient with biopsy-proven idiopathic pulmonary fibrosis shows numerous large cystic radiolucencies (honeycombing) involving both lungs. Although most of the lung parenchyma of the lower lobes is involved, the cystic process is more prominent in the subpleural regions.

idiopathic pulmonary fibrosis and bronchiolitis obliterans. The distinct onset of a flu-like illness with a nonproductive cough is the most common presentation. Fever, malaise, weight loss, and fatigue are usually present for 2 to 4 months prior to the onset of dyspnea. Patients have often been unsuccessfully treated with multiple courses of antibiotics. Rales are common, but wheezing is rare. A restrictive defect with a reduction in DL_{CO} is present in a majority of patients. An obstructive defect is present in 20% of patients, most of whom are current or past smokers. Chest radiography reveals bilateral diffuse alveolar opacities with normal lung volumes. Infiltrates may be peripheral, as seen in chronic eosinophilic pneumonia, or migratory. Reticulonodular infiltrates and honeycombing are rare. In selected instances the diagnosis can be made by transbronchial biopsy, but thoracoscopic or open lung biopsy is usually required to confirm this diagnosis. Honeycombing and diffuse alveolar wall fibrosis are not features of BOOP. Corticosteroid therapy is the most common treatment and results in recovery in two thirds of patients. Clinical improvement is rapid (days to a few weeks) in some individuals, but relapse may occur when steroids are withdrawn; retreatment is often successful. Cyclophosphamide has been used to treat patients with progressive disease.

LYMPHOCYTIC INTERSTITIAL PNEUMONIA. Lymphocytic interstitial pneumonia is an uncommon cause of ILD. It must be differentiated from other lymphocytic infiltrations of the lung, including primary lymphomas and lymphomatoid granulomatosis. This disorder is sometimes idiopathic but is frequently associated with other conditions such as hypogammaglobulinemic or hypergammaglobulinemic states, acquired immunodeficiency syndrome (AIDS), systemic rheumatic disorders, and bone marrow transplantation. Infectious complications occur in patients with AIDS and hypogammaglobulinemia. Corticosteroid therapy is successful in approximately 50% of patients, although some patients progress to end-stage lung disease or lymphoma.

HISTIOCYTOSIS X (see Chapter 173). Histiocytosis X is a term that encompasses three systemic diseases (eosinophilic granuloma, Letterer-Siwe disease, and Hand-Schüller-Christian disease) that have in common an abnormal proliferation of a mononuclear cell, the Langerhans cell. "Langerhans' cell granulomatosis" has been proposed as an alternate term to histiocytosis X because current evidence suggests that the histiocytes are Langerhans' cells. "Pulmonary Langerhans' cell granulomatosis" has been proposed as an alternative to eosinophilic granuloma of the lung. Most new patients are 20 to 40 years old, with an equal gender distribution. A history of cigarette smoking is obtained in more than 90% of patients. Patients present with nonproductive cough and exertional dyspnea. Hemoptysis, fever, weight loss, and wheezing are occasionally noted. Pleuritic chest pain and acute dyspnea secondary to

spontaneous pneumothorax occur in 25% of patients. Cystic bone lesions (skull, ribs, pelvis) accompany the pulmonary disease in 10% of cases. Diabetes insipidus complicates 10% of cases and indicates poor prognosis. HRCT demonstrates multiple thin-walled cysts (dilated small bronchi and bronchioles or destroyed parenchyma) and nodules (peribronchiolar granulomas) in the upper and midlung zones. Pulmonary function studies demonstrate a mixed obstructive and restrictive pattern. DL_{CO} is reduced, and hypoxemia is present at rest or with exercise.

Definitive diagnosis requires a thoracoscopic or open lung biopsy. Morphologically, a granulomatous reaction develops in a bronchocentric distribution but also involves the walls of blood vessels and the interstitium. Langerhans' cells, monocytes, eosinophils, and lymphocytes are present in these lesions. A granulomatous vasculitis may also be noted. Langerhans' cells may be detected by their characteristic X body or Birbeck's granule and/or by monoclonal antibody staining for the CD1a (T6) surface antigen. The clinical course of histiocytosis X is variable; spontaneous remission, stabilization, and disease progression may all occur. Corticosteroids have been reported to be effective in some cases.

LYMPHANGIOLEIOMYOMATOSIS. Lymphangioleiomyomatosis is a rare disorder occurring only in women of child-bearing age. It is characterized by smooth muscle cells proliferating in the lymphatic, peribronchial, perivascular, and interstitial tissues of the lung. Very little inflammation is present, but in most cases, the alveolar walls are eventually destroyed. Patients present with dyspnea, chylous pleural effusions (secondary to obstruction of the pleural lymphatics), and recurrent pneumothorax (due to rupture of emphysematous cysts). Coarse reticular infiltrates with areas of cystic dilation are noted on chest radiography. HRCT is superior to chest radiography in discerning the cystic nature of this disease. Numerous thin-walled cysts are distributed diffusely without a predilection for specific regions or lobes. Nodules, interstitial fibrosis, and irregular lung pleural interfaces, features that are observed in other chronic interstitial lung diseases, are absent. Pleural effusions or recurrent pneumothoraces may be the sole radiographic manifestation. Thoracoscopic or open lung biopsy is required to make the diagnosis. Most patients die of respiratory failure within 10 years of onset of symptoms. Hormonal influences are thought to be important in the pathogenesis because lymphangioleiomyomatosis occurs predominantly in premenopausal women and is accelerated during pregnancy, the postpartum period, and exogenous estrogen therapy. Progesterone (10 mg/day) or tamoxifen (20 mg/day) are the drugs of choice. Lung transplantation has been successful in patients with lymphangioleiomyomatosis.

INTERSTITIAL LUNG DISEASE ASSOCIATED WITH SYSTEMIC RHEUMATIC DISORDERS

The association between systemic rheumatic diseases and ILD is well established, and all systemic rheumatic disorders are associated with ILD (Table 78-4). The airways, alveoli, vascular system, and pleura are all variably affected. ILD associated with systemic rheumatic diseases accounts for 1600 deaths/year, which constitutes 25% of all mortality associated with ILD and 2% of all respiratory deaths.

RHEUMATOID ARTHRITIS (see Chapter 286). Although rheumatoid arthritis is more common in women (female-to-male ratio, 2:1 to 4:1), rheumatoid arthritis associated with ILD is more common in men (male-to-female ratio, 3:1) and occurs in patients with late-onset rheumatoid arthritis. The majority of cases occur between ages 50 and 60 years. Symptoms are similar to those seen with idiopathic pulmonary fibrosis. Tachypnea and bibasilar rales are common. Associated pleural rubs may be heard, and clubbing occurs in as many as 75% of cases. Pulmonary symptoms most often follow the onset of arthritis, but simultaneous onset of ILD and arthritis may occur. In one-fifth of cases, ILD precedes joint manifestations. Pleural disease accompanies ILD in 20% of patients. The physiologic abnormalities of rheumatoid ILD are identical to those of other fibrosing lung diseases. Bronchoalveolar lavage reveals an increase in macrophages and neutrophils. A subset of patients with rheumatoid arthritis but without clinical lung disease have lymphocytosis on BAL. Open lung biopsy early in the course

Table 78–4 ■ PULMONARY MANIFESTATIONS OF SYSTEMIC RHEUMATIC DISORDERS

RHEUMATOID ARTHRITIS
Interstitial lung disease (ILD)
Pleural disease (pleuritis with or without effusion, empyema, pyopneumothorax)
Bronchiolitis obliterans with or without organizing pneumonia
Caplan's syndrome
Pulmonary vascular disease
Apical fibrobullous disease
Central airway obstruction secondary to cricoarytenoid arthritis

SYSTEMIC LUPUS ERYTHEMATOSUS
Pulmonary infection
ILD—acute, chronic
Pleuritis with or without effusion
Pulmonary hemorrhage
Pulmonary vascular disease, thromboembolic disease
Bronchiolitis obliterans
Diaphragmatic dysfunction
Central airway obstruction

SYSTEMIC SCLEROSIS (SCLERODERMA)
ILD
Pulmonary hypertension
Aspiration pneumonia (gastroesophageal reflux)
Bronchogenic carcinoma (scar carcinoma)

POLYMYOSITIS/DERMATOMYOSITIS
Aspiration pneumonia (pharyngeal/esophageal disorder)
ILD
Bronchiolitis obliterans organizing pneumonia (BOOP)
Respiratory muscle dysfunction (pneumonia, atelectesis, hypoventilation, respiratory failure)
Malignancy (primary, metastatic)

SJÖGREN'S SYNDROME
ILD
Lymphocytic interstitial pneumonitis
BOOP
Lymphoma
Chronic bronchitis
Recurrent pneumonia

MIXED CONNECTIVE TISSUE DISEASE
ILD
Pleuritis with or without effusion
Pulmonary hypertension
Aspiration pneumonia (esophageal disorder)

ANKYLOSING SPONDYLITIS
Upper lobe fibrobullous disease
Pleural disease (pleural thickening, pneumothorax)
Mycobacterial infections (tuberculous and nontuberculous)
Aspergillomas
Abnormal chest wall mobility
Bronchogenic carcinoma (scar carcinoma)

of the disease reveals interstitial pneumonitis with perivascular, peribronchiolar, and interstitial infiltration by lymphocytes, plasma cells, and macrophages. This prominent lymphocytic infiltrate, which may contain germinal follicles adjacent to vessels and airways, is useful in differentiating rheumatoid ILD from idiopathic pulmonary fibrosis. The presence of rheumatoid nodules, pleural fibrosis, and adhesions is also helpful diagnostically. Rheumatoid ILD appears to be more indolent and less severe than idiopathic pulmonary fibrosis; prolonged periods of symptomatic and clinical stability may occur. Gold salts and methotrexate, common therapies for rheumatoid arthritis, can also induce ILD. It is difficult to distinguish between drug-induced and rheumatoid-induced ILD, except that the drug-induced disease may reverse when the drug is discontinued.

Progressive bronchiolitis obliterans is also associated with rheumatoid arthritis. Clinical manifestations include the abrupt onset of dyspnea and dry cough associated with rales and midinspiratory squeaks, occurring particularly in middle-aged women with seropositive rheumatoid arthritis. Pulmonary function studies reveal airflow obstruction, arterial hypoxemia, and respiratory alkalosis. The predominant lesion is bronchiolitis with lymphoplasmacytic infiltration of the small airway walls and obliteration of the bronchiolar airspace with granulation tissue. The prognosis is poor because treatment is ineffective. BOOP, which has also been described in patients with rheumatoid arthritis, has a more favorable prognosis than obliterative bronchiolitis alone.

SYSTEMIC LUPUS ERYTHEMATOSUS (see Chapter 289). Acute lupus pneumonitis is characterized by the acute or subacute onset of tachypnea, tachycardia, dyspnea, cough, and cyanosis. Fever is common, hemoptysis is infrequent, and clubbing is absent. In 50% of patients with acute lupus pneumonitis, the acute pneumonitis is the presenting manifestation of SLE. An evolution from acute to chronic ILD likely occurs in some individuals because persistent disease can occur after an acute onset. Clubbing is seen in some of these patients, but less frequently than in rheumatoid ILD. The overall impact of ILD on mortality in SLE appears small; acute and chronic ILD causes death in 2.5% of cases of SLE. Strong consideration should be given to the possibility of pulmonary infections in patients with acute infiltrates in SLE, because infections outnumber SLE pneumonitis by a ratio of more than 30:1. High doses of corticosteroids are indicated in severely ill patients with acute pneumonitis; azathioprine can be added for refractory cases.

SYSTEMIC SCLEROSIS (see Chapter 290). ILD is the most common pulmonary manifestation of scleroderma. Morphologic changes are found in 90% of patients at autopsy, and radiographic evidence of ILD has been noted in 14 to 67% of cases. Clinical manifestations include dyspnea, initially with exertion and later at rest, but this symptom may be denied because of marked limitation of physical activity. Cough is usually present. Primary pulmonary hypertension may occur in the absence of pulmonary fibrosis and is often the cause of cor pulmonale. In general, correlation between the severity of pulmonary and cutaneous manifestations in scleroderma is poor. Pulmonary symptoms may antedate either cutaneous changes or Raynaud's phenomenon by intervals as long as 14 years. Reticulonodular densities may be noted on chest radiographs in both CREST syndrome (*c*alcinosis, *R*aynaud's phenomenon, *e*sophageal involvement, *s*clerodactyly, and *t*elangiectasia) and diffuse scleroderma, but ILD is much less common in the former. A strikingly high incidence of calcified pulmonary granulomas (65%) has been noted in the CREST syndrome. A restrictive ventilatory defect with impaired DL_{CO} is found on pulmonary function testing. Bronchoalveolar studies of scleroderma have demonstrated an alveolitis in a significant proportion of patients, with or without ILD. Pulmonary function abnormalities have significant prognostic implications: patients with normal function have a greater than 90% 5-year survival, whereas those with restrictive spirometry have a 58% 5-year survival. Patients with a DL_{CO} of less than 40% predicted have a dismal 9% 5-year survival rate. No consistently effective treatment exists for scleroderma ILD. No data support a favorable long-term effect of corticosteroid therapy. D-Penicillamine may diminish the rate of visceral disease, but no data show improvement in lung function.

A significant association exists between the development of bronchogenic carcinoma and chronic pulmonary fibrosis in scleroderma. The majority of bronchogenic carcinomas are either bronchoalveolar cell or adenocarcinoma.

POLYMYOSITIS/DERMATOMYOSITIS (see Chapter 296). The clinical presentation includes progressive dyspnea on exertion, nonproductive cough, and basilar rales, but a rapidly progressive syndrome (Hamman-Rich) may occur. Lung disease may precede muscle complaints by months to years or be superimposed on established muscular disease. No correlation exists between the severity or duration of the muscular disease and the ILD. Interstitial pneumonitis and BOOP are the most common histologic patterns identified in patients with polymyositis/dermatomyositis. Active inflammation on lung biopsy, especially BOOP, predicts a good therapeutic response. Corticosteroids have stabilized and improved symptoms and physiologic abnormalities in up to 40% of patients. Methotrexate and azathioprine have been used as therapies; both can cause ILD.

SJÖGREN'S SYNDROME (see Chapter 291). Diffuse ILD is the most common lung abnormality identified in patients with primary Sjögren's syndrome. Malignant lymphomas may occur in primary Sjögren's syndrome and are usually fatal. Corticosteroids and immunosuppressive drugs are used in patients with extraglandular involvement. Lymphocytic interstitial pneumonia or BOOP may be present and often responds well to corticosteroid or immunosuppressive therapy.

MIXED CONNECTIVE TISSUE DISEASE (see Chapter 290). Evidence of pulmonary dysfunction has been reported in as many as 80% of patients with mixed connective tissue disease. A proliferative vasculopathy with intimal thickening and medial muscular hypertrophy affects pulmonary arteries and arterioles and is usually more prominent than the associated interstitial fibrosis. Although early detection and treatment of the ILD with corticosteroid therapy and/or immunosuppressive therapy has been advocated, prevention of irreversible pulmonary fibrosis has not been documented.

ANKYLOSING SPONDYLITIS (see Chapter 287). Upper lobe fibrobullous disease, the most common pulmonary manifestation of ankylosing spondylitis, is found in patients with advanced disease. The disease is usually bilateral, and the chest radiograph commonly shows diffuse reticulonodular infiltrates in the upper lung zones with cyst formation as a result of parenchymal destruction. Patients with ankylosing spondylitis appear to be predisposed to typical and atypical tuberculosis. Additionally, aspergillomas are a late complication of colonization of the apical fibrobullous cavities. No therapy is available for the apical fibrobullous disease.

DRUG-INDUCED INTERSTITIAL LUNG DISEASE

More than 100 drugs are known to alter the structure or function of the lower respiratory tract (Table 78–5). Most drug-induced ILD is reversible if it is recognized early and the responsible drug is discontinued. Drugs can cause acute, subacute, or chronic ILD. Acute and subacute forms of drug-induced ILD usually present with fever and cough and may be mistakenly treated as bacterial pneumonia. Rales, tachypnea, tachycardia, and, occasionally, cyanosis are noted. A diffuse reticulonodular infiltrate, perhaps accompanied by a pleural effusion, is noted on the chest radiograph. Blood eosinophilia is frequent. Pulmonary function studies reveal a restrictive defect, and arterial blood gas analysis reveals hypoxemia and hypocarbia. The chronic form of drug-induced ILD is more difficult to associate with a specific causative agent because of the insidious nature of this disease. Mild, nonproductive cough is the most common symptom. Fever and eosinophilia are less common. The pathogenesis of most drug-induced reactions is poorly understood.

ANTIBIOTICS. Nitrofurantoin-induced ILD is one of the most commonly reported drug-induced pulmonary diseases. Both acute and chronic ILD occur. The mechanisms of acute and chronic ILD secondary to nitrofurantoin appear to be different, and chronic reactions can occur without previous acute ILD. The acute ILD begins 2 hours to 10 days after the onset of therapy and does not appear to be dose related. A reticulonodular or alveolar infiltrate, most prominent at the bases, is noted. The infiltrate may be asymmetrical; a pleural effusion (usually unilateral) is present in one-third of patients. Discontinuing the drug is the only treatment required. Chronic nitrofurantoin-induced ILD mimics idiopathic pulmonary fibrosis. Dyspnea and nonproductive cough begin 6 months to several years after initiating therapy. In these cases, fever, eosinophilia, and pleural effusion are unusual. A diffuse interstitial process with lower zone predominance is noted on chest radiograph. A restrictive pattern is present on pulmonary function testing. Discontinuation of the drug is important, but function can be permanently lost. Corticosteroid therapy can be used if no improvement occurs after 2 months, but data regarding its use are scanty. Chronic nitrofurantoin-induced ILD is fatal in approximately 8% of cases.

ANTI-INFLAMMATORY DRUGS. Methotrexate causes granulomatous pneumonitis in 5% of patients on low-dose methotrexate for rheumatoid arthritis or other chronic inflammatory conditions. Most patients present with dyspnea, fever, rales, and hypoxemia. Hilar lymphadenopathy is seen in 10 to 15% of patients, and pleural effusion is present in 10%. When methotrexate is used in low doses, granulomatous pneumonitis is usually noted after administration of approximately 10 mg/week for an average of 80 weeks. BAL reveals a marked lymphocytosis. Most patients respond favorably to discontinuing methotrexate; corticosteroids may also be helpful, but deaths have been associated with this pneumonitis.

Table 78–5 ■ DRUG-INDUCED INTERSTITIAL LUNG DISEASE

ANTIBIOTICS
Nitrofurantoin
Cephalosporins
Sulfonamides
Penicillin
Isoniazid

ANTI-INFLAMMATORY AGENTS
Methotrexate
Gold
Penicillamine
Phenylbutazone
Nonsteroidal anti-inflammatory agents

CARDIOVASCULAR DRUGS
Amiodarone
Tocainide
β-blockers (propranolol, practolol, pindolol, acebutolol)
Hydralazine
Procainamide
Hydrochlorothiazide

ANTI-NEOPLASTIC AGENTS
Bleomycin
Busulfan
Cyclophosphamide
Methotrexate
Nitrosoureas (BCNU, CCNU, methyl-CCNU, DCNU)
Melphalan
Chlorambucil
Mercaptopurine
Mitomycin
Procarbazine

CENTRAL NERVOUS SYSTEM DRUGS
Phenytoin
Carbamazepine
Chlorpromazine
Imipramine

ORAL HYPOGLYCEMIC AGENTS
Tolbutamide
Tolazamide
Chlorpropamide

ILLICIT DRUGS
Heroin
Propoxyphene
Methadone

OXYGEN
RADIATION

CARDIOVASCULAR DRUGS. Amiodarone, an antiarrhythmic drug used predominantly for treating refractory ventricular dysrhythmias, causes ILD in 5 to 10% of patients. Risk factors include maintenance doses greater than 400 mg/day and previous pulmonary disease. The combination of amiodarone with general anesthesia, cardiopulmonary bypass, or pulmonary angiography is synergistic for development of acute lung injury.

Two clinical patterns exist. The most common presentation includes the insidious development of dyspnea, cough, fever, and malaise accompanied by weight loss. Pleuritic chest pain occurs in 10 to 20% of patients. Histologic findings include phospholipid-laden lamellar inclusions within lung parenchymal cells. These distinctive histologic findings may be seen in any patient receiving amiodarone and do not prove a drug-induced lung injury. Diffuse reticulonodular infiltrates are present on chest roentgenograph. Other patients may present with a more abrupt onset of an acute illness characterized by fever and localized alveolar infiltrates. This clinical presentation may strongly mimic infectious pneumonia or, in severe cases, adult respiratory distress syndrome (ARDS). Multiple, nodular pulmonary infiltrates with necrotizing pneumonia and cavities have also been reported. Amiodarone-induced ILD is unlikely in the absence of a 15% decline in DL_{CO}. If reasonable alternative therapy is available (see Chapters 51 through 54), amiodarone should be withdrawn if ILD is present. The same is true for patients with ventricular arrhythmias. If no alternative is available but to continue the drug, a trial of corticosteroid therapy is reasonable.

ANTINEOPLASTIC AGENTS (see Chapter 198). Chemotherapeutic drug–induced ILD is a major cause of morbidity and mortality in immunocompromised patients and patients with malignancies. In these patients, drug toxicity may be the cause of 20% of diffuse pulmonary infiltrates. The diagnosis of chemotherapeutic drug-induced ILD is one of exclusion. Dyspnea occurs within the first few weeks of treatment, followed by cough and intermittent fever. Auscultation reveals dry rales; clubbing has not been reported. Symptoms frequently precede chest radiographic findings. An asymmetrical infiltrate limited to a single lobe may be the initial radiographic presentation, but the infiltrate generally becomes diffuse and uniform in distribution. Pulmonary function studies invariably show a restrictive pattern with a reduction in DL_{CO}.

Bleomycin-induced lung disease is common. Ten per cent of patients develop parenchymal lung disease; the mortality rate approaches 50%. The incidence of pulmonary reactions to bleomycin increases in the presence of risk factors such as age (>70 years), oxygen therapy, radiation therapy, multidrug regimens, and a cumulative dose of more than 450 units. Busulfan-induced ILD occurs in 2 to 3% of patients and frequently develops a year after onset of therapy. The ILD usually does not respond to withdrawal of the drug or to administration of corticosteroids. Cyclophosphamide-induced lung disease, which can begin a few weeks to 6 years after initiating therapy, has a variable course; both steroid-responsive and nonresponsive disease has been reported. Nitrosourea (BCNU and methyl-CCNU)-induced ILD has been reported in as many as 50% of patients who have received doses of more than 1500 mg/m². These agents may have a synergistic effect with cyclophosphamide. Procarbazine causes acute ILD with peripheral and pulmonary eosinophilia and pleural effusions.

ENVIRONMENTAL/OCCUPATIONAL-ASSOCIATED INTERSTITIAL LUNG DISEASE (see Chapter 80)

Alveolar Filling Disorders

Alveolar filling diseases occur when air spaces distal to the terminal bronchiole are filled with blood, lipid, protein, water, or inflammatory cells. An acinar infiltrate characterized roentgenographically by small nodular densities with ill-defined margins is noted. Virtually all of the alveolar filling disorders can ultimately result in interstitial lung disease.

GOODPASTURE'S SYNDROME (see Chapter 106). Goodpasture's syndrome is characterized by diffuse pulmonary hemorrhage, progressive glomerulonephritis, circulating anti–glomerular basement membrane (anti-GBM) antibodies, anti–alveolar basement membrane (anti-ABM) antibodies, and ILD. Goodpasture's syndrome occurs primarily in young men between ages 18 and 35 years. The most common presenting symptoms are hemoptysis, dyspnea, cough, and fatigue. Hemoptysis may be modest, but it can be massive and life-threatening. Gross hematuria, nausea, and vomiting are present in 50% of patients. Fever and weight loss are noted in approximately one fourth of patients. Hypochromic, microcytic anemia is characteristic of Goodpasture's syndrome. Bilateral symmetrical alveolar or acinar infiltrates are present on chest radiographs. When active bleeding stops, the alveolar infiltrates fade within 48 hours, leaving residual reticulonodular infiltrates. The DL_{CO} increases during intrapulmonary bleeding due to CO uptake by the intra-alveolar erythrocytes. An increase in DL_{CO} ($>30\%$) is highly suggestive of diffuse hemorrhage. The differential diagnosis of Goodpasture's syndrome includes SLE, Wegener's granulomatosis, Henoch-Schönlein syndrome, polyarteritis nodosa, and cryoglobulinemia. Serologic assays for anti-GBM antibodies are positive in 95% of patients. The diagnosis is confirmed by immunofluorescent studies of renal tissue in some patients; lung biopsy is seldom necessary.

Spontaneous remissions can occur but are rare. The severity of the renal involvement best predicts the outcome. Therapy consists of corticosteroids and cytotoxic drugs together with plasmapheresis until circulating anti-GBM antibodies have been removed.

IDIOPATHIC PULMONARY HEMOSIDEROSIS. Idiopathic pulmonary hemosiderosis is a rare disorder characterized by intermittent, diffuse alveolar hemorrhage without evidence of vasculitis, inflammation, granulomas, necrosis, circulating anti-GBM antibodies, elevated pulmonary venous pressure, or systemic disease. Iron deficiency anemia and ILD frequently accompany this disorder. Although predominantly a disease of children, about 20% of patients with idiopathic pulmonary hemosiderosis are adults, usually younger than age 30 years. There is a 2:1 male predominance in adults. Respiratory symptoms include cough, fatigue, substernal chest pain, and malaise due to anemia. Tachycardia, tachypnea, fever, and hepatosplenomegaly (20%) may be found. Roentgenographic examination usually reveals diffuse, bilateral, acinar infiltrates. Following repeated episodes, a chronic interstitial infiltrate, infrequently associated with hilar and mediastinal adenopathy, remains. Systemic corticosteroids appear to be beneficial in improving the immediate outcome of acute exacerbations, but a long-term beneficial effect has not been demonstrated.

PULMONARY ALVEOLAR PROTEINOSIS. Pulmonary alveolar proteinosis is characterized by the accumulation of an acellular, periodic acid-Schiff–positive, lipoproteinaceous material within alveoli. Approximately half of patients with alveolar proteinosis have been exposed to various dusts or solvents, including silica, asbestos, tin, cadmium, molybdenum, or cement dust. Pulmonary alveolar proteinosis has been associated with hematologic abnormalities (10% of cases), including myeloblastic leukemia, chronic myelocytic leukemia, paraproteinemia, and Fanconi's anemia. Melanoma metastatic to the lung, dermatomyosis, and busulfan-induced ILD have also been associated with alveolar proteinosis. Alveolar proteinosis may present with (1) an abnormal chest roentgenogram in an asymptomatic patient; (2) the abrupt onset of cough, fever, and chest discomfort due to a superimposed infection; or (3) the insidious onset of cough and dyspnea related to accumulation of large amounts of intra-alveolar lipoproteinaceous material. Roentgenographic findings include diffuse, bilateral, symmetrical lower lobe alveolar infiltrates associated with air bronchograms. Secondary opportunistic infections are associated with pulmonary alveolar proteinosis in 15% of patients; specific organisms include *Nocardia* (most common), *Cryptococcus, Aspergillus, Histoplasma, Mycobacterium, Pneumocystis,* and cytomegalovirus (CMV). The diagnosis of alveolar proteinosis can often be established by bronchoscopic transbronchial lung biopsy. Open lung biopsy may be required in some instances. The treatment of choice is therapeutic whole-lung lavage using 40 to 60 L of fluid via a double-lumen endotracheal tube while the patient is under general anesthesia. The clinical course in alveolar proteinosis is highly variable and may include (1) a progressive disease with superimposed pulmonary infection despite frequent, repeated lavages; (2) stable, recurrent disease requiring repeated lavage (every 6 to 24 months); (3) improvement without relapse; or (4) development of severe ILD.

CHRONIC EOSINOPHILIC PNEUMONIA. A wide spectrum of clinical illness may be seen at presentation, ranging from no symptoms to respiratory failure. Cough, fever (as high as 40°C), dyspnea, weight loss, malaise, and night sweats are the most common symptoms. Wheezing is part of the syndrome in one-third to half of patients, but some patients never wheeze. Peripheral blood eosinophilia is present in 85% of patients during the course of chronic eosinophilic pneumonia, but it may be absent at initial presentation in as many as one-third of patients. The proportion of eosinophils in peripheral blood may be as high as 65%, although it is more commonly 10 to 40%. BAL eosinophils may be greater than 40% during exacerbations. The abnormalities on chest roentgenograms are variable, but a classic, almost pathognomonic, group of findings occurs in about 25% of cases: peripheral, nonsegmental alveolar infiltrates that resolve within 2 to 4 days after treatment with corticosteroids but recur in the same distribution with clinical relapses. The dense peripheral infiltrates have been characterized as the "photographic negative of pulmonary edema." Dense apical or axillary peripheral infiltrates, lobar consolidation, patchy perihilar infiltrates, nodules with cavities, and bilateral reticulonodular infiltrates also have been described. Although the diagnosis of chronic eosinophilic pneumonia often can be made with enough certainty to justify a therapeutic trial of corticosteroids, transbronchial biopsy and BAL should be performed unless contraindications exist. Open lung biopsy is rarely required. Administration of corticosteroids almost universally leads to rapid improvement in chronic eosinophilic pneumonia; failure to improve with corticosteroids should raise doubts about the accuracy of the diagnosis. Improvement often occurs within hours, and chest roentgenograms usually clear in 2 to 4 days. Prolonged therapy is often required (6 to 12 months), and the rate of relapse is high, even after a year of corticosteroid therapy.

INTERSTITIAL LUNG DISEASE ASSOCIATED WITH PULMONARY VASCULITIS

The pulmonary vasculitic syndromes are a diverse, rare group of diseases with overlapping clinical and pathologic manifestations. Although ILD is not a common presenting feature of the pulmonary vasculitides, most patients ultimately develop significant pulmonary fibrosis.

WEGENER'S GRANULOMATOSIS (see Chapter 294). Wegener's granulomatosis is a systemic disease in which granulomatous, necrotizing vasculitis involves the upper and lower respiratory tracts and kidneys. All patients have respiratory tract involvement, but certain patients with a limited form of the disease have no apparent renal disease. Chest radiographs usually reveal multiple nodular or cavitary infiltrates, but single nodules may be found. Patients in whom Wegener's granulomatosis is expected should be tested for antineutrophil cytoplasmic antibody (ANCA), but a negative ANCA does not exclude Wegener's granulomatosis. An open lung biopsy is the procedure of choice for establishing the diagnosis. Cyclophosphamide (1 to 2 mg/kg/day, orally) in conjunction with oral corticosteroids (prednisone, 60 mg/day) is the standard initial therapy for Wegener's granulomatosis. After clinical manifestations have subsided, the prednisone dose can be decreased. Initial remission occurs in more than 90% of patients. Relapses occur in 25 to 30% of patients after a successful course of therapy or during the period of corticosteroid dose reduction. Trimethoprim-sulfamethoxazole (one double-strength tablet twice a day) can be used to treat early, predominantly granulomatous disease if systemic vasculitis is absent. Patients with disease confined to the upper respiratory tract or lungs or both may respond to as little as 10 days of therapy with trimethoprim-sulfamethoxazole, but 8 weeks of treatment is often required. If this therapy fails, conventional therapy as outlined above should be given. The serum C-ANCA is a useful monitor of disease activity.

CHURG-STRAUSS SYNDROME (ALLERGIC ANGIITIS AND GRANULOMATOSIS) (see Chapter 293). This systemic necrotizing vasculitis affects the upper and lower respiratory tracts and is almost invariably preceded by allergic manifestations such as asthma, allergic rhinitis, or a drug reaction. Chest radiographs reveal bilateral patchy, fleeting infiltrates, diffuse nodular infiltrates without cavitation, or diffuse reticulonodular disease. Open lung biopsy provides definitive histologic evidence of Churg-Strauss syndrome.

INHERITED DISORDERS

ILD may result from a group of rare inherited disorders. Both autosomal dominant and recessive disorders may be associated with ILD.

FAMILIAL IDIOPATHIC PULMONARY FIBROSIS. This is an autosomal dominant disease with clinical, roentgenographic, physiologic, and morphologic features that are indistinguishable from nonfamilial idiopathic pulmonary fibrosis. Symptoms begin between ages 20 and 40 years. Evidence of alveolar inflammation is usually present in clinically unaffected family members.

NEUROFIBROMATOSES (see Chapter 456). ILD occurs in 20% of patients with neurofibromatosis, usually between ages 35 and 60 years. Dyspnea is the predominant symptom. The ILD has histologic features similar to those of idiopathic pulmonary fibrosis. There is no known therapy.

TUBEROUS SCLEROSIS (see Chapter 456). Hamartomas, which are the characteristic histologic lesion, may be found in the lungs (1% of patients), central nervous system, bones, eyes, kidneys, skin, and heart. The clinical, physiologic, radiographic, and pathologic features strongly resemble those of lymphangioleiomyomatosis.

AUTOSOMAL RECESSIVE DISEASES. ILD has been described in several autosomal recessive diseases, including Gaucher's disease, Niemann-Pick disease (see Chapter 208), and Hermansky-

Pudlak syndrome (partial oculocutaneous albinism, a hemorrhagic defect due to platelet dysfunction, and accumulation of ceroid in the reticuloendothelial system).

Cooper JAD Jr: Drug-induced pulmonary disease. Clin Chest Med 2:1, 1990. *Reviews the clinical findings and pathogenesis of drug-induced interstitial lung disorders.*

Gay SE, Kazerooni EA, Toews GB, et al: Idiopathic pulmonary fibrosis: Predicting response to therapy and survival. Am J Respir Crit Care Med 157:1063, 1998. *Defines the role of high-resolution CT and lung biopsy in predicting response to therapy and survival in idiopathic pulmonary fibrosis.*

Hunninghake GW, Kalica AR: Approaches to the treatment of pulmonary fibrosis. Am J Respir Crit Care Med 151:915, 1995. *A report of a consensus conference on therapy for pulmonary fibrosis.*

Katzenstein AA: Idiopathic pulmonary fibrosis: Clinical relevance of pathologic classification. Am J Respir Crit Care Med 157:1301, 1998. *A review of the pathology of interstitial lung diseases.*

Keane MP, Belperio JA, Moore TA, et al: Neutralization of the CXC chemokine, macrophage inflammatory protein–2, attenuates bleomycin-induced pulmonary fibrosis. J Immunol 162:5511–5518, 1999. *Mechanism of this drug-induced toxicity.*

Muller NL, Ostrow DN: High resolution computed tomography of chronic interstitial lung diseases. Clin Chest Med 12:97, 1991. *Reviews the use of high-resolution CT in chronic interstitial lung diseases.*

79 OCCUPATIONAL PULMONARY DISORDERS

Jonathan M. Samet

Interstitial lung diseases (ILDs) damage the pulmonary interstitium by disrupting alveolar structures and the small airways. Occupational diseases affecting the pulmonary interstitium include primarily the pneumoconioses, or dust diseases of the lung (Table 79–1), and hypersensitivity pneumonitis. The principal pneumoconioses—asbestosis, coal workers' pneumoconiosis, and silicosis—typically occur after sustained exposures to dust concentrations that are no longer legally permissible in many developed countries, including the United States. Although these diseases are declining, cases still occur in locales where industries have been historically associated with high dust exposures and as "sentinel" cases, signaling unsuspected and uncontrolled occupational exposures. Beryllium, originally linked to lung disease in workers making fluorescent lamps, now has widespread usage in high-technology applications. New agents introduced into the workplace may also cause unanticipated diseases. People with occupational ILD may present to health care providers through diverse paths. Physicians may evaluate previously undiagnosed patients with occupational ILD who present with dyspnea or unexplained radiographic infiltrates or previously diagnosed patients who present for assessment of the extent of associated physiologic impairment, often in the context of a legal proceeding or a claim for disability. Current or former workers exposed to agents causing lung disease may also present for screening for adverse effects.

The occupational ILDs result from inhaling and retaining dusts that induce inflammation and fibrosis. Dust particles in the respirable size range are generated in workplaces by diverse processes; power-driven equipment, such as drills and grinders, place their operators at risk for diseases caused by dust, and nearby workers, even if not working directly with the materials, may be secondarily exposed. The lung is defended against dust particles by a system that includes the physical barrier posed by the upper airway that filters out larger particles, the mucociliary escalator that removes

Table 79–1 ■ PRINCIPAL PNEUMOCONIOSES CAUSED BY MINERAL DUSTS

AGENT	DISEASE	RADIOGRAPHIC APPEARANCE
Asbestos	Asbestosis	Reticular, basilar predominance
Coal dust	Coal workers' pneumoconiosis	Nodular, upper lobe predominance
Cobalt	Hard metal disease	Reticular, basilar predominance
Silica	Silicosis	Nodular, upper lobe predominance
Talc	Talcosis	Rounded, irregular, or both

inhaled particles, and the alveolar macrophages that scavenge inhaled and deposited particles in the small airways and alveoli. Particle size determines the likelihood and site of deposition in the respiratory tract. During quiet breathing, most particles larger than 10 μm in aerodynamic diameter are deposited in the upper respiratory tract, although some particles in this size range may enter the lung during exertion. Particles between approximately 3 and 10 μm tend to deposit in the larger airways of the lung, whereas smaller particles down to about 0.1 μm are preferentially deposited in the small airways and alveoli.

Inflammation and subsequent fibrosis are central in the pathogenesis of the occupational ILDs, although the mechanisms underlying the distinctive pathologic responses found in the different pneumoconioses are still not characterized. Present concepts of pathogenetic mechanisms for the pneumoconioses emphasize the roles of alveolar macrophages in the initial response to dust inhalation, of cytokine release, and of interactions among macrophages, lymphocytes, neutrophils, and fibroblasts. Hypersensitivity pneumonitis reflects cell-mediated immune responses to inhaled antigens.

Preventing these diseases rests largely on controlling exposures in the workplace through regulations that limit exposures to levels considered to be safe and that specify respiratory protection. Medical screening for early evidence of disease represents a complementary but secondary control approach. In the United States, the standard-setting agencies are the Occupational Safety and Health Administration (OSHA) and the Mine Safety and Health Administration (MSHA). Physicians who make a diagnosis indicating a failure of control measures should follow through by contacting relevant agencies, and with permission and possibly preservation of confidentiality, the employer or the union, as appropriate. The burden of respiratory morbidity and mortality in workers at risk for occupational lung disease can also be reduced by preventing and stopping smoking (see Chapter 13). For the nonmalignant occupational lung diseases, the adverse effects of cigarette smoking on lung function appear additive to those of the occupational agents, whereas for lung cancer, synergism with smoking has been found for most occupational carcinogens. New genetic approaches may eventually provide strategies for identifying workers with the greatest susceptibility; however, prevention will continue to be based on workplace controls for the foreseeable future.

For patients with clinically significant impairment, supportive treatment, as for other chronic lung diseases, is warranted. Patients should receive pneumococcal and influenza vaccines and oxygen therapy, as needed. Physical activity should be encouraged, and a comprehensive pulmonary rehabilitation program may benefit some patients. As for other patients with advanced chronic lung diseases, lung transplantation may be a consideration (see Chapter 89).

EVALUATING THE PATIENT WITH SUSPECTED OCCUPATIONAL INTERSTITIAL LUNG DISEASE

GENERAL APPROACH. Diagnosis of an occupational ILD is based on an appropriate clinical picture and documentation of exposure, related in a temporally appropriate fashion to the occurrence of the disease. In addition to the exposure history, chest radiography, lung function testing, and high-resolution computed tomography (HRCT) are the key components of the diagnostic evaluation (Fig. 79–1). As indicated, evaluation may also be needed to exclude other disorders associated with a comparable clinical picture. For example, in an elderly man with a history of underground mining and of cigarette smoking, a lung nodule might represent complicated silicosis or a primary cancer of the lung. The clinical history should cover the cardinal respiratory symptoms— cough, phlegm production, dyspnea, and wheezing; emphasis should be placed on quantifying the degree of dyspnea. Graded questions should be used for this purpose that inquire, for example, about having dyspnea while hurrying on the level ground or walking up a slight hill, about walking slower on level ground than same-age peers, about stopping for breath after walking about 100 yards, and about having dyspnea during such routine activities as dressing and bathing. On physical examination, the physician should look for finger clubbing or cyanosis, indicative of advanced disease. On examining the chest, the physician should note the quality of the breath sounds and the timing (early or late) and the type (fine or coarse) of any crackles (see Chapter 72).

HISTORY. A comprehensive occupational history should be

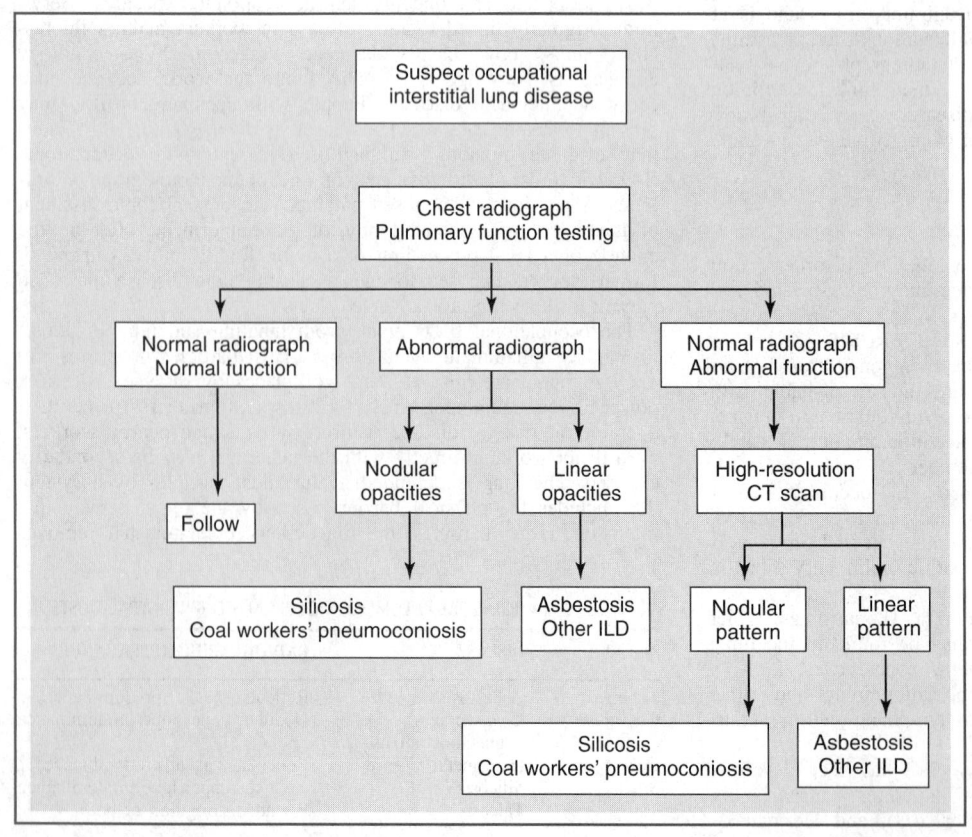

FIGURE 79–1 ■ Diagnostic approach to occupational interstitial lung disease (ILD). CT = computed tomography.

taken from all patients with suspected occupational disease. The history needs to cover each job systematically, describing the industry in which the patient worked, the specific occupation and job duties, materials handled, required and actual use of respiratory protective equipment, and occurrence of disease in fellow workers. Seasonal, part-time, and temporary jobs should not be omitted, as such jobs may have a greater likelihood of hazardous exposure. The dates of specific jobs may also be relevant because exposures for many agents were higher during past decades. Although the frequency of the more common pneumoconioses is now declining, some exposures (e.g., beryllium) are still widespread, and newer exposures may cause ILD. The history should inquire about specific materials (e.g., asbestos) and also about exposure through hobbies and the jobs of family members. A temporal association between entering the workplace and symptoms may indicate an exposure that triggers hypersensitivity pneumonitis.

The history should also cover cigarette smoking and other tobacco use (see Chapter 13). Chronic bronchitis and chronic airflow obstruction associated with smoking may explain cough and dyspnea or complicate the diagnosis of a distinct occupational lung disease.

IMAGING OF THE CHEST. In addition to a comprehensive occupational history, the diagnostic evaluation of patients with suspected occupational ILD also includes imaging of the lungs to establish the presence of disease and the characteristics of any infiltrates. All patients suspected of having an occupational ILD need to have standard posteroanterior (PA) and lateral radiographs. Most patients with a pneumoconiosis have an abnormal chest radiograph, but 10 to 20% do not. The type of infiltrates, nodular or reticular, and the distribution provide an indication of the underlying disease (see Table 79–1). The International Labour Organization has developed a standardized system for classifying the abnormalities found on the PA radiograph in pneumoconioses. Although intended for use in epidemiologic research, the scheme is now widely applied clinically. In this system, small parenchymal opacities are classified by shape (irregular or rounded), size, distribution, and profusion or concentration. The profusion, scored on a 12-point scale, is indicative of the degree of histopathologic derangement. The pneumoconiosis is termed "simple" if all opacities are less than 1 cm in diameter and "complicated" if opacities of 1 cm or greater are present.

HRCT is increasingly used to evaluate patients with ILD, including occupational diseases. The narrow slice thickness of 1 to 2 mm provides visualization of fine parenchymal detail and detects interstitial changes and emphysema. For example, in berylliosis, the chest radiograph shows hilar adenopathy and extensive infiltrates, whereas the HRCT documents extensive air-space destruction and infiltration (Fig. 79–2). In silicosis, the typical nodular opacities are evident in the chest radiograph, whereas the HRCT shows the nodules as well as airspace enlargement (Fig. 79–3). Although the role of HRCT is still evolving, it should be considered for patients who have a normal chest radiograph but are suspected of having an occupational ILD. HRCT may also prove valuable for quantifying the degree of abnormality and the extent of coexisting emphysema, but it cannot be recommended for these purposes at present.

PULMONARY FUNCTION TESTING. Spirometry should be performed on all patients at risk for an occupational ILD and the results compared with predicted values based on gender, race, age, and height (see Chapter 73). If the results are within the limits of normal, further testing is not indicated except for patients complaining of dyspnea or having roentgenographic abnormalities indicative of pneumoconiosis. Those patients, as well as patients with abnormal spirometry, should have measurements of the single breath diffusing capacity for carbon monoxide and lung volumes (total lung capacity [TLC] and residual volume). Exercise testing with measurement of blood gases and gas exchange parameters may be needed to evaluate dyspnea and to quantitate exercise impairment.

INVASIVE DIAGNOSTIC MEASURES. Invasive procedures are rarely indicated to establish the diagnosis of an occupational ILD, although biopsy may be warranted on clinical grounds to exclude alternative diagnoses. Bronchoalveolar lavage, the least invasive approach, provides fluid that can be analyzed for dusts and fibers and for cell populations; it is primarily a research tool at present. Transbronchial lung biopsy specimens obtained via the fiberoptic bronchoscope may yield a specific diagnosis, and the specimens can be analyzed for dusts and fibers, as can those obtained by open lung biopsy. Polarized light microscopy, which is routinely available, can detect crystals, and ferruginous bodies—ferritin-coated fibers—can be identified with routine optical microscopy. More sophisticated techniques can be used to quantify and identify particles in lung tissue if needed for medicolegal purposes.

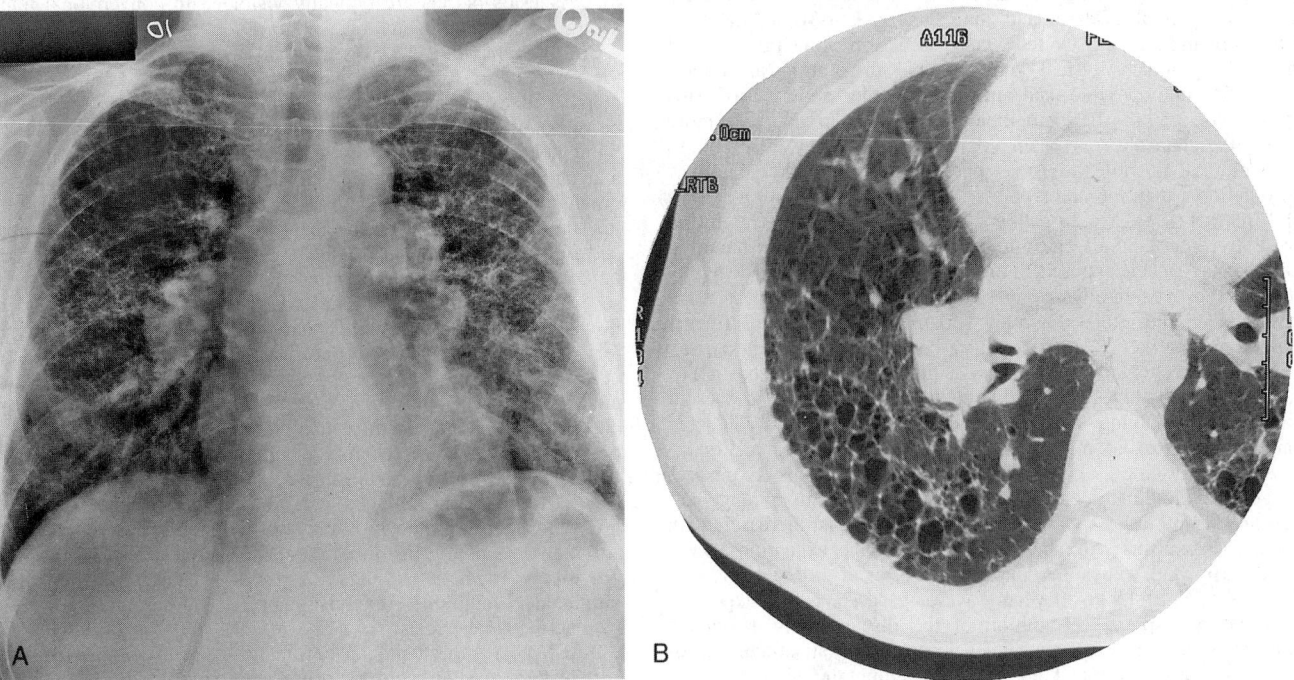

FIGURE 79-2 ■ PA chest radiograph (*A*) and high-resolution computed tomography (HRCT) scan (*B*) from a patient with berylliosis. The chest radiograph demonstrates hilar adenopathy and extensive infiltrates, and the HRCT shows extensive air-space destruction and infiltrates.

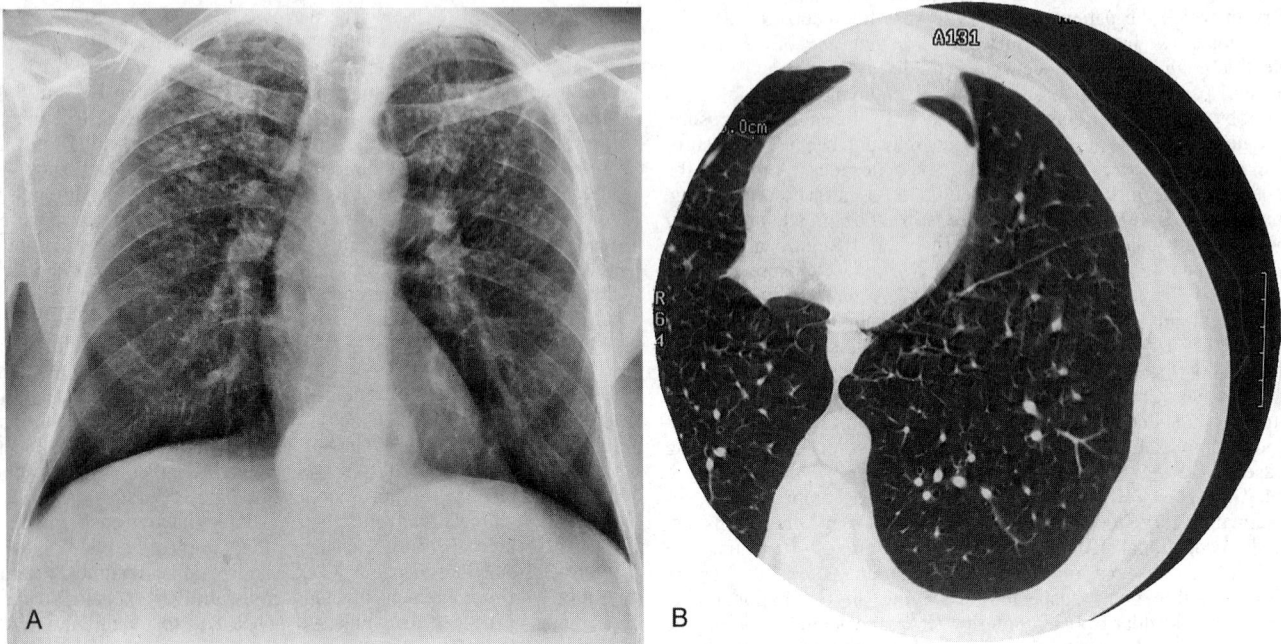

FIGURE 79–3 ■ PA chest radiograph (*A*) and high-resolution computed tomography (HRCT) scan (*B*) from a patient with silicosis. The chest radiograph demonstrates the typical nodular opacities, and the HRCT shows the nodules as well as air-space enlargement.

PNEUMOCONIOSES

ASBESTOSIS. DEFINITION. Asbestosis refers to fibrosis of the lung parenchyma and not to the pleural fibrosis and plaques that are frequently found in asbestos-exposed workers. Asbestos exposure is also associated with mesothelioma of the pleura and peritoneum, lung cancer, laryngeal cancer, and, possibly, gastrointestinal cancers.

ETIOLOGY. Asbestos refers to several fibrous silicate minerals having unique physical-chemical properties that make them effective for insulation, reinforcing materials, friction products, and other purposes. All types of asbestos fibers are associated with asbestosis, pleural disease, and lung cancer. Chrysotile, the type principally used in the United States, is a serpentine mineral that undergoes gradual physical and chemical dissolution in tissues. Crocidolite, anthophyllite, and amosite, the other principal asbestos types used, are in the amphibole mineral group and are more needle-like than the curly chrysotile fibers and not as prone to dissolution. Chrysotile asbestos appears to be a weaker cause of mesothelioma than the amphiboles.

EPIDEMIOLOGY. Asbestos fibers have been widely used during the 20th century, and large numbers of workers directly handling asbestos have been exposed, along with indirectly exposed nearby workers and even family members exposed to fibers brought home on clothing. The exposed worker groups include asbestos miners and millers, workers manufacturing asbestos products such as textiles and brake linings, and workers using asbestos products such as insulators, and other construction trades. With a large number of buildings now having asbestos-containing materials, custodial and maintenance workers may also be exposed, as may workers involved in removing asbestos and demolishing buildings. Exposures for general building occupants are quite low and in a range not associated with asbestosis. The risk of asbestosis increases with cumulative exposure to asbestos fibers; with the exception of extraordinarily high exposures, manifestations of disease are not usually present until 15 to 20 years have elapsed since first exposure. With the widespread recognition of the disease risks associated with asbestos, exposures have been lowered and substitutes introduced in many developed countries, including the United States. The cohort of workers at greatest risk for asbestosis comprises workers exposed through the early 1970s, and the incidence of asbestosis should diminish as these workers age.

PATHOLOGY. In experimental models of asbestosis, the earliest lesions are found in the alveolar ducts and peribronchiolar regions, where deposited asbestos fibers attract alveolar macrophages. The lungs of asbestos-exposed workers show an inflammatory and fibrotic lesion of the small airways, termed "mineral dust–induced small airways disease." As disease progresses, the fibrotic process becomes more extensive and may ultimately involve the entire lung. In advanced cases, extensive fibrosis may destroy the normal architecture of the lung to cause honeycombing, cystic spaces bounded by fibrosis. In advanced disease, the lungs are small and stiff with macroscopically visible fibrosis and honeycombing. Asbestos bodies are typically visible with conventional microscopy.

CLINICAL MANIFESTATIONS. Patients with asbestosis present with the same clinical picture found in other interstitial lung diseases: cough and exertional dyspnea. Some cases of asbestosis may also be detected by screening of exposed worker populations. Bibasilar fine crackles are heard on auscultation of the chest in most patients, and clubbing may be present in advanced cases. The chest radiograph shows irregular opacities that are typically most prominent in the lung bases; pleural disease, particularly in the form of localized and often calcified plaques, is often present as well. The degree of physiologic impairment on lung function testing varies with the severity of the asbestosis. The small airways lesions produce airflow obstruction, manifest by changes in the shape of the expiratory flow-volume curve, with corresponding reduction of flow rates at lower lung volumes. Airflow obstruction cannot be readily attributed to asbestos exposure in individual patients who have smoked cigarettes. In patients with clinically significant dyspnea, spirometry typically shows a reduced forced vital capacity (FVC) with preservation of the ratio of the forced expiratory volume in 1 second (FEV₁) to FVC, and reduced TLC and diffusing capacity; however, this typical physiologic profile is not invariably observed, and obstruction secondary to smoking may complicate interpretation of pulmonary function findings. Progressive exercise testing shows pulmonary limitation of exercise capacity and desaturation in many patients with asbestosis.

DIAGNOSIS. Asbestosis can be diagnosed with confidence if there is a history of significant exposure to asbestos; radiographic, clinical, and physiologic evidence of ILD compatible with asbestosis; and no indication of another disease process associated with a comparable clinical picture of interstitial lung disease, e.g., scleroderma (see Chapter 290). The exposure should have started at least 15 years before the disease developed. Pleural plaques provide a strong indication of past asbestos exposure. In patients with biopsy-proven ILD without a firm history of exposure, the presence of asbestos bodies should increase suspicion for asbestosis. More formal counting of asbestos bodies or of fibers may be warranted.

TREATMENT. At present, no effective treatment for asbestosis is available, other than oxygen therapy as needed. Lung transplantation may be considered for selected patients. Because of the increased risk of asbestos-exposed individuals for lung cancer, perhaps particularly those with asbestosis, smoking cessation should be emphasized.

PROGNOSIS. The course of radiographically identified asbestosis is variable, with some cases showing progression, whereas others remain static. Factors influencing progression are not well established but appear to include the cumulative exposure to asbestos, the duration of exposure, and the type of asbestos exposure. The extent of radiographic fibrosis is a strong predictor of mortality.

COAL WORKERS' PNEUMOCONIOSIS. **DEFINITION.** Coal workers' pneumoconiosis is the parenchymal lung disease caused by inhaling coal mine dust. The disease is termed "simple" if all radiographic opacities are less than 1 cm in diameter. Progressive massive fibrosis complicates simple coal workers' pneumoconiosis if any nodular opacities of 1 or greater cm are present on the chest radiograph. Exposure to coal mine dust is also associated with industrial bronchitis and loss of lung function at a rate beyond that associated with aging; these consequences of such exposure are not considered coal workers' pneumoconiosis, although they do contribute to the respiratory morbidity experienced by coal miners. The group of lung diseases caused by coal mine dust are commonly referred to as "black lung."

ETIOLOGY. Coal refers to a group of carbonaceous materials characterized by the hardness or "rank," ranging from peat, the softest, to anthracite, the hardest. Inhaling coal dust causes coal workers' pneumoconiosis, but inhaling more pure carbon materials—lamp-black and carbon black—has also been associated with a comparable lung disease. Silica in the coal dust may also contribute to the development of coal workers' pneumoconiosis. Determinants of progression from simple coal workers' pneumoconiosis to progressive massive fibrosis, other than coal rank and coal mine dust exposure, have not been identified.

EPIDEMIOLOGY. Extensive epidemiologic information shows that the risk of coal workers' pneumoconiosis increases with dust level in the mine and cumulative exposure to coal mine dust. Risk also increases with the rank of the coal, being greatest for the harder coals. In studies of the mortality of underground coal miners, progressive massive fibrosis increases risk of death, whereas simple coal workers' pneumoconiosis has a lesser adverse effect. Reduced exposures for US miners since the passage of the Coal Mine Health and Safety Act of 1969 should reduce risks for those recently starting to mine.

PATHOLOGY. The characteristic lesion of coal workers' pneumoconiosis is the coal macule, an inflammatory lesion consisting of focal collections of coal mine dust–laden macrophages surrounding respiratory bronchioles. The coal macule may extend to the alveoli and be accompanied by fibrosis of the small airways and alveoli and by focal emphysema. Larger "coal nodules," which are grossly firm and contain dust-filled macrophages in collagen and reticulin, may develop. Progressive massive fibrosis is diagnosed pathologically if nodules reach at least 2 cm, although the radiographic definition is based on opacities of at least 1 cm. These lesions are also collagen-containing and tend to disrupt the lung's architecture. In Caplan's syndrome, or rheumatoid pneumoconiosis, multiple lung nodules, ranging from 1 to 5 cm, are present, typically in the periphery.

CLINICAL MANIFESTATIONS. Coal mine dust–exposed miners may present with cough and sputum production reflecting industrial bronchitis and dyspnea associated with pulmonary function impairment, whether secondary to progressive massive fibrosis involving the parenchyma or accelerated loss of ventilatory function related to dust-induced airways disease. Other than characteristic radiographic findings, there are no specific clinical manifestations of simple coal workers' pneumoconiosis; despite widespread radiographic abnormalities, many miners are asymptomatic or have only mild adverse changes in lung function, whereas some may have significant impairment with little or no radiographic abnormality. In

simple disease, the chest radiograph typically shows small nodules that tend to predominate in the upper lung zones. Reticular opacities may also be present, more often in cigarette smokers.

Progressive massive fibrosis is associated with progressive dyspnea, pulmonary hypertension, and even respiratory failure. The chest radiograph shows the characteristic nodules of progressive massive fibrosis, often with contraction of the affected lung, typically upper lobes, and compensatory hyperinflation, typically lower lobes. The nodules may cavitate and produce melanoptysis. In progressive massive fibrosis, lung function is typically impaired, particularly if larger nodules are present. Both airflow obstruction (reduced FEV_1 and FEV_1/FVC ratio) and lung restriction (reduced TLC) can occur. The single-breath diffusing capacity for carbon monoxide is also reduced, and resting hypoxemia or desaturation with exercise may be present. Caplan's syndrome should be considered in miners with multiple peripheral nodules; this uncommon syndrome may develop in miners with rheumatoid arthritis or with circulating rheumatoid factor without arthritis (see Chapter 286).

DIAGNOSIS. Coal workers' pneumoconiosis is diagnosed on the basis of an appropriate history of exposure and characteristic radiographic abnormalities. In patients with probable progressive massive fibrosis, consideration should be given to alternative causes of lung masses, including lung cancer.

TREATMENT. No effective treatment is currently available for coal workers' pneumoconiosis. Appropriate supportive care and rehabilitation should be provided for those with impaired lung function.

PROGNOSIS. Total coal mine dust exposure and increasing severity of simple pneumoconiosis predict the development of progressive massive fibrosis, which is associated with more severe morbidity and increased overall mortality. Simple pneumoconiosis alone does not increase mortality.

SILICOSIS. **DEFINITION.** Silicosis refers to the parenchymal lung diseases associated with crystalline silica exposure, including acute, accelerated, and chronic or classic silicosis. These entities are distinguished by their clinical pictures and time course in relation to silica exposure. In acute silicosis, an alveolar filling process follows heavy exposure within a few years. Accelerated silicosis occurs within 5 to 10 years of exposure and has a clinical picture comparable to that of chronic silicosis, which develops after a longer latent period.

ETIOLOGY. Crystalline silicon dioxide, the causal agent, is abundant and ubiquitous in the earth's crust and is used in a variety of industrial applications. Quartz is the most common form. Consequently, large numbers of workers, probably millions in the United States, are still exposed (Table 79–2).

EPIDEMIOLOGY. As for the other pneumoconioses, the risk of developing disease increases with the level and duration of exposure. Although the hazard posed by silica exposure has long been recognized and exposure standards have been promulgated, new cases continue to occur, even of acute silicosis, which has been recently reported in sandblasters, ground silica workers, and rock drillers.

PATHOLOGY. Like coal workers' pneumoconiosis, chronic silicosis occurs in a simple form and as progressive massive fibrosis. The earliest lesions are collections of dust-laden macrophages in the peribronchiolar and paraseptal or subpleural areas. The silicotic nodule has an acellular core composed of collagen surrounded by a cellular capsule with macrophages, lymphocytes, and fibroblasts. Silicotic nodules may also involve the hilar lymph nodes. Silicotic nodules coalesce to form the lesions of progressive massive fibrosis, masses of dense hyalinized connective tissue with little inflammation. Accelerated silicosis progresses rapidly to progressive massive fibrosis, whereas acute silicosis has a distinct pattern with few

Table 79–2 ■ **PRINCIPAL OCCUPATIONS ASSOCIATED WITH SILICON EXPOSURE**

Abrasives workers	Silica flour workers
Foundry workers	Silica millers
Glass makers	Stone workers
Pottery workers	Surface mine drillers
Quarriers	Underground miners
Sandblasters	

or no nodules and alveolar filling with proteinaceous material. Polarized light microscopy may show birefringent particles indicative of silica in the lungs of silica-exposed persons, including those with silicosis.

CLINICAL MANIFESTATIONS. Chronic silicosis without progressive massive fibrosis is associated with little physiologic impairment. Cough and sputum production may reflect underlying bronchitis related to dust exposure or cigarette smoking. As in coal workers' pneumoconiosis, progressive massive fibrosis can be associated with significant impairment on lung function testing and clinically significant dyspnea. Both airflow obstruction and lung restriction may be present. Acute silicosis presents with rapidly progressive dyspnea. Persons with silicosis are at increased risk for mycobacterial infection (see Chapter 358), and they may present with manifestations of infection such as fever and weight loss.

In chronic silicosis, the chest radiograph shows small nodules that tend to predominate in the upper lobes (Fig. 79–3). Calcification of the nodules is rare, as is so-called eggshell calcification of enlarged hilar nodes. In progressive massive fibrosis, the mass lesions are typically in the upper lobes and are often associated with compensatory hyperinflation of the lower lobes. Widespread consolidation is present on the chest radiograph in acute silicosis. Caplan's syndrome may also occur in silica-exposed workers, but it is rare.

DIAGNOSIS. The diagnosis of chronic silicosis is made on the basis of characteristic radiographic findings and history of employment in a job associated with exposure to silica-containing dust. Before accepting a diagnosis of progressive massive fibrosis in a silica-exposed worker, other causes of lung masses should be considered, including, specifically, lung cancer and mycobacterial infection. Acute silicosis should be considered in heavily exposed individuals with a diffuse consolidating process. Unless the epidemiologic features of the case make the diagnosis of acute silicosis certain, lung biopsy may be indicated to establish the diagnosis and to exclude other diseases.

TREATMENT. As in any chronic lung disease, supportive therapy, oxygen, and rehabilitation may be indicated. One report suggested possible short-term benefits of corticosteroid therapy, but steroid therapy cannot be recommended at present. Because of the increased risk of mycobacterial diseases, particularly *Mycobacterium tuberculosis,* all persons with silicosis should receive yearly tuberculin skin tests and evaluation for active tuberculosis if the test is positive. Isoniazid prophylaxis is recommended if the test is positive and active disease is not present. Some studies indicate that prolonged antituberculous therapy may be indicated in patients with silicosis and active tuberculosis (see Chapter 358).

PROGNOSIS. The prognosis of accelerated and acute silicosis is poor; both are associated with progressive loss of function, and acute silicosis may be rapidly fatal. Progressive massive fibrosis has a more variable course, which may also lead to progressive impairment and respiratory failure. Factors determining progression from chronic silicosis to progressive massive fibrosis are uncertain.

OTHER PNEUMOCONIOSES. Inhaling other minerals and metals may also cause pneumoconioses (see Table 79–1). Silicates other than asbestos have been linked to interstitial lung disease, including talc, kaolinite, mica, and vermiculite. Benign pneumoconioses are associated with inhaling forms of barium (baritosis) and tin (stannosis). Hard-metal disease occurs in workers exposed to cobalt in applications involving its use in alloys and abrasives. This diffuse interstitial disease, which can be associated with clinically significant impairment, should be considered in workers in foundries and in industries involving grinding of metals, gems, and other materials. Some workers exposed to man-made fibers develop small opacities, but a distinct pneumoconiosis has not yet been identified from exposure to these newer fibers. Mixed-dust pneumoconiosis is a nonspecific label often used for the presence of both rounded and irregular opacities on the chest radiograph of a worker with exposure to several types of dust. Typically, there is exposure to silica and to an additional mineral.

BERYLLIUM DISEASE. Beryllium disease is a granulomatous lung disease that results from inhaling beryllium, a rare metal now widely used in high-technology applications (Table 79–3). The

Table 79–3 ■ CURRENT INDUSTRIES USING BERYLLIUM

Aerospace	Foundries
Beryllium extraction, fabrication, smelting	Nuclear reactors Nuclear weapons
Ceramics	Plating
Dental alloys and prostheses	Telecommunications
Electronics	Tool and die

typical cases currently observed present with gradual onset and are referred to as chronic beryllium disease; a more acute form was reported with past higher levels of exposure. When first recognized, the disease was found in workers who extracted and produced beryllium and in workers making fluorescent lamps containing a beryllium phosphor. Cases have been reported in bystanders not working directly with the metal and in persons residing in the vicinity of beryllium processing plants. More contemporary industries place a large number of workers at risk. In a study of nuclear weapons workers, about 5% of exposed workers were shown to be sensitized to beryllium.

Advances in understanding of the pathogenesis of beryllium disease have provided both a screening test for sensitization and a marker for individual susceptibility. The beryllium lymphocyte transformation test can be used to establish sensitization to the metal and as a workplace screening tool. In this in vitro assay, blood lymphocytes or lung lymphocytes obtained by bronchoalveolar lavage are exposed to beryllium salts; cells from sensitized individuals show proliferation. A genetic marker for susceptibility to beryllium disease has been identified. A strong association has been reported between a specific phenotype associated with the major histocompatibility complex (MHC) HLA-DPβ1 (see Chapter 278) and beryllium disease. This marker may eventually prove useful to identify workers at greatest risk and to better understand the pathogenesis of beryllium disease.

The lymphocyte transformation test can confirm beryllium exposure, but the metal can also be measured in tissue specimens and urine. Patients with beryllium disease may have both respiratory and systemic symptoms and chest radiograph findings ranging from normal to diffuse interstitial infiltrates and hilar adenopathy. Corticosteroid therapy may be beneficial, but life-long treatment is needed.

HYPERSENSITIVITY PNEUMONITIS. Hypersensitivity pneumonitis, typically a granulomatous ILD, results from inhaling diverse environmental antigens and chemicals. Although interstitial fibrosis is classically considered to be a granulomatous disorder, some patients may have interstitial fibrosis without granulomas. If granulomas are present in lung or other tissue specimens, the differential diagnosis includes sarcoidosis and hypersensitivity pneumonitis. Hypersensitivity pneumonitis may present as an acute illness, but it may also present in a chronic form with pulmonary fibrosis. The workplace is often a site of exposure to antigens generated by microbial contaminants of heating, ventilating, and air conditioning systems or other moist devices or materials. Chemical agents associated with hypersensitivity pneumonitis include isocyanates and trimellitic anhydride. The diagnosis is made on the basis of the clinical picture, exposure history, and demonstration of precipitating antibodies to antigens.

Kreiss K, Miller F, Newman LS, et al: Chronic beryllium disease: From the workplace to cellular immunology, molecular immunogenetics, and back. Clin Immunol Immunopathol 71:123–129, 1994. *This is a review of pathogenesis and clinical implications.*

Markowitz SB, Morabia A, Lilis R, et al: Clinical predictors of mortality from asbestosis in the North American insulation cohort, 1981 to 1991. Am J Resp Crit Care Med 156:101, 1997. *Describes predictors of mortality.*

Rom WN: Environmental and Occupational Medicine, 3rd ed. Philadelphia, Lippincott-Raven, 1998. *This comprehensive text reviews the full scope of occupational medicine, touching on workplace assessment, clinical evaluation, and specific agents and disease entities.*

Rosenman KD, Reilly MJ, Kalinowski DJ, Walt FC: Silicosis in the 1990s. Chest 111: 779, 1997. *Provides a picture of silicosis in Michigan, 1987–1995.*

Satini C, et al: Immunogenetics of environmental lung disease: Lessons from the berylliosis model. Eur Respir J 12:1463–1475, 1998. *An HLA marker has been identified in patients who develop berylliosis.*

Wagner GR: Asbestosis and silicosis. Lancet 349:1311–1315, 1997. *A succinct review of clinical aspects and prevention.*

80 PHYSICAL, CHEMICAL, AND ASPIRATION INJURIES OF THE LUNG

Claude A. Piantadosi

PHYSICAL AND CHEMICAL INJURIES OF THE LUNG

The lung's large and delicate surface area is protected from toxic substances in the environment by extensive defense mechanisms. Normally, inspired gas is fully humidified and warmed to body temperature, and all large particulate substances are cleared by the upper airways. These normal defenses are not adequate to handle exposure to many physical and chemical substances that cause lung injury, so lung disorders may be initiated by inhalation or aspiration of injurious chemicals or by exposure to potentially harmful physical environments.

Thermal Injuries and Smoke Inhalation

ETIOLOGY. After major burns, about one-third of patients have pulmonary complications; these complications account for the majority of burn-related deaths. Smoke inhalation sufficient to cause respiratory injury may also occur without external burns. Thermal injury to the lung is associated with four groups of complications: (1) *immediate reaction*–direct thermal injury to upper airways leading to upper airway obstruction; (2) carbon monoxide and cyanide poisoning; (3) *acute respiratory distress syndrome* (ARDS) developing 24 to 48 hours after the thermal injury; and (4) *late-onset pulmonary complications,* which include pneumonia, atelectasis, thromboembolism, and, in case of thoracic burns, chest wall restriction.

The constituents of smoke are by-products of pyrolysis and incomplete combustion. Many of these products are potent mucosal irritants and bronchoconstrictors and contribute to both upper and lower lung injury. Certain constituents of smoke have been identified consistently as contributors to respiratory injury (Table 80–1). Smoke inhalation rarely causes thermal injury to the lung parenchyma; the large capacity of the upper airways to humidify and modify the temperatures of inhaled air protects the alveolar tissue from heat. Exceptions are steam burns and explosions in an enclosed space.

CLINICAL MANIFESTATIONS. The initial signs and symptoms of smoke inhalation are tachypnea, cough, dyspnea, wheezing, cyanosis, hoarseness, and stridor (an ominous sign). Facial burns may provide a clue to smoke inhalation and thermal injury to the upper airway. During the 12 to 48 hours after the injury, the patient can manifest increasing hypoxemia, and lung compliance may decrease owing to noncardiogenic pulmonary edema. Roentgenograms of the chest may reveal a pattern of diffuse, patchy infiltrates. A major complication is infection, often caused by *Pseudomonas aeruginosa* or *Staphylococcus aureus.* The lung defenses against infection are compromised by thermal and chemical injury to the airway epithelium as well as by the presence of an endotracheal or tracheostomy tube. The pathway for infection is either by inhaling airborne organisms or by hematogenous spread from cutaneous burns.

ARDS may develop 24 to 48 hours after the initial injury. The causes of ARDS are controversial in burn patients, but possibilities include chemical pneumonitis from constituents in smoke, a circulating burn toxin, disseminated intravascular coagulation, microembolism, and neurogenic pulmonary edema. The extent of surface thermal injury does not correlate with the degree of respiratory distress that occurs subsequently.

TREATMENT AND PROGNOSIS. The most immediate life-threatening complications in the patient presenting with major burns or with a history of smoke inhalation are upper airway obstruction and carbon monoxide (CO) poisoning. The patient should be closely observed for evidence of these complications. Laryngeal and tracheobronchial inflammation may be detected by fiberoptic bronchoscopy. Arterial blood gases should be measured; prompt intubation or tracheostomy should be performed if there is evidence of significant airway obstruction. Corticosteroids may help treat edema of the upper airways, but they must be used with caution, because infection is a major concern for managing both skin and pulmonary injury. Prophylactic antibiotics are of no value in preventing pneumonia and may predispose to infection with resistant organisms. Careful pulmonary toilet, humidification, and sterile suctioning should be used to reduce the risk of pneumonia. Serial bronchoscopy may be necessary to remove mucus plugs and thereby prevent segmental atelectasis and postobstructive infection. Late-onset pulmonary burn complications include atelectasis (see Chapter 86), thromboembolism (see Chapter 84), and pneumonia (see Chapter 82).

Carbon Monoxide Poisoning

ETIOLOGY. Smoke inhalation is invariably accompanied by the body taking up CO. In some fires, CO exposure is complicated by cyanide poisoning from the combustion of plastic compounds. CO poisoning also is encountered frequently after exposure to automobile exhaust and in the winter, when victims are exposed to fumes from faulty furnaces. As a result, CO is the leading cause of accidental poisoning in the United States.

CO toxicity is a consequence of tissue hypoxia created by the displacement of oxygen from hemoglobin. CO competes with oxygen for binding at the iron-porphyrin centers of hemoglobin. These centers bind CO reversibly, but with an affinity more than 200 times greater than that for oxygen. The oxygen affinity of heme not occupied by CO is also increased in the presence of carboxyhemoglobin (HbCO). This HbCO-related increase in oxygen affinity shifts the oxyhemoglobin dissociation curve to the left and impairs the release of oxygen to the tissues. These two effects of CO on hemoglobin decrease the partial pressure of oxygen in the tissues. Tissue hypoxia has serious functional consequences for organ systems that require a continuous supply of oxygen, such as the brain and the heart. In addition, when tissue partial pressure of oxygen (PO_2) is low, CO binds to intracellular hemoproteins, such as myoglobin and cytochrome *c* oxidase, inhibiting their functions.

CLINICAL MANIFESTATIONS. The clinical features of acute CO poisoning are diverse but are most often related to the central nervous system. In normal non-smoking individuals, symptoms may appear when HbCO levels reach 10%. Patients with chronic obstructive pulmonary disease (COPD) and coronary artery disease are more sensitive to the effects of HbCO. Smokers often maintain HbCO levels of 3 to 10%, and they may tolerate slightly higher levels without symptoms. Common symptoms of CO poisoning include headache, nausea, vomiting, confusion, and visual disturbances. More severe CO poisoning can produce seizures, transient unconsciousness, coma, and death. Metabolic acidosis, pulmonary edema, and rhabdomyolysis may also accompany serious CO poisoning. The "classic" clinical findings of cherry red lips and nail beds are rare.

DIAGNOSIS. The diagnosis is based on the history of exposure and an elevated HbCO level in the blood. The differential diagnosis includes drug overdoses, other poisonings (e.g., cyanide), and cerebrovascular accidents. The clinical diagnosis is confirmed by an elevated blood HbCO level measured by CO-oximetry. The severity of the clinical illness, however, correlates better with the duration and extent of the exposure than with HbCO level.

TREATMENT AND PROGNOSIS. Symptoms of mild CO poisoning generally subside within minutes to a few hours after removing the patient from the noxious environment. Patients with more se-

Table 80–1 ■ TOXIC BY-PRODUCTS OF SMOKE IMPLICATED IN RESPIRATORY INJURY

SOURCE	BY-PRODUCTS
Cotton, paper, wood	Acrolein, CO, acetaldehyde
Petroleum products	Acrolein, CO, benzene
Polyvinyl chloride (PVC)	Hydrocyanic acid, CO, chlorine, phosgene
Nylon, silk, wool	Hydrocyanic acid, ammonia
Nitrocellulose	Oxides of nitrogen
Sulfur compounds	Sulfur dioxide

CO = carbon monoxide.

vere CO intoxication benefit from inspiring high concentrations of oxygen to hasten the removal of CO from hemoglobin. In obtunded or comatose patients, 100% oxygen should be administered via endotracheal tube until the HbCO level is less than 5%. Pure oxygen reduces the half-time for eliminating HbCO from the body from approximately 240 minutes to 60 minutes. Patients with loss of consciousness or other neurologic impairment, cardiac symptoms or signs, or HbCO levels greater than 25% should receive hyperbaric oxygen if it is available. Hyperbaric oxygen at 2.5 atmospheres absolute (ATA) reduces the HbCO half-life to approximately 20 minutes. Oxygen dissolved in plasma under hyperbaric pressure also avoids problems with oxyhemoglobin dissociation and hastens removal of CO from tissue stores. As a result, potentially serious neurologic sequelae may be averted if the therapy can be instituted promptly. Adjunctive therapy, such as administration of corticosteroids, hyperventilation, administration of mannitol, and hypothermia, has been recommended for treating serious cases of CO poisoning, but benefit from these modalities is unproved.

Neurologic recovery in patients with mild to moderate CO poisoning is good. The prognosis after severe CO poisoning is variable and correlates with the extent and duration of the insult. Short-term memory impairment, depression, and syndromes related to lesions of the basal ganglia are well described. A syndrome of delayed neurologic deterioration occurs in about 10% of victims of serious CO intoxication. Risk factors for the delayed syndrome include age older than 40 years, prolonged exposure, and abnormalities of the brain on computed tomography (CT). Hyperbaric oxygen therapy has been reported to decrease the incidence of the delayed syndrome.

Other Toxic Inhaled Gases

A large number of gases and chemicals, to which exposures most frequently occur in an industrial setting, can acutely and sometimes chronically injure the respiratory system. A few agents cause an "asthma-like" reaction with cough, chest pain, and wheezing. Toluene diisocyanate and other isocyanates (liberated as a gas in making polyurethane foams), aluminum soldering flux, and platinum salts are typical examples. Reaginic and precipitating antibodies against platinum salts and soldering flux have been found in symptomatic individuals, suggesting an immunologic basis for the reaction. An allergic basis has not been demonstrated for the reaction to toluene diisocyanate. The symptoms usually subside after removal from exposure; however, chronic lung injury may occur if the exposure is prolonged.

ETIOLOGY. A number of highly irritating gases cause *acute chemical pneumonitis*. Such gases include chlorine (used in the chemical and plastics industries and to disinfect water), ammonia (used in refrigeration), sulfur dioxide (used in making paper and smelting sulfide-containing ores), ozone (generated in welding and in photochemical smog), nitrogen dioxide (released from decomposed corn silage), and phosgene (used in producing aniline dyes).

Different mechanisms are involved in the injury caused by irritant gases. Most of them cause injury by acting as a strong acid, a strong base, or an oxidant. Gases of chemicals that are strong acids or bases in water solution, such as hydrogen chloride, sulfuric acid, sulfur dioxide, and ammonia, tend to react more in the upper airways.

The clinical response caused by irritant gases varies but appears to be closely related to the degree of acute irritation and to the water solubility of the gas. The less irritating gases, such as ozone and the oxides of nitrogen, phosgene, mercury, and nickel carbonyl, can be inhaled for prolonged periods and thereby cause injury throughout the respiratory system. Highly irritating and soluble gases, such as ammonia and hydrochloric acid, are less likely to be inhaled deeply and tend to result in immediate injury to the upper airways and have potential for obstruction secondary to mucosal edema. Less-soluble substances, such as chlorine, cadmium, zinc chloride, osmium tetroxide, and vanadium, can cause injury to the entire tracheobronchial tree and generally do not produce upper airway obstruction as the initial presentation. Bronchiolitis and pulmonary edema are common, ultimately leading to bronchiolitis obliterans. Long-term consequences vary with the gas. Cadmium, for example, can cause diffuse emphysema and severe airway obstruction but only minimal fibrosis.

CLINICAL MANIFESTATIONS. A typical syndrome occurs in silo-filler's disease (nitrogen dioxide). During the exposure, no symptoms may be present, tracheobronchitis with cough and shortness of breath may be noted, or immediate acute pulmonary edema may occur. Signs of ocular and oropharyngeal mucous membrane irritation may be present. The symptoms can progress rapidly, but commonly the initial symptoms resolve and are followed by a period of minimal symptoms (cough) lasting up to 48 hours. Fever, myalgias, dyspnea, and progressive hypoxemia then occur, and the radiographic picture is that of pulmonary edema. These severe symptoms can resolve, only to recur 2 to 5 weeks later and lead to progressive bronchiolitis obliterans.

TREATMENT AND PROGNOSIS. The initial step of removing the victim from the noxious environment is usually sufficient to treat mild exposures. The prognosis for more severe toxic gas exposures varies with duration and extent of exposure. Bronchodilators and supplemental oxygen may be necessary. In silo-filler's disease, treatment with corticosteroids (prednisone, 1 mg/kg/day) for 4 to 6 weeks can dramatically improve the acute illness. Because improvement after the initial exposure may be temporary, close observation for 48 hours after the exposure is advisable.

Pulmonary Oxygen Toxicity

ETIOLOGY AND PATHOGENESIS. Oxygen is toxic to the lungs when used in high concentrations for prolonged periods. This toxicity occurs clinically in patients in intensive care units who are on mechanical ventilators. The toxic effects of hyperoxia are believed to result from excessive generation of superoxide, an unstable free radical produced by the single electron reduction of oxygen. Superoxide is produced as a normal by-product of oxidative metabolism and scavenged by the protective enzymes, the superoxide dismutases, that catalyze its dismutation to hydrogen peroxide (Fig. 80–1). If it is not scavenged enzymatically, superoxide anion can donate an electron to hydrogen peroxide in the presence of transition metals (e.g., iron) to form hydroxyl radical (OH·). Hydroxyl radical is highly reactive and can initiate lipid peroxidation and oxidize protein and nucleic acids.

In the adult, the major sites of oxygen injury are the alveolar epithelium and the capillary endothelium. Pathologically, the lungs are atelectatic, congested, and edematous. Hyaline membranes are often present. Oxidant injury attracts inflammatory cells to the lung, including neutrophils. Advanced injury destroys the capillary bed with resultant interstitial and alveolar edema, hypoxemia, and sometimes death. Other pathologic changes include hyperplasia of type II cells, and histologic changes have been found in the ciliated epithelium and Clara cells of the small airways.

CLINICAL MANIFESTATIONS. Oxygen toxicity usually occurs in acutely ill patients who are receiving oxygen in high concentrations and mechanical ventilation for lung injuries that obscure the onset of pulmonary toxicity. Lung compliance progressively falls; the alveolar-arterial oxygen gradient gradually widens, and increasing concentrations of oxygen are needed to maintain adequate oxygenation of arterial blood. This cycle progresses to pulmonary edema, respiratory failure, and death.

The earliest symptoms of oxygen toxicity are those of acute tracheobronchitis. A dry, hacking cough and substernal pain may occur after 6 to 12 hours of breathing pure oxygen. Vital capacity decreases, and respiratory rate increases. The flow of tracheal mucus decreases after short exposures to excess oxygen, probably reflecting functional injury of airway epithelium. These patients are therefore more susceptible to mucus impaction and to infection caused by failure to clear inhaled pathogens adequately.

TREATMENT AND PROGNOSIS. The only proven therapy is to prevent the insult by judicious use of high oxygen concentrations. The physician often faces a dilemma in that increasing concentrations of oxygen are needed to save the patient immediately but can eventually kill the patient. Alternative methods to enhance arterial oxygen content should be used whenever possible; these methods include a number of maneuvers based on strategies related to mechanical support of ventilation (see Chapter 93) and transfusion of packed red cells to maintain the hematocrit near 30%. Cardiac output should be maintained and accompanied by measures to decrease the tissue oxygen demand by reducing fever or agitation.

The safe maximal concentration of oxygen is not known. Little or no injury occurs in normal animals or human volunteers breathing oxygen concentrations of 40 to 50% for prolonged peri-

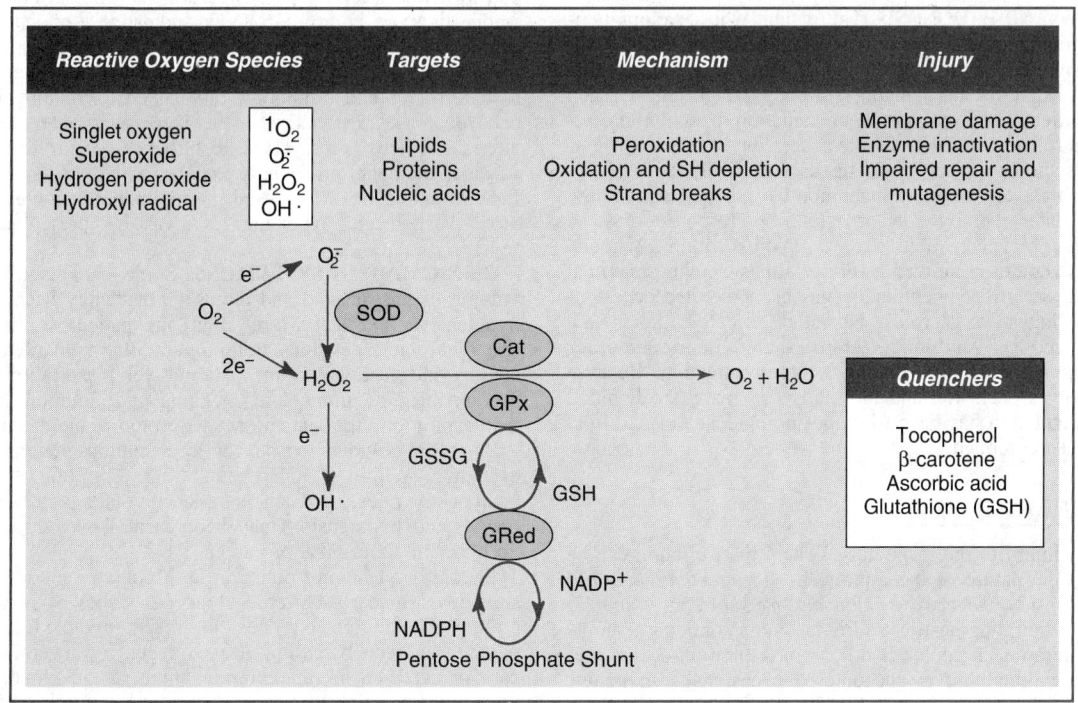

FIGURE 80-1 ■ Reactive oxygen species and antioxidant defenses. When oxygen (O_2) is reduced incompletely, toxic oxygen species are formed such as singlet oxygen ($^1O_2$), superoxide anion (O_2^-), and hydrogen peroxide (H_2O_2). H_2O_2 in the presence of iron (Fe^{2+}) or other reduced transition metals can generate highly reactive hydroxyl radical ($OH\cdot$). Reactive oxygen species can oxidize lipids (lipid peroxidation), proteins, and nucleic acid (DNA strand breaks). Quenchers react with reactive oxygen species or with oxidized cellular molecules to prevent further oxidation. The enzymatic antioxidant defenses consist of the superoxide dismutases (SOD), catalase (Cat), and the glutathione peroxidase-reductase system (GPx and GRed). These enzymes detoxify O_2 and H_2O_2 to prevent undesirable biologic oxidations. NADPH is required both for reduction of glutathione and for pathways for repair of oxidant damage. Glucose-6-phosphate dehydrogenase determines availability of NADPH because it is the rate-limiting step in the pentose phosphate shunt.

ods. The diseased lung, however, may be more susceptible to oxygen injury. A rational therapy is to use only enough oxygen to provide adequate arterial blood saturation, (e.g., an SaO_2 of 90%). Corticosteroids have no benefit and may actually worsen the lung injury caused by hyperoxia. If the patient survives oxygen toxicity, some residual damage to the lung parenchyma may remain, with septal fibrosis replacing areas where the pulmonary capillary bed was destroyed by the hyperoxia.

Radiation Lung Injury (see Chapter 19)

ETIOLOGY AND PATHOGENESIS. Ionizing radiation produces oxidant lung injury related to the degree of the radiation exposure. The clinical occurrence of radiation pneumonitis is determined by the total radiation dose, the number of fractions, and the duration of time over which the radiation is given. Chemotherapeutic drugs that produce oxidant-based lung toxicity, such as bleomycin, may potentiate lung injury from radiation. A total lung dose of less than 2000 cGy generally is not associated with severe radiation pneumonitis, whereas a total dose in excess of 4000 cGy, even if distributed over as many as 30 fractions, has virtually a 100% risk of radiation pneumonitis.

The reaction of the lung to radiation injury can be divided into three phases. (1) An *acute phase,* occurring 1 to 2 months after radiation exposure, is characterized by vascular damage, congestion, edema, and mononuclear cell infiltration. Alveolar type II cells and alveolar macrophages are increased in number. (2) A *subacute phase* occurs 2 to 9 months later. The alveolar walls become infiltrated with mononuclear inflammatory cells and fibroblasts. (3) The *chronic* or *fibrotic phase* generally occurs more than 9 months after irradiation. Alveolar fibrosis and capillary sclerosis are its predominant histologic features.

CLINICAL MANIFESTATIONS. Signs of bronchial irritation (e.g., cough) may appear immediately after radiation therapy, followed shortly thereafter by esophagitis. Some patients may have no symptoms for 6 to 12 weeks. If large volumes of lung have been irradiated, or if high radiation doses have been given over short periods, the patient can develop dyspnea, tachypnea, and fever. These symptoms can either progress to severe dyspnea and death or gradually subside, leaving varying degrees of respiratory impairment due to lung fibrosis. Permanent fibrosis takes 6 to 24 months to evolve, and it then usually remains stable if no further exposure occurs. Auscultation of the chest is usually normal, although rales, signs of consolidation, and pleural rubs may be found. Clubbing does not develop after radiation injury. Laboratory findings include a mild leukocytosis and an increased erythrocyte sedimentation rate. If the irradiated area is extensive, arterial hypoxemia may develop. Radiographic changes generally appear 1 to 3 months after treatment. The affected areas are generally demarcated by a "straight edge" defining the margins of the radiation portal, and they have a "ground-glass appearance"—a hazy increase in density with indistinct pulmonary markings. In the later phases of the radiation injury, fibrosis and contraction of the irradiated region are the predominant radiographic findings. Pulmonary function tests do not change until clinical symptoms appear, and then pulmonary restriction may be noted. Capillary sclerosis is associated with a decrease in blood flow to the affected region and a decrease in CO diffusing capacity.

DIAGNOSIS. The diagnosis of acute radiation pneumonitis may be difficult to establish because of coincidental disease. The clinical picture is often complicated by the immunocompromised state of many of the patients, resulting in increased risk of bacterial or opportunistic pneumonias (e.g., those caused by *Pneumocystis carinii*) or by the signs and symptoms of the original neoplasm. Radiation pneumonitis in parts of the lung outside the radiation portal has been suspected in a few patients on the basis of typical clinical and radiographic features. Complications of radiation pneumonitis include small pleural effusions and, occasionally, spontaneous pneumothorax.

TREATMENT AND PROGNOSIS. The patient who develops radiation pneumonitis requires supportive care, including cough suppression, antipyretics, and supplemental oxygen for hypoxemia. Corticosteroids (prednisone, 1 mg/kg of body weight) have been advocated for treating severe cases of radiation pneumonitis, although no controlled clinical trials have been undertaken. No evidence supports the purely prophylactic use of corticosteroids, but using them at the very onset of pneumonitis appears to be more effective than later therapy. On occasion, the response may be dramatic, with complete resolution of symptoms within 24 hours. Corticosteroids should be tapered carefully after achieving maximal clinical benefit. Recurrent pneumonitis has been reported occasionally after withdrawal of steroids. No other effective therapeutic strategies are known. Antibiotic therapy should be reserved for patients in whom the clinical findings suggest infection. Because the lesion involves occlusion and thrombosis of many small blood vessels, anticoagulation has been tried, but no evidence of its effectiveness has been compiled.

ASPIRATION-RELATED INJURIES

ETIOLOGY. Injury to the respiratory system by aspiration can be categorized by the nature of the aspirate as (1) *infectious material* (see Chapter 82), (2) *chemical* or *inflammatory substances,* and (3) *inert material.* Aspirating gastric acid is the most common example of chemical aspiration in adults; hydrocarbon aspiration occurs predominantly in children but is encountered occasionally in adults. Both of these injuries can cause fulminant illness. By contrast, lipids (mineral oil, vegetable and animal fats) most often provoke a chronic inflammatory reaction. Aspirating inert material such as water causes injury (e.g., drowning), predominantly by asphyxia. Food particles can cause a fibrotic, granulomatous lesion or, if large enough to occlude the larynx or trachea, sudden death by asphyxiation ("café coronary").

Aspiration Pneumonitis

Aspiration pneumonitis refers to pulmonary injury caused by acidic stomach contents. This condition is in contrast to "aspiration pneumonia," an infectious process caused by oropharyngeal flora contaminating the tracheobronchial tree. Aspiration of gastric acid can occur during vomiting or regurgitation, and in the latter instance the event may go unnoted (i.e., "silent aspiration"). The normal protective mechanisms of the upper airway include epiglottic closure during deglutition, glottic closure on contact with solids or fluids, the cough reflex, and esophageal sphincters. Altered states of consciousness, anesthesia and surgery, neuromuscular disease, gastrointestinal disease, and medical devices (nasogastric tubes or tracheostomy tubes) impair these defenses. Protecting the airway is a major concern in these high-risk situations. Using low-pressure, high-volume cuffs on endotracheal tubes reduces the extent of aspiration of gastric contents in patients at risk.

ETIOLOGY AND PATHOGENESIS. The main factors determining the extent of illness caused by gastric acid aspiration are as follows:

1. *The pH of the aspirate.* The acidity of the material is the single most important contributor to lung injury. A pH of 2.5 or less has been proposed as a critical value for inducing severe pneumonitis from acid aspiration.
2. *The presence of food particles.* Aspiration of gastric food substances causes a severe pneumonitis and peribronchial inflammatory reaction in the absence of acid.
3. *Volume of the aspirate.* Aspirating as little as 30 mL of gastric acid is sufficient to cause pneumonitis in the adult.
4. *Distribution of the aspirate.* Many patients who aspirate immediately begin to cough, which may partially protect the lung from injury or may enhance dispersion of the acid over a greater area and create a diffuse injury.

Acid in the trachea is rapidly distributed in the lungs and can reach the pleura in 12 to 18 seconds. It is rapidly neutralized by bronchial secretions; in less than 30 minutes, the pH at the bronchial surface returns to normal. Acid causes chemical burns of the bronchi, bronchioles, and alveolar walls, with subsequent exudation of fluid into the lungs. Plasma volume may decrease by as much as 35% in severe injury without fluid replacement, and cardiac output and systemic arterial blood pressure may fall. Pulmonary capillary wedge pressure is normal or low, indicating a nonhydrostatic cause of the pulmonary edema. The characteristics of phospholipids in the alveolar surface lining layer (surfactant) are altered, increasing surface forces and promoting early alveolar collapse. Lung compliance decreases secondary to the increase in interstitial fluids and altered surface forces. These disturbances of airways, alveoli, and vascular elements profoundly unbalance the normal ventilation-perfusion relationships. Increased intrapulmonary shunting is also common. As a result, hypoxemia is invariably present and is usually severe.

CLINICAL MANIFESTATIONS. Some patients aspirate a large volume of gastric acid and almost immediately become apneic and hypotensive and die. More often, the patient survives the initial crisis but later develops a fulminant illness marked by dyspnea, cough, and frothy sputum. Alternatively, aspiration may not be accompanied by immediate coughing and agitation. After such silent aspiration, the patient may develop acute respiratory failure without an obvious reason for a precipitous deterioration in gas exchange. Within 1 to 5 hours after aspiration of gastric acid, tachypnea, rales, and rhonchi occur, and wheezing, cyanosis, cough, and hypotension may be present. Fever occurs in the first 36 hours in about 50% of patients.

Laboratory tests are nonspecific. Moderate leukocytosis with left shift develops early. Arterial blood gases show hypoxemia, and the arterial oxygen tension does not reach predicted levels after the patient has been breathing 100% oxygen for several minutes, indicating increased intrapulmonary shunting of blood. The arterial PCO_2 may be slightly elevated, normal, or mildly reduced. Abnormalities on chest roentgenograms are extremely variable, and no characteristic pattern is present. Radiographic abnormalities do not correlate with clinical outcome, although about 50% of patients have changes consistent with pneumonitis. The acid is sometimes distributed preferentially to dependent areas, but usually the radiographic abnormalities are diffuse, presumably from enhanced dispersion of the acid during coughing. Pleural effusions and cavitation of infiltrates are not seen in uncomplicated cases. Bronchoscopic findings are diagnostic if food particles or other gastric contents are seen in the trachea or bronchi.

The diagnosis of aspiration pneumonitis begins with a high index of suspicion in patients with abrupt respiratory deterioration, especially patients with conditions that predispose to gastric acid aspiration. The differential diagnosis includes cardiogenic pulmonary edema, pulmonary embolism, bacterial pneumonia, and many of the causes of ARDS, such as sepsis and hypotension.

TREATMENT. Treatment of the individual whose aspiration was witnessed begins with promptly establishing an adequate airway. The airway should be suctioned to remove any particulate matter. Supplemental oxygen is given to maintain a PaO_2 of more than 60 mm Hg. Bronchodilators (intravenous aminophylline) may be helpful. Associated pulmonary edema is noncardiogenic in origin and is usually associated with intravascular volume depletion. General supportive measures include judicious replacement of fluids.

The prophylactic use of antibiotics for acid aspiration is not indicated because they do not reduce morbidity or mortality and may increase the risk of subsequent infection with a resistant organism. The acid-damaged respiratory tract is more susceptible to bacterial infection, and one-third of patients with significant aspiration develop bacterial pneumonia. Such patients undergo new deterioration after 2 or 3 days, with increasing fever, leukocytosis, production of purulent sputum, worsening hypoxemia, and new infiltrates on the chest radiograph.

Systemic corticosteroids should not be used routinely in aspiration pneumonitis. As for other forms of ARDS, use of corticosteroids is controversial and may increase the rate of infection.

Positive-pressure ventilation (see Chapter 93) is helpful after severe cases of aspiration to improve arterial oxygen tension. Other measures useful to treat ARDS, such as maintaining a normal pulmonary capillary wedge pressure, are beneficial after aspiration injury of the lung. PEEP is commonly used to improve oxygenation in patients with gastric acid aspiration. Caution should be used in applying PEEP because it can produce a marked increase in extravascular water content in the acid-injured lung.

Aspiration pneumonitis carries a high mortality rate despite treatment; because it largely occurs in a defined population at increased risk, efforts should be made at prevention. Elevating the head of the bed retards regurgitation. In intubated patients, placement of a nasogastric tube should be considered to keep the stomach decompressed. Aspiration may occur even in the presence of a cuffed endotracheal tube. Elective general anesthesia should be given with the stomach empty, after at least a 12-hour fast. Preoperatively, the pH of gastric contents can be raised by a single dose of an H_2-receptor blocker given 2 hours before surgery.

PROGNOSIS. Mortality from aspiration pneumonitis is high, reaching 30 to 60%. Factors associated with highest mortality are age older than 50 years, the early development of shock or apnea, severe and prolonged hypoxemia, very low pH of gastric contents at the time of aspiration, and the development of secondary bacterial pneumonia. Most patients survive the early moments but deteriorate over 12 to 24 hours. Some then show steady improvement, with radiographic resolution within a week. Others have a second episode of deterioration, an event that should suggest a new problem, such as bacterial infection, pulmonary embolism, heart failure, or another aspiration. Still others pursue a relentlessly worsening course to death. Few data exist regarding long-term clinical follow-up, but pulmonary fibrosis of varying degrees may occur in some of the survivors.

Hydrocarbon Pneumonitis

ETIOLOGY. Hydrocarbon pneumonitis results from the direct toxic effects of volatile hydrocarbons on the respiratory epithelium and vasculature. It occurs in individuals who, having ingested the hydrocarbons, aspirate them into the respiratory tract. The problem occurs most often in children, particularly those younger than 5 years. It is an uncommon problem in adults, occurring most often in industrial accidents, in patients attempting suicide, in siphoning of gasoline, and in alcoholics seeking an ethanol substitute.

Different hydrocarbons cause respiratory injury of varying extent, depending on the viscosity and volume of the aspirate. The lower the viscosity or the larger the volume, the worse the lesion. As lipid solvents, these compounds are directly toxic to respiratory tissues. The lungs of children dying of hydrocarbon pneumonitis demonstrate hemorrhage, pulmonary edema, atelectasis, hyaline membrane formation, and necrosis of airway epithelium and alveolar septa. These compounds also have systemic toxicity, and in fatal cases, degenerative changes have been seen in the liver and kidneys.

CLINICAL MANIFESTATIONS. Aspiration usually occurs when hydrocarbons are ingested, and a history of vomiting after ingestion is obtained in fewer than half the patients. Dyspnea, tachypnea, tachycardia, and high fever quickly ensue. Sputum may be bloody. Lethargy is common, but more severe disturbances of consciousness also occur, such as confusion, coma, and seizures. Auscultation is frequently normal, but rales and rhonchi may be present.

Laboratory tests give nonspecific results. Moderate leukocytosis with left shift is common. Arterial hypoxemia of various degrees develops owing to shunting and to ventilation-perfusion mismatching. The chest radiograph is particularly helpful, as infiltrates may occur within 20 to 30 minutes after aspirating some types of hydrocarbons. The multiple, fluffy, ill-defined infiltrates favor dependent areas of the lungs. Some patients present a picture of bilateral perihilar infiltrates, a pulmonary edema pattern. Pleural effusions, pneumothorax, and pneumomediastinum occur but are uncommon. Pneumatoceles can form later, especially in children.

DIAGNOSIS. The differential diagnosis is that of sudden respiratory distress. Frequently, the patient has an impaired sensorium at presentation. The adult patient is often an alcoholic. Gastric acid aspiration, cardiogenic pulmonary edema, pulmonary embolism, and acute bacterial pneumonia can all manifest similarly. The correct diagnosis requires the history of hydrocarbon ingestion or aspiration. The diagnosis is also suggested by the odor of the patient's breath and by extensive radiographic abnormalities in a patient with a clear chest on auscultation.

TREATMENT. Emesis to remove residual hydrocarbons is contraindicated. Gastric lavage by nasogastric tube may cause vomiting in the patient who has recently ingested a large volume of hydrocarbons and should be performed only after placing a cuffed endotracheal tube. Supplemental oxygen should be given to maintain a PaO_2 greater than 60 mm Hg. Mechanical ventilation and PEEP may be necessary. No data support the routine use of antibiotics. Systemic corticosteroids (prednisone, 1 mg/kg/day) during the acute

illness have been suggested by anecdotal reports of improvement after their use in children and adults.

PROGNOSIS. Hydrocarbon pneumonitis in adults is rare, so that estimates of morbidity and mortality are not available. In children, death occurs in about 10% of cases, but most children have a prompt clinical recovery. Bronchiectasis, recurrent bronchitis, and/or pulmonary fibrosis develop in an unknown portion of cases. After recovery, children frequently have normal chest examinations and radiographs, although pulmonary function abnormalities suggestive of small airway (<2 mm in diameter) disease have been found in asymptomatic patients as late as 8 to 14 years after hydrocarbon pneumonitis.

Lipoid Pneumonia

Lipoid pneumonia is a chronic inflammatory reaction of the lungs to the presence of lipid substances. Exogenous lipoid pneumonia results from the aspiration of vegetable, animal, or (most commonly) mineral oils. This material differs greatly from the excessive accumulation of endogenous lipids in the lungs occurring in fat embolism, cholesterol pneumonitis, pulmonary alveolar proteinosis, and the lipid storage diseases (endogenous lipoid pneumonia).

ETIOLOGY. The most frequently implicated agent is mineral oil used as a laxative and to reduce dysphagia, either in clear liquid form or as petroleum jelly. Mineral oil is bland and, when introduced into the pharynx, can enter the bronchial tree without eliciting the cough reflex. It also mechanically impedes the ciliary action of the airway epithelium. The risk of mineral oil aspiration is increased in debilitated or senile patients, in those with neurologic disease that interferes with deglutition, and in patients with esophageal disease. Mineral oil taken as nose drops to relieve nasal dryness has caused lipoid pneumonia and was a frequent cause of the illness years ago. Inhalation of mineral oil mist by airplane and automobile mechanics has also been implicated as a cause of the problem.

Mineral oils, which cannot be hydrolyzed in the body, provoke a chronic inflammatory reaction that may not become clinically overt until years later. In the alveolar spaces, macrophages accumulate and phagocytize the emulsified oil. Some macrophages disintegrate, releasing their lysosomal enzymes and oil. The alveolar septa become thickened and edematous, containing lymphocytes and lipid-laden macrophages. Oil droplets are seen in the pulmonary lymphatics and hilar nodes. Later, fibrosis develops, and the normal lung architecture is effaced. It is usual in a single specimen to find both the early inflammatory and the later fibrotic picture, in keeping with repetitive aspirations over many months or years. If nodular, the lesion may grossly resemble tumor and is called a paraffinoma.

CLINICAL MANIFESTATIONS. Most patients are asymptomatic, coming to the physician's attention because of an abnormal chest radiograph. When patients are symptomatic, cough and exertional dyspnea are the most frequent complaints. Chest pain (sometimes pleuritic), hemoptysis, fever (usually low grade), chills, night sweats, and weight loss may occur. The physical examination may be completely normal, or fever, tachypnea, dullness on percussion of the chest, bronchial or bronchovesicular breath sounds, rales, and rhonchi may be found. Clubbing and cor pulmonale are rare.

In mild lipoid pneumonia, arterial blood gas values may be normal with the patient at rest but may show hypoxemia after exercise. In more severe disease, resting hypoxemia, hypocapnia, and mild respiratory alkalosis develop. Pulmonary function testing reveals a restrictive ventilatory defect; lung compliance is decreased. The only specific laboratory finding is the presence in sputum of macrophages with clusters of vacuoles 5 to 50 μm in diameter that stain deep orange with Sudan IV and of extracellular droplets that stain similarly.

Radiographically, the earliest abnormalities are air-space infiltrates; these infiltrates may be unilateral or bilateral, localized or diffuse, but most often occur in the dependent portions of the lung. Air bronchograms may be seen. Hilar adenopathy and pleural reaction are rare. As fibrosis develops, volume loss occurs and linear and nodular infiltrates appear. A solid lesion that closely resembles bronchogenic carcinoma may develop.

DIAGNOSIS. The differential diagnosis is extensive, particularly in the late phase, when multiple other causes of pulmonary fibrosis must be considered. The key to the correct diagnosis before biopsy is the history of chronic oral or intranasal use of an oil- or a lipid-based product, or an occupational exposure to oil mists. The presence of lipid-laden macrophages in the sputum confirms the diagnosis. The diagnosis also can be confirmed by a computed tomographic scan showing fat within a mass or area of consolidation.

TREATMENT AND PROGNOSIS. Once the diagnosis has been made and the aspiration stopped, the subsequent course is variable. Some patients have no change in symptoms. Others improve in some or all parameters, whereas a few patients deteriorate, with worsening pulmonary function and cor pulmonale. Because the only way the lung can dispose of mineral oil is by expectoration, the patient should be instructed in coughing exercises to be performed many times each day for months. Expectorants have not been shown to help. Systemic corticosteroids are recommended by some on the basis of improvement seen in a few uncontrolled reports. The rationale has been that the cellular reaction, rather than the oil itself, is the destructive factor. Because of the well-recognized side effects of systemic corticosteroids, their use for lipoid pneumonia should be limited to patients who have significant symptoms, and then for as brief a period as possible.

Near-Drowning

Drowning is one of the three leading causes of accidental death in children and young adults. In adults, alcohol consumption and shallow water blackout during breath-hold diving are common aggravating factors. Pathophysiologically, drowning can be of two types: (1) "wet" drowning, or initial laryngospasm but early relaxation and subsequent aspiration of copious amounts of fluid; and (2) "dry" drowning, or asphyxiation secondary to intense glottic spasm that persists beyond the point of apnea, so that when the muscles relax, little or no water is aspirated; this latter type accounts for 10 to 20% of drownings. The immediate cause of death in many victims of drowning is cardiac arrhythmia. Victims who survive the initial episode frequently develop ARDS a few hours to a few days after the event (secondary drowning).

PATHOGENESIS. The most important consequences of near-drowning are attributed to asphyxia. Asphyxia results in severe hypoxemia, hypercarbia, and metabolic acidosis. The metabolic consequences of drowning in fresh water or salt water appear to differ little except for drowning in water with very high mineral content (e.g., the Dead Sea). In both cases, hypoxemia is caused by the occlusion of airways with water and particulate debris, by changes in surfactant activity, by direct injury to the alveolar septa, and by bronchospasm. Right-to-left shunting is markedly increased, and physiologic dead space is increased. Life-threatening electrolyte disturbances caused by water aspiration in humans are rare. Cardiac arrhythmias, central nervous system abnormalities, and renal insufficiency often occur after near-drowning. Brain anoxia is usually global anoxia, and if it is of sufficient duration and magnitude, it leads to diffuse cerebral edema.

Autopsies of drowned persons demonstrate wet, heavy lungs with varying amounts of hemorrhage and edema and some disruption of alveolar walls. In about 70% of victims, vomitus, sand, mud, and aquatic vegetation are aspirated. Specimens from victims dying of secondary drowning show desquamation of alveolar epithelial cells, hemorrhage, hyaline membrane formation, acute inflammatory infiltrates, and foreign body reactions to particulate matter. Cerebral edema and diffuse neuronal injury are seen. Acute tubular necrosis is common in the kidneys.

CLINICAL MANIFESTATIONS. The initial appearance of the patient can vary widely, from coma to agitated alertness. Cyanosis, coughing, and the production of frothy pink sputum are common. Tachypnea, tachycardia, and a low-grade fever in the first few hours are seen if the patient did not become hypothermic during submersion. Rales, rhonchi, and, less often, wheezes are heard. Neurologic signs vary and can fluctuate in any given patient, but they usually derive from diffuse cerebral dysfunction. Signs of associated trauma to the head and neck should be sought.

Laboratory studies reveal mild hypokalemia, hypernatremia, and hyperchloremia. Moderate leukocytosis may be present. Hematocrit

and hemoglobin usually are normal at first measurement; in fresh water aspiration, the hematocrit may fall slightly in the first 24 hours owing to hemolysis. An isolated increase in serum-free hemoglobin without a change in hematocrit is more common. Occasionally, the clinical picture of disseminated intravascular coagulation occurs in near-drowning. Arterial blood gas values, usually obtained after preliminary resuscitation, show severe hypoxemia and metabolic acidosis. The most common electrocardiographic changes are sinus tachycardia and nonspecific ST-segment and T-wave changes, which revert to normal within hours; however, other, more ominous abnormalities may occur, such as ventricular arrhythmias, complete heart block, or myocardial infarction. The chest radiograph may be normal initially despite severe respiratory disturbances; however, it often shows patchy infiltrates, and sometimes a classic pattern of pulmonary edema is seen.

TREATMENT. Treatment of the near-drowning victim begins with establishing an adequate airway and, if necessary, emergency cardiopulmonary resuscitation. Oxygen in high concentrations is necessary, because hypoxemia is present in essentially all victims. Even the patient who quickly becomes apparently normal should be hospitalized for 24 hours to watch for a subsequent clinical picture of ARDS. During transportation to a hospital, supplemental oxygen should be continued and precautions taken for potential head and neck injuries and other serious trauma.

In the hospital, therapy is dictated largely by the arterial blood gas values and the degree of respiratory failure. Continuous positive airway pressure or PEEP is particularly helpful for managing hypoxemia (see Chapter 93). Bronchospasm should be treated with nebulized β-agonists. Patients with persistent localized atelectasis or localized wheezing should undergo bronchoscopy to exclude a foreign body as the cause. Prophylactic antibiotics have not been shown to be beneficial, although many victims of near-drowning develop pneumonia, sometimes caused by unusual microorganisms. No controlled human studies are available to support the use of corticosteroids for the pulmonary lesions of near-drowning; animal models and retrospective studies in humans have failed to demonstrate any benefit.

The therapeutic approach to brain resuscitation after near-drowning is also controversial. If evidence of cerebral edema exists, intracranial pressure (ICP) monitoring may be useful to guide therapy. In the event of increased ICP, PEEP should be minimized because it may increase ICP. Hyperventilation to maintain a $PaCO_2$ of 25 to 30 mm Hg decreases ICP at the expense of cerebral blood flow. Mannitol may decrease cerebral edema; it should be used to maintain the serum osmolarity near 300 mOsm/L. Corticosteroids are used widely (e.g., dexamethasone, 10 mg given intravenously initially, and then 4 to 6 mg given intravenously every 4 hours), but they are not of proven benefit for the brain injury. Seizures should be treated with anticonvulsants. Shivering or random, purposeless movements can increase ICP and should be controlled. If these maneuvers fail to lower ICP, then barbiturate coma for 24 to 48 hours has been recommended, although its benefit is questionable.

PROGNOSIS. Outcome in near-drowning is best judged by the neurologic status (i.e., the presence or absence of coma). The shorter the interval between recovery from the water to first spontaneous gasp, the better the prognosis for recovery. The absence of spontaneous respiration after resuscitation from near-drowning is an ominous sign associated with severe neurologic sequelae. Permanent neurologic sequelae persist in about 20% of comatose victims. Common sequelae include minimal brain dysfunction, spastic quadriplegia, extrapyramidal syndromes, optic and cerebral atrophy, and peripheral neuromuscular damage. Survival without neurologic damage is best in children who are hypothermic when recovered and may occur even after 40 minutes of submersion. Similar reports of survival after prolonged immersion in adults are very rare.

DISORDERS CAUSED BY ALTERED BAROMETRIC PRESSURE

Significant alterations in environmental pressure are encountered by humans during ascent to altitude and during underwater diving. As altitude increases, barometric pressure falls from approximately 760 mm Hg at sea level to 380 mm Hg (0.5 ATA) at 18,000 feet. In seawater, the pressure of the water column increases by an amount equal to the barometric pressure for every 33 feet of depth.

Hence, at 33 feet of seawater, the absolute pressure is doubled (2 ATA). As a result, participants in activities such as mountaineering and scuba diving are often exposed to extremes of environmental pressure. Rapid pressure changes produce notable physiologic effects related to the behavior of atmospheric gases in the lungs and body tissues.

Diseases of High Altitudes

At high altitudes, the low barometric pressure causes physiologic effects due primarily to the decrease in the partial pressure of inspired oxygen. Physiologic changes, characterized primarily by hyperventilation, appear at 8000 to 10,000 feet. At altitudes above 10,000 feet, the physiologic responses become more pronounced owing to the shape of the oxygen-hemoglobin dissociation curve, which has a steep downslope below a PO_2 of approximately 60 mm Hg. A small drop in PO_2 below this level results in a relatively large decrease in arterial saturation. At 10,000 feet (3048 m), the alveolar PO_2 is approximately 60 mm Hg, and some individuals manifest impairment of memory, judgment, and the ability to perform complex calculations. At 18,000 feet (5486 meters), the alveolar PO_2 is 40 mm Hg, and unacclimatized individuals develop serious neurologic signs and symptoms.

Exposure to high altitude occurs most commonly in commercial aviation. In general, aircraft cabins are maintained at a pressure equal to or greater than that encountered at 8000 feet, so that supplemental oxygen is not required. Some patients with reduced cardiac reserve or with COPD may have difficulty tolerating even a small drop in arterial oxygen saturation and may require oxygen during flights. Aircraft regulations require that the flight crew receive supplemental oxygen when the cabin pressure drops below that at 10,000 feet, and that passengers receive supplemental oxygen should the cabin pressure drop below that at 15,000 feet.

ACUTE MOUNTAIN SICKNESS (AMS). Ascent to high altitude produces a wide spectrum of illness that depends on factors such as the absolute altitude, the rate of ascent, the length of stay, and individual susceptibility (Table 80–2). The acute syndromes probably reflect a common pathophysiology initiated by a relatively abrupt lack of oxygen, although the precise mechanisms remain uncertain. The ventilatory response to hypoxia and poor physical conditioning may play a role in susceptible individuals. The most common malady is AMS, and self-limited symptoms of headache, anorexia, malaise, and disturbed sleep may appear within a few hours of arriving at altitudes above 8000 feet. Symptoms may become worse with exercise owing in part to further oxygen desaturation of arterial blood. AMS may affect half of unacclimatized visitors to 14,000 feet. At altitudes above 9500 feet, AMS may be severe and followed sometimes by the more serious conditions of high-altitude pulmonary edema (HAPE) and high-altitude cerebral edema (HACE), which frequently coexist. High-altitude retinal hemorrhages (HARH) are prevalent above 14,000 feet and probably share a similar pathophysiology with cerebral edema. Retinal hemorrhages are not significant unless they produce visual symptoms; the latter circumstance usually indicates involvement of the macula and mandates immediate descent. The more serious forms of AMS are discussed below.

HIGH-ALTITUDE PULMONARY EDEMA (HAPE). Acute pulmonary edema is a potentially fatal complication of rapid ascent to altitudes above 9500 feet. HAPE occurs by noncardiogenic mechanisms, although pulmonary hypertension appears to be involved in its pathogenesis. Symptoms begin after 6 to 36 hours at high altitude and may follow an episode of AMS. Dyspnea at rest, tachypnea, and crackles are characteristic features of HAPE. Cyanosis, orthopnea, and hemoptysis commonly develop in more advanced cases.

At autopsy, the lungs are typically heavy, congested, and edematous and have hyaline membranes in small airways and alveoli. Hemodynamic studies have shown elevated pulmonary artery pressure with normal pulmonary venous pressure. The pulmonary edema may be due to an increase in pulmonary capillary pressure in small regions of the pulmonary capillary bed or to increased permeability in lung capillaries.

HIGH-ALTITUDE CEREBRAL EDEMA (HACE). HACE is relatively uncommon, occurring in perhaps 1.5% of individuals affected by AMS. Hypoxemia produces cerebral vasodilation and increased cerebral blood flow, which may lead to mild brain edema and produce the symptoms of AMS. Cerebral edema may also be aggravated by hypoxic inhibition of the adenosine triphosphate (ATP)–dependent sodium pump. By factors yet to be defined, the brain edema may progress and become life threatening. Signs and symptoms of HACE include severe, progressive headache, ataxia, confusion, anxiety, hallucinations, and coma. Papilledema and meningeal signs occur. Examining the cerebrospinal fluid reveals high opening pressures and perhaps hemorrhage or leukocytosis. Pathologically, the pattern of cerebral edema appears to be heterogeneous, and focal areas of capillary damage, red cell sludging, and platelet aggregation are seen.

TREATMENT OF ACUTE HIGH-ALTITUDE DISEASE. The simplest approach to preventing and treating acute altitude illness is to ascend to altitude gradually and to descend when troubling symptoms appear. Gradual ascent allows time for the body to adapt. If possible, the rate of ascent should be limited to approximately 1000 feet/day between altitudes of 8000 and 10,000 feet. Slower ascent (500 feet/day) is recommended for altitudes above 10,000 feet. If slow ascent is impractical, prophylactic treatment with acetazolamide is effective in preventing AMS. Acetazolamide increases renal bicarbonate excretion and lessens the degree of respiratory alkalosis. The drug is administered (250 mg) every 12 hours the day before, during, and for 1 day after the ascent. The use of twice-daily acetazolamide minimizes dehydration and potassium depletion over the 3 days. Other diuretics have not proved to be effective, and in practice, liberal water intake appears to hasten bicarbonate excretion and prevent hemoconcentration. Dexamethasone also reduces the incidence and early symptoms of AMS; however, its prophylactic use is not recommended because of potential side effects.

Management consists of rest, mild analgesics, alcohol avoidance, and adequate hydration. The symptoms usually abate within a few days. The definitive treatment for HAPE, HACE, and severe HARH is oxygen administration and descent to lower altitude. High-altitude pulmonary edema may improve dramatically with a descent of only a few thousand feet. If the descent is delayed, the combination of oxygen with PEEP or continuous positive airway pressure, or placing the victim in a pressurized bag or chamber, is effective. Nifedipine and dexamethasone also have been reported to ameliorate serious AMS when descent is not feasible.

CHRONIC MOUNTAIN SICKNESS (MONGE'S DISEASE). Chronic mountain sickness occurs in people living at high altitudes,

Table 80–2 ■ HIGH-ALTITUDE SYNDROMES

SYNDROME	CLINICAL DESCRIPTION
Acute mountain sickness (AMS)	Common, self-limited; characterized by headache, anorexia, and malaise after ascent to altitudes >8000 ft; "normal puna"
High-altitude pulmonary edema (HAPE)	Noncardiac pulmonary edema recognized by dyspnea and tachypnea at rest, cough, and bibasilar crackles; usually at altitudes >9500 ft; "pulmonary puna"
High-altitude cerebral edema (HACE)	Uncommon, severe central nervous system dysfunction following AMS, characterized by severe headache, memory loss, ataxia, hallucinations, and confusion; may progress to coma and death; "nervous puna"
High-altitude retinal hemorrhages (HARH)	Dilated retinal vessels and peripheral flame-shaped or dot hemorrhages, which occasionally cause visual symptoms
Chronic mountain sickness (Monge's disease)	Cor pulmonale with minimal lung disease in long-term residents of high altitude

usually over 14,000 feet, for many years. These "highlanders" have a blunted respiratory drive in response to hypoxia and have a lower minute ventilation at high altitudes than do those who normally reside at lower altitudes. Chronic mountain sickness is characterized by an exaggerated response to hypoxia resulting in cor pulmonale. Physiologic responses include erythrocytosis with hemoglobin levels as high as 25 g/dL, a decreased minute ventilation with an elevated PCO_2, hypoxemia, and impaired sensitivity of the respiratory center to hypoxia. Clinical manifestations are similar to those of polycythemia rubra vera and include cyanosis, dyspnea, cough, palpitations, headache, giddiness, muscular weakness, pain in the extremities, sensory and motor changes, and episodic stupor. The only therapy is to move the patient to a lower altitude. Subacute forms of this illness, in which cyanosis and alveolar hypoventilation are absent, also occur. A similar syndrome, brisket disease, has been described in cattle.

Decompression Illness

Rapid ascent to a high altitude or from underwater toward the surface can cause decompression illness (DCI). Ambient pressure changes outside the body must be reflected across the lungs by proportional changes in the partial pressures of various gases dissolved in the tissues of the body. This condition is a consequence of the physical behavior of gases and their interactions with solutions. Because the quantity of gas dissolved in tissue varies directly with atmospheric pressure, changes in gas concentrations in the body are most pronounced during diving with compressed air, when, in order for divers to expand their lungs, the pressure of the breathing gas must be increased in proportion to the column of water around them. Nitrogen uptake is most important in this respect because it comprises 80% of the atmosphere and, unlike oxygen, it is inert (not metabolized). Inert gases like nitrogen must be eliminated from the body after a decrease in ambient pressure, e.g., return from a compressed air dive or rapid ascent to high altitude. The process of eliminating inert gas is called decompression.

During decompression, inert gas dissolved in the tissues may come out of physical solution if environmental pressure falls too rapidly. Bubbles of inert gas form within the tissues and venous blood and produce various clinical manifestations known as DCI, or Caisson's disease. DCI, however, is not entirely explained by gas bubbles in blood and tissue, and not all bubbles cause symptoms. Bubbles produce a number of secondary manifestations attributed to surface activity at the interface between the bubble and the blood or tissue. These secondary effects, such as activation of complement, platelet aggregation, and release of vasoactive mediators, may lead to ischemia and some of the manifestations of DCI.

CLINICAL MANIFESTATIONS. DCI can occur during decompression after diving to more than 25 feet of seawater (1.75 ATA) or during rapid ascent from sea level to 18,000 feet (0.5 ATA). DCI is most commonly encountered in compressed air (or gas) divers after prolonged or repetitive dives or after severe exercise and in divers with excessive body fat, poor physical conditioning, and increasing age. The signs and symptoms of DCI usually appear within a few minutes to a few hours after the end of the dive. Historically, DCI has been classified as either mild (type 1) or serious (type 2) (Table 80–3). This distinction is somewhat arbitrary, because both mild and serious manifestations of DCI occur simultaneously in about one-third of patients. Type 2 DCI usually involves the nervous system, although in its most serious form, abnormal gas exchange and hemodynamic compromise occur.

TREATMENT AND PROGNOSIS. The first step in treating DCI is administering high concentrations of oxygen by face mask. Prompt recompression in a hyperbaric chamber with 100% oxygen usually relieves symptoms in a matter of minutes. If recompression therapy is delayed for more than a few hours, the illness is more difficult to treat. The rationale for recompression is based on (1) enhancing the dissolution of gas bubbles by compression and (2) lowering the concentration of inert gas in venous blood with oxygen, thus increasing the rate of nitrogen removal from body tissues and bubbles. With prompt treatment, complete recovery is to be expected. If therapy is delayed for more than 24 hours, the outcome is less

certain, although many patients, even those with serious neurologic disease, respond to recompression after delays of 1 or more days.

Pulmonary Barotrauma and Arterial Gas Embolism

Pulmonary barotrauma and arterial gas embolism (AGE) may occur in compressed air divers when they ascend to the surface, particularly with failure to exhale normally. They are also encountered during explosive decompression at high altitude and in blast injury of the thorax. Under these circumstances, ambient hydrostatic or barometric pressure decreases rapidly, and gas within the lungs expands reciprocally according to Boyle's law. Under water near the surface, small decreases in depth result in large increases in gas volume. If the expanding gas is not allowed to escape, it may create a pressure gradient exceeding the compliance of lung tissue. This positive-pressure gradient between alveolar gas and the pulmonary interstitium may lead to alveolar disruption and pulmonary interstitial emphysema and then to soft tissue or mediastinal emphysema, pneumothorax, or pneumopericardium. This condition is known as pulmonary barotrauma. Free gas may also enter pulmonary venous blood and travel through the left side of the heart to the systemic circulation. Air can be embolized throughout the arterial system, including the cerebral, coronary, and renal arteries. Air in the systemic circulation is more common in persons with intra-cardiac shunts, including a previously undetected patent foramen ovale, which may be present in about 15% of the normal population.

CLINICAL MANIFESTATIONS. The clinical manifestations of AGE usually occur within minutes after the diver surfaces. Signs and symptoms that suggest distribution of gas to the carotid arteries frequently develop. This condition leads to acute cerebral dysfunction characterized by severe headache, blindness, loss of consciousness, seizures, or paralysis. Depending on the amount of pulmonary barotrauma, the quantity of embolized gas may be very large. This serious complication of ascent can occur in compressed air diving after very brief exposures or at very shallow depths, when DCI is not a diagnostic consideration.

TREATMENT AND PROGNOSIS. Severe central nervous system deficits from AGE are more likely to be permanently disabling or lethal in the absence of adequate treatment than is DCI. Recompression therapy should commence within minutes if good neurologic recovery is to be ensured. The management is similar to that of DCI, but the magnitude, length, and number of recompression treatments are generally greater. If treatment is delayed more than 24 hours, the benefit from recompression therapy is likely to be small.

Berg BW, Saenger JS: Images in clinical medicine: Exogenous lipoid pneumonia. N Engl J Med 338:512, 1998. *Radiographic and pathologic images of lipoid pneumonia.*

Bove AA: Diving Medicine: Section IV. Diving Related Disorders, 3rd ed. Philadelphia, WB Saunders, 1997, pp 115–204. *A comprehensive text on diving-related medical problems.*

Golden FS, Tipton MJ, Scott RC: Immersion, near-drowning, and drowning. Br J Anaesth 79:214–225, 1997. *A review of the pathophysiology, clinical manifestations, and treatment of these conditions.*

Klocke DL, Decker WW, Stepanek J: Altitude-related illnesses. Mayo Clin Proc 73:988–993, 1998. *A review of altitude-related syndromes, including high-altitude pulmonary edema.*

Table 80–3 ■ CLASSIFICATION OF DECOMPRESSION ILLNESS (DCI)

ORGAN SYSTEM	SIGNS AND SYMPTOMS
Mild DCI (Type 1)	
Skin	Pruritus, mottling, urticaria
Musculoskeletal	Pain (bends), usually in the joints; numbness; edema
Serious DCI (Type 2)	
Central nervous system	
Cerebral	Loss of consciousness, ataxia, vertigo, aphasia, hemiparesis
Audiovestibular	Vertigo, nystagmus, auditory symptoms
Spinal cord	Back pain, paraparesis, bladder and bowel dysfunction
Cardiopulmonary	Cough, substernal pain, tachypnea, asphaxyia (chokes)
Systemic	Extreme fatigue, hypovolemic shock

81 SARCOIDOSIS

Steven E. Weinberger

DEFINITION. Sarcoidosis is a disease of unknown cause and is characterized by the presence of non-caseating granulomas in one or more organ systems. Although the lungs and the lymph nodes in the mediastinum and hilar regions are the most common sites of involvement, the disorder is considered a systemic disease, and a variety of other organ systems or tissues may be the source of either primary or concomitant clinical manifestations and morbidity. The clinical course is quite variable, ranging from asymptomatic disease with spontaneous resolution to progressive disease with organ system failure and even death.

EPIDEMIOLOGY. Although sarcoidosis has a worldwide distribution, its reported incidence and prevalence vary considerably in different geographic areas and among disparate population subgroups. However, the accuracy and the comparability of available data are suspect, based on a high frequency of asymptomatic cases and widely differing methods of case identification.

Sarcoidosis appears to be relatively common in northern Europe (especially Scandinavia, Ireland, and Great Britain), North America, and Japan, whereas countries with a reportedly low incidence include China, Africa, India, and Russia. Even in these presumed low-incidence countries, it is likely that more cases of sarcoidosis have been present but have been misdiagnosed, especially as tuberculosis or leprosy. In a number of countries, such as Italy and Japan, the incidence of the disease is significantly greater in the northern than the southern part of the country, raising the possibility that climate affects the likelihood of the disease.

The peak age incidence of sarcoidosis is in the 20s and 30s, and women are affected slightly more often than men. Approximately 50% of patients are younger than age 30 at the time of presentation, and approximately 75% are younger than age 40. In some countries, such as Sweden and Japan, a second peak in incidence has been noted in middle age, especially in women.

In the United States, sarcoidosis is more frequent in blacks than in whites, with age-adjusted annual incidences reported as 35.5 and 10.9 per 100,000, respectively. However, worldwide nearly 80% of affected patients are white.

ETIOLOGY. The cause of sarcoidosis is unknown. A substantial body of information has suggested that immune mechanisms are important in disease pathogenesis, and it has been presumed that one or more causal antigens trigger a cascade of immunologic events. Genetic factors may also contribute in determining susceptibility.

Several observations have suggested that an exogenous agent may be responsible for sarcoidosis:

1. Identification of case clusters of sarcoidosis (e.g., in nurses, firefighters, and in specific geographic regions) supports the possibility of either person-to-person transmission of an infectious agent or shared exposure to an environmental agent.
2. The disease berylliosis, which is due to exposure to beryllium, produces a histologic pattern and a clinical presentation that are quite similar to those seen with sarcoidosis.
3. Recurrence of disease can occur in the transplanted lung of patients who receive a transplant for end-stage sarcoidosis. In addition, sarcoidosis has been reported to develop in the transplant recipient of tissue from a donor with sarcoidosis.

A variety of exogenous agents, both infectious and non-infectious, have been hypothesized as possible causes of sarcoidosis. Proposed infectious causes include mycobacteria (both *Mycobacterium tuberculosis* and non-tuberculous mycobacteria), cell wall–deficient mycobacteria (called L-forms), fungi, spirochetes, and the agent associated with Whipple's disease. Although the diagnosis of sarcoidosis depends on the absence of organisms that are known to be associated with granuloma formation (e.g., mycobacteria and fungi on stain or culture), the possibility remains that sarcoidosis may represent a variant host response to an infectious agent and that the organism may not be readily identifiable or recoverable at the time of disease presentation. For example, a number of studies have used the polymerase chain reaction in an attempt to identify mycobacterial DNA from biologic specimens obtained from patients with sarcoidosis, but results are inconclusive.

Environmental or occupational exposure to non-infectious agents has been an important alternative theory of the etiology of sarcoidosis. Based on the model provided by berylliosis, it has been suggested that an exogenous agent induces immunologic sensitization, perhaps by acting as a "hapten" that binds to peptides or alters major histocompatibility complex molecules. Non-infectious agents proposed to be causally related to sarcoidosis have included beryllium and other metals, organic antigens (e.g., pine pollen, peanut dust), and inorganic dusts (e.g., clay). However, the weight of evidence does not adequately support any of these agents as a primary cause of sarcoidosis.

PATHOGENESIS. It is believed, although not proved, that genetic factors may influence the development of sarcoidosis by affecting the nature of the cellular and immune response to the exogenous agent(s). Familial sarcoidosis, in which an individual with sarcoidosis is found to have a first- or second-degree relative with the disease, has been noted in approximately 15% of patients and appears to be more common in blacks than in whites. However, the relative role of genetics versus shared environmental exposure in explaining these findings has not yet been defined, and studies of human leukocyte antigen associations in sarcoidosis have not been conclusive.

Despite the lack of definitive evidence about intrinsic and extrinsic factors that initiate sarcoidosis, a substantial body of information has been accumulated about the intermediate pathogenesis of the disease (i.e., the role played by cellular responses, immune mechanisms, and elaboration of cytokines). Antigen processing by macrophages is believed to trigger an oligoclonal expansion of CD4 (helper-inducer) lymphocytes of the T_H1 phenotype, with production of IL-2 and IFN-γ. IL-2 causes the proliferation of more CD4 cells, which elaborate cytokines that recruit macrophages into the granuloma. A variety of cytokines, adhesion molecules, and growth factors are released from both lymphocytes and macrophages, with amplification of the inflammatory response and the potential to induce fibrosis.

Although B lymphocytes do not appear to play a primary role in the disease, their function is altered secondarily by mediators released from activated T lymphocytes. Polyclonal hyperglobulinemia results, with formation of antibodies reactive against a variety of microbial agents and self-antigens.

CLINICAL MANIFESTATIONS. Sarcoidosis is notable for its protean manifestations and variable course. Not only can almost any organ system be affected, but the clinical presentation and natural history of disease affecting a particular organ system are also quite variable. The respiratory system is most commonly affected, with approximately 90% of patients demonstrating intrathoracic involvement on a chest radiograph. Patients can develop extrathoracic disease either with or without concomitant intrathoracic involvement. Extrathoracic disease can be the predominant component of the clinical picture or alternatively can be either subclinical or less problematic than intrathoracic disease.

Thirty to 60 per cent of patients have no symptoms at the time of presentation, and the disease is identified because of abnormalities on a chest radiograph. Alternatively, patients commonly present with respiratory symptoms, such as dyspnea and cough, which may or may not be accompanied by constitutional symptoms, such as fever and malaise. Ten to 20 per cent of patients present with a syndrome of bilateral hilar adenopathy and erythema nodosum, a constellation of findings that is called *Löfgren's syndrome*; fever and/or arthralgias may also accompany this form of presentation. Presentations related primarily to extrathoracic involvement are less common; specific signs and symptoms depend on the particular organ system(s) involved.

RESPIRATORY SYSTEM DISEASE. Intrathoracic nodal involvement and parenchymal lung disease are the two most common ways in which sarcoidosis affects the respiratory system. Both hilar and mediastinal lymph nodes may be affected; involvement of the hilar nodes is usually bilateral and relatively symmetrical. The pulmonary parenchyma demonstrates well-defined, non-caseating granulomas within the pulmonary interstitium, typically in a pattern that preferentially follows bronchovascular bundles. Upper lobes of the lung tend to be more involved than the lower lobes. The granulomatous inflammation is often accompanied by non-specific mononuclear cell infiltration; in severe disease, parenchymal involvement may progress to irreversible fibrosis and honeycombing. Cystic lesions may be complicated by colonization with *Aspergillus* and the development of intracavitary aspergillomas.

Granulomatous involvement of the airways (i.e., endobronchial sarcoidosis) is common and may lead to bronchostenosis in a small proportion of cases. The upper respiratory tract may be affected by sarcoidosis, with involvement taking the form of nasal mucosal, nasal bone, or laryngeal disease. Pleural disease is relatively infrequent, with effusions occurring in fewer than 5% of patients.

Dyspnea and cough, typically non-productive, are the primary symptoms that accompany either pulmonary parenchymal or endobronchial sarcoidosis. Examination of the chest can reveal crackles resulting from parenchymal lung involvement, although the examination is often notable for the paucity or even absence of findings despite the extent of radiographic changes. Wheezing may be present in a small proportion of cases, resulting either from endobronchial involvement or airway distortion as a consequence of end-stage fibrotic disease.

Pulmonary function tests in the presence of parenchymal lung disease often demonstrate a pattern of restrictive disease, with a relatively symmetric decrease in lung volumes, although they can remain normal despite parenchymal changes on chest radiograph. The diffusing capacity of the lung for carbon monoxide may be either normal or abnormal and does not necessarily follow the presence or absence of abnormal lung volumes.

SKIN DISEASE. Cutaneous manifestations of sarcoidosis resulting from granulomatous involvement of the skin affect 15 to 20% of patients. A variety of lesions can be seen, including papules, plaques, nodules, infiltration of old scars, and lupus pernio. Old scars or tattoos often become infiltrated with granulomas, so that previously atrophic scars develop an appearance of keloid formation. *Lupus pernio* is a chronic, violaceous, often disfiguring lesion primarily affecting the nose, cheeks, and ears. It tends to affect women older than 40 years of age, especially those from the West Indies.

Erythema nodosum commonly occurs in combination with bilateral hilar adenopathy as part of Löfgren's syndrome. These raised, red, tender, nodular lesions, generally but not exclusively on the anterior surface of the lower leg, do not represent granulomatous involvement of the skin. Rather, the histopathology is primarily that of a panniculitis, with cellular inflammation and edema of the deep dermis and subcutaneous tissue, especially involving connective tissue septa of adipose tissue.

EYE DISEASE. Ocular sarcoidosis can take a number of forms, including anterior or posterior uveitis, conjunctival involvement, and papilledema. Overall, 15 to 25% of patients have some form of ocular involvement. Anterior uveitis, the most common form of ocular sarcoidosis, is often associated with the relatively acute onset of a red eye, photophobia, and ocular discomfort. *Heerfordt's syndrome*, or uveoparotid fever, is a form of sarcoidosis in which anterior uveitis is accompanied by parotid gland enlargement and often fever and facial palsy. Posterior uveitis, which may be obscured on examination by anterior chamber involvement, can present with vitreous infiltrates, choroidal nodules, periphlebitis, retinal hemorrhage, and papilledema. Conjunctival involvement can produce small, pale yellow nodules that demonstrate granulomatous inflammation on biopsy.

CARDIAC DISEASE. The frequency of cardiac sarcoidosis is difficult to ascertain, but 5 to 10% of patients have significant cardiac involvement (see Chapter 64). Potential clinical consequences of such involvement include conduction defects (e.g., first-, second-, or third-degree heart block or a bundle branch block), ventricular or supraventricular arrhythmias, and heart failure.

NEUROLOGIC DISEASE. Five to 10% of patients with sarcoidosis develop neurologic complications of their disease. Virtually any part of the nervous system can be involved, including cranial nerves, peripheral nerves, meninges, cerebrum, spinal cord, and the hypothalamic-pituitary axis. The most common form of clinically apparent neurologic involvement is unilateral facial nerve palsy, but other clinical consequences include seizures, meningitis, peripheral neuropathy, and psychiatric symptoms. Involvement of the hypothalamic-pituitary axis can cause hyperprolactinemia and diabetes insipidus.

OTHER EXTRATHORACIC DISEASE. Although granulomas are commonly found on histologic examination of the liver in patients with sarcoidosis, symptoms related to hepatic involvement are uncommon, and clinical evidence is usually limited to abnormalities in one or more hepatic enzymes. In addition to intrathoracic lymph node involvement, peripheral lymph nodes may be enlarged because of granulomatous infiltration, but they rarely produce important clinical consequences. Parotid gland enlargement, lacrimal gland infiltration, bone lesions, splenomegaly, and myopathy due to granulomas within muscle tissue may also be seen.

BIOCHEMICAL CHANGES. Biochemical changes noted in many patients with sarcoidosis include alterations in calcium metabolism and elevations in the level of angiotensin-converting enzyme (ACE). Hypercalcemia, a potentially important complication of sarcoidosis, occurs in fewer than 10% of patients and is thought to be due to elevated levels of 1,25-dihydroxyvitamin D (calcitriol), which is produced by macrophages within the granulomas. As a result, calcium absorption from the intestine is increased, leading to hypercalciuria with or without hypercalcemia.

ACE, which catalyzes breakdown of the decapeptide angiotensin I to the octapeptide angiotensin II, is normally found in the lung. Elevated levels of ACE occur relatively frequently in sarcoidosis, with estimates varying widely but usually in the range of 40 to 90%. This elevation in ACE is believed to be due to production of the enzyme by epithelioid cells and macrophages within the granulomas. Although it was initially proposed that measurement of serum ACE might be a useful diagnostic and prognostic test in sarcoidosis, subsequent experience has shown its lack of diagnostic specificity and poor prognostic value in identifying patients with progressive disease.

DIAGNOSTIC EVALUATION. The initial consideration of sarcoidosis is usually based on the clinical and/or chest radiographic findings. When intrathoracic disease is the primary mode of presentation, the differential diagnosis generally depends on the radiographic presentation. Hilar and/or mediastinal adenopathy, either with or without associated parenchymal lung disease, can also be produced by lymphoma, mycobacterial or fungal infection, and selected pneumoconioses, such as berylliosis and silicosis. When interstitial lung disease is present in the absence of intrathoracic lymphadenopathy, a much broader differential diagnosis is raised, including idiopathic pulmonary fibrosis, pulmonary fibrosis associated with systemic rheumatic disease (e.g., scleroderma, rheumatoid arthritis, polymyositis), and disease due to a broad range of inorganic dusts (i.e., pneumoconiosis), organic antigens (i.e., hypersensitivity pneumonitis), and drugs (e.g., cancer chemotherapeutic agents).

The diagnosis of sarcoidosis is confirmed by the finding of well-formed non-caseating granulomas in one or more affected organ systems or tissues, with appropriate additional studies to exclude other causes of granulomas. Special stains and cultures must be performed for mycobacteria and fungi, and specimens should be examined under polarized light to identify foreign, potentially granulomagenic material. In patients with symmetrical bilateral hilar lymphadenopathy, either in association with erythema nodosum (Löfgren's syndrome) or in the absence of any symptoms, physical findings, or screening laboratory data that might indicate another cause, many clinicians believe that a clinical diagnosis of sarcoidosis can be made without needing histologic confirmation.

CHEST RADIOGRAPHY AND OTHER IMAGING PROCEDURES. The plain chest radiograph is an important component of the diagnostic evaluation of patients with sarcoidosis; the diagnosis is frequently suspected initially based on the radiographic abnormalities, either in the presence or absence of symptomatic disease. The major abnormalities seen on the chest radiograph include lymphadenopathy, usually involving both hila in a relatively symmetrical fashion as well as the right paratracheal region, and involvement of the pulmonary parenchyma (Fig. 81–1). Although the pattern of parenchymal involvement is typically described as interstitial, alveolar and nodular patterns may also be seen. A commonly used radiographic staging system considers the pattern of involvement seen on the chest radiograph (Table 81–1).

Computed tomography (CT) of the chest is not generally indi-

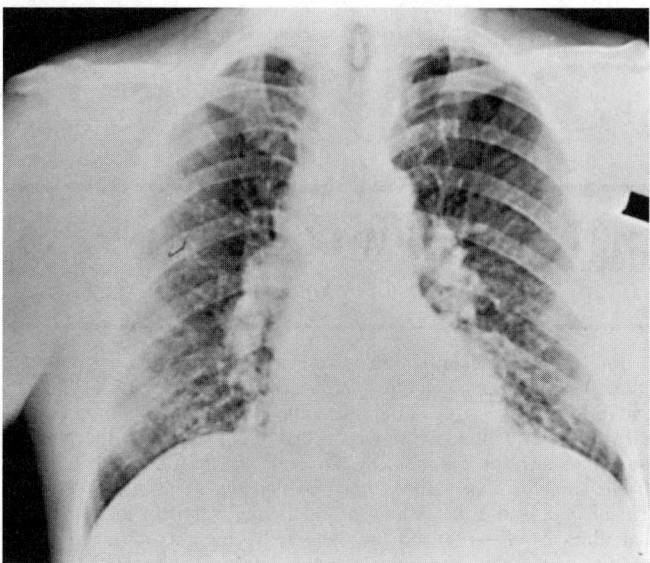

FIGURE 81–1 ■ Chest radiograph shows characteristic features of stage II sarcoidosis: bilateral hilar adenopathy and diffuse interstitial lung disease. In stage I sarcoidosis (not shown), patients have hilar adenopathy without interstitial lung disease, whereas in stage III sarcoidosis (not shown), patients have diffuse interstitial lung disease without hilar adenopathy. (From Weinberger SE: Principles of Pulmonary Medicine. Philadelphia, WB Saunders, 1998, p 161.)

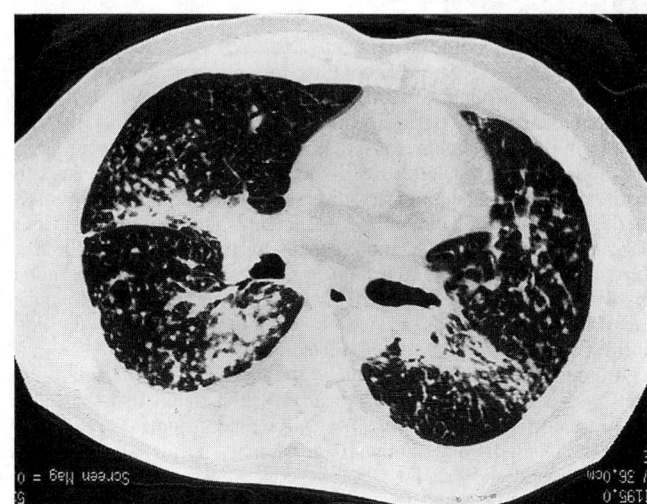

FIGURE 81–2 ■ High-resolution chest CT scan in a patient with pulmonary parenchymal involvement by sarcoidosis. There are numerous small nodules in a predominantly bronchovascular distribution. (Courtesy of Dr. David Levin.)

cated in the evaluation of suspected sarcoidosis, especially when typical findings are seen on plain chest radiography. However, when the findings are atypical or if there is a need for better definition of mediastinal lymph node involvement, CT may be beneficial. In addition to bilateral hilar lymphadenopathy, the chest CT scan commonly shows much more mediastinal involvement than was suspected on the chest radiograph, especially involving right paratracheal, subcarinal, and aortopulmonary lymph nodes. High-resolution CT commonly demonstrates that pulmonary parenchymal involvement is localized around bronchovascular structures, producing an appearance resembling budding branches on a tree (Fig. 81–2).

Scanning with gallium citrate-67 may demonstrate uptake of this isotope in regions involved with granulomatous inflammation, probably reflecting a combination of increased capillary permeability as well as uptake of tracer by activated macrophages. However, because tracer uptake is non-specific and because the correlation with other indices of disease activity or involvement is not particularly good, gallium scanning is not generally recommended as part of the routine evaluation of patients with suspected sarcoidosis.

TISSUE BIOPSY. Non-caseating granulomas found on biopsy of an affected organ or tissue are generally well formed, consisting of a localized collection of epithelioid histiocytes surrounded by a rim of variable numbers of lymphocytes. Multinucleated giant cells are typically present within the granulomas. Additional findings of a mononuclear cell alveolitis and variable amounts of fibrosis are diagnostically non-specific. Although non-caseating granulomas may also be seen in hypersensitivity pneumonitis, the granulomas are generally less discrete and well formed than in sarcoidosis.

The pulmonary parenchyma, intrathoracic lymph nodes, and skin are the most common sites of diagnostic biopsy in sarcoidosis.

Flexible bronchoscopy with transbronchial lung biopsy is particularly useful, with a yield of 60 to 95%, depending on the radiographic stage of the disease and the number of biopsy specimens. Interestingly, even when pulmonary parenchymal involvement is not grossly visible on plain chest radiography (e.g., in radiographic stage I disease), transbronchial lung biopsy is positive in approximately 60% of patients.

Mediastinoscopy is sometimes performed in the presence of isolated mediastinal adenopathy without parenchymal lung disease, when another diagnosis such as lymphoma is being strongly considered. Thoracoscopic lung biopsy is sometimes used when a broader differential diagnosis of parenchymal lung disease has been raised, and more tissue is believed to be necessary than can be obtained by transbronchial lung biopsy.

Biopsy of tissue other than the lung or mediastinal lymph nodes is performed primarily based on clinical evidence of involvement. Skin biopsy, a relatively non-invasive procedure, is useful when findings suggestive of cutaneous sarcoidosis are present. Similarly, biopsy of peripheral lymph nodes, liver, conjunctiva, parotid glands, skeletal muscle, and myocardium can be performed in selected cases.

NATURAL HISTORY AND PROGNOSIS. The natural history of sarcoidosis is quite variable, ranging from spontaneous resolution to either smoldering or progressive disease. Patients who present with Löfgren's syndrome tend to have a good prognosis characterized by spontaneous resolution of disease. The chest radiographic stage of disease is also helpful (see Table 81–1). Patients with progressive disease can become disabled from significant organ system involvement, particularly respiratory failure from severe interstitial lung disease.

Assessment of functional involvement of an organ and its course over time provides the general framework for monitoring the natural history of disease. For pulmonary disease, monitoring includes symptoms, pulmonary function tests, and chest radiographs; conversely, gallium scanning, bronchoalveolar lavage (using lavage

Table 81–1 ■ RADIOGRAPHIC STAGING OF INTRATHORACIC SARCOIDOSIS

STAGE	HILAR ADENOPATHY	PARENCHYMAL DISEASE	PERCENT AT ONSET	PERCENT WITH RESOLUTION
0	No	No	<10	NA
1	Yes	No	50	65 (<10% progress to parenchymal disease)
2	Yes	Yes	30	20–50
3 or 4	No	Yes (with fibrosis in stage 4)	10–15	<20

NA = not applicable.

lymphocytosis as a marker of alveolitis), and measurement of serum ACE level are not recommended.

TREATMENT. Because sarcoidosis follows such a variable natural history, it is often difficult to decide whether and when therapy should be instituted. Serial evaluation can assess whether the disease is improving spontaneously. Whenever there is significant ocular, myocardial, or neurologic involvement, treatment is generally instituted early. For pulmonary disease, intrathoracic nodal involvement is not an indication for treatment, but parenchymal lung disease is a potential indication, depending on its effects on pulmonary function and symptoms, not on the severity of radiographic involvement. Presentation with Löfgren's syndrome does not warrant therapy, except as needed for symptoms (e.g., non-steroidal anti-inflammatory drugs for associated joint symptoms).

Although corticosteroids acutely suppress the manifestations of the disease, it has never been clearly demonstrated that they alter its long-term natural history. Typically, prednisone is started at a dose of 0.5 mg/kg/day, although occasionally up to 1.0 mg/kg/day, and continued at that dose for several weeks in an attempt to suppress the disease acutely. The dose can then be tapered, with the goal of using the lowest possible dose that keeps the disease under adequate control. Many clinicians taper to 10 to 30 mg every other day. Patients requiring systemic corticosteroid therapy for hypercalcemia can often be treated with relatively low doses of prednisone even initially, such as 10 to 20 mg/day.

The optimal overall duration of therapy is not known and needs to be customized for each patient depending on the response to therapy and the effect of drug tapering. Treatment durations of 6 to 12 months are typical, and premature discontinuation of therapy may lead to recurrence of symptomatic and functional disease. Patients must be advised about and monitored for the myriad potential side effects observed with systemic corticosteroids (see Chapter 28).

Alternative agents when systemic corticosteroids are ineffective or not tolerated include methotrexate, generally at a dose of 10 to 15 mg/week, or other immunosuppressive or cytotoxic agents. Although methotrexate has been used most as a corticosteroid-sparing agent, it can be used as the sole agent, particularly for musculoskeletal or cutaneous sarcoidosis. Hydroxychloroquine has been used for serious and disfiguring cutaneous sarcoidosis. Topical corticosteroid preparations are used for anterior uveitis, but refractory disease may require treatment with systemic corticosteroids. Clinical experience with cyclosporine has been disappointing. In patients with severe, end-stage pulmonary disease refractory to therapy, lung transplantation is an important option, but the disease may recur in the allograft.

British Thoracic Society: The diagnosis, assessment and treatment of diffuse parenchymal lung disease in adults. Thorax 54(Suppl. 1):S1, 1999. *A recent position paper from the British Thoracic Society with recommendations regarding the evaluation and management of diffuse parenchymal lung disease in general and several specific causes, including sarcoidosis.*

Newman LS, Rose CS, Maier LA: Sarcoidosis. N Engl J Med 336:1224, 1997. *An excellent review of possible causes and pathogenesis as well as clinical aspects of the disease.*

Sharma OP (ed): Sarcoidosis. Clin Chest Med 18:663, 1997. *Multiple articles within this monograph provide an excellent review of the spectrum of issues relating to sarcoidosis.*

82 OVERVIEW OF PNEUMONIA

Waldemar G. Johanson, Jr.

Pneumonia is a term used to indicate inflammation of the distal lung: terminal airways, alveolar spaces, and interstitium. To improve the precision of communication, the term pneumonia is usually further qualified with words that imply a cause, mechanism, anatomic site, or clinical course. Thus, descriptors such as *viral bronchopneumonia, aspiration pneumonia, chronic interstitial pneumonia,* and *acute bacterial pneumonia* serve to identify clinical illnesses characterized by signs and symptoms of lung inflammation in a variety of clinical situations (see Chapters 319 to 323).

PATHOPHYSIOLOGY

Bacterial pneumonia results when host defense mechanisms fail to contain a bacterial challenge presented to the lungs (Fig. 82–1). The sources of bacteria may be endogenous or exogenous. Bacteria are introduced into the lungs by any of four routes: by microaspiration, by inhalation, via the blood stream, or by direct extension (Table 82–1). The blood stream may transport to the lung organisms that may produce pneumonia, but the originating site of infection and the severe systemic effects of sepsis usually outweigh the importance of the resulting pneumonia. Direct extension from a focus of infection adjacent to the lungs is uncommon, and the initial site of infection is always more important.

USUAL ROUTES OF INOCULATION

Aspiration of contaminated oropharyngeal secretions containing organisms that have colonized the upper airways is the most common route of lung inoculation. The term *aspiration* is often mistakenly equated with inhalation of large volumes of material into the tracheobronchial tree, an event that occurs only in patients with depressed consciousness or seriously deranged swallowing mechanisms. However, normal individuals aspirate small quantities of oropharyngeal secretions during sleep, and the frequency and amount of aspiration are increased in patients with altered consciousness. Because the concentration of aerobic bacteria in upper respiratory tract secretions is about 10^8 organisms per milliliter, and that of anaerobic bacteria is about 10 times greater, aspiration of even small quantities of oropharyngeal secretions introduces an enormous bacterial challenge to the lungs. Bacteria aspirated in

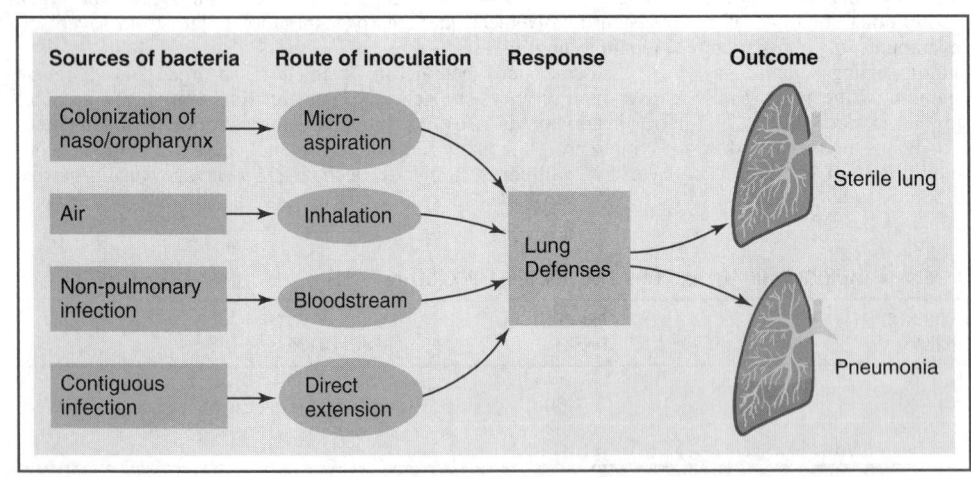

FIGURE 82–1 ■ Overview of the pathophysiology of bacterial pneumonia.

Table 82–1 ■ ROUTES OF BACTERIAL INOCULATION OF THE LUNGS

ROUTE	EXAMPLES
Microaspiration of oropharyngeal secretions	Most bacterial pneumonias, anaerobic pleuropulmonary infections
Inhalation of airborne organisms	*Mycobacterium tuberculosis, Legionella* sp., many viruses, including influenza
Blood stream	Staphylococcal endocarditis, septic emboli
Direct extension	Amebic liver abscess

oropharyngeal secretions colonize the respiratory tract primarily by adhering to selective cell-surface receptors that bind only certain species of bacteria to mucosal cells; these receptors are major determinants of the resident flora, which may include highly pathogenic organisms even in normal humans. The chemical nature of receptors for different species of bacteria is highly variable, and the site of the receptor may be either an integral part of the cell surface or contained in proteins attached to the cell. The availability of epithelial receptors and therefore susceptibility to colonization vary with the underlying disease, antimicrobial therapy, or concurrent viral infections. In contrast, pathogenic respiratory viruses do not establish chronic colonization of the airways.

Organisms present in ambient air are highly selected by environmental conditions and must survive aerosolization, drying, temperature changes, and ultraviolet irradiation. Further, because few if any microorganisms are inhaled with each breath, only organisms capable of causing infection with a very small inoculum can produce disease by the airborne route. Most pathogenic bacteria are not sufficiently virulent, but the infecting dose of *Mycobacterium tuberculosis* may be as low as a single organism, and many viruses are transmitted by the airborne route. However, the list of bacteria capable of being transmitted by this route is short and includes only organisms that are unusually invasive, such as the plague and anthrax bacilli, and organisms that are present in large numbers in contaminated air in confined spaces, such as *Legionella* organisms. Organisms capable of airborne transmission often produce outbreaks of infection when groups of susceptible people are exposed; examples include *Legionella,* influenza, and anthrax.

HOST DEFENSES

The anatomy of the upper air passages (see Chapter 73) is an important aspect of defense against inhaled particulates, including bacteria. Droplets that exceed 10 μm in diameter are deposited by inertial impaction in the upper airways, a process that is promoted by the angulation of these structures. About 90% of particles 5 to 10 μm in diameter are deposited along the tracheobronchial tree, whereas particles 0.5 to 3 μm in diameter are deposited in the alveoli. Smaller particles behave like gas molecules and are largely exhaled rather than retained. *Droplet nuclei* is the term applied to particles about 1 to 3 μm in diameter containing a single bacterium, the likely infecting unit for organisms transmitted by the airborne route.

The first line of defense against bacteria deposited in the lungs is the mucociliary escalator, an integrated multifaceted system consisting of the ciliated cells lining the airways, the secretory cells (goblet cells and submucosal glands), and the secretions. Cilia beating 10 to 20 times per second propel the secretions toward the mouth. However, the effectiveness of this activity depends on maintaining the depth and viscosity of secretions and coordination of ciliary activity. Processes that impair ciliary movement, cause excessive secretion of respiratory mucus, or change the viscosity of

secretions may hinder the effectiveness of this transport system (Table 82–2).

Bacteria that penetrate to the distal airways or alveoli are killed in situ by phagocytic cells. Nonspecific opsonization, which aids phagocytosis, may be provided by lung surfactant or fibronectin. Alveolar macrophages that reside in the lungs can ingest and kill enormous numbers of nonpathogenic bacteria, such as most of the normal oropharyngeal flora, without eliciting an inflammatory response. For bacteria that are more pathogenic, the situation is more complicated; some species promptly recruit neutrophils, and bacterial killing appears to depend much more upon the availability of neutrophils than on the presence of alveolar macrophages. Clearance of these organisms from the lung is enhanced by the presence of specific antibody. Immunoglobulin (Ig) G is the predominant immunoglobulin in the alveolus, comprising about 10 to 15% of the protein in alveolar fluid.

If viable bacteria persist, an inflammatory response swiftly develops and is characterized by interstitial and alveolar edema as well as an influx of neutrophils. The chemoattractants responsible for the latter include a variety of molecules including bacterial products, C5a, interleukins-8 and -12 (IL-8, IL-12), tumor necrosis factor-alpha (TNF-α), interferon-γ, and several chemokines (see Chapters 171 and 271). Countering the pro-inflammatory mediators are a variety of molecules that modulate and inhibit one or another aspect of the inflammatory response, such as IL-10, which deactivates polymorphonuclear leukocytes and macrophages. As neutrophils and bacteria accumulate, the milieu becomes acidic and hypoxic, and bacterial ingestion and killing are remarkably retarded. Spreading edema and inflammation at the periphery of the lesion continue until specific antibody appears (days 5 to 7) or effective antibiotic therapy is initiated.

Community-acquired pneumonias are usually due to a single organism, an observation that appears to contradict the aspiration mechanism that necessarily includes multiple species. However, the susceptibility of individual bacterial species to lung defenses varies widely, so the lung's defenses and other clinical factors determine the organism (or organisms) that will cause pneumonia—the species most capable of evading phagocytosis and killing (Table 82–3).

Organisms gain access to the systemic circulation early in the development of pneumonia. For example, pneumococci introduced into the lungs of dogs can be recovered from hilar lymph nodes within 15 minutes. Bacteremia and positive cultures of spleen and liver occur when the lung bacterial burden exceeds 10^4 bacteria per gram of lung tissue. Successful host defense against the systemic spread of infection requires a functioning reticuloendothelial system, opsonins, and adequate numbers of neutrophils. Patients who present with overwhelming sepsis due to pneumonia generally lack one or more of these defenses.

SIGNS AND SYMPTOMS

The signs and symptoms associated with bacterial pneumonia vary widely depending on the offending pathogen and the state of the host. At one extreme is the previously healthy person with pneumococcal pneumonia. Such patients complain of a brief prodromal upper respiratory illness followed by fever, a single shaking chill, pleuritic chest pain, and a cough productive of purulent or "rusty" sputum. Physical examination reveals signs of consolidation, which are readily confirmed by chest radiography. At the other extreme might be an elderly, confused patient who presents with only deterioration in mental function. Physical examination

Table 82–2 ■ FACTORS THAT IMPAIR MUCOCILIARY FUNCTION

FACTOR	MECHANISM	EXAMPLES
Genetic	Altered secretions	Cystic fibrosis
	Ciliary dysfunction	Dysmotile cilia syndromes
Environmental	Mucus hypersecretion, epithelial cell injury	Cigarette smoke, irritant gases, dust
Bacterial infection	Decreased ciliary beating, cell injury	*Pseudomonas aeruginosa, Bordetella pertussis, Mycoplasma pneumoniae*
Viral infection	Epithelial cell injury	Influenza

Table 82-3 ■ COMMON ETIOLOGIC AGENTS OF COMMUNITY-ACQUIRED PNEUMONIA IN APPROXIMATE ORDER OF FREQUENCY

OUTPATIENT MANAGEMENT (AGE <60 YR, NO UNDERLYING DISEASE)	HOSPITALIZED PATIENT	SEVERE PNEUMONIA, ICU CARE
Streptococcus pneumoniae	*S. pneumoniae*	*S. pneumoniae*
Mycoplasma pneumoniae	*Haemophilus influenzae*	*Legionella* sp.
Respiratory viruses	Aerobic gram-negative bacilli	Aerobic gram-negative bacilli
Chlamydia pneumoniae	*Legionella* sp.	*M. pneumoniae*
Miscellaneous, including *Legionella* sp.	Miscellaneous, including *M. pneumoniae,* viruses	Respiratory viruses

Adapted from American Thoracic Society: Guidelines for the initial management of adults with community-acquired pneumonia: Diagnosis, assessment of severity, and initial antimicrobial therapy. Am Rev Respir Dis 148:1418, 1993.

reveals only rhonchi without signs of consolidation, and the chest radiograph shows only bilateral lower lobe interstitial infiltrates that might represent acute or chronic changes.

The physician should explore the presence of risk factors, including chronic illnesses, recent acute illnesses, illness in family members, use of alcohol or other drugs, and possible exposures to infectious agents. A thorough physical examination, posteroanterior and lateral chest radiographs, and blood leukocyte count with differential cell count should be performed. On the basis of the data available from these steps, it is usually possible to conclude that pneumonia is present. The remaining task is to determine its cause.

MICROBIOLOGIC DIAGNOSIS

Controversy exists over the proper microbiologic evaluation of the patient with pneumonia because of questions of sensitivity, specificity, cost, and benefit. Further, because most patients with pneumonia respond satisfactorily to simple, relatively nontoxic antibiotic regimens, the need to document the precise cause of the process is uncertain.

Sputum should be examined microscopically. The portion chosen should be purulent and contain fewer than 10 squamous cells and more than 25 leukocytes per low-power field. A well-done Gram stain discloses whether one species of organism predominates. Often, such specimens contain a vast preponderance of a single species, and if these are encapsulated gram-positive cocci (pneumococci) or small pleomorphic gram-negative coccobacilli (*Haemophilus*), a presumptive diagnosis can be made. Problems arise when a predominant organism is less apparent, when enteric gram-negative bacilli are present, or when an adequate specimen cannot be obtained.

Aerobic culture of expectorated sputum suffers from a lack of sensitivity (organisms causing pneumonia are not detected) and specificity (organisms are present that did not cause pneumonia); both sensitivity and specificity are only about 50%. The results may be improved by microscopic screening of the specimen prior to culture. Although some authorities have recommended that sputum cultures be abandoned except in unusual cases, others argue that the increasing incidence of antimicrobial resistance among agents causing community-acquired pneumonias mandates continued surveillance through routine cultures.

Contamination of expectorated sputum during passage through the mouth can be avoided by collecting the specimen distal to the larynx. Needle aspiration through the trachea (transtracheal aspiration) or of the lung through the chest wall (transthoracic lung aspiration) have been largely replaced by fiberoptic bronchoscopy, which has far fewer complications. Both the protected specimen brush and bronchoalveolar lavage techniques can be used; the former provides a small (0.001 mL) specimen of uncontaminated distal airway secretions, the latter a large volume suitable for special stains as well as cultures. A further advantage of bronchoscopy is that transbronchial lung biopsies can be obtained at the same time if a tissue diagnosis is needed. Invasive sampling approaches are certainly not needed in most patients with pneumonia but are indicated when a delay in accurate diagnosis may have serious consequences, such as in immunocompromised patients or patients whose conditions have worsened on empirical antimicrobial therapy.

Immunologic techniques, such as immunofluorescence, enzyme-linked immunosorbent assay, and DNA hybridization, hold great promise for determining the cause of pneumonia. However, compared with conventional cultures, these techniques are expensive and relatively insensitive; they should be considered only when specific organisms are strongly suspected on clinical grounds. Uncontaminated specimens obtained via bronchoscopy or transtracheal or transthoracic aspiration provide better materials for immunodiagnosis than expectorated sputum.

Cultures of the blood or pleural fluid, if positive, are highly specific, but only about 30% of patients with bacterial pneumonia have bacteremia. About the same percentage of pleural fluid aspirates are positive in the absence of antibiotic therapy, but only 10 to 15% of patients with pneumonia have pleural effusion. Blood cultures should be obtained in patients with serious illness due to pneumonia, and diagnostic thoracentesis should be performed if an effusion is large enough to be aspirated safely.

In most patients, the history, physical examination, radiographic studies, and evaluation of the sputum by Gram stain provide all the required data. Additional procedures should be reserved for those patients in whom a delay in making an accurate diagnosis will have serious consequences or those in whom therapy cannot be reasonably planned on the basis of simpler approaches.

RADIOGRAPHIC PATTERNS

Posteroanterior (PA) and lateral chest radiographs are an invaluable adjunct in diagnosis and should be part of the evaluation of every patient with suspected pneumonia. Although a specific microbiologic diagnosis is seldom, if ever, possible on the basis of radiographic data alone, important clues to the cause of pneumonia and its distribution and severity may be gained by this technique (Table 82-4).

Lobar or segmental consolidation suggests a bacterial cause for pneumonia, especially *Streptococcus pneumoniae* or *Klebsiella pneumoniae.* Consolidation may obscure the borders between the lung and adjacent structures (e.g., heart border or diaphragm). This obliteration is termed the *silhouette sign* and is very useful to localize infiltrates. Less well-defined and inhomogeneous radiographic densities, often described as "patchy" or "streaky" infiltrates, may be observed in bronchopneumonia caused by a variety of organisms, including bacteria and viruses. Diffuse pulmonary infiltrates are most commonly caused by infection with viruses (such as cytomegalovirus or influenza), *Legionella pneumophila,* or

Table 82-4 ■ COMMON RADIOGRAPHIC PATTERNS OF PNEUMONIA AND ASSOCIATED PATHOGENS

PATTERN	PATHOGENS
Lobar or segmental consolidation	*Streptococcus pneumoniae, Klebsiella pneumoniae, Haemophilus influenzae,* other gram-negative bacilli
Inhomogeneous infiltrates (patchy or streaky opacities)	*Mycoplasma pneumoniae,* viruses, *Legionella* sp.
Diffuse interstitial infiltrates	*Legionella* sp., viruses, *Pneumocystis carinii*
Cavitary infiltrates	*Mycoplasma tuberculosis,* gram-negative bacilli, *Staphylococcus aureus* (multiple nodules)
Pleural effusion plus infiltrate	*S. pneumoniae, S. aureus,* anaerobes, gram-negative bacilli, *Streptococcus pyogenes*

opportunistic pathogens such as *Pneumocystis carinii*. Cavitary infiltrates generally suggest the presence of a necrotizing infection from organisms such as *Staphylococcus aureus*, gram-negative bacteria, anaerobes, and *M. tuberculosis*.

The chest radiograph may also yield valuable information about infectious involvement of structures outside the parenchyma of the lung, including the pleural surface and thoracic lymph nodes. Pleural effusions, which occur in a variety of respiratory infections, are best documented by lateral decubitus radiographs; thoracentesis can then identify complicated parapneumonic effusions or empyema, which may require drainage (see Chapters 82 and 86). Enlargement of mediastinal and hilar lymph nodes is rare in acute bacterial infection and suggests infection by fungi or mycobacteria or the presence of an underlying lung cancer. Loss of volume of a pulmonary segment or lobe (partial or complete atelectasis) should raise suspicion of an obstructing endobronchial lesion with distal infection.

American Thoracic Society: Guidelines for the initial management of adults with community-acquired pneumonia: Diagnosis, assessment of severity, and initial antimicrobial therapy. Am Rev Respir Dis 148:1418, 1993. *A well-referenced guide to diagnosis and initial therapy of patients with community-acquired pneumonia. A patient-stratifying scheme is suggested that uses age, underlying disease, and severity to modify therapy.*

Bartlett JG, Breiman RF, Mandell LA, File TM Jr: Community-acquired pneumonia in adults: Guidelines for management: The Infectious Diseases Society of America. Clin Infect Dis 26:811–838, 1998. *This clinical practice guideline for pneumonia was created by experts in infectious diseases and offers a concise summary of recommendations for diagnosis and/or treatment. It differs from earlier guidelines published by others in the reliance on laboratory findings and in its specific recommendations for antimicrobial therapy.*

Cate TR: Impact of influenza and other community-acquired viruses. Semin Respir Infect 13:17–23, 1998. *The evidence that antecedent viral respiratory infections play an important role in the pathogenesis of pneumonia is reviewed in this article. Influenza has been implicated for many years, but recent studies have shown that respiratory syncytial virus infection is an important predisposing factor as well.*

Rubins JB, Janoff EN: Community-acquired pneumonia: Tailoring management of adult patients according to risk category. Postgrad Med 102:45–62, 1997. *Current concepts of management according to the patient's presentation and underlying risk factors.*

Standiford TJ, Hufnagle GB: Cytokines in host defense against pneumonia. J Invest Med 45:335–345, 1997. *An up-to-date discussion of the complex interactions between various components of the immune response to infectious agents in the lungs.*

83 LUNG ABSCESS

Sydney M. Finegold

DEFINITION

Lung abscess is a cavity containing pus and necrotic debris. Although mycobacterial, fungal, and parasitic infections can cause cavitary lesions, the term *lung abscess* is usually reserved for other bacterial infections and is distinguished from empyema, which is a collection of pus within the pleural space rather than the lung parenchyma. Many different microorganisms may produce lung abscess, and a number of conditions may simulate it radiographically (Table 83–1). Lung abscess formation usually reflects infection with an unusual microbial burden (e.g., acute aspiration), an especially virulent organism (e.g., *Staphylococcus aureus*), and/or a failure in microbial clearance mechanisms (e.g., bronchial obstruction).

ETIOLOGY

Conditions that predispose to lung abcesses include any cause of aspiration or reduced ciliary action, such as reduced levels of consciousness, alcoholism, seizure disorders, general anesthesia, cerebrovascular accidents, drug addiction, dysphagia, esophageal reflux, and mechanical interference with the cardiac sphincter such as caused by nasogastric tubes and endotracheal intubation. Periodontal disease, gingivitis, sinus infection, and bronchiectasis provide a source for anaerobic infection and are other important background factors. Another cause of lung abscess is septic pulmonary embolism, most commonly with *S. aureus* and most commonly in intra-

Table 83–1 ■ ORGANISMS AND CONDITIONS WITH THE RADIOGRAPHIC APPEARANCE OF LUNG ABSCESS

Infectious
Bacterial aspiration/pneumonia
  Anaerobes: pigmented and non-pigmented *Prevotella*, *Fusobacterium*, *Peptostreptococcus*, *Bacteroides fragilis*, and *Clostridium perfringens*
  Aerobes: streptococci, *Staphylococcus aureus*, Enterobacteriaceae, *Pseudomonas aeruginosa*, *Klebsiella pneumoniae*, *Legionella* spp., *Nocardia asteroides*, *Haemophilus influenzae*, *Eikenella corrodens*, *Salmonella* spp., *Burkholderia pseudomallei*, *B. mallei*, *Rhodococcus equi*
Bacterial embolic
  S. aureus, *P. aeruginosa*
Mycobacteria (often multifocal)
  M. tuberculosis, *M. avium* complex, *M. kansasii*, other mycobacteria
Fungi
  Aspergillus spp., Mucoraceae, *Histoplasma capsulatum*, *Pneumocystis carinii*, *Coccidioides immitis*, *Blastomyces dermatitidis*, *Cryptococcus neoformans*
Parasites
  Entamoeba histolytica, *Paragonimus westermani*, *Stronglyoides stercoralis* (post-obstructive)
Empyema (with air-fluid level)
Septic embolism (endocarditis)
Predisposing Conditions
Fluid-filled cysts or bullae
Infarction without infection
  Pulmonary embolism
  Vasculitis
    Goodpasture's syndrome
    Wegener's granulomatosis
    Polyarteritis nodosa
Bronchiectasis
Post-obstructive pneumonia (neoplasm, foreign body)
Pulmonary sequestration
Pulmonary contusion
Neoplasm

venous drug users. Unlike lung abscesses related to aspiration, which are usually solitary, the lung abscesses seen with septic pulmonary emboli are commonly multiple or are associated with other septic embolic lesions in various stages of development. Any necrotizing pneumonia can also present with areas of abscess, which are commonly small and multiple and less likely to be defined clearly as abscesses by chest radiograph than by pathologic specimen. When bronchial obstruction develops distal to a pulmonary neoplasm, drainage is difficult and abscess formation is common. For all causes of abscess, however, diabetes, malignancy, and other immunocompromising conditions are common predisposing factors.

Ninety per cent of cases involve anaerobic bacteria; half include aerobes as well. The principal anaerobes are pigmented and nonpigmented *Prevotella*, *Fusobacterium*, and *Peptostreptococcus*. *Bacteroides fragilis* group strains are found in 7% of cases. Among the aerobes, streptococci, staphylococci, and gram-negative bacilli are prominent.

INCIDENCE AND PREVALENCE

The incidence of lung abscess has decreased since the advent of antimicrobial therapy, but larger hospitals see 10 to 25 cases per year.

EPIDEMIOLOGY

Most lung abscesses involve the indigenous flora of the oropharynx. Abscesses involving *S. aureus* or gram-negative bacilli are most often nosocomial. *Nocardia* and *Rhodococcus* are found almost exclusively in immunocompromised hosts. Septic pulmonary emboli are usually due to *S. aureus*, primarily in intravenous drug abusers with tricuspid valve endocarditis. Lung abscesses due to *Paragonimus westermani* and melioidosis are usually acquired in the Far East or Indonesia.

PATHOGENESIS

Small numbers of oropharyngeal bacteria are commonly aspirated during sleep but are readily cleared by host defense mechanisms. Defense mechanisms are not as efficient in handling larger numbers of aspirated bacteria.

Counts of anaerobes in oral flora are lower than usual in edentulous subjects and higher in patients with periodontal disease. Alcoholics and patients who are acutely or chronically ill (especially if hospitalized) often demonstrate oropharyngeal colonization with aerobic or facultative gram-negative bacilli and *S. aureus.* Among the anaerobes, organisms more likely to cause infection as sole agents are *Fusobacterium nucleatum, F. necrophorum, B. fragilis,* and *Clostridium perfringens.* Both the size of the bacterial inoculum and the role of associated organisms and host defenses are important. Organisms such as *S. aureus* and *K. pneumoniae,* which produce extracellular toxins or enzymes, often produce abscesses.

The various types of aspiration-related pleuropulmonary infections—pneumonitis (the initial stage), necrotizing pneumonia (multiple excavations < 2 cm in diameter), lung abscess (one or more cavities ≥ 2 cm in diameter communicating with a bronchus), and empyema—should be considered as one process with a continuum of changes. A predilection for infection in dependent segments is seen, particularly the posterior segments of the upper lobes and the superior segments of the lower lobes, but the location of the abscess depends on gravity and the position of the subject (Fig. 83–1). Normally, the aspirated material is handled effectively by ciliary action, cough, and alveolar macrophages. Endotracheal tubes impair coughing, impede pulmonary clearance mechanisms, and allow leakage of oropharyngeal secretions into the tracheobronchial tree. Thick or particulate matter and foreign bodies are not easily removed and can produce bronchial obstruction and atelectasis. In pneumonia following aspiration of gastric contents, gastric acid and enzymes are the primary offending agents. Subdiaphragmatic infection may extend to the lung by way of lymphatic vessels, directly through the diaphragm, or by way of the blood stream.

CLINICAL MANIFESTATIONS

A relatively insidious onset of infection is seen in many patients; additional clues are involvement of dependent segments of lung, predisposition to aspiration, and, often, periodontal disease. After 1 to 2 weeks, tissue necrosis, with abscess formation or empyema, occurs. Following cavitation, putrid sputum is noted in 50% or more of patients, and hemoptysis may be seen. Weeks to months of malaise and low-grade fever may be associated with cough, weight loss, and anemia. Neoplasia is a serious diagnostic consideration in such patients. On occasion, the picture is acute, with fever, malaise, cough, and, pleurisy. Patients with lung abscess due to *S. aureus* or gram-negative bacilli and those with secondary lung abscess due to septic pulmonary emboli may have a more fulminant course. In

edentulous persons with intact oropharyngeal function, lung abscesses are uncommon and suggest the presence of an obstructing lesion of the bronchus (carcinoma or other) or pulmonary embolus.

DIAGNOSIS

The classic radiographic appearance of lung abscess is a cavity with an air-fluid level, with or without surrounding infiltrate; in some patients, however, repeat chest radiographs or computed tomographic (CT) scanning may be needed to detect the cavity. A similar radiographic appearance can be seen with a variety of conditions other than bacterial lung abscess (see Table 83–1), so definitive bacterial confirmation is required. Radiography occasionally reveals mediastinal lymphadenopathy, making the differential diagnosis include tuberculosis, fungal infection, and lung cancer. Infected cysts or bullae and pulmonary sequestration are often evident with radiography. CT can readily distinguish between lung abscess and an air-fluid level in an empyema cavity.

The spectrum of organisms causing lung abscess has widened as patients present with more complex medical and surgical conditions. Antibiotic resistance has emerged and the number of immunocompromised persons has increased. Thus, microbiologic studies are increasingly desirable to guide therapy. Expectorated sputum cannot be used for anaerobic culture because large numbers of anaerobes are present in the indigenous flora. Even for infection with *S. aureus* and gram-negative bacilli, use of expectorated sputum is a problem because of frequent oropharyngeal colonization with such organisms in institutionalized patients. Bacteremia is uncommon in aspiration pneumonia, and all organisms involved in the lung abscess may not be recovered in blood cultures. Empyema fluid constitutes an excellent source for anaerobic (and aerobic) culture. Transtracheal aspiration bypasses the normal flora of the upper respiratory tract, but contamination with indigenous flora can be a problem, and the procedure is now seldom performed. Two approaches that are preferable to transtracheal aspiration are the use of a protected specimen brush and the use of bronchoalveolar lavage. The protected specimen brush procedure involves sampling with a bronchial brush protected within a telescoping plugged double-catheter via a fiberoptic bronchoscope. It is essential that the technique be used exactly as described and that cultures be done quantitatively. For the protected specimen brush procedure, 10^3 to 10^4 or more colony-forming units per milliliter is significant. The small volume of material obtained and the difficulty in anaerobic transport are concerns. Quantitative culture of fluid obtained by bronchoalveolar lavage, during or without bronchoscopy, also provides reliable results. Counts of 10^4 or more organisms per milliliter are considered significant. Demonstration of bacteria intracellularly in at least 3 to 5% of cells in bronchoalveolar lavage fluid is good evidence of pneumonia, and the morphology of those bacteria is extremely useful in directing therapy. Specimens must be placed under anaerobic conditions immediately after being obtained. Bronchoscopy also is often important to exclude cavitating or obstructing malignancy or presence of a foreign body.

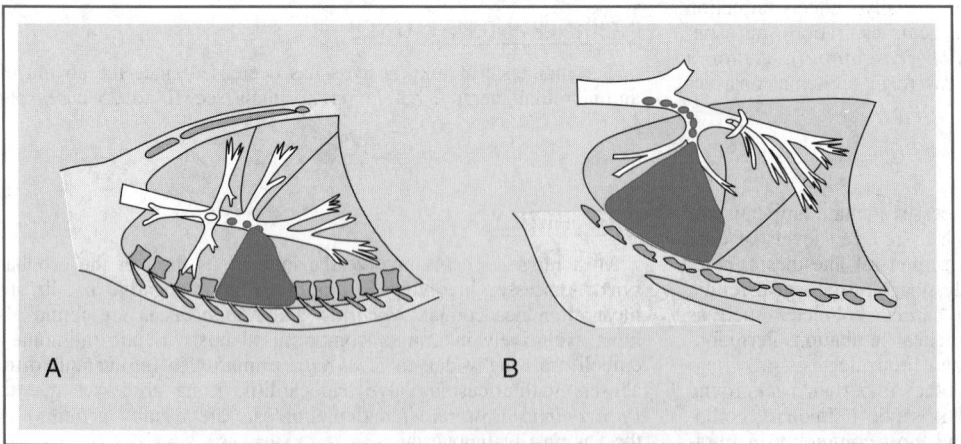

FIGURE 83–1 ■ Relationship between posture and location of lung abscess. With patient lying on back (*A*), aspiration occurs into the superior segment of the lower lobe. With patient lying on side (*B*), aspiration occurs into the posterior segment of the lower lobe. (From Brock RC: Lung Abscess. Oxford, Blackwell, 1952.)

TREATMENT

Antimicrobial therapy and drainage are the keystones of treatment; identification and treatment of underlying or primary processes is also important. Prolonged therapy is important to prevent relapse; the actual duration of treatment must be individualized, but periods of 1 to 3 months or more may be required. The approach to a specific patient is based on the clinical status of the patient as well as the microbiologic features of the infection. The initial choice of antimicrobial agents is empiric but should be guided by the Gram stain and the likely bacteriologic source of the infection, and then it should be adjusted as culture and susceptibility data become available. A small to moderate-sized abscess in an otherwise healthy person may respond to conservative management with antimicrobial therapy and postural drainage. A rapidly expanding pulmonary abscess in an immunocompromised host (e.g., due to one of the Mucoraceae) requires urgent lung resection in addition to antimicrobial therapy. Secondary lung abscesses may require more intensive antimicrobial therapy.

Therapy for infections due to aerobic bacteria (see Chapter 82), mycobacteria (see Chapter 358), fungi (see Chapter 343), and parasites (see Chapter 420) is based on their sensitivities to specific agents. Anaerobic agents, which include *Prevotella* and *Bacteroides* species, fusobacteria, anaerobic cocci, clostridia, and *B. fragilis,* and which predominate in bacterial lung abcesses, produce β-lactamases and demonstrate resistance to penicillin G in up to 40% of cases. Clindamycin, given initially at a dose of 600 mg every 6 hours intravenously, then when the patient is afebrile and improved, 300 mg orally every 6 hours, is more effective than penicillin. When penicillin is used, it should be used in high dosage (12 million units/day intravenously in average-sized adults with normal renal function) and in combination with clindamycin or metronidazole (2 g/day intravenously in four divided doses). Metronidazole alone may be ineffective because of resistance of aerobic bacteria, *Actinomyces,* and some anaerobic streptococci. After improvement, one option is to give ampicillin or amoxicillin plus metronidazole orally, each in a dose of 500 mg every 6 to 8 hours. Imipenem or meropenem and β-lactam/β-lactamase inhibitor combinations such as ticarcillin and clavulanic acid are active against essentially all anaerobes and many of the aerobes important in nosocomial aspiration pneumonia. If a specific anaerobe or set of anaerobes is identified in the lung abscess, antibiotic therapy can be targeted on the basis of general sensitivity characterisitics (Table 83–2) while awaiting local sensitivity testing results.

Postural drainage is important in therapy of lung abscess. Bronchoscopy may help in effecting good drainage, removal of foreign bodies, and diagnosis of tumor. Experience dictates caution with the bronchoscopic drainage of closed cavities; spillage of cavity contents into other lung segments may occur and be catastrophic.

Persistence of bacteremia or high-grade fever after 72 hours, or the absence of change in sputum production or character or in radiographic images during a period of 7 to 10 days, suggests undiagnosed obstruction, empyema, or resistant organisms. Progression of pulmonary infiltrates may occur after the initiation of appropriate therapy, reflecting poorly ventilated and underperfused infected lung tissue. Surgical resection of necrotic lung may occasionally be needed if the response to antibiotics is poor or if airway obstruction limits drainage. In patients who are poor surgical risks, percutaneous drainage via catheters may be useful.

PROGNOSIS

At present the mortality rate is 5 to 10%. Patients with large abscesses (>6 cm), progressive pulmonary necrosis, obstructing lesions, aerobic bacterial infection, immune compromise, old age, and systemic debility, and those in whom major delays have occurred in seeking medical attention have a higher mortality and a higher incidence of complications. The most common complication is empyema, with or without bronchopleural fistula. Spillover of pus from a large lung abscess sometimes leads to spread of infection and even to asphyxiation. Other complications, which are now rare, include brain or other distal abscesses, generalized infection, severe hemorrhage, and pulmonary gangrene. Superinfection by other bacteria or by fungi can occur in relation to antimicrobial therapy. In chronic lung abscess, chronic bronchitis, localized emphysema, or bronchiectasis may be present, with subsequent recurrences of acute pneumonitis in the involved area.

PREVENTION

Precautions should be taken to minimize aspiration, particularly in feeding feeble or confused patients and patients with swallowing difficulties. In the case of gross aspiration, immediate clearing of the airway by postural drainage and suctioning, preferably by bronchoscopy, is important. Proper treatment of periodontal disease and gingivitis and early treatment of pneumonia minimize the risk of bacterial lung abscess.

Bartlett JG: Anaerobic bacterial infections of the lung and pleural space. Clin Infect Dis 16 (suppl 4):S248, 1993. *An excellent review of the author's extensive experience with 193 carefully studied cases of anaerobic pleuropulmonary infection, including 83 cases of lung abscess.*
Civen R, Jousimies-Somer H, Marina M, et al: A retrospective review of cases of anaerobic empyema and update of bacteriology. Clin Infect Dis 20 (suppl 2):S224, 1995. *The most thorough and up-to-date bacteriologic study of anaerobic pleuropulmonary infection, based on 46 cases of empyema (9 with lung abscess).*
Hoffer FA, Bloom DA, Colin AA, Fishman SJ: Lung abscess versus necrotizing pneumonia: Implications for interventional therapy. Pediatr Radiol 29:87, 1999. *In children, percutaneous aspiration of lung abscess contents was well tolerated and yielded positive Gram stains and cultures in virtually all cases; in contrast, percutaneous aspiration led to a significant incidence of pneumatoceles and bronchopleural fistulae in patients with necrotizing pneumonia and was not very useful diagnostically.*
Rubin SA, Winer-Muram HT, Ellis JV: Diagnostic imaging of pneumonia and its complications in the critically ill patient. Clin Chest Med 16:45, 1995. *Includes good discussion of radiographic and CT scan findings in lung abscess, empyema, and aspiration pneumonia.*

Table 83–2 ■ DRUGS OF CHOICE FOR ANAEROBES INVOLVED IN LUNG ABSCESS*

Principal Pathogens
Prevotella: Metronidazole, clindamycin, β-lactam/β-lactamase inhibitor combinations, carbapenems
Fusobacterium: As for *Prevotella*
Peptostreptococcus: β-Lactam/β-lactamase inhibitor combinations, carbapenems, penicillin (high dosage)
Streptococcus (anaerobic, microaerophilic strains): penicillin (high dosage), β-lactam/β-lactamase inhibitor combinations, carbapenems
Less Common Pathogens
Bacteroides: Metronidazole, β-lactam/β-lactamase inhibitor combinations, carbapenems
Clostridium: Metronidazole, β-lactam/β-lactamase inhibitor combinations, carbapenems, penicillin
Actinomyces: Penicillin (high dosage), clindamycin
Eikenella corrodens (microaerophilic): Penicillin, β-lactam/β-lactamase inhibitor combinations, carbapenems
Unknown Bacteriology
Metronidazole plus penicillin, β-lactam/β-lactamase inhibitor combinations, carbapenems

*Drugs listed for each group of organisms are roughly comparable in activity and are the drugs that are most active. Other drugs (for example, cefoxitin or clindamycin, alone or with penicillin) may be useful in patients with abscess of unknown bacteriologic origin who are only mildly to moderately ill.

84 | PULMONARY EMBOLISM

Victor F. Tapson

DEFINITIONS

Pulmonary embolism refers to exogenous or endogenous material that travels to the lungs and causes a potential spectrum of consequences, including dyspnea, chest pain, hypoxemia, and sometimes death. Although thrombus from the deep veins of the lower extremities is the most common material to embolize to the lungs, other substances such as neoplastic cells, air bubbles, carbon dioxide, intravenous catheters, fat droplets, and even talc in intravenous drug abusers are potential sources of emboli. Deep venous thrombosis (see Chapter 69) and pulmonary embolism represent a continuum of one disease entity (venous thromboembolism).

INCIDENCE

Both deep venous thrombosis and pulmonary embolism, which in this chapter will refer to thromboemboli arising from the deep leg veins, frequently are clinically unsuspected, leading to significant diagnostic and therapeutic delays and accounting for substantial morbidity and mortality. Although thromboembolism is diagnosed and treated in as many as 260,000 patients annually in the United States, more than half of the cases that actually occur are not diagnosed antemortem. In addition, effective prophylaxis remains dramatically underutilized. Many patients who die from acute pulmonary embolism have coexisting terminal illnesses, but this disease entity is nevertheless responsible each year for the preventable deaths of 50,000 to 100,000 patients with an otherwise good prognosis.

PATHOPHYSIOLOGY

One or more components of Virchow's triad (stasis, hypercoagulability, and intimal injury) is present in nearly all patients who develop deep venous thrombosis (see Chapter 69) and subsequent pulmonary embolism. The incidence of venous thromboembolism is especially high in hospitalized patients, particularly in the postoperative setting, and the risk appears to increase with age. More than 95% of pulmonary emboli arise from the proximal deep veins in the lower extremities (including and above the popliteal veins), but calf vein thrombi can sometimes embolize to the lung. Emboli may emanate from axillary-subclavian vein thrombosis in patients with central (subclavian) vein catheters, particularly those with malignancies, and in patients with effort-induced upper extremity thrombosis (Paget-Schroetter syndrome).

Gas Exchange and Hemodynamic Alterations

Hypoxemia occurs in the majority of patients with acute pulmonary embolism. The resulting tachypnea acutely increases minute ventilation. The predominant factor explaining hypoxemia in acute pulmonary embolism is the mismatch between pulmonary blood flow and regional alveolar ventilation: the obstruction of blood flow creates regions with maintained or increased ventilation and high ventilation-perfusion ratios as well as regions through which poorly oxygenated blood is shunted due to maintained perfusion of atelectatic lung tissue. In addition, the release of vasoactive substances such as serotonin from platelets appears to contribute to the elevation of pulmonary vascular resistance. The finding that heparin blocks an increase in airway resistance and a decrease in lung compliance after pulmonary embolism suggests that bronchoconstriction due to mediators from thrombi may also contribute to ventilation-perfusion mismatching.

When emboli obstruct a substantial portion of the pulmonary arterial bed, profound hemodynamic alterations occur. The impact of the embolic event depends on the extent of reduction of the cross-sectional area of the pulmonary vasculature as well as on the presence or absence of underlying cardiopulmonary disease. Submassive emboli in normal individuals may augment cardiac output: hypoxemia stimulates an increase in sympathetic tone with systemic vasoconstriction, augmentation of venous return, and an increase in stroke volume. With massive emboli, cardiac output is initially diminished, but then it may be sustained as the mean right atrial pressure increases. The ensuing increase in pulmonary vascular resistance impedes right ventricular outflow and reduces left ventricular preload. In the absence of underlying cardiopulmonary disease, occlusion of 25 to 30% of the pulmonary vascular bed by emboli is associated with a significant rise in pulmonary artery pressure. With increasing pulmonary vascular obstruction, hypoxemia worsens, stimulating vasoconstriction and a further rise in pulmonary artery pressure. More than 50% obstruction of the pulmonary arterial bed is usually required before substantial elevation of the mean pulmonary artery pressure is seen. When the extent of obstruction of the pulmonary circulation approaches 75%, the right

ventricle usually must generate a systolic pressure in excess of 50 mm Hg and a mean pulmonary artery pressure of greater than 40 mm Hg to preserve pulmonary perfusion. The normal right ventricle is unable to achieve such pressures acutely, and right ventricular failure develops. In patients with underlying cardiopulmonary disease, the deterioration in cardiac output is even more substantial. A depressed cardiac output *without* elevation of the right atrial pressure suggests cardiac dysfunction superimposed on pulmonary embolism. Although supportive measures may sustain a patient with massive embolism, any additional increment in embolic burden may be fatal.

PATHOLOGY

The pathologic findings of pulmonary embolism vary depending on the age and extent of the emboli. Both lungs are affected in the majority of cases, and the lower lobes are involved more often than the upper lobes. An embolus generally has blunt, non-tapering ends and may be folded over on itself. When unfolded, emboli may be "Y" shaped from branch points of the veins from which they formed, and they may contain imprints of venous valve cusps. In cases of massive embolism with rapid deterioration and death, the autopsy may reveal large emboli obstructing the main pulmonary artery or the pulmonary artery bifurcation. Smaller, more peripheral emboli of differing ages and various stages of organization usually indicate prior pulmonary emboli.

The dual pulmonary circulation, which includes both the pulmonary and bronchial arteries, prevents most emboli from causing pulmonary infarction. However, pulmonary infarction, characterized histologically by intra-alveolar hemorrhage and necrosis of alveolar walls, may be evident in areas of the peripheral lung supplied by smaller vessels and is more common in patients with pre-existing heart failure. Because patients dying from acute pulmonary embolism die with right ventricular failure, a dilated right ventricle is commonly found at autopsy.

CLINICAL MANIFESTATIONS

The history and physical examination are notoriously insensitive and nonspecific for both deep venous thrombosis (see Chapter 69) and pulmonary embolism. The most common symptom of acute pulmonary embolism is dyspnea, which is often sudden in onset (Table 84–1). Pleuritic chest pain and hemoptysis occur more commonly with pulmonary *infarction* due to smaller, peripheral emboli. Palpitations, cough, anxiety, and lightheadedness are all symptoms of acute pulmonary embolism, but they may also result from a number of other entities. Syncope and/or sudden death may occur with massive pulmonary embolism. Pulmonary embolism should always be considered whenever unexplained dyspnea, syncope, or hypotension is present.

Table 84–1 ■ SYMPTOMS AND SIGNS IN 117 PATIENTS WITH ACUTE PULMONARY EMBOLISM WITHOUT PRE-EXISTING CARDIAC OR PULMONARY DISEASE

SYMPTOMS	% OF PATIENTS	SIGNS	% OF PATIENTS
Dyspnea	73	Tachypnea (≥20/min)	70
Pleuritic pain	66	Rales (crackles)	51
Cough	37	Tachycardia (>100/min)	30
Leg swelling	28	Fourth heart sound	24
Leg pain	26	Increased pulmonary component of second sound	23
Hemoptysis	13		
Palpitations	10	Deep venous thrombosis	11
Wheezing	9	Diaphoresis	11
Angina-like pain	4	Temperature >38.5°C	7
		Wheezes	5
		Homans' sign	4
		Right ventricular lift	4
		Pleural friction rub	3
		Third heart sound	3
		Cyanosis	1

Adapted from Stein PD, Terrin ML, Hales CA, et al: Clinical, laboratory, roentgenographic and electrocardiographic findings in patients with acute pulmonary embolism and no pre-existing cardiac or pulmonary disease. Chest 100:598, 1991.

Table 84–2 ■ DIFFERENTIAL DIAGNOSIS OF ACUTE PULMONARY EMBOLISM

Myocardial infarction
Pericarditis
Congestive heart failure
Pneumonia
Asthma
Chronic obstructive pulmonary disease
Pneumothorax
Pleurodynia
Pleuritis from collagen vascular disease
Thoracic herpes zoster ("shingles")
Rib fracture
Musculoskeletal pain
Primary or metastatic intrathoracic cancer
Infradiaphragmatic processes (e.g., acute cholecystitis, splenic infarction)
Hyperventilation syndrome

Tachypnea and tachycardia are the most common signs of pulmonary embolism, but they are also nonspecific. Other physical findings that may occur include fever, wheezing, rales, a pleural rub, and cardiac findings such as a loud pulmonic component of the second heart sound, a right-sided fourth heart sound, and a right ventricular lift.

The diagnosis of pulmonary embolism may not be suspected clinically because dyspnea, tachypnea, and hypoxemia occurring in patients with concomitant cardiopulmonary disease, such as heart failure, pneumonia or chronic obstructive pulmonary disease, may be blamed on the underlying disease, when in reality they are the result of acute pulmonary embolism. Pulmonary embolism must always be seriously considered in the patient with any symptoms or signs consistent with the diagnosis, particularly in the setting of significant risk factors for venous thromboembolism such as concomitant heart failure, malignancy, coagulation disorders, immobility, or the postoperative state.

DIAGNOSIS

The differential diagnosis for acute pulmonary embolism depends on the clinical presentation and the presence of concomitant disease. When patients present with dyspnea and/or chest pain, the differential diagnosis includes pneumonia, a flare of asthma or chronic obstructive lung disease, anxiety with hyperventilation, pneumothorax, heart failure, angina or myocardial infarction, musculoskeletal pain, pericarditis, pleuritis from collagen vascular disease, herpes zoster, rib fracture, intrathoracic cancer, and, occasionally, intra-abdominal processes such as acute cholecystitis (Table 84–2). Assessment of risk factors together with the history and physical examination can help place patients into groups according to probability of pulmonary embolism and help guide further diagnostic testing (Fig 84–1).

Laboratory Testing

Hypoxemia is common in acute pulmonary embolism. Some individuals, particularly young patients without underlying lung disease, may have a normal arterial oxygen tension (PaO_2) and, even rarely, a normal alveolar-arterial difference. A sudden decrease in the PaO_2 or in the oxygen saturation in a patient unable to communicate an accurate history (e.g., a mechanically ventilated patient) may be evidence of acute pulmonary embolism.

The diagnostic utility of plasma measurements of circulating D-dimer (a specific derivative of cross-linked fibrin) in patients with pulmonary embolism has been extensively evaluated. A normal enzyme-linked immunosorbent assay (ELISA) appears sensitive in excluding pulmonary embolism. When the D-dimer level is 500 μg/L or greater, the sensitivity for pulmonary embolism may be as high as 96 to 98%, but the specificity is much lower. The sensitivity of the plasma D-dimer appears to remain high up to 1 week after presentation. Thus, increased levels of cross-linked fibrin

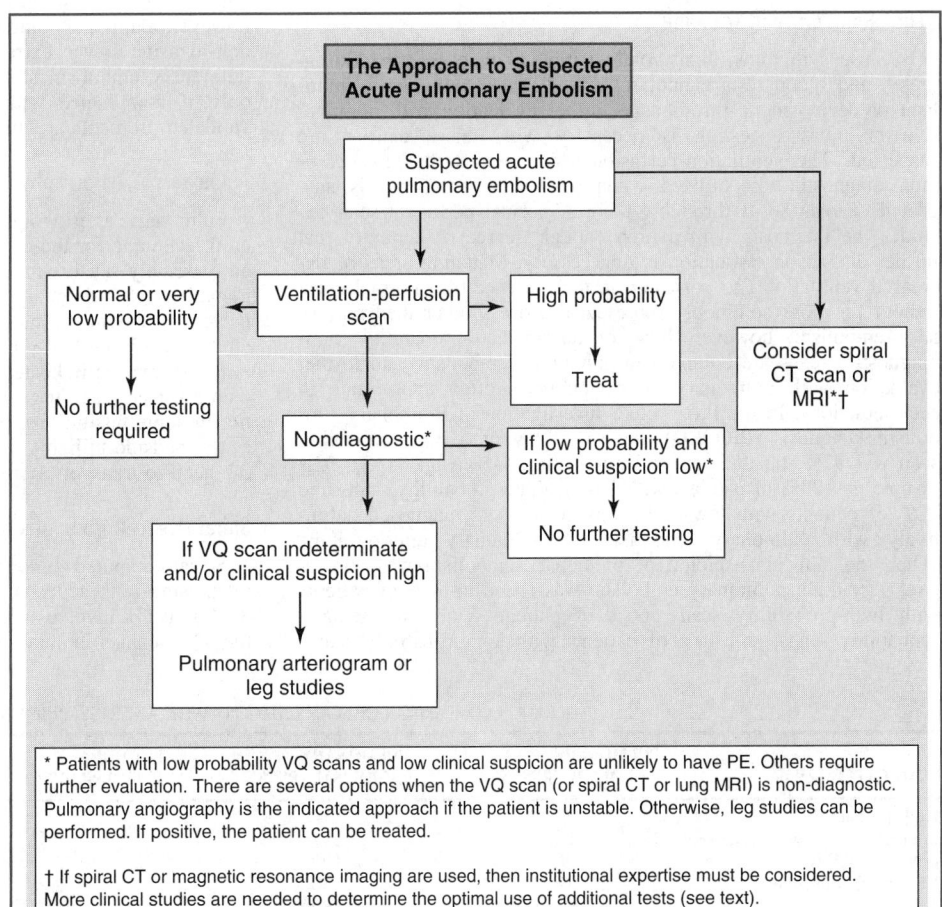

FIGURE 84–1 ■ An algorithm for the diagnostic approach to suspected acute pulmonary embolism. CT = computed tomography; MRI = magnetic resonance imaging; VQ = ventilation perfusion; PE = pulmonary embolism.

The Approach to Suspected Acute Pulmonary Embolism

Suspected acute pulmonary embolism

Ventilation-perfusion scan

Normal or very low probability → No further testing required

High probability → Treat

Consider spiral CT scan or MRI*†

Nondiagnostic* → If low probability and clinical suspicion low* → No further testing

If VQ scan indeterminate and/or clinical suspicion high → Pulmonary arteriogram or leg studies

* Patients with low probability VQ scans and low clinical suspicion are unlikely to have PE. Others require further evaluation. There are several options when the VQ scan (or spiral CT or lung MRI) is non-diagnostic. Pulmonary angiography is the indicated approach if the patient is unstable. Otherwise, leg studies can be performed. If positive, the patient can be treated.

† If spiral CT or magnetic resonance imaging are used, then institutional expertise must be considered. More clinical studies are needed to determine the optimal use of additional tests (see text).

degradation products are an indirect but non-specific marker of intravascular thrombosis in addition to being indicative of fibrinolysis. As this diagnostic test becomes more readily available, it may prove increasingly useful in excluding acute pulmonary embolism, particularly when other diagnostic tests support its absence.

Electrocardiography

In acute pulmonary embolism, electrocardiographic (ECG) findings are present in the majority of patients and include T-wave changes, ST-segment abnormalities, and left- or right-axis deviation. Only one third of patients with massive or submassive emboli have manifestations of acute cor pulmonale, such as the $S_1Q_3T_3$ pattern, right bundle branch block, P-wave pulmonale, or right-axis deviation. Unfortunately, all of these findings are nonspecific as well as insensitive. ECG is more useful in excluding alternative diagnoses, such as myocardial infarction, rather than in establishing or excluding pulmonary embolism.

Chest Radiography

The chest radiograph is often abnormal in patients with acute pulmonary embolism, but it is nearly always nonspecific. Common radiographic findings include pleural effusion, atelectasis, pulmonary infiltrates, and mild elevation of a hemidiaphragm. Classic findings of pulmonary infarction, such as Hampton's hump or decreased vascularity (Westermark's sign), are suggestive of the diagnosis, but are seen infrequently. A normal chest radiograph in the setting of severe dyspnea and hypoxemia without evidence of bronchospasm or anatomic cardiac shunt is strongly suggestive of pulmonary embolism. Although exclusion of other processes such as pneumonia, pneumothorax, or rib fracture is possible, pulmonary embolism may frequently coexist with other underlying lung diseases. As a result, under most circumstances the chest radiograph cannot be used conclusively to diagnose or exclude pulmonary embolism.

Ventilation-Perfusion Scanning

Because symptoms, signs, radiographic findings, electrocardiography, and blood tests cannot reliably diagnose pulmonary embolism or deep venous thrombosis, further evaluation with noninvasive or invasive testing is necessary when these entities are suspected. The ventilation-perfusion scan remains the most common diagnostic test utilized when pulmonary embolism is suspected (Tables 84–3 through 84–5). A normal perfusion scan excludes the diagnosis with a high enough degree of certainty that further diagnostic evaluation is unnecessary. Matching areas of decreased ventilation and perfusion in the presence of a normal chest radiograph more commonly represent a process other than pulmonary embolism; however, low- or intermediate-probability (nondiagnostic) scans are common in pulmonary embolism, and further evaluation with pulmonary arteriography is often appropriate in such situations. In the Prospective Investigation of Pulmonary Embolism Diagnosis (PIOPED), the specificity of a high-probability scan was 97%, but the sensitivity was only 41% (Fig. 84–2). It is of note that 33% of patients with intermediate-probability scans and 12% of patients with low-probability scans were diagnosed definitively with pulmonary embolism by pulmonary arteriography. When the clinical suspicion of pulmonary embolism was considered very high, pulmonary embolism was found in 96% of patients with high-probability scans, 66% of patients with intermediate-probability scans, and 40% of patients with low-probability scans.

Table 84–3 ■ INTERPRETATION OF VENTILATION-PERFUSION (V̇/Q) LUNG SCANS

CATEGORY	PATTERN
Normal	No perfusion defects
Low probability	Small V̇/Q mismatches
	V̇/Q matches without corresponding roentgenographic changes
	Perfusion defect substantially smaller than roentgenographic density
Intermediate probability	Marked, diffuse obstructive pulmonary disease with perfusion defects
	Perfusion defect of same size as roentgenographic change
	Single segmental mismatch*
High probability	Two or more segmental mismatches*
	Perfusion defect substantially larger than roentgenographic density

*Controversy exists regarding the importance of a single segmental mismatch, which has been considered either of high or intermediate probability. The more conservative interpretation, that is, intermediate probability, has been used in this table.

Adapted from Biello DR: Radiological (scintigraphic) evaluation of patients with suspected pulmonary thromboembolism. JAMA 257:3257, 1987.

Thus, the diagnosis of pulmonary embolism should be rigorously pursued, even when the lung scan indicates a low or intermediate probability, if the clinical setting suggests the diagnosis. Even when the ventilation-perfusion scan is non-diagnostic, it may serve as a guide for selective pulmonary arteriography and thus minimize the contrast dye load and reduce the likelihood of complications from the procedure.

Stable patients with suspected acute pulmonary embolism, nondiagnostic lung scans, and adequate cardiopulmonary reserve (absence of hypotension or severe hypoxemia) may undergo noninvasive lower extremity testing in an attempt to diagnose deep venous thrombosis and hence avoid pulmonary arteriography. For example, positive compression ultrasound or impedance plethysmography (see Chapter 69) in this setting is adequate to require treatment without further testing. If the lower extremity test is negative, however, pulmonary angiography is an appropriate option. *Serial non-invasive lower extremity testing in the setting of suspected pulmonary embolism should be performed instead of angiography only if compliance with follow-up is absolutely certain and if validated protocols are utilized.*

Pulmonary Arteriography

Pulmonary arteriography has remained the accepted gold standard technique for the diagnosis of acute pulmonary embolism. It is an extremely sensitive and specific test and is relatively safe. Complications of pulmonary arteriography among 1111 patients suspected of having pulmonary embolism in the PIOPED study included death in 0.5% and major nonfatal complications in 1%. Arteriography is indicated when the diagnosis of pulmonary embolism must be made urgently and prior tests have been non-diagnostic. In some institutions, pulmonary arteriography can be performed at the bedside utilizing a pulmonary artery catheter so as to avoid the need to transport a critically ill patient.

Spiral (Helical) Computed Tomography

Spiral computed tomographic (CT) scanning is another option for diagnosing both acute and chronic pulmonary embolism (Fig. 84–3). Spiral CT involves continuous movement of the patient through the CT scanner and allows concurrent scanning by a constantly

Table 84–4 ■ COMPARISON OF SCAN CATEGORY WITH ANGIOGRAPHIC FINDINGS

SCAN CATEGORY	PULMONARY EMBOLISM PRESENT	PULMONARY EMBOLISM ABSENT	PULMONARY EMBOLISM UNCERTAIN	NO ANGIOGRAM	TOTAL NO.
High probability	102	14	1	7	124
Intermediate probability	105	217	9	33	364
Low probability	39	199	12	62	312
Near-normal/normal	5	50	2	74	131
Total	251	480	24	176	931

From PIOPED Investigators: Value of the ventilation/perfusion scan in acute pulmonary embolism: Results of the Prospective Investigation of Pulmonary Embolism Diagnosis (PIOPED). JAMA 263:2753–2759, 1990.

Table 84–5 ▪ PIOPED: POSITIVE PREDICTIVE VALUE OF PE AT ANGIOGRAPHY BASED ON LUNG SCAN CATEGORY AND CLINICAL LIKELIHOOD OF PE

LUNG SCAN CATEGORY	CLINICAL PROBABILITY			
	80–100% No. of PE/No. of Pts. (%)	20–79% No. of PE/No. of Pts. (%)	0–19% No. of PE/No. of Pts. (%)	0–100% No. of PE/No. of Pts. (%)
High	28/29 (96)	70/80 (88)	5/9 (56)	103/118 (87)
Intermediate	27/41 (66)	66/236 (28)	11/68 (16)	104/345 (30)
Low	6/16 (40)	30/191 (16)	4/90 (4)	40/296 (14)
Very low	0/5 (0)	4/62 (6)	1/61 (2)	5/128 (4)
Total	61/90 (68)	170/569 (30)	21/228 (9)	252/887 (28)

PIOPED = Prospective Investigation of Pulmonary Embolism Diagnosis; PE = pulmonary emboli; Pts. = patients.
Adapted from PIOPED Investigators: Value of the ventilation/perfusion scan in acute pulmonary embolism. Results of the Prospective Investigation of Pulmonary Embolism Diagnosis (PIOPED). JAMA 263:2757, 1990.

rotating gantry and detector system. This technique enables rapid scanning with continuous volume acquisitions obtained during a single breath. Retrospective reconstructions can be performed. A contrast bolus is required for imaging of the pulmonary vasculature. The several apparent limitations of spiral CT scanning for acute pulmonary embolism include poor visualization of the peripheral areas of the upper and lower lobes and difficulty imaging horizontally oriented vessels in the right middle lobe and lingula. Lymph nodes may result in false-positive findings, but multiplanar reconstructions in coronal or oblique planes may aid in differentiating lymph nodes from emboli.

In at least one clinical trial, spiral CT has been associated with greater than 95% sensitivity and specificity. Spiral CT has the greatest sensitivity for emboli in the main, lobar, or segmental pulmonary arteries. For subsegmental emboli, spiral CT appears less accurate, although the importance of emboli of this size have been questioned. The use of thinner sections as well as techniques such as multiplanar two-dimensional reformation may enhance the usefulness of spiral CT for diagnosing pulmonary emboli. An advantage of spiral CT over ventilation-perfusion scanning and arteriography includes the ability to define nonvascular structures and to establish alternative diagnoses such as lung tumors, emphysema, and other parenchymal abnormalities as well as pleural and pericardial disease. A second advantage of spiral CT over other diagnostic methods is the rapidity (10 to 15 minutes) with which a study can be performed. Contrast-enhanced electron-beam CT also appears useful in diagnosing acute pulmonary embolism and shares many advantages and limitations with spiral CT.

Magnetic Resonance Imaging

Magnetic resonance imaging (MRI) has several attractive advantages, including excellent sensitivity and specificity for the diagnosis of deep venous thrombosis together with the potential for performing lung imaging. This technique may ultimately allow the simultaneous and accurate detection of both pulmonary embolism and venous thrombosis. Disadvantages include the potential difficulty in performing MRI on critically ill patients.

Echocardiography in Acute Pulmonary Embolism

Echocardiography (see Chapter 43), which can often be obtained more rapidly than either lung scanning or pulmonary arteriography, may reveal abnormalities of right ventricular size or function that strongly support hemodynamically significant pulmonary embolism. Unfortunately, because patients with suspected pulmonary emboli often have underlying cardiopulmonary disease, neither right ventricular dilation nor hypokinesis can be used reliably even as indirect evidence of pulmonary emboli. In the setting of documented pulmonary embolism, however, echocardiographic evidence of right ventricular dysfunction has been suggested as a guide for which patients may be likely to benefit from thrombolytic therapy. Such cases need to be individualized, and no firm recommendations can be made about this approach at present. Intravascular ultrasound, which may be performed at the bedside, can image large emboli, but the technique remains investigational at this time.

TREATMENT

Options for treatment of acute pulmonary embolism include treatment with heparin or related compounds, thrombolytic agents, or interruption of the inferior vena cava. Each approach has advantages and disadvantages.

Anticoagulation with Heparin and Related Compounds

By accelerating the action of antithrombin III, heparin exerts a prompt antithrombotic effect that prevents thrombus extension (see

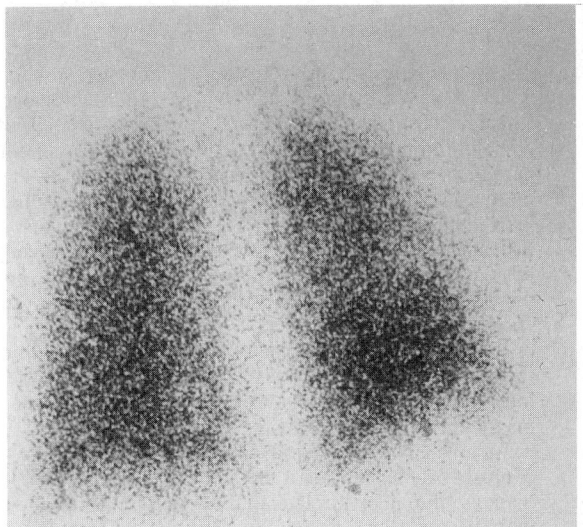
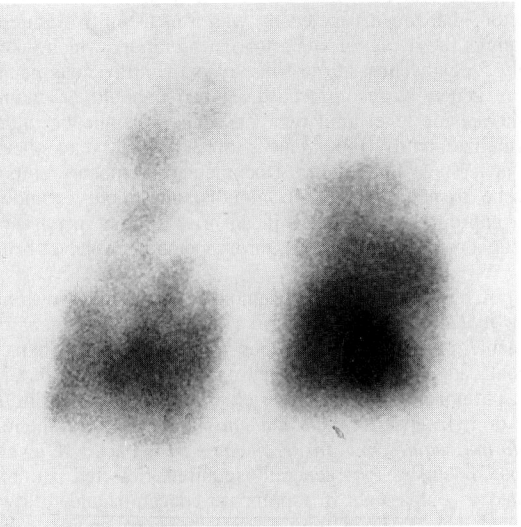

FIGURE 84–2 ▪ A lung ventilation-perfusion scan that indicates a high probability for pulmonary embolism. In the first panel (ventilation scan), it is evident that ventilation is minimally altered. The perfusion scan reveals multiple bilateral perfusion defects.

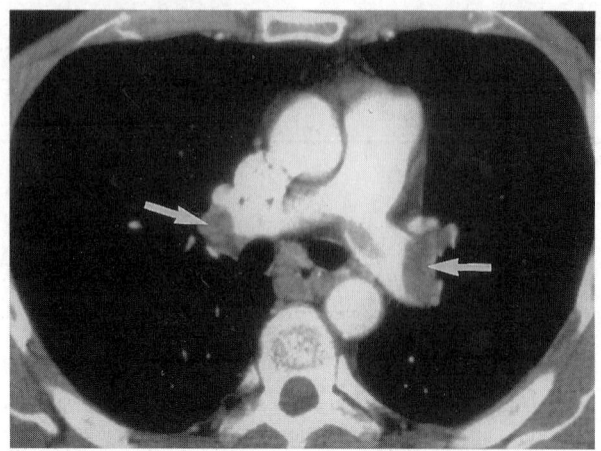

FIGURE 84–3 ■ Spiral CT image of acute pulmonary emboli in both main pulmonary arteries in a postoperative patient with the sudden onset of dyspnea, hypoxemia, and hypotension.

Chapters 69 and 188). Although it does not directly prevent the development of acute pulmonary embolism or dissolve thrombus, heparin allows the fibrinolytic system to proceed unopposed and more readily reduce the thromboembolic burden. Although thrombus growth can be prevented, early recurrence can develop even in the setting of therapeutic anticoagulation. Anticoagulation has been proven to reduce mortality in acute pulmonary embolism. When deep venous thrombosis or pulmonary embolism is diagnosed, heparin therapy (see Chapter 188) should be instituted immediately unless contraindications are present. If the risk of anticoagulation appears to be low, it is appropriate and often absolutely indicated to initiate therapy in patients with highly probable acute pulmonary embolism, even while confirmatory diagnostic testing is under way; confirmatory diagnostic testing should be arranged as soon as possible if anticoagulation is to be continued.

For standard heparin, the activated partial thromboplastin time (APTT) should be followed at 6-hour intervals until it is consistently in the therapeutic range of 1.5 to 2.0 times control values. This range corresponds to a heparin level of 0.2 to 0.4 U/mL as measured by protamine sulfate titration. Achieving a therapeutic APTT within 24 hours after pulmonary embolism has been documented to reduce the recurrence rate. Heparin should be administered as an intravenous bolus of 80 U/kg followed by 18 U/kg/hour; further adjustment should also be weight-based (see Table 69–5). Warfarin therapy may be initiated as soon as the APTT is in a therapeutic range (which should be within the first 24 hours). Earlier initiation of warfarin may intensify hypercoagulability and increase the clot burden due to the short-half life of anticoagulation factors that are dissipated by warfarin. Definitive anticoagulation requires the depletion of factor II (thrombin), which takes approximately 5 days. Thus, at least five days of intravenous heparin therapy is generally recommended. Heparin should be maintained at a therapeutic level until two consecutive therapeutic international normalized ratio (INR) values of 2.0 to 3.0 have been documented at least 24 hours apart. Documented pulmonary embolism should be treated for 3 to 6 months, and more extended treatment is appropriate when significant risk factors persist or when previous episodes of venous thromboembolism have been documented.

A number of clinical trials have demonstrated the efficacy and safety of *low-molecular-weight heparin (LMWH)* for treatment of established acute proximal deep venous thrombosis (see Chapter 69), and recent data suggest the efficacy of these agents for certain patients with pulmonary embolism as well. LMWHs can be administered once or twice per day *subcutaneously,* even at therapeutic doses, *and do not require monitoring of the APTT.* Factor X levels may prove useful but are not generally required. Selected patients may be treated as outpatients if appropriate education and follow-up are arranged. One LMWH (enoxaparin) has been approved by the Food and Drug Administration to treat deep venous thrombosis with or without pulmonary embolus, and LMWH is quickly becoming the usual approach for uncomplicated patients.

Although heparin is the most closely studied antithrombin agent, it works indirectly and requires antithrombin III as a co-factor. Hirudin is a direct thrombin inhibitor that has several potential advantages over heparin, including efficacy against fibrin clot-bound thrombin. This drug, derived from the saliva of the medicinal leech (*Hirudo medicinalis*), does not require co-factors and is not inactivated by platelet factor 4 or plasma proteins. As with heparin, these direct thrombin inhibitors have very narrow therapeutic indices. Inogatran (a selective, active-site inhibitor of thrombin), napsagatran (a synthetic direct thrombin inhibitor), argatroban (a direct thrombin inhibitor), tick anticoagulant peptide (a selective factor Xa inhibitor), and tissue factor pathway inhibitor are also under investigation.

Bleeding is the major complication of heparin and warfarin therapy (see Chapter 188). The rates of major bleeding in recent trials using heparin by continuous infusion or high-dose subcutaneous injection are less than 5%. Heparin-induced thrombocytopenia (defined as a platelet count less than 150,000/mm³) typically develops 5 or more days after the initiation of heparin therapy, and occurs in 5 to 10% of patients (see Chapter 188); the syndrome is caused by heparin-dependent immunoglobulin (Ig) G antibodies that activate platelets via their Fc receptors. If heparin therapy is instituted for venous thromboembolism and the platelet count progressively decreases to 100,000/mm³ or less, heparin therapy should be discontinued. LMWHs may be considered in this setting because the formation of heparin-dependent IgG antibodies and the risk of thrombocytopenia appears to be lower with this form of heparin. For example, danaparoid (a heparinoid) has been approved for use in the setting of heparin-induced thrombocytopenia.

Bleeding related to warfarin therapy increases with intensity and duration of therapy (see Chapter 188). Warfarin-induced skin necrosis is a rare but serious complication that mandates immediate cessation of the drug; it is related, at least in some patients, to protein C or S deficiency. Warfarin crosses the placenta and may cause fetal malformations if used during pregnancy.

Vena Cava Interruption

If a patient cannot be given anticoagulants, inferior vena cava (IVC) filter placement can be performed to prevent lower extremity thrombi from embolizing to the lungs. The primary indications for filter placement include contraindications to anticoagulation, recurrent embolism while receiving adequate therapy, and significant bleeding complications during anticoagulation. Filters are sometimes placed in the setting of massive pulmonary embolism when it is believed that any further emboli might be lethal, particularly if thrombolytic therapy is contraindicated. A number of filter designs exist, but the Greenfield filter has been most widely used. Filters can be inserted via the jugular or femoral vein. These devices are usually effective, and short-term complications are unusual. Recurrent deep vein thrombosis is more common in patients treated with IVC filters alone, so anticoagulants should also be given if no contraindications exist.

Thrombolytic Therapy

Thrombolytic agents activate plasminogen to form plasmin, which then results in fibrinolysis as well as fibrinogenolysis (see Chapter 188). Because anticoagulants do not actively cause lysis of emboli, thrombolytic agents are considered in certain settings to hasten the reduction in thromboembolic burden. In the 160-patient multicenter, prospective, randomized, Urokinase Pulmonary Embolism Trial, thrombolysis was accelerated in the first 24 hours in patients receiving urokinase compared with those receiving heparin, but thereafter the difference between the two groups diminished; by day 5, the improvement in each group was similar, and no difference was noted in the frequency of recurrent pulmonary embolism or mortality within 2 weeks of treatment. Subsequent clinical studies have led to the approval of streptokinase, urokinase, and recombinant tissue-type plasminogen activator (t-PA) for the treatment of massive pulmonary embolism (see Table 188–1).

Although no data are available from prospective, randomized, clinical trials to indicate a reduction in mortality from thrombolytic therapy, thrombolytic therapy is often recommended in patients with hemodynamic instability (hypotension) or severely compromised oxygenation. An argument can also be made for thrombolytic therapy when the perfusion defect by lung scan or pulmonary arteriogram is extensive (defect approaching the equivalent of one-

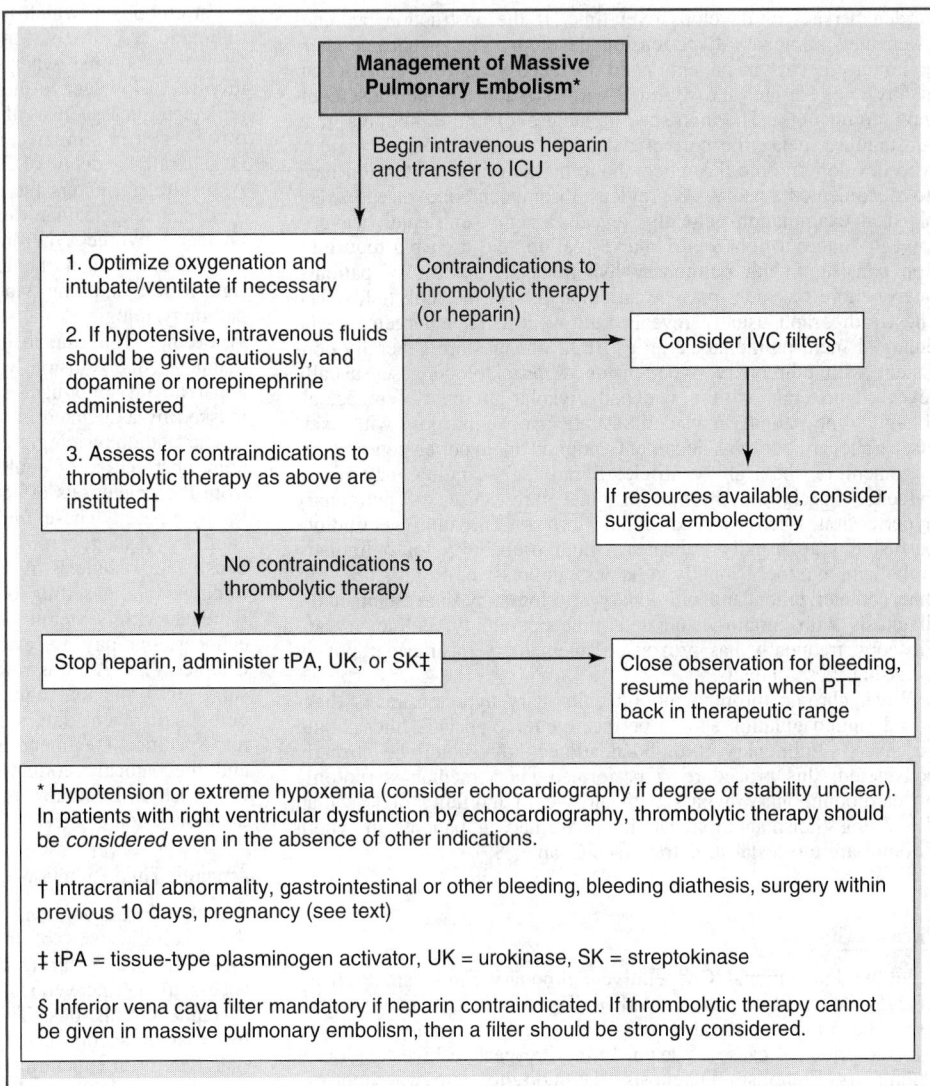

Figure 84–4 ■ An algorithm for the approach to the patient with massive acute pulmonary embolism. ICU = intensive care unit; IVC = inferior vena cava.

half of the pulmonary vascular bed), even without clear hemodynamic instability. Although thrombolytic therapy may result in more rapid improvement of right ventricular function in patients with acute pulmonary embolism, controversy remains as to whether or not patients with echocardiographic right ventricular dysfunction without hypotension or severe hypoxemia should receive this form of treatment. Thrombolytic therapy may also be considered when extensive deep-vein thrombosis accompanies a submassive pulmonary embolism.

Coagulation assays are unnecessary during thrombolysis because the approved regimens are administered as fixed doses. Heparin should be withheld until the thrombolytic infusion is completed. The APTT is then determined, and heparin is initiated without a loading dose if this value is less than twice the upper limit of normal. If the APTT exceeds this value, the test is repeated every 4 hours until it is safe to proceed with heparin administration. Catheter-directed administration of intra-embolic thrombolytic therapy has been utilized in small clinical studies, but data are currently inadequate to recommend this approach.

Hemorrhage is the primary adverse effect associated with thrombolytic therapy. Both lysis of hemostatic fibrin plugs and fibrinogenolysis can lead to bleeding complications, which commonly occur at sites of invasive procedures such as pulmonary arteriography or arterial line placement. If possible, invasive procedures should be minimized. The most devastating complication associated with this form of treatment is the development of intracranial hemorrhage, which occurs in fewer than 1% of patients. Retroperitoneal hemorrhage may result from a vascular puncture above the inguinal ligament and may be life-threatening. Absolute contraindications to systemic thrombolytic therapy include intracranial surgery or other intracranial pathologic processes and active or recent internal bleeding, whereas relative contraindications include bleeding diathesis/thrombocytopenia, uncontrolled severe hypertension, recent cardiopulmonary resuscitation, surgery within the previous 10 days, and pregnancy.

Hemodynamic Management of Massive Pulmonary Embolism

Massive pulmonary embolism should always be suspected in the setting of the sudden onset of hypotension, extreme hypoxemia, electromechanical dissociation, or sudden cardiac arrest. Once massive pulmonary embolism associated with hypotension and/or severe hypoxemia is suspected, supportive treatment is initiated immediately (Fig. 84–4). Intravenous saline should be infused rapidly but cautiously, because right ventricular function is often markedly compromised. Dopamine or norepinephrine appear to be the best vasoactive agents and should be administered if the blood pressure is not rapidly restored. Because death in this setting results from right ventricular failure, dobutamine may be useful to augment right ventricular output. Oxygen therapy is administered, and thrombolytic therapy should be strongly considered. Intubation and institution of mechanical ventilation are undertaken as needed to support respiratory failure. Pulmonary embolectomy may be appropriate if patients with massive embolism cannot receive thrombolytic therapy.

CHRONIC THROMBOEMBOLIC PULMONARY HYPERTENSION
(see Chapter 56)

Although the vast majority of acute pulmonary emboli resolve with therapy, occasionally a substantial residual thromboembolic burden persists or develops over time. If the obstruction becomes extensive, pulmonary hypertension develops. This syndrome most commonly occurs in patients aged 40 to 70 years, but it can occur at any age. Fatigue and dyspnea with exertion are the most common complaints. The non-specific nature of these findings may substantially delay the correct diagnosis. At least 50% of patients who develop chronic thromboembolic pulmonary hypertension have no documented history of previous thromboembolic disease. The physical examination generally reveals a right ventricular heave, a loud P_2 sound, a right ventricular S_3 gallop, and tricuspid regurgitation consistent with pulmonary hypertension. In 20% of patients, one or more murmurs may be auscultated over the lung fields. The chest radiograph usually reveals right ventricular enlargement and enlarged main pulmonary arteries. ECG changes are generally consistent with pulmonary hypertension. Arterial blood gases usually reveal hypoxemia with a widened alveolar-arterial difference, although some patients may demonstrate hypoxemia only with exercise. Echocardiography documents pulmonary hypertension and enlargement of the right ventricle. Spiral CT scanning may reveal evidence of chronic thrombi or other rare causes of pulmonary hypertension, such as mediastinal fibrosis. The lung ventilation-perfusion scan usually indicates a high probability for pulmonary embolism, but occasionally it is less impressive. Right-sided cardiac catheterization and pulmonary arteriography can establish the diagnosis with certainty and determine operability. Pulmonary angioscopy frequently has proven complementary to arteriography in assessing these patients.

When chronic thromboembolic pulmonary hypertension is diagnosed, anticoagulation should be instituted and an IVC filter should be placed. Pulmonary thromboendarterectomy should be strongly considered; this procedure is performed via a median sternotomy on cardiopulmonary bypass with an overall mortality of less than 5%. Lung transplantation can be performed in patients in whom thrombi are too distal to extract (see Chapter 89).

PROGNOSIS

In the International Cooperative Pulmonary Embolism Registry of 2454 consecutive patients with a diagnosis of pulmonary embolism, the 3-month mortality was 17.5% and pulmonary embolism was the principal cause of death. In the Prospective Investigation of Pulmonary Embolism Diagnosis, the mortality rate was approximately 15%, but only 10% of deaths during the first year of follow-up were attributed to pulmonary embolism. Mean 1-month mortality rates of treated and untreated pulmonary embolism have been estimated at 8% and 30%, respectively.

Although a small percentage of patients with acute pulmonary embolism ultimately develop chronic dyspnea and hypoxemia due to chronic thromboembolic pulmonary hypertension, most patients who survive the acute episode have no long-term pulmonary sequelae. However, chronic leg pain and swelling from deep venous thrombosis (postphlebitic syndrome) (see Chapter 69) may result in significant morbidity.

PREVENTION

Every hospitalized patient should be assessed for the need for interventions to prevent venous thromboembolic disease. Patients can be stratified according to deep venous thrombosis risk (see Table 69–3), and certain prophylactic measures are more appropriate for some patients than for others (see Table 69–4). Appropriate prophylaxis can greatly reduce this potentially devastating complication.

NON-THROMBOTIC PULMONARY EMBOLI

By virtue of venous blood return to the lungs, the pulmonary vascular bed is exposed to a wide variety of potentially obstructing and detrimental substances. These substances, which may be exogenous or endogenous in origin, may result in a number of consequences, including dyspnea, chest pain, hypoxemia, and, sometimes, death.

Fat Embolism

Fat embolism, which most commonly occurs in the setting of the traumatic fracture of long bones, is generally a more impressive clinical syndrome when larger bones and multiple fractures are involved. However, orthopedic procedures and trauma to other fat-replete tissues such as the liver or subcutaneous tissue can sometimes result in similar consequences. After the inciting event, there is generally a delay of 24 to 48 hours before symptoms develop. As neutral fat enters the vascular system, a characteristic syndrome of dyspnea, petechiae, and mental confusion often develops. It is unclear why the syndrome develops in some patients and not in others, even when the extent of injury is comparable. However, right-to-left shunting via a patent foramen ovale may be a key pathophysiologic explanation for the systemic manifestations of the syndrome. The diagnosis of fat embolism syndrome remains a diagnosis of exclusion and is based on clinical criteria. Clinically apparent fat embolism syndrome is uncommon, and it may be masked by associated injuries in more severely injured patients.

The pathophysiologic consequences of fat embolism derive from both obstruction of multiple vessels by neutral fat particles and from the deleterious effects of free fatty acids released from neutral fat by lipases. These free fatty acids cause diffuse vasculitis with capillary leakage from cerebral, pulmonary, and other vascular beds. The diagnosis is made from the clinical and radiographic findings in the setting of risk factors such as surgery or trauma. Patients with systemic signs or symptoms should have contrast echocardiography to evaluate a possible intracardiac shunt (see Chapter 43). Although fat droplets (made evident by oil red O stain) in bronchoalveolar lavage fluid may be suggestive of fat embolism, recent data suggest that this finding is neither sensitive nor specific. Treatment is generally supportive, including oxygen and mechanical ventilation, and the prognosis is generally good. Corticosteroid therapy remains controversial, but steroid prophylaxis has been suggested by some for high-risk patients.

Amniotic Fluid Embolism

Although uncommon, amniotic fluid embolism represents one of the leading causes of maternal death in the United States. This syndrome occurs during or after delivery when amniotic fluid gains access to uterine venous channels and then to the pulmonary and systemic circulations. The delivery may be either spontaneous or by cesarean section and usually has been without complication. No risk factors are identifiable in either the patient or the baby. The syndrome is heralded by the sudden onset of severe respiratory distress; hypotension and death frequently result. The primary mechanism of injury appears to involve the thromboplastic activity of amniotic fluid, with extensive fibrin deposition in the pulmonary vasculature and sometimes in other organs. A severe consumptive coagulopathy ensues, with marked hypofibrinogenemia. After the acute event, an enhanced fibrinolytic state often develops. Left ventricular dysfunction may result, and a potential role has been suggested for the myocardial depressant effect of amniotic fluid. The resulting pulmonary edema may be both hydrostatic and noncardiogenic. The differential diagnosis includes pulmonary thromboembolism, septic and hemorrhagic shock, venous air embolism, aspiration pneumonia, heart failure (from acute myocardial infarction or other causes), abruptio placentae, and ruptured uterus. The diagnosis may be suspected on the basis of the clinical picture. Examination of the pulmonary arterial blood may or may not reveal the amorphous fragments of vernix caseosa, squamous cells, or mucin. Although administration of heparin and antifibrinolytic agents (e.g., aminocaproic acid and cryoprecipitate) has been suggested, the primary treatment is supportive, with oxygen and mechanical ventilation.

Air Embolism

The consequences of venous air embolism range from none to death. The incidence of this entity reflects the variety of invasive surgical and medical procedures now available, the frequent use of indwelling venous and arterial catheters, and the frequency of thoracic and other forms of trauma. With venous embolism in the setting of a patent foramen ovale, embolization to the coronary or cerebral circulation is of most concern. In the absence of a patent foramen ovale, the lungs can filter modest amounts of air, but large single or continuous episodes of air embolism can still gain access to the systemic arterial circulation. Symptoms and signs are dependent on the severity of the episode. Air in the systemic circulation may be difficult to recognize because only small quantities may cause significant symptoms, and intravascular air clears quickly. Dyspnea, wheezing, chest pain, cough, agitation, confusion, tachycardia, and hypotension may be evident. A "mill-wheel murmur" (air in the right ventricle) may sometimes be auscultated. Hypoxemia and hypercapnia are present in severe cases, and the chest radiograph may reveal pulmonary edema or air-fluid levels. The treatment of venous air embolism includes immediate placement of the patient in the Trendelenburg or left lateral decubitus position and administration of 100% oxygen. If a central venous catheter is in place near the right atrium, air aspiration should be attempted. Occasionally, hyperbaric oxygen is indicated. The head should be elevated at 30 degress to prevent further air from reaching the brain and coronary circulation. Anticonvulsants are administered in the presence of seizures.

Schistosomiasis (see Chapter 431)

This parasitic disorder causes severe pulmonary vascular obstruction and pulmonary hypertension via both anatomic obstruction by the organism itself and an inflammatory vasculitic response to the organism. In endemic areas (e.g., Egypt), schistosomal disease is a common cause of cor pulmonale. The liver is always involved, usually quite extensively, before pulmonary involvement occurs. The disease is refractory to treatment unless it is detected prior to the development of extensive hepatic and pulmonary inflammation.

Septic Embolism (see Chapters 17 and 326)

Until intravenous drug abuse became common, septic embolism was nearly always a complication of septic pelvic thrombophlebitis due to both septic abortion and postpartum uterine infection. Intravenous drug abuse is now by far the most common cause. Infections secondary to indwelling intravenous catheters are increasingly common as well. Subcutaneous injections can cause local infections that subsequently invade veins.

Other Emboli

The lung may be embolized on occasion by a variety of other substances. Cancer cells may enter and adhere to pulmonary vessels, occasionally mimicking pulmonary embolism. Brain tissue has been discovered in the lungs after head trauma, and liver cells can be seen after abdominal trauma. Bone marrow has been reported in lung tissue after cardiopulmonary resuscitation.

Noninfectious vasculitic-thrombotic complications also occur in intravenous drug users (see Chapter 17). Materials such as talc, and occasionally the drugs themselves, may provoke vascular inflammation and secondary thrombosis. Perfusion scans occasionally demonstrate segmental or smaller defects. Distinguishing these from emboli due to deep venous thrombosis can be difficult. Occasionally, repetitive insults lead to chronic pulmonary hypertension.

Dalen JE, Hirsh J (eds): Fourth American College of Chest Physicians Consensus Conference on antithrombotic therapy. Chest 108:225S–522S, 1995. *Guidelines for prophylaxis and treatment of venous thromboembolism using an evidence-based approach.*

Fedullo PF, Auger WR, Channick RN, et al: Chronic thromboembolic pulmonary hypertension. *In* Tapson VF, Fulkerson WJ, Saltzman HA (eds): Clinics in Chest Medicine: Venous Thromboembolism. Philadelphia, WB Saunders, 1995, pp 353–374. *A comprehensive overview of the complexities of the diagnosis and management of this entity.*

Goldhaber SZ: Pulmonary embolism. N Engl J Med 339:93, 1998. *A superlative overview.*

Remy-Jardin MJ, Remy J, Deschildre F, et al: Diagnosis of acute pulmonary embolism with spiral CT: Comparison with pulmonary angiography and scintigraphy. Radiology 200:699, 1996. *This group of investigators has extensive experience with spiral CT scanning for acute pulmonary embolism, and they found a sensitivity of 91% and specificity of 78% for this technique, using pulmonary arteriography as the gold standard test.*

Simonneau G, Sors H, Charbonnier B, et al: A comparison of low-molecular-weight heparin with unfractionated heparin for acute pulmonary embolism. N Engl J Med 337:663–669, 1997. *More than 600 patients in a series were randomized to either standard heparin or low-molecular-weight heparin. Mortality, recurrence rate, and major bleeding were equal. Newer agents are being successfully explored for the treatment of pulmonary embolism.*

Stein PD, Dalen JE, Goldhaber SZ, et al: Opinions regarding the diagnosis and management of venous thromboembolic disease (opinion statement II). Chest 113:499–504, 1998. *Addresses difficult issues regarding acute venous thromboembolism.*

The American Thoracic Society Consensus Statement: Clinical practice guidelines. Am J Resp Crit Care Med, in press.

85 ■ PULMONARY NEOPLASMS
York E. Miller

DEFINITION

Lung cancer is the leading cause of cancer death in both men and women in the United States. More than 99% of malignant lung tumors arise from the respiratory epithelium and are termed *bronchogenic carcinoma*. For practical purposes, bronchogenic carcinoma can be divided into two subgroups: small cell lung cancer (SCLC) and non–small cell lung cancer (NSCLC), which includes the subtypes adenocarcinoma, squamous cell carcinoma, and large cell carcinoma (Table 85–1). A correct tissue diagnosis is crucial, because SCLC has a high response rate to chemotherapy and radiation and is appropriately treated by surgery only in rare situations. Conversely, NSCLC can be cured by surgery in certain stages and is not curable by chemotherapy alone. The overall 5-year survival rate for lung cancer is a disappointing 14%. Smoking is the major risk factor for development of lung cancer (see Chapters 13 and 193).

INCIDENCE AND PREVALENCE

In the first decade of the 20th century, lung cancer was a rare disorder. In 1998, approximately 171,000 new cases of lung cancer were seen in the United States, with approximately 160,000 deaths. Lung cancer is now the most common cause of cancer death for both genders and accounts for 28% of the overall cancer death rate. In terms of both cancer deaths and years of life lost, the effect of lung cancer is greater than that of breast, prostate, colon, and rectal cancer combined. Lung cancer incidence for middle-aged white men recently peaked and is now declining slightly. However, trends for women show a continued increase, and in the past decade, lung cancer surpassed breast cancer as the leading cause of cancer death in women. On a worldwide basis, lung cancer will continue to be a major problem into the 21st century, due to cases in ex-smokers, the increasing incidence of smoking in teenagers, and the marketing of cigarettes to developing countries.

EPIDEMIOLOGY

Modifiable Risk Factors

TOBACCO PRODUCTS. Tobacco smoking causes approximately 87% of cases in men and 85% in women, with a dose-dependent relationship of both duration and intensity of smoking with mortality from lung cancer. SCLC has the strongest association with smoking, with attributable fractions of 97% and 91% for men and women, respectively. Smoking cessation causes a gradual drop in lung cancer risk, but not a complete normalization of risk, over a number of years. Cigarette smoke contains a number of active carcinogens and procarcinogens, and the pattern of mutations (transversions versus transitions) seen in oncogenes and tumor suppressor genes isolated from smokers with lung cancer is that expected from the mechanism of action of the major cigarette smoke carcinogens (see Chapter 191).

Table 85–1 ■ MALIGNANT PULMONARY NEOPLASMS

	INCIDENCE (%)
Common	99
Non–small cell lung cancer	~75
Adenocarcinoma	~35
Squamous cell carcinoma	~30
Large cell carcinoma	~10
Small cell lung cancer	~20
Carcinoids	~5
Rare	<1
Lymphoma, carcinosarcoma, mucoepidermoid carcinoma, malignant fibrous histiocytoma, melanoma, sarcoma, blastoma	

PASSIVE SMOKE EXPOSURE. The Environmental Protection Agency has classified passive smoke exposure as carcinogenic. In support of this association, increased levels of carcinogens are measurable in the blood of passive smokers. A number of studies have shown increased risk for lung cancer in the spouses of smokers. The tobacco smoke exposure of a smoker's child is greater than that of a spouse. Exposure to 25 smoker-years in childhood approximately doubles the risk of lung cancer in a non-smoker.

OCCUPATIONAL AND OTHER EXPOSURES (see Chapter 79). In addition to its association with mesothelioma, asbestos exposure also increases the risk for all histologic subtypes of lung cancer. The relative risk of lung cancer in a non-smoking asbestos worker is approximately 5. The effect of smoking and asbestos exposure is synergistic, with a risk ratio of between 50 and 100. Common sources of asbestos exposure include the shipbuilding industry, nautical engine rooms, automotive (particularly brake-lining) work, painting, and the construction industry. Exposures that may seem trivial can be significant; for example, cases of mesothelioma have been reported in the spouses and children of asbestos workers who brought their workclothes home to be washed. Exposure to asbestos fibers is now closely regulated. Because risk from asbestos exposure and smoking is synergistic, the most important intervention in an individual with both exposures is to stop smoking.

The association between ionizing radiation (see Chapter 19) and lung cancer was made in classic studies of uranium miners exposed to radon daughters. Other miners in areas of significant subterranean radioactivity can also be exposed. Some home environments also have significant levels of radon, especially because modern insulation practices lead to increased radon levels. It is estimated that between 5000 and 15,000 excess lung cancer deaths, mostly in smokers, are caused annually in the United States by radon. As with asbestos and smoking, the risks of ionizing radiation exposure and smoking are synergistic. Other environmental or occupational lung carcinogens include arsenic, chromium, chloromethyl ethers, mustard gas, nickel, polycyclic hydrocarbons, vinyl chloride, and possibly silica and certain man-made fibers (see Chapter 21).

AIR POLLUTION. Air pollution is associated with a variety of respiratory disorders and has long been suspected as a possible pulmonary carcinogen. A number of studies demonstrate an increased incidence of lung cancer in urban versus rural environments, but other factors could also explain these differences.

CHRONIC OBSTRUCTIVE PULMONARY DISEASE. The presence of chronic obstructive pulmonary disease (COPD), defined as either airflow obstruction on pulmonary function testing or symptoms of chronic bronchitis, increases the risk of lung cancer several-fold. COPD is a risk factor by itself and is not just a reflection of the number of cigarettes smoked.

DIET (see Chapter 11). Epidemiologic studies demonstrate increased risk for lung cancer in individuals with a diet low in fruits and vegetables. The effect of dietary intervention by increasing fruit and vegetable intake on risk for lung cancer has not been determined.

Nonmodifiable Risk Factors

GENDER AND RACIAL DIFFERENCES. The largest factor in gender differences in incidence of lung cancer is differences in cigarette smoking habits. The predominant lung cancer incidence and mortality in the United States is currently seen in men, but the incidence rates for women are rising rapidly, whereas those for middle-aged men are reaching a plateau. However, given the same exposures, women may be more susceptible to lung cancer than men. Black men have the highest incidence of lung cancer, but racial differences are confounded by differences in socioeconomic status and smoking behavior. One study has concluded that black men and black women have higher rates of lung cancer than do whites, after adjustment for differences in these factors.

GENETIC SUSCEPTIBILITY. A segregation analysis has demonstrated that lung cancer incidence within families is consistent with mendelian inheritance of a major autosomal gene governing susceptibility (see Chapter 31). It is estimated that segregation at this locus accounts for 69%, 47%, and 22% of lung cancers diagnosed at ages 50, 60, and 70 years, respectively.

Major categories of genes that potentially determine susceptibility to lung cancer (see Chapter 191) include proto-oncogenes, tumor suppressor genes, genes encoding enzymes that metabolize procarcinogens to active carcinogens (typified by the p450 enzymes), and genes that detoxify carcinogens (typified by glutathione S transferase μ). Although kindreds with germ line abnormalities of either the p53 or the retinoblastoma tumor suppressor genes have higher incidences of lung cancer, these abnormalities do not appear to be a common mechanism in the general population. Two isozymes, CYP2D6 and CYP1A1, of the P-450 enzyme system, which metabolizes and in many cases activates carcinogens, have been implicated in susceptibility to lung cancer. Glutathione S-transferase μ has a common null allele that confers an increased risk for lung cancer in some populations. Combinations of susceptibility genes appear to increase lung cancer risk significantly.

PATHOGENESIS

The respiratory epithelium develops as an outpouching from the endoderm of the primitive foregut. All respiratory epithelial cells differentiate from the primitive respiratory epithelium. Animal studies demonstrate that in the airway epithelium, both the secretory and basal cells can dedifferentiate and subsequently redifferentiate into the various epithelial subtypes. In the alveolar epithelium, the type II cell is the proliferative stem cell. All histologic subtypes of bronchogenic carcinoma are believed to be derived from the respiratory epithelium. The different histologic subtypes are a reflection of the differentiation pathway taken by a particular tumor. The plasticity of this differentiation is demonstrated by the occurrence of mixed tumors expressing differentiation markers for more than one histologic subtype. In addition, experimental expression of specific oncogenes in lung cancer cell lines can alter their differentiation characteristics.

Premalignant Biology

Currently, the favored model for the development of bronchogenic carcinoma is that of multistep carcinogenesis with the successive accumulation of mutations in a number of genes involved in regulating growth. Premalignant lesions have been described and widely accepted only for squamous cell carcinoma. Microdissection of bronchial epithelium has allowed the identification of genetic lesions including chromosome 3p deletion, chromosome 9p deletion, and p53 gene mutations in premalignant lesions. The usual order of occurrence and prognostic import of these genetic alterations is not yet known.

Increased cellular proliferation is also necessary for carcinogenesis. It is likely that growth factors, derived from inflammatory cells, epithelial cells, and neuroendocrine cells, may be elevated in tobacco smokers and play a role in pathogenesis of lung cancer.

Tumor Biology

GENETIC ALTERATIONS. Bronchogenic carcinomas (see Chapter 191) have highly abnormal tumor karyotypes, but certain consistent chromosomal abnormalities have been noted both in SCLC and NSCLC, including deletions involving chromosomes 3p, 5q, 9p, 11p, 13q, and 17p (Table 85–2). These abnormalities typically result in loss of heterozygosity but not homozygous deletion of a region. The deleted regions are likely the loci of tumor suppressor genes. Indeed, several tumor suppressor genes, Rb (13q14), p53 (17p13), CDKN2A (9p21) and CDKN2B (9p21) have been assigned to regions typically deleted in lung cancer and are fre-

Table 85–2 ■ CHARACTERISTIC CHROMOSOMAL DELETIONS COMMON IN LUNG CANCER

CHROMOSOMAL REGION DELETED	TUMOR SUPPRESSOR GENES INACTIVATED
3p14-25	Unknown, probably multiple, ?FHIT
5q	?APC, MCC
9p21	CDKN2A, CDKN2B, possibly others
13q14	Rb (~100% SCLC, ~20% NSCLC)
17p13	p53 (~90% SCLC, ~60% NSCLC)

FHIT = fragile histidine triad; APC = adenomatous polyposis coli; MCC = mutated in colon carcinoma; Rb = retinoblastoma; SCLC = small cell lung cancer; NSCLC = non-SCLC (see Chapter 191).

Table 85-3 ■ ONCOGENE ABNORMALITIES

ONCOGENE	ABNORMALITY	
	SCLC	NSCLC
Ki-ras	0	30–50% of adenocarcinomas (activating mutation)
H-ras	0	Rare mutation; overexpression occurs
N-ras	0	Rare mutation; overexpression occurs
myc (c, L, N)	Majority	Gene amplification and overexpression
her2/neu	—	30% (overexpression)
c-kit	Overexpression	—
bcl-2	?	Overexpression
cyclin D1 (prad)	—	Overexpression

SCLC = small cell lung cancer; NSCLC = non-SCLC.

quently inactivated. For other regions, such as the short arm of chromosome 3, candidate tumor suppressor genes, such as FHIT, have been identified. Although Rb and p53 mutations are found in both SCLC and NSCLC, the incidence of both is significantly higher in SCLC.

Transforming oncogenes can be activated by a number of mechanisms, including point mutation, gene amplification, and overexpression (Table 85–3). Abnormalities of the Ki-ras, her2/neu, and myc family oncogenes have been described and reported in small studies to affect prognosis adversely. Cyclin D1 overexpression is common in NSCLC and, in conjunction with inactivation of the cyclin-dependent kinase inhibitors CDK2NA and CDK2NB, represents a nonmutation mechanism inactivation of Rb that leads to loss of cell cycle control. Bcl-2 oncogene overexpression has been reported to have a favorable effect on prognosis. Because abnormalities in tumor suppressor and proto-oncogenes in lung cancer may have prognostic significance, it is likely that in the future treatment plans will be altered on the basis of these abnormalities.

AUTOCRINE GROWTH FACTORS. Bronchogenic carcinomas produce a variety of autocrine growth factors. Multiple neuropeptide growth factors, exemplified by the bombesin-like peptides, acting through G protein–coupled receptors (characterized by possession of seven transmembrane-spanning domains), are particularly dominant in SCLC, although they also drive proliferation in NSCLC. Other autocrine growth factors expressed by bronchogenic carcinomas include insulin-like growth factor 1, transforming growth factor-alpha, the c-kit ligand (stem cell growth factor), and the heregulins. Clinical trials are under way in humans using strategies either to disrupt stimulation by autocrine growth factors or to bias postreceptor signal transduction pathways to lead to apoptosis rather than proliferation.

Pathology

NON–SMALL CELL LUNG CANCER. Adenocarcinoma has increased in incidence and is now the most frequent histologic subtype. Adenocarcinomas may be derived from either the periphery of the lung or the central airways. Approximately half of adenocarcinomas exhibit markers for type II or Clara cells, such as mRNA for the surfactant proteins A, B, and C. The hallmark of adenocarcinomas is the tendency to form glands. Special stains demonstrate that the tumor cells contain mucins. Bronchoalveolar carcinoma, a subcategory of adenocarcinoma, arises in the periphery and tends to spread in a lepidic fashion along pre-existing alveolar septa. Peripheral adenocarcinomas are sometimes associated with pulmonary scars; in a few cases the carcinoma likely arose from the scar, and in most the carcinoma probably caused the scar, either by producing a localized infarct or by instituting a desmoplastic cellular reaction. Precursor lesions for adenocarcinomas have not been well described.

Squamous cell carcinoma tends to originate in the central airways. Histologically, squamous cell carcinomas are characterized by keratinization with keratin "pearl" formation (i.e., flattened cells surrounding central cores of keratin). Squamous carcinomas are also characterized by predominant desmosomes that can be visualized on histologic sections as intercellular bridges.

Large cell carcinoma, often referred to as large cell undifferentiated carcinoma, is a group of carcinomas undifferentiated at the light microscopic level. Large cell carcinomas may exhibit neuroendocrine or glandular differentiation markers when studied by immunohistochemistry or electron microscopy. Two rare subtypes of large cell carcinomas are the giant cell carcinomas, associated with peripheral leukocytosis, and clear cell carcinomas, which resemble renal cell carcinomas.

Bronchial carcinoids are well-differentiated neuroendocrine tumors that often cause localized bronchial obstruction and present in young persons (see Chapter 245). Although carcinoids tend not to metastasize widely, they can exhibit a spectrum of biologic behavior.

SMALL CELL LUNG CANCER. SCLC is characterized by small, dark-staining cells with little cytoplasm. The nuclear chromatin is finely distributed, and nucleoli are inconspicuous. Biopsies frequently exhibit a "crush artifact," in which the tumor cells are compressed and distorted. Rarely, SCLC tumors comprise a combination of cells with SCLC and NSCLC features and are termed combined small cell carcinomas in the recent World Health Organization/International Association for the Study of Lung Cancer classification. When SCLC recurs after chemotherapy, NSCLC elements often increase. The diagnosis of SCLC is not usually difficult to make, but in certain situations, such as fine-needle aspirations of lymph nodes, immunohistochemical markers can be helpful.

CLINICAL MANIFESTATIONS

Lung cancer is clinically silent for most of its course. The presence of symptoms is usually accompanied by late disease, and prognosis is worse than with a carcinoma that presents as an asymptomatic radiographic abnormality. Symptoms can be divided into four categories: (1) those caused by tumor growing locally, (2) those caused by tumor invading adjacent structures, (3) those caused by metastatic disease, and (4) paraneoplastic syndromes.

LOCAL. Either a new cough or a change in the nature of a chronic cough is the most common presenting symptom of bronchogenic carcinoma. This symptom in a smoker should always cause concern. Cough productive of copious thin secretions, often with a salty flavor, has been described as classically occurring in bronchoalveolar carcinoma, but it occurs in only a minority of cases. Hemoptysis, either gross or minor, commonly occurs when mucosal lesions ulcerate. Although the most common cause of hemoptysis is bronchitis, this symptom in a high-risk individual should lead to prompt investigation. Tumors that obstruct major airways can produce wheezing, and unilateral wheezing suggests a localized obstruction. Airway obstruction can result in atelectasis or postobstructive pneumonia. Bronchogenic carcinomas are often associated with cavitation and lung abscess formation, due either to airway obstruction with postobstructive pneumonia or to necrosis of a large tumor mass. Clinical signs particularly indicative of malignancy-associated lung abscess include chronicity of symptoms, lack of high fever, and lack of leukocytosis.

LOCAL INVASION. Local invasion can produce chest pain, dyspnea from pleural effusion, and symptoms referable to nerves, heart, and great vessels. Malignant pleural effusions occur in approximately 10 to 20% of patients at the time of diagnosis and are most frequently a sign that the tumor is not surgically resectable. Invasion of the pericardium can lead to cardiac tamponade as well as to arrhythmias.

A number of syndromes have been described in locally invasive disease. The superior vena cava syndrome is characterized by facial suffusion and swelling due to blockage of the superior vena cava by either tumor or associated thrombosis. Although this syndrome is no longer considered a medical emergency, it should be treated promptly. Horner's syndrome results from disruption of the cervical sympathetic nerves and is characterized by unilateral facial anhidrosis, ptosis, and miosis in its full-blown form. Hoarseness can occur from invasion of the recurrent laryngeal nerve, usually by either tumor directly extending into the mediastinum or by adjacent malignant lymph nodes. The symptom of hoarseness is important because vocal cord paralysis denotes that the tumor is not resectable. The Pancoast syndrome occurs in tumors involving the apex and superior sulcus of the lung and results from local invasion into the brachial plexus as well as the cervical sympathetic nerves.

Clinical manifestations are dominated by shoulder and arm pain and may include Horner's syndrome. The tumor may not be readily apparent on plain radiographs, and computed tomographic (CT) scanning or magnetic resonance imaging (MRI) may be necessary for diagnosis.

METASTATIC DISEASE. Common sites of metastases of bronchogenic carcinomas include brain, bone, adrenal, and liver. In smokers who present with space-occupying lesions in these sites, the possibility of bronchogenic carcinoma should be immediately considered. In addition, metastatic carcinoma is a frequent cause of cervical and supraclavicular lymphadenopathy. Metastases to skin are relatively rare but are important to recognize clinically because of the ease of making a diagnosis by biopsy.

PARANEOPLASTIC SYNDROMES. Paraneoplastic syndromes occur in approximately 10% of patients with bronchogenic carcinoma and occasionally are the presenting symptom. Paraneoplastic manifestations can be divided into systemic, endocrine, neurologic, cutaneous, hematologic, and renal categories. Systemic manifestations are often nonspecific and can include weight loss, anorexia, and fever. The endocrine and neurologic manifestations of bronchogenic carcinoma are more specific (see Chapter 194).

Digital clubbing is seen in a variety of pulmonary conditions but occurs most commonly in association with bronchogenic carcinoma. Clubbing is caused by soft tissue subungual thickening that most commonly involves the fingernails, resulting in loss of the normal angle between the fingernail and nail bed. In addition, the fingernails are easily compressed against the nail bed and have a spongy feel. Hypertrophic pulmonary osteoarthropathy (see Chapter 194) is often associated with clubbing and commonly presents with exquisite tenderness over the long bones. Hypercoagulable states can result from bronchogenic carcinoma. Invasion of the bone marrow can produce anemia or leukocytosis with a leukoerythroblastic reaction.

ASYMPTOMATIC RADIOGRAPHIC ABNORMALITY. High-risk individuals (i.e., smokers with COPD) receive frequent chest radiographs for a variety of indications. A significant number of lung cancers are initially detected as an asymptomatic radiographic abnormality, especially a solitary pulmonary nodule (see Chapter 72). Lack of symptoms should not delay evaluation, as these patients are the most likely to be cured by appropriate therapy.

DIAGNOSIS AND STAGING

General Principles

In many cases the decision of whether or not to investigate a patient aggressively for lung cancer is obvious (Fig. 85–1). In other situations, such as when a relatively low-risk patient presents with an asymptomatic radiographic abnormality, the decision to initiate an evaluation is less clear. A variety of factors must be considered, including the patient's age, smoking history, exposure to other environmental carcinogens, family history of lung cancer, exposure to fungal and other infectious diseases that might cause pulmonary nodules, general health and operative risk, and personality and tolerance for uncertainty regarding a diagnosis. Once a decision to investigate is made, a firm diagnosis should be obtained. Usually, diagnosis requires a tissue biopsy. Positron-emission tomographic (PET) scanning can often reliably discriminate between benign and malignant nodules, but it is available only at a limited number of centers. It is imperative that the clinicians directing the patient's evaluation consult closely with the pathologist who is interpreting tissue biopsy and cytologic results. When the cell type is in doubt, additional tissue should be obtained for pathologic study.

IMAGING STUDIES. The chest radiograph is the most important radiologic study to diagnose lung cancer. When an abnormality is visualized on a chest radiograph, it is extremely helpful to obtain old chest radiographs if available. The stability of the lesion over time can be very helpful in suggesting either a benign or malignant diagnosis (see Fig. 72–2). Doubling times of less than 6 weeks or more than 18 months strongly suggest a benign diagnosis (doubling is calculated on the basis of volume, i.e., proportional to the cube of the radius of a lesion). Another reliable sign of benignity is the presence of heavy calcification within a lesion, particularly when present in a concentric, solid, or popcorn pattern. It must be kept in mind, however, that carcinomas can arise adjacent to calcified granulomas; therefore, if a lesion that contains a significant amount of calcium enlarges over time, it should be considered likely to be malignant. CT scanning of the thorax is now frequently undertaken in patients with suspicious nodules. In many cases, dense or diffuse calcification (suggesting a high likelihood that the lesion is a granuloma) or fat (suggesting a hamartoma) can be detected. CT scans also reliably detect enlarged lymph nodes, although biopsy is required to determine whether the lymphadenopathy is due to metastatic tumor. The CT scan can easily be extended to include the liver and adrenals to assess common sites of metastatic disease. MRI studies are particularly useful to detect vertebral, spinal cord, and mediastinal invasion in selected patients.

PATHOLOGIC DIAGNOSIS. Sputum cytology is the least invasive means to establish a tissue diagnosis. Sputum cytology is approximately 60 to 70% sensitive for central lesions but much less accurate for small peripheral lesions. In some instances, the diagnosis of cell type can be difficult on sputum cytologic analysis, and many clinicians believe that it is preferable to obtain biopsies of a tumor if at all possible. Other relatively noninvasive means of establishing a diagnosis include pleural fluid cytologic analysis, biopsy or aspiration cytologic analysis of enlarged cervical and supraclavicular lymph nodes, and biopsies of skin lesions. More invasive means of establishing a tissue diagnosis include either bronchoscopy, needle biopsy, video-assisted thoracoscopy, cervical mediastinoscopy, and thoracotomy. Flexible fiberoptic bronchoscopy to visualize all the central, lobar, segmental, and subsegmental airways (see Color Plate 3F) can be performed on awake patients with local sedation; it has a low morbidity and mortality and is highly accurate, with a sensitivity of approximately 95% for diagnosing lesions that can be directly visualized. The sensitivity of fiberoptic bronchoscopy for peripheral lesions is lower than for directly visualized airway lesions, with a sensitivity dependent on size and location of the lesion. Peripheral nodules can also be biopsied with fluoroscopic guidance. Bronchoscopy also provides important staging information by allowing inspection of potential resection margins for endobronchial tumor and by allowing detection of occult second primary lesions, which are present in 1 to 3% of patients presenting with lung cancer. All patients in whom a resection of a carcinoma is planned should undergo a bronchoscopic examination, either at the time of surgery or prior to it. Needle biopsy of suspicious pulmonary masses under either fluoroscopic or CT guidance is highly accurate, with a sensitivity of 90 to 95%. Video-assisted thoracoscopy is increasingly used to diagnose pulmonary nodules and provides excellent tissue specimens. Lesions that lie close to the visceral pleura are most easily accessible by this technique. Cervical mediastinoscopy with sampling of lymph nodes is also highly accurate in selected patients with lymphadenopathy. Finally, thoracotomy with biopsy of a lesion is often appropriately used when the pretest probability of a malignancy is high, such as when a peripheral nodule has been demonstrated to increase in size on serial chest radiographs.

Staging

Accurate staging of lung cancer is necessary to predict prognosis and determine the appropriate therapy. The staging systems for NSCLC and SCLC are different: in NSCLC a TNM (tumor-node-metastasis) staging system is used, whereas in SCLC, patients are divided into those with limited and extensive disease (Tables 85–4 through 85–6).

All patients with lung cancer should have a thorough history and physical examination with attention to symptoms of metastatic disease, such as weight loss and bone pain, and signs such as lymphadenopathy and neurologic abnormalities. Laboratory studies include a complete blood cell count, liver function tests, and serum calcium assay. Routine radiographic studies include a chest radiograph with posteroanterior and lateral views. In most patients, chest CT with extension through the liver and adrenals is useful. In subsets of patients, such as those with obvious contralateral hilar or

Table 85–4 ■ STAGING OF SMALL CELL LUNG CANCER

Limited	Tumor confined to chest plus supraclavicular nodes, but excluding cervical, axillary nodes
Extensive	Tumor outside of above confines

Table 85-5 ■ STAGING DEFINITIONS FOR NON-SMALL CELL LUNG CANCER

Tumor

T0	No tumor
TX	Primary tumor cannot be assessed; or positive cytology, no apparent tumor
Tis	Carcinoma in situ
T1	Tumor <3 cm diameter; no visceral pleural or main bronchial involvement
T2	Tumor >3 cm diameter, visceral pleural or main bronchial involvement >2 cm from carina; atelectasis extending to hilum but not involving whole lung
T3	Direct extension to chest wall, diaphragm, mediastinal pleura, parietal pericardium or <2 cm from carina, but not involving carina; atelectasis involving whole lung
T4	Invades heart, great vessels, esophagus, trachea, carina, vertebrae, malignant pleural or pericardial effusion, or satellite tumor nodules within the ipsilateral primary tumor lobe of lung

Nodes

N0	No involvement
NX	Cannot assess regional lymph nodes
N1	Ipsilateral peribronchial or hilar nodal involvement and intrapulmonary nodes involved by direct extension
N2	Ipsilateral mediastinal or subcarinal nodal metastasis
N3	Contralateral mediastinal or hilar nodal metastasis; any supraclavicular or scalene nodal metastasis

Metastasis

M0	None detected
M1	Any distant metastasis

From Mountain CF: Chest 111:1710, 1997.

mediastinal adenopathy on the plain chest radiograph, chest CT may not be necessary. CT of the brain and abdomen is frequently ordered in asymptomatic patients with SCLC because of the high incidence of metastases.

Intrathoracic lymph nodes that exceed 1 cm in size have a high likelihood of harboring metastatic disease. However, a variety of benign conditions including pneumonia, healed tuberculous and fungal infection, silicosis, and sarcoidosis, can cause significant lymphadenopathy, so the specificity of lymph node enlargement for metastasis is as low as 60%. Therefore, enlarged intrathoracic lymph nodes should always undergo biopsy, and metastatic disease should be proven before therapy is planned in patients with NSCLC. Cervical mediastinoscopy is the most common option; needle biopsy (either transbronchial or transthoracic), video-assisted thoracoscopy, and mediastinal exploration at thoracotomy are also useful in certain patients.

The presence of metastatic disease outside the chest predicts a poor prognosis, and these patients are almost never referred for surgery. In the absence of any symptoms, clinical signs, or laboratory abnormalities suggesting metastasis, routine brain, liver, and bone scans are not cost-effective for detecting occult metastases. Bone scans are complicated by a high rate of false-positive results due to old fractures. CT of the upper abdomen is often performed

Table 85-6 ■ STAGE GROUPING AND SURVIVAL FOR NON-SMALL CELL LUNG CANCER

		5-YR SURVIVAL (%)	
STAGE	DEFINITION	Clinical Staging	Pathologic Staging
0	Carcinoma in situ		
IA	T1N0M0	60	67
IB	T2N0M0	38	57
IIA	T1N1M0	34	55
IIB	T2N1M0, T3N0M0	22–24	38
IIIA	T3N1M0, T1N2M0 T2N2M0, T3N2M0	9–13	25
IIIB	T4, any N, M0 T1–3, N3, M0	3–7	
IV	Any T, any N, M1	1	

T = tumor; N = node; M = metastasis.

in asymptomatic patients to detect occult metastases, particularly silent metastasis involving the adrenal gland. However, a high incidence of adrenal adenomas occurs in the normal population, so the rate of false-positive findings is high; most adrenal lesions in patients without clinical signs of metastatic disease should be histologically confirmed to be metastatic disease before altering treatment plans.

PHYSIOLOGIC ASSESSMENT FOR RESECTION. Before considering a patient for surgical resection of a bronchogenic carcinoma, it must be determined that adequate pulmonary reserve exists to permit this therapy. Simple spirometry and an arterial blood gas measurement are the only tests routinely required. Patients with a forced expiratory volume in 1 second (FEV_1) of greater than 60% predicted or more than 2.0 L will likely tolerate a pneumonectomy. When pulmonary function does not appear to be evenly distributed between right and left lungs, perfusion scanning, which correlates well with regional pulmonary function, may help estimate postoperative pulmonary function. CO_2 retention on arterial blood gas analysis, unless solely on the basis of a low respiratory drive, is a predictor of poor postoperative outcome, but hypoxemia is not a strong indicator of poor outcome. The roles of exercise testing and pulmonary artery pressure measurement are unclear.

With the advent of lung-sparing operations, including sleeve-and-wedge resections, many patients who previously would not have been considered surgical candidates are now undergoing pulmonary resection. Close collaboration between internists and thoracic surgeons is necessary to determine whether marginal candidates are indeed appropriate for surgical therapy.

TREATMENT

Non-Small Cell Lung Cancer Therapy

SURGICAL. Surgery offers the best chance for curing appropriately staged patients with NSCLC. Patients with stages I through IIIA NSCLC are routinely considered for surgery, with 5-year survival rates ranging from 60 to 80% for patients with stage I disease to 15 to 25% for selected patients with stage IIIA disease. Since the late 1960s, operative mortality has dropped from 10 to 20% to approximately 3%. The incidence of "fruitless thoracotomy," in which a lesion is discovered to be inoperable at the time of thoracotomy, has decreased from 25% to approximately 5%. The increased use of lung-sparing resections including sleeve lobectomy, segmentectomy, wedge resection, and thoracoscopic wedge resection has allowed surgical therapy to be applied to a group of patients with less pulmonary reserve than in the past. Although a prospective trial comparing conventional lobectomy with wedge resection has demonstrated that local recurrence rates are higher with the latter procedure, wedge resection is still an acceptable alternative in patients with diminished pulmonary reserve.

Before a decision for surgical therapy is made in a given patient, three questions must be addressed (Fig. 85-1). (1) Is the cell type NSCLC? With the exception of peripheral solitary pulmonary nodules without hilar or mediastinal lymphadenopathy, a firm tissue diagnosis should almost always be obtained prior to surgical therapy. Owing to the rarity with which SCLC presents with stage I disease and the likelihood that surgical therapy benefits stage I patients, it may not be necessary to obtain tissue diagnosis for all patients in this group prior to surgical therapy. (2) Is the patient physiologically capable of tolerating resectional surgery? General medical criteria, such as absence of a recent myocardial infarction, should be applied. In addition, physiologic assessment should determine whether the planned resection will leave the patient with adequate pulmonary reserve. (3) Can the lesion be completely resected? This answer requires adequate staging with detection of both distant metastases and local lymph node involvement. As surgical therapy provides the best hope for long-term survival in NSCLC, physiologic assessment and staging should be accurate and objective.

RADIATION THERAPY. Radiation therapy of NSCLC often effectively controls local disease. Significant physiologic impairment does result, however, so most patients who might be considered for curative radiation therapy are also candidates for curative surgical therapy. Although few trials of radiation therapy have been undertaken in early-stage lung cancer, an estimated 10 to 20% of localized lesions can be cured by radiation. Radiation therapy is often

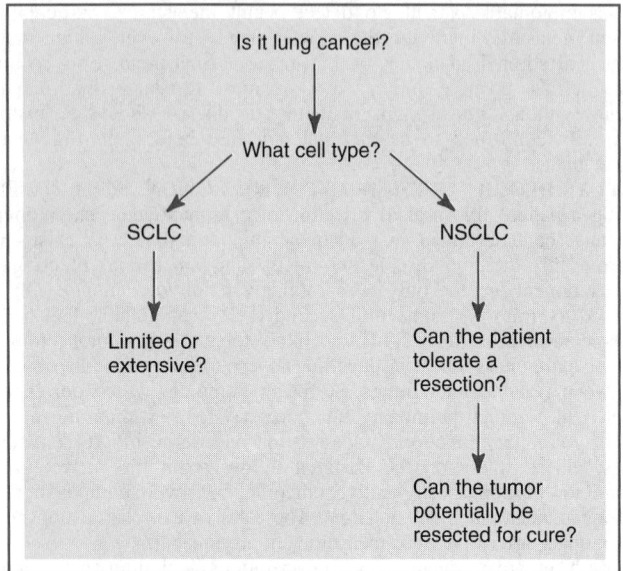

FIGURE 85-1 ■ Questions to determine therapy for lung cancer.

used to palliate symptoms; endobronchial symptoms, including hemoptysis and obstruction, frequently respond to radiation. Distant metastases also are frequently treated primarily with radiation. Radiation therapy is an important component of combined modality therapy of NSCLC.

CHEMOTHERAPY. A number of drugs are frequently used: cisplatin, carboplatin, paclitaxel, mitomycin, vinca alkaloids, ifosfamide, and etoposide. Newer regimens, such as carboplatin and paclitaxel, have improved activity over the regimens with which most controlled trials have been performed. Trials comparing chemotherapy with best supportive care for stage IV NSCLC have yielded conflicting results; however, several recent trials and meta-analyses suggest a small (several weeks to months increased survival) benefit from chemotherapy, and the costs of the chemotherapy option are less than the best supportive care because of lower utilization of palliative treatments. Several trials treating stage IIIB patients with chemotherapy plus radiation have demonstrated a longer survival with chemoradiotherapy than with radiation alone. Further trials are under way.

In selecting patients with NSCLC for chemotherapy, several factors should be kept in mind. Survival is reduced and side effects of chemotherapy are increased in patients who are not fully ambulatory; benefits to this group are likely to be minimal. Response to therapy must be ascertainable. Patients must be fully informed of the limitations of chemotherapy in NSCLC; many physicians discontinue treatment if no clinical response occurs after two or three cycles of chemotherapy. Most patients with NSCLC are not cured by surgery and eventually die with stage IV disease; the disappointing response to chemotherapy for this subgroup emphasizes the major need for new agents and approaches.

MULTIMODALITY THERAPY. In patients with resectable stage II or III NSCLC, surgical therapy often fails because of local, mediastinal, or distant metastatic recurrence; adding adjuvant radiation therapy decreases the risk of mediastinal recurrence but does not improve overall survival. Several trials have demonstrated increased disease-free survival in stage II and III NSCLC patients treated after resection either with chemotherapy or with radiation therapy plus chemotherapy; again, however, overall survival has not increased. Induction chemotherapy, followed by surgery, has shown survival benefit in two relatively small phase III trials and is being evaluated further.

Therapy of Small Cell Lung Cancer

Before the development of effective chemotherapy for SCLC, the median survival was approximately 6 to 12 weeks for extensive disease and approximately 6 months for limited-stage SCLC; the overall 5-year survival rate was <1%. With optimal therapy, current median survival for limited-stage SCLC exceeds 1 year, and for extensive-stage disease it is approximately 10 months. The 5-year survival rate has increased to between 5 and 10%.

Chemotherapy is the cornerstone of treatment for both limited- and extensive-stage SCLC. A variety of agents have activity. Many experts believe that regimens containing etoposide and either carboplatin or cisplatin offer the best combination of efficacy and lack of toxicity.

A number of trials have examined whether increased duration or intensity of chemotherapy for SCLC is beneficial. At the present time, no data support the efficacy of more than four to six cycles of chemotherapy. Increasing dose intensity above standard results in increased toxicity and is not currently supported.

In patients with limited-stage SCLC, the most frequent site of recurrence is the primary lesion. Therefore, at the present time, either concurrent or alternating chest radiation therapy with chemotherapy is preferred in patients with limited-stage disease. No evidence indicates that prophylactic cranial irradiation improves survival, but it is associated with increased central nervous system morbidity. In patients with extensive-stage SCLC, radiation therapy is generally not used in the initial management because chemotherapy produces initial palliation in 80% or more of cases. The addition of radiation therapy does not seem to increase survival, but it does increase toxicity. Radiation therapy is used as palliation in patients in whom initial chemotherapy fails.

A small proportion (<1%) of patients with SCLC present with stage I disease. This rare subset of patients has a 5-year survival of 50 to 70% if treated by surgery followed by chemotherapy with or without radiation therapy. Surgery for patients with SCLC, with the exception of rare stage I disease, is not indicated.

PROGNOSIS

The overall prognosis for patients with lung cancer remains grim, with a 5-year survival rate of 14%. Owing to the high incidence of bronchogenic carcinoma, this 14% survival rate represents a large number of patient years that are potentially salvageable, however. Certain subgroups, including patients with stage I and II NSCLC treated by surgery, have a 40 to 85% 5-year survival rate, making it critical for the physician to recognize and appropriately diagnose and treat these individuals. Long-term survivors of both NSCLC and SCLC are a high-risk group for second primary lung cancers, with an incidence of 3 to 5% per year.

PREVENTION

The most important preventive measure is deterring young individuals from starting to smoke (see Chapter 13). This public health issue is mainly a social, economic, and political problem. Increasing the cost of tobacco products, through increased taxes, is an effective strategy for keeping people from starting this habit. Negative advertising and measures that make it less socially acceptable and glamorous to smoke are also effective.

Smoking cessation is also an important strategy and results in a gradual decrease in risk for lung cancer over 10 to 15 years. Approximately 5 to 20% of patients who enter a smoking cessation program are successful long term. Physician input is crucial in this process.

Large trials in the 1970s that examined the value of early detection efforts using sputum cytology and chest radiographs as screening tools failed to show a benefit in terms of long-term survival. A shortcoming of these trials is that women and high-risk smokers were not studied. It is possible that early detection may become a viable strategy, especially if improved screening tests are developed and high-risk groups targeted.

Chemoprevention of lung cancer may be possible. The use of 13-*cis*-retinoic acid in patients with laryngeal cancer has been shown to decrease the incidence of second primary lesions in the aerodigestive system. However, toxicity associated with high doses of this compound is significant. Vitamin A and its derivatives have potent effects on the differentiation of the respiratory epithelium and are logical agents for chemoprevention studies, but several trials have demonstrated that dietary supplementation with β-carotene alone or in combination with vitamin A or vitamin E actually increased rates of lung cancer in a susceptible population. These unexpected results emphasize the need for further controlled trials. Additional micronutrients, including selenium, vitamins C and E, and low dose 13-*cis*-retinoic acid, may have protective effects. Owing to the large reservoir of smokers and ex-smokers at risk, chemoprevention has considerable potential.

American Thoracic Society/European Respiratory Society: Pretreatment evaluation of non-small cell lung cancer. Am J Respir Crit Care Med 156:320, 1997. *A well-referenced and broad review of the field, containing much information on efficient, cost-effective work-up and staging.*

Lee JD, Ginsberg RJ: The multimodality treatment of stage IIIA/B non-small cell lung cancer. Hematol/Oncol Clin North Am 11:279, 1997. *Concise review of a rapidly evolving area.*

Miller YE, Franklin WA: Molecular events in lung carcinogenesis. Hematol/Oncol Clin North Am 11:215, 1997. *Reviews molecular genetic alterations in lung cancer and premalignant bronchial epithelium.*

Mountain CF: Revisions in the international system for staging lung cancer. Chest 111:1710, 1997. *Outlines the new staging system and describes prognosis of various stage groupings.*

86 DISEASES OF THE DIAPHRAGM, CHEST WALL, PLEURA, AND MEDIASTINUM

Bartolome R. Celli

THE DIAPHRAGM

The diaphragm, the most important muscle of respiration, is shaped like a thin dome and separates the thoracic and abdominal cavities. It has two components—the central non-contractile tendon and the muscle fibers that arise from it and radiate down and outward to insert distally in the circumferential caudal limits of the rib cage. There is a hiatus for the structures that pass from thorax to abdomen. The diaphragm is neurologically controlled by the phrenic nerve, the motor neurons of which arise in the cervical spinal cord at levels C3 to C5. The anatomic arrangement of the diaphragm and its coupling to the rib cage/abdomen explain its mechanical action. Diaphragmatic contraction displaces the abdominal contents downward and raises the ribs outward, resulting in the negative intrapleural inspiratory pressure. Like the heart, the diaphragm and, to a lesser degree, the other respiratory muscles must intermittently contract throughout a person's life. Unlike the heart, it has no intrinsic contractile mechanism, and the respiratory cycle is regulated by a complex set of centrally organized neurons and several peripheral feedback mechanisms that synchronize the diaphragm with many other muscles. The diaphragm serves other non-respiratory functions such as speech, defecation, and parturition. The blood supply to the diaphragm is rich and is arranged to minimize interruption during contraction. Nevertheless, the muscle itself is highly oxygen dependent.

DYSFUNCTION AND FATIGUE. Diaphragmatic dysfunction is most frequently caused by lung hyperinflation—acute as in asthma or chronic as in chronic obstructive pulmonary disease. Hyperinflation shortens the diaphragm and changes its shape to a flatter one in which the horizontal fibers do not generate the normally expanding action on the thorax but rather an inward retraction of the lower rib cage (i.e., Hoover's sign in chronic obstructive pulmonary disease). These changes, coupled with increased airways resistance and decreased lung and chest wall compliance, result in increased work of breathing. If the increased energy demand outstrips the energy supply, the muscle fatigues and ventilation may fail.

Diaphragmatic fatigue can be determined by using pressure measurements across the diaphragm (transdiaphragmatic pressure) or by the more elaborate power spectrum analysis of electromyographic signals. Both correlate well with the simpler clinical signs of increased respiratory rate with progressively shallow breathing. As fatigue progresses, ventilation is maintained by intermittent expansions of rib cage and abdomen (respiratory alternans) and then paradoxical inward abdominal motion during inspiration (abdominal paradox). A number of strategies can improve diaphragmatic function in impending fatigue (Table 86–1); if fatigue results in hyper-

Table 86–1 ■ THERAPEUTIC MODALITIES TO IMPROVE DIAPHRAGMATIC FUNCTION

Reduce mechanical load
1. Decrease airways resistance (administer bronchodilators, treat infection, decrease inflammation).
2. Reduce hyperinflation.
3. Decrease ventilatory requirement (administer oxygen, control fever, avoid caloric loads).
Improve respiratory muscle contractility and endurance
1. Administer oxygen therapy.
2. Improve nutrition.
3. Improve cardiovascular performance.
4. Correct electrolytes (sodium, potassium, calcium, phosphorus).
5. Administer drugs that improve contractility (theophylline, β_2-agonist, caffeine).
6. Check for hypothyroidism or drugs that impair contractility (aminoglycosides).
7. Give ventilatory muscle training.
Improve respiratory muscle coordination and energy conservation
Rehabilitation
Respiratory muscle resting

capnia and acidosis, the respiratory muscles must be rested with mechanical ventilation for at least 1 to several days.

DISORDERS OF DIAPHRAGMATIC MOTION. Unilateral diaphragmatic paralysis is usually secondary to phrenic nerve involvement by a tumor, with bronchogenic carcinoma being the most frequent. Paralysis may result from neurologic diseases such as myelitis, encephalitis, poliomyelitis, and herpes zoster; from trauma to the thorax or cervical spine; or from compression by benign processes such as a substernal thyroid, aortic aneurysm, and infectious collections. With the advent of cardiac surgery, paralysis secondary to phrenic nerve cooling has increased. Occasionally, the paralysis may be idiopathic. The diagnosis is suspected when, on the chest radiograph, the diaphragmatic leaflet is elevated and is confirmed fluoroscopically by observing paradoxical diaphragmatic motion on sniff and cough. In patients with normal lungs, unilateral paralysis is usually asymptomatic and rarely requires treatment. Irreversible symptomatic unilateral paralysis may be treated with surgical plication of the affected hemidiaphragm. Bilateral paralysis usually results from high cervical trauma (C3 to C5), neuropathies, or myopathies. The myopathy may be generalized (muscular dystrophy, polymyositis, hypothyroidism) or limited, primarily affecting the diaphragm (acid maltase deficiency, collagen vascular disorders). In many cases the cause remains unknown. Patients become symptomatic early. The dyspnea is characteristically worsened by the supine position because abdominal contents displace the diaphragm into the thorax, resulting in a significant (>500 mL) drop in the vital capacity and in oxygen saturation. Fluoroscopy is not reliable because the flaccid diaphragm may lag behind the rib cage expansion when accessory muscles contract, thus giving the impression of diaphragmatic contraction. The diagnosis is suspected by the presence of inspiratory abdominal paradoxical retraction. It is confirmed by measuring transdiaphragmatic pressure with and without electromyographic recording. Phrenic nerve conduction establishes the diagnosis of neuropathy. Treatment of ventilatory failure secondary to bilateral paralysis consists of intermittent mechanical ventilation. In some cases, such as cardiac surgery, the paralysis recovers, and ventilation may be discontinued. In permanent paralysis with intact muscle function (e.g., high quadriplegic), diaphragmatic pacing has been lifesaving.

Hiccup (singultus) is a disorder produced by spasm of the diaphragm followed by closure of the glottis during an inspiratory effort. Hiccups are usually self-limited but may persist for days or weeks. In most patients a cause is never found, but hiccups may occasionally be a sign of serious disease such as a central nervous system disorder (encephalitis, stroke, tumor), uremia, herpes zoster, and pleural or abdominal processes that irritate the diaphragm. Prolonged hiccups are sometimes psychogenic. In general, hiccups subside spontaneously or when the initiating disease improves. When hiccups are chronic or debilitating, local anesthesia or phrenic nerve crushing may be required (permanent paralysis may occur with the latter). Diaphragmatic flutter is a rare disorder in which rhythmic contractions of the diaphragm occur at a rate of 1 to 8/sec; the cause and treatment are similar to those of hiccups.

Diaphragmatic hernias occur through congenitally weak or incompletely fused areas of the diaphragm, through the esophageal hiatus (>70% of all hernias), or because of traumatic rupture of the muscle. Anterior hernias occur through the foramina of Morgagni, are rare, and tend to occur in obese patients; they usually show as a rounded density in the right cardiophrenic angle. Posterior hernias through the foramina of Bochdalek are more common, especially in infants; they occur more frequently on the left. Traumatic diaphragmatic hernias may result from penetrating injuries or abdominal compression. Diaphragmatic hernias usually contain omentum but may also contain stomach, bowel, or liver anteriorly or kidney and spleen posteriorly.

Symptom severity depends on the extension of abdominal contents into the thorax and the presence of strangulation. Hernias may be asymptomatic for several years before respiratory and abdominal symptoms occur.

Eventration may resemble a hernia but consists of a localized elevation of the diaphragm resulting from impaired muscle development or weakness. Eventration is more frequent in the right anteromedial portion and tends to occur in middle-aged obese persons; once differentiated from neoplasm, it rarely requires surgical treatment.

A diaphragmatic hernia is suspected on chest radiography and in some cases when there is borborygmus over the chest. Computed tomographic (CT) scans, gastrointestinal contrast films, radioisotope scan of the liver, and induction of a pneumoperitoneum with a follow-up film help establish the diagnosis. In infants, large hernias may compromise ventilation, requiring immediate surgical correction. In the asymptomatic adult with previous evidence of a hernia, observation is indicated. Surgery may be needed for diagnosis or to relieve strangulation of sac contents.

Celli BR, Grassino A: Respiratory muscles: Functional evaluation. Semin Respir Crit Care Med 19:367–381, 1998. *Comprehensive, up-to-date review covering the clinical aspects and practical application of respiratory muscle function.*

Jasmer RM, Luce JM, Matthay MA: Noninvasive positive pressure ventilation for acute respiratory failure. Chest 111:1672–1678, 1997. *This article reviews the reasoning for mechanical ventilation as a treatment for fatiguing respiratory muscles. It analyzes non-invasive ventilation, an area of renewed interest, and has a good solid list of references.*

THE CHEST WALL

The chest wall, an integral part of the ventilatory pump, consists of the bony thoracic cage (ribs, sternum, and vertebrae) and the various muscles of respiration. Besides the diaphragm, the intercostals and scaleni are active even during quiet breathing in normal persons. Other muscles such as the sternocleidomastoid, pectoralis minor and major, serratus anterior, latissimus dorsi, and trapezius partake in respiration during increased ventilatory demand. Even the abdominal muscles can participate in ventilation, by contracting during exhalation. The thoracic cage is a major determinant of ventilation and of static and dynamic lung volumes. Diseases that disrupt the system alter the ventilation and ventilation-perfusion relationship, thus causing hypoxemia or hypercapnia. Primary disorders of the chest wall may occur from impairments of the neuromuscular apparatus or the bony thoracic cage. Alterations in the neuromuscular apparatus are dealt with in different parts of the text, whereas primary alterations of the bony thoracic cage are dealt with in this section.

Diseases of the bony thoracic cage (Table 86–2) are all linked by a similar pathophysiologic process: (1) changes in chest wall compliance, (2) variable lung compression, (3) ventilation-perfusion imbalance, (4) alveolar hypoventilation, and (5) pulmonary hypertension and cor pulmonale. Clinical symptoms include dyspnea without significant cough, sputum, or pain. Physical examination usually establishes the diagnosis and helps determine the presence of cor pulmonale.

KYPHOSCOLIOSIS. Deformities of the dorsolumbar spine are the most common causes of symptomatic derangements of the chest wall. Scoliosis consists of lateral angulation and rotation of the spine and is categorized as right (most frequent) or left according to the direction of the convexity of the curvature. Kyphosis is less important and consists of anteroposterior angulation of the spine.

The severity of scoliosis is quantified by measuring the angle (Cobb's angle) between the upper and lower portions of the spinal curve on a radiograph. Only when this angle exceeds 70 degrees is any abnormality of respiratory function detectable. When the angle is more than 120 degrees, dyspnea and respiratory failure are expected. The ribs over the convex side are separated and rotated posteriorly, giving rise to the kyphoscoliotic hump. On the concave side, the ribs are crowded and displaced anteriorly, combined with decreased thoracic height. These abnormalities produce forward bulging of the anterior wall.

Kyphoscoliosis is usually idiopathic and begins in childhood. Ventilatory failure may result in death in the fourth to sixth decade. If the scoliosis is not severe and progressive, life expectancy may be normal. Static lung volumes, chest wall, and, to a lesser degree, lung compliance are also decreased. Ventilation-perfusion imbalances result in hypoxemia. When the mechanical load, caused by progressive scoliosis or superimposed infection, is such that the muscles fail, the hypoxemia may be associated with hypercapnia. Blood gases may worsen during sleep and cause the frequent worsening of some patients with otherwise stable kyphoscoliosis.

Several therapeutic approaches are available. Surgical correction includes traction, plasters, and rods; the effects are mostly cosmetic, and improvement in pulmonary function is usually minimal. In hypoxemic patients, oxygen is beneficial. Intermittent positive-pressure ventilation increases tidal volume, temporarily improving compliance and lung volumes. In chronic ventilatory failure, night-time ventilatory assistance is beneficial. Efforts must be made to induce the patient to stop smoking. Bronchospasm and respiratory infections must be treated aggressively. If obese, the patient should lose weight.

ANKYLOSING SPONDYLITIS. This inflammatory disease results in fusion of costotransverse and vertebral joints but may also involve sternomanubrial and clavicular joints (see Chapter 287). With relative fixation of the rib cage in an inspiratory position, most of the ventilatory movement is performed by the diaphragm-abdomen, which is already placed in a mechanical disadvantage because of a normal or increased functional residual capacity. In contrast to kyphoscoliosis, cor pulmonale and ventilatory failure are rare. Some patients may develop upper lobe fibrosis with minimal alterations in gas exchange.

PECTUS EXCAVATUM. This congenital deformity of the lower portion of the sternum produces symmetrical bowing of the anterior ribs. In infants it tends to occur with multiple abnormalities and is associated with high mortality. It may also be associated with mitral valve prolapse. With severe deformity, the heart and mediastinal structures are laterally displaced. Although some patients may fail to increase cardiac output normally during exercise, functional impairment is usually mild. Surgical correction is mainly cosmetic.

THORACOPLASTY. Surgical procedures used from 1940 to 1950 to treat tuberculosis included resection of several ribs with collapse of the underlying lung. This procedure results in paradoxical retraction of that portion of the chest wall. Thoracoplasty was originally thought to have minimal physiologic consequences, but the incidence of cardiorespiratory failure is increased in these patients.

FIBROTHORAX. Resulting from pleural diseases such as hemothorax or asbestosis, fibrothorax is also considered a primary disease of chest wall because the lung itself may not be affected. It may result in ventilatory and cardiac failure. The treatment is similar to that for kyphoscoliosis. Occasional pleurectomy may help patients with fibrothorax secondary to pleural fibrosis.

FLAIL CHEST. Flail chest is produced by double fractures of three or more adjacent ribs or by combined sternal and rib fractures. The flail segment paradoxically moves inward during inspiration. The inefficient ventilation increases the work of breathing, which may worsen ventilation owing to the frequent association with neuromuscular impairment. Flail chest occurs most frequently with accidental chest trauma and/or after cardiopulmonary resuscitation. Ventilation-perfusion mismatch and lung contusion cause hypoxemia. In most cases, supportive care with attention to oxy-

Table 86–2 ■ MOST IMPORTANT RIB CAGE DERANGEMENTS

Spine
Scoliosis (idiopathic, congenital, paralytic)
Kyphosis
Ankylosing spondylitis
Sternum, Ribs, or Pleura
Pectus excavatum
Thoracoplasty
Fibrothorax

genation, clear airways, and infection prevention is the preferred therapy. Artificial ventilation should be reserved for patients with ventilatory failure. When the flail segment is large, chest fixation may be considered.

Goldstraw P, Taggart D: Surgery of the chest wall. *In* Roussos C (ed): The Thorax. New York, Marcel Dekker, 1995, p 2701. *Excellent review of the pathophysiologic changes in respiratory function secondary to chest deformities, trauma, and surgery.*

THE PLEURA

ANATOMY AND PHYSIOLOGY. The pleura consists of a layer of mesothelial cells with a smooth semitransparent appearance. It is supported by a network of connective and fibroelastic tissue, lymphatics, and vessels. The mesothelial cells are rich in microvilli, and their most important function is to deliver glycoproteins rich in hyaluronic acid to decrease friction between lung and chest wall. The parietal pleura covers the surface of the chest wall, diaphragm, and mediastinum; it is supplied with blood from the systemic circulation, and contains sensory nerves. The visceral pleura covers the surface of the lungs, including the interlobar fissures; its blood supply arises from the low-pressure pulmonary circulation and has no sensory nerves. The two layers are separated by a virtual cavity, which is lubricated by 5 to 10 mL of fluid, facilitates lung expansion, and helps maintain lung inflation by coupling it with the chest wall.

Pleural fluid has a low protein concentration (<2 g/dL) with a pH and glucose similar to that of blood. Pleural fluid is formed primarily from the parietal pleura, and part of its turnover depends on the same Starling forces that govern vascular and interstitial fluid exchange. The parietal pleura has a hydrostatic pressure similar to that of the systemic circulation (30 cm H_2O), whereas that of the visceral pleura depends on the pulmonary circulation (10 cm H_2O). Oncotic pressure is similar in both (25 cm H_2O), but the pressure within the pleural cavity is affected by the gravity gradient. Thus, the pleural space is heterogeneous with a non-dependent portion where Starling forces favor outpouring of fluid to the cavity and into parenchymal capillaries. The stomas, or "lacuna," present over the parietal surface of the low mediastinum, low chest wall, and diaphragm, seem to empty into lymphatics. These subpleural lymphatics represent the major pathway for liquid and solute drainage. Alterations of this formation-resorption mechanism frequently result in the accumulation of pleural fluid. Increases in hydrostatic forces or decreases in oncotic pressures result in low protein "transudates." Increased outpouring by capillaries or cells and/or blocking of lymphatics results in high-protein "exudates" (Table 86–3).

DIAGNOSTIC PROCEDURES. HISTORY AND PHYSICAL EXAMINATION. Although suggestive, a patient's history of pain, dyspnea, or cough is neither sensitive nor specific. These symptoms may be absent in some large effusions and in critically ill patients. When present, the pain is usually unilateral and sharp and worsens with inspiration or cough. It may radiate to the shoulder, neck, or abdomen. Dyspnea may result from compression of lung tissue and from mechanical alterations in the respiratory muscles as the fluid changes their length-tension relationship. The degree of dyspnea relates to fluid volume and intrathoracic pressure and their effect on mechanics and gas exchange. Pleural effusions in patients with minimal lung compromise are well tolerated, whereas similar effusions in patients with lung disease may cause ventilatory failure. The physical examination shows decreased breath sounds and excursions in the affected hemithorax (splinting). Percussion shows dullness with absent tactile fremitus over the area. Frequently there are E to A changes (egobronchophony) at the upper fluid border where underlying lung parenchyma is compressed.

RADIOLOGIC EXAMINATION. An effusion is suspected when there is blunting and medial displacement of the sharp costophrenic an-

Table 86–3 ■ MECHANISMS THAT LEAD TO ACCUMULATION OF PLEURAL FLUID

1. Increased hydrostatic pressure in microvascular circulation (congestive heart failure)
2. Decreased oncotic pressure in microvascular circulation (severe hypoalbuminemia)
3. Decreased pressure in the pleural space (complete lung collapse)
4. Increased permeability of the microvascular circulation (pneumonia)
5. Impaired lymphatic drainage from the pleural space (malignant effusion)
6. Movement of fluid from peritoneal space (ascites)

Table 86–4 ■ CHARACTERISTICS OF PLEURAL FLUID TRANSUDATES

	ABSOLUTE VALUE	PLEURAL FLUID/ SERUM VALUE
Protein	<3 g/dL	<0.5
Lactate dehydrogenase	<200 IU/L	<0.6
Glucose	>60 mg/dL	1.0
White blood cell count	$<1000/mm^3$	—
Cholesterol	<45 mg/dL	

gle. Fluid accumulation between the lung and the diaphragm (subpulmonic effusion) is suspected when there is apparent elevation of the hemidiaphragm or widening of the shadow between the gascontaining stomach and the lower left lung margin. Up to 300 mL of fluid may fail to be seen in a posteroanterior chest radiograph, whereas as little as 150 mL may be seen in a lateral decubitus view. A supine film (frequent in patients in intensive-care units) may obscure the diagnosis as the fluid layers posteriorly. A pseudotumor occurs when fluid loculates in an interlobar fissure, most commonly in the minor fissure, and gives the radiologic appearance of a tumor; a clue to the diagnosis is the presence of pleural fluid elsewhere and a biconvex lenticular configuration of the mass. A collection of pleural air and fluid (hydropneumothorax) usually produces horizontal and not concave margins. A pneumothorax is identified by the contrast between the water density of the visceral pleura centrally and the gas lucency without vascular markings laterally. Small pneumothoraces may be harder to diagnose, but an expiratory film may help outline them. Pleural plaques may be seen when calcified or may be detected when viewed tangentially but not en face. Ultrasonography and CT scans may provide better definition of pleural and parenchymal abnormalities.

THORACENTESIS AND PLEURAL FLUID ANALYSIS. Thoracentesis may be performed for diagnosis or therapy. A thoracentesis is diagnostic in approximately 75% of patients, and even when not diagnostic it helps exclude other important diagnoses, such as empyema. Diagnostic thoracentesis requires a relatively small amount of material (30 to 50 mL). As a rule, newly discovered effusions should be tapped. Although there are no absolute contraindications to a diagnostic thoracentesis, relative contraindications include a bleeding diathesis, anticoagulation, a small volume, mechanical ventilation, and low benefit-to-risk ratio. Therapeutic thoracentesis involves removing larger amounts of fluid (no more than 1000 to 1500 mL at one time because edema may occur in the re-expanded underlying lung, especially in cases of tension effusions).

Although the classification of "transudate" or "exudate" is not absolute, the distinction is helpful in suggesting further evaluation and possible diagnoses. To differentiate transudates and exudates, it is cost effective to obtain total protein, lactate dehydrogenase (LDH), white blood cell count with differential, and either glucose or pH (Table 86–4). *Transudates* are due to imbalances in hydrostatic and oncotic pressures such as seen in heart failure or hypoalbuminemia; they may result from movement of fluid from the peritoneum to the pleural space. *Exudates* (Table 86–5) are defined by the presence of at least one of the following criteria: (1) pleural fluid/serum protein ratio greater than 0.5; (2) pleural fluid/serum LDH ratio of more than 0.6; and (3) pleural fluid LDH greater than 200 IU/L. A fluid cholesterol level greater than 45 mg/dL may also be helpful.

The diagnoses that can be established by thoracentesis include malignancy, empyema (pus), tuberculosis (positive acid-fast bacillus in smear or cultures), fungal infection (positive potassium hydroxide stains or culture), lupus pleuritis (LE cells), chylothorax (high triglycerides or presence of chylomicrons), urinothorax (pleural fluid/serum creatinine ratio >1), and esophageal rupture (increased pleural fluid amylase and pH around 6.0). Because many diagnoses produce overlapping values, acid-fast and Gram stains, aerobic and anaerobic cultures, cell count and differential, and cytologic analysis should be included in the study of these effusions. A predominance of polymorphonuclear leukocytes (PMNs) is most compatible with bacterial infection, whereas lymphocytes (particularly with paucity of mesothelial cells) suggest tuberculosis. Lymphocytes are also seen in lymphoma and leukemic effusions. Eosinophils are

Table 86–5 ■ CORRELATION OF PLEURAL FLUID EXUDATE FINDINGS AND CAUSATIVE DISEASE

TESTS	DISEASE(S)
pH <7.2	Empyema, malignancy, esophageal rupture; rheumatoid, lupus, and tuberculous pleuritis
Glucose (<60 mg/dL)	Infection, rheumatoid pleurisy, tuberculous and lupus effusions, esophageal rupture
Amylase (>200 μ/dL)	Pancreatic disease, esophageal rupture, malignancy, ruptured ectopic pregnancy
Rheumatoid factor, antinuclear antibody, LE cells	Collagen vascular diseases
Complement (decreased)	Lupus erythematosus, rheumatoid arthritis
Red blood cells (>5000/μL)	Trauma, malignancy, pulmonary embolus
Chylous effusion (triglycerides >110 mg/dL)	Violation of thoracic duct (trauma, malignancy)
Biopsy (+)	Malignancy, tuberculosis

non-specific and suggest long-standing fluid or air, sometimes even in small amounts, as from a prior thoracentesis. A bloody effusion not due to trauma is most likely due to malignancy or pulmonary infarction. A white effusion suggests either chyle, cholesterol, or lymphoma. Black fluid suggests aspergillosis. A yellow-green color may be seen in rheumatoid pleurisy. A putrid odor is diagnostic of anaerobic empyema, whereas an ammonia odor suggests urinothorax. The value of other diagnostic markers such as adenosine deaminase, β_2-microglobulin, pleural/serum cholinesterase, and lysozyme remain to be determined. The complications of thoracentesis include pain, bleeding (local, pleural, or abdominal), pneumothorax, infection, and spleen or liver puncture. With therapeutic thoracentesis, up to 50% of patients experience a temporary fall in PaO$_2$ of as much as 20 mm Hg.

PERCUTANEOUS PLEURAL BIOPSY. Biopsy is indicated to evaluate patients with undiagnosed exudative effusion (particularly those with lymphocytic predominance) because the most frequently diagnosed disease is malignancy or tuberculosis (TB). The procedure is performed under local anesthesia using a hook-type needle (Cope or Abrams). The contraindications are a small or loculated pleural effusion, an uncooperative patient, and anticoagulation or bleeding diathesis including azotemia with abnormal bleeding time. Because pleural seeding may not be uniform, multiple samples are needed. The overall diagnostic yield is about 60% for malignancy and 75% for TB.

EXPLORATION OF THE PLEURA. In most of the 5 to 10% of patients with undiagnosed effusion, the effusion itself disappears spontaneously or the cause becomes evident. When it is considered necessary to make a diagnosis, a biopsy can be obtained through thoracoscopy (introducing a rigid scope with a cold light source). Thoracoscopy may be performed under local anesthesia and has a high yield (> 85%). In some cases, it is necessary to perform an open pleural biopsy under general anesthesia. The main advantage is the possibility of obtaining larger specimens and concomitant lung tissue.

TRANSUDATIVE EFFUSION. Heart failure that results in biventricular failure with venous hypertension, is the most common cause of a transudative effusion. Effusions are often bilateral, usually larger on the right, and on the chest radiograph are associated with vascular congestion and cardiomegaly. In chronic heart failure (months), the total protein may be more than 3 g/dL. Thoracentesis is indicated if the patient is febrile, the effusion is large and unilateral, or there is pain or unexplained hypoxemia. Transudates occur in 5 to 10% of patients with liver cirrhosis, secondary to movement of ascitic fluid through diaphragmatic defects or lymphatic channels; the effusion is more frequent on the right (70%). If in doubt, radioactive tracer injected in the ascitic fluid appears in the chest. The effusion often improves with improvement of the ascites. Occasionally, chemical pleurodesis has effectively relieved symptomatic, recurrent effusions. A transudate is seen in up to 20% of patients with nephrotic syndrome due to decreased oncotic pressure (hypoalbuminemia) and increased hydrostatic forces; fre-

quently bilateral, it improves by correcting the protein-losing nephropathy. Peritoneal dialysis and atelectasis may also cause transudative effusions. Urinothorax is a rare ipsilateral pleural transudate that occurs with urinary system obstruction. The effusion has the characteristic odor of urine, and relief of the obstruction promptly resolves the effusion.

EXUDATIVE EFFUSIONS. INFECTIONS. Parapneumonic effusion (pleural fluid associated with pneumonia or lung abscess) is the most common cause of exudates. They may be uncomplicated and resolve spontaneously with antibiotics or may be complicated and require drainage. Complicated effusions are rich in white blood cells (empyema) and/or have positive Gram stains or cultures. Uncomplicated effusions are usually small and contain moderate amounts of PMNs, a glucose similar to blood, a pH greater than 7.30, and an LDH level less than 500 U/L. In contrast, complicated effusions have large numbers of PMNs, often more than 100,000/mm^3, pH less than 7.20, glucose less than 40 g/dL, and LDH greater than 1000 U/L. If the effusion is also purulent and has bacteria, immediate drainage is necessary and is best achieved with a chest tube. If a fever persists for more than 48 to 72 hours in patients with complicated effusions, either the drainage is inadequate (such as when fluid becomes loculated), the antibiotic is inappropriate, or the diagnosis is wrong. If drainage is not effective because of loculation, inserting an additional tube or instilling intrapleural streptokinase may be effective. Poorly treated empyemas may result in communications with the bronchial tree (bronchopleural fistula) or skin (bronchopleurocutaneous fistula) and require open drainage with rib resection, decortication, and extensive reconstruction. In some patients with uncontrolled pleural sepsis, a thoracotomy with drainage and decortication may be lifesaving. Pleural involvement by non-bacterial, non-tuberculous infection is uncommon and, when present, is usually small. Fungal diseases rarely affect the pleura except for coccidioidomycosis, which may cause a hypersensitivity pleuritis.

OTHER INFECTIVE-INFLAMMATORY DISORDERS. Exudative effusions may result from subdiaphragmatic processes such as upper abdominal abscess, of which a subphrenic site is the most common location. Frequently postoperative in origin, subphrenic abscesses may result from hepatic diseases and gastrointestinal perforations. Patients are usually febrile and dyspneic and manifest an elevated hemidiaphragm with ipsilateral splinting. Abscesses may also arise in the liver or spleen. Antibiotics alone may not be sufficient; drainage may be necessary.

Pancreatitis and pancreatic pseudocyst can cause pleural effusions, more often on the left or bilaterally. The amylase level is higher than that in the serum, and the exudates may be blood tinged; the exudate tends to resolve as the pancreatic problem improves.

Esophageal rupture is an urgent cause of pleural effusion. Close to half of cases are secondary to endoscopy or esophageal dilatation, whereas others are secondary to a foreign body or trauma or occur spontaneously (Boerhaave's syndrome). Patients complain of chest pain, dyspnea, and dysphagia. Fever is universal, and half have subcutaneous emphysema. The radiograph may confirm the emphysema and may show pneumothorax, more frequent on the left. Pleural effusion occurs in 75% of patients, with the findings depending on the time of thoracentesis. Early on the exudate has abundant PMNs, followed by high concentrations of salivary amylase. Later, anaerobic mouth organisms seed the space, and the pH approaches 6.0. The diagnosis is established by using barium sulfate or water-soluble compounds (see Chapter 124). Early diagnosis and prompt surgical correction result in more than 90% survival. If surgical closure is delayed, antibiotics for anaerobes, parenteral nutrition, and mediastinal and pleural drainage are necessary.

TUBERCULOSIS (see Chapter 358). Pleural effusion occurs in most cases of pulmonary TB but is frequently inapparent. The effusion may accompany the primary infection, in which case it is an exudate, is commonly unilateral, and results from a hypersensitivity phenomenon. These patients, who usually are febrile, may recover without treatment, but close to two thirds develop active TB within 5 years. A second form occurs when a subpleural focus of *Mycobacterium tuberculosis* ruptures into the pleural space. The clinical presentation simulates an acute pneumonia (60% of cases) with fever, non-productive cough (80%), chest pain (75%), or a subacute or chronic fever. Chest radiography shows small to moderate effusion (4% are large), with parenchymal disease seen in one third of cases. Intermediate-strength purified protein derivative (PPD) testing is positive in 70% of patients; and if repeated after 6 to 8 weeks it may become positive in those with a prior negative test. The fluid is usually rich in protein (>4 g/dL), with a leukocyte count about 5000 cells/mm^3 (90 to 95% lymphocytes). A PMN predominance may occur the first few days after the bacillus reaches the pleural space. The glucose level may be low, but rarely lower than 20 mg/dL. The pH ranges between 7.00 and 7.30, with pH more than 7.40 virtually excluding TB. The fluid is characteristically free of mesothelial cells. Recently, the presence of adenosine deaminase and lysozyme has been found to correlate with TB. An enzyme-linked immunosorbent assay or polymerase chain reaction to demonstrate mycobacterial antigen may be helpful diagnostically and provide more rapid diagnosis in the more than 90% of cases in which acid-fast bacilli are not seen on smear. Multiple samples from a closed pleural biopsy are positive in 50 to 80% of cases, whereas positive cultures range from 30 to 70%. With all methods combined, the yield is close to 95%. The fever usually resolves within 2 weeks after instituting treatment but may persist for 6 or 8 weeks. The effusion usually resolves by 6 weeks but may persist for 3 to 4 months. Very ill patients may be helped by short-term corticosteroid treatment. Rarely, surgical drainage or decortication may be necessary.

OTHER INFECTIOUS EFFUSIONS. Actinomycosis (see Chapter 354) caused by the anaerobic organism *Actinomyces israelii* may cause purulent effusions that may bulge the thoracic wall and drain through the chest. Sulfur granules (whitish yellow or brown interwoven filaments) can be identified in the fluid. Pleural effusions are also common in *Nocardia* infection (see Chapter 355); the effusion is usually purulent with abundant PMNs, and sulfonamides are the treatment of choice. Aspergillosis (see Chapter 401) of the pleura is uncommon, but an inflammatory, thickened pleura is frequently seen in progressive invasive aspergillosis. Pleural effusions due to parasitic diseases are uncommon but increasing among Third World immigrants. Paragonimiasis (see Chapter 432) causes pleural thickening or effusion in up to 48% of patients; the effusion has a triad of low glucose (<10 g/dL), high LDH (>1000 U/L), and low pH (<7.10); complement-fixation antibodies greater than 1:64 are diagnostic. Amebiasis and echinococcosis are rare causes of pleural effusions.

HEMOTHORAX. Frank blood in the pleural space (hematocrit >20%) is usually the result of trauma, hematologic disorders, pulmonary infarction, or pleural malignancies. Left-sided pneumothorax, particularly with a widened mediastinum, may indicate rupture of the aorta. Pleural blood often does not clot and can be readily removed by lymphatics if the volume is small. Larger effusions require tube drainage. Persistent bleeding requires surgical correction.

CHYLOTHORAX. Leakage of the lymph (chyle) from the thoracic duct most commonly results from mediastinal malignancy (50%), especially lymphoma. Chylothorax may also result from thoracic surgery (20%) or trauma (5%). The triad of slow-growing yellow nails, lymphedema, and pleural effusion (yellow-nail syndrome) is due to hypoplastic or dilated lymphatics. Because chyle collects within the posterior mediastinum, the chylothorax may not appear for days, until the mediastinal pleura ruptures. The usual milky appearance of the effusion may be confused with a cholesterol effusion or an effusion with many leukocytes. The best diagnostic criterion for chylothorax is the presence of a triglyceride concentration greater than 110 mg/dL, with rare instances of values between 50 and 110 mg/dL. The major complications are malnutrition and immunologic compromise, as fat, protein, and lymphocytes are depleted with repeated thoracentesis or chest tube drainage. Treatment should include drainage of the pleural space and attempts to decrease chyle formation by intravenous hyperalimentation, decreased oral fat intake, and intake of medium-chain triglycerides, which are absorbed directly into the portal circulation. For traumatic effusions, thoracic duct ligation should be considered; when due to tumor, treatment should focus on the primary cause.

IMMUNOLOGIC CAUSES OF PLEURAL EFFUSIONS. Clinical pleurisy occurs in close to 5% of patients with *rheumatoid arthritis* (see Chapter 286), even though autopsy studies suggest up to 50% involvement. It has a male predominance and appears within 5 years after onset of the disease; nevertheless, effusions have occurred up to 20 years before the onset of articular disease. The fluid is an exudate with low glucose (<30 mg/dL), low pH, and high LDH. The complement level is usually low, with high titers of

rheumatoid factor. The patient may complain of pleuritic pain or dyspnea. Fever is not common, in contrast with lupus pleuritis. The effusion does not resolve quickly but rather over months and occasionally persists over years. The major complication is fibrosis with lung trapping. Anti-inflammatory agents and corticosteroids are recommended therapy. Pleuritic pain or effusion can be the presenting manifestation in 5% of patients with *systemic lupus erythematosus* and occurs at some point in the course in up to 50% of patients. Pain (86%), cough (64%), dyspnea (50%), pleural friction rub (71%), and fever (57%) are common. The effusions are exudates that in the majority of cases have normal pH and glucose. Hemolytic complement, especially C3 and C4 components, is low, and classic LE cells may be present. Lupus pleuritis is likely if the antinuclear antibody ratio in the fluid is more than 1:160. Spontaneous resolution of lupus pleuritis is uncommon, but it usually disappears within 2 weeks after beginning therapy with corticosteroids. Sarcoidosis, Wegener's granulomatosis, Sjögren's syndrome, and immunoblastic lymphadenopathy are rare causes of pleural effusions.

OTHER CONDITIONS. Asbestosis (see Chapter 78) is frequently associated with pleural disease; the effusion is often unilateral, small, and serosanguineous. The cell count is less than 6000 cells/mm^3, with either PMNs or mononuclear predominance. Eosinophilia to up to 50% of the white blood cell count has been described. The diagnosis is suspected with known exposure. Exclusion of malignant mesothelioma in the presence of pleural plaques may be difficult and requires follow-up every 2 to 3 years. The effusion tends to resolve in 1 month to 1 year, leaving a blunted costophrenic angle in more than 90% of patients and diffuse pleural thickening in about 50%. Calcification of the plaques occurs late (20 to 40 years after exposure). About 5% of patients may have underlying pulmonary parenchymal asbestosis.

Meigs' syndrome is the triad of benign fibroma or other ovarian tumors with ascites and large pleural effusions (usually on the right side). Most commonly seen after menopause, the symptoms are malaise, chest pain, and increased abdominal girth. Fluid moves from the abdomen through small diaphragmatic defects or lymphatics. The fluid is usually an exudate with a paucity of mononuclear cells. When suspected, the pelvic examination or abdominal-pelvic CT scan documents the ovarian tumor. Removal of the tumor resolves the effusion within 2 to 3 weeks.

Uremia causes a polyserositis and usually a bloody pleural exudate that resolves with treatment of the uremia. The diagnosis must be distinguished from a urinothorax or a hydrothorax caused by the nephrotic syndrome. Repeated thoracentesis may be needed if the patient is symptomatic (dyspnea, cough, chest pain).

Other causes of inflammatory effusions include radiation therapy, esophageal sclerotherapy, enteral feeding misplacement, and drug-induced pleural disease from medications such as nitrofurantoin, dantrolene, methysergide, methotrexate, procarbazine, amiodarone, mitomycin, bleomycin, and minoxidil. Pleuritis with a lupus-like syndrome has been associated with procainamide, hydralazine, isoniazid, and quinidine; signs and symptoms usually resolve after discontinuing the medicine but may occasionally require corticosteroids.

MALIGNANCY. Malignant effusions probably are the most common cause of exudate in patients older than age 60. Invasion by lung cancer is the most frequent, whereas spread from liver metastasis or chest wall lymphatic invasion is the most frequent mechanism in breast cancer. Ovarian and gastric cancer represent close to 5% of cases, whereas 7% may have an unknown primary lesion at time of diagnosis. Patients may be asymptomatic or develop cough, pain, and dyspnea. The effusion is an exudate with abundant red cells (30,000 to 50,000/mL) and mononuclear cells (lymphocytes >50%). Occasionally (5 to 10%) they are transudative, and about one third may have pH less than 7.3 or glucose value less than 60 mg/dL. Cytology is positive in close to 60% of cases, but biopsy increases the yield only to 70%. Thoracentesis should be repeated if the diagnosis is still suspected. Malignant pleural effusion carries a very poor prognosis, with the exception of breast and small cell carcinoma of the lung, both of which may respond temporarily to therapy. The best method, short of pleurectomy or pleural abrasion, to control recurrent malignant effusion is to instill tetracycline, talc, or medroxyprogesterone intrapleurally after chest tube drainage.

Lymphomas, especially non-Hodgkin's lymphoma, may cause exudative effusions because of tumor spread to the pleura. Mediastinal invasion with lymphatic blockage and effusion is more common with Hodgkin's lymphoma. Although the prognosis is unsure when lymphoma causes pleural effusion, patients frequently respond to chemotherapy.

MALIGNANT MESOTHELIOMA. Asbestos exposure precedes 80 to 90% of malignant mesotheliomas. Patients may present with dyspnea, cough, weight loss, and pain. Smoking is not a risk factor. The tumors often encase the underlying lung. The effusion may be massive and is often bloody; in 70% of cases, the pH is less than 7.30. Cytology is controversial because even when positive it may be difficult to differentiate mesothelioma from metastatic carcinoma. Elevated levels of hyaluronic acid and special stains and electron microscopy of biopsy tissue may help in the diagnosis. Median survival is 8 to 12 months after diagnosis. Malignant mesotheliomas may be confused with benign mesothelioma, which has the histology of a fibroma. Benign mesotheliomas may reach a large size and be pedunculated (migrating with position changes); they are often associated with hypertrophic pulmonary osteoarthropathy and clubbing. Treatment of mesothelioma involves surgical removal and, in malignant cases, chemotherapy.

PNEUMOTHORAX. Pneumothorax is defined as an accumulation of gas in the pleural space. It may be caused by (1) perforation of the visceral pleura and entry of gas from the lung; (2) penetration of the chest wall, diaphragm, mediastinum, or esophagus; or (3) gas generated by microorganisms in an empyema. When gas originates in the lung, the rupture may occur in the absence of known disease (simple pneumothorax) or as a result of parenchymal disease (secondary pneumothorax).

Simple spontaneous pneumothorax occurs most commonly in previously healthy men aged 20 to 40 and is due to spontaneous rupture of subpleural blebs at the apex of the lungs. The right lung is more frequently involved, and recurrence is frequent (30% ipsilateral, 10% contralateral). Patients usually present with acute pain, dyspnea (related to size of pneumothorax), and cough. Physical examination shows decreased breath sounds and tactile fremitus with ipsilateral hyperresonance. The chest radiograph classically shows the visceral pleural line, but small pneumothoraces may become evident only with an expiratory or lateral decubitus film. Small amounts of fluid (sometimes blood) are present in 25% of patients. *Tension pneumothorax* (caused by increased positive pressure through a "ball-valve" air leak) can cause mediastinal shift and compromise circulation. For a small pneumothorax (<20% of the hemithorax) in an asymptomatic patient, observation may suffice because the air may reabsorb in 7 to 14 days. Larger pneumothoraces can be treated with air aspiration. A chest tube, which can be connected to suction or placed under water seal, is required for a pneumothorax that occupies more than 50% of the hemithorax, for symptomatic patients, or for a tension pneumothorax. The tube should be left in for 2 to 4 days until the leak seals. Because of frequent recurrences, chemical pleurodesis or surgical correction may be necessary.

Secondary or complicated pneumothorax results from trauma or pulmonary diseases. Widespread emphysema is the most common cause, but rupture of an abscess with spillage of pus into the pleural space can cause a pyopneumothorax. Less frequent underlying conditions are asthma, certain interstitial lung diseases (idiopathic fibrosis, eosinophilic granulomatosis, sarcoidosis, tuberous sclerosis), neoplasms (sarcoma, bronchogenic carcinoma), some rare diseases such as Marfan and Ehlers-Danlos syndromes, and endometriosis (catamenial pneumothorax). Iatrogenic injuries (e.g., insertion of central lines) and barotrauma are frequent causes in the intensive-care unit. The patient should be hospitalized and a chest tube inserted because spontaneous expansion is rare and the decreased reserve resulting from the pneumothorax may cause ventilatory compromise. Surgery must not be taken lightly because the rate of complications is high, but it may be lifesaving in some patients. In patients on ventilatory support, a pneumothorax is always under tension and requires immediate insertion of a chest tube. If a bronchopleural fistula persists, a portion of the minute ventilation exits through it; hence, it is necessary to increase ventilation to compensate for this loss. For severe leak, high-frequency low-pressure ventilation or synchronized chest tube occlusion may be helpful. Frequent complications of chest tube insertion include re-expansion pulmonary edema, lung trauma or infarction, subcutaneous emphysema, bleeding, and infection.

Aisner J: Current approach to malignant mesothelioma of the pleura. Chest 1995; 107(Suppl 6):332S–344S. *Excellent review of the treatment options for pleural mesothelioma.*

Light RW: Management of spontaneous pneumothorax. Am Rev Respir Dis 148:245–251, 1993. *Reviews the pathogenesis and treatment of pneumothorax. Summarizes the results of a VA study with a total of 118 patients.*

Veena BA (ed): Diseases of the pleura. Clin Chest Med 19:229–417, 1998. *This issue of the Chest Clinics is entirely devoted to the pleura. It covers all the important aspects of pleural anatomy, function, and pathology. Excellent single source for in-depth information.*

MEDIASTINUM

The mediastinum is the anatomic space that lies in the midthorax and separates the two pleural cavities. It is limited by the diaphragm below and the suprasternal thoracic outlet above. The mediastinum contains several vital structures in a small space, so mediastinal abnormalities can produce important symptoms. For clinical purposes, it is convenient to divide the mediastinum into anterior, middle, and posterior compartments (Fig. 86–1). The anterior compartment contains the thymus, substernal extensions of the thyroid and parathyroid glands, blood vessels, pericardium, and lymph nodes. The middle compartment contains the heart, great vessels, trachea, main bronchi, lymph nodes, and phrenic and vagus nerves. The posterior compartment contains the vertebrae, descending aorta, esophagus, thoracic duct, azygous and hemizygous veins, lower portion of the vagus, sympathetic chains, and posterior mediastinal nodes.

SIGNS AND SYMPTOMS. Most patients with mediastinal masses are asymptomatic, and the finding is incidental on a chest radiograph obtained for another reason. The most common symptoms are chest pain, cough, hoarseness, and dyspnea, whereas stridor, dysphagia, and Horner's syndrome are less frequent. Occasionally, some syndromes are associated with a primary mediastinal lesion. Myasthenia gravis is seen in nearly 50% of patients with thymoma. Hypoglycemia has been seen in patients with mesotheliomas, fibrosarcomas, and teratomas. Parathyroid tumors may induce hypercalcemia, whereas neurogenic tumors may cause neurologic symptoms. The physical examination is usually non-specific. The mass may produce superior vena caval obstruction with facial edema, dilated veins, and arm edema. The masses may erode the trachea, esophagus, and great vessels with life-threatening consequences.

DIAGNOSIS. Most mediastinal masses are detected on a plain chest radiograph (Figs. 86–2 and 86–3). Chest CT is the initial procedure of choice (Fig. 86–4) because it provides good definition of mediastinal structures. If the patient is asymptomatic and the non-invasive information obtained by CT, with and without contrast medium enhancement, suggests a benign process, careful follow-up is justified. The radiologic evaluation may include angiography and an esophagogram. The role of magnetic resonance imaging is being investigated, specifically for evaluating vessels and blood flow without the need for contrast medium enhancement. In some

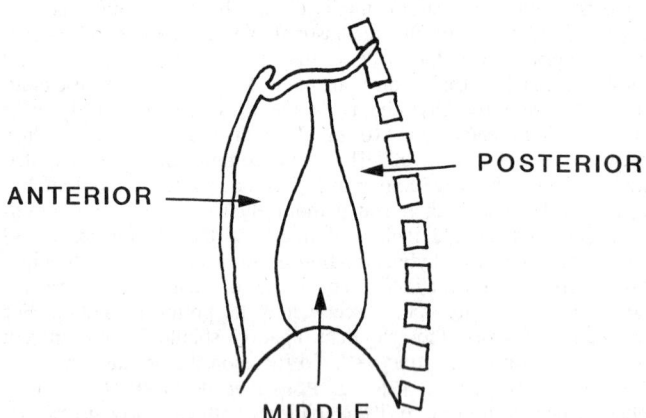

FIGURE 86–1 ■ Anatomic compartments of the mediastinum. The anterior compartment is bound posteriorly by the pericardium, ascending aorta, and brachiocephalic vessels and anteriorly by the sternum. The middle compartment extends from the posterior limits of the anterior compartment to the posterior pericardial line. The posterior compartment extends from the pericardial line to the dorsal chest wall.

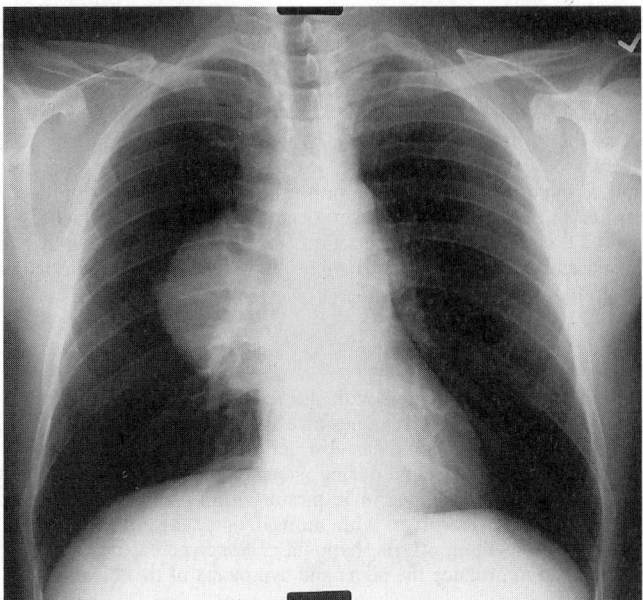

FIGURE 86-2 ■ Posteroanterior radiograph of a patient with a mass in the anterior mediastinum.

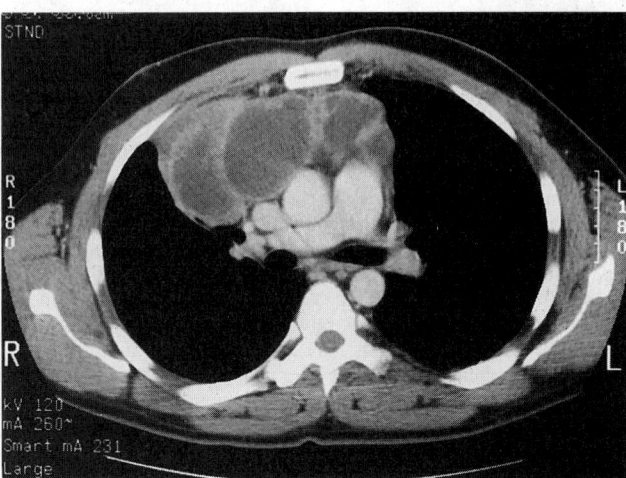

FIGURE 86-4 ■ CT of same patient as in Figures 86-2 and 86-3. The mass proved to be a dermoid cyst. (Courtesy of Paul Palefsky, MD, and Barbara Balkin, MD, Department of Radiology, St. Elizabeth's Medical Center, Boston.)

patients it may be necessary to obtain tissue for histologic diagnosis. Classically, anterior and middle compartment lesions are reached through mediastinoscopy or mediastinotomy. Thoracotomy may be needed for middle and posterior compartment lesions or when surgery is the treatment of choice for the suspected lesion (i.e., lung cancer). Direct sampling using CT-guided needle aspiration has proven useful and has become the procedure of choice in many centers.

SPECIFIC DISEASES. TUMORS (Table 86-6). The most common cause of a mediastinal mass in older patients is a metastatic carcinoma (most commonly bronchogenic carcinoma). In young adults, primary mediastinal pathology is more frequent.

In the posterior mediastinum, neurogenic tumors are most common (20%). Non-specific chest pain and non-productive cough with occasional compression of intercostal nerves, trachea, and bronchi are the most frequent symptoms. Most tumors are benign, originating in the nerve sheath (neurilemoma, neurofibroma) or sympathetic

ganglion cells (ganglioneuroma). Neuroblastoma (malignant tumor of sympathetic ganglion cells) has a better prognosis than the same tumor occurring in the adrenals. Neurofibromas may occur in association with von Recklinghausen's disease. Ganglioneuromas and neuroblastomas may secrete hormones that cause flushing, diarrhea, and hypertension. Pheochromocytomas may occasionally arise in the mediastinum. Neurogenic tumors should be resected; neuroblastomas require postoperative radiation.

LYMPHORETICULAR. Thymomas account for 20% of mediastinal tumors and are located in the superior portion of the anterior mediastinum. Two thirds of them are malignant. Myasthenia gravis is seen in 40% of cases, and other paraneoplastic syndromes such as Cushing's syndrome, refractory anemia, and hypogammaglobulinemia have been reported. All thymomas should be regarded as malignant, and surgical resection should be followed with radiation. Lymphatic tumors (17%) also arise in the anterior mediastinum. Hodgkin's lymphoma is the most frequent and carries the best prognosis. Non-Hodgkin's lymphoma, plasmacytomas, and angiomatous lymphoid hamartomas with similar clinical presentation carry a worse prognosis. Teratomatous tumors, also located in the anterior compartment, comprise 10% of mediastinal tumors, and one third of them are malignant. They are embryologically and histologically linked to the thymus. Cystic teratomas are more frequent and may contain squamous cells, hair follicles, sweat glands, cartilage, and linear calcifications. Intrathoracic goiter (10%) is usually a benign nodular or follicular enlargement of the thyroid gland. Three quarters of patients present with stridor, cough, and dyspnea. Most frequently located in the anterior mediastinum, intrathoracic goiters occasionally cause superior vena cava syndrome. Benign cysts are usually asymptomatic and occur as an incidental radiographic finding. Bronchogenic cysts develop around the paratracheal area or carina and are seen in the middle and posterior compartments; they are filled with liquid and are lined with respiratory epithelium and cartilage but do not communicate with the tracheobronchial tree. Pericardial cysts occur in the anterior compartment and cardiophrenic angle; they contain clear liquid and flattened endothelial or mesothelial lining with a bland fibrous wall. Enteric cysts are located in the posterior mediastinum and are lined

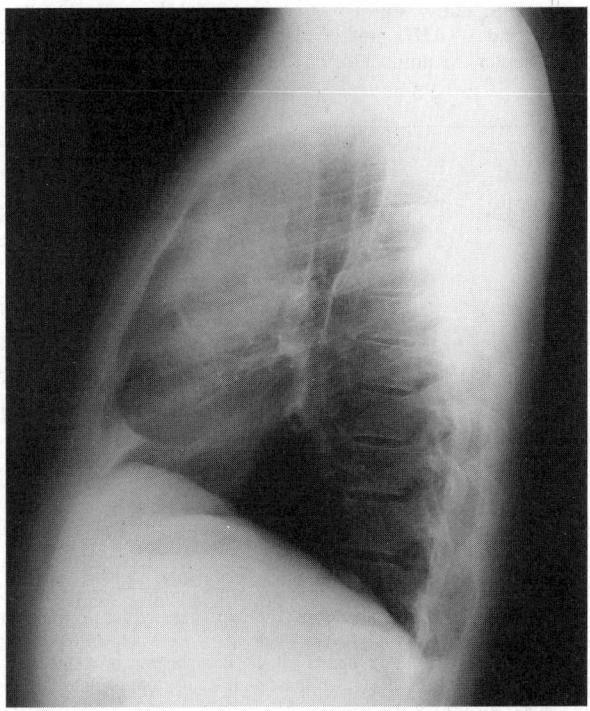

FIGURE 86-3 ■ Lateral chest radiograph of same patient as in Figure 86-2.

Table 86-6 ■ **MOST FREQUENT CAUSES OF MEDIASTINAL MASSES**

ANTERIOR	MIDDLE	POSTERIOR
Thymoma	Lymphoma	Neurogenic tumors
Lymphoma	Cancer	Enteric cysts
Teratogenic tumors	Cysts	Esophageal lesions
Thyroid	Aneurysms	Aneurysms
Parathyroid aneurysms	Hernia (Morgagni)	Diaphragmatic hernias (Bochdalek)

by gastric or intestinal epithelium. All cysts may become infected, bleed, or rupture into the mediastinum or pleural cavity.

Vascular tumors may originate primarily in the mediastinum. The vascular hamartomas, lymphangiomas, and hemangiomas are benign tumors, whereas hemangiopericytomas are malignant. Mesenchymal benign (lipoma) or malignant (liposarcoma, mesothelioma, rhabdomyosarcoma, and mesenchymoma) tumors rarely cause mediastinal masses.

Hernias through the diaphragm may also present as mediastinal masses. They may be retrosternal through the foramen of Morgagni, posterolateral through the foramen of Bochdalek, or most commonly through the esophageal hiatus. When gas is contained in the herniated organ, the presumptive diagnosis is easily made.

PNEUMOMEDIASTINUM. Air may enter the mediastinum through a tear in the esophagus or tracheobronchial tree or as dissecting air from ruptured alveoli. Tears in the esophagus and tracheobronchial tree commonly have a traumatic origin, whereas alveolar rupture may occur spontaneously or as a complication of artificial ventilation. Air may track to the neck and the body, producing subcutaneous emphysema and/or pneumothorax. The patient complains of retrosternal pain and dyspnea. Subcutaneous emphysema may cause classic crepitus. Auscultation may reveal a crunching sound synchronous with the heartbeat (Hamman's sign). Rarely, cardiac function is compromised. A lateral chest radiograph is usually diagnostic. Simple spontaneous pneumomediastinum usually resolves without treatment. When severe or resulting from organ rupture, surgical drainage and repair are required.

SUPERIOR VENA CAVA SYNDROME. Obstruction of blood flow through the superior vena cava causes dilatation of collateral veins of the upper thorax and neck and edema and congestion of the face; patients may have headache, dyspnea, dysphagia, and wheezes. Malignancy is the most frequent cause of this syndrome, with bronchogenic carcinoma responsible for more than 70% of cases and lymphoma a distant second (see Chapter 199). Fibrosing mediastinitis after granulomatous diseases such as histoplasmosis or tuberculosis or associated with methysergide ingestion can also be seen. Aortic aneurysm and retrosternal thyroid are relatively benign causes of superior vena cava syndrome. Because of vessel dilatation, invasive procedures are contraindicated. An effort must be made to obtain tissue elsewhere, and irradiation or chemotherapy should be begun before attempts are made to obtain mediastinal tissue.

Cohen A, Thompson L, Edwards F, Bellamy R: Primary cysts and tumors of the mediastinum. Ann Thorac Surg 51:378–384, 1991. *Review of 230 cases. It provides an excellent framework for the proper understanding of the relative frequency of mediastinal masses according to their anatomical location.*

Moore EH: Radiologic evaluation of mediastinal masses. Chest Surg Clin North Am 2: 1–16, 1992. *In-depth review of the basis and radiologic evaluation of mediastinal masses.*

87 OBSTRUCTIVE SLEEP APNEA-HYPOPNEA SYNDROME

Kingman P. Strohl

DEFINITIONS

Obstructive sleep apnea-hypopnea syndrome is a sleep disorder characterized by a constellation of neurobehavioral symptoms with recurrent episodes of partial and/or complete closure of the upper airway during sleep. The disorder resolves when the sleep-induced upper airway instability is eliminated.

During *obstructive apnea*, respiratory efforts persist, but airflow is absent at the nose and mouth. *Central* or *non-obstructive apnea* occurs when both airflow and respiratory efforts are absent. Obstructive and central apnea are not necessarily unrelated. Many adult patients exhibit *mixed apnea*, in which both central and ob-

structive patterns occur. In a single apneic episode, a period may be noted in which no efforts occur, followed by the appearance of respiratory efforts, also without airflow. In addition, patients may have central, mixed, and obstructive apnea in the same night.

Hypoventilation (*hypopnea*) arises by mechanisms similar to those that produce apnea, and it leads to increased arterial CO_2 and decreased arterial O_2 levels as well as arousals from sleep; like apnea, hypopnea may result from either a reduction in respiratory efforts or partial upper airway obstruction. Snoring, which is a form of partial airway obstruction, results in flow limitation and increased respiratory efforts; it may produce hypoventilation and/or arousals from sleep.

ETIOLOGY

Sleep and its interaction with the respiratory control system destabilize the ability of the upper airway to conduct air to and from the lungs. Partial or complete obstruction of the nasopharynx, oropharynx, or both occurs during sleep (Fig. 87–1). Obstruction causes exaggerated swings in inspiratory efforts and a reduction in gas exchange; it resolves with arousal or change in sleep state. Obstructed breathing efforts, hypoxia and/or hypercapnia, and sleep fragmentation produce the signs and symptoms of this disorder.

INCIDENCE AND PREVALENCE

Overall prevalence is approximately 2 to 4% with a male predominance of 2 to 4:1. Furthermore, the prevalence of excessive daytime sleepiness associated with sleep apnea (2 to 4%) is very high compared with the prevalence of narcolepsy (0.02 to 0.06%).

Clinical surveys find higher rates (20%) in the elderly, but these estimates are confounded by co-morbidity and concomitant administration of medications. The extremely healthy elderly have few sleep complaints or abnormalities. Rates are as high as 85% in obese persons. Sleep apnea-hypopnea is also associated with hypertension, stroke, and heart disease (see below).

EPIDEMIOLOGY

Healthy volunteers exhibit obstructive apnea at sleep onset or during periods of sleep. Apneic episodes are usually less than 10 to 15 seconds in duration and are not repetitive. Occasionally, longer periods of apnea last up to 30 seconds, particularly during rapid-eye-movement (REM) sleep. These episodes are not usually accompanied by arousal or sleep-state changes. No gender differences are seen in the appearance of brief episodes of sleep apnea in healthy subjects.

In one U.S. study, 9% of women and 27% of men had an apnea-hypopnea index (AHI) greater than 5 (see Sleep Monitoring, later in this chapter), a number often quoted as a "threshold value" for

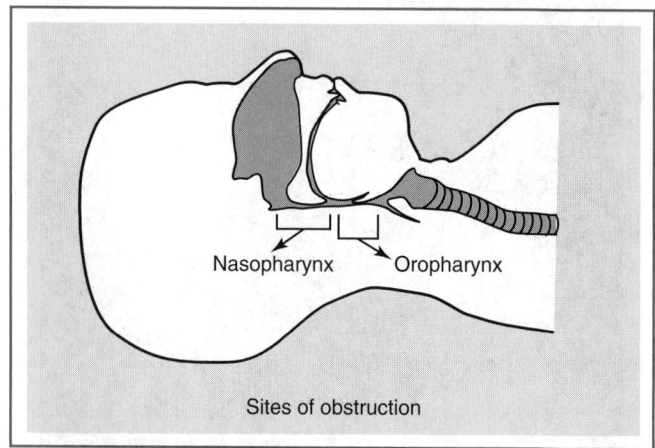

FIGURE 87–1 ▪ Potential sites for airway closure during sleep are indicated. Patients with a normal examination of the upper airway during wakefulness exhibit functional narrowing (heavy snoring or obstructive hypopnea) or complete closure (obstructive apnea) of the nasopharynx or oropharynx, or both. Relief of airway closure comes with activation of muscles, often accompanied by arousal from sleep.

normality; however, many people with an AHI greater than 5 have no symptoms or apparent illness. Community-based studies, however, suggest that subjects with an AHI greater than 5 *and* with symptoms (about 2% of women and 4% of men) have higher rates of accidents, disability, and high blood pressure.

Snoring is believed to be a predisposing feature in the development of obstructive sleep disease. Snoring increases markedly with age, so that approximately 45% of men and 30% of women older than 65 years snore. Hypertension is twice as common among persons who snore, even after age and obesity are taken into account. A history of heavy snoring is reported in more than 70% of adult patients with obstructive sleep apnea syndrome.

Symptoms relating to apnea are present with two to six times greater frequency in family members of affected patients than in age-, sex-, and socioeconomically matched control families. However, this familial effect is not sufficient to recommend screening of asymptomatic family members.

MECHANISMS AND PATHOGENESIS

The rhythmic cycle of a breath depends on interactions among groups of neurons located in the medulla: a dorsal group located in the vicinity of the nucleus tractus solitarius and a ventral group consisting of neurons in the nucleus retro-ambigualis and para-ambigualis, the nucleus retrofacialis, and nucleus ambigualis. Efferent activity of the cranial nerves that supply upper airway muscles is adjusted by nucleus ambigualis activity and the neural discharge to the chest-wall muscles by dorsal medullary nuclei. The activity of these medullary groups of respiratory neurons can be altered by descending pathways from pontine and suprapontine areas and can be affected by the sleep-wake cycle, in particular the waxing and waning of the median raphe, or reticular activating system.

The respiratory controller influences the activity of upper airway as well as chest wall muscles. The electrical activity of upper airway muscles often seems to be entrained to the respiratory rhythm, and phasic increases and decreases in the activity of many upper airway muscles can be discerned. The amplitude of these phasic changes can be altered by the same stimuli (e.g., CO_2 and hypoxia) that affect diaphragm and intercostal muscle activity. Sleep may depress the sensitivity of upper airway muscles to chemical stimulation even more than the diaphragm.

An essential feature of the obstructive sleep apnea-hypopnea syndrome is the presence of recurrent apneic episodes during sleep. The causes of an apneic event include reduced excitatory stimulation; active suppression of breathing from inhibitory reflexes arising from the cardiovascular system, the lungs, and the chest wall or via other somatic and visceral afferents; and loss of reflexes that normally ensure the maintenance of ventilation and do not depend on chemical drive. Recurrent apnea results from instability in the feedback control of breathing, which causes ventilation to cycle rather than to maintain a constant level. Upper airway instability will occur in response to the cyclic changes in drive or if the mechanical outputs of chest-wall muscles and upper airway muscles are not identical either in phase or in amplitude.

Negative pressures produced by the chest-wall muscles during

inspiration tend to collapse the semirigid tissues surrounding the oropharynx and nasopharynx. The mechanical features of small airstream size and a collapsible airway wall are essential in the pathogenesis of obstructive apnea (Fig. 87–2). Inspiratory efforts against an obstruction produces instability in cardiac output and blood pressure.

CLINICAL MANIFESTATIONS

The essential features of the obstructive sleep apnea-hypopnea syndrome include loud disruptive snoring, nocturnal choking or gasping, daytime fatigue, and impaired concentration (Table 87–1). Excessive daytime sleepiness is subdivided into the following three categories:

MILD. Sleep episodes are present only during times of rest or when little attention is required. Examples include sleepiness that is likely to occur while lying down in a quiet room, watching television, reading, or traveling as a passenger. Symptoms produce incidental impairment of social or occupational function.

MODERATE. Sleep episodes occur during activities that require some attention. Examples include sleep episodes that occur while attending activities such as concerts, meetings, or presentations. Symptoms produce impairment of social or occupational function, to the extent that people take efforts to avoid situations where sleep is likely to occur.

SEVERE. Sleep episodes are present during activities that require at least moderate attention. Examples include uncontrollable sleepiness while eating or during conversation, walking, or driving. Symptoms produce marked impairment in social or occupational function. Families are highly aware, perhaps more aware than the person, of adverse consequences of this level of sleepiness.

Restless sleep and observed apnea are sensitive and relatively specific indications of recurrent apnea. Both sleep complaints and daytime sleepiness are very roughly related to the number and length of nocturnal arousals. Family members, rather than the patient, are often the first to recognize the sleep disturbance (e.g., periods of absent breathing, loud snoring, or thrashing movements during sleep). Patients occasionally present with complaints of fatigue or decreased alertness, and sleepiness symptoms should be elicited by direct questioning and distinguished from fatigue.

A number of associated features should suggest the diagnosis of obstructive sleep apnea-hypopnea syndrome (Table 87–2). Nearly half of patients with the sleep apnea syndrome are not obese, and the suspicion that the syndrome is present should not be limited to the fat patient or to those with characteristics previously called the pickwickian syndrome.

DIAGNOSIS

Routine laboratory examinations are generally not helpful. Likewise, pulmonary function tests will reveal no abnormality except those caused by associated obesity (somewhat diminished lung capacities, with greater reduction in the expiratory reserve volume). In the patient without upper airway or respiratory complaints, the flow-volume loop is unhelpful. A pattern consistent with variable extrathoracic obstruction (i.e., a decreased inspiratory flow relative to expiratory flow at 50% of vital capacity) has been described in

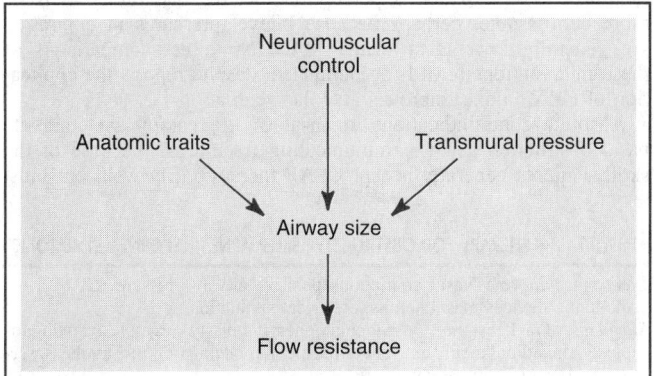

FIGURE 87–2 ■ Three factors determine patency of the upper airway, one or more of which can lead to a reduction in airway size and to high upper airway resistance (snoring) or obstruction (apnea).

Table 87–1 ■ **DEFINITION OF OBSTRUCTIVE SLEEP APNEA-HYPOPNEA SYNDROME**

Episodes of upper airway obstruction during sleep result in recurrent arousals associated with:
  Excessive daytime sleepiness, unexplained by other factors, and two or more of the following:
    Loud disruptive snoring
    Nocturnal choking/gasping/snort
    Recurrent nocturnal awakening
    Unrefreshing sleep
    Daytime fatigue
    Impaired concentration
                    AND
Overnight sleep monitoring documenting
>5 episodes of hypopnea and apnea per hour

Table 87–2 ■ FEATURES COMMONLY ASSOCIATED WITH OBSTRUCTIVE SLEEP APNEA-HYPOPNEA SYNDROME

Obesity
Mandibular/maxillary hypoplasia
Systemic hypertension
Pulmonary hypertension
Tonsillar hypertrophy
Sleep fragmentation
Sleep-related arrhythmias
Nocturnal angina
Gastroesophageal reflux
Impaired quality of life

sleep apnea, but it is not predictive of the illness nor by itself helpful in directing therapy.

Patients with heart and lung disease also may have the obstructive sleep apnea-hypopnea syndrome; however, no convincing epidemiologic evidence has been offered to verify that sleep apnea occurs more frequently in patients with cardiopulmonary impairment. Obstructive sleep apnea-hypopnea syndrome should be considered in patients with hypercapnia that is disproportionate to abnormalities in the mechanical function of the lungs. Hypercapnia rarely occurs with obstructive lung disease unless forced expiratory volume in 1 second (FEV_1) is reduced to less than 50% of predicted. Patients with unexplained right-sided heart failure or pulmonary hypertension should be questioned for the presence of sleep-disordered breathing. Finally, some patients with the syndrome may be mistakenly treated for primary heart disease because cardiac arrhythmias have been detected during sleep, whereas the respiratory disturbances have not. Certain tests, such as arterial blood gas analyses, thyroid function testing, echocardiogram, and chest roentgenogram, are electively indicated if signs of hypoxic exposure are present.

SLEEP MONITORING

The definitive diagnostic test is the monitoring of the patient during sleep with continuous measurements of breathing and gas exchange. Sleep staging requires monitoring of the electroencephalogram (EEG) (usually with two or three leads), the chin electromyogram (activity decreases in REM), and the electro-oculogram (EOG) to detect REM. It is also useful to record the electrocardiogram (ECG) to see if arrhythmias occur with the apneic episodes.

Other variables recorded may include noninvasive oximetry (looking for falls in excess of 3% from baseline values), muscle activity from the limbs (looking for non-respiratory causes for arousal), and body position (looking for expression of apneas only in the supine position). In some instances it may be necessary to measure esophageal pressure to identify transient episodes of inspiratory flow limitation leading to arousals or producing a fall in oxygen saturation of more than 3%.

A common summary measure used to describe respiratory disturbances during sleep is the AHI, the total number of episodes of apnea and hypopnea during sleep divided by the hours of sleep time. AHI values can be computed for the different stages of sleep. Another term used is the respiratory disturbance index (RDI), which most often refers to the number of times per hour that oxygen saturation falls more than 3%. If EEG measures are performed, an arousal index (AI) is computed. The number of arousals per hour of sleep may be correlated with AHI or RDI; however, some episodes (approximately 20%) of apnea or hypopnea are not accompanied by arousals and/or other causes for arousals are present. The number of arousals during sleep or respiratory disturbances per se is not a good indicator of disease, and symptoms of sleepiness are better predictors of treatment success.

DIFFERENTIAL DIAGNOSIS

Reports from sleep clinics suggest that sleep apnea should be considered in any patient referred for complaints of sleepiness. The most common factor producing mild and moderate degrees of sleepiness is sleep restriction (a reduction in nocturnal sleep length) as a result of lifestyle issues. Narcolepsy and restless leg syndrome are two disorders that also present with moderate and severe sleepi-

ness. Cardiovascular, respiratory, or metabolic disturbances or their therapy (e.g., diuretics, insulin) may predispose the patient to restless sleep. Drug addiction or depression may masquerade as sleep apnea. In the elderly, in whom reports of snoring are high and a number of episodes of apnea during sleep may be considered "normal," sleepiness can be secondary to a lifestyle or medication effect. A careful sleep history is the key to recognizing sleep apnea as well as these other diseases.

TREATMENT

Therapy is directed at sleep fragmentation and hypoxic exposure. Initially, a review should be undertaken for the presence of anatomic or medical conditions whose reversal would ameliorate or eliminate breathing disturbances during sleep. Because respiratory depressants seem to increase the appearance of respiratory disturbances during sleep, perhaps by elevating the CO_2 threshold, withdrawal of respiratory depressants such as major tranquilizers, antihistamines, or alcohol is indicated.

Treatment should be tailored to the individual patient and to the degree to which he or she is disabled by the breathing disturbances during sleep (Table 87–3). Thyroid hormone replacement reverses the sleep apnea and clinical symptoms in myxedema. Treatment of hypertension will modestly decrease apneic activity. Patients with sleep apnea and cardiac or respiratory disease, such as heart failure or asthma, should be placed on maximal therapy for the concomitant disease, because decreased circulation time and/or increased oxygenation may decrease the incidence or severity of respiratory disturbances during sleep. In the patient with recent stroke, time may be all that is needed before respiratory stability is restored.

ELECTROMECHANICAL DEVICES

Nasal continuous positive airway pressure (CPAP) is effective in the long-term treatment of obstructive sleep apnea and in the prevention of snoring. The effect is dependent on the level of positive pressure applied to the upper airway, and the optimal levels of pressure differ among patients. In general, though, at lower levels of pressure (3 to 6 cm H_2O), apneic episodes are eliminated, but episodes of partial upper airway obstruction (snoring) persist. At higher levels of pressure (5 to 15 cm H_2O), regular breathing tends to be restored. Positive pressures must be present over the entire respiratory cycle for nasal CPAP to be effective.

If CPAP is withdrawn, symptoms recur gradually over several days, so short interruptions of therapy for surgery or acute medical illnesses are usually well tolerated. Late failures of nasal CPAP occur occasionally: some are due to poor application of the mask, so that pressure is lost; some are due to too low a pressure; and some are due to an increase in the pressure required to prevent apnea. Factors such as alcohol use, hypothyroidism, and obesity may worsen airway stability.

Bilevel ventilation for obstructive apnea is the application of an inspiratory assist over and above the expiratory pressure required to keep the pharyngeal airway open. One indication for this approach is a concomitant finding of chronic hypoventilation in addition to obstructive apnea. Titration and chronic use of bilevel ventilation is facilitated by the patient's perception that the inspiratory assist is more comfortable, perhaps because bilevel pressures in expiration are generally lower than with CPAP. No direct comparisons of these interventions have been published, despite reports the application of CPAP alone improves alveolar ventilation.

Absolute contraindications to nasal CPAP therapy are complete nasal obstruction and a communicating fracture of the base of the skull. Patients generally accept CPAP therapy fairly well, but most

Table 87–3 ■ THERAPY FOR OBSTRUCTIVE SLEEP APNEA-HYPOPNEA SYNDROME

Electromechanical: Nasal continuous positive airway pressure (CPAP), orthodontic devices, nasal splints, electrical simulation
Surgical: Tracheostomy, uvulopalatopharyngoplasty, hyoplasty, linguoplasty, mandibular advancement; plastic remodeling of the uvula (laser-assisted or radiofrequency ablation)
Medical: Vasoconstrictive anti-inflammatory nasal sprays,* weight-loss medications,* oxygen, and miscellaneous agents (e.g., progesterone, serotonin receptor blockade, acetazolamide, methylxanthines*)

*Not formally approved for obstructive sleep apnea-hypopnea syndrome.

large series indicate that some patients (30% or so) do not. Side effects of therapy include feelings of suffocation, nasal drying or rhinitis, ear pain, and conjunctivitis. Inner ear and eye problems are said to resolve spontaneously and do not recur with continued CPAP therapy. Pulmonary function does not deteriorate with nasal CPAP, and patients with lung disease apparently have no adverse effects.

Intraoral appliances are gaining wider acceptance in the treatment of both snoring and obstructive apnea. Some devices are designed to tug the tongue forward and others to protrude the mandible or, at the very least, prevent the mandible from retruding with sleep. Experience with this therapy is limited, but it may be an attractive alternative if CPAP is not tolerated. Indications and cost-effectiveness are not yet well developed.

SURGICAL INTERVENTIONS

Tracheostomy bypasses the site of obstruction during sleep and is the most effective therapeutic maneuver for obstructive apnea. The tracheostomy may be technically difficult owing to morphologic features such as obesity, a short neck, or a short mandible. Problems with stomal infection and granulation tissue often occur, and it may take a year or more before the tracheal site is well healed.

Surgical correction directed at a specific, pathologic narrowing of the upper airway caused by enlarged tonsils, nasal polyps, macroglossia, or micrognathia is reported to improve signs and symptoms of sleep apnea. In prospective studies in which tonsillectomy has been performed for sleep apnea, obstructive apnea may persist, but the frequency is greatly diminished.

Extensive excision of soft tissue in the oropharynx, termed *uvulopalatopharyngoplasty*, may improve pharyngeal function during sleep. The procedure involves a submucosal resection of redundant tissue from the tonsillar pillars to the arytenoepiglottic folds. The indications for the procedure are the same as for a tracheostomy. In one series, the success rate was approximately 60%, but success has varied considerably from center to center. Most patients report symptomatic improvement; however, objective reduction in the number or magnitude of respiratory disturbances during sleep is often absent. Patients with massive obesity or with anatomic narrowing of the airway may not show success with uvulopalatopharyngoplasty, whereas patients who snore but do not have frank obstructive apnea may do well. Potential complications of the procedure include speech and swallowing difficulties, in particular regurgitation of food. Some patients may have an increased number of respiratory disturbances during sleep after the procedure, but recognition of the disturbances is obscured because snoring is absent. These "silent obstructions" may be as severe as apneic episodes prior to surgical intervention.

Newer procedures, such as laser-assisted uvuloplasty and radiofrequency tissue ablation, are designed and promoted as outpatient treatments for loud snoring. Outcome studies show some short-term (70 to 80% at 2 to 6 months) reductions in snoring loudness; however, long-term success rates at 1 year are 50% and continue to decline at 2 years. Sleep apnea syndrome should be excluded before either procedure is contemplated, because apnea may increase after these procedures and because use of these procedures may delay more definite treatments.

The concept of two-stage surgical management of obstructive sleep apnea is based on the fact that a uvulopalatopharyngoplasty is often not curative, as defined by a resolution of symptoms along with a reduction in AHI below some threshold (usually 10). Additional procedures include expansion hyoplasty, a procedure directed at moving the hyoid arch forward by placing a prosthetic device in the hyoid arch, and midline glossectomy. A second procedure would include mandibulomaxillary advancement. Success across centers in large series of unselected patients remains to be determined.

MEDICAL TREATMENT

Case reports have been published of successful treatment of obstructive apnea during sleep using nasal vasoconstrictive sprays. Consequently, a trial of nasal (vasoconstrictive and anti-inflammatory) decongestants is warranted in the patient in whom nasal obstruction is present.

Even a 5 to 10% decrease in body weight can be accompanied by clinical and objective remission of sleep apnea syndrome in obese subjects. Few investigators, however, are enthusiastic about the long-term efficacy of dietary strategies, perhaps because adherence to dietary restrictions is difficult in the sleepy patient. Better treatments for obesity would have an immediate and major impact on the management and prevention of sleep apnea.

A beneficial effect of oxygen on upper airway obstruction during sleep cannot be found in every patient. Indeed, in some patients with obstructive sleep apnea syndrome, oxygen administration provokes respiratory acidosis. At present, it is not possible to predict which patients will respond to oxygen therapy.

Various drugs have been used in an attempt to stimulate upper airway muscles, to increase respiratory neural drive, or to increase both upper airway and chest-wall muscle activation. Although this kind of therapy would seem optimal, it has not yet shown much success.

PSYCHOLOGICAL FACTORS IN TREATMENT

Sleepiness compromises the patient's ability to solve problems at work or at home or to perform even simple tasks. Family members may suffer injury from automobile accidents caused by the patient's falling asleep at the wheel. Patients who are sleepy limit their social activities out of embarrassment. Family conflicts may result in personal and financial losses before a diagnosis is sought or made.

If the patient and family feel reasonably informed of therapeutic alternatives, they will be better able to cope with a treatment strategy, including tracheostomy in cases refractory to other treatment. Supervised meetings of patient and family with other patients and their families who have faced the same problem may be helpful.

After effective treatment, changes in family dynamics may occur as the patient becomes a more active person. With successful treatment, the patient can return to full employment and duties.

PROGNOSIS

The natural history of sleep apnea syndrome is largely unknown. Although patients present in clinical categories of mild, moderate, and severe sleepiness, little evidence exists that progression from health to severe disease occurs according to these categories. Few longitudinal studies have been undertaken in untreated patients with sleep apnea syndromes, but disease progression is generally slow.

Death and sleep apnea are associated, but the nature and strength of causality have not been satisfactorily studied. Early reports of patients with the pickwickian syndrome noted a high in-hospital mortality due to cardiorespiratory failure, pulmonary embolus, and renal failure. From case reports only, death has been reported to result from preoperative medications and spinal anesthesia. The risk in regard to conscious sedation remains to be defined. Moreover, it is the impression of some that automobile accidents related to excessive daytime sleepiness may have a greater impact on morbidity and mortality than cardiovascular complications or other non-accidental sudden death.

PREVENTION

Obstructive sleep apnea-hypopnea syndrome is not rare, and those with the syndrome have a chronic illness. Modifiable risk factors include obesity, use of sedatives and respiratory depressants, inadequate sleep, and, possibly, hypertension.

Preoperative sedation and intubation is a time of risk for lethal respiratory disturbances. The patient should be advised to inform the anesthesiologist of his or her diagnosis prior to undergoing any elective surgical procedure. In addition, the excessively sleepy untreated patient should not operate a motor vehicle or engage in activities during which sleep attacks would be hazardous. The risk of serious injury or death from accidents is reduced by behavioral measures and by direct treatment of obstructive events during sleep.

American Thoracic Society: Statement of Health Outcomes Research in Sleep Apnea.

Am J Respir Crit Care Med 157:335–341, 1998. *This working group report references and critiques current information on cardiovascular risk, neurobehavioral sequelae, medical utilization, and cost relevant to sleep apnea and suggests avenues for future research.*

Bresnitz EA, Goldberg R, Kosinski RM: Epidemiology of obstructive sleep apnea. Epidemiol Rev 16:210–227, 1994. *This review contains many of the key references on sleep apnea and its potential impact on human health.*

Loube DI, Gay PC, Strohl KP, et al: Indications for positive airway pressure treatment of adult obstructive sleep apnea patients: A consensus statement. Chest 115:863–6, 1999. *This document delineates prudent criteria for reimbursement of positive airway pressure costs in the treatment of obstructive sleep apnea. Recommendations are based on peer-reviewed studies and accepted clinical practice.*

Redline S, Tishler PV, Williamson J, et al: The familial aggregation of sleep apnea. Am J Respir Crit Care Med 151:682–687, 1995. *Some 40 to 50% of the variability in apneic activity during sleep in the population can be attributed to familial factors. This original article quantifies risk.*

Strohl KP, Redline SA: Recognition of sleep apnea. Am J Respir Crit Care Med 154: 279–289, 1996. *Review of those factors of concern in the identification of sleep apnea by health care providers.*

Strohl KP, Bonnie RJ, Findley L, et al: Sleep apnea, sleepiness, and driving risk. Am J Respir Crit Care Med 150:1463–1473, 1994. *This committee report examines the evidence and makes recommendations for assessment of driving risk.*

Wright J, Johns R, Watt I, et al: Health effects of obstructive sleep apnea and the effectiveness of continuous positive airways pressure: A systematic review of the research evidence. Br Med J 314:851–860, 1997. *A critical, but selective, appraisal of the literature emphasizing current gaps in evidence-based treatments for sleep apnea.*

88 RESPIRATORY FAILURE

Warren R. Summer

Respiratory failure, whether acute or chronic, is a frequently encountered medical problem and a major cause of death in the United States. For example, mortality from chronic obstructive lung disease (COPD see Chapter 75), which ends in death from respiratory failure, continues to increase. More than 70% of the deaths in patients with pneumonia (see Chapter 82) are attributed to respiratory failure. About one third of patients in critical care units in the United States, about 500,000 persons, receive mechanical ventilation each year. For acute respiratory failure not preceded by additional lung disease or systemic illness, short-term survival is more than 85%; healthy independent elderly persons (older than 80 years) do nearly as well. However, multisystem organ failure or pre-existing renal, liver, or chronic gastrointestinal disease with malnutrition substantially worsens outlook. About 17% of patients placed on mechanical ventilation require assistance for more than 14 days. Among those requiring this amount of mechanical ventilation, elderly patients have a 9% survival and younger patients a 36% survival (Table 88–1).

Respiratory failure is a functional acute or chronic disorder caused by any condition that severely affects the lungs' ability to maintain arterial oxygenation or carbon dioxide (CO_2) elimination. Both acute and chronic respiratory failure may be divided into two main categories: a *failure of gas exchange* manifested preponderantly or entirely by hypoxemia, or a *failure of ventilation* manifested by hypercapnia or inability to exhale adequate quantities of CO_2. Differentiating *hypoxic (gas exchange)* from *hypercapnic-hypoxic (ventilatory)* respiratory failure is a convenient if somewhat artificial way to group conditions with related pathophysiology or common clinical presentations and related therapeutic strategies (Table 88–2).

ACUTE RESPIRATORY FAILURE

DEFINITION. *Hypoxic respiratory failure* may be defined as any condition that severely reduces arterial oxygen tension ($PaO_2 < 50$ mm Hg) and that cannot be corrected by increasing the inspired oxygen concentration to >50% ($FIO_2 > 0.5$). Although both $PaO_2 < 50$ mm Hg and $FIO_2 > 0.5$ are arbitrary levels, they represent critical physiologic landmarks. At a PaO_2 level of 50 mm Hg, hemoglobin is about 80% saturated, and further small reductions in the PaO_2 produce significant reductions in arterial oxygen (O_2) content (see Fig. 92–4). Under those circumstances, the O_2 reserve is minimal and patients become symptomatic. An FIO_2 of 0.5 is probably the highest level that can be readily achieved in a patient's airway without requiring a closed system (intubation) or specialized non-rebreathing masks, both of which generally require management in an intensive care unit (ICU) (see Chapters 91 to 93). In addition, an FIO_2 of 0.5 usually corrects the hypoxemia associated with hypercapnic-hypoxic respiratory failure and nearly all conditions in which anatomic or physiologic right-to-left shunting is not the dominant clinical problem. In hypoxic respiratory failure, the low PaO_2 is due to a large right-to-left shunt in well-perfused but poorly oxygenated lung tissue; PaO_2 therefore increases minimally with increasing FIO_2 so that the alveolar-arterial gradient increases markedly at increasing levels of FIO_2. The exact PaO_2 depends on the amount of blood that bypasses the gas-exchanging portion of the lung, the alveolar O_2 tension, and the mixed venous oxygen tension (PvO_2). In the presence of a large right-to-left shunt, small changes in PvO_2 caused by decreases in cardiac output or increases in metabolism can result in a major reduction in PaO_2. The calculated right-to-left shunt is usually between 25 and 50% in most patients.

Hypercapnic-hypoxic respiratory failure may be defined as a life-threatening condition with inadequate CO_2 excretion. CO_2 retention, and thus $PaCO_2$, are inversely related to the alveolar ventilation (VA), i.e., $PaCO_2 = kVCO_2/VA$, where VCO_2 is the amount of steady-state CO_2 produced each minute as determined by the patient's metabolic rate. A rise in the $PaCO_2$ level signifies reduced alveolar ventilation or hypoventilation. The mechanism for the failure in CO_2 excretion varies, but it is usually associated with severe airflow obstruction such as is seen in COPD or asthma. Hypercapnia may also occur in normal lungs, if the control of breathing is

Table 88-1 ■ CHARACTERISTICS OF PATIENTS AND CIRCUMSTANCES ASSOCIATED WITH RESPIRATORY FAILURE

MEAN AGE (YR)	MALE (%)	ASSISTED VENTILATION	HOSPITALIZATION
60	54	3 days, median; 10 days, mean	14 days, median; 26 days, mean

COMMON ETIOLOGY*	FREQUENCY (%)	SURVIVAL (%)
ARDS†	7	60
Cardiogenic pulmonary edema	16	60
Cardiopulmonary arrest	10	20
COPD	12	65
CNS: trauma, stroke, hemorrhage, seizures	11	60
Drug overdose	7	95
Metabolic coma	8	30
Neuromuscular disease‡	8	36
Pneumonia	10	38
Asthma	<1	90
Other§	10	50

*A large portion of patients have more than one condition leading to respiratory failure.

†Overlaps with other causes: sepsis, pneumonia, renal failure. Includes cardiac patients and those undergoing various hospital procedures. Does not represent patients already critically ill in an ICU.

‡Guillain-Barré syndrome, myasthenia gravis, tetanus, amyotrophic lateral sclerosis, etc.

§Multiple cause of respiratory failure: hard to define single reason; multisystem organ failure (MOSF) and sepsis common.

Table 88–2 ■ FEATURES OF HYPOXIC AND HYPERCAPNIC-HYPOXIC ACUTE RESPIRATORY FAILURE

FEATURE	CONDITION	
	Hypoxic	Hypercapnic-Hypoxic
Physiologic	Large right-to-left intrapulmonary shunt; hyperventilation usual	COPD: hypoventilation due to marked wasted (dead space) ventilation; minute ventilation normal to increased; $\dot{V}/Q$ imbalance with increased A-a gradient. Neuromuscular and overdose: hypoventilation due to decreased minute ventilation, normal A-a gradient
Anatomic	Extensive edema; atelectasis or consolidation; hyaline membranes	Mucous gland hyperplasia (bronchitis); alveolar wall destruction (emphysema); hypertrophied bronchial muscle and mucous impaction (asthma); upper airway obstruction (fixed or variable); normal
Clinical Presentation		
Age	Any	Any; bronchitis and emphysema >55 yr
Medical history	Well; hypertension; heart disease	Chronic shortness of breath; history of depression; weakness and wheezing
Present illness	Acute shortness of breath temporally related to some serious event (e.g., car accident, sepsis, worsening blood pressure, chest pain)	Recent upper respiratory tract infection; gradual worsening of shortness of breath, increased cough, sputum, and wheezing; drug overdose; new or increased muscle weakness
Physical examination	Evidence of acute illness, tachypnea (>35/min); tachycardia; hypotension; diffuse crackles; signs of consolidation	Tachypnea (<30/min); tachycardia; prolonged expiration; decreased breath sounds; wheezing; pedal edema; reduced strength; altered consciousness
Laboratory Examination		
Chest roentgenogram	Small, white lungs; multiply patchy, diffuse infiltrates; lobar atelectasis or consolidation	Hyperinflation; large black lungs, bullae; wide interspaces; prominent bronchovascular marking with COPD or asthma; hypoinflation, small black lungs; with overdose or neuromuscular disease
Electrocardiogram	Sinus tachycardia; acute myocardial infarction; left ventricular hypertrophy	Right ventricular hypertrophy; "P" pulmonale; low voltage; clockwise rotation; normal
Laboratory	Nonspecific; hemoglobin low to normal; respiratory alkalosis; metabolic acidosis; raised BUN	Hemoglobin normal to high; respiratory acidosis; mixed metabolic and respiratory acidosis; low potassium

$\dot{V}/Q$ = ventilation/perfusion; A-a = alveolar-arterial.

altered (e.g., sedative drug overdose) or if the neuromuscular apparatus is inadequate (see Chapter 90).

A $PaCO_2$ > 55 mm Hg is generally considered hypercapnic-hypoxic respiratory failure in patients with known COPD and previously normal $PaCO_2$ values. By contrast, a $PaCO_2$ > 45 mm Hg has greater importance in patients suffering from acute asthma, drug overdose, or neurologic weakness. No $PaCO_2$ value indicates with certainty the extent of deterioration in a patient with known chronic hypercapnia. Because of renal compensation and the development of base excess, the arterial pH does not always reflect the rate at which $PaCO_2$ rose (see Chapter 92). About 25% of patients with acute respiratory failure on admission have a compensated pH resulting from transient increases in alveolar ventilation.

During hypoventilation under ambient conditions, the PCO_2 and PO_2 levels change in opposite directions by nearly the same amount, with no significant increase above normal in alveolar-arterial O_2 gradient. For example, normal $PaCO_2$ (40 mm Hg) + PaO_2 (90 mm Hg) = 130 mm Hg. If the change in $PaCO_2$ can account for the change in PaO_2 ($PaCO_2$ 60 mm Hg + PaO_2 70 mm Hg = 130 mm Hg), no additional cause of hypoxia other than pure

Table 88–3 ■ CLINICAL MANIFESTATIONS OF HYPOXIA AND HYPERCAPNIA

HYPOXEMIA*	HYPERCAPNIA*
Tachycardia	Somnolence
Tachypnea	Lethargy
Anxiety	Restlessness
Diaphoresis	Tremor
Altered mental status	Slurred speech
Confusion	Headache
Cyanosis	Asterixis
Hypertension	Papilledema
Hypotension	Coma
Bradycardia	
Seizures	
Lactic acidosis†	

*Listed in order of development with progressive alteration in PaO_2 or $PaCO_2$.
†Usually requires additional reduction in oxygen delivery due to inadequate cardiac output, severe anemia, or redistribution of blood flow.

hypoventilation is present. By contrast, the primary mechanism of hypoxemia in hypercapnic-hypoxic respiratory failure secondary to COPD and asthma is perfusion of poorly ventilated lung units or ventilation-perfusion ($\dot{V}/Q$) mismatch ($PaCO_2$ 60 mm Hg + PaO_2 40 mm Hg = 100 mm Hg). Low $\dot{V}/Q$ ratios can be recognized by the ability of 100% oxygen to provide the expected rise in arterial PaO_2 (>500 mm Hg); because the degree of $\dot{V}/Q$ mismatch varies, the increase in PaO_2 with low levels of supplemental O_2 cannot be predicted, and the targeted PaO_2 must be reached by trial and error.

CLINICAL MANIFESTATIONS. The clinical presentation is dictated primarily by the condition causing the functional impairment (see Table 88–2), by the level of arterial PaO_2, and by any resulting tissue hypoxia (Table 88–3). Arterial hypoxemia increases ventilation by stimulating carotid body chemoreceptors. The degree of ventilatory response depends on the ability to sense hypoxemia and the capacity of the respiratory system to respond. Activity of the sympathetic nervous system increases with secondary vasoconstriction and elevated cardiac output. Severe hypoxia impairs mental performance and may progress to myocardial ischemia and permanent brain damage. Manifestations of hypoxic respiratory failure are more pronounced in the presence of underlying hematologic or circulatory abnormalities.

Acute hypercapnia depresses central nervous system activity but does so primarily by lowering the cerebrospinal fluid pH. Thus, low pH, rather than absolute levels of CO_2, best correlates with altered mental status. Although hypercapnia stimulates ventilation in normal subjects, the mechanism leading to hypercapnia often impairs or depresses any effective increases in minute ventilation. Symptoms of hypercapnia may overlap those of hypoxemia. Precipitating neurologic disorders, overmedication with sedatives, myxedema, or head trauma may mask the physiologic effect of both hypercapnia and hypoxemia.

ACUTE HYPOXIC RESPIRATORY FAILURE

Several relatively common diseases or conditions cause respiratory failure in a small percentage of affected patients but, because they are so common, account for a substantial number of cases in aggregate (Table 88–4). Different underlying diseases require specific therapies in addition to control of the severe hypoxemia itself.

Table 88-4 ■ CAUSES OF HYPOXIC RESPIRATORY FAILURE

Adult respiratory distress syndrome
Pneumonia: lobar, multilobar (see Chapter 82)
Pulmonary emboli (massive) (see Chapter 84)
Atelectasis (acute lobar) (see Chapter 77)
Cardiogenic pulmonary edema or shock (see Chapters 48 and 95)
Lung contusion or hemorrhage: trauma, Goodpasture's disease, idiopathic
  pulmonary hemosiderosis, systemic lupus erythematosus (see Chapter 78)

ADULT RESPIRATORY DISTRESS SYNDROME
(see Chapters 92 and 93)

Adult respiratory distress syndrome (ARDS), which is a form of acute lung injury often seen in previously healthy patients, is characterized by rapid respiratory rates and a sensation of profound shortness of breath. The consensus definition includes severe hypoxemia not responsive to supplemental oxygen ($PaO_2/FIO_2 < 200$) and widespread pulmonary infiltrates (involvement of three of six lung regions) not explained by cardiovascular disease or volume overload. The functioning lung tends to be small, as is indicated by a diminished thoracic gas volume and a reduction in the amount of air that can enter the lung at usual pressures (low compliance of <40 mL of air per cm H_2O, where normal approximates 100 mL/cm H_2O). Each year 100,000 cases of ARDS are seen in the United States. ARDS can result from a diverse array of systemic and pulmonary insults (Table 88-5), but 80% of cases are associated with systemic or pulmonary infection, severe trauma, or aspiration of gastric contents. The likelihood of development of ARDS is highest in patients with severe sepsis or septic shock (30%) (see Chapter 96), increases in the presence of multiple risk factors, and often occurs as part of multisystem organ failure (see Chapter 91). The generic term ARDS belies the non-uniformity of possible mechanisms and diverse precipitating events.

PATHOGENESIS. Despite the many risk factors and different initiating processes, the crucial stimulus seems to be an inflammatory response to distant or local tissue injury. The initial insult causes release of cytokines, mediators from cell membranes (arachidonic

Table 88-5 ■ DISORDERS ASSOCIATED WITH ADULT
RESPIRATORY DISTRESS SYNDROME

Aspiration
  Gastric contents
  Fresh and salt water
  Hydrocarbons
Central nervous system
  Trauma
  Anoxia
  Seizures
  Increased intracranial pressure
Drug overdose or reactions
  Acetylsalicylic acid
  Heroin
  Hydroxychloroquine (Plaquenil)
  Propoxyphene
  Paraquat
Hematologic alterations
  Disseminated intravascular coagulation
  Massive blood transfusion
  Leukoagglutination reactions
Infection
  Sepsis (gram-positive or -negative)
  Pneumonia: bacterial, viral, fungal
  Tuberculosis
Inhalation of toxins
  Oxygen
  Smoke
  Corrosive chemicals (NO_2, Cl_2, NH_3, phosgene)
Metabolic disorders
  Pancreatitis
  Uremia and diabetes mellitus seem to contribute to other risk factors
Shock (rare in cardiogenic or embolic; uncommon in pure hemorrhagic)
Trauma
  Fat emboli (long bones usually)
  Lung contusion
  Non-thoracic (severe)
  Cardiopulmonary bypass

acid and platelet-activating factor), and activation of a number of cascades (complement, coagulation, and kinin) with injury to the pulmonary endothelium. Neutrophils activating and adhering to endothelial cells with release of oxygen radicals and proteases may contribute to endothelial cell damage over several hours or days. Although ARDS is usually defined by a level of hypoxemia ($PaO_2/FIO_2 < 200$), the spectrum of *acute lung injury* includes less severe cases, which frequently can be identified by PaO_2/FIO_2 less than 300. The extent of injury depends on the magnitude of initial damage and repeated insults, such as persistent septicemia or retained necrotic and inflamed tissue. Experimental and clinical evidence shows that some cases of ARDS resolve rapidly (e.g., postictal, heroin overdose), whereas others progress relentlessly through several stages to severe fibrosis and lead to death from persistent respiratory failure. The correlations among PaO_2 levels, measurements of extravascular lung water, and extent of chest radiographic densities are surprisingly poor.

DIFFERENTIAL DIAGNOSIS. Although several generalized and focal disease processes can result in severe hypoxemia, in most cases the differential diagnosis is primarily between hydrostatic or cardiogenic pulmonary edema versus non-cardiogenic pulmonary edema from increased pulmonary capillary permeability (i.e., ARDS) (Table 88-6). Because reliable historical information may be absent, and physical and non-invasive laboratory findings may overlap, clinical distinctions can be accurate in only 60 to 80% of cases. If accurate indices of volume status and cardiac function are unavailable, right-sided hemodynamics by heart catheterization can be diagnostic. However, high left-sided filling pressures may fall rapidly after resolution of an acute episode of left ventricular ischemia or after vasodilator and diuretic therapy; by comparison, the intrapulmonary edema may take several days to clear roentgenographically. Echocardiography to assess ventricular function can help in making a diagnosis and in guiding subsequent therapy.

TREATING ACUTE HYPOXIC RESPIRATORY FAILURE. The predisposing condition producing the diffuse lung injury and pulmonary capillary leak should be identified and treated, because removal of ongoing inflammatory stimuli limits further injury and allows gradual resolution (Fig. 88-1). No therapies have been proved to repair endothelial and alveolar permeability or increase removal of alveolar and interstitial fluid.

Corticosteroids and non-steroidal anti-inflammatory agents have been evaluated in clinical trials and have shown no effect on lung mechanics, gas exchange, or outcome in early established ARDS. *Surfactant levels* are reduced in patients with ARDS, and their bronchoalveolar lavage fluid has diminished surface tension–reducing properties. Direct instillation of surfactant in animal models and neonates with respiratory distress syndrome produces rapid and impressive improvements in gas exchange as well as radiographic clearing. In adults with ARDS, however, surfactant has not improved outcome, perhaps because current aerosol techniques do not deliver sufficient amounts of surfactant to the alveoli most in need. Antibodies or receptor blockers to endotoxin, tumor necrosis factor-alpha (TNF-α), and interleukin-1 during established sepsis have also been unsuccessful, and a number of recent clinical trials with prostaglandin E_1 and nitric oxide have been disappointing. Preliminary data in patients with sepsis-induced ARDS have shown an encouraging reduction in the number of organs developing dysfunction and a trend toward improvement in survival after administering or upregulating *free-radical scavengers*. Alternatively, the outcome in many of these patients may be primarily influenced by multisystem organ failure and not the lung injury itself.

SUPPORTIVE THERAPY. Major energy and attention should be directed to supportive therapy. The primary goals of treatment are to relieve respiratory distress, to maintain adequate PaO_2 levels and O_2 transport while avoiding lung damage, and to prevent complications such as O_2 toxicity, fluid overload, gastrointestinal bleeding, local or systemic infection, thromboembolism, malnutrition, and ventilator-associated problems (Table 88-7) (see Chapter 93). Convincing data from randomized clinical trials indicate that a low tidal volume is superior to larger tidal volumes. Several other principles (Table 88-8) also should guide the use of mechanical ventilation in patients with ARDS (see Chapter 93). Clinicians should always choose the ventilator mode with which they are familiar and not switch to newer modes until data are clear and both physicians and staff are trained and prepared.

OUTCOME. Survival in ARDS is 60% and is highest when it occurs as an isolated event ($>85\%$) and lowest when it is part of

Table 88–6 ■ FEATURES DIFFERENTIATING NON-CARDIOGENIC AND CARDIOGENIC PULMONARY EDEMA

NON-CARDIOGENIC (ARDS)	CARDIOGENIC/VOLUME OVERLOAD
Prior History	
Younger	Older
No history of heart disease	Prior history of heart disease
Appropriate fluid balance (difficult to assess after resuscitation from shock, trauma, etc.)	Hypertension, chest pain, new onset palpitations; positive fluid balance
Physical Examination	
Flat neck veins	Elevated neck veins
Hyperdynamic pulses	Left ventricular enlargement, lift, heave, dyskinesis
Physiologic gallop	3rd and 4th heart sounds; murmurs
Absence of edema	Edema: flank, sacrum, legs
Electrocardiogram	
Sinus tachycardia, non-specific ST-T wave changes	Evidence of prior or ongoing ischemia, supraventricular tachycardia; left ventricular hypertrophy
Chest Radiograph	
Normal heart size	Cardiomegaly
Peripheral distribution of infiltrates	Central or basilar infiltrates; peribronchial and vascular congestion
Air bronchogram common (80%)	Septal lines (Kerley lines), air bronchograms (25%); pleural effusion
Hemodynamic Measurements	
Pulmonary artery wedge pressure <15 mm Hg; cardiac index >3.5 L/min/m²	Pulmonary capillary wedge pressure >18 mm Hg; cardiac index <3.5 L/min/m² with ischemia; may be >3.5 with volume overload

multisystem organ failure (30%). Nosocomial pneumonia significantly increases mortality. In the majority of patients who survive to extubation, lung damage completely resolves (60%); only a small percentage of patients are left with significant functional impairment.

ACUTE HYPERCAPNIC-HYPOXIC RESPIRATORY FAILURE

Acute hypercapnic-hypoxic respiratory failure is a physiologic derangement that results from many pathologic events. It may occur in previously healthy persons without specific lung injury or in persons with underlying pulmonary disease. In the presence of severe COPD, a minor event may precipitate acute decompensation. The presentation and treatment of hypercapnic-hypoxic respiratory failure can be divided into conditions in which the hypercapnia results from decreased minute ventilation (Table 88–9, categories I through III and IVa) and those in which the increased PaCO₂ results from severe ventilation-perfusion mismatch and increased

dead space despite high minute ventilation (Table 88–9, category IVb). Categories V and VI usually result from varying degrees of decreased tidal volume but maintained minute ventilation due to chest wall abnormalities; their clinical presentation is similar to that of category IVb. About half of the clinical cases of hypercapnic-hypoxic respiratory failure are category IVb.

SECONDARY TO DECREASED MINUTE VENTILATION. The diseases or conditions that may present with hypercapnic-hypoxic respiratory failure secondary to decreased minute ventilation are numerous. Each entity has characteristic signs and symptoms that initially or ultimately point to the primary pathogenesis (see Chapters 476, 482, and 497 to 511).

The disease presentation varies from a sudden onset, as seen in high cervical cord trauma or botulism, to a subacute course, as seen in polyneuritis or myasthenia gravis. An even slower onset is observed in hypothyroidism and muscular dystrophy. Kyphoscoliotic cardiopulmonary disease and obesity-hypoventilation syndrome are generally present for decades before respiratory failure

Table 88–7 ■ SUPPORTIVE MANAGEMENT OF ADULT RESPIRATORY DISTRESS SYNDROME

PRINCIPLE	GOAL	STRATEGY
Improve PaO₂	PaO₂ >60 mm Hg, SaO₂ >90%; accept PaO₂ <60 mm Hg, especially in young	Initiate therapy with 100% O₂; usually requires intubation; monitor pulse oximetry
Prevent O₂ toxicity	FIO₂ <0.6	Recruit lung units by adding PEEP, increasing mean airway pressure or periodic prolonged inflation >20 sec
Provide adequate O₂ transport	Normalize blood pressure, pulse pressure, and organ perfusion; maintain cardiac index >3.5 L/min/m²; hemoglobin ±9 g/dL	Fluid replacement for adequate venous return following increased PEEP; vasoactive drugs to maintain blood pressure and organ perfusion; measure cardiac index if uncertain
Optimize fluid status	Lowest tolerated filling pressures; keep dry	Limit extraneous IV fluids, follow intake and output; diurese empirically; measure pulmonary capillary wedge pressure if fluid status unclear
Meet ventilatory demands	Reduce work of breathing and O₂ consumption of respiratory muscles; eliminate CO₂	Assisted ventilation, sedation, rarely paralysis; follow arterial blood gases; permit hypercapnia, 60–70 mm Hg
Avoid gastrointestinal bleeding	Gastric pH >4; protect gastric lining	H₂-blockers, sucralfate, proton pump inhibitors
Prevent thromboembolism	Reduce clotting and venous stasis	Pneumatic and elastic compression stockings, subcutaneous heparin
Supply adequate nutrition	Replace resting energy expenditure	25–30 kcal/kg, 1.5 g of protein/kg; enteral feeding preferred, total parenteral nutrition if gut dysfunctional. Some diets may improve outcome.
Prevent respiratory and system infection	Maintain sterile techniques, promote gastric emptying, minimize lung congestion and atelectasis, limit antibiotic use	Handwashing and good respiratory therapy technique, elevate bed 30 degrees, enteral feeding, frequent or continuous turning, oral endotracheal tubes
Weaning and extubation	Remove from ventilator and extubate ASAP	Take every opportunity to reduce PEEP and do not prolong weaning or extubation any longer than absolutely necessary
Minimize anxiety, pain, discomfort	Keep sedated but easily aroused	Regular intermittent sedation, anticipate analgesic needs as clinically dictated, try to communicate frequently with patient

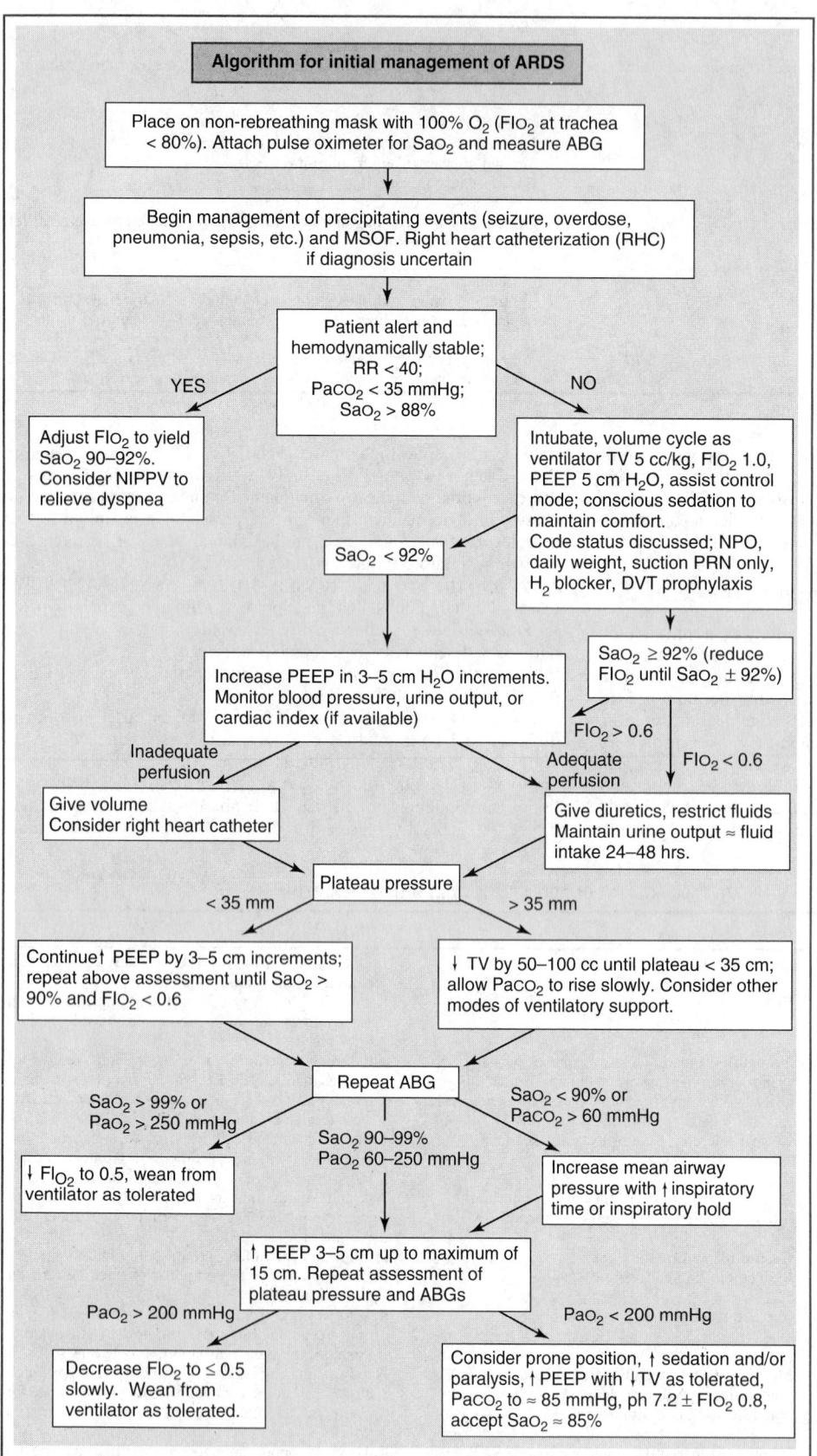

Algorithm for initial management of ARDS

Place on non-rebreathing mask with 100% O_2 (FIO_2 at trachea < 80%). Attach pulse oximeter for SaO_2 and measure ABG

Begin management of precipitating events (seizure, overdose, pneumonia, sepsis, etc.) and MSOF. Right heart catheterization (RHC) if diagnosis uncertain

Patient alert and hemodynamically stable; RR < 40; $PaCO_2$ < 35 mmHg; SaO_2 > 88%

YES

Adjust FIO_2 to yield SaO_2 90–92%. Consider NIPPV to relieve dyspnea

NO

Intubate, volume cycle as ventilator TV 5 cc/kg, FIO_2 1.0, PEEP 5 cm H_2O, assist control mode; conscious sedation to maintain comfort. Code status discussed; NPO, daily weight, suction PRN only, H_2 blocker, DVT prophylaxis

SaO_2 < 92%

$SaO_2 \geq 92\%$ (reduce FIO_2 until $SaO_2 \pm 92\%$)

Increase PEEP in 3–5 cm H_2O increments. Monitor blood pressure, urine output, or cardiac index (if available)

FIO_2 > 0.6

FIO_2 < 0.6

Inadequate perfusion

Adequate perfusion

Give volume
Consider right heart catheter

Give diuretics, restrict fluids
Maintain urine output ≈ fluid intake 24–48 hrs.

Plateau pressure

< 35 mm

> 35 mm

Continue↑ PEEP by 3–5 cm increments; repeat above assessment until SaO_2 > 90% and FIO_2 < 0.6

↓ TV by 50–100 cc until plateau < 35 cm; allow $PaCO_2$ to rise slowly. Consider other modes of ventilatory support.

Repeat ABG

SaO_2 > 99% or PaO_2 > 250 mmHg

SaO_2 90–99% PaO_2 60–250 mmHg

SaO_2 < 90% or $PaCO_2$ > 60 mmHg

↓ FIO_2 to 0.5, wean from ventilator as tolerated

Increase mean airway pressure with ↑ inspiratory time or inspiratory hold

↑ PEEP 3–5 cm up to maximum of 15 cm. Repeat assessment of plateau pressure and ABGs

PaO_2 > 200 mmHg

PaO_2 < 200 mmHg

Decrease FIO_2 to ≤ 0.5 slowly. Wean from ventilator as tolerated.

Consider prone position, ↑ sedation and/or paralysis, ↑ PEEP with ↓TV as tolerated, $PaCO_2$ to ≈ 85 mmHg, ph 7.2 ± FIO_2 0.8, accept SaO_2 ≈ 85%

FIGURE 88–1 ■ An algorithm for the initial management of adult respiratory distress syndrome (ARDS). ABG = arterial blood gas analysis; CO_2 = carbon dioxide; DVT = deep venous thrombosis; FIO_2 = inspired oxygen concentration; MSOF = multisystem organ failure; NIPPV = non-invasive intermittent positive-pressure ventilation; O_2 = oxygen; $PaCO_2$ = arterial partial pressure of carbon dioxide; PaO_2 = arterial partial pressure of oxygen; PEEP = positive end-expiratory pressure; RR = respiratory rate; SaO_2 = arterial oxygen saturation; VT = tidal volume.

Table 88–8 ■ VENTILATOR GUIDELINES TO MAXIMIZE EFFICIENCY AND MINIMIZE COMPLICATIONS

PARAMETER	TARGET
FIO_2	<0.5; balance against PEEP, relative risk problematic
PEEP	12–16 cm H_2O, can increase to recruit a majority of alveolar units and to maintain FIO_2 <0.8
Tidal volume	5–8 mL/kg; may allow $PaCO_2$ to rise
Plateau pressure*	<35 cm (and preferably <30 cm) H_2O end inspiration during respiratory hold
Flow rate†	>90 L/min
Sensitivity	−0.5 to 21.5 cm H_2O
Respiratory rate‡	Assist-control at 10–15/min or 5/min below patient's rate

*Usually measured by inducing a brief inspiratory hold. Pressure falls from peak inspiratory pressure but often only 5 to 10 cm H_2O, depending on inspiratory flow rate and degree of airway resistance secondary to endotracheal tube and small airways reactivity.

†Increase in mean airway pressure best achieved with an inspiratory hold or prolonged plateau.

‡In spontaneously breathing patients, rate is determined by inspiratory drive and/or ventilatory demand. Select inspiratory flow and resulting inspiratory-expiratory ratio to meet air flow demands and prevent hemodynamic compromise and air trapping. Reductions in tidal volume or patient sedation may be necessary to achieve these goals.

develops. In many chronic neuromuscular or musculoskeletal conditions, a minor acute respiratory insult may precipitate sudden respiratory failure by worsening the underlying neuromuscular condition (as in myasthenia gravis) or abruptly reducing pulmonary function (as with aspiration pneumonia in parkinsonism).

In conditions that alter control of respiration, the degree of respiratory failure may not correlate with the level of consciousness. For example, barbiturate overdoses often result in coma without elevated $PaCO_2$, whereas morphine overdoses produce profound hypercapnia with only moderate reductions in the level of consciousness. Respiratory failure should be suspected in all unconscious or obtunded patients and in all patients with neuromuscular insults; the diagnosis is established by evaluating arterial blood gases. In addition, patients with marked neuromuscular diseases should be followed with frequent measurements of their vital capacity and negative inspiratory force; when the vital capacity is less than 1 L or the inspiratory force cannot exceed 15 cm H_2O, acute respiratory failure should be anticipated and patients should be transferred to an ICU for close monitoring.

Early intubation is indicated for potentially reversible causes of acute respiratory failure. Methods of artificial ventilatory support without intubation, such as external negative pressure ventilation or nasal/face mask continuous or intermittent positive-pressure ventilation (CPAP and BIPAP), may suffice in some patients but are often unreliable due to poor upper airway control and aspiration of secretions (see Chapter 93). Hypoxemia should always be corrected. Inspiratory O_2 greater than 30% is necessary only in such superimposed conditions as atelectasis, pneumonia, or pulmonary embolism.

Good airway toilet is essential. Postural drainage may help clear

Table 88–9 ■ COMMON CAUSES OF HYPERCAPNIC-HYPOXIC RESPIRATORY FAILURE

I. Altered control
  a. Primary intracranial disease (tumor, hemorrhage)
  b. Trauma and raised intracranial pressure
  c. Drugs, poisons, and toxins
  d. Central hypoventilation
  e. Excess oxygen administration in hypercapnic patient
II. Neuromuscular disease
  a. Spinal cord lesions (trauma, tumor, vascular)
  b. Acute polyneuritis
  c. Myasthenia gravis
  d. Polymyositis, dermatomyositis
  e. Parkinson's disease
III. Metabolic derangements
  a. Severe acidosis
  b. Severe alkalosis
  c. Hypokalemia
  d. Hypophosphatemia
  e. Hypomagnesemia
IV. Lungs and airway disease
  a. Upper airway disease (fixed, variable, or sleep-dependent)
  b. Lower airway disease (COPD, asthma)
V. Musculoskeletal alterations
  a. Kyphoscoliosis
  b. Ankylosing spondylitis
VI. Obesity-hypoventilation syndrome

secretions and atelectasis. Minor episodes of aspiration pneumonia are frequent; however, transient low-grade fevers or minor leukocytosis without pulmonary infiltration should be treated by increased respiratory toilet alone and raise the suspicion of a non-pulmonary infection. Left lower lobe infiltrates often elude detection in patients in ICUs because routine chest roentgenograms are usually obtained by portable anteroposterior techniques. Right and left lateral decubitus films are helpful in excluding suspected left lower lobe pneumonia.

Recovery from hypercapnic-hypoxic respiratory failure with decreased minute ventilation depends on the underlying condition and the supportive care. Some patients with neuromuscular disease may require prolonged or even permanent assisted ventilation. After extubation, long-term nocturnal ventilatory assistance with CPAP or BIPAP (see Chapter 93) may support patients with moderate daytime hypoventilation. Electrophrenic pacing of both diaphragms has helped in some central hypoventilation syndromes. A long-term commitment to respiratory support with an artificial ventilator should be avoided in patients with progressive neuromuscular disease who do not have an acute reversible cause of respiratory failure.

SECONDARY TO LOWER AIRWAY DISEASE. COPD and asthma represent the major causes of acute hypercapnic-hypoxic respiratory failure. In COPD, minute ventilation is usually high with increased absolute dead space; by comparison, in asthma, tidal volume is reduced, and wasted ventilation results from rebreathing anatomic dead space (see Chapters 74 and 75). Examination usually reveals an anxious person in severe respiratory distress. Breathing is labored, and the rate is moderately increased. Accessory muscles are active. If respiratory depressant drugs are given (e.g., for agitation or insomnia), respiratory rate and depth may not seem abnormal, and the patient may appear calm; this particular clinical presentation is characteristic of patients who have received high inspiratory O_2 en route to the hospital. Cyanosis may be obvious, but its absence does not exclude severe hypoxemia. Papilledema is occasionally seen, most often in comatose patients but occasionally as the only impressive finding of respiratory failure. Supraventricular arrhythmias and signs of right ventricular failure are common in patients with severe COPD.

A chest radiograph may reveal the presence of obvious chronic lung disease or superimposed acute pulmonary infiltrates; however, the chest roentgenogram may not be helpful except to eliminate competing diagnoses. Leukocytosis suggests infection, but severe leukoerythroblastic responses may follow the stress of severe hypoxemia.

Table 88–10 ■ RECOMMENDED INITIAL FIO_2 BY VENTI MASK OR NASAL O_2 BY CANNULA TO ACHIEVE PaO_2 >60 mm Hg

INITIAL PaO_2 ON ROOM AIR (mm Hg)	VENTI MASK FIO_2 (%)	NASAL CANNULA (L/min)
50	24	1
45–49	28	2
40–44	32	3
<40	35	4

Table 88–11 ▪ INDICATIONS FOR ICU ADMISSION OF PATIENTS WITH ACUTE COPD EXACERBATION

Severe dyspnea unresponsive to initial emergency therapy
Confusion, lethargy, or respiratory muscle fatigue (the last characterized by paradoxical diaphragmatic motion)
Worsening hypoxemia despite supplemental oxygen or worsening respiratory acidosis (pH <7.30)
Assisted mechanical ventilation is requiring endotracheal tube

Adapted from: ATS Committee Statement. Inpatient Management of COPD. Am J Respir Crit Care Med 152:S97–S106, 1995.

TREATMENT SECONDARY TO CHRONIC OBSTRUCTIVE LUNG DISEASE. Principles of patient care that apply to most cases include applying immediate life-saving measures; determining the precipitating factors; treating the airways dysfunction; and monitoring. Appropriate life-saving measures for acute respiratory failure center on the immediate correction of hypoxemia, need for emergency intubation or assisted ventilation, and adequate circulatory support. If, as in most cases, the patient is alert or only minimally confused and has a stable cardiovascular status, low-flow O_2 is the principal therapy. Adequate oxygenation is nearly always achieved; however, it may take serial elevations in inspiratory FIO_2 to as high as 0.5 (Table 88–10). The patient should be transferred to an ICU (Table 88–11) or other appropriate setting for continuous monitoring of vital signs and pulse oximetry. Minute ventilation is usually maintained in COPD patients with O_2 therapy. The expected modest rise in $PaCO_2$ is attributed largely to increased dead space ventilation secondary to O_2-induced changes in $\dot{V}/\dot{Q}$ mismatch and is generally of little concern unless $PaCO_2$ continues to rise to extremely high levels (>75 mm Hg) or obtundation develops. A new steady state usually takes several hours. Reducing FIO_2 under these circumstances is dangerous. The physician must closely follow blood gas measurements (Table 88–12), systemic arterial pressure, respiratory rate, vital capacity, cardiac rhythm, urinary output, hemoglobin levels, and serum electrolyte levels.

Most patients with COPD in whom hypercapnic-hypoxic respiratory failure develops have a reversible precipitating factor that decreases alveolar ventilation; the most common is increased bronchospasm associated with a change in weather, minor infection, or failure to take medication. Infection may also increase bronchial secretions, reduce functional pulmonary parenchyma, or increase CO_2 production, and thus overwhelm an already-limited respiratory system. Occasionally, inadvertent or surreptitious sedative consumption or factors such as pneumothorax, cardiac arrhythmias, left ventricular failure, or dehydration may contribute. If adequate oxygenation can be maintained without major worsening of respiratory acidosis, conservative measures can usually be applied to reverse all of these precipitating conditions (Table 88–13, Fig. 88–2). Respiratory stimulants are rarely effective to reduce hypercapnia because minute ventilation is normal or increased and mechanical work is already excessive.

ASSISTED VENTILATION. Most patients hospitalized with hypercapnic-hypoxic respiratory failure improve after conservative therapy without needing artificial ventilatory support. If a patient continues to deteriorate, however, assisted ventilation is indicated. Arterial blood gas values are of limited use in making this judgment. High respiratory rates (>36 per minute), excessive use of accessory muscles, paradoxical thoracoabdominal movement, a subjective sense of exhaustion, and even minor mental status changes should be considered probable indications. In approximately one-third of patients, face mask or nasal noninvasive intermittent positive-pressure ventilation (NIPPV) (see Chapter 93) are effective in sustaining or augmenting alveolar ventilation and reducing the work of breathing; they allow time for specific therapy to improve airway dysfunction without intubation.

If hypoventilation cannot be effectively reversed by mechanical assistance of some type, an endotracheal tube must be inserted. Intubation results in laryngeal and tracheal irritation, loss of effective cough, and increased risk of infection. It is also a source of discomfort in the conscious and alert patient. With careful handling, endotracheal tubes may be kept in place for at least 2 weeks (see Chapter 93). When artificial ventilation is required for more than 2 weeks, a tracheostomy is often required. The most important indication for early tracheostomy is the presence of copious, tenacious secretions that cannot be adequately removed through the endotracheal tube. Tracheostomy carries some risk of bleeding, pneumothorax, and local infection and an increased incidence of aspiration.

Short-term outcome following acute hypoxic respiratory failure is generally good (see Table 88–1). The long-term prognosis is dictated by underlying disease and the functional impairment before acute respiratory failure developed. Only 25% of COPD patients survive 2 years after an episode of acute respiratory failure.

CHRONIC RESPIRATORY FAILURE

Any process that affects the airways, lung parenchyma, chest wall, or neuromuscular system can evolve into chronic respiratory failure. The condition leading to lung failure is usually obvious. If historical information is not available, however, a specific diagnosis may be difficult, because many end-stage primary lung diseases overlap clinically. Obstruction can be separated from restriction (see Chapter 72), although patients may not be able to perform the necessary rigorous pulmonary function tests. At times, superimposed infection, pleural disease, or previous surgery also blurs these distinctions. In the most severe cases of chronic hypoxic respiratory failure, progressive lung destruction also impairs ventilation, and hypercapnia develops.

Many patients with chronic hypoxic respiratory failure have end-stage fibrosis (honeycomb lung) (see Chapter 78). Supportive care includes oxygen for severe hypoxia and diuretics for excessive edema. About two-thirds of delivered O_2 per breath escapes into the environment. Various O_2-conserving devices are available and may allow for more cost-effective supplementation and longer periods away from home. If patients are younger than 60 years and have no other significant problems, lung transplantation (see Chapter 89) should be considered.

A variety of diseases lead to chronic hypercapnic respiratory failure (see Chapters 74 and 75). Progressive elevation in PCO_2 levels indicates a poor prognosis. Application of periodic negative- and positive-pressure devices with a nasal or full face mask may reduce respiratory work, relieve dyspnea, and lower daytime PCO_2. Using these devices during sleep may improve quality of life and prolong survival, especially in patients with neuromuscular diseases. The major contraindication to NIPPV (see Chapter 93) is a swallowing dysfunction, because aspiration is likely. Transtracheal

Table 88–12 ▪ SUGGESTED MODIFICATIONS OF TREATMENT (WITHOUT INTUBATION) BASED ON FOLLOW-UP ARTERIAL BLOOD GAS ANALYSES

FOLLOW-UP PaO_2 (mm Hg)	FOLLOW-UP $PaCO_2$ (mm Hg)	FOLLOW-UP pH	THERAPEUTIC RECOMMENDATION
>60	<55	>7.30	No change in O_2; follow SaO_2 with pulse oximetry
>60	>55–<65	7.25	No change in O_2; repeat ABG in 3–4 hr or SaO_2 >96%
>60	>65	<7.25 >7.20	No change in O_2; repeat ABG in 1 hr
>60	>80	<7.20 >7.05	Add NIPPV
<60	<55	Unchanged	Increase nasal O_2 flow 1 L/min
<60	>55	>7.25	Increase nasal O_2 flow until SaO_2 85%; check ABG in 1 hr

ABG = arterial blood gas analysis; NIPPV, non-invasive intermittent positive-pressure ventilation.

Table 88–13 ■ THERAPY FOR ACUTE HYPERCAPNIC-HYPOXIC RESPIRATORY FAILURE SECONDARY TO AIRWAY DISEASE

CONDITION	THERAPY	ROUTE	DOSE	EXPECTED RESPONSE OR TARGET	ADVANTAGE/COMMENT
Hypoxia	O_2	Nasal prongs	2–3 L/min	Pa_{O_2} >55 mm Hg	Reduces pulmonary hypertension and airway resistance, improves diuresis
		Venti mask	FIO_2, 0.24–0.3	Lower initial PaO_2, lower initial target	Low FIO_2 reduces $PaCO_2$ increase
Airway obstruction	Albuterol	MDI and spacer	400–600 μg q1–4h	Improve FEV_1 or peak flow	Cost-effective; use only when patient alert, cooperative, coordinated
		Aerosol solution	2.5–7.5 mg q1–4h	Same as above	More reliable than MDI when patient cannot take deep breath; when intubated, deep breath improves deposition of either MDI or aerosol; maximum dose determined by response and toxicity
	Ipratropium	MDI and spacer	80–120 μg q4–6h	Same as above	Little to no toxicity, slower onset than albuterol; drug of choice with any cardiac arrhythmia
		Aerosol solution	500 μg q4–6h	Same as above	Effective in acute failure
	Theophylline	IV	5.6 mg/kg load, 0.3–0.6 mg/kg/hr	Same as above; may improve air trapping, shorten hospital stay	Not first-line; add if patient not improving, keep blood levels <15 mg/L; clearance influenced by numerous other drugs, diseases, age
Anti-inflammatory	Methylprednisolone	IV	40–80 mg q8–12h	Reduced inflammation; improved FEV_1	Recommend in all patients; takes hours to days for response
Infection	2nd-generation cephalosporin	IV	Depends on preparation	Resolve pneumonia more quickly, improve bronchitis, fewer relapses	Usually concerned about *Streptococcus pneumoniae* and *Haemophilus influenzae*
	Newer fluoroquinolones	PO	Varies		
	Ampicillin/clavulanate	PO	150 mg bid		Use with productive sputum, temperature, presumed acute bronchitis, suspected pneumonia
Prevention of deep venous thrombosis and pulmonary embolism	Heparin	SC	500 U	Reduce clotting, decrease morbidity	Graduated elastic stockings of additional value, encourage leg movement
Gastrointestinal bleeding	H_2-blocker	IV or PO; various compounds	q12h	Gastric pH >4	Not all patients have low pH; standard dose achieves target in only 80%
	Sucralfate	PO	1 g qid	Protect mucosal lining	Must be placed in stomach if patient not eating
Agitation	Lorazepam	IV	1–3 mg q3–4h	Mild sedation and amnesia	Only when patient on ventilator
Arrhythmias	Improve respiratory failure, reduce theophylline or β_2 agonists, correct K, Mg, alkalosis			If symptomatic supraventricular tachycardia, treat with diltiazem, adenosine, or digoxin	Usually more of a nuisance than a real problem; do not be distracted; avoid β-blockers, especially in patients with asthma
Dehydration	0.45 normal saline	IV	100 mL/hr	Volume expansion; better cardiac output	Better slightly wet; especially in patients on ventilator; 1+ edema safe
Volume overload	Diuretics (furosemide)	IV	40 mg q8–12h	Improvement in gas exchange	Have impaired capacity to excrete water load; assisted ventilation reduces atrial natriuretic factor, increases SIADH
Electrolytes	KCl, etc. as detected	IV	K^+ 40 mEq in 100 mL as needed	Normalize serum K^+, prevent alkalosis	Patients often hypokalemic, total body stores may be depleted, even with normal values
Thick secretions	Correct dehydration, treat infection, postural drainage, vibration, percussion		q4–12h as tolerated	Improved expectoration; improved FEV_1	Encourage cough, nasotracheal suction; monitor O_2 saturation with drainage or suction; continue therapy only if cough is productive

MDI = metered-dose inhaler.

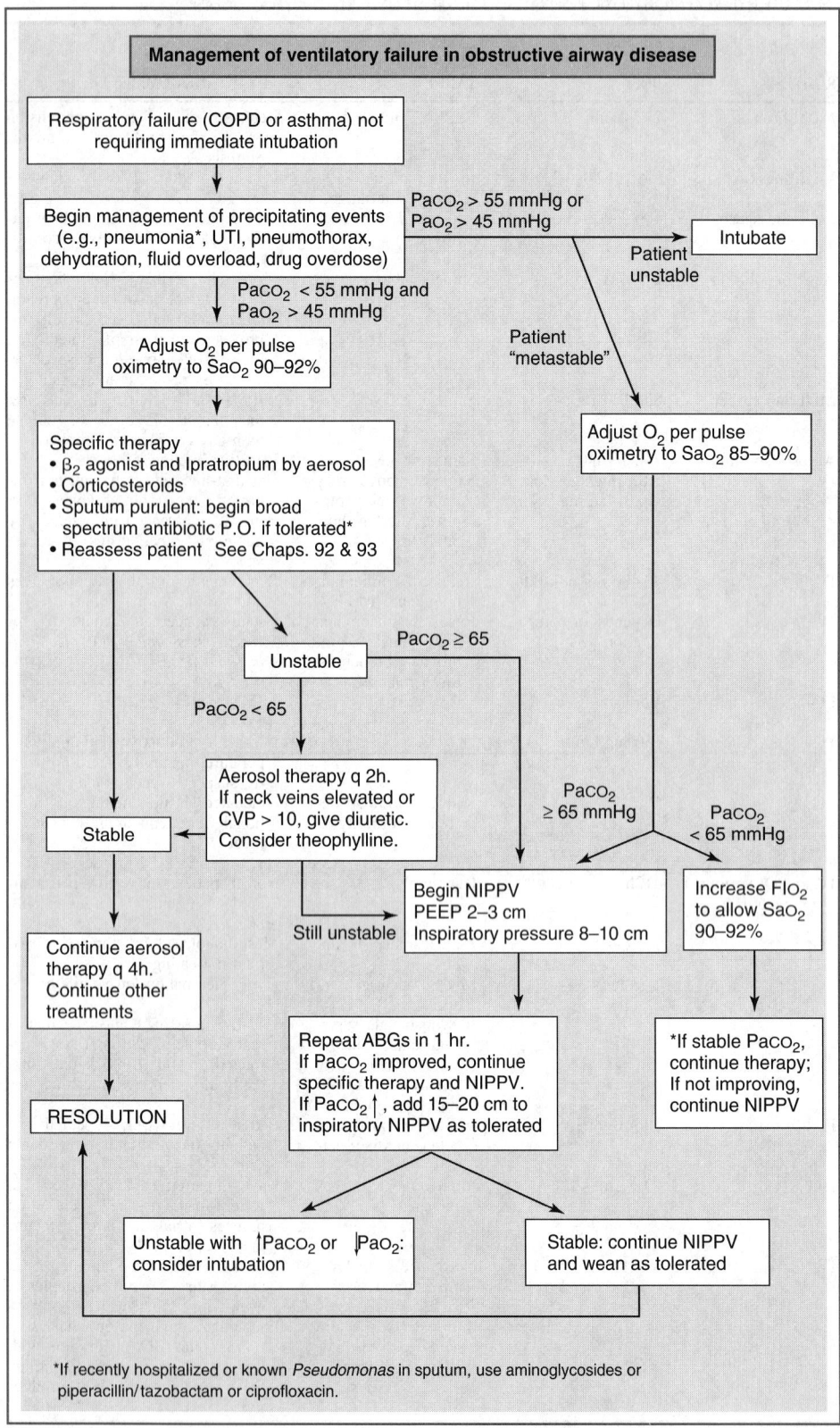

FIGURE 88–2 ■ An algorithm for the management of ventilatory failure in a patient with obstructive airway disease. CVP = central venous pressure; HRF = hypoxic respiratory failure; UTI = urinary tract infection. (See Fig. 88–1 legend for key to other abbreviations.)

O_2 may decrease the work of breathing, improve dyspnea, and reduce costs of O_2 therapy. Younger patients with α_1-antitrypsin deficiency (see Chapter 75), cystic fibrosis (see Chapter 76), and other causes of bronchiectasis (see Chapter 77) are good candidates for lung transplantation (see Chapter 89). Quality of life is always an issue for elderly patients, and relief of suffering may be the major therapeutic goal of both patient and physician.

Artigas A, Bernard GR, Carlet J, et al: The American-European consensus conference on ARDS: 2. Am J Respir Crit Care Med 157:1332–1347, 1998.

Block ER: Pulmonary endothelial cell pathobiology: Implications for acute lung injury. Am J Med Sci 304:136, 1992. *Excellent review of the chemical and cellular insults that may lead to ARDS.*

Dhand R, Tobin MJ: Inhaled bronchodilator therapy in mechanically ventilated patients. Am J Respir Crit Care Med. 156:3–10, 1997.

Hillberg RE, Johnson DC: Noninvasive ventilation. N Engl J Med. 337:1746–1752, 1997. *An excellent review.*

Pingleton SK, Hall JB: Prevention and early detection of complications of critical care. Principles Crit Care 218:587, 1992. *Recent compendium of this perplexing problem.*

Pittet JF, Mackersie RC, Martin TR, et al: Biological markers of acute lung injury: Prognostic and pathogenetic significance. Am J Respir Crit Care Med 155:1187–1205, 1997.

Table 89–2 ■ CONTRAINDICATIONS TO LUNG TRANSPLANTATION

Absolute contraindications
Major organ dysfunction (other than lung)
Recent active malignancy
Infection with HIV
Hepatitis B antigen positivity
Hepatitis C with histologic evidence of active liver disease
Active substance abuse (including cigarettes)
Severe musculoskeletal disease affecting the thorax
Relative contraindications
Poor nutritional status (<70% or >130% ideal body weight)
Symptomatic osteoporosis
Colonization with fungi, atypical mycobacteria or pan-resistant bacteria
Requirement for invasive ventilation
Psychosocial problems likely to affect outcome adversely
High-dose (>20 mg of prednisone daily) corticosteroid use

From Joint Statement of American Society of Transplant Physicians/American Thoracic Society/International Society of Heart and Lung Transplantation: International Guidelines for the Selection of Lung Transplant Candidates. Am J Respir Crit Care med 158:335–339, 1998.

89 SURGICAL APPROACH TO LUNG DISEASE

John J. Reilly, Jr. ■ *Steven J. Mentzer*

The role of surgery in the diagnosis and therapy of lung disease has expanded greatly as lung transplantation has gained acceptance as a therapeutic option for selected patients with advanced lung disease. In addition, the concept of surgery to reduce lung volume in patients with emphysema has been reintroduced and is an area of active clinical investigation. Minimally invasive thoracic surgery has also created new options for lung biopsy and pulmonary resection.

LUNG TRANSPLANTATION

Historical Background

Human lung transplantation was first attempted in the 1960s but little success was achieved until the availability of more effective immunosuppressive drugs (cyclosporine) and improved surgical techniques in the early 1980s. The annual number of lung transplant procedures increased steadily from 1982 through 1993, but it has recently remained constant at 1300 to 1400 patients annually because of limited donor availability.

Transplant Types

Currently, four types of lung transplantation procedures are performed. *Single lung transplantation* is typically performed through a posterolateral thoracotomy incision and requires three anastomoses: mainstem bronchus, pulmonary artery, and pulmonary veins/left atrium. The contralateral lung is not removed, so single lung transplantation is not performed in patients with bilaterally infected lungs (e.g., patients with cystic fibrosis).

Bilateral lung transplantation was initially performed as an en bloc procedure but is currently performed in a sequential fashion that is functionally equivalent to two single lung transplants done during a single operation, most commonly through a transverse

sternotomy ("clamshell") incision. It requires six anastomoses: both mainstem bronchi, both pulmonary arteries, and both sets of pulmonary veins. It is the procedure of choice for patients with bilaterally infected lungs and is also performed in certain patients with emphysema, primary pulmonary hypertension, and other diseases.

Heart-lung transplantation was initially the most common type of lung transplant procedure but is now performed infrequently. It is an en bloc procedure, with right atrial, aortic, and distal tracheal anastomoses. It is performed in patients with advanced lung disease and coexistent cardiac disease, such as those with Eisenmenger's syndrome (see Chapter 57) who have uncorrectable intracardiac defects, end-stage lung disease, and irreversible cor pulmonale, or patients who have advanced lung disease and left ventricular dysfunction due to coronary artery disease.

The most recently introduced lung transplant procedure is *living donor lobar transplantation*. This procedure involves the removal of a lower lobe from each of two living donors, with the implantation of one in each hemithorax of the recipient in a manner similar to bilateral lung transplantation.

Diseases Treated with Lung Transplantation

The most common indications for transplantation are diseases or conditions that share the following common features: they produce extreme disability in affected patients, they are unresponsive to medical therapy, and they are responsible for limited life expectancy in affected patients (Table 89–1). With the exception of a small number of cases of sarcoidosis and lymphangioleiomyomatosis, the original lung disease does not recur after lung transplantation.

Considerations in the Evaluation of Potential Transplant Recipients

The ideal candidate for lung transplantation has lung disease unresponsive to medical therapy but is in otherwise good health. In contrast to cardiac transplantation (see Chapter 71), patients who are critically ill are usually not appropriate candidates for lung transplantation. Patients who experience critical illness due to lung disease often have poor nutritional status, coexistent major organ dysfunction, refractory infection, or other contraindications to transplantation (Table 89–2). Older patients have a higher mortality after transplant, leading to the current recommendations that single

Table 89–1 ■ INDICATIONS FOR LUNG TRANSPLANTATION

SINGLE LUNG TRANSPLANT	% OF PATIENTS	DOUBLE LUNG TRANSPLANT	% OF PATIENTS
Emphysema	44	Cystic fibrosis	34
Idiopathic pulmonary fibrosis	21	Emphysema	18
α_1-Antitrypsin deficiency	11	α_1-Antitrypsin deficiency	11
Primary pulmonary hypertension	5	Primary pulmonary hypertension	10
Other	19	Other	27

From the Registry of the International Society for Heart and Lung Transplantation. See Figure 89–1.

Table 89–3 ■ GUIDELINES FOR LUNG TRANSPLANT REFERRAL

DISEASE	PULMONARY FUNCTION	ARTERIAL BLOOD GAS VALUES	NYHA CLASS	OTHER CONSIDERATIONS
Chronic obstructive lung disease	FEV$_1$ <25% predicted	Pco$_2$ >55 mm Hg		Pulmonary hypertension; progressive deterioration
Cystic fibrosis	FEV$_1$ <30% predicted or rapid decline	Pco$_2$ >50 mm or Po$_2$ <55 mm Hg		Increasing admissions or rapid deterioration
Idiopathic pulmonary fibrosis	Vital capacity <60% predicted or D$_L$CO <50% predicted	Exertional desaturation		Lack of response to therapy
Pulmonary hypertension			Functional class III or IV despite vasodilator therapy	CI, <2 L/min/m²; RAP, >15 mm Hg; mean PAP, >55 mm Hg
Eisenmenger's syndrome			Functional class III or IV	

NYHA = New York Heart Association; FEV$_1$ = forced expiratory volume in 1 second; VC = vital capacity; CI = cardiac index; RAP = right atrial pressure; PAP = pulmonary artery pressure.

Adapted from Joint Statement of American Society of Transplant Physicians/American Thoracic Society/International Society of Heart and Lung Transplantation: International Guidelines for the Selection of Lung Transplant Candidates. Am J Respir Crit Care Med 158:335–339, 1998.

lung transplant recipients should be younger than 65 years and bilateral transplant recipients should be younger than 60 years; nevertheless, policies concerning age limits vary from program to program. The specific recommendations for referral for transplant evaluation vary depending on the underlying disease (Table 89–3). As waiting times for transplantation lengthen because of the expansion of the potential number of recipients, patients will likely need to be referred earlier to have a reasonable chance of surviving until transplantation.

Issues after Lung Transplantation

Most of the medical issues that patients and physicians face after lung transplantation are the consequence of the transplant and post-transplant medication, rather than the underlying disease for which the transplant was performed. Examples include immunosuppression, infections and their prophylaxis, acute allograft rejection, chronic allograft rejection, and nonpulmonary complications of transplantation.

IMMUNOSUPPRESSION. The standard chemotherapeutic regimen for immunosuppression after lung transplantation consists of cyclosporine, azathioprine, and corticosteroids. Use of tacrolimus instead of cyclosporine may result in fewer episodes of acute rejection in the first year after transplantation. Some centers add an antilymphocyte antibody preparation in the first days after transplantation, but the effect of this practice on rates of acute and chronic rejection are unknown. Experience with mycophenolate mofetil is limited, and its role remains to be defined.

INFECTIONS AND PROPHYLAXIS AFTER LUNG TRANSPLANTATION. Lung transplant recipients are at high risk for bacterial, viral, fungal, and protozoal infections; infections are the leading causes of death during the early post-transplant period. Predisposing factors include the allograft's susceptibility due to ventilator-induced damage, the severing of the lymphatic drainage at the time of the procedure, and ischemia and/or reperfusion injury. Additionally, patients are pharmacologically immunosuppressed, are in a catabolic state, have impaired defenses as the result of endotracheal intubation, and have arterial and central venous catheters, chest tubes, and a large surgical incision.

In the first 3 months after transplantation, bacterial infections are responsible for the majority of deaths. Approximately one-third of patients are diagnosed with pneumonia in the first weeks after transplantation, with gram-negative organisms as the etiology in 75% of cases. Patients with chronic rejection often develop colonization and recurrent infections, usually with Pseudomonas species.

Among potential viral pathogens, cytomegalovirus (CMV) is the most important in lung transplant recipients. Seronegative patients who receive an allograft from a seropositive donor are at particularly high risk for the development of a clinically significant CMV infection. Seronegative patients who have a seronegative donor are at low risk for infection, provided they are treated with seronegative blood products. The CMV syndrome includes fever, bone mar-

row suppression, hepatitis, enteritis, and pneumonitis. Most programs now use prophylactic ganciclovir in patients at risk, although the optimal dosing regimen and duration of treatment are as yet undetermined.

Epstein-Barr virus (EBV) has been associated with the development of post-transplant lymphoproliferative disorder (PTLD). Herpes simplex infections are relatively unusual, in part due to the standard use of prophylactic antiviral medication (ganciclovir or acyclovir). There are reports of paramyxovirus and respiratory syncitial virus (RSV) infections after lung transplant.

Aspergillus species are the most common cause of invasive fungal infection. Predisposing factors for such infection include preoperative colonization with Aspergillus, stenotic airways, or the presence of an airway stent.

Due to the nature of the immunosuppressive chemotherapeutic regimen used, patients are at high risk for infection by the protozoan Pneumocystis carinii. The use of trimethoprim-sulfamethoxazole prophylaxis has virtually eliminated Pneumocystis pneumonia.

ACUTE REJECTION. Histologically, the initial manifestation of acute rejection is a lymphocyte-predominant inflammatory response, usually centered around blood vessels and/or airways. The vascular inflammation is accompanied by endothelial inflammation, and the lymphocyte infiltration can progress to involve alveolar walls. By convention, acute rejection is graded from 0 (normal) to 4 (severe), with subclasses defined by the presence or absence of airway inflammation.

The risk of acute allograft rejection is highest in the early months after transplant and declines with time. Multiple episodes of acute rejection are the major risk factor for the subsequent development of chronic rejection. Because up to 25% of surveillance bronchoscopies reveal asymptomatic rejection, some programs perform surveillance biopsies at regular intervals with the goal of reducing the incidence of chronic rejection; however, the efficacy of this approach has not been established.

Clinically, patients may present with fever, cough, and exertional dyspnea. Evaluation may demonstrate rales or rhonchi on chest examination, a decline in pulmonary function by spirometry, leukocytosis, opacities on chest radiography, and exertional desaturation. The clinical presentation is often indistinguishable from infectious pneumonia, and the clinical impression is accurate in only 50% of cases. Bronchoscopy with bronchoalveolar lavage and/or transbronchial biopsy is commonly needed to clarify the diagnosis.

Treatment of acute rejection most often consists of high-dose corticosteroids administered intravenously for 3 days. In patients with persistent or recurrent acute rejection, therapeutic strategies include antilymphocyte antibodies, changing maintenance immunosuppressive drugs, and other attempts to augment immunosuppression.

CHRONIC REJECTION. The bronchiolitis obliterans syndrome is thought to be a manifestation of chronic rejection. Risk factors for the development of the syndrome include the number of acute rejection episodes and, in some series, prior symptomatic CMV

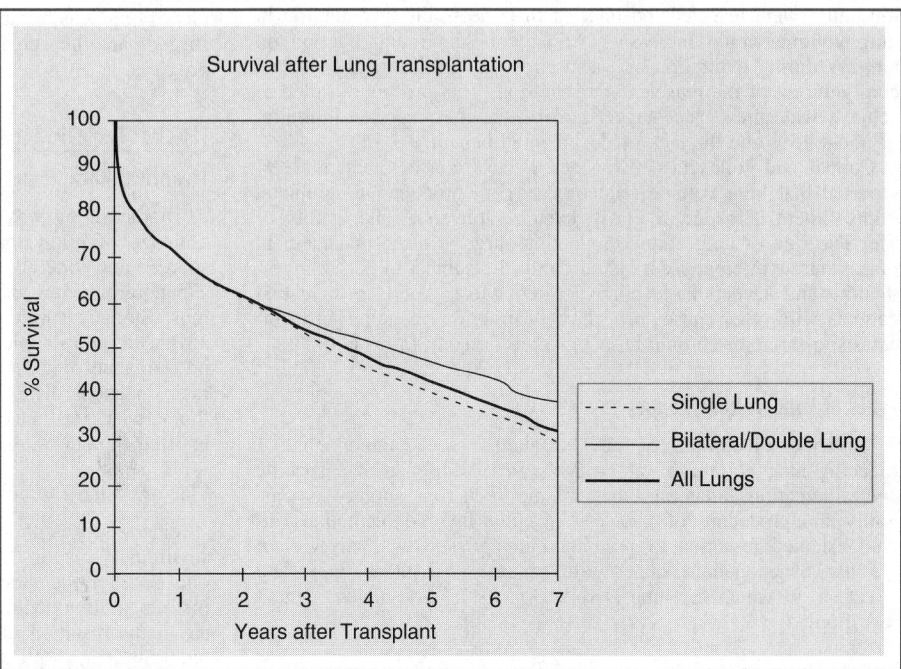

Survival after Lung Transplantation

FIGURE 89-1 ■ Survival after lung transplantation. (Data from International Society of Heart and Lung Transplantation, 15th Annual Data Report. Available at www.ishlt.org/registry.html.)

infection. Evidence supporting the conclusion that it is a manifestation of chronic rejection includes the association with the number of acute rejection episodes, the association with donor and/or recipient HLA locus mismatch, the similarity to the syndrome seen after bone marrow transplantation (graft versus host disease), and laboratory evidence of donor-specific alloreactivity in certain allograft recipients.

Pathologically, "early" lesions demonstrate inflammation and disruption of the epithelium of small airways followed by growth of granulation tissue into the airway lumen, resulting in complete or partial obstruction. The granulation tissue then organizes in a stereotypical pattern with resultant fibrosis that obliterates the lumen of the airway.

Clinically, bronchiolitis obliterans presents with nonspecific symptoms. Patients typically develop progressive exertional breathlessness, and pulmonary function testing usually demonstrates evidence of progressive airflow obstruction. Bronchiolitis obliterans is classified according to the forced expiratory volume in one second (FEV_1): 0 (no significant abnormality) if FEV_1 is greater than 80% of baseline; 1 (mild) if FEV_1 is 65 to 80% of baseline; 2 (moderate) if FEV_1 is 50% to 65% of baseline; and 3 (severe) if FEV_1 is 50% or less of baseline. In early stages, chest radiography is notable only for hyperinflation, but it may show bronchiectasis as the syndrome progresses. Later stages of bronchiolitis obliterans may include a syndrome of bronchiectasis with chronic productive cough and airway colonization with *Pseudomonas* species.

The diagnosis of bronchiolitis obliterans is made both on clinical and pathologic grounds. Transbronchial biopsy has a low yield for demonstrating histologic evidence of bronchiolitis obliterans; but when such evidence is seen, it is diagnostic. In patients with a compatible clinical syndrome, the exclusion of anastomotic stenosis and occult pulmonary infection is sufficient to establish the diagnosis.

A variety of types of therapy have been tried, including pulse corticosteroids, antilymphocyte antibodies, total lymphoid irradiation, photopheresis, and nebulized cyclosporine, but none is clearly effective. Most patients with bronchiolitis obliterans experience a progressive decline in pulmonary function despite augmentation of immunosuppression. Bronchiolitis obliterans is the leading cause of late mortality after lung transplantation.

NONPULMONARY MEDICAL COMPLICATIONS OF LUNG TRANSPLANTATION. Most of the nonpulmonary medical complications that arise in patients after lung transplantation are the result of immunosuppressive therapy. Virtually all lung transplant recipients develop one or more of these complications.

Osteoporosis is common owing to the chronic use of corticosteroids and cyclosporine. Bone density should be monitored periodically, and pharmacologic therapy should be instituted if excessive bone loss is identified (see Chapter 257).

Chronic renal insufficiency is common and is the result of therapy with cyclosporine or tacrolimus, both of which affect afferent vascular tone in the kidneys and result in an average 50% drop in the glomerular filtration rate in the 12 months after lung transplantation. Hypertension is also common and is caused by corticosteroids and cyclosporine. Calcium-channel blockers, which are often used to treat hypertension, raise serum cyclosporine levels; appropriate monitoring and dose adjustment are needed when starting such therapy. Both corticosteroids and tacrolimus contribute to the development of diabetes mellitus and hyperlipidemia.

Organ transplantation is associated with an increased incidence of malignancy, thought to be due to pharmacologic immunosuppression and alteration in immune surveillance. Patients are at increased risk for lymphoproliferative malignancies and other types of cancer. *Post-transplant lymphoproliferative disorders* occur in about 4% of patients after organ transplantation; most are associated with Epstein-Barr virus. These syndromes can be polyclonal or monoclonal. Reduction in immunosuppression is sometimes therapeutic in those with polyclonal disease. The prognosis in patients with monoclonal disease is poor, with little response to modification of immunosuppression or antineoplastic chemotherapy. Patients are also at increased risk for skin, cervical, anogenital, and hepatobiliary malignancy after solid organ transplantation.

Outcomes after Lung Transplantation

A comparison of survival data in lung transplants done before 1990 with those done between 1991 and 1993 shows that 1-year survival rates improved significantly (64.2% versus 70.5%), but little subsequent change was noted in 1994 through 1997 (72.1%). The subsequent rate of decline in survival (~8 to 10% annually) has not changed and largely reflects the effects of bronchiolitis obliterans on patient survival. Median survival after lung transplantation is approximately 4 years (Fig. 89-1).

LUNG VOLUME REDUCTION SURGERY

Historical Background

The concept that surgery to reduce lung volume may provide symptomatic and demonstrable physiologic benefit in patients with emphysema was first advanced by Dr. Otto Brantigan in the 1950s. He proposed a procedure in which peripheral areas of emphysematous lung were resected, postulating that the resulting reduction in lung volume would increase elastic recoil and radial traction on airways during expiration and also allow restoration of the normal configuration of the muscles of respiration. This procedure failed to achieve widespread acceptance, largely due to a reported mortality of about 15% and the lack of documented benefit.

Cooper and colleagues reconsidered these concepts and in 1994 reported that lung volume reduction surgery produces a significant improvement in expiratory flow, exercise tolerance, and quality of life. The role of lung volume reduction surgery in the management of patients with emphysema is currently the subject of active investigation and several large clinical trials. Most experts believe that patients with other causes of airflow obstruction, including bronchiectasis, asthma, or chronic bronchitis, are unlikely to benefit.

Types of Lung Volume Reduction Surgery

A variety of approaches may be taken in the common goal of reducing lung volume by about 30%. In the absence of a specific contraindication, bilateral lung volume reduction surgery is currently the procedure of choice. Currently favored techniques include stapled resection of peripheral lung tissue, with or without the use of exogenous material to buttress the suture lines, and plication, in which the lung is rolled on itself and stapled without resection.

Considerations in the Evaluation of Potential Candidates for Lung Volume Reduction Surgery

The evaluation of candidates for lung volume reduction surgery can be viewed as both an assessment of risk and an attempt to identify those most likely to benefit from the procedure. Few of the criteria used to select or exclude patients have been subject to prospective validation.

In general terms, the principles of evaluation are similar to those before lung transplantation. In addition, pulmonary hypertension and marked deconditioning are contraindications to lung volume reduction surgery. The ideal candidate has severe airflow obstruction due to emphysema but is otherwise in good health. Patients undergo computed tomographic scanning, pulmonary function testing (with lung volumes by plethysmography), echocardiography to assess pulmonary artery pressure, and some form of noninvasive screening for significant coronary artery disease. If a candidate appears suitable for lung volume reduction surgery, most programs require completion of a 6 to 10 week course of pulmonary rehabilitation prior to surgery.

The ideal candidate for this experimental procedure has anatomic evidence of emphysema; severe obstruction not reversed by bronchodilators on spirometry; no significant cardiac, hepatic, or renal disease; a pulmonary artery systolic pressure less than 45 mm Hg; does not smoke cigarettes; has completed pulmonary rehabilitation; and has no significant pleural disease or prior thoracic surgery. Contraindications include severe deconditioning (6-minute walk <150 m); use of parenteral corticosteroids (e.g., prednisone >20 mg/day); clinically significant bronchiectasis; a pulmonary artery systolic pressure greater than 45 mm Hg; or a need for invasive mechanical ventilation. Hypercarbia, age greater than 75 years, marked anatomic deformity of the thorax, or marked pleural scarring are relative contraindications. Patients who seem most likely to benefit at present are those with emphysema that is primarily in the upper lobe or is heterogeneously distributed, with evidence of dynamic airway collapse rather than fixed airway disease, and with an elevated residual volume/total lung capacity ratio.

Outcomes of Lung Volume Reduction Surgery

The available data show that most patients attain significant improvements in exercise tolerance, expiratory flow rates measured by spirometry, and self-reported quality of life; however, about 30% do not benefit from the procedure. The average improvement in FEV_1 is approximately 50% at about 6 months after surgery. On average, arterial oxygen levels improve, but some patients show no improvement. The operative mortality is 5 to 10%.

The limited data available suggest that some patients may experience a decline in pulmonary function after experiencing improvement over the first 12 months after surgery. Criteria for reliably identifying which patients will benefit from lung volume reduction surgery are the subject of several large clinical trials currently in progress.

THORACOSCOPY AND VIDEO-ASSISTED THORACIC SURGERY

Historical Background

Thoracoscopy was originally limited to pleural biopsies and the drainage of empyemas or pleural effusions. With improved light sources and video-optic instrumentation, the thoracoscope provides a panoramic view of the hemithorax and has been integrated into most thoracic surgical procedures. The coincident development of advanced endoscopic surgical instrumentation has facilitated the performance of these operations through "minimally invasive" thoracic incisions. The widespread application of the thoracoscope in thoracic surgery has led to the more inclusive term of "video-assisted thoracic surgery."

Video-Assisted Thoracic Surgery Procedures

Video-assisted thoracic surgery generally involves at least three small incisions or "access ports" placed in any intercostal space: one port for the video-thoracoscope and two ports for endoscopic instrumentation. Although the access ports are small, the rigid instruments result in trauma to the intercostal nerves and rib periosteum that can result in substantial postoperative discomfort.

Incisions can be expanded, depending on the goals of the procedure and the anatomic findings at the time of exploration. Unexpected pleural symphysis or incomplete lobar fissures may require extension of the incision to facilitate visualization as well as the use of more standard instrumentation. In patients undergoing anatomic resection, such as segmentectomy or lobectomy, at least one of the incisions is extended to permit extraction of the lung from the hemithorax. For most video-assisted thoracic procedures, the operation requires single lung ventilation. The requirement for selective ventilation excludes many patients with severe pulmonary hypertension or acute respiratory failure. In contrast, many patients with chronic respiratory insufficiency and preserved ventilation-perfusion matching will tolerate periods of selective lung ventilation. The ability of many patients with severe emphysema to tolerate selective ventilation has led to the application of thoracoscopy for lung volume reduction surgery. Obliteration of the pleural space, either from infection or previous surgery, is a relative contraindication for thoracoscopic surgery.

Diseases in which Video-Assisted Thoracic Surgery Plays a Role in Treatment

BENIGN LUNG DISEASE. A variety of benign lung diseases present as focal parenchymal lesions that require a tissue biopsy for diagnosis. The traditional approach to lung biopsy has been a limited thoracotomy and wedge resection. As an alternative to limited thoracotomies, thoracoscopy has proven to be an effective approach to the diagnosis of localized disorders of the lung. Thoracoscopy can provide a more complete view of the ipsilateral hemithorax, including the visceral, parietal, and mediastinal pleura. Additional subpleural nodules that were not imaged by preoperative radiography can be examined, and representative biopsies can be obtained.

Diffuse lung diseases can often be diagnosed clinically on the basis of history, characteristic chest radiographs, physical findings, and pulmonary function testing. In cases that require histopathologic confirmation, lung tissue can be obtained by transbronchial biopsy. Thoracoscopy plays a limited role in diffuse lung disease but may be helpful when a large pathologic sample is required.

BULLOUS LUNG DISEASE. Most patients with chronic obstructive lung disease (COPD) (see Chapter 75) have diffuse parenchymal disease. A small number of patients with COPD can develop heterogeneous disease with dominant bullae and relatively preserved lung parenchyma. In some cases, the rapid expansion of these bullae can be associated with a substantial increase in respiratory symptoms and a decrease in expiratory air flow. Chest radiographs of patients with acute respiratory symptoms frequently demonstrate compression of surrounding lung tissue. Alternatively, patients with bullous lung disease occasionally present with an infected bulla and require drainage prior to definitive surgery.

The indications for thorascopic bullectomy are similar to lung volume reduction surgery for emphysema. Patients who benefit most from surgery are those who have rapidly progressive symptoms associated with the expansion of a single bullous lesion and radiographic demonstration of compression of the surrounding lung parenchyma. Either excision or plication can remove the bullous lesion.

RECURRENT SPONTANEOUS PNEUMOTHORAX. Primary spontaneous pneumothorax (see Chapter 86) is caused by rupture of subpleural blebs of the lung. In more than 95% of cases, the blebs are located at the apex of the lung. In approximately 5% of cases, associated subpleural blebs are found at the margin of the lower lobe, usually in the superior segment. In an otherwise healthy patient with less than a 20% pneumothorax, the uncomplicated pneumothorax can be observed without intervention. In patients with larger pneumothoraces, a tube may be necessary to evacuate the pleural air and re-expand the lung. Most cases of primary spontaneous pneumothorax heal from the inflammation associated with pleural rupture and are free of ongoing air leak after re-expansion of the lung.

Although most spontaneous pneumothoraces are uncomplicated, 3 to 20% of patients with pneumothoraces develop complications such as tension pneumothorax, persistent air leaks, or recurrent pneumothoraces. Patients who develop a second pneumothorax have a 70 to 80% chance of a third recurrence within 2 years. The surgical approach to the treatment of recurrent pneumothoraces has been the removal of subpleural blebs. These blebs can be effectively removed using a thoracoscopic approach or through a more traditional axillary incision.

SOLITARY PULMONARY NODULES. Solitary pulmonary nodules or "coin lesions" are defined as spherical lesions, less than 3 cm in diameter, present in the outer one-third of the lung (see Chapter 72). Although most solitary pulmonary nodules do not represent cancer, the diagnosis must be considered in all patients, especially those with a smoking history.

Transthoracic needle biopsy has a low morbidity: fewer than 10% of normal patients and a slightly higher percentage of patients with emphysema will develop a postprocedure pneumothorax. However, a small but tangible false-negative rate occurs with transthoracic needle biopsies. Furthermore, in the absence of a malignant diagnosis, transthoracic needle biopsies rarely are able to establish a benign diagnosis.

Thoracoscopic resection of the solitary pulmonary nodule is an alternative to transthoracic needle biopsy. Because thoracoscopic resection excises the entire nodule, there are no false-negative diagnoses. Further, thoracoscopy can positively establish a diagnosis of benign disease. The disadvantage of thoracoscopic resection is that it requires general anesthesia; however, the hospital stay will generally be less than 24 hours.

ANATOMIC LUNG RESECTIONS. In most cases of primary lung cancer, a standard anatomic resection is indicated to decrease the incidence of local recurrence. Patients who can tolerate general anesthesia and single lung ventilation for the thoracoscopic resection are generally able to tolerate the segmentectomy or lobectomy. Although thoracoscopic resections of primary lung cancers have not been studied in a randomized setting, the available evidence indicates that a parenchymal margin within 2 cm results in a 20% incidence of local recurrence. In addition, a recent Lung Cancer Study Group report demonstrated a 2.5-fold increase in local recurrence rates with limited resection. Another disadvantage to limited parenchymal wedge resection is that the peripheral wedge resection does not provide segmental or lobar nodal staging. In patients with isolated regional metastases, this staging information could provide important information to guide possible adjuvant therapy.

Anatomic resections can be performed with a variety of techniques, including video-assisted surgical techniques. The difference between standard lobectomy and a thoracoscopic lobectomy has become less distinct in recent years. Thoracoscopic instruments have become commonplace in the resection of a lobe of the lung, even when performed through a standard thoracotomy. The improved visualization and smaller instruments have resulted in smaller incisions and less morbidity.

Arcasoy SM, Kotloff RM: Lung transplantation. N Engl J Med 340:1081, 1999. *Comprehensive, updated review.*

DeCamp MM Jr, Jaklitsch MT, Mentzer SJ, et al: The safety and versatility of video-thoracoscopy: A prospective analysis of 895 consecutive cases. J Am Coll Surg 181: 113, 1995. *This article is a comprehensive study of the morbidity and mortality of thoracoscopy applied to a range of lung diseases.*

Ginsberg RJ, Rubinstein LV: Randomized trial of lobectomy versus limited resection for T1 N0 non-small cell lung cancer: Lung Cancer Study Group. Ann Thorac Surg 60:615, 1995. *A widely cited randomized study reporting the higher local recurrence rate of lung cancer with limited (wedge) resection when compared with anatomic lobectomy.*

Joint Statement of American Society of Transplant Physicians/American Thoracic Society/European Respiratory Society/International Society of Heart and Lung Transplantation: International Guidelines for the Selection of Lung Transplant Candidates. Am J Respir Crit Care Med 158:335–339, 1998. *Recently released consensus statement concerning guidelines for evaluation and listing of patients considered for transplantation.*

Trulock EP: Lung tansplantation. Am J Respir Crit Care Med 155:789–818, 1997. *A comprehensive review with an extensive bibliography of lung transplantation. Extensive discussion of medical management after transplantation.*

90 DISORDERS OF VENTILATORY CONTROL

Steven A. Shea ■ *David P. White*

NORMAL VENTILATORY CONTROL SYSTEM

The human ventilatory control system (Fig. 90–1) determines the neural output to the respiratory muscles thereby dictating the quantity and pattern of ventilation in an attempt to maintain arterial blood gas values within fairly tight constraints despite substantial alterations in metabolic rate (exercise), the work of breathing (underlying cardiopulmonary or chest wall disease), or disease of the respiratory muscles. Although the respiratory rhythm emerges primarily from neurons in the medulla and pons, these neurons receive afferent input from a number of sources that provide constant information about blood gases (e.g., arterial oxygen partial pressure [PaO_2], arterial carbon dioxide partial pressure [$PaCO_2$]), lung/chest wall inflation, and respiratory muscle function. The principal sources of this afferent input include the carotid bodies (responsive to changes in PaO_2, $PaCO_2$, and pH), the medullary chemoreceptor ($PaCO_2$ and pH), muscle spindles and Golgi tendon organs (responsive to respiratory muscle activity and chest wall inflation), and receptors located in the airways and lungs (responsive to temperature, stretch, and pressure). During wakefulness, ventilation is also substantially influenced by behavioral activities such as speech, swallowing, and anxiety. The principal focus of this chapter is disorders of the chemoreceptor mechanisms (PaO_2, $PaCO_2$), because these are more common and clinically important.

Awake

In awake resting individuals, $PaCO_2$ is generally stable, varying by less than 2 to 4 mm Hg (slightly more in premenopausal adult women, because progesterone stimulates breathing during the luteal phase of the menstrual cycle). Ventilation increases briskly if $PaCO_2$ is acutely elevated above this resting level but does not decline significantly if $PaCO_2$ falls. This "dog-leg" appearance on the hypercapnic ventilatory response (Fig. 90–2) has led to the concept of a "wakefulness drive to breathe" that persists in the absence of chemoreceptive ($PaCO_2$, PaO_2) stimulation of breathing. Similarly, decreases in PaO_2 from 500 mm Hg to approximately 65 mm Hg have a negligible effect on breathing; below 65 mm Hg, a hyperbolic relationship occurs between decreasing PaO_2 and increasing ventilation. Within the normal physiologic range, the fairly weak chemical control system permits relatively unfettered behavioral control of breathing. However, should the $PaCO_2$ rise above about 42 mm Hg or the PaO_2 fall below about 65 mm Hg, ventilation increases rapidly. Because of the shapes of the ventilatory response curves relative to those of normal blood gases, hypercapnia rather than hypoxia stimulates the response to hypoventilation and thereby normalizes blood gases. In clinical situations in which

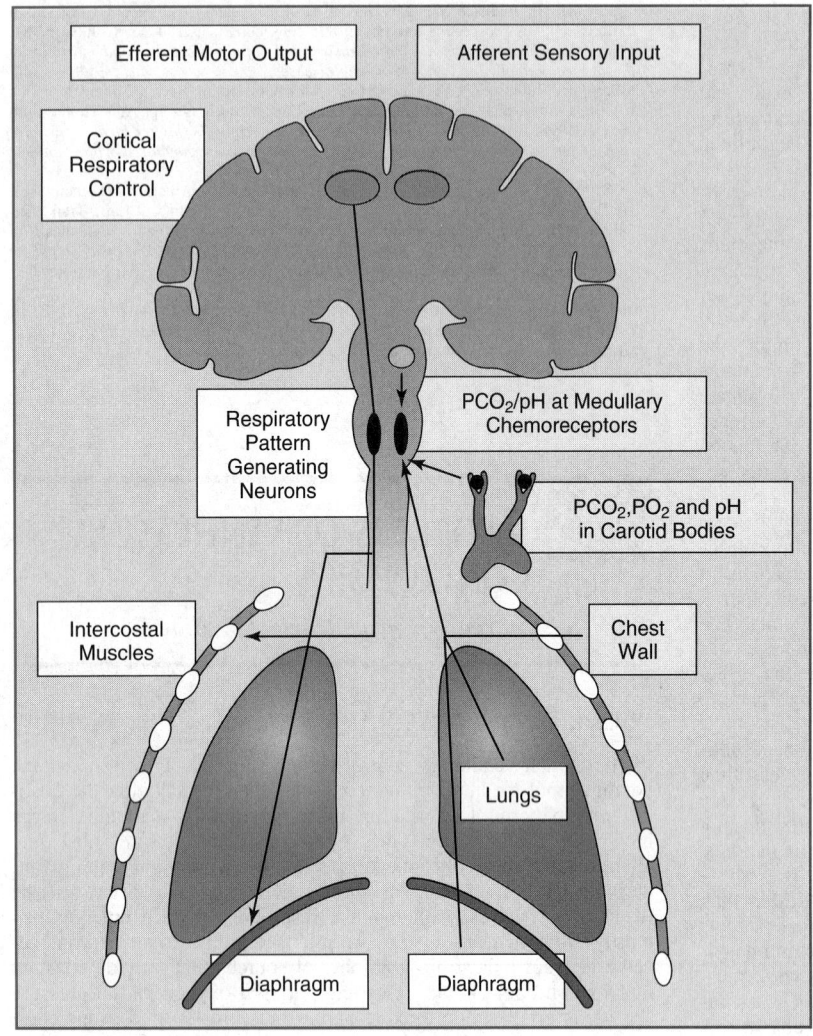

FIGURE 90–1 ■ A simplified diagram of the principal efferent (*left*) and afferent (*right*) respiratory control pathways. A section through the brain, brain stem, and spinal cord is shown (with pertinent respiratory areas indicated by shading), as are the central nervous system links with the respiratory apparatus.

$PaCO_2$ and PaO_2 change simultaneously, however, hypoxia accentuates the ventilatory response to hypercapnia in a synergistic fashion.

During mild exercise, ventilation normally increases in direct proportion to CO_2 production, such that $PaCO_2$ does not change. Surprisingly, the chemoreceptive feedback system seems unlikely to be responsible for such tight $PaCO_2$ control, as no detectable change in $PaCO_2$ or PaO_2 is generally noted during mild exercise. Other proposed mechanisms that may contribute to hyperpnea during exercise include stimulation of breathing via afferents in the moving limbs, afferents from receptors detecting CO_2 flow to the lungs, mixed venous chemoreceptors, and conditioned responses.

However, ventilatory control during exercise remains poorly understood.

Asleep

Numerous important changes occur in respiratory control on falling asleep. During non–rapid eye movement (NREM) sleep, both wakeful and behavioral influences on respiration are largely lost, leaving the chemoreceptive (primarily $PaCO_2$) metabolic system to control breathing. Despite its importance during sleep, the responsiveness to changes in $PaCO_2$ is altered in several ways. First, the entire ventilation-$PaCO_2$ curve is shifted to the right, such that higher $PaCO_2$ levels are required to stimulate breathing, allowing $PaCO_2$ to rise during sleep. Second, if $PaCO_2$ falls below a certain level, ventilation is substantially inhibited, so that apnea commonly occurs at $PaCO_2$ values near the waking level (as may occur at altitude where hypoxia leads to hyperventilation and hypocapnia). Finally, the slope of the ventilatory response to $PaCO_2$ is also mildly reduced. In addition, during NREM sleep, the resistance to airflow through the upper airway commonly rises due to falling pharyngeal dilator muscle activity (see Chater 87). This increase is likely important because, unlike during wakefulness, the respiratory control system during sleep does not compensate well for increased resistive work. As a result, ventilation generally falls in response to this increased upper airway resistance. During REM sleep, a further decrement is seen in ventilatory responsiveness to $PaCO_2$ but behavioral influences on breathing return. Breathing may become quite erratic during REM sleep. These changes in ventilatory control during sleep are important clinically. As there is less robust ventilatory control during sleep, many disorders that ultimately lead to clinically important hypoventilation manifest themselves during sleep well before they can be detected during wakefulness.

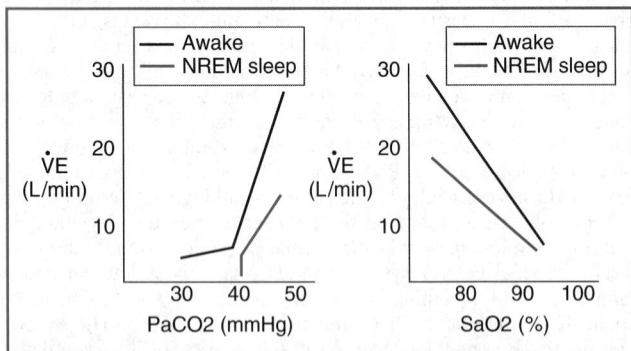

FIGURE 90–2 ■ Typical ventilatory responses to hypercapnia (*left*) and hypoxia (*right*). Compared with wakefulness, the ventilatory responses decline during non–rapid eye movement (NREM) sleep and decline even further during REM sleep (not shown). $\dot{V}E$ = expired minute ventilation.

Relationship to Respiratory Failure

Ventilatory control disorders that cause respiratory failure are more commonly hypercapnic than hypoxic. First, the development of hypercapnic respiratory failure generally reflects an interaction between ventilatory control (often quantified by the slope of the hypoxic and hypercapnic ventilatory responses) and the work of breathing (increments in work of breathing are usually a product of parenchymal lung disease or chest wall disease, including obesity). When chemoresponsiveness is markedly diminished or absent, hypercapnia may develop in an individual with a normal respiratory apparatus and normal work of breathing. Conversely, when the work of breathing is extraordinarily high (as might occur with severe chronic obstructive pulmonary disease [COPD]), respiratory failure may develop despite normal or robust ventilatory control. Therefore, although low or diminished chemoresponsiveness may predispose an individual to hypercapnia, the work required to maintain ventilation will often determine when hypercapnia actually occurs. Second, individual variability in chemoresponsiveness is substantial, with slopes varying sixfold or sevenfold from one individual to another because of genetic differences, previous neurologic disease (e.g., encephalitis, meningitis), prolonged exposure to hypoxia and hypercapnia, and other poorly understood influences. Regardless of the cause, low chemoresponsiveness in combination with increased work of breathing contribute to the development of hypercapnic respiratory failure. Finally, the speed of development of respiratory failure is variable. Acute changes in blood gas values (over hours), such as occur with a respiratory infection, can generally be detected quickly by a patient (e.g., by sensing shortness of breath) and lead to effective early treatment. Conversely, with diminished ventilatory control, hypercapnia and hypoxia may develop slowly, with little sensation of dyspnea, making the early detection of respiratory failure difficult.

Hypoventilation Associated with "Pure" Control of Breathing Abnormalities (without Cardiopulmonary Disease)

Hypoventilation can develop in an individual with quite normal lungs and respiratory muscle function but with a markedly diminished ability to respond to hypoxia or hypercapnia. The most common such disorder in adults is acquired central alveolar hypoventilation, which is defined by markedly diminished ventilatory chemoresponsiveness, normal respiratory apparatus (normal pulmonary function), and an absence of obesity or chest wall disease. Due to their decreased chemoresponsiveness, these patients have arterial blood gas values that are quite labile when awake and that worsen substantially with sleep. Ventilation also may deteriorate during respiratory infections, even if the work of breathing rises only minimally. Therefore, most of these individuals are chronically hypoxic and hypercapnic, often with cor pumonale. Despite these severe blood gas abnormalities, patients rarely complain of dyspnea or respiratory discomfort and can often correct the hypercapnia with voluntary hyperventilation. Some, but not all, patients with acquired central hypoventilation have previously documented neurologic disease as the explanation for their diminished chemoresponsiveness.

Hypoventilation with Increased Work of Breathing

Hypercapnia may also develop in patients with increased work of breathing in whom chemoresponsiveness may be diminished but is not necessarily absent; the most common example is COPD. As airflow obstruction worsens (increasing work of breathing), the incidence of respiratory failure rises, although the relationship between pulmonary function and rising $PaCO_2$ is certainly not linear. Such patients are sometimes classified as either "pink puffers" (high chemoresponsiveness and a general maintenance of blood gas homeostasis) or "blue bloaters" (low chemoresponsiveness and frequent respiratory failure), implying an important role for individual variability in chemosensitivity. However, overlap between groups is considerable, and hypercapnia in COPD has a multifactorial etiology.

The obesity hypoventilation ("pickwickian") syndrome is characterized by morbid obesity, diminished to absent ventilatory chemoresponsiveness during wakefulness, hypoxia and hypercapnia during wakefulness, absence (generally) of parenchymal lung disease, and severe obstructive sleep apnea (see Chapter 87). Although the diminished responsiveness to hypoxia and hypercapnia almost certainly contributes to the blood gas abnormalities when the patient is awake and asleep, the cause of this abnormal ventilatory control is controversial. Some argue that genetically diminished chemoresponsiveness leads to the entire syndrome, whereas others contend that the obstructive apnea desensitizes the chemoreceptors and ultimately culminates in waking hypercapnia.

Hypoventilation with Neuromuscular Disease

Hypoventilation is also commonly observed in patients with neuromuscular weakness (e.g., motor neuron disease, muscular dystrophy, myasthenia gravis, poliomyelitis, Guillain-Barré syndrome, and quadriplegia). In these patients, the neural output from the brain-stem respiratory center cannot always fully compensate for the defects in neuromuscular function, particularly during REM sleep, when chemoreceptor responsiveness is substantially reduced and a general loss of accessory respiratory muscle activity occurs (skeletal hypotonia characterizes this stage of sleep). Therefore, REM sleep becomes a potentially vulnerable time for patients with diaphragmatic dysfunction. Other rare neurologic disorders that influence ventilatory control include *Ondine's curse* (patients lack the ability to breathe automatically but are able to breathe voluntarily) and the *locked-in syndrome* (patients lack the ability to breathe voluntarily but are able to breathe automatically).

TREATMENT (Table 90-1)

Treatments for ventilatory control disorders include (1) reducing the work of breathing (e.g., with bronchodilators or weight loss); (2) using ventilatory stimulants, such as acetazolamide or progesterone; (3) providing supplemental oxygen; and (4) using assisted ventilation. Reducing the work of breathing is always advisable but not always possible. Ventilatory stimulants are often of only limited effectiveness, particularly in patients with central neural de-

Table 90-1 ■ APPROACHES TO THERAPY OF THE MOST COMMON DISORDERS OF VENTILATORY CONTROL

DIAGNOSIS	APPROACH	SPECIFIC THERAPY	TIME UNTIL RESPONSE
COPD "blue bloaters"	Reduce work of breathing	Bronchodilators	Hours to days
		Nocturnal ventilation	Days to weeks
	Improve oxygenation	O_2 supplementation	Immediate
	Ventilatory stimulants*	Rarely used	
Central alveolar hypoventilation	Improve oxygenation	O_2 supplementation	Immediate
	Nocturnal ventilation	Nasal ventilator	Days to weeks
		Diaphragmatic pacers	Days to weeks
	Ventilatory stimulants*	Progesterone (20 mg tid)	~1 wk
		Acetazolamide (250 mg qid; 500 mg bid)	~1 wk
Obesity hypoventilation	Reduce work of breathing	Weight loss	Months
		Nasal CPAP	Days to weeks
		Nocturnal ventilation	Days to weeks
	Improve oxygenation	O_2 supplementation	Immediate
	Ventilatory stimulants*	Progesterone (20 mg tid)	~1 wk
		Acetazolamide (250 mg qid; 500 mg bid)	~1 wk

*Note: Ventilatory stimulants, although used occasionally in the disorders listed, are generally of limited efficacy, particularly when compared to nocturnal ventilation.

fects. Supplemental oxygen may improve oxygenation but rarely corrects hypercapnia; in some situations, oxygen may actually worsen hypercapnia. Assisted ventilation is most often the treatment of choice, particularly for patients with central neural defects and neuromuscular disease. Positive-pressure assisted ventilation is usually applied noninvasively via a nose-mask, but it may be administered via tracheotomy, depending on the clinical situation. Currently, positive-pressure ventilation is predominantly adminis-tered during sleep, so the patient can have a more normal waking existence; however, improved nocturnal ventilation also often leads to diminished daytime hypercapnia, which suggests a role for nocturnal hypoventilation in the development of waking hypercapnia.

Shea SA: Behavioural and arousal-related influences on breathing in humans. Exp Physiol 81:1–26, 1996. *A review of the efficacy of behavioral and arousal-related influences on breathing in humans in the absence of chemoreceptive control.*

Shneerson JM: Techniques in mechanical ventilation: Principles and practice. Thorax 51:756–61, 1996. *A review of long-term treatments of respiratory pump failure, including mechanical ventilation.*

PART IX

CRITICAL CARE MEDICINE

91 APPROACH TO THE PATIENT IN A CRITICAL CARE SETTING

John M. Luce

CHARACTERISTICS OF CRITICAL CARE MEDICINE

Many kinds of patients require critical care, mostly because of dysfunction or failure of one or more organ systems. Circulatory and respiratory failures are most common, and patients who manifest dysfunction or failure of two or more organ systems are said to have multiple organ dysfunction syndrome (MODS).

The parent boards of internal medicine, anesthesiology, surgery, and pediatrics provide certification of special competence in critical care medicine, and many hospitals require such certification of physicians who direct or practice in critical care units. The Joint Commission on Accreditation of Healthcare Organizations has mandated that critical care units have medical directors to assure that quality is improved and proper utilization is maintained.

Although physicians usually manage the care of critically ill patients, critical care medicine is a team approach that involves nurses, respiratory care practitioners, nutritionists, biomedical technologists, and other health care professionals. Also essential are mental health experts, clergy, social workers, and other persons who serve as counselors to patients and families and sources of support for the critical care team.

ATTRIBUTES OF CRITICAL CARE UNITS

Critical care units were first developed in the 1950s for patients who required mechanical ventilation because they had poliomyelitis or were recovering from anesthesia. Currently, critical care units are defined by their ability to provide the environment, facilities, and personnel for the care of severely ill patients (Table 91–1).

Critical care units may have a general orientation, treating all kinds of severely ill patients, or be more specialized, accepting only specific categories of patients as defined by the type of illness (e.g., burn units), organ system involved (e.g., coronary and acute neurologic care units), specialty service designation (e.g., medical and surgical units), or the patient's age (e.g., neonatal and pediatric units). Specialized units provide medical personnel specifically skilled in the unit's areas of care and have available particular forms of technology.

Because of the severity of the illness of their patients, critical care units require clear delineation of administrative and medical lines of authority and responsibility. Critical care units must also have general guidelines for admission and discharge, specifically described roles for nurses and respiratory therapists, standing orders, critical pathways and clinical guidelines for management of common disorders, and programs of continuing staff education and

quality assurance. Such policies and guidelines reduce the apparent ambiguity often inherent in the difficult environment of a critical care unit and enable prompt decision making by health care professionals.

APPROACH TO THE CRITICALLY ILL PATIENT

Patients are admitted to critical care units from a variety of settings, including the emergency department, medical or surgical service, or operating room. Although a few patients may be admitted for simple monitoring purposes, such as the on-line measurement of pulse and blood pressure, these admissions have become less prevalent because of the relative scarcity of critical care beds and the development of "step-down" units, where patients can be monitored noninvasively and at lower cost. Thus, most critical care patients are, by definition, acutely and severely ill, commonly with dysfunction or failure of more than one organ system.

Due to the nature of critical illness, the initial assessment of the critically ill patient must be rapid and focus on real or potentially life-threatening processes that require immediate diagnostic and/or therapeutic intervention (Table 91–2). As a result, history taking, physical examination, and the gathering of laboratory information should be abbreviated. An example of this rapid approach is the resuscitation of a patient with cardiopulmonary arrest, which may take place elsewhere in the hospital but continue in the critical care unit. The pace of resuscitation is necessarily quick; physical examination may be restricted initially to the central nervous (CNS), cardiovascular, and respiratory systems, and interventions may be limited to the essential ABCs of *a*irway, *b*reathing, and *c*irculation.

After initial resuscitation, or in lieu of this step if the patient has not experienced cardiopulmonary arrest or another major catastrophe, time should be available to form a broader and more comprehensive diagnostic and therapeutic plan. The history taking (often from family, friends, or onlookers) should be more detailed and the physical examination more complete. Laboratory tests, such as radiographic studies, should be obtained, monitoring should be initiated, and treatment should be started. For example, the cause of the cardiopulmonary arrest should be ascertained in the previously mentioned patient, if it is not known already. Continuous external electrocardiographic monitoring and measurement of blood pressure with a sphygmomanometer should commence; invasive monitoring of vascular pressures with systemic arterial and pulmonary arterial catheters may be useful; and diuretics, vasoactive drugs, and other appropriate agents should be administered if the cause is heart failure.

Management of the critically ill patient should be based primarily on an understanding of physiology and pathophysiology. Although the contributions of cell and molecular biology to critical care medicine are substantial, the critical care unit resembles somewhat a physiology laboratory, wherein variables such as heart rate and blood pressure are measured in an online fashion, and the effects of interventions such as vasoactive drugs can be directly observed. Although the benefit of the critical care unit is related to the availability of these physiologic data, practitioners must exer-

---

Table 91–1 ■ FEATURES OF CRITICAL CARE UNITS

High nurse-to-patient ratio
Ready accessibility of physicians
Ability to provide invasive cardiovascular and respiratory monitoring
Availability of respiratory support techniques
Ability to provide supervised continuous infusion of pharmacologic agents
Ability to provide humane end-of-life care

Table 91–2 ■ APPROACH TO THE CRITICALLY ILL PATIENT

Rapid initial assessment and intervention
Formulation of a broader and more comprehensive diagnostic and treatment plan
Management based on understanding of physiology and pathophysiology
Appreciation of organ-system interdependence
Directed and dynamic management approach

cise clinical judgment and avoid the temptation to collect data for their own sake.

Consistent with this pathophysiologic approach, the interdependence of organ systems must be kept in sharp focus in critical care practice. Limited attention to one component of an illness, even if it is predominant, will frequently yield a therapeutic approach that is detrimental to the patient as a whole. For example, treatment directed toward reducing intravascular volume in a patient with MODS to improve respiratory function may adversely affect renal and CNS function. Conversely, increasing intravascular volume to raise cardiac output in a patient with left ventricular infarction may result in noncardiogenic pulmonary edema if pre-existent parenchymal lung injury is present. One of the major challeges of critical care is that physicians caring for severely ill patients must synthesize an overall management strategy that supports several organ systems and often incorporates the view of numerous consultants.

Finally, the management should be directed and dynamic. Diagnostic studies should be performed for good reasons, not just because the results are intellectually interesting, and treatments should be initiated with specific end points in mind. Although many such treatments constitute therapeutic trials, both their potential benefits and adverse effects should be appreciated. Practitioners also should appreciate that critically ill patients frequently (and often swiftly) change, and that such change must be explained and addressed. Thus, although standing orders may be appropriate in many circumstances, other orders should be revised regularly. Similarly, while making rounds, critical care physicians should review not only the patient's overall course, but also the functioning of all organ systems, preferably several times a day.

PROGNOSIS OF CRITICALLY ILL PATIENTS

Critical care units have been used in more or less their present form since approximately the late 1960s, yet their contribution to health care has not been well quantified. For example, the outcome of patients with bacteremic pneumococcal pneumonia has not been appreciably improved by critical care. Cardiopulmonary resuscitation (CPR), when performed on hospitalized patients or persons older than 70 years out of the hospital, may be successful less than 10% of the time. The survival rate of patients with three or more organ failures after 5 days in a critical care unit approached zero in one large investigation. And the mortality rate of patients with cardiogenic shock in the absence of coronary revascularization remains approximately 75% despite pulmonary artery catheterization, a finding that has led to questions regarding the value of this monitoring technique. Indeed, in a recent observational study of a wide variety of critically ill patients, after adjustment for treatment selection bias, pulmonary artery catheterization was associated with increased mortality as well as increased cost.

Data such as these imply that critical care is of little or no value in several categories of illness. Yet patients in the postoperative period and patients with cardiac arrhythmias, narcotic and sedative drug overdose, reversible neuromuscular disease, hypovolemic shock, and asthma and chronic obstructive pulmonary disease clearly benefit from critical care. Furthermore, the prognoses in certain diseases seem to be improving. For example, 90% of patients with a severe form of the acute respiratory distress syndrome (ARDS) died in a series from the 1970s compared with fewer than 50% of comparable patients in a series from 1983 through 1993. Given the lack of therapeutic breakthroughs in the treatment of ARDS since the 1970s, the most likely explanation for the better outcome of patients with this disorder over time is improved supportive care.

Establishing prognosis is difficult in critically ill patients because such patients are heterogeneous and their prognosis changes over time. In recent years, a number of prognostic scoring systems based on the findings from large groups of patients have been developed to help quantify the severity of illness and determine whether individual patients will survive to hospital discharge. For example, the Acute Physiology and Chronic Health Evaluation (APACHE) III system uses major medical and surgical disease categories, acute physiologic abnormalities, age, pre-existing functional limitations, major co-morbidities, and treatment location prior to critical care

admission for these purposes. Mortality estimated by APACHE III is comparable to that estimated by physicians in most circumstances, and this and other systems are increasingly used as adjuncts to clinical judgment in critical care medicine.

ETHICAL ISSUES IN CRITICAL CARE MEDICINE

Despite their potential usefulness, prognostic scoring systems such as APACHE are rarely used to restrict admission to critical care units. This is because most clinicians who treat severely ill patients hope that the patient may survive, and they therefore request critical care almost regardless of the likely prognosis. One reason for this clinical approach is that statistical prediction is difficult in individual patients despite data derived from groups. Another is that patients and their families usually desire critical care if it will prolong life, assuming that self-awareness and social interaction are maintained. A third reason is that physicians may respond to what has been called the technologic imperative: the desire to do everything possible despite the ratio of benefit to cost.

Critical care is extraordinarily expensive. The issue of who should be admitted to critical care units and how aggressively they should be treated is a social, as well as medical, concern. This concern is likely to increase as society grapples with limited medical resources and adopts approaches such as managed care to reduce health care costs. Nevertheless, one major professional group recently published a statement asserting that although marginally beneficial critical care can be restricted on the basis of high cost relative to benefit, decisions to limit care should be made only by explicit institutional policies that reflect a social consensus in support of such limitations. Furthermore, patients and the public should be informed of any potential financial incentives for physicians or health care institutions to limit care.

Until this issue of allocation of critical care resources is resolved at a societal level, physicians should base decisions regarding critical care primarily on the wishes of well-informed, mentally capable patients or their surrogates. Certainly physicians are not obligated to provide care they consider nonbeneficial, but patients and surrogates who request critical care should receive it if they can benefit and if space in the unit permits. Conversely, the wishes of mentally capable patients who choose against therapies, such as endotracheal intubation and mechanical ventilation, should be respected, as should the wishes of the surrogates who speak for them.

Orders not to initiate CPR, which are also called "do-not-attempt-resuscitation" or "DNAR" orders, may be written at the request of patients or may be initiated by physicians when, to the best of their knowledge, CPR will not be successful in the broad sense of restoring meaningful life. In most instances, such decisions should be discussed with the patient and, when appropriate, with his or her family. The order should then be written in standard fashion on the order sheet, and a note describing the basis for the order and the decisions that took place should be included in the chart. Such orders clarify the ambiguity that surrounds the decisions concerning critical care for patients with irreversible illnesses, and they relieve nurses or uninvolved physicians from the responsibility of deciding not to initiate CPR.

Some patients with pre-existing DNAR orders may still benefit from critical care. Treatment of airway obstruction, metabolic abnormalities, or arrhythmias may at least temporarily improve the patient's condition and make the existence of prior DNAR orders moot. Nevertheless, when written in a critical care unit, DNAR orders usually represent the start of a pattern of witholding or withdrawing life support. Currently the majority of patients who die in critical care units do so during the forgoing of life-sustaining therapy; death results from the patient's underlying disease. In such instances, the withholding and withdrawal of life support generally is accompanied by the administration of sedatives and analgesics to reduce pain and suffering and by other aspects of what might be called intensive palliative care (see Chapter 3). The ability to provide humane end-of-life care to patients who are unlikely to recover is as important a feature of critical care units as is the ability to provide potentially life-saving monitoring and medical interventions to patients who are likely to live.

American Thoracic Society: Fair allocation of intensive care unit resources. Am J Respir Crit Care Med 156:1282–1301, 1997. *This statement, from a major professional group, provides guidelines for allocating resources in an era of managed care.*

Brody H, Campbell ML, Faber-Langendoen K, Ogle KS: Withdrawing intensive life-sustaining treatment—recommendations for compassionate clinical management. N Engl J Med 336:652–656, 1997. *Guidelines for providing humane end-of-life care to critically ill patients.*

Connors AF Jr, Speroff T, Dawson NV, et al: The effectiveness of right heart catheterization in the initial care of critically ill patients: SUPPORT investigators. JAMA 276:889–897, 1996. *This observational study suggests that pulmonary artery catheterization is associated with increased patient mortality and increased use of critical care resources.*

Milberg JA, Davis DR, Steinberg KP, Hudson LD: Improved survival of patients with acute respiratory distress syndrome (ARDS): 1983–1993. JAMA 273:306–309, 1995. *Using the same criteria for ARDS, the authors demonstrated an improved outcome in one institution over a 10-year period.*

Prendergast TJ, Claessens MT, Luce JM: A national survery of end-of-life care for critically ill patients. Am J Respir Crit Care Med 158:1163–1167, 1998. *Withholding and withdrawal of life support are common practices in American intensive care units, but there is wide practice variation.*

92 RESPIRATORY MONITORING IN CRITICAL CARE

John M. Luce

RESPIRATION

The word *respiration* describes the exchange of oxygen (O_2) and carbon dioxide (CO_2) between humans (or other animals) and the environment. Human respiration may be divided into the following four processes: (1) *ventilation,* in which O_2 is inhaled and CO_2 is excreted into the atmosphere; (2) *arterial oxygenation,* in which O_2 is transferred from the alveoli into mixed venous blood in the pulmonary capillaries in exchange for CO_2; (3) *oxygen transport* or *delivery,* in which O_2 is carried in systemic arterial blood to the tissues; and (4) *oxygen extraction* and *utilization,* in which the tissues take up O_2 from the blood and give up CO_2, which is transported in venous blood to the lungs.

ASSESSMENT OF VENTILATION

Physical Examination

Ventilation requires the rhythmic use of the respiratory muscles to pump gases in and out of the lungs. Measurement of the respiratory rate is particularly important in assessing the adequacy of ventilation. The respiratory rate at rest usually ranges from 12 to 22 breaths/min; a respiratory rate substantially less than 12 breaths/min suggests that ventilation is inadequate to meet metabolic needs, whereas a respiratory rate substantially greater than 22 breaths/min may reflect incipient ventilatory failure. In fact, patients may require mechanical ventilation if their respiratory rate exceeds 35 breaths/min over a prolonged period.

Whereas respiratory rate can be easily measured by direct obser-

vation, tidal volume, which is the amount of gas that enters and leaves the lungs with each breath, can only be approximated. Such approximation may be useful, for example when the respiratory rate and tidal volume are so low or high that ventilation must be impaired and medical intervention is necessary. Nevertheless, clinicians should avoid using words like hypoventilation and hyperventilation for patients whose respiratory rates and tidal volumes appear low or high, because these words refer to specific abnormalities in the systemic arterial CO_2 tension ($PaCO_2$) that can be diagnosed only by blood gas analysis.

In the presence of increased airway resistance or decreased lung or chest-wall compliance, patients must expend more respiratory muscle work to achieve adequate ventilation. The work of breathing in such patients is the product of the tidal volume and the pressure required to generate that tidal volume. This pressure, the transpulmonary pressure, is the difference between airway and pleural pressure. Transpulmonary pressure cannot be measured on physical examination. Recession of the suprasternal and intercostal spaces during inspiration suggests a greater than normal negative swing in pleural pressure and hence an increase in the work of breathing. Another manifestation of increased breathing effort is the forceful contraction of the sternocleidomastoid muscles.

Finally, a marked increase in the work of breathing, along with probable ventilatory inadequacy, may be suggested by certain abnormal breathing patterns. The first, an asynchrony between the peak excursions of the chest wall and abdomen, is called respiratory muscle asynchrony (Fig. 92–1). The second, respiratory muscle paradox, is seen when the abdomen moves inward rather than outward during inspiration, indicating that the chest-wall muscles are being recruited more than the diaphragm.

Systemic Arterial Blood Gas Analysis

Samples of systemic arterial blood may be obtained from repeated percutaneous arterial punctures or from indwelling arterial catheters for measurement of $PaCO_2$, pH, arterial O_2 tension (PaO_2), and bicarbonate (HCO_3^-) concentration. Miniature intra-arterial sensors may also be placed through the catheters for continuous analysis of blood gases, although this technology is not sufficiently accurate for clinical use.

The $PaCO_2$ is used to assess the adequacy of ventilation and to diagnose hypercapneic respiratory failure, also called failure of ventilation. At sea level the $PaCO_2$ normally ranges from 35 to 45 mm Hg. Hyperventilation and respiratory alkalosis are said to be present if the $PaCO_2$ is less than 35 mm Hg. Hypoventilation, hypercapnia, and respiratory acidosis are present if the $PaCO_2$ is greater than 45 mm Hg, and ventilatory failure exists when the $PaCO_2$ exceeds 50 mm Hg.

The pH and HCO_3^- concentration measurements can be used to determine whether hypercapnia and hypocapnia and respiratory acidosis and respiratory alkalosis are acute or chronic. Such determination is based on the Henderson-Hasselbalch equation for the HCO_3^- buffer system:

$$pH = 6.1 + \log [HCO_3^-]/0.003 \ PaCO_2 \qquad (1)$$

In keeping with this equation, acute increases or decreases in $PaCO_2$ cause the pH to fall or rise until the kidneys gradually retain or release HCO_3^- to buffer the fall or rise in pH.

The pH normally ranges from 7.35 to 7.45. An acute increase in $PaCO_2$ causes the pH to fall below 7.35, a condition called acute respiratory acidosis. If the $PaCO_2$ is increased, the pH is below normal, and the HCO_3^- concentration is increased, the patient has either a chronic respiratory acidosis with a compensatory metabolic alkalosis or a respiratory acidosis of unknown duration with a concurrent but not compensatory metabolic alkalosis.

Conversely, an acute decrease in $PaCO_2$ causes the pH to rise above 7.45, creating an acute respiratory alkalosis. If the $PaCO_2$ is decreased, the pH is above normal, and the HCO_3^- concentration is decreased, the patient has either a chronic respiratory alkalosis with a compensatory metabolic acidosis or a respiratory alkalosis of unknown duration with a concurrent metabolic acidosis.

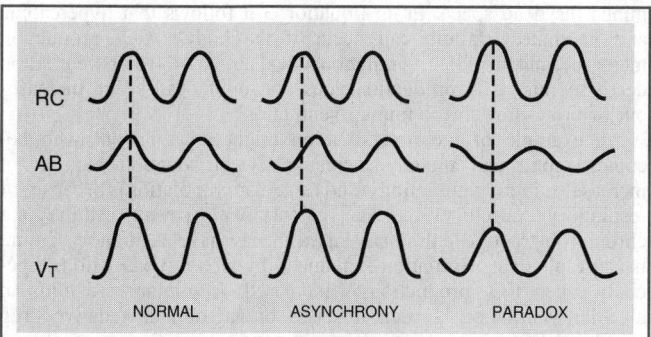

FIGURE 92–1 ■ Tracings of the movements of the rib cage (RC), the abdomen (AB), and their sum (VT) recorded by inductance plethysmography. The dashed lines are drawn at the time of maximum inspiratory volume. (From Dantzker DR, Tobin MJ: Monitoring respiratory muscle function. Respir Care 30:422–428, 1985, with permission.)

$$V_D/V_T = (Pa_{CO_2} - PE_{CO_2})/Pa_{CO_2} \qquad (2)$$

Measurement of Transcutaneous Carbon Dioxide Tensions

The Pa_{CO_2} can be estimated by measuring the transcutaneous CO_2 tension through an electrode placed on the skin. Because the electrode is heated, this value is generally higher than the Pa_{CO_2}, although the transcutaneous CO_2 tension can be adjusted to obtain a close approximation of the Pa_{CO_2}. In contrast to transcutaneous O_2 values, the transcutaneous CO_2 tension is relatively insensitive to alterations in skin perfusion and does not change significantly with age. Transcutaneous monitoring of the CO_2 tension is performed most commonly in neonates in whom percutaneous arterial punctures and arterial catheters are impractical.

Measurement of End-Tidal Carbon Dioxide Tensions

In intubated patients of all ages, the Pa_{CO_2} may be approximated by measuring the end-tidal CO_2 tension in expired gas. The end-tidal CO_2 tension can be measured either by a capnometer, which displays its value breath by breath, or by a capnograph, which also displays its wave form.

The capnogram (Fig. 92–2) reflects the sequential measurement of CO_2 tensions from several dead space compartments that do not participate in CO_2 exchange—apparatus, anatomic, and alveolar—in addition to the CO_2 tension in alveolar gas that is in equilibrium with end-capillary blood. When a plateau is reached, indicating the presence of CO_2 in alveolar gas and minimal amounts of gas from areas of dead space, the end-tidal CO_2 tension should be similar to the Pa_{CO_2}, albeit usually 1 to 5 mm Hg less. If the CO_2 tensions in samples of systemic arterial blood and end-tidal gas obtained simultaneously are measured, the correlation of CO_2 tensions can be known.

In the presence of ventilation and perfusion inhomogeneities, there may not be a plateau on the capnogram, and as a result, there will be a difference between the Pa_{CO_2} and the end-tidal CO_2 tension of as much as 10 to 20 mm Hg or more. Although the end-tidal CO_2 tension no longer reflects the Pa_{CO_2} in this circumstance and cannot be used to estimate it, trends in the end-tidal CO_2 tension and the difference between it and the Pa_{CO_2} may be followed to determine the evolution of a patient's dead space.

Measurement of Dead Space

Dead space is usually expressed as a fraction of tidal volume. The ratio of dead space to tidal volume (V_D/V_T) per breath can be calculated in patients whose Pa_{CO_2} and mean expired P_{CO_2} (PE_{CO_2}) are known, using the modified Bohr equation:

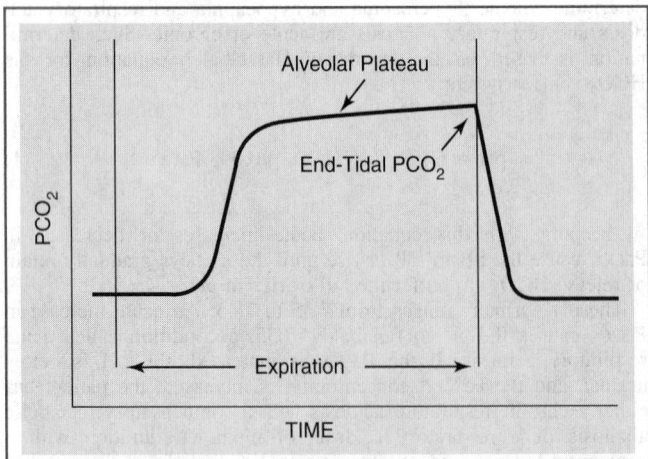

FIGURE 92–2 ■ Illustration of a normal capnogram, in which the carbon dioxide tension (P_{CO_2}) rises as dead-space gas from the apparatus, the airways, and the alveoli is supplanted by alveolar gas with a high concentration of CO_2. The high point of this "alveolar plateau" represents the end-tidal P_{CO_2}. See text for further discussion.

The ratio of dead space to tidal volume is usually 0.30 to 0.40 in healthy persons breathing spontaneously. In patients with normal lungs being ventilated mechanically, it approaches 0.50 because gas is stored transiently in compressible portions of the ventilator circuit. The ratio of dead space to tidal volume may rise to values of 0.7 or more in patients with significant respiratory disease.

Measurement of Ventilatory Variables

Ventilatory variables such as respiratory rate and tidal volume may be measured by respiratory inductance plethysmography, which uses wire coils imbedded in bands that fit around the chest and abdomen to detect movements in these areas. These variables may also be measured with a pneumotachograph or other types of spirometers in patients who are breathing through endotracheal tubes. In healthy persons, tidal volume is approximately 400 mL. A patient with a tidal volume of less than 300 mL or 5 mL/kg during spontaneous breathing is unlikely to be weaned from mechanical ventilation.

The product of respiratory rate and tidal volume is the minute ventilation. Minute ventilation is approximately 6 L/min in normal adults (at rest) and is usually increased in critically ill patients due to increases in CO_2 production, increases in the ratio of dead space to tidal volume, or both. Values in excess of 10 L/min are difficult to maintain without mechanical ventilatory support.

The ratio of respiratory rate to tidal volume increases as patients breathe rapidly and shallowly. This breathing pattern is inefficient in excreting CO_2 when the ratio of dead space to tidal volume is normal and is associated with CO_2 retention when this ratio is increased. Recent studies have demonstrated that weaning from mechanical ventilation is unlikely in patients whose ratio of respiratory rate to tidal volume exceeds 105 breaths/min/L (see Chapter 93), and that a low tidal volume is superior to a larger tidal volume.

Measurement of Carbon Dioxide Production

The body's CO_2 production can be measured in patients breathing spontaneously or receiving mechanical ventilation by closed systems that compare the difference in CO_2 in inspired (with virtually no CO_2) and expired gases. Newer systems such as indirect calorimeters allow rapid calculation of CO_2 production at the bedside. The CO_2 production of a healthy adult is approximately 200 mL/min, and it varies with body temperature and metabolism.

Use of the Alveolar Ventilation Equation

Although measurement or approximation of the Pa_{CO_2} helps determine the adequacy of ventilation, the explanation of why ventilation is inadequate in a given patient can be derived only by using the alveolar ventilation equation:

$$Pa_{CO_2} = (K)\ \dot{V}_{CO_2}/\dot{V}_A \qquad (3)$$

where K is a constant, $\dot{V}_{CO_2}$ is the body's CO_2 production, and $\dot{V}_A$, the alveolar ventilation, is equal to the minute ventilation minus the dead space. From Equation 3 it follows that hypercapnia and ventilatory failure can occur if the body's CO_2 production increases and alveolar ventilation does not, if alveolar ventilation decreases and CO_2 production does not, or if dead space increases out of proportion to the minute ventilation.

An example of the first situation might be a patient who becomes septic and thereby increases CO_2 production but cannot increase minute ventilation (and alveolar ventilation) because of respiratory muscle weakness. Patients with severe asthma and chronic obstructive pulmonary disease may have ventilatory failure because alveolar ventilation is reduced by airway obstruction, especially when CO_2 production is increased. A primary reduction in alveolar ventilation is seen in cases of narcotic or sedative drug overdose. Diseases such as the acute respiratory distress syndrome (ARDS) and pulmonary embolism, in which dead space may increase because of vascular obstruction in the lungs, can cause ventilatory failure if patients cannot increase alveolar ventilation; for example, because of oversedation.

Measurement of Respiratory Mechanics

Vital capacity (VC) is the greatest amount of gas that can be exhaled after a maximum inspiration. The normal VC is approximately 70 mL/kg. VC is reduced in most obstructive and restrictive respiratory diseases, and a VC of less than 10 mL/kg is generally associated with inadequate ventilation. VC can be measured by a variety of spirometers in intubated or non-intubated patients.

The volume change per unit of pressure change across the lungs and chest cavity is termed the compliance of the respiratory system. When determined in a patient who is being mechanically ventilated, effective respiratory system compliance (CEFF) is tidal volume divided by the maximum or peak airway pressure (PMAX) required to deliver a given tidal volume (VT) minus the amount of positive end-expiratory pressure (PEEP) the patient is receiving. Thus,

$$\text{CEFF} = \text{VT}/(\text{PMAX} - \text{PEEP}) \qquad (4)$$

Because it is a dynamic measurement made when gas is flowing, CEFF includes the resistance to gas flow in the airways and ventilator tubing, as well as the volume and pressure characteristics of the lungs and chest wall. Normal CEFF is 50–80 mL/cm H_2O; it will be decreased by airway obstruction, secretions, and a small-diameter endotracheal tube.

Static respiratory system compliance (CSTAT) is a measure of the airway pressure required to distend the lungs and chest wall and maintain the increase in volume after a VT has been delivered and gas is not flowing in or out of the lungs. This pressure is called the plateau pressure or static recoil pressure (PSTAT) and is measured while temporarily occluding the expiratory port of a mechanical ventilator for approximately 2 seconds (Fig. 92–3). The amount of PEEP should be subtracted from the PSTAT. Thus,

$$\text{CSTAT} = \text{VT}/(\text{PSTAT} - \text{PEEP}) \qquad (5)$$

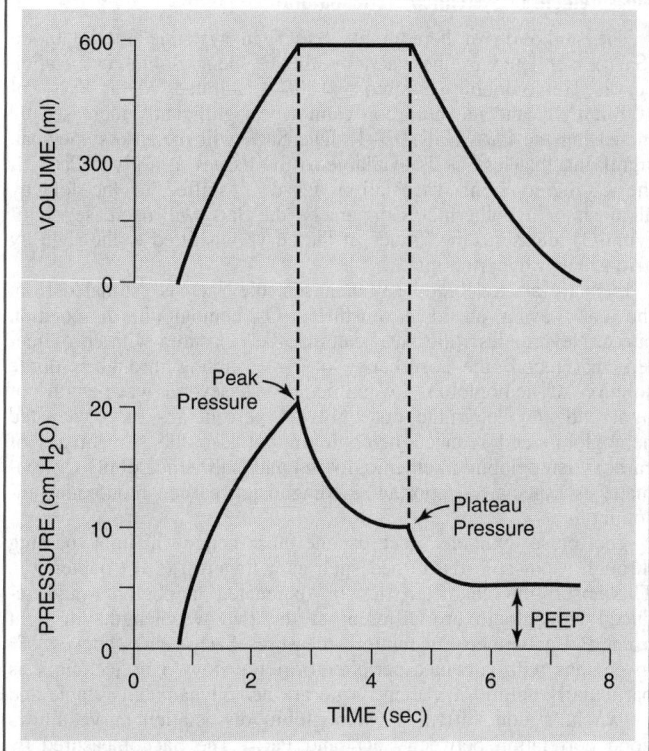

FIGURE 92–3 ■ Relationship between tidal volume and airway pressure in a mechanically ventilated patient. The peak pressure is used to calculate effective respiratory system compliance, whereas the plateau pressure is used to calculate static compliance. (From Tobin MJ: Respiratory monitoring in the intensive care unit. Am Rev Respir Dis 138:1625–1642, 1988, with permission.)

Because it is a static measurement, CSTAT reflects the compliance of the lungs and chest wall and is not affected by resistance to gas flow. It will be decreased (normal level is 60–100 mL/cm H_2O) by conditions, such as ARDS, that decrease lung volume. Weaning from mechanical ventilation is difficult if CSTAT is less than 25 mL/cm H_2O.

Intrinsic or auto-PEEP occurs in patients with airway obstruction and other disorders who fail to complete expiration either during spontaneous breathing or on a mechanical ventilator. The result is air trapping that produces positive pressure at end-expiration. The positive pressure in turn can decrease cardiac filling and increase vascular pressures in the chest, as intentional PEEP can. Auto-PEEP can be measured in mechanically ventilated patients by stopping airflow at end-expiration just before the next breath, allowing pressure in the airways and the ventilator tubing to equilibrate, and reading the pressure from the ventilator manometer. Auto-PEEP should be taken into account when calculating effective respiratory system compliance and CSTAT.

Measurement of Ventilatory Drive

The drive to breathe is responsible in large part for the sensation of dyspnea and determines how avidly patients attempt to achieve adequate ventilation. Ventilatory drive can be estimated in intubated patients by measuring the inspiratory pressure developed in the first 100 ms of surreptitious airway occlusion. This measurement provides only an estimate because the inspiratory pressure developed in the first 100 ms of surreptitious airway occlusion, which is normally less than 2 cm H_2O, is influenced somewhat by respiratory muscle strength and, hence, lung volume. Values of greater than 4 cm H_2O are thought to reflect the need for ventilatory support, and values of less than 4 cm H_2O are associated with successful discontinuation of ventilatory support.

Measurement of Respiratory Muscle Strength

Respiratory muscle strength can be assessed by measuring with a manometer the maximum airway pressures developed during inspiration from a low lung volume and expiration from a high lung volume. Healthy adults have a maximum inspiratory pressure greater than 100 cm H_2O and a maximum expiratory pressure greater than 150 cm H_2O. A maximum inspiratory pressure that is less negative than -30 cm H_2O suggests the need for ventilatory support, whereas a value that is more negative than -30 cm H_2O, especially if it can be sustained for 3–5 seconds, correlates with successful weaning from mechanical ventilation.

Measurement of the Work of Breathing

As noted earlier, the work of breathing is the product of the transpulmonary pressure (the difference between airway and pleural pressure) multiplied by the tidal volume (the VT). Although pleural pressure is impractical to measure and varies regionally, it can be approximated by measuring pressure in the esophagus with a balloon. Changes in this pressure can be used to compute the work of breathing in spontaneously breathing and mechanically ventilated patients.

ASSESSMENT OF ARTERIAL OXYGENATION

Physical Examination

Cyanosis of the tongue and oral mucosa, which is called central cyanosis, provides a crude estimation of the adequacy of arterial oxygenation. Central cyanosis reflects the presence of 3 g/dL or more of reduced, that is, deoxygenated, hemoglobin. However, the blue discoloration of tissues caused by deoxygenated hemoglobin also may be caused by dyshemoglobins such as sulfhemoglobin. Furthermore, clinicians vary in their ability to detect cyanosis when it actually occurs.

Arterial Blood Gas Analysis

The systemic arterial O_2 tension (PaO$_2$) obtained by arterial blood gas analysis is the standard for assessing the adequacy of arterial oxygenation. The normal PaO$_2$ at sea level is approximately

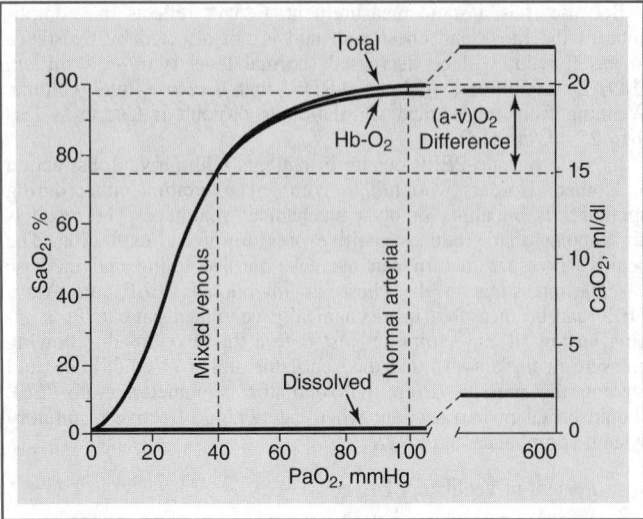

FIGURE 92-4 ■ Normal oxyhemoglobin dissociation curve showing the relationship between the systemic arterial O_2 saturation (SaO_2), tension (PaO_2), and content (CaO_2). See text for further discussion.

100 mm Hg (Fig. 92–4). However, the PaO_2 is inversely correlated with age, as expressed in the following equation:

$$\text{Normal } PaO_2 = 100 \text{ mm Hg} - (0.3) \text{ age in years} \qquad (6)$$

However, Equation 6 does not correct for the effects of barometric pressure.

Measurement of Transcutaneous Oxygen Tensions

As with CO_2, the transcutaneous tension of O_2 can be measured by a heated electrode on the skin. However, the correlation between PaO_2 and transcutaneous tension of O_2 is affected by both age and perfusion status, which is not the case with the correlation between $PaCO_2$ and transcutaneous CO_2 tension.

Use of the Alveolar Gas Equation

Although the alveolar O_2 tension (PAO_2) cannot be measured directly, it can be calculated from the alveolar gas equation:

$$PAO_2 = FIO_2 (PB - 47) - PaCO_2/R \qquad (7)$$

where FIO_2 is the fraction of inspired O_2 (normally 0.21), PB is barometric pressure, 47 is the vapor pressure of water at 37° C, and R is the respiratory exchange ratio, which represents the ratio of CO_2 production to O_2 consumption (usually assumed to be 0.8). Normally a difference or gradient of 10 mm Hg or less exists between the PAO_2 and PaO_2. This difference, the P (A − a) O_2, increases to 30 mm Hg with age and increases further with respiratory disease.

The word hypoxemia is used to describe a PaO_2 of less than normal; hypoxemic respiratory failure, also called failure of arterial oxygenation, exists when the PaO_2 is below 50–60 mm Hg. As indicated by the alveolar gas equation and the relationship between PaO_2 and PAO_2, hypoxemia can be caused by a decrease in FIO_2, as might result from breathing air in a fire where O_2 has been consumed; a decrease in barometric pressure, as occurs at altitude; an increase in $PaCO_2$, as might happen during a drug overdose; or an increase in the alveolar-arterial gradient of oxygen as caused, for example, by a mismatch of ventilation and perfusion in the lungs.

Even if the PaO_2 of a patient with hypoxemic respiratory failure is normalized by the administration of supplemental O_2, O_2 exchange in the lungs may remain abnormal. In this situation, the inadequacy of O_2 exchange will be reflected by an increased alveolar-arterial gradient of oxygen, which remains a helpful indicator of respiratory function at all but the highest levels of FIO_2, where it may change unpredictably.

Other Indicators of Arterial Oxygenation

The arterial to alveolar PO_2 ratio (PaO_2/PAO_2) can be calculated using the alveolar gas equation. The PaO_2/PAO_2 is relatively stable with changing levels of FIO_2 and can be used to predict the expected PaO_2 when the FIO_2 is altered. The normal PaO_2/PAO_2 is 0.9. The PaO_2 to FIO_2 ratio (PaO_2/FIO_2) is easier to calculate because it does not require use of the alveolar gas equation. The normal PaO_2/FIO_2 is 460. Although the PaO_2/FIO_2 does not account for changes in $PaCO_2$, this limitation is not important at high levels of FIO_2.

Measurement of Venous Admixture and Shunt Fraction

Venous admixture ($\dot{Q}VA/\dot{Q}T$) is the fraction of mixed venous blood that does not become oxygenated as it courses through the lungs. It can be calculated with the equation:

$$\dot{Q}VA/\dot{Q}T = (C'cO_2 - CaO_2) / (C'cO_2 - C\bar{v}\,O_2) \qquad (8)$$

where $\dot{Q}T$ is the cardiac output, and $C'cO_2$, CaO_2, and $C\bar{v}\,O_2$ are the O_2 contents of end-capillary, arterial, and mixed venous blood, respectively. Although end-capillary blood cannot be sampled routinely, the end-capillary O_2 content can be calculated by assuming that the tension of end-capillary blood is the same as PaO_2.

The normal $\dot{Q}VA/\dot{Q}T$ is ≤0.07; increases in $\dot{Q}VA/\dot{Q}T$ are caused by ventilation-perfusion mismatching or right-to-left intrapulmonary shunting ($\dot{Q}s/\dot{Q}T$). Equation 8 can be used to calculate $\dot{Q}s/\dot{Q}T$ in patients receiving an FIO_2 of 1.0 because this FIO_2 eliminates areas of ventilation-perfusion mismatch in the lungs. A simpler but less precise way of estimating $\dot{Q}s/\dot{Q}T$ is to divide the P (A − a) O_2 by 20. The PaO_2 can rarely be improved by increasing FIO_2 if $\dot{Q}s/\dot{Q}T$ exceeds 0.25.

Measurement of Systemic Arterial Saturation

The saturation of hemoglobin by O_2 in systemic arterial blood (SaO_2) is related to the PaO_2 by the O_2 hemoglobin dissociation curve. Hemoglobin is almost 100% saturated at a PaO_2 of 100 mm Hg, and its saturation cannot be significantly increased by increasing the PaO_2 (Fig. 92–4). The SaO_2 will increase somewhat, signifying that less O_2 is available to the tissues at a given PaO_2, if the O_2 hemoglobin dissociation curve is shifted to the left by alkalosis or hypothermia. Conversely, the SaO_2 will decrease, signifying O_2 release to the tissues, if the curve is shifted to the right by acidosis or hyperthermia.

In many arterial blood gas analyses, the SaO_2 is estimated from the PaO_2 using an ideal, unshifted O_2 hemoglobin dissociation curve. Nevertheless, the SaO_2 can also be measured with co-oximeters that record the absorbency of light passing through a dilute solution of hemoglobin. Co-oximeters use several wavelengths of light and can determine not only the percentages of oxygenated hemoglobin and reduced hemoglobin but also the percentages of carboxyhemoglobin, methemoglobin, and sulfhemoglobin. Co-oximetry is especially important in diagnosing carbon monoxide poisoning.

The pulse oximeter records the absorbency of light passing through a pulsatile tissue bed such as a fingertip (see Chapter 91). The absorption characteristics of oxgenated hemoglobin and reduced hemoglobin are different at the two wavelengths of light used. Pulse oximetry accurately measures SaO_2 values above 80% in persons with adequate peripheral arterial flow. This technique is particularly helpful in patients who are hemodynamically stable and in whom a non-shifted O_2 hemoglobin dissociation curve allows good correlation between SaO_2 and PaO_2. The SaO_2 measured by pulse oximetry does not account for hemoglobin that is saturated by substances other than O_2, such as carbon monoxide; because of this, the SaO_2 is falsely elevated in patients with carbon monoxide poisoning. In addition, the SaO_2 provides no information about $PaCO_2$ or pH. Nevertheless, the accuracy, ease, and low expense of pulse oximetry make it a useful substitute for analysis of PaO_2 in many situations.

Physical Examination

The adequacy of O_2 delivery and utilization may be appreciated by examination of the skin. For example, the presence of normal skin color and warmth suggest an adequate peripheral flow of oxygenated blood in some circumstances. Such adequacy is also suggested by normal capillary refill, in which skin color returns to baseline 2–3 seconds after the skin is blanched. Nevertheless, although these findings may help exclude significant hypovolemia or impairment of cardiac output, which are associated with increased systemic vascular resistance, they do not exclude sepsis and other processes in which systemic vascular resistance is decreased.

When skin findings are unreliable, O_2 delivery and utilization may be assessed in other organs where blood supply is maintained despite hypoperfusion elsewhere. In this regard, the onset of confusion or obtundation in a previously healthy patient may signify a significant decrease in cerebral oxygenation. Similarly, a decrease in urine output below 0.5 mL/kg/h may result from a reduction in renal blood flow from sepsis and other causes.

Measurement of Oxygen Delivery

The amount of O_2 delivered to the tissues ($\dot{D}O_2$) is the product of cardiac output ($\dot{Q}T$) and the content of O_2 in systemic arterial blood (CaO_2). Thus,

$$\dot{D}O_2 = (\dot{Q}T)(CaO_2) \qquad (9)$$

The CaO_2 (mL O_2/dL blood) can be calculated from the following equation:

$$CaO_2 = (1.39)\,(Hb)\,\frac{(SaO_2)}{100} + (0.003)\,(PaO_2) \qquad (10)$$

where 1.39 is the oxygen-carrying capacity of hemoglobin in mL O_2/g, and 0.003 is the solubility coefficient of O_2 in plasma. Most of the O_2 in blood is bound to hemoglobin (Fig. 92–4), although additional O_2 can be dissolved in blood if the PaO_2 is raised to supranormal levels. At a normal SaO_2 of approximately 100%, a PaO_2 of 100 mm Hg, and a hemoglobin concentration of 14 g, the CaO_2 is 20 mL O_2/dL of blood.

Cardiac output can be measured with the thermodilution technique using a pulmonary artery catheter. With this technique, a bolus of cold liquid, usually dextrose in water, is rapidly injected into the right atrium through the proximal catheter port, causing the negative heat to be diluted by mixing with blood as it passes into the pulmonary artery. A thermistor senses the temperature of blood on passing the distal catheter port, and the temperature change is used to compute cardiac output, which averages 5 L/min in healthy persons. If arterial O_2 content is normal, the amount of O_2 delivered to the tissues normally averages 1000 mL O_2/min.

Measurement of Mixed Venous Oxygen Saturation

Placement of a pulmonary artery catheter allows the collection of samples for determination of the O_2 tension, saturation, and content of mixed venous blood. The saturation can also be measured continuously with an oximetric pulmonary artery catheter containing fiberoptic bundles that transmit and receive light from the catheter tip.

Normal persons have a mixed venous O_2 saturation of approximately 75%, which corresponds to a mixed venous O_2 tension of 40 mm Hg on an unshifted O_2 hemoglobin dissociation curve. Reductions in mixed venous O_2 saturation to below 60%, corresponding to mixed venous O_2 tension values of less than 28 mm Hg, are associated with a severely impaired amount of O_2 delivered to the tissues. Indeed, anaerobic metabolism commonly develops when the mixed venous O_2 saturation falls below 50%.

Although a low mixed venous O_2 saturation may be clinically alarming, inadequate O_2 transport and utilization may exist in the face of normal or supranormal values. For example, a mixed venous O_2 saturation >80% may be seen in sepsis, when the tissues either cannot extract O_2 from the blood or perform aerobic metabolism, or when blood is redistributed to metabolically inactive organs such as the skin.

Measurement of Oxygen Consumption

Total body O_2 consumption, which reflects the amount of O_2 utilized during aerobic metabolism, can be measured in closed systems by comparing the difference in O_2 in inspired and expired gases, which is difficult to accomplish in patients with a high minute ventilation and FIO_2. Alternatively, total body O_2 consumption can be measured by indirect calorimetry, which can be calculated using Fick's equation.

Use of Fick's Equation

The Fick equation holds that total body O_2 consumption ($\dot{V}O_2$) is equal to the product of cardiac output ($\dot{Q}T$) and the amount of O_2 extracted by the tissues, which is the difference in O_2 contents in systemic arterial (CaO_2) and mixed venous ($C\bar{v}O_2$) blood. Thus,

$$\dot{V}O_2 = (\dot{Q}T)(CaO_2 - C\bar{v}O_2) \qquad (11)$$

The mixed venous O_2 content is normally 15 mL O_2/dL of blood. Because the mixed arterial content is usually 20 mL/dL, the normal difference is 5 mL O_2/mL blood. With this value and a cardiac output of 5 L/min, total body O_2 consumption averages 250 mL O_2/min in healthy persons.

In addition to allowing calculation of total body O_2 consumption, Fick's equation provides insights into physiologic function during stress and exercise. It reveals, for example, that normally only 25% of the O_2 in systemic arterial blood is extracted by the tissues, leaving a large O_2 reserve. Patients characteristically call on this reserve when the amount of O_2 delivered to the tissues decreases because of a fall in cardiac output, a fall in the content of O_2 in systemic arterial blood (and its major components, SaO_2 and hemoglobin), or both. Nevertheless, a shift to anaerobic metabolism generally occurs when more than 50% of the O_2 is extracted, and lactic acidosis may result.

Measurement of Other Indicators of Oxygen Transport and Utilization

Clinicians commonly monitor serum lactate levels as a sign of the development and progression of anaerobic metabolism. This approach is supported by studies demonstrating that lactate levels above 2 mEq/L correspond to a mixed venous O_2 tension less than 28 mm Hg with an increased mortality rate among critically ill patients. Nevertheless, elevated lactate levels may result from decreased lactate degradation rather than increased production, and they should be interpreted with caution.

Assessment of oxygenation of the gastrointestinal tract may provide an early indication of inadequate tissue perfusion in the critically ill. Such assessment can be derived from measurement of gastric intramucosal pH by a saline-filled balloon passed into the lumen of the stomach. After approximately 30 minutes, the gastric CO_2 tension equilibrates with the CO_2 tension in the balloon; the equilibrated CO_2 tension can then be combined with the HCO_3^- concentration in blood to calculate intramucosal gastric pH using the Henderson-Hasselbalch equation.

Recent studies have suggested that a gastric intramucosal pH of less than the normal level of 7.35 correlates with a high mortality rate in patients admitted to a critical care unit and that such mortality can be reduced by therapy designed to restore intraluminal pH to normal. Nevertheless, this approach has not been verified in large groups of patients. In fact, it is not clear whether any method of assessing O_2 delivery and utilization is superior to monitoring urine output and changes in the physical examination.

Gattinoni L, Brazzi L, Pelosi P, et al: A trial of goal-oriented hemodynamic therapy in critically ill patients. N Engl J Med 333:1025, 1995. *A large study in which normalization of the mixed venous O_2 saturation did not improve outcome.*

Guttierez G, Palizas F, Doglio G, et al: Gastric intramucosal pH as a therapeutic index of tissue oxygenation in critically ill patients. Lancet 339:195, 1992. *The first major trial to indicate that changes in intramucosal pH may reflect tissue oxygenation.*

Jubran A, Mathru M, Dries D, Tobin MJ: Continuous recordings of mixed venous oxygen saturation during weaning from mechanical ventilation and the ramifications thereof. Am J Respir Crit Care Med 158:1763–1769, 1998. *Patients who fail weaning develop a progressive decrease in mixed venous oxygen saturation because of increased oxygen extraction by the tissues and the inability to increase oxygen transport.*

Tobin MJ: Respiratory monitoring in the intensive care unit. Am Rev Respir Dis 138: 1625, 1988. *This article remains the best short review of respiratory monitoring in critical care.*

93 VENTILATOR MANAGEMENT IN THE INTENSIVE CARE UNIT

John M. Luce

MECHANICAL VENTILATION

Indications for Mechanical Ventilation

The term mechanical ventilation is used to describe the artificial support of ventilation in which oxygen (O_2) is inhaled and carbon dioxide (CO_2) is excreted. Mechanical ventilation may be necessary for patients who have inadequate ventilation as reflected in a high systemic arterial CO_2 tension ($PaCO_2$), inadequate arterial oxygenation as reflected in a low arterial O_2 tension (PaO_2), or both (Table 93–1). Furthermore, severe airway obstruction caused by asthma and chronic obstructive pulmonary disease (COPD) or parenchymal disease caused by disorders such as the acute respiratory distress syndrome (ARDS) may increase the work of breathing to levels that cannot be maintained by spontaneous breathing. Finally, mechanical ventilation may be required for clinically unstable patients such as those in shock and for patients who require hyperventilation to decrease cerebral blood flow and intracranial pressure.

Ventilatory support supplied through endotracheal intubation is called invasive mechanical ventilation. Noninvasive ventilation can be provided by devices that apply intermittent negative extrathoracic pressure or furnish intermittent positive pressure through a tight-fitting nasal or face mask without an artificial airway in place. Both types of ventilation can create a closed system for delivering O_2 at a high inspired fraction (FIO_2) and for furnishing positive end-expiratory pressure (PEEP). Noninvasive positive-pressure ventilation has become increasingly popular for treating acute ventilatory failure, especially that caused by exacerbations of COPD, in critical or intensive care units. Nevertheless, its use is restricted for the most part to patients who are conscious, cooperative, hemodynamically stable, and not in need of airway protection. Hence, most mechanical ventilation requires the use of endotracheal intubation, which is discussed later in this chapter.

Kinds of Mechanical Ventilation

Negative-Pressure Ventilation

Ventilation can be supported by devices that generate a negative pressure around the chest during inspiration to substitute for the negative pleural and airway pressures normally created by contraction of the respiratory muscles. Negative-pressure ventilation can be achieved by including the entire body except the head in an iron lung, by encompassing the thorax in a garment or poncho wrap, or by fitting a cuirass to the anterior chest. Negative-pressure ventila-

Table 93–1 ■ INDICATIONS FOR MECHANICAL VENTILATION

Acute increase in $PaCO_2$ to >50 mm Hg with a decrease in pH to <7.30
Respiratory rate >35 breaths/min for prolonged period
Tidal volume <5 mL/kg body weight
Ratio of respiratory rate (breaths/min) to tidal volume (L) >105
Minute ventilation >10 L/min
Vital capacity <10 mL/kg body weight
Maximum inspiratory pressure between 0 and −20 cm H_2O
Dead space to tidal volume fraction 0.60 or more
Acute hypoxemia (PaO_2 <60 mm Hg or SaO_2 <90%, especially if inspired oxygen fraction is 0.4 or more, or $P(A - a)O_2$ >300 mm Hg on inspired FIO_2 of 1.0)
Clinical instability
Need for hyperventilation therapy

$PaCO_2$ = systemic arterial carbon dioxide tension
PaO_2 = systemic arterial oxygen tension
SaO_2 = systemic arterial oxygen saturation
$P(A - a)O_2$ = systemic alveolar to arterial oxygen pressure difference
FIO_2 = fraction of inspired oxygen

tors are best suited for stable patients with neuromuscular diseases whose lungs are normal and who do not require O_2 at a high FIO_2.

Positive-Pressure Ventilation

Due to the limitations of negative-pressure ventilation, positive-pressure ventilation is the kind of mechanical ventilation most widely used today for both invasive and noninvasive ventilation. With positive-pressure ventilation, gas is delivered under positive pressure into the airways and the lungs. In contrast to negative-pressure ventilation, positive-pressure ventilation produces a positive airway pressure during inspiration. This pressure overcomes the impedance to gas flow and the elastance (reciprocal of the compliance, which is the change in volume with a given change in pressure) of the respiratory system and thereby inflates the alveoli, providing both ventilation and arterial oxygenation while reducing the work of breathing.

Most positive-pressure ventilators regulate gas delivery to maintain a constant pressure (pressure limited) or volume (volume limited) during inspiration. The first approach allows establishable limits on the peak and plateau pressures used for lung inflation but allows tidal volume, and hence minute ventilation, to vary, depending on the impedance of the respiratory system. Alternatively, the ventilators may deliver a preset tidal volume at whatever pressure is required to inflate the lungs, which guarantees minute ventilation but may increase peak and plateau pressures. Maintenance of airway pressure and lung volume is usually achieved by ventilator manipulation of gas flow.

When positive-pressure ventilation was first introduced, clinicians generally hoped to achieve a tidal volume in the range of 10 to 15 mL/kg of ideal body weight at whatever peak and plateau pressures were required or resulted, yielding a normal $PaCO_2$ in patients unless hyperventilation was desired. However, increasing concerns about ventilator-induced lung injury, as discussed later, have led clinicians today to seek a lower tidal volume (6 to 10 mL/kg) and low plateau pressure (less than 35 cm H_2O) in many patients. Because this approach may lead to an increase in $PaCO_2$, the strategy is called permissive hypercapnia or intentional hypoventilation. A strategy using 6 mL/kg compared with 12 mL/kg has been shown to improve mortality rates in patients with asthma and with the acute respiratory distress syndrome (ARDS).

With most modes of positive-pressure ventilation, an inspiratory-to-expiratory ratio of 1:3 or less is generally used to achieve an inspiratory time of 0.8 to 1.0 second and allow adequate time for expiration. This helps avoid air trapping, which may cause intrinsic or auto-PEEP. Auto-PEEP is most common in patients with COPD and other causes of airways obstruction. In addition, inspiratory flow rates of about 60 L/min are usually selected unless a higher flow rate is used to achieve a more rapid inflation and hence more time for exhalation, as might be desirable in patients with COPD. Flow can be delivered either with a square wave (constant flow) or a decelerating pattern; the latter may allow for a more uniform transpulmonary pressure throughout inspiration, which may be desirable in patients with ARDS.

MODES OF POSITIVE-PRESSURE VENTILATION. Perhaps the simplest mode of positive-pressure ventilation is *controlled mechanical ventilation,* in which the ventilator delivers gas at a preset respiratory rate and inspiratory time and either a preset peak pressure or tidal volume (Fig. 93–1 and Table 93–2). A square wave flow pattern is customarily used with controlled mechanical ventilation. In volume-limited controlled mechanical ventilation, the ventilator adjusts inspiratory flow over time to ensure stable tidal volume delivery. For example, as impedance increases during a breath, the resulting decreases in flow output are detected, and the ventilator's inspiratory valve opens wider to increase flow and maintain a constant tidal volume. Volume-limited controlled mechanical ventilation is most often used for patients who are unconscious due to illness or drugs, who are being intentionally hyperventilated, or who are recovering from anesthesia. Because patients receiving controlled mechanical ventilation cannot increase their minute ventilation voluntarily, their ventilatory status must be followed closely. Thus, the advantage of controlled mechanical ventilation—complete control of ventilatory function—is also its major limitation, and this mode is rarely used today.

Assisted mechanical ventilation is a positive-pressure ventilation mode in which the patient triggers the ventilator to deliver a preset

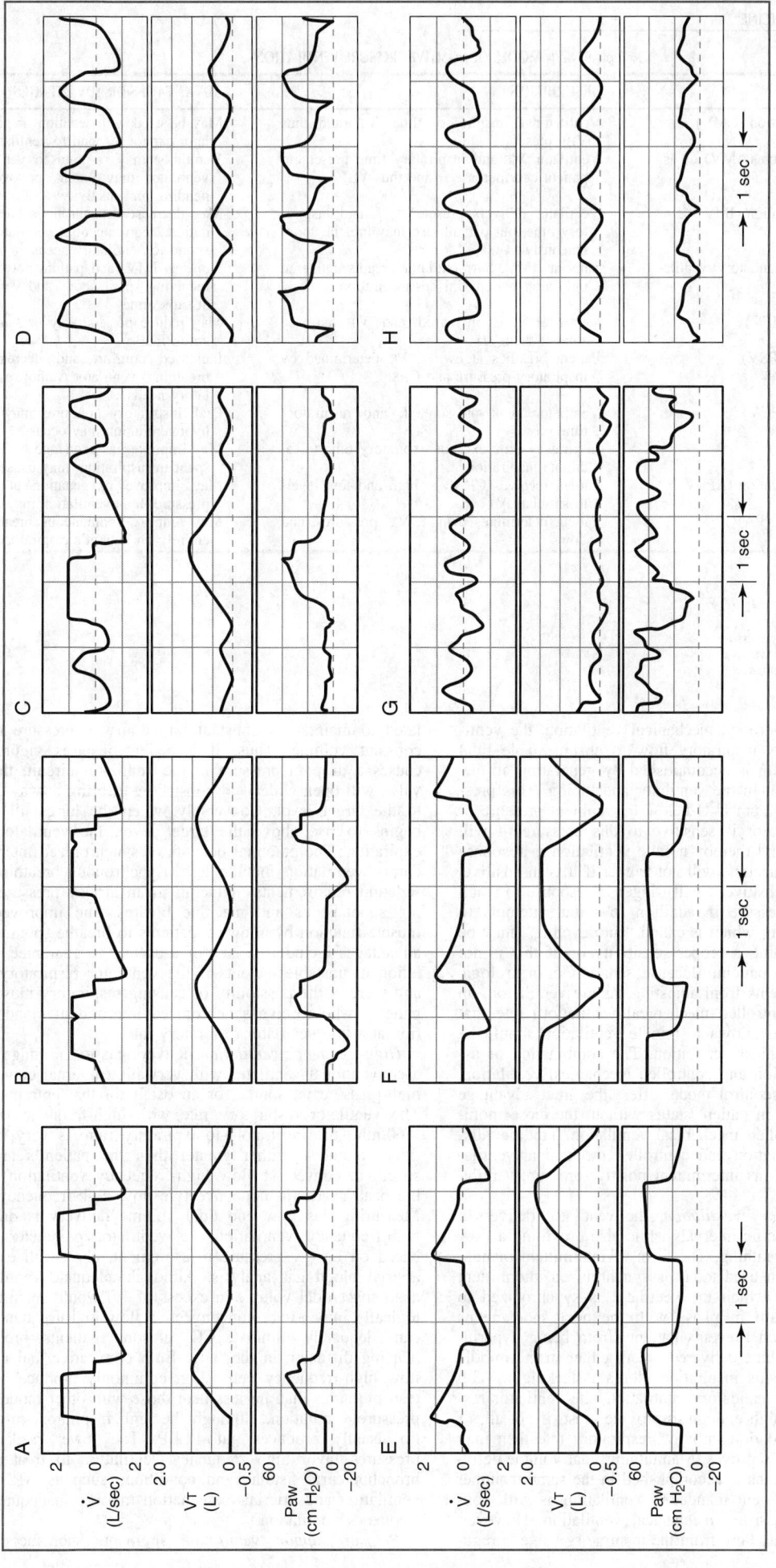

FIGURE 93–1 ■ Tracings drawn from a lung model illustrating gas flow ($\dot{V}$ in L/sec), tidal volume (V_T in L), and airway pressure (Paw in cm H_2O) during (A) controlled mechanical ventilation (CMV), (B) assisted volume-limited mechanical ventilation (AMV), (C) synchronized intermittent mandatory ventilation (SIMV), (D) pressure support ventilation (PSV), (E) pressure control ventilation (PCV), (F) pressure control ventilation with inverse ratio ventilation (PCV-IRV), (G) airway pressure release ventilation (APRV), and (H) continuous positive airway pressure (CPAP). Positive end-expiratory pressure (PEEP) is applied during all modes so that Paw does not return to 0 at end-expiration.

Table 93–2 ■ MODES OF POSITIVE PRESSURE VENTILATION

MODE	DESCRIPTION	ADVANTAGES/DISADVANTAGES
Controlled mechanical ventilation (CMV)	Ventilator f, inspiratory time, V_T (and thus $\dot{V}_E$), preset	May be used with sedation or paralysis; ventilator cannot respond to ventilatory needs
Assisted mechanical ventilation (AMV) or assist/control	Ventilator V_T and inspiratory time preset but patient can increase f (and thus $\dot{V}_E$)	Ventilator may respond to ventilatory needs; ventilator may under- or over-trigger, depending on sensitivity
Intermittent mandatory ventilation (IMV)	Ventilator delivers preset V_T, f, and inspiratory time, but patient also may breathe spontaneously	May decrease asynchronous breathing and sedation requirements; ventilator cannot respond to ventilatory needs
Synchronized intermittent mandatory ventilation (SIMV)	Same as IMV, but ventilator breaths delivered only after patient finishes inspiration	Same as IMV, and patient not overinflated by receiving spontaneous and ventilator breaths at same time
High-frequency ventilation (HFV)	Ventilator f is increased and V_T may be smaller than V_D	May reduce peak airway pressure; may cause auto-PEEP
Pressure-support ventilation (PSV)	Patient breathes at own f; V_T determined by inspiratory pressure and C_{RS}	Increased comfort and decreased work of breathing; ventilator cannot respond to ventilatory needs
Pressure-control ventilation (PCV)	Ventilator peak pressure, f, and respiratory time preset	Peak inspiratory pressures may be decreased; hypoventilation may occur
Inverse ratio ventilation (IRV)	Inspiratory time exceeds expiratory time to facilitate inspiration	May improve gas exchange by increasing time spent in inspiration; may cause auto-PEEP
Airway pressure release ventilation (APRV)	Patient receives CPAP at high and low levels to simulate V_T	May improve oxygenation at lower airway pressure; hypoventilation may occur.
Proportional assist ventilation (PAV)	Patient determines own, f, V_T, pressures, and flows	May amplify spontaneous breathing; depends entirely on patient's respiratory drive.

f = respiratory rate
V_T = tidal volume
$\dot{V}_D$ = dead space
$\dot{V}_E$ = minute ventilation
PEEP = positive end-expiratory pressure
CPAP = continuous positive airway pressure
C_{RS} = respiratory system compliance

tidal volume. As with controlled mechanical ventilation, the ventilator monitors and adjusts inspiratory flow to ensure stable tidal volume delivery. Triggering is accomplished by generating an airway pressure less than that in the ventilator and tubing. This pressure is usually set at 1 to 2 cm H_2O below the ambient pressure or PEEP level. If the ventilator is sensitive to this pressure, it will increase respiratory rate and thereby minute ventilation in response to patient demands. The machine will not trigger if it is insensitive, however, and if unduly sensitive it will trigger in response to small fluctuations in airway pressure in addition to actual attempts to breathe. The latter problem, which is called "auto cycling," may be circumvented by establishing a proper sensitivity or, if this is not possible, by sedating the patient. Because sedation or neurologic changes may prevent patients from adjusting minute ventilation, an obligatory backup (or controlled mechanical ventilation) rate that will provide the minimum allowable minute ventilation should be used with assisted mechanical ventilation. The combination of assisted mechanical ventilation and controlled mechanical ventilation, which is called the assist/control mode, offers the great advantage of responding to changes in patient status without the close monitoring needed with controlled mechanical ventilation. Traditionally, assisted mechanical ventilation and controlled mechanical ventilation have been referred to as intermittent positive-pressure ventilation.

In *intermittent mandatory ventilation,* the ventilator delivers a preset tidal volume at specific intervals while also providing a flow of gas for spontaneous breathing. The form of intermittent mandatory ventilation most often used today is synchronized intermittent mandatory ventilation, in which the ventilator is synchronized to deliver a mandatory breath in phase with the next spontaneous effort. This synchronization prevents patients from being hyperinflated by receiving a machine-delivered breath either in the middle or the end of a spontaneous inspiration ("breath stacking"). With synchronized intermittent mandatory ventilation, the ventilator respiratory rate may be set high enough to provide most, if not all, of the patient's minute ventilation initially; respiratory rate then may be lowered as the patient improves. Maintaining tidal volume delivery during mandatory breaths is accomplished in the same mannner with synchronized intermittent mandatory ventilation as with controlled mechanical and assisted mechanical ventilation. However, during spontaneous breaths, flow from the inspiratory valve is regulated to maintain a constant target airway pressure rather than a constant volume. Thus, if a patient inspires vigorously, which causes a drop in pressure in the ventilator circuit, the inspiratory valve will open wider and boost flow to bring airway pressure back to the target level. Conversely, when the lungs fill and pressure begins to rise above the target level, the ventilator cycles into expiration. The potential benefits of synchronized intermittent mandatory ventilation include less asynchronous breathing and lower sedation requirements, reducing mean airway pressure by combining spontaneous and machine breaths, and improved respiratory muscle function by allowing patients to breathe spontaneously. Disadvantages include the lack of a backup to guarantee minute ventilation in unstable patients if the ventilator respiratory rate is low, and there is the possibility of causing respiratory muscle fatigue in patients who receive synchronized intermittent mandatory ventilation at a low ventilator respiratory rate.

High-frequency ventilation delivers gas to the lungs by means of a conventional ventilator with very high internal compressibility, a high-pressure jet source, or an oscillator that entrains ambient air. The ventilator respiratory rate with high-frequency ventilation is >60/min, the inspiratory-to-expiratory ratio is very high, and the tidal volume is either greater than the patient's anatomic dead space (in convective flow high-frequency ventilation) or less than the dead space (in nonconvective flow high-frequency ventilation). Measuring gas flow and tidal volume delivery is difficult during high-frequency ventilation, so ventilator parameters are usually based on airway pressure measurement, chest-wall expansion, and arterial blood gas analysis. Although adequate ventilation with a dead space/tidal volume in excess of 1.0 would seem to be physiologically impossible, nonconvective flow high-frequency ventilation can adequately eliminate CO_2 in some patients, probably by enhancing diffusion in the lung. Both convective and nonconvective flow high-frequency ventilation commonly produce peak and plateau pressures that are less than those with other modes of positive-pressure ventilation, although the high inspiratory-to-expiratory ratio usually produces auto-PEEP. The lower peak and plateau pressures favor high frequency ventilation to treat patients with bronchopleural fistulae and conditions such as ARDS. However, ventilation and arterial oxygenation may be inadequate with high-frequency ventilation.

Pressure-support ventilation augments spontaneous ventilatory efforts with a level of positive airway pressure that is preset to achieve a desired tidal volume. With pressure-support ventilation, the ventilator senses when the patient initiates a breath, and inspiratory flow is regulated to maintain a constant airway pressure. As impedance increases during a breath, the resulting increases in airway pressure are sensed, and the inspiratory valve narrows to decrease flow and thereby achieve the desired pressure. The ventilator then terminates the flow and pressure when it detects a fall in the inspiratory flow rate to approximately 25% of the peak flow achieved during that breath. The initial pressure-support ventilation level is set to the plateau pressure level needed to achieve the tidal volume used during assisted mechanical ventilation or synchronized intermittent mandatory ventilation, or the pressure-support ventilation level is arbitrarily set around 25 cm H_2O. Pressure-support ventilation allows patients to set their own respiratory rate, timing of breaths, and peak flow, which may be more comfortable than other modes of positive-pressure ventilation. Pressure-support ventilation is also useful in overcoming the work of breathing through an endotracheal tube. Inasmuch as patients must initiate breaths with pressure-support ventilation, it should not be used in unstable patients and is most applicable during discontinuation of mechanical ventilation.

With *pressure-control ventilation,* gas is not delivered at a constant tidal volume. Instead, inspiratory flow is regulated to maintain a constant peak pressure during inspiration, and the patient's minute ventilation is determined by the preset peak pressure, ventilator rate, and inspiratory time. Monitoring and control of ventilator function is the same with pressure-control ventilation as with pressure-support ventilation, except that pressure-control ventilation is time-cycled rather than flow-cycled to expiration. As with pressure-support ventilation, peak pressure is usually set at the plateau pressure needed to achieve the tidal volume used during assisted mechanical ventilation or synchronized intermittent mandatory ventilation, or it can be set to the level considered safe in patients with ARDS (less than 35 cm H_2O). Advocates of pressure-control ventilation believe that barotrauma is reduced because peak pressure and plateau pressure are reduced. Nevertheless, the theoretical benefits of pressure-control ventilation in reducing barotrauma have not been documented conclusively. In addition, pressure-control ventilation may not provide a minute ventilation that is sufficient to prevent hypoventilation, assuming that hypoventilation is not desired.

In *inverse ratio ventilation,* the inspiratory-to-expiratory ratio is increased above the normal level of 1:3 or less to 1:1 or more. The rationale for this approach is that the longer duration of inspiratory positive-pressure will open stiff or fluid-filled alveoli, and the shorter expiratory time will not allow these alveoli to collapse. Peak pressure also may be lower than with other modes of positive-pressure ventilation, although the increase in inspiratory-to-expiratory time probably increases auto-PEEP. It has been argued that inverse ratio ventilation improves oxygenation primarily by such an increase in auto-PEEP. Inverse ratio ventilation is usually used in conjunction with pressure-control ventilation to allow a limited peak pressure. One drawback to inverse ratio ventilation is that it is often uncomfortable and usually requires sedation or paralysis of the patient. The discomfort stems in part from the long inspiratory time with inverse ratio ventilation; if patients try to exhale during this period, they will perform Valsalva's maneuver because the expiratory valve on the ventilator will remain closed.

With *airway pressure release ventilation,* a high level of continuous positive airway pressure (12 to 20 cm H_2O) is maintained for 2 to 4 seconds. The pressure is then released to a lower level of continuous positive airway pressure (2 to 5 cm H_2O) for 0.5 to 1.5 seconds. With the release of pressure, lung volume decreases, and CO_2 is excreted. The number of cycles/min to the lower pressure levels is titrated to the desired $PaCO_2$ and generally does not exceed 20 cycles/min. As the patient's spontaneous breathing ability improves, the number of cycles is decreased, and as the patient's oxygenation improves, the high level of continuous positive airway pressure is decreased. As with pressure-support ventilation and pressure-control ventilation, inspiratory flow is regulated with airway pressure release ventilation to maintain a constant airway pressure. In addition, the ventilator may contain an "open circuit" whereby both the inspiratory and expiratory valves are potentially open during all phases of a breath. As a result of this feature, pressure overshoot during inspiration is attenuated because excess flow is vented through the expiratory valve. Airway pressure re-

lease ventilation has the potential advantage of maintaining oxygenation at lower airway pressures, but it has not been fully investigated in large clinical trials.

Proportional assist ventilation is a new mode in which the positive pressure delivered to the airways increases in direct proportion to the patient's instantaneous effort. Respiratory system resistance and elastance are calculated from a passive ventilator breath, and the ventilator tidal volume and flow are set to achieve 80% of these values. Proportional assist ventilation is described by its proponents as providing greater patient comfort, lower airway pressure, less need for sedation and paralysis, and less likelihood for overventilation. However, these attributes have not been widely demonstrated, and rapid changes in resistance and elastance may cause ventilator "runaway" with large tidal volumes. In addition, initiation of gas flow during proportional assist ventilation is entirely dependent on a patient's drive to breathe.

COMPLICATIONS OF POSITIVE-PRESSURE VENTILATION. One possible result of positive-pressure ventilation is that inflating lungs at high pressure may damage them. Such damage has been described traditionally as barotrauma, implying that it is the consequence of pressure changes. However, because alveolar distention occurs as a result of changes in pressure and because such distention is probably responsible for lung damage, "volutrauma" may be a more accurate term. Pneumothorax is a common kind of barotrauma, but subcutaneous and mediastinal emphysema, parenchymal lung cysts, and systemic air embolism may also occur. Recent studies suggest that positive-pressure ventilation at high pressures and volumes also cause bronchopulmonary dysplasia and diffuse alveolar damage that is identical to ARDS; this damage is now referred to as ventilator-induced lung injury.

In addition to these respiratory effects, positive-pressure ventilation may also compromise the cardiovascular system, because the positive airway pressure during inspiration reduces venous return to the chest and may depress cardiac output. This effect may be increased if PEEP is intentionally added to positive-pressure ventilation, or if auto-PEEP is unintentionally produced. Conversely, this effect may be decreased if adequate time is allowed for airway and alveolar pressure to return to or close to ambient levels during exhalation.

DISCONTINUING POSITIVE-PRESSURE VENTILATION. Mechanical ventilatory support can generally be discontinued when there is complete or near-complete resolution of the patient's disease process, whether or not it involves the lungs. Such resolution should be reflected in clinical stability and a return of $PaCO_2$ to less than 50 mm Hg, a respiratory rate to less than 35 breaths/min, tidal volume to greater than 5 mL/kg, respiratory rate/tidal volume to less than 105 (breaths/min/L), peak pressure to more negative than -20 cm H_2O, dead space/tidal volume to below 0.6, PaO_2 to greater than 60 mm Hg on an FIO_2 of 0.4, and alveolar-arterial gradient of oxygen to less than 300 mm Hg on an FIO_2 of 1.0.

Discontinuing assisted mechanical ventilation and other modes of positive-pressure ventilation may be accomplished by connecting the endotracheal tube to a piece of tubing, called a T-piece, which is connected to a source of O_2 that is diluted with air to create the desired FIO_2. The patients then may breathe spontaneously through the T-piece at their own respiratory rate and tidal volume until they meet some or all of the weaning criteria just described. Otherwise healthy persons recovering from anesthesia or drug overdoses may be put on a T-piece when they wake up and may be extubated after a brief (15 to 30 minutes) period. Chronically ventilated patients may be put on a T-piece for a few minutes each hour or a few hours each day; 2-hour trials have been used in most clinical studies. When their respiratory muscles are less fatigued and patients can tolerate longer periods on a T-piece, discontinuation of the ventilator may be appropriate.

To discontinue synchronized intermittent mandatory ventilation, it is recommended that the ventilator respiratory rate be reduced until the patient can maintain an adequate minute ventilation by breathing spontaneously; reduction rates of 2 to 4 breaths/min, 2 or more times daily, have been used in clinical studies. Synchronized intermittent mandatory ventilation can usually be discontinued if patients tolerate a ventilator rate of less than 4 per minute for 2 hours. In discontinuing pressure-support ventilation, the pressure-support ventilation level may be reduced in increments of

2 to 5 cm H_2O every 2 to 4 hours or so until patients tolerate a level of 5 cm H_2O for 2 hours.

Large studies to date have shown that mechanical ventilation can be discontinued more rapidly in patients using T-piece trials and pressure-support ventilation than with synchronized intermittent mandatory ventilation. These studies differed somewhat in how the three techniques were used, and most clinicians would agree that all three can be effective if they are used aggressively. One approach would be to subject stable patients to daily testing to determine whether the indications for mechanical ventilation are no longer present. Patients who perform satisfactorily on these tests should then undergo 2-hour trials on either a T-piece with or without 5 cm H_2O of continuous positive airway pressure or 5 cm H_2O of pressure-support ventilation. In a recent investigation, when patients passed such trials, and their physicians were aware of these results, there was a striking reduction in positive-pressure ventilation and its complications.

Extracorporeal Ventilation

Mechanical ventilation can also be extracorporeal, in that gas exchange takes place entirely, or in part, outside the body. With extracorporeal membrane oxygenation (ECMO), venous blood is circulated through a CO_2 scrubber and membrane oxygenator and returned to the body as arterial blood with the desired $PaCO_2$ and PaO_2. Low-frequency positive-pressure ventilation with extracorporeal CO_2 removal also uses an extracorporeal circuit to remove CO_2 from venous blood, but oxygenation is achieved by insufflating O_2 into the lungs at high flow rates while the lungs are inflated with positive-pressure ventilation at a low rate and held open with small amounts of PEEP to recruit alveoli. Both ECMO and extracorporeal CO_2 removal are used only occasionally, primarily in neonates and occasionally in patients with severe ARDS. In a randomized trial of patients with ARDS, extracorporeal CO_2 removal did not prove to be superior to more conventional forms of positive-pressure ventilation.

POSITIVE END-EXPIRATORY PRESSURE

Indications for Positive End-Expiratory Pressure

PEEP improves arterial oxygenation by recruiting alveoli for gas exchange. It should be noted that PEEP does not improve ventilation; in fact, the $PaCO_2$ may increase because PEEP increases dead space/tidal volume by distending the airways and alveoli in normal lung units. PEEP also does not reduce extravascular lung water. Rather, PEEP either opens alveoli that would otherwise remain collapsed at end-expiration or acts as a counterforce mechanism that prevents or reverses compression atelectasis caused by extravascular fluid in the lungs.

One indication for PEEP is to prevent or reverse atelectasis (Table 93–3). For example, low levels such as 5 cm H_2O of PEEP commonly are given to intubated patients who are supine in bed. Some investigators believe that low levels of PEEP facilitate weaning from mechanical ventilation by maintaining higher lung volumes while patients breathe through an endotracheal tube; these investigators therefore continue PEEP during T-piece trials and when patients are receiving synchronized intermittent mandatory ventilation at a low ventilator respiratory rate or pressure-support ventilation.

Another major indication for PEEP is to improve arterial oxygenation in patients with diffuse parenchymal lung disorders such as ARDS. Because their hypoxemia is primarily due to intrapulmonary shunt, such patients often cannot be oxygenated adequately even at an FIO_2 of 1.0. Administered in levels in excess of 5 cm H_2O, PEEP usually improves the PaO_2 of these patients. It also allows the FIO_2 to be reduced to levels of 0.6 or less, thereby minimizing the risk of O_2 toxicity.

Finally, PEEP (usually in levels of less than 10 cm H_2O) may be used to decrease the work of breathing related to triggering the ventilator in patients on assisted mechanical ventilation, synchronized intermittent mandatory ventilation, or pressure-support ventilation who have significant amounts of auto-PEEP. In this setting, the patients have to reduce airway pressure from a positive pressure to below 0 to trigger the ventilator. However, if PEEP is added intentionally, only a small downward reduction in pressure from the auto-PEEP level is necessary to provide inspiratory flow.

Modes of Positive End-Expiratory Pressure

PEEP may be administered to spontaneously breathing patients through either a tight-fitting face mask or an endotracheal tube, in which case it is called continuous positive airway pressure (CPAP). PEEP may also be combined with intermittent positive mechanical ventilation to create what is called continuous positive-pressure ventilation (CPPV). The improvement in oxygenation that may be produced by these two modes of PEEP depends on the increase in mean airway pressure. The increase in mean airway pressure is generally greater with CPPV than with CPAP; hence, patients who have merely atelectasis often may be managed solely with CPAP. However, because they also have pulmonary edema and because their ventilatory needs are greater, patients with diffuse parenchymal lung disease generally receive CPPV or bilevel CPAP in the form of airway pressure release ventilation.

Complications of Positive End-Expiratory Pressure

As with its benefits, the complications of PEEP are related to lung volume and airway pressure. Delivering gas at high pressure to achieve an increase in lung volume throughout the ventilatory cycle is more likely to cause barotrauma or "volutrauma" than is delivering pressurized gas solely during inspiration. It also is more likely to decrease venous return to the chest and thereby depress blood pressure and cardiac output. Although the incidence of complications due to PEEP has not been well studied, these complications appear to be significant if levels higher than 12 cm H_2O are used.

Discontinuing Positive End-Expiratory Pressure

Patients who receive low levels of PEEP for atelectasis can usually be discontinued from PEEP without difficulty. However, premature withdrawal or reduction of PEEP from patients with diffuse parenchymal lung disorders can worsen oxygenation and cause clinical deterioration that requires hours or days of therapy to reverse. For this reason, PEEP should be withdrawn slowly, in small (2 to 5 cm H_2O) increments, with close monitoring of PaO_2 or systemic arterial saturation (SaO_2) in such patients. Prematurely reduced PEEP can be avoided if the disease process for which PEEP was initiated has resolved or is substantially improved, if the PaO_2 is ≥ 80 mm Hg on an $FIO_2 \leq 0.4$, and if these conditions have been present for several hours.

ENDOTRACHEAL INTUBATION

Indications for Intubation

Humidified O_2 at an FIO_2 higher than 0.40 is most reliably delivered through the closed system provided by an endotracheal tube. Although intubation (Table 93–4) often precedes mechanical ventilation, it should be stressed that the indications for these two therapies and their timing are not necessarily the same. For example, some patients who are intubated to prevent aspiration of gastric contents never require mechanical ventilation.

Table 93–3 ■ INDICATIONS FOR POSITIVE END-EXPIRATORY PRESSURE (PEEP)

To prevent or reverse atelectasis
To facilitate weaning from mechanical ventilation
To improve arterial oxygenation at a low inspired oxygen fraction
To reduce trigger-related work of breathing in patients with auto-PEEP

Table 93–4 ■ INDICATIONS FOR ENDOTRACHEAL INTUBATION

To provide a closed system for mechanical ventilation or oxygen delivery, especially at a high fraction of inspired oxygen
To prevent or reverse upper airway obstruction
To protect against aspiration of gastric contents
To facilitate tracheobronchial toilet

Kinds of Intubation

Endotracheal intubation may be performed either via the translaryngeal route through the nose or mouth or via a tracheotomy. Tracheotomy tubes once were used routinely in patients requiring intubation for longer than 1 or 2 days. However, the development of low-pressure and high-compliance cuffs that limit tracheal damage from nasal or oral tubes demonstrates that such tubes can be left in place for weeks and even months without severe sequelae, and documentation of complications after tracheotomy has led to a preference for nasotracheal or orotracheal intubation over tracheotomy in all but a few patients. Such patients include those with laryngeal fractures and those who will require intubation for longer than 3 weeks. Tracheotomy tubes generally are more comfortable than translaryngeal tubes; they also are easier to suction through, and talking may be made possible by fitting the tubes with a device that directs a stream of air retrograde through the larynx above the cuff site.

Nasal intubation provides good support for the endotracheal tube and often allows patients to swallow their secretions better than when the tube passes orally. Oral intubation may allow passage of a tube with a larger diameter (8 mm or more) than the nostril will accommodate and is usually the preferred route during emergency intubations. Whichever route is chosen, the tube diameter should be sufficient to seal the trachea without cuff pressures greater than 25 mm Hg, which exceeds capillary pressures in the trachea. These pressures should be monitored regularly. Tube position should be determined by chest radiograph or bronchoscopy immediately following insertion and on a regular basis thereafter. Intubation of the right mainstem bronchus, which extends from the trachea at less of an angle than the left mainstem bronchus, must be avoided.

Complications of Intubation

Many patients receiving endotracheal intubation suffer adverse consequences. Excessive cuff pressure requirements (>25 mm Hg), self-extubation, and inability to seal the airway are the most common complications with nasotracheal and orotracheal tubes. Problems associated with tracheotomy include stomal hemorrhage, excessive cuff pressure requirements, and subcutaneous emphysema. Follow-up studies of patients receiving intubation and mechanical ventilation reveal a higher incidence of tracheal stenosis after tracheotomy as compared with translaryngeal intubation, although laryngeal complications are more common with nasal and oral tubes.

Discontinuing Intubation

In general, endotracheal tubes may be removed when the original indications for their insertion are no longer present. For example, extubation frequently follows the return of consciousness and an adequate gag reflex in previously comatose patients or restored adequate ventilation and arterial oxygenation in patients with acute respiratory failure. If an endotracheal tube has been in place only briefly, it may be removed after secretions have been suctioned from above the cuff site and the patient has been seated upright. However, patients with previous neck surgery, laryngeal trauma, vocal cord paralysis, or infections of the neck or mouth may be at risk for upper airway obstruction following extubation. Obstruction at the tracheal level is unlikely if less than 10 cm H_2O of positive airway pressure is required to cause a leak of air around the endotracheal tube when the tube cuff is deflated. Obstruction is also unlikely if the patient can breathe around the tube when the cuff is deflated and the proximal end of the tube is blocked. Direct or indirect laryngoscopy may be helpful in evaluating potential obstruction at the pharyngeal level.

Amato MBP, Barbas CSV, Mederios DM, et al: Effect of a protective-ventilation strategy on mortality in the acute respiratory distress syndrome. N Engl J Med 338: 347, 1998. *A strategy incorporating low tidal volume breaths with a level of positive end-expiratory pressure associated with high respiratory system compliance improved outcome.*

Antonelli M, Conti G, Rocco M, et al: A comparison of noninvasive positive-pressure ventilation and conventional mechanical ventilation in patients with acute respiratory failure. N Engl J Med 339:429, 1998. *Noninvasive ventilation, which has been shown to be effective in patients with acute respiratory failure due to airflow obstruction, also is effective in some patients with parenchymal lung disease.*

Tobin MJ: Mechanical ventilation. N Engl J Med 330:1056, 1994. *Reviews the indications for kinds of complications from and discontinuation of mechanical ventilatory support.*

Yang KL, Tobin MJ: A prospective study of indexes predicting the outcome of trials of weaning from mechanical ventilation. N Engl J Med 324:1445, 1991. *The ratio of respiratory frequency to tidal volume proved to be a helpful indication of the need for mechanical ventilation in this study.*

94 APPROACH TO THE PATIENT WITH SHOCK

Joseph E. Parrillo

Shock is a very serious medical condition that results from a profound and widespread reduction in effective tissue perfusion leading to cellular dysfunction and organ failure. Unless it is promptly corrected, this circulatory insufficiency will become irreversible. The most common clinical manifestations of shock are hypotension and evidence of inadequate tissue perfusion. A number of diseases can result in shock, and the specific clinical characteristics of these diseases usually accompany the shock syndrome.

To understand the definition of shock, it is important to comprehend the meaning of *effective* tissue perfusion (Table 94–1). Certain forms of shock result from a global reduction in systemic perfusion (low cardiac output), whereas other forms produce shock due to a maldistribution of blood flow or a defect of substrate utilization at the subcellular level. These latter forms of shock have normal or high global flow to tissues, but this perfusion is not effective due to abnormalities at the microvascular or subcellular levels.

CLASSIFICATION

It is valuable to classify different forms of shock according to etiology and cardiovascular physiology (Fig. 94–1 and Table 94–2) because such a classification results in appropriate patient management. *Hypovolemic shock* results from blood and/or fluid loss and is due to a decreased circulating blood volume leading to reduced diastolic filling pressures and volumes. The result is inadequate cardiac output, hypotension, and shock. *Cardiogenic shock* is caused by a severe reduction in cardiac function due to direct myocardial damage or a mechanical abnormality of the heart; the cardiac output and blood pressure are reduced. *Extracardiac obstructive shock* results from obstruction to flow in the cardiovascular circuit, leading to inadequate diastolic filling or decreased systolic function due to increased afterload; this form of shock results in inadequate cardiac output and hypotension. The cardiovascular abnormality of *distributive shock* is more complex than the other shock categories. Distributive shock is characterized by vasodilata-

Table 94–1 ■ DETERMINANTS OF EFFECTIVE TISSUE PERFUSION

Arterial Pressure
Cardiac Performance
Cardiac function
  Preload
  Afterload
  Contractility
  Heart rate
Venous return
Vascular Performance
Distribution of cardiac output
  Extrinsic regulatory systems
    Sympathetic nervous system
    Adrenal hormone release
  Intrinsic regulatory systems
  Anatomic vascular disease
  Exogenous vasoactive agents
Microvascular Function
  Pre- and post-capillary sphincter function
  Capillary endothelial integrity
  Microvascular obstruction
Cellular Function
Oxygen unloading and diffusion
  RBC 2, 3 DPG
  Blood pH
  Temperature
Cellular energy generation/substrate utilization
  Citric acid (Krebs) cycle
  Oxidative phosphorylation
  Other energy metabolism pathways

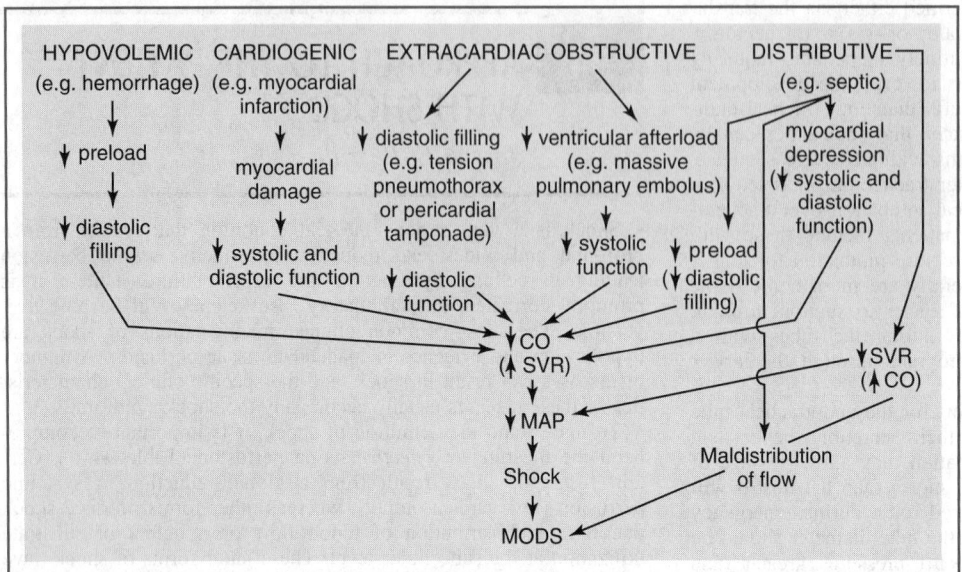

FIGURE 94–1 ■ A classification of shock showing interrelationships among the different forms of shock. CO = cardiac output, SVR = systemic vascular resistance, MAP = mean arterial pressure, MODS = multiple organ dysfunction syndrome.

tion: the venodilatation leads to a decrease in preload, which can be corrected with fluid administration, and the arterial vasodilatation leads to hypotension with a normal or elevated cardiac output. Myocardial depression frequently accompanies distributive shock. The most characteristic pattern is decreased vascular resistance, normal or elevated cardiac output, and hypotension. Distributive shock, which results from mediator effects at the microvascular and cellular levels, may produce inadequate blood pressure and multiple organ system dysfunction without a decrease in cardiac output.

Although many patients develop pure forms of shock as classified above, others may manifest characteristics of several forms of shock, termed *mixed shock*. For example, septic shock is considered to be a distributive form of shock; however, prior to resuscitation with fluids, a substantial hypovolemic component may exist due to venodilatation. Also, septic shock patients have a cardiogenic component due to myocardial depression. Patients with severe hemorrhage, classified as hypovolemic shock, may manifest significant myocardial depression. Thus, although these four catego-

Table 94–2 ■ CLASSIFICATION OF SHOCK

Hypovolemic	**Extracardiac Obstructive**
Hemorrhagic	Impaired diastolic filling (decreased ventricular preload)
Trauma	Direct venous obstruction (vena cava)
Gastrointestinal	Intrathoracic obstructive tumors
Retroperitoneal	Increased intrathoracic pressure
Fluid depletion (nonhemorrhagic)	Tension pneumothorax
External fluid loss	Mechanical ventilation (with excessive pressure or volume depletion)
Dehydration	Asthma
Vomiting	Decreased cardiac compliance
Diarrhea	Constrictive pericarditis
Polyurea	Cardiac tamponade
Interstitial fluid redistribution	Impaired systolic contraction (increased ventricular afterload)
Thermal injury	Right ventricle
Trauma	Pulmonary embolus (massive)
Anaphylaxis	Acute pulmonary hypertension
Increased vascular capacitance (venodilatation)	Left ventricle
Sepsis	Aortic dissection
Anaphylaxis	**Distributive**
Toxins/drug	Septic (bacterial, fungal, viral, rickettsial)
Cardiogenic	Toxic shock syndrome
Myopathic	Anaphylactic, anaphylactoid
Myocardial infarction	Neurogenic (spinal shock)
Left ventricle	Endocrinologic
Right ventricle	Adrenal crisis
Myocardial contusion (trauma)	Thyroid storm
Myocarditis	Toxic (e.g., nitroprusside, bretylium)
Cardiomyopathy	
Postischemic myocardial stunning	
Septic myocardial depression	
Pharmacologic	
Anthracycline cardiotoxicity	
Calcium channel blockers	
Mechanical	
Valvular failure (stenotic or regurgitant)	
Hypertropic cardiomyopathy	
Ventricular septal defect	
Arrhythmic	
Bradycardia	
Tachycardia	

ries are valuable for classifying the hemodynamics of shock, patients may manifest combinations of these categories.

PATHOGENESIS AND PATHOPHYSIOLOGY

Adequate, effective tissue perfusion of organs must be maintained for survival. Perfusion is dependent on a number of variables that are carefully regulated by the body's compensatory mechanisms.

Control of Arterial Pressure

One excellent physiologic and clinical measure of perfusion is arterial pressure, which is determined by cardiac output and vascular resistance and can be defined by the following equation:

$$\text{Mean arterial pressure (MAP)} - \text{Central venous pressure (CVP)}$$
$$= \text{Cardiac output (CO)} \times \text{Systemic vascular resistance (SVR)}$$

Because the mean arterial pressure and cardiac output can be measured directly, these two variables are used to describe tissue perfusion, although systemic vascular resistance can be calculated as a ratio of mean arterial pressure minus central venous pressure divided by cardiac output.

The arterial pressure is regulated by changes in cardiac output and/or systemic vascular resistance. These regulatory mechanisms consist of neural and hormonal reflexes and local factors. Blood flow to the heart and brain is carefully regulated and maintained over a wide range of blood pressure (from a mean arterial pressure of 50 to 150 mm Hg); this autoregulation results from reflexes in the local vasculature and ensures the perfusion of these especially vital organs. Failure to maintain the minimal arterial pressure required for autoregulation during shock indicates a severe abnormality that may produce inadequate coronary perfusion and a further reduction in cardiac function due to myocardial ischemia.

Cardiac Performance

Cardiac output is a product of heart rate and stroke volume. The stroke volume is determined by preload, afterload, and contractility, whereas preload is dependent on adequate venous return (see Chapter 40).

Vascular Performance

Effective perfusion requires appropriate resistance to blood flow to maintain arterial pressure. Resistance to flow of blood in a vessel is proportional to the vessel's length and the viscosity of blood and inversely proportional to the vessel's radius raised to the fourth power. Therefore, the cross-sectional area of a vessel is by far the most important determinant of resistance to flow. In the systemic vasculature, the major (>80%) site of resistance is at the arteriolar sphincter, and regulation of this arteriolar tone constitutes the major determinant of vascular resistance.

Arteriolar smooth muscle tone is regulated by extrinsic and intrinsic factors. The extrinsic factors consist of sympathetic nervous system innervation of arterioles, which are largely regulated by arterial and cardiopulmonary baroreceptors. Circulating epinephrine and norepinephrine are released into the circulation by stimulation of the adrenal medulla. The intrinsic mechanisms include a vascular smooth muscle (myogenic) response in which blood vessels relax or constrict in response to changes in transmural vessel pressure to maintain vessel blood flow at a constant level despite changes in perfusion pressure. Other intrinsic mechanisms are a metabolic response that results from release of vasodilators in response to increased metabolic activity and an oxygen tension response that results in vasodilatation with low oxygen tensions. Vasodilators released locally and systemically include nitric oxide (formerly known as endothelial-derived relaxing factor), prostacyclin, eicosanoids, kinins, and adenosine. Vasoconstrictor molecules include endothelin 1, renin, angiotensin II, thromboxane, vasopressin, and oxygen-free radicals.

In addition to vascular tone, the microvasculature also affects perfusion by obstruction to microvascular flow. In shock, this obstruction can be caused by adhesion of leukocytes or platelets to the endothelium, with sludging and occlusion of microvessels. Activation of the coagulation system with fibrin deposition and mi-

crothrombi may contribute to this process. Shunting around these occluded vessels may occur. Decreased red or white cell deformability may also aggravate this microvascular dysfunction.

Microvascular permeability to fluids or other substances may also be altered by vasoactive mediators, activated leukocytes, and damaged endothelial cells. Because intravascular and extravascular fluid is determined by a balance between hydrostatic pressure and colloid osmotic pressure, damage to the endothelium may cause increased extravasation of fluid into the interstitial space and result in tissue edema. This fluid accumulation may further worsen organ dysfunction.

Cellular Function

At the cellular level, a number of factors regulate the unloading of oxygen and other substrates to cells. Shock produces cellular dysfunction through three major mechanisms: cellular ischemia, inflammatory mediators, and free radical injury. Cellular ischemia is probably the major cause of cell damage in shock with a low cardiac output. In hypovolemic shock, inadequate perfusion and the resultant lack of oxygen lead to increasing dependence on anaerobic glycolysis, which produces only 2 adenosine triphosphate (ATP) molecules during breakdown of 1 glucose molecule as opposed to 36 ATP molecules produced by aerobic metabolism through the citric acid (Krebs) cycle; the result is depletion of ATP and intracellular energy reserves. Intracellular acidosis occurs, and anaerobic glycolysis leads to accumulation of lactate. Lack of adequate energy leads to failure of energy-dependent ion transport pumps and the inability to maintain normal transmembrane gradients of potassium, chloride, and calcium; the result is mitochondrial dysfunction, abnormal carbohydrate metabolism, and failure of many energy-dependent enzyme reactions. Ultrastructural changes in mitochondria ensue, and the cell dies.

One important but controversial hypothesis regarding cellular ischemia in shock is the role of oxygen supply dependency. In normal humans, oxygen delivery to tissues (cardiac output × oxygen content of arterial blood) is maintained at a high level so that tissue oxygen consumption [cardiac output × (oxygen content of arterial blood − oxygen content of mixed venous blood)] is not altered or dependent on changes in oxygen delivery. However, if systemic flow drops below a critical value of oxygen delivery, tissues must switch from aerobic metabolism to the less efficient anaerobic metabolism. This deficiency of energy production may lead to multiple organ system dysfunction and death. Below this critical value (estimated at 8 to 10 mL of oxygen/min/kg in anesthetized humans), oxygen consumption is dependent on oxygen delivery (or supply), a relationship termed *physiologic oxygen supply dependency*. This process is believed to be an important mechanism of cellular damage in forms of shock that are characterized by low oxygen delivery due to inadequate cardiac output, low oxygen saturation, or decreased hemoglobin concentration. The controversy regarding this mechanism stems from the hypothesis that a *pathologic oxygen supply dependency* exists in patients with sepsis, trauma, or adult respiratory distress syndrome (ARDS). These patients have oxygen delivery in the normal or elevated range but manifest lactate production and organ dysfunction. Some animal and human studies suggest the presence of a pathologic oxygen supply dependency because they demonstrate an increase in oxygen consumption with increases in oxygen delivery even at elevated levels of oxygen delivery. This suggests dependency of consumption on delivery over a wide range of delivery values. Proponents argue that inadequate oxygen delivery is occurring in these forms of shock due to microvascular and cellular abnormalities. This hypothesis has led to the argument that the management of sepsis, trauma, and ARDS patients should include methods to maximize cardiac output and oxygen delivery. In general, these studies have been inconclusive, and the hypothesis of pathologic oxygen supply dependency remains controversial.

Inflammatory mediators are a major cause of cell injury in shock due to sepsis and trauma and may play a significant role in other forms of shock. These mediators may exert their influence on the vasculature to produce inadequate perfusion, or they may produce direct injury to cells in a number of organs. The cytokines, especially tumor necrosis factor (TNF) and interleukin-1 (IL-1), can produce dysfunction of transmembrane ion gradients similar to that described with cellular ischemia. Administration of TNF to animals produces a cardiovascular state indistinguishable from septic shock. TNF can also stimulate release of many other mediators, including other cytokines, platelet activating factor, leukotrienes, prostaglandins, and thromboxane.

It should be appreciated that the inflammatory response is a physiologic, homeostatic mechanism designed to respond to injury or infection. Release of inflammatory mediators usually provides beneficial effects such as activating host defense systems and enhancing blood flow to damaged tissues. With a self-limited insult, the inflammatory reaction is carefully controlled by counter-regulatory, anti-inflammatory mechanisms. In shock, the inflammatory response becomes excessive and unregulated, and it contributes to cell injury and tissue damage.

Free radicals are highly reactive oxygen intermediates that can occur after ischemia with subsequent reperfusion. Cellular ischemia and intracellular calcium accumulation can result in formation of xanthine oxidase, which can oxidize purines with the formation of the highly toxic superoxide radical. These oxygen products can inactivate proteins, damage DNA, induce lipid peroxidation of cell membranes, and lead to cell lysis and tissue injury.

Altered gene expression may also play a role in the cellular dysfunction during shock. For example, generation of cytokines, adhesion proteins, and inducible nitric oxide synthase enzymes represents up-regulation of gene expression. The heat shock proteins may be an especially important genetic response in shock. These proteins are involved in the genetic program of cell death known as *apoptosis,* a physiologic mechanism that normally functions to remove senescent cells. During shock, the induction of heat shock proteins may interfere with cell synthetic pathways and may initiate a heightened activation of programmed cell death. Inappropriate initiation of this mechanism may be an important contributor to cell demise in shock.

COMPENSATORY MECHANISMS

With the onset of hemodynamic dysfunction in shock, homeostatic compensatory mechanisms attempt to maintain effective tissue perfusion, and many of the manifestations of shock represent the body's attempt to correct abnormalities. Most compensatory mechanisms are dependent on various sensing mechanisms designed to recognize hemodynamic or metabolic dyshomeostasis (Table 94–3). The sensing mechanisms consist of pressure receptors located in the cardiovascular system (right atrium, pulmonary artery, aortic arch, carotid, and splanchnic baroreceptors) and the kidney (juxtaglomerular apparatus) as well as chemoreceptors sensitive to concentrations of carbon dioxide or oxygen and located in the central nervous system (mostly in the medulla).

The compensatory responses in shock are designed to maintain mean circulatory pressure, maximize cardiac performance, redistribute perfusion to the most vital organs, and optimize the unloading of oxygen to tissues. These effects are produced by stimulation of the sympathetic nervous system, release of hormones (angiotensin II, vasopressin, epinephrine, and norepinephrine), and creation of a local tissue environment that enhances the unloading of oxygen to tissues due to acidosis, pyrexia, and increased red blood cell 2,3-diphosphoglycerate (RBC 2,3 DPG). The magnitude of these compensatory mechanisms is dependent on the severity of hemodynamic or metabolic derangements. Compensation will be effective at restoring tissue perfusion for a period during shock; however, if the initiating process is not reversed during this period, shock will become irreversible due to widespread cellular damage.

MULTIPLE ORGAN DYSFUNCTION SYNDROME

The clinical presentation of shock is quite variable and depends on the initiating cause and the response of multiple organs (Table 94–4). Different organs may be affected minimally, mildly, moderately, or severely. This leads to multiple organ dysfunction syndrome (MODS) (see Fig. 94–1), which is one of the major causes of death in shock.

Table 94–3 ■ CARDIOVASCULAR AND METABOLIC COMPENSATORY RESPONSES TO SHOCK

Maintain mean circulatory pressure (venous pressure)
Volume
  Fluid redistribution to vascular space
    From interstitium (Starling's effect)
    From intracellular space (osmotic)
  Decrease renal losses
    $\downarrow$ Glomerular filtration rate
    $\uparrow$ Aldosterone
    $\uparrow$ Vasopressin
Pressure
  Decrease venous capacitance
    $\uparrow$ Sympathetic activity
    $\uparrow$ Circulating (adrenal) epinephrine
    $\uparrow$ Angiotensin
    $\uparrow$ Vasopressin
Maximize cardiac performance
Increase contractility
  Sympathetic stimulation
  Adrenal stimulation
Redistribute perfusion
Extrinsic regulation of systemic arterial tone
Dominant autoregulation of vital organs (heart, brain)
Optimize oxygen unloading
  $\uparrow$ RBC 2,3 DPG
Tissue acidosis
Pyrexia
  $\downarrow$ Tissue PO_2

$\uparrow$ = Increases
$\downarrow$ = Decreases

Central Nervous System

The most frequent findings are alterations in the level of consciousness ranging from confusion to coma. Autoregulation protects the ischemia-sensitive neurons by maintaining adequate blood flow down to a mean arterial pressure of approximately 50 to 60 mm Hg. Below this level, however, tissue ischemia ensues. Acid-base and electrolyte abnormalities also contribute to neuronal damage. Sepsis-related central nervous system dysfunction may occur at a higher mean arterial pressure due to the effects of inflammatory mediators.

Table 94–4 ■ ORGAN SYSTEM DYSFUNCTION IN SHOCK

ORGAN SYSTEM	MANIFESTATIONS
Central nervous system	Encephalopathy (ischemic or septic)
	Cortical necrosis
Heart	Tachycardia, bradycardia
	Supraventricular tachycardia
	Ventricular ectopy
	Myocardial ischemia
	Myocardial depression
Pulmonary	Acute respiratory failure
	Adult respiratory distress syndrome
Kidney	Prerenal failure
	Acute tubular necrosis
Gastrointestinal	Ileus
	Erosive gastritis
	Pancreatitis
	Acalculous cholecystitis
	Colonic submucosal hemorrhage
	Transluminal translocation of bacteria/endotoxin
Liver	Ischemic hepatitis
	"Shock" liver
	Intrahepatic cholestasis
Hematologic	Disseminated intravascular coagulation
	Dilutional thrombocytopenia
Metabolic	Hyperglycemia
	Glycogenolysis
	Gluconeogenesis
	Hypoglycemia (late)
	Hypertriglyceridemia
Immune system	Gut barrier function depression
	Cellular immune depression
	Humoral immune depression

Heart

Many of the clinically apparent manifestations of cardiac involvement in shock result from sympathoadrenal stimulation, with tachycardia being the most sensitive indicator that shock is present. As in the brain, autoregulation assures good coronary perfusion down to a mean arterial pressure of approximately 50 mm Hg. In low cardiac output forms of shock, myocardial ischemia is prominent and produces a vicious cycle in which ischemia produces further reduction in cardiac output, which further aggravates ischemia. This cycle is believed to be important in producing the high mortality (70 to 90%) rate of cardiogenic shock (see Chapter 95).

Shock produces complex effects on myocardial contractility. Although sympathoadrenal stimulation should lead to increases in contractility due to adrenoreceptor stimulation, there is strong evidence for myocardial depression (decreased ejection fraction) and compliance abnormalities, especially in septic and hypovolemic shock. Septic myocardial dysfunction has been linked to cytokine-induced (specifically, TNF and IL-1) depression of myocardial contraction; this cytokine mechanism produces much of its effect via nitric oxide and cyclic guanosine monophosphate. In addition, there is evidence decreased of β-receptor function. Similar depressant mechanisms may also contribute to myocardial dysfunction in hypovolemic and cardiogenic shock.

Lungs

Acute lung injury causes impaired gas exchange, decreased compliance, and shunting of blood through underventilated areas. The pathologic findings are fibrin-neutrophil aggregates within the pulmonary microvasculature, inflammatory damage to the interstitium and alveoli, and exudation of proteinaceous fluid into the alveolar space; the result is severe hypoxemia with bilateral pulmonary infiltrates, a condition termed adult respiratory distress syndrome (see Chapter 88). The work of breathing is increased, and respiratory muscle fatigue and ventilatory failure ensue, often requiring mechanical ventilation.

Kidney

Acute renal failure is a major complication of shock and is associated with a high mortality rate. Hypoperfusion of the renal vasculature occurs frequently in shock, in part due to preferential direction of blood flow to the brain and heart. Initially, vasoconstriction may maintain glomerular perfusion, but when this compensatory mechanism fails, acute tubular necrosis and renal insufficiency occur. An important clinical challenge is to differentiate between acute tubular necrosis and hypovolemia, because both present with oliguria (see below).

Gastrointestinal Tract and Liver

Typical clinical manifestations of gut involvement during shock include ileus, erosive gastritis, pancreatitis, acalculous cholecystitis, and submucosal hemorrhage. Some studies suggest that gut barrier integrity may be compromised, leading to translocation of bacteria and their toxins into the blood stream.

The most common manifestation of liver involvement in shock is mild increase in transaminases and lactate dehydrogenase. With severe hypoperfusion, shock liver may be manifested by massive transaminase elevations and extensive hepatocellular damage. With an acute insult that resolves, these transaminase elevations will peak in 1 to 3 days and resolve by 10 days. Decreased levels of clotting factors and albumin may occur and reflect decreased synthetic function. In septic shock, significant elevations of bilirubin may be seen with only modest transaminase increases because of dysfunction of bile canaliculi due to inflammatory mediators or bacterial toxins.

Hematologic

Thrombocytopenia can occur due to dilution during volume repletion or may result from immunologic platelet destruction, which is especially common during septic shock. Activation of the coagulation cascade can lead to disseminated intravascular coagulation, which results in thrombocytopenia, decreased fibrinogen, elevated fibrin split products, and microangiopathic hemolytic anemia.

Immune System

Widespread dysfunction of the immune system has been described especially during hypovolemic and traumatic shock. Abnormalities of function in macrophages, T and B lymphocytes, and neutrophils have been described. These abnormalities are not thought to produce immediate effects but may contribute significantly to late mortality, which is frequently due to complicating infection.

Metabolic

Early in shock, hyperglycemia usually occurs due to glycogenolysis and gluconeogenesis mediated by increases in adrenocorticotropic hormone, glucocorticoids, glucagon, and catecholamines as well as decreases in insulin. Hypertriglyceridemia may also occur. Later in shock, hypoglycemia may occur due to glycogen depletion or failure of glucose synthesis in the liver. Also, protein catabolism ensues, resulting in negative nitrogen balance; this catabolism may be an important determinant of late mortality in shock, and some studies suggest nutritional supplementation is important in shock therapy.

SPECIFIC FORMS OF SHOCK

Inadequate tissue perfusion results from a low cardiac output in hypovolemic, cardiogenic, and extracardiac obstructive forms of shock. In distributive shock, although a low cardiac output may occur infrequently due to inadequate preload or myocardial depression, most commonly a low systemic vascular resistance and maldistribution of blood flow lead to low blood pressure and shock despite normal or increased cardiac output.

Hypovolemic Shock

This form of shock is characterized by fall in ventricular preload, resulting in decreased ventricular diastolic pressures and volumes, decreased stroke volume and cardiac output, and reduced blood pressure. Patients manifest pale, cool, clammy skin; tachycardia; decreased jugular venous pulse; decreased urine output; and altered mental status. The severity of hypovolemic shock is clearly associated with both the magnitude and the rate of fluid loss. Acute loss of 10% of circulating blood volume results in tachycardia and increased systemic vascular resistance with maintenance of blood pressure. Compensatory mechanisms begin to fail with a 20 to 25% volume loss: mild to moderate hypotension and decreased cardiac output occur, systemic vascular resistance is markedly increased, and lactate production may begin. With loss of 40% of circulating blood volume, severe hypotension develops with signs of shock; cardiac output and tissue perfusion are severely decreased. If this shock state persists for more than 2 hours, sufficient tissue damage will have occurred so that adequate fluid repletion will no longer be effective in reversing shock; that is, the shock will be irreversible.

If the volume loss is produced at a slower rate, the compensatory mechanisms are more effective, and similar amounts of volume depletion are better tolerated. Furthermore, a patient's underlying disease, especially a limited cardiac reserve, also influences the response to a hypovolemic insult.

Cardiogenic Shock

Cardiogenic shock results from failure of the heart as a pump, due to myocardial, valvular, or structural abnormalities. Hemodynamically, ventricular filling pressures and volumes are increased; cardiac output, stroke volume, and mean arterial pressure are reduced. Patients manifest signs of peripheral hypoperfusion coupled with evidence of ventricular failure (see Chapters 47 and 95).

Extracardiac Obstructive Shock

This form of shock results from an obstruction to flow in the cardiovascular circuit. Pericardial tamponade and constrictive pericarditis impair diastolic filling of the right ventricle. Massive pulmonary emboli may result in shock due to a severe increase in afterload. The hemodynamic pattern is similar to other low output

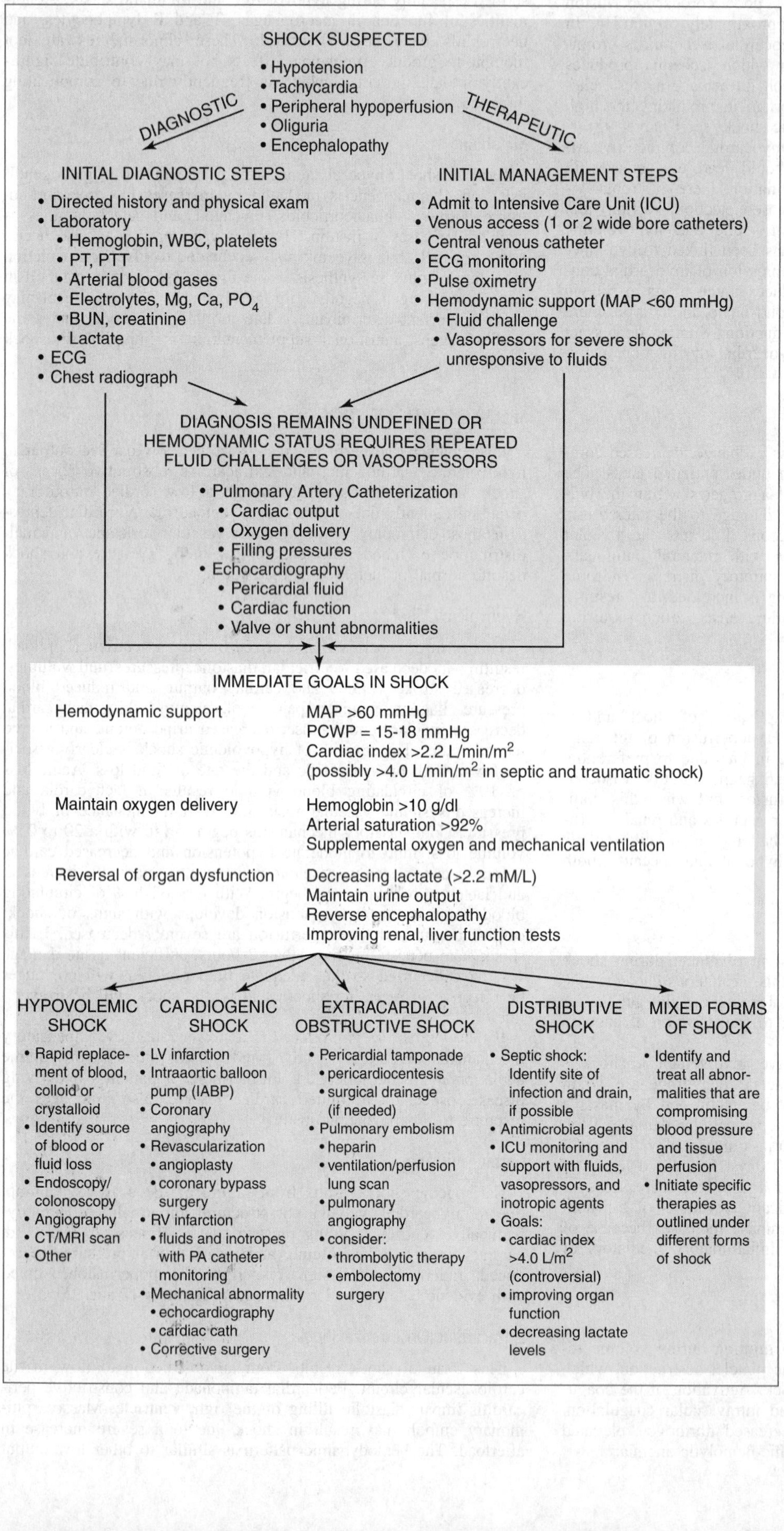

SHOCK SUSPECTED
- Hypotension
- Tachycardia
- Peripheral hypoperfusion
- Oliguria
- Encephalopathy

DIAGNOSTIC   *THERAPEUTIC*

INITIAL DIAGNOSTIC STEPS
- Directed history and physical exam
- Laboratory
  - Hemoglobin, WBC, platelets
  - PT, PTT
  - Arterial blood gases
  - Electrolytes, Mg, Ca, PO_4
  - BUN, creatinine
  - Lactate
- ECG
- Chest radiograph

INITIAL MANAGEMENT STEPS
- Admit to Intensive Care Unit (ICU)
- Venous access (1 or 2 wide bore catheters)
- Central venous catheter
- ECG monitoring
- Pulse oximetry
- Hemodynamic support (MAP <60 mmHg)
  - Fluid challenge
  - Vasopressors for severe shock unresponsive to fluids

DIAGNOSIS REMAINS UNDEFINED OR HEMODYNAMIC STATUS REQUIRES REPEATED FLUID CHALLENGES OR VASOPRESSORS
- Pulmonary Artery Catheterization
  - Cardiac output
  - Oxygen delivery
  - Filling pressures
- Echocardiography
  - Pericardial fluid
  - Cardiac function
  - Valve or shunt abnormalities

IMMEDIATE GOALS IN SHOCK

Hemodynamic support	MAP >60 mmHg PCWP = 15-18 mmHg Cardiac index >2.2 L/min/m^2 (possibly >4.0 L/min/m^2 in septic and traumatic shock)
Maintain oxygen delivery	Hemoglobin >10 g/dl Arterial saturation >92% Supplemental oxygen and mechanical ventilation
Reversal of organ dysfunction	Decreasing lactate (>2.2 mM/L) Maintain urine output Reverse encephalopathy Improving renal, liver function tests

HYPOVOLEMIC SHOCK
- Rapid replacement of blood, colloid or crystalloid
- Identify source of blood or fluid loss
- Endoscopy/colonoscopy
- Angiography
- CT/MRI scan
- Other

CARDIOGENIC SHOCK
- LV infarction
- Intraaortic balloon pump (IABP)
- Coronary angiography
- Revascularization
  - angioplasty
  - coronary bypass surgery
- RV infarction
  - fluids and inotropes with PA catheter monitoring
- Mechanical abnormality
  - echocardiography
  - cardiac cath
- Corrective surgery

EXTRACARDIAC OBSTRUCTIVE SHOCK
- Pericardial tamponade
  - pericardiocentesis
  - surgical drainage (if needed)
- Pulmonary embolism
  - heparin
  - ventilation/perfusion lung scan
  - pulmonary angiography
  - consider:
    - thrombolytic therapy
    - embolectomy surgery

DISTRIBUTIVE SHOCK
- Septic shock: Identify site of infection and drain, if possible
- Antimicrobial agents
- ICU monitoring and support with fluids, vasopressors, and inotropic agents
- Goals:
  - cardiac index >4.0 L/m^2 (controversial)
  - improving organ function
  - decreasing lactate levels

MIXED FORMS OF SHOCK
- Identify and treat all abnormalities that are compromising blood pressure and tissue perfusion
- Initiate specific therapies as outlined under different forms of shock

FIGURE 94–2 ■ An approach to the diagnosis and treatment of shock. MAP = mean arterial pressure, PCWP = pulmonary capillary wedge pressure.

Table 94–5 ■ DIAGNOSIS OF SHOCK ETIOLOGY USING PULMONARY ARTERY CATHETERIZATION

DIAGNOSIS	PULMONARY CAPILLARY WEDGE PRESSURE	CARDIAC OUTPUT (CO)	MISCELLANEOUS COMMENTS
Cardiogenic shock			
Cardiogenic shock due to myocardial dysfunction	↑↑	↓↓	Usually occurs with evidence of extensive myocardial infarction (40% of LV infarcted), severe cardiomyopathy, or myocarditis.
Cardiogenic shock due to a mechanical defect			
Acute ventricular septal defect	↑	LVCO ↓↓ and RVCO >LVCO	Predominant shunt is left to right, pulmonary blood flow is greater than systemic blood flow: oxygen "step-up" occurs at RV level.
Acute mitral regurgitation	↑↑	Forward CO ↓↓	V waves in pulmonary capillary wedge pressure tracing.
Right ventricular infarction	Normal or ↓	↓↓	Elevated RA and RV filling pressures with low or normal pulmonary capillary wedge pressures.
Extracardiac obstructive forms of shock			
Pericardial tamponade	↑	↓ or ↓↓	RA mean, RV end-diastolic, pulmonary capillary wedge mean pressures are elevated and within 5 mmHg of one another.
Massive pulmonary embolism	Normal or ↓	↓↓	Usual finding is elevated right-sided pressures.
Hypovolemic shock	↓↓	↓↓	
Distributive forms of shock			
Septic shock	↓ or normal	↑ or normal, rarely ↓	
Anaphylactic shock	↓ or normal	↑ or normal	

Adapted from JE Parrillo, SM Ayres (eds): Major Issues in Critical Care Medicine. Baltimore, Williams & Wilkins, 1984.

shock states with decreased cardiac output, stroke volume, and mean arterial pressure. Other hemodynamic variables will depend on the site of the obstruction. With pericardial tamponade, patients usually develop increased and equalized right and left heart ventricular diastolic pressures. Constrictive pericarditis may produce a similar pattern. Acute pulmonary embolism will result in right heart failure with elevated pulmonary artery and right heart pressures and low or normal left heart filling pressures.

The tempo of the result influences the clinical manifestations. With pericardial tamponade due to myocardial rupture following myocardial infarction, for example, immediate tamponade and shock can occur within minutes with as little as 150 mL of blood in the pericardium. Survival requires immediate drainage and surgery. Patients with malignant or inflammatory causes of pericardial tamponade develop fluid accumulation more slowly, and 1 or 2 L of fluid may be necessary to produce shock.

Distributive Shock

The major feature of distributive shock is decreased peripheral resistance. Although anaphylaxis, drug overdose, neurogenic insults, and Addisonian crisis can produce this form of shock, the most important and prevalent cause is septic shock (see Chapter 84). In this form of shock, tissue hypoperfusion results from either microvascular abnormalities (maldistribution or shunting of blood flow) or a mediator-induced metabolic block that prevents cells from adequately utilizing oxygen and other nutrients delivered via the vasculature.

Early in distributive shock, venodilation and leakage of fluid from the microvasculature will lead to an inadequate intravascular volume and reduced preload. Volume resuscitation will correct this preload abnormality and produce the usual hemodynamic pattern of distributive shock: a normal or elevated cardiac output, normal stroke volume, tachycardia, decreased systemic vascular resistance, and decreased mean arterial pressure. Left and right heart filling pressures are variable and depend on the amount of fluid resuscitation.

In addition, most patients with distributive shock also manifest myocardial depression, which is characterized by a decreased stroke work response to volume loading, biventricular reduction in ejection fraction, and ventricular dilatation. The dilatation allows patients to compensate for a depressed ejection fraction and maintain stroke volume, which combined with a high heart rate leads to an elevated cardiac output. In approximately 10 to 15% of septic shock patients, the myocardial dysfunction is dominant and severe, and it results in a hypodynamic, low cardiac output form of shock (see Fig. 94–1).

CLINICAL APPROACH TO SHOCK

Shock is a life-threatening emergency. Diagnosis, evaluation, and management must often occur simultaneously, and speed in the evaluation is important to a good outcome. The clinical approach must balance two important goals: (1) the need to initiate therapy before shock causes irreversible damage to organs; and (2) the need to perform a diagnostic evaluation to determine the cause of shock (see Fig. 94–2). A reasonable approach is to make a rapid clinical evaluation initially based on a directed history and physical examination and to initiate diagnostic tests aimed at determining cause. In severe shock, therapy should be initiated based on the initial clinical impression. Certain symptoms and signs are similar to all forms of shock. Most patients have hypotension, tachycardia, cool extremities, oliguria, and a clouded sensorium. In general, a mean arterial pressure less than 60 mm Hg in an adult is considered hypotension. However, blood pressure must be evaluated in terms of previous chronic blood pressures. A patient with chronic hypertension may experience shock pathophysiology at higher blood pressures. A decrease of 50 mm Hg or more from chronic elevated levels is frequently sufficient to produce tissue hypoperfusion. Conversely, some patients with chronically low blood pressure may not develop shock until the mean arterial pressure drops below 50 mm Hg.

Other clinical manifestations may be useful in differentiating the etiology of shock. Hypovolemic shock patients frequently manifest evidence of gastrointestinal hemorrhage, bleeding from another site, or evidence of vomiting or diarrhea. Patients with cardiogenic shock may have manifestations of heart disease with prior angina or myocardial infarction and often have elevated filling pressures, cardiac gallops, or pulmonary edema. Cardiac murmurs may suggest mechanical causes of cardiogenic shock. Elevated jugular venous pressure and a quiet precordium suggest pericardial tamponade. A site of infection with prominent fever should raise the possibility of septic shock.

Even though a brief history and physical examination are directed at potential causes and signs of shock, blood should be

Table 94–6 ■ RELATIVE POTENCY OF VASOPRESSORS AND INOTROPIC AGENTS IN SHOCK

AGENT	DOSE	CARDIAC		PERIPHERAL VASCULAR		
		Heart Rate	Contractility	Vasoconstriction	Vasodilation	Dopaminergic
Dopamine	1–4 μg/kg/min	1+	1+	0	1+	4+
	4–20 μg/kg/min	2+	2–3+	2–3+	0	2+
Norepinephrine	2–20 μg/min	1+	2+	4+	0	0
Dobutamine	2.5–15 μg/kg/min	1–2+	3–4+	0	2+	0
Isoproterenol	1–5 μg/min	4+	4+	0	4+	0
Epinephrine	1–20 μg/min	4+	4+	4+	3+	0
Phenylephrine	20–200 μg/min	0	0	3+	0	0
Amrinone	0.75 mg/kg bolus; then 5–15 μg/kg/min	1+	3+	0	2+	0
Milrinone	37.5–75 μg/kg bolus; then 0.375–0.75 μg/kg/min	1+	3+	0	2+	0

The 1 to 4 + scoring system is an arbitrary system to allow a judgment of comparative potency among these vasopressor agents. Adapted from JE Parrillo, SM Ayres (eds): Major Issues in Critical Care Medicine. Baltimore, Williams & Wilkins, 1984.

drawn to evaluate hemoglobin, platelets, coagulation, oxygenation and ventilation, electrolytes, kidney function, and blood lactate levels. An electrocardiogram and chest radiograph should be taken.

Simultaneously, venous access with one or two large-bore catheters should be established, and central venous and arterial catheters should be inserted (see Fig. 94–2). Electrocardiographic monitoring and continuous pulse oximetry are usually valuable. If the mean arterial pressure is less than 60 mm Hg or evidence of tissue hypoperfusion is present, a fluid challenge with 500 to 1000 mL of crystalloid or colloid should be given intravenously (if hemorrhage is likely, blood should be the volume replacement). If the patient remains hypotensive, vasopressors such as dopamine and/or norepinephrine should be administered to restore an adequate blood pressure while the diagnostic evaluation continues. The shock patient should be admitted to an intensive care unit.

If the diagnosis remains undefined or the hemodynamic status requires repeated fluid challenges or vasopressors, a flow-directed pulmonary artery catheter should be placed (Table 94–5), and echocardiography should be performed. Echocardiography is valuable in identifying the presence of pericardial fluid, tamponade physiology, ventricular function, valvular heart disease, and intracardiac shunts. Based on these data, patients can usually be classified and managed according to the specific form of shock.

MANAGEMENT AND THERAPY

In all forms of shock, restoration of blood pressure and tissue perfusion are critical goals and commonly require fluids, vasopressors, inotropic agents (Table 94–6), mechanical ventilation, and repeated monitoring.

Hypovolemic Shock

The major goal is to infuse adequate volume to restore perfusion before the onset of irreversible tissue damage without raising cardiac filling pressures to a level that produces hydrostatic pulmonary edema, which usually begins at a pulmonary capillary wedge pressure >18 mm Hg. In hemorrhagic shock, restoration of oxygen delivery is achieved by transfusion of packed red blood cells with the goal of maintaining hemoglobin concentration >10 g/dL. Restoration of intravascular volume must be accompanied by aggressive evaluation to identify a bleeding source and treatment to prevent further bleeding.

In other forms of hypovolemic shock, crystalloid solutions such as normal saline or Ringer's lactate are conventionally employed. Some authors advocate use of colloid solutions, such as albumin or hetastarch, because they may produce faster restoration of intravascular volume, especially in traumatic shock where volume losses can be large. However, no convincing evidence demonstrates clear superiority of colloids over crystalloids in restoring volume depletion. Because colloids are more expensive, most physicians favor crystalloids unless serum albumin is low and requires repletion. Hypertonic saline, which can provide volume repletion with small volumes of fluid, may be therapeutically useful in burns and head trauma, in which limitation of free water is often important.

Cardiogenic Shock

In hypotensive patients with cardiogenic shock, pulmonary capillary wedge pressure should be maintained at 14 to 18 mm Hg, and medications should be used to try to restore mean arterial pressure to >60 mm Hg and the cardiac index (cardiac output divided by body surface area in meters squared) to >2.2 L/min/m^2 (see Chapters 40 and 47). Appropriate patients will benefit from an intra-aortic balloon pump, emergent coronary revascularization, or surgical correction of valvular abnormalities or septal defects.

Extracardiac Obstructive Shock

In pericardial tamponade, blood pressure can be maintained using fluids and vasopressors in a fashion similar to the method employed in cardiogenic shock. However, these are only temporizing measures, and one should move quickly to drain pericardial fluid using needle pericardiocentesis or surgery (see Chapter 65).

In severe pulmonary embolism (see Chapter 84) producing right ventricular failure and shock, thrombolytic therapy should be considered in addition to conventional anticoagulation with heparin and warfarin. If thrombolysis is contraindicated, emergency surgical pulmonary embolectomy can sometimes produce a successful outcome.

Distributive Shock

For septic shock (see Chapter 96), principles of management include eliminating the nidus of infection with surgical drainage and antimicrobial therapy; restoring blood pressure using fluids and vasopressor agents; and maintaining adequate tissue perfusion using fluids, inotropic agents, and other supportive measures.

Gattinoni L, Brazzi L, Pelosi P, et al for the SVO2 Collaborative Group: A trial of goal-oriented hemodynamic therapy in critically ill patients. N Engl J Med 333: 1025, 1995. *A randomized, prospective trial demonstrating that supranormal oxygen delivery does not improve survival in critically ill patients.*

Task Force of the American College of Critical Care Medicine, Society of Critical Care Medicine: Practice parameters for hemodynamic support of sepsis in adult patients in sepsis. Crit Care Med 27:639, 1999. *Updated, evidence-based guidelines.*

Kumar A, Parrillo JE: Shock: Classification, pathophysiology, and approach to management. In Parrillo JE, Bone RC (eds): Critical Care Medicine: Principles, Diagnosis and Management. St. Louis, Mosby-Year Book, 1995, pp 355–374. *Provides a detailed review of pathogenesis and management of different forms of shock.*

Kumar A, Venkateswarlu T, Dee L, et al: Tumor necrosis factor and interleukin-1 are responsible for in-vitro myocardial cell depression induced by human septic shock serum. J Exp Med 183:949, 1996. *Demonstrates that cytokines are the cause of myocardial depression in human septic shock.*

95 CARDIOGENIC SHOCK

David R. Holmes

In 1912, Herrick described a very early case of cardiogenic shock in which a 55-year-old man in good health was seized with severe pain in the lower pericordial region an hour after a moderately full meal. On evaluation he was described as "cold, nauseated, small rapid pulse (140), cyanosis, scant of urine, and coarse, moist rales."

Cardiogenic shock describes tissue hypoperfusion in the setting of an acute ischemic event, which is usually either an ST-segment elevation or ST-segment depression myocardial infarction (MI). Cardiogenic shock can be defined by clinical parameters alone, including the manifestations of a low cardiac output state with peripheral hypoperfusion and cool, clammy extremities, cyanosis, oliguria, and altered central nervous system functions. An obligate requirement is the presence of hypotension. The degree of hypotension required to fulfill the criteria of shock has varied but is usually systolic blood pressure less than 90 mm Hg; an alternative definition is a systolic blood pressure more than 30 mm Hg *below* the patient's basal level. In addition to clinical manifestations and a systolic blood pressure less than 90 mm Hg, other prominent hemodynamic manifestations are elevated left ventricular filling pressures greater than 15 mm Hg and a reduction in cardiac index to less than approximately 2.2 L/minute/m^2.

ETIOLOGY

In the setting of an acute ischemic event, cardiogenic causes of shock must be distinguished from noncardiogenic causes including hypotension caused by medications such as nitrates or streptokinase, hemorrhage from anticoagulant or thrombolytic drugs, or, as the precipitating cause of the acute ischemic event, pulmonary embolism or hypovolemia.

Cardiogenic causes are also diverse. The classic etiology is pump failure secondary to extensive left ventricular damage, but right ventricular infarction may also lead to cardiogenic shock if associated posterior left ventricular infarction is present (see Chapter 60). The differential diagnosis of cardiogenic shock also includes the mechanical causes of mitral regurgitation from papillary muscle rupture or dysfunction, rupture of the left ventricular free wall, and ventricular septal defect. Shock may also result from co-morbid cardiac conditions such as aortic stenosis (see Chapter 63) or cardiac tamponade (see Chapter 65), the latter of which may be the result of an ascending aortic dissection that propagates in a retrogade fashion, shearing off the right coronary artery and then creating a rupture into the pericardium. Cardiac arrhythmias, such as atrial fibrillation with a rapid ventricular response or ventricular tachycardia, may contribute to hypotension. Identifying the specific etiology is important as it may mandate a different treatment strategy and may affect prognosis.

INCIDENCE AND EPIDEMIOLOGY

The incidence of cardiogenic shock after an acute MI has varied from 5 to 19%. The incidence may be underreported because some reports may exclude patients with shock on admission or may not represent the full spectrum of the patient population with both ST elevation and ST-segment depression MIs. Compared with patients with ST elevation, patients with ST depression have approximately one-half the incidence of cardiogenic shock. The incidence of cardiogenic shock has also varied over time; earlier recognition of the symptoms of MI and earlier presentation for medical care may affect the incidence.

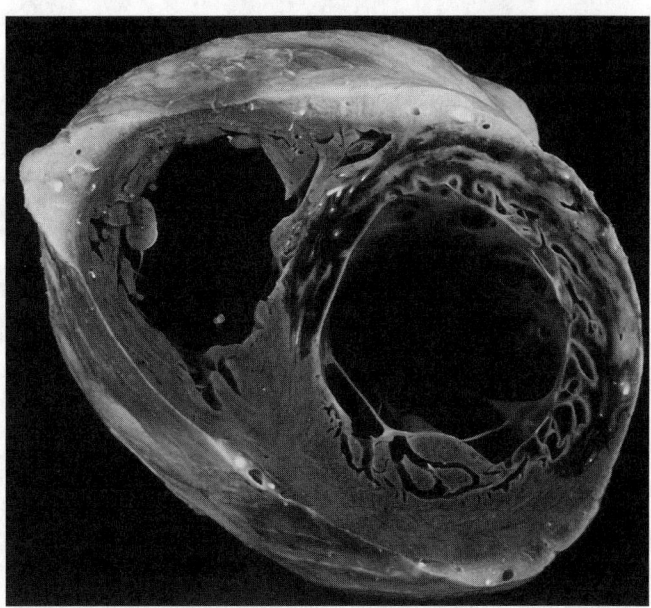

FIGURE 95–1. ■ Postmortem autopsy specimen from a patient who died of cardiogenic shock from acute myocardial infarction. Extensive necrosis is evident. (Courtesy of William D. Edwards.)

Typically, only a minority of patients with shock—approximately 10 to 15%—have it on admission. Shock develops in the majority of patients within the next 48 hours. When cardiogenic shock develops in patients without ST-segment elevation, it usually develops relatively later, commonly due to reinfarction.

As might be expected, prior MI, older age, diabetes mellitus, female gender, and a history of angina pectoris, stroke, or peripheral vascular disease have been associated with increased incidence of cardiogenic shock, but the discriminatory power of these variables in individual patients is limited. Patients with pre-existing left ventricular dysfunction are also at higher risk. Coronary angiographic documentation of multivessel disease or the location of the infarct-related arterial stenosis may be helpful. The prevalence of left main coronary artery disease appears to be increased in patients with shock (Table 95–1).

PATHOGENESIS

Cardiogenic shock is typically the result of an extensive MI associated with damage to 40% or more of the left ventricular myocardium (Fig. 95–1). It does not appear to matter whether this loss of left ventricular myocardium is the result of a single ischemic insult, with occlusion of a single artery that supplies a large region of myocardium, or a series of multiple prior MIs. However, autopsy and angiographic studies have documented that multivessel disease is almost universally present, particularly involving the left anterior descending (LAD) coronary artery.

Infarct extension or reinfarction is common in patients with shock and is often the mechanism responsible for shock. Among

Table 95–1 ■ **RISK FACTORS AND CARDIOGENIC SHOCK**

FACTORS ASSOCIATED WITH DEVELOPMENT OF SHOCK	FACTORS ASSOCIATED WITH INCREASED MORTALITY FROM SHOCK
Older age	Older age
Diabetes mellitus	Prior infarction
History of prior MI, stroke, or peripheral vascular disease	Altered sensorium
Female gender	Peripheral vasoconstriction
Reinfarction	Baseline systolic blood pressure
Initial EF <35%	Lower cardiac output
Lack of compensatory hyperkinesis in remote segments	Higher heart rate

MI = myocardial infarction; EF = ejection fraction.

the multiple factors that may be involved in infarct extension or expansion are impaired collateral flow, increased myocardial oxygen consumption, and passive collapse or vasoconstriction at a second site within the coronary circulation due to low coronary perfusion pressure during diastole. In patients with hypertensive cardiovascular disease and left ventricular hypertrophy or aortic stenosis, the hypotension and elevated left ventricular end-diastolic pressure may cause or aggravate diffuse subendocardial ischemia.

The mechanical complications of mitral regurgitation, ventricular septal defect, or rupture of left ventricular myocardium account for up to 15% of cases of cardiogenic shock. The underlying MI may be only small or moderate in size but may involve critical structures such as the interventricular septum or papillary muscle. Free wall rupture accounts for 10% of all deaths from MI and is typically associated with an ST-elevation anterior MI. Rupture of the interventricular septum may result in a single direct perforation or a number of complex serpentine tracts; this defect also is seen with ST-elevation anterior MI. Partial or complete rupture of one of the papillary muscles may result in severe mitral regurgitation; the posteromedial papillary muscle is more frequently involved than the anterolateral papillary muscle because the former usually receives its blood supply from just one source, the posterior descending coronary artery.

Cardiogenic shock is a distinct and well-recognized complication of a right ventricular MI, which is always associated with posterobasal infarction of the left ventricle. With occlusion of the proximal right coronary artery, right ventricular pump function decreases and the right ventricle dilates, leading to a decrease in left ventricular preload and subsequent hypotension.

CLINICAL MANIFESTATIONS AND ASSESSMENT

Cardiogenic shock is manifest as tissue hypoperfusion in the setting of an acute ischemic event. Hypotension is usually defined as systolic blood pressure less than 90 mm Hg or a decrease in systolic blood pressure from baseline by more than 30 mm Hg, although the latter criterion includes a larger group of patients who may not actually have shock or who have a milder form of shock. Hypoperfusion is recognized by altered sensorium, cyanosis, oliguria, and cool, clammy extremities. Attendant dyspnea and ongoing ischemic chest pain may be present. This constellation of findings may be present at initial presentation with acute MI, but it more frequently develops somewhat later, up to 48 hours following the onset of MI. Either bradycardia, usually a manifestation of the Bezold-Jarisch reflex, or tachycardia may be present.

On physical examination, findings are variable. Typically, the venous pressure is elevated. The finding of a low venous pressure identifies a group of patients who usually have hypovolemia rather than cardiogenic shock as a predominant cause; correction by fluid administration may lead to improved outcome. Concomitant pulmonary edema may be present, which in the hypotensive patient establishes the diagnosis of cardiogenic shock. In patients with a mechanical complication resulting in shock, the physical findings may not be typical of the underlying cause. For example, patients with acute mitral regurgitation may not have a systolic murmur because of equalization of the pressures between the left ventricle and left atrium; in these patients, a high index of suspicion is required so that appropriate tests (e.g., left ventricular angiography or echocardiography) can be performed to make the definitive diagnosis. In patients with a ventricular septal defect, the systolic murmur may be at the lower left sternal border without a thrill. Patients with a free wall rupture commonly present with electromechanical dissociation, which is almost uniformly fatal.

In patients with circulatory collapse, an initial electrocardiogram (ECG) is essential, and it will be abnormal in cardiogenic shock. ST-segment elevation is most common, although cardiogenic shock can occur without it. Given the predominant finding of left anterior descending artery involvement, an anterior wall injury pattern is most common. The ECG also provides information on prior MI and rhythm disorders. Isolated elevation in aVR in a patient with acute MI and shock suggests the possibility of left main coronary artery involvement. In patients in whom a right ventricular MI is suspected, a modified right precordial lead is very helpful.

Echocardiography is used with increasing frequency and is an extremely important tool; it can make the diagnosis of a mechanical complication, such as a ruptured papillary muscle or a ventricular septal defect. In addition, echocardiography can provide assessment of overall left ventricular function, including compensatory hyperkinesis of noninfarcted segments. Patients with cardiogenic shock from a large MI can be expected to have severe regional wall motion abnormalities. If severe regional wall motion abnormalities are not present, then another etiology for the hemodynamic compromise may be present. In patients in whom rupture is suspected, echocardiography can document a pericardial effusion.

Hemodynamic monitoring, which can provide extremely important information, is often underutilized. Right-sided heart catheterization with flow-directed catheters can aid in diagnosis, for example, by documenting low left ventricular filling pressures in hypovolemic shock or right ventricular infarction, giant V waves in a patient with unsuspected severe mitral regurgitation, or an oxygen saturation gradient in a patient with a ventricular septal defect. Monitoring of left-sided heart pressures with periodic wedge recordings also aids in optimizing filling pressures during the initial attempts at stabilization.

Although findings such as altered sensorium and peripheral vasoconstriction are important predictors of prognosis, cardiac output and wedge pressure measurements add important independent information regarding prognosis and increase the ability to identify patients at greatest risk of dying with cardiogenic shock. Using data derived from clinical, laboratory, and right-sided heart catheterization, mortality for cardiogenic shock can be predicted (Table 95–2).

TREATMENT

The prognosis of patients with cardiogenic shock remains grim. The optimal treatment strategies have not yet been identified in scientifically controlled, randomized trials. Supportive measures, such as maintenance of adequate oxygenation and treatment of arrhythmias are essential, and documentation of volume status is extremely important. Attempts to improve blood pressure are essential to break the vicious cycle of progressive hypotension with further myocardial ischemia. If left ventricular pressures are elevated as assessed by either hemodynamic monitoring or the presence of pulmonary edema, then further volume expansion is not beneficial and may be harmful. If volume status is uncertain, a trial of volume expansion is warranted with careful monitoring. Right ventricular pressure monitoring improves assessment of filling pressures. As is true in all patients with acute MI, aspirin and heparin are extremely important and serve as baseline treatments.

Vasopressor therapy to improve cardiac performance carries some risks, including aggravation of arrhythmias and, even more importantly, increase in myocardial oxygen demand; it is, however, essential for stabilization. Dopamine, 5 to 10 μg/kg/minute, is usually the initial drug given, and it can result in increasing systemic pressure and cardiac output. Dobutamine, 2 to 8 μg/kg/minute, may be used in combination with dopamine to augment cardiac output further, but it does not usually increase arterial pressure further. In patients with very severe hypotension or those with resistant hypotension, norepinephrine, 0.04 to 0.4 μg/kg/minute, is usually used, and it may be effective. In general, vasopressive agents should be titrated to the lowest dose required to optimize blood pressure and maintain adequate cardiac output; myocardial oxygen demand can be minimized in this manner. Vasodilators such as intravenous nitroglycerine or nitroprusside are usually not used initially because they can aggravate hypotension; however, they may be used later in combination with vasopressors and inotropic agents.

Thrombolytic drugs have been widely used for acute MI, but the majority of trials have not included patients with cardiogenic shock. The benefit of thrombolysis has been equivocal, with some trials showing no benefit and others showing a small benefit. Thrombolysis may reduce the subsequent development of shock after admission, due either to a decrease in reinfarction or to a limitation of the size of the initial infarct. Thrombolytic efficacy is decreased with hypotension, so vigorous attempts to augment blood pressure appear to be important.

Other pharmacologic approaches are aimed at altering myocardial metabolism. L-Carnitine, which has been studied experimentally in

Table 95–2 ▪ SCORING SYSTEM PREDICTING 30-DAY MORTALITY RATES BASED ON DEMOGRAPHIC, CLINICAL, AND HEMODYNAMIC VARIABLES AS WELL AS RIGHT HEART CATHETERIZATION DATA

1. FIND POINTS FOR EACH PREDICTIVE FACTOR

Age		Mean Arterial Pressure During Shock		Heart Rate During Shock		Lowest Cardiac Output		Highest Pulmonary Capillary Wedge Pressure	
Yr	Points	mm Hg	Points	bpm	Points	L/min	Points	mm Hg	Points
20	0	20	20	20	5	2	42	10	31
30	11	40	38	40	11	4	13	20	0
40	22	60	35	60	16	6	0	30	24
50	33	80	17	80	22	8	7	40	26
60	44	100	19	100	27	10	13	50	25
70	56	120	25	120	33	12	20	60	24
80	67	140	32	140	38	14	27		
90	78	160	38	160	43	16	33		
100	89	180	44	180	49	18	40		

Miscellaneous Risk Factors			
Factor	Points	Factor	Points
Killip class		Prior infarction	15
I	7	Altered sensorium	15
II	26	Cold, clammy skin	15
III	25	Oliguria	23
IV		Ventricular septal defect	38

2. SUM POINTS FOR ALL PREDICTIVE FACTORS

3. LOOK UP RISK CORRESPONDING TO TOTAL POINTS

Points	Probability of 30-Day Mortality (%)
138	10
160	20
175	30
188	40
199	50
210	60
223	70
238	80
260	90

From Hasdai D, Holmes DR Jr, Califf RM, et al. for the GUSTO investigators: Cardiogenic shock complicating acute myocardial infarction: Predictors of mortality. Am Heart J 138:21–31, 1999.

small series of patients, is potentially an important adjunct. Adenosine can improve myocardial salvage in patients with acute MI, but its use is limited by the attendant hypotension.

MECHANICAL SUPPORT. Insertion of an intra-aortic balloon pump (IABP) for counterpulsation increases diastolic coronary artery perfusion pressure, decreases left ventricular afterload, improves cardiac output, and decreases myocardial oxygen demand. Although an IABP can stabilize hemodynamics in patients with shock, early studies documented a persistently high mortality, particularly if revascularization either was not possible or was not performed. More recent studies have confirmed improved survival at 30 days and 1 year when patients with cardiogenic shock have been treated with IABP. Other devices, such as percutaneous partial cardiopulmonary bypass, are also available but are used infrequently because of the need for specialized equipment and large catheters; nevertheless, these devices decrease myocardial oxygen demand while maintaining or augmenting perfusion and so may provide an important adjunctive approach to myocardial salvage.

REVASCULARIZATION. Assessment of the role of revascularization in patients with cardiogenic shock has been very problematic. Selection of patients to undergo angiography or revascularization may identify a lower risk group of shock patients; in contrast, conservative therapy may be selected in higher-risk patients who are thought to be in the process of dying. This problem was illustrated in some studies in which patients who underwent angiography alone had a better outcome than patients who did not. A second confounding problem is that revascularization is often bundled with other aggressive interventions, any of which may add incremental benefit.

Despite these problems, the importance of restoration of flow in the infarct-related artery has been emphasized repeatedly, and coronary blood flow is improved more with primary percutaneous transluminal coronary angioplasty (PTCA) than with thrombolysis. As a result, studies have identified almost a 50% reduction in early mortality, which is sustained at 1 year, in patients treated with urgent PTCA after shock develops. It is of note that an aggressive strategy, including PTCA, often includes other adjunctive therapies, such as IABP.

From a technical standpoint, PTCA is more complex in shock patients. An IABP should be placed prior to treatment. Typically, only the infarct-related artery has been treated at the initial PTCA, unless the patient has multivessel disease with other critical lesions and PTCA of the infarct-related artery does not improve the clinical situation. With the use of coronary stents (see Chapter 61), it may be possible to treat all significant stenoses and provide more complete revascularization. Adjunctive therapy with class IIb/IIIa agents may be very helpful, although these drugs may complicate the situation by increasing the potential for bleeding in patients in whom surgery is required.

The role of coronary artery bypass grafting (CABG) is even more controversial. The same issues of whether patient selection biases outcome are even more important for CABG than for PTCA. CABG has potential major advantages, including the ability to achieve complete revascularization and the opportunity to vent the ventricle and cool the heart with cardioplegia so as to limit ongoing ischemia and reduce myocardial oxygen consumption dramatically.

In patients with mechanical complications, surgery may provide

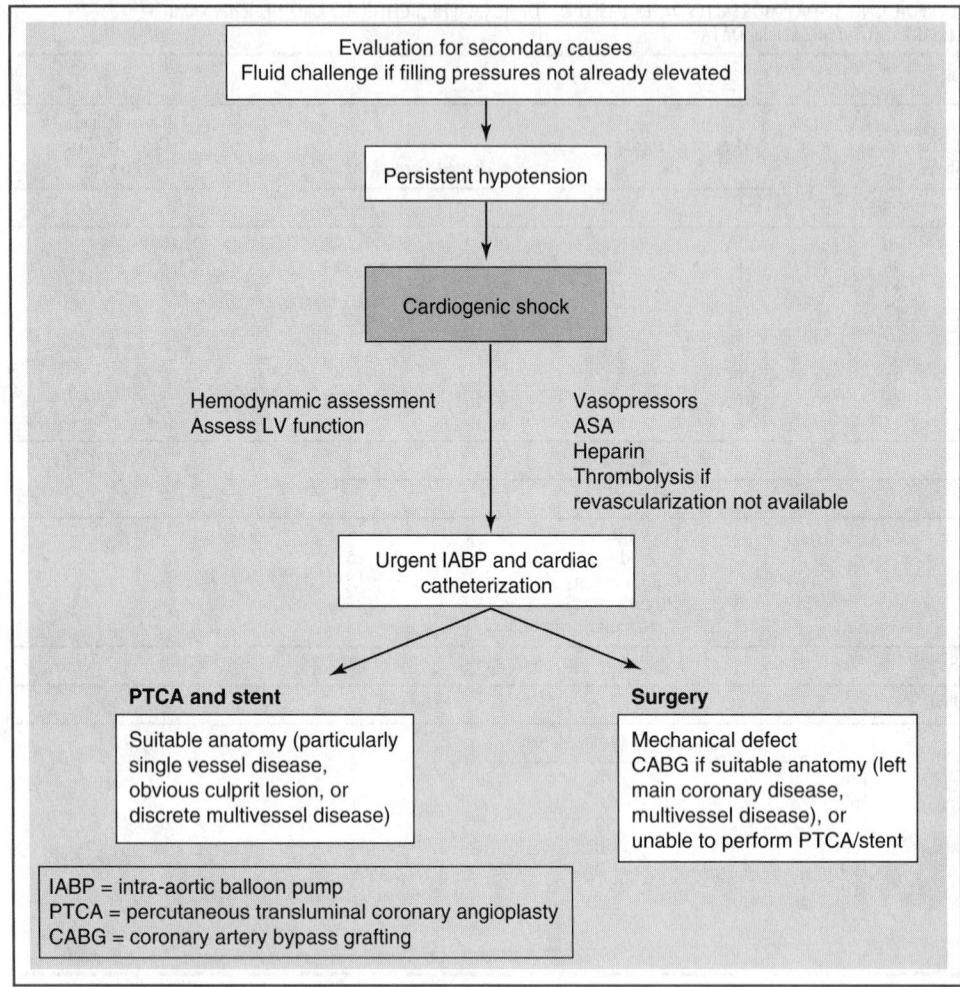

FIGURE 95–2. ■ Acute myocardial infarction with hypotension: an aggressive approach.

the only approach to resolve the problem. If possible, these patients should be stabilized prior to surgery, often with an IABP. In patients with a ventricular septal defect or severe mitral regurgitation, surgery can dramatically improve outcome despite high operative mortality rates. Free-wall rupture commonly presents with electromechanical dissociation and is almost always fatal. Subacute rupture with false aneurysm formation is extremely infrequent, but it can be treated surgically with suture or patch closure when it is diagnosed in time.

RECOMMENDED CURRENT APPROACH. At present, an aggressive approach appears to have the most potential to improve outcome (Fig. 95–2). Management requires rapid evaluation of the multiple potential causes of shock in parallel with supportive therapy designed to improve perfusion and optimize right and left ventricular pressures. An IABP and right-sided heart catheterization are very helpful if available, in terms of both stabilization and facilitation of diagnosis. Revascularization with either emergent PTCA or CABG appears to confer early and longer-term survival benefits in eligible patients, although the problem of selection bias and its effect on outcome must be kept in mind.

PROGNOSIS

Cardiogenic shock now accounts for the majority of all fatalities related to acute MI. Prior to the era of reperfusion, mortality from cardiogenic shock approximated 80%. In the larger thrombolytic trials, mortality rates remain at 51% to 70%. In selected series of shock patients, an aggressive strategy with placement of an IABP

followed by revascularization, either with PTCA/stent or CABG, may reduce 30-day mortality to 30 to 40%.

The outlook in patients who survive for 1 month is quite good; among 1-month survivors, 85 to 90% remain alive at 1 year. This survival rate is favorably affected by coronary revascularization, compared with the rate in patients who did not undergo revascularization.

Berger PB, Holmes DR Jr, Stebbins AL, et al: Impact of an aggressive invasive catheterization and revascularization strategy on mortality in patients with cardiogenic shock in the GUSTO I trial. Circulation 96:122–127, 1997. *Data to support an aggressive invasive strategy to improve outcome in patients with cardiogenic shock.*

Berger PB, Tuttle RH, Holmes DR Jr: One year survival among patients with acute myocardial infarction complicated by cardiogenic shock and the impact of early revascularization: Results from the GUSTO I trial. Circulation 99:873–878, 1999. *This 1-year outcome study supports the longer-term benefit of aggressive interventions.*

Goldberg RJ, Samad NA, Yarzebski J, et al: Temporal trends in cardiogenic shock complicating acute myocardial infarction. N Engl J Med 340:1162–1168, 1999. *Over a 23-year period, the incidence of cardiogenic shock following acute MI has not changed, but the short-term survival rate has improved coincident with the increased use of coronary reperfusion strategies.*

Hasdai D, Holmes DR, Califf RM, et al: Cardiogenic shock complicating acute myocardial infarction: Predictors of mortality. (In press.) *The largest prospectively defined shock population allows identification of patients who might benefit from the most intensive treatments.*

Holmes DR Jr, Califf RM, Van de Werf F, et al: Difference in countries' use of resources and clinical outcome for patients with cardiogenic shock after myocardial infarction: Results from the GUSTO trial. Lancet 349:75–78, 1997. *This study reveals striking differences in resource utilization and clinical outcome in patients with cardiogenic shock in different countries.*

Leor J, Goldbourt U, Reicher-Reiss H, et al: Cardiogenic shock complicating acute myocardial infarction in patients without heart failure on admission: Incidence, risk factors, and outcome: SPRINT Study Group. Am J Med 94:265–273, 1993. *Excel-*

lent multicenter data on factors that identify patients at risk for development of cardiogenic shock.

Stone GW, Marsalese D, Brodie BR, et al: A prospective, randomized evaluation of prophylactic intra-aortic balloon counterpulsation in high risk patients with acute myocardial infarction treated with primary angioplasty: Second Primary Angioplasty in Myocardial Infarction (PAMI-II) Trial Investigators. J Am Coll Cardiol 29:1459–1467, 1997. *The role of intra-aortic balloon counterpulsation in higher risk patients.*

Webb JG, Carere RG, Hilton JD, et al: Usefulness of coronary stenting for cardiogenic shock. Am J Cardiol 79:81–84, 1997. *Coronary stents can improve flow and reduce recurrent ischemia in cardiogenic shock.*

96 SHOCK SYNDROMES RELATED TO SEPSIS

Joseph E. Parrillo

Sepsis refers to the systemic response to serious infection. Patients with sepsis usually manifest fever, tachycardia, tachypnea, leukocytosis, and a localized site of infection. Microbiologic cultures from blood or the infection site are frequently, though not invariably, positive. When this syndrome results in hypotension or multiple organ system failure, the condition is called *septic shock.*

INCIDENCE AND EPIDEMIOLOGY

The incidence of sepsis and septic shock has been increasing since the 1930s, and all recent evidence suggests that this rise will continue. The reasons for this increasing incidence are many: increased use of invasive devices such as intravascular catheters; widespread use of cytotoxic and immunosuppressive drug therapies for cancer and transplantation; increased lifespan of patients with cancer and diabetes, who are prone to develop sepsis; and increase in infections due to antibiotic-resistant organisms. Septic shock is the most common cause of death in intensive care units, and it is the 13th most common cause of death in the United States. The precise incidence of the disease is not known because it is not reportable; however, a reasonable annual estimate for the United States is 400,000 bouts of sepsis, 200,000 cases of septic shock, and 100,000 deaths from this disease.

ETIOLOGY

Gram-negative and gram-positive organisms as well as fungi can cause sepsis and septic shock. Certain viruses and rickettsiae probably can produce a similar syndrome. Compared with gram-positive organisms, gram-negative bacteria are somewhat more likely to produce septic shock. Culture-positive gram-negative bacteremia produces shock in approximately 50% of infections, whereas gram-positive bacteremia produces shock in about 25% of infections.

Any site of infection can result in sepsis or septic shock. Frequent causes of sepsis are pyelonephritis, pneumonia, peritonitis, cholangitis, cellulitis, meningitis, or abscess formation at any site. Many of these infections are nosocomial and occur in patients hospitalized for other medical problems. In patients with normal host defenses, a site of infection is identified in most patients. In neutropenic patients, however, a clinical site of infection is found in less than 50% of septic patients, probably because small, clinically inapparent infections in skin or bowel can lead to blood stream invasion in patients with inadequate circulating neutrophils.

DEFINITIONS

Considerable effort has been directed toward identifying septic patients early in their clinical course, when therapies are most likely to be effective. Definitions have incorporated manifestations of the systemic response to infection (fever, tachycardia, tachypnea, and leukocytosis) as well as evidence of organ system dysfunction (cardiovascular, respiratory, renal, hepatic, central nervous system,

hematologic, or metabolic abnormalities). The most recent definitions (Table 96–1) use the term *systemic inflammatory response syndrome* (SIRS) to emphasize that sepsis is one example of the body's inflammatory responses that can be triggered not only by infections but also by noninfectious disorders, such as trauma and pancreatitis (Fig. 96–1).

Sepsis is severe and has a poorer prognosis when it is associated with organ dysfunction, hypoperfusion (lactic acidosis, oliguria, or altered mental status), or hypotension (septic shock). Septic shock is defined as sepsis-induced hypotension that persists despite adequate fluid resuscitation and is associated with hypoperfusion abnormalities or organ dysfunction. In clinical practice, many patients with these signs and symptoms are receiving vasopressor and/or inotropic agents and are no longer hypotensive when they manifest hypoperfusion abnormalities or organ dysfunction, but they still are considered to be experiencing septic shock.

PATHOGENESIS

Microorganisms proliferate at a nidus of infection; they may invade the blood stream, resulting in positive blood cultures, or they may grow locally and release their structural components, such as teichoic acid antigens from staphylococci, endotoxins from gram-negative organisms, or exotoxins (e.g., toxic shock syndrome toxin-1, or TSST-1) synthesized and released by the microorganisms (Fig. 96–2). These organism-derived products can stimulate the release of a large number of endogenous host-derived mediators from plasma protein precursors or cells (monocytes-macrophages, endothelial cells, neutrophils, and others).

The endogenous mediators can produce profound physiologic effects on the vasculature and organ systems. When released in small amounts, these mediators result in beneficial effects such as regulating immune function, killing bacteria, and detoxifying bacterial products. However, an exaggerated response can result in harmful effects. Some of these effects stem from direct mediator-induced injury to end organs. However, a portion of the organ

Table 96–1 ■ DEFINITIONS OF SEPSIS

Infection: A microbial phenomenon characterized by an inflammatory response to the presence of microorganisms or the invasion of normally sterile host tissue by those organisms.

Bacteremia: The presence of viable bacteria in the blood.

Systemic inflammatory response syndrome: The systemic inflammatory response to a variety of severe clinical insults. The response is manifested by two or more of the following conditions:
  Temperature >38° C or <36° C
  Heart rate >90 beats/min
  Respiratory rate >20 breaths/min or PaCO$_2$ <32 mm Hg (<4.3 kPa)
  White blood cell count >12,000 cells/mm^3, <4000 cells/mm^3, or >10% immature (band) forms

Sepsis: The systemic response to infection. This systemic response is manifested by two or more of the following conditions as a result of infection:
  Temperature >38° C or <36° C
  Heart rate >90 beats/min
  Respiratory rate >20 breaths/min or PaCO$_2$ <32 mm Hg (<4.3 kPa)
  White blood cell count >12,000 cells/mm^3, 4000 cells/mm^3, or >10% immature (band) forms

Severe sepsis: Sepsis associated with organ dysfunction, hypoperfusion, or hypotension. Hypoperfusion and perfusion abnormalities may include, but are not limited to, lactic acidosis, oliguria, or an acute alteration in mental status.

Septic shock: Sepsis with hypotension, despite adequate fluid resuscitation, along with the presence of perfusion abnormalities that may include, but are not limited to, lactic acidosis, oliguria, or an acute alteration in mental status. Patients who are on inotropic or vasopressor agents may not be hypotensive at the time that perfusion abnormalities are measured.

Hypotension: A systolic blood pressure <90 mm Hg or a reduction >40 mm Hg from baseline in the absence of other causes for hypotension.

Multiple organ system failure: Presence of altered organ function in an acutely ill patient such that homeostasis cannot be maintained without intervention.

Adapted from American College of Chest Physicians Society of Critical Care Medicine Consensus Conference: Definitions for sepsis and organ failure and guidelines for the use of innovative therapies in sepsis. Crit Care Med 20:864, 1992.

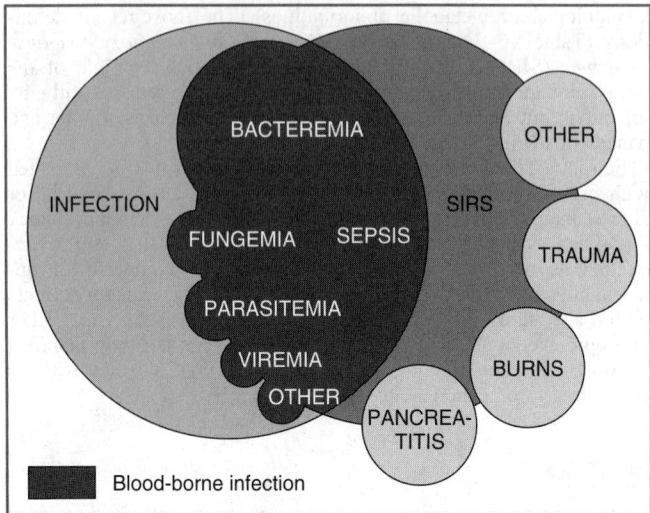

FIGURE 96–1 ■ Interrelationships among systemic inflammatory response syndrome (SIRS), sepsis, and infection. (From American College of Chest Physicians Society of Critical Care Medicine Consensus Conference: Definitions for sepsis and organ failure and guidelines for the use of innovative therapies in sepsis. Crit Care Med 20:864, 1992.)

dysfunction is probably due to mediator-induced abnormalities in vasculature, resulting in abnormalities of systemic and regional blood flow. Although certain mediators are undoubtedly more important than others in producing sepsis, probably dozens of organism- and host-derived mediators interacting, accelerating, and inhibiting one another are responsible for the pathogenesis of septic shock.

Approximately 50% of patients who have hypotension secondary to sepsis and who are admitted to an intensive care unit survive; the other 50% develop refractory hypotension or multiple organ system failure and die from progressive septic shock. Early and throughout the course of most of these patients, cardiovascular evaluation reveals a low systemic vascular resistance and a high cardiac output—the hyperdynamic response to sepsis. Despite this elevated cardiac output, cardiac performance is abnormal, with a decreased ventricular ejection fraction and a dilated ventricle. In approximately 20% of patients, progressively diminished cardiac performance results in an abnormally low cardiac output. In non-survivors, organ system dysfunction progresses to multiple organ system failure, manifested by further myocardial dysfunction, adult respiratory distress syndrome (ARDS), acute renal failure, hepatic failure, and disseminated intravascular coagulation (DIC). Death results from progressive hypotension or complete failure of one or more organ systems.

MICROORGANISM-DERIVED MEDIATORS. A number of molecules can initiate the pathway leading to septic shock. Certain microorganisms synthesize and release exotoxins that can activate the cascade. Examples include toxin A produced by *Pseudomonas aeruginosa* and TSST-1 produced by staphylococci. More frequently, the structural components of the microorganism initiate the sequence. The polysaccharide surface of *Candida albicans,* the teichoic acid antigens of staphylococci, and the polysaccharide capsule of *Streptococcus pneumoniae* can all initiate the sepsis pathway.

However, endotoxin—the distinctive lipopolysaccharide (LPS) associated with the cell membrane of gram-negative organisms—represents the classic example of an initiator of the septic shock pathogenetic cascade. The endotoxin molecule consists of an outer core with a series of oligosaccharides that are antigenically and structurally diverse, an inner oligosaccharide core that has similarities among common gram-negative bacteria, and a core lipid A that is highly conserved across bacterial species. The lipid A, which is responsible for many of the toxic properties of endotoxin, has been the focus of attempts to synthesize nonactive analogues or develop inhibitors to interfere with the septic process.

Administering endotoxin to a variety of animals results in a cardiovascular response very similar to human septic shock. Administering a very small dose of purified endotoxin to normal humans results in fever, mild constitutional symptoms, and a cardiovascular pattern qualitatively similar to that of spontaneous sepsis: tachycardia, decreased systemic vascular resistance, and depressed ventricular ejection fraction. In septic patients, detectable plasma levels of endotoxin are correlated with positive blood cultures, decreased systemic vascular resistance, depressed ventricular ejection fraction, and lactic acidemia. In patients with positive blood cultures and septic shock, detectable plasma endotoxin is associated with increased mortality (39% versus 7% for those without endotoxemia). Thus, endotoxin is an important mediator in many (though not all) septic shock patients; however, routine measurement of circulating plasma endotoxin is not prognostically reliable enough to be used clinically.

CYTOKINES. The monocyte-macrophage plays an important role in the body's response to infection or endotoxin. Endotoxin can stimulate monocytes to produce tumor necrosis factor (TNF), interleukin-1 (IL-1), and other cytokines. Serum contains a protein, the LPS-binding protein, that can bind the lipid A portion of endotoxin. When complexed with this protein, LPS can bind the CD14 receptor and stimulate the monocyte to produce cytokines at concentrations far below those required for stimulation by LPS alone.

Cytokines are 15- to 30-kD polypeptides that have profound immune regulatory and physiologic effects. Considerable evidence suggests that cytokines can enhance host defense mechanisms (e.g., stimulating lymphocyte progenitor cells, enhancing neutrophil oxidative burst) but also can produce harmful effects. In animal models, administering TNF results in a cardiovascular pattern of shock that is very similar to clinical sepsis. Anti-TNF antibodies have prevented shock and death from endotoxin and live organism challenge in animals. TNF produces vascular dilation and myocardial cell depression in biologic models, suggesting its involvement in these sepsis-associated physiologic abnormalities. Although TNF probably has a central role in mediating sepsis-induced injury, it most likely does not work alone. TNF and IL-1 have been shown to work synergistically to produce hypotension in animals, and additive or synergistic actions among a number of cytokines probably account for many sepsis-associated abnormalities.

MYOCARDIAL DEPRESSION. A number of animal models suggest the presence of a circulating myocardial depressant as the possible cause of ventricular dysfunction during sepsis. Human studies have documented the presence of circulating myocardial depressant activity that correlates temporally with the reduced ventricular ejection fraction (Table 96–2). Recent data suggest that this depression may result from a synergistic effect of TNF and IL-1 on myocardial cell contraction.

ENDOTHELIAL CELLS AND NEUTROPHILS. A number of mediators, including LPS and TNF, can cause endothelial cells to express adhesion receptors (selectins) and can activate neutrophils to express ligands for these receptors. Neutrophils must stick to the endothelial cell surface for their adherence, margination, and migration into foci of inflammatory tissue. Blockage of the adhesion process with monoclonal antibodies prevents tissue injury and improves survival in certain animal models of septic shock.

NITRIC OXIDE. In response to LPS, TNF, and other mediators, endothelial cells and macrophages can release nitric oxide, which causes smooth muscle cell relaxation and potent vasodilation. Inhibition of nitric oxide production with competitive inhibitors of nitric oxide synthase increases blood pressure in animals with endotoxin shock, suggesting that nitric oxide is partially responsible for the hypotension associated with sepsis. Although inhibition of nitric oxide restores blood pressure, such inhibition may also reduce tissue blood flow.

COMPLEMENT, KININ, AND THE COAGULATION SYSTEM. Endotoxin can activate the complement cascade, usually via the alternative pathway, and result in the release of the anaphylotoxins C3a and C5a, which can induce vasodilation, increased vascular permeability, platelet aggregation, and activation and aggregation of neutrophils. These complement-derived mediators may be responsible in part for the microvascular abnormalities associated with septic shock. Endotoxin can also result in the release of bradykinin via the activation of factor XII (Hageman factor), kallikrein, and kininogen. Bradykinin is a potent vasodilator and hypotensive agent. LPS activation of factor XII also leads to intrinsic and (through macrophage and endothelial cell release of tissue factor)

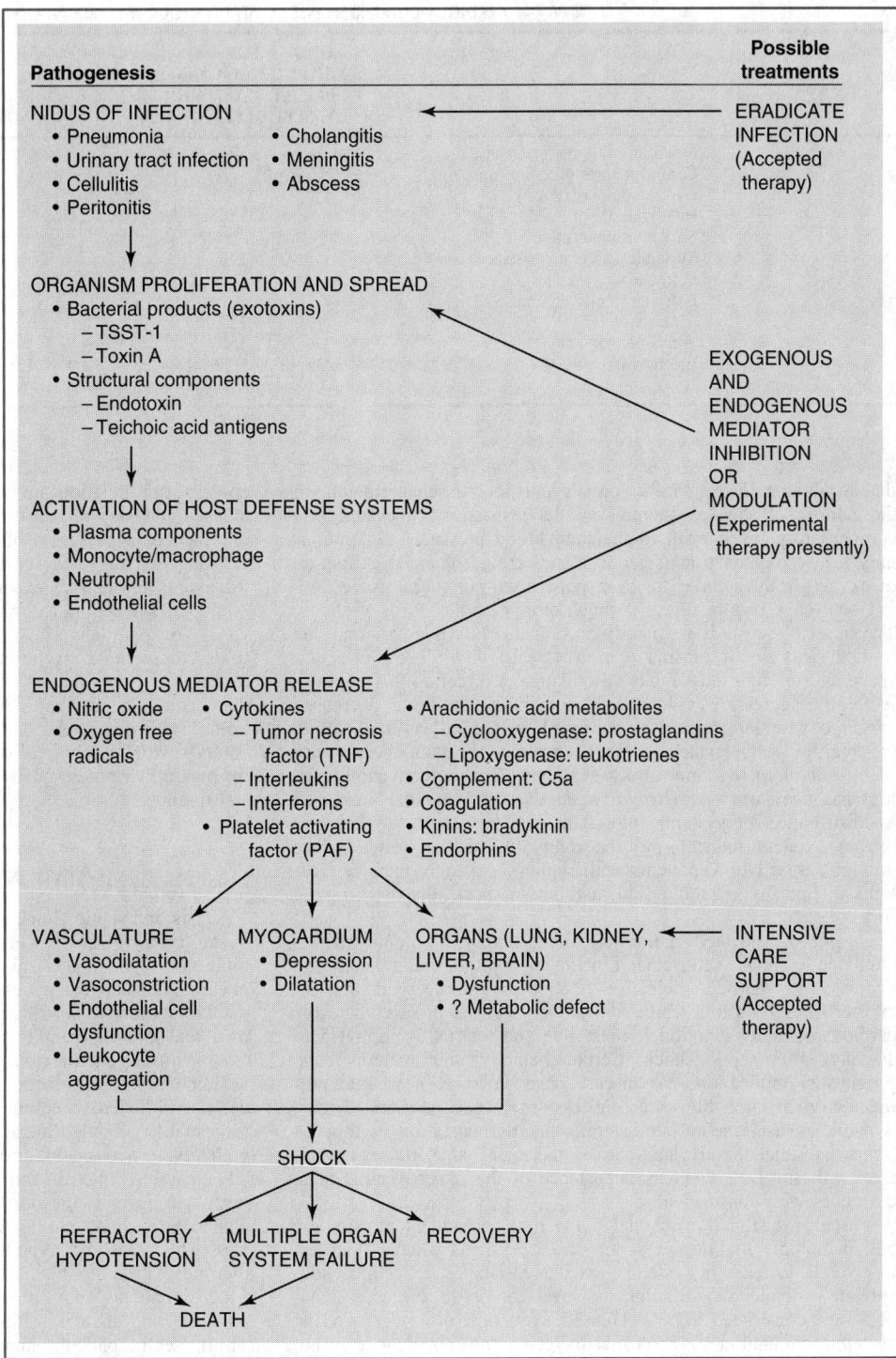

Pathogenesis

Possible treatments

NIDUS OF INFECTION
- Pneumonia
- Urinary tract infection
- Cellulitis
- Peritonitis
- Cholangitis
- Meningitis
- Abscess

ERADICATE INFECTION (Accepted therapy)

ORGANISM PROLIFERATION AND SPREAD
- Bacterial products (exotoxins)
  - TSST-1
  - Toxin A
- Structural components
  - Endotoxin
  - Teichoic acid antigens

EXOGENOUS AND ENDOGENOUS MEDIATOR INHIBITION OR MODULATION (Experimental therapy presently)

ACTIVATION OF HOST DEFENSE SYSTEMS
- Plasma components
- Monocyte/macrophage
- Neutrophil
- Endothelial cells

ENDOGENOUS MEDIATOR RELEASE
- Nitric oxide
- Oxygen free radicals
- Cytokines
  - Tumor necrosis factor (TNF)
  - Interleukins
  - Interferons
- Platelet activating factor (PAF)
- Arachidonic acid metabolites
  - Cyclooxygenase: prostaglandins
  - Lipoxygenase: leukotrienes
- Complement: C5a
- Coagulation
- Kinins: bradykinin
- Endorphins

VASCULATURE
- Vasodilatation
- Vasoconstriction
- Endothelial cell dysfunction
- Leukocyte aggregation

MYOCARDIUM
- Depression
- Dilatation

ORGANS (LUNG, KIDNEY, LIVER, BRAIN)
- Dysfunction
- ? Metabolic defect

INTENSIVE CARE SUPPORT (Accepted therapy)

SHOCK

REFRACTORY HYPOTENSION   MULTIPLE ORGAN SYSTEM FAILURE   RECOVERY

DEATH

FIGURE 96-2 ■ Pathogenesis and possible treatment strategies in sepsis and septic shock. TSST-1 = toxic shock syndrome toxin-1.

extrinsic coagulation pathway activation, which may result in consumption of coagulation factors and DIC. TNF also activates the extrinsic pathway and may contribute to these coagulation abnormalities.

ARACHIDONIC ACID METABOLITES. Different metabolites of the arachidonic acid cascade are known to cause vasodilation (prostacyclins), vasoconstriction (thromboxanes), platelet aggregation, or neutrophil activation. In experimental animals, inhibition of cyclooxygenase or thromboxane synthase has protected against endotoxin shock. Elevated levels of thromboxane B_2 (TBX$_2$) and 6-ketoprostaglandin F_{1a} (the end product of prostacyclin metabolism) are present in patients with sepsis. A number of cytokines can cause release of these arachidonic acid metabolites from endothelial cells or leukocytes. In addition to nitric oxide, some arachidonic

acid products are partially responsible for the vasodilation that is characteristic of septic shock.

OPIOID PEPTIDES. In certain animal models of endotoxin challenge, administering an endogenous opioid antagonist, such as naloxone, can reverse hypotension. The role of endogenous opioids in clinical septic shock is unclear.

CARDIOVASCULAR DYSFUNCTION

Shock is classically defined as inadequate perfusion of tissues that results in cell dysfunction and, if prolonged, cell death. This definition adequately describes shock due to the hypovolemic, cardiogenic, and vascular obstructive mechanisms (see Chapter 94)

Table 96–2 ■ CARDIOVASCULAR RESPONSE TO SEPTIC SHOCK: A REPRESENTATIVE EXAMPLE

	ACUTE PHASE (HYPOTENSION AND REDUCED SYSTEMIC VASCULAR RESISTANCE)	RECOVERY PHASE (NORMOTENSION)
Mean arterial pressure (mm Hg)	40	75
Central venous pressure (mm Hg)	2	5
Cardiac output (L/min)	11.25	5.25
Heart rate (bpm)	150	70
Stroke volume (mL)	75	75
Systemic vascular resistance (dyne·sec·cm^{-5})	270	1067
Left ventricular volumes (mL):		
Diastole	225	125
Systole	150	50
Ejection fraction (%)	$\dfrac{225\ mL\ -\ 150\ mL}{225\ mL} = 33$	$\dfrac{125\ mL\ -\ 50\ mL}{125\ mL} = 60$

that result in reduced cardiac output and poor tissue perfusion. In these forms of shock, systemic vascular resistance is elevated as a compensatory mechanism to maintain blood pressure, and pulmonary artery oxygenation is reduced, reflecting enhanced extraction of oxygen from erythrocytes by hypoperfused peripheral tissues.

However, sepsis results in a much more complex form of shock. The onset of sepsis is frequently accompanied by hypovolemia due to both leakage of plasma (capillary leak) into the intravascular space and arterial and venous vasodilation. Correcting this hypovolemia by aggressive volume replacement results in a decreased systemic vascular resistance, increased or normal cardiac output, tachycardia, and elevated oxygen content in the pulmonary artery blood—the hyperdynamic shock syndrome. This hemodynamic pattern has been termed *distributive shock* to indicate the presumed maldistribution of systemic blood flow leading to the high blood oxygen content returning to the right side of the heart. Before volume resuscitation, patients with septic shock may manifest features of both hypovolemic and distributive shock, that is, a mixed form of shock.

Despite the elevated or normal cardiac output in volume-resuscitated septic shock, ventricular function is abnormal, as reflected by decreases in ventricular ejection fraction and stroke work and increases in end-diastolic and end-systolic volumes. In survivors, this cardiovascular dysfunction is reversible and returns to normal 5 to 10 days after septic shock. Certain hemodynamic patterns have prognostic implications. At disease onset, a lower heart rate predicts survival, probably reflecting less severe disease. Serial hemodynamic measurements demonstrate that normalization (within 24 hours) of either the elevated cardiac index or tachycardia is associated with survival, whereas persistence of the hyperdynamic state correlates with nonsurvival.

Vascular dysfunction is one of the most prominent physiologic and pathologic findings in septic shock. Patients usually manifest an overall decrease in systemic vascular resistance, reflecting widespread systemic vasodilation; however, some localized vascular beds are constricted. The decreased extraction of oxygen in the systemic circulation suggests that oxygen is not reaching or is not being used by cells. One hypothesis argues that vascular abnormalities (vasodilation, vasoconstriction, leukocyte aggregation, and endothelial cell dysfunction induced by complex interactions among the mediators summarized previously) result in decreased tissue perfusion. A second hypothesis argues that a direct mediator-induced cellular metabolic abnormality causes the failure of oxygen uptake. A central question in the pathogenesis of sepsis is whether decreased perfusion due to microvascular dysregulation is a primary cause or only an associated event in sepsis-induced organ failure.

Another method of judging whether a vascular perfusion abnormality is important in septic shock is to evaluate the relationship between oxygen delivery and oxygen consumption. In patients with cardiogenic or hypovolemic shock, when tissue hypoperfusion clearly occurs, increases in oxygen delivery result in increased consumption until hypoperfusion is reversed and oxygen consumption plateaus. Some investigators have argued that septic shock (especially with ARDS) is characterized by a pathologic delivery-

consumption relationship in which consumption continues to increase (and not plateau) with increased delivery, suggesting the presence of a perfusion abnormality that can be overcome by increasing delivery to a supranormal range. This observation is controversial, and animal experiments have yielded conflicting results. Although some initial clinical studies reported improved outcomes when oxygen delivery was increased, subsequent larger clinical trials comparing conventional strategies with strategies designed to increase oxygen delivery to a supranormal range have failed to demonstrate a survival advantage for the supranormal approach. Some studies suggest that pretreatment of critically ill surgical patients with supranormal oxygen delivery may provide some benefit, but further studies will be necessary to resolve these controversial findings.

CLINICAL MANIFESTATIONS AND DIAGNOSTIC EVALUATION

Sepsis and septic shock produce three categories of clinical manifestations (Fig. 96–3). First, the patient usually manifests symptoms and signs related to the primary focus of infection. If it is pneumonia, then the patient usually has cough, dyspnea, and productive sputum; if a urinary tract infection is the focus, then flank pain and dysuria would be expected. A careful history, physical examination, and directed imaging and laboratory studies will reveal the probable infectious focus in most patients. However, elderly, debilitated, and immunosuppressed patients may not exhibit the usual localizing clinical signs. In some patients, especially those with severe neutropenia, no site is identified. Second, patients usually manifest one or more signs of the systemic inflammatory response. Fever is the most characteristic and is frequently accompanied by shaking chills. A significant proportion of patients (perhaps 15%) will be hypothermic (<36.5°C or 97.6°F) or normothermic, especially the elderly, debilitated, or immunosuppressed. Elderly patients may present with tachypnea-induced respiratory alkalosis and mental status changes as the only signs of sepsis. Third, septic patients may develop evidence of shock, such as hypotension, lactic acidemia, and progressive organ system dysfunction. A variety of organs will show characteristic dysfunction (see Fig. 96–3).

The diagnosis of sepsis is confirmed by culturing pathogenic organisms from blood or from the likely site of infection. Blood cultures are positive in only 40 to 60% of patients with clinical manifestations of septic shock, probably owing to the intermittent nature of the bacteremia and the high incidence of prior antibiotic administration. A Gram stain from an abscess, empyema, or other usually sterile site can provide invaluable early diagnostic information.

TREATMENT

Septic shock can be managed effectively at three points along the pathogenetic sequence. First, the infection site can be eradicated with antimicrobials, surgical drainage, or both. Second, the serious disturbances in cardiovascular, respiratory, and other organ system

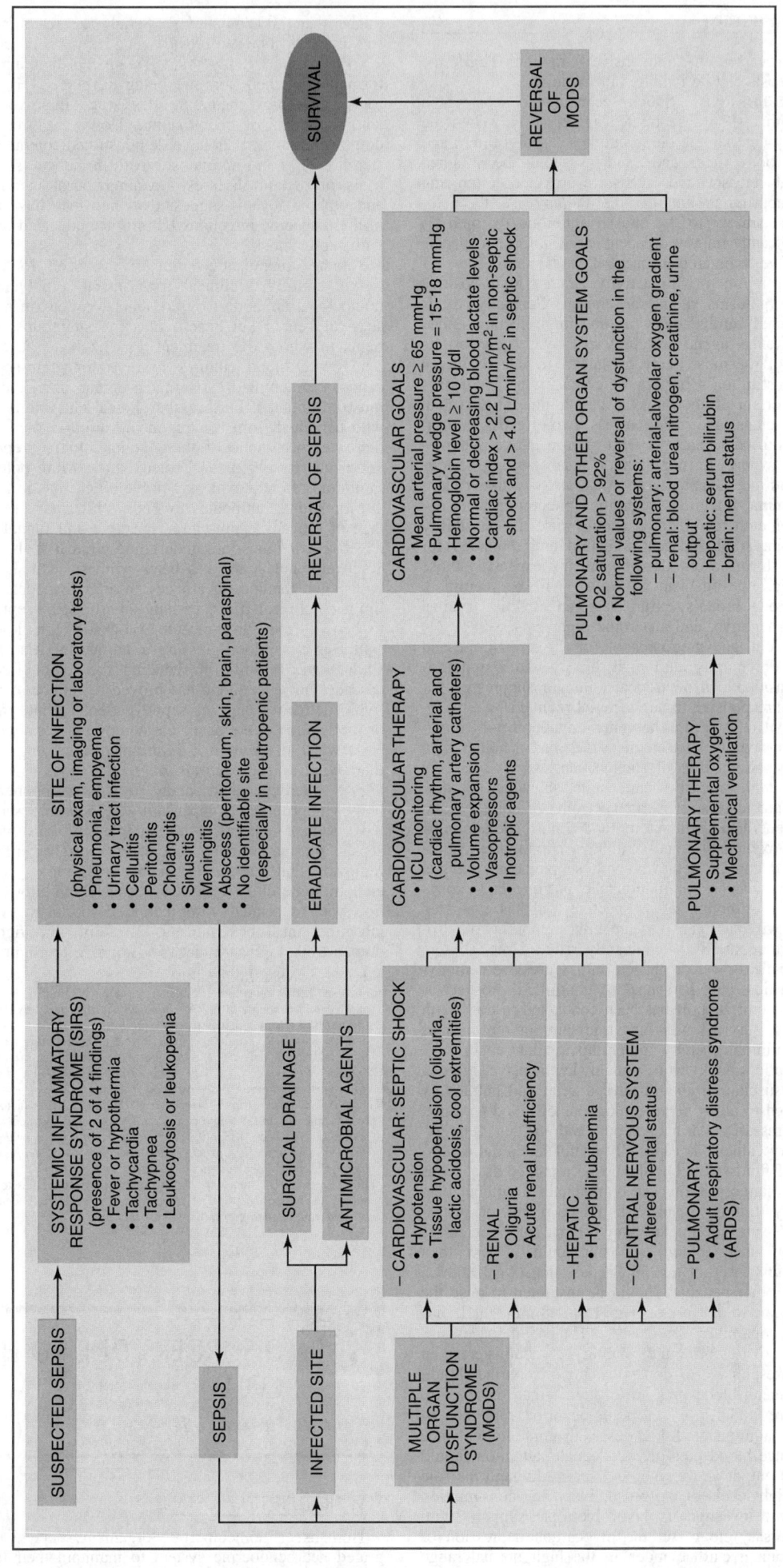

FIGURE 96–3 ■ Algorithm for diagnostic evaluation and management of sepsis and septic shock.

physiology can be reversed in an intensive care unit. Third, the toxic mediators of sepsis can be inhibited or modulated.

ANTIMICROBIAL THERAPY. Shock secondary to sepsis is a very major disease that should be treated aggressively. When the diagnosis is seriously entertained, blood cultures (usually three) and cultures of relevant body fluids and exudates should be obtained rapidly. Several large retrospective trials have provided convincing evidence that early appropriate antimicrobial therapy (i.e., the pathogen has in vitro sensitivity to the chosen antibiotic regimen) is associated with significantly improved patient survival. Once a specific pathogen is isolated, the antimicrobial spectrum can be narrowed.

A broad-spectrum regimen with activity against gram-positive and gram-negative organisms should be chosen. Generally, drugs should be administered intravenously at maximum recommended dosages, and bactericidal agents are preferred over bacteriostatic agents. Knowledge of the most likely organisms to infect a given site and the local institution's bacteriologic sensitivity and resistance patterns is important in choosing the best initial antimicrobial regimen. Many physicians favor using at least two effective antimicrobial agents in neutropenic patients with gram-negative pneumonia and a two-drug synergistic combination when treating serious enterococcal infection (see Chapter 314). Anaerobes are likely pathogens in intra-abdominal infections, aspiration pneumonia, and abscesses. Intravascular catheter infection should raise the possibility of methicillin-resistant staphylococcal infection and the need for vancomycin therapy. In up to one third of patients, especially those who are neutropenic, no organism or source will be identified. Such patients require a broad-spectrum regimen effective against gram-positive, gram-negative, and anaerobic organisms such as (1) vancomycin, gentamicin, and metronidazole or (2) ceftazidime and gentamicin. The need for early antifungal therapy with amphotericin B should be considered in neutropenic, immunosuppressed patients and in those unresponsive to antibacterial regimens.

THERAPY FOR SHOCK. Before the general availability of intensive care units, gram-negative bacteremic shock had a higher than 90% mortality. Now, about 50% of such patients survive, largely because of treatment in intensive care units, in which cardiac rhythm, blood pressure, cardiac performance, oxygen delivery, and metabolic derangements can be monitored and abnormalities can be corrected. Adequate oxygenation and ventilatory support are critical goals of therapy and can be achieved with supplemental oxygen and, if necessary, mechanical ventilation and positive end-expiratory pressure (PEEP). Although no prospective trial has evaluated outcomes with and without intensive care unit support, two retrospective studies have reported a significantly reduced mortality in septic shock when patients were managed with aggressive hemodynamic support by critical care personnel. A controlled, prospective trial of intensive care unit support has been conducted in dogs with gram-negative sepsis; survival was increased only in the animals that received both antibiotic therapy and cardiovascular support.

Patients with septic shock who remain hypotensive after a 1- or 2-L volume resuscitation should have arterial and pulmonary artery catheters placed to allow serial evaluations of blood pressure, ventricular filling pressures, cardiac output, and oxygen delivery. The pulmonary artery catheter is especially useful for initial assessment and titration of fluid status but should be removed as soon as the patient's hemodynamic stability can be maintained without it in the pulmonary artery. Initial emphasis should be placed on restoring mean blood pressure to greater than 65 mm Hg. Aggressive volume resuscitation using blood (if hemoglobin is less than 10 g/100 mL), colloid (if serum albumin is less than 2 g/100 mL), or crystalloid (in all other patients) should be instituted to raise the pulmonary artery mean wedge pressure to 15 to 18 mm Hg. If hypotension persists, dopamine (low-dose and then, if necessary, higher doses up to 20 μg/kg/minute) should be administered. In patients who are unresponsive to dopamine, norepinephrine should be infused to raise mean blood pressure to higher than 65 mm Hg. Patients who require high doses of norepinephrine may benefit from concomitantly administered low-dose dopamine to enhance renal blood flow. Once blood pressure is adequate, attention should be turned to cardiac output and oxygen delivery. Although the role of achieving very high levels of oxygen delivery and consumption is controversial, most investigators favor inotropic support (with dobutamine, if necessary) to offset the myocardial depression of sepsis and to maintain a cardiac index in the high normal range

(higher than 4.0 L/minute/m²). Serial measures of lactate, urine output, and organ function can provide good measures of patient prognosis.

MEDIATOR INHIBITORS. Treatments that inhibit the action or formation of mediators are being developed. High-dose corticosteroids can inhibit mediator release and improve survival in some animal models of endotoxemia. However, three prospective, randomized clinical trials have demonstrated convincingly that corticosteroids do not improve survival in human septic shock. Small trials in certain diseases—meningococcal meningitis in children and typhoid fever—suggest that they may have a therapeutic role in these specific infections but are not indicated in the usual patient with septic shock.

Another therapeutic strategy has been to inhibit endotoxin. Large, controlled clinical trials using a polyclonal antisera and monoclonal antibodies raised against endotoxin revealed no overall survival benefit but benefit in some subgroups. However, the patients in whom the treatment was likely to be effective (e.g., patients with blood cultures positive for gram-negative organisms) cannot be identified early in the course of infection, when therapy must be initiated. Further, the clinical characteristics of the patients who benefited from the treatment varied in the different trials. For these reasons, none of these antiendotoxin preparations has been approved for use in the United States. More potent pharmacologic inhibitors of endotoxin may prove efficacious in future trials.

Monoclonal antibodies to TNF, which have the theoretic advantage of efficacy against gram-positive and fungal as well as gram-negative infections, are undergoing clinical trials at present. An IL-1 receptor antagonist has been synthesized in large quantities and has shown therapeutic efficacy in animal models of sepsis; in preliminary clinical trials, certain subgroups of septic patients appear to benefit from IL-1 receptor blockade. Inhibitors of nitric oxide synthesis raise blood pressure in animal models of septic shock and show some promise in reducing the toxic effects of the sepsis cascade; however, none has proved to reduce mortality in prospectively defined groups of septic patients. Thus, mediator inhibition or modulation is not accepted therapy of sepsis and septic shock.

A word of caution is warranted regarding mediator inhibitor therapy. The pathogenesis of septic shock is very complex and highly interdependent; many of the components represent the body's appropriate compensatory response to sepsis and therefore have salutary effects. For example, in dogs with gram-negative sepsis, plasma exchange increases mortality, presumably because removal of all circulating mediators is more harmful than beneficial. In some clinical trials using TNF inhibitors, high-dose inhibition was associated with increased mortality. All these mediator inhibitors must be evaluated carefully with rigorous animal and human trials to ensure that they improve morbidity and mortality.

Fisher CJ Jr, Agosti JM, Opal SM, et al: Treatment of septic shock with the tumor necrosis factor receptor: Fc fusion protein. N Engl J Med 334:1697, 1996. *A multicenter clinical trial of TNF inhibitor therapy in sepsis demonstrating the potential harmful effects of excessive TNF inhibition.*

Kumar A, Kosuri R, Kandula P, et al: Effect of epinephrine and amrinone on contractility and cyclic adenosine monophosphate generation of tumor necrosis factor α exposed myocytes. Crit Care Med 27:286, 1999. *Data demonstrating important differences among inotropic/vasopressor agents in sepsis.*

Kumar A, Venkateswarlu T, Dee L, et al: Tumor necrosis factor and interleukin-1 are responsible for in-vitro myocardial cell depression induced by human septic shock serum. J Exp Med 183:949, 1996. *Recent convincing evidence that a synergistic effect of TNF and IL-1 produces the myocardial cell depressant activity present in blood of septic shock patients.*

Zeni F, Freeman B, Natanson C: Anti-inflammatory therapies to treat sepsis and septic shock: A reassessment. Crit Care Med 25:7, 1997. *A concise summary of our present understanding of antimediator therapies in sepsis.*

97 DISORDERS DUE TO HEAT AND COLD

Ernest Yoder

TEMPERATURE HOMEOSTASIS

Humans as homeothermic organisms depend on a highly integrated neuroendocrine system to maintain their thermal homeostasis. Equilibrium between heat gained and lost must be maintained to prevent the organism from becoming either hyperthermic or hypothermic. Thus, body temperature is normally maintained at $36.5 \pm 0.7°$ C ($97.7 \pm 1.3°$ F). Mechanisms of heat transfer to the environment, largely dependent on a temperature gradient between the body and its milieu, are radiation, conduction, convection, and evaporation.

Information from peripheral and central receptors is integrated by the hypothalamus, which effects changes in autonomic tone and endocrinologic function to maintain stable body temperature. Voluntary responses, also important in preventing hypo- and hyperthermia, include moving to a cooler or warmer environment, removing or adding clothing, decreasing or increasing activity level, and increasing or decreasing exposed skin areas.

HYPERTHERMIC SYNDROMES

Hyperthermia is present when core body temperature is higher than $37.2°$ C. Heat injury syndromes may result in body temperatures higher than $40°$ C ($104°$ F) (Table 97–1). When temperatures are above $41°$ C, enzymes are denatured, mitochondrial function is disturbed, cell membranes are destabilized, and oxygen-dependent metabolic pathways are disrupted. Multisystem failure regularly occurs concomitantly with heat injury syndromes, along with significant associated morbidity and mortality. Patients with these syndromes usually require admission to the intensive care unit.

Painful spasm of major muscle groups is the hallmark of *heat cramps.* Typically seen in young, unacclimatized athletes or laborers who exert themselves excessively in a hot climate, heat cramps are related to excessive losses of sodium, chloride, and water. Patients complain of nausea, vomiting, and fatigue in addition to muscle cramps, with the onset of symptoms typically occurring several hours after ceasing strenuous activity.

Heat exhaustion, the most common heat injury syndrome seen in athletes, may be preceded by heat cramps and is due to severe dehydration and electrolyte loss. In the young, heat exhaustion usually occurs following strenuous activity by unacclimatized individuals in a hot, humid environment. In the elderly, the problem is usually related to inadequate cardiovascular response to heat with disruption of normal compensatory mechanisms. Patients frequently complain of cramps, headache, fatigue, nausea, and vomiting. They appear listless, with pallor of the skin and profuse sweating. Other clinical findings include orthostatic hypotension, core temperatures of 37.5 to $39°$ C (99.5 to $102.2°$ F), altered mental status, incoordination, and diffuse weakness.

Heatstroke, classified as *exertional* or *nonexertional,* is a syndrome due to acute disruption of thermoregulatory mechanisms that is manifested by central nervous system depression, hypohidrosis, core temperatures of $41°$ C or higher, and severe physiologic and biochemical abnormalities. Exertional heatstroke occurs in people working or exercising in a warm environment with an over-

Table 97–1 ■ FACTORS PREDISPOSING TO HYPERTHERMIA

Patient factors	Medical conditions
Lack of acclimatization	Alcoholism
Dehydration	Neurologic lesions/events
Exercising when poorly trained	Cardiovascular disease
Fever/infection	Skin/sweat gland diseases
Obesity	Diabetes mellitus
Fatigue/exhaustion	Thyrotoxicosis
Excessive clothing	Hypokalemia
Advanced age	Chronic obstructive pulmonary
Living or working on upper	disease
floors of buildings	Psychiatric illness
Environmental factors	**Drugs**
High ambient temperature	Amphetamines
High humidity	Anticholinergics
Lack of wind	Antidepressants
	Antihistamines
	Anti-Parkinson's drugs
	Barbiturates
	β-Blockers
	Butyrophenones
	Diuretics
	Ethanol
	Hallucinogens
	Phenothiazines

Table 97–2 ■ INITIAL DIAGNOSTIC STUDIES: HYPERTHERMIC AND HYPOTHERMIC STATES

Electrocardiogram (ECG)
Chest radiograph
Complete blood count (CBC) with differential
Platelet count
Serum studies
   Lactate dehydrogenase
   Transaminases
   Alkaline phosphatase
   Bilirubin
   Creatine kinase
   Blood urea nitrogen
   Creatinine
   Phosphate
   Calcium
   Glucose
   Electrolytes
   Uric acid
   Lactate*
   Cortisol*
   Thyroid-stimulating hormone (TSH), T_3, T_4*
   Prothrombin time (PT) and partial thromboplastin time (PTT)
Fibrin split products
Fibrinogen
Arterial blood gases
Urinalysis
Toxicology screen

*Necessary only in hypothermic states.

whelmed but unimpaired central thermoregulatory center. Nonexertional heat stroke occurs most frequently in elderly, debilitated, schizophrenic, intoxicated, or paralyzed individuals. These people have impaired central and/or peripheral thermoregulatory mechanisms (physiologic or drug-induced autonomic impairment), impaired awareness of or inability to leave a hot environment, poor acclimatization, and inadequate ability to increase cardiac output in response to heat.

Severe hypothermia associated with rhabdomyolysis, consumption coagulopathy, and acute renal failure may be related to ingestion of amphetamines, amphetamine cogeners (ecstasy), and cocaine. Presentation of such patients may mimic heat stroke. *Neuroleptic malignant syndrome* is a complex of extrapyramidal muscular rigidity (see Chapters 459 to 464), high core temperature, altered level of consciousness, and elevated creatine kinase levels occurring as an acute or subacute reaction to therapy with neuroleptic medications.

Malignant hyperthermia (see Chapter 508) is a hypermetabolic, myopathic syndrome that is chemically or stress induced and is manifested by an abrupt rise in core temperature, vigorous muscle contractions, metabolic and respiratory acidosis, and ventricular arrhythmias. It usually occurs when inducing anesthesia.

Consequences of heat-induced cell damage are rhabdomyolysis, heart failure, cardiac arrhythmias, vasodilation, cytotoxic cerebral edema, hypotension, acute renal failure, adult respiratory distress syndrome, gastrointestinal hemorrhage, and acute hepatic failure. Concomitant laboratory abnormalities include hyperkalemia, hypocalcemia, hyperphosphatemia or hypophosphatemia, rising creatinine, hemoconcentration, stress leukocytosis, thrombocytopenia, consumptive coagulopathy, lactic acidosis, hypoglycemia, proteinuria, and an active urinary sediment. Arterial blood gas values should be corrected for hyperthermia. PaO_2 values are incorrectly low and should be increased by 6% for each degree centigrade above 37; $PaCO_2$ is also lower and should be increased by 4.4% for each degree centigrade above 37; and pH is high and should be reduced by 0.015 unit for each degree centigrade above 37. These corrections are approximate, and nomograms provide the most precise corrections. The expected abnormalities guide the recommended laboratory evaluation of patients with pathologic states of altered core temperature (Table 97–2).

MANAGEMENT

The primary goal of therapy is rapid cooling. Three initial steps include removal from the hot environment, inhibition of thermoge-

Table 97–3 ■ MANAGEMENT OF HYPERTHERMIA

1. Protect the airway
2. Insert at least two large-bore intravenous lines
3. Monitor core temperature
   a. Pulmonary artery
   b. Rectal probe
   c. Esophageal probe
4. Actively cool the skin until core temperature reaches 39° C
   a. Exposure to cool environment
   b. Wetting with water (avoid alcohol rubs)
   c. Continuous fanning
   d. Ice baths/immersion (22° C)
   e. Axillary/perineal ice packs
   f. Infusion of room-temperature saline
   g. Gastric/colonic iced saline lavage
   h. Peritoneal lavage with cool saline
5. If shivering occurs, administer chlorpromazine, 10 to 25 mg intramuscularly
6. Monitor for seizures
7. Monitor electrocardiogram for dysrhythmia
8. Obtain serial diagnostic studies (see Table 97–2)

nesis, and active cooling (Table 97–3). The severity of the patient's clinical condition dictates the aggressiveness of cooling techniques.

Heat cramps and heat exhaustion rarely result in permanent sequelae. Mild to moderate neurologic, hepatic, and renal dysfunction seen in heatstroke usually resolves after return to normothermia. Muscle weakness may persist for several months when rhabdomyolysis has been severe. The greater the severity of injury, the greater the likelihood of permanent sequelae. Heatstroke mortality may approach 50% and is usually associated with advanced age and severe organ failure.

HYPOTHERMIC SYNDROMES

Hypothermia, defined as a core body temperature lower than 35° C (95° F), is classified as *accidental* (primary) or *secondary.* The accidental form is defined as a spontaneous decrease of core temperature to lower than 35° C, usually in a cold environment, often but not necessarily associated with an acute medical problem, and without a primary disturbance of the temperature-regulating center.

Secondary hypothermia is characterized by dysfunction of hypothalamic thermoregulation. An underlying illness or drug is often the predisposing factor (see Table 97–4).

Hypothermia affects virtually every body system owing to generalized slowing of enzymatic activity, peripheral vasoconstriction, and uncoupling of oxygen-dependent metabolism. Alterations in cardiovascular physiology include an early catecholamine-mediated increase in heart rate, cardiac output, and mean arterial pressure.

Later, negative inotropic and chronotropic effects of hypothermia and decreased effective blood volume cause diminished cardiac output and tissue perfusion.

Patients may present with tachypnea, but as hypothermia becomes pronounced, there is depression of the respiratory center. Shivering increases oxygen consumption. Because alveolar ventilation is decreased, PaO_2 may decline to subnormal levels. Hypoxemia also may result from aspiration pneumonia, pulmonary edema, or adult respiratory distress syndrome. Arterial blood gas values should be corrected for hypothermia. PaO_2 values are incorrectly high and should be decreased by 4.4% for each degree centigrade below 37; $PaCO_2$ is also higher and should be decreased by 3.5% for each degree centigrade below 37; and pH is lower and should be increased by 0.015 unit for each degree centigrade below 37. These corrections are approximate, and nomograms provide the most precise corrections.

The electrocardiogram may demonstrate sinus bradycardia and slowing of conduction with atrioventricular block, prolonged QT interval, widened QRS complex, and T-wave inversion. P waves may be absent. When core temperature declines to 32° C, the classic Osborne (or J) wave appears (Fig. 97–1). The cold heart is highly irritable, and any physical stimulation may lead to ventricular fibrillation.

Owing to enzyme damage, renal concentrating ability is lost, resulting in very dilute (cold diuresis) urine and systemic hyperosmolarity. Later, with decreased perfusion, acute tubular necrosis may develop. Laboratory abnormalities include metabolic acidosis, hyperkalemia, hyponatremia, hyperglycemia, and hyperphosphatemia. Complications of hypothermia also include rhabdomyolysis, gastric dilation, ileus, upper gastrointestinal bleeding, acute pancreatitis, and severe hepatic dysfunction. Hematologic alterations include hemoconcentration, increased blood viscosity, thrombocytopenia, granulocytopenia, and consumptive coagulopathy. Infection is a frequent sequela of hypothermia.

Hypothermia should be considered in the differential diagnosis of any hypotensive, comatose patient. Initial evaluation (see Table 97–2) should be directed toward identifying predisposing conditions (see Table 97–4).

MANAGEMENT

The goals of management depend on the severity of the hypothermia but in all cases are to prevent further heat loss, increase core temperature, and anticipate and prevent complications (Table 97–5). If the person is without vital signs, cardiopulmonary resuscitation should be initiated and continued until the patient is normothermic.

Because of liver impairment and cardiac irritability, all drugs must be used with caution. Digitalis should be avoided. If myxedema or panhypopituitarism is suspected, proper hormonal replacement therapy should be initiated. Dysrhythmias can be treated safely with lidocaine, propranolol, and bretylium. Electrocardioversion is rarely successful. Vasoactive agents may be required for

Table 97–4 ■ FACTORS PREDISPOSING TO HYPOTHERMIA

Patient factors	Medical conditions
Inadequate clothing	Alcoholism
Extremes of age	Burns, severe
Mental impairment	Cancer chemotherapy
Immobility	Cardiac failure
Altered level of consciousness	Central nervous system lesions/events
Debility and exhaustion	Dementia
Wet clothing	Encephalopathy
Drugs	Diabetes
Alcohol	Hypoadrenalism
Anesthetics	Hypoglycemia
Antidepressants	Hypopituitarism
Antithyroid agents	Malnutrition
Cannabis	Myxedema
Hypoglycemic agents	Prolonged cardiopulmonary resuscitation
Major tranquilizers	Prolonged surgery
Narcotics	Sepsis
Paralyzing agents	Shock
Sedative/hypnotics	Uremia

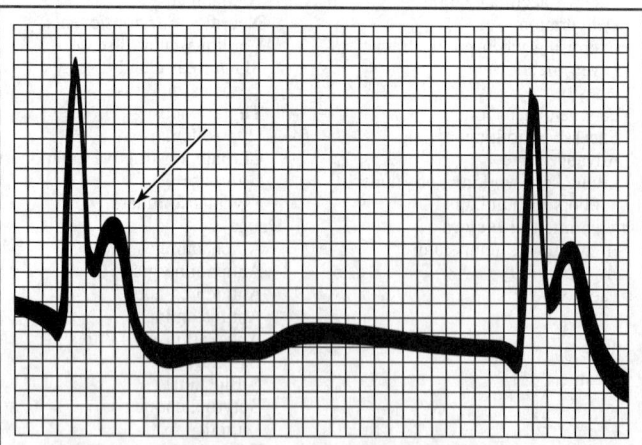

FIGURE 97–1 ■ J (Osborne) wave.

Table 97–5 ■ MANAGEMENT OF HYPOTHERMIA

Mild hypothermia (34–36° C)

1. Remove from cold environment, replace wet clothing, cover with blankets or equivalent, use gentle passive rewarming techniques.
2. Give warm oxygen through a mask or an endotracheal tube.
3. Give warm dextrose/saline intravenous fluids.
4. Warm the environment (thermostat, overhead lights).
5. Monitor electrocardiogram, respiratory status, core temperature.
6. Obtain initial diagnostic studies (see Table 97–2).

Moderate to severe hypothermia (≤33° C)

1. Admit to intensive care unit.
2. Peripheral active rewarming: heating blankets, heating pads, hot-water bottles, warming lights, warm water immersion.
3. Actively warm central core: inhale heated, humidified oxygen, gastric lavage, colonic irrigation, and warmed intravenous fluids.
4. Consider special beds, and protect against pressure necrosis.
5. If core temperature is not rising 0.5 to 1.0° C per hour, consider peritoneal dialysis, bladder lavage, hemodialysis, or bypass.
6. Anticipate multiorgan dysfunction and secondary infection.

severe hypotension. Intravenous sodium bicarbonate should be used only in severe acidosis (pH lower than 7.1) and with extreme caution.

Lloyd EL: Accidental hypothermia. Resuscitation 32:111, 1996. *A critical review of hypothermia research with emphasis on management.*

Loke J, MacLennan D: Malignant hyperthermia and central core disease: Disorders of Ca++ release channels. Am J Med 104:470–486, 1998. *The biologic explanation for this disorder.*

Simon HB: Hyperthermia. N Engl J Med 329:483, 1993. *A complete review of hyperthermia, including pathophysiology, clinical presentation, and details of management.*

98 ACUTE POISONING

Lester M. Haddad

Poisoning is defined as "to injure or kill with poison, a chemical substance that usually kills, injures, or impairs an organism." The terms *poisoning* and *drug overdose* often are used interchangeably, especially with prescription drugs, although, by definition, a drug overdose does not produce poisoning unless it causes clinical symptoms.

Defining the extent of human poisoning is not easy, because the three major sources of data have different viewpoints and surely overlap. The Toxic Exposure Surveillance System (TESS) of the American Association of Poison Control Centers records more than 2 million exposures and more than 700 deaths annually. Ninety-nine per cent of all patients who have experienced significant poisoning present directly to hospital emergency departments, which record more than 8,000 drug abuse deaths annually, the most common of which involves cocaine. The National Center of Health Statistics reviews primarily medical examiner death certificates and reports carbon monoxide (CO) as the leading cause of death. Analgesics remain a leading cause of poisoning, and calcium channel blocker overdose has surpassed digitalis as the most common cause of cardiovascular drug death.

DIAGNOSIS AND EMERGENCY MANAGEMENT

The general approach to the poisoned patient may be divided into seven phases: (1) emergency management; (2) clinical evaluation; (3) elimination of poison from the gastrointestinal tract, skin, and eyes or removal from the site of exposure in inhalation poisoning; (4) administration of an antidote; (5) elimination of any absorbed substance; (6) supportive therapy; and (7) observation and disposition.

EMERGENCY MANAGEMENT. Because overdose patients often present moribund, resuscitation with airway establishment, adequate ventilation and perfusion, and restoration of all vital signs (including temperature) must be accomplished first. Continuous cardiac and pulse oximetry monitoring is essential. Rapid-sequence intubation may be indicated. Naloxone, 2 mg intravenously (IV); thiamine, 100 mg IV; and 50% glucose, 50 mL IV (if the patient is

hypoglycemic by Dextrostix), are given to all adult patients in coma after inserting an intravenous line and drawing appropriate blood samples. Maintenance of blood pressure and tissue perfusion may require adequate volume replacement, correction of acid-base disturbances, antidotal therapy (Table 98–1), and pressor agents. Cardiac arrhythmias and seizures should be treated appropriately if possible.

CLINICAL EVALUATION. Any patient presenting with multisystem involvement should be suspected of poisoning until proven otherwise. A thorough history and physical examination are essential. Although the initial manifestations of poisoning are legion, a patient with acute poisoning often presents with coma, cardiac arrhythmia (Table 98–2), seizures (Table 98–3), metabolic acidosis, or gastrointestinal disturbances, either together as symptom complexes or as isolated events. Symptom complexes, or toxic syndromes, may give clues to an unknown poisoning. For example, a patient with a history of depression who presents in coma with seizures, a widened QRS complex or dysrhythmia on electrocardiogram (ECG), and dilated pupils suggests tricyclic antidepressant overdose. Hepatic, renal, respiratory, and hematologic disturbances are generally delayed manifestations of poisoning. The physical examination may provide important clues (Table 98–4), and laboratory studies help guide diagnosis and therapy.

ELIMINATION OF POISON. In the event of inhalation (e.g., smoke, carbon monoxide, hydrogen sulfide, or chlorine gas), the patient should be removed from the site of exposure, and 100% oxygen should be administered. Caustic alkalis, acids, and other chemicals should be removed from the eye with copious irrigation by normal saline, which should be continued for at least 30 minutes. For caustic alkalis, irrigation should continue for at least 30 minutes, and emergency ophthalmologic consultation must be obtained; skin exposure requires 30-minute irrigation as well.

The majority of poisoning occurs via the gastrointestinal tract. Gastric decontamination is indicated to reduce absorption of the poisonous substance. Principal modalities in historical order include syrup of ipecac, gastric lavage, activated charcoal, and whole-bowel irrigation. Controversy has raged over which therapy is most effective, because with each individual patient the exact amount ingested and the exact amount remaining after each procedure is never known. However, it is becoming apparent that the availability of multiple options allows the clinician to individualize treatment for each particular situation.

Syrup of ipecac is still indicated for home use. Dosage recommendations include 10 mL for ages 6 to 12 months, 15 mL for ages 1 to 12 years, and 30 mL for ages 12 years to adulthood. Contraindications to the use of syrup of ipecac include caustic or petroleum distillate ingestion, impending or frank coma, and seizures. Because both gastric lavage and activated charcoal have each demonstrated superiority over ipecac in recent studies, ipecac is seldom used in the hospital emergency setting today, although it is still useful in the child who will not drink charcoal and whose parents will not allow a nasogastric tube.

Gastric lavage has been shown to be effective within the first hour of ingestion; with proper airway management, it is indicated for the critically ill patient with a recent life-threatening ingestion such as tricyclic antidepressants, calcium channel blockers, digoxin, salicylate, theophylline, or unknown substances. The largest-bore tube possible, such as a 36 French Ewald with gravity drainage should be used. Gastric lavage is contraindicated in caustic ingestion.

Activated charcoal is clearly the single most important intervention that can be provided to an overdose patient. Activated charcoal is considered safe and adequate treatment for all but a few overdoses (Table 98–5) and is especially useful for patients who are awake or have ingested only a mildly toxic substance. Activated charcoal is often administered during field transport, may be beneficial before lavage, and is definitely indicated after lavage. The dose is 1 g/kg, or 50 to 100 g in an adult. Commercial preparations of charcoal usually include sorbitol as a cathartic; however, charcoal alone should be used for young children. Serially administered activated charcoal (50 g every 4 hours) has a role in the inpatient management of overdose of drugs that enter the hepatobiliary circulation (tricyclic antidepressants, digitoxin, glutethimide) or diffuse into the gastrointestinal lumen (theophylline and phenobarbital).

Table 98-1 ■ COMMON EMERGENCY ANTIDOTES

POISON	ANTIDOTE	ADULT DOSAGE*	COMMENTS
Acetaminophen	N-acetylcysteine	140 mg/kg initial oral dose, followed by 70 mg/kg q 4 hr for 17 doses	Most effective within 16 hr; may be useful up to 24 hr; IV N-acetylcysteine protocols available.
Atropine	Physostigmine	Initial dose 0.5–2 mg (IV) Children: 0.02 mg/kg	Can produce convulsions, bradycardia, and asystole.
Benzodiazepines	Flumazenil	0.2 mg (2 mL) (IV) over 15 sec; repeat 0.2 mg (IV) every minute as necessary; initial dose not to exceed 1 mg	Recommended only for reversal of pure benzodiazepine sedation.
β-Blockers	Glucagon	1 mg/mL ampule; 5–10 mg (IV) initially	Stimulates cyclic adenosine monophosphate synthesis; increases myocardial contractility.
Calcium channel blockers	Calcium	Calcium chloride 10%, 1 g (10 mL) (IV) over 5 min as initial dose; repeat as necessary in critical patients	Each syringe contains 1 g or 10 mL of 10% calcium chloride; each milliliter contains 100 mg of calcium chloride or 1.4 mEq of calcium.
Carbon monoxide	Oxygen	Hyperbaric oxygen in critical patients	
Cyanide	Amyl nitrate	Pearls every 2 min	
	Sodium thiosulfate	25% solution 50 mL (IV) over 10 min; 1.65 mL/kg for children	Forms harmless sodium thiocyanate.
	Sodium nitrite	10 mL of 3% solution over 3 min (IV); 0.33 mL (10 mg 3% solution)/kg initially for children	Methemoglobin-cyanide complex causes hypotension; dosage assumes normal hemoglobin.
Digitalis	Digibind FAB antibodies (antigen-binding fragments)	IV dose of Digibind in critical patients with unknown ingestion: 800 mg (20 vials); dosage if serum digoxin and patient's weight (in kg) are known: the number of vials to administer = [concentration (in ng/mL) × 5.6 × kg]/600	IV dose of Digibind should be equimolar to total body load of digoxin; one vial Digibind contains 40 mg of FAB fragments, which neutralize 0.6 mg of digoxin. The number of mg of digoxin ingested divided by 0.6 is the number of vials required; indicated for life-threatening cardiac arrhythmias, hyperkalemia, serum digoxin level >10 ng/mL in adults or 4 ng/mL in children.
Hydrofluoric acid	Calcium	Calcium gluconate gel or calcium carbonate paste; 10% calcium gluconate 10 mL in 40 mL D₅W via intra-arterial infusion over 4 hr may be indicated for significant digital hydrofluoric acid burns	An intra-arterial infusion of 10 mL 10% calcium gluconate (1 syringe) provides 4.65 mEq of elemental calcium to bind fluoride ion, preventing cellular injury and tissue necrosis.
Iron	Deferoxamine	Initial dose: 40–90 mg/kg (IM) not to exceed 1 g; 15 mg/kg/hr (IV)	Deferoxamine mesylate forms excretable ferrioxamine complex.
Lead	Dimercaptosuccinic acid (succimer)	5-d course of 30 mg/kg/d in 3 divided doses; then 14-day course of 20 mg/kg/d divided in 2 doses	Succimer 100 mg capsule; oral congener of chelator dimercaprol, indicated for blood lead levels >45 μg/dL.
Mercury Arsenic Gold	Dimercaprol	5 mg/kg (IM) as soon as possible	Each milliliter of dimercaprol-in-oil has dimercaprol, 100 mg, in 210 mg (21%) benzyl benzoate and 680 mg peanut oil; forms stable, nontoxic, excretable cyclic compound.
Methyl alcohol Ethylene glycol	Ethyl alcohol	1 mL/kg of 100% ethanol initially in glucose solution; dilute ethanol to 10%; maintain blood level of 100 mg/dL; maintenance dose 0.15 mL/kg/hr (double during dialysis)	Ethyl alcohol competes for alcohol dehydrogenase, prevents formation of formic acid in methanol toxicity and of oxalates in ethylene glycol poisoning.
Nitrites	Methylene blue	0.2 mL/kg of 1% solution (IV) over 5 min	Often exchange transfusion is needed for severe methemoglobinemia.
Opiates, Darvon, Lomotil	Naloxone	2.0 mg (IV); 0.1 mg/kg (IV) for children; repeat as needed	Naloxone; no respiratory depression (0.4 mg/1 mL amp).
Organophosphates	Pralidoxime (2-PAM) (Protopam Chloride)	Initial dose: 1 g (IV); Children: 25–50 mg/kg (IV)	Specific: breaks alkyl phosphate-cholinesterase bond; up to 500 mg every hour may be necessary in the critical adult patient.
	Atropine	Initial dose: 0.5–2 mg (IV) 0.05 mg/kg (IV) initially for children	Physiologic: blocks acetylcholine. Cardiac monitoring and proper oxygenation are indicated.
Tricyclic antidepressants	Sodium bicarbonate	Sodium bicarbonate 1–2 ampules (IV); (1 mEq/kg) (IV) bolus for initial dose; (IV) drip to maintain arterial pH of 7.5	One ampule of 50 mL sodium bicarbonate contains 50 mEq NaHCO₃ in 50 mL or 1 molar sodium bicarbonate; IV bolus for life-threatening cardiac arrhythmias.

*Dosages listed may require modification according to specific clinical conditions.
Updated and adapted from Haddad LM: Acute poisoning. In Bennett JC, Plum F (eds): Cecil Textbook of Medicine, 20th ed. Philadelphia, WB Saunders, 1996; and the American College of Emergency Physicians poster on poisoning, Dallas, Texas, 1980.

Whole-bowel irrigation with a nonabsorbable osmotically active compound such as polyethylene glycol (GoLYTELY) is a new means of catharsis. In adults, 240 mL by mouth or nasogastric tube every 10 to 15 minutes is given until the gallon container is emptied or the rectal effluent becomes clear. Whole-bowel irrigation is probably useful for awake, functional patients who have ingested iron tablets, sustained-release preparations such as theophylline or calcium channel blockers, or "crack" vials or cocaine packets.

ADMINISTRATION OF AN ANTIDOTE. With the development of sophisticated new antidotes and the changing spectrum of clinical poisoning, the use of emergency antidotes is becoming the primary treatment method in clinical toxicology (see Table 98–1). With known poisoning, early use is indicated to provide emergency

Table 98-2 ■ COMMON TOXIC CAUSES OF CARDIAC ARRHYTHMIA

Tricyclic antidepressants*
Arsenic
β-Blockers
Calcium channel blockers
Carbon monoxide
Chloral hydrate
Clonidine
Cocaine
Succinylcholine
Cyanide
Digitalis
Phenothiazines
Phosphorus
Physostigmine
Quinine

*Tricyclic antidepressants are listed first, as they remain the number one cause of prescription drug death; the list then follows alphabetically.

Table 98-4 ■ IMPORTANT CLUES ON PHYSICAL EXAMINATION

CLINICAL FINDING	DIAGNOSTIC EXAMPLE
Needle tracks	Intravenous drug abuse
Characteristic odor of breath	Gasoline
Destruction of nasal mucosa/cartilage	Cocaine
New significant heart murmur	Infective endocarditis
Pulmonary edema	Heroin
Boardlike abdomen	Black widow spider bite
Changes in neurologic status	Organophosphates

stabilization, often within the first hour. Admission to an intensive care unit is generally indicated following antidotal therapy.

ELIMINATION OF ABSORBED SUBSTANCE. Specific methods are indicated to eliminate certain absorbed substances (Table 98–6). Hemodialysis is also indicated for any drug overdose patient who has severe intractable metabolic acidosis, severe electrolyte abnormalities, or renal failure.

SUPPORTIVE CARE. Observation and prudent medical care are the mainstays of therapy for the poisoned patient and may be all that is necessary for the majority of patients. The indiscriminate use of drugs, antidotes, and gastric lavage should be avoided. Hospitalization in an intensive care unit is often indicated for serious poisoning.

OBSERVATION AND DISPOSITION

The disposition of the patient with intoxication may involve medical and psychiatric care as well as sound follow-up. All patients admitted to the hospital with intentional overdose warrant close observation and the institution of suicide precautions.

SPECIFIC AGENTS

Acetaminophen is one of the three leading over-the-counter analgesics (Tylenol, Panadol, and Tempra) and is one of the leading causes of drug overdose in the United States as well as the leading cause in the United Kingdom. It is also a leading cause of liver failure. Acetaminophen is metabolized in the liver and is relatively safe in therapeutic doses. A small fraction of each administered dose is converted to a reactive metabolite, N-acetyl-p-benzoquino-neimine (NAPQI), by the cytochrome P-450–dependent mixed-function oxidase hepatic enzymes. With therapeutic doses, glutathione stores can detoxify NAPQI by conjugation. Glutathione stores are depleted in overdoses, however, and NAPQI covalently binds to cellular proteins, producing hepatocellular necrosis.

The therapeutic dose of acetaminophen is 10 to 20 mg/kg every 4 hours. Toxicity is likely to occur after a minimum acute ingestion of 140 mg/kg, or about 10 g in an adult. Acetaminophen poisoning clinically produces only nausea, vomiting, and anorexia 12 to 24 hours after ingestion. Hepatic coma and coagulopathy do not occur until 48 to 96 hours after ingestion, after irreversible hepatic necrosis has occurred.

N-acetylcysteine (Mucomyst) is the drug of choice for acetaminophen overdose. N-acetylcysteine effectively prevents hepatotoxic-ity if given within 8 hours; it is strongly effective if given within 16 hours and may be effective up to and perhaps beyond 24 hours. N-acetylcysteine therapy should be instituted with a 4-hour acetaminophen level of 150 μg/mL, an 8-hour level of 75 μg/mL, or a 12-hour level of 37.5 μg/mL. Because this therapy may be effective 24 hours after ingestion, the presence of any measurable acetaminophen or biochemical evidence of hepatic injury at 24 hours is an indication to start N-acetylcysteine therapy. Tylenol (Arthritis Extended Relief) has a different pharmacokinetic configuration and causes toxicity *below* standard toxic levels; liberal use of N-acetylcysteine therapy is indicated. Because the P-450 enzyme system is present in the fetus by the 14th week of pregnancy, acetaminophen is highly toxic to the fetus, and N-acetylcystein therapy should be given to the pregnant patient as soon as possible. The oral dose is 140 mg/kg initially and then 70 mg/kg every 4 hours for 17 doses. Both 20- and 48-hour intravenous N-acetylcysteine protocols are available but are under investigation at present.

The *salicylates* (aspirin) remain a leading cause of analgesic drug overdose. The association of Reye's syndrome with aspirin and the introduction of the safety cap have produced a dramatic fall in use and accidental poisoning in the pediatric age group. Salicylates inhibit the cyclooxygenase enzyme of the prostaglandin synthetase complex, uncouple oxidative phosphorylation, and produce respiratory alkalosis and a high anion gap metabolic acidosis. Salicylates are metabolized by first-order kinetics and are conjugated with glycine and glucuronic acid; as plasma concentrations rise in overdose and glycine stores are depleted, zero-order kinetics prevail, and renal excretion of salicylate becomes prominent.

Clinical presentation includes tinnitus, hearing loss, diaphoresis, facial flushing, hyperpyrexia, and hyperventilation. With severe salicylate poisoning, patients progressively develop dehydration, hypernatremia, pulmonary edema, purpura, gastrointestinal bleeding, and death. A plasma salicylate level of more than 30 mg/dL indicates salicylate toxicity, and a level of 80 to 100 mg/dL indicates critical salicylate poisoning.

The treatment of choice for salicylate poisoning is an alkaline diuresis with sodium bicarbonate. Fluid, electrolyte, and acid-base disturbances must be corrected, vitamin K supplementation should be given, and supportive care is paramount. Hemodialysis is indicated for patients whose salicylate level is higher than 80 to 100 mg/dL, patients who do not respond to a trial of bicarbonate therapy, or patients whose condition is critical.

Ibuprofen is the leading nonsteroidal anti-inflammatory drug (NSAID) and has become a common prescription and over-the-counter product. Although a common cause of overdose, ibuprofen and similar NSAIDs produce only mild toxicity in acute overdose, primarily gastritis. Supportive care is all that is generally indicated.

The incidence of *anticholinergic* poisoning has dramatically decreased since atropine, scopolamine, and hyoscyamine have been

Table 98-3 ■ COMMON TOXIC CAUSES OF SEIZURES

Amoxapine	LSD
Anticholinergics	Oral hypoglycemics
Camphor	Parathion
Carbon monoxide	Phencyclidine
Cocaine	Phenothiazines
Ergotamine	Propoxyphene
Insulin	Propranolol
Isoniazid	Strychnine
Lead	Theophylline
Lindane	Tricyclic antidepressants
Lithium	

Table 98-5 ■ TOXINS NOT EFFECTIVELY ABSORBED BY CHARCOAL

Acids
Heavy metals
Alcohols
Hydrocarbons
Alkalis
Iron
Carbamates
Lithium
Cyanide
Organophosphates
Ethylene glycol

Table 98–6 ■ TREATMENT METHODS FOR ELIMINATION OF ABSORBED SUBSTANCE

Alkaline diuresis
    Phenobarbital
    Salicylate
Hemodialysis
    Ethylene glycol
    Lithium
    Methanol
    Salicylates
    Theophylline
Hemoperfusion
    Barbiturates
    Theophylline

removed from over-the-counter sleep medications. Overdoses of benztropine, amantadine, and prescription sinus, gastrointestinal, and eye medications are still seen occasionally, as is abuse of Jimson weed, the plant *Datura stramonium*. The classic anticholinergic syndrome is produced by blockade of acetylcholine with central and peripheral effects: psychosis, delirium, seizures, flushing, dry mucous membranes and skin, hyperpyrexia, dilated pupils, and urinary retention. The antidote physostigmine should be reserved for severe cases of pure anticholinergic poisoning. Physostigmine should not be used for agents with only some anticholinergic properties, such as tricyclic antidepressants. The initial dose of physostigmine is 0.5 to 2 mg IV slowly in adults and 0.02 mg/kg in children. The maximum dose is not to exceed 4 mg in 30 minutes in adults. Cardiac monitoring is essential, because physostigmine has caused asystole, bradycardia, and seizures.

Barbiturates still constitute a major source of overdose and mortality. Largely replaced as prescription sleep medication by the benzodiazepines, barbiturates are still present in headache prescriptions such as butalbital (Fiorinal and Esgic), and sleep medications such as secobarbital (Seconal) remain common drugs of abuse. Phenobarbital is one of the leading anticonvulsant medications. Thiopental is used as an intravenous anesthetic for in-hospital rapid-sequence intubation or as a sedative before cardioversion and surgery. Phenobarbital is excreted primarily unchanged by the kidney, whereas most other barbiturates are metabolized by the liver. Overdose is associated with depression of the central nervous system (CNS) and cardiovascular system, coma, hypotension, loss of reflexes, hypothermia, respiratory arrest, and death. A characteristic of a barbiturate overdose is the persistence of the pupillary light reflex even with stage IV coma. Bullous skin lesions often occur over pressure areas. Treatment of the critically ill patient involves mechanical ventilation, resuscitation of cardiovascular status, gastric lavage and activated charcoal (after securing the airway), and supportive care in an intensive care unit. An alkaline diuresis with sodium bicarbonate is specifically indicated for phenobarbital, which is a weak acid that is excreted unchanged in the urine. Multiple-dose activated charcoal every 4 to 6 hours is also specifically indicated for phenobarbital, as it diffuses into the gastrointestinal lumen. Charcoal hemoperfusion and hemodialysis have a role in barbiturate overdose for critical patients who do not respond to conservative therapy.

The *benzodiazepines* have become extremely popular and have virtually replaced other sedative-hypnotics. All benzodiazepines are effective anxiolytics and sedatives, and they have varying properties as muscle relaxants, anticonvulsants, and amnestics. In addition, diazepam (Valium), lorazepam (Ativan), and midazolam (Versed) have major therapeutic roles as intravenous drugs for in-hospital use as anticonvulsants, preanesthetics, and sedatives. Although the benzodiazepines are common agents involved in overdose, they generally cause only coma and ataxia; mortality is rare, and supportive care is all that is usually necessary. The new antidote flumazenil is reserved only for reversing pure in-hospital benzodiazepine sedation. Flumazenil may also serve as an antidote in reversing coma in zolpidem (Ambien) overdose. Its use in the general overdose patient or in a patient with head injury or coma of unknown etiology is not recommended, because flumazenil has been reported to cause seizures in patients who have co-ingested benzodiazepines and cyclic antidepressants and has caused increased intracranial pressure in patients with head injury.

The *calcium channel blockers* are among the most common antihypertensive agents in the United States and are now the most common cause of cardiovascular drug death by overdose. A special problem is presented by the sustained-release preparations, which allow for continued absorption. Persistent hypotension, bradycardia with atrioventricular block (especially with verapamil), coma, pulmonary edema, and cardiac arrest may constitute the clinical picture. Treatment must be aggressive if these patients are to survive. Whole-bowel irrigation with polyethylene glycol is indicated if sustained-release preparations have been ingested. An intravenous 10% calcium chloride 1-g bolus (over 5 minutes) may be lifesaving, and 1 gram IV every 15 minutes over the first hour may be necessary in critically ill patients, followed by 10% calcium chloride via continuous intravenous infusion (the dosage and rate depending on the clinical condition) until blood pressure stabilizes. For patients who do not respond to high-dose calcium therapy, dopamine, dobutamine, amrinone, epinephrine, and/or glucagon have been employed with varying results. Glucagon is indicated in patients with concomitant β-blocker overdose. Pacing may be necessary, especially with verapamil overdose. Symptomatic patients and patients who have ingested sustained-release preparations should be admitted to the critical care unit for continuous ECG monitoring for at least 24 hours after stabilization.

Carbon monoxide is the leading cause of death from poisoning in the United States. CO is a colorless, odorless, tasteless gas produced by incomplete combustion of carbon materials. CO has a 200 times greater affinity for hemoglobin than oxygen and thus produces cellular hypoxia and death. Fires, smoke, wood-burning stoves, gas space heaters, and engine exhaust are sources of unintentional poisoning. Because the heart and brain are the most sensitive to hypoxic insult, clinical presentation usually involves CNS or cardiac symptoms—headache, altered mental status, convulsions, chest pain, cardiac arrhythmia, and/or acute myocardial infarction. Mild CO poisoning often is mistaken for influenza, as both occur primarily in the winter months and cause headache and gastrointestinal symptoms. Because most patients receive oxygen in an ambulance on the way to the hospital, the carboxyhemoglobin level is usually an unreliable indicator of the extent of poisoning. In general, the deeper the level of coma, the greater the chance of neuropsychiatric sequelae. CO poisoning is treated with oxygen: Breathing room air, it takes a patient 6 hours to halve his or her carboxyhemoglobin level ($T_{1/2}$); breathing 100% oxygen, the CO $T_{1/2}$ is 90 minutes; with hyperbaric oxygen at 2.5 atmospheres of pressure absolute (ATA), the CO $T_{1/2}$ is less than 1 hour. Hyperbaric oxygen therapy reduces the incidence of neurologic sequelae and has become the standard of care for treating CO-poisoned patients with coma and altered mental status (Table 98–7).

Caustic alkali ingestion became far less of a problem because of a reduction of the lye concentration in liquid products to less than 5%. Accidentally swallowing button batteries larger than 20 mm in diameter and intentional ingestion of alkali substances are the major causes of morbidity. Because solid crystals adhere to the tongue and cause burning, they uncommonly produce esophageal burn. Although the extent of burn cannot be determined by symptoms, drooling in children and inability to swallow are highly suggestive. Mouth burns are also suggestive, but the absence of mouth burns does not exclude esophageal burn. Milk is the only possible home antidote, but it must be given immediately. To detect significant burns, some suggest upper gastrointestinal esophagoscopy within 12 hours, whereas others prefer to wait 24 to 72 hours following ingestion. A 3-week course of methylprednisolone, 2.5 mg/kg/day, to prevent esophageal stricture has been the mainstay of therapy, but its efficacy has been questioned. Esophageal dilation and, if necessary, gastric tube esophageal replacement are indicated for treating esophageal stricture.

Cocaine (see Chapter 17) is the leading cause of death from

Table 98–7 ■ CARBON MONOXIDE POISONING: SPECIFIC INDICATIONS FOR HYPERBARIC OXYGEN THERAPY

All comatose patients
Patients with neurologic impairment by examination or psychometric testing
Patients with carboxyhemoglobin levels >40%
Cardiovascular involvement (chest pain, ECG changes, arrhythmias)
Pregnant patients with carbon monoxide levels >15%
Patients who do not respond to 100% oxygen
Patients with recurrent symptoms up to 3 weeks after exposure

illicit drug abuse in the United States. Cocaine alkaloid benzolymethylecgonine is metabolized to benzoylecgonine and ecgonine methyl ester and is excreted in the urine for 24 to 36 hours following administration. In overdose, cocaine induces primarily cardiac, neurologic, and psychophysiologic effects. Cardiac effects include palpitations, chest pain, ischemia, acute myocardial infarction, cardiac arrhythmia, and/or cardiac arrest. Neurologic events include altered mental status, seizures that often progress to status epilepticus, focal neurologic signs, and ischemic stroke. Suicide attempts and violent behavior are often part of the acute cocaine experience. Cocaine toxicity should be suspected in all young patients who present to the emergency department with chest pain, palpitations, cardiac arrhythmia, or cardiac arrest; altered mental status, seizures, or other neurologic signs; or any bizarre illness inappropriate for the patient's age. Patients with mild cocaine toxicity frequently present with palpitations, supraventricular tachycardia, hypertension, and excitability; treatment of the patient with no evidence of coronary artery disease includes observation; sedation, generally with benzodiazepines; and the occasional judicious use of labetalol, which has both α- and β-blocking effects, or the short-acting β-adrenergic blocker esmolol for control of heart rate. β-Adrenergic blockers should not be used in cocaine-associated myocardial ischemia. Emergency management of patients with serious cocaine toxicity consists of cardiac monitoring, supportive therapy, and management of complications. Patients with chest pain are often admitted because they may have either coronary vasospasm or acute myocardial infarction. Nitrates and/or calcium channel blockers may be warranted if angina is present. Coronary reperfusion therapy (see Chapter 60) may be indicated for acute myocardial infarction. Grand mal seizures are common, and standard therapy with intravenous benzodiazepines, phenytoin, or phenobarbital may be unsuccessful because these patients often progress to status epilepticus. Should status epilepticus occur, paralysis with rapid-sequence intubation and thiopental-induced coma with electroencephalographic (EEG) monitoring may be warranted. Correction of the high anion gap metabolic acidosis is indicated, and observation and treatment for rhabdomyolysis may be necessary. In addition to psychiatric follow-up, patients who used cocaine intravenously must be screened for hepatitis, human immunodeficiency virus, and other complications of intravenous drug use. *Amphetamines* and *phenylpropanolamine* are stimulants that produce effects clinically similar to those of cocaine but generally more benign and of shorter duration.

Cyanide poisoning most commonly is due to smoke inhalation. One public source is acetonitrile in the form of acrylic nail remover. Hydrogen cyanide gas is a fumigant rodenticide. Prolonged administration of nitroprusside can result in elevated cyanide levels. Cyanide poisoning produces cellular hypoxia by binding with the ferric iron of mitochondrial cytochrome oxidase and disrupting the electron transport chain and the ability of cells to use oxygen. Patients who inhale cyanide rapidly develop coma, shock, seizures, lactic acidosis, and respiratory and cardiac arrest. Mild exposures following smoke inhalation may be difficult to diagnose. Emergency administration of antidote may be life-saving. Cyanide poisoning should be suspected in patients who have inhaled smoke and who have evidence of lactic acidosis. The cyanide antidote kit manufactured by Eli Lilly Company contains amyl nitrite pearls, 12.5-g ampules of sodium thiosulfate, and 300-mg ampules of sodium nitrite. The body has a natural enzyme, rhodanese, that can complex cyanide and sulfur to form thiocyanate, which is only mildly toxic. Intravenous administration of 12.5 g of sodium thiosulfate provides the sulfur necessary to produce thiocyanate and is relatively safe. Because sodium nitrite causes hypotension and methemoglobinemia, its use is reserved for the most critical cases. The new antidote hydroxocobalamin (initial adult dosage 5 g IV), not yet approved, is a safer alternative for cyanide poisoning.

Digitalis intoxication is still common. Patients who suffer yellow or blurred vision, nausea or vomiting, and sinus bradycardia may improve simply by stopping the drug. Significant digitalis intoxication is heralded by hyperkalemia and a variety of major cardiac arrhythmias. Digoxin-specific Fab antibodies (Digibind) offer a definitive means of therapy and are indicated for life-threatening cardiac arrhythmia, hyperkalemia, a serum digoxin level of 10 ng/mL, or a massive overdose of 10 mg or greater in adults or 4 mg in children (see Table 98–1). Antidotal therapy should be instituted before conventional therapy in life-threatening situations.

Common drugs of abuse are *alcohol*, the leading cause of drug-

related emergency department visits; marijuana; cocaine (see Chapter 17); and the opiates (see Chapter 17). The legal definition of intoxication by alcohol (see Chapter 16) is a blood level of 100 mg/dL, although impairment may be seen at lower levels, particularly in children. A lethal blood level is 500 mg/dL. However, because of tolerance to alcohol, the patient's mental state may not correlate with the alcohol level. Supportive therapy for acute alcohol intoxication includes restoring fluid, electrolyte, and acid-base balance, as well as thiamine and magnesium replacement.

Marijuana is a well-documented cause of motor vehicle accidents and resultant trauma because of its adverse effect on complex motor functions and driving performance. Marijuana interferes with cognitive function; short-term memory performance continues to be impaired even several hours after a marijuana user no longer feels high.

Respiratory arrest and noncardiogenic pulmonary edema are common presentations of intravenous abuse of *heroin* (see Chapter 17) and other opiates. The antidote to opiate toxicity is naloxone, which is relatively safe and should be administered to all patients who present in coma of unknown etiology. The adult dose is 2 mg IV, repeated as needed up to a total of 10 mg. It is effective against all opiate derivatives, including codeine, propoxyphene, methadone, fentanyl, and diphenoxylate. When the duration of action of the opiate, such as methadone, exceeds that of naloxone, naloxone by continuous infusion may be indicated.

Hallucinogens (Table 98–8) include lysergic acid diethylamide (LSD), which can produce a full-scale "trip" with as little as 50 to 100 μg. LSD is not addictive, but it can produce "flashbacks." Phencyclidine (PCP), commonly known as "angel dust," was first produced as a human anesthetic but, because of emergent hallucinosis, was restricted to veterinary use; its milder analogue ketamine is now used for human anesthesia. Street preparations usually use 1 to 2 mg PCP to produce the desired hallucinogenic effects. Although LSD trips are usually self-limiting, phencyclidine and its many synthetic derivatives in overdose cause a serious clinical picture, including nystagmus, hypertensive crisis, sensory anesthesia, hyperpyrexia, seizures, and respiratory arrest. The designer amphetamine drugs MDMA, or "ecstasy," and MDEA, or "eve," also can produce hallucinosis. The diagnosis of natural hallucinogen abuse, such as psilocybin mushrooms, peyote and mescaline, morning glory seeds, and nutmeg, can usually be ascertained by obtaining a careful history from either the patient or friends (Table 98–9). Treatment of the hallucinating patient involves placing him or her in a quiet room, "talking down" the patient, and sedating the patient with benzodiazepines. Haloperidol may be necessary for prolonged toxic psychosis. Although acidification with ascorbic acid markedly increases excretion of phencyclidine, acidification in the presence of rhabdomyolysis can precipitate renal failure and is now discouraged. Intensive supportive care is required for the critically ill phencyclidine patient.

The introduction of *hydrofluoric acid* into commercial products such as rust removers and car products such as chrome and wire-wheel cleaners has made clinical exposures commonplace. In addition to producing corrosive burns, the ability of hydrofluoric acid to penetrate intact skin into deeper tissues is unique among inorganic acids. With industrial exposures to hydrofluoric acid in concentrations greater than 20%, hydrofluoric acid in deeper tissues complexes with calcium and magnesium to form insoluble salts and produce hypocalcemic tetany, hypomagnesemia, disruption of electrical membrane function, cellular injury, and death. The initial

---

Table 98–8 ■ **HALLUCINOGENS**

LSD (lysergic acid diethylamide)
PCP (phencyclidine)
DMT (dimethyltryptamine) (*Piptadenia peregrina*)
Jimson weed (*Datura stramonium*)
Mescaline (the active chemical from the peyote cactus)
Nutmeg
Psilocybin (mushrooms)
Psychotomimetic amphetamines
   MDMA (3,4-Methylenedioxymethamphetamine)
   MDEA (3,4-Methylenedioxyethamphetamine)
THC (Δ-9-tetrahydrocannabinol)
Woodrose and the morning glory plants

Table 98–9 ■ CLINICAL EFFECTS OF HALLUCINOGEN ABUSE

	LSD-25	MDMA	PCP
Street name	Acid	Ecstasy	Angel dust
Pharmacologic effect	Hallucinogenic	Sympathomimetic	Hallucinogenic
Preparation	Blotter paper	Gelatin capsule	Cigarette
Half-life (hr)	3	7–34	24
Pupils	Dilated	Dilated	Pinpoint, may be dilated
Nystagmus	No	No	Yes
Anesthesia and analgesia	No	No	Yes
Hypertension	No	Yes	Yes
Social behavior	Contemplative or bizarre	Outgoing and energetic	Violent, agitated

presentation begins with intense and excruciating pain at the site of exposure, progresses with time as hydrofluoric acid penetrates to bone, and generally, but not always, is accompanied by local erythema and edema. Symptoms may be delayed up to 12 hours with exposure to home products. Tissue necrosis then occurs, and systemic fluoride poisoning develops with major exposures (Table 98–10). The first-line treatment of local burns is topical application of calcium gluconate gel or calcium carbonate paste. Intra-arterial calcium gluconate is indicated for patients with severe burns that are unresponsive to topical therapy or for those who develop systemic signs of fluoride poisoning (Fig. 98–1).

Iron poisoning has a direct corrosive action on the stomach and proximal small bowel; once absorbed, iron produces shock, metabolic acidosis, liver failure, and death. Initially, gastrointestinal symptoms prevail with persistent vomiting, abdominal pain, and hemorrhage. A quiescent phase may be observed, followed by shock, coma, metabolic acidosis, and liver failure. Laboratory data may reveal leukocytosis, hyperglycemia, and radiopaque tablets on a flat plate of the abdomen. A serum iron level should be determined (during peak levels) at 2 to 4 hours after ingestion: higher than 300 μg/dL indicates mild intoxication, and higher than 500 μg/dL indicates serious intoxication, but a serum iron level in excess of the total iron-binding capacity does not serve as a useful predictor of iron poisoning. Management of iron poisoning includes gastric lavage with normal saline. Whole-bowel irrigation may be indicated after ingestion of sustained-release capsules. The treatment of choice is the antidote deferoxamine, which chelates free serum iron in the plasma to form ferrioxamine, which is readily excreted and imparts a vin rosé color to the urine. Deferoxamine is indicated for all critical patients who present with coma, shock, or hemorrhage, for all patients with a serum iron level higher than 500 μg/dL, and for patients who are symptomatic with a serum iron level higher than 300 μg/dL. Intravenous deferoxamine at a rate of 15 mg/kg/hour is the preferred initial rate of administration; up to 6 g may be given in 24 hours. Chelation therapy should continue until the patient becomes stable for at least 24 hours, until the vin rosé urine (when present) becomes clear, and until the serum iron level has fallen below 300 μg/dL. Exchange transfusion may be indicated for the unusual patient who is critically ill and does not respond to chelation therapy.

Lithium intoxication may occur from either acute overdose or long-term administration of lithium carbonate in manic depressive psychosis. Lithium has a narrow therapeutic index, and patients who do not have serial blood levels determined during treatment

Table 98–10 ■ ACUTE FLUORIDE POISONING

Metabolic
   Hypocalcemia
   Hypomagnesemia
   Hyperkalemia
Neuromuscular
   Tetany
   Seizures
   Central nervous system depression
   Respiratory depression and paralysis
Cardiopulmonary
   Tachycardia
   Hypotension
   Pulmonary edema
   Ventricular fibrillation

frequently become toxic. Lithium displaces sodium, potassium, magnesium, and calcium in that order. Lithium intoxication produces altered mental status, parkinsonism, and ataxia; gastroenteritis following acute overdose; hypotension, cardiac arrhythmia, and myocarditis; nephrogenic diabetes insipidus; and renal insufficiency. Treatment involves withdrawing the drug and correcting fluid and electrolyte abnormalities in mild intoxication (serum lithium level of 1.5 to 2.5 mEq/L). Gastric lavage with sodium polystyrene sulfonate is indicated for acute lithium overdose. Patients with moderate acute lithium intoxication (2.5 to 3.5 mEq/L) who have normal renal function and are asymptomatic may respond to an intravenous infusion of normal saline to reduce the lithium level. Because lithium is the most dialyzable toxin known, the treatment of choice for lithium intoxication is hemodialysis. Hemodialysis should be used for patients with a serum lithium level higher than 3.5 mEq/L, for patients who are symptomatic or have impaired renal function and whose level may be 2.5 mEq/L, and for patients whose condition clinically warrants such treatment.

Methanol and *ethylene glycol* poisoning constitute true medical emergencies. Methanol is most commonly found as the active ingredient in windshield washer fluid, and ethylene glycol constitutes antifreeze; both are also found in many commercial and marine products. Methanol, or wood alcohol, is converted by alcohol dehydrogenase to formaldehyde and then to formic acid. Signs and symptoms develop over a 24-hour period (Table 98–11) and may include infarction of the putamen. Severe high anion gap metabolic acidosis occurs with an increase in the osmolal gap. Treatment emphasizes intravenous ethanol, sodium bicarbonate, and hemodialysis. The diagnosis of ethylene glycol poisoning in adults, commonly from antifreeze, is generally, but not always, evident from the history. Metabolism of ethylene glycol by alcohol dehydrogenase causes poisoning by producing severe metabolic acidosis due to aldehyde, glycolate, and lactate formation and the deposition of oxalate crystals in the lungs, heart, and kidneys (see Table 98–11). Fomepizole (4-methylpyrazole) inhibits alcohol dehydrogenase and may be an alternative to intravenous alcohol for the treatment of ethylene glycol poisoning. Hemodialysis is the treatment of choice for ethylene glycol poisoning and should be instituted as early as possible once the diagnosis is made.

Isopropanol, or rubbing alcohol, is a common source of ingestion. Approximately 15% of isopropyl alcohol is converted by alcohol dehydrogenase to acetone; clinical manifestations are similar to those of ethanol ingestion. Diagnosis is usually by history, and patients who become symptomatic will exhibit a "fruity odor" to their breath, characteristic of acetone. Treatment is generally conservative. Although both isopropanol and acetone are readily dialyzable, hemodialysis is seldom necessary in management.

The *organophosphates* are highly popular insecticides because they are effective, disintegrate within days of application, and do not persist in the environment (Table 98–12). Even minute quantities can penetrate the skin and be lethal, as evidenced by the use of organophosphate nerve gases sarin, soman, tabun, and VX in chemical warfare.

The organophosphates irreversibly inhibit acetylcholinesterase, resulting in an overabundance of acetylcholine at synapses and the myoneural junction. The acetylcholine initially excites and then paralyzes the CNS, the parasympathetic nerve endings, and the sweat glands (muscarinic effects), as well as the somatic nerves and ganglionic synapses of autonomic ganglia (nicotinic effects). Initial symptoms resemble a flulike syndrome with abdominal pain, vom-

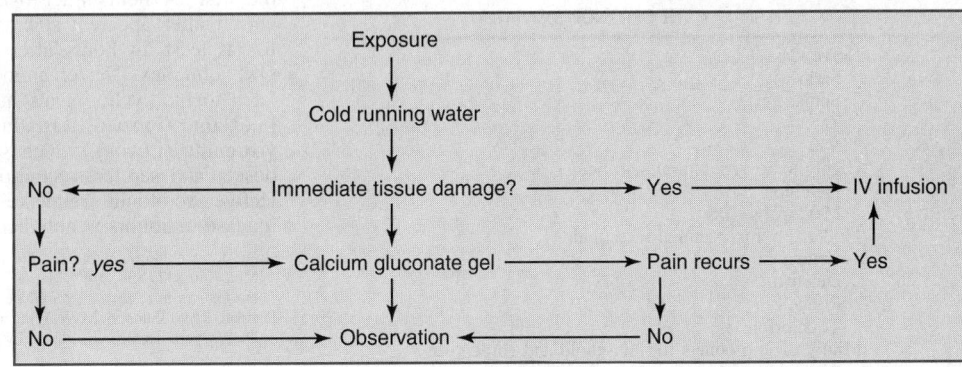

FIGURE 98–1 ■ Algorithm for the treatment of acute hydrofluoric acid burns.

iting, headache, and dizziness. The full-blown picture generally develops by 24 hours and includes coma, convulsions, confusion, or psychosis; fasciculation and weakness or paralysis; dyspnea, cyanosis, and pulmonary edema; and sometimes pancreatitis. Torsades de pointes has also been described. Emergency management includes decontamination of the skin, if necessary, and removal of clothes; establishing an airway and ensuring proper ventilatory support and cardiac monitoring; and administering the specific antidote pralidoxime and the physiologic antidote atropine. A 25% reduction in red blood cell cholinesterase confirms organophosphate poisoning. Atropine should be given as a physiologic antidote (see Table 98–1) to reverse the muscarinic effects and to dry the excessive pulmonary secretions seen in patients with respiratory distress. Atropine use requires cardiac monitoring and proper oxygenation. Pralidoxime is the treatment of choice for organophosphate poisoning and should be begun on clinical grounds before return of any blood studies. To be effective, pralidoxime must be given in the first 48 hours before irreversible binding of acetylcholinesterase occurs. The initial dose is 1 g IV given over 15 to 30 minutes; the effect may be dramatic. Pralidoxime by continuous infusion of up to 500 mg/hour may be necessary in critically ill patients. Pralidoxime may obviate the need for high-dose atropine therapy and reduce the incidence of late-onset paralysis.

The carbamate insecticides include carbaril, methomyl, and propoxur and are reversible cholinesterase inhibitors. They produce clinical effects similar to those of the organophosphates but without CNS signs; they are considerably more benign and of much shorter duration. Atropine is the drug of choice for carbamate poisoning. Pralidoxime is not indicated because the carbamate-cholinesterase complex is quite reversible.

Paraquat, a bipyridyl herbicide, is a highly lethal concentrate that accounts for roughly 1000 deaths a year in Japan alone. Paraquat reduces oxygen to form superoxide radicals that cause alveolar cell injury and death. Extensive pulmonary fibrosis ensues, prevent-

ing gas exchange and causing subsequent hypoxic death. Patients who ingest more than 30 mg/kg die within a few hours to days of multiple organ system failure. Smaller amounts produce esophagitis with possible perforation, pulmonary edema with subsequent development of pulmonary fibrosis, and renal failure. Aggressive intervention within the first 2 hours following ingestion may be the only hope of preventing severe toxicity. If the patient arrives within the first hour, gastric lavage should be performed immediately. Paraquat is absorbed by a 15% solution of Fuller's earth or a 7% solution of bentonite, the diatomaceous clays. Soil or clay in a slurry of water may be substituted at home if the patient is found within minutes of ingestion. Activated charcoal and kayexalate also may be effective. Other than early gastric decontamination, supportive care may be all that is available. Because oxygen is converted to superoxide radicals by paraquat to produce cellular injury, oxygen is withheld until it becomes mandatory.

Theophylline intoxication and mortality from both plain theophylline and sustained-release preparations occur from acute overdose and long-term unintentional intoxication. Vomiting is often the first symptom, and sinus tachycardia is the most common sign in both acute and chronic toxicity. Seizures may be common when the serum concentration is higher than 40 μg/mL in chronic toxicity or higher than 80 to 100 μg/mL in acute overdose. Likewise, cardiac arrhythmia, cardiovascular collapse, and respiratory arrest are seen infrequently unless the concentration is higher than 50 μg/mL in chronic toxicity or higher than 100 μg/mL in acute overdose. Profound hypokalemia, hyperglycemia, and metabolic acidosis are also seen. Serum theophylline concentrations are considerably higher in acute overdose compared with those in chronic toxicity. Treatment of theophylline toxicity includes withdrawing the drug, cardiac monitoring, and supportive care. Gastric lavage and activated charcoal are indicated for acute overdose. The serum half-life of theophylline can be reduced by serial administration of activated charcoal, because theophylline diffuses into the gastroin-

Table 98–11 ■ POISONING WITH METHANOL OR ETHYLENE GLYCOL

Methanol	
Signs and symptoms	Altered mental status; coma; seizures; gastrointestinal disturbance with abdominal pain; pancreatitis in some; visual disturbances: blurred vision, diplopia, photophobia, sensation of "being in a snowstorm," blindness (end result).
Treatment	Aggressively prevent methanol conversion by infusing IV ethanol (see Table 98–1 for dose).
	Correct metabolic acidosis with sodium bicarbonate;
	Hemodialysis to remove methanol/metabolites—indicated for patients with visual disturbance, serum methanol >50 mg/dL, or with intractable metabolic acidosis.
Ethylene Glycol	
Signs and symptoms	*Early*
	Altered mental status; seizures; hypocalcemic tetany
	12 hr after ingestion
	Congestive heart failure
	24–72 hr after ingestion
	Profound renal failure
Treatment	Treat ethylene glycol with:
	aggressive gastric lavage;
	ethanol infusion or 4-methylpyrazole,
	sodium bicarbonate to correct metabolic acidosis,
	Correct hypocalcemia with calcium chloride,
	Hemodialysis

Table 98–12 ■ THE ORGANOPHOSPHATES

Nerve Gas
  Sarin
  Soman
  Tabun
  VX
Highly toxic agricultural insecticides
  Parathion
  Mevinphos
Moderately toxic animal insecticides
  Coumaphos
  Dursban
  Ronnel
  Trichlorfon
Mildly toxic products for household and garden use
  Acephate
  Diazinon
  Malathion

testinal lumen; dosage is 1g/kg every 4 hours. Whole-bowel irrigation may be indicated for ingestion of sustained-release capsules. Cardiac arrhythmias are often difficult to manage but may respond to intravenous propranolol. Correction of hypokalemia, metabolic acidosis, and fluid-electrolyte balance is indicated. Although seizures may respond to intravenous diazepam, status epilepticus and rhabdomyolysis may occur and generally signify a poor outcome. Charcoal hemoperfusion is the treatment of choice for significant theophylline toxicity. Because of newer high-flux machines capable of increasing theophylline clearance rates to greater than 200 mL/minute, hemodialysis is becoming an option equal to charcoal hemoperfusion. Charcoal hemoperfusion is most beneficial for patients with a serum theophylline concentration of more than 80 to 100 μg/mL in acute overdose or more than 40 μg/mL in chronic toxicity (especially in the elderly or patients with hepatic disease or other conditions that delay theophylline clearance) or patients in critical condition.

Tricyclic (or cyclic) antidepressant overdose is still the leading cause of prescription drug death in the United States. Cardiovascular toxicity (primarily cardiac arrhythmia and hypotension), CNS effects (especially coma and seizures), and anticholinergic signs are seen with tricyclic overdose. The cardiotoxic effects are seen with ingestion of 1 g (10 to 20 mg/kg) and account for the high mortality rate. The hallmark of tricyclic toxicity on ECG is prolongation of the QRS complex. A QRS complex longer than 100 ms is a sign of severe toxicity and, generally correlates with a plasma drug level higher than 1000 ng/mL. Although sinus tachycardia and anticholinergic signs are evident with mild toxicity, QRS complex prolongation is associated with the development of ventricular arrhythmias, seizures, and death. Ventricular tachycardia is the most common ventricular rhythm, although ventricular bigeminy, slow ventricular rhythms, and torsades de pointes ventricular tachycardia also have been described. Ventricular fibrillation and sudden cardiac arrest are not uncommon.

The treatment of choice for tricyclic overdose is intravenous sodium bicarbonate. Alkalinization of blood via continuous infusion to maintain a blood pH of 7.5 appears to reduce the incidence of cardiac arrhythmia, and an intravenous bolus of sodium bicarbonate (1 to 2 mEq/kg) is the treatment of choice for the sudden onset of ventricular tachycardia, ventricular fibrillation, and cardiac arrest. Sodium bicarbonate also may be useful for correcting hypotension, although vasopressors may be necessary. Airway establishment, proper oxygenation and ventilation, fluid replacement at maintenance levels (to avoid pulmonary edema), gastric lavage with serially administered activated charcoal, and supportive therapy are indicated. Phenytoin (Dilantin) has been reported to reverse QRS complex prolongation in tricyclic overdose, but it is generally reserved for managing seizures. Prophylactic intravenous phenytoin (15 mg/kg) before the onset of seizures may be given in cases of amoxapine overdose, which has a high incidence of status epilepticus. Diazepam is quite effective in controlling seizures, although intensive therapy including thiopental and rapid-sequence intubation may be necessary to manage status epilepticus. Physostigmine is no longer used in tricyclic overdose, because by itself it can cause

seizures, bradycardia, and asystole. Death generally occurs within the first 24 hours after overdose. Because sudden death has occurred after apparent stabilization, cardiac monitoring is indicated for at least 24 hours after stabilization and normalization of the QRS complex. Newer antidepressants that are not structurally related to the cyclic agents include the serotonin reuptake inhibitors fluoxetine (Prozac), sertraline (Zoloft), paroxetine (Paxil), and fluvoxamine (Luvox), which generally cause only sedation in overdose. Fatal serotonin syndrome from concomitant overdose of *selective serotonin reuptake inhibitors* (SSRIs) and monoamine oxidase inhibitors is now being reported.

Brent J, et al: Fomepizole for the treatment of ethylene glycol poisoning. N Engl J Med 340:832–838, 1999. *A new approach to preventing renal injury by inhibiting the formation of toxic metabolites.*
Haddad LM, Shannon MW, Winchester JE: Clinical Management of Poisoning and Drug Overdose, 3rd ed. Philadelphia, WB Saunders, 1998. *A comprehensive text.*

99 RHABDOMYOLYSIS

Juha P. Kokko

Rhabdomyolysis is a syndrome that results from destruction of skeletal muscle. It is usually diagnosed from laboratory findings that are characteristic of myonecrosis. Once thought to be rare, rhabdomyolysis now is recognized with increased frequency, in part as a consequence of increased awareness of its potential presence in clinical settings that may predispose to muscle necrosis (e.g., exercise, hypophosphatemia, hypokalemia, alcoholism, sepsis, drug overdoses) and in part because of increased availability of routine tests for measurement of creatine kinase (CK) and myoglobin. For example, in a 3-month period at one hospital with predominantly economically disadvantaged individuals, 498 patients had nontraumatic elevations of CK to more than 1000 IU/L, and 46 patients had CK levels higher than 10,000 IU/L. Although there are no standard CK values that establish the diagnosis of rhabdomyolysis, elevations above 10,000 IU/L are usually indicative of clinically significant rhabdomyolysis; by comparison, with exercise to near exhaustion and its associated morphologic changes of muscle injury, CK rises only to about 1000 IU/L. However, studies have also shown that there is a poor correlation between CK elevations and the morphologic degree of muscle damage.

CLINICAL PRESENTATION

A careful history is critically important in evaluating patients with rhabdomyolysis. Although the approach to patients in the acute phase of rhabdomyolysis may be similar except in the extreme cases of malignant hyperthermia and neuroleptic malignant syndrome, the long-term preventive approach to these patients is quite variable depending on the underlying reason and classification of rhabdomyolysis (Table 99–1). A functionally useful approach is to classify patients into three broad categories: patients who have pure exertional rhabdomyolysis, those who have exertional precipitation of rhabdomyolysis in a setting of genetic defect in the synthesis of adenosine triphosphate (ATP), and those who have a precipitating cause that may or may not be associated with exercise (Table 99–2).

It is not surprising that the most common clinical symptoms of rhabdomyolysis are muscle weakness, pain, swelling, and cramps. However, some patients may be entirely asymptomatic, and the diagnosis may be established only from a laboratory profile. In patients who present with muscular signs and symptoms, the most

Table 99–1 ■ CLASSIFICATION OF RHABDOMYOLYSIS

Pure exertional rhabdomyolysis
Genetically transmitted defect leading to rhabdomyolysis
Nonhereditary, nonexertional rhabdomyolysis

Table 99–2 ■ PRECIPITATING FACTORS LEADING TO NON-HEREDITARY, NONEXERTIONAL RHABDOMYOLYSIS

Alcoholism
Phosphate deficiency
Potassium deficiency
Various bacterial and viral infections
Drugs (e.g., cocaine, amphetamines, neuroleptics)
Toxins (e.g., tetanus, snake venom, toluene)
Direct injury (e.g., crush, electric shock, burns)
Ischemic injury (compression, sickle cell disease*)

*Listed as nonhereditary because the mechanism of injury is not related to a genetic defect in the synthesis of adenosine triphosphate.

commonly affected muscles are those that were involved with exercise. Some patients, especially those without a history of exercise, may present with diffuse weakness and pain in all of their striated muscles. Usually the symptoms of rhabdomyolysis are self-limited because the muscle has a remarkable ability to repair itself completely. In the most severe cases of rhabdomyolysis, however, the muscle may swell sufficiently to cause compression of vessels and nerves and result in irreversible necrosis unless surgical decompression and fasciotomy are performed. The most common extramuscular complications are metabolic abnormalities and acute renal failure.

Striated muscle fibers are generally of two principal types. Type I are myoglobin-rich "red" muscles that use aerobic mechanisms to generate ATP, whereas type II are "white" muscles that use anaerobic (glycolytic) pathways to form ATP. The former muscles, which are better developed for endurance and are fatigue-resistant, are found, for example, in ducks; the latter, which are commonly used for intermediate sources of strength and are easily fatiguable, are found, for example, in chickens. Humans have both types of muscle fibers, and individuals who are conditioned for endurance exercise have a higher percentage of red muscle fibers. However, each of these fibers has similar intracellular constituents, and interruption of their sarcolemmal membrane causes these constituents to leak into the plasma, which produces the expected abnormalities of rhabdomyolysis (Fig. 99–1). For example, necrosis of only 100 gm of muscle is roughly equivalent to the acute infusion of 10 to 15 mEq of potassium into the circulation. Whether this influx of potassium or other intracellular constituents can be measured as a metabolic abnormality is highly dependent on circulatory and renal status.

PURE EXERTIONAL RHABDOMYOLYSIS. Relatively heavy exercise to 80% of maximum for only three periods of 15 minutes each on an exercise bicycle is consistently associated with a rise in CK values as well as light microscopy evidence of muscle fiber damage, especially in untrained and older individuals. Therefore, it is not surprising to see patients who have no presumptive inciting factors for rhabdomyolysis other than exercise. Most of these patients have no major laboratory findings except for CK elevations and marked myoglobinuria. Because myoglobin has a low molecular weight of roughly 17,800, it is filtered into urine rapidly and can be detected with a urine dip stick only up to 6 hours after muscle injury. Conversely, CK has a much higher molecular weight of more than 80,000 and takes several days to several weeks to return to normal levels. However, in the absence of volume contraction or renal failure, individuals with rhabdomyolysis from exercise usually do not develop the full laboratory picture of severe rhabdomyolysis.

GENETICALLY TRANSMITTED DEFECTS LEADING TO RHABDOMYOLYSIS. ATP is the intracellular currency of life; it is used for muscular contractions, to maintain the integrity of the cell membrane, and for many other vital functions. ATP is generated by two primary mechanisms: oxidative fatty acid oxidation and anaerobic glycolysis (Fig 99–2). Failure in either of these pathways can lead to ATP depletion and thus can lead to muscle necrosis. The integrity of each of these pathways is dependent on a number of different enzymes, and defects in these enzymes can cause rhabdomyolysis that is associated with depletion of ATP during exercise (Table 99–3). Of these defects, carnitine palmitoyltransferase deficiency is the most common hereditary aerobic disorder causing rhabdomyolysis, and myophosphorylase deficiency (McArdle's disease) is the most common anaerobic disorder causing rhabdomyolysis.

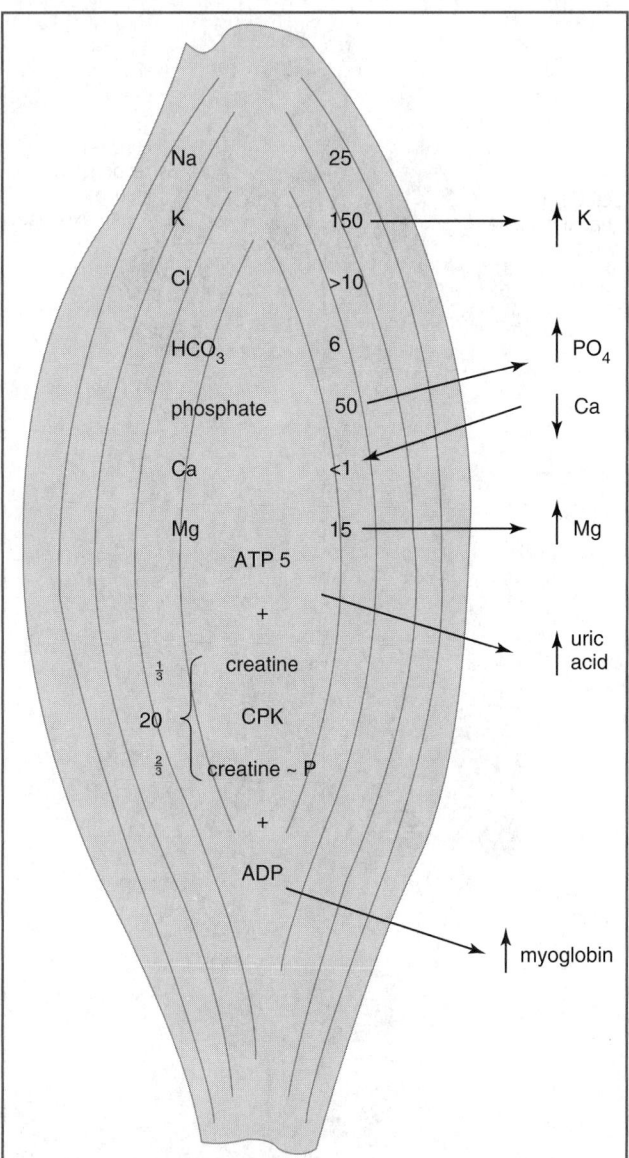

FIGURE 99–1 ■ Values within the depicted striated muscle cell reflect concentration (in mm/L of water) of various intracellular constituents. The values outside of the cell reflect increases (↑) or decreases (↓) that are characteristic of rhabdomyolysis, whereby intracellular constituents leak into the plasma through injured muscle membranes.

Many patients who previously were thought to have "idiopathic" rhabdomyolysis instead have an inherited enzyme defect in ATP synthesis. The clinical suspicion for an enzymatic defect should be heightened if the patient has more than one episode of rhabdomyolysis or a positive family history of rhabdomyolysis. About 50% of patients with recurrent rhabdomyolysis have a metabolic inability to generate ATP rapidly enough to keep up with the demands. If patients develop symptoms of rhabdomyolysis after some dura-

Table 99–3 ■ ENZYME DEFECTS IDENTIFIED* AS A CAUSE OF MYOGLOBINURIA

Carnitine palmitoyltransferase
Myophosphorylase
Phosphofructokinase
Phosphorylase kinase
Phosphoglycerate kinase
Phosphoglycerate mutase
Lactate dehydrogenase
Myoadenylate deaminase

*Most likely, other defects will be identified in the future.

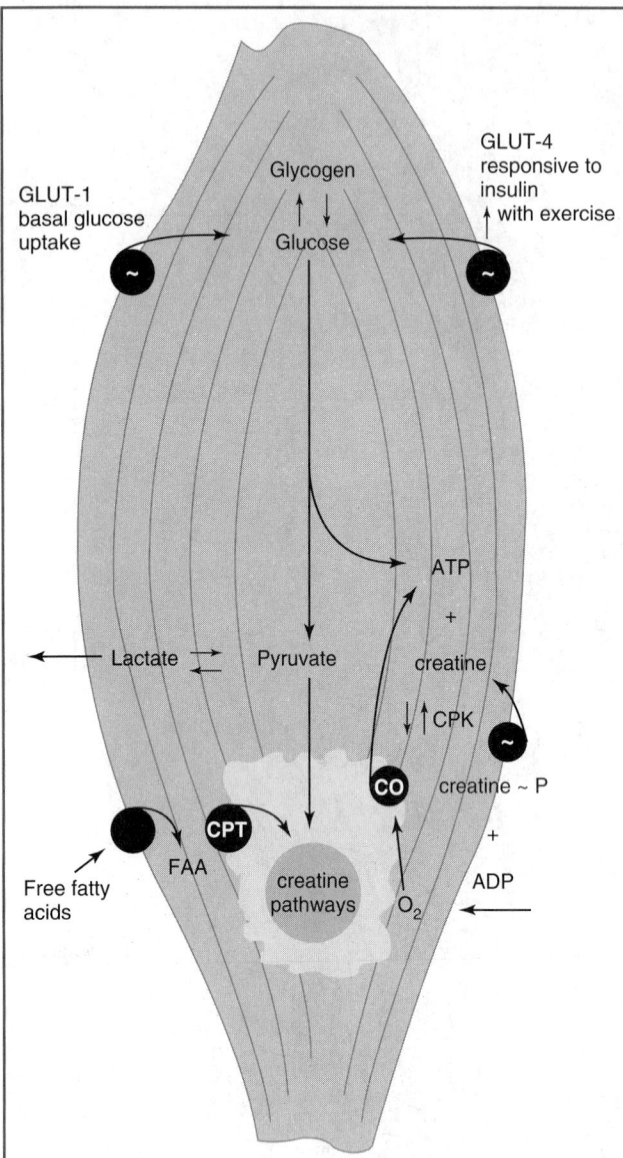

FIGURE 99–2 ■ ATP is the major energy for muscle. It is generated by the anaerobic metabolism of glycogen or the oxidative metabolism of fatty acids. Glucose uptake in turn comes across two primary pumps: GLUT-1 that reflects basal glucose uptake and GLUT-4 that can be increased with exercise and in response to insulin. The up-regulation of GLUT-4 protein formulates the basis why exercise improves glucose metabolism in diabetes as well as increases glycogen formulation in well-conditioned humans.

tion of strenuous exercise, a defect in fatty acid metabolism should be suspected; by comparison, an abnormality in the glycolytic pathways usually becomes apparent in the earlier phases of exercise. It is important to differentiate between these pathways because alteration of dietary habits can be palliative.

NONHEREDITARY CAUSES OF RHABDOMYOLYSIS. Acquired rhabdomyolysis may occur in response to a number of precipitating factors including drugs, toxins, or infections. Each of these factors may be the only precipitating cause, but often they are associated with exercise. Among the most common causes of rhabdomyolysis is exercise in patients who are alcoholic (especially if they have an associated potassium and phosphate deficiency) or patients who have ingested cocaine.

Patients with nonhereditary rhabdomyolysis are most likely to develop the laboratory abnormalities of the syndrome (see Fig 99–1), including hyperuricemia, hyperkalemia, and hypocalcemia. These findings are especially more frequent in the setting of myoglobinuric acute renal failure.

TREATMENT

Treatment of the acute phase of rhabdomyolysis must be highly individualized depending on the patient's presentation. If a patient complains of myalgias after strenuous exercise, if that exercise has occurred without nephrotoxic cofactors, if the urinary sediment is reasonably clear, and if the metabolic profile is otherwise normal, patients can be treated on an outpatient basis, despite a significant CK elevation. These patients should be instructed to take ample oral fluids at home and should be seen again in follow-up within 2 days. However, if any of the classic metabolic findings of rhabdomyolysis are present (see Fig 99–1), the patient should be admitted and treated aggressively (Table 99–4).

One of the most feared complications of rhabdomyolysis is the development of myoglobinuric acute renal failure. Although no large-scale prospective studies exist, the general consensus is that aggressive and early intravenous (IV) fluid therapy is the cornerstone for preventing acute renal failure. If the cardiovascular status permits (and most patients with rhabdomyolysis are in the younger age group), it is not unreasonable to administer between 6 to 12 L of IV fluids in the acute phase of myoglobinuria while monitoring the urine output so the rate of infusion can be individualized as dictated by the clinical circumstances. The aggressive infusion rate dilutes the various intraluminal constituents that otherwise might precipitate within the nephron, especially myoglobin, hemoglobin, and uric acid. Because all of these compounds have progressively increased solubility as the pH of the urine is increased, some authorities have suggested alkalinizing the urine by adding sodium bicarbonate IV fluids; however, this approach can increase precipitation of calcium into soft tissues. A possible alternative if the plasma bicarbonate concentration is above 13 to 15 mEq/L is to use carbonic anhydrase inhibitors (such as acetazolamide [Diamox] 250 mg orally, three times a day) to increase the alkalinity of the urine without inducing systemic alkalosis.

The duration of treatment also must be individualized because of the great variability among patients. Although no well-controlled studies exist to guide hospital length of stay, patients are often discharged from the hospital with an elevated CK, provided the CK has shown a steady drop for the previous 48 hours; there are no significant metabolic abnormalities; and the patient feels quite well, is compliant, and will return for an out-patient follow-up visit within a week. Myoglobinuric acute renal failure generally is self-limiting and starts to improve within 10 to 14 days of treatment if the release of myoglobin into the circulation has ceased.

Correction of the other metabolic abnormalities in rhabdomyolysis is no different from correction of these same abnormalities when they occur in other settings (see Chapters 100 and 102). However, management of hypocalcemia, which is common in rhabdomyolysis, especially in association with acute renal failure, requires special consideration because of deposition of calcium phosphate in muscle and other soft tissues early in the course of rhabdomyolysis. The greater the muscle damage, the greater the ectopic calcification. The hypocalcemia often coexists with hyperphosphatemia that in part is due to phosphate leak from injured muscle and in part due to diminished phosphaturia in acute renal failure. Thus, it is imperative that *IV calcium generally should not be given to patients with rhabdomyolysis and hypocalcemia* because it could worsen ectopic calcification. The only indications for IV calcium in patients with rhabdomyolysis are severe symptoms of hypocalcemia or severe hyperkalemia.

Patients with ectopic calcifications are at increased risk of devel-

Table 99–4 ■ **TREATMENT OF RHABDOMYOLYSIS**

1. Fluid replacement—be aggressive
2. Urine alkalinization—controversial. Benefit: Increased solubility of uric acid, myoglobulin. Harmful: HCO_3 could promote calcium deposition
3. Correct hyperkalemia
4. Management of hypocalcemia—avoid IV calcium unless tetany is present
5. Management of hypercalcemia—prevention is key. IV fluid, furosemide
6. Correction of hypoalbuminemia—usually not necessary
7. Disseminated intravascular coagulation—usually resolves spontaneously
8. Dialysis—if necessary
9. Hyperphosphatemia—oral binders, dialysis
10. Fasciotomy—relief of compartment syndromes

oping hypercalcemia during the diuretic phase of recovery. A number of hypotheses for the etiology of hypercalcemia have been advanced; the most important of these is dissolution of previous ectopic calcification. The rise in serum calcium can be very high, but fortunately it is usually self-limited. The treatment is aggressive volume repletion (to the degree that the recovering renal failure will allow) coupled with administration of a loop diuretic such as furosemide or bumetanide (see Table 99–4).

Poels PJE, Gabreëls FJM: Rhabdomyolysis: a review of the literature. Clin Neurol Neurosurg 95:175, 1993. *Comprehensive review of pathophysiology, clinical presentation, and treatment of rhabdomyolysis.*

Sinert R, Kohl L, Rainone T, Scalea T: Exercise-induced rhabdomyolysis. Ann Emerg Med 23:1301, 1994. *Nice clinical study calling attention to the fact that exercise-induced rhabdomyolysis is rarely associated with acute renal failure unless it occurs in a setting with other nephrotoxic cofactors.*

Slater MS, Mullins RJ: Rhabdomyolysis and myoglobinuric renal failure in trauma and surgical patients: A review. J Am Coll Surg 186:693, 1998. *Comprehensive review of rhabdomyolysis that focuses on the mechanism and treatment of rhabdomyolysis most relevant to the practice of surgery. However, many of the principals apply to internal medicine. The review has a nice introductory section on pathophysiology of muscle injury.*

Tonin P, Lewis P, Servidei S, DiMauro S: Metabolic causes of myoglobinuria. Ann Neurol 27:181, 1990. *Large study on 77 consecutive patients with myoglobinuria, demonstrating that roughly 50% of these patients have an underlying metabolic defect in synthesizing ATP in striated muscle.*

Zager RA: Rhabdomyolysis and myohemoglobinuric acute renal failure (editorial). Kidney Inter 49:314, 1996. *Comprehensive review of the pathophysiology of myoglobinuric renal injury.*

PART X

RENAL AND GENITOURINARY DISEASES

100 APPROACH TO THE PATIENT WITH RENAL DISEASE

Juha P. Kokko

A comprehensive history and physical examination are crucial in the approach to the patient with renal disease. Although it is well accepted that significant variability exists in the presentation of patients with renal disease, there nevertheless are historical, physical and laboratory findings that require emphasis.

Historically, it should be recognized that patients may be relatively asymptomatic for long periods even though they may have relatively far advanced renal disease. On the other hand, less advanced but rapidly progressive renal disease may be associated with severe symptoms. When taking a history from a patient with renal disease, specific emphasis should be placed on history of gross hematuria, dysuria, polyuria, the presence and nature of flank pain, nocturia, and signs and symptoms of uremia (see Chapter 104).

Likewise, the physical examination needs to be complete, but emphasis should be placed on carefully measuring the blood pressure in both the supine and upright positions, evaluating both the circulatory and interstitial blood volume status, examining the cardiovascular system, palpating the kidneys together with listening for potential renovascular bruits, and palpating potentially enlarged bladder or prostate gland.

Certain minimal laboratory evaluations are necessary, including a complete urinalysis, hematocrit and hemoglobin, and an SMA-6 determination that includes measuring serum levels of sodium, potassium, chloride, bicarbonate, glucose, and serum creatinine or blood urea nitrogen (BUN). The history, physical examination, and the laboratory findings will provide sufficient initial information to determine if any additional examinations are necessary for complete evaluation of a patient with renal disease.

APPROACH TO RENAL FAILURE

For the kidney to maintain normal volume, electrolyte, and acid-base homeostasis, it is necessary that it receive normal amounts of substrate (normal blood flow) to form urine, has normal glomerular filtration rate (GFR) and tubular function to form urine, and has a normal excretory path for urine. Thus, renal failure may be broadly classified as prerenal (those conditions in which the kidney does not receive adequate blood flow), renal (those conditions in which components of the kidney per se do not function normally), and postrenal (those processes that impair normal excretion of urine after it has been formed) (Table 100–1). Renal failure is also classified according to the rate of progression of functional abnormality as being either *acute* (see Chapter 103) or *chronic* (see Chapter 104). "Acute" generally refers to states in which an identifiable decrease in function occurs within days (often reversible), whereas "chronic" is a more insidious process in which the decline in GFR is progressive over weeks or months, often progressing through years to end-stage renal disease (ESRD) that requires dialysis or transplantation (see Chapters 105.1 and 105.2).

"Prerenal failure" refers to a state in which the kidney is underperfused. In the broadest terms, this is the result of either contraction of true circulatory volume or decrease in effective arterial blood volume (EABV). The term *effective arterial blood volume* is a dynamic concept that cannot be measured directly but reflects the amount of blood reaching volume-sensitive organs, mainly the kidney and hypothalamus. Often the true circulatory volume may be increased, as measured by red cell dilution techniques such as in congestive heart failure, but the blood flow reaching the kidney is actually decreased. Thus, in these states the homeostatic mechanisms sense that the circulation is decreased (states referred to as decrease in EABV), whereas the true circulatory volume is actually increased. Other examples of decrease in EABV besides congestive heart failure include states with decreased systemic vascular resistance, as seen in sepsis and vascular shunts, hepatorenal syndrome, and bilateral renal artery stenosis, thrombosis, or renal vasoconstriction and, occasionally, as seen in circumstances in which prostaglandin synthesis is inhibited. Measures of decrease in EABV include increases in antidiuretic hormone, renin, or aldosterone, but, clinically, the most useful measure of decrease in EABV is a decrease in fractional excretion of sodium (FE_{Na}) to values of less than 1%.

Renal failure is a term reserved for those conditions that are associated with abnormalities of the renal parenchyma. These may be primarily glomerular diseases (states with decreased GFR or increased protein leakage or both), primarily tubular lesions, or disease processes of the interstitium (interstitial nephritis). These abnormalities may occur as discrete events, but often the abnormalities are combined involvements of the aforementioned renal components. However, it is convenient to consider renal diseases either as primarily glomerular, tubular, or interstitial, because then it is easier to consider various causes and therapeutic approaches that are common to these renal components.

Postrenal failure is a term that refers to structural and/or functional impairment to normal urine flow that may be due to intrinsic obstruction of the ureter or urethra or secondary to extrinsic obstruction of multiple causes to compress the upper or lower urinary tract. By far the most common of these diseases are benign prostatic hyperplasia and ureteral calculi. Although there may be multiple causes of postrenal failure, many patients present with hydronephrosis and pain. Anuria is not a feature of urinary obstruction unless there is complete bilateral ureteral obstruction. Similarly, functional acute renal failure secondary to obstruction does not occur unless there is bilateral ureteral obstruction or unless unilateral obstruction is superimposed on pre-existing parenchymal renal failure.

STUDIES OF RENAL FUNCTION

URINALYSIS. Urinalysis is an inexpensive, often informative laboratory procedure that should be a component of any initial

Table 100–1 ■ MAJOR GROUPINGS OF RENAL FAILURE

Prerenal	(see Chapter 103)
Renal	
Acute	(see Chapter 103)
Chronic	(see Chapter 104)
Postrenal	(see Chapter 108)

evaluation. A number of important parameters may be measured. These will be described sequentially.

SPECIFIC GRAVITY. Specific gravity is the weight of an equal volume of urine to water. It, therefore, is a measure of the weight of solutes in water. Thus, urine with a specific gravity of 1.010 is 1.0% heavier than water. In practical terms, clinicians have used specific gravity of urine to estimate urine osmolality and thus the patient's state of hydration. This is especially important to pediatricians, whose patients can change their volume status rapidly. Indeed, low urine specific gravity (<1.015) always indicates hypotonic urine with corresponding urine osmolalities below 220 mOsm/kg H_2O. However, values above this do not necessarily reflect normal concentrating ability, because substances such as glucose, protein, and radiocontrast material highly increase the specific gravity. Thus, in adult patients with episodes of albuminuria and glucosuria, specific gravity has less limited significance than in pediatric patients. However, a real limitation of measuring specific gravity in pediatric patients is that using a hydrometer requires more urine than often is available. Therefore, alternate measures of urinary specific gravity have been developed. These include using a refractometer that measures the refractive index of urine and various reagent strips that change color in response to ionic (electrolyte) strengths of urine and not to undissociated solutes (mainly urea). However, the strip tests do not reflect urine concentration accurately and are mainly useful if the specific gravity is less than 1.015 (see Table 100–2). Under these conditions, urine has been found to be hypotonic. The refractometer is more useful and a better index of urinary osmolality, but it is mainly accurate at both extremes. Values less than 1.008 predict hypo-osmolality, whereas values greater than 1.020 predict hyperosmolality. Still the most accurate measure of urine concentration is measuring urine osmolality by freezing-point depression or by vapor-pressure techniques, but, unfortunately, these measurements require a technician and more complex equipment.

URINE pH. Calorimetric pH reagent strips measure urine pH in freshly voided specimens with satisfactory accuracy for clinical use. The more cumbersome glass electrodes with special techniques to collect urine are necessary to evaluate renal tubular acidosis or other abnormalities of acid-base metabolism that require sophisticated evaluation of urinary acid excretion. Urinary pH does not measure net acid excretion but only the unbuffered ion concentration. This, in turn, is affected by many variables, including diet.

GLUCOSE. Glucose oxidase reagent strips measure urinary glucose (see Table 100–2). Once the serum glucose concentration exceeds 160 to 200 mg/dL, then it is routine to exceed renal capacity to reabsorb glucose with resultant glycosuria. Glucose measured in

Table 100–2 ■ FACTORS INTERFERING WITH URINE DIPSTICK INTERPRETATION*

FACTOR	FALSE-NEGATIVE RESULT	FALSE-POSITIVE RESULT	COMMENTS
Glucose	Elevated urinary ascorbate concentrations	Oxidizing agents in urine containers	Ketone bodies reduce sensitivity of test Reactivity of test decreases as specific gravity increases Newer preparations minimize false-negative result with ascorbate
Bilirubin	Elevated urinary ascorbate concentrations	Phenazopyridine Etodolac	Sensitivity lowered by ascorbate Sensitivity lowered by elevated urine nitrite Indoxyl sulfate interferes with both negative and positive
Ketone		Pigmented urine (trace or less) Large amount levodopa metabolites in urine 2-Mercaptoethane sulfonic acid (MESNA)	No reaction with β-hydroxybutyrate or acetone Colors red to red-orange with phenylketone or phthalein compounds, distinguishable from ketone color
Specific gravity		Significant glycosuria Radiocontrast media	Note some new indicators not affected as previously by nonionic particles or radiocontrast Very alkaline urine may read low Elevated values may occur with significant proteinuria (>100 mg/dL)
Blood	Formalin urine preservation	Oxidizing agents in urine container Microbial peroxidase with UTI	
pH			False lowering of pH if urine spills from protein region of dipstick
Protein	Bence Jones protein, globulin not detected	Highly alkaline urine Urine contamination with quaternary ammonium compounds (skin cleansers, chlorhexidine) Phenazopyridine Polyvinylpyrrolidone infusion (blood substitute) Gross hematuria	
Urobilinogen	Formalin	p-Aminosalicylic acid, sulfonamides, PABA Phenazopyridine (with non-Ehrlich reagent)	The absence of urobilinogen cannot be determined with this test
Nitrite	Infecting organisms lacking nitrate → nitrite reductase Short bladder transit time limiting nitrate → nitrite reduction Ascorbate concentrations ≥25 mg/dL	Medications discoloring urine red or which make red in acid medium	
Leukocytes	High urine tetracycline levels		Decreased activity with high glucose concentration (>3 g/dL), high specific gravity, high oxalic acid concentration Interference from nitrofurantoin, gentamicin, cephalexin, and high albumin concentrations (>500 mg/dL)

*This table incorporates data drawn from several commercially available dipsticks. Individual preparations may differ in terms of test reagents used; therefore, clinical settings in which false or ambiguous readings occur may vary. The package insert always should be reviewed in each individual instance.

Data from Ames, Multistix reagent strips, tests for glucose, bilirubin, ketone, specific gravity, blood, pH, protein, urobilinogen, nitrite, and leukocytes in urine; Boehringer Mannheim Diagnostics, Chemstrip, urinalysis tests for leukocytes, nitrite, pH, protein, glucose, ketones, urobilinogen, bilirubin, and blood in urine; and Rose BD: Pathophysiology of Renal Disease. New York, McGraw-Hill, 1986.

urine is used as a presumptive indicator of diabetes mellitus except in rare cases of renal glycosuria.

PROTEIN. Urinary protein concentrations are commonly measured by calorimetric reagent strips (see Table 100–2). These are quite qualitative but can measure concentrations as low as 10 mg/dL (trace) to values greater than 500 mg/dL (4+). Clearly, the measurement of 24-hour urinary protein excretion rate correlates better with disease processes than urinary concentration; however, using reagent strips can alert the physician that further studies are needed if the rest of the clinical picture so dictates.

Normal urinary protein excretion rates are less than 40 mg/24 hr. However, many nephrologists have accepted protein excretions of up to 150 mg/24 hr as "normal" in non-diabetic patients. The reason for this more liberal upper limit is that in the absence of any other disease processes these patients generally do not develop progressive renal disease. Consensus exists that urinary excretion rates greater than 150 mg/24 hr are abnormal and reflect either renal or extrarenal causes (see Table 100–3). *Overflow proteinuria* refers to those conditions in which increased quantities of low-molecular-weight protein are present in the circulation and the amount that is filtered exceeds the tubular capacity to reabsorb it (e.g., light chain proteinuria of multiple myeloma). *Selective proteinuria* refers to a primary increase in albumin excretion, with the predominant pathophysiologic change being the loss of a negative charge from the endothelial surface of the glomerular basement membrane that would normally reject the permeation of negatively charged albumin (e.g., "minimal-change" nephrotic syndrome). *Non-selective glomerular proteinuria* refers to proteinuria with severe disruption of the glomerular capillary wall. In these cases, the urinary proteins reflect the concentrations of circulating proteins to a first approximation. A typical example of this type of proteinuria is diabetic nephropathy. *Tubular proteinuria* refers to conditions with a defect in normal endocytic reabsorption of filtered protein. In these conditions, the urine contains a disproportionate amount of low-molecular-weight proteins, such as β_2-microglobulin, in contrast to albumin. An example of this is various heavy metal poisons or tubular interstitial diseases. *Functional proteinuria* refers to common sources of proteinuria that do not indicate primary renal disease (e.g., high fever, exercise, congestive heart failure, and orthostatic proteinuria). It is for these reasons that urine collections should be done under standardized conditions. Although 24-hour urine collections without undue exercise are preferable, it is acceptable to collect a shorter 8-hour urine if it is done overnight. Functional proteinuria usually is transient and reversible.

All patients with abnormal excretion of protein must be evaluated. Indeed, persistent microalbuminuria in a 24-hour urinary specimen of a diabetic has prognostic significance and suggests development of diabetic nephropathy in the future. If proteinuria is noted, then one should consider obtaining two or three 24-hour urinary protein excretion rates because the coefficient of variance between these 24-hour samples can be quite high. If these measurements document that proteinuria is persistent, then efforts should be made to establish the etiology. The degree of proteinuria is only of limited value. However, the protein excretion rates seldom exceed 2 g/24 hr in interstitial nephritis, whereas protein excretion rates vary widely in primary glomerular diseases. Protein excretion rates greater than 3.5 g/24 hr/m² are known as "nephrotic-range protein-

uria" and almost always reflect primary glomerular disease. Patients with significant and persistent proteinuria greater than 150 mg/24 hr are at risk for developing functional renal insufficiency without appropriate therapy. Thus, these patients must undergo a thorough investigation (described later in this chapter), including further blood studies for evidence of specific systemic disease, urinary electrophoresis to determine the nature of proteinuria, various radiologic studies, and/or renal biopsy in those patients in whom there is reasonable chance of obtaining therapeutically relevant information. There exists some difference of opinion as to how aggressively a patient should be evaluated if he or she is non-diabetic and has a protein excretion rate between 40 and 150 mg/24 hr. A reasonable approach is to observe these patients on an annual basis if urinalysis is otherwise normal ("isolated proteinuria") and they do not have evidence of any systemic disease. Although an occasional patient is at increased risk of developing hypertension and renal disease in the future, in most, the long-term prognosis is good and does not justify further evaluation by a renal biopsy.

MICROSCOPIC. HEMATURIA. Hematuria may be macroscopic (red in color) or microscopic (more than two to three cells per high-power field in a button of sediment over a 12-mL spun urine sample). Although the quantitative count of microscopic hematuria is of little or no value, it is important to differentiate between glomerular hematuria, renal non-glomerular hematuria, and extrarenal causes of hematuria. In general, red cells in glomerular hematuria tend to be spiculated and have many sizes and shapes, whereas in non-glomerular hematuria the red blood cells are non-spiculated and uniform in size. It should be recognized, however, that in very dilute urine with specific gravities of less than 1.006, the red blood cells of any origin may be hemolyzed.

PYURIA. A number of techniques have been developed to establish the presence of pyuria: calculating excretion rate of leukocytes, examining the button of a spun sediment, using a hemocytometer on an unspun urine specimen, and using the leukoesterase dipstick method. One of the simplest is the routine microscopic examination of a spun specimen, or even more simple is the leukoesterase dipstick method. More than three white blood cells per high-power field and a positive leukoesterase dipstick measurement are abnormal values. These observations are a cost-effective way (with a relatively high degree of sensitivity) to suggest the presence of a urinary tract infection. However, it is important to recognize that wide variation in specificity in leukoesterase determination has been reported. This variation is due in part to spectrum bias of the patient population and in part to variations in test performance. The test must be done according to the directions that are provided with the specific dipsticks. Indeed, it is reasonable to initiate treatment for cystourethritis in non-complicated sexually active females without cultures based simply on the finding of more than three white blood cells per high-power field or leukoesterase-positive urine if symptoms of urinary tract infection exist. However, the more costly urine cultures are necessary if patients are diabetic, elderly, pregnant, or have recurrent urinary tract infections. Not all patients with pyuria have bacteriuria and this may reflect tuberculosis, viral infections, or fungal or other non-bacterial pathogens. Also, the presence of significant eosinophiliuria may suggest allergic interstitial nephritis.

Urine also should be examined microscopically for bacteria, yeasts, fungi, crystals, casts, and other components in the sediment that may be of diagnostic importance.

Table 100–3 ■ TYPES OF PROTEINURIA*

TYPE	MECHANISM	QUANTITY†	MOLECULAR WEIGHT	EXAMPLES
Overflow	Increased filtration of abnormal plasma proteins across normal glomeruli	Variable (0.2 to >10 g)	Low (<40,000)	Bence Jones proteinuria, myoglobinuria
Glomerular‡	Defective glomerular retention of normal plasma proteins			
Selective		>3 g	60,000	Minimal-change nephrotic syndrome
Nonselective		>3–5 g	High (>68,000)	Glomerulonephritis, diabetes
Tubular	Defective reabsorption of normally filtered plasma proteins	<2 g	Low (<40,000)	Interstitial nephritis, antibiotic injury, heavy metals
Hemodynamic	Increased filtration and possibly decreased reabsorption	<2 g	Variable (20,000–68,000)	Transient proteinuria, congestive heart failure, fever, seizures, exercise

*Values > 150 mg per 24 hours.
†Quite variable—values given are characteristic.
‡Molecular weight of proteinuria is a function of impairment of change and structural integrity.

Once the urine has been examined, then further laboratory testing of renal function becomes an important component of nephrologic evaluation. However, the physician must be aware of sensitivity, specificity, and predictive values of each test. Table 100–2 lists circumstances in which certain clinical situations cause false-positive and false-negative results. Evaluating volume, electrolyte, and acid base homeostasis is covered in Chapters 102.1 through 102.4, but a routine SMA-6 that includes measurements of sodium, potassium, chloride, bicarbonate, glucose, and either BUN or creatinine will offer useful information concerning metabolic abnormalities caused by abnormal renal function. Many of the just-mentioned variables are highly dependent on GFR.

GLOMERULAR FILTRATION RATE. Although many sophisticated techniques for measuring GFR exist, such as inulin clearance and radioactive iothalamate clearance tests, in most clinical circumstances the endogenous creatinine clearance is a sufficient estimate of a patient's GFR. Because there is some creatinine secretion, the creatinine clearance actually overestimates GFR as measured by more exact techniques. Also, drugs such as cimetidine, trimethoprim, triamterene, spirolactone, and amiloride inhibit tubular secretion of creatinine and therefore may cause a falsely low estimate of GFR. Nevertheless, measuring GFR by collecting a 24-hour urine specimen is adequate in most circumstances and can give a good estimate by

$$C_{Cr} = \frac{U_{Cr} \cdot V}{P_{Cr}}$$

where C_{Cr} is a measure of creatinine clearance, U_{Cr} is urinary concentration of creatinine, V is urine volume for 24 hours, and P_{Cr} is plasma concentration of creatinine.

Serum creatinine is a much better index than BUN of renal function. Indeed, isolated measurements of BUN should not be used because synthetic rates of urea (primary end-products of protein metabolism) are influenced by protein intake as well as liver function, and urea excretion rates from the kidney are influenced by renal tubular flow rates. In conditions with decreased tubular flow rates such as exist in prerenal failure, there is increased tubular reabsorption of urea and therefore a disproportionate rise in BUN with respect to creatinine. In these cases, the high BUN might falsely suggest a lower than actual GFR, whereas anorexia with poor protein intake with a low BUN would actually suggest the presence of a higher GFR. BUN is at best a rough index of renal function.

URINARY ELECTROLYTES. The significance of urinary electrolyte measurement has recently become more apparent. Measuring urinary sodium or chloride excretion is especially useful in attempting to differentiate between causes of hyponatremia, as seen in volume contraction (whether a decrease in total circulatory volume or a decrease in effective arterial blood volume) versus conditions associated with increased salt loss, as seen with the syndrome of inappropriate antidiuretic hormone secretion (SIADH), salt-losing nephropathy, or adrenal insufficiency. If metabolic alkalosis is present in its early-generation phase, as seen with vomiting, then urinary chloride, as is discussed later, becomes a more important measure of volume status than urinary sodium. A measure of urinary potassium is also important to differentiate between causes of both hypokalemia and hyperkalemia.

Measuring the 24-hour urine excretion rate of electrolytes is cumbersome and does not provide as much significant information as a spot urinary measurement of fractional secretion of these ions. The reason for this is that the 24-hour urine excretion rate reflects total intake in a steady-state condition (higher sodium intakes are associated with higher sodium excretion rates), whereas fractional excretion of ions reflects the sum of regulatory factors on a more acute basis. Fractional excretion (FE) does not depend on accurate timed volume collections and is easy to calculate:

$$FE_x = \frac{U_x/P_x}{U_{Cr}/P_{Cr}} \cdot 100$$

where urinary (U) to plasma (P) concentrations of given electrolytes (X) are measured and divided by simultaneously measured urinary and plasma concentration of creatinine.

FE_{Na} generally has a value of less than 1 in prerenal failure,

Table 100–4 ■ URINARY FINDINGS IN OLIGURIC* PRERENAL VERSUS ACUTE PARENCHYMAL RENAL FAILURE

	PRERENAL	PARENCHYMAL
U_{osm}† (mOsm/kg H_2O)	>500	<350
Urine sodium (mEq/L)	<20	>40
FE_{Na}	<1	>1

*Urinary indices are of less significance in non-oliguric renal failure, though U_{Na} and FE_{Na} tend to be lower in non-oliguric versus oliguric acute intrinsic renal failure.

†Significant amount of overlap exists between these two groups if urine osmolality is between 350 and 500 mOsm/kg or urine Na is between 20 and 40 mEq/L for these indices to be of diagnostic significance.

From Miller TR, Anderson KJ, Linas SL, et al: Urinary diagnostic indices in acute renal failure: A prospective study. Ann Intern Med 89:47, 1978.

whereas in SIADH, acute tubular necrosis, or salt-losing nephropathy the values are greater than 1% and tend to be greater than 3% (Table 100–4). The clinical utility of values in the intermediate range is less, but in general, values greater than 1 suggest disease processes, other than states in which the kidney is underperfused. Exceptions to this are those pure glomerular diseases, especially acute poststreptococcal glomerular nephritis, in which tubular function and renal blood flow are well maintained but the tubule has low flow rates as a result of an isolated decrease in GFR. In these cases, the FE_{Na} also will be decreased, as it will occasionally with radiocontrast-induced nephropathy, but in general, FE_{Na} less than 1 indicates renal underperfusion, whether secondary to decreases in EABV or due to true volume depletion. A decrease in FE_{Na} is especially useful in patients who have increases in total-body fluid volume but decreases in EABV. Examples include congestive heart failure and hypoalbuminemic states, whether secondary to renal or hepatic causes.

There is one clinical scenario worthy of special comment in which volume contraction is associated with a high FE_{Na}—the generation phase of metabolic alkalosis related to vomiting. As a patient develops metabolic alkalosis with vomiting, the plasma bicarbonate concentration rises to levels that exceed renal capacity for reabsorption, and, therefore, urinary bicarbonate concentration rises. This bicarbonate must be associated with a cation, either sodium or potassium. In these circumstances, the urine sodium excretion is elevated, but it is essentially free of chloride. FE_{Cl} thus becomes a better index of volume status than FE_{Na}. However, without increases in nonreabsorbable anion in the urine, the FE_{Na} is a good index of functional status of renal perfusion.

FE_K normally rises with decreases in renal function (Figure 100–1). It is thus important to interpret the significance of FE_K in this context. FE rates below normal indicate aldosterone deficiency or renal tubular defects for potassium secretion, whereas values above normal suggest increased concentration of aldosterone or other factors that stimulate potassium secretion. However, one of the most important uses of FE_K is determining the etiology of hypokalemia. Extrarenal losses or a decrease in dietary intake of potassium is associated with low FE_K, whereas renal losses are associated with an increase in FE_K. Generally, a U_K of 40 mEq/L or greater suggests renal losses of potassium, as seen with primary aldosterone secretion, diuretics, Bartter's syndrome, renal artery stenosis, and other causes with increased stimulus for potassium secretion.

Once the history, physical examination, and laboratory values have been interpreted, there are certain patients who require further evaluation to determine fully the nature of abnormalities in renal function. The next section describes the indications, use, and predictive value of various additional studies.

RADIOLOGIC STUDIES

Modern departments of radiology have a number of different diagnostic techniques that are useful in evaluating patients with renal abnormalities.

ULTRASOUND EXAMINATION. Ultrasonography (US) is a noninvasive, relatively inexpensive diagnostic tool that does not depend on renal function and gives information in "real-time" format. It has no complications and can be done at the bedside if necessary. In this technique, the US transducer is both a transducer and

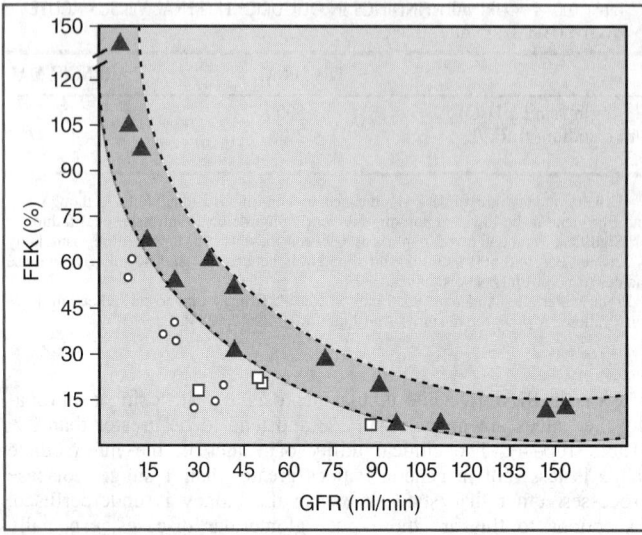

FIGURE 100-1 ■ The relationship between fractional excretion of potassium (FE$_K$) and glomerular filtration rate (GFR) in patients with normal adaptive increase in FE$_K$ with progressive decrease in GFR (area inside broken lines with individual patients depicted with solid triangles). The open circles and squares refer to patients with renal tubular secretory defects and aldosterone deficiency, respectively. (Reprinted with permission from Batlle DC, Arruda JAL, Kurtzman NA: Hyperkalemic distal renal tubular acidosis associated with obstructive uropathy. N Engl J Med 304:373, 1981. Copyright, the Massachusetts Medical Society.)

a receiver in which images are created from differences in acoustic impedance of different tissues containing various quantities of water, fat, collagen, and other substances. High-frequency sound waves are transmitted through solid tissues and water but not through air or calcified structures. Thus, collections of air (lungs, bowel gas, and bones) severely impair penetration of sound waves and result in poor-resolution imaging. In general, more aqueous media have better sound wave transmission and appear darker, whereas less aqueous tissues appear less dark. The white hyperechogenic images arise from calcified structures or free air.

Although US often contributes to a correct diagnosis, its main use diagnostically is to rule out hydronephrosis and polycystic renal disease (Table 100-5). In circumstances of anuria, with resultant acute renal failure, US can be used rapidly to determine whether hydronephrosis exists—either unilaterally or bilaterally. US is not sensitive to causes of hydronephrosis, but it may suggest the diagnosis of benign prostatic hypertrophy, nephrolithiasis, or any extrinsic or intrinsic cause of obstruction. In hydronephrosis, the central calyceal system is dilated and appears darker because it is filled with fluid (see Fig. 100-2).

US can be used to help differentiate between benign and malignant cysts. Benign cysts have smooth walls without internal septa or mural nodules. Classically, benign cysts do not need further evaluation, but cysts that do not meet these criteria need additional work-up. However, US is not particularly sensitive nor specific in evaluating solid renal masses. US is gaining more acceptance in evaluating the renal parenchyma. A small, echogenic kidney would indicate chronic renal disease (thus a renal biopsy would not be indicated), whereas large echogenic kidneys are seen with amyloidosis, human immunodeficiency virus infection, and acute glomerulonephritis. Asymmetrical kidney size suggests renal vascular disease. Primary renal carcinomas, renal metastases, lymphomas, and various benign tumors are not uniformly picked up until they are larger than 3 cm, and then their echogenicity is highly variable. US also is not very helpful in post-transplant evaluations, with the exception of ruling out hydronephrosis, but the technique is very

Table 100-5 ■ INDICATIONS FOR RENAL ULTRASONOGRAPHY

Rule out hydronephrosis
Define the nature of renal cysts
Localize calculi
Guide needles

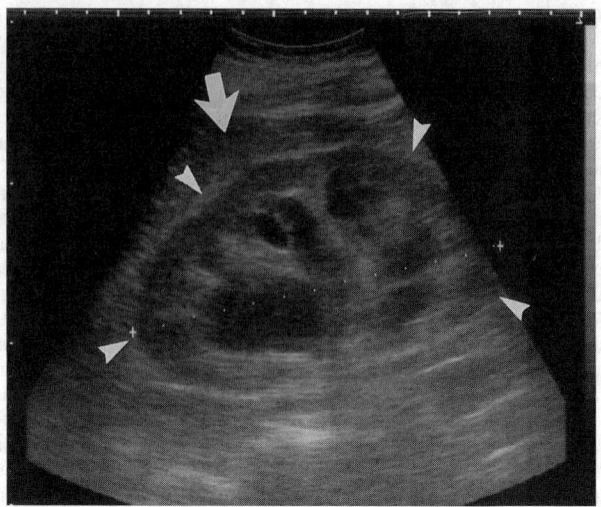

FIGURE 100-2 ■ Ultrasonography of a hydronephrotic right kidney. Small arrowheads indicate renal capsule beneath liver (arrow). Cortex appears as dark rim underlying capsule, surrounding bright sinus fat. Dilated collecting system appears as dark areas within the sinus fat.

beneficial for guiding diagnostic needles into appropriate anatomic spaces.

INTRAVENOUS PYELOGRAPHY. Intravenous pyelography (IVP) is used predominantly to evaluate anatomic features of the renal excretory system. After preliminary plain x-ray films, the radiologist injects one of various types of iodinated contrast materials, followed by serial x-rays. The contrast material is filtered by the glomeruli, after which it follows the normal flow of urine. Initial films (≤1 minute) after injecting the dye are known as "nephrograms," in which general radiopacity of the kidney is seen. Nephrograms initially can be used to measure the size of the kidney by measuring the maximum distance from the cephalad to the caudad margins. However, plain nephrotomography also can be used to estimate renal size without having to administer contrast material. The left kidney is normally somewhat larger than the right, with normal kidneys being somewhere between 11.5 to 12.5 cm. However, because of size differences in patients, some investigators believe that expression of renal size with respect to vertebral height is a more accurate measure of normal renal size. In adults, mean kidney length to height of the second lumbar spine is 3.7. After the nephrogram, calyces, pelvis, ureters, and bladder are sequentially viewed. The radiologist needs to be flexible to modify views and timing of the IVP to tailor the approach to suspected findings. IVP can be helpful in the kidney to define scars, cysts, and other anatomic abnormalities, whereas in the renal pelvis it is used to evaluate hydronephrosis, calyceal deformities, and stones; in the ureter it is used to evaluate obstruction, dilation, and abnormal course due to extrinsic factors; in the bladder it can be used to examine for intrinsic or extrinsic masses that cause either filling defects or extrinsic displacement of bladder opacification.

Special note should be taken with respect to radiocontrast-induced nephropathy. The incidence of radiocontrast nephropathy is most frequent in patients with chronic renal failure, diabetes mellitus, or multiple myeloma. Incidences as high as 50% have been reported in some patients receiving high doses of radiocontrast material for cardiac catheterization, but the incidence of renal failure secondary to IVP is relatively rare if the patient is adequately volume expanded. Regretfully, there are no proven methods to prevent prophylactically radiocontrast-induced nephropathy except volume repletion and good clinical judgment with respect to patients with risk factors for acute renal failure (see Chapter 103).

RETROGRADE PYELOGRAPHY. If adequate definition of the urinary collecting system is not achieved by IVP, then the physician may consider a retrograde pyelogram. It should be recognized that indications for retrograde pyelography are steadily decreasing with improvements in IVP technology. In this technique, the ureters are catheterized by cystoscopy, and contrast material is injected. This technique does not give information concerning the renal parenchyma but is used to define anatomically the calyces, renal pelvis, and remainder of the excretory system.

RENAL ARTERIOGRAPHY. Renal arteriography may be performed by a skilled radiologist, introducing vascular catheters percutaneously into the femoral artery and advancing them above the renal arteries to indicate their exact number and takeoff points. Subsequently, the catheters may be selectively advanced into a specific renal artery under fluoroscopic control. Contrast dye then is injected into the renal artery, and the branches subsequently will be opacified. A number of magnification techniques can be used to improve visualization, and vasoconstrictive agents occasionally will be helpful to define normal vessels that constrict to epinephrine from tumors or inflammatory changes that are not as vigorously constricted by epinephrine. Renal arteriography is especially useful for defining the extent and type of fibromuscular dysplasia and is diagnostically helpful in differentiating other stenotic lesions such as arteriosclerosis, arteriodissections, emboli, thromboses, various types of vasculitides, and effects of trauma. There are no well-accepted criteria for choosing patients for renal arteriography, but the technique should be considered in those in whom therapeutically useful information is reasonably expected: patients with moderately severe hypertension, especially if they are young and have renal bruits on physical examination, and patients in whom renal arteriography can help define the nature of suspected tumors or help in the differential diagnosis of specific types of vasculitis.

A modification of traditional renal arteriography is intravenous digital subtraction arteriography. In this technique, radiocontrast material is injected into either the inferior or superior vena cava, and digital subtraction imaging and filming are done later when the radiocontrast material circulates over the renal arteries. The technique has the advantage of using a lower contrast material dose, but the disadvantage is that it is mainly useful for diseases of the main renal artery and not its subsequent segments.

COMPUTED TOMOGRAPHY. Since the introduction of computed tomography (CT) technology in the mid-1970s, the technique has undergone significant advances to the point where the contrast and spatial resolutions have enormous diagnostic utility. The principle of this technique is that a computer constructs images mathematically from multiple x-ray absorption measurements from different projections of the body. To enhance the renal image, the studies are usually done with the aid of contrast material, except in circumstances in which the nature of renal calculi is being evaluated. Although CT scanning is not a primary modality to evaluate the kidney, it is especially useful to evaluate renal masses, study perirenal anatomy, and evaluate a non-functioning kidney; it is being used more and more frequently in the biopsy of renal masses, in which exact localization of small lesions is mandatory.

MAGNETIC RESONANCE IMAGING. Although nuclear magnetic resonance has been a routine tool of the chemist since the 1950s, magnetic resonance imaging (MRI), which uses the principles of nuclear magnetic resonance, has only recently become a routine diagnostic tool for the clinician. However, although MRI is an excellent tool in neuroimaging, the current generation of MRI should be considered only as an expensive and complementary modality to examine the kidney.

In the simplest phenomenologic terms, the signal in the MRI is produced by protons that flip from a lower energy state to a higher one and again return to the lower energy state. Protons can be considered as small magnets with a north and a south pole that rotate about a static magnetic field (as applied by an MRI machine). These protons can absorb energy at only a very specific combination of local magnetic strength and the applied radiofrequency. Once the applied radiofrequency is stopped, the protons (small magnets) return to their previous lower-energy orientation in the magnetic field. The process of changing magnetic vector orientation (relaxation) creates a small electric current that is interpreted by the receiving coils. The signal is dependent on unique magnetic surroundings of protons in tissue, and the ultimate image is constructed by complicated computer technology from evaluating the proton signals in three separate magnetic field axes. The resulting images from tissues of given characteristics form images of differing brightness. The organs are well outlined by differences in the magnetic environment of capsules and surrounding tissues. Indeed, differences in magnetic homogeneity of flowing blood in contrast to thromboses are easily picked up by MRI technology.

However, the principal advantage of MRI at the present time is that it does not require radiocontrast material, nor does it expose the patient to radioactive compounds. The process of MRI is not associated with any known complications, but it is expensive, re-

quires enormous technical support, and at present gives more sensitive soft tissue contrast than CT. Nevertheless, it cannot differentiate the nature of renal masses such as abscess versus carcinoma. The current technology also does not give metabolic information, but the future development of MRI technology that is coupled with simultaneous phosphate imaging may overcome some of these limitations.

RADIONUCLIDE STUDIES. Radionuclide activity can be measured as counts per volume of fluid by appropriate counters or by number of energy emissions as detected by a gamma camera (alpha and beta emittors do not have long enough penetration to be of use clinically). The principal use of the former method is to measure GFR and renal blood flow, whereas the latter technology is used for imaging and estimating relative renal function.

GLOMERULAR FILTRATION. GFR may be measured by clearance techniques or by disappearance rates of radiotracer from blood. In each case, an ideal tracer is one that is only cleared from the body by glomerular filtration.

The clearance of radionuclide is much easier to measure than the time-honored measure of GFR by clearing inulin. In this technique, stable blood concentrations of radionuclide must be achieved by either continuous infusion techniques or by single subcutaneous injections with suitable equilibration periods (usually 40 to 60 minutes). Urine must be collected for a known time period, and GFR can be calculated as

$$GFR = \frac{U_X \cdot V}{P_X}$$

where U_X and P_X are counts per minute and per milliliter of radionuclide in urine and plasma, respectively, and V is the volume of urine per minute. Many centers use the single subcutaneous method because of its ease. There are a number of good tracers for measuring GFR, and one currently in favor is iodine-125 iothalamate. If the rate of disappearance of radiotracer from blood is used to estimate GFR, a radioactive material is injected and samples of blood are obtained at fixed intervals (e.g., 3, 4, 5, and 24 hours). The GFR may then be calculated from disappearance rates of the compound from blood. Although the technique is not easy, it is useful in situations in which collecting urine is difficult, such as in pediatric populations or patients with urinary diversions.

RENAL BLOOD FLOW. Renal blood flow is measured by the same technology as GFR except in this case the patient is injected with a radiotracer that is extracted as completely as possible by a single pass through the kidney. Clinically, the most effective compound that is available is radiolabeled *p*-aminohippurate, which has an extraction efficiency of 87%. Other compounds have been developed with both lower and higher extraction efficiencies. The renal blood flow can be calculated from the clearance of radioactive nuclide from blood at short intervals up to 2 hours. The renal blood flow can be calculated from the rate of decrease of the compound from blood and corrected for the extraction efficiency.

RADIONUCLIDE IMAGING. Radiopharmaceuticals may be used to obtain general images of the kidney. These are only rough estimates of renal anatomy but have some advantage in that allergic reactions or induced nephropathy is essentially non-existent to radioactive compounds as compared with radiocontrast materials. In this technique, radiopharmaceuticals that are taken up by the kidney are injected. Images are then collected at 30-second intervals for 2 minutes and then at 5-minute intervals. The technique is useful to compare the function of one kidney versus the other and gives a general outline of renal size and shape.

RELATIVE RENAL FUNCTION. One of the most important uses of radionuclides in nephrology is to measure the function of one kidney relative to that of the other when nephrectomy is considered. The technique is similar to imaging, but in this circumstance the uptake of radiopharmaceuticals by one kidney is compared with that of the other. It is important to start images only after adequate mixing of radionuclide has occurred in circulation—usually within $2\frac{1}{2}$ to 3 minutes.

RENAL BIOPSY. If the preceding approaches fail to give a diagnosis or are not indicated for clinical reasons, then one might consider the potential of a renal biopsy. In broadest terms, renal biopsy is indicated for diagnostic information and as an aid in a

Table 100–6 ■ INDICATIONS FOR RENAL BIOPSY

Nephrotic syndrome
Systemic disease
    Systemic lupus erythematosus
    Goodpasture's syndrome*
    Wegener's granulomatosis*
    Diabetes mellitus only if atypical course
Hematuria if persistent for >6 months
Acute renal failure†
Transplanted kidney‡

*If etiology of process cannot be determined with a renal biopsy.
†If unknown cause and not acute tubular necrosis.
‡To help manage post-transplant state.

rational approach to treatment. It is of limited prognostic use, and only rarely is it indicated for monitoring progression of renal disease. Table 100–6 lists the indications for renal biopsy, but it should be recognized that wide variations exist among nephrologists for indication of a renal biopsy, and therefore, it often becomes a matter of personal preference. However, each patient should be evaluated carefully to choose those patients in whom diagnostic yield is thought to be high while complication rates are minimized. In general, it is rare that a renal biopsy is indicated in chronic renal failure with small kidneys. Similarly, renal biopsy is not required to confirm diabetic nephropathy if the presentation of diabetic nephropathy is classic. However, in cases of persistent hematuria (if glomerular), proteinuria, acute renal failure, and various systemic diseases with renal failure and after renal transplant in patients with unexplained deterioration of renal function, a renal biopsy is indicated to obtain a diagnosis or to initiate or modify therapy. However, renal biopsy should not be done if the patient cannot cooperate, if he or she has bleeding abnormalities with platelets that are below 60,000/mm^2 and a prothrombin time greater than 3 seconds from control, and/or if bleeding time is prolonged. Also, renal biopsy should not be done if a solitary kidney exists or before diastolic blood pressure has been brought to less than 90 mm Hg.

The biopsy may be performed percutaneously or by open technology. The percutaneous approach is much more inexpensive and, when performed by a skilled nephrologist, yields adequate tissue in more than 90% of cases. Open biopsy should be reserved for uncooperative patients and those who are at risk for uncontrolled bleeding or have solitary kidneys. Clearly, in the latter case, the index of suspicion for therapeutically relevant information must be high. Adequately sized samples should be obtained for electron microscopy, immunofluorescence, and light microscopy. If minimal tissue is present, then electron microscopy should be done alone, followed by electron microscopy and immunofluorescence, and both of these should be done with light microscopy if adequate tissue is present. Although renal biopsy gives only histologic information, it nevertheless often will allow a correct clinical diagnosis that could not be made otherwise when interpreted in the context of other clinical information.

Blum RN, Wright RA: Detection of pyuria and bacteriuria in symptomatic ambulatory women. J Gen Intern Med 7:140, 1992. *Evaluating accuracy and cost-effectiveness of dipstick urinalysis and standard microscopic urinalysis to predict significant bacteriuria.*
Gottlieb RH, Weinberg EP, Rubens DJ, et al: Renal sonography: Can it be used more selectively in the setting of an elevated serum creatine level? Am J Kidney Dis 29:362–367, 1997. *Nice discussion on the indications and role of renal ultrasonography in evaluating patients who are suspected of having urinary tract obstruction and in patients with a rise in serum creatinine levels.*
Lachs MS, Nachamkin I, Edelstein PH, et al: Spectrum bias in the evaluation of diagnostic tests: Lessons from the rapid dipstick test for urinary tract infection. Ann Intern Med 117:135, 1992. *A careful determination of sensitivities and specificities of leukocyte esterase and bacterial nitrate dipstick tests for urinary tract infections.*
Madaio MP: Renal biopsy. Kidney Int 38:529, 1990. *A complete discussion of indications, safety, and value of renal biopsy.*
Miller TR, Anderson RJ, Linas SL, et al: Urinary diagnostic indices in acute renal failure: A prospective study. Ann Intern Med 89:47, 1978. *A nice prospective analysis of the significance in fractional excretion of filtered sodium as a predictor of a prerenal versus a renal cause of azotemia.*
Rowe MI, Lloyd DA, Lee M: Is the refractometer specific gravity a reliable index for pediatric fluid management? J Pediatr Surg 21:580, 1986. *A study to examine the accuracy of the refractometer to determine the osmolarity of urine in pediatric patients.*

101 STRUCTURE AND FUNCTION OF THE KIDNEYS

C. Craig Tisher

The complex multicellular composition of the kidney reflects the complicated nature of its functional properties. This organ is responsible for maintaining both the volume and ionic composition of the body fluids; excreting fixed or non-volatile metabolic waste products such as creatinine, urea, and uric acid; and eliminating exogenous drugs and toxins. The kidney is a major endocrine organ, because it produces renin, erythropoietin, 1,25-dihydroxy-cholecalciferol, prostaglandins, and kinins; and it also serves as a target organ for many hormones. The kidney also catabolizes small-molecular-weight proteins and is responsible for a host of metabolic functions (e.g., ammoniagenesis and gluconeogenesis).

DEVELOPMENT. The kidney originates from two sources: (1) the ureteral bud, which gives rise to the ureter, pelvis, calyces, and collecting ducts; and (2) the metanephric blastema, which gives rise to the glomerulus and tubules. During embryogenesis, three successive sets of excretory organs develop: the pronephros, mesonephros, and metanephros. The permanent kidney evolves from the metanephros. Cellular and molecular mechanisms that underlie renal morphogenesis include cell proliferation, expression of nuclear proto-oncogenes and homeobox genes, the actions of peptide growth factors, and alterations in both cell adhesion and the composition of the extracellular matrix.

GROSS ANATOMY. The kidneys are located in the retroperitoneal space and extend from the twelfth thoracic vertebra to the third lumbar vertebra. The right organ usually is more caudad, whereas the left organ tends to be slightly larger. Each adult human kidney weighs 115 to 170 g, measures approximately 11 × 6 × 2.5 cm, and is surrounded by a tough, fibroelastic capsule.

The cut surface of a bisected kidney reveals a darker inner region, the medulla, and a pale outer region approximately 1 cm in thickness, the cortex. The human kidney has a multipapillary configuration in which the medulla is divided into 8 to 18 striated conical masses called *pyramids* (Fig. 101–1). The base of each pyramid is positioned at the corticomedullary junction, and the apex extends toward the renal pelvis, forming a papilla. On the tip of each papilla there are numerous small openings that represent the distal ends of the collecting ducts (of Bellini). Extending downward between the pyramids are portions of cortex, the septa of Bertin. Close examination of the cut surface reveals fine longitudinal striations, the medullary rays (of Ferrein), which extend into the cortex. Despite their name, the medullary rays actually represent

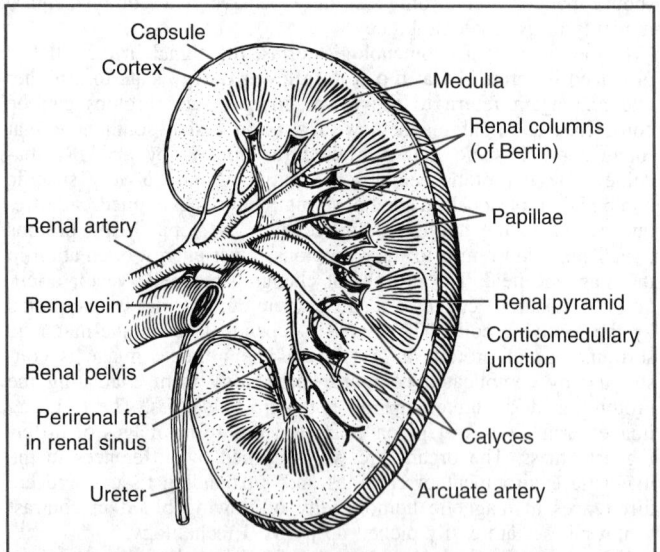

FIGURE 101–1 ■ Sagittal section of human kidney illustrating gross anatomic features.

part of the cortex and are formed by the straight segments of the proximal tubule, the thick ascending limbs, and the collecting ducts.

The renal pelvis is the saclike dilatation of the upper ureter. Two or three major calyces extend from the pelvis and divide into the minor calyces that surround individual papillae.

THE NEPHRON. Each human kidney contains about 0.8 to 1.2 $\times$ 10^6 nephrons—the functional units of the kidney. A nephron consists of the glomerulus or renal corpuscle, the proximal tubule, the thin limbs of Henle, and the distal tubule, all of which originate from the metanephric blastema (Fig. 101–2). The connecting tubule, a transitional segment also derived from the metanephric blastema, joins the nephron to the collecting duct system. Although not anatomically precise, the term *nephron* is commonly used to also include the entire collecting duct.

ARCHITECTURE. In the renal cortex, two architectural regions can be distinguished, the *cortical labyrinth* and the *medullary rays* (see Fig. 101–1). The cortical labyrinth is a continuous zone of parenchyma that surrounds the medullary rays. Glomeruli, proximal and distal convoluted tubules, connecting tubules, initial collecting tubules, interlobular veins, and a rich capillary network are located in the cortical labyrinth. Ascending connecting tubules of juxtamedullary nephrons fuse to form arcades within the cortical labyrinth. The medullary rays contain the proximal and distal straight tubules and collecting ducts that all enter the medulla.

In the medulla, specific nephron segments are found at precise levels and divide the medulla into an inner and an outer zone, with the latter subdivided into an inner and an outer stripe (see Fig. 101–2). In the outer stripe of the outer medulla are the terminal portions of the proximal straight tubules, the thick ascending limbs, and the collecting ducts. The thicker inner stripe of the outer medulla contains thin descending limbs, thick ascending limbs, and collecting ducts. The thin descending and thin ascending limbs of long loops and the collecting ducts are located in the inner medulla. This intricate arrangement of the parenchyma in the cortex and medulla provides an anatomic basis for integration of many of the complex functions of the kidney.

VASCULATURE. STRUCTURE. The kidney has an extensive vasculature that accommodates 20 to 25% of the cardiac output. The main renal artery branches to form anterior and posterior divisions, which in turn divide into five segmental arteries. The *segmental arteries* traverse the renal sinus to divide into the *interlobar arteries*. The latter pierce the parenchyma and course toward the cortex along the septa of Bertin between adjacent renal pyramids (see Fig. 101–1). At the corticomedullary junction, the interlobar arteries branch into the *arcuate arteries*, which follow a gently curved course along the base of the pyramids. The arcuate arteries give rise to the *interlobular arteries* that ascend in the cortex toward the renal surface.

Afferent arterioles are branches of the interlobular arteries, and each supplies a single glomerulus (renal corpuscle) (Fig. 101–3). The *efferent arterioles* exit the glomeruli and divide to form an intricate peritubular microcirculation. The capillary networks formed by the efferent arterioles of superficial and midcortical glomeruli supply the cortical labyrinth and medullary rays, while the efferent arterioles of the juxtamedullary glomeruli are responsible for the entire medullary blood supply. In the outer stripe of the outer medulla these vessels divide to form the *descending vasa recta,* which are located in vascular bundles. At various levels in the medulla the descending vasa recta exit the bundles to form capillary networks. The *ascending vasa recta* drain the medulla.

FUNCTION. In a 70-kg person, renal blood flow (RBF) amounts to one fourth to one fifth of the resting cardiac output or 1.2 L/min. The renal cortex receives 85 to 90% of this flow compared with 10% for the outer medulla and 1 to 2% for the inner medulla including the papilla. With one kidney removed, blood flow to the remaining kidney will nearly double within a few weeks.

RBF and glomerular filtration rate (GFR) remain relatively constant over a wide range of perfusion pressures, a process that is termed *autoregulation.* An intrinsic property of smooth muscle cells in the renal vasculature—the myogenic reflex—permits instantaneous alterations in the tone of the vessel wall to maintain RBF and GFR constant over a pressure range of 80 to 180 mm Hg.

There are a host of hormonal and neural factors that can alter RBF. Renal vasoconstrictors that reduce RBF include endothelin, angiotensin II, thromboxane, stimulation of the α-adrenergic system, vasopressin, and catecholamines. Vasodilating agents include the prostaglandins PGI_2 and PGE_2 and atrial peptides, bradykinin, and endothelial-derived relaxing factor or nitric oxide.

GLOMERULUS. STRUCTURE. The anatomically correct name for the glomerulus is the *renal corpuscle*. However, because of com-

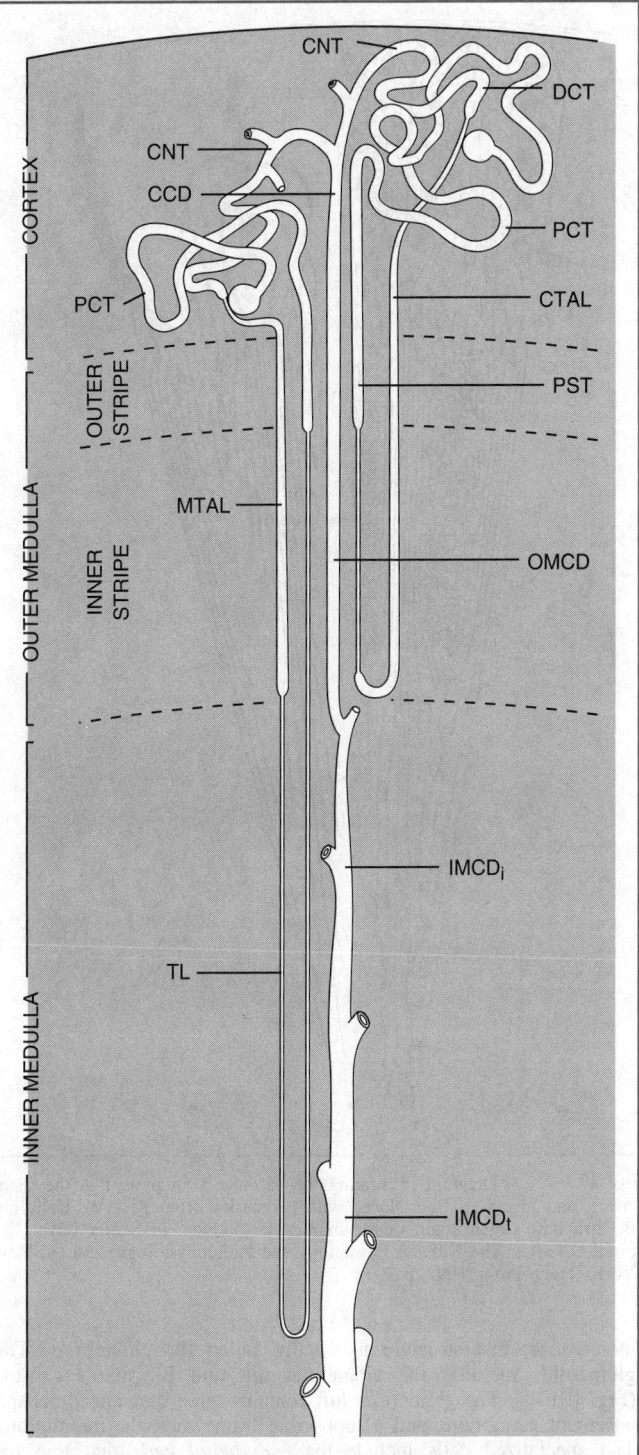

FIGURE 101–2 ■ Diagram illustrating superficial and juxtamedullary nephrons. PCT = proximal convoluting tubule; PST = proximal straight tubule; TL = thin limb of Henle's loop; MTAL = medullary thick ascending limb; CTAL = cortical thick ascending limb; DCT = distal convoluted tubule; CNT = connecting segment; CCD = cortical collecting duct; OMCD = outer medullary collecting duct; $IMCD_i$ = initial inner medullary collecting duct; and $IMCD_t$ = terminal inner medullary collecting duct. (Modified from Madsen KM, Tisher CC: Structural-functional relationships along the distal nephron. Am J Physiol 250:Fl, 1986.)

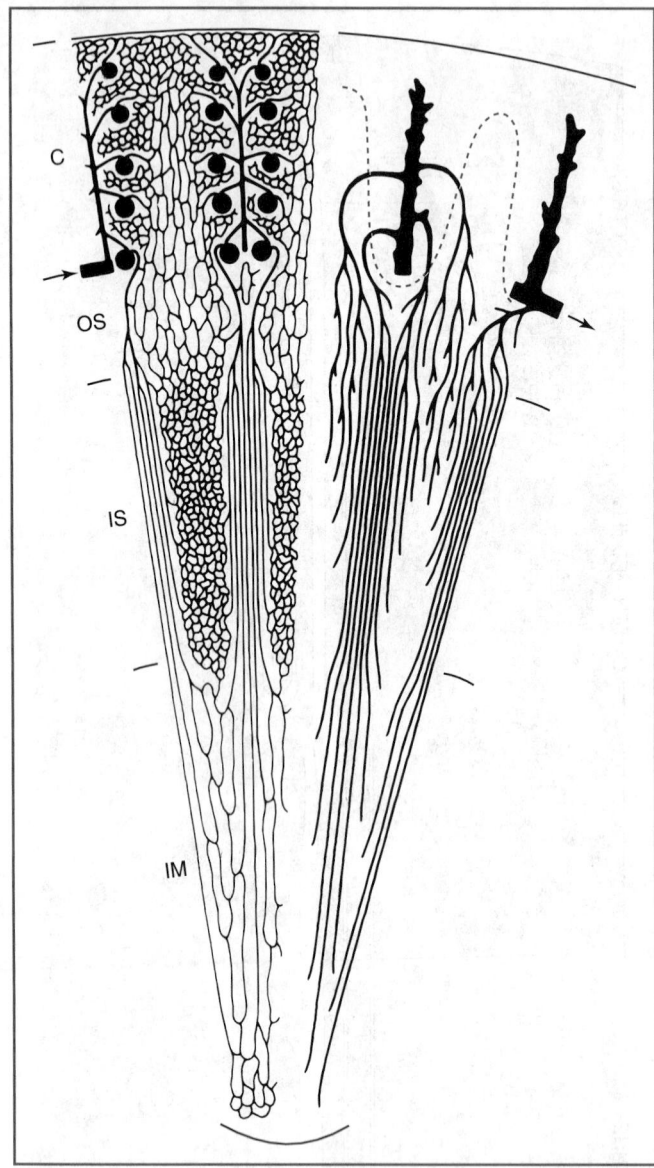

FIGURE 101–3 ▪ Diagram illustrating the vascular arrangement in the renal cortex and medulla. (Reproduced with permission from Kriz W, Kaissling B: Structural organization of the mammalian kidney. *In* Seldin DW, Giebisch G [eds.]: The Kidney: Physiology and Pathophysiology. 2nd ed. New York, Raven Press, 1992, p 709.)

mon usage, this structure is usually called the *glomerulus.* The glomerulus includes the glomerular tuft and Bowman's capsule (Fig. 101–4). The glomerular tuft contains three specialized cells, a basement membrane, and a supporting framework, the mesangium. The specialized cells include the *endothelial cells* that line the lumina of the capillaries, the *mesangial cells* located in the centrilobular region of the glomerular tuft, and the *visceral epithelial cells* that are situated on the outer surfaces of the capillaries (Fig. 101–5). A fourth cell type, the *parietal epithelial cell,* lines Bowman's capsule. At the vascular pole where the afferent and efferent arterioles enter and exit the glomerulus, respectively, the visceral epithelium is continuous with the parietal epithelium. Thus the glomerulus resembles an epithelial-lined sac invaginated by a tuft of capillaries. Bowman's space, also called the "urinary space," represents the area between the visceral epithelial cells and the parietal epithelial layer lining Bowman's capsule. It receives the glomerular filtrate, which exits Bowman's space at the urinary pole to enter the proximal tubule (see Fig. 101–4). A filtration barrier is formed between the blood and the urinary space by the fenestrated endothelium lining the capillary loops, the peripheral glomerular basement membrane (GBM), and the overlying visceral epithelial

cell (Fig. 101–6). In humans, the mean area of the filtration surface per glomerulus is approximately 0.136 sq mm.

FUNCTION. Ultrafiltration. In a 70-kg person, the kidney forms approximately 180 L of glomerular filtrate each day through a process termed *ultrafiltration.* This represents the initial step in urine formation. The driving force to move fluid from the glomerular capillaries across the glomerular capillary wall to the urinary space (Bowman's space) is derived from the hydraulic pressure that is generated by the pumping action of the heart. Each glomerulus has a filtration rate (single nephron glomerular filtration rate [SNGFR]) of 60 nL/min, which is much higher per unit surface area than other capillary beds in the body. The rate of filtration is proportional to the net ultrafiltration pressure (P_{UF}) that is present across the glomerular capillary wall and is determined by the balance of hydraulic (P) and oncotic (Π) pressures (Starling forces) that are operative between the glomerular capillary lumen and Bowman's space. The intrinsic water permeability of the capillary wall (k) and the surface area (A), which together define the ultrafiltration coefficient (K_f), are also important determinants of ultrafiltration. Thus

$$\begin{aligned} SNGFR &= K_f \cdot \overline{P}_{UF} \\ &= K_f \cdot [(\overline{P}_{GC} - P_T) - (\Pi_{GC} - \Pi_T)] \\ &= k \cdot A(\overline{\Delta P} - \overline{\Delta \Pi}) \end{aligned}$$

where GC and T refer to glomerular capillary and Bowman's space, respectively, and the overbar denotes mean values.

Because under normal circumstances there is virtually no protein in the ultrafiltrate, the oncotic pressure in the urinary space (Π_T) approaches zero and therefore does not affect ultrafiltration. Increasing the oncotic pressure in the glomerular capillary (as in multiple myeloma with its characteristic hyperproteinemia), increasing the hydraulic pressure in Bowman's space (via ureteral obstruction), and lowering glomerular capillary hydraulic pressure (as in hypotension) all reduce SNGFR.

GLOMERULAR BASEMENT MEMBRANE. Structure. The GBM is a hydrated gel containing cross-linked molecules that form a complex, three-dimensional lattice-like network (see Fig. 101–6). Biochemical and immunocytochemical studies have revealed that the GBM is composed of type IV and type V collagen, laminin, heparan sulfate proteoglycans, and nidogen or entactin, as well as other components. Type IV collagen is the main component in the *lamina densa,* whereas in the *laminae rarae* other proteins predominate. The polyanionic character of the heparan sulfate proteoglycans is largely responsible for the net negative charge of the GBM.

FUNCTION. Physiologic and ultrastructural studies have established that the GBM is both a *size-selective* and a *charge-selective* barrier to the passage of macromolecules. The GBM, along with the endothelium, serves as the principal functional barrier to the passage of circulating polyanions across the glomerular capillary wall. The size-selective properties of the GBM allow molecules such as inulin, with a radius of about 1.4 nm, to pass freely from the capillary lumen to the urinary space. Because the concentration of inulin in both the plasma water and the fluid in the urinary space is identical, the fractional clearance of inulin is equal to 1. As the radii of macromolecules increase above 2.0 nm, their passage is restricted across the GBM, and molecules with a radius greater than 4.2 nm are completely restricted. Thus their fractional clearance approaches zero under normal circumstances.

In addition to size, the charge of a molecule can greatly affect its ability to cross the glomerular capillary wall. The size- and charge-selective properties of the GBM are summarized in Figure 101–7.

JUXTAGLOMERULAR APPARATUS. STRUCTURE. The juxtaglomerular apparatus is located at the vascular pole of the glomerulus (see Figs. 101–4 and 101–5). In the wall of the afferent arteriole there are modified smooth muscle cells, the so-called myoepithelial cells, which secrete renin.

The macula densa is a plaque-like configuration of specialized cells within the cortical thick ascending limb of Henle that is in contact with the extraglomerular mesangium (see Figs. 101–4 and 101–5).

FUNCTION. The juxtaglomerular apparatus is believed to be responsible for *tubuloglomerular feedback,* in which the composition of tubular fluid delivered to the macula densa changes the filtration

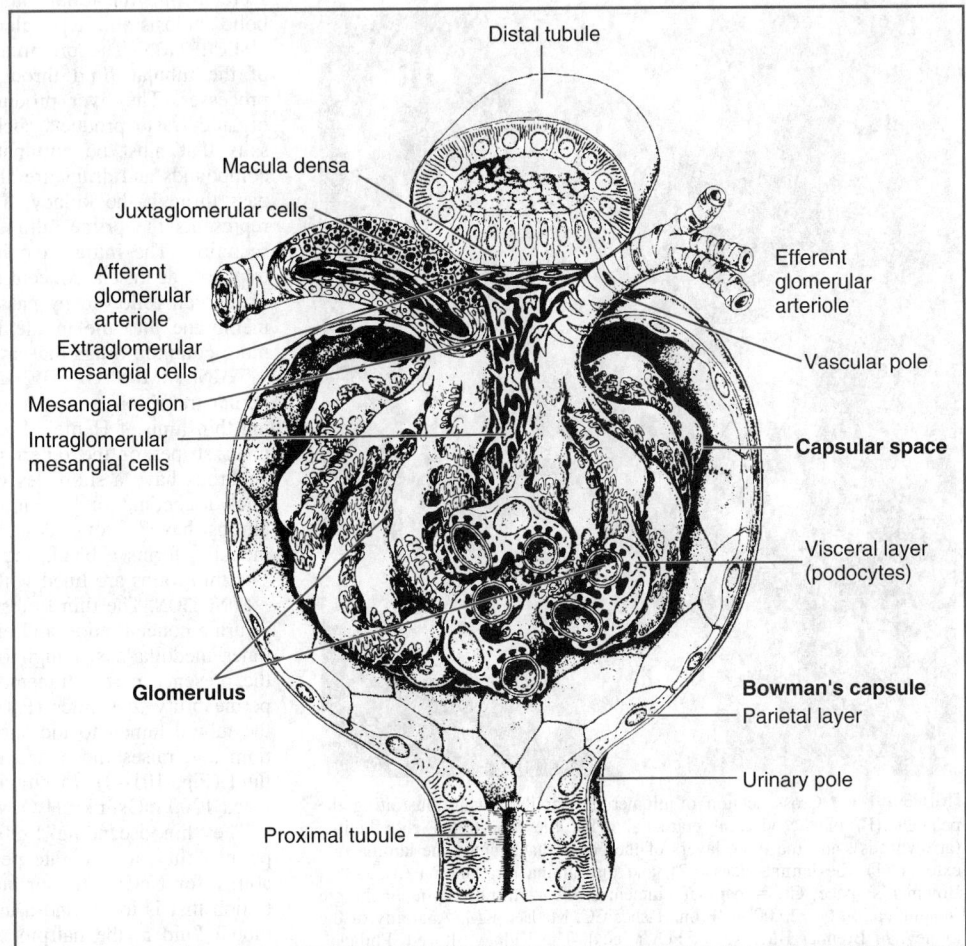

FIGURE 101–4 ■ Schematic three-dimensional depiction of the glomerulus. (From Bargmann W: Histologie und Mikroscopische Anatomie des Menschen. Stuttgart, Georg Thieme Verlag, 1977, p 86.)

rate of the associated glomerulus, presumably by altering renin secretion, which ultimately regulates glomerular hemodynamics.

PROXIMAL TUBULE. STRUCTURE. The proximal tubule includes an initial convoluted portion, the *pars convoluta,* located in the cortical labyrinth, and a straight portion, the *pars recta,* located in the medullary ray. Proximal tubule cells are tall and possess a

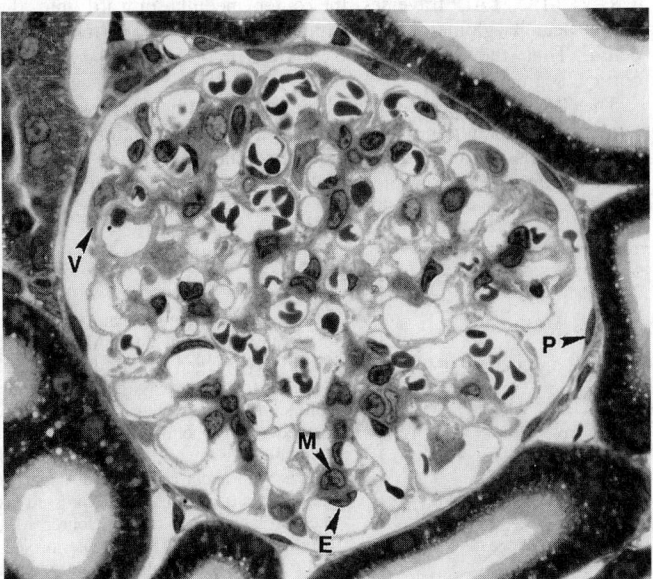

FIGURE 101–5 ■ Cross-sectional view of glomerulus depicting endothelial cells (E), mesangial cells (M), visceral epithelial cells (V), and parietal epithelial cells (P). (magnification × 480)

prominent brush border that markedly increases the surface area of the luminal membrane. The cells contain a well-developed endocytic-lysosomal apparatus that has an important role in the absorption and degradation of macromolecules such as albumin from the glomerular filtrate.

The basolateral plasma membranes are markedly amplified due to extensive interdigitations of basal and lateral cytoplasmic processes between adjacent cells. The localization of Na^+,K^+-ATPase (the sodium pump) to the basolateral membranes explains the active transport of sodium characteristic of this tubule segment. Numerous elongated mitochondria are located close to the interdigitating basolateral membrane processes, providing a source for the cellular energy required for active transport. There is an excellent correlation along the length of the proximal tubule between the elaborate basolateral membrane expressed as surface area, the high Na^+,K^+-ATPase activity localized to this membrane, and the capacity to transport sodium and other ions. Therefore, the intrinsic rates at which solutes and fluid are transported decrease along the length of the proximal tubule.

FUNCTION. The proximal tubule is the first component of the nephron that modifies the volume and ionic composition of the glomerular ultrafiltrate. Through isosmotic fluid reabsorption, fluid volume is reduced by 60% or more under normal conditions. The principal driving force for the reabsorption of solutes is Na^+,K^+-ATPase located along the basolateral plasma membrane. By maintaining a low intracellular sodium concentration, there is passive entry of sodium into the cell across the luminal plasma membrane and down its electrochemical gradient. In the early proximal tubule this leads to a small electrical potential difference (PD) that is lumen negative. Sodium is pumped out of the cell actively at the basolateral surface via Na^+,K^+-ATPase. This process also creates a slight osmotic gradient that facilitates the reabsorption of fluid. The balance between osmotic and hydraulic pressures (Starling forces) in the peritubular capillaries and the surrounding interstitium deter-

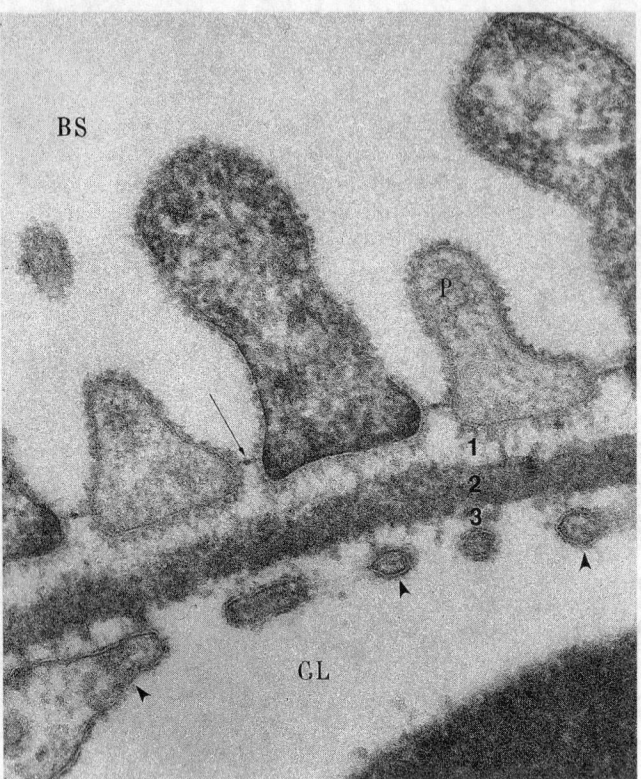

FIGURE 101-6 ▪ Cross section of glomerular capillary wall illustrating the pedicels (P) of the visceral epithelial cells, the fenestrated endothelium (arrowheads), and the three layers of the GBM that include the lamina rara externa (1), the lamina densa (2), and the lamina rara interna (3). BS = Bowman's space; CL = capillary lumen; arrow = filtration slit diaphragm (magnification × 120,000). (From Tisher CC, Madsen KM: Anatomy of the kidney. *In* Brenner BM, Rector FC Jr [eds]: The Kidney. 4th ed. Philadelphia, WB Saunders, 1991, p 14.)

mines the extent of the backleak of sodium and water to the tubule lumen via the intercellular space through the non-occluding tight junction and thus the net reabsorption of sodium and water and other solutes. Water permeability of the proximal tubule is due largely to the presence of a transmembrane protein, aquaporin 1, that functions as a molecular water channel and is located in the luminal and basolateral membranes.

Reabsorption of glucose, amino acids, citrate, lactate, acetate, and phosphate also occurs early in the proximal tubule by sodium-coupled active transport processes. Other transported ions are listed in Table 101–1.

The critical elements of bicarbonate reabsorption are depicted in Figure 101–8.

The proximal tubule is also an important site for *ammoniagenesis* in which glutamine serves as the substrate. Ammonia combines with protons, forming the ammonium ion (NH_4^+), which is then secreted into the tubule lumen. This process is enhanced in metabolic acidosis and hypokalemia.

SECRETION. The proximal tubule also modifies the composition of the tubular fluid through a number of well-defined secretory processes. The liver produces a number of cationic and anionic organic waste products such as urate, hippurate, oxalate, and bile salts that must be eliminated by the kidney. Certain exogenous compounds and drugs are also removed from the plasma in a single pass through the kidney. The S_2 segment of the proximal tubule represents the prime, although not exclusive, site for organic ion secretion. The initial step in the secretory process involves active transport against a concentration gradient at the basolateral surface of the cell followed by passive diffusion across the luminal plasma membrane into the tubule fluid. Table 101–2 lists several of the more common drugs that are secreted by the proximal tubule.

THIN LIMBS OF HENLE'S LOOP. STRUCTURE. There is an abrupt transition from the terminal proximal tubule to the descending thin limb of Henle's loop at the junction between the outer and inner stripes of the outer medulla (see Fig. 101–2). Short-looped nephrons have a short descending thin limb that continues into the thick ascending limb near the bend in the loop. Long-looped nephrons have a long descending thin limb that enters the inner medulla, forms a bend, and returns as a long ascending thin limb. The thin limbs are lined with a low-lying simple epithelium.

FUNCTION. The thin limbs of Henle's loop play an important role in urine concentration and dilution. The thin descending limb in the inner medulla has a high osmotic water permeability (L_p) due to the presence of the transmembrane protein aquaporin 1 but a low permeability to solutes (P_s). This facilitates transfer of water from the tubule lumen to the surrounding hypertonic medullary interstitium and raises the concentration of NaCl and urea in the tubule fluid (Fig. 101–9). In humans, the tonicity of the tubule fluid can reach 1200 mOsm/kg H_2O with severe water restriction.

The thin ascending limb of Henle has a low osmotic water permeability, a moderate permeability for urea, and a high permeability for NaCl. The surrounding interstitium has a NaCl concentration that is lower and a urea concentration that is higher than the tubule fluid at the hairpin turn. These characteristics favor formation of a dilute tubule fluid, because the passive movement of NaCl out of the tubule exceeds the passive entry of urea into the tubule. Thus, at any given level in the inner medulla, the tonicity of the surrounding interstitial fluid is greater than that of the tubule fluid in the thin ascending limb of Henle (see Fig. 101–9). Overall, the thin limbs of the loop of Henle reabsorb about 15% of the glomerular ultrafiltrate and up to 25% of the sodium and chloride.

DISTAL TUBULE. STRUCTURE. The distal tubule includes two morphologically distinct segments: the *thick ascending limb* (TAL) of Henle's loop and the *distal convoluted tubule* (DCT) (see Fig. 101–2). The TAL traverses the outer medulla upward into the cortex near its glomerulus of origin to end just beyond the macula densa. Thus the TAL can be divided into a medullary and a cortical segment.

The TAL is composed of cuboidal cells with extensive basolateral plasma membrane invaginations and interdigitations between adjacent cells that enclose elongated mitochondria. These ultrastructural features are typical of epithelial cells involved in active solute

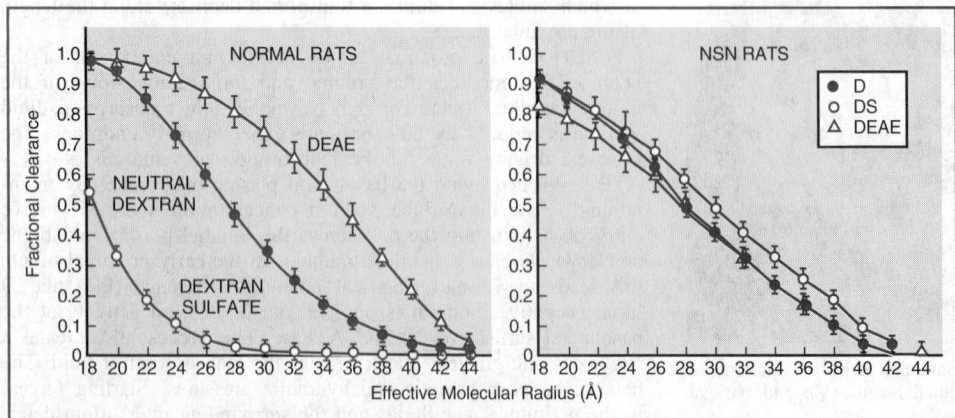

FIGURE 101-7 ▪ Fractional clearances of diethylaminoethyl (DEAE) dextran (positively-charged molecule), neutral dextran (neutral charge), and dextran sulfate (negatively-charged molecule), plotted as a function of effective molecular radius in normal rats (left) and in rats with nephrotoxic serum nephritis (NSN, right). Values are expressed as means ± 1 SEM. (From Bohrer MP, Baylis C, Humes HD, et al: Permselectivity of the glomerular capillary wall: Facilitated filtration of circulating polycations. J Clin Invest 61:72, 1978, by copyright permission of the American Society for Clinical Investigation.)

Table 101-1 ■ TRANSPORT OF IONS IN THE PROXIMAL TUBULE

ION	PRINCIPAL SITE OF TRANSPORT	PROCESS
Potassium	Early proximal tubule	Freely filtered by the glomerulus; up to 70% reabsorbed by a passive process that parallels sodium and water and is regulated in part by the transepithelial potential difference
Bicarbonate	Early proximal tubule	Filtered by the glomerulus; up to 90% of the 4500 mEq filtered each day is reabsorbed secondary to proton secretion
Hydrogen	Proximal convoluted tubule	Approximately 65% secreted via Na^+/H^+ antiporter; 35% secreted by an electrogenic sodium-independent H^+-ATPase
Chloride	S_2 segment of proximal tubule	Coupled to active transport of sodium; passive transport driven by favorable lumen-to-peritubular concentration gradient for Cl^-
Calcium	Entire proximal tubule	Can exit tubule lumen through paracellular pathway via passive voltage-dependent diffusion; active transport via a Na^+-Ca^{2+} exchange and Ca^{2+}-ATPase

transport. The *macula densa* is a specialized region of the cortical TAL that is in contact with the extraglomerular mesangium (see Figs. 101-4 and 101-5).

The DCT represents the terminal part of the distal tubule and begins at a variable distance beyond the macula densa. The cells of the DCT resemble those of the TAL.

FUNCTION. The TAL actively reabsorbs NaCl, which is mediated by an Na^+-K^+-$2Cl^-$ co-transport mechanism in the apical plasma membrane (see Fig. 101-9). The energy for this process is provided by the Na^+,K^+-ATPase localized on the basolateral plasma membrane. The principal function of the medullary TAL is to generate and maintain a hypertonic medullary interstitium that permits a maximally concentrated urine to form, while the cortical segment continues to dilute the tubule fluid, permitting the formation of a maximally dilute urine. Thus the tubule fluid that exits the cortical TAL has an osmolality of less than 150 mOsm/kg H_2O. At this point, the total volume of the original glomerular ultrafiltrate in the nephron has been reduced by 85%.

The TAL also reabsorbs *calcium* from the tubular fluid. Throughout the TAL, a significant component of calcium transport is passive and driven by the transepithelial potential difference (PD_1). Active transport has been identified in the cortical TAL, which is independent of Ca^{2+}-ATPase activity, sodium transport, and anaerobic metabolism. Calcium transport is enhanced in the cortical TAL by parathyroid hormone (PTH) and cyclic adenosine monophosphate and in the medullary TAL by calcitonin and cyclic adenosine monophosphate.

Bicarbonate transport is present along the entire TAL through a sodium-coupled HCO_3^- transport mechanism located on the basolateral plasma membrane. Active and passive transport of NH_4^+ out of the lumen and into the interstitium for subsequent transport in the form of NH_3 into the lumen of the collecting duct also occurs

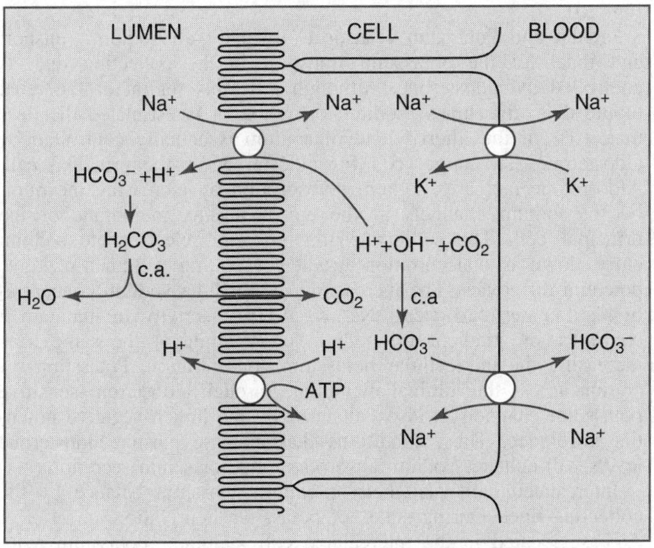

in the TAL. Thus this region of the nephron also plays a role in acidification of the tubule fluid.

The cortical TAL is a major site for reabsorbing *magnesium*. The passive component of magnesium transport is facilitated by the Na^+-K^+-$2Cl^-$ co-transport mechanism that establishes a favorable lumen-positive electrochemical gradient, whereas the active magnesium transport mechanism is incompletely understood.

In the DCT, *sodium chloride* continues to be reabsorbed through a ouabain-sensitive Na^+,K^+-ATPase-driven active transport process. Because the DCT is also impermeable to water, there is further dilution of the tubule fluid to an osmolality of approximately 100 mOsm/kg H_2O. This segment is also a site for *calcium* reabsorption stimulated by calcitonin and PTH.

CONNECTING TUBULE. STRUCTURE. The connecting tubule or connecting segment joins the DCT with the collecting duct system (see Fig. 101-2). Representing a transitional segment in the human kidney, the connecting tubule is composed of four specific cell types resulting from an intermixing of cells from the adjacent DCT and the initial collecting tubule (ICT). The most characteristic cell type is the connecting tubule cell, which is intermediate in appearance between the DCT cell and the principal cell of the collecting duct. Intercalated cells involved in proton and bicarbonate transport vary considerably in structure in the connecting tubule.

FUNCTION. PTH affects *calcium* transport in this segment, whereas vasopressin (antidiuretic hormone) has no effect on adenylate cyclase activity or water permeability. This segment is responsible for reabsorbing *sodium* and secreting *potassium*. The latter is believed to be at least partially controlled by mineralocorticoids. The connecting segment is also involved in *proton* and *bicarbonate* transport and is a major site for kallikrein production and secretion in the kidney.

COLLECTING DUCT. STRUCTURE. The collecting duct begins in the cortex and descends through the medulla to the tip of the papilla. It can be divided into cortical, outer medullary, and inner medullary segments (see Fig. 101-2). There is remarkable cellular heterogeneity along the collecting duct.

The *cortical collecting duct* (CCD) can be subdivided into the ICT and the medullary ray portion. The CCD is composed of both principal cells and intercalated cells. The principal cells, which represent approximately two thirds of the total cell population, have a light-staining cytoplasm and relatively few organelles but prominent infoldings of the basal plasma membrane. The intercalated or "dark" cells comprise approximately one third of the cells in the CCD.

There is evidence for the presence of two distinct configurations

FIGURE 101-8 ■ Diagram depicting the major mechanism for bicarbonate reclamation in the proximal convoluted tubule. c.a. = carbonic anhydrase.

Table 101-2 ■ COMMON DRUGS SECRETED BY THE PROXIMAL TUBULE

CATIONIC	ANIONIC
Cimetidine	Penicillin
Paraquat	Furosemide
Quinine	Probenecid
Morphine	Salicylates
Trimethoprim	Acetazolamide
Atropine	Chlorothiazides
Epinephrine	Cephalothin
	Ethacrynic acid

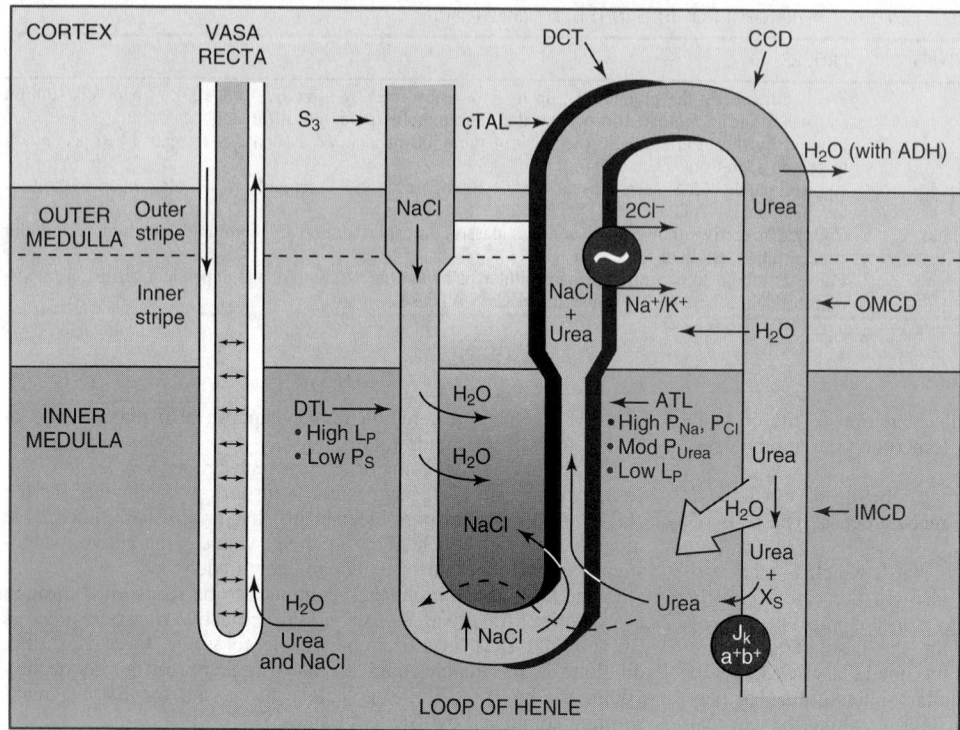

FIGURE 101–9 ■ Diagram illustrating the essential components of the countercurrent multiplication and exchange systems in the kidney (see text for explanation). The heavy black line indicates water-impermeable segments of the nephron, and shading denotes progressive increase in tonicity of the medullary interstitium. S_3 = third segment of proximal tubule; DTL = descending thin limb; ATL = ascending thin limb; cTAL = cortical thick ascending limb; DCT = distal convoluted tubule; CCD = cortical collecting duct; OMCD = outer medullary collecting duct; IMCD = inner medullary collecting duct; L_p = osmotic water permeability; P_S, P_{Na}, P_{Cl}, P_{ure} = permeability to solutes, Na^+, Cl^-, and urea, respectively; X_S = nonreabsorbable solutes; and $J_Ka^+b^+$ = Kidd antigen and urea transporter. (Modified from Brenner BM, Coe FL, Rector FC Jr [eds]: Renal Physiology in Health and Disease. Philadelphia, WB Saunders, 1987, pp 53 and 160.)

of intercalated cells, type A and type B, in the CCD. Type A cells have prominent microprojections on the apical plasma membrane and extensive tubulovesicular structures in the apical cytoplasm. Type B cells have a denser cytoplasm, more mitochondria, more spherical vesicular structures in the cytoplasm, and a larger basolateral membrane surface area. The type B cell is localized to the CCD.

The *outer medullary collecting duct* (OMCD) is lined by principal cells and intercalated cells. The latter comprise one third of the cells in the OMCD and resemble the type A cells in the CCD.

The *inner medullary collecting duct* (IMCD) is subdivided into two regions: the initial IMCD, located in the outer third of the inner medulla, and the terminal IMCD, situated in the distal two thirds of the inner medulla (see Fig. 101–2). The initial IMCD is composed mainly of principal cells and a few intercalated cells, whereas the terminal IMCD is composed of one cell type, the IMCD cell.

FUNCTION. The collecting duct represents the final site in the renal tubule that modifies the volume and solute composition of the tubule fluid.

Water Transport. Aquaporins (AQP)-2, -3, and -4 function as molecular water channels in the collecting duct. AQP-2 is located predominantly in the apical plasma membrane of all principal cells and IMCD cells, whereas AQP-3 is found in the basolateral membrane throughout the collecting duct system from cortex to papillary tip. AQP-4 is limited to the basolateral plasma membrane of principal cells in the inner stripe of the outer medulla and the outer third of the inner medulla. In all segments of the collecting duct the osmotic water permeability is controlled largely by vasopressin. In the absence of vasopressin, only the papillary collecting duct manifests some residual permeability. With vasopressin, the principal cells and all cells in the terminal IMCD are highly permeable to water (see Fig. 101–9). However, in vasopressin-induced antidiuresis, the bulk of the tubule fluid is reabsorbed in the CCD.

Proton and Bicarbonate Transport. The entire collecting duct is involved in proton transport and hence the fine tuning of acid secretion by the kidney. The presence of high levels of carbonic anhydrase II in the intercalated cells suggested initially that they were involved in urine acidification. Immunocytochemical studies have localized a vacuolar type H^+-ATPase in the apical membrane and a Cl^-/HCO_3^- exchanger in the basolateral membrane of type A intercalated cells (Fig. 101–10A). These findings implicate the type

A cell in proton or hydrogen ion secretion in the CCD. The immunolocalization of H^+-ATPase to the basolateral membrane of type B cells and the functional evidence for an apical Cl^-/HCO_3^- exchanger in these cells provide evidence that type B intercalated cells are involved in bicarbonate secretion (see Fig. 101–10B).

The intercalated cells in the OMCD are responsible for hydrogen ion secretion, which is an active mineralocorticoid-stimulated, sodium-independent process driven in part by H^+-ATPase. The IMCD is also involved in urine acidification. Acid-secreting intercalated cells are present in the initial IMCD. Microcatheterization studies have documented a decrease in luminal pH along the IMCD.

Urea Transport. The cortical and outer medullary segments of the collecting duct are largely impermeable to urea in both the presence and absence of vasopressin. In the terminal IMCD, urea reabsorption occurs by means of a vasopressin-sensitive, phloretin-inhibitable, facilitated transport pathway that helps to maintain a high urea concentration in the deep inner medulla to facilitate urea recycling, which is important for maximum urine concentration (see Fig. 101–9).

Sodium and Potassium Transport. Virtually all sodium transport and much of the potassium transport in the collecting duct is controlled by aldosterone. Although it is this region of the renal tubule that "fine tunes" sodium excretion, it is estimated that less than 10% of the filtered load of sodium is actually controlled by aldosterone. The target cell for aldosterone is the principal cell. Aldosterone increases sodium reabsorption by increasing the number of sodium channels in the apical plasma membrane of the principal cell. The sodium channels permit electrogenic sodium entry down a concentration gradient, creating a lumen-negative potential difference. The increase in intracellular sodium concentration stimulates basolateral Na^+,K^+-ATPase activity to maintain a concentration gradient for sodium entry while at the same time increasing the intracellular potassium concentration. Potassium secretion across the luminal membrane through aldosterone-sensitive potassium channels is also enhanced by the lumen-negative potential difference. Thus, conditions that increase plasma aldosterone levels will enhance sodium absorption and potassium secretion.

Intercalated cells also help maintain potassium balance by the collecting duct. During states of potassium deprivation, an H^+,K^+-ATPase located in the intercalated cell facilitates potassium reabsorption in exchange for hydrogen ions throughout the CCD and OMCD.

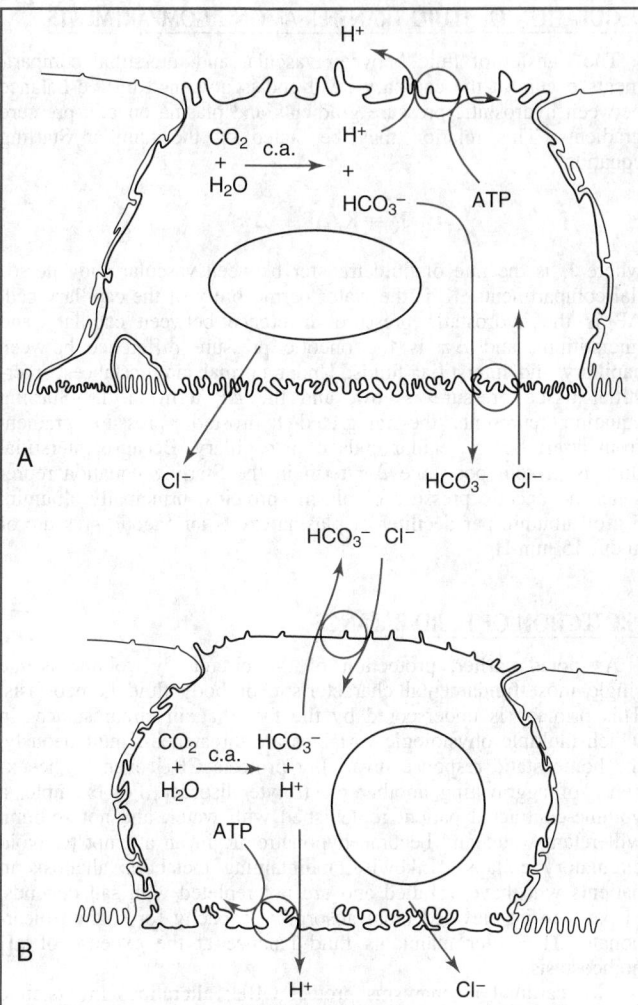

FIGURE 101-10 ■ Diagrams illustrating transport characteristics of type A (above) and type B (below) intercalated cells of the CCD. (Used with permission from Madsen KM, Verlander JW, Kim J, Tisher CC: Morphological adaptation of the collecting duct to acid-base disturbances. Kidney Int 40[Suppl 33]:S57, 1991.)

INTEGRATION OF NORMAL NEPHRON FUNCTION. SODIUM HOMEOSTASIS. Each day approximately 25,000 mEq of sodium (140 mEq/L × 180 L) is filtered, whereas less than 1% is actually excreted in the urine by a euvolemic individual. Thus, the bulk of filtered sodium is reabsorbed along the nephron. Normally, about 65% of the filtered sodium is reabsorbed by the proximal tubule, 20% by the TAL, 7 to 10% by the DCT, and the remainder by the collecting duct. With a salt load, there is a progressive increase in urine sodium excretion until a new steady state is achieved where output matches intake. Until a steady state is attained, however, the individual goes into positive sodium balance, retains water, and gains weight. Restricting sodium intake will produce the opposite effect until the kidney fully compensates over a 3- to 5-day period.

Several factors influence normal sodium balance. For instance, the kidney is extremely sensitive to changes in effective arterial blood volume. Dehydration or acute volume depletion secondary to blood loss leads to a fall in RBF and GFR secondary to a decrease in cardiac output, activation of the renin-angiotensin-aldosterone system, and an increase in renal sympathetic nerve activity. As the filtered load of sodium decreases, the proximal tubule increases sodium reabsorption. Because the vasoconstrictive effect of angiotensin II affects the efferent glomerular arteriole to a greater degree than the afferent arteriole, the filtration fraction is increased, thereby increasing the oncotic pressure in the peritubular capillaries. This, in turn, enhances proximal tubule sodium and fluid reabsorption. An increase in the plasma level of aldosterone from activation of the renin-angiotensin-aldosterone system stimulates sodium reabsorption in the collecting duct. Expansion of the effective

arterial blood volume, as occurs with excessive sodium intake or administering intravenous saline, has the opposite effect.

Other factors also control renal sodium excretion. Several hormones lead to retention of sodium by acting at the tubular level (e.g., growth hormone, cortisol, insulin, and estrogen). On the other hand, PTH, progesterone, and glycogen inhibit the tubular reabsorption of sodium. Atrial natriuretic peptide—a 28-amino acid peptide produced in the atria of the heart and released in the circulation in response to atrial stretch from, for example, expansion of the central blood volume—also enhances sodium excretion, in part by inhibiting sodium reabsorption by the collecting duct.

POTASSIUM HOMEOSTASIS. The kidney is chiefly responsible for maintaining potassium homeostasis. The total-body potassium content of a 70-kg individual is estimated at approximately 3500 mEq, 98 to 99% of which resides in the intracellular compartment at a concentration of 125 mEq/L. The concentration of potassium in the extracellular fluid ranges between 3.5 and 4.5 mEq/L. Each day approximately 720 mEq of potassium (4.0 mEq/L × 180 L) is filtered, whereas only 10 to 15% is excreted in the urine by an individual with normal body potassium stores. In general, potassium excretion equals potassium ingestion. With a normal potassium intake of approximately 100 mEq/d, the kidney will excrete all but about 10 mEq. Approximately 70% of the filtered load of potassium is reabsorbed in the proximal tubule and another 15 to 20% in the loop of Henle. The kidney can respond quickly to increase potassium excretion as much as 10-fold when potassium intake is increased. However, with potassium deprivation, it takes up to 14 days to reach a new steady state, a period of time sufficient to develop a considerable potassium deficit.

It is the collecting duct that is responsible for "fine tuning" potassium excretion. In general, the principal cells secrete potassium under the control of mineralocorticoids, whereas intercalated cells reabsorb potassium. Most of the potassium that appears in the urine is secreted by the collecting duct. Several factors influence renal potassium secretion. These include the rate of distal tubule fluid flow, acid-base balance, aldosterone, and the electronegativity of the distal tubule. The flow dependence of potassium secretion in the collecting duct is well documented. With an increase in flow (such as that induced by diuretics), there is a parallel increase in sodium delivery to the collecting duct, which facilitates sodium reabsorption and potassium secretion. With metabolic acidosis, and to a lesser extent with respiratory acidosis, potassium secretion is suppressed. An opposite effect is observed in metabolic alkalosis. With an increase in the circulating aldosterone level (such as that induced by hyperkalemia), there is a parallel increase in the exchange of sodium for potassium by the principal cells, leading to enhanced potassium secretion. Finally, an increase in the lumen-negative potential, a decrease in the luminal potassium concentration, an increase in the intracellular potassium concentration, and an increase in the luminal membrane permeability to potassium all favor potassium secretion by the principal cell.

The kidney also can protect against hypokalemia. The presence of H^+,K^+-ATPase has been documented in the intercalated cell of the collecting duct, and data suggest that with potassium deprivation there is enhanced reabsorption of potassium in exchange for protons in these cells.

ACID-BASE BALANCE. See Chapter 102.4.

CALCIUM, PHOSPHORUS, AND MAGNESIUM HOMEOSTASIS. See Chapters 261 and 262.

URINE CONCENTRATION AND DILUTION. See Chapter 102.1.

Alpern RJ, Rector FC Jr: Renal acidification mechanisms. *In* Brenner BM (ed): The Kidney, 5th ed. Philadelphia, WB Saunders, 1996, p 408. *A detailed and up-to-date review of acidification in the kidney.*

Clapp WL, Abrahamson DR: Development and gross anatomy of the kidney. *In* Tisher CC, Brenner BM (eds): Renal Pathology With Clinical and Functional Correlations, 2nd ed. Philadelphia, JB Lippincott, 1994, pp 3–59. *One of the most detailed and current discussions of kidney development.*

Gonzalez-Campoy JM, Knox FG: Integrated responses of the kidney to alterations in extracellular fluid volume. *In* Seldin DW, Giebisch G (eds): The Kidney: Physiology and Pathophysiology, 2nd ed. New York, Raven Press, 1992, pp 2041–2098. *An elegant presentation of the mechanisms that control sodium excretion by the kidney.*

Knepper MA, Wade JB, Terris J, et al: Renal aquaporins. Kidney Int 49:1712–1717, 1996. *A detailed description of the distribution and function of aquaporins in the kidney.*

Tisher CC, Madsen KM: Anatomy of the kidney. *In* Brenner BM (ed): The Kidney, 5th ed. Philadelphia, WB Saunders, 1996, p 3. *A detailed and lucid review of kidney structure.*

102 FLUIDS AND ELECTROLYTES

Juha P. Kokko

102.1 Volume Disorders

PHYSIOLOGIC CONSIDERATIONS

Considering that total body water is distributed into distinct compartments, the volumes of these compartments can be measured relatively accurately. However, to understand fluid homeostasis, one must recognize the significance of the term *effective arterial blood volume (EABU)*. This is discussed in Chapter 100, but in its broadest sense it refers to the volume of blood delivered to the volume-sensitive organs, predominantly brain and kidney.

The Body Fluid Compartments

In healthy adults, body water constitutes about 60% of body weight and exists in two compartments: the intracellular fluid (ICF) contains two thirds of body water, or 40% of body weight; the extracellular fluid (ECF) contains the remaining one third of total body water; and total circulatory blood volume (CBU), that is, plasma plus formed elements, constitutes one third of the total ECF volume. This "rule of thirds" for the body fluid compartments is useful in assessing most clinically encountered fluid and electrolyte disorders. Thus, in a healthy 70-kg man, total body water is about 40 L, of which 25 L is intracellular. The functional ECF volume is 15 L, 5 L of which is blood, and because the normal hematocrit is 40 to 45%, total plasma volume is 2.75 to 3.0 L (Fig. 102–1).

More than 95% of total body sodium is extracellular, and sodium and its associated anions, primarily chloride and bicarbonate, constitute the principal solutes of the ECF. Albumin and other macromolecules present in plasma are restricted to the vascular bed and constitute 5% of plasma volume, so plasma is about 95% water. Because capillaries are freely permeable to water and small solutes, interstitial fluid is a protein-poor, but not entirely protein-free, ultrafiltrate of plasma.

Principal anions of ICF vary among different cells, and Figure 102–1 summarizes the approximate concentrations of various intracellular and extracellular cation and anion concentrations.

Intracellular Water (2/3)		Extracellular Water (1/3)	
		Interstitial (2/3)	Blood (1/3)
±25	Na	140	
±150	K	4.5	
±15	Mg	1.2	
±0.01	Ca	2.4	
±2	Cl	100	
±6	HCO₃	25	
±50	Phos	1.2	

FIGURE 102–1 ■ Relative volumes of various body fluid compartments. In a normally built individual, the total-body water content is roughly 60% of body weight. Because adipose tissue has a low concentration of water, the relative water to total body weight ratio is lower in obese individuals. The intracellular electrolyte concentrations are in millimoles per liter and are typical values obtained from muscle.

REGULATION OF FLUID TRANSFER AMONG COMPARTMENTS

The transfer of fluid between vascular and interstitial compartments occurs at the capillary level and is governed by the balance between hydrostatic pressure gradients and plasma oncotic pressure gradients. This relation may be stated by the familiar Starling equation:

$$J_v = K_f(\Delta P - \Delta \pi)$$

where J_v is the rate of fluid transfer between vascular and interstitial compartments, K_f is the water permeability of the capillary bed, ΔP is the hydrostatic pressure difference between capillary and interstitium, and $\Delta \pi$ is the oncotic pressure difference between capillary and interstitial fluids. Under normal circumstances, interstitial tissue pressure is low, and the ΔP term in the Starling equation represents the integrated hydrostatic pressure gradient from arteriolar to venular ends of a capillary. Because interstitial fluid is protein poor, the $\Delta \pi$ term in the Starling equation represents the oncotic pressure of plasma proteins, principally albumin; 5 g of albumin per deciliter of plasma exerts an oncotic pressure of about 15 mm Hg.

PROTECTION OF FLUID BALANCE

As noted earlier, protection of the circulatory volume is the single most fundamental characteristic of body fluid homeostasis. This primacy is underscored by the fact that, in circumstances in which multiple physiologic variables are threatened simultaneously, the homeostatic response invariably protects CBU even at the expense of aggravating another electrolyte disorder. For example, a volume-contracted patient replenished with water, and not sodium, will retain water and become hyponatremic in an attempt to avoid circulatory collapse. Likewise, maintaining metabolic alkalosis in patients who have vomited and are not repleted with salt depends, in part, on an elevated renal absorptive capacity for sodium bicarbonate. The latter maintains fluid balance at the expense of pH homeostasis.

Two cardinal mechanisms protect CBU: alterations in systemic hemodynamic variables and alterations in external sodium and water balance. Both mechanisms maintain filling of the arterial tree and consequently are activated by external fluid losses, by inability to transfer fluid from the interstitium to the venous system, for example, in ascites, or by impaired fluid transfer from venous to arterial systems, for example, in congestive heart failure, pericardial tamponade, or constrictive pericarditis.

The combination of alterations in systemic hemodynamic variables and alterations in external water and solute balance has been termed the *integrated volume response* (Table 102–1). Increases in pulse rate and blood pressure are modulated not only by antidiuretic hormone (ADH), catecholamines, and angiotensin II but also by a series of factors derived from vascular endothelial cells. These factors include endothelin-1, a 21-residue peptide with potent vasoconstrictor properties, and thromboxane A_2 and prostaglandin H_2, both derived from the cyclooxygenase pathway in vascular endo-

Table 102–1 ■ THE INTEGRATED VOLUME RESPONSE

	SYSTEMIC HEMODYNAMIC CHANGES	EXTERNAL SALT AND WATER BALANCE
Response	Tachycardia ↑ Peripheral resistance ↓ Venous capacitance	Thirst Renal Na⁺, water retention
Onset	Minutes	Hours
Major activators	Catecholamines ADH Angiotensin II Endothelin-1 Prostaglandin H_2 Thromboxane A_2	Catecholamines Aldosterone ADH
Major inactivators	Prostaglandin E_2 Atriopeptin Nitric acid	Prostaglandin E_2 Atriopeptin

ADH = Antidiuretic hormone.

thelial cells. The major inactivators of these systemic hemodynamic changes include prostaglandin E_2 and atriopeptin, both of which are discussed later, and nitric oxide, an endogenous vasodilator released by vascular endothelial cells.

There are differences in the two response systems, indicated in Table 102–1. Tachycardia, peripheral arteriolar vasoconstriction, and peripheral venoconstriction occur within minutes of external fluid losses, whereas renal salt and water conservation lags behind by 12 to 24 hours. The sensitivities of the two limbs also differ. For example, a 2 to 3% decrease in ECF volume, which amounts to the loss of 40 to 60 mEq of sodium, results in the virtual elimination of sodium from the urine but produces negligible changes in systemic hemodynamic factors, such as heart rate, blood pressure, or systemic vascular resistance. Because there is 2500 to 3000 mEq of exchangeable sodium in the ECF, the system for conserving renal sodium is remarkably sensitive.

RENAL VOLUME REGULATION

Figure 102–2 provides a schematic summary of the renal factors regulating volume homeostasis. In general, the system is characterized by a positive limb, activated by volume contraction, and by negative feedback, activated by volume repletion. The separate details of this mechanism are as follows.

SENSING AND EFFECTOR ELEMENTS. Changes in effective ECF volume that exceed acceptable physiologic limits are sensed by baroreceptors located in both the high- and the low-pressure regions of the circulation. The low-pressure baroreceptors are located primarily in the left atrium and in major thoracic veins, whereas the arterial high-pressure baroreceptors are located in the sinus body and aortic arch. Both sets of baroreceptors respond to pressure and stretch stimuli associated with changes in ECF volume. Activation of these extrarenal baroreceptors by slightly reducing effective circulating volume results in increased sympathetic nerve activity and in rises in plasma catecholamine activity.

This catecholamine response raises blood pressure by increasing arteriolar resistance and heart rate while simultaneously decreasing venous capacitance. Increases in arteriolar resistance also reduce capillary hydrostatic pressure and therefore promote fluid transfer from interstitial fluid to the vascular compartment. Within the kidney this increase in arteriolar resistance results in renal hypoperfusion. Moreover, adrenergic nerve terminals are in direct contact with proximal renal tubular epithelial cells and direct stimulation of renal sympathetic nerves increases proximal tubular sodium absorption.

A second effector mechanism activated by stimulation of extrarenal baroreceptors is release of ADH. When blood volume is isotonically contracted by more than 8 to 10%, afferent stimuli carried by the ninth and tenth cranial nerves result in non-osmotic ADH release by the neurohypophysis. In turn, ADH enhances renal water conservation and, because the hormone also has potent vasoconstrictor activity, reduces renal perfusion.

In addition to these extrarenal baroreceptors, the renal juxtaglomerular apparatus serves as an intrarenal baroreceptor system. Sympathetic nerve stimulation, reductions in afferent arteriolar blood pressure, or reductions in the rates of distal tubular sodium delivery enhance renin release by the juxtaglomerular apparatus. Renal renin release into plasma accelerates the formation of angiotensin II according to the following general scheme:

$$\begin{array}{c} \textit{Renin Substrate} \\ \downarrow \text{ renin} \\ \textit{Angiotensin I} \\ \downarrow \text{ pulmonary converting enzyme} \\ \textit{Angiotensin II} \\ \downarrow \text{ circulating angiotensinase} \\ \textit{Angiotensin III} \end{array}$$

The octapeptide angiotensin II has three major effects on volume conservation: (1) It is a potent pressor agent; on a molar basis, angiotensin II is a more potent vasoconstrictor than norepinephrine; (2) angiotensin II is the major stimulus to aldosterone secretion and consequently is a key factor modulating renal sodium conservation; (3) the angiotensin II formed in the central nervous system (CNS) is a potent stimulus to thirst. Recently it has become evident that angiotensin II may be synthesized locally in the vessels. The heptapeptide angiotensin III is also a potent vasoconstrictor but is not as potent a stimulator of aldosterone secretion as is angiotensin II; angiotensin III also stimulates thirst.

Finally, as indicated in Table 102–1, factors produced and released by vascular endothelial cells also play a major role in modulating systemic hemodynamics. The vasoconstricting factors include the potent vasoconstrictor peptide endothelin-1. Moreover, endothelin-1 is also released from the posterior pituitary and may play a role in modulating ADH release. The vasoconstrictor agents derived from the cyclooxygenase pathway in vascular endothelial cells include thromboxane A_2 and prostaglandin H_2. Nitric oxide produced by vascular endothelial cells is the major endogenous nitrovasodilator.

RENAL ELEMENTS. The kidneys respond to slight reductions in ECF volume by increasing the rate of proximal tubular sodium absorption without disturbing either the glomerular filtration rate

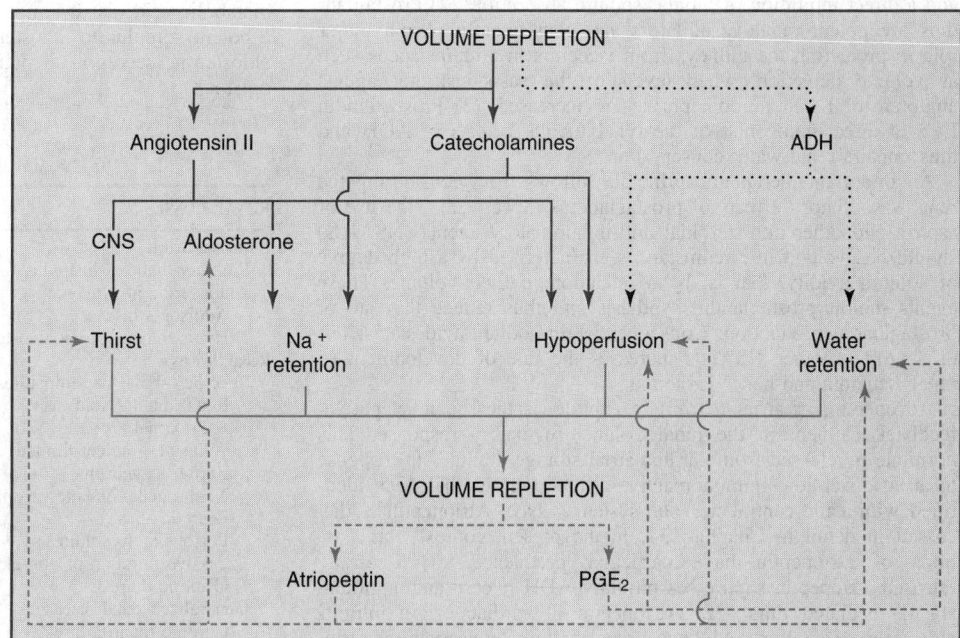

FIGURE 102–2 ■ The volume repletion reaction. The solid and dotted lines originating from "volume depletion" indicate positive mechanisms activated when volume depletion is either modest or severe, respectively. The dashed lines originating with "volume repletion" indicate negative feedback mechanisms.

(GFR) or osmoregulatory mechanisms. In normal circumstances, approximately 70% of filtered sodium is absorbed by the proximal nephron. As long as euvolemia persists, the fractional rate of proximal sodium absorption remains constant when the GRF is varied; this constant relation is referred to as *glomerulotubular balance.*

A number of factors modulate glomerulotubular balance in association with changes in ECF volume. In empirical terms, this modulation includes a downsetting of glomerulotubular balance in volume-expanded states and an increase in the rate of fractional proximal sodium absorption when arterial tree filling is impaired. Among these factors, the hemodynamic regulation of oncotic pressure in peritubular capillaries seems to have a dominant role. At relatively low concentrations, angiotensin II has a vasoconstricting effect on efferent, but not afferent, glomerular arterioles. Therefore, this agent, by increasing the glomerular filtration fraction, can increase peritubular capillary oncotic pressure and thereby enhance proximal tubular rates of sodium absorption. At high concentrations, angiotensin II, like norepinephrine, produces afferent glomerular arteriolar constriction, resulting in reductions in GFR and in renal ischemia.

The kidney responds to modest sodium depletion by increasing the rate of tubular sodium absorption without altering the GFR. Glomerulotubular balance is reset upward so that a greater fraction of glomerular filtrate is absorbed in the proximal nephron; both direct stimulation of renal nerves and the effect of angiotensin II on efferent glomerular arterioles contribute in part to this resetting of glomerulotubular balance. Angiotensin II also provides a second mechanism for conserving renal sodium by increasing the rate of aldosterone secretion, which enhances sodium absorption in the cortical collecting tubule. When volume contraction becomes severe, the vasoconstrictive effects of high levels of norepinephrine and angiotensin II tend to reduce both the GFR and the rate of renal sodium excretion.

NEGATIVE FEEDBACK. As indicated in Figure 102–2, atriopeptin and E series prostaglandins constitute the principal negative-feedback elements of the renal volume regulatory response. The major features of these negative feedback mechanisms are as follows.

Prostaglandins, particularly of the E series, are potent vasodilators. Within the kidney, two cardinal loci of prostaglandin E_2 production include renal glomeruli, where angiotensin II activates eicosanoid production and release, and renal medullary interstitial cells, which produce and release prostaglandin E_2 in response to increases in medullary osmolality.

As indicated in Figure 102–2, E series prostaglandins suppress renal volume conservation by at least three effects. (1) These agents are natriuretic due to both changes in renal hemodynamics and a direct inhibition of tubular sodium absorption. (2) Prostaglandins are potent renal vasodilators and consequently play a major role in protecting the kidneys from ischemia in circumstances such as volume depletion, when levels of the vasoconstrictor agents angiotensin II and norepinephrine are increased. (3) Prostaglandin E_2 is a direct antagonist of the renal tubular effects of ADH and thus impairs renal water conservation.

An important therapeutic principle follows from considering the renal vasodilatory effects of prostaglandins. Specifically, the use of aspirin and other non-steroidal anti-inflammatory agents (NSAIDs) should be avoided in circumstances characterized by a high degree of sodium avidity, that is, by a reduction in ECF volume. These agents inhibit prostaglandin synthesis and thus reduce the rate of prostaglandin production. Consequently, in sodium-avid states, use of aspirin or other NSAIDs increases the rate of development of renal ischemia and hence azotemia.

Atriopeptin, or atrial natriuretic peptide, is the second negative-feedback element in the renal volume regulatory response. This hormone is released from cardiac atrial storage granules in response to atrial distention; immunoreactive atriopeptin also has been identified within the central nervous system (CNS). Atriopeptin is discussed in detail in Chapter 234. In the present context, three actions of atriopeptin have particular pertinence. (1) Centrally released atriopeptin suppresses pituitary ADH release and angiotensin II–mediated thirst. (2) Atriopeptin of cardiac origin inhibits aldosterone secretion and hence renal sodium conservation; atriopeptin also may block collecting duct sodium and water absorption

directly. (3) Atriopeptin is a potent vasodilator that increases renal blood flow strikingly. The last-named effect also accounts in part for the natriuretic effects of this peptide.

SUMMARY. When considered in an overall context, two features of the volume repletion reaction illustrated in Figure 102–2 are noteworthy. First, redundant mechanisms protect CBU. Thus angiotensin II release, catecholamine release, and ADH release all produce overlapping results. Second, the magnitude of the volume repletion reaction varies depending on the degree of volume contraction. In modestly volume-contracted states, peripheral vasoconstriction and renal sodium conservation occur, but renal blood flow, GFR, and osmoregulation are unaffected. When volume contraction becomes advanced, non-osmotic ADH release, angiotensin II–mediated thirst, and reductions in the rate of salt delivery to the loop of Henle act in concert to produce hyponatremia. Finally, when catecholamine release and angiotensin II release become sufficiently great that renal blood flow is compromised beyond autoregulatory limits, prerenal azotemia ensues.

VOLUME DEPLETION

DEFINITION. A true hypovolemic state is one in which there is reduced total body water; it occurs when the rate of salt and water intake is less than the combined rates of renal plus extrarenal volume losses. In chronic volume-contracted states, input and output may be equal.

ETIOLOGY AND PATHOGENESIS. True volume contraction occurs as a consequence of decreased intake of fluid or increased loss of fluid. Increased loss may be conveniently considered as renal (either as a consequence of altered hormones or defective renal mechanisms) or extrarenal (Table 102–2).

HORMONAL DEFICIT. Volume contraction can occur whenever there is loss of ADH or aldosterone. Untreated *diabetes insipidus,* either pituitary or nephrogenic, produces profound volume contraction and hypertonic encephalopathy in patients denied free access to water. The obligatory loss of solute-free water in diabetes insipidus may be as high as 10 to 18 L daily. Both forms of diabetes insipidus are discussed in Chapter 238.

Addison's disease may impair aldosterone production and hence lead to renal sodium wasting. A second major cause of aldosterone lack occurs in *hyporeninemic hypoaldosteronism,* which may accompany interstitial renal disease. Disorders that damage the renal interstitium, such as hypertension, diabetes mellitus, gout, sickle cell disease, chronic ingestion of lead-containing illicit alcohol, and analgesic abuse, can suppress the ability of the juxtaglomerular apparatus to produce renin. In turn, the low rate of renin secretion results in low rates of aldosterone secretion. Thus, hyporeninemic hypoaldosteronism represents a disorder in which impaired aldosterone production results in renal salt wasting, hyperkalemia, and metabolic acidosis. It is not yet known why hyperkalemia, which is a potent stimulus to aldosterone secretion, fails to enhance rates of aldosterone secretion in patients with hyporeninemic hypoaldosteronism.

Table 102–2 ■ MAJOR CAUSES OF VOLUME DEPLETION

RENAL LOSSES	EXTRARENAL LOSSES
Hormonal Deficit	**Hemorrhage**
Pituitary diabetes insipidus	**Cutaneous Losses**
Aldosterone insufficiency	Sweating
Addison's disease	Burns
Hyporeninemic hypoaldosteronism	**Gastrointestinal Losses**
Renal Deficits	Vomiting
Specific tubular nephropathies:	Diarrheal disorders
Renal tubular acidosis	Gastrointestinal fistulas
Proximal	Tube drainage
Distal, gradient-limited	
Bartter's syndrome	
Nephrogenic diabetes insipidus	
Diuretic abuse	
Postobstructive diuresis	
Excessive filtration of non-electrolytes:	
Osmotic diuresis	
Generalized renal disease:	
Chronic renal failure	
Interstitial nephritis	

RENAL DEFICITS. A number of disorders impairing renal tubular sodium or water conservation can lead to volume contraction. For convenience, these derangements may be grouped into three classes. First, various tubular nephropathies are characterized by specific deficits in salt or water absorption. As mentioned earlier, nephrogenic diabetes insipidus and interstitial renal disease may produce water or sodium wasting, respectively. Because interstitial renal disease often results in hyperchloremic, hyperkalemic metabolic acidosis, the term *renal tubular acidosis, type IV* is often applied to this disorder. However, the general term *renal tubular acidosis* also includes other sodium-wasting disorders accompanied by hyperchloremic acidosis, such as proximal tubular acidosis, a specific proximal defect in bicarbonate reabsorption, and gradient-limited distal renal tubular acidosis, a specific defect in distal tubular sodium bicarbonate regeneration (see Chapter 107).

Alternatively, Bartter's syndrome is a specific tubular nephropathy that results in failure of sodium chloride absorption by the thick ascending limb of the nephron; the disorder is accompanied by excessive production of prostaglandins by the renal medullary interstitium and is characterized by sodium chloride wasting, juxtaglomerular hyperplasia, high renin levels, and secondary hyperaldosteronism; the last-named results in hypokalemic metabolic alkalosis.

Inhibition of tubular sodium absorptive processes due to *chronic diuretic abuse* also may lead to salt wasting, volume contraction, and specific metabolic acid-base abnormalities. These abnormalities are discussed later in this chapter.

Profound but reversible defects in tubular salt and water absorption may occur during *postobstructive diuresis,* that is, shortly after relief of partial or complete urinary tract obstruction. Salt and water losses also may occur in the *diuretic phase* of acute tubular necrosis. However, profound salt and water losses associated with the diuretic phase of acute tubular necrosis are seen uncommonly if CBU is carefully controlled during oliguric acute tubular necrosis.

Third, glomerular filtration of large amounts of non-electrolytes may produce volume deficits by overwhelming renal tubular reabsorptive capacity for salt and water; in this instance, water losses predominate so that hypernatremia generally occurs. This phenomenon, termed *osmotic diuresis* or *solute diuresis,* occurs in diabetic ketoacidosis, hyperglycemic hyperosmolar coma, or hyperalimentation with large glucose loads in chronically debilitated patients; in patients with burns, in whom there are abnormally high rates of urea production; and during mannitol or glycerol administration to those with CNS disorders requiring reductions of intracranial pressure.

EXTRARENAL LOSSES. In addition to hemorrhage, two other classes of extrarenal losses account for volume contraction. Simple dehydration may result from increased insensible water loss in *excessive sweating* due to high ambient temperatures or to fever. Because sweat usually contains less than 50 mEq/L of sodium, the ICF and the ECF share the water loss, and body water osmolality rises while ECF volume loss is modest. *Burns* allow the loss of large amounts of plasma and interstitial fluid through affected areas and therefore can lead rapidly to profound ECF losses.

Finally, gastrointestinal volume losses occur when portions of the 8 to 10 L of normal gastrointestinal secretions are lost, particularly in secretory diarrheas. Volume depletion is most commonly the consequence of vomiting, gastric drainage, or diarrhea but may occur with any type of bowel fistula. Loss of hydrochloric acid from the stomach may produce metabolic alkalosis, whereas loss of sodium bicarbonate from pancreatic secretions lost through the lower gastrointestinal tract, as in diarrhea, may produce metabolic acidosis.

CLINICAL MANIFESTATIONS. The clinical findings in states of true volume contraction are due both to underfilling of the arterial tree and to the subsequent renal and hemodynamic responses. In mild or partially compensated volume contraction, particularly when the latter has occurred gradually, the patient may exhibit nothing more than mild postural giddiness, postural tachycardia, and weakness, whereas in severe volume contraction, life-threatening circulatory collapse may occur. The lack of physical findings does not exclude the presence of mild to moderate volume contraction in a given patient. In the postoperative period, 7 to 10% blood volume losses in patients are often accompanied by normal vital signs and by only slight decreases in the central venous pressure or the pulmonary capillary wedge pressure. Skin turgor and the moistness of mucous membranes are valuable indices to the volume of body water in infants but are unreliable in adults. In young adults, reductions in skin turgor do not occur unless profound volume contraction is present, and normal loss of skin elasticity makes skin turgor difficult to assess in older patients. Similarly, mouth breathing and other factors affect the oral mucosa independently of external volume balances.

The signs and symptoms of volume contraction, regardless of cause, are referable to a reduction in ECF volume. Consequently, the clinical findings in volume contraction depend primarily on the interplay among four major factors: (1) the magnitude of the volume loss; (2) the rate of volume loss; (3) the nature of the fluid loss, that is, whether the fluid loss is primarily water, a combined sodium plus water loss, or a blood loss; and (4) the responsiveness of the vasculature to volume reduction. Some simple considerations illustrate these relations.

The clinical manifestations of volume contraction are obviously related intimately to the volume and rate of fluid loss. For example, an acute gastrointestinal hemorrhage of 1 L of blood can easily result in oliguria, coupled with the signs and symptoms of circulatory collapse, while the hematocrit remains constant. In other words, the hemorrhage is sufficiently acute that fluid flux from the interstitial to the vascular bed makes a negligible contribution to expanding the vascular bed. However, the same amount of gastrointestinal blood loss occurring more slowly (e.g., over a 1-day period) permits a partial transfer of fluid from the interstitium to the vascular bed and consequently produces a fall in hematocrit; but because the CBU is at least partially restored by this fluid shift, the volume of urine flow and the hemodynamic response to volume contraction may be minimally affected.

Second, the kind of fluid loss significantly affects the clinical findings in volume contraction. Consider, for example, a 1-L loss of different kinds of body fluids in a 70-kg man with a total body water of 40 L and a hematocrit of 45%. The acute loss of 1 L of predominantly solute-free water, as in diabetes insipidus, reduces the blood volume by 2.5%; urine flow and systemic hemodynamics are minimally affected. The acute loss of 1 L of predominantly ECF reduces blood volume by 6.6%, because sodium is confined to the ECF; in this circumstance, modest oliguria and tachycardia while the patient is recumbent ensue. Lastly, the acute loss of 1 L of blood by hemorrhage reduces blood volume by 20%, thus resulting in profound oliguria and near circulatory collapse.

Finally, peripheral vasoconstriction and tachycardia represent important physiologic responses to volume losses. Consequently, even modest signs and symptoms of volume contraction are amplified appreciably in patients with diminished myocardial reserve or reduced sympathetic nervous system function. The former occurs commonly in cardiomyopathies of any cause or in pericardial tamponade or pericardial constriction. The latter occurs commonly in patients on prolonged bed rest, in diabetic patients with autonomic neuropathy, and as a consequence of therapy with certain antihypertensive drugs.

DIAGNOSIS. The pulse, blood pressure, and changes of these variables with position, together with a clinical estimate of the venous pressure and skin temperature, provide an initial assessment of circulatory dynamics. Wide variations exist in blood pressure and pulse changes to orthostatic measurements. A decrease in orthostatic diastolic blood pressure of 10 mm Hg is considered to be the most reliable indicator of significant volume depletion. Even then, a physician cannot be certain, and it is useful to consider a fluid challenge to evaluate patients in whom a volume deficit is thought to contribute to a reduced cardiac output. A convenient way of achieving this goal is to administer 500 mL of normal saline over 1 to 3 hours.

In patients with a normal cardiac reserve, the effect of a fluid challenge may be monitored safely by evaluating the pulse, blood pressure, and urine flow. In patients with impaired cardiac function, using a flow-directed Swan-Ganz catheter to measure the pulmonary capillary wedge pressure or cardiac output, as estimated by thermal dilution, provides a more precise indicator to early volume overload secondary to a fluid challenge. Because volume contraction is associated with vasoconstriction, both in the venous and the arterial circuits, transient changes in the pulmonary capillary wedge pressure may not accurately reflect volume status. During volume expansion, the wedge pressure rises and subsequently falls. The initial pressure elevation is due to fluid infusion into a vasoconstricted, low-capacity vascular bed and should not be misinterpreted to indicate adequacy of volume repletion. The subsequent reduction in wedge pressure coincides with decreases in arterial resistance coupled with increases in venous capacitance. Finally, central venous pressure measurements provide unreliable estimates of pulmonary vascular volume.

The cardinal laboratory findings associated with volume contraction follow directly from the volume repletion mechanism summarized in Figure 102–2. The kidney initially responds to a decrease in effective circulating blood volume by reducing urine volume and sodium excretion. Severe degrees of volume contraction also reduce filtration rate and result in prerenal azotemia and a decrease in fractional excretion of sodium (see Chapter 100).

TREATMENT. The major goal of treating volume contraction is to expand the CBU by replacing fluid deficits. The type of fluid, the route and rate of fluid administration, and the total amount of fluid to be given will vary with the particular circumstance. For example, a mild, non-persisting upper gastrointestinal hemorrhage may be treated appropriately by infusing normal saline, whereas a major, persisting upper gastrointestinal hemorrhage will generally require replacement with whole blood.

The degree to which a given volume of crystalloid solution expands the CBU depends on solution composition. If glucose metabolism is normal, infusing 5% dextrose in water (D_5W) is equivalent to administering solute-free water, which distributes uniformly in total body water. Because less than 10% of total body water is in the intravascular compartment, infusing 1 L of D_5W expands the intravascular volume by 75 to 100 mL, that is, by about 2%. Thus, expansion of CBU by D_5W cannot be suggested except when used principally in hypertonic volume-contracted states such as diabetes insipidus and excessive sweating.

Solutions containing sodium as the principal solute preferentially expand the ECF volume. Infusing 1 L of a normal saline solution increases blood volume by about 300 mL, or about 6%; the remaining portion is distributed in the interstitial compartment. Hypotonic sodium-containing salt solutions expand intravascular volume in a manner intermediate between that of D_5W and normal saline. Sodium-containing crystalloid solutions are indicated primarily in volume-contracted states secondary to renal or gastrointestinal sodium losses (see Table 102–2). They are also useful adjuncts to therapy in burns and in hemorrhage.

Colloid-containing solutions, such as iso-oncotic albumin solutions and plasma, preferentially expand the intravascular compartment, because large molecules like albumin are mainly restricted to the intravascular space. This kind of fluid replacement is most helpful in burns, in which cutaneous protein losses are appreciable, and in circulatory collapse, in which rapid intravascular expansion is critical. In most other instances of volume contraction, using colloid-containing solutions is difficult to justify, since the half-life of infused albumin in ill patients is relatively short, only 4 to 6 hours, and the cost of colloid solutions such as iso-oncotic albumin is more than 50 times greater than that of an equal volume of crystalloid solution.

Finally, blood—which contains formed elements—is the most potent expander of the intravascular space. A unit of packed red blood cells will remain entirely in the vascular bed. In most hemorrhagic situations, the combination of packed red blood cells with either normal saline solutions or colloid solutions is adequate for volume replacement. Few circumstances occur in modern practice, with the possible exception of massive hemorrhagic shock, in which whole-blood therapy for volume expansion is used.

CIRCULATORY COMPROMISE WITHOUT EXTERNAL FLUID LOSSES

DEFINITION. In the preceding section we considered those disorders characterized by inadequate filling of the arterial tree that occurred because of true volume deficits. Clearly, the cardinal signs and symptoms of these disorders are referable to responses accompanying the integrated volume repletion reaction (see Fig. 102–2). There are also disorders in which inadequate arterial filling occurs

in the absence of external fluid losses and which indeed are often associated with increased total body water. However, the signs and symptoms of these disorders mimic closely those that characterize true volume contraction.

ETIOLOGY AND PATHOGENESIS. Table 102–3 lists three commonly encountered classes of derangements that may manifest clinically with tachycardia, acute hypotension, oliguria, azotemia, and a reduced fractional excretion of sodium.

IMPAIRED CARDIAC OUTPUT. A profound collapse of cardiac output, due to acute myocardial infarction with pump failure (cardiogenic shock) or to acute pericardial tamponade, may clearly result in circulatory collapse. In this instance, failure to fill the arterial tree and to maintain an EABU volume occurs because the heart fails to translocate blood adequately from venous to arterial beds.

INCREASED VASCULAR CAPACITANCE. Circulatory collapse with its attendant signs and symptoms occurs when there is a sudden increase in the capacitance of the vascular bed, most notably in the venous part of the circulation. This kind of increase in ratio of vascular capacitance to vascular volume occurs most commonly in sepsis and cirrhosis with increased arteriovenous shunts and decreased systemic vascular resistance. Increased vascular capacitance also may be seen in circumstances in which peripheral vasodilators, particularly those having a postarteriolar locus of action, are administered injudiciously.

VASCULAR-INTERSTITIAL FLUID SHIFTS. Profound hypotension, tachycardia, progressive oliguria, and azotemia are also encountered when there is a translocation of fluid from vascular to interstitial compartments, presumably because of a sudden, profound increase in the permeability characteristics of peripheral capillaries or when there is decreased circulatory oncotic pressure such as in any disease process with hypoalbuminemia. Some common causes of increased translocation of vascular fluid without hypoalbuminemia having an etiologic role include infarction of the small or large intestine, extensive tissue trauma, acute pancreatitis, and rhabdomyolysis. An analogous mechanism—namely, a marked increase in the permeability of pulmonary capillaries—is also presumed to account for the formation of non-cardiogenic pulmonary edema in the adult respiratory distress syndrome.

DIAGNOSIS AND THERAPY. The diagnosis and therapy of acute myocardial infarction with circulatory collapse and of acute pericardial tamponade are considered in detail in Part VII. It is, however, worth citing certain factors particularly germane to managing fluid therapy in such patients. In individuals affected either by right ventricular infarction or by pericardial tamponade, maintaining adequate filling of the systemic arterial tree depends critically on providing a relatively high venous preload to the right side of the heart. Attempts at volume contraction in patients with right ventricular infarcts or pericardial tamponade may exacerbate systemic hypotension. Thus, treating these disorders generally requires concomitant hemodynamic monitoring with a flow-directed Swan-Ganz catheter to avoid excessive preload to the left side of the heart.

In patients with left ventricular infarction and systemic hypotension, particular attention should be directed to excluding the possibility that antecedent true volume depletion—for example, with prolonged diuretic therapy and salt restriction before the myocardial infarction—may be a significant contributor to what otherwise

Table 102–3 ■ CIRCULATORY COMPROMISE WITHOUT EXTERNAL FLUID LOSSES

I. Impaired Cardiac Output
 Acute myocardial infarction
 Pericardial tamponade
II. Increased Vascular Capacitance
 Septic shock
 Cirrhosis
III. Vascular → Interstitial Fluid Shifts
 A. Hypoalbuminemia
  Nephrotic syndrome
  Liver failure
  Malnutrition
  Cytokine-mediated
 B. Normal plasma albumin
  Acute pancreatitis
  Bowel infarction
  Rhabdomyolysis
  Non-cardiogenic pulmonary edema

might be mistaken for true cardiogenic shock. The combined findings of acute left ventricular infarction, systemic arterial hypotension, the absence of pulmonary edema on the chest radiography, a reduced pulmonary capillary wedge pressure, and an antecedent history of prolonged diuretic therapy, when taken together, indicate that improved systemic hemodynamics may be achieved by cautious attempts to expand volume while also measuring—serially—the cardiac output and the pulmonary capillary wedge pressure.

The distinction between hypotension as being due either to true volume contraction or to an increase in the capacitance/volume ratio of the vascular bed, as occurs in sepsis, is often difficult. This distinction is particularly difficult in individuals who have been in intensive care units for prolonged periods of time and in those at high risk for developing sepsis, such as cancer patients treated with potent chemotherapeutic agents. A useful clue to the presence of septic circulatory collapse is the occurrence of warm extremities coupled with hypotension and oliguria, because true hypovolemia, particularly when advanced, is ordinarily accompanied by profound peripheral vasoconstriction and hence cool and often cyanotic extremities.

True hypovolemia and sepsis also may coexist. In such a circumstance, invasive hemodynamic monitoring may be helpful. Both in true hypovolemia and in sepsis, the pulmonary capillary wedge pressure is reduced, but in septic circulatory collapse, the calculated systemic vascular resistance falls, because of peripheral vasodilation, whereas in true hypovolemia, peripheral vasoconstriction ordinarily raises the systemic vascular resistance. The diagnosis of disorders producing rapid transfer of fluids from the vascular bed to the interstitium, such as trauma, acute pancreatitis, or rhabdomyolysis, is generally evident from clinical appraisal.

Treating patients with sepsis and an increased vascular capacitance/volume ratio, as well as those with rapid vascular to interstitial fluid shifts, has as a mainstay the administration of sufficient sodium-containing fluids, generally isotonic saline, to permit adequate filling of the arterial tree. This therapy necessarily expands total body water, particularly in the vascular and interstitial compartments. Consequently, during recovery from the underlying disorder, care must be taken to avoid unnecessary expansion of the vascular bed and consequently the risk of volume-mediated cardiac decompensation.

VOLUME EXCESS

DEFINITION. Volume-expanded states are characterized by an increase in total body water, which is usually accompanied by an increase in total body sodium. Total body salt and water may be increased while the CBU is decreased. In other words, certain volume-expanded states are characterized by dissociation between total body salt and water and the CBU.

ETIOLOGY AND PATHOGENESIS. Volume expansion occurs whenever the rate of salt or water intake exceeds the rate of renal plus extrarenal losses; in chronic volume expansion, the external salt and water balance may be normal. A convenient way of considering volume-expanded states is to view them in the context of three different classes of physiologic explanations (Table 102–4).

DISTURBANCES IN STARLING FORCES. The most common diseases encountered in which both volume expansion and edema occur are those in which derangements in the Starling forces regulating fluid transfer between capillaries and interstitium tend to expand the interstitial compartment at the expense of the CBU. Consequently, renal sodium retention and edema occur. By definition, this group of disorders is characterized by increases in capillary hydrostatic pressure, by decreases in capillary oncotic pressure, or by a combination of these two factors.

Four groups include most edematous states characterized by abnormal Starling forces (see Table 102–4). First, the systemic venous pressure may be increased because of primary cardiac disorders, such as right-sided heart failure or constrictive pericarditis. Second, local elevations in pulmonary or systemic venous pressure may occur, as in left-sided heart failure, vena caval obstruction, or portal vein obstruction. Third, a reduction in plasma oncotic pressure, and consequently a net increase in the tendency for fluid to transudate from capillaries to interstitium, accounts plausibly for edema formation in the nephrotic syndrome. Circulatory albumin concentrations of less than 3.2 g/dL are usually insufficient to pre-

Table 102–4 ■ DISORDERS OF VOLUME EXCESS

I. Disturbed Starling Forces	II. Primary Hormone Excess
(Reduced effective circulating volume; edema formation)	(Increased effective circulating volume)
Systemic venous pressure increases	Primary aldosteronism
Right-sided heart failure	Cushing's syndrome
Constrictive pericarditis	SIADH
Local venous pressure increases	**III. Primary Renal Sodium Retention**
Left-sided heart failure	(Increased effective circulating volume)
Vena cava obstruction	Renal failure
Portal vein obstruction	
Reduced oncotic pressure	
Nephrotic syndrome	
Decreased albumin synthesis	
Combined disorders	
Cirrhosis	

SIADH = Syndrome of inappropriate antidiuretic hormone production.

vent transudation of fluid across capillary beds. Finally, a combination of these factors may be responsible for edema. For example, both hypoalbuminemia and portal hypertension are major contributory factors to developing ascites in hepatic cirrhosis.

Plasma renin activity and aldosterone concentrations in these disorders tend to be elevated, although the results also tend to be variable. In advanced cases of disorders characterized by increases in local or systemic venous pressure, most notably in severe congestive heart failure and in cirrhosis, hyponatremia may occur; this finding represents an ominous prognostic sign. Finally, edema formation due to such derangements of Starling forces may result in the "third space" phenomenon, namely, large volumes of interstitial fluid sequestered in regions such as the pleural or peritoneal cavities.

PRIMARY HORMONAL EXCESS. These disorders include those disturbances with unregulated production of mineralocorticoids or ADH. The volume expansion that occurs in states of mineralocorticoid excess, such as primary hyperaldosteronism, is due to sodium retention and is accompanied by a primary, preferential expansion of the ECF and consequently by hypertension. The serum sodium level is generally normal. In the syndrome of inappropriate ADH production (SIADH), primary water retention occurs. Consequently, the volume expansion involves both the ICF and ECF; dilutional hyponatremia is the hallmark of SIADH, whereas hypertension is uncommon. Edema is not characteristic in either of these two disorders. Instead, patients with primary aldosteronism or SIADH reach a volume-expanded steady state in which output equals input.

PRIMARY RENAL SODIUM RETENTION. The kidneys also may retain sodium abnormally when the ECF volume is normal and there is no effector excess. For example, in acute glomerulonephritis, unidentified renal mechanisms are primarily responsible for edema. Patients with acute glomerulonephritis retain salt and water and become hypertensive without reductions in the GFR or in ECF volume. Furthermore, sodium retention and edema may develop when intake exceeds renal capacity for excretion with a decrease in GFR of any cause.

DIAGNOSIS AND TREATMENT. The recognition and management of volume-expanded states depend on proper identification and treatment of the underlying disorder. Clearly, the cornerstones of therapy in volume-expanded states characterized by sodium excess include salt restriction and diuretics. Table 102–5 provides a summary of some of the major diuretics used commonly and certain of their properties, whereas Figure 102–3 summarizes the sites of action of the various families of diuretics. For convenience, these drugs have been classified according to their sites of action in the nephron.

PROXIMAL TUBULE DIURETICS. The cardinal example of a proximal tubule diuretic is acetazolamide, a carbonic anhydrase inhibitor that blocks proximal reabsorption of sodium bicarbonate. Consequently, prolonged use of acetazolamide may lead to hyperchloremic acidosis, in contrast to all other diuretics that act at loci prior to the late distal nephron. Metolazone, a congener of the thiazide

Table 102–5 ■ CHARACTERISTICS OF COMMONLY USED DIURETICS

DIURETIC	PRIMARY EFFECT	SECONDARY EFFECT	COMPLICATIONS
I. Proximal Diuretics			
Acetazolamide	↓ Na^+/H^+ exchange	↑ K^+ loss, ↑ HCO_3^- loss	Hypokalemic, hyperchloremic acidosis
Metolazone	↓ Na^+ absorption	↑ K^+ loss, ↑ Cl^- loss	Hypokalemic alkalosis
II. Loop Diuretics			
Furosemide			
Bumetanide	↓ $Na^+:K^+: 2Cl^-$ absorption	↑ K^+ loss, ↑ H^+ secretion	Hypokalemic alkalosis
Ethacrynic acid			Hearing deficits, hypomagnesemia
III. Early Distal Diuretics			
Thiazide	↓ NaCl absorption	↑ K^+ loss, ↑ H^+ secretion	Hypokalemic alkalosis
Metolazone			Hyperglycemia, hyperuricemia
IV. Late Distal Diuretics			
Aldosterone antagonists			
Spironolactone			
Non-aldosterone antagonists	↓ Na^+ absorption	↓ K^+ loss, ↓ H^+ secretion	Hyperkalemic acidosis
Triamterene			
Amiloride			

class of diuretics, blocks sodium chloride absorption in two ne-phron sites by unknown mechanisms. Specifically, in addition to an action on the early distal tubule, metolazone also inhibits proximal tubular sodium chloride absorption. Because the major locus for phosphate absorption is in the proximal nephron, the phosphaturia accompanying metolazone administration exceeds considerably that observed with other thiazide class diuretics.

Proximal tubule diuretics are rarely used as primary diuretic therapy in modern practice. More commonly, these diuretics, partic-ularly metolazone, are used as supplements to loop diuretics in instances in which loop diuretics alone are ineffective in producing diuresis.

Mannitol also inhibits proximal tubule reabsorption. It is mainly used to prevent acute tubular necrosis.

LOOP DIURETICS. Loop diuretics, such as furosemide, bumeta-nide, and ethacrynic acid, produce diuresis by inhibiting the cou-pled entry on Na^+, Cl^-, and K^+ across apical plasma membranes in the thick ascending limb of Henle. The latter is responsible for the reabsorption of approximately 25% of filtered sodium. The natri-uretic dose-response characteristics of these diuretic agents are con-siderably more linear than those of all other currently used diuret-ics. Consequently, the loop diuretics are, for practical purposes, the most potent diuretics currently available; therefore, these drugs are commonly referred to as "high-ceiling" diuretics.

DISTAL TUBULE DIURETICS. Distal tubule diuretics, such as thia-zide and metolazone, interfere primarily with sodium chloride ab-sorption in the earliest segments of the distal convoluted tubule. The thiazide diuretics appear to exert their effect by blocking the NaCl co-transport mechanism across apical plasma membranes.

With the exception of acetazolamide (which impairs bicarbonate absorption), hypokalemia and metabolic alkalosis may complicate the administration of proximal diuretics, loop diuretics, and distal tubular diuretics. This occurs because the rate of sodium delivery to the collecting duct, in which a significant fraction of potassium and proton secretion occurs, is a major factor promoting these two processes. Consequently, increase in salt delivery to the late distal nephron, occasioned by inhibition of sodium reabsorption in the proximal tubule, the ascending limb of Henle, or the distal tubule and collecting duct, leads to accelerated rates of proton and potas-sium secretion and consequently to hypokalemia and metabolic alkalosis.

In general, distal tubule diuretics are used for the same circum-stances as loop diuretics. The major exception occurs in chronic renal failure and in disorders of calcium metabolism. Loop diuret-ics are calciuric and therefore are valuable for managing acute hypercalcemia. In contrast, thiazide diuretics promote hypocalciuria and calcium retention and are therefore useful in managing hyper-calciuric states, but not hypercalcemia. Loop diuretics are much more effective in chronic renal failure than are thiazide diuretics.

COLLECTING DUCT DIURETICS. Finally, a group of agents inhibit

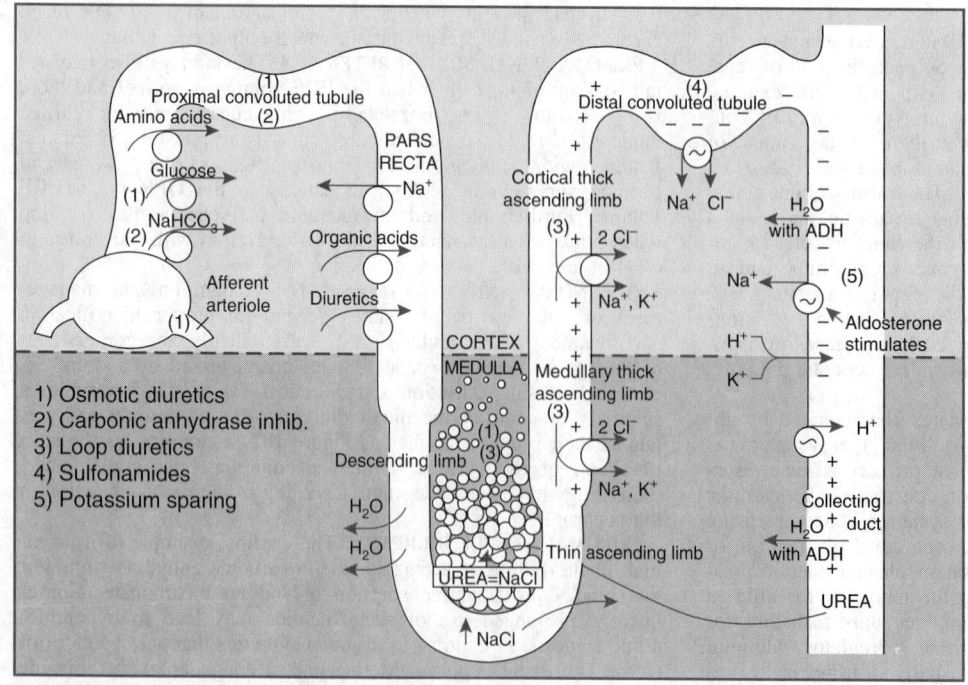

FIGURE 102–3 ■ Major transport processes along the nephron segment and the pri-mary sites of action of the diuretics. The numbers next to diuretics in the insert refer to sites of action along the nephron. (From Kokko JP: Diuretics. In Alexander RW, Schlant RC, Fuster V [eds]: The Heart, 9th ed. New York, McGraw-Hill, 1998. With permission of The McGraw-Hill Companies.)

sodium absorption in the collecting duct and concomitantly suppress indirectly potassium secretion and proton secretion. Spironolactone competes with aldosterone; the primary use of this agent is restricted to conditions of aldosterone excess, either primary or secondary. Alternatively, both triamterene and amiloride operate independently of aldosterone. These agents directly block sodium uptake by collecting duct cells and concomitantly suppress indirectly both potassium and proton secretion. Accordingly, hyperkalemic, hyperchloremic metabolic acidosis may complicate the injudicious use of spironolactone, triamterene, or amiloride. These diuretics are useful especially in managing disorders characterized by secondary hyperaldosteronism, such as cirrhosis with ascites, and in promoting diuresis in hypokalemic patients.

One factor common to treatment of disorders with reduced CBU and with expanded ECF volumes merits particular consideration. A major factor in edema formation is an increase in the Starling forces promoting fluid translocation from the vascular to interstitial spaces. When potent diuretics are given to patients with portal hypertension or with hypoalbuminemia, urinary sodium excretion may exceed the rate at which salt and water are transferred from the interstitium to the vascular bed. As a result, vigorous diuretic therapy may result in volume contraction, reduced salt delivery to diluting segments, non-osmotic ADH release, and consequently hyponatremia. Hyponatremia occurs most commonly with the thiazide group of diuretics, because these diuretics inhibit free water formation. In advanced cases of diuretic abuse, hypotension, hemoconcentration, and azotemia also occur.

Azizi M, Guyene TT, Chatellier G, Menard J: Pharmacological demonstration of the additive effects of angiotensin-converting enzyme inhibition and angiotensin II antagonism in sodium depleted healthy subjects. Clin Exp Hypertens 19:937–951, 1997. *A well-conducted crossover study in mildly sodium depleted normotensive volunteers showing more complete blockade of hemodynamic effects of renin-angiotensin system achieved by combination of ACE inhibitors and angiotensin receptor blockers than could be achieved by either alone.*

Dzau VJ: Circulating versus local renin-angiotensin system in cardiovascular homeostasis. Circulation 77(Suppl. 1):1, 1988. *A comprehensive review demonstrating that renin and angiotensinogen genes are expressed in many tissues. Studies also have shown that cardiac vascular cells can synthesize angiotensin II in vitro. Current data further suggest that angiotensin antagonists affect vascular contractility by their effects on angiotensin produced by either the kidney or local vascular mechanisms.*

Kokko JP: Diuretics. In Alexander RW, Schlant RC, Fuster V, et al (eds): Hurst's The Heart, 9th ed. New York, McGraw Hill, 1998, pp 783-798. *Complete overview of site of action, indications, and complications of diuretics.*

Koziol-McLain J, Lowenstein SR, Fuller B: Orthostatic vital signs in emergency department patients. Ann Emerg Med 20:606–610, 1991. *A well-conducted study in an emergency department setting evaluating the significance of blood pressure and pulse changes in response to postural changes from lying to standing positions. It demonstrates that changes in diabetic blood pressure, in contrast to changes in systolic blood pressure or pulse, should receive priority in evaluating patients' volume status.*

Nonoguchi H, Sands JM, Knepper MA: ANF inhibits NaCl and fluid absorption in cortical collecting duct of rat kidney. Am J Physiol 256(Renal Fluid Electrolyte Physiol 25):F179, 1989. *Carefully conducted in vitro study examining how atrial natriuretic factor increases urinary sodium and excretion.*

102.2 Osmolality Disturbances

PHYSIOLOGIC CONSIDERATIONS

In normal individuals, the serum osmolality as determined by freezing-point depression is virtually constant from day to day. It is useful to define *effective ECF osmolality,* because the osmoregulatory mechanisms that adjust water balance in normal individuals are determined primarily by changes in cell volume that result from variations in effective ECF osmolality. Effective ECF osmolality is that osmolality that is "sensed" across a specific membrane. In dilutional states, the measured and effective ECF osmolalities are approximately equal, because ECF dilution also produces ICF dilution and, at least acutely, cell swelling. Osmoregulatory mechanisms are activated when ECF hypertonicity is due to a solute that is excluded from cells and therefore produces, at least acutely, cell shrinkage; in this case, the measured and effective ECF osmolalities are approximately equal. If the ECF osmolality is increased by solutes, such as urea, which penetrate cell membranes, acute cell shrinkage does not occur to the degree predicted from freezing-point osmolality and osmoregulatory mechanisms are not fully activated. In this case, the measured ECF osmolality is greater than the effective ECF osmolality.

The freezing-point serum osmolality can be approximated from the following formula:

$$\text{Osmolality} = 2[Na^+] + \frac{glucose}{18} + \frac{BUN}{2.8}$$

where the glucose and blood urea nitrogen (BUN) concentrations are expressed as milligrams per deciliter and the serum sodium concentration is expressed as milliequivalents per liter. In normal circumstances, glucose contributes 5.5 mOsm/kg H_2O to the serum osmolality. When hyperglycemia occurs, the effective ECF osmolality rises because glucose entry into cells is limited.

Cell Volume Regulation

Starling forces regulate fluid transfer between the ICF and the ECF. Because plasma membranes cannot tolerate even small hydrostatic gradients, the operational Starling forces between ICF and ECF are almost entirely osmotic. Significant changes in cell volume, particularly in the CNS, are by themselves potentially lethal. Thus the goals of fluid transport between the ECF and ICF are to maintain constancy of cell volume and to maintain a negligible hydrostatic pressure gradient between cells and the ECF. Because most cell membranes are freely permeable to water, these two goals are achieved when the ECF osmolality is normal and intracellular and extracellular osmolalities are identical.

Because cell membranes are partially permeable to sodium and potassium, there is a tendency for sodium to leak into cells and for potassium to leak out of cells. Because impermeant macromolecules account for a large fraction of intracellular anions, passive sodium and potassium movements tend toward a Donnan distribution, in which total intracellular cations would exceed total interstitial cations, in precise analogy to the way in which total plasma water cations exceed total interstitial cations. If these passive cation movements across cell membranes were unopposed, osmotic water movement into cells would tend to produce cell lysis. Consequently, active transport mechanisms are required to balance intracellular and interstitial cation concentrations.

Specifically, both sodium leakage from the ECF into cells and potassium leakage out of cells into the ECF are counterbalanced exactly by active outward sodium transport coupled to active inward potassium transport. These active transport events maintain the intracellular cation (and therefore osmolar) content equal to that of extracellular fluid and also maintain the predominant extracellular and intracellular distributions of sodium and potassium, respectively. Thus, because cellular cation pumps balance cellular cation leaks, cells are *operationally* impermeable to sodium and to potassium. Active sodium efflux coupled to active potassium influx is mediated by membrane-bound Na^+, K^+-ATPase, and the activity of these cellular cation pumps accounts for more than 50% of the basal calorie consumption.

Cation transport mediated by Na^+, K^+-ATPase is the major factor regulating cell volume when the effective ECF osmolality is normal. When the effective ECF osmolality is increased or decreased, additional processes are required to maintain the constancy of cell volume. These auxiliary mechanisms are particularly important in minimizing potentially lethal changes in brain volume because of osmotic water shifts into or out of brain cells.

In chronic hypotonic disorders, cell swelling is offset by the loss of potassium chloride from cells. This potassium chloride efflux mechanism appears to be activated by small increases in cell volume produced by ECF dilution. In chronic hypernatremia, brain shrinkage is minimized by the accumulation of additional solutes within brain cells. These latter solutes, often called "idiogenic osmoles," include amino acids and other solutes, including myoinositol betaine, and urea. As is discussed in the section on treatment, these auxiliary transport processes affect significantly the therapeutic approach to patients with osmoregulatory failure.

Water Balance

The key elements regulating water balance are summarized in Figure 102–4. The osmoreceptors, both for ADH release and for thirst, respond to small changes in effective ECF osmolality, whereas baroreceptors respond to changes in CBU. As little as a

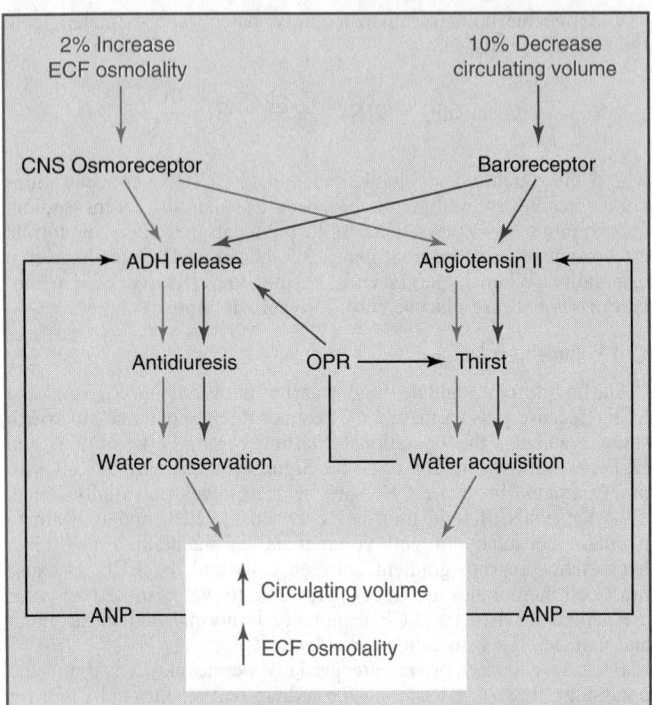

FIGURE 102–4 ■ The water repletion reaction. The white lines are positive water conservation processes activated by osmolality. The red lines are water conservation processes that are volume activated. The black lines indicate negative feedback. OPR = oropharyngeal reflex. (From Reeves WB, Andreoli TE: The posterior pituitary and water metabolism. *In* Wilson JD, Foster DW [eds]: Williams Textbook of Endocrinology, 8th ed. Philadelphia, WB Saunders, 1992.)

2% increase in effective ECF osmolality shrinks osmoreceptor cells and stimulates both ADH release from the posterior pituitary and thirst. A second way of stimulating both ADH release and thirst involves volume-mediated stimuli that can operate independently of changes in plasma osmolality. When the CBU is reduced by approximately 10%, these volume-dependent mechanisms stimulate ADH release.

SENSORS AND EFFECTORS. Three kinds of *sensor* elements adjust water balance. Two of these, osmoreceptors and the thirst center, respond to small changes in effective ECF osmolality, whereas baroreceptors respond to changes in CBU. The osmoreceptors are situated in the supraoptic and paraventricular nuclei of the hypothalamus, whereas the thirst center is in the organum vasculosum of the anterior hypothalamus. As little as a 2% increase in effective ECF osmolality produced by solutes such as sodium chloride, but not urea, shrinks osmoreceptor cells and thirst center cells. The osmoreceptors stimulate the release of the *effector* hormone ADH from storage sites in the posterior pituitary gland. The stimulation of thirst by the thirst centers depends on centrally produced angiotensin II.

Endothelin-1 is also released from the posterior pituitary in response to water deprivation. Moreover, administered endothelin-1 increases plasma ADH levels. Thus, endothelin-1 may have a central role in modulating ADH release.

When the CBU is reduced by more than 10%, volume-dependent blood produces afferent signals, carried by the ninth and tenth cranial nerves, which result in non-osmotic ADH release. Volume contraction also acts as a potent stimulus to thirst by means of angiotensin II.

THE ANTIDIURETIC RESPONSE. The cardinal characteristics of the antidiuretic response depend primarily on the integrated activity of two nephron regions: the medullary thick ascending limb of Henle, which concentrates the medullary interstitium, and the collecting duct, which, with ADH present, allows water reabsorption from this segment.

The medullary thick ascending limb absorbs much (possibly as much as 25%) of the filtered load of sodium. Some of this reabsorbed sodium is trapped in the renal medullary interstitium, thus accounting largely for the hypertonicity of the renal medullary interstitium. However, the medullary thick limb of Henle is also impermeable to water. Consequently, salt abstraction from the thick limb of Henle accounts simultaneously for the development of medullary hypertonicity, thus permitting—in the presence of ADH—maximal antidiuresis, and the appearance of maximally dilute urine in early distal convolutions, thus permitting—in the absence of ADH—maximal water diuresis.

In normal individuals, approximately 18 L/d of tubular fluid reaches the early distal tubule; the osmolality of this fluid is quite dilute, approximately 50 mOsm/kg H$_2$O. Thus, in the total absence of ADH and volume contraction, maximal rates of water diuresis include a urinary volume of 18 L/d having an osmolality of 50 mOsm/kg H$_2$O. During antidiuresis, ADH increases the water permeability of collecting ducts (see Chapter 238). Tubular fluid equilibrates osmotically with the hypertonic medullary interstitium, reducing urinary volume, concentrating the urine, and conserving body water. When ADH is absent, the water permeability of collecting ducts is low, and absorption of tubular fluid is reduced, so it escapes unchanged as hypotonic urine.

Finally, because collecting ducts are partially permeable to water in the absence of ADH, a reduced volume of hypotonic fluid reaching collecting ducts equilibrates partially with the medullary interstitium, thereby limiting the ability to dilute urine maximally.

NEGATIVE FEEDBACK. Water repletion activates a negative feedback of water conservation by at least two systems, atriopeptin and the oropharyngeal reflex (see Fig. 102–2). Immunoreactive atriopeptin is released both within the CNS and by secretory granules in cardiac atria. The centrally released atriopeptin can suppress by ADH release and thirst. Oropharyngeal stimulation by water suppresses both ADH release and thirst before absorbing water or producing a fall in plasma osmolality. This oropharyngeal reflex probably depends on neural traffic between the oropharynx and the CNS.

Finally, intrarenal prostaglandin E$_2$ suppresses the effects of ADH on nephron segments. Prostaglandin E$_2$ is produced by renal interstitial cells in response to increases in medullary osmolality. In turn, prostaglandin E$_2$ impairs water conservation by inhibiting the actions of ADH on nephron segments involved in the antidiuretic response, namely, the medullary thick ascending limb and the collecting duct.

HYPOTONIC DISORDERS

DEFINITION. In a hypotonic disorder, the ratio of solutes to water in body fluids is reduced, and the serum osmolality and serum sodium are both reduced in parallel. True hypotonicity must be distinguished from disorders in which the *measured* serum sodium is low while the measured serum osmolality is either normal or increased.

The distinction among these disorders is listed in Table 102–6. The measured serum sodium concentration can be reduced either because there is an increased concentration of small, non-sodium solutes restricted to the ECF or because of a laboratory artifact. In hyperglycemia or excessive mannitol administration, these solutes, which are restricted to the ECF, draw water from the cellular

Table 102–6 ■ DISTINCTION BETWEEN APPARENT AND REAL HYPOTONICITY

CONDITION	MEASURED SERUM (NA)	MEASURED SERUM OSMOLALITY
True hypotonicity	↓	↓
Increased non-sodium ECF solutes		
Hyperglycemia	↓	↑
Mannitol administration	↓	↑
Increased non-sodium ECF and ICF solutes		
Ethanol	Normal	↑
Ethylene glycol	Normal	↑
Methanol	Normal	↑
Isopropyl alcohol	Normal	↑
Laboratory artifact		
Hyperlipemia	↓	Normal
Hyperproteinemia	↓	Normal

compartment. The serum sodium level is therefore reduced, even though the serum osmolality may be increased. When a small, non-sodium solute is distributed in total body water, as in ethanol intoxication or in azotemia, the serum osmolality rises but the serum sodium concentration remains normal, resulting in an "osmolar gap." The latter is a useful diagnostic aid in intoxication with the different alcohols shown in Table 102–6.

Instances of spurious hyponatremia due to hyperlipemia or hyperproteinemia are becoming less common as more laboratories use ion-selective electrodes to measure the serum sodium concentration.

ETIOLOGY AND PATHOGENESIS. Hyponatremia and simultaneous body water hypotonicity develop whenever water intake exceeds the sum of renal plus extrarenal water losses; in chronic hyponatremia, the net water intake and net water output may be equal. Thus, hyponatremia and body fluid hypotonicity occur when there is a primary increase in water ingestion, when the ability of the kidney to dilute urine maximally is limited, or when a combination of these factors is operative.

The kidney regulates serum sodium concentration by increasing or decreasing free water excretion. The term *free water* refers to that amount of solute-free water that has to be added or subtracted from urine to leave it isosmolar to blood. Thus, adding free water to blood, either by failure to generate free water or by increased reabsorption of free water, will decrease serum sodium concentration. Free water is generated by the kidney across the diluting segments by absorbing salt without water. Thus, free water is formed and excreted. Failure to generate free water occurs in those clinical circumstances in which less salt is delivered to the diluting segments.

Free water is absorbed in the collecting duct. The rate of free water reabsorption is regulated in large part by ADH. Thus, the higher the ADH concentration, the greater is the rate of free water reabsorption, assuming that other driving forces for water reabsorption remain constant. Conditions with increased ADH concentrations are generally associated with hyponatremia. The collecting duct can maintain large osmotic gradients; however, this capacity is limited, and the minimal osmolality of the urine is approximately 50 mOsm/kg H_2O. If more dilute fluid is delivered to the collecting duct, this water will be reabsorbed even in the absence of ADH, as occurs in psychogenic polydipsia and in beer potomania. These conditions are described next.

REDUCED SOLUTE DELIVERY TO DISTAL NEPHRON SEGMENTS. These disorders may occur because of decreased sodium delivery to the diluting segment or decreased solute delivery to the collecting duct. Decreased sodium delivery generally occurs in a setting of decreased effective arterial blood volume (e.g., congestive heart failure, hypoalbuminemic states, and decreases in systemic vascular resistance), as in sepsis and cirrhosis. These conditions often are also associated with ADH increases.

An example of decreased solute delivery to the collecting duct is *beer potomania.* Without beer, a normal individual on a normal diet produces roughly 1000 mOsm of solute for urinary excretion. Because maximally dilute urine is 50 mOsm/kg, each 50 mOsm of solute can capture no more than 1 L of free water. Thus, on a normal diet, an individual can consume up to 20 L of fluid without becoming hyponatremic. However, beer has a low concentration of salts and other solutes, except it has a relatively high carbohydrate content that prevents metabolic generation of solutes by preventing protein catabolism. Indeed, it has been estimated that total urinary osmolal clearance is no more than 200 mOsm. Thus, beer drinkers who get most of their calories from beer cannot drink more than 4 L of free water (most of which will be consumed as beer) without becoming hyponatremic.

Hyponatremia due to reduced solute intake is not restricted to individuals with beer potomania but may occur during starvation, when intake may be dramatically reduced without parallel reductions in water intake. This form of hyponatremia occurs with increasing frequency in elderly patients in nursing homes who are inadequately supervised.

PRIMARY EFFECTOR ADH EXCESS. The Syndrome of Inappropriate ADH Production (SIADH). In SIADH, hyponatremia occurs as a result of sustained endogenous production and release of ADH or ADH-like substances; the ECF volume is normal or increased, and there are no other physiologic or pharmacologic stimuli to ADH release. Table 102–7 lists the major causes of SIADH. A similar

Table 102–7 ■ MAJOR CAUSES OF SIADH

Malignant Neoplasia
Carcinoma: bronchogenic, pancreatic, duodenal, ureteral, prostatic, bladder
Lymphoma and leukemia
Thymoma and mesothelioma
Central Nervous System Disorders
Trauma
Infection
Tumors
Porphyria
Pulmonary Disorders
Tuberculosis
Pneumonia
Fungal infections
Lung abscesses
Ventilators with positive pressure
Drug Induced
Desmopressin
Oxytocin
Vincristine
Chlorpropamide
Nicotine
Cyclophosphamide
Morphine
Amitriptyline
Selective serotonin reuptake inhibitors

process may account in part for the hyponatremia seen in myxedema.

ADH, or a peptide having comparable biologic activity, is produced by tumors. Increased ADH levels, estimated by either bioassay or radioimmunoassay, also have been noted in patients with cranial disorders such as skull fractures, subdural hematomas, subarachnoid hemorrhage, and brain tumors; in acute intermittent porphyria; and possibly in myxedema. Four different patterns of plasma ADH concentrations have been described in patients with SIADH. Figure 102–5 illustrates three of these patterns; the shaded area in the figure illustrates the normal relation between plasma ADH levels and serum osmolality. The pattern denoted "erratic ADH release" in Figure 102–5 accounts for about 37% of patients with SIADH; the hormone is released completely independently of osmotic control. About one third of patients with SIADH have a "reset osmostat"; there is an abnormally low

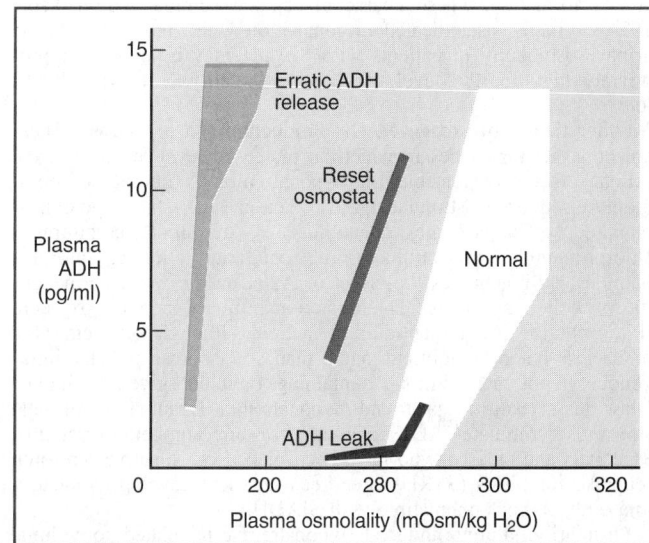

FIGURE 102–5 ■ The patterns of serum ADH abnormalities in SIADH. The shaded areas indicate the normal relation between increases in effective extracellular osmolality and ADH levels; the normal osmotic threshold is lower than the normal serum osmolality. The three shaded areas indicate ADH patterns in SIADH. (Adapted from Zerbe R, Strope L, Robertson G: Vasopressin function in the syndrome of inappropriate diuresis. Annu Rev Med 31:315, 1980.)

Table 102–8 ■ MAJOR CHARACTERISTICS OF SIADH

Hyponatremia
Volume expansion without edema
Natriuresis
Hypouricemia
Normal or reduced serum creatinine level
Normal thyroid and adrenal function

threshold for ADH secretion, but if sufficiently hyponatremic, these patients with SIADH can produce a maximally dilute urine. About 16% of patients with SIADH exhibit the "ADH leak" pattern, namely, sustained ADH production below the osmotic threshold, and normal increases in serum ADH levels with osmotic challenge (see Fig. 102–5). Finally, about 14% of patients with SIADH have no detectable abnormality in ADH levels; they fail, for reasons not yet understood, to dilute urine maximally.

The typical features of SIADH are listed in Table 102–8. The cardinal results of the sustained water conservation in SIADH are twofold: hyponatremia and volume expansion. In fact, patients with SIADH who are allowed free access to water generally gain about 3 kg in water weight or, in other words, nearly 10% of body water. In that respect, patients with SIADH differ from those with hyponatremia secondary to salt depletion, Addison's disease, or diuretic excess, because patients with the latter disorders are volume contracted. However, patients with SIADH, although volume expanded, do not develop edema and thus differ in that respect from patients with congestive heart failure or cirrhosis.

When total body water is expanded by about 10% by water conservation in SIADH, a natriuresis occurs even with hyponatremia. Thus, the patient with SIADH reaches a steady state when body water is expanded by water retention and when natriuresis, even with hyponatremia, prevents edema formation.

The causes for the natriuresis that is characteristic of SIADH are multiple. First, volume expansion will result in enhanced release of atriopeptin, which enhances urinary sodium wasting both by enhancing glomerular filtration and by suppressing tubular sodium absorption. Second, the volume expansion of SIADH also reduces the rate of proximal tubular sodium absorption, as well as the rate of proximal uric acid absorption.

In short, SIADH is a disorder in which hormone-stimulated water conservation results in hyponatremia, volume expansion, and consequently an increased GFR, tubular sodium wasting, and reduced net tubular absorption of creatinine and uric acid, but no edema formation. These characteristics are summarized in Table 102–8. Finally, as indicated in connection with Figure 102–5, the urinary osmolality in patients with SIADH may be either inappropriately high for the level of serum osmolality or maximally dilute.

Other Causes of Excessive ADH Production and/or Release. There are other circumstances in which an increased level of ADH is the primary factor responsible for hyponatremia. A number of commonly used drugs stimulate ADH release: vincristine, cyclophosphamide, carbamazepine, phenothiazines, morphine, barbiturates, chlorpropamide, amitriptyline, thiothixene, and clofibrate. Chlorpropamide also potentiates the effect of ADH on the water permeability of collecting ducts. The posterior pituitary peptide oxytocin (Pitocin) also has an antidiuretic action, although oxytocin is a much less potent antidiuretic agent than is vasopressin. Thus, intravenous hypotonic solutions containing oxytocin given to induce labor may result in profound hyponatremia. Trauma or surgical stress also stimulates ADH release. Increasing numbers of patients, especially the elderly, who have been placed on selective serotonin reuptake inhibitors (SSRIs) have been noted to develop hyponatremia with findings compatible with SIADH.

Ordinarily, diuretic-induced hyponatremia is related to volume contraction; this kind of body fluid dilution is discussed later. Chronic severe potassium depletion induced by diuretics can also result in ADH release, although the mechanisms by which potassium depletion stimulates ADH release are unknown.

MIXED DISORDERS. Hyponatremia occurs commonly in true volume contraction and in edematous states when filling of the arterial tree is impaired. The former disorders include patients in whom both ECF and total body water are reduced; the latter group com-

prises those patients with deranged Starling forces, notably local or systemic increases in venous pressure, which result in inadequate filling of the arterial tree. In both sets of disorders, two factors contribute, individually or in unison, to the pathogenesis of hyponatremia: non-osmotic, volume-mediated ADH release and reductions in the rate of sodium delivery to the diluting segment.

Volume contraction is a potent non-osmotic stimulus to ADH release. Figure 102–6 shows the relations between osmotic and non-osmotic, volume-mediated stimuli and plasma ADH levels in experimental animals; entirely comparable responses occur in humans. Increases in plasma osmolality are related linearly to increases in plasma ADH levels. The relation between blood volume depletion and plasma ADH levels is non-linear. However, with depletion of more than 7 to 10% blood volume, plasma ADH levels rise sharply and produce an antidiuretic effect even when the plasma osmolality is reduced below normal. In other words, volume-mediated, non-osmotic ADH release occurs primarily when circulatory dynamics are moderately to severely advanced; in that circumstance, volume-mediated stimuli override osmotically mediated ADH release, and hyponatremia ensues.

A second factor that accounts for hyponatremia in volume-contracted states is an inability to dilute urine maximally because the rate of sodium delivery to diluting segments in the thick ascending limb is reduced. This situation occurs because increased rates of proximal tubular sodium absorption are stimulated by reduced sodium intake or by inadequate filling of the arterial tree in conditions with combined ECF volume expansion and reduced arterial tree filling.

Hyponatremia is a common feature of untreated Addison's disease and occurs because of a combination of circumstances. In mineralocorticoid deficiency, ECF volume contraction, glomerular filtration reduction, enhanced proximal tubular salt absorption, and volume-mediated, non-osmotic ADH release appear to be the major

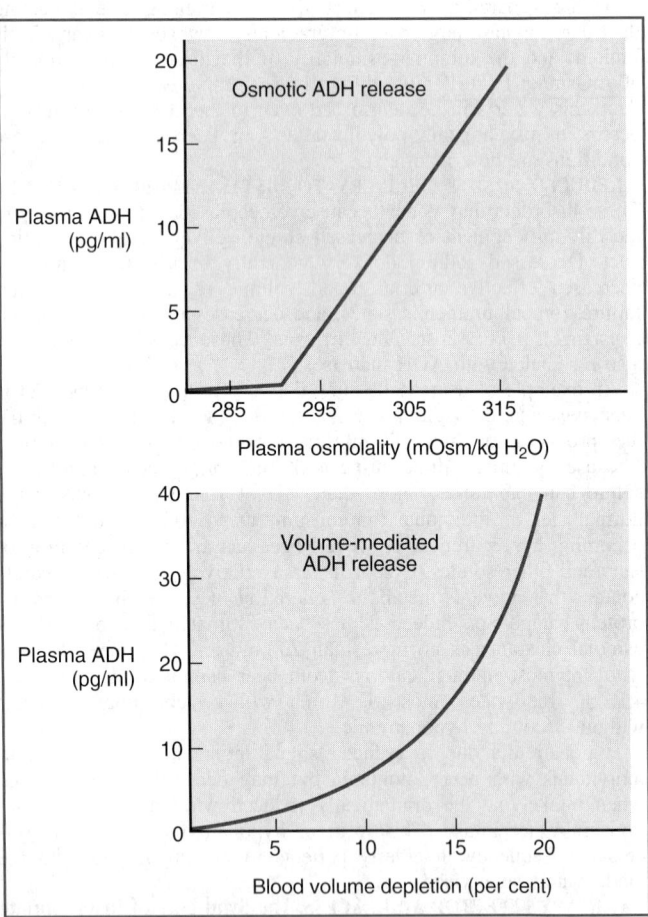

FIGURE 102–6 ■ Relation between plasma ADH concentrations and either effective extracellular fluid osmolality (upper plot) or the percentage of blood volume depletion (lower plot). (Adapted from Dunn FL, Brennan TJ, Nelson AE, et al: The role of blood osmolality and volume in regulating vasopressin secretion in the rat. J Clin Invest 52:3212, 1973, by copyright permission of the American Society for Clinical Investigation.)

factors responsible for an inability to excrete water loads. Gluco-corticoid deficiency also impairs the ability to excrete water loads. One of the factors responsible for water retention in Addison's disease is non-osmotic ADH release, which results from impaired cardiac function.

Hyponatremia occurs commonly in advanced stages of disorders characterized by edema formation and a reduced EABU, particularly in intractable heart failure and advanced hepatic cirrhosis with ascites. Reduced rates of salt delivery to diluting segments of the renal tubule clearly contribute to impaired water excretion in these disorders. In patients with heart failure or severe ascites, the plasma concentrations of ADH tend to be inappropriately high with respect to plasma osmolality so that non-osmotic ADH release secondary to contraction of the effective arterial blood volume may contribute to the development of hyponatremia in these disorders. Furthermore, since non-osmotic ADH release occurs only with profound reductions in blood volume (see Fig. 102–6), the occurrence of hyponatremia in congestive heart failure or cirrhosis indicates profound arterial underfilling. This observation correlates well with the ominous prognosis of hyponatremia in these disorders.

CLINICAL MANIFESTATIONS. The clinical manifestations of hyponatremia are produced by brain swelling and are primarily a function of the rate of fall of serum sodium concentration and not the absolute level. The early symptoms include lethargy, weakness, and somnolence, which proceed rapidly to seizures, coma, and death as hyponatremia worsens. Untreated acute water intoxication is nearly uniformly fatal and represents a medical emergency. In chronic hyponatremia, CNS manifestations are far less common, even when the serum sodium concentration is as low as 100 mEq/L, because the loss of brain solutes, principally potassium chloride, minimizes brain cell swelling for a given reduction in body water osmolality.

DIAGNOSIS. Hyponatremia should be considered whenever there is a sudden deterioration in CNS function, particularly in circumstances such as intractable heart failure, hepatic cirrhosis with ascites, or when large volumes of intravenous fluids are administered. The hyponatremic patient should be evaluated to determine the underlying condition that produced body fluid dilution. This evaluation should include a careful history and physical examination; measurement of the serum creatinine, BUN, and electrolyte levels; measurement of the urinary sodium concentration, or the fractional excretion of sodium; measurement of serum and urinary osmolalities; and, when appropriate, evaluation of thyroid and adrenal function.

The history and physical examination are generally adequate for recognizing disorders such as beer potomania or compulsive water ingestion or for noting the ingestion of drugs that stimulate ADH release or enhance ADH action. The presence of edema is characteristic of individuals in whom hyponatremia occurs because of a reduced effective arterial blood volume coupled to ECF volume expansion. In myxedema or Addison's disease, the typical clinical or laboratory findings of these disorders are generally present (see Chapters 239 and 240).

The most difficult differential diagnosis among hyponatremic disorders involves the distinction between patients who are modestly volume contracted and those who have SIADH. In both circumstances, the serum sodium and the serum osmolality are reduced, whereas the urinary osmolality is inappropriately high with respect to the reduced serum osmolality. Non-osmotic water conservation in SIADH and in volume contraction is recognized by the presence of a urinary osmolality greater than 120 to 150 mOsm/kg H_2O in association with a reduced serum osmolality. The distinction between the two disorders therefore depends on a clinical and laboratory assessment of effective arterial blood volume.

Patients who are volume contracted may provide a history of volume losses or of diuretic ingestion and may exhibit the signs of ECF volume contraction discussed previously in the section on volume depletion. When the volume losses are due to extrarenal causes, the urinary sodium concentration is less than 10 to 15 mEq/L and the fractional excretion of sodium is generally less than 1%. Uric acid concentration is influenced by volume status of the patient. In volume expansion, there is increased urinary excretion of uric acid and therefore a tendency toward hypouricemia. Conversely, the presence of hyperuricemia suggests effective arterial volume contraction. Prerenal azotemia may occur if the volume contraction is severe. Patients with SIADH are generally normovolemic or slightly volume expanded and therefore exhibit

Table 102–9 ■ DISTINGUISHING FEATURES OF APPROPRIATELY VERSUS INAPPROPRIATELY INCREASED ADH CONCENTRATIONS

Appropriate		Inappropriate
↓	Plasma sodium	↓
↑	Urine osmolality	↑
↓	Urine sodium	↑
↑	Plasma uric acid	↓

none of the signs of volume contraction. The serum BUN and creatinine levels are normal, and the serum uric acid level is generally reduced. The urinary sodium concentration is usually greater than 30 mEq/L, and the fractional excretion of sodium is greater than 1%. Tests of adrenal function yield normal results (Table 102–9).

The previous studies usually discriminate between SIADH and extrarenal volume contraction. When ECF volume contraction is due to renal salt wasting, urinary sodium losses generally persist unless volume contraction is profound. Moreover, as noted previously (see Volume Depletion), the blood pressure and pulse may be normal in states of modest volume contraction. A useful diagnostic and therapeutic maneuver in this situation is to observe the results of water restriction. When water intake is restricted to 600 to 800 mL/d, patients with SIADH exhibit a highly characteristic response: a 2- to 3-kg weight loss is accompanied by correction of hyponatremia and cessation of salt wasting, usually over 2 to 3 days. If weight loss fails to correct both hyponatremia and urinary sodium wasting simultaneously, the diagnosis of SIADH is doubtful. Rather, renal sodium wasting with ECF volume contraction, due to Addison's disease or the other renal salt-losing disorders listed in Table 102–2, is the more probable diagnosis.

TREATMENT. Neurologic symptoms secondary to osmotic swelling of the brain are much more common when hyponatremia develops rapidly in menstruant women and prepubescent children (i.e., age, gender, and hormonal status of patients are important factors in predisposing to symptoms of hyponatremia), but the most severe neurologic complications of acute treatment of hyponatremia are more common if existing hyponatremia is of long standing and developed chronically. Patients with CNS manifestations of hyponatremia require immediate therapy to prevent death, whereas too-rapid hyponatremia correction may be associated with osmotic demyelination syndrome, which is the result of the selective loss of myelin (with sparing of neurons and axial cylinders). These histologic findings may occur in any part of the brain but are more common in the central areas of the pons. The symptoms of osmotic demyelinating syndrome often occur several days after too-rapid hyponatremia correction and include behavioral disturbances, fluctuating levels of consciousness, ataxia, pseudo-bulbar palsy, difficulty in speaking, and other varying features. In non-fatal cases, the recovery is slow, often taking weeks, and recovery may not be complete with residual sequelae. Thus, differing opinions exist as to the ideal rate for correcting hyponatremia. The rate and magnitude of this correction can be considered conveniently as a two-step process: acute correction of symptomatic hyponatremia and chronic correction of asymptomatic or residual hyponatremia. Although the development of osmotic demyelination syndrome is quite rare, failure to correct symptomatic hyponatremia is associated with unacceptable morbidity and mortality rates.

ACUTE CORRECTION OF HYPONATREMIA. Acute hyponatremia associated with a serum sodium concentration less than 120 mEq/L and with CNS manifestations requires immediate therapy. In volume-contracted states, the treatment of choice is to raise the serum sodium concentration by 10 mEq/L or to levels of 120 to 125 mEq/L over a 6-hour interval by administering hypertonic 3 to 5% saline. As was discussed, elevating serum sodium too quickly to values more than 125 mEq/L may be hazardous. Because the desired effect is to correct total body water osmolality, the amount of sodium administered must be sufficient to raise total body water osmolality to approximately 250 mOsm/kg H_2O, that is, to approximately twice the desired serum sodium concentration. A convenient formula for calculating this sodium requirement is as follows:

$$[125 - \text{measured serum Na}^+] \times 0.6 \text{ body weight}$$
$$= \text{required mEq of Na}^+$$

The serum sodium level is in milliequivalents per liter, and the body weight is in kilograms. Because 60% of body weight is water, the formula allows an estimate of the amount of sodium required to raise total body water osmolality to 250 mOsm/kg H_2O. However, if one cannot remember this formula, a useful practice is to administer 250 mL of either 3 or 5% saline over 4 to 6 hours. This will usually raise the serum sodium concentration by 10 to 15 mEq/L and abate the neurologic symptoms. Once the acute corrective phase of hyponatremia is complete, one can initiate the principle of chronic correction of hyponatremia.

CHRONIC CORRECTION OF HYPONATREMIA. The most important aspect in managing asymptomatic, non–volume-depleted hyponatremia is to restrict electrolyte-free water intake. If water intake is restricted to less than 1 L/d, the serum sodium concentration will rise regardless of its cause. Fluid intake restriction should be coupled with high dietary salt intake. Because this approach is clinically unacceptably slow in certain patients, an alternative is to use normal saline in combination with a loop diuretic. The diuretic induces urinary salt loss and therefore reduces the risk of ECF volume expansion. It should be emphasized that isotonic saline infusion without a loop diuretic may actually lower the serum sodium concentration in patients with SIADH. Thus, one must use a loop diuretic with intravenous saline if this approach is taken.

Another approach to correcting chronic hyponatremia in SIADH is to use lithium carbonate or demeclocycline. These two compounds block the effect of ADH at the level of the collecting duct and, therefore, increase the excretion of free water. However, both these drugs may have complications and should only be used if the patient cannot adequately comply with water restriction and high dietary salt intake. Specific inhibitors of ADH-V_2 receptors may have a role in the future in treatment of hyponatremia.

HYPERTONIC DISORDERS

DEFINITION. A hypertonic disorder is one in which the ratio of solutes to water in total body water is increased. All hypernatremic states are hypertonic. In some hypertonic disorders, such as uncontrolled hyperglycemia, the increase in effective ECF osmolality is due to non-sodium solutes.

ETIOLOGY AND PATHOGENESIS. Hypernatremia develops whenever water intake is less than the sum of renal and extrarenal water losses; in chronic hypertonic states, net water balance may be zero. The most common causes of clinically significant hypernatremia occur as a consequence of three pathogenic mechanisms: impaired thirst, solute or osmotic diuresis, excessive losses of water, either through the kidneys or extrarenally, and combinations of these derangements. These disorders are grouped in Table 102–10 according to the primary pathogenic mechanism. There is also a group of miscellaneous disorders, such as hypokalemia, hypercalcemia, and interstitial renal disease, as well as chronic renal failure, which either partially impair renal urinary concentrating ability or partially blunt the responsiveness of collecting ducts to ADH. These disorders rarely cause significant hypernatremia and are not discussed further.

INADEQUATE INTAKE OF WATER. This problem occurs in patients who are comatose or who are otherwise unable to communicate thirst. Because of the exquisite sensitivity of thirst mechanisms to

Table 102–10 ■ MAJOR CAUSES OF HYPERNATREMIA

I. **Impaired Thirst**
Coma
Essential hypernatremia
II. **Solute Diuresis**
Osmotic diuresis: diabetic ketoacidosis, non-ketotic hyperosmolar coma, mannitol administration
III. **Excessive Water Losses**
Renal
Pituitary diabetes insipidus
Nephrogenic diabetes insipidus
Extrarenal
Sweating
IV. **Combined Disorders**
Coma plus hypertonic nasogastric feeding

changes in effective body water osmolality, hypernatremia due to inadequate water intake is rare in conscious patients allowed free access to water. Rarely, patients will have a primary thirst deficiency. Patients with Cushing's syndrome or primary hyperaldosteronism commonly have slight elevations in the serum sodium level for unknown reasons.

Finally, "essential hypernatremia" is characterized by a slightly elevated serum sodium level that occurs in the conscious state. The defect in patients with essential hypernatremia appears to be an insensitivity of thirst centers and osmoreceptors to osmotic stimuli. However, both thirst and antidiuresis occur when these patients are volume contracted. Consequently, it has been inferred that volume-mediated stimuli to thirst and ADH release are intact in patients with essential hypernatremia. This disorder may be either congenital or acquired, sometimes in association with histiocytic infiltration of the CNS.

OSMOTIC DIURESIS. This is another mechanism for producing renal water losses in excess of sodium losses and, therefore, hypertonicity. Osmotic diuresis occurs commonly in uncontrolled glycosuria and may occur when mannitol is given. Because these solutes are restricted to the ECF, the serum sodium level is generally reduced in the early stages of osmotic diuresis, and the effective ECF osmolality is increased primarily by the impermeant non-sodium solute. In prolonged osmotic diuresis, net water losses may be sufficiently great that hypernatremia develops. In this circumstance, the increase in effective ECF osmolality is due to the combined effects of hypernatremia and the non-sodium solute. Hypernatremia due to an osmotic urea diuresis can occur if large amounts of protein and amino acids are administered by nasogastric tube, or if tissue catabolism is great, as in burns. In this circumstance, hypernatremia is entirely responsible for the increased effective ECF osmolality.

Hypernatremia also may complicate use of normal saline solutions when the endogenous osmolar solute load is high and renal concentrating ability is limited. Patients with diabetic ketoacidosis, who are generally young, have sufficient urinary concentrating ability that hypernatremia does not occur when normal saline solutions are used to treat ketoacidosis. In contrast, the non-ketotic hyperglycemic syndrome generally occurs in elderly patients, who can have partial impairment of urinary concentrating power. In this setting, hypernatremia can occur during therapy with normal saline solutions. This complication can be avoided by treating with half-normal saline and thus providing sufficient solute-free water for urinary elimination of the osmolar glucose load.

EXCESSIVE WATER LOSSES. Impairment of ADH production, release, or action, as occurs in pituitary or nephrogenic diabetes insipidus, respectively, can lead to profound water deficits and to hypernatremia. In such circumstances, the urine volumes are large, the urinary osmolality is low, and the net rate of solute excretion is low, in contrast to individuals undergoing osmotic diuresis, in whom rates of urinary solute excretion are elevated. The diabetes insipidus syndromes are considered in detail in Chapter 238.

Striking water losses also may occur with excessive sweating, particularly during rigorous physical activity by untrained individuals exercising in high humidity. This phenomenon plays a major role in the evolution of heat stroke.

COMBINED DISORDERS. Finally, hypertonic dehydration may occur as a combination of these events. A common example in modern clinical practice involves injudiciously administering large amounts of carbohydrate or amino acids by nasogastric tube, coupled with limited amounts of water, to stroke patients unable to communicate thirst.

CLINICAL MANIFESTATIONS AND DIAGNOSIS. Because two thirds of body water is intracellular, primary water losses tend to have modest effects on circulating volume unless fluid losses are profound. Rather, the clinical manifestations are produced by brain shrinkage that results from increases in effective ECF osmolality. Thus, the symptoms of hypertonicity produced either by hypernatremia or by impermeant non-sodium solutes such as glucose are referable to the CNS and range from somnolence and confusion to coma, respiratory paralysis, and death. The degree of symptomatology varies with the degree of hypertonicity and with the rate at which hypertonicity develops. In acute hypertonicity, symptoms generally appear when the effective ECF osmolality exceeds 320 to 330 mOsm/kg H_2O, and coma and respiratory arrest may occur when the ECF osmolality exceeds 360 to 380 mOsm/kg H_2O.

Chronic hypertonicity generally produces fewer CNS manifestations, because brain cells accumulate idiogenic osmoles, which minimize the tendency for brain shrinkage.

TREATMENT. To treat acute hypernatremia, normal saline solutions are initially given intravenously. These factors should be considered when treating acute hypernatremia. In the highly volume-contracted patient with severe hypernatremia, administering isotonic saline solutions has two advantages. It provides fluid resuscitation in impending cardiovascular collapse. Moreover, the isotonic salt solution, which is hypotonic with respect to the hypertonic patient, avoids an unnecessary rapid fall in the serum sodium level.

Rapid correction of hypertonicity to a normal serum osmolality is hazardous. Because accumulation of idiogenic osmoles by brain cells is a compensatory mechanism for preserving brain volume in hypertonic disorders, a normal serum osmolality may be relatively hypotonic to brain cells that have accumulated idiogenic solutes. Hence, if the serum osmolality is reduced rapidly, CNS damage due to brain swelling may occur. A useful guide to circumventing this difficulty is to reduce the serum sodium level by no more than 1 mEq/L during every 2 hours of the first 2 days of treatment.

Cheng J-C, Zikos D, Skopicki HA, et al: Long-term neurologic outcome in psychogenic water drinkers with severe symptomatic hyponatremia: The effect of rapid correction. Am J Med 88:561, 1990. *Study of patients with hyponatremia secondary to compulsive water drinking demonstrating that it is safe to reverse the neurologic sequelae by rapid correction of serum sodium level by 15 mEq/kg H₂O followed by more gradual correction of the remaining hyponatremia.*

De Vita MV, Michelis MF: Perturbations in sodium balance. Clin Lab Med 13:135, 1993. *Discusses the pathophysiology, assessment, and treatment of hyponatremia and hypernatremia syndromes.*

Fraser CL, Arieff AI: Epidemiology, pathophysiology, and management of hyponatremic encephalopathy. Am J Med 102:67–77, 1997. *Nice review of pathogenesis of hyponatremia and hyponatremic encephalopathy. Authors call attention to increased morbidity and mortality with hyponatremia especially in children and menstruant women. Easy to understand therapeutic approach is given to asymptomatic and symptomatic hyponatremia.*

Goldman MB, Luchins DJ, Robertson GL: Mechanisms of altered water metabolism in psychotic patients with polydipsia and hyponatremia. N Engl J Med 318:397, 1988. *An account of factors causing hyponatremia in hospitalized patients with affective disorders.*

Lauriat SM, Berl T: The hyponatremic patient: Practical focus on therapy. J Am Soc Nephrol 8:1599–1607, 1997. *Clear discussion on potential complicating factors in formulating a therapeutic plan for treatment of hyponatremia.*

Liu BA, Mittmann N, Knowles SR, Shear NH: Hyponatremia and the syndrome of inappropriate secretion of antidiuretic hormone associated with the use of selective serotonin reuptake inhibitors: A review of spontaneous reports. Can Med Assoc J 15:519–527, 1996. *Clinicians have noted an increased incidence of hyponatremia and SIADH with the use of selective serotonin reuptake inhibitors—especially in the elderly. This often can be quite serious, but is usually reversible. This manuscript summarizes and reviews a large number of these cases.*

Sonnenblick M, Friedlander Y, Rosin AJ: Diuretic-induced severe hyponatremia: Review and analysis of 129 reported patients. Chest 103:601, 1993. *Literature review of severe diuretic-induced hyponatremia showing that severity of hyponatremia as well as too-rapid correction was associated with higher mortality. Thiazide diuretics were associated with severe hyponatremia much more frequently than loop diuretics.*

Tang WW, Kaptein EM, Feinstein EI, Massry SG: Hyponatremia in hospitalized patients with the acquired immunodeficiency syndrome (AIDS) and the AIDS-related complex. Am J Med 94:169, 1993. *A well-conducted prospective study showing that hyponatremia is common in AIDS patients and is usually associated with gastrointestinal losses with hypovolemia, but euvolemia with SIADH was also a common association. Hyponatremia of either cause was associated with increased morbidity and mortality.*

102.3   Disturbances in Potassium Balance

PHYSIOLOGIC CONSIDERATIONS

Hypokalemia ($K^+ < 3.5$ mEq/L) and hyperkalemia ($K^+ > 5.5$ mEq/L) are common in the practice of medicine. Whereas the plasma potassium concentration is influenced by total body potassium stores, it should be recognized that factors influencing the distribution of potassium between extracellular and intracellular spaces are important determinants of plasma potassium concentration.

Transfer Between ICF and ECF

The intracellular compartment acts as a large potassium reservoir in series with the small ECF potassium pool. In potassium-depleted states with normal acid-base status, a 1 mEq/L fall in the serum potassium level reflects the loss of about 300 mEq of potassium; hence, the bulk of external potassium loss comes from the cellular

compartment. Conversely, if large amounts of potassium are administered acutely, the rise in serum potassium level is less than would be expected if the administered potassium were distributed solely in the ECF. In this situation, cellular uptake of potassium obviously occurs and prevents greater increases in the serum potassium concentration. This ability of cells to accumulate potassium can be enhanced strikingly by chronic administration of high-potassium diets.

A number of *effector* mechanisms regulate the partition of potassium between the ICF and ECF. These include active and passive ionic transcellular transport processes.

ACTIVE TRANSPORT PROCESSES. The cardinal transport process regulating K^+ distribution between the ICF and ECF is cell membrane–bound Na^+, K^+-ATPase, which actively transports potassium into cells and therefore counterbalances the passive leak of potassium from cells into interstitial fluid. Insulin is a second effector that promotes potassium transfer from ECF to ICF. This hormone promotes cellular uptake of potassium independently of cellular glucose uptake by increasing Na^+, K^+-ATPase activity. Insulin also reduces sodium permeability; the resultant cellular hyperpolarization of cells produces a passive driving force for potassium accumulation within cells. Furthermore, hyperkalemia augments insulin release. Thus, hyperkalemia may be the sensor that stimulates release of insulin, which then serves as an effector for potassium entry into cells. β-Adrenergic agents, particularly β_2 agonists such as terbutaline, also promote cellular potassium uptake by enhancing Na^+, K^+-ATPase activity; it is not yet known whether hyperkalemia can provoke β-agonist release, as it does for insulin release. Finally, mineralocorticoids such as aldosterone, in addition to enhancing renal potassium excretion (see later), also enhance cellular potassium uptake; the mode of aldosterone action in the latter instance is not understood.

PASSIVE TRANSPORT PROCESSES. A number of passive effector mechanisms also regulate the partition of potassium between the ICF and the ECF. First, alterations in the pH of ECF reproducibly shift potassium between the ICF and the ECF. Systemic acidosis, whether metabolic or respiratory, promotes potassium efflux from cells, whereas systemic alkalosis, either metabolic or respiratory, promotes cellular potassium uptake. As a general rule, a reduction in plasma pH of 0.1 unit in metabolic acidosis raises the serum potassium level by 0.6 mEq/L, whereas a plasma pH increase of 0.1 unit produces a similar reduction in serum potassium. The magnitude of transcellular potassium shifts is not as great in response to acid-base balance changes due to respiratory causes as it is in those due to metabolic causes.

Second, cellular shrinkage produced by increases in effective ECF osmolality raises the intracellular potassium concentration and thereby increases the driving force for passive potassium leakage from the ICF to the ECF. This leakage may result in hyperkalemia when large glucose loads are administered to insulin-deficient diabetic patients who also have hyporeninemic hypoaldosteronism; the insulin lack limits cellular re-entry of potassium, and the aldosterone deficiency limits renal potassium excretion. Increases in cellular potassium concentrations produced by cellular shrinkage also contribute significantly to the hyperkalemia of diabetic ketoacidosis, because hyperglycemia raises cellular potassium levels by cell shrinkage and insulin lack prevents accelerated potassium re-entry into cells.

Finally, brain cells and renal tubular cells lose potassium when exposed to chronic ECF hypotonicity. However, muscle cells, which are the largest component of ICF potassium, do not appear to participate in this process. Consequently, hypotonic disorders, by themselves, have little effect on the serum potassium level or on external potassium balance.

Renal Handling of Potassium

The kidney is responsible for the excretion of approximately 90% of dietary potassium. Although the stool potassium concentration is quite high (75 to 90 mEq/L of stool water) under normal circumstances, only roughly 10% of dietary potassium is excreted by the gastrointestinal tract. Thus, factors that cause an increase in renal excretion of potassium are of importance (Table 102–11).

Almost all the potassium excreted in urine gains access to the

Table 102–11 ■ **FACTORS CAUSING INCREASED URINARY LOSS OF POTASSIUM**

Increased mineralocorticoids
Increased delivery of Na$^+$ to collecting duct
Increased fluid flow to distal tubule
Metabolic and respiratory alkalosis
Increased excretion of non-reabsorbable solutes

urinary space by secretory mechanisms that are located across distal convoluted and collecting duct segments. These transport processes are described in Chapter 101, but for the purposes of this chapter, it is important to identify these factors in clinical situations that cause increased excretion of potassium. Of the factors listed in Table 102–11, increased plasma aldosterone is most important, with a higher resultant kaliuresis occurring by the other factors if they are superimposed on a baseline of higher aldosterone concentration. The rate of urinary potassium excretion in any given clinical circumstance depends on the interplay between these factors.

The rate of renal tubular adaptation to factors regulating urinary excretion of potassium is relatively slow. However, the renal adaptation to excess loads occurs over a 24- to 36-hour period, and, therefore, hyperkalemia from the ingestion of large oral potassium loads is uncommon in normal individuals. But the renal response to dietary potassium restriction is more sluggish and requires 7 to 10 days for full development. Even under the latter circumstances, urinary potassium losses are rarely less than 20 mEq/d.

HYPOKALEMIA AND POTASSIUM DEPLETION

DEFINITION. Chronic hypokalemia generally reflects a reduction in total body potassium. A 1-mEq reduction in serum potassium level generally implies the net loss of 300 mEq of potassium from the body. In extreme body potassium depletion, the serum potassium level may be as low as 1.5 to 2.0 mEq/L. Acute reductions in serum potassium level without parallel reductions in total body potassium occur when potassium is shifted from the ECF to the ICF.

ETIOLOGY AND PATHOGENESIS. Hypokalemia and simultaneous potassium depletion occur whenever renal plus extrarenal potassium losses exceed potassium intake. In advanced body potassium depletion, intake and output of potassium may be equal. The four major causes for hypokalemia are given in Table 102–12.

EXCESSIVE RENAL LOSSES. Many of the causes for renal potassium wasting can be analyzed in terms of factors that modulate the common effector system for potassium secretion. *Mineralocorticoid excess* accelerates distal tubular potassium secretion. Consequently, hypokalemia occurs regularly in primary hyperaldosteronism, in Cushing's syndrome, and in secondary hyperaldosteronism. *Chronic European licorice ingestion* produces a syndrome that mimics primary hyperaldosteronism, because glycyrrhizic acid, a component of licorice extract, has physiologic properties similar to those of aldosterone.

Table 102–12 ■ **MAJOR CAUSES OF HYPOKALEMIA**

I. Excess Renal Loss	II. Gastrointestinal Losses
Mineralocorticoid excess	Vomiting
Bartter's syndrome	Diarrhea, particularly secretory
Diuresis	diarrheas
Diuretics with a pre-late	III. ECF → ICF Shifts
distal locus	Acute alkalosis
Osmotic diuresis	Hypokalemic periodic paralysis
Chronic metabolic alkalosis	Barium ingestion
Antibiotics	Insulin therapy
Carbenicillin	Vitamin B$_{12}$ therapy
Gentamicin	Thyrotoxicosis (rarely)
Amphotericin B	IV. Inadequate Intake
Renal tubular acidosis	
Distal, gradient-limited	
Proximal	
Liddle's syndrome	
Gitelman's syndrome	
Acute leukemia	
Ureterosigmoidostomy	

The primary pathophysiologic defect in Bartter's syndrome is incomplete reabsorption of NaCl by the thick ascending limb of Henle. This causes increased delivery of Na$^+$ to the collecting duct and net salt wastage. The resulting volume contraction results in increased renin and aldosterone concentrations. These hormonal changes, together with increased delivery of Na$^+$ to the collecting duct, cause increased excretion of potassium.

Most diuretics having a locus of action before the late distal tubule (see Fig. 102–3) increase urinary potassium losses. Enhanced sodium delivery to distal nephron segments is the major factor responsible for the kaliuresis produced by these diuretics, and sodium restriction or volume depletion tends to minimize diuretic-induced potassium losses. Carbonic anhydrase inhibitors such as acetazolamide inhibit proximal bicarbonate absorption and thereby accentuate potassium losses. Distal tubular segments are relatively impermeable to bicarbonate, consequently, increased delivery of bicarbonate to distal nephron regions has an impermeant anion effect that increases luminal electronegativity in these nephron regions.

Osmotic diuresis is commonly associated with increased renal potassium losses, because increased tubular flow rates enhance net potassium secretion. In diabetic ketoacidosis, renal potassium losses are common. Yet patients with diabetic ketoacidosis and a reduced total body potassium concentration commonly present with hyperkalemia because metabolic acidosis tends to promote potassium shifts from the ICF to the ECF. Consequently, profound hypokalemia may develop if body potassium is not replenished concomitantly with insulin therapy and ECF volume expansion (see Chapter 242).

Potassium depletion is seen frequently in *chronic metabolic alkalosis*. When the alkalosis is associated with volume contraction, secondary hyperaldosteronism results in renal potassium losses. Potassium depletion in chronic metabolic alkalosis is also enhanced if bicarbonaturia is present, because of the impermeant anion effect produced by bicarbonate delivery to collecting duct segments. In fact, the hypokalemia associated with upper gastrointestinal fluid losses, as in vomiting or nasogastric suction, is primarily the result of the renal potassium losses produced by secondary hyperaldosteronism or bicarbonaturia or both. The potassium losses from the upper gastrointestinal tract are small, because upper gastrointestinal tract fluid contains only about 10 mEq of potassium per liter.

Hypokalemia may develop during therapy with certain *antibiotics*. Carbenicillin or other penicillin-like antibiotics exist as sodium or potassium salts of impermeant anions and promote kaliuresis because they increase net sodium excretion and because of an impermeant anion effect. Amphotericin B increases the permeability of luminal membranes to potassium and therefore promotes potassium secretion. Gentamicin produces potassium losses by unknown mechanisms.

Hypokalemia and potassium depletion are common findings in both type II proximal tubular acidosis and type I *distal, gradient-limited renal tubular acidosis* (see Chapter 107). Increased distal sodium delivery and the impermeant anion effect produced by bicarbonate wasting account for most of the potassium losses seen in proximal renal tubular acidosis. Consequently, salt restriction, which enhances the rate of proximal sodium bicarbonate absorption in this disorder, also tends to correct potassium depletion. In gradient-limited distal renal tubular acidosis, hypokalemia may be accentuated by volume losses and secondary hyperaldosteronism. Other factors, not yet understood, also contribute to hypokalemia in this disorder. Hyperkalemia, rather than hypokalemia, commonly accompanies the hyperchloremic acidosis of interstitial disease (type IV acidosis) or of voltage-dependent renal tubular acidosis (see later).

Liddle's syndrome is a rare inherited tubular disorder characterized by hypokalemia, metabolic alkalosis, hypertension, and subnormal aldosterone secretion rates. Therapy with triamterene or amiloride, but not with aldosterone antagonists such as spironolactone, ameliorates the disorder. These findings suggest that collecting duct sodium avidity and potassium secretion independent of aldosterone are major factors in the pathogenesis of Liddle's syndrome. Indeed, recent studies have shown that collecting duct sodium channels are mutated in such a manner as to be "open" even with subnormal aldosterone concentrations (aldosterone normally opens sodium channels in the collecting duct to increase sodium absorption). Thus, in operational terms, Liddle's syndrome may be described as distal nephron hyperfunction, in regard to Na$^+$ absorption and H$^+$ and K$^+$ secretion.

GASTROINTESTINAL LOSSES. These provide the major route for potassium depletion, other than the kidney. As indicated earlier, potassium depletion associated with vomiting is referable primarily to renal potassium losses. Diarrhea produces significant potassium losses, because normal stool water potassium concentration is 70 to 90 mEq/L and voluminous diarrheal fluid contains 30 mEq/L of potassium. The most striking diarrheal potassium losses occur in secretory diarrheas, such as with non-beta islet cell tumors of the pancreas, which produce vasoactive intestinal polypeptide, and in laxative abuse. In both secretory diarrheas and chronic laxative abuse, hypokalemia is probably caused by increased rates of K^+ secretion through apical membrane K^+ channels. Villous adenomas of the colon produce potassium depletion because of excessive colonic K^+ secretion from the adenoma. Hypokalemia is uncommonly seen in inflammatory bowel disease.

ECF-ICF SHIFTS. Acute hypokalemia with a normal total body potassium may occur because of *potassium shifts* from the ECF to the ICF. In *hypokalemic periodic paralysis*, acute shifts of potassium from the ECF to the ICF produce limb and trunk paralysis. The periodic attacks are often precipitated by high-carbohydrate meals. Patients with the disorder often can abort attacks by exercising affected muscles. The chronic use of acetazolamide can prevent attacks. A condition resembling hypokalemic periodic paralysis occurs with the ingestion of *barium salts* and is endemic in China, where the disorder is referred to as *Pa-Ping.* Barium appears to produce hypokalemia by blocking K^+ channels in skeletal muscle and thus blocking efflux of potassium from the ICF to the ECF. *Insulin* therapy and *vitamin B_{12}* therapy also promote potassium shifts from the ECF to the ICF. Hypokalemia also can result rarely from thyrotoxicosis, especially in Asian males, for reasons that are unclear.

INADEQUATE INTAKE. Reduced potassium intake may result in potassium depletion and hypokalemia because maximal renal conservation of potassium requires, as indicated previously, 7 to 10 days. During this interval, the net renal potassium loss may be as much as 150 to 200 mEq.

CLINICAL MANIFESTATIONS. The clinical effects of potassium deficiency are manifest in one or more organ systems, including skeletal muscle, heart, kidneys, and the gastrointestinal tract. The most serious disturbances are those affecting the neuromuscular system. At serum potassium concentrations in the range of 2.0 to 2.5 mEq/L, muscular weakness is likely to occur, with more severe hypokalemia, the patient may develop areflexic paralysis, in which case respiratory insufficiency is an immediate threat to survival. The severity of the neuromuscular disturbance tends to be proportional to the speed with which the potassium level has declined.

Losses of large amounts of potassium from skeletal muscle may contribute to the development of rhabdomyolysis and myoglobinuria. Hence, rhabdomyolysis sometimes occurs in athletes and in military recruits subject to severe exercise, sweating, and ECF volume contraction. The secondary hyperaldosteronism that follows excessive salt loss produces urinary potassium wasting and, consequently, potassium depletion. Potassium and phosphate depletion secondary to malnutrition and alcoholism is also a pathogenic mechanism in the development of rhabdomyolysis in these conditions.

The electrocardiographic abnormalities of potassium depletion, shown in Figure 102–7, affect primarily repolarization segments of the electrocardiogram, in keeping with the effects of hypokalemia on the action potential. The common electrocardiographic manifestations of hypokalemia include sagging of the ST segment, depression of the T wave, and elevation of the U wave. With marked hypokalemia, the T wave becomes progressively smaller and the U waves show increasing amplitude. In some cases the merging of a flat or positive T wave with a positive U wave may erroneously be interpreted as a prolonged QT interval. Ordinarily, there are no serious clinical consequences from the abnormalities in cardiac excitation. In patients treated with digitalis, hypokalemia may precipitate serious arrhythmias.

Long-standing potassium depletion may produce renal tubular damage, referred to as "hypokalemic nephropathy." Potassium deficiency also affects smooth muscle of the gastrointestinal tract and can result in paralytic ileus.

TREATMENT. The treatment of potassium depletion involves replacement therapy with potassium salts and attempts to correct the underlying disorder. It is useful to remember that a decrease in

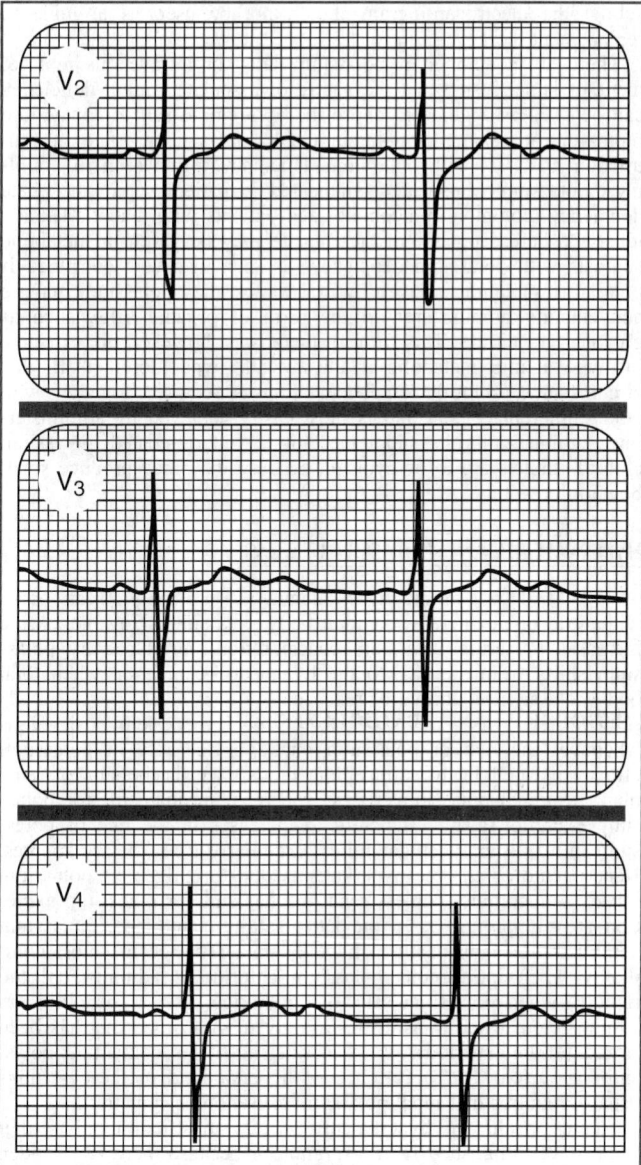

FIGURE 102–7 ■ The electrocardiographic manifestations of hypokalemia. The serum potassium was 2.2 mEq/L. Note that the ST segment is prolonged, primarily because of a U wave following the T wave, and that the T wave is flattened.

plasma potassium concentration of 1 mEq/L with normal acid-base balance is roughly equivalent to 300 mEq of total body potassium deficiency.

Except in extreme circumstances, oral rather than parenteral potassium replacement is prudent. However, when gastrointestinal function is impaired, or when neuromuscular manifestations of hypokalemia are present, parenteral therapy with potassium may be advisable. Because potassium deficits involve both the ICF and the ECF, their correction requires the transfer of administered potassium from the ECF into the ICF. The major problem in parenteral therapy is to avoid intravenous administration of potassium at rates sufficiently great to produce hyperkalemia. A prudent protocol to follow is to add potassium chloride to intravenous solutions at a final concentration of 40 to 60 mEq/L and to administer no more than 10 to 20 mEq of potassium per hour. Except in unusual circumstances, the total amount of potassium administered daily should not exceed 200 mEq. The serum potassium level should be monitored at appropriate intervals, the frequency of monitoring should be determined by the patient's clinical condition, by the initial serum potassium, by the rate at which the serum potassium changes in a given patient, and by the patient's renal function. Because the electrocardiographic manifestations of hypokalemia are subtle, the electrocardiogram should not be used as a guide to replacement therapy.

There are a number of potassium salts for intravenous replacement. It is suggested that the nature of associated anion deficiency can be used as a guide to chose the appropriate salt for potassium repletion. For example, potassium chloride is appropriate in contraction alkalosis with potassium deficiency (often seen in vomiting); potassium phosphate is indicated in patients with phosphate deficiency (common in alcoholics and patients with diabetic ketoacidosis); whereas potassium bicarbonate may be given in metabolic acidosis with potassium deficiency (as seen in severe diarrhea). If potassium repletion is given by oral routes, then potassium may be conveniently administered in the form of organic salts, such as gluconate or citrate. This form of therapy is, however, not effective in hypokalemic metabolic alkalosis with hypochloremia. In this circumstance, chloride supplementation is required together with potassium replacement and is most easily achieved by administering sodium chloride supplementation. Enteric-coated potassium chloride tablets are to be avoided, because they may produce small bowel ulcerations.

HYPERKALEMIA AND POTASSIUM EXCESS

DEFINITION. Chronic hyperkalemia (> 5.5 mEq/L) can occur with little or no increase in total body potassium. However, acute increases in serum potassium concentrations, produced by potassium shifts from the ICF to the ECF, can occur even when total body potassium is normal or reduced.

ETIOLOGY AND PATHOGENESIS. Hyperkalemia develops whenever the rate of potassium intake or the rate of potassium efflux from cellular to extracellular fluids exceeds the sum of renal plus extrarenal potassium losses. The renal mechanisms for potassium excretion adapt efficiently to increases in the rate of potassium influx to extracellular fluid, particularly from dietary sources. Hence acute or chronic hyperkalemia due to exogenous potassium intake is uncommon, unless renal mechanisms for potassium excretion are compromised. In the latter setting, injudicious potassium administration may result in hyperkalemia. This occurs most commonly when intravenous potassium chloride is administered too rapidly, when potassium salts of antibiotics such as pencillin are administered, when transfusions are given with blood that has been stored for long periods, or when salt substitutes containing potassium are used. The occurrence of hyperkalemia in these settings usually requires that renal potassium excretion be impaired.

Acute or chronic hyperkalemia occurs most commonly either because of diminished *renal excretion* or because there is a sudden *transcellular shift* of potassium from the ICF to the ECF. The major causes for hyperkalemia listed in Table 102–13 follow this format.

DIMINISHED RENAL EXCRETION. Hyperkalemia may occur in *acute oliguric renal failure* of any cause. In *chronic renal failure,* hyperkalemia generally does not occur until the GFR has reached markedly low levels, usually not until the GFR is less than 15 mL/min. Hyperkalemia may be precipitated in chronic renal

failure, however, either by the development of acidosis or, as indicated earlier, by the injudicious administration of potassium salts. Hyperkalemia also occurs with little or modest reduction in the GFR, if there is impairment of potassium secretion by collecting duct segments. This occurs in *Addison's disease,* in *hyporeninemic hypoaldosteronism,* and with injudiciously administering *potassium-sparing diuretics,* such as trimaterene or spironolactone. Hyperkalemia also may be seen with NSAIDs and angiotensin-converting enzyme (ACE) inhibitors. Although mild hyperkalemia is relatively common, occurring in some 10% of patients taking ACE inhibitors, severe hyperkalemia is rare in patients with normal renal function.

Hyperkalemia also characterizes *voltage-dependent renal tubular acidosis.* The latter is a specific defect in sodium transport of distal nephron segments. This blockade of distal sodium absorption reduces luminal electronegativity and consequently impairs both proton secretion and potassium secretion. Thus, voltage-dependent renal tubular acidosis, like hyporeninemic hypoaldosteronism, is characterized by sodium wasting and hyperkalemia. In hyporeninemic hypoaldosteronism, the urine is acidic, and plasma levels of aldosterone are reduced even during volume contraction, whereas in voltage-dependent renal tubular acidosis there is impaired urinary acidification but a normal plasma aldosterone response to volume contraction.

Finally, in each of the disorders characterized by diminished renal potassium excretion, hyperkalemia can be aggravated by ECF volume contraction, which reduces sodium delivery to collecting duct segments, or by acidosis, which promotes cellular potassium efflux.

TRANSCELLULAR SHIFTS. The second class of disorders causing acute hyperkalemia includes situations when there is an abrupt shift of potassium from the ICF to the ECF. This shift occurs in acidosis or in circumstances that result in *cell destruction;* in the former, the serum potassium level rises by 0.6 mEq/L with a metabolic decrease in plasma pH of 0.1 unit, whereas the latter occurs commonly with tissue trauma, burns, rhabdomyolysis, or hemolysis, as well as with lysis of large masses of tumor cells. As indicated previously, hypokalemia predisposes to rhabdomyolysis. Thus, the sudden occurrence of hyperkalemia in potassium-depleted patients is a diagnostic clue to the development of rhabdomyolysis.

Hyperkalemic periodic paralysis is an autosomal dominant disorder in which sudden increases in the serum potassium level result in muscle paralysis. The hyperkalemia is often provoked by excessive dietary potassium intake or by exercise. Myotonia occurs commonly in the disorder and appears either between attacks or immediately preceding attacks. The pathogenesis of the disorder is not understood. The acute paralytic attack can be treated by intravenous administration of calcium gluconate or glucose and insulin. Chronic treatment with diuretics such as acetazolamide minimizes the frequency of attacks.

Paradoxical hyperkalemia occurs when *sudden hyperglycemia* develops in insulin-dependent diabetics who also have interstitial renal disease and associated hyporeninemic hypoaldosteronism. The sudden increase in ECF osmolality draws water from cells, raises intracellular potassium concentrations, and therefore promotes passive potassium efflux from cells. The insulin lack minimizes cellular re-entry of potassium, and the aldosterone deficiency blunts renal potassium excretion. Insulin therapy promptly corrects the hyperkalemia. Also, therapy with β-adrenergic blockers can increase plasma concentration. The rise in plasma potassium concentration can be as high as 1 mEq/L in dialysis patients but usually is in the range of 0.1 to 0.2 mEq/L in patients with normal renal function. Finally, anesthetic agents or other drugs that cause a *depolarizing muscle paralysis,* such as succinylcholine, promote potassium efflux from muscle cells. The loss of cell electronegativity in this situation increases passive potassium efflux from muscle cells.

Hyperkalemia also occurs in patients treated with trimethoprim-sulfamethoxazole. Essentially all patients on this drug combination increase their plasma potassium concentration within a few days of initiation of the therapy. The hyperkalemia is reversible with cessation of the drug and occurs as a consequence of inhibition of distal tubule potassium secretion.

Pseudohyperkalemia may occur in thrombocytosis or leukocytosis, because clotting of blood promotes potassium release from these cells and may be identified by noting that the *serum* potassium level is elevated while the *plasma* potassium level is normal.

Table 102–13 ■ MAJOR CAUSES OF HYPERKALEMIA

I. Diminished Renal Excretion	II. Transcellular Shifts
Reduced glomerular filtration rate	Acidosis
Acute oliguric renal failure	β-Adrenergic blockade
Chronic renal failure	Cell destruction
Reduced tubular secretion	Trauma, burns
Addison's disease	Rhabdomyolysis
Hyporeninemic hypoaldosteronism	Hemolysis
Potassium-sparing diuretics	Tumor lysis
Voltage-dependent renal tubular acidosis	Hyperkalemic periodic paralysis
Trimethoprim-sulfamethoxazole	Diabetic hyperglycemia
Angiotensin converting enzyme inhibitors	Insulin dependence plus aldosterone lack
	Depolarizing muscle paralysis
	Succinylcholine

This kind of artifact occurs most commonly in patients with myeloproliferative disorders.

CLINICAL MANIFESTATIONS. The most important clinical manifestations of hyperkalemia relate to alterations in cardiac excitability. For this reason, the electrocardiogram is the single most important guide in appraising the threat posed by hyperkalemia and in determining how aggressive a therapeutic approach is necessary.

The electrocardiographic manifestations of hyperkalemia, shown in Figure 102–8, follow directly from the effects of hyperkalemia on cardiac action potentials. The earliest manifestation of hyperkalemia is the development of peaked T waves, which become evident when the serum potassium level exceeds 6.5 mEq/L. This peaking of the T waves is a manifestation of the accelerated repolarization of the cardiac action potential produced by hyperkalemia. When the potassium concentration exceeds 7 to 8 mEq/L, diminished cardiac excitability results in prolongation of the PR interval, followed by a loss of P waves and widening of the QRS complex. These changes indicate progressive inexcitability of cardiac muscle and are referable to hyperkalemia-induced inactivation of sodium permeability during the initial spike of the action potential. When the serum potassium level exceeds 8 to 10 mEq/L, the electrocardiogram may develop a sine wave pattern and cardiac standstill can occur.

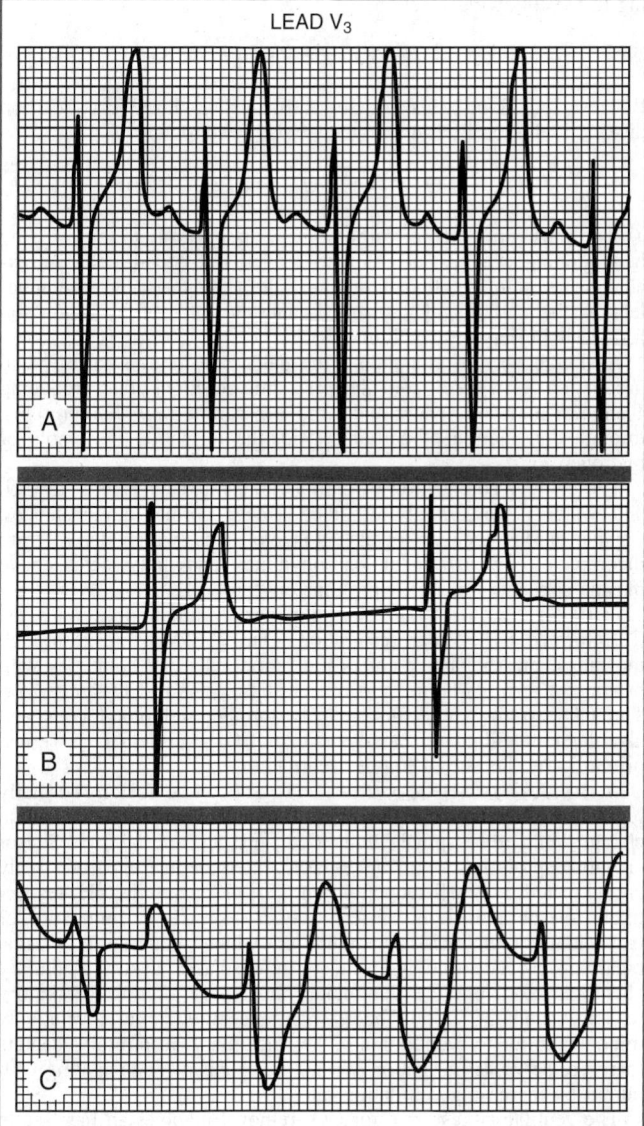

LEAD V$_3$

FIGURE 102–8 ■ The effects of progressive hyperkalemia on the electrocardiogram. All of the illustrations are from lead V$_3$. *A,* Serum K$^+$ = 6.8 mEq/L; note the peaked T waves together with normal sinus rhythm. *B, C,* Serum K$^+$ = 8.9 mEq/L; note the peaked T waves and absent P waves. *C,* Serum K$^+$ > 8.9 mEq/L; note the classic sine wave with absent P waves, marked prolongation of the QRS complex, and peaked T waves.

The correlation between serum potassium concentrations and electrocardiographic abnormalities is approximate at best; in a given patient, progression from peaked T waves to a sine wave pattern may occur rapidly, particularly if the serum potassium concentration rises rapidly. Therefore, the development of peaked T waves in conjunction with hyperkalemia should be viewed as a serious disorder; more advanced electrocardiographic manifestations of hyperkalemia should be treated as life-threatening medical emergencies.

TREATMENT. Three kinds of maneuvers are used to treat hyperkalemia: (1) agents such as glucose plus insulin, sodium bicarbonate, or β agonists, which promote the transfer of potassium from the ECF to the ICF; (2) maneuvers that enhance potassium elimination from the body, such as diuretics, exchange resins, or dialysis; and (3) the use of calcium, which does not alter serum potassium concentrations but counteracts the effects of hyperkalemia on cardiac excitability.

Both insulin and sodium bicarbonate promote potassium entry into cells. Administering 25 g of glucose, together with 10 units of regular insulin, is an effective way of reducing the serum potassium level rapidly. The glucose should be administered over 30 minutes as a 10% solution. Using a 50% glucose solution may actually worsen the hyperkalemia transiently if given rapidly. Insulin promotes potassium entry into cells, and glucose is administered to prevent hypoglycemia. In insulin-dependent diabetic patients in whom sudden hyperglycemia has precipitated the hyperkalemia, insulin administration alone suffices to reduce the serum potassium concentration.

Administering 40 to 150 mEq of sodium bicarbonate intravenously over a 30- to 60-minute interval also promotes potassium entry into cells, particularly if acidosis is also present. This maneuver should be used with caution in patients with compromised renal function because of the risks of hypernatremia and of ECF volume overload.

Potassium shifts from extracellular to intracellular fluids also may be enhanced by using aerosolized specific β$_2$ agonists; albuterol is a commonly used agent of this kind. Agents such as albuterol are most helpful in managing mild hyperkalemia in chronic disorders such as chronic renal failure and hyperkalemic periodic paralysis.

In settings of extreme hyperkalemic cardiotoxicity, when P waves are absent and the QRS complexes are widened, calcium gluconate, 10 to 30 mL of a 10% solution given over a 10- to 20-minute interval, may be lifesaving. This approach should be undertaken with constant electrocardiographic monitoring and should be used with extreme caution in patients who have received digitalis. In the latter circumstance, calcium administration may unmask digitalis intoxication, especially if other agents are used simultaneously to reduce the serum potassium level. Calcium salts should not be added to bottles of intravenous fluids containing bicarbonate, because water-insoluble calcium salts will form.

The influence of calcium salts in minimizing the cardiotoxic effects of hyperkalemia may be understood by noting that depolarization of excitable tissues by elevating serum K$^+$ concentrations inactivates sodium channels and that the extracellular sides of these sodium channels are electronegative. Divalent cations such as calcium provide a remarkably effective way of screening these electronegative sites. Thus, calcium salts raise the voltage gradient across sodium channels by screening electronegative surface charges of these channels on their extracellular fluid sides and consequently restoring the voltage-dependent excitability of these channels.

None of the maneuvers described removes potassium from the body. Gastrointestinal potassium losses may be produced by the use of cation exchange resins in the sodium cycle, such as sodium polystyrene sulfonate (Kayexalate), or by agents that induce secretory diarrhea. Each gram of the resin contains approximately 1 mEq of sodium and exchanges for about 1 mEq of potassium. This stoichiometry is not precise, since the sodium form of the resin also exchanges for other cations in gastrointestinal secretions, including calcium. In chronic hyperkalemia, 20 g of Kayexalate may be given three or four times a day in a 70% solution of sorbitol. The sorbitol creates an osmotic diarrhea and enhances resin passage through the gastrointestinal tract. It must be stated that use of resin-cathartic therapy is relatively unpleasant for the patient. Kayexalate may also be administered by enema, generally as 100 g of resin suspended in 200 g/mL of 20% sorbitol. The effect of single dose Kayexalate on fecal potassium output is minimal when compared to non-cation exchange agents that induce secretory diarrhea, however Kayexalate may be of benefit in management of hyperkalemia when given more chronically. The use of chronic Kayexalate therapy in patients with chronic renal failure carries with it the risk of sodium overload.

Finally, acute hemodialysis or peritoneal dialysis provides another mechanism for potassium removal from the body. This approach is particularly advantageous in acute renal failure, when patients are volume expanded and sodium administration may produce congestive heart failure, or when there is a continued efflux of large amounts of potassium from the ICF to the ECF, as in burns or rhabdomyolysis.

Alappan R, Perazella MA, Buller GK: Hyperkalemia in hospitalized patients treated with trimethoprim-sulfamethoxazole. Ann Intern Med 124:316–320, 1996. *Study shows that standard-dose trimethoprim-sulfamethoxazole therapy consistently increases peak serum potassium concentrations. The rise of serum potassium above 5.5 mEq/L occurred in 21.2% of patients. This antibiotic blocks sodium channels in a manner similar to amiloride.*

Kupin WL, Narins RG: The hyperkalemia of renal failure: Pathophysiology, diagnosis and therapy. Contrib Nephrol 102:1, 1993. *Pathophysiology and treatment of patients with hyperkalemia and renal failure.*

Reardon LC, Macpherson DS: Hyperkalemia in outpatients using angiotensin-converting enzyme inhibitors. Arch Intern Med 158:26–32, 1998. *Reviews 1818 patients using ACE inhibitors and shows that mild hyperkalemia is common; however, severe hyperkalemia is uncommon unless patients are elderly and/or have significant decrease in renal function.*

Weiner ID, Wingo CS: Hypokalemia: Consequences, causes, and correction. J Am Soc Nephrol 8:1179–1188, 1997. *Nice article that discusses the reasons and mechanisms in management of hypokalemia.*

Whang R, Whang DD, Ryan MP: Refractory potassium repletion: A consequence of magnesium deficiency. Arch Intern Med 152:40, 1992. *Data review showing that refractory K⁺ repletion is often associated with total body Mg²⁺ deficiency.*

Wingo CS, Cain BD: The renal H-K-ATPase: Physiological significance and role in potassium homeostasis. Annu Rev Physiol 55:323, 1993. *Reviews the role of the collecting duct and renal H⁺, K⁺-ATPase on potassium homeostasis.*

102.4 Disturbances in Acid-Base Balance

PHYSIOLOGIC CONSIDERATIONS

Much of the confusion and apparent complexity in understanding disturbances in acid-base balance comes from failure to appreciate basic terminology in the field and is due to a lack of understanding of the simple principles of the Henderson-Hasselbalch equation.

Acidemia and *alkalemia* refer to blood hydrogen concentration and therefore to the pH of the blood. These terms do not refer to the mechanism by which a disturbance in pH is reached. *Acidosis* and *alkalosis,* on the other hand, refer to the mechanism by which a given acid-base disturbance is reached. *Primary* refers to the initiating process of acid-base disturbance, whereas *secondary* refers to a compensatory process. Mixed acid-base disturbances are combinations of two or more primary acid-base disturbances. These terms are defined early in this chapter for the sake of clarity and are developed in more detail later.

The pH of arterial blood and interstitial fluid normally ranges between 7.38 and 7.42 despite wide variations in dietary intake of acids or alkali. The arterial pH range over which cardiac function, metabolic activity, and CNS function can be maintained is narrow; the widest range of pH values compatible with life is from 6.8 to 7.8, or an interval of 1 pH unit.

The major buffer system in ECF is the bicarbonate–carbonic acid pair. The relation between pH, bicarbonate, and carbonic acid concentrations in ECF may be expressed according to the familiar Henderson-Hasselbalch equation:

$$pH = pK + \log \frac{HCO_3^-}{H_2CO_3}$$

where pK is the carbonic acid dissociation constant, HCO_3^- is the plasma bicarbonate concentration, and H_2CO_3 is the plasma carbonic acid concentration. The H_2CO_3 concentration is given by $\alpha PaCO_2$, where α is the CO_2 solubility constant and has a value of

0.0301 and $PaCO_2$ is the arterial carbon dioxide tension. Therefore, the Henderson-Hasselbalch equation becomes

$$pH = 6.1 + \log \frac{HCO_3^-}{0.03 \, PCO_2}$$

Primary changes in the numerator (blood bicarbonate concentration) refer to primary metabolic changes, whereas primary changes in the denominator (blood carbon dioxide tension) refer to primary respiratory changes.

Proton shifts between the ECF and ICF stabilize the plasma pH against acute fluctuations. However, the ultimate maintenance of pH balance requires that input of acid or base into the body be matched by output of acid or base so that the HCO_3^-/H_2CO_3 ratio and the total bicarbonate content in the ECF remain constant. The cardinal systems involved in these external processes are the kidneys, for bicarbonate balance, and the lungs, for CO_2 balance.

Carbon Dioxide Production and Elimination

VOLATILE ACID INPUT. The largest source of endogenous acid production is from combustion of glucose and fatty acids to carbon dioxide and water or, in other words, to a volatile acid. During aerobic glycolysis, that is, cellular respiration, glucose oxidation involves oxygen utilization and carbon dioxide production according to the following reaction:

$$C_6H_{12}O_6 + 6O_2 \longrightarrow 6CO_2 + 6H_2O$$

Because red blood cells contain carbonic anhydrase (c.a.), carbon dioxide hydration in erythrocytes yields the following:

$$CO_2 + H_2O \overset{c.a.}{\rightleftharpoons} H_2CO_3 \rightleftharpoons H^+ + HCO_3^-$$

The protons formed from carbonic acid dissociation are buffered by hemoglobin, whereas bicarbonate leaves red blood cells in exchange for chloride. In other words, the CO_2 generated is equivalent to the carbonic acid formed, and the bulk of hydrogen ion formed is buffered intracellularly.

A simple way of calculating the daily rate of non-volatile acid production is to note, from the preceding reactions, that producing 1 mole of metabolic water and 1 mole of carbon dioxide represents, through dissociation of carbonic acid, the formation of 1 mole of hydrogen ions.

The cellular combustion of carbohydrates and fatty acids to CO_2 and water is remarkably efficient. Under normal circumstances, organic anions such as lactate and keto acids, which derive from incomplete combustion of carbohydrates and fatty acids, have plasma concentrations of approximately 5 mEq/L.

VOLATILE ACID OUTPUT. Pulmonary ventilation excretes the CO_2 formed by cellular respiration. During blood transit through the lungs, bicarbonate re-enters red blood cells and combines with protons to form carbonic acid, which dissociates to CO_2 and water. The CO_2 so formed diffuses freely through red blood cells and alveolar epithelium so that the rate of CO_2 excretion is governed primarily by the rate of minute ventilation.

MODULATION OF RESPIRATION. The prime factors normally regulating alterations in the rate of minute ventilation are subtle changes in cerebrospinal fluid (CSF) pH or arterial pH. Sensor chemoreceptors in central medullary centers or in the carotid body are activated by small reductions in CSF pH or arterial pH, respectively; the pH reduction can result either from CO_2 accumulation or from non-volatile acid accumulation, which reduces the plasma bicarbonate concentration. In most circumstances, central medullary chemoreceptors provide the major impetus to altering ventilatory response, and the carotid body chemoreceptors serve as relatively minor stimuli to ventilation. The medullary respiratory centers therefore serve as the major *effector* mechanism for regulating CO_2 output by increasing ventilation rate.

The ventilatory response for CO_2 removal involves an increase in both tidal volume and respiratory rate. On average, for every 1 mEq/L reduction in plasma bicarbonate produced by metabolic acidosis, increased minute ventilation will produce a 1.0 to 1.2 mm Hg fall in the $PaCO_2$. In most circumstances, the maximum reduction in $PaCO_2$ produced by the hyperventilatory response to severe metabolic acidosis is to a $PaCO_2$ in the 10 to 12 mm Hg range, but hyperventilation to $PaCO_2$ values less than 10 mm Hg in severe chronic metabolic acidosis is rare but may occur. Conversely, an increase in arterial pH reduces the rate of minute ventilation and therefore results in CO_2 retention. For increases in plasma bicarbonate concentrations to 35 mEq/L, the $PaCO_2$ usually remains less than 50 mm Hg. When profound metabolic alkalosis occurs, the $PaCO_2$ may rise farther but virtually never exceeds 65 mm Hg.

Renal Bicarbonate Processing

In addition to volatile acid production due to CO_2 formation, cellular metabolism also results in the formation of a number of non-volatile acids. The major source for non-volatile acid production is the metabolism of sulfur-containing amino acids, such as cysteine and methionine, which results in sulfuric acid formation. Consequently, the daily rate of non-volatile acid production is closely related to dietary protein intake and to the rate of endogenous protein catabolism. Non-volatile acids also derive from oxidation of phosphoproteins and phospholipids, which results in phosphoric acid formation; nucleoprotein degradation, which yields uric acid; and incomplete combustion of carbohydrates and fatty acids, which produces lactic acid and the keto acids.

The daily rate of non-volatile acid production under normal conditions is about 1 mEq/kg of body weight. Thus, daily non-volatile acid production would consume the total body fluid buffering capacity in about 2 weeks, were it not for the fact that the kidneys excrete non-volatile acids and, in so doing, regenerate bicarbonate. Because the minimal urinary pH ordinarily attainable is 5.0 and the amount of non-volatile acid to be excreted is about 70 mEq/d, renal hydrogen ion excretion, which is equivalent to renal bicarbonate regeneration, occurs mainly as protons trapped in an undissociated form by urinary buffers.

The kidneys also filter large quantities of bicarbonate daily: for a normal plasma bicarbonate concentration of 24 mEq/L and a glomerular filtration of 180 L/d, the net amount of bicarbonate filtered daily is approximately 4300 mEq, or about four times the total body buffering capacity. Thus, in addition to generating new bicarbonate, the renal tubules must also absorb filtered bicarbonate.

BICARBONATE REABSORPTION. Virtually all filtered bicarbonate is absorbed, together with sodium, by the proximal tubule. Within renal tubular cells, CO_2 is hydrated to H_2CO_3. Apical membrane Na^+ exchange permits H^+ secretion into urine and Na^+ entry into cells, with subsequent absorption of sodium bicarbonate to blood.

The rate of proximal bicarbonate reabsorption is modulated by the same *effectors* that regulate proximal sodium absorption. Among these, the ECF volume exerts a central effect. Volume expansion, which resets glomerulotubular balance downward, reduces the fractional rate of proximal bicarbonate reabsorption. Conversely, volume contraction raises the bicarbonate threshold by increasing the fractional rate of proximal tubular sodium bicarbonate reabsorption.

Two other *effectors* regulate, in operational terms, the rate of bicarbonate reabsorption. One of these is the $PaCO_2$: High $PaCO_2$ values raise the apparent bicarbonate threshold, whereas low $PaCO_2$ values reduce the rate of bicarbonate reabsorption. This factor accounts for the compensatory increase in plasma bicarbonate concentrations in respiratory acidosis. Second, hypokalemia also increases the rate of bicarbonate reabsorption, presumably by raising the intracellular hydrogen ion concentration. This factor accounts for the fact that in hypokalemic, hypochloremic metabolic alkalosis associated with volume contraction, alkalosis can persist after volume deficits are restored. In this circumstance, correcting potassium deficits is required to correct the alkalosis.

BICARBONATE REGENERATION. The excretion of non-volatile acids and the simultaneous renal regeneration of bicarbonate occur principally in distal nephron segments. Distal renal tubular cells hydrate CO_2 to carbonic acid, which dissociates to protons, which are secreted into urine, and bicarbonate anions, which are absorbed into blood. The major mode of proton secretion in terminal nephron segments, particularly collecting tubules, involves an apical membrane proton–ATPase.

The secreted protons titrate urinary buffers, principally phosphate, while sodium is absorbed. Thus the overall reaction is as follows:

$$Na_2HPO_4 + H^+ + HCO_3^- \longrightarrow NaH_2PO_4 + NaHCO_3$$
$$\text{(filtered)} \qquad\qquad \text{(excreted)} \quad \text{(absorbed)}$$

Titratable acid formation normally accounts for about one third of renal acid excretion. The remaining two thirds of acid excretion is accounted for by ammonia (NH_3) secretion by the following sequence:

$$NaR + NH_3 + H^+ + HCO_3^- \longrightarrow NaHCO_3 + NH_4R$$
$$\text{(filtered)} \qquad\qquad\qquad\qquad \text{(reabsorbed)} \quad \text{(excreted)}$$

where NaR is the filtered sodium salt of a non-volatile acid. NH_3 is ammonia produced by renal tubular cells, and the protons and bicarbonate come from CO_2 hydration by tubular cells.

Distal acid excretion and bicarbonate absorption are accompanied by sodium absorption. Consequently, *effector* systems that enhance distal sodium absorption, such as aldosterone or increased rates of sodium delivery to terminal nephron segments, also promote terminal nephron hydrogen ion excretion. Three other *effector* mechanisms also increase the rate of hydrogen ion excretion. (1) Delivery of sodium to terminal nephron segments in association with impermeant anions such as sulfate favors proton movement from tubular cells to lumen. (2) Hypokalemia enhances hydrogen ion excretion, particularly in sodium-acquisitive states, presumably because hypokalemia is accompanied by a fall in intracellular pH. (3) Acidosis stimulates ammoniagenesis by renal tubular cells; consequently, in metabolic acidosis, increases in the rate of renal acid excretion are referable primarily to increased rates of ammonium excretion. These three last-named effector systems enhance renal acid excretion by creating a favorable situation for proton transfer from tubular cells to urine. Conversely, aldosterone deficiency, alkalosis, or reduced rates of salt delivery to terminal nephron segments reduce renal capacity for acid excretion.

pH Disequilibria Between Plasma and CSF

Central rather than arterial chemoreceptors are the prime sensors for pH-mediated changes in respiration. The ventilatory responses to pH changes mediated by respiratory processes or by metabolic processes therefore differ. The blood-brain barrier is freely permeable to CO_2. Consequently, pH changes produced exclusively by hyperventilation or hypoventilation occur almost simultaneously in arterial plasma and in the CSF, and the respiratory response to primary increases or decreases in $PaCO_2$ occurs almost instantaneously. The blood-brain barrier imposes a lag, however, in the rate at which arterial bicarbonate equilibrates with the CSF. Thus, in metabolic acidosis, the arterial pH and bicarbonate concentration fall more rapidly than they do in the CSF, and in metabolic alkalosis, the CSF pH and bicarbonate concentration rise more slowly than they do in arterial plasma. Consequently, in the early stages of acute metabolic acidosis, there may be a 1- to 3-hour delay in the development of a maximal hyperventilatory response. Conversely, when metabolic acidosis is corrected rapidly, hyperventilation may persist for a few hours because of a delay in the rise of CSF pH.

An unusual situation relating to this effect occurs in diabetic ketoacidosis and in certain other metabolic acidoses associated with impaired CNS function. In these situations, carotid body chemoreceptors, rather than central medullary chemoreceptors, provide the major stimulus to respiration driven by a reduced arterial pH. The rapid correction of ECF acidosis by administering bicarbonate reduces the rate at which carotid body chemoreceptors drive ventilation. When this occurs, $PaCO_2$ levels in plasma and in the CSF rise almost simultaneously, but because of a lag in the rate of bicarbonate entry into the CSF, the CSF bicarbonate/carbonic acid ratio tends to fall. In severe diabetic ketoacidosis, this situation can result in an actual fall in CSF pH simultaneously with a rise in arterial pH produced by intravenous bicarbonate administration.

DEFINITION OF ACID-BASE ABNORMALITIES

The arterial pH is determined by the ratio of the bicarbonate/carbonic acid buffer system, as expressed in the Henderson-Hasselbalch equation. These data also provide an index to total-body acid-base balance, because, as indicated in the preceding section, the majority of body buffering occurs within cells. As stated earlier, acid-base disturbance can therefore occur either by altering the serum bicarbonate concentration, referred to as a "metabolic" disorder, or by altering arterial CO_2 tension, referred to as a "respira-

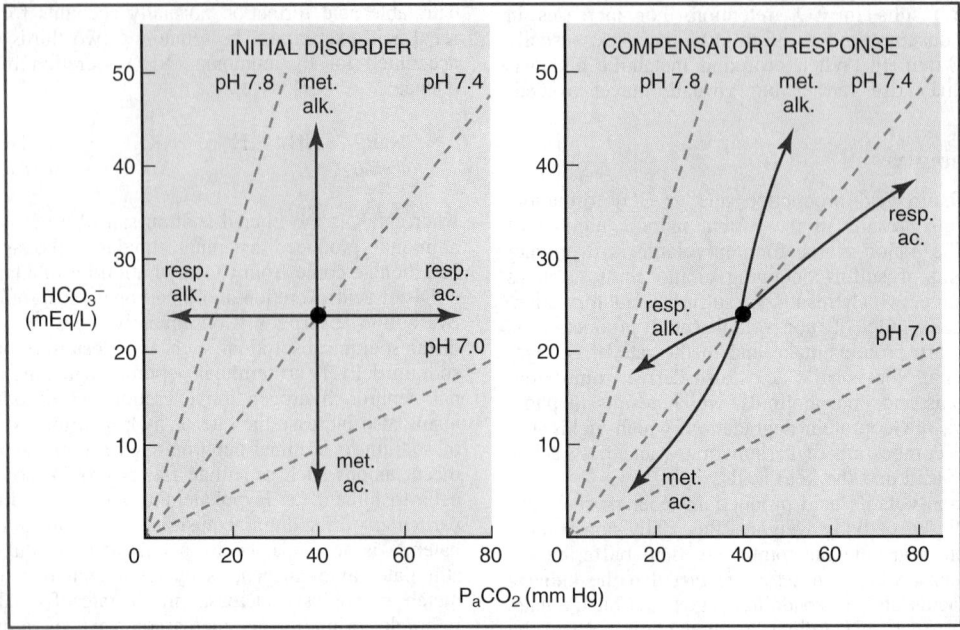

FIGURE 102–9 ■ Schematic frame of reference for considering acid-base disturbances. The dotted lines are the pH isobars for pH values of 7.8, 7.4, and 7.0 computed from the Henderson-Hasselbalch equation for given combinations of arterial bicarbonate (HCO_3^-) values (vertical axes) and arterial carbon dioxide ($PaCO_2$) tensions (horizontal axes). The graph on the left shows the initial derangement in HCO_3^- concentrations in metabolic acidosis and metabolic alkalosis and the initial $PaCO_2$ derangement in respiratory acidosis and respiratory alkalosis. Note that each of the four changes in either HCO_3^- or $PaCO_2$ tends to displace the arterial pH from the pH 7.4 isobar. The graph on the right, labeled compensatory response, indicates the general trend of pH. HCO_3^- and $PaCO_2$ changes were actually observed in the four primary acid-base disturbances: respiratory acidosis, respiratory alkalosis, metabolic acidosis, and metabolic alkalosis. Respiratory acidosis and alkalosis are accompanied by compensatory renal bicarbonate retention and loss, respectively. Metabolic acidosis and alkalosis are accompanied by compensatory hyperventilation and hypoventilation, respectively. Note that the compensatory response in each of the four acid-base disorders tends to restore arterial pH values toward the pH 7.4 isobar.

tory" disorder. A convenient way for considering these disturbances is illustrated in Figure 102–9, which illustrates pH isobars (for pH 7.0, 7.4, and 7.8) calculated according to the Henderson-Hasselbalch equation for the bicarbonate concentrations and $PaCO_2$ values listed on the ordinate and abscissa, respectively.

TYPES OF ACID-BASE ABNORMALITIES. The left-hand panel in Figure 102–9 shows the directional changes in $PaCO_2$, and bicarbonate concentrations that initiate the four primary types of acid-base abnormalities. *Respiratory acidosis* results from hypoventilation and reduces pH by raising the $PaCO_2$. *Respiratory alkalosis* results from hyperventilation and raises pH by reducing the $PaCO_2$. *Metabolic alkalosis* occurs when increases in the plasma bicarbonate concentration raise pH, and *metabolic acidosis* occurs when reductions in plasma bicarbonate decrease pH.

Any of these initial acid-base disturbances activates *compensatory responses,* illustrated in the right-hand panel of Figure 102–9, that tend to minimize the pH changes produced by the initial acid-base abnormality. By comparing the directional arrows in the left- and right-hand panels of Figure 102–9, it becomes evident that the initial disturbance in any of these four acid-base abnormalities tends to displace the arterial pH away from the pH 7.4 isobar and that the compensatory response partially restores arterial pH values toward the pH 7.4 isobar. The arterial pH, $PaCO_2$, and plasma bicarbonate concentrations illustrated in the right-hand panel of Figure 102–9 are the values usually observed clinically in the four primary acid-base disturbances.

THE COMPENSATORY RESPONSES. Renal and pulmonary mechanisms aggressively protect the body from changes in pH of arterial blood and interstitial fluid against primary acid-base disturbances that would threaten the optimal activity of various pH-dependent organ functions. These are known as "compensatory mechanisms" that blunt the effect of the initial insult or pH homeostasis (see Fig. 102–X). Although the magnitude and rate of the compensatory responses vary among individual patients and do not provide complete compensation for the initiating abnormality, they nevertheless are relatively predictable. The predicted compensatory responses to the primary acid-base disturbances are listed in Table 102–14.

THE SERUM ANION GAP. Sodium is the principal cation in extracellular fluids. The sum of plasma chloride plus bicarbonate concentrations is less than the serum sodium concentration; the remaining anions required for electroneutrality, generally not reported with routine serum electrolyte measurements, are referred to as unmeasured anions, or as the serum anion gap. A convenient formula for calculating the serum anion gap is the following:

$$\text{Serum anion gap} = Na^+ - (Cl^- + HCO_3^-)$$

where Na^+, Cl^-, and HCO_3^- are the serum sodium, chloride, and bicarbonate concentrations, respectively. The anion serum gap includes primarily phosphates and sulfates derived from tissue metabolism, lactate and keto acids arising from incomplete combustion of carbohydrates and fatty acids, and negatively charged protein molecules, principally albumin. The normal value for unmeasured an-

Table 102–14 ■ **RELATIONSHIPS BETWEEN HCO_3^- AND PCO_2 IN SIMPLE ACID-BASE DISORDERS**

CONDITION	PRIMARY DISTURBANCE	PREDICTED RESPONSE
Metabolic acidosis	↓ HCO_3^-	ΔPCO_2 (↓) = 1–1.4ΔHCO_3^-*
Metabolic alkalosis	↑ HCO_3^-	ΔPCO_2 (↑) = 0.4–0.9ΔHCO_3^-*
Respiratory acidosis	↑ PCO_2	Acute: ΔHCO_3^- (↑) = 0.1ΔPCO_2 Chronic: ΔHCO_3^- (↑) = 0.25–0.55ΔPCO_2
Respiratory alkalosis	↓ PCO_2	Acute: ΔHCO_3^- (↓) = 0.2–0.25ΔPCO_2 Chronic: ΔHCO_3^- (↓) = 0.4–0.5ΔPCO_2

*After at least 12 to 24 hours.
From Hamm L: Mixed acid-base disorders. *In* Kokko JP, Tannen RL (eds): Fluids and Electrolytes, 3rd ed. Philadelphia, WB Saunders, 1996, p 344.

ions, or the serum anion gap, is 10 to 12 mEq/L; albumin and other proteins normally account for about half the anion gap.

An *increased* serum anion gap generally indicates the presence of metabolic acidosis. The factors responsible for this kind of metabolic acidosis are discussed in the next section.

A *reduced* serum anion gap provides an index to certain other disorders. The anion gap will be reduced if the sodium concentration falls while the chloride plus bicarbonate concentrations are unchanged or, in other words, when the concentration of another cation in serum is increased while the serum osmolality remains normal. This may occur in multiple myeloma of the immunoglobulin G (IgG) variety if the myeloma proteins are cationic at pH 7.4. Hyperviscosity syndromes also may result in a reduced anion gap because of a laboratory artifact: when serum is excessively viscous, automatic pumps deliver decreased volumes of serum to a flame photometer, producing artifactual reductions in sodium concentrations. Rarely, lithium intoxication, hypermagnesemia, and hypercalcemia raise non-sodium cation concentrations sufficiently high to reduce the anion gap.

The serum anion gap also will be decreased if the serum sodium concentration remains normal while the serum chloride plus bicarbonate concentrations are increased. This situation occurs most commonly in hypoalbuminemia. A low serum anion gap also occurs in bromide intoxication, since colorimetric techniques for serum chloride determinations give spuriously high values for chloride plus bromide when bromide is present in relatively high concentrations in serum.

THE URINARY ANION GAP. The urinary anion gap, defined as

$$\text{Urinary anion gap} = (Na^+ + K^+) - Cl^-$$

is useful in evaluating patients with hyperchloremic acidosis. The test provides an approximate index to urinary NH_4^+ excretion, as measured by a negative urinary anion gap, that is, urinary $Na^+ + K^+$ is less than urinary Cl^-. Thus, in hyperchloremic metabolic acidosis, a normal renal response would be a negative urinary anion gap, generally in the range of 30 to 50 mEq/L. In such an instance, the hyperchloremic acidosis is probably due to gastrointestinal losses rather than a renal lesion. In contrast, a positive urinary anion gap implies a renal tubular disorder, as is discussed below.

URINARY RESPONSE TO ORAL FUROSEMIDE. The urinary response to oral furosemide loading is another useful test for evaluating tubular acidifying capability. The rationale for the test is that in normal individuals blockade of sodium absorption in diluting segments by furosemide increases sodium delivery to distal nephron segments where potassium and protons are secreted (see earlier) and increases the excretion rate of the latter two moieties. Consequently, the oral administration of 40 to 80 mg of furosemide should be followed, in a subsequent 4- to 6-hour urinary collection, by an increase in urinary sodium excretion and fractional sodium excretion, an increase in urinary potassium excretion and fractional potassium excretion, and a reduction in urinary pH. In some renal tubular acidosis syndromes, proton and/or potassium excretion is impaired (Table 102–15).

METABOLIC ACIDOSIS

ETIOLOGY AND PATHOGENESIS. A convenient way to consider the metabolic acidoses is to divide them into two groups: normal anion gap and increased anion gap metabolic acidoses (Table 102–16). The pathogeneses of these two groups differ appreciably.

NORMAL ANION GAP METABOLIC ACIDOSIS. The metabolic acidoses having a *normal anion gap* result whenever there are abnormally high net bicarbonate losses. This situation may occur because the kidneys fail to reabsorb or regenerate bicarbonate,

Table 102–16 ■ MAJOR CAUSES OF METABOLIC ACIDOSIS

NORMAL ANION GAP	INCREASED ANION GAP
I. Renal Causes	**I. Endogenous Causes**
A. Bicarbonate loss	A. Uremic acidosis
Proximal RTA, type II	B. Lactic acidosis
Dilutional acidosis	C. Ketoacidosis
Carbonic anhydrase inhibitors	D. β-Hydroxybutyric
Primary hyperparathyroidism	acidosis
B. Failure of bicarbonate regeneration	**II. Exogenous Causes**
Distral RTA, type I	A. Salicylates
Distal RTA, type IV	B. Paraldehyde
Diuretics: amiloride, spironolactones, triamterene	C. Methanol
	D. Ethylene glycol
II. Gastrointestinal Causes	
Diarrheal states	
Small bowel drainage	
Ureterosigmoidostomy	
III. Acidifying Salts	
Ammonium chloride	
Lysine hydrochloride	
Arginine hydrochloride	
Parenteral hyperalimentation	

because there are extrarenal losses of bicarbonate, or because excessive amounts of substances yielding hydrochloric acid have been administered.

RENAL CAUSES. BICARBONATE LOSSES. *Renal bicarbonate wasting* occurs in *proximal renal tubular acidosis* type II, either alone or as part of Fanconi's syndrome (see Chapter 109). The apparent threshold for bicarbonate in this disorder is set below the normal value of 26 mEq of bicarbonate per deciliter of glomerular filtrate and may be as low as 15 to 20 mEq of bicarbonate per deciliter of glomerular filtrate. Consequently, bicarbonate wasting occurs whenever the plasma bicarbonate level is raised above the apparent renal threshold for bicarbonate.

Attempts to correct the acidosis of proximal renal tubular acidosis by bicarbonate administration are generally unrewarding, because increases in the plasma bicarbonate level produced by administering bicarbonate salts are accompanied by corresponding increases in bicarbonaturia. A promising approach to this disorder involves reducing the ECF volume by sodium restriction. This maneuver exploits the fact that ECF contraction resets glomerulotubular balance upward and consequently increases the fractional rate of sodium, and hence bicarbonate, reabsorption by the proximal tubule.

A converse of this situation is sometimes referred to as "dilutional acidosis." Individuals who are volume expanded reduce the fractional rate of sodium bicarbonate absorption by the proximal tubule and consequently develop mild reductions in plasma bicarbonate concentrations. Also, *carbonic anhydrase inhibitors* such as acetazolamide inhibit proximal sodium bicarbonate absorption, resulting in metabolic acidosis. *Primary hyperparathyroidism* also reduces the apparent bicarbonate threshold in the proximal tubule; mild degrees of hyperchloremic acidosis are commonly noted in patients with this disorder.

FAILURE OF BICARBONATE REGENERATION. The second major group of disorders producing hyperchloremic acidosis includes those disorders in which the ability of the distal nephron to regenerate bicarbonate is impaired. Three different tubular disorders account for the majority of cases of renal hyperchloremia encountered clinically. *Classic gradient-limited renal tubular acidosis type I* is a tubular disorder in which proton secretion may be normal, but because the collecting duct is unable to maintain a steep urine to

Table 102–15 ■ CHARACTERISTICS OF DISTAL RENAL TUBULAR ACIDOSIS (RTA) SYNDROMES

CONDITION	URINARY pH	SERUM K^+	URINARY ANION GAP	RESPONSE TO FUROSEMIDE		ALDOSTERONE SECRETION
				Urinary pH	Urinary K^+	
Gradient-limited RTA	>5.5	↓	Positive	Unchanged	↑	Normal
Hyporeninemic hypoaldosteronism	<5.5	↓	Positive	↓		Reduced
Voltage-dependent RTA	>5.5	↑	Positive	Unchanged	Unchanged	Normal

blood proton concentration gradient, secreted protons are recycled back to blood. Administering large quantities of phosphate salts permits the excretion of large amounts of titratable acid in this disorder, because the pH of the phosphate buffer system is 6.8 (i.e., relatively high). Potassium wasting and hypokalemia are common in distal gradient-limited renal tubular acidosis owing at least in part to secondary hyperaldosteronism stimulated by sodium wasting.

In *hyporeninemic hypoaldosteronism* type IV renal tubular acidosis, which generally occurs in association with interstitial disease and diabetes mellitus, the distal tubular derangements include diminished rates of sodium absorption and diminished rates of proton and potassium secretion. Aldosterone secretion is impaired. Consequently, sodium wasting and hyperkalemic, hyperchloremic acidosis are the hallmarks of this disorder. Diuretics such as *triamterene, spironolactone,* and *amiloride,* which interfere with distal tubular sodium absorption, proton secretion, and potassium secretion, also result in hyperkalemic, hyperchloremic metabolic acidosis.

Finally, *voltage-dependent renal tubular acidosis,* also known as *hyperkalemic tubular acidosis,* is characterized by an impaired ability of the distal nephron to absorb sodium and by an inability to secrete either potassium or protons. The latter two secretory deficits appear to be secondary to the defect in sodium absorption, which diminishes the magnitude of the lumen-negative transepithelial voltage in those nephron segments. Aldosterone secretion is normal.

Table 102–15 provides a summary of the distinguishing features of the three renal tubular acidosis syndromes. When hyporeninemic hypoaldosteronism is associated with extensive interstitial disease, the ability to increase urinary potassium excretion or decrease urinary pH in response to furosemide may be blunted.

Gastrointestinal bicarbonate wasting can occur in several circumstances. First, because stool water is rich in bicarbonate, diarrheal states result in significant bicarbonate losses. Both pancreatic and small bowel secretions are rich in bicarbonate; pancreatic fluid, for example, has a pH of approximately 8.0. Hence *ileal drainage* also can result in significant bicarbonate losses. *Ureterosigmoidostomy* results in metabolic acidosis because the colon can secrete bicarbonate in exchange for chloride. Thus, in these patients, urine reaching the colon is alkalinized by bicarbonate exchange for chloride, thereby producing a net bicarbonate loss.

GASTROINTESTINAL CAUSES. ACIDIFYING SALTS. The third major group of conditions producing hyperchloremic acidosis includes those that result from administering *acidifying salts,* such as ammonium hydrochloride, lysine hydrochloride, or arginine hydrochloride. In each instance, metabolism of the ammonium or of the amino acids leads to hydrochloric acid formation. *Parenteral hyperalimentation* without administering adequate amounts of bicarbonate or bicarbonate-yielding solutes (such as lactate or acetate) also can produce hyperchloremic metabolic acidosis. The acidosis occurs because the synthetic amino acids used in hyperalimentation mixtures contain positively charged amino acids, such as arginine, lysine, and histidine, which yield proton equivalents when metabolized.

INCREASED ANION GAP METABOLIC ACIDOSIS. Metabolic acidoses characterized by an increased anion gap occur either because the kidneys fail to excrete organic acids, such as phosphate or sulfate, or because there is net accumulation of organic acids (see Table 102–16).

REDUCED ACID EXCRETION. Renal failure, either acute or chronic, results in metabolic acidosis with an increased anion gap due to retention of sulfates and phosphates. In chronic renal failure, metabolic acidosis occurs because the net amount of ammonium excreted daily falls as functional renal mass diminishes. The plasma bicarbonate concentration in most patients with chronic renal failure ranges between 16 and 20 mEq/L. Although this degree of acidosis appears relatively modest, the daily acid load is buffered by bone salts; this buffering may contribute to the osteopenia of chronic renal failure (see Chapter 104). In acute tubular necrosis, acidosis occurs because of generalized tubular dysfunction, including impaired net acid excretion. The plasma bicarbonate level generally remains above 16 mEq/L unless sepsis, profound hypoxia, or extensive tissue necrosis complicates the disorder. In chronic renal failure, the anion gap generally does not exceed

22 to 24 mEq/L. Thus, if the anion gap exceeds this value, then other superimposed causes of metabolic acidosis must be sought.

ORGANIC ACID ACCUMULATION. Accumulation of organic acids represents the second major cause for metabolic acidosis with an increased anion gap and is the most common cause for acute metabolic acidosis. Normally, the complete combustion of carbohydrates and fatty acids to CO_2 and water is highly efficient and results in the production of approximately 22,000 mEq of hydrogen ion per day. Thus, the lungs eliminate, as expired CO_2, more than 300 times as much acid as the 70 mEq of fixed acid excreted daily by the kidneys as titratable acid plus ammonia. Processes that impair cellular respiration and therefore result in non-volatile rather than volatile acid production lead to profound metabolic acidosis. In these circumstances, the interplay of four cardinal factors determines the magnitude of the anion gap acidosis.

The first two of these factors are insulin and glucagon and the interplay between these two hormones. In disorders such as diabetic ketoacidosis or starvation, insulin lack accelerates lipolysis whereas aerobic glycolysis is impaired. Concomitantly, glucagon increases augment ketogenesis by the liver.

The third variable is the rate of cellular respiration, which in practical terms is determined by the rate of tissue perfusion with oxygen and the functional state of mitochondria. Lactic acidosis due to hypoperfusion or phenformin thereby is an anion gap acidosis caused by impaired cellular respiration.

The last factor determining the magnitude of the anion gap for such conditions is the extent of renal perfusion, which, in turn, regulates the proximal renal tubular threshold for organic acid excretion. Thus, in diabetic ketoacidosis, volume expansion with normal saline can convert a large anion gap acidosis to a normal anion gap acidosis, not by correcting the underlying metabolic derangement, which requires insulin, but simply by increasing the rate of renal organic acid excretion.

The syndrome of *lactic acidosis* results from impaired cellular respiration. Lactic acid is produced in muscle, red blood cells, and other tissues as a consequence of anaerobic glycolysis. Lactic acid oxidation involves reduction of nicotine adenine dinucleotide (NAD) by lactic acid dehydrogenase (LDH) according to the following reaction:

$$\text{Lactate} + \text{NAD} \underset{\longleftarrow}{\overset{\text{LDH}}{\longrightarrow}} \text{pyruvate} + \text{NADH}$$

Cellular respiration involves mitochondrial oxidation of pyruvate and NADH to CO_2 and water. When lactic acidosis occurs because of impaired cellular respiration, the lactate/pyruvate ratio rises, as does the NADH/NAD ratio. Thus, glycolysis in a setting of impaired cellular respiration results in increased production of nonvolatile lactic acid. Lactic acidosis should not be confused with states in which serum lactate levels are elevated with normal lactate/pyruvate and NADH/NAD ratios, as, for example, in vigorous exercise. Lactic acidosis is also characterized by negative serum nitroprusside (Acetest) reactions, because Acetest tablets react only with ketone bodies such as acetoacetic acid and acetone, but not with lactic acid or β-hydroxybutyric acid. β-Hydroxybutyric acid does not have a ketone group and therefore does not react in nitroprusside reactions. In lactic acidosis the β-hydroxybutyric acid/acetoacetic acid ratio is elevated in parallel with the increased NADH/NAD ratio.

Lactic acidosis occurs most commonly in disorders characterized by inadequate oxygen delivery to tissues, such as shock, septicemia, and profound hypoxemia. Drug-induced lactic acidosis may occur with phenformin therapy and isoniazid toxicity; in both circumstances, oxygen utilization by tissues is thought to be impaired. Lactic acidosis also occurs in association with leukemia and diabetes mellitus. There is also a spontaneous, idiopathic form of lactic acidosis in debilitated patients, which is almost uniformly fatal.

A second group of disorders characterized by an anion gap metabolic acidosis includes those disorders in which cellular respiration may not be impaired but accelerated rates of organic acid production, particularly from lipolysis, result in an increased anion gap. *Alcoholic ketoacidosis* occurs in patients with chronic alcoholism and a recent history of binge drinking, little or no food intake, and recurrent vomiting. Hypoglycemia may be present. The major pathogenic mechanism for alcoholic ketoacidosis is accelerated lipolysis and hepatic ketoacid production because of relative de-

FIGURE 102-10 ■ Pathophysiology of alcoholic ketoacidosis. Hypoglycemia develops due to decreased nicotine adenine dinucleotide (NAD)-dependent gluconeogenesis. This results in hypoglycemia and a compensatory decrease in insulin and an increase in glucagon concentrations. Decreased insulin activates free fatty acid formation by increasing lipolysis from adipose tissue. Free fatty acids in turn are transported into mitochondria for ketogenesis by carnitine acyltransferase (CAT), which is activated in part by increased glucagon content. Alcohol also may increase ketogenesis directly by being metabolized to acetate and thus providing substrate for ketogenesis.

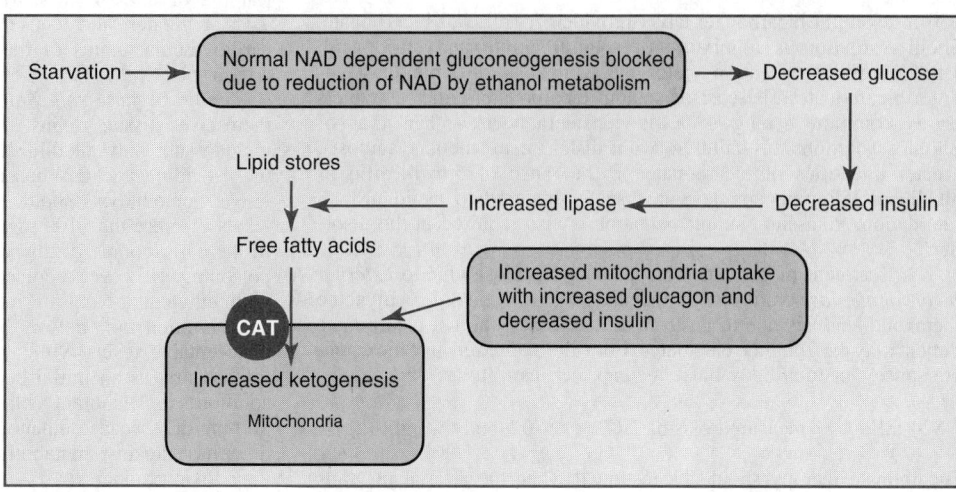

creases and increases in the secretion rates for insulin and glucagon, respectively (Fig. 102–10). The Acetest reaction is variably positive, and the β-hydroxybutyrate/acetoacetate ratio is elevated. Lactate utilization is diminished in this disorder. Patients with alcoholic ketoacidosis have β-hydroxybutyric acid, rather than lactic acid, as the principal non-volatile acid. *Diabetic ketoacidosis* is the most common cause of metabolic acidosis with an increased anion gap and occurs because of increased rates of ketogenesis due to insulin lack and inadequate carbohydrate combustion. *Starvation* produces metabolic acidosis by essentially the same mechanism: increased hepatic ketogenesis with reduced caloric intake. Thus, in a general sense, alcoholic ketoacidosis, diabetic ketoacidosis, and starvation share at least one common feature: accelerated lipolysis and ketogenesis due to a relative insulin lack coupled with a relative glucagon excess.

Finally, a number of ingested substances result in severe metabolic acidosis with a large anion gap. *Salicylism* produces a complex set of acid-base abnormalities. Salicylates stimulate ventilation through central mechanisms; the decrease in $PaCO_2$ then results in reductions in plasma bicarbonate concentrations. Because salicylate is a relatively strong acid, the ingestion of large quantities of salicylate can, by itself, contribute to metabolic acidosis and an increased anion gap. Salicylates also interfere with mitochondrial function. As a consequence, a number of as yet unidentified organic acids accumulate in serum and are the major factors responsible for the anion gap acidosis of salicylism.

A number of other agents, including *paraldehyde, methanol,* and *ethylene glycol,* also produce severe metabolic acidosis with organic acid accumulation. In methanol poisoning, formic acid (an end-product of methanol metabolism) accounts in large part for the reduction in serum bicarbonate concentration. In ethylene glycol intoxication, glycolic and lactic acid accumulation accounts for the majority of the reduction in plasma bicarbonate level; however, oxalate deposition in tissues is clearly a major factor in ethylene glycol toxicity. The organic acids responsible for an increased anion gap in paraldehyde intoxication have not been identified.

DIAGNOSIS AND TREATMENT. The diagnosis of metabolic acidosis requires analyzing serum electrolytes and measuring arterial pH and $PaCO_2$. A cardinal clinical manifestation of metabolic acidosis is hyperventilation, which, when severe, is manifest as Kussmaul's respiration. In patients with chronic metabolic acidosis, however, hyperventilation may be difficult to detect clinically.

Severe metabolic acidosis exerts a negative inotropic effect on the heart, which depends, at least in part, on the fact that acidosis diminishes tissue responsiveness to catecholamines. Thus, in lactic acidosis, negative inotropy sets the stage for a potentially lethal chain of events: poor tissue perfusion → lactic acidosis → decreased cardiac function → further reduction in tissue perfusion.

Acidosis also affects the delivery of oxygen to tissues. In acidosis, the Bohr effect shifts the oxyhemoglobin dissociation curve to the right. This compensatory mechanism permits oxygen delivery to inadequately perfused tissues. However, the protective characteristics of the Bohr effect may be offset by the effect of pH variation

on red blood cell 2,3-diphosphoglycerate (2,3-DPG). Increases in red cell 2,3-DPG also shift the oxyhemoglobin dissociation curve to the right. However, acidosis tends to reduce red blood cell 2,3-DPG; this may offset partially the compensatory Bohr effect and therefore aggravate inadequate tissue oxygenation in acidosis. Other major adverse consequences of severe acidemia are noted in Table 102–17.

Because metabolic acidosis is a manifestation of a variety of different diseases, the treatment of metabolic acidosis varies, depending on the underlying process and on the acuteness and severity of the acidosis. Certain general principles serve as useful guidelines for therapy. Those disorders characterized by *failure of bicarbonate regeneration* or *reduced excretion of inorganic acids* represent acidoses in which the kidneys fail to excrete a normal load of non-volatile acid or, in other words, fail to regenerate approximately 70 mEq of bicarbonate daily. Thus, the treatment of these metabolic acidoses requires administering relatively modest amounts of bicarbonate. In chronic renal failure, alkali therapy is generally not required unless the plasma bicarbonate level falls below 16 to 18 mEq/L. If the acidosis is more severe, bicarbonate supplementation in the form of Shohl's solution (see later) may be instituted. Caution should be exercised to avoid sodium overload or the appearance of tetany, if overalkalinization occurs.

In distal, gradient-limited renal tubular acidosis, administering 30 to 60 mEq of bicarbonate daily, either as sodium bicarbonate tablets or as Shohl's solution, usually corrects the acidosis. A

Table 102–17 ■ MAJOR ADVERSE CONSEQUENCES OF SEVERE ACIDEMIA

Cardiovascular
  Impairment of cardiac contractility
  Arteriolar dilatation, venoconstriction, and centralization of blood volume
  Increased pulmonary vascular resistance
  Reductions in cardiac output, arterial blood pressure, and hepatic and renal blood flow
  Sensitization to re-entrant arrhythmias and reduction in threshold of ventricular fibrillation
  Attenuation of cardiovascular responsiveness to catecholamines
Respiratory
  Hyperventilation
  Decreased strength of respiratory muscles and promotion of muscle fatigue
  Dyspnea
Metabolic
  Increased metabolic demands
  Insulin resistance
  Inhibition of anaerobic glycolysis
  Reduction in adenosine triphosphate synthesis
  Hyperkalemia
  Increased protein degradation
Cerebral
  Inhibition of metabolism and cell-volume regulation
  Obtundation and coma

650-mg sodium bicarbonate tablet provides 7.7 mEq of bicarbonate. Shohl's solution is a mixture of sodium citrate and citric acid; 1 mL of Shohl's solution yields the equivalent of 1 mmol of sodium bicarbonate. The cost of sodium bicarbonate, either as tablets or as common baking soda, is considerably less than that of Shohl's solution. In children with distal renal tubular acidosis, greater quantities of bicarbonate, in the range of 5 to 14 mEq of alkali per kilogram per day, are usually required to avoid growth retardation. Potassium supplementation is also required in the disorder.

The treatment of patients with metabolic acidosis due to *external bicarbonate loss* varies with the nature of the disorder. In acute metabolic acidosis due to gastrointestinal losses, the net bicarbonate deficit may be roughly calculated from the reduction in "bicarbonate space," or total body buffering capacity, as follows:

$$(24 \text{ mEq/L} - \text{measured plasma HCO}_3^-) \times 0.6 \text{ body weight (kg)}$$

Bicarbonate therapy should be instituted when the arterial pH falls below 7.1. It is prudent to administer sufficient sodium bicarbonate intravenously to raise the plasma bicarbonate concentration to 16 mEq/L over a 12- to 24-hour interval, rather than to repair the entire bicarbonate deficit. Calculating the bicarbonate deficit in this manner is valid only if there are no further bicarbonate losses. If the latter persist, as in cholera or other types of secretory diarrhea, the daily amount of bicarbonate given to maintain the plasma bicarbonate concentration in the range of 16 mEq/L may actually exceed the calculated bicarbonate space.

The treatment of acidoses due to *accumulation of organic acids* varies with the disorder. In *lactic acidosis,* therapy should be directed toward improving tissue perfusion. Because the disorder results from a failure of lactic acid and other organic acids to convert to CO_2 and water, large amounts of sodium bicarbonate, sometimes in excess of 1000 mEq per 24-hour period, have been used in attempts to avoid lethal acidosis.

The treatment is complicated by the fact that the response to alkali therapy is not predictable. In experimental lactic acidosis, dichloroacetate can raise arterial pH by suppressing endogenous lactic acid production, but bicarbonate therapy worsens the disorder by increasing the rate of splanchnic bed lactate production. Moreover, large amounts of sodium bicarbonate (in the form of ampules containing 44.5 mmol of sodium bicarbonate per 50 mL) can produce cellular shrinkage due to hypertonicity and circulatory overload due to ECF volume expansion. Finally, in controlled clinical trials in patients with lactic acidosis, sodium bicarbonate therapy has failed to improve circulatory dynamics when compared with equimolar sodium chloride therapy.

The treatment of *alcoholic ketoacidosis* generally requires only administering saline solutions and glucose. Because blood insulin values are generally decreased in alcoholic ketoacidosis–associated hypoglycemia, insulin is contraindicated in this condition because it may induce life-threatening hypoglycemia. Alkali therapy should not be used unless the metabolic acidosis is in the lethal range. The same considerations apply to starvation ketosis. The insulin release provoked by administering glucose suppresses lipolysis and consequently the overproduction of keto acids.

In *diabetic ketoacidosis,* insulin therapy promotes glucose utilization and, consequently, complete oxidation of keto acids; simultaneously, ketogenesis is reduced. Therefore, alkali therapy is ordinarily not required in the disorder. Furthermore, because the hyperventilatory response to acidosis in some diabetic patients is governed by arterial rather than central medullary chemoreceptors, intravenous sodium bicarbonate administration may result in arterial alkalinization, a reduction in the rate of minute ventilation, and a fall in CSF pH.

However, there is no consensus that a transient fall in CSF pH may change mental status or otherwise be detrimental. Also, it has been postulated that bicarbonate therapy may adversely affect the oxygen-releasing capacity of hemoglobin. Furthermore, some authors have noted that late metabolic alkalosis may develop with vigorous use of bicarbonate, once the ketone bodies are metabolized to bicarbonate. Thus, although good reasons exist to administer bicarbonate with severe depression of arterial pH, there also are reasons to not administer bicarbonate. It seems prudent to give parenteral bicarbonate to all diabetics in ketoacidosis with an arterial pH of 6.95 or less, to not give bicarbonate if arterial pH is 7.15 or greater, and to use clinical judgment, largely based on the cardiovascular status of the patient, in those with an intermediate arterial pH.

Finally, because *salicylates, methanol,* and *ethylene glycol* are by themselves tissue toxins, appropriate therapy for these disorders includes not only alkalinization but also hemodialysis for removing the offending agent. When the blood levels are at potentially lethal range, hemodialysis should be used to treat patients with salicylate levels of more than 100 mg/dL, and hemodialysis may be beneficial in the early course of all patients with ethylene glycol or methanol poisoning. However, hemodialysis should be performed on all those with ethylene glycol or methenol poisoning if the serum HCO_3^- concentration falls below 15 mEq/L, because mortality rates rise to unacceptable levels without hemodialysis. Also, ethanol should be infused first as an initial bolus of 0.6 g/kg and then as a sustaining solution to maintain blood alcohol levels at approximately 100 mg/dL, because ethanol competes effectively for alcohol dehydrogenase against metabolism of ethylene glycol and methanol to their toxic products.

METABOLIC ALKALOSIS

ETIOLOGY AND PATHOGENESIS. Maintaining the plasma bicarbonate concentration depends on renal bicarbonate reabsorption and renal bicarbonate regeneration (i.e., net acid excretion). Consequently, although metabolic alkalosis may be *initiated* by hydrogen ions lost from the body, e.g., during gastric drainage, the *maintenance* of a sustained metabolic alkalosis requires that the net rate of renal bicarbonate reabsorption or renal bicarbonate generation, or both, be greater than normal. In other words, a steady-state elevation of plasma bicarbonate concentrations to levels greater than 24 mEq/L requires increased activity of one or more of the effector mechanisms regulating bicarbonate handling by renal tubules. In normal individuals it is therefore difficult to produce metabolic alkalosis by simple alkali loading.

Table 102–18 lists the major clinical causes of increased serum bicarbonate concentrations. The table includes three disorders in which the apparent threshold for proximal bicarbonate reabsorption is increased, namely, volume contraction, potassium depletion, and increased $PaCO_2$, and disorders that increase net bicarbonate regeneration, including increased rates of distal salt delivery and mineralocorticoid excess, either primary or as a consequence of volume contraction. All factors that increase serum bicarbonate concentrations in Table 102–18 are associated with metabolic alkalosis except increased $PaCO_2$, in which the rise in serum bicarbonate concentration is a compensatory mechanism for increased $PaCO_2$. The latter is included in Table 102–18 for the sake of completeness, even though the arterial pH is acidemic with rises in $PaCO_2$.

Volume contraction can sustain metabolic alkalosis because of an increase in the apparent rate of bicarbonate reabsorption by the proximal tubule. The most common cause for initiating this kind of alkalosis is hydrochloric acid loss because of vomiting or gastric suction. In the early stages of gastric fluid losses, there is a modest sodium bicarbonate diuresis, but urinary sodium chloride excretion is reduced. As volume contraction becomes increasingly severe, sodium conservation occurs and potassium bicarbonate is excreted in an attempt to maintain pH homeostasis. Finally, when potassium depletion becomes severe, urinary sodium plus potassium excretion is sharply reduced and paradoxical aciduria occurs: the urine is acidic whereas the plasma bicarbonate level and pH are both elevated. *Contraction alkalosis* is a frequently misunderstood term; the designation should be reserved for those patients in whom metabolic alkalosis has developed and volume contraction maintains the alkalosis by increasing the apparent proximal tubular threshold for

Table 102–18 ■ **MAJOR CAUSES FOR INCREASED PLASMA BICARBONATE CONCENTRATION**

ECF volume contraction
Potassium depletion
Hypercapnia
Increased distal salt delivery
Mineralocorticoid excess

bicarbonate reabsorption. Thus, contraction alkalosis is a mirror image of dilutional acidosis.

Potassium depletion from any cause, when sufficiently severe, can sustain metabolic alkalosis initiated by acid loss, for example, during gastric drainage. Presumably, potassium loss from cells is accompanied by increased hydrogen ion concentrations within cells, including renal tubular cells. Thus, potassium depletion, when sufficiently severe, can raise the rate of renal tubular bicarbonate reabsorption and hence maintain a metabolic alkalosis. Consequently, when serum potassium concentrations are reduced to about 2 mEq/L, metabolic alkalosis due to gastric fluid loss becomes saline resistant but responsive to potassium chloride administration.

Acute increases in $PaCO_2$ initiate renal compensatory mechanisms almost immediately, whereby the kidney increases acid excretion and thereby increases bicarbonate regeneration. The cumulative effect of these renal responses is increased net bicarbonate addition to the circulation. Although the compensatory changes begin immediately, they are not complete for several days.

Situations in which there occurs *enhanced delivery of sodium chloride* to terminal nephron segments enhance renal acid excretion and therefore lead to metabolic alkalosis by increasing the rate of renal bicarbonate generated. This effect occurs with loop diuretics such as furosemide, ethacrynic acid, or bumetanide, and with the proximal tubular diuretic metolazone. These diuretics also contribute to the maintenance of metabolic alkalosis by contracting ECF volume and by promoting potassium depletion. Salt wasting is common in *Bartter's syndrome;* metabolic alkalosis due to renal bicarbonate generation is therefore a common feature of the disorder. Administering large amounts of *impermeant anions* such as carbenicillin also favors distal hydrogen ion secretion. Thus, carbenicillin therapy is one of the few circumstances in which an increased anion gap and metabolic alkalosis can be produced simultaneously by the same agent.

Mineralocorticoid excess, either primary or secondary, also can result in metabolic alkalosis because of renal bicarbonate generation. The disorder can occur in volume-expanded patients, as, for example, in primary hyperaldosteronism, in which the alkalosis is unresponsive to sodium chloride loading, and in patients with a reduced ECF volume and secondary hyperaldosteronism. The alkalosis of mineralocorticoid excess occurs primarily because of increased generation of bicarbonate by collecting duct segments (or, in other words, by increased renal acid excretion) and is clearly accentuated by potassium depletion. *Liddle's syndrome* is a disorder that is due to collecting duct sodium channels being more conductive. This syndrome is characterized by metabolic alkalosis, hypokalemia, and hypertension that occurs because of an increase in sodium avidity by collecting duct segments, which can be blocked by triamterene therapy. This disorder metabolically simulates a mineralocorticoid excess state but one in which aldosterone measurements are normal.

In normal circumstances it is nearly impossible to produce metabolic alkalosis by increasing dietary alkali intake. In certain situations, however, *bicarbonate loading* can produce either a transient or a steady-state alkalosis. One such circumstance is *post-hypercapnic alkalosis.* Patients with chronic hypercapnia develop compensatory increases in plasma bicarbonate concentrations: on an average, chronic hypoventilation results in a 0.3 to 0.5 mEq/L rise in serum bicarbonate level for each 1.0 mm Hg in excess of a $PaCO_2$ of 40 mm Hg. If ventilatory status is improved acutely, the $PaCO_2$ will fall quickly but the plasma bicarbonate level will remain elevated, particularly if the patient is salt acquisitive because of congestive heart failure or ECF volume contraction. A common way to accentuate post-hypercapnic alkalosis is to maintain patients on ventilators having high positive end-expiratory pressures, which causes a central tourniquet effect that reduces cardiac output.

Delayed conversion of *accumulated organic acids* is a second mechanism for producing transient metabolic alkalosis. This may occur after insulin therapy for diabetic ketoacidosis, during the recovery phase of lactic acidosis, and following high-efficiency hemodialysis. In the last-named circumstance, acetate in the dialysis bath is taken up rapidly during dialysis. The accumulated acetate, which represents "potential bicarbonate," is then converted to bicarbonate after dialysis has been completed. Prolonged metabolic alkalosis because of alkali loading is a common feature of the *milk-alkali syndrome.* The alkalosis occurs because of prolonged ingestion of absorbable alkali in patients with impaired renal function due to hypercalcemic nephropathy. Frequent vomiting and attendant ECF volume contraction may also contribute to alkalosis in this disorder.

CLINICAL FEATURES AND DIAGNOSIS. There are no specific signs or symptoms of metabolic alkalosis. Relatively severe metabolic alkalosis can result in cardiac arrhythmias. Severe metabolic alkalosis also can result in severe hypoventilation, especially in patients with reduced renal function. Tetany and increased neuromuscular irritability, which are quite common in acute respiratory alkalosis, are very rare in chronic metabolic alkalosis. Rather, since hypokalemia generally accompanies metabolic alkalosis, muscular weakness and hyporeflexia are often seen in chronic metabolic alkalosis.

The diagnosis is inferred in most cases by routine measurements of serum electrolytes and can be confirmed by arterial blood gas analysis. Hypokalemia is generally present.

The urinary chloride concentration is a useful index for distinguishing metabolic alkalosis due to volume contraction from that due to primary mineralocorticoid excess. In volume-contracted states, the urinary chloride concentration is generally less than 10 mEq/L. Volume-contracted patients with Bartter's syndrome or volume-contracted patients taking diuretics generally have elevated urinary chloride concentrations. The combination of postural hypotension, hypokalemic metabolic alkalosis, and a urinary chloride concentration more than 20 mEq/L is therefore suggestive of diuretic abuse or Bartter's syndrome.

TREATMENT. Some authorities have classified metabolic alkalosis patients by response to treatment. Two broad classifications are chloride-responsive patients, who have urinary chlorides less than 10 mEq/L, and chloride-resistant patients, with urinary chlorides greater than 20 mEq/L.

Examples of chloride-responsive patients include those with gastric fluid loss, after diuretic therapy, and after hypercapnia. Treatment in these patients should focus on intravenously administering 0.9% NaCl at rates sufficient to correct tachycardia and hypotension. Many are also potassium deficient, so simultaneous repletion with potassium salts is indicated. If the metabolic alkalosis is sufficiently severe that significant hypoventilation is present ($PaCO_2 >$ 60 mm Hg), it may be necessary to administer dilute hydrochloric acid or other acidifying salts, such as lysine hydrochloride or arginine hydrochloride. The use of these amino acid salts carries with it the risk of hyperkalemia that is in excess of that expected simply from the change in arterial pH, presumably because these agents promote potassium efflux from cells. Ammonium chloride, lysine hydrochloride, or arginine hydrochloride should not be used in patients with significant liver disease.

Chloride-resistant alkaloses are characterized by urinary chloride concentrations greater than 20 mEq/L and normal or expanded ECF volume. Patients with excessive mineralocorticoid states are common examples, although other causes include Bartter's syndrome, Liddle's syndrome, hypercalcemia, and selective dietary potassium depletion. Metabolic alkalosis in these circumstances is best handled by treating the underlying disease process.

MIXED METABOLIC DISORDERS

Mixed metabolic derangements occur commonly. Consequently, the evaluation of metabolic acid-base abnormalities depends on history and physical examination with a simultaneous assessment of the anion gap, serum electrolytes, and, when appropriate, arterial blood gases. Electroneutrality requires that the sum of the principal anions in serum ($Cl^- + HCO_3^- +$ anion gap) equals the serum sodium level. Thus, unless the serum sodium level changes, a change in the serum concentration of one or more of these principal anions necessitates a reciprocal change in the remaining anions.

Table 102–19 indicates the pattern of serum anion concentrations in single and mixed acid-base disorders. In the single acid-base disturbances, the change in the concentration of one anion is usually balanced by a reciprocal change in one other anion. For example, in hyperchloremic acidosis, the increase in chloride concentration equals the decrease in bicarbonate concentration.

In mixed disorders, the anion patterns are more complex. In a

Table 102–19 ■ ANION PATTERNS IN METABOLIC ACID-BASE DISORDERS

CONDITION	SERUM ANION CONCENTRATIONS		
	HCO_3^-	Cl^-	Anion Gap
Simple Disorders			
Hyperchloremic acidosis	↓	↑	nl
Anion gap acidosis	↓	nl	↑
Metabolic alkalosis	↑	↓	nl
Mixed Disorders			
Metabolic alkalosis + anion gap acidosis	nl, ↑, or ↓	↓	↑
Anion gap acidosis + hyperchloremic acidosis	↓	↑	↑
Metabolic alkalosis + hyperchloremic acidosis	nl	nl	nl

nl = normal

mixed metabolic alkalosis combined with an anion gap acidosis (e.g., diabetic ketoacidosis complicated by vomiting), the identifying pattern is an increased anion gap offset partially or entirely by a reduction in chloride; the serum bicarbonate level is variable. In an anion gap plus hyperchloremic acidosis, the reduction in bicarbonate is offset by increases in both chloride and the anion gap. Finally, in metabolic acidosis combined with hyperchloremic acidosis (e.g., vomiting combined with interstitial nephritis), offsetting changes in serum bicarbonate and chloride concentrations may result in normal anion concentrations.

RESPIRATORY ACIDOSIS

ETIOLOGY AND PATHOGENESIS. Respiratory acidosis occurs whenever the rate of alveolar ventilation is impaired. CO_2 elimination involves the following sequence: transfer of CO_2 from tissues to the lungs in the form of venous bicarbonate, formation of CO_2 within red blood cells, perfusion of the lungs with systemic venous blood, diffusion of CO_2 from pulmonary capillaries to alveoli, and alveolar ventilation. Under normal circumstances, the rate of CO_2 hydration within red blood cells and the rate of CO_2 diffusion from pulmonary capillaries into alveoli are sufficiently rapid that CO_2 accumulation is virtually synonymous with hypoventilation.

Acute respiratory acidosis may result from a number of different causes in which the common denominator is failure of pulmonary excretion of CO_2. In the broadest terms, these causes may be classified into three general categories: primary failure in the CNS drive to ventilation (e.g., anesthesia, sleep apnea, or sedative overdose), primary failure in transport of CO_2 from alveolar space (e.g., obstructive defects, restrictive defects or neuromuscular defects as in myasthenic crises, severe hypokalemia, Guillain-Barré syndrome), and primary failure in the transport of CO_2 from tissues to alveoli (e.g., severe heart failure).

Chronic respiratory failure may occur essentially from the same causes except that the duration of CO_2 retention is longer and thus the renal compensation in plasma bicarbonate concentrations may be to higher levels.

These concepts are also useful in evaluating the possibility of mixed acid-base disorders occurring in association with respiratory acidosis. For example, because the rate of compensatory bicarbonate retention is delayed in acute respiratory acidosis, the presence of an elevated plasma bicarbonate concentration in a setting of acute CO_2 retention should be an index to the simultaneous occurrence of acute respiratory acidosis and metabolic alkalosis. Similarly, because renal bicarbonate reabsorption is an effective compensatory mechanism for chronic CO_2 retention, plasma bicarbonate concentrations below 28 to 30 mEq/L in patients having chronic $PaCO_2$ values greater than 50 mm Hg should alert one to the possible coexistence of acute metabolic acidosis and chronic respiratory acidosis.

Because hypercapnia is synonymous with alveolar hypoventilation, patients with CO_2 retention are invariably hypoxemic. A compensatory polycythemia occurs commonly in chronic hypercapnic states.

CLINICAL MANIFESTATIONS. The clinical manifestations of respiratory acidosis vary, depending on the severity of the disorder and on the rate at which CO_2 retention has occurred. Acute increases in $PaCO_2$ values result in somnolence, in confusion, and ultimately in *CO_2 narcosis*. Asterixis may also be present. Because CO_2 is a cerebral vasodilator, the blood vessels in the optic fundi are often dilated, engorged, and tortuous; in severe hypercapnic states, frank papilledema may occur.

TREATMENT. The only practical treatment for acute respiratory acidosis involves treating the underlying disorder and ventilatory support. The possibility of drug abuse should always be considered in otherwise healthy patients who suddenly develop acute respiratory depression; consequently, naloxone (Narcan) therapy should be considered in all comatose patients seen in the emergency department in whom no apparent cause for respiratory depression can be identified.

In patients with chronic hypercapnia who develop sudden increases in $PaCO_2$ values, attention should be directed toward identifying factors such as pneumonia that may have aggravated the underlying disorder. Oxygen therapy in patients with chronic hypercapnia should be instituted with extreme caution and in the lowest possible concentration to avoid serious tissue hypoxia, because hypoxemia may be the primary stimulus to respiration in this setting. Consequently, in such patients, sudden increases in the arterial $PaCO_2$ produced by oxygen administration may result in cessation of respiration. Under such severe circumstances, mechanically assisted ventilation should be considered. Care must be exercised to prevent post-hypercapnic alkalosis. Administering alkalinizing salts has no place in the management of chronic respiratory acidosis.

RESPIRATORY ALKALOSIS

ETIOLOGY AND PATHOGENESIS. Respiratory alkalosis occurs when hyperventilation reduces the arterial $PaCO_2$ and consequently increases arterial pH. There are divergent causes. Acute respiratory alkalosis generally is a consequence of increased stimulation of the CNS or secondary to tissue hypoxia. Increased CNS stimulation may be voluntary, as in anxiety hyperventilation syndrome, or involuntary, as occurs secondary to neurologic disorders (e.g., trauma, infections, CNS malignancies, or cerebrovascular accidents), pharmacologic agents (e.g., salicylates, nicotine, methylxanthines), or various heat-related causes (e.g., heat stroke, fever, or sepsis). Chronic respiratory alkalosis may have the same causes in addition to being a commonly associated finding in pregnancy, hepatic encephalopathy, severe anemia, and chronic exposure to high altitudes.

The predicted changes in plasma bicarbonate concentrations in response to acute and chronic decreases in $PaCO_2$ are listed in Table 102–14. It is difficult to achieve $PaCO_2$ values of less than 15 to 17 mm Hg acutely, whereas $PaCO_2$ values of less than 10 mm Hg may be achieved in young individuals as a compensatory response to chronic metabolic acidosis, such as diabetic ketoacidosis.

CLINICAL MANIFESTATIONS AND TREATMENT. Chronic hyperventilation may be asymptomatic. The acute hyperventilation syndrome is characterized by light-headedness, paresthesias, circumoral numbness, and tingling of the extremities. Tetany occurs in severe cases. Both the acute respiratory alkalosis and the resultant reduction in ionized calcium and magnesium contribute to the increased neuromuscular excitability.

The treatment of acute respiratory alkalosis involves correcting the underlying disorder. When severe anxiety provokes the hyperventilation syndrome, air rebreathing with a paper bag generally terminates the acute attack. If this maneuver fails, sedation may also be required. If an individual is to be exposed to high altitude, 2 days of pretreatment with acetazolamide, 500 mg daily, will produce a mild metabolic acidosis that will offset the initial respiratory alkalosis on exposure to high altitude and thus minimize symptoms due to hyperventilation on initial exposure to high altitude.

Adrogué HJ, Madias NE: Management of life-threatening acid-base disorders: I and II. N Engl J Med 338:26–34, 107–111, 1998. *Comprehensive review of major adverse consequences of acid-base disorders with special focus on risks and benefits of various therapeutic alternatives. Table 102–17 is reproduced from this manuscript.*
Adrogué HJ, Rashad MN, Gorin AB, et al: Assessing acid-base status in circulatory

failure: Differences between arterial and central venous blood. N Engl J Med 320: 1312, 1989. *A comparison of arterial blood gases with central venous blood measurements.*

Bailey JL: Metabolic acidosis and protein catabolism: Mechanisms and clinical implications. Miner Electrolyte Metab 24:13–19, 1998. *Nice paper reviewing the pathophysiology and adverse effects of uremic metabolic acidosis. Study suggests methods and reasons for aggressive treatment of acidosis.*

Batlle DC, Hizon M, Cohen E, et al: The use of the urinary anion gap in the diagnosis of hyperchloremic metabolic acidosis. N Engl J Med 318:594, 1988. *An account of the urinary anion gap in renal tubular disorders. The data in Table 102–15 are adapted in part from this paper.*

Cooper DJ, Walley KR, Wiggs BR, et al: Bicarbonate does not improve hemodynamics in critically ill patients who have lactic acidosis. Ann Intern Med 112:492; 1990. *This paper compares the effects of sodium chloride versus sodium bicarbonate on pH balance and hemodynamics in critically ill patients with lactic acidosis.*

DuBose TD: Hyperkalemic hyperchloremic metabolic acidosis: Pathophysiologic insights. Kidney Int 51:591–602, 1997. *Excellent discussion of various causes of hyperkalemic metabolic acidosis. Focus is especially placed on commonly used drug-induced causes of hyperkalemia.*

Haber RJ: A practical approach to acid-base disorders. West J Med 155:146, 1991. *Shows that acid-base disturbances are easy to analyze if approached systematically.*

Preuss HG: Fundamentals of clinical acid-base evaluation. Clin Lab Med 13:103, 1993. *Excellent review on evaluating disturbances in acid-base homeostasis.*

103   ACUTE RENAL FAILURE

William E. Mitch

Many serious problems associated with kidney failure arise from the patient's limited capacity to achieve a balance between the intake and excretion of water and minerals and the accumulation of metabolic by-products (chiefly from protein) that cause the symptoms of uremia. These two limitations cause the serious complications of acute renal failure (ARF), including pulmonary edema, hyponatremia, hyperkalemia, acidosis, hyperphosphatemia, anorexia, nausea, vomiting, and other uremic symptoms. The severity of these complications depends on how much function is lost and on how successfully the treatment plan keeps a patient close to a zero balance between intake and excretion. When compared with chronic renal failure (see Chapter 104), the consequences of ARF are invariably more severe because patients with ARF have not had time to activate adaptive mechanisms to blunt the consequences of accumulated waste products.

SCOPE OF THE PROBLEM

Some degree of ARF can be found in about 5% of hospitalized patients, usually as a complication of other illnesses, surgery, or both. How serious is ARF? It is associated with a 35 to 65% mortality depending mainly on the presence of other diseases or complications. Despite the almost universal availability of dialysis, only in obstetric patients with ARF has a sharp decline in mortality to about 1.2% been achieved. The reason for persistently high mortality is unknown, but it cannot be blamed on loss of kidney function because dialysis can replace the excretory capacity of the kidney. Undoubtedly, illnesses associated with ARF (e.g., sepsis) and especially the degree of hypercatabolism are important factors; mortality rates are higher in older patients and in those with more severe renal damage or serious underlying disorders (e.g., infection, cancer).

A SYSTEMATIC APPROACH TO DIAGNOSIS

Diagnosing the cause of an acute decline in kidney function is crucial because some conditions are remediable (Table 103–1). The diagnosis should be approached systematically, and it must be remembered that patients with ARF have impaired function of *both* kidneys (unless the patient initially has only one functioning kidney). This concept is emphasized because few or no clinical signs of renal insufficiency are seen in subjects with only one kidney or those who have donated a kidney for transplantation.

The steps in a systematic approach are shown in Table 103–2. After a urine sample is collected to evaluate renal function (Tables 103–3 and 103–4), a bladder catheter should be placed to exclude

Table 103–1 ■ CAUSES OF ACUTE RENAL FAILURE

PRIMARY DISORDER	CLINICAL EXAMPLES
	Pre-renal
Hypovolemia	Hemorrhage, skin losses (burns, sweating), gastrointestinal losses (diarrhea, vomiting), renal losses (diuretics, glycosuria), extravascular pooling (peritonitis, burns)
Ineffective arterial volume	Congestive heart failure, cardiac arrhythmias, sepsis, anaphylaxis, liver failure
Arterial occlusion	Bilateral arterial thromboembolism, thromboembolism of a solitary kidney, aortic or renal artery aneurysm
	Post-renal
Ureteral obstruction	Bilateral or in a solitary kidney (calculi, neoplasm, clot, retroperitoneal fibrosis, iatrogenic)
Urethral obstruction	Prostatitis, clot, calculus, neoplasm, foreign object
Venous occlusion	Bilateral or a solitary kidney (renal vein thrombosis, neoplasm, iatrogenic)
	Intrarenal/Intrinsic
Vascular	Vasculitis, microangiopathy, malignant hypertension, vasopressors, eclampsia, hyperviscosity states, hypercalcemia, iodinated radiocontrast agents
Glomerulus	Acute glomerulonephritis
Tubuluar injury	
Ischemia	Profound hypotension, post–renal transplant, vasopressors, microvascular constriction, sepsis
Endogenous proteins	Hemoglobinuria, myoglobinuria, light chain myeloma
Intratubular crystals	Uric acid, oxalate, sulfonamides, pyridium
Tubulointerstitial inflammation	Interstitial nephritis caused by drugs, infection, radiation
Nephrotoxins	Antibiotics (aminoglycosides, cephaloridine, amphotericin B); metals (mercury, bismuth, uranium, arsenic, silver, cadmium, iron, antimony); solvents (carbon tetrachloride, ethylene glycol, tetrachloroethylene); iodinated contrast agents; antineoplastic agents (bleomycin, cisplatin)

obstructing lesions in the urethra or bladder. The urine is obtained first to avoid diagnostic problems caused by catheter-induced urethral or bladder trauma (e.g., hematuria). A systematic approach is necessary so that ARF can be assigned to one of three causes: prerenal obstruction, post-renal obstruction, or intrarenal intrinsic damage. Understanding the pathophysiology of each cause helps establish the diagnosis.

PRE-RENAL ACUTE RENAL FAILURE. Causes of renal insufficiency not associated with histologic damage to the kidney are referred to as "pre-renal" or "pre-renal azotemia" (azotemia means the accumulation of nitrogenous waste products). Pre-renal azotemia from various causes (see Table 103–1) is characterized by decreased perfusion of the kidney leading to an accumulation of water and minerals (i.e., positive balance) because of a reduced

Table 103–2 ■ SYSTEMATIC APPROACH TO DIAGNOSING THE CAUSE OF ACUTE RENAL FAILURE

1. Medical history: Clinical setting, medications
2. Physical examination: Evaluation of hemodynamic status, skin rash, signs of systemic diseases
3. Urinalysis with evaluation of sediment
4. Chemical analysis of blood and urine: Serum bicarbonate, potassium, uric acid, calcium, phosphorus, urine osmolality, urine and serum urea, creatinine, sodium
5. Bladder catheterization
6. Fluid-diuretic challenge
7. Radiologic studies to exclude obstruction:
   Ultrasonography
   CT scan
   Retrograde pyelography
8. Renal biopsy

Table 103–3 ■ URINARY INDICES IN ACUTE RENAL FAILURE

LABORATORY TEST	PRE-RENAL	ACUTE TUBULAR INJURY
Urinary osmolality (mOsm/kg H$_2$O)	>500	<350
Urinary sodium (mEq/L)	<20	>40
Urinary/plasma creatinine ratio	>40	<20
Fractional sodium excretion*	<1	>1

$$* \frac{\text{Urine [Na]/serum [Na]}}{\text{Urine [creatinine]/serum [creatinine]}} \times 100.$$

glomerular filtration rate and limited excretory capacity. The crucial point is that pre-renal ARF is potentially reversible because no histologic kidney damage has occurred. Fortunately, it is unusual for pre-renal ARF to progress to intrinsic kidney damage if perfusion of the kidney is restored. Protection against intrinsic damage is afforded by autoregulation, a response that preserves renal blood flow despite systolic blood pressure as low as 70 to 80 mm Hg. Although autoregulation depends on relaxation of the pre-glomerular arterioles, the exact mechanism of this phenomenon is still debated.

In conditions termed "ineffective perfusion" or "ineffective arterial volume" (e.g., heart or liver failure), extracellular fluid volume is, in fact, normal or expanded (such patients usually have edema, ascites, or both), but the kidneys respond as though the blood volume were inadequate. In fact, kidneys from patients with terminal ARF from liver failure function normally when transplanted into chronically uremic patients. In such conditions, histologic kidney damage is unusual, but certain pre-renal conditions can progress to histologic kidney damage (e.g., sepsis, anaphylaxis). Bilateral renal artery occlusion from emboli originating in the heart or from atheromas in the aorta (especially after difficult surgical procedures) can also cause pre-renal ARF. In this setting, severe, sudden compromise of renal blood flow causes histologic damage to the kidney because of ischemia.

The term *pre-renal azotemia* is applied when the blood urea nitrogen (BUN) concentration relative to the serum creatinine concentration exceeds 10 to 1. The BUN is excessively high because tubular function is unimpaired, and the avid reabsorption of filtered sodium and water creates a high concentration of urea in tubular fluid, thereby raising urea reabsorption. These responses decrease urea clearance. The pathophysiology of pre-renal azotemia, then, includes reduced perfusion of the kidney, with high plasma levels of renin, aldosterone, and antidiuretic hormone resulting in avid tubular reabsorption of water and ions. The urine is concentrated and contains small amounts of sodium. The latter finding has been refined by correcting sodium excretion for the amount of functioning renal tissue (i.e., the fraction of filtered sodium that is excreted [FE$_{Na}$]). When tubular function is intact, FE$_{Na}$ is low (<1%) (see Tables 103–3 and 103–4).

Because no histologic damage to the tubules is present, no erythrocytes, inflammatory cells, or granular casts should be present in the urine. Although a strict definition of pre-renal ARF excludes patients with damaged renal tubules, reduced renal perfusion from heart failure can decrease renal function in patients with established renal disease and lead to a diagnosis of "acute-on-chronic renal failure."

Table 103–4 ■ CONDITIONS ASSOCIATED WITH FRACTIONAL SODIUM EXCRETION LESS THAN 1% DESPITE INTRINSIC RENAL DAMAGE

Intense Intrarenal Vasoconstriction
Liver disease
Congestive heart failure
Norepinephrine administration
Severe burns, sepsis
Non-steroidal anti-inflammatory drugs
Acute bilateral ureteral obstruction
Iodinated radiocontrast agents
Vascular Inflammation
Acute glomerulonephritis
Acute vasculitis
Renal transplant rejection

POST-RENAL OBSTRUCTION. Bilateral ureteral obstruction is caused by blood clots, calculi, or necrotic papillae (e.g., with diabetes or analgesic nephropathy); neoplasms closing both ureters (e.g., retroperitoneal lymphoma); and iatrogenic factors affecting both of the ureters and/or the urethra. In obstructive nephropathy, urine flow may decrease rapidly or cease, but this event is unusual for the following reasons: (1) if only one kidney is obstructed, the other kidney will compensate for the loss; and (2) even if a solitary kidney is obstructed (or both kidneys are obstructed simultaneously), filtration continues and tubular pressure rises to overcome the obstruction and increase urine flow.

The causes of post-renal ARF are listed in Table 103–1. In hospitalized patients with indwelling urinary catheters, the catheter should always be checked for correct placement and patency. Obstruction, such as in pre-renal ARF, does not make the urine sediment abnormal unless a coexisting infection produces pyuria and bacteria. Because obstruction has no characteristic features, it should be excluded in all patients with ARF by ultrasonography (see Chapter 108).

INTRARENAL HISTOLOGIC DAMAGE. The different types of acute vasculitis and glomerulonephritis fall in this category, as do scleroderma, malignant hypertension, eclampsia, and microangiopathies. Vascular damage leads to infarction and/or ischemic damage to glomeruli. Glomerular inflammation (i.e., acute glomerulonephritis, see Chapter 106) can cause ARF by the sharp reduction in blood flow to glomeruli and hence the reduced function of glomeruli. Finally, ischemic glomerular damage can result from the infusion of α-adrenergic agonists (e.g., norepinephrine) or the use of non-steroidal anti-inflammatory drugs or iodinated radiocontrast agents (especially in patients with pre-existing renal vasoconstriction associated with hypovolemia).

Whenever glomerular damage occurs, it will be reflected by abnormalities in clinical function and by urinalysis. Clinical abnormalities in renal function include a high BUN-to-creatinine ratio and a concentrated urine that contains very little sodium, presumably because the tubules are less severely damaged. Urinalysis reveals proteinuria, generally with hematuria; in classic cases, red cell casts are seen. Proteinuria and hematuria result from loss of the barrier function of the glomerular basement membrane. Interestingly, urinary erythrocytes may appear to be irregular or crenated because their membranes are damaged and hemoglobin is lost as erythrocytes pass through the inflamed glomerular capillaries.

Casts result from an aggregation of Tamm-Horsfall protein secreted by cells of the ascending limb of the loop of Henle (plus protein filtered through the damaged glomerulus). Normal subjects constantly excrete Tamm-Horsfall protein, but when pre-renal azotemia and a low urine flow coexist, Tamm-Horsfall proteins aggregate to form casts of the tubule lumen and are excreted as hyaline casts. Hyaline casts do not signify pathology because they do not arise from histologic damage to the kidney. With ischemic glomerular damage from vasculitis involving smaller arteries, arterioles, or capillaries (see Chapters 106 and 112) or with glomerulonephritis, erythrocytes filtered through the glomerulus are trapped in the aggregating Tamm-Horsfall protein and produce red cell casts that are excreted when tubular fluid flow increases to flush them into the urine.

ARF can also be caused by disorders damaging renal tubules. This most common clinical form of ARF is often designated *acute tubular necrosis*. Clinically, urine flow slows dramatically or ceases, and casts containing damaged tubular cells are formed. If casts remain in the kidney for only a short period, they appear as tubular cell casts, but more commonly the cells are partly degraded to form "coarsely granular casts" (Fig. 103–1). Because of the severity of injury, it is not surprising that red cells and inflammatory cells are also present in the urine.

Ischemic injury to tubules occurs with hypotension during sepsis or surgery (especially in elderly patients) and produces loss of tubular cells (especially in the loop of Henle) or even irreversible necrosis of the kidney cortex. Cells in the loop of Henle appear to be especially prone to ischemic damage because blood flow to this region is low and the cells have a high adenosine triphosphate requirement. Other causes of ischemic damage include powerful vasoconstrictors (e.g., norepinephrine) and sepsis. In acute tubular necrosis, it has been suggested that tubule cell damage results from loss of cell membrane integrity because of insufficient adenosine triphosphate and/or the excessive production of reactive oxygen

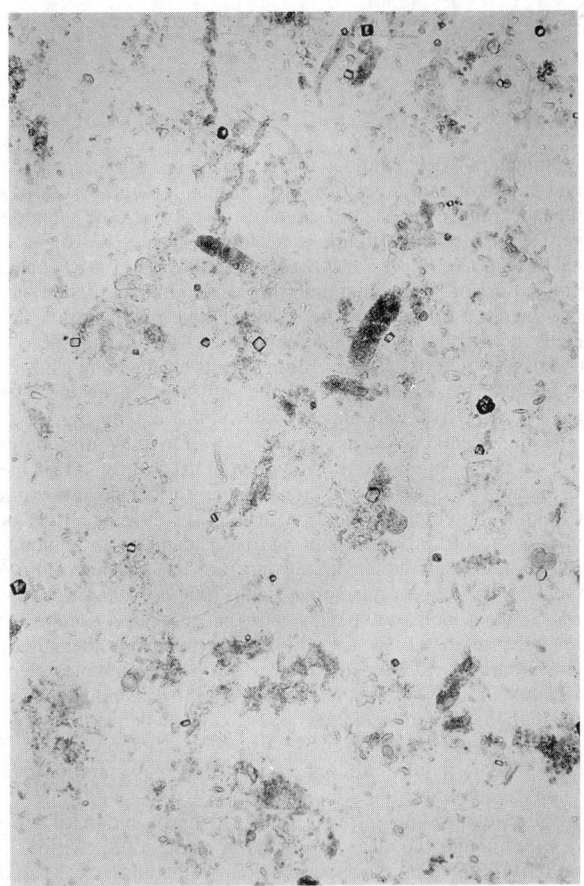

FIGURE 103-1 ■ The urine sediment of a patient with acute intrinsic renal failure from sepsis. Pigmented coarsely and finely granular casts of different size plus erythrocytes and clumps of cells are seen. The larger cells are probably renal tubular cells and the crystals are talc from gloves worn to protect the examiner.

metabolites or "free radicals" released during oxidative processes. Free radicals are implicated because they can damage cell membranes directly.

It is interesting that acute tubular necrosis does not occur more frequently in view of the number of patients who experience hypotension from heart disease or during surgery. Presumably, the autoregulatory response protects the kidney. Alternative explanations are that tubular cell damage does occur but is not clinically important because reserve capacity is sufficient to achieve water and mineral balance and excrete waste products. It is also possible that hypovolemia and/or hypotension by themselves are not sufficient to cause kidney damage unless one or more vasoactive agents that depress renal blood flow profoundly are released concomitantly. The need for a "second insult" is consistent with the widely held notion that acute tubular injury is not usually clinically significant except in susceptible patients (e.g., the elderly or patients with infection or other serious illnesses).

Besides ischemia, renal tubular cells are susceptible to injury from nephrotoxic drugs, chemicals, and high levels of endogenous proteins that are filtered after hemolysis or muscle damage (i.e., hemoglobinuria and myoglobinuria, respectively) or certain proteins produced by multiple myeloma (i.e., the κ and γ light chains). Damage to renal tubules can also occur following occlusion of tubules by uric acid, oxalate, sulfonamide, or phenazopyridine hydrochloride (Pyridium) crystals. Filtration of toxic proteins or endogenous compounds causes more severe renal damage in patients who are hypotensive or hypovolemic.

Nephrotoxic compounds are concentrated in tubular fluid when water is reabsorbed, thereby establishing a concentration gradient to reabsorb the toxins by a passive process, or transport mechanisms may actually lead to toxin reabsorption to increase their uptake into tubule cells. Exogenous nephrotoxic agents include heavy metals (e.g., lead), certain antibiotics (e.g., aminoglycosides, cephaloridine, amphotericin), and chemotherapeutic drugs (e.g., cisplatin). Gener-

ally, nephrotoxicity occurs only with high blood levels (from high doses or with a "usual dose" in a patient with impaired drug clearance). However, lower doses of certain compounds can damage renal tubules when they are given in combinations (e.g., aminoglycosides and certain cephalothin drugs). Likewise, the nephrotoxic potential rises when two classes of drugs are given simultaneously (e.g., cisplatin plus an aminoglycoside). Nephrotoxic damage is more frequent in hypotensive or hypovolemic patients and in patients with impaired kidney function from other diseases. Radiocontrast agents are more likely to damage the kidneys of patients with diabetic nephropathy, systemic lupus erythematosus, or multiple myeloma.

Interstitial nephritis also falls into the intrarenal damage classification. Inflammatory cells (lymphocytes, mononuclear cells, and/or eosinophils) are present in the kidney interstitium when ARF results from immunologic or allergic damage. Whenever clinical findings suggest a hypersensitivity reaction (e.g., ARF associated with a rash following treatment with methicillin or allopurinol) or kidney infection, acute interstitial nephritis is likely to be present. Acute interstitial nephritis can cause a urinary sediment similar to that in Figure 103-1; more commonly, abundant polymorphonuclear leukocytes and especially eosinophils are found in the urine. Whenever acute interstitial nephritis is suspected, it has been suggested that a Hansel stain rather than a Wright stain of the urine sediment be made because it detects eosinophils more easily.

CLINICAL MANIFESTATIONS

After initiation of ARF, four factors depress renal function (Fig. 103-2): vasoconstriction, decreased glomerular permeability, tubular obstruction, and backleak of filtrate. Clinical evidence of recovery may not be observed for days or weeks (average, 10 to 14 days). Recovery of function is generally better in younger individuals who have no serious complicating disease.

The most common problems in ARF are positive sodium and water balance causing weight gain and edema. Kidney pain is uncommon (except with acute pyelonephritis, urolithiasis, or tumors). Although serum creatinine and urea nitrogen rise steadily, their ratio should remain at 10:1 unless pre-renal ARF is present or the patient has gastrointestinal bleeding, hypercatabolism, and/or excessive protein intake (or infusion of amino acids in hyperalimentation regimens). If renal function is stable, these possibilities can be resolved by urinalysis and a 24-hour urine collection. In the urine of patients in the pre-renal classification, inflammatory cells, erythrocytes, or casts should not be present (Table 103-5). The 24-hour urine is used to measure urea and creatinine clearance. The ratio of urea-to-creatinine clearance should be about 0.6, and patients in the pre-renal category have a ratio of 0.3 or less, which results in a high BUN–to–serum creatinine ratio because of a

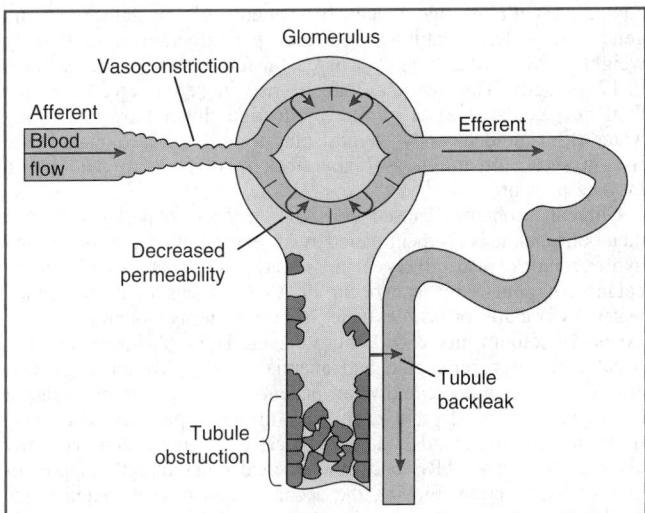

FIGURE 103-2 ■ Potential mechanisms causing oliguria in patients with acute renal failure.

Table 103–5 ■ DIAGNOSTIC CLUES TO THE CAUSE OF ACUTE RENAL FAILURE

PRIMARY DISORDER	URINALYSIS	CLINICAL FINDINGS
Pre-renal		
Hypovolemia	Hyaline casts, no RBC, or WBC, low FE_{Na}	Rapid weight loss, postural hypotension
Ineffective arterial volume	Hyaline casts, no RBC, or WBC, low Fe_{Na}	Weight gain, edema, normal or low blood pressure
Arterial occlusion	Hyaline casts, rare to many RBCs	Occasional flank or low back pain
Post-renal		
Ureteral obstruction	WBCs if infected, crystals or RBCs	Flank pain radiating into the groin
Urethral	WBCs and RBCs	Urethral pain
Venous occlusion	Proteinuria, hematuria	Occasional flank pain
Renal		
Vascular	Granular casts, proteinuria, RBCs and WBCs	Systemic illness suggesting vasculitis, hypertension
Glomerulus	RBC casts, granular casts, RBCs, WBCs, proteinuria	Systemic illness, hypertension
Tubular	Granular casts, tubular cells, RBCs, WBCs	Hypotension, sepsis

FE_{Na} = fractional sodium excretion.

selective increase in fractional urea reabsorption. The 24-hour excretion of urea nitrogen is useful because it will be less than nitrogen intake. If such is not the case, the extra nitrogen must have come from gastrointestinal bleeding or hypercatabolism. In short, a high BUN-to-serum creatinine ratio should always prompt a search for other causes inasmuch as the diagnosis of prerenal ARF is made only by excluding other causes.

It is often said that the serum creatinine should rise at a rate of about 1.0 to 2.0 mg/dL/day in ARF and that a more rapid rise means that the patient has myoglobinuric ARF. It is not wise to accept this guideline because the 1- to 2-mg/dL/day rise is based on results obtained from Vietnam war patients who had varying degrees of kidney damage. In fact, the rise in serum creatinine depends on both the creatinine clearance and the rate of creatinine production. If renal failure is stable (i.e., body weight and serum creatinine are relatively constant), the 24-hour production rate of creatinine can be estimated from urinary creatinine excretion and compared with average values for patients of the same age and gender: in males, creatinine production per kilogram of ideal body weight is $28 - (0.2 \times age)$, whereas in females the value is $22 - (0.17 \times age)$. The maximal rate of rise in serum creatinine can then be calculated as creatinine production divided by total body water ($[0.6 \times$ ideal body weight] plus weight from edema). If the rise in serum creatinine is higher than this value, myoglobinuria may be present.

Clinical problems caused by ARF include hyperkalemia and metabolic acidosis from impaired renal excretion of potassium and hydrogen ions, respectively. If no attention is given to maintaining balance, hyponatremia can occur in ARF patients given too much water by mouth or as dextrose in water intravenously, whereas excessive sodium intake will cause edema. Hyperphosphatemia, hypocalcemia, hyperuricemia, and anemia usually develop after several days—or more rapidly in patients with rhabdomyolysis or hemolysis. Hypercalcemia can occur in some patients recovering from myoglobinuric ARF, and hypercalcemia associated with any disease can cause ARF because hypercalcemia directly depresses glomerular function. Finally, the accumulation of unexcreted waste products can cause the uremic syndrome, which affects virtually every organ and is manifested by progressive anorexia, nausea, vomiting, nervous irritability, hyperreflexia, asterixis, seizures, and coma. Disorders of coagulation can cause ecchymoses and gastric hemorrhage.

TREATMENT

Treatment of ARF includes correction of reversible causes, prevention of additional injury, use of metabolic support during the maintenance and recovery phases of the syndrome, and attempts to convert oliguric to non-oliguric renal failure (Table 103–6).

CORRECTION OF REVERSIBLE CAUSES. In all ARF patients, administration of drugs that interfere with renal perfusion or are directly nephrotoxic should be stopped and radiocontrast agents avoided. In fact, dosages of all drugs should be adjusted according to guidelines for renal failure; plasma drug levels should be monitored because the guidelines provide only average dosing recommendations. For hypovolemic, hypotensive patients in the pre-renal classification, blood pressure should be restored by discontinuing the use of antihypertensive drugs and administering blood (if bleeding or anemia is present) or isotonic saline to expand the extracellular volume. In elderly patients with long-standing hypertension, a blood pressure of 100/70 may in fact be inadequate to maintain the GFR. If doubt exists about the adequacy of the plasma volume, an intravenous challenge of isotonic saline (250 to 500 mL) is warranted. Saline should not be given to patients with edema and/or ascites because in these cases the low perfusion of the kidney is due to intrarenal vasoconstriction, which is not counteracted by intravenous fluids. Moreover, the presence of edema and ascites means that the patient is in positive sodium balance, and the infused saline will merely increase the edema and/or ascites. Obstructed patients require urologic consultation plus careful attention to maintenance of zero fluid balance.

Not all patients with intrinsic kidney damage and ARF are oliguric, even though the clearance function of the kidney is low. The physiologic basis for non-oliguric ARF is not understood; it may represent a milder form of tubular damage, but these patients do not necessarily regain renal function more rapidly. It is worthwhile to attempt to convert oliguric patients to the non-oliguric state of ARF because fluid balance in non-oliguric patients is more easily managed. In conditions (see Table 103–4) associated with low FE_{Na} and no edema, a challenge with 500 mL of saline combined with 40 to 80 mg of intravenous furosemide may reverse an oliguric to a non-oliguric state and, in some cases, even prevent progressive tubular damage. A trial of 80 to 100 mg furosemide can be used in edematous patients to attempt conversion of oliguric to non-oliguric renal failure. If urine flow does increase to exceed 20 to 30 mL/hour, furosemide can be used to achieve fluid balance. Infusion of low doses (1 to 3 $\mu g/kg/minute$) of dopamine has become popular because it can cause renal vasodilatation, but dopamine does not hasten the recovery of renal function and may cause cardiac arrhythmias. If urine flow increases within hours of beginning dopamine, furosemide, or both, use of the drugs can be continued. If not, dopamine or furosemide administration should not be continued to prevent complications.

GENERAL SUPPORT. Indwelling urinary catheters should be avoided in uncomplicated cases; intermittent catheterization using sterile technique usually suffices even in oliguric obtunded patients and reduces the risk of infection. In all patients, maintaining fluid balance is crucial. The simplest and most accurate estimate of fluid balance is a compulsive daily weight measurement; fluid intake and output records are more cumbersome and less accurate. To approximate the required fluid intake, patients can be given fluids (water, tea, etc.) equal to 500 mL plus the amount of urine excreted in the preceding 24 hours. In febrile patients this limit can be increased as long as weight does not increase.

Table 103–6 ■ GUIDELINES FOR TREATING ACUTE RENAL FAILURE

General	Avoid drugs that reduce renal blood flow (e.g., NSAIDs) and/or are nephrotoxic (e.g., radiocontrast agent)
Pre-renal	Restore blood pressure and vascular volume
Post-renal	Urologic evaluation
Intrinsic	Prevent hypotension and try to convert oliguria to non-oliguria; if edematous, try 80–100 mg furosemide, but if non-edematous, try 500 mL saline intravenously

Extra sodium, potassium, and chloride besides that in food should not be given to patients with ARF. If weight increases, sodium should be restricted, but as long as the serum sodium concentration is normal, water restriction is unnecessary. If serum sodium levels decrease, water should be restricted. Dietary protein should be limited to 0.8 g/kg of body weight per day unless the patient is hypercatabolic, and energy intake (carbohydrates plus fats) should supply 35 kcal/kg/day. In patients who cannot eat, an intravenous infusion of essential amino acids and glucose may be necessary. On the other hand, this approach entails considerable fluid intake and may lead to the need for dialysis.

Besides daily weight, serial determinations of blood pressure (supine and upright), serum electrolytes, creatinine, BUN, and hematocrit are needed. Hyperkalemia exceeding 6 mEq/L is potentially serious and can be treated by ingesting sodium polystyrene sulfonate exchange resin (20 to 30 g) in a solution containing sorbitol to ensure excretion of potassium polystyrene resin. Electrocardiographic abnormalities such as widened QRS complexes or atrioventricular dissociation demand immediate treatment with intravenous calcium gluconate or calcium chloride because such treatment is the most rapidly acting method of correcting the cardiac conduction abnormality. Glucose and insulin (0.5 U of regular insulin per kg per hr with 3 mL of 20% glucose per kg per hr) or hypertonic sodium bicarbonate (for acidotic patients) can reduce the serum potassium concentration within 30 to 60 minutes. However, none of these measures removes excess potassium, and dialysis is usually required. (See Chapter 102.3 for a discussion of hyperkalemia.)

Hemodialysis should be considered for hyperkalemia that is unresponsive to polystyrene exchange resins or if electrocardiographic abnormalities are present. Hemodialysis is also required for severe metabolic acidosis that cannot be managed by sodium bicarbonate; hemodialysis is necessary to treat pulmonary edema, progressive azotemia (urea nitrogen concentration greater than 100 mg/dL), encephalopathy, seizures, bleeding, pericarditis, and/or uremic enteropathy. Peritoneal dialysis may be the most suitable method of treatment for patients with severe heart failure because it avoids the rapid shifts in blood volume and blood components that occur with hemodialysis. However, it is not suitable if the patient does not require rapid removal of potassium or waste products. Moreover, anticoagulants are not needed for peritoneal dialysis.

RECOVERY OF RENAL FUNCTION. ARF secondary to pre-renal causes is potentially reversible if the underlying disease is treated. In post-renal, obstructive ARF, renal function may be expected to stabilize or improve significantly after the obstruction is relieved. Intrarenal, intrinsic ARF has a variable outcome. Glomerulonephritis and vasculitis may respond to immunosuppressive therapy with complete recovery of renal function. Renal tubular injury from ischemia or toxins is usually reversible; recovery to nearly normal renal function seems to be more likely in non-oliguric than in oliguric patients. Whereas a major improvement in renal function usually appears in the second week, mild defects in renal function can persist for months or years after acute tubular injury.

PREVENTION

Every effort should be made to prevent ARF. Patients should be given intravenous saline before receiving iodinated radiocontrast material and before surgical procedures, especially patients with poor kidney function or those in whom renal blood flow will be interrupted (e.g., repair of abdominal aortic aneurysm). Intravenous saline is also given with cisplatin and other nephrotoxic drugs. Pretreatment with allopurinol can decrease uric acid production when leukemia or massive tumors are being treated. Non-steroidal anti-inflammatory drugs should be avoided in patients with renal disease, and nephrotoxic antibiotics should be avoided or carefully monitored in patients with ARF.

Alejandro V, Scandling JD, Sibley RK, et al: Mechanisms of filtration failure during postischemic injury of the human kidney: A study of the reperfused renal allograft. J Clin Invest 95:820, 1995. *The initial hemodynamic influence of ischemia in the kidney reduces the pressure required for glomerular filtration and predisposes the tubular cells to ischemic damage.*

Druml W: Nutritional support in acute renal failure. *In* Mitch WE, Klahr S (eds): Handbook of Nutrition and the Kidney. Philadelphia, JB Lippincott, 1998, pp 213–236. *A review of metabolic abnormalities associated with acute renal failure that affect nutritional therapy. Guidelines for providing adequate nutrition are presented.*

Faber MD, Kupin WL, Krishna GG, et al: The differential diagnosis of acute renal

failure. *In* Lazarus JM, Brenner BM (eds): Acute Renal Failure. New York, Churchill Livingstone, 1993, pp 133–192. *A comprehensive discussion of clinical abnormalities associated with acute renal failure and the interpretation of commonly used tests of kidney function.*

104 CHRONIC RENAL FAILURE
Robert G. Luke

DEFINITION AND EPIDEMIOLOGY

Chronic renal failure (CRF) is a progressive disease characterized by an increasing inability of the kidney to maintain normal low levels of the products of protein metabolism (such as urea), normal blood pressure and hematocrit, and sodium, water, potassium, and acid-base balance. Renal function is clinically monitored by measurement of serum creatinine and blood urea nitrogen (BUN) and by urinalysis. Once serum creatinine in an adult reaches about 3 mg/dL and no factors in the pathogenesis of the renal disease are reversible, the renal disease is highly likely to progress to end-stage renal disease (ESRD) over a very variable period (from a few years to as many as 20 to 25). Unless contraindications are present such as terminal irreversible disease in another organ system(s) or the patient does not wish it, almost all patients in industrialized nations then receive renal replacement therapy (RRT). These modalities of treatment, dialysis and transplantation, are discussed in Chapters 105.1 and 105.2.

It is useful for the physician to regard CRF and RRT as a continuum of the same disease process. Chronic hemodialysis is equivalent, for example, to only about 10 to 15% of normal renal function. Preserving endogenous renal function as long as possible above that level is better for the patient than hemodialysis and, in slowly progressive renal disease, especially in an older patient, may avoid hemodialysis. The mean age of patients now entering RRT is 60 years, and the major cause of death in patients receiving RRT is cardiovascular. Patients with progressive renal disease, including but not limited to patients with diabetes mellitus, must be regarded as "vasculopaths" and cardiovascular risk factors sought and treated vigorously. Treatment of such risk factors as hypertension, hyperlipidemia, and hyperhomocystinuria must begin early in the treatment of CRF to prevent long-term morbidity and mortality. In patients with an elevated serum creatinine level (1.5 to 3.0 mg/dL), the term *chronic renal insufficiency* is useful and implies that progression to CRF and ESRD is not inevitable.

In the United States, about 220,000 patients are presently undergoing dialysis and another 80,000 are living with a functioning renal transplant. It is *estimated* that about seven times these numbers, i.e., about 2 million people, are in various stages of CRF and chronic renal insufficiency. Because of the progressive nature of chronic renal disease and our increasing ability to slow this progression, the association with worsening hypertension, and the predilection of these patients for cardiovascular disease, we should recognize and carefully monitor such patients.

ETIOLOGY

We know the causes of ESRD very well, but because of varying rates of progression, we are less sure of the prevalence and relative frequency of the different types of chronic renal disease. Systemic diseases frequently involve and potentially destroy the kidneys (Table 104–1).

There is now good evidence that essential hypertension is caused by renal genetic mechanisms and that the propensity for the development of renal disease in response to renal injury may also, and separately, be partly genetically determined. For almost all causes except polycystic kidney disease, progressive renal disease is more common in African-American than white individuals by a factor of about 2 to 3:1. Indeed, in the 30- to 40-year-old group, hyperten-

Table 104–1 ■ CAUSES OF CHRONIC RENAL FAILURE

Diabetic glomerulosclerosis*
Hypertensive nephrosclerosis*
Glomerular disease
   Glomerulonephritis
   Amyloidosis, light chain disease*
   SLE, Wegener's granulomatosis*
Tubulointerstitial disease
   Reflux nephropathy (chronic pyelonephritis)
   Analgesic nephropathy
   Obstructive nephropathy (stones, BPH)
   Myeloma kidney*
Vascular disease
   Scleroderma*
   Vasculitis*
   Renovascular renal failure (ischemic nephropathy)
   Atheroembolic renal disease*
Cystic diseases
   Autosomal dominant polycystic kidney disease
   Medullary cystic kidney disease

*Systemic disease involving the kidney.
SLE = systemic lupus erythematosus; BPH = benign prostatic hypertrophy.

sive nephrosclerosis is as much as 25 times more likely to cause ESRD in the African-American than the white population.

Although most of the diseases causing CRF are discussed in detail elsewhere, the relationship to progressive renal disease is emphasized here. CRF develops in about 30% of type I and type II diabetics, with a peak incidence at about 15 years after the development of diabetes mellitus. Predictors of the development of diabetic glomerulosclerosis are hypertension, poor glycemic control, microalbuminuria, and the development of proliferative retinal vascular disease. The drug of choice for diabetic patients with hypertension and/or microalbuminuria or fixed proteinuria is an angiotensin-converting enzyme (ACE) inhibitor. If treatment commences at the stage of microalbuminuria and before fixed albuminuria (300 mg/24 hours) develops, especially if combined with improved glycemic control, progression to diabetic glomerulosclerosis may be prevented. Even after fixed albuminuria has developed, ACE inhibitors can markedly delay progression of the decline in the glomerular filtration rate (GFR) to about 2 mL/minute/year. Untreated, the GFR in diabetic glomerulosclerosis progresses downward at a rate of about 10 to 12 mL/minute/year.

About 50 million Americans have hypertension, but each year ESRD develops in only 20,000 of them because of hypertensive nephrosclerosis. Evidence is increasing that microalbuminuria (>30 mg/24 hours) is a harbinger of hypertensive nephrosclerosis and that progression to fixed albuminuria may be diminished by some, but probably not all, antihypertensive drugs. Microalbuminuria is certainly well documented as a cardiovascular risk factor, and that alone justifies intensifying antihypertensive treatment in such patients. It has not yet been established whether normalization of blood pressure can delay or stop progression once the serum creatinine concentration is elevated and/or fixed albuminuria has developed. Nor it is yet known which is the best antihypertensive to use in such clinical circumstances; a large trial is in progress.

The primary care physician has a vital role in the prevention of ESRD, especially for patients with diabetes mellitus and hypertension. Without a fall in the present 7% annual rate of growth in patients with ESRD, at least 500,000 patients in the United States will be undergoing RRT by the year 2010.

Very large cysts, onset of the disease at an early age, and hypertension are associated with progression in polycystic kidney disease, and intense study is also ongoing to determine how to stop progression in that disease. The relevant causative genes are known, but how the defective protein product of these genes contributes to progressive renal cyst formation and loss of renal function has not yet been elucidated. Treatment of hypertension is best initiated by an ACE inhibitor.

Focal glomerulosclerosis and membranoproliferative glomerulonephritis are the most likely chronic glomerulonephrides to progress quickly in adults. No therapy has yet been proved to consistently prevent progression in these glomerular diseases in randomized controlled studies.

A considerable decrease has been noted in the proportion of patients with lupus nephritis progressing to ESRD because of improved treatment of this disease. Scleroderma, Wegener's granulomatosis, and other vasculitides also now less often progress to ESRD, especially if detected and treated before severe renal impairment has developed.

Just as coronary artery disease has benefited from coronary artery bypass and coronary angioplasty, bilateral renal arterial stenoses or unilateral disease in a single functioning kidney can sometimes be prevented from progressing to ESRD by similar techniques applied to the renal arteries. The frequency of renovascular renal failure as a cause of ESRD has not yet been established, but some experts believe that it is a significant and preventable cause of ESRD, especially in elderly white males who smoke and have diffuse atherosclerotic vascular disease.

The listed tubulointerstitial diseases offer a chance for amelioration or normalization of renal function if, for example, obstruction can be relieved before too much renal function has been lost. Cessation of analgesic abuse is likewise potentially beneficial, especially if the patient is still in the stage of chronic renal insufficiency.

CLINICAL MANIFESTATIONS

Patients are often not seen until late in the course of the disease, when much of their kidney function has already been lost (Table 104–2). All CRF patients with the exception of those with medullary cystic kidney disease (see Chapter 115) have fixed proteinuria (>200 mg/24 hours). Because many transient and benign causes of proteinuria are possible, population screening is not justified at present. Insurance companies, however, routinely require testing for proteinuria because of the morbidity and mortality associated with CRF.

The syndrome may also come to attention because of an elevated BUN or serum creatinine concentration in laboratory testing done for a variety of reasons. Only unusually is CRF initially manifested by urinary tract symptoms, and most patients with such symptoms as dysuria, frequency, and polyuria do not have CRF. Occasionally, patients with primary tubulointerstitial disease may have polyuria and nocturia because impaired renal concentrating ability is an early feature secondary to predominant damage to the renal medulla.

Patients with progressive primary glomerular disease may have nephrotic syndrome (e.g., membranous glomerulopathy), recurrent nephritic syndrome (e.g., membranoproliferative or mesangioproliferative glomerulonephritis), or recurrent gross hematuria (e.g., IgA nephropathy). Patients with systemic disease potentially involving the kidney must be regularly checked for proteinuria and abnormal urinary findings on microscopy. Examples include diabetes mellitus, hypertension, Wegener's granulomatosis, and systemic lupus erythematosus. As noted, diabetics should also be routinely monitored for microalbuminuria before the development of fixed proteinuria.

Screening for hypertension is cost-effective, and all patients with hypertension should be screened by urinalysis. If a patient with

Table 104–2 ■ FEATURES OF CHRONIC RENAL FAILURE

Early
Hypertension
Proteinuria; elevated BUN or SCr
Nephrotic syndrome
Recurrent nephritic syndrome
Gross hematuria
Late (GFR < 15 mL/min, BUN > 60 mg/dL) ("Uremia")
Cardiac failure
Anemia
Serositis
Confusion, coma
Anorexia
Vomiting
Peripheral neuropathy
Hyperkalemia
Metabolic acidosis

BUN = blood urea nitrogen; SCr = serum creatinine; GFR = glomerular filtration rate.

what is believed to be essential hypertension is, or becomes, resistant to therapy and requires multiple drugs to control blood pressure, underlying renal or renovascular disease is the probable cause. Hypertension develops in 95% of patients with CRF before ESRD does, and 5% of all hypertensives have an elevated blood pressure secondary to CRF or an underlying kidney disease before the development of azotemia. (Azotemia means an elevation of BUN above normal, but uremia implies the presence of symptoms secondary to renal nitrogen retention.) Examples of parenchymal renal diseases in which hypertension is commonly present before azotemia include polycystic kidney disease, type II diabetes mellitus, and focal glomerulosclerosis.

Initial presentation of patients who already have features of CRF such as uremic symptoms (see Table 104–2) is common because the kidney adapts so well to progressive loss of nephrons and can maintain constancy of the internal environment until about 75% of renal function has been lost. Patients with uremic manifestations, the pathophysiology of which is discussed later, can have a myriad of different complaints referable to almost any organ system. Initial misdiagnosis is common, especially for anemic, gastrointestinal, and cardiovascular manifestations. In some specific renal diseases, other symptoms may call the causative disease into question. Polycystic kidney disease can be characterized by recurrent acute pain in renal cysts and/or gross hematuria. Patients with reflux nephropathy may come to attention with recurrent pyelonephritis or persistent hypertension after what is believed to have been preeclamptic toxemia of pregnancy.

PATHOPHYSIOLOGY OF CHRONIC RENAL FAILURE

Regardless of the primary cause of nephron loss, some usually survive or are less severely damaged (Fig. 104–1). These nephrons then adapt and enlarge, and clearance per nephron markedly increases. If the initiating process is diffuse, sudden, and severe, such as in some patients with rapidly progressive glomerulonephritis (crescentic glomerulonephritis), acute or subacute renal failure may ensue with the rapid development of ESRD. In most patients, however, disease progression is more gradual and nephron adaptation is possible. This process has been studied extensively in animal models, especially in rats with bilateral segmental renal infarction or a 1⅔ nephrectomy. Glomerular hypertrophy, a marked

increase in glomerular plasma flow and single-nephron GFR, and increased capillary pressure are noted. Focal glomerulosclerosis develops in these glomeruli, and they eventually become non-functional. At the same time that focal glomerulosclerosis develops, proteinuria markedly increases and systemic hypertension worsens. Some antihypertensive drugs, especially ACE inhibitors, slow this process and diminish proteinuria; even at the same level of blood pressure control, other drugs such as β-blockers, hydralazine, and dihydropyridine calcium channel blockers do not. It is now believed that a similar pathophysiology occurs in humans and that ACE inhibitors and probably angiotensin II receptor blockers are also protective by mechanisms that depend on both a reduction in systemic blood pressure and a fall in intraglomerular pressure.

Other mechanisms of progression that are probably important in the sclerosis of adapted glomeruli include glomerular coagulation, hyperlipidemic effects, and mesangial cell proliferation. The pathophysiology of focal glomerulosclerosis has been compared with that of atherosclerosis. It is likely that tubulointerstitial fibrosis contributes to nephron failure in the process of nephron adaptation. This result is in part secondary to the potential of proteinuria to cause proximal tubule atrophy; the release of transforming growth factor β, endothelin, and angiotensin II secondary to tubular injury; and nephron ischemia secondary to arteriosclerosis.

This process of nephron adaptation has been termed the "final common path." The ability of nephrons to adapt by enlarging and increasing function has beneficial effects in maintaining whole-kidney GFR, as well as rates of sodium potassium, phosphate, acid, and solute excretion, especially the end products of protein metabolism that cause the uremic syndrome. Adapted nephrons enhance the ability of the kidney to postpone uremia, but ultimately the adaptation process leads to the demise of these nephrons. Much of the present experimental work is aimed at maintaining adaptation but without deleterious effects on the nephron by blocking the effects of angiotensin II, endothelin, and transforming growth factor β, which promote mesangial proliferation, fibrogenesis, and vasculopathic changes.

If these processes are, initially at least, important in postponing ESRD, it is clear that monitoring renal function only by changes in serum creatinine is, at the least, insensitive to nephron dropout

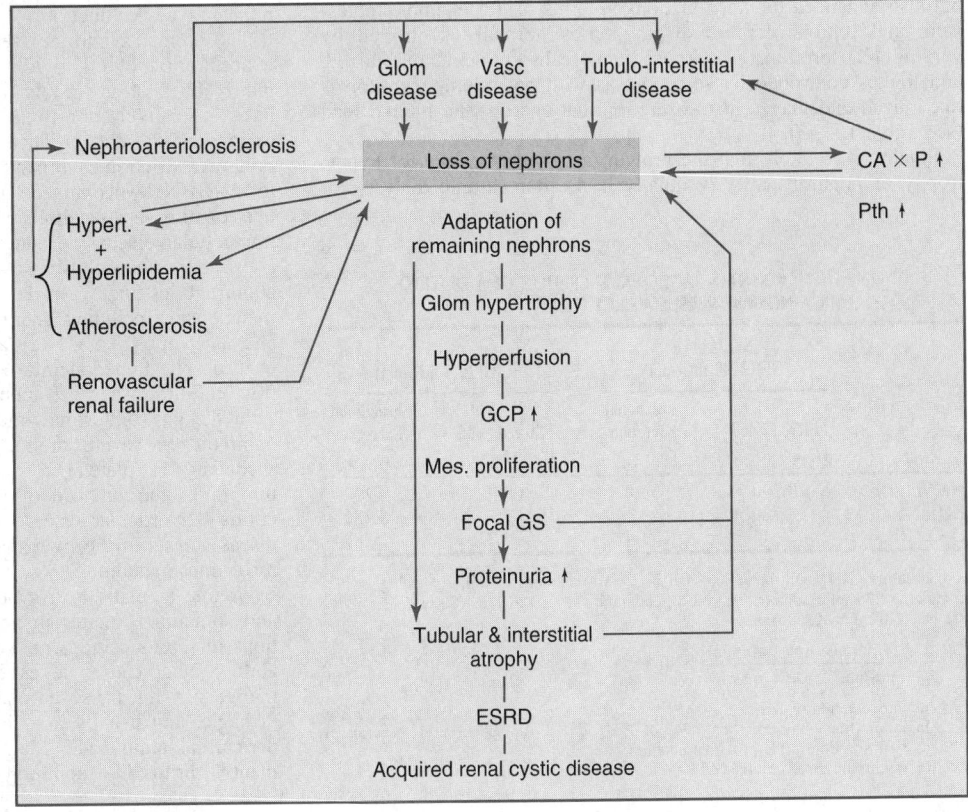

FIGURE 104–1 ■ Pathogenesis of the "final common path" in patients with chronic renal failure. It is assumed that all primary etiologies have been appropriately treated. The best-documented intermediate agents for these deleterious processes are angiotensin II, endothelin, and transforming growth factor. At least experimentally, blockers of these hormones/cytokines have slowed or prevented the further loss of nephrons. In humans, the value of the use of angiotensin-converting enzyme (ACE) inhibitors is well documented.

because whole-kidney GFR can be maintained by increasing single-nephron GFR in surviving adapted nephrons. Quantitation of urinary protein excretion, the use of urinary microscopy, and perhaps in the future, measurement of potentially harmful urinary and blood cytokines may all be important. Whenever possible, primary continuing injury must also be treated, as in immunosuppressive therapy for lupus nephritis, reduction of blood pressure in hypertensive nephrosclerosis, and control of blood sugar and the use of ACE inhibitors in diabetic glomerulopathy.

Two other important concepts in understanding progression of CRF are the intact-nephron hypothesis and the trade-off hypothesis. The first states that in general, adapted nephrons behave like normal nephrons. Some of the failure to regulate sodium and water relates to increased solute excretion per nephron—in effect, an osmotic diuresis of the remaining nephrons that impairs sodium and water conservation, especially in states of extracellular fluid volume depletion. Thus renal concentrating ability is lost, as well as the ability of the remaining nephrons to adjust to low and high intake of sodium, water, potassium, and other dietary solutes because these nephrons are functioning at maximum capacity even with normal intake of these substances (Table 104–3). If the maximum concentrating ability is 300 mOsm and daily urinary solute excretion is 600 mOsm/kg, 2 L of urine is required to maintain excretion, whereas only 500 mL is needed in normal subjects with a renal concentrating ability of 1200 mOsm/kg.

Renal handling of solute is influenced by hormonal effects. For example, as serum phosphate levels rise secondary to a fall in GFR, plasma calcium decreases, serum parathormone levels increase, thereby decreasing tubular reabsorption of phosphate, and serum phosphate returns to normal. The latter in turn contribute to the pathogenesis of renal osteodystrophy. The "trade-off" is increased renal excretion of phosphate with serum levels maintained, but at the expense of elevated parathormone levels. Similarly, normal serum potassium levels can be maintained at the expense of elevated aldosterone secretion.

The progressive drop in GFR, osmotic diuresis of the remaining nephrons, and elevated hormone levels all contribute to restrict the flexibility of the kidney to adapt to low and high intake of various solutes (see Table 104–3). Chronic renal failure is thus associated with progressive loss of the ability of the kidney to maintain a constant internal environment in the face of substantial changes in solute intake. Adapted nephrons have not only an enhanced GFR but also enhanced tubular functions in terms of, for example, potassium and proton secretion. If an ion is normally controlled by varying reabsorption, as with sodium, reabsorption is minimized, and if it is controlled by secretion, as with potassium, secretion is maximized and may lead to excretion that exceeds the filtered load (see Table 104–3).

Finally, it is likely that the growth factors responsible for hypertrophy of nephrons also eventually lead, after chronic dialysis for some years, to acquired renal cyst formation; these cysts are believed to be pre-malignant.

PATHOPHYSIOLOGY OF THE UREMIC SYNDROME

The mechanisms of sodium and potassium retention and how the failing kidney adapts to loss of nephrons by increased excretion of these ions per remaining functional nephron have already been discussed. Progressive metabolic acidosis develops with CRF. The major cause of the failure to excrete enough acid is diminished renal ammonia production and excretion. Although the metabolic acidosis of CRF is commonly referred to as an anion gap acidosis, this gap does not develop until the serum creatinine concentration approaches 5 to 6 mg/dL. Before this stage, serum chloride initially rises as the serum bicarbonate level falls. High serum parathormone levels and extracellular fluid volume lead to proximal tubular acidosis but do not seem to fully account for the early hyperchloremic metabolic acidosis of CRF. Patients who have hyperkalemic distal (type 4) renal tubular acidosis (e.g., in hyporeninemic hypoaldosteronism, common in diabetics) because of tubulointerstitial disease have a much more severe non–anion gap metabolic acidosis relative to the stage of progression of CRF.

Hypertension complicating CRF is due to retention of NaCl, inappropriately high renin levels for the status of expended extracellular fluid volume, sympathetic stimulation via afferent renal reflexes, and impaired renal endothelial function with deficient nitric oxide and enhanced endothelin production. If untreated, this type of hypertension is much more likely to enter the malignant phase than is essential hypertension.

Other cardiovascular risk factors include high parathormone levels, vascular and myocardial calcification, left ventricular hypertrophy, hyperlipidemia (characterized by hypertriglyceridemia and elevated lipoprotein Lp[a] levels), hyperhomocystinemia, increased insulin resistance (even in non-diabetic patients), and smoking. All these factors must be vigorously managed as soon as possible. Acute cardiovascular events, especially stroke and myocardial infarction, account for about half of the deaths occurring in dialysis patients and also deaths after the first year post-transplantation. Heart failure is common and is due to sodium and water retention, acid-base changes, hypocalcemia and hyperparathyroidism, hypertension, anemia, coronary artery disease, and diastolic dysfunction secondary to increased myocardial fibrosis with oxalate and urate deposition and myocardial calcification. Uremia itself may also impair myocyte function.

The uremic syndrome (see Table 104–2) is rare before a BUN concentration of 60 mg/dL is achieved, but it occurs more commonly but not invariably when BUN exceeds 100 mg/dL. Urea itself is relatively non-toxic but is a good surrogate measure of the toxicity of the end products of protein metabolism. If very severe protein restriction is imposed, the uremic syndrome may occur at lower BUN levels. In addition to accumulation of the toxic products of nitrogen metabolism, uremia is caused by extracellular and intracellular electrolyte and acid-base disturbances, by inhibitors of Na,K-adenosinetriphosphatase (ATPase), and by various hormonal abnormalities that contribute to defects in cellular function and metabolism, including energy production, cell membrane function, and ion pumps. Total body and cell potassium may actually be low even despite hyperkalemia because of impaired Na,K-ATPase function and diminished cell membrane potential.

In the gastrointestinal tract, anorexia and morning vomiting are common. In severe uremia, gastrointestinal bleeding may occur secondary to platelet dysfunction and diffuse mucosal erosions throughout the gut. Bloody diarrhea can occur secondary to uremic colitis. Diverticular disease is more frequent in polycystic kidney disease; cysts in the liver may cause hepatic pain, more often after renal transplantation.

Uremic serositis is a syndrome of pericarditis, pleural effusion, and sometimes ascites in any combination. These fluid accumulations in serous cavities are secondary to defects in capillary permeability; other causes of exudative effusions such as infection and malignancy must also be considered. Pericarditis is fibrinous, hemorrhagic, and usually associated with a mild fever and may cause pericardial tamponade. Maintenance by dialysis leads to improvement. Pruritus is a common and troublesome complication of ure-

---

Table 104–3 ■ RENAL FRACTIONAL EXCRETION OF A FILTERED LOAD IN A NORMAL VERSUS A CRF PATIENT*

	NORMAL (GFR, 100 mL/min)		CRF (GFR, 5 mL/min)	
	Filtered Load (24 hr)	Fractional Excretion (%)	Filtered Load (24 hr)	Fractional† Excretion (%)
Na (mEq)	20,160	1.0	1080	20
K (mEq)	720	14	36	278‡
H₂O (L)	144	1.4	7.2	28§

*Sodium, water, and potassium balance was maintained while ingesting a diet containing 200 mEq sodium, 100 mEq potassium, and 2 L of fluid. Serum electrolytes are Na, 140 mEq; K, 5.0 mEq.

$$\dagger \frac{U_{Na} \ (mEq/mL) \times V \ (mL/min)}{P_{Na} \ (mEq/mL) \times GFR \ (mL/min)} \times 100.$$

‡Tubular secretion of K.

§Maximum fractional excretion rates of Na and H₂O are about 20% because of obligatory absorption in the proximal nephron.

CRF = chronic renal failure; GFR = glomerular filtration rate.

mia that is only partially explained by hyperparathyroidism and a high Ca × P product with increased microscopic calcification of subcutaneous tissues. In some patients, pruritus remains troublesome even after chronic hemodialysis is instituted.

Renal osteodystrophy (see Chapter 266) is characterized by secondary hyperparathyroidism, which is due to hyperphosphatemia, hypocalcemia, marked parathyroid hypertrophy, and bony resistance to the action of parathormone; by inadequate formation of 1,25-dihydroxyvitamin D in the kidney resulting in osteomalacia in adults and rickets in children; and for as yet obscure reasons, by areas of osteosclerosis. Tertiary hyperparathyroidism is said to exist when high parathormone levels persist despite normal or high levels of serum calcium. This condition is secondary to the marked increase in parathyroid mass with abnormal and inadequate suppression of parathormone secretion. Metabolic acidosis also contributes to the bone disease by titration of protons for calcium in bone matrix. High parathormone levels and high cytosol calcium concentrations probably contribute to uremic encephalopathy, myocyte dysfunction, and an impaired bone marrow response to erythropoietin. Severe syndromes termed *calciphylaxis* include metastatic calcification in soft tissues and small blood vessels and ischemic necrosis of skin and muscle. In such circumstances, partial parathyroidectomy—removal of 3½ glands—may be required, but secondary hyperparathyroidism is best prevented. Adynamic renal bone disease, which is associated with much-diminished bone turnover, is now being seen and requires bone biopsy for diagnosis. It may reflect skeletal resistance to the action of parathormone. Other joint diseases include secondary gout and pseudogout, which may be associated with chondrocalcinosis.

Endocrine function is diffusely abnormal in patients with uremia and CRF secondary to diminished renal degradation of polypeptides, receptor dysfunction, changes in protein binding, and abnormal endocrine feedback control. Patients in late CRF often appear hypothyroid and thyroid function tests may be abnormal, despite normal free levothyroxine; free triiodothyronine levels are low and binding of levothyroxine to thyroxine-binding globulin is diminished. Thyroid-stimulating hormone testing is useful, and the incidence of hypothyroidism is not increased in CRF. Most women are amenorrheic—although occasionally menorrhagia can occur—and infertile, at least in the later stages of CRF. Impotence and oligospermia are common in men. Follicle-stimulating hormone and luteinizing hormone levels are high, and hyperprolactinemia is present; gonadal resistance to hormones and complicated hypothalamic-pituitary disturbances contribute to these abnormalities. Although renal erythropoietin and 1,25-dihydroxyvitamin D production is severely impaired with progressive renal disease, renin secretion is enhanced; histologic study of kidneys with ESRD often shows prominent juxtaglomerular apparatuses. Diabetic patients commonly require less exogenous insulin as CRF progresses because of diminished degradation by renal insulinase. Non-diabetic patients demonstrate uremic pseudodiabetes secondary to peripheral insulin resistance, especially in muscle; fasting hyperglycemia is rarely severe, and this abnormality improves with dialysis. Oral hypoglycemic agents should be used with great caution in patients with CRF because of the prolonged half-life of both the drugs, which are in whole or part excreted by the kidney, and the resulting endogenous insulin produced.

As uremia progresses, subtle mental and cognitive dysfunction develops and, if untreated, progresses to coma. These changes respond to dialysis, which may be required to differentiate uremia from other causes of encephalopathy or dementia. Neuromuscular abnormalities with asterixis and muscle twitching are common, as are muscle cramps. The restless legs syndrome is a manifestation of sensory peripheral neuropathy. Motor neuropathy is a late phenomenon in uremia.

Progressively more severe normochromic, normocytic anemia develops as the GFR and renal erythropoietin secretion decrease. In most patients, the hematocrit reaches about 20 to 25% by the time that ESRD develops. Uremic coagulopathy is secondary to a defect in platelet function, as well as abnormal Factor VIII function. It is characterized by a prolonged bleeding time but usually normal prothrombin and partial thromboplastin times, platelet count, and clotting time. The platelet dysfunction responds to dialysis and to infusion of desmopressin. Epistaxis, menorrhagia, bruising, and purpura, as well as gut bleeding, may all occur.

Uremic patients should be regarded as immunocompromised, and infection is an important cause of death in CRF and dialysis patients. The leukocyte count, but not polymorphonuclear function, is commonly normal with a normal differential, as are total immunoglobulin and complement levels. Cellular immune function is depressed, however. Antibody responses to hepatitis B and influenza immunization, for example, are less than in normal subjects, but protection is still indicated and feasible.

DIFFERENTIAL DIAGNOSIS

It is sometimes difficult to differentiate between acute and chronic renal failure when a patient with azotemia and an elevated serum creatinine concentration is recognized for the first time. A diagnosis of CRF is supported by a history of nephrotic or nephritic syndrome, long-standing nocturia, findings of renal osteodystrophy, very severe renal anemia in the absence of blood loss, and the presence of bilaterally small kidneys with increased echogenicity on renal ultrasonography. Evidence of long-standing hypertensive disease in the cardiovascular system is supportive but not diagnostic of chronicity. Acute-on-chronic renal failure is a common circumstance, and reversible factors should always be sought when a diagnosis of CRF is made or when a patient with CRF shows unexpectedly rapid deterioration in renal function. A list of such reversible factors is shown in Table 104–4. A hypercatabolic state as in trauma, sepsis, or severe gastrointestinal bleeding can precipitate uremia even if the GFR is stable.

Because of the limited ability of a chronically damaged kidney to either conserve or excrete sodium in response to dietary changes or in response to gastrointestinal losses of salt and water, pre-renal failure is a common reversible factor in patients with CRF. Cardiac failure responds to the usual therapy, and non-steroidal anti-inflammatory drugs and ACE inhibitors can cause (hemodynamic) pre-renal failure in such patients, as well as in CRF patients with normal renal function. Renal stones and benign prostatic hypertrophy are the most common causes of superimposed obstruction.

A careful review of all ingested drugs is mandatory. Renally excreted drugs may either accumulate and reach nephrotoxic levels (aminoglycosides) or cause superimposed acute interstitial nephritis (penicillins). Vascular diagnostic procedures can cause radiocontrast agent–induced renal failure or cholesterol emboli in the kidney as well as elsewhere, including the skin. Unilateral or bilateral renal artery stenosis can complicate CRF and lead to deteriorating renal function and worsening hypertension. Renal vein thrombosis can cause increased proteinuria and a falling GFR in patients with nephrotic syndrome. Hypercalcemia is commonly caused by the

Table 104–4 ▪ **POTENTIALLY REVERSIBLE FACTORS IN CHRONIC RENAL FALIURE**

Pre-renal Failure
  ECF volume depletion
  Cardiac failure
  NSAIDs, ACE inhibitors
Post-renal Failure
  Obstructive uropathy
Intrinsic Renal Failure
  Severe hypertension
  Acute pyelonephritis
  Drug nephrotoxicity (ATN, AIN, vasculitis)
  Acute interstitial nephritis
  Radiocontrast agents (ATN)
  Hypercalcemia
Vascular
  Renovascular
  Renal vein thrombosis*
  Atheroembolism
Miscellaneous
  Hypoadrenalism
  Hypothyroidism

*In nephrotic syndrome.
ECF = extracellular fluid; NSAIDs = non-steroidal anti-inflammatory drugs; ACE = angiotension-converting enzyme; ATN = acute tubular necrosis; AIN = acute interstitial nephritis.

combination of 1,25-dihydroxyvitamin D and calcium carbonate, which is used to treat or prevent renal osteodystrophy.

SPECIFIC DIAGNOSIS

A history of nephrotic syndrome suggests primarily previous glomerular disease as a cause of the CRF. Recurrent gross hematuria may accompany IgA nephropathy or membranoproliferative glomerulonephritis. A careful personal and family history for hypertension and diabetes mellitus should be obtained, including information on any family members in whom ESRD developed. It now appears that some families have a genetic predisposition not only for essential hypertension and diabetes mellitus but also for the development of renal disease secondary to these systemic diseases. A history of recurrent renal stones or obstructive uropathy, including prostatism, or excessive mixed analgesic intake may suggest primarily tubulointerstitial disease. The family history is also very helpful in the diagnosis of autosomal dominant polycystic kidney disease—although in about 30% a spontaneous mutation occurs—familial glomerulonephritis (Alport's syndrome), IgA nephropathy, and medullary cystic kidney disease.

On physical examination, signs of hypertensive (left ventricular hypertrophy and hypertensive retinopathy) or diabetic disease (peripheral neuropathy, diabetic retinopathy) are important. Knobby, bilaterally enlarged kidneys support a diagnosis of polycystic kidney disease, and a palpable bladder or large prostate suggests obstructive uropathy and is an indication for measurement of residual urinary volume after voiding. Gouty tophi and a history of gout may be relevant. Signs and symptoms of polyarteritis nodosa, systemic lupus erythematosus, Wegener's granulomatosis, scleroderma, and essential mixed cryoglobulinemia should be sought because these systemic diseases often involve the kidney. The findings of rheumatoid arthritis are important because this disease is now the most common cause of systemic amyloidosis, which often involves the kidneys. Hepatosplenomegaly and macroglossia also suggest renal amyloidosis.

Laboratory studies should include measurement of serum electrolytes, calcium, phosphorus, alkaline phosphatase, and albumin. Careful urinalysis and urinary microscopy should be performed, as well as measurement of 24-hour urine protein excretion. Marked proteinuria with an abundance of red blood cell, white blood cell, and granular casts suggests a proliferative type of glomerulonephritis, whereas membranous glomerulopathy and focal glomerulosclerosis are associated with less active findings on urinary microscopy. Predominant pyuria occurs in analgesic abuse nephropathy, polycystic kidney disease, and renal tuberculosis, even without superimposed bacterial urinary tract infection.

Urinary protein excretion of over 3 g/24 hours suggests primary glomerular disease. Serum complement and antinuclear antibodies should then be measured because of the association of hypocomplementemia with membranoproliferative glomerulonephritis and lupus nephritis. Serologic screens for hepatitis B and C are important because of their respective associations with membranous and membranoproliferative glomerulonephritis. Human immunodeficiency virus–associated glomerulopathy is an important cause of focal glomerulosclerosis. Antineutrophil cytoplasmic antibodies are often positive in Wegener's granulomatosis.

Renal ultrasound is a useful noninvasive test that can demonstrate cortical scarring (consistent with reflux nephropathy or segmental infarction), renal stones, hydronephrosis, ureteric obstruction, or polycystic kidney disease. Medical kidney disease may be associated with symmetrically diminished size and increased echogenicity; these findings are otherwise non-specific. Asymmetry of renal size raises a question of renovascular renal failure or previous obstruction from a stricture or stone. A more severe degree of anemia than would be anticipated for the degree of renal failure suggests myeloma kidney; serum and urine immunoelectrophoresis should be performed to detect monoclonal antibodies. If a monoclonal antibody is found, bone marrow examination is usually necessary to confirm the diagnosis.

If the diagnosis remains obscure and kidney size is normal or only slightly reduced, renal biopsy should be considered for diagnosis after control of blood pressure and, if necessary, dialysis.

TREATMENT

Once it is determined that a patient has CRF, careful and regular follow-up is mandatory (Fig. 104–2). It is best if the primary care physician and the nephrologist cooperate closely in the management of such patients. Blood pressure, status of extracellular fluid volume, and a careful history and examination for early signs and symptoms of the complications of CRF and the uremic syndrome (e.g., peripheral neuropathy) are essential. Serum electrolytes, BUN and serum creatinine, calcium, phosphorus, hematocrit and mean corpuscular volume, 24-hour urinary protein excretion, and in some patients, urinary microscopy are obtained at regular intervals. In the later stages of CRF and in all patients with nephrotic syndrome, serum albumin is also measured to help to assess nutritional status. The patient should be advised to consult about any intake of over-the-counter or prescribed medications and should avoid non-steroidal anti-inflammatory drugs.

Treatment of hypertension is the most important measure to slow progression of CRF and reduce cardiovascular morbidity and mortality. Unlike essential hypertension, hypertension secondary to CRF usually progresses and causes a vicious circle of worsening hypertension and renal function (see Fig. 104–1), so any chronic elevation in blood pressure above normal should usually be treated. If the patient is African-American or has proteinuria of more than 1 g/24 hours, blood pressure should be reduced to a mean of less than 95 mm Hg (125/75) unless relative contraindications such as significant coronary artery disease or cerebrovascular disease are present. Patients with lesser degrees of proteinuria should have blood pressure reduced to a mean level of 102 mm Hg (135/85) or less. If proteinuria greater than 1 g/24 hours is present, ACE inhibitors should generally be used. The degree of reduction in proteinuria produced by ACE inhibitors predicts the degree of slowing of the decrease in GFR in that patient. Virtually all patients with CRF require a loop diuretic as part of their antihypertensive treatment. Thiazides are no longer efficacious in patients with CRF, except when used together with loop diuretics. The use of ACE inhibitors requires surveillance for hyperkalemia and hemodynamic pre-renal failure. Hyperkalemia develops in only about 10% of patients while taking ACE inhibitors until very late in the course of CRF. The presence of type 4 hyperkalemic renal tubular acidosis, not uncommon in diabetic glomerulosclerosis, usually prevents their use. The most common side effect associated with ACE inhibitors is chronic cough, which can be treated with angiotensin II receptor blockers such as losartan.

Long-acting calcium channel blockers are usually the next anti-

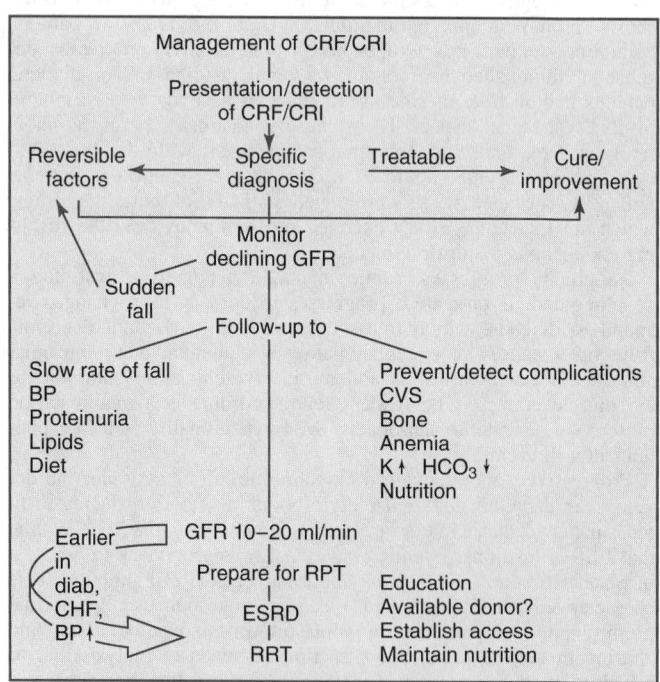

FIGURE 104–2 ■ Outline of management of patients in the various stages of chronic renal failure.

hypertensive to be added, and they have synergistic effects with ACE inhibitors and loop diuretics. Some would use these agents as the first antihypertensive in patients with hypertensive nephrosclerosis or renovascular renal failure. Patients with CRF often require multiple drug therapy for treatment of hypertension. Centrally acting α_2-blockers such as clonidine or peripheral α-blockers such as prazosin are good next choices. Minoxidil may also be required, and usually this drug mandates an increased diuretic dose and a β-blocker if reflex tachycardia occurs; both of these side effects occur in response to the profound vasodilatation produced by minoxidil. β-Blockers are used in patients who have had myocardial infarction. Other cardiovascular risk factors such as hyperlipidemia and hyperhomocystinuria should be treated appropriately.

When hypertension or edema develops, sodium intake should be reduced to 2 g (5 g NaCl). Potassium restriction is not usually needed until late in the course of CRF, although the use of ACE inhibitors or β-blockers for hypertension may necessitate restriction sooner. Care should be exercised to avoid high potassium intake, as with potassium-containing salt substitutes. Modest dietary phosphate restriction is also indicated but is difficult to implement because of its presence in so many foods. Magnesium-containing antacids and laxatives should be avoided because of the dangers of hypermagnesemia.

Protein restriction should be instituted to reduce or forestall symptoms of uremia, which are secondary to accumulating products of protein metabolism at any given low GFR, and to reduce the rate of fall in GFR, even in nephrotic syndrome, caused by progressive glomerular disease. Protein restriction must always be accompanied by adequate caloric intake (35 kcal/kg) to avoid catabolism of endogenous protein. A high-protein diet accelerates the rate of loss of GFR and actually increases proteinuria. Protein restriction to 0.7 to 0.8 g/kg body weight per day is indicated. If proteinuria is greater than 5 g/24 hours, that amount should be added to the protein intake. Dietary protein restriction also has the advantage of reducing potassium and phosphate intake and proton production from sulfur- and phosphorus-containing amino acids. The metabolism of each gram of protein yields 1/3 g urea and 1 mmol/L of hydrogen ion. Nitrogen balance can be maintained by a protein intake of 0.6 g/kg body weight per day, but a margin of safety is preferred. Patients who enter RRT in negative nitrogen balance have diminished survival and an increased complication rate. Uremia itself induces reduced intake of nitrogenous foods, and a vicious circle can ensue and must be terminated by initiating RRT. Protein catabolism in nephrotic syndrome is much greater than suggested by the loss of protein in urine—many times more protein is catabolized in the proximal tubule after passing through the glomerular capillaries. This process is now thought to also invoke tubular atrophy and tubulointerstitial fibrosis (see Fig. 104–1). Measurement of the BUN–serum creatinine ratio helps monitor the patient's dietary compliance with protein restriction. The ratio should be less than 10 in a stable patient with CRF who is ingesting 0.7 to 0.8 g/kg protein per day. The latter can also be estimated more accurately by periodically measuring 24-hour urinary urea nitrogen. Dietary protein intake (grams) = 6.25 (urinary urea nitrogen + 0.031 × body weight in kilograms) + urinary protein (if 5 g/24 hours or more). The 0.031 factor accounts for other sources of nitrogen loss in feces, skin, etc. A multivitamin preparation is usually given and hyperhomocystinemia treated by oral folic acid and vitamin B_{12} and B_6 tablets.

Metabolic acidosis leads to increased protein catabolism via the ubiquitin degradation pathway and should be treated by maintaining serum bicarbonate at normal levels with small doses of sodium bicarbonate (0.6 g three times daily gives 22 mmol/L bicarbonate). Metabolic acidosis should also be avoided because it contributes to renal bone disease; excess protons are buffered in the apatite of bone, with release of calcium. Oral calcium carbonate or acetate used as a phosphate binder also provides a base intake to counteract metabolic acidosis. It is obviously difficult to manage the dietary changes just mentioned without good patient compliance and expert dietetic help.

To avoid renal osteodystrophy, calcium carbonate is used with meals to reduce dietary phosphate absorption as soon as serum phosphate rises to the upper limit of normal. If serum calcium levels remain low despite calcium carbonate or if renal bone disease is already detectable, small doses of 1,25-dihydroxyvitamin D (0.25 to 1 μg) are added with continued monitoring of serum

calcium and phosphate to avoid hypercalcemia. Serum parathormone should also be monitored and is best maintained at twice normal because some resistance to its effect on bone is noted in patients with CRF. Patients who are initially seen late in the course of uremia may already have renal osteodystrophy as manifested by bone pain, pathologic fractures, elevated alkaline phosphatase, hypocalcemic hyperphosphatemia, radiologic evidence of hyperparathyroidism (e.g., erosion of the margins of the proximal phalanges and the outer third of the clavicle), and soft tissue and vascular calcification. To avoid the latter, the product of calcium × phosphate, with both measured in milligrams per deciliter (the "solubility product"), should be less than 65. Aluminum hydroxide is now best avoided as a phosphate blocker because of the danger of aluminum toxicity, especially in brain and bone. Its use for short periods may still be required, however, in severe and resistant cases of hyperphosphatemia because it is still the most potent phosphate binder available.

Anemia can be treated by the administration of subcutaneous erythropoietin (50 to 70 U/kg) one to three times weekly. The dose is carefully titrated against the hematocrit. Some of the so-called uremic symptoms are in fact due to anemia. The hematocrit should be maintained around 30 to 35%. Erythropoietin often causes an increase in blood pressure, which should be treated in the same way as discussed before. Avoiding a low hematocrit appears to also help prevent left ventricular hypertrophy, an independent risk factor for cardiovascular morbidity. Failure to respond to erythropoietin indicates a search for deficiencies of iron, folic acid, or vitamin B_{12} or the presence of an inflammatory or immunologic process.

When the serum creatinine reaches 4 to 6 mg/dL in women and 6 to 8 mg/dL in men, planning for RRT should begin. If 24-hour creatinine clearance is being monitored, it must be remembered that as the GFR falls, creatinine clearance progressively overestimates the true GFR because of increasing secretion of creatinine. The goal of the primary care physician and nephrologist must be to initiate RRT at the ideal time, just before or at the very onset of uremic symptomatology, which requires a combination of good clinical judgment and monitoring of the parameters already noted. Any suggestion of declining appetite and commencing negative nitrogen balance should be taken as an indication to proceed to RRT. If the patient has a willing and acceptable live donor, transplantation can sometimes be initiated without prior hemodialysis or peritoneal dialysis. All the modalities discussed in the next chapter must be carefully explained to the patient, and it is very helpful for the patient to meet other patients who have experienced the various RRT modalities. The relative indications for hemodialysis, peritoneal dialysis, and renal transplantation are discussed in Chapter 105. Although not universally agreed, most nephrologists initiate RRT somewhat earlier in patients with diabetes, especially if evidence of other diabetic complications is present. Diabetic and uremic peripheral neuropathy and retinopathy tend to compound the effects of one another.

In some patients, hypertension, congestive heart failure, or anemia may indicate initiation of RRT sooner than otherwise would be expected. In patients who have continued to work, an inability to do so may be an indication for RRT. The uremic syndrome is variable in onset and in character in different patients, but subtle signs of anorexia, cognitive impairment, and sensory peripheral neuropathy must be searched for carefully. The development of pericarditis, acute pulmonary edema, or motor peripheral neuropathy, for example, is a clear indication that RRT has been delayed too long. It is now evident that if RRT is delayed too long, its initiation is associated with a longer hospital stay, increased cost, and increased morbidity. When done appropriately, RRT can be initiated on an outpatient basis.

Vascular or peritoneal access should usually be established about 2 months before the probable requirement for hemodialysis. This practice gives the best chance of creating a viable arteriovenous (often radiocephalic) fistula in the nondominant forearm. Venipuncture should be avoided in that arm before and after fistula formation. Fistula survival is much greater than the survival of synthetic grafts, which are, however, still the most commonly used. Placement of a fistula too early in the course of CRF, however, can lead to thrombosis, whereas late CRF is associated with a hypocoagulable state. When patients are initially seen with frank uremia and no reversible factors are present, emergency dialysis may be required. As in acute renal failure, access can be obtained quickly via the internal jugular vein. In general, the subclavian vein is now avoided because of the development of subclavian stenosis and subsequent venous hypertension in the arm, which complicates the formation of a forearm fistula. Femoral vein access can also be used, but a semipermanent catheter is much more difficult to maintain and much more likely to become infected at that site. If the BUN is very high (above 120 mg/dL), the initial hemodialysis should be done only for a short period and at relatively low blood flow rates to avoid the dialysis disequilibrium syndrome (discussed in Chapter 105). Great care must be taken with anticoagulation for hemodialysis if pericarditis is present; if possible, heparin administration should be avoided.

The physician must be alert to neuropsychiatric and other complications of CRF that may be prematurely diagnosed as uremia secondary to ESRD. These complications include hyponatremia secondary to the much-diminished free water clearance as the GFR falls and to excess fluid intake, which is sometimes unfortunately iatrogenic. Hypernatremia may result from obligatory polyuria if free water intake is not maintained, as during surgery. Hypoxia associated with heart failure or pneumonia may cause confusion, especially in elderly patients with CRF. Symptoms may be caused by retention of drugs, the dosage of which has not been modified appropriately as the GFR falls, especially sedatives and tranquilizers excreted in whole or part by renal mechanisms. Digoxin toxicity may cause nausea, vomiting, and arrhythmias. It is most unwise to perform dialysis on a patient who is uremic because of superimposed pre-renal failure; hypovolemic patients tolerate hemodialysis very poorly, and extracellular fluid volume must be repleted before initiation of hemodialysis. Often, if pre-renal factors are corrected, dialysis can be postponed. Hyperkalemia is an unusual single cause for initiation of hemodialysis and can usually be managed by potassium restriction, restoration of urinary flow rates by correction of pre-renal failure, sodium polystyrene sulfonate (Kayexalate) retention enemas, intravenous glucose and insulin, and treatment of severe metabolic acidosis with sodium bicarbonate.

Giatras I, Lau J, Levey AS: Effect of angiotensin-converting enzyme inhibitors on the progression of nondiabetic renal disease: A meta-analysis of randomized trials. Ann Intern Med 127:337, 1997. *A summary of all randomized studies of ACE inhibitor treatment in this population. The beneficial effects are probably due to both nonspecific antihypertensive effects and specific antiproteinuria mechanisms.*
Kurtzman NA (ed): Semin Nephrol 16(3), 1996. *In-depth reviews of the pathogenesis of the major components of uremic syndrome, including effects on immune responses and the cardiovascular system.*
Lazarus MJ, Bourgoignie JJ, Buckalew VM, et al: Achievement and safety of a low blood pressure goal in chronic renal disease. Hypertension 29:641, 1997. *These data indicate that a lower than usual blood pressure is achievable in the majority of patients with either moderate or advanced renal disease (GFR between 13 and 55 mL/minute/1.73 m²) and that reduction of elevated blood pressure to levels lower than usually regarded as standard practice is safe, at least in patients without a history of cardiovascular and cerebrovascular disease.*
Remuzzi G, Ruggenenti P, Benighi A: Understanding the nature of renal disease progression. Kidney Int 51:2, 1997. *Discusses the evidence that non-selective proteinuria itself contributes to the progression of renal disease, probably through cytotoxic effects on the proximal tubule, perhaps via increased renal endothelin and transforming growth factor β production.*

105 TREATMENT OF IRREVERSIBLE RENAL FAILURE

John J. Curtis

105.1 Dialysis

As early as 1861, chemists applied the techniques of dialysis to remove solutes from solution. Indeed, the first solution used for dialysis in the 1800s was urine—from which urea could be extracted. Nearly a century passed, however, before dialysis moved from the chemistry laboratories into clinical medicine. Two seemingly unrelated events occurred. Heparin was discovered by workers not focused on dialysis, and cellophane was invented for use in the meat packing industry. These developments and the genius of men such as Abel, Thalheimer, and Kolff resulted in applying dialysis as a treatment—first for poison ingestion and ultimately for acute and chronic renal failure (see Chapters 103 and 104). It was humanity's first attempt at simulating the function of a then vital organ system. *It worked!* In 1960, in Seattle, Washington, the first patient was treated for chronic renal failure with long-term dialysis.

Today, there are more than 200,000 chronic renal failure patients treated with dialysis in the United States, and the number grows each year (more rapidly than expected). Much to the chagrin of health care planners, no plateau in the number of patients is in sight. Many of these patients have survived without natural kidney function for more than 20 years. In 1972, the Congress of the United States was approached with a trial of dialysis. Physicians performed hemodialysis on a renal failure patient in front of the legislators. This clinical trial convinced Congress that the therapy of dialysis worked. The performance won Medicare financial coverage for end-stage renal failure patients in the United States. Nephrology is the only medical subspecialty that has dealt with a "single-payer" reimbursement system since 1973. It has been both a good and a bad experience. It is impossible to separate the clinical aspects of dialysis from its unique (in the United States) form of financing.

ARTIFICIAL KIDNEYS. The dialysis procedure is based on two scientific principles—diffusion and ultrafiltration. Diffusion is *not* how the normal kidney works, yet it plays a critical role in dialysis. Ultrafiltration (which is more akin to normal kidney function) plays a less crucial role in dialysis.

Small particles of differing concentrations in two different solutions will, with time, equalize their concentration when separated by a thin, semipermeable membrane. Cellophane is the classic semipermeable membrane. The peritoneal membrane is a natural semipermeable membrane. The smaller the particle, the more brownian movement there is, and the more quickly it will move across the semipermeable membrane. The direction of net movement the particle (or solute) takes is from the solution of higher concentration to the solution of lower concentration. Larger particles will move across the membrane, but more slowly. Particles larger than the pores in the membrane will not move. The cellophane membranes were replaced by cuprophan or cuprophane, which, like cellophane, is derived from cellulose. Moreover, synthetic membranes (e.g., polymethyl methacrylate, polycarbonate) are in use in newer dialysis devices. Human blood is exposed to a solution in a hollow-fiber dialyzer (Fig. 105–1). This device allows blood and solution (dialysate) to be separated by a large surface area of semipermeable membrane.

Important, then, in dialysis by diffusion are the membrane (its pore number and size), the time that solutions are exposed to the membrane, and the concentration of the particles in the solutions. Small molecules, such as urea, are effectively cleared by diffusion. The difference in concentration gradient between blood and the dialysate is important, and thus the flow rate of blood and dialysate consequentially influences clearance of small molecules. Rapid flow ensures a large concentration difference. Larger molecules are not as sensitive to flow rates of blood and dialysate. They require more time for diffusion. The normal kidney does not employ diffusion and is quite effective in removing both small molecules such as urea and larger molecules. If larger molecules are responsible for uremia, this may be a problem in assessing how well artificial kidneys function.

Ultrafiltration, on the other hand, depends on pressure to move particles or water across a membrane. The pressure is either hydrostatic or osmotic in nature. In the normal kidney, pressure generated by the heart is transmitted to the glomerular capillary and, with the proper resistance, can force fluid across the capillary into Bowman's space. This forced fluid moves (drags) small and relatively large molecules (up to a point) equally well. In dialysis, pressure from the heart and specially designed extracorporeal blood pumps (Fig. 105–2) can be used to move fluid and solutes out of the circulation and across membranes. Large particles that move slowly or not at all across the semipermeable membrane attract water to move in their direction. This is osmotic pressure, which,

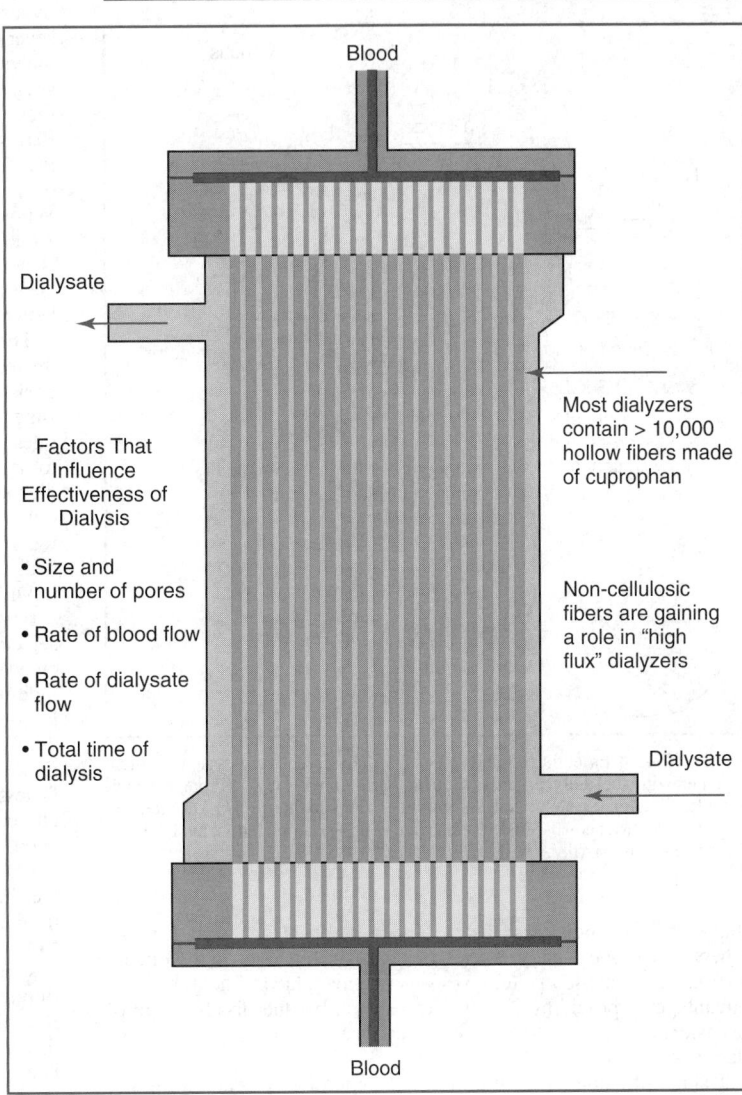

Blood

Dialysate

Factors That
Influence
Effectiveness of
Dialysis

• Size and
  number of pores

• Rate of blood flow

• Rate of dialysate
  flow

• Total time of
  dialysis

Most dialyzers
contain > 10,000
hollow fibers made
of cuprophan

Non-cellulosic
fibers are gaining
a role in "high
flux" dialyzers

Dialysate

Blood

FIGURE 105–1 ■ Most dialyzers in clinical use today are hollow-fiber types. Some use of parallel-plate dialyzers continues, but coil dialyzers have almost disappeared from clinical use.

like the pressure generated by pumps, can be used in dialysis (especially peritoneal dialysis) to produce ultrafiltration.

The normal kidney, however, does more than ultrafilter. It reclaims from the ultrafiltrate exactly those solutes that are needed and excretes (and secretes) those that are toxic and not needed. This is critical. Without the tubular function of reclamation, we would all quickly die of ultrafiltration. Just how the kidney "knows" what to keep and what to discard is the question that has created the entire branch of medicine called "nephrology."

REMOVING SUBSTANCES THAT CAUSE UREMIA. It is not known for certain, however, what substances are responsible for the uremic syndrome and uremic death when the kidneys fail (see Chapter 104). Without this knowledge, it might seem that an artificial kidney would be impossible to develop—even with an understanding of diffusion and ultrafiltration and their ability to remove and replace solutes and water. The genius of the early pioneers of dialysis was their ability to put aside (for the moment) the unknown but to continue the thought process. Without knowing the toxic substance(s), one can make a non-toxic solution with the known concentration of solutes in a normal person's serum. Dialysis of this solution against a solution with unknown toxic substances should result in moving these unknown toxic substances into the normal solution. This assumes that the toxic substances are small enough to pass the membrane pores, not tightly bound to huge proteins, and located in the blood. The clinical success of dialysis suggests that the assumptions are correct.

The solutions (dialysate) that are usually used in hemodialysis and peritoneal dialysis are described in Table 105–1. Before dialysis, neither solution has urea, creatinine, or the toxic substances

associated with uremia. At the end of dialysis, these solutions have urea, creatinine, and presumably many of the toxic substances of uremia. They are discarded. The patient has lost urea, creatinine, and many of the toxic substances associated with uremia, and the uremic symptoms disappear.

Two points need to be made about the dialysate solutions. First, note that neither solution contains bicarbonate (the solutions have a low pH of approximately 5). This is unlike human plasma, which has a pH of 7.4 and a bicarbonate concentration of 22 to 25 mmol/L. The reason that some dialysate solutions do not contain bicarbonate is to keep calcium and magnesium in solution. At the concentrations listed, they could precipitate out of solution, combining with bicarbonate. Dialysate without bicarbonate has a low pH and is bacteriostatic. Acetate and lactate are often used as substitutes for bicarbonate because they are quickly converted by the liver into bicarbonate. Quickly is sometimes not fast enough—especially with newer high-efficiency (large surface areas) and high-flux dialyzers (dialyzers with special membranes designed to be exceptionally porous). In some patients, acetate has been associated with dialysis hypotension. In the last few years, high-efficiency dialysis machines have used "bicarbonate dialysis" with water and concentrate of dialysate mixed with complex-proportioning units to prevent calcium bicarbonate insolubility. Bicarbonate dialysis has advantages for some patients. It is believed to cause less hypotension; clinical problems associated with severe metabolic acidosis are often better managed with bicarbonate dialysis. Now bicarbonate dialysis is almost universally used and the use of acetate is rare.

Second, note that the solution for peritoneal dialysis contains considerable glucose—more than 10 times that of hemodialysis

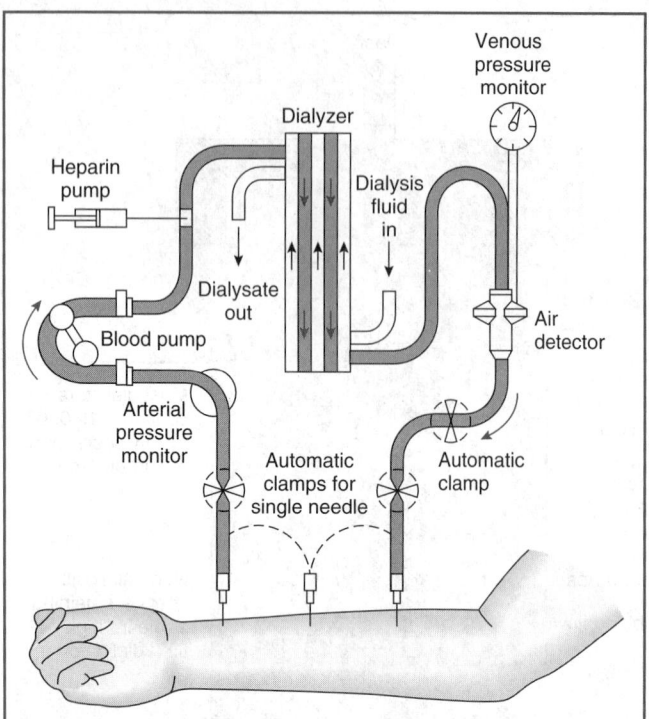

FIGURE 105–2 ■ Essential components of a dialysis delivery system, which, together with the dialyzer, makes up an "artificial kidney." (From Keshaviah PR, Shaldon S: Hemodialysis monitors and monitoring. *In* Drukker W, Parsons FM, Maher FJ [eds]: Replacement of Renal Function by Dialysis, 3rd ed. Boston, Martinus Nijhoff Publishers, 1988.)

dialysate. Hemodialysis uses blood pumps for ultrafiltration, whereas peritoneal dialysis uses the osmotic forces of high concentrations of glucose to remove water. This glucose load has the advantage of providing nutrition to patients but the disadvantage of occasionally leading to severe hyperglycemia and hypertriglyceridemia.

Using diffusion and ultrafiltration, nephrologists had made life without kidneys possible. Blood urea nitrogen (BUN) and creatinine levels could be corrected and the uremic toxins removed. Patients who ingested water and sodium in excess of their losses from residual kidney function could have them removed. Serum electrolytes could be kept normal, and death from hyperkalemia (a common event before dialysis) was almost never seen. Several problems remained, however, that the artificial kidney (by itself) did not correct. Anemia, bone disease, and nerve damage were not corrected and had to await further advances in knowledge. Several new clinical problems were seen—aluminum intoxication, accelerated atherosclerosis, acquired cystic disease, and dialysis amyloidosis. These will be covered later.

TYPES OF DIALYSIS. Dialysis can be performed for either acute or chronic renal failure and is done either by employing an artifi-

cial membrane system using extracorporeal blood (hemodialysis) or by using the peritoneal membrane (peritoneal dialysis). There are several types of hemodialysis (e.g., home, in-center) and peritoneal dialysis (Table 105–2). The ample assortment of types of dialysis suggests that no one form is superior. Hemodialysis is considered more efficient, and peritoneal dialysis is seen as simpler to deliver. Peritoneal dialysis can be learned easily by the patient, allowing the patient to have some control over therapy. Clearing toxins (especially small molecules) is more efficient with hemodialysis. With peak clearance rates (rates often greater than the normal kidney) spaced between long periods of no clearance, hemodialysis is less physiologic than the "smoother," although less efficient, clearing peritoneal dialysis. Moreover, peritoneal dialysis may be better at clearing larger molecules.

The vast majority (80%) of patients in the United States are treated with in-center hemodialysis. Home hemodialysis has decreased in popularity in recent years, even though most studies suggested that this form of dialysis had the best patient survival rates. Chronic ambulatory peritoneal dialysis (CAPD) has increased to nearly 12% of patients on chronic dialysis. Patients on peritoneal dialysis are slightly younger than those on hemodialysis. They have fewer co-morbid conditions. On the other hand, patients whose renal failure is due to diabetes mellitus often are placed on peritoneal dialysis because insulin delivery can be simplified by infusing it with the dialysate. There are no controlled trials that compare survival rates between hemodialysis and peritoneal dialysis. Patient selection for these two different forms of treatment is usually decided by special needs of the patient and the nephrologist's clinical judgment of which treatment will be best tolerated. There is more long-term experience with hemodialysis, and clearly, many patients who start peritoneal dialysis switch to hemodialysis before they finish a year of treatment. Nonetheless, CAPD currently is the fastest growing form of dialysis. Decisions based primarily on clinical judgment, of course, will result in differences of opinion about the relative merits of peritoneal and hemodialysis.

RECENT ADVANCES IN DIALYSIS. Advances in access to both the vascular circulation and the peritoneal cavity have been made in the past decade. Indeed, new medical industries have grown from these technical advances. Using arteriovenous (AV) fistulas is best for hemodialysis patients. It requires the nephrologist's skilled timing to have a functioning AV fistula placed at the proper time. If it is constructed (surgical connection of the radial artery to the forearm venous system) too soon, it may clot; if constructed too late, however, the patient may need dialysis before the fistula is ready to use. A good AV fistula may make the difference between long-term success and failure of dialysis. Using longer-lasting temporary access procedures (e.g., subclavian catheters) has helped make timing slightly easier. Artificial grafts (polytetrafluoroethylene, bovine) have been used with success when AV fistulas cannot be placed. Permanent peritoneal catheters also have advanced in construction. Those with double cuffs seem to provide the best protection against peritonitis. Tubing connectors (another new

Table 105–1 ■ COMPARISON OF TYPICAL MAKEUP OF DIALYSATE USED IN DIALYSIS

SOLUTES	HEMODIALYSIS (mEq/L)	PERITONEAL DIALYSIS (mEq/L)
Sodium	135	132
Potassium	0–4.0	0
Calcium	2.5–3.5	3.5
Magnesium	0.5–1.0	1.5
Chloride	100–119	102
Acetate or lactate	35–38 acetate	35–40 lactate
Bicarbonate	0	0
Dextrose	200 mg/dL	1.5% (1500 mg/dL) or 2.5% (2500 mg/dL) or 4.25% (4500 mg/dL)
Urea-creatinine-toxins	0	0

Table 105–2 ■ TYPES OF DIALYSIS IN CLINICAL PRACTICE

Hemodialysis ↓	Peritoneal Dialysis ↓	
Acute chronic ↓	Acute chronic ↓	} Two major forms of dialysis in clinical use
Home	Chronic ambulatory peritoneal dialysis—CAPD	
In-center for profit in-hospital	Chronic cycling peritoneal dialysis—CCPD Intermittent peritoneal dialysis—IPD	} Different subgroups of hemodialysis and peritoneal dialysis
More time efficient	More physiologic—fewer peaks and valleys in clearance	
Greater long-term clinical experience and follow-up		} Advantages
	Procedure simple to learn	

growth industry) also have reduced infections for the patient on peritoneal dialysis.

Replacing only the excretory functions of the kidney ignores the fact that the kidney also manufactures and adds substances to the systemic circulation. Thus the kidney plays a major role in blood and bone production, and lack of normal kidney function can lead to anemia and bone disease (see Parts XIII and XIX). Recently, the complication of anemia in dialysis patients has been nearly resolved by the development of recombinant human erythropoietin, and most dialysis patients now receive erythropoietin regularly. The quality of life for dialysis patients has improved as their anemias have diminished. Recent work suggests that correcting anemia also had an unexpected beneficial effect on neurologic problems in dialysis patients.

Nephrologists have advanced the knowledge of bone disease greatly in the past decade. Bone disease in dialysis patients is much better understood and relates in part to another product that is created (not excreted) by the kidney, 1,25-dihydroxyvitamin D (see Chapter 266). Impaired production of this vitamin increases the production of parathyroid hormone (PTH). Now, most patients can have secondary hyperparathyroidism controlled medically by supplementing 1,25-dihydroxyvitamin D (which results in decreases in PTH and increases in calcium absorption) and adjusting serum calcium and phosphate levels. The bone disease of renal failure, however, is not entirely due to secondary hyperparathyroidism. Aluminum poisoning (which may be due to trace quantities of aluminum in the dialysate and aluminum antacids) may be responsible for some portion of the bone disease. Bone biopsy has become a common procedure to assess the type and degree of bone disease in dialysis patients.

Newer, more efficient membranes have been made—"high-flux" and "high-efficiency" dialyzers. These newer membranes have allowed nephrologists to remove more urea and water in shorter time periods. High-flux membranes remove larger-molecule toxins more efficiently. The newer machines allow careful control of ultrafiltration and use of bicarbonate dialysis. Thus artificial kidneys now are more efficient in replacing the kidney's excretory and fluid-control functions. The failed kidney's inability to produce erythropoietin and 1,25-dihydroxyvitamin D has been overcome. Advances in vascular and peritoneal access have been dramatic.

BETTER TECHNOLOGY BUT DECLINING SURVIVAL. Despite these modern techniques, new drugs, and extra emphasis on urea kinetics, a rather worrisome trend toward decreased patient survival has been noted in the United States that has not been seen elsewhere. Convincing arguments have been made that the reason for this difference has to do (at least in part) with the method of financing dialysis in the United States and thus the amount of time that patients are dialyzed.

The federal program that finances dialysis grossly underestimated the numbers of patients and thus the cost of chronic dialysis. A program that was estimated to cost $100 million (at most) when first proposed now is estimated to cost $7 billion. To hold down expenditures of tax money, the cost of a dialysis procedure has not increased since 1972—it is the only medical procedure that has decreased in cost (nearly a 50% decrease when inflation is considered) over the past 15 years. Today, a dialysis procedure in the United States costs less than in a number of other countries. This cost consciousness has been responsible (in part) for two widely practiced procedures in the United States that are not seen elsewhere: (1) reuse of dialyzers and (2) shorter dialysis time with fewer, less experienced staff.

Most do not believe that reusing dialyzers has been harmful. Even without the cost savings, most nephrologists would favor reusing dialyzers to eliminate the so-called first-use syndrome. This is a syndrome of chest and back pain seen immediately after onset of dialysis with a new dialyzer. It has, on occasion, been more severe, with an anaphylactic type of clinical picture. This is rare, but it appears to be eliminated by reusing dialyzers. Nonetheless, reuse is not standard procedure in Europe and Japan.

Shorter dialysis has been correlated with decreasing reimbursement. Although efforts to maintain urea kinetics with high-efficiency dialysis have been instituted, it is possible that larger molecules (those more affected by time of treatment) are the more important measure of adequacy of dialysis and that the 20 to 25% longer times that patients spend on dialysis in Europe are responsible for better survival. In Japan, reimbursement for dialysis (which

is also higher than U.S. reimbursement) is linked to time of dialysis. If dialysis lasts less than 4 hours per treatment, reimbursement is decreased. In the United States, time of treatment averages 3 hours. Many people believe that the failure of some U.S. patients "to thrive on dialysis" is due to underdialysis. It is, of course, possible that all the difference seen in dialysis survival in the United States and other countries is due to patient selection. At any rate, decreasing patient survival rates have resulted in a re-examination of both dialysis prescription and the means of dialysis reimbursement in the United States.

NEW CLINICAL PROBLEMS UNCOVERED WITH LONG-TERM DIALYSIS. Nephrologists with large numbers of patients surviving on dialysis therapy have called attention to four disease concepts that were previously unknown. Dialysis dementia, or aluminum intoxication, was seen in nearly epidemic proportions in some dialysis units. Its pathogenesis was debated at first, but now, all agree that both aluminum from the dialysate and that used for phosphate binders are responsible. The syndrome usually occurs in patients who have been on dialysis for a number of years. It is characterized by intermittent speech disturbance, stuttering, personality changes, seizures, myoclonus, and auditory and visual hallucinations. The symptoms progress until patients become mute and unable to perform useful motions—followed by coma and death. Patients dying of dialysis dementia were found to have elevated levels of brain aluminum. Epidemiologic studies demonstrated that those dialysis units with high rates of dialysis dementia also had high concentrations of aluminum in the water used for their dialysate. Removing aluminum using deionizers and reverse-osmosis devices from dialysate water halted dialysis dementia. Understanding that dialysis dementia is caused by aluminum intoxication has decreased the incidence in patients. Nonetheless, it is seen occasionally in dialysis units, and aluminum bone disease (see Chapter 266) remains a common complication.

Myocardial infarction and cerebrovascular accidents account for nearly 50% of deaths in dialysis patients. This rate and the age of deaths are strikingly different from those of the general population. Some nephrologists have even suggested that chronic dialysis *per se* may cause a syndrome of "accelerated atherosclerosis." Hypertension, which is common in dialysis patients, is a major risk factor for cardiac problems. Left ventricular hypertrophy is also common and can lead to cardiac arrhythmias. Anemia, increased cardiac preload, and AV fistulas all lead to increased cardiac output that may contribute to left ventricular hypertrophy. Abnormal lipid metabolism also has been incriminated (heparin may lead to the high rates of hypertriglyceridemia seen in dialysis patients) as increasing cardiac risks. Hyperparathyroidism may induce vascular calcification. Acetate in the dialysate may be toxic to the myocardium. All these factors then might contribute to the high rate of cardiac mortality seen in dialysis. On the other hand, it has been suggested that the dialysis procedure may not have any deleterious effects on atherosclerosis but that chronic renal disease results in patients arriving at dialysis settings with well-established cardiac and cerebrovascular disease. The kidney transplantation experience (of high mortality from the same vascular events) supports this view.

Although it occurs with chronic renal failure (before dialysis), acquired cystic disease was first noted in long-term dialysis patients. The number of patients who have cysts develop in their kidneys increases with time on dialysis and total time of uremia. The presence of at least four cysts in each native kidney is usually used to diagnose acquired cystic kidney disease. It is easily differentiated from polycystic kidney disease because the kidneys are small and there is no family history of cystic disease. Unlike polycystic kidney disease, the cysts are limited to the kidneys. The clinical importance of this new entity is that some have reported that 2 to 10% of patients will have malignant tumors develop in the acquired cysts. On the other hand, death from renal malignancies does not appear to be greater for dialysis patients than for the non-dialysis population. There remains controversy about the need to screen for the problem of acquired cystic disease.

The fourth new complication is hemodialysis-related amyloidosis. β_2-Microglobulin is an amyloid material that becomes deposited in the bones and joints of long-term dialysis patients. It can cause carpal tunnel syndrome and the severe problem of erosive spondyloarthropathy. Amyloidosis is becoming an increasingly difficult

Table 105–3 ■ DIALYSIS COMPLICATIONS

PERITONEAL DIALYSIS	HEMODIALYSIS
Peritonitis	Hypotension
Abdominal hernias	Hypoxia
Diminished peritoneal ultrafiltration	Nausea, vomiting, and headache
Hyperglycemia	Air embolism
Protein malnutrition	Trace metal intoxication

COMPLICATIONS COMMON TO BOTH TYPES OF DIALYSIS
Hepatitis, infection, osteodystrophy, heart disease

problem for long-surviving patients on hemodialysis—by 20 years on dialysis, the majority of patients have evidence of amyloidosis (see Chapter 297).

Along with the new clinical problems that long-term survival of patients with end-stage renal disease (ESRD) on dialysis has created, both hemodialysis and peritoneal dialysis have their own set of specific complications and share a set of long-term complications that are quite similar (Table 105–3). It is interesting that the long-term difficulties of both forms of dialysis and of long-surviving transplant patients are similar, involving vascular disease and infections.

Ahmad S, Blagg CR, Scribner BH: Center and home chronic hemodialysis. *In* Schrier RW, Gottschalk CW (eds): Diseases of the Kidney, 5th ed. Boston, Little, Brown 1993, p 3031. *This is an in-depth chapter written by authors who were responsible for many of the clinical successes of dialysis.*

Nuhad I, Hakim RM, Oreopoulos DG, et al: Renal replacement therapies in the elderly: I. Hemodialysis and chronic peritoneal dialysis. Am J Kidney Dis 22:759, 1993. *This report is an in-depth review of dialysis and the changes in the demographics of the end-stage population in the United States.*

United States Renal Data System. USRDS 1993 Annual Data Report. Bethesda, MD, U.S. Department of Health and Human Services, National Institutes of Health, National Institute of Diabetes and Digestive and Kidney Diseases, August 1993. *This is the best source of data concerning dialysis outcome available in the United States.*

105.2 Renal Transplantation

In the 1920s, Alexis Carrel developed the technique of vascular anastomoses. This momentous surgical breakthrough made possible David Hume's and Joseph Murray's human allograft attempts in the early 1950s. Similarly, Willem Kolff fashioned dialysis techniques and machinery that set the stage for George Thorn's group at Harvard Medical School to advance clinical dialysis to a viable and familiar therapy. Both accomplishments eventually joined, with synergistic results, to effect truly dramatic changes in managing chronic renal disease.

Those involved in other forms of organ transplantation envy the advantages produced by combining dialysis techniques with allograft transplantation. Because of the combination of these two effective renal replacement therapies, the volume of kidney transplant operations is vastly greater than that of other transplantation procedures. Patients can freely move back and forth between dialysis and transplantation so that life does not depend on only one form of treatment. Kidney transplantation leads the field of organ replacement therapies by a large and growing margin.

Other advances in knowledge flow from these milestone developments. Peter Medawar's description of second-set reactions and his insights into cellular immunology were pre-eminent advances in thinking. Both ideas are still actively advancing our understanding of human life. The close collaboration of pharmaceutical companies and clinical researchers resulted in azathioprine, which made kidney transplantation possible in non-related individuals.

IMMUNOLOGIC ASPECTS OF KIDNEY TRANSPLANTATION. In kidney transplantation, the translation of understanding of the human immune system into clear-cut clinical advances is dramatic. Small lymphocytes are central to the problem of kidney allograft rejection. Both T and B lymphocytes are important players in kidney allograft rejection. B lymphocytes make circulating antibodies. The T lymphocyte, however, is critical. Acute rejection depends on the presence of T lymphocytes.

T lymphocytes constitute a heterogeneous group (see Chapter 270): helper, suppressor, cytotoxic, and natural-killer (NK) T lym-

phocytes are recognized by the presence of characteristic antigens on their cell membranes. The helper T lymphocyte is required for the rejection process. It participates in initial recognition of foreign antigen on transplanted tissue. Foreign antigens stimulate the T helper lymphocyte to release lymphokines that produce both growth and differentiation of other T and B lymphocytes.

Newly developed immunosuppressive agents target T lymphocytes and the lymphokines they produce. These new agents may be both more potent and more specific than those used in the past. Further understanding of the methods by which foreign antigens are presented to lymphocytes and the lymphokine communication network (in which the T helper cell is central) will yield more specific immunosuppression.

The major histocompatibility complex (MHC) (see Chapter 278), which in humans is on chromosome 6, codes for two classes of antigens (class I [A, B, and C] and class II [D, DR, DQ, DP, and DO]) on cell membranes. Inheritance of these cell antigen markers is co-dominant. Each parent transmits one set of HLA antigens (haplotype) to his or her child. Nearly all cells, except red blood cells, express class I antigens, whereas B lymphocytes, monocytes, and endothelial cells express class II antigens. These antigens are pivotal in the rejection process.

Transplantation usually succeeds if all known class I and class II antigens between donor and recipient are identical. Unfortunately, from a matching perspective, the MHC is the most polymorphic coding system known in human biology. Most donors and recipients cannot be matched perfectly for MHC-coded antigens unless the organ comes from a close family member. Figure 105–3 shows that siblings of a given patient with end-stage renal disease (ESRD) may be either two-haplotype matches (25% likelihood), one-haplotype matches (50% likelihood), or zero-haplotype matches (25% likelihood). True parents are usually a one-haplotype match. As noted in Figure 105–3, ABO blood groups also must be compatible to ensure successful transplantation.

In animals and human recipients of kidney allografts, matching for both class I and class II antigens correlates with successful graft outcomes. The source of most human kidney transplants, however, is a cadaveric donor (a donor who has died but whose kidneys are still viable). Finding a good HLA match is more difficult from cadavers than from blood relatives. Although retrospective analysis of cadaveric transplantation data shows the benefit of class I and class II matching, the benefit is not as dramatic as for kidneys from relatives. Recently, new methods of identifying cell antigens using "DNA typing" have shown that the previous typing was not as accurate as thought.

Transplantation centers in the United States currently follow a policy of mandatory sharing of six-antigen (both class I and class II) matches for cadaveric kidneys. Organ banks consider other factors besides HLA match (e.g., the patient's age and length of time on a waiting list) in distributing cadaveric kidneys. Living-unrelated donors have been used at an increasing rate in the United States and seem to have better outcomes than cadaveric donors despite poor HLA matching.

Unquestionably important for both living-related transplantation and cadaveric transplantation is the "crossmatch" test. Tissue-typing laboratories perform this test before all kidney transplant operations. Technicians incubate leukocytes from the potential donor (living-related or cadaveric) with serum from the potential recipient and serum complement. If the serum of the recipient destroys the membranes of the leukocyte of the potential donor, the laboratory reports the test as positive.

The surgeon usually cancels the transplant operation if the cross match is positive. Such a result signifies circulating antibodies against the HLA antigens. A positive crossmatch predicts nearly immediate and severe ("hyperacute") allograft rejection if the transplant is done. Investigators are testing modifications of the cross matching procedure to find a more sensitive yet more specific test. The current tests, however, have all but eliminated hyperacute rejections. More sensitive tests could decrease other types of early rejection ("accelerated rejections").

Currently, many patients on waiting lists for kidney transplants have developed broad anti-HLA sensitization. Exposure to blood transfusions, failed previous transplants, or pregnancy causes such sensitization to HLA antigens. Nearly one third of patients awaiting transplantation fall into this "highly sensitized," difficult-to-transplant category. Such patients benefit from receiving the best HLA antigen match possible.

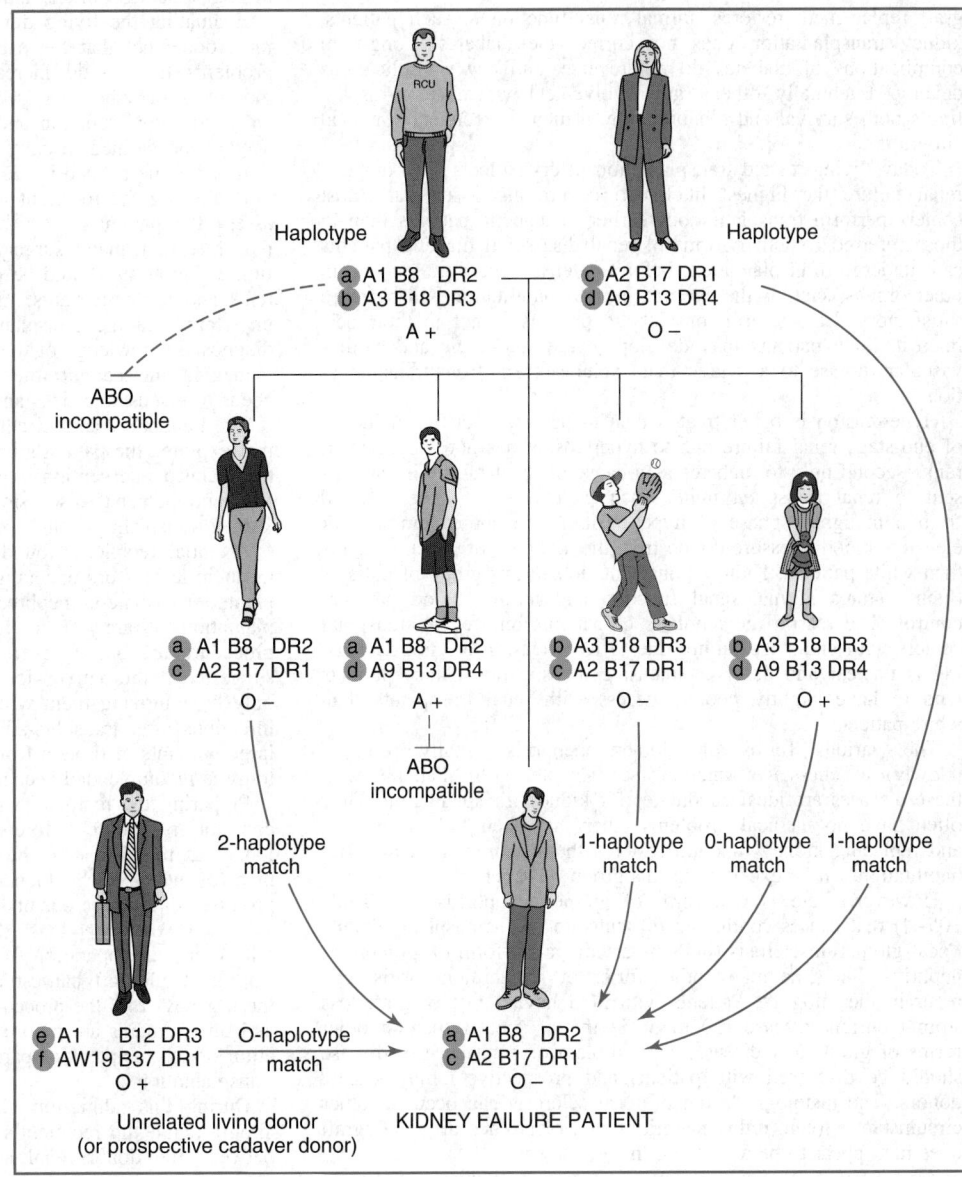

FIGURE 105–3 ■ Family tree of HLA genotypes and unrelated HLA genotype.

Physicians have tried other strategies such as plasmapheresis and extracorporeal immunoadsorption to find a suitable method of overcoming the problem of circulating preformed antibodies. These trials offer promise but are not yet established practice. The more common use of erythropoietin in patients awaiting transplantation will reduce the exposure to blood transfusions. Introducing this new therapy to dialysis promises to decrease the rate of development and degree of circulating antibodies in patients with ESRD.

INDICATIONS FOR KIDNEY TRANSPLANTATION. The most common diseases that result in referring patients for transplantation are (1) diabetes mellitus with renal failure, (2) hypertensive renal disease, and (3) glomerulonephritis. These three causes of ESRD account for nearly 75% of candidates.

No specific cause of intrinsic and irreversible renal failure is considered a contraindication to kidney transplantation. Nonetheless, all patients still should have reversible causes of renal dysfunction excluded (e.g., incomplete obstruction) before considering renal replacement therapy. Most patients undergo a period of chronic dialysis before receiving an allograft. Table 105–4 lists select diseases that can cause renal failure and need special consideration before choosing renal transplantation as a therapy. The listed diseases are not contraindications for transplantation; yet the outcome may be less satisfactory for patients with these diseases as compared with other renal diseases.

Patients with renal failure induced by diabetes (Kimmelstiel-Wilson disease) make up the greatest population of patients cur-

rently referred for transplantation. In the past such patients were not routinely considered for kidney transplantation, but today many nephrologists consider this the treatment of choice. The change in medical practice for this condition has resulted in a major extension of the life expectancy of patients whose kidneys fail from diabetes.

The long-term outcome for patients with diabetes is less likely to result in full rehabilitation than for patients with forms of renal disease that do not have other organ involvement. Although allo-

Table 105–4 ■ FACTORS LIMITING SUCCESS OF RENAL TRANSPLANTATION IN CERTAIN DISEASES

DISEASE	COMMENT
Hemolytic uremic syndrome	Disease can recur and cause graft failure rapidly; cyclosporine may increase the risk of recurrence.
Sickle cell disease	Improved hematocrit can result in increased incidence of sickle crises.
Scleroderma	Long-term vascular and gastrointestinal problems of scleroderma can limit rehabilitation.
Oxalosis	Recurrence of stone disease can be severe.
Cystinosis and Fabry's disease	Disease activity continues.
Focal glomerulosclerosis	Graft loss from recurrence is common.

graft replacement restores normal renal function to such patients, kidney transplantation does not correct the diabetes. Long-term complications of diabetes do not reverse, and new complications develop. Eventually, other organ involvement with diabetic disease limits both survival and rehabilitation in diabetic recipients of renal allografts.

Today, living-related transplantation offers patients with diabetic renal failure the highest likelihood of prolonged survival. Most centers perform transplantations earlier in diabetic patients than in those referred for other forms of renal disease. If diabetic patients can undergo transplantation before extensive damage occurs in other organs, such as the eye and heart, rehabilitation will be more satisfactory. Late referral of diabetic patients is not in their best interest. Such patients may develop severe neurologic and cardiovascular disease to a degree that excludes them from transplantation.

Hypertension is better treated than in the past, yet the incidence of end-stage renal failure due to hypertension has not decreased. It ranks second only to diabetes as a cause of renal failure in patients sent to renal transplant units. Such patients often have suffered from a malignant phase of hypertension. It is more common for elevated blood pressure to destroy the kidneys of black patients than white patients. Kidney transplantation in this group of patients often restores normal renal function and normal blood pressure control. The reason the numbers of patients referred to transplant centers with end-stage failure due to hypertension are not decreasing is unclear and deserves intensive investigation. Black patients tend to have slightly poorer success with renal transplants than white patients.

The various forms of glomerulonephritis usually progress (slowly) to end-stage function (see Chapter 106). Patients with these diseases are ideal candidates for kidney transplantation. They often have no medical problems other than their kidney disease, and replacing kidney function restores them to normal health. Rehabilitation can be excellent in this group of patients.

However, there is one form of glomerulonephritis (see Table 105–4) that causes continuing difficulty in renal transplant centers. Focal glomerulosclerosis (FGS) is an idiopathic form of glomerulonephritis that (like many other forms of glomerulonephritis) can recur in the allograft. Patients with FGS have a rate of graft loss from recurrent disease (20 to 30%) that is greater than in other forms of glomerular disease. The problem of recurrence of disease should be discussed with patients and prospective family kidney donors. The histologic lesion of focal sclerosis can occur in other circumstances (e.g., reflux nephritis), and recurrence in the allograft does not appear to be a problem in such cases.

Age is never an absolute contraindication for kidney transplantation. Although infants have had successful transplantations, most centers maintain infants on dialysis until body size is increased to 10 to 20 kg. Older patients are becoming more numerous in transplant clinics. Older age (> 65 years) never precludes transplantation, but it increases the risk of complications. Transplant centers usually encourage older patients who have multiple medical problems (rather than isolated kidney failure) to remain on dialysis. On both ends of the age spectrum, however, transplantation is becoming more common.

Malignancy is considered a contraindication for kidney transplantation, as is severe atherosclerotic or pulmonary disease. Patients with active liver disease are also usually excluded. Both hepatitis B and C can result in eventual liver failure in some patients after transplantation. How best to screen patients infected with these agents and who to avoid transplanting are problems currently under active investigation. Infection with the human immunodeficiency virus is a relative contraindication. Case reports suggest that such patients progress more rapidly from carrier status to clinical acquired immunodeficiency syndrome when given immunosuppressive therapy. Social circumstances (inability to take medications or arrange follow-up) also can make kidney transplantation an impossibility.

EVALUATING THE DONOR AND RECIPIENT OF THE KIDNEY TRANSPLANT. The transplant team that will perform the surgery and follow-up should evaluate the donor (living-related) and potential recipient of the transplant. This is best done at the transplant center before the actual transplantation date. The evaluation team

usually includes a transplant surgeon, nephrologist, transplant nurse, urologist, social worker, and psychiatrist.

Evaluating the living donor focuses on three issues. Physicians must document that the patient does not have significant medical problems that would increase the risk of surgery. The donor's motives should be appraised to ensure that they are altruistic. Finally, the renal function and anatomy of the donor's renal arteries need to be defined, usually with a renal arteriogram. This evaluation is best performed in the hospital.

Evaluating the recipient also has three goals. Physicians should assess the patient's overall medical status, because the recipient may face both major surgery and potent immunosuppression in the future. Emphasis should be placed on the recipient's cardiovascular risks and urologic status. The recipient's original disease often is uncertain, and the transplant center should attempt to clarify the diagnosis. Knowledge of the original kidney disease is important in managing the patient after the transplant. Finally, the recipient needs to discuss the risks and benefits of transplantation surgery.

The patient's social circumstances need evaluation. A discussion that explores the patient's understanding of the disease process and the planned intervention is part of the evaluation. Both audiovisual aids and personal discussions with nurses, physicians, and other kidney transplant patients are key to preparing the patient.

Potential recipients found to have correctable cardiovascular or urologic lesions are encouraged to have them repaired before transplantation. Bilateral nephrectomy of native kidneys before transplantation is rarely done. In the past, this was a more common procedure to control severe hypertension. A nephrectomy is also suggested if the native kidneys are infected in such a fashion that only by removing them will the patient be protected from serious infections after transplantation. Occasionally, patients excrete such large amounts of protein from diseased native kidneys that nephrectomy is recommended because of protein malnutrition.

Preparing the recipient with deliberate blood transfusions was a common procedure before routine use of cyclosporine. It is no longer as popular as in the past. An understanding of the mechanism by which such blood transfusions altered rejection, however, promises to increase our understanding of immune responses.

THE ADMISSION FOR KIDNEY TRANSPLANTATION. Cadaveric transplant operations are more "planned" than in the past. Improved allograft harvesting has removed some (but not all) of the urgency from the procedure. It is not elective surgery, however, and time remains an important factor. The pretransplantation evaluation of the recipient prepares the patient for the actual day of the transplantation.

During this admission, the transplant surgeon places a kidney allograft into the recipient's iliac fossa. An anastomosis is created between the donor renal artery and the hypogastric artery. The surgeon also must connect the donor renal vein to the iliac vein and implant the ureter to the recipient's bladder. These three connections all have variations, and all need skillful surgical technique.

On return from the operating room, three issues face the patient. If the kidney is not working immediately ("immediate non-function"), the reasons need to be identified. If the kidney is working, careful observation for possible rejection is begun. In either case, a new immunosuppressive regimen starts.

Immediate non-function of the allograft is less common with improvement of techniques for procurement and storage. It is due, most often, to an acute tubular necrosis (ATN)-like syndrome in which there is reversible ischemic damage to the allograft that will heal, given time. Evidence suggests that this phenomenon, although similar to classic ATN, differs in that the immune system plays a role.

Obstruction, vascular thrombosis, and ureteral compression from hematoma should be considered in cases of primary non-function. Renal scans and ultrasound tests, as well as the patience of the managing physician, are indicated. Occasionally, immediate return to the operating room is required. Most patients with immediate non-function, however, have reversible renal impairment that does not require surgical intervention.

Allografts that work immediately after releasing the vascular clamps engender immediate optimism. Observation is key in the postoperative management. It is usually in the first 3 months after transplantation that reversible acute rejections occur. Many of these rejections will occur during the initial hospital stay. All patients should have daily assessment of renal function, and when physicians notice impairment, a rapid diagnosis of cause (rejection versus other causes) is in order. Despite pressures to cut costs, early discharge is not in the best interest of the kidney transplant patient.

During the first hospital stay, patients are given potent immunosuppressive agents. Immunosuppressive regimens remained stable from the 1960s through the early 1980s. Azathioprine and prednisone were the two drugs used. Physicians became experienced with these two agents and with their predictable complications.

The Food and Drug Administration (FDA) approved cyclosporine in 1983. Since then, the transplant community has developed a frenzy for new and different immunosuppressive protocols. Transplant centers often change to new protocols before research groups test the older protocols with controlled, randomized trials. Nonetheless, as transplant groups have experimented with new and different immunosuppressive agents, results have improved markedly over the results seen in previous years. However, changes other than the new drugs (e.g., flow cytometry) may have added to improved allograft survival.

Currently, many centers in the United States use sequential or "induction" therapy. Initially, either antilymphocyte globulin (ALG) or monoclonal antibody (OKT3) is given as the primary immunosuppressant agent. These anti-T lymphocyte agents are continued until the allograft functions well. Then, cyclosporine, azathioprine, and prednisone are added, and ALG or OKT3 is discontinued shortly thereafter. Recently, humanized anti–T cell agents have been approved by the U.S. Food and Drug Administration and may increase use of "induction" therapy. They also hold the promise of less toxicity than OKT3. Other groups begin with a regimen of cyclosporine, azathioprine, and prednisone immediately preceding the transplant operation ("triple-drug therapy"). Some groups believe that a combination of cyclosporine and prednisone or cyclosporine alone is adequate therapy.

Adding cyclosporine and routinely using anti–T lymphocyte agents, although credited with improved allograft success rates, makes management more complex. Cyclosporine can result in impaired renal function that is difficult to distinguish from rejection.

Cyclosporine has revolutionized organ transplantation. Transplant groups have achieved a 10 to 15% improvement in initial and long-term allograft survival rates with cyclosporine. Some investigators believe that the added immunosuppression of this agent overcomes the risks of rejection with poorly matched allografts. Others suggest that preparing recipients with pretransplant blood transfusions is no longer necessary.

Unfortunately, one of cyclosporine's major side effects is nephrotoxicity. Investigators have shown acute, "reversible," and chronic kidney damage. Cyclosporine slows recovery from ATN and potentiates nephrotoxicity due to other substances. The drug is difficult to monitor, and clinical toxicity is common even in experienced hands. Besides nephrotoxicity, cyclosporine commonly causes tremor, palmar and plantar paresthesia, hyperglycemia, hepatotoxicity, hypertrichosis, gingival hypertrophy, and hyperkalemia.

Tracolimus impairs the immune system in a manner that is similar to that of cyclosporine, but it has a side-effect profile that is different from cyclosporine. The availability of two interleukin-2 inhibitors with different side-effect profiles is a major advantage for transplant physicians and the patients.

Mycophenolic acid has replaced azathioprine in many units and is believed to be less toxic and more immunosuppressive. Acute rejection rates have decreased dramatically with this addition and the addition of a new formulation of cyclosporine that gives better absorption.

OUTPATIENT FOLLOW-UP. If the transplant admission is uncomplicated, it is possible for patients to be discharged as early as a week after surgery. Unless arrangements can be made for daily outpatient visits after discharge, however, most centers keep patients in the hospital for longer periods. Complications can lengthen this first admission to months. Geography, financial resources of patients, facilities of the center, and clinical judgment of physicians involved result in initial hospital stays that vary markedly in length. Nonetheless, whether patients are in the hospital or are outpatients, the two major problems faced are infection and rejection.

Two forms of rejection have been alluded to previously: hyperacute rejection and accelerated rejection. Both, by definition, occur before the end of the first week. Hyperacute rejection is rare with current crossmatch techniques. Accelerated rejections are less well understood, are more common, and often do not respond to therapy. More sensitive crossmatch techniques might decrease the frequency of accelerated rejections.

Acute and chronic rejections are more common. These episodes usually occur after the first week and can occur at any time, even years after the transplant. Mediated by T lymphocytes, such rejections are often associated with marked cellular infiltration of the allograft with edema. Kidney vascular lesions also occur and suggest a poor prognosis.

Most acute rejection episodes, if diagnosed early, will respond to therapy with increased dosages of immunosuppressive agents. Diagnosis is suggested by a sudden impairment of function. Confirmation of acute rejection is obtained with renal scans and allograft biopsies.

Chronic rejection is a phenomenon less well understood than acute rejection. Most cadaveric allografts eventually show histologic changes of rejection. These changes are vascular and are similar to the histology of nephrosclerosis. Eventually, the allograft develops fibrosis and glomerular lesions that appear secondary to ischemia. There is neither a good understanding of chronic rejection nor an accepted effective therapy.

Serial "flowsheet" measurements of serum creatinine concentration reveal a gradual trend for slow but progressive impairment of allograft function. The renal scan reveals a more marked loss of renal blood flow than of glomerular filtration rate (GFR), and renal biopsy reveals fibrosis and vascular narrowing. Patients are generally asymptomatic. Recurrence of original kidney disease and cyclosporine toxicity are two other causes of allograft impairment that can mimic chronic rejection.

Renal scans and isotope measurements of renal blood flow (^{131}I-orthoiodohippurate) and GFR (^{99m}Tc-diethylenetriamine) are used frequently to provide additional assessment of renal function. Ultrasound has proven useful to visualize the structure of the allograft and to rule out obstruction. Arteriography of the transplant renal artery is useful to diagnose stenosis. Although an invasive procedure, an arteriogram of the allograft also can provide information about the small vessels of the allograft in a more global fashion than renal biopsy. Biopsy of the allograft is also an invasive procedure. Transplant physicians believe that it gives the most useful assessment of the allograft and helps differentiate the causes of allograft dysfunction. When other clinical assessment leaves considerable doubt in the mind of the managing physician concerning the cause of impaired function, a biopsy is indicated.

Infections during the first few weeks after transplantation cause fever and can impair allograft function. They may be confused with rejection. Wound, intravenous line, and catheter-related infections are common and not usually due to opportunistic organisms when they occur within a few weeks of transplantation.

Opportunistic infections usually occur a month or more after the transplant operation. Whereas *Aspergillus, Nocardia,* and *Toxoplasma* were once common, newer immunosuppressive protocols have resulted in a change in the spectrum of opportunistic infections. Viral infections, especially cytomegalovirus, have become dominant. Many investigators believe this is a result of using more specific anti–T lymphocyte preparations, such as OKT3. Infection with cytomegalovirus can be asymptomatic or can be so severe as to cause coma and death. Fortunately, most of these infections after transplantation, characterized by spiking fevers, leukopenia, and general malaise, last only 1 to 2 weeks and then resolve without sequelae.

Immunosuppressed kidney transplant patients believed to be infected should be hospitalized and aggressively managed. Infections in this group are the leading early cause of mortality, and aggressive management can reverse the process without need of sacrificing the allograft.

LONG-TERM FOLLOW-UP. Long-term immunosuppression is surprisingly well tolerated by most kidney transplant recipients. Nonetheless, it is this therapy that accounts for most of the posttransplant morbidity and mortality. Vascular disease, infections, malignancy, and chronic liver disease pose the most serious problems for recipients of kidney transplants. Immunosuppressive agents either cause or aggravate these four medical problems. Table 105–5 lists some of the more common medical problems that are seen in kidney transplant clinics.

Table 105–5 ■ MEDICAL COMPLICATIONS AFTER KIDNEY TRANSPLANTATION

Cardiovascular Events
Myocardial infarction
Cerebrovascular accident
Hypertension
Stenosis of transplant renal artery
Native kidney–induced
Drug-induced
Renal impairment of the allograft
Malignancies
Skin carcinomas
Lymphomas
Erythrocytosis
Induced by native kidneys (?)
Thromboembolic disease
Bone Disease
Osteoporosis
Aseptic necrosis
Persistent hyperparathyroidism
Infections
Listeria monocytogenes
Pneumocystis carinii
Cryptococcus
Aspergillus
Nocardia
Toxoplasma
Mycobacterium
Legionella pneumophila
Cytomegalovirus (CMV)
Herpes simplex virus (HSV)
Varicella-zoster virus (VZV)
Hepatitis viruses
Papovaviruses
Human immunodeficiency virus (HIV)
Epstein-Barr virus (EBV)
Gastrointestinal Problems
Peptic ulcer
Pancreatitis
Diverticulitis
Hepatitis
Glucocorticoid-induced Complications
Obesity
Cataracts
Hyperglycemia
Myopathy
Endocrine and Metabolic Disorders
Secondary hyperparathyroidism
Proximal and distal types of renal tubular acidosis
Asymptomatic hyperuricemia and gout
Mild hyperkalemia
Glycosuria without an increased serum glucose concentration
Hypophosphatemia
Miscellaneous
Idiopathic polyarthritides
Hirsutism
Lymphocele
Warts
Psychiatric affective disorders

Like the general population, kidney transplant patients are most likely to die of atherosclerotic vascular disease. Kidney transplant patients, however, die of myocardial infarctions and cerebrovascular accidents at an earlier age. The reason for this precocious onset of vascular disease is not understood.

Kidney transplant patients experience a high incidence of hypertension, which is multifactorial. Some immunosuppressive drugs (cyclosporine and prednisone) can cause hypertension, as does kidney disease. Even if the allograft is normal, the diseased native kidneys can maintain elevated blood pressure. Stenosis of the artery of the transplanted kidney is another cause of such hypertension. Abnormal lipid profiles in kidney transplant patients are a risk factor for atherosclerotic death. These abnormal lipid patterns are believed to be an effect of the immunosuppressive drugs. Besides hypertension and abnormal lipid profiles, there is convincing evidence that renal transplant patients usually have vascular disease even before the transplant. This vascular disease is associated with their chronic renal failure.

Most successful recipients of renal transplants enjoy a quality of life superior to that achieved on dialysis. Women frequently give birth after transplantation, and men can father children. It is unusual for patients with successful transplants not to return to employment. Many return to a lifestyle similar to that preceding the onset of kidney disease. On the other hand, the experience of chronic disease, frequent hospitalizations, disability financing, and fear of allograft failure with long-term complications of transplant immunosuppression limit full rehabilitation for some patients.

In the United States in 1995, the average 1-year allograft survival rate was 88% for recipients of cadaveric kidneys. This is a remarkable advance compared with survival rates of 50% for cadaveric kidneys just a few years ago. Mortality and morbidity continue to decrease as allograft survival rates increase. It seems likely that even these rates of success will improve in the near future.

Success can create problems. The number of patients on waiting lists for kidney transplantation is growing faster than the number of transplant operations that are possible. The shortage of donor kidneys is the most consequential limitation of kidney transplantation.

Alexander JW: The cutting edge: A look to the future of transplantation. Transplantation 49:237, 1990. *A review of the growth of kidney transplantation and predictions about future growth.*
Class FHJ, van Rood JJ: The hyperimmunized patient: From sensitization toward treatment. Transplant Int 1:53, 1988. *The reasons that patients develop antibodies against HLA antigens and current strategies for dealing with this problem are reviewed.*
Combined Report on Regular Dialysis and Transplantation in Europe. XIX, 1988. Nephrology Dialysis Trans 4(Suppl 4):5, 1989. *A review of recent trends in immunosuppressive regimens in Europe.*
Kahan BD: Cyclosporine. N Engl J Med 321:1725. 1989. *A detailed description of cyclosporine from pharmacology to future prospects.*
Shapiro ME, Reed MH, Strom TB, et al: The role of a primate model of renal transplantation in the development of new monoclonal antibodies. Am J Kidney Dis 14(Suppl 2):58. 1989. *A brief description of testing of new monoclonal antibodies.*

106 GLOMERULAR DISORDERS

Gerald B. Appel

Glomerular diseases (see Color Plate 4*A* to *I*) affect many millions of persons in the United States and worldwide. By 1998 in the United States more than 280,000 persons were in end-stage renal disease (ESRD) programs, largely as a result of renal involvement by glomerular diseases. Diabetic renal damage alone affects millions of persons and is the major cause of ESRD in the United States, with an annual cost to the government of billions of dollars. Worldwide, glomerular diseases associated with infectious agents such as malaria and schistosomiasis are major health problems. In both the United States and elsewhere the emergence of glomerular diseases linked to viral causes, such as human immunodeficiency virus (HIV) and hepatitis B and C, has focused new attention on the patterns and mechanisms of glomerular injury. The manifestations of glomerular injury range from asymptomatic microhematuria and albuminuria to abrupt oliguric renal failure. Some patients develop massive fluid retention with peripheral and periorbital edema as presenting symptoms and signs of glomerular damage, whereas still others present only with the slow insidious signs and symptoms of chronic renal failure.

The mechanisms of the glomerular injury are quite varied. Although certain common mechanisms may underlie the hematuria and proteinuria (e.g., loss of the glomerular charge barrier), the nature of the processes initiating this damage differs. In some glomerular disorders, such as diabetes and amyloidosis, there are structural and biochemical alterations of the glomerular capillary wall. In others, there is immune-mediated renal injury, whether through deposition of circulating immune complexes, through localization of anti–glomerular basement membrane (GBM) antibodies, or by other mechanisms.

The Normal Glomerulus (see also Chapters 100 and 101)

Each glomerulus, the basic filtering unit of the kidney, consists of a tuft of anastomosing capillaries formed by the branchings of the afferent arteriole. Approximately 1 million glomeruli comprise about 5% of the kidney weight and provide almost 2 square meters of glomerular capillary filtering surface. The GBM provides both a size- and charge-selective barrier to the passage of circulating macromolecules.

Histopathologic Terms

Renal processes involving all glomeruli are called *diffuse* or *generalized;* if only some glomeruli are involved, the process is called *focal.* When dealing with the individual glomerulus, a process is *global* if the whole glomerular tuft is involved and *segmental* if only part of the glomerulus is involved. The modifying terms *proliferative, sclerosing,* and *necrotizing* are often used (e.g., focal and segmental glomerulosclerosis; diffuse global proliferative lupus nephritis). Extracapillary proliferation or crescent formation is caused by the accumulations of macrophages, fibroblasts, proliferating epithelial cells, and fibrin within Bowman's space. In general, crescent formation in any form of glomerular damage conveys a serious prognosis.

Clinical Manifestations of Glomerular Diseases

Several findings indicate the presence of a glomerular origin of any parenchymal renal disease. They include erythrocyte casts and/or dysmorphic erythrocytes in the urinary sediment and the presence of large amounts of albuminuria. Urinary excretion of more than 500 to 1000 erythrocytes per milliliter is abnormal, and dysmorphic erythrocytes deformed in passage through the glomerular capillary wall and tubules indicate glomerular damage. Red blood cell casts, formed when erythrocytes pass the glomerular capillary barrier and become enmeshed in a proteinaceous matrix in the lumen of the tubules, are indicative of glomerular disease.

In a normal person, the urinary excretion of albumin is less than 50 mg/day. Although increases in urinary protein excretion may come from the filtration of abnormal circulating proteins (e.g., light chains in multiple myeloma) or from the deficient proximal tubular reabsorption of normal filtered small-molecular-weight proteins (e.g., β_2-microglobulin), the most common cause of proteinuria, and specifically albuminuria, is glomerular injury. Proteinuria associated with glomerular disease may range from several hundred milligrams to more than 30 g daily. In some diseases, such as minimal change nephrotic syndrome, albumin is the predominant protein found in the urine. In others, such as focal sclerosing glomerulonephritis and diabetes, the proteinuria, although still largely composed of albumin, contains many larger molecular weight proteins as well and is said to be *non-selective.*

THE NEPHROTIC SYNDROME

The nephrotic syndrome is classically defined by albuminuria in amounts of more than 3 to 3.5 g/day accompanied by hypoalbuminemia, edema, and hyperlipidemia. In practice, many clinicians refer to "nephrotic range" proteinuria regardless of whether their patients have the other manifestations of the full syndrome because the latter are consequences of the proteinuria.

Hypoalbuminemia is partly a consequence of urinary protein loss. It is also due to the catabolism of filtered albumin by the proximal tubule as well as to redistribution of albumin within the body. This, in part, accounts for the inexact relationship between urinary protein loss, the level of the serum albumin, and other secondary consequences of heavy albuminuria.

The salt and volume retention in the nephrotic syndrome may occur through at least two different major mechanisms. In the classic theory, proteinuria leads to hypoalbuminemia, a low plasma oncotic pressure, and intravascular volume depletion. Subsequent underperfusion of the kidney stimulates the priming of sodium-retentive hormonal systems such as the renin-angiotensin-aldosterone axis, causing increased renal sodium and volume retention. In the peripheral capillaries with normal hydrostatic pressures and decreased oncotic pressure, the Starling forces lead to transcapillary fluid leakage and edema. In some patients, however, the intravascular volume has been measured and found to be increased along with suppression of the renin-angiotensin-aldosterone axis. An animal model of unilateral proteinuria shows evidence for primary renal sodium retention at a distal nephron site, perhaps due to altered responsiveness to hormones such as atrial natriuretic factor. Here only the proteinuric kidney retains sodium and volume and at a time when the animal is not yet hypoalbuminemic. Thus, local

factors within the kidney may account for the volume retention of the nephrotic patient as well.

Recent epidemiologic study clearly defines an increased risk of atherosclerotic complications in the nephrotic syndrome. Most nephrotic patients have elevated levels of total and low density lipoprotein (LDL)-cholesterol with low or normal high density lipoprotein (HDL)-cholesterol. In addition to hyperlipidemia, many nephrotic patients have additional cardiovascular risk factors, including hypertension, smoking, and left ventricular hypertrophy.

Initial evaluation of the nephrotic patient includes laboratory tests to define whether the patient has primary, idiopathic nephrotic syndrome or a secondary cause related to a systemic disease. Common screening tests include the fasting blood sugar and glycosylated hemoglobin tests for diabetes, an antinuclear antibody test for collagen vascular disease, and the serum complement, which screens for many immune complex–mediated diseases (Table 106–1). In selected patients, cryoglobulins, hepatitis B and C serology, antineutrophil cytoplasmic antibodies, anti-GBM antibodies, and other tests may be useful. Once secondary causes have been excluded, treating the adult nephrotic patient often requires a renal biopsy to define the pattern of glomerular involvement. In adults, the nephrotic syndrome is a common condition leading to renal biopsy. In many studies, patients with heavy proteinuria and the nephrotic syndrome have been a group highly likely to benefit from renal biopsy in terms of a change in specific diagnosis, prognosis, and therapy. Selected adult nephrotic patients such as the elderly have a slightly different spectrum of disease, but once again the renal biopsy is the best guide to treatment and prognosis (Tables 106–2 and 106–3).

Idiopathic Nephrotic Syndrome

MINIMAL CHANGE DISEASE. Minimal change disease, also known as *nil disease* and *lipoid nephrosis,* is the most common pattern of nephrotic syndrome in children and comprises from 10 to 15% of idiopathic nephrotic syndrome in adults. A similar histologic pattern may be seen as an adverse reaction to certain medications (non-steroidal anti-inflammatory drugs [NSAIDs], lithium) and associated with certain tumors (Hodgkin's disease and leukemias). Patients typically present with periorbital and peripheral edema related to the proteinuria, which is usually well into the nephrotic range. Additional findings in adults are hypertension and microscopic hematuria, each in about 30% of patients. However, active urinary sediment with erythrocyte casts is not found. Many adult patients have mild to moderate azotemia, which may be related to hypoalbuminemia and intravascular volume depletion. Complement levels and serologic test results are normal.

In true minimal change disease, histopathology typically reveals no glomerular abnormalities on light microscopy (LM). The tubules may show lipid droplet accumulation from absorbed lipoproteins (hence the older term *lipoid nephrosis*). Immunofluorescence staining (IF) and electron microscopy (EM) (Fig. 106–1) show no immune-type deposits. By EM the GBM is normal, and effacement or "fusion" of the visceral epithelial foot processes is noted along virtually the entire distribution of every capillary loop.

The course of minimal change nephrotic syndrome is often one of remissions and relapses and responses to additional treatment.

Table 106–1 ■ SERUM COMPLEMENT LEVELS IN GLOMERULAR DISEASES

Diseases with a Reduced Complement Level
Post-streptococcal glomerulonephritis
Subacute bacterial endocarditis/visceral abscess/shunt nephritis
Systemic lupus erythematosus
Cryoglobulinemia
Idiopathic membranoproliferative glomerulonephrits
Diseases Associated with a Normal Serum Complement
Minimal change nephrotic syndrome
Focal segmental glomerulosclerosis
Membranous nephropathy
IgA nephropathy
Henoch-Schönlein purpura
Anti-GBM disease
Pauci-immune rapidly progressive glomerulonephritis
Polyarteritis nodosa
Wegener's granulomatosis

Table 106–2 ■ CAUSES OF THE NEPHROTIC SYNDROME

IDIOPATHIC OR PRIMARY NEPHROTIC SYNDROME	INCIDENCE (%)
Minimal change disease	10–15
Focal segmental glomerulosclerosis	20–25
Membranous nephropathy	25–30
Membranoproliferative glomerulonephritis	5
Other proliferative and sclerosing glomerulonephritides	15–30

When treated with corticosteroids for 8 weeks, 90 to 95% of children experience a remission of the nephrotic syndrome. In adults, the response rate is somewhat lower, with 75 to 85% of patients responding to regimens of daily (60 mg) or alternate-day (120 mg) prednisone therapy, tapered after 2 months of treatment. The time to clinical response may be slower in adults, and they should not be considered steroid-resistant until they have failed to respond to 16 weeks of treatment. Tapering of the steroid dose after remission should be gradual over 1 to 2 months. Both children and adults are likely to have a relapse of their minimal change disease once corticosteroids have been discontinued. Approximately 30% of adults experience relapse by 1 year, and in 50% it occurs by 5 years. Most clinicians treat the first relapse similarly to the initial episode of nephrotic syndrome. Patients who relapse a third time or who become corticosteroid dependent (unable to tolerate decrease in the prednisone dose beyond a certain level without proteinuria recurring) may be treated with a 2-month course of an alkylating agent. Cyclophosphamide at a dose of up to 2 mg/kg/day has been used successfully, as has chlorambucil. Up to 50% of these patients have a prolonged remission of the nephrotic syn-

Table 106–3 ■ NEPHROTIC SYNDROME ASSOCIATED WITH SPECIFIC CAUSES ("SECONDARY" NEPHROTIC SYNDROME)

Systemic Diseases
Diabetes mellitus
Systemic lupus erythematosus and other collagen diseases
Amyloidosis (amyloid AL or AA associated)
Vasculitic-immunologic diseases (mixed cryoglobulinemia, Wegener's granulomatosis, rapidly progressive glomerulonephritis, polyarteritis, Henoch-Schönlein purpura, sarcoidosis, Goodpasture's syndrome)
Infections
Bacterial (post-streptococcal, congenital and secondary syphilis, subacute bacterial endocarditis, shunt nephritis)
Viral (hepatitis B, hepatitis C, HIV infection, infectious mononucleosis, cytomegalovirus infection)
Parasitic (malaria, toxoplasmosis, schistosomiasis, filariasis)
Medication-Related
Gold, mercury, and the heavy metals
Penicillamine
Non-steroidal anti-inflammatory drugs
Lithium
Paramethadione, trimethadione
Captopril
"Street" heroin
Others—probenecid, chlorpropamide, rifampin, tolbutamide, phenindione
Allergens, Venoms, and Immunizations
Associated with Neoplasms
Hodgkin's lymphoma and leukemia-lymphomas (with minimal change lesion)
Solid tumors (with membranous nephropathy)
Hereditary and Metabolic Disease
Alport's syndrome
Fabry's disease
Sickle cell disease
Congenital (Finnish type) nephrotic syndrome
Familial nephrotic syndrome
Nail-patella syndrome
Partial lipodystrophy
Other
Pregnancy-related (includes preeclampsia)
Transplant rejection
Serum sickness
Accelerated hypertensive nephrosclerosis
Unilateral renal artery stenosis
Massive obesity–sleep apnea
Reflux nephropathy

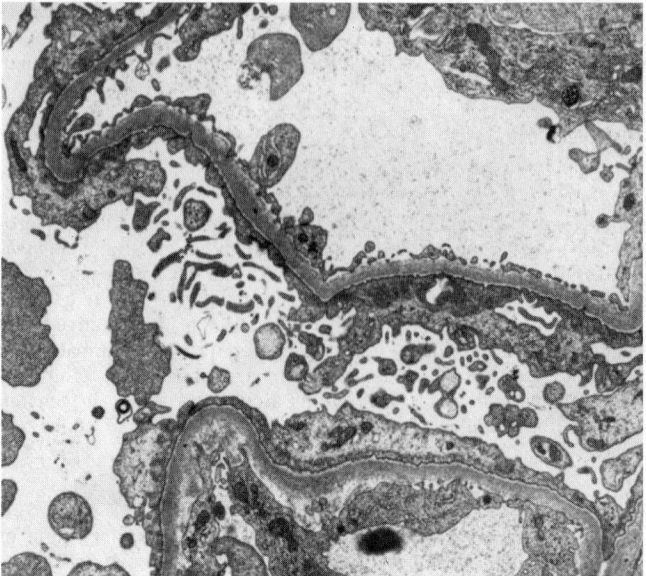

FIGURE 106–1 ■ Minimal change disease. Electron micrograph shows widespread effacement of foot processes with microvillous transformation of the visceral epithelium. No electron-dense deposits are present (uranyl acetate, lead citrate, ×6000).

drome (at least 5 years). The response rate is lower in corticosteroid-dependent patients. An alternative to an alkylating agent is low-dose cyclosporine (4 to 6 mg/kg/day for 4 months), but this carries the risk of nephrotoxicity and a higher relapse rate.

FOCAL SEGMENTAL GLOMERULOSCLEROSIS. From 20 to 25% of adults with idiopathic nephrotic syndrome are found on biopsy to have focal segmental glomerulosclerosis (FSGS). FSGS is the most common form of idiopathic nephrotic syndrome in blacks. This histologic diagnosis may be either idiopathic or secondary to a number of different causes (e.g., heroin abuse, HIV infection, sickle cell disease, obesity, reflux of urine from the bladder to the kidneys, and lesions associated with single or remnant kidneys).

Patients with idiopathic FSGS typically present with either asymptomatic proteinuria or edema. Although the nephrotic syndrome is present in two thirds of patients at presentation, proteinuria may vary from less than 1 to 30 g/day and is typically nonselective. Hypertension is found in 30 to 50%, and microscopic hematuria occurs in about one half of these patients. The glomerular filtration rate (GFR) is decreased at presentation in 20 to 30% of patients. Complement levels and other serologic test results are normal.

By LM, initially only some glomeruli have areas of segmental scarring. As renal function declines, repeat biopsy specimens show more glomeruli with segmental sclerosing lesions and increased numbers of globally sclerotic glomeruli. By IF staining, IgM and C3 are commonly trapped in the areas of glomerular sclerosis.

The course of untreated FSGS is usually one of progressive proteinuria and declining GFR. Only a minority of patients experience a spontaneous remission of proteinuria, and eventually most untreated patients develop ESRD in 5 to 20 years from presentation.

The therapy for FSGS is controversial. There have been few randomized, controlled trials, and newer studies with promising results remain uncontrolled. In general, patients with a sustained remission of their nephrotic syndrome are unlikely to progress to ESRD whereas those with unremitting nephrotic syndrome are likely to progress. Recent studies using more intensive and more prolonged immunosuppressive regimens (6 to 12 months) with corticosteroids and cytotoxics have achieved up to a 40 to 60% remission rate of the nephrotic syndrome with preservation of long-term renal function. Low-dose cyclosporine (4 to 6 mg/kg/day for 4 to 6 months) has also been used with success even in patients who have been corticosteroid and cytotoxic unresponsive.

MEMBRANOUS NEPHROPATHY. Membranous nephropathy is the most common pattern of idiopathic nephrotic syndrome in white Americans. It may also be associated with infections (lues, hepatitis B and C), with systemic lupus, with certain medications (gold salts), and with certain tumors (solid tumors and lymphomas). It typically presents as proteinuria and edema. Hypertension and microhematuria are not infrequent findings, but renal function and GFR are usually normal at presentation. Despite the finding of complement in the glomerular immune deposits, serum complement levels are normal. Membranous nephropathy is the most common pattern of the nephrotic syndrome to be associated with a hypercoagulable state and renal vein thrombosis. The presence of sudden flank pain, deterioration of renal function, or symptoms of pulmonary disease in a patient with membranous nephropathy should prompt an investigation for renal vein thrombosis and pulmonary emboli.

On LM, the glomerular capillary loops often appear rigid or thickened, but there is no cellular proliferation. EM shows subepithelial electron-dense deposits all along the glomerular capillary loops (Fig. 106–2).

In most large series, renal survival is more than 75% at 10 years. There is also a spontaneous remission rate of 20 to 30%. Both the slow progression and spontaneous remission rate have confounded clinical treatment trials. A number of older studies using corticosteroids to treat membranous nephropathy have given conflicting results. A more recent controlled trial of alternating monthly corticosteroids and monthly oral chlorambucil over 6 months has given a greater number of total remissions and better preservation of renal function. Recent controlled studies using only corticosteroids for 6 months have shown similar beneficial results. Although others believe that the good results in the treatment arms are not significantly better than the natural history of the disease, recent meta-analyses have found beneficial results from the use of cytotoxic agents in idiopathic membranous nephropathy. Finally, several uncontrolled studies suggest that patients with membranous nephropathy who are progressing to renal failure may benefit from cyclophosphamide plus corticosteroids with a reversal of progressive renal failure and remission of heavy proteinuria.

Membranoproliferative Glomerulonephritis

Membranoproliferative or mesangiocapillary glomerulonephritis (MPGN) is an uncommon glomerular disease that comprises only a small percentage of renal biopsies. By LM, similar patterns of glomerular damage have been seen in association with certain infectious agents (hepatitis C), autoimmune disease (systemic lupus erythematosus [SLE]), and diseases of intraglomerular coagulation. All of these stimuli have been proposed to incite the glomerular mesangial cells to grow out along the capillary wall and split the GBM. Type II MPGN, dense deposit disease, has been called an

autoimmune disorder with an autoantibody (an IgG, C3 nephritic factor) directed against C3bBb, the alternate pathway C3 convertase (see Chapter 271). By preventing degradation of the enzyme, there is increased activation and consumption of complement noted in dense deposit disease.

Most adults with MPGN present with proteinuria or the nephrotic syndrome. A low serum complement level is found intermittently in type I MPGN, whereas the C3 level is always reduced in type II MPGN. Most studies have found a similar course and prognosis for the various patterns of MPGN. Attempts to treat MPGN have included using corticosteroids and other immunosuppressive medications as well as anticoagulants and antiplatelet agents. No therapy has proven to be effective in adults with MPGN.

ACUTE GLOMERULONEPHRITIS

Pathophysiology

Known inciting causes of acute glomerulonephritis include a variety of infectious agents such as streptococcal infections and bacteria causing endocarditis, as well as the deposition of immune complexes in autoimmune diseases such as SLE, or the damaging effect of circulating antibodies directed against the GBM as in Goodpasture's syndrome. Regardless of the inciting cause, acute glomerulonephritis is characterized on LM by hypercellularity of the glomerulus. This may be secondary to infiltrating inflammatory cells, proliferation of resident glomerular cells, or both. Both invading inflammatory neutrophils and monocytes, as well as resident cells, can damage the glomerulus through a number of mediators, including a host of oxidants, chemoattractants, proteases, cytokines, and growth factors. Some factors, such as transforming growth factor-β, have been related to eventual glomerulosclerosis and chronic glomerular damage.

Patients with acute glomerulonephritis often present with a nephritic picture characterized by a decreased GFR and azotemia, oliguria, hypertension, and an active urinary sediment. The hypertension is caused by intravascular volume expansion, although renin levels may not be appropriately suppressed for the degree of volume expansion. Patients may note dark, smoky, or cola-colored urine in association with the active urinary sediment. This sediment is composed of erythrocytes, leukocytes, and a variety of casts, including erythrocyte casts, because damage to the glomerular capillaries allows cellular elements to exit into Bowman's space and the proximal tubule. Although many patients with acute glomerulonephritis have proteinuria, sometimes even in the nephrotic range, most patients have lesser degrees of albumin leakage into the urine, especially when the GFR is markedly reduced.

IgA Nephropathy

IgA nephropathy was originally thought to be an uncommon and benign form of glomerulopathy (Berger's disease). It is now recognized as the most frequent form of idiopathic glomerulonephritis worldwide (comprising 15 to 40% of primary glomerulonephritides in parts of Europe and Asia) and clearly can progress to ESRD. In geographic areas where renal biopsies are commonly performed for milder urinary findings, a higher incidence of IgA has been noted. In the United States, some centers report this diagnosis in up to 20% of all primary glomerulopathies. Males outnumber females, and the peak occurrence is in the second to third decades of life.

The diagnosis of IgA nephropathy is established by finding glomerular IgA deposits either as the dominant or co-dominant immunoglobulin on IF microscopy. Deposits of C3 and IgG are also often found. The LM picture varies from mild mesangial proliferation to crescentic glomerulonephritis. The most common picture is mesangial hypercellularity. By EM, immune-type dense deposits are typically found in the mesangial and paramesangial areas. In IgA nephropathy the predominant antibody appears to be composed of polymeric IgA1 originating in the secretory-mucosal system, but the antigen—whether viral, dietary, or other—to which it is directed is unknown in the vast majority of cases.

IGA nephropathy often presents either as asymptomatic microscopic hematuria and/or proteinuria (most common in adults) or as episodic gross hematuria following upper respiratory tract and other

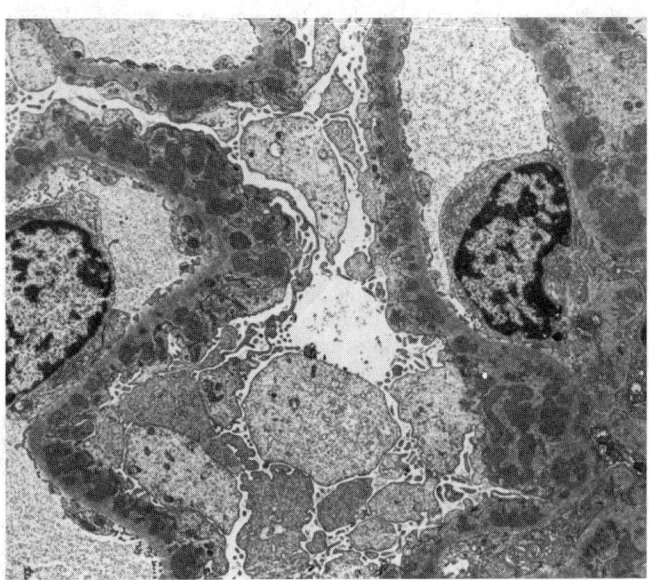

FIGURE 106–2 ■ Membranous glomerulopathy. On ultrastructural examination, there are numerous, closely apposed epimembranous electron-dense deposits separated by basement membrane spikes (uranyl acetate, lead citrate, ×2500).

infections or exercise (most common in children). The course of IgA nephropathy is variable, with some patients showing no decline in GFR over decades and others developing the nephrotic syndrome, hypertension, and renal failure. Hypertension is present in 20 to 50% of all patients. Increased serum IgA levels, noted in one third to one half of cases, do not correlate with the course of the disease.

Factors predictive of a poor outcome in IgA nephropathy have included (1) older age at onset, (2) absence of gross hematuria, (3) hypertension, (4) persistent and severe proteinuria, (5) being male, (6) an elevated serum creatinine level, and (7) the histologic features of severe proliferation and sclerosis and/or tubulointerstitial damage and crescent formation. Renal survival is estimated at 85 to 90% at 10 years and 75 to 80% at 20 years. A significant percentage of patients transplanted have a morphologic recurrence in the allograft, but graft loss due to the disease is uncommon.

Because the pathogenesis of IgA nephropathy is thought to involve abnormal antigenic stimulation of mucosal IgA production and subsequent immune complex deposition in the glomeruli, treatment has been directed at these sites. Efforts to treat the disease by preventing antigenic stimulation, including broad-spectrum antibiotics (e.g., doxycycline), tonsillectomy, and dietary manipulations (e.g., gluten elimination), have been generally unsuccessful. The benefit of glucocorticoids and cytotoxic agents is far from clear; however, they have been recommended for some patients with the nephrotic syndrome and those with crescentic IgA nephropathy. Recent trials with fish oils have given conflicting results. With no proven therapy, many physicians choose to treat only those patients at highest risk for progression to renal failure.

Henoch-Schönlein Purpura

Henoch-Schönlein purpura (HSP) is characterized by a small-vessel vasculitis with arthralgias, skin purpura, and abdominal symptoms along with a proliferative acute glomerulonephritis that has similar histopathologic features to IgA nephropathy. HSP is predominantly a disease of childhood, although cases do occur in adults. Despite the finding of circulating IgA-containing immune complexes, no infectious agent or allergen has been defined as causative.

The renal histopathology of HSP is similar to that of IgA nephropathy. In the skin there is a small vessel vasculitis, a leukocytoclastic angiitis with immune deposition of IgA.

The clinical manifestations of HSP (see Chapter 292) include dermatologic, gastrointestinal, rheumatologic, and renal findings. Skin involvement typically starts with a macular rash on the ankles that extends to the legs and occasionally the arms and buttocks. The macules darken and coalesce into purpuric lesions that are often palpable. Gastrointestinal symptoms include cramps, diarrhea, and, less frequently, nausea and vomiting. Melena and bloody diarrhea are present in the most severely involved cases. Although arthralgias of the knees, wrists, and ankles are common, true arthritis is uncommon. Symptoms of different organ system involvement may occur concurrently or separately, and recurrent episodes during the first year are not uncommon.

Like IgA nephropathy, HSP has no proven therapy. Episodes of rash, arthralgias, and abdominal symptoms usually resolve spontaneously. Some patients with severe abdominal findings have been treated with short courses of high doses of corticosteroids. Patients with severe glomerular involvement may benefit by modalities used to treat patients with severe IgA nephropathy. Although most patients with HSP recover fully, patients with a more severe nephritic or nephrotic presentation and more severe glomerular damage on renal biopsy have an unfavorable long-term prognosis.

Post-Streptococcal Glomerulonephritis

Acute post-streptococcal glomerulonephritis (PSGN) may present as an acute nephritic syndrome or with isolated hematuria and proteinuria. It may occur in either an epidemic form or as sporadic cases. PSGN is largely a disease of childhood, but well-documented cases of severe disease do occur in adults. The disease is most common in winter after episodes of pharyngitis, but it can occur after streptococcal infections at any site, and subclinical cases greatly outnumber clinical cases.

PSGN is an immune complex disease in its acute phase and is characterized by the formation of antibodies against streptococcal antigens and the localization of immune complexes with complement in the kidney. PSGN occurs only after infection with certain nephritogenic strains of group A β-hemolytic streptococci. Typical nephritogenic strains, characterized by antibodies to antigenic M components of their cell wall, include M types 1, 2, 4, 12, 18, 25, 49, 55, 57, and 60.

On LM, glomeruli are markedly enlarged and often fill Bowman's space. They exhibit hypercellularity due to both an infiltration of monocytes and especially polymorphonuclear cells during the early weeks of the disease and a proliferation of the glomerular cellular elements. The capillary lumina are often compressed by the glomerular hypercellularity. Some cases demonstrate extracapillary proliferation with crescent formation. By IF microscopy there is coarse granular deposition of IgG, IgM, and complement, especially C3, along the capillary wall. EM shows the classic dome-shaped, electron-dense subepithelial deposits resembling the humps of a camel at isolated intervals along the GBM.

Most cases are diagnosed by detecting hematuria, proteinuria, and hypertension and only some of the findings of the nephritic syndrome after a latency period of 10 days to several weeks after a streptococcal pharyngitis or a longer interval after a streptococcal skin infection. Throat cultures and skin cultures of suspected sites of streptococcal involvement may often not be positive for group A β-hemolytic streptococci. A variety of antibodies (e.g., antistreptolysin O[ASLO]), antihyaluronidase [AHT]), and a streptozyme panel of antibodies against streptococcal antigens (which includes ASLO, AHT, antistreptokinase, and anti-DNAse) often show high titers, but a change in titer over time is more indicative of a recent streptococcal infection. More than 95% of patients with PSGN secondary to pharyngitis and 85% of patients with streptococcal skin infections have positive antibody titers. The serum total hemolytic complement levels and C3 levels are decreased in more than 90% of patients during the episode of acute glomerulonephritis.

In the classic case of an acute nephritic episode after a latency period after a streptococcal infection and associated with both a change in streptococcal antibody titer and a depressed serum complement level, a renal biopsy adds little to the diagnosis. In other cases, a biopsy may prove necessary to confirm or refute the diagnosis. In most patients, PSGN is a self-limited disease, with recovery of renal function and disappearance of hypertension in several weeks. Proteinuria and hematuria may resolve more slowly over months. Therapy is symptomatic and directed at controlling the hypertension and fluid retention with antihypertensives and diuretics.

Glomerulonephritis with Endocarditis and Visceral Abscesses

Various glomerular lesions have been found in patients suffering from acute and chronic bacterial endocarditis (see Chapter 63). Although embolic phenomena can lead to glomerular ischemia and infarcts, a common finding is an immune complex pattern of glomerular damage. In the preantibiotic era with most cases of endocarditis due to *Streptococcus viridans,* both focal and diffuse proliferative glomerulonephritides were seen in many patients. More recently, the incidence of acute endocarditis associated with *Staphylococcus aureus* has markedly increased, especially in the drug-addicted population. From 40 to 80% of patients with staphylococcal endocarditis have clinical evidence of a proliferative glomerulonephritis. Glomerulonephritis is now more common with acute rather than subacute bacterial endocarditis, and the duration of illness is not an important determinant of the renal disease.

Patients often have hematuria and erythrocyte casts in urinary sediment, proteinuria ranging from less than 1 g/day to nephrotic levels, and progressive renal failure. Serum total complement and C3 levels are usually reduced. Renal insufficiency may be mild and reversible with appropriate antibiotic therapy or progressive, leading to dialysis and irreversible renal failure.

A proliferative glomerulonephritis with similar pathology has also been noted in patients with deep visceral bacterial abscesses and infections such as empyema of the lung and osteomyelitis. With appropriate antibiotic therapy most patients' glomerular lesions heal and they recover renal function. Immune complex forms of acute glomerulonephritis have also been noted in patients with pneumonias associated with many bacterial organisms as well as

Primary
Type I: Anti–glomerular basement membrane antibody disease (with pulmonary disease—Goodpasture's syndrome)
Type II: Immune complex mediated
Type III: Pauci-immune (usually antineutrophil cytoplasmic antibody-positive)
Secondary
Membranoproliferative glomerulonephritis
IgA nephropathy—Henoch-Schönlein purpura
Post-streptococcal glomerulonephritis
Systemic lupus erythematosus
Polyarteritis nodosa, hypersensitivity angiitis

Mycoplasma. Patients with chronically infected cerebral ventriculoatrial shunts for hydrocephalus have also had renal damage associated with immune deposits in the glomeruli. Many have nephrotic-range proteinuria and only mild renal dysfunction.

Rapidly Progressive Glomerulonephritis

Rapidly progressive glomerulonephritis (RPGN) comprises a group of glomerulonephritides that have in common progression to renal failure in a matter of weeks to months and the presence of extensive extracapillary proliferation (i.e., crescent formation). RPGN thus includes renal diseases with different causes, pathogeneses, and clinical presentations (Table 106–4). Patients with primary RPGN have been divided into three patterns defined by immunologic pathogenesis: type I, with anti-GBM disease (e.g., Goodpasture's syndrome); type II, with immune complex deposition (e.g., SLE, post-streptococcal); and type III, without immune deposits or anti-GBM antibodies, so-called pauci-immune. Most of the last group fall into the category of antineutrophil cytoplasmic antibody (ANCA)-positive RPGN. In the past, with the exception of postinfectious RPGN, prognosis was generally poor for most patients regardless of pathogenesis. This prognosis has dramatically changed for some patterns of RPGN.

Anti-GBM Disease

Anti-GBM disease (Table 106–5) is caused by circulating antibodies directed against the noncollagenous domain of type 4 collagen that damages the GBM. This leads to an inflammatory response, breaks in the GBM, and the formation of a proliferative and often crescentic glomerulonephritis. If the anti-GBM antibodies cross-react with and damage the basement membrane of pulmonary capillaries, the patient develops pulmonary hemorrhage and hemoptysis. The association of anti-GBM antibody–mediated damage to the kidneys and lungs is called Goodpasture's syndrome (see Chapter 78). The disease most commonly affects young adults, and males are far more commonly affected than females. The patient presents with a nephritic picture. Renal function may deteriorate from normal to dialysis-requiring levels in a matter of days to weeks. Patients with pulmonary involvement may have life-threatening hemoptysis. The course of the disease, once it has progressed to renal failure, is usually one of permanent renal dysfunction. If treatment is started early in the course of the disease, patients may regain considerable kidney function.

Table 106–5 ■ COMMON RENAL DISEASES WITH ASSOCIATED PULMONARY DISEASES

DISEASE	MARKER
Goodpasture's syndrome	+Anti–glomerular basement membrane antibodies
Wegener's granulomatosis, polyarteritis	+Antineutrophil cytoplasmic antibodies
Systemic lupus erythematosus	+Anti-DNA antibodies, low complement
Nephrotic syndrome, renal vein thrombosis, pulmonary embolus	+Lung scan
Pneumonia with immune complex glomerulonephritis	−Low complement, circulating immune complexes
Uremic lung	−Elevated blood urea nitrogen and creatinine levels

The pathology of anti-GBM disease shows a proliferative glomerulonephritis, often with severe crescentic proliferation in Bowman's space. There is linear deposition of immunoglobulin along the GBM by IF, but EM does not show any electron-dense deposits.

The treatment of anti-GBM disease is unproven, with no significant controlled trials of this least-common form of crescentic glomerulonephritis. For patients with pulmonary hemorrhage, high-dose oral or intravenous corticosteroids have successfully halted the pulmonary bleeding. They have usually not proven effective in treating the renal lesions. Intensive therapy to reduce the production of anti-GBM antibodies (immunosuppressive agents such as cyclophosphamide and corticosteroids) combined with plasmapheresis to remove circulating anti-GBM antibodies has proven effective for the renal lesion in many cases. Rapid intensive therapy is necessary to prevent irreversible renal damage.

Immune Complex RPGN

Type II RPGN is associated with immune complex–mediated damage to the glomeruli and may occur with primary glomerulopathies such as IgA nephropathy and MPGN or diseases of known origin such as postinfectious glomerulonephritis and SLE. The therapy for IgA nephropathy and MPGN was discussed previously. Most cases of crescentic postinfectious glomerulonephritis resolve with successful treatment of the underlying infection. The treatment of severe SLE is considered later.

Pauci-immune RPGN and Vasculitis-Associated RPGN

Pauci-immune type III RPGN includes patients with and without evidence of systemic vasculitis. A large retrospective analysis found no difference in prognosis between the patients with or without small artery or medium-sized renal artery vasculitis along with crescentic and focal segmental necrotizing glomerulonephritis (polyarteritis-like) (see Chapters 292 and 293). Patients often present with progressive renal failure and a nephritic picture. Many patients have circulating antibodies directed against components of neutrophil primary granules, ANCA. Patients who are P-ANCA positive (antibodies usually directed against granulocyte myeloperoxidase) more often have a clinical picture akin to microscopic polyarteritis with arthritis, skin involvement with leukocytoclastic angiitis, and constitutional and systemic signs. Patients who are C-ANCA positive (antibodies usually directed against a granulocyte serine proteinase) more likely have granulomatous disease associated with their glomerulonephritis as in Wegener's granulomatosis (see Chapter 294). There is considerable overlap between these groups. As in all forms of RPGN, renal function may deteriorate rapidly. Oral cyclophosphamide in addition to corticosteroids has led to markedly improved patient and renal survival rates in patients with Wegener's granulomatosis and polyarteritis nodosa. For example, in a series of 158 patients with Wegener's granulomatosis, more than 90% experienced marked improvement and 75% experienced a complete remission. These excellent results include patients with true crescentic glomerulonephritis. More recently, steroids plus cytotoxic agents have produced successful results in both oliguric and dialysis-dependent patients.

ASYMPTOMATIC URINARY ABNORMALITIES

Some patients have the asymptomatic urinary abnormalities of microhematuria and/or proteinuria discovered through routine evaluations. Microscopic hematuria associated with deformed erythrocytes and/or erythrocyte casts is likely to be glomerular in origin. Levels of proteinuria less than the nephrotic range may be due to orthostatic proteinuria, hypertension, and tubular disease as well as glomerular damage.

In patients with a glomerular cause for their asymptomatic urinary abnormality, the underlying glomerular lesion is either the early phase of one of the progressive glomerular diseases (discussed in other sections) or due to a benign, non-progressive glomerular lesion. Most such patients have a lesion with mild proliferation limited to the mesangial areas of the glomeruli. Some patients have mesangial IgA immune deposits and hence IgA nephropathy, whereas others have deposition of IgM or complement only. Some patients, often with a history of similar findings in siblings and other relatives, have a hereditary nephritis. One form of hereditary nephritis is associated with areas of focal thinning of the GBM, so-called thin basement membrane disease. Another hereditary form of glomerulonephritis that often presents as asymptomatic urinary findings is Alport's syndrome, an X-linked condition associated with high-pitched hearing loss and abnormalities of the lens of the eye. In males, this disease can lead to progressive glomerulosclerosis and ESRD. In general, for patients with less than 1 g of proteinuria daily and/or glomerular microhematuria if the GFR (as measured by the creatinine clearance) is normal, most clinicians would not proceed to a renal biopsy to confirm a diagnosis. Because the vast majority of these patients need no therapy, they prefer to follow the patient closely and perform biopsy only on patients with progressive increasing proteinuria or evidence of a decreasing GFR.

GLOMERULAR INVOLVEMENT IN SYSTEMIC DISEASES

Systemic Lupus Erythematosus

Renal involvement may greatly influence the course and therapy of SLE (see Chapter 289). The incidence of clinically detectable renal disease varies from 15 to 75%. Histologic evidence of renal involvement by immune deposits is found in the vast majority of biopsy specimens, even in the absence of clinical renal disease.

The World Health Organization (WHO) classification of lupus nephritis has been used successfully for both clinical and research activities (Table 106–6). It has the advantages of using LM, IF, and EM to classify each biopsy specimen rather than only one form of microscopy; of separating the milder mesangial disease from the true focal and diffuse proliferative lupus nephritis; and of using well-defined criteria allowing different groups to compare results (Fig. 106–3). The WHO classes correlate well with the clinical picture and subsequent course of patients with SLE.

In general, all patients with class IV lesions on biopsy deserve vigorous therapy for their lupus nephritis. Many class III patients (especially those with active necrotizing lesions and large amounts of subendothelial deposits) also would benefit from such therapy. The optimal therapy for class V patients is less clear; some clinicians treat all membranous lupus nephritis patients vigorously, whereas others reserve such therapy for those with serologic activity or more severe nephrotic syndrome. Vigorous lupus nephritis therapy may include corticosteroids, plasmapheresis, azathioprine, or cyclophosphamide, as well as newer immunosuppressive medications such as cyclosporine, gamma globulin, and mycophenolate mofetil. Plasmapheresis, reported to be successful anecdotally, has recently proven unsuccessful in improving renal or patient survival in a major clinical controlled trial. A series of well-performed studies of patients with lupus nephritis randomized to treatment protocols of either oral prednisone, oral azathioprine, oral cyclophosphamide, oral azathioprine plus oral cyclophosphamide, or every-third-month high doses of intravenous cyclophosphamide (1 g/m²) found patients treated with any of the cytotoxic agents had less renal failure at 10 years than those who had corticosteroid treatment. Extended follow-up at 20 years showed the azathioprine group to be no different from the prednisone groups. Intravenous cyclophosphamide appeared to be an effective therapy with fewer side effects than oral cyclophosphamide. Recent studies document the superiority of regimens with monthly high-dose intravenous cyclophosphamide therapy over monthly pulse methylprednisolone in preventing renal progression and flares of disease. Although a controlled trial proved that combination therapy with monthly cyclophosphamide along with methylprednisolone was more effective in preventing renal failure than either drug regimen alone, the combination therapy had the highest incidence of side effects. At present, for severe lupus nephritis many clinicians use a regimen of monthly pulses of intravenous cyclophosphamide with low doses of corticosteroids given for 6 months followed by every-third-month pulses of the cytotoxic agent for up to 2 years.

Many patients with lupus nephritis (40 to 50%) produce autoantibodies against certain phospholipids, including anticardiolipin antibodies and lupus anticoagulants. Some of these patients have coagulation in the glomeruli and arterioles and require treatment

Table 106–6 ■ WORLD HEALTH ORGANIZATION CLASSIFICATION OF LUPUS NEPHRITIS

CLASS	CLINICAL FEATURES
I. Normal glomeruli (LM, IF, EM)	No renal findings
II. (a) Mesangial disease normal by LM with mesangial deposits by IF and/or EM (b) Mesangial hypercellularity with mesangial deposits	Mild clinical renal disease; minimally active urinary sediment; mild to moderate proteinuria (never nephrotic) but may have active serology.
III. Focal proliferative glomerulonephritis	More active sediment changes; often active serology; increased proteinuria (about 25% nephrotic); hypertension may be present; some evolve into class IV pattern.
IV. Diffuse proliferative glomerulonephritis	Most severe renal involvement with active sediment, hypertension, heavy proteinuria (frequent nephrotic syndrome), often reduced glomerular filtration rate; serology very active.
V. Membranous glomerulonephritis	Significant proteinuria (often nephrotic) with less active lupus serology

LM = light microscopy; IF = immunofluorescence; EM = electron microscopy.

with anticoagulation and/or antiplatelet agents as well as immunosuppressive medications.

Diabetes Mellitus

Diabetic nephropathy is the most common form of glomerular damage seen in developed countries. In 1998, forty per cent of all new patients with ESRD in the United States had diabetes (see Chapter 110) as their primary etiology. From 20 to 30% of all patients with type I or type II diabetes develop nephropathy, with a much higher percentage of those with type I disease progressing to ESRD. However, because of the much greater prevalence of type II disease, the majority of the diabetics starting dialysis have this form of the disease.

The histopathologic changes in the kidneys of diabetics involve all components of the kidney, including the glomeruli, vessels, tubules, and interstitium. In the glomeruli there are thickening of the GBM, mesangial sclerosis, nodular intercapillary glomerulosclerosis (the so-called Kimmelstiel-Wilson, or KW, nodules), lesions due to insudation of plasma proteins along the glomerular capillary walls, and microaneurysms of the glomerular capillaries.

A current goal of treatment in diabetics is to prevent diabetic

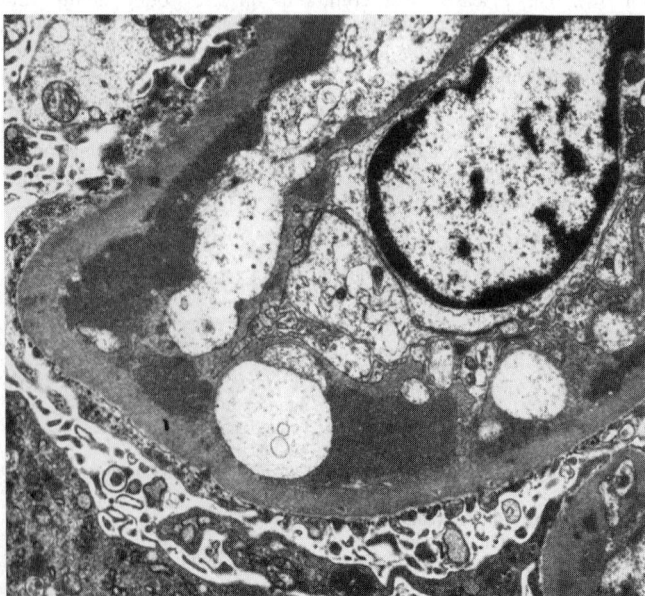

FIGURE 106–3 ■ Lupus nephritis. At the ultrastructural level, wire-loop deposits correspond to large subendothelial electron-dense deposits (uranyl acetate, lead citrate, ×5000).

nephropathy by controlling hyperglycemia and blood pressure and reducing intracapillary glomerular pressures. The superiority of angiotensin-converting enzyme (ACE) inhibitors over other antihypertensives in preventing the progression of renal disease and renal morbidity and mortality in type I diabetics has been documented in controlled trials. In type II diabetics with microalbuminuria, ACE inhibitors also prevent the appearance of clinical proteinuria and progression of renal dysfunction. Current studies focus on the efficacy of ACE inhibitors and angiotensin II receptor antagonists in the prevention of renal disease progression in type II diabetics. Survival in diabetics with renal transplantation may approach that of the non-diabetic population.

Amyloidosis

Renal amyloid deposits—whether due to AL or to AA amyloid—are predominantly found within the glomeruli, often appearing as amorphous eosinophilic extracellular nodules (see Chapter 297). They stain positively with Congo red stain and, under polarized light, display apple-green birefringence. Under EM, amyloid appears as non-branching rigid fibrils 8 to 10 nm in diameter.

Although almost 80% of patients with AL amyloid have renal disease, amyloidosis is a disease with multisystemic involvement, and hence patients may present with symptoms referable to cardiac or neural involvement as well as with renal symptoms. Diagnosis may be made from organ biopsy other than the kidney (e.g., gingival biopsy, rectal biopsy, or fat pad biopsy). Common renal manifestations are albuminuria and renal insufficiency found in almost one half of patients. Approximately 25% of patients with AL amyloid present with the nephrotic syndrome, and this is eventually found in up to one half of patients. Amyloid is rarely found in association with light chain cast nephropathy. Treatment strategies for renal amyloidosis have focused on combined therapy with melphalan, prednisone, and colchicine or marrow transplantation and ablative therapy to destroy the clone of abnormal plasma cells leading to the amyloid production.

Light Chain Deposition Disease

Light chain deposition disease (LCDD), like AL amyloidosis, is a systemic disease caused by the overproduction and extracellular deposition of a monoclonal immunoglobulin light chain (see Chapter 181). However, the deposits do not form β-pleated sheets, do not stain with Congo red, and are granular rather than fibrillar. Most patients with LCDD have a lymphoplasmacytic B-cell disease similar to multiple myeloma. On LM, most glomeruli have eosinophilic mesangial glomerular nodules. Others are either normal or have sclerosing or proliferative features. By IF, a single class of immunoglobulin light chain (kappa in 80% of cases) stains in a diffuse linear pattern along the GBMs, in the nodules, and along the tubular basement membranes with little or no staining for complement components.

Moderate albuminuria is common, and the nephrotic syndrome is found in one half at presentation, often accompanied by hypertension and renal insufficiency. The treatment for most patients with LCDD is chemotherapy similar to that for myeloma, which has led to significant renal and patient survival.

Fibrillary Glomerulopathy–Immunotactoid Glomerulopathy

Some patients with renal disease have glomerular lesions with deposits of non-amyloid fibrillar proteins ranging in size from 12 to 49 nm. In the past, these lesions were called fibrillary glomerulopathy, immunotactoid glomerulopathy, amyloid-like glomerulopathy, Congo red–negative amyloid-like glomerulonephritis, and non-amyloiditic fibrillary glomerulopathy. Recently, patients with these lesions have been divided into two groups: those with fibrillary glomerulonephritis with fibrils of 20 nm in diameter and those with immunotactoid glomerulonephritis, a rare disease in which the fibrils are much larger (30 to 50 nm). Proteinuria is found in almost all patients, and hematuria, the nephrotic syndrome, and renal insufficiency are eventually found in the majority. There is no proven therapy for fibrillary glomerulopathy at this time.

HIV Nephropathy

Infection with HIV (see Chapter 417) has been associated with a number of patterns of renal disease, including acute renal failure and a unique form of glomerulopathy now called HIV nephropathy.

The most common precipitating factors for acute renal failure include medications (pentamidine, aminoglycosides, trimethoprim-sulfamethoxazole, NSAIDs), and pyrexia and dehydration superimposed on sepsis hypotension respiratory failure.

Several histologic patterns of glomerulopathy seen in HIV-infected patients have included minimal change pattern, mesangial hyperplasia, glomerulopathies associated with immune complex deposition and/or IgA deposition, and, most importantly, HIV nephropathy. HIV nephropathy is a unique pattern of glomerulopathy characterized by heavy proteinuria and rapid progression to renal failure. Studies suggest use of ACE inhibitors and antiviral agents may slow this progression to renal failure.

Both clinical and histologic data suggest that HIV nephropathy differs from the older entity of heroin nephropathy. The latter is a form of FSGS, occurring in intravenous heroin users associated with proteinuria and often the nephrotic syndrome and renal insufficiency. HIV nephropathy may occur in non-addicted patients and has a more fulminant course to renal failure than heroin nephropathy. The pathology of HIV nephropathy also shows several distinct features from classic FSGS. In HIV nephropathy on LM, diffuse global glomerular sclerosis and glomerular collapse are common. There are severe tubulointerstitial changes with interstitial inflammation, edema, microcystic dilatation of tubules, and severe tubular degenerative changes. On EM, tubuloreticular inclusions are prevalent in the glomerular endothelium.

Mixed Cryoglobulinemia

Cryoglobulinemia is caused by the production of circulating immunoglobulins that precipitate on cooling and resolubilize on warming. Cryoglobulinemia may be found associated with many types of diseases, including infections, collagen-vascular disease, and lymphoproliferative diseases such as multiple myeloma and Waldenström's macroglobulinemia (see Chapter 181). Recently, many patients with what was originally described as glomerulonephritis due to essential mixed cryoglobulinemia have been found to have hepatitis C–associated renal disease. Some patients develop an acute nephritic picture with acute renal insufficiency. Most patients have proteinuria, and about 20% present with the nephrotic syndrome. The majority with renal disease have a slow, indolent renal course characterized by proteinuria, hypertension, hematuria, and renal insufficiency. Hypocomplementemia, especially of the early components Clq–C4, is a characteristic and often helpful finding in cryoglobulinemic glomerulonephritis.

Thrombotic Microangiopathies

A number of systemic diseases including hemolytic-uremic syndrome, thrombotic thrombocytopenic purpura, and the antiphospholipid syndrome (see Chapter 184), as well as microangiopathy associated with drugs such as mitomycin and cyclosporine are characterized by microthromboses of the glomerular capillaries and small arterioles. The renal findings may be dominant or only part of a more generalized picture of microangiopathy.

The histologic findings in all of the microangiopathies resemble each other. Glomerular capillary thromboses are noted in some glomeruli, whereas others downstream from thrombosed arterioles may show only ischemic damage. Arterioles and small arteries show intimal proliferation with luminal narrowing by thrombus. The renal manifestations of the thrombotic microangiopathies may include gross or microscopic hematuria, proteinuria that is typically less than 2 g/day but may reach nephrotic levels, and renal insufficiency. Patients may have oliguric or non-oliguric acute renal failure. Treatment of the thrombotic microangiopathies includes correcting hypovolemia, controlling hypertension, and use of dialytic support for those with severe renal failure. In the antiphospholipid syndrome, anticoagulation with heparin and then warfarin (Coumadin) has been useful.

Renal Vasculitis—Polyarteritis, Wegener's Granulomatosis, Hypersensitivity Angiitis

A number of systemic vasculitic disease processes can involve the kidney. In many cases of polyarteritis nodosa, hypersensitivity angiitis, and Wegener's granulomatosis (see Chapters 293 and 294), renal involvement is predominant and overshadows other manifestations of the systemic vasculitis. The renal lesions of these disorders typically range from focal and segmental necrotizing glomerulonephritis to severe necrotizing crescentic glomerulonephritis. Therapy for the microscopic form of polyarteritis and Wegener's granulomatosis is discussed under the therapy for RPGN.

Appel GB: Focal segmental glomerulosclerosis. *In* Greenberg A (ed): Primer on Kidney Disease. New York, Academic Press, 1998, pp 160–164. *A review of the epidemiology, pathogenesis, clinical features, course, and treatment of this increasing form of idiopathic nephrotic syndrome.*

Bakris GL, Copley JB, Vicknair N, et al: Calcium channel blockers versus other antihypertensive therapies on progression of NIDDM-associated nephropathy: Results of a 6-year study. Kidney Int 50:1641–1650, 1996. *A controlled trial of certain calcium channel blocking antihypertensives versus ACE inhibitors and β-blockers in adult-onset diabetics with nephrotic syndrome.*

D'Agati V, Appel GB: HIV infection and the kidney. J Am Soc Nephrol 8:138–152, 1997. *A review of the clinical features, course, pathogenesis, and treatment of HIV nephropathy.*

Gourley MF, Austin HA, Scott D, et al: Methylprednisolone and cyclophosphamide, alone or in combination, in patients with lupus nephritis. Ann Intern Med. 125:549–557, 1996. *A controlled trial of three treatment regimens for lupus nephritis emphasizing renal survival as an outcome and the side effects of therapy.*

Johnson RJ, Gretch DR, Yamabe H, et al: Renal manifestations of hepatitis C infection. Kidney Int 46:1255–1263, 1994. *A review of the patterns of kidney involvement by hepatitis C including data on therapy with interferon.*

Kyle RA, Gertz MA, Greipp PR, et al: A trial of three regimens for primary amyloidosis: Colchicine alone, melphalan and prednisone, and melphalan, prednisone, and colchicine. N Engl J Med 336:1202–1207, 1997. *An analysis of clinical features and response to therapeutic regimens of 220 patients with primary amyloidosis.*

Maschio G, Alberti D, Janin G, et al: Effect of the angiotensin-converting enzyme inhibitor benazepril on the progression of chronic renal insufficiency. N Engl J Med. 334:939–945, 1996. *A randomized multicenter trial showing ACE inhibition leads to less renal failure than other antihypertensives in patients with renal diseases.*

Nachman PH, Hogan SL, Jennette JC, et al: Treatment response and relapse in ANCA-associated microscopic polyangiitis and glomerulonephritis. J Am Soc Nephrol 7: 23–32, 1996.

Orth SR, Ritz E: The nephrotic syndrome. N Engl J Med 338: 1202–1211, 1998. *A review of the features, pathophysiology, and treatment of the various patterns of the nephrotic syndrome.*

Savin VJ, Arturo M, Sharma R, et al: Circulating factor associated with increased glomerular permeability to albumin in recurrent focal segmental sclerosis. N Engl J Med 334:878–882, 1996. *A study showing that the presence of a circulating permeability factor correlates with recurrences of the nephrotic syndrome due to FSGS in renal transplant patients, and that removal of the substance by plasmapheresis is associated with improvement of these patients' course.*

Schieppati A, Mosconi L, Perna A, et al: Prognosis of untreated patients with idiopathic membranous nephropathy. N Engl J Med 329:85, 1993. *A long-term follow-up of idiopathic membranous nephropathy showing favorable prognosis without specific immunosuppressive therapy.*

107 TUBULOINTERSTITIAL DISEASES AND TOXIC NEPHROPATHIES

Garabed Eknoyan

TUBULOINTERSTITIAL NEPHROPATHY

At their onset, diseases of the kidney primarily affect the glomeruli, the vasculature, or the other two components of the renal parenchyma, the tubules and the interstitium. The tubules and interstitium of the kidney are separate structural and functional compartments that are intimately related, and any injury initially involving either of them will inevitably be associated with damage to the other, hence the term *tubulointerstitial diseases*. A constant histologic feature of these diseases is an inflammatory cell infiltrate. The clinicopathologic syndrome that results from these disorders is commonly termed *tubulointerstitial nephropathy*. The abbreviation TIN will be used in this chapter to refer synonymously to tubulointerstitial nephritis and tubulointerstitial nephropathy.

As a rule, TIN is categorized as being *primary* or *secondary* in origin. *Primary* TIN is defined as injury that affects the tubules and interstitium without significant involvement of the glomeruli or renal vasculature, at least in the early stages of the disease. *Secondary* TIN is defined as tubulointerstitial injury caused by diseases that initially affect the glomeruli or renal vasculature, with the subsequent superimposition of TIN. The presence of secondary TIN has come to be identified as an important determinant of reduced

renal function and its progression to renal failure, both of which correlate better with the extent of secondary TIN than they do with the severity of the glomerular or vascular lesions that were the cause of the original kidney disease.

Clinically, TIN will pursue an *acute* (ATIN) or *chronic* (CTIN) course. Primary ATIN accounts for some 15 to 20% of patients with acute renal failure, and primary CTIN, for 20 to 30% of those with chronic renal failure who progress to end-stage renal disease (ESRD). The clinical and social implications of the primary forms of TIN are especially important since more than half of these cases are the result of a toxic nephropathy produced by a drug or an environmental toxin. As such, potentially they are either preventable or treatable if recognized early, before the onset of irreversible renal failure.

More broadly defined and inclusive of both its primary and secondary forms, TIN is a component of all cases of acute and chronic renal failure. The World Health Organization classification of the pathology of diseases of the kidney lists acute tubular necrosis (ATN) as a form of ATIN. Both are associated with tubulointerstitial injury; however, necrosis is more prominent in ATN, whereas interstitial inflammatory cellular infiltrates and edema are more prominent in ATIN (Table 107–1). In fact, their pathologic features may overlap sufficiently to make differentiation of ATN and ATIN difficult on morphologic examination of kidney tissue. Clinically, both result in acute renal failure and must be considered in the differential diagnosis of acute deterioration in renal function. By the same token, most forms of primary glomerular or vascular kidney diseases that become chronic and progress to ESRD are associated with secondary TIN. As such, apart from its importance as a primary cause of renal disease, TIN is the common pathway of all forms of progressive chronic renal failure.

CLINICAL MANIFESTATIONS. In all cases of primary ATIN and in the majority of cases of primary CTIN, renal insufficiency occurs in conjunction with or subsequent to the tubulointerstitial injury, and the earliest manifestations of the disease are usually those of tubular dysfunction. Whenever such dysfunction is detected clinically, removal of the toxic cause of injury or correction of the underlying disease can result in reversal of injury or preservation of residual renal function.

The pattern of tubular dysfunction encountered clinically depends on the site of the lesions of TIN (Fig. 107–1), and their severity depends on the extent of interstitial infiltrates and tubular injury. Essentially, TIN affects either the cortex or the medulla of the kidney. Cortical lesions affect either the proximal or the distal

Table 107–1 ■ **MORPHOLOGIC FEATURES OF ACUTE AND CHRONIC TUBULOINTERSTITIAL NEPHRITIS**

MORPHOLOGY	ATN	ATIN	CTIN
Gross Features			
Size	Enlarged	Enlarged	Small
Surface	Normal	Normal	Scarred
Echogenicity	Normal	Normal	Increased
Microscopic Features			
Interstitium			
Edema	$+\rightarrow++$	$+\rightarrow++++$	$\pm\rightarrow++$
Fibrosis	None	Unusual	Severe
Cell infiltrates	Few	Prominent	Modest
Tubules			
Cells	Necrotic	Injured	Atrophy/ hypertrophy
Basement membrane	$\pm\rightarrow++$	$+\rightarrow+++$	Thickened
Shape	Preserved	Preserved	Atrophy/ dilatation
Glomeruli			
Capillaries	Normal	Normal $\rightarrow$ MCD	Sclerosis
Capsule	Normal	Normal	Thickened/ fibrosed
Vasculature			
Endothelium	Normal $\rightarrow$ swollen	Normal	Normal
Wall	Normal	Normal	Variable sclerosis

ATN = acute tubular necrosis; ATIN = acute tubulointerstitial nephritis; CTIN = chronic tubulointerstitial nephritis; MCD = minimal change disease; + indicates presence, and the greater the number of + symbols, the more severe the morphologic feature.

tubule. Proximal tubular lesions result in bicarbonaturia (plasma CO_2 content, ≤ 20 mEq/L), glucosuria (with normal blood glucose), uricosuria (normal or low serum urate levels, particularly relative to the level of azotemia), and ß$_2$-microalbuminuria and aminoaciduria (Fanconi's syndrome). Distal tubular lesions result in reduced hydrogen secretion or distal tubular acidosis (urine pH, >6.0; plasma CO_2 content, ≤ 20 mEq/L), either without or with coexistent impairment of distal tubular potassium secretion (hyperkalemia, type IV renal tubular acidosis). Medullary lesions result in a reduced ability to achieve the hypertonicity essential for concentrating urine and in impaired responsiveness of the distal tubule to antidiuretic hormone (nephrogenic diabetes insipidus), effects manifested clinically by polyuria and nocturia. On occasion, concomitant injury to several tubular segments may occur, and in fact, as the disease progresses, this pattern becomes the norm in most forms of primary TIN, in which case simultaneous cortical and medullary tubular dysfunction will be present in the same patient.

Because epithelial cell sodium transport is a principal function of the entire tubule, some degree of reduced sodium reabsorption will occur independent of the tubular segment affected by TIN (see Fig. 107–1). This phenomenon accounts for the absence of the clinical features of sodium retention (hypertension, edema) in primary CTIN, an extremely useful clinical feature in the differential diagnosis of primary CTIN from its secondary forms caused by glomerular or vascular diseases, in which hypertension and edema are almost always present when renal failure supervenes.

PATHOGENESIS. The mechanism by which TIN is mediated remains to be elucidated. Tubular epithelial cell injury appears to be pivotal in initiation of the process. The initial injury may be direct cytotoxicity (drugs, environmental toxins) or indirect damage secondary to an inflammatory reaction (systemic diseases, autoimmune disorders). Studies in experimental models and humans provide compelling evidence for a role of immune mechanisms in subsequent progression of the process, which for purposes of clarification has been arbitrarily classified into three phases: antigen expression or recognition, integrative or regulatory, and effector or mediator.

In the first phase, either the injured tubular epithelial cells or the stimulated interstitial dendritic cells, both of which express the class II major histocompatibility complex, function as antigen-presenting cells. The second, or integrative or regulatory, phase determines the subsequent course of renal involvement. In this poorly

deciphered phase, the recruited infiltrating and antigenically activated T lymphocytes play a central role. In the final, or effector or mediator, phase, humoral factors released by the infiltrating cells and by the injured epithelial cells cause further recruitment of inflammatory cells and the initiation of fibrogenesis. Cytokines, which have chemoattractant, pro-inflammatory, and cytotoxic properties and are actually operative in all three phases, assume a greater role in the perpetuation of this final phase.

Each of the individual phases of this immune response is usually part of a recuperative process to repair injury. It is the apparent loss of their regulatory mechanisms or continuous exposure to the causative injury that accounts for progressive injury.

PATHOLOGY. Although the clinical history and laboratory evidence of tubular dysfunction will strongly suggest the possibility of tubulointerstitial disease, a diagnosis of TIN can be established only from morphologic examination of kidney tissue (see Table 107–1). As a rule, it is the extent of the lesions of TIN, whether focal or diffuse, that correlates with the degree of impairment in renal function.

Interstitial cellular infiltrates are present in all forms of TIN but are a more prominent feature of ATIN. They are composed mostly of activated lymphocytes and macrophages, but other types of inflammatory cells (polymorphonuclear leukocytes, fibroblasts, histiocytes) and even granulomatous reactions may be present. In all cases, the cortical tubules, which are normally very closely approximated, are separated by an expanded interstitium as a result of edema in ATIN and fibrosis in CTIN. Consequently, the edematous kidneys of patients with ATIN are enlarged, whereas the fibrosclerotic kidneys of those with CTIN are small, contracted, and scarred. The shape of the tubules is well preserved in ATIN, but focal loss of tubular basement membrane and epithelial cell injury by infiltrating mononuclear cells may be present. By contrast, a principal feature of CTIN is tubular atrophy and dilatation. These changes are patchy in distribution, with areas of atrophic, chronically damaged tubules adjacent to dilated tubules displaying compensatory hypertrophy. In general, the glomeruli are normal in ATIN and in the early stages of CTIN, but they ultimately become sclerosed in CTIN and severe periglomerular fibrosis develops. The vasculature is normal in ATIN and early CTIN, but in progressive CTIN the vasculature will demonstrate arteriosclerotic changes,

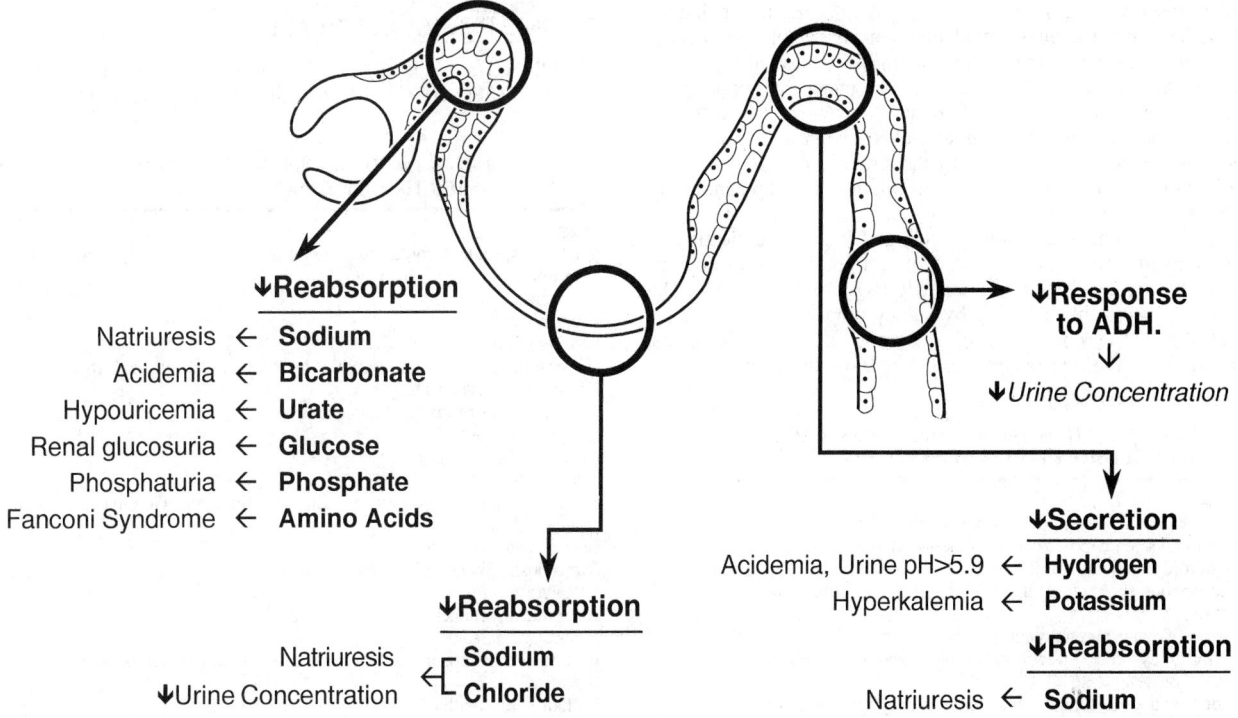

FIGURE 107–1 ■ Schematic presentation of the principal sites of injury and patterns of tubular dysfunction in tubulointerstitial diseases. Heavy set lettering indicates a functional abnormality, and lighter lettering, its consequent clinical manifestation. Arrows indicate the directional change of the abnormality.

even in the absence of elevated blood pressure. Immunofluorescent studies for immune deposits are unrevealing and in general are negative. In the few instances in which they are positive, no definite diagnostic pattern is evident, except in the rare instance of TIN caused by anti–tubular basement membrane antibodies, in which case the characteristic linear immunofluorescence of the tubular basement membrane is diagnostic.

ACUTE TUBULOINTERSTITIAL DISEASES

DRUGS. Drugs have emerged as the most common cause of ATIN (Table 107–2).

Drug-induced ATIN is a hypersensitivity reaction that is not dose related, appears anywhere between 2 to 40 days after the initiation of treatment, and can occur in the absence of any systemic manifestations of hypersensitivity. Also termed *acute allergic interstitial nephritis*, ATIN is actually a rare complication of drugs. It is the increased frequency with which drugs are used that accounts for their emergence as a major cause of ATIN. The absence of previous reactions to an incriminated drug does not preclude the development of ATIN, although a previous systemic reaction to a drug should always suggest its causative role in the diagnosis. Recurrent episodes, often more severe and sudden in onset, can occur upon re-exposure to the same drug or one of its structural analogues (see Chapter 26).

Systemic manifestations indicative of a hypersensitivity reaction are more common with antibiotics. They are transient and may be mild enough to go undetected. In antibiotic-induced ATIN, fever occurs in the majority (60 to 100%); a fleeting skin rash of erythematous, pruritic, maculopapular lesions develops in 30 to 50% of cases; and eosinophilia is present in 30 to 60%. Elevated serum levels of IgE are detected in up to half of these patients. A history of non-specific arthralgias (15 to 20%) and flank pain (variable) secondary to the distended renal capsule of the edematous kidney may be elicited. Hematuria, proteinuria, and pyuria are present in over 80% of cases. The hematuria, which is microscopic in 90% of cases, can be gross and be the initial symptom in some. The proteinuria is tubular in origin and generally mild (<2 g/day). The pyuria is non-specific, except when eosinophils constitute 5% of the urinary white blood cells. Although the presence of eosinophiluria supports a diagnosis of ATIN, it does not establish it, just as its absence does not exclude it.

Sudden onset of renal insufficiency is generally the first evidence of ATIN. The impairment in renal function is variable and occurs with or without oliguria. The increments in blood urea nitrogen and serum creatinine develop at a time when the patient is non-oliguric or even polyuric because of the tubular defect in concentrating ability. Oliguria develops if the tubular dysfunction and mild azotemia go undetected and exposure to the drug is continued. Renal failure is more severe in those in whom oliguria develops and more common in older individuals.

A renal ultrasound scan showing enlarged kidneys, indicative of interstitial edema, and a positive gallium scan, indicative of interstitial inflammatory cell infiltrates, are only suggestive of ATIN. The diagnosis can be established only by kidney biopsy.

TREATMENT. The cornerstones of therapy are early diagnosis, identification of the responsible drug, and discontinuation of its use. Each of these steps is equally important because early diagnosis is essential if severe renal failure is to be avoided, recognition of the responsible drug is important because patients are often taking several drugs that can cause ATIN, and discontinuation of therapy with the incriminated drug is crucial because this measure can result in complete recovery of renal function. Those in whom severe renal failure develops will require supportive therapy and, if oliguric, will require dialysis.

In cases of severe renal failure or in those with progressive renal failure after discontinuation of therapy with the drug, a renal biopsy is indicated to establish the diagnosis and rule out the ATN that occurs in the same prevailing clinical conditions of acutely ill hospitalized patients. It is in such cases that a short course of steroids (60 mg prednisone per day for 10 to 14 days or 1 g methylprednisolone per day intravenously for 3 days) can expedite recovery. The duration of steroid therapy should be guided by the response noted and should never exceed 2 to 4 weeks.

NON-STEROIDAL ANTI-INFLAMMATORY DRUGS. ATIN associated with non-steroidal anti-inflammatory drugs (NSAIDs) is unique because of the accompanying massive proteinuria and the absence of evidence of a hypersensitivity reaction (fever, skin rash, eosinophilia). The proteinuria is insidious in onset and often precedes the onset of renal failure. In some cases, either nephrotic-range proteinuria (10%) or renal failure (15%) may be the only initial feature. Although ATIN has been reported to occur with most NSAIDs, the propionic acid derivatives (ibuprofen, naproxen, fenoprofen) account for the majority of cases encountered clinically.

Unlike the situation with other drugs, usually the patient has a long history of exposure to NSAIDs (weeks to months) before the onset of ATIN, and recovery is slow (months to a year) after withdrawal of the inciting agent. Steroids do not seem to hasten the course of recovery from NSAID-induced ATIN and probably should not be used.

OTHER CAUSES. ATIN may complicate the course of several systemic diseases and infections (see Table 107–2). In about 15 to 20% of cases of ATIN, no etiology can be identified. Prominent among these are cases associated with an idiopathic bone marrow granulomatous reaction and cases with associated uveitis. In the latter, ocular symptoms may precede, accompany, or develop subsequent to clinical evidence of ATIN. Both the renal and ocular changes show a favorable and rapid response to a short course of steroid therapy.

CHRONIC TUBULOINTERSTITIAL DISEASES

CTIN is the unifying feature of an assorted group of diverse diseases (Table 107–3). By definition, chronic renal involvement is

---

Table 107–2 ■ PRINCIPAL CONDITIONS ASSOCIATED WITH ACUTE TUBULOINTERSTITIAL DISEASE

Drugs
Antibiotics (penicillins, cephalosporins, rifampin)
Sulfonamides (cotrimoxazole, sulfamethoxazole)
Non-steroidal anti-inflammatory drugs (propionic acid derivatives)
Miscellaneous (phenytoin, thiazides, allopurinol, cimetidine)
Infections
Invasion of renal parenchyma
Reaction to systemic infections (streptococcal, diphtheria, Hantavirus)
Systemic Diseases
Immune mediated (lupus, transplanted kidney, cryoglobulinemias)
Metabolic (urate, oxalate)
Neoplastic (lymphoproliferative diseases)
Idiopathic

Table 107–3 ■ CONDITIONS ASSOCIATED WITH CHRONIC TUBULOINTERSTITIAL DISEASE

Drugs
Analgesics, non-steroidal anti-inflammatory drugs, cisplatin, cyclosporine, lithium
Heavy metals
Lead, cadmium
Vascular Diseases
Hypertension, vasculitis, embolic disorders, radiation nephritis
Urinary Tract Obstruction
Vesicoureteral reflux, mechanical
Metabolic Disorders
Urate, oxalate, cystinosis
Immune Diseases
Systemic lupus erythematosus, allograft rejection, Goodpasture's syndrome, amyloidosis
Granulomatous Diseases
Sarcoidosis, Wegener's granulomatosis
Infections
Bacterial, mycobacterial, viral, fungal
Hematologic Diseases
Plasma cell dyscrasias, sickle hemoglobinopathies, lymphomas
Endemic
Balkan nephropathy
Hereditary
Cystic diseases, Alport's syndrome
Idiopathic

insidious in onset in these cases, and in most it will go undetected unless specifically sought. Documentation requires testing for tubular dysfunction (see Fig. 107–1) and, if necessary, confirmation by renal biopsy (see Table 107–1). The more common causes of primary CTIN are potentially treatable or preventable.

ANALGESIC NEPHROPATHY. The weight of the available clinical evidence indicates that lesions of analgesic nephropathy develop in those who use analgesic combinations (aspirin and acetaminophen, with or without caffeine) regularly and over extended periods. The extent of injury is related to the quantity of analgesic ingested chronically over the years. In those with severe renal failure, the average dose consumed has been estimated to be about 10 kg over a mean period of 13 years. The minimum amount of drug consumption that is associated with detectable renal impairment is unknown. It has been estimated to be a cumulative dose of 3 kg, or the daily ingestion of 1 g of the index agent for 3 years or longer.

The intrarenal distribution and metabolism of analgesics provide a basis for the location of the renal lesions and their mechanism of injury. Both acetaminophen and aspirin attain significant concentrations in the medulla and papilla of the kidneys. In experimental studies it has been shown that the state of hydration determines the intrarenal concentrations attained and that intrarenal concentrations can be abolished by forced diuresis, which actually results in protection from injury. The intrarenal oxidation of acetaminophen results in the generation of toxic reactive metabolites that are normally reduced by substances such as glutathione. Aspirin uncouples oxidative phosphorylation and reduces the ability of epithelial cells to generate reducing substances. Thus agents that attain sufficient renal medullary concentration to exert a local detrimental effect on their own tend to magnify the degree of renal injury when they are used together.

The initial site of injury is the papilla, where analgesics attain their highest concentration, and patchy necrosis is the first sign of injury. With continued exposure, lesions extend to the outer medulla, increase in severity and extent, and begin to calcify as larger necrotic foci develop. Ultimately, the entire papilla becomes necrotic and may slough or remain in situ, where it shrinks and calcifies. Cortical atrophic scars develop over the necrotic medullary segments, with adjacent areas of compensatory hypertrophy imparting a characteristic cortical nodularity. Visualization of these configurational changes (reduced size, nodularity, calcification) by computed tomography can be extremely useful in the diagnosis of analgesic nephropathy (Fig. 107–2). A decrease in kidney size combined with bumpy contours of both kidneys provides a diagnostic sensitivity of 90% and a specificity of 95%. The additional finding of evidence of papillary necrosis increases the specificity to 97%, with a positive predictive value of 92%.

The lesions of analgesic nephropathy are patchy and slowly progressive, remain asymptomatic, and will usually go undetected until the onset of azotemia. They should be considered in anyone with sterile pyuria, reduced concentrating ability, and a distal tubular acidifying defect, effects that are evident at levels of mild renal insufficiency and gradually become more pronounced and clinically evident as renal function deteriorates. Proximal tubular function is preserved in those with mild renal insufficiency, but it becomes abnormal with advanced renal failure. A tendency toward impaired sodium conservation is common. The presence of any tubular dysfunction, even with normal blood urea nitrogen and serum creatinine levels, should always lead to careful questioning about analgesic use and possible urinary screening for analgesic metabolites.

Analgesic nephropathy is more common in women, in those who are 30 to 50 years old, and in regions where over-the-counter sale of analgesic mixtures is high. Certain personality features (dependency, moodiness) and clinical complaints (headache, musculoskeletal pain, arthralgias) characterize individuals prone to analgesic use. Anemia and peptic ulcer symptoms caused by the gastrointestinal effects of analgesics are common findings and may be the initial complaint in some.

THERAPY. The primary goal of therapy should be discontinuation of analgesic use. In most of those who do, renal function will stabilize or even improve. Those who do not discontinue analgesic

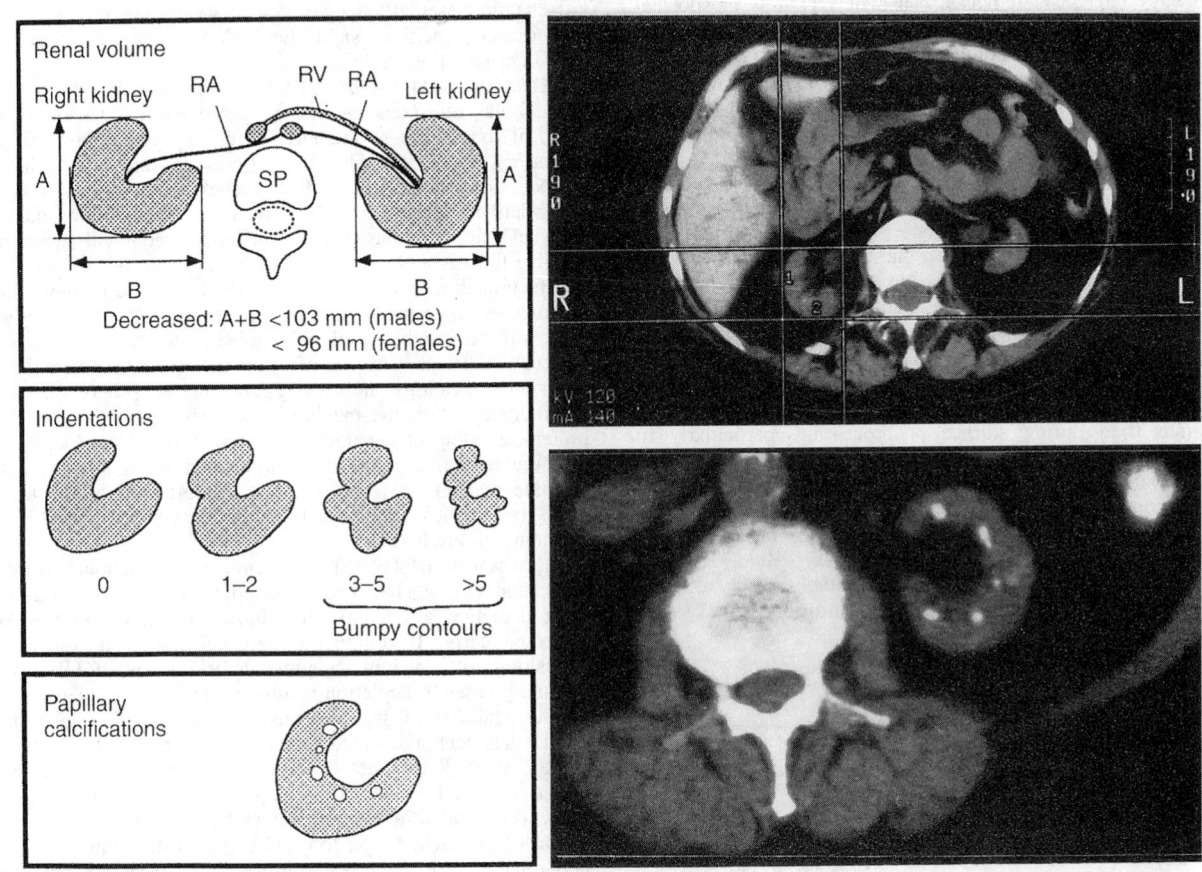

FIGURE 107–2 ▪ Configurational changes (reduced volume, nodularity, calcification) observed on computed tomographic scanning of the kidney in analgesic nephropathy. (Used with permission from *Kidney International* 48:1316, 1995.)

use should be encouraged to increase fluid intake, which reduces the intramedullary concentration of analgesics, and to avoid dehydration or the use of diuretics and laxatives, which increases their medullary concentration. Psychological support and guidance can be useful in discontinuing analgesic use. Monitoring for uroepithelial malignancies is important, even after analgesic discontinuation, because as many as 10% of chronic analgesic users are prone to this otherwise rare form of cancer.

Although discontinuation of chronic analgesic use is important, avoidance of their use in combination is by far more essential. In countries in which over-the-counter sale of analgesic mixtures has been banned, a reduced incidence of analgesic nephropathy has been noted. Aspirin alone in therapeutic doses does not impair renal function in patients with normal renal function. The majority of studies fail to demonstrate an increased risk of ESRD associated with the habitual use of aspirin as a single agent in therapeutic doses. However, aspirin overdosage may impair renal function, especially in those with renal disease. Clinical evidence suggesting that the habitual use of acetaminophen alone causes the clinical entity of classic analgesic nephropathy is negligible. Acetaminophen has been preferentially recommended to patients with renal failure because of the bleeding complications associated with aspirin in these individuals. As such, its association with renal failure may well be an epiphenomenon rather than one of causal association. There is no evidence that the occasional use of acetaminophen causes renal injury or is detrimental to those with renal disease.

OTHER DRUGS. Drugs that have been associated with CTIN include a number of therapeutic medications, antineoplastic agents, and immunosuppressive drugs (see Table 107–3).

LITHIUM. The most common side effect of lithium is vasopressin-resistant nephrogenic diabetes insipidus, which is often accompanied by additional evidence of distal tubular dysfunction, such as a mild form of distal renal tubular acidosis and sodium wasting. CTIN develops in some of these cases, especially in patients with a history of prolonged exposure and recurrent episodes of lithium overdose.

CYCLOSPORINE. Of the immunosuppressive drugs, cyclosporine should always be considered as a cause of CTIN. Cyclosporine-mediated vasoconstriction of the microvasculature accounts for a characteristic occlusive arteriolopathy and subsequent tubular epithelial cell injury. The lesions are characteristically patchy in their early stage and reversible after cessation of therapy, but they can result in more diffuse involvement and irreversible CTIN with prolonged use of the drug.

ANTINEOPLASTIC AGENTS. A principal side effect of antineoplastic agents is direct tubular toxicity with the clinical features of acute renal failure. An invariable concern in all such cases is the consequently prolonged half-life of the agents administered and their increased tendency to systemic toxicity. CTIN will result in some patients, especially after cisplatin and nitrosourea.

HEAVY METALS. Exposure to heavy metals results in different forms of renal toxicity, including CTIN (Table 107–4). Of these agents, the more common and clinically relevant is lead.

Major sources of lead exposure are lead-based paints, lead leached into food during storage or processing, particularly in home-brewed illegal alcoholic beverages (moonshine), and increasingly, environmental exposure (gasoline, industrial fumes). This insidious accumulation of lead has been implicated in the etiology of a syndrome of hyperuricemia, hypertension, and progressive renal failure. Gout occurs in over half of these cases. Blood levels of lead are usually normal. The diagnosis is established by demonstrating increased levels of urinary lead after infusion of the chelat-

Table 107–4 ■ HEAVY METAL NEPHROTOXICITY

Chronic Tubulointerstitial Disease
Bismuth, cadmium, chromium, copper, iron, lead, lithium, mercury, platinum, silicon, uranium
Acute Renal Failure
Arsenic, bismuth, cadmium, chromium, copper, gold, iron, lead, mercury, silver, uranium
Nephrotic Syndrome
Bismuth, gold, mercury, nickel

ing agent calcium disodium ethylenediaminetetraacetic acid (EDTA). EDTA has also been used in the treatment of such cases but appears to be of limited value in mobilizing the total body load of lead or in reversing renal failure.

The renal lesions of lead nephropathy are those of CTIN. Patients examined early, before the onset of ESRD, show primarily focal tubular epithelial cell accumulation of lead with relatively little interstitial cellular infiltrates. In more advanced cases, the kidneys are fibrotic and shrunken and on microscopy show diffuse lesions of CTIN. As might be expected from its association with elevated blood pressure, hypertensive vascular changes are a prominent feature of the kidney in these cases.

Acute lead intoxication is rare but may be encountered after accidental ingestion, usually by children. Its principal manifestations are abdominal colic, hemolytic anemia, and encephalopathy. Acute renal failure secondary to ATIN has been described but is rare.

Of the other heavy metals associated with CTIN (see Table 107–4), cadmium is a relatively more common source of renal toxicity. Exposure to cadmium results in the preferential accumulation of cadmium in the proximal tubule, where it is retained with a rather long biologic half-life of at least 10 years. Its local toxic effect results in CTIN whose principal manifestations are those of proximal tubular dysfunction—aminoaciduria, glucosuria, uricosuria, bicarbonaturia, and hypercalciuria. Urinary calculi occur in one fourth of these cases.

The other heavy metals are rarely a cause of CTIN, and their features mimic those of cadmium. Enough experimental data and some weak epidemiologic evidence suggest a possible role of organic solvents as a cause of CTIN.

VASCULAR DISEASE. Tubular degeneration, interstitial fibrosis, and mononuclear cell infiltration are central components of injury to the kidney by vascular diseases that affect the intrarenal circulation. In rare instances in which the onset of the vascular disease is sudden and severe, such as fulminant vasculitis, the kidney lesions are those of infarction and are associated with acute renal failure. More commonly, they are slow to develop and will go undetected until renal insufficiency supervenes. It is this chronic form of TIN that accounts for the renal insufficiency of hypertensive individuals.

Ischemic vascular changes contribute to the CTIN of patients with diabetes mellitus, sickle hemoglobinopathy, cyclosporine toxicity, and radiation nephritis.

URINARY TRACT OBSTRUCTION. Tubular injury and interstitial cellular infiltrates are some of the earliest responses to any physical impedance to the flow of urine (see Chapter 108). With persistent obstruction, fibrosis becomes prominent and changes of CTIN set in within weeks. Early relief of the obstruction, within this relatively short period, can result in stabilization and reversal of renal failure. Persistence of the obstruction will result in irreversible fibrosis and progressive renal failure.

Infection is a usual, but not invariable feature of most forms of obstructive nephropathy. In fact, with few exceptions, urinary infection will ultimately develop in most patients with urinary tract obstruction. In such cases, infection will contribute significantly to the symptomatology and will aggravate the progression to renal insufficiency. Pressure-mediated extravasation of Tamm-Horsfall protein, a lining of the thick ascending limb of the loop of Henle, into the interstitium has been implicated in mediating an altered immune reaction that contributes to progression of the lesions of CTIN in obstructed individuals, particularly when caused by severe vesicoureteral reflux.

METABOLIC DISORDERS. A number of metabolic disorders are associated with CTIN. Those caused by hypercalcemia and potassium depletion are mainly functional in nature and reversible if corrected early. If prolonged, hypercalcemia can result in focal deposition of calcium (nephrocalcinosis) and CTIN. Whether chronic potassium depletion results in persistent tubular dysfunction is not certain, although a propensity to microcystic dilatation of the tubules has been associated with prolonged potassium depletion.

URIC ACID. The kidneys are the major organs of urate excretion and a principal target of its abnormal metabolism (see Chapter 299). The renal lesions result either from the intratubular crystallization of uric acid in the low pH of the distal tubules (acute urate nephropathy, uric acid nephrolithiasis) or from the deposition of amorphous tophi of sodium urate in the renal parenchyma (chronic urate nephropathy).

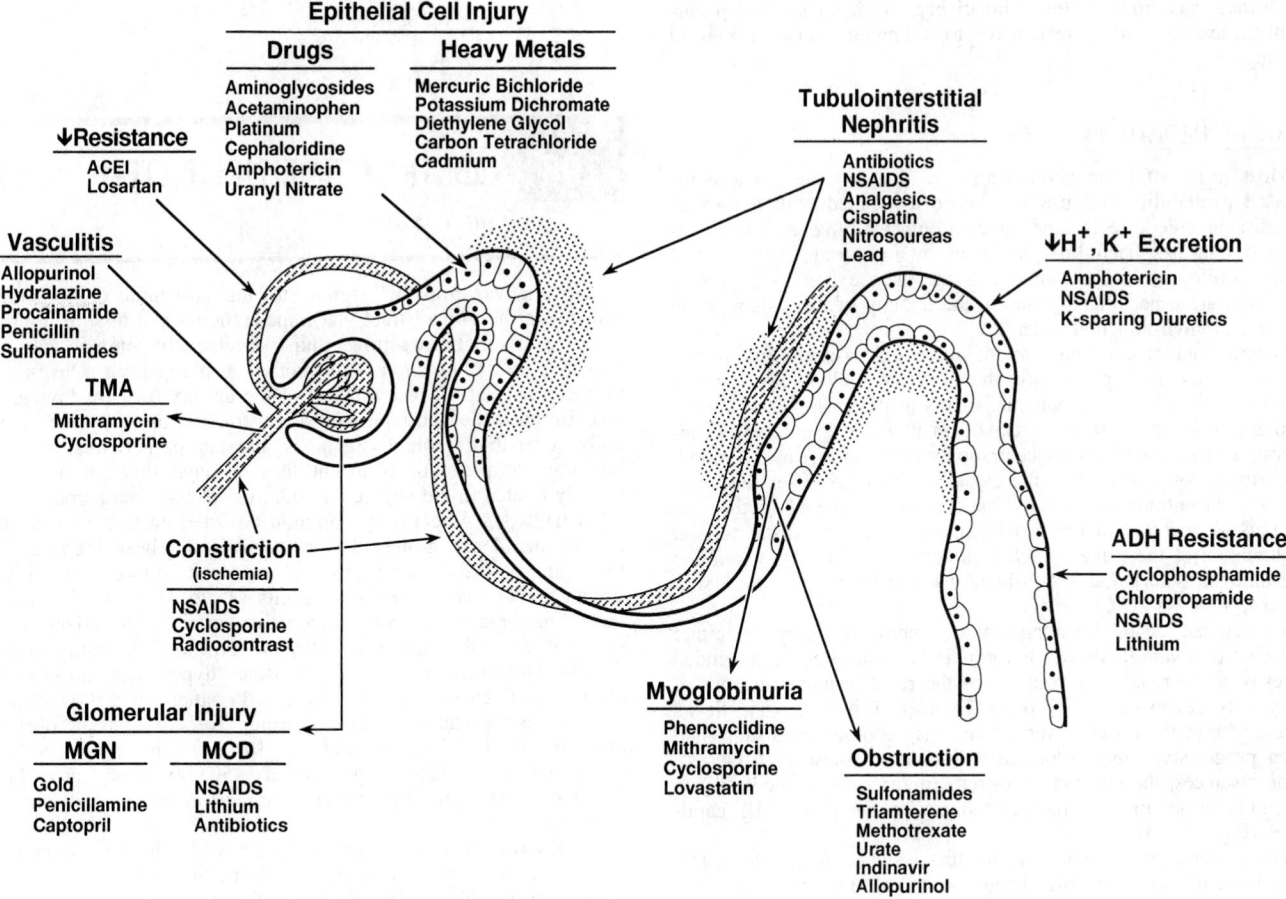

FIGURE 107-3 ■ Schematic presentation of the nephronal sites and mechanism of injury of the principal nephrotoxic agents. The heavy set arrows indicate the directional changes observed. ACEI = angiotensin-converting enzyme inhibitor; ADH = antidiuretic hormone; MCD = minimal change disease; MGN = membranous glomerulopathy; NSAIDs = non-steroidal anti-inflammatory drugs; TMA = thrombotic microangiopathy.

Acute urate nephropathy develops when nucleoprotein release following massive cell injury (tumor lysis syndrome, rhabdomyolysis) in a setting of volume depletion causes a sudden overproduction of urate that results in an acute progressive deterioration in renal function and oliguria. The serum urate concentration is usually greater than 20 mg/dL, and the ratio of the concentration of uric acid to that of creatinine is greater than 1 in a spot urine sample. Hyperphosphatemia, hyperkalemia, and hypocalcemia are common in these patients. The hyperphosphatemia and hyperkalemia are the result of the cell necrosis that also accounts for the hyperuricemia. The hypocalcemia is consequent to the precipitation of calcium at sites of injury where in situ concentrations of the released intracellular phosphate are high. Treatment consists of volume replacement sufficient to maintain a high urine flow rate, which washes out urate precipitates and reduces the urinary concentration of urate; alkalinization of the urine, which increases the solubility of uric acid; and reduction of the excreted urate load by blocking its production with allopurinol.

Chronic urate nephropathy results in CTIN from the deposition of urate microtophi in the renal parenchyma or the precipitation of uric acid in the collecting ducts. The latter form is more common in overproducers of uric acid and in those who have a defect in their ability to increase ammonia production in response to an acid load. *Uric acid nephrolithiasis* is common in these individuals, whose urinary excretion of uric acid is elevated even in the presence of normal blood levels. Intratubular uric acid precipitates can be also a nidus for calcium oxalate stones, which are common in these individuals. This propensity for nephrolithiasis, with its consequent obstructive effect and susceptibility to urinary tract infections, accounts for the CTIN that ultimately sets in.

Renal failure as a result of intrarenal gouty tophi is rare but can occur in those with chronically elevated serum urate levels of more than 10 mg/dL in women and 13 mg/dL in men.

OXALATE. Increased renal excretion of the metabolic end product oxalate results in its intratubular precipitation as calcium oxalate. The hyperoxaluria may be primary or acquired. The former is a rare recessive disorder. Acquired forms of hyperoxaluria are secondary to ingestion or exposure to oxalate precursors (ethylene glycol, methoxyflurane anesthesia, ascorbic acid, pyridoxine deficiency) or increased intestinal absorption of oxalate (regional enteritis, small bowel resection).

Sudden massive hyperoxaluria, such as after ethylene glycol poisoning or prolonged methoxyflurane anesthesia, will be manifested as acute renal failure. The more common chronic forms of hyperoxaluria will result in CTIN, with a propensity for recurrent calcium oxalate nephrolithiasis.

IMMUNE DISEASES. CTIN is a feature of several immune disorders such as immune suppression required for kidney transplantation, Sjögren's syndrome, systemic lupus erythematosus, amyloidosis, mixed cryoglobulinemia, and Goodpasture's syndrome. Except in the latter, immune deposits are not always present in the kidneys of such patients and immunofluorescent studies are either non-specific or negative. Linear deposits of anti–tubular basement membrane antibodies are characteristic of Goodpasture's syndrome.

GRANULOMATOUS DISEASES. Interstitial granulomatous reactions are a rare but characteristic hallmark of certain forms of TIN such as tuberculosis, Wegener's granulomatosis, berylliosis, and other chronic inflammatory diseases. By far, the most common of these diseases is *sarcoidosis*. Granulomatous infiltrates of varying extent are present in as many as 40% of patients with sarcoidosis. Renal insufficiency is rare, except when the lesions are extensive, but distal tubular dysfunction (inability to acidify and concentrate the urine) is common. Almost invariably, the renal lesions of sarcoidosis are exquisitely responsive to a limited course of steroid therapy.

TOXIC NEPHROPATHIES

Most forms of toxic nephropathy are due to drugs, whose increased availability and use have been associated with a host of undesirable side effects, and to environmental toxins, whose increased risk has been brought about by industrial exposure and urban development. The kidneys, as the main excretory organs of the body, are especially exposed to the toxicity of these therapeutic agents and environmental hazards.

Several factors contribute to the increased susceptibility of the kidney to toxicity, specifically, the high renal blood flow, which increases the delivery of potential toxins to the kidney; the tubular epithelial cell transport and metabolism of most agents, which increases their intracellular concentration relative to that in the blood; the urinary concentration in the medulla, which increases the intratubular concentration of agents that have been filtered in the glomerulus or secreted in the proximal tubule; and the distal tubular acidification of the urine, which facilitates intratubular precipitation of some substances and non-ionic back-diffusion of other substances.

The course of the resultant toxic nephropathy may be either *acute* or *chronic*. In its *acute* form, it is manifested as a sudden onset of acute renal failure in which the renal lesions are those of potentially reversible ATN or ATIN (see Table 107–1). In its *chronic* form, the onset of renal failure is insidious, persistent, and often progressive, and its principal lesions are those of CTIN. In some instances, the mechanism of renal injury may be secondary to vasculitis or an immune-mediated injury to the glomerular capillaries (Fig. 107–3).

The principal toxic nephropathies that result in ATIN and CTIN have been discussed in this chapter, and those that result in ATN are covered in the chapter on acute renal failure (Chapter 103) and will not be reconsidered. One mechanism of injury illustrated in Figure 107–3 deserves special comment—that of drug-induced, intrarenal hemodynamic changes, with a potential to cause ischemic tubular injury. Prominent among those are NSAIDs, angiotensin-converting enzyme (ACE) inhibitors, and angiotensin II blockers.

The ability of NSAIDs to inhibit prostaglandin synthesis results in an acute reduction in renal perfusion, which is of negligible import in normal individuals but, in subjects who are volume depleted, will result in acute renal failure. The renal failure is often reversible with early drug withdrawal, but it can progress to ATN and necessitate dialysis with continued exposure. ACE inhibitors exert their effect by inhibiting the angiotensin-mediated efferent vasoconstriction necessary to maintain the glomerular intracapillary pressure essential for filtration. This mechanism, which comes into play in conditions of volume depletion, renders such individuals particularly susceptible to the inhibition of angiotensin. Each of these two broad category of agents, NSAIDs and ACE inhibitors, has been estimated to account for some 15 to 20% of cases of acute renal failure in hospitalized patients, and they are a leading cause of overt acute renal failure, equal in prevalence to the acute renal failure from aminoglycoside nephrotoxicity. Proper evaluation for evidence of intravascular volume (blood pressure and pulse changes in response to tilting) is essential before their use in any hospitalized, acutely ill patient, particularly the elderly and those taking potent diuretics for congestive heart failure, cirrhosis of the liver, or the nephrotic syndrome.

Bennet W (ed): Nephrotoxicity of clinically relevant drugs. Miner Electrolyte Metab 20:169, 1994. *A series of authoritative articles on the most common nephrotoxic drugs encountered in clinical practice; particularly valuable for their focus on diagnosis and management.*

DeBroe ME, Elsevier MM: Analgesic nephropathy. N Engl J Med 338:446, 1998. *A well-referenced review of the evidence for and diagnosis of analgesic nephropathy.*

Eknoyan G: Acute tubulointerstitial nephritis (Chapter 49); Chronic tubulointerstitial nephropathies (Chapter 72). *In* Schrier RW, Gottschalk CW (eds): Diseases of the Kidney, 6th ed. Boston, Little, Brown, 1997, pp 1249–1272, 1983–2015. *In-depth review of the subject matter of this chapter for the specialist; extensively referenced.*

Palmer BF: The renal tubule in the progression of chronic renal failure. J Invest Med 45:346, 1997. *A good review of the central role of the tubular epithelial cells in the pathogenesis of chronic renal failure; 172 references.*

Strutz F, Mueller GA (eds): Symposium on Renal Fibrosis: Prevention and Progression. Kidney Int 49(Suppl. 54):1, 1996. *A series of relatively brief state-of-the-art*

articles on the cell biology of interstitial fibrogenesis, which accounts for the progressive nature of renal failure to end-stage renal disease.

108 OBSTRUCTIVE UROPATHY

Saulo Klahr

"Obstructive uropathy" refers to the structural or functional changes in the urinary tract that impede the normal flow of urine. It occurs in a variety of settings and is a relatively common cause of impaired renal function (obstructive nephropathy). Obstructive uropathy may also cause dilation of the urinary tract (hydronephrosis). Because the consequences of obstructive uropathy are potentially reversible, prompt diagnosis and appropriate treatment are important to prevent permanent loss of renal function, which is directly related to the degree and duration of the obstruction.

INCIDENCE. A relatively common disorder, obstructive uropathy is seen in all age groups. Hydronephrosis has been found at autopsy in 3.5 to 3.8% of adults and in 2% of children. Urolithiasis occurs predominantly in young adults (25 to 45 years old) and is three times more common in men than women. In patients older than 60 years, obstructive uropathy is seen more frequently in men than in women owing to benign prostatic hyperplasia and prostatic carcinoma. Each year, approximately 166 patients per 100,000 population are hospitalized with a presumptive diagnosis of obstruction, and about 387 patient visits per 100,000 population are related to obstructive uropathy. Approximately 450,000 surgical procedures for benign prostatic hyperplasia are performed annually in the United States.

ETIOLOGY. Obstruction can occur anywhere in the urinary tract from the renal tubules (uric acid nephropathy) to the urethral meatus (phimosis) (Table 108–1). Clinically, it is helpful to divide the causes of obstruction into *upper urinary tract* causes (lesions located above the ureterovesical junction) and *lower urinary tract* causes (below the ureterovesical junction). The causes of upper urinary tract obstruction can be divided into *intrinsic* (intraluminal or intramural) and *extrinsic* (see Table 108–1). Intraluminal obstruction is due to stones, clots, or sloughed papillary tissue. Intramural causes are either anatomic (tumors, strictures) or functional (defects in peristalsis: pyeloureteral or vesicoureteral junctions). Extrinsic causes of obstruction can be classified according to the system of origin of the obstructing lesion (see Table 108–1).

Clinically, the age and gender of the patient are helpful in narrowing the differential diagnosis. In children, congenital causes of obstructive uropathy are common (stenosis at the ureteropelvic or ureterovesical junction, urethral valves, and so on). In middle-aged women, cervical cancer is a common cause of extrinsic ureteral or ureterovesical junction obstruction. In elderly men, benign prostatic hyperplasia and prostatic carcinoma are frequent causes of obstruction.

PATHOLOGY AND PATHOPHYSIOLOGY. The effects of obstructive uropathy on renal function are due to several factors with complex interactions. After the onset of obstruction, pressures in the renal pelvis and tubules increase and result in dilatation of these structures. Renal damage is probably initiated by high intraureteral and high intratubular pressures. Decreases in renal blood flow cause ischemia, cellular atrophy, and necrosis. In addition, parenchymal infiltration by macrophages and T lymphocytes may cause scarring of the kidney. Superimposed infection may accelerate kidney destruction in this setting.

Normal urine flow from the renal pelvis to the bladder depends on ureteral peristalsis and a progressive decrease in hydrostatic pressure from Bowman's space to the renal pelvis. Impaired urine flow in the urinary tract leads to a rise in the pressure and volume of urine proximal to the obstruction. In this setting, the high intraureteral pressures transmitted to the kidney result in increased intratubular pressure. The rise in intratubular pressure without a similar rise in intraglomerular pressure decreases the net hydrostatic filtration pressure across glomerular capillaries and thereby results in a fall in the glomerular filtration rate (GFR) (Fig. 108–1).

After the onset of complete obstruction, transient renal vasodila-

Table 108-1 ■ CAUSES OF URINARY TRACT OBSTRUCTION

UPPER URINARY TRACT	LOWER URINARY TRACT
Intrinsic Causes	1. Phimosis, meatal stenosis, paraphimosis
1. Intraluminal	2. Urethra: strictures, stones, diverticulum, posterior or anterior urethral valves, periurethral abscess, urethral surgery
a. Intratubular deposition of crystals (uric acid, acyclovir)	3. Prostate: benign hyperplasia, abscess, carcinoma
b. Ureter: stones, clots, renal papillae	4. Bladder
2. Intramural	a. Neurogenic bladder: spinal cord defect or trauma, diabetes, multiple sclerosis, cerebrovascular accidents, Parkinson's disease
a. Ureteropelvic or ureterovesical junction dysfunction	b. Bladder neck dysfunction
b. Ureteral valve, polyp, stricture, or tumor	c. Bladder calculus
Extrinsic Causes	d. Bladder cancer
1. Vascular system	5. Trauma
a. Aneurysm: abdominal aorta, iliac vessels	a. Straddle injury
b. Aberrant vessels: ureteropelvic junction	b. Pelvic fracture
c. Venous: retrocaval ureter	6. Drugs: spinal anesthesia, anticholinergics, smooth muscle depressants
2. Reproductive system	
a. Uterus: pregnancy, prolapse, tumors, endometriosis	
b. Ovary: abscess, tumors, ovarian remnants	
c. Gartner's duct cyst, tubo-ovarian abscess	
3. Gastrointestinal tract: Crohn's disease; diverticulitis; appendiceal abscess; tumors; pancreatic tumor, abscess, or cyst	
4. Retroperitoneal disease	
a. Retroperitoneal fibrosis (idiopathic, radiation, drugs)	
b. Inflammatory: tuberculosis, sarcoidosis	
c. Hematomas	
d. Primary tumors (lymphoma, sarcoma, and so on)	
e. Metastic tumors (cervix, bladder, colon, prostate, and so on)	
f. Lymphocele	
g. Pelvic lipomatosis	

tation occurs and is followed by progressive vasoconstriction of the renal circulation. This vasoconstriction leads to a decrease in renal blood flow, a fall in intraglomerular pressure, and a decrease in the GFR (see Fig. 108–1). The vasoconstriction is mediated by angiotensin II and thromboxane A_2. These two compounds, through their effects on mesangial cell contraction, may also decrease the glomerular surface area available for filtration, which may explain the greater decrease in GFR than in renal plasma flow observed in obstruction.

Because of increased intrarenal levels of angiotensin II, the synthesis of prostaglandin E_2 and prostacyclin is augmented. These eicosanoids are vasodilatory substances that also antagonize the effects of angiotensin II on mesangial cell contraction. Hence in the setting of obstruction, the increased synthesis of both prostaglandin E_2 and prostacyclin tends to prevent the GFR and renal blood flow from decreasing further. After the obstruction is released in experimental animals, administering inhibitors of prostaglandin synthesis, such as non-steroidal anti-inflammatory agents or inhibitors of nitric oxide, decreases the GFR and renal blood flow.

Partial obstruction of the urinary tract may also decrease renal blood flow and the GFR. In addition, functional tubular defects are prominent. An inability to concentrate the urine and decreased excretion of hydrogen ions and potassium are noted. The concentrating defect is due in part to decreased osmolality of the renal medulla, probably related to decreased sodium reabsorption in the thick ascending limb of Henle's loop, and to the removal of medullary solutes (sodium, urea) as a consequence of the initial increase in medullary blood flow seen in obstruction. A decrease in the hydro-osmotic response of the cortical collecting duct to vasopressin because of down-regulation of aquaporin-2 (a permeable water channel) also contributes to the concentrating defect. The decreased hydrogen ion and potassium excretion is due to impaired secretion of these ions in distal segments of the nephron, presumably as a consequence of diminished response to the action of aldosterone.

CLINICAL MANIFESTATIONS. The clinical manifestations of obstructive uropathy depend on the location (upper or lower urinary tract), degree (complete or partial), and duration (acute or chronic) of the obstruction (Table 108–2).

The symptoms of upper and lower urinary tract obstruction differ. Patients with acute complete obstruction may have acute renal

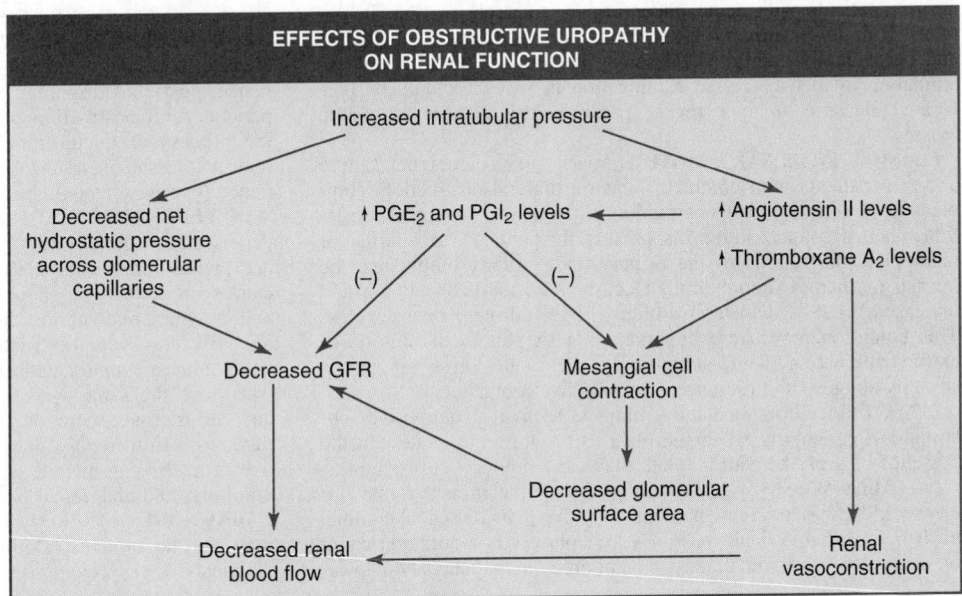

FIGURE 108–1 ■ Increased levels of prostaglandin E_2 (PGE_2) and prostacyclin (PGI_2) tend to antagonize (−) the effects of angiotensin II and thromboxane A_2 on mesangial cell contraction and renal vasoconstriction. Hence they tend to prevent the glomerular filtration rate from decreasing further.

EFFECTS OF OBSTRUCTIVE UROPATHY ON RENAL FUNCTION

Table 108-2 ■ CLINICAL MANIFESTATIONS AND LABORATORY FINDINGS IN URINARY TRACT OBSTRUCTION

1. No symptoms (chronic hydronephrosis)
2. Intermittent pain (chronic hydronephrosis)
3. Elevated levels of BUN and serum creatinine with no other symptoms (chronic hydronephrosis)
4. Renal colic (usually due to utereral stones or papillary necrosis)
5. Changes in urinary output
   a. Anuria or oliguria (acute renal failure)
   b. Polyuria (incomplete or partial obstruction)
   c. Fluctuating urinary output
6. Hematuria
7. Palpable masses
   a. Flank (hydronephrotic kidney, usually in infants)
   b. Suprapubic (distended bladder)
8. Hypertension
   a. Flank (hydronephrotic kidney, usually in infants)
   b. Suprapubic (distended bladder)
9. Hypertension
   a. Volume dependent (usually due to chronic bilateral obstruction)
   b. Renin dependent (usually due to acute unilateral obstruction)
10. Repeated urinary tract infections or infection that is refractory to treatment
11. Hyperkalemic, hyperchloremic acidosis (usually due to defective tubular secretion of hydrogen and potassium)
12. Hypernatremia (seen in infants with partial obstruction and polyuria)
13. Polycythemia (increased renal production of erythropoietin)
14. Lower urinary tract symptoms: hesistancy, urgency, incontinence, postvoid dribbling, decreased force and caliber of urinary stream, nocturia

BUN = blood urea nitrogen.

failure. Patients with chronic partial obstruction (chronic hydronephrosis) may be asymptomatic, may have intermittent pain, or may have symptoms and laboratory findings of impaired renal function, including an inability to concentrate the urine manifested as nocturia and/or polyuria, with or without elevated levels of blood urea nitrogen and serum creatinine.

PAIN AND RENAL COLIC. Pain caused by distention of the bladder or stretching of the collecting system or the renal capsule is a common initial symptom in obstructive uropathy, particularly in patients with ureteral calculi. Classic "renal colic" is a steadily increasing severe pain located in the flank (in the case of stones lodged in the upper third of the ureter) or radiating to the labia, testicles, or groin (stones in the lower two thirds of the ureter) and may be associated with sweating and vomiting. The acute attack may last less than 30 minutes or as long as a day. Pain radiating into the flank during micturition is said to be pathognomonic of vesicoureteral reflux. Chronic partial obstruction may cause intermittent flank pain. Pain may be elicited in some of these patients by the administration of diuretics and/or excessive fluid intake. Physical examination may be normal or may reveal flank tenderness in patients with acute upper urinary tract obstruction. In patients with lower urinary tract obstruction, a distended, palpable, and occasionally painful bladder may be found. Careful rectal examination in men or pelvic examination in women should be performed because it may reveal prostatic enlargement or pelvic masses.

CHANGES IN URINARY OUTPUT. Anuria and acute renal failure occur in patients with complete bilateral ureteral obstruction, complete lower urinary tract obstruction, or unilateral ureteral obstruction when a solitary kidney is present. In patients with partial or incomplete obstruction of the urinary tract, urinary output may be normal or increased (polyuria). Occasionally, marked polyuria and increased thirst (a diabetes insipidus–like syndrome) may develop. This condition may cause hypernatremia. A pattern of oliguria or anuria alternating with polyuria or the acute onset of anuria strongly suggests the presence of obstructive uropathy.

HEMATURIA. Gross hematuria may be seen in patients with obstruction, particularly when the obstruction is due to stones. In the presence of gross hematuria, clots may cause ureteral obstruction.

PALPABLE MASSES. Long-standing obstructive uropathy may increase kidney size. Such patients may have increased abdominal girth or a palpable flank mass. Hydronephrosis is a common cause of a palpable abdominal mass in children. In patients with lower

urinary tract obstruction, particularly obstruction secondary to benign prostatic hyperplasia, a suprapubic mass may be caused by a distended bladder. This part of the physical examination should not be neglected in patients with anuria and suspected obstructive uropathy. This type of obstruction is readily reversed by placing a catheter in the bladder.

HYPERTENSION. Hypertension is commonly associated with renal disease of diverse causes. Patients with obstructive uropathy may have hypertension from (1) fluid retention and expansion of the extracellular fluid volume, (2) increased renin secretion, and (3) possibly decreased synthesis of medullary vasodepressor substances. In some patients with obstructive uropathy, hypertension may be coincidental and occur in about one third of patients with acute unilateral obstruction and is usually, but not always, renin dependent. Release of the acute obstruction should alleviate the hypertension when the two are causally related.

In patients with chronic bilateral obstruction, the hypertension is usually due to impaired sodium excretion and expansion of the extracellular fluid volume (volume-dependent hypertension). In such patients, circulating levels of renin are usually suppressed.

URINARY TRACT INFECTIONS OR INFECTION THAT IS REFRACTORY TO TREATMENT. Repeated urinary tract infections without apparent cause suggest obstruction. Infection is more common in patients with lower urinary tract obstruction, possibly because of decreased bacterial "washout" and increased bacterial adherence to the mucosa of the bladder. Moreover, in the presence of obstruction, eradicating the infection is difficult. In non-instrumented patients, the finding of unusual organisms (Proteus, Pseudomonas) in urine cultures should suggest the presence of underlying obstruction. Thus in patients with repeated urinary tract infections or persistent infection refractory to treatment, the possibility of underlying obstructive uropathy should be considered.

INCREASED LEVELS OF BLOOD UREA NITROGEN AND SERUM CREATININE. Obstructive uropathy is a potential cause of impaired renal function and end-stage renal disease and should be considered in the differential diagnosis, particularly in patients with a normal urinary sediment and no previous history of renal disease. Obstruction of the urinary tract may occur in patients with established renal parenchymal disease and cause an acceleration in the rate of progression.

HYPERKALEMIC, HYPERCHLOREMIC METABOLIC ACIDOSIS. A hyperkalemic, hyperchloremic (non–anion gap) metabolic acidosis may be present in patients with obstructive uropathy. It is seen more frequently in elderly individuals. The abnormality is due to decreased hydrogen ion and potassium secretion by distal segments of the nephron and may be caused by decreased aldosterone production and/or refractoriness of the distal tubule to the actions of this mineralocorticoid. Hyperchloremic metabolic acidosis may occur in the absence of hyperkalemia and results from a selective defect in hydrogen ion secretion.

POLYCYTHEMIA. Polycythemia that subsides after obstruction is relieved is a rare manifestation of urinary tract obstruction. Increased renal production of erythropoietin, presumably due to ischemia, may account for the development of polycythemia.

LOWER URINARY TRACT SYMPTOMS. Symptoms such as decreased force and caliber of the urine stream, intermittency, incontinence, post-void dribbling, hesitancy, and urgency may develop in patients with obstruction of the lower urinary tract. Alterations in the process of micturition because of neurogenic bladder disease may also result in urgency, frequent urination, and urinary incontinence (overflow incontinence).

DIFFERENTIAL DIAGNOSIS. The differential diagnosis varies depending on the clinical signs and symptoms. Patients with anuria and acute renal failure should be evaluated for other potential causes of acute renal failure (see Chapter 103). Partial obstruction and polyuria may mimic the entity of nephrogenic diabetes insipidus. Patients with obstruction manifested as hyperchloremic, hyperkalemic metabolic acidosis should be distinguished from patients who have the same syndrome on the basis of low levels of renin and aldosterone secretion. Gastrointestinal pathology may mimic flank pain from renal stones. In children, manifestations of obstructive uropathy can include gastrointestinal symptoms such as nausea, vomiting, and abdominal pain.

DIAGNOSTIC APPROACH. The presence of obstructive uropathy may not be obvious. Definitive tests are needed to exclude this diagnosis in suspected cases. Early diagnosis and prompt treatment are essential because the degree of renal impairment resulting from obstructive uropathy is related to its severity and duration. The diagnostic approach to obstructive uropathy depends on the symptoms and the clinical findings of patients with asymptomatic renal insufficiency, renal colic, or acute renal failure and anuria (Fig. 108–2).

When obstruction is suspected, the history may be of value: previous urinary tract infections, drugs ingested, and the presence of lower urinary tract symptoms (see above). In the hospital setting, the pattern of urinary output can be ascertained from input and output records. The physical examination may yield some clues: tenderness in the costovertebral angle, a mass in the flank area, and muscle rigidity over the kidney area. Abdominal distention and diminished peristalsis accompany acute renal colic. A suprapubic mass may be due to bladder outlet obstruction. Urinalysis may yield important clues: hematuria, bacteriuria, or a urinary pH greater than 7.5 indicative of stones and/or infection with urea-splitting organisms. The urinary sediment should be examined carefully for the presence of crystals (uric acid, cystine, and so forth). Laboratory studies should include an assessment of renal function (blood urea nitrogen, serum creatinine).

Tests used to diagnose obstructive uropathy are summarized in Table 108–3. Ultrasound is a noninvasive diagnostic test used as the initial procedure in suspected obstruction. The main finding detected by ultrasound is dilation of the urinary tract. In a few instances, ultrasound may give false-negative results because dilation does not occur as a consequence of dehydration or too recent an onset of obstruction (see Fig. 108–2). *Plain films of the abdomen (kidneys, ureter, bladder)* are particularly useful in patients with renal colic because ureteral calculi may be visualized (see Fig. 108–2). They also provide information on renal and bladder morphology, such as size differences between the two kidneys or an enlarged bladder that suggests outlet obstruction. The *intravenous pyelogram* is used to investigate acute renal colic (see Fig. 108–2). Excretion of contrast media may be delayed in patients with a low GFR because of a decrease in the filtered load of dye. In such patients, the procedure should be extended until the collecting sys-

Table 108–3 ■ DIAGNOSTIC TESTS USED IN OBSTRUCTIVE UROPATHY

Upper Urinary Tract Obstruction
Sonography (ultrasound)
Plain films of the abdomen (KUB)
Excretory or intravenous pyelography
Retrograde pyelography
Isotopic renography
Computed tomography
Magnetic resonance imaging
Pressure flow studies (the Whitaker test)
Lower Urinary Tract Obstruction
Some of the tests listed above
Cystoscopy
Voiding cystourethrogram
Retrograde urethrography
Urodynamic tests
  Debimetry
  Cystometrography
  Electromyography
  Urethral pressure profile

KUB = Kidneys, ureter, bladder.
Reproduced by permission from Klahr S: Obstructive uropathy. *In* Jacobson HR, Striker GE, Klahr S (eds): The Principles and Practice of Nephrology. Toronto, BC Decker, 1991, pp 432–441. By permission of Mosby–Year Book.

tem and the site of obstruction are identified. This identification may require delayed films. Intravenous pyelography is not useful in patients with compromised renal function, particularly those with serum creatinine levels greater than 3 to 4 mg/dL. It also has the risk of potential nephrotoxicity. *Retrograde pyelography* requires the retrograde injection of radiocontrast material and is used to visualize the ureter and collecting system when intravenous pyelography cannot be done or is not justified because of a history of allergic reaction to contrast material or other contraindications. This

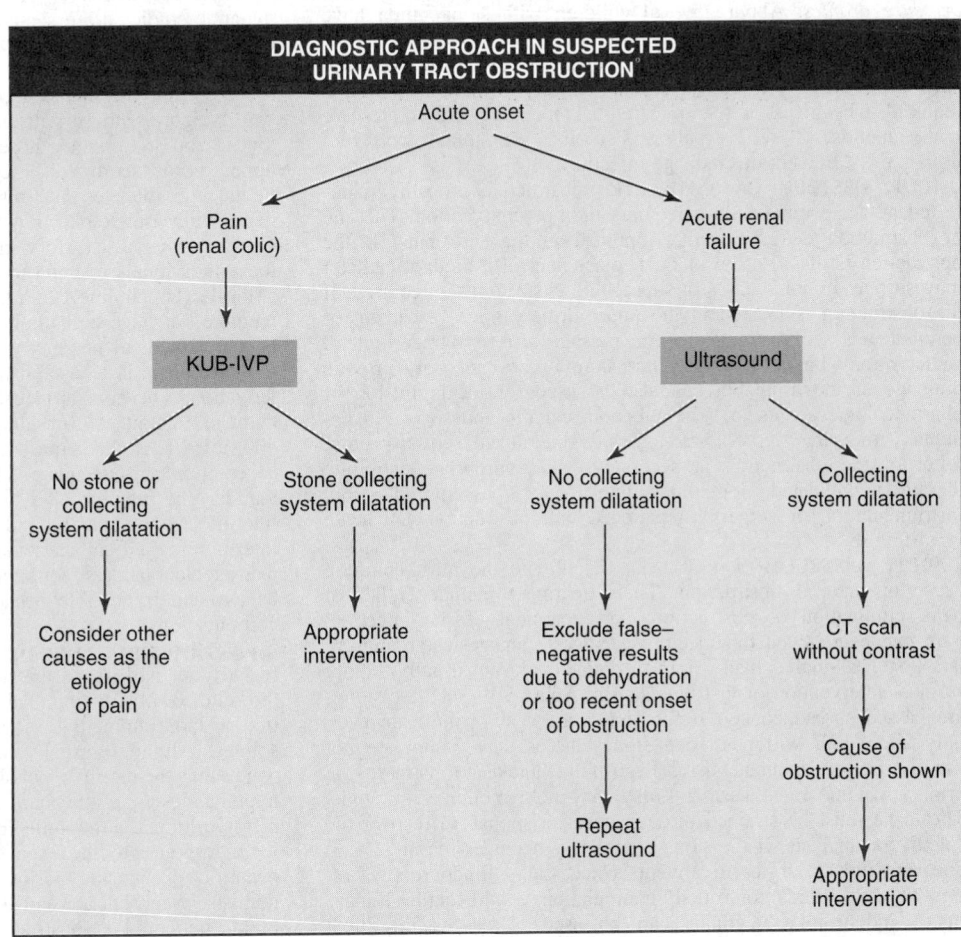

FIGURE 108–2 ■ Scheme of a diagnostic approach to urinary tract obstruction. KUB (kidney, ureter, bladder) = a flat film of the abdomen without contrast material; IVP = intravenous pyelography; CT = computed tomography.

procedure can identify both the site and the cause of the obstruction. Isotopic renography can be used to diagnose upper urinary tract obstruction. It requires the intravenous injection of a radionuclide and subsequent imaging with a gamma scintillation camera. This imaging can be combined with intravenous furosemide administered 20 to 30 minutes after the isotope is injected. Other diagnostic procedures for obstructive uropathy include computed tomography and magnetic resonance imaging. *Computed tomography* is particularly useful for *diagnosing causes of obstruction*. Occasionally, upper urinary tract obstruction is difficult to diagnose with the techniques described above, and *pressure-flow studies* (the Whitaker test) may be required. This test consists of measuring pressure differences between the renal pelvis and the bladder during the infusion of fluid at a known rate into the renal pelvis.

A number of tests are useful in diagnosing lower urinary tract obstruction, including *voiding cystourethrography*, which is used to investigate the presence of vesicoureteral reflux as a cause of dilation of the urinary tract. *Cystoscopy* allows visual inspection of the entire urethra and bladder during the same procedure. However, this test requires the use of anesthesia in children and young adults. The anterior urethra can be assessed by *retrograde urethrography*, which is performed by occluding the urethral meatus with a syringe or catheter and injecting contrast medium. However, a retrograde urethrogram is not adequate to evaluate the posterior urethra. This anatomic area is best examined by an *excretory or retrograde cystogram*. The two tests combined usually provide a complete study of the urethra. *Urodynamic tests* with measurement of the urine flow rate per unit time are useful for evaluating bladder outlet obstruction. Measurement of the *urine flow rate (debimetry)* is a noninvasive test that examines the interplay between the expulsive force of the detrusor muscle and urethral resistance. *Cystometrography* can be used to assess the force of the detrusor muscle in the bladder, and it quantifies the pressure-volume relationships of this organ. "Dyssynergy" of the bladder sphincter refers to the inability of the sphincter to relax during contraction of the detrusor muscle and is seen in patients with neurologic disorders. This type of resistance is better analyzed by *electromyography* and *urethral pressure profiles*. About 25% of children with spina bifida have detrusor sphincter dyssynergia at birth.

TREATMENT. After establishing a diagnosis of obstructive uropathy, it is necessary to decide whether surgery or instrumentation is required. The goals of therapy are to (1) restore and/or preserve renal function, (2) relieve pain and/or other symptoms of obstruction, and (3) prevent or eradicate infection.

ACUTE OBSTRUCTION (COMPLETE). Obstructive uropathy manifested as acute renal failure requires prompt intervention. The site of obstruction determines the approach in these patients. If the obstruction is distal to the bladder, placement of a urethral catheter may suffice. In some cases, a suprapubic cystostomy is required. If the obstruction is located in the upper urinary tract, placement of percutaneous nephrostomy tubes or passage of a retrograde ureteral catheter may be necessary. Nephrostomy tubes not only provide drainage of the urine but can also be used for local infusion of pharmacologic agents to treat infection, calculi, and so on. In patients with urinary tract infection and generalized sepsis, prompt relief of the obstruction is necessary, and appropriate antibiotic therapy is indicated. Sometimes dialysis may be required before instrumentation or surgery in patients with obstruction and acute renal failure.

ACUTE OBSTRUCTION (PARTIAL). Calculi are the most common cause of ureteral obstruction. Their treatment includes relief of pain, elimination of obstruction, and treatment of the infection. Pain can be relieved by injecting a narcotic analgesic intramuscularly. Stones smaller than 5 mm in diameter do not usually require surgical intervention or instrumentation. About 90% of these stones are passed spontaneously. If the stones are 5 to 7 mm, however, only about half will pass, and stones larger than 7 mm are not usually passed spontaneously. High fluid intake to increase the urinary volume to at least 2 L/day may help mobilize the stone. The urine must be strained through a gauze sponge to recover the calculi for analysis. If the stone completely occludes the ureter and does not move, surgical treatment is necessary. "Endourology" refers to the closed, controlled manipulation of the entire urinary tract. Endourologic methods can be used to successfully treat

stones obstructing the ureter in about 98% of patients. In addition, this approach shortens the hospital stay to 3 to 4 days and the convalescence period to only 4 to 7 days. Extracorporeal shock wave or ultrasound lithotripsy involves the focusing of electrohydraulic or ultrasonically generated shock waves to disintegrate the stone. The method is effective for ureteral calculi of 7 to 15 mm that lie above the pelvic brim. The stone is disintegrated in 90% of patients, and all particulate matter passes within a 3-month period. Morbidity is low. However, all patients should be monitored for stone recurrence and should be given preventive therapy. In addition, post-treatment hypertension may occur and requires follow-up. In selected individuals, the procedure can be done on an outpatient basis, and most patients are back at work 2 to 3 days after shock wave therapy. Calculi located distal to the pelvic brim can be approached from below. Antibiotics are useful when infections complicate renal calculi, with the choice of antibiotic depending on appropriate urine cultures and sensitivity studies.

CHRONIC PARTIAL OBSTRUCTION. Surgical intervention can sometimes be delayed for weeks or even months in patients with low-grade obstruction or partial chronic obstruction. However, prompt relief of partial obstruction is indicated when (1) repeated episodes of urinary tract infection occur, (2) the patient has significant symptoms (dysuria, voiding dysfunction, flank pain), (3) urinary retention exists, or (4) evidence of recurrent or progressive renal damage is present.

LOWER URINARY TRACT OBSTRUCTION. Urethral and bladder neck obstruction requires surgery in patients with recurrent infections who are ambulatory, particularly when reflux, renal parenchymal damage, marked urinary retention, repeated bleeding, or other symptoms are present. Obstruction secondary to benign prostatic hyperplasia is not always progressive. Therefore, patients with minimal symptoms, no infection, and a normal upper urinary tract may be monitored safely until the patient and physician agree that surgery is desirable. Urethral strictures in men can be treated by dilation or internal urethrotomy via direct vision. The incidence of bladder neck and urethral obstruction in women is low. Hence urethral dilation, internal urethrotomy, meatotomy, and revision of the bladder neck in women are seldom indicated.

When obstruction is the result of neuropathic bladder function, dynamic studies are essential to determine therapy. The main goals of therapy should be to (1) establish the bladder as a urine storage organ without causing renal injury and (2) provide a mechanism for bladder emptying that is acceptable to the patient. Patients fall into two categories, those with atonic bladders secondary to lower motor neuron injury and those with unstable bladder function from upper motor neuron disease. The neurogenic bladder seen in patients with diabetes mellitus is usually the result of lower motor neuron disease. Requesting these patients to void at regular intervals achieves satisfactory emptying of the bladder. Occasionally, these individuals respond to cholinergic agents such as bethanechol chloride (Urecholine). α-Adrenergic blockers relax urethral sphincter tone but have only limited success because of side effects. The best treatment of patients with significant residual urine and recurrent urosepsis is to establish clean, intermittent, regular self-catheterization. The goal is to catheterize four or five times per day so that the amount of urine drained from the bladder does not exceed 400 mL. This technique may be successful but requires patient acceptance and adequate training. In patients with a hypertonic bladder, the major goal is to improve its storage function. Anticholinergic agents may be indicated. Occasionally, long-term, clean, intermittent self-catheterization is necessary. In all patients with neurogenic bladders, long-term use of indwelling catheters should be avoided if possible because of the risk of infection and other complications.

POST-OBSTRUCTIVE DIURESIS. "Post-obstructive diuresis" refers to the marked natriuresis and diuresis that occasionally follow the relief of obstruction. This diuresis is characterized by the excretion of large amounts of sodium, potassium, magnesium, and other solutes. Although usually self-limited, the losses of solutes and water may result in hypokalemia, hyponatremia or hypernatremia, hypomagnesemia, and marked volume depletion. In many patients, a brisk diuresis after relief of obstruction may represent a physiologic response to the expansion in extracellular fluid volume that occurred during the period of obstruction. This post-obstructive diuresis is appropriate and does not compromise the volume status of the patient. Post-obstructive diuresis in this setting can be prolonged by overzealous replacement of salt and water after the relief of obstruction.

Fluid replacement is justified only when excessive losses of sodium and water are inappropriate for the volume status of the patient and are presumably due to an intrinsic tubular defect in sodium and water reabsorption. Fluid replacement in these patients is guided in large part by what is excreted. Intravenous fluid administration may be necessary, but urinary losses should be replaced only to the extent necessary to prevent extracellular fluid volume contraction or electrolyte imbalance.

PROGNOSIS. The return of renal function after relieving obstruction is variable and influenced by the severity and duration of the obstruction. Other events that condition the degree of recovery of renal function include the presence of infection, stones, pre-existing renal disease, and/or the underlying cause of the obstruction. Renal cortical thickness is a prognostic indicator of residual renal function in patients with chronic hydronephrosis. Patients with a very thin cortex have lost considerable renal function.

Klahr S: Obstructive nephropathy; pathophysiology and management. *In* Schrier RW (ed): Renal and Electrolyte Disorders, 5th ed. Philadelphia, Lippincott-Raven, 1997, pp 544–589. *A chapter with major emphasis on the pathophysiology of obstructive nephropathy.*

Klahr S: Obstructive uropathy. *In* Kassirer JP, Greene HL (eds): Current Therapy in Adult Medicine, 4th ed. St Louis, CV Mosby, 1997, pp 1135–1140. *Discusses the therapeutic approach to patients with obstructive uropathy.*

Klahr S: Urinary tract obstruction. *In* Schrier RW, Gottschalk CW (eds): Diseases of the Kidney, 6th ed. Boston, Little, Brown, 1997, pp 709–738. *A detailed chapter on pathogenesis and clinical and diagnostic issues in obstructive nephropathy; numerous references.*

109 SPECIFIC RENAL TUBULAR DISORDERS

Russell W. Chesney

Renal tubular disorders represent a group of conditions in which the renal tubular reabsorption of either ions or organic solutes is diminished, resulting in excessive amounts of either substance in the urine. The defect can be characterized by the nephron segment affected. The functions of each segment will influence the type of substance lost as well as the rate of loss. As noted in Chapter 101, the proximal nephron is responsible for reclaiming most of the filtered glucose, amino acids, uric acid, phosphate, bicarbonate, and low-molecular-weight proteins. Henle's loop reabsorbs over half the filtered sodium chloride as well as divalent cations. The distal nephron (including the cortical and medullary collecting ducts), under the influence of aldosterone, reabsorbs the final amount of sodium and secretes hydrogen and potassium ions. The terminal collecting ducts are influenced by antidiuretic hormone to permit water reabsorption and hence lead to urinary concentration.

Many tubular disorders are inherited and appear to involve the loss or formation of a defective transport protein ("carrier") and represent an inborn error of transport. Because many of these transporter proteins and channels have been cloned, the precise genetic defect of many of these conditions can now be understood more completely. Acquired conditions also can perturb transport function (Table 109–1). These conditions include (1) a single selective transport defect, (2) a class-specific defect (e.g., dibasic amino acids in cystinuria), or (3) those solutes whose transport is influenced by a specific hormone, which can arise from hormone deficiency or resistance (e.g., in hypoaldosteronism or diabetes insipidus). Perturbation of tubular energy production or direct structural alteration is more likely to result in a global disorder, such as the generalized tubular dysfunction found in Fanconi's syndrome. Luminal, intracellular, or peritubular components of the net transport process can be affected in each situation. Several of the more usual transport defects of individual nephron segments are described here.

DISORDERS OF THE PROXIMAL TUBULE FUNCTION

The proximal tubule is the site of reabsorption of 80 to 99% of filtered solutes, including glucose, amino acids, and phosphates.

Urinary wastage of bulk quantities of these solutes implies a disorder of proximal tubular function.

RENAL GLYCOSURIAS. The renal glycosurias are caused by inherited or acquired defects in proximal tubule glucose reabsorption such that glycosuria is evident at normal serum glucose concentrations.

PATHOPHYSIOLOGY. D-Glucose is actively reabsorbed across the luminal surface of the proximal tubule by a stereospecific carrier that requires sodium. The quantity of glucose reabsorbed changes, depending on the filtered glucose load, until a maximal reabsorptive capacity, or Tm, is achieved. Before saturation, glucose reabsorption is incomplete and a "splay" is evident (Fig. 109–1). The initial point in the splay represents that filtered glucose concentration (the "threshold") at which reabsorption no longer equals filtration and glucose appears in the urine. Normally, the threshold concentration, 200 to 240 mg/dL, is far above the plasma values; thus, scant glucose (<125 mg/day) appears in the urine. The kinetics of D-glucose reabsorption have been compared with classic enzyme kinetics. The T_m is likened to the V_{max}, whereas the degree of splay represents the K_m. In the two main forms of renal glucosuria, either the capacity (type A, V_{max}, or K_m mutation) or the affinity (type B, K_m, or extent-of-splay mutation) of glucose reabsorption is affected. Consistent with this view, the genes encoding the high affinity (*SGLT1*) and low affinity (*SGLT2*) are found on different chromosomes: *SGLT1* is on chromosome 22q13.1, and *SGLT2* is on chromosome 16. *SGLT1* alone also transports galactose and is present in the intestine. A defect in *SGLT1* has been found in families with glucose-galactose malabsorption. Mutations in *SGLT2* account for familial glucosuria. In either form, the threshold is influenced so that glucose is lost in the urine at a normal plasma glucose concentration. Glucosuria becomes marked after intravenous infusion of D-glucose.

SYMPTOMS AND CAUSES. Renal glucosuria is uncommon, with a prevalence of 0.2 to 0.6%. Inheritance is autosomal recessive, and heterozygotes have more marked glucosuria. Usually, but not always, V_{max} and K_m variants are inherited separately, as would be anticipated with two separate genes. Renal biopsy samples reveal no consistent pathologic features. Unlike the aminoacidurias, no intestinal transport defects are found. Renal glucosuria is completely asymptomatic.

Intermittent glucosuria is not uncommon during the third trimester of pregnancy (see Chapters 110 and 253) and in terminal chronic renal insufficiency. In each instance, the functional change in glucose transport kinetics relates to an increase in tubular flow rate from an increase in total single-nephron glomerular filtration rate (GFR). In a rare disorder in children, markedly decreased *SGLT1* results in both gut and renal malabsorption of both glucose and galactose, which results in diarrhea and mellituria.

DIAGNOSIS AND TREATMENT. Diagnosis should be based on finding glucosuria of more than 500 mg/24 hr (on a diet containing 50% carbohydrate) without hyperglycemia (serum glucose <140 mg/dL). To confirm the excreted sugar as glucose, the glucose oxidase method should be used; this will exclude other mellituric conditions (pentosuria, fructosuria, sucrosuria, maltosuria, galactosuria, and lactosuria). Appropriate tests should be performed to exclude coexistent tubular transport defects (of amino acids, bicarbonate, phosphorus, and uric acid) such as Fanconi's syndrome, as well as diabetes. If desired, differentiation of the V_{max} or K_m variants can be made by glucose loading (see Fig. 109–1).

This condition is completely benign, and therapy is unnecessary.

RENAL AMINOACIDURIAS. The renal aminoacidurias represent inborn errors of renal tubular transport in which a single or group of amino acids is hyperexcreted and is often accompanied by intestinal malabsorption of the same amino acid(s) (see Table 109–1).

GENERAL CHARACTERISTICS. The 20 L-amino acids are predominantly reabsorbed by the proximal tubule at a rate of reabsorption exceeding 95 to 98% of the filtered load. Stereospecific amino acid transport occurs across the luminal membrane of the proximal tubule, accompanied by sodium and driven by the lumen-to-cell sodium concentration gradient. Reabsorptive kinetics are similar to those of D-glucose. Amino acid transport systems for at least five groups or classes of amino acids have been described: (1) *basic*—lysine, arginine, ornithine, and cystine; (2) *acidic*—aspartic and

Table 109–1 ■ CLINICAL SYNDROMES ASSOCIATED WITH NEPHRON TRANSPORT DEFECTS

PROXIMAL NEPHRON

I. *Selective Transport Defects*
  A. Renal glycosurias
    1. Primary
    2. Combined
      a. Glucose/galactose malabsorption
      b. Glucoglycinuria
  B. Renal aminoacidurias
    1. Basic aminoacidurias
      a. General: cystinuria (cystine, lysine, arginine, ornithine)
      b. Specific: hypercystinuria, dibasic aminoaciduria (lysine, arginine, ornithine), lysinuria
    2. Neutral aminoacidurias
      a. General: Hartnup disease
      b. Specific: methioninuria, tryptophanuria, histidinuria
    3. Iminoglycinuria
      a. General (proline, hydroxyproline, glycine)
      b. Specific: glycinuria
    4. Dicarboxylic aminoaciduria
      a. General (glutamic, aspartic acids)
  C. Proximal renal tubular acidosis
    1. Primary: idiopathic or genetic
    2. Transient (infants)
    3. Carbonic anhydrase deficiency, inhibition, alteration
      a. Drugs: acetazolamide, sulfanilamide, mafenide acetate
      b. Idiopathic?
  D. Renal uric acid disorders (see Chapter 299)
  E. Phosphate and calcium disorders (see Chapter 261)
II. *Non-selective Transport Defects: Fanconi's Syndrome*
  A. Primary: idiopathic or genetic
  B. Genetically transmitted systemic diseases
    1. Cystinosis
    2. Lowe's syndrome
    3. Wilson's disease
    4. Tyrosinemia
    5. Hereditary carboxylase deficiency
    6. Pyruvate carboxylase deficiency
  C. Dysproteinemic states
    1. Multiple myeloma
    2. Monoclonal gammopathy
  D. Secondary hyperparathyroidism with chronic hypocalcemia
    1. Vitamin D deficiency or resistance
    2. Vitamin D dependency
  E. Drugs and toxins
    1. Outdated tetracycline
    2. Methyl-3-chromone
    3. Streptozotocin
    4. Glue
    5. Gentamicin
    6. Ifosfamide
  F. Heavy metals
    1. Lead
    2. Cadmium
    3. Mercury
  G. Tubulointerstitial diseases
    1. Sjögren's syndrome
    2. Medullary cystic disease
    3. Renal transplantation
  H. Other diseases
    1. Nephrotic syndrome
    2. Amyloidosis
    3. Osteopetrosis
    4. Paroxysmal nocturnal hemoglobinuria

LOOP OF HENLE

I. *Bartter's Syndrome*
II. *Drugs*
  A. Furosemide
  B. Bumetanide
  C. Ethacrynic acid

DISTAL NEPHRON

I. *Selective Transport Defects*
  A. Classic distal renal tubular acidosis
    1. Primary: genetic or idiopathic
    2. Genetically transmitted systemic diseases
      a. Ehlers-Danlos syndrome
      b. Hematologic disorders: hereditary elliptocytosis, sickle cell anemia, carbonic anhydrase I deficiency or alteration
      c. Medullary cystic disease
      d. With nerve deafness
      e. Glycogenosis type III
    3. Autoimmune diseases
      a. Hypergammaglobulinemia: hyperglobulinemic purpura, cryoglobulinemia, familial
      b. Sjögren's syndrome
      c. Thyroiditis
      d. Pulmonary fibrosis
      e. Chronic active hepatitis
      f. Primary biliary cirrhosis
      g. Systemic lupus erythematosis
    4. Diseases associated with nephrocalcinosis
      a. Primary hyperparathyroidism
      b. Vitamin D intoxication
      c. Hyperthyroidism
      d. Hypercalciuria: idiopathic or genetic
      e. Hereditary fructose intolerance
      f. Medullary sponge kidney
      g. Fabry's disease
      h. Wilson's disease
    5. Drug or toxic nephropathies
      a. Amphotericin B
      b. Toluene
      c. Glue
      d. Analgesics
      e. Cyclamate
    6. Tubulointerstitial diseases
      a. Chronic pyelonephritis secondary to urolithiasis
      b. Obstructive uropathy
      c. Renal transplantation
      d. Leprosy
      e. Hyperoxaluria
    7. Miscellaneous
  B. Renal tubular acidosis of glomerular insufficiency
  C. Hypermineralocorticoid and other potassium secretory disorders (see Chapter 240)
II. *Non-selective Transport Defects: Generalized Distal Renal Tubular Acidosis, Hyperkalemia, and Renal Salt Wasting*
  A. Primary mineralocorticoid deficiency (see Chapter 240)
  B. Hypoangiotensinemia
    1. Converting-enzyme inhibitors: captopril, enalapril
    2. Angiotensin receptor blockers
  C. Hyporeninemic hypoaldosteronism
    1. Diabetic nephropathy
    2. Tubulointerstitial nephropathies
    3. Nephrosclerosis
    4. Non-steroidal anti-inflammatory agents
    5. Acquired immunodeficiency syndrome
  D. Mineralocorticoid-resistant hyperkalemia
    1. Without salt wasting: genetic
    2. With salt wasting
      a. Childhood forms
      b. Tubulointerstitial nephropathies: methicillin, obstructive nephropathy, transplantation, sickle cell disease, cyclosporine
      c. Other drugs: spironolactone, amiloride, triamterene

LOOP AND MEDULLARY COLLECTING DUCTS

I. *Diabetes Insipidus* (see Chapter 238)
II. *Syndrome of Inappropriate Secretion of Antidiuretic Hormone* (see Chapter 102)
III. *Other Concentrating and Diluting Disorders*

glutamic acid; (3) *neutral amino group*—glycine, proline, hydroxyproline, and sarcosine; (4) *neutral (Hartnup) group*—alanine, serine, threonine, valine, leucine, isoleucine, phenylalanine, glutamine, histidine, asparagine, tyrosine, tryptophan, and citrulline; and (5) *β-amino acids*—taurine, β-alanine, and β-aminoisobutyrate. Inherited dysfunction of a carrier results in urinary loss of the entire amino

acid group: cystinuria (basic aminoaciduria), dicarboxylic aminoaciduria, Hartnup disease (neutral aminoaciduria), and iminoglycinuria. There are at least 25 selective amino acid carriers that transport a single or few numbers of a given amino acid group. Human disorders of these carriers result in even more selective aminoaciduria: hypercystinuria, histidinuria, and lysinuria.

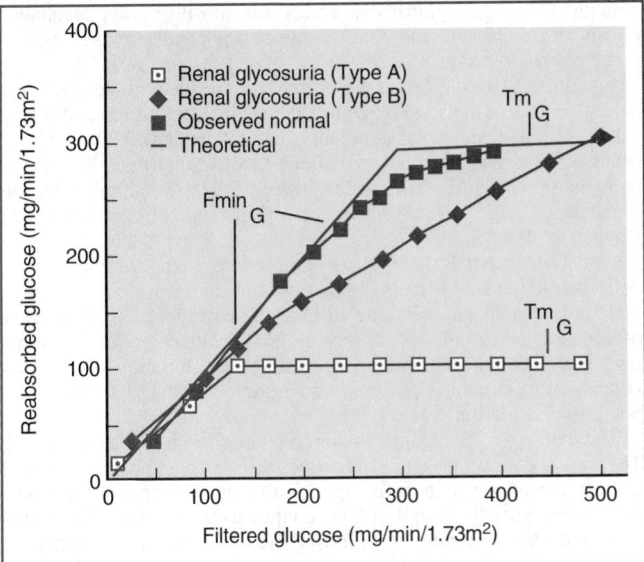

FIGURE 109–1 ■ Glucose titration curves demonstrating the maximal transport rate (Tm G) on the ordinate and the venous plasma threshold (FminG) on the abscissa. This depicts both the normal pattern and the pattern in the two variants of renal glucosuria (type A and type B).

Many proximal nephron amino acid carriers are also expressed within the luminal (brush border) membrane of gastrointestinal epithelial cells. Defective gut absorption occurs concomitantly with renal hyperexcretion of the amino acid(s) in question. Di- and tripeptides can be absorbed normally by the gut; hence nutritional problems arising from amino acid malabsorption are unusual.

To diagnose a renal aminoaciduria, an elevated plasma level of the amino acids must be excluded. Whenever the filtered load of an amino acid exceeds the transport capacity of the renal tubule, an "overload" or "prerenal" aminoaciduria can occur. Most inborn errors of amino acid metabolism exhibit this type of aminoaciduria because the plasma concentration of individual amino acids that are poorly metabolized rises sharply. By contrast, the renal aminoacidurias are associated with low or normal levels of plasma amino acid concentrations, because the aminoaciduria is due to an inborn error of proximal tubule transport.

CYSTINURIA. *Cystinuria* is the term used to designate a group of renal transport disorders that have in common the excessive excretion of the highly insoluble amino acid cystine and the formation of urinary calculi. An autosomal recessive disease, it is estimated to affect 1 in 7000 individuals (between 1 in 1000 and 1 in 20,000, depending on the population examined). Urinary losses of lysine, arginine, and ornithine are asymptomatic. The gene defect in classic cystinuria involves single point or deletion mutations of COLA, the dibasic amino acid transporter. This transporter is known as SLC 3A1 and is found on chromosome Z. Cystine loss leads to cystine urolithiasis, which accounts for 1 to 2% of all urinary calculi. Stone formation usually becomes evident during the second and third decades of life, although presentation may occur from infancy to the ninth decade, and males are more severely affected. Cystine stones are radiopaque, can create staghorn calculi, and often form a nidus for calcium oxalate stone formation. Symptoms include renal colic, which may be associated with obstruction or infection or both. Evidence associating cystinuria with central nervous system (CNS) disorders has been tenuous. A more general discussion of nephrolithiasis can be found in Chapter 114.

The diagnosis of cystinuria should be considered in any patient with renal calculus, even if the stone is composed primarily of calcium oxalate. Typical hexagonal crystals may be recognized by urinalysis, particularly in a concentrated, acidic, early-morning specimen. A useful screening test is the cyanide-nitroprusside test, which detects a cystine concentration of more than 75 to 150 mg/L. Because of false-positive test results, a definitive diagnosis requires thin-layer or ion-exchange chromatography. Excretion ratios in an adult of more than 18 mg of cystine per gram of creatinine confirm the diagnosis. Homozygous individuals usually excrete more than 250 mg of cystine per gram of creatinine.

Medical therapy for cystinuria is aimed at reducing the urinary concentration below the solubility limit of 300 mg of cystine per liter. The production of a high-volume alkaline urine (pH >7.5) will increase the solubility of cystine to this level. Because cystine excretion may be as high as 1 g/24 hr, a total of 4 L of water should be ingested. The most effective means of converting cystine to a more soluble compound follows the therapeutic administration of D-penicillamine, which by way of a disulfide exchange reaction produces cysteine-penicillamine. Pyridoxine also should be given, because penicillamine can deplete this cofactor. The compound mercaptopropionylglycine (XMPG) has proven to be more efficacious, because it is more effective in disulfide exchange reactions and its side effects appear to be fewer than those of D-penicillamine.

HARTNUP DISEASE. Hartnup disease, a neutral aminoaciduria, is a rare autosomal recessive disorder (1 in 26,000 births) in which the clinical presentation is dominated by nicotinamide deficiency. Because up to 50% of nicotinamide is normally supplied by metabolism of tryptophan, malabsorption and renal loss of tryptophan contribute to nicotinamide deficiency, especially when dietary nicotinamide is insufficient. Hence, this disorder demonstrates the importance of both the intestinal and renal transport defects. Clinical evidence of nicotinamide deficiency is intermittent and often worse in children and includes pellagra in sun-exposed areas, cerebellar ataxia, and sometimes psychiatric disturbances.

Hartnup disease should be suspected in a patient with pellagra or cerebellar symptoms without a history of niacin deficiency. The diagnosis can be confirmed by chromatography of the urine. Siblings of an affected individual should be examined for heterozygosity. Supplemental nicotinamide (40 to 250 mg per day) will prevent pellagra and neurologic problems.

OTHER AMINOACIDURIAS. Less common aminoacidurias that are asymptomatic include iminoglycinuria, isolated hypercystinuria (without hyperexcretion of other basic amino acids), isolated glycinuria, and dicarboxylic aminoaciduria. Mental retardation predominates in the rare disorders of hyperdibasic aminoaciduria, isolated lysinuria, histidinuria, and methioninuria.

PROXIMAL RENAL TUBULAR ACIDOSIS (RTA). Proximal (type II) RTA is a hyperchloremic, hypokalemic metabolic acidosis caused by a selective defect in proximal acidification and defined by a normally acidic urine during acidosis but marked bicarbonate wasting after normalization of plasma bicarbonate concentrations.

PATHOPHYSIOLOGY. Between 85 and 90% of the filtered bicarbonate load occurs in the proximal nephron, mainly by Na^+/H^+ exchange and the degradation of H_2CO to CO_2 plus H_2O by carbonic anhydrase (Fig. 109–2). Interference with a normal Na^+/H^+ exchange or carbonic anhydrase activity results in excessive delivery of bicarbonate to the distal nephron. Because of limited bicarbonate reabsorptive capacity, excessive bicarbonate is wasted into the urine. The loss of 15% or more of filtered bicarbonate at a normal plasma bicarbonate concentration is pathognomonic of proximal RTA. Excess delivery of bicarbonate to the distal nephron also results in accelerated potassium secretion and hypokalemia with defective proximal bicarbonate reabsorption. The plasma bicarbonate concentration and filtered load fall, and absolute bicarbonate delivery to the distal nephron decreases progressively. After a certain time, usually when plasma bicarbonate is between 15 and 18 mm, the distal nephron can cope with excessive delivery from the proximal nephron. At this point, bicarbonaturia ceases, urinary pH can be lowered normally, and net acid excretion equals endogenous acid production. Acid-base homeostasis is re-established at the expense of metabolic acidosis.

SYMPTOMS AND ETIOLOGIES. Clinical features of proximal RTA are related to acidemia (growth failure, anorexia and malnutrition, volume depletion), hypokalemia and potassium depletion (muscular weakness, polyuria, nocturia, polydipsia), and disordered mineral, parathyroid, and vitamin D metabolism (osteomalacia and rickets). Proximal RTA is quite rare, usually due to defective carbonic anhydrase activity or in association with the complete Fanconi syndrome (see Table 109–1).

DIAGNOSIS AND TREATMENT. Laboratory evidence of proximal RTA consists of a hyperchloremic, hypokalemic metabolic acidosis. When the patient is acidemic, the urine is acidic and net acid excretion equals endogenous acid production. If bicarbonate is in-

PROXIMAL TUBULE

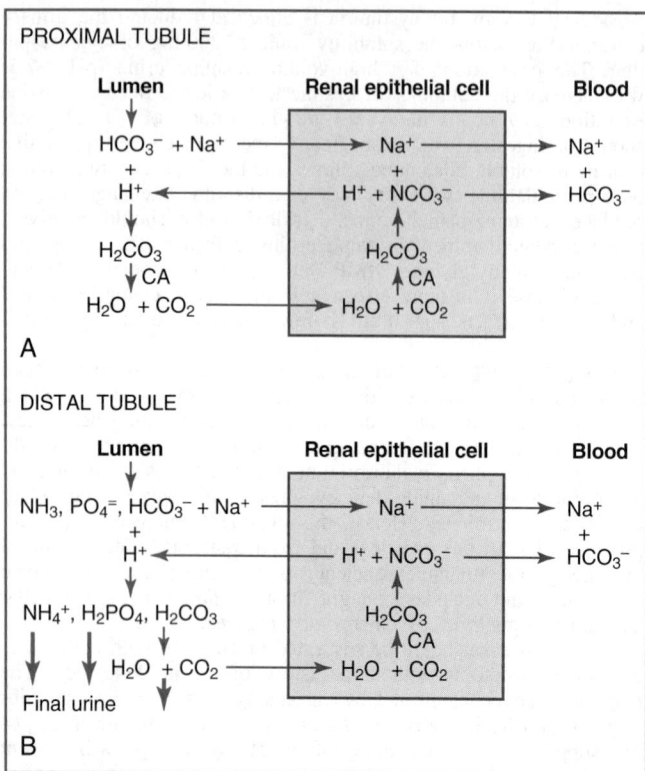

FIGURE 109–2 ■ *A,* Proximal tubule bicarbonate reabsorption. A sodium hydrogen exchange acts to exchange Na for hydrogen ion to form H_2CO_3, which is rapidly broken down to $H_2O + CO_2$ by the enzyme carbonic anhydrase (CA). $H_2O + CO_2$ are both translocated into the proximal tubule, where carbonic anhydrase rapidly catalyzes the reverse reaction to form H_2CO_3 and then $H^+ + HCO_3^-$. Na^+ and HCO_3^- are then returned to the circulation. *B,* Distal tubule secretion of hydrogen ion occurs by means of sodium-dependent and voltage-dependent transport processes. The absence of carbonic anhydrase on the luminal membrane of the distal tubule results in a delay in the formation of $H_2O + CO_2$ from H_2CO_3. CO_2 is "trapped" in the urine, raising the urinary P_{CO_2}. H^+ is also excreted in the form of titratable acids such as H_2PO_4 or NH_4^+. The process does result in the regeneration of some bicarbonate, which is ultimately returned to the circulation.

fused to normalize plasma bicarbonate concentrations, massive bicarbonaturia ensues ($\geq 15\%$ of the filtered load). Proximal RTA is not usually an isolated diagnosis but part of Fanconi's syndrome. Therapy for the underlying disease should be undertaken if possible (e.g., multiple myeloma) or offending drugs or toxins removed (e.g., heavy metals). When this is not feasible, proximal RTA is treated with large quantities of sodium and potassium bicarbonate. Potassium wasting is enhanced as plasma bicarbonate rises after therapy, which raises the requirement for potassium supplements because bicarbonate alone cannot correct the disorder. Volume contraction using diuretics (particularly thiazides) is also attempted to stimulate fractional proximal bicarbonate reabsorption. Therapy with vitamin D analogues is indicated when clinically relevant.

GENERALIZED PROXIMAL TUBULE DYSFUNCTIONS: FANCONI'S SYNDROME. In Fanconi's syndrome, the entire panoply of proximal tubule transport functions is impaired, resulting in glucosuria, generalized aminoaciduria, proximal RTA phosphaturia, and uricosuria. The lumen-to-cell sodium gradient provides the driving force in the proximal tubular epithelium for the reabsorption of these respective compounds. Collapse of the sodium gradient could arise by several mechanisms: a primary disturbance of the Na^+, K^+-ATPase, increased permeability of the cell to sodium, or reduced metabolic energy due to an abnormality in the redox potential or in the intracellular phosphate supply. Recently, Fanconi's syndrome has been associated with depletion of mitochondrial DNA, particularly in a mitochondrial myopathy associated with generalized tubulopathy. The gene responsible for Lowe's syndrome, *OCRL1,* has also been identified and mutations have been detected in many

patients. This gene normally codes for inositol polyphosphate-5 phosphatase, an enzyme that removes 5-phosphate from inositol (1, 4, 5)-triphosphate.

In addition to the solutes previously described, there exist impaired reabsorption and frequently reduced serum concentrations of calcium, magnesium, citrate, and low-molecular-weight (<50 kd) proteins. Because the proximal tubular mitochondria is the site of conversion of 25(OH) vitamin D to 1,25(OH)$_2$ vitamin D, the circulating value of this latter compound may be reduced (see Chapter 262).

SYMPTOMS AND ETIOLOGIES. As a result of the complex disorders of mineral and vitamin D metabolism, the most frequent clinical finding is metabolic bone disease, either rickets in children or osteomalacia in adults (see Chapter 263). Nausea, episodic vomiting, anorexia, and marked growth failure are common in children. Other features include polyuria and muscle weakness secondary to potassium depletion.

The causes of Fanconi's syndrome are listed in Table 109–1. The most common is the inherited disease cystinosis, in which cystine accumulates in cells, specifically in lysosomes of the kidney, liver, gut, lymphoid tissue, conjunctivae, thyroid gland, cornea, and bone marrow. Cystinosis may be present as Fanconi's syndrome after the first birthday or with renal failure in childhood (infantile nephropathic form) or during adolescence. An adult form, which is generally benign, may involve corneal and conjunctival cystine crystal deposition. The defect represents a failure in the lysosomal cystine efflux process. A form of Fanconi's syndrome that can be induced by diet is hereditary fructose intolerance due to a deficiency of fructose aldolase B (see Chapter 204). Ingestion of fructose by affected patients causes acute symptoms, including nausea, vomiting, abdominal pain, and neurologic dysfunction, as well as profound hypophosphatemia. Mutations in *GLUT2,* the gene for the facilitative diffusion liver-type glucose transporter, are found in patients with Fanconi-Bikel syndrome. Patients with this variant of Fanconi's syndrome also have hepatorenal glycogen storage and impaired vitalization of glucose and galactose. In adults, acquired Fanconi's syndrome is most often due to dysproteinemias, heavy metal exposure (especially chronic cadmium or acute lead), and immunologic disorders (see Table 109–1). An older adult presenting with Fanconi's syndrome should be assumed to have multiple myeloma unless proven otherwise.

DIAGNOSIS AND TREATMENT. Diagnosis is established by finding evidence for global tubular dysfunction. Underlying causes of Fanconi's syndrome should be sought. Serum and urine electrophoresis are indicated in adults.

Therapy includes sodium and potassium supplements (up to 10 to 15 mEq/kg/day) and potassium, phosphate, magnesium, and vitamin D analogues. Therapy for the underlying disorder is also important. Efficacy has been shown for cysteamine in cystinosis, D-penicillamine in Wilson's disease (see Chapter 220), fructose restriction in hereditary fructose intolerance, and removal of heavy metals by environmental changes or chelation (for lead).

DISORDERS OF FUNCTION OF THE ASCENDING LIMB OF THE LOOP OF HENLE

The thick ascending limb of the loop of Henle reabsorbs sodium chloride by means of a luminal Na^+-K^+-$2Cl^-$ system. A lumen-positive potential difference and parallel transport system affect potassium, calcium, and magnesium reabsorption. Defective reabsorption by the thick ascending limb of Henle occurs during diuretic therapy or in Bartter's syndrome.

BARTTER'S SYNDROME. Bartter's syndrome includes hypokalemia, metabolic alkalosis, and hyper-reninemic hyperaldosteronism. Hypertension and edema are absent.

PATHOPHYSIOLOGY. Recent advances have elucidated at least three gene defects responsible for Bartter's syndrome: (1) a loss of function mutations of the gene encoding the bumetanide-sensitive Na^+-K^+-$2Cl^-$ co-transporter of the medullary thick ascending limb of Henle's loop; (2) a defect in the chloride channel CLCNKB; and (3) a defect in the gene for the inwardly rectifying potassium channel ROMK1 in the neonatal form. Mild extracellular volume depletion causes hyper-reninemic hyperaldosteronism and the juxtaglomerular hyperplasia evident in renal biopsy. Enhanced sodium chloride delivery to the collecting duct stimulates potassium secretion (exacerbated by concurrent hyperaldosteronism), resulting in marked hypokalemia.

SYMPTOMS AND ETIOLOGY. Bartter's syndrome usually presents during childhood. Inheritance is autosomal recessive with males affected more often. Adult cases are described. Presenting features relate mainly to hypokalemia, including growth failure, muscle weakness, and vasopressin-resistant polyuria consisting of polyuria, nocturia, and enuresis. Divalent cation (calcium and magnesium), wasting, and metabolic alkalosis may result in hypocalcemia with Trousseau's and Chvostek's signs. These electrolyte abnormalities also can present as paralytic ileus or growth failure in children.

DIAGNOSIS AND TREATMENT. Other conditions associated with hypokalemia, metabolic alkalosis, and secondary hyper-reninemic hyperaldosteronism must be excluded before making the diagnosis of Bartter's syndrome. Surreptitious vomiting, chronic diarrheal states, or surreptitious diuretic or laxative abuse can cause symptoms and laboratory findings indistinguishable from those of Bartter's syndrome. The diagnosis must be preceded by determination that urinary chloride concentration is more than 20 mmol/L and by negative screening test results for diuretics in the urine and for laxatives in the stool (phenolphthalein test). In general, other states of primary hyper-reninism or hypermineralocorticoidism can be readily excluded, because they are normally associated with hypertension.

Therapy involves amelioration of hypokalemia by disrupting the renin-angiotensin-aldosterone and the kinin-prostaglandin axes. Potassium supplementation, magnesium repletion, propranolol, spironolactone, prostaglandin inhibition (in the form of aspirin or indomethacin), and captopril have all been used.

DISORDERS OF DISTAL NEPHRON FUNCTION

Distal nephron, including the distal convoluted tubule and collection ducts, absorbs the final quantity of sodium in the tubular fluid and is the site for potassium and hydrogen ion secretion. Inherited and acquired defects exist for selected and combined disorders of sodium, potassium, and acid-base regulation.

GITTLEMAN VARIANT OF BARTTER'S SYNDROME. The hypocalciuric-hypomagnesemic variant described by Gitelman is due to a gene defect in the distal convoluted tubule thiazide-sensitive Na^+-Cl^- co-transporter and hence is a distal tubule disorder. Its clinical features, in general, are less severe than the neonatal variant or adult Bartter's syndrome.

CLASSIC DISTAL RTA. Classic distal (type I) RTA (see Chapter 101) is a hypokalemic, hyperchloremic metabolic acidosis related to a selective defect in distal acidification.

PATHOPHYSIOLOGY. The distal nephron (especially the cortical and medullary collecting ducts) usually can lower the urinary pH fully 2 to 3 pH units below that of blood in order to hydrate the filtered buffers (mainly phosphate) to form titratable acids and endogenously produced ammonia to form ammonium (see Fig. 109–2). If the distal nephron is incapable of lowering the luminal pH below 5.5 after challenge by metabolic acidosis, classic distal RTA is present. Due to the inappropriately high urinary pH, net acid excretion (titratable acid plus ammonium minus bicarbonate) is reduced and is below total acid production by the body. Enhanced potassium secretion occurs, presumably because there is reduced competition by proton secretion for the electrochemical driving forces in the distal nephron. The acidification defect may result from an insufficient number of proton-secreting pumps in the distal nephron. Alternately, a back leak of acid across the luminal membrane may exist so that establishment of a pH gradient is prevented even when proton secretion is normal. A gene defect in AE-1, the chloride-bicarbonate anion exchanger, is also a possible cause of distal RTA.

SYMPTOMS AND CAUSES. Distal RTA is evident in infants, children, and adults; symptoms are those of acidosis or hypokalemia, as noted earlier. Nephrocalcinosis and nephrolithiasis are common, either as a cause or result of classic distal RTA. However, bone disease is not as frequent as in proximal RTA. Classic distal RTA also may be genetic (usually autosomal dominant) or due to autoimmune diseases, drugs and toxins, and various tubulointerstitial diseases (see Table 109–1).

DIAGNOSIS AND TREATMENT. The findings of hyperchloremic, hypokalemic metabolic acidosis with an inappropriately high urine pH (>5.5) and diminished net acid excretion confirm the diagnosis. Diagnosis is facilitated by measuring the urinary anion gap (defined as urinary sodium plus potassium minus chloride, which is proportionate to the negative value of urinary ammonium [NH_4^+]). Diarrhea has a large, negative urinary anion gap and hence a high urinary ammonium concentration (accounting for the high urinary pH), whereas classic distal RTA has a zero or positive anion gap and a low urinary ammonium concentration due to impaired acidification. In subjects with a normal plasma bicarbonate concentration, the failure to lower urinary pH to less than 5.5 after an acute acid challenge with NH_4Cl defines the syndrome of incomplete classic distal RTA. Treatment with alkali is generally very effective. The daily dose of alkali in adults is 1 to 3 mEq/kg, to compensate for the normal acid production by the body plus a small amount of urinary bicarbonate wastage. In distinction to proximal RTA, urinary potassium wasting is ameliorated with alkali therapy.

RTA OF GLOMERULAR INSUFFICIENCY. Moderate renal insufficiency may be associated with a normokalemic, hyperchloremic metabolic acidosis (glomerular filtration rate of 20 to 30 mL/min) due to insufficient ammonia delivery. It is characterized by an appropriately low urine pH but subnormal urinary net acid (ammonium) excretion.

NON-SELECTIVE DISTAL NEPHRON DYSFUNCTION: GENERALIZED DISTAL RTA, HYPERKALEMIA, AND RENAL SALT WASTING. These disorders derive from global dysfunction of the distal nephron due to aldosterone deficiency or antagonism and are typified by hyperkalemic, hyperchloremic (type IV) metabolic acidosis caused by subnormal net acid excretion and often by salt wasting.

PATHOPHYSIOLOGY. Aldosterone influences distal sodium reabsorption to the extent that urinary sodium is less than 10 mEq/L. Sodium reabsorption creates a lumen negative potential difference that favors secretion of potassium and hydrogen ions. Disruption of sodium reabsorption and of potassium and hydrogen ion secretion may be ascribable to a defect in the integrity of the distal nephron cell, reduced aldosterone production or action, diminished sodium reabsorption, or blunting of the lumen negative potential by enhanced chloride reabsorption. Any of these processes can diminish total hydrogen and potassium excretion, resulting in hyperkalemic metabolic acidosis. This hyperkalemia also serves to depress renal ammoniagenesis independently, which enhances the defect in renal acidification. The ability of the distal nephron to lower urine pH remains intact.

DIAGNOSIS AND TREATMENT. Generalized distal RTA is unique among the hyperchloremic metabolic acidoses in being a hyperkalemic disorder (Table 109–2). The glomerular filtration rate is in-

Table 109–2 ■ **RENAL TUBULAR ACIDOSES**

TYPE	RENAL DEFECT	GFR	PLASMA [K^+]	PROXIMAL ACIDIFICATION HCO$_3^-$ Reabsorption (During HCO$_3^-$ Loading)	DISTAL ACIDIFICATION Minimal Urinary pH (During Acidosis)	DISTAL ACIDIFICATION UAG ≈ − Urine [NH_4^+] (During Acidosis)
Proximal (type II)	⇓ Proximal acidification	N	⇓	⇓	<5.5	0 or +
Classic distal (type I)	⇓ Distal pH gradient	N	⇓	N	>5.5	0 or +
Glomerular insufficiency	⇓ NH$_3$ production	⇓	N	N	<5.5	0 or +
Generalized distal (type IV)	⇓ Aldosterone action	⇓	⇑	N	<5.5	0 or +

N = normal; UAG = urinary anion gap = [Na^+] + [K^+] − [Cl^-] ≈ −[NH_4^+]; GFR = glomerular filtration rate.

variably reduced in hyporeninemic or tubulointerstitial nephropathy but may be at levels (≥30 mL/min) above those typically found in the RTA of glomerular insufficiency. Treatment of the hyperkalemia and generalized distal RTA is effected with 9α-fluorocortisone, 0.1 mg/day, when mineralocorticoid is deficient. When hyporeninemia is the cause, high doses of the synthetic mineralocorticoid are necessary (up to 0.5 mg/day) because of associated mineralocorticoid resistance. Hypertension can be precipitated with this treatment. A loop diuretic (furosemide or ethacrynic acid) is also useful, especially when hypertension precludes administration of mineralocorticoid, because it augments urinary potassium excretion even when endogenous aldosterone is reduced. Useful adjuncts to diuretic therapy include dietary potassium restriction (<50 mEq/dL), alkali therapy to compensate for daily acid generation (sodium bicarbonate, 1 to 3 mEq/kg/day), and sometimes short-term use of cation-exchange resin.

Chesney RW, Jones DP: Renal tubular disorders. *In* Gonick H (ed): Current Nephrology, vol 19. Chicago, Mosby–Year Book, 1996, pp 1–34. *This review relates recent progress made in the understanding of renal proximal tubular disorders.*

Chesney RW, Novella AC: Defects of renal tubular transport. *In* Massry SG, Glassock R (eds): Textbook of Nephrology, 4th ed, Baltimore, Williams and Wilkins, 1998. *This is a comprehensive review of renal tubular disorders and their clinical features.*

Saner R, Schneppenheim R, Dombrowski A, et al: Mutations in *GLUT2*, the gene for the liver-type glucose transporter, in patients with Fanconi-Bickel syndrome. Nutr Genet 17:324, 1997. *A description of defining the genetic defect in a form of Fanconi's syndrome.*

Vollmer M, Kochrer M, Topaloglu R, et al: Two novel mutations of the gene of Kir 1.1 (*ROMK*) in neonatal Bartter syndrome. Pediatr Nephrol 12:69–71, 1998. *A good discussion of the variants and gene defects in Bartter's syndrome.*

110 ▪ DIABETES AND THE KIDNEY

Thomas H. Hostetter

Diabetes is the leading cause of chronic renal failure in the United States, which is one of the most serious long-term complications for the individual diabetic patient. Approximately one third of patients who develop chronic renal failure in the United States do so because of diabetes. At present, about half these patients have long-standing insulin-dependent diabetes mellitus (IDDM) and the other half have non–insulin-dependent diabetes mellitus (NIDDM), at least in the initial presentation of their metabolic disorder. However, not all patients with diabetes develop serious

renal complications. Although the fraction of patients with IDDM who develop renal failure seems to have been declining over the past several decades, between 20 and 40% still suffer this complication. On the other hand, for patients with NIDDM, a somewhat lower fraction, perhaps as low as 10 to 20%, develop uremia due to diabetes; and therefore their nearly equal contribution to the total number of diabetic patients developing kidney failure results from the much larger total number of patients with NIDDM than IDDM (5- to 10-fold more cases of the former than the latter). The lower cumulative incidence of renal failure and NIDDM may reflect different aspects of the disease but also likely reflects the more advanced age of these patients and their susceptibility to death from other cardiovascular events, such as myocardial infarction and stroke, before renal failure occurs.

NATURAL HISTORY. Whereas the renal disease of IDDM and NIDDM is in many regards similar, the natural history follows somewhat different paths. After the initial polyuria and ketoacidosis that usually announce the abrupt onset of IDDM, by clinical standards renal function is generally normal. However, careful measurements of the glomerular filtration rate (GFR) have demonstrated that a substantial fraction (25 to 50%) of patients with IDDM will have a GFR well in excess of the normal range (Fig. 110–1). In addition, in the early phases of IDDM, patients tend to have enlarged kidneys commensurate with the heightened filtration rate. This hyperfiltration depends somewhat on the degree of glycemic control. Over the succeeding several years, renal function by standard laboratory testing as well as arterial pressure tends to be no different than that for age-matched normal individuals. However, beginning toward the end of the first decade of IDDM, a certain fraction of patients will begin to demonstrate urinary abnormalities that bespeak the underlying structural and functional renal alterations of early diabetic nephropathy. The earliest finding is usually a small but abnormal amount of urinary albumin detectable only by sensitive antibody-based techniques. This "microalbuminuria" precedes the later development of larger rates of albumin excretion detectable by standard dipstick technology or other chemical assays. The lag time between the appearance of microalbuminuria and full-blown proteinuria is typically in the range of 1 to 5 years. However, recent advances in therapy seem likely to prolong this interval, forestalling the appearance of the more overt phases of the disease (see later). In addition to serving as an early marker for the nephropathic complications, the presence of microalbuminuria also marks those patients who are more likely to develop serious extrarenal cardiovascular disease as a consequence of IDDM. Without effective treatment (see later), the albuminuria tends to progressively worsen, and arterial hypertension usually supervenes in this subgroup during the transition between microalbuminuria and greater degrees of proteinuria. Finally, with the presence of dipstick-positive proteinuria and arterial hypertension, GFR begins to

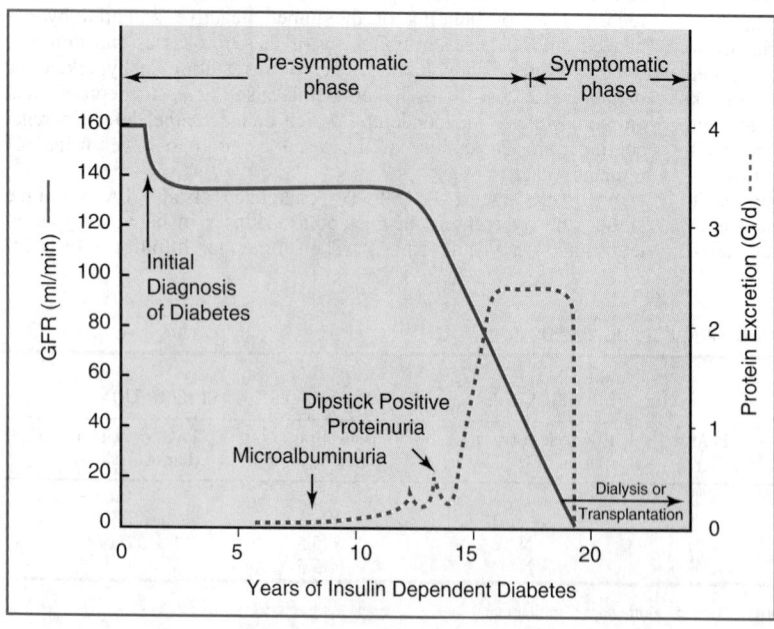

FIGURE 110–1 ▪ Course of diabetic nephropathy.

decline below normal values and serum creatinine rises. Before effective intervention, the rate of decline in filtration rate in these individuals was quite variable but averaged about 1 mL/min of GFR per month. Thus, from the first evidence of standard dipstick-positive proteinuria and numerically only modest elevations of serum creatinine above the normal range, the time to end-stage renal disease has been 3 to 8 years.

As with IDDM, patients with NIDDM also tend to have elevated GFR in the early period after being diagnosed with diabetes. The degree of increase in GFR is usually not so striking, however. In contrast to the IDDM patients, those with NIDDM have a higher prevalence of microalbuminuria and arterial hypertension when their diabetes is first identified. As many as 10 to 25% will have such abnormalities. The apparently earlier appearance of these abnormalities in NIDDM probably reflects a longer period of asymptomatic hyperglycemia before the formal diagnosis of NIDDM, rather than any fundamental difference in pathogenesis. Nevertheless, microalbuminuria in NIDDM also reflects an underlying predisposition to developing progressive kidney disease as well as serving as a marker of predilection for generalized cardiovascular disease. The progression of the renal complications in NIDDM generally thereafter essentially follows the same course as for IDDM.

CLINICAL PRESENTATION. During the period of declining GFR, patients often remain asymptomatic until they have lost 70 to 90% of their normal filtration rate. However, during this interval, arterial hypertension is prevalent, if asymptomatic, and protein excretion rates can rise to the levels of a nephrotic syndrome with the usual clinical and biochemical consequences of edema, hypoalbuminemia, and hypercholesterolemia. When the decay in filtration rate reaches the last 10 to 30% of baseline levels, uremic symptoms begin to appear. However, as with other progressive renal diseases, considerable individual variability exists in the development and severity of uremic symptoms. Furthermore, several elements of diabetes and its complications may exacerbate uremic symptoms or be indistinguishable from them. The nausea and vomiting that mark the uremic phase may be complicated by diabetic autonomic neuropathy with poor gastric emptying due to gastroparesis. Distinguishing between gastroparesis and uremic nausea and vomiting is often difficult. Furthermore, diabetic peripheral neuropathy in its sensory disturbance may to some degree mimic uremic neuropathy, although in general the painful and hypesthetic neuropathic symptoms are more attributable to long-standing diabetes than to uremia in most patients. The presence of autonomic neuropathy also may make it harder to manage arterial hypertension in some patients. Specifically, the propensity to orthostatic hypotension with certain drugs may be exaggerated in the presence of autonomic neuropathy; and for some patients, their arterial pressure may be quite elevated when supine but below normal when standing. Diabetic retinopathy is nearly universally present in patients with IDDM who develop renal disease; but for patients with NIDDM, a sizable fraction, perhaps as large as 30 to 40%, manifests significant renal dysfunction without retinopathy. Cardiovascular complications commonly accompany renal disease both for NIDDM and IDDM, although they are generally more severe in the patients with NIDDM. However, for both categories of diabetes, myocardial infarction, stroke, and progressive peripheral vascular disease often requiring amputation seem to occur disproportionately in diabetic patients with renal failure compared with those spared from kidney disease.

PATHOLOGY. The heightened filtration and an enlarged overall renal size of early diabetes are matched by increases in glomerular and tubular size. With microalbuminuria and yet greater degrees of proteinuria and hypertension, the more characteristic glomerular changes become ever more prominent (Fig. 110–2). Increases in the mesangial compartment of the glomerulus are produced by increases in matrix and probably in the number of mesangial cells. These expansions can manifest as diffuse enlargement of this portion of the glomerulus as well as nodular increases in extracellular matrix material. These latter lesions have been termed *Kimmelstiel-Wilson nodules* but probably represent simply a different geometric arrangement of the generalized mesangial expansion. As the mesangium expands, the density of capillaries and their area for filtration progressively decline, and these abnormalities are thought to play an important role in the falling filtration rate. The glomerular basement membrane also progressively thickens, although this change

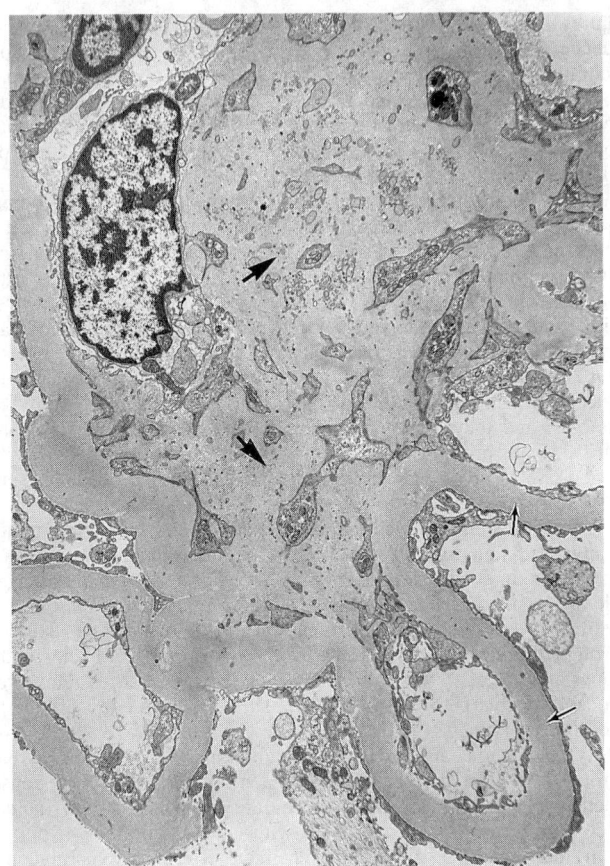

FIGURE 110–2 ■ Electron photomicrograph of a portion of a glomerulus from a patient with proteinuric, diabetic glomerulopathy (magnification ×5000). A striking increase in collagenous components has resulted in (1) widening of the basement membrane of peripheral capillary loops (small arrows) and (2) expansion of the matrix of the glomerular mesangium (large arrows). The latter alteration is responsible for compressing and ultimately obliterating the glomerular capillary network.

does not clearly bear a relationship to the decline in filtration. Hyaline-like material (a presumed protein of uncertain type) can deposit in the arterioles about the glomerulus as well as in droplets along the capillary loops themselves. As with most progressive renal diseases, a prominent tubulointerstitial pathology develops pari passu with the glomerular abnormalities. The tubular basement membranes thicken, and occasional glycogen droplets appear in tubular epithelium. However, these tubulointerstitial abnormalities have few particular diagnostic features for diabetes but may be important in occluding vascular and tubular structures and contributing to the demise of renal function. In the main, the tubulointerstitial lesions comprise progressive fibrosis and mononuclear cell infiltrates surrounding atrophic tubules, some containing proteinaceous casts. These lesions are essentially identical in IDDM and NIDDM patients sustaining renal complications. However, roughly similar patterns of nodular expansion can develop in the glomerulus in non-diabetic renal disease.

Amyloidosis, membranoproliferative glomerulonephritis type II, and light chain nephropathy may all demonstrate nodular patterns; and specific staining and other histologic techniques, as well as clinical data, are necessary to distinguish them from diabetes. In addition to glomerular and non-specific tubular disease, diabetic patients will more rarely develop sufficient compromise of the circulation to the medullary regions to cause papillary necrosis. This abnormality, although potentially serious, is relatively unusual compared with the progressive glomerular and tubular interstitial lesions of the cortex.

PATHOGENESIS. The degree of glycemic control determines the appearance of diabetic nephropathy. Multiple lines of evidence indicate that better glucose control leads to a lower incidence of this complication. The mechanism whereby poorly controlled diabetes injures the kidney is less certain, however. The chemical consequences of an elevated glucose level have received the most consideration. Glucose reacts with amino groups on proteins to form covalently bonded glycated products. An example of such a product is the glycated hemoglobin used to monitor the long-term control of glucose in patients with diabetes. However, multiple other circulating and structural proteins also are modified.

Glycation by itself can substantially alter functions of numerous proteins, including changing their permeability through vascular walls and reducing their rates of normal catabolism. The simple glycation product is nevertheless reversible such that with better glucose control the glucose is removed from the protein. However, with sustained hyperglycemia, further and more complicated reactions occur, yielding what are generally termed *advanced glycosylation end-products*. These complex compounds often include several glucose or glucose-derived products that are covalently bound to proteins, and they also can encompass the binding of several proteins through bridging glucose products. These advanced glycosylation products are nearly irreversibly formed and, hence, once created, respond very little to improvements in metabolic control.

As with simple glycation, these alterations can importantly change the functions of the affected proteins, and such products may even interact with receptors on cells such as macrophages, which can in turn liberate cytokines and other factors that scar or restructure the renal parenchyma. Glucose reduced to sorbitol through the aldose reductase pathway also may perturb the oxidation states of cells with pathophysiologic consequences. However, blockers of this pathway have as yet shown only modest effects on the diabetic kidney.

Hyperglycemia also activates protein kinase C, perhaps in part through shifts in the redox environment of the cells. The consequences of activation of this pathway are complex but may include excess production of matrix and vascular proliferation.

In addition to the more direct chemical effects of hyperglycemia on renal structures, diabetes is associated with renal vasodilation early in the course of the disease, leading to the heightened GFR in a subset of diabetic patients, as noted earlier. Studies in experimental animals have demonstrated that this hyperfiltration is associated with elevations in glomerular capillary pressures, and such elevations also may occur in non-renal capillaries as well. The elevations in glomerular capillary pressure may in their own right, or perhaps through interacting with the effects of glycation or the structural glomerular enlargement, induce pathologic glomerular capillary changes, including mesangial proliferation matrix expansion and basement membrane thickening. Maneuvers designed to reduce these capillary pressures in experimental animals, and more recently in clinical reports, have successfully mitigated damage to the kidney.

In addition to the renal hemodynamic alterations that lead to hyperfiltration and glomerular capillary hypertension, patients with overt diabetic nephropathy (dipstick-positive proteinuria and decreasing GFR) generally develop systemic hypertension. Hypertension is an adverse factor in all progressive renal diseases and seems especially so in diabetic nephropathy. The deleterious effects of hypertension are likely directed at the vasculature and microvasculature. Furthermore, the renal vasodilation noted earlier allows for greater transmission of systemic elevations in pressure to the glomerulus and may further exaggerate the glomerular capillary hypertension.

In addition to the hemodynamic and metabolic factors contributing to the appearance of diabetic nephropathy, familial or perhaps even genetic factors also appear to play a role. Evidence for this possibility derives from studies demonstrating familial clustering of diabetic nephropathy such that siblings who are both diabetic are more likely to either be concurrent for this renal complication or to avoid it entirely. Furthermore, certain ethnic groups, particularly American blacks, Hispanics, and Native Americans, may be particularly disposed to renal disease as a complication of diabetes. Obviously, their ethnic and familial risks also may include a complex set of social and economic factors.

Efforts to identify specific genes and their alleles that predispose to nephropathy have focused on those associated with the renin-angiotensin system. Some evidence has accrued for a polymorphism in the gene for the angiotensin-converting enzyme in either predisposing to nephropathy or accelerating its course. However, definitive, strong genetic markers have yet to be located.

TREATMENT. Prevention of diabetic nephropathy has not yet been achieved but may be possible by use of several approaches. First, control of glucose by careful insulin administration diminishes the risk of nephropathy in patients with IDDM. Whether assiduously maintaining near euglycemia would be equally effective in NIDDM is less certain but seems a highly desirable goal. Because animal experiments suggest that maintaining euglycemia could prevent the renal complications, it seems likely that the nearer to euglycemia a patient can be reasonably maintained, the better. In addition to glycemic control, antihypertensive treatment is a crucial element in preventing diabetic nephropathy or at least in forestalling its progression. Indeed, initiating converting enzyme inhibitors at the stage of microalbuminuria, even without significant arterial hypertension, appears to delay and perhaps prevent more substantial degrees of proteinuria. Whether such therapy will prevent the decline in the filtration rate is yet uncertain. Nevertheless, patients with IDDM should be screened regularly for microalbuminuria with antibody-based tests that either use special antibody-impregnated dipsticks or immunoassays for albumin on urine collection. If there are abnormal rates of albumin excretion even before the standard dipstick is positive, converting enzyme inhibitors should be prescribed. Even though such patients are often normotensive, they do not suffer adverse hemodynamic consequences of treatment with a converting enzyme inhibitor. With more advanced degrees of nephropathy and dipstick-positive proteinuria and a diminution in GFRs reflected in even modest elevations in creatinine, arterial hypertension is more frequently present. Therapy with converting-enzyme inhibition has proven more effective than other types of antihypertensive agents in slowing the progression of renal disease at this point as well. The efficacy of this class of antihypertensives has been extended to patients with both IDDM and NIDDM. However, particularly in the latter group, special care must be exercised to ensure that hyperkalemia does not occur in the first few days to weeks of converting enzyme inhibition. Also, because of the potential for renal artery stenosis, particularly in the older NIDDM group, careful monitoring of serum creatinine level in the first 1 to 2 weeks of a converting enzyme inhibitor regimen is necessary to screen for the occasional patient who may have a serious decline in GFR based on renal vascular disease. The level of blood pressure sought is not entirely certain, but probably levels of less than 130 mm Hg systolic and less than 90 mm Hg diastolic would be desirable using a regimen based on converting enzyme inhibitors. Dietary protein also should be restricted at this stage of disease. The value to the kidney of intensified glycemic control and lipid-lowering agents in these more advanced phases is unknown. But because of the high rates of extrarenal cardiovascular disease in this group, such efforts seem justified.

For those patients who either progress despite therapy or are noted at advanced stages of their diabetic nephropathy, the criteria used to initiate dialysis or recommend transplantation do not differ substantially from those used for patients with other types of chronic progressive renal diseases. However, because of their propensity to multiple other systemic lesions, particularly those of the cardiovascular and autonomic nervous systems, patients with diabetic nephropathy may tolerate uremia less well than patients with isolated kidney diseases of other sorts. For example, hyperkalemia may supervene more rapidly because of the predisposition to hyporeninemic hypoaldosteronism. Symptoms of gastroparesis and uremic gastrointestinal disturbance may adversely interact. As yet another example, patients with ischemic or diabetic cardiomyopathies may tolerate hypertension and extracellular fluid volume overload less readily than do non-diabetic uremic patients. For these sorts of reasons, patients with diabetes may often require treatment for their end-stage renal disease at somewhat earlier phases in the decline of GFR than do other subjects. However, as with chronic renal disease in general, the decision to initiate such therapy is generally based on the patients' symptoms rather than on the biochemical indices of uremia per se.

Patients with diabetes do less well with both transplantation and dialysis than non-diabetic patients. The poorer outcomes with therapy of end-stage renal disease rest mainly on the associated cardiovascular mortality, with stroke, myocardial infarction, and peripheral vascular disease that requires amputation representing significant co-morbid risks. However, efforts to prevent, screen for, and prophylactically treat these other complications seem to be rewarded by improved outcomes for these patients.

Simultaneous kidney and pancreas transplantation is often considered for IDDM patients with renal failure who qualify for a kidney transplant. Systematic controlled studies of this combined approach are lacking, and a small increase in mortality may occur with the more extensive procedure, especially in patients with pre-existing cardiovascular disease. However, patients with serious hypoglycemic unawareness and those with difficult management may benefit substantially from a functioning pancreas. Presently, for most patients, no solid guidelines can direct the choice between the combined procedure and a kidney transplant alone.

The Euclid Study Group. Randomised placebo-controlled trial of lisinopril in normotensive patients with insulin-dependent diabetes and normoalbuminuria or microalbuminuria. Lancet 349:1787–1792, 1997. *This large clinical trial extends previous studies in demonstrating efficacy of ACE inhibition at a very early stage of IDDM.*

King GL, Brownlee M: The cellular and molecular mechanisms of diabetic complications. Endocrinol Metab Clin Am 25:255–270, 1996. *These authors review current thinking about the cellular pathophysiology of diabetic vascular injury.*

O'Bryan GT, Hostetter TH: The renal hemodynamic basis of diabetic nephropathy. Semin Nephrol 17:93–100, 1997. *This publication considers in detail the renal hemodynamic abnormalities in diabetes.*

Parving HH, Tarnow L, Rossing P: Genetics of diabetic nephropathy. J Am Soc Nephrol 7:2509–2517, 1996. *The authors review the epidemiology and familial studies and then concentrate on studies of the polymorphism of the ACE gene.*

Ravid M, Brosh D, Levi Z, et al: Use of enalapril to attenuate decline in renal function in normotensive, normoalbuminuric patients with type 2 diabetes mellitus: A randomized, controlled study. Ann Intern Med 128:982–988, 1998. *This study provides evidence for the use of ACE inhibitors at a relatively early stage of NIDDM.*

111 URINARY TRACT INFECTIONS AND PYELONEPHRITIS

Calvin M. Kunin

DEFINITION. *Urinary tract infection* (UTI) is a broad term that encompasses both asymptomatic microbial colonization of the urine and symptomatic infection with microbial invasion and inflammation of urinary tract structures. The epithelial surfaces of the urinary tract are contiguous and extend from the renal post-glomerular filtrate to the urethral meatus. In the absence of infection, these structures are bathed in a common stream of sterile urine. The infectious process may involve the kidney, renal pelvis, ureters, bladder, and urethra, as well as adjacent structures such as the perinephric fascia, prostate, and epididymis. Bacteria are by far the most common invading organisms, but yeasts, fungi, and viruses may also produce UTI. *Invading microbe(s) and inflammatory cells in the urine are the laboratory hallmarks of the disease.* Urine may be sterile when the infection site does not contact the stream (such as when the ureter is blocked by a stricture or stone, during treatment with an antimicrobial drug, soon after metastatic infection to the kidney, or with perinephric or prostatic abscesses).

The concept of *significant bacteriuria* distinguishes colonization and growth of microorganisms in the urine from contaminants collected during voiding, particularly in females. The standard criterion of 10^5 or more colony-forming units (CFU) per milliliter takes into account that most microorganisms that cause UTI grow well in urine. The quantitative count is an excellent guide to diagnosis and evaluation of therapy because infection may persist even when symptoms are no longer present. Lower counts of 10^3 to 10^4 CFU per milliliter (with "uropathogens"; see definition below) may be clinically meaningful when voided specimens are obtained from males, under conditions of brisk diuresis and suppressive antimicrobial therapy, and for relatively slowly growing organisms such as staphylococci. Suprapubic aspiration of urine from the bladder is considered the diagnostic "gold standard." Suprapubic aspiration may also detect transient colonization in the bladder by commensal urethral and vaginal microbes without true infection. Low bacterial counts with "uropathogens" are found in about a third to a half of females with pyuria and dysuria. This condition, termed the "pyuria/dysuria (urethral) syndrome," appears to be an early phase of

UTI. It is often clinically indistinguishable from urethritis caused *by Chlamydia trachomatis, Neisseria gonorrhoeae,* or herpes simplex.

Asymptomatic bacteriuria is a common condition, particularly in females, in which large numbers of bacteria are present in the urine despite a lack of symptoms. It is considered to be an *asymptomatic infection* when accompanied by pyuria. Clinical conditions such as *urethritis, cystitis, prostatitis,* and *pyelonephritis* reflect the symptomatology manifested by the involved organ, but the infection may be more widespread.

Acute pyelonephritis is a pyogenic, focal infection of the renal parenchyma usually involving one or more wedge-shaped segments of the kidney accompanied by local and systemic symptoms of infection. "Chronic pyelonephritis" refers to the pathologic and radiologic findings of chronic cortical scarring, tubulointerstitial damage, and deformity of the underlying calyx. Chronic pyelonephritis may be *active,* with persistent infection, or *inactive,* with focal sterile scars of a past infection.

Non-infectious diseases can produce renal lesions that mimic chronic pyelonephritis. Identical changes on radiographic studies may be seen in patients who suffered severe vesicoureteral reflux during childhood. The entity "reflux nephropathy" refers to the radiologic triad of intrarenal reflux, vesicoureteral reflux, and scarring with loss of parenchymal mass. In the absence of infection it can lead to end-stage renal failure with scarred, shrunken kidneys. Some evidence suggests that reflux nephropathy may result from autoimmune renal damage rather than bacterial infection of the kidney. Because reflux is usually detected by radiologic studies in patients with recent infection, it may be difficult to determine whether renal scarring was produced by reflux alone or in combination with infection. Sensitive methods such as radionuclide scanning may help resolve these issues. Long-standing *hypertension* may produce renal cortical scars similar to pyelonephritis, and *analgesic nephropathy* may produce papillary necrosis.

ETIOLOGY. The nature of the invading microbe depends, for the most part, on the history of infection, underlying host factors, receipt of antimicrobial drugs, and instrumentation of the urinary tract. The term *uropathogen* is commonly used to describe the microorganisms found most frequently in patients with UTI. These organisms include Enterobacteriaceae, *Pseudomonas* species, *Staphylococcus* species, enterococci, and other gram-negative and gram-positive bacteria and yeasts that grow well in urine. *Lactobacillus,* α-hemolytic streptococci, and anaerobes are considered to be contaminants if found in voided urine.

The clinical distinction between uncomplicated and complicated UTI is of paramount importance. Host factors are the key in determining the invasive properties of the microorganisms and localization of the infection; determining the extent of renal damage, bacteremia, and dissemination; forming therapeutic and prophylactic strategies; anticipating the development of resistant microorganisms; and determining the ultimate prognosis.

Uncomplicated infections occur in otherwise healthy individuals with intact voiding mechanisms, most often females. Evidence suggests that susceptibility to infection is related to several blood group antigens (see Chapter 170), including Lewis nonsecretor status (Le[a+b−] and Le[a−b−]), P1, and B, rather than personal hygiene. Patients may suffer considerable morbidity from recurrent symptomatic infections, but renal failure almost never develops. Acute, uncomplicated pyelonephritis may produce transient functional abnormalities and leave residual renal scars but rarely leads to permanent renal damage. The most common invading microorganism is *Escherichia coli,* which is present in about 80 to 90% of cases. *Staphylococcus saprophyticus* may account for as many as 10 to 20% of cases in young adult women that occur during the late summer and fall. Occasionally, other members of the family Enterobacteriaceae, such as *Klebsiella, Enterobacter, Proteus,* and rarely, *Salmonella* and *Shigella,* may be causative organisms. Gram-positive bacteria other than *S. saprophyticus* are relatively uncommon but may include group B and D streptococci (*Enterococcus faecalis* and *Enterococcus faecium*). Most uncomplicated infections readily respond to antimicrobial agents.

Complicated infections occur in individuals of both sexes who have structural or functional abnormalities of the voiding mechanism (Table 111–1). Complicated infections are exceedingly diffi-

Table 111–1 ■ CHARACTERISTICS OF COMPLICATED URINARY TRACT INFECTIONS

Host Factors
Structural abnormalities of the voiding mechanism
    Calculi (renal, bladder, or prostatic)
    Strictures (urethra or ureter)
    Prostatic obstruction (benign or neoplastic)
    Vesicoureteral reflux
    Neurogenic bladder (diabetics, paraplegics)
    Indwelling urinary catheters
Common underlying diseases
    Diabetes mellitus
    Sickle cell anemia
    Polycystic renal disease
    Renal transplantation
Common microorganisms*
Gram-negative bacteria
    Escherichia coli
    Klebsiella pneumoniae
    Enterobacter aerogenes
    Proteus mirabilis
    Pseudomonas aeruginosa
    Acinetobacter species
    Serratia marcescens
    Providencia stuartii and *rettgeri*
Gram-positive bacteria
    Staphylococcus aureus
    Coagulase-negative staphylococci
    Groups B and D streptococci (enterococci)
    Corynebacterium urealyticum
Yeasts
    Candida albicans

*See the text.

cult to eradicate without correcting the underlying defect or removing a foreign body. Patients with complicated infections are at increased risk for severe renal damage, bacteremia, sepsis, and increased mortality. The organisms tend to be less susceptible to antimicrobial drugs (see Table 111–1). *Candida albicans* and even *Cryptococcus neoformans* and other *opportunistic fungi* may be significant and produce disease in diabetics, those with acquired immune deficiency syndrome, and patients treated with corticosteroids or immunosuppressive agents.

INCIDENCE AND PREVALENCE. UTIs are among the most common conditions encountered in office practice, hospitals, and extended care facilities. About 6,200,000 physician office visits are made each year (about two thirds are females) for acute symptomatic infection. About 40 to 50% of adult women report that they have had a UTI at some time. UTIs are important complications in pregnancy, diabetes, polycystic renal disease, renal transplantation, and structural and neurologic conditions that interfere with urine flow. UTIs are the leading cause of gram-negative sepsis in hospitalized patients. About half of all hospital-acquired infections originate in the urinary tract in association with the urinary catheter and urologic procedures. Urinary catheters are used in about 10% of patients admitted to hospitals and long-term care facilities. Catheter-associated UTIs have been shown to increase mortality threefold in a general hospital and to be an independent risk factor for death in long-term care facilities.

EPIDEMIOLOGY. The quantitative bacterial count has proved useful for detecting asymptomatic infections and defining the frequency of underlying infection in large populations. The frequency of bacteriuria is about 1 to 2% in newborns, as determined by suprapubic aspiration or meticulously clean urine samples. Newborn males are more often infected than newborn females, and uncircumcised males are at higher risk. After the first year of life, infections are more common in females. During the ages 5 to 18 years, the prevalence is 1.2% in girls and 0.03% in boys. The incidence in girls is 0.4% per year, is linear with time throughout the school years, and is unaffected by menarche. The cumulative frequency of asymptomatic infection in girls during the school years is about 5%. Bacteriuria in girls is independent of socioeconomic status and race and is not increased in diabetics. The prevalence of bacteriuria in females rises about 1% per decade and may be as high as 10% in elderly women. Women with asymptomatic bacteriuria appear to be prone to symptomatic infections when they become sexually active or pregnant. The frequency of bacteriuria

during pregnancy varies from 2 to 6%, depending on age, parity, and socioeconomic group. Detecting and treating bacteriuria early in pregnancy prevent acute pyelonephritis during the third trimester.

ROLE OF INSTRUMENTATION. After a single catheterization, persistent bacteriuria will develop in about 1 to 2% of healthy individuals; the risk is increased at the time of delivery, in debilitated patients, or in males with prostatic obstruction. With open indwelling catheter drainage, infection will develop in more than 90% of patients within 3 to 4 days. Catheter-associated infection may be prevented by avoiding *instrumentation of the urinary tract* whenever possible, removing the catheter when it is no longer needed, and using aseptic closed drainage.

PATHOGENESIS. The urinary tract is ordinarily sterile except at the distal end of the urethra and the meatus. These regions are colonized by staphylococci, diphtheroids, and other commensal organisms that do not grow well in urine. In contrast, in females prone to recurrent infections, the urethra and vaginal introitus are more likely to be colonized with small numbers of enteric gram-negative bacteria, which do grow well in urine. Urine is a variable culture medium. High concentrations of urea, low pH, hypertonicity, and dietary organic acids produce unfavorable conditions for bacterial growth. Enteric gram-negative bacteria overcome hypertonic conditions by taking up the osmoprotectants glycine betaine and proline betaine that exist in urine. Important defense mechanisms include the dynamics of urine flow (washout) and the antibacterial properties of the membrane lining the urinary tract.

Urinary infections arise most commonly by an ascending route. Gram-negative enteric bacilli and other microorganisms normally present in the large bowel colonize the distal segment of the urethra, enter the bladder intermittently, and become established when conditions are favorable. The bladder defense mechanism is usually highly effective. Most women suffer only an occasional episode, and infection rarely develops in men spontaneously. The higher rate of urinary infections in females appears to be due to their shorter urethra. Homosexual males who engage in anal intercourse are at increased risk. The role of sexual intercourse in acquiring urinary infection in females is controversial but may be important for a subpopulation prone to recurrent infections. Vaginal diaphragms and *spermicidal jellies* increase the risk of UTI apparently by mechanical effects and by altering the vaginal flora. *Transmission of uropathogens between sex partners may occur, but sexual transmission of UTI from female to male is rare.*

Other less common pathways include the hematogenous and possibly the lymphatic routes. Staphylococcal bacteremia from a distant site can produce multiple microabscesses in the kidney (renal carbuncles), which may extend to the perinephric fascia and produce perinephric abscesses. A similar but more insidious process may occur with tuberculosis. Disseminated *C. albicans* infections in an immunocompromised, leukopenic host can involve the kidney. Occasionally, bacteremia arising from an infected kidney may produce metastatic abscesses to bone and back to the kidney. Septic emboli, particularly in the setting of infective endocarditis, can produce extensive infection in the kidney. A rare but striking finding in diabetics is the occurrence of pneumaturia, or urinary flatulence, from the production of gas by fermentation.

Hematogenous infection in experimental models requires antecedent structural damage to the kidney. The renal medulla is much more susceptible to infection than the cortex is. In experimental pyelonephritis, as few as 10 to 100 *E. coli* can produce infection in the medulla, whereas 100,000 are required to infect the cortex. The increased susceptibility of the renal medulla is thought to be due to its unique hypertonicity, which impairs leukocyte mobilization and phagocytosis. Ascending infections begin in the renal fornices and extend in segmental fashion to the papilla, medulla, and cortex.

Microbial virulence factors are also important (see Chapter 311). Strains of *E. coli* isolated from patients with pyelonephritis are more likely to contain capsular polysaccharides (K antigens), which resist phagocytosis, and to possess P fimbriae (pili). These fimbriae are hair-like surface structures with a lectin at their tip that recognizes complementary structures on the surface of host epithelial cells. P-fimbriated strains bind to α-D-Gal-(-4)-β-D-Gal (P blood group) receptors on urothelial cells and are more commonly recovered from the blood and urine of patients with acute uncomplicated pyelonephritis. Type I (mannose sensitive) fimbriae appear to help initiate infection in the bladder. They are recognized by phagocytic cells and bound by Tamm-Horsfall mucoprotein in the urine. Fimbriated *E. coli* convert to nonfimbriated forms (phase variation), possibly to avoid recognition by phagocytic cells. Other less well established virulence factors include the O antigens and production of hemolysin and aerobactin. Virulent strains are found more often in patients with uncomplicated rather than complicated infections, presumably because of the greater need to overcome host resistance. Urease-producing bacteria such as *Proteus, Providencia, Morganella, S. saprophyticus,* and *Corynebacterium urealyticum* are particularly virulent because they can produce ammonia, which is toxic to the kidney, and form infection (struvite) stones, which may block the urinary tract and urinary catheters.

CLINICAL MANIFESTATIONS. Symptoms and laboratory findings in acute urinary infection and pyelonephritis are shown in Table 111–2. It is not usually possible to distinguish on clinical grounds whether the patient has urethritis, cystitis, or the pyuria/dysuria syndrome. Otherwise healthy females may have an occasional isolated episode of uncomplicated UTI, but some suffer from highly recurrent infections. Recurrence is usually due to reinfection with a new bacterial strain rather than relapse with the same strain. *In approximately one third to one half of cases the same strain is reintroduced from an extraurinary tract reservoir.*

Acute pyelonephritis is easy to recognize and is seldom confused with any other renal disease. Renal colic and hematuria from the passage of urinary calculi may mimic pyelonephritis, but patients are usually afebrile. Pyelonephritis is at times characterized by symptoms that do not point to the urinary tract. Dysuria and fever may be absent. Headache may be the only symptom, with no demonstrable flank tenderness. Some patients have pain in either the upper or the lower part of the abdomen, together with symptoms of disturbed gastrointestinal function. Others complain only of general fatigue. Clues to the diagnosis include a history of infection, underlying host abnormalities such as diabetes, the presence of a urinary catheter, fever of uncertain etiology, and unexplained pyuria, bacteriuria, and gram-negative bacteremia. Uroradiographic studies are often helpful in demonstrating a specific lesion. Usually no changes are found in renal function other than a transiently decreased ability to concentrate urine, and secondary hypertension is unusual.

A number of tests have been developed to differentiate "upper" (kidney) from "lower" (bladder) infection. Ureteral catheterization and bladder washout maneuvers are considered research studies. The antibody-coated bacteria test has insufficient sensitivity and specificity for clinical use. The most useful guide is clinical assessment. Patients with complicated infections are more likely to have upper tract infection.

The symptoms and signs of acute, uncomplicated pyelonephritis usually resolve within several days after instituting adequate antimicrobial therapy. More severe forms of pyelonephritis or urinary tract obstruction should be suspected if fever, leukocytosis, and flank pain persist. Diabetics are prone to widely destructive, emphysematous pyelonephritis and renal papillary necrosis. Other conditions that should be considered are renal carbuncle or perinephric abscess, xanthogranulomatous pyelonephritis, and metastatic abscess in the vertebrae. Surgical drainage may be required for perinephric and large renal abscesses. Patients with chronic active py-

elonephritis may have persistent smoldering infections and gradual progression to end-stage renal failure. This process may persist for many years and be complicated by generalized debility, anemia of chronic infection, and secondary amyloidosis and eventually result in proteinuria and severe hypertension and its complications.

Patients subjected to urethral instrumentation, especially an indwelling catheter, are at increased risk for bacteremia and acute pyelonephritis. The urinary catheter is an independent risk factor for about a three-fold increase in mortality among patients in short-term general hospitals and extended care facilities. The infectious process is often subclinical, but in some individuals it may take a sudden fulminating course, with bacteremia, septic shock, and death. Gram-negative sepsis and bacteremic shock are described in Chapter 96.

DIAGNOSIS. MICROSCOPIC AND DIPSTICK METHODS. Rapid diagnostic methods include examination of a Gram stain of unsedimented urine with an oil immersion lens or examination of the centrifuged urinary sediment with the high-dry objective under reduced light, with or without the addition of methylene blue. The presence of one or more organisms on the Gram stain correlates about 90% with quantitative culture (10^5 CFU per milliliter). Examining the unstained sediment is very helpful and can be done with the routine examination for formed elements. The criterion is the presence of many (preferably more than 20) obvious bacteria regardless of motility. "Pyuria" is usually defined as 10 or more leukocytes per high-powered field in a centrifuged specimen or 5 or more when uncentrifuged. The leukocyte esterase test correlates well with chamber counts of greater than 10 to 20 leukocytes per cubic millimeter. "Sterile pyuria" may be due to vaginal leukorrhea. The nitrite test is highly specific but relatively insensitive unless performed on a first morning urine. Microscopic hematuria is common in acute infections, but proteinuria is rare.

UROLOGIC AND RADIOLOGIC INVESTIGATIONS. Searching for important structural abnormalities such as urethral valves (in male infants), severe vesicoureteral reflux, malformations, and obstructive and neurogenic lesions is indicated for young children of both sexes. Urologic studies are rarely productive in adult females, even with recurrent infections. Ultrasonography of the kidneys with bladder-voiding studies and radionuclide examinations have reduced the need to routinely use more invasive procedures such as intravenous urography, cystoscopy, and voiding cystourethrography. Computed tomography is particularly helpful for detecting renal abscesses. It is not usually necessary to repeat normal studies. Cystoscopy should be reserved for demonstrating anatomic defects, interstitial cystitis, and bladder tumors and should not be used as a guide to measure response to therapy.

MANAGEMENT. The goals are to eradicate bacteria from the urinary tract, relieve symptoms, prevent renal damage, and diminish the likelihood of spreading infection to other sites. Prophylaxis is used to prevent recurrent symptomatic infection. Suppression, although rarely effective, may be used to diminish the number of bacteria in the urine or tissues. Indications for therapy depend on the potential of infection to produce symptoms or damage the urinary tract and the likelihood that treatment will be effective.

ASYMPTOMATIC BACTERIURIA. Asymptomatic bacteriuria need not be treated in otherwise healthy or elderly females without underlying structural or neurologic lesions because the likelihood of renal damage is slight and the toxicity and expense of therapy often outweigh the risk of disease. Furthermore, reinfection is common following successful eradication of bacteriuria, and little is accomplished in the long term. Urease-producing bacteria (see above) should be eradicated whenever possible because of their potential to produce urinary calculi. *Antimicrobial therapy is usually ineffective in patients with indwelling catheters and should not be used unless the patient is in a septic state. It will result in superinfection with more resistant microorganisms.*

Treatment is recommended for patients who are at high risk for symptomatic infections or patients who have complicating conditions. Such patients include those with diabetes, polycystic kidneys, or anatomic or neurologic abnormalities or those scheduled for urologic procedures or renal transplantation. Treating asymptomatic bacteriuria early in pregnancy quite successfully prevents acute pyelonephritis in the third trimester.

Table 111–2 ■ COMMON MANIFESTATIONS OF URINARY TRACT INFECTIONS

CLINICAL	LABORATORY
1. Urethritis or cystitis	Leukocyte esterase test positive
Frequent urination	Nitrite test may be positive
Burning on urination	Gram stain of uncentrifuged urine
Suprapubic discomfort	Leukocytes (≥5/hpf)
Lassitude	Gram-negative rods or gram-positive cocci (≥1/hpf)*
Cloudy or blood-tinged urine	
Occasional low-grade fever	Urine culture (≥10^5 CFU/mL*)
	Low-count bacteriuria* (10^3–10^4 CFU/mL*)
2. Acute pyelonephritis	Same findings as above *plus*
Sudden onset of fever	Leukocytosis
Shaking chills	Blood cultures positive (about 20%)
Flank pain (may radiate)	Minimal effect on serum creatinine
Urinary symptoms may be absent	Decreased concentration ability

*See the text.
hpf = high-power field; CFU = colony-forming unit.

ACUTE SYMPTOMATIC URINARY TRACT INFECTION. The initial attack of UTI is usually by *E. coli.* Treatment should be started before the results of susceptibility tests are available. The choice of drug is based on the likelihood that the organism will be susceptible. The choice of an oral or parenteral agent depends on the severity of the infection and the patient's ability to take the oral agent. Drugs are selected on the basis of cost, side effects, and antibacterial spectrum.

Microscopic examination of urine and urine cultures ensure an accurate diagnosis of UTI. Pre-treatment urine cultures are desirable, but not essential in young women with acute dysuria and pyuria, in whom the probability of uncomplicated bacterial cystitis is high. These patients usually respond to short-course therapy. Response to therapy can be determined by the disappearance of bacteria on microscopic examination by 24 to 48 hours, but pyuria may persist for up to a week. It is important to recognize bacteriologic failure early and to change antibiotics. Pre-treatment urine cultures should be obtained in symptomatic infants, children, men, and the elderly; patients with suspected pyelonephritis or complicated infection; patients with *recurrent* infections; those with *symptomatic* catheter- or instrument-associated nosocomial infection; and pregnant women.

Acute uncomplicated episodes of symptomatic infection (bacterial cystitis or urethritis) are treated most effectively with a short course of oral therapy (Table 111–3). Three-day treatment is recommended because it is more effective than single-dose therapy and is as effective as 7 to 10 days of treatment. Single-dose therapy usually fails to eradicate either renal bacteriuria or complicated infections and, if used, should be started early in the course of infection. Patients with complicated infections should be treated for 7 to 14 days or even longer, provided that the drug is effective in eradicating bacteriuria (Fig. 111–1). Effective drugs are listed in Table 111–3. Symptomatic urethritis caused by *C. trachomatis* should respond to azithromycin (1 g orally in a single dose) or oral doxycycline (100 mg twice daily) or tetracycline (500 mg four times per day) for 7 days.

Acute uncomplicated pyelonephritis should be treated for 7 to 14 days. Parenteral agents such as trimethoprim-sulfamethoxazole, a cephalosporin, a fluoroquinolone, or an aminoglycoside may be required when the patient is too ill to receive an oral agent. *Ampicillin and amoxicillin with or without β-lactamase inhibitors are not recommended, unless the organisms are shown to be susceptible, because of the high frequency of resistant strains.* Usually, no more than one drug is needed. Oral agents may be used on an outpatient basis, provided that the patient is not nauseated. Patients treated with parenteral agents should convert to oral therapy as

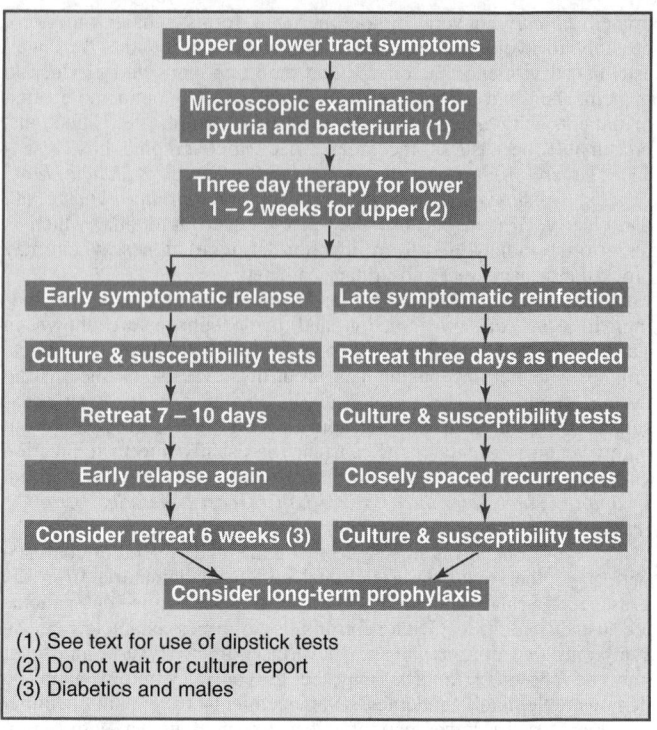

FIGURE 111–1 ■ Management of urinary tract infections.

soon as they are stable. Patients with active chronic pyelonephritis may not respond to antimicrobial therapy, even when the organism is susceptible, unless an obstruction or foreign body is removed or an abscess is drained. Hematogenous pyelonephritis requires specific therapy directed at the invading organism. A follow-up culture 1 week after completion of antimicrobial therapy is recommended to document a cure.

RECURRENT INFECTIONS. Recurrent infection within a week or two after treatment is usually due to persistence of the same focus, whereas recurrence after several weeks is more often a result of reinfection, especially in women. Relapses in diabetics, transplant recipients, and elderly men should be treated for up to 4 to 6 weeks. Frequently recurrent infections may be managed either by repeated short courses for each symptomatic episode (these can be self-administered by reliable patients) or by long-term prophylaxis with trimethoprim, trimethoprim-sulfamethoxazole, nitrofurantoin, *or a low dose of a fluoroquinolone* as a single bedtime dose or following intercourse. Resistant strains infrequently emerge with these drugs. Prophylaxis, when given for 6 months or longer, is highly effective for recurrent infections. The risk of recurrence is still high once prophylaxis is stopped, and it may need to be resumed. Urinary antiseptics such as methenamine mandelate or hippurate require an acidic urine, preferably at pH 5.5, and are relatively ineffective unless given with agents that consistently lower urinary pH such as a high-protein diet, ammonium chloride, or methionine. Methenamine and its salts may be used for prophylaxis when no other drug is active. Infection should be eradicated first by a more potent drug before beginning prophylaxis with these drugs.

Some women take high volumes of fluids when acute urinary symptoms develop. This approach may be helpful at times, but antimicrobial drugs are much more effective. Double voiding in patients with vesicoureteral reflux is recommended. Voiding after sexual intercourse is believed by some to decrease the chance of recurrent infection, *but this practice is unproved.* Post-coital use of prophylactic agents is far more effective.

COMPLICATED INFECTIONS. Complicated urinary infections are exceedingly difficult to eradicate. The key to management is to relieve obstruction and remove foreign bodies, in addition to the use of effective antimicrobial drugs. It is important to recognize failure early and not to continue using an ineffective drug, which will only lead to superinfection with more resistant microorganisms and increase costs unnecessarily. It is often best to leave the infection untreated except to manage acute episodes. Suppressive ther-

Table 111–3 ■ ORAL ANTIMICROBIAL DRUGS FOR UNCOMPLICATED URINARY TRACT INFECTIONS*

DRUG	DOSE	COMMENTS
Trimethoprim	100 mg every 12 hr†	About equally effective
Trimethoprim-sulfamethoxazole	80/400 mg every 12 hr†	
Nitrofurantoin	100 mg every 8 hr‡	Take with food
Cefixime	400 mg daily	Expensive
Cefuroxime axetil	250 mg every 12 hr	Expensive
Cefpodoxime	200 mg every 12 hr	Expensive
Norfloxacin	400 mg every 12 hr	Expensive§
Ciprofloxacin	100 mg every 12 hr	Expensive§
Ofloxacin	200 mg every 12 hr	Expensive§
Lomefloxacin	400 mg once daily	Expensive§
Enoxacin	200 mg every 12 hr	Expensive§
Carbenicillin indanyl	Two 382-mg tablets every 6 hr	For *Pseudomonas* species
Fosfomycin	3 g, single dose	Expensive‖

*Ampicillin, amoxicillin, cephalexin, or a tetracycline may be used if the bacteria are susceptible, but resistance to these drugs is common.

†Many clinicians prefer to use a double dose of these drugs.

‡Contraindicated in patients with elevated serum creatinine levels. The monohydrate/macrocystal form is administered as 100 mg every 12 hours.

§Bacteria resistant to one quinolone are usually resistant to all others.

‖See the text for a discussion of single-dose therapy versus 3-day therapy.

apy should be abandoned unless it can be shown that the bacterial populations in the urine are markedly reduced.

Kunin CM: Urinary Tract Infections, Detection, Prevention and Management, 5th ed. Baltimore, Williams & Wilkins, 1997. *A comprehensive, single-author text that describes the pathogenesis, management, and prevention of urinary tract infections.*

Mobley HLT, Warren JW (eds): Urinary Tract Infections, Molecular Pathogenesis and Clinical Management. Washington, DC, ASM Press, 1996. *A multiauthored text that deals with the clinical and microbiologic aspects of urinary tract infection with special emphasis on microbial pathogenesis.*

Ronald A: Sex and urinary tract infections. N Engl J Med 335:511, 1996. *A short, thoughtful review of a controversial subject.*

Sheinfeld J, Schaeffer AJ, Corrdon-Cardo C, et al: Association of the Lewis blood-group phenotype with recurrent urinary tract infections in women. N Engl J Med 320:773, 1989. *An explanation for the remarkable susceptibility of some women to recurrent urinary tract infections.*

Stamey TA, Timothy M, Miller M, et al: Recurrent urinary tract infections in adult women. Calif Med 115:1, 1971. *A classic paper that describes the remarkable resistance of the vagina and urethra to colonization with uropathogens in healthy women without urinary tract infections and selective colonization in women with recurrent infections.*

112 VASCULAR DISORDERS OF THE KIDNEY

Thomas D. DuBose, Jr.

The fact that the kidneys depend on systemic blood pressure to maintain normal renal blood flow, glomerular filtration rate (GFR), and tubular function underscores the vulnerability of the kidneys to diseases involving the renal vasculature. Renal vessels may be involved by thrombosis, emboli, atherosclerosis, inflammation, or hypertension. Renal vascular disease can be classified according to anatomic location: arteries, arterioles and microvasculature, and renal veins.

ARTERIES

Thromboembolic Occlusion of the Renal Arteries

DEFINITION AND ETIOLOGY. Thrombosis of the renal arteries and segmental branches may arise as a result of intrinsic pathology of the renal arteries or as a complication of embolization of thrombi arising in distant vessels. In situ thrombosis occurs as a complication of progressive atherosclerosis in elderly patients and may be an important cause of progressive renal insufficiency in this population. In patients younger than 60 years, traumatic thrombosis is the most common etiology. Blunt trauma and deceleration injuries may cause acute thrombosis. Trauma to the renal pedicle may result in an intimal tear with thrombosis in the middle third of the renal artery. Thrombosis may arise in the setting of dissection of the renal artery or as a complication of renal arteriography, angioplasty, or stent placement. Finally, thrombosis may occur as a consequence of inflammatory disorders that involve the large arteries (Takayasu's arteritis, syphilis, systemic vasculitides, and thromboangiitis obliterans), as well as structural lesions of the renal arteries such as fibromuscular dysplasia or renal artery aneurysm. Embolization is a more common cause of renal artery occlusion than in situ thrombosis is and is usually unilateral (bilateral in 15 to 30%). Total infarction of the kidney is much less common than is segmental infarction or ischemia. Approximately 90% of thromboemboli to the renal arteries originate in the heart, and a common cause is left atrial thrombi in patients with atrial fibrillation. Valvular heart disease, bacterial endocarditis, non-bacterial (aseptic) endocarditis, and atrial myxomas are other sources of emboli originating in the heart. The diverse causes of occlusion of the renal artery or its segmental branches are summarized in Table 112–1.

CLINICAL MANIFESTATIONS. The manifestations of thromboembolic occlusion of the renal arteries depend on the extent and time course of the occlusive event, as well as the pre-existing status of the renal circulation. Occlusion of a primary or secondary branch of the renal artery in a patient with pre-existing disease and established collateral circulation, such as long-standing renal artery

Table 112–1 ▪ CAUSES OF RENAL ARTERY OCCLUSION

Thrombosis
Progressive atherosclerosis
Trauma, blunt
Aortic or renal artery aneurysm
Aortic or renal artery dissection
Aortic or renal artery angiography
Superimposed on inflammatory disorders
  Vasculitis
  Thromboangiitis obliterans
  Syphilis
Superimposed on structural lesions
  Fibromuscular dysplasia
Thromboembolism
Atrial fibrillation
Mitral stenosis
Mural thrombus
Atrial myxoma
Prosthetic valve
Septic or aseptic valvular vegetations
Paradoxical emboli
Tumor emboli
Fat emboli
Atheroemboli (Cholesterol Embolization)
Elderly patients with advanced atherosclerosis
Abdominal aortic surgery
Trauma, blunt
Angiographic catheters
Angioplasty or stent placement
Excessive anticoagulation

stenosis, may produce little or no infarction and minimal symptoms. Acute thrombosis and infarction may result in sudden onset of flank pain (which resembles renal colic), fever, nausea, vomiting, and, on occasion, hematuria. Pain may be localized to the abdomen or back or even the chest, but in more than half of cases, pain is absent. If infarction occurs, leukocytosis usually develops, and serum enzyme levels may be elevated (aspartate aminotransferase, lactate dehydrogenase, and alkaline phosphatase); urinary lactate dehydrogenase and alkaline phosphatase may also increase. Urinalysis usually reveals microscopic hematuria. The blood urea nitrogen and creatinine levels typically increase transiently with unilateral infarction, but more severe and protracted renal dysfunction may follow bilateral renal infarction or infarction of a solitary kidney. Hypertension, which usually occurs with infarction, is the result of release of renin from the ischemic renal parenchyma.

DIAGNOSIS. The diagnosis of renal artery occlusion is most reliably established by renal arteriography. The advantage of conventional arteriography is that the anatomy, even of subsegmental occlusion, can be most reliably established. Computed tomography (CT), especially spiral acquired-volume CT scans, magnetic resonance (MR) angiography, and duplex ultrasound scanning can be used reliably as screening tests for the diagnosis of acute arterial thrombosis. MR angiography is superior to CT scanning and duplex ultrasound scanning. In embolic renal artery occlusion, the presence of an intracardiac thrombus must be sought by echocardiography.

MANAGEMENT. Managing acute arterial thrombosis usually includes surgical revascularization, control of hypertension, adequate hydration, anticoagulation, and acute renal replacement therapy when needed. Alternative approaches such as intra-arterial thrombolytic therapy are being used more frequently, especially for iatrogenic occlusion of the renal artery as a result of angiographic manipulations or angioplasty. Obviously, atheroemboli should not be treated by fibrinolysis. Surgery is also the treatment of choice for traumatic renal artery thrombosis, which is associated with poor salvage of renal function unless surgery is accomplished immediately. The warm ischemia time beyond which recovery of renal function would not be anticipated is no more than several hours.

PROGNOSIS. Mortality is high in these conditions, particularly because of the severity of underlying and associated conditions. The mortality rate of patients undergoing surgical revascularization for complete acute renal artery occlusion is 11 to 25%. Hypertension may develop as a late sequela of renal artery occlusion and may be treated by angiotensin-converting enzyme (ACE) inhibitors, angiotensin receptor antagonists, or non-dihydropyridine calcium channel blockers or, if refractory, by balloon angioplasty. Chronic renal replacement therapy may be necessary.

Renal Artery Stenosis and Azotemic-Ischemic Renal Disease

DEFINITION AND ETIOLOGY. The prevalence of renal artery stenosis as the etiology of hypertension in the general population is only 2 to 4%. In selected subgroups of patients (accelerated hypertension with renal insufficiency), the prevalence increases to 30 to 40%. Atherosclerosis causes approximately 60 to 70% of cases in middle-aged and elderly patients. In younger women, renal artery stenosis is usually the result of fibromuscular dysplasia. Atherosclerosis of one or both renal arteries is being recognized more frequently among the elderly, in whom it may or may not be associated with hypertension. It is often associated with generalized atherosclerotic peripheral vascular disease and may progress to cause progressive loss of renal function with or without renal infarction. This entity has been referred to as "azotemic," or "ischemic," renal disease. A striking association has been noted between the number of peripheral vessels involved (more than five) with peripheral vascular disease and the presence of renal artery stenosis. Renal artery stenosis secondary to atherosclerosis is more prevalent among heavy smokers and those with high cholesterol levels.

CLINICAL MANIFESTATIONS. Renal artery stenosis should be suspected when hypertension develops in a previously normotensive patient older than 55 or younger than 30 years or when accelerated hypertension develops in a patient with previously established, controlled hypertension. Features that suggest renal artery stenosis include persistent hypokalemia, metabolic alkalosis, symptoms or signs of peripheral vascular disease, unexplained progression of renal insufficiency, recurrent pulmonary edema, disparate renal size, and the presence of an epigastric bruit on physical examination. Azotemic-ischemic nephropathy should be considered in all patients older than 60 years with unexplained progression of renal insufficiency, with or without hypertension.

DIAGNOSIS. The captopril renal scintigram (scan) is an excellent noninvasive function test for screening patients with suspected renal artery stenosis. It has been most useful in patients with unilateral renal artery stenosis associated with hypertension and relative preservation of renal function (serum creatinine, <2.0 mg/dL). This test is based on the assumption that angiotensin II–dependent constriction of the efferent arteriole is a physiologic prerequisite for maintaining GFR and renal blood flow in significant renal artery stenosis. ACE inhibition is usually associated with decreased uptake of the nuclide, prolonged retention, or a longer peak uptake on the affected side. Three-dimensional phase-contrast MR angiography compares favorably with conventional arteriography (sensitivity and specificity of 94 and 98%, respectively, for stenoses greater than 50%) and offers significant advantages over the captopril renal scintigram in the face of renal insufficiency. Duplex scanning or Doppler flowmetry relies on combined techniques to localize the renal arteries and estimate blood flow, but it is less reliable. Intravenous urography no longer plays a role in the investigation of hypertension or chronic renal failure. Although no single screening test is sufficiently sensitive and specific, in patients in whom stenosis is suspected, renal arteriography may be required to confirm the diagnosis and define the vascular anatomy before surgical or nonsurgical intervention. The risk for contrast nephropathy, as well as the risks of catheterization, must be considered, especially in older patients with renal insufficiency. Peripheral vein renin determinations are not helpful in the diagnosis or management of renal artery stenosis. Renal vein renin determinations are not usually helpful for screening or diagnosis but may assist with planning the approach to therapy. In unilateral renal artery stenosis, the expected finding for clinically significant disease is a ratio of renin from the affected side to renin from the contralateral renal vein of greater than 1.5. A reasonable diagnostic approach is to screen with a captopril scintigram when the creatinine is below 2.0 and with MR angiography when it is above 2.0 mg/dL. If either test is normal and in the absence of a very high degree of clinical suspicion, arteriography is not usually requested.

MANAGEMENT. The goal of therapy for renal artery stenosis is to control the blood pressure and stabilize renal function by restoration of renal perfusion. Because considerable controversy surrounds the issue of how best to treat presumed renal artery stenosis, patients should be managed cooperatively by a nephrologist, vascular surgeon, and interventional radiologist. Therapeutic options include percutaneous transluminal renal angioplasty (PTRA), surgical revascularization, and conservative medical management. Conservative medical management, as primary therapy, is clearly inferior to either form of interventional therapy and should be reserved for patients with definite contraindications to surgery or PTRA. Nevertheless, conservative medical management is a critical component of the continuing care of all patients with atherosclerotic renal artery disease after surgery or PTRA. Medical management includes cessation of smoking, weight loss, exercise, strict blood pressure control with skillful agent selection, and lipid-lowering agents. PTRA is generally considered to be the initial treatment of choice for both fibromuscular dysplasia and atherosclerotic renal artery stenosis.

PROGNOSIS. PTRA is clearly the initial treatment of choice for hypertension caused by fibromuscular dysplasia inasmuch as the initial success rate for PTRA is high and the re-stenosis rate is low. PTRA is less effective in atherosclerotic renal artery stenosis if normalization of blood pressure is the outcome to be achieved. Fifty per cent or more of patients benefit to some extent by improvement in blood pressure. Moreover, PTRA is associated with improved renal function in a significant percentage of patients with sufficient residual renal mass. The progressive nature of atherosclerotic renal artery disease must be taken into consideration when outcomes are assessed. Stabilization or improvement in renal function has been observed in patients with both unilateral and bilateral renal artery stenosis. Prevention of loss of renal function seems more important than recovery from renal insufficiency that has already developed. An aggressive attitude in the diagnosis and treatment of atheromatous renal disease to protect from progressive renal insufficiency seems warranted. In the event that angioplasty fails, surgical revascularization should be considered, but the patient's age and suitability as a surgical candidate must be considered. The risk of surgical reconstruction in younger patients, such as those with fibromuscular dysplasia, is very low. Operative mortality, which is limited to patients with atherosclerosis, has been reported to be as low as 2% but as high as 7%. Not surprisingly, the risk of surgery is highest in older patients with azotemia, generalized atherosclerosis, and cerebrovascular and cardiac disease.

ARTERIOLES AND MICROVASCULATURE

Atheroembolic Disease of the Renal Arteries

DEFINITION AND ETIOLOGY. Embolization of cholesterol crystals as a cause of renal artery occlusion occurs almost exclusively in elderly patients with widespread atherosclerosis. Atheroemboli may also occur as a complication of abdominal aorta or renal artery manipulation or surgery or as a consequence of angiography or transluminal angioplasty. This entity may be overlooked because patients at risk for this complication often have other chronic illnesses associated with renal failure, hypertension, and atherosclerosis.

CLINICAL MANIFESTATIONS. Renal insufficiency, hypertension, or both disorders occur regularly with atheroembolization to the renal vasculature. Evidence of cholesterol embolization in the retina, muscles, or skin (associated with livedo reticularis) can be helpful and obviate the need for a renal biopsy. Evidence of embolization to other organs resulting in cerebrovascular events, acute pancreatitis, ischemic bowel, and gangrene of the extremities may be noted. Urinalysis may not be helpful because cholesterol crystals are not usually present, but mild proteinuria, eosinophiluria, and increased cellularity are more often observed.

MANAGEMENT. Therapy for this disorder is often disappointing inasmuch as cholesterol embolization leads to structural changes in the microvasculature without inflammation. Anticoagulants have not proved to be of value and may delay healing of ulcerating atherosclerotic lesions. Dialysis, treating the hypertension with attention to avoiding hypotension, and adequate hydration are the mainstays of treatment.

PROGNOSIS. With adequate blood pressure control for several months or years, renal function may recover sufficiently, even in patients requiring chronic renal replacement therapy, to allow nondialytic conservative management.

Hypertensive Arteriolar Nephrosclerosis

DEFINITION AND ETIOLOGY. Although autoregulation of renal blood flow and GFR occurs throughout a wide range of systemic blood pressure, the renal vasculature is exquisitely sensitive to damage incurred by systemic hypertension when it is transmitted to the glomerular capillary bed (see Chapter 101). Unopposed or sustained increases in glomerular capillary hydrostatic pressure eventually result in sclerosis. In *benign nephrosclerosis,* the kidney is the victim of the adverse effects of chronic hypertension over a prolonged period and does not appear to participate in the pathogenesis of the disorder. The vascular injury in the kidney is non-specific but more pronounced than vascular changes observed systemically. When advanced, such changes can result in end-stage renal disease (ESRD). In *malignant* or *accelerated hypertension,* the vascular changes are unique and severe and lead to renal ischemia, renin production, and exacerbation of the disease, which may terminate in acute renal failure and, if not treated successfully, ESRD. In contrast to benign nephrosclerosis, in which the principal lesion is in the media of the vessels, malignant or accelerated hypertension is characterized by a unique lesion of the intima. Renal vascular lesions similar to those seen in malignant hypertension are also observed in scleroderma, thrombotic microangiopathy, and renal transplant rejection.

CLINICAL MANIFESTATIONS. Patients with benign hypertensive nephrosclerosis have been hypertensive for many years (more than 10 to 15 years). Kidney size is usually reduced, and the urine sediment is unremarkable except for proteinuria, which is usually less than 1.5 g/day. The sudden development of malignant or accelerated hypertension, in either patients with previously established mild to moderate hypertension or patients in whom hypertension had not previously been diagnosed, is manifested by an abrupt increase in blood pressure (diastolic usually greater than 130 mm Hg). Papilledema may develop, and renal function may decline rapidly. The kidneys may be enlarged, or the urinary sediment may be active, with gross or microscopic hematuria, and proteinuria is often in the nephrotic range. Microangiopathic hemolytic anemia may be present. Abnormalities in the central nervous system are usually evident and range from headaches to generalized seizures to coma. Malignant hypertension may coexist with cerebral vascular accidents.

The availability of effective antihypertensive medication has sharply reduced the occurrence of this devastating disorder. However, both benign and malignant hypertensive renal disease and the sequelae of these disorders appear to be more prevalent in blacks.

MANAGEMENT. For either benign or malignant hypertension, the primary goal is to control the blood pressure. In benign hypertensive nephrosclerosis, the renal outcome is dependent on timely initiation of effective therapy, patient compliance, and careful follow-up by a nephrologist. Inadequate treatment may result in irreversible glomerular sclerosis, as well as end-organ damage in the cardiovasculature and central nervous system. Antihypertensives that provide renal protection usually include ACE inhibitors or angiotensin receptor antagonists and non-dihydropyridine calcium channel blockers. Malignant hypertension, by contrast, is a medical emergency and must be approached aggressively. Controlling the blood pressure can reverse the major manifestations in most patients, including the renal functional impairment. Parenteral antihypertensives, such as nitroprusside infused in the critical care setting, may be necessary initially. Blood pressure should be controlled smoothly and gradually but be into the normal range by 36 to 48 hours. Antihypertensive medications should be continued even if renal function continues to deteriorate and renal replacement therapy is required. Some patients experience partial reversal of vascular lesions and return of renal function to levels compatible with non-dialytic, conservative management.

PROGNOSIS. With skillful selection of antihypertensive agents and obsessive control of blood pressure, progression of renal disease can be avoided. Hypertension with nephrosclerosis is the second most common cause of ESRD in the United States. The importance of early recognition and aggressive treatment cannot be overemphasized.

Hemolytic-Uremic Syndrome and Thrombotic Thrombocytopenic Purpura

DEFINITION AND ETIOLOGY. Renal failure is a common consequence of both hemolytic-uremic syndrome (HUS) and thrombotic thrombocytopenic purpura (TTP). For additional information, see Chapters 103 and 104. These conditions are characterized by platelet and fibrin thrombi within the renal microvasculature, accompanied by thrombocytopenia and microangiopathic hemolytic anemia. Although the vascular lesions are identical, central venous system involvement predominates in TTP, whereas renal involvement is predominant in HUS.

CLINICAL MANIFESTATIONS. TTP is suggested by the co-occurrence of hemolysis, thrombocytopenia, fever, purpura, and alternating mental status changes. HUS may be associated with acute renal failure, thrombocytopenia, and microangiopathic hemolytic anemia, most commonly in children after an acute diarrheal illness. Either disorder may be observed in the setting of cancer and infection and while administering chemotherapeutic agents.

MANAGEMENT AND PROGNOSIS. Acute implementation of renal replacement therapy has significantly improved survival. The oliguria and degree of renal failure, as well as the severity of hypertension, are more pronounced in HUS. Early diagnosis and initiation of dialysis, antihypertensives, supportive transfusions, and control of seizures are essential to a good outcome. Up to 85% of children with typical HUS recover with supportive care. In TTP, plasma exchange combined with antiplatelet therapy is recommended and may be required for 1 to 2 weeks.

Scleroderma

CLINICAL MANIFESTATIONS. The clinical features and progression of scleroderma are highly variable. The various limited skin and systemic manifestations of scleroderma are considered in more detail in Chapter 290. Although it is widely appreciated that the mortality associated with scleroderma increases as a function of the number of organ systems involved, significant renal involvement (which has been reported in 50% of patients with systemic sclerosis of 20 or more years' duration) is the most dreaded complication and is associated with the poorest prognosis. When the kidneys are involved, the typical manifestation is intimal proliferation, medial thinning, and increased collagen deposition in the adventitial layer of small renal arteries. An increase in vasomotor tone at the level of the renal vasculature is probably a renal manifestation of Raynaud's phenomenon and contributes to the reduction in renal blood flow, hypertension, and progressive renal functional impairment. The increase in renin and angiotensin II elaboration contributes to the development of worsening hypertension and hypertensive nephrosclerosis. Most patients with renal scleroderma display mild proteinuria with or without hypertension. Once azotemia develops, hypertension may become more difficult to manage, and dialysis is required within 1 to 2 years. Conversely, patients may initially come to medical attention with a "renal crisis" manifested by the abrupt onset of malignant hypertension and renal failure. This manifestation, which occurs in 10 to 25% of patients with type 3 scleroderma, usually of several years' duration, is a medical emergency requiring aggressive antihypertensive therapy.

MANAGEMENT AND PROGNOSIS. Therapy in patients with scleroderma and renal involvement should be directed primarily toward controlling hypertension in an attempt to slow progression of the renal failure. Referral to a nephrologist is highly recommended. Adequate control may require several drugs in combination, such as ACE inhibitors or angiotensin II receptor antagonists, non-dihydropyridine calcium channel blockers, and vasodilators (such as minoxidil) and other agents. For patients with manifestations of a "renal crisis," intravenous antihypertensive therapy in the critical care setting may be indicated because of the high mortality without therapy. With aggressive management, particularly with ACE inhibitors, progression to ESRD may be slowed significantly. Indeed, even in the event that long-term maintenance dialysis is required, there is evidence that with continued aggressive management of hypertension, a small but significant percentage of patients will regain sufficient renal function to allow cessation of renal replacement therapy.

Sickle Cell Nephropathy

ETIOLOGY. The hypoxemic and hypertonic environment of the renal medulla (vasa recta) encourages the sickling of red blood cells circulating through this region (see Chapter 169). When sickle hemoglobin desaturates, polymerization of hemoglobin can impair or interrupt capillary flow. The major manifestations of sickle cell nephropathy can all be explained by the development of papillary infarction.

CLINICAL MANIFESTATIONS. A defect in urinary concentration resulting in a tendency toward volume depletion is one of the best-characterized abnormalities in sickle cell nephropathy. Obliteration of the vasa recta compromises the operation of the medullary countercurrent system and impairs the ability to generate and maintain medullary solute gradients. The concentrating defect is also observed in sickle trait. A defect in urinary acidification is common and manifested as distal renal tubular acidosis with hyperkalemia and hyperchloremic metabolic acidosis (type 4 renal tubular acidosis). The acidification defect is not usually observed in patients with sickle trait. Painless gross hematuria has been estimated to occur in up to 50% of patients with sickle cell nephropathy. It also occurs in patients with Hb SA or Hb SC. With recurrent papillary infarction, papillary necrosis can occur and progress. Sickle cell "crisis," dehydration, hypoxemia, and the use of non-steroidal anti-inflammatory drugs predispose to papillary necrosis. Renal papillary necrosis is often "silent," but it may progress to chronic renal insufficiency and predispose the patient to repeated urinary tract infections. Nephrotic syndrome may occur in approximately 4% of patients with sickle glomerulopathy. Findings on renal biopsy usually indicate membranoproliferative glomerulopathy with segmental and global sclerosis. As this disorder progresses, glomerulopathy results in sclerosis and progressive loss of glomerular function, whereas papillary infarction can result in persistent hematuria.

MANAGEMENT. Volume depletion should be corrected by isotonic or hypotonic saline intravenously, as dictated by the serum sodium concentration. Hyperkalemia may require potassium exchange resin (sodium polystyrene, Kayexalate) per rectum or orally. When acidosis accompanies the hyperkalemia, alkali may help correct the hyperkalemia and the acidosis. Long-term administration of Shohl solution or sodium bicarbonate tablets may be necessary, and loop diuretics may be helpful. Potassium-sparing diuretics, non-steroidal anti-inflammatory drugs, or potassium supplements should be strictly avoided. Attempts to increase medullary blood flow and reduce medullary tonicity, including the use of distilled water, sodium bicarbonate, and diuretics such as mannitol or loop diuretics, may alleviate the hematuria. Rarely, small doses of ϵ-aminocaproic acid may be necessary for life-threatening hematuria but can result in thrombosis or ureteral obstruction.

RENAL VEINS

Renal Vein Thrombosis

ETIOLOGY. Unilateral or bilateral thrombosis of the major renal veins or their segments is a common but often subtle disorder that may develop in a variety of conditions. The serious risk for thromboembolic complications and vascular occlusion underscores the need for accurate and timely diagnosis and therapy. The disparate causes of renal vein thrombosis are outlined in Table 112–2. The reported incidence of renal vein thrombosis in patients with nephrotic syndrome is striking, ranging from 5 to 62%. Although some series emphasize a stronger association with membranous nephropathy, a prospective study of 26 patients with nephrotic syndrome demonstrated an association of renal vein thrombosis with a variety of glomerulopathies, including membranoproliferative, membranous, and proliferative glomerulonephritis and focal glomerular sclerosis. Renal vein thrombosis has also been reported in patients with sickle cell nephropathy, amyloidosis, diabetic nephropathy, renal vasculitis, and lupus nephritis, as well as allograft rejection. Predisposing factors include abnormalities in coagulation

Table 112–2 ■ CAUSES OF RENAL VEIN THROMBOSIS

Nephrotic syndrome
Renal cell carcinoma with renal vein invasion
Pregnancy or estrogen therapy
Volume depletion (especially in infants)
Extrinsic compression (lymph nodes, tumor, retroperitoneal fibrosis, aortic aneurysm)

or fibrinolysis, and attention has focused on components of clotting parameters in the blood or urine of patients with nephrotic syndrome. Antithrombin III levels are depressed as a result of loss of antithrombin III in the urine of nephrotic patients, and the association between low antithrombin III levels and renal vein thrombosis has been reported in some but not all studies. Circulating levels of proteins S and C may also be altered in nephrotic syndrome and contribute to the tendency toward thromboembolic complications. Renal vein thrombosis in infancy usually occurs in the setting of severe volume depletion and impaired renal blood flow. Extrinsic compression from retroperitoneal sources such as lymph nodes, retroperitoneal fibrosis, abscess, aortic aneurysm, or tumor may lead to renal vein thrombosis as a result of sluggish renal venous flow. Acute pancreatitis, trauma, and retroperitoneal surgery may also predispose to renal vein thrombosis. Renal cell carcinoma characteristically invades the renal vein and compromises venous flow, thereby resulting in renal vein thrombosis.

CLINICAL MANIFESTATIONS. The manifestations of renal vein thrombosis depend on the extent and rapidity of the development of renal venous occlusion. Patients with acute renal vein thrombosis may have nausea, vomiting, flank pain, leukocytosis, hematuria, renal function compromise, and an increase in renal size. Adult nephrotic patients with chronic renal vein thrombosis may have more subtle findings such as a dramatic increase in proteinuria or evidence of tubule dysfunction such as glycosuria, aminoaciduria, phosphaturia, and impaired urinary acidification.

DIAGNOSIS. Supportive data may be provided by non-invasive studies such as MR angiography. Doppler ultrasonography is not adequately sensitive for segmental thrombosis. The diagnosis is established by selective renal venography. Evidence of parenchymal edema, stretching of calyces, and notching of the ureters on intravenous pyelography is much less reliable.

MANAGEMENT. The most widely accepted form of therapy for both acute and chronic renal vein thrombosis is anticoagulation with heparin, which can be converted to oral warfarin (Coumadin) after 7 to 10 days and maintained long term. Therapy is usually continued for at least 1 year. In patients with recurrence or continued risk factors, anticoagulation might be continued indefinitely. In a pediatric patient with volume depletion and acute renal vein thrombosis, attention to restoration of fluid and electrolyte balance is essential. Fibrinolytic therapy might be considered in patients with acute renal vein thrombosis associated with acute renal failure.

Breyer JA, Jacobson HR: Ischemic nephropathy. Curr Opin Nephrol Hypertens 2:216, 1993. *Emphasizes "ischemic nephropathy" as an important cause of progressive renal failure, particularly in elderly patients with atherosclerotic peripheral vascular disease.*

Missouris CG, Buckenham T, Cappuccio FP, et al: Renal artery stenosis: A common and important problem in patients with peripheral vascular disease. Am J Med 96: 10, 1994. *Demonstrates the strong association between peripheral vascular disease and renal artery stenosis.*

Novick AC, Scoble J, Hamilton G: In Novick AC, et al (eds): Renal Vascular Disease. Philadelphia, WB Saunders, 1996, pp 1–529. *This text represents the most complete, albeit narrowly focused, compendium available on this topic. Recommended for the reader who wishes to evaluate, in depth, the most recent diagnostic and therapeutic measures in renal artery diseases.*

Pickering TG, Blumenfeld JD, Laragh JH: Renovascular hypertension and ischemic nephropathy. *In* Brenner BM (ed): Brenner and Rector's The Kidney, 5th ed. Philadelphia, WB Saunders, 1996, p 2106. *An authoritative and practical review of the causes of renovascular disease and management.*

113 HEREDITARY CHRONIC NEPHROPATHIES: GLOMERULAR BASEMENT MEMBRANE DISEASES

Manuel Martinez-Maldonado

This chapter will discuss three disorders: Alport's syndrome, the nail-patella syndrome (NPS), and benign familial hematuria, or thin-basement-membrane nephropathy, all of which are or may be caused by defects in type IV collagen. Some hereditary disorders of renal tubular function are described in Chapter 109. Other genetic

Table 113–1 ■ MOLECULAR GENETICS OF ALPORT'S SYNDROME

INHERITANCE	LOCUS	AFFECTED GENE PRODUCT
X-linked dominant	COL4A5	α5(IV)
X-linked dominant + leiomyomatosis	COL4A5 + COL4A6	α5(IV) + α6(IV)
Autosomal recessive	COL4A3	α3(IV)
	COL4A4	α4(IV
Autosomal dominant*	COL4A3†	α3(IV)†
	COL4A4†	α4(IV)†

*Small number of patients.
†Not fully worked out.

disorders that may be associated with renal disease are listed in Table 113–1 and discussed in the section on Metabolic Diseases (Part XV).

ALPORT'S SYNDROME

DEFINITION. Alport's syndrome, or "chronic hereditary nephritis," is characterized by the familial occurrence in successive generations of a progressive nephritis that is more severe in males, manifested invariably by hematuria, and frequently associated with a sensorineural hearing deficit.

GENETICS. The mode of *transmission* in most kindreds is consistent with X-linked dominant inheritance; mutations in COL4A5, a gene located in Xq22 that codes for the α5 chain of type IV collagen, are responsible (see Table 113–1 for further details). Deletions also occur and tend to result in more severe renal disease and more severe hearing loss. Alport's disease is termed "juvenile" when early onset occurs in males and termed "adult" when renal failure occurs in middle age. Juvenile kindreds tend to be small and frequently arise from new mutations; adult kindreds are large and exhibit few new mutations.

INCIDENCE AND PREVALENCE. Several hundred kindreds of all races and geographic origins exist. With an incidence of approximately 1 in 5000 people, Alport's syndrome accounts for nearly 5% of patients with end-stage renal disease.

PATHOLOGY AND PATHOGENESIS. Normal or large kidneys may exist at the onset, but they shrink with progression of the disease. Although glomeruli may be normal (light microscopy), hypertrophy of epithelial cells and an increase in mesangial matrix may be seen (Table 113–2).

The etiology of Alport's syndrome appears to be the absence of a 28-kd peptide component of the non-collagenous (NC1) domain of the α3 chain of type IV collagen in the glomerular basement membrane. This peptide is also known as the Goodpasture antigen (see below).

CLINICAL MANIFESTATIONS. The disease is discovered in 70% of patients by the age of 6 years, the rest of the cases being discovered at any age thereafter up to and well into adulthood. Persistent or intermittent microscopic hematuria, sensorineural hearing loss, and ocular disorders are typical of the syndrome (see Table 113–2).

DIAGNOSIS. Progressive renal disease in a patient with hematuria, proteinuria (may be absent), azotemia, or hypertension and the presence of sensorineural hearing loss form the basis for the diagnosis of Alport's syndrome. If all of the above occur in a family member—other than the proband—or in a relative younger than 50 years, the diagnosis is probable. The differential diagnosis is shown in Table 113–3.

TREATMENT. No specific treatment is available for Alport's syndrome, nor will any therapy alter its course. Control of hypertension is necessary. Conventional management of progressive renal disease (peritoneal dialysis or hemodialysis) and related or cadaveric donor kidney transplantation have been used with degrees of success that match the results obtained in other renal disorders. Improvement of the hearing deficit and no recurrence of the renal lesion have been observed following transplantation. In several patients, Goodpasture's syndrome has developed in the renal graft from an antibody directed against the basement membrane antigen that is absent in Alport's syndrome (see above). Genetic counseling may be useful but is complicated in view of the genetic heterogeneity of Alport's syndrome.

NAIL-PATELLA SYNDROME

Also known as osteo-onychodysplasia, NPS is characterized by atrophic or absent fingernails, hypoplasia or aplasia of the patella,

Table 113–2 ■ CLINICAL AND GENETIC CHARACTERISTICS OF THE INHERITED GLOMERULAR BASEMENT MEMBRANE DISEASES

CHARACTERISTIC	AS	NPS	TBMN
Inheritance	85% X-linked; ~15% autosomal dominant; autosomal recessive (rare)	Autosomal dominant	Autosomal dominant
Clinical findings	Hematuria (100%)*—dysmorphic RBCs are common, especially after exercise or respiratory infection; proteinuria (70%), nephrotic range, 30–40%; sensorineural hearing loss,† anterior lenticonus, perimacular flecks (15–40%); thrombocytopathia (rare): thrombocytopenia with giant platelets, bruising, epistaxis, GI bleeding, prolonged bleeding time; leiomyomatosis (rare)	Hematuria (33%)* proteinuria (42%), nail hypoplasia (98%); patellar aplasia/hypoplasia (90%); "iliac horns" (80%); elbow deformities (90%); Lester's sign (50%)‡	Hematuria (100%), proteinuria (60% to 71%); hypertension (not documented)
Histology	Thickened GBM with splitting of the lamina densa ("basket weave" appearance) by electron microscopy. Glomerular crescents may be found in the juvenile form	Light microscopy shows glomerular, cellular proliferation, mesangial sclerosis, and basement membrane thickening. Electron microscopy reveals areas of rarefaction in the lamina densa of the GBM filled with bundles of curvilinear fibrils having the typical periodicity of collagen (moth-eaten appearance)	Thin GBM with attenuation of the lamina densa
Clinical course	Males: all progress to ESRD, hypertension, azotemia; predilection for those with massive proteinuria Females: usually do not progress to ESRD, some may exhibit decline in renal function during pregnancy	28% reach ESRD by age 33 yr	Rarely progresses to ESRD

*Prevalence of clinical finding.
†May require audiometric testing and may progress to clinical deafness; high-frequency range, 4000 to 8000 Hz, 40 to 60% of patients, predominantly in males (81% male; 19% female). Tinnitus is present in some cases.
‡Lester's sign: heterochromia of the iris. The pale appearance of the outer zone of the iris in contrast to a darker central portion results in a "cloverleaf" arrangement.
AS = Alport's syndrome; NPS = nail-patella syndrome; TBMN = thin-basement-membrane nephropathy; RBCs = red blood cells; GI = gastrointestinal; GBM = glomerular basement membrane; ESRD = end-stage renal disease.

Table 113–3 ■ DIFFERENTIAL DIAGNOSIS OF ALPORT'S SYNDROME

CONDITION	CHARACTERISTICS
Benign familial hematuria	Non-progressive disorder, uniformly thin glomerular basement membrane
Berger's disease	IgA nephropathy; mesangial proliferative glomerulonephritis with mesangial deposits of IgA and variable amounts of C3, IgM, or IgG; strong IgA immunofluorescence in mesangial regions

and other bone anomalies. Table 113–2 summarizes the mode of inheritance and the clinical findings in NPS. In 40% of patients, kidney involvement is manifested by proteinuria (mild to nephrotic range) and, rarely, hematuria. Progression to renal failure may be observed. The *COL5A1* gene, which encodes the pro $\alpha 1(V)$ chain of fibrillar type V collagen, has been located within the segment 9q34.2 to 9q34.3, which places the gene near the NPS locus, which also maps to 9q34; it is not clear whether the *COL5A1* gene is aberrant in NPS. No specific therapy exists for this disorder. Renal transplantation has been carried out without evidence of recurrence of the disease in the transplanted organ. Reports suggest that an enzyme deficient in NPS (e.g., adenylate kinase) may be replenished by transplantation inasmuch as dystrophic nails have completely grown back post-transplant.

BENIGN FAMILIAL HEMATURIA

Also known as thin-basement-membrane nephropathy, benign familial hematuria is characterized by thinning of the basement membrane and normal renal function. Genetic and clinical characteristics are listed in Table 113–2. A glycine–to–glutamic acid substitution has been identified in the collagenous region of the *COL4A4* gene. Moreover, patients with benign familial hematuria can be carriers of autosomal recessive Alport's syndrome.

Bodziak KA, Hammond WS, Molitoris BA: Inherited diseases of the glomerular basement membrane. Am J Kidney Dis 23:605, 1994. *A good review of the inherited diseases of the glomerular basement membrane, including the nail-patella syndrome.*

Kashtan CE, Michael AF: Alport syndrome. Kidney Int 50:1445, 1996. *An excellent review of the biochemical defect and genetic transmission of Alport's syndrome.*

Lemmink HH, Nillesen WN, Mochizuki T, et al: Benign familial hematuria due to mutation of the type IV collagen α4 gene. J Clin Invest 98:1114, 1996. *First demonstration of a genetic defect of type IV collagen in thin-basement-membrane disease.*

114 RENAL CALCULI (NEPHROLITHIASIS)

Keith Hruska

EPIDEMIOLOGY. Nephrolithiasis is a common disorder defined as the development of stones within the urinary tract. It is a major cause of morbidity in the United States, and it is becoming an increasingly greater problem in Western Europe and Japan. Approximately 12% of the population of the United States will have a kidney stone at some time. The economic impact of the morbidity associated with kidney stones is more than $2 billion per year; most of the costs relate to surgical extraction or fragmentation and loss of productivity. Kidney stones are two to three times more common in men than women and are distinctly uncommon in African Americans and Asians. There is also a geographic distribution of nephrolithiasis, with the highest incidence in the southeastern United States.

GENERAL CLINICAL CONSIDERATIONS. The pain associated with passing a kidney stone is referred to as *renal colic*. It begins suddenly and quickly becomes an unbearable pain that may cause

nausea and vomiting. The distribution of the pain resembles that of the path of the stone to the bladder, beginning in the flank and curving anteriorly toward the groin. Urinary frequency and dysuria occur as the stone reaches the ureterovesical junction. When the stone passes into the bladder or moves in the ureter to decompress the urinary system, the pain vanishes. Unique symptoms develop when the stone passes into the urethra.

Hematuria from nephrolithiasis is common and disturbing to patients. Occasionally, the hematuria is associated with flank pain without detectable obstruction. Nephrolithiasis may be associated with obstructive uropathy (see Chapter 108), especially if the stone is not painful and remains undetected for long periods. Obstruction predisposes to infection, especially in women.

Radiologic techniques are used to diagnose stone disease. The radiographic appearance of stones may help identify stone type and guide further evaluation. Calcium phosphate and calcium oxalate stones are radiodense, and struvite (magnesium ammonium phosphate), when it complexes with calcium carbonate or phosphate, is also visible. Cystine stones are usually poorly visualized, and uric acid stones are radiolucent, requiring computed tomography (CT), ultrasonography, or intravenous urography for detection.

Intravenous urography is usually the first step in evaluating patients with renal colic, although there is concern regarding use of this test in patients with renal insufficiency. It is the most useful test to define the degree and extent of urinary tract obstruction. Renal ultrasonography, which is the safest approach, is useful to rule out significant hydronephrosis or hydroureter; however, it may not detect stones unless they are relatively large. Ultrasonography does not delineate the site of obstruction. Retrograde pyelography allows visualization of the urinary tract without intravenously administering contrast dye. This test requires cystoscopy and is usually performed during endourologic procedures or when intravenous pyelography is contraindicated (i.e., in patients with renal insufficiency or contrast dye allergy).

CT is the modality most useful for defining radiolucent stones not detectable by other means. Pure uric acid stones and, in some cases, cystine stones can be identified by CT with or without contrast material.

TREATING RENAL COLIC. Treatment should focus on relieving pain and urinary tract obstruction. A stepwise scheme for management of patients with renal colic is presented in Figure 114–1. Careful analgesic therapy, hydration, and radiologic assessment are the cornerstones. If significant obstruction is detected, the patient is observed during hydration for movement of the stone. If evidence does not suggest that the stone will pass within 2 to 3 days, urologic intervention is indicated. Stones lodged in the ureteropelvic junction or in the proximal ureter are best pushed into the renal pelvis and disrupted by extracorporeal shock wave lithotripsy (ESWL). Moving the stone backward requires cystoscopy and passing a catheter up the ureter. If the stone cannot be pushed back, it can be bypassed with a stent to provide drainage and disrupted in situ with ESWL. Percutaneous nephrolithotomy is required if lithotripsy fails. Surgical ureterolithotomy is largely an operative procedure of the past.

Stones that are smaller than 2 cm but larger than 5 mm in diameter are best treated with ESWL alone. Stones larger than 2 cm, or those larger than 1 cm and in the lower poles, may be best treated with percutaneous nephrostolithotomy, because with lithotripsy alone residual stones are left in 35 to 50% of cases. Percutaneous nephrostolithotomy succeeds in most cases. Asymptomatic kidney stones smaller than 5 mm in diameter should be left untreated. The guidelines for ESWL and percutaneous nephrostolithotomy hold for struvite and uric acid stones. Because lithotripsy disrupts cystine stones poorly, percutaneous nephrostolithotomy is often required.

PREVENTING RECURRENT NEPHROLITHIASIS. Careful correlation of stone counts with the clinical history and information from hospital emergency department and past office records determines whether a stone is a new episode or the passage of an existing stone. Nephrolithiasis prevention is a multistep process beginning with accurate diagnosis of the cause of nephrolithiasis (Table 114–1). Diagnosis requires crystallographic analysis of the stones and a battery of urine and blood tests that are begun after the patient has fully recovered from an episode of renal colic and has resumed normal activity and diet for approximately 2 weeks. Because of inherent day-to-day variation, repeated sampling of 24-hour urine specimens from patients on their normal diets and after

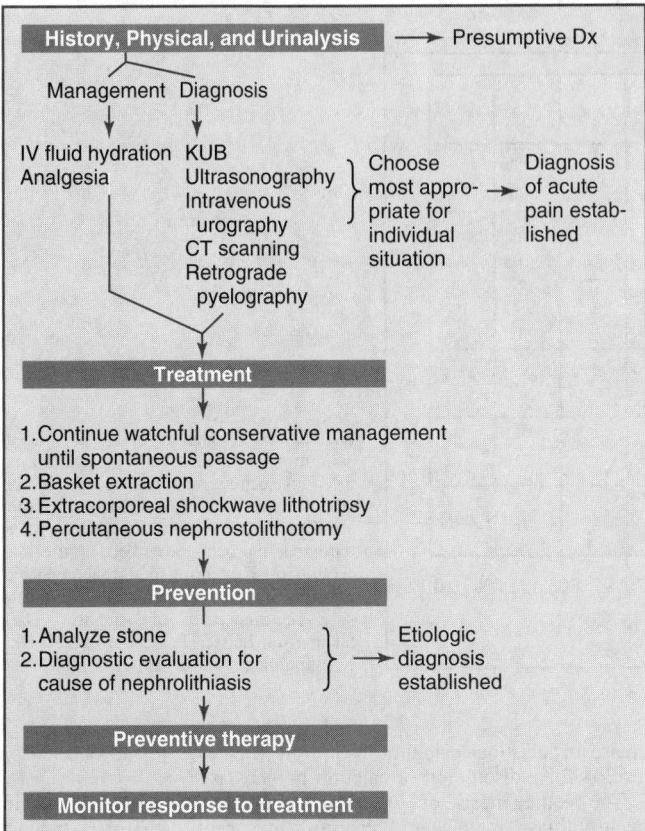

FIGURE 114–1 ■ Flow diagram for management of renal colic. See text for the description of the approach to patients with acute stone episodes.

test diets is required. The most useful test diet is a 400-mg calcium diet used for 1 week before a calcium challenge test to carefully define hypercalciuria. The analyses performed on urine specimens include determining volume, pH, calcium, magnesium, potassium, sodium, ammonia, phosphorus, citrate, oxalate, chloride, sulfate, uric acid, urinary urea nitrogen, and creatinine. Measuring the full panel allows calculation of relative supersaturation for calcium oxalate, apatite, brushite, urate, and struvite. The addition of exogenous calcium oxalate or phosphate helps determine formation products for various crystal nucleation events. Cystine screening should be performed on all patients. Blood samples should be assayed for electrolytes (sodium, potassium, chloride, and bicarbonate), calcium, phosphorus, parathyroid hormone, and calcitriol.

The analyses performed on blood specimens should include electrolytes, calcium, phosphorus, parathyroid hormone, and calcitriol levels. The stone, urine, and blood analyses are pooled to make a diagnosis of stone pathogenesis, and treatment recommendations are based on the diagnoses. Follow-up includes repeat urianalyses and assessment of compliance. Compliance parameters in the 24-hour urine specimen include the volume, creatinine, sodium, urea nitrogen, sulfate, and potassium that can be used to monitor adherence to therapy. The assumption of therapy is that normalization of the metabolic abnormalities detected in reaching the diagnosis will result in prevention of stone recurrence. This assumption has been shown to be true in the vast majority of cases.

The report of a 1989 National Institutes of Health consensus conference recommends limited evaluation after the first stone episode. However, more recent studies indicate that recurrence of nephrolithiasis is common in patients with a first stone and detectable metabolic abnormalities. Because repeated stone episodes cause pain, morbidity, and time loss from work, prevention is clearly the recommended approach (see later), and it should be applied to all stone formers.

PATHOGENESIS. STONE COMPOSITION. Stone composition should be analyzed in every patient, because it is the cornerstone of the diagnostic approach to preventive therapy. About three fourths of all kidney stones are composed of calcium oxalate: 35% of stones are pure calcium oxalate (calcium oxalate monohydrate or calcium oxalate dihydrate or both); 40% are calcium oxalate with hydroxyapatite or carbonate apatite; and 1% are calcium oxalate with uric acid. Four per cent of all stones are apatite or hydroxyapatite $[Ca_{10}(PO_4)_6(OH)_2]$, and 1% are brushite ($CaHPO_4\ 2H_2O$). The non–calcium-containing crystal types are struvite and comprise 8% of all stones, although carbonate apatite is always intermixed in the struvite stone. Eight per cent of all stones are composed of uric acid and 2% are composed of cystine. Rarely, stones composed of acid ammonium urate or xanthine or proteinaceous matrix of potentially insoluble drugs are observed. Determining the composition of stones requires polarization microscopy, radiologic diffraction, or infrared spectrometry. The latter two procedures surpass microscopy in precision and sensitivity but are more costly.

PHYSICAL AND CHEMICAL FACTORS IN RENAL STONE FORMATION. Formation of kidney stones results from (1) initial formation of crystals (nucleation), (2) reduced effects of normal urinary constituents that inhibit crystal growth and aggregation, (3) the presence of substances promoting crystal growth and aggregation, and (4) the processes that determine crystal attachment to the surface of renal papillary epithelial cells. Attachment allows time for crystal growth and/or aggregation to the size of a clinically symptomatic stone in high urinary solute concentrations. Much of the current approach to evaluating, treating, and preventing nephrolithiasis is centered on identifying excessive urinary excretion of salts that precipitate (nucleate) when units of metastable supersaturation are exceeded (Table 114–2). Supersaturation can result from (1) too little urine output; (2) an absolute increase in the amount of stone constituent excreted over a period of time, such as calcium, oxalate, or uric acid; or (3) altered urine pH. Low urinary pH (<5.5) decreases solubility of uric acid, whereas high urinary pH decreases that of calcium phosphate and magnesium ammonium phosphate.

DEFICIENT URINARY INHIBITORS. Although most recurrent stone formers tend to have an increased risk of nucleation, 1% or more of stone formers exhibit no detectable abnormality. Many healthy subjects, patients with cancer, and normal pregnant women exhibit hypercalciuria but do not form kidney stones. Thus, factors beside supersaturation are crucial in the pathogenesis of kidney stones. Macromolecular inhibitors of crystal growth and aggregation, particularly the growth and aggregation of calcium oxalate, have been identified (see Table 114–2). Nephrocalcin is a powerful inhibitor of calcium oxalate crystal growth and appears to act by binding to crystal surfaces. This substance is apparently defective when isolated from the urine of calcium stone formers. Urinary osteopontin (uropontin) is perhaps the most potent calcium oxalate crystal growth inhibitor, and its post-translational modifications may be affected in nephrolithiasis because its rate of excretion appears normal. Tamm-Horsfall mucoprotein may inhibit crystal growth but at times promotes calcium oxalate crystal aggregation. Some patients with recurrent nephrolithiasis produce Tamm-Horsfall mucoprotein that self-aggregates and loses its ability to inhibit aggregation of calcium oxalate crystals.

CRYSTAL ATTACHMENT. Crystal attachment to epithelial surfaces is also crucial for forming at least some stones. Normal subjects often have crystalluria without forming stones. Crystal binding appears to depend on the physicochemical structure of urothelial cell surfaces because the chemically injured urinary bladder binds more

Table 114–1 ■ OUTLINE OF STONE PREVENTION PRACTICE

- Stone analysis
- Urinalysis
- Blood analysis
- Diagnoses
- Treatments
- Follow up/compliance assessment
- Outcomes/continuous quality control

Table 114–2 ■ ETIOLOGY OF CALCIUM STONES

High urinary solute concentration	↑ Ca, ↑ Ox, ↓ UV
Deficient inhibitor	Citrate, uropontin, nephrocalcin
Excess promoter	Uric acid
Crystal attachment	Epithelial crystal receptors

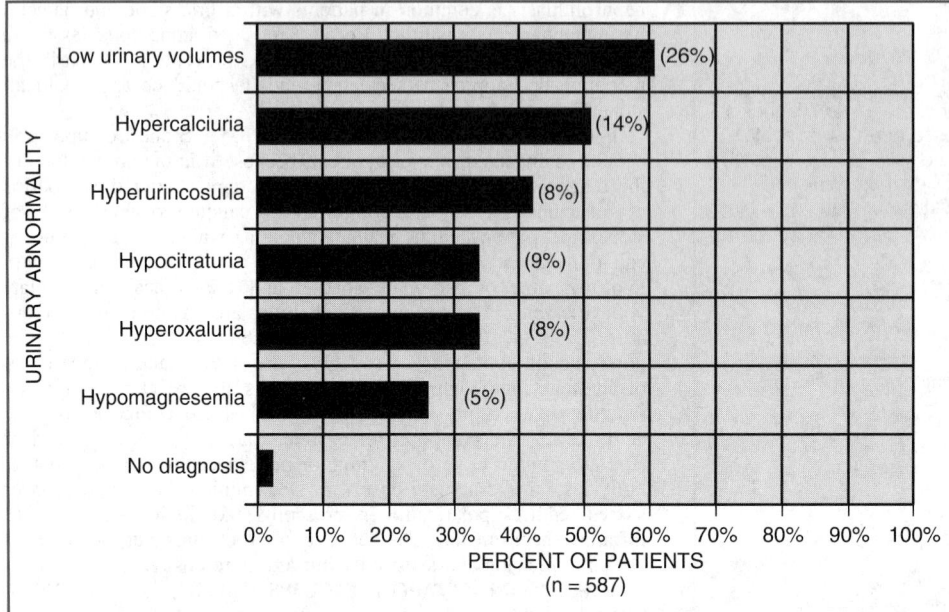

FIGURE 114-2 ■ Causes of urinary supersaturation in patients with nephrolithiasis: 587 consecutive patients seen in the stone center of St. Louis, Missouri, from 1987 to 1992 were evaluated with a standardized approach described in the text section on preventing recurrent nephrolithiasis. Numbers in parentheses indicate sole occurrence of abnormality. (Data taken from Seltzer J, Winborn K, Hruska K [unpublished observation].)

calcium oxalate than the uninjured bladder. In addition, there exist specific calcium oxalate crystal receptors on renal tubular epithelial cells.

PATHOGENESIS OF CALCIUM OXALATE AND APATITE STONES. HYPERCALCIURIA. After low urinary volumes, hypercalciuria is the most frequently observed abnormality of the urine from stone formers (Fig. 114-2). The definition of hypercalciuria varies with body size and diet. In general, the normal upper limit for urinary calcium is 4 mg of calcium per kilogram of body weight per day (280 mg/day, males; 240 mg/day, females) on a diet containing 1000 mg of calcium per day. Total excretion may drop to 200 mg/day on a diet of 400 mg of calcium and 100 mEq or less of sodium. Dietary sodium is important because calcium reabsorption parallels that of sodium in the proximal nephron, such that high rates of sodium excretion are calciuric. Hypercalciuria can result from (1) enhanced absorption from dietary intake; (2) primary renal transport defects leading to excess calcium excretion and secondary enhanced calcium absorption; (3) excessive resorption from storage in bone; or (4) a combination of the above (Table 114-3).

Since the late 1980s, a consensus has emerged that the hypercalciuria of nephrolithiasis is a more uniform defect than was previously thought. The basis for this change is the fact that hypercalciuria is the most frequent abnormality found in patients with a family history of nephrolithiasis, suggesting a genetic basis for hypercalciuria. In addition, it has been found that fasting hypercalciuria, observed in 20 to 30% of patients who have nephrolithiasis and hypercalciuria, is not due to a renal transport defect (renal leak) as previously thought. True renal hypercalciuria is uncommon (Table 114-4). The source of fasting hypercalciuria has been shown to be bone and in many patients is associated with a decrease in bone mineral density. This presumed increase in skeletal remodeling is a transient defect associated with, and in addition to, absorptive hypercalciuria. Increased skeletal remodeling does not persist throughout the clinical course of nephrolithiasis. Patients with nephrolithiasis and hypercalciuria uniformly exhibit an increase in intestinal calcium absorption. (See Fig. 114-3 and Chapter 264 for a discussion of calcium homeostasis.)

The pathogenesis of intestinal hyperabsorption of calcium in nephrolithiasis is unclear. Thirty to 40 per cent of the patients have abnormally high 1,25(OH)$_2$ vitamin D$_3$ levels compared with a population of non-stoneformers. In the other patients, data suggest that abnormalities in the vitamin D receptor do not play a role in intestinal calcium hyperabsorption and that the intestinal calcium hyperabsorption is independent of vitamin D action.

The finding of hypercalciuria that persists on a low-calcium diet or the presence of fasting hypercalciuria increases the likelihood of associated reductions in bone mineral density with nephrolithiasis. Hence, the wisdom of low-calcium diets in nephrolithiasis is most certainly questioned by the observed reductions in bone mineral density associated with the disease.

The discovery that X-linked nephrolithiasis, which is characterized by absorptive hypercalciuria, is caused by a mutation in a chloride channel of the proximal tubule. Furthermore, recent studies have reported the discovery that some patients have multiple defects in proximal tubular ion transport, including tubular proteinuria, which has returned the focus of calcium neprolithiasis back to the nephron. In this paradigm, absorptive hypercalciuria is produced by abnormal regulation of calcitriol production by the kidney.

HYPOCITRATURIA. Reductions in urinary citrate excretion are a common trait among patients who form stones. This hypocitraturia may be (1) idiopathic; (2) due to defective urinary acidification; (3) due to small bowel malabsorption; (4) due to hypokalemia, especially iatrogenic; or (5) due to metabolic acidosis. Hypocitraturia, defined as less than 300 mg/day in women and less than 250 mg/day in men, was observed in 30 to 40% of patients with nephrolithiasis (see Fig. 114-2). More women than men exhibited hypocitraturia. Hypocitraturia often overlaps with hypercalciuria, owing to the high prevalence of idiopathic hypercalciuria in nephrolithiasis. In patients who do not spontaneously acidify urine (es-

Table 114-3 ■ POTENTIAL MECHANISMS OF HYPERCALCIURIA

Increased intestinal calcium absorption
   Direct
   Excess 1,25(OH)$_2$ vitamin D$_3$
Decreased renal mineral reabsorption
   Calcium
   Phosphorus
Enhanced bone demineralization

Table 114-4 ■ PATHOGENESIS OF HYPERCALCIURIA IN NEPHROLITHIASIS

	FREQUENCY (%)
Idiopathic absorptive ± skeletal remodeling defect	95
Primary hyperparathyroidism	3
Sarcoidosis	<1
Renal tubular transport defects	
Calcium	1–2
Phosphorus	<1

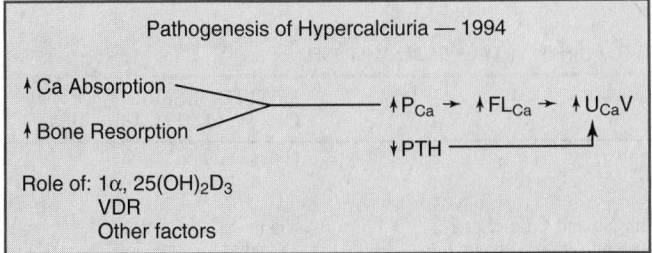

FIGURE 114–3 ▪ Current concepts of the pathogenesis of idiopathic hypercalciuria link intestinal hyperabsorption and transient elevations of skeletal remodeling as the basis of hypercalciuria, accounting for the approximately 20% of patients who exhibit fasting hypercalciuria during evaluation.

pecially in the early morning) to pH 5.5 or less, an ammonium chloride load test should rule out an acidification defect as the cause of hypocitraturia. The hypocitraturia associated with small bowel malabsorption is due to a metabolic acidosis and stimulation of citrate transport in the proximal nephron. The metabolic acidosis stems from bicarbonate lost in the stool. Treating nephrolithiasis with thiazides may induce hypokalemia and a secondary hypocitraturia. The metabolic acidosis associated with excess consumption of sulfur and phosphorus-containing protein may also cause hypocitraturia by stimulating citrate transport in the proximal tubule.

HYPEROXALURIA. Dietary Hyperoxaluria. Oxalate is the anion most frequently associated with calcium in the precipitation of salts leading to crystal formation, growth, and retention and stone formation. Normal people excrete 20 to 40 mg (222 to 444 μm) of oxalate daily. A reasonable upper limit of excretion is 45 mg (500 μm) daily for men and 40 mg for women. A simple dietary excess of oxalate from foods such as spinach, rhubarb, Swiss chard, cocoa, beets, peppers, wheat germ, pecans, peanuts, okra, chocolate, and lime peel commonly increases urinary oxalate to 50 to 60 mg (556 to 667 μm) daily. This form of hyperoxaluria is frequently observed in nephrolithiasis (see Fig. 114–2), and treatment consists of altering the diet to avoid an excess of oxalate. However, no clinical trials have proven the efficacy of avoiding oxalate for treating nephrolithiasis.

Enteric Hyperoxaluria. Malabsorption by the small bowel from any cause, including resection, intrinsic disease, and jejunal ileal bypass, often leads to hyperoxaluria. The pathogenesis is exposure of the colonic mucosa to detergents—in the form of bile salts—and fatty acids, which non-selectively increase the permeability to numerous molecules, including oxalate. These detergents also bind calcium and magnesium, making oxalate more available for transport. The hyperoxaluria from small bowel malabsorption often exceeds 100 mg (1111 μm) daily, provoking frequent stone formation and even tubulointerstitial renal disease from intrarenal calcifications. A consistent metabolic pattern is observed in the urine of patients with enteric hyperoxaluria, consisting of low urinary volumes, a tendency toward hypocalciuria, hypocitraturia, and hyperoxaluria. Treatment includes reducing dietary oxalate and fat; taking oral calcium supplements, cholestyramine, and oral citrate supplements; and high fluid intake (see later).

Primary Hyperoxaluria. Two genetic disorders lead to hyperoxaluria (see Chapter 205). Type I primary hyperoxaluria, an autosomal recessive trait, results from molecular abnormalities that reduce the activity of hepatic peroxisomal alanine glyoxylate aminotransferase, thereby increasing the availability of glyoxylate, which is irreversibly converted to oxalic acid. The second form (type II), resulting from a deficiency of D-glycerate dehydrogenase or glyoxylate reductase, is much rarer than type I. Both forms cause a high level of oxalate production and corresponding urinary oxalate excretion above 135 to 270 mg (1523 μmol) daily. Stone formation often begins in childhood, but tubulointerstitial nephritis progressing to renal failure is the more important and dominant expression of the disease.

HYPERURICOSURIA. Hyperuricosuria (see Chapter 299) is a common finding associated with hypercalciuria in patients with calcium oxalate nephrolithiasis. The relationship between hyperuricosuria and calcium oxalate precipitation remains controversial. Some evidence suggests that urate crystals increase the nucleation of calcium oxalate by the process of heterogeneous nucleation and epitaxial

growth. However, urate crystals are uncommon in urine compared with the frequency of calcium oxalate crystallization, and the epitaxial theory remains to be proven. However, well-controlled studies demonstrate that allopurinol, a drug that decreases urate synthesis, significantly reduces the rate of recurring calcium oxalate stones. Because allopurinol has no direct effect on calcium oxalate crystallization, it is likely that this effect was produced by reduced urinary uric acid excretion. Because an excess of purine in the diet causes hyperuricosuria, normal levels of dietary purine should also be protective.

NEW PROTEIN INHIBITORS OF CALCIUM OXALATE STONE FORMATION. See the discussion of various inhibitors of calcium oxalate stone formation in the section on the physical chemistry of nephrolithiasis.

RENAL STRUCTURAL ABNORMALITIES. Were they not retained within the kidney, the forming and passing of crystalline particles would be no more than a common urologic curiosity. Crystal adherence promoting crystal growth and aggregation, especially in areas of relatively diminished urinary flow, is crucial in the development of urinary stones. Little is known regarding the process of crystal growth attachment. The role of urinary stasis has not been quantified. Other structural abnormalities, such as medullary sponge kidney, ectopic kidney, polycystic kidney, and horseshoe kidneys, may be associated with nephrolithiasis. Medullary sponge kidney probably is a process that occurs or develops as a result of nephrocalcinosis. It is probably not a specific disease in itself but a process associated with acidification defects and other causes of calcium oxalate nephrolithiasis, especially hypercalciuria. The other structural abnormalities pose a major risk for stones due to urinary stasis and infection.

TREATMENT OF CALCIUM OXALATE OR APATITE STONES. The first tenet of therapy for preventing nephrolithiasis is an increase in the urinary volume (Table 114–5). Urinary volumes between 2 and 3 L must be maintained. Helpful clues to assist the patient with increasing urinary volume include avoiding urinary concentration at night and taking a metered amount of water to the workplace.

DIET. With careful attention to diet, most calcium oxalate stones could be prevented, but long-term dietary compliance is essential (see Table 114–5). Recurrent calcium nephrolithiasis should be considered a disease of dietary excess superimposed on the genetic predispositions produced by hypercalciuria, renal tubular acidosis, gout, and cystinuria. In patients with calcium oxalate stones, reduced sodium and calcium diets may be effective. In patients with idiopathic hypercalciuria, diets containing 700 to 800 mg of calcium contain sufficient calcium to prevent further bone loss during therapy.

THIAZIDE DIURETICS. Thiazide diuretics are the mainstay of the pharmacologic approach to preventing nephrolithiasis. They lower urinary calcium excretion by increasing calcium reabsorption in the proximal nephron due to volume contraction. They also directly stimulate calcium reabsorption through their actions on the luminal Na^+/Cl^- transporter of the diluting segment of the nephron. The relative importance of the two actions is heavily weighted toward the proximal nephron/volume contraction effects. Thus, an adequate response to thiazide diuretics requires controlling sodium intake. Retention of calcium by the kidney results in a secondary suppression of intestinal calcium hyperabsorption. Some reports suggest that this secondary action on the intestine is lost after a period of 2 to 3 years on therapy. This may result in thiazide resistance during long-term treatment of absorptive hypercalciuria. Thiazide diuretics tend to improve calcium balance, and the result is observed as an increase in bone mineral density due to increased bone formation (see Table 114–5).

ORAL PHOSPHATE. In patients with absorptive hypercalciuria, 1500 mg of neutral potassium phosphate per day in three to four divided doses lowered urinary calcium excretion in some trials as effectively as thiazide diuretics. However, compliance is more difficult to achieve related to frequency of dosing and intestinal side effects such as diarrhea and bloating. Studies estimating efficacy of oral phosphate therapy (see Table 114–5) reported relapses of 9% and 25%. A new slow-release formulation has been developed, avoiding many of the side effects and dosing frequency required of earlier preparations. This new agent is in clinical trials.

Table 114–5 ■ SUMMARY OF TREATMENT OPTIONS FOR DIFFERENT TYPES OF RENAL STONES*

INDICATION	TREATMENT	EXPECTED RESULTS (90% SUCCESSFUL TREATMENT)
All stones	High fluid intake	Unknown
Calcium oxalate and brushite (CaOx/CaHPO$_4$) stones		
Idiopathic hypercalciuria	1) Controlled protein Na and Ca diets	Unknown
	2) Thiazide diuretics and related drugs	85–90%
	3) Oral phosphate	Unknown
	4) Na cellulose phosphate	Low
Hypocitraturia	Potassium citrate	88%
Renal tubular acidosis	Potassium citrate	Unknown
Ileostomy or small bowel malabsorption	Potassium citrate	Unknown
Hyperoxaluria		
Dietary	Reduced oxalate diet	Unknown
Enteric	Low fat diet, calcium supplement, cholestyramine	Unknown
Primary	Pyridoxine	Only in a small fraction
Hyperuricosuria	Allopurinol	86%
	Potassium citrate	Unknown
Uric acid stones	Allopurinol	Unknown
	Potassium citrate	88%
Struvite stones	ESWL or percutaneous nephrostolithotomy	30–40% with stones < 2 cm
	Acetohydroxamic acid	Control of stone growth if tolerated
Cystine stones/cystinuria	Tiopronin	Unknown
	Penicillamine	Unknown

*Each type of renal stone is listed under indication and the expected success rate per 100 patients is listed under expected results and described in the text.
ESWL = Extracorporeal shock wave lithotripsy.

SODIUM CELLULOSE PHOSPHATE. A calcium-binding resin, sodium cellulose phosphate, reduces calcium absorption when taken with meals. This approach has not demonstrated a high success rate, possibly due to reflex hyperoxaluria. In addition, a negative calcium balance may lead to additional bone mineral loss.

TREATMENT OF HYPOCITRATURIA. Because citrate lowers calcium oxalate supersaturation by binding calcium and, to some extent, by reducing calcium excretion, correcting hypocitraturia should reduce the recurrence of nephrolithiasis. No carefully controlled trials of citrate therapy have been reported. Uncontrolled studies suggest an efficacy of approximately 88% over a 2-year period (see Table 114–5). Citrate therapy may be very useful for patients who demonstrate hypocitraturia as a result of thiazide diuretic therapy. Furthermore, in patients with inflammatory bowel disease or renal tubular acidosis, citrate therapy seems a very rational replacement for the losses of alkali. Because of the volume expansion effects, sodium bicarbonate or sodium citrate does not have the required actions of potassium citrate to lower urinary calcium and improve calcium balance.

TREATING HYPEROXALURIA. Dietary. Normal people excrete 20 to 40 mg (222 to 444 μm) of oxalate daily. A simple dietary excess of oxalate from foods may increase urinary oxalate, and a low-calcium diet may further increase excretion. Treating this mild form of dietary hyperoxaluria associated with calcium oxalate stones consists of altering the diet to avoid foods that contain high concentrations of oxalate. However, no carefully controlled trials have proven the efficacy of this approach.

Enteric. Hyperoxaluria observed in patients with inflammatory bowel disorders and intestinal bypass is usually associated with hypocitraturia. Patients exhibiting hypocalciuria should be treated with a low-fat diet in addition to calcium supplements. Cholestyramine, a non-resorbable resin that binds fatty acids, bile acids, and oxalate (4 to 16 g/day in four divided doses with meals), oral citrate supplements, and high fluid intake are the mainstays of therapy. These patients may also exhibit magnesium deficiency and hypomagnesuria. Magnesium replacement may be important to increase urinary citrate excretion in response to exogenous potassium alkali.

Primary Hyperoxaluria. Type I primary hyperoxaluria occasionally responds to pyridoxine supplement (2 to 200 mg/day). High urinary volume and supplemental citrate, thiazide diuretics, and possibly oral phosphate supplements can also be used. After renal transplantation, a special protocol is required to avoid accelerated renal oxalosis. Liver transplantation restores the missing enzymes, and many patients with hyperoxaluria have been treated in this manner.

HYPERURICOSURIA. Because an excess of purine in the diet causes hyperuricosuria, normal levels of dietary purine should prevent stones. However, careful studies documenting a response to low purine diets are not available. Compelling evidence that hyperuricosuria contributes to the formation of calcium oxalate stones comes from a prospective double-blind trial that demonstrated a reduction in stone formation with allopurinol compared with placebo (see Table 114–5).

TREATMENT OF URIC ACID STONES. A persistently acid urine decreases the solubility of fully protonated uric acid. Half of the uric acid is fully protonated at pH 5.35, making uric acid supersaturation inevitable at normal excretion rates of 600 to 800 mg (3.6 to 4.8 mM) because the solubility of fully protonated uric acid in urine is 96 mg/L. Acidic urine is a common finding in patients with uric acid stones, and many of these patients also have gout. Attempts to alkalinize the urine by raising urinary pH to 6 to 6.5 with potassium alkali salts may be effective. However, avoidance of temporary periods of acidification sufficient to nucleate uric acid or uric acid and calcium oxalate is difficult. Because of the general tolerance and safety of allopurinol, which is very effective in reducing urinary uric acid excretion rates, it is the mainstay of therapy.

TREATMENT OF STRUVITE STONES. Struvite, or magnesium ammonium phosphate, crystals are produced when the urinary tract is colonized by bacteria, producing high concentrations of ammonia. *Proteus, Pseudomonas,* and enterococci usually cause struvite stones. Patients who produce only struvite stones generally present with large stones that cause bleeding, obstruction, and infection without stone passage. These patients rarely have idiopathic hypercalciuria and often have reduced renal function. Patients who pass struvite stones have a higher frequency of idiopathic hypercalciuria because the stone is usually a calcium stone that became secondarily infected, resulting in the struvite. Contralateral spread of struvite stones due to urinary tract infection is frequent.

Struvite stones must be removed. ESWL and percutaneous nephrostolithotomy are used to reduce the damage incurred by growth and spread of these stones. Prolonged use of antibiotics in patients with struvite stones amounts to treatment of an infected foreign body. Once patients are free of stones, they benefit from antibiotics directed against the predominant urinary organism, although no controlled studies support this reasonable approach. Acetohydroxamic acid has limited use because of patient intolerance of side effects.

CYSTINE STONES. Approximately 2% of patients attending renal stone clinics exhibit a hereditary defect of amino acid transport leading to excessive amounts of cystine in the urine. Cystine is the disulfide of cysteine, which is soluble in the urine to the level of only 20 to 48 mg/dL (1 to 2 mM/L). The rate of cystine excretion in patients with cystinuria ranges from 480 to 3600 mg/day (2 to 15 mM/day) so that high fluid intake can prevent stones in only some patients. Most patients require treatment with penicillamine or tiopronin. Both combine with cysteine to form a soluble salt that reduces, through competition, the formation of cystine. The ability of these treatments to reduce stone frequency is not quantitatively known, although they are effective. However, they exhibit a high rate of intolerance due to severe side effects, which require careful surveillance.

Consensus Conference: Prevention and treatment of kidney stones. JAMA 260:977, 1988. *An NIH conference establishing standards to consider in the approach to nephrolithiasis.*

Fanus MJ, Coe FL: Idiopathic hypercalciuria and nephrolithiasis. In Feldman D, Glorieux FH, Pike JW (eds): Vitamin D. New York, Academic Press, 1997, pp 867–881. *Very good review by an established leader in nephrolithiasis, on the pathogenesis of hypercalciuria, low bone mineral density in nephrolithiasis, and treatment options.*

Hruska KA, Seltzer JR, Grieff M: Nephrolithiasis. In Schrier RW, Gottschalk CW (eds): Diseases of the Kidney, 6th ed. Boston, Little, Brown & Company, 1997, pp 739–765.

115 CYSTIC DISEASES OF THE KIDNEY

Jared J. Grantham

DEFINITIONS. Cystic diseases are among the few disorders that cause the kidneys to enlarge. Individual renal cysts, which derive from segments of the renal tubule and glomerular capsule, are composed of a single layer of tubular epithelium encapsulating a fluid-filled cavity. *Solitary* cysts visible to the naked eye are the most common structural abnormalities observed in the kidneys. Generalized cystic diseases are typified by cysts scattered throughout the cortex and the medulla of one or both kidneys. *Polycystic* is a term reserved for conditions in which innumerable cysts are diffusely scattered throughout the renal cortex and medulla. In *medullary cystic diseases* the lesions occur primarily in the medulla and papilla. The major types of renal cystic disease are listed in Table 115–1.

AUTOSOMAL DOMINANT POLYCYSTIC KIDNEY DISEASE

ETIOLOGY. Autosomal dominant polycystic kidney disease (ADPKD) is caused by mutations in at least three different genes that lead to manifestations of the disease that are clinically indistinguishable given current diagnostic methods. The most common mutation (~85%) leading to *PKD1* is found in a segment of chromosome 16q13.3 that encodes a 4303–amino acid integral membrane glycoprotein, polycystin-1. *PKD2* (~15%) is caused by a mutation located in chromosome 4q21-23 that encodes a 968–amino acid integral membrane protein, polycystin-2. A third ADPKD gene has been implicated as a rare cause of the disease but has not been mapped.

PREVALENCE AND INCIDENCE. ADPKD affects between 1 in 500 and 1 in 1000 live births in all racial groups worldwide, and approximately 6000 new cases are recognized annually. ADPKD is usually recognized in adults between the third and fourth decades of life. The diagnosis is occasionally made in utero during routine fetal ultrasound monitoring or on the discovery of palpable kidneys shortly after birth of a child with a family history of ADPKD.

PATHOGENESIS. The development of renal cysts in ADPKD is illustrated in Figure 115–1. In an affected individual, each renal tubule cell carries a single copy of a mutated gene, which in itself is not sufficient to cause cysts to form. A second somatic mutation, or "hit," is required to initiate the process. The nature of the somatic mutation is not known, but it has been suggested that certain segments of DNA within the gene may be unusually susceptible to acquired mutations. This process occurs within a relatively few solitary renal tubule cells and leads to increased epithelial proliferation. This sustained proliferation causes enlargement of the tubule, which is eventually recognized as a "microcyst." When microcysts exceed about 2 mm in diameter, about 70% of them become disconnected from the tubule segments from which they arose. In these solitary sacs of liquid, cyst growth continues as a consequence of the steady cellular proliferation and the secretion of NaCl and water under the influence of growth factors, hormones, and intracellular cyclic adenosine monophosphate. The expanding cysts remodel the tubular basement membranes and other interstitial structures, similar to invading benign cellular tumors, and in approximately 50% of patients this cyst-interstitium interaction leads to profound tubulointerstitial fibrosis that ultimately compromises renal function.

Although cysts develop in fewer than 1% of the renal tubules and glomerular capsules, polycystic kidneys are strikingly enlarged. The cysts are scattered diffusely throughout the kidneys and vary in size from a few millimeters to several centimeters in diameter. The cysts are lined by epithelium that in most cases appears relatively undifferentiated with respect to the tubule site of origin. In the early stage of development the cysts are filled with a urine-like fluid, but in more advanced cases the fluid may be blood tinged or dark amber and relatively thick because of bleeding or the shedding and accumulation of tubule epithelial cells within the cyst cavity. Interstitial fibrosis is a late consequence of the disease that is preceded in the earlier stages by foci of inflammation and the deposition of type I and type IV collagen around expanding cysts.

CLINICAL MANIFESTATIONS. All patients with ADPKD have renal cysts, but in addition, cysts may be found in the liver, pancreas, spleen, and brain with lesser frequency. Affected individuals have a relatively high rate of cardiac valvular abnormalities, especially mitral valve prolapse, and abdominal and inguinal hernias are

Table 115–1 ■ CHARACTERISTICS OF RENAL CYSTIC DISORDERS

CHARACTERISTIC	POLYCYSTIC		CYSTIC		MEDULLARY	
	Dominant	**Recessive**	**Simple**	**Acquired**	**Sponge Kidney**	**Cystic**
Prevalence	1:500–1:1000	1:16,000	Common	End-stage renal diseases	1:1000–1:5000	Rare
Symptoms	Common	Common	Rare	Occasional	Occasional	Common
Inherited	Yes	Yes	No	No	Unknown	Yes
Kidney size	Large	Large	Normal	Small to large	Normal	Small
Hypertension	Common	Common	Rare	Common	Rare	Rare
Hematuria	Common	Common	Occasional	Occasional	Unusual	Rare
Azotemia	Common	Common	No	Always	Rare	Common
Liver disease	40–60%	100%	No	No	No	No
Cranial aneurysm	5–20%	No	No	No	No	No
Differential diagnosis	ARPKD	ADPKD	Tumor	ADPKD	Medullary cystic kidney	End-stage renal disease
	Tuberous sclerosis	Medullary sponge kidney	Diverticula of the renal pelvis	Simple cysts	Renal tubular acidosis	Medullary sponge kidney
	Multiple simple cysts			Hippel-Lindau disease	Idiopathic nephrocalcinosis	

ARPKD = autosomal recessive polycystic kidney disease; ADPKD = autosomal dominant polycystic kidney disease.

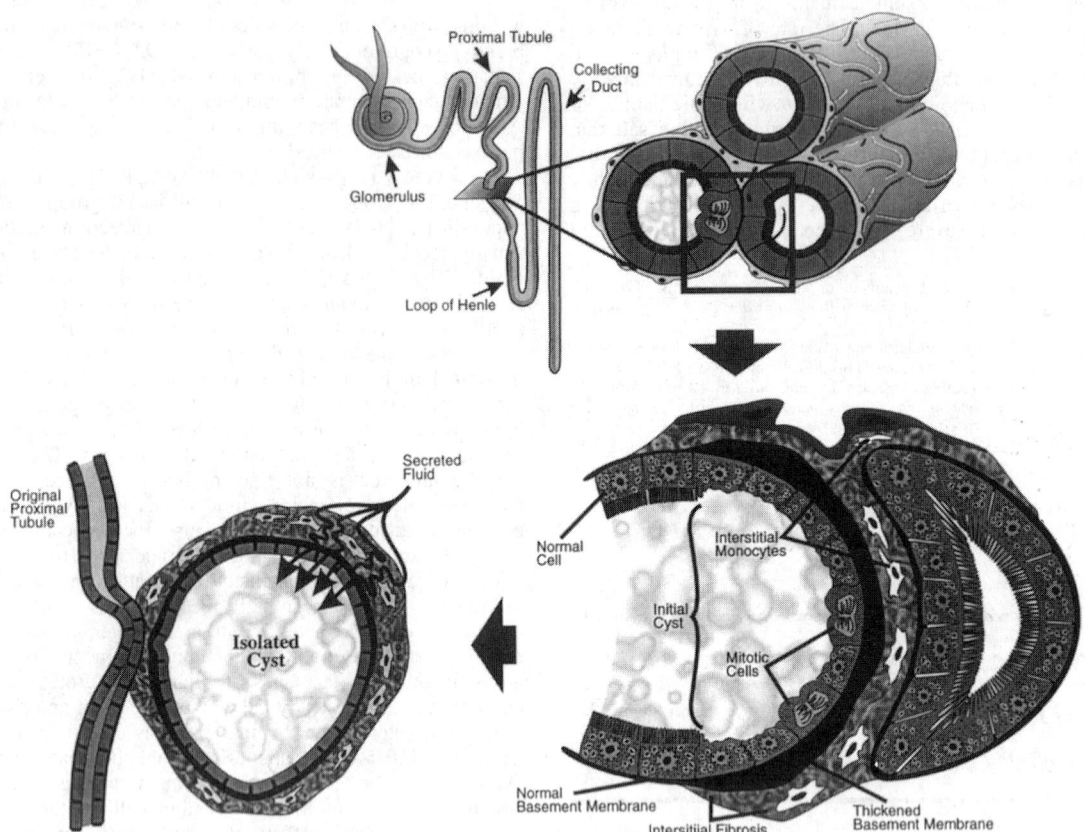

FIGURE 115–1 ■ Evolution of cysts in renal tubule segments (see the text).

relatively common. *Intracranial aneurysms* occur in approximately 5% of patients with ADPKD overall, but the prevalence increases to 20% in individuals with a family history of brain aneurysm. ADPKD is clearly a systemic disorder with major manifestations in the kidneys.

Abdominal pain and *hematuria* are the most common initial symptoms in patients with ADPKD. Infected renal cysts are also relatively common. *Hypertension* occurs in over 50% of patients with ADPKD and often precedes diagnosis of the disease. *Renal insufficiency* occurs relatively late in this disorder and is not usually an initial feature. No distinguishing laboratory features of the disease are noted other than mild degrees of proteinuria and the appearance of urinary lipid bodies in approximately 60% of individuals with moderately advanced disease.

DIAGNOSIS. The kidneys are frequently palpable by abdominal examination. Confirmation of the diagnosis of ADPKD with ultrasound in patients older than 20 years is expeditious and relatively inexpensive and does not use ionizing radiation or contrast agents. A diagnosis can confidently be made when more than five cysts total are found distributed between both kidneys in a patient with an unequivocal family history of ADPKD. Computed tomography (CT) with contrast enhancement or "single-breath" magnetic resonance imaging (MRI) are even more definitive tests that can be used in cases that remain equivocal after sonography. In patients with a creditable family history of ADPKD, a diagnosis can be made if one of the radiologic tests shows diffuse cysts in both kidneys and cysts in the liver, pancreas, or brain. Gene linkage studies can be done with a high degree of certainty, but this test requires at least two affected and willing family members and is only performed in a relatively few centers. Currently, no genetic test is available for clinical use that defines specific mutations in patients at risk for ADPKD.

ADPKD can be differentiated from multiple simple cysts on CT and MRI scans by establishing that the vast majority of parenchyma contains no cysts. Tuberous sclerosis may demonstrate bilateral polycystic lesions, but this disease can be distinguished from ADPKD by its involvement of the lung, skin, and brain and by

demonstrating angiomyolipomas within the kidneys. Medullary cystic diseases typically affect children, and when encountered in adults, the kidneys are not enlarged and the cysts are limited to the medulla. Acquired cystic kidney disease (ACKD) develops as a consequence of renal failure, whereas in ADPKD, the cysts precede the development of renal failure. Autosomal recessive polycystic kidney disease (ARPKD) may be present in young adults with typical polycystic kidneys; however, these patients exhibit hepatic fibrosis and have no family history of polycystic kidneys.

TREATMENT. The clinical course of ADPKD is highly variable. Approximately half of patients with ADPKD live a normal life span with adequate renal function. By contrast, the remainder progress to end-stage renal failure at highly variable rates. Several risk factors have been identified that accelerate the rate of progression, including the *PKD1* versus the *PKD2* genotype, male gender, hypertension, hematuria, proteinuria, multiple pregnancies, and clinical expression of the disease in childhood.

Presently, no specific treatment is available to preserve renal function in ADPKD. Stringent restriction of dietary protein in patients with advanced disease is of little benefit, although moderate limitation of protein (0.6 to 0.8 g/kg/day) may be beneficial if initiated before extensive renal fibrosis has supervened. Uncontrolled *hypertension* has been shown to be associated with a more rapid rate of functional decline than in patients without hypertension. Although a controlled study has not yet been done to show that treatment of hypertension is beneficial to the kidneys over the long term, it is strongly recommended that the hypertension be treated sufficiently to keep the blood pressure within the range of normal for age and gender. Control of blood pressure is also indicated to prevent secondary effects on the entire cardiovascular system. The hypertension of ADPKD involves the renin-angiotensin system, but a volume-dependent component is also present. Salt restriction and long-acting diuretics in conjunction with angiotensin inhibitors and calcium blocking agents have been found to control the hypertension in most cases. Hypokalemia should be avoided. *Urinary tract infections* must be treated promptly and aggressively. Once the cysts become infected, eradication of the infection can be difficult. For uncomplicated lower urinary tract infections, generally accepted treatment programs can be initiated, with a clear urine sediment and a negative urine culture used as satisfactory therapeutic end points. On the other hand, parenchymal infection as revealed by urinary pus casts, fever, leukocytosis, and a kidney(s) tender to palpation is best treated with bactericidal antibiotics specifically targeted to the organism cultured from the blood or urine. Treatment should be continued until the renal pain has subsided completely and the urine has been cleared of pus cells. In some cases, treatment may be required for several months. If oral antibiotic therapy fails to reverse the train of symptoms, parenteral administration of an antibiotic that penetrates cysts is indicated, including ciprofloxacin, chloramphenicol, or trimethoprim-sulfamethoxazole. Gross *hematuria* is usually due to a ruptured cyst, and the bleeding ordinarily subsides in a day or two with bed rest and hydration. Renal *calculi* composed of urate or calcium oxalate are relatively common and are treated by conventional measures, including lithotripsy. Renal *adenocarcinoma*, although no more common than in the population at large, can be difficult to diagnose. CT and MRI are useful when cancer is suspected. *Cranial aneurysms* occur with sufficient frequency to warrant consideration in all patients. In the absence of a family history of aneurysm and no symptoms or signs of intracranial disease, no diagnostic radiographic tests are currently recommended. On the other hand, even in an individual with no intracranial signs or symptoms, a family history of cerebral aneurysm is an indication for angio-MRI. All patients with ADPKD and new-onset headache or signs of intracranial disease should be evaluated for aneurysm expeditiously. *Chronic renal failure* is treated with hemodialysis or peritoneal dialysis and renal transplantation.

Patients with established ADPKD should be advised that they can expect each of their children to have a 50-50 chance of inheriting the defective gene. It is common practice to defer diagnostic testing in children at risk until they reach the age of majority, which in most states is 18 years, unless a family history of aneurysm is present or the child has hypertension or other signs of renal disease.

PROGNOSIS. Life-threatening renal insufficiency develops in approximately 50% of patients with ADPKD. The status of renal function can be monitored by repeated measurement of the serum creatinine concentration. Levels consistently above 1.5 mg/dL usually indicate that the disease has entered the progressive phase of renal insufficiency. Risk factors that accelerate progression include the *PKD1* genotype, male gender, hypertension, hematuria, proteinuria, and multiple pregnancies. Although no specific treatment is at hand to slow or prevent the development and progressive enlargement of polycystic kidneys, adherence to diets limited in protein and salt, control of hypertension with pharmacologic agents, and avoidance of nephrotoxic drugs appear to be lengthening the functional duration of kidneys destined for failure. Aspiration of fluid by surgical or laparoscopic decompression of hundreds of cysts within the kidneys has not proved to slow progression, although renal discomfort is usually improved by these procedures. Patients with ADPKD do as well or better with hemodialysis, peritoneal dialysis, and renal transplantation than patients with other nephropathies.

AUTOSOMAL RECESSIVE POLYCYSTIC KIDNEY DISEASE

ARPKD is usually recognized in infants at or shortly after birth. The diagnosis is occasionally made in utero during routine fetal ultrasound monitoring. ARPKD is found in approximately 1 in 16,000 live births and is caused by a mutation in chromosome 6p21. This gene has not been cloned and the gene product is unknown. Neither parent is aware that they carry a copy of the mutant gene until they have had an affected child. Each subsequent child has a 1 in 4 chance of inheriting the disease and a 50-50 chance of being a gene carrier.

ARPKD may lead to death shortly after birth because of renal insufficiency and pulmonary maldevelopment. Occasionally, the massive kidneys must be removed in infants because of their effect of compromising respiration. Approximately half of affected children will live to adulthood with moderately enlarged cystic kidneys. These patients usually exhibit hepatic fibrosis, often severe enough to cause portal hypertension and hypersplenism.

No specific treatment is known for ARPKD in children or adults. Supportive care is given with attention to the treatment of hypertension and urinary tract infections. Extrarenal manifestations other than hepatic fibrosis are not commonplace. Renal and hepatic transplantation has been performed when these organs fail to function adequately.

MEDULLARY CYSTIC DISORDERS

Medullary cystic kidney disease, an inherited, rare disorder, has also been called nephronophthisis, cystic medullary complex, and renal-retinal dysplasia (because of the coincidence of retinitis pigmentosa in some families). Both autosomal dominant and recessive forms (chromosome 2q13) of medullary cystic disease have been described. The kidneys are moderately small and exhibit medullary cysts and severe tubulointerstitial inflammation and fibrosis. A history of polyuria and polydipsia, pallor, lethargy, and growth retardation is frequently obtained. The disease may progress to the end stage before the age of 20 years, but abnormalities have been described in the seventh decade of life. Renal salt wasting is an impressive feature in some patients. Diagnosis is difficult, but in some cases the medullary cysts can be seen well enough by sonography to be definitive. Open renal biopsy may be needed to establish a definite diagnosis in patients without clear-cut medullary cysts. No specific treatment is available.

Medullary sponge kidney is encountered most frequently in the course of a work-up for nephrolithiasis. This condition has no known hereditary predisposition or gender preference. It has been described in association with parathyroid adenoma and hyperparathyroidism. The collecting ducts demonstrate ectatic segments in which calcium deposits may collect. The kidneys exhibit a spongy quality on cut section, which accounts for the name used to describe this condition. The disease is usually noticed in the fourth or fifth decade of life, when it may be associated with microscopic hematuria or nephrolithiasis. The disease seldom progresses to end-stage renal failure, and only then as a consequence of infectious or surgical complications related to nephrolithiasis. The collecting ducts of these patients may have a defect in the capacity to concentrate urine and secrete protons.

The diagnosis is made by intravenous urography, which shows the typical striations in the papillary portions of the kidney produced by the accumulation of contrast material in the dilated collecting ducts. On plain films of the abdomen, calcium precipitates may also be observed in the papillary regions of the kidney. No specific therapy is known, and treatment is usually directed at control of urinary lithiasis.

SOLITARY OR SIMPLE CYSTS

Solitary or "simple" cysts are derived primarily from distal tubules, are commonly seen in patients older than 50 years, and are usually clinically silent. They are frequently discovered as an incidental finding during abdominal ultrasound, CT, or MRI studies. Asymptomatic renal cysts, which appear on CT and MRI scans to have sharp margins, liquid contents, and no internal structure, do not require further study inasmuch as they have not been found to be forerunners of renal cancer or indicative of other renal or systemic diseases. Occasionally, renal cysts may be associated with flank pain, hematuria, or fever, and in these cases additional radiographic and urologic studies, including cyst aspiration, may be performed to exclude tumors or infection. Renin-dependent hypertension has occasionally been attributed to a renal cyst that stretches intrarenal arteries. Medullary cysts have been associated with severe chronic potassium depletion.

ACQUIRED CYSTIC KIDNEY DISEASE

ACKD is an exaggerated manifestation of otherwise simple cysts that develop in patients with chronic glomerulonephritis, tubulointerstitial nephritis, diabetes mellitus, and Alport's syndrome that has progressed to the end stage. The cysts are thought to develop in renal tubules that have survived the underlying nephropathy and have undergone compensatory hypertrophy. Tubule cell hyperplasia develops in some of these enlarged tubules and results in cystic expansion. This process occurs in sufficient numbers of tubules that the atrophied kidneys begin to enlarge as the individual cysts expand. In some cases, overall kidney size may be large enough to make distinction between ACKD and genetically defined polycystic kidney disease difficult.

ACKD is usually diagnosed by ultrasound or CT in patients with long-standing, progressive renal disorders and severe azotemia. The cystic process continues to progress in over 50% of patients after the initiation of hemodialysis or peritoneal dialysis treatments. Major complications of ACKD include urinary tract or retroperitoneal hemorrhage and renal stone formation with ureteral colic. Cancer develops in these kidneys at a higher rate than in the population at large.

Grantham JJ: The etiology, pathogenesis and treatment of autosomal dominant polycystic kidney disease: Recent advances. Am J Kidney Dis 28:788, 1996. *A discussion of polycystic kidney disease written for those who seek more in-depth understanding of its etiology and pathogenesis.*

Martinez JR, Grantham JJ: Polycystic kidney disease: Etiology, pathogenesis and treatment. Dis Mon 41:693, 1995. *A discussion of polycystic kidney disease written especially for practicing clinicians.*

Watson ML, Torres VE (eds): Polycystic Kidney Disease. Oxford, Oxford University Press, 1996. *The most comprehensive textbook in English on polycystic and other cystic renal conditions.*

116 ANOMALIES OF THE URINARY TRACT

Jay Bernstein

Developmental abnormalities of the urinary tract are relatively common and are believed to affect 10% of newborns and to account for almost one third of all congenital malformations. Many are asymptomatic and inconsequential, but major malformations are important causes of early infantile death and later morbidity and renal failure. The congenital malformations that cause renal and urinary tract disease in adolescents and adults are the subject of this chapter.

RENAL PARENCHYMAL DEFICIENCY. *Renal agenesis* is a failure of embryogenesis that, when unilateral, results in a solitary kidney. *Renal hypoplasia* signifies a small kidney with otherwise normally formed renal parenchyma that results from deficient nephrogenesis or reduced postnatal growth, whereas *renal dysplasia*, regardless of renal size, indicates abnormal metanephric differentiation resulting in abnormally and incompletely differentiated renal elements and in abnormal renal architecture. Small dysplastic kidneys are commonly referred to as "aplastic." Large dysplastic kidneys are often cystic, the most common type being *multicystic dysplasia.*

RENAL AGENESIS. Unilateral agenesis occurs in approximately 1 in 1000 births. Males predominate by approximately 2:1. More than one third of patients with unilateral agenesis have other congenital defects, e.g., cardiovascular and gastrointestinal. Almost 70% have genital anomalies. Because renal agenesis is a developmental field defect, unilateral agenesis is commonly associated with müllerian defects in women (e.g., absent ipsilateral oviduct) and with wolffian defects in men (e.g., absent ipsilateral ductus deferens), which are sometimes clues to the renal abnormality. A solitary kidney is not ordinarily at increased risk of acquired disease, except that one serious, but uncommon complication is compensatory hypertrophy with hyperfiltration, glomerular sclerosis, and eventual renal insufficiency.

Unilateral agenesis in adults occurs as a component of several heritable disorders, e.g., Kallmann's syndrome of anosmia and hypogonadotropic hypogonadism (see Chapter 246), which is caused by mutation of the *KAL* gene at Xp22.3. Another syndrome is *hereditary renal adysplasia*, an autosomal dominant condition with variable penetrance. Unilateral and bilateral renal agenesis, renal

dysplasia, and congenital hydronephrosis may all occur in a kindred, and the recurrence risk is for any of the defects. First-degree relatives of infants with bilateral renal agenesis carry a 12% risk of hereditary renal adysplasia, and conversely the offspring of either affected or obligate heterozygotes carry a 15 to 20% empirical risk of bilateral renal maldevelopment.

RENAL HYPOPLASIA. Bilateral hypoplasia, in which small kidneys contain a reduced complement of nephrons and in which the glomeruli and tubules individually undergo hypertrophy, has been called *oligoméganéphronie* or *oligonephronic hypoplasia*. Patients typically survive into the second decade with slowly progressive renal insufficiency and are good candidates for renal transplantation. The abnormality is characterized by the early onset of a urinary concentrating defect, often with salt wasting, and hypertension occurs late if at all. This abnormality is a sporadic, usually isolated maldevelopment, although renal hypoplasia has recently been identified as a component of the optic nerve coloboma–renal syndrome associated with *PAX2* mutations. Renal hypoplasia must be differentiated from acquired renal atrophy, particularly segmental atrophy in reflux nephropathy, and from nephronophthisis–medullary cystic disease. Unilateral hypoplasia is recognized in imaging studies that show unirenicular and birenicular kidneys, often with contralateral hypertrophy.

RENAL DYSPLASIA. Unilateral dysplasia may be asymptomatic well into adult life. Small aplastic and large multicystic dysplastic kidneys are non-functioning, but modern imaging studies differentiate these abnormalities from renal agenesis. The ipsilateral ureter is typically atretic, and contralateral malformations, among them obstruction and reflux, are common and increase morbidity if left untreated. Unilateral multicystic kidneys involute over time and sometimes disappear almost completely and become indistinguishable from renal agenesis. Unilateral aplasia and multicystic dysplasia may, as noted above, be manifestations of the hereditary renal adysplasia syndrome.

RENAL AND URETERAL DUPLICATION AND ECTOPY. Duplex kidneys with partial ureteral duplication are harmless, relatively common abnormalities. Renal duplication with complete ureteral duplication, on the other hand, is a more serious malformation because of associated ureteral ectopy (Fig. 116–1). The ureter arising from the cephalad portion of the duplicated kidney typically enters the bladder below the normal position, e.g., in the lower part of the trigone or the proximal end of the urethra, where it often terminates in an ectopic ureterocele—a cyst-like dilatation of the terminal ureter in the bladder submucosa. Stenosis of the ectopic ureteral orifice results in varying degrees of urinary obstruction. High-grade obstruction causes maldevelopment and non-function of the upper part of the kidney, and enlargement of the ureterocele compresses and mildly obstructs the lower-pole ureter. This malformation, commonly discovered during childhood because of reflux and urinary tract infection, may not become symptomatic until adulthood, also because of urinary tract infection.

Simple ureteral ectopy in the urethra or vagina is associated with incontinence and an increased risk of ascending infection. Ectopic ureters in the seminal vesicle become symptomatic at the onset of sexual activity. The ipsilateral kidney in these circumstances is commonly small and dysplastic.

Renal ectopy is often unilateral, e.g., a pelvic kidney located at the pelvic brim with its blood supply from pelvic or iliac vessels. Pelvic kidneys are occasionally injured during parturition and are susceptible to infection and lithiasis because of stasis and reflux. Bilateral renal ectopia is often associated with fusion of the two kidneys, the most common type being a horseshoe kidney (Fig. 116–2). It occurs in about 0.25% (1 in 400) of the population, with a 2:1 male preponderance. Crossed ectopia occurs with and without fusion. Supernumerary (extra) kidneys are also ectopic and vary in location.

CONGENITAL LOWER URINARY TRACT OBSTRUCTION AND MALDEVELOPMENT. Ureteropelvic obstruction in an adult is less often congenital and more often acquired as a result of ureteritis and pyelitis. Extrinsic ureteropelvic and upper ureteral obstruction has sometimes been attributed to aberrant blood vessels that appear to kink and constrict the ureter, but intrinsic ureteral abnormalities may underlie this association. Hydrocalycosis, secondary to infundibular stenosis, and caliceal diverticula in early life are probably congenital, although the same abnormalities later in life are of uncertain pathogenesis. Both become symptomatic because of in-

---

Note: Jay Bernstein retains copyright to his original illustrations.

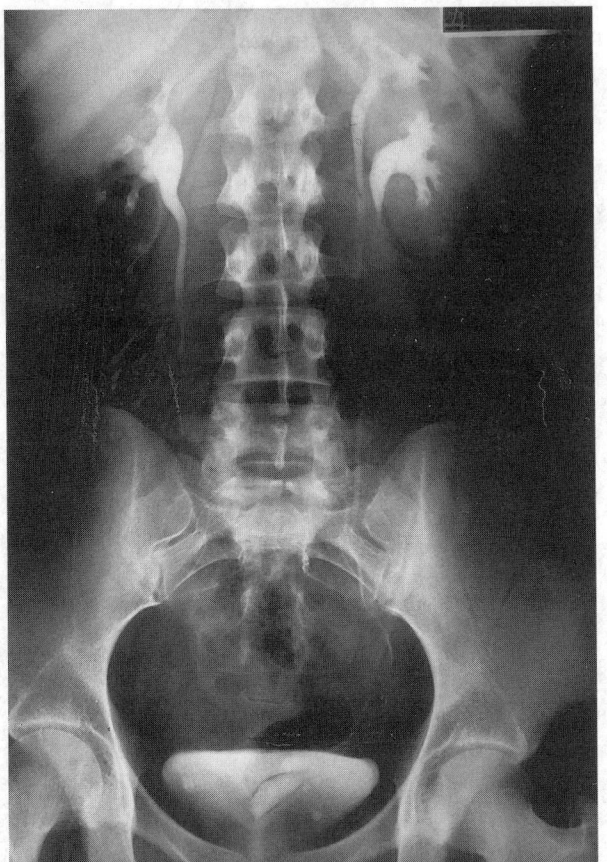

FIGURE 116-1 ■ Urographic demonstration of left renal duplication with an ectopic ureterocele in the bladder. (Copyright Jay Bernstein, M.D.)

fection and lithiasis. Diverticula and mucosal folds and valves are rare, presumably congenital causes of low ureteral obstruction.

Abnormal insertion of the ureter into the bladder is arguably the basis of vesicoureteral reflux. Nonetheless, reflux gradually diminishes in frequency and severity during childhood. Extreme ureteral dilation in association with severe vesicoureteral reflux (refluxing megaureter) is linked with obstructive maldevelopment of the lower urinary tract, e.g., posterior urethral valves, functional bladder outlet obstruction, and prune-belly syndrome. Some boys with posterior urethral valves and reasonably functioning urinary tracts survive into adulthood with little impairment in renal function. Posterior urethral valves are only occasionally familial. The *prune-belly syndrome* consists of a distended abdominal wall with deficient abdominal musculature, cryptorchidism, dilated bladder and

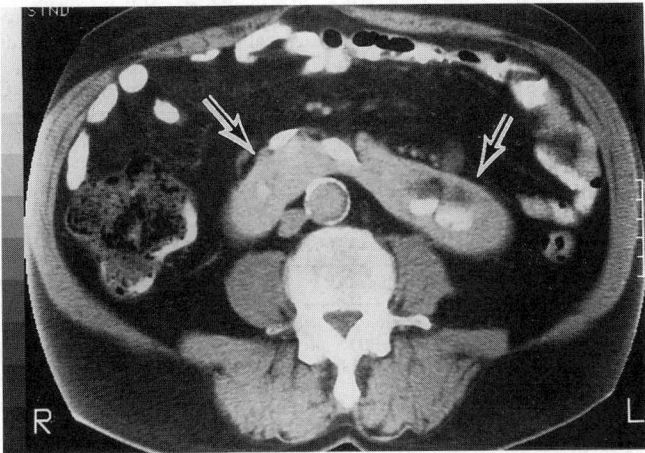

FIGURE 116-2 ■ A horseshoe kidney, fused across the midline (arrows), is demonstrated by enhanced computed tomography. The pelvis of the right kidney faces anteriorly. (Copyright Jay Bernstein, M.D.)

ureters, and hypoplastic prostate. The major factor in survival is preservation of renal function. The lax, wrinkled anterior abdominal wall, from which the syndrome derives its name, smoothes out with growth into a prominent potbelly. Only about 3% of such patients are female. Siblings are at some risk of developing the abnormality; surviving males have been sterile. Anterior urethral diverticula related to mucosal folds that function as flap valves partially obstruct the urethra and become complicated by local infection and lithiasis. In megalourethra, the penile urethra distends during micturition because of partial or complete absence of the corpus spongiosum. Severe forms of the abnormality are usually accompanied by other malformation, but milder forms involve only the distal end of the urethra.

Vesical exstrophy and epispadias are ordinarily treated in early childhood and rarely neglected into adolescence. Late repair of exstrophy is associated with a greatly increased risk of bladder cancer. Repair may be followed by vesicoureteral reflux, and inguinal hernias are commonly present in males. Although complete epispadias causes incontinence, the less severe balanic and penile forms are usually continent. Hypospadias with a short and curved penis (chordee) is rarely allowed to persist into adulthood. Urethral duplication and vesical septation are rare abnormalities.

Bauer SB, Perlmutter AD, Retik AB: Anomalies of the upper urinary tract. *In* Walsh PC, Retik AB, Stamey TA, Vaughan ED (eds): Campbell's Urology, 6th ed. Philadelphia, WB Saunders, 1992, pp 1357–1442. *A comprehensive urologic discussion of renal and upper urinary tract malformations.*

Bernstein J, Gilbert-Barness E: Congenital malformations of the kidney. *In* Tisher C, Brenner B (eds): Renal Pathology, 2nd ed. Philadelphia, JB Lippincott, 1994, pp 1355–1386. *A clinicopathologic evaluation of renal maldevelopment.*

Woolf AS: Clinical impact and biological basis of renal malformations. Semin Nephrol 15:361, 1995. *Emerging knowledge of cell biology and molecular mechanisms.*

117 TUMORS OF THE KIDNEY, URETER, AND BLADDER

Charles L. Shapiro ■ *Marc B. Garnick* ■ *Philip W. Kantoff*

RENAL CELL CARCINOMA

EPIDEMIOLOGY AND ETIOLOGY. Renal cell carcinoma is typically diagnosed during the sixth and seventh decade. The male-to-female ratio is 3:2. Approximately 29,900 new cancers are diagnosed annually, and annual cancer deaths number 11,600. Risk factors for renal cell carcinoma include cigarette smoking, obesity, excessive ingestion of phenacetin analgesics, acquired cystic kidney disease in dialysis patients, adult polycystic kidney disease, exposure to Thorotrast contrast medium, and occupational exposure to asbestos, cadmium, leather tanning, and petroleum products. Rare familial forms of renal cell carcinoma include von Hippel-Lindau (VHL) disease. VHL is an autosomal dominant disorder characterized by the development of multiple tumors of the central nervous system, pheochromocytomas, and bilateral renal cell carcinomas.

A putative tumor suppressor gene for renal cell cancer has recently been identified. More than 90% of nonhereditary renal cell carcinomas and renal cell carcinomas occurring in patients with VHL disease are associated with structural deletions or alterations of 3p, the short arm of chromosome 3. A gene for VHL was mapped to the 3p region using genetic linkage studies and has recently been cloned and partially sequenced. Loss of one copy of the VHL gene through deletion and a mutation in the remaining copy of the gene has been found in the majority of nonhereditary renal cell carcinomas. These data suggest that the loss of the function of the VHL gene is a crucial step in the development of renal cell carcinoma.

PATHOLOGY. Renal cell carcinomas arise from the proximal renal tubular epithelium. Although most are solitary, 7% are multicentric. The histopathologic subtypes of renal cell carcinoma are the clear cell, the granular cell, and the spindle cell or sarcomatoid variant. The clear cell subtype is the most common form (75% of cases), and the less frequent sarcomatoid variety (1 to 6% of cases) is associated with a poorer prognosis. Oncocytomas are rare variants of renal cell carcinoma thought to arise from the distal tubule. These are well differentiated tumors of low malignant potential. In contrast to the common forms of renal cell carcinoma, 3p deletions are not found in oncocytomas. In the past, renal cell carcinomas were divided pathologically into a classification that considered cell type and growth pattern. The former included clear cell, spindle cell, and oncocytic varieties, whereas the latter included acinar papillary or sarcomatoid varieties. Recently this classification has undergone a transformation that more accurately reflects the morphologic, histologic, and genetic characteristics of these tumors. Based on recent studies, five distinct categories have been identified. These include clear cell, chromophilic, chromophobic, oncocytic and collecting duct varieties. Table 117–1 summarizes this information and more accurately reflects the increased knowledge of the genetic abnormalities of these lesions.

CLINICAL MANIFESTATIONS AND DIAGNOSIS. Hematuria is the most frequent presenting symptom of renal cell carcinoma. Pain and an abdominal mass are also common, but the "classic triad" of hematuria, pain, and abdominal mass occurs in fewer than 10% of patients. Systemic symptoms, including fever, weight loss, anemia, polycythemia, hypercalcemia, and nonmetastatic hepatic dysfunction, occur frequently in patients with renal cell carcinoma and may represent the sole manifestation of the cancer. Cytokines and hormones, such as interleukin-6, transforming growth factor-alpha (TGF-α), erythropoietin-like substances, and parathyroid hormone-like substances, are produced by renal cell carcinomas and may be responsible for some systemic symptoms. Systemic symptoms may be relieved by surgical removal of the primary tumor.

Routine use of computed tomography (CT) and ultrasonography (US) has led to increased detection of incidental renal masses. The majority of these are benign and include cysts, inflammatory process, pseudotumors, and benign tumors. Cysts are the most frequent renal masses, and several radiographic features help to distinguish benign renal cysts from renal cell carcinomas. The thickness and contour of the wall, the presence and thickness of septa, the extent and location of calcifications, the density of the fluid, and the presence of solid components are used to categorize lesions into those that are benign and do not require surgical evaluation and those in which the suspicion of carcinoma is high and surgery is required.

An algorithm for the work-up of an incidental renal mass is presented in Figure 117–1. US is particularly useful to determine whether masses imaged on excretory urography are either cystic or solid. If the US appearance suggests a complex or solid mass, contrast-enhanced CT is the most sensitive imaging method for renal cell carcinoma. CT also provides important information regarding perirenal tumor extension, regional nodal involvement, renal vein involvement, and local and regional spread of cancer. In comparative studies, magnetic resonance imaging (MRI) provides information similar to that provided by CT. Although controversial, selective renal arteriography is generally not necessary unless nephron-sparing surgery is planned (see below).

A variety of tumors may spread to the kidney, the most common

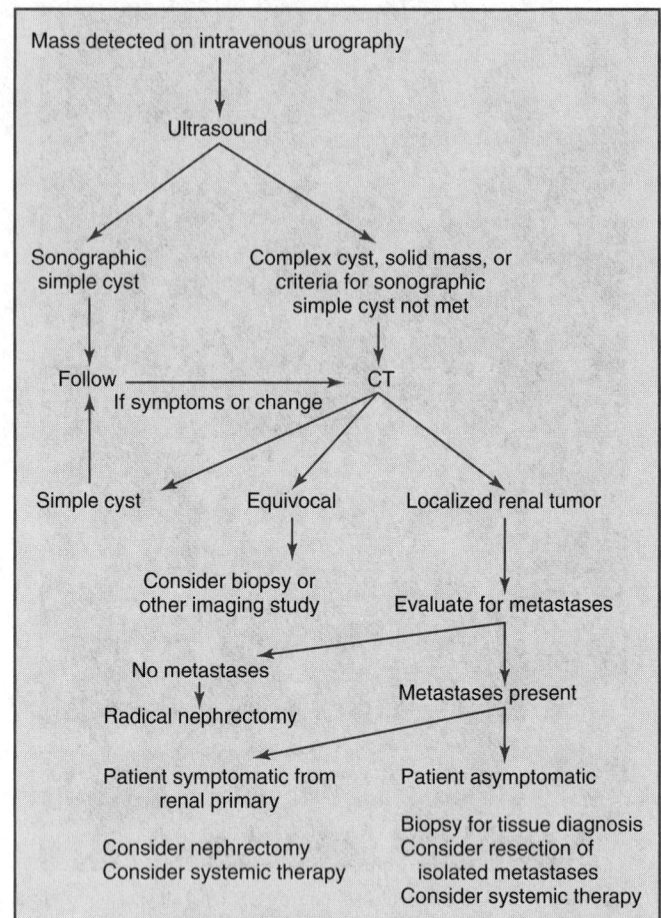

FIGURE 117–1 ■ Algorithm for work-up of incidental renal mass.

being lung cancer. Metastases to the kidney are often multiple and typically occur in the setting of other disseminated disease. A solitary renal mass in a patient with a prior history of malignant disease without evidence of metastases suggests a new primary renal cell carcinoma and should prompt a diagnostic evaluation. Lymphoma of the kidney usually is found with other evidence of systemic lymphoma and often occurs with multiple masses or more diffuse infiltration of the kidney.

STAGING AND PROGNOSIS. The Robson and TNM (tumor/nodes/metastasis) staging systems for renal cell carcinoma are described in Table 117–2. Renal vein invasion per se does not adversely affect prognosis, and tumor thrombus in the vena cava that can be completely removed also does not adversely affect prognosis, even if the thrombus extends above the diaphragm. About 18% of patients with surgically staged renal cell carcinoma have regional lymph node metastases. Regional nodal metastases provide direct evidence of the metastatic potential of the tumor, and virtually all such patients have subsequent development of overt metastases. Other prognostic factors include nuclear grade, tumor size,

Table 117–1 ■ PATHOLOGICAL CLASSIFICATION OF RENAL-CELL CARCINOMA

| CARCINOMA TYPE | GROWTH PATTERN | CELL OF ORIGIN | CYTOGENETIC CHARACTERISTICS | | INCIDENCE (%) |
			Major	Minor	
Clear-cell	Acinar or sarcomatoid	Proximal tubule	3p-	+5, +7, +12, −6q, −8p, −9, −14q, −Y	75–85
Chromophilic	Papillary or sarcomatoid	Proximal tubule	+7, +17, −Y	+12, +16, +2, −4	12–14
Chromophobic	Solid, tubular, or sarcomatoid	Intercalated cell of cortical collecting duct	Hypodiploid	—	4–6
Oncocytic	Typified by tumor nests	Intercalated cell of cortical collecting duct	Undetermined	—	2–4
Collecting-duct	Papillary or sarcomatoid	Medullary collecting duct	Undetermined	—	1

Motzer RJ, Barnder NH, Nanus DM: Renal cell carcinoma. N Engl J Med 1996, 335:865–875. Copyright 1996, Massachusetts Medical Society. All rights reserved.

ROBSON STAGE	ROBSON DESCRIPTION	TNM STAGE	N	N	M	5-YR SURVIVAL (%)
I	Tumor confined to renal parenchyma	I II	T1 T2	N0	M0	66–88
II	Tumor invades perinephric fat	III	T3a	N0, 1	M0	47–68
IIIa	Tumor invades renal vein or vena cava	III	T3b	N0, 1	M0	35–60
IIIb	Tumor in regional lymph nodes	III	T1–3	N1–3	M0	15–30
IV	Tumor in adjacent or distant organs	IV	T4 Any T	N1–3 Any N	M0 M1	2–13

Modified from Robson, CJ, Churchill BM, Anderson W: The results of radical nephrectomy for renal cell carcinoma. J Urol 101:297, 1969; and Linehan WM, Shipley WU, Longo DL: Cancer of the kidney and ureter. In Devita VT, Hellman S, Rosenberg SA (eds): Principles and Practice of Oncology. Philadelphia, JB Lippincott, 1993, pp 1023–1051.

histologic pattern, and flow cytometric parameters, but currently these have little impact on routine clinical decisions.

One-third of patients with renal cell carcinoma have distant metastases at the time the primary tumor is diagnosed. The most common sites are the lung (50%), bone (49%), skin (11%), liver (8%), and brain (3%). In patients with newly diagnosed renal cell carcinoma, radiographic staging evaluation with chest radiograph or CT and bone scan must be done to determine whether metastases are present before definitive surgical treatment of the primary tumor is undertaken.

TREATMENT. The standard treatment for localized renal cell carcinoma is radical nephrectomy, including removal of the kidney, Gerota's fascia, the ipsilateral adrenal gland, and, often, the regional hilar nodes. The value of extended regional lymph node dissection is unproven, and it cannot be routinely recommended. Removal of the ipsilateral adrenal gland may not be necessary unless the primary renal tumor is located in the mid- or upper pole of the kidney. Radiation therapy, either before or after nephrectomy, is of no proven benefit.

Indications for nephron-sparing surgery, which removes the tumor and leaves the rest of the normal kidney, include situations in which a radical nephrectomy would result in a patient's being anephric and requiring dialysis. Examples include bilateral renal cell carcinomas and renal cell carcinoma in a solitary functioning kidney. In carefully selected patients with stage I renal cell carcinomas, the long-term prognosis after nephron-sparing surgery is favorable and exceeds that of patients after nephrectomy and dialysis. Experience with nephron-sparing surgery in patients who would otherwise be candidates for radical nephrectomy or in patients with stage IV renal cell carcinoma is more limited.

The definitive indication for nephrectomy in patients with documented stage IV disease is symptom palliation. Pain, hemorrhage, and systemic symptoms may be relieved after nephrectomy. In the asymptomatic stage IV patient, a so-called adjunctive nephrectomy is controversial. It has been suggested that nephrectomy improves patient survival or increases the possibility of response to immunotherapy. However, it is not possible to separate the therapeutic benefits of nephrectomy from the patient selection factors for nephrectomy, which are likely to identify patients with inherently more favorable prognoses or greater chances of responding to immunotherapy. Prospective, randomized, controlled trials of the value of adjunctive nephrectomy in stage IV patients are under way. Except for a clinical trial, nephrectomy cannot be routinely recommended for asymptomatic patients with stage IV renal cell carcinoma.

Patients with renal cell carcinoma may have a solitary metastasis at the time of the initial diagnosis, or it may develop after nephrectomy. After resection of a solitary metastasis, particularly in the lung, long-term disease-free survival has been observed in some patients. This approach may be advocated for selected patients.

Following nephrectomy, no role has been established for additional systemic forms of therapy (called adjuvant therapy) to reduce the risks of relapse. Treatment options for patients with stage IV disease include immunotherapy and chemotherapy and, in selected

patients, surgical removal of metastatic deposits. Interferons possess limited activity in renal cell carcinoma, with objective tumor regressions of 12 to 14%. Recombinant human interleukin-2 (rhIL-2) induces partial tumor regression in about 13% of patients and complete tumor regression in 7%. Occasionally, patients experiencing complete tumor regression have remained free of disease for more than 5 years. Toxic response to rhIL-2 can be severe. The vascular leak syndrome, characterized by a generalized increase in capillary permeability, fluid retention, and hypotension, can be life-threatening. Lowering the dose of rhIL-2 may lessen toxicity but preserve antitumor activity.

Adding lymphokine-activated killer cells (LAK) to rhIL-2 does not provide additional benefits over rhIL-2 alone. Outpatient combinations of rhIL-2 and interferon appear to offer benefits similar to those seen with rhIL-2 alone, although the toxicity of outpatient regimens may be lower. Tumor-infiltrating lymphocytes isolated from primary renal cell carcinomas can be expanded and activated ex vivo and reinfused into the patient. Too few patients with renal cell carcinoma have been treated with tumor-infiltrating lymphocytes to determine whether this therapy is superior to rhIL-2 alone. New therapeutic approaches for metastatic renal cell carcinoma, including autologous tumor vaccines and new cytokines such as IL-12, are being evaluated in the clinic.

Most chemotherapy drugs have little or no activity in renal cell carcinoma. Two drugs with limited activity are vinblastine and floxuridine, which induce objective tumor regression in about 10 and 16% of patients respectively. Normal proximal tubules and renal cell carcinomas express high levels of the p-glycoprotein, which mediates multidrug resistance. Calcium-channel blockers and other drugs that interfere with the function of the p-glycoprotein are being tested in clinical trials. The hormones medroxyprogesterone acetate and tamoxifen induce objective tumor regression in 1 to 2% and fewer than 10% of renal cell carcinoma patients, respectively.

WILMS' TUMOR (NEPHROBLASTOMA). Wilms' tumors are rare malignant tumors of the kidney occurring predominantly in children younger than 4 years. A gene located on chromosome 11 is abnormally mutated in Wilms' tumor. Signs and symptoms of Wilms' tumor, in decreasing order of frequency, are abdominal mass, pain, hematuria, hypertension, and fever. CT or MRI is useful in identifying the tumors and assessing the extent of disease. In 5% of patients, the tumors are bilateral, and in 15% of patients, metastases are present at the time of the initial diagnosis. The most common sites of metastases are the lungs and liver. Neuroblastoma, another common malignant pediatric tumor that may involve the kidney, may be distinguished from Wilms' tumor by the production of urinary vanillylmandelic acid and homovanillic acid, levels of which are increased in more than 90% of patients with neuroblastoma. Treatment involves surgical excision of the tumor, followed by multiagent chemotherapy for all patients and radiation for patients with tumor in a more advanced stage. In selected instances, bone marrow transplantation may be used. The combined-method treatment approach cures nearly 90% of patients.

BLADDER CANCER AND OTHER UROTHELIAL CANCERS

EPIDEMIOLOGY AND ETIOLOGY. Tumors that arise from the transitional cell lining of the urinary tract are referred to as urothelial cancers. More than 90% of these tumors are transitional cell carcinomas; the remainder are squamous cell carcinomas and adenocarcinomas. These tumors may arise from any location where urothelium exists, including the collecting system of the kidney (i.e., the calyces and renal pelvis), the ureter, the bladder, and the urethra, and from within the urothelium-lined ducts of the prostate. The most common malignant urothelial tumor is bladder cancer, accounting for 54,400 new cases and 12,500 deaths in 1998. Urothelial cancers arising in the renal pelvis are histologically and clinically distinct from the more common renal parenchymal tumors. The latter tumors, called renal cell carcinomas, are usually adenocarcinomas. Similarly, the rare transitional cell carcinomas that arise from within the prostate are distinct from the much more common prostatic adenocarcinomas.

Urothelial cancers have long been recognized as being attributa-

Table 117–3 ■ STAGING OF BLADDER CANCER

	MARSHALL-JEWETT	TNM*
Confined to mucosa	0	Ta
Carcinoma in situ	0	Tis
Infiltration of submucosa	A	T1
Infiltration of superficial muscle	B1	T2
Infiltration of deep muscle	B2	T3a
Perivesical infiltration	C	T3b
Adjacent organ		
Prostate	D1	T4a
Uterus/vagina	D1	
Fixed to pelvic or abdominal wall	D1	T4b
Nodes positive (pelvic only)	D1	T (any), N+
Distant metastases or nodes positive above aortic bifurcation	D2	T (any), N (any), M1

*TNM = tumor/node/metastasis.

ble to environmental toxins (see Chapter 18). Studies 100 years ago determined that exposure to aromatic amines caused an increased likelihood of development of transitional cell carcinomas of the bladder. Workers within the dye industry in Germany, particularly those who distilled 2-naphthylamine, had a strikingly high incidence of bladder cancer. Since that time, numerous other aromatic amines have been associated with bladder cancer, as have the industries in which these chemicals are used, such as the rubber, electric, cable, paint, and textile industries. In today's workplace the relative risk of development of urothelial cancers due to environmental exposures is low. Tobacco use, however, is probably the most important etiologic factor with respect to bladder cancer in the United States; it may account for half of the cases currently diagnosed (see Chapter 13). Worldwide, infection with *Schistosoma haematobium* (*Bilharzia*) accounts for a large proportion of bladder cancer cases, particularly in endemic areas such as the Nile River delta in Egypt (see Chapter 43). Bladder cancer occurring as a result of *S. haematobium* frequently is squamous cell carcinoma, although transitional cell carcinomas may occur. Two other factors associated with an excess risk of urothelial cancers are long-term administration of cyclophosphamide, an alkylating agent used in treating many malignant diseases, and chronic excessive use of the analgesic phenacetin. Transitional cell carcinoma of the renal pelvis and ureters is more likely to occur with analgesic abuse.

Our understanding of the molecular basis of bladder cancer over the past few years has increased. Chromosome 9 abnormalities, particularly monosomy, is a common early event in bladder cancer, and abnormalities of 11p and 17p, including mutations in the p53 gene, may be found in more advanced tumors.

The majority of urothelial cancers are confined to the transitional cell epithelial layer and do not invade into the lamina propria or muscularis layers. Such tumors tend to be polypoid in appearance and papillary in configuration. With invasion beyond the transitional cell layer, the potential for metastatic spread increases dramatically. Higher-grade cancers tend to have a greater propensity for invasion and metastatic spread, as do tumors that possess p53 mutations. Urothelial cancers have a high propensity for multifocality (i.e., multiple simultaneous tumors) and polychronotropism (i.e., recurrence over time). Tumors arising in the bladder most commonly recur elsewhere in the bladder and rarely in the renal pelvis or ureter, whereas tumors that arise from the renal pelvis or ureter frequently (25% of the time) recur in the bladder. Recent studies have supported the concept that these multifocal and polychronotropic tumors are clonal in origin, suggesting a common malignant stem cell abnormality and/or reimplantation of tumor cells as a dominant mechanism for tumor recurrence. Although tumors confined to the epithelial layer may recur and require treatment because of bleeding or other problems, it is the tumors that invade the deeper layers of the wall that may compromise survival.

Bladder Cancer

PATHOLOGY AND STAGING. Bladder cancer, the most common urothelial malignant tumor, is diagnosed three times as frequently in men as in women. Death occurs in a fraction of patients

and is largely attributable to the uncontrolled growth of metastatic deposits of tumor. Fortunately the majority of patients with bladder cancer have superficial bladder tumors confined to the transitional cell layer, which have low potential for metastatic spread. One particularly troublesome type of superficial bladder cancer is carcinoma in situ (CIS), a multifocal disease that can persist despite treatment. If persistent, CIS may progress to invasive bladder cancer. Although superficial tumors are very common, few patients ultimately succumb to the disease. The staging of bladder cancer is shown in Table 117–3.

CLINICAL MANIFESTATIONS AND DIAGNOSIS. Hematuria and irritative bladder symptoms, such as dysuria or urinary frequency, are the most common presenting symptoms of bladder cancer. Most patients have hematuria, which is frequently gross but occasionally microscopic. The hematuria can be episodic. Irritative urinary symptoms, such as urgency, dysuria, and frequency without hematuria, particularly in the absence of infection, should lead to an evaluation for bladder cancer. Larger tumors may cause bladder outlet obstruction or ureteral obstruction resulting in hydronephrosis. Bilateral ureteral obstruction leading to azotemia is rare. Bladder tumors may cause pelvic pain by infiltrating regional nerves or bone, may cause lymphedema as a result of lymphatic obstruction from lymph node metastasis, or may present as manifestations of metastatic disease to bone, lungs, or liver. If bladder cancer is suspected, an intravenous pyelogram (IVP) should be undertaken to locate filling defects in the bladder and in the upper tracts. In addition, cystoscopy should be performed to locate the tumor and to facilitate biopsy for pathologic confirmation and to determine depth of invasion. Urinary cytologic analysis is a useful adjunct in the initial assessment and follow-up evaluation. Newer tests including an evaluation of the urine for bladder cancer antigens, such as bladder tumor antigen and nuclear matrix protein 22, and the genetic "fingerprinting" of exfoliated cells is under study. Evaluation of metastatic sites is essential, including abdominal pelvic CT, chest radiograph, and bone scan.

TREATMENT AND PROGNOSIS. Bladder tumors confined to the transitional cell layer are generally treated only with transurethral excision. These tumors tend to recur, and current practice dictates frequent cystoscopy and removal of recurrent tumors, although the value of this practice is uncertain. Higher-grade tumors confined to the transitional cell layer and high-grade flat tumors, so-called CIS, may be treated with intravesical chemotherapy or immunotherapy with bacille Calmette-Guérin (BCG), because use of intravesical agents may deter or prevent the development of more deeply invasive cancers that have greater metastatic potential. Bladder tumors that invade into the deeper layers of the bladder wall, in general, require more definitive therapy. The preferred treatment is radical cystectomy (i.e., total removal of the bladder), with urinary diversion in the form of an ileal loop, a continent reservoir, or an orthotopic neobladder. Alternative strategies include attempts to preserve bladder function with either partial cystectomy or chemotherapy coupled with radiation therapy. Such treatments may be appropriate for a subset of patients. For patients with tumors that have invaded into the deeper layers of the bladder wall, the likelihood of occult distant spread and future recurrence at metastatic sites is quite high and may be diminished with the use of chemotherapy after cystectomy. For patients with metastatic bladder cancer, polyagent chemotherapy may be life-prolonging and, under rare circumstances, curative.

Transitional Cell Carcinomas of the Renal Pelvis, Calyces, and Ureter

Similar to bladder tumors, upper tract tumors frequently present with gross or microscopic hematuria. However, these tumors may present with ureteral obstruction and pain due to renal colic. The diagnosis is strongly suspected with the finding of a filling defect in a calyx, infundibulum, renal pelvis, or ureter, but cystoscopy with retrograde pyelography with cytologic analysis or ureteroscopy may be required to document the lesion.

TREATMENT AND PROGNOSIS. Many of these lesions are superficial in nature (i.e., they are confined to the transitional cell layer and are low grade). Selected cases may be treated with less radical therapy (i.e., segmental resection), particularly in patients with a solitary kidney. Higher-grade tumors and/or those that invade more deeply into the wall of the ureter or renal pelvis are associated with a greater likelihood of metastatic spread. With definitive treatment, which is nephroureterectomy and removal of a cuff of bladder, the prognosis with such tumors is excellent. The role of chemotherapy as an adjunct to surgery in such cases is less well documented. Before surgery, it is essential to evaluate other areas in the urothelium by IVP, cystoscopy, and retrograde pyelography, because of the high likelihood of contralateral kidney involvement and simultaneous or subsequent bladder involvement. Invasive transitional cell carcinomas of the renal pelvis, calyces, and ureter have a high propensity for metastatic spread. The pattern of spread is similar to that of bladder cancer to lymph nodes, liver, lung, and bone. Multiagent chemotherapy under such circumstances may be of benefit.

Renal Cell Carcinoma

Latif F, Tory K, Gnarra J, et al: Identification of the von Hippel-Lindau disease tumor suppressor gene. Science 28:1317, 1993. *The cloning of the von Hippel-Lindau gene.*

Motzer RJ, Bander NH, Nanus DM: Renal cell carcinoma. N Engl J Med 335:865–875, 1996. *Excellent, up-to-date review of clinical and basic science issues.*

Pizzo PA, Horowitz ME, Poplack DG, et al: Solid tumors of childhood. *In* Devita VT, Hellman S, Rosenberg SA (eds): Principles and Practice of Oncology. Philadelphia, JB Lippincott, 1993, p 1744. *A review of Wilms' tumor.*

Rosenberg SA, Yang JC, Topalian SL, et al: Treatment of 283 consecutive patients with metastatic melanoma or renal cell cancer using high-dose bolus interleukin 2. JAMA 271:907, 1994. *A large experience with high-dose interleukin-2 treatment of renal cell carcinoma and melanoma.*

Storkel S, van den Berg E: Morphologic classification of renal cancer. World J Urol 13:153–158, 1995. *Elaborates the basis for new renal cell carcinoma classification.*

Bladder Cancer and Other Urothelial Cancers

Kantoff PW, Zietman AL, Wishnow K: Bladder cancer. *In* Holland JF, Bast RC, Morton, et al (eds): Cancer Medicine, 4th ed. Philadelphia, Lea & Febiger, 1997, p 2105. *Multidisciplinary view of treatment of bladder cancer.*

Kaufman DS, Shipley WU, Griffin PP, et al: Selective bladder preservation by combination treatment of invasive bladder cancer. N Engl J Med 329:1377, 1993. *Documents utility of chemotherapy used with radiation for invasive bladder cancer.*

Richie JP, Kantoff PW: Neoplasms of the renal pelvis and ureter. *In* Holland JF, Bast RC, Morton, et al (eds): Cancer Medicine, 4th ed. Philadelphia, Lea & Febiger, 1997, p 2097. *Comprehensive review of these rare cancers.*

Sternberg CN, Yagoda A, Scher HI, et al: M-VAC (methotrexate, vinblastine, doxorubicin and cisplatin) for advanced transitional cell carcinoma of the urothelium. J Urol 139:461, 1988. *Describes utility of combination chemotherapy in urothelial cancers.*

118 DISEASES OF THE PROSTATE

Alan W. Partin

The prostate, the largest of the human male accessory sex tissues, normally weighs approximately 20 g in a young adult male. At present, little is known regarding the specific biologic function of the prostate in adult men. The prostate requires continued support of a functioning testis for its development, growth, and maintenance. Anatomically, the prostate is situated in the male pelvis and surrounds a significant portion of the posterior male urethra. The prostate lies deep within the male pelvis between the rectum and pubic bone, where it is situated between the bladder superiorly and the urethra inferiorly. Embryologically, the prostate develops from the urogenital sinus under the influence of dihydrotestosterone produced from fetal testosterone through the action of the enzyme 5α-reductase. Histologically, the prostate is composed of numerous acini and collecting ducts originated by an arborization process branching from the urethra. Prostatic epithelial cells secrete a slightly acidic fluid containing high concentrations of citric acid, polyamines (spermine and spermidine), acid phosphatase, serum protease (prostate-specific antigen [PSA]), and electrolytes (potassium, zinc, calcium, and sodium). Testosterone, secreted by the testes under control of luteinizing hormone from the pituitary gland, is the principal circulating androgen in the adult male. Testosterone is converted to dihydrotestosterone and is thus available as the principal intracellular androgen within the prostate. Other androgens such as adrenal androstenedione are also believed to play a minor role in humans but are not capable of stimulating and maintaining prostate growth (see also Chapter 247).

The immense medical problems caused by the prostate gland are increasing at a most alarming rate, and the full magnitude and impact of these diseases have only recently been established. Pathologic growth in the form of benign prostatic hyperplasia (BPH) or adenocarcinoma and infections of the human prostate gland together combine to yield one of the most common and costly combinations of disease entities occurring in males. In fact, the National Kidney and Urological Disease Advisory Board estimate that within the United States alone, 4.4 million physician visits and over 800,000 hospitalizations led to nearly 40,000 deaths and a cost of over $3 billion for the treatment of prostatic diseases. Unfortunately, most men with prostate disease(s) do not have complaints specifically referable to disorders of prostatic function. In practice, most men have inflammatory, congestive, or cancerous processes of the prostate that give rise only to abnormalities in urination. For this reason, most men are often unaware of the existence of their prostate gland until one of these disorders develops, which for the majority of men, could be in the fourth through eighth decade of life. Starting at puberty, the prostate increases in mass from approximately 4 g to 20 g by 20 years of age. For the next several decades, prostatitis is the most common prostatic disorder. Beyond the age of 50, BPH and carcinoma of the prostate are the predominant diseases of the prostate.

CARCINOMA OF THE PROSTATE

INCIDENCE, PREVALENCE, AND EPIDEMIOLOGY. At present, prostate cancer is the most common cancer diagnosed in men in the United States and the second most common cause of cancer-related death in males. Prostate cancer will develop in approximately 9% of white and 11% of black men in the United States in their lifetimes. Furthermore, it has been calculated that a newborn U.S. male has an approximately 3 to 4% chance of dying of prostate cancer. Over the past decade, major advances have been achieved in the diagnosis and treatment of this disorder. The common use of digital rectal examination (DRE), PSA testing, and improved techniques for biopsy have made it possible to diagnose prostate cancer in more men at an earlier curable stage. Similar to BPH, carcinoma of the prostate likewise does not develop in men who are castrated before puberty. Unlike BPH, no evidence suggests a direct relationship between serum hormone levels and the development of prostate cancer. Likewise, very little evidence can be found to link the development of BPH and prostate cancer. The prevalence of prostate cancer continues to increase with age. Like BPH, after 50 years of age, both the incidence and the mortality rate for prostate cancer increase exponentially. Both family history and race (African-American) are definitive risk factors for the development of carcinoma of the prostate. Other potential risk factors for the development of prostate cancer include excessive dietary fat intake and a diet low in selenium.

PATHOLOGY. Ninety-five per cent of all prostatic carcinomas are adenocarcinomas. Prostatic tumors are multifocal in more than 80% of cases, which suggests a multifocal rather than a single site of molecular origin. Prostatic carcinoma can metastasize by lymphatic or hematogenous dissemination. Prostatic carcinoma can spread locally into the urethra, the bladder neck, the seminal vesicles, or the bladder trigone. The most common sites of lymphatic metastasis are the obturator, hypogastric, iliac, presacral, and periaortic lymph nodes. Bone metastases constitute the most common form of hematogenous spread. The most frequent sites of bony metastatic involvement are the pelvis, lumbar spine, femora, thoracic spine, and ribs. Although uncommon, visceral metastases can be identified in the lung and the liver. Prostatic intraepithelial neoplasia (PIN) is an architecturally benign prostatic acinus or duct lined by cytologically atypical cells. It is now well recognized that high-grade PIN is a premalignant lesion for prostate cancer. When high-grade PIN is found on needle biopsy, the chance of detecting carcinoma on subsequent biopsies is 30 to 50%. Transrectal ultrasound-guided methods are the usual and preferred means of obtaining prostate tissue for histologic diagnosis. The histologic diagnosis of prostate cancer is made, in the majority of cases, by transrectal ultrasound-guided needle biopsy. Prostate cancer rarely causes symptoms until advanced disease is evident. Thus a suspicion of prostate cancer resulting in a recommendation for prostatic biopsy is often raised through abnormalities found on DRE or elevations

Table 118–1 ■ CARCINOMA OF THE PROSTATE

STAGE (TNM)	DEFINITION OF STAGE
T1	Not palpable, found following TURP or biopsy
T1a	Focal, <5% of tissue, not high grade
T1b	Diffuse, >5% of tissue, and/or high grade
T1c	Biopsy for PSA elevation only
T2	Palpable disease limited to the prostate
T2a	Disease $< \frac{1}{2}$ of one lobe
T2b	Disease $> \frac{1}{2}$ of one lobe but < 1 lobe
T2c	Disease > 1 lobe
T3	Palpable disease beyond the prostate
T3a	Unilateral disease beyond the capsule
T3b	Bilateral disease beyond the capsule
T3c	Spread to seminal vesicles
T4	Metastatic spread to adjacent organs (e.g., bladder, pelvic sidewall)

TURP = transurethral resection of the prostate; PSA = prostate-specific antigen.

in serum PSA (>4.0 ng/mL). Although controversial, it has been demonstrated that an early diagnosis of prostate cancer is best achieved through a combination of DRE and PSA measurements. The prognosis of men with prostate cancer correlates well with the histologic grade and stage of the tumor (Table 118–1): Stage T1 disease represents non-palpable prostate cancer detected on pathologic examination of prostatic tissue following prostatectomy for BPH (T1a and T1b) or needle biopsy for PSA elevation (T1c) or an abnormal DRE. Stage T1 is subdivided into three biologically meaningful subclasses: Stage T1c (biopsy for PSA elevation only) is the most common clinical stage at diagnosis of prostate cancer in the 1990s. Stage T2 prostate cancer is palpable disease limited to the prostate on DRE and is likewise further subdivided into three clinically meaningful categories based on the size and location of the palpable lesion. Stage T3 represents tumor extending beyond the prostatic capsule, including invasion into the seminal vesicles. Like other tumors, carcinoma of the prostate has a nodal and metastatic category as well. N0 disease represents no evidence of lymph node involvement; N1 through N3 represents greater involvement of either a single regional lymph node (N1) or multiple large-volume lymph node metastases (N3). Similarly, subdivisions of the M category are based on the extent of metastasis.

CLINICAL MANIFESTATIONS AND DIAGNOSIS. Prostate cancer rarely causes symptoms early in the course of disease because the majority of adenocarcinomas arise in the periphery of the gland distant to the urethra and other pelvic organs. The presence of symptoms as a result of prostate cancer suggests locally advanced or metastatic disease. Growth of prostate cancer into the urethra or bladder neck may result in obstructive or irritative voiding symptoms (e.g., hesitancy, decreased force of the urinary stream, and intermittency). In addition, irritative voiding symptoms (e.g., frequency, nocturia, urgency, urge incontinence) may develop from advanced prostate cancer. Local progression of disease and obstruction of the ejaculatory ducts may result in hematospermia and decreased ejaculate volume. Impotence can likewise be a rare manifestation of prostate cancer that has spread outside the prostatic capsule to involve the branches of the pelvic plexus responsible for innervation of the corpora cavernosa. On DRE, carcinoma of the prostate characteristically has a hard consistency. A nodular dense region of induration within the substance of the prostate suggests a suspicious lesion that should undergo biopsy. Other causes of prostatic induration include BPH, prostatic calculi, granulomatous prostatitis, prostatic infarction, and changes after transurethral resection of the prostate (TURP). Approximately 50% of palpable prostatic nodules are malignant. Thus prostate biopsy is recommended for all men who have DRE abnormalities, regardless of the PSA level. DRE and serum PSA are the most useful screening tests for assessing the risk of prostate cancer in an individual.

PSA is a serum protease secreted in the seminal fluid in high concentrations by prostatic epithelial cells and is responsible for liquefaction of the seminal coagulum. PSA is normally found in low concentrations in the sera (<4.0 ng/mL). Disruption of prostatic architecture as seen in development of adenocarcinoma often leads to "leakage" of PSA into the circulation. Although PSA as a single test has the highest positive predictive value for prostate cancer detection, the most effective method of early detection of prostate cancer is the combined use of DRE and PSA. Various methods for optimizing the usefulness of serum PSA (e.g., PSA velocity, PSA density, age-specific PSA reference ranges, and measurement of the molecular forms of PSA) have been introduced to improve the specificity of the PSA test while maintaining adequate sensitivity for prostate cancer detection. At present, these methods are primarily investigational and require further evaluation before widespread use.

After the diagnosis of adenocarcinoma of the prostate has been histologically confirmed, an accurate assessment of stage—or extent—of disease should be made. The goals of staging prostate cancer are two-fold: (1) to predict prognosis and (2) to rationally direct therapy based on the extent of disease. Methods commonly used for assessing the extent of prostate cancer include DRE, serum tumor markers, histologic grade, radiologic imaging, and surgical lymphadenectomy. A combination of DRE, PSA, and grade on biopsy best predicts stage. In the PSA era, prostatic acid phosphatase has a limited role in staging because of the closer relationship between PSA and disease extent. In addition, radionuclide bone scintigraphy, magnetic resonance imaging, and computed tomography offer little staging information for patients in whom clinically localized adenocarcinoma of the prostate is routinely diagnosed. Men with a serum PSA level greater than 10 ng/mL should undergo a radionuclide bone scan and/or pelvic magnetic resonance imaging for further evaluation of the extent of disease. When used alone, the prognostic value of any clinical criterion used to predict stage is limited for individual patients with newly diagnosed prostate cancer. The staging accuracy of prostate cancer can be significantly enhanced through the combination of parameters of local disease extent (clinical T stage by DRE), serum PSA level, and Gleason grade from the prostate biopsy specimen. Probability nomograms based on these three preoperative parameters give an accurate description of the probability of organ-confined disease before therapeutic decision making.

TREATMENT. Considerable debate is ongoing concerning the best mode of therapy for each particular stage of carcinoma of the prostate. The rational selection of treatment options often places the patient and treating physician in the dilemma of attempting to maintain quality of life while increasing the duration of survival. Many older men with carcinoma of the prostate have other comorbid illnesses that may pose a greater threat than prostate cancer to their overall survival. Present therapeutic options for the treatment of clinically localized prostate cancer include (1) watchful waiting/deferred therapy; (2) definitive local therapy, radical prostatectomy, and external-beam radiation therapy; or (3) investigational interstitial seed radiation therapy and cryosurgery. Only a paucity of clinical trials have directly compared the relative efficacy of these various forms of therapy. Each form of therapy is associated with undesirable risks and side effects. Rational selection of treatment must include an understanding and decision process that take into account the benefits and risks of the treatment options for each individual patient to arrive at a proper balance between efficacy and morbidity.

The decision regarding definitive therapy should be based on a patient's co-morbidity, life expectancy, and more importantly, possibility of cure. Clinically localized prostate cancer is best cured with definitive therapy when disease is confined to the prostate. However, not all potentially curable, clinically localized prostate cancers in fact need therapy. When low-grade, low-volume disease is detected in a man with a life span of less than 10 years, watchful waiting or deferred therapy is a valid option for treatment. Watchful waiting protocols consist of serial DREs and PSA measurements with yearly prostate biopsies to ensure lack of progression of disease. This approach is still investigative and it is unknown whether it will place men at undue risk of uncontrolled disease progression during the watchful waiting period. Men with clinical stage T1b, T1c, and T2 prostatic cancer who have greater than a 15-year life expectancy and no significant co-morbid disease are ideal candidates for definitive therapy, either in the form of radical prostatectomy or external-beam radiation therapy. Large clinical series have demonstrated that the majority of these tumors are confined on pathologic analysis and are thus potentially curable. Long-term survival for these men, when correctly treated, is presently excellent. The complications of definitive therapy should be emphasized and include the possibility of urinary incontinence and impotence. In the hands of an experienced surgeon or radiation oncologist, however, the incidence of these complications should be low. Increased public awareness of prostate cancer and widespread use of DRE and serum PSA for screening have markedly decreased the number of men first seen with stage T3–T4 and N1–N3 prostate cancer. At present, combined use of total androgen deprivation therapy for a period and a formal course of external-beam radiation therapy is recommended as the best form of therapy for stage T3 prostate cancer. The preferred modality for initial treatment of men with soft tissue or bony metastasis from prostate cancer remains an area of major controversy. Although androgen deprivation therapy is the best form of palliative therapy for this stage of advanced disease, the timing and type of therapy delivery are controversial.

Androgen deprivation therapy in the form of either orchiectomy or treatment with endogenous estrogens or luteinizing hormone–releasing hormone (LHRH) analogues alone or coupled with antiandrogens produces regression of prostate cancer cells through suppression of serum testosterone levels. All forms of therapy appear to be effective in that castrate levels of androgens can be induced. Secondary to untoward cardiovascular side effects, routine use of estrogen therapy has been supplanted by orchiectomy or treatment with either LHRH analogues alone or a combination of an LHRH analogue with an antiandrogen. No compelling evidence has proved that total androgen ablation (LHRH or orchiectomy and antiandrogens) is better than LHRH or orchiectomy alone.

The controversy stemming from the proper timing of endocrine therapy centers around "early" or "delayed" treatment. One study demonstrated that the survival rates of men with stage T3–T4 and greater than N0 prostate carcinoma treated initially at diagnosis with androgen deprivation therapy were identical to the survival rates of men whose androgen deprivation therapy was delayed until symptoms appeared. Therefore, it would seem that delaying hormonal therapy until men are symptomatic has no adverse effect on survival. In addition, the side effects associated with LHRH analogue therapy are bothersome and quite significant. Studies comparing bilateral orchiectomy with either an LHRH analogue alone or combined LHRH analogue and antiandrogen therapy demonstrated no difference in survival as well. When disease becomes androgen insensitive following initial successful treatment with androgen deprivation therapy, attempts at further endocrine therapy have been uniformly disappointing. At present, investigational gene-based and immunomodulatory-based therapies, as well as combined use of various chemotherapeutic agents, offer the only hope for advanced androgen-insensitive disease. Several large-scale clinical studies to evaluate combinations of these newer agents for the treatment of metastatic carcinoma are in progress.

Carter HB, Partin AW: Diagnosis and staging of prostate cancer. *In* Walsh PC, Retik AB, Vaughan ED, Wein AJ (eds): Campbell's Urology, 7th ed. Philadelphia, WB Saunders, 1998, pp 2519–2537. *This chapter provides a comprehensive review of the important aspects related to the diagnosis and staging of clinically localized prostate cancer.*

Partin AW, Kattan MW, Subong EN, et al: Combination of prostate-specific antigen, clinical stage, and Gleason score to predict pathological stage of localized prostate cancer. A multi-institutional update. JAMA 277:1445, 1997. *This article provides clinically useful nomograms for combining clinical stage, serum PSA, and biopsy histologic grade to predict the pathologic extent of disease to aid physicians and patients in rational treatment decisions for clinically localized prostate cancer.*

Walsh PC: The natural history of localized prostate cancer: A guide to therapy. *In* Walsh PC, Retik AB, Vaughan ED, Wein AJ (eds): Campbell's Urology, 7th ed. Philadelphia, WB Saunders, 1998, pp 2539–2546. *This chapter provides a clear understanding of the natural history of localized prostate cancer and compares watchful waiting and radical prostatectomy as forms of therapy for clinically localized disease.*

BENIGN PROSTATIC HYPERPLASIA

INCIDENCE AND PREVALENCE. BPH is the most common non-neoplastic disease process in men directly associated with aging. Although BPH has traditionally been a term used to refer to non-malignant enlargement of the prostate gland resulting from hyperplasia of the prostatic epithelium and subsequent urinary outflow obstruction, recent studies have suggested that prostatic enlargement and histologic hyperplasia are only one facet of a larger syndrome consisting of both irritative and obstructive lower urinary tract symptoms, diminished urinary flow rate, and bladder dysfunction. Histologic evidence of BPH has been demonstrated in men as young as 40 years; however, microscopic nodular hyperplasia associated with irritative symptoms or outlet obstruction is more com-

monly seen in men aged 50 to 70. The frequency of symptomatic BPH is variable yet increases between the fifth and eighth decade of life. Although the frequency of BPH is equal in all races and cultures, the mean age of detection for whites (65 years) differs from that of African-Americans (60 years). In addition, between 200,000 and 250,000 surgical procedures (TURP) are performed annually in the United States. TURP is a common operation performed in older men and accounts for an immense cost to the American health care system each year.

ETIOLOGY AND PATHOGENESIS. Increasing age and a normal androgen-related hormonal axis (presence of the testes) are the most well known etiologic risk factors for the development of BPH. With the exception of a lower prevalence of both microscopic and macroscopic evidence of BPH in the Asian population, no documented racial differences in the prevalence of BPH have been detected. Other studies investigating the relationship between smoking, obesity, alcohol consumption, liver dysfunction, and vasectomy have likewise failed to reveal clear risk factors accounting for the high prevalence of BPH. In addition, it has been well documented that androgens do not initiate the development of BPH. Yet the development and maintenance of BPH require the presence of both testosterone and dihydrotestosterone during puberty and aging. Consequently, great interest has been directed at identifying the role of androgens in the etiology of BPH. Several key elements strongly support the hypothesis that the development and passive maintenance of BPH in men are under profound endocrine control: (1) BPH is not seen either histologically or microscopically in men castrated before puberty, (2) regression of both pathologic and clinical symptoms of BPH has been documented following castration, (3) lack of prostate development is seen in men with 5α-reductase deficiency, and (4) animal studies (canine) have demonstrated that histologic BPH can be produced with hormonal treatment. Unlike other androgen-dependent organs, the prostate maintains its ability to respond to testicular androgens throughout life. This property may in part be due to induction of increased androgen receptor levels associated with aging or to increased sensitivity of the receptors to androgens with aging. In addition, age-related increases in estrogen (aromatized from testosterone) may support further prostatic growth or a decrease in cell death within the aging prostate. Present medical approaches to the management of BPH are focused on these hormonal relationships. In addition, substantial evidence now suggests that BPH has an inheritable genetic component. An individual in whom BPH develops at a young age (<55 years), who has a large prostate, and who has a first-degree male relative requiring surgery for significant BPH has a 4.2-fold increased risk of significant BPH requiring surgery within his lifetime. Segregation analysis has also demonstrated an autosomal dominant inheritance pattern for familial BPH, with about 9% of men undergoing prostatectomy before age 60 predicted to have this familial risk. However, specific genetic alterations in familial BPH remain to be elucidated.

CLINICAL MANIFESTATIONS. The symptom complex often referred to as BPH can be better characterized as lower urinary tract symptoms. The majority of initial lower urinary tract symptoms are the result of secondary effects seen in the urethra, the bladder, and the kidneys. These symptoms can be arbitrarily divided into obstructive and irritative. *Obstructive symptoms* consist of abdominal straining, intermittency, post-void dribbling, weak stream, hesitancy, and sensations of incomplete bladder emptying. *Irritative symptoms* consist of dysuria, nocturia, urgency, frequency, and possibly, urge incontinence. These symptoms are by no means exclusive to either BPH or lower urinary tract sources, and non-prostatic causes of these symptoms must be excluded with a detailed history, physical examination, and urinalysis.

INITIAL EVALUATION AND DIFFERENTIAL DIAGNOSIS. In general, it is not very difficult to establish the diagnosis of BPH or lower urinary tract symptoms with a detailed medical history, physical examination, and urinalysis. The medical history should focus on the urinary tract, previous pelvic surgical procedures, and general health issues such as hypertension and diabetes. The physical examination should consist of a careful DRE and examination of the external genitalia. The estimated size of the prostate by DRE should be considered when deciding on the necessity or type of treatment if administration of a 5α-reductase inhibitor is contemplated. For the most part, however, prostatic size correlates poorly with the degree of urinary obstruction, treatment outcome, and degree of symptom severity in the population of older men in whom these symptoms develop. Hyperplasia of the prostate usually produces a smooth, broad, firm, and elastic enlargement of the prostate. Some patients have prostatic enlargement of the intravesical median lobe portion only, which is not palpable by standard DRE. Urinalysis (both the dipstick test and microscopic examination of spun sediment) is used to rule out urinary tract infection and hematuria that might suggest non–lower urinary tract pathology such as bladder infection, a bladder stone, or carcinoma. Men with severe irritative symptoms should have urine cytologic studies performed to rule out carcinoma in situ of the bladder. In addition to urinalysis, a urine culture and serum creatinine measurement should be performed to screen for infection and renal insufficiency, respectively. Elevated serum creatinine is an indication for imaging studies such as ultrasound or intravenous urography to evaluate the upper urinary tract. Serum PSA assay should also be offered to men older than 50 years after the risks and benefits associated with early detection of prostate cancer have been discussed. Men at high risk for carcinoma of the prostate (positive family history and African-American race) should be offered a serum PSA assay beginning at age 40. Finally, a symptom assessment score such as the Internal Prostate Symptom Score (IPSS) or the American Urological Association Symptom Index is recommended as a "yardstick" to compare baseline lower urinary tract symptom severity with symptom severity after therapy. In general, symptoms (decreased force of stream, nocturia, urgency, frequency, incomplete emptying, hesitancy, and intermittency graded from 0 to 5) are summed and classified as mild (0 to 7), moderate (8 to 19), or severe (20 to 35). Cystourethroscopy should be reserved for the evaluation of men in whom surgical therapy is contemplated or for those who have hematuria. Cystoscopic examination can confirm the presence of bladder neck obstruction, bladder neck contracture, and the degree of detrusor muscle hypertrophy and exclude the presence of concomitant bladder tumors. In addition, cystourethroscopy can confirm prostatic size and shape before therapeutic planning. Included in the differential diagnosis of lower urinary tract symptoms are conditions such as bladder neck contracture, carcinoma of the prostate, bladder calculus, carcinoma of the bladder, chronic and acute prostatitis, prostatodynia, neurogenic bladder, and urethral stricture.

TREATMENT AND PROGNOSIS. At present, treatment of BPH can be divided into four categories: (1) watchful waiting or deferred therapy, (2) medical management, (3) minimally invasive techniques, and (4) surgical prostatectomy. Recommendations regarding the optimal form of therapy for lower urinary tract symptoms should be determined on the basis of symptom severity, the efficacy and durability of the therapy, and the morbidity associated with treatment. For example, TURP is the most efficacious therapy for BPH at present. However, TURP is associated with the highest morbidity. Conversely, medical therapy is a somewhat less efficacious mode of therapy for BPH but has less associated morbidity. Present indications for surgical intervention include urinary retention, azotemia with hydronephrosis, severe hematuria, recurrent urinary tract infection secondary to high post-void residuals, bladder calculi, overflow incontinence, and severe symptoms (IPSS: 20 to 35). Medical therapies for BPH include phytotherapy (saw palmetto), α-adrenergic antagonists (e.g., prazosin, 1 mg at bedtime; terazosin [Hytrin], 5 to 10 mg at bedtime; doxazosin [Cardura], 4 to 8 mg at bedtime; or tamsulosin [Flomax], 0.4 mg g/day), or 5α-reductase inhibition (finasteride [Proscar], 5 mg/day). Minimally invasive techniques include hyperthermia, microwave therapy, needle ablation techniques, laser prostatectomy, and transurethral electrovaporization. Standard surgical techniques include TURP, transurethral incision of the prostate, and for markedly enlarged prostates (>80 g), open simple retropubic or suprapubic prostatectomy. A majority of men are now being seen early in the evolution of the disease, and symptoms are mild to moderate. Many men, curious about the natural history of the disease, can be reassured that watchful waiting or deferred therapy is a strong therapeutic option in that they can expect little change in their symptoms for many years. With this in mind, it is advisable to examine men periodically to observe the natural history of the disease and anticipate the development of strong indications for intervention.

Bluestein DL, Oesterling JE: Hormonal therapy in the management of benign prostatic hyperplasia. In Lepor H, Lawson RK (eds): Prostate Diseases. Philadelphia, WB Saunders, 1993, pp 183–198. A concise discussion of the hormonal and endocrine factors involved in the management of benign prostatic hyperplasia.

McConnell JD: Epidemiology, etiology, pathophysiology, and diagnosis of benign prostatic hyperplasia. In Walsh PC, Retik AB, Vaughan ED, Wein AJ (eds): Campbell's Urology, 7th ed. Philadelphia, WB Saunders, 1998, pp 1429–1452. A comprehensive review of all aspects relative to the etiology, clinical evaluation, and epidemiology of benign prostatic hyperplasia.

Sanda MG, Beaty TH, Stutzman RE, et al: Genetic susceptibility of benign prostatic hyperplasia. J Urol 152:115, 1994. A discussion of recent evidence documenting genetic susceptibility and familial predisposition to benign prostatic hyperplasia.

PROSTATITIS

Prostatitis, which can be defined as a condition associated with prostatic inflammation, is one of the most common yet most imprecise diagnoses in all of urology. National Health Center for Health Statistics studies have demonstrated that 25% of all visits to urologists are associated with prostatitis. The medical manifestations of prostatitis range from asymptomatic to acute life-threatening symptoms. The hallmark of diagnosis centers on the microbiologic and microscopic examination of prostatic fluid. Prostatitis can be classified into several forms: (1) acute and chronic bacterial prostatitis, (2) non-bacterial prostatitis, and (3) prostatodynia.

ETIOLOGY AND PATHOGENESIS. Bacterial prostatitis is caused by organisms similar to those most frequently associated with urinary tract infections. Escherichia coli and other members of the family Enterobacteriaceae are the typical causative agents in older men. Prostatitis infections involving other organisms (e.g., Pseudomonas and Enterococcus faecalis), as well as infections involving two or more different strains or classes of microorganism(s), are less common. Recent data have also suggested that unprotected anorectal insertive intercourse can cause prostatitis or acute epididymitis from previously unidentified coliform bacteria. The routes of infection leading to bacterial prostatitis include (1) ascending urethral infection resulting from meatal inoculation during sexual relations, (2) reflux of infected urine into prostatic ducts entering into the posterior urethra, (3) invasion of colonic bacteria through either direct extension or lymphatic spread, and (4) hematogenous seeding of prostatic tissue. Efforts to identify unusual pathogens (e.g., anaerobic bacteria, Mycoplasma, Ureaplasma, viruses, or other protozoans) as a cause of non-bacterial prostatitis have been uniformly unsuccessful. The most controversial agent thought to be associated with non-bacterial prostatitis is Chlamydia trachomatis. Although initially believed to play a major role in the development of prostatitis, C. trachomatis has recently been shown with advanced molecular techniques to play an insignificant role in the etiology of prostatitis.

CLINICAL MANIFESTATIONS, DIAGNOSIS, AND DIFFERENTIAL DIAGNOSIS. Much of the confusion concerning the etiology, diagnosis, and classification of prostatitis may be attributed to imprecise methods of diagnosis. Most male patients seeing a physician for genitourinary complaints often attribute their multiple genitourinary difficulties to the prostate. For the most part, the medical history (e.g., fever, chills, perineal pain) and physical findings (e.g., tender prostate on examination) do not significantly aid in the differential diagnosis of the type of prostatitis. In addition, isolated cultures of urine offer little diagnostic assistance. Since its introduction in 1968 by Meares and Stamey, the two most useful tools for creating a differential diagnosis of prostatitis have been microbiologic and microscopic examination of expressed prostatic secretions (EPSs) and quantitative bacterial localization cultures.

Collection of segmented specimens, immediate culturing after collection, and the application of bacteriologic techniques capable of quantifying small numbers of bacteria are mandatory for the proper differential diagnosis of bacterial prostatitis from non-bacterial prostatitis. To perform this technique, sequential quantitative bacteriologic cultures of the urethra, bladder urine, and prostatic secretion must be aseptically obtained. Figure 118–1 demonstrates the segmental collection technique for localizing lower urinary tract infections in a male. In summary, the voided urine is partitioned into urethral (VB-1—voided bladder 1, which represents the first 5 to 10 mL of voided urine), bladder (VB-2—voided bladder 2 or midstream urine collection), and post-prostatic massage urine collection (VB-3—voided bladder 3, the first voided 10 mL following prostatic massage). In addition, collection and culture of EPS are useful when the VB-1 and VB-3 urine specimens yield equivalent

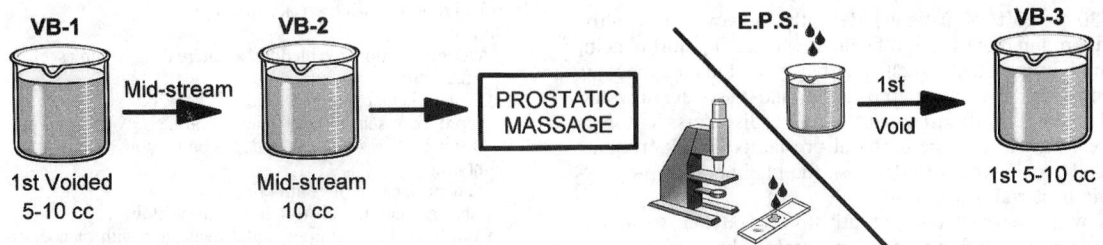

FIGURE 118–1 ■ Segmental culture technique for localizing urinary infections in the male to the urethra or the prostate. (Modified from Meares EM, Stamey TA: Bacteriologic localization of patterns in bacterial prostatitis and urethritis. Invest Urol 5:492, 1968, Williams & Wilkins Co., with permission.)

bacterial counts. The presence of more than 20 white blood cells per high-power field in the EPS is abnormal and usually suggestive of an inflammatory process. In addition, it is not uncommon to see lipid-laden macrophages (oval fat bodies) within the EPS on microscopic examination. All specimens (VB-1, VB-2, VB-3, and EPS) must be quantitatively cultured onto both blood and either eosin–methylene blue or MacConkey agar plates. Interpretation of these culture results depends heavily on the number of bacteria in each specimen. To avoid the necessity for repeat collection of samples, it is advisable to alert the microbiology laboratory regarding the need for quantitative colony counts. The diagnosis of bacterial prostatitis is confirmed when the quantitative bacterial colony counts of the prostatic secretion (EPS and VB-3) significantly exceed those of the urethral (VB-1) and bladder (VB-2) specimens by at least 1 logarithm. When the bacterial counts in the urethral specimen (VB-1) exceed those of either the EPS or the VB-3 specimen, bacterial urethritis is present. High bacterial counts in the VB-2 (bladder) specimen are indicative of a urinary tract infection that must be treated with an antibacterial agent such as nitrofurantoin or penicillin before repeat analysis. These microscopic and microbiologic diagnostic maneuvers can further aid in the classification of prostatitis into four categories: (1) acute bacterial prostatitis, (2) chronic bacterial prostatitis, (3) non-bacterial prostatitis, and (4) prostatodynia.

ACUTE BACTERIAL PROSTATITIS. Acute bacterial prostatitis is an acute febrile illness characterized by chills, low back and perineal pain, urinary urgency and frequency, voiding symptoms such as nocturia and dysuria, and often bladder outlet obstruction. Rectal examination, although usually disclosing a markedly tender prostate that is swollen, firm, and warm, is not recommended because of the possibility of inducing sepsis. The infecting pathogen can usually be identified simply through culture of the voided urine. In addition, transurethral instrumentation and catheterization should be avoided in the acute stages of bacterial prostatitis. When complete urinary retention is present, a catheter should be placed for temporary diversion. Acute bacterial prostatitis often responds dramatically to intravenous antibiotic therapy.

CHRONIC BACTERIAL PROSTATITIS. Chronic bacterial prostatitis is a non-acute infection of the prostate usually caused by one or more specific bacteria similar to those seen in acute bacterial prostatitis. The course of chronic bacterial prostatitis is usually that of a relapsing, recurring urinary tract infection in men. The initial symptoms are similar but less dramatic than those seen in acute bacterial prostatitis and include irritative as well as obstructive voiding symptoms. The discomfort associated with chronic bacterial prostatitis can often be debilitating and focuses around the suprapubic, perineal, lower sacral, scrotal, and penile area. DRE often discloses no specific or characteristic finding. The diagnosis is usually based on quantitative bacterial localization cultures as previously described. EPS culture often identifies the offending microorganism, and treatment usually consists of an extended course of antibiotics. Men who fail several extended courses of antibiotic therapy (1 to 2 months) for chronic bacterial prostatitis may rarely be candidates for TURP. Transurethral prostatectomy is only curative if the infectious etiology (stone or tissue) has been completely removed. Reinfection of the prostate and reappearance of symptoms often occur after surgery.

NON-BACTERIAL PROSTATITIS/PROSTATODYNIA. Non-bacterial prostatitis/prostatodynia is an inflammatory process of the prostate of indeterminate cause. Non-bacterial prostatitis is the most common of the prostatitis syndromes, yet its etiology remains unknown. Although men with non-bacterial prostatitis have increased numbers of inflammatory cells in their prostatic secretions, no causative infectious agent can usually be found by culture or other means. Earlier reports have classified prostatodynia as a "special type" of non-bacterial prostatitis; however, the symptoms, differential diagnosis, and therapy for both entities are similar. As early as 1986, Meares and colleagues were the first to suggest that there is no reason to distinguish prostatodynia from non-bacterial prostatitis. Furthermore, their work with video-urodynamics has recently revealed similar functional findings in men with prostatodynia and men with non-bacterial prostatitis. Typically, the symptoms, physical findings, and microscopic and microbiologic findings of segmented cultures of the lower urinary tract are similar for both of these disease entities. Patients with non-bacterial prostatitis, however, do not have a history of a documented urinary tract infection. The differential diagnosis of non-bacterial prostatitis and prostatodynia requires the exclusion of fungal, anaerobic bacterial, trichomonal, and viral causative agents as the etiology of the symptoms. One pathophysiologic hypothesis explaining the symptoms thought to be due to non-bacterial prostatitis/prostatodynia is smooth muscle spasm of the bladder neck and prostatic urethra. These spasms elevate pressure in the prostatic urethra and thereby result in intraprostatic and ejaculatory duct urinary reflux causing chemical prostatitis and the ensuing symptom complex. Regardless of the actual etiology of the non-bacterial prostatitis/prostatodynia complex, the symptoms are most likely the result of failure of the internal urinary sphincter to relax and failure of the pelvic floor striated musculature to function properly, either alone or in combination. Elevated prostatic urethral pressures and intraprostatic urinary reflux may initiate an inflammatory response and induce a chemical irritation within the prostatic ducts.

The majority of men with significant lower urinary tract symptoms require urologic evaluation. The differential diagnosis of men with lower urinary tract irritative symptoms should include consideration of transitional cell carcinoma, carcinoma in situ, or the presence of calculi in the bladder. Examination of the urethra for urethral stricture disease and urethral carcinoma may also need to be performed. Cystoscopic examination of the lower urinary tract may rule out prostatic obstruction as a cause of the symptoms. Other differential diagnoses include perirectal abscess, neurogenic bladder, diabetes mellitus, detrusor-sphincter dyssynergia, and both self-inflicted and iatrogenic trauma. Because the symptoms of men with non-bacterial prostatitis are similar to those with flat "in situ" carcinoma of the bladder, a urinary cytology study and cystoscopic examination should be routinely performed to exclude the presence of malignancy.

TREATMENT. Both acute and chronic bacterial prostatitis is treated with antibacterial agents routinely. The choice of antibacterial agent is based on bacterial sensitivities and factors that limit diffusion into prostatic fluid. Theoretic factors limiting diffusion into prostatic fluid include lipid solubility, pKa, protein binding, and molecular size and molecule shape. Traditional antibiotics such as trimethoprim, which fulfills all theoretic criteria, has been useful for the majority of patients with prostatitis in the past. The usual dosage is one double-strength tablet (160 mg trimethoprim, 800 mg sulfamethoxazole orally twice daily). The optimal duration of therapy remains uncertain, and this treatment produces a cure in approximately 30 to 40% of patients. Recently, however, the introduction of fluoroquinolones (ciprofloxacin, enoxacin, norfloxacin, and ofloxacin) has provided excellent efficacy in the treatment of both acute and chronic bacterial prostatitis, and they are now the antibiotics of choice for the treatment of these disorders. The recommended treatment of chronic bacterial prostatitis is a fluoroquinolone twice daily for 6 weeks to decrease the likelihood of progression to chronic bacterial disease.

In patients with non-bacterial prostatitis/prostatodynia, treatment with an α-adrenergic blocking agent may relax the bladder neck and prostate and improve voiding dysfunction, thus eliminating the urinary reflux and improving the symptoms associated with this complex. Once-a-day dosing of an α-adrenergic agent provides few adverse side effects. In addition, counseling the patient about the non-infectious and non-contagious nature of this disease is important. Dietary restrictions are unnecessary unless offending foods and beverages seem to cause or aggravate the symptoms. Prostatic massage is not therapeutic and is not recommended. Acute bouts of pain and discomfort can be treated with short courses of anti-inflammatory agents. Severe irritative bladder dysfunction will often respond to anticholinergic drugs. Men responding poorly to the medical management of non-bacterial prostatitis/prostatodynia should be referred to a psychologist or psychiatrist for stress management.

Meares EM Jr: Prostatitis and related disorders. *In* Walsh PC, Retik AB, Vaughan ED, Wein AJ (eds): Campbell's Urology, 7th ed. Philadelphia, WB Saunders, 1998, pp 615–630. *A comprehensive evaluation and review of the basic clinical and surgical aspects dealing with the diagnosis and management of prostatitis and its related disorders.*

119 URINARY INCONTINENCE

Joseph G. Ouslander

DEFINITION AND SCOPE OF THE PROBLEM. Urinary incontinence is defined as involuntary loss of urine of sufficient severity to be a health and/or social problem. Although it is commonly hidden and not discussed with health professionals, urinary incontinence is a prevalent, morbid, and expensive condition. Up to half of young and middle-aged women experience urinary incontinence, often in association with childbirth. Urinary incontinence is a common manifestation of benign and malignant prostate enlargement in middle-aged and older men. The prevalence and incidence of urinary incontinence are higher in women and increase with age. Among relatively healthy community-dwelling adults 60 years and older, about one third of women and close to 20% of men have some degree of urinary incontinence. Close to 10% of both sexes have frequent (at least weekly) episodes and/or use protective padding. The prevalence is close to 40% in hospitalized older adults and is as high as 70 to 80% in long-term care institutions.

Urinary incontinence causes considerable physical and psychosocial morbidity and health care costs. The condition is uncomfortable and predisposes to skin problems and falls in older patients rushing to the bathroom. It is a social stigma and can lead to embarrassment, isolation, and depression. Urinary incontinence is commonly an important precipitating factor in the decision to enter a long-term care facility. The annual health care costs of managing urinary incontinence and its complications have been estimated to be well over $10 billion.

PATHOGENESIS. Continence requires effective lower urinary tract functioning; adequate mobility, dexterity, cognition, and motivation to be continent; and absence of environmental and iatrogenic barriers (Table 119–1). From a lower urinary tract standpoint, incontinence results from (1) failure to store urine because of bladder overactivity and/or low urethral resistance, (2) failure to empty the bladder because of anatomic or physiologic obstruction and/or inadequate bladder contractility, or (3) a combination of these factors.

Aging per se does not cause urinary incontinence, but age-related

Table 119–1 ■ REQUIREMENTS FOR CONTINENCE

1. Effective lower urinary tract function
   Storage
   　Accommodation by bladder of increasing volumes of urine under low
   　　pressure
   　Closed bladder outlet
   　Appropriate sensation of bladder fullness
   　Absence of involuntary bladder contractions
   Emptying
   　Bladder capable of contraction
   　Lack of anatomic obstruction to urine flow
   　Coordinated lowering of outlet resistance with bladder contractions
2. Adequate mobility and dexterity to use toilet or toilet substitute and to
   manage clothing
3. Adequate cognitive function to recognize toileting needs and to find a
   toilet or toilet substitute
4. Motivation to be continent
5. Absence of environmental and iatrogenic barriers such as inaccessible
   toilets or toilet substitutes, unavailable caregivers, or drug side effects

From Kane RL, Ouslander JG, Abrass IB: Essentials of Clinical Geriatrics, 4th ed. New York, McGraw-Hill, 1998. Copyright © by McGraw-Hill, Inc. Used by permission of McGraw-Hill Book Company.

changes can predispose to it. Among women, urethral resistance declines because of diminished estrogen effects and weakened periurethral and pelvic muscles. Among men, urethral resistance increases and the urine flow rate decreases in association with prostatic enlargement. In both sexes the bladder tends to become overactive and is affected by involuntary detrusor contractions (more so in men than women). At the same time, in many older individuals impaired bladder contractility develops and can result in a condition termed "DHIC" (detrusor hyperactivity with impaired contractility). Finally, age-related declines in renal concentrating mechanisms and loss of the normal diurnal rhythm of arginine vasopressin can predispose older patients to nocturnal polyuria and incontinence.

Several potentially reversible factors may cause or contribute to urinary incontinence, especially in geriatric patients (Table 119–2). The common reversible factors can be remembered by the mnemonic "DRIP" (delirium; restricted mobility; retention; infection, inflammation, impaction; and polyuria and pharmaceuticals).

CLINICAL MANIFESTATIONS. Urinary incontinence may have a sudden onset. In geriatric patients a sudden onset is commonly associated with an acute medical illness and/or one or more potentially reversible factors (see Table 119–2). More commonly, urinary incontinence is a chronic problem and patients often wait years after its onset before discussing it with a health professional. For this reason, it is helpful to periodically ask screening questions specifically about bladder control problems.

Persistent types of urinary incontinence can be categorized into four basic types (Table 119–3). *Stress* incontinence is far more common in females than males, among whom it occurs only after sphincter damage from surgery or radiation. *Urge* incontinence is the most common and bothersome symptomatic type in the geriatric population and is usually associated with other symptoms of bladder overactivity such as daytime frequency (voiding every 2 hours or more often) and nocturia (voiding two or more times during normal sleeping hours). The symptoms and signs of *overflow* incontinence are non-specific and may mimic those of the stress and urge types. Men, diabetics, and patients with neurologic disorders are at highest risk for this type of urinary incontinence. *Functional* incontinence refers to patients whose involuntary urine loss is predominately related to impaired mobility and/or cognition. These basic types of urinary incontinence commonly coexist. For example, a substantial proportion of women have symptoms of *both* urge and stress incontinence (generally referred to as a "*mixed*" type). Frail geriatric patients commonly have urge incontinence with bladder overactivity, as well as functional impairments that contribute to their incontinence problem.

DIAGNOSIS. The basic evaluation of incontinent patients includes a focused history (which can be enhanced by a voiding diary), a targeted physical examination, urinalysis, and a post-void residual determination (Table 119–4). Post-void residual determination is essential in almost all patients because the symptoms of overflow incontinence are non-specific and the physical examination alone is not sensitive in detecting significant urinary retention

Table 119-2 ■ REVERSIBLE CONDITIONS THAT CAUSE OR CONTRIBUTE TO URINARY INCONTINENCE

CONDITION	MANAGEMENT
Conditions Affecting the Lower Urinary Tract	
Urinary tract infection (symptomatic with frequency, urgency, dysuria, etc.)	Antimicrobial therapy
Atrophic vaginitis/urethritis	Topical estrogen
Post-prostatectomy, postpartum	Behavioral interventions. Further evaluation if condition does not resolve over a few months
Stool impaction	Disimpaction; appropriate use of stool softeners, bulk-forming agents, and laxatives if necessary; high fiber intake; adequate exercise and fluid intake
Drug Side Effects	
Diuretics	Discontinue or change therapy if clinically appropriate. Dosage reduction or modification (e.g., flexible scheduling of rapid-acting diuretics) may also help
Anticholinergics	
α-Adrenergic agents	
Psychotropics	
Narcotics	
Increased Urine Production	
Metabolic (hyperglycemia, hypercalcemia)	Better control of diabetes mellitus. Therapy for hypercalcemia depends on the underlying cause
Excess fluid intake	Reduction in intake of caffeinated beverages
Volume overload	
Venous insufficiency with edema	Support stockings
	Leg elevation
	Sodium restriction
	Diuretic therapy
Congestive heart failure	Medical therapy
Impaired Ability or Willingness to Reach a Toilet	
Delirium	Diagnosis and treatment of underlying cause(s) of acute confusional state
Chronic illness, injury, or restraint that interferes with mobility	Regular toileting
	Environmental alterations (e.g., bedside commode, urinal)
Psychological	Pharmacologic and/or non-pharmacologic treatment

From Kane RL, Ouslander JG, Abrass IB: Essentials of Clinical Geriatrics, 4th ed. New York, McGraw-Hill, 1998. Copyright © by McGraw-Hill, Inc. Used by permission of McGraw-Hill Book Company

(i.e., post-void residual greater than 200 mL). A portable ultrasound device is available that can non-invasively provide an accurate estimate of bladder volume. The objectives of this basic evaluation are to (1) identify potentially reversible factors (see Table 119-1); (2) determine, if possible, the most likely type(s) and underlying cause(s) (see Table 119-2); and (3) identify patients who may require further evaluation.

Selected patients may benefit from one or more of the additional diagnostic procedures listed in Table 119-4. For example, patients with sterile hematuria should be considered for urine cytology and cystoscopy. Women with severe pelvic prolapse should be referred to a gynecologist for consideration of pessary placement or surgery. Patients with significant urinary retention, those with a neurologic disorder that may underlie the incontinence, and patients who fail initial treatment interventions should be considered for urodynamic evaluation. The urodynamic tests listed in Table 119-4 can assist in determining the precise underlying lower urinary tract pathophysiology and in targeting specific treatment based on the findings.

TREATMENT. The most common method of managing urinary incontinence is adult diapers and pads. Although many of these products are well designed and helpful, they are non-specific and expensive. Many patients cannot afford these products and design their own, often poorly hygienic solutions. Use of adult diapers and pads may serve to simply hide a curable or potentially serious problem or foster dependency in frail geriatric patients. Thus these products should generally be used as adjuncts to more specific interventions, and patients should be encouraged to undergo at least a basic evaluation of their condition.

Reversible factors identified by the basic evaluation outlined above should be treated (see Table 119-1). In some patients, the urinary incontinence will resolve after treating one or more of these factors. Primary therapies for persistent types of urinary incontinence are listed in Table 119-3. A variety of behavioral therapies have been shown in randomized, controlled clinical trials to be highly effective for targeted patients. Functional, motivated patients with stress, urge, and mixed incontinence generally respond well to behavioral interventions. Such interventions include education, self-monitoring with a voiding diary, modifications of fluid intake, various bladder training techniques (such as timed voiding and strategies to manage urgency), and pelvic muscle exercises. Many patients have difficulty isolating the appropriate pelvic muscles and benefit from adjunctive techniques such as biofeedback (using surface electromyography of sphincteric and abdominal muscles),

Table 119-3 ■ BASIC TYPES AND CAUSES OF PERSISTENT URINARY INCONTINENCE

TYPE	CLINICAL MANIFESTATIONS	COMMON CAUSES	PRIMARY TREATMENTS
Stress	Involuntary loss of urine (usually small amounts) with increases in intra-abdominal pressure (e.g., cough, laugh, exercise)	Weakness of pelvic floor musculature and urethral hypermobility Bladder outlet or urethral sphincter weakness	Pelvic muscle exercises and other behavioral interventions. α-Adrenergic agonists (phenylpropanolamine, 75 mg bid) Periurethral injections Surgical bladder neck suspension or sling
Urge	Leakage of urine (variable but often larger volumes) because of inability to delay voiding after sensation of bladder fullness is perceived	Detrusor overactivity, isolated or associated with one or more of the following: Local genitourinary condition such as tumors, stones, diverticuli, or outflow obstruction CNS disorders such as stroke, dementia, parkinsonism, spinal cord injury	Bladder training and other behavioral interventions Bladder relaxants (tolterodine, 2 mg bid; other anticholinergics)
Overflow	Leakage of urine (usually small amounts without warning) resulting from mechanical forces on an overdistended bladder or from other effects of urinary retention on bladder and sphincter function	Anatomic obstruction by prostate, stricture, cystocele Acontractile bladder associated with diabetes mellitus or spinal cord injury Neurogenic (detrusor-sphincter dyssynergy), associated with multiple sclerosis and other suprasacral spinal cord lesions	Surgical removal of obstruction Intermittent or chronic catherization
Functional	Urinary accidents associated with inability to toilet because of impairment of cognitive and/or physical functioning, psychological unwillingness, or environmental barriers	Severe dementia and other neurologic disorders Psychological factors such as depression and hostility	Prompted voiding and other behavioral intervention Absorbent padding Drug treatment for bladder overactivity (selected patients)

From Kane RL, Ouslander JG, Abrass IB: Essentials of Clinical Geriatrics, 4th ed. New York, McGraw-Hill, 1998. Copyright © by McGraw-Hill, Inc. Used by permission of McGraw-Hill Book Company.

Table 119–4 ■ COMPONENTS OF THE DIAGNOSTIC
EVALUATION OF PERSISTENT URINARY INCONTINENCE

All Patients
History, including bladder record or voiding diary
Physical examination
Urinalysis
Post-void residual determination
*Selected Patients**
Laboratory studies
   Urine culture
   Urine cytology
   Blood glucose, calcium
   Renal function tests
   Renal ultrasound
Gynecologic evaluation
Urologic evaluation
Cystourethroscopy
Urodynamic tests
   Simple
      Observation of voiding
      Cough test for stress incontinence
      Simple (single-channel) cystometry
   Complex
      Urine flowmetry
      Multichannel cystometrogram
      Pressure-flow study
      Leak point pressure
      Urethral pressure profilometry
      Sphincter electromyography
      Videourodynamics

*See the text.
From Kane RL, Ouslander JG, Abrass IB: Essentials of Clinical Geriatrics, 4th ed. New York, McGraw-Hill, 1998. Copyright © by McGraw-Hill, Inc. Used by permission of McGraw-Hill Book Company.

vaginal weights, and electrical stimulation (which can both help identify and exercise pelvic muscles and help inhibit bladder activity, depending on the frequency of the stimulus). For some mobility and/or cognitively impaired patients in long-term care institutions and at home, prompted voiding (or some other form of systematic toileting assistance) can be highly effective in managing urinary incontinence during the daytime.

Pharmacologic treatment is also effective and may be combined with behavioral interventions. For stress incontinence in women, α-adrenergic medications enhance the contraction of periurethral smooth muscle. These drugs may be combined with estrogen. Estrogen alone is not effective for stress incontinence, and topical estrogen appears to be more effective than oral estrogen for lower urinary tract symptoms. Bladder relaxant medications can be effec-

tive in managing urge incontinence, but they are often limited by their anticholinergic side effects (especially dry mouth). Tolterodine, the newest approved bladder relaxant, may have fewer bothersome side effects than other anticholinergics. α-Adrenergic blockers have been shown to improve irritative voiding symptoms, including frequency and urgency, in men with prostatic enlargement. New approaches to the pharmacologic management of urge incontinence, including alternative delivery systems and new classes of drugs, are under development. Pharmacologic treatment of an underactive bladder associated with chronic urinary retention and overflow incontinence is not generally effective.

Surgical treatment can be highly effective in women with stress incontinence, at least over a 1- to 5-year period. Women with intrinsic sphincter weakness (as opposed to urethral hypermobility) may benefit from periurethral injections of collagen.

PREVENTION. No strategies have proved effective in preventing urinary incontinence. Three approaches may, however, be of some benefit and are worthy of brief consideration. First, general education about bladder health and the behavioral and dietary factors that can affect it can help people understand that urinary incontinence and related urinary problems are not normal and that when such symptoms do occur, they should seek evaluation and treatment. Second, pelvic muscle exercises may be an effective preventive measure. Whether patients will comply and the long-term effectiveness of this intervention are currently under investigation. Finally, estrogen replacement for the prevention of osteoporosis, heart disease, and perhaps Alzheimer's disease may also have a preventive effect on the development of incontinence. Analysis of data from large-scale trials of estrogen therapy in postmenopausal women should shed some light on this issue in the future.

Abrams P, Wein AJ (eds): The overactive bladder. Basic Science to Clinical Management Consensus Conference. Urology 50(Suppl. 6A), 1997. *State-of-the-art symposium on the pathophysiology and management of the overactive bladder.*
Elbadawi A, Yalla SV, Resnick: Structural basis of geriatric voiding dysfunction. I. Methods of a prospective ultrastructural/urodynamic study and an overview of the findings. J Urol 150:1650, 1993. *One of a series of elegant studies that relate the basic pathology of the bladder to clinical and urodynamic characteristics of incontinent older patients.*
Fantl JA, et al: Urinary Incontinence in Adults: Acute and Chronic Management. Clinical Practice Guidelines No. 2, 1996 Update. Rockville, MD, US Department of Health and Human Services, Public Health Service, Agency for Health Care Policy and Research, AHCPR Publication No. 96-0682, 1996. *An evidence-based guideline that includes a diagnostic algorithm and treatment guidelines.*
Kane RL, Ouslander JG, Abrass IB: Essentials of Clinical Geriatrics, 4th ed. New York, McGraw-Hill, 1998. *Chapter 7 of this text is a comprehensive review of urinary incontinence in the geriatric population. The chapter contains numerous tables, figures, and relevant references.*
Ouslander JG (ed): Aging and the lower urinary tract. Am J Med Sci, October 1997. *Comprehensive series of articles reviewing aging and the lower urinary tract. Several of the articles provide specific information on the diagnosis and management of urinary incontinence.*
Ouslander JG, Schnelle JF: Incontinence in the nursing home. Ann Intern Med 122: 438, 1995. *Comprehensive review of the etiology and management of urinary incontinence in the setting in which it is most prevalent.*

PART XI

GASTROINTESTINAL DISEASES

120 APPROACH TO THE PATIENT WITH GASTROINTESTINAL DISEASE

Don W. Powell

EPIDEMIOLOGY

Diseases of the gastrointestinal tract and liver together account for about 10% of the total burden of illness in the United States. Digestive diseases account for over 50 million office visits annually and nearly 10 million hospital admissions. Colorectal cancer is the second most common cause of cancer in men and women, and, when all of the gastrointestinal organs are combined, gastrointestinal malignancies are the most common of any organ system. As a group, gastrointestinal diseases probably cost the American public up to $100 billion dollars per year, and the cost of diagnosis and management of gastrointestinal diseases consumes up to one fourth of a managed-care organization's capitation payment to the primary care physician. Finally, gastrointestinal diseases as a group account for approximately 10% of all deaths each year. Thus, the practicing physician must understand the various functional and anatomic diseases of the gastrointestinal tract and provide cost-effective and successful management.

OVERVIEW OF THE GASTROINTESTINAL TRACT

The major function of the gastrointestinal tract is to process and absorb nutrients while food moves physically from mouth to colon, where non-absorbable wastes are stored for periodic elimination. Dysfunction of the epithelial absorptive process and of the smooth muscle contractile process causes the major pathologic processes related to the gastrointestinal tract. The epithelial lining of the gastrointestinal tract is a huge surface area, greater than that of a tennis court; it interacts with the external environment's food, water, and xenobiotics and also with the intestinal microflora. The epithelium allows the absorption of fluid, electrolytes, and nutrients in health and the secretion of huge volumes of fluid and electrolytes in disease. The rapid turnover of the epithelial cells, which have a life span of 3 to 7 days, allows environmental interaction with genes that may lead to the development of neoplasia. The common diseases affecting the muscular layers are disorders of integrated function controlled by secreted hormones, paracrine mediators, and the enteric nervous system. Disruption of this neuroendocrine control of the gastrointestinal tract is much more likely to cause symptom-complexes (e.g., functional diseases such as irritable bowel syndrome and non-ulcer dyspepsia) than anatomically defined disease.

However, it would be a mistake to view the gastrointestinal tract only as a muscular tube with an epithelial lining. The enteric nervous system contains between 10 and 100 million neurons, a conglomerate equal to the total number in the spinal cord. If the total number of enteroendocrine cells were put together into a single organ, it would probably be the largest endocrine gland in the body. The gastrointestinal tract's immune cells, which make up the gastrointestinal-associated lymphoid system (GALT), constitute the largest immune organ of the body. These three systems allow the smooth integration of the function of this complex organ, but they also represent points of dysfunction, which can cause both local and even systemic disease.

The enteric nervous system is, for all intents and purposes, an independent nervous system. A growing body of evidence suggests that interaction of the sensory nerves with the spinal cord and brain causes functional gastrointestinal disorders. Current lack of understanding of the enteric nervous system may compromise the management of the 15 to 20% of the population who present with irritable bowel syndrome and/or non-ulcer dyspepsia (see Chapter 131).

The enteroendocrine system of the gastrointestinal tract is unique because it responds to intraluminal stimuli as well as to systemic stimuli presented to it from either the nervous system or the blood. The secretions of these endocrine cells not only affect epithelial, smooth muscle and vascular function, but also have poorly understood effects on distal organs such as the liver, pancreas, and brain.

The GALT is part of a common mucosa-associated lymphoid tissue (MALT) that exists also in the lung, the breast, and the genitourinary tract. The major function of the GALT is to recognize the myriad of antigens presented to the gastrointestinal tract, differentiating between those that should be ignored (e.g., the proteins of nutrients and commensal microflora) and those that should excite a major immune response (e.g., the proteins of pathogenic bacteria). The enteric immune system may play a role in systemic autoimmune diseases and in the development of immune tolerance.

CLINICAL APPROACH TO GASTROINTESTINAL DISEASE

The diagnosis of gastrointestinal diseases derives predominantly from the patient's history and, to a lesser extent, from the physician's physical examination. Laboratory tests and imaging studies can provide objective evidence for or against a given disease among those included in the differential diagnosis raised by an accurate and expert history and physical examination. Diagnoses arise out of specific symptoms (e.g., dysphagia) or from pairing gastrointestinal complaints (e.g., diarrhea) with extraintestinal symptoms or physical findings (e.g., the arthritis of inflammatory bowel disease or the flushing of carcinoid syndrome). However, gastrointestinal symptoms arise not only from disease or dysfunction of the gastrointestinal tract but also through the brain-gut axis and blood stream and from dysfunction or disease of other organs, especially the central nervous system (CNS). For example, nausea and vomiting are just as likely to result from stimuli that affect the CNS as from stimuli arising in the gastrointestinal tract.

NAUSEA AND VOMITING. To understand nausea and vomiting, it is first necessary to differentiate these symptoms from closely related phenomena such as hunger, appetite, satiety, and anorexia. Both hunger and appetite refer to the desire to eat. The determinants of *hunger* are usually physiologic mechanisms from the complex interaction between adrenergic receptors in the medial hypothalamus of the CNS and the serotoninergic, dopaminergic, and β-adrenergic receptors in the lateral hypothalamus. *Appetite* is closely related to hunger, but it is thought to be influenced predominantly by the environmental and psychological processes (i.e., the aroma, appearance and taste of food, as well as the patient's mood). *Satiety* refers to the gratification of hunger and appetite, mediated in part by cholecystokinin and bombesin, which appear to act both peripherally through the vagus nerve and centrally in the hypothalamic satiety center. The discovery of the Ob gene and its peptide hormone leptin in adipocytes has improved our understanding of the homeostasis of body mass. Leptin and insulin act on the hypothalamus to inhibit release of anabolic substances such as neuropeptide Y and peptides called orexins that promote feeding and weight gain. Leptin also stimulates release of catabolic substances such as melanocortin and corticotropin-releasing factor, which reduce feeding behavior. *Anorexia* is a clinical symptom characterized by the absence of hunger or appetite. It may be caused by CNS, systemic or gastrointestinal disease, or by emotional processes that initiate functional disorders.

Satiety and anorexia must be differentiated from *nausea*, which is the unpleasant feeling that one is about to vomit, and *vomiting* (or *emesis*), which is the forceful ejection of contents of the upper gut through the mouth. In contrast, *retching* involves coordinated, voluntary muscle activity of the abdomen and thorax—in effect, a forced respiratory inspiration against a closed mouth and glottis without discharge of gastric contents from the mouth. *Regurgitation* is the effortless return of gastric or esophageal contents into the mouth without nausea, and it occurs without spasmodic, abdominal, thoracic, or gastrointestinal muscular contractions. *Rumination* (merycism) is the effortless but purposeful regurgitation of food from the stomach into the mouth, where it is rechewed and reswallowed, often several times during or after a meal.

The coordinated events that allow the process of vomiting (see Chapter 132) begin in the reticular areas of the medulla and include the dorsal vagal complex nuclei, which was formerly called the "vomiting center." More recent investigations indicate that multiple brain stem sites mediate emesis, and there is no single "vomiting center." Indeed, several brain stem nuclei are necessary to integrate the various responses of the gastrointestinal, respiratory, pharyngeal, and somatic systems in the act of vomiting. The brain stem control of nausea and vomiting has sensory input from at least four additional areas: (1) the chemoreceptor trigger zone, (2) the vestibular nucleus mediating input from the inner ear and through the cerebellum; (3) the gastrointestinal tract itself, as well as other viscera within the peritoneal cavity; and (4) the upper cortical regions of the CNS. These four areas, through various neurons and receptors of the serotoninergic (5-HT$_3$), dopaminergic (D$_2$), histaminergic (H$_1$), muscarinic (M$_1$), and vasopressinergic (V$_1$) type, respond to environmental and internal stimuli to signal and then activate the vomiting center(s).

The chemoreceptor trigger zone is in the area postrema in the floor of the fourth ventricle. This area lacks a tight blood-brain barrier, so blood-borne agents can penetrate it. The chemoreceptor trigger zone also receives neural input from the upper centers of the brain and the peripheral nerves, and it responds to certain systemic medications and to metabolic diseases. Motion sickness and inner ear disease, such as Ménière's disease (see Chapter 517), act through the vestibular nucleus, which contains H$_1$ and M$_1$ receptors. The vagus and sympathetic nerves, via the nodosum ganglion and the nucleus tractus solitarius, mediate nausea that arises from gastric irritants such as salicylates or staphylococcal enterotoxin; gastric, small intestinal, colonic, or bile duct distention; and inflammation or ischemia of bowel, liver, pancreas, and peritoneum. Higher cortical centers also may affect the vomiting center and mediate nausea and vomiting induced by intense emotions or stress, as well as the classic anticipatory nausea and vomiting seen with administration of cancer chemotherapy.

To understand the causes of nausea and vomiting, stimuli arising from the CNS must be differentiated from those originating in the gastrointestinal tract. Historical information concerning the duration, precipitation, and pattern of nausea and vomiting as well as the nature of the vomitus is not sufficient; the physician must also seek signs and symptoms of gastrointestinal diseases (e.g., abdominal pain, diarrhea, constipation, or weight loss) and of CNS diseases (e.g., headache, changes in mental status, change in neuromuscular function, symptoms related to the inner ear, drug ingestion, or a history of emotional or environmental stress).

Medications are among the most common causes of nausea and vomiting. Apomorphine, opiates, digitalis, levodopa, bromocriptine, and anticancer drugs act on the chemoreceptor trigger zone. Drugs that frequently cause nausea through other mechanisms include non-steroidal anti-inflammatory drugs, erythromycin, cardiac antiarrhythmic medications, antihypertensive drugs, diuretics, oral antidiabetic agents, oral contraceptives, and gastrointestinal medications such as sulfasalazine. Chemotherapeutic agents most likely to induce vomiting are cisplatin, nitrogen mustard, and dacarbazine. *Gastrointestinal and systemic infections,* both viral and bacterial,

are probably the second most common cause of nausea and vomiting. Infections may be at fault through the release of bacterial enterotoxins or the inflammation initiated by the pathogen. *Obstruction* of the gastrointestinal tract or organs—stomach, small intestine, colon, pancreas, or biliary tract—and ischemia or inflammation of these organs or the liver or peritoneum are the third most common cause. In addition to *labyrinthine disorders* (motion sickness, space sickness, viral labyrinthitis, acoustic tumors, and Ménière's disease), a major CNS cause of nausea and vomiting is diseases that increase intracranial pressure. *Emotional responses* to unpleasant smells or taste and severe psychogenic stress are additional CNS causes. *Metabolic causes* such as uremia, diabetic ketoacidosis, hypercalcemia, hypoxemia, hyperthyroidism, Addison's disease, and radiation therapy cause nausea by stimulating the chemoreceptor trigger zone. The first trimester of *pregnancy* causes vomiting in approximately 70% of pregnant women. *Postoperative nausea and vomiting* complicate up to 40% of surgical operations.

Effective drugs for nausea and vomiting include those that block the major receptors of (1) the area postrema (D$_2$, 5-HT$_3$, H$_1$, and M$_1$ receptor antagonists), (2) the H$_1$ and M$_1$ receptors of brain stem nuclei that receive input from the vestibular nucleus, (3) the vagus, (4) the sympathetic nerves, and (5) the vomiting center itself. Phenothiazines act on D$_1$, H$_1$, and M$_1$ receptors; the benzamides such as metoclopramide, domperidone, and cisplatin affect 5-HT$_3$ and 5-HT$_4$ receptors; scopolamine is an M$_1$-receptor antagonist; and diphenhydramine (Dramamine) and cyclizine (Marezine) are H$_1$ antagonists. The most effective of the antinausea drugs for chemotherapy-induced vomiting are the 5-HT$_3$ receptor antagonists such as ondansetron.

ABDOMINAL PAIN. This symptom-complex arises from intra-abdominal, nociceptive impulses that are variously modulated by input from the spinal cord and the CNS. Abdominal pain is either acute or chronic; when chronic, it may be intermittent (e.g., recurrent biliary colic), unrelenting (e.g., chronic pancreatitis or pancreatic cancer), or intractable but of unclear cause (e.g., the functional abdominal pain syndromes).

In the gastrointestinal tract, nociceptive pain receptors are present in the walls (lamina propria and muscle layers) of the hollow organs, in serosal structures (the visceral peritoneum and the capsules of the solid organs), and within the mesentery that supports and surrounds the abdominal organs. These receptors respond to distention, contraction, traction, compression, torsion, and stretch; to transmitters such as bradykinin, substance P, serotonin, histamine, and prostaglandins; and to chemicals such as hydrochloric acid, potassium chloride, and hypertonic saline. These receptors do not respond to classic nociceptive stimuli such as pinching, burning, stabbing, or cutting or to electrical or thermal stimulation. As a result, the gastroenterologist can biopsy or thermally coagulate the gastrointestinal mucosa with impunity yet a patient notes severe pain with contraction or distention of the viscera or with traction and pulling on the mesentery and abdominal organs. The cell bodies of the sensory receptors of the gut and viscera are in the dorsal root ganglion of the spinal cord. These neurons synapse in the dorsal horn and then either cross the cord to ascend in the contralateral spinal thalamic tract or ascend in the contralateral posterior column to reach the reticular formation of the brain stem or the thalamus, where they synapse and project to the limbic system and frontal lobe or to the somatosensory cortex, respectively.

In the embryo, the gut and organs are present in the midline and receive innervation from both sides of the spinal canal. Thus, stimuli arising in the gastrointestinal tract (e.g., from inflammation, ischemia) are often perceived as midline pain until the process (e.g., appendicitis or cholecystitis) extends to the adjacent parietal peritoneum, where laterally localizing nerves project the pain to the brain.

The synapses of the pain fibers from the viscera and the dorsal horn of the spinal cord allow the CNS and somatic nerves to modulate the perception of visceral pain. Descending inhibitory neurons arising in the CNS, when activated, stimulate interneurons in the cord, which inhibit the firing of the second-order and visceral pain neurons, which travel up the cord to the brain. The balance of these excitatory and inhibitory forces determines the degree to which the nociceptive information is transmitted to the CNS. This process is called the gate control theory of pain; it explains how acupuncture might inhibit the perception of visceral pain. The location of painful sensations is determined by the spinal

PLATE 1 CARDIOVASCULAR AND GASTROINTESTINAL DISEASES

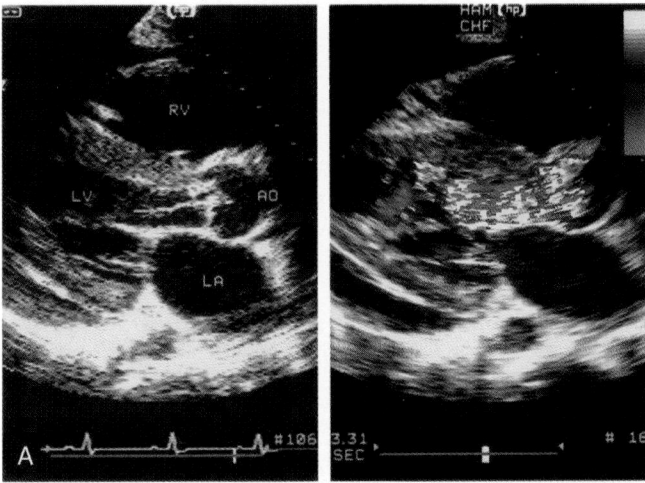

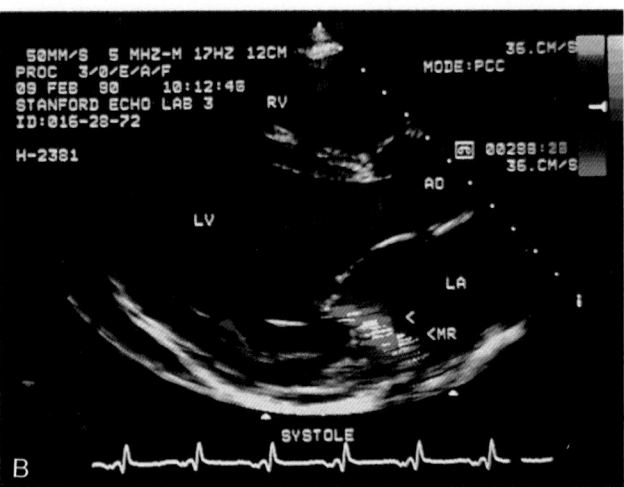

A, Echocardiogram of a patient with aortic regurgitation due to infectious endocarditis. The left panel shows a linear vegetation (arrow) prolapsing into the left ventricular outflow tract from the aortic valve leaflet in diastole. The right panel is a color flow Doppler exhibiting turbulent blood flow filling the left ventricular outflow tract during diastole. (Courtesy Dr. Anthony DeMaria.)

B, A two-dimensional echocardiogram with Doppler flow mapping superimposed on a portion of the image. The color information is represented in the sector of the imaging plane extending from the apex of the triangular plane to the two small arrows at the bottom of the image plane. Mitral regurgitation (MR) is indicated (open arrows), extending from the mitral valve leaflets toward the posterior aspect of the left atrium (LA) during systole. The mosaic of colors representing the mitral regurgitant signal is typical of high-velocity turbulent flow. The low-intensity orange-brown signal represents flow directed away from the transducer on the chest wall, and the blue shades represent blood in the left ventricular outflow tract moving toward the transducer. (AO = aorta; LV = left ventricle; RV = right ventricle.)

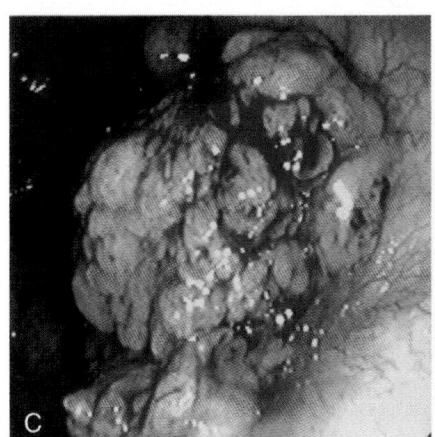

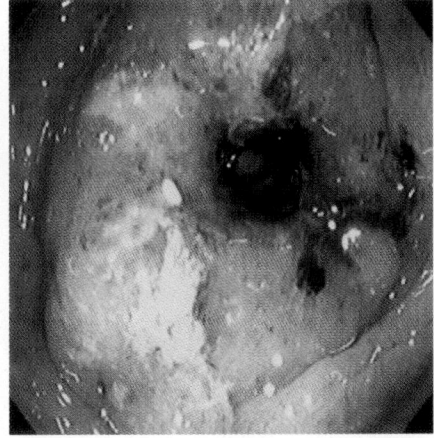

C, Two manifestations of colorectal cancer. *Left*, Exophytic growth within the lumen. *Right*, "Stricturing" (apple-core) lesion.

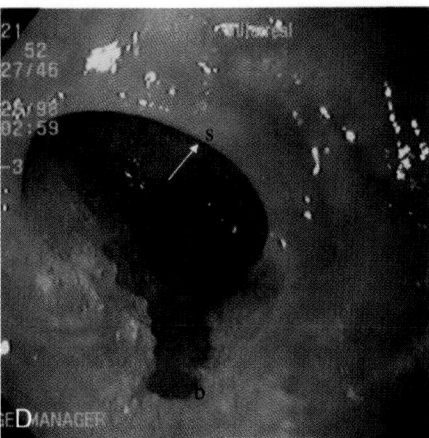

D, Endoscopic view of the distal esophagus from a patient with gastroesophageal reflux disease showing a tongue of Barrett's mucosa (b) and a Schatzki's ring (s) (arrow).

PLATE 2 GASTROINTESTINAL DISEASES

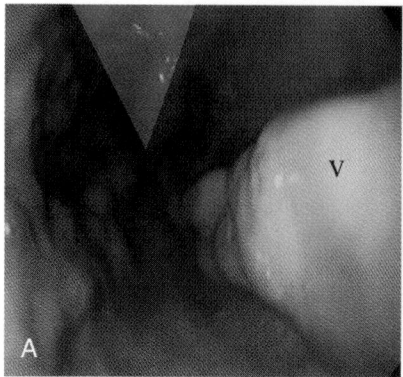
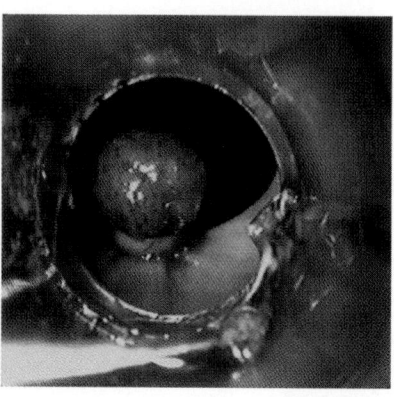

A, Endoscopic view of esophageal varices *(left)* in the wall of the esophagus (V). *Right,* Image of a varix that has been endoscopically ligated with a band.

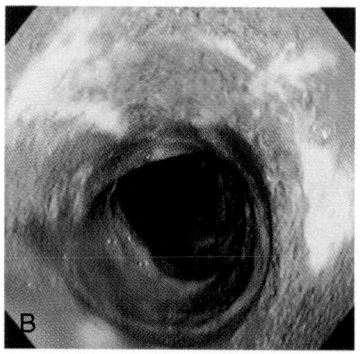

B, Endoscopic view of the colonic mucosa in a patient with idiopathic ulcerative colitis, showing a very friable mucosa, extensive ulceration, and exudates.

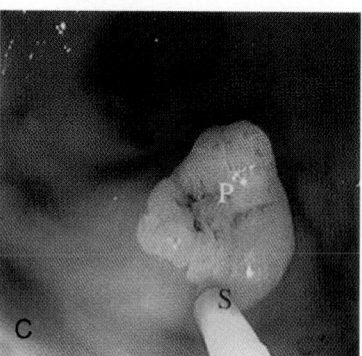
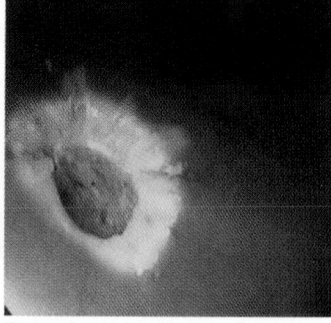

C, Endoscopic polypectomy. *Left,* A snare (S) has been passed through the endoscope and positioned around the polyp (P). *Right,* Subsequently, cautery was applied and the polyp guillotined, leaving behind a clean mucosal defect.

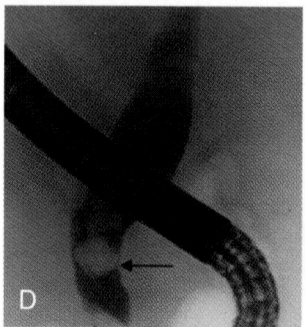
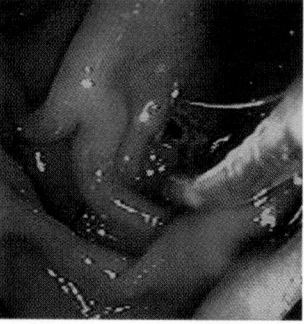
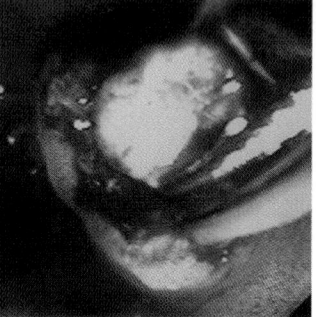

D, Biliary sphincterotomy and stone removal from the bile duct. *Left,* Endoscopic retrograde cholangiographic image showing stones (arrow) in the distal common bile duct. *Center,* Endoscopic image of a sphincterotome in the bile duct with the wire cutting the roof of the ampulla (sphincter). *Right,* A stone is being removed from the bile duct using an endoscopically passed basket.

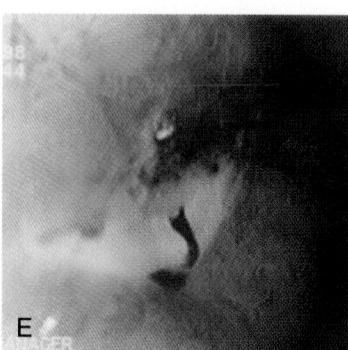
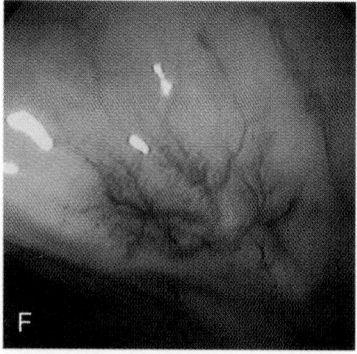
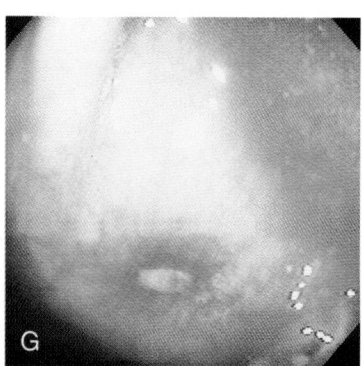

E, Gastric ulcer (white base) with bleeding vessel.

F, Mucosal telangiectasia (arteriovenous malformation, or AVM) in the colon. The patient presented with hematochezia. The lesion was subsequently cauterized endoscopically.

G, A single aphthous ulcer, the earliest endoscopic finding in Crohn's disease.

PLATE 3   GASTROINTESTINAL AND RESPIRATORY DISEASES

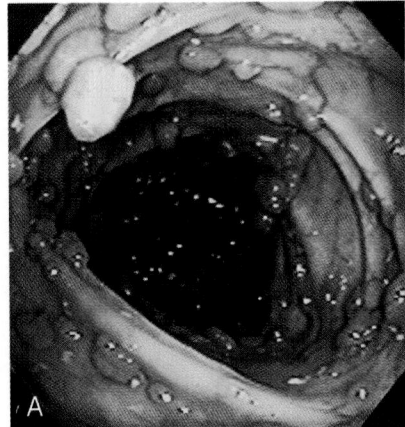

A, Endoscopic view of colon of patient with familial adenomatous polyposis.

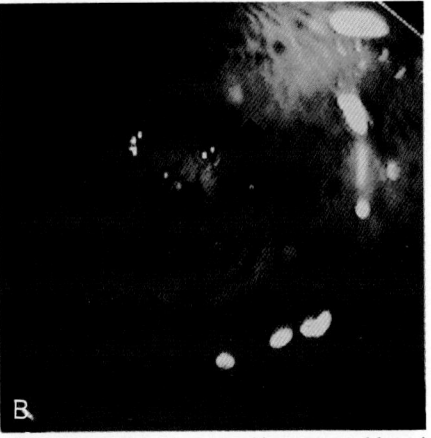

B, Duodenal bulbar ulcer. A white excavated base is noted just inside the pylorus (large arrows) containing a dark red central artery oozing blood (small arrow).

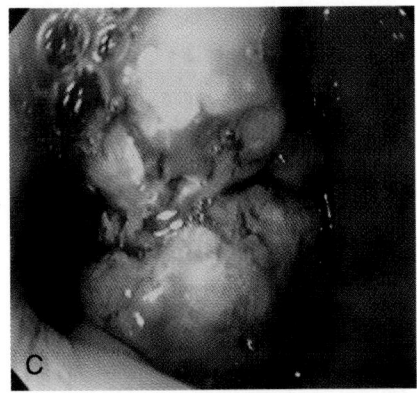

C, Large malignant mass at the gastroesophageal junction as seen endoscopically.

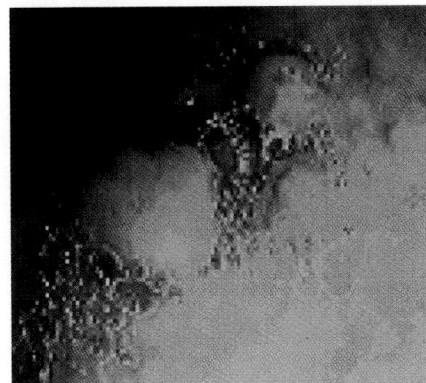
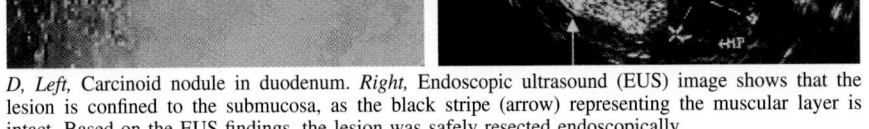

D, Left, Carcinoid nodule in duodenum. Right, Endoscopic ultrasound (EUS) image shows that the lesion is confined to the submucosa, as the black stripe (arrow) representing the muscular layer is intact. Based on the EUS findings, the lesion was safely resected endoscopically.

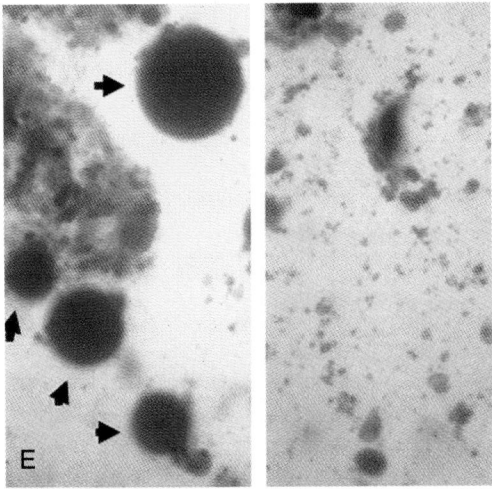

Positive   Negative

E, Sudan stain of stool for fat. The positive stain (left) shows large globules of unabsorbed fat (arrows).

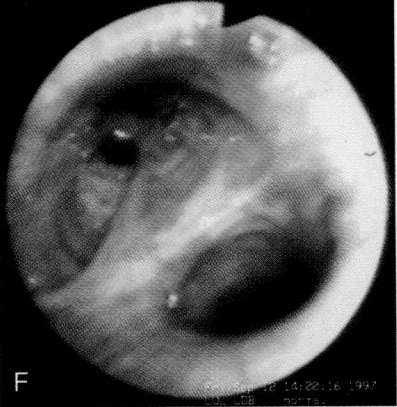
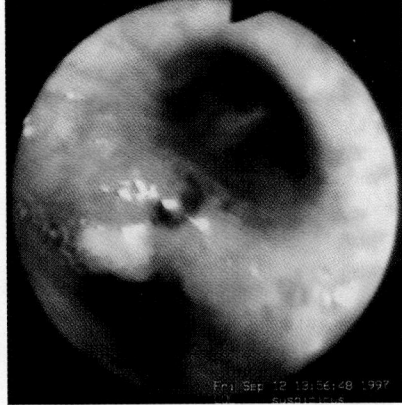

F, Left, Carina between lingula and upper division bronchus of left upper lobe. Note well-defined, sharp features of carina. Right, Carina between left upper and lower lobes in same patient. Note swollen, red and infiltrated appearance of mucosa, and white, exophytic lesion. In addition, there is subepithelial hemorrhage. Biopsy specimen demonstrated squamous cell carcinoma. The patient presented with increased sputum production, positive sputum cytology, and nonlocalizing chest radiograph and CT scan.

PLATE 4   RENAL AND NUTRITIONAL DISEASES

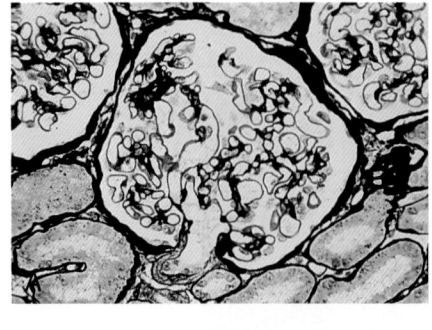
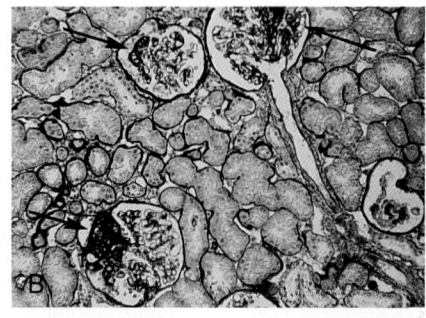

A, Minimal change disease. The glomeruli demonstrate no abnormalities at the light microscopic level (Jones methenamine silver, ×260).

B, Focal segmental glomerulosclerosis. The glomerular capillary lumina are segmentally obliterated by basement membrane material (arrows). The adjacent glomerular lobules are unremarkable (Jones methenamine silver, ×100).

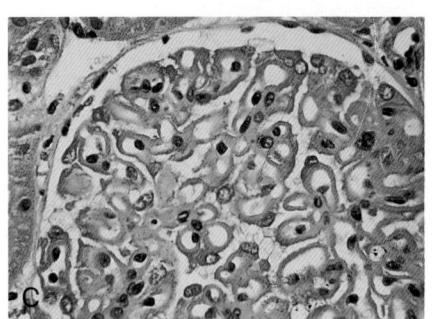
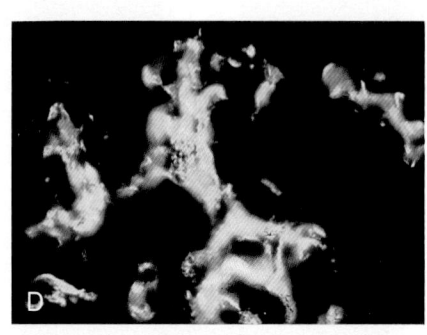

C, Membranous glomerulopathy. The glomerular basement membranes are uniformly thickened and rigid. There is no hypercellularity of the glomerular tuft (H & E, ×400).

D, IgA nephropathy. Fluorescence micrograph shows intense staining of the mesangium with antisera to IgA (×600).

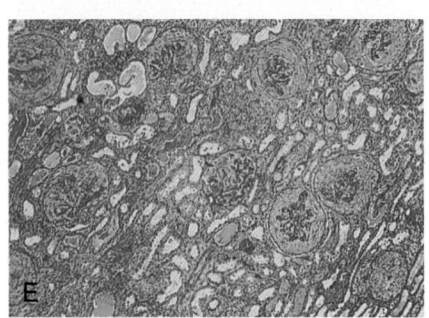
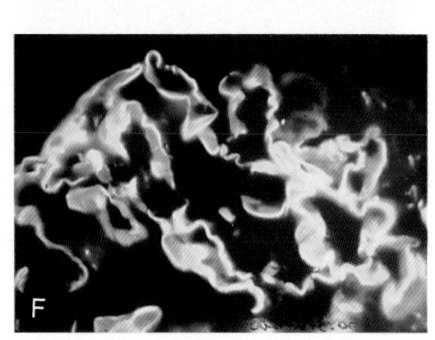

E, Anti-glomerular basement membrane disease. Low-power micrograph showing diffuse involvement of the glomeruli by crescents, which compress the glomerular tuft (PAS, ×40).

F, Anti-glomerular basement membrane antibody disease. Fluorescence micrograph showing intense linear reactivity of the glomerular basement membranes with antisera to IgG (×600).

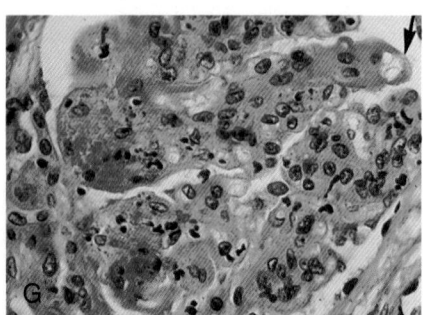
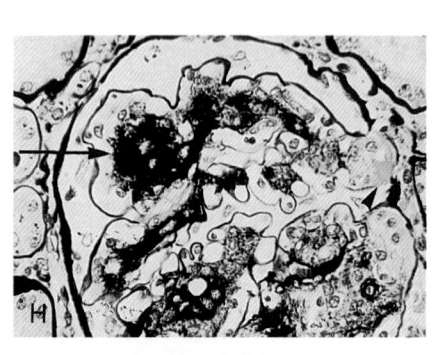
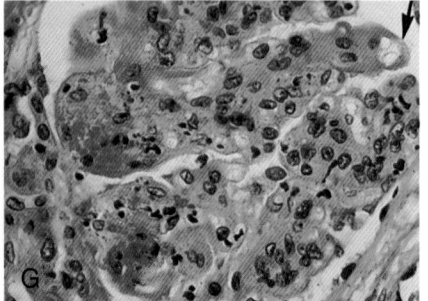
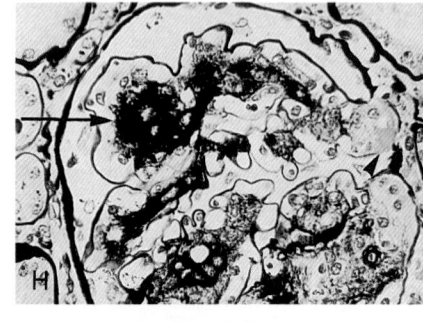

G, Lupus nephritis. Diffuse proliferative lupus nephritis showing global occlusion of the glomerular capillary lumina by endocapillary and mesangial proliferation. There are numerous infiltrating mononuclear and polymorphonuclear leukocytes with focal pyknosis and karyorrhexis. The arrow denotes a "wire-loop" deposit (H & E, ×400).

H, Nodular diabetic glomerulosclerosis. The mesangium is expanded by matrix material forming nodules (arrow). The glomerular basement membranes are diffusely thickened. Intramembranous hyaline deposits are also present (arrowhead) (Jones methenamine silver, ×400).

I, Amyloidosis. The glomerular tuft is segmentally infiltrated by amorphous eosinophilic material with a hyaline appearance (H & E, ×260).

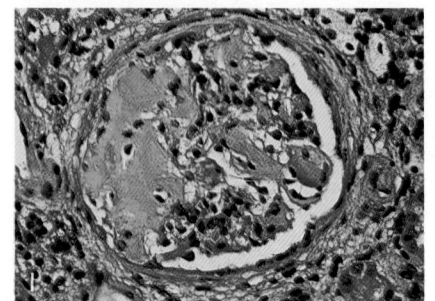
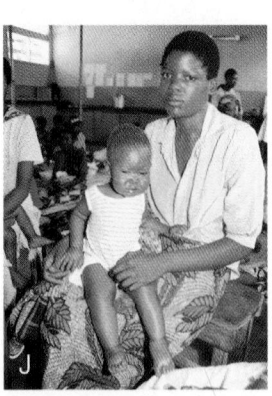

J, A child with kwashiorkor in Blantyre, Malawi, manifests some of the classic features of the disease, including leg edema, reddish-blond hair discoloration, and irritability. (Courtesy of Mark Manary, M.D.)

segments in which the afferent nerves from the abdominal viscera enter the spinal cord. For example, foregut structures, such as the esophagus, stomach, proximal duodenum, liver, biliary tree, and pancreas, are innervated at T5 to T9; pain from these structures is perceived between the xiphoid and the umbilicus. Pain from midgut structures, such as the small intestine, appendix, and ascending and proximal two thirds of the transverse colon, is transmitted from T8 to L1 and is perceived as periumbilical. Pain from hindgut structures, which include the distal one third of the transverse colon, the descending colon, and the rectosigmoid, is transmitted from T11 to L1 and is perceived between the umbilicus and the pubis. Referred pain is pain perceived in the skin or muscle in the same cutaneous dermatomes as those nerve roots where the innervation of the abdominal organ enters the spinal cord. Referred pain is a helpful phenomenon to diagnose the cause of acute abdominal pain: gallbladder pain may be perceived in the right shoulder or scapula, and pain from retroperitoneal processes such as pancreatitis is referred to the back.

In addition to the location of pain and the presence of referred pain, the character of the pain (burning, steady, or colic), its duration, its time to reach peak intensity, and its relieving and aggravating factors (such as eating or passing gas or stool) are helpful components of the medical history. Esophagitis is classically described as substernal burning pain relieved by antacids and aggravated by lying down. Peptic ulcer pain occurs when the stomach is empty (often 4 A.M.), and it is relieved by eating or taking antacids. Gallbladder colic is perceived either in the midline or right upper quadrant, reaches a peak intensity within minutes to an hour, and usually persists for 1 to 4 hours. In contrast, the pain of cholecystitis and pancreatitis reaches its peak more slowly, becomes sustained, and lasts for days. Intestinal obstruction causes colicky pain that waxes and wanes over the course of minutes and is usually periumbilical.

Chronic intermittent abdominal pain may be due to obstructed viscera, such as in recurrent cholelithiasis or intestinal obstruction; to metabolic or genetic diseases, such as acute intermittent porphyria or familial Mediterranean fever; to neurologic diseases, such as diabetic reticulopathy, abdominal migraine, or vertebral nerve root compression; or to miscellaneous inflammatory diseases, such as Crohn's disease, endometriosis, lead poisoning, and mesenteric ischemia. Functional abdominal pain, which is common but of less clear pathophysiology, includes three major types: (1) irritable bowel syndrome, in which recurrent abdominal pain is accompanied by changes in gastrointestinal function (constipation, diarrhea, or alternating constipation and diarrhea); (2) non-ulcer dyspepsia, which is defined as ulcer-like symptoms in the absence of endoscopically definable anatomic or histologic evidence of inflammation; and (3) chronic, intractable abdominal pain, in which pain is not accompanied by other symptoms of organ dysfunction. These functional diseases are quite common and may account for up to 50% of patients who present to either the primary care physician or gastroenterologist with gastrointestinal symptoms.

PHYSICAL EXAMINATION. In acute abdominal pain, the physical examination is targeted quite differently than in patients with chronic gastrointestinal complaints. The goal of the examination in acute abdominal pain is to determine the presence of surgical disease. Observation of facial expression is key to determining the presence and severity of pain. Distention, particularly if tympanic, suggests bowel obstruction, but simple obesity and ascites are more likely causes of distention without tympany. The character of bowel sounds (absent in peritonitis, high-pitched tinkles in intestinal obstruction) can be important, but any bowel sounds that are hypoactive, hyperactive, or present in one quadrant or another are of little consequence. The most useful part of the examination is palpation, which gives clues to the presence of severe peritoneal inflammation, as manifested by involuntary guarding, abdominal rigidity, or rebound tenderness; when these symptoms are accompanied by absent bowel sounds, perforation and peritonitis must be suspected. Palpation with the stethoscope rather than with the hand can sometimes differentiate true abdominal rebound tenderness from a response that is either feigned or imagined.

In the patient with chronic gastrointestinal complaints, the goal of the physical examination is to determine the presence or absence of other systemic findings that might suggest the underlying disease, to determine the size of the abdominal viscera, and to detect any abnormal masses. For example, the presence of jaundice and

spider telangiectasia suggests liver disease and perhaps varices as a cause of gastrointestinal bleeding. Large joint arthritis and aphthous ulcers of the mouth might suggest celiac disease or inflammatory bowel disease. The abdominal examination might reveal epigastric, right upper quadrant, right lower quadrant, or left lower quadrant tenderness to complement a compatible history for peptic ulcer disease, cholecystitis, Crohn's disease, or diverticulitis, respectively. An epigastric mass might suggest a pancreatic neoplasm or pseudocyst, whereas right lower quadrant and left lower quadrant masses suggest abscess due to inflammatory bowel disease and diverticulitis, respectively, or colonic cancer. Examination of the liver (see Chapter 144) should focus primarily on its breadth and consistency. Auscultation is useful to determine the presence of bruits indicative of vascular disease or friction rubs that suggest pancreatic or hepatic cancer.

The physical examination is not complete without a digital rectal examination. The examiner should not forget to sweep the finger posteriorly to search for anorectal carcinoma and masses in the pouch of Douglas and also anteriorly to determine the size and consistency of the prostate. Tenderness and masses laterally can occur in appendicitis, inflammatory bowel disease, or diverticulitis, as well as abdominal cancers. The character and color of the stool and the presence of fecal occult blood should be assessed.

LABORATORY TESTS AND IMAGING PROCEDURES A complete blood cell count, liver chemistries, and erythrocyte sedimentation rate can be useful screening tests in assessing gastrointestinal disease. The choice of endoscopy versus barium contrast radiographs depends on the acuteness of the gastrointestinal disease and the diseases being sought (see Chapters 121 and 122). Although endoscopy is relatively expensive and should never be used indiscriminately, it often can expedite definitive diagnosis and provide definitive therapy.

Feldman M, Scharschmidt BE, Sleisenger MH: Sleisenger and Fordtran's Gastrointestinal and Liver Disease: Pathophysiology, Diagnosis, Management, 6th ed. Philadelphia, WB Saunders, 1998. *Section II of this textbook, "Approach to Patients with Symptoms and Signs," is directed toward common gastrointestinal diseases and symptoms and gives much useful information.*
Yamada T, Alpers DH, Owyang C, et al: Textbook of Gastroenterology, 3rd ed. Philadelphia, Lippincott Williams & Wilkins, 1999. *Part II of this textbook, a section entitled "Approaches to Common Gastrointestinal Problems," gives authoritative information on the common gastrointestinal diseases and can be very useful reading for physicians hoping to improve their mastery of the common diseases and symptoms of the gastrointestinal tract.*

121 DIAGNOSTIC IMAGING PROCEDURES IN GASTROENTEROLOGY

Gerhard R. Wittich

Long-established techniques, such as plain film radiography and barium studies, continue to play an important role as efficient and cost-effective imaging methods in gastroenterology. In addition, ultrasonography (US), computed tomography (CT), and magnetic resonance imaging (MRI) have greatly improved gastroenterologic diagnosis and have stimulated a number of image-guided interventions.

PLAIN FILM RADIOGRAPHY

Plain film radiography remains a valuable tool for the diagnosis of several abdominal disorders. The *acute abdominal series*, consisting of supine and upright films of the abdomen, readily provides information regarding abnormal gas patterns. Demonstration of gas/fluid levels within dilated loops of bowel may suggest obstruction or adynamic ileus. This technique is a reliable method to confirm or exclude the presence of intraperitoneal bowel perforation, since as little as 5 mL of air can be detected with proper radiographic technique. Plain film radiography of the abdomen is also useful to detect abnormal calcifications such as calcified gallstones (see Chapter 157), pancreatic calcifications (see Chapter 141), calcified aneurysms, and calcified hydatid cysts of the liver.

BARIUM STUDIES

Barium studies of the upper gastrointestinal tract allow diagnosis of inflammatory, neoplastic, and motility disorders and of lesions that cause stenosis or obstruction. In the hands of experienced investigators who take advantage of the diagnostic capabilities of optimized single- and double-contrast studies, the sensitivity of barium studies for detection of gastric ulcers or esophageal or gastric neoplasms approaches that of endoscopic examination. In the esophagus, barium studies cannot quite match the almost 100% sensitivity of diagnostic endoscopy. However, the lower cost of barium studies and their non-invasive nature make them excellent initial tests for many suspected disorders of the upper gastrointestinal tract. For example, in a subgroup of immunocompromised patients with dysphagia, double-contrast evaluation of the esophagus allows detection of *Candida* esophagitis (see Chapter 124), characterized by a granular mucosa and plaquelike lesions, in about 90% of cases. Alternatively, barium study of the esophagus may reveal ulcerative changes suggesting herpes esophagitis or infection with cytomegalovirus or human immunodeficiency virus. Although endoscopy is more sensitive and may allow a specific diagnosis by obtaining samples for microbial cultures, it may be more economical to reserve endoscopy for patients with equivocal or negative radiographic studies. In patients with symptoms of reflux esophagitis (see Chapters 124 and 131), double-contrast barium examination demonstrates ulcerations and possible stricture formation in advanced cases, but barium studies are inferior to endoscopy in the earlier stages of the disease.

High-quality double-contrast techniques remain a reasonable alternative as initial imaging studies for the evaluation of the stomach and duodenum, because the vast majority of gastric and duodenal ulcers (see Chapter 126) are readily displayed radiographically, and barium studies are safer and less expensive than endoscopy. An indication for primary endoscopic evaluation is acute upper gastrointestinal hemorrhage: whereas barium studies may reveal the source of bleeding in 70 to 80% of cases, the ability to control hemorrhage by endoscopic intervention clearly makes it the preferred method (see Chapter 123).

Because routine endoscopy of the small bowel is not feasible, the most common techniques to visualize this organ are the small bowel follow-through study with intermittent fluoroscopic evaluation and *enteroclysis*, which is intubation of the proximal jejunum with infusion of contrast material. Enteroclysis, which should be restricted to patients with a high level of suspicion of small bowel disease, has several advantages over the small bowel follow-through study. It is independent of the activity of the pylorus, so a high-quality study can usually be completed in less than 30 minutes. Double-contrast enteroclysis, which includes the use of barium and methylcellulose, allows complete evaluation of all loops of small bowel, including ileal loops that often are superimposed on one another within the pelvis. Common indications for enteroclysis include partial mechanical small bowel obstruction, suspected peritoneal neoplasms (see Chapter 139), suspected radiation enteritis (see Chapter 136), unexplained, intermittent lower gastrointestinal bleeding (see Chapter 123), Crohn's disease being considered for surgery (see Chapter 135), and malabsorption possibly due to small bowel disease (see Chapter 134).

Endoscopic and radiographic studies play a complementary role in evaluation of the colon. Single-contrast studies are sufficient for documentation of large colon carcinomas, but double-contrast enemas are required for detection of more subtle lesions, such as small polyps or early mucosal changes in patients with inflammatory bowel disease (see Chapters 135 and 139). With meticulous double-contrast technique, the detection rate of colonic polyps is approximately 90% and approaches the sensitivity of colonoscopy (Fig. 121–1). Typical indications for barium enemas include symptoms of colon carcinoma (see Chapter 139), diverticular disease (see Chapter 136), and inflammatory bowel disease (see Chapter 135). In addition, double-contrast barium enema is part of one of

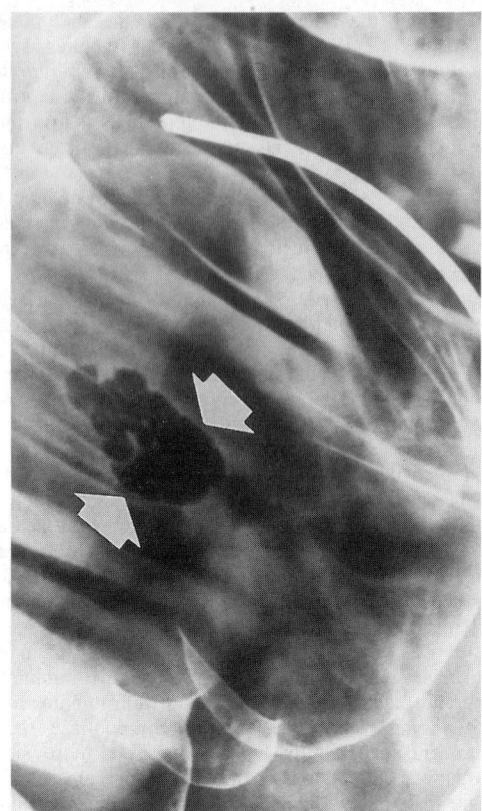

FIGURE 121–1 ■ Graded compression during double-contrast barium enema demonstrates a small, lobulated, sessile polyp (arrows) on the posterior wall of the ascending colon.

the alternate strategies to screen asymptomatic patients for colon cancer (see Chapter 139).

ULTRASONOGRAPHY

Ultrasonography has many applications in patients with gastroenterologic disorders, but a disadvantage is its inability to penetrate gas-filled structures. For example, US can yield exquisite images of the pancreatic parenchyma and the pancreatic duct in thin patients, but it may be difficult to evaluate this retroperitoneal organ in obese patients with a large amount of bowel gas within the transverse colon and stomach.

The sensitivity of US for detection of gallbladder stones is greater than 90% (see Fig. 157–7). In the jaundiced patient (see Chapter 146), US allows quick differentiation of obstruction of the intrahepatic and extrahepatic bile ducts (Fig. 121–2) from other causes of jaundice, such as hepatitis. Both the level of obstruction and its cause often can be determined. For example, lesions in the pancreatic head or the porta hepatis or a stone within the common bile duct can be detected.

Because of its anatomic position posterior to the pancreatic head, the distal common bile duct may be obscured by gas within the duodenum, transverse colon, or gastric antrum. Additional studies such as MR cholangiography, endoscopic retrograde cholangiopancreatography (ERCP), or percutaneous transhepatic cholangiography (PTC) may be necessary.

Ultrasound is also an excellent imaging tool for the evaluation of the hepatic parenchyma. It allows detection of fatty liver as well as textural changes of cirrhosis, and it has a sensitivity between 80% and 90% for detection of hepatic neoplasms (see Chapter 156). Cystic lesions within the liver and hepatic abscesses are readily detected.

The spleen is readily imaged by US to determine its size as well as to visualize intrasplenic or perisplenic fluid collections or mass lesions. Doppler and color Doppler studies can evaluate portal venous flow in patients with portal hypertension before and after placement of a transjugular intrahepatic portosystemic shunts (TIPS).

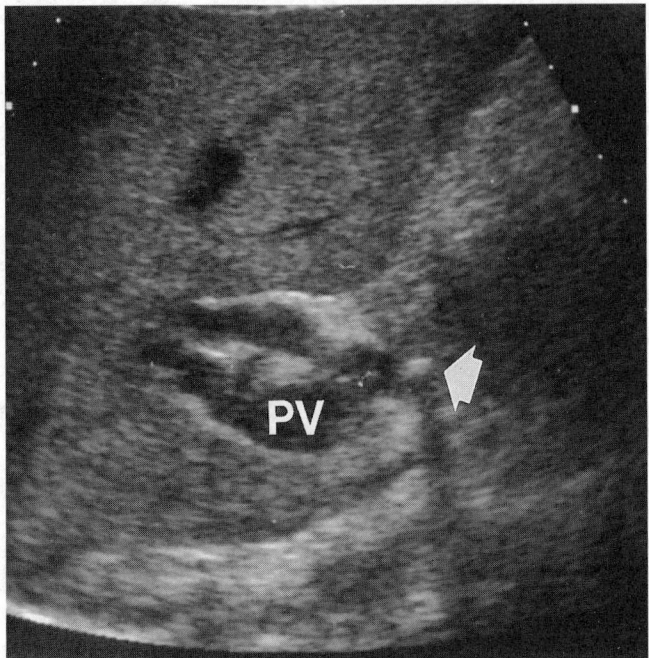

FIGURE 121–2 ■ Choledocholithiasis. Sagittal scan through the porta hepatis demonstrates a dilated common bile duct anterior to the portal vein (PV). Note the obstructing stone within the distal portion of the common bile duct (arrow).

COMPUTED TOMOGRAPHY

The development of fast CT scanners that use spiral, or helical, scanning techniques has enhanced the role of CT for evaluation of abdominal organs. Single images can be obtained in 100 to 1000 msec (depending on the scanner), and the entire liver can be imaged in a single breath-hold in less than 30 seconds. This speed permits optimal utilization of contrast material. For example, the entire liver can be imaged during the arterial phase after injection of a contrast bolus to detect hypervascular lesions such as hepatomas (see Chapter 156) that typically enhance more than normal hepatic parenchyma during the arterial phase (Fig. 121–3). Less vascular lesions such as metastases from a colon carcinoma can typically be detected as low-density lesions during the portal venous phase because they receive significantly less blood than normal parenchyma through the portal system.

An additional benefit of rapid-sequence CT scanning is the possi-

bility to use specialized software for three-dimensional display of organ systems such as the vascular system. CT angiography is of particular value for the non-invasive evaluation of liver transplant recipients (see Chapter 155). Application of this technique to the colon has been termed *virtual colonoscopy* and may become useful as a non-invasive screening test for colonic polyps.

CT is also an essential tool for evaluating and staging abdominal mass lesions; for diagnosis of hepatic, pancreatic, and splenic abscesses; and for detecting abscesses associated with disorders of the bowel such as appendicitis, diverticulitis, or Crohn's disease (see Chapters 135 and 136). In patients with biliary obstruction, CT is very useful to determine the cause of obstruction, including carcinoma of the pancreatic head or the ampulla (see Chapters 140 and 157), particularly when ultrasound evaluation remains inconclusive. Another important use of CT is to guide abdominal interventions such as percutaneous needle aspiration of mass lesions or abnormal fluid collections, placement of needles and probes for percutaneous tumor ablation, and drainage of abdominal abscesses.

MAGNETIC RESONANCE IMAGING

The more water and hence the more protons a specific tissue contains, the greater is its signal intensity. This property results in a contrast resolution that is superior to that of CT and US. Additional advantages of MRI include its non-invasiveness, the absence of ionizing radiation, and the ability to obtain images in multiple planes such as cross-sectional, sagittal, and coronal displays.

Drawbacks of MRI compared with US and CT are the significantly higher cost of equipment, the longer imaging times, the need to exclude patients with ferromagnetic intracranial metallic clips or cardiac pacemakers, and the tunnel-like gantry design of conventional scanners that causes some patients to become claustrophobic. Low- and mid-field scanners (0.5 to 1.0T) have reduced the cost of equipment and provide good quality images, albeit still at relatively long scanning times.

MR cholangiography is evolving as an alternative to diagnostic ERCP or PTC. MR angiography, which can image the vascular supply of the liver, is of particular value in liver transplant patients (see Chapter 155).

MRI is often used when US or CT is inconclusive. For example, MRI can differentiate cavernous hemangiomas (see Chapter 156) from other liver lesions owing to their very long T2 value. The use of contrast agents such as gadolinium-diethylenetriaminepenta-acetic acid (Gd-DTPA) gives MR a high sensitivity for detecting hepatic tumors, but its specificity has not reached a level that would obviate the need for percutaneous biopsies, except in certain lesions such as hemangiomas.

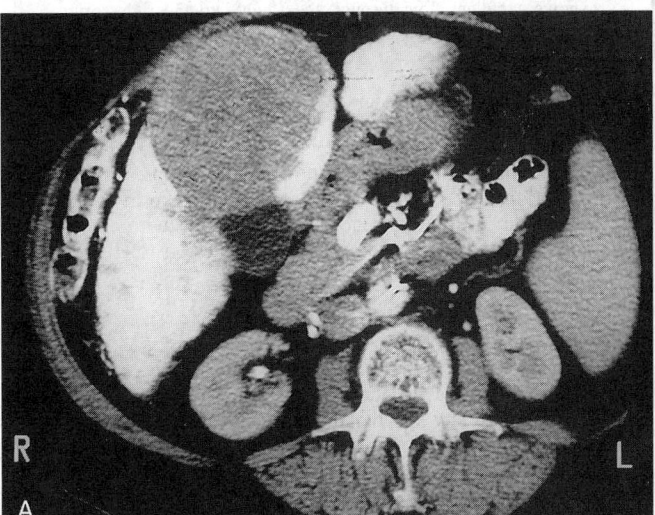
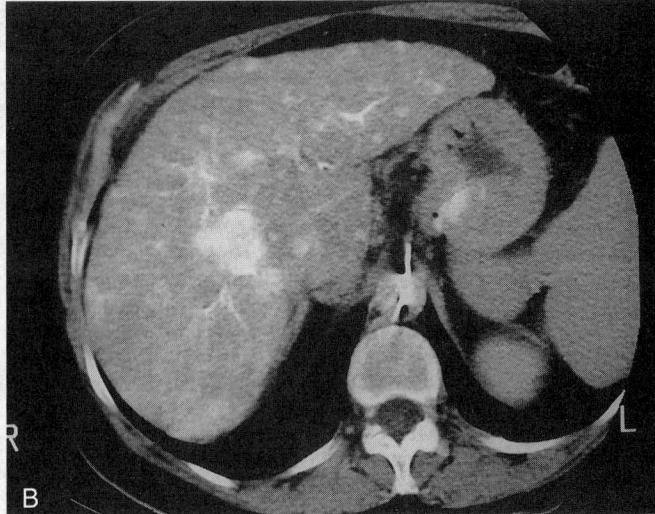

FIGURE 121–3 ■ *A*, Computed tomography (CT) scan through the lower portion of the liver obtained during the portal venous phase shows a single large hypodense lesion. Percutaneous biopsy confirmed a hepatoma. *B*, CT scan through the cranial portion of the liver during the arterial phase demonstrates multiple additional hypervascular lesions, suggesting an unresectable, multicentric hepatoma.

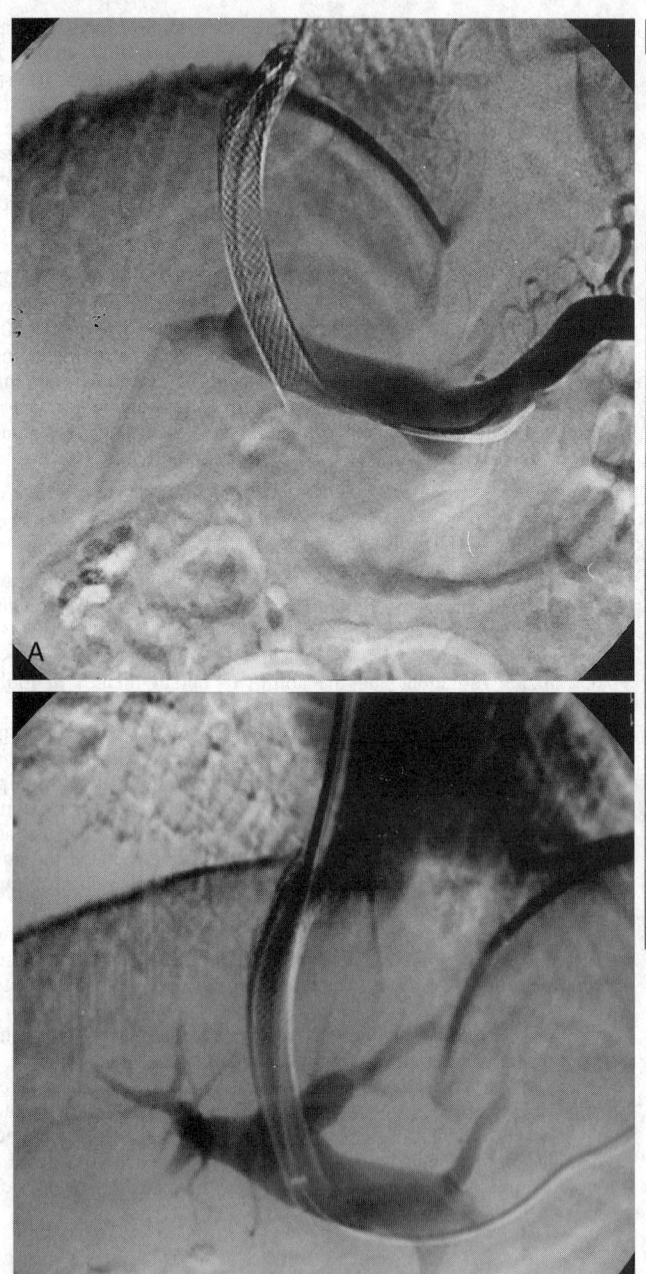

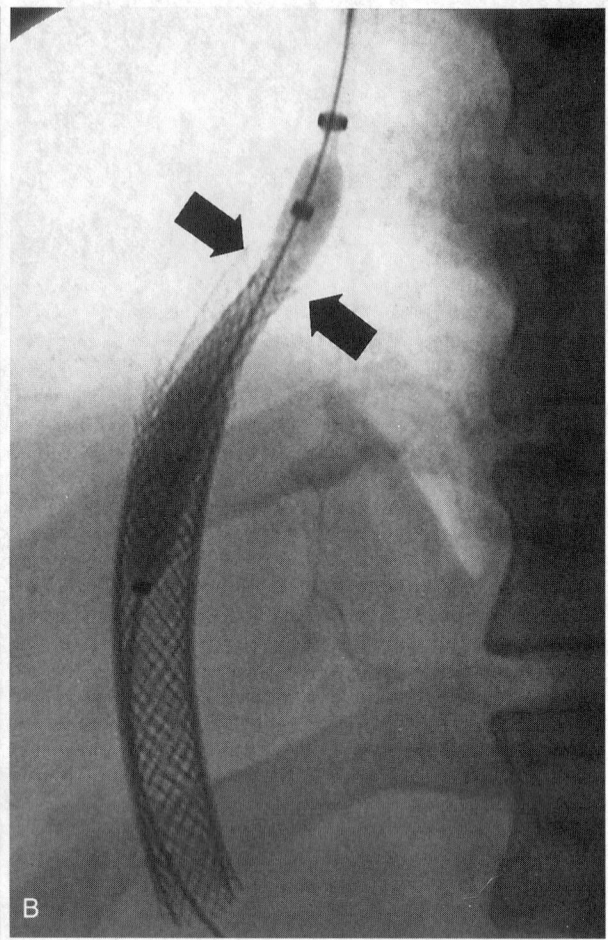

FIGURE 121–4 ■ Transjugular intrahepatic portosystemic shunt (TIPS) revision in a patient with recurrent variceal bleeding 3 years after a successful TIPS procedure. *A,* With the use of a transjugular approach a guidewire has been advanced through the occluded stent. Contrast medium injection demonstrates a patent splenic and portal vein but no flow through the shunt. The portal venous pressure was elevated to 21 mm Hg. *B,* Balloon dilatation of occluded shunt. The waist of the balloon (arrows) was completely abolished after inflation to 15 atmospheres. *C,* Contrast medium injection into the portal vein now shows excellent flow through the shunt into the right atrium. The pressure gradient between portal vein and right atrium was reduced to 10 mm Hg.

RADIONUCLIDE IMAGING

Scintigraphic studies are rarely used as the primary method to image abdominal disorders, but they are indicated to solve certain diagnostic problems. Cavernous hemangiomas (see Chapter 156), which are found in 1 to 7% of autopsies, must be differentiated from hepatomas, metastases, or other lesions. Technetium-99m (^{99m}Tc)–labeled red blood cell studies represent a non-invasive, economic method to diagnose a cavernous hemangioma. The sensitivity for detection of small lesions (less than 2 cm) has been increased with the introduction of single-photon emission computed tomography. ^{99m}Tc pertechnetate allows detection of ectopic gastric mucosa in symptomatic Meckel's diverticulum, particularly in pediatric patients. Of clinical importance is localization of the source of gastrointestinal hemorrhage (see Chapter 123) with labeled red cell scintigraphy; this study is often indicated before angiography for patients in whom endoscopy has failed to localize and control the bleeding source.

Biliary scintigraphy with ^{99m}Tc-HIDA is often useful in patients with clinical symptoms of acute cholecystitis (see Chapter 157). In a normal patient, radionuclide uptake can be seen in the liver, bile ducts, gallbladder, and the bowel within 60 minutes after intravenous injection. The absence of radionuclide uptake in the region of the gallbladder despite presence of radionuclide within the remainder of the biliary system suggests cystic duct obstruction and supports the diagnosis of acute cholecystitis.

VASCULAR INTERVENTIONS

Although non-invasive imaging by US, CT, or MRI has largely replaced angiography for the diagnostic evaluation of hepatic and pancreatic masses, angiography remains valuable for tumor therapy (see Chapter 156). Catheter delivery systems are useful for chemoembolization to palliate unresectable primary or secondary liver tumors.

Selective angiography of the celiac and mesenteric vessels has long been important for the management of acute gastrointestinal hemorrhage (see Chapter 123); it should be considered when endoscopic attempts to control gastroduodenal bleeding fail. Selective embolization of arteries feeding bleeding sources in the stomach and duodenum is highly effective in controlling active hemorrhage with low risk of tissue infarction. The role of angiography in acute and massive lower gastrointestinal hemorrhage is primarily for precise preoperative localization of the bleeding source and possibly to temporize for surgery by local infusion of a vasoconstrictor. Bleeding is controlled in more than 70% of patients, thereby making them candidates for elective rather than more risky emergency surgery. In a subgroup of patients who remain at high risk for surgery, selective embolization may be considered. This method is also highly effective in controlling lower gastrointestinal hemorrhage but carries about a 10% risk of bowel infarction.

Patients with coagulopathy should be considered for *transjugular liver biopsy* if a tissue diagnosis is required for proper management. Refinements in biopsy devices allow retrieval of adequate tissue samples in more than 90% of cases with minimal morbidity.

TIPS has rapidly evolved as standard treatment for patients with complications of cirrhosis (see Chapters 153 and 154), such as refractory ascites or hemorrhage from esophageal varices after failure of endoscopic sclerotherapy. The technical success rate of this method is more than 90%, and its morbidity and mortality are lower than those of emergency surgical portacaval shunts. Although the long-term success of this method is currently somewhat limited by shunt stenosis or occlusion, close surveillance with periodic visits and color Doppler US can often discover shunt stenosis before recurrent episodes of bleeding. Angiographic reintervention may be required to maintain portal decompression (Fig. 121–4). Although the primary patency rate of TIPS at 1 year is approximately 50%, reinterventions such as balloon dilatation of stenotic shunts can result in a secondary patency rate of more than 90% after 1 year and more than 80% after 3 years.

NON-VASCULAR INTERVENTIONS

Percutaneous US- or CT-guided biopsy of hepatic, pancreatic, or other abdominal mass lesions has become standard practice. The sensitivity of fine needle biopsy of abdominal neoplasms is more than 90%, with a complication rate that is less than 1%. Similar techniques can be used for nerve blocks, such as celiac ganglion blocks in patients with intractable pain secondary to advanced pancreatic carcinoma (see Chapter 140) or chronic pancreatitis (see Chapter 141). Percutaneous tumor ablation may be indicated in patients who are poor candidates for surgical resection. Investigational techniques that show promise for tissue ablation include percutaneous alcohol injection and tissue ablation with radiofrequency, laser, or cryotherapy probes.

Percutaneous drainage of abscesses and other abnormal fluid collections under US or CT guidance also has become a standard radiologic procedure. More than 90% of simple abdominal abscesses can be drained by percutaneous catheter drainage. The success rates with more complicated abscesses, such as those in the pancreas or those associated with underlying bowel disorders, are in the range of 70 to 90%. Definitive surgery may be required in this subgroup of patients.

Percutaneous biliary interventions (see Chapter 157) under fluoroscopic control are complementary to endoscopic and surgical procedures. Transhepatic techniques are of particular value when endoscopic techniques fail or are contraindicated, such as in patients with prior surgical interventions in the biliary system that make endoscopic access impossible. Transhepatic insertion of an indwelling expandable metallic prosthesis is well established as palliation for malignant biliary obstructions and may avoid endoscopic treatment or palliative surgery. Emergency percutaneous biliary drainage may be necessary in patients with acute cholangitis. Transhepatic stone removal is useful in patients with hepatolithiasis. Transhepatic balloon dilatation has a greater than 70% long-term success rate in patients with benign biliary strictures. Percutaneous cholecystostomy is useful for initial decompression of the gallbladder in patients with acute calculous or acalculous cholecystitis, particularly if patients are considered to be at high risk for emergency surgery, and permits subsequent elective cholecystectomy. Alternatively, percutaneous methods can be used for fragmentation and removal of stones from the gallbladder in patients who remain at high risk for surgery.

Gastrointestinal interventions such as balloon dilatation of benign strictures of the esophagus or placement of an endoprosthesis for palliative treatment of malignant obstructions of the esophagus (see Chapter 124) or colon (see Chapter 139) can be performed by interventional endoscopists or interventional radiologists. Similarly, percutaneous gastrostomy has a high success rate because high-grade or complete esophageal obstruction is not a contraindication to this method.

Birnbaum BA, Jeffrey RB Jr: CT and sonographic evaluation of acute right lower quadrant abdominal pain. AJR 170:361–371, 1998. *Review of the role of imaging in the management of patients with acute abdominal pain.*

Lewis BS: Radiology versus endoscopy of the small bowel. Gastrointest Endosc Clin N Am 9:13–27, 1999. *Neither approach is ideal.*

van Sonnenberg E, Wittich GR, Chon K, et al: Percutaneous radiologic drainage of pancreatic abscesses. AJR 168:979–984, 1997. *This article summarizes results and limitations of percutaneous management of patients with pancreatic abscesses.*

Zerhouni EA, Rutter C, Hamilton SR, et al: CT and MR imaging in the staging of colorectal carcinoma: Report of the Radiology Diagnostic Oncology Group II. Radiology 200:4432, 1996. *Excellent description of the role of CT and MR for diagnosis and staging of colon cancer.*

---

122 GASTROINTESTINAL ENDOSCOPY
Pankaj Jay Pasricha

Technologic advances in radiologic and endoscopic imaging have transformed medicine in the past few decades. With its remarkable accessibility, the gastrointestinal tract, perhaps more than any other organ system, has particularly benefited from the endoscopic approach. The major advantages of endoscopy over contrast radiography in evaluation of diseases of the alimentary tract include direct visualization, resulting in a more accurate and sensitive evaluation of mucosal lesions; the ability to obtain biopsy specimens from superficial lesions; and the ability to perform therapeutic interventions. These advantages make endoscopy the procedure of choice in most cases in which mucosal lesions or growths are suspected. Conversely, contrast radiography is more useful when anatomic information may be required, such as in patients with suspected volvulus, intussusception, or subtle strictures; patients with complicated postsurgical changes; or parts of the small bowel that are relatively inaccessible to endoscopy. For most upper gastrointestinal lesions, however, the sensitivity (about 90%) and specificity (nearly 100%) of endoscopy are far higher than for barium radiography (about 50% and 90%, respectively).

Diagnostic endoscopy (Table 122–1) is usually a remarkably safe and well-tolerated procedure. However, complications do occur and need to be carefully explained to the patient as part of the informed consent process; patients also must be appropriately prepared to reduce complication rates (Table 122–2). Although not listed in the table, some of the new diagnostic modalities that are already in clinical trials include endoscopic magnetic resonance imaging, endoscopic spectroscopy, and optical coherence tomography. Potential new therapeutic modalities include endoscopic antireflux surgery (using endoscopic "sewing machines") and photodynamic therapy.

LUMINAL ENDOSCOPY: SPECIFIC INDICATIONS

Most indications for gastrointestinal endoscopy are based on the presenting symptoms of the patient (e.g., dysphagia, bleeding, diarrhea). In other instances, endoscopy is required to evaluate specific lesions found by other diagnostic imaging, such as a gastric ulcer or colon polyp discovered by barium radiography. Finally, screening endoscopy is often performed in asymptomatic individuals based on their risk for commonly occurring and preventable conditions such as colon cancer (see later).

Implicit in the decision to perform endoscopy (or any other medical procedure for that matter) is the assumption that it will have a bearing on future management strategy. Although this is intuitively accepted by most physicians, rigorous evidence supporting this assumption may not always be readily available, particularly for the "softer" indications for endoscopy such as evaluation

Table 122–1 ■ TYPES OF DIAGNOSTIC ENDOSCOPY

PROCEDURE	THERAPEUTIC APPLICATIONS
Luminal Endoscopy	
Common Procedures	Hemostasis, luminal restoration (dilation, ablation, stenting), lesion removal (e.g., polypec-
Esophagogastroduodenoscopy (upper endoscopy)	tomy), percutaneous endoscopic gastrostomy
Colonoscopy	
Flexible sigmoidoscopy	
Less Common Procedures	
Enteroscopy	
Pancreatobiliary Imaging	
Endoscopic retrograde cholangiopancreatography	Sphincterotomy, stone removal, relief of obstruction (stenting), pseudocyst drainage
Transluminal Imaging	
Endoscopic ultrasonography	Staging of tumors

of unexplained chronic abdominal pain. In dealing with the evaluation of gastrointestinal symptoms, several questions therefore need to be addressed by the referring physician and the endoscopist: *Which* patients need endoscopy? *When* should the endoscopy be done? *What* is the endoscopist looking for? What *endoscopic therapy,* if any, should be planned?

GASTROESOPHAGEAL REFLUX (see Chapters 124 and 131). Gastroesophageal reflux disease (GERD) is an extremely common condition in the general population. Fortunately, its cardinal symptom, heartburn, is relatively specific; because of the safety of most antireflux medications, an empirical approach is appropriate for many patients with GERD. However, the presence of certain symptoms or signs in a patient with reflux-like symptoms should lead to an early endoscopy: dysphagia or odynophagia, weight loss, gastrointestinal bleeding, or frequent vomiting. These symptoms imply either the development of a GERD-related complication (e.g., stricture, Barrett's esophagus, or adenocarcinoma) or another disorder masquerading as GERD (e.g., squamous cell cancer or a gastric/duodenal lesion such as cancer or peptic ulcer). Because endoscopy is the most accurate method to detect and grade esophagitis, it can be helpful to triage patients with GERD into a low-risk group (managed symptomatically) and those at high-risk for complications (who will require a more aggressive regimen). Patients with severe, persistent, or frequently recurrent symptoms may have significant esophagitis and are therefore appropriate candidates for endoscopy (see Fig. 124–1). Finally, most experts recommend some form of periodic surveillance endoscopy for patients with Barrett's esophagus, a subset of patients with GERD who may be at risk for the development of adenocarcinoma (Color Plate 1*D*).

The overall sensitivity of endoscopy in GERD is only about 70%. Thus, although the presence of esophagitis is very specific, milder cases of GERD are not necessarily detected by endoscopy, and a negative endoscopy does not rule out the diagnosis of GERD. If necessary, further evaluation with ambulatory pH monitoring may be indicated to establish the diagnosis.

Heartburn in immunocompromised patients often indicates an esophageal infection. The most common causes in patients with human immunodeficiency virus infection are *Candida,* cytomegalovirus, herpesvirus, and idiopathic esophageal ulcers. Because most patients with the acquired immunodeficiency syndrome and esophagitis will have candidiasis, an empirical 1- to 2-week course of antifungal therapy may be justified. Those who fail this approach, however, should almost always have an endoscopy and biopsy because each of the common causes requires specific therapy.

DYSPHAGIA (see Chapter 124). Dysphagia can often be categorized as oropharyngeal based on the clinical features of nasal regurgitation, laryngeal aspiration, or difficulty in moving the bolus out of the mouth. Conversely, the most common causes of esophageal dysphagia include malignant lesions, benign processes (peptic strictures secondary to reflux, Schatzki's rings), and motility disturbances of the esophageal body or the lower esophageal sphincter. Although endoscopic examination is considered mandatory in all patients with dysphagia, barium radiography can guide an endoscopy that is anticipated to be difficult (e.g., a patient with a complex stricture), suggest an underlying disturbance in motility, and occasionally detect subtle stenoses that are not appreciated on endoscopy (the scope diameter is typically 10 mm or less, whereas some symptomatic strictures can be as wide as 18 mm).

Endoscopic treatment options are available for many causes of esophageal dysphagia. Tumors may be dilated mechanically, ablated by thermal means (cautery or laser), or stented with prosthetic devices; metallic expandable stents have become the palliative procedure of choice for most patients with symptomatic esophageal cancer. Benign lesions of the esophagus, such a strictures or rings, can also be dilated endoscopically, usually with excellent results (Color Plate 1*D*). Finally, some motility disturbances such as achalasia are best approached endoscopically with the use of large balloon dilators for the lower esophageal sphincter or sometimes with the local injection of botulinum toxin.

DYSPEPSIA (see Chapter 131). Dyspepsia, which is chronic or recurring pain or discomfort centered in the upper abdomen, is seen in approximately 25% of the population and accounts for 2 to 5% of all family practice consultations. Up to 40% of patients with dyspepsia will have a structural lesion such as peptic ulcer (15–25%), reflux esophagitis (5–15%), and, rarely, gastric or esophageal cancer (<2%). Other structural lesions such as gallstones, pancreatic diseases, infiltrative diseases of the stomach or intestines (e.g., eosinophilic gastritis or Crohn's disease), space-occupying lesions of the liver, or ischemic diseases of the bowel are rarely found in these patients. The majority (up to 60%) of patients with chronic (>3 months) dyspepsia belong to the so-called functional

Table 122–2 ■ ENDOSCOPIC COMPLICATIONS, PREPARATION, PRECAUTIONS, AND PROPHYLAXIS

Complications of Endoscopy
General Complications
Complications related primarily to sedation (cardiovascular and respiratory depression, aspiration)
Perforation
Bleeding
Complications Associated with Specialized Procedures
Pancreatitis (ERCP)
Cholangitis (ERCP)
Wound infections (PEG)
Preparation
Upper endoscopy: nothing orally (solids: 6 hours; liquids: 4 hours)
Colonoscopy: bowel purge the day before; optional enemas before the procedure
Sigmoidoscopy: 1–2 enemas before the procedure
Precautions and Prophylaxis
Hemodynamic and respiratory stabilization
Prophylactic antibiotics
Prevention of endocarditis, if indicated (patients with artificial valves, pulmonary-systemic shunts, previous history of endocarditis [see Chapter 326])
Prevention of cholangitis (patients with biliary obstruction)
Prevention of wound infection (PEG)
Prevention of pancreatic infection (patients undergoing therapeutic pancreatic procedures)
Patients on Anticoagulants
Diagnostic procedure only: no adjustment required
High-risk procedure: discontinue anticoagulants 3–5 days before endoscopy and resume after the procedure. In patients at high risk for thromboembolism, heparin may be considered while the INR is subtherapeutic (discontinue heparin for 4–6 hours before the procedure).

ERCP = endoscopic retrograde cholangiopancreatography; PEG = percutaneous endoscopic gastrostomy; INR = international normalized ratio.

category in which there is no definite structural or biochemical explanation for the symptoms; although *Helicobacter pylori* gastritis is found frequently in these patients, there is no definite evidence to prove a cause-and-effect between these two findings.

The optimal diagnostic approach to dyspepsia is somewhat controversial and is still evolving (see Fig. 131–2). In recent years there has been a move toward empirical approaches to dyspepsia because only a minority of patients with dyspepsia have peptic ulcers and gastric cancer is extremely rare in Western countries. However, dyspepsia is a recurrent condition, and patients who fail to respond to empirical therapy will commonly undergo endoscopy. If a diagnostic test is to be performed, endoscopy, sometimes with biopsies to detect *H. pylori,* is clearly the procedure of choice with an accuracy of about 90% (compared with about 65% for double-contrast radiography).

UPPER GASTROINTESTINAL BLEEDING (see Chapter 123). Upper gastrointestinal (UGI) bleeding is a major health care problem, and bleeding peptic ulcers alone account for more than 100,000 admissions per year in the United States. Acid-peptic disease (including ulcers, erosions, and gastritis) as a group accounts for the majority (50–75%) of all cases of UGI bleeding (Color Plate 2*E*), followed by variceal bleeding (10% or more) and Mallory-Weiss tears (5–10%). Vascular malformations are a less common but important cause and include angiomas or the rarer Dieulafoy's lesion (a superficial artery that erodes through the gut mucosa). Finally, upper gastrointestinal cancers are occasionally associated with significant bleeding.

Endoscopy is mandatory in essentially all patients with UGI bleeding, with the rare exception being the terminally ill patient in whom the outcome is unlikely to be affected. Endoscopy is able to detect and localize the site of the bleeding in 95% of cases and is clearly superior to contrast radiography (with an accuracy of only 75 to 80%). The endoscopic appearance of bleeding lesions can also help predict the risk of rebleeding, thus facilitating the triage and treatment process. Finally, and perhaps most importantly, bleeding can be effectively controlled during the initial endoscopy itself in the majority of cases.

In general, endoscopy should be performed only after adequate stabilization of hemodynamic and respiratory parameters. The role of gastric lavage before endoscopy is controversial; some endoscopists prefer that it be done, occasionally even using a large-bore tube, whereas others avoid such preparation because of the fear of producing artifact. The timing of subsequent endoscopy is dependent on two factors: the severity of the hemorrhage and the risk status of the patient (see Fig. 123–1). Patients with active, persistent, or severe bleeding (>3 units of blood) will require urgent endoscopy. Endoscopy in these patients is best performed in the intensive-care unit because they are at particular risk for aspiration and may require emergent intubation for respiratory protection and ventilation. Patients with slower or inactive bleeding may be evaluated by endoscopy in a "semi-elective" manner (usually within 12–20 hours), but a case can be made to perform endoscopy very early even in these stable patients (perhaps in the emergency department itself) to allow triage decisions to be made more confidently.

Most bleeding from upper gastrointestinal lesions can be effectively controlled endoscopically. The endoscopist considers factors such as age (older patients have a higher risk of rebleeding) and the severity of the initial hemorrhage (which has a direct correlation with the risk of rebleeding) in addition to the appearance of the lesion when determining the need for endoscopic therapy. Nonvariceal bleeding vessels can be treated with a variety of means including injections of various substances (epinephrine, saline, sclerosants) or thermal coagulation (laser or electrocautery). In the United States, the most popular approach to a bleeding peptic ulcer lesion is a combination of injection with dilute epinephrine and electrocoagulation. Initial hemostasis can be achieved in 90% or more of cases; rebleeding, which may recur in up to 20% of cases, will respond about half of the time to a second endoscopic procedure. Patients who continue to bleed (typically patients with large ulcers in the posterior wall of the duodenal bulb) are usually managed angiographically (with embolization of the bleeding vessel) or surgically.

Variceal bleeding is also effectively managed endoscopically, with a similar success rate as with bleeding ulcers (Color Plate 2*A*). Hemostasis is achieved using either band ligation (Fig. 122–1), sclerotherapy, or a combination of both. Increasingly, patients who

do not respond to endoscopic treatment are then considered candidates for a transjugular intrahepatic portosystemic shunt; traditional shunt surgery for bleeding varices is rarely performed. Even if initial endoscopic hemostasis is successful, long-term prevention of rebleeding requires a program of ongoing endoscopic sessions until variceal obliteration is complete. Ligation is the preferred approach in this setting because it is associated with fewer side effects.

ACUTE LOWER GASTROINTESTINAL BLEEDING (see Chapter 123). The most common cause of acute lower gastrointestinal bleeding is angiodysplasia, followed by diverticulosis, neoplasms, and colitis. In about 10% of patients presenting with hematochezia, a small bowel lesion may be responsible. In contrast to upper gastrointestinal bleeding, there is no single best test for acute lower gastrointestinal bleeding (see Fig. 123–1). In young patients (<40 years) with minor bleeding, features that are highly suggestive of anorectal origin (e.g., blood on the surface of the stool or on the wipe) may warrant only a flexible sigmoidoscopy. Conversely, patients presenting with hemodynamic compromise may need an upper endoscopy first to exclude a lesion in the upper gastrointestinal tract (typically post-pyloric) that is bleeding so briskly that it presents as hematochezia (which may be seen in 10% or more of acute upper gastrointestinal bleeding). Colonoscopy has traditionally been recommended after bleeding has slowed or stopped and the patient has been given an adequate bowel purge. However, a disadvantage of delaying endoscopy is that when a pathologic lesion such as an arteriovenous malformation (Color Plate 2*F*) or diverticulum is found, it may be impossible to implicate it confidently as the site

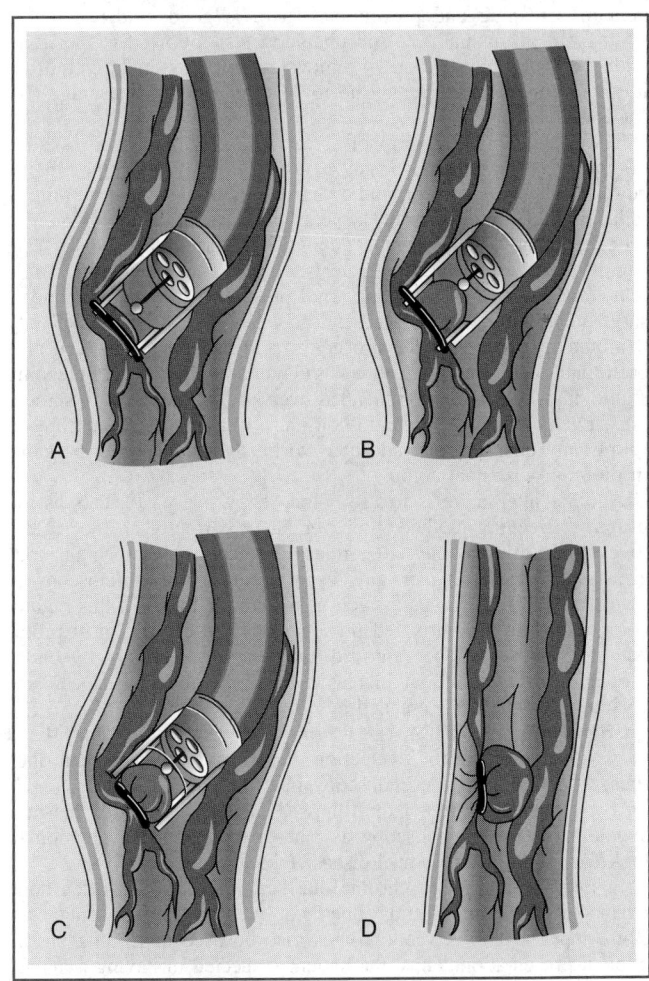

FIGURE 122–1 ▪ Endoscopic variceal ligation technique. *A,* The endoscope, with attached ligating device, is brought into contact with a varix just above the gastroesophageal junction. *B,* Suction is applied, drawing the varix-containing mucosa into the dead space created at the end of the endoscope by the ligating device. *C,* The trip-wire is pulled, releasing the band around the aspirated tissue. *D,* Completed ligation.

of bleeding (complementary information by radiography or scintigraphy becomes particularly important in this situation). Some experts therefore recommend an urgent diagnostic endoscopy with little or no preparation for acute lower gastrointestinal hemorrhages and have reported success rates of 50%.

OCCULT GASTROINTESTINAL BLEEDING OR IRON-DEFICIENCY ANEMIA (see Chapter 123). Normal fecal blood loss is usually less than 2 to 3 mL/day. Most standard fecal occult blood tests will detect blood loss of 10 mL/day or more. Therefore, even if this test is negative, patients with iron-deficiency anemia and no other obvious source of blood loss should always undergo aggressive gastrointestinal evaluation, which will uncover a gastrointestinal lesion in the majority of cases. Although most lesions that cause overt gastrointestinal bleeding can also cause occult blood loss, occult bleeding should almost never be ascribed to diverticulosis or hemorrhoids. Endoscopy is always preferable to radiographic studies for evaluation of occult blood loss or iron-deficiency anemia because of its ability to detect flat lesions, particularly vascular malformations, which may be found in 6% or more of patients. If both upper and lower endoscopy are negative, a small bowel radiographic series to look for gross lesions often completes the evaluation. However, if the patient continues to have symptomatic bleeding, enteroscopy (the use of a very long upper endoscope to intubate the small bowel) may be helpful to detect small bowel angiomata.

COLORECTAL NEOPLASMS (see Chapter 139). Colonoscopy is the most accurate test for detecting mass lesions of the large bowel that are suspected on clinical or radiologic grounds. However, the greatest impact of endoscopy on colorectal neoplasia may be in the area of screening and prevention. There is good evidence that a strategy of an annual fecal occult blood test followed (if positive) with a colonoscopy and polyp removal significantly reduces mortality from colorectal cancer by up to 33% in patients at average risk for colon cancer.

The second popular form of screening is sigmoidoscopy with a 60-cm scope that should detect 40 to 60% of all adenomas in the colon. Three case-control studies have shown an almost two-thirds reduction in mortality from cancers within reach of the sigmoidoscope compared with matched controls. Its advantages over fecal occult blood test include a greater sensitivity and specificity; it is a relatively simple and straightforward procedure that requires only a short preparation. Experienced endoscopists take an average of only 8 minutes to complete the procedure, and non-physicians can also be trained to do this procedure with comparable efficacy. Screening sigmoidoscopies are recommended every 4 to 5 years. Any screening strategy utilizing sigmoidoscopy also requires a colonoscopy to follow any positive sigmoidoscopy to look for synchronous lesions in the more proximal colon.

Another alternative is to use colonoscopy every 10 years as the primary screening method; however, there currently are no studies to evaluate this strategy. Regardless of the initial screening strategy, a positive finding on any test warrants a full colonoscopy to detect all possible polyps as well as to remove them. In this regard, colonoscopy is the unrivaled procedure of choice, and most protuberant growths can be removed safely and effectively by endoscopic means. Patients at increased risk for colorectal cancer (see Chapter 139) are best screened by colonoscopy.

CHRONIC DIARRHEA (see Chapter 133). Endoscopy may be a very valuable aid in the evaluation of patients with persistent diarrhea. The timing of the endoscopy in these patients often depends on the clinical features of the illness. Patients with bloody diarrhea should have lower endoscopy as part of their initial evaluation to look for inflammatory bowel disease (see Chapter 135).

In most patients with chronic diarrhea, endoscopy is often done when initial routine testing does not yield a specific diagnosis. Both upper and lower endoscopies may be used depending on the clinical presentation. Thus, the patient suspected of having a malabsorptive process may require an upper endoscopy with jejunal or duodenal biopsies to look for celiac sprue or rarer lesions such as lymphoma or Whipple's disease (endoscopic biopsy has largely replaced blind intestinal biopsies for these conditions). Conversely, patients suspected to have a secretory cause of diarrhea will require a colonoscopy with biopsies to look for subtle forms of inflammatory bowel disease that may have a normal endoscopic appearance,

such as microscopic colitis, and the diagnosis is made only after careful examination of the biopsy specimens.

The endoscopic approach to diarrhea in immunocompromised patients, such as those with human immunodeficiency virus infection, is guided by the degree of immunosuppression and the need to find treatable infections. When routine stool tests are negative, patients with CD4 counts of less than 100/mm^3 should undergo endoscopic evaluation to detect pathogens such as cytomegalovirus, *Mycobacterium avium-complex,* and microsporidiosis. Small-volume stools with tenesmus suggest a proctocolitis, for which sigmoidoscopy (rather than a full colonoscopy) with biopsies is usually adequate. In patients with upper gastrointestinal symptoms (large-volume diarrhea, bloating, and dyspepsia), an upper endoscopy with biopsy may be attempted first.

MISCELLANEOUS INDICATIONS. The upper endoscope has provided a relatively quick and non-invasive means for removal of accidentally or deliberately ingested foreign bodies. Timing is critical for removal, however, because objects are usually beyond endoscopic retrieval once they reach the small bowel. Any foreign object that is causing symptoms should be removed, as should potentially dangerous devices such as batteries or sharp objects. In general, objects greater than 2.5 cm in width or 13 cm in length are unlikely to leave the stomach and so should also be removed.

Because of the relatively poor correlation between oropharyngeal lesions and more distal visceral injury, upper endoscopy is usually recommended urgently in patients with *corrosive ingestion* (see Chapter 98). Endoscopy allows patients to be triaged into high- or low-risk groups for complications, with institution of appropriate monitoring and therapy.

Among the myriad causes of *nausea and vomiting,* a few, such as mucosal lesions or unsuspected reflux disease, are particularly amenable to endoscopic diagnosis. Patients with new-onset *constipation* (see Chapter 132), particularly those who are older than 40 years of age, should also undergo a colonoscopic evaluation to exclude an obstructing carcinoma. Colonoscopy is also useful in patients with pseudo-obstructive (non-obstructive) colonic dilation or *Ogilvie's syndrome* (see Chapter 132); such patients are at risk for colonic rupture at diameters above 9 to 12 cm, and colonoscopic decompression is often required, sometimes on an emergent basis.

A major advance in enteral feeding has been the introduction of percutaneous endoscopic gastrostomy (PEG), a relatively quick, simple, and safe endoscopic procedure that has virtually eliminated surgical placement of gastric tubes. A variation of PEG is the percutaneous endoscopic jejunostomy (PEJ), in which a long tube is passed through the gastric tube, past the pylorus, and into the jejunum. The most common indication for these procedures is the need for sustained nutrition in patients with neurologic impairment of swallowing or with head and neck cancers. Patients with very short life expectancy are not suitable candidates for PEG and can be managed by nasoenteral tubes. PEJ was originally introduced to prevent aspiration, but it does not prevent this complication; the major indication for PEJ is significant impairment of gastric emptying. Retrograde tube migration with PEJ is quite common, however, and PEJ may require frequent replacement.

PANCREATOBILIARY ENDOSCOPY (IMAGING)

Endoscopic retrograde cholangiopancreatography (ERCP), involves a special side-viewing endoscope (the duodenoscope) that is used to gain access to the second part of the duodenum. A small catheter is then introduced into the bile or pancreatic duct, and radiographic contrast medium is injected under fluoroscopic monitoring. Successful cannulation and imaging can be achieved in up to 95% of cases. ERCP is perhaps the technically most demanding of gastrointestinal endoscopic procedures, and it is associated with the highest risk of serious complications, notably pancreatitis in about 5% of cases. The technique should be performed only by experts, in part because of the frequent need to provide urgent therapy.

SUSPECTED BILIARY PATHOLOGY (see Chapters 144 and 157). The diagnostic approach to patients with cholestasis begins with an attempt to differentiate obstructive from hepatocellular causes. The most common causes of obstructive jaundice are common bile duct stones and tumors of the pancreatic and bile duct. Less invasive conventional imaging with ultrasonography, computed tomography, or magnetic resonance imaging will demonstrate dilated bile ducts and mass lesions but are not very sensitive or specific in detecting or delineating pathology in the distal common bile duct and pancreas, two regions where the majority of obstructing lesions are found. Furthermore, there are some biliary diseases, such as sclerosing cholangitis, that do not result in dilated ducts but have a characteristic appearance on cholangiography. Finally, the ability to use devices such as cytology brushes and biopsy forceps during cholangiography provides an additional aid in the diagnosis of biliary lesions.

Cholangiography by means of injection of contrast material (either percutaneously or endoscopically) is therefore almost always indicated in patients suspected of biliary obstruction or those with a cholestatic pattern of abnormal liver function tests. Both techniques are associated with a high rate of success in experienced hands, but the endoscopic approach allows visualization of the ampullary region and the performance of sphincterotomy, and it also avoids the small risk of a biliary leak associated with puncturing of the liver capsule.

Of the approximately 600,000 patients undergoing cholecystectomy in this country, 5 to 10% may present with bile duct stones before or after the surgery. Endoscopic stone removal is successful in 90% or more of these cases and usually requires a sphincterotomy (Color Plate 2D). The sphincter of Oddi is a band of muscle that encircles the distal common bile duct and pancreatic duct in the region of the ampulla of Vater; cutting of this muscle, or sphincterotomy, is one of the mainstays of endoscopic biliary treatment and is accomplished using a special tool called a papillotome or sphincterotome. This procedure is often sufficient for the treatment of small stones in the bile ducts, but larger stones may require additional procedures, such as mechanical, electrohydraulic, or laser lithotripsy, all of which can be performed endoscopically. In addition to stone disease, sphincterotomy can also be curative for patients with papillary stenosis or muscle spasm (termed *sphincter of Oddi dysfunction*). Finally, by enlarging the access to the bile duct, sphincterotomy also facilitates the passage of stents and other devices into the bile duct. Sphincterotomy carries an additional small risk of bleeding, but its morbidity is about one-third that of surgical exploration, and its cost is only about 20% as high.

Endoscopic therapy has also revolutionized the palliative approach to malignant biliary obstruction. The technique, which requires the placement of indwelling stents, is superior to both radiologic and surgical techniques. Plastic stents have been the mainstay of treatment, but metal stents last longer and are perhaps preferred in patients with longer life expectancies.

PANCREATIC DISEASE (see Chapters 140 and 141). ERCP is also useful in patients with pancreatic diseases that do not present with obstructive jaundice, such as pancreatic cancer and, less commonly, chronic pancreatitis. It is also indicated in patients with acute or recurrent pancreatitis without any obvious risk factors on history or routine laboratory evaluation. Imaging of the pancreatic duct may delineate anatomic abnormalities that may be responsible for the pancreatitis, such as congenital variants (pancreas divisum, annular pancreas), intraductal tumors, or possibly sphincter of Oddi dysfunction. In such cases, bile can also be collected from the bile duct for microscopic examination for crystals (so-called microlithiasis) that can result in pancreatitis in some patients even in the absence of macroscopic stones. In patients with chronic pancreatitis, which is most often due to excessive alcohol intake, pancreatography can confirm the diagnosis, provide useful information about the severity of the disease, and identify ductal lesions that potentially may be amenable to therapy by either endoscopic (see later) or surgical means. In more subtle cases, collection and analysis of pancreatic juice after stimulation with secretin may be useful in establishing exocrine impairment and hence in confirming chronic pancreatic injury.

ERCP also has a role in some patients with *acute* pancreatitis (see Chapter 141) that is likely caused by obstructing biliary stones. Patients presenting with severe biliary pancreatitis may benefit from an urgent ERCP early in their course, with the intention of detecting and removing stones from the common bile duct. Similarly, patients who have smoldering acute pancreatitis that does not appear to be improving satisfactorily on conservative treatment may require ERCP to identify and treat any obstructing lesions in the pancreatic or distal biliary duct.

Therapeutic endoscopy for pancreatic disease is still evolving.

Relief of ductal obstruction (e.g., by endoscopic removal of pancreatic stones or dilation of strictures) can provide short to intermediate pain relief in some patients with chronic pancreatitis. Endoscopic pseudocyst drainage by a variety of techniques is now technically feasible, with results that appear to be comparable with those of surgical or radiologic techniques. Patients with ductal disruptions (e.g., those with pancreatic ascites) can often be treated with endoscopic stent placement. Pancreatic papillotomy may also be useful for selected cases of recurrent pancreatitis, such as those with pancreas divisum or sphincter of Oddi dysfunction. Although the ability to approach these difficult clinical entities by the relatively less-invasive endoscopic techniques represents a major accomplishment, the exact role of the various treatment modalities (surgical, radiologic, and endoscopic) in the treatment of pancreatic diseases remains to be determined.

TRANSLUMINAL IMAGING: ENDOSCOPIC ULTRASONOGRAPHY

The development of endoscopic ultrasonograpy (EUS), or endosonography, has been a major technological achievement in gastroenterology. The incorporation of an ultrasonic transducer into the tip of a flexible endoscope or the use of "stand-alone" ultrasound probes has now made it possible to obtain images of gastrointestinal lesions that are not apparent on superficial views, including lesions within the wall of the gut as well those that lie beyond (e.g., pancreatic or lymph node lesions). A further role of EUS is to guide fine-needle aspiration, which often provides pathologic confirmation of suspicious lesions. In many cases, this approach appears to be even more accurate than conventional radiologic techniques such as abdominal ultrasound or computed tomography. Thus, EUS is probably the single best test for diagnosing pancreatic tumors (see Chapters 130 and 140), particularly the small endocrine varieties, with sensitivities approaching 95%. It is also the procedure of choice for imaging submucosal and other wall lesions of the gastrointestinal tract (overall accuracy of 65–70%) as well as for staging of a variety of gastrointestinal tumors (overall accuracy of 90% or more). Preoperative staging is a critical element in the management strategy of tumors such as esophageal and pancreatic cancer, and EUS can complement more conventional radiologic tests to help determine the resectability and curative potential of surgery in these cases.

American Gastroenterological Association Medical Position Statement: Evaluation of dyspepsia. Gastroenterology 114:579–581, 1998. *An authoritative review of the clinical approach to patients with dyspepsia with useful practice guidelines.*

American Society of Gastrointestinal Endoscopy: The role of endoscopy in the management of non-variceal acute upper gastrointestinal bleeding: Guidelines for clinical application. Gastrointest Endosc 38:760–764, 1992. *Summary of the usefulness of endoscopy in patients with bleeding ulcers and other non-variceal lesions.*

Byers T, Levin B, Rothenberger D, et al: (for the American Cancer Society Detection and Treatment Advisory Group on Colorectal Cancer): American Cancer Society guidelines for screening and surveillance for early detection of colorectal polyps and cancer: Update 1997. CA Cancer J Clin 47:154–160, 1997. *Practical guidelines from the American Cancer Society.*

Folsch UR, Nitsche R, Ludtke R, et al, and the German Study Group on Acute Biliary Pancreatitis: Early ERCP and papillotomy compared with conservative treatment for acute biliary pancreatitis. N Engl J Med 336:237–242, 1997. *An important clinical trial studying the usefulness of early endoscopic intervention in patients with acute biliary pancreatitis.*

Winawer SJ, Fletcher RH, Miller L, et al: Colorectal cancer screening: Clinical guidelines and rationale. Gastroenterology 112:594–642, 1997. *A review of suggested guidelines for colorectal cancer screening and the underlying rationale.*

123 GASTROINTESTINAL HEMORRHAGE AND OCCULT GASTROINTESTINAL BLEEDING

John P. Cello

Bleeding from the gastrointestinal tract is one of the most common reasons for admission to the hospital. Although the number of patients admitted for peptic ulcer disease has gradually decreased, the overall mortality for gastrointestinal tract hemorrhage (8–10%) has remained largely unchanged over the past several decades. Whereas the specific bleeding lesion and pathophysiology of hemorrhage may vary considerably (Tables 123–1 and 123–2), the initial therapeutic and diagnostic approach to the bleeding patient remains largely the same.

Gastrointestinal tract hemorrhage usually produces dramatic clinical signs and symptoms and brings patients promptly to the attention of physicians. *Hematemesis* is vomiting of gross blood. Usually, vomiting of bloody material indicates bleeding from the upper gastrointestinal tract, but blood entering the gastrointestinal tract from anywhere proximal to the ligament of Treitz (duodenojejunal junction) can be vomited by the patient. Hematemesis most frequently follows bleeding from the esophagus, stomach, or duodenum, but occasionally gingival, nasopharyngeal, pulmonary, and even pancreaticobiliary bleeding can be manifested initially by hematemesis. *Melenemesis,* or "coffee grounds" vomiting, occurs when blood is in contact with gastric acid for at least 1 hour. Patients who vomit "coffee grounds" material are usually bleeding at a slower rate than those who have grossly bloody emesis, but the same sources may present as either type of bleeding. *Melena,* usually noted by patients with bleeding from the proximal gastrointestinal tract, is characterized by dark black, liquid, tarry, metallic-smelling stools. Melenic stools usually indicate upper gastrointestinal tract bleeding, but not infrequently mid- to distal small bowel and even slow proximal colonic bleeding can be manifested by dark black, liquid stools. *Hematochezia,* the passage of bright red stools, is usually a sign of distal small bowel or brisk colonic hemorrhage, with the majority, particularly those without orthostatic signs or symptoms, bleeding from superficial mucosal lesions in the sigmoid, rectum, or anorectal junction. However, up to 10% of patients with hemodynamically significant hematochezia are actively bleeding from an upper, not lower, gastrointestinal tract lesion and have accelerated gastrointestinal transit times. Patients with hemodynamically significant gastrointestinal tract bleeding from any site often have lightheadedness, dizziness, diaphoresis, or frank syncope if hypovolemia has occurred. Patients with chronic gastrointestinal tract bleeding have signs and symptoms of profound iron-deficiency anemia, including pallor, dyspnea, angina, and exertional weakness.

Patients with gastrointestinal tract bleeding must be assessed for the hemodynamic significance of the blood loss and appropriately resuscitated. The most accurate non-invasive indicator of the severity of acute blood loss is the presence of shock or postural changes in vital signs. Shock indicates an acute blood volume loss of at least 15 to 20%. Postural vital sign changes (e.g., upright tachycardia, widening of the pulse pressure, and/or upright systolic hypotension) indicate acute intravascular volume loss of at least 10 to 15%. It is essential to determine the blood pressure and pulse in both the supine and upright positions in patients who report signs and symptoms of gastrointestinal tract bleeding, unless supine hypotension precludes such an evaluation.

Brisk hemorrhage with hematemesis and/or "coffee grounds" emesis is usually associated with increasing stool frequency, hyperactive bowel sounds, and a change in the color of the stools from dark black to dark red color. With bleeding from a duodenal ulcer, relatively small amounts of blood may be vomited or lavaged by nasogastric tube, whereas most blood passes distally into the gastrointestinal tract and presents as melena. Nasogastric lavage is helpful but highly inaccurate in estimating the severity of upper gastrointestinal tract bleeding, particularly duodenal bleeding. The absence of significant blood by nasogastric lavage (particularly when the lavage does not contain bile) does not exclude upper gastrointestinal tract bleeding. With profuse hematemesis, the return of large amounts of clots or bright red blood obviously indicates vigorous active upper gastrointestinal tract hemorrhage. With acute hemorrhage, the hematocrit and hemoglobin levels are not reliable indicators of the severity of bleeding. For the hematocrit to fall, the blood plasma must have equilibrated with extracellular fluid or with administered intravenous fluids, and this equilibration may require 24 to 48 hours to occur. Exsanguination can occur with a relatively normal hematocrit, and patients with extremely low hematocrits can be hemodynamically quite stable. For these reasons, one should avoid relying too heavily on the initial hemoglobin concentration or hematocrit, particularly in patients with other manifestations of brisk gastrointestinal tract hemorrhage.

INITIAL EVALUATION AND TREATMENT

Regardless of the site or cause of hemorrhage, all patients with significant active blood loss from the gastrointestinal tract should be evaluated in a similar manner (Fig. 123–1). Initially, vital signs, including supine and upright blood pressure and pulse, must be measured to assess the hemodynamic severity of blood loss. If blood loss is significant by hemodynamic assessment, intravenous fluids must be started immediately to restore intravascular volume. Saline or other balanced electrolyte solutions are most readily available, but there is no substitute for packed red blood cells in patients who are bleeding briskly.

After the initial evaluative and resuscitative measures, the history of the bleeding episode and of any previous gastrointestinal tract hemorrhage should be obtained rapidly. A personal or family history of gastrointestinal tract illness particularly from peptic ulcers, cancer, or vascular ectasias (e.g., Osler-Weber-Rendu syndrome), is helpful, as is a history of previously documented gastrointestinal tract disease as determined by radiography, endoscopy, or surgery.

Table 123–2 ■ **ETIOLOGY OF HEMATOCHEZIA IN 72 HOSPITALIZED PATIENTS***

SOURCE OF HEMORRHAGE	PERCENTAGE
Colonic cancer	7
Colonic polyps	11
Diverticula	23
Colitis	11
Vascular ectasia	1
Large hemorrhoids only	12
Ulcer tear (rectum)	10
Upper gastrointestinal or small bowel source	10
No site identified	15
	100

*Patients undergoing colonoscopy (and endoscopy if colonoscopy was negative) at San Francisco General Hospital.

Table 123–1 ■ **ETIOLOGY AND SEVERITY OF UPPER GASTROINTESTINAL TRACT HEMORRHAGE***

SOURCE OF HEMORRHAGE	SEVERITY OF HEMORRHAGE	
	Mild–Moderate (246 Patients)	Severe (140 Patients)
Esophagus		
Esophagitis	12%	7%
Ulcer	2%	2%
Mallory-Weiss tear	5%	19%
Esophageal varices	5%	31%
Total esophagus	24%	59%
Stomach		
Gastric ulcer	15%	14%
Prepyloric ulcer	2%	4%
Pyloric channel ulcer	4%	2%
Gastric erosions	2%	0
Gastritis	7%	0
Varices	1%	2%
Portal-hypertensive gastropathy	2%	0
Gastric cancer	2%	0
Polyp	0	2%
Dieulafoy lesion	0	0
Total stomach	35%	24%
Duodenum		
Ulcer	30%	15%
Duodenitis	8%	0
Aortoenteric fistula	0	2%
Pancreatic pseudocyst	2%	0
Post-sphincterotomy	1%	0
Total duodenum	41%	17%
	100%	100%

*All patients underwent diagnostic endoscopy at San Francisco General Hospital over 3 years.

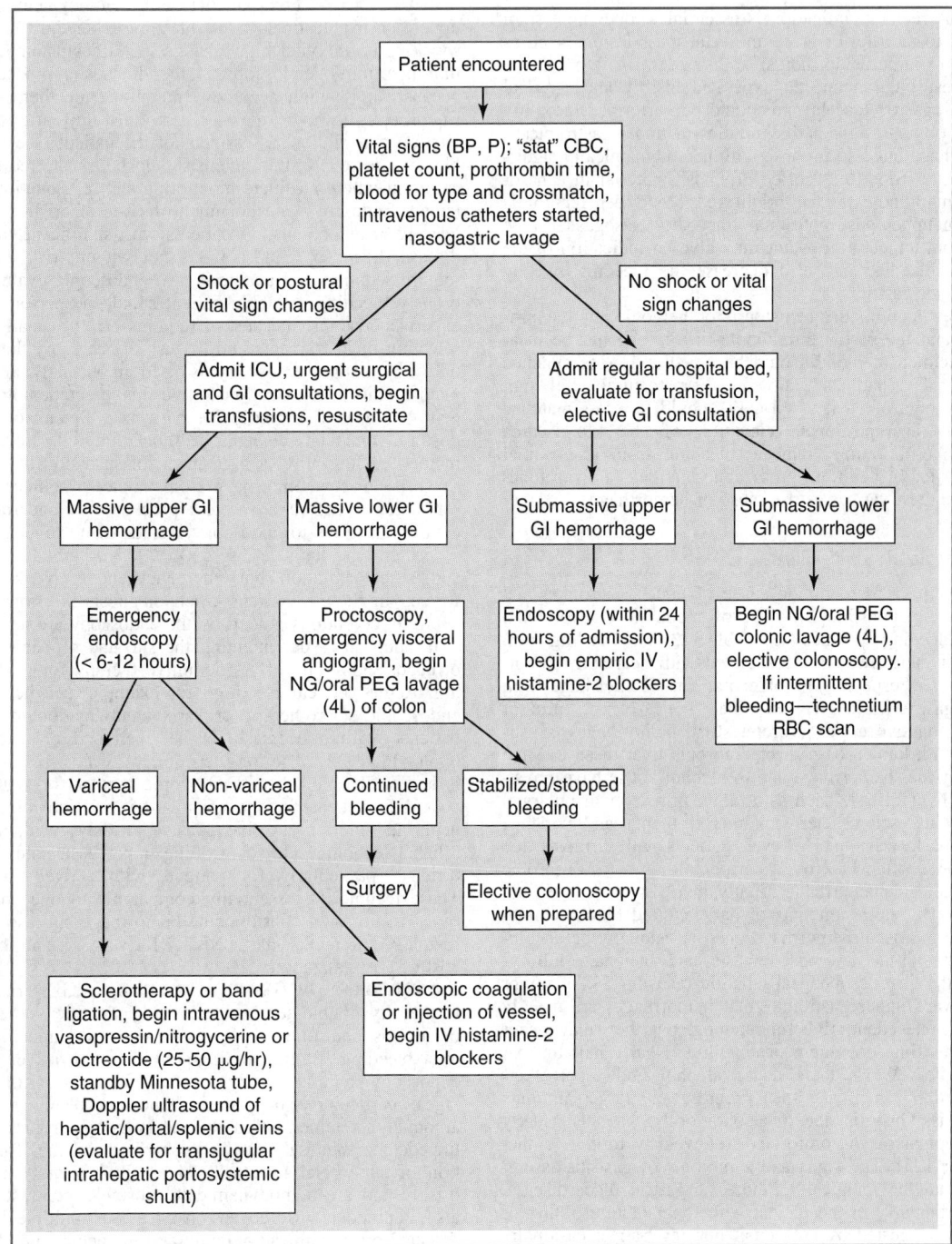

FIGURE 123–1 ■ Approach to the patient with gastrointestinal hemorrhage.

Patients with a history of alcohol abuse or known or suspected chronic liver disease may present with painless hematemesis from esophageal varices (see Chapter 153). Substernal burning pain, regurgitation, or reflux symptoms may indicate long-standing reflux esophagitis. Patients with forceful, dry retching or multiple episodes of vomiting of food before the onset of hematemesis may be bleeding from Mallory-Weiss tears of the gastroesophageal junction. A history of epigastric burning pain promptly relieved by food or antacids or nocturnal pain suggests peptic ulcer disease, particularly duodenal ulcer (see Chapter 126). However, as many as one third of patients presenting with bleeding from peptic ulcers have no antecedent dyspepsia. Use of nonsteroidal anti-inflammatory drugs (NSAIDs), which predispose to both gastric and duodenal ulcers, should be ascertained.

A history of known diverticular disease supports the possibility of colonic diverticular hemorrhage in patients with brisk hemato-

chezia (see Chapter 136). Colorectal malignancy is often suggested by a history of gradual weight loss, intermittent blood in the stools, or altered bowel habits (see Chapter 139). Patients with idiopathic inflammatory bowel disease often have long-standing mucous and bloody diarrhea (see Chapter 135). Hemorrhoidal bleeding is often suggested by the presence of bright red blood surrounding well-formed, normal-appearing stools (see Chapter 143).

The physical examination is sometimes helpful in suggesting the cause of hemorrhage. Patients with stigmata of chronic liver disease (e.g., spider angiomata, ascites, gynecomastia) and upper gastrointestinal tract bleeding often bleed from esophageal varices, but almost half are found to be bleeding from lesions other than varices. Localized epigastric tenderness to palpation may indicate peptic ulcer disease or gastritis. Occasionally, patients with lower gastrointestinal tract bleeding from a malignancy have a palpable lower abdominal mass, hepatomegaly, signs of obvious weight loss, or adenopathy. A rectal examination is essential to document stool color as well as to palpate for gross anorectal mass lesions such as polyps, cancers, or large hemorrhoids.

After rapid resuscitation and an expedited history and physical examination, nasogastric tube lavage should be performed, not only in patients with obvious signs and symptoms of upper gastrointestinal tract hemorrhage but also in those with hemodynamically significant hematochezia. Blood or "coffee grounds" material in a nasogastric lavage may indicate that bright red blood per rectum is coming from an upper gastrointestinal tract site. Nasogastric tube lavage using room temperature water may give an indication of the rate of ongoing bleeding and also decrease the bleeding rate by constricting smaller gastric vessels.

After initial evaluation, the hematocrit or hemoglobin, the prothrombin time, and the partial thromboplastin time should be measured and a specimen of blood should be typed and cross-matched for transfusions. For patients with shock or postural vital sign changes, 4 to 6 units of packed red cells should be cross-matched immediately. A disproportionate elevation of the blood urea nitrogen:creatinine ratio may indicate bleeding from a proximal gastrointestinal site. In addition, gross abnormalities of liver function tests may suggest varices as the cause of hemorrhage.

Upper Gastrointestinal Tract Bleeding

Ulcer disease, the most common cause of upper gastrointestinal tract bleeding, is responsible for 50% of moderately severe and 35% of severe bleeding episodes (see Table 123–1). Bleeding from peptic ulcers may not always be associated with heartburn or epigastric burning pain, especially in older patients. Hemorrhage from esophageal or gastric varices (responsible for nearly one third of the episodes of massive upper gastrointestinal hemorrhage) is usually associated with known or suspected chronic liver disease. Most patients with variceal hemorrhage due to alcohol abuse have physical stigmata of liver disease such as a large, firm liver or enlarged spleen, gross ascites, scleral icterus, palmar erythema, and evidence of peripheral muscle wasting. However, patients with cirrhosis due to hepatitis B or C often lack overt peripheral stigmata of chronic liver disease. Variceal hemorrhage usually involves brisk bleeding, with regurgitation of large amounts of dark, clotted blood without emesis. However, variceal hemorrhage may occasionally be accompanied by only "coffee grounds" emesis and melena. Mallory-Weiss tears of the gastroesophageal junction (causing 5% of minor and 20% of severe upper gastrointestinal hemorrhage) are usually associated with antecedent, forceful retching, but they may occur after forceful sneezing, coughing, or singultus. Nearly half the patients with Mallory-Weiss tears abuse alcohol and report "dry heaves" followed by small and then progressively larger amounts of bloody emesis. Gastritis due to alcohol or NSAIDs is usually manifested by epigastric discomfort not relieved by food or antacids (see Chapter 125). The signs and symptoms of gastritis-associated bleeding may be identical to those of gastric ulcer disease. Esophagitis, particularly in the patient with long-standing reflux or regurgitation, is suggested by substernal burning pain occasionally relieved by ingestion of food or antacids (see Chapter 124). Alcohol abusers or patients with prolonged recumbency may sometimes have brisk bleeding from esophagitis or esophageal ulcers without any antecedent substernal burning. Gastrointestinal tract malignancies, such as esophageal and gastric cancer or carcinoma of the ampulla of Vater, rarely cause hemodynamically significant upper gastrointestinal tract bleeding. Rare causes of upper gastrointestinal tract bleeding include aortoduodenal fistulas in patients with atherosclerotic aneurysms of the abdominal aorta, usually after prosthetic grafting; chronic renal disease and acquired vascular ectasias; and ectasias associated with other systemic conditions, such as hereditary hemorrhagic telangiectasias (Osler-Weber-Rendu syndrome). Patients with trauma to the liver or with pancreatic pseudocysts may have signs and symptoms that suggest upper gastrointestinal tract bleeding but are actually bleeding from adjacent organs. Ectatic superficial arteries (Dieulafoy lesions), duodenal diverticula, and certain conditions related to the acquired immunodeficiency syndrome (cytomegalovirus infection–related ulcers, Kaposi's sarcoma, and lymphoma) are occasionally encountered by clinicians.

Diagnostic and Therapeutic Approach

ENDOSCOPY. For patients with hemodynamically significant upper gastrointestinal tract bleeding (bleeding associated with shock, postural vital sign changes, or transfusion requirements of multiple units), endoscopy is the diagnostic procedure of choice because of its high accuracy and immediate therapeutic potential. Endoscopy, however, must be performed only after adequate resuscitation and clinical assessment of the patient (see Fig. 123–1). If bleeding is severe, the patient should be transferred to an intensive care unit where adequate monitoring and resuscitation can be maintained. Endoscopy can document the site of brisk hemorrhage in at least 95% of patients. In patients with significant cardiopulmonary disease, however, endoscopy is not without risk, because it does require sedation and analgesia. An endoscopic evaluation of a vigorously bleeding, unstable patient should be performed only by an expert endoscopist because it requires careful sedation, lavage, and selection of instruments and the use of accessory therapeutic procedures. Although endoscopy is used in virtually all patients with manifestations of acute gastrointestinal tract hemorrhage, it is urgently indicated primarily for patients with any of the following: postural vital sign changes or shock, multiple transfusions, a hematocrit below 30%, a high index of suspicion of variceal hemorrhage, recurrent hemorrhage from unknown sources, and high risk for surgery (before a surgical procedure is undertaken). Relative contraindications to endoscopy include acute myocardial infarction, severe chronic lung disease ($SO_2 \leq 90\%$), hemodynamic instability, and patient agitation, but emergency endoscopy is commonly performed in these situations when diagnosis is critical and/or therapeutic interventions guided by the endoscopy are needed.

In addition to documenting the site and probable cause of hemorrhage, endoscopy offers definitive therapy for most active bleeding. Acute variceal bleeding, for example, can be controlled with endoscopic sclerotherapy or varix band ligation in nearly 90% of patients, with a decrease in the likelihood of recurrent bleeding (Color Plate 2A). The long-term effect of this treatment on survival is less well established. Endoscopic bipolar (or "BICAP") electrocoagulation, heater probe coagulation, and injection of dilute epinephrine solution are inexpensive, widely available, and highly reliable techniques for controlling upper gastrointestinal tract hemorrhage, particularly for patients with actively bleeding ulcers. These techniques, essentially comparable to one another in effectiveness, not only control acute hemorrhage but also decrease transfusion requirements, the necessity for surgery, and the duration and cost of hospitalization.

BARIUM RADIOGRAPHY. An "upper GI series," when performed by double-contrast technique, identifies at least 70 to 80% of lesions confirmed to be associated with upper gastrointestinal tract bleeding. Barium radiography is noninvasive, costs less than endoscopy, and is readily available but has significant disadvantages, particularly in patients who are bleeding briskly. Large amounts of retained blood or food in the upper gastrointestinal tract impede the mucosal coating by barium and therefore the localization of superficial mucosal lesions. In patients who are bleeding briskly and are hemodynamically unstable, contrast radiography is also impractical. Moreover, on occasion, multiple lesions may be detected by barium radiography and the actual site of bleeding may be difficult to assess. Barium contrast radiography is an acceptable alternative for diagnosing upper gastrointestinal lesions in patients who have not bled excessively, who have no stigmata of chronic liver disease, and who are not in need of endoscopic hemostasis.

ANGIOGRAPHY. In those infrequent instances when the site of upper gastrointestinal tract bleeding is missed on endoscopy, angiography may localize the bleeding. In addition, selective infusion with vasopressin or coil embolization of actively bleeding arteries may control bleeding. In most instances, angiography localizes the bleeding site but does not establish its cause. Bleeding must also be active (>30 mL/h) because angiography detects only extravasation of contrast medium into the gastrointestinal tract. Angiography is expensive, time-consuming, and invasive and requires transporting the patient to a specialized unit, but it is particularly helpful if bleeding is brisk in the face of a negative evaluation of the upper or lower gastrointestinal tract.

NUCLEAR SCINTIGRAPHY. For patients with less active blood loss, technetium red cell nuclear scintigraphy ("red cell scan") can localize the site of bleeding, with adequate sensitivity maintained with as little as 3 mL of blood loss per hour. Scintigraphy is non-invasive and can be performed with portable gamma cameras. As with angiography, the sensitivity of technetium scintigraphy is limited, because active hemorrhage is needed; therefore, frequent repeat scanning is necessary. Technetium red cell scanning is often performed before any angiographic evaluation to prove the presence of active bleeding and to assist in the localization of the bleeding focus.

Lower Gastrointestinal Tract Bleeding

Colonic diverticula are responsible for nearly one fourth of all episodes of hemodynamically significant bleeding from the lower gastrointestinal tract (see Table 123–2). Diverticular hemorrhage is nearly always painless and associated with acute large-volume hematochezia. Patients with clinical diverticulitis rarely bleed significantly (see Chapter 136). Colonic cancers and polyps often present as hematochezia, particularly with lesions in the distal sigmoid colon and rectum. Colonic neoplasms cause nearly 20% of lower gastrointestinal bleeding episodes. Proximal colonic polyps and cancers, however, cause iron deficiency anemia and frequently dark black or bloody stools. Patients with idiopathic ulcerative colitis and Crohn's colitis commonly present with bloody diarrhea and tenesmus, and they usually present with a long-standing history of inflammatory bowel disease (see Chapter 135). Significant lower gastrointestinal tract bleeding also occurs from abnormal, superficial vessels called vascular ectasias (Color Plate 2F); up to 10% of cases of hemodynamically significant hematochezia are caused by bleeding from upper gastrointestinal sites, particularly from duodenal bulbar ulcers (see Table 123–2). Other uncommon causes of "lower" gastrointestinal blood loss include aortoenteric fistulas, Meckel's diverticulum of the ileum, and mesenteric varices.

Diagnostic and Therapeutic Approach

PROCTOSCOPY. Proctoscopy, whether by rigid or flexible instruments, and careful evaluation of the anorectal junction are the initial diagnostic step for all patients with hematochezia. The anus and anorectal junction must be carefully examined for hemorrhoids or lacerations, because documented brisk bleeding from one of these sources can obviate the need for further invasive or non-invasive imaging. Blood from a very distal site in the rectum may reflux proximally into the colon and appear to come from above the maximal depth of insertion of the proctoscope or sigmoidoscope. Diverticula, rectal lacerations, colitis, and many polyps and cancers are found within reach of a flexible sigmoidoscope.

If blood loss is modest (as evidenced by a normal hematocrit and vital signs), sigmoidoscopy may be followed by double-contrast barium radiography, which is highly accurate for detecting even smaller polyps and superficial mucosal abnormalities such as colitis. If signs and symptoms indicate lower gastrointestinal tract hemorrhage together with anemia, colonoscopy should be performed. The colon can be rapidly cleansed within a few hours, using oral polyethylene glycol–based electrolyte solutions. Colonoscopic evaluation not only allows the site of hemorrhage to be determined accurately but also allows biopsy of suspicious mass lesions, polypectomy for modest-sized polyps, and the use of coagulation techniques to control bleeding from vascular ectasias. Upper endoscopic evaluation should be performed in all patients with hematochezia who also have "coffee grounds" nasogastric lavage, in patients with known or suspected ulcer disease, and when brisk bleeding continues to cause profuse hematochezia.

When bleeding is brisk, however, colonoscopy is usually not possible. Technetium red blood cell scintigraphy can detect active bleeding at a rate of at least 3 to 10 mL/hr. Frequent repeat scanning may be needed over the first several hours. Technetium red cell scintigraphy usually localizes the site but not the cause of active hemorrhage. If bleeding continues at a rate exceeding 30 to 50 mL/hr, angiography can be extremely helpful in localizing the site of hemorrhage. In addition, angiographic therapy is possible with vasopressin or embolization techniques. An obvious advantage for technetium scintigraphy or angiographic localization is that surgical resection of the site of hemorrhage, regardless of cause, is usually very effective.

SURGERY. Although therapeutic endoscopy, interventional radiology, potent antisecretory medications, and the treatment of *Helicobacter pylori* infection have dramatically reduced the need for emergency surgery, the clinician must consult surgical colleagues early. Approximately 10% of patients undergoing endoscopic coagulation or injection therapy continue to bleed despite repeated attempts at endoscopic hemostasis and need operative intervention. An upper limit should be set on the number of units of blood transfused (perhaps as low as 6 to 8) and the number of sessions of therapeutic endoscopy (realistically no more than two) before surgery is undertaken, particularly for patients with peptic ulcers, colonic neoplasms, or diverticular hemorrhage, all of which are easily amenable to standard surgical therapy with low morbidity and mortality when performed in low-risk patients by skilled surgeons.

Occult Gastrointestinal Tract Hemorrhage

In approximately 5% of patients evaluated for gastrointestinal hemorrhage, a definitive site of bleeding cannot be detected by routine endoscopy and/or colonoscopy. In the further evaluation of patients with "occult" gastrointestinal blood loss, the clinician must be mindful that the adequacy of the endoscopic visualization is only as good as the equipment, the patient preparation, and the training and experience of the endoscopist. Patients with occult gastrointestinal tract hemorrhage can be classified into three general categories: (1) patients with overt signs of "upper" gastrointestinal tract hemorrhage (i.e., hematemesis or melenemesis but a "negative" upper endoscopy), (2) patients with overt signs of apparent "lower" intestinal tract hemorrhage (i.e., hematochezia but a "negative" colonoscopy), and (3) patients presenting with positive fecal occult blood testing with or without iron deficiency anemia and negative routine upper *and* lower endoscopies.

For patients with overt signs suggestive of an upper gastrointestinal tract lesion but without initial detection of a clear-cut site of bleeding by endoscopy, uncommon lesions must be considered (see Table 123–4), including proximal gastric varices, Dieulafoy lesions, antral or duodenal varices, vascular ectasias, and bleeding from duodenal or gastric diverticula. Pancreaticobiliary bleeding into the duodenum via the papilla of Vater is also extremely difficult to diagnose. Bleeding from an aortoduodenal fistula is rarely diagnosed at the time of standard endoscopy because the fistula is usually quite small and the site of fistula is usually in the third portion of the duodenum, just out of reach of the standard upper gastrointestinal endoscopes. Lesions of the third and fourth portions of the duodenum, such as vascular ectasias, and malignancies such as lymphoma, adenocarcinoma, or Kaposi's sarcoma are very difficult to diagnose unless a colonoscope or a small bowel enteroscope is used for upper gastrointestinal endoscopy.

Occasionally, patients with apparent *lower* gastrointestinal tract hemorrhage (i.e., those presenting with hematochezia) do not have a definitive diagnosis after an initial colonoscopy and follow-up upper endoscopy. The most common problem is inadequate colonic preparation, failure to pass the colonoscope proximal to the hepatic flexure, or bleeding from a site distal to the inferior duodenal angle but proximal to the ileocecal valve. Lesions of the mid–small bowel that present in this fashion include adenocarcinoma, lymphoma, sarcomas, metastases (lung, breast, or melanoma), and vascular malformations such as ectasias or Dieulafoy lesions. On rare instances, small bowel diverticula including Meckel's diverticulum can present with dramatic signs or symptoms of apparent lower gastrointestinal tract hemorrhage and are, of course, undetected by standard endoscopic procedures.

Because many of the lesions associated with lower gastrointestinal tract hemorrhage are flat and/or superficially erosive, a small amount of blood or fecal coating of the mucosa can obscure lesions. The most common causes of "occult" lower gastrointestinal tract hemorrhage are unseen colonic diverticula, vascular ectasias, shallow ulcerations, and small vascular tumors of the colon.

Iron deficiency anemia with occult blood loss can be caused by colonic polyps or neoplasms, but a substantial minority have non-neoplastic lesions of upper and/or lower gastrointestinal tract. In one study of iron deficiency anemia, for example, 26% of patients had lower gastrointestinal tract lesions on colonoscopy (including colon cancer and large neoplastic polyps), but upper gastrointestinal tract lesions (including duodenal ulcer, esophagitis, gastritis, and gastric ulceration) were diagnosed after negative colonoscopy in 37% of patients (Table 123–3).

Table 123–3 ■ GASTROINTESTINAL LESIONS FOUND IN 100 PATIENTS WITH IRON DEFICIENCY ANEMIA*

SOURCE OF HEMORRHAGE	PERCENTAGE
Colon	
Cancer	11
Polyp	5
Vascular ectasia	5
Colitis	2
Cecal ulcer	2
Parasites	1
Total colonic	26
Upper gastrointestinal tract	
Duodenal ulcer	11
Esophagitis	6
Gastritis	6
Gastric ulcer	5
Vascular ectasia	3
Anastomotic ulcer	3
Gastric cancer	1
Portal hypertensive gastropathy	1
Adenomatous polyp	1
Total upper gastrointestinal tract	37

*Patients evaluated by colonoscopy followed by upper endoscopy under the same conscious sedation.

The designation of "occult GI hemorrhage" (Table 123–4) mandates first and foremost adequate endoscopic visualization of the upper gastrointestinal tract from the esophagus through the inferior duodenal angle and the colon from ileocecal valve through anorectum. Furthermore, it also depends on a careful consideration of other potential sites of unexplained hemorrhage where blood ultimately passes into the gastrointestinal tract. For patients whose blood loss approximates 1 unit every 1 to 6 hours, mesenteric angiography may be diagnostic. For patients whose blood loss is intermittent and/or minimal with transfusion requirements of less than 1 unit every 12 hours, technetium red cell scintigraphy is indicated. For patients in whom red cell scintigraphy is unrevealing and/or not practical, thought must be given to small bowel enteroclysis with barium contrast and/or small bowel enteroscopy. With the latter technique, 3-meter endoscopes can visualize the upper

Table 123–4 ■ SOURCES OF "OCCULT" GASTROINTESTINAL HEMORRHAGE

"Occult" Bleeding with Signs of "Upper Gastrointestinal" Hemorrhage
Epistaxis
Hemoptysis
Gingival/glossal/pharyngeal bleeding
Ingestion of blood—human or animal
Gastric cardia varices
Antral/duodenal varices
Dieulafoy lesions
Pancreaticobiliary bleeding
  Pancreatic pseudoaneurysm
  Hepatic neoplasms/trauma
Aortoduodenal fistula
Duodenal diverticulum
Vascular ectasias
"Occult" Bleeding with Signs of "Lower Gastrointestinal" Hemorrhage
Briskly bleeding duodenal ulcers
Small bowel Dieulafoy lesions
Vascular ectasias of colon
Meckel's diverticulum—distal ileum
Aortocolonic or arteriocolonic fistula
Solitary colonic ulcers
Colorectal varices
Blood Loss without Signs/Symptoms of Either Upper or Lower Bleeding
Small bowel neoplasms
  Adenocarcinoma
  Sarcoma, leiomyoma
  Lymphoma
  Metastases—breast, lung, melanoma
Vascular ectasias
Crohn's disease of small bowel
Dieulafoy lesions
Small bowel varices

gastrointestinal tract for approximately 1.5 meters distal to the ligament of Treitz.

In the evaluation of the patients with apparent "occult" gastrointestinal hemorrhage, the primary care physician must personally consult with the endoscopist to be sure that adequate visualization of the upper gastrointestinal tract from the cricopharyngeus to the inferior duodenal angle has been obtained and that visualization of the colon from the ileocecal valve to the anorectum has been achieved. If there is any question about the adequacy of the visualization, then the appropriate endoscopic procedures should be repeated after adequate patient preparation.

Lau JYW, et al: Endoscopic treatment compared with surgery in patients with recurrent bleeding after initial endoscopic control of bleeding ulcers. N Engl J Med 340: 751–756, 1999. *Endoscopic retreatment reduced the need for surgery and reduced the complication rate.*

124 DISEASES OF THE ESOPHAGUS

Sidney Cohen ■ *Henry P. Parkman*

Antegrade esophageal flow is achieved by the act of swallowing with the initiation of primary peristalsis. Gastroesophageal reflux is prevented by the physiologic lower esophageal sphincter (LES).

Abnormalities in esophageal transport may be due to disruption of peristalsis by a neuromuscular disorder or by an organic obstructing lesion. The physiologic LES may contribute to transport disorders when relaxation of its tonically elevated pressure is impaired. Disorders of peristaltic function, such as achalasia, may occur together with abnormalities in sphincter relaxation. When the LES fails to function as an effective barrier to reflux, gastroesophageal reflux develops, with the associated complications of mucosal inflammation (reflux esophagitis).

The symptoms of esophageal disease relate closely to the abnormality in function. Disorders in transport lead to difficulty in swallowing or dysphagia. Abnormal esophageal contractions may cause chest pain. Gastroesophageal reflux leads to heartburn and postural regurgitation of food into the mouth.

The esophagus and its sphincters function through complex neural, humoral, and myogenic mechanisms. The pharynx, upper esophageal sphincter, and upper third of the esophagus are composed of skeletal muscle. Timing of upper esophageal events during swallowing is controlled by the central nervous system (CNS). The lower two-thirds of the esophagus and the LES are smooth muscle. Disorders of skeletal muscle, such as polymyositis, affect the upper portions of the swallowing mechanism. Disorders of smooth muscle, such as scleroderma, affect the distal esophagus and the LES.

The neurohumoral control of the esophagus is incompletely understood. The initiation of peristalsis by swallowing involves both cholinergic and noncholinergic neural pathways as well as myogenic mechanisms. The relaxation of the LES during swallowing is initiated by nonadrenergic, noncholinergic inhibitory nerves in the vagus. These nerves may release vasoactive intestinal peptide (VIP) and/or nitric oxide. The role of excitatory peptides and hormones, such as cholecystokinin, gastrin, substance P, and motilin, in the physiologic control of the sphincter is not clear, but they may cause the fluctuations in sphincter pressure that follow a meal.

DYSPHAGIA

The sensation of food bolus arrest during swallowing is dysphagia; even if transient, it indicates esophageal dysfunction. The patient usually uses the term "sticks," "pauses," or "hangs up," and often points to the subjective site of arrest with a finger. The sensation of a substernal lump (globus), present one-half hour after eating, is not dysphagia.

Dysphagia is never an expression of a purely psychiatric disorder nor a manifestation of hysteria. However, some patients with well-established esophageal disease, such as achalasia, may report that their dysphagia is worse during severe emotional tension.

"Transfer dysphagia" occurs when the bolus cannot be propelled from the mouth or hypopharynx into the esophagus. This type of dysphagia is most commonly related to neurologic disease or to pharyngeal muscle weakness.

The sensation of dysphagia is localized to the suprasternal notch or substernal region, but the location of the sensation is of little use in localizing the actual site of bolus arrest. Dysphagia for a liquid bolus usually indicates an esophageal motor disorder. Dysphagia for solids can occur either with an organic obstruction (stricture or cancer) or with esophageal motor disorders. The patient's response to dysphagia can also provide useful information about the cause of dysphagia. If the bolus must be regurgitated, and if an attempt to force the bolus down with water is met by a sudden return of the fluid, then an organic obstruction should be suspected. If the patient is able to force the bolus down by changing their posture, by performing a Valsalva maneuver, by repeated swallowing, or by ingesting fluid, then a motor disorder is more likely. Progressive worsening of dysphagia over weeks to months usually signals the presence of organic narrowing, caused by either a lumen-obliterating carcinoma or a stricture from ongoing reflux esophagitis.

ODYNOPHAGIA

Pain on swallowing, odynophagia, is another cardinal symptom that indicates esophageal disease, but it can be due to a variety of underlying disorders. Bolus arrest producing dysphagia can sometimes progress to a sensation of pain as esophageal obstruction continues. However, odynophagia usually occurs during the transit of the bolus and disappears once the swallowed material has left the esophagus. It can be of such intensity that the patient refuses to swallow any solids or liquids and expectorates saliva, or it may be mild in intensity, so that the patient is merely aware of the location of the swallowed bolus, as often occurs in patients with reflux disease. Odynophagia can be seen after involvement of the mucosa by reflux, radiation, or viral or fungal infections. Odynophagia can be an uncommon manifestation of carcinoma or of a localized ulcer caused by a lodged tablet.

HEARTBURN (PYROSIS)

Heartburn or pyrosis is the most common manifestation of esophageal disease and may occur in up to 20% of the population. The term "burning" rather than "pain" is usually used, although heartburn can increase in intensity until it is perceived as chest pain. Patients often illustrate heartburn with a movement of the open hand up and down the sternum, as compared with the stationary, tightly clenched fist of angina pectoris. Heartburn is usually relieved, even if only temporarily, by taking antacids. A constant burning unrelieved by antacids may well be of esophageal origin, but it does not represent heartburn. Heartburn is often worse after recumbency or lifting and may follow overeating or alcoholic indiscretion.

REGURGITATION

Regurgitation of fluid contents into the mouth often accompanies heartburn. Sometimes regurgitation is associated with eructation; often it accompanies bending over, lifting, or lying down at night. The bitter regurgitated fluid is often described as yellow-brown or green. Regurgitation at night may lead to stridor or to wheezing, a hoarse voice, and other respiratory symptoms from unrecognized reflux. Less commonly, regurgitated fluid is not from the stomach or duodenum but from fluid retained in an achalasic esophagus or in a large pharyngeal diverticulum. An uncommon process that can be confused with regurgitation is rumination. In this condition, recently eaten food is propelled back into the mouth from the stomach by a strong contraction of the abdominal wall musculature. The food commonly is rechewed, reswallowed, and again returned to the stomach (see Chapter 227).

SPONTANEOUS ESOPHAGEAL CHEST PAIN

In addition to the discomfort from severe reflux, which can advance from heartburn into pain, abnormal contractile activity of the esophageal muscle can cause severe chest pain that is clinically

indistinguishable from angina pectoris in terms of intensity, radiation, relationship to exercise, and even response to nitroglycerin (see Chapter 38). Chest pain of esophageal origin can radiate directly through to the back and is often found in patients who also have dysphagia. Esophageal chest pain can last from several seconds to many hours.

HEMATEMESIS

Although vomiting blood is less specific for esophageal disease than are many of the symptoms listed above, hematemesis can signal the presence of esophageal varices, of mucosal ulceration resulting from esophageal reflux, of a mucosal tear in the lower esophagus, or, uncommonly, of an ulcerating carcinoma or leiomyoma of the esophagus (see Chapter 123). Although nonvariceal bleeding from the esophagus may be life-threatening, more often it is a slow ooze, usually caused by esophageal reflux disease, which may present clinically as an iron deficiency anemia or occult blood–positive stool.

GASTROESOPHAGEAL REFLUX DISEASE

DEFINITION. Gastroesophageal reflux disease (GERD) refers to the varied clinical manifestations of reflux of stomach and duodenal contents into the esophagus and is preferable to the term "reflux esophagitis." Although GERD may be associated with a sliding hiatal hernia, the term "symptomatic hiatal hernia" tends to emphasize an anatomic entity and not the underlying pathophysiology. GERD can be characterized by any combination of symptoms and radiologic, endoscopic, or pathologic changes. In its milder manifestations, it is a common disease; its most florid state is uncommon but may be life-threatening.

PATHOGENESIS. Several factors must work in concert to produce clinical effects of esophageal reflux. Normal subjects may have a few short-duration reflux episodes postprandially and in the upright position. Those in whom reflux has produced symptoms or pathologic changes will demonstrate more frequent and prolonged episodes of reflux, which also tend to occur at night. The factor or factors that cause this difference are not entirely known. However, important differences between persons with and without reflux might help explain these findings.

The LES is a specialized bundle of circular muscle at the lower end of the esophagus with different physical and pharmacologic characteristics when compared with the circular muscle above and below it. Although mean LES pressure is significantly lower in subjects with GERD than in normal persons, much overlap occurs between the groups; LES pressure is not very useful in predicting whether reflux is present in an individual patient unless the pressure is very low. The most common event associated with reflux appears to be a transient relaxation of the LES unassociated with either swallowing or the distention of the esophageal body by refluxed fluid. Thus, two abnormalities of LES may be associated with reflux: a sphincter with very low tone, as measured by LES pressure, or inappropriate relaxation of a normally competent sphincter.

Several factors are important in removing refluxed material from the esophagus. The upright position facilitates esophageal emptying by gravity. Peristaltic waves initiated by swallowing or by esophageal distention help remove the refluxed material. Acid placed within the esophagus is cleared less well by patients with GERD than by normal subjects, although the manometric tracings seen in both groups seem identical. Clearing of acid regurgitation occurs in two phases: the bulk of the fluid is returned to the stomach by a peristaltic contraction, and the remaining acid film clinging to the esophageal wall is neutralized by swallowed saliva.

The composition and perhaps the quantity of the refluxed material also play a role in the production of GERD. Gastric acid and pepsin seem clearly important in the pathogenesis of GERD. Bile salts, and possibly pancreatic enzymes, may be responsible in patients in whom acid is absent. The combination of bile salts plus acid is more injurious to the esophagus than either agent alone. Other less well-studied factors, such as altered or abnormal esophageal mucus, swallowed saliva of high bicarbonate content, and diminished resistance of the esophageal mucosa to digestion, may be important in determining the amount of mucosal damage in GERD.

Esophageal squamous epithelium reacts to reflux by an increase in the basal cell or germinative layer. The dermal pegs are increased in height and may become more vascular. If the process becomes more severe, the epithelial layer is destroyed, with the appearance of micro-ulcers and classic signs of inflammation in the lamina propria, such as infiltration with polymorphonuclear leukocytes and edema. Even deeper lesions cause first submucosal and then muscular inflammation and fibrosis, resulting in an esophageal stricture. Why reflux is so common, yet inflammation and stricture formation are relatively uncommon, is not known.

Reflux during pregnancy, once thought to be due to the increased abdominal pressure from the fetus, may be due mainly to diminished LES strength caused by increased estrogen and progesterone. Weight gain also tends to aggravate reflux through an unknown mechanism. Resection of the lower esophageal area for cancer or myotomy for achalasia can lead to severe postoperative reflux. Gastroesophageal reflux with stricture formation is especially severe in patients with progressive systemic sclerosis.

The crural diaphragm usually wraps around the gastroesophageal junction to augment the intrinsic LES. In a hiatal hernia, an anatomic displacement of the LES and crural diaphragm is seen. Although hiatal hernias may be associated with reflux, the presence of a hiatal hernia is now considered to be much less of a factor in GERD than previously thought, because it is present in a large percentage of normal subjects. It is not appropriate to spend time trying to define whether a hiatal hernia is present or absent in dealing with most patients with GERD; rather, the focus should be on the symptoms of reflux.

SYMPTOMS. Heartburn, the most common manifestation of GERD, can vary from an occasional mild burning after overeating to an ever-present, severe discomfort that markedly limits a patient's lifestyle. It may be accompanied by regurgitation of gastric contents, either into the mouth or into the respiratory tree. The latter group of patients may complain of nocturnal wheezing, coughing, hoarseness, a need to clear the throat repeatedly, or a sensation of deep pressure at the base of the neck. This group of symptoms may be the primary clinical presentation and more prominent than the classic symptoms of GERD.

Dysphagia is often present in patients with significant GERD. Although dysphagia may be severe and even mark the onset of stricture formation, it usually is mild and must be carefully sought. Dysphagia of GERD is for solids, and the dysphagia is usually overcome by swallowing repeatedly or by washing the bolus down with water. Many patients with GERD do not complain of bolus arrest, but rather of being aware of the location of each solid morsel as it travels down the esophagus.

Blood loss may result from esophageal erosions and shallow ulcers. The erosions rarely produce life-threatening hemorrhage and are much more likely to weep quietly over a prolonged period of time, producing iron deficiency anemia. Some of these patients have very few other clinical manifestations of GERD, and the condition is discovered by endoscopy during evaluation of occult gastrointestinal bleeding. Persons who vigorously and repeatedly abuse alcohol seem prone to develop severe erosive esophagitis with bleeding; in these patients abstinence from alcohol is the important therapy.

DIAGNOSIS. The history and clinical manifestations of GERD are the most important diagnostic aids; objective testing can quantify the extent and severity of the process. In the vast majority of patients, typical symptoms of GERD and the response to initial gastric acid suppressive therapy make the diagnosis relatively easy. Diagnostic evaluation becomes important when symptoms are atypical and/or do not respond to therapy.

DOCUMENTING REFLUX. Reflux during a barium swallow in adults is uncommon unless vigorous provocative maneuvers are employed. When spontaneous reflux of barium is seen, it usually denotes free reflux. The absence of reflux seen radiographically does not, however, imply that the patient does not have GERD.

The 24-hour monitoring of esophageal pH can be performed with a portable unit, which allows the patient to follow an almost normal lifestyle. During the prolonged monitoring period, the relationship between symptoms (heartburn, chest pain, wheezing) and episodes of acid reflux can be ascertained, and calculations can be made of the number of episodes of reflux and the amount of time the esophagus is acidified (pH < 4). A small amount of reflux, especially in the postprandial period, can be seen normally. Repeated and prolonged bursts of acid exposure suggest that abnormal gastroesophageal reflux is present.

In children and infants, reflux can be measured noninvasively by scanning the esophageal area with a gamma-camera after placing a solution of ^{99m}Tc sulfur colloid in the stomach. An abdominal binder is used to increase intra-abdominal pressure and to stress the gastroesophageal junction if free reflux is not seen.

LINKING REFLUX TO SYMPTOMS. If pain is the predominant symptom, rather than heartburn, a Bernstein test may be performed using the same catheter as is used for esophageal manometry. After a 5-minute period of dripping normal saline in the mid-esophagus, the infusion is changed to 0.1 N hydrochloric acid. Reproduction of the symptoms during acid infusion (usually 4 to 5 minutes into the infusion), followed by rapid symptom disappearance after returning to a saline infusion, suggests an esophageal cause of the discomfort.

As another approach, the patient is asked to signal the time of discomfort during prolonged pH monitoring of the esophagus. If the patient signals discomfort at the same time that acid reflux is demonstrated by the pH probe, then a causal relationship is more likely.

ASSESSING THE EFFECT OF REFLUX ON THE ESOPHAGEAL MUCOSA. A barium swallow detects gross changes, such as stricture formation or a deep esophageal ulcer, but misses the much more common shallow ulcerations and erosions, which are detected by endoscopy. Only discrete lesions such as erosions and ulcerations should be taken as proof of esophageal damage, because endoscopic findings, such as erythema, edema, or friability, are subject to wide interobserver variation. In approximately one-half of patients with moderate to severe symptoms of GERD, the mucosa appears absolutely normal, but a biopsy may demonstrate the histologic changes of reflux.

APPROACH TO THE PATIENT (FIG. 124–1). Endoscopy is generally indicated if hematemesis is present, if symptoms are prolonged and do not respond to empiric treatment, or if systemic manifestations, such as weight loss, anemia, and occult blood–positive stool are present. If the appearance of the esophageal mucosa is normal during endoscopy, biopsies can also be obtained to search for objective evidence of microscopic esophagitis. If dysphagia is present, a barium swallow is appropriate. Uncommonly, reflux is demonstrated, a stricture found, or a deep ulcer seen, which leads to immediate endoscopy for more complete evaluation. After first evaluation, it may be appropriate to begin empiric therapy (see Treatment, below). If the response to therapy is poor, esophageal pH monitoring can confirm the diagnosis. At the same time, esophageal manometry may be performed to estimate LES pressure and to determine the presence or absence of peristaltic waves.

COMPLICATIONS. ESOPHAGEAL STRICTURE. Of the many who complain of symptoms of GERD, only a few develop esophageal strictures, usually at the lower end of the esophagus, but sometimes migrating over years to the mid-esophagus or higher. Presumably, patients who develop strictures have had deep circumferential ulceration of the esophageal mucosa due to reflux damage. Instead of healing with only minimal submucosal and muscular fibrosis, these patients develop esophageal obstruction with a narrowed esophageal lumen. If reflux can be controlled, these strictures may disappear.

Dysphagia is the clinical hallmark of esophageal stricture formation. Unlike the relatively mild dysphagia seen in uncomplicated GERD, the dysphagia in patients with strictures tends to be constant and slowly progressive, causing the patient to alter the type of food taken.

Strictures are most easily evaluated by barium swallow. Sometimes the extent of the strictured area is overestimated unless the esophagus below the stricture can be fully distended by barium. For mild strictures, the ingestion of barium-soaked bread or a marshmallow bolus can draw attention to slight luminal narrowing where the bolus is impacted. Endoscopy with biopsy and/or brush cytology is required to make certain that the stricture is benign.

ESOPHAGEAL ULCER. In addition to the more common shallow erosions, deep esophageal ulcers may complicate severe GERD. These ulcers, which retain barium and usually project outside the wall of the esophagus, characteristically produce severe and unre-

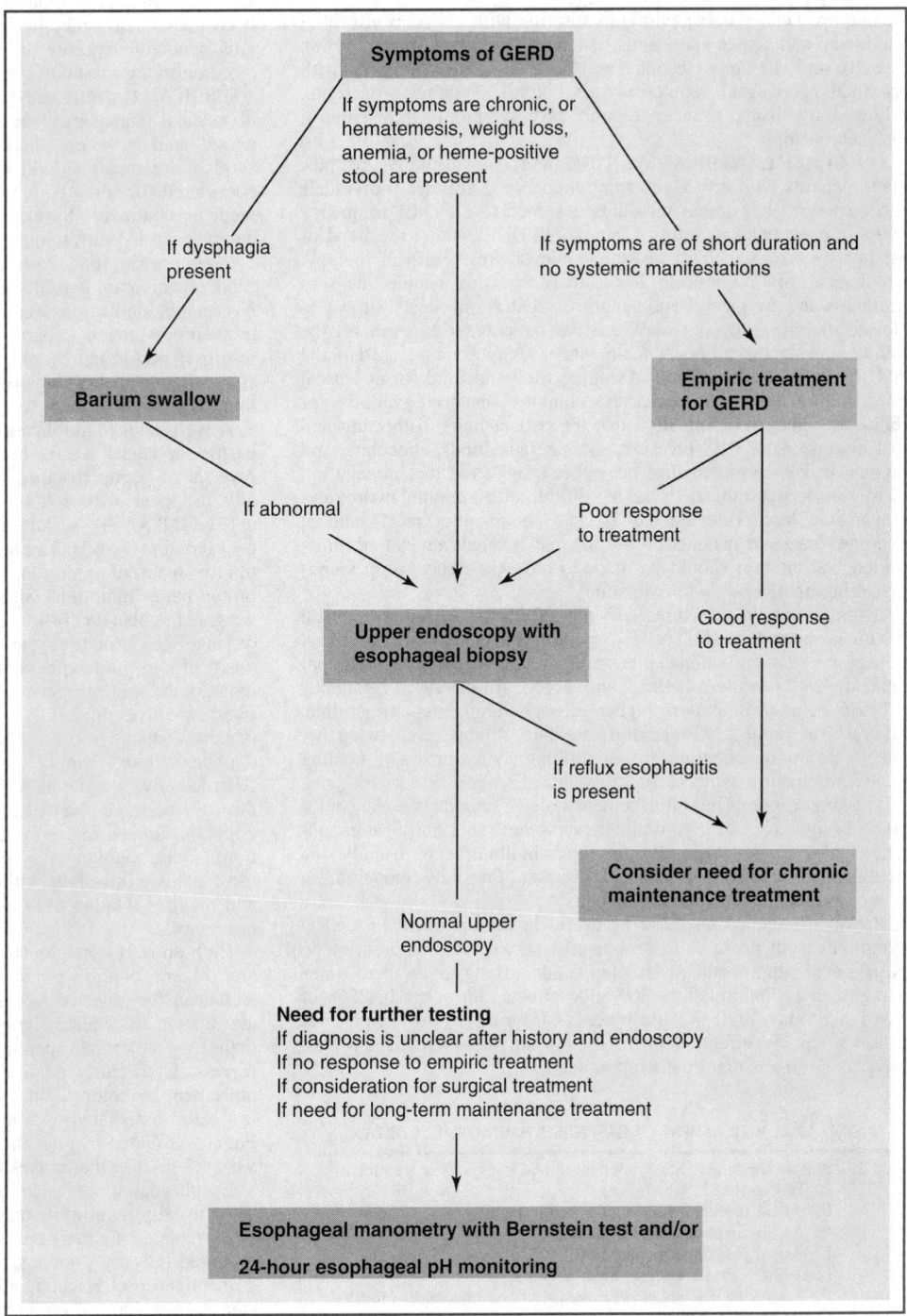

Symptoms of GERD

If symptoms are chronic, or hematemesis, weight loss, anemia, or heme-positive stool are present

If dysphagia present

If symptoms are of short duration and no systemic manifestations

Barium swallow

Empiric treatment for GERD

If abnormal

Poor response to treatment

Good response to treatment

Upper endoscopy with esophageal biopsy

If reflux esophagitis is present

Consider need for chronic maintenance treatment

Normal upper endoscopy

Need for further testing
If diagnosis is unclear after history and endoscopy
If no response to empiric treatment
If consideration for surgical treatment
If need for long-term maintenance treatment

Esophageal manometry with Bernstein test and/or
24-hour esophageal pH monitoring

FIGURE 124–1 ■ Diagnosis and evaluation of patients with possible gastroesophageal reflux disease (GERD).

lenting pain, often with radiation of the pain to the back. Brisk hemorrhage may be caused by erosion through to an esophageal artery. The presence of an ulcer can be suspected on a barium swallow and confirmed endoscopically. The ulcer usually is in columnar (Barrett's) epithelium.

BARRETT'S ESOPHAGUS (COLUMNAR EPITHELIUM). In some patients with chronic reflux esophagitis, the healing epithelium may be replaced not with squamous epithelium, but with a specialized columnar epithelium with intestinal metaplasia. The junctional zone between squamous and columnar (Barrett's) epithelium can progress upwards over years (Color Plate 1*D*). Barrett's esophagus is defined as the presence on biopsy of specialized columnar epithelium with goblet cells in the esophagus. It is usually identified endoscopically as salmon-pink (gastric-appearing) mucosa above the lower esophageal sphincter. Barrett's epithelium is often found at and below mid-esophageal strictures and around deep esophageal

ulcers. The major clinical importance of Barrett's epithelium is not only as a marker for severe reflux, but also as a precursor to adenocarcinoma of the esophagus (see Esophageal Tumors).

PULMONARY ASPIRATION. If material refluxes above the upper esophageal sphincter, it may easily spill into the larynx and tracheobronchial tree. Some patients react to such a spill with intense respiratory stridor. Others seem to tolerate the presence of refluxed material in the larynx and tracheobronchial tree with milder laryngeal or respiratory symptoms. It is even possible that the gastric contents do not have to reach the larynx; instilling acid in the esophagus of susceptible individuals can be shown to cause closure of small bronchial airways by a vagal reflex.

None of the clinical features of pulmonary aspiration, such as wheezing, hoarseness, or coughing, is pathognomonic, but together they may point toward reflux and aspiration as a possible etiology. Diagnostic proof of the relationship may be difficult with current techniques. Dual esophageal pH monitoring with pH probes in both the lower and upper esophagus can help determine if acid reflux ascends into the upper esophagus. Correlation of symptoms with proximal esophageal reflux may be helpful. Treatment of reflux followed by disappearance of pulmonary symptoms may confirm the relationship.

TREATMENT. MEDICAL MANAGEMENT. Most mildly symptomatic patients with reflux and some moderately afflicted individuals can be helped by simple measures designed to alter the frequency or type of esophageal reflux (Table 124–1). Elevating the head of the bed by 6 to 8 inches is a simple and effective form of therapy. Esophageal pH monitoring has shown that this simple measure decreases the frequency and length of reflux episodes. Pillows to elevate the thorax do not work well, as patients tend to roll off the pillows during the night. A foam rubber wedge can be used if the bed frame cannot be moved. Avoiding food and fluid for at least 3 hours before retiring decreases the amount of material available for reflux at night. Avoiding food that the patient finds distressing and that may decrease LES pressure, such as fatty foods, chocolate, and onions, makes sense but has never been subjected to clinical trial. Acid can be neutralized by taking 30 mL of aluminum hydroxide-magnesium hydroxide antacid 1 and 3 hours after meals and at bedtime, but most patients do not tolerate frequent antacid administration. An attempt should be made to have the patient stop smoking, drinking alcohol, and overeating.

If these simple measures are not effective, systemic medical treatment is indicated. The H_2-receptor antagonists in the usual dosage range for duodenal ulcer and titrated to the individual patient improve heartburn better than placebo. An increased frequency of administration and/or higher dosage regimens—cimetidine, 800 mg; ranitidine, 300 mg; or famotidine, 40 mg (each twice per day)—are more effective for controlling symptoms and healing peptic esophagitis, which usually requires 12 weeks.

The proton-pump inhibitors omeprazole (20 mg/day) or lansoprazole (30 mg/day) can give dramatic symptom relief and heal esophagitis in 4 to 8 weeks. Proton-pump inhibitors are usually the treatment of choice for mucosal disease, especially moderate to severe esophagitis seen endoscopically.

Prokinetic agents may also be useful in the treatment of GERD symptoms with no to mild esophagitis, occasionally in addition to gastric acid suppressants. Metoclopramide, 10 mg given three times a day, can be helpful, but CNS side effects can occur in 25% of cases and may limit its usefulness. Cisapride 10 mg given four times a day, is effective primarily for nocturnal GERD and has fewer side effects than metoclopramide.

Table 124–1 ■ **TREATMENT OF GASTROESOPHAGEAL REFLUX DISEASE**

Step 1. Simple measures (lifestyle changes and nonsystemic treatment)
    A. Elevate head of bed
    B. Avoid food and fluid intake before bedtime
    C. Avoid cigarettes, coffee, alcohol
    D. Avoid chocolate, peppermint
    E. Avoid tight clothing around the waist
    F. Take antacids 1 hour after meals, at bedtime, and as needed
    G. Reduce fat in diet
    H. Lose weight
Step 2. Measures for resistant cases (systemic treatment)
Step 2a. H_2-receptor antagonists
    A. Cimetidine, 300 mg q.i.d.*
    B. Ranitidine, 150 mg b.i.d.*
    C. Famotidine, 20 mg b.i.d.*
    D. Nizatidine, 150 mg b.i.d.*
Step 2b. Prokinetic agents
    A. Metoclopramide, 10 mg q.i.d.*
    B. Cisapride, 10 mg q.i.d.*
    C. Bethanechol, 10 mg q.i.d.*
Step 3. Measures for patients with GERD resistant to H_2-receptor antagonists
    A. Proton pump inhibitor: omeprazole, 20 mg/day, or lansoprazole, 30 mg/day*
Step 4. Measures for patients with GERD resistant to steps 1, 2, and 3 or patients who need long-term maintenance treatment
    A. Surgical fundoplication

*Higher doses or more frequent administration of an H_2-antagonist, proton-pump inhibitor, or prokinetic agent may be required in some cases

Once healing of esophagitis has been achieved with either an H_2-antagonist or a proton-pump inhibitor, recurrence rates exceed 80% if no maintenance therapy is used. Maintenance therapy for esophagitis generally requires full dosage of an H_2-receptor antagonist or a proton-pump inhibitor.

SURGICAL MANAGEMENT. In a patient in whom an adequate trial of medical management has not brought good results in a 6-month period, and in whom there is good objective evidence of reflux, surgical treatment should be considered. Surgery should also be considered for some patients who may need long-term maintenance medical treatment. Surgical therapy attempts to restore sphincter competence by surrounding the lower end of the esophagus with a cuff of gastric fundal muscle, completely in the case of Nissen fundoplication or partially in the case of Hill-Belsey repairs. The Nissen fundoplication seems to provide the most satisfactory long-term improvement. Laparoscopic techniques appear to have similar results if performed by experienced surgeons. This minimally invasive surgery makes laparoscopic fundoplication an alternative to long-term medical therapy.

A well-done fundoplication can restore a competent LES, reduce gastroesophageal reflux, heal peptic esophagitis, and even lead to reversal of peptic stricture. The columnar epithelium does not usually disappear in Barrett's esophagus.

TREATMENT OF COMPLICATIONS. Mildly symptomatic esophageal strictures can be handled by careful attention to dietary intake, improvement of dentition, and use of medical therapy, primarily proton-pump inhibitors. Short, simple strictures can be dilated with weighted rubber or Teflon dilators (e.g., Hurst-Maloney). Tortuous or angulated strictures are more easily approached over a previously placed guidewire passed through an endoscope or under radiographic control (Savary dilators). Graded-steel olives (Eder-Puestow olive dilators), a dilator with graded increases of size (Celestin dilator), or a balloon with a fixed maximal diameter (Cooke balloon) can be passed over the previously placed wire. Alternatively, a balloon of fixed maximal diameter can be passed through the large channel of an endoscope during diagnostic endoscopy and dilated under direct vision (through-the-scope [TTS] dilation). Once the lumen is restored to a diameter of 13 to 15 mm, most patients swallow without difficulty. If the stricture is stable and requires dilation only every 4 to 6 months, no other therapy is necessary.

High-dose H_2-antagonists or, preferably, proton-pump inhibitors and dilation of the stricture can lead to healing of the mucosa and less need for repeated stricture dilation. Patients who do not tolerate dilation or require vigorous dilation every 3 to 4 weeks need a definitive antireflux operation, following which the stricture may regress. If strictures persist after antireflux surgery, esophageal replacement by colon, jejunum, or stomach is a surgical maneuver of last resort associated with a relatively high morbidity and mortality. Patients afflicted by strictures may have significant lung and cardiovascular disease that makes them unsuitable operative candidates.

Esophageal ulcers also represent a major therapeutic problem. They usually require treatment with a proton-pump inhibitor.

Barrett's (columnar) epithelium may be premalignant and can be removed only by esophageal resection. Adequate antireflux therapy with high-dose H_2-antagonists or with a proton-pump inhibitor causes regression of columnar epithelium in some patients. Patients with Barrett's epithelium should be followed up with periodic endoscopic biopsies every 1 to 3 years to look for dysplasia and early changes of adenocarcinoma. The persistence of confirmed high-grade dysplasia is an indication for esophagectomy, because high-grade dysplasia may progress to carcinoma and because coexistent carcinoma may be undetected on biopsy. If low-grade dysplasia is present, the patient is treated medically with proton-pump inhibitors and undergoes biopsy every 6 to 12 months. Experimental endoscopic ablation therapies using photodynamic therapy, laser, or multipolar electrocoagulation are being tried to remove the columnar epithelium with the hope of subsequent growth of the normal squamous epithelium, primarily in patients with low-grade dysplasia or in patients with high-grade dysplasia who are not surgical candidates. Following these new ablation techniques, either long-term gastric acid suppression or laparoscopic Nissen fundoplication is needed to control the reflux and prevent recurrence of Barrett's epithelium.

Treatment of the pulmonary complications of reflux in adults relies on improved night posture, gastric acid suppressants, and prokinetic agents. Caution is advised before recommending esophageal surgery in patients with reflux and predominant pulmonary problems, because the cause-and-effect relationship may be uncertain in individual patients.

MOTOR DISORDERS OF THE ESOPHAGUS

DEFINITION AND PATHOGENESIS. The muscular tube of the esophagus is guarded at both ends by specialized bundles of muscle, the upper esophageal sphincter (UES) and LES. Material from the oropharynx is propelled at a high velocity (in the case of liquids), and precise coordination is required to link the muscles of the oropharynx, UES, body of the esophagus, and LES into a functional unit. Failure of any or all of these components results in an esophageal motor disorder. The oropharyngeal and UES units can fail because of either primary muscle disease, such as myotonic dystrophy and dermatomyositis, or neurologic lesions involving the innervation of these muscle groups, such as brain-stem infarcts, multiple sclerosis, and amyotrophic lateral sclerosis.

The pathogenesis of motor abnormalities of the esophageal body is less well understood. The striated muscle that constitutes the upper to one-third of the body can be affected by primary muscle disease, such as myotonic dystrophy, or by metabolic disease affecting muscle function, such as hypothyroidism. The smooth muscle seems more resistant to muscular disease, but the intrinsic nervous network can be involved in Chagas' disease and achalasia. In the latter disorder, Auerbach's plexus is infiltrated with lymphocytes, or the neuron cell bodies in the myenteric plexus may disappear.

The motor disorders of the body of the esophagus have historically been classified as achalasia or diffuse spasm (Table 124-2). In achalasia, dysphagia and esophageal retention predominate; the radiograph shows a dilated esophagus with distal tapering at the gastroesophageal junction, and manometry reveals high LES pressure with no or incomplete relaxation and simultaneous smooth muscle and striated muscle contractions. Diffuse spasm may cause esophageal chest pain, dysphagia, or both; segmental contractions are seen on radiography, and the manometric picture is of peristaltic waves interspersed with periods of simultaneous esophageal contractions. Many variations of these "classic" diseases occur; diffuse spasm can progress to achalasia, and many nonspecific motor disorders do not fit either of these syndromes. For example, a common manometric abnormality is high-amplitude, long-duration waves that are peristaltic and can be associated with either esophageal chest pain or dysphagia or both (nutcracker esophagus). Occasionally the nonspecific motor abnormalities may be secondary manifestations of gastroesophageal reflux.

SYMPTOMS. Weakness of the oropharyngeal musculature may cause transfer dysphagia—the inability to propel a solid or liquid bolus from the pharynx to the esophagus. Patients are aware that they cannot begin the act of deglutition. Solids are usually more trouble than liquids. Palatal weakness may lead to nasal regurgitation of fluids or to laryngeal aspiration because of muscular failure to seal off the larynx. Such weakness may be signaled by a nasal quality of the voice.

Incoordination of UES relaxation with pharyngeal contraction has been suggested as a cause of transfer dysphagia and for Zenker's diverticulum. Transfer dysphagia can be accompanied by a prominent cricopharyngeal impression on a barium swallow ("cricopha-

Table 124-2 ■ **MANOMETRIC CLASSIFICATION OF ESOPHAGEAL MOTOR DISORDERS**

Achalasia
Diffuse esophageal spasm
Scleroderma
Isolated lower esophageal sphincter dysfunction
  High pressure with normal relaxation
  Normal pressure with impaired relaxation
Nonspecific esophageal motor disorder
  High-amplitude peristaltic esophageal contractions ("nutcracker esophagus")
  Reptitive esophageal contractions
  Nontransmitted esophageal contractions
  Low-amplitude esophageal contractions

ryngeal achalasia"); however, no defect in relaxation or in timing of contractions is seen with modern manometric methods.

Motor disorders in the body of the esophagus produce dysphagia, pain, or both. This transport dysphagia may be intermittent or continuous, and it may occur with both solids and liquids. It is rare for the arrested material to be regurgitated; often, assuming a particular posture (e.g., throwing the shoulders back and extending the neck) or performing a Valsalva maneuver helps the material pass into the stomach.

Chest pain is the other major clinical presentation of esophageal motor disorders. The pain is usually substernal, described as a feeling of pressure or aching, which radiates to the back as well as to the neck, jaw, and arms. It can range in intensity from a transient discomfort to an overwhelming, agonizing pain similar to that of a major myocardial infarction or dissecting aortic aneurysm. The pain may last for only several seconds or may be present for hours. The differentiation between angina pectoris and esophageal chest pain may be impossible on clinical grounds; both may be related to exercise, have the same intensity and distribution, and respond to sublingual nitroglycerin. In some patients with esophageal spasm, microvascular coronary spasms may contribute to chest pain and make it difficult to separate cardiac from esophageal etiologies (see Chapter 38).

Abnormalities of the LES may present as two separate symptom complexes. If the sphincter fails to relax on deglutition (as occurs in achalasia), dysphagia occurs, and contents are retained in the body of the esophagus. This failure, coupled with loss of peristalsis (achalasia), leads to marked esophageal retention, regurgitation, and overflow of esophageal contents into the tracheobronchial tree. If primary muscle failure of the sphincter occurs, as is seen in scleroderma, massive reflux and the consequences of GERD follow.

DIAGNOSIS. A careful history is essential in choosing the correct diagnostic tools for evaluating esophageal motor disorders (Fig. 124-2). If the difficulty is thought to be in the oropharynx and UES, a videoesophagram may reveal incoordination of tongue and palate, unilateral pharyngeal weakness, or aspiration of small amounts of barium into the trachea with swallowing. Air double-contrast examinations of the pharynx can elucidate an unsuspected hypopharyngeal carcinoma or a diverticulum or prominence of the cricopharyngeal muscle. Manometric examination of the hypopharynx and UES can also aid in diagnosis.

Radiology of the esophageal body offers the best chance of diagnosis when motor disorders are associated with relatively static changes. In achalasia, the body of the esophagus commonly dilates with retention of food, secretions, and barium (Fig. 124-3). Special attention can be paid to the terminal end of the esophagus, which has a smooth, tapering beak. Any irregularity of this beak should lead to a vigorous search for an infiltrating neoplasm of the cardia, which can mimic achalasia clinically and radiologically.

If the esophageal muscle is atonic, as is seen in far-advanced scleroderma (see Chapter 290), barium and even air are retained for long periods of time when the patient is in the supine position. Assuming the upright position rapidly clears the barium from the esophagus and leaves a double-contrast view of a dilated esophagus.

When the motor abnormality is more intermittent, simultaneous contractions can be occasionally detected fluoroscopically. Such a radiologic appearance is not always evidence for a clinically important motor disorder; elderly patients often show similar radiologic findings and yet are totally asymptomatic (presbyesophagus).

Manometric examination allows more prolonged evaluation of esophageal motor function and is the only method that allows LES function to be determined directly. Normally, a swallow causes a peristaltic wave to be detected sequentially by pressure detectors spaced along the esophagus. Aperistalsis (no peristaltic response to a swallow), simultaneous single or multiple contractions, prolonged contractions of high amplitude and low velocity, and spontaneous activity not related to swallowing can be recorded (Fig. 124-4).

Manometric examination is especially helpful to evaluate chest pain when the patient has an attack during the examination. If the chest pain is simultaneously accompanied by abnormal motor activity, the diagnosis of an esophageal origin of chest pain is established. Similarly, if pH is being simultaneously monitored and the episodes of chest pain correlate closely with drops in intra-

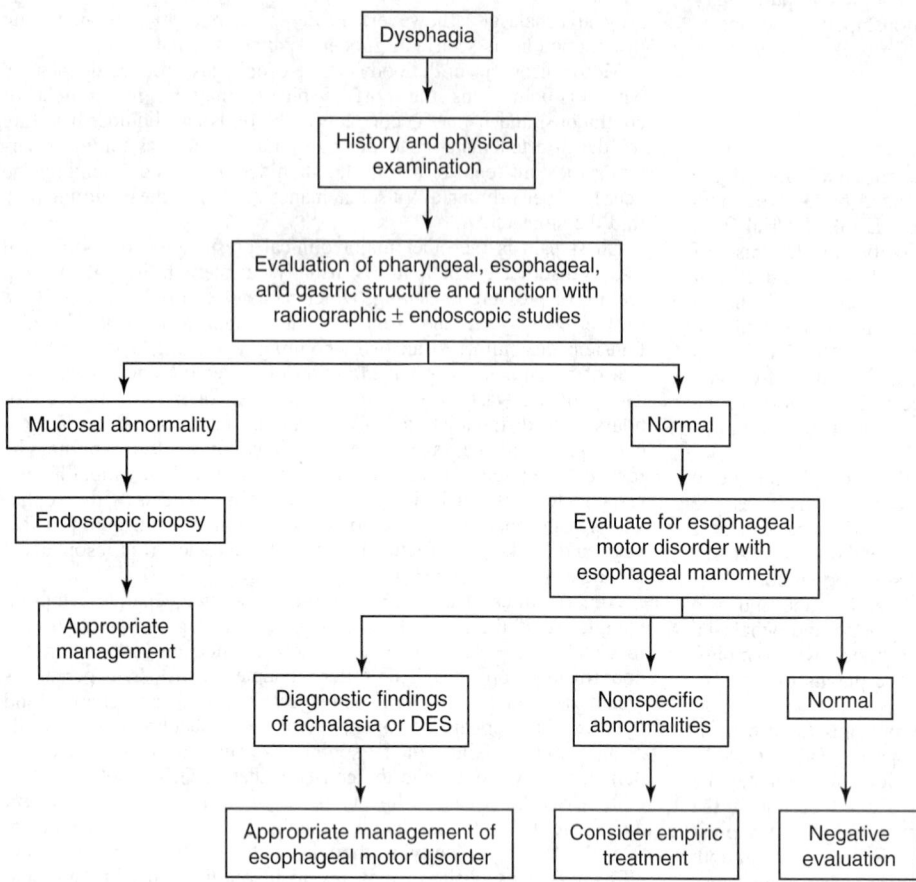

FIGURE 124–2 ■ Diagnostic evaluation of patients with dysphagia.

esophageal pH, an esophageal origin of pain is likely. Conversely, if typical chest pain occurs but no change in motor activity or pH is seen, an esophageal cause of pain is unlikely. Unfortunately, such definitive statements can be made only for a small minority of the patients examined. Pharmacologic stimulation of the esophagus with short-acting edrophonium (Tensilon) is safe and can provoke chest pain and simultaneous esophageal contractions; such testing is sometimes helpful in patients with normal baseline esophageal manometry.

Prolonged esophageal pH monitoring and pH/motility monitoring may help correlate symptoms of dysphagia or chest pain to reflux episodes or motility abnormalities. Endoscopy is useful for evaluating motor disorders, for inspecting the cardia with a retroflexed view from the stomach (to exclude an infiltrating carcinoma), and for excluding inflammatory disorders. Therapeutic trials with a proton-pump inhibitor may also help establish gastroesophageal reflux as a cause of chest pain.

TREATMENT. Achalasia is the most treatable esophageal motor disorder; all forms of therapy are directed at relieving obstruction. Short-term improvement in clinical symptoms and in scintigraphic esophageal emptying may occur with isosorbide dinitrate or nifedipine, but pharmacologic treatment usually is not successful for long-term management. Dilation with a pneumatic bag under radiographic control is the preferable initial therapy for almost all patients. It should be performed by an expert, because perforation, even in good hands, may occur in about 5% of patients.

Surgery is reserved for patients in whom bag dilation fails or for patients who do not wish to be exposed to the risk of perforation. Direct section of the LES muscle (myotomy) is performed, sparing some gastric muscle fibers to prevent postoperative reflux (Heller esophagomyotomy). Postoperative gastroesophageal reflux with esophagitis and peptic stricture of the esophagus may occur if the myotomy abolishes all LES pressure and if no fundoplication is performed, so many surgeons combine a partial fundoplication with the Heller myotomy. Heller myotomy can be performed laparoscopically.

Botulinum toxin, which reduces acetylcholine release and LES pressure, can be injected into the LES from an endoscopic ap-

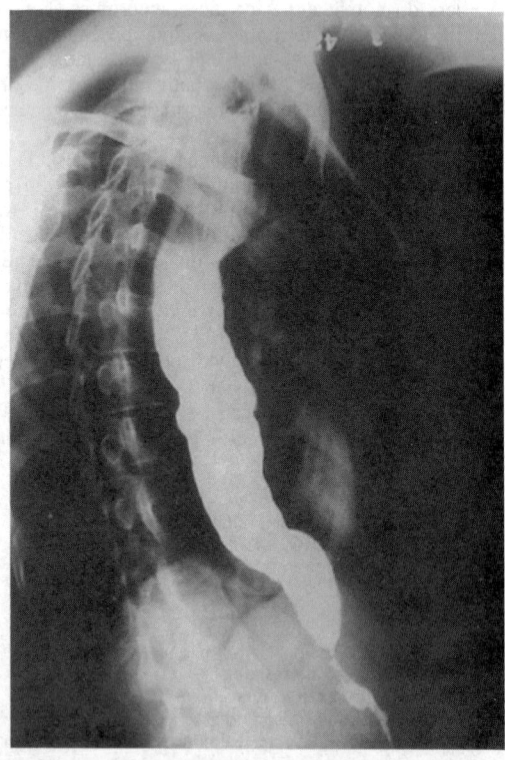

FIGURE 124–3 ■ Radiologic appearance of achalasia. The esophageal body is dilated and terminates in a narrowed segment. (Courtesy of Dr. F.E. Templeton. From Pope CE II: Motor disorders. *In* Sleisenger MH, Fordtran JS [eds]: Gastrointestinal Disease, 3rd ed. Philadelphia, WB Saunders, 1983.)

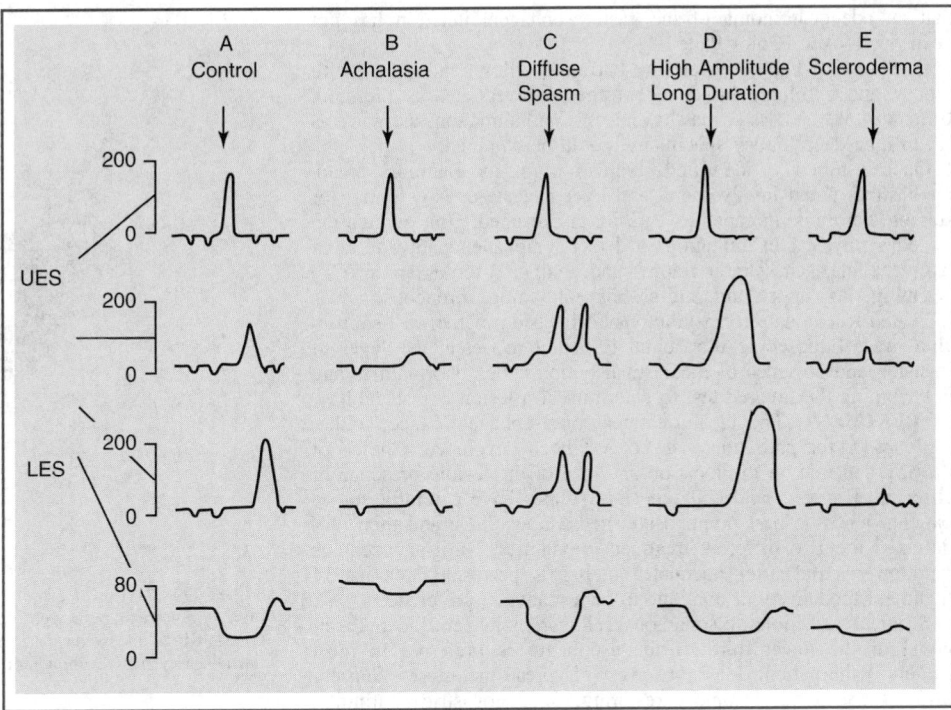

FIGURE 124-4 ■ Idealized manometric patterns. *A,* The normal swallow consists of a progressive wave with a wave of short duration and rapid rise time in the striated upper esophagus. The lower esophageal sphincter (LES) shows a fall in pressure coincident with swallowing. *B,* In achalasia, the striated muscle sometimes, but not always, produces a typical wave. The smooth muscle portion of the esophagus has a simultaneous low-amplitude contraction that follows the striated muscle contraction. The elevated pressure in the LES shows either incomplete or no relaxation. *C,* Diffuse spasm shows an elevation of the baseline after swallowing, on top of which are superimposed repetitive simultaneous contractions. LES pressure may be high and relaxation may terminate prematurely. *D,* High-amplitude, long-duration waves (nutcracker esophagus). The wave is peristaltic but of high amplitude. Duration is increased and velocity of propagation may be decreased. *E,* Scleroderma. Striated muscle contraction is normal, but the amplitude of contraction in the smooth muscle is reduced, or contraction may be absent. Sphincter pressure is low.

proach to improve symptoms for several months. It is used in patients at high risk for complications during dilation or surgery; its role in idiopathic achalasia is controversial owing to the incomplete and short-lived responses it evinces.

Treatment of most other motor disorders is more difficult. Patients with diffuse spasm can be given nitroglycerin, anticholinergics, or calcium-channel antagonists. Balloon dilation of the LES may be of benefit in diffuse spasm and in patients with abnormal lower esophageal function or high basal tone with impaired relaxation.

Treatment of other nonspecific motor disorders, such as nutcracker esophagus associated with chest pain, can be equally frustrating. Sublingual nitroglycerin may help and may predict the success of long-acting nitrate therapy. Anticholinergic drugs benefit only a few. Calcium-channel antagonists reduce the force of the esophageal contractions and may relieve pain. Meperidine (Demerol) has been useful but is not a good long-term solution to the problem. Some patients respond to gastric acid suppression, indicating that some of these nonspecific motility disorders may be caused by gastroesophageal reflux.

The treatment of scleroderma and other conditions marked by aperistalsis revolves mostly around the associated reflux. If no obstruction exists at the lower end of the esophagus—either as a result of malfunctioning sphincter or as a result of organic narrowing—aperistalsis is amazingly well tolerated, usually with only mild dysphagia for solids. Antireflux surgery should be offered with caution to patients with scleroderma, as a tight fundoplication without any peristalsis in the body of the esophagus leads to severe dysphagia. Additionally, fundoplication has poor results because the disease progresses to severe muscle atrophy and collagen deposition in the esophageal wall.

ESOPHAGEAL TUMORS

ETIOLOGY AND PATHOGENESIS. Carcinoma of the esophageal epithelium, both squamous cell and adenocarcinoma, is by far the most common and important tumor of the esophagus. Benign neoplasms (leiomyoma, papilloma, and fibrovascular polyps) are rarer and are usually discovered incidentally. Esophageal cancer is more common in men than in women by a 3 : 1 ratio. Squamous cell cancer has an incidence of 5 per 100,000 in men in the United States, rising to 130 per 100,000 in North China. It is less common in women. It is associated with both alcohol intake and tobacco

smoking. Esophageal cancer occurs more commonly in patients with squamous cancers of the head and neck, in those with lye strictures, and in patients with untreated or inadequately treated achalasia.

Adenocarcinoma of the esophagus arises in columnar (Barrett's) epithelium and appears to represent malignant degeneration in the metaplastic columnar tissue that arises in response to chronic inflammation from GERD. The actual incidence of adenocarcinoma in a patient with columnar epithelium is probably less than the original estimate of 10 to 15%, but the tumor still represents a significant problem. The incidence of esophageal adenocarcinoma has been increasing in frequency over the last several decades.

SYMPTOMS. In Western countries, the most common clinical symptom of carcinoma is progressive dysphagia over a several-month period until only liquids can be taken. The obstruction reflects circumferential involvement of the esophageal wall by tumor and does not occur until the cancer is biologically far advanced. The dysphagia may be accompanied by a steady, boring pain, which often signals mediastinal involvement and inoperability. Unexplained persistent chest pain should always be investigated by a careful double-contrast radiographic view of the esophagus or by endoscopy.

More advanced lesions manifest themselves with halitosis and weight loss. Coughing after drinking fluid may be caused either by nearly complete esophageal lumen obstruction, with overspill into the larynx, or by the development of a tracheoesophageal fistula. Hoarseness from involvement of the recurrent laryngeal nerve by tumor and hematemesis are unusual symptoms. Nail bed clubbing can be seen with both benign and malignant tumors.

Because dysphagia is the most common presenting symptom of neoplasm of the esophagus, the physician must be sure that cancer is not the cause of dysphagia. Early diagnosis affords the only chance for cure.

DIAGNOSIS. The clinical suspicion of cancer of the esophagus should lead immediately to an esophagogram, possibly with double-contrast techniques. Any irregularity, especially if it narrows the lumen, mandates further evaluation. If dysphagia is present, the radiologist should give a bolus of barium-soaked bread or marshmallow to discover any possible sites of arrest.

In the presence of suspicious symptoms and normal barium swallow results, endoscopy with biopsy and brushing of any suspicious lesion is indicated. The endoscopist should always obtain a good retroflexed view of the cardia from below, to make certain that an adenocarcinoma of the gastroesophageal junction has not been overlooked (Color Plate 3*C*).

If narrowing has been seen by barium swallow, endoscopy with biopsy and cytologic brushings of the involved area is required. Biopsy of visible tissue may reveal only inflammation; as many as six to nine deep biopsy specimens should be obtained.

Once a tumor is identified, evaluation for local tumor spread, mediastinal nodal involvement, and liver metastases is essential for staging before a therapeutic decision is reached. This evaluation includes physical examination to detect lymphadenopathy, tests of liver enzymes, chest radiography, and computed tomographic (CT) scanning. For upper and mid-esophageal tumors, bronchoscopy is indicated to evaluate for asymptomatic invasion of the tracheobronchial tree. Endoscopic ultrasound is useful to detect the level of invasion and presence of mediastinal lymph node abnormalities and is becoming the favored test to determine if a lesion is resectable.

TREATMENT. The ideal treatment of esophageal cancer, either for cure or for palliation, has not yet been developed. Choice of therapy depends on the location and size of the lesion, presence or absence of spread, and cell type. No studies have carefully staged patients with the best noninvasive methods available and then randomized them to different treatment modalities. Until an adequate randomized trial after adequate staging is performed, choice of treatment modality will continue to be a matter of preference.

Surgical resection of squamous cell carcinoma and adenocarcinoma of the lower third of the esophagus is preferred in most centers if the patient does not have widespread metastases. Surgery offers the benefit of rapidly restoring esophagogastric continuity. Perhaps only a quarter of all patients have a resectable tumor; of these patients, 10 to 20% do not survive the operative period, and 5-year survival is only 5 to 20%, even with extensive resection. Long-term survival cannot be predicted in the individual case by the operative findings. There is growing enthusiasm for palliative resection with restoration of gastrointestinal continuity with stomach or colon.

Radiation therapy alone or in combination with surgery or chemotherapy has been a mainstay for squamous cell carcinoma, but adenocarcinomas are relatively radioinsensitive. Radiotherapy has little hospital mortality, but some short-term and long-term morbidity. Patients treated with definitive radiation therapy (50 to 80 Gy) alone have a 1-year survival of 18 to 40% and a 5-year survival of 6 to 14%; the values are dependent on the initial stage of the tumor. Combination of preoperative and postoperative radiation with resective therapy has been employed, but no good evidence has demonstrated that such combined therapy is better.

Chemotherapy with cisplatin-containing combinations has demonstrated objective tumor response. Preliminary evidence suggests that multimodality treatment with radiation therapy plus chemotherapy with cisplatin and fluorouracil is superior to radiation therapy alone.

When obvious extraesophageal spread is present, palliation may be achieved with bougienage to restore and maintain an adequate esophageal lumen. If performed with a guidewire under fluoroscopic guidance, such therapy is not hazardous in skilled hands. If dilation does not offer lasting relief, then a Silastic tube or metal stent can be placed perorally to relieve esophageal obstruction. Such tubes are also greatly beneficial in treating malignant tracheoesophageal fistula. Destruction of intraluminal tumor and restoration of an adequate lumen may be performed by endoscopic laser therapy, intraluminal heat-coagulating probe, or photodynamic therapy.

OTHER CONDITIONS

Rings and Webs

During early development, the lumen of the esophagus becomes completely obliterated and then is recanalized to form the adult hollow viscus; failure of this process leads to atresia or a residual web. Such webs usually occur in the upper esophagus, often with eccentric openings; occasionally they are multiple. An acquired web located in the postcricoid area is sometimes associated with iron deficiency anemia (Plummer-Vinson syndrome). A much more common ring is located in the terminal esophagus, has a symmetri-

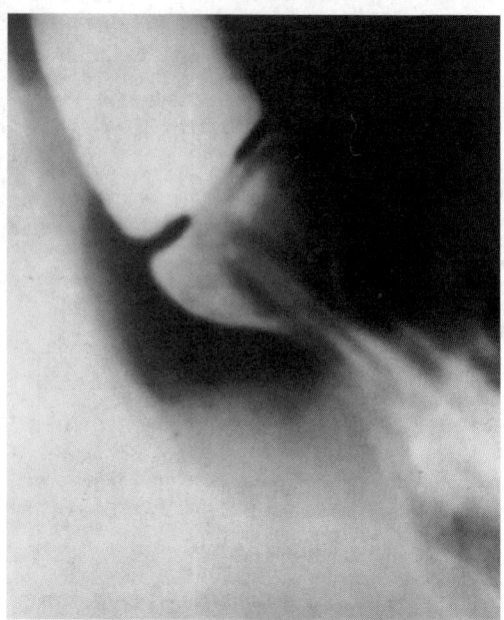

FIGURE 124–5 ■ Lower esophageal ring (Schatzki's ring). This ring consists of a symmetrical, thin web located in the terminal esophagus. (From Pope CE II: Rings and webs. *In* Sleisenger MH, Fordtran JS [eds]: Gastrointestinal Disease, 3rd ed, Philadelphia, WB Saunders, 1983.)

cal opening, and is usually at the junction between squamous and normal transitional or columnar epithelium of the stomach (Fig. 124–5). This latter ring (Schatzki's ring) can be demonstrated in many individuals if video studies of the lower esophageal zone are used (Color Plate 1*D*).

All webs or rings can cause dysphagia for solids, and the impacted bolus usually has to be regurgitated. The lower esophageal ring (Schatzki's ring) has a characteristic clinical presentation that allows the diagnosis to be made by history. Every 3 to 4 months, after a bolus of meat or bread, the patient complains of dysphagia and total inability to swallow solids or liquids. The bolus is regurgitated, and then the patient can continue to eat normally. Lower esophageal rings may be dilated using a TTS balloon or a bougie.

Symptomatic webs require mechanical disruption with either a dilator or an endoscope. Treatment of iron deficiency anemia may cause the postcricoid webs to disappear. Only very rarely is a surgical approach to a web or ring necessary.

Diverticula of the Esophagus

Zenker's diverticulum of the pharynx is not actually anatomically an esophageal diverticulum, as its neck is above the UES muscle. An epiphrenic diverticulum usually occurs on the right side of the esophagus just above the LES. Other diverticula are at the level of the carina and are known as traction diverticula, although traction by scar tissue is rarely demonstrated. Scleroderma is occasionally associated with numerous wide-mouthed diverticula scattered along the length of the esophagus. Large-amplitude motor waves have been associated with midbody diverticula, and achalasia or motor incoordination can occur with epiphrenic diverticula.

Symptoms vary widely; many diverticula are found incidentally during barium examination of the esophagus. If a patient with dysphagia is found to have a diverticulum, it is often difficult to determine whether the diverticulum or the associated motor disorder is the cause. Zenker's diverticulum often has a classic symptom complex, particularly when it becomes large. It retains saliva and food particles, which may either be aspirated or cause repeated postprandial throat clearing with production of liquid and food particles. Patients with this type of diverticulum can often press on the neck and empty the diverticulum. The pouch can become so large that it can compress the esophagus anteriorly and obstruct it. In the presence of diverticula, great caution must be exercised in passing tubes or endoscopes into the esophagus or stomach. Zenker's diverticulum is a special problem, because tubes naturally enter it rather than the esophageal opening, and the risk of perforation into the mediastinum is great.

Traction and epiphrenic diverticula do not require treatment. Zenker's diverticulum, if large, may require diverticulectomy or diverticulopexy with section of the cricopharyngeus muscle. If the diverticulum is small, it may regress after section of the cricopharyngeus.

Infections of the Esophagus

Infections afflicting the esophagus are usually fungal (*Candida*) or viral (cytomegalovirus [CMV], herpes simplex virus [HSV]). Although both are most common in immunocompromised hosts, such as those receiving corticosteroids, undergoing cancer chemotherapy, or afflicted with AIDS (see Chapter 413), either or both can infect apparently healthy hosts. All can be found incidentally at autopsy or during endoscopy for other indications. Most commonly, infection of the mucosa leads to marked odynophagia. Dysphagia for both solids and liquids usually accompanies the odynophagia and can be of such intensity that weight loss is rapid. Herpes esophagitis may present with hematemesis.

Although barium radiography occasionally reveals a shaggy mucosa, or even a stricture in candidal esophagitis, endoscopy is the best method of detecting and confirming infectious involvement. *Candida* infection can present as isolated white plaques, which can be confused with glycogenic acanthosis or progress to form confluent ulcerations with an overlying membrane. Herpesvirus tends to produce vesicles or isolated superficial ulcers, but extensive involvement can produce confluent ulcerations. CMV lesions initially appear as serpiginous ulcers, but they may coalesce to form giant ulcers. Biopsy of the ulcerated area usually shows either invasive hyphae of *Candida* or characteristic nuclear changes of the squamous cells when herpesvirus is present. Cytologic washings occasionally demonstrate the same change. Viral cultures of esophageal biopsies or brushings are useful for diagnosing HSV.

Treatment depends on correct identification of the etiologic agent. For mild, noninvasive candidal disease, topical therapy with nystatin (250,000 units every 2 hours) or clotrimazole (dissolved in the mouth 5 times per day) suffices. For more serious infections, systemic treatment with oral fluconazole or occasionally ketoconazole is used. Fluconazole (100 mg/day, given orally for 10 to 14 days) is generally preferred over topical treatment in patients with AIDS. Low-dose intravenous amphotericin may be needed for patients who do not respond to oral treatment and those unable to swallow medications. Herpesvirus infection is treated with parenteral acyclovir. Ganciclovir or foscarnet can be tried for CMV infection.

Esophageal Injuries

Caustic Ingestion

Caustic burns of the esophagus occur in children by accident; adults usually suffer such burns because of suicide attempts. Lye crystals, and especially liquid lye preparations for drain cleaning, detergents, and bleach are the most common causes (see Chapter 98). The speed of lye injury is so great that attempts to neutralize the caustic are futile. The history is all-important, but the degree of esophageal injury must be assessed emergently by endoscopy. Significant esophageal damage has been seen even without oral burns; conversely, oral burns do not necessarily mean that the material has reached the esophagus. If no esophageal reaction is present after apparent caustic ingestion, further care directed toward the esophagus will not be necessary. Circumferential burns and ulcers in the esophagus may result in delayed perforation over several days or in stricture formation.

The goals of therapy are to prevent perforation and to avoid progressive fibrosis and stricture of the esophagus. However, the accepted therapy of a definite lye or caustic burn remains unsupported by clinical trials. For burns with solid lye or other solid agents, corticosteroids have been recommended at an initial dose of 80 mg/day, tapering to 20 mg/day until the esophagus heals. Most clinicians also use broad-spectrum antibiotics. For liquid lye, serious consideration should be given to emergent esophagogastrectomy because lesser measures have met with unacceptably high mortality.

Damage by Medication

Ingested pills may lodge in the esophagus and damage the mucosa in a localized area. Tetracycline, doxycycline, potassium tablets, ascorbic acid, quinidine, and nonsteroidal anti-inflammatory agents are the principal medications that cause pill-induced esophagitis, but the list is long. For example, the bisphosphonates, such as alendronate, also cause esophageal injury. Normal individuals can retain small capsules in the esophagus even when swallowing in the upright position. The clinical syndrome consists of steady burning or chest pain accompanied by local odynophagia occurring 4 to 6 hours after ingesting one of the offending capsules or tablets. Endoscopy usually shows a localized mucosal ulcer, which may heal without scar or lead to a stricture requiring dilation. Symptomatic therapy is adequate, but prophylaxis is better. Pills should be taken by the patient in the upright position, with several swallows of water taken both before and after pill ingestion.

Esophageal Trauma

The esophagus is well protected by the thoracic cage, but it can be involved either by blunt trauma (e.g., automobile accidents) or by penetrating missiles (e.g., gunshots or knife wounds). Often the surgeon's attention is directed toward more life-threatening damage to heart, lungs, or major blood vessels, and a rent in the esophagus may be overlooked and may be followed by mediastinitis. Iatrogenic perforation with an endoscope, dilator, or, very rarely, nasogastric tube can lead to similar complications.

Vomiting itself can cause esophageal injury, either mucosal (Mallory-Weiss) or through-and-through rupture (Boerhaave's syndrome). The mucosal lesion first described by Mallory and Weiss has been recognized much more frequently since the advent of emergency fiberoptic endoscopy. Classically, the patient has repeated attacks of retching, at first producing gastric contents and later bright red blood. One quarter of patients shown to have a Mallory-Weiss tear have no prior history of vomiting. The tear is usually in the gastric mucosa just below the gastroesophageal junction, although it can extend through the junction and up into the esophageal mucosa. Diagnosis is almost always made at endoscopy; the rent is usually seen as the endoscope is being withdrawn from the stomach into the esophagus. The majority of such lesions heal with conservative therapy, and angiographic or surgical therapy is necessary in fewer than 5% of cases. Bleeding can be stopped during endoscopy by directly applying electrocoagulation or by injecting epinephrine.

Vomiting can also cause a complete tear in the esophageal wall. Unlike the Mallory-Weiss lesion, the tear in Boerhaave's syndrome is located above the gastroesophageal junction on the left side. It usually follows vomiting, but other marked increases in intra-abdominal pressure, such as from lifting a heavy weight or straining at stool, have been associated with this syndrome. The clinical diagnosis can be extremely difficult; often, patients with esophageal rupture are thought to have a myocardial infarction, pneumothorax, perforated viscus, or pancreatitis. Air in the mediastinum or the rapid appearance of a pleural effusion on the left usually leads to the correct diagnosis.

The diagnosis of esophageal perforation can usually be established by a cautious radiographic examination with water-soluble material. Barium should be used only if a tear is not demonstrated by the water-soluble agent. Immediate surgical repair is the accepted method of treatment of esophageal perforation. In those too ill for surgery, treatment consists of nasogastric suction, administration of antibiotics, and subsequent mediastinal drainage if necessary.

Axelrad AM, Fleisher DE: Esophageal tumors. *In* Feldman M, Scharschmidt BF, Sleisinger MH: Sleisinger and Fordtran's Gastrointestinal Disease, 6th ed. Philadelphia, WB Saunders, 1998.

Clouse RE, Diamant NE: Motor physiology and motor disorders of the esophagus. *In* Feldman M, Scharschmidt BF, Sleisinger MH: Sleisinger and Fordtran's Gastrointestinal Disease, 6th ed. Philadelphia, WB Saunders, 1998.

Kahrilas PJ: Gastroesophageal reflux disease and its complications. *In* Feldman M, Scharschmidt BF, Sleisinger MH: Sleisinger and Fordtran's Gastrointestinal Disease, 6th ed. Philadelphia, WB Saunders, 1998.

Richter JE: Dysphagia, odynophagia, heartburn, other esophageal symptoms. *In* Feldman M, Scharschmidt BF, Sleisinger MH: Sleisinger and Fordtran's Gastrointestinal Disease, 6th ed. Philadelphia, WB Saunders, 1998.

Baehr PH, McDonald GB: Esophageal infections: Risk factors, presentation, diagnosis and treatment. Gastroenterology 106:509, 1994. *Review of esophageal infections.*

Castell DO, Richter JE (eds): The Esophagus. 3rd ed. Philadelphia, Lippincott Williams & Wilkins, 1999. *This is a new edition of an excellent textbook on the esophagus.*

125 GASTRITIS AND *HELICOBACTER PYLORI*

Andrew H. Soll

The normal gastric mucosa has a remarkable ability to resist acid-peptic injury (see Chapter 126). Although *gastritis* was first interpreted to be an effect of aging and lifelong exposure to various insults, it is now clear that the most common cause of this inflammatory condition is infection with *Helicobacter pylori* (HP). Gastritis can be most readily classified by cause (Table 125–1). The term *non-erosive* is no longer used because the most common form, HP gastritis, can also be associated with erosions and peptic ulcers. Three conditions (severe physiologic stress, alcohol, and non-steroidal anti-inflammatory agents) that cause erosive or hemorrhagic damage have been traditionally included among disorders causing gastritis. However, these three disorders cause little, if any, inflammation; when inflammation is present, it is associated with HP infection.

HELICOBACTER PYLORI–INDUCED GASTRITIS

HP, a gram-negative microaerophilic organism, appears to be the cause of the most common worldwide human infection. This organism has three attributes that allow it to fill a unique ecologic niche (Table 125–2). The inflammation associated with HP is usually superficial, found in the foveolar or gastric pit region and upper portion of the lamina propria, and characterized by infiltration with polymorphonuclear leukocytes. Therefore, the gastritis is called

Table 125–1 ■ CLASSIFICATION OF "GASTRITIS" AND GASTROPATHY

Helicobacter pylori—induced gastritis (superficial, forms a spectrum from antral predominant, type "B" gastritis to pangastritis, type "AB")
Atrophic gastritic
  Pernicious anemia (fundal gland predominant, type "A," autoimmune markers)
  Atrophic pangastritis (involving antrum and fundal gland region, probably end-stage form of *H. pylori* gastritis
Erosive hemorrhagic gastropathy
  Non-steroidal anti-inflammatory drug (NSAID) gastroenteropathy
  Stress-related mucosal disease
  Alcohol gastropathy
Unusual or specific forms of gastritis
  Phlegmonous gastritis
  Infections, usually in immunocompromised hosts
    Viral (cytomegalovirus, herpes)
    Fungal (*Candida*, *Histoplasma*)
    Tuberculosis, syphilis
  Chronic erosive (diffuse varioliform) gastritis
  Postoperative alkaline reflux gastropathy
  Gastric ischemia
  Radiation-induced gastritis
  Ingestion of corrosive substances
  Ménétrier's disease (giant hypertrophic gastritis)
  Eosinophilic gastritis
  Granulomatous gastritis
  Vascular ectasia: watermelon stomach (antral vascular ectasia)
  Portal congestive gastropathy
  Lymphocytic gastritis

Table 125–2 ■ FEATURES OF THE UNIQUE ECOLOGIC NICHE FOR *HELICOBACTER PYLORI*

Colonization
  Motility
  Urease (and catalase)
  Adhesion to surface epithelial cells
Virulence (non-invasive, due to release of bacterial factors)
  Epithelial cytolysis and tight junction disruption by cytotoxins
  Induction of inflammatory immune response: chemotaxins, lipopolysaccharide, immune modulators, antigenic stimulation, induction of epithelial cytokines
Persistence
  Inaccessibility
  Immune evasion

chronic active. The antrum is consistently involved, whereas inflammation in the acid-secreting, fundic or oxyntic gland mucosa (gastric body and fundus) is more variable (see later). Four arguments establish that this antral-predominant, superficial gastritis (type B) is due to HP: (1) HP is present in virtually all patients with superficial gastritis, (2) the gastritis resolves once the infection is cured, (3) gastritis has been induced in a few subjects by inadvertent or self-administration of HP, and (4) the epidemiologic and geographic patterns for the occurrence of HP and superficial gastritis are identical.

EPIDEMIOLOGY. No reservoir other than the human gastric mucosa has been identified for HP. The epidemiology of HP reflects a pattern typical of fecal-oral transmission and is similar to hepatitis A or polio, with high prevalence at a young age in developing countries and in impoverished subpopulations in developed countries. Poor hygiene and poor sanitation are important variables. Transmission is most likely by a fecal-oral route or by exposure to gastric juice of infected individuals *(oral-gastric).* Transmission has also occurred with contaminated nasogastric tubes and endoscopes. Water-borne infection has been documented, but not in the United States. The *prevalence* of HP infection increases with age at an average rate of about 1% per year, but infection is usually acquired in childhood or in families with young children. A large component of the increase in prevalence with age reflects an *age cohort* effect whereby older individuals, especially those older than 60, acquired the infection at a young age. In the United States and other developed countries, HP infection is decreasing in parallel with the decrease in the incidence of peptic ulcer and cancer of the gastric body and antrum.

ACUTE HP GASTRITIS. With acute HP infection, superficial gastritis develops in association with epigastric pain, nausea, and vomiting. Two outbreaks of HP have been reported after common source exposure; despite the absence of glandular gastritis and the presence of histologically robust parietal cells, acid secretion was markedly reduced, suggesting release of a factor inhibiting acid secretion. Occasionally, sporadic acute HP gastritis can be recognized.

DISTRIBUTION AND PROGRESSION: RELATION TO PEPTIC ULCER AND GASTRIC CANCER. In the era before HP was recognized, gastritis involving predominantly the antrum was common in "normal" younger subjects. Follow-up over subsequent decades revealed progressive involvement of the fundic or body gland mucosa, resulting in pangastritis (type AB). In contrast to this progressive involvement from antrum to acid-secreting mucosa, simultaneous involvement of both the antrum and fundic gland regions has been observed in some young individuals, particularly in geographic regions with high endemic rates and early onset of HP infection and a high risk of gastric cancer. A different pattern occurs in HP-positive duodenal ulcer patients: although modest to moderate superficial antral gastritis is invariably found (see Chapter 126), involvement of the fundic gland mucosa is usually minimal, and progression occurs at a slower rate than in non-ulcer subjects. The clinical correlate is that duodenal ulcer patients secrete acid at high-normal or high rates and have a lower risk of gastric cancer. In contrast to duodenal ulcer, patients with gastric ulcer tend to have more severe antral gastritis, more involvement with superficial fundic gland gastritis, and low-normal acid secretory rates. The variability in the distribution and progression of HP gastritis among individuals is probably due to age at acquisition of HP infection, as well as host and environmental factors.

With time and increasing severity of pangastritis, fundic gland atrophy can occur and cause a decrease in maximal acid secretion with age. Atrophy of antral glands can also occur, often accompanied by pseudopyloric metaplasia (the parietal and chief cells of fundic glands are replaced by mucous glands indistinguishable from normal antrum) and intestinal metaplasia (mucin-containing goblet cells, absorptive cells, and occasionally rudimentary villi). Dysplastic epithelial change can develop subsequent to this metaplasia as part of the progression to gastric cancer (see Chapter 138) induced by HP gastritis.

OTHER PATHOGENIC FACTORS. In the pre-HP era, many other factors were considered in the pathogenesis of chronic gastritis, including chronic trauma, gastric bacteria, toxins, thermal insult, dietary factors (including dietary nitrosamines), and reflux of bile and pancreatic enzymes. Because curing HP infection rapidly resolves superficial gastritis, it is unlikely that these factors are etiologic on their own, although they may affect progression to chronic atrophic gastritis, intestinal metaplasia, or gastric cancer.

DETECTING HP (see Chapter 126). HP can be detected using "non-invasive" modalities: serology with an enzyme-linked immunosorbent assay (ELISA) for IgG or IgA antibodies and ^{13}C- or ^{14}C-urea breath tests after an oral urea load. Invasive testing includes biopsy for histologic examination, urease test on antral biopsies, or culture (which is not routinely available). The optimal method depends on circumstances, local expertise, and availability. All tests have good sensitivity and specificity, but false determinations occur. In tests that depend on the number of organisms (testing breath and gastric biopsies for urease activity, histology, and culture), false-negative results occur especially when the organism has been suppressed by antibiotics, proton pump inhibitors (omeprazole or lansoprazole), or bismuth. Therapy may need to be discontinued for several weeks before these tests become positive.

CLINICAL PRESENTATION AND TREATMENT. Individuals with gastritis are usually asymptomatic; the relation of pathologic gastritis to dyspepsia is mired in the vagaries of visceral sensation (see Chapter 126). However, HP gastritis is found in patients with dyspepsia more frequently than in age-matched controls. In contrast to the clear indication for antibiotic therapy with HP-positive peptic ulcer, the causal relation and proper approach to HP in the setting of "non-ulcer" dyspepsia is controversial (see Chapter 131). Non-ulcer dyspepsia is frequently due to functional disorders that are independent of HP; therefore, it is not surprising that curing infection often does not eliminate symptoms in many patients. Although benefit over placebo has not been established in controlled studies, some individuals with HP gastritis and upper abdominal symptoms improve once HP infection is cured. Because antibiotic therapy for HP (see Chapter 127) is less expensive and probably safer than additional diagnostic studies and long-term continuous anti-acid therapy, cure of HP infection is a reasonable option for patients with persisting symptoms who do not respond to or require continued treatment. HP testing and treatment are also appropriate for new-onset or previously undiagnosed dyspepsia (see Chapters 126 and 131).

ATROPHIC GASTRITIS

ATROPHIC PANGASTRITIS DUE TO HP. The adhesion molecule for HP is present on the apical membrane of normal and metaplastic gastric-type but not intestinal-type cells. HP-associated pangastritis can progress to fundic and antral gland atrophy, but HP is frequently absent when hyposecretion of acid disrupts HP's unique ecologic niche in the acidic stomach and allows overgrowth of other bacteria. IgG and IgA antibodies to HP usually begin to fall within months after loss of the organism (but it may take years for the titers to return to the normal range). Autoimmune markers are generally absent from HP pangastritis, and only a small (and undefined) proportion of subjects develop secondary vitamin B_{12} deficiency. The contribution of other factors to pathogenesis and the overlap with autoimmune gastritis and pernicious anemia remain to be established.

PERNICIOUS ANEMIA (see Chapter 163). This immune gastritis (type A) predominantly involves the fundic gland mucosa, is deep

(encompassing the gastric glands that contain parietal and chief cells), and usually is atrophic (with decreased or absent glandular elements and mucosal thinning). Superficial inflammation is minimal, and deep inflammatory changes usually are most prominent along the greater curvature of the fundus and body. Once glandular atrophy develops, the inflammatory infiltrate may be minimal. Even with sufficient fundic gland atrophy to produce histamine-fast achlorhydria, some patchy nests of parietal and chief cells may persist. The relative absence of glandular atrophy in the antrum accounts for the ability of many of these patients to develop marked hypergastrinemia when there is no feedback inhibition of acid on gastrin release.

Immunologic mechanisms appear operative in pernicious anemia but not HP gastritis. About 90% of patients with pernicious anemia have antibodies against parietal cells. Antibodies reacting with intrinsic factor block the vitamin B_{12} binding site, leading to depleted serum levels and body stores of vitamin B_{12} and a megaloblastic anemia (see Chapter 163). Pernicious anemia is also associated with other immunologic disorders (e.g., Hashimoto's thyroiditis, hyperthyroidism, insulin-dependent diabetes mellitus, and vitiligo). Genetic factors are important in pernicious anemia; family members of patients have an increased incidence of atrophic gastritis, achlorhydria, vitamin B_{12} malabsorption, and antibodies to parietal cells and intrinsic factor.

CLINICAL PRESENTATION. Patients with pernicious anemia may develop symptoms secondary to vitamin B_{12} deficiency. Macroscopic endoscopic findings (erythema, petechiae, nodularity, pallor, and atrophy) are generally non-specific. Diagnosis requires multiple biopsies because the histopathology may be patchy. The ratio of pepsinogen I (present in fundic chief cells) to pepsinogen II (present in both chief cells and surface epithelial cells) falls in proportion to glandular atrophy.

Enterochromaffin-like cells undergo hyperplasia in atrophic gastritis because the elevated gastrin levels exert trophic effects on them. These endocrine cells in the fundic gland mucosa contain histamine and are distinguished by characteristic granules and silver staining properties. Enterochromaffin-like cells can form carcinoid tumors in atrophic gastritis. Enterochromaffin-like cell hyperplasia also occurs in Zollinger-Ellison (gastrinoma) syndrome (see Chapter 130), but carcinoid tumors are largely restricted to patients with multiple endocrine neoplasia (MEN) type I. Enterochromaffin-like cells do not contain serotonin, and thus these tumors do not produce the classic carcinoid syndrome found with tumors composed of serotonin-containing enterochromaffin cells (see Chapter 245). Enterochromaffin-like carcinoids associated with hypergastrinemia can be metastatic, but they are usually indolent, multifocal tumors that may respond to antrectomy and local excision. In contrast, gastric carcinoids found without hypergastrinemia are solitary, aggressive tumors.

MANAGEMENT. Other than replacing vitamin B_{12}, no specific therapy exists for pernicious anemia. It is reasonable to evaluate family members for gastritis and vitamin B_{12} deficiency. *Gastric adenocarcinomas* (see Chapter 138) have been reported to occur with increased frequency with pernicious anemia, but the assessment of increased risk is variable, ranging from none to threefold in different series. At the time of an initial diagnosis, endoscopic biopsy is usually recommended to obtain sufficient antral and fundic gland tissue to assess the severity of intestinal metaplasia and epithelial dysplasia; although imperfect, these features are the best indicators of the cancer risk. Using this approach, only those patients with dysplasia warrant close follow-up and/or surgical intervention. Otherwise, no recommendations regarding screening have been established.

EROSIVE-HEMORRHAGIC GASTROPATHY

NON-STEROIDAL ANTI-INFLAMMATORY DRUG (NSAID) GASTROENTEROPATHY. See Chapter 126.

STRESS-RELATED MUCOSAL DAMAGE AND ULCERS. See Chapter 126.

ALCOHOL GASTROPATHY. Characteristic subepithelial (intramucosal) hemorrhages, with the endoscopic appearance of "blood under a plastic wrap," are commonly found in individuals who abuse alcohol. Termed *hemorrhagic gastritis*, these lesions are composed of hemorrhage and edema in the interstitial space under the surface epithelium, without inflammation. Usually the bleeding is mild. If more severe bleeding is found, associated lesions, such as portal hypertension, peptic ulcer, or a Mallory-Weiss tear, should be sought (see Chapter 123).

UNUSUAL OR SPECIFIC FORMS OF GASTRITIS. PHLEGMON-OUS GASTRITIS. This rarely encountered, purulent process involves the gastric submucosa and wall. α-Hemolytic streptococci, staphylococci, *Escherichia coli*, and *Proteus* have been implicated. The course is usually fulminant, and medical management is generally ineffective; surgery is usually unavoidable.

OTHER INFECTIONS. Herpes simplex virus type I has been implicated as a cause of ulcer disease in normal hosts (see Chapter 126). The *Ascaris*-like larva, *Anisakis* (see Chapter 433), present in raw fish, may infect the normal gastric mucosa, producing pain and dyspepsia. *Strongyloides stercoralis* (see Chapter 433) usually involves the small intestine but can also involve the stomach.

A variety of infectious causes of gastritis occur in the immunocompromised host. Gastric tuberculosis, diagnosed by caseating granulomas and positive cultures, occurs in the acquired immunodeficiency syndrome (AIDS). Secondary syphilis may involve the stomach with thickened folds and erosions. Cytomegalovirus can also involve the stomach. Whether *Candida* causes gastric ulcers remains controversial. Mycelia may occur at the ulcer margin, but ulcer healing does not appear to be impaired, and antifungal therapy does not accelerate healing, suggesting colonization rather than an initial infectious etiology.

CHRONIC EROSIVE (DIFFUSE VARIOLIFORM) GASTRITIS. In this condition, lesions are multiple and consist of gastric erosions on top of small nodules, usually involving the body and fundus more than the antrum. The multiplicity and chronicity distinguish this entity from occasional isolated antral erosions found without symptoms. The entity can be considered only after HP and use of NSAIDs and alcohol have been excluded. Symptoms are non-specific and include abdominal pain, nausea, vomiting, anorexia, weight loss, and sometimes bleeding. Lymphocytic gastritis may be associated with these lesions.

POSTOPERATIVE ALKALINE GASTRITIS. Macroscopic gastropathy with a dramatic red color may develop rapidly after gastric resection or pyloroplasty, but this endoscopic appearance does not correlate with symptoms, bile reflux, or histologic inflammation. In fact, inflammation is minimal to absent. The characteristic histologic picture is reactive gastropathy, with elongation of the glands in the pit region resulting in a corkscrew appearance (foveolar hyperplasia). Importantly, this abnormality can be confused with dysplasia, which it is not. The occurrence of this difficult-to-treat complication of surgery for peptic ulcer (see Chapter 128) is another rationale for avoiding surgery or doing the least physiologically disruptive operation (i.e., highly selective vagotomy), whenever possible.

GASTRIC ISCHEMIA. Ischemic gastric injury is rarely recognized, although erosive changes have been reported with vasculitis and atheromatous embolization. Whether chronic gastric ulcers have an ischemic component remains speculative.

MÉNÉTRIER'S DISEASE. Ménétrier's disease is defined by four features: (1) giant folds in the gastric fundus and body, (2) diminished acid secretory capacity, (3) hypoalbuminemia secondary to protein-losing gastropathy, and (4) histologic features of foveolar hyperplasia (gastric pit region) and a marked increase in mucosal thickness combined with gland atrophy and cystic dilation. Tortuous gastric folds may resemble the cerebral cortex. Hypochlorhydria is generally present, but a hypersecretory variant (which may be an unrelated entity) has been described. Symptoms are variable and may include abdominal pain, nausea, vomiting, weight loss, and edema. The disease is more common in men than in women and generally presents after age 50, although a childhood form exists. Typically, biopsies confirm the diagnosis, but variant patterns warrant the less specific diagnosis of idiopathic hypertrophic

gastropathy. Variant cases that do not include all of the typical features are more common than classic cases. The differential diagnosis includes gastrinoma syndrome, infiltrating carcinoma, lymphoma, and amyloidosis. Large gastric folds and a picture of hypertrophic gastritis may be associated with HP infection. If present, the organism should be treated, but the impact on gastric protein loss has not been established. Accompanying ulcers and erosions usually respond to standard antiulcer therapy if HP is not present. No increased risk of cancer has been established.

EOSINOPHILIC GASTRITIS. Eosinophils may infiltrate the gastrointestinal mucosa and muscular layers, especially with antral involvement. Thickening of gastric mucosal folds and wall rigidity are common. Antral motility may be altered, leading to gastric retention. Patients may present with eosinophilia, nausea, vomiting, or pain. Rarely, serosal involvement results in ascites. Milk-sensitive enteropathy of infancy, connective tissue disorders, and parasitic infections should be excluded. Glucocorticoid therapy may be useful, and surgery may be needed if mechanical outlet obstruction occurs.

GRANULOMATOUS GASTRITIS. Granulomas may occur in the gastric mucosa with generalized diseases such as sarcoidosis, Crohn's disease, or infections. Crohn's disease (see Chapter 135) may involve the duodenum, pylorus, antrum, and gastric body (in that order), usually in association with disease in the small intestine or colon. Mucosal granulomas may occur in eosinophilic granulomas or in isolated, idiopathic granulomatous gastritis or may be incidental findings. Involved portions of the stomach may be rigid or narrow or have thickened folds on radiographic examination; these findings must be distinguished from malignancy. The antrum is most often involved, and granulomas may occur in all layers of the stomach. Ulcerated lesions may perforate. Patients are often operated on because of the difficulties in differentiating this entity from malignancy. Once the diagnosis is made, it is important to exclude potentially curable diseases (e.g., tuberculosis, histoplasmosis, syphilis) or treatable processes (e.g., sarcoidosis, Crohn's disease). If malignancy and associated diseases have been excluded, the patient can be observed and not treated because spontaneous resolution has been reported.

WATERMELON STOMACH. This entity, also known as gastric antral vascular ectasia, represents another non-gastritic condition. At endoscopy, the antrum has erythematous folds or linear angioid streaks, the latter converging at the pylorus in a pattern reminiscent of a watermelon. Biopsy can be diagnostic, demonstrating dilated antral vasculature with intravascular fibrin thrombi and fibromuscular hyperplasia. This uncommon lesion can present with either acute gastrointestinal bleeding or chronic iron-deficiency anemia. Corticosteroid therapy has been tried with uncertain success. Antrectomy is effective in eliminating bleeding; however, success has also been reported with repeated coagulation using endoscopic laser or heater probes. No relation to HP has been reported.

CONGESTIVE GASTROPATHY. Subepithelial hemorrhage and vascular ectasia can occur in portal hypertension due to cirrhosis. Endoscopic abnormalities include distinct red spots in the antrum and a mosaic pattern in the body, which is an exaggeration of the normal gastric surface morphology. Mucosal vascular congestion appears to be the operative mechanism in susceptible hosts, although no definitive studies have been performed and histologic correlation with congestion is poor.

LYMPHOCYTIC GASTRITIS. The histologic appearance of the mucosa resembles celiac disease or lymphocytic colitis. A superficial small cell infiltrate is present. There is a relation to other forms of gastritis (varioliform gastritis, Ménétrier's, and celiac disease) but no obvious relation to HP gastritis.

Lewin KJ, Riddell RH, Weinstein WM: Stomach and proximal duodenum: Inflammatory and miscellaneous disorders. *In* Gastrointestinal Pathology and Its Clinical Implications. New York, Igaku-Shoin, 1992, p 506. *Definitive reference on gastritis and related conditions.*

Weinstein WM: Gastritis and gastropathies. *In* Feldman M, Scharshmidt BF, Sleisenger MH (eds): Sleisenger and Fordtran's Gastrointestinal Disease, 6th ed. Philadelphia, WB Saunders, 1998, p 711. *Detailed discussion of the common forms of gastritis.*

126 PEPTIC ULCER DISEASE: EPIDEMIOLOGY, PATHOPHYSIOLOGY, CLINICAL MANIFESTATIONS, AND DIAGNOSIS

Andrew Soll ■ *Jon Isenberg*

EPIDEMIOLOGY

THE PROBLEM. Peptic ulcer diseases (gastric and duodenal ulcer) represent serious medical problems due in large part to their frequency and high economic costs. Each year in the United States there are approximately 500,000 new cases and 4 million recurrences with direct costs (i.e., physician visits, hospitalizations, medications) that are estimated in excess of $10 billion and equivalent indirect costs (principally due to time lost from work). The annual mortality rate due to ulcer disease is low (<15,000). Deaths are due to ulcer complications, principally hemorrhage (see Chapter 128). Peptic ulcer disease related to infection with *Helicobacter pylori* (HP) and independent of non-steroidal anti-inflammatory drugs (NSAIDs) tends to be chronic, with a high recurrence rate (60–90% per year) unless HP is eradicated. In patients with NSAID-induced ulcer disease, recurrences are diminished substantially if NSAID intake is discontinued. On a worldwide basis, HP infection is widespread across all age groups, whereas NSAIDs are used primarily by the elderly and others to relieve the pain due to degenerative joint diseases, musculoskeletal problems, and other chronic pain syndromes.

INCIDENCE, PREVALENCE, AND RELATIVE RISK. The bedside diagnosis of ulcer disease is not precise. Furthermore, large endoscopic surveys of random U.S. populations have not been conducted. Thus, estimates of the incidence (number of new cases per unit time, usually yearly) and prevalence (the total number of cases at a given point in time within the population under study) within the Unites States lack precision. By comparison, ulcer complications (see Chapter 128) require hospitalization, so their frequency can be assessed with greater accuracy.

Before 1900, gastric ulcer was more common than duodenal ulcer. The incidence of duodenal ulcer began to increase in the early 1900s, reached a peak in about the 1950s, and progressively decreased thereafter. The reasons for the greater prevalence of duodenal ulcer in the cohort born during the latter decades of the last century and first decade of this century is not fully understood, but it may be due in part to poor sanitation with increased transmission of HP.

The overall lifetime prevalence for peptic ulcer (combined gastric and duodenal ulcer) is estimated at approximately 12% in males and about 9% in females; the 1-year "point prevalence" (percentage of the population with ulcer) in the United States is about 1.8%. In the mid-1950s, the male:female ratio for deaths due to duodenal ulcer was 5:1, but this ratio has decreased to about 1.3:1 because of a decrease in males and little change in females for unclear reasons. Gastric ulcer tends to occur with equal frequency in males and females. Onset for duodenal ulcer is most commonly between the ages of 25 and 55, whereas gastric ulcer is most frequent between ages 40 and 70, likely due to increased use of NSAIDs.

The daily use of NSAIDs significantly increases the risk of ulcer disease (relative risk = 10- to 20-fold), because of the suppression of prostaglandin synthesis. However, a new class of potentially less damaging NSAIDs termed *cyclooxygenase-2 or COX-2 inhibitors* (see Chapter 29) has been developed. These agents have only a modest inhibitory effect on the constitutively expressed cyclooxygenase-1 (COX-1) and instead inhibit the inducible form of cyclooxygenase-2 that is produced by macrophages, fibroblasts, and synovial and endothelial cells in areas of inflammation. Thus, the "COX-2 inhibitors" have only a modest effect in suppressing the generation of the constitutive prostaglandins (i.e., those regulated by COX-1 and that have a defensive effect on the stomach and

duodenum by stimulating blood flow, mucosal bicarbonate, and mucus secretion), whereas they suppress the production of the proinflammatory prostaglandins that results in inflammation and pain. The clinical efficacy and side-effect profile of the COX-2 inhibitors is under investigation. If they or the recently developed NSAIDs bound to nitric oxide are indeed effective in relieving arthritic pain and have fewer untoward gastrointestinal effects than conventional NSAIDs, they would be a major therapeutic advance.

HP increases the risk of developing duodenal ulcer disease by fivefold to sevenfold. In addition, cigarette smoking decreases duodenal bicarbonate production and increases the risk of ulcer disease about twofold.

GENETICS. Genetic factors appear to play a role in ulcerogenesis. For example, in monozygotic twins in whom one twin develops ulcer, the concordant twin has about a 50% chance of developing an ulcer. Also, first-degree relatives of ulcer patients have about a threefold greater chance of developing ulcer. Duodenal ulcer and gastric ulcer occur independently in families. It is possible that some of the presumed genetic linkage is instead due to early familial infection with HP. Rare genetic syndromes associated with duodenal ulcer include multiple endocrine neoplasia (MEN) type 1, gastrin-secreting pancreatic tumor associated with another endocrine tumor (e.g., hyperparathyroidism), and systemic mastocytosis (increased circulating levels of histamine) (see Chapter 130).

PATHOPHYSIOLOGY

Peptic ulcers are holes extending through the mucosa into the muscularis propria of the esophagus, stomach, or duodenum. Schwarz, who was credited with the "no acid: no ulcer" dictum, recognized in 1910 that peptic ulcer was a product of self-digestion, resulting from an excess of autopeptic power in gastric juice over the defensive power of gastric and intestinal mucosa. Three lines of defense functioning at pre-epithelial, epithelial, and post-epithelial levels preserve mucosal integrity (Table 126–1). When these defenses are overwhelmed, the intrinsic epithelial repair mechanisms have the potential to restore mucosal integrity. However, when the defense and repair processes are overwhelmed and wounds form in the basement membrane, classic wound healing processes remodel the basement membrane and permit epithelial regrowth. Thus, peptic ulcers are a failure of normal wound healing. In the past decade it has become apparent that, with rare exception, these mucosal defense, repair, and healing mechanisms fail only when disrupted by exogenous factors. The two most common forms of peptic ulcer are associated with HP infection and use of aspirin and other NSAIDs (Table 126–2). In the absence of these factors, ulcers would be a rare disease.

ULCERS DUE TO *H. PYLORI*. Even in the era before the HP revolution, peptic ulcer in the absence of NSAIDs was recognized to be consistently associated with diffuse, chronic antral-predominant inflammation. Duodenal ulcer is also associated with duodenitis, but the distribution is patchy and variable. The significance of this inflammation remained unknown until Marshall and Warren recognized that the very common superficial, antral-predominant

---

Table 126–1 ■ **THE MULTIPLE LINES OF MUCOSAL DEFENSE, REPAIR, AND HEALING**

Lines of Defense
First line: mucus and bicarbonate
  Adherent mucous layer excludes pepsin
  Bicarbonate output creates pH gradient stabilized by mucous layer
Second line: Epithelial cell mechanisms
  Barrier function of apical plasma membrane
  Intrinsic cell defense (e.g., glutathione and heat shock protein)
  Extrusion of "back-diffused" H^+ via basolateral carriers
Third line: Mucosal blood flow (removal of "back-diffused" H^+ and supply of energy substrate)

Lines of Repair and Healing
First line: Epithelial cell restitution (sliding of adjacent cells to fill gaps created by sloughed cells)
Second line: Epithelial cell replication
Third line: Classic wound healing (formation of granulation tissue, angiogenesis, and remodeling of basement membrane permitting ingrowth of epithelial cells)

Table 126–2 ■ CAUSES AND ASSOCIATIONS OF PEPTIC ULCER

Common Forms of Peptic Ulcer
Helicobacter pylori-associated
NSAID-associated
Stress ulcer
Uncommon Specific Forms of Peptic Ulcer
Acid hypersecretion
   Gastrinoma: inherited—multiple endocrine neoplasia I, sporadic
   Increased mast cells/basophils
      Mastocytosis: inherited and sporadic
      Basophilic leukemias
   Antral G-cell hyperfunction/hyperplasia
Other infections
   Viral infection: herpes simplex virus type I, cytomegalovirus
   ? Other infections
Duodenal obstruction/disruption (congenital bands, annular pancreas)
Vascular insufficiency: crack cocaine–associated perforations
Radiation-induced
Chemotherapy-induced (hepatic artery infusions)
? Rare genetic subtypes
   ? Amyloidosis type III (Van Allen–Iowa)
   ? Tremor-nystagmus-ulcer syndrome of Neuhauser

Modified from Soll AH: Gastric, duodenal, and stress ulcer. *In* Sleisinger M, Fordtran J (eds): Gastrointestinal Disease, 5th ed. Philadelphia, WB Saunders, 1993, p 580.

(type B) form of gastritis was linked to HP (see Chapter 125). Two lines of evidence established HP as a crucial causal factor for development of both duodenal ulcer and gastric ulcer: (1) the large majority of duodenal and gastric ulcers are associated with HP, and (2) well-designed, controlled studies have consistently indicated that successfully eradicating the HP infection predicts a markedly reduced rate of ulcer recurrence. Although studies from Europe and Australia indicated that more than 90% of duodenal ulcers were associated with HP, studies from the United States indicate that the prevalence of HP in duodenal ulcer is somewhat less, at about 75%.

The challenging aspect of this pathophysiology is that HP is the most common infection in the world yet only a small percentage (10–20%) of infected subjects develop peptic ulcer during a lifetime of infection. The ulcer diathesis that separates the few subjects destined to develop peptic ulcer disease from those with HP infection without ulcer disease has not been defined. Organisms from duodenal ulcer patients have been distinguished from those occurring in non-ulcer subjects by genetic homology and cytotoxin production, but no single pathogenic factor has been identified that is consistently and selectively associated with ulcer formation. Once the HP infection is cured, inflammation rapidly resolves and ulcer recurrence is infrequent, making it unlikely that autoimmunity contributes to pathogenesis.

ARE PEPTIC ULCERS STILL PEPTIC? Schwarz recognized that acid-peptic activity is an indispensable component of ulcer pathogenesis. The persisting validity of this generalization is supported by the observation that very potent antisecretory agents heal the large majority of peptic ulcers.

ACID SECRETION. Maximal gastric acid output is elevated in about one third of duodenal ulcer patients and in the high-normal range in the remaining patients. Duodenal ulcer virtually does not occur with a maximal gastric output less than about 12 mEq/hour, and acid secretion is consistently high-normal or elevated in duodenal ulcer. No agreement exists regarding whether these changes are due to an increase in the number of acid-secreting parietal cells ("secretory mass"), defective inhibitory mechanisms, or increased basal (neural and/or hormonal) drive to acid secretion. About 80% of duodenal ulcer subjects also have an increased nocturnal acid secretion; this increased rate of acid secretion between 4 P.M. and midnight probably reflects an exaggeration of a normal circadian rhythm.

HP and the Secretion of Gastrin, Somatostatin, and Acid. Both ulcer and non-ulcer subjects infected with HP demonstrate enhanced secretion of gastrin in response to food and other stimuli. Abnormalities of gastric somatostatin cells have also been identified in HP-infected subjects. Despite the elevation in serum gastrin and the decrease in the paracrine (locally acting) inhibitor somatostatin, acid secretion is usually normal in non-ulcer, HP-infected subjects. The normal or increased acid secretion found in duodenal ulcer

subjects appears to be a feature of the ulcer diathesis rather than of the HP infection per se. Three hypotheses are probably true regarding duodenal ulcer and acid secretion: (1) in *some* duodenal ulcer subjects, acid secretion is decreased after successful cure of the HP infection, suggesting in this subset that acid secretion may be increased by either HP-induced hypergastrinemia or the perturbed inhibitory mechanisms; (2) in another subset of duodenal ulcer subjects, acid hypersecretion appears to reflect a predisposing condition that is independent of HP infection; and (3) duodenal ulcer subjects may be "selected" from non-duodenal ulcer HP-infected subjects by the relative sparing of the gastric body from gastritis, thereby preserving acid secretion.

DUODENITIS, GASTRIC METAPLASIA, AND DUODENAL ULCER. Gastric metaplasia of the duodenum occurs principally in the duodenal bulb when the normal intestinal epithelium is replaced by cells with the staining properties of gastric surface mucous cells. This change may be a key pathogenic step toward ulcer formation. The importance of this metaplasia in the duodenum probably reflects the fact that HP binds only to a glycoprotein receptor on the surface of these gastric-type cells; gastric metaplasia therefore appears to be the carpet on which HP resides in the duodenum. Present evidence suggests that gastric metaplasia occurs as a function of exposure to the acid-peptic activity in gastric juice. Another consistent pathogenic feature present in about 80% of duodenal ulcer subjects is a decrease in duodenal bicarbonate secretion. Studies have indicated that cure of HP infection causes return of depressed bicarbonate secretion to normal, suggesting that this effect may be an important consequence of HP infection leading to duodenal ulcer.

THE FOCAL AND RECURRENT NATURE OF ULCER PATHOGENESIS. Many features of peptic ulcer remain enigmatic. No pathophysiologic variables have been identified to correlate with the tendency of ulcers to heal and recur spontaneously. Ulcer disease is a focal process, and ulcers tend to recur in the same region; whereas ulcers persist, nearby areas readily heal.

ULCERS DUE TO NSAIDs. The second common form of ulcer disease is related to use of NSAIDs. One-half to 4 per cent of patients taking NSAIDs develop gastrointestinal complications during the course of a year of continued use. Because all of the subjects taking NSAIDs are exposed to the same damaging effects, a fascinating, unanswered question is why only a small number of affected subjects develop clinically significant ulcer disease.

INHIBITION OF PROSTAGLANDIN PRODUCTION. There is considerable evidence that ulcers develop as a result of NSAID inhibition of endogenous prostaglandin production, resulting in impaired prostaglandin-dependent mucosal defense and repair mechanisms. All NSAIDs inhibit the enzyme cyclooxygenase that catalyzes the formation of the prostaglandin precursor endoperoxide from arachidonic acid that is derived from cell membrane phospholipids. In animal models, ulcers are also produced by antibodies to prostaglandins but not to inactive prostaglandin analogues, further supporting the conclusion that endogenous prostaglandins are important elements in mucosal defense.

ROUTE OF DELIVERY. NSAIDs can be delivered to the gastroduodenal mucosa by topical, systemic, or enterohepatic delivery. Although each of these routes may be important, parenterally administered ketorolac (Toradol) produces ulcer complications within a few days, leaving no doubt that the systemic route is sufficient for ulcerogenesis. Use of enteric coating will reduce local toxic exposure and may reduce symptoms. However, because systemic effects are unperturbed, the ulcer risk is unchanged.

HP VS. NSAID ULCERS. There is no question that NSAIDs cause clinically relevant ulcers in patients who do not have HP. However, a subset of subjects with NSAID ulcers are also infected with HP. Studies have demonstrated that curing HP infection reduces the risk of endoscopic ulcers during subsequent NSAID therapy, although the interaction between NSAIDs and HP remains highly controversial.

CLINICAL ULCERS VS. ENDOSCOPIC ULCERS AND SUPERFICIAL INJURY. It is important to distinguish among three types of NSAID-induced lesions (Table 126–3): (1) superficial injury, which includes erosions and petechiae (punctate intramucosal hemorrhage); (2) "endoscopic ulcers," which are found in 10 to 25% of subjects taking NSAIDs; and (3) "clinical ulcers," which present as bleeding, perforation, or obstruction at a rate of 1 to 2% per patient-year of NSAID use. Intramucosal hemorrhages are frequent but of little clinical significance. Erosions, unlike ulcers, are small, superficial

Table 126-3 ■ THREE TYPES OF NSAID-ASSOCIATED MUCOSAL LESIONS

FEATURE	SUPERFICIAL MUCOSAL INJURY	ENDOSCOPIC ULCERS	CLINICAL ULCERS
Onset	Acute (onset in minutes)	Subacute (onset days to months)	Chronic (persist for days to years)
Site	Fundus > antrum	Antrum > fundus	Antrum, duodenum > fundus
Depth	Involves mucosa only	Often indeterminate	Penetrate submucosa
Mode	Topical contact, pH partition	Probably systemic, secondary to decreased prostaglandins	Probably systemic, secondary to decreased prostaglandins
Size	Smaller	Arbitrary (>3, >5 mm)	Big enough
Enteric coating	Decreases acute injury	Probably some decrease	May not decrease ulcer incidence
Clinical importance	Usually trivial	A few probably evolve to clinical ulcers	Sometimes cause complications
Healing	Rapid	Probably rapid, little chronic change	Slower or slow
Adaptation	Occurs, especially at low doses	Uncertain	Probably not: ulcers reflect failed adaptation
Prostaglandin cytoprotection	Yes	Yes	Probable partial prevention

breaks that do not extend deeper than the mucosa itself and therefore do not cause perforation or significant bleeding. However, superficial gastric lesions from NSAID ingestion may uncommonly lead to iron-deficiency anemia from chronic blood loss or to active bleeding due to widespread involvement or anticoagulation. NSAIDs also can cause very significant intestinal damage, ulceration, and weblike strictures presenting as chronic gastrointestinal blood loss, obstruction, or perforation.

Most of the clinical investigation of the pathogenesis and prevention of NSAID ulcers has been based on endoscopic and not clinical ulcers. The definition of endoscopic ulcers varies among studies and is usually based on size alone. There is little doubt that flat lesions less than 5 mm have a different natural history and response to therapeutic intervention than do lesions larger than 5 mm with visible depth. Furthermore, these endoscopic lesions are likely to behave quite differently than are chronic deep ulcers with surrounding fibrosis.

THE RISK OF GASTROINTESTINAL COMPLICATIONS WITH NSAIDs. NSAID use is reported in 40 to 60% of patients presenting with the ulcer complications of bleeding and perforation. Although the magnitude of the risk of complications from NSAIDs is controversial, in a controlled study, aspirin (1 g/day) caused a 9- to 10-fold increased risk of hospitalization for both duodenal ulcer and gastric ulcer. The risk begins within days after treatment, is highest within the first 3 months of therapy, but persists for years. Ulcer risk also appears to be increased with one aspirin tablet (325 mg) daily; mucosal prostaglandin production is decreased with doses as low as a "baby" ASA tablet (82 mg) daily, and the risk of bleeding is increased even with this low dose. Although gastrointestinal bleeding from NSAIDs is often linked to ulcers, an important component of bleeding, especially with aspirin, is platelet dysfunction due to inhibition of thromboxane production. A thorough evaluation is appropriate with any patient who bleeds while on NSAID therapy because the probability of finding lesions other than ulcers (see Chapter 29) is at least as high as in subjects who are not taking NSAIDs.

RISK FACTORS FOR NSAID ULCERS. Compared with the general population, the risk of NSAID-associated ulcer complications is higher in elderly women, probably because of the increased consumption of NSAIDs by this group and the poor tolerance to complications because of associated diseases. However, a randomized study comparing 1 g of aspirin daily to placebo indicated that age is an independent risk factor for hospitalizations due to ulcer complications. Corticosteroids alone cause little risk of ulcer disease, but when they are combined with NSAIDs their added risk is significant. Anticoagulant co-therapy also increases the risk of gastrointestinal complications.

The most important risk factor for NSAID ulcers is a history of prior peptic ulcer disease, either due to HP or to NSAIDs. This finding justifies curing HP infection whenever it is encountered in a subject with NSAID-associated ulcers.

SUPERPEPTIC ULCERS. Acid secretion has to be markedly inhibited to promote rapid healing of gastric ulcers in the presence of continued NSAID use. This observation underlines the point that NSAID ulcers are "super-peptic" ulcers, probably with increased sensitivity to the gastric acid-peptic activity. However, it should

also be emphasized that NSAIDs must be considered along with cancer and HP infection as a cause of ulcers in patients with achlorhydria. The ability of NSAIDs to cause intestinal ulcers leaves no question about their ulcerogenesis independent of acid-peptic activity.

GASTRINOMA. This uncommon form of ulcer disease is caused by excessive secretion of gastrin by a tumor and gastric acid hypersecretion (see Chapter 130).

RETAINED ANTRUM. This is an unusual complication of peptic ulcer surgery (see Chapter 129).

ANTRAL G-CELL HYPERFUNCTION. This is a rare form of duodenal ulcer disease in which acid hypersecretion is caused by enhanced secretion of antral gastrin. Fasting gastrin levels are usually only modestly elevated, but the response to a meal is greatly exaggerated. In contradistinction to patients with gastrinoma, intravenous secretin does not elevate gastrin secretion. Although controversial, this entity appears both in an HP-independent form and as the end of the spectrum of HP-induced hypergastrinemia and acid hypersecretion.

MASTOCYTOSIS AND BASOPHILIC LEUKEMIA. These unusual conditions can be associated with peptic ulcer as the result of release of the acid secretagogue histamine from the malignant cells.

CONGENITAL DISORDERS OF THE DUODENUM. Disorders such as annular pancreas and congenital bands have been associated with duodenal ulcer and acid hypersecretion. The mechanisms accounting for these associations remain to be established.

"VIRO-PEPTIC" ULCERS. The presence of herpes simplex virus type 1 (HSV-1) has been documented in the mucosa near ulcers in a small proportion of ordinary peptic ulcer patients with normal immunocompetence. Although the studies are intriguing, causality in ulcer pathogenesis has not been established.

STRESS ULCERS. Superficial mucosal damage (petechiae and erosions) is found in most patients hours after major operations or within 24 hours of the onset of major multisystem illness. However, this damage remains silent in the large majority of these patients and rarely results in clinically significant acute bleeding unless complicated by severe coagulopathy. Major bleeding in the setting of severe and prolonged physiologic stress occurs with discrete ulcers rather than from superficial mucosal lesions.

No association has been established between HP and stress ulcers. Several risk factors have been identified and constitute the indications for preventive intervention with antiulcer agents. Mechanical ventilation for more than 5 days and coagulopathy are the clearest predictors of major hemorrhage. Prolonged hospitalizations with hepatic or renal failure, sepsis, and shock are important predictors of stress ulcer risk, especially when complicated by prolonged, multisystem failure. Acute stress ulcers also occur in characteristic clinical settings, such as with extensive third-degree burns ("Curling's ulcers") and after head trauma ("Cushing's ulcers"). The rates of stress ulcer complications have dramatically decreased, for example, from about 30% in serious burn patients 30 years ago to less than 1 to 2% today, reflecting improved overall management (e.g., control of sepsis and respiratory care) and rapid institution of enteral or, when necessary, parenteral nutrition. Patients with stress ulcer–induced gastrointestinal bleeding have greatly increased mortality, in part because of the severity of their underlying disease and superimposed multiorgan failure, which simultaneously increase both mortality and the risk of stress ulcer bleeding.

A great deal of pharmacologic "fire power" and resources have gone into preventing stress ulcers with antacids, sucralfate, H₂-receptor antagonists, and now proton pump inhibitors. In unselected patients in the intensive-care unit, risks are so low that this intervention does not sufficiently improve outcomes to justify routine use. However, preventive therapy is appropriate in high-risk patients or in patients with a history of peptic ulcer or gastrointestinal bleeding when exposed to severe, prolonged physiologic stress. There has been concern over increased rates of nosocomial pneumonia in patients placed on H₂-receptor blockers; the data are conflicting, and the effects are probably modest, at most.

CLINICAL MANIFESTATIONS

ABDOMINAL PAIN. Classically, an ulcer was considered likely when pain was located in the epigastric area, was burning in quality, occurred on an empty stomach 2 to 4 hours after meals and/or at night, was relieved by antacids and/or meals, and tended to wax and wane over months. This pattern has been called "acid dyspepsia" because it occurs when acid is unbuffered by food and is relieved with neutralizing acid or inhibiting acid secretion. It has been assumed that most patients with ulcer disease had epigastric abdominal distress. However, with the availability of upper gastrointestinal endoscopy, it is now recognized that the majority of patients (approximately 70%) with epigastric distress ("dyspepsia") do not have evidence of active ulcer disease; conversely up to 40% of patients with an active ulcer crater deny abdominal pain (Table 126–4). In addition, patients can present with an ulcer-related complication, particularly hemorrhage in chronic NSAID users, without antecedent symptoms. Nevertheless, despite being both insensitive and non-specific, the symptom of epigastric abdominal pain, particularly burning after meals and at night and relieved with food or antacid, suggests the possibility of ulcer disease.

The dissociation between organic pathology and symptoms highlights the marked individual variation in visceral sensitivity. Patients with high visceral sensitivity may have one or more manifestations of functional bowel disease (see Chapter 131): (1) gastroesophageal reflux (including upright and supine reflux and non-cardiac chest pain); (2) "acid" dyspepsia; (3) indigestion or functional dyspepsia (symptoms of indigestion occurring with or shortly after eating and characterized by epigastric fullness and discomfort, belching, bloating, nausea, early satiety, and specific food intolerances); and (4) the irritable bowel syndrome. When visceral sensation is low, organic disease, such as peptic ulcer, may present "silently," even with life-threatening complications. If visceral sensation is high, the presentation may be confounded by the other functional manifestations such as functional bowel disease. For example, about one half of the patients evaluated for peptic ulcer also have symptoms indicative of gastroesophageal reflux, functional dyspepsia, or irritable bowel syndrome, suggesting the presence of an "irritable gut." Somatic hyperalgesia may also be a confounding factor of peptic ulcer. Patients who have undergone surgery for "intractable" ulcer disease have a high recurrence of ulcer-type symptoms in the absence of recurrent ulcer, suggesting

that the symptoms represent other manifestations of visceral hyperalgesia. With the availability of endoscopy to confirm the presence or absence of a crater, antibiotics for curing HP infection, and potent antiulcer therapies to heal virtually all ulcers, symptoms due to an active crater can be separated from symptoms due to other causes, thereby permitting appropriate clinical decisions.

PHYSICAL EXAMINATION. Physical examination is of limited value in patients with uncomplicated ulcer. For epigastric tenderness on deep palpation, the sensitivity, specificity, and positive and negative predictive value are all approximately 50% or less. Furthermore, many patients with non-ulcer diseases also have epigastric tenderness on physical examination (see later). However, in patients with free perforation or ulcer penetration into the pancreas, findings of peritonitis are usually present, whereas in those with gastric retention who have been fasting for a few hours, a succussion splash (produced by auscultating the abdomen while rocking the patient back and forth) suggests retained gastric contents.

DIFFERENTIAL DIAGNOSIS. Epigastric abdominal pain can be caused by a number of processes, including, most frequently, non-ulcer dyspepsia ("visceral hypersensitivity"), gastroesophageal reflux, biliary tract disease, pancreatitis, coronary and/or mesenteric vascular insufficiency, intra-abdominal neoplasms (particularly gastric, pancreatic, and hepatic), functional bowel syndrome, inflammatory bowel disease, and others. Symptoms of indigestion can be associated with gastric dyskinesia (gastroparesis, slow gastric emptying) or with gastric dysesthesia (hypersensitivity to gastric distention or specific foods). Delayed gastric emptying can be secondary to diabetic neuropathy, drugs, or connective tissue diseases, although it is most commonly part of the spectrum of functional bowel disorders.

DIAGNOSIS

ENDOSCOPY VS. RADIOGRAPHY. The diagnosis of ulcer disease can only be suspected based on the history and physical examination. Diagnostic confirmation requires either upper gastrointestinal endoscopy (Color Plate 3B) or barium contrast gastrointestinal radiography. Endoscopy has a greater accuracy for establishing the diagnosis than conventional radiography, but it also has a greater cost and a small risk of untoward events (<1 in 1000 procedures) (see Chapters 121 and 122). In centers with highly skilled radiologists, air-contrast radiography may be as accurate as endoscopy. There is no justification for routinely using one procedure followed by the other, but there are situations when a lesion observed on radiography (e.g., gastric ulcer) requires endoscopic biopsies (see later Color Plate 2E).

Duodenal ulcers are almost never malignant and do not require biopsies or repeat endoscopy to ensure healing. However, ulcerating lesions within the stomach may be due to gastric cancer, and approximately 4% of those that appear to be benign even by endoscopy are in fact malignant; therefore, under almost all circumstances it is imperative to obtain multiple biopsy specimens of gastric ulcers. There is controversy regarding the necessity of repeat endoscopy to ensure complete healing after 8 to 12 weeks of medical treatment. Repeat endoscopy will have a very low yield if the initial endoscopy revealed a benign-appearing ulcer *and* adequate biopsy specimens (4 jumbo or 6–7 regular) were carefully reviewed and found to be negative for malignancy. Repeated endoscopy is also unnecessary in young patients (<40 years old) with an adequately biopsied gastric ulcer in the setting of regular NSAID intake.

IS A PRECISE DIAGNOSIS OF ULCER REQUIRED? One of the major tenets of medicine has been to establish a precise diagnosis and thereby apply the appropriate and specific therapy. This principle has come into question for ulcer disease. Most patients with dyspepsia who undergo endoscopy do not have active ulcer disease but instead have either "non-ulcer dyspepsia" or evidence of esophagitis, gastritis, or duodenitis (see Chapter 131). The American College of Physicians recommended that patients with uncomplicated dyspepsia be empirically treated with a short (4–8 week) course of antiulcer medication and observed to assess their symptomatic response. Further evaluation was recommended only in patients who were unresponsive to this therapeutic trial or whose symptoms recurred after its discontinuation. This approach is preferred in patients younger than age 40 with mild, intermittent symptoms and no ulcer-related complications. The American Gas-

Table 126–4 ■ **DIAGNOSIS OF ULCER DISEASE BY SYMPTOMS ALONE IS IMPRECISE**

SYMPTOM	PREVALENCE (%)		
	Duodenal Ulcer	Gastric Ulcer	Non-Ulcer Dyspepsia
Epigastric pain	~70	~70	~70
Nocturnal pain	50–80	30–45	25–35
Food causes pain relief	20–65	5–50	5–30
Episodic pain	50–60	10–20	30–40
Belching/bloating	30–65	30–70	40–80

Ulcers occur without symptoms (10–40%), and ulcer symptoms occur without ulcer (30–60%).

Modified from Isenberg JI, Walsh JH, Johnson LR: Peptic Ulcer Diseases. AGA Undergraduate Teaching Project—Unit 23. Timonium, MD, Milner-Fenwick, Inc, 1991.

Table 126–5 ■ DIAGNOSTIC TESTS FOR *HELICOBACTER PYLORI*

TEST	SENSITIVITY	SPECIFICITY	COMMENTS
Rapid urease test	89–98%	93–98%	Requires endoscopy
Histology	93–99%	95–99%	Requires endoscopy
Culture	77–92%	97–100%	Requires endoscopy
Serologic tests			
ELISA	88–99%	86–95%	Unsuitable for follow-up
Quick office test	94–96%	88–95%	Inexpensive, rapid
^{14}C- or ^{14}C-urea breath test	90–100%	89–100%	Good for diagnosis and follow-up

ELISA = enzyme-linked immunosorbent assay.
Modified from Walsh JH, Peterson WL: Treatment of *Helicobacter pylori* infection in the management of peptic ulcer disease. N Engl J Med 333:984–991, 1995.

troenterological Association recommends that patients with *uncomplicated* dyspepsia have HP serologic testing and that patients with positive results be treated to eradicate HP. However, in patients requiring NSAIDs on a regular basis or with persistent or systemic symptoms (e.g., anorexia, weight loss, back pain), the diagnosis should be established, preferably by endoscopy. Endoscopy not only permits a firm diagnosis but also provides opportunity for biopsies of the lesion and/or gastric antrum to test for HP.

MEASURING SERUM GASTRIN AND GASTRIC SECRETORY TESTING. Determination of fasting and secretin-stimulated serum gastrin is indicated in patients who have intractable ulcer disease, those who will undergo elective duodenal ulcer surgery, and those in whom a diagnosis of Zollinger-Ellison (gastrinoma) syndrome is a consideration (see Chapter 130). There is a marked overlap in resting and histamine- or gastrin-stimulated gastric acid secretory rates in normal and ulcer patients. Overall, gastric ulcer patients tend to secrete less gastric acid, both basal and stimulated, than do normal subjects; and duodenal ulcer patients have acid secretion that is either elevated or in the high-normal range (>12 mEq/hour). HP-infected duodenal ulcer patients tend to have increased basal and meal-stimulated gastric acid secretion and serum gastrin levels that return toward normal after eradication of HP. Because of the lack of clinical utility of gastric secretory testing, it has become obsolete as a diagnostic tool except in patients with hypergastrinemia or in whom gastrinoma or another cause of acid hypersecretion is considered (see Chapter 130).

DIAGNOSTIC TESTS FOR HP. Because HP produces large amounts of urease, its presence can be determined by breath tests (^{14}C- or ^{13}C-urea), by release of ammonia (NH_3) from gastric mucosal biopsies, or by histologic identification of the microorganism or culture. Because HP induces immunologic responses, it can also be diagnosed by enzyme-linked immunosorbent assay or a rapid serologic test. The urea breath test is the most convenient method to monitor successful HP cure; however, the patient should be off all drugs that suppress HP (antibiotics, bismuth, and proton pump inhibitors) for at least 4 weeks. Even then, the test is only 90% sensitive. Although antibody levels fall after successful cure, serial HP serologies have not been proven to be a reliable way to establish cure. (Table 126–5).

An important initial treatment alternative for patients with new onset or previously undiagnosed dyspepsia is to perform serologic tests for HP. Patients who are HP positive should then be considered for antibiotic therapy to cure HP (see Chapter 127). Although this strategy has not been tested rigorously in clinical trials, several decision analyses support the cost effectiveness of this strategy, and the American Gastroenterological Association has also issued guidelines to support this approach (see Chapter 131).

HP TESTING IN ULCER PATIENTS. The National Institutes of Health Consensus Conference on HP concluded that only those ulcer patients (with duodenal ulcer and/or gastric ulcer) in whom HP has been diagnosed by one of the sensitive and specific tests should be treated to eradicate the microorganism. Such a policy mandates that all ulcer patients undergo HP testing. When it was assumed that more than 90% of duodenal ulcer patients harbored HP, an argument was made for empirically prescribing anti-HP therapy rather than routinely performing HP testing. However, the prevalence of HP in duodenal ulcer in the United States is probably closer to 75%, so that testing for HP is indicated to avoid unnecessary treatment of a substantial number of patients. Approximately 65% of gastric ulcer patients are infected with HP, and NSAIDs are incriminated as causative in most of the remainder. Because

endoscopy is performed in almost all gastric ulcer patients because of the potential for gastric cancer, it is appropriate to determine the HP status at the time of endoscopy. Those who harbor HP, even those with a history of NSAID intake, should be treated to cure HP (see Chapter 127).

HP TESTING IN PATIENTS WITH NON-ULCER DYSPEPSIA. The pathogenesis and management of "non-ulcer dyspepsia" (i.e., is it a single disease or a manifestation of more than one disease?) remains controversial. In general, most studies indicate that eradicating HP in patients with non-ulcer dyspepsia fails to alter dyspeptic symptoms significantly (see Chapter 131). However, there may be a subgroup of patients with chronic dyspeptic symptoms related to HP infection and chronic active gastritis. Therefore, in patients unresponsive to routine treatment for non-ulcer dyspepsia, testing for HP is reasonable.

Agreus L, Talley NJ: Dyspepsia: Current understanding and management. Ann Rev Med 49:475–493, 1998. *A recent review of non-ulcer dyspepsia that deals with the interaction of HP and abdominal pain.*
American Gastroenterological Association: American Gastroenterological Association medical position statement: Evaluation of dyspepsia. Gastroenterology 114:579–581, 1998. *Comprehensive coverage of the guidelines regarding the management of dyspepsia.*
Cook DJ, Guayatt GH, Marshall J, et al: A comparison of sucralfate and ranitidine for the prevention of upper gastrointestinal bleeding in patients requiring mechanical ventilation. N Engl J Med 338:791, 1998. *In this large study, H_2 receptor blockers reduced clinically significant bleeding to a greater extent than sucralfate. The risk of pneumonia was comparable.*
Griffin MR: Epidemiology of nonsteroidal anti-inflammatory drug-associated gastrointestinal injury. Am J Med 104:23S–29S, 1998. *This article assesses the frequency, costs, and risk factors that contribute to NSAID-induced mucosal damage and complications.*
Ofman JJ, Etchason J, Fullerton S, et al: Management strategies for HP-seropositive patients with dyspepsia: Clinical and economic consequences. Ann Intern Med 126:280–291, 1997. *A decision analysis reviewing the role of HP in management of new-onset dyspepsia.*
Peterson WL, Graham DY: HP. *In* Feldman M, Scharschmidt, BF, Sleisenger, MH (eds): Sleisenger & Fordtran's Gastrointestinal Disease, 6th ed. Philadelphia, WB Saunders, 1998, p 604. *Detailed discussion of HP epidemiology, diagnosis, and therapy.*
Raff T, Germann G, Hartmann B: The value of early enteral nutrition in the prophylaxis of stress ulceration in the severely burned patient. Burns 23:313, 1997. *This study demonstrated the benefit of enteral nutrition compared with cimetidine in reducing the incidence of gastrointestinal bleeding.*
Soll AH: Peptic ulcer and its complications. *In* Feldman M, Scharschmidt BF, Sleisenger MH (eds): Sleisenger & Fordtran's Gastrointestinal Disease, 6th ed. Philadelphia, WB Saunders, 1998, p 620. *Detailed reference for peptic ulcer pathogenesis and therapy.*
Terdiman JP, Ostroff JW: Gastrointestinal bleeding in the hospitalized patient: A case-controlled study to assess risk factor, causes, and outcome. Am J Med 104:349, 1998. *This study identifies risk factors for stress ulcer bleeding and provides a good reference list.*

127 PEPTIC ULCER DISEASE: MEDICAL THERAPY

David Y. Graham

Although traditional therapies that neutralize or suppress gastric acid are effective in accelerating ulcer healing, they do not change the natural history of the disease; and ulcers recur soon after ther-

Table 127–1 ■ CLUES SUGGESTIVE OF SPECIFIC CAUSES OF PEPTIC ULCER

	HELICOBACTER PYLORI	NSAIDs	ZOLLINGER-ELLISON SYNDROME
One or more:			
Serology	Positive	Negative	Negative
Urea breath test	Positive	Negative	Negative
Histology	Positive	Negative	Negative
NSAID use			
History	Absent	Positive	Absent
Elevated serum salicylate	Absent	Positive	Absent
Unusual location	Absent	Absent	Present
Severe esophagitis	Absent	Absent	Present
Diarrhea	Absent	Absent	Present

NSAIDs = non-steroidal anti-inflammatory drugs.

apy is discontinued. The current recommendation is to tailor therapy to the cause of the disease.

The two most common causes of peptic ulcer are infection with *Helicobacter pylori* (HP) and use of non-steroidal anti-inflammatory drugs (NSAIDs). HP infection is the more common cause, accounting for more than 75 to 90% of duodenal ulcers and 60 to 90% of gastric ulcers. NSAID use makes up the bulk of the remainder, with pathologic hypersecretory diseases such as the Zollinger-Ellison syndrome (see Chapter 130) and other less common causes accounting for less than 1%. Specific clues may point to one of these causes (Table 127–1).

A variety of methods are available to determine whether an HP infection is present (see Table 126–5). HP infection is generally acquired in childhood; because it is often lifelong, detection of IgG antibodies against HP is often the simplest and least expensive diagnostic method, but tests for IgA or IgM antibodies often provide inaccurate and misleading results. One caveat is that a number of poor tests are commercially available; it is prudent to use only tests that are approved by the U.S. Food and Drug Administration (FDA). Because antibody titers remain elevated long after successful treatment, serologic tests cannot be used to follow the course of treatment for individual patients.

Urea breath tests provide data about active HP infection and are useful not only for diagnosis of the presence of the infection but also for assessing the results of antimicrobial therapy. If an ulcer is diagnosed at endoscopy, biopsy of normal-appearing gastric mucosa will provide definitive proof of HP infection because histologically normal mucosa excludes the infection. Some NSAID users will also have HP infection, and it may be impossible to distinguish which is the cause.

Gastric ulcers still remain a special challenge because 1 to 5% of endoscopically benign gastric ulcers are gastric cancers. Endoscopy still has a major role to play in excluding cancer in gastric ulcer patients and at the same time can assess HP status (Table 127–2).

ULCER THERAPY

The goals of ulcer therapy are to relieve symptoms, to heal the ulcer, and to cure the disease (HP ulcers) and/or prevent recurrence (NSAID ulcers). Treatment should be aimed at curing HP infection, if it is present, or at neutralizing acid with antisecretory agents such as H$_2$-receptor antagonists, anticholinergics, proton pump in-

Table 127–2 ■ FACTORS INFLUENCING THE DECISION FOR EARLY ENDOSCOPY IN GASTRIC ULCER DISEASE

EARLY ENDOSCOPY	DELAYED ENDOSCOPY
Advanced age	Young patient
Long history	Short history
Weight loss	No weight change
Anorexia	Normal appetite
UGI bleeding/anemia	Normal blood cell count
Significant vomiting	No vomiting
No ulcerogenic drugs	NSAID use and positive *Helicobacter pylori* serology
Equivocal UGI series	Unequivocal UGI series

UGI = upper gastrointestinal; NASID = non-steroidal anti-inflammatory drug.

hibitors, or prostaglandins. Antacids and surface active agents such as sucralfate are outmoded as primary therapy for ulcer disease.

Antisecretory Drugs

Antisecretory therapy will accelerate healing of ulcers regardless of cause. The H$_2$-receptor antagonists available in the United States include cimetidine (Tagamet), ranitidine (Zantac), famotidine (Pepcid), and nizatidine (Axid). The main difference is potency, not effectiveness. The clinically equivalent doses when administered with the evening meal are 800 mg of cimetidine, 300 mg of ranitidine or nizatidine, and 20 mg of famotidine. Choice should be based on cost. Cimetidine is associated with prolongation of the metabolism of warfarin, theophylline, and phenytoin, and the dosage of those drugs may have to be adjusted if they are administered with cimetidine.

Proton pump inhibitors omeprazole (Prilosec, 20 to 40 mg/day) and lansoprazole (Prevacid, 30 mg/day) are the most effective antisecretory agents and work by inhibiting the hydrogen-potassium adenosine triphosphatase responsible for acid secretion. The main disadvantage of the acid-pump inhibitors is their high cost.

Misoprostol is the only synthetic prostaglandin available in the United States. It is a relatively weak antisecretory drug; 200 μg of misoprostol is slightly less potent as an antisecretory drug than 300 mg of cimetidine. Misoprostol is not a first-line therapy for treating peptic ulcers. The primary role of misoprostol is to prevent ulcer and ulcer complications in NSAID users.

Antimicrobial Therapy

Helicobacter pylori is a gram-negative spiral bacterium that is sensitive in vitro to a variety of antimicrobial agents. A number of effective regimens are available, and several have been approved by the FDA. The best results have been obtained with combination therapies using three or four drugs (Table 127–3). Antimicrobial agents used in combination therapies include bismuth subsalicylate, ranitidine bismuth citrate, tetracycline, metronidazole, amoxicillin, and clarithromycin. One cannot substitute doxycycline for tetracycline or other macrolides (e.g., erythromycin) for clarithromycin. Tinidazole can substitute for metronidazole. Proton pump inhibitors also have some in vivo anti-HP activity and have a potential benefit over H$_2$-receptor antagonists in that they more effectively control pH and may also have some anti-HP activity. One reason to include antisecretory therapy with the antimicrobial agents is to control pH because many antibiotics become increasingly less effective as the pH falls below 7.4.

Treating the *Helicobacter pylori* Ulcer Patient

The goals are to relieve symptoms, heal the mucosal defect, and cure the disease. Antibiotic therapy should not be prescribed to ulcer patients who do not have an infection because such treatment presents only risks without possible benefits. The steps in the treatment of ulcer patient's HP infection are test, treat, and confirm cure. The widespread availability of non-invasive testing (e.g., serologic or urea breath tests) have made pretreatment testing easy. The minimal duration of antibiotic therapy is unknown. Studies in the US and in Europe have generally shown that 14 days of therapy provide better cure rates than therapies of either 7 or 10 days' duration. The simplest approach for HP-related ulcers is to combine

Table 127–3 ■ ANTIMICROBIAL THERAPIES SUCCESSFUL FOR TREATMENT OF *HELICOBACTER PYLORI* INFECTION

THERAPY	*H. PYLORI* DRUGS			NOTES	SUCCESS
	Drug 1	Drug 2	Drug 3		
Triple (3–4x/d)	Tetracycline, 500 mg qid	Metronidazole, 250 mg tid or qid or amoxicillin 750 mg tid, or clarithromycin, 500 mg tid	Bismuth subsalicylate* 2 tablets qid	With meals for 14 days plus an H₂ blocker	~90%
Quadruple†	Tetracycline, 500 mg qid	Metronidazole, 500 mg tid, or clarithromycin 500 mg tid	Bismuth subsalicylate, 2 tablets qid	With meals for 14 days plus a PPI‡ (bid)	~90%
Triple	Amoxicillin, 500 mg qid	Clarithromycin, 500 mg tid	Bismuth subsalicylate, 2 tablets qid	With meals for 14 days plus an H₂ blocker	~90%
MPpiC Triple	Metronidazole, 500 mg bid	PPI‡ bid	Clarithromycin, 250–500 mg bid	With meals for 14 days	~90%
APpiC Triple	Amoxicillin, 1000 mg bid	PPI‡ bid	Clarithromycin, 500 mg bid	With meals for 14 days	~90%
RBC Triple	RBC,§ 400 mg bid	Clarithromycin or metronidazole, 500 mg bid	Tetracycline, 500 mg bid	With meals for 14 days	~90%
Approved but not recommended	Clarithromycin, 500 mg tid	Omeprazole, 40 mg every A.M.		With meals for 14 days	70–80%
Approved but not recommended	RBC,§ 400 mg bid	Clarithromycin, 500 mg tid		With meals for 14 days, then RBC alone for 14 days	70–80%
Approved but not recommended	PPI‡ bid	Amoxicillin, 1000 mg tid			20–70%

*Bismuth subcitrate can be substituted.
†Possibly also effective with metronidazole resistant *H. pylori.*
‡PPI; lansoprazole and omeprazole can be used interchangeably.
§RBC = ranitidine bismuth citrate.

antisecretory therapy with antimicrobial therapy for 2 weeks. Antisecretory therapy provides rapid relief of pain, accelerates ulcer healing, and, with many drug combinations, improves the cure rate. Antisecretory therapy can then be discontinued unless the patient has a history of prior ulcer complications, in which case H₂-receptor antagonists would be continued until cure of the infection was confirmed.

A number of combination therapies are available that will reliably cure *Helicobacter pylori* infection. Single drug and dual-drug combination therapies are not recommended because they have lower than desired cure rates and failure is associated with development of antibiotic resistance. The major factors reducing effectiveness of therapy are the presence of antibiotic-resistant HP and poor compliance with the regimens. The best therapies combine a bismuth or proton pump inhibitor with two antibiotics.

Confirmation of the Results of Therapy

Evaluation of the results of treatment of the HP infection must be delayed until any remaining bacteria have had an opportunity to repopulate the stomach. It has been determined that reliable results can be obtained 4 or more weeks after ending antimicrobial therapy. Urea breath testing is the preferred test for evaluation of the outcome of therapy unless there is a compelling reason for endoscopy, such as the need to re-evaluate a "suspicious" gastric ulcer or the status of pyloric stenosis. Because proton pump inhibitors inhibit HP growth, they must be discontinued at least 1 week before testing to see whether therapy was successful. H₂-receptor antagonists do not have a detrimental effect on culture, histology, or the ¹³C-urea breath test and can be continued, if necessary, throughout the follow-up period. H₂-receptor antagonists adversely affect the ¹⁴C-urea breath test and must be discontinued if that test is chosen to confirm cure.

Although few disagree that it is important to confirm the presence of infection before institution of antibiotic therapy for peptic ulcer disease, the role of post-therapy testing remains somewhat controversial. The decision about whether to test should be made with the patient's input. The decision not to confirm cure should include discussion of the options, costs, and outcomes of failed therapy. Failure to cure the infection in a patient with peptic ulcer will be associated with return of symptoms, recurrent ulcer disease, continuing risk of development of ulcer complications, and the need for more tests and additional treatment for peptic ulcer; the patient will also remain a reservoir for transmission of the infection to others in the environment, especially family members. If the patient declines post-therapy testing, the discussion should be recorded in the chart to protect the physician if ulcer complications should occur.

Treatment Failure

Failure of therapy to cure the infection is an increasing problem. In general, failure to cure means that the organism was, or has become, resistant to one of the major antibiotics used (e.g., clarithromycin or metronidazole). A drug combination that does not use the suspect drug should be given. For example, if the combination of a proton pump inhibitor, clarithromycin, and amoxicillin failed, the next attempt would avoid clarithromycin. Ideally, pretreatment culture and sensitivity testing would be used to choose the best therapy, but this approach requires biopsy and is rarely available. Salvage therapy, or therapy for patients who have failed more than two attempts, is best handled by referral to a specialized center. Alternately, quadruple therapy with a proton pump inhibitor, tetracycline (500 mg qid), metronidazole (500 mg tid), and bismuth (e.g., bismuth subsalicylate 2 tablets qid) for 14 days can be tried. The rate of success, even in the face of metronidazole resistance, is high.

NSAID ULCERS

The available data suggest that continued NSAID use delays ulcer healing. The approach is therefore to stop the NSAID and use antisecretory therapy to heal the ulcer. Patients who are NSAID users and who are also infected with HP should also receive therapy for HP infection. Many elderly patients with osteoarthritis receive potent NSAIDs when they actually require only analgesia. Stopping the NSAID provides a reverse therapeutic challenge that allows the physician to assess whether the NSAID was actually needed. In many instances, the patient will do just as well using acetaminophen or low doses of less potent over-the-counter NSAIDs such as 200 mg of ibuprofen. For patients with rheumatoid arthritis who require active anti-inflammatory therapy, prednisone (5 to 10 mg/day) can be given without apparently adversely affecting ulcer healing. After ulcer healing, required NSAID therapy can be restarted with concomitant misoprostol or with a proton pump inhibitor. Head to head comparison studies have shown that 600 and 800 µg of misoprostol per day are approximately equal for prevention of NSAID ulcers, and both are superior to 400 µg/day, which in turn is superior to placebo. Omeprazole, 20 mg/day, has also been shown to be equivalent to 400 μg of misoprostol for prevention of ulcer relapse in true NSAID ulcers (i.e., HP negative). There is no evidence to suggest that higher doses of a proton pump inhibitor provide additional benefit. Thus, for the patient who cannot take misoprostol, it is reasonable to prescribe omeprazole, 20 mg, or lansoprazole, 30 mg, as co-therapy with the NSAID.

PREVENTING ULCER RECURRENCE

Curing HP infection cures HP ulcers; maintenance antisecretory therapy is not needed. For patients with resistant infections, antisecretory therapy can be continued at approximately one half of the healing dose to reduce ulcer recurrence and prevent ulcer complications. Patients who have experienced NSAID ulcers and require continuation of NSAID therapy should receive co-therapy with misoprostol, 200 μg two to four times a day, or with a proton pump inhibitor once daily.

SPECIAL SITUATIONS

Patients with a history of ulcer complications such as bleeding have a high probability of having another complication. It is important not to discontinue antisecretory therapy until it has been confirmed that the HP infection has been cured. Very large ulcers, especially those that have recently bled, ulcers after balloon dilatation of gastric outlet obstruction, or ulcers in very old frail individuals with major co-morbid disease are special cases in which proton-pump inhibitors (e.g., omeprazole, 40 to 60 mg/day, or lansoprazole, 60 mg in divided doses) are preferred until ulcer healing occurs.

Graham DY: Editorial: Can therapy ever be denied for HP infection? Gastroenterology 113:S113–S117, 1997. *Review of the data supporting the premise that HP infection has a worse outcome than asymptomatic tuberculosis or syphilis and that therapy is required in almost every instance when the infection is confirmed to be present.*

Graham DY: Nonsteroidal anti-inflammatory drugs, HP, and ulcers: Where we stand. Am J Gastroenterol 91:2080–2086, 1996. *Review of the relationship between NSAID use and peptic ulcer disease.*

Howden CW, Hunt RH: Guidelines for the management of *Helicobacter pylori* infection. Ad Hoc Committee on Practice Parameters of the American College of Gastroenterology. Am J Gastroenterol. 93:2330–2338, 1998. *Excellent review of the approach to treating HP in the United States.*

van der Hulst RWM, Keller JJ, Rauws EA, Tytgat GNJ: Treatment of HP infection in humans: A review of the world literature. Helicobacter 1:6–19, 1996. *Excellent comprehensive review of drug therapies for HP infection.*

128 COMPLICATIONS OF PEPTIC ULCER

David Y. Graham

Patients with ulcer disease are at risk of developing ulcer complications such as bleeding, perforation, or obstruction. The risk for patients who have never suffered a complication is in the range of 1% per year; the likelihood of a complication sometime during the life history of peptic ulcer disease is in the range of 20 to 30%. Once a complication has occurred, the risk of a subsequent complication increases to approximately 1% per month.

INTRACTABILITY

Intractability, which is now defined as failure of an ulcer to heal despite successful treatment of HP infection and adequate antisecretory therapy, is rare and suggests a complicating factor such as Zollinger-Ellison syndrome (see Chapter 130), concomitant, and often covert, non-steroidal anti-inflammatory drug (NSAID) use, or another disease, such as Crohn's disease, masquerading as a peptic ulcer. Evaluation should include a determination of the serum gas-

trin and calcium levels and requestioning about drug use, especially that of over-the-counter medications that contain aspirin. Assessment of gastric secretory function (see Chapter 130) with a gastric analysis may occasionally be necessary to exclude hypersecretory states. This problem is infrequent enough that referral to a gastroenterologist with particular interest in peptic ulcer disease is probably indicated. Ultimately, surgery may be necessary (see Chapter 129).

HEMORRHAGE

For major upper gastrointestinal bleeding (see Chapter 123), the incidence rate is 150 per 100,000 population; the mortality rate remains in the range of 5 to 10%, in part because of bleeding in older and sicker patients. Peptic ulcer disease remains the most common cause of major upper gastrointestinal bleeding; between 15% and 20% of ulcer patients will experience hemorrhage during the course of their disease. Use of NSAIDs has become responsible for an increasingly large percentage of upper gastrointestinal bleeding because of the increasing use of these drugs and the fall in prevalence of HP infection.

Approximately 80% of patients will relate a history of symptomatic ulcer disease before the onset of bleeding, about one third will have suffered a previous hemorrhage, and about 10% of patients will have bled more than once. At presentation, hematemesis, melena, or a combination of both will be evident in more than 95%; 15% will present in shock. Clinical features that suggest a poor outcome are age older than 60 years, hematemesis, the presence of shock, severe bleeding requiring multiple transfusions, and/or the presence of clinically active co-morbid disease (particularly that of cardiovascular, respiratory, hepatic, or malignant origin). Physical examination should assess circulatory status, determine the presence of co-morbid disease, and search for features suggesting the other causes of hemorrhage, such as the presence of chronic liver disease or cutaneous telangiectasia.

MANAGEMENT

The management steps are resuscitation, diagnosis, therapy, and a plan for long-term management (see also Chapter 123). Outcome is best if initial management is in an intensive-care unit and decisions are made by a team experienced in managing gastrointestinal hemorrhage. Resuscitation takes precedence over diagnosis, and one of the first steps for the patient with significant bleeding is to restore the vascular and the oxygen-carrying capacity of the blood. A systolic blood pressure less than 100 mm Hg or pulse greater than 100 beats per minute is suggestive of volume depletion of 20% or more. A positive tilt test (defined as a systolic blood pressure drop more than 10 mm Hg or an increase in pulse rate of more than 20 beats per minute on standing or sitting) suggests an acute blood loss of more than 1 L. An intravenous line should be inserted in all patients, and 0.9% saline should be infused as rapidly as the patient's cardiopulmonary status will allow. Blood should be obtained for a complete blood cell count, assessment of coagulation status, and determination of serum electrolyte, blood urea nitrogen (BUN), and creatinine levels. In most instances, it is also prudent to send blood for typing and crossmatching. Transfusions should generally be given to maintain the hemoglobin at about 10 g/dL; overtransfusion should be avoided. The response of the blood pressure to postural changes will usually provide a reasonably reliable indication of whether the intravascular volume is unstable. The hematocrit is not reliable after acute hemorrhage. The presence of an elevated BUN concentration and a normal serum creatinine value in the presence of melena strongly suggests a significant upper gastrointestinal site of bleeding. The rate of normalization in the BUN is a useful gauge of the effectiveness of volume replacement because correction of the deficit in the vascular volume will result in a rapid return of the BUN to normal. Most clinicians would insert a nasogastric tube to ascertain whether there is fresh blood or clots within the stomach. Lavage of the stomach with ice water is no longer thought to be of value and is not recommended.

Bleeding from a peptic ulcer is usually self-limited; about 5% do not stop bleeding. Rebleeding occurs in 20 to 25%, with 80 to 90% of rebleeding episodes occurring within 48 hours of presentation. After the patient's condition has stabilized, attention can focus on the site of bleeding. Endoscopy provides rapid diagnosis, and endoscopically applied therapy has become the method of choice for initial management of upper gastrointestinal bleeding. All patients with clinical evidence of major bleeding, such as hemodynamic instability, need for transfusions, or decreasing hematocrit should undergo early endoscopy; those with endoscopic evidence of active bleeding, adherent clot, or visible vessel should receive endoscopic therapy. Most would also begin ulcer therapy with an H_2-receptor antagonist administered intravenously by continuous infusion or with oral administration of a proton pump inhibitor. Endoscopy is increasingly being used to triage patients into subgroups who can be sent home, as compared with those who require a regular medical-surgical bed or intensive care.

Management After Bleeding

Patients who have bled should be investigated for HP status and for NSAID use. Maintenance antisecretory therapy will reduce the incidence of subsequent complications and should not be withdrawn until it has been confirmed that the HP infection has been treated successfully. If the patient was receiving NSAIDs and does not have HP infection, such medications should be prohibited in the future, if at all possible. If NSAIDs are required, a newer selective COX2 inhibitor may be tried or the lowest possible dose of a conventional NSAID should be used, and co-therapy with a proton pump inhibitor (e.g., omeprazole, 20 mg/day, or lansoprazole, 30 mg/day, in divided doses) or the synthetic prostaglandin misoprostol (200 μg bid to qid) should be prescribed. H_2-receptor antagonists and sucralfate are ineffective prophylaxis against NSAID-induced bleeding and are not recommended. For cardiovascular indications, newer antiplatelet medications (see Chapter 188) should be substituted for aspirin if possible; if not, the dose of aspirin should be as low as possible, preferably no more than 30 to 50 mg/day.

The recognition that HP peptic ulcer disease can be cured has eliminated gastric surgery as an acceptable first-line therapy. Ulcer surgery for bleeding should be restricted as a second-line form of homeostasis. If an operation is required to control hemorrhage, simple oversewing of the ulcer and, if possible, a highly selective vagotomy is the treatment of choice (see Chapter 129). Gastrectomy should be avoided whenever possible.

Perforation

The incidence of ulcer perforation is 7 to 10 per 100,000 population per year. Perforation is more common in men than in women (4–8:1), although that ratio appears to be changing as the frequency of gastric perforation is increasing in association with NSAID use in elderly women. The most common presentation is an abrupt onset of severe abdominal pain followed rapidly by signs of peritoneal inflammation. The typical patient will appear to be acutely and seriously ill, lying immobile in bed with grunting and shallow respiration. Abdominal tenderness is usually most pronounced in the epigastrium; spasm of the abdominal musculature usually approaches boardlike rigidity. Loss of hepatic dullness, if present, is a valuable clue to the correct diagnosis. The possibility of a perforated viscus should be the differential diagnosis in any patient with unexplained shock.

Leukocytosis appears rapidly. The blood chemistries are usually normal, with the exception of the serum amylase value, which may be slightly increased. The suspected diagnosis can be confirmed by the identification of free intraperitoneal air, which is demonstrable in about 80% of cases and is best seen on erect chest radiograph or a left decubitus film of the abdomen rather than a plain abdominal film. When the diagnosis is suspected and the radiographs are negative, it is worthwhile to repeat the radiographic evaluation after several hours. The diagnosis may be confirmed by an upper gastrointestinal series using Gastrografin, especially if it is combined with computed tomography to enhance the ability to identify the perforation and exclude other pathology.

Initial management is to prepare the patient for presumed surgery (see Chapter 129). The steps include resuscitation by correction of fluid and electrolyte abnormalities, treatment of complications, continuous nasogastric suction, parenteral administration of broad-spectrum antibiotics (ampicillin-sulbactam and gentamicin) and, if a tension pneumoperitoneum is present, needle aspiration of the peritoneal cavity. Nasogastric suction is one of the mainstays of therapy, and it is important to confirm that the aspirating ports of the nasogastric tube are positioned in the most dependent portion of the stomach. A randomized trial comparing non-operative treatment to emergency surgery showed that an initial period of non-operative observation yielded similar outcome, and the decision not to operate immediately could be based on the age and clinical condition of the patient. If there is evidence of increasing peritoneal irritation after 6 hours of treatment, it is best to declare non-operative therapy a failure and to proceed to surgery. Alternatively, surgery may be chosen immediately in any patient in whom there is not good evidence that the perforation has sealed. Simple closure of the perforation and proximal selective gastric vagotomy is the preferred operation.

The long-term plan for a patient who survived a perforation and is ready to be discharged from the hospital depends on whether the patient received a definitive ulcer operation, had simple closure of the perforation, or was managed with conservative medical therapy, as well as whether the perforation was a complication of concomitant NSAID use. HP status should be determined and, if present, the infection should be treated even if the patient received a definitive ulcer operation. Because treatment of HP infection cures peptic ulcer disease, it is likely that it will also prevent the complication from recurring. Recommendations regarding future NSAID and aspirin use are the same as for patients who have survived an ulcer hemorrhage (see earlier).

Obstruction

Approximately 2% of ulcer patients develop gastric outlet obstruction; 90% are caused by previous or coexistent duodenal or channel ulcers. Inflammatory swelling surrounding the ulcer, muscular spasm associated with nearby ulcer, or cicatricial narrowing with fibrosis are the factors responsible for the obstruction. The mainstay of initial resuscitation and therapy is conservative medical management with decompression of the obstructed stomach; correction of fluid, electrolyte, and acid-base abnormalities; plus intravenous H_2-receptor antagonist therapy. Endoscopic balloon dilatation and treatment of HP infection have reduced the need for surgery to relieve obstruction. Resuscitation and antisecretory therapy usually provide rapid relief for most patients in whom the obstruction is functionally related to edema. For those with stricture, endoscopic balloon dilatation of the pylorus combined with anti-secretory therapy (e.g., omeprazole 40 to 60 mg/day) and followed by treatment of the HP infection is usually effective. For patients in whom the stricture rapidly recurs, missed gastric cancer becomes a likely diagnosis, and endoscopic biopsy is required and is often followed by surgery.

Boey J, Wong J: Perforated duodenal ulcers. World J Surg 11:319–324, 1987. *A scoring system has been devised to separate those with essentially no risk from those with a high risk of dying. Those with all three risk factors have a very high risk of dying; it "denotes such a critical state that it is problematic whether any form of early operative intervention will be tolerated, much less beneficial."*

Crofts TJ, Park KGM, Steele RJC, et al: A randomized trial of nonoperative treatment for perforated peptic ulcer. N Engl J Med 970–973, 1989. *A randomized trial of non-operative treatment versus emergency surgery showed that an initial period of non-operative treatment with careful observation yielded similar outcome.*

Howden CW, Hunt RH: Guidelines for the management of *Helicobacter pylori* infection. Ad Hoc Committee on Practice Parameters of the American College of Gastroenterology. Am J Gastroenterol. 93:2330–2338, 1998. *Good review of treatment options and rational therapy for HP-related diseases.*

Laine LA. HP and complicated ulcer disease. Am J Med 100:52S–57S, 1996. *Review of the role of HP in complicated ulcer disease and the data showing that cure of the infection largely eliminates recurrence of complications.*

129 PEPTIC ULCER DISEASE: SURGICAL THERAPY

Haile Debas ▪ *Susan Orloff*

The overall role of surgery in ulcer therapy has declined over the past two decades because of a decrease in the natural incidence of peptic ulcer disease; the advent of effective pharmacologic therapies; the understanding of the central role of *Helicobacter pylori* (HP) in the etiology of peptic ulcer disease; and the dramatic reduction of ulcer recurrence after HP eradication. However, the rate of emergent surgery for complications of peptic ulcer (bleeding and perforation) has not changed. Part of the explanation for this may be that the use of non-steroidal anti-inflammatory drugs (NSAIDs), which are an important and growing cause of peptic ulcer and its complications, has been on the rise (see Chapter 126). Perhaps as a result, the average age of patients with perforation has increased from 40 to 50 years two decades ago to 60 to 70 years now. Thus, many of the gains in ulcer treatment obtained from eradication of HP may have been offset by the greater role of NSAIDs as a cause of ulcer disease.

INDICATIONS

Today elective surgical treatment for peptic ulcer is exceedingly rare. The only indication is intractable ulcer disease despite total eradication of HP and several courses of pharmacologic therapy (see Chapter 128). Indications for emergent or urgent operative intervention are more common and include perforation, bleeding, and gastric outlet obstruction.

A patient clearly needs surgery if there is acute peritonitis due to a perforated peptic ulcer. In the patient with equivocal signs of peritonitis, some have advocated examination of the upper gastrointestinal tract with water-soluble contrast medium followed by conservative management if the studies show that the perforation is sealed. When patients present more than 48 hours after a perforation, non-operative management is indicated provided that the perforation is sealed and the patient is not septic. Otherwise, an operative approach is recommended.

In more than 90% of the patients admitted with bleeding duodenal ulcer, the bleeding stops spontaneously; in some clinical situations, however, emergent surgical intervention is required (Table 129–1). In older patients or patients with more life-threatening bleeding, a surgical consultation should be obtained promptly.

| Perforation |
| Bleeding |
| Exsanguinating hemorrhage |
| Bleeding >6 units of blood |
| "Visible vessel," especially if bleeding |
| Rebleeding on medical therapy or after endoscopic hemostasis |
| Slow, persistent bleeding over days |
| Age older than 65 years |
| Ulcer >2 cm |
| Gastric outlet obstruction unresponsive to medical therapy |

OPERATIVE PROCEDURES

Over the past few decades, gastric resection procedures have rarely been used, and the most appropriate and commonly used procedure is highly selective vagotomy (Fig. 129–1). Truncal vagotomy and pyloroplasty should be reserved for elderly or high-risk patients in whom expediency is desirable. For ulcers that cause gastric outlet obstruction, the most common procedure is vagotomy and antrectomy with gastroduodenal (Billroth I) or gastrojejunal (Billroth II) anastomosis.

LAPAROSCOPIC ULCER SURGERY

A major recent advance in the surgical treatment of peptic ulcer disease is the use of laparoscopic techniques (Table 129–2). This minimally invasive surgery has the advantages of reduced postoperative pain, a shortened hospital stay (1 to 3 days), earlier return to work (7 to 10 days), and avoidance of a large scar.

CHOICE OF OPERATIVE PROCEDURE

Elective surgical therapy is rarely required for peptic ulcer because failure to heal is unusual and because most cases of gastric cancer are diagnosed at the original endoscopy (Fig. 129–2).

Duodenal Ulcer

ELECTIVE SURGERY. The elective procedure of choice for intractable duodenal ulcer is highly selective vagotomy, which has

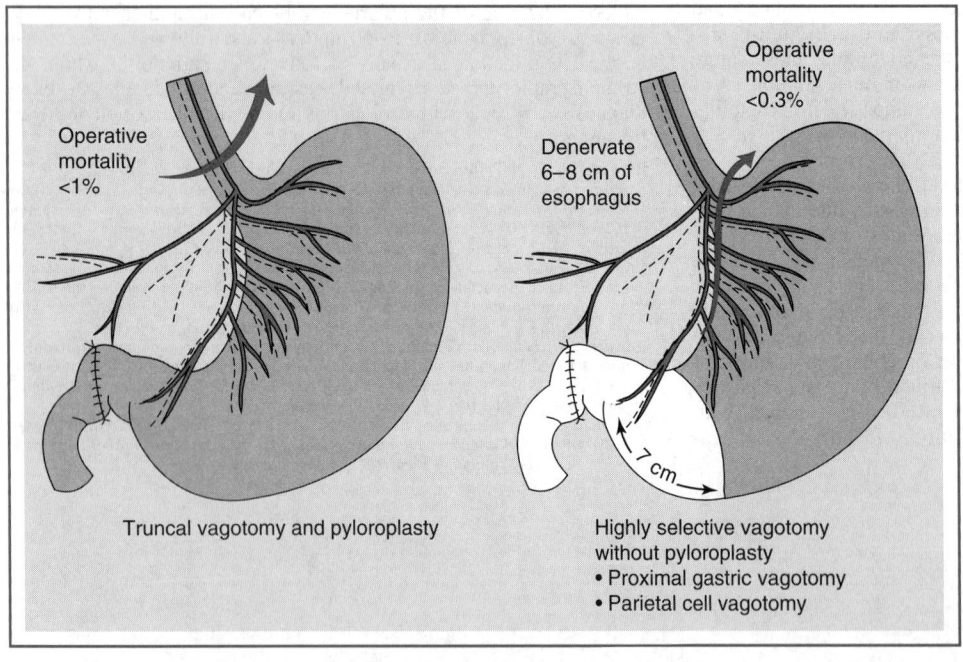

Operative mortality <1%

Truncal vagotomy and pyloroplasty

Operative mortality <0.3%

Denervate 6–8 cm of esophagus

7 cm

Highly selective vagotomy without pyloroplasty
• Proximal gastric vagotomy
• Parietal cell vagotomy

FIGURE 129–1 ▪ Model illustrating the most common surgical procedures used for peptic ulcer disease.

Table 129–2 ■ LAPAROSCOPIC SURGICAL PROCEDURES

PROCEDURE	COMMENTS
Laparoscopic closure of perforated peptic ulcer	Closure, omental patching, peritoneal toilet. Gastric ulcers must be sampled in four quadrants
Laparoscopic suture ligation of bleeding peptic ulcer	Gastric ulcers must be sampled in four quadrants
Posterior truncal vagotomy and anterior highly selective vagotomy or seromyotomy (Taylor II)	Widely used, adequate results
Highly selective vagotomy	Best elective antiulcer procedure, 4–11% recurrence rate

minimal morbidity (1 to 2% dumping and diarrhea), a mortality rate that approaches 0%, and a recurrence rate of 4 to 11%. This procedure may be done either open or laparoscopically, depending on the surgeon's preference and experience. The combination of truncal vagotomy and pyloroplasty, which should rarely be used in the elective setting, is reserved for those elderly or otherwise high-risk patients in whom a shorter operative procedure is advised.

EMERGENT/URGENT SURGERY. PERFORATION. The primary goal of surgery is to close the perforation and prevent continuing peritoneal contamination and infection (Fig. 129–3). Prospective, randomized clinical trials have shown that adding routine highly selective vagotomy is associated with a significant decrease in ulcer recurrence and subsequent need for operation but no increase in morbidity or mortality. However, some authors now advocate patching of the perforation combined with postoperative therapy to eradicate HP rather than an operative procedure to reduce acid.

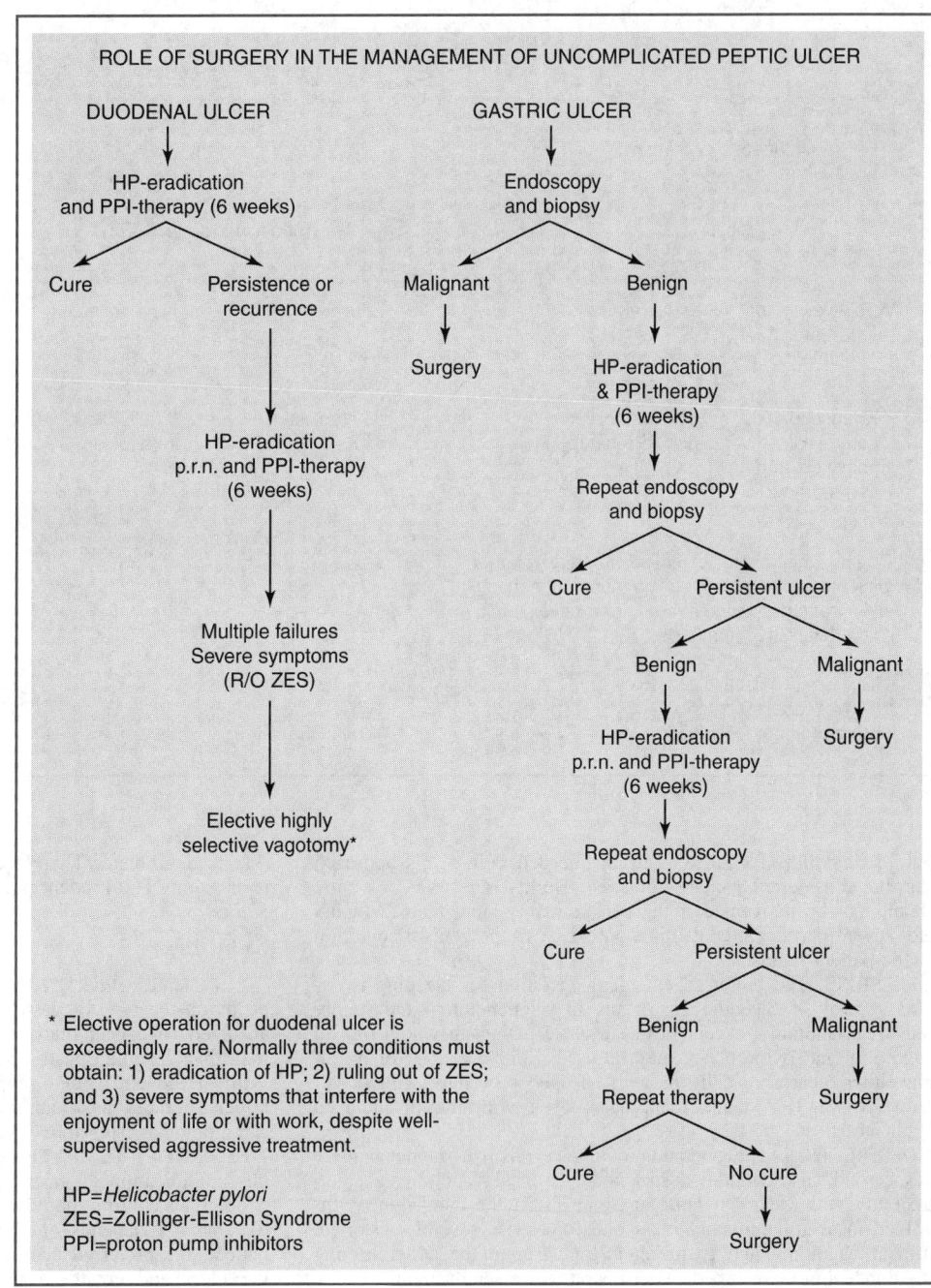

FIGURE 129–2 ■ Role of surgery in the management of uncomplicated ulcer.

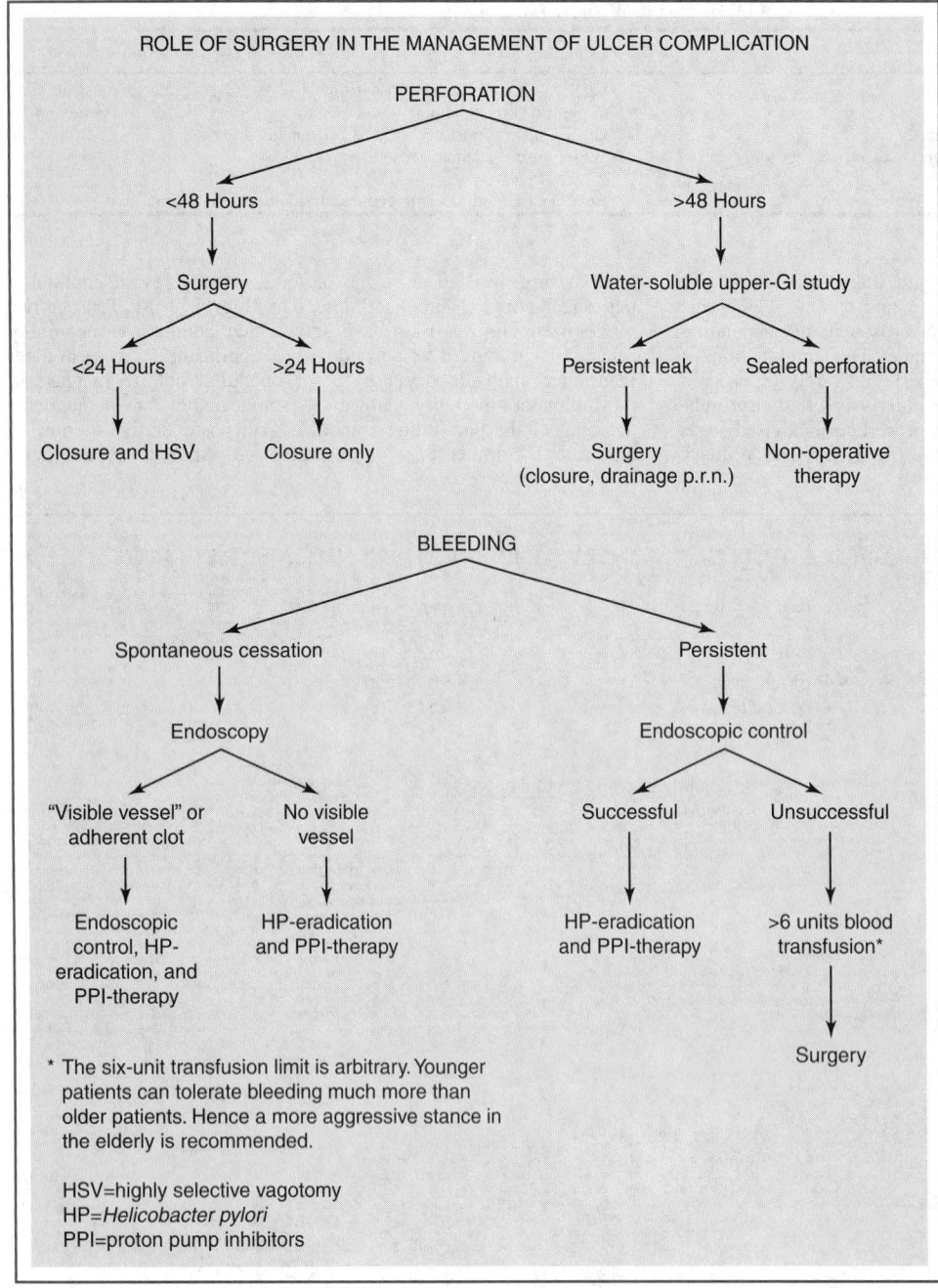

ROLE OF SURGERY IN THE MANAGEMENT OF ULCER COMPLICATION

PERFORATION

<48 Hours → Surgery
- <24 Hours → Closure and HSV
- >24 Hours → Closure only

>48 Hours → Water-soluble upper-GI study
- Persistent leak → Surgery (closure, drainage p.r.n.)
- Sealed perforation → Non-operative therapy

BLEEDING

Spontaneous cessation → Endoscopy
- "Visible vessel" or adherent clot → Endoscopic control, HP-eradication, and PPI-therapy
- No visible vessel → HP-eradication and PPI-therapy

Persistent → Endoscopic control
- Successful → HP-eradication and PPI-therapy
- Unsuccessful → >6 units blood transfusion* → Surgery

* The six-unit transfusion limit is arbitrary. Younger patients can tolerate bleeding much more than older patients. Hence a more aggressive stance in the elderly is recommended.

HSV=highly selective vagotomy
HP=Helicobacter pylori
PPI=proton pump inhibitors

FIGURE 129–3 ■ Role of surgery in the management of ulcer complication.

Future randomized clinical trials are needed before this approach can be considered standard practice. Highly selective vagotomy should not be performed if the perforation is more than 24 hours old, severe peritoneal contamination exists, or the general condition of the patient is unstable.

BLEEDING. The preferred emergent operation for bleeding is suture control of bleeding by means of duodenotomy and highly selective vagotomy, except in the unstable patient in whom truncal vagotomy and pyloroplasty may be used. Simple control of bleeding either laparoscopically or with an open procedure without vagotomy is not a standard approach, even with the potential to eradicate HP.

OBSTRUCTION. The operation of choice when a duodenal ulcer has caused gastric outlet obstruction is truncal vagotomy and antrectomy with gastroduodenal anastomosis. If the duodenum is involved in an inflammatory mass or is otherwise severely distorted, truncal vagotomy and gastrojejunostomy should be done, leaving the duodenum undisturbed. After operation for long-standing gastric outlet obstruction, postoperative delay in gastric emptying presents

a serious problem. Therefore, the addition of a temporary feeding jejunostomy is a prudent practice.

Gastric Ulcer

ELECTIVE OPERATION. The choice of elective operation depends on the type of gastric ulcer (Table 129–3). The problem of an ulcerated cancer masquerading as a benign ulcer is more common than a benign gastric ulcer degenerating into a malignant one. With the advent of endoscopy, fewer patients diagnosed as having a benign ulcer have an ulcerated cancer. In the United States, carcinoma has been found in only 3% of resected gastric ulcers.

EMERGENT OPERATION. BLEEDING. Bleeding is a more serious complication in gastric ulcers than in duodenal ulcers. Initial endoscopic control should be attempted before surgery. The operative therapy depends on the condition of the patient. In a stable patient, the preferred procedure is distal gastrectomy that removes the ulcer and creates a gastroduodenal (Billroth I) anastomosis. Excision of the ulcer combined with a highly selective vagotomy is

Table 129–3 ■ SURGICAL OPTIONS FOR GASTRIC ULCERS

TYPE	LOCATION	INCIDENCE	TREATMENT OF CHOICE	COMMENTS
I	Body (lesser curve)	55–60%	Antrectomy (Billroth I)	Ulcer resected with specimen. Mortality/recurrence rate of 2%. Highly selective vagotomy and ulcer excision is a less optimal approach.
II	In association with duodenal ulcer	20–25%	Vagotomy and antrectomy	Acid reduction and ulcer excision accomplished
III	Prepyloric	20%	Vagotomy and antrectomy	Behaves like duodenal ulcer
IV	High-lying near gastroesophageal junction	<5%	Resection and esophagogastrojejunostomy (Csendes)	More common in South America

another approach, but this procedure is associated with very high recurrence rates in two types of gastric ulcers: those associated with duodenal ulcer and those located in the prepyloric area. In the less stable patient, ulcer excision alone or with vagotomy and pyloroplasty is recommended. If the ulcer cannot be excised, bleeding should be controlled by suture ligation; biopsy may be obtained if deemed safe or it may be postponed to subsequent endoscopy. Laparoscopic techniques have been used for all of the previous approaches and can be considered as dictated by the surgeon's experience and technical ability with laparoscopy. For ulcers in the body of the stomach, some advocate that bleeding be controlled either by the combination of biopsy and oversewing of the ulcer or by excising the ulcer. In either case, the patient then needs postoperative treatment to eradicate HP. The efficacy of this form of therapy has not been substantiated by published reports.

PERFORATION. In the stable patient the preferred and definitive procedure is distal gastrectomy with Billroth I anastomosis. Definitive operation should be avoided if the perforation is older than 24 hours, if the patient is frail or unstable, or if there is severe peritoneal contamination. In these circumstances, a lesser procedure may be considered, such as ulcer excision with vagotomy and pyloroplasty. In extremely ill patients, the ulcer should be sampled in four quadrants and patched with omentum, without the addition of an acid-reducing procedure. Future prospective studies are necessary to determine if this latter approach combined with a postoperative HP eradication regimen can be considered in all patients.

Recurrent Ulcer after Surgery

Before the introduction of H_2-receptor antagonists and proton pump inhibitors, recurrent postoperative ulcer was considered a surgical disease. However, H_2-receptor antagonists and proton pump inhibitors have been shown to be effective in treating recurrent ulcer, particularly after previous vagotomy (Fig. 129–4). With the increased understanding of the role of HP in peptic ulcer disease, indications for surgical treatment of recurrent ulcer have further declined. In recurrent ulcers, the incidence of HP positivity has been reported to range from 5 to 50% (compared with 75 to 90%

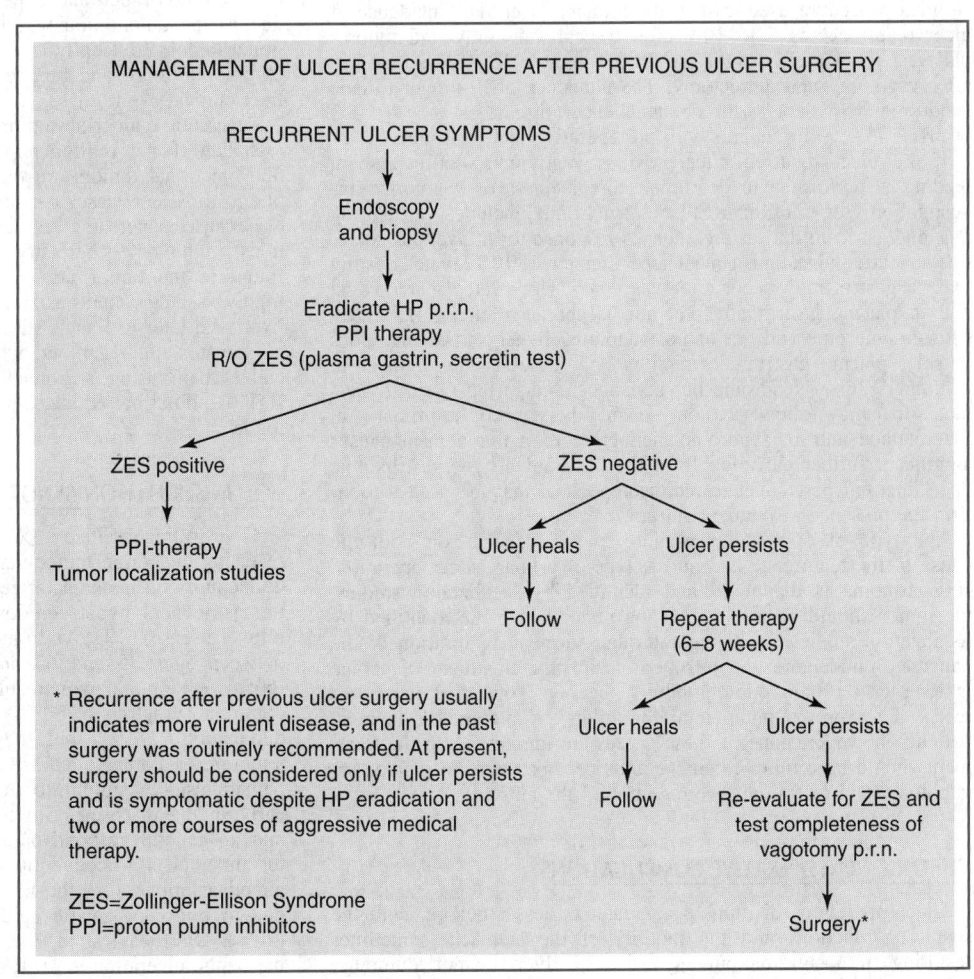

FIGURE 129–4 ■ Management of ulcer recurrence after previous ulcer surgery.

Table 129–4 ▪ CAUSES OF POSTOPERATIVE ULCER RECURRENCE

Persistent *Helicobacter pylori* infection
Inappropriate primary operation
  Highly selective vagotomy for gastric and prepyloric ulcer
Inadequate operation
  Incomplete vagotomy
  Inadequate drainage
  Inadequate resection
  Retained antrum
Hypersecretory states
  Gastrinoma
  Multiple endocrine neoplasia I syndrome
  G-cell hyperplasia
  Hypercalcemia
Ulcerogenic drugs
  Non-steroidal anti-inflammatory drugs
  Steroids
  Reserpine

incidence in primary ulcer disease). In the absence of a surgically treatable cause of the recurrence (retained antrum, gastrinoma), medical therapy should be attempted; surgery should be considered only if medical therapy fails.

The first step in the management of recurrent ulcer is to assess for the presence of HP and, if present, to eradicate it with appropriate therapy. If ulcer recurrence persists despite HP eradication and aggressive therapy with proton pump inhibitors, reoperative intervention may be appropriate.

The clinical presentation of recurrent ulcer includes pain (95%), hemorrhage or anemia due to occult bleeding (20–63%), obstruction (5–19%), and free perforation (1–9%). Endoscopy with multiple biopsies is the most useful method of establishing the diagnosis; the cause of the recurrence must be identified (Table 129–4).

Ulcers recurring after peptic ulcer surgery depend on both the type of the primary ulcer (i.e., duodenal or gastric) and the type of surgical procedure used to treat the primary ulcer. The incidence of ulcer recurrence is 5 to 10% after truncal vagotomy and pyloroplasty, 4 to 11% after highly selective vagotomy, and less than 1% after vagotomy and antrectomy. The incidence of Zollinger-Ellison syndrome in patients with duodenal ulcer disease is only 1:1000 but rises to 1:50 in patients with postoperative recurrent ulcer.

If the ulcer recurred after previous vagotomy, modified sham feeding is performed to determine completeness of vagotomy. Investigation for Zollinger-Ellison syndrome includes measuring plasma gastrin in the fasting state, in response to intravenous secretin, and after ingesting a meal (see Chapter 130). Elevated fasting plasma gastrin may occur after vagotomy. However, a paradoxical rise in plasma gastrin after secretin is characteristic of Zollinger-Ellison syndrome and not of postvagotomy hypergastrinemia. Conversely, plasma gastrin elevation is only modest after a meal in Zollinger-Ellison syndrome but is exaggerated in the G-cell hyperplasia that may follow vagotomy or may very rarely be primary. In the retained antrum syndrome, neither secretin nor a meal causes significant further elevation from the basal level hypergastrinemia. A technetium pertechnetate radioisotope scan may be used to confirm the presence of retained antrum.

The type of operative procedure to use depends on both the cause of the recurrence and on the type of primary ulcer operation. If gastrinoma is diagnosed and identified by localization studies, the tumor should be resected. If the tumor cannot be identified by localization studies, including thorough surgical exploration of the pancreas, duodenum, and retroperitoneum, the treatment of choice is long-term proton pump inhibitor therapy. Total gastrectomy is reserved for proton pump inhibitor failure or intolerance. In most patients, however, none of these causes are identified and the treatment should be a more extensive antiulcer operation, to include revagotomy and resection or re-resection of the antrum.

CHRONIC POSTOPERATIVE COMPLICATIONS

Ulcer operations disrupt, to a greater or lesser degree, both the secretory functions and the motility of the stomach, sometimes resulting in postgastrectomy syndromes, which include dumping, diarrhea, alkaline reflux gastritis, and maldigestion. All these complications are associated with truncal vagotomy and/or gastric resection. Highly selective vagotomy, which is the elective operation of choice, avoids these complications.

Casas AT, Gadacz TR: Laparoscopic management of peptic ulcer disease. Surg Clin North Am 76:515, 1996. *A complete review of the rationale and development of vagotomy for peptic ulcer disease and the role and outcomes of laparoscopic techniques in the treatment of peptic ulcer disease.*
Druart ML, Van Hee R, Etienne J, et al: Laparoscopic repair of perforated duodenal ulcer: A prospective multicenter clinical trial. Surg Endosc 11:1017–1020, 1997. *A clinical trial of laparoscopic repair of perforated peptic ulcer demonstrates that the procedure is technically feasible and carries an acceptable morbidity and mortality rate compared with conventional surgery.*
Lau JYW, Sung JJY, Lam Y, et al: Endoscopic retreatment compared with surgery in patients with recurrent bleeding after initial endoscopic control of bleeding ulcers. N Engl J Med 340:751–756, 1999. *Endoscopic retreatment was preferred.*

130 PANCREATIC ENDOCRINE TUMORS

Robert T. Jensen

Pancreatic endocrine tumors, also called islet tumors or islet cell tumors, can also occur outside the pancreas. The eight pancreatic endocrine tumors (Table 130–1) are classified as APUDomas (*a*mine *p*recursor *u*ptake and *d*ecarboxylation), sharing cytochemical features with carcinoid tumors, melanomas, and a number of other endocrine tumors (pheochromocytomas, medullary thyroid cancer). Except for insulinomas, each is frequently malignant. All appear similar histologically, with chromogranin immunoreactivity.

Pancreatic endocrine tumors frequently are classified as functional or non-functional depending on whether a clinical syndrome due to the autonomously released hormone is present. Non-functional tumors frequently release pancreatic polypeptide, neurotensin, chromogranin A, and breakdown products, but these cause no distinct clinical syndromes.

Pancreatic endocrine tumors are uncommon, with a prevalence of less than 10 per million population. Insulinomas, gastrinomas, and non-functional tumors are the most common, with an incidence of one to three new cases per million population.

Because pancreatic endocrine tumors synthesize multiple peptides, immunocytochemistry alone cannot establish which peptides found in the tumor are clinically important. The tumors are all highly vascular, metastasizing first to regional lymph nodes, then to liver, and later to bone. All except insulinomas have a high density of somatostatin receptors, which are now increasingly used to localize them using radionuclide detection after injection of [111]In-[DTPA-DPhe[1]]octreotide, a synthetic radiolabeled somatostatin analogue.

ZOLLINGER-ELLISON SYNDROME (GASTRINOMAS)

The Zollinger-Ellison (ZE) syndrome is caused by a gastrin-releasing endocrine tumor that is usually located in the pancreas or duodenum and is characterized by clinical symptoms and signs due to gastric acid hypersecretion (ulcer disease, diarrhea, esophageal reflux disease). ZE syndrome occurs most frequently in persons between ages 35 and 65 and is slightly more common in men (60%). Abdominal pain resulting from a peptic ulcer is the most common symptom (>80%). The majority of ulcers occur in the duodenum (>85%), but they can occur in the postbulbar area, jejunum, or stomach and are occasionally in multiple locations. The pain is usually similar to that of typical peptic ulcers, especially early in the disease. With time, the symptoms become persistent and, in general, respond poorly to conventional doses of H_2-receptor antagonists, to conventional surgical treatments, or to treatments aimed at eliminating the bacterium *Helicobacter pylori*. Heartburn due to reflux of gastric acid into the esophagus is also common (20%). Diarrhea (60 to 70%) occurs frequently and may precede the peptic ulceration in 10 to 20% of patients.

Table 130-1 ■ PANCREATIC ENDOCRINE TUMORS

NAME OF TUMOR	NAME OF SYNDROME	MAIN SIGNS OR SYMPTOMS	LOCATION (%)	MALIGNANCY (%)	HORMONE CAUSING SYNDROME
Gastrinoma	Zollinger-Ellison syndrome	Abdominal pain Diarrhea Esophageal symptoms	Pancreas (30%) Duodenum (60%) Other (10%)	60–90	Gastrin
Insulinoma	Insulinoma	Hypoglycemic symptoms	Pancreas (100%)	5–15	Insulin
Glucagonoma	Glucagonoma	Dermatitis Diabetes/glucose intolerance Weight loss	Pancreas (100%)	60	Glucagon
VIPoma	Verner-Morrison Pancreatic cholera WDHA	Severe watery diarrhea Hypokalemia	Pancreas (90%) Other (10%) (neural, adrenal, periganglionic tissue)	80	Vasoactive intestinal peptide (VIP)
Somatostatinoma	Somatostatinoma	Diabetes mellitus Cholelithiasis Diarrhea	Pancreas (56%) Duodenum/jejunum (44%)	60	Somatostatin
GRFoma	GRFoma	Acromegaly	Pancreas (30%) Lung (54%) Jejunum (7%) Other (13%) (adrenal, foregut, retroperitoneum)	30	Growth hormone–releasing factor
ACTHoma	ACTHoma	Cushing's syndrome	Pancreas (4–16% all ectopic Cushing's)	>95	Adrenocorticotropic hormone (ACTH)
Nonfunctioning	PPoma Nonfunctional	Weight loss Abdominal mass Hepatomegaly	Pancreas (100%)	60–90	None (pancreatic polypeptide or chromogranin released but no known symptoms due to hypersecretion)

WDHA is the acronym for *watery diarrhea, hypokalemia and achlorhydria.*

Twenty to 25 per cent of patients have ZE syndrome as part of the multiple endocrine neoplasia type 1 (MEN-1) syndrome, an autosomal dominant inherited disease. These patients have hyperplasia or tumors of multiple endocrine glands, most commonly parathyroid hyperplasia (>90%), pituitary tumors (60%), and pancreatic endocrine tumors (80%). Patients typically first develop renal stones due to hypercalcemia from hyperparathyroidism or have elevated prolactin levels due to pituitary tumors and only later develop the ZE syndrome.

PATHOLOGY AND PATHOPHYSIOLOGY. In older studies, gastrinomas were found primarily in the pancreas, but in recent large surgical series, they were found more frequently in the duodenum. Duodenal gastrinomas are generally smaller (<1 cm) than pancreatic gastrinomas. Occasionally, the ZE syndrome is due to a gastrinoma in the splenic hilum, mesentery, stomach, heart, or only in a lymph node or to a gastrin-releasing tumor of the ovary. Approximately one third of patients have metastatic liver disease at presentation, but less than 20% of the remainder will develop metastatic disease to the liver during a 10-year follow-up period. As with other pancreatic endocrine tumors, malignancy can be reliably determined only by presence of metastatic disease because no light microscopic or ultrastructural finding can clearly establish malignant behavior. Up to 5% of patients with ZE syndrome develop Cushing's syndrome due to ACTH secretion by the gastrinoma.

Gastrin stimulates parietal cells to secrete acid and also has a growth effect (trophic) on cells of the gastric mucosa, leading to increased gastric mucosal thickness, prominent gastric folds, and increased numbers of parietal cells and gastric enterochromaffin-like cells. Almost all of the symptoms are due to the effects of gastric acid hypersecretion, but late in the disease cachexia, weight loss, and pain can be due to the extensive tumor metastasis. In contrast to patients with routine peptic ulcers (see Chapter 126), *H. pylori* appears not to be important. Diarrhea is due to the large volume of gastric acid output, leading to small intestinal structural damage (inflammation, blunted villi, edema), interference with fat transport, inactivation of pancreatic lipase, and precipitation of bile acids. These same mechanisms, if prolonged, can lead to steatorrhea. If acid hypersecretion is controlled either medically, surgically, or with nasogastric suction, the diarrhea will stop at once.

DIAGNOSIS AND DIFFERENTIAL DIAGNOSIS. The ZE syndrome may be suspected because of peptic ulcer disease that is recurrent; is non-healing despite treatment; is not associated with *H. pylori* infection; is complicated by bleeding; causes obstruction

or esophageal stricture; is multiple or in unusual locations; or is associated with a pancreatic tumor or diarrhea. It should also be suspected in patients with chronic watery diarrhea, especially in patients with hypercalcemia, or in patients with large gastric folds on radiography or endoscopy. The initial measurement is a fasting serum gastrin level, which is elevated in 99 to 100% of patients with ZE syndrome. However, other causes of hypergastrinemia include a physiologic response to achlorhydria or hypochlorhydria because of pernicious anemia, atrophic gastritis, renal failure, *H. pylori* infection, or use of the H+, K+-ATPase inhibitors (omeprazole, lansoprazole), which suppress acid for up to 1 week after discontinuation. If the serum gastrin level is elevated, the fasting gastric pH should be determined. If the serum gastrin level is greater than 1000 pg/mL (normal, <100) and the pH is less than 2.5, then the patient almost certainly has ZE syndrome.

A secretin stimulation test can exclude *H. pylori* infection, retained gastric antrum syndrome, antral G cell hyperfunction/hyperplasia, chronic renal failure, and gastric outlet obstruction that may mimic ZE syndrome. Normal individuals show an increase in serum gastrin level to less than 200 pg/mL after intravenous secretin, whereas 87% of patients with ZE syndrome and a fasting gastrin value less than 10-fold above normal have a positive test. No false-positive results have been reported except in patients with achlorhydria. In all patients with the ZE syndrome, evaluation must exclude hyperparathyroidism and pituitary adenomas.

TREATMENT. Therapy is directed at controlling both the gastric acid hypersecretion and the gastrinoma itself. H₂-receptor antagonists are effective, but frequent dosing (every 4 to 6 hours) and high doses are needed. H+, K+-ATPase inhibitors, either omeprazole or lansoprazole (starting at 60 mg/day), are now the drugs of choice. Because of their long duration of action, acid hypersecretion can be controlled in all patients with once- or twice-a-day dosing. In 30% of patients, higher doses are needed, particularly in patients with MEN-1, previous gastric surgery, or a history of severe esophageal reflux. Patients must be treated indefinitely unless they are surgically cured. Long-term therapy appears safe, with patients treated with omeprazole for up to 9 years without loss of efficacy but with decreasing vitamin B₁₂ levels after prolonged treatment. Total gastrectomy is now performed only for patients who cannot or will not take oral antisecretory medications. Selective vagotomy effectively reduces acid secretion, but many patients continue to require a low dose of drug. Parathyroidectomy should be performed in patients with hyperparathyroidism, ZE syndrome, and MEN-1 because it markedly reduces acid secretion and increases the sensitivity to antisecretory drugs.

All patients should have imaging studies to localize the tumor. Somatostatin receptor scintigraphy (SRS) using single-photon emission computed tomography after injection of ^{111}In-[DTPA-DPhe^1]octreotide is the localization method of choice. SRS will identify 60% of primary gastrinomas and more than 90% of patients with metastatic disease in the liver and is equal in sensitivity to all conventional imaging studies combined. For pancreatic gastrinomas, endoscopic ultrasound is particularly sensitive. Small duodenal gastrinomas (<1 cm) are frequently not detected by any imaging modality but can be found at surgery if routine duodenotomy is performed.

Tumors can be identified in 95% of patients. Surgical exploration for cure is now recommended in all patients without liver metastases, MEN-1, or complicating medical conditions limiting life expectancy. Surgical resection decreases the metastatic rate and results in a 5-year cure rate of 30%. Patients with metastatic gastrinoma in the liver have a poor prognosis with a 5-year survival rate of 30%. If the metastatic disease is increasing in size or is symptomatic, chemotherapeutic agents (streptozotocin, 5-fluorouracil, doxorubicin) are usually the first treatment. Treatment with interferon alfa or octreotide is reported to be effective in a small percentage of patients if chemotherapy fails. Liver transplantation is occasionally used in the rare patient with metastases limited to the liver.

GLUCAGONOMAS

Glucagonomas are endocrine tumors of the pancreas that ectopically secrete glucagon, which causes a clinical syndrome whose cardinal features are a distinct dermatitis (necrolytic migratory erythema) (70–90%), diabetes mellitus or glucose intolerance (40–90%), weight loss (70–96%), anemia (30–85%), hypoaminoacidemia (80–90%), thromboembolism (10–25%), diarrhea (15–30%), and psychiatric disturbances (0–20%). The characteristic rash is usually found at intertriginous and periorificial sites, especially in the groin and buttocks. It is initially erythematous and becomes raised with central bullae that erode and become crusty. Healing occurs with hyperpigmentation.

PATHOLOGY AND PATHOPHYSIOLOGY. Glucagonomas are generally large when discovered (mean size, 5–10 cm), most frequently in the pancreatic tail (>50%); liver metastases are usually present at diagnosis (45–80%). Excess glucagon explains the glucose intolerance. The etiology of the rash is unclear, but it may be related to zinc deficiency in some patients. The hypoaminoacidemia is thought secondary to the effect of glucagon on amino acid metabolism by altering gluconeogenesis.

DIAGNOSIS AND DIFFERENTIAL DIAGNOSIS. The diagnosis is established by demonstrating elevation of plasma glucagon levels. Normal levels are 150 to 200 pg/mL; in patients with glucagonomas, levels usually (>90%) are more than 1000 pg/mL. However, in some recent studies up to 40% of patients had plasma glucagon values of 500 to 1000 pg/mL. Increased plasma glucagon levels are reported in renal insufficiency, acute pancreatitis, hypercortisolism, hepatic diseases, severe stress (trauma, exercise, diabetic ketoacidosis), prolonged fasting, and familial hyperglucagonemia. In these conditions the level does not usually exceed 500 pg/mL except in patients with hepatic diseases such as cirrhosis or familial hyperglucagonemia.

TREATMENT. Subcutaneous administration of the synthetic long-acting somatostatin analogue octreotide controls the rash in 80% of patients and improves weight loss, diarrhea, and hypoaminoacidemia but usually does not improve the diabetes mellitus. Zinc supplementation or infusion of amino acids can diminish the severity of the rash. After tumor localization, surgical resection is preferred, and even debulking the tumor may be of benefit. For residual disease, chemotherapy with dacarbazine or streptozotocin and doxorubicin, hepatic embolization, or chemoembolization may help control symptoms.

VIPOMAS

The VIPoma syndrome (also called the Verner-Morrison syndrome, pancreatic cholera, and WDHA syndrome [for *watery diar-*rhea, *h*ypokalemia, *a*chlorhydria]) is due to an endocrine tumor, usually in the pancreas, that ectopically secretes vasoactive intestinal peptide (VIP). The cardinal clinical feature is severe, large-volume, watery diarrhea (>1 L/day) (100%), which is secretory and occurs during fasting. Hypokalemia (80–100%) and dehydration (83%) commonly occur because of the volume of the diarrhea. Achlorhydria was originally reported, but hypochlorhydria is more usually found (54–76%). Flushing occurs in 20% of patients, hyperglycemia in 25 to 50%, and hypercalcemia in 25 to 50%. Steatorrhea is uncommon (16%) despite the volume of diarrhea.

PATHOLOGY AND PATHOPHYSIOLOGY. VIPomas in adults are in the pancreas in 80 to 90% of cases, with rare cases due to intestinal carcinoids, ganglioneuromas, ganglioneuroblastomas, or pheochromocytomas. VIPomas are usually large and solitary; 50 to 75% occur in the pancreatic tail and 40 to 70% have metastasized at diagnosis. VIPomas frequently secrete both VIP and peptide histidine methionine, but VIP is responsible for the symptoms. VIP is a potent stimulant of secretion in both the small and large intestine, and this action is responsible for the cardinal features of the syndrome. VIP also relaxes gastrointestinal smooth muscle, and this often causes dilated loops of bowel as well as a dilated, atonic gallbladder. Hypochlorhydria is thought to be due to the inhibitory effect of VIP on acid secretion; flushing is due to the vasodilatory effects of VIP; and hyperglycemia is due to the glycogenolytic effect of VIP. The mechanism of the hypercalcemia remains unclear.

DIAGNOSIS AND DIFFERENTIAL DIAGNOSIS. Because the diarrhea of VIPomas characteristically persists during fasting and is large in volume (>3 L/day, 70–80%), the diagnosis is excluded when fasting stool volume is less than 700 mL/day. To differentiate VIPomas from other causes of large-volume, fasting diarrhea, fasting plasma VIP levels should be determined. The normal value in most laboratories is less than 190 pg/mL, and elevated levels are present in 90 to 100% of patients in various series. The differential diagnosis of large-volume, fasting diarrhea (>700 mL/day) includes the ZE syndrome, diffuse islet-cell hyperplasia, surreptitious use of laxatives, the pseudopancreatic cholera syndrome, and, rarely, human immunodeficiency virus infections.

TREATMENT. The symptoms of the VIP can be controlled in more than 85% of patients by octreotide, but increased doses may be required over time. Tumor localization studies with somatostatin receptor scintigraphy and surgical resection are preferred if possible; chemotherapy with streptozotocin and doxorubicin, hepatic chemoembolization, or hepatic embolization may benefit patients with unresectable or residual tumor.

SOMATOSTATINOMAS

Somatostatinomas are endocrine tumors in the pancreas or upper small intestine that ectopically secrete somatostatin, which causes a distinct clinical syndrome of diabetes mellitus, gallbladder disease, diarrhea, steatorrhea, and weight loss. These symptoms occur three to four times more commonly (80–95% of all cases) in patients with pancreatic than in patients with intestinal somatostatinomas. Duodenal somatostatinomas are frequently reported in patients with von Recklinghausen's disease and are usually asymptomatic. Although these von Recklinghausen tumors are commonly called somatostatinomas because of the immunocytochemical finding of somatostatin in the tumor, the plasma somatostatin level is not usually elevated, and they are not clinical somatostatinomas.

PATHOLOGY AND PATHOPHYSIOLOGY. Sixty per cent of somatostatinomas occur in the pancreas and 40% occur in the duodenum/jejunum. Pancreatic somatostatinomas occur in the pancreatic head in 60 to 80% of cases, 70 to 92% have metastasized at diagnosis, and they are usually large (mean, 5 cm), solitary tumors. In contrast, duodenal somatostatinomas are smaller (mean, 2.4 cm), are frequently associated with psammoma bodies on histologic examination, and less frequently have metastases at diagnosis (30–40%). Duodenal somatostatinomas without von Recklinghausen's disease have elevated plasma somatostatin levels in 70% of cases. In the gastrointestinal tract, somatostatin inhibits basal and stimulated gastric acid secretion, pancreatic secretion, intestinal absorption of amino acids, gallbladder contractility, and release of numerous hormones, including cholecystokinin and gastrin.

DIAGNOSIS AND DIFFERENTIAL DIAGNOSIS. Somatostatinomas are usually found by accident, particularly at exploratory laparotomy for cholecystectomy, during endoscopy, or on imaging studies. The diagnosis requires the demonstration of increased plasma and tumor concentrations of somatostatin-like immunoreactivity, which is also found with endocrine tumors outside the pancreas or intestine, including small cell lung cancer, medullary thyroid carcinoma, pheochromocytomas, and paraganglioma.

TREATMENT. Treatment is difficult, and octreotide is of little benefit. Somatostatinomas can be imaged using somatostatin receptor scintigraphy or, if needed, other conventional imaging studies to assess tumor location and extent. Surgery, if possible, or chemotherapy, hepatic chemoembolization, or hepatic embolization may be of value.

GRFOMAS

GRFomas are endocrine tumors that frequently originate in the pancreas but also occur in other extrapancreatic locations and ectopically release growth hormone-releasing factor (GRF), which causes acromegaly that is clinically indistinguishable from that due to a pituitary adenoma. GRFomas are an uncommon cause of acromegaly, occurring in none of 177 unselected patients with acromegaly in one study. The intra-abdominal features of GRFoma are due to its metastases and are typical of any malignant pancreatic endocrine tumor.

PATHOLOGY AND PATHOPHYSIOLOGY. GRFomas most commonly occur in the lung (54%), with most of the remainder occurring in the gastrointestinal tract, including 30% in the pancreas. Pancreatic GRFomas are usually large (mean, 6 cm), 39% are metastatic at diagnosis, 40% occur in combination with the ZE syndrome, and 33% occur in patients with MEN-1.

DIAGNOSIS AND DIFFERENTIAL DIAGNOSIS. Any patient with acromegaly with abdominal complaints, acromegaly without a pituitary tumor, or acromegaly with hyperprolactinemia (which occurs in 70% of persons with GRFomas) should be suspected of having a GRFoma. The diagnosis is confirmed by performing a plasma assay for GRF and growth hormone.

TREATMENT. The effects of the GRF can be controlled with octreotide in more than 90% of patients. Treatment should be directed at the GRFoma per se, as described earlier for the pancreatic endocrine tumors.

NON-FUNCTIONAL PANCREATIC ENDOCRINE TUMORS

Non-functional pancreatic endocrine tumors originate in the pancreas and either secrete no peptides or their secreted products do not cause clinical symptoms. The symptoms and signs are due to the tumor per se and include abdominal pain, hepatosplenomegaly, cachexia, and jaundice. In 20% of asymptomatic patients, tumors are found incidentally at surgery.

PATHOLOGY AND PATHOPHYSIOLOGY. More than 60% of the tumors have metastasized to the liver at presentation. Most are large (70% > 5 cm), and 70% occur in the pancreatic head. Frequently secreted, non-functional peptides include chromogranin A (100%), chromogranin B (100%), pancreatic polypeptide (60%), and the α-subunit (40%) and β-subunit of human chorionic gonadotropin. Immunocytochemically, the tumors contain these peptides as well as insulin (50%), glucagon (30%), and somatostatin (13%).

DIAGNOSIS AND DIFFERENTIAL DIAGNOSIS. Non-functional pancreatic endocrine tumors are frequently diagnosed only late in the disease course after the patient presents with symptoms or signs of metastatic disease, and a liver biopsy reveals a metastatic neuroendocrine tumor. Any patients with a long survival (>5 years) after a diagnosis of metastatic pancreatic adenocarcinoma should be suspected of having a non-functional pancreatic endocrine tumor. An elevated plasma chromogranin A or pancreatic polypeptide level or positive somatostatin receptor scintigraphy are strong evidence that a pancreatic mass is a pancreatic endocrine tumor.

TREATMENT. Tumor localization, surgical resection, and chemotherapy with streptozotocin and doxorubicin, hepatic embolization, or chemoembolization are useful, as described earlier.

ACTHOMAS AND OTHER UNCOMMON PANCREATIC ENDOCRINE TUMORS

Pancreatic endocrine tumors ectopically secreting adrenocorticotropic hormone (ACTH) explain 4 to 16% of cases with ectopic

Cushing's syndrome. Cushing's syndrome occurs in 5% of cases of the ZE syndrome and invariably reflects metastatic disease to the liver. Occasional cases benefit from the use of octreotide, but prognosis is poor even with chemotherapy.

Paraneoplastic hypercalcemia can result from a pancreatic endocrine tumor that releases parathormone-related peptide or an unknown hypercalcemic substance. Tumors are generally large and metastatic to the liver at diagnosis. Octreotide may help control the hypercalcemia, but surgery, chemotherapy, hepatic embolization, or chemoembolization are the mainstays of therapy.

Jensen RT: Gastrin-producing tumors. Cancer Treat Res 89:293–334, 1997. *Summary of recent advances in gastrinoma with emphasis on the tumor biology.*

Jensen RT, Norton JA: Endocrine neoplasms of the pancreas. *In* Yamada T, Alpers DH, Owyang C, et al (eds): Textbook of Gastroenterology, 3rd ed. Philadelphia, Lippincott Williams & Wilkins, 1999. *A general chapter covering all aspects of pancreatic endocrine tumors.*

O'Shea D, Bloom SR (guest eds): Gastrointestinal endocrine tumours. Bailliere's Clinical Gastroenterology 10:571–766, 1996. *Covers recent advances of the pathology and surgical and medical management of all pancreatic endocrine tumors with individual sections on VIPomas, insulinomas, glucagonomas, gastrinomas, and carcinoids.*

131 FUNCTIONAL GASTROINTESTINAL DISORDERS: IRRITABLE BOWEL SYNDROME, NON-ULCER DYSPEPSIA, AND NON-CARDIAC CHEST PAIN

Nicholas J. Talley

In clinical practice, the majority of patients who present with chronic or recurrent gastrointestinal symptoms do not have a structural or biochemical explanation identified by routine diagnostic tests. These patients are labeled as having a functional gastrointestinal disorder. Functional does not imply a psychiatric disturbance or absence of disease but rather a known or suspected underlying disorder of gut function. Based on clinical and epidemiologic studies, the functional gastrointestinal disorders have been classified according to the presumed anatomic site of the disorder (Table 131–1). The most widely recognized functional gastrointestinal disorders are the irritable bowel syndrome, functional (or non-ulcer) dyspepsia, and functional (or non-cardiac) chest pain.

IRRITABLE BOWEL SYNDROME

DEFINITION. In the past, most patients with unexplained abdominal pain or bowel dysfunction were labeled as having irritable bowel syndrome, but irritable bowel syndrome is now considered to be characterized by chronic or recurrent abdominal pain and an erratic disturbance of defecation. Bloating is also common.

EPIDEMIOLOGY. Symptoms consistent with irritable bowel syndrome are reported by one in six Americans, and similar prevalence rates have been found in Europe, Australia, and Asia. The prevalence is greater in women but is similar in whites and blacks; it is lower in people older than age 60 years. Approximately 30% of persons with irritable bowel syndrome become asymptomatic over time.

Only about one third of persons with irritable bowel syndrome consult a physician, but the condition still accounts for about 12% of primary care visits. The first presentation is typically between the ages of 30 and 50 years. Those who seek care for irritable bowel syndrome tend to have more severe abdominal pain, a greater frequency and severity of non-gastrointestinal symptoms, such as headache, fatigue, or menstrual pain, and greater psychological distress.

PATHOGENESIS. Accumulating evidence suggests that irritable

Table 131–1 ■ ROME CLASSIFICATION OF FUNCTIONAL GASTROINTESTINAL DISORDERS AND ESTIMATED PREVALENCE IN THE UNITED STATES*

DISORDER	APPROXIMATE U.S. PREVALENCE (%)
Functional bowel disorders	
Irritable bowel syndrome	15
Abdominal pain or discomfort, relieved with defecation or associated with a change in the frequency or consistency of stools, and	
An irregular pattern of defecation (at least 25% of the time) consisting of two or more of the following: altered stool frequency, altered stool form, mucus, bloating, or feeling of distention	
Functional abdominal bloating	30
Functional constipation	<5
Functional diarrhea	<5
Functional gastroduodenal disorders	
Functional (non-ulcer) dyspepsia	15*
Chronic or recurrent pain or discomfort centered in the upper abdomen (i.e., epigastrium)	
Endoscopy fails to identify a definite structural cause	
Aerophagia	20
Functional esophageal disorders	
Non-cardiac chest pain	15
Rumination syndrome	10
Globus	10
Functional abdominal pain	<5
Functional biliary pain (biliary dyskinesia)	<1
Functional anorectal disorders	
Functional incontinence	5
Functional anorectal pain	
Levator syndrome	5
Proctalgia fugax	10
Pelvic floor dyssynergia	10

*Assumes one third with dyspepsia have a structural explanation and are excluded.

bowel syndrome represents a true disorder of function. The symptoms are neither imagined nor the result of a psychiatric disorder.

ABNORMAL MOTOR FUNCTION. Irritable bowel syndrome is associated with a generalized disorder of smooth muscle function; the colon, small bowel, and upper gastrointestinal tract as well as the gallbladder and urinary tract may be affected. Basal colonic motility is normal in irritable bowel syndrome, but these patients tend to have an abnormally responsive colon to meals, drugs, gut hormones (e.g., cholecystokinin), and stress. The motility of the distal colon after meals (the gastrocolonic response) is augmented in patients with irritable bowel syndrome and may explain why postprandial cramps or discomfort is common. Increased fasting colonic contractions and rapid colonic transit in the proximal colon has been linked to diarrhea, whereas a reduction of high-amplitude propagated contractions in the left colon has been linked to constipation (see Chapter 132).

Abdominal pain in irritable bowel syndrome has been associated with an exaggerated ileal response with high postprandial pressure waves (prolonged propagated contractions). Fasting clusters of jejunal pressure waves (discrete clustered contractions) occur in some patients with irritable bowel syndrome, appear to coincide with abdominal pain, and disappear during sleep.

DISTURBED SENSATION. The vagal (and spinal) afferent nerves conduct sensory information from the gut through the dorsal horn neurons to the brain. Abnormal perception of gut sensation (visceral hypersensitivity) is a characteristic finding in irritable bowel syndrome. In response to rectal or colonic distention by a balloon, a subset of patients with irritable bowel syndrome will sense the distention at lower volumes and/or pressures than healthy persons. Many patients complain of unsatisfactory defecation or incomplete rectal emptying, which may be a direct result of excess rectal sensitivity. Moreover, repetitive rapid sigmoid distentions induce rectal hypersensitivity in patients with irritable bowel syndrome but not in healthy controls. The mechanisms that lead to increased gut visceral sensitivity are unclear, and patients with irritable bowel

syndrome do not have generalized lower pain thresholds in other parts of their bodies.

CENTRAL NERVOUS SYSTEM. The brain modulates gut sensory and motor function, and vice versa. Normal subjects activate the anterior cingulate gyrus (the part of the limbic system that may help reduce sensory input) in response to rectal distention, but patients with irritable bowel syndrome do not. Such abnormalities may help to explain why patients with irritable bowel syndrome have visceral hypersensitivity.

A high proportion of patients with a diagnosis of irritable bowel syndrome in tertiary referral centers (40–60%) have coexisting psychiatric disease, including depression or panic disorder, or a history of sexual or physical abuse. However, patients seen by primary care physicians and those with irritable bowel syndrome who do not seek medical help have a lower prevalence of psychiatric comorbidity. Stressful life events, personality, level of social support, and childhood experiences influence how a patient responds to a chronic illness such as irritable bowel syndrome.

INFECTION. Approximately 20% of patients with irritable bowel syndrome identify a history of traveler's diarrhea or gastroenteritis (e.g., *Salmonella*) preceding the onset of symptoms. Prospective studies of patients who develop gastroenteritis suggest that up to a fourth will continue to have chronic bowel symptoms and one in eight will develop irritable bowel syndrome. *Candida* does not cause irritable bowel syndrome.

DIET. True food allergy appears to be very rare, but food intolerance may be more important. Lactase deficiency may coexist with irritable bowel syndrome, and lactose intolerance may exacerbate symptoms. Excess ingestion of sorbitol or fructose may induce diarrhea and bloating. Short-chain fatty acids may stimulate prolonged propagated contractions in the ileum. Dietary exclusion has resulted in symptomatic improvement in approximately 50% of patients with functional diarrhea (in whom pain is not a prominent feature), but a response is probably less frequent in diarrhea-predominant irritable bowel syndrome. No single food group has been implicated, although foods high in amines and salicylates may be most important.

CLINICAL FEATURES. Chronic or recurrent abdominal pain is always a feature of irritable bowel syndrome. The pain commonly occurs in the lower abdomen but may occur at any location and tends to be somewhat variable in quality, severity, and duration. Classically, the pain is cramplike or aching and occurs in episodes. The pain of irritable bowel syndrome is relieved by defecation or is associated with a change in stool frequency or consistency. Pain from irritable bowel syndrome rarely awakens the patient from sleep. Pain related to exercise, urination, or menstruation is unlikely to be due to irritable bowel syndrome. Chronic unremitting pain for more than 6 months unrelated to defecation is never due to irritable bowel syndrome but most often represents a chronic pain syndrome (functional abdominal pain).

An irregular disturbance of defecation (predominant constipation or diarrhea, or an alternating bowel pattern) is also a key feature of irritable bowel syndrome and its absence excludes the diagnosis. Constipation may refer to a decreased frequency of stools, passage of hard stools or lumps, excessive straining, or an inability to empty the rectum adequately. Diarrhea may mean loose or watery stools, an increased stool frequency, the passage of mucus, urgency, or even fecal incontinence.

Bloating is a common symptom in the irritable bowel syndrome. Typically, there is visible abdominal distention so patients can see that their abdomen is distended or feel that they have to loosen their clothes. Sometimes, women complain that they look pregnant.

Symptoms of gastroesophageal reflux (heartburn or acid regurgitation) are reported by up to one third of patients with irritable bowel syndrome. Up to one third of patients also report dyspepsia (epigastric pain or discomfort). Nausea, usually without vomiting, is a common complaint. Some patients will report difficulty swallowing, but the complaint is most often the sensation of a lump in the throat between meals (globus). Urinary frequency, dysuria, nocturia, and urinary urgency may occur, as may dyspareunia and dysmenorrhea. Fatigue, headache, and back pain are also common. However, none of these extraintestinal symptoms is helpful diagnostically.

Transient bowel symptoms should not be confused with irritable bowel syndrome. Patients who have recently had to rest in bed, had a surgical procedure, or lost weight may become constipated. Similarly, patients who have been under acute stress may develop "nervous diarrhea." Pregnancy, various dietary indiscretions, traveler's diarrhea, food poisoning, and viral or bacterial gastroenteritis may all cause temporary bowel disturbances.

Physical examination is useful to exclude organic disease. Patients with irritable bowel syndrome may have abdominal scars due to their higher rates of cholecystectomy, appendectomy, and hysterectomy, in part because of a failure to recognize the condition. Abdominal tenderness is a common and a non-specific finding; localized abdominal tenderness that persists after tensing the abdominal wall muscles (e.g., by asking the patient to do a half sit up) usually indicates abdominal wall pain (e.g., from nerve entrapment, muscle strain, or myositis), which should not be confused with functional gastrointestinal pain and typically responds to infiltration with a local anesthetic and/or steroid.

DIAGNOSIS. It is important to make a positive clinical diagnosis of irritable bowel syndrome by careful history and physical examination. Investigations should be undertaken selectively to exclude important diseases that may be confused with irritable bowel syndrome (Fig. 131–1); exhaustive testing before making irritable bowel syndrome the diagnosis of exclusion should be discouraged. Flexible sigmoidoscopy is needed to exclude ulcerative colitis. Biopsy specimens may be obtained in patients with predominant

diarrhea to exclude collagenous or microscopic colitis, but the yield is very low and unlikely to be cost effective. In patients older than 50 years of age with new-onset symptoms, either a colonoscopy or a double-contrast barium enema with flexible sigmoidoscopy is indicated. Weight loss, bleeding, anemia, steatorrhea, fever, vomiting, or a family history of colon cancer require appropriate investigation.

The yield from laboratory tests is low in the presence of typical symptoms. A thyroid-stimulating hormone level should be measured if there is any suspicion of hyperthyroidism (diarrhea) or hypothyroidism (constipation). Lactose intolerance causes diarrhea and bloating and is common in certain racial groups (e.g., blacks, Asians, Native Americans, or persons of Jewish descent); a substantial amount of lactose usually needs to be ingested to induce symptoms. A resolution of symptoms with a 2-week trial of a lactose-free diet suggests clinically relevant lactase deficiency; the diagnosis can be confirmed with a lactose hydrogen breath test.

If severe pain is predominant, a plain abdominal radiograph is indicated during an acute episode to exclude bowel obstruction or other pathologic process. Gynecologic examination may detect

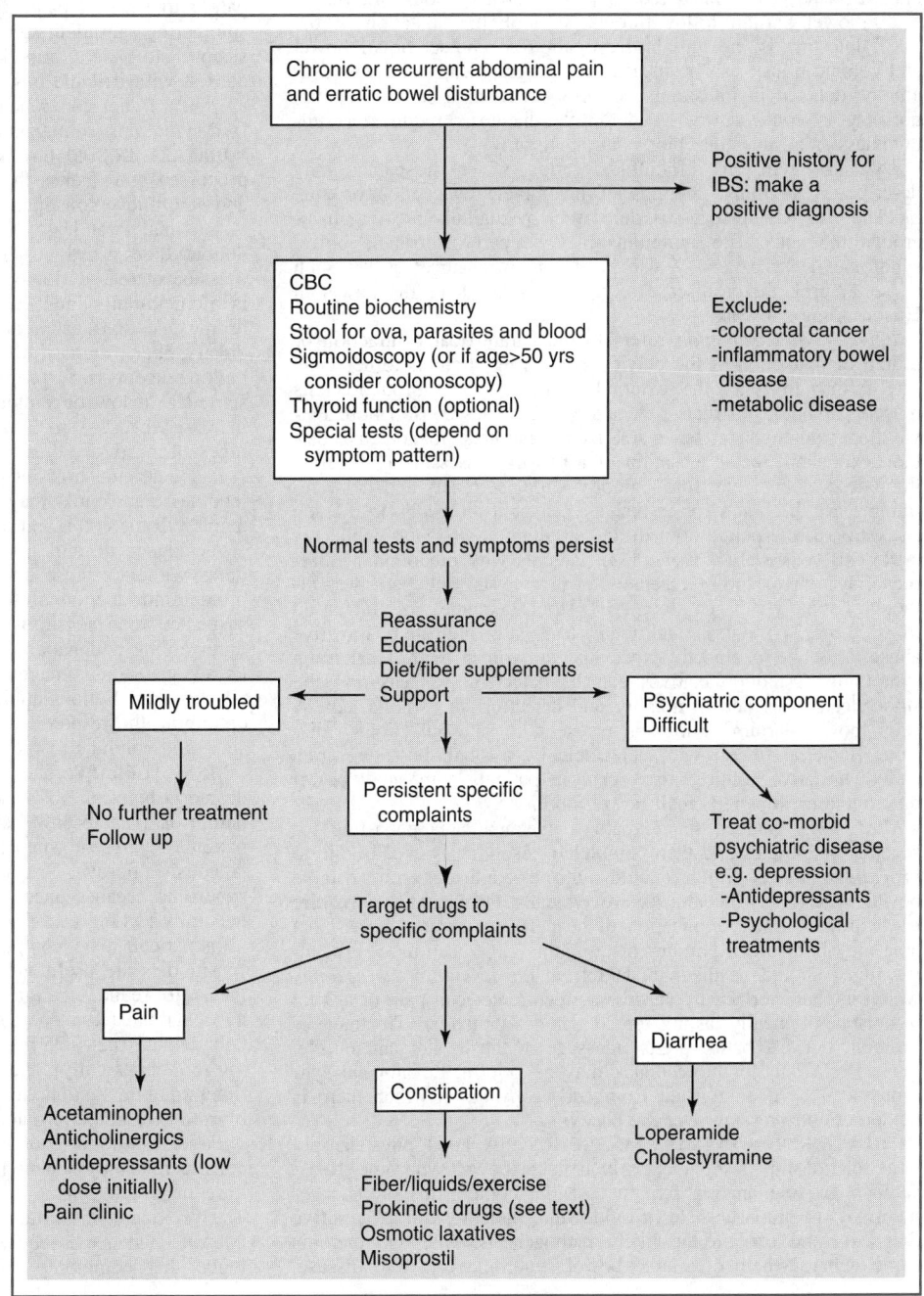

FIGURE 131–1 ■ Algorithm for the evaluation of suspected irritable bowel syndrome (IBS). ESR = erythrocyte sedimentation rate.

evidence of diseases such as endometriosis or fibroids. Endometriosis classically causes mid–menstrual cycle pain that can be associated with disturbed defecation; pelvic ultrasonography is a helpful screening test, but laparoscopy is often required. Pelvic inflammatory disease should be considered if a vaginal discharge is present.

Once a firm diagnosis has been made, subsequent testing has an extremely low yield and should not be undertaken unless symptoms have changed.

DIFFERENTIAL DIAGNOSIS. CONSTIPATION (see also Chapter 132). *Colonic inertia* is characterized by the passage of stools once a week or less and may be diagnosed by a radiopaque marker study, such as having the patient ingest 24 radiopaque markers on three separate days and obtaining a single plain abdominal radiograph on the fourth day. By counting the number of markers retained, total colonic transit can be calculated by multiplying by 1.2. A total colonic transit time greater than 72 hours is grossly abnormal and suggests colonic inertia.

Patients with *chronic idiopathic intestinal pseudo-obstruction* typically present with recurrent abdominal pain, visible distention, vomiting, and either constipation (because of colonic and/or small bowel inertia) or diarrhea (because of bacterial overgrowth). This diagnosis must be considered in patients with colonic inertia. A small bowel barium follow-through to look for dilatation of the small intestine is the initial investigation of choice. Small bowel and colonic transit can be measured scintigraphically and will usually be delayed in intestinal pseudo-obstruction. Small bowel manometry is confirmatory. A definitive diagnosis requires a full-thickness small intestinal biopsy at laparotomy.

Dyschezia refers to difficult defecation, which the patient may describe as straining, feelings of incomplete evacuation or anal blockage, or having to assist defecation by digitally pressing in or around the anus. The symptoms may be part of irritable bowel syndrome. Dyschezia may also be due to mechanical causes such as rectal prolapse or disease (e.g., aganglionosis of the bowel in Hirschsprung's disease).

Pelvic floor dysfunction refers to the paradoxical contraction or failure of relaxation of the pelvic floor during attempts to defecate. The failure to relax the external anal sphincter or puborectalis muscle, or both, obstructs defecation and causes constipation. Pelvic floor function can be evaluated by anorectal manometry, balloon expulsion, rectal sensation of a balloon, assessment of pelvic floor descent, and electromyography. Stool softeners and habit retraining are the first steps in management, but biofeedback to teach relaxation of the pelvic floor during straining is also worthwhile.

DIARRHEA (see also Chapter 133). Patients with predominant diarrhea must have stools screened for ova, cysts, and parasites, although the yield is low. If stool volume is increased (> 400 mL/24 hours), additional tests are indicated. Laxative abuse must be excluded, especially in women with recalcitrant symptoms. Osmotic laxatives can be detected by measuring the stool electrolytes and osmolality and detecting an osmotic gap. A small bowel barium radiograph is useful to rule out Crohn's disease. Bacterial overgrowth, detectable by a small bowel aspirate and quantitative culture, may occur in patients with small bowel diverticula or impaired small bowel motility.

ANAL PAIN. Sudden severe pain in the anal area persisting for seconds or minutes and then completely resolving is usually due to *proctalgia fugax,* which should not be confused with irritable bowel syndrome. The attacks are typically infrequent and require no treatment. Local application of heat or pressure to the perianal area may be of help. Nitrates or quinidine have been used. Proctalgia fugax should be distinguished from the *levator ani syndrome,* which is characterized by chronic or recurrent rectal pain or aching in episodes typically lasting for 20 minutes or longer. Treatment is difficult, but sitz baths, digital massage of the levator ani muscle, muscle relaxants, or biofeedback may be helpful. Levator ani syndrome can be distinguished from *coccygodynia,* in which there is tenderness on pressing over the coccyx.

TREATMENT. GENERAL MANAGEMENT. A good physician-patient relationship is therapeutic in irritable bowel syndrome. Reassurance and explanation remain essential components of management. It is important to provide the patient with a positive diagnosis and explain the likely pathogenesis. Although there is some debate whether irritable bowel syndrome is a real disease,

most clinicians accept that it is and patients should be so advised. It is important to tell the patient that the symptoms are real. Patients need to be advised that irritable bowel syndrome is not life threatening and does not cause cancer. Although symptoms may be life long, they tend to come and go, sometimes with prolonged remissions. Physicians who order an extensive battery of tests without explanation and then tell their patients that they do not believe there is a serious underlying disease are likely to engender confusion and bewilderment.

A change in medications may improve symptoms, and unnecessary drugs should be avoided. Constipation may be aggravated by anticholinergics, opiates, psychotropics, aluminium-containing antacids, bile-acid binding resins, calcium channel blockers, or nonsteroidal anti-inflammatory drugs. Diarrhea may be exacerbated by magnesium-containing antacids, sorbitol-containing cough syrups, antibiotics, and laxatives. Heavy alcohol use and caffeine or decaffeinated products may precipitate symptoms. Those who drink excess diet drinks or chew gum may ingest enough sorbitol to induce symptoms. Reduction of stress may be helpful.

Fear of serious disease or coexistent psychiatric disease frequently precipitates the decision to seek medical attention and must be identified and addressed. Panic disorder is characterized by abrupt discrete episodes of extreme fear or apprehension associated with other symptoms that may include abdominal pain, nausea, palpitations, chest pain, dyspnea, dizziness, flushing, a choking or smothering sensation, sweating, and fainting. Depression may cause sleep disturbances, mood alterations, and weight loss, and may coexist with irritable bowel syndrome. If gastrointestinal symptoms are but a minor component in patients with a multitude of generalized symptoms, somatization disorder should be considered.

DIETARY RECOMMENDATIONS. Increasing dietary fiber with unprocessed bran makes the stools bulkier, softer, and easier to pass and can relieve constipation. Urgency may also improve. The effect is maximal if at least 30 g of fiber is taken daily, approximately double the normal American dietary fiber intake. Fiber content must be increased slowly to reduce the bloating and flatulence that is often initially induced. Some patients with irritable bowel syndrome and diarrhea or abdominal pain also improve on increased dietary fiber, whereas others may get worse. Many patients prefer a bulking agent (e.g., psyllium fiber supplement), which should be started at a low once-daily dose of approximately 5 g and slowly increased every 1 to 2 weeks until a total of 15 to 20 g is being ingested in divided doses two to three times per day.

Fad diets and high-fat diets should be avoided. Cabbage, beans, legumes, and lentils may be worth avoiding because they are fermented in the colon and may increase flatus.

Avoidance of milk products may be helpful even in some patients without lactose intolerance. An elimination diet and double-blind reintroduction of foods may be undertaken in patients with suspected food sensitivity and diarrhea, but this approach is often unrewarding and patient compliance is poor. Regular exercise and an adequate fluid intake is important in patients with predominant constipation. Follow up in 3 to 6 weeks allows the physician to determine the response to initial therapy, reassess psychosocial issues, and continue to support the patient.

DRUG THERAPY. The placebo response in irritable bowel syndrome is between 40% and 70%, in part because of the fluctuating nature of irritable bowel syndrome symptoms, and the tendency for patients to present when their symptoms are worse and then spontaneously improve. Drugs must be used sparingly in irritable bowel syndrome because unequivocal evidence of benefit over placebo is generally lacking (see Fig. 131–1).

In patients who complain of postprandial abdominal pain, antispasmodics are useful when administered 30 to 60 minutes before meals to reduce the gastrocolonic response. Alternatives include hyoscyamine (e.g., one to two timed-release capsules twice daily), belladonna (0.2–0.75 mL four times daily), dicyclomine (20–40 mg four times daily), and propantheline bromide (7.5 or 15 mg four times daily). Anticholinergic side effects including dry mouth, blurred vision, and urinary retention may require dose reduction.

Patients who do not respond to dietary fiber for treatment of constipation may benefit from lactulose or milk of magnesium, the dose of which can be titrated depending on the clinical response. The prokinetic cisapride (10 mg four times daily) may also help, but the evidence is equivocal. Misoprostil, the prostaglandin analogue that commonly induces diarrhea, is empirically useful in severe cases. Metoclopramide and domperidone are not useful in constipation. Stimulant laxatives such as phenolphthalein, bisacodyl, senna, and docusate should be avoided because of potential harmful effects such as water and electrolyte loss and, theoretically, long-term damage to the colonic myenteric plexus.

The pharmacologic agent of choice for predominant diarrhea is loperamide at a dose of 2 to 4 mg three to four times per day. Loperamide slows intestinal transit and increases intestinal water absorption; it should be taken to prevent diarrhea and not after the event. A bile acid–sequestering agent such as cholestyramine (4 g four times daily) may be helpful, particularly in post-cholecystectomy patients with refractory diarrhea caused by idiopathic bile acid malabsorption. Patients who have fecal incontinence may respond to loperamide or biofeedback treatment depending on the underlying cause.

Simethicone is not helpful for bloating. Activated charcoal can reduce flatus after a lactulose challenge in normal persons, but whether it is of benefit in irritable bowel syndrome is not established. α-D-Galactosidase may be helpful in some patients after a vegetable meal. Prokinetics such as cisapride may reduce postprandial bloating. Treatment of constipation may also reduce bloating.

Some patients will fail to respond to any approach. Shotgun testing should be avoided, while the physician emphasizes positive, realistic goals with brief, regular visits to provide key psychosocial support. Such patients should be encouraged to join a local irritable bowel syndrome support group.

The majority of patients with functional gastrointestinal complaints do not wish to see a psychiatrist. If referral to a mental health professional is contemplated, patients should be reassured that this is part of a team approach to promote patient motivation. Relaxation therapy, hypnosis, cognitive behavioral therapy, and short-term psychotherapy appear to be of value particularly in patients with moderate symptoms who are motivated and who can identify a link between emotional difficulties or stressful events and their symptoms. Diarrhea and abdominal pain generally respond better than abdominal distention or constipation. Conversely, patients with chronic, constant pain for many years and patients who are resistant to the idea that psychological factors are related to their illness are unlikely to respond.

Tricyclic antidepressants are particularly useful in resistant patients or patients with chronic pain because of their anticholinergic effects and/or central modulation of sensation. Benefits may occur within 3 to 4 weeks even in patients without symptoms of depression. Tricyclic antidepressants should be started at a low dose in the evening (e.g., amitriptyline, desipramine, or imipramine— 10 or 25 mg). If this dose fails, the dose can be slowly titrated upward, although the drugs may worsen constipation. Amitriptyline causes a high incidence of anticholinergic side effects, whereas desipramine causes fewer anticholinergic problems. Although there is less experience with selective serotonin reuptake inhibitors (e.g., fluoxetine, paroxetine, sertraline) in irritable bowel syndrome, these drugs may be useful when begun once daily in the morning; side effects are less than with tricyclic antidepressants but include nausea, diarrhea, and weight loss. If antidepressant therapy is successful, it should usually be continued for 3 to 12 months and then the dose should be tapered.

Anxiolytics may induce a rebound effect on withdrawal, are potentially habituating, and interact with other drugs and alcohol; they should be avoided in most patients. Leuprolide acetate, a gonadotropin-releasing hormone analogue, initially appeared to improve symptoms in women with severe functional gastrointestinal complaints, but in clinical practice the drug has been disappointing.

PROGNOSIS. Once a positive diagnosis of irritable bowel syndrome has been made, it is rarely altered later. The majority of patients continue to be intermittently symptomatic. The life expectancy of patients with irritable bowel syndrome is no different than that of the background population.

FUNCTIONAL (NON-ULCER) DYSPEPSIA

DEFINITION. Dyspepsia refers to persistent or recurrent epigastric pain or subjective upper abdominal discomfort that may be characterized by early satiety, postprandial fullness, or bloating. Heartburn is distinct from dyspepsia. Dyspepsia is not restricted to meal-related symptoms because patients with peptic ulcer disease

will often report pain unrelated to meals. With the widespread availability and use of endoscopy, it has become evident that a structural explanation is found in a minority of persons with new-onset dyspepsia, and most patients have functional (or non-ulcer) dyspepsia (see Table 131–1).

EPIDEMIOLOGY. Population-based studies from around the world indicate that the prevalence of dyspepsia is about 25%. In the United States, however, only one in four persons suffering from dyspepsia seeks medical care.

PATHOGENESIS. MUCOSAL INFLAMMATION AND *HELICOBACTER PYLORI*. *H. pylori* infection is the most common cause of histologic gastritis in humans and is causally linked to peptic ulcer disease and gastric cancer (see Chapters 136 and 138). Symptoms in patients with functional dyspepsia are indistinguishable from the symptoms encountered in patients with peptic ulcer disease. *H. pylori* gastritis is found in 30 to 60% of patients with functional dyspepsia but is also common in totally asymptomatic subjects in the general population, so a link between *H. pylori* and functional dyspepsia is not established, although it may be important in a small subgroup of patients.

GASTRIC ACID. Basal and peak acid output is normal in patients with functional dyspepsia, but acid secretion in response to gastrin-releasing peptide may be significantly higher in *H. pylori*–positive patients with functional dyspepsia. Overall, up to 50% of infected patients with functional dyspepsia may have a similar disturbance of stimulated acid secretion as observed in duodenal ulcer. Whether the mucosa is more sensitive to acid in patients with functional dyspepsia is unknown.

DISTURBED MOTOR FUNCTION. Up to 50% of patients seen at tertiary referral centers with functional dyspepsia have delayed gastric emptying for solids, and a similar number have antral hypomotility after meals. The prevalence of gastric motility disturbances in patients with functional dyspepsia seen in primary care is unknown but may be lower. Reflux of bile into the stomach is not more frequent in functional dyspepsia than in healthy controls.

In patients with otherwise unexplained nausea, slow and rapid sequences of gastric slow waves with either a regular or an irregular rhythm have been observed. Gastric arrhythmias occur in some patients with functional dyspepsia and have also been documented in patients with severe nausea caused by gastroesophageal reflux disease.

DISTURBED SENSORY FUNCTION. Patients with functional dyspepsia have a decreased pain threshold during balloon distention of the stomach. No significant differences in sensory thresholds between *H. pylori*–positive and *H. pylori*–negative patients with functional dyspepsia have been observed. Sensory thresholds are lower after intraduodenal lipid, but not glucose infusion, which may explain why fatty meals induce symptoms in some patients with functional dyspepsia. Lowered duodenal sensory thresholds also occur, as do abnormal rectal and esophageal sensory thresholds in some patients with functional dyspepsia.

CENTRAL NERVOUS SYSTEM DISTURBANCES. In general, patients who present for medical care with functional dyspepsia are more anxious and depressed than healthy controls and have higher neuroticism and somatization scores. The prolactin response to buspirone, an azaspirone that stimulates central serotoninergic-1(A) receptors, may be greater in patients with functional dyspepsia compared with healthy controls.

Acute stress may result in decreased gastric contractility, but it is not known whether chronic dyspeptic symptoms are explained by such mechanisms. Indeed, patients with functional dyspepsia with or without antral hypomotility have normal autonomic and humoral responses to acute experimental stressors. The role of major life stress such as bereavement or divorce in the pathogenesis of functional dyspepsia remains controversial.

DIET AND ENVIRONMENTAL FACTORS. Some patients with functional dyspepsia complain of specific food intolerances, but a convincing relationship between diet and chronic dyspepsia remains to be demonstrated. Coffee may induce symptoms in approximately 50% of patients with functional dyspepsia compared with one in five healthy controls, perhaps because coffee acts as a direct irritant, stimulates acid secretion, or precipitates gastroesophageal reflux.

Aspirin and other non-steroidal anti-inflammatory drugs cause asymptomatic mucosal lesions in 30 to 60% of chronic users and can cause acute dyspepsia. Smoking and alcohol are not important risk factors for functional dyspepsia.

CLINICAL FEATURES. It has been suggested that patients with functional dyspepsia can be subdivided into those with typical ulcer symptoms, such as epigastric pain related to meals or waking the patient from sleep (ulcer-like dyspepsia), and symptoms suggestive of gastric stasis, such as postprandial bloating or early satiety (dysmotility-like dyspepsia). Dyspepsia is often associated with classic reflux symptoms, in particular heartburn; if reflux symptoms dominate, the diagnosis is symptomatic gastroesophageal reflux disease until proven otherwise. Although this categorization is used in

clinical practice, standardized symptom questionnaires have demonstrated considerable overlap among categories.

DIFFERENTIAL DIAGNOSIS. The major organic causes to consider are chronic peptic ulcer disease, gastroesophageal reflux (with or without esophagitis), and, rarely but importantly, malignancy (Fig. 131–2).

PEPTIC ULCER. The most important condition to exclude is peptic ulcer disease because definitive therapy is now available. Unfortunately, the type or pattern of symptoms discriminates very poorly between peptic ulcer disease and functional dyspepsia. In clinical practice, peptic ulcer disease must be excluded by upper gastrointestinal endoscopy before functional dyspepsia can be firmly diagnosed (see Chapter 126).

GASTROESOPHAGEAL REFLUX (see Chapter 124). Gastroesophageal

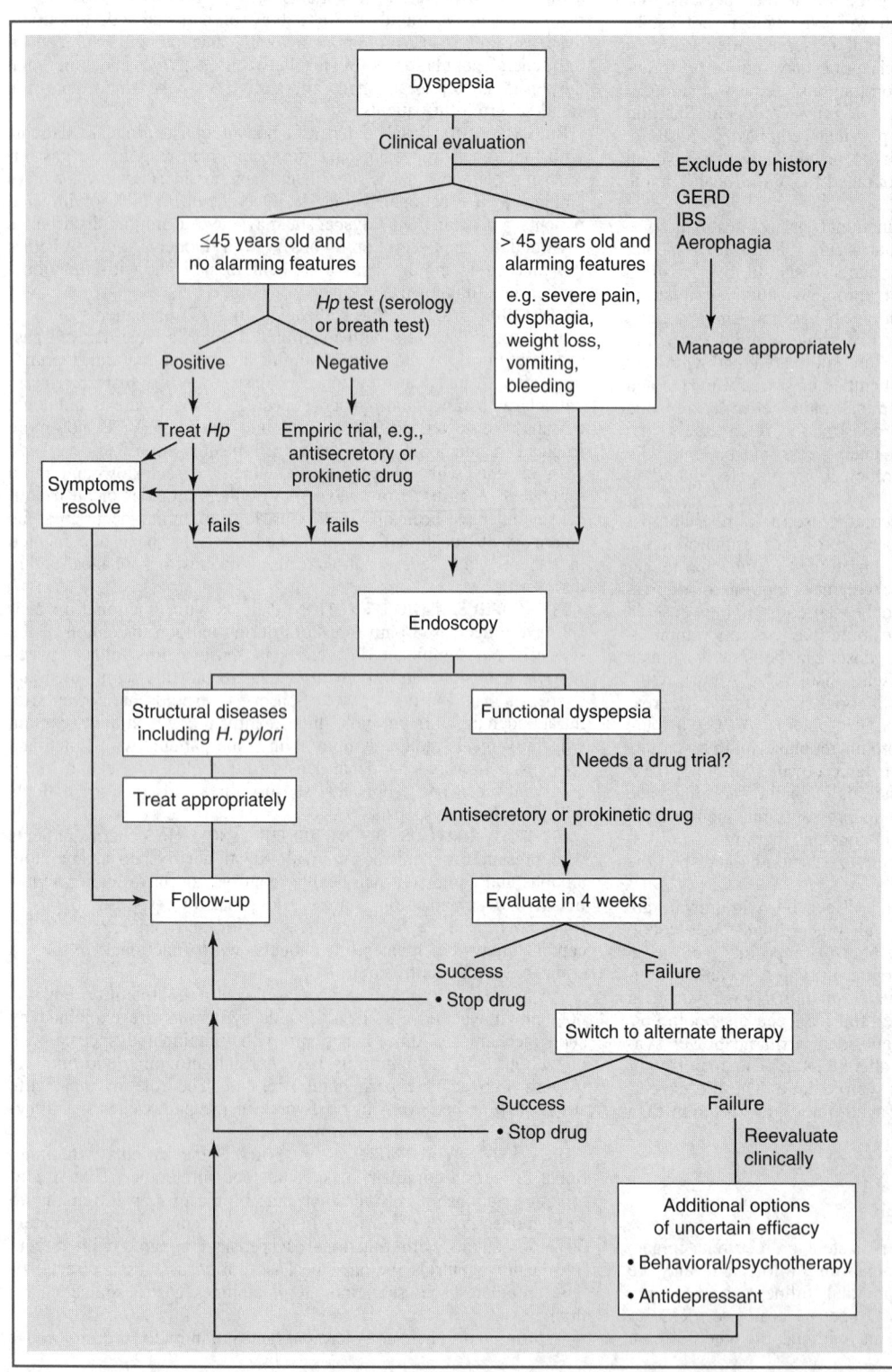

FIGURE 131–2 ■ Algorithm for the evaluation of dyspepsia. *Hp* = *Helicobacter pylori;* GERD = symptomatic gastroesophageal reflux disease; IBS = irritable bowel syndrome.

reflux should be strongly suspected in patients with predominant epigastric or retrosternal burning pain or discomfort that radiates up toward the throat and is relieved by antacids at least transiently. Over 50% of patients with pathologic gastroesophageal reflux confirmed by 24-hour esophageal pH testing have no visible esophagitis at endoscopy; these patients should not be misclassified as having functional dyspepsia.

GASTRIC AND ESOPHAGEAL CANCER (see Chapters 124 and 138). In persons younger than 55 years of age in most Western countries, cancer is an extremely rare cause of dyspepsia; overall, gastric cancer is found in only about 1% of patients with new-onset dyspepsia. Nevertheless, a neoplasm must be considered as a possible cause of dyspepsia because delayed diagnosis can adversely affect prognosis.

BILIARY TRACT DISEASE (see Chapter 157). Cholelithiasis causes biliary pain, which is typically severe, constant pain in the epigastrium or right upper quadrant that persists for hours and occurs episodically. In the absence of characteristic biliary pain, there is no evidence that gallstones are linked to dyspepsia. At ultrasonography, gallstones may be found in 1% to 3% of cases with chronic dyspepsia but are usually incidental. The prevalence of incidental gallstones increases with age; they are three times more prevalent in women. Biliary dyskinesia also causes biliary-type pain and is due to a motility disorder of the sphincter of Oddi. It is usually recognized after cholecystectomy.

PANCREATIC DISEASE. Chronic pancreatitis or pancreatic carcinoma (see Chapters 140 and 141) may cause symptoms that are occasionally confused with functional dyspepsia. However, these patients tend to have severe pain that is persistent and often radiates through to the back; they may have a history of risk factors for pancreatitis, such as excess alcohol use.

DRUG-INDUCED DYSPEPSIA. Drugs that may produce upper abdominal symptoms include iron or potassium supplements, digitalis, theophylline, and oral antibiotics, especially erythromycin and ampicillin. Reducing the dose or discontinuing drug therapy usually relieves the dyspepsia.

OTHER DISORDERS. Diabetes mellitus can cause postprandial fullness, early satiety, nausea, and vomiting in the presence or absence of gastroparesis (see Chapter 242). Furthermore, diabetic radiculopathy of the thoracic nerve roots can cause upper abdominal pain. Metabolic disturbances (e.g., hypothyroidism, hypercalcemia) can produce upper gastrointestinal distress. Ischemic heart disease sometimes presents as upper abdominal pain induced by exertion. Intestinal angina (chronic mesenteric ischemia) should be considered in older patients, particularly smokers; it typically presents as postprandial pain that is associated with a fear of eating and significant weight loss (see Chapter 137). Colon cancer, gastric lymphoma or sarcoma, and ampullary cancer rarely cause upper abdominal distress that may initially be confused with functional dyspepsia. Infiltrative diseases of the stomach, including eosinophilic gastritis, Crohn's disease, sarcoidosis, tuberculosis, and syphilis, may also very rarely produce dyspepsia. Abdominal wall pain can be confused with functional dyspepsia.

AEROPHAGIA. Air swallowing with postprandial belching is normal and occurs up to three to four times per hour. Aerophagia is characterized by excessive unconscious swallowing of air that results in abdominal distention or bloating; patients usually report transient improvement of symptoms after belching. The diagnosis of aerophagia is suggested by a specific history and can be confirmed by observing excessive air swallowing between meals and repetitive belching. Because excessive gas is probably not present, either disturbed upper gastrointestinal tract motility or psychopathology probably explains the symptoms.

TREATMENT. GENERAL MANAGEMENT OF FUNCTIONAL DYSPEPSIA. In patients with documented functional dyspepsia after endoscopy, a positive clinical diagnosis and firm reassurance remain the key steps in management. Not all patients want or require medication for functional dyspepsia after a confident diagnosis has been made. A careful explanation of the meaning of the symptoms and their benign nature can have very positive therapeutic effects; some patients lose their symptoms spontaneously after a positive diagnosis. It is useful to ask the patient with long-standing functional dyspepsia symptoms why he or she decided to present for care on this occasion; allaying the patient's unwarranted fears is effective therapy. Patients with functional dyspepsia may improve by eating low-fat meals or by ingesting more frequent but smaller meals throughout the day.

DRUG THERAPY. There is a considerable response to placebo in functional dyspepsia, ranging from 30 to 60%. This placebo response, however, may not reflect a non-specific effect of treatment but rather spontaneous regression of the disease. Indeed, the course of functional dyspepsia is typically characterized by relapsing and remitting symptoms, but over a 1-year period more than 70% will continue to be symptomatic.

Antacids and Acid Inhibitors. Antacids are commonly used by patients with functional dyspepsia, but randomized controlled studies have all failed to show a significant benefit over placebo. The results of controlled trials testing full-dose H_2-receptor antagonists have been conflicting. A meta-analysis suggested an approximately 20% benefit of H_2-receptor antagonists over placebo, but only selected trials could be included. These drugs should be prescribed twice daily (e.g., ranitidine or nizatidine, 150 mg, or famotidine, 20 mg) initially; the value of over-the-counter H_2 blockers is unknown. Reports have described promising improvement of ulcer-like dyspepsia during treatment with a proton pump inhibitor (e.g., omeprazole, 20 mg/day, or lansoprazole, 30 mg/day) compared with placebo.

Prokinetics. The dopaminergic receptor blockers metoclopramide (and domperidone) and the serotonin type 4 receptor agonist cisapride are widely used in functional dyspepsia, and convincing evidence from randomized controlled trials demonstrates that these prokinetics are superior to placebo. Up to 80% of patients with uninvestigated dyspepsia in primary care may respond to cisapride (10 mg four times a day). The prokinetics, and in particular cisapride, have an excellent safety profile, but life-threatening arrhythmias may occur very rarely with cisapride, especially if blood levels are high (e.g., if used in combination with a macrolide). Metoclopramide can induce side effects, owing to its central antidopaminergic effects, including dystonic reactions, drowsiness, and increased prolactin levels. Rarely, tardive dyskinesia may occur, particularly in the elderly, and in some cases it is not reversible.

Cytoprotection. Sucralfate and bismuth subsalicylate may be useful for intermittent dyspepsia but are not clearly superior to placebo. Misoprostil is not efficacious in functional dyspepsia.

Treatment Targeting *H. pylori*. Several large trials have assessed the long-term outcome of *H. pylori* eradication therapy with mixed results. Up to one in five patients may respond, but the placebo response is similar in some studies. *H. pylori* eradication may be considered for patients who do not respond to initial therapy.

Antispasmodics. Theoretically, anticholinergic agents might be of value in patients with pyloric or antral spasm, but these disturbances have not been documented in functional dyspepsia. Anticholinergic drugs have been formally evaluated in small studies, but neither dicyclomine nor trimebutine was more efficacious than placebo.

Antinausea Drugs. In addition to prokinetics, antinausea drugs include antihistamines, phenothiazines (e.g., prochlorperazine), and others with an uncertain mechanism of action (e.g., trimethobenzamide). Benzodiazepines may also help reduce nausea by their sedative effects. The 5-hydroxytryptamine type 3 receptor antagonist ondasetron and other similar agents are not of established value but may be worth a trial in difficult cases.

Antidepressants. There are a lack of formal randomized placebo-controlled trials on the effects of antidepressants in functional dyspepsia, but anecdotally this class of drugs may be of value in patients with resistant symptoms.

MANAGEMENT GUIDELINES. New-Onset (Uninvestigated) Dyspepsia. The medical history is key (Fig. 131–2). The physician should inquire about typical reflux symptoms; if heartburn or acid regurgitation is the predominant complaint, then a diagnosis of gastroesophageal reflux should be made and appropriate treatment instituted. If there is uncertainty, a short trial of high-dose proton pump inhibitor therapy (e.g., omeprazole 20 mg twice daily for 14 days) is useful as a diagnostic test for distinguishing reflux, in which symptoms are typically abolished, from other causes of upper gastrointestinal symptoms (see Chapter 124). Similarly, if bowel dysfunction is directly linked to the epigastric pain or discomfort, a diagnosis of irritable bowel syndrome should be considered.

Older patients (> 45 years) with new, unexplained dyspepsia and those with alarming symptoms or on non-steroidal anti-inflammatory drugs have an increased risk of organic disease and should undergo prompt upper endoscopic evaluation. In younger patients without alarming features, management depends on the degree of uncertainty that both patient and physician are willing to accept. Utilization of a locally validated non-invasive *H. pylori* test (serology or breath test) and initiation of anti–*H.pylori* treatment in infected subjects is a reasonable initial approach as an alternative to routine endoscopy. Such an approach should relieve symptoms in most patients with peptic ulcer disease (see Chapter 127).

In *H. pylori*–negative patients, who are most likely to have functional dyspepsia, the major first-line drugs are a prokinetic, a proton pump inhibitor, or an H_2 blocker. Some clinicians prefer initially to treat ulcer-like dyspepsia with an antisecretory and dysmotility-like dyspepsia with a prokinetic. Therapy can be switched if there is no benefit after 1 month. Patients require endoscopy if they fail to respond within 8 weeks or relapse rapidly.

Refractory Patient with Documented Functional Dyspepsia. Failure to respond to treatment raises the possibility that the diagnosis of functional dyspepsia was incorrect or that the chosen treatment was suboptimal. Combination therapy (e.g., cisapride and domperidone or an antisecretory plus a prokinetic) is not established to be beneficial but may be worth a trial in patients with documented refractory functional dyspepsia. In patients who need continuous therapy to avoid incapacitating or unremitting symptoms, drug holidays can confirm that the therapy is still of value. Another option is to initiate low-dose antidepressant treatment.

Aerophagia. Treatment of excessive unconscious air swallowing is difficult. Stress reduction and dietary modifications (avoiding sucking sweets or chewing gum, eating slowly, encouraging small swallows at meal time, and avoiding diet beverages) may occasionally help. Simethicone and activated charcoal are not of established value. Tranquilizers or prokinetics may sometimes be of benefit.

PROGNOSIS. A firm diagnosis of functional dyspepsia after endoscopy generally excludes ulcer or other structural disease, reduces a patient's fears, and may improve the prognosis. Some patients may then be free of symptoms for years. Patients seen at tertiary centers for functional dyspepsia represent a subgroup with more intractable symptoms, and spontaneous remissions are less common.

NON-CARDIAC (FUNCTIONAL) CHEST PAIN

One third to one half of patients presenting to an emergency department with chest pain do not have coronary artery disease. Angina-like chest pain in these patients is most often caused by gastroesophageal reflux and occasionally by motor disorders of the esophagus. Musculoskeletal chest pain and psychiatric disease (e.g., panic attacks) are also important causes to consider (see Chapter 38).

Clinical evaluation should be directed initially at excluding cardiac causes of chest pain (see Chapter 38). The history should screen for psychiatric disease and especially panic disorder, which may present as recurrent chest pain. Pain aggravated by movement may be musculoskeletal and can be confirmed by reproducing the patient's typical pain with palpation of the sternum or chest wall.

In patients who do not have cardiac, musculoskeletal, or psychiatric disease, the possibility of esophageal disease must be evaluated (see Chapter 124). Ambulatory 24-hour esophageal pH monitoring, endoscopy, or acid perfusion (Bernstein) tests may be useful in diagnosing reflux. In the remaining patients, esophageal manometry may be considered but the yield is low. Manometry will rule out achalasia (<1% of patients with chest pain) as well as esophageal spasm (<5% of patients with chest pain). "Nutcracker esophagus" refers to very high amplitude distal contractions (mean >180 mm Hg) with normal peristalsis. Other less common, non-specific motor abnormalities include a hypertensive lower esophageal sphincter or exaggerated esophageal body contractions. Whereas 30% of patients with chest pain will have a non-specific motor abnormality, they rarely coincide with spontaneous chest pain, and the relevance of the manometric disturbances remains highly questionable.

Treatment relies on reassurance and explanation. An aggressive trial of acid suppression with proton pump inhibitors should be prescribed if there is any suspicion of reflux, with the dose doubled if there is no response after 1 to 2 weeks (see Chapter 124).

Calcium channel blockers such as nifedipine (10 to 20 mg four times daily) or diltiazem (30 to 60 mg four times daily) may be tried in unexplained cases, but their efficacy is questionable; use of nitrates (both short and long acting) and anticholinergic agents has been disappointing. Antidepressants are of particular value, in part because a subset of patients have esophageal hypersensitivity. Behavioral therapy is of value in patients with and without panic disorder who have unexplained chest pain.

Achen SR, Kolts BE, Macmath T, et al: Effects of omeprazole versus placebo in treatment of noncardiac chest pain and gastroesophageal reflux. Dig Dis Sci 42: 2138–2145, 1997. *The proton pump inhibitor omeprazole significantly improved chest pain (81%) compared with placebo (6%) in patients with documented abnormal 24-hour esophageal pH studes and non-cardiac chest pain.*

Agreus L, Talley NJ: Dyspepsia—current understanding and management. Annu Rev Med 49:175–193, 1998. *Up-to-date review of management options.*

Drossman DA: Diagnosing and treating patients with refractory functional gastrointestinal disorders. Ann Intern Med 123:688–697, 1995. *Excellent review of management options for this difficult group of patients.*

Drossman DA, Whitehead WE, Camilleri M: Irritable bowel syndrome—a technical review for practice guideline development. Gastroenterology 112:2120–2137, 1997. *Comprehensive overview with very detailed references.*

Kahrilas PJ, Clouse RE, Hogan WJ: American Gastroenterological Association technical review on the clinical use of esophageal manometry. Gastroenterology 107: 1865–1884, 1994. *A clear and comprehensive overview of the clinical utility of esophageal manometry, and the lack of clinical relevance of non-specific esophageal motor abnormalities.*

Talley NJ, Silverstein M, Agreus L, et al: AGA technical review: Evaluation of dyspepsia. Gastroenterology 114:582–595, 1998. *Describes and evaluates current management strategies for dyspepsia.*

132 DISORDERS OF GASTROINTESTINAL MOTILITY

William J. Snape, Jr.

NORMAL MOTILITY IN STOMACH, SMALL INTESTINE, AND COLON

Motility of the gastrointestinal tract regulates the orderly movement of ingested material through the gut to ensure adequate absorption of nutrients, electrolytes, and fluid. Transit of intraluminal contents through the stomach, small intestine, and colon depends on the coordination of regional control of intraluminal pressure. Sphincters, interposed at several discrete areas along the length of the bowel, not only regulate the forward movement of intraluminal contents but impede the retrograde flow of intestinal contents. Coordinated gastrointestinal motility depends on neural and hormonal control of sphincter and longitudinal and circular smooth muscle contraction and relaxation.

SMOOTH MUSCLE. Movement of luminal contents from the stomach to the distal colon requires coordination between phasic and tonic contractions and relaxation of the intrinsic smooth muscle tone (peristaltic reflex), because luminal contents move from a high-pressure zone to a lower one. Myoelectric activity, including slow waves and spike potentials, coordinates regional intestinal smooth muscle contractions by controlling their frequency and by electrically linking neighboring smooth muscle cells (Fig. 132–1). The slow wave frequency of a smooth muscle cell is intrinsic to the cell, but it can be modified by the activity in neighboring cells. A pacemaker region sets the dominant frequency of each region of the gastrointestinal tract. Interstitial cells of Cajal, spontaneously active cells recognized by the presence of the proto-oncogene c-*kit* that codes for a tyrosine kinase receptor, may serve as pacemakers for the different regions of the gastrointestinal tract.

Tight electrical coupling of gastric smooth muscle cells is responsible for progressive propagation of the slow waves, oral to caudal, along the proximal to distal slow wave gradient. A higher contraction frequency elevates mean pressure, stimulating movement of intraluminal contents distally into the lower pressure area. Higher intraluminal pressure in the descending colon creates a pressure gradient that regulates the movement of intraluminal contents back to the transverse colon and forward to the sigmoid

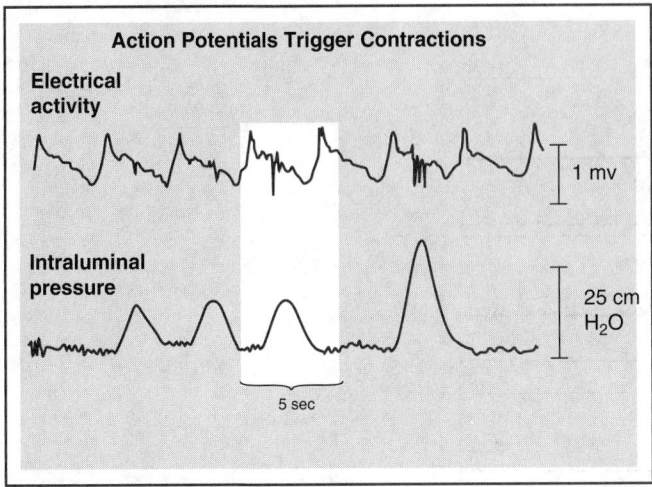

Action Potentials Trigger Contractions

Electrical activity

Intraluminal pressure

1 mv

25 cm H₂O

5 sec

FIGURE 132–1 ■ Simultaneous electrical and mechanical activity in the canine jejunum. The electrical signal was recorded from an extracellular electrode in the tunica muscularis; it shows a regular cycle of depolarization-repolarization at 12 to 14 cycles/min. Superimposed on some of these cycles (basic electrical rhythm, slow wave, or pacesetter potential) are more rapid oscillations (fast waves, spikes). When spiking occurs, the smooth muscle contracts, causing intraluminal pressure to rise (lower tracing).

Table 132–1 ■ ENTERIC NEUROTRANSMITTERS AND PEPTIDES AFFECTING GASTROINTESTINAL MOTILITY

EXCITATORY	INHIBITORY
Acetylcholine	Vasoactive inhibitory polypeptide
Neurokinins	Nitric oxide
Gastrin-releasing peptide	Calcitonin gene–related peptide
Neurotensin	Adenosine triphosphate
Enkephalin	Neurotensin
Cholecystokinin	Enkephalin
5-Hydroxytryptamine	Somatostatin (high dose)
Somatostatin (low dose)	Neuropeptide Y
	Peptide YY

gastric muscle and stimulates small intestinal and colonic muscles). Nitric oxide (NO), produced by myenteric neurons, smooth muscle cells, and the cells of Cajal, is likely the final mediator of gastrointestinal smooth muscle relaxation by inducing intracellular cyclic guanosine monophosphate.

The intrinsic enteric neurons of the gastrointestinal tract have numerous interconnections (Fig. 132–2). Input comes from the central nervous system, internuncial neurons, and interaction with afferent neurons by means of the prevertebral ganglia. Sympathetic and cholinergic fibers, which originate in the central nervous system and travel in the vagus, splanchnic, lumbar colonic, or sacral nerves, regulate the output of neurotransmitters from the myenteric plexus. Control of the myenteric plexus is mediated by intestinal afferent neurons and central nervous system neurons, interacting in the celiac, superior mesenteric, and inferior mesenteric ganglia. The interaction of interneurons within the myenteric plexus controls

colon. Therefore, a pressure amplitude gradient, rather than a frequency gradient, determines colonic transit. In the colon the dominance of contractions in the proximal descending colon and splenic flexure mixes the intraluminal contents and is responsible for a storage area in the transverse colon. Another motility pattern, the propagating contraction, is under neural control and propagates the fecal content distally from the transverse colon for further storage in the sigmoid colon.

Circular contractions throughout the gut segment the lumen, mixing the contents to expose the mucosa to continually different contents. The longitudinal muscle shortens the bowel, moving intraluminal contents forward.

Sphincters are high-pressure zones interposed through the gastrointestinal tract. The upper esophageal and external anal sphincters are localized bands of skeletal muscle. The lower esophageal sphincter is not an anatomically distinct structure; in contrast, the pylorus is a localized collection of smooth muscle. The ileocecal valve, a valvelike structure separating the colon and the ileum, responds like a sphincter. The internal anal sphincter is a localized collection of circular smooth muscle surrounded by the external anal sphincter. Sphincter contraction or relaxation is controlled by enteric neurotransmitters or by circulating peptide hormones in response to changes in pressure in the surrounding bowel or physiologic stimuli, such as eating and emotional stress.

Contraction of gastrointestinal smooth muscle requires an increase in the intracellular calcium concentration, which is necessary to phosphorylate the myosin light chain that is required to form cross-bridges with actin. When receptors are activated, inositol triphosphate is produced and releases calcium from the sarcoplasmic reticulum or stimulates opening of voltage-dependent or receptor-operated calcium channels. The rapid actin-myosin cross-bridge formation is associated with a rapid increase in the velocity of smooth muscle shortening.

Relaxation of smooth muscle is equally important for transporting intraluminal contents through the gastrointestinal tract. Cyclic adenosine monophosphate production, initiated by ligand activation of receptors on the smooth muscle cell membrane, decreases intracellular calcium concentration by moving calcium into sarcoplasmic reticulum or out of the cell.

ENTERIC NERVOUS SYSTEM. Enteric neurons contain many different excitatory and inhibitory neurotransmitters (Table 132–1), and the complex interaction among inhibitory and excitatory neurotransmitters coordinates bowel activity. Although some neurotransmitters are generally stimulating (e.g., acetylcholine) and others inhibitory (e.g., vasoactive intestinal polypeptide [VIP]), some neurotransmitters may control the motility pattern through different effects on nerve and muscle (opiates stimulate muscle and inhibit acetylcholine release) or by different regional effects (neurotensin relaxes

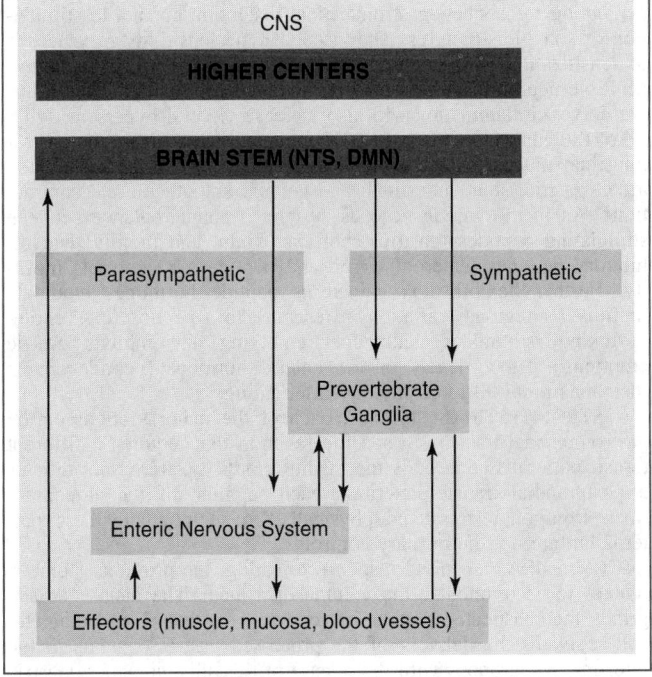

CNS

HIGHER CENTERS

BRAIN STEM (NTS, DMN)

Parasympathetic

Sympathetic

Prevertebrate Ganglia

Enteric Nervous System

Effectors (muscle, mucosa, blood vessels)

FIGURE 132–2 ■ Schematic diagram showing control levels for neural regulation of gastrointestinal effector function. The enteric nervous system integrates information from the periphery and the central nervous system and modulates effector function. In prevertebral ganglia, afferent inputs from the gut and descending inputs through the sympathetic branch of the autonomic nervous system are integrated into output that has primarily inhibitory effects on gut motility. Autonomic nuclei of sympathetic and parasympathetic nerves located in the brain stem integrate inputs from the periphery and the cortex. Output reaches the gut through the parasympathetic and sympathetic nerves. NTS = nucleus tractus solitarius; DMN = dorsal motor nucleus. (Adapted from Mayer EA, Raybould H: Role of neural control in gastrointestinal motility and visceral pain. *In* Snape WJ Jr. [ed]: Pathogenesis of Functional Bowel Disease. New York, Plenum, 1989, pp 13–35.)

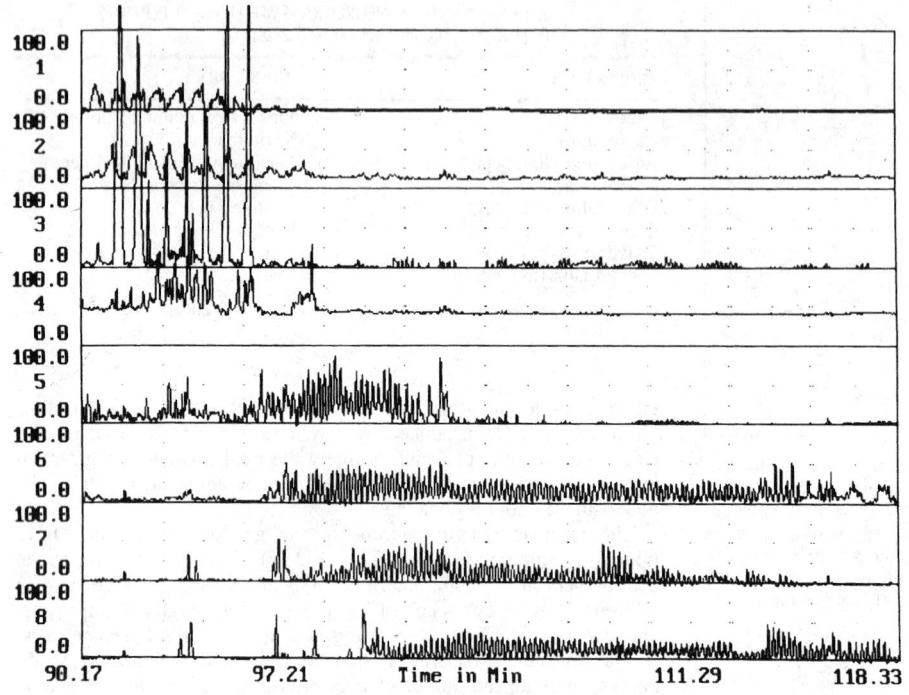

FIGURE 132-3 ■ An antroduodenal motility recording in a normal subject during fasting. The proximal three ports are in the antrum, port 4 is in the pylorus with contractions at the gastric and duodenal frequencies, and ports 5 through 8 are in the duodenum. A phase 3 migrating motor complex progresses from the stomach (3 cycles/min) down the duodenum (11 cycles/min). (From Snape WJ Jr: Role of motility measurements in managing upper gastrointestinal dysfunction. Gastroenterologist 6:44–59, 1998.)

neural output to the gut. Each site of neural interconnection may be a potential target for future therapeutic intervention.

Afferent sensory nerves play a large role in the symptoms of abdominal pain or bloating in patients with gastrointestinal motility disorders. Patients with functional gastrointestinal diseases (Chapter 131) have a heightened awareness and decreased threshold for pain perception to esophagogastrointestinal distention but not to stimulation of somatic structures. The visceral hypersensitivity may be due to sensitization of the neurons in the gut, dorsal horn, or thalamus. Multiple neurotransmitters may be involved in sensitizing the afferent nerves. Inflammation will also increase visceral hypersensitivity.

ENTERIC PEPTIDE HORMONES. Peptides, released from the gastrointestinal mucosa into the blood after eating, act as hormones and affect gastric, small intestinal, and colonic smooth muscle contractions. As in the enteric nervous system, a counterbalance between stimulating peptides (gastrin, cholecystokinin, and motilin) and inhibitory peptides (enteroglucagon and peptide YY) controls motility. Further flexibility is gained as peptide hormones modulate motility by regional variation in response to a peptide (e.g., cholecystokinin stimulates gallbladder emptying and inhibits gastric emptying). Blood levels of the enteric hormonal peptides reach their maximum 30 to 60 minutes after eating.

GASTROINTESTINAL TRANSIT. Each of the major sections of the gastrointestinal tract has a specific function that requires a different transit pattern. Eating ends the fasting motility pattern and initiates a postprandial transit pattern in each segment of the alimentary tract. Emotional stress and physical exercise modulate these patterns but are not the primary controls.

STOMACH. As an initial response to eating, the proximal stomach relaxes to accommodate the volume of a meal. The distal stomach grinds the masticated chunks of food to less than 1 mm diameter and regulates the delivery of the processed gastric contents to the intestine synchronous with the release of digestive enzymes. Gastric emptying adjusts to the different physical and chemical characteristics of the food. Liquids are emptied faster (T_{12} = 15 minutes) than solids (T_{12} = 45 to 90 minutes). Gastric emptying of glucose solutions is regulated so that approximately 2 kcal of glucose is emptied per minute; an equiosmolar solution of saline empties more rapidly. The gastric fundal tone regulates liquid emptying, whereas antral contractions control the rate of solid food emptying.

SMALL INTESTINE. The small intestine slowly moves the chyme distally, allowing mixing of the contents with digestive enzymes and absorption of the nutrients, electrolytes, and water. The transit time for material to move through the small intestine and appear in the cecum is 40 to 180 minutes. In addition to controlling the distal transit of nutrients, the small intestine must clear extruded dead cells and bacteria. The migrating motor complex (Fig. 132–3), which occurs during fasting and removes indigestible luminal contents, consists of three different phases: phase 1 is a period of inactivity; phase 2 is a period of intermittent phasic contractions similar to the postprandial pattern; and phase 3 is a continuous period of contractions that propels the remaining intestinal contents during fasting.

COLON. Regulation of colonic transit allows the colon to absorb additional water and electrolytes and to store the fecal waste for elimination. Eating stimulates back and forth mixing of the luminal contents and allows greater time for absorption by the colonic mucosa. The transverse and rectosigmoid colons are separate sites of storage. Propagating contractions transport the luminal contents distally and appear necessary for normal bowel movements. The transit time is 40 to 60 hours for excretion of the colonic content.

CLINICAL ASSESSMENT OF GASTROINTESTINAL MOTILITY

HISTORY AND CLINICAL EXAMINATION. Although symptoms can originate from disturbances of any part of the gastrointestinal tract, particular symptoms may suggest dysfunction of a specific site. In motility disturbances of each of the distinct organs (stomach, small intestine, colon), cramping abdominal pain occurs frequently, often after eating. The pain location can indicate the most likely source—epigastric for stomach, periumbilical or generalized for small intestine, or lower quadrants for the colon. However, pain referred from the anatomic location of the colon may occur in any of the abdominal quadrants. Colonic pain resolves after a bowel movement or passing flatus.

Early satiety, nausea, and postprandial vomiting occur in patients with delayed transit through the stomach and upper small bowel. These symptoms can also result from organic non-motility disorders (Table 132–2). Postprandial vomiting caused by an obstructed gastric outlet is characteristically voluminous and may not occur until after eating several meals. When disturbed motility causes these symptoms, the pathophysiologic defect may be caused by reduced receptive relaxation, a low threshold for sensory nerve recognition of gastric distention, or uncoordinated antroduodenal contractions. The vomiting center in the lateral reticular formation and the chemoreceptor trigger zone in the area postrema in the floor of the fourth ventricle are stimulated by visceral afferent nerves from the upper gut. The chemoreceptor trigger zone, not protected by the blood-brain barrier, is influenced by substances in the plasma and initiates vomiting through the vomiting center. Acute, non-specific vomiting can be treated with antiemetics such

Gastroenteritis
Gastritis/gastric ulcer
Motion sickness
Gastroparesis
Gastric outlet obstruction
Small bowel obstruction (usually above mid jejunum)
Systemic illness (high fever/severe pain)
Peritonitis
Pregnancy (including hyperemesis gravidarum or acute fatty liver of pregnancy)
Drugs or toxins (including chemotherapy)
Increased intracranial pressure
Psychogenic vomiting/eating disorder

as prochlorperazine or trimethobenzamide. If the patient has a disturbance in motility, a prokinetic agent such as cisapride or metoclopramide can be helpful. Rapid gastric emptying causes symptoms of the "dumping syndrome," which include sweating, weakness, occasional orthostasis, tachycardia, and diarrhea.

Vomiting is a common symptom of intestinal pseudo-obstruction, acute ileus, and a high anatomic obstruction. If the obstruction is in the distal small intestine, distention is a more prominent complaint than vomiting. In distal obstructions the vomitus, when present, has a feculent odor. An abdominal radiograph usually shows a cut-off between dilated and non-dilated bowel in a true obstruction. In acute ileus or pseudo-obstruction, the bowel is dilated throughout, with air visible in the rectum.

With massive gastric retention (> 750 mL), findings include a soft mass in the left upper quadrant. In a fasting patient, recovery of more than 150 mL of gastric contents through a nasogastric tube, especially if old food is present, suggests gastric retention. An abdominal radiograph shows a large fluid-filled viscus in the left upper quadrant. If the patient is vomiting acutely, nasogastric suction should be initiated and the hypovolemia and metabolic alkalosis should be treated.

Abdominal distention and pain occur in both anatomic and functional disorders of the gastrointestinal tract. In patients with pseudo-obstruction, distention is an objective physical sign, whereas in patients with irritable bowel syndrome, a bloating sensation without an increase in bowel gas may be caused by a defect in sensory recognition (see Chapter 131). In patients with obstruction, bowel sounds are loud with high-pitched rushes. If the obstruction has been present for a long time, bowel sounds are quieter or absent. In acute ileus or pseudo-obstruction, bowel sounds are quiet but usually present. If the ileus is associated with a severe abdominal insult, such as peritonitis or surgery, bowel sounds are absent.

An alteration in bowel habit (diarrhea or constipation) is the cardinal symptom of motor disorders of the gastrointestinal tract, but these alterations do not specifically identify the pattern of motility. In the absence of a defect in mucosal absorption, diarrhea results from more rapid transit of intestinal contents through either the small intestine or the colon (see Chapter 133). The mechanism of rapid transit through the small intestine is unclear, but diarrhea due to altered colonic motility is associated with an increased frequency of propagating contractions. Constipation generally results from slow colonic transit due to either colonic inertia or increased segmenting contractions, which impede the forward movement of the intraluminal contents. Propagating contractions are markedly decreased or absent in patients with constipation.

The frequency, character, and volume of bowel movements should be carefully defined in each patient. More than three bowel movements a day defines excessive frequency. Stool volume is increased in small bowel-mediated diarrhea, whereas low-volume stools result from disordered colonic motility. Stools may vary in consistency from liquid to merely soft. Constipation is defined as fewer than three bowel movements each week. The constipated stool generally has a lower volume (weight) and is firmer than normal stools, since more water has been absorbed. These strict definitions may exclude the patient who complains of constipation and who has stools of normal size and consistency but who strains to defecate. The patient who has only increased straining may have a functional anal outlet obstruction (Chapter 143).

MOTILITY TESTS. In addition to identifying the motility disturbance responsible for the patient's symptoms, standardized motility tests allow objective assessment of response to treatment. *Gastric emptying* of liquids and solids must be measured independently to provide a full description of the organ's function. Gastric emptying can be performed simultaneously using different radionuclides to tag the liquid and the solid phases. Bedside assessment of the gastric transit of a bolus of isotonic saline may be a useful and inexpensive screening test. After 30 minutes, the residual should be less than 40% of an oral volume of 750 mL administered. Estimating gastric emptying from an upper gastrointestinal barium study often does not provide useful information. A breath test measures both liquid and solid gastric emptying using non-radioactive isotopes of carbon (^{13}C or ^{14}C) bound to octanoic acid. A serum test measuring acetaminophen can monitor gastric emptying. Correlation of the results of the radionuclide emptying with measurement of antroduodenal motility provides an estimate of the duodenum's contribution to slow gastric emptying. With an enteric neuropathy, the migrating motor complex is absent, whereas with a myopathy, contractions are present but their amplitude is decreased.

Small intestinal transit can be measured by breath tests to estimate small intestinal transit by reflecting the bacterial metabolism of non-absorbable carbohydrate marker to H_2, or the bacterial release of a radionuclide label from a bile salt conjugate, both of which increase in the breath after the substrates reach the colon. These tests are invalid if the patient has small intestinal bacterial overgrowth resulting from the motility dysfunction or a blind loop of intestine, because the bacteria release the marker proximal to the ileocecal valve. The appearance in the right lower quadrant (cecum) of a radionuclide-labeled non-absorbable marker ingested with a meal also provides an estimate of small intestinal transit.

Intraluminal pressures measured in the small intestine may document abnormalities in the fasting migrating motor complex and the postprandial motility response. As in the stomach, concomitant use of transit and manometric studies allows the contribution of the enteric nerves and smooth muscle to the motility disorder to be estimated objectively.

Global colonic transit can be easily measured by orally administering radiopaque markers and measuring the distribution of the markers throughout the colon 5 days later. If no markers are then present within the colon, the patient probably is not constipated. In the constipated patient, localization of the markers to the rectosigmoid region suggests a rectoanal outlet dysfunction. If the markers are distributed throughout the colon, a colonic motility disturbance exists. Regional emptying times can be calculated from this test. Once the motility defect has been localized to the colon, more specific transit and motility tests, measuring increases in intraluminal pressure and segment transit times with radionuclide markers, are available in specialized centers. The absence of a postprandial increase in segmenting contractions suggests a neural lesion, whereas low amplitude or absent postprandial contraction suggests disturbed smooth muscle function. Anorectal manometry shows whether the anal sphincter contributes to outlet dysfunction.

DISORDERS OF GASTRODUODENAL MOTILITY

Delayed Gastric Emptying

Chronic delayed gastric emptying (gastroparesis) is caused most often by an intrinsic disturbance in gastric or upper gastrointestinal motility and requires specific therapy of the underlying neuromuscular disorder. Acute gastroparesis, which is most frequently associated with an electrolyte disturbance, ketoacidosis, systemic infection, or an acute abdominal insult, is managed by treating the underlying disease, not the gastric motility disorder.

Delayed gastric emptying may be associated with other systemic diseases or may be due to a primary dysfunction of the stomach (Table 132-3). The typical symptoms of delayed gastric emptying include early satiety, nausea, and vomiting. Phytobezoars sometimes occur in these patients as well, especially if the migrating motor complex is absent.

DELAYED GASTRIC EMPTYING COMPLICATING GASTRIC SURGERY. Vagotomy, with the exception of the highly selective vagotomy (parietal cell vagotomy), decreases fundic relaxation, antral contractions, and coordinated relaxation of the pylorus (Chapter 129). The expected physiologic response to vagotomy is rapid emptying of liquids, possibly predisposing the patient to dumping

Table 132-3 ■ GASTRIC MOTILITY DISORDERS

DELAYED GASTRIC EMPTYING	RAPID GASTRIC EMPTYING
Postvagotomy	Dumping syndrome
Diabetes mellitus	Pancreatic insufficiency
Viral infections	Celiac sprue
Reflux esophagitis	Zollinger-Ellison syndrome
Brain stem lesions	Duodenal ulcer
Anorexia nervosa	
Tachygastria	

syndrome, and slow emptying of solids. Although most often patients have no gastric symptoms after abdominal vagotomy, 5 to 10% have delayed gastric emptying. This complication is more likely to occur if the patient had gastric outlet obstruction caused by a primary disease.

Metoclopramide improves symptoms in many patients with delayed gastric emptying after a vagotomy. The usual dose of metoclopramide (10 mg orally, four times a day) can cause anxiety, fatigue, or sedation or dyskinesia in about 15% of patients. Domperidone, also a dopamine antagonist, does not cross the blood-brain barrier and has fewer central nervous system side effects but is investigational in the United States. Cisapride, which releases acetylcholine from the enteric neurons, may be useful in gastroparesis. Erythromycin, a macrolide antibiotic, initiates phase 3 in the stomach, improving gastroparesis symptoms. New analogues with no antibiotic activity are being clinically tested.

Roux-en-Y anastomoses after gastric resection occasionally cause poor gastric emptying, especially of solids. The migrating motor complex and the postprandial motor response are abnormal in the roux limb. Delayed gastric emptying of solids is the major functional disturbance; liquid gastric emptying may be normal. Patients with severe vomiting can be treated with subcutaneous bethanechol, further gastric resection, or elimination of the roux loop. Leuprolide may reduce symptoms, and some patients may benefit from a near-total gastrectomy.

DIABETIC GASTROPARESIS. Delayed gastric emptying complicating diabetic hyperglycemia or ketoacidosis resolves as the patient's metabolic status improves, but the stomach is sometimes massively distended, exhibits mucosal bleeding, and may require decompression by nasogastric tube (Chapter 242). Chronic delayed gastric emptying, associated with long-standing insulin-dependent diabetes mellitus, is a greater clinical problem. Such patients have frequent episodes of nausea and vomiting, which affect food intake and complicate insulin requirements. Retinopathy, nephropathy, peripheral neuropathy, and other complications are commonly present. Absence of the gastric migrating motor complex, necessary for emptying of non-digestible material more than 1 mm, predisposes the diabetic patient to bezoars, causing abdominal discomfort, early satiety, and vomiting. Vagal neuropathy is thought to be the pathogenesis of gastric stasis in diabetes mellitus, although a demonstrable autonomic neuropathy is not always present.

Metoclopramide improves the symptoms of gastric stasis in patients with diabetes mellitus both by increasing gastric emptying and decreasing the central nervous system recognition of nausea and distention. Bethanechol also stimulates an increase in gastric motility and improves symptoms in patients with diabetic gastric stasis. Erythromycin improves symptoms of gastroparesis by increasing antral contractions and fundal tone. Clonidine can improve gastric emptying and symptoms.

ANOREXIA NERVOSA. The gastric emptying of solids, but not of liquids, is slowed in patients with anorexia nervosa (see Chapter 227), but not in patients with bulimia. The delayed gastric emptying is associated with antral dysrhythmia, fundal hypotonia, decreased postprandial plasma concentrations of norepinephrine and neurotensin, and impaired autonomic function (decreased resting diastolic blood pressure and skin conductance). Patients with equal weight loss but without the psychiatric disorder do not have delayed gastric emptying.

Repleting the patient's calories improves gastric emptying in the absence of prokinetic medicine. Reversal of the underlying psychiatric disturbance appears necessary for complete resolution of symptoms.

MISCELLANEOUS CAUSES. Delayed gastric emptying in progressive systemic sclerosis may exacerbate problems with esophageal reflux. Parvovirus-like agents (Norwalk or Hawaii viruses) can slow gastric emptying. The decreased gastric emptying associated with an acute viral infection usually resolves quickly. Up to 25% of patients with reflux esophagitis, associated with an incompetent lower esophageal sphincter, have delayed gastric emptying, which must be corrected to treat the reflux esophagitis adequately. Lesions such as tumors, infarction, or viral encephalitis that affect the vagal complex in the medulla can delay gastric emptying. There is no evidence that infection with *Helicobacter pylori* affects gastric emptying.

Rapid Gastric Emptying

Rapid gastric emptying occurs in some patients with duodenal ulcer disease and Zollinger-Ellison syndrome as a result of duodenal insensitivity to an acid load (Chapter 130). Rapid liquid emptying occurs in patients with pancreatic insufficiency (Chapter 141) and possibly with celiac sprue because of poor feedback inhibition of gastric motility by fat due to a maldigestion or malabsorption. Rapid emptying that occurs in the dumping syndrome is not affected by octreotide, even though symptoms are improved.

DISORDERS OF SMALL INTESTINAL MOTILITY

Small intestinal motility may be hypoactive, hyperactive, or uncoordinated (Table 132-4). Decreased intestinal motility reflects either absent or fewer contractions of phase 3 of the migrating motor complex during fasting or a minimal increase in postprandial motility in the different regions of the small bowel. Conversely, increased motility is reflected in increased numbers of fasting migrating motor complexes or an augmented intraluminal pressure response to eating. Uncoordinated intestinal motility can be caused by retrograde migrating motor complexes and clustered contractions.

In patients with motility disorders, qualitatively similar transit patterns may result in different symptoms. For example, patients with constipation may have delayed small intestinal transit. In contrast, a patient with pseudo-obstruction may have a greater delay in intestinal transit that results in diarrhea due to bacterial overgrowth. Therefore, symptoms may not be helpful in determining the cause of a disease.

Diarrhea is generally the result of rapid intestinal transit because of decreased time of contact of the luminal contents with the mucosa. Patients also may have maldigestion and malabsorption due to poor mixing of the dietary material with the digestive enzymes and bile salts. Accentuated borborygmi may also disturb the patient.

Patients with slow intestinal transit tend to complain of nausea, vomiting, abdominal distention, and periumbilical abdominal cramps. Although constipation can occur with delayed intestinal

Table 132-4 ■ SMALL INTESTINAL MOTILITY DISORDERS

Decreased Motility
Hollow visceral myopathy (primary intestinal pseudo-obstruction)
Progressive systemic sclerosis (late)
Amyloidosis
Muscular dystrophy
  Duchenne
  Myotonic
Hypothyroidism
Jejunal diverticulosis
Jejunoileal bypass
Increased or Uncoordinated Motility
Primary visceral neuropathy
Carcinoma-associated visceral neuropathy
Progressive systemic sclerosis (early)
Irritable bowel syndrome
Diabetes mellitus
Infectious diarrhea
Mass lesion of brain stem
Amyloidosis
Hyperthyroidism
Carcinoid syndrome
Shy-Drager syndrome

transit, diarrhea is more common. Phase 3 of the migrating motor complex—in which bacteria and sloughed, dead epithelial cells are propelled from the small intestine into the colon—is often absent or severely deranged by an enteric neuropathy. Bacterial overgrowth due to a diminished number of migrating motor complex contractions deconjugates bile salts, causing steatorrhea and diarrhea. The absence of postprandial motility impedes the normal transit through the small intestine.

Decreased Intestinal Motility

HOLLOW VISCERAL MYOPATHY (PRIMARY INTESTINAL PSEUDO-OBSTRUCTION). This disorder, which is the prototype for myopathic diseases of the small intestine, generally displays vacuolized and degenerated smooth muscle in the circular or longitudinal layers, separately or together, without affecting the enteric nerves. Defective slow wave generation or actin-myosin crossbridge formation may cause the decreased muscle contraction. The contractions are decreased in amplitude and number, but usually the migrating motor complex is present because the nerves are unaffected (Fig. 132–4). The migrating motor complex may function poorly, however, because of the low-amplitude contractions. The motility pattern differs from that associated with a partial small bowel obstruction, in which 3 to 10 clustered contractions occur regularly, separated by 1-minute intervals of quiescence.

Patients usually present with symptoms and signs of small intestinal stasis without evidence of an anatomic obstruction or of a secondary cause for pseudo-obstruction (see Table 132–3). Hollow visceral myopathy is familial, but random, non-familial cases are probably more common. With familial primary intestinal pseudo-obstruction, parts of the urinary system (bladder, renal pelvis) may also be dilated as a result of abnormal smooth muscle contraction. Familial visceral myopathy is also associated with a high incidence of intestinal malrotation.

Anatomic bowel obstruction or acute ileus must be excluded before the diagnosis of pseudo-obstruction is made. Acute adynamic ileus occurs most frequently after abdominal surgery, peritonitis, intra-abdominal vascular accidents, or a severe electrolyte imbalance. Ileus or obstruction can cause hypovolemia or third-space accumulation of fluid. The signs and symptoms of acute ileus are similar to those of chronic disorders of decreased intestinal motility, but, in contrast, treatment of the initiating cause resolves the symptoms. Acute ileus or obstruction is treated by decompression with a nasogastric tube, replacement of fluid volume, and correction of electrolyte and acid-base imbalances.

The therapy for hollow visceral myopathy is generally highly unsatisfactory. The newer prokinetic agent cisapride shows promise for treating severe small intestinal motility disorders, especially in those patients with postprandial hypomotility but a normal fasting pattern. Intestinal bypass surgery should be avoided in patients with pseudo-obstruction. Occasionally, antibiotics may be of help if a blind loop syndrome with bacterial overgrowth is present.

PROGRESSIVE SYSTEMIC SCLEROSIS (see Chapter 290). This is the most common "collagen vascular disease" to cause disordered intestinal motility, although polymyositis and systemic lupus erythematosus may rarely do so. Approximately 40% of patients with progressive systemic sclerosis have defects in both neural and smooth muscle function of the intestine. Early in the course of the disease, signs of neuropathy predominate; when collagen later replaces smooth muscle, myopathy becomes the major component. In symptomatic patients, postprandial motility is usually markedly reduced. Because a neuropathy is often present, the migrating motor complexes are absent. In general, patients become symptomatic only after extensive replacement of the smooth muscle with collagen. In contrast to hollow visceral myopathy, muscle cells in progressive systemic sclerosis are decreased in number but morphologically normal. Because the number of functional smooth muscle cells is decreased, pharmacologic stimulation with prokinetic drugs is generally unsuccessful. However, low doses of the somatostatin analogue octreotide stimulate phase 3 of the migrating motor complex and improve symptoms in systemic sclerosis.

OTHER CONDITIONS. *Amyloidosis* (Chapter 297) of the small intestine may cause either a myopathy or a neuropathy, depending on its distribution. Several of the *muscular dystrophy* syndromes (Chapter 506) may affect the intestinal smooth muscle in addition to skeletal and cardiac muscle. *Hypothyroidism* (Chapter 239) decreases the slow wave frequency and amplitude of contraction of the intestine, which may result in atony. *Jejunal diverticulosis* is caused by pseudo-obstruction, which predominantly involves the small intestine. The histologic pattern is similar to that of progressive systemic sclerosis in most patients, although some patients have neuropathy.

Increased or Uncoordinated Motility

VISCERAL NEUROPATHY. Intestinal motility can be increased, as well as uncoordinated, in patients with visceral neuropathy because of a decrease in neural inhibition. The hallmarks of visceral neuropathy are a patchy loss of nerve tracts, a decreased number of neurons, or fragmentation and dropout of axons. Specialized silver stains are needed for the accurate histologic diagnosis of an enteric neuropathy.

Familial cases may be associated with other neural lesions, in-

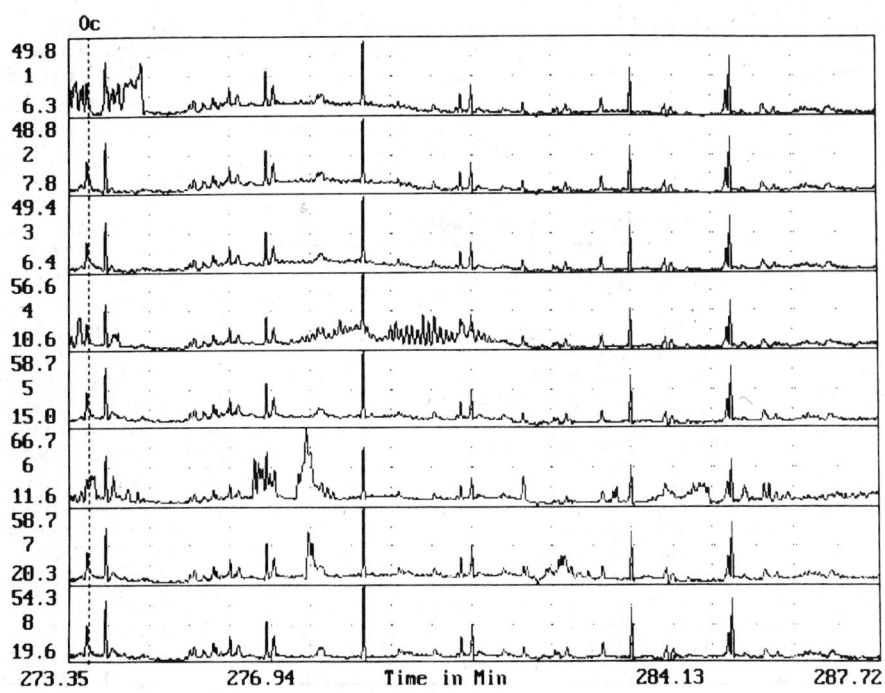

FIGURE 132–4 ■ An antroduodenal motility recording from a patient with myopathic pseudo-obstruction. The proximal two ports record pressure from the stomach, and the distal six ports are in the duodenum. Octreotide (Oc) stimulates recognizable contractions only in lead 4. These contractions have a low amplitude (10 mm Hg). (From Snape WJ Jr: Role of motility measurements in managing upper gastrointestinal dysfunction. Gastroenterologist 6:44–59, 1998.)

cluding mild autonomic insufficiency, mental retardation, altered sensory recognition of position, and absent deep tendon reflexes. Random cases may be caused by injury from a viral infection, an environmental toxin, or carcinomatous neuropathy (see Chapter 195). During fasting, a neuropathy generally disrupts either the propagation or configuration of the migrating motor complex. In some patients the migrating motor complex may be absent. Eating may initiate no contractions or uncoordinated contractions, or it may fail to inhibit migrating motor complexes in patients with neuropathy.

FUNCTIONAL (NON-ULCER) DYSPEPSIA (see Chapter 131). Midepigastric postprandial abdominal pain with concomitant nausea and occasionally vomiting may be associated with abnormal motility in the stomach and small intestine. Two patterns of contractions, "discrete clustered contractions" and "prolonged propagated contractions," are associated with abdominal pain more frequently in patients with the irritable bowel syndrome than in healthy control subjects. In many patients with non-ulcer dyspepsia, antral motility is decreased after eating a meal compared with non-symptomatic control subjects.

DIABETES MELLITUS. The diarrhea associated with diabetes mellitus is most likely due to small intestinal motility disturbances. Abnormal manometric patterns in diabetics with gastroparesis include decreased motility or uncoordinated bursts of small intestinal contractions. The migrating motor complexes can be present, deranged, or absent in diabetic patients. Patients with the central autonomic nervous system disturbance Shy-Drager syndrome (see Chapter 451) have similar findings to patients with diabetes. Diabetic diarrhea may respond to treatment with clonidine.

OTHER DISORDERS. *Infectious diarrhea* (e.g., due to enterotoxigenic *Escherichia coli* or *Shigella*) initiates a significant motility disorder, characterized experimentally by powerful migrating contractions (Chapter 339). *Amyloid* (Chapter 297) can affect the enteric nerves of the small intestine as well as replace smooth muscle. *Hyperthyroidism* (Chapter 239) increases the slow wave frequency of the bowel, which is a possible cause of the frequently associated diarrhea. *Carcinoid syndrome* (Chapter 245) with increased 5-hydroxytryptamine production increases the migration velocity of the migrating motor complex and increases the cycling frequency.

DISORDERS OF COLON MOTILITY (Table 132–5)

Orderly transit of contents through the colon "fine tunes" the absorption of salt and water. If the transit is too slow, the mucosa can extract too much water and the stool becomes hard, resulting in constipation. Rapid transit causes frequent, soft stools. Diarrhea caused by colonic motility disorders is low in volume (<400 mL/day), because most intestinal fluid is absorbed in the small intestine (see Chapter 133). Many of the systemic diseases that affect gastric and small intestinal motility also alter colonic motility.

Either increased or decreased segmenting contractions can slow transit through the colon. A functional partial obstruction results

---

Table 132–5 ■ PATHOGENESIS OF COLONIC MOTILITY DISORDERS

Slow Transit
Increased segmenting contraction
  Primary constipation
  Irritable bowel syndrome (spastic)
  Diverticular disease
  Anal outlet obstruction
    Congenital—Hirschsprung's disease
    Acquired
Decreased segmenting contractions
  Irritable bowel syndrome (inertia)
  Primary colonic pseudo-obstruction
  Ogilvie's syndrome
  Diabetes mellitus
  Progressive systemic sclerosis
  Spinal cord injury
Rapid Transit
Functional diarrhea
Bile salt diarrhea
Surreptitious abuse of laxatives

---

from increased segmenting contractions, because the segmentation impedes movement of colonic contents. The colonic contents also move slowly if colonic segmenting activity is decreased (colonic inertia). Propagating contractions are invariably absent in patients with slow colonic transit and constipation, suggesting that these contractions are necessary for net forward movement of feces into the distal rectosigmoid.

Patients with diarrhea and rapid colonic transit have decreased colonic segmenting contractions and increased numbers of contractions propagating into the rectum. As a result, intraluminal contents are rapidly transported distally. When these powerful contractions carry the colonic contents into the rectum, the patient experiences urgency.

Cramping abdominal pain referable to the colon occurs predominantly in the lower abdominal quadrants, but it can be felt anywhere over the anatomic distribution of the colon. This pain is characteristically relieved by flatus or a bowel movement. Although patients feel bloated, ascribed to increased gastrointestinal gas, they actually have normal amounts of bowel gas. Tenesmus, a feeling of incomplete evacuation, is associated with rectosigmoid spasm.

Slow Colonic Transit with Increased Segmenting Contractions

PRIMARY CONSTIPATION. Most people experience brief periods of constipation during their lives; treatment is usually not necessary unless the symptoms last for several months. Infrequent bowel movements (less than every other day) result in hard fecal pellets, which require straining to eliminate, because of slow colonic transit and the ensuing desiccation of the stool. Patients do not complain of abdominal pain but rather have non-specific symptoms of bloating, increased flatus, and mild malaise. Fecal impactions, which rarely occur except in elderly or sedentary patients, may cause overflow diarrhea or bleeding from stercoral rectal ulcers.

Although the pathophysiology of primary constipation is poorly understood, most patients respond quickly to increased fiber and water in their diets. The chronic use of stimulant laxatives has the potential to damage the myenteric plexus, causing an unresponsive "cathartic colon."

IRRITABLE BOWEL SYNDROME (SPASTIC COLON) (see Chapter 131). Patients with constipation-predominant irritable bowel syndrome may have alterations in both smooth muscle and myenteric nerve function. Propagating contractions are generally absent in the constipated patients. In approximately 40% of patients with constipation-predominant irritable bowel syndrome, there is no postprandial increase in segmenting contractions. Therapy is aimed at improving colonic motility and decreasing the visceral hypersensitivity (see Chapter 131).

ACQUIRED DIVERTICULAR DISEASE OF THE COLON. Diverticular disease, mucosal outpouchings through the colonic wall that occur with aging, results in a spectrum of abnormalities extending from no symptoms to diverticulitis. Acquired diverticula, which occur most frequently in the left colon, result from increased intraluminal pressure pushing sleeves of mucosa through perivascular weaknesses in the wall of the colon juxtaposed to the taeniae coli (Chapter 136). The predilection for the left colon is because of the decreased colonic diameter and resulting increased pressures, as predicted by Laplace's law: intraluminal pressure is directly correlated with wall tension and inversely correlated with bowel diameter. Decreased dietary fiber and distal colonic smooth muscle hypertrophy contribute to elevation in distal colonic intraluminal pressure.

The symptoms of painful colonic diverticular disease are similar to those of irritable bowel syndrome but are more likely to be localized in the left lower quadrant. When diverticulitis occurs as a complication, the patient may have fever, left lower quadrant mass, leukocytosis, and occult blood in the stool (see Chapter 136). Physical exercise decreases the incidence of symptomatic diverticular disease. Gross hematochezia is more frequent in asymptomatic patients with diverticula. Diverticula can be diagnosed by barium enema or colonoscopy. Muscular hypertrophy gives a saw tooth pattern visible on barium enema. Narrowing due to diverticular inflammation can be difficult to differentiate from carcinoma of the colon.

Painful diverticular disease of the colon is best treated by decreasing the intraluminal pressure, similar to the therapy for the irritable bowel syndrome. Narcotics, especially morphine, should be avoided because of an exaggerated increase in smooth muscle contraction.

FUNCTIONAL ANAL OUTLET OBSTRUCTION. Constipation may result from a disturbance in the elimination of stool through the anal sphincter. Elimination normally begins by the involuntary relaxation of the internal anal sphincter after distention of the rectum. Voluntary controls open the rectoanal angle and relax the external anal sphincter. A disturbance of any component of this mechanism leads to constipation.

Hirschsprung's disease is the congenital absence of enteric neurons in the submucosal and myenteric plexuses, owing to an arrest of the embryonic caudal migration of the enteric neurons along the gut. Several studies have localized the genetic defect to the chromosomal loci *ret* proto-oncogene, endothelin B, and endothelin 3. The aganglionic segment remains contracted, dilating the proximal normal bowel. Absence of nitric oxide synthase and the consequent absence of the inhibitory mediator nitric oxide may cause the constant contraction of the affected bowel. The severity of symptoms and the age at diagnosis are related to the length of the aganglionic segment. Involvement of the entire rectum or additional parts of the colon results in constipation or obstipation in infancy, requiring emergent resection of the aganglionic bowel and a pull-through anastomosis to the anus. If a short segment of the distal rectum is aganglionic, the patient may not present with symptoms until adolescence or even adulthood.

Abnormalities in anal physiology are a significant cause of constipation; impaired anal sphincter relaxation occurs relatively frequently in adults. The absent rectoanal reflex may be secondary to a short aganglionic segment (short-segment Hirschsprung's disease), to chronic distention with a fecal impaction, or to an insufficient distention stimulus due to an enlarged rectal vault. In acquired megacolon, relaxation of the internal anal sphincter may be impaired if a large volume is not used to distend the rectum. Some patients have subtle histologic abnormalities in the myenteric plexus, suggesting that an acquired neuropathy may also account for the abnormal sphincter response. In the spastic pelvic floor syndrome (animus), the external anal sphincter and the puborectalis relax poorly or the levator ani contracts poorly, leading to impaired opening of the rectoanal angle (Chapter 143). This acquired condition, which occurs more often in multiparous women, can prevent normal stool evacuation. Impaired internal anal sphincter relaxation in an adult may respond to a posterior anal sphincter myomectomy.

Slow Transit with Decreased Segmenting Contractions

Patients with decreased segmenting contractions after stimulation have symptoms similar to those in patients with increased contractions. The colonic inertia form of the irritable bowel syndrome and primary colonic pseudo-obstruction may be a similar pathophysiologic disturbance. Postprandial increases in colonic motility are absent in both, but the colon is dilated in primary intestinal pseudo-obstruction, explaining the increased incidence of abdominal distention. Constipation is a major symptom in both conditions. Ogilvie's syndrome is a form of primary colonic pseudo-obstruction that often is paraneoplastic.

Constipation is present in many patients with chronic, insulin-requiring diabetes mellitus, progressive systemic sclerosis, or thoracic spinal cord lesions. There is no postprandial increase in colonic motility in these patients. In patients with diabetes or spinal cord lesions, colonic smooth muscle can be stimulated with exogenous drugs, suggesting a neural lesion, not a myopathy. In progressive systemic sclerosis, the colon cannot increase intraluminal pressure after drug stimulation.

It is difficult to treat patients with decreased colonic motility. In patients with neuropathy and normal smooth muscle function, prokinetic drugs have had some success. In myopathy, pharmacologic stimulation usually has no effect. Colonic resection with an ileoanal anastomosis has successfully treated patients with colonic inertia who do not have motility disorders in the upper gastrointestinal tract.

Rapid Transit

FUNCTIONAL DIARRHEA. Some patients have functional, painless diarrhea with fecal urgency but with no associated anatomic or histologic abnormality of the gastrointestinal tract. These patients present with small frequent stools, consistent with a large bowel

diarrhea; fecal incontinence is relatively frequent because their anal sphincters cannot retard evacuation of liquid stool. Lactose intolerance must be excluded either by history or by specific tests of lactose intolerance. The diarrhea is greater than that in the spastic irritable colon syndrome, and abdominal pain may be absent.

Segmenting postprandial contractile activity is decreased in functional diarrhea. Propagating contractions are increased and propagate into the rectum, possibly accounting for the increased urgency and fecal incontinence in these patients. The lack of segmenting contractions to impede forward movement or transit may exacerbate the urgency. Increased concentrations of fecal bile salts contribute to the functional diarrhea by irritating colonic sensory nerves.

In treating functional diarrhea, antidiarrheal agents such as the opioid analogues, loperamide, and diphenoxylate decrease symptoms. Fecal continence improves as the stool consistency becomes firmer. Some patients may require biofeedback training to maintain continence. If excess bile salts contribute to the diarrhea, low doses of cholestyramine may decrease the diarrhea. Microscopic and collagenous colitis may respond to 5-aminosalicylic compounds.

SURREPTITIOUS LAXATIVE ABUSE. Surreptitious laxative abuse is a common but difficult to diagnose cause of functional diarrhea (see Chapter 227). Oxyphenisatin and bisacodyl stimulate increased numbers of propagating contractions and diarrhea. Patients may take these or other laxatives as a manifestation of a psychiatric disorder.

ULCERATIVE COLITIS (see Chapter 135). Rapid transit of colonic contents and increased mucosal secretion occur in patients with active ulcerative colitis. As in the other colonic causes of diarrhea, propagating contractions are increased in number and propagate into the rectum, accounting for the significant incidence of fecal incontinence. The rapid transit improves as the mucosal inflammation decreases after therapy for the underlying inflammation.

DRUGS THAT AFFECT GASTROINTESTINAL MOTILITY

Drugs that stimulate motility may indiscriminately increase smooth muscle contractions or increase a specific motility function, such as migrating motor complex initiation (Table 132–6). When some of these drugs are used to treat other systemic diseases, they may precipitate gastrointestinal symptoms as a side effect.

Excitatory Agents

Drugs that excite the gastrointestinal tract should be used to treat decreased motility when the smooth muscle can functionally contract. In general, patients who benefit from these agents have an enteric neuropathy with decreased release of endogenous stimulatory neurotransmitters or an increased release of inhibitory neurotransmitters. When the smooth muscle is absent or severely damaged, the prokinetic drugs are rarely helpful. Acetylcholine analogues, such as bethanechol, stimulate both longitudinal and circular gastrointestinal smooth muscle by directly binding to the M_2 muscarinic receptor to release inositol triphosphate or to open receptor-operated or voltage-dependent calcium channels. Drugs that block acetylcholinesterase increase endogenous acetylcholine concentration at the myoneural junction. These drugs have a theoretical advantage in regulating as well as in increasing motility, because the distribution of acetylcholine release is predetermined by the autonomic nervous system.

Dopamine antagonists can variably increase motility throughout the gastrointestinal tract. Metoclopramide, a centrally and peripherally acting dopamine antagonist, increases gastric emptying and transit through the small intestine and the colon; it is useful in diabetic gastroparesis and constipation but has little therapeutic value in symptomatic patients with progressive systemic sclerosis or in many patients with pseudo-obstruction. Domperidone, a peripherally acting dopamine antagonist, mainly increases gastric emptying and has little therapeutic effect in small intestinal or colonic motility disorders.

Cisapride may stimulate motility through agonism of a serotonin 5-HT$_4$ receptor in the bowel. It stimulates gastric emptying, increases small intestinal transit, and stimulates colonic contractility. Cisapride may improve symptoms in patients with decreased gastric emptying, small intestinal pseudo-obstruction, or colonic inertia.

Table 132-6 ■ EFFECTS OF DRUGS ON SMALL AND LARGE INTESTINAL CONTRACTILITY

DRUG	EFFECT ON STOMACH	EFFECT ON SMALL INTESTINE	EFFECT ON COLON	MECHANISM OF ACTION
Acetylcholine analogues	Excitatory	Excitatory	Excitatory	Agonist of muscarinic receptors on muscle cells
Neostigmine	Excitatory	Excitatory	Excitatory	Acetylcholine esterase inhibitor
Metoclopramide	Excitatory	Excitatory	Excitatory	Dopamine antagonist (central, peripheral)
Domperidone	Excitatory	Excitatory	No effect	Dopamine antagonist (peripheral)
Cisapride	Excitatory	Excitatory	Excitatory	5-HT$_4$ agonist
Macrolide antibiotics	Excitatory	Excitatory	?	Binds to motilin receptor
Octreotide (low dose)	No effect	Excitatory	?	Possible block of inhibitory neurons
Leuprolide acetate	?	Excitatory	?	Reduces progesterone and relaxin
Atropine	Inhibitory	Inhibitory	Inhibitory	Antagonist of muscarinic receptor
Secoverine	?	Inhibitory	Inhibitory	Antagonist of M$_2$ muscarinic receptors on muscle cells
Papaverine	?	?	Inhibitory	Unknown
Calcium channel blockers	Inhibitory	Inhibitory	Inhibitory	Blocks voltage-operated calcium channels
Nitrate compounds	?	Inhibitory	Inhibitory	Blockade of receptor-operated calcium channels; increase of intracellular cGMP
Peppermint oil	?	Inhibitory	Inhibitory	Possible block of calcium channels
Cholecytokinin antagonists	?	?	?	Blocks CCK receptors

Erythromycin stimulates migrating motor complex activity, which is absent in many patients with neuropathic pseudo-obstruction, by binding at the motilin receptor on the small intestinal smooth muscle cell. Low dose octreotide (<100 μg) initiates phase 3 of the migrating motor complex, which also makes it useful in patients with pseudo-obstruction.

Leuprolide acetate may improve symptoms secondary to functional disturbances of small intestinal motility. This drug is believed to work by decreasing the concentrations of the smooth muscle inhibitory hormones progesterone and relaxin.

Inhibitory Agents

Inhibitory drugs should be most useful for treating patients whose symptoms result from increased motility, which causes uncoordinated movement of the intestinal contents. The inhibitory drugs may block the receptors for excitatory neurotransmitters or block the increase in intracellular calcium necessary for normal smooth muscle contraction.

Anticholinergic drugs, which inhibit muscarinic receptor stimulation, are sometimes effective for the small intestinal or colonic variants of the irritable bowel syndrome. The anticholinergics must be used with care in patients who may develop urinary retention (e.g., prostatism) or glaucoma.

Several classes of calcium channel blockers, including verapamil and the dihydropyridines, such as nifedipine, inhibit the increase in intracellular calcium that is necessary for smooth muscle contraction and hence decrease smooth muscle contraction. These may be used in some patients with increased small intestinal or colonic motility. Nitrate compounds inhibit smooth muscle contraction, probably by increasing the intracellular concentration of cyclic guanosine monophosphate and decreasing calcium influx into the smooth muscle cell.

Peppermint oil relaxes smooth muscle, which improves symptoms in some patients with the irritable bowel syndrome. Cholecystokinin antagonists may prove useful for treating multiple gastrointestinal motility disorders.

Bueno L, Fioramonti J, Delvaux M, Frexinos J: Mediators and pharmacology of visceral sensitivity: From basic to clinical investigations. Gastroenterolgy 112:1714–1743, 1997. *Comprehensive review of the pathophysiology of increased visceral pain; can serve as a guide to therapy for abdominal pain.*

Camilleri M, Hasler WL, Parkman HP, et al: Measurement of gastrointestinal motility in the GI laboratory. Gastroenterology 115:747–762, 1998. *Excellent review of techniques used in patients with disease.*

Camilleri M, Ford MJ: Colonic sensorimotor physiology in health, and its alteration in constipation and diarrheal disorders. Aliment Pharmacol Ther 12:287–302, 1998. *A review article on sensorimotor physiology.*

DiLorenzo C: Pseudo-obstruction: Current approaches. Gastroenterology 116:980–987, 1999. *A helpful review.*

Koch KL, Stern RM: Functional disorders of the stomach. Semin Gastrointest Disord 7:185–195, 1996. *Excellent review of motility disorders of the upper gastrointestinal tract with explanation of work-up.*

Noor N, Small PK, London MA, et al: Effects of cisapride on symptoms and postcibal small-bowel motor function in patients with irritable bowel syndrome. Scand J Gastroenterol 33:605–611, 1998. *Cisapride has a therapeutic effect on patients with bowel dysmotility associated with symptoms of the irritable bowel syndrome.*

Snape WJ Jr: Role of motility measurement in managing upper gastrointestinal dysfunction. Gastroenterologist 6:44–59, 1998. *Discussion of techniques for measuring motility in symptomatic patients.*

133 APPROACH TO THE PATIENT WITH DIARRHEA

Don W. Powell

DEFINITIONS

Normal stool frequency ranges from three times a week to three times a day. Although individuals rarely cite increases in frequency alone as the definition of diarrhea, a decrease in stool consistency (increased fluidity) and stools that cause urgency or abdominal discomfort are likely to be termed *diarrhea. Consistency* is defined as the ratio of fecal water to the water-holding capacity of fecal insoluble solids, which are made up of bacterial mass and dietary fiber. One half of the dry weight of stool is bacteria. Because it is very difficult to measure stool consistency and because stool is predominantly (60–85%) water, stool weight becomes a reasonable surrogate of consistency.

Physicians often define diarrhea as a physical sign, 24-hour stool excretion by weight or volume, rather than as a symptom. Daily stool weights of children and adults are less than 200 g, and greater stool weights are an objective definition of diarrhea; however, this definition will miss 20% of diarrheal symptoms in patients with loose stools below this daily weight.

Acute diarrheas are defined as those of less than 2 to 3 weeks', and rarely 6 to 8 weeks', duration. The most common cause of acute diarrheas are infectious agents. *Chronic diarrheas* are those of at least 4 and, more usually, greater than 6 to 8 weeks' duration. There are three categories of chronic diarrheas: osmotic (malabsorptive) diarrhea, secretory diarrhea, and inflammatory diarrhea.

EPIDEMIOLOGY

More than 3 million deaths occur each year from acute diarrhea in infants and children in developing nations, where two thirds of the world's population live in extreme poverty with inadequate sewage disposal and water supplies, insufficient food, lack of refrigeration, poor education, and lack of access to health care. The incidence of infant and child diarrheal deaths in the United States decreased by 75% between 1968 and 1991 but remains more than 500 deaths each year. The acute diarrheal death rate for children and young adults in the United States is 2 to 3/100,000 persons, but it is 15/100,000 for persons older than age 74. In the United

States, diarrheal diseases are frequent and severe enough to result in over 300,000 hospital admissions, 6 million visits to physicians, and 48 million episodes that last at least one full day and result in loss of time from school or work. Although improvement in sanitation and education in the United States has decreased rates for infectious parasitic diarrheas, diarrheas resulting from person-to-person contact (e.g., rotavirus) and from food-borne transmission (e.g., *Salmonella* or *Campylobacter*) have doubled in the past 10 years.

The appropriate population studies have not been performed to determine the incidence or prevalence of chronic diarrhea. The best estimate is that chronic diarrhea occurs in approximately 5% of the U.S. population.

PATHOPHYSIOLOGY

Abnormalities of Fluid and Electrolyte Transport

Diarrhea was once thought to be caused principally by abnormal gastrointestinal motility. It is now clear, however, that most diarrheal conditions are due primarily to alterations of intestinal fluid and electrolyte transport and less to smooth muscle function.

Each 24 hours 8 to 10 L of fluid enters the duodenum with 800 mEq sodium (Na^+), 700 mEq chloride (Cl^-), and 100 mEq potassium (K^+). The diet supplies 2 L of this fluid; the remainder comes from salivary, stomach, liver, pancreatic, and duodenal secretions. The small intestine normally absorbs 8 to 9 L of this fluid and presents 1.5 L to the colon for absorption. Of the remaining fluid, the colon absorbs all but approximately 100 mL, which contains 3, 8, and 2 mEq of Na^+, K^+, and Cl^-, respectively. Diarrhea can result from decreased absorption or increased secretion by either the small intestine or the colon. If either deranged electrolyte transport or the presence of non-absorbable solutes in the intestinal lumen reduces the absorptive capacity of the small intestine by 50%, the volume of fluid (50% of 10 L, or 5 L) presented daily to the normal colon would exceed its maximum daily absorptive capacity of 4 L. Stool excretion of 1000 mL would result, which by definition is diarrhea. Alternatively, if the colon is deranged so that it cannot absorb even the 1.5 L normally presented to it by the small intestine, then a stool volume of greater than 200 mL/24 hours would result, again defined as diarrhea.

At the cellular level, excess intraluminal fluid volumes occur when there is a derangement of electrolyte transport capabilities of the small or large intestine or when osmotic solutes in the bowel lumen create an adverse osmotic gradient that the normal electrolyte absorptive mechanisms cannot overcome. Na^+ transport by the epithelium from lumen to blood (by Na^+:H^+ exchange proteins in the small intestine and proximal colon and by amiloride-sensitive Na^+ channels in the distal colon) create a favorable osmotic gradient for absorption. Na^+ absorption in the small intestine can be enhanced by the glucose and galactose or by amino acids in the lumen because of the presence of Na^+-coupled sugar and amino acid transporters in the small bowel epithelium. Oral rehydration solutions, which are used extensively to replace diarrheal fluid and electrolyte losses, are effective because they contain Na^+, sugars, and, often, protein (amino acids). If unabsorbable solutes (e.g., lactose in lactase-deficient individuals, polyethylene glycol in colon-cleansing solutions, or magnesium [Mg^{2+}] citrate in cathartics) are present in the lumen, the Na^+-absorbing mechanisms are incapable of creating an osmotic gradient favorable for absorption; as a result, fluid remains in the lumen and is the basis of osmotic or malabsorptive diarrhea.

Active Cl^- secretion or inhibited Na^+ absorption also creates an osmotic gradient favorable for the movement of fluids from blood to lumen and is the basis of the secretory diarrheas. Agents that increase enterocyte cyclic adenosine monophosphate, cyclic guanosine monophosphate, or intracellular ionized calcium (Ca^{2+}) all inhibit Na^+ absorption and stimulate Cl^- secretion (Table 133–1).

Classification of Diarrhea

To understand the three general categories of diarrhea—malabsorption (osmotic diarrheas), secretory diarrheas, and inflammatory diarrheas—it is necessary to understand how the normal intestine handles fluid and solutes in health and disease.

Regardless of whether a subject ingests a hypotonic meal, such as a steak, or a hypertonic meal, such as milk and doughnut, the

Table 133–1 ■ AGENTS THAT CAUSE INTESTINAL SECRETION

Laxatives
  Phenolphthalein, anthraquinones, bisacodyl, oxyphenisatin, senna, aloe, ricinoleic acid (castor oil), dioctyl sodium sulfosuccinate; endogenous laxatives such as dihydroxy bile acids and long-chain fatty acids
Medications/drugs
  Diuretics (furosemide, thiazides), coffee, tea, or cola (caffeine and other methylxanthines); asthma medication (theophylline)
  Cholinergic drugs, glaucoma eye drops and bladder stimulants (acetylcholine analogues or mimetics); myesthenia gravis medication (cholinesterase inhibitors); cardiac drugs (quinidine and quinine); gout medication (colchicine); antihypertensives (ACE inhibitors); H_2 blocker (ranitidine); antidepressants (selective serotonin reuptake inhibitors)
  Prostaglandins (misoprostol); di-5-aminosalicylic acid (azodisalicylate); gold (may also cause colitis)
Toxins
  Metals (arsenic); plant (mushroom, e.g., *Amanita phalloides*); organophosphates (insecticides and nerve poisons); seafood toxins (ciguatera, scombroid poisoning, paralytic, diarrhetic or neurotoxic shellfish poisoning); monosodium glutamate
Bacterial enterotoxins
  Vibrio cholerae, toxigenic *Escherichia coli* (heat-labile and heat-stable toxins), *Campylobacter, Yersinia, Klebsiella, Clostridium difficile, Staphylococcus aureus* (toxic shock syndrome); *Clostridium perfringens* and *C. botulinum, Bacillus cereus*
Hormone-producing tumors
  Vipoma and ganlioneuromas; medullary carcinoma of thyroid (calcitonin and prostaglandins); mastocytosis (histamine), villous adenoma (prostaglandins)
Inflammatory conditions
  Allergy and anaphylaxis (histamine, serotonin, platelet-activating factor, prostaglandins); infection (reactive oxygen metabolites, platelet-activating factor, prostaglandins, histamine); idiopathic inflammation, inflammatory bowel disease, celiac disease
Ischemic colitis

Adapted from Powell DW: Approach to the patient with diarrhea. *In* Yamada T, Alpers DH, Owyang C, et al (eds): Textbook of Gastroenterology, 3rd ed. Philadelphia, Lippincott–Raven, 1999.

volume of the meal is augmented by gastric, pancreatic, biliary, and duodenal secretions. The very permeable duodenum then renders the meal approximately isotonic with an electrolyte content similar to plasma by the time it reaches the proximal jejunum. As the chyme moves toward the colon, the Na^+ concentrations in the luminal fluid remain constant, but Cl^- is reduced to 60 to 70 mmol/L, and bicarbonate (HCO_3^-) is increased to a similar concentration as the result of the Cl^- and HCO_3^- transport mechanisms in the enterocyte. In the colon, K^+ is secreted, and the amiloride-sensitive Na^+ transport mechanism of the colonocyte and the low epithelial permeability extract Na^+ and fluid from the stool. As a result, the Na^+ content of stool drops to 30 to 40 mmol/L, K^+ increases from 5 to 10 mmol/L in the small bowel to 75 to 90 mmol/L, and poorly absorbed divalent cations such as Mg^{2+} and Ca^{2+} are concentrated in stool to values of 5 to 100 mmol/L. The anion concentrations in the colon change drastically because bacterial degradation of carbohydrate (i.e., unabsorbed starches, sugars, and fiber) creates short-chain fatty acids that attain concentrations of 80 to 180 mmol/L. At colonic pH, these are present as organic anions such as acetate, propionate, and butyrate. These fatty acids/anions may decrease stool pH to 4 or lower. The osmolality of stools is approximately that of plasma (280 to 300 mOsm) when it is passed.

With ingestion of either unabsorbable solute (i.e., Mg^{2+} or polyethylene glycol) or unabsorbed carbohydrate (i.e., lactulose or, in lactase-deficient individuals, lactose), a considerable proportion of the osmolality of stool results from the non-absorbed solute. This gap between stool osmolality and the sum of the electrolytes in the stool causes osmotic diarrhea.

Inflammatory diarrheas are characterized by enterocyte damage and death, villous atrophy, and crypt hyperplasia. The enterocytes on rudimentary villi of the small intestine are immature cells with poor disaccharidase and peptide hydrolase activity, reduced or absent Na^+-coupled sugar or amino acid transport mechanisms, and reduced or absent NaCl absorptive transporters. Conversely, the hyperplastic crypt cells maintain their ability to secrete Cl^- (and perhaps HCO_3^-). If the inflammation is severe, immune-mediated vascular damage or ulceration allows protein to leak (exudate) from capillaries and lymphatics and contribute to the diarrhea. Lymphocyte and phagocyte activation releases various inflammatory mediators that induce intestinal secretion. Interleukin-1 and tumor necrosis factor are also released into the blood.

ACUTE DIARRHEAS

Sporadic and Food/Water-Borne Infectious Diarrhea

Most infectious diarrheas are acquired through fecal-oral transmission from water, food, or person-to-person contact (Table 133–2). Patients with infectious diarrhea often complain of nausea, vomiting, and abdominal pain and have either watery, malabsorptive, or bloody diarrhea and fever (dysentery) (see Chapters 339–348). Many of the short-lived watery diarrheas ascribed to "viral gastroenteritis" are likely to be mild, sporadic, food-borne bacterial infections. In addition to enteric infections, certain systemic infections (e.g., hepatitis, listeriosis, and legionellosis) may cause substantial diarrhea.

The incidence of food-borne illness in the United States is estimated to be 6 to 80 million cases per year, including at least 9000 deaths annually. The incidence may be underestimated because most patients present with sporadic diarrhea rather than as part of a clear epidemic, and most epidemic diarrheas are not reported. Emerging food-borne diseases in the United States include the *enteritides* serotype of *Salmonella, Campylobacter jejuni, Escherichia coli* O157:H7, and *Cyclospora* infections. Fish can become contaminated in their own environment (especially the filter-feeding bivalve molluscs such as mussels, clams, oysters, and scallops) or by food handlers. Organisms that are specific for seafood include *Vibrio parahemolyticus,* which causes either watery or bloody diarrhea, and *V. vulnificus,* which causes watery diarrhea and, especially in those with liver disease, a fatal septicemia.

Food- and Water-Borne Poisonings

Food poisoning occurs with environmental chemicals such as monosodium glutamate (used in Asian food), heavy metals (arsenic from rat poison), or insecticides and with natural toxins found in mushrooms and seafood (fin fish or shellfish). Most of these toxins cause varying combinations of gastrointestinal and neurologic symptoms. Arsenic also induces cardiovascular collapse at higher, acute doses; and one form of mushroom (*Amanita*) poisoning can cause acute liver and kidney failure.

Diarrhea and neurologic symptoms (tingling and burning around the mouth, facial flushing, sweating, headache, palpitations, and dizziness) of seafood poisoning may be caused by histamine release from the decaying flesh of blood fish (mahi-mahi, tuna, marlin, or mackerel) after it is caught. This form of seafood poisoning is called *scomboid.* Plankton, algae, or dinoflagellates ingested by tropical fish (amberjack, snapper, grouper, or barracuda) produce a toxin (ciguatoxin) that causes seafood poisoning known as ciguatera. Fish from the Albermarle-Pamlico estuary ingest toxic dinoflagellates that cause *Pfisteria piscicida* poisoning. The dinoflagellate toxins cause nausea, vomiting, abdominal pain, diarrhea, and neurologic symptoms such as weakness, pruritus, circumoral paresthesias, temperature reversal (hot drinks taste cold and vice versa) and even psychiatric abnormalities and memory loss. Shellfish poisonings are also due to algae or dinoflagellates ingested by bivalve mollusks; these different toxins may cause predominantly and occasionally severe neurologic symptoms (paralytic, neurotoxic or amnestic shellfish poisonings) or predominantly gastrointestinal symptoms (diarrhetic shellfish poisoning). Puffer fish poisoning (tetrodotoxin) causes neurologic symptoms, respiratory paralysis, or even death.

High-Risk Groups

ANTIBIOTIC-ASSOCIATED DIARRHEAS. Diarrhea may occur in up to 20% of patients receiving broad-spectrum antibiotics; only half or less of these diarrheas are due to *Clostridium difficile* colitis (pseudomembranous colitis). Non–*C. difficile* diarrhea is mild and self-limited, and it clears spontaneously or in response to cholestyramine therapy. *C. difficile* colitis, however, can cause severe diarrhea and may have a relapsing course after seemingly successful therapy with metronidazole or vancomycin.

TRAVELERS' DIARRHEA. North American travelers to developing countries and travelers on airplanes and cruise ships where errors in food preparation occur are at high risk for acute infectious diarrhea. Bacterial agents account for 85% of travelers' diarrhea.

SEXUALLY TRANSMITTED AND AIDS DIARRHEAS. Homosexuals and prostitutes develop infectious diarrhea through the oral-fecal route. The incidence of infectious diarrhea among homosexuals (gay bowel syndrome) has markedly decreased, but the decline has been more than offset by the high incidence and seriousness of enteric infections in the acquired immunodeficiency syndrome (AIDS) (see Chapter 413).

DAY CARE DIARRHEA. Over 6 million children in the United States attend day care, and diarrhea from organisms that colonize at a low inoculum dose (e.g., *Shigella, Giardia, Cryptosporidium*) or those that are spread easily (e.g., rotavirus, astrovirus, adenovirus) is extremely prevalent in this setting. The secondary attack rate for parents and siblings is 10 to 20%.

Diagnosis of Acute Infectious Diarrhea (Fig. 133–1; see also Chapters 339–348)

The differential diagnosis of acute watery diarrhea includes food toxins, drugs, medications, and diseases (see Table 133–1). The use of the laboratory to make the diagnosis of infectious diarrhea

---

Table 133–2 ■ EPIDEMIOLOGY OF ACUTE INFECTIOUS DIARRHEA AND INFECTIOUS FOOD-BORNE ILLNESS

VEHICLE	CLASSIC PATHOGEN
Water (including foods washed in such water)	*Vibrio cholerae,* Norwalk agent, *Giardia* and *Cryptosporidium*
Food	
Poultry	*Salmonella, Campylobacter,* and *Shigella* species
Beef, unpasteurized fruit juice	Enterohemorrhagic *Escherichia coli*
Pork	Tapeworm
Seafood and shellfish (including raw sushi and gefilte fish)	*V. cholerae, parahaemolyticus,* and *vulnificus;* Salmonella and Shigella species; hepatitis A and B; tapeworm; and anisakiasis
Cheese, milk	*Listeria* species
Eggs	*Salmonella* species
Mayonnaise-containing foods and cream pies	Staphylococcal and clostridial food poisonings
Fried rice	*Bacillus cereus*
Fresh berries	*Cyclospora* species
Canned vegetables or fruits	*Clostridium* species
Animal-to-person (pets and livestock)	*Salmonella, Campylobacter, Cryptosporidium,* and *Giardia* species
Person-to-person (including sexual contact)	All enteric bacteria, viruses, and parasites
Day care center	*Shigella, Campylobacter, Cryptosporidium,* and *Giardia* species; viruses, *Clostridium difficile*
Hospital, antibiotics or chemotherapy	*C. difficile*
Swimming pool	*Giardia* and *Cryptosporidium* species
Foreign travel	*E. coli* of various types; *Salmonella, Shigella, Campylobacter, Giardia,* and *Cryptosporidium* species; *Entamoeba histolytica*

Adapted from Powell DW: Approach to the patient with diarrhea. *In* Yamada T, Alpers DH, Owyang C, et al (eds.): Textbook of Gastroenterology, 3rd ed. Philadelphia, Lippincott–Raven, 1999.

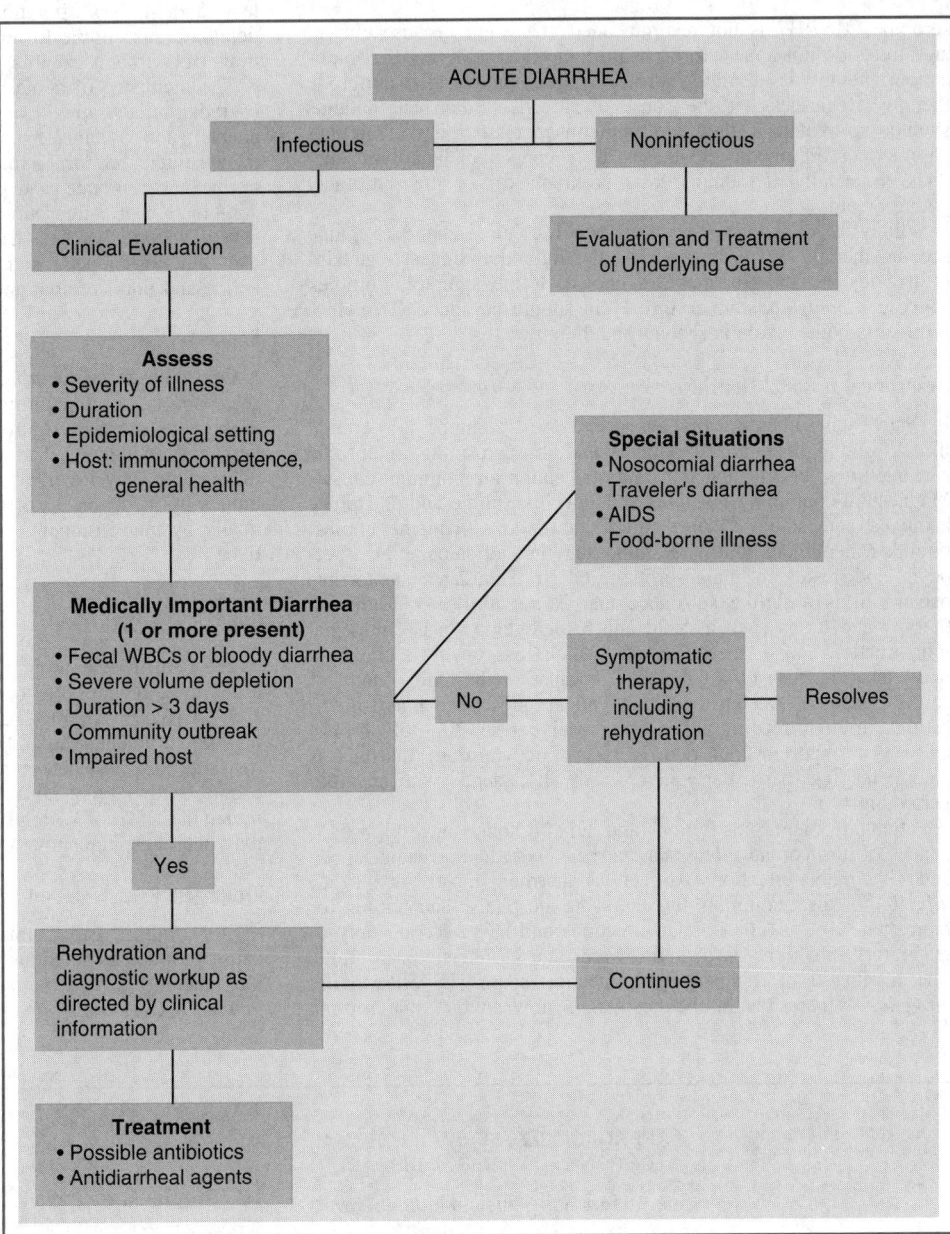

FIGURE 133–1 ■ Algorithm for the diagnostic approach to acute diarrhea. (Adapted from Parks SI, Giannella R: Approach to the patient with acute diarrhea. Gastroenterol Clin North Am 22: 483, 1993.)

can be reduced if the evaluation focuses on *Campylobacter, Salmonella, Shigella,* and *C. difficile* and if only liquid stools are cultured. Organisms that can cause diarrhea and that are not routinely sought by most clinical microbiology laboratories unless specifically requested include *Yersinia, Plesiomonas,* enterohemorrhagic *E. coli* serotype O157:H7, *Aeromonas, Cryptosporidium, Cyclospora, Microsporidia,* and non-cholera *Vibrio.* Parasites such as *Giardia* as well as *Strongyloides* and enteroadherent bacteria may be difficult to detect in stool but may be diagnosed by intestinal biopsy. Even with the use of all available laboratory techniques, the cause of 20% to 40% of all acute infectious diarrheas remains undiagnosed.

Treatment of Acute Infectious Diarrhea

The treatment of diarrhea can be symptomatic (fluid replacement and antidiarrheal agents) and/or specific (antimicrobial therapy). Because death in acute diarrhea is caused by dehydration, an important principle is to assess the degree of dehydration and replace fluid and electrolyte deficits. Severely dehydrated individuals should be rehydrated with intravenous Ringer's lactate or saline solutions to which additional K^+ and $NaHCO_3^-$ may be added as necessary. Alert patients should be given oral replacement solutions. In mild to moderate dehydration, oral replacement solutions

can be given to infants and children in volumes of 50 to 100 mL/kg over a period of 4 to 6 hours; adults may need to drink up to 1000 mL/hour. After the patient is rehydrated, oral replacement solutions are given at rates equaling stool loss plus insensible losses until the diarrhea ceases.

Bismuth subsalicylate (Pepto-Bismol) is safe and efficacious in bacterial infectious diarrheas, whereas kaolin-pectin preparations are only minimally effective. Because of the possibility of worsening the colonization or invasion of infectious organisms by paralyzing intestinal motility and because of evidence that the use of motility-altering drugs may prolong microorganism excretion time, neither opiates nor anticholinergic drugs are recommended for infectious diarrheas. However, loperamide can be both useful and safe in acute or travelers' diarrhea, provided it is not given to patients with dysentery (high fever, with blood or pus in the stool), and especially when administered concomitantly with effective antibiotics. Anxiolytics and antiemetics that decrease sensory perception may make symptoms more tolerable and are safe.

Certain infectious diarrheas should be treated with antibiotics: shigellosis, cholera, travelers' diarrhea, pseudomembranous enterocolitis, parasitic infestations, and sexually transmitted diseases. Antibiotics are not usually indicated in viral diarrhea and cryptosporidiosis because there is no effective therapy. Treatment of *E. coli* serotype O157:H7 is not recommended at present because current antibiotics do not appear to be helpful and the incidence of complications (hemolytic-uremic syndrome) may be greater after antibiotic therapy. Regardless of the cause of infectious diarrhea, patients should be treated if they are immunosuppressed; have valvular, vascular, or orthopedic prostheses; have congenital hemolytic anemias (especially if salmonellosis is involved); or are extremely young or old.

While the clinician is awaiting stool culture results to guide specific therapy (see Chapter 339), the fluoroquinolones (e.g., ciprofloxacin) are the treatment of choice. If the symptom-complex suggests *Campylobacter*, erythromycin should be added. Trimethoprim-sulfamethoxazole is second-line therapy.

Nosocomial Hospital Diarrheas

Diarrhea is either the first or second most common nosocomial illness among hospitalized patients and those residing in chronic care facilities. Fecal impaction and medication are common causes. Magnesium-containing laxatives and antacids, sulfate and phosphate laxatives, and lactulose cause osmotic diarrheas. Colchicine, cholestyramine, neomycin, and para-aminosalicylic acid damage the enterocyte and result in malabsorption. Olestra simulates steatorrhea because it is a fatlike substance that is not absorbed. Radiation therapy and drugs such as gold and α-methyldopa cause intestinal inflammation and diarrhea. Liquid formulations of any medication may cause diarrhea (elixir diarrhea) because of the high content of sorbitol used to sweeten the elixir. Patients prescribed liquid medications through feeding tubes may receive over 20 g of sorbitol daily. An important but poorly understood cause of diarrhea is enteral feeding, particularly in critically ill patients, who may develop diarrhea.

Patients in mental institutions and nursing homes have high incidences of nosocomial infectious diarrheas (e.g., hemorrhagic *E. coli* and *C. difficile* infections). Infectious diarrhea (mostly due to *C. difficile*) is also common in acute-care hospitals, accounting for more than 20% of nosocomial infections and being second only to respiratory infections on pediatric wards and in intensive care units. The likelihood of a nosocomial infection caused by *Salmonella*, *Shigella*, or parasites in the hospital is now so rare that routine evaluation for these agents is not cost effective if diarrhea begins at least 3 or 4 days after hospital admission. Immunosuppressed patients are susceptible to nosocomial diarrhea, especially viral infections (rotavirus, astrovirus, adenovirus, and coxsackievirus).

The incidence of acute, mild diarrhea with cancer chemotherapy or radiation therapy is quite high, approaching 100% with some agents such as amsacrine, azacitidine, cytarabine, dactinomycin, daunorubicin, doxorubicin, floxuridine, 5-fluorouracil, 6-mercaptopurine, methotrexate, and plicamycin. Interleukin-2 therapy and the combination of 5-fluorouracil plus leucovorin are frequent causes of severe watery diarrhea. Current treatment for both chemotherapy- and radiation-induced diarrhea is symptomatic and includes loperamide and non-steroidal anti-inflammatory drugs (NSAIDs).

Runner's Diarrhea

Gastrointestinal disturbances including anorexia, heartburn, nausea, vomiting, cramps, urgency, and diarrhea occur in 10 to 25% of those who exercise vigorously, particularly women marathon runners and triathletes. The pathophysiology in runner's diarrhea is unclear but may involve release of intestinal secretogogues or hormones by ischemia. Loperamide and NSAIDs are taken prophylactically by many runners, but it is not clear whether they are effective.

CHRONIC DIARRHEA

The goal in evaluating a patient with chronic diarrhea is to make a definitive diagnosis as quickly and inexpensively as possible (Fig. 133–2). In 25 to 50%, expert history and physical examination may be sufficient. The addition of stool culture and examination for ova and parasites, determination of stool fat, and flexible sigmoidoscopy with biopsy raises the diagnostic rate to about 75%. The remaining 25% of patients with severe or elusive chronic diarrhea may need hospitalization and extensive testing.

Prolonged, Persistent, and Protracted Infectious Diarrheas

Stool culture and examination may detect organisms that often cause protracted infectious diarrhea in adults: enteropathogenic (enteroadherent) *E. coli*, *Giardia*, *Entamoeba*, *Cryptosporidium*, *Aeromonas*, and *Yersinia enterocolitica*. If none of these organisms is

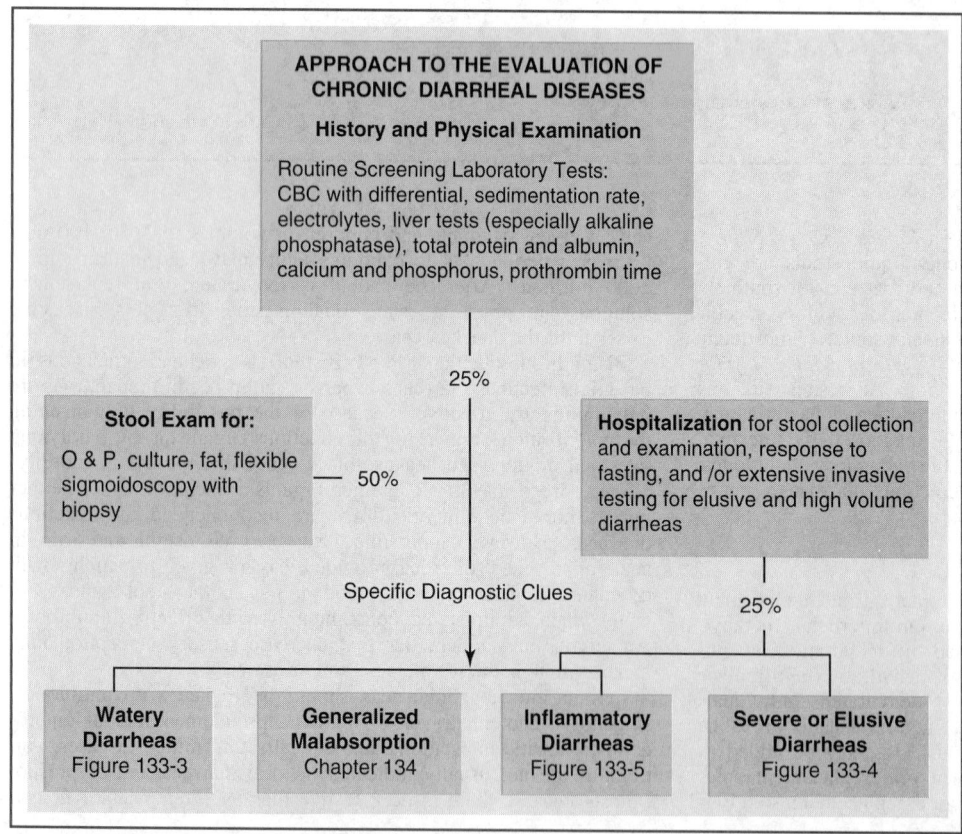

FIGURE 133–2 ■ Approach to the evaluation of malabsorption. O & P = ova and parasites. (Adapted from Powell DW: Approach to the patient with diarrhea. *In* Yamada T, Alpers DH, Owyang C, et al [eds]: Textbook of Gastroenterology, 3rd ed. Philadelphia, Lippincott–Raven, 1999.)

found, a therapeutic trial of metronidazole or trimethoprim-sulfamethoxazole may be indicated. Persistent infectious diarrhea lasting more than 3 to 4 weeks occurs in up to 3% of returned travelers; if trimethoprim-sulfamethoxazole or the fluoroquinolones have been unsuccessful, tetracycline or metronidazole should be tried.

Up to 25% of patients will experience pain, bloating, urgency, a sense of incomplete evacuation, and loose stools for 6 months or longer after documented infectious diarrhea. This syndrome of infectious diarrhea-induced irritable bowel syndrome, also called Brainerd's diarrhea, is a prolonged, often severe diarrhea initiated by unidentified organisms. Some patients respond to cholestyramine.

Visitors residing in the tropics for as short a time as 1 to 3 months may develop tropical sprue (see Chapter 134). A severe postinfectious diarrhea syndrome (severe protracted diarrhea) may develop in infants and children in developing nations and can occur in milder forms (post-enteritis syndrome) in infants and children in developed countries. Malnutrition and death (mortality up to 50%) can occur in severe disease. Treatment includes dietary lactose exclusion in mild disease or total parenteral nutrition in those severely affected. Metronidazole, tetracycline, trimethoprim-sulfamethoxazole, and folic acid therapy may also help.

STEATORRHEA (MALABSORPTIVE DISEASES)

Fat malabsorption can be divided into three broad categories: intraluminal maldigestion, mucosal malabsorption, and postmucosal malabsorption related to lymphatic obstruction (see Chapter 134).

WATERY DIARRHEAS (Figs. 133–3 and 133–4)

Ingestion of Nonabsorbable Solutes: Magnesium and Sodium Phosphate/Sulfate Diarrheas

Individuals ingesting significant amounts of Mg^{2+}-based antacids or high-potency multimineral/multivitamin supplements, or those surreptitiously taking Mg^{2+}-containing laxatives or non-absorbable anion laxatives such as Na_2PO_4 (neutral phosphate) or Na_2SO_4 (Glauber's or Carlsbad salt) may develop significant osmotically induced, watery diarrhea.

Carbohydrate Malabsorption

SORBITOL AND FRUCTOSE DIARRHEA. Chewing gum and elixir diarrhea can result from the chronic ingestion of dietetic foods, candy, chewing gum, or medication elixirs that are sweetened with unabsorbable carbohydrates such as sorbitol. Excessive consumption of pears, prunes, peaches, and apple juice, which also contain sorbitol and fructose, results in diarrhea as well. Fructose may be malabsorbed if ingested in high concentrations, and an occasional patient may have diarrhea related to ingestion of large volumes of fruit juice or soft drinks that are sweetened with fructose-containing corn syrup.

RAPID INTESTINAL TRANSIT. Approximately 25% of the normal 200 g carbohydrate diet may be unabsorbed by the normal small intestine. When passed into the colon, it is metabolized to osmotically active short-chain fatty acids by colonic flora. Diets

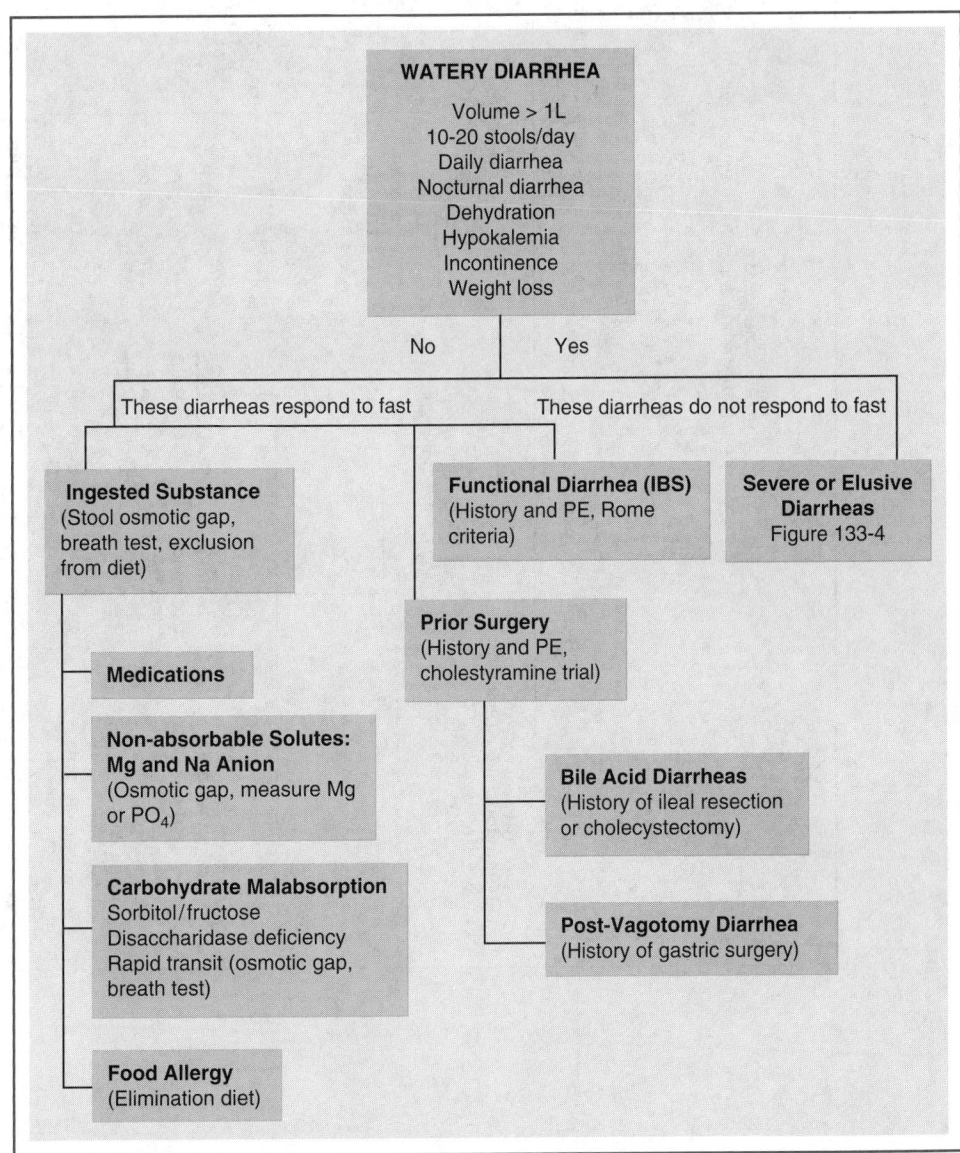

FIGURE 133–3 ■ Approach to the evaluation of watery diarrheas. IBS = irritable bowel syndrome. (Adapted from Powell DW: Approach to the patient with diarrhea. *In* Yamada T, Alpers DH, Owyang C, et al [eds]: Textbook of Gastroenterology, 3rd ed. Philadelphia, Lippincott–Raven, 1999.)

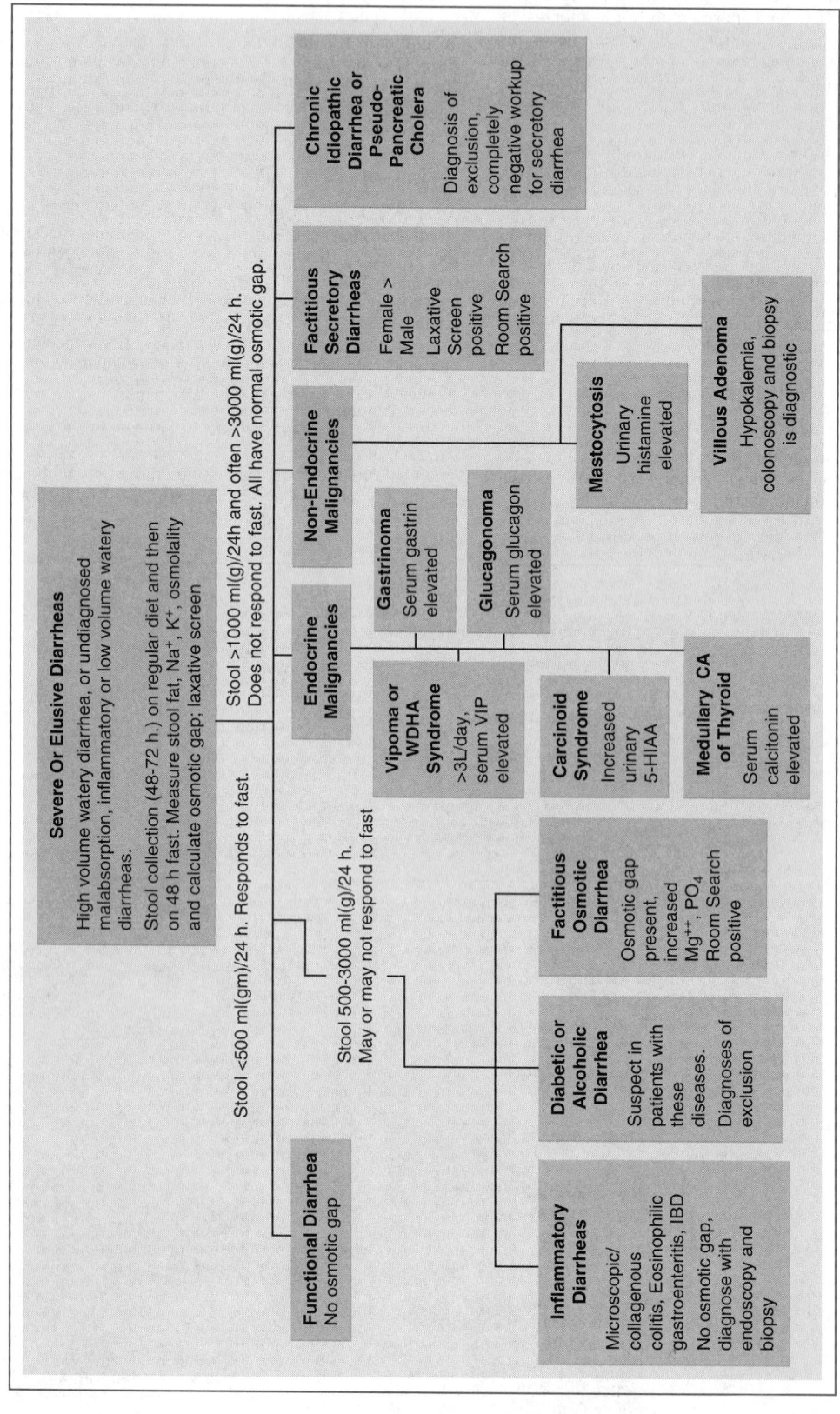

FIGURE 133-4 ■ Approach to the evaluation of severe or elusive diarrheas. CA = cancer; IBD = inflammatory bowel disease; VIP = vasoactive intestinal polypeptide; WDHA = watery diarrhea hypokalemia achlorhydria. (Adapted from Powell DW: Approach to the patient with diarrhea. *In* Yamada T, Alpers DH, Owyang C, et al [eds]: Textbook of Gastroenterology. 3rd ed. Philadelphia, Lippincott–Raven, 1999.)

high in carbohydrate and low in fat may allow rapid gastric emptying and rapid small intestine motility, leading to carbohydrate malabsorption and osmotic diarrhea. Rapid orocecal transit time also occurs in thyrotoxicosis. Because carbohydrate is metabolized also to H_2 and CO_2 by colonic bacteria, the symptoms of excess flatus, abdominal bloating, and cramping abdominal pain may be important clues to the diagnosis of carbohydrate malabsorption.

GLUCOSE-GALACTOSE MALABSORPTION AND DISACCHARIDASE DEFICIENCIES. Lactase deficiency and congenital absence of enterocyte brush border carbohydrate hydrolases and transport proteins may cause diarrheas (see Chapter 134). Lactase deficiency should be considered in cases of unexplained watery diarrhea, especially if accompanied by abdominal cramps, bloating, and flatus.

Prior Surgery

BILE ACID DIARRHEA. There are three types of bile acid–induced diarrhea. Type 1 results from severe disease (e.g., Crohn's disease), resection, or bypass of the distal ileum, which allows dihydroxy bile salts to escape absorption. If concentrations higher than 2 mmol are attained in the colon, secretory diarrhea ensues. Bile acid diarrhea must be differentiated from fatty acid diarrhea, which occurs when such a large segment of ileum (>100 cm) is resected that hepatic synthesis cannot maintain an adequate intraluminal bile salt pool; as a result, steatorrhea ensues, and fatty acid–induced intestinal secretion synergizes with the bile acid–induced secretion. Bile acid diarrhea responds to bile salt binders such as cholestyramine, but the diarrhea of fatty acid malabsorption may worsen with such therapy.

Type 2 bile acid diarrhea, or primary bile acid malabsorption, may be congenital or acquired. This form of diarrhea often responds to cholestyramine. Type 3 bile acid diarrhea is caused by measured increases in fecal bile acids in patients with postcholecystectomy diarrhea. It is unclear why interruption of gallbladder storage would lead to increased bile acid wastage. Although many patients respond to cholestyramine, some do not. Another cause of type 3 bile acid diarrhea is truncal vagotomy combined with a drainage procedure (post-vagotomy diarrhea), after which 20 to 30% of patients develop diarrhea. Many patients do not respond to cholestyramine, but motility-altering drugs (opiates and anticholinergics) may be of benefit. Celiac sprue also may first appear after gastric surgery or vagotomy.

Functional Watery Diarrheas (Irritable Bowel Syndrome)

About 25% of patients with irritable bowel syndrome have a symptom complex of predominantly painless diarrhea (see Chapter 131), but many such patients are discovered to have other conditions, such as occult lactose intolerance, collagenous or microscopic/lymphocytic colitis, rapid transit with carbohydrate-wasting diarrhea, malabsorption of fructose or sorbitol, or even primary bile acid malabsorption (type 2).

TRUE SECRETORY DIARRHEAS (Fig. 133–4)

Endocrine Tumor Diarrheas

CARCINOID SYNDROME. Patients with metastatic carcinoid tumors of the gastrointestinal tract or, rarely, primary non-metastatic carcinoid tumors of the bronchial epithelium may develop a watery diarrhea and cramping abdominal pain in addition to these other symptoms (see Chapter 245). Because up to one third of these patients do not have other symptoms at the time the diarrhea begins, carcinoid should be considered in patients with secretory diarrhea.

GASTRINOMA. Diarrhea occurs in up to one third of patients with Zollinger-Ellison's syndrome (see Chapter 130), may precede the ulcer symptoms, and in about 10% of patients may be the major pathophysiologic manifestation. The diarrhea is caused by high volumes of HCl secretion (it can be reduced by nasogastric aspiration or effective antisecretory therapy) and by maldigestion of fat due to pH inactivation of pancreatic lipase and precipitation of bile acids.

VIPOMA OR WATERY DIARRHEA-HYPOKALEMIA-ACHLORHYDRIA (WDHA) SYNDROME. Non–beta cell pancreatic adenomas may secrete various peptide secretagogues, including vasoactive intestinal polypeptide (VIP) that produces all of the symptoms

of this disease (see Chapter 130). Patients with this syndrome have secretory diarrhea, with 70% of patients having more than 3 L of stool per day and virtually all having more than 700 mL/day. Stool electrolyte losses account for the dehydration, hypokalemia, and acidosis that give this syndrome its name.

MEDULLARY CARCINOMA OF THE THYROID. This cancer may present in sporadic form, or it may present as part of the multiple endocrine neoplasia (MEN II) syndrome with pheochromocytomas and hyperparathyroidism in 25 to 50% of cases. Watery (secretory) diarrhea is caused by the secretion of calcitonin by the tumor; however, these tumors also elaborate other secretagogues, such as prostaglandins, VIP, and serotonin. By the time watery diarrhea occurs, the tumor has metastasized, and this symptom portends a poor prognosis.

Non-endocrine Malignancies

VILLOUS ADENOMAS. Large (4–10 cm) villous adenomas of the rectum or rectosigmoid may cause a secretory form of diarrhea of 500 to 3000 mL/24 hours with hypokalemia. Secretagogues such as prostaglandins have been found in both the tumor and rectal effluent of such patients, and indomethacin administration reduces the diarrhea in some.

SYSTEMIC MASTOCYTOSIS. The diarrhea of systemic mastocytosis may be malabsorptive, secondary to mast cell infiltration of the mucosa with resulting villus atrophy, or intermittent and secretory. Histamine or another mast cell mediator may be the secretagogue responsible for these symptoms and for the secretory diarrhea, by either stimulating gastric acid secretion (such as in Zollinger-Ellison syndrome) or by having a secretory effect on the intestine. Antihistaminics (H_1 blockers), H_2 blockers, and cyclooxygenase inhibitors may be helpful. Blockade of mast cell degranulation with disodium cromoglycate may reduce all the symptoms and the diarrhea but not the steatorrhea.

Factitious Diarrhea

Approximately 15% of patients referred for diarrhea to secondary or tertiary centers and 25% of patients with proven secretory diarrheas are found to be ingesting either laxatives or diuretics surreptitiously. These patients present with severe chronic watery, often nocturnal, diarrhea, and may also have abdominal pain, weight loss, nausea, vomiting, hypokalemic myopathy, acidosis, or protein-losing enteropathy. Patients may have up to 10 to 20 bowel movements per day, with 24-hour stool volumes in the range of 300 to 3000 mL. Phenolphthalein, now removed from the market, bisacodyl, and anthraquinone (senna, cascara, aloe, rhubarb, frangula, and danthron) ingestion, and osmotic laxatives (neutral-phosphate, epsom salts, and magnesium citrate) can cause this syndrome. Because there is no readily available assay for the stool softener dioctyl sodium sulfosuccinate (the docusate salts), one of the more common laxatives, it is unclear how often it contributes. Some patients ingest large quantities of diuretics, such as furosemide or ethacrynic acid.

More than 90% of the patients are women, and two different clinical syndromes are most common: (1) women younger than 30 years of age in whom eating disorders such as anorexia nervosa or bulimia may be part of the psychic abnormality and (2) middle-aged to elderly women who have extensive medical histories and are more likely to be health care workers. Factitious diarrhea is sufficiently common to warrant laxative screening to exclude this syndrome before initiating extensive medical evaluation for the other causes of diarrhea.

Chronic Idiopathic Diarrhea and Pseudopancreatic Cholera Syndrome

Patients in whom extensive evaluation for a cause of secretory diarrhea is negative are said to have either chronic idiopathic diarrhea or pseudopancreatic cholera syndrome, depending on whether the fasting stool volumes are less than or greater than 700 mL/24 hours, respectively. If no diagnosis is revealed after thorough testing and a search for surreptitious laxative abuse, a therapeutic trial with bile salt–binding drugs, NSAIDs, or opiates is warranted. Follow-up studies suggest that the diarrhea is usually self-limited and disappears spontaneously in 6 to 24 months.

Diabetic Diarrhea

Up to 20% of young to middle-aged diabetics, particularly men between 20 and 40 years of age whose diabetes has been poorly controlled for more than 5 years, may have a profuse watery, urgent diarrhea, often occurring at night with incontinence. These patients usually have concomitant neuropathy, nephropathy, and retinopathy. Exocrine pancreatic insufficiency is sometimes the cause, and bacterial overgrowth occasionally is present because of the motility disturbance of the autonomic neuropathy. Diabetic patients must have an appropriate evaluation to exclude other causes of diarrhea. If no other cause is found, clonidine may be helpful. Patients with neuropathy frequently have impaired anal sphincter function, and high-dose loperamide may improve the incontinence.

Alcoholic Diarrhea

Binge drinking of alcohol causes a brief episode of diarrhea that usually lasts less than 1 day. Chronic alcoholics often have a severe watery diarrhea that persists for days or even weeks after hospitalization. Various physiologic abnormalities have been described in alcoholics as a cause of diarrhea but none have been proven. With abstinence, renourishment, and replenishment of vitamin deficiencies, the diarrhea slowly improves.

INFLAMMATORY DIARRHEAS

Inflammatory Bowel Disease (see Chapter 135)

Patients with Crohn's disease or ulcerative colitis have diarrhea with stool volumes usually less than 1 L/24 hours. Occasional patients with severe ulcerative colitis may have more severe diarrhea with water and electrolyte secretion in the unaffected small intestine, suggesting the presence of circulating secretagogues originating from the inflamed colon.

Eosinophilic Gastroenteritis

Infiltration of various layers of the gastrointestinal tract with eosinophils is a recognized clinical entity that is accompanied by diarrhea in 30% to 60% of such patients. Peripheral eosinophilia is present in 75% of these patients. The disease may involve the entire gastrointestinal tract from esophagus to anus, or it may be isolated to a segment. Abdominal pain, nausea, vomiting, weight loss, steatorrhea, and protein-losing enteropathy are other prominent signs and symptoms of this disease. The cause of this disease is unknown, but approximately 50% of patients have atopic (allergic) histories, and food allergy is suspected. Corticosteroids remain the mainstay of therapy; sodium cromoglycate may be useful.

Milk and Soy Protein Intolerance and Food Allergy

Intolerance to cow's milk and soy protein is a well-established cause of enterocolitis in infants. Approximately 50% of the patients who are allergic to one of these proteins are also allergic to the other. However, the role of food allergy in causing diarrhea in adults is less clear. Commonly suspected allergens include milk, eggs, seafood, nuts, artificial flavors, and food coloring.

Collagenous and Microscopic Colitis

These two conditions may or may not be the same or variants of the same disease. Microscopic (lymphocytic) colitis is equally prevalent in men and women, whereas collagenous colitis occurs 10 times more often in middle-aged or elderly women. These diseases may be categorized as either inflammatory or secretory diarrheas. An epidemiologic relation to chronic NSAID use has been reported, and increased luminal prostaglandin levels may cause the diarrhea. Either food hypersensitivity or intraluminal bile has been proposed as a trigger for prostaglandin release from lymphocytes. The disease disappears with fecal stream diversion. Bismuth subsalicylate therapy was successful in a small series.

Protein-Losing Enteropathy

Severe protein loss through the gastrointestinal tract caused by ulceration, obstructed lymphatics, and immune-related vascular in-

jury occurs in a variety of disease states: bacterial or parasitic infection, gastritis, gastric cancer, collagenous colitis, inflammatory bowel disease, congenital intestinal lymphangiectasia, sarcoidosis, lymphoma, mesenteric tuberculosis, Ménétrier's disease, sprue, eosinophilic gastroenteritis, systemic lupus erythematosus, or food allergies. The condition usually responds to corticosteroids or immunosuppressive therapy.

Chronic Radiation Enterocolitis

Patients receiving pelvic radiation for malignancies of the female urogenital tract or the male prostate may develop chronic radiation enterocolitis 6 to 12 months after total doses of radiation greater than 40 to 60 Gy. The diarrhea may be caused by bile acid malabsorption if the ileum is damaged, by bacterial overgrowth if radiation causes small intestine strictures, or by radiation-induced chronic inflammation of the small intestine and colon. Anti-inflammatory drugs such as sulfasalazine and corticosteroids have been tried with little success. Cholestyramine and NSAIDs may help, as may opiates.

Miscellaneous Diseases

Although acute mesenteric arterial or venous thrombosis presents as an acute bloody diarrhea, chronic mesenteric vascular ischemia may present as watery diarrhea. Gastrointestinal tuberculosis and histoplasmosis present as diarrhea that may either be bloody or watery, as do certain immunologic diseases such as Behçet's syndrome or Churg-Strauss syndrome. All of these diseases may be misdiagnosed as inflammatory bowel disease. Diarrhea, the hallmark of acute graft-versus-host disease after allogeneic bone marrow transplantation, presents as the triad of dermatitis, hepatic cholestasis, and enteritis. Neutropenic enterocolitis, an ileocolitis occurring in neutropenic leukemic patients, is sometimes caused by *C. difficile* infection.

History and Physical Examination

A detailed history, physical examination, and certain screening tests can lead to a diagnosis in 75% of patients with watery diarrheas (see Figs. 133–2, 133–3, and 133–4), whereas the approach to malabsorptive diarrheas is different (see Chapter 134). A history of 10 to 20 bowel movements per day suggests secretory diarrhea. A history of peptic ulcer should suggest gastrinoma or systemic mastocytosis. Physical examination is helpful only if the thyromegaly of medullary carcinoma, the cutaneous flushing of the neuroendocrine tumors and systemic mastocytosis, the dermatographism of systemic mastocytosis, or the migratory necrolytic erythema of glucagonoma is evident. Scars from previous surgery may suggest postvagotomy diarrhea or terminal ileal resection with bile acid diarrhea as a diagnosis. Autonomic dysfunction (e.g., postural hypotension, impotence, gustatory sweating) is almost invariably present in diabetic diarrhea.

The important clinical manifestations of inflammatory diarrheas are the signs and symptoms of inflammation and/or the effects of severe chronic protein loss (Fig. 133–5). Diarrhea in these inflammatory diseases may be meager (e.g., the pseudodiarrhea of proctitis), or it may be fairly severe (e.g., as in graft-versus-host disease). Systemic manifestations of inflammatory bowel disease include oral aphthous ulcers, polymigratory arthritis, uveitis, erythema nodosum, pyoderma gangrenosum, and the palpable purpura of vasculitis.

Screening Laboratory Examinations

Blood levels (see Fig. 133–2) of iron, folate, vitamin B_{12}, vitamin K, or vitamin D help evaluate malabsorption. Although serum carotene levels may be low simply from poor intake, values less than 50 μg/dL suggest malabsorption. Peripheral blood findings of leukocytosis, eosinophilia, elevated erythrocyte sedimentation rate, hypoalbuminemia, or low total serum proteins suggest inflammatory diarrheas, whose hallmark is the presence of blood, either gross or occult, and leukocytes in the stool. There are no bedside screening tests to establish the diagnosis in watery diarrheas.

Radiography

Radiology should be viewed as an adjunct to the diagnosis of diarrheal diseases and not a primary test. Malabsorption may be

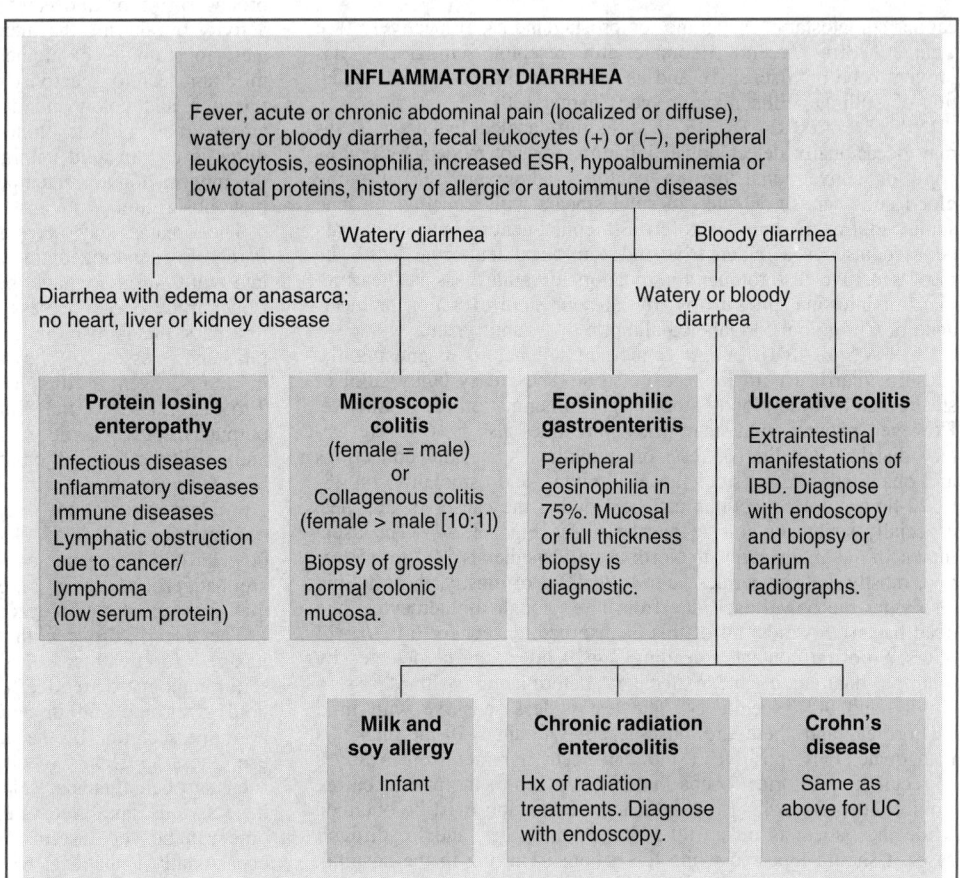

FIGURE 133–5 ■ Approach to the evaluation of inflammatory diarrheas. IBD = inflammatory bowel disease; UC = ulcerative colitis. (Adapted from Powell DW: Approach to the patient with diarrhea. *In* Yamada T, Alpers DH, Owyang C, et al [eds]: Textbook of Gastroenterology, 3rd ed. Philadelphia, Lippincott–Raven, 1999.)

suggested by a flat plate of the abdomen that demonstrates pancreatic calcification. Some diseases (e.g., previous gastric surgery, gastrocolic fistulas, blind loops from previous intestinal anastomoses, small intestine strictures, multiple jejunal diverticula, and abnormal intestinal motility that could lead to bacterial overgrowth) may be demonstrated by an upper gastrointestinal series with small intestine follow-through or by an enteroclysis examination. Certain diseases may present radiographically as uniform thickening of the intestinal folds (e.g., amyloidosis, lymphoma, Whipple's disease); others such as lymphoma or lymphangiectasia demonstrate uniform or patchy abnormalities. Patients with sprue show dilatation of the small intestine, with little mucosal abnormality, and segmentation of the barium column as a result of precipitation or flocculation of the barium. Routine contrast radiographs of the gastrointestinal tract are not usually helpful in the diagnosis of watery diarrheas, unless they show a previous vagotomy, extensive small bowel resection or cholecystectomy, the presence of a tumor (carcinoid or villous adenoma), or a bowel filled with fluid (endocrine tumor). Contrast radiographic examination may show diagnostic evidence of inflammatory bowel disease or changes suggestive of eosinophilic gastroenteritis or radiation enterocolitis. Early or mild gut inflammation may be missed entirely by radiography.

Endoscopy and Biopsy

Upper endoscopy with distal duodenal biopsy should be undertaken if the presence of steatorrhea and diagnostic clues suggest small bowel mucosal malabsorption. Patients with severe watery or elusive diarrhea should have a flexible sigmoidoscopy or, preferably, a colonoscopy to exclude villous adenomas of the rectosigmoid and biopsy to exclude microscopic or collagenous colitis, mastocytosis, or early inflammatory bowel disease. Colonoscopy and biopsy may also reveal melanosis coli secondary to chronic anthracene laxative use. Terminal ileal biopsy may give an indication of inflammatory bowel diseases.

Laboratory Testing

MALABSORPTION. Certain tests can help determine the cause of steatorrhea (see Chapter 134).

WATERY DIARRHEA. *Breath tests* to measure the respiratory excretion of labeled CO_2 after oral administration and metabolism of radioactive carbon–labeled substrates or of H_2 after administration of carbohydrates can assess fat, carbohydrate, and bile salt malabsorption or bacterial overgrowth. CO_2 breath tests are based on the principle that either intraluminal (bacterial) or cellular (intermediary) processes convert the substrate into CO_2, which is excreted in expired air. Hydrogen breath tests can be used to study carbohydrate malabsorption or bacterial overgrowth of the small intestine. The sole source of H_2 in the mammal is bacterial fermentation; bacteria in the small bowel and unabsorbed carbohydrate that makes its way to colonic bacteria will yield excess breath H_2. To test for lactase deficiency in individuals in whom a therapeutic trial of carbohydrate-restricted free diet is inconclusive, breath hydrogen testing may be indicated. In lactase deficiency, small intestine mucosal disease, or pancreatic insufficiency the peak of increased hydrogen comes between 3 and 6 hours after ingestion, when the carbohydrate reaches the colonic bacteria. The increase in hydrogen excretion by patients with pancreatic insufficiency can be reduced by concomitant administration of pancreatic enzymes. To test for lactose intolerance, a lactose dose of 25 g is given after an overnight fast. A rise of over 20 ppm in exhaled hydrogen over baseline values within the first 3 to 8 hours of ingestion is diagnostic. Bacterial overgrowth of the small bowel may cause an early peak of increased hydrogen production within 2 hours after a carbohydrate meal.

The diagnosis of endocrine tumors such as carcinoids, gastrinoma, VIPoma, medullary carcinoma of the thyroid, glucagonoma, somatostatinoma, and systemic mastocytosis is made by demonstrating elevated blood levels of serotonin or urinary 5-hydroxyindole acetic acid and serum levels for gastrin, VIP, calcitonin, glucagon, somatostatin, histamine, or prostaglandins, respectively (see Chapter 130). Recently, somatostatin receptor scintigraphy has proven to be both sensitive and useful in the diagnosis and evaluation of Zollinger-Ellison syndrome (Chapter 130).

INFLAMMATORY DIARRHEA. Indium-labeled leukocyte scans may occasionally detect bowel inflammation not evident by endoscopy or conventional barium contrast radiography. Fecal white blood cells can be detected in stool smears with a methylene blue stain. Stool excretion of lactoferrin (a constituent of leukocytes) can be used also as a quantitative index of fecal leukocyte loss. The most sensitive test for certain inflammatory diarrheas is measurement of intestinal protein loss by 24-hour stool excretion or clearance of Chromium-51–labeled albumin or α_1-antitrypsin.

ELUSIVE DIARRHEA. An important adjunct to diagnosing the cause of diarrhea is to look at the stool. The greasy bulky stool of steatorrhea and the bloody stool of gut inflammation are distinctive. However, patients with steatorrhea sometimes also have severe watery diarrhea. Qualitative tests on outpatient spot stool collections and quantitative tests (stool fat, electrolytes, and osmolality) on 48- to 72-hour stool collections can help define the causes of diarrhea, especially severe or elusive diarrheas (see Fig. 133–4). The usual intake of fat in the typical North American diet is 100 to 150 g/ day, mostly as triglycerides, and 40 to 50 g of mostly phospholipid also enter the bowel each day from bile, sloughed enterocytes, and dead bacteria. Almost all of this is absorbed, except for 6 to 7 g/24 hours. Stool fat content exceeding 7 g/24 hours can be detected by a simple qualitative (Sudan) fecal fat determination with 90% sensitivity and 90% specificity. The test is less sensitive with mild steatorrhea, and there are false-negative findings if fat intake is inadequate. False-positive results can occur if mineral oil laxatives or rectal suppositories (cocoa butter) are given to the patient before stool collection. A 48- to 72-hour stool collection must be obtained while the patient is on a 100-g fat (normal) diet, and for difficult cases it should repeated while the patient is fasting in the hospital. Stool collections can be analyzed for appearance, weight, quantitative fecal fat, electrolytes (Na^+, K^+, and, if thought necessary, Cl^-, PO_4^{2-} and Mg^{2+}), osmolality, fecal pH, and laxative screen.

Carbohydrate malabsorption will lower stool pH because of colonic fermentation of carbohydrate to short-chain fatty acids. Stool pH less than 5.3 usually means pure carbohydrate malabsorption, whereas in generalized malabsorptive diseases, stool pH is above 5.6 and usually above 6.0.

Stool or urine can be analyzed for emetine (a component of ipecac), bisacodyl, castor oil, or anthraquinone. Stool SO_4, PO_4^{2-}, and Mg^{2+} analysis detects factitious diarrheas caused by osmotic cathartics.

The normal stool osmotic gap, which is the difference between stool osmolality (or 290 mOsm) and twice the stool Na^+ and K^+ concentrations, is 50 to 125. In secretory diarrheas, the solutes causing the movement of water from blood to bowel lumen are the secreted Na^+ and K^+ molecules; stool Na^+, concentrations are usually greater than 90 mmol/L, and the osmotic gap is less than 50. In osmotic diarrhea, the ingestion of non-absorbable (or non-absorbed) solutes displaces Na^+ from the stool and causes the osmotic gap and the diarrhea (see section on Pathophysiology); stool Na^+ is less than 60 mmol/L, and the osmotic gap is greater than 125. Stools with Na^+ concentration between 60 and 90 mmol/L and calculated osmotic gaps between 50 and 100 can result from either secretory or malabsorptive abnormalities. Patients with Mg^{2+}-induced diarrhea can be diagnosed by fecal Mg^{2+} values above 50 mmol/L. Sodium anion-induced diarrheas mimic secretory diarrhea because the stool Na^+ content is high (>90 mmol/L), and there is no osmotic gap; this diarrhea can be diagnosed by determining stool Cl^- concentration because these anions displace stool Cl^-, and the resulting stool Cl^- value is usually less than 20 mmol/L.

ANTIDIARRHEAL THERAPY

Antidiarrheal agents are of two types: agents useful for mild to moderate diarrheas and those helpful in secretory and other severe diarrheas. The bulk-forming agents (kaolin-pectin, psyllium, and methylcellulose) increase the consistency of stool and have no antisecretory activity. Other antidiarrheal agents have only mild proabsorptive or antisecretory action, and most have antidiarrheal activity by altering the intestinal motility. Bismuth salicylates, opiates, loperamide, clonidine, phenothiazine, and somatostatin have mild antisecretory activity but also cause dilatation of the small intestine and colon and decrease peristalsis. The opiates also increase anal sphincter tone. The therapeutic mechanism of these drugs is to trap fluid within the intestine and put it in contact with the mucosa for a greater period of time, thus allowing more complete absorption.

The opiates may be symptomatically useful in mild diarrheas. Paregoric, deodorized tincture of opium, codeine, and diphenoxylate with atropine have been largely supplanted by loperamide. Loperamide does not pass the blood-brain barrier and has a high first-pass metabolism in the liver; it has a high therapeutic/toxic ratio and is essentially devoid of addiction potential. It is quite safe in adults, even in total doses of 24 mg/day. The usual dose is 2 to 4 mg, two to four times daily. When giving opiates, stool output is not a reliable gauge for replacing fluid losses because the antimotility effects of opiates will cause fluid to sequester in the bowel lumen (third space). Furthermore, the antimotility effects are a problem in infectious diarrheas because stasis may enhance bacterial invasion and delay clearance of the microorganisms from the bowel, thus increasing carriage time. Opiates and anticholinergics are dangerous also in severe inflammatory bowel disease, where they may precipitate megacolon.

The use of drugs with potentially serious side effects can be justified for treatment of severe secretory diarrheas. The somatostatin analogue octreotide has its major antisecretory effect in carcinoid syndrome and in neuroendocrine tumors because it inhibits hormone secretion by the tumor. Octreotide may be of only limited usefulness in short bowel syndrome and AIDS diarrhea. Agents such as phenothiazine, calcium channel blockers, or clonidine can have serious side effects but may be tried if octreotide fails. Clonidine can be very useful in the diarrhea of opiate withdrawal and occasionally in patients with diabetic diarrhea. Indomethacin, a cyclooxygenase blocker that inhibits prostaglandin production, may occasionally be useful in neuroendocrine tumors, irritable bowel, and food allergy and is most useful in patients with diarrhea due to acute radiation, AIDS, and villous adenomas of the rectum or colon. Cyclooxygenase blockers may be harmful in inflammatory bowel disease. Glucocorticoids reduce prostaglandin and leukotriene production in inflammatory bowel disease and have a proabsorptive effect on the intestine that is demonstrable by 5 hours after administration.

Blaser MJ, Smith PD, Ravdin JI, et al (eds): Infections of the Gastrointestinal Tract. New York, Raven Press, 1995. *This book contains a current description of enteric infections and food poisonings.*

Fine KD: Diarrhea. *In* Feldman M, Scharschmidt BF, Sleisenger MH (eds): Sleisenger and Fordtran's Gastrointestinal and Liver Disease: Pathophysiology, Diagnosis, Management, 6th ed. Philadelphia, WB Saunders, 1998, pp 128–152. *This is another excellent general chapter on diarrhea.*

Fine KD, Schiller LR: American Gastroenterological Association technical review on the evaluation and management of chronic diarrhea. Gastroenterology 116:1464–1486, 1999. *This is an up-to-date review of diagnosis and treatment of chronic diarrhea.*

Powell DW: Approach to the patient with diarrhea. *In* Yamada T, Alpers DH, Owyang C, et al (eds): Textbook of Gastroenterology, 3rd ed. Philadelphia, Lippincott-Raven, 1999. *This is an expanded and detailed version of the chapter presented here.*

134 MALABSORPTION SYNDROMES

Carol E. Semrad ■ *Eugene B. Chang*

Malabsorption is caused by a number of different diseases, drugs, or nutritional products that impair intraluminal digestion, mucosal absorption, or nutrient delivery to the systemic circulation. Individuals can present with classic gastrointestinal symptoms such as diarrhea and weight loss, indicative of significant fat, carbohydrate, and protein malabsorption, or with symptomatic anemia, bone disease, or coagulopathy, indicative of vitamin or mineral malabsorption. A careful history is critical in guiding further testing to confirm the suspicion of malabsorption and to make a specific diagnosis. The goals of treatment are to correct or treat the underlying disease and to replenish water, electrolyte, and nutritional losses.

PRINCIPALS OF NORMAL NUTRIENT ABSORPTION

Fat, Carbohydrate, and Protein Absorption

The digestion and absorption of dietary carbohydrate, fat, and protein begins with the action of salivary amylase on starch, gastric lipase on fat, and hydrochloric acid and pepsin on protein. Hydrochloric acid also aids in the liberation of cobalamin from food proteins and the solubilization of calcium and iron salts. The majority of nutrient digestion and absorption occurs in the small intestine (Fig. 134–1).

INTRALUMINAL DIGESTION. Amino acids and fatty acids cause the release of cholecystokinin (CCK) from the upper small intestinal mucosa. CCK stimulates the release of digestive enzymes (amylase, lipase, colipase, and proteases) from pancreatic acinar cells, and it contracts the gallbladder and relaxes the sphincter of Oddi, resulting in the release of bile into the intestinal lumen. Pancreatic proteases (trypsinogen, chymotrypsinogen, proelastase, and procarboxypeptidases) are secreted from cells in inactive forms. The cleavage of trypsinogen to trypsin by the duodenal brush border peptidase enteropeptidase (enterokinase) allows trypsin to cleave the remaining trypsinogen and other proteases to their active form. Gastric acid causes the release of secretin from the upper small intestinal mucosa, which in turn stimulates bicarbonate secretion from pancreatic ductular cells. Acetylcholine and CCK enhance secretin's stimulatory effect. Neutralization of acid in the small intestinal lumen by bicarbonate is physiologically important, as pancreatic enzyme activity and bile salt micelle formation is optimal at a luminal pH of 6 to 8.

Dietary lipids (long-chain triglycerides, cholesterol, phosphatidylcholine [lecithin], and fat-soluble vitamins) are insoluble in the aqueous milieu of the intestinal lumen and must undergo lipolysis and incorporation into mixed micelles before they can be absorbed. Pancreatic lipase, in the presence of its cofactor, colipase, cleaves long-chain triglycerides into fatty acids and monoglycerides. The products of lipolysis interact with bile salts and phospholipids to form mixed micelles, which also incorporate cholesterol and fat-soluble vitamins in their hydrophobic centers. Although long-chain fatty acids form lamellar structures that can be slowly absorbed intact, cholesterol and the fat-soluble vitamins can be absorbed only via mixed micelles. Failure of micelle formation leads to deficiencies of fat-soluble vitamins (D, A, K, E).

Carbohydrates and most dietary proteins are water-soluble and readily digested by pancreatic enzymes. Starch is digested by amylase into oligosaccharides, whereas dietary proteins are digested by proteases to larger oligopeptides, tripeptides, dipeptides, and amino acids. Oligosaccharides and larger oligopeptides must be further digested by brush border hydrolases before being absorbed.

MUCOSAL ABSORPTION. Water and electrolytes are absorbed by both the small intestine and colon. Nutrients are absorbed along the entire length of the small intestine with the exception of iron and folate, which are absorbed predominantly in the duodenum and proximal jejunum, and bile salts and cobalamin, which can only be absorbed in the distal ileum. The efficiency of nutrient uptake at the mucosa is influenced by the number of villus absorptive cells, the presence of functional hydrolases and specific nutrient transport proteins on the brush border membrane, and transit time. Transit time determines the contact time of luminal contents with the brush border membrane and thereby influences the efficiency of nutrient uptake across the mucosa.

Most luminal lipids, including the fat-soluble vitamins, diffuse to the brush border membrane of villus epithelial cells in the form of mixed micelles. Long-chain fatty acids are transported across the microvillus membrane after first binding to fatty acid–binding proteins. The mechanism of monoglyceride, cholesterol, and fat-soluble vitamin uptake is poorly understood. In the epithelial cell, long-chain fatty acids are resynthesized into triglycerides and combine with cholesterol ester, fat-soluble vitamins, phospholipid, and apoproteins to form chylomicrons. The bile salts from mixed micelles remain in the intestinal lumen. Protonated forms of bile salts, which at physiologic pH are at very low concentrations, are absorbed passively across the small intestinal mucosa. The majority of bile salt uptake occurs in the distal ileum by sodium-dependent cotransport.

Oligosaccharides and larger oligopeptides are further hydrolyzed by enzymes present in the brush border membrane of villus epithelial cells before they are absorbed. The oligosaccharides maltose, maltotriose, and alpha-limit dextrins (products of starch digestion) are hydrolyzed into glucose monomers by maltase and isomaltase. Sucrose is hydrolyzed by sucrase into fructose and glucose; lactose by lactase to glucose and galactose. Glucose and galactose are taken up at the apical epithelial cell membrane by the sodium-glucose ligand transporter (SGLT1) and fructose by the facilitative glucose transporter (GLUT5). Oligopeptides are hydrolyzed into

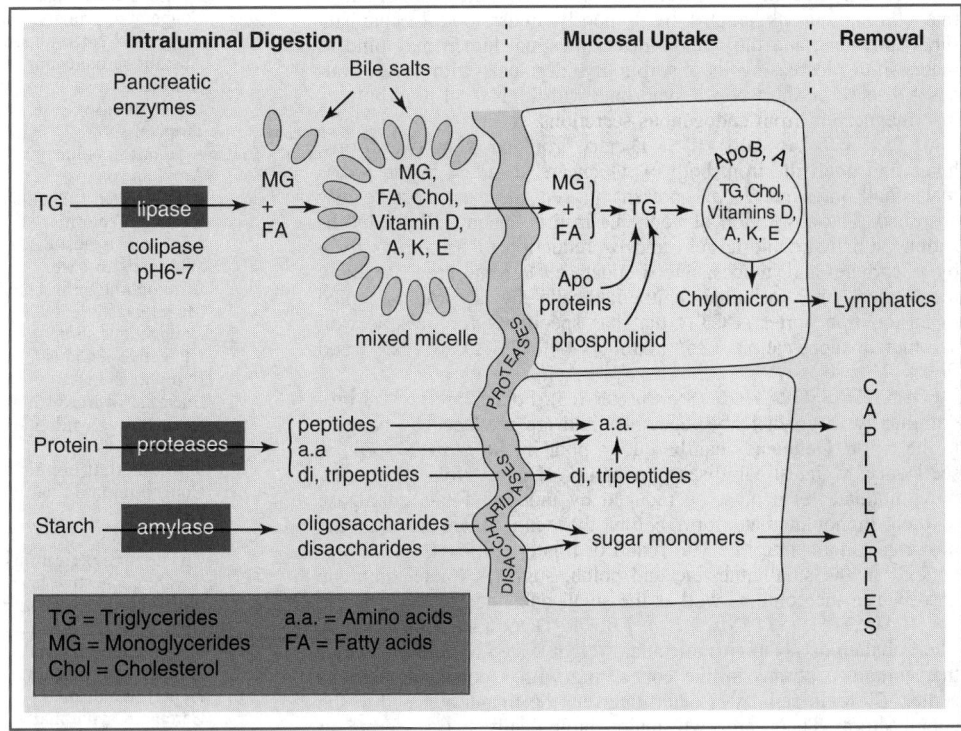

FIGURE 134–1 ■ Phases of intestinal digestion and absorption of dietary fat, protein, and carbohydrate.

dipeptides and tripeptides and amino acids by peptidases on the brush border membrane. Several different sodium-dependent amino acid carriers, some with overlapping substrate specificities, transport cationic, anionic, and neutral amino acids into epithelial cells. In addition, dipeptides and tripeptides are transported into epithelial cells by a hydrogen-coupled oligopeptide carrier, PepT1, which is driven by luminal hydrogen ions generated by the epithelial sodium hydrogen exchanger. Defects in amino acid uptake in Hartnup's disease and cystinuria are characterized by renal and intestinal malabsorption of neutral and basic amino acids, respectively. In the intestine, such defects can be offset by the absorption of amino acids as dipeptides and tripeptides.

DELIVERY OF NUTRIENTS TO THE SYSTEMIC CIRCULATION. Insoluble lipids (present in chylomicrons) are exocytosed across the basolateral membrane of epithelial cells into the intestinal lymphatics. From there, they enter the mesenteric lymphatics and then the general circulation via the thoracic duct. Sugar monomers, amino acids, and medium-chain fatty acids are transported across the basolateral membrane of intestinal epithelial cells into capillaries and then into the portal circulation. Sugar monomers are transported across the basolateral membrane by the facilitative glucose transporter isoform (GLUT2) and amino acids by facilitative amino acid carriers.

Absorption of Calcium, Magnesium, Metals, and Vitamins

CALCIUM ABSORPTION. Dairy products are the main source of dietary calcium. Calcium is absorbed in the small intestine by a poorly understood vitamin D–dependent uptake process. Transport across the epithelial cell is facilitated by the calcium-binding protein calbindin. Calcium exits the cell at the basolateral membrane by a Ca^{2+}-ATPase and a Na-Ca exchanger. The active form of vitamin D, $1,25(OH)_2$ vitamin D_3, increases the calcium uptake mechanism, calbindin synthesis, and the synthesis of the Ca^{2+}-ATPase, resulting in increased calcium absorption. Calcium absorption is also facilitated by hydrochloric acid, which solubilizes calcium salts. Intraluminal compounds, such as oxalate, phytates, and long-chain fatty acids, precipitate with calcium to form insoluble complexes and hence decrease calcium absorption.

MAGNESIUM ABSORPTION. Magnesium is most abundant in green vegetables, unrefined grains, and nuts. In addition, magnesium is secreted into the intestinal lumen in biliary, gastric, and pancreatic juices. About 50% of dietary magnesium and all of the endogenously secreted magnesium is absorbed by the small intestine (throughout its length) by a poorly understood mechanism. Fiber, phytates, and fatty acids in the intestinal lumen may bind to magnesium, decreasing its absorption. Individuals with severe mucosal disease or short bowel syndrome with high fecal fluid outputs lose magnesium from endogenous secretions.

METAL ION ABSORPTION. Dietary iron exists in two forms, heme and nonheme iron, both of which are absorbed in the proximal small intestine. Heme present in red meat is most readily absorbed. The absorption of nonheme iron is enhanced by solubilization with hydrochloric acid and by reduction to its ferrous form by ascorbate and mucosal ferrireductase. Ferrous iron is likely transported into intestinal epithelial cells by a proton-coupled metal-ion transporter (DCT1) that has specificity for Fe^{2+} as well as other divalent cations (Zn^{2+}, Mn^{2+}, Co^{2+}, Cd^{2+}, Cu^{2+}, Ni^{2+}, and Pb^{2+}).

FOLATE ABSORPTION (See Chapter 163). Folates are present predominantly in green leafy vegetables and are produced by bacteria in the colon. Deficiency can be due to poor intake or malabsorption secondary to intestinal disease or drugs. Dietary folates in their polyglutamate form must be reduced by mucosal folate conjugase to their monoglutamate form before they can be absorbed in the proximal small intestine. A reduced folate carrier (RFC1), expressed in the small intestine and colon, suggests folate might be absorbed in the colon as well as the small intestine.

COBALAMIN (VITAMIN B_{12}) ABSORPTION (See Chapter 163). The cobalamins are high molecular weight water-soluble molecules that contain a porphyrin-like corrin ring with a cobalt atom in its center. Biologic activity is determined by the ligand attached to the cobalt atom. There are two major biologically active forms in human tissues: one contains a methyl group attached to the cobalt atom and the other a 5-deoxyadenosyl group. The supplemental form contains a cyanide group attached to the cobalt atom; hence, the name cyanocobalamin (vitamin B_{12}). The cobalamins are readily abundant in foods containing animal proteins (e.g., meat, seafood, eggs, and milk), so cobalamin deficiency in industrialized countries is rarely due to poor dietary intake but rather reflects the inability to absorb cobalamin in the intestine. Large amounts of cobalamin are present in the liver (2 to 5 mg), and cobalamin is reabsorbed from bile via the enterohepatic circulation, limiting daily losses to only 0.5 to 1 μg. It usually takes 10 to 12 years for cobalamin deficiency to develop when it is eliminated from the diet, but deficiency can occur more rapidly (2 to 5 years) with malabsorptive syndromes.

A number of proteins are necessary for the normal absorption of cobalamin from food. Initially, cobalamin must be liberated from food proteins by acid-peptic hydrolysis. Both R-proteins and intrinsic factor (IF) are secreted in the stomach. At the low pH in the stomach, about 95% of free cobalamin binds to R-proteins. In the small intestine, pancreatic proteases degrade R-proteins and allow the freed cobalamin to bind to IF. The cobalamin-IF complex then travels to the ileum, where it binds to specific receptors in the brush border membrane and is then taken up by the ileal epithelial cell. Inside the epithelial cell, IF is degraded, perhaps by cathepsin L, and the released cobalamin binds to transcobalamin II (TC II). The cobalamin–TC II complex is then transported across the basolateral membrane of ileal epithelial cells into the circulation, from which it is delivered to the liver, bone marrow, and nervous system.

Table 134–1 ■ **CAUSES OF MALABSORPTION**

Conditions that impair mixing
  Partial gastrectomy with gastrojejunostomy
Conditions that impair lipolysis
  Chronic pancreatitis
  Pancreatic cancer
  Congenital pancreatic insufficiency
  Congenital colipase deficiency
  Gastrinoma
Conditions that impair micelle formation
  Severe chronic liver disease
  Cholestatic liver disease
  Bacterial overgrowth
  Crohn's disease
  Ileal resection
  Gastrinoma
Conditions that impair mucosal absorption
  Congenital, primary, and secondary lactase deficiency
  Congenital enterokinase deficiency
  Abetalipoproteinemia
  Giardiasis
  Celiac disease
  Tropical sprue
  Agammaglobulinemia
  Amyloidosis
  AIDS-related (infections, enteropathy)
  Radiation enteritis
  Graft versus host disease
  Whipple's disease
  Eosinophilic gastroenteritis
  Megaloblastic gut
  Collagenous sprue
  Ulcerative jejunitis
  Lymphoma
  Bacterial overgrowth
  Short bowel syndrome
  Mastocytosis
Conditions that impair nutrient delivery
  Congenital intestinal lymphangiectasia
  Lymphoma
  Tuberculosis
  Constrictive pericarditis
  Severe congestive heart failure
Conditions in which the mechanism of malabsorption is unknown
  Hypoparathyroidism
  Adrenal insufficiency
  Hyperthyroidism
  Carcinoid syndrome

Table 134–2 ■ DRUGS AND DIETARY PRODUCTS THAT IMPAIR NUTRIENT ABSORPTION

DRUG	MECHANISM	NUTRIENT MALABSORBED
Cholestyramine	Bile salt binder	Iron and cobalamin
High fiber, phytates	Chelator	Iron, calcium, magnesium
Tetracycline	Chelator	Calcium
Antacids	Chelator	Calcium, phosphate ions
Olestra	Nonabsorbable fat (lipophile)	Fat-soluble vitamins
Orlistat	Lipase inhibitor	Fat, fat-soluble vitamins
Metformin	?Mechanism	Glucose, cobalamin, folate
Acarbose	Competitive inhibitor of intestinal α-glucosidases	Carbohydrates
Colchicine	?Altered membrane trafficking	Carbohydrates, fat, cobalamin
Neomycin	Inhibitor of protein synthesis Binds bile salts	Carbohydrates, fat, protein
Methotrexate	Villus blunting	Carbohydrates, fat, protein
Phenytoin	Decreases folate absorption	Folate
Sulfasalazine	Inhibits folate hydrolase ?Inhibits folate transporter	Folate

Cobalamin deficiency impairs DNA synthesis and affects especially the bone marrow (megaloblastic anemia), tongue (glossitis), intestinal mucosa, and nervous system (paresthesias, ataxia, dementia). The most common cause of cobalamin deficiency, which is the lack of IF due to destruction of parietal cells by autoimmune chronic atrophic gastritis, is present in about 10% of middle-aged or elderly adults. When lack of gastric acid alone causes food-cobalamin malabsorption, treatment with oral cyanocobalamin is curative. Cobalamin deficiency can also be due to the uptake of cobalamin by anaerobic bacteria when they proliferate in the small intestinal lumen (blind loop syndrome) or to malabsorption due to mucosal destruction or resection of the ileum. Rare congenital deficiencies or abnormal forms of IF, TC II, or the ileal IF-cobalamin receptor can also cause cobalamin malabsorption. The diagnosis of cobalamin deficiency is made by demonstrating a low serum cobalamin level (see Chapter 163).

CLINICAL MANIFESTATIONS OF MALABSORPTION

Many diseases (Table 134–1) and drugs (Table 134–2) can cause malabsorption by impairing various aspects of luminal digestion, mucosal absorption, or nutrient delivery to the systemic circulation. Patients can present with a variety of gastrointestinal or extraintestinal manifestations (Table 134–3). Significant malabsorption of fat and carbohydrate usually causes chronic diarrhea, abdominal cramps, gas, bloating, and weight loss. Steatorrhea (fat in the stool) manifests as oily, foul smelling stools that are difficult to flush down the toilet. Individuals with malabsorption can also present with manifestations of vitamin and mineral deficiencies. Dyspnea can be due to anemia from iron, folate, or vitamin B_{12} deficiency. Cheilosis and angular stomatitis can be due to riboflavin, iron, cobalamin, or folate deficiency. Skin rash can be a manifestation of zinc, vitamin A, or essential fatty acid deficiency. Dermatitis herpetiformis is a blistering, burning, itchy rash on the extensor surfaces and buttocks associated with gluten intolerance and celiac disease. Manifestations of calcium, magnesium, or vitamin D malabsorption include paresthesias and tetany due to hypocalcemia or hypomagnesemia and bone pain due to osteomalacia or osteoporosis-related fractures. Paresthesias and ataxia are manifestations of cobalamin and vitamin E deficiency.

EVALUATION FOR MALABSORPTION

Evaluation for malabsorption begins with a careful history regarding bowel habits, weight loss, travel, food or milk tolerance, underlying gastrointestinal or liver diseases, abdominal surgery, radiation or chemotherapy treatments, family history, and drug and alcohol use. If diarrhea is the presenting symptom, a stool for ova and parasites should be obtained. If *Giardia* infection is suspected, a stool antigen capture enzyme-linked immunosorbent assay (ELISA) test for *Giardia* should be obtained (Fig. 134–2). A stool test for fat is the best available screening test for malabsorption

(Table 134–4). If the fecal fat test result is negative, selective carbohydrate malabsorption or other causes of diarrhea should be considered. If the fecal fat test result is positive (Color Plate 3*E*), further testing should be based on clinical suspicion for particular diseases. If pancreatic insufficiency is suspected, imaging studies of the pancreas should be performed. If proximal mucosal damage is suspected, multiple small intestinal biopsies should be undertaken. If there are no clues as to the cause of malabsorption, a D-xylose test should be obtained to distinguish mucosal disease from pancreatic insufficiency. The D-xylose test result can also be abnormal in individuals with bacterial overgrowth; if this condition is suspected, culture of an intestinal aspirate or a breath test should be obtained (see Table 134–4). A small bowel barium study is useful in detecting ileal disease and structural abnormalities that predispose to bacterial overgrowth. Some individuals with celiac disease present

Table 134–3 ■ CLINICAL CONSEQUENCES OF NUTRIENT AND WATER AND ELECTROLYTE MALABSORPTION

NUTRIENT MALABSORBED	CLINICAL MANIFESTATION
Protein	Wasting
	Edema
Carbohydrate and fat	Diarrhea
	Abdominal cramps and bloating
	Weight loss/growth retardation
Fluid and electrolytes	Diarrhea
	Dehydration
Iron	Anemia
	Cheilosis
	Angular stomatitis
Calcium/vitamin D	Bone pain
	Fractures
	Tetany
Magnesium	Paresthesias
	Tetany
Vitamin B_{12}/folate	Anemia
	Glossitis
	Cheilosis
	Paresthesias
	Ataxia (vitamin B_{12} only)
Vitamin E	Paresthesias
	Ataxia
	Retinopathy
Vitamin A	Night blindness
	Xerophthalmia
	Hyperkeratosis
Vitamin K	Ecchymoses
Riboflavin	Angular stomatitis
	Cheilosis
Zinc	Dermatitis
	Hypogeusia
Selenium	Cardiomyopathy
Essential fatty acids	Dermatitis

Table 134–4 ■ TESTS FOR THE EVALUATION OF MALABSORPTION*

GENERAL TESTS OF ABSORPTION	COMMENTS
Quantitative stool fat test	• Gold standard test of fat malabsorption with which all other tests are compared. Requires ingestion of a high-fat diet (100 g) for 2 d before and during the collection. Stool is collected for 3 d. Normally less than 7 g/24 hr is excreted on a high-fat diet. Borderline abnormalities of 8–14 g/24 hr may be seen in secretory or osmotic diarrheas that are not due to malabsorption
Qualitative stool fat test	• Sudan stain of a stool sample for fat. Many fat droplets (larger than the size of a red blood cell) per medium power (40×) field constitutes a positive test result. The test is dependent on an adequate fat intake (100 g/d). High sensitivity (90%) and specificity (90%) with fat malabsorption of >10 g/24 hr. Sensitivity drops with stool fat in the range of 6–10 g/24 hr.
^{14}C-triolein breath test	• A test of fat absorption. Normally, 99% of triglycerides ingested are absorbed, and the labeled fat is metabolized to $^{14}CO_2$, which appears in the breath. With fat malabsorption, there is a reduction in $^{14}CO_2$ in the breath. Sensitivity and specificity are 85–95% when compared with the quantitative fecal fat test. False-positive test results are often recorded in the irritable bowel syndrome, which limits its usefulness.
D-xylose test	• A test of small intestinal mucosal absorption, which is used to distinguish mucosal malabsorption from malabsorption due to pancreatic insufficiency. An oral dose of D-xylose (25 g/500 mL water) is administered and D-xylose excretion is measured in a 5-hr urine collection. Normally >4 g of D-xylose is excreted in the urine over 5 hr. The test may also be positive in bacterial overgrowth owing to metabolism of D-xylose by bacteria in the intestinal lumen. False-positive test results occur with renal failure, ascites, and an incomplete urine collection. Blood levels at 1 and 2 hr improve sensitivity. May be normal with limited mucosal disease.
Hydrogen breath test	• Most useful in the diagnosis of lactase deficiency. An oral dose of lactose (1 g/kg body weight) is administered following measurement of basal breath hydrogen levels. A *late peak* (within 3–6 hr) of >20 ppm of exhaled hydrogen following lactose ingestion is suggestive of lactose malabsorption. Absorption of other carbohydrates (e.g., sucrose, glucose, fructose) can be tested as well.

SPECIFIC TESTS FOR MALABSORPTION	
Tests for Pancreatic Function Secretin stimulation test	• The gold standard test of pancreatic function with which all other tests are compared. Requires duodenal intubation with a double lumen tube and collection of pancreatic juice in response to IV secretin. Allows measurement of HCO_3^- and pancreatic enzymes. A sensitive test of pancreatic function, but labor intensive and invasive.
Tests for Bacterial Overgrowth Quantitative culture of small intestinal aspirate	• Gold standard test for bacterial overgrowth. Greater than 10^5 colony-forming units/mL in the jejunum suggests bacterial overgrowth. Requires special anaerobic sample collection, rapid anaerobic and aerobic plating, and care to avoid oropharyngeal contamination. False-negative results occur with focal jejunal diverticula or when overgrowth is distal to the site aspirated.
^{14}C-D-xylose breath test	• Diagnostic sensitivity and specificity is comparable to or better than quantitative culture for the diagnosis of bacterial overgrowth except perhaps in those with motility disorders. Following an oral dose of ^{14}C-D-xylose (1 g), overgrowth of gram-negative bacteria metabolizes D-xylose with release of $^{14}CO_2$, which is absorbed and exhaled. An increase of breath $^{14}CO_2$ at 30 min is most indicative of a positive test. Cannot be used in pregnant women or children. Development of a nonradioactive ^{13}C-D-xylose breath test is under way.
Hydrogen breath test	• Has a lower sensitivity and specificity when compared with intestinal culture and the D-xylose breath test. The nonabsorbable sugar lactulose (1 g/kg body weight) or glucose is administered orally. When bacterial overgrowth is present, increased hydrogen is excreted in the breath. An *early peak* (within 2 hr) of >20 ppm of exhaled hydrogen is suggestive of bacterial overgrowth.
Tests for Mucosal Injury Small bowel biopsy	• Often obtained for a specific diagnosis when there is a high index of suspicion for small intestinal disease or when a D-xylose test result is abnormal. Several biopsies (4–5) must be obtained to maximize the diagnostic yield. Duodenal biopsies are usually adequate for diagnosis, but occasionally enteroscopy with jejunal biopsies is necessary. Small intestinal biopsy provides a specific diagnosis in some diseases, e.g., intestinal infection, Whipple's disease, abetalipoproteinemia, agammaglobulinemia, lymphangiectasia, lymphoma, and amyloidosis. In other conditions such as celiac disease and tropical sprue, the biopsy shows characteristic findings but the diagnosis is made on improvement after treatment.
Permeability studies	• A test of mucosal integrity. These tests are gaining favor as a screening test for small intestinal disease and to follow response to treatment. The study is performed by administering an oral dose of nonabsorbable markers, e.g., mannitol/lactulose, or lactulose/^{51}Cr-EDTA, and measuring urinary excretion. Currently a research tool.
Tests of Ileal Function Schilling test	• A test of vitamin B_{12} absorption. Performed as part I, followed by parts II, III, and IV if needed. **Part I:** A saturating dose (1 mg IM) of vitamin B_{12} is given followed by an oral dose of radioactive cyanocobalamin (0.5–2 μg). Urine is collected for 24 hr because of a poorly understood delay in the passage of cobalamins across ileal cells. Part I is abnormal in all individuals with vitamin B_{12} deficiency except those with dietary deficiency and food-cobalamin malabsorption. **Part II:** The test is repeated with a dose of intrinsic factor (IF). Distinguishes lack of IF from other causes of vitamin B_{12} malabsorption. **Part III:** The test is repeated with pancreatic enzymes. Can be used as a test for pancreatic insufficiency. In such individuals, administration of exogenous enzymes frees cyanocobalamin from R-proteins, reverting the Schilling test to normal. **Part IV:** The test is repeated with antibiotics. When parts I and II are low, bacterial overgrowth can be distinguished from ileal disease by repeating the test after a 5-d course of antibiotics.

*Not all of these tests are readily available. A strong suspicion for any disease may warrant foregoing an extensive work up and obtaining the test with highest diagnostic yield. In some cases, empiric treatment, such as removing lactose from the diet of an otherwise healthy individual with lactose intolerance, is warranted without any testing.

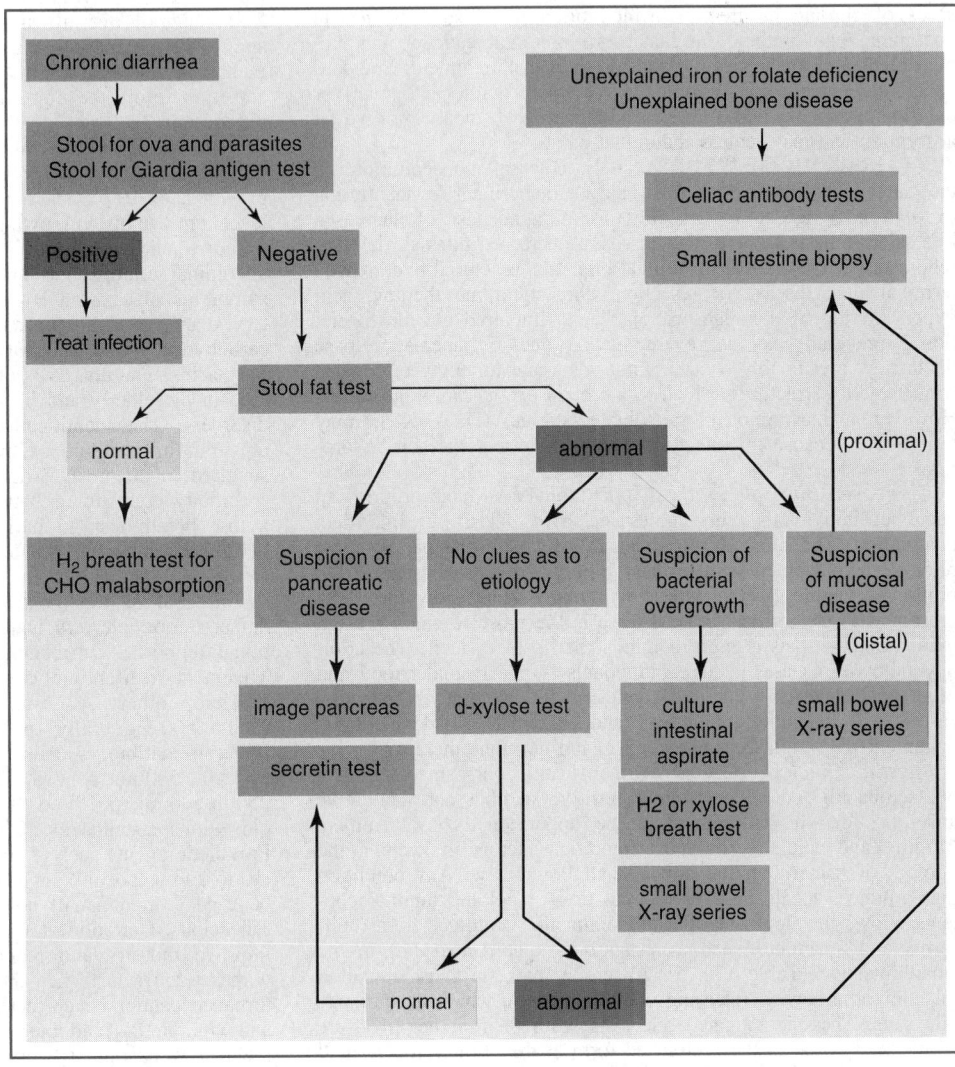

FIGURE 134–2 ■ Strategy for obtaining a diagnosis when malabsorption is suspected.

with selective nutrient deficiencies without diarrhea. When this is suspected, antibody tests (see later discussion) and intestinal biopsy should be performed. When malabsorption is suspected in patients hospitalized for severe diarrhea or malnutrition, a more streamlined evaluation usually includes a stool for culture, ova and parasites, and fat; an abdominal imaging study; and a biopsy of the small intestine.

MALABSORPTIVE SYNDROMES

Conditions That Impair Intraluminal Digestion

IMPAIRED MIXING. Surgical alterations such as partial gastrectomy with gastrojejunostomy (a Billroth II anastamosis) result in the release of biliary and pancreatic secretions into the intestine at a site remote from the site of entry of gastric chyme into the jejunum. This imbalance can result in impaired lipolysis and impaired micelle formation, with subsequent fat malabsorption. Rapid transit through the jejunum contributes to the malabsorption of nutrients. Individuals with these conditions also have surgical anastamoses that predispose to bacterial overgrowth.

IMPAIRED LIPOLYSIS. A deficiency in pancreatic lipase can be due to the congenital absence of pancreatic lipase or due to destruction of the pancreatic gland from alcohol-related pancreatitis, cystic fibrosis, or pancreatic cancer. Pancreatic lipase can also be denatured by excess secretion of gastric acid (e.g., Zollinger-Ellison syndrome).

Chronic pancreatitis (see Chapter 141) is the most common

cause of pancreatic insufficiency and impaired lipolysis. In the United States, chronic pancreatitis is most commonly due to alcohol abuse; in contrast, tropical (nutritional) pancreatitis is most common worldwide. Malabsorption of fat does not occur until more than 90% of the pancreas is destroyed. Individuals typically present with steatorrhea, abdominal pain, and diabetes, although some present with diabetes in the absence of gastrointestinal symptoms. Weight loss, when it occurs, is usually due to decreased oral intake to avoid abdominal pain or diarrhea and less commonly to malabsorption. Fat malabsorption due to chronic pancreatitis usually causes bulky, fat-laden stools. These individuals have more than 30 g/day of fat loss in the stool. Stools are not usually watery because undigested triglycerides form large emulsion droplets with little osmotic force and, unlike fatty acids, do not stimulate water and electrolyte secretion in the colon. Deficiency of fat-soluble vitamins is seen only rarely, presumably because gastric and residual pancreatic lipase generates enough fatty acids for some micelle formation. Clinical manifestations of carbohydrate and protein malabsorption are also rare in pancreatic insufficiency. However, in severe disease, subclinical protein malabsorption, manifested by the presence of undigested meat fibers in the stool, and subclinical carbohydrate malabsorption, manifested by gas-filled, floating stools, can occur. About 30 to 40% of individuals with chronic pancreatitis due to alcohol abuse have calcifications on abdominal radiographs. A qualitative or quantitative test for fecal fat will be positive in individuals whose pancreas is more than 90% destroyed. There are no convenient laboratory tests for the diagnosis of milder cases of chronic pancreatitis, which often manifest with chronic abdominal pain without fat malabsorption. Pancreatic enzyme replacement and analgesics are the mainstays of treatment. Standard pancreatic enzyme preparations (6 to 8 tabs with each meal) or enteric-coated enzymes (three capsules with each meal) improve fat absorption and may reduce abdominal pain.

IMPAIRED MICELLE FORMATION. Bile salt concentrations in the intestinal lumen can fall below the critical concentration (5 to 15 mM) needed for micelle formation because of decreased bile salt synthesis (severe liver disease), decreased bile salt delivery (cholestasis), or removal of luminal bile salts (bacterial overgrowth, terminal ileal disease or resection, cholestyramine therapy, acid hypersecretion). Fat malabsorption due to impaired micelle formation is generally not as severe as that due to pancreatic lipase deficiency, presumably because fatty acids and monoglycerides can form lamellar structures, which to a certain extent can be absorbed. However, malabsorption of fat-soluble vitamins (D, A, K, E) may be marked because micelle formation is required for their absorption.

Decreased Bile Salt Synthesis and Delivery: Malabsorption can occur in individuals with cholestasic liver disease or bile duct obstruction. The clinical consequences of malabsorption are most often seen in women with primary biliary cirrhosis because of the prolonged nature of the illness. Although these individuals can present with steatorrhea, bone disease is the most common presentation. Osteoporosis is more common than osteomalacia. The etiology of bone disease in these individuals is poorly understood and often not related to vitamin D deficiency. Treatment of bone disease is with calcium supplements (and vitamin D if a deficiency is documented), weight-bearing exercise, and hormone therapy.

Intestinal Bacterial Overgrowth: In health, only small numbers of lactobacilli, enterococci, gram-positive aerobes, or facultative anaerobes can be cultured from the upper small bowel lumen. Motility and acid are the most important factors in keeping the number of bacteria in the upper small bowel low. Any condition that produces local stasis or recirculation of colonic luminal contents allows development of a predominantly "colonic" flora (coliforms and anaerobes such as *Bacteroides* and *Clostridia*) in the small intestine (Table 134–5). Anaerobic bacteria cause impaired micelle formation by releasing cholyl-amidases, which deconjugate bile salts. The unconjugated bile salts, with their higher pKa, are more likely to be in the protonated form at the normal upper small intestinal pH of 6 to 7 and can therefore be absorbed passively. As a result, the concentration of bile salts decreases in the intestinal lumen and can fall below the critical micellar concentration to cause fat and fat-soluble vitamin malabsorption. Vitamin B_{12} deficiency and carbohydrate malabsorption can also occur with generalized bacterial overgrowth. Anaerobic bacteria ingest vitamin B_{12} and release proteases that degrade brush border disaccharidases. Lactase is the disaccharidase normally present in lowest abundance and is therefore the first affected. Although anaerobic bacteria utilize vitamin B_{12}, they synthesize folate. Therefore, individuals with bacterial overgrowth usually have low serum vitamin B_{12} levels but normal or high folate levels, which help distinguish bacterial overgrowth from tropical sprue—in which both vitamin B_{12} and folate levels are usually low owing to decreased mucosal uptake.

Individuals with bacterial overgrowth can present with diarrhea, abdominal cramps, gas and bloating, weight loss, and signs and symptoms of vitamin B_{12} and fat-soluble vitamin deficiency. Watery diarrhea occurs because of the osmotic load of unabsorbed carbohydrates and stimulation of colonic secretion by unabsorbed fatty acids. The diagnosis of bacterial overgrowth should be considered in the elderly and in individuals with predisposing underlying disorders. The identification of greater than 10^5 colony-forming units/mL in a culture of small intestinal aspirate remains the gold standard in diagnosis. The noninvasive test with a sensitivity and specificity equal to or better than intestinal culture is the [^{14}C]D-xylose breath test; in individuals with low vitamin B_{12} levels, a Schilling test before and after antibiotic therapy can be diagnostic (see Table 134–4).

The goal of treatment is to correct the structural or motility defect if possible, eradicate offending bacteria, and provide nutritional support. Acid-reducing agents should be stopped if possible. Treatment with antibiotics should be based on culture results when possible; otherwise, empiric treatment is given. Tetracycline (250 to 500 mg orally [po] four times a day [qid]) or a broad-spectrum antibiotic against aerobes and enteric anaerobes (ciprofloxacin, 500 mg po twice a day [bid], amoxicillin/clavulanic acid, 250 to 500 mg po three times a day [tid], cephalexin, 250 mg po qid, with metronidazole, 250 mg tid) should be given for 14 days. Prokinetic agents such as metoclopramide (10 mg po qid), cisapride (10 to 20 mg po qid), or erythromycin (250 to 500 mg po qid) can be tried to treat small bowel motility disorders but often are not efficacious. Octreotide (50 μg subcutaneously every day [qd]) may improve motility and reduce bacterial overgrowth in individuals with scleroderma. When the structural abnormality or motility disturbance cannot be corrected, patients are at risk for malnutrition and vitamin B_{12} and fat-soluble vitamin deficiencies. Cyclic treatment (1 week out of every 4 to 6 weeks) with rotating antibiotics may be required in these patients to prevent recurrent bouts of bacterial overgrowth. If supplemental calories are needed, medium-chain triglycerides should be given, as they are not dependent on micelle formation for their absorption. Monthly treatment with vitamin B_{12} should be considered, along with supplemental vitamins D, A, K, and E and calcium.

Ileal Disease or Resection: Disease of the terminal ileum is most commonly due to Crohn's disease (which may also lead to ileal resection) but can also be caused by radiation enteritis, tropical sprue, tuberculosis, *Yersinia* infection, and idiopathic bile salt malabsorption. These diseases cause bile salt wasting. Bile salt losses of up to 3 g/day can be offset by increased hepatic synthesis.

The clinical consequences of bile salt malabsoption are directly related to the length of the diseased or resected terminal ileum. In an adult, if less than 100 cm of ileum is diseased or resected, watery diarrhea results owing to stimulation of colonic fluid secretion by unabsorbed bile salts. Fat absorption remains normal because increased bile salt synthesis in the liver compensates for bile salt losses, and micelle formation is preserved. Such individuals can be treated with cholestyramine (2 to 4 g taken at breakfast, lunch, and dinner), an antimotility agent (loperamide or diphenoxylate hydrochloride), and a multiple vitamin and mineral supplement. When more than 100 cm of ileum is diseased or resected, bile salt losses in the colon exceed the capacity for increased bile salt synthesis in the liver; the bile salt pool shrinks, micelle formation is impaired, and steatorrhea and diarrhea develop. Individuals with these conditions can be treated with a low-fat diet, vitamin B_{12} injections, dietary supplements of calcium, and a multiple vitamin-mineral supplement. An antimotility agent should be administered for diarrhea. The patient should be screened for fat-soluble vitamin deficiencies (vitamins A and E, 25-(OH) vitamin D, and prothrom-

Table 134–5 ■ **ABNORMALITIES CONDUCIVE TO BACTERIAL OVERGROWTH**

STRUCTURAL
Surgical
    Afferent loop dysfunction following gastrojejunostomy
    Ileocecal valve resection
    Surgical loops (end-to-side intestinal anastomoses)
Anatomic
    Duodenal and jejunal diverticula
    Obstruction
        Strictures (Crohn's disease, radiation enteritis)
        Adhesions (postsurgical)
    Gastrojejunocolic fistulas
MOTOR
Scleroderma
Diabetes mellitus
Idiopathic pseudo-obstruction
HYPOCHLORHYDRIA
Acquired immune deficiency syndrome
Atrophic gastritis
Proton pump inhibitors
Acid-reducing surgery for peptic ulcer disease
MISCELLANEOUS
Immunodeficiency states
Pancreatitis
Cirrhosis

bin time) and bone disease (bone densitometry, serum calcium, and intact parathyroid hormone).

Malabsorption in Crohn's disease also can be due to bacterial overgrowth from strictures or enterocolic fistula. Gastrocolic or enteroenteric/colic fistulas can also bypass segments of small intestine and significantly decrease the surface area available for absorption.

Three long-term complications of chronic bile salt wasting and fat malabsorption are renal stones, bone disease (osteoporosis and osteomalacia), and gallstones. Oxalate renal stones occur as a consequence of excess free oxalate absorption in the colon. Free oxalate is generated when unabsorbed fatty acids bind luminal calcium, which is then unavailable for binding oxalate. Renal oxalate stones can sometimes be avoided with a low-fat, low-oxalate diet and calcium supplements. Bone disease is due to impaired micelle formation with a resulting decrease in absorption of vitamin D; year-round sun exposure reduces this complication. Vitamin D and calcium supplements should be given to susceptible individuals, but vitamin D levels and urinary calcium should be monitored for response to treatment because excess vitamin D can be toxic. The mechanism of gallstone formation in these individuals is unclear; pigmented gallstones are most common.

Diseases That Impair Mucosal Absorption

Mucosal malabsorption can be caused by specific (usually congenital) brush border enzyme or nutrient transporter deficiencies or by generalized diseases that damage the small intestinal mucosa or result in surgical resection or bypass of small intestine. The nutrient(s) malabsorbed in these general malabsorptive diseases depend on the site of intestinal injury (proximal, distal, or diffuse) and the severity of damage. The main mechanism of malabsorption in these conditions is a decrease in surface area available for absorption. Some conditions (infection, celiac disease, tropical sprue, food allergies, and graft versus host disease) are characterized by intestinal inflammation and villus flattening; other conditions by ulceration (ulcerative jejunitis, nonsteroidal anti-inflammatory drugs), infiltration (amyloidosis), or ischemia (radiation enteritis, mesenteric ischemia).

LACTASE DEFICIENCY. Acquired lactase deficiency is the most common cause of selective carbohydrate malabsorption. Most individuals, except those of northern European descent, begin to lose lactase activity by the age of 5 years. The prevalence of lactase deficiency is highest (85 to 100%) in Asians, African blacks, and Native Americans. In most individuals, lactase deficiency is due to decreased synthesis of the enzyme. In some, however, intracellular transport and glycosylation of lactase is defective. Adults with lactase deficiency typically complain of gas, bloating, and diarrhea after the ingestion of milk or dairy products but do not lose weight. Unabsorbed lactose is osmotically active, drawing water followed by ions into the intestinal lumen. On reaching the colon, bacteria metabolize lactose to short-chain fatty acids, carbon dioxide, and hydrogen gas. Short-chain fatty acids are transported with sodium into colonic epithelial cells, facilitating the reabsorption of fluid in the colon. If the colonic capacity for the reabsorption of short-chain fatty acids is exceeded, an osmotic diarrhea results (see Chapter 133).

The diagnosis of lactase deficiency can be made by empirical treatment with a lactose-free diet, which results in resolution of symptoms, or by the hydrogen breath test after oral administration of lactose. A number of intestinal diseases cause secondary reversible lactase deficiency, such as viral gastroenteritis, celiac disease, giardiasis, and bacterial overgrowth.

CONGENITAL ENTEROPEPTIDASE (ENTEROKINASE) DEFICIENCY. Enteropeptidase is a brush border protease that cleaves trypsinogen to trypsin, thereby triggering the cascade of pancreatic protease activation in the intestinal lumen. The rare congenital deficiency of enteropeptidase results in the inability to activate all pancreatic proteases and leads to severe protein malabsorption. It manifests in infancy as diarrhea, growth retardation, and hypoproteinemic edema.

ABETALIPOPROTEINEMIA. Formation and exocytosis of chylomicrons at the basolateral membrane of intestinal epithelial cells are necessary for the delivery of lipids to the systemic circulation. One of the proteins required for assembly and secretion of chylomicrons is the microsomal triglyceride transfer protein, which is mutated in individuals with abetalipoproteinemia. Children with this disorder suffer from fat malabsorption and, in particular, from the consequences of vitamin E deficiency (retinopathy and spinocerebellar degeneration). Biochemical tests show low plasma levels of apoprotein B, triglyceride, and cholesterol. Membrane lipid abnormalities result in red blood cell acanthosis ("burr cells"). Intestinal biopsy is diagnostic and characterized by engorgement of epithelial cells with lipid droplets. Calories are provided by treatment with a low-fat diet containing medium-chain triglycerides. Medium-chain fatty acids are easily absorbed and released directly into the portal circulation, thereby bypassing the defect of abetalipoproteinemia. Poor absorption of long-chain fatty acids can sometimes result in essential fatty acid deficiency. High doses of fat-soluble vitamins, especially vitamin E, are often needed.

CELIAC DISEASE. Celiac disease, also called celiac sprue, nontropical sprue, and gluten-sensitive enteropathy, is an inflammatory condition of the small intestine precipitated by the ingestion of wheat, rye, and barley in individuals with certain genetic predispositions. The prevalence of celiac disease in the United States, based on the number of individuals presenting with typical gastrointestinal symptoms, is estimated at 1:4500. However, recent screening studies for the antigliadin and antiendomysial antibodies that are associated with celiac disease suggest a much higher prevalence in Northern Ireland (1:122), as well as in Europe and the United States (about 1:250). High-risk groups for celiac disease include first-degree relatives and individuals with type I diabetes mellitus and autoimmune thyroid disease. Virtually 100% of individuals with dermatitis herpetiformis have gluten-sensitive enteropathy.

Both environmental and genetic factors are important in the development of celiac disease. The alcohol-soluble protein fraction of wheat gluten, the gliadins, and similar prolamins in rye and barley trigger intestinal inflammation in susceptible individuals. Oat grains, which have prolamins rich in glutamine but not proline, appear to be less toxic. The specific peptide sequence or sequences responsible for triggering intestinal inflammation and the processes leading to villus flattening remain unknown.

Approximately 15% of first-degree relatives of affected individuals are found to have celiac disease. Predisposition to gluten sensitivity has been mapped to the HLA-D region on chromosome 6. Ninety per cent of individuals with celiac disease have the DQ2 heterodimer encoded for by alleles DQA1*0501 and DQB1*0201 compared with 20 to 30% of controls. The DQ2 protein is expressed on antigen-presenting cells, but the site on DQ2 that interacts with gliadin and host T-cell receptors, thereby sensitizing the intestine to gluten, has not been identified.

The diagnosis of celiac disease is made by characteristic changes found on small intestinal biopsy and improving when a gluten-free diet is instituted (Figs. 134–3 and 134–4). Mucosal flattening can be observed endoscopically as reduced duodenal folds or duodenal scalloping. Characteristic features found on intestinal biopsy include the absence of villi, crypt hyperplasia, increased intraepithelial lymphocytes, and infiltration of the lamina propria with plasma cells and lymphocytes.

Serologic markers for celiac disease are useful in supporting the diagnosis, in screening first-degree relatives, and in following the response to a gluten-free diet. Antigliadin IgG and IgA antibodies are sensitive but not specific. Antiendomysial IgA antibodies (antibodies against tissue transglutaminase) are highly sensitive (90%) and specific (90 to 100%) for active celiac disease in skilled laboratory testing. Antiendomysial and antigliadin IgA antibodies will be negative in the small percentage of individuals with selective IgA deficiency.

Celiac disease usually manifests early in life at about 2 years of age, after wheat has been introduced into the diet, or later in the third or fourth decades of adult life. Individuals with significant mucosal involvement present with watery diarrhea, weight loss or growth retardation, and the clinical manifestations of vitamin and mineral deficiencies. All nutrients, most notably carbohydrate, fat, protein, electrolytes, fat-soluble vitamins, calcium, magnesium, iron, folate, and zinc, are malabsorbed. Cobalamin malabsorption is rare, as the disease most often affects the proximal small intestine more than the distal. Some individuals also have impaired pancre-

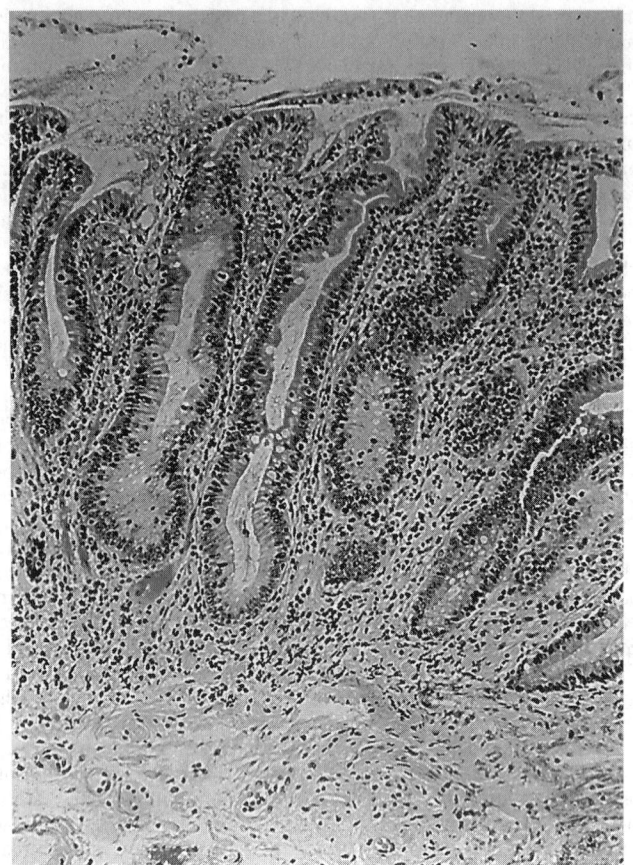

FIGURE 134–3 ▪ Intestinal biopsy appearance of flattened villi and hyperplastic crypts. (Courtesy of Heidrun Rotterdam, MD.)

atic enzyme secretion owing to impaired release of CCK and secretin from the diseased intestinal mucosa. Diarrhea is due to a number of mechanisms, including a decreased surface area for water and electrolyte absorption, the osmotic effect of unabsorbed luminal nutrients, and the stimulation of intestinal fluid secretion by inflammatory mediators and unabsorbed fatty acids.

A significant number of adults with celiac disease present with anemia or osteoporosis without gastrointestinal symptoms. These individuals likely have proximal disease that impairs iron, folate, and calcium absorption but an adequate surface area in the remaining intestine for absorption of other nutrients. Other extraintestinal manifestations of celiac disease include rash (dermatitis herpetiformis), neurologic disorders (myopathy, epilepsy), psychiatric disorders (depression, paranoia), and reproductive disorders (infertility, spontaneous abortion).

Treatment consists of a lifelong gluten-free diet. Wheat, rye, and barley grains should be excluded from the diet. Rice and corn grains are tolerated, and a moderate amount of oat grain (if not contaminated by wheat grain) may be tolerated as well. Early referral to a celiac support group is often helpful in maintaining dietary compliance. Owing to secondary lactase deficiency, a lactose-free diet should be recommended until symptoms improve. All individuals with celiac disease should be screened for vitamin and mineral deficiencies and have bone densitometry. Seventy per cent of individuals with celiac disease have osteopenia. Documented deficiencies of vitamins and minerals should be replenished (Table 134–6), and women of childbearing age should take folic acid supplements.

Up to 90% of patients with celiac disease treated with a gluten-free diet experience symptomatic improvement within 2 weeks. The most common cause of a poor dietary response is continued ingestion of gluten. Other possibilites include an overlooked intestinal infection, other food allergies (cow's milk, soy protein), ulcerative jejunitis, or intestinal lymphoma. In a small percentage of individuals, collagen deposition is found beneath the surface epithelium

(collagenous sprue), or a hypoplastic mucosa demonstrates both villus and crypt atrophy; individuals with these conditions characteristically have severe disease refractory to a gluten-free diet. Although some with collagenous sprue respond to steroid treatment, a hypoplastic mucosa is indicative of irreversible (end-stage) intestinal disease. Individuals with celiac disease are at increased risk for intestinal T-cell lymphoma and carcinomas; a strict gluten-free diet for life may lessen this risk. Lymphoma should be suspected in individuals who have abdominal pain and a recurrence of symptoms despite a gluten-free diet.

TROPICAL SPRUE. Tropical sprue is an inflammatory disease of the small intestine associated with the overgrowth of predominantly coliform bacteria. It occurs in residents or travelers to the tropics, especially India and Southeast Asia. Individuals classically present with diarrhea as well as megaloblastic anemia due to vitamin B_{12} and folate deficiency, but some have anemia only. Intestinal biopsy characteristically shows subtotal and patchy villus atrophy in the proximal and distal small intestine, which may be due to the effect of bacterial toxins on gut structure or to the secondary effects of vitamin B_{12} deficiency on the gut (megaloblastic gut). Diagnosis is based on history, documentation of vitamin B_{12} and/or folate deficiency, and the presence of an abnormal small intestinal biopsy report. Treatment is a prolonged course of broad-spectrum antibiotics, oral folate, and vitamin B_{12} injections until symptoms resolve. Relapses occur mainly in natives of the tropics.

INFECTION. *Giardia lamblia,* the most common protozoal infection in the United States, can cause malabsorption in individuals infected with a large number of trophozoites, especially the immunocompromised or IgA-deficient host. Malabsorption occurs when a large number of organisms cover the epithelium and cause mucosal inflammation, which results in villus flattening and a decrease in absorptive surface area. Stool for ova and parasites at this stage of infection is often negative because of the attachment of organisms

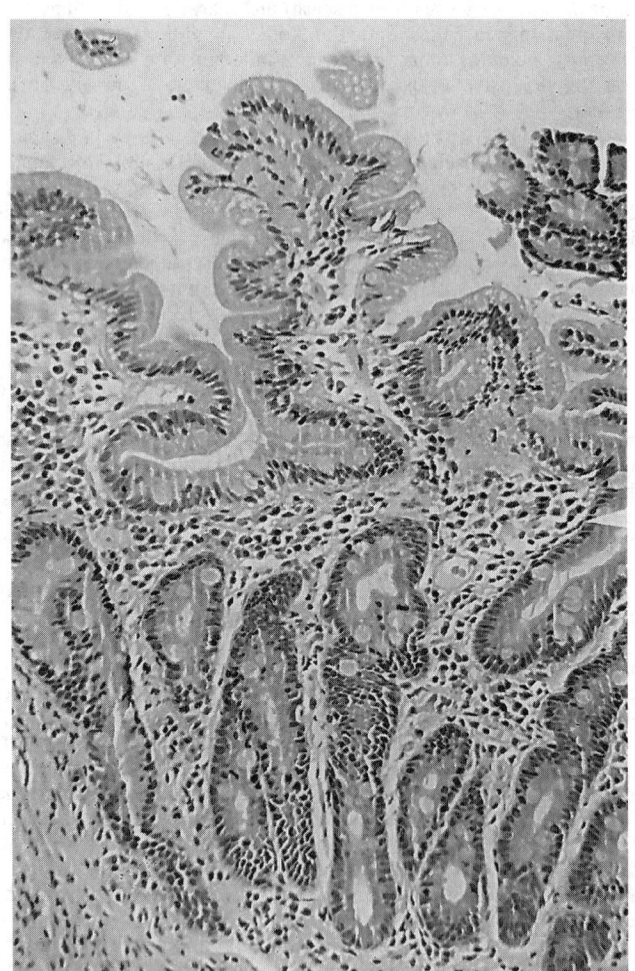

FIGURE 134–4 ▪ Regeneration of villi 4 weeks after initiation of a gluten-free diet. (Courtesy of Heidrun Rotterdam, MD.)

Table 134–6 ▪ VITAMIN AND MINERAL DOSES USED IN THE TREATMENT OF MALABSORPTION

	ORAL DOSE	PARENTERAL DOSE
Vitamin A*	Water-soluble A 25,000 U/d§	
Vitamin E	Water-soluble E 400–800 U/d§	
Vitamin D†	25,000–50,000 U/d	
Vitamin K	5 mg/d	
Folate	1 mg/d	

Calcium‡	1500–2000 mg elemental calcium/d
	    Calcium citrate, 500 mg calcium/tab§
	    Calcium carbonate, 500 mg calcium/tab§	

Magnesium	Liquid magnesium gluconate§
	    1–3 tbsp (12–36 mEq magnesium) in 1–2 L of
	    ORS or sports drink sipped throughout the day
		2 mL of a 50% solution (8 mEq)
		both buttocks IM

Zinc	Zinc gluconate§ 20–50 mg elemental zinc/d‖	

Iron	150–300 mg elemental iron/d
	    Polysaccharide-iron complex§
	    Iron sulfate or gluconate
		Iron dextran as calculated for
		anemia (IV or IM)

B-complex vitamins	1 megadose tab/d	
Vitamin B$_{12}$	2 mg/d	1 mg IM or SC/month#

IM = intramuscular; IV = intravenous; ORS = oral rehydration solution; SC = subcutaneous.
*Monitor serum vitamin A level to avoid toxicity, especially in those with hypertriglyceridemia.
†Monitor serum calcium and 25-OH vitamin D levels to avoid toxicity.
‡Monitor 24-hr urine calcium to assess adequacy of dose.
§Form best absorbed or with least side effects.
‖If intestinal output is high, additional zinc should be given.
#For vitamin B$_{12}$ deficiency 1 mg IM or SC twice a week for 4 weeks, then once a month.

in the proximal small intestine. Diagnosis can be made by a stool antigen capture ELISA test but may require duodenal aspiration and biopsies.

Diarrhea, malabsorption, and wasting are common in individuals with the acquired immune deficiency syndrome (AIDS) but are seen less frequently with improved anti-retroviral therapy (Chapter 413). Malabsorption is usually due to infection with cryptosporidia, *Mycobacterium avium-intracellulare* complex (MAC), *Isospora belli*, and microsporidia. AIDS enteropathy (a term used when no organism is identified) can also cause malabsorption. An organism can be identified by stool examination or intestinal biopsy about 50% of the time. In individuals with AIDS and diarrhea, fecal fat and D-xylose absorption study results are frequently abnormal. Serum albumin, vitamin B$_{12}$, and zinc levels are often low. Low serum levels of vitamin B$_{12}$ have been reported in human immunodeficiency virus (HIV)–infected individuals without AIDS as well. Vitamin B$_{12}$ deficiency is mainly due to ileal disease, but low IF and decreased TC II may be contributing factors. Management of malabsorption should focus on restoring the immune system by treating the underlying HIV infection with antiviral therapy. When possible, the offending organism should be treated with antibiotics. If the organism cannot be eradicated, chronic diarrhea and malabsorption will result; treatment in such cases consists of antimotility agents and a lactose-free, low-fat diet. If supplemental calories are needed, liquid oral supplements that are predigested and high in medium-chain triglycerides are best tolerated. Vitamin and mineral deficiencies should be screened for and treated.

Whipple's disease, a rare cause of malabsorption, manifests with gastrointestinal complaints in association with systemic symptoms such as fever, joint pain, or neurologic manifestations. Occasionally, individuals present with ocular or neurologic disease without gastrointestinal symptoms. The organism responsible for causing Whipple's disease is a gram-positive actinomycete, *Tropheryma whippelii.* The HLA-B27 gene is more common in Whipple's disease patients. Small intestinal biopsy shows villus blunting and infiltration of the lamina propria with large macrophages that stain positive with the periodic acid–Schiff method and are filled with the organism. It is important to distinguish these macrophages from macrophages infected with MAC, which stain positive on acid-fast staining and are found in individuals with AIDS. Treatment is with a prolonged course of broad-spectrum antibiotics. Relapses are common.

RADIATION ENTERITIS. Gastrointestinal dysfunction is common after radiation treatment to the pelvis or abdomen. Most individuals have an increased frequency of bowel movements for life. Diarrhea and abdominal cramps can develop up to 20 years after radiation treatment. Radiation damage to the intestine, characterized histologically by an obliterative endarteritis of the small vessels, can result in intestinal ulceration, strictures, and fistula formation. A small number of individuals develop malabsorption due to bacterial overgrowth, intestinal bypass, or bile salt wasting. Rapid transit may also contribute to malabsorption and diarrhea. Treatment is often unsatisfactory. Antimotility agents, cholestyramine, antibiotics, steroids, and sulfasalazine can be tried.

GRAFT VERSUS HOST DISEASE (GVHD). Diarrhea occurs frequently after allogeneic bone marrow or stem cell transplantation. Immediately after transplant, diarrhea is due to the toxic effects of cytoreductive therapy on the intestinal epithelium. At 20 to 100 days after transplant, diarrhea is usually due to GVHD or infection. Individuals with GVHD present clinically with a skin rash, buccal mucositis, anorexia, nausea, vomiting, abdominal cramps, and diarrhea. The diagnosis of GVHD in the gastrointestinal tract can be made on biopsy of the stomach, small intestine, or colon. In mild cases, the mucosa appears normal on inspection at endoscopy, but apoptosis of gastric gland or crypt cells can be found on biopsy. In severe cases, denuding of the intestinal epithelium results in diarrhea and malabsorption and often requires parenteral nutritional support. Octreotide (50 to 250 μg subcutaneous tid) may be helpful in controlling voluminous diarrhea. Treatment of GVHD is with steroids and antithymocyte globulin combined with parenteral nutrition support until intestinal function returns.

SHORT BOWEL SYNDROME. Malabsorption due to small bowel resection or surgical bypass is referred to as the short bowel syndrome. The most common causes in the United States are Crohn's disease, radiation enteritis, and mesenteric ischemia. The severity of malabsorption depends on the site and extent of resection, the capacity for bowel adaptation, and the function of the residual bowel. Adaptive changes to enhance absorption in the remaining bowel include hyperplasia, dilation, and elongation. Mechanisms of malabsorption after small bowel resection include a decreased absorptive surface area, decreased luminal bile salt concentration, rapid transit, and bacterial overgrowth. Limited jejunal resection is usually best tolerated because bile salt and vitamin B$_{12}$ absorption remain normal. Ileal resection is less well tolerated because of the consequences of bile salt wasting and the limited capacity of the jejunum to undergo adaptive hyperplasia.

When fewer than 100 cm of jejunum remain, the colon takes on an important role in caloric salvage and fluid reabsorption. Malabsorbed carbohydrates are digested by colonic bacteria to short-chain fatty acids, which are absorbed in the colon. Parenteral nutrition may be avoided by a diet rich in complex carbohydrates, oral rehydration solution, and an antimotility agent. In comparison, individuals with fewer than 100 cm of jejunum and no colon have high jejunostomy outputs and often require intravenous fluids or parenteral nutrition to survive. These individuals waste sodium, chloride, bicarbonate, magnesium, zinc, and water in their ostomy effluent. Diet modifications should include a high-salt, nutrient-rich diet given in small meals and taken separately from fluids. An oral rehydration solution with a sodium concentration greater than 90 mmol is best absorbed. Oral vitamin and mineral doses higher than the usual U.S. recommended daily allowances are required (see Table 134–6). Vitamin B_{12} should be given parenterally. Magnesium deficiencies are often difficult to replenish with oral magnesium because of its osmotic effect in the intestinal lumen. A liquid magnesium preparation added to an oral rehydration solution and sipped throughout the day may minimize magnesium-induced fluid losses. Potent antimotility agents such as tincture of opium are often needed to slow transit and maximize contact time for nutrient absorption. High-volume jejunostomy outputs can be lessened by inhibiting endogenous secretions with a proton pump inhibitor and, in severe cases, octreotide (50 to 100 μg subcutaneous tid). The benefit of octreotide may be offset by its potential to inhibit intestinal adaptation and impair pancreatic enzyme secretion. In the most severe cases, supplemental calories must be provided by nocturnal tube feeding or parenteral nutrition. Long-term complications include bone disease, renal stones (oxalate stones if the colon is present, urate stones with a jejunostomy), gallstones, bacterial overgrowth, fat-soluble vitamin deficiencies, essential fatty acid deficiency, and D-lactic acidosis. Small bowel transplantation should be considered in individuals who require parenteral nutrition to survive and then develop liver disease or venous access problems.

DISEASES THAT IMPAIR NUTRIENT DELIVERY TO THE GENERAL CIRCULATION

IMPAIRED LYMPHATIC DRAINAGE. Diseases that cause intestinal lymphatic obstruction, such as primary congenital lymphangiectasia (malunion of intestinal lymphatics), or those that result in secondary lymphangiectasia (lymphoma, tuberculosis, Kaposi's sarcoma, retroperitoneal fibrosis, constrictive pericarditis, severe heart failure) result in fat malabsorption. The increased pressure in the intestinal lymphatics leads to leakage and sometimes rupture of lymph into the intestinal lumen with the loss of lipids, gamma globulins, albumin, and lymphocytes. The diagnosis of lymphangiectasia can be made by intestinal biopsy, but the specific cause may be more difficult to identify. Individuals with lymphangiectasia malabsorb fat and fat-soluble vitamins and have protein loss into the intestinal lumen. The most common presentation is hypoproteinemic edema. Nutritional management includes a low-fat diet and supplementation with medium-chain triglycerides, which are absorbed directly into the portal circulation. Fat-soluble vitamins should be given if deficiencies develop.

PROTEIN-LOSING ENTEROPATHY. Protein-losing enteropathy can result from a variety of inflammatory diseases and some as yet ill-defined mechanisms (see Chapter 133).

Feldman M, Scharschmidt BT, Sleisenger MH (eds): Sleisenger and Fordtran's Gastrointestinal and Liver Disease, 6th ed. Philadelphia, WB Saunders, 1998, Chaps. 16, 26–28, 48, 86–89, 91–94, 100, 101. *Comprehensive discussion of diseases that cause maldigestion and malabsorption, including pathophysiology, diagnosis, and management.*

Murray JA: The widening spectrum of celiac disease. Am J Clin Nutr 69:354, 1999. *Excellent review of pathophysiology, genetics, immunology, and clinical diagnosis and management.*

135 INFLAMMATORY BOWEL DISEASE

William F. Stenson

DEFINITION. Inflammatory bowel diseases (IBD), including ulcerative colitis and Crohn's disease, are chronic inflammatory diseases of the gastrointestinal tract. They are diagnosed by a set of clinical, endoscopic, and histologic characteristics, but no single finding is absolutely diagnostic for one disease or the other. Moreover, some patients have a clinical picture that falls between the two diseases and are said to have indeterminate colitis.

The inflammatory response in ulcerative colitis is largely confined to the mucosa and submucosa, but in Crohn's disease the inflammation extends through the intestinal wall from mucosa to serosa. Ulcerative colitis is confined to the colon, and colectomy is a curative procedure. Crohn's disease, in contrast, can involve any part of the gastrointestinal tract, although the distal small bowel and the colon are most commonly involved. Resection of the inflamed segment is not curative in Crohn's disease, and inflammation is likely to recur.

EPIDEMIOLOGY. The incidence and prevalence of Crohn's disease and ulcerative colitis vary with geographic location; the highest rates are for white populations in northern Europe and North America, where the incidence for each disease is about 5 per 100,000 and the prevalence is about 50 per 100,000. Rates in central and southern Europe are lower, and in South America, Asia, and Africa lower still. Crohn's disease and ulcerative colitis are both more common in Jews than non-Jews. In the United States, the incidence of IBD in the black population has been one fifth to one half that in the white population, but in recent years that gap has narrowed. In northern Europe and North America, the incidence of ulcerative colitis has leveled off but that of Crohn's disease is still increasing. For both diseases, the incidence is equal in men and women. The peak age at onset is between 15 and 25 years of age, with a second, lesser peak between 55 and 65 years of age. Both diseases occur in childhood, although the incidence before 15 years of age is low.

The risk of developing ulcerative colitis is increased among both non-smokers and former smokers compared with current smokers. Whether initiation of smoking improves symptoms is unclear, although success has been reported with nicotine patches. In contrast, the incidence of smoking is higher among Crohn's disease patients than the general population, and patients who continue to smoke may be less likely to respond to medical therapy.

ETIOLOGY AND PATHOGENESIS. The most important risk factor for IBD is a positive family history. Approximately 15% of IBD patients have affected first-degree relatives, and the incidence among first-degree relatives is 30 to 100 times that of the general population. The best estimates of the lifetime risk of developing IBD among first-degree relatives of affected individuals is 3 to 9%. The increased incidence among first-degree relatives contrasts to the absence of an increased incidence in spouses of patients. Dizygotic twins have the same rate of concordance as would be expected for siblings, whereas monozygotic twins have higher rates of concordance for both diseases. A susceptibility locus for Crohn's disease has been mapped to chromosome 16.

In IBD, the lamina propria is infiltrated with lymphocytes, macrophages, and other cells of the immune system. An intensive search for the antigens that trigger the immune response has yet to identify a specific microbial pathogen. Anticolon antibodies of unclear significance have been identified in the sera of ulcerative colitis patients. IBD may also be related to a failure to suppress (or "down-regulate") the normal, finely tuned, low-grade chronic inflammation of the intestinal lamina propria in response to its chronic exposure to luminal antigens.

Whatever the antigenic trigger, activated lamina propria T cells are involved in the pathogenesis of IBD. In Crohn's disease, the activated lymphocytes appear to be primarily Th1 lymphocytes that produce interferon (IFN)-γ. Proinflammatory cytokines including interleukin (IL)-1 and tumor necrosis factor (TNF)-α amplify the immune response. Intravenous infusion of an antibody to TNF-α is clinically effective in Crohn's disease. Large numbers of neutrophils enter the inflamed mucosa attracted by chemotactic agents including IL-8 and leukotriene B_4. Epithelial injury in IBD appears to be due to reactive oxygen species from neutrophils and macrophages, as well as to cytokines including TNF-α and IFN-γ.

Mice develop colitis when the genes for IL-2, IL-10, or TGFβ1 are knocked out or when there are certain T-cell receptor mutants, and transgenic rats develop colitis if the human HLA-B27 gene has been introduced. If the same animals are raised in a germ-free environment, colitis does not develop.

PATHOLOGY. Ulcerative colitis and Crohn's disease each have a characteristic pathologic appearance, but in any given case the

	ULCERATIVE COLITIS	CROHN'S DISEASE
Pathology		
Rectal involvement	Always	Common
"Skip lesions"	Never	Common
Transmural involvement	Rare	Common
Granulomas	Occasional	Common
Perianal disease	Never	Common
"Cobblestone" mucosa	Rare	Common
Radiology		
"Collar button" ulcers	Common	Occasional
Small intestinal involvement	Never	Common
Discontinuous involvement	Never	Common
Fistulas	Never	Common
Strictures	Occasional	Common
Endoscopy		
Aphthous ulcers	Never	Common
Discontinuous involvement	Never	Common
Rectal sparing	Never	Common
Linear or serpiginous ulcers	Never	Common
Ulcers in terminal ileum	Never	Common

pathologic picture may not be specific enough to distinguish between them or to differentiate them from other diseases such as infectious colitis or ischemic colitis (Table 135–1). In IBD, the pathologic assessment of disease activity may not correlate with the clinical and endoscopic assessments.

In ulcerative colitis, inflammation begins in the rectum, extends proximally a certain distance, and then abruptly stops, with a clear demarcation between involved and uninvolved mucosa. In mild disease, there are superficial erosions, whereas in more severe disease, ulcers may be large but superficial, penetrating the muscularis mucosa only in very severe disease. Inflammatory polyps or pseudopolyps may be present. Most of the pathologic findings in ulcerative colitis are limited to the mucosa and submucosa; the muscularis propria is affected only in fulminant disease. Active ulcerative colitis is marked by neutrophils in the mucosa and submucosa and clumps of neutrophils in crypt lumens (crypt abscesses). There is mucus depletion, mucosal edema, and vascular congestion with focal hemorrhage. In addition to signs of acute activity, there are also signs of chronicity, with lymphoid aggregates, plasma cells, mast cells, and eosinophils in the lamina propria.

In Crohn's disease, the bowel wall is thickened and stiff. The mesentery, which is thickened, edematous, and contracted, fixes the intestine in one position. Transmural inflammation may cause loops of intestine to be matted together. All layers of the intestine are thickened, and the lumen is narrowed. "Skip lesions" with two involved areas separated by a length of normal intestine suggest Crohn's disease. Colonic inflammation with rectal sparing is more consistent with Crohn's disease than with ulcerative colitis. The earliest lesion of Crohn's disease is the aphthous ulcer, which typically occur over Peyer patches in the small intestine and over lymphoid aggregates in the colon. As the disease progresses, aphthous ulcers enlarge and become stellate or serpiginous. Eventually, the stellate ulcers coalesce to form longitudinal and transverse linear ulcers. The remaining islands of non-ulcerated mucosa give a cobblestone appearance. Fissures develop from the base of ulcers and extend down through the muscularis to the serosa. Lymphoid aggregates are found in the submucosa and external to the muscularis propria. Granulomas are common in Crohn's disease but not in ulcerative colitis.

ULCERATIVE COLITIS: CLINICAL FINDINGS AND NATURAL HISTORY. The dominant symptom in ulcerative colitis is diarrhea, which is usually associated with blood in the stool (Table 135–2). Bowel movements are frequent but small in volume as a result of irritability of the inflamed rectum. Urgency and fecal incontinence

Table 135–2 ■ CRITERIA FOR SEVERITY IN INFLAMMATORY BOWEL DISEASE

Mild:	Fewer than four bowel movements per day with little or no blood, no fever, and sedimentation rate less than 20 mm/hr.
Moderate:	Between mild and severe.
Severe:	Six or more bowel movements per day with blood, fever, anemia, and sedimentation rate greater than 30 mm/hr.

may limit the patient's ability to function in society. Other symptoms include fever and pain, which may be in either lower quadrant or in the rectum. Systemic features—fever, malaise, and weight loss—are more common if all or most of the colon is involved and may have a greater effect than diarrhea on the patient's ability to function. Some patients, especially elderly persons, complain of constipation rather than diarrhea because rectal spasm prevents the passage of stool. The initial attack of ulcerative colitis may be fulminant with bloody diarrhea, but more commonly the disease begins indolently, with non-bloody diarrhea progressing to bloody diarrhea. Ulcerative colitis can present initially with any extent of anatomic involvement, from disease confined to the rectum to pancolitis. Most commonly, ulcerative colitis follows a chronic intermittent course with long periods of quiescence interspersed with acute attacks lasting weeks to months; however, a significant percentage of patients suffer a chronic continuous course.

In ulcerative colitis of mild to moderate severity, there may be tenderness over the affected area of the colon, and rectal examination may reveal tenderness or blood on the glove. In severe disease the patient is more likely to be febrile and tachycardic.

Anemia and an elevated leukocyte count and erythrocyte sedimentation rate are useful in confirming severe disease and in following the clinical course of a severe exacerbation. Electrolyte disorders, particularly hypokalemia, are seen with severe diarrhea.

CROHN'S DISEASE: CLINICAL FINDINGS AND NATURAL HISTORY. Crohn's disease presents with one of three major patterns: (1) disease in the ileum and cecum (40% of patients); (2) disease confined to the small intestine (30%); and (3) disease confined to the colon (25%). Much less commonly, Crohn's disease involves more proximal parts of the gastrointestinal tract—the mouth, the tongue, the esophagus, the stomach, and the duodenum.

The predominant symptoms are diarrhea, abdominal pain, and weight loss; any of these three symptoms may be most prominent in a given individual. The initial presentation may not be dramatic; patients may complain for months or years with vague abdominal pain and intermittent diarrhea before the diagnosis is considered. Diarrhea occurs in almost all those with Crohn's disease, but the pattern varies with the anatomic location of the disease. In patients with colonic disease, especially with rectal involvement, diarrhea is of small volume and associated with urgency and tenesmus. Inflammation in the rectum causes a loss of distensibility; the entry of even a small amount of stool into a non-distensible rectum causes an immediate and urgent need to defecate. Prolonged inflammation and scarring in the rectum can leave it so rigid and non-distensible that the patient is incontinent. In disease confined to the small intestine, stools are of larger volume and not associated with urgency or tenesmus. Patients with severe involvement of the terminal ileum and those who have had surgical resections of the terminal ileum may have bile salt diarrhea or steatorrhea.

The location and pattern of pain correlate with disease location. In patients with ileal disease, cramping right lower quadrant pain occurs after eating and is related to partial intermittent obstruction of a narrowed intestinal lumen. Abdominal distention, nausea, and vomiting may accompany the pain. Weight loss of some degree, which occurs in most patients with Crohn's disease irrespective of anatomic location, is a product of malabsorption or diminished intake because of pain, diarrhea, or anorexia. Fever and chills often accompany disease activity; a low-grade fever may be the patient's first warning sign of a flare. Induction of remission by drugs or surgery is invariably associated with increased energy and a sense of well-being. Crohn's disease, like ulcerative colitis, is a relapsing and remitting disease. About 30% of placebo-treated patients with Crohn's disease of mild to moderate activity go into remission within 4 months. Conversely, of patients in remission and on no therapy, about 30% will relapse within 1 year and 50% at 2 years.

Physical findings in Crohn's disease vary with the distribution and severity of the disease. Aphthous ulcers of the lips, gingiva, or buccal mucosa are common. The abdomen may be tender, typically over the area of disease activity. Thickened bowel loops, thickened mesentery, or an abscess may cause a mass, often in the right lower quadrant. The presence of perianal disease is suggested by fistulous openings, induration, redness, or tenderness near the anus.

Laboratory findings are largely non-specific. Anemia may result from chronic disease, blood loss, or nutritional deficiencies (of iron, folate, or vitamin B_{12}). A modestly elevated leukocyte count is indicative of active disease, but a marked elevation suggests the presence of an abscess or other suppurative complication. The erythrocyte sedimentation rate has been used to follow disease activity, and it tends to be higher in colonic disease than ileal disease. Hypoalbuminemia is an indication of malnutrition. Ileal disease or resection of more than 100 cm of ileum results in a diminished serum vitamin B_{12} level because of malabsorption.

EXTRAINTESTINAL MANIFESTATIONS. Although IBD primarily involves the bowel, it is associated with manifestations in other organ systems. The extraintestinal manifestations (e.g., sclerosing cholangitis or ankylosing spondylitis) may be more problematic than the bowel disease. The extraintestinal manifestations can be divided into two major groups: (1) those in which the clinical activity follows the activity of the bowel disease and (2) those in which the clinical activity is unrelated to the clinical activity of the bowel disease.

The most common extraintestinal manifestation of IBD is arthritis, including colitic arthritis and ankylosing spondylitis. Colitic arthritis, a migratory arthritis that affects knees, hips, ankles, wrists, and elbows, parallels the course of the bowel disease; successful treatment of the intestinal inflammation results in improvement in the arthritis. Ankylosing spondylitis (see Chapter 287) presents with morning stiffness, low-back pain, and stooped posture; it can be relentlessly progressive and crippling. Patients with ulcerative colitis have a 30-fold increase in the incidence of ankylosing spondylitis compared with the general population. Non-steroidal anti-inflammatory drugs reduce inflammation and pain but do not halt the progression of the disease. Medical treatment of the IBD and colectomy are not helpful in managing ankylosing spondylitis. Sacroiliitis, which is inflammation of the joint between the sacrum and the ilium, occurs in conjunction with ankylosing spondylitis but is more often seen alone. In ulcerative colitis, 15% of patients have radiographs consistent with sacroiliitis but most are asymptomatic.

The hepatic complications of IBD include fatty liver, pericholangitis, chronic active hepatitis, and cirrhosis. The biliary tract complications are sclerosing cholangitis (ulcerative colitis) and gallstones (Crohn's disease). Cholesterol gallstones occur in patients with ileal disease or ileal resections because of malabsorption of bile salts and the resultant decrease in the size of the bile salt pool. Pericholangitis is the most common hepatic complication of IBD; patients with pericholangitis are usually asymptomatic. Elevations of alkaline phosphatase are seen frequently; elevations of bilirubin are less common.

Sclerosing cholangitis (see Chapter 157) is a chronic cholestatic liver disease marked by fibrosing inflammation of the intrahepatic and extrahepatic bile ducts. While it occurs in only 1 to 4% of patients with ulcerative colitis and with lower frequency in Crohn's disease, the majority of patients with sclerosing cholangitis have IBD. Colectomy and medical therapy of the bowel disease do not ameliorate the course; sclerosing cholangitis is now one of the most common indications for liver transplantation (see Chapter 155) in adults.

The two common dermal complications of IBD are pyoderma gangrenosum (see Chapter 522) and erythema nodosum (see Chapter 522). The lesions of pyoderma gangrenosum almost always develop during a bout of acute colitis and usually resolve with control of the colitis by oral corticosteroids or with intradermal corticosteroids; in rare cases, colectomy is required. The activity of erythema nodosum, which is seen particularly in association with Crohn's disease in children, follows the activity of the bowel disease.

The ocular complications of IBD are uveitis and episcleritis (see Chapter 512). Local therapy with corticosteroids and agents that dilate the pupil helps to prevent scarring and blindness.

RADIOGRAPHY. In both ulcerative colitis and Crohn's disease, radiographic findings may not correlate well with disease activity. The patient's clinical response or endoscopic findings are more useful for this purpose.

In early ulcerative colitis, the barium enema may be normal or there may be limited distensibility of the involved segment, resulting in a narrowed, shortened, and tubular form of the lumen. The haustral markings disappear, and the normally tortuous appearance

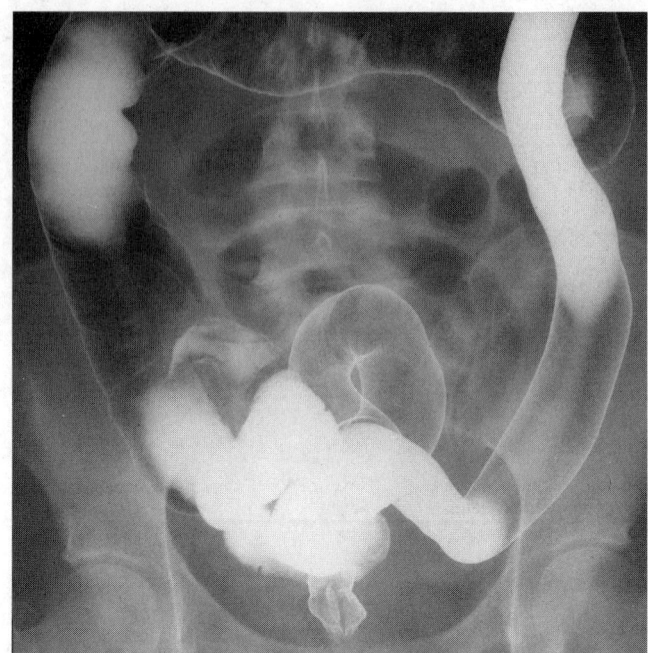

FIGURE 135–1 ▪ Air contrast barium enema demonstrating luminal narrowing and loss of haustral markings in the sigmoid and descending colon in a patient with ulcerative colitis.

of the colon is straightened (Fig. 135–1). Air contrast examination reveals a fine granular appearance to the mucosa, with a slightly irregular surface. In more severe disease, the granularity becomes coarser and eventually nodular; ulcers penetrate through the mucosa and can be seen in profile as small collar-button collections of barium extending beyond the colonic lumen.

The earliest form of Crohn's disease detectable by air contrast barium enema is marked by the presence of aphthous ulcers, which appear as small discrete collections of barium surrounded by radiolucent halos of inflammatory infiltrate. These small ulcers are usually multiple, and the intervening mucosa is normal. As Crohn's disease becomes more severe, the aphthous ulcers enlarge, deepen, and connect with one another to form linear ulcers; the intervening mucosa develops a nodular appearance on a radiograph, a process termed *cobblestoning*. Progressive deepening of ulcers can lead to abscess formation or fistulization. Contrast studies are more likely than endoscopic studies to identify fistulas. Transmural inflammation and fibrosis lead to limited distensibility, with decreased luminal diameter and stricture formation. Like fistulas, strictures are more easily appreciated on radiographic studies than by endoscopy. Transmural inflammation and fibrosis result in thickening of the bowel wall, with wide gaps between the barium-filled lumens of loops of inflamed small bowel (Fig. 135–2). Small bowel Crohn's disease can be evaluated by small bowel follow-through or by enteroclysis. Computed tomography and ultrasonography are useful in identifying abscesses and other fluid collections and in assessing the thickness of the bowel wall.

ENDOSCOPY. The earliest endoscopic manifestations of ulcerative colitis are the development of diffuse erythema and loss of the fine vascular pattern seen in the normal rectal mucosa (Color Plate 2B). Erythema is usually accompanied by mucosal edema, which is manifested endoscopically by blunting of the rectal valves, loss of normal vasculature, and development of granular-appearing mucosa. Inflammation is associated with the presence of yellowish exudate on the mucosa. The inflamed mucosa bleeds easily if touched with the endoscope; this easy bleeding is termed *friability*. In more severe disease, the mucosa bleeds spontaneously and small ulcerations appear. An important aspect of the endoscopic findings in ulcerative colitis is their distribution: inflammation begins in the rectum, extends proximally a certain distance, and then stops; all the mucosa proximal to that point is normal, and all the mucosa distal to it is abnormal.

The earliest endoscopic manifestation of Crohn's disease is the aphthous ulcer, a small discrete ulcer a few millimeters in diameter surrounded by a thin red halo of edematous tissue (Color Plate

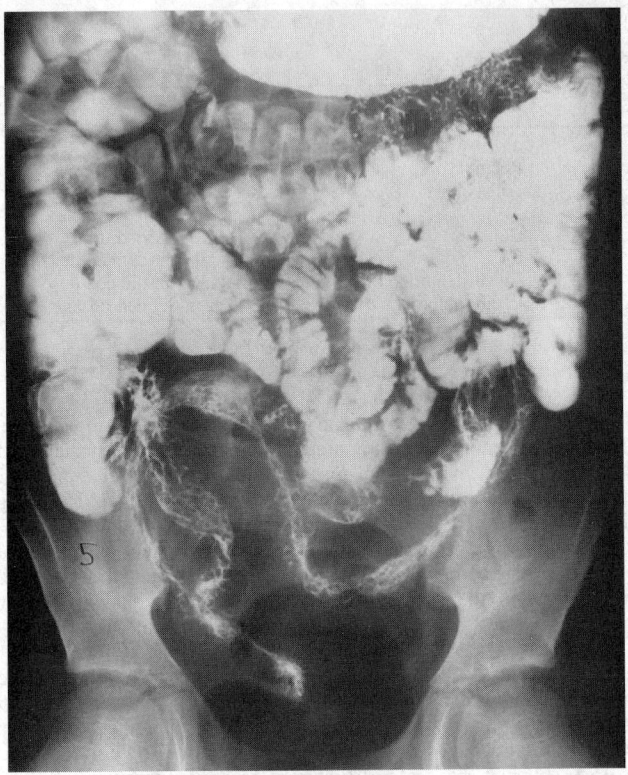

FIGURE 135–2 ■ Small bowel follow-through in a patient with Crohn's disease of the ileum demonstrating luminal narrowing, mucosal ulceration, and separation of the barium-filled loops due to thickening of the bowel wall.

2*G*). Ulcers may be rounded or long and serpiginous. Longitudinal and transverse ulcers may intersect to form a grid with intervening cobblestone-like areas of non-ulcerated mucosa. Large, deep, penetrating ulcers can be surrounded by areas of normal-appearing mucosa. The diffuse mucosal irregularities of erythema, edema, and granularity, which are prominent in ulcerative colitis, occur less commonly and later in the course of Crohn's disease. The rectum may or may not be involved in Crohn's disease. Areas of involvement are typically interspersed with normal "skip" areas.

DIFFERENTIAL DIAGNOSIS. For many therapeutic decisions, it is not particularly important to know whether the patient has ulcerative colitis or Crohn's disease. However, when surgery is contemplated, the distinction is important. For example, a colectomy and ileoanal anastomosis could be recommended as a curative procedure if the physician were confident the patient had ulcerative colitis rather than Crohn's colitis.

The anatomic distribution of the inflammatory response may be helpful in distinguishing ulcerative colitis from Crohn's disease. In ulcerative colitis, inflammation is seen in the rectum and extends proximally for some distance; in extensive disease, inflammation extends to the cecum. Although ulcerative colitis does not involve the small intestine, there may be a few centimeters of inflamed mucosa without ulceration in the terminal ileum. If the rectum is spared or if there are areas of uninflamed mucosa (skip areas) between areas of inflamed mucosa, then Crohn's colitis is more likely. Ulcerative colitis is not only continuous along the longitudinal axis of the colon, but the degree of inflammation is also consistent and symmetric circumferentially at any level. In contrast, in Crohn's colitis, deep linear ulcers may be separated by areas of normal mucosa. A major distinguishing mark in favor of Crohn's disease is the presence of transmural inflammatory changes; in ulcerative colitis, inflammation is confined to the mucosa and submucosa. Extensive perianal involvement with fistulas and abscesses point to Crohn's disease. The presence of non-caseating granulomas suggests Crohn's disease, but even in Crohn's disease, most patients have no granulomas on biopsy. Despite all these differences, there is a small but significant number of patients with IBD who cannot be assigned with confidence to one disease category or the other; these patients are considered to have indeterminate colitis.

Infections with *Shigella, Amoeba, Giardia, Escherichia coli*

O157:H7, and *Campylobacter* organisms can present with bloody diarrhea, cramps, and an endoscopic picture identical to ulcerative colitis (Chapter 339). An important distinction between these infectious diseases (excepting amebiasis) and IBD is that the diarrhea in the infectious diseases tends to be limited to a period of days to a few weeks, whereas the diarrhea of IBD is typically of longer duration. Stool cultures for bacterial pathogens and serologic tests for amebiasis help distinguish infectious diarrhea from IBD. In patients who present with prolonged diarrhea, other protozoal diseases, such as giardiasis, must be considered. Pseudomembranous colitis presents as profuse watery diarrhea and may last from a few days to months; the presence of small membranous plaques adherent to the mucosa on sigmoidoscopy is pathognomonic. As part of the initial evaluation of patients with acute exacerbation of IBD, it is appropriate to check the stool for *C. difficile* toxin, especially if there has been recent antibiotic exposure.

Mild ulcerative colitis, in which rectal bleeding is the primary manifestation, can be confused with hemorrhoids or anal fissures (Chapter 143). The presence of urgency or diarrhea is more consistent with ulcerative colitis. Sigmoidoscopy should easily differentiate ulcerative colitis from these perianal problems.

Collagenous colitis is a chronic inflammatory disease marked pathologically by the presence of a thick collagen deposition in the subepithelial layer of the colonic mucosa (Chapter 133). The typical clinical presentation is chronic watery diarrhea in a middle-aged woman. Endoscopically, the mucosa appears mildly inflamed or, more commonly, absolutely normal; biopsy with histology provides the diagnosis. Ischemic colitis is part of the differential diagnosis of the initial bout of IBD and should be considered in elderly persons or others at particular risk for ischemic disease (Chapter 137). Diverticulitis, which may be difficult to separate from acute Crohn's colitis, tends to be a more acute problem without a chronic inflammatory state (Chapter 136). Intestinal lymphoma can mimic the symptoms of Crohn's disease; in lymphoma, small bowel radiographs may show diffuse involvement with masses in the bowel wall. If Crohn's disease has a long, indolent course with relatively mild symptoms, it may be difficult to differentiate from irritable bowel syndrome, and some patients may have both (Chapter 131).

DRUGS USED IN IBD. GENERAL SUPPORTIVE THERAPY. Antidiarrheal agents, usually loperamide or diphenoxylate, are useful in patients with mild IBD to reduce the number of bowel movements and to relieve rectal urgency. Anticholinergics (tincture of belladonna, clidinium, propantheline bromide, and dicyclomine hydrochloride) may reduce cramps, pain, and rectal urgency. An especially effective combination of an antidiarrheal and an antispasmodic is powdered opium (25 mg) and belladonna (15 mg). Antidiarrheal agents and antispasmodics are contraindicated in severe colitis because of the risk of precipitating toxic megacolon. The chronic use of narcotics for pain should not be part of the management of IBD. Sometimes antidepressants can be helpful. Non-steroidal anti-inflammatory drugs can exacerbate the clinical activity of IBD and should be used cautiously.

Nutritional management plays only a small role in ulcerative colitis. Patients should avoid specific foods (typically high-fiber foods) that worsen their symptoms. Nutritional management plays a much larger role in Crohn's disease, in which many patients have diminished caloric intake and vitamin B_{12}, vitamin D, calcium, magnesium, zinc, and iron may be malabsorbed. Both total parenteral nutrition and elemental enteral diets can decrease intestinal inflammation by reducing the antigen load in the lumen.

AMINOSALICYLATES. Sulfasalazine is composed of 5-aminosalicylic acid (5-ASA) joined by an azo bond to sulfapyridine (Table 135–3). Colonic bacteria split the azo bond to release 5-ASA, the active ingredient, into the colonic lumen. 5-ASA is not absorbed from the colon; it appears to have a local therapeutic effect by acting intraluminally. Sulfasalazine has been used successfully as a single agent in mild to moderate acute attacks of ulcerative colitis and Crohn's colitis; it is the drug of choice in mild cases. Success rates with sulfasalazine are dose related, with better success rates at doses of 4 g/day or more. Patients who respond to sulfasalazine usually do so in 2 to 3 weeks, although some take 4 weeks or longer to respond. Dose-related toxic effects (headache, nausea, vomiting, and abdominal discomfort) are related to serum sulfapyridine levels, but hypersensitivity reactions (rash, fever, aplastic ane-

Table 135–3 ■ PREPARATIONS OF 5-AMINOSALICYLIC ACID

PREPARATION	DELIVERY	DISTRIBUTION	DOSE*
Topical			
Mesalamine suppository	Direct	Rectum	500 mg once or twice a day
Mesalamine enema	Direct	Left colon	4 g in 60 mL at bedtime
Oral			
Sulfasalazine	Bacterial azo reductase	Colon	4–6 g in divided doses
Dipentum	Bacterial azo reductase	Colon	1.5–3.0 g in divided doses
Asacol	Release at pH > 7	Distal ileum, colon	2.4–4.8 g in divided doses
Pentasa	Time-release ethyl cellulose microgranules	Ileum, colon	3–4 g in divided doses

*Doses given are for active disease; similar doses can be given for maintenance therapy, although some practitioners use lower doses for maintenance.

mia, pancreatitis, lupus-like rash, nephrotoxicity, hepatitis, agranulocytosis, and autoimmune hemolysis) are not. Sulfasalazine commonly causes changes in sperm morphology and number, leading to reversible infertility. Sulfasalazine inhibits folic acid absorption and is a competitive inhibitor of folate conjugase in the jejunal brush border; folic acid supplementation of 1 to 2 mg/day is commonly recommended.

If 5-ASA alone is administered orally, it is rapidly absorbed, and significant luminal concentrations are not achieved. 5-ASA is available in the United States as an enema and as a suppository. Several oral formulations provide 5-ASA to the colon by binding two 5-ASAs through an azo linkage, by coating 5-ASA in granules that dissolve at pH 7 or above in the colon and terminal ileum, or by encapsulating 5-ASA in a semipermeable membrane that releases 65% of its 5-ASA in the colon and 35% in the small intestine.

CORTICOSTEROIDS. Oral corticosteroids are effective in mild to moderate ulcerative colitis and Crohn's disease. Parenteral therapy is reserved for moderate to severe disease. The typical initial dose of prednisone is 40 mg/day in moderate to severe disease. The patient is left on high doses of corticosteroids until symptoms begin to diminish, after which the dose is gradually reduced. If an inadequate initial dose of prednisone is used because of the fear of side effects, the likelihood of a positive response diminishes. In some patients, disease activity flares when the dose of prednisone is reduced below a certain level (steroid dependence). For most patients, administration of oral prednisone in a single morning dose is as effective as divided doses. Corticosteroids should not be used in patients with undrained abscesses or when symptoms are due to a stricture or fibrotic process. Maintenance therapy with corticosteroids is ineffective to prevent recurrences in ulcerative colitis or Crohn's disease in remission. The many side effects of corticosteroids (see Chapter 28) are the major factor limiting their use in IBD.

IMMUNOMODULATORS. Immunomodulator drugs act by blocking lymphocyte proliferation, activation, or effector mechanisms. There is extensive experience with azathioprine and its metabolite 6-mercaptopurine (6-MP) to treat IBD and lesser experience with cyclosporine and methotrexate. Azathioprine and 6-MP are effective in treating active Crohn's disease and in maintaining remission; their roles in ulcerative colitis are less clear. Typical initial doses are 1 to 1.5 mg/kg for 6-MP and 2.0 to 2.5 mg/kg for azathioprine. The delay between the initiation of therapy and the clinical response is typically 3 to 6 months. These drugs are used in patients who have active disease that is unresponsive to corticosteroids (refractory patients) and in corticosteroid-dependent patients. In these patients, 6-MP or azathioprine is added to corticosteroid therapy; then after 3 or 4 months, when the 6-MP and azathioprine are likely to have taken effect, the dose of corticosteroids is gradually tapered. Most clinicians maintain patients on 6-MP or azathioprine for several years if remission is induced by these drugs. The major limiting factor in the use of 6-MP and azathioprine is their toxicity; both commonly cause leukopenia, may cause pancreatitis, and may increase the risk of lymphoma. Methotrexate, given either orally or parenterally, is effective in active Crohn's disease. Cyclosporine, given intravenously, is effective in reducing inflammation in patients with severe ulcerative colitis who are facing colectomy.

ANTIBIOTICS. Except in cases of overt sepsis, there is little role for antibiotics in the management of ulcerative colitis. Antibiotics do not affect the remission rate; moreover, the risk of inducing antibiotic-associated pseudomembranous colitis must be considered.

Antibiotics play a larger role in Crohn's disease; they are used in the management of the suppurative complications, especially abscess formation and perianal disease, although surgical drainage is the primary therapy for abscesses. Metronidazole (10 to 15 mg/kg/day) is effective in perianal Crohn's disease and is as effective as sulfasalazine in Crohn's colitis. The major side effect of metronidazole is peripheral neuropathy, which is dose dependent and usually resolves when the drug is discontinued. Ciprofloxacin at 500 mg twice a day for a few weeks is also effective in some patients.

MEDICAL MANAGEMENT OF ULCERATIVE COLITIS (Fig. 135–3). **PROCTITIS.** For active ulcerative proctitis, a relatively effective and rapidly-acting approach is the nightly administration of 5-ASA retention enemas or suppositories, often supplemented with an oral aminosalicylate. Corticosteroid enemas can also be used. Either 5-ASA suppositories or corticosteroid foam is appropriate for disease of up to 20 cm of distal colon; 5-ASA or corticosteroid retention enemas can be used for active disease, involving up to 60 cm of distal colon. Another approach to proctitis or distal colitis is an oral aminosalicylate, although a response may not be evident for 3 to 4 weeks.

EXTENSIVE COLITIS. For patients with colitis of mild to moderate activity and extension proximal to the sigmoid colon, the initial drug of choice is an oral aminosalicylate; efficacy increases with increasing doses. For patients with more active disease (>5–6 bowel movements per day), patients in whom a more rapid response is desired, or patients who have not responded to 3 to 4 weeks of aminosalicylates, the treatment of choice is oral prednisone. Patients with severe diarrhea, systemic symptoms, or significant amounts of blood in the stool should be started on 40 mg/day; most patients respond to oral corticosteroids within a few days. After the symptoms are controlled, prednisone can be gradually tapered by 5 to 10 mg every 1 to 2 weeks. Patients who respond to oral prednisone and can be fully withdrawn from it should be maintained on an aminosalicylate.

For patients who do not respond to corticosteroids (steroid-refractory) or who do respond but whose disease flares whenever the corticosteroids are withdrawn (steroid-dependent), options include indefinite corticosteroids, an immunomodulator (azathioprine or 6-MP), or colectomy. Continuation of high-dose corticosteroid therapy for too long a time is the most common serious error in the management of ulcerative colitis. If the patient is on a substantial dose (>15 mg/day of prednisone) for more than 6 months, a trial of an immunomodulator or colectomy should be given serious consideration.

The most common reason for hospitalization is intractable diarrhea, although blood loss is also a common problem. Patients with severe active ulcerative colitis should be evaluated for toxic megacolon. Anticholinergics and antidiarrheal agents are contraindicated in severe ulcerative colitis because of the risk of precipitating toxic megacolon. The mainstays of therapy for severe ulcerative colitis are bed rest, rehydration with intravenous fluids, and intravenous corticosteroids (hydrocortisone 300 mg/day; prednisolone, 60–80 mg/day, or methylprednisolone, 48–60 mg/day). Total parenteral nutrition may be necessary if there is malnutrition. Patients with peritoneal signs or signs of systemic infection should be treated with parenteral antibiotics. Patients who do not improve in 7 to 10 days should be considered for either colectomy or a trial of intravenous cyclosporine.

MAINTENANCE THERAPY. Aminosalicylates reduce the incidence of recurrences in patients with ulcerative colitis; almost all patients

TREATMENT ALGORITHM FOR ULCERATIVE COLITIS

CONDITION	TREATMENT
PROCTITIS	5-ASA enemas or 5-ASA suppositories or oral 5-ASA drugs or corticosteroid enemas —*Continued activity*→ Prednisone or immunomodulators —*Continued activity*→ Colectomy
MILD TO MODERATE PANCOLITIS	Oral 5-ASA drugs —*Continued activity*→ Prednisone —*Continued activity or Steroid dependence*→ Immunomodulators or colectomy
SEVERE OR FULMINANT PANCOLITIS	Parenteral steroids —*Continued activity*→ Cyclosporine or colectomy
DISEASE IN REMISSION	Maintenance with oral 5-ASA drugs

ASA=aminosalicylic acid

FIGURE 135-3 ■ Treatment algorithm for ulcerative colitis.

should receive maintenance therapy. The efficacy of sulfasalazine at 3 to 4 g/day is greater than the efficacy of 2 g/day even though 2 g/day is the usual recommended maintenance dose. Corticosteroids are not effective as maintenance therapy and should not be used. Most of the experience with 6-MP as maintenance therapy in ulcerative colitis is in patients whose acute disease has been brought under control with 6-MP; withdrawal of 6-MP from these patients results in a high incidence of exacerbation.

MEDICAL MANAGEMENT OF CROHN'S DISEASE (Fig. 135-4). **GENERAL APPROACH.** It is difficult to develop generally applicable guidelines for the management of Crohn's disease because of the great variety of anatomic locations, clinical presentations, and gastrointestinal complications such as fistulas, abscesses, strictures, and perforations. Response to therapy is monitored by empiric clinical assessment directed at the problem that is most troublesome for the patient.

A common problem in the management of Crohn's disease is a marked discrepancy between the severity of the patient's symptoms and the objective signs of disease activity. Patients with severe pain and diarrhea may have minimal findings on endoscopy or radiographic studies. Patients who have undergone ileal resections may have significant diarrhea on the basis of their surgery alone.

ACTIVE DISEASE. For colonic or ileocolic Crohn's disease with mild to moderate activity, an aminosalicylate is a reasonable first therapy. Pentasa, an oral 5-ASA preparation with greater availability of 5-ASA in the ileum than sulfasalazine or Asacol, may be a better choice for patients with ileitis or ileocolitis. Metronidazole, given by mouth at a dose of 10 to 15 mg/kg/day, is an alternative to aminosalicylates for Crohn's colitis. Prednisone is the drug of choice for patients who have failed to respond to aminosalicylates or metronidazole, for patients with ileal disease, and for patients with highly active colonic or ileocolic disease. The response to prednisone is usually more rapid than that to aminosalicylates. Before corticosteroids are given to a Crohn's disease patient with abdominal pain, fever, and a high leukocyte count, an abdominal computed tomographic scan should be obtained to exclude an abscess.

For patients who have been brought into clinical remission on corticosteroids, the rate at which the dose is tapered is arbitrary and not defined by controlled trials. Usually the prednisone dose can be tapered from 40 mg/day to 20 mg/day relatively rapidly (5–10 mg/1–2 weeks) without inducing a flare of disease activity. If the patient has not been on a 5-ASA preparation, one should be added to increase the likelihood of a successful corticosteroid withdrawal. Once the dose of prednisone has reached 20 mg/day, the taper is

slowed to 5 mg every 10 to 14 days; if symptoms flare, the dose of prednisone is increased. At this point, the best approach for most patients is a trial of an immunomodulator, either 6-MP or azathioprine; corticosteroid therapy is continued for 3 to 4 months and then tapered gradually. Approximately 60% of corticosteroid-dependent patients will be able to withdraw from corticosteroids using this approach; the alternative is surgery if there is a stricture or a focal area of involvement.

The approach to severe Crohn's disease is similar to the approach to severe ulcerative colitis. The patient is hospitalized, given nothing by mouth, rehydrated with intravenous fluids, and given parenteral corticosteroids. Patients who respond to parenteral corticosteroids are switched to high-dose oral corticosteroids (prednisone 40 mg/day), and the dose of prednisone is gradually reduced. Patients with severe Crohn's disease who do not respond to parenteral corticosteroids within a week should be considered for surgery. A course of total parenteral nutrition may be useful as adjunctive therapy.

MAINTENANCE THERAPY. Maintenance therapy with aminosalicylates is recommended for those brought into remission on corticosteroids or with surgery; however, the efficacy of aminosalicylates as maintenance therapy is less well established in Crohn's disease than in ulcerative colitis. Maintenance with 6-MP or azathioprine is recommended for patients brought into remission on those drugs or who were corticosteroid dependent and then converted to those drugs. There is no role for corticosteroids as maintenance therapy.

SURGERY. Twenty to 25 per cent of patients with extensive ulcerative colitis eventually undergo colectomy, usually because their disease has not responded adequately to medical therapy. In ulcerative colitis, colectomy is a curative procedure. Emergency colectomy may be required in toxic megacolon or in a severe fulminant attack without toxic megacolon. The standard operation for ulcerative colitis is a proctocolectomy and Brooke's ileostomy. The most popular alternative operation is the proctocolectomy and ileoanal anastomosis; in this procedure, a pouch is constructed from the terminal 30 cm of ileum, and the distal end of the pouch is pulled through the anal canal. The decision for or against colectomy is influenced by the patient's age, social circumstances, and duration of disease. The risk of developing malignancy enters into the equation when considering colectomy in those with long-standing ulcerative colitis; if the other indications are equivocal, the risk of malignancy may push the balance in favor of colectomy.

Within 10 years of diagnosis, approximately 60% of patients with Crohn's disease undergo surgery for their disease. Because surgical resection is not curative in Crohn's disease and recurrences

TREATMENT ALGORITHM FOR CROHN'S DISEASE	
CONDITION	**TREATMENT**
COLITIS OR ILEOCOLITIS	Oral 5-ASA drug or metronidazole → *Continued activity* → Prednisone → *Continued activity or* → Immunomodulator → *Continued activity* → Surgery; *Steroid dependence*
ILEITIS	Prednisone → *Continued activity* → Immunomodulator → *Continued activity* → Surgery
FISTULA	TPN or immunomodulator → *Failure to close* → Surgery
ABSCESS	Antibiotics, drainage, and resection
OBSTRUCTION DUE TO INFLAMMATION	IV fluids, nasogastric suction, parenteral steroids → *Failure to respond* → Surgery
OBSTRUCTION DUE TO SCARRING	IV fluids, nasogastric suction → *Failure to respond* → Surgery
PERIANAL DISEASE	Antibiotics and surgical drainage
DISEASE IN REMISSION	Maintenance with oral 5-ASA drugs or immunomodulators
ASA=aminosalicylic acid IV=intravenous TPN=total parenteral nutrition	

Figure 135–4 ■ Treatment algorithm for Crohn's disease.

are likely, the approach is more conservative in terms of the amount of tissue removed. Failure of medical management is a common cause for resection in Crohn's disease, as it is in ulcerative colitis, but complications (e.g., obstruction, fistula, abscess) are often indications for resection in Crohn's disease. Surgery is also performed to allow patients to stop taking medications (usually corticosteroids). For small bowel Crohn's disease, the most common surgical procedure is segmental resection for obstruction or fistula. The incidence of recurrence severe enough to need repeat surgery after ileal or ileocolic resection is about 50% after 10 years and 75% after 15 years. Endoscopic and histologic surgical approaches to Crohn's colitis include segmental resection, subtotal colectomy with ileoproctostomy, and total colectomy with ileostomy. For patients with extensive colonic disease including the rectum, the procedure of choice is total proctocolectomy with a Brooke's ileostomy. Total colectomy with ileoanal anastomosis is not appropriate in Crohn's colitis because recurrence of Crohn's disease in the ileal segment forming the new pouch would require a repeat operation and loss of a long segment of ileum.

COMPLICATIONS. The most severe complication of ulcerative colitis is toxic megacolon, that is, dilatation of the colon to a diameter of greater than 6 cm associated with a worsening of the patient's clinical condition and the development of fever, tachycardia, and leukocytosis. Physical examination may reveal postural hypotension, tenderness over the distribution of the colon, and absent or hypoactive bowel sounds. Antispasmodics and antidiarrheal agents are likely to initiate or exacerbate toxic megacolon. Medical therapy is designed to reduce the likelihood of perforation

and to return the colon to normal motor activity as rapidly as possible. The patient is given nothing by mouth, and nasogastric suction is begun. Intravenous fluids should be administered to replete water and electrolytes, broad-spectrum antibiotics are given in anticipation of peritonitis resulting from perforation, and parenteral corticosteroids are given at a dose equivalent to more than 40 mg of prednisone per day. Signs of improvement include a decrease in abdominal girth and the return of bowel sounds. Deterioration is marked by the development of rebound tenderness, increasing abdominal girth, and cardiovascular collapse. If the patient does not begin to show signs of clinical improvement during the first 24 to 48 hours of medical therapy, the risk of perforation increases markedly, and surgical intervention is indicated.

Abscesses and fistulas, which are common complications in Crohn's disease, are products of the extension of a mucosal fissure or ulcer through the intestinal wall and into extraintestinal tissue. Leakage of intestinal contents through a fissure into the peritoneal cavity results in an abscess. Extension of the inflammatory process through the wall of adjacent viscera or through the abdominal wall to the exterior results in a fistula. Abscesses occur in 15% to 20% of patients with Crohn's disease and are especially common in the terminal ileum. The typical clinical presentation of intra-abdominal abscess is fever, abdominal pain, tenderness, and leukocytosis. Abdominal abscess is most often diagnosed by computed tomography. Broad-spectrum antibiotic therapy, including anaerobic coverage, is indicated. Percutaneous drainage of abscesses in patients with Crohn's disease may improve the clinical picture but will not provide adequate therapy because of persistent communication between the abscess cavity and the intestinal lumen. Resection of the portion of involved intestine containing the communication is usually required for definitive therapy. The prevalence of fistulas is 20% to 40% in Crohn's disease. Most fistulas are enteroenteric or enterocutaneous, with smaller numbers that are enterovesical or enterovaginal. Total parenteral nutrition or immunomodulator therapy may induce fistula closure; however, the fistulas often recur after the total parenteral nutrition or immunomodulator is stopped. Surgical therapy includes resection of the segment involved with active disease.

Obstruction is a common complication of Crohn's disease, particularly in the small intestine, and is a leading indication for surgery. Small bowel obstruction in Crohn's disease may be caused by mucosal thickening from acute inflammation, by muscular hyperplasia and scarring as a result of previous inflammation, or by adhesions. Obstruction may also occur because of impaction of a bolus of fibrous food in a stable, long-standing stricture. Obstruction presents with cramping abdominal pain and diarrhea that worsen after meals and resolve with fasting. Strictures may be evaluated by oral contrast studies, barium enema, or colonoscopy, depending on anatomic location. Corticosteroids are useful if acute inflammation is an important component of the obstructive process, but not if the obstruction is due to fibrosis. A common error in the management of Crohn's disease is treatment with long courses of corticosteroids in patients who have obstructive symptoms from fixed anatomic lesions. If the obstruction does not resolve with nasogastric suction and corticosteroids, surgery is necessary.

Perianal disease is an especially difficult complication of Crohn's disease. A complex of problems is caused by ulcers in the anal canal and the resulting fistulas. The fistulous openings are most commonly in the perianal skin but can be in the groin, the vulva, or the scrotum. Fistulas present as drainage of serous or mucous material. If the fistula does not drain freely, there is local accumulation of pus (perianal abscess) with redness, pain, and induration. The pain of perianal abscesses is exacerbated by defecation, sitting, or walking. The typical physical presentation of abscess is redness with tenderness on digital examination. Adequate evaluation of perianal disease usually requires proctoscopic examination under anesthesia. Computed tomography is useful in defining the presence and extent of perianal abscesses. The goals of therapy in perianal disease are relief of local symptoms and preservation of the sphincter. Limited disease can be approached with sitz baths and metronidazole, but in most cases adequate external drainage is also required. Persistent severe perianal Crohn's disease can result in destruction of the anal sphincter and fecal incontinence.

COLON CANCER, DYSPLASIA, AND COLONOSCOPIC SURVEILLANCE. Patients with extensive ulcerative colitis have a markedly increased risk for colon cancer compared with the general population beginning 8 to 10 years after diagnosis and increasing with time. The risk of malignancy is also a function of the anatomic extent of the disease; the risk is much greater with pancolitis than with left-sided disease. Patients with long-standing ulcerative colitis are at risk for developing cancer even if their symptoms have been relatively mild; that is, colon cancer is seen in patients whose disease has been quiescent for 10 to 15 years. In ulcerative colitis, colon cancers are frequently submucosal and may be missed at colonoscopy. Colon cancer in ulcerative colitis is associated with dysplastic changes in the mucosa at other sites in the colon. Dysplasia cannot be identified by visual inspection; microscopic examination of biopsy specimens is required. Some practitioners perform surveillance colonoscopies with random biopsies in patients with long-standing ulcerative colitis beginning 8 to 10 years after the onset of disease and repeated every 1 to 2 years. If the specimens show dysplasia, the patient is sent for colectomy. Although it is clear that dysplasia is associated with colon cancer in ulcerative colitis, the utility of surveillance colonoscopy has not been firmly established. The risk of colon cancer in Crohn's colitis is less than in ulcerative colitis but greater than in the general population. The utility of surveillance in Crohn's colitis is unproven.

PREGNANCY AND INFLAMMATORY BOWEL DISEASE. Fertility in women with IBD is normal or only minimally impaired, and the incidences of prematurity, stillbirth, and developmental defects in IBD are similar to those of the general population. The incidence of fetal complications may be somewhat higher in cases in which the mother's disease is clinically active, irrespective of drug therapy. Previous proctocolectomy or the presence of an ileostomy

is not an impediment to the successful completion of a pregnancy. Many women have taken sulfasalazine throughout the course of pregnancy, and there is no evidence for its causing harm to the fetus. Pregnant women have an increased requirement for folic acid, and sulfasalazine interferes with folate absorption. Therefore, women taking sulfasalazine who are pregnant or considering pregnancy should receive folate supplementation (1 mg twice daily) to ensure that the fetus receives amounts adequate for normal development. The use of corticosteroids by pregnant women with IBD is not associated with an increased rate of fetal complications. In general, it appears that the risks to the pregnancy of treatment with sulfasalazine or corticosteroids are less than the risks of allowing disease activity to go untreated. Most of the data on azathioprine and 6-MP in pregnancy come from the transplant literature and involve higher doses than are commonly used in IBD. Reported fetal effects in the transplant population include congenital malformations, immunosuppression, prematurity, and growth retardation; risks in the IBD population are not known. The effects of pregnancy on IBD depend on disease activity. If the patient's disease is inactive at the time of conception, it is likely that it will remain inactive during the course of the pregnancy. If the disease is active at the time of conception, the course is harder to predict. Ulcerative colitis that is active at the time of conception tends to worsen. In two thirds of Crohn's disease cases that are active at conception, the degree of activity remains the same; among the other third, some improve clinically and others deteriorate.

Hanauer SB: Drug therapy: Inflammatory bowel disease. N Engl J Med 334:841, 1996. *A useful summary of drug therapy in IBD.*

Jewell DP: Ulcerative colitis. *In* Feldman M, Scharschmidt BF, Sleisenger MH (eds): Gastrointestinal and Liver Disease, 6th ed. Philadelphia, WB Saunders, 1997, p 1735. *A comprehensive overview of ulcerative colitis.*

Kirsner JB, Shorter RG (eds): Inflammatory bowel disease, 4th ed. Philadelphia, Lea & Febiger, 1995. *A multi-authored textbook on IBD.*

Kornbluth A, Sachar D, Salomon P: Crohn's disease. *In* Feldman M, Scharschmidt BF, Sleisenger MH (eds): Gastrointestinal and Liver Disease, 6th ed. Philadelphia, WB Saunders, 1997, p 1708. *A comprehensive overview of Crohn's disease.*

Stenson WF: Inflammatory bowel disease. *In* Yamada T (ed): Textbook of Gastroenterology, 3rd ed. Philadelphia, Lippincott–Raven, 1999. *A comprehensive overview of IBD, including pathogenesis and treatment.*

136 MISCELLANEOUS INFLAMMATORY DISEASES OF THE INTESTINE

C. Mel Wilcox

ACUTE APPENDICITIS (INCLUDING THE ACUTE ABDOMEN)

DEFINITION. Appendicitis is an acute inflammatory disorder of the vermiform appendix. It is uncommon at the extremes of age, with the highest incidence in the 2nd and 3rd decades. Because of its prevalence, varied manifestations mimicking other intra-abdominal diseases, and curability, appendicitis provides a framework for an understanding of the causes and approach to the acute abdomen.

ETIOLOGY AND PATHOGENESIS. Although not demonstrable in all cases, obstruction of the appendiceal lumen by a fecalith is the usual inciting event. Less common causes include neoplasms (carcinoid tumors, adenocarcinoma, Kaposi's sarcoma) and infections (*Enterobius vermicularis*, cytomegalovirus). With appendiceal obstruction, normally secreted mucus becomes impacted and causes appendiceal distention, thrombosis, and subsequently, bacterial invasion of the wall; the end result is gangrene and perforation.

CLINICAL FINDINGS. The clinical manifestations follow a stereotypic course paralleling these pathologic events. Almost invariably, abdominal pain is the first manifestation. Initially, mild pain may be discounted as indigestion. It is often poorly localized to the periumbilical area or epigastrium; appendiceal distention results in this poorly localized visceral type of periumbilical discomfort. The pain is at first colicky, then steady, and increases in severity as the inflammatory process progresses. When the parietal peritoneum becomes inflamed, usually hours after the initial onset of symptoms, the pain becomes localized in the right iliac region. Right iliac pain is typical of appendicitis; however, pelvic pain (pelvic appendix) or right upper quadrant pain may result, depending on the location of the appendix. Anorexia is frequent, and the urge to eat argues against the diagnosis of appendicitis. Vomiting is not a prominent symptom.

PHYSICAL EXAMINATION. Physical findings depend on the stage of the inflammatory process, location of the appendix, and in some cases, the age of the patient. Acute abdominal conditions have notoriously atypical manifestations in the elderly and in patients receiving corticosteroid therapy. The most consistent physical finding is tenderness in the right iliac region at McBurney's point (one fingerbreadth from the anterosuperior iliac spine toward the umbilicus). The area of tenderness, however, corresponds to the location of the inflamed appendix. With a retrocecal appendix, tenderness may be mild. Rectal examination may disclose tenderness anteriorly with a pelvic appendix or a bulge in the pelvic wall from an abscess. An inflamed parietal peritoneum results in localized rebound tenderness and rigidity. Only with generalized peritonitis are diffuse rebound tenderness and peritoneal signs elicited. Rarely, a mass is palpable in the right lower quadrant. Rotating a flexed right hip when supine (obturator sign) or raising a straightened leg against resistance (psoas sign) may elicit pain. Bowel sounds can be heard unless peritonitis and ileus are present. Fever occurs only in the later stages of inflammation; fever at the onset of abdominal pain should suggest another diagnosis.

LABORATORY STUDIES. Leukocytosis with increased polymorphonuclear leukocytes is a consistent finding only in the later stages of appendicitis. Urinalysis is usually normal. Standard abdominal radiography is frequently normal, although it may demonstrate localized loops of bowel, obliteration of the psoas shadow, or a soft tissue mass; however, these latter findings represent abscess formation. Fewer than 10% of patients have a calcified fecalith seen in the region of the appendix by abdominal imaging.

DIFFERENTIAL DIAGNOSIS OF APPENDICITIS AND THE ACUTE ABDOMEN. Although the differential diagnosis of acute appendicitis and acute abdomen is broad, a systematic history and physical examination, combined with selected laboratory tests and abdominal imaging studies, in most cases lead to a diagnosis. For an acutely ill patient, early surgical consultation is mandatory. Although a firm diagnosis before laparotomy is the rule today, surgical exploration when the appendix is normal is entirely acceptable given the increase in morbidity and mortality with appendiceal rupture. Indeed, 5 to 10% of patients with suspected acute appendicitis have a normal appendix at the time of laparotomy.

A variety of disorders cause a subacute to acute right lower quadrant pain syndrome mimicking acute appendicitis (Table 136–1). In young children, bacterial infections may result in a mesenteric adenitis or terminal ileitis or involve the right colon. Crohn's ileitis or ileocolitis frequently masquerades as acute appendicitis (see Chapter 135). Meckel's or cecal diverticulitis may be impossible to distinguish from acute appendicitis. Special consideration should be given to female patients. Pelvic inflammatory disease is infrequently unilateral but may mimic appendicitis. Ectopic pregnancy, ruptured endometrioma, or torsion of an ovarian cyst may cause unilateral pain. A ruptured graafian follicle would occur in

Table 136–1 ■ CAUSES OF RIGHT LOWER QUADRANT PAIN SYNDROMES

INFLAMMATORY DISORDERS	NEOPLASMS	OTHER
Appendicitis	Carcinoid	Gynecologic disorders
Crohn's ileitis/colitis	Lymphoma	
Cecal diverticulitis	Cecal adenocarcinoma	
Meckel's diverticulitis	(perforated)	
Yersinia ileocolitis		
Amebic colitis		
Tuberculous colitis		

mid-cycle without fever and leukocytosis. Appendicitis may be difficult to diagnose during pregnancy because the appendix moves toward the right upper quadrant.

CHARACTERISTICS OF PAIN. Acute severe abdominal pain most often results from perforation of an abdominal viscus (peptic ulcer), small bowel obstruction, choledocholithiasis, nephrolithiasis, or rupture and dissection of an abdominal aortic aneurysm. Subacute onset of pain is more typical of intestinal ischemia, cholecystitis, pancreatitis, diverticulitis, Crohn's disease, and appendicitis. Pain of a constant nature is seen with cholecystitis, pancreatitis, intestinal ischemia, and other inflammatory disorders (see Chapters 137, 141, and 157). Colicky pain occurs with nephrolithiasis or intestinal obstruction. Although more typical of nephrolithiasis, pain radiating to the groin may rarely be seen in appendicitis. Radiation of pain to the back suggests pancreatitis, peptic ulcer disease, or biliary tract disease. Shoulder pain results from diaphragmatic irritation (pancreatitis, cholecystitis). Significant vomiting is seen with pancreatitis or obstruction of the stomach or small bowel.

PHYSICAL EXAMINATION. Careful observation of the patient may provide clues to the cause. With peritonitis, the patient attempts to lie quietly. In contrast, patients with intermittent visceral-type pain (nephrolithiasis or choledocholithiasis) are restless during the attack. Tachycardia is non-specific. Hypotension suggests bleeding (ruptured aneurysm), sepsis, or severe pancreatitis. Low-grade fever occurs with any inflammatory process, including acute pancreatitis. Abdominal inspection should include attention to scars that may suggest hernias or to masses (aneurysm, abscess). Absence of bowel sounds suggests ileus, whereas "rushes and tinkles" occur with small bowel obstruction. Abdominal palpation should begin opposite the point of subjective pain to minimize voluntary guarding, which may limit the examination. Coughing may cause local pain with peritonitis. Diffuse abdominal rigidity, unequivocal rebound tenderness, or severe localized tenderness with rebound represents generalized peritonitis and indicates a need for urgent surgical exploration. Involuntary guarding or referred rebound suggests a focal peritoneal process. Abdominal ischemia causes subjective pain disproportionate to the findings on examination until infarction and perforation occur. Abdominal distention and tympany are found with dilation of either the large or small bowel. Femoral artery or abdominal bruits suggest vascular disease (ischemic disease or aneurysms). Rectal and pelvic examinations may help evaluate for a pelvic appendix and peritonitis or gynecologic disorders.

LABORATORY STUDIES. In patients with an acute abdomen, the following studies should be performed: complete blood cell count with differential, serum electrolytes, blood urea nitrogen and creatinine, serum amylase, liver chemistry tests, urinalysis, and a pregnancy test in women of childbearing potential. An elevated polymorphonuclear leukocyte count points to infection (appendicitis, cholecystitis), tissue necrosis (bowel infarction), or other inflammatory processes (pancreatitis). Anemia may result from gastrointestinal bleeding secondary to carcinoma or peptic ulcer. Pyuria and bacteriuria indicate a urinary tract infection, and microscopic or gross hematuria suggests nephrolithiasis. Fecal white blood cells or blood in the stool is seen with colitis (ischemia, inflammatory bowel disease, infection); fecal white cells are not present in acute appendicitis. Mildly elevated serum amylase (less than two times the upper limit of normal) is non-specific and occurs with a variety of intra-abdominal disorders (see Chapter 141).

ABDOMINAL IMAGING. Radiographic films of the chest and supine/upright abdominal series are useful to evaluate for free peritoneal air, bowel gas pattern, and the presence of calculi (nephrolithiasis, 80%; gallstones, 15%; appendicolith, 5%; or pancreatic calcification). Pneumonia or another basilar pulmonic process may mimic an abdominal syndrome. Abdominal sonography may demonstrate gallstones and a thickened gallbladder wall (acute cholecystitis), a dilated common bile duct (choledocholithiasis), or pancreatic calcifications (chronic pancreatitis). Recent studies suggest that in experienced hands, sonography has a sensitivity and specificity of greater than 90% in diagnosing acute appendicitis.

Abdominal computed tomographic (CT) scanning has been invaluable in the evaluation of patients with an acute abdomen. Localized inflammatory processes of the right lower quadrant may suggest appendicitis or possibly Crohn's disease if the terminal ileum and/or right colon is thickened; however, overlap between these two entities may occur. CT also helps exclude diverticulitis, acute pancreatitis, biliary obstruction, luminal disorders such as small bowel or colonic infarction, and aortic dissection, as well as unsuspected processes of the liver and spleen. Because of its ability to evaluate essentially all intra-abdominal organs, CT has become the imaging modality of choice in patients with an acute abdomen. Helical CT with both oral and intravenous contrast, if no contraindications are present, has the highest diagnostic yield.

A variety of other non-surgical conditions may cause an acute abdominal pain syndrome. Disorders "above the diaphragm" include myocardial infarction, bacterial pneumonia, and acute pericarditis. Severe right heart failure and a distended liver may cause mild to moderate right upper quadrant pain. Acute hepatitis rarely results in severe abdominal pain and should be suspected by marked elevations of serum aminotransferase concentrations. Marked transient elevations in serum aminotransferases, however, are commonly seen with acute biliary obstruction (choledocholithiasis). Systemic disorders with abdominal manifestations include sickle cell crisis, acute intermittent porphyria, diabetic neuropathy, heavy metal poisoning, and cutaneous herpes zoster.

TREATMENT. Surgical therapy is curative. Mortality is minimal when the diagnosis is rapidly established and appendectomy performed. Mortality rates increase significantly with frank perforation, particularly in the elderly. For patients with a typical history, no confirmatory studies may be necessary before surgical exploration. When the diagnosis is in doubt, careful observation for 6 to 12 hours may be diagnostic. Broad-spectrum antibiotics directed toward gram-negative rods and anaerobes should be given before surgery or at the time of CT-guided drainage. In some patients, acute appendicitis resolves with localized perforation alone; however, subsequent relapse is frequent (chronic appendicitis), so elective appendectomy should be performed.

DIVERTICULITIS OF THE COLON

Colonic diverticula are mucosal outpouchings occurring where arteries penetrate the muscularis to reach the submucosa and mucosa. Because these areas are inherently weak and under stress, prolapse of mucosa and submucosa may occur. Diverticula form throughout the entire colon, although more commonly in the left colon, particularly the sigmoid. Diverticulitis results when a fecalith becomes impacted in a diverticulum, with erosion through the serosa resulting in perforation.

CLINICAL FINDINGS. Diverticulitis of the colon typically affects patients 50 years and older because the prevalence of diverticulosis increases with age. The pain is usually subacute and constant and located in the left lower quadrant (sigmoid diverticulitis). However, the location of pain depends on the colonic segment involved. Fever is almost invariably present. High-grade fever and sepsis occur when the perforation is not contained or when the peritonitis is generalized. Constipation or loose stools may be reported. Rectal bleeding is distinctly unusual.

DIFFERENTIAL DIAGNOSIS. Constant left lower quadrant pain and fever in the elderly are highly suggestive of acute diverticulitis. Lower abdominal pain, fever, and bloody diarrhea suggest a bacterial colitis (*Shigella, Salmonella, Campylobacter*), ischemic colitis, or other inflammatory bowel disease (see Chapters 135, 137, and 339). With generalized peritonitis, the differential diagnosis becomes that of the acute abdomen (see above). Gynecologic disorders may be localized to the left lower quadrant and should always be considered in females.

DIAGNOSTIC STUDIES. Leukocytosis is common, although nonspecific. Urinalysis may demonstrate non-specific findings such as protein or rare white blood cells. If significant diarrhea is reported, fecal leukocytes should be searched for.

Abdominal radiographs may indicate a displaced colon, extraluminal gas, or colonic mucosal abnormalities. These studies are probably more helpful in excluding other potential causes of left lower quadrant pain.

Diagnostic barium enema has been used for many years and is safe when carefully performed. Typical findings include spiculation of the mucosa, spasm, or frank perforation and abscess. These findings are relatively specific for acute diverticulitis but may be difficult to differentiate from carcinoma. Abdominal CT, which has become the test of choice, may demonstrate bowel wall thickening, abscess formation, and diverticula (Fig. 136–1). Barium enema and CT are complementary because neither is 100% sensitive and specific.

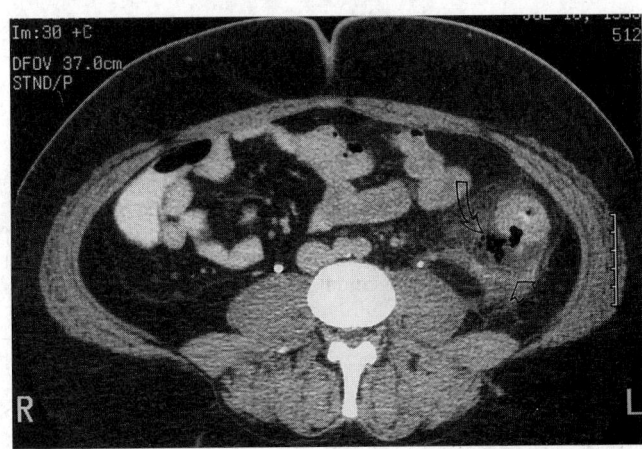

FIGURE 136–1 ■ CT scan showing marked thickening of the distal end of the descending colon with surrounding inflammatory changes (straight arrow) and extraluminal gas (curved arrow) diagnostic of diverticulitis.

Endoscopic examination is contraindicated with diverticulitis given the theoretic potential to exacerbate perforation; however, when carcinoma or inflammatory bowel disease is highly suspected, sigmoidoscopy is appropriate.

TREATMENT. Initial therapy includes broad-spectrum antibiotics such as a 3rd-generation cephalosporin combined with anaerobic coverage (metronidazole). For mild disease, oral antibiotics and bowel rest can be used in the outpatient setting. Early surgical consultation is important, especially in the presence of more significant pain or an acute abdomen. If a large abscess is identified by CT imaging, percutaneous catheter drainage can be a temporary measure before subsequent definitive surgical therapy.

Complications of diverticulitis include colonic stricture, bleeding, or fistula formation to the small bowel, colon, bladder, or vagina.

RADIATION ENTEROCOLITIS

Although radiation is commonly used to palliate abdominal and pelvic malignancies, clinically significant radiation injury in the gastrointestinal tract is unusual. Injury usually develops when the total dosage exceeds 50 Gy.

PATHOGENESIS. Given the high turnover rate of gastrointestinal epithelium, it is not unexpected that the gut, particularly replicating cells in the crypts, would be affected by radiation. If the dose of radiation does not exceed 50 Gy, minor mucosal injury (edema, erosions) may be temporary. With more intense therapy, damage to submucosal blood vessels results in an arteritis and, secondarily, mucosal ischemia. Late complications include fibrosis, strictures, and diffuse vascular ectasia in the affected segments.

CLINICAL FINDINGS. During the early phases of radiation therapy, patients may report nausea, vomiting, and diarrhea, which may be bloody. Symptoms caused by the complications of high-dose radiation are not seen for months or even years following therapy (intestinal ulcerations with bleeding, obstruction from fibrosis and stricture, fistulas to other pelvic organs or abscesses, or chronic gastrointestinal bleeding and anemia from vascular ectasia). If a significant amount of small bowel is in the radiation field, malabsorption may be noted.

DIAGNOSIS. In the appropriate setting, the diagnosis is relatively straightforward. Symptoms early in the course of therapy suggest acute injury. Endoscopic features include mucosal edema, ulceration (early), and diffuse vascular ectasia and stricture (late). Although non-specific, barium enema may demonstrate mucosal edema, fistula formation, and strictures. In an older patient with a stricture, carcinoma must be excluded.

TREATMENT. Treatment options are limited. Iron deficiency anemia from bleeding (vascular ectasia) should be treated with chronic iron therapy. For symptomatic distal colonic strictures, dilation may be attempted, although surgery is usually required. Diarrhea can be treated with antimotility agents. Abscess and fistula formation requires surgical resection. Surgery should be performed only when necessary given the potential for further complications after anastomosis owing to the involvement of adjacent bowel segments.

INTESTINAL AND COLONIC ULCERATION

Small intestinal and colonic ulceration is uncommon. Ulcerations may be isolated or diffuse and may be located anywhere throughout the small bowel. The location of disease and the character of the ulcers suggest the underlying cause. Isolated proximal small bowel ulcerations are most commonly caused by medications such as slow-release potassium pills or non-steroidal anti-inflammatory drugs (NSAIDs). Other disorders include infections, collagen-vascular diseases (Behçet's disease, systemic lupus erythematosus), and ulcerated neoplasms. Multiple ulcers may be caused by Zollinger-Ellison syndrome and have been associated with celiac disease. In some cases they are idiopathic.

Because of their small size, these ulcers are difficult to identify by routine small bowel barium radiographs. Enteroclysis (see Chapter 121) is more sensitive in defining these abnormalities. Small bowel enteroscopy is time consuming and not widely available, although it is the best method to visualize the proximal end of the small bowel directly. Diffuse processes (celiac sprue, lymphoma, or Crohn's disease) are more reliably identified by these radiographic studies.

Ulceration(s) in the right colon has recently been documented to result from NSAIDs. These ulcerations may result in one or multiple circumferential strictures, termed diaphragms, and may also appear in the small bowel. Infections such as tuberculosis, amebiasis, or rarely bacterial infections may produce right colonic ulceration. Ischemia usually produces diffuse segmental ulceration. Distal colonic ulcers result from ischemia, infections, or inflammatory bowel disease, particularly Crohn's colitis. Rectal ulcers, when solitary, may be seen with chronic constipation (stercoral ulcer) or trauma or may be idiopathic.

Barium enema may suggest Crohn's disease or ischemia. Colonoscopy with ulcer biopsy may demonstrate characteristic histopathologic changes in Crohn's disease or the solitary rectal ulcer syndrome.

Anderson RE, Hugander AP, Ghazi SH, et al: Diagnostic value of disease history, clinical presentation, and inflammatory parameters of appendicitis. World Surg 23: 133, 1999. *This prospective study documents the diagnostic utility of the history, physical examination, and parameters of inflammation in suggesting the diagnosis of appendicitis.*

Choi YH, Fischer E, Hoda SA, et al: Appendiceal CT in 140 cases: Diagnostic criteria for acute and necrotizing appendicitis. Clin Imaging 22:252, 1998. *The overall accuracy of CT was 98% and it had a 90% positive predictive accuracy for necrotizing appendicitis.*

Hellberg A, Rudberg C, Kullman E, et al: Prospective randomized multicentre study of laparoscopic versus open appendectomy. Br J Surg 86:48, 1999. *Laparoscopic appendicectomy is as safe as open appendicectomy and has the advantage of allowing a quicker recovery.*

137 VASCULAR DISORDERS OF THE INTESTINE

Lawrence J. Brandt

Vascular disorders may present either with ischemic damage consequent to insufficient blood flow or by bleeding caused by a focal or diffuse increase in vascularity. The development of sophisticated radiologic imaging techniques has expanded the spectrum of clinically relevant vascular disorders.

ISCHEMIC DISORDERS

Three major vessels supply almost all of the blood to the gastrointestinal tract, albeit with incredible variation in anatomy. The *celiac axis* and its branches supply the liver, biliary tract, spleen, stomach, duodenum, and pancreas; the *superior mesenteric artery* (SMA) gives off branches to the duodenum and pancreas and then supplies the entire small intestine as well as the ascending colon and a part of the transverse colon; the *inferior mesenteric artery* (IMA) delivers blood to the rectum and descending colon and then anastomoses with the superior mesenteric artery to supply the transverse colon. In some areas such as the stomach, duodenum, and rectum, collateral circulation is abundant and ischemia is unusual, whereas in other regions, such as the splenic flexure and sigmoid, anastomoses are more limited and segmental ischemic damage is common. Ischemic injury of the bowel is influenced by the health of the cardiovascular system; the potential for collateral flow; the response of the vasculature to autonomic stimuli and circulating vasoactive substances; local modulation of blood flow; and a host of exogenous agents causing vasoconstriction (digitalis glycosides, vasopressin, and α-adrenergic agonists) or vasodilation (β-adrenergic agonists, papaverine, calcium channel blockers, aminophylline).

The types of intestinal ischemia and their approximate incidences are colonic (60%), acute mesenteric (30%), focal segmental (5%), and chronic mesenteric (5%). Ischemic injury may be occlusive (due to an anatomic obstruction to blood flow) or non-occlusive (mediated by vasoconstriction), but these two processes often coexist. When a major vessel is suddenly occluded, collaterals open immediately in response to the fall in arterial pressure. Increased blood flow through these collaterals continues as long as the pressure in the vascular bed distal to the obstruction remains below systemic pressure. However, after several hours of ischemia, vasoconstriction develops in the involved vascular bed, elevating its pressure and reducing collateral flow. If the ischemia and vasoconstriction are prolonged, the vasoconstriction can persist even after the cause of the ischemia is corrected. The bowel may tolerate a remarkable reduction in blood flow without damage. Normal oxygen consumption can be maintained with only 20 to 25% of normal blood flow, but below this critical level, oxygen consumption falls because increased oxygen extraction can no longer compensate for diminished blood flow.

Acute Mesenteric Ischemia

Intestinal ischemia can be acute or chronic and of venous or arterial origin. Acute mesenteric ischemia is much more common than chronic mesenteric ischemia, and ischemia of arterial origin is much more frequent than venous disease. Acute mesenteric ischemia is caused by superior mesenteric arterial embolus (50%), non-occlusive mesenteric ischemia (25%), superior mesenteric artery thrombosis (10%), focal segmental ischemia (5%), and acute mesenteric venous thrombosis (10%).

ARTERIAL FORMS OF ACUTE MESENTERIC ISCHEMIA. SMA emboli usually originate from a left atrial or ventricular thrombus and lodge distal to the origin of a major branch. Many patients with SMA emboli have had previous peripheral emboli, and approximately 20% have synchronous emboli to other arteries. Non-occlusive mesenteric ischemia usually results from splanchnic vasoconstriction hours to days after some cardiovascular event (e.g., acute myocardial infarction, heart failure, arrhythmia, or shock). Patients with chronic renal diseases, especially those requiring hemodialysis and those undergoing major cardiac or intra-abdominal operations, are also at risk. SMA thrombosis occurs at severe atherosclerotic narrowings, most often at the SMA origin. The acute episode is commonly superimposed on chronic ischemia, and 20 to 50% of these patients have a history suggesting intestinal angina during the weeks to months preceding the acute event.

CLINICAL ASPECTS OF SEVERE ACUTE MESENTERIC ISCHEMIA. Sudden severe abdominal pain developing in a patient with heart disease and arrhythmias, long-standing and poorly controlled heart failure, recent myocardial infarction, or hypotension should suggest the possibility of acute mesenteric ischemia. Early on, the pain is accompanied by a paucity of physical findings. Increasing abdominal tenderness and muscle guarding indicate infarcted bowel. Right-sided abdominal pain associated with maroon or bright red blood in the stool, although characteristic of colonic ischemia, also can suggest acute mesenteric ischemia because the blood supply to both the right colon and small bowel originates from the SMA.

Leukocytosis, metabolic acidemia, and elevations of serum phosphate, amylase, lactate dehydrogenase, creatine kinase, and intestinal alkaline phosphatase are seen with advanced ischemic bowel injury. Early in the course of disease, plain films of the abdomen usually are normal. Later, formless loops of small intestine, ileus, or "thumbprinting" of the small bowel or right colon due to submucosal hemorrhage may develop. Duplex ultrasonography of the celiac axis and SMA may demonstrate partial or complete occlusion of these vessels but is not reliable to evaluate peripheral blood flow. Abdominal computed tomography (CT) is helpful in some cases, especially those caused by mesenteric venous thrombosis, but early signs are non-specific and later signs develop only with necrosis and gangrene. Selective mesenteric angiography is the mainstay of diagnosis and initial treatment of both occlusive and non-occlusive acute mesenteric ischemia.

The approach to diagnosing and managing acute mesenteric ischemia is based on several observations: (1) if the diagnosis is not made before intestinal infarction, the mortality rate is 70 to 90%; (2) both occlusive and non-occlusive forms can be diagnosed by angiography; (3) vasoconstriction may persist even after the initial cause of the ischemia is corrected; and (4) vasoconstriction can be relieved by vasodilators infused into the SMA. Early and liberal use of angiography and the incorporation of intra-arterial papaverine are therefore the cornerstones in the treatment of both occlusive and non-occlusive mesenteric ischemia.

Initial management of patients suspected of having acute mesenteric ischemia includes resuscitation, abdominal plain films, and selective angiography. Resuscitation includes relieving acute heart failure and correcting hypotension, hypovolemia, and cardiac arrhythmias. Mesenteric blood flow cannot be improved if low cardiac output, hypovolemia, or hypotension persists. Broad-spectrum antibiotics are begun immediately. Plain films of the abdomen are obtained, not to establish the diagnosis of acute mesenteric ischemia but to exclude other causes of abdominal pain. A normal plain film does *not* exclude acute mesenteric ischemia. If no alternative diagnosis is made on the abdominal films, selective SMA angiography is performed. Based on the angiographic findings and the presence or absence of peritoneal signs, treatment can be planned (Fig. 137–1).

Even when the decision to operate has been made based on clinical grounds, a preoperative angiogram should be obtained. Relief of mesenteric vasoconstriction is essential in treating emboli, thromboses, and "low flow" states and is accomplished by infusing papaverine at 30 to 60 mg/hour through the indwelling SMA angiography catheter (Fig. 137–2).

Laparotomy is performed in acute mesenteric ischemia to restore arterial flow after an embolus or thrombosis, to resect irreparably damaged bowel, or both. Except in the case of mesenteric venous thrombosis, heparin should not be used immediately postoperatively. However, late thrombosis after embolectomy or arterial reconstruction occurs frequently enough that anticoagulation 48 hours postoperatively is advisable. Survival is in the range of 55%; 90% of patients with acute mesenteric ischemia diagnosed angiographically before the development of peritonitis survive.

MESENTERIC VENOUS THROMBOSIS. Mesenteric venous thrombosis accounts for 5 to 10% of intestinal ischemia. Underlying causes have been identified in more than 80% of patients and include antithrombin III, protein S and C deficiencies, and hypercoagulable states associated with polycythemia vera, myeloproliferative disorders, pregnancy, and neoplasms. Oral contraceptives account for less than 10% of cases. As many as 60% of patients have a history of peripheral vein thromboses. Mesenteric venous thrombosis can have an acute, subacute (weeks to months), or chronic onset; the latter is unaccompanied by symptoms unless and until late complications occur. *Acute mesenteric venous thrombosis* resembles arterial forms of acute mesenteric ischemia because it presents as abdominal pain that, early on, is typically out of proportion to the physical findings. However, the tempo of illness is slower than that with arterial ischemia, and the mean duration of pain before hospital admission is 5 to 14 days. Nausea and vomiting are common, and lower gastrointestinal bleeding or hematemesis indicating bowel infarction is found in 15%. Abdominal plain film signs of mesenteric venous thrombosis are similar to those of other forms of acute mesenteric ischemia and almost always reflect the presence of infarcted bowel. Characteristic findings on small bowel series include luminal narrowing from congestion and edema of the bowel wall, separation of loops due to mesenteric thickening, and "thumbprinting" due to submucosal hemorrhage and

edema. Selective mesenteric arteriography can differentiate venous thrombosis from arterial forms of ischemia, but ultrasonography, CT, and magnetic resonance imaging (MRI) are more commonly used to demonstrate thrombi in the superior mesenteric vein (SMV) and portal vein. If patients with suspected acute mesenteric ischemia have features suggesting mesenteric venous thrombosis, a contrast medium–enhanced CT scan is obtained before SMA angiography; a history of deep vein thrombosis or a family history of an inherited coagulation defect also suggest CT as the initial imaging study. In the few patients with no physical findings of intestinal infarction in whom a diagnosis of mesenteric venous thrombosis is made by ultrasonography, CT, or MRI, a trial of anticoagulant or thrombolytic therapy is worthwhile. All other patients should have prompt laparotomy, resection of non-viable bowel, and heparinization. The mortality of acute mesenteric venous thrombosis is lower than that of the other forms of acute mesenteric ischemia, varying from 20 to 50%. Recurrence rates of 20 to 25% fall to 13 to 15% if heparin is begun promptly.

Subacute mesenteric venous thrombosis is a condition in which patients have abdominal pain for weeks to months but have no intestinal infarction. It is caused by either extension of thrombosis at a rate rapid enough to cause pain but slow enough to allow collaterals to develop before infarction occurs or by acute thrombosis of a sufficiently small portion of the venous drainage system to permit recovery from ischemic injury. Diagnosis usually is made on imaging studies done for other suspected diagnoses. Non-specific abdominal pain usually is the only symptom, and physical examination and laboratory tests are normal. In *chronic mesenteric venous thrombosis,* there usually are no symptoms at the time of thrombosis, and the patient may remain asymptomatic or may develop gastrointestinal bleeding. If the portal vein is involved, physical findings are those of portal hypertension, but if only the SMV is involved, there may be no abnormal findings. Laboratory studies may show hypersplenism with pancytopenia or thrombocytopenia. Treatment of chronic mesenteric venous thrombosis is aimed at controlling bleeding, which is usually from esophageal varices. No treatment is indicated for patients with asymptomatic chronic mesenteric venous thrombosis. The natural history of chronic mesenteric venous thrombosis is not known, but from postmortem studies it appears that almost 50% of patients do not have bowel infarction and most are without symptoms.

Focal Segmental Ischemia of the Small Bowel

Vascular insults to short segments of small bowel produce a broad spectrum of clinical features without the life-threatening complications associated with more extensive ischemia. Focal segmental ischemia usually is caused by atheromatous emboli, strangulated hernias, vasculitis, blunt abdominal trauma, radiation, or oral contraceptives. With focal segmental ischemia there usually is adequate collateral circulation to prevent transmural infarction, and patients present with one of three clinical patterns: (1) acute enteritis often simulating appendicitis (see Chapter 136), (2) chronic enteritis resembling Crohn's disease (see Chapter 135), and (3) intestinal obstruction often with bacterial overgrowth and a "blind loop" syndrome. Treatment is resection of the involved bowel.

Colon Ischemia

Colon ischemia is the most common ischemic injury to the gastrointestinal tract. A spectrum of colon ischemic injury is recognized, including reversible colopathy (submucosal or intramural hemorrhage) (at least 30 to 40%); transient colitis (at least 15–20%); chronic ulcerating colitis (20–25%); stricture (10–15%); gangrene (15–20%); and fulminant universal colitis (<5%). In most cases, no specific cause is identified, and what finally triggers the presenting episode is usually unknown. However, colonic blood flow is lower than that of any other intestinal segment, decreases with functional motor activity, and is greatly affected by autonomic stimulation—a combination that may make the colon especially susceptible to ischemia. More than 90% of patients are older than age 60, although colon ischemia has been documented in young individuals with vasculitis (especially systemic lupus erythematosus), sickle cell disease, coagulopathies, medication-induced reactions (estrogens, danazol, vasopressin, gold, psychotropic drugs),

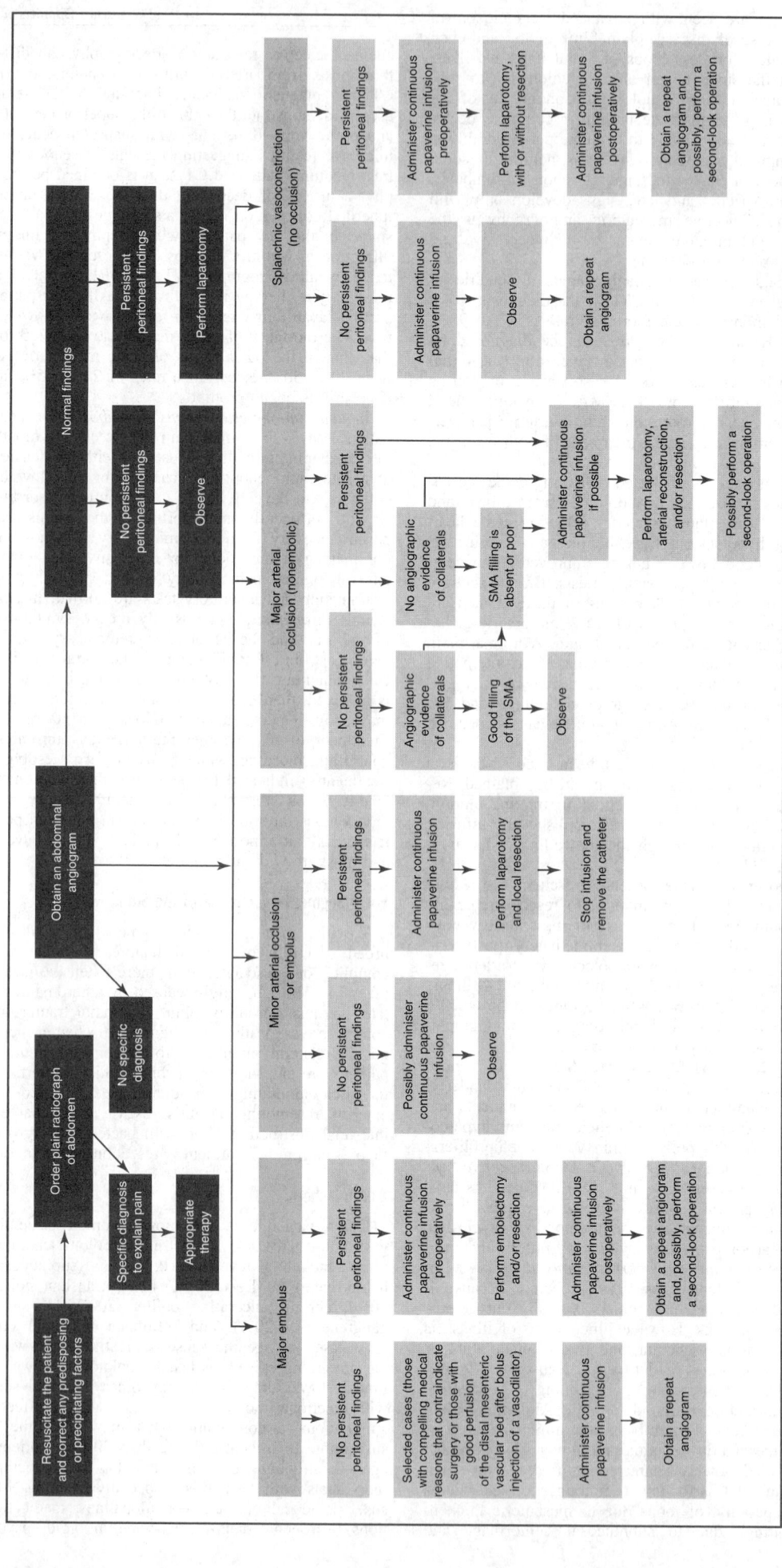

FIGURE 137–1 ■ Algorithm for managing patients with suspected acute mesenteric ischemia.

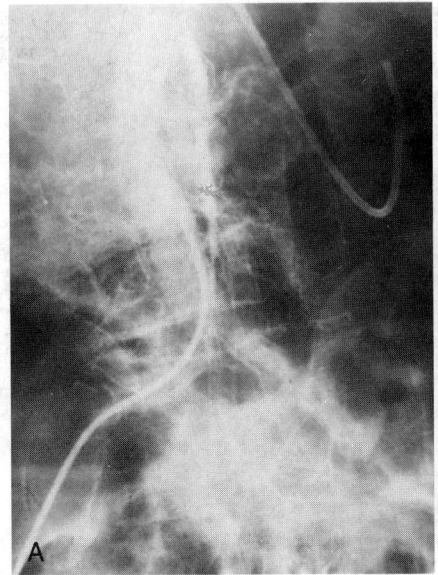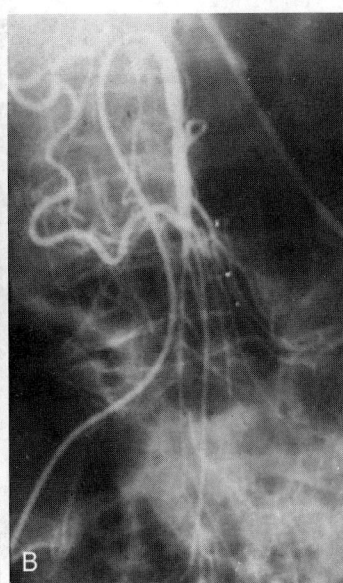

FIGURE 137–2 ■ Selected films from a superior mesenteric angiogram. *A,* Diffuse vasoconstriction characteristic of non-occlusive mesenteric ischemia. *B,* Intra-arterial infusion of papaverine (30 to 60 mg/hr) resulted in vasodilation.

cocaine abuse, and long distance running. Five to 10 per cent of patients with colon ischemia have had a distal and potentially obstructing colonic or rectal lesion, including carcinoma, diverticulitis, stricture, or fecal impaction. Colon ischemia is a complication of elective aortic surgery in 1 to 7% of cases, but after surgery for ruptured abdominal aortic aneurysm it may be as high as 60%.

Pathologic abnormalities are varied. Mildest changes include mucosal and submucosal hemorrhage and edema with or without partial mucosal necrosis. Hemorrhages are subsequently resorbed or the overlying mucosa sloughs, forming an ulcer. Multiple ulcers manifest clinically as a transient segmental colitis. With more severe injury, the mucosa and submucosa are replaced by granulation tissue. Later, the mucosa may regenerate over the edematous submucosa, which contains granulation and fibrous tissue and iron-laden macrophages. Moderately severe colon ischemia can produce chronic ulcerations separated by normal bowel, a picture that mimics inflammatory bowel disease. With more severe and prolonged ischemia, the muscularis propria is damaged and replaced by fibrous tissue, thus forming a stricture. The most severe cases show transmural infarction with gangrene and perforation.

In contrast to acute mesenteric ischemia, most colon ischemia is not associated with either a major vascular occlusion or a period of low cardiac output. Colon ischemia usually presents with sudden, crampy, mild, left lower abdominal pain, an urge to defecate, and passage of bright red or maroon blood mixed with the stool within 24 hours. Bleeding is not vigorous, and blood loss requiring transfusion suggests another diagnosis. Physical examination usually reveals only mild to moderate abdominal tenderness over the involved segment of bowel. Any part of the colon may be affected, but the splenic flexure and sigmoid are most commonly involved. Systemic low flow states usually involve the right colon; local non-occlusive ischemic injuries involve the "watershed" areas of the colon (i.e., the splenic flexure and rectosigmoid), whereas ligation of the inferior mesenteric artery produces changes in the sigmoid.

If colon ischemia is suspected and the patient has no signs of peritonitis and an unrevealing abdominal plain film, colonoscopy or the combination of sigmoidoscopy and a gentle barium enema should be performed on the unprepared bowel within 48 hours of the onset of symptoms; colonoscopy is more sensitive in diagnosing mucosal abnormalities, and biopsy specimens may be obtained. Hemorrhagic nodules seen at colonoscopy represent submucosal bleeding and appear as filling defects called "thumbprints" on barium enema examination (Fig. 137–3). The initial diagnostic study should be performed within 48 hours, because thumbprinting disappears as the submucosal hemorrhages are resorbed or the overlying mucosa sloughs. Studies performed 1 week after the initial study should reflect evolution of the injury: normalization of the colon or replacement of the thumbprints with segmental ulceration. Mesenteric angiography usually is *not* indicated in colon ischemia, be-

cause by the time of presentation colonic blood flow has returned to normal. Angiography may be indicated, however, when the clinical presentation does not allow a clear distinction between colon ischemia and acute mesenteric ischemia or if only the right side of the colon is involved, a situation indicating disease in the distribution of the SMA and thus implying coincident acute mesenteric ischemia. In such situations, because untreated acute mesenteric ischemia rapidly becomes irreversible and because optimal management requires angiography, acute mesenteric ischemia must be excluded before barium studies, which would preclude an adequate angiographic examination.

In general, symptoms of colon ischemia subside within 24 to 48 hours, and healing is seen within 2 weeks. Two thirds of patients with reversible disease exhibit intramural and submucosal hemorrhage (reversible colopathy), whereas one third manifest a transient colitis. More severe reversible damage may take up to 6 months to resolve. Irreversible damage results in less than 50% of patients, of whom approximately two thirds develop gangrene with or without perforation. The prognosis of patients with colon ischemia complicating shock, heart failure, myocardial infarction, or severe dehydration is particularly poor, perhaps due to associated acute mesenteric ischemia.

When physical examination does not suggest gangrene or perforation, the patient is treated expectantly. The bowel is placed at rest, broad-spectrum antibiotics are given, cardiac function is optimized, and medications that cause mesenteric vasoconstriction are withdrawn if possible. Serial roentgenographic or endoscopic evaluations of the colon and continued monitoring of the hemoglobin, white blood cell count, and electrolytes are performed. Increasing abdominal tenderness, guarding, rising temperature, and paralytic ileus indicate colonic infarction and mandate expedient laparotomy and colon resection. If, as usual, colon ischemia completely resolves within 1 to 2 weeks, no further therapy is indicated. When segmental colitis develops, corticosteroid therapy does not appear to be beneficial and may predispose to perforation. Asymptomatic patients with evidence of persistent disease should have frequent examinations to determine if the colon is healing, has persisting inflammation, or is developing a stricture. Recurrent fevers, leukocytosis, and septicemia in otherwise asymptomatic patients with unhealed segmental colitis usually are caused by the diseased bowel, and elective resection is indicated. Because patients with diarrhea or rectal bleeding for more than 2 weeks usually develop irreversible disease, often with colonic perforation, resection might be indicated. Colon ischemia may not produce symptoms during the acute insult but cause a chronic colitis frequently misdiagnosed as inflammatory bowel disease. Involvement is segmental, resection is not followed by recurrence, and the response to corticosteroid therapy usually is poor. Ischemic strictures that produce no symptoms should be observed; some disappear over 12 to 24 months

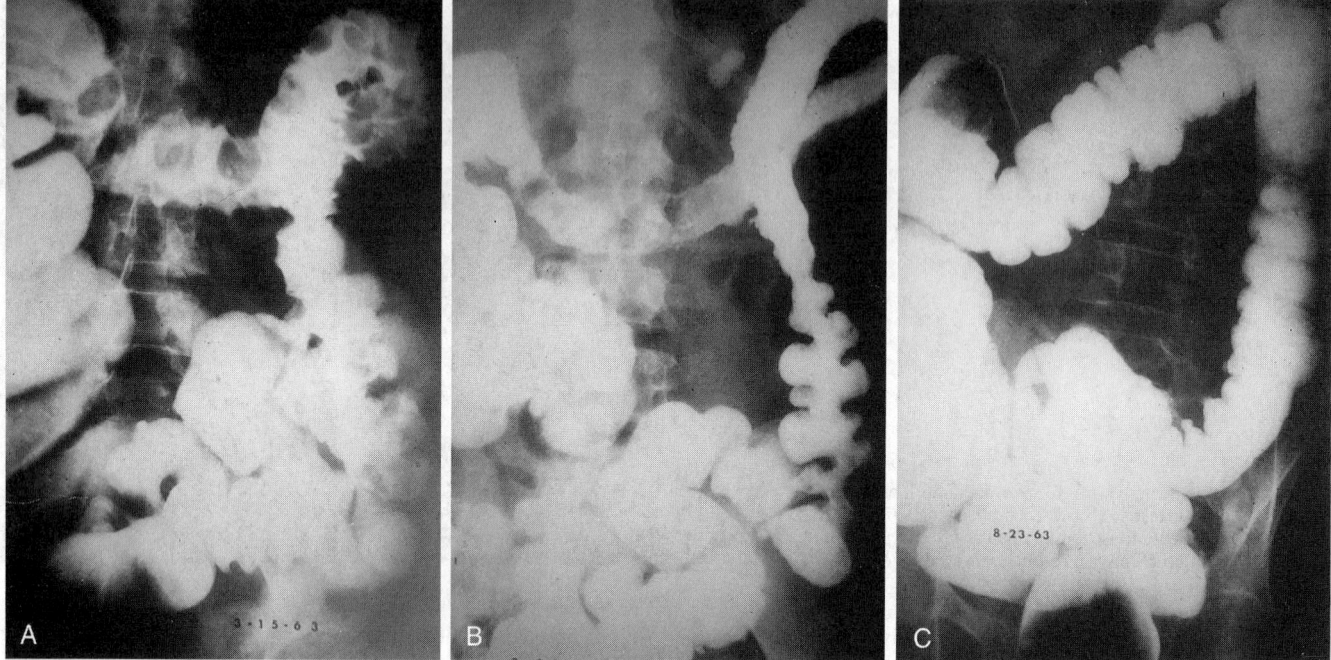

FIGURE 137–3 ■ Ischemic changes in the transverse colon and splenic flexure. *A,* Initial study shows dramatic thumbprints throughout the involved area. *B,* Eleven days later thumbprints have resolved and a segmental colitis has developed. *C,* Five months after onset there is complete return to normal. Patient was asymptomatic 3 weeks after her illness. (From Boley SJ, Schwartz SS, Williams FL [eds]: Vascular Disorders of the Intestine. New York, Appleton-Century-Crofts, 1971.)

with no specific therapy, but resection is required for those that cause obstruction. For the rare form of fulminant colon ischemia involving all or most of the colon and rectum, management is similar to that of other fulminant colitides.

Chronic Mesenteric Ischemia

Atherosclerosis is almost always the cause of chronic mesenteric ischemia or "abdominal angina." Abdominal pain probably results from a meal-induced increase in gastric blood flow that, in the presence of a fixed splanchnic arterial inflow, "steals" blood from the small bowel and makes it ischemic. Although autopsy and angiographic studies frequently demonstrate partial or complete occlusions of the major splanchnic vessels, chronic mesenteric ischemia is rare; many patients with occlusion of two or even all three of these vessels remain asymptomatic. Hence, the clinical significance of an angiogram demonstrating an occlusion of one or more of these vessels in an individual patient varies. The lack of available and reliable means to determine the inadequacy of intestinal blood flow before morphologic changes of ischemia occur has been the major obstacle to identifying patients with chronic mesenteric ischemia.

The one consistent clinical feature of chronic mesenteric ischemia is abdominal discomfort or pain, which most commonly occurs 10 to 30 minutes after eating, gradually increases in severity, reaches a plateau, and then slowly abates over 1 to 3 hours. The pain is usually dull, gnawing, or cramping and is located periumbilically or in the epigastrium. Initially the pain only follows a large meal but characteristically increases in frequency and severity, so the patient reduces the meal size ("small meal syndrome"), becomes reluctant to eat, and often loses significant weight. Bloating, flatulence, constipation, and diarrhea are not infrequent. Physical findings are limited and non-specific. Patients with advanced disease appear chronically ill with marked weight loss. The abdomen is usually soft and non-tender even during episodes of pain. A systolic bruit is usually present in the upper abdomen but is nonspecific. Many patients have cardiac, cerebral, or peripheral vascular insufficiency.

There is no specific reliable diagnostic test for abdominal angina,

so the diagnosis is based on clinical symptoms, arteriographic demonstration of splanchnic arterial occlusions, and the exclusion of other gastrointestinal disease. Conventional examinations of the gastrointestinal tract usually are unremarkable. Studies for malabsorption often show increased fecal fat and decreased D-xylose excretion. Duplex ultrasound can detect a 70% stenosis of the celiac axis or SMA with a sensitivity of 97% and 87%, respectively. Angiographic evaluation includes flush aortography and selective injections of the SMA, celiac axis, and, if possible, the IMA. The presence of stenosis of a major vessel with prominent collateral vessels indicates that the stenosis is hemodynamically significant and chronic. However, *stenosis or occlusion of one or two or all of the major vessels does not by itself establish the diagnosis of chronic mesenteric ischemia, and patients with even three occluded vessels may be asymptomatic.* Techniques to measure the effect of eating on mesenteric blood flow are Duplex ultrasound of the celiac axis and SMA, MRI of blood flow in the SMA and SMV, and balloon tonometry to determine intestinal intramural pH. Intestinal blood flow normally increases after eating, whereas in patients with intestinal ischemia, it does not; intramural pH decreases in patients with intestinal ischemia when postcibal blood flow becomes insufficient.

A patient with typical pain and unexplained weight loss, whose diagnostic evaluation has excluded other GI disease and whose angiogram shows occlusion of at least two of the three major arteries, should have the benefit of surgical revascularization. Tests of the adequacy of blood flow may identify patients who should have mesenteric angiography and who may benefit from revascularization procedures. The infrequency of fatal acute mesenteric infarction after a successful revascularization operation suggests that such procedures may prevent a major intestinal ischemic episode.

VASCULAR LESIONS

Through the widespread use of endoscopy and angiography, vascular lesions of the gastrointestinal tract are being recognized with increasing frequency as causing hemorrhage. They may be solitary or multiple, exist as isolated abnormalities, or be part of a syndrome or systemic disorder.

Colonic vascular ectasia (angiodysplasia) is the most common vascular abnormality of the gastrointestinal tract. These degenerative lesions are associated with aging and are not associated with other cutaneous or visceral lesions. They almost always are confined to the cecum or ascending colon, are usually multiple, and rarely can be identified at operation or on routine histologic sections; they usually can be diagnosed by angiography or colonoscopy.

Colonic vascular ectasias are one of the most common causes of recurrent lower gastrointestinal bleeding in the elderly. Patients may have bright red blood, maroon-colored stools, and melena on separate occasions. Bleeding is usually low grade, but about 15% of patients present with massive hemorrhage; in 20 to 25% of episodes, only tarry stools are passed. In 10 to 15% of patients, bleeding is evidenced only by iron-deficiency anemia with stools that are intermittently positive for occult blood. In more than 90% of instances, bleeding stops spontaneously.

Approximately 50% of patients with bleeding colonic vascular ectasias have evidence of cardiac disease, and up to 25% have been reported to have aortic stenosis. However, the interrelationships of aortic stenosis, gastrointestinal bleeding, and colonic vascular ectasias are obscure. Histologic identification of colonic vascular ectasia is difficult without special techniques. Colonic vascular ectasias consist of dilated, distorted, thin-walled veins, venules, and capillaries. The earliest abnormality noted is the presence of a dilated, tortuous, submucosal vein, which often exists in areas where the mucosal vessels are normal. More extensive lesions show increasing numbers of dilated and deformed vessels involving the mucosa until, in the most severe lesions, the mucosa is replaced by a maze of distorted, dilated vascular channels.

Studies using special injection and clearing techniques indicate that colonic vascular ectasias are degenerative lesions associated with aging, probably caused by intermittent, low-grade obstruction of submucosal veins, where they pierce the colonic muscle layers of the cecum. Dilation and tortuosity of the submucosal vein, and later the venules and capillaries of the mucosal units draining into it, lead to a small arteriovenous fistula, which is responsible for the "early filling vein" that was the original angiographic hallmark of this lesion. The prevalence of colonic vascular ectasias in the right colon has been attributed to the greater tension in the cecal wall than in other parts of the colon.

Angiography was formerly the primary method to identify ectasias, but currently colonoscopy is preferable (Color Plate 2*F*). The endoscopist's ability to diagnose the specific nature of a vascular lesion, however, is limited by the similar appearance of many disparate lesions (e.g., spider angiomata, hereditary hemorrhagic telangiectasia, angiomas, and the focal hypervascularity of various colitides). Biopsies of vascular lesions obtained during endoscopy usually are non-specific, and the risk of biopsy is not justified. The appearance of vascular lesions is influenced by the patient's blood pressure, blood volume, state of hydration, and medications (e.g., meperidine) administered during colonoscopy. Colonic vascular ectasias may not be evident in patients with severely reduced blood volumes or those who are in shock, so accurate evaluation may not be possible until red blood cell and volume deficits are corrected. Angiography can determine the site and nature of lesions during active bleeding and can identify colonic vascular ectasias even when bleeding has ceased if a slowly emptying and tortuous vein, a vascular tuft, or an early filling vein is present.

The natural history of colonic vascular ectasias is not known precisely. It has been estimated that less than 10% of patients with such lesions eventually bleed, data that further support the recommendation not to treat incidental colonic vascular ectasias. Although some colonoscopists remain eager to treat colonic vascular ectasias, almost half the patients may not bleed again after the initial episode. Laser therapy, sclerosis, electrocoagulation, and the argon plasma coagulator heater probe all have been used to ablate colonic vascular ectasias. None has been established as superior, but the heater probe and bipolar coagulation are most commonly used. Moreover, no data prove that endoscopic ablation of colonic vascular ectasias changes their natural history. Under emergent conditions, angiographic methods have been used to arrest bleeding from colonic vascular ectasias, and intra-arterial (SMA) vasopressin infusions stop hemorrhage in more than 80% of patients in whom extravasation is demonstrated. Right hemicolectomy is performed if the bleeding continues and an experienced endoscopist is not available or endoscopic ablation has been unsuccessful. The extent of colonic resection is not altered by the presence or absence of diverticulosis in the left colon; only the right half of the colon is removed. Because up to 80% of bleeding diverticula are located in the right side of the colon, the risks of leaving a left colon containing diverticula are far outweighed by the increased morbidity and mortality of the larger procedure, a subtotal colectomy. Recurrent bleeding can be expected in up to 20% of patients so treated. Subtotal colectomy should be performed only as a last resort: that is, in the patient in whom active colonic bleeding persists, the angiogram is completely normal, and colonoscopy either yields negative findings or is not helpful.

HEREDITARY HEMORRHAGIC TELANGIECTASIA (OSLER-WEBER-RENDU DISEASE). This autosomal dominant familial disorder is characterized by telangiectasias of the skin and mucous membranes and recurrent gastrointestinal bleeding. The gene for hereditary hemorrhagic telangiectasias, localized to chromosome 9q3, is the gene for endoglin, a membrane glycoprotein that binds transforming growth factor β (TGF-β). Perturbation of one or more of the processes modulated by TGF-β may cause the vascular dysplasia. Lesions are frequently noticed in the first few years of life, and recurrent epistaxis in childhood is characteristic. By age 10, about one half of patients have some gastrointestinal bleeding, but severe hemorrhage is unusual before the fourth decade and has a peak incidence in the sixth decade. In most patients, bleeding presents as melena; hematochezia and hematemesis are less frequent. Lesions are usually present on the lips, oral and nasopharyngeal membranes, tongue, or periungual regions. Telangiectasias occur in the colon but are more common in the stomach and small bowel, where they are also more likely to cause significant bleeding. Telangiectasias are easily seen on endoscopy as millet seed–sized cherry-red hillocks, although, in the presence of severe anemia and blood loss, they may transiently become invisible or subtle. Angiography may be normal or may demonstrate arteriovenous communications, conglomerate masses of abnormal vessels, phlebectasias, and aneurysms. Pathologically, the major changes involve the capillaries and venules, but arterioles also may be affected. Lesions consist of irregular ectatic tortuous blood spaces lined by a single layer of endothelial cells and supported by a fine layer of fibrous connective tissue. No elastic lamina or muscular tissue is present in these vessels, so they cannot contract, perhaps explaining why they tend to bleed. Arterioles show intimal proliferation, often with thrombi. Many forms of treatment have been recommended for bleeding telangiectasias, including estrogens, endoscopic ablation, and resection of involved bowel.

PROGRESSIVE SYSTEMIC SCLEROSIS (see Chapter 290). Vascular lesions are a prominent feature of progressive systemic sclerosis, especially in the CREST variant with calcinosis, Raynaud's phenomenon, esophageal dysmotility, scleroderma, and telangiectasia. These lesions may be the source of occult or clinically significant bleeding and are best treated, if possible, by endoscopic ablation.

WATERMELON STOMACH. This term describes an unusual vascular lesion of the gastric antrum consisting of tortuous dilated vessels radiating outward from the pylorus like spokes from a wheel and resembling the dark stripes on the surface of a watermelon. It produces both acute and chronic occult bleeding, but its cause is unknown; gastric peristalsis may cause prolapse of the loose antral mucosa with consequent elongation and ectasia of the mucosal vessels. The lesion is seen particularly in middle-aged or older women and is associated with achlorhydria, atrophic gastritis, and cirrhosis. The cirrhosis and portal hypertension found in almost half of the reported cases of watermelon stomach suggest an association with portal gastropathy. Microscopic features include dilated capillaries with focal thrombosis, dilated tortuous submucosal venous channels, and fibromuscular hyperplasia. Corticosteroid treatment is unsuccessful, and antrectomy or preferably transendoscopic therapy are more likely to be successful.

DIEULAFOY'S ULCER. An increasingly diagnosed cause of massive gastrointestinal hemorrhage, this lesion is usually found in the stomach and sometimes in the small or large bowel. Dieulafoy's lesion is twice as common in men as in women and presents at a mean age of 52. The abnormality is the presence of an artery of extramural caliber in the submucosa and, in some instances, the mucosa, typically with a small overlying mucosal defect. It is believed that focal pressure from this large "caliber-persistent" vessel erodes the overlying mucosa, destroying the exposed vascular wall and resulting in hemorrhage. There is sudden onset of massive hematemesis or melena, usually followed by intermittent bleeding over several days. The bleeding site is usually 6 cm distal to the cardioesophageal junction, where the arteries are largest. The mortality rate for elderly patients with this lesion has been high. However, with present angiographic and endoscopic techniques to localize and treat bleeding lesions, thus decreasing the need for emergent surgery, prognosis for this lesion is likely to improve.

HEMANGIOMAS. These occur throughout the gastrointestinal tract and are the second most common vascular lesions of the colon. Hemangiomas may be of cavernous, capillary, or mixed types. Most are small and appear as polypoid, reddish purple mounds, ranging from a few millimeters to 2 cm; larger lesions occur, especially in the rectum, where they may be associated with phleboliths. Bleeding from hemangiomas is usually slow, producing occult blood loss with anemia or melena. Hematochezia is less common, except in large cavernous hemangiomas of the rectum. Diagnosis is best established by endoscopy, including enteroscopy, because roentgenologic studies, including angiography, are frequently normal. Small hemangiomas that are solitary or few and can be approached endoscopically are locally ablated. Large or multiple lesions usually require resection of either the hemangioma alone or the involved segment of colon.

BLUE RUBBER BLEB NEVUS SYNDROME. This term describes a particular type of cutaneous vascular nevus associated with intestinal lesions and gastrointestinal bleeding. A familial history is infrequent, although a few cases of autosomal dominant transmission have been reported. The lesions are distinctive: blue and raised, varying from 0.1 to 5.0 cm, and leaving a characteristic wrinkled sac when the contained blood is emptied by direct pressure. Lesions may be single or innumerable and are usually found on the trunk, extremities, and face but not on mucous membranes; they are most common in the small intestine. They are infrequently detected by barium or angiographic studies and are seen best by endoscopy. These lesions are cavernous hemangiomas composed of clusters of dilated capillary spaces lined by cuboidal or flattened endothelium with connective tissue stroma. Resection of the involved segment of bowel is recommended for recurrent hemorrhage. Endoscopic laser coagulation may be dangerous because these lesions may involve the full thickness of the bowel wall.

CONGENITAL ARTERIOVENOUS MALFORMATIONS. These developmental anomalies are found mainly in the extremities but potentially are located anywhere in the vascular tree. They may be small and resemble ectasias or large and involve a long segment of bowel. Arteriovenous malformations are persistent communications between arteries and veins located primarily in the submucosa. Characteristically, there is "arterialization" of the veins (i.e., tortuosity, dilatation, and thick walls with smooth muscle hypertrophy) and intimal thickening or sclerosis. Angiography is the primary means of diagnosis. Patients with significant bleeding should have resection of the involved segment.

KLIPPEL-TRENAUNAY-WEBER SYNDROME. This syndrome consists of a vascular nevus involving the lower limb, varicose veins limited to the affected side and appearing at birth or in childhood, and hypertrophy of all tissues of the involved limb (especially the bones), probably due to local venous hypertension and stasis. Edema of the involved leg is common; and if the thigh is involved, a variety of lymphatic abnormalities may be present (e.g., chylous mesenteric cysts, chyloperitoneum, and protein-losing enteropathy). Symptomatic gastrointestinal or genitourinary involvement is rare and manifests as hemorrhage. Bleeding may be mild or severe, and it may be recurrent. It is usually due to a rectal or vaginal hemangioma, localized rectovaginal varices due to an obstructed internal iliac system, or portal hypertension with varices. Physical examination is diagnostic, and a variety of imaging techniques are used to define the anatomy and to plan surgical repair. Plain films showing calcified pelvic phleboliths in a child suggest pelvic hemangiomatosis.

Schwartz LB, Gewertz BL: Mesenteric ischemia. Surg Clin North Am 77:2, 1997. *An entire volume devoted to gastrointestinal ischemia, including pathophysiology, pathology, radiographic diagnosis, clinical presentations, and therapies.*

138 NEOPLASMS OF THE STOMACH

Anil K. Rustgi

Gastric neoplasms are predominantly malignant, and nearly 90 to 95% of cases are adenocarcinomas. Less frequently observed malignancies include lymphomas, especially non-Hodgkin's lymphoma, as well as sarcomas, such as leiomyosarcoma. Benign gastric neoplasms include leiomyomas, carcinoid tumors, and lipomas.

ADENOCARCINOMA OF THE STOMACH

Epidemiology

There is great geographic variation in the incidence of gastric cancer worldwide, strongly indicating that environmental factors influence the pathogenesis of gastric carcinogenesis. Further support for this notion comes from observations that groups emigrating from high-risk to low-risk areas, e.g., Japanese moving to Hawaii and Brazil, acquire the low-risk of the area into which they emigrate, presumably because of adoption of the endogenous lifestyle and exposure to different environmental factors.

Gastric adenocarcinoma was the most frequently observed malignancy in the world until the mid-1980s, and it remains extremely common among males in certain regions, such as tropical South America, some parts of the Caribbean, and Eastern Europe. Regardless of gender, it remains the most common malignancy in Japan and China. It was the first-ranked malignancy in the United States in the 1930s to 1940s, but it has rapidly declined in recent decades, approaching an incidence rate of less than 10 cases per 100,000. While gastric adenocarcinoma localized to the distal stomach has declined, the incidence rate of proximal gastric and gastroesophageal adenocarcinomas has been steadily increasing in the United States, perhaps reflecting differences in pathogenic factors.

Etiology

Risk factors for the development of gastric adenocarcinoma can be divided into environmental and genetic factors as well as precursor conditions (Table 138–1). For example, *Helicobacter pylori* infection is significantly more common in patients with gastric cancer than in matched control groups. Epidemiologic studies of high-risk populations have also suggested that genotoxic agents such as *N*-nitroso compounds may play a role in gastric tumorigenesis. *N*-nitroso compounds can be formed in the human stomach by nitrosation of ingested nitrates, which are common constituents of the diet. High nitrate concentrations in the soil and drinking water have been observed in areas with high death rates from gastric cancer. In one human model of gastric tumorigenesis, chronic

Table 138–1 ■ CONDITIONS PREDISPOSING TO OR ASSOCIATED WITH GASTRIC CANCER

Environmental
  Helicobacter pylori infection
  Dietary: excess of salt (salted pickled foods), nitrates/nitrites, carbohydrates; deficiency of fresh fruit, vegetables, vitamins A and C, refrigeration
  Low socioeconomic status
  Cigarette smoking
Genetic
  Familial gastric cancer (rare)
  Associated with hereditary non-polyposis colorectal cancer
  Blood group A
Predisposing conditions
  Chronic gastritis, especially atrophic gastritis with or without intestinal metaplasia
  Pernicious anemia
  Intestinal metaplasia
  Gastric adenomatous polyps (>2 cm)
  Post-gastrectomy stumps
  Gastric epithelial dysplasia
  Ménétrier's disease (hypertrophic gastropathy)
  Chronic peptic ulcer

atrophic gastritis, occurring naturally or due to predisposing factors such as pernicious anemia or *H. pylori,* leads to achlorhydria, which in turn favors the growth of bacteria capable of converting nitrates to nitrites. The nitrosamine MNNG (*N*-methyl-*N'*-nitro-*N*-nitrosoguanidine) causes a high rate of induction of adenocarcinoma in the glandular stomach of rats.

Genetic

Recent advances in molecular genetics have uncovered a large number of structurally altered genes in clonal human tumors that are presumed to play important roles in carcinogenesis. It has been very difficult from the study of human gastric tumors alone to determine the true order of events and, in particular, to demonstrate a causal function for each genetic alteration at a specific stage of tumor development. Nonetheless, it is clear that genetic factors do play a role. For example, blood group A is associated with a higher incidence rate of gastric cancer, even in nonendemic areas. There is a threefold increase in gastric cancer among first-degree relatives of gastric cancer patients. Furthermore, germline or inherited mutations in the E-cadherin gene have been described in familial gastric cancer. In addition, in hereditary nonpolyposis colorectal cancer (HNPCC) type II, there are associated extracolonic cancers, including gastric cancer.

Predisposing Conditions

Atrophic gastritis with or without intestinal metaplasia is seen in association with gastric cancer (see Table 138–1), especially in endemic areas. Pernicious anemia is associated with a several-fold increase in gastric cancer. Atrophic gastritis and gastric cancer share a number of common environmental risk factors. It is likely that atrophic gastritis and intestinal metaplasia represent intermediary steps to gastric cancer. At the same time, most patients with atrophic gastritis do not develop gastric cancer, suggesting that neither atrophic gastritis nor achlorhydria alone is responsible.

Benign gastric ulcers do not appear to predispose patients to gastric cancer. However, patients who have a gastric remnant after subtotal gastrectomy for benign disorders have a 1.5 to 3.0 relative risk of gastric cancer by 15 to 20 years after surgery.

Incidence and Prevalence

Whereas gastric cancer was the most common cancer in the United States in the 1930s, its annual incidence rate has steadily decreased; the annual incidence is now fewer than 20,000 new cases per year. The age-adjusted mortality rate for males and females decreased by 25% from 1973 to 1985. Typically, gastric cancer occurs between ages 50 to 70 years and is uncommon before age 30 years. The rates are higher in males than females by 2 to 1. Five-year survival is less than 20%.

Pathology and Pathogenesis

Gastric adenocarcinomas can be divided into two types: intestinal and diffuse. The intestinal type is typically in the distal stomach with ulcerations, is often preceded by premalignant lesions, and is declining in incidence in the United States. In contrast, the diffuse type involves widespread thickening of the stomach, especially in the cardia, and often affects younger patients; this form may present as "linitis plastica," a nondistensible stomach with absence of folds and narrowed lumen due to infiltration of the stomach wall with tumor. The prognosis is generally worse in the diffuse type. The classification of gastric cancer into these two types is helpful in considering the causes of gastric cancer.

Key histopathologic features of gastric cancer include degree of differentiation, invasion through the gastric wall, lymph node involvement, and presence or absence of signet-ring cells within the tumor itself. Other pathologic manifestations include a polypoid mass, which may be difficult to distinguish from a benign polyp. Early gastric cancer, a condition that is not uncommon in Japan and that has a relatively favorable prognosis, consists of superficial lesions with or without lymph node involvement.

A number of potential mechanisms have been postulated to explain how *H. pylori* predisposes to gastric cancer. The leading hypothesis is that the increased cancer risk is due to the induction of an inflammatory response, which itself is genotoxic. Chronic inflammatory states have been associated with a number of gastrointestinal malignancies, such as ulcerative colitis with colon cancer, Barrett's esophagus with adenocarcinoma, and chronic hepatitis/cirrhosis with liver cancer. It is also possible that chronic *H. pylori* infection leads to chronic atrophic gastritis with resulting achlorhydria, which in turn favors bacterial growth that can convert nitrates (dietary components) to nitrites. These nitrites, in combination with genetic factors, promote abnormal cellular proliferation, genetic mutations, and eventually cancer.

It now appears several genetic mechanisms are important in gastric cancer: oncogene activation, tumor suppressor gene inactivation, and DNA microsatellite instability. For example, loss of heterozygosity of the *APC* (adenomatous polyposis coli) gene has been observed in gastric cancers. The *p53* tumor suppressor gene product regulates the cell cycle at the G1/S phase transition and likely also functions in DNA repair and apoptosis (programmed cell death). The *p53* gene is mutated not only in gastric cancer but also in gastric precancerous lesions, suggesting that mutation of the *p53* gene is an early event in gastric carcinogenesis. Microsatellite DNA alterations or instability in dinucleotide repeats that were originally identified in HNPCC also occur frequently in sporadic gastric carcinoma. Mutations in oncogenes and tumor suppressor genes may accumulate as a result of DNA microsatellite instability.

Clinical Manifestations (Table 138–2)

In its early stages, gastric carcinoma may often be asymptomatic or have only nonspecific symptoms, thereby making early diagnosis difficult. Later symptoms include bloating, dysphagia, epigastric pain, or early satiety. Early satiety or vomiting may suggest partial gastric outlet obstruction, although gastric dysmotility may contribute to the vomiting in nonobstructive cases. Epigastric pain, reminiscent of peptic ulcer, occurs in about one fourth of patients; but in the majority of patients with gastric cancer, the pain is not relieved by food or antacids. Pain that radiates to the back may indicate that the tumor has penetrated into the pancreas. When dysphagia is associated with gastric cancer, this symptom suggests a more proximal gastric tumor at the gastroesophageal junction or in the fundus.

Signs of gastric cancer include bleeding, which can result in anemia that produces the symptoms of weakness, fatigue, and malaise as well as more serious cardiovascular and cerebral consequences. Perforation due to gastric cancer is unusual. Metastatic gastric cancer to the liver can lead to right upper quadrant pain, jaundice, and/or fever. Lung metastases can cause cough, hiccups, and hemoptysis. Peritoneal carcinomatosis can lead to malignant ascites unresponsive to diuretics.

In the earliest stages of gastric cancer, the physical examination may be unremarkable. At later stages, patients become cachectic, and an epigastric mass may be palpated. If the tumor has metastasized to the liver, then hepatomegaly with jaundice and ascites may

Table 138–2 ▪ TNM STAGING OF GASTRIC CANCER

TUMOR

T1: Tumor confined to the mucosa or submucosa
T2: Tumor extending into the muscularis propria
T3: Tumor extending through the serosa without involving contiguous structures
T4: Tumor extending through the serosa and involving contiguous structures

NODES

N0: No lymph node metastases
N1: Regional lymph node involvement within 3 cm of the tumor along the greater or lesser curvature
N2: Regional lymph node involvement more than 3 cm from the primary tumor
N3: Involvement of other intra-abdominal lymph nodes not removable at surgery

METASTASES

M0: No distant metastases
M1: Distant metastases

be present. Portal or splenic vein invasion can cause splenomegaly. Lymph node involvement in the left supraclavicular area is termed Virchow's node, and periumbilical nodal involvement is called Sister Mary Joseph's node. The fecal occult blood test may be positive.

Paraneoplastic syndromes may precede or occur concurrently with gastric cancer. Examples include Trousseau's syndrome (see Chapter 197), which is recurrent migratory superficial thrombophlebitis indicating a possible hypercoagulable state; acanthosis nigricans, which presents in flexor areas with skin lesions that are raised and hyperpigmented; neuromyopathy with involvement of the sensory and motor pathways; and central nervous system involvement with altered mental status and ataxia.

Laboratory studies may reveal iron deficiency anemia. Predisposing pernicious anemia can progress to megaloblastic anemia. Microangiopathic hemolytic anemia has been reported. Abnormalities in liver function tests generally indicate metastatic disease. Hypoalbuminemia is a marker of malnourishment. Protein-losing enteropathy is rare but can be seen in Ménétrier's disease (see Chapter 125), another predisposing condition. Serologic test results, such as those of carcinoembryonic antigen and CA 72.4, may be abnormal. Although these tests are not recommended for original diagnosis, they may be useful for monitoring disease after surgical resection.

Diagnosis

On upper gastrointestinal barium contrast studies, a benign gastric ulcer is suggested by a smooth, regular base. In contrast, a malignant ulcer is manifested by a surrounding mass, irregular folds, and an irregular base. The location of the ulcer does not necessarily help to predict benign versus malignant disease because there is about equal frequency of malignancy on the greater and lesser curvatures. It is important for the radiologist to assess for rigidity, poor distensibility, ragged contour, and lack of peristalsis that suggest an ulcer is malignant. Extensive infiltration of the stomach wall may result in linitis plastica. For modern diagnosis, an upper endoscopy with biopsy and cytology is mandatory whenever a gastric ulcer is found on the radiologic study, even if the ulcer has benign characteristics.

The diagnostic accuracy of upper endoscopy with biopsy and cytology is far greater than upper gastrointestinal series, approaching 95 to 99% for both types of gastric cancer. Cancers may present as small mucosal ulcerations, a polyp, or a mass (Color Plate 3C). Staging of gastric cancer, and at times diagnosis, has been greatly enhanced by the advent of endoscopic ultrasound. The extent of tumor, including wall invasion and local lymph node involvement, can be assessed by endoscopic ultrasonography (Fig. 138-1), which provides complementary information to computed tomographic (CT) scans. Endoscopic ultrasonography can help guide aspiration biopsies of lymph nodes to determine their malignant features, if any. CT scans of the chest and abdomen should be performed to document lymphadenopathy and extragastric organ (especially lung and liver) involvement. In some centers, staging of gastric cancer will entail bone scans because of the proclivity of gastric cancer to metastasize to bone.

Treatment

The only chance for cure of gastric cancer remains surgical resection, assuming no evidence of distant metastatic disease. Complete resection is possible in only 25 to 30% of cases, however. If the tumor is confined to the distal stomach, subtotal gastrectomy is performed with resection of lymph nodes in the porta hepatis and in the pancreatic head. In contrast, tumors of the proximal stomach merit total gastrectomy to obtain an adequate margin and to remove lymph nodes; distal pancreatectomy and splenectomy are usually also performed as part of this procedure, which carries with it higher mortality and morbidity rates. Limited gastric resection is necessary for patients with excessive bleeding or obstruction. If cancer recurs in the gastric remnant, then limited resection may again be necessary for palliation. Most recurrences in both types of gastric cancer are in the local or regional area of the original tumor.

Gastric cancer is one of the few gastrointestinal cancers that is somewhat responsive to chemotherapy. Single-agent treatment with

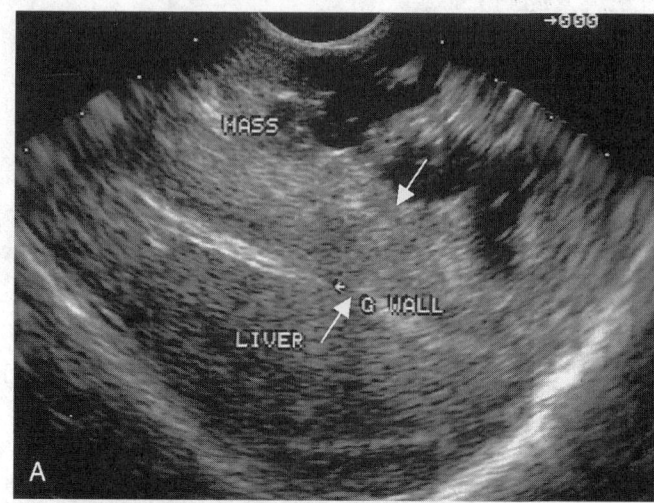

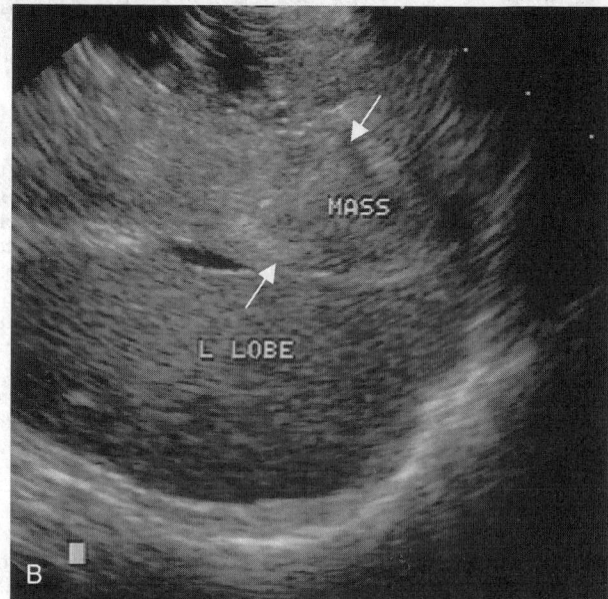

FIGURE 138–1 ■ Endoscopic ultrasound depicting a large gastric mass that is compressing the liver and gallbladder wall *(A)* and, on a different view, the left lobe of the liver *(B)*.

5-fluorouracil, doxorubicin, mitomycin-C, or cisplatin provides partial response rates of 20 to 30%. When used in combination, certain chemotherapeutic regimens, such as doxorubicin and mitomycin-C, doxorubicin and cisplatin, or doxorubicin and high-dose methotrexate, yield partial response rates of 35 to 50%. However, it is not clear if combination chemotherapy translates into prolonged survival. Postoperative adjuvant chemotherapy after curative intent does not currently offer any survival advantage. Radiation therapy is ineffective and generally employed only for palliative purposes in the setting of bleeding, obstruction, or pain. The combination of chemotherapy with radiation therapy or intraoperative radiation therapy has yet to be supported by prospective clinical trials. Gene therapy or immune-based therapy are currently only investigational in animal models.

Implicit in the management of the patient with gastric cancer is meticulous attention to nutrition (jejunal enteral feedings or total parenteral nutrition), correction of metabolic abnormalities that arise from vomiting or diarrhea, and treatment of infection from aspiration or spontaneous bacterial peritonitis. To maintain lumen patency, endoscopic laser treatment or prosthesis placement can be utilized in a palliative fashion.

Prognosis

Approximately one third of patients who undergo a curative resection are alive after 5 years. In the aggregate, the overall 5-year survival rate of gastric cancer is less than 10%. Prognostic factors include anatomic location and nodal status (see Table 138–2); distal gastric cancers without lymph node involvement carry a better prognosis compared with proximal gastric cancers with or without lymph node involvement. Other prognostic factors include depth of penetration and tumor cell DNA aneuploidy. Linitis plastica and infiltrating lesions carry a much worse prognosis than polypoid disease or exophytic masses. In the subset of mostly Japanese patients with the entity of early gastric cancer that is confined to the mucosa and submucosa, surgical resection may be curative and definitely improves the 5-year survival rate to more than 50%. In fact, when early gastric cancer is confined only to the mucosa, studies are investigating the adequacy of endoscopic resection.

LYMPHOMA OF THE STOMACH

Gastric lymphoma represents about 5% of all malignant gastric tumors and is increasing in incidence. The majority of gastric lymphomas are non-Hodgkin's lymphomas, and the stomach is the most common extranodal site for non-Hodgkin's lymphomas. Patients with gastric lymphoma are generally younger than those with gastric adenocarcinoma but retain the male predominance. Patients commonly present with symptoms and signs similar to those of gastric adenocarcinoma. Lymphoma in the stomach can be a primary tumor or can be due to disseminated lymphoma.

B-cell lymphomas of the stomach are most commonly large cell with a high-grade type. Low-grade variants are noted in the setting of chronic gastritis and are termed mucosa-associated lymphoid tissue (MALT). MALT lesions are strongly associated with *H. pylori* infection.

Radiographically, gastric lymphoma usually presents as ulcers or as exophytic masses; a diffusely infiltrating lymphoma is more suggestive of secondary lymphoma. Thus, upper gastrointestinal barium studies usually show multiple nodules and ulcers for a primary gastric lymphoma and typically have the appearance of linitis plastica with secondary lymphoma. As with gastric adenocarcinoma, however, upper endoscopy with biopsy and cytology are required for diagnosis and have an accuracy of nearly 90%. Apart from conventional histopathologic analysis, immunoperoxidase staining for lymphocyte markers is helpful in diagnosis. As for gastric adenocarcinoma, proper staging of gastric lymphoma involves endoscopic ultrasonography, chest and abdominal CT scans, and bone marrow biopsy as needed.

Treatment of large cell gastric lymphoma is best pursued with subtotal gastrectomy followed by combination chemotherapy (see Chapter 179), especially where there is lymph node involvement. In this context, 5-year survival rates of 40 to 60% have been reported. Trials of chemotherapy alone or radiation therapy alone are in progress. Prognosis is better if the lymphoma contains small lesions limited to the stomach, is well-differentiated, does not have lymph node involvement, and is associated with only superficial penetration of the gastric wall. In contrast, HIV-associated gastric lymphoma and disseminated gastric lymphoma carry a poor prognosis. For MALT lesions, early data suggest that eradication of *H. pylori* infection with antibiotics induces regression of the tumor, but longer-term follow-up will be needed to be confident that such therapy is sufficient. The efficacy of combined chemotherapy and radiation therapy is not yet established for MALT lesions.

OTHER MALIGNANT TUMORS OF THE STOMACH

Leiomyosarcomas, which constitute about 1% of all gastric cancers, usually present as an intramural mass with central ulceration. Symptoms may include bleeding accompanied by a palpable mass. Leiomyosarcomas are often relatively indolent; surgical resection yields a 5-year survival rate of about 50%. Metastasis can occur to lymph nodes and the liver. Other gastric sarcomas include liposarcomas, fibrosarcomas, myosarcomas, and neurogenic sarcomas. Recently, some gastrointestinal stromal tumors have been associated with activating mutations in the *c-kit* gene. Carcinoid tumors may begin in the stomach and are curable by removal if they have not yet spread to the liver.

Primary tumors can also spread to the stomach. In addition to lymphomas, other tumors found in the stomach include primary lung and breast cancers as well as malignant melanoma.

LEIOMYOMAS AND BENIGN TUMORS

Leiomyomas, which are smooth-muscle tumors of benign origin, occur with equal frequency among men and women and are typically located in the middle and distal stomach. Leiomyomas can grow into the lumen with secondary ulceration and resulting bleeding. Alternatively, they can expand to the serosa with extrinsic compression. On upper gastrointestinal series, leiomyomas are usually smooth with an intramural filling defect, with or without central ulceration. Endoscopy may reveal a mass that has overlying mucosa or mucosa replaced by ulceration. However, benign leiomyomas can be difficult to distinguish from their malignant counterparts radiographically or endoscopically; tissue diagnosis is imperative. Symptomatic leiomyomas should be removed, but those without associated symptoms do not require therapy.

Other benign gastric tumors include lipoma, neurofibroma, lymphangioma, ganglioneuroma, and hamartoma, the latter associated with Peutz-Jeghers syndrome or juvenile polyposis (restricted to the stomach).

ADENOMAS

Gastric adenomas and hyperplastic polyps are unusual but may be found in middle-aged and elderly patients. Polyps may be sessile or pedunculated and are also found in nearly 50% of patients with familial adenomatosis polyposis or Gardner's syndrome. Gastric adenocarcinoma arising in the antrum has been described in such patients. Although isolated gastric adenomatous polyps are generally asymptomatic, some patients may have dyspepsia, nausea, or bleeding. Gastric adenomas and hyperplastic polyps are smooth and regular on upper gastrointestinal series, but the diagnosis must be confirmed by upper endoscopy with biopsy. Pedunculated polyps that are >2 cm or that have associated symptoms should be removed by endoscopic snare cautery polypectomy, whereas large sessile gastric adenomatous polyps may merit segmental surgical resection. If polyps progress to an intermediary stage of severe dysplasia or culminate in cancer, the treatment is the same as for gastric adenocarcinoma.

Agboola O: Adjuvant treatment in gastric cancer. Cancer Treat Rev 20:217, 1994. *This article provides an overview on different therapeutic modalities for gastric cancer.*

Fuchs C, Mayer R: Gastric carcinoma. N Engl J Med 333:32, 1995. *An excellent comprehensive overview of gastric cancer.*

Muir CS, Harvey JC: Cancer of the stomach. GI Cancer 1:213, 1996. *This review concentrates on epidemiologic features of gastric cancer.*

Rustgi AK: GI cancers: Biology, diagnosis, and therapy. Philadelphia, Lippincott-Raven, 1995. *The section on gastric cancer encompasses individual chapters on clinical manifestations, pathology, biology, surgery, and chemotherapy/radiation therapy.*

139 NEOPLASMS OF THE LARGE AND SMALL INTESTINES

Bernard Levin

NEOPLASMS OF THE LARGE INTESTINE

Cancer of the large bowel (colon and rectum) is the most common malignancy of the gastrointestinal tract, and together with breast and lung cancer it is one of the three most frequent malignancies in the United States. With more than 570,000 new cases each year, it is also a worldwide health problem of great importance, particularly in Western countries. Approximately 131,000 cases of cancer of the colon and rectum were diagnosed in the United States in 1998; only half of patients survive 5 years or longer. During the period 1973 to 1989, colorectal cancer mortality in the United States decreased by 20% in white women and by 8.5% in white men; in contrast, mortality increased in black men by 22.5% and by 2.6% in black women. The reasons for this disparity are not clear, although it may be attributable in part to late diagnosis and less access to appropriate medical care. Incidence trends also show substantial increases for black men and women but substantially lower incidence rates for white men and women. New insight into the genetics and molecular biology of this neoplasm has been gained since the late 1980s; advances have also been made in methods of prevention, diagnosis, and treatment.

The large bowel also may be involved by other malignant tumors. These include anal carcinoma (squamous or transitional cell types), lymphoma, leiomyosarcoma, malignant carcinoid tumor, and Kaposi's sarcoma. The large bowel may also be involved through direct invasion by malignancies from adjacent sites, such as prostate, ovary, uterus, and stomach. The most frequent tumors that occur in the large intestine are benign polyps. Except for lipomas of the ileocecal valve, other benign tumors are very unusual.

Polyps of the Colon

A polyp is any lesion that arises from the surface of the gastrointestinal tract and protrudes into the lumen. Polyps in the large intestine, whether noted at sigmoidoscopy, colonoscopy, or during barium enema, may be single or multiple, pedunculated or sessile, and sporadic or part of an inherited syndrome. Polyps become clinically significant because of bleeding or because of their potential for malignant transformation.

PATHOLOGY. In addition to adenocarcinoma, which may present as a polypoid mass, three distinct types of benign polyps arise from colonic epithelium: hyperplastic (metaplastic), inflammatory, and neoplastic (adenomatous). Hyperplastic polyps, which tend to be small and asymptomatic, account for about one-fifth of all polyps in the colon and for most of the polyps in the rectum and distal sigmoid colon. They are not considered neoplastic. Inflammatory polyps occur in chronic ulcerative colitis and also are not neoplastic (see Chapter 135). Juvenile polyps, which are hamartomas of the lamina propria, may be single or multiple and occur most commonly in the rectum. They are susceptible to hemorrhage and autoamputation.

Adenomatous Polyps

PREVALENCE AND DISTRIBUTION. The incidence of colonic adenomas increases with age in countries with a high or intermediate risk for colorectal cancer, occurring in 30% to 40% of individuals older than 60 years in the United States. Adenomas are uncommon in areas where the incidence of cancer is low; for example, the prevalence of adenomas varies from almost zero among black South Africans to 10% in Japan and Colombia. The low incidence of cancer in some countries, such as Japan, is probably related to the small number of large adenomas as well as to the total number of adenomas. The presence of adenomas does not necessarily convey a high risk because the propensity for neoplastic transformation is related to size and histologic characteristics (dysplasia).

MACROSCOPIC AND MICROSCOPIC APPEARANCE. Adenomas may be separated into tubular, villous, and intermediate tubulovillous types. The typical tubular adenoma is small and spherical and has a stalk. Its surface is roughly separated into lobules by intercommunicating clefts. In contrast, the villous adenoma may be large and sessile with a velvety surface. Histologically the tubular adenoma consists of closely packed tubular glands that divide and branch. In the villous adenoma, finger-like projections of neoplastic epithelium project toward the bowel lumen. The tubulovillous lesions consist of a mixture of tubular and villous patterns. About 60% of adenomas are tubular, 20 to 30% are tubulovillous, and about 10% are villous. All adenomas are dysplastic, and dysplasia in adenomas may be graded into mild, moderate, and severe. This classification is based on the presence of cytologic (mainly nuclear) abnormalities and glandular architectural changes.

DEVELOPMENT. In the normal adult, the epithelial tissue of the colon actively renews itself with a turnover period of about 3 to 8 days. DNA synthesis occurs primarily in cells in the lower one-third of crypts. Normally cells replicate and migrate up the crypt, subsequently to be exfoliated from the mucosal surface. In adenomas, immature cells are found higher up the colonic crypt than normal and are associated with unrepressed DNA synthesis, which represents abnormal cell renewal along the surface of the crypt and

the entire length of the crypt. DNA-synthesizing cells can accumulate on the luminal surface, thus forming new adenomatous tissue.

RELATIONSHIP OF COLONIC ADENOMAS TO CANCER. Colonic adenomas appear to have malignant potential: (1) the epidemiology of adenomas and carcinoma is similar; (2) adenocarcinomas and adenomas occur in the same anatomic distribution in the colon; (3) residual adenomatous tissue is observed quite commonly in small cancers; (4) the incidence of cancer increases as the size of the adenoma increases; (5) the adenoma-to-cancer transition has been observed in familial polyposis, hereditary nonpolyposis colorectal carcinoma, and in experimental animals treated with a carcinogen; (6) the risk for colorectal cancer is higher in patients with a history of adenomas and is significantly lessened if the adenoma is removed; (7) a period of approximately 5 years elapses between the diagnosis of adenoma and the development of carcinoma.

Fewer than 5% of adenomas develop into carcinomas. Several important factors in this transformation can be identified, especially size, histologic type, and epithelial dysplasia. The frequency of cancer in adenomas under 1 cm is 1 to 3%; in those between 1 to 2 cm, 10%; and in those over 2 cm, more than 40%. The highest malignancy rate is associated with a villous growth pattern. Invasive neoplasm has been found in 40% of the villous tumors, in fewer than 5% of the tubular adenomas, and in 23% of the tubulovillous variety. The malignant potential of adenomas also increases with increasing degrees of dysplasia. Most adenomas smaller than 1 cm show only mild dysplasia and have a low malignant potential. With severe dysplasia, the rate of malignant transformation rises to 27%.

Cancer in adenomas is usually well differentiated and occurs most commonly in the tip of a pedunculated adenoma without invasion of the muscularis mucosae. These lesions are usually satisfactorily treated by polypectomy. Occasionally cancers in adenomas invade the muscularis mucosae, grow down the stalk, invade lymphatic vessels and adjacent lymph nodes, and metastasize. The roles of autocrine factors, tumor suppressor genes, and oncogenes in the development of adenomas and their malignant transformation are currently under study.

CLINICAL MANIFESTATIONS. Most adenomatous polyps are asymptomatic, but they may cause hematochezia. Some adenomatous polyps are diagnosed after the detection of occult blood loss in asymptomatic individuals who are screened for colon cancer. Adenomas may also be detected by fiberoptic sigmoidoscopy or colonoscopy or by double-contrast barium enema examination.

MANAGEMENT AND FOLLOW-UP. Because of the association of adenomas with the development of adenocarcinomas, colonic polyps should usually be removed or destroyed. In individual clinical circumstances (e.g., age of patient, location of lesion) this rule may rarely have to be modified. Pedunculated polyps, even if large, can be removed by electrocautery snare, whereas small sessile polyps (1 to 8 mm) should be biopsied and destroyed with the "hot biopsy" forceps. For sessile polyps with a wide-based attachment to the colonic wall, several electrocautery sessions may be required for complete excision. Endoscopic removal may not be safe or possible if a lesion is in a relatively inaccessible location. The endoscopic appearances that suggest carcinomatous invasion include ulceration, an irregular surface contour, firm consistency, and friability. If a diagnosis of malignancy is made after polypectomy, a decision has to be made about the adequacy of the polypectomy. In the presence of poorly differentiated histologic features, penetration of the muscularis mucosa, vascular or lymphatic invasion, or a resection margin containing cancer, the risk of regional lymph node involvement is approximately 5%. The mortality from surgical resection is less than 2% in patients aged 50 to 69 years and 4.4% for those older than 70 years, so any decision to recommend surgical resection must take into account individual operative risk.

FOLLOW-UP AFTER COLONOSCOPIC POLYPECTOMY. Ideally, all adenomas should be removed from the colon at the time of the initial colonoscopy. A follow-up colonoscopy is appropriate at 3 years to evaluate for the presence of any lesions missed at the previous procedure or to discover new lesions. If the colon is free of polyps at this examination, an interval of 3 years is appropriate before the next colonoscopy. Chemopreventive strategies aimed at preventing adenoma recurrence are being studied, including diet, nonsteroidal anti-inflammatory drugs (NSAIDs), supplemental calcium, folic acid, and ursodeoxycholic acid.

Inherited Polyposis Syndromes

Recent advances in genetics and molecular biology have accentuated our interest in the inherited risk of colorectal cancer. The polyposis syndromes account for approximately 1% of colorectal cancer, whereas the nonpolyposis inherited conditions may be responsible for up to 6%.

ADENOMATOUS POLYPOSIS SYNDROMES. The adenomatous polyposis syndromes include familial adenomatous polyposis and Gardner's syndrome; in both hereditary disorders, hundreds to thousands of colonic adenomas are present (Color Plate 3A). The adenomas begin to appear early in the second decade of life. Gastrointestinal symptoms occur in the third or fourth decade. Almost all patients with familial polyposis develop carcinoma of the colon by age 40 years if the colon has not been removed. Some cases occur without a family history and may represent spontaneous mutations.

Gardner's syndrome differs from familial adenomatous polyposis in that affected individuals exhibit benign extraintestinal growth, including osteomas (especially mandibular) and soft tissue tumors (lipomas, sebaceous cysts, fibrosarcomas). Other associated features include supernumerary teeth, desmoid tumors, and mesenteric fibromatosis (Figs. 139–1 and 139–2). The colonic adenomas are similar to those of familial adenomatous polyposis and have the same potential for malignancy.

In both familial adenomatous polyposis and Gardner's syndrome, upper gastrointestinal polyps are commonly found. Multiple gastric "fundic gland polyps" are found in 50 to 100% of affected individuals. Adenomatous duodenal polyps are present in up to 80% of individuals with familial adenomatous polyposis or Gardner's syndrome, and periampullary cancer develops in approximately 10%. Adenomas occur in the small bowel distal to the duodenum but rarely undergo malignant transformation.

Familial adenomatous polyposis and Gardner syndrome are inherited as autosomal dominant disorders with incomplete penetrance. The mutant gene for both conditions is on the long arm of chromosome 5. Different mutations at that locus may account for the phenotypic differences between the syndromes. The APC (adenomatous polyposis coli) gene mutations lead to the formation of a truncated protein. Gene abnormalities can be detected by a blood test in 87% of affected individuals, thereby enabling screening within affected families to be much more accurate. Genetic counseling should always precede and accompany genetic testing.

SCREENING RECOMMENDATIONS. Flexible proctosigmoidoscopy should be performed annually in all first-degree relatives, from age 12 years until age 40 years, and every 3 years thereafter. Screening is appropriate for those with the mutant gene. Because gene markers are not yet 100% specific and sensitive, screening is also indicated for those without the mutant gene, although considerably less often. Surveillance with a side-viewing endoscope for gastric and duodenal polyps should begin when the diagnosis of colonic polyposis is made and should continue every 2 to 3 years thereafter, and possibly yearly if prominent lesions are apparent in the duodenum.

MANAGEMENT. Surgery is the primary management option in FAP. Total proctocolectomy with conventional ileostomy or ileal pouch–anal anastomosis is more often used as opposed to the older procedure of subtotal colectomy with ileo-rectal anastomosis. Pharmacologic interventions such as the use of cyclooxygenase-2 inhibitors are under study.

Hereditary Nonpolyposis Colorectal Cancer

Hereditary nonpolyposis colorectal cancer (HNPCC) is caused by germline mutations in DNA nucleotide mismatch repair genes (hMLH, hMSH2, PMS, PMS2, and GTBP) located on chromosome 2, 3, or 7, and is inherited in a highly penetrant autosomal dominant fashion. HNPCC has been classically defined as colorectal cancer in three or more family members, two of whom are first-degree relatives of the third, and involving people in at least two generations, with at least one person diagnosed with colorectal cancer before age 50 years. This definition may be too restrictive, and other variants of this classic pedigree exist.

Several adenomas may be present despite the name of the syndrome, but diffuse adenomatosis is not found. The average age at diagnosis of cancer is the mid-40s, and it is characteristic to find multiple synchronous cancers with a majority of lesions proximal to the splenic flexure. Individuals with genetic mutations that can lead to HNPCC are also at high risk for cancers of the ovary, uterus, ureter, pancreas, and stomach. Genetic tests are now available to detect the major mutations that lead to HNPCC, and these should be considered after appropriate counseling for individuals with a suggestive family history. Individuals in families with HNPCC who have a positive genetic test or in whom genetic testing has not been performed, should undergo colonoscopy every

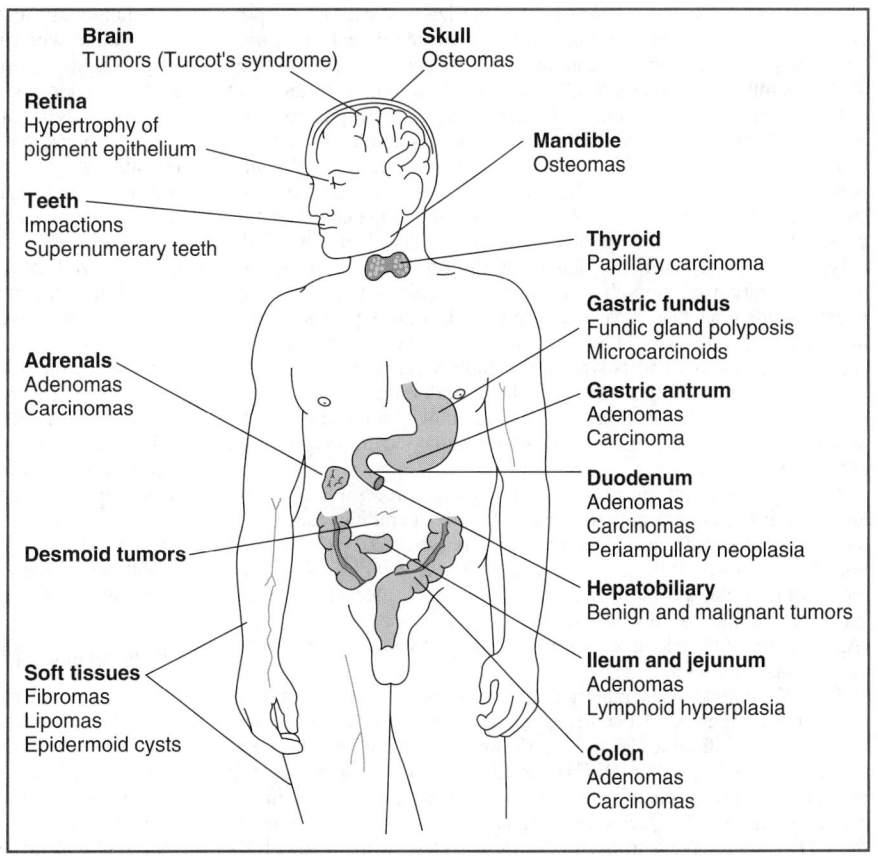

FIGURE 139–1 ■ Schematic representation of the intestinal and extraintestinal manifestations of familial adenomatous polyposis (FAP) and Gardner's syndrome. The primary features of Gardner's syndrome consist of a triad of colonic polyposis, bone tumors (particularly in the skull and mandible), and soft tissue tumors, but the phenotypic overlap between FAP and Gardner's syndrome is considerable. (From Itzkowitz SH, Kim YS: *In* Feldman M, Scharschmidt BF, Sleisinger MH [eds]: Sleisinger and Fordtran's Gastrointestinal and Liver Disease, 6th ed. Philadelphia, WB Saunders, 1998, p 1844.)

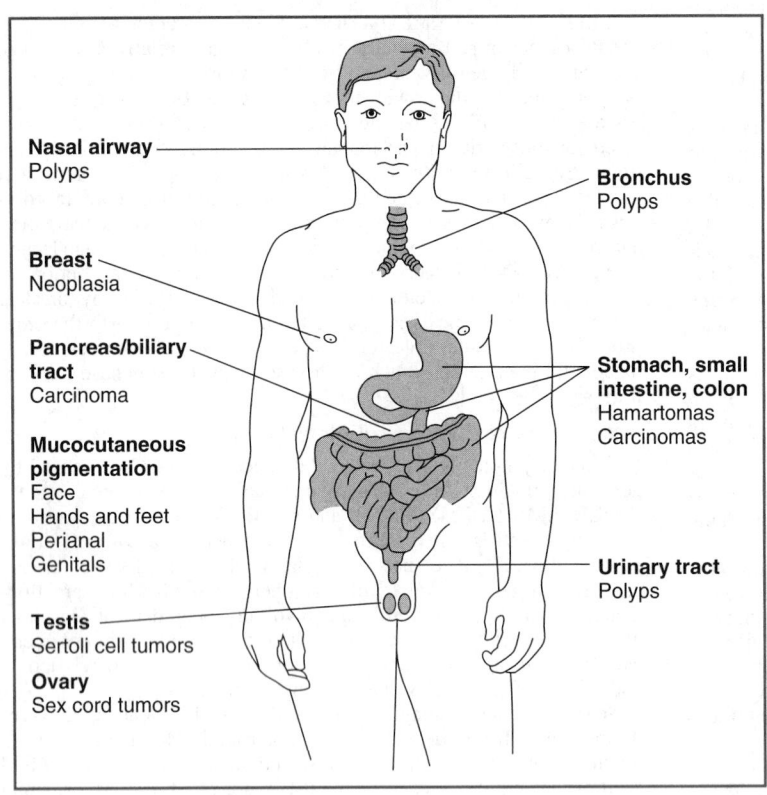

FIGURE 139–2 ■ Schematic representation of Peutz-Jeghers syndrome. Mucocutaneous pigmentation and benign gastrointestinal polyposis are the primary features of the syndrome. (From Itzkowitz SH, Kim YS: *In* Feldman M, Scharschmidt BF, Sleisenger MH [eds]: Sleisinger and Fordtran's Gastrointestinal and Liver Disease, 6th ed. Philadelphia, WB Saunders, 1998, p 1844.)

2 years from ages 21 to 40 years, then annually thereafter. In asymptomatic women from families with HNPCC who are found by gene testing to be HNPCC gene carriers or who have not undergone genetic testing, pelvic examinations should be performed every 1 to 3 years beginning at age 18 years; at age 25 years, women should have annual pelvic examination and transvaginal ultrasonography. Endometrial biopsy may also be necessary.

The *Peutz-Jeghers syndrome* is characterized by melanotic spots on the lips, buccal mucosa, and skin, and by multiple hamartomatous polyps throughout the gastrointestinal tract from the stomach to the rectum. It is inherited in an autosomal dominant fashion but it has a variable expressivity. Recently, the gene responsible has been localized to chromosome 19p, where mutations in a novel *serine-threonine* gene (*STKII*) are believed to be causative. Usually polyps are fewer in number than in familial adenomatous polyposis. Microscopically, these polyps consist of elongated branching glands lined by benign epithelium native to the location of the polyps. The most distinctive feature is the presence of an arborizing proliferation of smooth muscle in the lamina propria. Rarely, intestinal malignancies have been described, with a preponderance in the small intestine. Other manifestations include ovarian sex cord stromal tumors and polyps of the gallbladder, ureter, and nose. Intestinal symptoms of recurrent, colicky abdominal pain may appear in adolescence, and intussusception may require surgical removal of a polyp. Gastrointestinal bleeding may occur, causing iron deficiency anemia.

Turcot's syndrome, inherited as an autosomal recessive or dominant condition, is rare and is characterized by hereditary adenomatous polyposis with a low number of polyps (20 to 300) and tumors of the central nervous system. These neoplasms include medulloblastoma, glioblastoma, and ependymoma. Recent evidence implicates abnormalities of both the adenomatous polyposis coli (APC) gene and nucleotide mismatch repair genes in the pathogenesis of this condition.

Juvenile polyposis is inherited as an autosomal dominant trait, with an occasional case occurring spontaneously. A subset of juvenile polyposis families carry germ line mutations in the gene SMAD4 (also known as DPC4) located on chromosome 18q21.1; this gene normally encodes a critical cytoplasmic mediator in the transforming growth factor-beta signaling pathway. Mutations in the PTEN gene have also been described. PTEN, which codes for a protein tyrosine phosphatase, is a tumor suppressor gene on chromosome 10q23. The number of polyps is less than in familial adenomatous polyposis, averaging 25 to 40. Polyps may be found throughout the gastrointestinal tract or may be restricted to the colon. Symptoms may begin in childhood or adolescence with rectal bleeding, anemia, abdominal pain, or intussusception. A variety of extraintestinal symptoms including congenital abnormalities, and pulmonary arteriovenous malformations have been described in association with juvenile polyposis. The hamartomas of juvenile polyposis are morphologically distinct from those found in Peutz-Jeghers syndrome. Foci of adenomatous epithelium may be present in these polyps, or adenomas may coexist. The true risk of malignancy in these patients is unknown, but carcinoma of the gastrointestinal tract has developed in 10% of reported patients with juvenile polyposis. Subtotal colectomy may occasionally be warranted in those with severely dysplastic adenomas.

Cronkhite-Canada syndrome is a nonfamilial disorder of adults characterized by diffuse gastrointestinal polyposis, alopecia, dystrophy of the fingernails, and cutaneous hyperpigmentation. The polyps resemble juvenile polyps and are in greatest density in the stomach and colon. Watery diarrhea, anorexia, abdominal pain, cachexia, protein-losing enteropathy, and carcinoma of the gastrointestinal tract (in up to 14% of cases) have been reported.

Cowden's syndrome (multiple hamartoma syndrome) is transmitted in an autosomal dominant manner and is characterized by multiple facial tricholemmomas, oral papillomas, keratoses of the hands and feet, and a high rate of associated systemic malignancies, particularly of thyroid and breast. The polyps are not dysplastic, and the risk of gastrointestinal malignancy is not increased. Mutations in the PTEN gene have recently been identified in Cowden's syndrome.

Adenocarcinoma of the Large Bowel

Carcinoma of the colon and rectum varies widely in frequency in different parts of the world. Large bowel cancers occur commonly in North America, northwestern Europe, and New Zealand, whereas in South America, southwest Asia, equatorial Africa, and India, the risk is much less. The incidence varies from 3.5 per 100,000 in India to 32.3 per 100,000 in Connecticut. Colorectal cancers display regional differences within the United States, with the highest incidence in the Northeast. Rectal cancer is more common in men in most, but not all, areas of the world. In the United States, rectal cancer incidence has declined during the past 50 years. Overall mortality from colorectal cancer has also declined in the United States during the past 20 years.

Migrants from parts of the world with a low incidence to regions with a higher risk, such as the United States or Canada, show a rapid increase in incidence. This change is also exemplified by the higher incidence in Puerto Ricans who have migrated to the mainland compared with those in Puerto Rico and in first- and second-generation Chinese and Japanese immigrants to Hawaii and the mainland United States compared with Japanese in Japan and Chinese in the Peoples' Republic of China.

ETIOLOGY. Both inherited predisposition and environmental factors seem to be implicated in carcinogenesis in the colon and rectum, but in ways yet to be clearly delineated. Of the environmental factors, diet has been the most extensively studied. Both the amount and type of fat intake correlate with the risk for colorectal cancer in many, but not all, studies. Consumption of saturated fat (with a high content of animal fat) has been reported to be correlated positively with colon cancer incidence. Other studies suggest that diets containing predominantly monounsaturated fats as a lipid source may exert a protective effect against the development of colorectal cancer, but other components of the diet may also play a role. In countries with a high incidence of colon cancer, the average fat content in the diet is about 40% of total calories, in contrast to the dietary fat content of 15 to 20% or less of total calories in countries with a low cancer incidence. If fat in the colon does promote cancer, the effect might be related to increased biliary sterol excretion leading to increased colonic epithelial proliferation, to modification of cell membranes, or to stimulation of the synthesis of prostaglandins that induce cellular proliferation. The possible role of *dietary fiber* in reducing colonic carcinogenesis has been suggested but has not been firmly established. Fiber is not a single chemical substance. Certain components of fiber found in vegetables, cereals, and fruits may be helpful in reducing the risk of cancer by diluting and binding carcinogens in the lumen, by modifying colonic bacterial flora, and by acidifying the colonic lumen because fiber is metabolized to short-chain fatty acids. Naturally occurring anticarcinogens found in fruits and vegetables (indoles, thioethers, dithiothiones, carotenoids) are being investigated. Other factors that have been postulated to play a role in colonic carcinogenesis are excess caloric intake, low physical activity level, obesity, and inadequate intake of calcium and vitamin D. Aspirin and other NSAIDs that modulate the formation of prostaglandins appear to protect against the development of colorectal neoplasms.

AGE. The risk of colorectal cancer begins to increase at the age of 50 years and rises sharply at age 60 years. With each succeeding decade the risk doubles, reaching a peak by age 75 years.

ASSOCIATION WITH INFLAMMATORY BOWEL DISEASE (see Chapter 135). Among all patients diagnosed as having a large bowel adenocarcinoma, only about 1% give an antecedent history of inflammatory bowel disease. In chronic ulcerative colitis, carcinoma of the colon occurs more commonly (approximately 10 to 20 times) than in the general population. The duration of disease and the extent of colonic involvement correlate with the subsequent development of colon cancer. Approximately 2 to 4% of all patients with chronic ulcerative colitis develop colorectal carcinoma, with a cumulative incidence of about 12% after 25 years. Patients with ulcerative proctitis have no increase in risk, and the risk for patients with left-sided colitis may be delayed until approximately 10 years later. In ulcerative colitis, mucosal dysplasia, defined as an unequivocal neoplastic alteration of the colonic epithelium, is the recognized precursor for development of carcinoma. Dysplastic epithelium may overlie an area of malignancy associated with direct invasion into the submucosa. The dysplastic area may be flat or proliferative, and the likelihood of carcinoma increases significantly in the presence of a dysplasia-associated lesion or mass. Whether routine colonoscopic surveillance is useful in patients with long-standing inflammatory bowel disease is still under evaluation. Nevertheless, many authorities favor periodic colonoscopy with multiple biopsies to diagnose dysplasia in individuals with more than 8 years of symptoms and extensive colonic involvement. The availability of newer surgical procedures, such as ileoanal pouches, favors a trend toward earlier colectomy in high-risk individuals. The demonstration of low- or high-grade dysplasia or a dysplasia-

associated lesion or mass, even in the presence of low-grade dysplasia, warrants prophylactic colectomy because the risk of an associated carcinoma may be as high as 50 or 60%. Newer epithelial biomarkers, such as flow cytometry, and oncogene and tumor suppressor gene mutations and deletions, are being studied in an attempt to define the biology of neoplastic transformation and to identify individuals at high risk before cancer develops.

Patients with Crohn's colitis (see Chapter 135) are also at higher risk (approximately four to seven times that of the general population) for the development of colorectal cancer, but this risk is probably lower than in ulcerative colitis. Colonic surveillance has not been widely used, but guidelines similar to those for surveillance of patients with chronic ulcerative colitis are applicable to patients with extensive colonic involvement.

HEREDITY AND COLONIC CANCER. Inherited risk is an important consideration in formulating screening guidelines. The adenomatous polyposis syndromes and hereditary nonpolyposis colorectal cancer together account for approximately 7% of colon cancers. The remainder of colon cancers are referred to as "sporadic," but this term is a misnomer. Population studies have demonstrated a twofold or threefold increased risk of colon cancer in first-degree relatives of individuals with colon cancer. A similar risk is present in first-degree relatives of individuals with adenomatous polyps. In fact, as many as 50% or more of "sporadic" adenomas and cancers may exhibit a partially penetrant autosomal dominant inheritance.

MOLECULAR GENETICS OF COLORECTAL CANCER. The genetic events surrounding the development of colorectal cancer are now understood with ever increasing sophistication (Fig. 139–3). The gene for familial adenomatous polyposis has been mapped to chromosome 5. Deletions of DNA sequences at the same locus are also frequently observed in adenocarcinomas from "sporadic" cases and may be the earliest change in the neoplastic process. *K-ras* mutations follow the chromosome 5 changes and are observed more commonly in larger adenomas and cancers. Chromosome 17 (p53 gene) and chromosome 18 (DCC gene) deletions are often present and may be important in malignant transformation. Mutations of the nucleotide mismatch repair genes have been identified in both inherited and sporadic colorectal cancers. The total accumulation of genetic changes (allelic deletions, oncogene mutations) may be more important than a particular sequence of events in the development of invasive cancer.

PATHOLOGY. The vast majority of colorectal cancers are adenocarcinomas. The tumors exhibit varying degrees of glandular differentiation and produce variable amounts of mucin. Gross morphologic features may be divided into two major groups: polypoid and annular constricting lesions. The polypoid type is most commonly found on the right side, and the annular constricting lesion is more common on the left side of the colon. Adenocarcinomas of the rectum may be sessile or polypoid. Approximately 75% of colorectal cancers occur in the descending colon, rectosigmoid, and rectum. Approximately 50% are within the reach of the 60-cm fiberoptic sigmoidoscope. The cecum and ascending colon are involved in 15% and the transverse colon in 10% (Fig. 139–4). Carcinoma of the colon spreads by direct extension through the wall of the bowel into the pericolonic fat and mesentery, by invasion of surrounding organs, by way of the lymphatics to the regional lymph nodes, and via the portal vein to the liver. Additionally, the tumor may spread throughout the peritoneal cavity and through the blood stream to the lungs and bones. Rectal cancers may directly invade the perirectal fat, vagina, prostate, bladder, ureters, and bony pelvis and may metastasize to the lungs and liver.

CLINICAL MANIFESTATIONS. The major symptoms of colorectal cancer are *rectal bleeding, pain,* and *change in bowel habit.* The clinical presentation in an individual patient is related to the size and location of the tumor. Those on the right side are often asymptomatic, and bleeding may be occult. Tumors of the cecum and ascending colon rarely obstruct early. Changes in bowel habit, with reduction in stool caliber or progressive constipation, and hematochezia are more common with left-sided lesions. Adenocarcinomas of the colon may present with a localized perforation and with signs of peritonitis. An abdominal mass or symptoms and signs of liver metastasis may be the earliest clinical manifestations of an underlying colorectal cancer.

Rectal or anal cancers may present with rectal bleeding, perineal

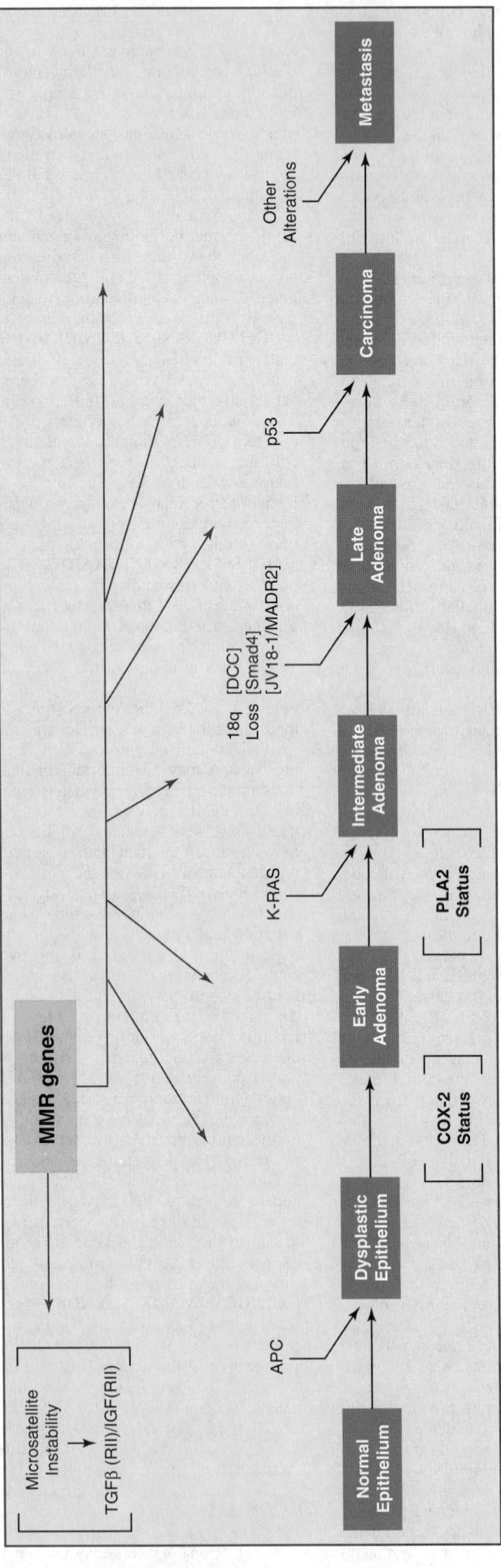

FIGURE 139–3 ■ Correlation between stages of progression of colorectal carcinoma and recognized mutational events affecting specific colon cancer-associated genes. MMR = mismatch repair genes; TGFIIR = tumor growth factor-β receptor II; IGF (RII) = insulin-like growth factor receptor II; APC = adenomatous polyposis coli tumor suppressor gene; DCC = deleted in colon cancer tumor suppressor gene; P53 = p53 tumor suppressor gene; ras = Ki-ras oncogene; COX-2 = cyclo-oxygenase 2; PLA2 = phospholipase A2; and SMAD = signaling components that control TGF-β mediated gene transcription. JV-18-1/MADR2 are tumor suppressor genes located on chromosome 18q (as are DCC and SMAD4). (Adapted from Powell SM: Genes driving the colonoscope. Energ. Technol Gastro Endosc 7:293–311, 1997.)

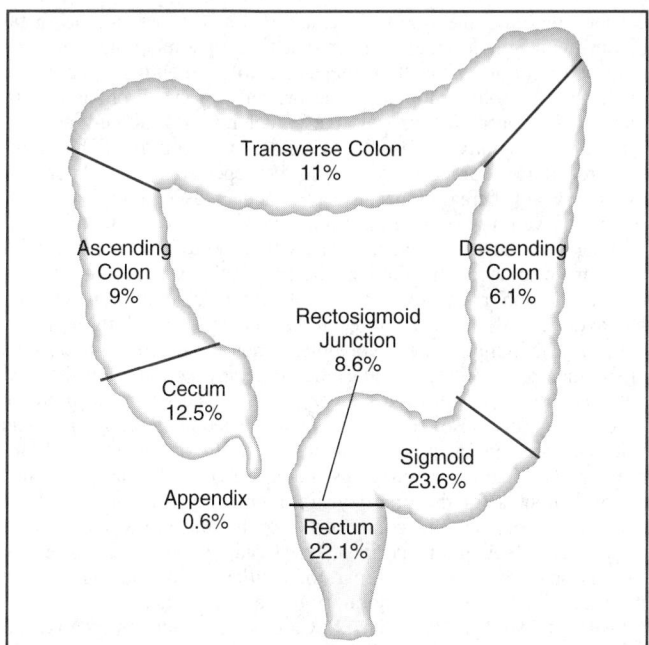

FIGURE 139–4 ▪ Distribution of large bowel cancer by anatomic segment according to the Third National Cancer Survey. (Data from Schottenfeld D, Fraumeni J Jr [eds]: Cancer Epidemiology and Prevention. Philadelphia, WB Saunders, 1982, p 703.)

pain, or change in bowel habit. Presenting symptoms may also include those referable to invasion of adjacent organs, including hematuria, renal insufficiency (obstructive uropathy), and vaginal fistulas.

Colorectal cancer must be suspected when patients present with rectal bleeding, a change in bowel habit, decrease in stool caliber, iron deficiency anemia, or unexplained abdominal pain. Rectal bleeding may be caused by other conditions, including hemorrhoids, angiodysplasia, diverticulosis, and other benign and malignant tumors (see Chapter 123). Beyond age 40 years, the frequency of neoplasia increases significantly. Unexplained iron deficiency in both older men and women always requires a thorough evaluation to exclude gastrointestinal cancer.

METASTATIC COLON CANCER. Metastases may be clinically apparent before or after resection of the primary colorectal cancer. Massive hepatomegaly may occur with pain due to distention of the liver capsule. Spread within the abdomen may cause small and large bowel obstruction and ascites. Pelvic spread may cause bladder dysfunction, sacral or sciatic nerve pain, and vaginal discharge or bleeding. Distant spread to lungs and bone may be silent until a very advanced stage is reached. Intestinal recurrences are uncommon and usually result from tumor implants, related to the original resection, growing from the serosa into the lumen.

DIAGNOSIS. A careful history, physical examination, and selected use of laboratory and radiologic tests facilitate the diagnosis of colorectal cancer. The history includes the patient's symptoms, prior removal of an adenoma or cancer, previous or present inflammatory bowel disease, or a family history of one of the inherited colorectal cancer syndromes. Special emphasis should be paid to first-degree relatives with a history of colorectal neoplasia. Physical examination may reveal evidence of Peutz-Jeghers or Gardner's syndrome and may provide substantiation of spread to lymph nodes, liver, or peritoneal cavity. A digital rectal examination is essential in determining the presence of a distal rectal cancer or of peritoneal or pelvic spread. A complete pelvic examination must be performed. Laboratory tests may reveal iron deficiency anemia or an abnormality of liver enzymes.

In evaluating patients with symptoms or signs of colorectal cancer, colonoscopy is now the generally preferred approach; the other option is flexible sigmoidoscopy followed by double-contrast barium enema (Fig. 139–5). In the patient with inflammatory bowel disease, a barium enema or even colonoscopy may be deferred briefly until acute inflammation has been controlled.

Colonoscopy is more sensitive than double-contrast barium en-

ema in detecting small adenomas and cancers (Color Plate 1*C*) and is also valuable for evaluating patients in whom an abnormality has been detected by barium enema. In addition, the presence or absence of synchronous cancers and adenomas can be determined. Colonoscopy can be used to remove adenomas (Color Plate 2*C*), to perform biopsy of suspected cancers, and to obtain brush biopsies of suspected malignancies and colonic strictures for cytologic examination.

Endoscopic ultrasonography is being used with increasing frequency to help in the staging of rectal cancers. Depth of invasion can often be accurately determined. Computed tomographic (CT) scanning of the abdomen and pelvis can help define the extent of tumor involvement and may be the initial mode of diagnosis in patients with abdominal pain or symptoms that could be caused by other conditions, such as diverticulitis. A chest radiograph will help evaluate the possibility of lung metastases; CT scanning can detect possible liver metastasis, especially in patients with abnormal liver enzyme levels.

MANAGEMENT. The modern approach to management is multidisciplinary and includes not only consideration of the immediate clinical problem but also a long-term approach to the patient, including preoperative and postoperative adjuvant treatment, future plans for assessment of local recurrence or distant metastasis, and attention to family members at increased risk.

SURGERY. The most important goal of treatment for primary malignancies of the colon and rectum is complete removal. Surgical resection of the affected segment, including omentum and lymph nodes, is performed. Laparoscopic resection is being used, although long-term follow-up data regarding its effectiveness are still being collected. Cancers of the right and left portions of the colon are treated by hemicolectomy; cancers of the sigmoid and upper rectum (above 6 cm from the anal verge) are resected anteriorly with removal of a margin of normal colon above and below the tumor. Stapling techniques have facilitated anastomoses within the pelvis. Although 3-cm proximal and distal margins have been previously emphasized, an adequate radial margin is equally important.

Lesions within 5 cm of the anal verge are usually treated by a combined abdominoperineal resection and permanent colostomy. Newer approaches for small, early rectal cancers include sphincter-saving procedures using local excision followed, in some instances,

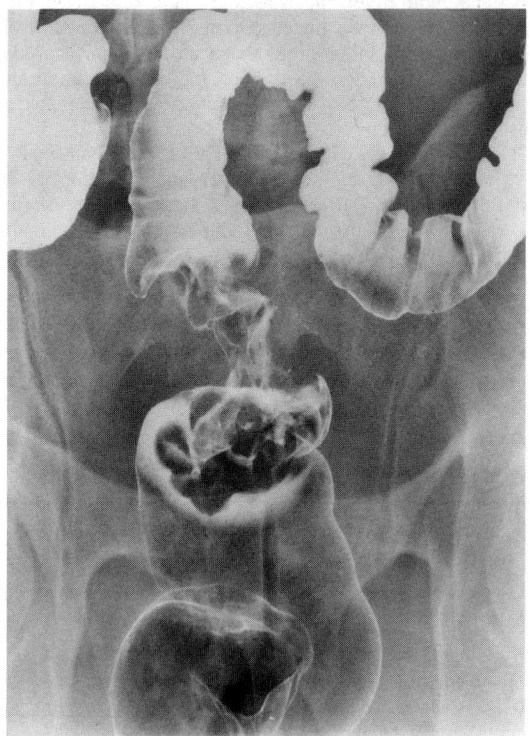

FIGURE 139–5 ▪ Annular constructing lesion of the rectosigmoid ("applecore") visualized on barium enema. (Adapted from DuBrow RA: Diagnostic Imaging. U.T. M.D. Anderson Cancer Center, Houston, 1998.)

by chemotherapy and radiation therapy to the pelvis. Preoperatively, combined radiation therapy and chemotherapy may facilitate resection, including sphincter-saving procedures.

For anal cancers the standard approach is to use a combination of radiation and chemotherapy, which usually shrinks or obliterates the cancer. HIV-infected patients or those with AIDS may be more susceptible to treatment-related toxicity. Surgical resection is now usually reserved for lesions that do not respond to chemoradiation and for those that recur.

Surgery may be required for palliation as well as for cure. Colonic obstruction may necessitate a palliative colostomy, although a primary resection and colostomy can often be accomplished at the same operation. A perforated carcinoma is usually managed by primary resection and colostomy with later closure of the colostomy. For selected medically fit patients with one to three hepatic metastases, surgical resection of part of the tumor-bearing liver is often possible. Careful preoperative radiologic staging and intraoperative ultrasonography of the liver facilitate these technically demanding procedures. Laser photoablation is being increasingly used to relieve colonic or rectal obstruction or to stop bleeding in patients with unresectable tumors or extensive metastatic disease.

RADIATION THERAPY. Radiation therapy plays an important role in the management of rectal cancer. Preoperative radiation therapy is often combined with fluorouracil and leucovorin in an effort to decrease local recurrence and distant spread. It may also be used to reduce tumor size and enable otherwise unresectable lesions to be resected. The postoperative administration of radiation (50 Gy) and chemotherapy is now standard therapy and has been shown to decrease local recurrence and distant metastasis. Biochemical modulation of fluorouracil by leucovorin is also being incorporated. Radiation therapy is useful in palliation of recurrent rectal cancer (pain or bleeding) or bone or brain metastases.

CHEMOTHERAPY. Patients with resected colonic cancer with lymph node spread have improved survival if treated with the combination of fluorouracil and leucovorin for 6 months. For patients with metastatic spread, the combination of fluorouracil and leucovorin increases tumor shrinkage compared with fluorouracil alone. New drugs such as topoisomerase I inhibitors (camptothecins) and oxaliplatin have therapeutic activity for palliation in patients with metastatic spread.

In patients with liver metastases, hepatic arterial therapy with implantable pumps or via injection ports using floxuridine alone or in combination with other drugs, such as leucovorin, produces an enhanced tumor shrinkage in the liver. Increased duration and quality of survival have not yet been convincingly demonstrated for this costly intervention.

PROGNOSIS AND FOLLOW-UP. The 10-year survival for patients with colorectal cancer after surgical resection is approximately 50%. Several histopathologic staging systems (e.g., the Dukes or TNM system) describe the extent of the malignancy (Table 139–1), and survival correlates well with the stage of the disease: 80 to 90% 10-year survival for cancer confined to the mucosa; 70 to 80% 10-year survival for cancer extending through all areas of the bowel wall; and 30 to 55% 10-year survival for

cancer involving the regional lymph nodes. Cancers of the distal rectum with lymph node involvement have a poorer prognosis.

Prior to surgical resection, the entire colon should be examined, preferably by colonoscopy, for the presence of synchronous adenomas. If not possible preoperatively, colonoscopy should be performed postoperatively, usually within 2 to 3 months of the surgical procedure. Colonoscopy should be repeated a year later and every 3 years thereafter because new adenomas require 3 years or more to develop into large adenomas with malignant potential.

After surgical resection, patients without known systemic metastases are evaluated for adjuvant therapy. Patients with colonic cancer and lymph node involvement should receive fluorouracil and leucovorin, and those with rectal cancer and spread through the wall or with lymph node involvement should receive radiation plus chemotherapy. While receiving chemotherapy or radiation therapy, patients should be followed up very carefully according to protocol guidelines. For those not receiving any specific therapy, periodic follow-up, including interim history, physical examination, and laboratory tests (e.g., liver enzymes, hematocrit), should be performed every 3 months for the first 3 years, then every 6 months until the fifth year. Considerable controversy exists concerning the cost-effectiveness of obtaining periodic chest radiographs or CT scans of the abdomen and pelvis as part of routine follow-up care in the absence of symptoms or laboratory test abnormalities.

CARCINOEMBRYONIC ANTIGEN. Carcinoembryonic antigen (CEA) levels in the blood may rise before symptoms or other laboratory test abnormalities are evident in patients with recurrent or metastatic colonic cancer. Some authorities favor periodic CEA determinations (e.g., every 3 months) after colorectal cancer resection, but this very expensive approach is helpful only in a minority of patients. Occasionally, a rising CEA level may detect a localized, surgically resectable metastasis. Certainly, its routine use should be confined to those individuals who do not have co-morbid conditions that would preclude subsequent resections of isolated liver or lung metastases. In conjunction with conventional radiologic techniques (CT scan, MRI, or PET scans), radiolabeled monoclonal antibodies to CEA may be helpful in localizing such metastases.

PREVENTION. Many colorectal cancers are first brought to medical attention by the patient's recognition of symptoms. For improved survival, the diagnosis should ideally be made earlier, in an asymptomatic phase. A greater emphasis is now being placed on preventive measures. Primary prevention is identification of factors, either genetic or environmental, responsible for colorectal cancers. Secondary prevention refers to identification and eradication of premalignant lesions and detection and resection of cancer while it is still curable.

Although definitive evidence of effectiveness is still lacking, the following dietary guidelines have been developed to try to reduce the risk of colorectal cancer: (1) reduce fat intake to fewer than 30% of calories; (2) increase dietary fiber to 20 to 30 g/day; (3) include a variety of vegetables and fruits in the diet; (4) avoid obesity; (5) consume alcohol in moderation, if at all; and (6) avoid cigarettes and tobacco. In addition, regular physical activity may also reduce risk. Chemopreventive measures such as aspirin or NSAIDs are being studied.

Implicit in the concept of secondary prevention is the need for improved techniques for screening for early cancer or premalignant adenomas. Effective screening requires the availability and application of simple and economic measures to a large number of asymptomatic individuals to identify those with these lesions.

Screening for colorectal cancer can be classified as general screening of patients at average risk and screening of patients in high-risk groups. Screening recommendations for patients at high risk because of ulcerative colitis, familial polyposis, HNPCC syndromes, or a personal history of colorectal adenomas or cancer have been discussed earlier in the chapter. For persons with a personal history of Crohn's colitis or a family history of sporadic colon cancer, recommendations vary and should include periodic evaluation of the entire colon.

AVERAGE-RISK PATIENTS. Currently, testing for fecal occult blood and flexible sigmoidoscopy in asymptomatic individuals are used for detecting early colorectal cancer. Testing for occult blood using guaiac-based methods detects lesions earlier in screened subjects compared with controls, and in three randomized controlled trials in the United States, Denmark, and the United Kingdom, colorectal mortality was significantly reduced (by 15 to 33%) by annual or bi-annual testing for fecal occult blood and appropriate

Table 139–1 ■ AMERICAN JOINT COMMITTEE ON CANCER: CLASSIFICATION OF COLON/RECTAL CANCER

Stage 0	Carcinoma in situ; the cancer does not extend beyond the smooth muscle that separates the mucosa from the submucosa (Tis, N0, M0)
Stage I	Cancer confined to the mucosa, submucosa, or external muscle; the cancer does not extend through the bowel wall (T1 or T2, N0, M0)
Stage II	Cancer that penetrates all layers of the bowel wall, with or without invasion of adjacent tissues (T3, N0, M0)
Stage III	Cancer involving regional lymph nodes or extending into nearby tissues or organs without spread to lymph nodes (any T, N1–N3, M0; or T4, N0, M0)
Stage IV	Cancer that has spread to distant sites, usually the liver or lungs (any T, any N, M1)

TNM = tumor/node/metastasis.

colonoscopic follow-up. Newer immunochemical tests for human hemoglobin in the stool, currently under clinical trial, are likely to be more specific. Randomized controlled trials of flexible sigmoidoscopy have not been performed on a large scale. Case-control studies have demonstrated significant effectiveness of flexible sigmoidoscopy in reducing mortality (by 70%) from distal colorectal cancer. Flexible sigmoidoscopy can identify and eradicate premalignant and malignant lesions in the area examined and also can identify individuals who may have more proximal synchronous adenomas and carcinomas.

Current guidelines include a number of options. One is to test for fecal occult blood annually after age 50 years; patients with abnormal findings require careful diagnostic evaluation, including colonoscopy. The American Cancer Society's recommendations include several alternatives. One is to test for fecal occult blood annually combined with flexible sigmoidoscopy every 5 years, both beginning at age 50 years. Patients with abnormal findings, e.g., positive fecal occult blood test or distal adenomas, should be referred for colonoscopic evaluation. Alternative screening approaches beginning at age 50 years include colonoscopy every 10 years or double contrast barium enema every 5 to 10 years.

NEOPLASMS OF THE SMALL BOWEL

Benign and malignant tumors of the lining epithelium and mesenchymal tissues may arise in the small intestine, or these areas may be secondarily involved by direct invasion from surrounding structures or by metastases. The small bowel represents almost 90% of the mucosal surface of the gut, but small intestinal cancers account for only 1 to 2% of all gastrointestinal neoplasms. Only about 2000 cases occur in the United States each year.

RISK FACTORS. Patients with regional enteritis, especially those who have had segments of intestine surgically bypassed, have an increased incidence of small bowel carcinoma. Individuals with Gardner's syndrome have an increased risk of periampullary adenocarcinoma. In patients with Peutz-Jeghers syndrome, the relative risk of small intestinal adenocarcinoma is 16 times that expected, with a lifetime incidence of 2%. Patients with celiac disease of long duration have an increased incidence of intestinal lymphoma, as do patients with AIDS and other immunodeficiency states. Mediterranean abdominal lymphoma (immunoproliferative small intestinal disease) has been widely reported among Arabs and Jews of Middle Eastern origin and also occurs sporadically throughout the world, including in blacks in southern Africa.

Why small bowel neoplasms, especially adenocarcinomas, are so uncommon compared with large bowel cancers is uncertain. It is possible that the rapid transit time with a resultant decreased exposure time to carcinogens, lower numbers of bacteria, and dilution of potential carcinogens by the large volume of enteric liquids may contribute.

PATHOLOGY. BENIGN. These lesions include adenomas, leiomyomas, lipomas, and angiomas. Brunner's gland adenomas are not neoplastic but represent hyperplasia or hypertrophy of submucosal duodenal glands; these lesions appear as small nodules in the duodenal mucosa detected at endoscopy or on barium radiographs.

MALIGNANT. Adenocarcinomas, carcinoids, lymphomas, and leiomyosarcomas account for more than 90% of malignant small bowel tumors. Adenocarcinomas are most common in the proximal small intestine, whereas lymphomas and carcinoids are most common in the distal small intestine.

CLINICAL MANIFESTATIONS. More than half of all benign bowel tumors remain asymptomatic and may be discovered only incidentally at laparotomy or autopsy. Lack of symptoms is attributable to the liquid contents of the small intestine and distensibility of the small intestine. Large tumors may lead to partial or complete mechanical obstruction from intussusception or volvulus.

Adenocarcinomas account for about half of the malignant tumors of the small intestine, with a peak incidence in the sixth and seventh decades. The duodenum is the most frequently affected site. When postbulbar in location, adenocarcinoma may simulate peptic ulcer disease; when in the periampullary region, it may cause obstructive jaundice. More distally, adenocarcinomas may remain silent until symptoms of intestinal obstruction or gastrointestinal hemorrhage occur.

Carcinoids are the most frequently occurring small intestinal neoplasm, with more than half found incidentally either at autopsy or at operation for other diseases. Small carcinoid tumors may be asymptomatic, but larger carcinoid tumors can obstruct the lumen or bleed (Color Plate 3D). Once metastasis occurs to the liver, features of the carcinoid syndrome become apparent (see Chapter 245).

Weight loss, intestinal obstruction, fever, bleeding, and evidence of malabsorption syndrome are features of lymphoma. Massive hemorrhage and intestinal perforation may be the presenting symptoms of large sarcomas.

SIGNS. Physical examination may be unremarkable in patients with benign tumors, unless the neoplasm is large enough to present with a mass. Loud borborygmi, visible peristalsis, and abdominal distention may be present in intestinal obstruction. In patients with malignant small bowel neoplasms, more obvious physical findings may be evident. Cachexia, hepatomegaly, ascites, and jaundice may be found. Peripheral lymphadenopathy or splenomegaly may be found in those with extensive lymphoma.

DIFFERENTIAL DIAGNOSIS. The initial symptoms may be vague and poorly defined. Once bleeding occurs, causes such as peptic ulceration, Meckel's diverticulum, and vascular anomalies need to be considered (see Chapter 137). Obstructive jaundice may occur with periampullary neoplasms, bile duct cancer, impacted common duct stones, pancreatitis, and pancreatic cancer (see Chapter 140). Intestinal obstruction may be due to adhesions, particularly in patients who have had prior abdominal operations, internal hernias, volvulus, or intussusception.

LABORATORY AND RADIOLOGIC STUDIES. Hypochromic, microcytic anemia is quite common. Elevation of alkaline phosphatase and bilirubin levels may occur if the ampulla of Vater is obstructed or if liver metastases are present. Elevated levels of plasma serotonin or urinary 5-hydroxyindoleacetic acid occur in the carcinoid syndrome (see Chapter 245). Dysproteinemia is a typical feature of Mediterranean lymphoma and is characterized by the presence of abnormal fragments of immunoglobulin A (Ig) A in the serum and urine that is devoid of light chains (see Chapter 179).

Upper gastrointestinal tract barium radiographs and selective nasoenteric intubation (enteroclysis), which permits the introduction of barium and air into a relatively localized segment, may be useful in localizing tumors. Abdominal ultrasonography and CT may determine the extent of hepatic involvement, aid in the work-up of jaundice, and assess intra-abdominal and retroperitoneal spread. Intestinal lymphoma may occasionally be diagnosed by peroral intestinal biopsy, but the disease mainly involves the lamina propria and usually requires a full-thickness surgical biopsy. A thorough staging of lymphoma involves bone marrow biopsy, laparotomy with splenectomy, and biopsies of regional lymph nodes and liver.

ENDOSCOPIC EVALUATION. Front-viewing and side-viewing fiberoptic endoscopes are used to examine the duodenum; suspicious lesions can be biopsied and brushed. Endoscopic ultrasound may be helpful in defining depth of involvement of a specific lesion. Periampullary lesions can be well visualized; the pancreatic and biliary trees can be studied by contrast radiography after endoscopic cannulation. The terminal ileum can also be viewed at colonoscopy. Small bowel enteroscopy is sometimes helpful in localizing a small bleeding lesion.

THERAPY. Treatment is primarily surgical for symptomatic benign tumors, adenocarcinomas, leiomyosarcomas, malignant carcinoids, and those with secondary involvement of the small intestine. Duodenal carcinomas or large villous adenomas are treated by pancreaticoduodenal resection (Whipple's procedure). In patients with localized lymphoma (stage I), surgical excision is recommended. Combination chemotherapy is used for more extensive lymphoma (see Chapter 179). Radiation therapy may be helpful for bulky tumors or localized recurrences.

PROGNOSIS AND PREVENTION. The prognosis for benign tumors of the intestine is good if surgical resection can alleviate bleeding and obstruction. The prognosis of small intestinal adenocarcinomas is generally poor. The prognosis for leiomyosarcomas and primary lymphomas is good if surgical resection is complete, but this is rarely possible. Patients with malignant carcinoid tumors may survive for long periods, even in the presence of extensive hepatic involvement.

Primary small intestinal lymphomas occurring in populations in the Middle East could possibly be decreased by public health measures that decrease parasitic infestation. Earlier diagnosis and adequate treatment of celiac disease (gluten-free diet) may reduce the frequency of malignancy. Surgical bypass should not be performed in patients with Crohn's disease. In patients with familial polyposis syndromes, duodenal and periampullary adenomas should be monitored periodically. Prophylactic endoscopic or surgical removal may be appropriate for large or dysplastic lesions.

Epidemiology

Potter JD: Epidemiologic, environmental and lifestyle issues in prevention and early detection of colorectal cancer. *In* Young GP, Rozen P, Levin B (eds): Prevention and Early Detection of Colorectal Cancer. Philadelphia, WB Saunders, 1996, p 23. *A concise but critical summary of current evidence.*

Schottenfeld D, Islam SS: Cancers of the small intestine. *In* Schottenfield D, Fraumeni JF Jr (eds): Cancer Epidemiology and Prevention, 2nd ed. New York, Oxford University Press, 1996, p 806. *An extensive discussion of current state of knowledge.*

Primary Prevention

Kelloff GH, Boone CW, Sigman CC, et al: Chemoprevention of colorectal cancer. *In* Young GP, Rozen P, Levin B (eds): Prevention and Early Detection of Colorectal Cancer. Philadelphia, WB Saunders, 1996, p 115. *The authors classify and describe the multiple natural and chemical compounds that are being evaluated in clinical trials and their mechanisms of action.*

Schatzkin A: Dietary prevention of colorectal cancer. *In* Young GP, Rozen P, Levin B (eds): Prevention and Early Detection of Colorectal Cancer. Philadelphia, WB Saunders, 1996, p 103. *The author reviews the evidence that dietary intervention can influence the development of adenomas and cancer.*

Screening and Early Detection

Byers T, Levin B, Rothenberger D, et al: American Cancer Society Guidelines for Screening and Surveillance for Early Detection of Colorectal Polyps and Cancer: Update 1997. CA Cancer J Clin 47:154, 1997. *A summary of current guidelines.*

Midgley R, Kerr D: Colorectal cancer. Lancet 353:391–399, 1999. *A concise review of the current state of clinical practice.*

Wagner JL, Tunis S, Brown M, et al: Cost-effectiveness of colorectal cancer screening in average-risk adults. *In* Young GP, Rozen P, Levin B (eds): Prevention and Early Detection of Colorectal Cancer. Philadelphia, WB Saunders, 1996, p 321. *The authors provide an extensive discussion about the cost-effectiveness of colorectal cancer screening.*

Winawer SJ, Fletcher RH, Muller L, et al: Colorectal cancer screening: Clinical guidelines and rationale. Gastroenterology 112:594, 1997. *A definitive, evidence-based analysis of the theoretical basis of screening measures and their practical application.*

Molecular Biology and Genetics

Bellacosa A, Genuardi M, Anti M, et al: Hereditary nonpolyposis colorectal cancer: Review of clinical, molecular genetics, and counseling aspects. Am J Med Genet 62: 353, 1996. *Reviews advances in molecular aspects of colorectal cancer.*

Lieters GJ, Tollenaar RA, Cleton-Jansen AM: Molecular staging of colorectal cancer: A step forward. Gastroenterology 116:769–770, 1999. *Utility of molecular markers to aid in estimating prognoses in colon cancer.*

Tomlinson I, Ilyas M, Novelli M: Molecular genetics of colon cancer. Cancer Metastasis Rev 16:67, 1997.

Adenomas and Their Management

Bond JH: Polyp guidelines: Diagnosis, treatment and surveillance for patients with non-familial colorectal cancer. Ann Intern Med 119:836, 1993. *An authoritative review of this topic with practical management guidelines.*

Zauber AG, Bond JH, Winawer SJ: Surveillance of patients with colorectal adenomas or cancer. *In* Young GP, Rozen P, Levin B (eds): Prevention and Early Detection of Colorectal Cancer. Philadelphia, WB Saunders, 1996, p 195. *An extensive discussion of the natural history and clinical approaches.*

Therapy

Cohen AM, Winawer SJ (eds): Cancer of the Colon, Rectum, and Anus. New York, McGraw-Hill, 1995. *A detailed multi-authored text that provides in-depth discussions of surgery, radiation therapy, and chemotherapy as well as newer experimental approaches.*

Small Intestine

Jones DV, Levin B, Salem P: Intestinal lymphomas, including immunoproliferative small intestinal disease. *In* Feldman M, Scharschmidt BF, Sleisenger MH (eds): Sleisenger and Fordtran's Gastrointestinal and Liver Disease, 6th ed. Philadelphia, WB Saunders, 1997, p 1844. *A summary of the pathogenesis, diagnosis, and management of intestinal lymphomas.*

Jones DV, Skibber J, Levin B: Adenocarcinoma and other small intestinal neoplasms, including benign tumors. *In* Feldman M, Scharschmidt BF, Sleisenger MH (eds): Sleisenger and Fordtran's Gastrointestinal and Liver Disease, 6th ed. Philadelphia, WB Saunders, 1997, p 1858. *A summary of the multidisciplinary approach to tumors of the small bowel.*

140 CARCINOMA OF THE PANCREAS

Eugene P. DiMagno

DEFINITION. Ductal adenocarcinoma, which accounts for 90% of pancreatic cancers, is a relentlessly progressive and fatal disease.

Most tumors are moderately well differentiated mucinous carcinomas arising from the cuboid epithelium of pancreatic ducts. The remaining 10% of pancreatic cancers are endocrine tumors (see Chapter 130); acinar cell, giant cell, and epidermoid cancers; adenoacanthomas; sarcomas; and cystadenocarcinomas.

INCIDENCE AND EPIDEMIOLOGY. In the past generation the incidence of pancreatic cancer has increased from fewer than 5 to between 11 and 12 per 100,000 population. Currently, pancreatic cancer kills more Americans than any other neoplasm except breast, colorectal, lung, and prostate cancers. Each year, pancreatic cancer develops in approximately 27,000 Americans and 25,000 die. The median survival after diagnosis is 4 to 8 months. The overall 5-year survival rate is less than 1%. Resecting the tumor improves median survival to 17 to 20 months, but the 5-year survival rate remains less than 10%.

Pancreatic cancer is associated with certain demographic characteristics and risk factors (Table 140–1). Pancreatic cancer occurs more frequently in men (1.5:1), and 80% occur between the ages of 60 and 80; the disease is unusual in people younger than 40 years. Patients with chronic pancreatitis and members of families with hereditary pancreatitis or the non-polyposis colon cancer syndrome are at increased risk. Patients with chronic pancreatitis have more than a nine-fold risk of pancreatic cancer, and the cumulative risk increases 2% per decade. Patients with hereditary pancreatitis have a cumulative risk of 40% by 70 years of age. Intraductal papillary mucinous tumor, which may mimic chronic pancreatitis clinically, carries a 50% risk of invasive cancer and is considered a pre-malignant neoplasm. Environmental factors are probably associated with an increased risk of pancreatic cancer, but coffee consumption, alcohol abuse, diabetes mellitus, and previous cholecystectomy or gastrectomy do not appear to increase the risk. Eliminating cigarette smoking and eating a diet low in cholesterol, with olive oil and fish as the main sources of fat, may reduce the risk.

The most common molecular abnormalities (>90%) in human pancreatic cancer are mutations in codon 12 of the K-*ras* gene, which is probably involved in cancer growth. A high proportion of pancreatic cancers also have deletions and mutations in the *p53* gene. Gene mutations result in loss of function, failure of inactivation, and intranuclear accumulation of the p53 protein. Epidermal growth factor and *erb*-b2 receptor pathways are also altered and may have a role in the pathogenesis of pancreatic cancer.

PATHOPHYSIOLOGY AND CLINICAL MANIFESTATIONS. In pancreatic ductal adenocarcinoma, well-differentiated to poorly differentiated duct glands are embedded in a dense network of fibrous tissue. As it extends into the pancreas and surrounding tissue, the tumor envelopes and fixes vessels and invades fat, lymph channels, and perineural areas. Symptoms and signs of pancreatic cancer are related to the location of the tumor within the gland and to extension of the tumor to the stomach, duodenum, bile duct, retroperitoneum, and porta hepatis.

Pain occurs in 90% of patients. It may be vague and rather nonspecific and may occur up to 3 months before the onset of jaundice. Early in the course the pain may be ignored by both the patient and the examining physician. The tumor most commonly extends to the retroperitoneal space and produces visceral pain variously described as persistent, disagreeable, aching, increased by

Table 140–1 ■ RISK FACTORS FOR PANCREATIC CANCER

Definite
  Age >60 yr
  Male sex
  Cigarette smoking
  Chronic pancreatitis
  Non-polyposis colon cancer syndrome
Probable
  High-cholesterol and high-fat diet with high linoleic acid content
  Chemical exposure (coal tar derivative, coke, benzidine, β-naphthylamine)
Unlikely
  Diabetes mellitus
  Coffee
  Alcohol
  Prior cholecystectomy, gastrectomy

Table 140–2 ■ DIAGNOSTIC ACCURACY (%) OF IMAGING TESTS IN DIAGNOSIS OF PANCREATIC CANCER

TEST	SENSITIVITY	SPECIFICITY	PREDICTIVE VALUE Positive	PREDICTIVE VALUE Negative
Ultrasonography	74	84	78	79
Computed tomography	79	64	76	78
Endoscopic retrograde cholangiopancreatography	95	90	87	97

lying supine or by eating, and causing the patient to awaken at night. Relief is sometimes obtained by bending forward, by lying on the side and drawing the knees to the chest or chin, and by crouching forward on all four extremities.

Jaundice caused by obstruction of the common bile duct occurs early in the course of the disease in 60 to 70% of carcinomas of the head of the pancreas. When carcinoma of the head of the pancreas arises in its central part or in the uncinate process, jaundice is not an early manifestation. In cancer of the body and tail, jaundice occurs late and may be caused by hepatic metastases or obstruction of the bile duct at the porta hepatis by lymphadenopathy. Painless jaundice is unusual.

Weight loss greater than 10% of ideal body weight, almost universal, is usually due to both malabsorption and decreased food intake. Seventy-five per cent of patients malabsorb fat, and 50% malabsorb protein. Malabsorption occurs in patients who have a carcinoma of the head of the pancreas that obstructs the pancreatic duct, thereby producing pancreatic exocrine insufficiency (see Chapters 134 and 141).

Glucose intolerance from increased plasma levels of islet amyloid polypeptide producing insulin resistance may be present in up to 80% of patients with pancreatic cancer, but in most patients the diabetes is mild. Fewer than 5% of patients have hyperphagia, polydipsia, and polyuria.

Other symptoms and signs include depression, light-colored stool (60% of patients with carcinoma of the pancreatic head), constipation, and emotional lability (27% of patients with carcinoma of the pancreatic tail). Vomiting and weakness occur in one third of patients. More rarely, patients exhibit superficial thrombophlebitis (Trousseau's syndrome) or gastrointestinal bleeding caused either by direct extension of the tumor into the stomach or duodenum or by varices secondary to splenic vein obstruction. Rarely, metastases from pancreatic cancer of the body and tail to the testicles, temporal bone, or esophagus may cause testicular enlargement and pain, sudden profound hearing loss, or dysphasia, respectively.

Hepatomegaly combined with jaundice is present in 80 and 30% of patients with carcinoma of the head and carcinoma of the body

Table 140–3 ■ DIFFERENTIAL DIAGNOSIS OF PANCREATIC CANCER

Benign Conditions
Chronic pancreatitis
Extrahepatic jaundice
  Common bile duct stones
  Bile duct stricture (secondary to previous biliary tract surgery or sclerosing cholangitis)
  Cholecystitis
Intrahepatic cholestatic jaundice
  Alcoholic hepatitis
  Toxins
  Cysts
  Abscess
Posterior penetrating duodenal or gastric ulcers
Depression
Functional bowel disorders
Malignant Conditions
Retroperitoneal lymphomas
Bile duct cancer
Ampullary cancer
Gynecologic malignancies
Carcinoma of the duodenum or small intestine

and tail, respectively. A palpable gallbladder (Courvoisier's sign) is present in 30% of patients with carcinoma of the head of the pancreas. An abdominal mass or ascites is present in fewer than 20% of patients. Ascites, splenomegaly, and peripheral edema may be caused by occlusion of the portal vein by tumor, whereas compression of the aorta or splenic artery may produce an abdominal bruit.

DIAGNOSIS. The preferred imaging test for diagnosing pancreatic cancer is a computed tomographic (CT) scan. If a tumor is highly suspected but not found by CT scan, the most sensitive test is endoscopic ultrasonography (US) (Table 140–2). Other imaging tests such as US or endoscopic retrograde cholangiopancreatography are not usually needed for diagnosis. As a group, patients with pancreatic cancer have higher values for serum lipase, amylase, and glucose than do other patients, but these tests do not distinguish between pancreatic cancer and pancreatitis. Similarly, serum alkaline phosphatase, aspartate aminotransferase, and bilirubin are commonly elevated, but these tests lack specificity to exclude hepatic disorders. Non-specific findings on the chest radiograph and abdominal films may be present in patients with pancreatitis or pancreatic cancer. Pancreatic calcifications have a sensitivity of 95% for diagnosing chronic pancreatitis, but primary ductal carcinoma, mucinous cystadenocarcinoma (curvilinear calcification), benign serous cystadenoma (central, "sunburst" calcification), and solid and papillary epithelial neoplasms can also calcify. If obvious pulmonary or bony metastases are found, further diagnostic tests may not be needed.

If the cancer is deemed resectable, endoscopic US or laparoscopy may be considered to determine whether vascular invasion and lymph node metastases are present or whether peritoneal seeding and small liver metastases have occurred, respectively. The availability of endoscopic US is increasing, and it may be as useful as laparoscopy in staging tumors preoperatively. When compared with traditional US, CT, and angiography, endoscopic US is more sensitive for detecting portal vein involvement and lymph node metastasis. Laparoscopy correctly identifies 85% of unresectable tumors. Aspiration cytology of the pancreatic mass with US or CT guidance is 90% sensitive but should not be performed unless the cancer is clearly unresectable because the procedure may cause intra-abdominal seeding of tumor cells.

New tests that have appeared in the last 5 to 10 years are magnetic resonance imaging, magnetic resonance cholangiopancreatography, and positron emission tomography. The role of these tests in the diagnosis of pancreatic cancer is evolving. Magnetic resonance imaging may be as accurate as CT but is not widely used.

No serologic marker (see Chapter 192) is sufficiently accurate to serve as a screening test for pancreatic cancer. CA 19-9 (the most commonly used marker), carcinoembryonic antigen, galactosyltransferase, pancreatic oncofetal antigen, and pancreatic cancer–associated antigen each have a sensitivity of 50 to 85%, but false-positive tests occur in up to 46% of patients with benign diseases and in up to 65% of those with other malignancies. Other markers such as plasma islet amyloid polypeptide and K-*ras* mutations in pancreatic secretions are under study.

DIFFERENTIAL DIAGNOSIS. The initial symptoms and signs of pancreatic cancer are non-specific (Table 140–3). Indeed, most patients with weight loss and abdominal pain, with or without jaundice, do not have pancreatic cancer. In patients without jaundice, the abdominal pain and weight loss of pancreatic cancer may be difficult to distinguish from many other disorders. In jaundiced patients, pancreatic cancer must be distinguished from potentially treatable benign conditions such as chronic pancreatitis obstructing the common bile duct and from causes of extrahepatic and intrahepatic cholestasis.

TREATMENT. Surgical resection of pancreatic cancer offers the only chance of cure. Unfortunately, only 10% of all pancreatic cancers are resectable, and the 5-year survival rate after resection is only 10%. Resection of tumors smaller than 2 cm in diameter is associated with a 20 to 37% 5-year survival rate. Pancreaticoduodenectomy is the surgical procedure of choice. In experienced hands, surgical mortality is 2 to 5%. Other surgical procedures such as total pancreatectomy and regional pancreatectomy are not commonly performed because of higher operative mortality and morbidity and 5-year survival rates that do not exceed those of pancreaticoduodenectomy. The pylorus-preserving pancreaticoduodenal resection may be performed in patients with a small cancer of the pancreatic head, but it does not improve nutrition when compared with standard pancreaticoduodenectomy. Adjuvant chemoradiation after resection prolongs survival, and preoperative neoadjuvant chemoradiation is under study.

Palliative procedures relieve symptoms of biliary obstruction, duodenal obstruction, or both. To relieve biliary obstruction, cholecystojejunostomy and a gastroenterostomy should be performed unless the cystic duct enters the common duct close to the tumor. In this case, choledochojejunostomy should be performed. To decompress the biliary tree, endoscopic stenting is as successful as surgical decompression and may have lower morbidity, but jaundice is more likely to recur late in the disease. An endoscopic stent should be placed if the patient has a high surgical risk or a short life expectancy (1 to 3 months). In contrast, cholecystojejunostomy and gastroenterostomy should be performed if an unresectable tumor is found at the time of surgery or if the patient has a life expectancy of 6 to 7 months because complete duodenal obstruction occurs in 5 to 15% of patients—usually as a pre-terminal event. Incomplete or functional gastric outlet obstruction occurs in 40 to 60% of patients; in such patients, the combination of a cholinergic (bethanechol, 25 mg three times per day) and a prokinetic agent (metoclopramide or cisapride, 10 mg four times per day) may alleviate the symptoms of gastric stasis by enhancing gastric emptying.

Gemcitabine is the only single agent that may prolong survival; it has a low response rate, but a small improvement in overall survival in comparison to 5-fluorouracil (5-FU) (5.7 versus 4.4 months and a 1-year survival rate of 18% versus 2%). No other single agent or combination of chemotherapeutic drugs prolongs or enhances the quality of life. 5-FU produces a partial response rate in 10 to 15% of patients, but its use is associated with a median survival of less than 20 weeks. Other agents have a similar effect (mitomycin), less effect (streptozotocin, doxorubicin, epirubicin, ifosfamide, methyl-CCNU [lomustine], and high-dose methotrexate), or no effect (actinomycin D, doxorubicin, BCNU [carmustine], standard-dose methotrexate, cisplatin, melphalan, and L-asparaginase).

The combination of external beam radiation with 5-FU or with streptozotocin, mitomycin, and 5-FU improves survival when compared with radiation or chemotherapy alone. Intraoperative electron beam radiation and ^{125}I implants do not improve survival in comparison to external beam radiation. These modalities may limit local tumor extension, but they do not control liver and peritoneal metastases.

Pain can usually be successfully managed if adequate doses of analgesics are prescribed on a regular basis and adjuvant drugs are used when necessary. Mild to moderate pain can be controlled with aspirin, acetaminophen, and non-steroidal anti-inflammatory agents. If these drugs fail to relieve pain, opioid analgesics should be used (see Chapter 27). Intraoperative or percutaneous neurolytic celiac plexus block is remarkably effective in controlling pain. If patients have intolerable pain, subcutaneous patient-controlled analgesia or epidural narcotics afford pain relief.

Malabsorption can be reasonably well controlled by ingesting eight tablets of pancrealipase with meals (the total dose of lipase should be 30,000 IU). Two tablets should be taken immediately after eating a few bites, two tablets at the end of the meal, and four tablets interspersed during the meal (see Chapter 141).

Burris HA, Moore HJ, Andersen J, et al: Improvements in survival and clinical benefit with gemcitabine as first line therapy for patients with advanced pancreatic cancer: A randomized trial. J Clin Oncol 15:2403, 1997. *First demonstration of a single agent that improves survival.*

Loftus EV, Olivares-Pazkad BA, Batts KP, et al: Intraductal papillary-mucinous tumors of the pancreas: Clinicopathological features, outcome, and nomenclature. Gastroenterology 110:1909, 1996. *IPMT is a dysplastic and pre-malignant lesion, separate from mucinous cystic neoplasm and often diagnosed as chronic pancreatitis, that if possible, should be treated with complete surgical excision because it is impossible to distinguish non-invasive IPMT from invasive cancer preoperatively.*

Urrutia R, DiMagno EP: Pancreatic cancer: Cellular and molecular mechanisms. *In* Bertino JR (ed): Encyclopedia of Cancer, vol 2 (G-Q). San Diego, Academic Press, 1996, pp 1201–1211. *A review of the molecular bases of pancreatic cancer.*

Yeo CJ, Cameron JL: Pancreatic cancer. Curr Prob Surg 36:59–152, 1999. *A useful review from the surgical perspective.*

141 PANCREATITIS

Konrad H. Soergel

ANATOMY AND PHYSIOLOGY OF THE PANCREAS

The pancreas first appears as ventral and dorsal budding evaginations of the primitive foregut at 5 weeks' gestation. The right portion of the ventral bud, including the common bile duct, migrates posteriorly with rotation of the duodenum. Both anlagen and their ducts fuse by the seventh week of gestation, with the ventral anlage forming the pancreatic head and uncinate process and the dorsal anlage forming the body and tail. Incomplete fusion results in two separate pancreatic ducts: the dorsal duct of Santorini draining through the minor papilla and a short ventral duct (Wirsung) ending at the major papilla of Vater. This anomaly, termed *pancreas divisum,* is present in 5 to 10% of the population. Fixation of the ventral bud while the duodenum rotates results in a band of pancreatic tissue encircling the descending duodenum, the resulting *annular pancreas* is very rare and may cause duodenal obstruction or pancreatitis.

The retroperitoneal location and the absence of a capsule surrounding the pancreas are important factors in understanding how pancreatitis evolves. Pancreatic inflammation and fibrosis may spread unimpeded by anatomic barriers to involve the spleen, the splenic artery and vein, the duodenum and distal common bile duct, the mesocolon and small bowel mesentery, the diaphragm and pararenal spaces, the lesser omental sac, and the celiac and superior mesenteric ganglia. The acinar cells of the exocrine pancreas synthesize approximately 20 digestive enzymes, colipase, a secretory trypsin inhibitor, and lithostathine S_{2-5}, a protein that inhibits the precipitation of $CaCO_3$ from pancreatic juice. These secretory proteins are sorted into condensing vacuoles, which then become zymogen granules. The granules fuse with the apical cell membrane and discharge their contents into the acinar lumen by exocytosis by a process controlled by cholecystokinin (CCK) which acts via central vagal pathways and gastropancreatic and enteropancreatic cholinergic reflexes. CCK is released from endocrine I cells in the duodenal and proximal jejunal mucosa during fat and protein digestion. All digestive enzymes, except α-amylase, lipase, ribonuclease, and deoxyribonuclease, are secreted as inactive zymogens. Trypsinogen is activated by enterokinase, which is secreted by the duodenum; trypsin then activates all other zymogens within the duodenal lumen. The centroacinar, ductular, and pancreatic duct epithelial cells represent a functional unit that exchanges HCO_3^- for Cl^-, with increasing flow rates of pancreatic secretion. This process involves the intracellular generation of carbonic acid by carbonic anhydrase and the actions of a Cl^-/HCO_3^- exchanger and a Cl^- channel, the cystic fibrosis transmembrane regulator (CFTR), at the luminal cell border. The excess intracellular H^+ ions are removed by a basolaterally located Na^+/H^+ exchanger. Secretion of alkaline, bicarbonate-rich pancreatic juice is stimulated by acetylcholine and by the hormone secretin, which is released from mucosal S cells when the duodenal pH decreases to ≤4.5. Premature activation of zymogens within the pancreas is the key event in the pathogenesis of acute pancreatitis. Protein and $CaCO_3$ precipitates within the pancreatic duct system play a major role in the development of chronic pancreatitis.

ACUTE PANCREATITIS

DEFINITIONS. Acute pancreatitis is an acute inflammatory process with variable involvement of adjacent and remote organs. Although pancreatic function and structure usually return to normal, the risk of recurrent attacks is 20 to 50% unless the precipitating cause is removed. The annual incidence of acute pancreatitis is close to 10 per 100,000 in the adult population. Initial manifestations and exacerbations of chronic pancreatitis may be indistinguishable from attacks of acute pancreatitis, and they should be treated as such. The inflammation begins in the perilobular and peripancreatic fatty tissue, manifested by edema and spotty fat necrosis. The disease may progress to the peripheral acinar cells,

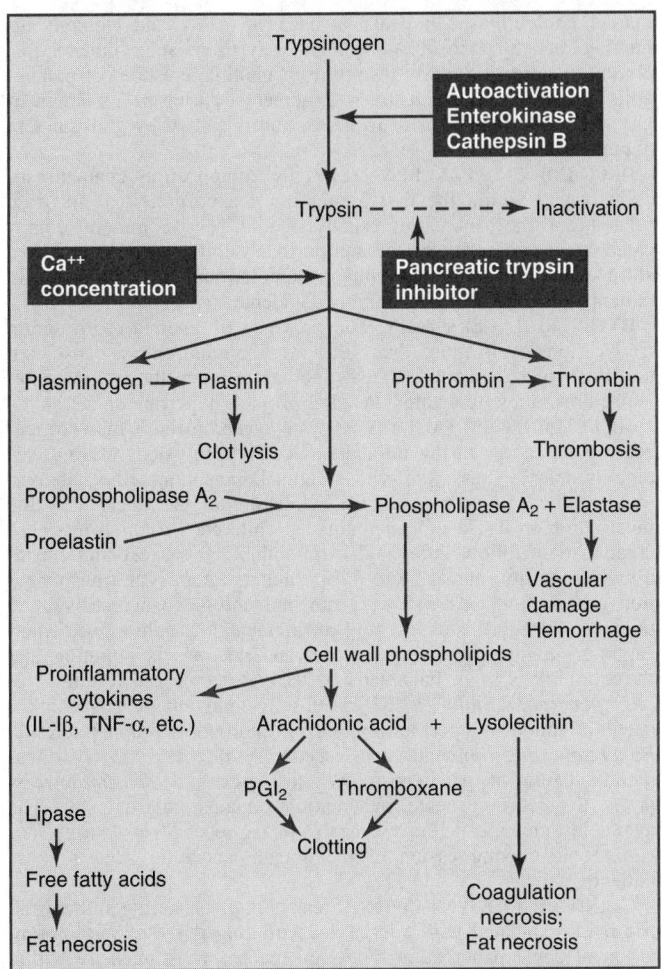

FIGURE 141–1 ■ The pathophysiology of pancreatic autodigestion. IL = interleukin; TNF = tumor necrosis factor. (Modified from Sleisenger MH, Fordtran JS [eds]: Gastrointestinal Disease, 5th ed. Philadelphia, WB Saunders, 1993, p 1631.)

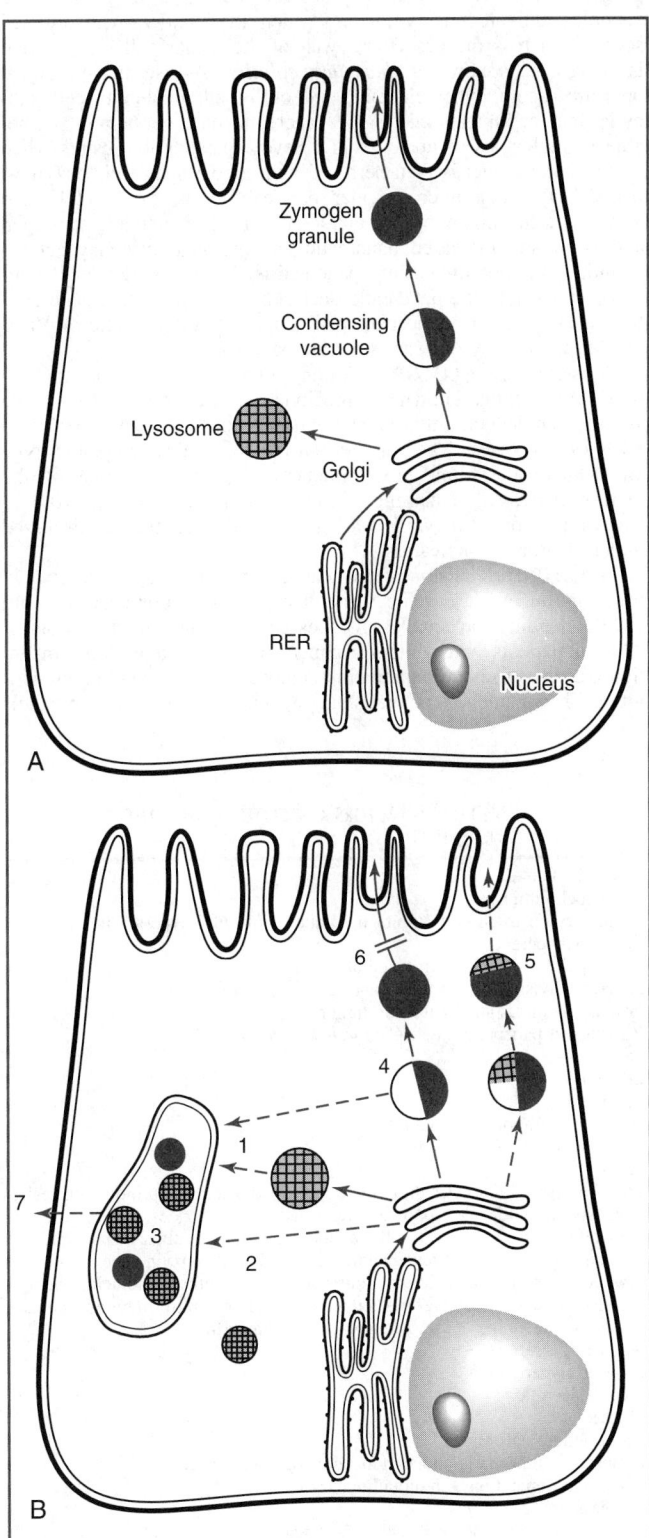

FIGURE 141–2 ■ Synthesis, sorting, and secretion of hydrolytic enzymes and zymogens in the pancreatic acinar cell. A, Normal. B, Abnormalities observed in various models of experimental pancreatitis: (1) crinophagy; condensing vacuoles and lysosomes coalesce; (2) absent compartmentalization; (3) autophagic vacuole; (4) autoactivation; (5) increased lysosomal hydrolase secretion; (6) exocytosis block; (7) secretion across basolateral cell wall. Interrupted lines indicate abnormal events. (From Sleisenger MH, Fordtran JS [eds]: Gastrointestinal Disease, 5th ed. Philadelphia, WB Saunders, 1993, p 1630.)

pancreatic ducts, blood vessels, and bordering organs. In severe cases, patchy areas of the pancreatic parenchyma become necrotic. *Local complication* are defined as (1) *acute fluid collections,* which are common and frequently multiple, occur early in the course, and lack a defined wall—the majority of these collections resolve spontaneously; (2) *pancreatic necrosis:* focal or diffuse necrosis of pancreatic parenchyma, frequently associated with peripancreatic fat necrosis—the necrotic tissue may be sterile or infected; and (3) *pancreatic abscess:* a rare complication that arises late in the course of acute pancreatitis. Ambiguous terms that should be discarded include *pancreatic phlegmon, acute* and *infected pseudocysts,* and *edematous* and *hemorrhagic acute pancreatitis. Severe pancreatitis* is defined as a local complication and/or organ failure generally associated with an APACHE II (Acute Physiology and Chronic Health Evaluation) score of 8 or more.

PATHOGENESIS. Premature activation of zymogens and the escape of activated enzymes from acinar cells and pancreatic ducts set the stage for the autodigestive process that represents acute pancreatitis (Fig. 141–1). Proteases released into the blood are inactivated by circulating inhibitors, including α_2-macroglobulin, α_1-antitrypsin, and the C_1-esterase inhibitor. In addition, trypsin activates kallikrein, a peptidase, which then cleaves several peptides, including bradykinin and kallidin, from their inactive precursors in blood plasma. These peptides, termed *kinins,* have various deleterious effects including vasodilatation, increased vascular permeability, pain, and neutrophil accumulation.

Two mechanisms may trigger pancreatic autodigestion. The first is *zymogen activation* within the pancreatic acinar cell (Fig. 141–2). The rate of exocytosis is decreased while acinar protein synthesis continues undiminished, leading to intracellular accumulation of zymogens. A variety of errors in intracellular traffic result in co-localization of zymogens and lysosomal enzymes in large autophagic vacules. Lysosomal enzymes and the acidic pH within these vacuoles activate the zymogens, which then undergo misdirected secretion across the basolateral wall of the acinar cell. The second is *increased pancreatic duct permeability*. A rise in intraductal pressure, acute hypercalcemia, and orally administered acetylsalicylic acid or ethanol makes the pancreatic duct epithelium permeable to molecules of up to 25 kD. Severe pancreatitis results when the pancreatic duct is then perfused with active pancreatic enzymes, particularly when microvascular permeability is increased by the actions of histamine or prostaglandins. Thus, pancreatic zymogen activation and increased pancreatic duct permeability may act sequentially in initiating acute pancreatitis. Reflux of duodenal contents or bile into the pancreatic duct does not cause acute pancreatitis but obstruction of the pancreatic duct near the ampulla of Vater may explain many episodes of acute pancreatitis.

ASSOCIATED FACTORS. Among clinical conditions, medications, and toxins known to precipitate acute pancreatitis (Table 141–1), choledocholithiasis and ethanol abuse account for 70 to 80% of all cases. The number attributed to the idiopathic type varies with the clinician's astuteness in identifying one of the factors listed. All remaining causes combined account for 10% or less of the total. *Alcoholic and familial* pancreatitis are discussed under "Chronic Pancreatitis."

GALLSTONES. Gallstones may cause pancreatitis by impacting in the ampulla of Vater. The stones usually pass spontaneously into the duodenum, and small gallstones can be found in the stools of 92% of patients with gallstone pancreatitis. Persistent stone impaction can cause severe pancreatitis combined with ascending cholangitis. The incidence of gallstone-associated pancreatitis parallels

Table 141–1 ■ FACTORS ASSOCIATED WITH ACUTE PANCREATITIS

Obstructive Causes
Choledocholithiasis
Ampullary obstruction by tumor or sphincter of Oddi hypertension
Choledochocele
Periampullary duodenal diverticulum
Pancreas divisum (?); annular pancreas
Primary or metastatic pancreatic tumor
Parasites in pancreatic duct: *Clonorchis, Ascaris*
Toxins
Ethanol
Methanol
Organophosphorus insecticides
Scorpion venom (*Tityus trinitatis*)
Drugs
Definite association: azathioprine/6-mercaptopurine; valproic acid; estrogens; metronidazole; loop diruetics, including thiazides, furosemide, bumetanide; pentamidine; sulfonamides, including sulfasalazine; methyldopa; L-asparaginase; tetracyclines, cytarabine, dideoxyinosine
Probable association: chlorthalidone; mesalamine; ethacrynic acid; phenformin; angiotensin-converting enzyme inhibitors; nitrofurantoin; cocaine and amphetamine abuse; acetaminophen, cimetidine.
Metabolic Causes
Hypertriglyceridemia
Hypercalcemia
Trauma
Blunt abdominal trauma
Endoscopic retrograde cholangiopancreatographic procedures
Abdominal operations, cardiopulmonary bypass
Infections
Viral; mumps, coxsackie B, hepatitis A and B
Bacterial: Mycoplasma, Salmonella, Campylobacter jejuni
Vascular
Shock-hypoperfusion
Vasculitis
Cholesterol emboli
Miscellaneous
Penetrating duodenal ulcer
Organ transplantation
Crohn's disease of duodenum
Familial pancreatitis
Idiopathic

that of cholelithiasis: it peaks at ages 50 to 70, and women outnumber men by 2 to 1. As with other types of acute pancreatitis, chronic pancreatitis rarely results from multiple episodes of pancreatitis associated with gallstones. Pancreatitis during *pregnancy* usually occurs during the third trimester and is caused by gallstones in approximately 90% of instances.

DRUG-INDUCED PANCREATITIS. This complication characteristically occurs within the first 2 months of exposure; it is not dose related, and the pancreatitis usually is mild. Most commonly implicated are azathioprine/6-mercaptopurine, valproic acid in children, sulfur-containing diuretics, and pentamidine and dideoxyinosine in patients with the acquired immunodeficiency syndrome.

HYPERTRIGLYCERIDEMIA. The presence of lipemia, with serum triglyceride levels more than 1000 mg/dL, represents a cause, not an effect, of pancreatitis. Causes include estrogen therapy, alcoholism, intravenous lipid infusions, and primary hyperlipidemias.

MISCELLANEOUS FACTORS. *Acute hypercalcemia* may trigger acute pancreatitis during intravenous calcium infusions, during cardiopulmonary bypass, and with vitamin D poisoning. Blunt abdominal *trauma* causes pancreatitis by disrupting the duct; it is the most common cause of pancreatitis in children. *Postoperative* pancreatitis may follow intra- and extra-abdominal surgery and carries a high mortality rate of 25 to 50%. Patients after organ transplantation are at increased risk of acute and chronic pancreatitis. It is unclear whether this is entirely attributable to azathioprine/6-mercaptopurine therapy; infected pancreatic necrosis is common and the mortality is high. Pancreatitis after *endoscopic retrograde cholangiopancreatography (ERCP)* is usually mild unless it is complicated by duodenal perforation during endoscopic sphincterotomy. *Pancreatic infections* are an exceedingly rare and poorly documented cause of pancreatitis. Whether *pancreas divisum* predisposes to recurrent acute pancreatitis remains controversial. The available evidence favors the decision to proceed with surgical or endoscopic decompression of the dorsal pancreatic duct in these patients.

CLINICAL PRESENTATION. Steady, dull, or boring midepigastric pain associated with nausea and vomiting is the classic presentation of acute pancreatitis. The pain reaches peak intensity within 15 minutes to 1 hour from onset, in contrast to the more abrupt onset of pain with a perforated viscus. It radiates straight to the midline of the lower thoracic vertebral region in about 50% of patients and is usually worse in the supine position. Painless acute pancreatitis is very rare but carries a grave prognosis because the patients frequently present in shock.

Initial physical examination reveals mild fever and tachycardia; hypotension is present in 30 to 40% of patients. There is marked tenderness to deep palpation of the upper abdomen, but signs of peritoneal irritation are absent. Paralytic ileus with abdominal distention may develop during the first few days, signifying extension of the inflammatory process into the small intestinal and colonic mesentery. One to 2 weeks after the onset, large ecchymoses rarely appear in the flanks (Grey Turner's sign) or the umbilical area (Cullen's sign); these represent blood dissecting from the pancreas along fascial planes. Similarly, inflammatory masses, large fluid collections, or a pancreatic abscess may become palpable later in the course of the disease.

DIAGNOSIS. The diagnosis of acute pancreatitis rests on a combination of clinical, laboratory, and radiologic findings, none of which is infallible. The goals of diagnostic studies are to exclude other acute conditions that may require urgent surgical management; to assess the prognosis; to detect local and systemic complications early; and to identify a precipitating cause.

LABORATORY TESTS. AMYLASE. Total serum amylase activity is the test most frequently used to diagnose acute pancreatitis. The level rises 2 to 12 hours after onset of symptoms and remains elevated for 3 to 5 days in most cases. Values more than five times the upper limit of normal are highly specific for acute pancreatitis but are found in only 80 to 90% of cases. The magnitude of the rise in serum amylase does not correlate with the severity of the attack, nor does prolonged hyperamylasemia indicate developing complications. Marked hypertriglyceridemia, sufficient to give the serum a lipemic appearance, masks elevations in serum amylase and lipase; dilution of these sera lead to a paradoxical rise in the measured enzyme values. Separation of total serum amylase into its pancreatic (P) and salivary (S) isoenzymes and measurements of urinary amylase output add little to the diagnostic information. The

Levels may be similar to those in acute pancreatitis
Chronic pancreatitis; pancreatic pseudocyst; carcinoma of the pancreas; perforation of stomach, duodenum, jejunum; mesenteric infarction; brain and spinal cord injury.
Minor amylase and lipase elevations
Acute cholecystitis; burn injury; end-stage renal disease; acute and chronic alcohol abuse.
Isolated amylase elevation
Salivary adenitis; ovarian neoplasm; tubal pregnancy; metabolic acidosis; admission to an intensive care unit; acute hepatitis; anorexia nervosa; upper gastrointestinal endoscopy; incidental finding.

amylase-creatinine clearance ratio (ACR) (the ratio of amylase concentration in urine over plasma, divided by the corresponding values for creatinine) is useful in diagnosing asymptomatic macroamylasemia, in which aggregates of circulating amylase escape glomerular filtration and the ACR is abnormally low. Serum amylase levels may be elevated in many other clinical conditions (Table 141–2), illustrating the fact that the diagnosis of acute pancreatitis should not be based only on laboratory results.

Lipase. Serum lipase assays, especially those using colipase, have similar specificity and sensitivity as serum amylase. The serum lipase levels tend to remain elevated longer than the amylase levels during the healing phase of pancreatitis.

Combinations of Serum Enzyme Tests. The combination of serum amylase and lipase determinations is more accurate than either test alone (Table 141–3). The diagnostic accuracy can be improved further by calculating cut-off values that lie above the upper limit of normal. Serum immunoreactive cationic trypsin, elastase, and phospholipase A_2 do not improve the diagnostic information obtained from serum amylase and lipase values. Measurements of trypsin activation peptide and serum anionic trypsinogen promise increased diagnostic accuracy but are not widely available.

Other Blood Tests. Leukocytosis of up to 25,000 cells/mm^3 is present in 80% of patients; the hematocrit is frequently elevated due to hemoconcentration. Hypocalcemia occurs in up to 30% of patients due to a combination of hypoalbuminemia and calcium precipitation in areas of fat necrosis. The ionized calcium concentration remains normal, and symptoms of tetany are extremely rare. Pre-existing hypercalcemia may, however, be obscured by the calcium-lowering effect of pancreatitis. Transient, mild hyperglycemia is common and does not require insulin treatment. Serum triglyceride levels should be obtained in all patients because of their etiologic implications and to help interpret unexpectedly normal serum amylase and lipase levels. Elevated alanine aminotransferase (ALT) and alkaline phosphatase values suggest gallstone-associated pancreatitis (see later). The serum aspartate aminotransferase (AST) is elevated in approximately 50% of patients, owing to alcoholic liver disease or to the pancreatic inflammation itself.

IMAGING TESTS. Plain Films of the Abdomen. Plain films should be obtained routinely to rule out the presence of free air caused by perforation of a viscus and "thumbprinting" of the intestinal wall, suggesting mesenteric infarction. Changes caused by pancreatitis include localized ileus of a loop of jejunum ("sentinel loop"), generalized paralytic ileus, spasm of the transverse colon with absent colonic gas beyond ("colon cut-off sign"), and calcifications indicating the existence of underlying chronic pancreatitis.

Chest Radiographs. Pleural effusion and basilar atelectasis indicate diaphragmatic involvement by acute pancreatitis but are not necessarily confined to the left side. Interstitial fluffy infiltrates are the hallmark of the adult respiratory distress syndrome (see later). Barium contrast studies of the upper gastrointestinal tract are of little diagnostic value.

Abdominal Ultrasonography (US) and Computed Tomography (CT). US is the method of choice for detecting cholelithiasis and for

determining the diameter of the extrahepatic and intrahepatic bile ducts. Dilatation of these ducts suggests recent or persisting impaction of a stone in the distal common bile duct or the ampulla of Vater. US also very accurately detects acute cholecystitis. For the *diagnosis* of acute pancreatitis, an abdominal CT scan should be obtained only when clinical impression and laboratory results are conflicting; but when the clinical diagnosis is made, the CT scan is far superior to US for assessing the extent and local complications of pancreatitis. With rapid intravenous bolus injection of contrast material, a dynamic CT scan will reveal extension of peripancreatic inflammation, involvement of adjacent organs, venous thrombosis, and fluid collections. Most important, pancreatic necrosis can be identified and quantitated by the lack of contrast medium enhancement after the bolus injection. The abdominal CT scan may be normal, however, in about 10% of patients with early, mild pancreatitis.

DIFFERENTIAL DIAGNOSIS. There is no single absolute criterion for the diagnosis of acute pancreatitis. The differential diagnosis should focus on other conditions presenting with acute upper abdominal pain that require specific therapy, including perforated peptic ulcer, acute cholecystitis, and mesenteric vascular occlusion. A gallstone impacted in the ampulla of Vater may not only delay the resolution of biliary pancreatitis but also cause complicating ascending cholangitis and obstructive jaundice. The combination of positive US findings (gallstones or bile duct dilatation) with a positive biochemical score is indicative of this situation. A positive score consists of three or more of the following tests exceeding the stated limit: (1) alkaline phosphatase greater than upper limit of normal (ULN); (2) total bilirubin greater than ULN; (3) gamma glutamyltransferase greater than two times ULN; (4) ALT greater than one and one-half times ULN; and (5) ALT/AST greater than 1.0.

PROGNOSTIC ASSESSMENT. Several scoring systems predict the morbidity and mortality of acute pancreatitis attacks (Table 141–4), based on clinical and laboratory observations obtained during the first 48 hours after admission to the hospital. Examples include the Ranson and the modified Glasgow criteria developed specifically for pancreatitis and the APACHE II (Acute Physiology and Chronic Health Evaluation) and SAPS (Simplified Acute Physiology) scores. These scoring systems are only 70 to 80% accurate in predicting a mild or a severe course. Their use cannot replace the careful observation of the individual patient. Recent reports indicate that elevation of serum C-reactive protein to more than 120 mg/L is an accurate predictor for the development of pancreatic necrosis.

CLINICAL COURSE AND THERAPY. MILD PANCREATITIS. Mild acute pancreatitis is defined by the absence of systemic and local

Table 141–4 ■ ADVERSE PROGNOSTIC FACTORS IN ACUTE PANCREATITIS

RANSON'S CRITERIA* MAINLY ETHANOL-INDUCED	GLASGOW CRITERIA† ALL CAUSES
On Admission:	**Within 48 hours:**
Age > 55	Age > 55
WBC > 16,000/mm^3	WBC > 15,000/mm^3
Glucose > 200 mg/dL‡	Glucose > 180 mg/dL‡
LDH > 350 IU/L	LDH > 600 IU/L
AST > 250 IU/L	BUN > 45 mg/dL
	Albumin < 3.2 g/dL
Within 48 hours:	Calcium > 8 mg/dL
Hematocrit decrease > 10%	Arterial PO$_2$ < 60 mm Hg
BUN rise > 5 mg/dL	
Calcium < 8 mg/dL	
Arterial PO$_2$ < 60 mm Hg	
Base deficit > 4 mEq/L	
Fluid deficit > 6 L	

Three or more positive criteria predict a complicated clinical course; mortality rises when ≥ 4 criteria are met.
*Ranson JHC, Rifkind KM, Turner JW: Prognostic signs and nonoperative peritoneal lavage in acute pancreatitis. Surg Gynecol Obstet 143:209, 1976.
†Blamey SL, Imrie CW, O'Neill WH, et al: Prognostic factors in acute pancreatitis. Gut 25:1340, 1984.
‡No pre-existing hyperglycemia.
LDH = lactic dehydrogenase; AST = aspartate aminotransferase; BUN = blood urea nitrogen.

Table 141–3 ■ DIAGNOSIS OF ACUTE PANCREATITIS BY SERUM ENZYME ELEVATIONS IN PATIENTS WITH ACUTE ABDOMINAL PAIN

	AMYLASE	LIPASE	EITHER	BOTH
Sensitivity	80–90%	90%	95%	—
Specificity	70%	70%	—	90%

complications. About 80% of patients belong to this category and require less than 1 week of hospitalization. Treatment consists of general supportive care and close monitoring for signs of systemic complications; local complications tend to manifest during the second and third weeks of illness. The intravascular volume deficit may exceed 30% due to peripancreatic fluid sequestration and vomiting. Volume restoration must be rapid and efficient to maintain regular monitored urine output of more than 40 mL/hr. The patient receives nothing by mouth, with the goal of resting the pancreas. Nasogastric aspiration is indicated in the presence of vomiting or developing ileus; it need not be initiated routinely. The patient should receive sufficient analgesic medications to alleviate pain. Opiates should not be withheld because of their potential for raising the sphincter of Oddi pressure. They may, however, cause or worsen paralytic ileus. Neither total parenteral nutrition nor routine prophylactic antibiotic therapy is indicated. Small feedings of a high carbohydrate diet are begun once the pain has subsided and bowel sounds have reappeared.

SYSTEMIC COMPLICATIONS. Most systemic complications (Table 141–5) occur during the first week of illness and are treated by standard medical measures. Close patient monitoring is the key to their timely recognition. *Circulatory shock* arises by a combination of volume depletion and hyperdynamic circulatory state with decreased peripheral vascular resistance (see Chapter 94). The management includes transfer to an intensive-care unit, volume replacement, and vasopressor substances. The occurrence of shock is frequently followed by pancreatic necrosis. *Acute renal failure* may be caused by circulatory shock and a selective increase in renal vascular resistance. The treatment is that of acute tubular necrosis arising in any setting (see Chapter 103). The leading cause of respiratory insufficiency during acute pancreatitis is the *adult respiratory distress syndrome,* although respiratory depression caused by opiate medications, pleural effusions, intravascular volume overload, and shallow respirations due to abdominal "splinting" may contribute. The pathogenesis probably involves damage to the pulmonary surfactant layer by circulating phospholipase A and free fatty acids. *Sepsis* is most commonly caused by infection of the bile ducts, of areas of pancreatic necrosis, or of peripancreatic fluid collections (see later).

LOCAL COMPLICATIONS. *Ascending cholangitis* and severe biliary pancreatitis present overlapping features and may coexist. Gram-negative bacteremia and spiking fevers are more common with infection of the biliary tract, whereas hyperbilirubinemia may be mild or absent in both situations. Appropriate antibiotic therapy should be instituted (e.g., gentamicin, ampicillin, and metronidazole) (see Chapter 157). The main therapeutic objective is to clear the gallstones without delay.

Pancreatic Necrosis. Pancreatic necrosis is found by dynamic CT in approximately 80% of patients (16% of the total) with clinically severe disease, usually during the second or third week of illness (Fig. 141–3) but is present in approximately 40% of patients within 4 days of symptom onset. Pancreatic necrosis resolves without incident in nearly 60% of patients who develop it. Therapy and prognosis of the severely ill patient depend crucially on whether the necrotic tissue is infected (Fig. 141–4). This question should be answered by fine-needle aspiration of necrotic areas under CT guidance. A Gram stain of the aspirate is more than 95% accurate in predicting the final results of bacterial cultures. The bacteria represent enteric flora that gained access to mesenteric lymphatics by

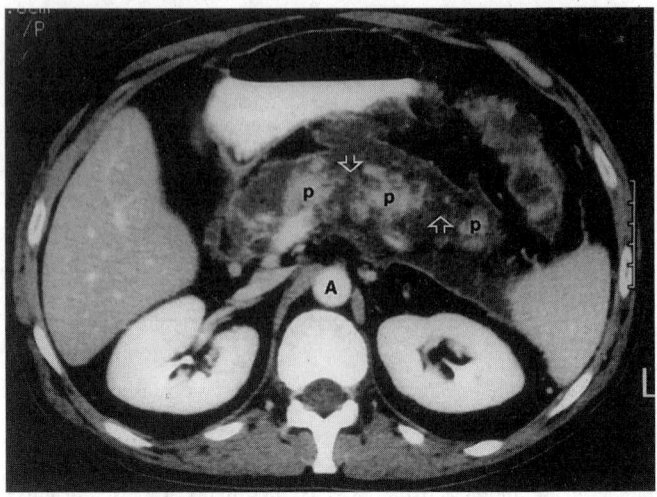

FIGURE 141–3 ■ Dynamic CT scan of patient with pancreatic necrosis. Interposed between normally perfused portions of the pancreas (p) are nonperfused necrotic areas (arrows). The pancreas is surrounded by fluid in the retroperitoneum, which extends into the small bowel mesentery. A = contrast medium–enhanced aorta. Failure of tissue enhancement during bolus injection with rapid scanning outlines areas of necrosis. (From Sleisenger MH, Fordtran JS [eds]: Gastrointestinal Disease, 5th ed. Philadelphia, WB Saunders, 1993, p 1642.)

translocating across the colonic mucosa. Antibiotics with high penetration into pancreatic tissue include the fluoroquinolones, imipenem/cilastatin, and metronidazole. The mortality of patients with *infected* pancreatic necrosis treated conservatively is 60 to 100%. Immediately removing necrotic tissue (necrosectomy), combined with continued lavage of the necrotic space, lowers the mortality to about 20%, but patients frequently require re-operation for continuing necrosis and other local complications, such as bleeding and fistula formation. The management of patients with *sterile* pancreatic necrosis remains controversial. Repeat CT with fine-needle aspiration reveals the later development of infection in over 40% of these patients. Prophylactic intravenous antibiotic therapy (e.g., ofloxacin, 200 mg twice daily plus metronidazole 500 mg twice daily) appears to decrease the risk of conversion to infected pancreatic necrosis and, thus, of mortality.

Fluid Collections. Fluid collections occur within or around the pancreas in up to 50% of patients with severe pancreatitis. The majority resolve spontaneously; collections that persist for more than 6 weeks develop a wall of granulation tissue and are then called pseudocysts (see "Chronic Pancreatitis"). Collections that continue to expand or become infected require percutaneous drainage. *Pancreatic abscesses* contain liquid pus and may be considered to represent infected fluid collections. The presence of extraluminal gas bubbles on radiographs or CT is a specific but rare clue

Table 141–5 ■ COMPLICATIONS OF ACUTE PANCREATITIS

SYSTEMIC	LOCAL
Circulatory shock	*Impacted common bile duct stones*
Respiratory insufficiency	Pancreatic necrosis ± *infection*
Acute renal failure	Fluid collections ± *infection*
Sepsis	*Pancreatic abscess*
Coagulopathy (DIC)	*Colonic necrosis*
Hyperglycemia	*Bleeding*
Hypocalcemia	Splenic vein thrombosis
	Splenic necrosis

Conditions in italics are life-threatening; they require prompt recognition and management.
DIC = disseminated intravascular coagulation.

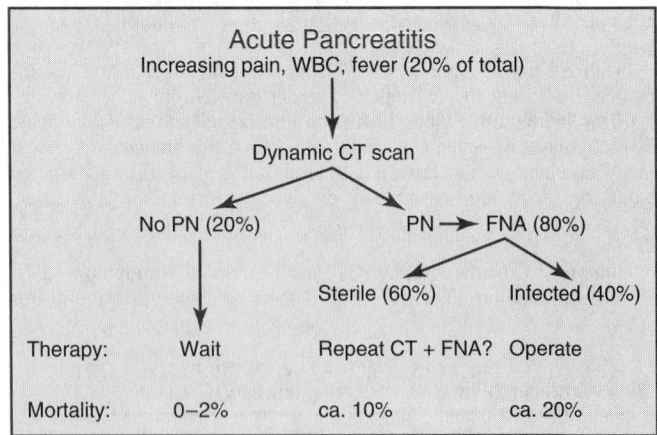

FIGURE 141–4 ■ Management and prognosis of severe acute pancreatitis. PN = pancreatic necrosis; FNA = fine-needle aspiration of necrotic areas under CT guidance with Gram stain and culture of aspirate.

to their presence. *Pancreatic ascites* reflects involvement of peritoneal surfaces by the inflammatory process and, rarely, the rupture of a pancreatic duct with pancreatic juice entering into the peritoneal cavity. There are several causes of *bleeding* during acute pancreatitis. Hemorrhage may occur into necrotic intrapancreatic and peripancreatic tissue and into fluid collections. Brisk hemorrhage occurs with erosion of the splenic or gastroduodenal arteries. At times, the blood gains access to a disrupted pancreatic duct and empties into the duodenum. Diffuse mucosal bleeding from the antrum and duodenum is common but rarely severe. Finally, bleeding may signal perforation of peripancreatic inflammation into any portion of the gastrointestinal tract from esophagus to colon. The spleen may become involved by direct extension of the inflammatory process or, secondarily, by splenic vein thrombosis. The latter complication leads to gastric fundic varices.

PREVENTING RECURRENCES. The search for the precipitating cause begins during the acute attack. Serum calcium and triglyceride levels are determined and the medication list is reviewed (see Table 141–1). An abdominal US examination is performed routinely. If gallstones are detected, the patient should undergo early cholecystectomy, preferably before discharge from the hospital. The absence of choledocholithiasis must be ascertained before or during this surgical procedure. At this stage, approximately 20% of patients are assumed to have idiopathic pancreatitis. After a second attack, ERCP with sphincter of Oddi manometry should be performed and will identify correctable obstructive causes of the pancreatitis attack in approximately one third of patients. Bile aspirated from the common bile duct or the duodenum from the remaining patients should undergo microscopic analysis. Cholesterol crystals, calcium bilirubinate granules, or microspheroliths may be detected, and the majority of these patients will develop biliary "sludge" or gallstones on serial US examinations. Treatment options include cholecystectomy, endoscopic papillotomy, or oral dissolution therapy with bile acids. This systematic search for obstructive causes of acute pancreatitis leaves only 5 to 10% of patients designated as having "idiopathic pancreatitis."

CHRONIC PANCREATITIS

DEFINITION AND PATHOGENESIS. Chronic pancreatitis is marked by progressive fibrosis, leading to loss of exocrine and endocrine (islets of Langerhans) tissue and irregular dilatation of pancreatic ductal structures (Table 141–6). Episodes of acute pancreatitis may be interspersed, especially during the early years of alcoholic pancreatitis. *Chronic calcifying pancreatitis* is the most common form, by far. It is characterized by irregular distribution within the gland with varying degrees of obstruction of the primary and secondary pancreatic ducts. The initiating event may be fibrillar proteins precipitating in small pancreatic duct branches; these protein plugs calcify by surface accretion. Later on, similar lamellar protein precipitates form in the major pancreatic duct and calcify as well. The plugs and concretions cause acinar atrophy, chronic inflammation with metaplasia of the ductal epithelium, periductal fibrosis, and irregular dilatation of major and secondary pancreatic ducts. The initiating event may be deficient acinar secretion of lithostathine, a protein that inhibits calcium precipitation from the supersaturated pancreatic juice. Alternatively, lithostathine may undergo proteolytic cleavage that yields an insoluble residue, LH_1, that forms fibrillar precipitates and no longer keeps calcium in solution. *Chronic obstructive pancreatitis* is caused by obstruction of the main pancreatic duct and leads to uniform dilatation of the duct system, rarely accompanied by protein plugs and intraductal calcifications.

ETIOLOGIC ASSOCIATIONS. ALCOHOL. Fully 70 to 80% of patients with chronic pancreatitis are chronic alcohol abusers. Alcoholic pancreatitis, even when it presents as an acute episode, is a chronic, progressive disease. Typically, the initial symptoms appear at ages 35 to 45, but some patients may experience their first attack before age 25. Alcoholic liver disease develops in 40 to 50% of patients and frequently becomes manifest 5 to 10 years after the onset of pancreatitis. Alcohol abstinence offers moderate and unpredictable benefits in terms of pain relief and the later development of diabetes mellitus but does not alter the progression of pancreatic fibrosis and exocrine insufficiency. The mechanism of alcohol-induced pancreatic injury remains unknown.

TROPICAL PANCREATITIS. Calcific chronic pancreatitis occurs in children and young adults in certain tropical areas, including southern India, Indonesia, and Central Africa. Although abdominal pain is common, the diagnosis is frequently made on the basis of newly discovered diabetes or pancreatic calcifications. Although malnutrition is suspected to play a role, this form of chronic pancreatitis is not found in other areas where malnutrition is equally common. There is no relationship to alcohol consumption.

HEREDITARY PANCREATITIS. Pancreatitis inherited as an autosomal dominant trait with 40 to 80% penetrance accounts for approximately 2% of patients with chronic pancreatitis. Episodes of abdominal pain usually start at ages 5 to 12. The *etiology* is amino acid substitutions in the cationic trypsin molecule. Families with hereditary pancreatitis have reduced degradation of trypsin, so active trypsin accumulates within the pancreas and causes repeated acute attacks and ultimately chronic pancreatitis.

SENILE PANCREATITIS/ATROPHY. Ten to 20% of patients with chronic pancreatitis are older than 60 at initial presentation. Pancreatic calcifications and malabsorption are common, but pain is commonly absent. Smoking and obesity, but not alcohol abuse, have been implicated. Senile atrophy and lipomatosis of the pancreas probably represent the same poorly understood entity. The clinical course is benign and generally non-progressive.

METABOLIC CAUSES. Chronic pancreatitis develops in up to 15% of patients with primary hyperparathyroidism and frequently is clinically silent. Hyperlipidemia and renal transplantation are rare causes of chronic pancreatitis.

OBSTRUCTION. Obstruction of the pancreatic duct by tumors, post-traumatic strictures, pancreatic duct calculi, or a "tight" minor papilla in patients with pancreas divisum may lead to chronic pancreatitis. The progression of the disease is halted when the obstructing lesion can be removed.

IDIOPATHIC. The remaining 10 to 25% of patients are in the "idiopathic" category. They present the full spectrum of the disease, from mild functional disturbances to advanced calcific disease. Notably, gallstone-associated acute pancreatitis is not a cause of chronic pancreatitis.

CLINICAL PRESENTATION AND COURSE. In approximately 40% of patients, chronic pancreatitis initially presents with episodes that are indistinguishable from acute pancreatitis. Insidious onset of pain heralds the disease in another 40%, and malabsorption, diabetes, or complications of chronic pancreatitis lead to the diagnosis in the remainder. Pain is minor or absent in 7 to 15% of patients during the course of the disease.

PAIN. Pain is intermittent or chronic; it is boring and dull, often accompanied by nausea and vomiting. It is perceived in the epigastrium and/or the left and right subcostal areas and radiates straight through to the back in approximately one half of patients. Pain may be aggravated by eating and on the day after a drinking bout. Pancreatic pain fibers pass through the celiac plexus and the paravertebral sympathetic ganglia. Events that may trigger the pain of chronic pancreatitis are raised intraductal and pancreatic parenchymal pressure due to ductal obstruction and perineural inflammation with fibrosis. Pain is the predominant symptom; it may keep the patient from work, impair social and family relationships, and frustrate attempts at abstaining from alcohol. Spontaneous pain relief occurs in approximately 60% of patients within 6 to 12 years after the onset of symptoms. Pancreatic calcifications, diabetes mellitus, and malabsorption frequently appear when the pain begins to diminish.

Table 141–6 ■ **ETIOLOGIC ASSOCIATIONS WITH CHRONIC PANCREATITIS**

Chronic Calcifying Pancreatitis
Chronic alcoholism
Tropical pancreatitis
Hereditary
Senile/pancreatic atrophy
Metabolic: hypercalcemia, hyperlipemia, post–renal transplant
Idiopathic
Obstructive Chronic Pancreatitis
Tumors
Duct strictures
Pancreas divisum (?)

Note: Hereditary isolated pancreatic enzyme deficiencies, congenital pancreatic insufficiency with neutropenia, and cystic fibrosis are separate nosologic entities.

WEIGHT LOSS. Weight loss is common during the course of the disease. Contributing causes include anorexia caused by pain or analgesics, funds being spent on alcohol rather than food, untreated diabetes, and malabsorption due to pancreatic exocrine insufficiency. Malabsorption develops in about 40% of patients, usually 5 to 10 years after the onset of pain. Most patients can compensate for weight loss due to malabsorption by increasing their food intake.

DIABETES MELLITUS. Progressive loss of islets of Langerhans eventually leads to diabetes in 70% of patients, half of whom require insulin treatment. Patients with chronic pancreatitis and diabetes are at increased risk of hypoglycemia because of concomitant glucagon deficiency, poor dietary habits, and the hypoglycemic effects of alcohol.

CARCINOMA. The incidence of adenocarcinoma of the pancreas is increased in chronic pancreatitis, particularly the hereditary type. Early diagnosis is rarely possible and the prognosis is dismal.

MORTALITY. The 10-year survival is 65% in alcoholics and 80% in patients with non-alcoholic chronic pancreatitis. Only 10 to 20% of deaths are directly related to the disease. Major contributors to the excess mortality are extrapancreatic and pancreatic carcinoma, hypoglycemia, and the effects of alcoholism.

DIAGNOSIS. IMAGING STUDIES. Plain anteroposterior and oblique views of the abdomen may reveal localized or diffuse intraductal calcifications of the pancreas. Abdominal CT may detect small calcifications missed on plain radiographs, dilatation of the main pancreatic duct, and pseudocysts. Differentiation from cancer of the pancreas may be difficult. Early in the course, ERCP may show blunting and dilatation of pancreatic duct branches, but the pancreatogram may be normal in up to 10% of patients. The main value of ERCP is to identify potentially correctable lesions, such as large ductal stones, pseudocysts, and duct strictures. Endoscopic US may detect early stages of the disease.

BLOOD TESTS. Serum amylase and lipase concentrations frequently remain normal during attacks of pain. Serum levels of pancreatic isoamylase and trypsin may be decreased, but these changes are not sufficiently reliable for the early diagnosis of chronic pancreatitis.

PANCREATIC FUNCTION TESTS. The so-called secretin test is the most sensitive test for chronic pancreatitis. Duodenal contents are aspirated after the intravenous administration of secretin ± cholecystokinin or cerulein. The calculated pancreatic output of bicarbonate and enzymes is decreased in approximately 85% of patients, and the test accuracy is 87%. In the simpler Lundh test, trypsin concentration is determined in the proximal jejunum after a liquid test meal. Both tests are time consuming, and neither is widely used.

OTHER TESTS. The bentiromide (NBT-PABA) test assesses intestinal tryptic activity by quantitating the urinary excretion of *p*-amino benzoic acid after oral dosing with the test compound. This test and measurement of stool chymotrypsin concentration are reliably abnormal only with advanced pancreatic insufficiency. Vitamin B_{12} absorption may be impaired due to decreased liberation of this vitamin bound to gastric R-proteins by duodenal trypsin (see Chapter 163). An abnormal Schilling test of vitamin B_{12} (cobalamin) absorption that corrects with administration of pancreatic enzymes is a specific, but not a sensitive, test for chronic pancreatitis. Clinical vitamin B_{12} deficiency develops rarely.

SEQUENCE OF TESTS. Diagnosis depends on symptoms, tests of pancreatic function, and radiologic studies, including ERCP. In general, the documentation of any two of these three manifestations is sufficient for making the diagnosis. An example is the presence of pancreatic calcifications on a plain film of the abdomen in a patient with chronic upper abdominal pain. Abdominal CT frequently provides additional information regarding the presence and possible complications of chronic pancreatitis. Two diagnostic dilemmas generally require expert consultation. The first is to rule out early, mild chronic pancreatitis. Because neither the duodenal secretin test nor the ERCP examination is 100% sensitive, both tests plus endoscopic US may have to be performed. The second is to differentiate chronic pancreatitis from adenocarcinoma or a cystic tumor of the pancreas. When imaging methods, cytologic testing of percutaneous aspirates from a pancreatic mass, and diagnostic

laparoscopy fail to provide the answer, surgical exploration and resection may be required.

THERAPY. PAIN. Control of abdominal pain is the most important and difficult task in treating chronic pancreatitis. Narcotics are frequently required and should not be withheld because of concerns about evolving addiction and concomitant alcoholism. Acute attacks of pain require hospitalization with no oral intake, parenteral analgesics, and renewed efforts at achieving abstinence from alcohol. The rationale for a trial of pancreatic enzymes is the inhibition of cholecystokinin release by intraduodenal trypsin, leading to decreased meal-stimulated pancreatic secretion. Non–enteric-coated preparations of pancrelipase should be used, such as Viokase, Cotazyme, or Ilozyme, at doses of 6 tablets per meal. Concomitant suppression of gastric acid secretion with an H_2-receptor blocker is advisable to minimize the destruction of the enzyme supplement at low gastric pH. Pain relief has been reported in some patients with mild non-alcoholic chronic pancreatitis, that is, without pancreatic calcifications or steatorrhea. Percutaneous destruction of the celiac plexus by alcohol or phenol injection reduces pain in approximately 60% of patients, but the effect is transient and the procedure has potential complications.

Patients with intractable chronic or intermittent pain should be considered for a surgical procedure based on ERCP and CT evaluation of the duct system. When the pancreatic duct is dilated to 8 mm or more in diameter, decompression may be attempted by endoscopic stent placement across the ampulla of Vater. Most patients, however, require permanent duct decompression by longitudinal pancreaticojejunostomy. In the absence of a dilated pancreatic duct, partial pancreatectomy, such as pancreaticoduodenectomy (Whipple procedure), can be performed when severe changes are confined to the head of the pancreas. When expertly performed and limited to patients who abstain from alcohol, these operations relieve pain in approximately 70% of patients.

MALABSORPTION. Malabsorption is a late manifestation of chronic pancreatitis and occurs when pancreatic secretion of digestive enzymes is reduced by 90% or more. Fat malabsorption due to lipase deficiency is the predominant abnormality. The condition is documented by a stool fat content of more than 7 g/d (steatorrhea). The indication for treatment is weight loss that cannot be corrected by increasing the caloric intake. Reducing or eliminating steatorrhea is difficult to achieve due to the low potency of available porcine pancreatic extracts and their irreversible denaturation at gastric pH values of less than 4. Enzymes can be taken as described earlier. Alternatively, enteric-coated enzyme preparations such as Pancrease or Creon, which are released only in the alkaline milieu of the duodenum, can be prescribed in doses of two to three capsules per meal.

COMPLICATIONS. PSEUDOCYSTS. Pancreatic pseudocysts contain high concentrations of pancreatic enzymes and are encapsulated by a rim of chronic inflammation and fibrosis; they are without an epithelial lining. Pseudocysts may represent fluid collections that developed during acute pancreatitis but failed to resolve over a period of 6 to 8 weeks. More commonly, they result from obstruction of small pancreatic ducts, a type of retention cyst formed during the course of chronic pancreatitis. Pseudocysts are located within or around the pancreas but may dissect retroperitoneally to the mediastinum or pelvis; pseudocysts in the head of the pancreas may compress the common bile duct. Pseudocysts can be diagnosed by abdominal US, CT, or endoscopic US, but their differentiation from rare uniloculated pancreatic cystic neoplasms is difficult. One or more pseudocysts appear in up to 60% of patients with chronic pancreatitis. Life-threatening but rare complications include infection, hemorrhage into the cystic space, and rupture of the pseudocyst. The contribution of a pseudocyst to the pain of chronic pancreatitis is difficult to assess. Treatment should be considered for large pseudocysts (>5 cm in diameter). Internal drainage into the stomach, duodenum, or jejunum yields excellent results. Successful treatment by percutaneous or endoscopic aspiration and drainage for several weeks has also been reported.

PANCREATIC ASCITES. Ascites and pleural effusions during the course of chronic pancreatitis are the result of leakage from a disrupted pancreatic duct. The amylase and lipase content is many times higher than in the blood. The majority of these patients require surgical correction of the leak by providing drainage into a loop of jejunum or by partial pancreatectomy.

OBSTRUCTION OF ADJACENT ORGANS. Several structures adjacent to the pancreas may become obstructed by fibrosis or a developing pseudocyst. *Common bile duct obstruction* with slowly developing jaundice requires a biliary-enteric drainage procedure to prevent the development of secondary biliary cirrhosis and ascending cholangitis. *Gastric outlet obstruction* can be bypassed by a gastrojejunostomy; a vagotomy should be added. *Compression or thrombosis of the splenic vein* leads to gastric fundic varices that may bleed; splenectomy is curative.

Fernandez-del Castillo C, Rattner DW, Makary MA, et al: Debridement and closed packing for the treatment of necrotizing pancreatitis. Ann Surg 228:676, 1998. *An account of the complexity and management problems presented by necrotizing acute pancreatitis.*

Gorry MC, Gabbaizedeh D, Furey W, et al: Mutations in the cationic trypsinogen gene are associated with recurrent acute and chronic pancreatitis. Gastroenterology 113: 1063, 1997. *Identification of the second single nucleotide mutation in families with hereditary pancreatitis. The mutations predict resistance of active trypsin to autodegradation within the pancreas.*

142 DISEASES OF THE PERITONEUM, MESENTERY, AND OMENTUM

Michael R. Lucey

PERITONEAL DISORDERS

Abdominal pain and ascites are characteristic clinical features in disorders of the peritoneum.

Ascites

Ascites, the accumulation of serous fluid in the peritoneal cavity, has many causes (Table 142–1). More than 90% of cases of ascites are due to portal hypertension, usually as a result of cirrhosis (see Chapter 153). Perhaps half of the remainder, i.e., 5% of all cases of ascites, are due to peritoneal disease.

CLINICAL FEATURES OF ASCITES. Increasing abdominal girth and rapid weight gain are the most common symptoms associated with new-onset ascites. Dullness in the flanks when the patient is supine, shifting dullness during percussion of the abdomen, and a fluid wave are useful clinical signs to detect ascites, but volumes smaller than 1500 mL are often clinically undetectable. When it is clinically important to confirm the presence of suspected ascites, sonography or computed tomographic (CT) scanning of the abdomen is advisable.

The investigation of new-onset ascites, especially if unexplained by standard clinical examination and tests, should always include paracentesis (Table 142–2). Ascitic fluid can be examined for biochemical content and cytology and sent for culture. In specific cases, such as suspected tubercular peritonitis, biopsy of the peritoneum during laparoscopy is valuable (see below).

The mechanism of ascites formation in portal hypertension is complex (see Chapter 153) and includes such factors as altered Starling forces in the portal circulation (increased portal venous hydrostatic pressure, reduced portal venous oncotic pressure), altered renal sodium handling, and increased hepatic and possibly splanchnic lymph formation. Portal oncotic pressure is reduced in cirrhotic patients because of hypoalbuminemia, which is due to hepatic synthetic failure. In contrast, obstructed outflow of normal lymphatics appears to be a principal causative factor in the development of ascites secondary to peritoneal carcinomatosis or malignant chylous ascites.

Medical management using diuretics and salt restriction is often effective in patients with portal hypertension. Conversely, ascites caused by peritoneal inflammation or malignancy alone does not respond to salt restriction and diuretics.

In the past, portal hypertensive ascites was distinguished from other forms of ascites by determining whether the ascitic fluid was a transudate or an exudate. This concept assumes that in portal hypertension, protein-poor ascitic fluid *transudes* from the normal peritoneal surface, whereas in peritoneal disease such as peritoneal

Table 142–1 ■ CAUSES OF ASCITES

CAUSES OF ASCITES	COMMENTS
Portal hypertension	
Cirrhosis	Accounts for 80% of ascites in the United States
Fulminant hepatic failure	Rarely causes ascites
Hepatic outflow obstruction	Ascites is a characteristic clinical feature of hepatic outflow obstruction
Congestive heart failure	
Constrictive/restrictive cardiomyopathy	
Budd-Chiari syndrome—hepatic vein and/or IVC occlusion	Most commonly associated with an underlying thrombotic disorder
Veno-occlusive disease	Important cause of ascites in bone marrow transplant recipients
Portal vein occlusion	Rarely causes ascites
Malignancy	Accounts for 10% of ascites in the United States. Peritoneal carcinomatosis causes 50% of malignant ascites
Infection	
Peritoneal tuberculosis	See Tables 142–6 and 142–7
Fitz-Hugh–Curtis syndrome	Perihepatitis associated with fibrous perihepatic exudate usually due to *Neisseria gonorrhoeae* or *Chlamydia trachomatis*
Infectious peritonitis in HIV-infected patients	
Renal	
Nephrotic syndrome	Covert cirrhosis should be excluded
Nephrogenous in hemodialysis recipients	Covert cirrhosis should be excluded
Endocrine	
Myxedema	
Meigs' syndrome	
Strauma ovarii	
Ovarian stimulation syndrome	
Pancreatic Ascites	Associated with pancreatitis, raised ascitic amylase concentration
Biliary Leak	Previous surgery, including laparoscopic cholecystectomy, gangrenous gallbladder, trauma, percutaneous liver biopsy
Urine ascites	Urinary leak into the peritoneum
Systemic lupus erythematosus	
Miscellaneous	Idiopathic chronic non-specific peritonitis in HIV-infected patients
Mixed causes	See text

IVC = inferior vena cava; HIV = human immunodeficiency virus.

inflammation or malignancy, protein-rich ascitic fluid *exudes* from the abnormal peritoneal surface. Consequently, ascitic fluid with a protein content greater than 2.5 g/dL was designated an exudate, and fluid with a protein content less than 2.5 g/dL was termed a transudate. However, the transudate-exudate characterization is flawed because many patients with spontaneous bacterial peritonitis (SBP), in which ascitic fluid is infected, nonetheless have low ascitic fluid protein rather than the expected high protein content (see below) and many samples of ascites from portal hypertension secondary to cardiac failure have a high protein content rather than the expected low protein content.

The preferred method to distinguish ascites associated with portal hypertension from other forms of ascites is the serum-ascites albumin gradient, which is calculated by subtracting the ascitic albumin concentration from the serum albumin concentration. Ascites associated with portal hypertension has a serum-ascites albumin gradient greater than 1.1 g/dL, whereas ascites caused by peritoneal inflammation or malignancy has a serum-ascites albumin gradient less than 1.1 g/dL (Table 142–3). Many patients have more than one potential cause of ascites, so-called mixed ascites, such as cirrhosis and peritoneal tuberculosis; the serum-ascites albumin gra-

Table 142–2 ■ DIAGNOSTIC TESTS IN ASCITES

FEATURE	DIAGNOSIS	ASCITIC WHITE BLOOD CELL COUNT (per mm³)	ASCITIC RED BLOOD CELL COUNT	CYTOLOGY (% POSITIVE NEOPLASTIC CELLS)	BIOCHEMICAL ANALYSIS	SERUM-ASCITES ALBUMIN GRADIENT (g/dL)	COMMENTS
Portal hypertension	Cirrhosis	<250 PMN	Few or none	0	Protein usually <2.5 g/dL	>1.1	—
	SBP	>250 PMN	Few or none	0	Albumin <1 g/dL	>1.1	—
	Cardiac ascites	<250 PMN	Few or none	0	Protein >2.5 g/dL	>1.1	—
Malignancy	Peritoneal carcinomatosis	75% have >500	Few or none	100	Protein usually >2.5 g/dL	<1.1	—
	MHM	Usually <500	Few or none	0	Protein variable	>1.1	Serum alkaline phosphatase ≥350 mU/mL
	Peritoneal carcinomatosis plus MHM	Variable, usually elevated	Few or none	~80	Protein content variable	>1.1	Serum alkaline phosphatase ≥350 mU/mL
	Malignant chylous ascites	Often >300	Few or none	0	Triglycerides >200 mg/dL	Usually <1.1	—
	Hepatoma plus ascites	Often >500	Commonly increased	0		>1.1	Elevated serum α-fetoprotein
Infection	Tuberculous peritonitis	80% >500, predominantly lymphocytes	Frequently present	0	Ascitic adenosine deaminase ≥32.3 U/L or LDH >90 μ/L	50% have >1.1 (i.e., may have cirrhosis)	See Table 142–6
Miscellaneous	Pancreatic ascites	Frequently increased		0	Ascitic amylase greatly increased	Variable	—

PMN = polymorphonuclear leukocytes; SBP = spontaneous bacterial peritonitis; MHM = massive hepatic metastases; LDH = lactate dehydrogenase.

dient usually reflects the presence of portal hypertension even when other causes of ascites are also present.

Portal hypertensive ascites that fails to respond to salt restriction and diuretics is termed refractory ascites. Serial large-volume paracentesis is the simplest approach to management. The value of intravenous infusions of albumin to counter the volume contraction caused by paracentesis is controversial but reasonable in patients with accompanying renal insufficiency, defined as a serum creatinine content greater than 1.5 mg/dL. Rapid removal of ascitic fluid occasionally results in peritoneal hemorrhage. Placement of a transjugular intrahepatic portosystemic shunt also improves ascitic control in cirrhotic patients with refractory ascites, albeit with the risks of encephalopathy and decompensation in hepatic function associated with this procedure.

MALIGNANT ASCITES. Malignant ascites constitutes a small fraction of all cases of ascites and represents a heterogeneous group of disorders and mechanisms. Peritoneal carcinomatosis, the most common form of malignant ascites, arises from primary peritoneal disease such as mesothelioma or from the metastatic spread of a wide variety of malignant processes (Table 142–4). On occasion, in addition to malignant studding of the peritoneum, a tumor also produces massive hepatic metastases sufficient to cause portal hypertension. Whenever ascites is due to malignant infiltration of the peritoneum, either alone or accompanied by massive hepatic metastases, shedding of malignant cells into the ascites is almost invariable (see Table 142–2). In contrast, massive hepatic metastases without peritoneal studding or multilocular primary hepatocellular carcinoma arising in a cirrhotic liver rarely cause shedding of malignant cells into the ascitic fluid. Thus cytologic analysis of the ascitic fluid is extremely valuable when attempting to identify peritoneal malignancy. Mesothelioma is an exception to this rule because it produces cytologic results that are often difficult to interpret.

The serum-ascites albumin gradient in malignant ascites reflects the presence or absence of portal hypertension. Therefore, the serum-ascites gradient is low in patients with peritoneal carcinomatosis and normal portal pressure, whereas ascites associated with massive hepatic metastases irrespective of peritoneal studding or with primary hepatocellular carcinoma arising in a cirrhotic liver is associated with a serum-ascites albumin gradient greater than 1.1 g/dL, which reflects the presence of portal hypertension. The underlying cause of malignant ascites is determined after a thorough clini-

Table 142–3 ■ CLASSIFICATIONS OF ASCITES BY SERUM-ASCITES ALBUMIN CONCENTRATION GRADIENT

HIGH GRADIENT (>1.1 g/dL)	LOW GRADIENT (<1.1 g/dL)
Cirrhosis	Peritoneal carcinomatosis
Alcoholic hepatitis	TB peritonitis (without cirrhosis)
Congestive restrictive heart failure	Pancreatic ascites (without cirrhosis)
Massive hepatic metastases	Bile leak
Fulminant hepatic failure	Nephrotic syndrome
Budd-Chiari syndrome	Systemic lupus erythematosus
Veno-occlusive disease	Bowel obstruction or infarction
Portal vein occlusion	
Acute fatty liver of pregnancy	
Myxedema	

TB = tuberculous.

Table 142–4 ■ CAUSES OF PERITONEAL CARCINOMATOSIS

Primary disorders of the peritoneum
 Mesothelioma
Metastatic spread from
 Gastrointestinal tumors
  Stomach
  Colon
  Pancreas
 Other intra-abdominal organs
  Ovary
  Pseudomyxoma peritonei
 Extra-abdominal primary tumors
  Breast
  Lung
 Hematologic malignancy
  Lymphoma

cal evaluation, which often includes laboratory tests and imaging procedures; for example, massive hepatic metastases are invariably associated with a marked elevation in serum alkaline phosphatase, usually greater than 350 IU/mL.

The presence of ascites with positive neoplastic cytologic findings indicating peritoneal carcinomatosis signifies an expected survival of 6 months or less. Therapy is palliative. In certain causes, such as mesothelioma, instilling antitumor agents into the peritoneal cavity may be part of a therapeutic program directed against the underlying tumor. Diuretics and salt restriction are ineffective in controlling ascites caused by peritoneal carcinomatosis. Serial paracentesis is the simplest method to control symptomatic malignant ascites. Occasionally, a peritoneovenous shunt may provide valuable, albeit temporary palliation. When malignant ascites is associated with portal hypertension, the prognosis is always poor. Salt restriction and diuretics may effectively control the ascites; when diuretics are ineffective, serial paracentesis is often the best method for rapid palliation.

CHYLOUS ASCITES. Chylous ascites is milky in appearance because of leakage of lymph into the peritoneal cavity; the triglyceride concentration is markedly elevated, always greater than 200 mg/dL and often greater than 1000 mg/dL. New-onset chylous ascites is most often due to underlying malignancy, especially lymphoma. Occasionally, chylous ascites occurs after trauma, intra-abdominal surgery, heart failure, and peritoneal infection such as tuberculosis (TB). Rarely, it occurs as an incidental unexplained finding in cirrhotic patients. Except in cases of known trauma, investigation is focused on identifying an underlying malignant process, even though malignant chylous ascites rarely contains malignant cells (see Table 142–2). Appropriate tests include abdominal CT or magnetic resonance imaging (MRI) and bone marrow aspiration. Lymphangiography does not identify intra-abdominal lymphadenopathy when CT or MRI has failed to do so. Chylous ascites, whether of malignant or benign origin, responds poorly to salt restriction or diuretics, except in rare idiopathic cases associated with cirrhosis and portal hypertension. Paracentesis offers simple palliative therapy. In the majority of cases, treatment is directed at the underlying lymphoma. Fat in the diet can be replaced with medium-chain triglycerides that are absorbed directly into the portal blood stream and bypass the lymphatics. Occasional patients may be placed on a regimen of total parenteral nutrition to reduce the formation of chylous ascites.

PANCREATIC ASCITES. Pancreatic ascites is due to leakage of pancreatic juice into the peritoneal cavity. It occurs in patients after pancreatitis when a pseudocyst ruptures into the peritoneum and causes pancreatic ascites (see Chapter 141). Because alcohol is a frequent cause of pancreatitis and is the most common cause of chronic liver failure, it may be difficult to distinguish pancreatic ascites secondary to alcoholic pancreatitis from ascites secondary to alcoholic cirrhosis in someone with concomitant alcoholic pancreatitis. Paracentesis reveals a high serum-ascites albumin gradient in the presence of portal hypertensive ascites, which suggests cirrhosis rather than pancreatitis as the source of ascites, or a very elevated amylase concentration, usually considerably greater than the serum level (see Table 142–2) in pancreatic ascites. In pancreatic ascites, the ascitic amylase concentration remains elevated even after the serum level declines toward normal. Endoscopic retrograde cholangiopancreatography is useful in pancreatic ascites, especially in trauma cases, to identify a disrupted pancreatic duct. Surgery to drain the pseudocyst and repair the duct is necessary in traumatic pancreatic ascites, but a conservative approach is often adopted in alcoholic and other non-traumatic cases.

ENDOCRINE ASCITES. In rare circumstances, ascites is a principal manifestation of an endocrine disorder. Examples include myxedema (which causes an elevated serum-ascites albumin gradient), struma ovarii, Meigs' syndrome (see Chapter 86) with ascites and pleural effusion caused by benign ovarian neoplasms, and ovarian overstimulation syndrome, which occurs in women receiving fertility-enhancing drugs such as clomiphene citrate, human chorionic gonadotropin, human menopausal gonadotropin, follicle-stimulating hormones, and luteinizing hormone–releasing hormone.

RENAL ASCITES. Nephrotic syndrome is a rare cause of ascites in the absence of liver disease when the serum albumin concentration falls below 2.0 g/dL. However, whenever this diagnosis is considered, a careful search for underlying liver disease is mandatory. Hepatitis B surface antigen and anti–hepatitis C antibodies

(see Chapters 149 and 150) should be measured because hepatitis B or C may produce glomerulonephritis as well as cirrhosis and the resulting ascites may be due to any combination of portal hypertension, poor albumin synthesis, and renal albumin wasting.

CONNECTIVE TISSUE DISORDERS. Occasionally, systemic lupus erythematosus is associated with the development of ascites in the absence of liver disease and portal hypertension. The ascites may respond to therapy for the underlying disease.

ASCITES IN HIV-INFECTED PATIENTS. When new-onset ascites occurs in patients with acquired immune deficiency syndrome (AIDS), causes of portal hypertension such as alcoholism or chronic viral hepatitis should be sought. Other sources of ascites in patients with AIDS include abdominal lymphoma, Kaposi's sarcoma, or peritoneal infection. Among the infections reported to cause ascites in human immunodeficiency virus (HIV)-infected patients are TB, *Mycobacterium avium* complex, cryptococcal disease, and coccidioidomycosis. Patients with a reduced peripheral CD4+ count may have ascites secondary to intestinal perforation or acute appendicitis without other more typical features of intestinal catastrophe. In addition, ascites develops in some HIV-infected patients as a result of a chronic non-specific peritonitis for which no infectious or malignant cause is identified.

Acute Peritonitis

DEFINITION. Acute peritonitis is inflammation of the peritoneum or peritoneal fluid from bacteria or intestinal contents (including gastric acid, gastrointestinal luminal contents, bile, or pancreatic juice) in the peritoneal cavity. Secondary peritonitis results from any definable cause, such as perforation of a viscus owing to acute appendicitis or diverticulitis, perforation of an ulcer (peptic ulcer, Crohn's disease, malignancy), and trauma, including iatrogenic intervention (e.g., surgery, needle biopsies). Primary peritonitis, including SBP, refers to peritonitis arising without a recognizable preceding cause. Tertiary peritonitis, which is persistent intra-abdominal sepsis without a discrete focus of infection, generally follows surgical treatment of prior severe peritonitis and occurs in severely ill patients in intensive care, especially patients who are immunosuppressed.

PROGNOSTIC FACTORS. Peritonitis after acute appendicitis or a perforated peptic ulcer occurring in an otherwise healthy patient is associated with a low mortality, whereas peritonitis after elective surgery, trauma, or pancreatitis has a high mortality irrespective of the patient's overall clinical setting. The prognosis for severe peritonitis has not changed in the past 50 years despite the advent of broad-spectrum antibiotics, critical care units, and radical approaches to eliminate bacterial contamination of the peritoneal cavity. The outcome in severe peritonitis is dictated by the patient's overall health, including nutritional status, immunocompetence, and systemic factors such as cardiac and renal function.

CLINICAL FEATURES. The classic features of acute peritonitis are abdominal pain, abdominal tenderness, and the absence of bowel sounds. Severe, sudden-onset abdominal pain suggests a ruptured viscus. The clinical signs of peritoneal irritation include abdominal tenderness, rebound tenderness, and eventually, abdominal rigidity. In florid cases, these signs and symptoms are accompanied by fever, hypotension, tachycardia, and acidosis. Although this clinical pattern is characteristic, acute peritonitis may frequently lack these features. For example, SBP arising in ascites is often very subtle in manifestation (see below). Acute peritonitis arising in elderly or immunosuppressed patients may lack the features of peritoneal irritation or systemic decompensation. Similarly, in patients with tertiary peritonitis, classic signs and symptoms may be absent or suppressed and the diagnosis suggested only by persistent leukocytosis or fever. In these atypical circumstances, a high index of suspicion is necessary.

DIAGNOSIS. Plain abdominal radiographs can determine the presence of free air in the abdominal cavity, a characteristic finding of a perforated viscus. CT and/or ultrasonography can identify the presence of free fluid or an abscess. When peritonitis is associated with ascites, paracentesis is mandatory (see Table 142–2).

THERAPY. The three key elements of therapy for acute peritonitis are resuscitation, laparotomy, and antibiotics. Resuscitation with intravenous fluids and correction of metabolic and electrolyte disturbances are the initial steps. Laparotomy is a cornerstone of therapy for secondary or tertiary acute peritonitis to identify and repair the cause of the acute catastrophe, to evacuate pus, and to irrigate the peritoneal cavity. In some patients, when biliary peritonitis is accompanied by little systemic disturbance, careful conservative management with intravenous fluids and broad-spectrum antibiotics is adequate, and laparotomy can be avoided. However, the threshold for proceeding to laparotomy should be low, even in these circumstances. Broad-spectrum systemic antibiotics are critical to cover bowel flora, including anaerobic species (see Chapter 157). When peritonitis persists despite all standard measures, antifungal agents (such as amphotericin B or fluconazole) are appropriate for possible candidal infections.

Spontaneous Bacterial Peritonitis

DEFINITION. SBP, which has no obvious precipitating cause, occurs almost exclusively in cirrhotic patients but may occasionally complicate acute hepatic failure. SBP is a marker of severe hepatic failure and usually occurs in patients with low ascitic protein content and elevated serum bilirubin. For example, SBP develops in approximately 25% of patients with an ascitic fluid total protein content of less than 1 g/dL during 3 years of subsequent observation. The mechanism of SBP development is related to deficient opsonic activity in ascitic fluid. The offending organisms are almost always enteric gram-negative aerobes such as *Escherichia coli* or *Klebsiella pneumoniae* or gram-positive aerobes, particularly *Streptococcus pneumoniae*. Anaerobic organisms rarely cause SBP.

CLINICAL FEATURES. The clinical manifestation of SBP is often subtle. It must be suspected not only whenever a cirrhotic patient has fever and abdominal pain more typical of acute peritonitis but also whenever a cirrhotic patient with ascites has a sudden deterioration in hepatic or renal function, worsening malaise, encephalopathy, or unexplained persistent leukocytosis, even in the absence of abdominal signs or symptoms typical of acute peritonitis. A high index of suspicion is also necessary whenever a patient with known established liver disease has features of sepsis or hepatic deterioration despite the absence of clinical ascites; small pockets of infected ascites may be present and detectable only by ultrasound or CT scan, and a presumptive diagnosis of SBP followed by empirical antibiotic therapy may be the wisest course.

DIAGNOSIS. The key to establishing SBP is diagnostic paracentesis in which the ascitic fluid is found to have 250 or more polymorphonuclear (PMN) cells per cubic millimeter. A very elevated PMN cell count in ascites (for example, >5000/mm³) suggests an intra-abdominal abscess or a secondary cause of peritonitis. Demonstrating an organism in the ascitic fluid is helpful but not required for diagnosis. The chances of identifying an organism in ascites are enhanced by directly transferring ascitic fluid to blood culture media bottles before incubation, but even then no organism is identified in 30 to 50% of cases. SBP is usually caused by a single species, so multiple organisms on ascitic culture suggest a perforated viscus. In addition to inspecting and culturing ascitic fluid, all patients suspected of having SBP should have blood cultures, chest radiography, and urine microscopy and culture to identify blood-borne sepsis and to look for additional sites of infection.

THERAPY. Antibiotics are the cornerstone of managing SBP, and laparotomy has no place in therapy for SBP. Three to 5 days of intravenous treatment with broad-spectrum antibiotics is usually adequate, at which time efficacy can be determined by estimating

Table 142–5 ■ **RISK FACTORS FOR INTRA-ABDOMINAL TUBERCULOSIS**

HIV infection
Immunosuppressive therapy
Advanced age
Intravenous drug use/alcoholism/cirrhosis
Immigration from an endemic area
Poverty
Incarceration/long-stay care
Peritoneal dialysis

Table 142–6 ■ **CLINICAL CHARACTERISTICS OF PERITONEAL TUBERCULOSIS* (%)**

Ascites	80–100
Abdominal swelling	65–100
Abdominal pain	36–93
Weight loss	37–87
Fever	56–100
Diarrhea	9–27
Abdominal tenderness	65–87
Anemia	46–68
Positive PPD test	55–100

PPD = purified protein derivative.

*The percentages represent the frequency with which these features have been observed in peritoneal tuberculosis. These data antedate studies of TB in HIV-infected persons.

the ascitic fluid PMN cell count; the use of intravenous antibiotics can be discontinued if the count is less than 250/mm³. The most important negative prognostic factors are the presence of renal failure, onset of SBP while in the hospital, and elevated serum aminotransferase levels.

SBP recurs in 70% of patients in the first year after their initial episode unless prophylactic antibiotics are used. The frequency of recurrence is greatest in patients with a low ascitic fluid total protein content and impaired hepatic synthetic function. The incidence of SBP can be markedly reduced, both in patients who are at risk for a first episode and in those who have already had SBP, with prophylactic antibiotics that cleanse the gut microflora, such as quinolones (norfloxacin once per day or ciprofloxacin once per week) or trimethoprim-sulfamethoxazole. Although prophylaxis reduces the incidence of SBP, mortality is related to the underlying hepatic dysfunction and is not affected.

Peritoneal Tuberculosis

TB is an important cause of peritonitis worldwide and, with advent of the AIDS epidemic, has re-emerged in the developed world (Table 142–5). Patients with peritoneal TB frequently have concomitant cirrhosis, which may incorrectly be implicated as the source of ascites and obscure the presence of tuberculous peritonitis. The serum-ascites albumin gradient is low in patients with peritoneal TB without portal hypertension or cirrhosis, but it is variably high or low in cirrhotic patients with TB. TB in HIV-infected patients is characterized by newly acquired infection rather than a recrudescence of quiescent infection, a high likelihood of TB among at-risk persons who are exposed to TB, a high rate of clinical rather than quiescent TB, rapidly progressive TB that frequently has extrapulmonary involvement, and, finally, the emergence of TB strains that are resistant to one or more of the standard antituberculous chemotherapeutic agents.

CLINICAL FEATURES. Ascites is almost invariable, whereas abdominal swelling and pain are common (Table 142–6). Many patients have accompanying systemic signs and symptoms such as fever, weight loss, and anemia.

DIAGNOSIS. Paracentesis reveals a lymphocytosis but rarely shows acid-fast bacilli on smear (Table 142–7). Culture of ascitic fluid has a somewhat higher diagnostic yield, but with a 4- to 6-week delay; the potential immediate value of molecular diagnostic

Table 142–7 ■ **DIAGNOSTIC TESTS OF PERITONEAL TUBERCULOSIS**

DIAGNOSTIC TEST	COMMENT
Paracentesis	
With smear	<3% positive
With culture	<20–80% positive
With ascitic ADA measurement	≥32.3 U/L. Low ascitic protein (i.e., cirrhosis) may cause false negatives. Not validated in U.S. patients
With LDH ≥90 U/L	
Laparoscopy with biopsy	Best test
	Up to 100% positive
Needle biopsy of the peritoneum	Largely replaced by laparoscopy
Diagnostic laparotomy	Should be considered if laparoscopy not available

ADA = adenosine deaminase; LDH = lactate dehydrogenase.

MESENTERY
Primary inflammatory diseases
   Mesenteric panniculitis
   Retractile mesenteritis
Mesenteric cysts
   Embryonic
   Traumatic/acquired
   Neoplastic
   Infective
Mesenteric tumors
   Benign: Lipoma, hemangioma, leiomyoma, ganglioneuroma, fibroma
      (Gardner's syndrome)
   Malignant: Various sarcomas; metastatic tumors
Mesenteric vascular insufficiency
   Acute
   Chronic
Tumor
   Benign: Fibroma, lipoma, hemangioma, neuroma, lymphangioma,
      leiomyoma, mesothelioma
   Malignant: Primary metastases—especially ovary, stomach, colon
Cysts
Vascular insufficiency
   Torsion
   Infarction
Inflammation: Usually secondary to peritonitis

methods has not yet been defined. An elevated ascitic concentration of adenosine deaminase, a marker of T-lymphocyte and macrophage activation, has been reported to be a sensitive and specific diagnostic test for tuberculous peritonitis in developing countries where laparoscopy and other diagnostic tests are scarce; however, the value of adenosine deaminase in diagnosing tuberculous peritonitis in the United States is less clear. An ascitic fluid lactate dehydrogenase level greater than 90 U/L may be a useful indicator of peritoneal TB irrespective of the presence of cirrhosis and portal hypertension. A definitive diagnosis of peritoneal TB is best made by laparoscopy and directed peritoneal biopsy. The occasional patient with fibroadhesive tuberculous peritonitis without ascites should not undergo laparoscopy.

THERAPY. Treatment of tuberculous peritonitis involves standard protocols using two or three drugs, usually for 9 months. All TB isolates must be tested for drug susceptibility. HIV-infected persons who are co-infected with a strain of TB that is susceptible to first-line chemotherapeutic agents usually respond well to standard therapeutic protocols, but HIV-infected persons with resistant strains have a high mortality.

Peritonitis in Continuous Ambulatory Peritoneal Dialysis

Infection in the washout dialysate is common in patients undergoing continuous ambulatory peritoneal dialysis, often unaccompanied by systemic disturbance and characterized by mild abdominal pain and low-grade fever. Cytologic analysis of the cloudy effluent shows a high white cell count. The great majority of causative organisms are gram-positive, especially *Staphylococcus epidermidis*, followed by *Staphylococcus aureus* and streptococci. Treatment should be begun promptly after recognizing a cloudy effluent even before culture results are available. Treatment consists of infusing broad-spectrum antibiotics into the peritoneum through the abdominal wall catheter; the catheter is not removed, and dialysis is not interrupted. For the minority of patients who fail to respond to prompt outpatient therapy, intravenous antibiotics and catheter removal are necessary.

Miscellaneous Forms of Peritonitis

In familial Mediterranean fever, the most common recurring feature is peritonitis, which affects more than 90% of symptomatic patients. It is manifested as episodic abdominal pain and fever. Colchicine may reduce the frequency and severity of attacks.

DISEASES OF THE MESENTERY AND OMENTUM

Mesenteric panniculitis and retractile mesenteritis (Table 142–8) may represent different manifestations of the same rare idiopathic disorder. Mesenteric panniculitis consists of diffuse fatty infiltration

of the mesentery, which is then replaced by fat necrosis, fibrosis, and calcification. Retractile mesenteritis is at the fibrotic end of this spectrum. Patients with these conditions have intermittent abdominal pain, abdominal swelling, and an abdominal mass. However, many patients are asymptomatic. The diagnosis is usually made at laparotomy; once recognized, surgical resection should not be undertaken unless the fibrosis is causing intestinal obstruction.

Cysts and tumors, including desmoid mesenteric fibromas that are part of Gardner's syndrome, are also rarely seen. Rare diseases of the omentum include mass lesions, acute vascular insufficiency from torsion or infarction, and inflammatory processes.

Ochs A, Rossle M, Haag K, et al: The transjugular intrahepatic portosystemic stent-shunt procedure for refractory ascites. N Engl J Med 332:1192, 1995. *A useful intervention in selected cases.*
Runyon BA: Care of the patient with ascites. N Engl J Med 330:337, 1994. *A superb clinical review of ascites management.*
Saab S, Rickman LS, Lyche KD: Ascites in the acquired immunodeficiency syndrome. Report of 54 cases. Medicine (Baltimore) 75:131, 1996. *Largest series to review ascites in patients with AIDS.*
Shakil AO, Korula J, Kanel GC, et al: Diagnostic features of tuberculous peritonitis in the absence and presence of chronic liver disease: A case control study. Am J Med 100:179, 1996. *A useful approach to the diagnostic challenge.*

143 DISEASES OF THE RECTUM AND ANUS

Theodore R. Schrock

ANATOMY

The rectum and anus fuse over a zone several centimeters long, and together these structures are termed the *anorectum* (Fig. 143–1). The distal anal canal is lined by modified skin (anoderm), the epithelium of the upper anal canal is columnar, and the transitional zone (cuboidal epithelium) lies between the two. The anoderm is exquisitely sensitive, but the upper anal canal is relatively insensitive.

At the dentate line, an important site of pathologic problems, anal papillae project into the lumen. Flaps of skin connecting anal papillae are termed *anal valves;* behind these valves lie anal crypts, each containing in its depths an anal gland.

The internal anal sphincter is the thickened lower portion of the circular smooth muscle layer of the gut. This involuntary muscle is encircled by skeletal muscle bundles comprising the external sphincters. The levators ani form the muscular floor of the pelvis. One of the levators, the puborectalis, passes around the rectum as a sling and is easily palpable posteriorly on digital rectal examination.

EXAMINATION OF THE ANORECTUM

The anorectum is examined with the patient in the left lateral decubitus position or in the prone jackknife position, if a special table is available for that purpose. Good lighting is essential. The buttocks are retracted to expose the anal orifice. Digital rectal examination is performed. Anoscopy is required to evaluate the anal canal thoroughly. Rigid or flexible sigmoidoscopy completes the examination in some patients, but others (e.g., those with bleeding) need colonoscopy or a barium enema.

HEMORRHOIDS

Hemorrhoids are masses of areolar tissue containing numerous small arteries and veins. These congenital vascular cushions are located above the dentate line and are termed *internal hemorrhoids*. External hemorrhoids are dilated vessels below the dentate line; they rarely cause symptoms by themselves, but they are enlarged in association with prolapsing internal hemorrhoids.

Intrarectal pressure pushes hemorrhoids downward, the anchoring

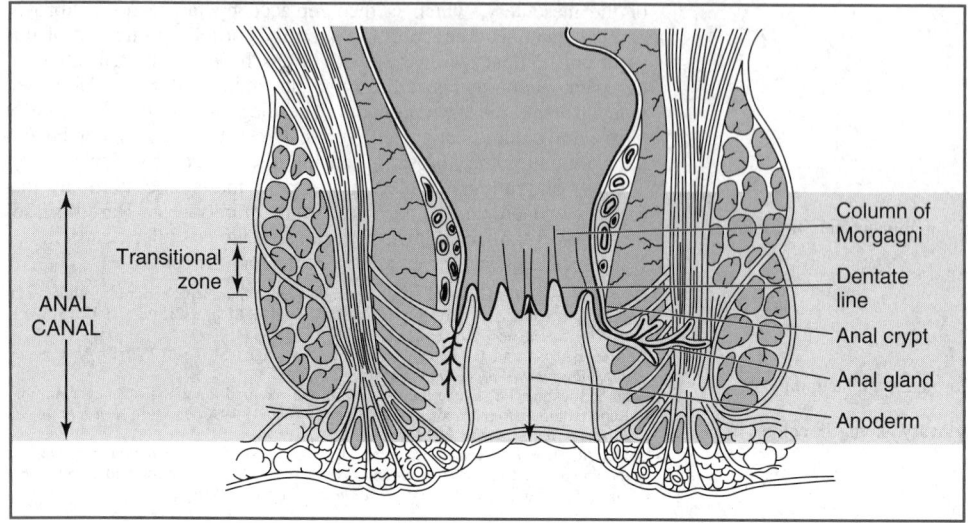

ANAL
CANAL

Transitional
zone

Column of
Morgagni

Dentate
line

Anal crypt

Anal gland

Anoderm

FIGURE 143–1 ■ The lining of the anal canal. (Redrawn from Goldberg SM, Gordon PH, Nivatvongs S: Essentials of Anorectal Surgery. Philadelphia. JB Lippincott, 1980. Used by permission.)

fibromuscular structures attenuate, and the tissues congest, bleed, and eventually prolapse. Small hemorrhoids that protrude a short distance into the anal canal are first-degree hemorrhoids. Second-degree hemorrhoids prolapse but reduce spontaneously. Third-degree hemorrhoids must be manually reduced, and fourth-degree hemorrhoids are irreducible. Internal hemorrhoids occur in three primary locations: right posterior, right anterior, and left lateral.

Bleeding and *prolapse* are the most common symptoms of internal hemorrhoids. Blood is typically bright red, and it may spurt or drip from the anus. Nonspecific discomfort is noted, but pain is usually caused by some other associated condition such as fissure or abscess.

Anoscopy reveals a mass of tissue above the dentate line; large hemorrhoids prolapse to the outside as the anoscope is withdrawn. Differential diagnosis includes skin tags, hypertrophied anal papillae, and rectal prolapse.

Acute prolapse with thrombosis of internal hemorrhoids is severely painful. The entire circumference of the anus appears to protrude, and there is extreme pain from the edema and inflammation.

Initial treatment of internal hemorrhoids involves a high-bulk diet and avoiding prolonged sitting at stool. Proprietary remedies have little benefit. Small bleeding hemorrhoids can be treated by a "fixation procedure" that promotes adherence of the vascular cushions to the underlying sphincter. These outpatient procedures require no anesthetic. One popular method is injecting a sclerosing agent (e.g., 5% phenol in oil) into the submucosa of the hemorrhoid above the dentate line. This painless injection evokes fibrosis and eventual adherence of the sliding mucosa. Another method is rubber band ligation, in which tiny bands are slipped over each internal hemorrhoid using a special instrument. The banded tissue sloughs and fixation results. Photocoagulation using an infrared device is also effective. Lasers can be used for the same purpose, but they are more expensive and more hazardous. Electrocoagulation with a bipolar electrode or a direct current device and thermocoagulation with a "heater probe" are alternatives. All of these procedures have the same objective and are similarly effective.

Fourth-degree hemorrhoids with large external components do not respond to fixation procedures, and if the symptoms warrant, hemorrhoidectomy is advised. Surgical excision can be performed in an outpatient setting. Results are good, although the operation is painful and there is loss of time from work. Complications are uncommon, and recurrences are unusual.

A *thrombosed external hemorrhoid* is a blood clot within a complex of subcutaneous external veins. This problem develops in young adults, often related to heavy exercise. A painful bluish mass is present at the anal verge. If pain does not subside after 48 hours, the thrombosed hemorrhoid can be excised under local anesthesia.

ANAL FISSURE

Anal fissure (fissure in ano, anal ulcer) is a tear in the anoderm just inside the anal verge. Acute fissures are common, but in some patients the tiny laceration does not heal and it becomes chronic. Severe pain with defecation and spots of blood on the toilet tissue are the symptoms.

The diagnosis is made by inspection. Pain is so severe that the patient may not tolerate digital rectal examination. Lateral traction on the buttocks exposes the fissure in nearly every instance. Acute fissures are red, but chronic fissures may have eroded completely through the anoderm to expose the white fibers of the internal sphincter in the base. The fissure triad seen in chronic lesions includes the fissure, an edematous sentinel tag at the anal verge, and a hypertrophied anal papilla at the dentate line.

Fissures are located in the posterior midline in 98% of men and 90% of women. The remaining fissures are in the anterior midline. A fissure off the midline should raise a suspicion of cancer, Crohn's disease, or a sexually transmitted infection.

Measures to improve bulk and softness of stools are important, and sitz baths are soothing. Acute fissures usually heal. Chronic fissures may require lateral subcutaneous internal anal sphincterotomy. This simple procedure reduces pressure in the anal canal and allows the fissure to heal. The long-term cure rate is greater than 95%. Topical application of nitroglycerine and injection of botulinum toxin (BoTox) are new and experimental terms of therapy.

ANORECTAL ABSCESS

Infections arising in anal glands at the dentate line may develop into abscesses in the adjacent tissue spaces (Fig. 143–2). Abscesses near the skin surface cause throbbing pain that is worse with walking. Deeper abscesses may produce insidious symptoms, including abdominal pain. Patients with large abscesses are febrile. An indurated tender mass is apparent on examination in a patient with a perianal or ischiorectal abscess, and the anus is pushed to one side. Intersphincteric abscesses are invisible on the outside, but they are palpable as a firm, tender area on digital rectal examination. Supralevator abscesses are also palpable.

Prompt surgical incision and drainage are required. A neglected abscess may extend, and necrotizing infections can be lethal. Abscesses in immunocompromised patients pose special problems, and standard treatment may not be appropriate. Pelvic computed tomography may be useful in assessing the extent of disease in these patients.

ANORECTAL FISTULAS

A hollow fibrous tract lined by granulation tissue develops after an anorectal abscess is spontaneously or surgically drained. The

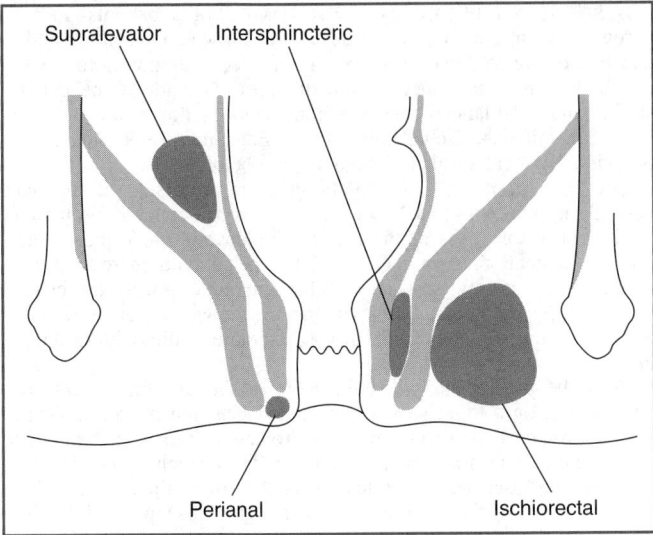

FIGURE 143-2 ■ Classification of anorectal abscesses. (Redrawn from Gordon PH: Management of anorectal abscesses and fistulous disease. *In* Kodner IJ, Fry RD, Roe JP [eds]: Colon, Rectal and Anal Surgery. St. Louis, CV Mosby, 1986.)

primary orifice is usually at the dentate line where the infection originated. The secondary orifice is most often external at the site of drainage. The patient has pus, blood, mucus, and discomfort. One or more reddish papules on the perianal skin mark the sites of secondary openings. Gentle pressure may produce a drop of pus from the orifice. A firm tract may be palpated with a well-lubricated finger as it travels from the secondary orifice toward the anal verge.

Anoscopy reveals the primary opening; a hooked probe confirms its patency. At times it is difficult to identify the primary orifice. Goodsall's rule describes the usual relationship of primary and secondary fistula orifices (Fig. 143–3). Crohn's disease, carcinoma, tuberculosis, and chlamydial infections should be considered in the differential diagnosis. Proctosigmoidoscopy is done routinely, and barium studies or even colonoscopy may be indicated in some cases.

Fistulas do not heal spontaneously, and an operation is required (fistulotomy). The tissue overlying the tract is incised and the base

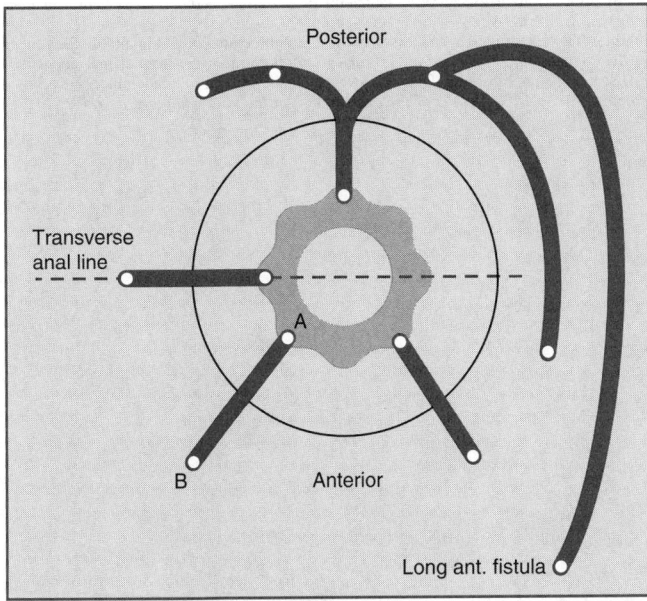

FIGURE 143-3 ■ Goodsall's rule indicates the usual relationship of primary (*A*) and secondary (*B*) fistula orifices. The long anterior fistula is an exception to the rule. (Redrawn from Schrock TR: *In* Fromm D [ed]: Gastrointestinal Surgery. New York, Churchill Livingstone, 1985. Used by permission.)

is curetted. The defect heals secondarily. High fistulas encompass important sphincters and require special techniques.

Rectovaginal fistulas most commonly result from childbirth injuries. Fecal incontinence may be associated. The patient complains of passage of flatus and occasionally feces through the vagina. Surgical repair is usually successful.

PRURITUS ANI

Pruritus ani is perianal itching. It is a symptom, not a diagnosis, and the causes are many and varied. Responsible conditions include anorectal diseases, dermatologic diseases, contact dermatitis, infections by bacteria or fungi, parasites, oral antibiotics, systemic diseases (e.g., diabetes), poor or excessively zealous hygiene, warmth and moisture, dietary intolerance (coffee, cola, tomatoes, chocolate), and psychological problems. Leakage of mucus or tiny amounts of stool onto the perianal skin is perhaps the most frequent cause of pruritus, and usually there is no significant sphincter defect.

A thorough history should be obtained. Examination may disclose no abnormality, or at the other extreme there may be moist, macerated, excoriated perianal skin. Dermatologic diseases should be looked for elsewhere on the trunk and extremities. Parasites are rare.

If a specific cause of pruritus is identified, appropriate therapy is given. Antibiotics should be stopped, topical agents discontinued, and diet modified. Cleansing after defecation should be accomplished with moist cotton followed by gentle drying. Non-medicated talcum powder is applied to combat moisture. A small bit of cotton applied to the anal verge may absorb excess moisture. More severe cases may require application of corticosteroid creams.

Other causes of anorectal pain are discussed in Chapter 131.

SEXUALLY TRANSMITTED DISEASES

Homosexually active men have a high incidence of anorectal infections, and women who practice anal intercourse also are at risk for developing these conditions.

CONDYLOMATA ACUMINATA. These warts are caused by human papillomaviruses, usually types 6 and 11. They are small, discrete excrescences on the perianal skin, on the anoderm, or just above the dentate line. In the last location they are pink and velvety, but on the skin they are pearly white. Pruritus and bleeding are common symptoms. Condylomata are treated by applying 25% podophyllin in tincture of benzoin, fulguration with electrocautery devices, or surgical excision.

GONOCOCCAL PROCTITIS. This involves the mucosa of the upper anal canal and rectum. Pain, frequent defecation, and purulent bloody discharge are symptoms. The rectal mucosa is edematous and friable with ulcerations and thick pus. Cultures confirm the diagnosis, but treatment may be warranted even if the cultures are negative (see Chapter 362).

SYPHILIS. The primary lesion of anorectal syphilis is an ulcer. Mild symptoms resolve as the lesion heals in a few weeks. Secondary lesions are multiple plaques with a white odorous discharge (see Chapter 365).

CHLAMYDIA TRACHOMATIS PROCTITIS. *Chlamydia trachomatis* is the most common sexually transmitted bacterial pathogen in the United States today (see Chapter 370). Three immuno-types of this organism cause lymphogranuloma venereum, which resembles Crohn's disease. Tetracycline is the treatment of choice after culture confirms the organism.

DISORDERS OF THE PELVIC FLOOR

Disorders of the pelvic floor are a group of conditions arising from abnormal structure or function of the levators ani and anal sphincters.

FECAL INCONTINENCE. Fecal incontinence has many causes (Table 143–1). Partial incontinence is occasional loss of flatus or loose stool, and major incontinence is abnormal control of stool of normal consistency. Thorough history should be obtained. The anus may be deformed and gaping, and an obvious anatomic defect may be visible and palpable. In other instances the structures seem

Table 143–1 ■ CAUSES OF FECAL INCONTINENCE

Normal sphincters and pelvic floor
   Diarrhea
   Fistula
Abnormal function of sphincters and/or pelvic floor
   Minor incontinence
      Deficient internal sphincter
         Trauma
         Rectal prolapse
         Third-degree hemorrhoids
      Fecal impaction
         Advanced age
         Neurologic disorders
      Minor external sphincter and pelvic floor denervation
   Major incontinence
      Congenital anomalies
      Trauma
      Complete rectal prolapse
      Rectal carcinoma
      Anorectal infection
      Idiopathic
      Drug intoxication
      Neurologic
      Upper motor neuron
         Cerebral
         Spinal
      Lower motor neuron

Modified from Henry MM, Swash M (eds): Coloproctology and the Pelvic Floor: Pathophysiology and Management, Boston, Butterworths, 1985.

intact but function is inadequate. Special investigations include anorectal manometry and electromyography.

The underlying systemic intestinal disorder, if any, should be treated. Loose stools are managed with bulk agents and constipating drugs. Elderly patients who soil because of fecal impaction may need regular laxatives and/or enemas. Biofeedback may be of benefit in patients with organic neuromuscular impairment. Surgical repair is successful for traumatically disrupted sphincters.

SOLITARY RECTAL ULCER SYNDROME. Solitary rectal ulcer syndrome is a chronic, benign condition characterized by anal pain, bleeding, mucous discharge, and obsessive straining to defecate. It affects mainly young women. Excessive straining forces the anterior rectal mucosa downward where it becomes traumatized.

On examination the anterior rectal mucosa 8 to 10 cm above the anal verge is indurated and may be grossly ulcerated. Biopsies confirm the diagnosis. Treatment should be directed toward avoiding straining by educating the patient and using bulk agents. Unfortunately, current methods of therapy are often disappointing, and patients must live with the chronic condition. Surgical repairs are unsatisfactory unless the patient has a true rectal prolapse.

DESCENDING PERINEUM SYNDROME. Some patients, mostly parous women, complain of a sense of incomplete evacuation and a constant desire to defecate. They are, in effect, attempting to evacuate their own rectal mucosa. The diagnosis is made if the patient strains and the plane of the perineum balloons downward below a line connecting the ischial tuberosities. Education, bulk agents, and occasionally local surgical procedures are helpful.

RECTAL PROLAPSE. Partial prolapse is protrusion of the mucosa alone, and complete rectal prolapse (procidentia) is protrusion of the entire thickness of the rectum. Prolapse is much more common in women than in men, and it appears with increasing frequency after age 40. Surgical or other traumatic injuries are causative in a few patients, but laxity of the pelvic musculature as a result of aging or neurologic disease is more commonly responsible.

With the patient sitting on the edge of the examining table or, even better, on a toilet seat, straining produces the prolapse. Mucosal prolapse is a small symmetrical projection 2 to 4 cm long with radial folds. True procidentia may protrude as much as 12 cm from the anus, and the mucosal folds are concentric. Palpation reveals a large mass of tissue anteriorly. Proctosigmoidoscopy and barium enema are required.

Procidentia must be repaired surgically to avoid further weakening of the anal sphincters. Repairs can be accomplished abdominally or through the perineum, depending on the circumstances. Mucosal prolapse is managed by fixation procedures or excision, as described for hemorrhoids.

MALIGNANT TUMORS OF THE ANUS

Epidermoid carcinomas of the anus are uncommon (2% of cancers of the large bowel). Human papillomavirus is etiologically linked to anal cancer. Anal carcinoma may extend directly into the sphincters, perianal tissues, vagina, or prostate, and it tends to metastasize to lymph nodes behind the rectum and in the groins. Bleeding, pain, and a mass are the usual complaints. Often symptoms are mistakenly attributed to hemorrhoids until examination reveals the lesion. Biopsy provides proof. A combination of radiation therapy and chemotherapy is the first line of treatment and is followed by local or radical surgical excision if the tumor is not controlled. Overall 5-year survival rates of 60% are expected.

Bowen's disease is chronic squamous cell carcinoma in situ. Local excision is required to prevent progression to invasive cancer. Extramammary *Paget's disease* is an intraepithelial mucinous adenocarcinoma. It is treated by wide local excision but tends to recur locally and can metastasize.

Mazies WP, Levier DH, Luchtefeld MA, Seragode AJ: Surgery of the Colon, Rectum, and Anus. Philadelphia, WB Saunders 1995. *Superb color plates and excellent descriptive text.*

Schrock TR: Examination and diseases of the anorectum. *In* Feldman M, Sleisenger MH, Schaeschmidt BF (eds): Sleisinger and Fordtran's Gastrointestinal and Liver Disease: Pathophysiology/Diagnosis/Management 6th ed. Philadelphia, WB Saunders, 1998, p 1460 *Details of the examination of the anorectum are described.*

PART XII

DISEASES OF THE LIVER, GALLBLADDER, AND BILE DUCTS

144 APPROACH TO THE PATIENT WITH LIVER DISEASES

D. W. Powell

The scope of practice of liver diseases has expanded dramatically in the past decade, primarily due to the success of liver transplantation, which now has a 1-year survival of 90% and 5-year survival of 75%, and the development of effective drug treatment for viral hepatitis. Diagnosis has been aided by safer techniques for sampling the liver and the advent of endoscopic therapeutic techniques for obstructive jaundice.

On the horizon is the full effect of the current epidemic of hepatitis C, which infected over 4 million people through contaminated blood transfusions (before its serologic identification) and injection drug use. Approximately 20% of these patients are destined to develop cirrhosis or hepatocellular carcinoma. As effective and simpler therapeutic approaches develop, the primary care physician is likely to play an increasingly important role.

The liver is an important metabolic factory for plasma proteins, blood glucose, and lipids. These roles become especially evident when the liver does not do its job (e.g., when vitamin K–dependent clotting factors are absent); when the absence of α_1-antitrypsin or ceruloplasmin leads to the development of emphysema, cirrhosis, or Wilson's disease; or when there is interference with the maintenance of normal fasting blood glucose by a biotoxin, such as occurs in alcoholic hypoglycemia. Similarly, the liver's role in lipid metabolism is brought to attention by the development of massive hepatomegaly owing to lipid accumulation in the liver in alcoholic liver diseases or diabetes mellitus or in the skin in the setting of chronic cholestatic liver disease.

The liver is also a major site for detoxification and excretion of drugs, hemoglobin metabolites, and ammonium ions. Its anatomic position as a filter of splanchnic blood flow makes it a critical determinant of the pharmacodynamics of drugs and crucial for the detoxification of absorbed metabolic poisons from the colon. When hepatic blood flow is obstructed, the shunting of mesenteric blood around the liver creates encephalopathy and hemorrhage from esophageal or gastric varices.

HISTORY

The recognition of liver disease is not difficult when the patient presents with classic manifestations, such as overt jaundice, or with the classic *stigmata of chronic liver disease,* such as ascites, spider angiomata, liver palms, and asterixis. However, the mettle of the physician is tested by the fact that liver disease can present with so many occult manifestations. Easy fatigability and malaise may be the only manifestations of chronic liver disease, and even these symptoms may be so mild that the patient is not aware of the illness until ascites, altered mental status, and even coma develop. Although *jaundice* may be the earliest manifestation of liver disease in some patients, it is often noticed by the patient or their family members as *scleral icterus* (yellow discoloration of the conjunctiva) or even similar discoloration of the gums and tongue. *Pruritus* may occur first in the course of obstructive jaundice (*cho-

lestasis*) because retention of bile salts can occur before significant retention of bilirubin. As jaundice progresses, patients develop light-colored stools and dark urine when the excretion of bile pigments is diverted from the gastrointestinal tract to the kidney.

Abdominal complaints may be absent or mild. An enlarging liver from inflammation or passive congestion may present only as mild right upper quadrant tenderness. Abdominal distention, due to the development of ascites, may be detected only by a change in belt size, and it may be intermittent, related to cyclic alcohol intake. As ascites progress, peripheral edema may develop.

Liver diseases may present as symptoms related to other systems. For example, early hepatic encephalopathy may manifest as changes in sleep pattern or mild alterations in personality long before confusion, combativeness, obtundation, and ataxia develop (see Chapter 154). Hepatitis C can present as glomerulonephritis or hemorrhagic skin lesions owing to the presence of cryoglobulinemia (see Chapter 149). Patients with hemochromatosis sometimes present with arthralgias, diabetes, or cardiac disease without the overt manifestations of hepatic involvement. Hemolytic anemias and psychic aberrations can be the presenting symptoms of Wilson's disease (see Chapter 220). Bleeding esophageal varices may be the first manifestation of cirrhosis. Surgical jaundice due to obstruction from common duct stones may present as atypical abdominal pain or even as silent jaundice, whereas the obstructive jaundice of pancreatic cancer may present as mental depression (see Chapter 140). In special settings such as pregnancy or diabetes mellitus, liver abnormalities may portend inconsequential or even dangerous hepatocyte lipid accumulation. Mild increases in aminotransferases in the asymptomatic patient may be the only manifestation of hepatitis C, whose ongoing inflammation silently destroys the liver. Silent cirrhosis may be discovered after the finding of asymptomatic thrombocytopenia caused by the congestive splenomegaly of portal hypertension. Thus, the effective physician must not only understand the classic presentations of the various liver diseases but also have a firm grasp on the atypical presentations.

In the United States, the two major epidemiologic settings for liver disease are alcohol ingestion and exposure to hepatitis virus. Thus, the medical history should seek the presence of occult alcoholism, even to the extent of questioning family members. Exposure to or contact with jaundiced persons or those with hepatitis is important to elicit. Hepatitis exposure from foreign travel, ingested shellfish, prior blood transfusions, and employment in the health care professions is not nearly as important as the history of injection drug use with even a single, one-time, experimental use of shared needles. Sexual promiscuity is unequivocally a risk factor for the viral hepatitides, particularly among the male homosexuals. Family history of liver diseases is a clue to genetic diseases such as Wilson's disease, hemochromatosis, or α_1-antitrypsin deficiency.

PHYSICAL EXAMINATION

The skin can be an important clue implicating liver disease. Spider angiomata occur on the upper trunk and face. Palmar erythema, except for the setting of pregnancy, may signal the presence of chronic liver disease. Scleral icterus and icterus of the gums or the tympanic membranes may be detected before bilirubin levels of 3 to 4 mg/dL are manifested by jaundice of the skin. Xanthomata and xanthelasmas are more common in lipid disorders than in obstructive jaundice but may be a sign of prolonged cholestasis. Chronic liver disease leads to changes in estrogen and testosterone metabolism, resulting in the development of gynecomastia, the loss of hair particularly on the shins, and reduction in the size or consistency of the testes. Chronic portal hypertension may lead to development of collateral circulation, which is manifested as caput medusa in the region of the umbilicus and epigastrium.

Abdominal examination should focus first on the presence or absence of ascites and then on the size and characteristics of the liver. Distention from ascites is difficult to differentiate from truncal obesity. Ascites can be determined most easily by the demonstration of flank dullness. By percussing first at the umbilicus, which is usually tympanic due to accumulated gas-filled loops of bowel, and then progressing radially toward the flanks, the fluid interface with the air-filled bowel loops can be detected as a ring of dullness in the flanks and lower abdomen at a uniform distance from the umbilicus. Shifting dullness and a fluid wave are more difficult to elicit and require more ascites. Ultimately, abdominal ultrasonography or computed tomography may be necessary to demonstrate small amounts of ascites.

Hepatomegaly is detected best by percussing hepatic breadth at the mid-clavicular line and demonstrating a size greater than 8 to 10 cm. How far the liver extends below the costal margin is of less importance, particularly in patients with emphysema and flattened diaphragms. Liver consistency can often be determined; the smooth liver with the sharp edge can be differentiated from the nodular liver of cirrhosis, the rock-hard liver of metastatic cancer, the tender liver of hepatitis or chronic passive congestion, and the pulsating liver of severe tricuspid insufficiency. Liver tenderness can be determined by having the patient inspire, which pushes the liver into the examining hand that is positioned below the liver, or by lightly punching a hand that is placed on the rib cage laterally over the right lobe of the liver. At times, a visible or palpable gallbladder, which may be somewhat tender, can be detected below the liver margin in patients with cystic or common bile duct obstruction. In pancreatic carcinoma with common bile duct obstruction, the presence of the palpable gallbladder in the jaundiced patient is known as Courvoisier's sign. When liver disease is expected, splenomegaly should be sought. Its presence is usually confirmation of portal hypertension.

Evaluation for possible hepatic encephalopathy is crucial in the physical examination in the patient with suspected liver disease. Early in the course of encephalopathy, manifestations are subtle and include personality change, mild confusion, and lethargy. At this point, a formal mental status examination and fine motor testing (e.g., drawing stars, connecting dots) may be necessary to show early mental aberration. Later, a flapping tremor (asterixis) develops. To elicit this neurologic sign, it is necessary to have the patient extend his or her hands against gravity and look for the release phenomenon that causes the flap. If the patient cannot follow this command, the patient can grasp two fingers of the examiner's hand and be asked to sustain the grasp; the release phenomenon might be thus elicited. Advanced encephalopathy presents as severe coma, often with decerebrate rigidity; but any neurologic presentation, including lateralization of signs, may be seen (see Chapter 154).

CLINICAL APPROACH TO DIAGNOSIS

In the setting of frank jaundice without stigmata of chronic liver disease, immediate diagnostic imaging (ultrasonography and computed tomography) is indicated to differentiate so-called surgical jaundice, which requires either operative or endoscopic intervention or even urgent transplantation, from medical jaundice, in which the diagnosis may be made from laboratory tests and/or biopsy and the management involves medications or watchful waiting. The approach to patients with abnormal liver tests or with signs and symptoms of cirrhosis is directed toward excluding medically treatable diseases, remembering that some diseases causing "surgical" jaundice can present this way as well (see Chapter 157).

The diagnosis of liver diseases will likely change in the future. The advent of improved imaging techniques such as nuclear magnetic resonance imaging of the biliary ducts may make conventional visualization of the hepatobiliary ducts by endoscopic retrograde cholangiopancreatography an archaic test. Such techniques, however, will not obviate the need for endoscopy as a mode to deliver therapy.

Schiff L, Schiff ER (eds): Diseases of the Liver, 8th ed. Philadelphia, Lippincott–Raven, 1998.
Zakim D, Boyer TD (eds). Hepatology: A Textbook of Liver Disease, 3rd ed. Philadelphia, WB Saunders, 1996.
Sherlock S, Dooley J: Diseases of the Liver and Biliary System, 10th ed. Cambridge, MA: Blackwell Science, 1997.
Three excellent hepatology textbooks that supply detail and clarity on liver diseases.

145 HEPATIC METABOLISM IN LIVER DISEASE

Richard A. Weisiger

The liver is the primary organ responsible for metabolism of carbohydrates, protein, and fat. Deranged hepatic metabolism is responsible for many of the features of end-stage liver disease, including malnutrition, muscle wasting, encephalopathy, and glucose intolerance.

CARBOHYDRATE METABOLISM

Except during the absorption of dietary carbohydrate, maintenance of normal blood glucose levels depends entirely on the liver. Two distinct mechanisms are involved: *glycogenolysis* and *gluconeogenesis.* In glycogenolysis, glucose is released from hepatic glycogen by activated glycogen phosphorylase. The process is triggered by the action of glucagon or epinephrine on liver cell surface receptors, which activate glycogen phosphorylase kinase by means of the calcium messenger system. Conversely, insulin stimulates the incorporation of glucose into hepatic glycogen. Normal hepatic glycogen stores are sufficient to sustain blood glucose levels for only about 24 hours. Beyond that time, maintenance of blood glucose in the fasting state depends entirely on hepatic gluconeogenesis: the de novo synthesis of glucose from precursors including lactate, pyruvate, and amino acids derived from catabolism of protein stores. Gluconeogenesis is stimulated by glucagon and epinephrine and is inhibited by insulin.

The normal liver continually responds to changes in its nutritional and hormonal milieu. In the fed state (relative excess of insulin and glucose), glucose production by gluconeogenesis and glycogenolysis is minimal. Instead, dietary glucose is either stored as glycogen or converted to fatty acids (lipogenesis), largely to be secreted from the liver in the form of triglyceride-rich lipoproteins and destined for storage in adipose tissue. In the fasting state the process is reversed, resulting in mobilization rather than storage of energy substrates. High glucagon levels relative to insulin trigger glycogenolysis and gluconeogenesis. The resulting glucose is no longer diverted to lipogenesis but released into the plasma. The decrease in fatty acid synthesis is associated with increased fatty acid oxidation, which becomes the principal energy source for the liver.

Failure of these homeostatic mechanisms in liver disease may produce *hypoglycemia* or *glucose intolerance.* Mild hypoglycemia (blood glucose concentrations between 45 and 60 mg/dL) occurs in about 50% of patients with uncomplicated acute viral hepatitis. As a rule, these patients are not hyperinsulinemic. Instead, hypoglycemia may reflect several metabolic abnormalities, including diminished glycogen stores, diminished glycogenolytic response to glucagon, diminished gluconeogenesis, and impaired repletion of hepatic glycogen during the fed state. In most cases, the hypoglycemia is not clinically significant, but in severe acute liver injury of any cause, such as fulminant hepatitis due to virus or drug toxicity, hypoglycemia may be profound and life threatening. Hypoglycemia may also occur in the absence of overt liver damage. For example, *alcoholic hypoglycemia* classically occurs in persons whose only important source of calories over a period of days is ethanol, which cannot be metabolically converted to glucose and may inhibit gluconeogenesis. Hypoglycemia should be considered in the differential diagnosis of altered mental status in any patient with significant acute liver disease or exposure to ethanol. Frequent monitoring of blood glucose is essential in all patients with fulminant hepatic failure, because hypoglycemic coma may be overlooked in patients with hepatic encephalopathy.

Conversely, *glucose intolerance* is more typically associated with chronic liver disease and cirrhosis. Plasma levels of insulin and many other hormones tend to rise in liver disease due to reduced hepatic hormone clearance, producing a state of *insulin resistance.* Both the number of insulin receptors and their binding affinity may be diminished in peripheral blood monocytes in liver disease, suggesting a generalized receptor defect. Insulin resistance may also reflect increased plasma glucagon concentrations and diversion of newly released insulin from the liver by portosystemic shunts. Regardless of the mechanism, the glucose intolerance associated with chronic liver disease is rarely of clinical significance. Occasionally, patients with chronic liver disease may also have other disorders such as *hemochromatosis* (see Chapter 221) and *chronic pancreatitis* (see Chapter 141), in which *diabetes mellitus* may contribute to glucose intolerance.

LIPID METABOLISM

The liver plays a central role in the metabolism of fatty acids and other lipids and lipoproteins. Of the total daily turnover of plasma non-esterified (free) fatty acids derived from adipose tissue, about one third enter the liver, where they are esterified to triglycerides or other esters, or undergo oxidation. The balance between esterification and oxidation is closely regulated, as is the rate of de novo fatty acid synthesis. In the fasting state, fatty acid synthesis is inhibited, whereas fatty acid oxidation is increased at the expense of the esterification pathways. In the fed state, de novo fatty acid synthesis and esterification are favored, whereas oxidation is diminished. Exclusive of dietary sources and de novo synthesis, a total of 60 to 70 g of plasma non-esterified fatty acid (> 200 mmol) is taken up by the liver each day in the average adult. These fatty acids provide the major energy source for the liver in the fasting state. Interference with hepatic fatty acid metabolism may either cause or be caused by clinically significant abnormalities of hepatic structure and function.

Fatty liver usually reflects excess accumulation of triglyceride, which may be deposited as a single large droplet displacing the nucleus, or as multiple small droplets surrounding a central nucleus. It usually reflects an imbalance between the rate of triglyceride biosynthesis and secretion into the plasma, primarily as very low density lipoproteins (VLDLs). This imbalance may result from many factors that can affect synthesis, secretion, or both. Conditions associated with large fat droplets in liver cells include obesity, protein-calorie malnutrition (e.g., kwashiorkor, jejunoileal bypass), diabetes mellitus, corticosteroid therapy, and ethanol ingestion (see Chapter 148). Small droplet fat accumulation (see later) is characteristic of acute fatty liver of pregnancy, Reye's syndrome, Jamaican vomiting sickness, and tetracycline and valproic acid hepatotoxicity but is occasionally ethanol related. Transient hepatic fat deposition is usually well tolerated. However, *nonalcoholic steatohepatitis* (see Chapter 148), which may progress to fibrosis and cirrhosis over many years, is a common cause of isolated aminotransferase elevations.

Interference with fatty acid oxidation at any of several stages may have profound consequences. For example, *alcoholic ketosis* is attributed to an ethanol- or acetaldehyde-mediated impairment of the tricarboxylic acid cycle, resulting in incomplete oxidation of the products derived from β-oxidation of fatty acids. Metabolites of hypoglycin, a low-molecular-weight compound present in the unripened fruit of the ackee tree and the cause of *Jamaican vomiting sickness*, are converted to coenzyme A thioesters and to carnitine derivatives. Because these cannot be metabolized further, they effectively sequester the cellular carnitine pool. Fatty acid oxidation is inhibited, and there is a corresponding decrease in adenosine triphosphate production and gluconeogenesis. Continuing fatty acid esterification under these conditions leads to a form of fatty liver characterized by *small-droplet fat deposition,* associated in severe cases with liver failure and hypoglycemia. This entity is clinically similar to *Reye's syndrome, obstetric fatty liver,* and *tetracycline* and *valproic acid hepatotoxicity,* but in none of these latter conditions has the pathogenesis been fully elucidated.

The liver is the major source of endogenously synthesized cholesterol (approximately 0.5 g/day). Together with cholesterol of dietary origin, this newly synthesized cholesterol enters a "metabolically active" hepatic cholesterol pool, from which is derived the cholesterol destined for secretion into bile or into plasma (in lipoproteins), for synthesis of liver cell membranes, and for conversion to bile acids. Bile acid synthesis accounts for the disposition of approximately half of the total daily turnover of cholesterol and, as such, is an important determinant of body cholesterol stores. Relative rates of secretion of bile acids, cholesterol, and phosphatidylcholine (lecithin) into bile are important factors in the pathogenesis of cholesterol gallstones (see Chapter 152), but the mechanism(s) by which the secretion of these substances is effected and controlled is incompletely understood. Hepatic secretion of lipoproteins and clearance of chylomicron remnants are reduced in chronic liver disease, in part reflecting the thickened subendothelial basement membrane that blocks passage of large particles to and from the plasma membrane.

AMINO ACID AND PROTEIN METABOLISM

Except for immunoglobulins, most plasma proteins, including albumin, clotting factors, transferrin, α_1-antitrypsin, and most lipoproteins are synthesized in the liver. Plasma protein synthesis totals 30 to 60 g/day and accounts for over 80% of all hepatic protein synthesis. The synthesis of each protein is controlled by specific regulatory mechanisms. In all cases, however, synthesis and secretion are dependent on the integrity of many aspects of cell function, including the transcriptional mechanisms in the nucleus, the translational mechanisms in the rough endoplasmic reticulum, the availability of amino acids, and the secretory mechanisms in the Golgi apparatus. Despite these common features, individual proteins are affected differently in liver disease. This variability may result from several factors such as the availability of an essential *nutritional* component (e.g., the vitamin K–dependent clotting factors), *hormonal* influences (e.g., VLDLs), *genetic* determinants (e.g., ceruloplasmin or α_1-antitrypsin), the effects of drugs or toxins (e.g., the warfarin-like anticoagulants or ethanol), or the response of selected proteins such as fibrinogen (and other "acute phase reactants," including C-reactive proteins, ceruloplasmin, haptoglobin, and transferrin) to inflammatory processes. In addition, the *kinetics* of synthesis and turnover of a particular protein are major determinants of the response of its plasma concentration to acute liver injury. In general, plasma concentrations of proteins with rapid turnover (e.g., clotting factors, with a plasma half-time of hours to days) are more likely to be depressed by severe acute liver injury than are those proteins that turn over more slowly (e.g., albumin, with a plasma half-time about 3 weeks). Finally, *catabolism* of certain plasma proteins may be accelerated (e.g., clotting factors in *disseminated intravascular coagulation,* or albumin in *protein-losing enteropathy*). For these reasons, although liver disease generally tends to depress the plasma concentration of proteins of hepatic origin, plasma concentrations of such proteins may not accurately reflect the severity of the liver disease in a given patient. Interpretation of the prothrombin time, partial thromboplastin time, and serum albumin concentrations are useful in the evaluation of liver disease (see Chapter 147).

Amino acids, in addition to their obvious importance in protein synthesis, also participate in other reactions in the liver. Of special significance is the role of certain amino acids as precursors for gluconeogenesis. Amino acids may undergo *transamination,* in which the α-amino group is transferred to an α-keto group, as in the alanine aminotransferase–mediated deamination of alanine to pyruvate; the resulting transfer of the amino group to α-ketoglutarate converts this acceptor to glutamate. Alternatively, amino acids may undergo *oxidative deamination.* In this case, an α-ketoacid is formed as the amino group is converted to ammonium ion and, ultimately, to urea (see later). The liver synthesizes all of the nonessential amino acids from their corresponding α-ketoacids. Severe liver disease is commonly associated with protein-calorie malnutrition, with relative plasma deficiency of branched-chain amino acids (leucine, isoleucine, and valine), and with accumulation of aromatic amino acids (phenylalanine and tyrosine).

BIOTRANSFORMATION AND DETOXIFICATION

The liver is the major site of chemical modification of a wide variety of exogenous drugs and toxins as well as endogenous substances such as hormones. The reactions potentially involved are numerous and, in many instances, involve the cytochrome P-450–dependent microsomal mixed function oxidase system. In addition to the basic principles of drug disposition (see Chapter 26), several aspects warrant special emphasis in the context of liver function and disease. First, although biotransformation of an endogenous or exogenous substance may *inactivate* it or render it more suitable for urinary or biliary excretion, there are many examples of compounds that are rendered toxic by this process. A number of clinically significant hepatotoxins are *activated* in this way, and some "idiosyncratic" drug reactions may reflect individual differences in drug metabolism rather than an immunologic response (see Chapter 148). Second, diseases of the liver may seriously impair the biotransformation of exogenous substances, thereby resulting in an *increased sensitivity* to certain drugs (e.g., sedatives and opiates), or may enhance the biologic effect of endogenous hormones (e.g., contributing to the feminizing effects of chronic liver disease) or toxins (e.g., diminished hepatic conversion of ammonia to urea in hepatic encephalopathy). Finally, one substance may significantly influence the hepatic biotransformation of another. Examples of this particular form of *drug-drug interaction* include the well-recognized induction of the microsomal drug-metabolizing system by prior administration of phenobarbital and its inhibition by various toxins.

A particularly important hepatic detoxification pathway converts *ammonium ion* to urea through the Krebs-Henseleit *urea cycle*, in which ornithine, citrulline, argininosuccinate, and arginine are intermediates and which involves both mitochondrial and cytosolic components. Glutamate, formed from NH_4^+ and α-ketoglutarate, is the principal NH_2 donor. Ammonium ion is produced in abundance in the intestinal tract, especially the colon, by the bacterial degradation of luminal proteins and amino acids and of endogenous urea, 25% of the daily production of which diffuses into the intestinal lumen. The NH_4^+ diffuses into the portal circulation and is transported to the liver, where it is converted to urea by the mechanism described earlier. *Hepatic encephalopathy,* which in part reflects the failure of this important detoxification process (and of analogous pathways for other endogenous and gut-derived toxins), may occur with either loss of functional liver cell mass or direct entry of portal blood into the peripheral circulation through spontaneous or surgically created portosystemic shunts (see Chapter 154).

Cicognani C, Malavolti M, Morselli-Labate AM, et al: Serum lipid and lipoprotein patterns in patients with liver cirrhosis and chronic active hepatitis. Arch Intern Med 157:792–796, 1997. *Lipoprotein abnormalities are common in liver disease and may predispose to vascular disease.*

Kondrup J, Muller MJ: Energy and protein requirements of patients with chronic liver disease. J Hepatol 27:239–247, 1997. *Review of altered nutritional needs in liver disease.*

Kondrup J, Nielsen K, Juul A: Effect of long-term refeeding on protein metabolism in patients with cirrhosis of the liver. Br J Nutr 77:197–212, 1997. *Cirrhotics need more protein to maintain hepatic synthesis and should not be placed on strict protein-restricted diets unless other measures to control encephalopathy have failed.*

146 BILIRUBIN METABOLISM, HYPERBILIRUBINEMIA, AND APPROACH TO THE JAUNDICED PATIENT

Bruce F. Scharschmidt

Jaundice, a yellow discoloration of the skin, sclerae, and mucus membranes, results from an elevated serum bilirubin concentration. It is the most visible manifestation of liver and biliary tract disease and has many causes.

BILIRUBIN METABOLISM

BILIRUBIN FORMATION. Bilirubin is a tetrapyrrole formed from the breakdown of heme (Fig. 146–1). Daily production in adults averages about 4 mg/kg. Most bilirubin (~70%) is derived from the heme moiety of hemoglobin in senescent erythrocytes that are sequestered and degraded in the mononuclear phagocytic cells of the spleen, liver, or bone marrow. The remainder results largely from the breakdown of non-hemoglobin hemoproteins in the liver, principally cytochrome P-450. A minor fraction results from ineffective erythropoiesis, that is, premature destruction of newly formed erythrocytes in the bone marrow or circulation.

The conversion of heme to bilirubin involves two steps. First, microsomal heme oxygenase, a heme-cleaving enzyme most abundant in the liver, spleen, and bone marrow, mediates conversion of heme to biliverdin. Next, biliverdin is reduced to bilirubin by cytosolic biliverdin reductase. Tinprotoporphyrin, a synthetic metalloporphyrin, is a potent competitive inhibitor of heme oxygenase and has shown promise in reducing bilirubin production and preventing kernicterus in selected infants with hyperbilirubinemia. Mammals, unlike birds, reptiles, and amphibia, convert non-toxic, water-soluble biliverdin to water-insoluble bilirubin. Biliverdin, unlike bilirubin, is not able to cross the placenta.

HEPATIC BILIRUBIN TRANSPORT AND CONJUGATION. Uptake of bilirubin and other substances tightly bound to protein is mediated by specific carrier proteins and facilitated by large fenestrations in the cells of the sinusoidal lining that permit plasma proteins to enter the space of Disse and directly contact the hepatocyte plasma membrane. Once inside the liver cell, bilirubin and other organic anions bind to cytoplasmic proteins and membranes.

Unconjugated bilirubin is virtually water-insoluble at physiologic pH and readily diffuses across biologic membranes such as the blood-brain barrier, placenta, and intestinal and gallbladder epithelium. Conjugation with glucuronic acid in hepatocytes by microsomal uridine diphosphate (UDP)-glucuronyl-transferase greatly enhances the aqueous solubility of bilirubin, thereby facilitating elimination from the body and preventing damage to the central nervous system. Exposure of unconjugated bilirubin to light causes the formation of polar photoisomers, which are excreted by the liver without conjugation; their formation is the mechanism by which phototherapy lowers serum bilirubin concentration in neonatal hyperbilirubinemia.

Secretion of conjugated bilirubin from the hepatocyte into the bile canaliculus occurs predominantly by means of an adenosine triphosphate (ATP)-dependent carrier, which also mediates the transport of other organic anions. Mutations in this carrier result in the *Dubin-Johnson syndrome.* Bilirubin diglucuronide predominates in human bile (70–80%), with the isomeric monoglucuronides present in small amounts.

ENTEROHEPATIC CIRCULATION. Absorption of conjugated bilirubin from the gallbladder and small intestine is negligible. In the terminal ileum and colon, conjugated bilirubin is hydrolyzed by bacterial enzymes to form unconjugated bilirubin, which is converted into colorless urobilinogens and related products, including urobilins. Most urobilinogen absorbed from the intestine is re-excreted in bile and ultimately in feces; a small fraction appears in urine. In addition to urobilins, the normal brown color of stool may reflect the presence of non-bilirubin pigments, perhaps of plant origin, which are also excreted in bile and undergo enterohepatic circulation.

BILIRUBIN IN SERUM. Unconjugated bilirubin is bound reversibly to albumin with high affinity. A variety of compounds, including certain sulfonamides, penicillin derivatives, furosemide, and radiographic contrast media, may displace bilirubin from its albumin-binding sites and increase the risk of kernicterus in neonates. Presumably because of its tight albumin binding and low water solubility, unconjugated bilirubin is not excreted in urine. Conjugated bilirubin is less tightly bound to albumin than is bilirubin. It is filtered to a greater extent at the glomerulus, is incompletely reabsorbed by the renal tubules, and therefore appears in the urine in small amounts in patients with conjugated hyperbilirubinemia.

In addition to the reversible binding to albumin, another bilirubin

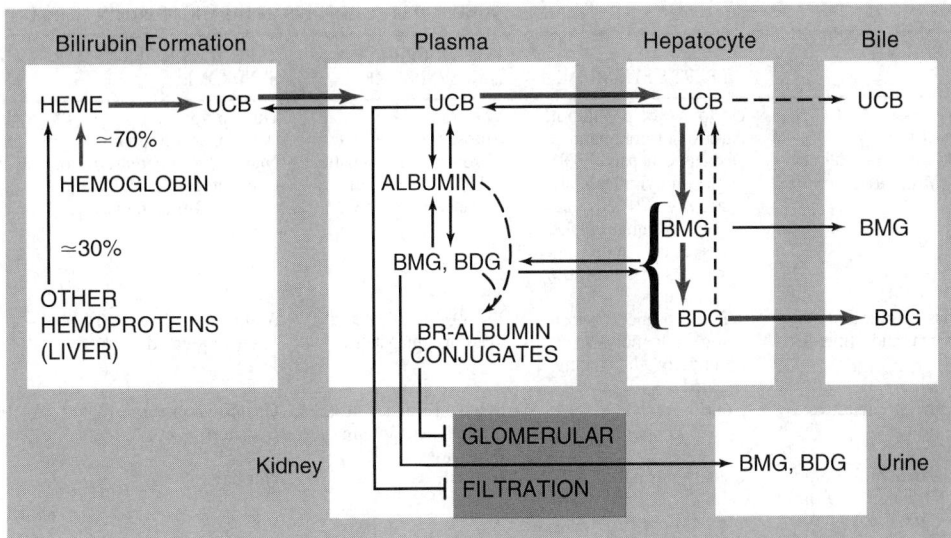

FIGURE 146–1 ■ Overview of bilirubin metabolism. Unconjugated bilirubin (UCB) formed from the breakdown of hemoglobin heme and other hemoproteins is transported in plasma reversibly bound to albumin and is converted in the liver to bilirubin monoglucuronide (BMG) and diglucuronide (BDG), the latter being the predominant form secreted in bile. BMG and BDG together normally account for less than 5% of serum bilirubin. In patients with hepatobiliary disease, BMG and BDG accumulate in plasma and appear in urine. Bilirubin glucuronides in plasma also react non-enzymatically with albumin and possibly other serum proteins to form protein conjugates, which do not appear in urine and have a plasma half-life similar to that of albumin.

Table 146–1 ■ DIFFERENTIAL DIAGNOSIS OF JAUNDICE

Isolated Disorders of Bilirubin Metabolism
Unconjugated hyperbilirubinemia
  Increased bilirubin production
    Examples: hemolysis, ineffective erythropoeisis, blood transfusion, resorption of hematomas
  Decreased hepatocellular uptake
    Examples: drugs (e.g., rifampin)
  Decreased conjugation
    Examples: Gilbert's syndrome, Crigler-Najjar syndromes, physiologic jaundice of the newborn
Conjugated or mixed hyperbilirubinemia
  Dubin-Johnson syndrome
  Rotor's syndrome
Liver Disease
Acute or Chronic Hepatocellular Dysfunction
  Acute or subacute hepatocellular injury
    Examples: viral hepatitis, hepatotoxins (e.g., ethanol, acetaminophen, *Amanita*), drugs (e.g., isoniazid, methyldopa), ischemia (e.g., hypotension, vascular occlusion), metabolic disorders (e.g., Wilson's disease, Reye's syndrome), pregnancy-related (e.g., acute fatty liver of pregnancy, pre-eclampsia)
  Chronic hepatocellular disease
    Examples: viral hepatitis, hepatotoxins (e.g., ethanol, vinyl chloride, vitamin A), autoimmune hepatitis, metabolic (Wilson's disease, hemochromatosis, α_1-antitrypsin deficiency)
Hepatic Disorders with Prominent Cholestasis
  Diffuse infiltrative disorders
    Examples: granulomatous diseases (e.g., mycobacterial infections, sarcoidosis, lymphoma, drugs, Wegener's), amyloidosis, infiltrative malignancy
  Inflammation of intrahepatic bile ductules and/or portal tracts
    Examples: primary biliary cirrhosis, graft-versus-host disease, drugs (e.g., chlorpromazine, erythromycin)
  Miscellaneous conditions
    Examples: benign recurrent intrahepatic cholestasis, drugs, estrogens, anabolic steroids, total parenteral nutrition, bacterial infections, uncommon presentations of viral or alcoholic hepatitis, intrahepatic cholestasis of pregnancy, postoperative cholestasis
Obstruction of the Bile ducts
Choledocholithiasis
  Cholesterol gallstones
  Pigment gallstones
Diseases of the bile ducts
  Inflammation/infection
    Examples: primary sclerosing cholangitis, AIDS cholangiopathy, hepatic arterial chemotherapy, postsurgical strictures
  Neoplasms
Extrinsic compression of the biliary tree
  Neoplasms
    Examples: pancreatic carcinoma, metastatic lymphadenopathy, hepatoma
  Pancreatitis
  Vascular enlargement (e.g., aneurysm, cavernous transformation of portal vein)

fraction binds very tightly, perhaps covalently, to albumin. It has been detected only in patients with conjugated hyperbilirubinemia, in whom it accounts for a varying (8–90%) fraction of total bilirubin (see later). This protein-bound fraction helps explain the occasionally slow resolution of hyperbilirubinemia in patients convalescing from hepatitis or in whom biliary obstruction has been relieved, as well as the disappearance of bilirubinuria in these patients before the resolution of jaundice.

Serum bilirubin concentration in normal adults is less than 1 to 1.5 mg/dL and varies directly with bilirubin production and inversely with hepatic bilirubin clearance. About 5% of circulating bilirubin in healthy adults is conjugated; circulating bilirubin in patients with hepatocellular or biliary tract disease consists predominantly of monoconjugates and diconjugates. A serum bilirubin value of 3 mg/dL is usually required for jaundice or scleral icterus to be clinically evident. Serum bilirubin is conventionally detected by the diazo reaction (van den Bergh reaction), whereby bilirubin is cleaved by compounds such as diazotized sulfanilic acid to form a colored azodipyrrole that can be assayed by spectrophotometry. Conjugated bilirubin reacts rapidly ("directly") with diazo reagents, whereas unconjugated bilirubin reacts slowly because the site of chemical cleavage is rendered inaccessible by internal hydrogen bonding. Thus, measurement of total bilirubin concentration requires the addition of an "accelerator" compound, such as ethanol or urea, which disrupts such hydrogen bonding and facilitates the reaction of unconjugated bilirubin with the diazo reagent. The concentration of the indirect bilirubin fraction is calculated by subtracting the direct bilirubin concentration (i.e., accelerator compound absent) from total (i.e., accelerator compound present). Although direct bilirubin and conjugated bilirubin are related, they are not equivalent. Similarly, indirect bilirubin is not equivalent to unconjugated bilirubin. Thus, reliance on direct and indirect bilirubin measurements can lead to errors in the diagnosis of isolated disorders of bilirubin metabolism (e.g., Gilbert's syndrome). In special cases, the diagnosis may require more sophisticated chromatographic techniques that measure the concentrations of unconjugated, monoglucuronidated, and diglucuronidated bilirubin as well as conjugated bilirubin-albumin complexes. However, these techniques are not widely employed. Moreover, even with such accurate techniques, measurement of conjugated and unconjugated bilirubin will not reliably distinguish between liver disease and biliary obstruction. Thus, measurement of direct and indirect bilirubin is of limited clinical utility.

DIFFERENTIAL DIAGNOSIS. Conditions that produce jaundice can be classified under the broad categories of isolated disorders of bilirubin metabolism, liver disease, or obstruction of the bile ducts (Table 146–1).

ISOLATED DISORDERS OF BILIRUBIN METABOLISM

INCREASED BILIRUBIN PRODUCTION. Disorders that cause increased bilirubin production include hemolysis, ineffective erythro-

Table 146–2 ■ HEREDITARY DISORDERS OF HEPATIC BILIRUBIN METABOLISM

	GILBERT'S SYNDROME	TYPE I CRIGLER-NAJJAR SYNDROME	TYPE II CRIGLER-NAJJAR SYNDROME	DUBIN-JOHNSON SYNDROME	ROTOR'S SYNDROME
Incidence	Up to 7% of population	Very rare	Uncommon	Uncommon	Rare
Inheritance	Autosomal dominant	Autosomal recessive	Autosomal dominant	Autosomal recessive	Autosomal recessive
Defect(s) in Bilirubin Metabolism	Decreased hepatic UDP-glucuronyl-transferase activity, (?) slow hepatic bilirubin uptake, associated mild hemolysis in up to 50% of patients	Absence of hepatic UDP-glucuronyl-transferase activity	Markedly decreased or undetectable UDP-glucuronyl-transferase activity	Impaired canalicular secretion of conjugated bilirubin	Impaired hepatic secretion or storage of conjugated bilirubin
Plasma bilirubin concentration (mg/dL)	≤3 in absence of fasting or hemolysis, essentially all unconjugated	17–50, usually >20, all unconjugated	6–45, usually >20, all unconjugated	1–25, usually <7, about 60% conjugated	1–20, usually <7, about 60% conjugated
Clinical manifestations	None	Death in infancy from kernicterus in almost all cases	Usually none, rarely kernicterus	Probably none	Probably none
Plasma sulfobromophthalein disappearance	Usually normal (<5%); mild 45-min (<15%) retention in some patients	Normal	Normal	Slow initial disappearance (retention <20% at 45 min) with frequent secondary rise at 1.5–2 hours	Very slow disappearance (45-min retention = 30–45%), no secondary rise
Oral cholecystography	Normal	Normal	Normal	Faint or nonvisualization	Usually normal
Hepatic histology (light microscopy)	Normal, occasionally increased lipofuscin	Normal	Normal	Coarse pigment in centrolobular cells	Normal
Other distinguishing features	Decreased bilirubin concentration with phenobarbital	No response to phenobarbital	Decreased bilirubin concentration with phenobarbital	Increased bilirubin concentration with estrogens, characteristic urinary coproporphyrin pattern	Urinary coproporphyrin pattern
Diagnosis	Clinical and laboratory findings, response to fasting occasionally helpful, liver biopsy not usually necessary	Clinical and laboratory findings, lack of response to phenobarbital	Clinical and laboratory findings, response to phenobarbital	Clinical and laboratory findings, sulfobromophthalein disappearance, urinary coproporphyrin excretion	Clinical and laboratory findings, sulfobromophthalein disappearance, urinary coproporphyrin excretion
Treatment	None available or necessary	Liver transplantation; other measures not uniformly effective	Phenobarbital if bilirubin concentration markedly elevated	None available or necessary; avoid estrogens	None available or necessary

UDP = uridine diphosphate.

poiesis, or resorption of a hematoma. Jaundice may occur in patients with hemolytic anemias of all types, megaloblastic anemia from either folate or vitamin B_{12} deficiency, iron-deficiency anemia, sideroblastic anemia, and polycythemia vera. With these disorders, bilirubin concentration does not generally exceed 4 to 5 mg/dL. Jaundice may follow massive transfusion, because the shortened lifespan of transfused erythrocytes leads to excessive bilirubin production. Patients who have suffered major trauma may also develop hyperbilirubinemia as a result of resorption of hematomas as well as from blood transfusions. Each of these disorders involves excessive delivery of unconjugated bilirubin to the liver. Consequently, indirect bilirubin concentration in serum is increased; other biochemical markers of liver function are normal.

DECREASED BILIRUBIN UPTAKE. The antituberculous agent rifampin has been shown competitively to inhibit bilirubin uptake by hepatocytes and may produce hyperbilirubinemia by this mechanism. Decreased bilirubin uptake may also contribute to the pathogenesis of the hereditary disorder Gilbert's syndrome, in which the predominant abnormality is an impairment of bilirubin conjugation due to reduced bilirubin UDP-glucuronyl transferase activity.

DECREASED BILIRUBIN CONJUGATION. Three familial disorders of unconjugated hyperbilirubinemia are attributable to diminished bilirubin conjugation. Gilbert's syndrome is the most common, occurring in up to 10% of white populations. It is entirely benign and rarely produces clinical jaundice. Serum bilirubin may rise two to threefold with fasting or dehydration but is generally below 4 mg/dL. Patients with Gilbert's syndrome commonly present during or after adolescence, when isolated hyperbilirubinemia is detected as an incidental finding on routine multiphasic biochemical screening. The pathogenesis of Gilbert's syndrome has been linked to a reduction in bilirubin *UGT-1* gene (*HUG-Br1*) transcription, resulting from a mutation in the promoter region.

Mutations in the coding region of HUG-Br1 appear to be responsible for Crigler-Najjar syndrome. In type I Crigler-Najjar syndrome, bilirubin UGT-1 activity is absent and the majority of patients die of kernicterus in the neonatal period (Table 146–2). Liver transplantation can be lifesaving. Patients with type II Crigler-Najjar syndrome have markedly reduced bilirubin UGT-1 activity, with serum bilirubin levels between those of Gilbert's syndrome and those of type I Crigler-Najjar syndrome. In contrast to type I Crigler-Najjar patients, patients with type II Crigler-Najjar syndrome experience a fall in serum bilirubin concentration to levels of 2 to 5 mg/dL with phenobarbital, which increases UDP-glucuronyl transferase activity. Such patients generally survive to adulthood without neurologic impairment. Delayed developmental expression of bilirubin *UGT-1* appears to be responsible for physiologic jaundice of the newborn, a transient disorder that rapidly resolves in the neonatal period.

Fasting increases the plasma concentration of unconjugated, indirect-reacting bilirubin, owing primarily to a decrease in hepatic bilirubin clearance (so-called fasting hyperbilirubinemia). This effect is particularly marked in patients with Gilbert's syndrome and the type II Crigler-Najjar syndrome. Both dietary composition and total caloric intake are important; a normocaloric but lipid-free diet produces a response similar to that observed with complete fasting, and the effect of complete fasting is reversed by feeding small amounts of lipid.

CONJUGATED OR MIXED HYPERBILIRUBINEMIA. A selective

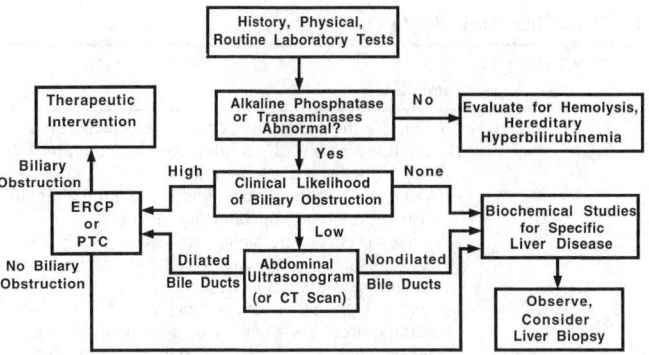

FIGURE 146-2 ■ Approach to the patient with jaundice. ERCP = endoscopic retrograde cholangiopancreatography; PTC = percutaneous transhepatic cholangiogram. (From Lidofsky SD, Scharschmidt BF: Jaundice. *In* Feldman M, Scharschmidt BF, Sleisenger MH [eds]: Gastrointestinal and Liver Disease, 6th ed. Philadelphia, WB Saunders, 1998, p 227.)

decrease in bilirubin secretion into the bile canaliculus may produce conjugated or mixed hyperbilirubinemia. Such a defect underlies two inherited disorders: Dubin-Johnson syndrome and Rotor's syndrome. Dubin-Johnson syndrome has been linked to an absence of canalicular expression of a multispecific organic anion transporter; the molecular basis of Rotor's syndrome is currently unknown. In each of these syndromes, the direct bilirubin level is elevated, but standard liver function tests are otherwise normal.

LIVER AND BILIARY DISEASE

Jaundice is a common feature of both acute and chronic generalized hepatic dysfunction. In contrast to isolated disorders of bilirubin metabolism, icteric liver disease is characterized by an increase in serum bilirubin concentration in association with abnormalities in other standard liver function tests.

Although an accurate diagnosis is possible in most patients based on clinical findings and biochemical studies (see later), certain hepatic disorders associated with cholestasis as their major manifestation may cause diagnostic confusion. These include infiltrative disorders, disorders that particularly affect the intrahepatic biliary tree, and certain other inflammatory or neoplastic conditions (see Table 146-1 and Chapters 152, 153, 156, and 157.)

Benign recurrent cholestasis is an autosomal recessive syndrome associated with intermittent and recurrent episodes of malaise, pruritus, and jaundice. Episodes of cholestasis last from days to months and are separated by asymptomatic periods with normal biochemical hepatic function. A single gene responsible both for benign recurrent cholestasis and one particular form of progressive cholestasis in infants has recently been identified; the function of this gene is under study.

Postoperative jaundice is multifactorial in origin, with both increased bilirubin production (e.g., breakdown of transfused erythrocytes, resorption of hematomas) and decreased hepatic clearance

(e.g., bacteremia, parenteral nutrition, perioperative or postoperative hypoxia) as contributing factors. Hyperbilirubinemia is the most prominent biochemical manifestation and may be accompanied by a severalfold elevation of alkaline phosphatase or γ-glutamyl transpeptidase. Aminotransferases are minimally elevated, and synthetic function is typically normal. The differential diagnosis includes biliary obstruction or liver disease due to shock, anesthetic injury, or post-transfusion hepatitis. Postoperative jaundice in the liver transplant patient presents a special problem, because the differential diagnosis also includes liver injury during organ preservation, rejection, and lymphoproliferative disorders. Postoperative jaundice per se does not pose a threat to the patient and typically resolves in 1 to 2 weeks as the overall condition of the patient improves.

Jaundice in pregnancy may present as a generally self-limited disorder of the first trimester, as intrahepatic cholestasis or as acute fatty liver, or in association with pre-eclampsia in the third trimester (see Chapter 152). *Obstruction of the biliary tree* can be caused by gallstones, neoplasms, inflammatory disorders, or extrinsic compression (see Chapters 153, 156, and 157).

DIAGNOSTIC APPROACH TO THE PATIENT WITH JAUNDICE

The diagnostic approach (Fig. 146-2) to the jaundiced patient begins with a careful history, physical examination, screening laboratory studies, and formulation of a differential diagnosis. The currently available tests for imaging the biliary tree represent a major advance and permit a definitive diagnosis in virtually all patients. However, if these tests are employed in an indiscriminate or redundant fashion, the patient is exposed to unnecessary discomfort, risk, and expense. The rational selection of these tests is based on the initial differential diagnosis and the likelihood that further evaluation will yield beneficial information.

HISTORY AND PHYSICAL EXAMINATION. The distinction between liver disease and extrahepatic obstruction is generally the most important aspect of the differential diagnosis (Table 146-3). Fever, rigors, and pain in the right upper abdominal quadrant suggest cholangitis and hence biliary obstruction, as do past biliary surgery or an abdominal mass. Certain causes of jaundice such as gallstone disease and malignant neoplasm are more common in the elderly. Risk factors for liver disease (e.g., hepatitis exposure, transfusions, intravenous drug use, alcohol use) or physical evidence of cirrhosis (e.g., spider angiomata, gynecomastia, ascites, splenomegaly) should all raise the possibility of intrinsic liver disease.

INITIAL LABORATORY STUDIES. Initial studies should include a complete blood cell count as well as measurement of serum bilirubin concentration, activities of alkaline phosphatase and alanine and aspartate aminotransferases, and prothrombin time. If hepatic tests other than bilirubin are normal, one should consider an isolated disorder of bilirubin metabolism, whereas certain patterns of abnormalities help distinguish intrinsic liver disease from biliary obstruction (see Table 146-3). However, many exceptions to these general patterns exist, and hepatic disorders associated with prominent cholestasis may mimic biliary obstruction. Both γ-glutamyl

Table 146-3 ■ OBSTRUCTIVE JAUNDICE VERSUS CHOLESTATIC LIVER DISEASE

	SUGGESTS OBSTRUCTIVE JAUNDICE	SUGGESTS CHOLESTATIC LIVER DISEASE
History	Abdominal pain Fever, rigors Prior biliary surgery Older age	Anorexia, malaise, myalgias, suggestive of viral prodrome Known infectious exposure Receipt of blood products, use of intravenous drugs Exposure to known hepatotoxin Family history of jaundice
Physical Examination	High fever Abdominal tendernesss Palpable abdominal mass Abdominal scar	Ascites Stigmata of liver disease (e.g., prominent abdominal veins, gynecomastia, spider angiomata, Kayser-Fleischer rings) Asterixis, encephalopathy
Laboratory Studies	Predominant elevation of serum bilirubin and alkaline phosphatase Prothrombin time that is normal or normalizes with vitamin K administration Elevated serum amylase	Predominant elevation of serum aminotransferase levels Prolonged prothrombin time that does not correct with vitamin K administration Blood tests indicative of specific liver disease

Table 146–4 ■ IMAGING STUDIES FOR THE EVALUATION OF JAUNDICE

TEST	SENSITIVITY (%)	SPECIFICITY (%)	MORBIDITY (%)	MORTALITY (%)	COMMENTS
Abdominal ultrasonography	55–91	82–95			*Advantages:* non-invasive, portable, least expensive *Disadvantages:* bowel gas may obscure common bile duct; difficult in obese individuals
Abdominal computed tomography	63–96	93–100	See comments		*Advantages:* non-invasive, higher resolution than ultrasonography, not operator-dependent *Disadvantages:* not portable, can visualize only calcified gallstones, intravenous contrast required (potential nephrotoxicity)
Endoscopic retrograde cholangiopancreatography	89–98	89–100	3	0.2	*Advantages:* provides direct imaging of bile ducts, permits direct visualization of periampullary region, and acquisition of tissue distal to bifurcation of hepatic ducts, potential for simultaneous therapeutic intervention, especially useful for lesions distal to bifurcation of hepatic ducts *Disadvantages:* cannot be performed if altered anatomy precludes endoscopic access to ampulla (e.g., Roux loop)
Percutaneous cholangiography	98–100	89–100	3	0.2	*Advantages:* provides direct imaging of bile ducts, potential for simultaneous therapeutic intervention, especially useful for lesions proximal to common hepatic duct *Disadvantages:* more difficult with non-dilated intrahepatic bile ducts

transpeptidase and alkaline phosphatase are typically elevated in patients with cholestasis; the combination of an elevated alkaline phosphatase and normal γ-glutamyl transpeptidase suggests that the alkaline phosphatase is from bone. Conversely, an isolated elevation of γ-glutamyl transpeptidase may result from certain drugs (e.g., phenytoin) or alcohol even in the absence of liver disease.

IMAGING STUDIES. If extrahepatic obstruction is suspected, further evaluation should determine its site and nature (Table 146–4; see Fig. 146–2). A reasonable next step is the use of a non-invasive study such as ultrasonography (US) or computed tomography (CT) to determine whether the intrahepatic and/or extrahepatic biliary system is dilated, thereby implying mechanical obstruction. Because of its lesser expense, lack of radiation exposure, portability and convenience, US is often the procedure of choice when obstruction is considered. CT may be preferred when precise definition of anatomic structure and information about the level of obstruction are desired. Both studies may occasionally fail to identify dilated ducts in obstructed patients with cirrhosis and poorly compliant hepatic parenchyma or in patients with primary sclerosing cholangitis. Conversely, the presence of dilated ducts in a patient who has previously undergone cholecystectomy does not necessarily signify obstruction.

If dilated ducts are identified, it is generally appropriate to visualize the biliary tree directly by endoscopic retrograde cholangiopancreatography (ERCP) or percutaneous transhepatic cholangiography (PTC). ERCP involves passing an endoscope into the duodenum, introducing a catheter into the ampulla of Vater, and injecting contrast medium into the distal common bile duct and or pancreatic duct. PTC involves percutaneous passage of a needle through the hepatic parenchyma and injection of contrast medium into the proximal biliary tree through a peripheral bile duct. The choice between these two procedures depends on the suspected location of the obstruction (proximal versus distal); the presence of a coagulation disorder or prior gastroduodenal surgery that might preclude, respectively, PTC or ERCP; anticipation of a therapeutic maneuver such as stent placement or endoscopic sphincterotomy; and the availability of skilled personnel.

SELECTION OF IMAGING TESTS. If the likelihood of obstruction is judged negligible (e.g., clinical findings and biochemical and serologic tests suggest viral hepatitis), no imaging studies are necessary. Conversely, if the likelihood of obstruction is judged to be very high (e.g., fever and rigors in a patient with recent biliary tract surgery), direct cholangiography may be an appropriate initial choice. If obstruction is considered possible but not highly likely, non-invasive imaging with US or CT is a reasonable first study.

Magnetic resonance imaging (MRI) can detect dilated ducts in patients with obstruction, but it has been studied less extensively than US or CT, is more expensive, and offers no clear advantage over these other techniques. Hepatobiliary scintigraphy, although occasionally helpful in the diagnosis of cholecystitis, is not sufficiently accurate to be used in most patients with suspected obstruction. Intravenous cholangiography and oral cholecystography have little or no role in the evaluation of biliary obstruction. Liver biopsy is not indicated in the routine evaluation of suspected ob-

Table 146–5 ■ MEDICAL THERAPY FOR CHOLESTASIS-ASSOCIATED PRURITUS

DRUG	REGIMEN	EFFICACY	ADVERSE EFFECTS
Antihistamines: Diphenhydramine Hydroxyzine	25–50 mg qid 25 mg tid	Rarely provide significant relief apart from sedation	Drowsiness
Cholestyramine	4–6 g 30 min before meals (may take double dose at breakfast and skip evening dose)	Beneficial in most patients	Fat malabsorption, decreased absorption of other medications, constipation
Phenobarbital	120 mg/d; dosage adjusted to maintain serum concentration between 10–40 μg/mL	Variable, not superior to placebo in controlled trials	Drowsiness, potent inducer of hepatic enzymes involved in drug metabolism
Ursodiol	13–15 mg/kg/d	Slows progression of primary biliary cirrhosis, inconsistent effect on pruritus, possibly effective in intrahepatic cholestasis of pregnancy	No major toxicity reported
Rifampin	300 mg bid	Beneficial in most but not all controlled trials to date	Inducer of hepatic enzymes involved in drug metabolism, potential hepatotoxicity, red-orange discoloration of secretions

struction, because findings diagnostic of obstruction are often absent even in the presence of biliary disease and the biopsy usually provides no information about the type or location of the obstruction. Liver biopsy should generally be reserved for the differential diagnosis of difficult or confusing cases of intrahepatic cholestasis.

TREATMENT

The treatment of hyperbilirubinemia depends on the cause. Apart from liver transplantation or phenobarbital for types I and II Crigler-Najjar syndrome, respectively, no specific therapy is available or necessary for hereditary disorders of bilirubin metabolism. Therapy in patients with increased bilirubin production should be directed at the underlying disorder, typically hemolysis. Apart from ursodeoxycholic acid for patients with primary biliary cirrhosis, little specific therapy is available for patients with cholestasis due to hepatic parenchymal disease. Offending agents such as drugs or alcohol should be withdrawn where appropriate, and transplantation should be considered for patients with progressive cholestasis and other complications of advanced liver disease.

In patients with prolonged cholestasis and fat malabsorption, orally or parenterally administered fat-soluble vitamins may be necessary, and dietary fat intake should emphasize medium-chain triglycerides. Pruritus (Table 146–5) can be a disabling manifestation of cholestasis and may be improved by bathing less frequently and using skin softeners; cholestyramine may be helpful in severe pruritus. The choleretic bile acid ursodeoxycholic acid produces biochemical improvement in patients with certain cholestatic disorders (e.g., primary biliary cirrhosis, possibly primary sclerosing cholangitis). Other agents (antihistamines, charcoal, rifampin, plasma exchange) are not of established benefit.

Bull LN, van Eijk MJT, Pawlikowska L, et al: Identification of a P-type ATPase mutated in two forms of hereditary cholestasis. Nat Genet 18:219–224, 1998. *Describes the cloning of a single gene responsible for the two allelic disorders: benign recurrent intrahepatic cholestasis and progressive familial intrahepatic cholestasis type 1.*

Lidofsky SD, Scharschmidt BF: Jaundice. *In* Feldman M, Scharschmidt BF, Sleisenger MH (eds): Gastrointestinal and Liver Disease, 6th ed. Philadelphia, WB Saunders, 1997, p 220. *Thoroughly referenced contemporary review.*

Muller M, Jansen PL: Molecular aspects of hepatobiliary transport. Am J Physiol 272: 1285, 1997. *Succinct summary of the cloning and function of membrane carriers mediating hepatic transport of bilirubin and other substances secreted in bile.*

Trauner M, Meier P, Boyer JL: Molecular pathogenesis of cholestasis. N Engl J Med 339:1217–1227, 1998. *An extensively referenced and nicely illustrated comprehensive review of the biology and molecular biology of bile formation as well as the pathophysiology of cholestasis.*

147 LABORATORY TESTS IN LIVER DISEASE AND APPROACH TO THE PATIENT WITH ABNORMAL TESTS

Richard A. Weisiger

Common liver tests fall into two categories: (1) tests that measure liver injury, such as release of hepatic enzymes (often incorrectly called liver function tests), and (2) true tests of liver function. Functions of the liver include clearance of toxic substances from the blood, synthesis of plasma proteins and lipoproteins, and intermediary metabolism (see Chapter 145). Depending on the particular disease, some of these functions may be highly compromised whereas others remain normal. Most liver tests provide only indirect evidence of hepatic integrity, and some may be abnormal for reasons other than liver disease. Liver tests must be carefully selected and interpreted within the total clinical context. Serial determinations are often required to assess the course of disease.

A number of disorders (including viral infection, drug or chemical toxicity, ischemia, biliary obstruction, and hepatic infiltration) can cause enzyme release. Because many hepatic enzymes are also found in other tissues, it may be necessary to confirm the hepatic origin of the enzyme when the underlying disease is uncertain. Three patterns of liver injury are seen: necrosis, cholestasis, and infiltration (Table 147–1). Necrosis accompanied by enzyme release is typically viral or toxic in origin and is characterized by elevated serum aminotransferase levels. Cholestasis reflects reduced biliary secretion of bile acids and bilirubin, due either to reduced bile formation by liver cells or to obstruction of bile flow at any level within the biliary tree. Chronic cholestasis is characterized by elevated alkaline phosphatase values. Infiltration of the liver by tumor or granulomas may also present as a predominant elevation of the alkaline phosphatase. Reduced hepatic synthesis (e.g., of clotting factors) typically occurs with severe acute necrosis and with any chronic liver disease that progresses to end-stage cirrhosis. Because these patterns may vary in individual cases, confirmatory studies (e.g., viral serologies, cholangiography) are typically required.

SERUM ENZYME TESTS

AMINOTRANSFERASES. Aminotransferases (transaminases) catalyze the transfer of the α-amino group from aspartate (aspartate aminotransferase [AST], formerly serum glutamic oxaloacetic transaminase [SGOT]) or alanine (alanine aminotransferase [ALT], formerly serum glutamic pyruvic transaminase [SGPT]) to the α-keto group of ketoglutarate. Serum levels are normally below 40 IU/L, but may exceed 1000 IU/L in acute viral or toxic injury. Isozymes of AST are present in liver cell mitochondria and cytoplasm, whereas ALT is confined to the cytoplasm. Aminotransferases are metabolized but are not cleared from the blood by excretion into urine or bile. Serum levels of AST and ALT are elevated in most hepatic diseases; the height of the aminotransferase activity in general reflects the current activity of the disease process. However, there are important exceptions. Even the most severe forms of alcoholic hepatitis rarely increase aminotransferase levels above 200 to 300 IU/L (see Chapter 153). In contrast, serum aminotransferase activities of 1000 IU/L or more are often present in mild acute viral hepatitis or shortly after acute biliary obstruction, as may occur during passage of a gallstone. Conversely, serum aminotransferase levels may fall during the clinical course of massive hepatic necrosis because the liver is so severely damaged that little enzyme activity remains (see Chapter 154).

Serum aminotransferase levels provide a relatively specific screening test for hepatobiliary disease. Although AST levels may be increased in diseases of other organs (e.g., myocardium and skeletal muscle), values more than ten times the upper limit of normal usually reflect hepatic or biliary pathology. In the context of other clinical and laboratory findings, identification of the source of increased serum aminotransferase activity is usually easy. Aminotransferase values are also useful in monitoring the activity of acute or chronic parenchymal liver disease after the diagnosis has been made. However, aminotransferase levels correlate poorly with prognosis and disease severity as assessed by liver biopsy, and they are often completely normal in advanced cirrhosis. Finally, aminotransferase levels may be useful diagnostically. It is distinctly uncommon for the AST to exceed 15 times the upper limit of normal in chronic bile duct obstruction without cholangitis, whereas AST levels more than 6 times normal are uncommon in alcoholic liver disease in the absence of other causes. In most liver diseases the ratio of AST to ALT is typically 1 or less. However, ratios of 2 or greater are common in alcoholic hepatitis, reflecting both increased secretion of mitochondrial AST into plasma and preferential loss of ALT activity due to pyridoxine deficiency, a common complication of alcoholism (see Chapter 153). Elevated ratios have also been reported in fulminant hepatitis due to Wilson's disease (see Chapter 220).

ALKALINE PHOSPHATASE. Alkaline phosphatases, present in many tissues (e.g., liver, bile ducts, intestine, bone, kidney, placenta, and leukocytes), catalyze the release of orthophosphate from ester substrates at alkaline pH. The normal serum activity in adults is 25 to 85 IU/L, although higher levels are normal in children and in pregnancy. The biologic function of alkaline phosphatase is unknown, except for an apparent role in the deposition of hydroxy-

Table 147–1 ■ TYPICAL LIVER TEST PATTERNS

TEST	HEPATOCELLULAR NECROSIS			BILIARY OBSTRUCTION			INFILTRATION (CHRONIC)
	Toxic or Ischemic	Viral	Alcohol	Chronic Complete	Chronic Partial	Acute Complete (First 24 hr)	
Aminotransferases	50–100x	5–50x	2–5x	1–5x	1–5x	1–50x	1–3x
Alkaline phosphatase	1–3x	1–3x	1–10x	2–20x	2–10x	May be normal	1–20x
Bilirubin	1–5x	1–30x	1–30x	1–30x	1–5x	Usually normal	1–5x
Prothrombin time	Prolonged in severe cases, unresponsive to vitamin K			May be prolonged, responsive to vitamin K	Usually normal	Usually normal	Usually normal
Albumin	Normal in acute illness, may be decreased in chronic disease			Usually normal, but may be decreased in biliary cirrhosis		Usually normal	Usually normal
Typical disorders	Acetaminophen toxicity, shock liver	Acute hepatitis A or B	Alcoholic hepatitis	Pancreatic carcinoma	Sclerosing cholangitis	Choledocholithiasis	Primary or metastatic carcinoma, *Mycobacterium avium-intracellulare* infection

Modified from Davern TJ, Scharschmidt B: Biochemical liver tests. *In* Feldman M, Scharschmidt BF, Sleisenger MH (eds): Sleisenger & Fordtran's Gastrointestinal and Liver Disease, 6th ed. Philadelphia, WB Saunders, 1998, pp 1112–1122.

apatite in osteoid to form bone. Normally, serum alkaline phosphatase activity reflects mainly the hepatic and bone isozymes, although the intestinal form may account for 20 to 60% of the total after a fatty meal, particularly in blood groups O and B. In the later stages of pregnancy, the placental contribution may be substantial. A less common variant, called the *Regan isozyme,* is associated with tumors (especially hepatoma and lung cancer) and appears identical to the placental form (see Chapter 156).

Serum alkaline phosphatase activity also may be increased in bone disorders (e.g., Paget's disease, osteomalacia, metastases to bone), later stages of pregnancy, rapid bone growth, chronic renal failure, and, occasionally, the presence of malignancy not involving bones or liver. In some cases, the source is obvious because of other clinical and laboratory findings. When the source is less apparent, methods such as heat stability and electrophoretic separation are available to differentiate hepatobiliary alkaline phosphatase from other isozymes. However, it is usually more practical to measure serum levels of γ-glutamyl transpeptidase (GGT) or 5′-nucleotidase, which tend to parallel levels of alkaline phosphatase in hepatobiliary disease but are not usually increased in bone disease. In liver disease, increased serum alkaline phosphatase activity, which reflects increased enzyme synthesis rather than decreased biliary excretion or leakage from damaged cells, may be triggered by high tissue bile salt concentrations in cholestasis. Because its half-life in serum is approximately 1 week, serum levels may remain elevated for days to weeks after resolution of biliary obstruction.

Slight to moderate increases in serum alkaline phosphatase activity (up to three times normal) occur in many parenchymal disorders of the liver such as hepatitis and cirrhosis. In the absence of bone disease, larger increases (3 to 10 times normal) usually indicate intrahepatic or extrahepatic obstruction of bile flow. Although the highest levels typically occur with common bile duct obstruction, very high levels may also be seen with intrahepatic cholestasis and with infiltrative or mass lesions (primary or metastatic cancer, lymphoma, leukemia, sarcoidosis, or *Mycobacterium avium-intracellulare* infection). A normal serum bilirubin in the setting of chronic elevation of the alkaline phosphatase suggests localized infiltrative disease or obstruction of a portion of the biliary tree due to stricture, tumor, or other localized lesions. Alkaline phosphatase is a relatively sensitive screening test for primary or metastatic tumors of the liver; however, up to one third of patients with isolated elevations of serum hepatobiliary alkaline phosphatase activity have no demonstrable liver or biliary disease.

OTHER HEPATIC ENZYMES. 5′-*Nucleotidase* (5′-NT) is a plasma membrane enzyme that cleaves orthophosphate from the 5′ position on the pentose sugar of adenosine or inosine phosphate whereas *leucine aminopeptidase* (LAP) is a ubiquitous cellular peptidase. The serum activity of both enzymes usually increases in cholestasis, and their major clinical value is to help determine if an elevated serum alkaline phosphatase activity originates from the liver. Both of these enzymes may be increased in normal late pregnancy.

γ-Glutamyl transpeptidase (GGT), present in many tissues, increases in serum not only in hepatobiliary disease but also after myocardial infarction, in neuromuscular diseases, in pancreatic disease (even in the absence of biliary obstruction), in pulmonary disease, in diabetes, and during the ingestion of ethanol and other inducers of microsomal enzymes. Because serum GGT levels are usually normal in bone disease, GGT may be helpful in confirming the hepatic origin of alkaline phosphatase. Measurement of GGT has been proposed as a sensitive screening test for hepatobiliary disease and for monitoring abstinence from ethanol, but its low specificity ensures that many who test positive will have no identifiable liver disease on further study. It offers no clear advantage over LAP or 5′-NT for identifying the source of increased serum alkaline phosphatase activity except in pregnancy. Serum GGT levels may be normal despite elevated hepatobiliary alkaline phosphatase levels in certain rare disorders, including benign recurrent intrahepatic cholestasis and Byler's disease (see Chapter 152).

Lactate dehydrogenase (LDH) levels are often elevated in liver disease but are usually not helpful in diagnosis because this enzyme is also found in most other body tissues.

TESTS BASED ON CLEARANCE OF METABOLITES AND DRUGS

A major function of the liver is to remove various metabolites and ingested toxins from the blood (see Chapter 148). In liver disease, clearance of these compounds may be impaired owing to loss of parenchymal cells, obstruction of bile flow, impaired cellular uptake or metabolism, or reduced or uneven hepatic blood flow. When a metabolite is produced at a relatively constant rate (as is usually true for bilirubin), its serum level can be a sensitive indicator of liver function. The removal rate of certain exogenous drugs and dye compounds from plasma can be used similarly.

BILIRUBIN. Serum bilirubin is usually elevated in significant liver disease, but it may be elevated in benign disorders such as Gilbert's syndrome (see Chapter 146), non-hepatic diseases such as hemolysis and ineffective erythropoiesis, and certain inherited disorders of bilirubin transport or metabolism (see Chapter 152). Higher plasma bilirubin levels are associated with a poorer prognosis in alcoholic hepatitis, primary biliary cirrhosis, and fulminant hepatic failure. Normal serum bilirubin is almost entirely unconjugated and reflects a balance between bilirubin production and hepatic elimination. Chronic hemolysis cannot produce elevations of serum bilirubin above 5 mg/dL in the absence of liver disease. Plasma conjugated bilirubin is elevated in liver disease owing to reflux from liver cells, but the level cannot reliably be used to distinguish parenchymal from obstructive causes. Because conjugated bilirubin is excreted in urine, plasma levels greater than 30 mg/dL are uncommon in the absence of renal failure. During the recovery phase of prolonged hepatitis or cholestasis, normalization of serum bilirubin may require much longer than other liver tests due to formation of poorly cleared albumin-bilirubin conjugates (the delta fraction).

AMMONIA. The liver clears ammonia from blood by converting it to urea by means of the Krebs-Henseleit cycle for excretion by the kidney (see Chapter 211). In the setting of severe hepatic dysfunction (e.g., fulminant hepatic failure) or portosystemic shunting, serum ammonia levels rise. The level of serum ammonia is widely used to confirm the diagnosis of hepatic encephalopathy and to monitor the success of therapy, but the correlation of the ammonia level with the degree of encephalopathy is only approximate (see Chapter 154). Elevated ammonia levels may also be seen when ammonia production is increased by intestinal flora (e.g., after a high protein meal or gastrointestinal bleeding), by the kidney (in response to metabolic alkalosis or hypokalemia), or in certain rare genetic diseases affecting the pathway of urea synthesis (see Chapter 211). Arterial or cerebrospinal levels of ammonia offer little advantage over venous levels.

DRUG CLEARANCE. The liver is primarily responsible for clearing many drugs from blood, and clearance of certain drugs can quantify this function. However, clearance tests are more expensive, invasive, and labor intensive than other equally or more useful liver tests and have not been shown to be superior in predicting survival.

SYNTHETIC FUNCTION TESTS

PROTHROMBIN TIME. The prothrombin time depends on the plasma concentration not only of prothrombin but also of other clotting factors synthesized in the liver, including Factors V, VII, and IX and fibrinogen. The test is abnormal in the setting of reduced synthesis (e.g., liver failure, vitamin K deficiency, warfarin administration), increased consumption (e.g., disseminated intravascular coagulation), or both.

All of the major coagulation factors are synthesized in the liver except for Factor VIII, which is made in vascular endothelium and reticuloendothelial cells. The prothrombin time measures the activity of several of these factors, including Factors I, II, V, VII, and X. Synthesis of prothrombin and Factors VII, IX, and X depends on an adequate supply of vitamin K, which activates certain hepatic polypeptides by stimulating the synthesis of the calcium-binding residue, γ-carboxyglutamic acid. An abnormal prothrombin time is commonly caused by vitamin K deficiency, liver disease, or both and may rarely be seen with inherited abnormalities. Vitamin K, a fat-soluble vitamin that is found in many foods, is also produced by intestinal bacteria (see Chapter 185). Deficiency is most commonly seen in malnutrition and malabsorption syndromes, including failure to absorb dietary fat due to biliary obstruction or other causes of cholestasis (see Chapter 185). It may also be seen with antibiotic suppression of intestinal bacteria, especially when the patient is receiving inadequate oral or parenteral vitamin K replacement.

Any acute or chronic liver disease may cause an abnormal prothrombin time by impairing the synthesis of essential clotting factors. Because the plasma half-life of these factors is typically less than one day, the prothrombin time responds rapidly to changes in hepatic synthetic function. This property makes the prothrombin time particularly useful for following the course of acute liver diseases; significant elevation often indicates an unfavorable prognosis.

An abnormal prothrombin time may be of diagnostic value in the evaluation of the jaundiced patient. In general, when it is prolonged on the basis of vitamin K deficiency alone (as in fat malabsorption due to cholestasis), it will usually normalize within 24 hours of parenteral administration of vitamin K. In contrast, when the synthesis of clotting factors is diminished because of parenchymal liver disease, response to vitamin K may be minimal or absent. Both factors may coexist, however. In severe liver failure, elevation of the prothrombin time may also reflect disseminated intravascular coagulation (see Chapter 185). Because of these complicating factors, the prothrombin time must be interpreted in the context of all available information.

The partial thromboplastin time is used to assess the "intrinsic" clotting mechanism and reflects the activity of all clotting factors except for platelet factor 3, Factor VII, and Factor XII. For this reason, the test is complementary to the prothrombin time and may indicate deficiencies of other clotting factors or the presence of a circulating anticoagulant (see Chapter 185).

ALBUMIN. Albumin, synthesized exclusively in the liver at a rate of 100 to 200 mg/kg/day, has a long half-life in plasma (about 3 weeks in healthy adults). The synthetic rate is influenced by many factors, including nutritional state, the presence of systemic and/or liver disease, thyroid and glucocorticoid hormones, plasma colloid osmotic pressure, and toxins such as alcohol and carbon tetrachloride. The normal mechanism of albumin turnover is not well understood, although losses are increased in nephrotic syndrome, protein-losing enteropathy, severe burns, exfoliative dermatitis, and gastrointestinal bleeding.

The serum albumin concentration reflects a balance between synthesis and loss and is therefore not specific for the functional state of the liver. Because the serum half-life is long, abnormalities are slow to develop and may persist for weeks after correction of the underlying problem. Only when other factors are excluded can hypoalbuminemia be used as an important indicator of chronic liver disease. In patients with cirrhosis and ascites, hypoalbuminemia commonly reflects diminished synthesis; but in some patients, synthesis is normal, and hypoalbuminemia is caused by a redistribution into ascitic fluid. Serum albumin may also be low after significant gastrointestinal blood loss as in variceal bleeding.

SERUM LIPIDS AND LIPOPROTEINS. Parenchymal liver disease and bile duct obstruction may produce significant abnormalities in serum lipids and lipoproteins. In acute parenchymal liver disease, the serum electrophoretic band of α_1-lipoprotein may be lost (altered high density lipoproteins) and transient hypertriglyceridemia may also occur (abnormal low-density lipoproteins rich in triglycerides). These changes appear attributable in part to deficient activity of plasma lecithin-cholesterol acyltransferase (LCAT), an enzyme of hepatic origin. With resolution of the acute liver injury, plasma lipids and lipoproteins return to their previous state.

The liver is primarily responsible for removing cholesterol from the body by its direct secretion into bile or its conversion to bile acids. In cholestasis, the serum concentrations of unesterified cholesterol and phospholipids increase, and xanthomas and xanthelasma may develop if these abnormalities are severe and sustained. A major fraction of the increased plasma unesterified cholesterol is accounted for by an abnormal low-density lipoprotein, designated LpX. LpX is not of value in the differential diagnosis of jaundice, but it may contribute to an elevated plasma cholesterol concentration in patients with liver disease.

IMMUNOLOGIC TESTS

GLOBULINS. Serum globulins are of limited diagnostic use in hepatobiliary diseases. Their concentration, as measured by serum protein electrophoresis or salt fractionation, may be influenced by a wide variety of hepatic and extrahepatic factors and disease states. An important exception is the finding by serum protein electrophoresis of a reduced concentration of the α_1-globulin fraction. Because approximately 85% of this fraction is α_1-antitrypsin, a decrease in its concentration suggests α_1-antitrypsin deficiency, an inherited disorder associated with neonatal hepatitis, cirrhosis, and pulmonary emphysema (see Chapter 75). The mechanism of the increased serum globulin concentration in liver disease is not fully understood. Elevated IgM concentrations are common in primary biliary cirrhosis, but other clinical, laboratory, and imaging procedures are of greater diagnostic value. Diffuse increases in globulin concentrations are commonly seen in cirrhosis and may be especially pronounced in chronic autoimmune hepatitis in the absence of active hepatitis B or C infection.

MITOCHONDRIAL ANTIBODY. In approximately 90% of patients with primary biliary cirrhosis, the serum contains antibodies directed against a lipoprotein component of the inner mitochondrial membrane (see Chapter 157). The antibodies are neither organ nor species specific. These antibodies include the three main immunoglobulin classes, are complement fixing, and bind to at least seven different components of the inner and outer mitochondrial membranes. In patients with primary biliary cirrhosis, the titer is not related to the increased level of serum IgM or the stage or severity of the disease. Of the several types of mitochondrial antibodies thus far identified, M_2 is the type usually found in primary biliary cirrhosis.

Mitochondrial antibodies are also present in up to 25% of patients with histologically active chronic hepatitis and postnecrotic cirrhosis and in 7 to 8% of asymptomatic relatives of patients with primary biliary cirrhosis, compared with only 0.4 to 0.7% of the general population. They are rarely present in extrahepatic biliary obstruction. Positive tests also occur in a small percentage of patients with non-hepatic diseases, including the collagen vascular disorders, thyroiditis, myasthenia gravis, Addison's disease, autoimmune hemolytic anemia, and chronic biologic false-positive reactions for syphilis.

A negative mitochondrial antibody renders the diagnosis of primary biliary cirrhosis unlikely, although it does not exclude it, and a positive result helps confirm parenchymal disease. Because the incidence of gallstones in patients with primary biliary cirrhosis is approximately 40%, a positive mitochondrial antibody test does not reliably exclude coexistent, clinically important extrahepatic obstruction.

ANTINUCLEAR AND SMOOTH MUSCLE ANTIBODIES. Either or both of these tests are positive in a variable percentage of patients with chronic non-viral hepatitis. These antibodies also occur in a minority of patients with primary biliary cirrhosis. As is true of the mitochondrial antibody, these factors are neither organ nor species specific. They probably do not play a role in pathogenesis. The presence of these antibodies in serum does not exclude bile duct obstruction.

TESTS FOR HEPATITIS VIRUS INFECTION. These tests and their clinical significance are discussed in Chapter 149.

EXAMINATIONS OF URINE AND STOOL

The presence of bilirubin in urine indicates that a significant fraction of plasma bilirubin is conjugated; it is strong evidence for hepatobiliary disease. Jaundice in the absence of bilirubinuria indicates an exclusively unconjugated hyperbilirubinemia, usually reflecting hemolysis, ineffective erythropoiesis, or an inherited disorder of bilirubin conjugation. Urine and fecal urobilinogen determinations rarely provide useful information. Fecal occult blood tests may provide the first evidence of an alimentary tract lesion related to hepatobiliary disease (e.g., tumors metastatic to liver, ulcerative colitis associated with sclerosing cholangitis) and may explain the onset or exacerbation of hepatic encephalopathy. In certain clinical circumstances, stool culture or examination for ova and parasites may provide important information.

HEMATOLOGIC TESTS IN LIVER DISEASE

Diseases of the liver may be associated with a wide variety of hematologic abnormalities. In acute liver disease not associated with liver failure, major changes in the formed elements are uncommon and consist primarily of mild anemia, reflecting either low-grade hemolysis or marrow depression. Slight leukopenia is not uncommon and is often associated with atypical lymphocytes. In other forms of acute liver disease, hematologic abnormalities such as marrow suppression may be caused by ethanol or drugs. Severe aplastic anemia may sometimes complicate acute viral hepatitis, especially after liver transplantation for fulminant hepatitis C infection. In the alcoholic, Zieve's syndrome (hemolytic anemia and hypertriglyceridemia) may rarely be found. Coagulopathy may complicate liver failure, owing to depressed hepatic synthesis of clotting factors and/or disseminated intravascular coagulation.

In chronic liver disease, especially with cholestasis, erythrocytic target cells result from an expansion of the cell membrane with relative preservation of the cholesterol-phospholipid ratio. Spur cells (acanthocytes), most often found in advanced alcoholic cirrhosis, reflect a more profound relative and absolute increase in membrane cholesterol. Red blood cells, white blood cells, and platelets may be decreased in patients with portal hypertension, primarily because of hypersplenism (see Chapter 178). Iron deficiency, megaloblastic anemias, and sideroblastic anemias may be caused by associated nutritional, pathologic, or pharmacologic influences.

LIVER BIOPSY

Liver biopsy is of value in the diagnosis of diffuse or localized parenchymal diseases, including cirrhosis, chronic hepatitis, and cancers. It is commonly performed by the blind percutaneous technique but may be guided by ultrasonographic or radiologic studies or performed under direct visualization during laparoscopy or laparotomy when specific areas must be sampled. Because the histologic changes in acute hepatitis or acute cholestatic jaundice are usually non-specific, the value of liver biopsy in this setting is primarily prognostic. Relative or absolute contraindications include the presence of biliary sepsis, high-grade biliary obstruction, ascites, coagulopathy, and right pleural disease.

IMAGING TECHNIQUES AND CHOLANGIOGRAPHY

These techniques are discussed in detail in Chapters 121 and 157.

APPROACH TO THE ASYMPTOMATIC PATIENT WITH ABNORMAL LIVER TESTS

The apparently healthy patient with an isolated abnormality of the aminotransferases or alkaline phosphatase requires careful evaluation to identify any underlying disease while avoiding unneeded testing. Often, no significant disease is found despite extensive evaluation. Common causes of abnormal enzyme tests include obesity, alcohol consumption, chronic hepatitis C, bone disease, and muscle injury.

ASYMPTOMATIC AMINOTRANSFERASE ELEVATION (FIG. 147–1). Incidental discovery of mild to moderate elevation of transaminases is common among blood donors and others subjected to routine screening. Approximately one third of such patients have no elevation on subsequent testing. Higher enzyme levels and the presence of other abnormal liver tests increase the probability of clinically significant liver disease. Further testing is generally indicated only in patients with persistent abnormalities. Initial screening

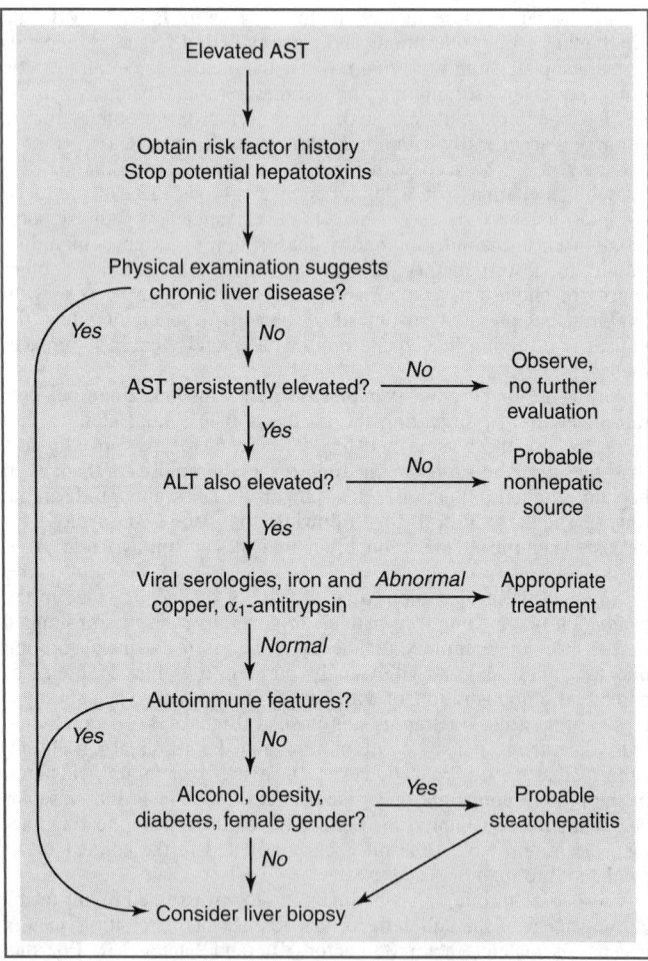

FIGURE 147–1 ■ Approach to the asymptomatic patient with isolated elevated levels of serum aspartate aminotransferase (AST). ALT = alanine aminotransferase.

should include a careful history of exposure to hepatotoxins (alcohol, prescription drugs, over-the-counter medications, herbs, chemicals, and occupational exposures) and their discontinuation. Hepatic origin should be confirmed using the ALT value; if the ALT level is normal, a muscle source is likely. If the ALT level is abnormal, the patient should be screened serologically for hepatitis A, B, and C. Older persons should be screened for hemochromatosis with an iron and transferrin level, whereas younger persons should be screened with a ceruloplasmin and urine copper for Wilson's disease. Malaria and schistosomiasis should be considered in appropriate settings. If these tests are negative, screening for α_1-antitrypsin deficiency is indicated. Younger women should also be screened for markers of autoimmune liver disease. A substantial fraction of patients have fatty liver associated with non-alcoholic steatonecrosis, which often responds to weight loss or improved diabetic control. AST abnormalities caused by alcohol-induced steatosis should normalize within several weeks of stopping ethanol. Fatty liver can often be diagnosed clinically. If the aminotransferase abnormality persists for 6 to 12 months in the absence of any apparent cause, liver biopsy may be warranted.

ASYMPTOMATIC ALKALINE PHOSPHATASE ELEVATION (FIG. 147–2). Many patients with isolated elevation of the alkaline phosphatase have non-hepatic causes, including bone disease, rapid bone growth, and pregnancy. An abnormal alkaline phosphatase should be confirmed with the patient fasting, because intestinal alkaline phosphatase may be elevated after a meal. An hepatic source may be inferred if the serum γ-glutamyl transpeptidase is abnormal or by fractionation of the alkaline phosphatase. Essentially all such patients should receive an hepatobiliary sonogram (or other imaging test). Demonstration of dilated intrahepatic or extrahepatic bile ducts should prompt retrograde or transhepatic cholangiography. Any suggestion of intrahepatic mass lesions should prompt an aggressive evaluation for possible malignancy. Because colon cancer often metastasizes to liver, colonoscopy or barium enema may be useful in appropriate cases. Infiltrative diseases,

including schistosomiasis and granulomatous hepatitis, should be considered. A careful history will identify patients at risk for intrahepatic cholestasis due to drugs or toxins. A positive antimitochondrial antibody test suggests primary biliary cirrhosis. Liver biopsy may be useful in those patients whose abnormality persists without any apparent cause.

Davern TJ, Scharschmidt B: Biochemical liver tests. *In* Feldman M, Scharschmidt BF, Sleisenger MH (eds) Sleisenger & Fordtran's Gastrointestinal and Liver Disease, 6th ed. Philadelphia, WB Saunders, 1998, pp 1112–1122. *A recent and comprehensive discussion of biochemical liver tests including their use in differentiating among liver and biliary diseases.*

Jalan R, Hayes PC: Review article: Quantitative tests of liver function. Aliment Pharmacol Ther 9:263–270, 1995.

148 TOXIC AND DRUG-INDUCED LIVER DISEASE

Nathan M. Bass

The central role of the liver in drug metabolism results in this organ being exposed to a large variety of potentially toxic chemical agents and metabolites, including naturally occurring plant alkaloids and mycotoxins, industrial chemicals, and, most commonly, pharmacologic agents used in treating disease. The manifestations of toxic and drug-induced liver disease constitute a spectrum of clinical, laboratory, and histopathologic changes and prognoses virtually as broad as the entire range of acute and chronic hepatobiliary disorders. The severity may range, at one extreme, from asymptomatic abnormalities in liver function tests to fatal, massive liver necrosis at the other. Viral hepatitis and biliary obstruction may be closely mimicked by hepatotoxic drug reactions, and exposure to certain agents may also lead to chronic hepatitis, cirrhosis, and liver tumors.

PATHOGENESIS

It is rare for a parent chemical to be directly responsible for chemically induced liver disease; more commonly a toxic metabolite(s) formed by the drug-metabolizing enzymes within the liver is the most immediate cause of damage. Drug biotransformation appears to be a common requirement for the expression of many different types of drug-induced liver injury. Individual susceptibility to the injury produced by some drugs varies considerably. Potentially hepatotoxic agents are therefore conventionally divided into two categories based on the predictability with which they produce liver disease: *intrinsic hepatotoxins* and *idiosyncratic hepatotoxins*.

Intrinsic hepatotoxins typically produce acute liver damage after a relatively brief latent period (usually a few days) in a predictable, dose-dependent fashion that is largely independent of host susceptibility factors and that is readily reproducible in experimental animals. Examples of this group include the industrial solvents carbon tetrachloride, 2-nitropropane, trichloroethane, the octapeptide toxins of the *Amanita* mushroom species, and the antipyretic acetaminophen. In most instances, toxic metabolites formed from the parent compound by the cytochrome P-450 drug-metabolizing enzymes (free radicals, electrophiles) produce liver damage by covalently modifying liver macromolecules or by generating reactive oxygen species and subsequent peroxidation of cell membrane lipids.

Idiosyncratic hepatotoxins, in contrast, produce liver disease in an infrequent, unpredictable fashion after a variable latent period, often only after several months of administration of the drug. A large number of therapeutic agents are capable of producing idiosyncratic hepatotoxic reactions in a small proportion of patients who receive them (e.g., halothane, isoniazid [INH], phenytoin, and chlorpromazine). Although severe liver disease occurs infrequently with these drugs, milder hepatic dysfunction may occur frequently (e.g., with INH and chlorpromazine), or toxic liver disease may be reproduced in animal models (e.g., halothane). Many of these

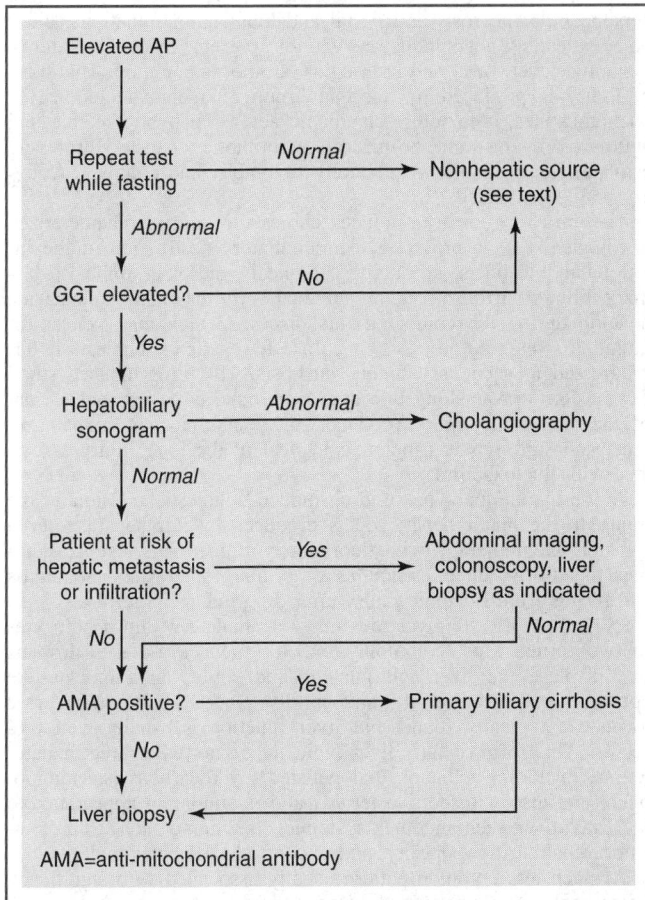

FIGURE 147–2 ■ Evaluation of isolated elevated levels of serum alkaline phosphatase (AP). GGT = γ-glutamyl transpeptidase.

agents may therefore be mild "intrinsic hepatotoxins" that lead to severe "idiosyncratic" liver disease in a few susceptible individuals, possibly because of variations in the pathways of drug biotransformation, immune-mediated hypersensitivity ("drug allergy"), or both. In a given individual, genetic polymorphism in drug-metabolizing enzymes may increase activity of enzyme pathways that form toxic metabolites and thereby increase the risk of severe toxicity from drugs that are processed in part through these pathways. In idiosyncratic drug-induced liver disease, fever, arthralgias, rash, and eosinophilia are often prominent, indicative of a hypersensitivity-based mechanism. Furthermore, in some cases of drug-induced hepatitis (e.g., halothane), antibodies that recognize liver cell macromolecules covalently modified by metabolites of the implicated drug antibodies have been detected. Adducts formed on the liver cell surface between drug metabolites and liver cell membrane proteins may therefore constitute neoantigens that can provoke immune-mediated liver damage.

Drugs and toxins produce a variety of pathologic lesions in the liver (Table 148–1). Some agents may injure the liver in more than one way. For example, INH may produce a non-specific focal hepatitis, an acute viral hepatitis-like lesion, or chronic active hepatitis, whereas oral contraceptives may cause cholestasis or liver cell adenoma and have been implicated in hepatic vein thrombosis and other vascular lesions.

ZONAL NECROSIS. Intrinsic hepatotoxins typically cause liver cell necrosis, largely confined within a particular zone of the liver lobule. Centrilobular necrosis, the most common pattern of zonal injury, is produced by carbon tetrachloride, acetaminophen, and *Amanita* toxins. This pattern of injury is explained in part by the greater abundance of cytochrome P-450 drug-metabolizing enzymes in the central region of the liver lobule and possibly also by the relative hypoxemia of the centrilobular region. Halothane, despite its classification as an idiosyncratic hepatotoxic agent, also frequently produces centrilobular necrosis. Periportal zonal necrosis, a much rarer lesion, is produced by allyl alcohol and yellow phosphorus. Extremely high elevations of serum aminotransferases usu-

ally accompany this type of liver injury; and, in severe cases, acute liver failure may result. Acute zonal necrosis is either fatal or is followed by complete recovery.

NON-SPECIFIC FOCAL HEPATITIS. Non-specific focal hepatitis consists of scattered foci of liver cell necrosis with mononuclear cell infiltrates, without the characteristic features of viral hepatitis. Non-specific hepatitis may result from many forms of drug injury, including the dose-dependent, intrinsic hepatotoxicity of aspirin and oxacillin. This lesion has an excellent prognosis and resolves completely when the responsible drug is discontinued.

VIRAL HEPATITIS–LIKE REACTIONS. Diffuse hepatocellular degeneration and necrosis with variable inflammatory infiltration and acidophil bodies, resembling the acute pathologic lesion and the clinical manifestations of viral hepatitis, is another common pattern of idiosyncratic injury. In severe cases this lesion may progress to bridging, submassive or massive liver necrosis, and fulminant liver failure. Drugs producing viral hepatitis–like reactions include halothane, INH, troglitazone, methyldopa, sulfonamides, and phenytoin. In some instances, the presence of fever, rash, and serum and tissue eosinophilia, as well as other evidence of immunologic dysfunction, are important clues in the diagnosis of drug-induced disease and also implicate a hypersensitivity-based mechanism. In other examples, such as halothane and INH, features of hypersensitivity are highly variable or distinctly rare.

CHOLESTASIS. Cholestasis is characterized clinically by symptoms of pruritus and jaundice and biochemically by elevated serum alkaline phosphatase levels and minimal or modest increases in serum aminotransferase levels. Four distinct forms of this common manifestation of drug-induced liver injury are recognized. In the first, caused principally by natural and synthetic estrogens and by 17α-substituted androgenic and anabolic steroids, there is usually little or no evidence of hepatocellular necrosis or inflammation. The injury is most simply viewed as the impaired secretion of bile by the liver cell, probably reflecting a direct steroid effect on the physical properties of cellular membranes or the function of canalicular proteins involved in bile secretion. The lesion is completely and rapidly reversible.

In the second form of cholestatic injury, there is significant hepatocellular necrosis and portal and lobular inflammation; acidophil bodies and eosinophils are variably present. Systemic features, including fever, rash, and arthralgias, are not uncommon. This form of injury is produced by a broad group of agents, including the phenothiazines, amoxicillin-clavulanic acid, oral hypoglycemic and antithyroid agents, and the macrolide antibiotics (e.g., erythromycin estolate). Its prognosis is generally favorable, and complete recovery may be expected.

The third form of drug-induced cholestatic injury is characterized histologically by a progressive inflammatory destruction of the interlobular bile ducts, producing a clinical syndrome similar to primary biliary cirrhosis. Deep jaundice, pruritus, and xanthelasma develop during the course of this disease, which may persist for months to years before resolving. In a few patients, cholestasis has progressed to secondary biliary cirrhosis. This drug-induced small duct lesion, or vanishing bile duct syndrome, is an unusual variant of the cholestatic injury produced by phenothiazines, carbamazepine, and sulfonylureas, but it is typical of the liver injury associated with flucloxacillin.

A fourth, unique type of drug-induced cholestatic lesion is the injury to the major hepatic ducts produced by intrahepatic arterial infusion chemotherapy with fluorodeoxyuridine. This lesion resembles the diffuse ductal strictures of primary sclerosing cholangitis and results from ischemic injury after drug-induced arteritis.

FATTY LIVER. Triglycerides may accumulate within hepatocytes in two forms. Most commonly, fat accumulates as large droplets that displace the liver cell nucleus and confer an adipocyte-like appearance. Hepatomegaly and mildly elevated aminotransferase levels are typically found, but liver function is usually well preserved. This form of fatty liver typically occurs with direct hepatotoxins, including ethanol, halogenated hydrocarbons, acetaminophen, and also with corticosteroids and is similar in appearance to the fatty liver seen in other systemic conditions, such as protein-calorie malnutrition, obesity, and uncontrolled diabetes mellitus.

A much less common pattern usually associated with significant, occasionally fatal, hepatic dysfunction, is seen in association with tetracycline or valproic acid hepatotoxicity, and occasionally with

Table 148–1 ■ CLASSIFICATION OF DRUG-INDUCED LIVER DISEASE

CATEGORY	EXAMPLES
Zonal necrosis	Acetaminophen, carbon tetrachloride, simvastatin
Non-specific hepatitis	Aspirin, oxacillin
Viral hepatitis–like reaction	Halothane, isoniazid, phenytoin, diclofenac
Chronic hepatitis	
Autoimmune hepatitis–like	Methyldopa, dantrolene, diclofenac
Viral hepatitis–like	Isoniazid, halothane
Cholestasis	
Non-inflammatory	Estrogens, 17α-substituted steroids
Inflammatory	Amoxicillin-clavulanate, piroxicam,
small duct injury (vanishing bile duct syndrome)	flucloxacillin, thiabendazole, haloperidol
Large duct injury (sclerosing cholangitis)	Fluorodeoxyuridine
Fatty liver	
Large droplet	Ethanol, corticosteroids
Small droplet	Tetracycline, valproic acid, didanosine
Phospholipidosis and steatohepatitis	Amiodarone, perhexiline maleate
Granulomas	Phenylbutazone, allopurinol
Fibrosis	Methotrexate, hypervitaminosis A
Tumors	
Adenoma	Estrogens
Angiosarcoma	Vinyl chloride
Vascular lesions	
Hepatic vein thrombosis	Estrogens
Veno-occlusive disease	Anticancer agents, azathioprine, *Senecio* alkaloids
Peliosis hepatis	Anabolic steroids, estrogens
Hepatic arteritis	Allopurinol, fluorodeoxyuridine
Nodular regenerative hyperplasia	Azathioprine, anticancer agents

alcoholic liver disease, and resembles that seen in Reye's syndrome, obstetric fatty liver, and Jamaican vomiting sickness. It consists of fat deposited in smaller droplets throughout the liver cell, with the nucleus remaining central. This pattern of liver injury, accompanied by profound, often fatal lactic acidosis, has been produced by several antiviral nucleoside analogues, including didanosine (ddI), fialuridine (FIAU), and zidovudine (azidothymidine [AZT]). Curiously, in the case of zidovudine, the hepatic morphologic lesion has been large-droplet rather than small-droplet fat. A distinctive type of hepatic lipid accumulation in the form of lysosomal phospholipid storage occurs as a direct effect of the drugs amiodarone and perhexiline maleate.

GRANULOMAS. Therapeutic agents are probably responsible for up to one third of cases of granulomatous hepatitis. Drug-induced granulomas are typically non-caseating and are often associated with extrahepatic granulomas and prominent systemic features of hypersensitivity. Responsible agents include phenylbutazone, quinidine, allopurinol, phenytoin, hydralazine, sulfonamides, and sulfonylurea derivatives.

CHRONIC HEPATITIS. Chronic hepatitis has been associated with an increasing number of drugs, including amiodarone, dantrolene, INH, methyldopa, nitrofurantoin, oxyphenisatin, troglitazone, phenytoin, propylthiouracil, sulfonamides, and diclofenac. Although these agents more often cause acute liver injury, prolonged use may occasionally result in a chronic progressive process, leading in some instances to cirrhosis. The histologic and clinical abnormalities usually resemble those seen in idiopathic autoimmune or viral chronic active hepatitis. In the case of amiodarone, a lesion strikingly similar to that of alcoholic hepatitis with prominent Mallory bodies may be produced. In many cases, the lesion is largely or completely reversible, but in severe cases resolution may require many months after the drug is discontinued. In some cases, progressive liver failure and death may ensue despite stopping the drug.

FIBROSIS. Chronic liver injury from some agents increases collagen deposition, often with minimal or absent evidence of hepatocellular necrosis or inflammatory response. This usually bland fibrosis may progress to cirrhosis and portal hypertension, although the latter may occur as a result of hepatic portal fibrosis even in the absence of cirrhosis. This type of injury may occur after the chronic administration of methotrexate, after exposure to inorganic arsenicals, and in hypervitaminosis A.

TUMORS. Tumors caused by drugs and other chemical agents may be of several types, including hepatic adenoma (and possibly hepatocellular carcinoma) associated with oral contraceptive use and angiosarcoma caused by prolonged exposure to vinyl chloride monomer or Thorotrast. The mechanisms by which these tumors are produced are not known, but their clinical and laboratory features generally resemble those of similar tumors occurring "spontaneously." A possible exception is the apparently greater size, vascularity, and tendency to sudden hemorrhage of hepatic adenomas associated with oral contraceptive use (see Chapter 156).

VASCULAR LESIONS. Vascular lesions of several kinds occasionally are caused by drugs. Oral contraceptives have been implicated as a cause of hepatic vein thrombosis. Hepatic veno-occlusive disease, a process that affects the smaller tributaries of the hepatic vein, has been associated with the use of antitumor agents, including 6-thioguanine, cytarabine, and azathioprine, as well as with ingestion of pyrrolizidine alkaloids, such as from plants of *Senecio* and *Crotalaria* species ("bush tea poisoning"). Antitumor drugs have also been implicated in causing non-cirrhotic portal hypertension from portal venular injury and fibrosis. Oral contraceptives and anabolic steroids have been identified as causes of peliosis hepatis, a condition in which the liver lobule contains extrasinusoidal blood-filled spaces; this lesion is also seen in certain chronic wasting neoplastic and inflammatory diseases.

PRINCIPLES OF DIAGNOSIS AND MANAGEMENT

A causal relationship between using a drug and liver injury may be difficult to establish. Drugs may produce abnormalities very similar to those of other common disorders such as viral hepatitis or biliary disease, and some drugs may produce more than one kind of lesion. A detailed drug history is essential, and information about past exposure and the response to a suspect agent may be of considerable value in diagnosis. Because a number of industrial chemicals are potential hepatotoxins, details of the patient's occupation and work environment should be routinely obtained. The diagnosis of drug-induced liver disease ultimately depends on (1) a history of exposure; (2) consistent clinical, laboratory, and occasionally liver biopsy findings; and (3) resolution of the liver injury after the presumed toxin is discontinued. In some instances, when only a single agent is involved and a characteristic histologic type of injury is found, the diagnosis based on laboratory and biopsy findings is relatively straightforward. Examples include the small-droplet fatty liver caused by tetracycline or the centrilobular necrosis produced by acetaminophen (usually associated with significant blood levels of the drug). Conditions are more complex when several drugs are being used, any one of which or even the underlying disorder for which the drugs were prescribed may be responsible for a non-specific or viral hepatitis–like liver injury. The causal role of a particular drug in idiosyncratic liver disease can usually be established through rechallenge with the drug. Rechallenge is rarely justified, however, because of the risk of a severe or even fatal outcome. Furthermore, it is not necessary to incriminate the drug unambiguously if alternative drugs are available.

Drug-induced liver disease is managed by discontinuing the implicated drug(s) and giving supportive care for acute hepatitis and hepatic failure as needed. In the case of severe, acute drug- or toxin-induced liver failure, urgent liver transplantation may be lifesaving (see Chapter 155). Specific pharmacologic intervention is generally limited to the administration of *N*-acetylcysteine in acetaminophen overdosage (see later). Corticosteroids have no established value in treating drug-induced liver disease, although they may suppress the serum sickness–like syndrome associated with certain idiosyncratic reactions.

SELECTED EXAMPLES OF DRUG-INDUCED LIVER DISEASE

ACETAMINOPHEN. This readily available analgesic and antipyretic is a classic example of an intrinsic, dose-dependent hepatotoxin causing zonal necrosis and acute liver failure, often associated with renal failure. Significant liver injury usually occurs with doses of more than 10 to 15 g, most frequently taken in a suicide attempt. Inadvertent therapeutic overdose has also occurred from frequent dosing with over-the-counter and prescription combination drugs that contain acetaminophen (e.g., Nyquil and Vicodin). Within a few hours, patients develop nausea, vomiting, and diarrhea. These initial symptoms soon subside and are followed by a relatively asymptomatic phase. Clinical and laboratory signs of liver damage become evident 24 to 48 hours after ingestion. Serum aminotransferase levels of more than 5000 U/L are common, whereas severe liver injury may lead to progressive liver failure, with encephalopathy, coagulopathy, hypoglycemia, and lactic acidosis.

The liver injury is caused by a toxic metabolite of acetaminophen formed by the cytochrome P-450–dependent drug-metabolizing system. Below threshold doses, this metabolite is efficiently detoxified by conjugation with glutathione. In the toxic dose range, glutathione stores are rapidly exhausted and the metabolite reacts with essential cellular constituents, leading to cell dysfunction and death. The rate at which reactive acetaminophen metabolites are formed is influenced not only by the dose ingested but also by the activity of the cytochrome P-450 enzymes (which may be stimulated by inducers such as phenobarbital and ethanol) and by the availability of glutathione, which may be reduced by fasting and ethanol. A combination of both enzyme induction and glutathione depletion may underlie the particular susceptibility of patients with chronic alcoholism to acetaminophen hepatotoxicity. In such individuals, doses of acetaminophen within the therapeutic range may produce severe liver damage.

The initial treatment of acetaminophen overdose consists of supportive measures and gastric lavage. *N*-Acetylcysteine should be administered to high-risk patients, in whom it may significantly reduce the severity of liver necrosis and its attendant mortality. The plasma level of acetaminophen is the most reliable means for assessing prognosis. Levels in excess of 200 mg/L at 4 hours, 100 mg/L at 8 hours, or 50 mg/L at 12 hours after ingestion are predictive of severe liver damage and are indications for treatment with *N*-acetylcysteine. This agent appears to act mainly by providing cysteine for glutathione synthesis and is most effective when given within 10 hours of acetaminophen ingestion. *N*-Acetylcysteine may afford some benefit after 10 hours, but its benefit after 24 hours is not established. Intravenous preparations have been used in Great Britain, but only the oral form of *N*-acetylcysteine is available in the United States. The recommended oral dose is 140 mg/kg initially, followed by maintenance doses of 70 mg/kg every 4 hours for 72 hours. Survivors of acute acetaminophen toxicity usually recover completely without progressive or residual liver damage.

AMIODARONE. A number of patients who receive amiodarone develop mild increases in serum aminotransferase levels, which may normalize despite continuation of therapy, accompanied by engorgement of lysosomes with phospholipid. Between 1 and 3% of patients receiving amiodarone develop a more severe liver injury that histologically resembles acute alcoholic hepatitis, with fat infiltration of hepatocytes, focal necrosis, fibrosis, polymorphonuclear leukocyte infiltrates, and Mallory bodies. This lesion, also known as *non-alcoholic steatohepatitis*, may progress to micronodular cirrhosis, with portal hypertension and liver failure. This pseudoalcoholic lesion and its progression to cirrhosis often occur in a clinically insidious manner, with minimal elevation of serum aminotransferases. Hepatomegaly may be found, but jaundice is rare. Evidence of hepatotoxicity may persist for several months after the drug is discontinued.

Liver biopsy is helpful in diagnosis and should be considered in patients receiving amiodarone who develop persistent or significant (greater than twofold) elevation of serum aminotransferase levels or hepatomegaly. The decision to discontinue amiodarone in the presence of histologic evidence of hepatotoxicity is often difficult in patients who have been treated with amiodarone after the failure of other, less toxic medications (see Chapters 51 through 54), especially if an automated implantable cardioverter/defibrillator is not appropriate.

AMOXICILLIN-CLAVULANIC ACID. Amoxicillin per se has little hepatotoxicity, but in combination with the β-lactamase inhibitor clavulanic acid (Augmentin) it has resulted in cholestatic liver injury that often is delayed for several weeks after treatment has ended. Elderly men are most frequently affected. Jaundice is a consistent feature, and liver histology shows cholestasis with minimal necrosis or inflammation. Hypersensitivity manifestations are unusual. The clinical course has been benign in the majority of cases, with complete recovery within 4 to 6 months.

ERYTHROMYCIN. A cholestatic reaction with components of inflammatory cell infiltration and liver cell necrosis may complicate the use of erythromycin. In most instances, this reaction has occurred with erythromycin estolate; other erythromycins including the ethylsuccinate and lactobionate have been less frequently implicated. Hepatotoxicity typically presents as an acute syndrome of right upper quadrant pain, fever, and variable cholestatic symptoms. The clinical picture may closely mimic acute cholecystitis or cholangitis and has prompted surgical exploration in some instances. The prognosis is uniformly excellent, but the reaction may recur within days of readministering the drug.

FLUCLOXACILLIN. The biliary epithelium is selectively targeted in the idiosyncratic cholestatic liver injury that has affected several hundred individuals treated with this semisynthetic penicillin. Older patients treated for longer than 2 weeks seem to be at greatest risk, with the onset of jaundice and pruritus usually between 1 and 3 weeks after therapy is completed. Although clinical symptoms usually resolve within 2 months, abnormalities in serum liver enzymes may persist for months to years. Furthermore, in a minority of patients, the injury has pursued a progressive course characterized by damage to and depletion of interlobular bile ducts (vanishing bile duct syndrome), with secondary biliary cirrhosis developing over a period of years.

HALOTHANE. This halogenated alkane anesthetic rarely causes a viral hepatitis–like reaction that, in severe cases, may progress to fatal massive hepatic necrosis. Susceptibility to halothane hepatitis appears to be increased in older persons, women, and obese individuals, and severe reactions usually occur after previous or multiple exposures to this anesthetic. Symptoms usually indistinguishable from viral hepatitis occur between 7 and 10 days after anesthesia, but this interval may shorten considerably after repeated exposure. Fever, which may be hectic, with chills and sweats, commonly precedes the onset of jaundice; rash and eosinophilia are less consistent features. The course may terminate fatally within days, or rapid and complete recovery may occur. Some patients run a more protracted course before either recovering or developing liver failure. Metabolites of halothane formed by the cytochrome P-450 system are clearly important in the mechanism of the hepatic injury. Some of these metabolites may be directly toxic; others may form haptens with cell membrane proteins, provoking an immune-mediated attack on the liver. Cross-sensitization may occur between halothane, methoxyflurane, and enflurane, although hepatic injury appears to be less common with the latter two anesthetic agents.

ISONIAZID. Among persons taking INH for single-drug chemoprophylaxis against tuberculosis, there is a 10 to 20% incidence of subclinical liver injury, which manifests during the first few weeks of therapy as a mild to moderate increase in serum aminotransferase levels. These laboratory abnormalities, which reflect a focal non-specific hepatitis, subside in the majority of patients despite continued administration of the drug. About 1% of patients receiving INH develop significant liver injury, which clinically and histologically resembles the wide spectrum of viral hepatitis. The liver disease may present as a relatively mild, acute process, a subacute or chronic hepatitis, or fatal massive liver necrosis. The onset usually occurs within 2 to 3 months after starting the drug, and initial symptoms are often non-specific, with malaise and anorexia preceding signs of liver disease. Clinical features of "drug allergy" are distinctly unusual. Age influences the incidence of severe INH liver injury, which increases significantly after age 35, and probably exceeds 2% among persons over age 50.

INH appears to injure the liver by forming a toxic metabolite, acetylhydrazine. The conversion of acetylhydrazine to the non-toxic diacetylhydrazine may be impaired in slow acetylators of the drug, thus favoring the formation of a toxic derivative of acetylhydrazine through the cytochrome P-450–dependent drug-metabolizing system. Induction of cytochrome P-450 enzymes by rifampin may account for occurrences of a precipitous and severe form of INH hepatitis in patients receiving both drugs.

Patients receiving INH should be followed at regular intervals and advised to report intercurrent symptoms. If these symptoms are associated with evidence of disturbed liver function, the drug should be discontinued, pending further evaluation. Because liver enzyme abnormalities are common early in the course of INH treatment and reflect, in the vast majority (especially in younger patients), a transient and self-limiting event, routine monitoring of liver function tests in patients taking INH is not generally recommended. The risk:benefit ratio of INH chemoprophylaxis rises rapidly after the age of 35, however, warranting a more conservative approach to instituting chemoprophylaxis in this group (see Chapter 358). A severalfold elevation in aminotransferase levels in a patient older than age 35, even in the absence of symptoms, should be regarded as potentially serious and may justify discontinuation of the drug.

METHYLDOPA. This antihypertensive drug is similar to INH in that minor and apparently inconsequential abnormalities in liver function occur in up to 6% of treated patients. Clinically overt hepatotoxicity is much less common and usually resembles acute viral hepatitis or chronic active hepatitis, as a rule developing within 20 weeks after methyldopa is started. The Coombs test is not infrequently positive in users of this drug but does not correlate with the occurrence of hepatic injury. Furthermore, clinical manifestations of drug hypersensitivity are unusual in methyldopa-induced liver disease, which may be mediated by a toxic drug metabolite. Hepatitis usually abates when the drug is discontinued, but full recovery may be delayed by months, and progression to a fatal outcome despite stopping the drug has occurred in some cases.

ORAL CONTRACEPTIVES. These hormonal agents produce several adverse effects on the hepatobiliary system: (1) hepatocellular cholestasis, (2) liver cell neoplasms, (3) increased predisposition to cholesterol gallstone formation, and (4) hepatic vein thrombosis (Budd-Chiari syndrome). In many cases of hepatic vein thrombosis associated with oral contraceptives, a latent myeloproliferative disorder appears to be present and undoubtedly predisposes to the thrombogenic disorder.

The cholestatic effects of oral contraceptives are largely attributable to the estrogenic component. Estrogens appear to affect directly several aspects of bile formation. Indeed, most users of oral contraceptives exhibit subtle disturbances in hepatic excretory function, as evidenced, for example, by impaired plasma clearance of sulfobromophthalein. A small number of patients develop clinical cholestasis with pruritus and jaundice in a matter of weeks to months after beginning taking oral contraceptives. Manifestations of drug hypersensitivity are absent, and, histologically, cholestasis is seen without inflammation or liver cell necrosis. This condition is highly analogous to the clinical syndrome of *intrahepatic cholestasis of pregnancy,* which manifests as subclinical to overt cholestasis in the later stages of gestation, resolving rapidly in the postpartum period. Women with either a personal or family history of cholestasis occurring during pregnancy are particularly susceptible to cholestasis induced by estrogenic preparations. A genetic predisposition to estrogen-induced cholestasis is also suggested by the high incidence of this disorder in certain populations (e.g., Scandinavian and Chilean women).

Treatment of oral contraceptive–induced cholestasis consists of discontinuing the drug and providing symptomatic support (e.g., cholestyramine for pruritus) as needed. Complete resolution within 2 to 3 months is the rule.

PHENYTOIN. This anticonvulsant has been rarely associated with a severe, viral hepatitis–like liver injury with pronounced hypersensitivity features. The onset, usually within 6 weeks of starting the drug, is characterized by malaise, marked fever, lymphadenopathy, and a striking rash. Leukocytosis may be marked, with atypical lymphocytosis and eosinophilia. Liver histology resembles that of acute viral hepatitis except with a greater abundance of eosinophils. In the most severe cases, progressive liver failure and death have ensued. Despite the marked serum sickness–like syndrome that characterizes phenytoin hepatotoxicity, a toxic metabolite may participate in its pathogenesis. Phenytoin is partly converted in the liver to highly reactive arene oxides. A genetically determined impairment in the ability to detoxify arene oxides may underlie individual susceptibility to toxicity from these metabolites through their covalent and hence immunologic modification of hepatic macromolecules.

SODIUM VALPROATE. This branched, medium-chain fatty acid used principally in the treatment of petit mal epilepsy may produce severe hepatotoxicity, most commonly in children younger than 10. Similar to INH, sodium valproate treatment is accompanied by a high incidence of transient, slight, and asymptomatic increases in serum aminotransferase activity, usually after several weeks of therapy. In rarer cases of severe liver injury, non-specific systemic and digestive symptoms are followed by jaundice and evidence of liver failure, including encephalopathy and coagulopathy. Rash and eosinophilia are absent. The liver injury is characterized histologically by centrilobular necrosis and small-droplet fat infiltration, and bile duct injury may also be evident. The clinical and histologic features of sodium valproate hepatotoxicity are, to a degree, reminiscent of Reye's syndrome, although the former is distinguished by a greater frequency of jaundice, bile duct injury, and liver necrosis. The mechanism of sodium valproate–induced liver disease is uncertain, but available evidence has implicated the impairment of mitochondrial oxidation of long-chain fatty acids by a metabolite of the drug. Underlying inherited abnormalities in mitochondrial β-oxidation and urea synthesis may also predispose to valproate hepatotoxicity. Spontaneous recovery after stopping sodium valproate is the rule; fatalities are rare.

Farrell GC: Drug-Induced Liver Disease. New York, Churchill Livingstone, 1994. *This comprehensive text on drug- and toxin-induced liver disease is meticulously researched and very readable.*

Garcia Rodriguez LA, Ruigomez A, Jick H: A review of epidemiologic research on drug-induced acute liver injury using the General Practice Research Database in the United Kingdom. Pharmacotherapy 17:721, 1997. *This review provides quantitative and qualitative information on acute liver toxicity associated with individual drugs through the use of a powerful epidemiologic tool, the General Practice Research Database (GPRD) in the United Kingdom. The results provide evidence of relative safety for commonly administered agents and point to a high prevalence of liver injury from chlorpromazine, INH, and amoxicillin-clavulanic acid.*

Lee WM: Drug-induced hepatotoxicity. N Engl J Med 333:1118, 1995. *An excellent, concise review with useful sections on acetaminophen toxicity and the diagnosis, treatment, and prevention of drug-induced liver disease.*

Zimmerman HJ, Ishak KG: General aspects of drug-induced liver disease. Gastroenterol Clin North Am 24:739, 1995. *A concise and lucid overview by two renowned*

authorities of the prevalence, mechanisms, diagnosis, and prevention of drug-induced liver disease.

149 ACUTE VIRAL HEPATITIS

Jay H. Hoofnagle
Karen L. Lindsay

Acute viral hepatitis is at least five different diseases caused by five or more distinct and unrelated viruses. The disease is characterized clinically by symptoms of malaise, nausea, poor appetite, vague abdominal pain, and jaundice; biochemically by marked increases in serum bilirubin and aminotransferase levels; serologically by the presence of a hepatitis viral genome in liver and serum followed by development of antibodies to viral antigens; and histologically by varying degrees of hepatocellular necrosis and inflammation. Acute viral hepatitis is typically self-limited and resolves completely without residual liver injury or viral replication. A proportion of some forms of hepatitis, however, can result in a persistent infection with chronic liver injury. The five forms of viral hepatitis are similar clinically but can be distinguished by serologic assays.

The five known causes of acute hepatitis are the hepatitis A (HAV), B (HBV), C (HCV), D or delta (HDV), and E (HEV) viruses (Table 149–1). All except hepatitis B are RNA viruses. Hepatitis A and E are forms of "infectious" hepatitis; they are spread largely by the fecal-oral route, are associated with poor sanitary conditions, are highly contagious, occur in outbreaks as well as sporadically, and cause self-limited hepatitis only. Hepatitis B, C, and D are forms of "serum" hepatitis; they are spread largely by parenteral routes and less commonly by intimate or sexual exposure; they are not highly contagious but instead occur sporadically, rarely causing outbreaks; and they are capable of leading to chronic hepatitis and, ultimately, to cirrhosis and hepatocellular carcinoma. Cases of an acute viral hepatitis–like syndrome that cannot be identified as being due to a known hepatitis virus occur and are termed acute non-A, non-B, non-C, non-D, non-E (non-A . . . E) hepatitis or as acute hepatitis of unknown cause.

The course of acute hepatitis is highly variable, ranging in severity from a transient, asymptomatic infection to a severe or fulminant disease. The disease can be self-limited and resolve, it can run a relapsing course, or it can lead to a chronic infection. In a typical clinically apparent course of acute resolving viral hepatitis (Fig. 149–1), the *incubation period* varies from 2 to 20 weeks, largely on the basis of viral etiology and dose of exposure. During this phase, virus becomes detectable in blood, but serum aminotransferase and bilirubin levels are normal, and antibody is not detected.

The *pre-icteric phase* of illness is marked by the onset of fatigue, nausea, poor appetite, and vague right upper quadrant pain. Viral specific antibody usually first appears during this phase, which typically lasts 3 to 10 days. In patients with subclinical or anicteric forms of acute hepatitis, this phase constitutes the entire course of illness. Viral titers are generally highest at this point, and serum aminotransferase levels start to increase. The onset of dark urine marks the *icteric phase* of illness, during which jaundice appears and symptoms of fatigue and nausea worsen. Typically, acute viral hepatitis is rarely diagnosed correctly before onset of jaundice. If jaundice is severe, stool color will lighten and pruritus may appear. Anorexia, dysgeusia, and weight loss of up to 20 pounds may also occur.

Physical examination usually shows jaundice and hepatic tenderness. In more severe cases, hepatomegaly and splenomegaly may be present.

Serum bilirubin levels (both total and direct) rise, and aminotransferase levels are usually greater than 10 times the upper limit of normal, at least at the onset. During the icteric, symptomatic phase, levels of hepatitis virus begin to decrease in serum and liver.

The duration of clinical illness is variable; it typically lasts 1 to

Table 149–1 ■ THE FIVE CAUSES OF ACUTE VIRAL HEPATITIS

HEPATITIS VIRUS	SIZE (nm)	GENOME	SPREAD	INCUBATION PERIOD (DAYS)	FATALITY RATE	CHRONIC RATE	ANTIBODY
A	27	RNA	Fecal-oral	15–45 mean = 25	1%	None	Anti-HAV
B	45	DNA	Parenteral Sexual	30–180 mean = 75	1%	2–7%	Anti-HBs Anti-HBc Anti-HBe
C	60	RNA	Parenteral	15–150 mean = 50	<0.1%	70–85%	Anti-HCV
D (delta)	40	RNA	Parenteral Sexual	30–150	2–10%	2–7% 50%	Anti-HDV
E	32	RNA	Fecal-oral	30–60	1%	None	Anti-HEV

3 weeks. Recovery is first manifested by return of appetite and is accompanied by resolution of the serum bilirubin and aminotransferase elevations and clearance of virus. *Convalescence,* however, can be prolonged before full degrees of energy and stamina return. Neutralizing antibodies usually appear during the icteric phase and rise to high levels during convalescence.

Complications of acute viral hepatitis include chronic infection, fulminant hepatic failure, relapsing or cholestatic hepatitis, and extrahepatic syndromes. Chronic hepatitis, usually defined as at least 6 months of illness, eventuates in approximately 5% of adults with hepatitis B but in 75% of those with hepatitis C. However, hepatitis B, C, and D can be confidently said to be chronic if viremia persists for more than 3 months after onset of symptoms.

Acute liver failure or fulminant hepatitis occurs in 1 to 2% of patients with symptomatic acute hepatitis, perhaps most commonly with hepatitis B and D, and least commonly with hepatitis C. The disease is called fulminant if hepatic encephalopathy appears; however, the initial symptoms (changes in personality, aggressive behavior, or abnormal sleep patterns) may be subtle or misunderstood. The most reliable prognostic factor in acute hepatic failure is the degree of prolongation of prothrombin time; other signs of poor prognosis are persistently worsening jaundice, ascites, and decreases in liver size. Serum aminotransferase levels and viral titers have little prognostic value and often decrease with worsening hepatic failure.

A proportion of patients with acute hepatitis develop a cholestatic pattern of illness, with prolonged and fluctuating jaundice and pruritus. Patients may have one or more clinical relapses. Patients may feel relatively well despite marked jaundice. Cholestatic hepatitis is generally benign and ultimately resolves.

Between 10 and 20% of patients develop a serum sickness–like syndrome during the pre-icteric phase of acute hepatitis, with variable combinations of rash, hives, arthralgias, and fever. This immune complex–like syndrome is often mistakenly attributed to other illnesses until the onset of jaundice, at which time the fever, hives, and arthralgias quickly resolve. Other extrahepatic manifestations of acute hepatitis are uncommon but include severe headaches, encephalitis, aseptic meningitis, seizures, acute ascending flaccid paralysis, nephrotic syndrome, and seronegative arthritis.

The pathogenesis of the liver injury in viral hepatitis is not well understood. None of the five agents appears to be directly cytopathic, at least at levels of replication found during typical acute and chronic hepatitis. The timing and histologic appearance of hepatocyte injury in viral hepatitis suggest that immune responses, particularly cytotoxic T-cell responses to viral antigens expressed on hepatocyte cell membranes, may be the major effectors of injury. Other proinflammatory cytokines, natural killer cell activity, and antibody-dependent cellular cytotoxicity may also play modulating roles in cell injury and inflammation during acute hepatitis virus infection. Recovery from hepatitis virus infections is usually

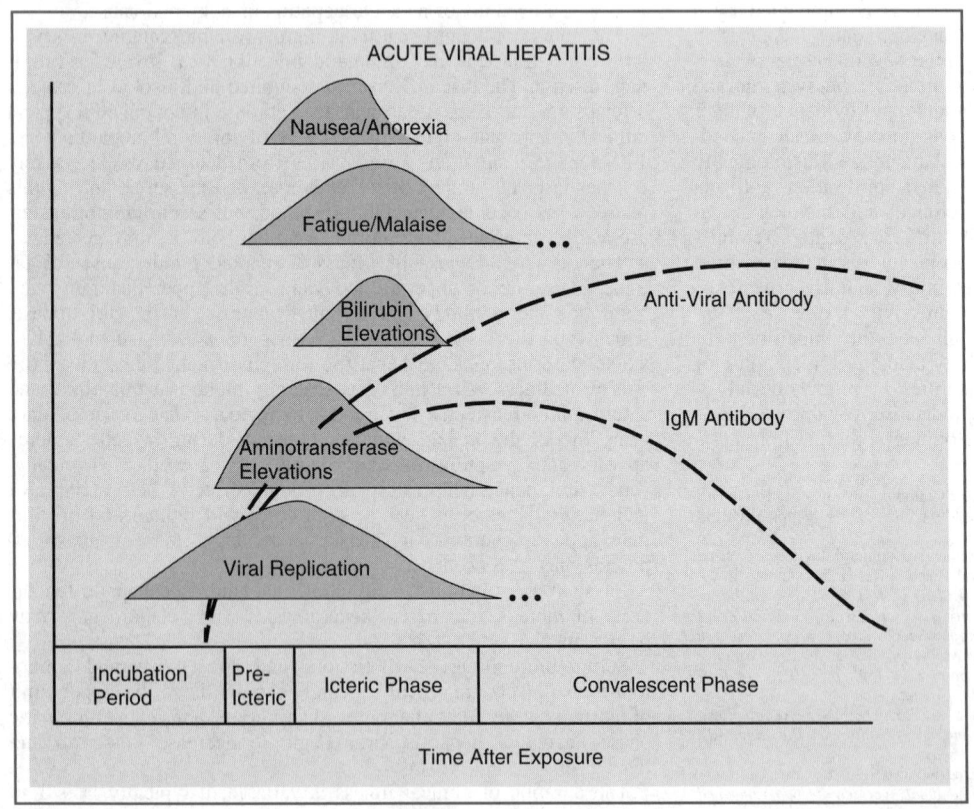

FIGURE 149–1 ■ The typical course of acute viral hepatitis.

accompanied by appearance of rising titers of antibody against envelope antigens, such as anti-HAV, anti-HBs, anti-HCV-E1 and anti-HCV-E2, and anti-HEV; these antibodies may provide at least partial immunity to reinfection.

Liver histology in acute viral hepatitis is characterized by widespread parenchymal inflammation and spotty necrosis. Inflammatory cells are predominantly lymphocytes, macrophages, and histiocytes. Fibrosis is absent. Immunohistochemical stains for hepatitis antigens are usually negative during acute disease, and there are no reliably distinctive features that separate the five viral forms of acute hepatitis from each other. Because serologic tests are usually adequate for diagnosis, liver biopsy is not recommended in acute hepatitis, unless the diagnosis remains unclear and a therapeutic decision is needed.

Acute viral hepatitis is a common disease, affecting between 0.5 and 1% of persons in the United States each year. The annual incidence of acute hepatitis fluctuates largely as a result of hepatitis A. Cases of hepatitis B and C have been decreasing since 1990. In recent population-based surveys, the viral causes of acute hepatitis were hepatitis A in 48%, hepatitis B in 34%, and hepatitis C in 15% of cases. Hepatitis D is quite rare in the United States (<1% of acute cases), where only imported cases of hepatitis E have been reported. In 3% of cases, the cause of hepatitis cannot be ascertained even after extensive testing. In clinical practice, other nonviral forms of acute hepatitis must be considered, especially mononucleosis, secondary syphilis, drug-induced liver disease, acute cholecystitis (or acute biliary obstruction), Wilson's disease, and various forms of ischemic, malignant, or toxic hepatic injury.

Although there are no specific therapies for the various forms of acute viral hepatitis, there are non-specific recommendations for all patients. Bed rest and sensible nutrition are recommended in the patient who is symptomatic and jaundiced. Alcohol should be avoided until convalescence. Sexual contacts should be limited until partners receive prophylaxis. In hepatitis A, all household contacts should be given immune globulin, and initiation of hepatitis A vaccination is appropriate. In hepatitis B, family members should be vaccinated; for recent sexual contacts, hepatitis B immune globulin should also be given. Patients who develop any signs of fulminant hepatic failure (prolongation of prothrombin time and/or personality changes or confusion) should be quickly evaluated for possible liver transplantation (see Chapter 155). The success of transplantation for severe, acute viral hepatitis often depends on

early referral and careful attention to all details of clinical management in the context of an experienced team of physicians. Follow-up of acute hepatitis should be adequate to demonstrate that resolution has occurred, particularly for patients with hepatitis C. Finally and importantly, all cases of acute hepatitis should be reported to the local or state health department as soon as possible after diagnosis.

HEPATITIS A

The hepatitis A virus is a small RNA virus that belongs to the family of Picornaviridae, genus Hepatovirus. The viral genome is 7.5 kb in length and has a single large open-reading frame that encodes a polyprotein with both structural and non-structural components. The virus replicates largely in the liver and is assembled in the hepatocyte cytoplasm as a 27-nm particle with a single RNA genome and an outer capsid protein (HAVAg). The virus is secreted into the bile and, to a lesser extent, the serum. Highest titers of virus are found in stool (10^6 to 10^{10} genomes per gram) during the incubation period and early symptomatic phase of illness.

Hepatitis A is highly contagious and is spread largely by the fecal-oral route especially when there are poor sanitary conditions. Hepatitis A has become the most common cause of acute hepatitis in the United States, occurring largely as sporadic, rather than epidemic cases. Investigation of the source of hepatitis A cases reveals that most are due to direct person-to-person exposure and, to lesser extent, to direct fecal contamination of food or water. Consumption of shellfish from contaminated waterways is a well-known but uncommon source of hepatitis A. Rare instances of spread of hepatitis A from blood transfusions and from pooled plasma products have been described. High-risk groups for acquiring hepatitis A include travelers to developing areas of the world, children in day-care centers (and secondarily their parents), promiscuous male homosexuals, injection drug users, hemophiliacs given plasma products, and persons in institutions.

The clinical course of typical acute hepatitis A (Fig. 149–2) begins with an incubation period that is typically 15 to 45 days (mean = 25 days). Jaundice occurs in 70% of adults infected with hepatitis A but in smaller proportions of children. Antibody to

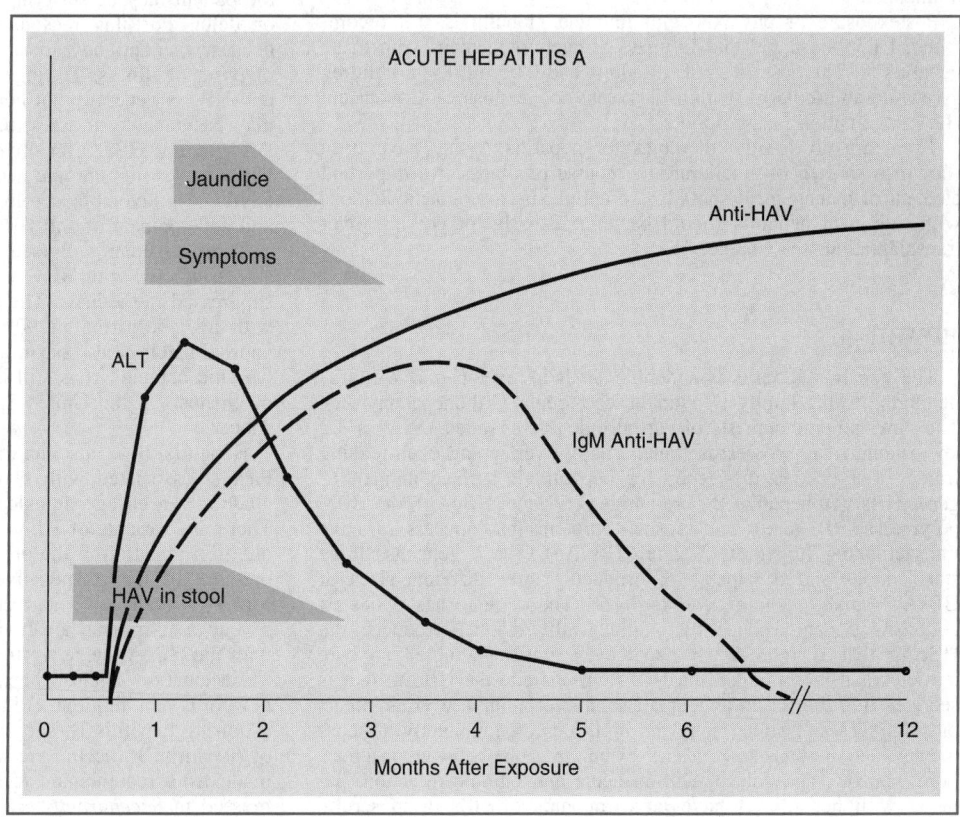

FIGURE 149–2 ■ The serologic course of acute hepatitis A.

HAV (anti-HAV), which appears in all patients infected with the virus, is first apparent shortly before the onset of symptoms, rises to high titer, and persists for life. Thus the finding of anti-HAV can indicate previous infection and immunity as well as ongoing acute hepatitis A. The diagnosis of acute hepatitis A can be made by testing for IgM-specific anti-HAV, which arises early in the disease and persists for 4 to 12 months. Acute hepatitis A is invariably a self-limited infection; the virus can persist for months, but it does not lead to a chronic infection, chronic hepatitis, or cirrhosis. Severe and fulminant cases of hepatitis A can occur, particularly in the elderly and in patients with pre-existing chronic liver disease. Hepatitis A is the most common cause of relapsing cholestatic hepatitis.

The diagnosis of acute hepatitis A can be made based on the finding of IgM anti-HAV in the serum of a patient with the clinical and biochemical features of acute hepatitis. Testing for total anti-HAV is not helpful in diagnosis but is a means of assessing immunity to hepatitis A.

A safe and effective hepatitis A vaccine is available and is recommended for patients at high risk of acquiring hepatitis A, including travelers to endemic areas of the world, children in communities with high rates of infection (such as Alaskan Natives or Native Americans on reservations), male homosexuals, injection drug users, and hepatitis and primate research workers. HAV vaccine is also recommended for all patients with chronic liver disease and recipients of pooled plasma products such as hemophiliacs. The universal use of HAV vaccine in childhood and in food handlers is still being evaluated.

Two formulations of HAV vaccine are available in the United States; both consist of inactivated hepatitis A antigen purified from cell culture. Havrix (SmithKline Beecham) is recommended as two injections 6 to 12 months apart in an adult dose of 1440 ELISA units (1.0 mL) and a pediatric (ages 2 to 18 years) dose of 720 units (0.5 mL). VAQTA (Merck) is recommended as two injections at least 6 months apart in an adult dose of 50 units (1.0 mL) and a pediatric dose (2 to 17 years) of 25 units (0.5 mL). Hepatitis A vaccines have an excellent safety record, with serious complications occurring in less than 0.1% of recipients. Seroconversion rates after HAV vaccine are greater than 90% but are lower in the elderly and in patients with chronic liver disease. Nevertheless, neither follow-up testing for anti-HAV nor booster inoculations are currently recommended.

Postexposure prophylaxis with immune globulin is still recommended for household and intimate contacts of persons with acute hepatitis A. The dose is 2 mL in adults and 0.02 mL/kg in children given intramuscularly within 2 weeks of exposure. Concurrent HAV vaccination is appropriate.

There are no specific therapies for hepatitis A that have been shown to shorten or ameliorate the course of illness. An important element of management should be prophylaxis for contacts. Persons with fulminant hepatitis should be referred early for possible liver transplantation (see Chapter 155).

HEPATITIS B

The hepatitis B virus is a double-shelled, enveloped DNA virus belonging to the family Hepadnaviridae (genus Orthohepadnavirus). The viral genome consists of partially double-stranded DNA, is 3.2 kb in length, and possesses four partially overlapping open-reading frames that encode the genes for hepatitis B surface antigen (S gene: HBsAg), hepatitis B core antigen (C gene: HBcAg), the HBV polymerase (P gene), and a small protein that appears to have transactivating functions (X gene: HBxAg). The S gene has three start codons and is capable of producing three different sizes of HBsAg (small, medium, and large S). The C gene has two start codons and can produce two antigenically distinct products: the HBcAg that is retained in hepatocytes until assembled as core particles and incorporated into HBV virions and the HBeAg that is secreted into the serum as a small soluble protein. The virus infects only humans and higher apes and replicates predominantly in hepatocytes and perhaps to a lesser extent in stem cells in pancreas, bone marrow, and spleen. During acute and chronic infection, patients with hepatitis B have large amounts of HBsAg in serum,

most in the form of incomplete 20-nm virus-like spherical and tubular particles. The intact virion is a double-shelled particle with an envelope of HBsAg, an inner nucleocapsid of HBcAg, and an active polymerase enzyme that is linked to a single molecule of double-stranded HBV DNA. Persons who produce large amounts of HBV in serum also typically produce HBeAg, making this a surrogate marker for high levels of viral replication.

Hepatitis B is spread predominantly by the parenteral route or by intimate personal contact. It is endemic in many areas of the world, such as Southeast Asia, China, Micronesia, and sub-Saharan Africa. Lesser rates occur in the Indian subcontinent and the Middle East. In the United States, hepatitis B is the second most common cause of acute hepatitis, and chronic infection affects approximately 0.5% of the population. Investigations of the source of hepatitis B reveal that most adult cases are due to sexual or parenteral contact. Hepatitis B is common among injection drug users and among heterosexuals and male homosexuals with multiple sexual partners. Blood transfusion and plasma products are now rarely infectious for hepatitis B because of the institution of routine screening of blood donations for HBsAg and antibody to HBcAg, anti-HBc. Maternal-infant spread of hepatitis B is another important mode of transmission not only in endemic areas of the world but also in the United States among immigrants from these endemic areas. Routine screening of pregnant women and prophylaxis of newborns are now recommended. Intrafamilial spread of hepatitis B can also occur, although the mode of spread in this situation is not well defined.

The typical course of acute, self-limited hepatitis B (Fig. 149–3) begins with an incubation period of 30 to 150 days (mean = 75 days). During the incubation period, HBsAg, HBeAg, and HBV DNA become detectable in serum and rise to high titers, with the virus reaching titers of 10^8 to 10^{11} virions/mL. By the onset of symptoms, anti-HBc arises, and serum aminotransferase levels are elevated. Jaundice appears in one third of adults with hepatitis B and lesser percentages of children. Generally, HBV DNA and HBeAg begin to fall at the onset of illness and may be undetectable at the time of peak clinical illness. HBsAg becomes undetectable and anti-HBs arises during recovery, several weeks to months after loss of HBeAg. Anti-HBs is a long-lasting antibody and is associated with immunity.

The diagnosis of acute hepatitis B can be made on the basis of finding HBsAg in the serum of a patient with the clinical and biochemical features of acute hepatitis. However, HBsAg may also be present as a result of chronic hepatitis B or the carrier state, and the patient may be suffering from a superimposed acute hepatitis A or delta. For this reason, testing for IgM anti-HBc is helpful, because this antibody arises early and is lost within 6 to 12 months of onset of illness. Testing for HBeAg, anti-HBe, HBV DNA, and anti-HBs is generally not helpful in the diagnosis of hepatitis B but may be valuable in assessing prognosis. Persons who remain HBV DNA and/or HBeAg positive 6 weeks after onset of symptoms are likely to develop chronic hepatitis B. Thus, loss of HBeAg or HBV DNA is a favorable serologic finding. Similarly, loss of HBsAg and development of anti-HBs denote recovery.

Chronic hepatitis B (see Chapter 150) develops in 2 to 7% of adults infected with HBV, more commonly in men and in immunosuppressed individuals. The risk of chronic infection also correlates with age, occurring in 90% of newborns infected with HBV, in approximately 30% of infants, but in less than 10% of adults. Chronic hepatitis B is still the third or fourth most common cause of cirrhosis in the United States and is an important cause of liver cancer.

Hepatitis B is also an important cause of fulminant hepatitis. Factors associated with severe outcomes of acute hepatitis B include advanced age, female sex, and perhaps some strains of virus. There are variants of HBV that lack the ability to produce HBeAg due to a mutation in the pre-core region of the viral genome. These pre-core or HBeAg-negative mutants are associated with atypical forms of both acute and chronic hepatitis B. Several clusters of severe or fulminant hepatitis B have been associated with infection with the HBeAg-negative forms of virus.

Vaccination against hepatitis B is now recommended for all newborns and children. Adults, especially in groups at high risk for acquiring hepatitis B, should also be vaccinated. Two formulations of hepatitis B vaccine are available in the United States; both are made from recombinant techniques using cloned HBV S gene expressed in Saccharomyces cerevisiae. For adults, the recommended

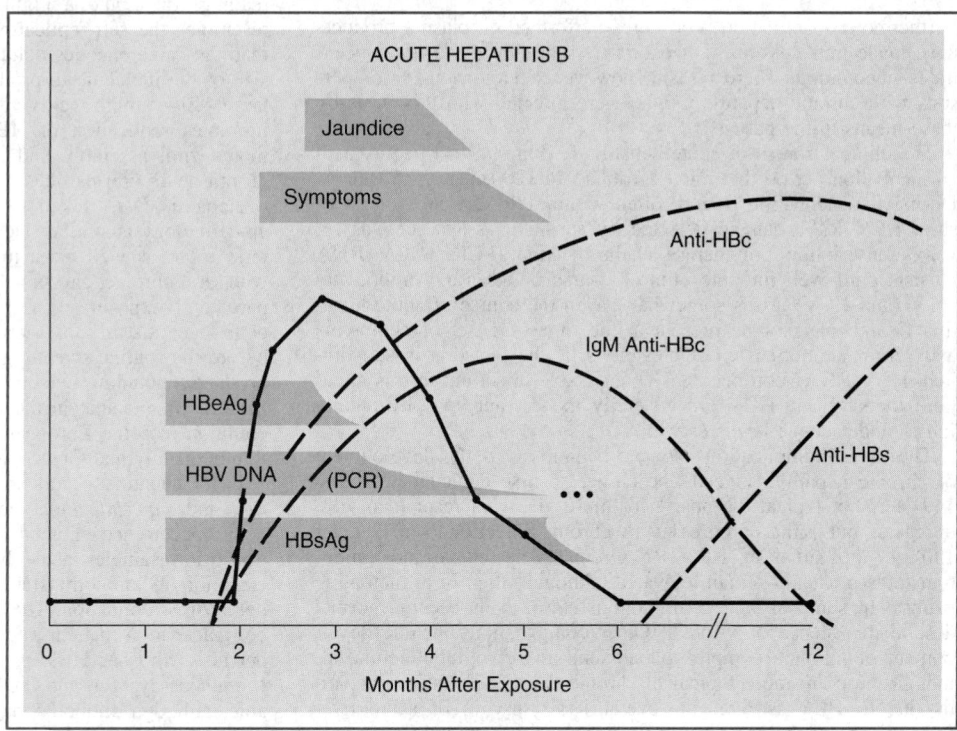

FIGURE 149–3 ■ The serologic course of acute hepatitis B.

regimen is three injections of 1.0 mL (10 μg of Energix-B [SmithKline Beecham] or 20 μg of Recombivax-HB [Merck]) given intramuscularly in the deltoid muscle at 0, 1 and 6 months. The dose in newborns, children, and adolescents is less (Table 149–2). The seroconversion rate is greater than 80% in adults but may be less in smokers, in the obese, in the elderly, and in patients who are immunocompromised, who may require higher doses and more injections. Pre-vaccination screening for anti-HBs is not recommended except for adult patients in high-risk groups (injection drug users or male homosexuals). In addition, post-vaccination testing for anti-HBs to document seroconversion is not routinely recommended except for persons who are at highest risk for continued exposures. At present, booster doses are not recommended, but they may be appropriate for high-risk individuals if titers of anti-HBs fall below what is considered protective (10 IU/mL).

Postexposure prophylaxis with hepatitis B immune globulin (HBIG) is recommended for newborns and patients with parenteral exposure to a patient with acute or chronic hepatitis B. A single dose of HBIG (0.5 mL in newborns, 2 mL in adults) should be given as soon as possible after exposure, and HBV vaccination should be started immediately. For patients with sexual or household contact with a patient with acute or chronic hepatitis B, vaccination alone may be appropriate, although HBIG is often recommended if the exposure is to a patient with acute hepatitis B.

There is no evidence that early therapy for acute hepatitis B with interferon-α or antiviral agents decreases the rate of chronicity or speeds recovery. Most patients with acute, icteric hepatitis B recover without residual injury or chronic hepatitis. Management of acute hepatitis B should focus on avoidance of further hepatic injury and prophylaxis of contacts. The patient should be followed with repeat testing for HBsAg and ALT levels 3 to 6 months later to determine whether chronic hepatitis B develops (see Chapter 150).

HEPATITIS C

The hepatitis C virus is an RNA virus that belongs to the family Flaviviridae and genus Hepacivirus. The virus was originally identified by molecular techniques, and the virus has not been visualized. Hepatitis C virus probably circulates as a double-shelled enveloped virus, 50 to 60 nm in diameter. The genome is a positively stranded RNA molecule, which is 9.5 kb in length and contains a single, large open-reading frame that encodes a large polyprotein that is post-translationally modified into three structural and several non-structural polypeptides. The structural proteins include two highly variable envelope antigens (E1 and E2) and a relatively conserved nucleocapsid protein (C). The HCV replicates largely in the liver and is detectable in serum in titers of 10^5 to 10^7 virions/mL during acute and chronic infection.

Hepatitis C is spread predominantly by the parenteral route. At highest risk are injection drug users and persons with multiple parenteral exposures. Sexual transmission of hepatitis C is rare. Maternal-infant spread occurs in approximately 5% of cases, usually to infants whose mothers have high levels of HCV RNA in serum. Other potential sources of hepatitis C are needlestick accidents, contamination and inadequate sterilization of re-useable needles and syringes, and sharing straws during intranasal cocaine use. Since the introduction of routine screening of blood for anti-HCV, post-transfusion hepatitis C (see Chapter 150) has become rare.

Table 149–2 ■ **HEPATITIS B VIRUS VACCINATION RECOMMENDATIONS**

GROUP	NO. DOSES	SCHEDULE (MONTHS)	RECOMBIVAX-HB	ENERGIX-B
Infants	3	0, 1, & 6	2.5 μg (0.25 mL)	10 μg (0.5 mL)
Infants born to HBsAg+ mother	3	0*, 1, & 6	5.0 μg (0.5 mL)	10 μg (0.5 mL)
Children (1–10 yr)	3	0, 1, & 6	2.5 μg (0.25 mL)	10 μg (0.5 mL)
Adolescents (11–19 yr)	3	0, 1, & 6	5.0 μg (0.5 mL)	20 μg (1.0 mL)
Adults	3	0, 1, & 6	10 μg (1.0 mL)	20 μg (1.0 mL)
Immunocompromised adults	3 or 4	0, 1, & 6 or 0, 1, 2, & 6	40 μg (1.0 mL)	40 μg† (2.0 mL)

*HBIG and initial vaccination should be given within 12 hours of birth.
†Another injection can be given at 2 months, giving a four-dose schedule.

Furthermore, inactivation procedures performed on plasma products have made transmission of hepatitis C from clotting factor concentrates uncommon. There remain, however, a large number of persons with chronic hepatitis C who were infected with this virus by these means in the past.

The clinical course of acute hepatitis C (Fig. 149–4) begins with an incubation period that ranges from 15 to 120 (mean = 50) days. During the incubation period, often within 1 to 2 weeks of exposure, HCV RNA can be detected by sensitive assays such as reverse-transcription polymerase chain reaction (PCR). HCV RNA persists until well into the clinical course of disease. Antibody to HCV (anti-HCV) arises somewhat late in the course of acute hepatitis C and may not be present at the time of onset of symptoms and serum aminotransferase elevations. If the hepatitis is self-limited, HCV RNA soon becomes undetectable in serum; in this situation, titers of anti-HCV are generally modest and may eventually fall to undetectable levels as well.

The major complication of acute hepatitis C is the development of chronic hepatitis. Indeed, the clinical course depicted in Figure 149–4 is not typical, because hepatitis C does not resolve in 70% of cases, but rather progresses to chronic infection (see Chapter 150). In this situation, HCV RNA remains detectable and aminotransferases usually remain elevated, although often in a fluctuating pattern. In some instances, aminotransferase levels become normal despite persistence of viremia. Other complications include development of immune complex phenomena and cryoglobulinemia, although these are more typical of chronic disease. Fulminant hepatitis due to HCV is rare; in several large surveys of acute liver failure, none of the cases could be attributed to hepatitis C.

The diagnosis of acute hepatitis C is generally made based on the finding of anti-HCV in serum in a patient with the clinical and biochemical features of acute hepatitis. However, some patients do not develop detectable levels of anti-HCV until weeks or months after onset of illness, so retesting for anti-HCV during convalescence or special tests for HCV RNA are necessary to exclude the diagnosis of acute hepatitis C in a patient who tests negative for all serologic markers. At present, the commercial tests for HCV RNA are not licensed or standardized, and their routine use cannot be recommended. When a test for HCV RNA is ordered, the physician should insist on laboratory documentation of the reliability of the assay and a sensitivity of at least 1000 genome-equivalents per milliliter.

At present there are no means of prevention of hepatitis C other than avoidance of high-risk behaviors and appropriate use of universal precautions. Injection drug use is currently the most common cause of newly acquired cases of hepatitis C. In this regard, needle exchange programs and education regarding the risks of drug use including intranasal cocaine and the role of reuseable equipment are important.

Accidental needlestick exposure is perhaps the most frequent issue in prevention of transmission. At present, neither immune globulin nor pre-emptive therapy with antiviral agents or interferon is recommended in this situation. Monitoring using aminotransferase levels, HCV RNA, and anti-HCV testing (at 1 and 6 months after exposure) is appropriate. This approach allows for early intervention and treatment.

There are no clear guidelines for treatment of acute hepatitis C. Because the majority of patients with acute disease progress to chronic infection, it is reasonable to treat patients during the acute phase rather than waiting for 6 months. However, interferon-α therapy with or without ribavirin entails subcutaneous injections for 6 to 12 months and is both expensive and not easily tolerated. For these reasons, therapy might best be delayed until proof that the disease is not self-limited by the monitoring of aminotransferase levels and/or HCV RNA for 2 to 3 months before initiation of therapy. Treatment should be the same as for chronic hepatitis C (see Chapter 150).

HEPATITIS D

The hepatitis delta virus is a unique RNA virus that requires the hepatitis B virus for replication. The viral genome is a short, 1.7-kb circular single-stranded molecule of RNA that has a single open-reading frame and a highly conserved non-translated region that resembles the self-replicating element of viroids. The single open-reading frame encodes delta antigen, and RNA editing can vary the size of the molecule to produce either a small (195 amino acids) or large (214 amino acids) delta antigen. The small delta antigen promotes replication of HDV RNA; the large delta antigen promotes viral assembly and secretion into the serum as the mature 36-nm delta viral particle.

Hepatitis D is linked to hepatitis B and, as a consequence, its epidemiology is similar. Delta hepatitis can be spread by the parenteral route as well as sexually. Persons at greatest risk are those who are chronic carriers of hepatitis B and who have repeated parenteral exposures. In the United States and Western Europe, delta hepatitis is most common among injection drug users and, before the routine screening of blood donations, recipients of blood products, including persons with hemophilia and thalassemia. Delta hepatitis is endemic in the Amazon basin and central Africa and is common in some European and Mediterranean countries, including Southern Italy and Greece, and in Eastern Europe.

Delta hepatitis occurs in two clinical patterns, termed *co-infection* and *superinfection*. Delta co-infection represents the simultaneous occurrence of acute delta and acute hepatitis B virus infections. It resembles acute hepatitis B but may manifest a second elevation in aminotransferase levels associated with the period of delta virus replication. The diagnosis of acute delta co-infection can be made in a patient presenting with clinical features of acute hepatitis who has HBsAg, anti-HDV, and IgM anti-HBc in serum. Immunoassays for anti-HDV are commercially available and reliable, although antibody may appear late during the illness. In patients suspected of having delta hepatitis, repeat testing for anti-HDV during convalescence is appropriate.

Acute delta superinfection represents the occurrence of acute HDV infection in a chronic HBsAg carrier. The diagnosis of acute delta superinfection can be made in a patient presenting with clinical features of acute hepatitis who has HBsAg and anti-HDV but no IgM anti-HBc in serum. Superinfection with HDV is more frequent than co-infection and is far more likely to lead to chronic delta hepatitis. Other tests that are helpful in making the diagnosis of ongoing HDV infection are serum HDV RNA (detectable by PCR) and HDV antigen (detectable by immunoblot); both of these tests are currently research assays and not standardized. Delta antigen can also be readily detected in liver biopsies using immunohistochemical stains.

Delta hepatitis tends to be more severe than hepatitis B alone and is more likely to lead to fulminant hepatitis as well as more likely to cause severe chronic hepatitis and ultimately cirrhosis. There are no specific means of therapy for acute delta hepatitis. Most cases of acute co-infection resolve; patients with superinfection should be treated once it is clear that chronic delta hepatitis has supervened.

Delta hepatitis can be prevented by preventing hepatitis B. The severity of delta hepatitis provides the rationale for routine hepatitis B vaccination in areas of the world where delta hepatitis is endemic. Unfortunately, there are no means of prevention of delta hepatitis in a person who is already an HBsAg carrier; in this situation, avoidance of further exposures is important.

HEPATITIS E

The hepatitis E virus (HEV) is a small non-enveloped, single-stranded RNA virus possibly belonging to the family Caliciviridae and genus Calcivirus. The viral genome is 7.5 kb in length and encodes three open-reading frames, the first (ORF1) for the nonstructural proteins responsible for viral replication, the second (ORF2) for the capsid protein (HEV antigen), and the third (ORF3) for a short protein of unknown function. The virus and HEV antigen can be detected in hepatocytes during acute infection. Highest levels of virus are detectable in the stool during the incubation period of disease.

Hepatitis E is responsible for both epidemic and endemic forms of "non-A, non-B" hepatitis that occur in lesser developed areas of the world. Large outbreaks have been described from India, Pakistan, China, Northern and Central Africa, and Central America. In

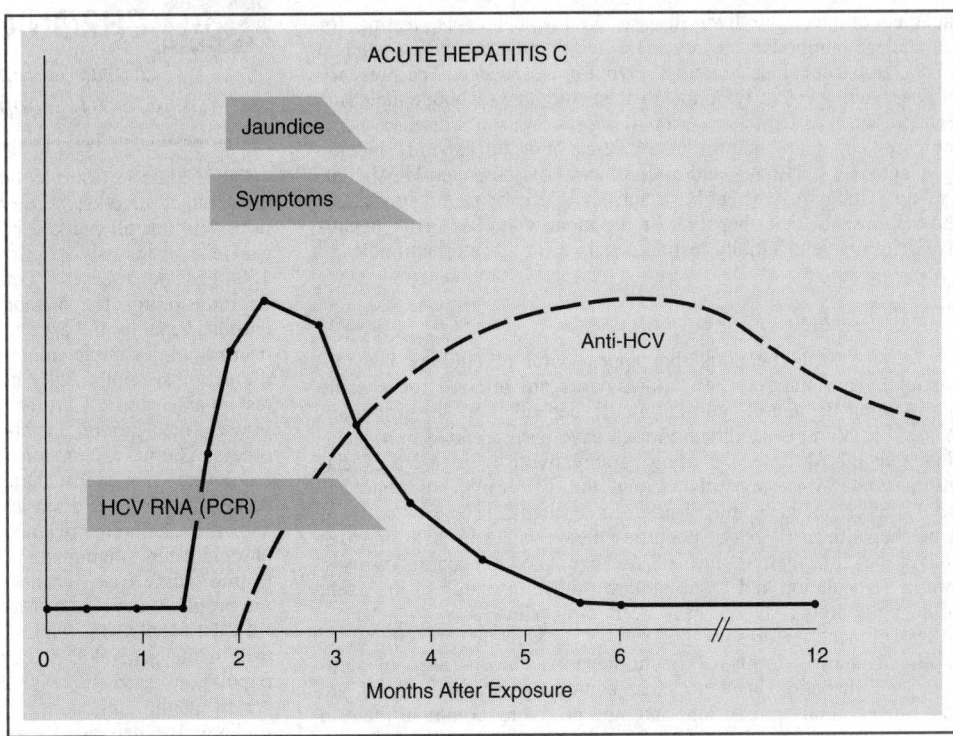

FIGURE 149–4 ■ The serologic course of acute hepatitis C.

studies from India and Egypt, hepatitis E has accounted for a high proportion of cases of sporadic acute hepatitis. In the United States and Western Europe, hepatitis E is very rare, with only imported cases being described in most Western countries. Hepatitis E is spread by the fecal-oral route, and most cases can be traced to exposure to contaminated water under poor hygienic conditions. Hepatitis E appears to be less contagious than hepatitis A, the other form of "infectious" hepatitis, and secondary cases are rare.

The clinical course of hepatitis E resembles that of other forms of hepatitis. The incubation period is 15 to 60 days (mean = 35 days). The disease is frequently "cholestatic," with prominence of bilirubin and alkaline phosphatase elevations. Hepatitis E also tends to be more severe than other forms of epidemic jaundice, with a fatality rate of 1 to 2% and a particularly high rate of acute liver failure in pregnant women. Hepatitis E virions and antigen can be detected in stool and liver during the incubation period and early symptomatic phase, but these tests are not practical means for diagnosis. Enzyme-linked immunoassays for IgM and IgG antibody to HEV (anti-HEV) have been developed and are reactive in at least 90% of patients at the onset of clinical illness. These tests, however, are not generally available nor standardized. In addition, anti-HEV is found in 1 to 2% of the normal population. It remains unclear, whether the finding of anti-HEV in persons without a history of hepatitis or travel to endemic areas represents evidence of previous infection or false-positive antibody reactivity. The recent discovery of HEV infection in domestic swine suggests a reservoir of infection and perhaps an explanation for finding antibody in non-endemic areas of the world.

The diagnosis of hepatitis E should be considered in a patient who presents with acute hepatitis and has recently traveled to an endemic area, particularly if tests for other forms of hepatitis are non-reactive. The finding of anti-HEV, particularly of the IgM subclass, is sufficient to make the diagnosis in this situation. However, hepatitis E is very rare in the United States and Western World, so testing for anti-HEV is rarely necessary.

There are no known means of prevention or treatment of hepatitis E. Immune globulin even when prepared from the plasma of populations with a high rate of hepatitis E does not appear to be effective. No specific means of treatment have been evaluated. Travelers to areas of the world (particularly pregnant women) where hepatitis E is endemic should be cautioned regarding drinking water and uncooked food.

DIFFERENTIAL DIAGNOSIS

The diagnostic approach to the patient with the clinical features of acute hepatitis (Table 149–3) begins with a careful history for risk factors and possible exposure, for medication use, including herbal and over-the-counter drugs, and for alcohol use. The onset and progression of symptoms may give clues to other causes of liver disease, such as alcohol or gallstones. Biochemical laboratory tests, including serum bilirubin, alanine and aspartate aminotransferases, alkaline phosphatase, lactic dehydrogenase, albumin, complete blood cell counts, and prothrombin time are valuable in defining whether the clinical picture is typical of acute hepatitis (high aminotransferases, normal or modest elevations in alkaline phosphatase and lactic dehydrogenase) or resembles that of obstructive

Table 149–3 ■ SEROLOGIC DIAGNOSIS OF ACUTE HEPATITIS

DIAGNOSIS	SCREENING ASSAYS	SUPPLEMENTAL ASSAYS
Hepatitis A	IgM anti-HAV	None needed
Hepatitis B	HBsAg, IgM anti-HBc	HBeAg, anti-HBe HBV DNA
Hepatitis C	Anti-HCV by EIA	HCV RNA by PCR; anti-HCV by Immunoblot
Hepatitis D	HBsAg	Anti-HDV
Hepatitis E	History	Anti-HEV
Mononucleosis	History, white blood cell differential counts	Monospot test
		Heterophile antibody
Drug-induced hepatitis	History	

jaundice or alcoholic liver disease. In atypical cases, testing for antinuclear antibodies to evaluate autoimmune hepatitis and a VDRL test to exclude secondary syphilis are needed. The presence of fever and atypical lymphocytosis should suggest mononucleosis. The presence of hemolysis should suggest Wilson's disease. Serologic tests that are helpful in all cases of acute hepatitis include IgM anti-HAV, HBsAg and/or IgM anti-HBc, and anti-HCV. Follow-up testing for anti-HDV or anti-HCV can be useful in making the diagnosis of delta hepatitis (in a patient with HBsAg) or hepatitis C (in a patient initially testing negative for all viral antibodies).

HEPATITIS NON-A . . . E

Cases of acute hepatitis that appear viral in etiology but that cannot be attributed to any known virus are referred to as acute non-A, non-B, non-C, non-D, non-E hepatitis, or hepatitis non-A . . . E. Various candidate viruses have been reported in association with this disease, including paramyxoviruses, togaviruses, flaviviruses (GBV-C, hepatitis G, and the TT virus), but none has been clearly linked to this disease. In serologic surveys of cases of acute hepatitis in Western countries, between 2 and 20% of cases cannot be attributed to any of the five known hepatitis viruses. Animal inoculation and tissue culture studies in search of the agent of hepatitis non-A . . . E have been unrevealing.

The clinical features of non-A . . . E hepatitis are similar to those of known forms of acute hepatitis. Most cases of non-A . . . E hepatitis have no clear source of exposure. Cases are rare after blood transfusion and are no more common than in control, non-transfused subjects. The absence of typical risk factors for viral hepatitis suggest that some cases of non-A . . . E hepatitis may be due to non-viral causes, such as an environmental exposure, drug, or autoimmune process.

The syndrome of non-A . . . E hepatitis has been particularly associated with the complications of acute liver failure and aplastic anemia. Hepatitis non-A . . . E is a more common cause of fulminant hepatic failure than hepatitis A or B combined, often accounting for 30 to 40% of cases. Approximately one third of patients with non-A . . . E hepatitis develop chronic hepatitis, and a small percentage ultimately develop cirrhosis.

Non-A . . . E hepatitis is a diagnosis of exclusion, usually made on the basis of an acute hepatitis occurring in a patient without anti-HAV, HBsAg, anti-HBc, or anti-HCV and without any other known cause of acute hepatic injury. Testing of serum during convalescence is helpful in excluding hepatitis C with delayed seroconversion. Tests for anti-HEV are generally not necessary unless there is a history of travel to an endemic area. The most important diagnoses to exclude are infectious mononucleosis and the non-viral causes of an acute hepatitis–like syndrome, most particularly drugs, over-the-counter medications, herbal preparations, toxins, alcoholic liver injury, acute cholecystitis, autoimmune hepatitis, and Wilson's disease. A careful history of exposure to drugs and toxins, along with an abdominal ultrasonography to exclude gallstone disease, and tests for antinuclear antibodies and ceruloplasmin (and urine copper if necessary) are helpful in fully defining a case of non-A . . . E hepatitis.

There are no means of either treatment or prevention of non-A . . . E hepatitis. A viral etiology of this syndrome is being actively investigated, particularly in the situation of acute liver failure and aplastic anemia.

Centers for Disease Control and Prevention: Prevention of hepatitis A through active or passive immunization: Recommendations of the Advisory Committee on Immunization Practices. MMWR 45:1–15, 1996. *Recommendations for hepatitis A vaccination and rationale for each.*

Lee WM: Hepatitis B virus infection. N Engl J Med 337:1733–1745, 1997. *A concise and accurate overview of the virology, immunology, clinical course, and outcome of acute and chronic hepatitis B.*

Lemon S, Thomas DL: Vaccines to prevent viral hepatitis. N Engl J Med 336:196–204, 1997. *An overview of present and potential future vaccines against hepatitis A and B.*

Major ME, Feinstone SM: The molecular virology of hepatitis C. Hepatology 25: 1527–1538, 1997. *A succinct overview of the virology of the hepatitis virus that provides the basis for understanding the epidemiology, clinical course, treatment, and prevention of hepatitis C.*

Villano SA, Vlahov D, Nelson KE, et al: Persistence of viremia and the importance of long-term follow-up after acute hepatitis C infection. Hepatology 29:908–914, 1999. *Among 43 injection drug users who developed anti-HCV during longitudinal follow up, 37 (85%) developed chronic infection. Lack of detectable HCV RNA on a single determination during the course of acute hepatitis C was not a reliable marker of recovery.*

150 CHRONIC HEPATITIS

Karen L. Lindsay
Jay H. Hoofnagle

DEFINITION. Chronic hepatitis comprises several diseases that are grouped together because they have common clinical manifestations and are all marked by chronic necroinflammatory injury that can lead insidiously to cirrhosis and end-stage liver disease (Table 150–1). The disease is defined as chronic if there is evidence of ongoing injury for 6 months or more. The strict definition of chronic hepatitis is based upon histologic features of hepatocellular necrosis and chronic inflammatory cell infiltration in the liver, but the diagnosis can usually be made from clinical features and blood test results alone. Chronic hepatitis has multiple causes including viruses, medications, metabolic abnormalities, and autoimmune disorders. The most common forms are chronic hepatitis B and C and autoimmune hepatitis. Drug-induced (Chapter 148) or metabolic (Chapter 152) liver diseases, alcoholic steatohepatitis (Chapter 153), and non-alcoholic steatohepatitis (Chapter 148) can also cause chronic necroinflammatory lesions of the liver. Despite extensive testing, some cases cannot be attributed to any known cause and are probably the result of as yet unidentified viruses.

EPIDEMIOLOGY. The incidence and prevalence of chronic hepatitis in the general U.S. population have not been well defined. In population-based surveys, 2.3% of Americans have elevations in serum alanine aminotransferase (ALT) level, 0.2% are seropositive findings for hepatitis B surface antigen (HBsAg), and 1.8% are reactive for anti–hepatitis C virus (anti-HCV). However, not all ALT elevations are due to chronic hepatitis and not all HBsAg-positive or anti-HCV-positive individuals have active liver disease. A fair estimate is that chronic hepatitis affects 2% of the population, but these diseases tend to occur mostly in high-risk groups rather than the general population. For hepatitis B, high-risk groups include recent immigrants from endemic areas of the world (Africa, Eastern Europe, Southeast Asia), male homosexuals and heterosexuals with multiple sexual partners, hemophiliacs, oncology and renal dialysis patients, and medical care workers. For hepatitis C, high-risk groups include recipients of blood or blood products before 1992, injection drug users, medical care workers, and perhaps persons with multiple sexual partners. Chronic hepatitis B and C probably cause 10,000 to 12,000 deaths yearly, and about another 1500 patients with this disease undergo liver transplantation annually for end-stage liver failure.

CLINICAL MANIFESTATIONS. The *clinical symptoms* of chronic hepatitis are typically non-specific, intermittent, and mild; a large proportion of patients have no symptoms of liver disease at all. The most common symptom is fatigue, which may be intermittent. Some patients have sleep disorders or difficulty in concentrating. Right upper quadrant pain, if present, is usually mild, intermittent, and achy in character. Indeed, in many cases, the diagnosis of chronic hepatitis is made after liver test result abnormalities are identified when blood is drawn for a routine health evaluation during assessment for an unrelated health problem or at the time of voluntary blood donation. Symptoms of advanced disease or an acute exacerbation include nausea, poor appetite, weight loss, muscle weakness, itching, dark urine, and jaundice. Once cirrhosis is present, weakness, weight loss, abdominal swelling, edema, ready bruisability, gastrointestinal bleeding, and hepatic encephalopathy with mental confusion may arise.

The clinical *signs* of liver disease in patients with chronic hepatitis are also usually minimal. The most common physical finding is

Table 150–1 ■ **MAJOR CAUSES OF CHRONIC HEPATITIS**

Chronic hepatitis B
Chronic hepatitis D
Chronic hepatitis C
Autoimmune hepatitis
Drug-induced chronic hepatitis
Wilson's disease
Cryptogenic hepatitis (non-A–E hepatitis)

liver tenderness. In patients with severe or advanced disease, other findings may include a firm liver or mild enlargement of the spleen, spider angiomata, and palmar erythema. Once cirrhosis is present, signs may include muscle wasting, ascites, edema, skin excoriations or bruises, and hepatic fetor.

Although symptoms and signs are not particularly useful in identifying chronic hepatitis, biochemical and hematologic blood test results are quite reliable. Most typical are elevations in ALT and aspartate aminotransferase (AST) levels with little or no elevation in alkaline phosphatase level. The elevations are usually in the range of 1 to 5 times the upper limit of normal, and the ALT level is generally somewhat higher than AST level unless cirrhosis is present. Serum aminotransferase levels can be normal when the disease is mild or inactive but can also be markedly elevated in the range typical of acute hepatitis (10 to 25 times the upper limit of normal) during acute exacerbations. Although there may be major discrepancies between the height of the liver enzyme elevations and the histologic estimates of activity as shown by liver biopsy, monitoring of these values over time generally provides a reasonable estimate of the severity of disease.

In general, alkaline phosphatase and γ-glutamyl transpeptidase elevations are mild in chronic hepatitis, unless cirrhosis is present. Creatine kinase (CK) and lactic dehydrogenase levels are normal. Serum bilirubin and albumin levels and prothrombin time are normal in patients with chronic hepatitis, unless the disease is severe or advanced. Any elevation in serum direct bilirubin level or decrease in albumin level should be considered evidence of serious disease activity or injury. Serum immunoglobulin levels are mildly elevated or normal in chronic viral hepatitis but may be strikingly elevated in chronic autoimmune hepatitis. Blood counts are normal in chronic hepatitis, unless cirrhosis or portal hypertension is present with associated decreases in white blood cell and platelet counts. Serial determinations of platelet counts may provide the earliest clinical evidence of progression of chronic hepatitis to cirrhosis.

Imaging with ultrasound can define hepatic texture and size, determine the presence of hepatic masses, assess the gallbladder and intrahepatic bile ducts, define the size of the spleen, and determine the presence of collateral vessels and portal venous flow. Computed tomography and nuclear magnetic imaging of the liver are not very helpful unless a mass or abnormality is found by ultrasound.

Hepatic histologic characteristics typically include spotty hepatocellular necrosis, chronic inflammatory cell infiltration in portal areas, and variable degrees of fibrosis. The hepatocellular necrosis is typically eosinophilic degeneration or ballooning degeneration. The necrosis is spotty throughout the parenchyma, but there is often most activity in the periportal area, which is referred to as "piecemeal" necrosis or interface hepatitis. The hepatocellular necrosis appears to be mediated largely by apoptosis in association with cytotoxic lymphocytes. Chronic inflammatory cells (CD4+ and CD8+ lymphocytes as well as plasma cells, histocytes, and macrophages) are found in the areas of necrosis and in sinusoids, but most prominently in portal areas. Fibrosis occurs insidiously during the course of chronic hepatitis and typically begins in the periportal

regions. Ultimately, bands of fibrosis can link up adjacent portal areas or portal and central areas, distort the hepatic architecture, and lead to cirrhosis and portal hypertension.

Hepatic histologic analysis is useful for grading the severity and for staging chronic hepatitis and is usually obtained to confirm the diagnosis made through the patient's history, physical exam, and blood test results. The hepatic histologic evaluation may help to confirm the diagnosis of autoimmune hepatitis and clarify the role of α_1-antitrypsin deficiency or Wilson's disease. Most importantly, liver histologic analysis can exclude other diagnoses that occasionally mimic chronic hepatitis clinically or cause similar patterns of liver enzyme level elevations, including fatty liver, alcoholic liver disease, steatohepatitis, drug-induced liver disease, sclerosing cholangitis, iron overload, and veno-occlusive disease.

The *grade* of chronic hepatitis refers to the activity of the disease in terms of necrosis and inflammation; the grade of disease fluctuates and is reversible. The *stage* of disease refers to how advanced the process is and whether cirrhosis is present; stages of disease are considered largely irreversible. The most commonly used system of grading and staging is the Histology Activity Index (HAI), in which the combined scores for periportal necrosis and inflammation (0 to 10), lobular necrosis and inflammation (0 to 4), and portal inflammation (0 to 4) define the grade or activity of disease. Disease stage is defined by scores between 0 and 4 for fibrosis, with 4 indicating cirrhosis.

DIFFERENTIAL DIAGNOSIS. Chronic hepatitis can be caused by several diseases that are similar clinically but that respond quite differently to therapy and must be managed individually. Patients with suspected chronic hepatitis should be carefully evaluated for fatty liver, alcohol- (Chapter 153) or drug-induced liver disease (Chapter 148), and metabolic liver diseases (Chapter 152), not only because these disorders mimic those that cause chronic hepatitis but also because they can coexist with the disorders that cause chronic hepatitis. After taking a history designed to elucidate risk factors for viral hepatitis, specific and appropriate serologic tests (Table 150–2) can be used to make the diagnosis. Liver biopsy with special stains is then used to confirm the diagnosis, assess the activity and severity of injury, and stage the disease. A treatment strategy should arise from a careful consideration of the diagnosis and grade and stage of disease. With the advances currently being made in the fields of antiviral and immunomodulatory therapeutics, it is anticipated that the considerable progress made in treating these diseases over the past decade will continue in the future.

CHRONIC HEPATITIS B

Chronic hepatitis B is caused by infection with the hepatitis B virus (HBV), a medium-sized DNA virus belonging to the family Hepadnaviridae (Chapter 149). The diagnosis of chronic hepatitis B is usually suspected on the basis of HBsAg in the serum of a patient with chronic hepatitis and confirmed by the finding of (HBV) DNA in serum or hepatitis B core antigen (HBcAg) in

Table 150–2 ■ DIFFERENTIAL DIAGNOSIS IN CHRONIC HEPATITIS

DIAGNOSIS	SCREENING TESTS	CONFIRMATORY TESTS	COMMENTS
Chronic hepatitis B	HBsAg	HBV DNA, HBeAg, or HBcAg in liver	
Chronic hepatitis C	Anti-HCV	HCV RNA (using PCR)	Immunoblot for anti-HCV can be used to confirm antibody reactivity
Chronic hepatitis D	Anti-HDV	HDV RNA or HDV antigen in liver	
Autoimmune hepatitis	ANA (Anti-LKM 1)	Exclusion of other causes and pattern of clinical disease	Suggested by raised IgG levels and by response to corticosteroid therapy
Drug-induced liver disease	History	Rechallenge if necessary	Medications most suspect include isoniazid, NSAIDs, methyldopa, nitrofurantoin
Wilson's disease	Ceruloplasmin	Urine and hepatic copper concentration	Suggested by hemolysis or severe chronic hepatitis in child or adolescent
Cryptogenic	Exclusion of other causes		Major differential is with autoimmune hepatitis and drug-induced liver disease

HBsAg = hepatitis B surface antigen; HCV = hepatitis C virus; HDV = hepatitis D virus; ANA = antinuclear antibody; LKM1 = liver-kidney microsomal 1 antibody; HBV = hepatitis B virus; HBeAg = hepatitis B e antigen; HBcAg = hepatitis B core antigen; IgG = immunoglobulin G; NSAIDs = non-steroidal anti-inflammatory drugs.

liver. Most patients with chronic hepatitis B also have hepatitis B e antigen (HBeAg) in serum, reflecting high levels of viral replication. Some patients have active liver disease with HBsAg and high levels of HBV DNA but no HBeAg in serum. These patients usually harbor a mutant HBV that replicates efficiently and is pathogenic but does not produce HBeAg.

In the typical course of chronic hepatitis B, HBsAg, HBeAg, and HBV DNA become detectable in serum during the incubation period and gradually rise in titer (Fig. 150–1). Symptoms appear 30 to 150 days after exposure (mean incubation period of 75 days), usually at the time of peak viral levels. Symptoms are mild and non-specific, and jaundice is rare. Indeed, appearance of jaundice during the course of acute infection is highly predictive of eventual recovery. In chronic hepatitis, serum ALT levels fall after the acute phase of infection but persist at levels between 1 and 10 times the upper limit of normal. HBsAg, HBeAg, and HBV DNA persist, generally in high levels; the finding of HBeAg more than 2 months after onset of symptoms is indicative of evolution to chronicity. Levels of HBV DNA are usually in the range of 10^7 to 10^{11} genome copies/mL, levels readily detectable by hybridization techniques.

The subsequent course of chronic hepatitis B is highly variable. Some patients continue to have active viral replication with high levels of HBV DNA and HBeAg in serum and progressive liver injury; cirrhosis and end-stage liver disease may soon develop. In other patients, the disease is more indolent, leading insidiously to cirrhosis in decades. However, in a large proportion of patients the outcome is more benign; the disease eventually goes into remission spontaneously, symptoms (if present) resolve, serum aminotransferase levels fall into the normal range, and liver histologic characteristics improve. Remission is often preceded by a transient flare of disease and can be quite precipitous, coinciding with a major fall in level of HBV DNA and seroconversion from HBeAg to anti-HBe. Strikingly, however, HBsAg persists in serum at levels somewhat lower than before this seroconversion, and HBV DNA can be detected at low levels (generally less than 10^5 genome copies/mL) if sensitive techniques such as the polymerase chain reaction (PCR) are used.

With the fall in viral levels and loss of HBeAg, the disease appears to go into remission, suggesting that there has been a transition from chronic hepatitis B to an "inactive" carrier state with no symptoms, normal serum aminotransferase levels, and inactive liver disease indicated by biopsy findings. The loss of HBeAg, however, is not always followed by permanent resolution of disease. In some patients, reactivation occurs with re-appearance of

HBeAg; in others an HBV mutant develops and replicates efficiently but cannot produce HBeAg. These patients with HBeAg-negative mutant-associated chronic hepatitis B can have severe disease and often suffer from multiple clinical relapses.

Chronic hepatitis B should be distinguished from the inactive (which has been somewhat inappropriately referred to as "healthy") HBsAg carrier state, in which HBsAg persists in serum without active liver disease or viral replication (Table 150–3); in the inactive carrier state, HBV DNA is not detectable in serum by using conventional hybridization assays sensitive to levels of 10^6 viral copies/mL. Testing for HBV DNA by PCR usually demonstrates low levels of viral genome in serum even in patients with the inactive carrier state, suggesting that the difference is quantitative rather than qualitative.

Liver injury and pathogenesis of chronic hepatitis B are believed to be immunologically mediated, so the severity and course of disease do not correlate well with the level of virus in serum or antigen expression in liver. Antigen-specific cytotoxic T cells are believed to mediate the cell injury in hepatitis B and account for ultimate viral clearance. Specific cytokines produced by cytotoxic and other T cells also have antiviral effects on hepatocytes, contributing to viral clearance without cell death. The progression of acute to chronic hepatitis B is attributed to lack of a vigorous cytotoxic T-cell response to hepatitis B antigens. Similarly, spontaneous seroconversion from HBeAg to anti-HBe during chronic hepatitis B may also be immunologically mediated, as is suggested from the transient flare of disease that often immediately precedes clearance of HBeAg. Viral factors may also affect outcome: Some HBV strains may be more pathogenic and more likely to lead to chronic infection, because they are less immunogenic or more resistant to T-cell attack. Furthermore, seroconversion may be due to spontaneous mutations in the predominant HBV species to forms that produce HBsAg without HBeAg (e-negative mutant) and that are less efficient in replication, and less pathogenic.

The extrahepatic manifestations of chronic hepatitis B include mucocutaneous vasculitis, glomerulonephritis, and polyarteritis nodosa. The glomerulonephritis of hepatitis B occurs more commonly in children than adults and is usually characterized by nephrotic syndrome with little decrease in renal function. Polyarteritis nodosa (see Chapter 293) occurs primarily in adults and is marked by sudden and severe onset of hypertension, renal disease, and systemic vasculitis with arteritis in vessels of the kidney, gallbladder, intestine, or brain.

TREATMENT. Non-specific recommendations for management of chronic hepatitis B include vaccination of all household and sexual contacts. Patients should be counseled on the modes of transmis-

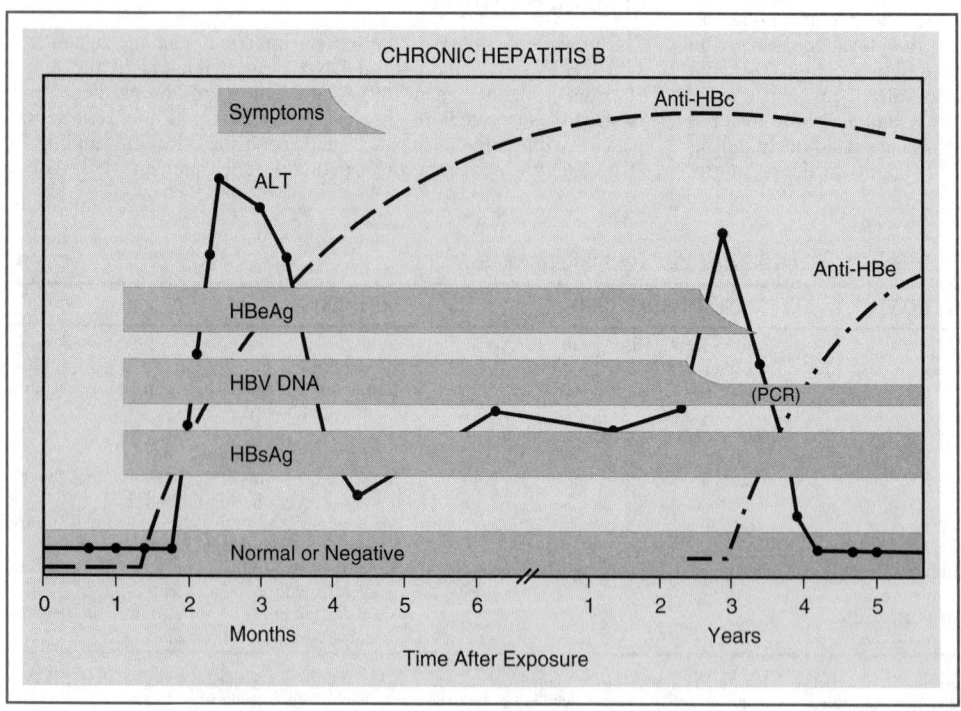

FIGURE 150–1 ■ The typical serologic course of chronic hepatitis B.

Table 150-3 ■ THREE FORMS OF CHRONIC HEPATITIS B VIRUS INFECTION

PATTERN	HBsAg	HBeAg	HBV DNA* (titer:range)	HBcAg IN LIVER	CHRONIC HEPATITIS
Typical chronic hepatitis B	Pos	Pos	Pos 10^7–10^{11}	Pos (nuclear)	Active
HBeAg-negative chronic hepatitis B	Pos	Neg	Pos 10^5–10^9	Pos (cytoplasmic)	Active (relapsing)
Inactive HBsAg carrier state	Pos	Neg	Pos 10^1–10^5	Neg	Inactive

*Positive or negative result by hybridization techniques (sensitive to a titer of 10^6 genome-equivalents/mL). Titers below 10^6 genome-equivalents/mL generally require polymerase chain reaction assays for detection. HBeAg = hepatitis B e antigen; HBsAg = hepatitis B surface antigen; Pos = positive result; Neg = negative result; HBV = hepatitis B virus; HBcAg = hepatitis B core antigen.

sion of hepatitis B and means of prevention of spread. Vaccination against hepatitis A is also recommended. Importantly, patients with hepatitis B should avoid all but the most necessary use of immunosuppressive medications. Severe flares of hepatitis B and even fatalities have followed short courses of corticosteroids or cancer chemotherapy.

The standard treatment of chronic hepatitis B is a 4- to 6-month course of α interferon given subcutaneously in doses of 5 million units (MU) daily or 10 MU thrice weekly, a regimen that results in clearance of HBeAg and HBV DNA (as detected by hybridization techniques) in 30 to 40% of patients and of HBsAg in 10% of patients. These are high doses of interferon, and therapy is often poorly tolerated. Therapy is indicated in patients who have chronic hepatitis B with HBsAg and HBV DNA in serum and elevations in serum aminotransferase levels. Therapy is contraindicated in patients with advanced cirrhosis, in solid organ transplantation recipients, in immunosuppressed patients, and in patients with other serious major illnesses. Therapy is not recommended in patients with normal or near-normal serum aminotransferase levels (even if HBeAg is present) largely because interferon therapy is usually ineffective in this situation. The major factors associated with response to α interferon in chronic hepatitis B are initial high levels of serum aminotransferases, low levels of HBV DNA, and absence of immunosuppression. The potential benefits as well as risks of interferon therapy should be thoroughly discussed before treatment. The major side effects of interferon include fatigue, muscle aches, fever, depression, and irritability; uncommon severe side effects include suicide, psychosis, renal and cardiac failure, bacterial infections, and induction of autoimmunity (see the discussion of treatment of chronic hepatitis C).

With initiation of treatment, levels of HBV DNA usually fall. In patients with a beneficial response (as defined by loss of HBeAg with treatment), there is typically a flare of disease with elevations of serum ALT to levels two to three times the baseline after 2 to 3 months of therapy coinciding with a precipitous fall in HBV DNA levels and loss of HBeAg. Serum aminotransferase levels fall to normal, and a proportion of patients lose HBsAg, often many months to several years after loss of HBeAg. Reactivation of disease with rises in aminotransferase levels and reappearance of HBeAg and high levels of HBV DNA occurs rarely.

More recently, oral nucleoside analogues including lamivudine (3-thiacytidine), famciclovir, adefovir dipivoxil (bis-POM-PMEA), lobucavir, and clevudine (L-FMAU) have shown potent effects against HBV. Lamivudine, which is currently the only one of these agents approved for use in the United States (see later), is given in a dose of 100 mg/day for 1 year. Initiation of therapy is followed rapidly by marked falls in level of HBV DNA, which is usually no longer detectable by hybridization tests (less than 106 genome copies/mL) within 1 to 3 months of starting therapy. Once HBV DNA level falls, serum aminotransferase levels begin to decrease and are usually normal or near normal within 3 to 6 months of starting treatment. Prolonged therapy (for 1 year or more) is associated with loss of HBeAg in 15 to 30% of patients. With loss of HBeAg and development of anti-HBe, lamivudine can be stopped; relapses are uncommon once seroconversion occurs. Most patients, however, remain HBeAg-positive despite improvements in HBV DNA and aminotransferase levels. Continued lamivudine therapy for more than a year is well tolerated but is associated with development of viral resistance in 14 to 32% of patients each year.

Viral resistance is marked by a rise of HBV DNA toward baseline levels followed by elevations in serum aminotransferase levels. Most patients in whom viral resistance develops harbor an HBV mutant with amino acid changes in the conserved region of the polymerase gene (YMDD mutates to either YIDD or YVDD). Typically patients with YMDD mutations have lower levels of HBV DNA and serum aminotransferases than were present before therapy, suggesting that the mutant HBV is less efficient in replication and less pathogenic than the wild-type virus. Approaches to treating patients with lamivudine resistance are now being developed, and the use of combination antiviral therapy (including combinations of lamivudine and interferon) is now being assessed.

At present, monotherapy with lamivudine should be limited to patients who have failed to respond to or cannot tolerate a course of α interferon. Because of the high rate of viral resistance, therapy should not be continued for more than 1 year in patients with typical, compensated chronic hepatitis B. Continuous, long-term therapy should be reserved for patients who are immunosuppressed and those who have severe disease. Monotherapy with lamivudine should not be used in patients with mild or minimal disease. The exception is the patient with chronic hepatitis B or the inactive carrier state who requires therapy with a pulse or short course of immunosuppression or corticosteroids, as with cyclic cancer chemotherapy. Such treatment is directed at preventing hepatitis re-activation, which can be severe and even life-threatening. These patients can be treated with lamivudine (100 mg/day) for the duration of the immunosuppressive therapy. Recommendations regarding indications and regimens as well as duration of therapy will change as more effective combination antiviral therapies are developed.

CHRONIC HEPATITIS D

Hepatitis D is caused by combined infection with hepatitis B and the hepatitis D virus (HDV), a defective RNA virus that replicates and spreads efficiently only in the presence of HBsAg (Chapter 149). Hepatitis D is the least common form of chronic viral hepatitis but is also the most severe. On average, cirrhosis develops in 70% of patients with chronic hepatitis D, generally at a younger age than in patients with hepatitis B alone.

The diagnosis of chronic hepatitis D is usually made on the basis of finding antibody to HDV (anti-HDV) in a patient with chronic hepatitis and HBsAg in serum. The diagnosis can be confirmed by the identification of HDV antigen in liver or by detection of HDV RNA in serum, a research test not generally available. Most patients with chronic hepatitis D have HBsAg without serologic markers of active viral replication: That is, they have a negative result for HBeAg and HBV DNA (at least as detected by hybridization assays). Replication of HDV appears to suppress that of HBV.

Therapy of hepatitis D is difficult. A prolonged course of rather high doses of alpha interferon (5 to 10 MU/day or thrice weekly) results in improvements in serum aminotransferase levels and liver histology in approximately one third of patients. With the exception of patients who become HBsAg-negative during treatment, however, most relapse when therapy is stopped. Corticosteroids are not helpful, nor is lamivudine or ribavirin. General management recommendations for hepatitis D are the same as for hepatitis B.

CHRONIC HEPATITIS C

Chronic hepatitis C is caused by infection with the hepatitis C virus (HCV), a small RNA virus classified in genus *Hepacivirus,* family Flaviviridae (Chapter 149). The diagnosis of chronic hepatitis C is usually based upon the finding of anti-HCV in a patient with serum aminotransferase elevations or chronic hepatitis on liver biopsy (Table 150–4). The typical test for anti-HCV is an enzyme immunoassay, which occasionally can yield a false-positive result. Recombinant immunoblot assay (RIBA) can be used to confirm anti-HCV reactivity. However, the diagnosis of hepatitis C is more aptly confirmed by a qualitative test for HCV RNA in serum using a sensitive assay such as a reverse-transcriptase PCR. If anti-HCV is present without HCV RNA, recovery from hepatitis C rather than persistent infection has probably occurred. In chronic hepatitis C, the quantitative serum level of virus is usually fairly constant and among different patients typically ranges from 10^3 to 10^7 viral copies/mL. The commercial virologic tests for hepatitis C have yet to be standardized; assays for viral level are particularly difficult to standardize and may not be reliable. Most patients with chronic hepatitis C have few if any symptoms; the diagnosis is often first made on the basis of blood tests taken during a routine medical examination or at the time of a blood donation.

Hepatitis C is spread largely by the parenteral route, most commonly as a result of injection drug use or receipt of blood transfusions before the introduction of routine screening of blood for anti-HCV (in 1992) or receipt of plasma products before the introduction of inactivation procedures (in 1987). Hepatitis C also occurs after accidental needle sticks and is an occupational hazard for medical care workers. In 10 to 30% of patients, a parenteral source of infection cannot be identified, even after careful questioning. These sporadic cases of hepatitis C may be related to sexual contact but are more likely related to "inapparent" parenteral spread. Hepatitis C is rarely spread between monogamous sexual partners. Maternal-infant spread of hepatitis C occurs in approximately 5% of cases of mothers with chronic hepatitis C. Neither breast-feeding nor type of delivery correlates with transmission.

In the typical course of chronic hepatitis C (Fig. 150–2), HCV RNA becomes detectable soon after exposure and remains present throughout the course of the acute illness and thereafter. Approximately one third of patients experience symptoms during the acute episode, and a similar percentage are jaundiced. Aminotransferase levels vary widely, but after the acute episode are usually less than 10 times the upper limit of normal. Indeed, in 30 to 50% of infected individuals, serum aminotransferase levels fall and remain in the normal range despite persistence of HCV RNA. These individuals, nevertheless, have chronic hepatitis indicated by liver biopsy. Anti-HCV arises somewhat after the onset of ALT elevations and symptoms, and it usually persists at high titers. Anti-HCV may not become detectable in patients who have renal failure, are immunosuppressed, or have hypo- or agammaglobulinemia.

The natural history of hepatitis C is highly variable. A proportion of patients have severe and progressive disease, and cirrhosis and end-stage liver disease develop within a few years; other patients have a benign outcome. In patients followed from the time of acute infection (such as after blood transfusion or receipt of contaminated blood products), approximately 75 to 85% have chronic infection, but cirrhosis develops in only 10 to 20% within the first 20 years. In these patients, there is little or no increase in hepatitis C–related mortality rate during the first two decades of infection. However, when patients with established chronic hepatitis C are followed prospectively from the time of initial presentation, 30 to 50% have cirrhosis, and morbidity and mortality rates are substantial, with development of end-stage liver disease or hepatocellular carcinoma, particularly in patients with cirrhosis or severe fibrosis indicated on initial liver biopsy. Interestingly, at the time of diagnosis the average patient has probably had the infection for 10 to 20 years (dating onset from time of suspected exposure).

Factors associated with the risk of development of cirrhosis in chronic hepatitis C include age, male sex, alcohol use, and coinfection with other hepatitis viruses. Factors associated with increased rate of development of hepatocellular carcinoma are cirrhosis or advanced fibrosis, indicated on liver biopsy; age; male sex; and alcohol abuse. In some retrospective studies, treatment with α interferon, even without a sustained virologic response, has been associated with a lower rate of development of liver cancer.

The pathogenesis of viral persistence and the cause of hepatic injury in chronic hepatitis C infection are unknown, but cytotoxic T-lymphocyte-mediated responses are probably important. In general, the degree of liver injury does not correlate with the level or genotype of virus but tends to increase with duration of infection. Nevertheless, there are some individuals who remain infected with HCV for decades yet have minimal changes indicated on liver biopsy. Alcohol ingestion and other hepatotoxic exposures (such as iron overload or concurrent hepatitis virus infection) may augment liver injury in chronic HCV infection.

The extrahepatic manifestations of chronic hepatitis C include cryoglobulinemia, glomerulonephritis, mucocutaneous vasculitis, non-Hodgkin's B-cell lymphoma, porphyria cutanea tarda, lichen planus, and perhaps fibromyalgia. Cryoglobulinemia, which is the most common and well-defined complication of hepatitis C, occurs in approximately 1% of adults with this infection. Typical manifestations are fatigue, myalgias, arthralgias, skin rash (purpura, hives, and leukocytoclastic vasculitis), neuropathy, and renal disease (glomerulonephritis). Laboratory testing reveals high levels of rheumatoid factor and of cryoglobulins containing anti-HCV and HCV RNA, with low levels of complement. Cryoglobulinemia can be severe and lead to end-stage renal disease or severe neuropathies.

The management of patients with chronic hepatitis C should include counseling to abstain from alcohol and evaluation for hepatitis A and B vaccination. The therapy of hepatitis C is rapidly evolving. α Interferons (recombinant and natural) have been used successfully to treat chronic hepatitis C for over a decade, but the overall sustained response rate to a course of α interferon is only 10 to 20%. More recently, the addition of ribavirin, an oral nucleoside analogue, to α interferon therapy has increased the sustained response rate substantially. The usual criteria used to define a beneficial response to therapy in chronic hepatitis C are (1) eradication of HCV RNA from serum, (2) normalization of serum aminotransferase levels, and (3) improvements in liver histologic characteristics. The single most accurate end-point in defining a beneficial response is absence of detectable HCV RNA (by a reliable and sensitive PCR technique) with treatment that persists for at least 6 months after stopping therapy. Thus a sustained virologic response at 6 months after treatment is highly predictive of long-term remission and resolution of disease, and it may indicate eradication of the infection.

With α interferon with or without ribavirin, serum aminotransferase and HCV RNA levels typically fall rapidly with onset of therapy and, in responders, become normal or undetectable within 1 to 3 months. In patients who relapse, HCV RNA and elevations in serum ALT level reappear soon after therapy is stopped. In nonresponders, ALT levels may decrease but rarely become normal, and HCV RNA remains detectable. However, exceptions to these pat-

Table 150–4 ■ INTERPRETATION OF SEROLOGIC MARKERS FOR HEPATITIS C

ANTI-HCV (EIA)	ANTI-HCV (RIBA)	HCV RNA (PCR)	ALT	INTERPRETATION
Pos	Pos	Pos	Elevated	Acute or chronic hepatitis C
Pos	Pos	Pos	Normal	Chronic hepatitis C
Pos	Pos	Neg	Normal	Resolved hepatitis C
Pos	Neg	Neg	Normal	False-positive EIA assay result

Anti-HCV = antibody to hepatitis C virus; EIA = enzyme immunoassay; RIBA = recombinant immunoblot assay; HCV RNA = hepatitis C viral RNA; PCR = polymerase chain reaction; ALT = alanine aminotransferase; POS = positive result; Neg = negative result.

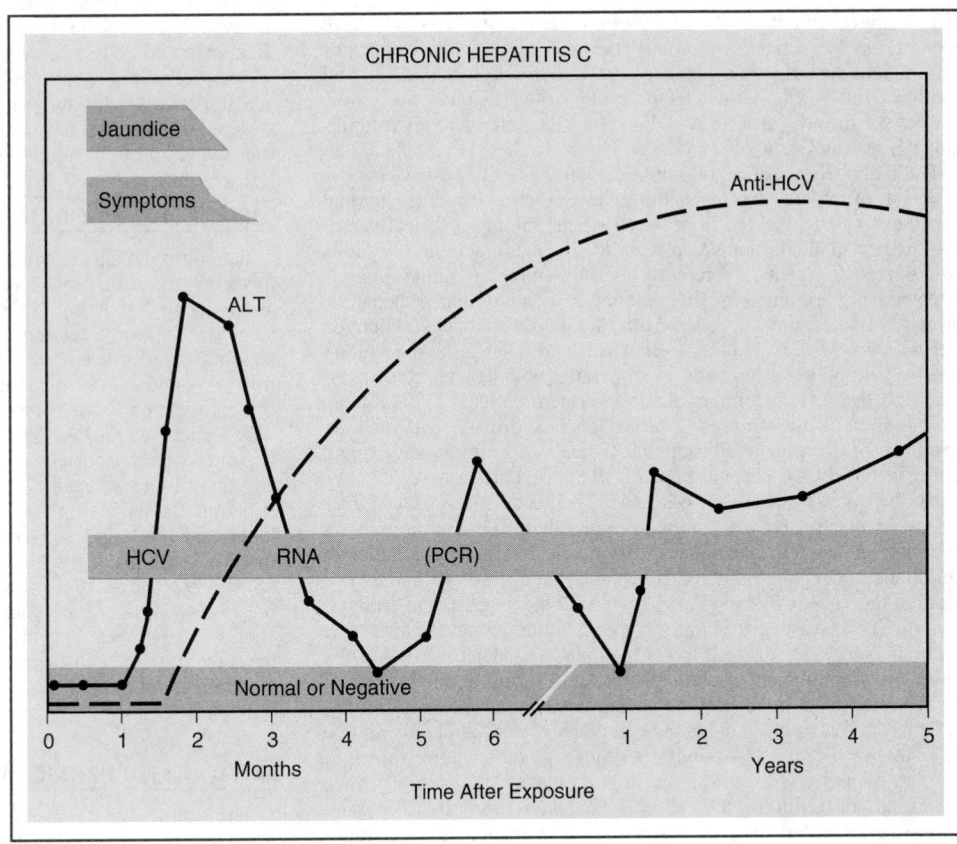

FIGURE 150–2 ■ The typical serologic course of chronic hepatitis C.

terns occur. In some instances, ALT levels become normal but HCV RNA is still detected; these individuals usually but not always relapse when therapy is stopped. In contrast, some patients become HCV RNA–negative during therapy but aminotransferase levels remain elevated; these patients often have a sustained response, and serum ALT levels may become normal only when interferon is stopped.

Pre-treatment factors associated with a beneficial response to α interferon include short duration of disease, lack of severe hepatic fibrosis or cirrhosis, low level of HCV RNA, and viral genotypes 2 and 3. In general, the virologic features are most strongly associated with a sustained response. Sustained responses also correlate with early clearance of HCV RNA (within 3 months of starting therapy) and with more prolonged courses of treatment. These predictive factors are interactive and can be used to guide therapy. Thus, the combination of α interferon and ribavirin for 48 weeks yields overall-sustained virologic response rates of 30 to 40%. However, rates of response vary greatly by genotype and by initial levels of viral RNA in serum. These differences are clinically important in determining the optimal regimen of treatment. Among patients with genotypes 2 and 3, the sustained response rates are 60 to 70%, and these rates are achieved by a 24-week course of therapy. In contrast, among patients with genotype 1, sustained responses are more common with a 48-week course of therapy (25 to 30%) than with a 24-week course (15 to 20%).

At present, therapy is recommended for patients with chronic hepatitis C with HCV RNA in serum, raised serum aminotransferases levels, chronic hepatitis of at least moderate severity indicated by liver biopsy (presence of fibrosis or moderate degrees of inflammation and necrosis), and no contraindications to treatment. The contraindications to α interferon therapy are advanced liver disease, renal failure, severe immunosuppression, solid organ transplantation, cytopenia, and active substance abuse. The combination of interferon and ribavirin is likely to become the recommended approach to therapy within the next year, with 24 weeks of treatment indicated for patients with HCV genotype 2 or 3 and 48 weeks for patients with genotype 1. Ribavirin therapy is contraindicated in patients with hemolysis, anemia, significant coronary or cerebrovascular disease, or renal insufficiency. As ribavirin is teratogenic, it is

essential that women practice adequate contraception during therapy and for at least 6 months thereafter. Similar precautions are also appropriate for men. The side effects of interferon and ribavirin must be reviewed carefully before starting therapy. Interferon induces an influenza-like syndrome with the first one to two doses. Thereafter, the major side effects are fatigue, malaise, depression, difficulty in concentrating, bone marrow suppression, and, in rare instances, bacterial infections or induction of autoimmune disease. Side effects of ribavirin include a dose-related hemolysis that usually results in a 5 to 15% decrease in hemoglobin level, mild itching, and nasal congestion.

Even with combination therapy, the sustained response rate to interferon treatment in hepatitis C is less than 50%, and many patients find the therapy difficult to tolerate. For patients with decompensated liver disease due to hepatitis C, liver transplantation (Chapter 155) is indicated. Potential future approaches include long-acting interferons, long-term continuous therapy with interferon or ribavirin, and specific inhibitors of HCV protease, helicase, and polymerase enzymes.

AUTOIMMUNE HEPATITIS

Autoimmune hepatitis is a chronic inflammatory disorder of the liver of unknown cause. It is characterized by presence of autoantibodies, high levels of serum immunoglobulins, and frequent association with other autoimmune diseases. The disease has been given a variety of names since it was first described in the 1950s, but in 1992 the International Autoimmune Hepatitis Group recommended the term *autoimmune hepatitis* and established diagnostic criteria. Two types of autoimmune hepatitis have been described: Type 1 or classic autoimmune hepatitis and Type 2 autoimmune hepatitis. Both forms are more common among women than men and have similar clinical and serum biochemical features. Type 2 autoimmune hepatitis is found largely in Europe and typically affects young women or girls.

Autoimmune hepatitis is one of the three major autoimmune liver diseases, along with primary biliary cirrhosis and primary sclerosing cholangitis. Also within this group of autoimmune liver diseases are variant forms of autoimmune hepatitis, which have been termed "overlap syndromes" because they share features of autoimmune hepatitis and another type of chronic liver disease, and "outlier syndromes," which have features of autoimmune hepatitis but do not to meet criteria established by the International Autoimmune Hepatitis Group.

The pathogenesis of autoimmune hepatitis is not known, but it is believed to be caused by autoimmune reactions against normal hepatocytes. The disease appears to occur among genetically predisposed individuals upon exposure to as yet unidentified noxious environmental agents, thereby triggering an autoimmune process directed at liver antigens. In patients with autoimmune hepatitis, primary associations are seen with the human leukocyte antigen (HLA) class I B8 and class II DR3 and DR52a loci. Among Asians, autoimmune hepatitis is associated with HLA-DR4, an association that is less common among Western patients.

Autoimmune hepatitis is a heterogeneous disease with a wide spectrum of clinical manifestations. It tends to be more severe and florid in onset than chronic hepatitis B or C. Furthermore, autoimmune hepatitis is usually progressive and leads to end-stage liver disease if not treated with immunosuppression. The disease is more common in women than men and typically has its onset either in childhood and young adulthood (between the ages of 15 and 25) or around the time of menopause (between the ages of 45 and 60 years). The disease, particularly Type 2 autoimmune hepatitis, can occur in young children. In some patients it is detected before the onset of symptoms and jaundice if elevated serum aminotransferase levels are found on a routine health evaluation. More typically, patients present with jaundice and fatigue. Abnormalities in routine liver test results are also similar to those found in other forms of chronic hepatitis with elevations in serum aminotransferase levels. Elevations in bilirubin or alkaline phosphatase levels indicate more severe or advanced disease. Perhaps most characteristic of autoimmune hepatitis are striking elevations in serum gamma globulin, and specifically in immunoglobulin (IgG), levels, accompanied by the autoantibodies directed at non–organ-specific cellular constituents, the detection of which forms the basis for the diagnosis of the disease.

The presence of serum autoantibodies is the basis for the diagnosis of the two types of autoimmune hepatitis: Type 1 (classic) autoimmune hepatitis is characterized by the detection of antinuclear (ANA), anti–smooth muscle (SMA), antiactin, and anti-asialoglycoprotein receptor antibodies. Type 2 autoimmune hepatitis is characterized by the detection of anti–liver-kidney microsomal 1 antibodies (anti-LKM1) and anti–liver cytosol 1 antibodies, as well as the absence of ANA or SMA. To meet criteria for the diagnosis of autoimmune hepatitis, these antibodies should be present in titers of at least 1:80 in adults and 1:20 in children.

Liver biopsy in patients with autoimmune hepatitis shows features characteristic of chronic hepatitis (as described earlier). Plasma cell infiltrates, which are rare in other forms of chronic hepatitis, are characteristic of autoimmune hepatitis.

Most typical of autoimmune hepatitis is a rapid clinical response to corticosteroid therapy, in terms of both resolution of clinical symptoms as well as improvements in serum aminotransferase and serum bilirubin elevations. Prednisone should be initiated in a dose of 20 to 30 mg/day. A biochemical response with fall of serum aminotransferase levels into the normal or near-normal range should occur within 1 to 3 months. A lack of biochemical or clinical response should lead to a re-evaluation of the diagnosis. To prevent the side effects of long-term prednisone therapy, azathioprine, 50 to 100 mg, can be combined with prednisone, starting at the same time or added later. In the typical patient, prednisone can be slowly tapered to a maintenance regimen of 5 to 10 mg/day combined with azathioprine 50 to 150 mg/day. In some patients, azathioprine alone, in a dose of 2 mg/kg body weight/day, can be used instead of prednisone as maintenance therapy. The long-term side effects of azathioprine (immune suppression, bone marrow suppression, and risk of cancer) need to be considered. Corticosteroid or immunosuppressive therapy is usually continued indefinitely; attempts can be made to withdraw therapy in some patients, but these trials should be monitored very carefully thereafter, be-

cause severe and even fatal flares of disease can occur weeks to months after stopping prednisone. Prognosis in this disease is generally related to the histologic stage of disease at the time of diagnosis and initiation of therapy, but patients whose disease responds to immunosuppressive therapy can do very well for many years. Patients with autoimmune hepatitis that progresses to end-stage liver disease have excellent survival rates following liver transplantation (Chapter 155).

VARIANT FORMS OF AUTOIMMUNE HEPATITIS

Patients who have features of autoimmune hepatitis but do not meet the criteria established by the International Autoimmune Hepatitis Group for definite or probable autoimmune hepatitis are considered to have a variant form of autoimmune hepatitis. These patients may have features associated with both autoimmune hepatitis and another type of chronic liver disease (overlap syndromes).

Three overlap syndromes are recognized: autoimmune hepatitis with concurrent features of primary biliary cirrhosis, autoimmune hepatitis with concurrent features of primary sclerosing cholangitis, and autoimmune hepatitis with concurrent features of chronic viral hepatitis. In each of these syndromes, the clinical manifestations, laboratory findings, and liver histologic characteristics share features of each of the two diseases. In general, treatment regimens are designed in relation to the more dominant of the two disorders. In another variant, *autoimmune cholangitis* (also called "anti–mitochondrial antibody–negative primary biliary cirrhosis"), patients have features of both hepatitis and cholangitis; both prednisone and ursodeoxycholic acid have been used to treat the disease with variable success.

CRYPTOGENIC CHRONIC LIVER DISEASE

The term *cryptogenic chronic liver disease* is generally reserved for patients with chronic hepatitis or cirrhosis of unknown cause. Cryptogenic hepatitis is a diagnosis of exclusion and should be made only after hepatitis B, C, and D; autoimmune hepatitis; and other causes of a chronic hepatitis–like syndrome are excluded (Table 150–1). It is most important to exclude drug-induced liver disease (Chapter 148) and inherited metabolic liver diseases (Chapter 152), such as Wilson's disease (by serum ceruloplasmin and, if necessary, urine and liver copper concentrations) and α_1-antitrypsin deficiency (by serum levels of α_1-antitrypsin and phenotyping if needed). Diseases that can resemble chronic hepatitis on blood test results but are readily excluded by liver biopsy histologic findings include alcoholic liver disease (Chapter 153), fatty liver, non-alcoholic steatohepatitis (NASH) (Chapter 148), hemochromatosis (Chapter 221), primary biliary cirrhosis (Chapter 157), and sclerosing cholangitis (Chapter 157).

Hoofnagle JH, Di Bisceglie AM: The treatment of chronic viral hepatitis. N Engl J Med 336:347–356, 1997. *A review of the various therapies of acute and chronic viral hepatitis, focusing largely on α interferon therapy of chronic hepatitis B, C, and D.*

Krawitt EL: Autoimmune hepatitis. N Engl J Med 334:897–903, 1996. *A concise overview of the pathogenesis, clinical features, natural history, and therapy of autoimmune hepatitis.*

Lai C-L, Chien R-N, Leung NWY, Chang T-T, Guan R, Tai D-I, Ng K-Y, Wu P-C, Dent J-C, Barber J, Stephenson SL, Gray DF, for the Asia Hepatitis Lamivudine Study Group: A 1-year trial of lamivudine for chronic hepatitis B. N Engl J Med 339:61–68, 1998. *Results of the large clinical trial comparing two doses (25 mg/day and 100 mg/day) of lamivudine to placebo treatment among 358 Chinese patients with HBeAg-positive chronic hepatitis B. A 1-year course of therapy with 100-mg/day dose of lamivudine improved aminotransferase levels in 72% and liver histology in 67% of patients. Side effects were minimal.*

Lee WM: Hepatitis B virus infection. N Engl J Med 337:1733–1745, 1997. *A concise and accurate overview on the virologic and immunologic features, clinical course, and outcome of acute and chronic hepatitis B.*

Management of Hepatitis C: Consensus Development Conference: Hepatology 26(Suppl. 1): S1–S156, 1997. *The proceedings of the 1997 National Institute of Health (NIH) Consensus Conference on hepatitis C with summaries on the virologic and epidemiologic characteristics, natural history, and therapy of hepatitis C as well as the Consensus Panel Statement regarding management.*

McHutchinson J, Gordon S, Schiff ER, Shiffman ML, Lee WM, Rustgi VK, Goodman Z, Ling M-H, Albrecht J, for the Hepatitis Interventional Therapy Group: Interferon alfa-2b monotherapy versus interferon alfa-2b plus ribavirin as initial treatment for chronic hepatitis C: Results of a U.S. multicenter randomized controlled trial. N Engl J Med 339:1485–1492, 1998. *Results of a U.S. multicenter trial comparing α interferon alone to the combination of α interferon and ribavirin in 912 patients with chronic hepatitis C. The combination improved the sustained response rate in all categories of patients. A 48-week course was superior to a 24-week course only among patients with HCV genotype 1.*

151 PARASITIC, BACTERIAL, FUNGAL, AND GRANULOMATOUS LIVER DISEASES

Willis C. Maddrey

The liver is affected by many local and disseminated infections, the frequency and types of which vary considerably around the world. For example, parasitic disorders are more prevalent in developing countries, especially those in tropical and subtropical regions. Infectious agents reach the liver through the portal or arterial blood or arrive directly by spread from neighboring organs. Hepatic involvement in an infectious process is often manifest only by mild to moderate elevations in aminotransferase and alkaline phosphatase levels. Occasionally, clinically apparent jaundice is noted. Jaundice may result from combinations of the effects of focal inflammation, endotoxemia, hemolysis, and bile duct obstruction. In patients with shock, hypoperfusion also contributes. The prognosis for infections involving the liver depends on the type of infection, the availability and early institution of appropriate therapy, and the underlying status of the patient. As would be expected, poor outcomes are more likely to occur in the elderly and in those with impaired immunocompetence.

PYOGENIC LIVER ABSCESS

DEFINITION. Pyogenic liver abscesses are focal areas of infection within the hepatic parenchyma. These abscesses may be single or multiple and result from liver invasion by a variety of bacteria.

ETIOLOGY. Pyogenic liver abscesses are more often found in individuals of middle age or older, especially those who have underlying biliary tract diseases with obstruction and bile stasis. In this setting, multiple abscesses are frequent. Pyogenic liver abscesses secondary to intestinal diseases are well recognized in patients with a variety of disorders, including Crohn's disease and diverticulitis. Penetrating wounds to the liver may also lead to abscesses. In many patients (up to one half), no definite cause for the abscess is found, and often the presumption is made that an episode of septicemia or occult biliary tract disease has occurred.

A remarkable array of bacteria cause liver abscesses, with gram-negative enteric bacteria, especially *Escherichia coli, Klebsiella pneumoniae, Streptococcus faecalis,* and *Proteus vulgaris* being the major contributors. Gram-positive staphylococci also cause abscess. Rarer causes include *Pasteurella multocida* and *Yersinia enterocolitica.* The role of anaerobic organisms, especially *Bacteroides* and *Clostridium,* has been increasingly recognized as culture techniques have improved. Infection by multiple organisms is frequent.

CLINICAL MANIFESTATIONS AND DIAGNOSIS. A bacterial liver abscess may be suspected when a patient develops fever, leukocytosis, and right upper quadrant abdominal pain. Often, especially in elderly patients, the presentation is subtle and involves an indolent process with loss of appetite, intermittent or low-grade fever, and dull abdominal pain.

Pyogenic liver abscess should be considered in any patient who has presumptive or definite evidence of septicemia in association with biochemical abnormalities of the liver. The liver is usually enlarged and is often tender when palpated. Most liver abscesses occur in the right lobe. If the abscess is high in the liver, the hemidiaphragm may be elevated and immobile (usually on the right), along with a pleural effusion. Rales and percussion dullness may be noted at the base of the compressed right lung.

Anemia and hypoalbuminemia are often present, especially in patients who have long-standing abscesses. Jaundice is unusual, but the alkaline phosphatase level is often elevated. Imaging studies, especially ultrasonography and computed tomography (CT), have shortened the time from suspicion of the presence of liver abscess to confirmation (Fig. 151–1). Ultrasonographic examination usually is reliable in differentiating liver abscess from hepatic cysts. Magnetic resonance imaging (MRI) shows characteristic findings of increased intensity on T2-weighted images with decreased intensity on T1-weighted images.

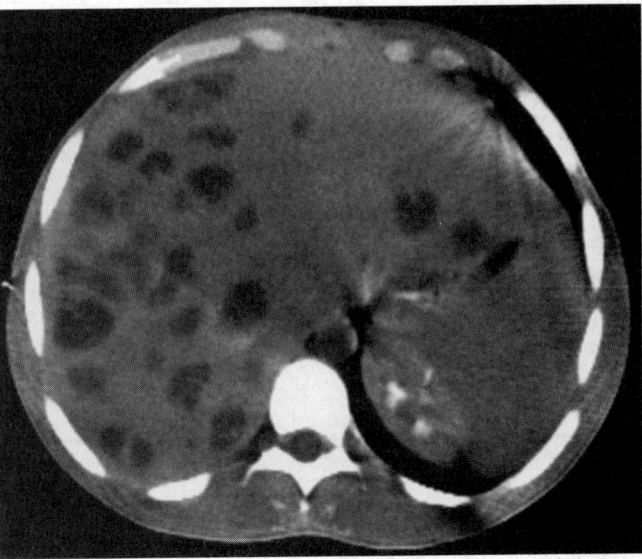

FIGURE 151–1 ■ CT scan demonstrating multiple pyogenic liver abscesses in a 25-year-old man.

Directed aspiration of the abscess with culture and cytologic examination usually accurately identifies the causative organism(s). Bacterial cultures of the aspirate are positive in 90% of patients if they include special attention to detection of anaerobic organisms. Endoscopic cholangiography can determine any underlying obstruction in the biliary tract.

TREATMENT. The cornerstones of treating bacterial liver abscesses are effective drainage and antibiotics. Occasionally, an indwelling drainage catheter is placed into a single abscess. Surgical drainage of liver abscesses is rarely required. If multiple abscesses are present, the larger accessible ones should be aspirated. Broad-spectrum antibiotics, including coverage for anaerobes, should begin immediately after aspiration, with later adjustments of treatment based on culture results. Metronidazole should be included in the initial therapeutic regimen if amebic abscess is being considered. Antibiotics may be required for several weeks or even months. Any biliary obstruction must be removed or drained because the ability to relieve obstruction largely determines how rapidly (or if) the abscesses resolve.

PROGNOSIS. The prognosis for patients with solitary bacterial liver abscesses is better than for those with multiple abscesses. The likelihood of complete recovery is influenced by the patient's underlying health status and age; the presence of immune compromising illnesses, including the acquired immunodeficiency syndrome (AIDS) and malignancy; the duration of the abscess before diagnosis; the effectiveness of draining the abscess; and, if necessary, relief of obstruction of the biliary tract.

ACTINOMYCOSIS

Actinomycosis (see Chapter 354) is a chronic suppurative bacterial infection that may involve the liver directly from adjacent infected organs or through the portal vein from cecal and appendiceal infection. Solitary or multiple intrahepatic masses develop, and sinus tracts from the liver and adherent viscera to the abdominal wall are frequent. The finding of characteristic sulfur granules containing branched filaments establishes the diagnosis. Once considered, the diagnosis is usually straightforward based on examining sinus tract drainage. The treatment is large doses of intravenously administered penicillin.

FUNGAL INFECTIONS OF THE LIVER

Histoplasmosis, coccidioidomycosis, North American blastomycosis, and cryptococcosis are the major fungal infections that affect the liver. A careful history emphasizing travel, places of residence, and lifestyle likely to affect immune status is often helpful for diagnosis. A variety of fungal infections have occurred in transplanted livers.

Granulomas are often found in patients with fungal infections. In immunosuppressed patients, candidiasis, aspergillosis, and mucormycosis are more likely to be found. Diagnosis of fungal diseases is based on identifying the organism on liver biopsy or occasionally from culture of the hepatic tissue. Serologic tests are generally not helpful. Treatment depends on the responsiveness of the underlying fungal agent and the immune status of the patient.

SPIROCHETAL DISEASES

SYPHILIS (see Chapter 365). The liver is involved in several stages of syphilis. In congenital syphilis, diffuse hepatitis occurs secondary to massive transplacental infection. In secondary syphilis, diffuse granulomatous changes are frequent. In tertiary syphilis, single or multiple gummas may be found. The treatment for all types of hepatic syphilis is penicillin.

PARASITIC DISEASES

Parasitic diseases often have distinctive geographic distributions. In part because of international travel and the occurrence of unusual infections in patients who are immunocompromised, clinicians need to be aware of the protean manifestations of these disorders (Table 151–1).

An array of helminths (see Chapters 430 to 434) with often complex life cycles affect the human liver either in larval or adult stages. The response to larvae is quite variable. In toxocariasis,

Table 151–1 ■ IMPORTANT PARASITIC DISEASES OF THE LIVER AND BILIARY TRACT

DISORDER (ORGANISM)	PREDISPOSITION TO INFECTION*	NATURE OF HEPATIC INVOLVEMENT		
		Pathophysiology	Manifestations	Diagnosis
Schistosomiasis (*Schistosoma mansoni, japonicum*) (flatworm)	Exposure to water in which appropriate snail hosts reside	Host immune response to ova delivered via portal vein, resulting in granulomas and fibrosis	*Acute:* eosinophilic infiltrate *Chronic:* hepatosplenomegaly, complications of portal hypertension, granuloma formation	Ova identified in stool or on liver biopsy
Echinococcosis (*Echinococcus granulosa, E. multilocularis*) (tapeworm)	Exposure to sheep, cattle, and dogs	Larval migration to liver leading to hydatid cyst	*Asymptomatic:* symptoms of hepatic mass lesions, biliary tract obstruction, cyst rupture	Serologic tests (indirect hemagglutination, ELISA); CT scans
Ascariasis (*Ascaris lumbricoides*) (round worm)	Eating raw vegetables	Larval migration via portal vein to liver; later adult invasion of biliary tract with egg production	Abdominal pain, fever, jaundice during larval migration; bile duct obstruction, cholangitis; granuloma may form around eggs	Ova or adult worm in stool; worms in duodenum on contrast studies or endoscopic examination. Demonstration of *Ascaris* in bile duct; may be calcified
Clonorchiasis (*Clonorchis sinensis*) (flatworm)	Ingesting raw freshwater fish	Worm migration through ampulla of Vater; eggs deposited in bile ducts	Bile duct obstruction, cholangitis, choledocholithiasis, cholangiocarcinoma	Ova in stool; multiple bile duct stones on ERCP
Fascioliasis (*Fasciola hepatica*) (flatworm)	Ingesting infected freshwater plants	Larval migration through liver, penetration of bile ducts	*Acute:* fever, abdominal pain, jaundice, hemobilia *Chronic:* asymptomatic hepatomegaly, choledocholithiasis	Eosinophilia; elevated liver tests; ova in stool; adult flukes in bile ducts on ERCP
Toxocariasis (*Toxocara canis, T. cati*) (round worm)	Contact with dogs and cats	Larval migration in hepatic parenchyma (visceral larva migrans)	Granulomas with eosinophilia	Larvae in tissue; serology; ELISA
Strongyloidiasis (*Strongyloides stercoralis*)	Immunodeficiency (AIDS, organ transplant, malignancy)	Penetration of larvae through intestinal wall into liver	Hepatomegaly, occasional jaundice, larvae in portal tract and liver lobule	Larvae in stool or duodenal aspirate; serologic tests not useful
Protozoan Disorders				
Amebiasis (*Entamoeba histolytica*)	Poor sanitation	Hematogenous spread with tissue invasion; abscess formation	Fever, right upper quadrant pain, peritonitis, elevated right hemidiaphragm, pleural effusion	Cysts in stool; serologic test (counterimmunoelectrophoresis, indirect hemagglutination); ultrasonography, CT scan
Malaria (*Plasmodium vivax, falciparum, ovale, malariae*)	Blood transfusion, parenteral drug use. Travel to endemic areas	Sporozoites cleared from circulation by hepatocytes; exoerythrocytic replication in liver	Tender hepatomegaly; rarely hepatic failure (*P. falciparum*)	Identification of organism on blood smear
Cryptosporidiosis (*Cryptosporidium*)	Immunodeficiency (AIDS)	Unknown; biliary tract involvement thus far only in immunodeficient patients	Fever, right upper quadrant pain	Elevated serum alkaline phosphatase; bile duct dilatation on ERCP
Toxoplasmosis (*Toxoplasma gondii*)	Intrauterine infection; immunodeficiency (AIDS, organ transplant)	Multiplication in liver causing necrosis and inflammation	Fever, hepatosplenomegaly	Aminotransferase elevation; isolation of organism from tissue; Sabin-Feldman dye test
Visceral leishmaniasis (*Leishmania donovani*)	Immunodeficiency (AIDS, organ transplant)	Infection of reticuloendothelial cells of liver	Fever, leukopenia, hepatosplenomegaly	Organism in bone marrow; immunoserologic tests
Trypanosomiasis (*Trypanosoma cruzi, T. rhodesiense, T. gambiense*)	*Acute:* parasites in reticuloendothelial cells of liver *Chronic:* passive congestion secondary to heart failure	*Acute:* fever, hepatosplenomegaly *Chronic:* hepatomegaly	Organisms in blood and/or tissue; immunofluorescent tests	

*Travel in endemic areas predisposes to specific infections.
ELISA = enzyme-linked immunosorbent assay; ERCP = endoscopic retrograde cholangiopancreatography.

for example, there is an intense inflammatory reaction (visceral larva migrans).

In ascariasis, the adult worm (*Ascaris lumbricoides*) may migrate into the common bile duct, become lodged, and obstruct the flow of bile. Some of the worms die in the bile duct and calcify. Occasionally, worm ova proceed up the bile duct, lodge in the liver, and lead to giant cells and granulomas. Effective treatment may require extracting the worms from the bile duct by endoscopic cholangiography and using piperazine citrate to kill any remaining worms.

SCHISTOSOMIASIS (see Chapter 431). Infections with several types of human blood flukes (schistosomiasis) are leading causes of liver disease worldwide, especially in the Far East, Middle East, and Africa. *Schistosoma mansoni* and *S. japonicum* regularly affect the liver. The life cycle of schistosomes is complex. Eggs excreted in human feces hatch in water to become swimming embryos that enter the body of an appropriate snail, where they develop into motile, fork-tailed cercariae that are then released into water. The cercariae penetrate human skin and migrate through the blood stream, taking up residence in the mesenteric capillaries. In the mesenteric vessels, the schistosomes reach adult status, then lay eggs that are delivered by means of portal blood to the small presinusoidal intrahepatic portal veins. The eggs elicit an immune response with a granulomatous reaction. Subsequently, fibrosis and portal hypertension with esophagogastric varices develop. Identifying eggs in a stool examination is the preferred method to diagnose schistosomiasis. Liver biopsy changes include granulomas (some containing remnants of ova) and fibrosis, which often contains arteriolar clefts. Cytokines released in the vicinity of the granulomas play an important role in eliciting fibrosis, which may progress to a characteristic pipe-stem cirrhosis. Antischistosomal drugs including praziquantel are available. Portosystemic shunt surgery may be required if bleeding from esophagogastric varices occurs.

CLONORCHIASIS. The Chinese liver fluke (*Clonorchis sinensis*) is a parasite affecting fish-eating mammals, including humans. Snails are intermediate hosts in which cercariae develop and are released to infect freshwater fish. The most important problems in humans with clonorchiasis are obstructed bile ducts and chronic cholangitis caused by flukes that have matured inside the bile ducts. Cholangiohepatitis and cholangiocarcinoma are known consequences. The diagnosis is based on finding characteristic eggs in the feces. Praziquantel has been used with varying success.

ECHINOCOCCOSIS (HYDATID DISEASE). Echinococcus granulosa is a tapeworm living in dogs that acquire the infection from eating infected sheep viscera. Humans, sheep, and cattle are intermediate hosts. The worms excrete ova that adhere to the dog's coat and may be passed to humans who have close contact with the dogs and ingest contaminated food. After the chitinous cover is broken down by gastric acid, the ova burrow into the intestinal mucosa and reach the liver through the portal vein. Complex cysts gradually develop in the liver (usually the right lobe) and other organs. The rim of the cyst may calcify. The echinococcal cyst may remain asymptomatic or continue to expand. In some patients, cysts rupture into bile ducts or the peritoneal cavity, lungs, and other organs. Indirect hemagglutination and enzyme-linked immunosorbent assays are helpful for diagnosis. Ultrasonography, CT, and MRI are useful to diagnose the presence of a cyst and may be highly suggestive of the echinococcal origin (Fig. 151–2). Diagnostic aspiration is dangerous and may lead to dissemination of the infection. If feasible, surgical removal of the cyst is indicated. Mebendazole or albendazole is of limited benefit.

PROTOZOAN INFECTIONS

Protozoa commonly infect the liver; some enter visceral reticuloendothelial cells (leishmaniasis and trypanosomiasis) and others enter the hepatocytes (toxoplasmosis and malaria). *Entamoeba histolytica* is one of the most important causes of liver abscess.

The clinical manifestations of protozoan infection are usually non-specific and may resemble viral hepatitis (e.g., in toxoplasmosis and malaria). Hepatosplenomegaly, anemia, emaciation, and many general symptoms may be encountered. In certain infections, extrahepatic manifestations predominate (e.g., cardiomyopathy with chronic trypanosomiasis). Extrahepatic features may be prominent

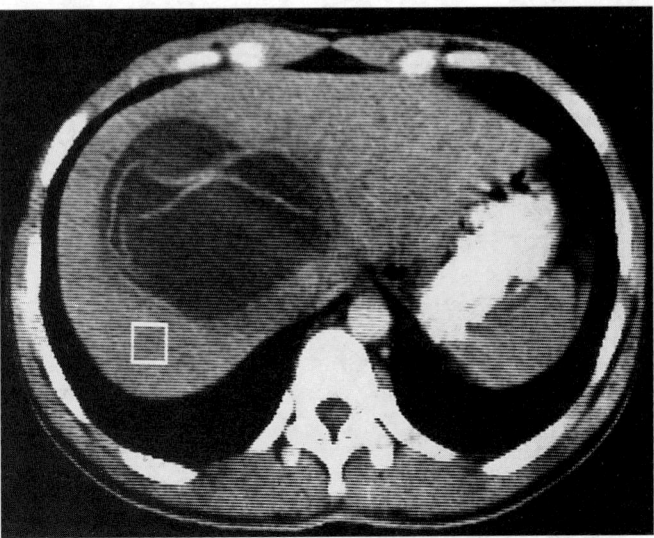

FIGURE 151–2 ■ CT scan of an echinococcal cyst in a 25-year-old man demonstrating the complex structure of the wall and the interior.

early in the course (e.g., amebic colitis), and hepatic symptoms predominate later (e.g., with hepatic abscess formation). Cryptosporidiosis has received increasing attention as an opportunistic infection in patients with AIDS; cholecystitis and bile duct changes that suggest sclerosing cholangitis are manifestations of this infection. Hepatic changes appear to be secondary to invasion of the biliary tract and gallbladder.

In contrast to helminthic infections, serologic tests are often useful in making a specific diagnosis in protozoan infections. In visceral leishmaniasis (kala-azar), the organisms may be identified in tissue or isolated in culture, with bone marrow a favored site.

AMEBIC LIVER ABSCESS

ETIOLOGY. *Entamoeba histolytica* (see Chapter 428) is an important worldwide cause of liver abscess, especially in tropical and subtropical regions. *E. histolytica* are ingested as cysts and pass to the colon where vegetative trophozoites enter the intestinal mucosa, causing colonic ulcers. Amebae then enter the portal vein and are swept to the liver. In the liver, the amebae block small portal radicles, release enzymes, and cause focal inflammatory lesions. This stage is called *amebic hepatitis*, although the term is a misnomer. Single or multiple abscesses may then be formed, although in most patients a single abscess is found. The preferred site for abscess formation is superoanteriorly in the right lobe of the liver (Fig. 151–3A). The right hemidiaphragm may be elevated and fixed. Pleural effusion is frequent (see Fig. 151–3B). For unknown reasons, amebic liver abscesses are far more likely to occur in males. There is scant correlation between the appearance of the liver abscess and evidence of active colonic infection. Long latent intervals have been documented between intestinal infection and the onset of an abscess.

CLINICAL MANIFESTATIONS AND DIAGNOSIS. The gradual onset of fever, malaise, and right upper quadrant abdominal pain is the usual presentation for a patient with an amebic abscess of the liver. If the abscess affects the hemidiaphragm, pain may be referred to the shoulder and may be worsened by deep breathing or coughing. Occasionally, the onset is abrupt with fever and repeated rigors. Almost all patients with amebic abscess have hepatic tenderness and dull aching right upper quadrant abdominal pain. Jaundice is unusual and, if present, suggests that the abscess has compressed a major bile duct. Only a few patients have concomitant evidence of amebic colitis, and cysts are found in the stool in a minority of patients. Leukocytosis and anemia may be present. Occasionally, the diagnosis is first suspected after intraperitoneal or intrathoracic rupture into the pleura or pericardium. Amebic abscesses should be considered in any patient who has resided in or traveled to an endemic area and in whom a hepatic filling defect is found on an

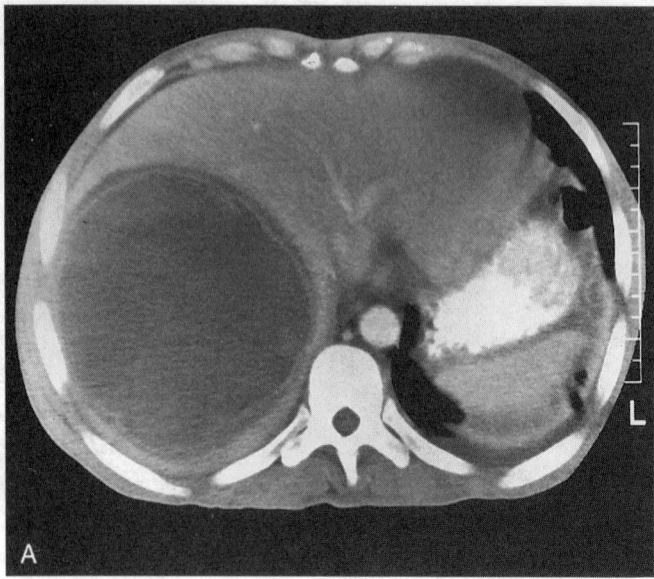

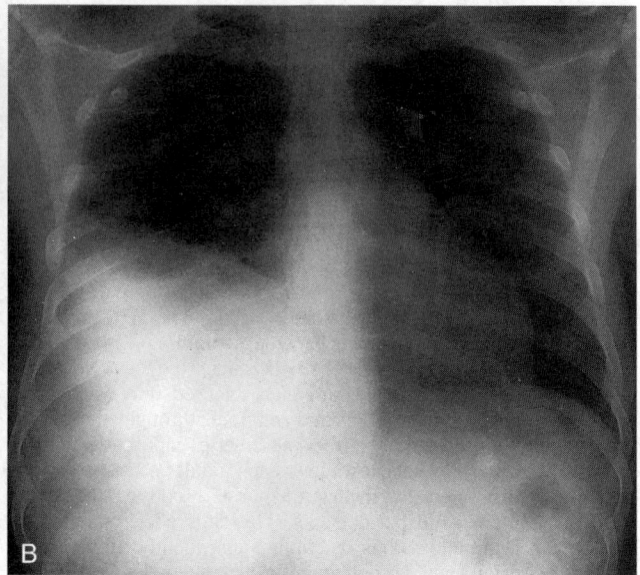

FIGURE 151-3 ■ *A*, CT scan of a large amebic liver abscess in a 36-year-old man. *B*, Chest radiograph demonstrating elevated right diaphragm with compression of the right lung and a pleural effusion.

imaging study. The indirect hemagglutination test indicates tissue invasion by amebae and is almost always indicative, although not diagnostic, of liver involvement. An elevated right hemidiaphragm and pleural effusion are often found. Aspiration is generally not required to establish the diagnosis.

TREATMENT. Metronidazole is the drug of choice. Aspiration may prove useful for patients who have large abscesses or those in whom there has been little response to 5 days of metronidazole therapy. Aspiration is also used if an abscess is likely to rupture. A course of an intestinal luminal amebicide such as iodoquinol may add to overall treatment.

GRANULOMATOUS LIVER DISEASE

ETIOLOGY. Granulomas represent a specialized type of inflammatory response of the mononuclear phagocytic system and are found in a wide variety of conditions. Granulomas of diverse causes may appear identical. Large, pale-staining epithelioid cells are characteristic. Evidence of caseation and perigranulomatous inflammation may also be found. Macrophages, the predominant cells in granulomas, often fuse to form characteristic multinucleated giant cells. Most granulomas are found in or near the portal tract. Granulomas have been found in 2 to 10% of all liver biopsy specimens, and often no specific cause is identified.

Major disorders in which hepatic granulomas are frequent include sarcoidosis, tuberculosis, histoplasmosis, and schistosomiasis (Table 151-2). There are considerable geographic variations in the causes of granulomas. Knowledge of a patient's profession, lifestyle, and travel may yield important clues. For example, coccidioidomycosis is a well-established cause of granulomas in the western United States. *Mycobacterium avium-intracellulare* has come to the fore as an important granulomatous disease in patients with AIDS. A variety of therapeutic drugs, including phenylbutazone, allopurinol, and carbamazepine, are well documented to cause granulomas. In addition, granulomas are characteristically found in the early stages of primary biliary cirrhosis and in sarcoidosis.

CLINICAL MANIFESTATIONS. In most patients, the presence of granulomas does not adversely affect the liver and may be detected when a liver biopsy is being performed for some other reason, especially during evaluation of an increase in serum alkaline phosphatase. Many patients with even extensive granulomatous inflammation in the liver are asymptomatic. Occasionally, however, the liver is enlarged and tender. Sometimes a chronic hepatitis—apparently related to the granuloma—can progress to cirrhosis with portal hypertension.

PATHOLOGY. Only occasionally are the histologic features of

the granulomas specific enough to help in the search for a cause. *Schistosoma* ova may be found within the granuloma. Special stains may identify *Mycobacterium tuberculosis* or *M. avium-intra-*

Table 151-2 ■ **MAJOR CAUSES OF HEPATIC GRANULOMAS**

DISEASE	DIAGNOSIS
Sarcoidosis	Paratracheal or hilar lymph node enlargement found on chest radiograph
	Elevated serum angiotensin-converting enzyme level
	Conjunctival granulomas
Tuberculosis (*Mycobacterium tuberculosis*)	Isolation/culture of sputum, bronchoalveolar lavage, bone marrow, liver
Mycobacterium avium-intracellulare	Tuberculin skin tests
	HIV positive
	Sputum cultures
Histoplasmosis	Complement fixation test (limited value)
	Chest radiograph
	Sputum cultures
Brucellosis	Agglutinin titer
	Blood culture
Lymphomas	Chest radiograph
Hodgkin's disease	CT scan
	Biopsy of lymph nodes
Schistosomiasis	Demonstration of parts of ova in granulomas
	Schistosomal eggs in rectal biopsy
Primary biliary cirrhosis	Antimitochondrial antibodies
	Female with cholestatic liver disease
Leprosy	Skin test for lepromin
	Country of origin
Drug reactions (allopurinol, procainamide, hydralazine, sulfonamides, phenylbutazone, carbamazepine, quinidine)	History of use of a drug known (or suspected) to cause granulomas
Berylliosis	Occupational exposure
	Chest radiograph
Q fever	Serologic tests
	Characteristic fibrinoid ring
Syphilis (secondary)	Serologic test
Lipogranulomas	Demonstration of mineral oil in a granuloma
Talc	Birefringent inclusions

cellulare. Occasionally, birefringent granules of starch are identified. A rather characteristic type of inflammation with a fibrinoid ring is characteristic of Q fever.

DIAGNOSIS. Granulomas in the liver often direct diagnostic attention toward a generalized disease process. Travel, profession, and lifestyle must all be considered. Even with exhaustive searching, the cause of granulomas often is not identified. Culture of liver tissue rarely yields the diagnosis.

TREATMENT. Because granulomas represent a reaction pattern rather than a disease, the treatment depends on the diagnosis established.

SARCOIDOSIS

Sarcoidosis, a granulomatous disease of unknown cause (see Chapter 81), almost always involves the liver. Most patients have no symptoms from the granulomas. A few patients develop a chronic cholestatic disease from bile duct obstruction that may progress to cirrhosis. There is no specific diagnostic test for sarcoidosis. Most patients have an elevated serum alkaline phosphatase level. There is no established treatment for sarcoidosis affecting the liver; corticosteroids do not reliably improve the liver disease.

INFECTIONS OF THE LIVER IN PATIENTS WITH AIDS

Patients who have AIDS are at high risk of acquiring hepatic infections, especially hepatitis B and hepatitis C. *M. avium-intracellulare* and *M. tuberculosis* both represent major problems in these immunocompromised patients (see Chapter 413). Other infections include cytomegalovirus, herpes simplex, *Cryptococcus neoformans*, coccidioidomycosis, histoplasmosis, and Epstein-Barr virus. Hepatotoxicity from one or more of the drugs used to treat AIDS and its complications may cause liver injury (see Chapter 148).

Huang CJ, Pitt HA, Lipsett PA, et al: Pyogenic hepatic abscess: Changing trends over 42 years. Ann Surg 223:600, 1996. *Excellent review of an evolving field.*

Maddrey WC: Granulomatous liver disease. *In* Schiff ER, Sorrell ML, Maddrey WC (eds): Diseases of the Liver Philadelphia, Lippincott–Raven, 1998. *Comprehensive review of pathogenesis and causes of granulomatous liver disorders.*

152 INHERITED, INFILTRATIVE, AND METABOLIC DISORDERS INVOLVING THE LIVER

Jacquelyn J. Maher

A variety of inherited, infiltrative, and metabolic diseases affect the liver and also involve multiple organs. In some cases the hepatic component dominates the clinical picture, and in other cases it plays a contributory or even relatively minor role.

α_1-ANTITRYPSIN DEFICIENCY

α_1-Antitrypsin (A_1AT) is a circulating glycoprotein whose primary function is to inhibit neutrophil elastase (see Chapter 75). This 52-kd protein, which comprises the α_1 globulin fraction of serum, is synthesized primarily by hepatocytes. Deficiencies in circulating A_1AT are caused by mutations in the A_1AT gene and lead either to single amino acid substitutions or more extensive frameshifts or deletions. A_1AT production is controlled by codominant alleles; thus, the protease inhibitor (Pi) phenotype of an individual is designated by the allelic pair. The normal allele is M, with the most common abnormal alleles being S and Z. Individuals who are PiMM have circulating levels of antitrypsin in the range of 200 mg/dL; those who are PiZZ have only 15% of this amount. Heterozygous combinations of 75 or more alleles permit a wide range of A_1AT levels in serum.

Pulmonary disease in patients with A_1AT deficiency is directly linked to the amount of functional A_1AT in the serum. Liver disease is not due to A_1AT deficiency but is instead related to accumulation of abnormal A_1AT within hepatocytes. Liver involvement occurs almost entirely in PiZZ homozygotes, who produce a protein that folds improperly and cannot pass from the endoplasmic reticulum to the Golgi apparatus. All PiZZ individuals exhibit impaired hepatocellular trafficking of A_1AT; however, only 10 to 15% of homozygotes actually develop liver disease. Homozygotes who escape liver disease are able to degrade retained A_1AT, whereas those who develop liver disease accumulate massive amounts of abnormal A_1AT in hepatocytes. The precise mechanism by which A_1AT causes hepatocyte injury is unknown.

Liver disease in infancy in PiZZ homozygotes typically presents as cholestasis. Roughly one in five PiZZ infants with neonatal cholestasis (or 2–3% of all PiZZ individuals) progresses to childhood cirrhosis. PiZZ homozygotes who escape liver disease in childhood have a 10% chance of developing cirrhosis as adults. Males are at higher risk for adult-onset cirrhosis than are females. Patients who develop liver disease have an unusually high incidence of liver cancer.

A_1AT deficiency should be suspected in adults with cirrhosis of unknown etiology. Emphysema need not be present to entertain the diagnosis. A_1AT deficiency can be detected by measuring the enzyme in serum or by directly analyzing protease inhibitor phenotype. Liver biopsy in individuals inheriting a Z allele reveals globular deposits of abnormal A_1AT within the rough endoplasmic reticulum of hepatocytes. Because the inclusions are present in heterozygotes as well as homozygotes, their presence alone is not pathognomonic of A_1AT-induced liver disease.

The only treatment for hepatic cirrhosis due to A_1AT deficiency is liver transplantation (see Chapter 155). After transplantation, the A_1AT in serum assumes the phenotype of the donor. Genetic strategies to prevent liver disease, such as the use of ribozymes to degrade RNA molecules that encode misfolded A_1AT, are under consideration.

WILSON'S DISEASE

Wilson's disease is an autosomal recessive disorder characterized by accumulation of copper in the liver and other organs (see Chapter 220). The disease is caused by several different mutations in the *WND* gene on chromosome 13. *WND* encodes a copper-transporting adenosine triphosphatase that is expressed predominantly in liver and kidney; affected patients exhibit impaired biliary excretion of copper and ineffective incorporation of copper into ceruloplasmin. The initial consequence of disease is accumulation of copper in the liver. In later stages, copper is released into the circulation, permitting deposition in the brain, cornea, and kidneys. Patients with Wilson's disease begin to accumulate hepatic copper in infancy but rarely develop symptoms before adolescence.

Symptoms of liver disease are the presenting complaint in roughly half of affected individuals. The most common syndrome is that of postnecrotic cirrhosis with hepatic dysfunction and portal hypertension. A small proportion (10–30%) of patients have chronic active hepatitis. Rarely, the disease manifests as fulminant hepatic failure; in patients with massive liver necrosis, coincident hemolysis may provide an important clue to the diagnosis.

No single biochemical test can establish the diagnosis. A serum ceruloplasmin value of less than 20 mg/dL is highly suggestive; however, up to 28% of patients with symptomatic Wilson's liver disease may have normal ceruloplasmin levels. Even Kayser-Fleischer rings are not pathognomonic, because they can occur in chronic cholestatic liver disease. For screening purposes, it is useful to test the copper levels in urine. All symptomatic patients with Wilson's disease should have abnormal urinary copper excretion in a 24-hour collection. Disease suspects identified by non-invasive testing should undergo liver biopsy to confirm and quantify hepatic copper accumulation. More than 250 μg of copper per gram of dry liver tissue is required to make the diagnosis. Genetic testing is also available, although the large number of mutations in the *WND* gene makes screening by genetic methods impractical.

Copper chelation (see Chapter 220) improves survival but does not reverse cirrhosis. Once initiated, therapy must be continued for life; discontinuation can result in rapid deterioration of liver function. In patients with fulminant hepatic failure or decompensated cirrhosis, liver transplantation provides effective therapy by correcting the primary metabolic defect.

HEMOCHROMATOSIS

Hereditary hemochromatosis (see Chapter 221) is an autosomal recessive disorder characterized by iron overload in the liver, heart, pancreas, pituitary gland, and joints. A gene for the disease, termed *HFE*, has been identified on chromosome 6 near the human leukocyte antigen-A (HLA-A) allele. About 80% or more of individuals with hereditary hemochromatosis are homozygous for a single mutation in *HFE* designated C282Y. The C282Y mutation itself is quite common, with a homozygote frequency of 1:200. Patients with hemochromatosis absorb excessive amounts of iron from the gut and deposit the metal in many organs, where it injures cells. Only homozygotes develop clinically significant hepatic iron overload; heterozygotes accumulate some hepatic iron but do not develop liver injury.

Iron accumulation is progressive from birth but rarely leads to symptoms before age 40. The onset of disease is delayed even further in females, because of loss of iron in menstrual blood and a lower intake of dietary iron. Presenting symptoms are often vague, with abdominal pain reported in as few as 16% or as many as 58% of patients. Despite the variability of symptoms, signs of liver disease (particularly hepatomegaly) can be found in more than 75% of patients.

Biochemical abnormalities that suggest hereditary hemochromatosis in symptomatic individuals include elevations in transferrin saturation ($> 62\%$ in males; $> 50\%$ in females) and ferritin (more than twice normal). However, both of these parameters are prone to false-positive elevations and must be interpreted with caution. Transferrin saturation can be falsely elevated in non-fasting patients, in those with active liver necrosis, and even in heterozygotes for hemochromatosis. Ferritin also increases non-specifically with hepatocellular necrosis and may cause particular confusion in patients with alcoholic liver disease. To diagnose hereditary hemochromatosis with certainty, experts recommend a liver biopsy with quantitation of total hepatic iron. Patients with hereditary hemochromatosis who have clinical evidence of liver disease will have a hepatic iron index (micromoles of hepatic iron per gram of dry tissue divided by age in years) greater than 1.9. Genetic testing can also be performed for the C282Y mutation in *HFE*, but treatment is generally reserved for patients with confirmed iron overload on liver biopsy.

Phlebotomy (see Chapter 221) is the mainstay of therapy and can prevent or even reverse hepatic fibrosis. Fully developed cirrhosis is not usually reversible, although phlebotomy can enhance the survival of patients with cirrhosis. Unfortunately, patients with cirrhosis are at high risk of developing hepatocellular carcinoma, whether or not they undergo iron depletion therapy. Hepatocellular carcinoma is currently the leading cause of death among patients with hereditary hemochromatosis.

Family members of probands are screened by genetic testing and by serial measurements of transferrin saturation and ferritin. Because of the high frequency of the genetic defect, screening the general population with iron studies or genetic tests is now recommended.

PROTOPORPHYRIA

Protoporphyria is an inherited disorder marked by a profound reduction in ferrochelatase, the final enzyme in the pathway of heme synthesis. The mode of inheritance is debated. The primary clinical features of protoporphyria are cutaneous photosensitivity and scarring of sun-exposed skin; patients can also develop pigment gallstones, frequently at a young age. Parenchymal liver disease has been reported in fewer than 30 patients.

Protoporphyria can be diagnosed by measuring elevated protoporphyrin levels in erythrocytes or feces. Patients with the highest levels of protoporphyrin (> 1000 $\mu g/dL$ in erythrocytes) may be predisposed to liver disease and should undergo liver biopsy. His-

tology reveals birefringent deposits of protoporphyrin in hepatocytes and Kupffer cells. Development of jaundice predicts rapid deterioration and demise.

Treatment of the liver disease of protoporphyria is aimed at reducing production and increasing excretion of protoporphyrin. Hematin appears to decrease protoporphyrin production and has been useful in selected patients. Both cholestyramine and activated charcoal bind protoporphyrin in the gut, preventing enterohepatic recirculation and promoting excretion. For patients with severe liver disease and jaundice, liver transplantation should be considered.

CYSTIC FIBROSIS

Cystic fibrosis (see Chapter 76) manifests rarely in infants as a syndrome of obstructive jaundice. Older children and adolescents are more likely to develop liver disease, although the reported prevalence varies from 2.2 to 16%. Patients usually have established hepatic fibrosis at the time of diagnosis. Biochemical tests often fail to predict liver injury; indeed, a catastrophe such as variceal hemorrhage is sometimes the first evidence for hepatic disease. Because chronic liver disease may be the initial manifestation of cystic fibrosis, the diagnosis should be considered in any child or adolescent with hepatic fibrosis of unknown cause. Therapy for portal hypertension follows that for other liver diseases.

GLYCOGEN STORAGE DISEASES

Most of the glycogen storage diseases (see Chapter 203) are accompanied by hepatic glycogen accumulation and hepatomegaly. Only four of these (types O, I, III, and IV) result in clinical liver disease. Type O (glycogen synthetase deficiency) is extremely rare. Type IV (α-1,4-glucan-6-glycosyltransferase deficiency) leads to mortality from cirrhosis in early childhood. Types I and III are the two most likely to be encountered in adults.

Type I glycogenosis (glucose-6-phosphatase deficiency) is characterized by hepatic glycogen accumulation and marked hepatic steatosis. Biochemical studies reveal profound hypoglycemia and hypertriglyceridemia. Hepatic aminotransferases are only mildly increased. Patients treated with a high glucose diet can survive to adulthood but are at extremely high risk for developing hepatic adenomas. Adenomas are present in 75% of patients by age 30; malignant transformation is rare. Rigorous therapy designed to maintain the blood glucose level above 75 mg/dL at all times may prevent or reverse adenoma formation.

Type III glycogenosis (debrancher enzyme deficiency) differs from type I in that hypoglycemia and hyperlipidemia are much milder. Liver biopsy does not reveal steatosis but frequently demonstrates fibrosis, which rarely progresses to cirrhosis or portal hypertension. Supplemental feedings are recommended for patients with progressive liver injury.

AMYLOIDOSIS

Hepatic involvement is common in patients with systemic amyloidosis (see Chapter 297). Localized disease in the liver is rare but has been reported. Features of hepatic amyloidosis include hepatomegaly and increased serum alkaline phosphatase, each of which are found in 60% of patients with biopsy-proven liver involvement; clinical liver disease, however, is rarely encountered. A small number of patients with hepatic amyloidosis develop severe intrahepatic cholestasis with jaundice. This syndrome portends a poor prognosis, although death results from extrahepatic (primarily renal) disease.

Liver biopsy is not required to confirm hepatic involvement in patients with known systemic amyloidosis. If the diagnosis is uncertain, liver biopsy may be useful and can be performed safely if clotting parameters are normal and any history of a bleeding disorder is excluded.

SARCOIDOSIS

Sarcoidosis is one of the most common granulomatous diseases affecting the liver. Hepatic granulomas can be identified in approximately two thirds of patients with sarcoidosis, placing the liver behind only the lung and lymph nodes as the primary sites of involvement (see Chapter 81). Nevertheless, clinical symptoms of liver disease are rare in sarcoidosis. Liver involvement is usually recognized because of hepatomegaly or an elevated alkaline phosphatase level. A small minority of patients can develop a cholestatic syndrome characterized by pruritus and jaundice or can have hepatic failure and portal hypertension in the event the disease progresses to cirrhosis.

Liver biopsy can be useful in establishing a diagnosis of sarcoidosis, because granulomas are so numerous as to be sampled even with a random needle core. Occasionally, portal granulomas can destroy intrahepatic bile ducts, mimicking primary biliary cirrhosis. The latter can be distinguished by the presence of antimitochondrial antibodies in serum. When sarcoidosis progresses to hepatic fibrosis, connective tissue deposition is more extensive than around the granulomas alone.

Corticosteroids alleviate the symptoms of sarcoidosis but have not been proven to alter liver histology or the tendency toward hepatic fibrosis. Therapy should therefore be reserved for symptomatic patients in whom tuberculosis and other infectious diseases have been excluded.

TOTAL PARENTERAL NUTRITION

The most common hepatobiliary complication of total parenteral nutrition (TPN) is hepatic steatosis. Fatty liver occurs in 25 to 100% of patients receiving TPN; the lesion is heralded by an increase in serum aminotransferase levels with a smaller increase in alkaline phosphatase. Enzymes peak at around 2 weeks of therapy and then decline even if TPN is continued without modification. Steatosis is completely reversible on cessation of the infusion.

Long-term TPN poses a risk of chronic liver injury in adults. The most common abnormality is steatohepatitis; cholestasis and hepatic fibrosis have also been observed. Because steatohepatitis and cholestasis can both progress to hepatic fibrosis, their development is considered by many an indication to discontinue therapy. Chronic liver injury may be prevented by avoiding caloric excess, by infusing TPN cyclically, and by providing small amounts of enteral nutrition when possible.

Adults receiving TPN for more than 30 days are at risk of forming biliary sludge and gallstones. Fifty per cent of patients develop sludge after 6 weeks, and virtually 100% of patients are affected after 3 months. Both acalculous and calculous cholecystitis can occur. Although the pathophysiology of sludge and stone formation in the setting of TPN is due in part to decreased bile flow, gallbladder stasis plays an important role. Stasis may be ameliorated by cholecystokinin, by pulsed infusions of amino acids, or by small enteral feedings.

LIVER DISEASE IN PREGNANCY

Pregnant women are susceptible to the full range of hepatic diseases. For the most part, pregnancy does not pose an increased risk of acute liver disease, nor does it alter the natural history of hepatic illnesses contracted during gestation. Notable exceptions are viral hepatitides caused by the herpes simplex, herpes zoster, and hepatitis E viruses. Herpes simplex hepatitis has a higher incidence in pregnant women than in the population at large. All three agents can provoke severe illness in pregnant women, with mortality rates as high as 20% in the case of hepatitis E.

LIVER DISEASES UNIQUE TO PREGNANCY (Table 152–1). Transient elevations in hepatic aminotransferase levels may accompany hyperemesis gravidarum. Biochemical cholestasis, defined as an increase in circulating bile acids, can be detected in as many as 10% of normal gestations. Symptomatic cholestasis occurs in only 1 to 5% of pregnant women and is generally confined to the second and third trimesters. Most patients complain only of pruritus (pruritus gravidarum); a minority exhibit a more severe syndrome with disabling pruritus, jaundice, and steatorrhea. The latter may have an inherited predisposition toward cholestasis, with women of South American Indian and Swedish descent being at high risk. Cholestasis of pregnancy is a self-limited syndrome that resolves spontaneously after delivery. Whereas mild disease poses no risk to either mother or fetus, severe disease places women at increased risk of premature delivery and fetal death. Symptoms of mild gestational cholestasis can be treated with antihistamines or cholestyramine. Severe disease warrants close monitoring and possible early delivery. Patients should be counseled that the syndrome often recurs with future pregnancies.

Acute fatty liver of pregnancy is characterized by microvesicular fat accumulation in hepatocytes and hepatic necrosis. It mimics diseases caused by impairment of mitochondrial fatty acid oxidation, and in some instances it has been linked to fetal long-chain 3-hydroxyacyl-CoA dehydrogenase (LCHAD) deficiency. The incidence is estimated from 1 in 6,000 to 1 in 13,000 gestations. Roughly half of affected women are primiparas. A specific diagnosis can be made only by demonstrating microvesicular fat droplets in hepatocytes; liver biopsy, however, is not essential for management and may be precluded by coagulopathy. Because acute fatty liver almost always resolves spontaneously post partum, prompt delivery of the fetus is the treatment of choice. Patients deteriorating despite delivery should be considered for liver transplantation. Fatty liver of pregnancy tends not to recur with subsequent gestations, although with fetal LCHAD deficiency the predicted recurrence rate is 25%.

HELLP syndrome is the name given to a disorder of pregnancy characterized by *h*emolysis, *e*levated *l*iver enzymes, and *l*ow *p*latelets. This microangiopathic disorder of the liver occurs in the setting of severe preeclampsia or eclampsia with a frequency of 2 to 12%. Older, multiparous patients are at increased risk of HELLP syndrome; of note is that the classic triad of hypertension, proteinuria, and edema need not be present to make the diagnosis. Patients can develop HELLP syndrome in the second or third trimester or even post partum. Symptoms are similar to those of acute fatty liver of pregnancy, including abdominal pain, nausea, and vomiting. In rare instances, subcapsular hematomas can occur and lead to hepatic rupture and circulatory collapse. Laboratory abnormalities are not specific but often include anemia (hematocrit <30%), increased aminotransferase levels, and depressed platelet count (<100,000/mm^3). Lactate dehydrogenase is commonly above 600 U/L. Prothrombin time, partial thromboplastin time, and fibrinogen are usually normal and may provide some distinction from acute fatty liver of pregnancy. Blood smear suggests intravascular hemolysis. Liver biopsy, when performed, reveals focal hepatocellular necrosis and fibrin deposits within the sinusoids.

Prompt delivery is the treatment of choice. In gestations of less than 34 weeks, corticosteroids can be given to promote fetal lung

Table 152–1 ■ LIVER DISEASES UNIQUE TO PREGNANCY

	TRIMESTER OF ONSET	SYMPTOMS	LABORATORY ABNORMALITIES	RECURRENCE WITH FUTURE PREGNANCIES
Hyperemesis gravidarum	1	Nausea, vomiting	Elevated AST/ALT (60–1000 U/L), occasionaly hyperbilirubinemia	
Cholestasis	2, 3	Pruritus	Bile acids >8 μM, elevated AST/ALT and bilirubin in more severe cases	Common
Acute fatty liver	3	Nausea, vomiting, abdominal pain	Elevated AST/ALT (100–1000 U/L), bilirubin >5 mg/dL, prolonged prothrombin time*	Rare
HELLP syndrome	2, 3, or post partum	Abdominal pain, nausea, vomiting	Elevated AST/ALT (60–1500 U/L), platelets <100,000/mm^3, LDH >600 U/L, microangiopathic anemia	3–25%

* Useful diagnostic distinction from HELLP syndrome, in which prothrombin time, partial thromboplastin time, and fibrinogen are usually normal.
AST = aspartate aminotransferase; ALT = alanine aminotransferase.

maturity and to permit delivery as early as practical. The syndrome usually resolves rapidly post partum; in patients with persistent thrombocytopenia, plasmapheresis may be successful. The recurrence rate of HELLP syndrome in two large series varied between 3 and 25%.

PREGNANCY WITH CHRONIC LIVER DISEASE. Fertility is reduced in women with chronic liver disease and particularly in those with cirrhosis. Nevertheless, pregnancies can occur in women with advanced liver disease and are encountered with some frequency in women with mild to moderate liver disease. In general, pregnancy does not alter the course of underlying liver disease. Nevertheless, severe underlying liver disease places the mother at risk of gestational complications such as variceal hemorrhage and fetal death. Prophylaxis of gastrointestinal bleeding is not warranted in patients with cirrhosis. Patients receiving specific medications, however, such as corticosteroids for autoimmune chronic active hepatitis or copper chelators for Wilson's disease, should continue them throughout gestation.

Cuthbert JA: Wilson's disease: A new gene and an animal model for an old disease. J Invest Med 43:323, 1995. *A comprehensive review of the disease and its genetics.*

Powell LW, George DK, McDonnell SM, Kowdley KV: Diagnoses of hemochromatosis. Ann Intern Med 129:925, 1998. *One of a series of articles on the detection and management of hemochromatosis.*

Teckman JH, Qu D, Perlmutter DH: Molecular pathognesis of liver disease in alpha₁-antitrypsin deficiency. Hepatology 24:1504, 1996. *An elegant summary that places new scientific information into cellular models of disease.*

Wolf JL: Liver disease in pregnancy. Med Clin North Am 80:1167, 1996. *Concise review with 86 references.*

---

153 ALCOHOLIC LIVER DISEASE, CIRRHOSIS, AND ITS MAJOR SEQUELAE

Scott L. Friedman

OVERVIEW

DEFINITION AND GENERAL FEATURES. Cirrhosis consists of fibrosis of the hepatic parenchyma resulting in nodule formation. It represents the consequences of a sustained wound-healing response to chronic liver injury from a variety of causes (Table 153–1), including toxins (e.g., alcohol), chronic viral infection, cholestasis, and metabolic disorders. The clinical manifestations of cirrhosis vary widely, from lack of symptoms to liver failure, and are determined by both the nature and severity of the underlying liver disease as well as the extent of fibrosis. Clinical manifestations can be broadly classified into those resulting from impaired hepatocellular function, such as jaundice and coagulopathy, and those that result from physical disruption of the parenchyma, such as gastroesophageal varices and ascites.

EPIDEMIOLOGY. Up to 40% of patients with cirrhosis are asymptomatic. In these individuals, cirrhosis may be discovered during routine examination or at autopsy. The overall incidence of cirrhosis in the United States is estimated at 360 per 100,000 population, or approximately 900,000 total patients. Of these, the large majority have either alcoholic liver disease or chronic viral infection.

Cirrhosis is the most common non-neoplastic cause of death among hepatobiliary and digestive diseases in the United States, accounting for approximately 30,000 deaths per year. An additional 10,000 deaths occur due to liver cancer, the majority of which involve underlying cirrhosis, and deaths due to liver cancer have increased in the past decade. Mortality in patients with alcoholic disease is considerably higher than in patients with other forms of cirrhosis. Death rates are also higher in men than in women. Since 1980, overall cirrhosis mortality has decreased by 25% in the United States, possibly reflecting decreasing alcohol consumption and, to a lesser extent, the advent of hepatitis B vaccination, improved supportive care, and availability of liver transplantation (see Chapter 155).

Table 153–1 ■ CLASSIFICATION OF HEPATIC FIBROSIS AND CIRRHOSIS

I. Presinusoidal fibrosis
  A. Schistosomiasis
  B. Idiopathic portal fibrosis
II. Parenchymal (sinusoidal) fibrosis (true cirrhosis)
  A. Drugs and toxins
    1. Alcohol
    2. Methotrexate
    3. Isoniazid
    4. Vitamin A
    5. Amiodarone
    6. Perhexiline maleate
    7. α-Methyldopa
    8. Oxyphenisatin
  B. Infections
    1. Chronic hepatitis B or C
    2. Brucellosis
    3. Echinococcosis
    4. Congenital or tertiary syphilis
  C. Autoimmune
    1. Autoimmune chronic hepatitis—types 1, 2, and 3
  D. Vascular abnormalities
    1. Chronic, passive congestion due to right-sided heart failure, pericarditis
    2. Hereditary hemorrhagic telangiectasias (Osler-Weber-Rendu)
  E. Metabolic/genetic diseases
    1. Wilson's disease
    2. Hemochromatosis
    3. α₁-Antitrypsin deficiency
    4. Carbohydrate disorders (e.g., fructose intolerance, galactosemia, glycogen storage diseases)
    5. Lipid disorders (e.g., Wolman's disease, abetalipoproteinemia)
    6. Urea cycle defects (e.g., ornithine transcarbamylase)
    7. Porphyria
    8. Amino acid disorders (e.g., tyrosinosis)
    9. Bile acid disorders (e.g., Byler's disease)
  F. Biliary obstruction
    1. Primary biliary cirrhosis
    2. Secondary ("mechanical") biliary obstruction
      a. Primary sclerosing cholangitis
      b. Neoplasm of bile ducts or pancreas
      c. Iatrogenic or inflammatory biliary stricture
    3. Cystic fibrosis
    4. Biliary atresia/neonatal hepatitis
    5. Congenital biliary cysts
  G. Idiopathic/miscellaneous
    1. Non-alcoholic steatonecrosis (including jejuno-ileal bypass, obesity)
    2. Indian childhood cirrhosis
    3. Granulomatous liver disease
    4. Polycystic liver disease
III. Post-sinusoidal fibrosis
  A. Veno-occlusive disease

CLASSIFICATION AND ETIOLOGY. Cirrhosis has traditionally been classified as either macronodular (> 3-mm nodules) or micronodular (<3 mm). There is, however, no etiologic, functional, or prognostic value to the nodule size. A rare exception is in the cirrhotic patient with a massive "regenerative" nodule, which must be distinguished from a neoplasm.

The chemical composition of the scar tissue in cirrhosis is similar regardless of etiology and consists of the extracellular matrix molecules, collagen types I and III (i.e., "fibrillar" collagens), sulfated proteoglycans, and glycoproteins. These scar constituents accumulate from a net increase in their deposition in liver and not simply collapse of existing stroma. Although the cirrhotic bands surrounding nodules are the most easily seen form of scarring, it is actually the early deposition of matrix molecules in the subendothelial space of Disse—so-called capillarization of the sinusoid—that more directly correlates with diminished liver function (Fig. 153–1).

Efforts to identify the cellular source of scar constituents in cirrhosis have established that the stellate cell is the main producer of matrix. In both human disease and animal models, these mesenchymal cells undergo characteristic activation from a resting perisinusoidal cell rich in vitamin A to a proliferating and fibrogenic cell type with reduced vitamin A content. Stellate cell activation is common to all forms of experimental liver injury studied to date, including chronic biliary obstruction. Increased matrix produced by stellate cells in liver injury results from increased cell numbers as well as enhanced matrix production per cell. Cell proliferation is

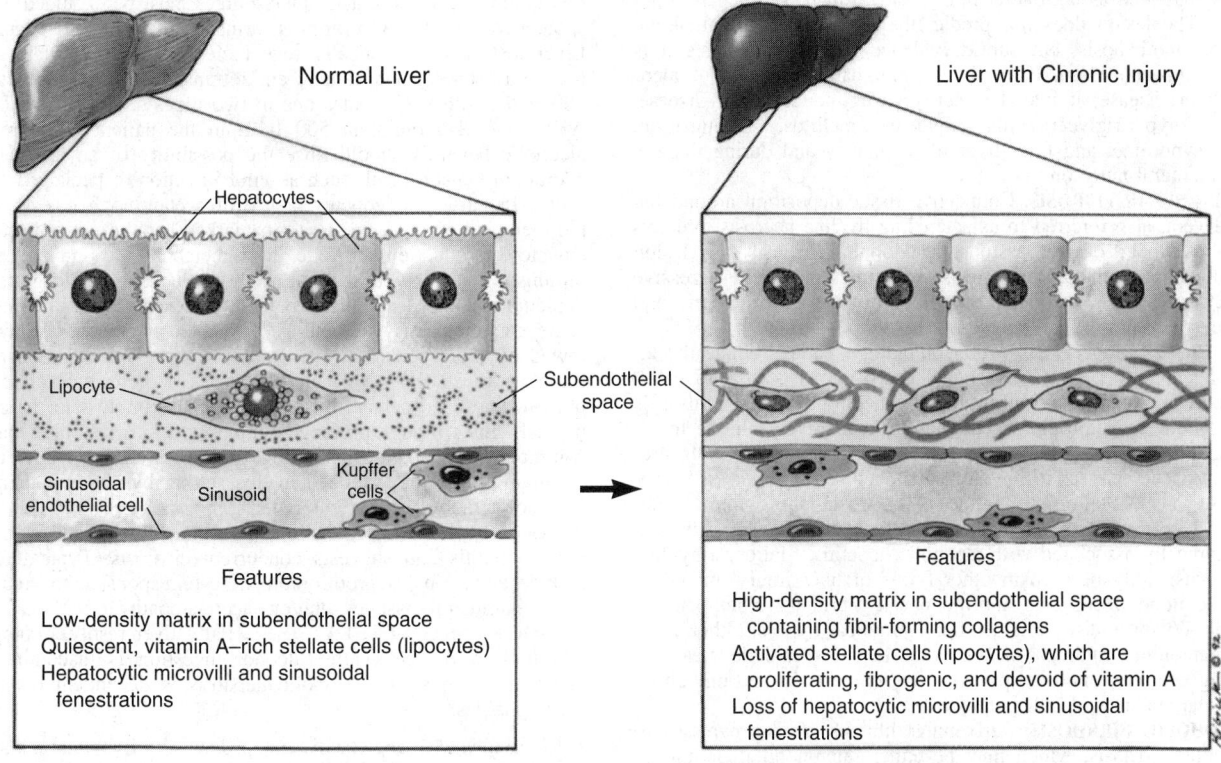

FIGURE 153–1 ■ Cellular and pathologic alterations in the hepatic sinusoid during chronic liver injury and fibrosis. (From Friedman SL: The cellular basis of hepatic necrosis. Reprinted by permission of the New England Journal of Medicine, 328:1829, 1993. Copyright 1993, Massachusetts Medical Society.)

regulated primarily by the cytokine platelet-derived growth factor (PDGF), whereas fibrogenesis is stimulated by transforming growth factor-β (TGF-β), whose messenger RNA levels are markedly increased in human cirrhosis. Activated stellate cells can also contract and secrete proteases, which can remodel the hepatic extracellular matrix. At present, there is no established treatment to arrest or reverse scar formation in chronic liver injury. Rather, removing the primary insult when possible remains the most effective way to prevent irreversible scarring.

DIAGNOSIS AND PROGNOSIS OF CIRRHOSIS. Liver biopsy remains the gold standard for documenting cirrhosis, identifying a cause, and assessing the extent of scar formation. Biopsy specimens should be large enough to identify portal tracts and central areas. Sections should be examined with both hematoxylin-eosin and a connective tissue stain such as Masson's trichrome or reticulin. Special stains may be appropriate as well to identify metals (e.g., iron, copper), lipids, carbohydrates, and/or protein accumulation associated with inborn errors of metabolism.

In the clinical setting, prognosis is best determined by the Pugh modification of the Child-Turcotte classification, which includes the variables of ascites, encephalopathy, serum albumin, serum bilirubin, and prothrombin time. Both the Child-Turcotte and Pugh classifications correlate closely with albumin synthesis rates. Several non-invasive markers of cirrhosis measure fragments of matrix molecules in serum (e.g., collagen propeptides), but these assays reflect inflammatory activity and may be falsely normal in established, quiescent cirrhosis. By reflecting inflammatory activity, these assays may indirectly have prognostic value but do not discriminate in all cases between different stages of injury and fibrosis.

ALCOHOLIC LIVER DISEASE

OVERVIEW, EPIDEMIOLOGY, AND RISK FACTORS. Alcoholic liver disease encompasses a spectrum of abnormalities ranging from fatty liver, a reversible consequence of acute ingestion, to irreversible cirrhosis (Laënnec's cirrhosis) (see Chapter 16). Although many patients who drink heavily develop hepatic enlargement and fatty accumulation, only a minority (~20%) of cases will progress to alcoholic hepatitis or cirrhosis. Risk factors for developing these more severe sequelae include the following:

1. *Duration and magnitude of alcohol ingestion.* An average total intake required for development of cirrhosis has been estimated as the regular consumption of 80 g of ethanol per day for 20 years, but the relative risk of chronic liver disease increases substantially with as little as 40 to 60 g/day (80 g of ethanol equals eight 12-oz beers, a liter of wine, or a half-pint of spirits). Only the total dose and not the type of alcoholic beverage or pattern of intake influences progression.

2. *Gender.* In females there is greater likelihood of progression to cirrhosis than in males ingesting the same relative amount of alcohol.

3. *Hepatitis B or C infection.* Concurrent liver disease of any type may be an accelerant to hepatic injury in the patient who drinks heavily. In particular, a strikingly high incidence of anti–hepatitis C virus (HCV) antibodies (10–40%) has been reported in patients with alcoholic cirrhosis; HCV acquired in this population is not solely explained by either prior transfusion or intravenous drug use, which are known risk factors for HCV infection.

4. *Genetic factors.* An inherited predisposition to alcoholism has been clearly established, but genetically determined increased susceptibility to liver damage in heavy drinkers is less certain. Increased susceptibility to organ injury may also be associated with certain isoenzymes of alcohol dehydrogenase, the principal metabolizing enzyme of ethanol.

5. *Nutritional status.* Protein-calorie malnutrition is extremely common in alcoholics. Malnutrition may be due not only to poor intake but also to abnormal nutrient metabolism. Whereas poor nutrition may contribute to the evolution of alcoholic liver disease, adequate nutrition does not prevent its development. In fact, studies suggest that obesity may be a risk factor.

PATHOLOGY. FATTY LIVER. Steatosis, or fatty liver, is a reversible short-term consequence of alcohol toxicity. Large fat droplets fill hepatocytes, distorting the nuclei and enlarging the acinus. The lesion occurs even in well-nourished alcoholics and results from enhanced production and decreased oxidation of fatty acids within the liver, as well as peripheral lipolysis with increased hepatic lipid uptake. The lesion does *not* predict the development of alcoholic hepatitis or cirrhosis, but subtle evidence of injury suggests it is not an innocent lesion. Fatty liver is not pathognomonic of alcoholic liver disease; it may be seen in drug-induced liver disease, obesity, hypertriglyceridemia, diabetes mellitus, malnutrition, Reye's syndrome, and fatty liver of pregnancy and during therapy with parenteral nutrition.

PERIVENULAR FIBROSIS. Connective tissue deposition around the central vein, also referred to as sclerosing hyaline necrosis, predicts a high likelihood of progression to panlobular cirrhosis. The lesion may develop in the absence of severe inflammation. Progressive perivenular fibrosis can lead to obliteration of central veins and postsinusoidal portal hypertension.

ALCOHOLIC HEPATITIS. Several obligatory features define the lesion of alcoholic hepatitis: liver cell necrosis, perivenular distribution, pericellular fibrosis, infiltration by neutrophils, and Mallory's hyaline bodies. Neutrophil accumulation is relatively unique to alcoholic injury (in most forms of hepatitis, mononuclear cells predominate) and may contribute to hepatocellular injury (see Pathogenesis, later). Mallory's hyaline is an eosinophilic intracellular inclusion composed of condensed cytoskeletal filaments. Although most typically associated with alcoholic hepatitis, Mallory's hyaline may occasionally be seen in other forms of liver injury, including Indian childhood cirrhosis, morbid obesity, primary biliary cirrhosis, and Wilson's disease, and after jejunoileal bypass. Other common pathologic findings of alcoholic hepatitis include steatosis, bridging necrosis, bile duct proliferation, cholestasis, and mitochondrial enlargement within hepatocytes.

ALCOHOLIC CIRRHOSIS. Perivenular fibrosis often progresses to panlobular cirrhosis, which may be either micronodular or macronodular. As scarring continues, the organ shrinks because of contraction of fibrous bands by activated stellate cells. At the ultrastructural level, loss of sinusoidal fenestrations may contribute to impaired nutrient exchange across the subendothelial space between sinusoidal blood and hepatocytes, contributing to the decay in liver function. In the cirrhotic patient who continues to drink, pathologic elements of both fatty liver and hepatitis may persist. It is unsettled whether hepatitis is a necessary precursor to cirrhosis.

PATHOGENESIS. The mechanism of alcoholic liver injury is not established. In fact, the most compelling evidence for an etiologic role of ethanol in alcoholic hepatitis is epidemiologic, not biochemical.

Theories of alcoholic liver injury invoke several complementary mechanisms:

1. *Centrilobular hypoxia*, which proposes that metabolism of ethanol acetaldehyde increases lobular oxygen consumption, leading to relative hypoxemia and cell damage in regions farthest from oxygenated blood (i.e., pericentral zones).
2. *Neutrophil infiltration/activity,* which may occur because of release of neutrophil chemoattractants by hepatocytes metabolizing ethanol. Tissue injury could ensue from neutrophils and hepatocytes releasing reactive oxygen intermediates, proteases, and cytokines.
3. *Formation of acetaldehyde-protein adducts,* which serve as neoantigens, generating sensitized lymphocytes and specific antibodies that attack hepatocytes bearing these antigens.
4. Free-radical generation by alternative pathways of ethanol metabolism, the so-called microsomal enzyme oxidizing system.

The pathogenesis of alcoholic fibrosis involves many of the cytokines prominent in other forms of liver injury, including tumor necrosis factor, interleukin-1, PDGF, and TGF-β. Acetaldehyde may have minor fibrogenic activity toward activated stellate cells but is not a major pathogenic factor in alcoholic fibrosis.

CLINICAL PRESENTATION. Fatty liver is associated with moderate to marked hepatomegaly and occasionally with right upper quadrant tenderness and epigastric discomfort. Liver test results are generally normal or only modestly elevated, and jaundice is unusual. The lesion may develop after a single binge of alcohol, in contrast to hepatitis, which requires more extensive alcohol intake.

Alcoholic hepatitis may lead to anorexia, fever, hepatomegaly, and jaundice. Alcoholic hepatitis generally requires several weeks to months of alcohol ingestion. Associated stigmas of chronic liver

disease (e.g., spider angiomas, palmar erythema, ascites) suggest underlying cirrhosis. The fever of alcoholic hepatitis is generally low grade ($<38.3°$ C), and other sources must be excluded, such as spontaneous bacterial peritonitis, urinary infection, and pneumonia. Liver tests characteristically reveal elevations of aspartate aminotransferase (AST) and alanine aminotransferase (ALT) to less than 500 IU/L, with AST values one to two times greater than ALT. An AST or ALT more than 500 IU/L in the patient with presumed alcoholic hepatitis should raise the possibility of an alternative or additional hepatic insult such as viral infection (especially HCV) or drugs. In particular, concurrent use of acetaminophen, even within the therapeutic range, may lead to marked hepatic injury because of enhanced production of toxic drug metabolites, combined with a diminished capacity to neutralize them due to hepatic glutathione depletion. In the hospitalized patient with acute alcoholic hepatitis, acute elevations of AST and ALT resolve over several days, followed by more persistent and sometimes marked elevation of bilirubin up to 20 times normal. Elevations of hepatic alkaline phosphatase may also persist, but to a lesser extent (two to three times normal). Even though prolonged cholestasis in alcoholic hepatitis is common, extrahepatic obstruction from common bile duct disease or tumor should be excluded in this setting by abdominal imaging (ultrasonography [US] or computed tomography [CT]).

Evidence of liver dysfunction is common in patients with alcoholic hepatitis and suggests concurrent cirrhosis. Typical features include elevations of prothrombin time unresponsive to vitamin K, hypoalbuminemia, ascites, and/or encephalopathy.

PROGNOSIS AND TREATMENT. Fatty liver resolves completely within 4 to 6 weeks after alcohol ingestion is discontinued. In contrast, prognosis of alcoholic hepatitis is dependent on at least four variables:

1. *Continued drinking.* Persistent, progressive liver disease and accelerated mortality are certain in the patient with alcoholic hepatitis who continues to drink. In contrast, in up to two thirds of patients who stop drinking, function will return to normal provided there is little underlying fibrosis.
2. *Degree of inflammation.* Peripheral leukocytosis in the absence of concurrent infection correlates with both increased tissue leukocytosis and mortality. Ten to 20% of cases with persistent blood leukocytosis (e.g., 15,000 to 25,000/mm³) progress to subfulminant hepatic failure despite withdrawal of alcohol.
3. *Perivenular fibrosis.* As noted earlier (see Pathology), this lesion portends likely progression to panlobular fibrosis.
4. *Indices of liver failure.* Evidence of coagulopathy, ascites, hepatorenal syndrome, or encephalopathy is a poor prognostic sign.

Abstinence is the crucial component in treating alcoholic hepatitis. Recognizing alcoholism and maintaining sobriety require family and social support. Ongoing studies are attempting to optimize strategies of behavioral and pharmacologic intervention (see Chapter 16).

In the hospitalized patient, sedation with benzodiazepines may be indicated if signs of withdrawal are present, such as tachycardia, hypertension, and agitation. Multivitamins (including thiamine, folate, vitamin K, and pyridoxine), fluids, and replacement of minerals (phosphate, magnesium) are usually warranted. In the patient with severe life-threatening alcoholic hepatitis, therapy with methylprednisolone (32 to 40 mg/day for 28 days) will lessen short-term mortality. Patients likely to respond to corticosteroids have evidence of liver failure with an elevated bilirubin level, prolonged prothrombin time, and encephalopathy. In one study, patients who benefited from corticosteroids were those with either spontaneous hepatic encephalopathy or a discriminant function value greater than 32, calculated by the formula: 4.6 (prothrombin time − control time) + [serum bilirubin (in micromoles per liter)/17.1]. The drug is not appropriate in patients with mild hepatitis or with either gastrointestinal bleeding or concurrent bacterial infection. Several other approaches have shown benefit in clinical trials but are not yet established for clinical practice, including propylthiouracil, invasive nutritional support, and androgenic steroids.

In patients with established cirrhosis, abstinence remains a crucial determinant of prolonged survival. In abstinent patients in whom there is progression to decompensated liver failure, orthotopic liver transplantation is a viable option (see Chapter 155). Survival of patients with alcoholic cirrhosis after transplantation is as high as for other forms of cirrhosis, and recidivism rates are less than 15% if patients have maintained documented abstinence for at least 6 months before surgery.

POSTVIRAL CIRRHOSIS

Chronic hepatitis B virus (HBV) and hepatitis C virus (HCV) infections are among the leading causes of cirrhosis in the Western World and the leading cause in Asia and Africa (see Chapter 150). The identification of HCV in 1989 as the major cause of "non-A, non-B" hepatitis has dramatically reduced the percentage of patients classified with truly "cryptogenic" cirrhosis.

In chronic HBV infection, the rate of progression to cirrhosis is influenced by the degree of inflammation and lobular distortion. These parameters in turn are determined by the replicative activity of the virus (i.e., e-antigen positive) and whether there has been superinfection by hepatitis delta virus (HDV). Concurrent liver injury from other causes (e.g., alcohol) may also amplify the degree of inflammation and hasten the onset of cirrhosis. Similarly, in chronic HCV, progression to cirrhosis is influenced by the degree of liver damage at initial biopsy, as well as the age of exposure and duration of infection. Although the development of cirrhosis in most patients with chronic HBV or HCV is insidious over many years, rapid progression within 1 year has been seen in cases with aggressive inflammation. The average progression rate from HCV infection to cirrhosis has been estimated at 30 years, with older age, male gender, and concurrent alcohol use identified as the major risk factors. Particularly rapid progression to cirrhosis has also been seen in patients with recurrent HBV or HCV after liver transplantation. Overall, at least 25% of cases of chronic HCV will progress to cirrhosis within 10 years.

PATHOLOGY. Although the extent of inflammation is a determinant of severity, distinguishing between chronic persistent and chronic active hepatitis is less meaningful in predicting progression to cirrhosis than previously thought. In either HBV or HCV, evidence of bridging necrosis and fibrosis is a harbinger of likely progression. As in other forms of cirrhosis, the activated stellate cell is likely to be responsible for fibrogenesis. Cirrhosis from HBV or HCV may be either micronodular or macronodular.

CLINICAL FEATURES AND ROLE OF BIOPSY. Clinical features in patients with postviral cirrhosis may span the spectrum from completely asymptomatic to liver failure. In general, typical hepatitis symptoms of fatigue, malaise, and anorexia correlate more closely with disease activity in chronic HBV than in HCV. It is not unusual for HCV to be first recognized by routine laboratory screening, yet biopsy will reveal marked inflammation and tissue distortion. Moreover, in chronic HCV, AST and ALT do not correlate well with the degree of inflammation on liver biopsy, so that modest elevations of laboratory test findings do not exclude the possibility of advanced liver disease. Thus, liver biopsy is an important tool to determine the type and extent of fibrosis. Biopsy may also determine the need and response to therapy. Improvement in liver histology after treatment with interferon-α is associated with diminished fibrosis and reduced tissue mRNA levels of fibrogenic cytokines. Once cirrhosis is well established in the patient with chronic viral infection, sequelae of liver failure are indistinguishable from other forms of end-stage liver disease.

CRYPTOGENIC CIRRHOSIS

Although HCV testing has substantially reduced the percentage of patients with unexplained cirrhosis, there remains a subset who develop progressive liver disease in the absence of viral infection, cholestasis, or genetic liver disease. This subset is a heterogeneous group of patients, about 75% of whom have features of autoimmunity (see Chapter 150). In autoimmune hepatitis, bridging necrosis and fibrosis predict a high likelihood of cirrhosis. Approximately 40% of patients with autoimmune hepatitis will develop cirrhosis within 10 years. Survival in cirrhotics with autoimmune hepatitis is 65%, which is greater than in those with cryptogenic cirrhosis lacking autoimmune features.

CIRRHOSIS IN GENETIC DISEASES

Several inborn errors of metabolism associated with accumulation of either metals or metabolites can lead to cirrhosis (see Chap-

ter 152). Mechanisms of cirrhosis are not well understood in these conditions. Abnormal accumulation of a metal or metabolite is the common link, yet inflammation is often minimal. Most common is hemochromatosis, in which the cirrhotic liver is greatly enlarged and stained reddish brown as a result of iron infiltration. Microscopically, late-stage liver disease is characterized by extensive pigmentation and dense fibrous septa progressing to complete nodule formation. Cirrhosis usually develops over decades. Early diagnosis is critical because removing excess iron in the precirrhotic stage prevents cirrhosis and its complications from developing. Wilson's disease often occurs with evidence of inflammatory liver disease or cirrhosis. Similar to hemochromatosis, cirrhosis can be averted by copper chelation with D-penicillamine in the precirrhotic phase. Onset of cirrhosis is generally more rapid and occurs at a younger age than in hemochromatosis. α_1-Antitrypsin deficiency is associated with cirrhosis as early as 2 weeks of age in homozygotes and as late as the ninth decade. In addition to these more common disorders, a large number of rarer genetic diseases are also associated with cirrhosis (see Table 153–1). These include errors in the metabolism of carbohydrates, amino acids, lipids, bile acids, or porphyrins.

BILIARY CIRRHOSIS

Biliary cirrhosis refers to nodular fibrosis due to bile duct obstruction, which may be intrahepatic or extrahepatic. *Primary biliary* cirrhosis is a well-defined inflammatory disease of intrahepatic bile ducts. *Secondary biliary cirrhosis* encompasses other causes of fibrosing biliary obstruction, including long-standing mechanical obstruction, sclerosing cholangitis, and genetic or developmental diseases in which cholestasis is prominent (e.g., cystic fibrosis, biliary atresia, and congenital biliary cysts).

PRIMARY BILIARY CIRRHOSIS. Primary biliary cirrhosis (PBC) is an immune-mediated disorder of unknown cause characterized by progressive destruction of intrahepatic bile ducts and the presence of antimitochondrial antibodies. The disease has a strong female preponderance (10:1). Although it is most common in whites from North America and Europe, cases have occurred in all races. The reason why prevalence appears to be increasing in Western populations is unknown. The disease is commonly associated with other autoimmune disorders, including sicca complex, CREST syndrome, rheumatoid arthritis, thyroiditis, pernicious anemia, and renal tubular acidosis.

PATHOLOGY. The pathologic progression of PBC is divided into four successive stages:

Stage I: Florid duct lesion, characterized by marked periductular inflammation and injury to septal and interlobular bile ducts. The inflammation is predominantly mononuclear cell and may be associated with granuloma formation. These pathognomonic features may be spotty and can coexist with features of later-stage disease.
Stage II: Ductular proliferation, marked by bile duct proliferation in portal tracts and early cholestasis, combined with periportal inflammation of the type also seen in chronic hepatitis.
Stage III: Fibrosis, marked by waning inflammation but increasing septal fibrosis and distortion of the normal architecture. Cholestasis may be prominent.
Stage IV: Cirrhosis; features possibly distinguishing PBC-related cirrhosis from other types include the absence of bile ducts, continued mononuclear cell infiltration, and cholestasis.

PATHOGENESIS. An autoimmune attack against the bile duct is probably an important pathogenetic element, but the precipitating event and contribution of genetic and environmental factors are not known. The antigens against which antimitochondrial antibodies (AMA) are directed have been recently identified as components of the E2 subunits of the 2-oxo-acid dehydrogenase enzyme family (M2 antigen). It appears increasingly likely that AMA play a pathogenic role and are more than simply an epiphenomenon of the illness.

CLINICAL FEATURES AND DIAGNOSIS. The disease typically occurs in middle-aged females, either as an incidental threefold to fourfold elevation of alkaline phosphatase or in evaluating complaints of fatigue and pruritus. Mild (twofold to threefold) elevation of transaminase levels is common. Identifying AMA in serum usually leads to liver biopsy, which establishes the diagnosis. Atypical presentations in several patterns may occur, including in patients with negative AMA but compatible biochemistry and biopsy (~5%), those with positive AMA and compatible biopsy but normal liver biochemistry (~15%), and disease in men (~10%).

Insidious onset of pruritus is the most characteristic symptom. Its etiology is uncertain, and it may appear at any stage of the disease. Fatigue is also common. Symptoms resulting from malabsorption of fat-soluble vitamins, including vitamin A, D, E, or K deficiency, may be evident. There may be symptoms attributable to other autoimmune diseases, especially dry eyes or mouth and arthritis. Physical findings are subtle in the patient with asymptomatic or early disease. As the disease progresses, however, jaundice develops, the skin becomes dry, xanthomas appear, and liver and spleen enlarge but are non-tender. Once cirrhosis develops, symptoms of portal hypertension and liver failure may predominate.

In addition to AMA, characteristic laboratory abnormalities include increased serum IgM (95%), hypercholesterolemia, and other autoantibodies, including rheumatoid factor (70%), anti–smooth muscle antibodies (65%), and thyroid-specific or antinuclear antibodies. Impaired sulfoxidation of sulfur-containing compounds is common (84%) in PBC, unlike in other forms of cirrhosis. Increasing prothrombin time and decreasing albumin characterize the late stages of disease.

The presence of AMA and a compatible biopsy establish the diagnosis of PBC. Extrahepatic ductal disease should be excluded with an abdominal imaging procedure, but endoscopic retrograde cholangiopancreatography is not required unless there are atypical laboratory or clinical features. Rare cases of progressive bile duct injury due to drugs may clinically resemble PBC but are distinguishable by the lack of AMA.

PROGNOSIS. PBC is a slowly progressive disease usually leading to liver failure over 5 to 10 years. Survival is impaired even in asymptomatic patients, emphasizing the need to consider therapy in hopes of delaying the onset of late-stage disease. Prognosis can be predicted more accurately than in most other types of chronic liver disease by using time-dependent multivariate analyses based on age, bilirubin level, serum albumin level, prothrombin time, presence of gastrointestinal bleeding, and severity of edema; biopsy findings also may be incorporated. Alternatively, a serum bilirubin value of more than 10 mg/dL by itself is a remarkably accurate indicator of impending liver failure. These indices are important for determining optimal timing for liver transplantation (see Chapter 155).

TREATMENT. Ursodeoxycholic acid (UDCA), a hydrophilic bile acid, has shown early success in slowing the progression of PBC (8 to 10 mg/kg/day), possibly by reducing the concentration of toxic bile acids in the hepatic pool. The drug is well tolerated. No specific antifibrotic effect of the UDCA has been observed, however. Although long-term follow-up (>4 years) is lacking, the drug clearly improves survival free of liver transplantation in patients with moderate or severe disease. Cyclosporine had shown early promise in a small controlled trial, but longer-term usage led to only modest efficacy combined with an adverse effect on renal function, which has dampened enthusiasm for its use. Other immunosuppressive agents have met with modest success in some patients, including azathioprine, methotrexate, chlorambucil, and prednisone. In addition to specific agents against the disease, management should include correcting vitamin A, D, E, and K deficiencies and using antipruritics, including cholestyramine (16 to 32 g/day). In rare cases of intractable pruritus, opioid antagonists and plasmapheresis may be beneficial. Liver transplantation offers excellent quality of life in most patients with end-stage disease. Although transplantation is usually curative, rare cases of disease have recurred after transplant.

SECONDARY BILIARY CIRRHOSIS. Secondary biliary cirrhosis occurs in response to chronic biliary obstruction from a variety of causes (see Chapter 157). Neither the mechanism of scarring nor the duration and severity of obstruction required for irreversible fibrosis are established. In general, at least 6 months of obstruction are required for cirrhosis to develop, but shorter intervals have been reported.

ETIOLOGY. Cholestasis may be intrahepatic or extrahepatic, the latter also referred to as "mechanical" cholestasis. Primary sclerosing cholangitis is the most common cause of intrahepatic cholestasis besides PBC (see Chapter 157). Cholestasis in this condition is incomplete but progressive and leads to cirrhosis in most patients within 10 years. Patients with associated inflammatory bowel disease who have undergone bowel resection may develop peristomal varices. In cystic fibrosis, intrahepatic cholestasis with focal biliary cirrhosis may complicate up to 25% of patients by the time of death, although liver disease is often asymptomatic. The precirrhotic lesion is marked by biliary proliferation and ductal occlusion. Cholestatic syndromes of infancy and childhood are frequently complicated by rapid progression of fibrosis within 10 to 12 weeks of birth even when recognized promptly. These disorders represent a spectrum of pathologic changes often involving atresia of either intrahepatic or extrahepatic ducts. There is overlap both clinically and histologically with neonatal hepatitis. Fibrosis often progresses even after successful biliary decompression and normalization of bilirubin, with biopsy specimens revealing a pattern resembling congenital hepatic fibrosis.

Extrahepatic cholestasis in adults most commonly results from structural or mechanical obstruction. Common lesions include choledocholithiasis, biliary or pancreatic cancer, iatrogenic stricture, or chronic pancreatitis. A variant form of cholangiohepatitis in Asians is characterized by intrahepatic obstruction from biliary sludge, which can lead to recurrent cholangitis and secondary cirrhosis; the cause is unknown.

PATHOLOGY. The progression of histologic changes in chronic cholestasis has been well characterized. Hepatocyte degeneration with formation of cellular rosettes and ductular proliferation may be followed by inflammatory biliary necrosis and early periductal fibrosis. Inspissated bile within ductal lumens, formation of bile lakes, and periductular bile infarcts are classic late features. Early ductular changes are reversible, but persistent obstruction ultimately leads to portal-central septa and nodule formation typical of irreversible fibrosis.

CLINICAL AND LABORATORY FEATURES. Clinical consequences of secondary biliary cirrhosis will initially be determined by the underlying disease. With progression, jaundice may become the prominent symptom. Pruritus is variable in severity. Fat malabsorption with steatorrhea and deficiencies of vitamins A, D, E, and K occur in long-standing obstruction. Osteomalacia or osteoporosis may occur because of vitamin D malabsorption and calcium deficiency.

Disproportionately increased hepatic alkaline phosphatase (fourfold to fivefold increase) relative to other liver tests is typical of secondary biliary cirrhosis. Other results of serum tests of biliary injury may be similarly elevated, including γ-glutamyl transpeptidase and 5′-nucleotidase. Aminotransferase levels are increased less than twofold. Hypercholesterolemia is common. Associated markers of immunologic disease or bacterial cholangitis may be evident in patients with sclerosing cholangitis or mechanical obstruction, respectively.

TREATMENT. Recognizing and treating the underlying cause of cholestasis is the mainstay of therapy. For extrahepatic obstruction, biliary decompression, either by surgical drainage or by placement of a biliary stent for neoplasms, is usually required. Intrahepatic cholestasis is less amenable to surgical drainage, with management limited to treating complications. Pruritus can be controlled with cholestyramine (16 to 32 g/day in two divided doses) or, in severe cases, opioid antagonists (e.g., naloxone, nalmefene). Calcium and vitamin D supplementation may be required for bone disease. Parenteral replacement of vitamins A, E, and K is sometimes required. Regular exposure to sunlight enhances the conversion of 7-dehydrocholesterol to vitamin D and can reduce the development of osteomalacia. Current single-agent medical therapy for primary sclerosing cholangitis is not effective. For example, UDCA improves biochemical parameters but does not retard disease progression; future approaches may use combination therapy (e.g., UDCA and methotrexate). Liver transplantation is highly successful in most patients with secondary biliary cirrhosis and deteriorating liver function (see Chapter 155).

VASCULAR DISORDERS ASSOCIATED WITH CIRRHOSIS

CHRONIC RIGHT-SIDED HEART FAILURE. Long-standing right-sided heart failure due to cardiomyopathy, tricuspid valve insufficiency, pulmonary disease, or pericardial constriction can lead to hepatic fibrosis; however, this late sequela is uncommon. The clinical picture is usually dominated by cardiac or pulmonary dysfunction. Liver abnormalities may be typical of hepatic congestion, with disproportionate elevation of bilirubin (up to 10-fold) and prothrombin time (2 to 6 seconds prolonged) yet modest aminotransferase elevations (less than threefold). Gross inspection of affected liver characteristically reveals focal areas of congestion (nutmeg liver).

HEPATIC VENO-OCCLUSIVE DISEASE. This syndrome occurs most commonly as a complication of bone marrow transplantation and/or pyrrolizidine alkaloid therapy and is characterized clinically by rapid onset of hepatomegaly, weight gain, and ascites. Hyperbilirubinemia and increased aminotransferase levels are typical. There is deposition of a fibronectin-rich matrix around terminal hepatic (central) veins, with evidence of endothelial cell injury. Because of its characteristic presentation, however, biopsy is rarely necessary to establish the diagnosis. The lesion is not a true cirrhosis, yet the clinical consequences are rapid and profound because the deposition of extracellular matrix occurs in a critical site of sinusoidal outflow.

BUDD-CHIARI SYNDROME. Like veno-occlusive disease, Budd-Chiari syndrome is not a true cirrhosis but rather an acute or subacute obstruction to hepatic venous outflow. Fibrous webs are one of the many causes of the disorder, but these are usually extrahepatic, and parenchymal fibrosis is uncommon.

MISCELLANEOUS DISORDERS ASSOCIATED WITH CIRRHOSIS

A variety of poorly understood chronic liver diseases are associated with cirrhosis. *Non-alcoholic steatonecrosis* is a clinicopathologic syndrome remarkably similar to alcoholic liver disease, but it occurs in the absence of alcohol use. The disorder, which is often identified incidentally, is found with several conditions, including diabetes mellitus, morbid obesity, jejunoileal bypass surgery, Weber-Christian disease, and abetalipoproteinemia. Amiodarone, diethylstilbestrol, perhexiline maleate, total parenteral nutrition, and synthetic estrogens have also been implicated. Cirrhosis develops in at least one third of patients if the precipitant is not removed. *Indian childhood cirrhosis* is a significant cause of preschool pediatric morbidity, occurring in up to 1 in 4000 live births in the Indian subcontinent. Marked hyaline accumulation, increased copper deposition, and extensive fibrosis are typical histologic features. The underlying defect is unknown. D-Penicillamine has been used to slow progression in some patients. *Polycystic liver disease* is usually associated with renal cysts and is characterized by macroscopic or microscopic hepatic cysts associated with fibrosis. *Granulomatous liver diseases,* including sarcoidosis (see Chapter 151), may progress to cirrhosis in some patients.

In addition to medications associated with non-alcoholic steatonecrosis, drug-induced hepatic fibrosis may also be seen in patients taking isoniazid or antimetabolites, especially methotrexate. The latter is associated with dose-dependent fibrosis in patients treated for psoriasis or rheumatoid arthritis for at least 2 years. Continuous therapy is more fibrogenic than intermittent dosing, and coexisting liver disease or heavy alcohol intake amplifies the risk of fibrosis. Surveillance liver biopsies are required in patients whose cumulative dose exceeds 1.5 to 2 g, because considerable fibrosis may develop in the absence of symptoms.

MAJOR SEQUELAE OF CIRRHOSIS (Table 153–2)

PORTAL HYPERTENSION. FEATURES OF THE PORTAL CIRCULATION AND CLASSIFICATION OF PORTAL HYPERTENSION. The portal circulation is a low-pressure system (<10 mm Hg) formed by the venous drainage from intraperitoneal viscera, including the luminal gastrointestinal tract, spleen, gallbladder, and pancreas. Veins collecting from these sites form the splenic vein and superior and inferior mesenteric veins, which, in turn, merge to create the portal vein. Portal hypertension occurs when portal venous pressure exceeds the pressure in the non-portal abdominal veins (e.g., inferior vena cava) by at least 5 mm Hg; portosystemic collateral vessels develop in an effort to equalize pressures between these two venous systems. These collateral vessels, or varices, most commonly develop in the esophagus and proximal stomach and can

Table 153–2 ▪ SEQUELAE OF CIRRHOSIS

1. Portal hypertension: bleeding from varices in esophagus/stomach (most common), duodenum, rectum, or surgical stomas; bleeding from congestive gastropathy; splenomegaly with hypersplenism
2. Ascites; spontaneous bacterial peritonitis; hepatic hydrothorax, abdominal hernia
3. Hepatorenal syndrome
4. Hepatic encephalopathy
5. Synthetic dysfunction/coagulopathy
6. Hepatopulmonary syndrome
7. Hepatocellular carcinoma
8. Feminization
9. Altered drug metabolism
10. Hepatic osteodystrophy

cause clinically significant bleeding. Altered portal hemodynamics can also lead to the development of ascites (see later) and contribute to hepatic encephalopathy (see Chapter 154).

Increased portal pressure in cirrhosis primarily results from increased resistance to blood flow through the shrunken, fibrotic liver. Increased intrahepatic resistance results both from fixed obstruction to flow by extracellular matrix and from dynamic organ and sinusoidal contraction by activated stellate cells (also referred to as myofibroblasts). Because pressure is a function of both resistance and flow, independent increases in portal inflow due to the hyperdynamic circulation of cirrhosis and splanchnic arteriolar vasodilation also contribute to portal pressure elevation.

In cirrhosis, which is the most common cause of portal hypertension, the lesion is intrahepatic and primarily sinusoidal. Portal hypertension may also arise from presinusoidal obstruction, either outside (e.g., portal vein thrombosis) or within (e.g., schistosomiasis) the liver. Similarly, lesions leading to portal hypertension may be postsinusoidal, either within the liver (e.g., veno-occlusive disease) or distal to it (e.g., Budd-Chiari syndrome, right-sided heart failure). In rare circumstances, portal hypertension can result in a normal liver from markedly increased inflow beyond the capacity of the compliant portal vessels to absorb. Examples include arterial-portal fistulas and massive splenomegaly due to infection or neoplasm.

CLINICAL PRESENTATION. The cirrhotic with portal hypertension will often have variceal hemorrhage (Fig. 153–2), ascites, encephalopathy, or some manifestation of hepatic dysfunction such as coagulopathy or infection. Splenomegaly and/or distention of abdominal wall veins (caput medusae) may be initial or associated findings. Patients with non-cirrhotic portal hypertension generally

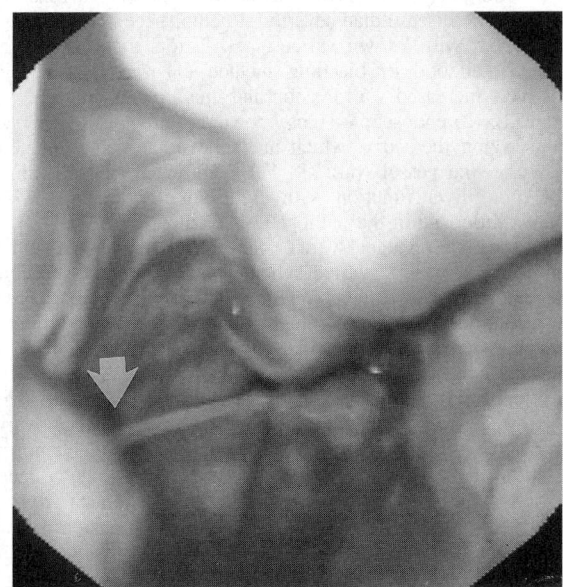

FIGURE 153–2 ▪ Active hemorrhage from an esophageal varix. An endoscopic view of hemorrhage in a patient with esophageal varices; a stream of blood across the esophageal lumen is evident (*arrow*). (Courtesy of Dr. Timothy Davern and Dr. Johannes Koch.)

have well-preserved liver function so that clinical manifestations primarily reflect altered hemodynamics. In patients with presinusoidal lesions such as schistosomiasis or portal vein thrombosis, variceal hemorrhage and splenomegaly are prominent. In postsinusoidal obstruction, such as veno-occlusive disease or Budd-Chiari syndrome, hepatomegaly and rapid onset of ascites and weight gain are typical presenting symptoms. When portal abnormalities are a manifestation of infection or neoplasm, there may be specific associated non-hepatic findings, such as a hypercoagulable state, anemia, or evidence of heart failure.

DIAGNOSIS. Portal hypertension should be suspected in any patient with ascites, splenomegaly, encephalopathy, or gastroesophageal varices. Assessment should include liver chemistry, prothrombin time, serum albumin, and complete blood cell count. Non-invasive abdominal imaging using US with Doppler probe can assess the hepatic parenchyma and patency/flow characteristics of the portal and hepatic veins. Varices may also be visualized using either this technique or abdominal CT or may be seen directly by upper endoscopy. It is important to remember that the presence of varices does not establish whether the lesion is intrahepatic or extrahepatic, because varices can develop with presinusoidal and postsinusoidal lesions. If abdominal US with Doppler is not conclusive, portal hemodynamics may be measured more directly by hepatic vein catheterization with a balloon-tipped catheter within the liver attached to a pressure transducer. When deflated, the catheter measures systemic venous (i.e., inferior vena cava [IVC]) pressure. When inflated within the liver, this "wedged" hepatic vein pressure (WHVP) reflects the pressure distal to the balloon (i.e., within the hepatic parenchyma). The differences between these two measurements (WHVP–IVC) or the wedged hepatic venous gradient (WHPG) is normally less than 5 mm Hg. Once this difference exceeds 12 mm Hg, variceal hemorrhage is possible; however, the risk of hemorrhage does not correlate with the extent of elevation beyond this threshold. Mesenteric angiography may be useful to visualize portal vessels directly, either when an extrahepatic cause of portal hypertension is suspected or in anticipation of elective short surgery in which definition of the anatomy is required.

VARICEAL HEMORRHAGE. Hemorrhage from gastroesophageal varices (see Chapter 123) is often the initial complication of portal hypertension (see Fig. 153–2). Less commonly, variceal hemorrhage occurs from other sites of portosystemic collateral vessels, including the duodenum, rectum, or sites of prior abdominal surgery.

Esophageal variceal hemorrhage typically occurs as painless, large-volume hematemesis or melena with minimal abdominal pain. Signs of significant volume depletion, including orthostasis and pallor, are common. Mortality from variceal hemorrhage is more a function of underlying liver disease than severity of hemorrhage per se.

In a patient with known varices, risk factors that correlate with increased likelihood of bleeding include (1) variceal size (large varices have increased wall tension and thus greater thinning of the vessel wall); (2) endoscopic signs known as red wales or cherry-red spots overlying the varix, which are believed to represent hemorrhage within the vessel wall; (3) WHPG greater than 12 mm Hg; and (4) poor liver function with ascites and/or jaundice. Gastric acid plays little role in the pathogenesis of bleeding.

Patients with esophageal varices may bleed from associated gastric varices. A gastric variceal hemorrhage is more difficult to diagnose than an esophageal one because gastric varices are not easily distinguished from prominent rugae. A rare cause of gastric variceal hemorrhage that should not be overlooked is splenic vein thrombosis due to pancreatic or retroperitoneal disease. In this setting, localized obstruction of short gastric veins leads to hemorrhage from gastric varices in the absence of esophageal varices. Splenectomy and splenic vein resection are curative. Hemorrhage from portal hypertensive gastropathy, also known as congestive gastropathy, refers to bleeding in the proximal stomach from submucosal veins engorged as a result of portal hypertension. Bleeding from this lesion is clinically indistinguishable from variceal hemorrhage and responds to portal decompression.

DIAGNOSIS AND TREATMENT (Table 153–3). Stabilizing blood pressure is the first requirement in suspected variceal hemorrhage. Replacing fluid and blood is essential in the orthostatic or hypotensive patient, but overexpanding volume with fresh-frozen plasma should

---

Table 153–3 ■ MANAGEMENT OF GASTROESOPHAGEAL VARICEAL HEMORRHAGE

1. Hemodynamic stabilization
2. Emergent diagnostic endoscopy
3. Initial control of hemorrhage (options)
   a. Endoscopic sclerotherapy
   b. Endoscopic variceal band ligation
   c. Intravenous vasopressin/nitroglycerin or octreotide
   d. Balloon tamponade
   e. Transjugular intrahepatic portacaval shunt (TIPS)
   f. Surgery: esophageal transection or non-selective portacaval shunt
4. Prevention of initial or recurrent variceal hemorrhage (options)
   a. Prophylactic β-blockers in high-risk patients who have not bled
   b. β-Blockers after initial bleeding episode
   c. Chronic obliterative endoscopic sclerotherapy or band ligation
   d. Portacaval shunt surgery
   e. Liver transplantation

---

be avoided in the stabilized individual, because it may increase portal pressure and accelerate hemorrhage. Endotracheal intubation to protect the airway is essential in the obtunded or inebriated patient to avoid aspiration and facilitate emergent endoscopy. Hemodynamic monitoring within the intensive-care unit may require placing intra-arterial or pulmonary artery catheters.

Once the patient's condition is stabilized, vigorous gastric lavage followed by emergent endoscopy is necessary to establish the source of hemorrhage, even if acute bleeding has subsided. Thirty to 50 per cent of bleeding episodes in patients with varices originate from non-variceal sources, particularly Mallory-Weiss tears, esophagitis, gastritis, or peptic ulcers. Bleeding from more than one lesion is not unusual.

INITIAL CONTROL OF VARICEAL HEMORRHAGE. Two thirds of variceal hemorrhage episodes will cease spontaneously, but rapid onset of rebleeding is significant. Thus, endoscopic hemostasis is required, either when varices are actively bleeding or when they display endoscopic evidence of recent bleeding (i.e., a visible punctum). Two endoscopic methods are equally effective in arresting active hemorrhage in more than 95% of patients: (1) direct or paravariceal injection with 1 to 2 mL of a sclerosant (ethanolamine oleate or sodium tetradecyl) or (2) band ligation, in which a rubber ligature is placed around the varix. Band ligation is associated with a lower incidence of esophageal ulceration and more rapid variceal obliteration than sclerotherapy.

Pharmacologic control of acute hemorrhage may be achieved using either a combination of intravenous vasopressin (0.2 to 0.4 units/minute) and nitroglycerin (5 μg/min, increased by 20-μg/min increments to a maximum of 200 μg/min) or a somatostatin analogue (octreotide, 50 μg bolus, then 50 μg/hour intravenously; this drug is not yet approved by the U.S. Food and Drug Administration for this indication). Although more costly, somatostatin analogues carry less systemic hemodynamic side effects than vasopressin (e.g., vasoconstriction) and may reduce the risk of rebleeding when used in conjunction with endoscopic hemostasis compared with endoscopic means alone.

In patients who continue to bleed after endoscopic or pharmacologic therapy, a Minnesota or Sengstaken-Blakemore tube can be used for balloon tamponade of vessels at the gastroesophageal junction. Intubation before placing the tube will reduce the risk of pulmonary aspiration. Only the gastric balloon should be inflated (250 mL for Sengstaken tube, 450 mL for Minnesota tube); inflating the esophageal balloon or using these devices in patients with hiatal hernias is associated with significant risk of esophageal perforation.

Emergent surgical portal decompression is an option in the rare patient in whom hemodynamic stabilization is not possible because of persistent hemorrhage. Optimal surgical options include esophageal staple-transection or portacaval shunt (end-to-side or mesocaval). Emergent abdominal surgery to control variceal hemorrhage should be undertaken with the recognition that subsequent liver transplantation may become much more technically difficult.

In the patient who is a potential candidate for liver transplantation, placing a transjugular intrahepatic portasystemic shunt (TIPS) is an attractive alternative to surgery. The shunt is placed under fluoroscopic guidance, creating an intrahepatic channel that decompresses the portal circulation non-selectively. TIPS is physiologically similar to a side-to-side surgical shunt. In experienced hands, placement is successful in more than 90% of patients, and bleeding is controlled in 90 to 95%.

PREVENTING INITIAL OR RECURRENT VARICEAL HEMORRHAGE.

In the patient with moderate or large varices and well-preserved liver function, prophylactic use of β-blockers (propranolol or nadolol) to reduce resting heart rate by 25% will lessen the risk of first variceal hemorrhage. β-Blockers will also reduce the risk of bleeding from congestive gastropathy and gastric varices associated with portal hypertension. Combined administration of β-blockers and nitrates (e.g., isosorbide-5-mononitrate) can reduce portal pressure to a greater extent than either drug alone and lead to a reduced risk of recurrent hemorrhage. Despite this efficacy in portal hypertension, the agents have no effect on mortality. In contrast to β-blockers, prophylactic sclerotherapy has not been shown consistently to reduce the likelihood of initial bleeding.

In patients who have already survived an episode of hemorrhage from varices or congestive gastropathy, β-blockers reduce the risk of rebleeding but are discontinued in up to 25% of patients because of adverse effects (e.g., bronchoconstriction, impotence, lethargy, heart failure). In those in whom β-blockers fail or who are intolerant of β-blockers, obliterating varices by endoscopic sclerotherapy is equally effective; multiple sessions are required to eliminate varices initially, followed by regular endoscopic surveillance every 3 to 6 months. There is no synergistic effect of β-blockers and long-term sclerotherapy. Studies using endoscopic band ligation suggest better efficacy than with β-blockers after short-term follow-up.

Elective portacaval shunt surgery is more effective at eliminating rebleeding than long-term sclerotherapy but is associated with higher initial transfusion requirement and cost. Like non-surgical treatments, there is no improvement in survival afforded by portacaval shunts. In experienced surgical hands, the optimal operation is a distal splenorenal shunt that selectively decompresses the short gastric veins draining the varices. The procedure is time consuming and usually requires preoperative angiography. Because portal flow is preserved, however, it is associated with a lower rate of encephalopathy and ascites. The role of TIPS is uncertain in long-term management of patients with variceal hemorrhage; TIPS is consistently more effective than sclerotherapy in reducing rebleeding in randomized trials, but it does not reduce overall morbidity, mortality, or health care costs. A significant risk of shunt occlusion or encephalopathy is emerging in longer follow-up of patients treated by TIPS, which may confine its use to those awaiting liver transplantation.

ASCITES. Ascites is the accumulation of excess fluid in the abdomen. Cirrhosis is the underlying cause in at least 80% of patients, but other etiologic factors in addition to liver disease must always be considered.

PATHOGENESIS. Multiple factors contribute to ascites formation in chronic liver injury:

1. *Sinusoidal hypertension,* which develops because of increased outflow resistance from matrix deposition and possibly stellate cell contraction. Initially, albumin traverses the porous sinusoidal endothelium along with fluid; but as fibrosis progresses, only protein-free fluid can escape the sinusoid, from where it enters hepatic lymphatics. Continued accumulation of lymph overcomes the capacity for lymphatic drainage, and the excess fluid "weeps" from the liver into the peritoneal cavity.
2. *Hypoalbuminemia,* which worsens with advancing liver dysfunction and decreases oncotic pressure.
3. *Fixed capacity to resorb ascites,* despite its increasing accumulation.
4. *Increased sodium reabsorption by the kidneys,* possibly due to humoral factors
5. *Splanchnic arteriolar vasodilation,* which may independently stimulate sodium and free water retention by increasing sympathetic tone.

The roles of antidiuretic hormone and atrial natriuretic peptide are not clearly established despite extensive study.

DIAGNOSTIC EVALUATION (Table 153–4). All patients with new-onset ascites or those requiring hospitalization should undergo diagnostic paracentesis with cell count, ascites albumin determination, Gram stain, and culture. US guidance may be necessary if ascites is minimal or fluid is loculated. Directly inoculating ascites into blood culture broth at the bedside is essential because the low bacterial count of infected ascites may otherwise lead to false-negative cul-

Table 153–4 ■ DIAGNOSTIC EVALUATION OF ASCITES

Paracentesis (see also Table 142–2)
1. Fluid analysis: cell count, albumin, Gram stain
2. Calculate serum-ascites albumin gradient (SAAG):
   SAAG ≥ 1.1 g/dL: portal hypertension very likely
   SAAG < 1.1 g/dL: suspect other causes
3. Direct bedside inoculation of ascites into blood culture broth
4. Optional: amylase, bilirubin, triglycerides, cytology, myobacterial culture

Abdominal Ultrasonography With Doppler
1. Assess patency/flow in portal, hepatic, and splenic veins
2. Examine hepatic and splenic parenchyma
3. Exclude neoplasm or peritoneal disease
4. Assess biliary ductal size

ture results. The status of all patients with new ascites should be evaluated by abdominal US.

The serum-ascites albumin gradient (SAAG), calculated by subtracting the ascites albumin concentration from the serum value, is the most accurate method to classify ascites. A SAAG value of greater than 1.1 g/dL predicts a portal hypertensive cause with more than 95% accuracy. Values less than 1.1 g/dL are associated with neoplasms, tuberculosis, pancreatitis, or bile leak. SAAG values less than 1.1 g/dL indicate the ascitic fluid needs additional testing, which may include amylase, cytology, and mycobacterial culture.

TREATMENT. Most patients with cirrhotic ascites respond to dietary sodium restriction (40 to 60 mEq/day) and a diuretic. Spironolactone should be started at 50 to 100 mg/day and can be advanced up to 400 mg to achieve a daily weight loss of 0.5 to 0.75 kg in patients without peripheral edema; more rapid weight loss is safe if peripheral edema is present. Furosemide can be used instead of or in combination with spironolactone, beginning at a dose of 40 mg/day, although there is a greater incidence of azotemia than with spironolactone. Patients treated with two diuretics must be monitored carefully because weight loss may be rapid, even when one diuretic alone has been ineffective. In patients with alcoholic liver disease, abstinence may be effective therapy if cirrhosis has not yet developed.

Ten per cent of patients with ascites fail to respond to standard therapy, either because fluid cannot be mobilized or there is associated prerenal azotemia. In these patients, therapeutic paracentesis is safe and can remove 4 to 6 L or more per visit in those with peripheral edema. In non-edematous patients, safe paracentesis requires infusing 6 to 8 g of albumin per liter of ascites removed. This option is quite costly; cost may be reduced by substituting for albumin with other plasma expanders such as dextran 70, although experience with non-albumin expanders is less extensive. Repeated paracentesis may increase the risk of bacterial peritonitis. Peritoneovenous shunting, performed by surgically placing a subcutaneous catheter between the superior vena cava and peritoneum, is as effective as therapeutic paracentesis in treating refractory ascites. However, low-grade disseminated intravascular coagulopathy, catheter infection, and shunt occlusion are frequent complications that reduce long-term efficacy substantially. Like other therapy for complications of portal hypertension, neither paracentesis nor peritoneovenous shunts prolong survival. Instead, survival is a function of the severity of liver disease. TIPS has been proposed as an alternative to the peritoneovenous shunt in treating refractory ascites. Preliminary results are encouraging in small numbers of patients, but long-term follow-up in larger study groups is required. Liver transplantation remains the most definitive therapy for liver disease underlying ascites and should be considered first when ascites develops. The urgency for transplantation is increased if complications of ascites appear, particularly spontaneous bacterial peritonitis.

COMPLICATIONS. Spontaneous bacterial peritonitis (SBP) is an ominous complication of late-stage liver disease because it portends a 2-year survival rate of less than 50%. The pathogenesis is uncertain but is believed to reflect altered gut wall permeability to bacteria, impaired capacity of hepatic and splenic macrophages to clear portal bacteremias, and/or the presence of a large volume of peritoneal fluid conducive to bacterial growth. The clinical presentation is subtle, and frank peritoneal pain or tenderness is uncommon. Thus, clinicians must have a high index of suspicion to recognize SBP before it is fatal. Typical findings include fever, signs of sepsis, or decompensation of previously stable liver function manifested by new encephalopathy or azotemia. Common causative organisms include *Escherichia coli, Pneumococcus, Klebsiella,* and anaerobes. Because ascites Gram stain is rarely positive, if ascites polymorphonuclear leukocyte count is greater than 250/mm³, a presumptive diagnosis should be made and empirical antibiotic therapy (e.g., cefotaxime, 1 to 2 g intravenously every 6 to 8 hours, or ceftriaxone, 500 to 1000 mg intravenously every 12 hours) given for 5 to 7 days. Adequate response to therapy should be documented by demonstrating a 50% reduction in ascites white blood cell (WBC) count. Culture-negative neutrophilic ascites (i.e., ascites WBC ≥ 250/mm³) is common, especially if ascites has not been promptly inoculated into blood culture broth; these patients should be treated for presumed SBP, and the response to antibiotics should be documented with repeat paracentesis. The recurrence rate of SBP is more than 70% in 1 year but can be reduced if patients are treated prophylactically with norfloxacin, 400 mg/day. Prophylaxis may be appropriate for high-risk patients even before the first episode of SBP (i.e., those with gastrointestinal bleeding or low-protein ascites), especially if the patient is a candidate for liver transplantation.

Other complications of ascites include hepatic hydrothorax, abdominal wall hernias with rupture, and tense ascites with leakage (especially after paracentesis). Conservative management consists of appropriate initial therapy for most of these except hernia rupture, which requires surgical reduction.

HEPATORENAL SYNDROME. Hepatorenal syndrome, also known as functional renal failure, is defined as renal failure associated with severe liver disease without an intrinsic abnormality of the kidney. Ascites is typically present. The cause is unknown, but reductions in renal blood flow, cortical perfusion, and glomerular filtration rate are consistent features. Elevated circulating levels of endothelin-1, a potent vasoconstrictor, may play an important role. The diagnosis is established in patients with cirrhosis by documenting very low urine sodium (<10 mEq/L) and oliguria in the absence of intravascular volume depletion. The syndrome must therefore be distinguished from prerenal azotemia by an empirical fluid challenge (1000 mL saline) or measurement of pulmonary wedge pressure. Other likely causes of renal failure must be excluded, such as acute tubular necrosis or renal impairment from aminoglycosides and contrast agents, although these typically lead to high sodium excretion. Patients with liver disease are especially sensitive to inhibition of renal vasodilation by non-steroidal anti-inflammatory drugs (NSAIDs). The prognosis of hepatorenal syndrome is very poor, in part because onset of the syndrome denotes end-stage liver disease. The most effective treatment for hepatorenal syndrome is to correct the underlying liver disease, by liver transplantation if appropriate. Treating any underlying infections and optimizing volume status are important adjunctive measures. Potentially nephrotoxic drugs, especially NSAIDs, should be withdrawn. Isolated responses to peritoneovenous shunt or TIPS have been reported, but no randomized trials have been conducted to confirm these treatments. There are no effective pharmacologic agents.

HEPATIC ENCEPHALOPATHY (See Chapter 154)

SYNTHETIC DYSFUNCTION AND COAGULOPATHY. Broad defects in protein synthesis and/or secretion characterize the cirrhotic liver. Clinically apparent defects include hypoalbuminemia, which can reduce oncotic pressure and accentuate edema formation, and reduced concentrations of plasma clotting factors. All clotting factors except Factor VIII are synthesized in the liver and may be defective both qualitatively and quantitatively. Fibrinolysis is also affected. In addition, Factors II, VII, IX, and X are vitamin K dependent and thus may have reduced activity if deficient because of cholestasis-related fat malabsorption. Thrombocytopenia can result from bone marrow hypoplasia induced by alcohol or due to hypersplenism associated with splenomegaly in portal hypertension. Platelet sequestration by the congested spleen often leads to significant thrombocytopenia, yet clinically significant bleeding almost never occurs; platelet transfusions are therefore not indicated in this setting unless there is an additional platelet defect. Similarly, portacaval decompression or splenectomy is usually curative but is not appropriate unless required to manage variceal hemorrhage.

HEPATOPULMONARY SYNDROME. Hepatopulmonary syndrome refers to the triad of liver disease, pulmonary vascular dilation, and reduced arterial oxygenation. Although marked manifestations of the syndrome are unusual in patients with chronic liver disease, more subtle abnormalities of oxygenation are common. The abnormalities have been attributed to right-to-left shunts through pulmonary arteriovenous fistulas and development of bronchial varices in association with pulmonary hypertension. The syndrome occurs in chronic liver disease of all types and is more common in those with severe liver disease (e.g., Child's C cirrhosis). As a result, the prognosis is poor, on the basis of both the pulmonary and hepatic disease. Affected patients complain of exertional dyspnea, with pulmonary function tests demonstrating normal lung volumes but markedly reduced diffusing capacity. Hypoxemia and dyspnea are usually worse in the standing than the supine position. Oxygen can improve symptoms but does not reverse the defects. Resolution of the syndrome has been seen in many patients after liver transplantation.

OTHER SEQUELAE. Feminization in men with end-stage cirrhosis is particularly common in alcoholics and has been associated with increased estrogen and diminished testosterone levels. Hypogonadism can be an independent consequence of alcohol abuse. *Altered drug metabolism* (see Chapter 148) is an important consideration in prescribing drugs to those with end-stage liver disease, either because of impaired clearance leading to enhanced activity or toxicity, reduced sulfoxidation, or decreased protein binding. *Bone disease* manifested as thinning and spontaneous fractures is a major complication of late-stage cholestatic or alcoholic liver disease, especially primary biliary cirrhosis. Hepatic osteodystrophy can be due to osteoporosis (see Chapter 257), osteomalacia (see Chapter 263), or both. Hepatocellular carcinoma (see Chapter 156) is often preceded by cirrhosis, which is usually but not always clinically apparent.

Cirrhosis—General

Caldwell SH, Oelsner DH, Iezzoni JC, et al: Cryptogenic cirrhosis: Clinical characterization and risk factors for underlying disease. Hepatology 29:664, 1999. *This is the most recent of several studies suggesting that many patients with "cryptogenic cirrhosis" have underlying nonalcoholic steatohepatitis (NASH).*
Poynard T, Bedossa P, Opolon P: Natural history of liver fibrosis progression in patients with chronic hepatitis C. Lancet 349:825, 1997. *Landmark study defining risk factors and natural history of progression to cirrhosis in patients with HCV infection.*

Alcoholic Liver Disease

McCullough AJ, O'Connor JF: Alcoholic liver disease: Proposed recommendations for the American College of Gastroenterology. Am J Gastroenterol 93:2022, 1998. *A thorough analysis of currently accepted criteria for diagnosis, clinical features, and therapy of alcoholic liver disease, including transplantation.*

Primary Biliary Cirrhosis

Angulo P, Batts KP, Therneau TM, et al: Long-term ursodeoxycholic acid delays histological progression in primary biliary cirrhosis. Hepatology 29:644, 1999. *The best long-term data to date showing a beneficial effect of ursodeoxycholic acid in primary biliary cirrhosis.*
Bassnedine MF, Jones DE, Yeaman SJ: Biochemistry and autoimmune response to the 2-oxoacid dehydrogenase complexes in primary biliary cirrhosis. Semin Liver Dis 17:49, 1997. *Review of our current knowledge about autoantigens in primary biliary cirrhosis.*

Variceal Hemorrhage

Rossle M, Haag K, Ochs A, et al: The transjugular intrahepatic portasystemic stent-shunt procedure for variceal bleeding. N Engl J Med 330:165, 1994. *Large trial demonstrating efficacy of TIPS to treat patients with cirrhosis and variceal hemorrhage; documents reduction in portal venous pressure gradient and cites incidence of complications.*
Sarin SK, Lamba GS, Kumar M, et al: Comparison of endoscopic ligation and propranolol for the primary prevention of variceal bleeding. N Engl J Med 340:988, 1999. *A trial suggesting increased efficacy of endoscopic ligation vs. propranolol in primary prevention of variceal hemorrhage. This conclusion remains controversial, as outlined in an accompanying editorial (p. 1033 of the same issue of N Engl J Med).*

Ascites—Diagnosis and Management

Martin PY, Gines P, Schrier RW: Nitric oxide as a mediator of hemodynamic abnormalities and sodium and water retention in cirrhosis. N Engl J Med 339:533, 1998. *A review of data implicating nitric oxide as a potential mediator of metabolic derangements associated with ascites formation.*
Runyon B: Care of patients with ascites. N Engl J Med 330:337, 1994. *Practical review of diagnostic and therapeutic issues in management of ascites.*

Hepatorenal Syndrome

Bataller R, Gines P, Guevara M, Arroyo V: Hepatorenal syndrome. Semin Liver Dis 17:233, 1997. *An excellent review.*
Guevara M, Gines P, Bandi JC, et al: Transjugular intrahepatic portosystemic shunt in hepatorenal syndrome: Effects on renal function and vasoactive systems. Hepatology 28:416, 1998. *Uncontrolled but carefully obtained data suggesting a potential role of TIPS in the treatment of hepatorenal syndrome.*

154 ACUTE AND CHRONIC LIVER FAILURE AND HEPATIC ENCEPHALOPATHY

Anna Mae Diehl

Liver failure is difficult to define because it implies an understanding of the most critical functions of the organ. The fact that no machine has been developed to save patients with liver failure indicates either that its most important functions are not well understood or that the liver performs so many complex vital functions that no single machine can replace all of them. Failure to complete one or more of these vital tasks can occur either due to massive destruction of liver cells or because liver cells become functionally "paralyzed" or "stunned," although they are not dead.

Acute liver failure can happen suddenly in patients without pre-existing liver disease. *Chronic liver failure* can also evolve gradually in individuals with various kinds of chronic liver problems. A key clinical benchmark to gauge the extent of globally deranged liver function is the impairment of brain function, or hepatic encephalopathy.

HEPATIC ENCEPHALOPATHY

DEFINITION. Hepatic encephalopathy is a poorly defined neuropsychiatric disorder that develops when certain products that are usually metabolized (detoxified) by the liver escape into the systemic circulation. Hepatic encephalopathy, which is potentially reversible, represents a spectrum of neurologic manifestations ranging from mild changes in personality to altered motor functions and/or level of consciousness. Clinical manifestations and treatment depend on whether hepatic encephalopathy is related to acute (fulminant) or chronic liver failure.

INCIDENCE AND PREVALENCE. Clinically overt hepatic encephalopathy is a universal feature of acute liver failure, whereas either subclinical or overt hepatic encephalopathy can be diagnosed in 50 to 70% of patients with chronic hepatic failure. However, the actual incidence and prevalence of hepatic encephalopathy are difficult to estimate because of differences in definition, diagnostic methods, and the types of patients studied.

PATHOGENESIS. The impairment of the central nervous system (CNS) in hepatic encephalopathy is probably multifactorial in origin. Several theories have been proposed, but none alone is adequate.

AMMONIA/GLUTAMINE NEUROTOXICITY. Ammonia, which is produced by colonic bacteria and by deamination of glutamine in the small bowel, is absorbed into the portal circulation and usually removed and deactivated by the liver. Hepatic failure or portosystemic shunting generally leads to an increase in the concentration of ammonia in the systemic circulation. Bleeding into the gastrointestinal tract exacerbates hyperammonemia because this heavy intestinal protein load increases ammonia production in the gut.

The permeability of the blood-brain barrier to ammonia is increased in patients with liver failure, probably explaining the imperfect correlation between plasma ammonia levels and the degree of hepatic encephalopathy in different patients. The ammonia/glutamine theory of hepatic encephalopathy is imperfect because some patients with liver failure develop hepatic encephalopathy despite normal blood ammonia levels; furthermore, ammonia is neuroexcitatory, whereas hepatic encephalopathy is generally characterized by CNS depression.

AMINO ACID IMBALANCE. Plasma levels of aromatic amino acids increase and those of branched-chain amino acids decrease in chronic liver disease, particularly in patients with hepatic encephalopathy. These two types of amino acids compete with each other for transport across the blood-brain barrier. Hence, increased plasma levels of aromatic amino acids may result in increased CNS levels of aromatic amino acids relative to branched-chain amino acids. Because aromatic amino acids may be precursors of "false" neurotransmitters (e.g., octopamine and phenylethanolamine), excess CNS levels of aromatic amino acids may cause relative depletion of "true" excitatory neurotransmitters and relative excess of

weaker (false) neurotransmitters. However, injection of octopamine into the brains of rats does not produce hepatic encephalopathy, and use of branched-chain amino acid–enriched formulations of amino acids to normalize plasma amino acid ratios in cirrhotic patients does not consistently improve hepatic encephalopathy.

SYNERGISM HYPOTHESIS. Neurotoxic metabolites of sulfur-containing amino acids (mercaptans), certain aromatic amino acids (phenols), and fatty acids (octanoic acid) are increased in patients with hepatic encephalopathy, and these substances might potentiate the neurotoxicity of ammonia. However, hepatic encephalopathy has not been noted in anecdotal reports of patients with inborn errors of metabolism that result in increased mercaptan levels.

γ-AMINOBUTYRIC ACID (GABA). GABA is the main inhibitory neurotransmitter. In some animal models of fulminant liver failure, serum GABA-like activity, expression of postsynaptic GABA receptors, and blood-brain GABA transfer are increased. These findings suggest that accumulation of GABA may be the cause of hepatic encephalopathy. In support of the GABA theory, gut flora produce GABA, and drugs with GABA-like activity cause visually evoked potentials that mimic those in patients with hepatic encephalopathy. However, actual plasma and CNS GABA levels are probably not increased in patients with hepatic encephalopathy, and the blood-brain barrier permeability of GABA is poor. Nevertheless, a substance or substances with GABA-like actions, rather than GABA itself, may be involved in the pathogenesis of hepatic encephalopathy.

BENZODIAZEPINE HYPOTHESIS. The postsynaptic GABA receptor is closely linked to the barbiturate (picrotoxin) receptor and the benzodiazepine receptor. Together, this complex of receptors controls chloride influx in the postsynaptic neuron and, hence, is responsible for the generation of inhibitory postsynaptic potentials. Stimulation of benzodiazepine and barbiturate receptors potentiates GABA-mediated neural inhibition. Antagonism of these receptors blocks chloride transport and the generation of postsynaptic inhibitory potentials. These data suggest that some (non-GABA) endogenous ligand of one of the members of the GABA/benzodiazepine/barbiturate receptor complex accumulates in the CNS of patients with liver disease and may be responsible for hepatic encephalopathy. In support of the benzodiazepine theory, both diazepam and desmethyldiazepam have been found in the brains of patients with hepatic encephalopathy who did not ingest benzodiazepines. Furthermore, treatment with flumazenil, a benzodiazepine receptor antagonist, sometimes reverses hepatic encephalopathy.

CLINICAL MANIFESTATIONS. In both acute and chronic liver failure, severity of neurologic dysfunction with hepatic encephalopathy is variable and can be graded symptomatically (Table 154–1). In acute liver failure, hepatic encephalopathy is strongly associated with the development of cerebral edema and it may present clinically as high fever, tachycardia, tachypnea, hyperventilation, intermittent hypertension, decerebrate posture, profuse sweating, or cardiac arrhythmias. Of note is that papilledema is often absent in cerebral edema owing to acute liver failure, even when cerebral edema is severe.

Hepatic encephalopathy associated with chronic liver failure can present as subclinical hepatic encephalopathy, a single acute episode or recurrent episodes of hepatic encephalopathy, chronic hepatic encephalopathy, hepatocerebral degeneration, or spastic paralysis. Subclinical hepatic encephalopathy presents as a mild alteration of cognition (stage 0–1 of hepatic encephalopathy) and is usually recognized only by psychometric testing; it occurs in the majority of patients with cirrhosis and may predispose them to vehicular or work-related accidents.

Acute hepatic encephalopathy presents as clinically overt changes of mental state (stages 1–4 of hepatic encephalopathy) and progresses at a variable rate. Most episodes are precipitated by identifiable factors, including gastrointestinal bleeding, excessive protein intake, constipation, overdiuresis, hypokalemia, hyponatremia or hypernatremia, azotemia (often due to constipation or gastrointestinal bleeding), infection, poor compliance with lactulose therapy, sedatives (benzodiazepines, barbiturates, antiemetics), hepatic insult (alcohol, drugs, viral hepatitis), surgery, or the development of hepatocellular carcinoma. Correction of the precipitating factor(s) typically permits gradual return to a subclinical stage of hepatic encephalopathy.

Table 154–1 ■ CLINICAL STAGING OF HEPATIC ENCEPHALOPATHY

STAGE	CONSCIOUSNESS	COGNITION	BEHAVIOR	MOTOR FUNCTION	PSYCHOMETRIC TESTS
0–1	Normal	Normal	Normal	Normal	Slow
1	Abnormal sleep	Decreased attention and calculation ability	Mood change, anxious, irritable, monotone voice	Dyscoordinated handwriting, tremor	Very slow
2	Lethargic, ataxia, dysarthria	Memory decreased, disoriented to time	Dysinhibition, inappropriate	Asterixis, ataxia, dysarthria, yawning, sucking, blinking, expressionless	Poor
3	Confusion, delirium, semistupor, incontinence	Disoriented, incoherent, amnesia, rigidity	Bizarre, anger, paranoia, seizures	Abnormal reflexes, nystagmus, Babinski reflex	Unable to perform
4	Coma	None	Absent	Oculocephalic or oculovestibular response, decorticate or decerebrate posture, dilated pupils	Unable to perform

Chronic recurrent or protein-intolerant hepatic encephalopathy also manifests itself as clinically overt hepatic encephalopathy (stages 1–4), but it develops despite maintenance therapy for hepatic encephalopathy and in the absence of excessive dietary protein intake. This type of hepatic encephalopathy is extremely difficult to manage because of its resistance to conventional therapy and diet restrictions.

Hepatocerebral degeneration is a chronic unremitting motor disorder of variable severity (tremor, rigidity, hyperreflexia, or signs of advanced pyramidal, extrapyramidal, and cerebral dysfunction) in addition to recurrent episodes of classic overt hepatic encephalopathy. This extremely rare disorder usually occurs in patients with massive portosystemic shunts (often surgically created); it responds poorly to therapy. Spastic paralysis, which is the least common presentation of hepatic encephalopathy, occurs only rarely in patients with chronic hepatic encephalopathy and/or hepatocerebral degeneration; it also is very difficult to treat.

DIAGNOSIS AND DIFFERENTIAL DIAGNOSIS. Hepatic encephalopathy is a diagnosis of exclusion. Therefore, if a patient with acute or chronic liver failure suddenly develops altered mental status, concomitant problems such as intracranial lesions (hemorrhage, infarct, tumor, abscess), infections (meningitis, encephalitis, sepsis), metabolic encephalopathies (hyperglycemia or hypoglycemia, uremia, acidosis, electrolyte imbalance), alcohol intoxication or withdrawal, Wernicke's encephalopathy, drug toxicity (sedatives and other psychoactive medications), postictal encephalopathy, and primary neuropsychiatric disorders must be excluded.

Preclinical and mild hepatic encephalopathy (stages 0–1, 1, 2) can be recognized by poor performance on psychometric tests (e.g., Reitan Trail Test, Number Connection Test, digital part of Wechsler Adult Intelligence Scale, or digit copying part of Kendrick battery). Clinically suspected hepatic encephalopathy may be objectively confirmed by prolonged reaction time to visual or auditory evoked potentials. Measurement of serum ammonia level is nonsensitive because hepatic encephalopathy can occur in patients with a normal blood ammonia level.

Advanced hepatic encephalopathy (stages 3–4) is not difficult to recognize clinically. Patients should be closely observed to detect frequently associated elevations in intracranial pressure (ICP). One alternative is to monitor ICP, with epidural monitoring being the safest approach in selected patients. Computed tomography cannot reliably predict elevations in ICP but may be useful to exclude other causes of altered mental status, such as intracranial abscess or hemorrhage.

TREATMENT. Consistent with the current theories about the pathogenesis of hepatic encephalopathy, there are four general targets/goals of therapy: (1) intestines: decrease production and absorption of possible toxins; (2) liver: improve liver function and clearance of toxins; (3) blood-brain barrier: prevent penetration of potential toxins into the brain; and (4) brain: correct abnormal neuronal activity.

INTESTINAL PRODUCTION AND ABSORPTION. The small and large intestines are the main sources of ammonia and the other toxins that may cause hepatic encephalopathy. *Lactulose* is a non-absorbable disaccharide; by causing acidification of intestinal contents and acting as a cathartic agent, it decreases the absorption of ammonia into the blood stream. Lactulose can be given orally, through a nasogastric tube, or rectally (less effective) in doses of 30 to 120 mL/day to produce two to four soft bowel movements per day. Some patients are not able to tolerate lactulose because of frequent side effects of flatulence, abdominal cramps, and its excessively sweet taste.

Poorly absorbed antibiotics, such as neomycin (initially 1–2 g orally four times a day), alter intestinal flora and thus decrease the production of nitrogenous substances by bacteria and reduce the release of ammonia into the blood. Because chronic neomycin can promote colonization with resistant organisms and may be absorbed systemically and cause nephrotoxicity and ototoxicity, neomycin should be used for short periods of time, and the dose should be decreased to 1 to 2 g/day after achievement of the desired clinical effect. Alternatively, metronidazole can be given at 250 mg orally three times a day alone or with neomycin; the most common side effects of chronic metronidazole are peripheral neuropathy and dysgeusia.

Dietary restriction of protein can decrease the production of ammonia by colonic bacteria. However, long-term dietary protein restriction can lead to malnutrition and can be harmful, especially in patients with decreased liver synthetic function. If tolerated, a positive nitrogen balance may improve hepatic encephalopathy by promoting hepatic regeneration and increasing the capacity of muscle to detoxify ammonia. Ideally, the diet should contain at least 1.2 g/kg/day of protein, and higher total calorie intake may improve the tolerance to protein. However, restriction of protein to 70 g/day may be necessary.

IMPROVEMENT OF LIVER FUNCTION. Clinical trials are currently evaluating the role of supplementary zinc, which is a cofactor of urea cycle enzymes, and ornithine-aspartate, which can reduce blood ammonia by stimulating ureagenesis and synthesis of glutamine in the liver. Benzoate, which conjugates with glycine to form hippuric acid, and phenylacetate, which conjugates with glutamine to form phenylacetylglutamine, can provide potential alternative pathways for the urinary excretion of nitrogen-containing molecules.

BLOOD-BRAIN BARRIER. Branched-chain amino acids (valine, leucine, isoleucine) given orally or parenterally can theoretically normalize the aromatic amino acid/branched-chain amino acid ratio and prevent excessive penetration of aromatic amino acids into the brain. However, clinical trials have failed to show major beneficial effects of branched-chain amino acid administration, and this treatment is not generally recommended.

BRAIN. Flumazenil may transiently improve the mental state in selected patients with hepatic encephalopathy. However, this drug is available only for intravenous injection and is not useful for the chronic therapy. Bromocriptine does not improve the level of consciousness in patients with hepatic encephalopathy, but it may be useful for treatment of extrapyramidal manifestations in selected patients with hepatocerebral degeneration or spastic paralysis.

PREVENTION. Prevention of clinically overt hepatic encephalopathy includes early identification and timely correction of reversible precipitating factors, strict adherence to the diet, prevention of constipation, improvement of liver function, and supportive therapy.

DEFINITION. Acute liver failure is a clinical syndrome caused by sudden, massive destruction of liver cells or by insults that severely inhibit the ability of hepatocytes to accomplish their normal functions. The duration of time that elapses between the clinical recognition of liver disease and the onset of hepatic encephalopathy (and/or impairment of liver functions) has been used to classify acute liver failure: within 2 weeks—fulminant liver failure; within 2 to 8 weeks—subfulminant liver failure; and within 8 to 24 weeks—late onset liver failure. Patients with a shorter interval from the onset of jaundice to the development of hepatic encephalopathy generally have a better prognosis, with a lower incidence of ascites but a greater incidence of cerebral edema compared with those who develop hepatic encephalopathy more slowly.

ETIOLOGY. A specific cause of acute liver failure can be identified in 60 to 80% of cases. In the United States the most common causes are hepatitis B virus (HBV) (see Chapter 149); non-A, non-B, non-C viral hepatitis (see Chapter 149); and exposure to certain drugs/toxins (see Chapter 148). Acetaminophen ingestion is responsible for 10% of acute liver failure cases in the United States. Massive liver cell necrosis from other drugs such as isoniazid, halogenated anesthetics, phenytoin, propylthiouracil, and sulfonamides accounts for another 10%; acute liver failure can also be induced by drug interactions, as seen with alcohol and acetaminophen, acetaminophen and isoniazid, and isoniazid and rifampin. A well-recognized cause of acute liver failure is ingestion of poisonous mushrooms (*Amanita phalloides*). Rare causes include infection with Epstein-Barr virus, herpes simplex virus, and cytomegalovirus; ischemic liver cell necrosis; Budd-Chiari syndrome (see Chapter 153); autoimmune liver disease; Wilson's disease (see Chapter 220); hyperthermia; primary graft non-function, and partial hepatectomy. Acute fatty liver of pregnancy, Reye's syndrome, and certain drugs (tetracycline, fialuridine, or valproate) can induce acute liver failure without provoking significant necrosis of hepatocytes.

INCIDENCE AND PREVALENCE. There are an estimated 2000 cases of acute liver failure in the United States yearly, representing 0.1% of all deaths and about 6% of liver-related deaths. Approximately 7% of all liver transplants are performed for acute liver failure.

PATHOGENESIS. Acute liver failure can be caused by liver cell death or serious dysfunction of living liver cells. Hepatocytes may die of necrosis or of programmed cell death (apoptosis). The former results from depletion of adenosine triphosphate, which prevents cells from maintaining membrane integrity. The molecular mechanisms that lead to liver cell apoptosis are not currently known and require further detailed experimental and clinical studies.

CLINICAL MANIFESTATIONS. Clinical features of acute liver failure may result directly from the loss of functioning hepatocytes (jaundice, coagulopathy, hypoglycemia, metabolic acidosis) or from multiple systemic manifestations (rapid development of infection, peripheral vasodilatation with hypotension, pulmonary edema, renal failure, disseminated intravascular coagulation, cerebral edema). Hepatic encephalopathy and the other extrahepatic manifestations of liver failure probably reflect the inability of the diseased liver to clear gut-derived bacterial products (ammonia, endotoxins, and endotoxin-inducible proinflammatory cytokines, such as tumor necrosis factor-α) from the blood.

Cerebral edema complicates stages 3 and 4 of hepatic encephalopathy in 50 to 85% of patients with acute liver failure and represents one of the most serious complications. Clinical signs of cerebral edema occur when the ICP exceeds 30 mm Hg. The earliest signs are systolic hypertension and increased muscle tone that progresses to decerebrate posturing.

DIAGNOSIS AND DIFFERENTIAL DIAGNOSIS. The diagnosis of acute liver failure is based on clinical findings (rapid onset of jaundice, decreased liver size, evidence of hepatic encephalopathy) and biochemical abnormalities (elevated aminotransferase levels, hyperbilirubinemia, hyperammonemia, hypoglycemia, coagulopathy) in a patient without prior history of chronic liver disease. Imaging studies (abdominal ultrasonography, computed tomography) can help in the evaluation of liver size and in detecting stigmata of portal hypertension (presence of ascites, varices, splenomegaly), which more often accompany chronic liver disease. Imaging studies may also detect space-occupying lesions or occlusion of major blood vessels. Blood serology and toxicologic screens are helpful in identifying patients with suspected viral hepatitis or poisoning. Liver biopsy may be necessary to document the characteristic histologic patterns in patients with vaso-occlusive diseases, graft-versus-host disease, and other less common causes of acute liver failure. However, biopsy is very risky in patients with acute liver failure because they generally have a serious coagulopathy.

TREATMENT. In general, treatment of acute liver failure should include prevention, early recognition, and treatment of the sequelae of hepatic encephalopathy, that is, elevated ICP, infection, coagulopathy, acute renal failure, and metabolic abnormalities (hypoglycemia, acidosis). Patients with acute liver failure usually require care in an intensive-care unit, especially when they develop stage 2 to 3 hepatic encephalopathy, serious bleeding, sepsis, or recurrent bouts of hypoglycemia; most such patients require a central venous pressure monitor, arterial line, urinary catheter, and nasogastric tube. For patients in stage 3 or 4 hepatic encephalopathy, endotracheal intubation is essential to prevent aspiration; liver transplant candidates may benefit from continuous monitoring of ICP.

Manipulations that increase ICP (e.g., Trendelenburg positioning) should be avoided in patients with documented ICP elevations. There is no evidence that elective hyperventilation is effective for decreasing ICP or controlling cerebral edema. Volume expansion with crystalloid or colloid solutions may be necessary in patients with hypotension, but it can exacerbate elevations of ICP. Therefore, fluid balance must be monitored carefully.

Mannitol (at a dose of 1 g/kg) may decrease ICP in selected patients with acute liver failure. Mannitol is usually given as a rapid intravenous infusion of a 20% solution to patients with documented ICP above 30 mm Hg. In the absence of ICP monitoring, mannitol should be considered only in patients with progressive cerebral edema. It is excreted in the urine, so urine output and plasma osmolality must be monitored carefully.

Some authors advocate barbiturates (thiopentone, 3–5 mg/kg IV infusion over 15 minutes) to resolve signs of intracranial hypertension and then to maintain ICP below 20 mm Hg. However, barbiturates may cause hemodynamic instability and mask clinical manifestations of cerebral edema; they should not be administered without ICP monitoring.

Prevention of hypoglycemia may require a continuous infusion of 5 or 10% glucose. Regular determination of peripheral blood glucose (every 4–6 hours) is recommended.

Coagulopathy is common in patients with acute liver failure due to decreased platelet count and inadequate synthesis of clotting factors. Vitamin K should be given to determine if it improves the coagulopathy. Patients with clinically significant bleeding and those who need invasive procedures (e.g., endoscopy, placement of central lines) should receive fresh frozen plasma for temporary correction of the coagulopathy.

Orthotopic liver transplantation (see Chapter 155) offers a definitive treatment for acute liver failure. However, this surgery is an option only for highly selected patients with hepatic failure (Table 154–2).

PROGNOSIS. Despite advances in medical therapy and intensive care, the survival rate of patients whose acute liver failure progresses to stages 3 to 4 of hepatic encephalopathy is still poor (10–40%). Survival depends on the age, time between the onset of hepatic failure and development of hepatic encephalopathy, the prothrombin time, and, most importantly, the cause of acute liver failure. With the introduction of orthotopic liver transplantation, survival rates have increased to 60 to 80%.

CHRONIC LIVER FAILURE

DEFINITION. Chronic liver failure, which is a progressive decline of multiple liver functions in patients with established chronic liver disease, is frequently associated with intermittent episodes of hepatic encephalopathy. Hepatic encephalopathy can occur in cirrhosis of any cause and typically signifies significant portal hypertension and end stage of chronic liver disease.

Patient with known chronic liver disease can also develop an acute decompensation of liver function usually caused by one or more potentially reversible precipitating events such as sepsis, worsening renal function, gastrointestinal bleeding, or superimposed

Table 154–2 ■ INDICATIONS FOR ORTHOTOPIC LIVER TRANSPLANATION IN PATIENTS WITH ACUTE LIVER FALIURE

GROUP OF PATIENTS	CLINICAL-BIOCHEMICAL CRITERIA
Acute liver failure due to acetaminophen poisoning	pH < 7.3 or INR > 5.5 and serum creatinine > 3.4 mg/dL
Acute liver failure not caused by acetaminophen poisoning	INR > 6.5 or any three of the following: Age < 10 or > 40 years Cause: non-A, non-B, non-C hepatitis; halothane hepatitis; idiosyncratic drug reaction; Wilson's disease, ischemia Duration of jaundice before encephalopathy < 7 days INR > 3.5 Serum bilirubin > 17.6 mg/dL

INR = International normalized ratio

acute hepatic necrosis due to drugs, alcohol, viral infections, or ischemia. It is important to distinguish reversible precipitating factors from the inexorable progression of chronic liver disease.

ETIOLOGY, INCIDENCE, AND PREVALENCE. The most common causes of end-stage liver disease include alcohol abuse, viral hepatitis (B, C, D) (see Chapter 150), primary biliary cirrhosis (see Chapter 153), primary sclerosing cholangitis (see Chapter 157), hemochromatosis (see Chapter 221), α_1-antitrypsin deficiency (see Chapter 152), Wilson's disease (see Chapter 220), Budd-Chiari syndrome, schistosomiasis, drugs and toxins (see Chapter 148), steatohepatitis, and cryptogenic liver cirrhosis. The exact prevalence of chronic liver failure is unknown, but chronic liver failure is much more common than acute liver failure and probably accounts for most liver-related deaths.

PATHOGENESIS. Loss of more than 70% of functioning liver cells results in the covert redistribution of splanchnic blood flow, an energy-deficient state, and the failure of multiple secondary organs. Chronic liver injury eventually results in the death of hepatocytes followed by the accumulation of fibrous tissue. The fibrous tissue distorts the architecture of the organ, causing portal hypertension and the development of portosystemic shunting.

CLINICAL MANIFESTATIONS. Clinical manifestations of chronic liver failure evolve over many months to years and eventually include recurrent episodes of hepatic encephalopathy, progressive metabolic derangements (hypoalbuminemia, osteodystrophy, hyponatremia, acidosis, hyperbilirubinemia, glucose intolerance, and hypoglycemia), worsening of portal hypertension and its life-threatening complications (variceal bleeding, ascites, spontaneous bacterial peritonitis), severe pruritus, hematologic abnormalities (coagulopathy, leukopenia, thrombocytopenia, anemia, folate deficiency, hemoptysis), altered metabolism of endogenous hormones and drugs, and the development of functional renal failure (i.e., the hepatorenal syndrome).

The Child-Pugh classification, which was developed to assess the severity of chronic liver failure, is based on five equally weighted clinical-laboratory parameters (encephalopathy, ascites, serum albumin, serum bilirubin, nutritional status) with a maximal possible score of 15 (Table 154–3). Patients with compensated chronic liver failure are Child-Pugh A (score 1–5), whereas those with advanced cirrhosis are Child-Pugh C (score 11–15).

DIAGNOSIS AND DIFFERENTIAL DIAGNOSIS. The distinction between chronic liver failure and acute liver failure is based on clinical evidence of chronic liver disease: the stigmata of portal hypertension (ascites, splenomegaly, spider angiomas, varices), palmar erythema, gynecomastia, Dupuytren's contractures, testicular atrophy, and malnutrition. Multiple laboratory abnormalities (e.g., coagulopathy, hyperbilirubinemia, hypoproteinemia, and hypoalbu-

minemia) help confirm the diagnosis and define the degree of liver impairment.

TREATMENT. Treatment of chronic liver failure includes identification and correction of potentially reversible factors that may precipitate liver failure in patients with chronic liver disease, such as sepsis, gastrointestinal bleeding, heavy loads of dietary protein, and unnecessary medications (e.g., diuretics, sedatives, analgesics). Hepatic encephalopathy (see earlier) and other complications of portal hypertension (see Chapter 153) must be treated appropriately, and orthotopic liver transplantation should be considered (see Chapter 155).

PROGNOSIS. Patients with recurrent hepatic encephalopathy, refractory ascites, hepatorenal syndrome, and/or recurrent variceal bleeding should be considered for possible liver transplantation (see Chapter 155). Currently, absolute contraindications for orthotopic liver transplantation include extrahepatic hepatobiliary malignancy, active sepsis outside the hepatobiliary system, and cardiopulmonary failure. Six-month survival after orthotopic liver transplantation in clinically stable patients with chronic liver failure is as high as 90%; for patients in intensive-care units at the time of transplantation, however, 6-month survival is only about 65%.

PREVENTION. Widespread administration of hepatitis B vaccine will significantly decrease the incidence of hepatitis B, which is one of the major causes of chronic liver failure worldwide. New therapeutic regimens for the hepatitis C virus may significantly retard development of end-stage liver disease. Treatment of alcoholism is critical. Detection of hereditary liver diseases, such as hemochromatosis and Wilson's disease, can permit removal of excessive iron and copper by phlebotomy or medications and prevent cirrhosis.

Chung RT, Jaffe DL, Friedman LS: Complications of chronic liver disease. Crit Care Clin 11:431–463, 1995. *A thorough review of the treatment of chronic liver failure.*
Cordoba J, Blei AT: Treatment of hepatic encephalopathy. Am J Gastroenterol 10: 1429–1439, 1997. *A review of the main principles of treatment and therapy of specific types of hepatic encephalopathy.*
Mas A, Rodes J: Fulminant hepatic failure. Lancet 349:1081–1085, 1997. *Extensive description of pathogenesis and management of acute liver failure.*
Shahil AO, Mazariegos GV, Kramer OJ: Fulminant hepatic failure. Surg Clin North Am 79:77–108, 1999. *A review of acute liver failure.*

Table 154–3 ■ CHILD-PUGH CLASSIFICATION OF LIVER CIRRHOSIS

PARAMETER/CLASS	A	B	C
Encephalopathy	Absent	Mild	Severe
Ascites	Absent	Moderate, easily treated	Severe, refractory to treatment
Serum albumin	>3.5	3–3.5	<3.0
Total bilirubin	<2.0	2.0–3.0	>3.0
Nutritional status	Good	Mild malnutrition	Severe malnutrition

155 LIVER TRANSPLANTATION

John P. Roberts

In the last 30 years, liver transplantation has moved from an experimental procedure to accepted medical therapy for patients with acute or chronic liver failure. About 4500 liver transplantations are performed annually in the United States, and the 1-year survival rate following liver transplantation is now 85 to 90% or better (Fig. 155–1). The procedure is currently underwritten by most states, private insurance companies, and Medicare. Although liver transplantation is still an expensive procedure, the cost has decreased such that it now offers a better outcome and lower cost than many treatments for acute and chronic liver failure.

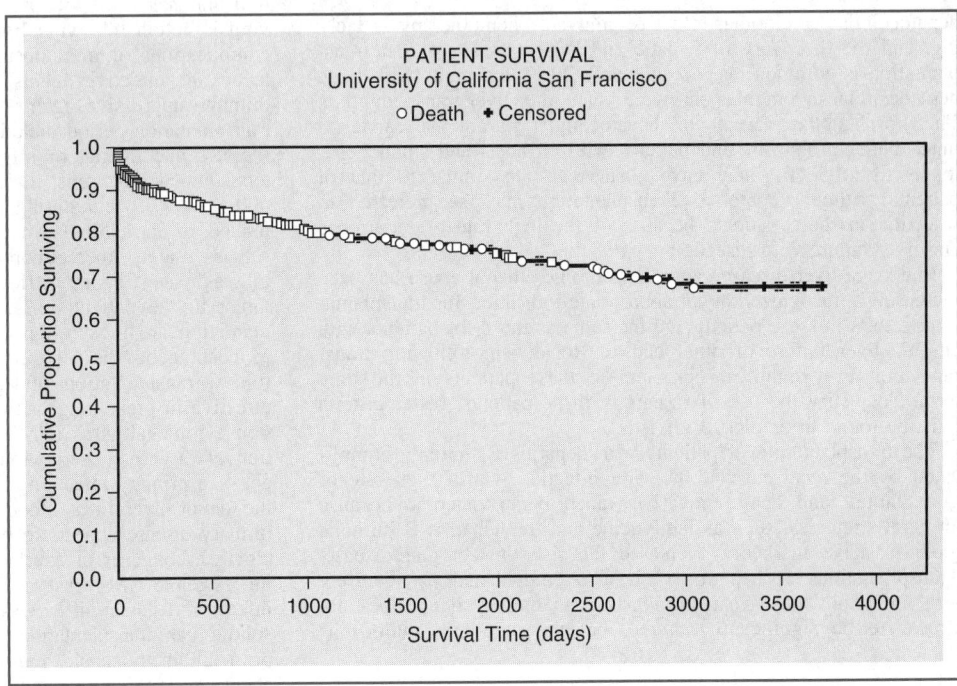

FIGURE 155-1 ■ UCSF liver transplantations: actuarial survival analysis.

The improvement in patient and graft survival following liver transplantation has resulted from changes in patient selection, operative techniques, and immunosuppressive regimens. As newer immnosuppressive medications become available, it appears likely that the morbidity and mortality rates and costs of liver transplantation will continue to decrease. With improvement in survival rate and with more patients undergoing liver transplantation, availability of donor organs has become the rate-limiting factor.

PATIENT SELECTION

The indications for liver transplantation have broadened with improved postoperative survival. Data are now available to predict the survival rate on the basis of the patient's native liver disease and pre-operative status. For example, an episode of spontaneous bacterial peritonitis suggests a 1-year survival rate of approximately 50%. It is also apparent that patients with stable cirrhosis, without decompensation or complications, are probably not well served by transplantation.

Liver transplantation has also altered the use of many of the procedures previously performed for complications of chronic liver disease, such as portal-systemic shunting for recurrent variceal hemorrhage, peritineovenous shunting for intractable ascites, and radical biliary tract surgery for patients with sclerosing cholangitis. These operations, which were once the only option for the patient with liver disease, are now assuming a secondary role. For example, portosystemic shunting has a poor outcome in patients with severe liver dysfunction, but these same patients can do well after liver transplantation. The use of portosystemic shunting (including the transhepatic portosystemic shunt [TIPS]) in the cirrhotic patient with well-preserved liver function is still indicated and more broadly used as organ shortages prolong the wait for transplantation.

Early referral for transplantation is extremely important for patients with fulminant *liver failure* (Chapter 154)—a diagnosis defined as evidence of hepatic failure, including stage III or IV encephalopathy, developing less than 8 weeks after the onset of signs or symptoms in a patient without known preexisting liver disease. Viral hepatitis is the most common cause of fulminant liver failure; other causes include toxins (e.g., *Amanita phalloides*), medications (e.g., acetaminophen), and metabolic disorders (e.g., fulminant Wilson's disease). These patients are at high risk for development of cerebral edema followed by brain herniation if not properly managed. Pre-transplantation management includes elevation of the head, careful monitoring of intracranial pressure, and aggressive therapy using mannitol, and sometimes even hyperventilation with barbiturate coma for increased intracranial pressure.

Transplantation is performed for a wide variety of causes of liver failure, with hepatitis C now the most common indication (Table 155–1). Contraindications to liver transplantation include systemic sepsis, active substance abuse (including ethanol), extrahepatic malignant disease, and advanced cardiopulmonary disease. Transplantation is generally not performed for cholangiocarcinoma because the survival rate of these patients following transplantation is poor.

Although liver transplantation seems to be logical therapy for

Table 155-1 ■ INDICATIONS FOR LIVER TRANSPLANTATION AND POSTOPERATIVE SURVIVAL*

DISEASE	(n)	ACTUARIAL PATIENT SURVIVAL (MONTHS)			
		12	24	60	120
Hepatitis C	138	90	79	63	63
Cryptogenic cirrhosis	105	87	82	67	65
Alcoholic liver disease	101	93	86	79	67
Primary biliary cirrhosis	69	89	89	82	53
Hepatitis C/alcoholic liver disease	68	91	87	82	67
Fulminant liver failure	60	90	90	90	76
Hepatitis B	58	74	69	69	61
Extrahepatic biliary atresia	48	91	88	88	88
Primary sclerosing cholangitis	47	93	93	87	66
Autoimmune hepatitis	36	92	92	89	89

*The 10 most common indications for liver transplantation based upon experience at University of California, San Francisco: February 1, 1988 to April 15, 1998.

hepatocellular carcinoma, effective adjuvant chemotherapy is lacking, and the discovery of hepatic and systemic cancer post transplantation is common; as a result, only 20% of patients with large hepatocellular carcinomas survive 3 years after liver transplantation. The fibrolamellar variant of hepatocellular carcinoma carries a much better prognosis, and patients with cirrhosis and small hepatomas (3 to 5 cm) may have a survival rate similar to that of patients without hepatoma. Transplantation may be preferred to resection in these patients because of the high rate of recurrence and liver failure with resection.

End-stage liver disease caused by chronic ethanol abuse has been increasingly recognized as an appropriate indication for transplantation; results in these patients are the same as those for patients with chronic liver failure of other causes. Recidivism following transplantation is a significant problem in these patients in the long term. To justify the use of organs in these patients, better criteria must be found to predict recidivism.

The transplantation of patients with hepatitis B, initially complicated by the recurrence of the viral infection with a high rate of graft failure and death, now has much better outcome because antiviral strategies, such as lamivudine and the hepatitis B immune globulin, have markedly decreased the risk of recurrent disease. Transplantation for hepatitis C is also complicated by recurrent viral infection; the 5-year survival rate in these patients does not appear to be significantly altered, but the long-term outlook is unclear.

DONOR SELECTION

Selection of the appropriate organ donor for liver transplantation is primarily based on ABO blood type and body size compatibility between donor and recipient. In general, donors for large non-O recipients tend to be more available than for small O recipients. This discrepancy reflects a higher accident rate for young adult males and the use of type O livers in recipients of other blood types. Priority for recipients is based on criteria that include the level of care that potential recipients currently require. Those in intensive care are assigned the highest priority; those at home, the lowest.

Because of the continuing shortage of organs for transplantation, there has been an interest in using portions of the liver from living donors and dividing cadaveric organs between two recipients. Living donor transplantation was first used in the situation in which a parent would donate the left lateral segment of the liver to a child. With the rapid acceptance of this technique for pediatric transplantation, interest turned to living-related transplantations between adults. Although these programs are in the early stages of development, it appears either the full left lobe or the full right lobe can provide adequate liver volume to the recipient. The division of a donor liver between the two recipients (split liver transplantation) has a similar rationale.

In auxiliary liver transplantation, the left lateral segment of the donor liver replaces the native left lateral segment, leaving the bulk of the native liver in place. This procedure is usually used in situations in which the recipient liver may be expected to recover, such as fulminant hepatic failure related to a toxin; the donor liver segment serves as a bridge until the patient recovers.

POST-TRANSPLATATION COMPLICATIONS

Complications of liver transplantation are primarily vascular (e.g., thrombosis of the anastomosed hepatic artery or portal vein), biliary (relating to reconstruction of the biliary tract), infectious, or related to organ rejection. Early post-operative hepatic artery thrombosis requires re-transplantation because it usually results in necrosis of the liver and/or biliary tree. Portal vein thrombosis can be asymptomatic or can present clinically as portal hypertension. Biliary tract complications usually appear as strictures within the biliary tree or as bile leaking from the biliary reconstruction. In the post-transplantation period, renal failure may result from preexisting renal dysfunction, intraoperative renal ischemia, postoperative cyclosporine toxicity, or a combination of these factors.

Postoperative infections are common (Chapter 314). The average patient experiences at least one episode of bacterial infection and has a 40 to 50% chance of development of a fungal or viral infection following liver transplantation. As one of the major complications of immunosuppression is infections, use of prophylactic anti-infective agents improves the therapeutic index of the immunosuppressive agents. Bacterial infections in the early post-transplantation period include biliary infections, intra-abdominal abscesses, pneumonia, or infections related to central venous catheters. Fungal infections, including systemic candidiasis (see Chapter 400), usually occur during the early transplantation period and are related to intravascular catheters or intra-abdominal candidal abscesses. Later, other opportunistic fungal infections, such as aspergillosis (see Chapter 401), predominate. All represent a serious threat to the patient's life. Viral infections following liver transplantation are most often caused by herpesviruses (Chapter 385). Mucocutaneous herpes simplex and varicella-zoster infections can follow transplantation, and prophylactic or therapeutic acyclovir is effective in preventing or treating these infections. Post-transplantation cytomegalovirus (CMV) infections represent either a reactivation of disease in a previously infected, immunosuppressed recipient or a primary infection arising from transmission of the agent via the donor liver or a blood transfusion (Chapter 386). In general, primary disease appears to be more serious than reactivation. Ganciclovir, a congener of acyclovir, is effective for preventing and treating systemic CMV disease in liver recipients. *Pneumocystis carinii* infection (Chapter 402) was previously a problem in all forms of solid organ transplantation, but with prophylactic use of trimethoprim-sulfamethoxazole, morbidity and mortality rates related to this agent have been eliminated in transplantation recipients.

IMMUNOSUPPRESSION

Immunosuppression in the liver transplantation recipient is currently based on the use of either cyclosporine or tacrolimus. Both drugs interfere with the production of interleukin 2 (IL-2) by T-helper cells and, as a result, prevent cell proliferation and the generation of cytotoxic T cells. Both drugs are usually started in the early post-transplantation period and are continued indefinitely. Both are metabolized by the cytochrome P-450-dependent monooxygenases, and therefore systemic levels can be decreased by drugs that induce this pathway, such as rifampin, barbiturates, or phenytoin. Major side effects of both drugs include neurotoxicity, manifested by headache and tremor; nephrotoxicity, manifested by increase in blood urea nitrogen (BUN) and creatinine levels; and by sensitivity to volume depletion; hyperkalemia; and glucose intolerance. Both drugs appear to increase the risk of post-transplantation lymphoproliferative disorders.

Prednisone is generally used in combination with cyclosporine or tacrolimus to prevent rejection. Prednisone reduces the release of interleukin 1 (IL-1) by macrophages and in this fashion inhibits amplification by IL-1 of IL-2 production. The complications of glucocorticoid therapy are well known (Chapter 28). In the liver transplantation recipient, a major issue is the exacerbation of the pre-transplantation bone loss that is associated with cholestatic liver disease by post-transplantation corticosteroids; significant disability may occur in the early post-transplantation period. Bisphosphonates may prove to be helpful in preventing steroid-induced bone disease in the transplantation recipient (Chapter 257).

Azathioprine, a third agent used for post-transplantation immunosuppression, blocks proliferation of white blood cells and thereby decreases the proliferative or amplification response of the rejection process. The major adverse effects of azathioprine are marrow depression and pancreatitis. Azathioprine likely will be replaced with the more powerful immunosuppressive agent mycophenolate mofetil, which inhibits synthesis of guanine nucleotides and appears to be more selective for lymphocytes. Randomized trials of mycophenolate mofetil have resulted in a 50% reduction in the incidence of acute rejection in recipients of renal transplantation; a similar reduction may be expected in liver transplantation recipients.

Another agent that holds promise is the humanized antibody against the IL-2 α chain receptor on the T cell. Studies in the renal transplantation population have demonstrated a 50% decrease in the rate of acute rejection with minimal toxicity.

The best long-term immunosuppressive regimen for the liver transplantation patient is unclear. With careful monitoring, prednisone probably can be safely withdrawn in most patients in the first year.

REJECTION

Rejection occurs commonly after liver transplantation, but with prompt diagnosis and treatment, it is becoming less important as a cause of graft loss. Histologic features include periportal infiltrate, bile duct epithelial damage, and endotheliitis. Treatment for rejection includes use of additional steroids or antilymphocyte preparations. A change from cyclosporine- to tacrolimus-based immunosuppression may result in an improved rate of salvage from ongoing rejection.

Lake JR, Martin P, McDiarmid SV, et al: Minimal criteria for placement of adults on the liver transplant waiting list: A report of a national conference organized by the American Society of Transplant Physicians and the American Association for the Study of Liver Diseases. Liver Transplant Surg 3:628–637, 1997. *This report describes the appropriateness of listing patients for transplantation on the basis of current knowledge of the natural-history of liver disease.*

Lo CM, Fan ST, Liu CL, et al: Applicability of living donor liver transplantation to high-urgency patients. Transplantation 65:73–77, 1999. *Describes the use of living donors for adult recipients.*

156 HEPATIC TUMORS

Michael Fallon

Tumors of the liver are relatively uncommon but are being increasingly recognized, often incidentally, owing to the frequent use of abdominal radiologic imaging techniques on which they present as space-occupying lesions. The appropriate diagnostic possibilities are best considered by determining the clinical setting in which the tumor is discovered (Table 156–1). Benign tumors are frequently found incidentally or present with local symptoms due to mass effect and may be influenced by gender and the use of oral contraceptives. Primary malignant tumors of the liver usually present in the setting of known chronic liver disease and may be associated with a deterioration in hepatic function. Metastatic liver tumors are most frequently found in patients who have documented primary extrahepatic tumors in the gastrointestinal tract, lung, or breast.

BENIGN HEPATIC TUMORS

HEMANGIOMA. Hemangiomas, which consist of ectatic dilated vascular spaces that usually measure less than 4 cm in diameter, are the most common benign hepatic tumors and do not have malignant potential. Autopsy studies show a prevalence of 2 to 7% in the general population. Because of hormonal factors, the preva-

lence is somewhat higher in females, in whom the lesions may also be larger. Most patients with hepatic hemangiomas are asymptomatic, and the tumors are usually discovered by chance. When symptomatic, abdominal pain may occur due to bleeding or thrombosis within the lesion or to stretching of Glisson's capsule. Hemoperitoneum can occur if a hemangioma near the surface of the liver ruptures, but this complication is so uncommon that prophylactic resection is not indicated. Rarely, disseminated intravascular coagulation with hypofibrinogenemia and thrombocytopenia (Kasabach-Merritt syndrome) is found in patients with large lesions. Imaging techniques can demonstrate characteristic findings that indicate a space-occupying lesion of the liver is a hepatic hemangioma: ultrasonography (US) generally reveals a well-circumscribed hyperechoic lesion; dynamic computed tomography (CT) with contrast medium enhancement shows peripheral enhancement early after contrast agent administration and homogeneous uptake on later images; and magnetic resonance imaging (MRI) shows a homogeneous high signal intensity lesion on T2-weighted images. However, technetium-99m–labeled human red cell scanning is the most specific test in lesions of more than 1.5 cm in diameter. Specific therapy is usually not necessary; in patients with symptoms or complications, surgical resection and/or hepatic artery ligation is recommended.

HEPATIC ADENOMA. Hepatic adenomas arise in normal livers from proliferation of normal-appearing hepatocytes that are arranged in cords or plates devoid of portal tracts. The estimated incidence is 4 per 1000. There is a strong association between the development of adenomas and the use of oral contraceptives, and 90% of these lesions are found in women of reproductive age during estrogen use. Uncommonly, adenomas have been reported in males using anabolic steroids and in patients with hemosiderosis or type I glycogen storage disease. The tumors are of variable size, usually single, and usually located in the right lobe. Patients frequently present with right upper quadrant fullness or pain, and the lesions are less commonly discovered incidentally. Patients may also present with severe abdominal pain and hypovolemic shock when the tumor ruptures and causes hemoperitoneum. This complication is particularly common during pregnancy and may have a high morbidity and mortality. Malignant transformation appears to be less common than previously thought, especially if stimulating factors are eliminated. The diagnosis should be suspected in females of child-bearing age using oral contraceptives. A combination of imaging modalities is frequently helpful: US often shows a hyperechoic lesion; CT and MRI demonstrate a solid tumor occasionally with areas of hemorrhage or necrosis; and sulfur colloid scanning demonstrates a filling defect due to the absence of Kupffer cells within the tumor. If the clinical and radiologic picture is consistent with hepatic adenoma, oral contraceptives should be discontinued and alternative birth control measures instituted to prevent pregnancy. Surgical resection should be considered for subcapsular lesions because of their increased risk of rupture, when

Table 156-1 ■ SELECTED FEATURES OF BENIGN AND MALIGNANT HEPATIC TUMORS

TUMOR	PATIENTS/RISK FACTORS	DIAGNOSIS	THERAPY
Benign			
Hemangioma	Healthy, incidental finding	Red blood cell–labeled scan	Observe; resect if symptoms
Adenoma	Young females on oral contraceptives	US/CT; sulfur-colloid scan: no uptake in lesion	Stop oral contraceptives; consider resection
Focal nodular hyperplasia	Middle-aged females, ± oral contraceptives	US/CT; sulfur-colloid scan: increased uptake in 60%	Stop oral contraceptives; observation
Focal fatty infiltration	Obesity, diabetes, corticosteroids, alcohol, weight changes, total parenteral nutrition	US/CT; sulfur-colloid scan: homogeneous uptake	Observation
Malignant			
Hepatocellular carcinoma	Cirrhosis, chronic viral hepatitis	US/three-phase CT; α-fetoprotein; biopsy	Resection, local ablation, liver transplantation
Fibrolamellar variant	Young, healthy, no risk factors	As above	As above
Cholangiocarcinoma	Sclerosing cholangitis, oriental cholangiopathies	US/CT/cholangiogram; carcinoembryonic antigen/CA 19-9	Resection, biliary drainage, chemotherapy/radiation
Metastatic	Extrahepatic malignancy (gastrointestinal, breast, lung)	US/CT, biopsy	Resection (colon cancer); treat underlying tumor
Angiosarcoma	Vinyl chloride, Thorotrast, arsenic exposure	US/CT/angiogram	Resection

US = ultrasonography; CT = computed tomography.

pregnancy is being contemplated, and when diagnostic uncertainty exists. In other patients, monitoring with serial imaging studies over a period of 6 to 12 months may be justified to document that there is no further increase in size or that the tumor has resolved after discontinuing oral contraceptive therapy.

FOCAL NODULAR HYPERPLASIA. Focal nodular hyperplasia is an uncommon hepatic pseudotumor thought to arise from hamartomatous change within the liver. Classically, there is a central scar with radiating bands of fibrosis surrounded by plates of hepatocytes associated with vessels and bile ducts. The lesion is more common in females and usually found incidentally between the ages of 20 to 50 years. There is no consistent association with the use of oral contraceptives, although estrogens do appear to have a trophic effect on focal nodular hyperplasia. The lesions are usually solitary, measure less than 5 cm, and are often located in the right hepatic lobe. Symptoms are reported by 10% of patients and usually consist of abdominal pain and/or right upper quadrant mass. Hemoperitoneum is rare. US, CT, and MRI detect focal nodular hyperplasia and may be diagnostic when the characteristic central scar is observed. Sulfur colloid scan demonstrates increased uptake in Kupffer cells in 60% of focal nodular hyperplasia lesions and thus may allow distinction from adenoma. Because focal nodular hyperplasia appears to lack malignant potential, asymptomatic lesions may be observed, with surgical intervention reserved for symptomatic or enlarging lesions or when there is diagnostic uncertainty.

BENIGN CYSTIC MASSES. Cystic lesions of the liver may be congenital or acquired. Most hepatic cysts are solitary and idiopathic, but multiple cysts presenting in adulthood as part of an autosomal dominant disorder involving the liver and kidney also occur. Idiopathic liver cysts are usually asymptomatic but may uncommonly cause right upper quadrant pain, abdominal fullness, and distention. Rare complications include spontaneous bleeding, rupture, or infection. Symptoms and complications are more commonly observed in inherited polycystic syndromes.

OTHER BENIGN TUMORS. A number of other uncommon benign lesions of the liver reported in adults arise from the biliary epithelium (adenomas), vascular endothelium (hemangioendothelioma, lymphangiomas), and mesenchymal cells (lipomas, leiomyomas). Other lesions that have been recognized on radiologic imaging and should be distinguished from true tumors in the liver include focal fatty infiltration and inflammatory pseudotumors.

MALIGNANT HEPATIC TUMORS

HEPATOCELLULAR CARCINOMA. DEFINITION. Hepatocellular carcinoma, or hepatoma, is an epithelial tumor arising from malignant transformation of the hepatocyte. It is the most common primary malignancy of the liver and is observed characteristically as a complication of chronic liver disease and cirrhosis, especially related to chronic viral infection with hepatitis B virus (HBV) and hepatitis C virus (HCV). Because early detection of hepatoma is difficult, the prognosis remains poor.

EPIDEMIOLOGY. Hepatocellular carcinoma is a leading cause of death from cancer throughout the world and is especially common in sub-Saharan Africa, Southeast Asia, Japan, and Korea, where its incidence (up to 500/100,000 per year) correlates with the prevalence of chronic HBV infection. In the United States, hepatoma is infrequent (annual incidence of 1–2 cases per 100,000) and commonly associated with liver disease caused by alcohol, HCV infection, hemochromatosis, or HBV infection. It occurs predominantly in males with a male:female ratio 2 to 4:1. The risk increases with age, and in Western countries hepatoma tends to appear in the fifth to seventh decades of life. In sub-Saharan Africa and Southeast Asia, hepatoma appears earlier and is likely related to vertical transmission of HBV infection. A rare fibrolamellar variant of hepatoma occurs in young patients without underlying liver disease and has a favorable prognosis because it often can be successfully resected.

PATHOGENESIS. Hepatocellular carcinoma usually arises in cirrhotic livers but may also develop rarely in patients without liver disease. The risk of hepatoma is highest in adult liver disease caused by HBV infection, HCV infection, and hemochromatosis. Cirrhosis results in cell proliferation and increased DNA synthesis in regenerating nodules; these processes may lead to aberrant rearrangements and altered regulatory protein function. Chronic HBV infection may predispose to hepatoma by integration of HBV DNA at sites within the human genome responsible for the control of the cell cycle, and thus lead to disruption of tumor suppresser genes or activation of oncogenes. The HBV gene product may also result in transactivation of oncogenes. Environmental factors are implicated in the development of hepatoma. The best understood is the ingestion of aflatoxins (especially aflatoxin B1) elaborated by Aspergillus molds, which frequently contaminate peanuts and grains. These toxins cause a mutation that impairs function of the p53 tumor suppresser gene. Other factors potentially important in the development of hepatoma include Thorotrast, a radionuclide used in angiographic procedures during the 1930s and 1940s, anabolic steroids and estrogens, and parasitic infection with Schistosoma, Clonorchis, Echinococcus, and Opisthorchis.

CLINICAL MANIFESTATIONS. Classically, hepatoma presents as abdominal pain, a palpable abdominal mass, and/or constitutional symptoms in patients with cirrhosis. More recently, tumors have been increasingly discovered during screening or incidentally during radiologic studies. Other symptoms and signs include fever, early satiety, anorexia, hepatomegaly, ascites, lower extremity edema, jaundice, and an hepatic arterial bruit or friction rub. Many signs and symptoms may be confused with progression of cirrhosis, and the diagnosis must be considered in cirrhotics with sudden decompensation or in those who develop bloody ascites. Hepatoma can also cause obstructive jaundice due to invasion or compression of the biliary tract or may bleed into the bile ducts. Hepatoma may also invade vascular structures and cause thrombosis of the portal or hepatic veins. Associated paraneoplastic syndromes include erythrocytosis, thrombocytosis, hypoglycemia, hypercholesterolemia, hypercalcemia, dysfibrinogenemia, cryofibrinogenemia, porphyria cutanea tarda, and hypertrophic osteoarthropathy. The tumor preferentially metastasizes to regional lymph nodes and lung.

DIAGNOSIS. Routine laboratory studies usually reflect abnormalities associated with the underlying chronic liver disease. The alkaline phosphatase may rise with tumor infiltration. α-Fetoprotein (AFP), an α_1-globulin produced in fetal, regenerating, and malignant hepatocytes, is a marker used in screening for hepatoma and for suggesting the diagnosis. It is elevated in 60 to 80% of patients, and the level is dependent, in part, on the size of the tumor. Levels of more than 400 to 500 ng/mL are virtually diagnostic when associated with a liver mass in a cirrhotic patient. Values over 20 ng/mL in cirrhosis have a sensitivity of 39 to 64% and a specificity of 64 to 91% for the presence of hepatoma. AFP levels may also rise during hepatic regeneration associated with inflammation, so the specificity of the test for the presence of tumor is lower in active hepatitis. Other proposed tumor markers are des-γ-carboxy prothrombin, plasma urokinase-like plasminogen activator, α-L-fucosidase, and transcobalamin I (patients with fibrolamellar variant). Imaging techniques that aid in the diagnosis include US, CT (especially three-phase tomography), and MRI. US generally shows a hypoechoic lesion. Dynamic CT with contrast characteristically demonstrates early diffuse enhancement of the lesion with rapid de-enhancement and a subsequent hypodense appearance relative to the surrounding parenchyma. T1-weighted MRI images may reveal high, low or isointense signals relative to surrounding parenchyma; the characteristic T2-weighted finding is a mosaic pattern of signal intensity within the lesion. Percutaneous fine-needle biopsy may not be needed to confirm the diagnosis in cirrhotic patients with an elevated AFP and a typical liver mass, but tissue diagnosis is reasonable in those without elevated tumor markers or when diagnostic uncertainty is present.

SCREENING. Screening and surveillance for hepatoma have been attempted in patients with cirrhosis in the hopes of detecting tumors at earlier and more treatable stages. Studies suggest that tumors of smaller size may be detected by surveillance and that the yield and efficacy of such strategies appear to be highest in areas with an increased prevalence of chronic viral liver disease. However, no controlled screening trials have been performed in the United States, and there is no consensus as to an appropriate surveillance schedule. Surveillance using US and AFP determinations at 6-month intervals is frequently used and is reasonable in high-risk patients for whom treatments are available and would be considered for use if a lesion were discovered.

TREATMENT. The prognosis of hepatoma is poor and is related to tumor size, residual liver function, and the presence of extrahepatic disease. For symptomatic unresectable disease, survival is less than 5% at 2 years. Treatment options include resection, transplantation, hepatic arterial chemo-embolization, intratumor injection of ethanol, and cryoablation. Systemic chemotherapy and radiation therapy are of limited value. The choice of a particular therapy must be individualized because no single therapy has emerged as a treatment of choice. Liver transplantation is reserved for patients with small tumors, no extrahepatic disease, and poor liver reserve.

CHOLANGIOCARCINOMA. DEFINITION AND EPIDEMIOLOGY. Cholangiocarcinoma is a rare malignant mucin-producing adenocarcinoma arising from the biliary epithelium. These tumors represent approximately 3% of all cancers, are most common in the Far East and Southeast Asia, and frequently present in the fifth to seventh decades of life. The major risk factor for the development of cholangiocarcinoma in the Far East and Southeast Asia is chronic biliary parasitic infestation (*Opisthorchis viverrini, Clonorchis sinensis*). In the United States, the most common risk factor is sclerosing cholangitis (9- to 21-fold increased risk). Other risk factors include biliary atresia and other developmental biliary abnormalities, intrahepatic cholelithiasis, and exposure to Thorotrast.

CLINICAL MANIFESTATIONS. Routine laboratory studies usually reveal evidence of biliary obstruction, including hyperbilirubinemia and elevations of alkaline phosphatase and γ-glutamyl transferase. The most common symptom is jaundice, which is present in 90 to 95% of patients. Other symptoms and signs include abdominal pain, pruritus, fever, weight loss, and a palpable abdominal mass. Purulent cholangitis occurs in up to 36% of patients. Two thirds of cholangiocarcinomas are located above the junction of the cystic duct and the hepatic duct, including intrahepatic or hilar (Klatskin) tumors. Cholangiocarcinomas spread by direct extension into contiguous structures, and lymphatic metastases are found in up to one third of patients. Hematogenous spread is rare.

DIAGNOSIS. When biliary obstruction is present, US and CT may allow localization of tumors as well as the identification of lobar atrophy. In the setting of sclerosing cholangitis, the development of cholangiocarcinoma may be extremely difficult to distinguish from progression of liver disease. Serum tumor markers including CA 19–9 and carcinoembryonic antigen, especially if used in combination, may be useful adjuncts in confirming the diagnosis. Invasive techniques, such as percutaneous transhepatic cholangiography and endoscopic retrograde cholangiopancreatography are often used to visualize the biliary tree and provide cytologic or biopsy specimens. Assessment of vascular involvement by angiography or Doppler ultrasound is often needed to determine resectability.

TREATMENT AND PROGNOSIS. Non-resectable disease is present at the time of diagnosis in more than 50% of patients with cholangiocarcinoma, and the median survival in this group is 6 months. Surgical resection in the remaining patients can achieve a 5-year survival rate of 37 to 44%. Palliation is generally achieved by percutaneous or endoscopic placement of stents to ensure passage of bile, with surgical drainage used in selected patients. Adjuvant therapy for cholangiocarcinoma has included radiation therapy (external-beam radiation or endoluminal brachytherapy) and chemotherapy with 5-fluorouracil, doxorubicin, and mitomycin-C; response rates for these modalities are approximately 20%.

ANGIOSARCOMA. Angiosarcoma is an extremely rare malignant endothelial tumor of the liver. It has been associated with exposure to vinyl chloride, Thorotrast, and arsenic compounds. The tumor usually presents as abdominal pain and a palpable right upper quadrant mass, but progressive liver failure and acute hemoperitoneum have been described. Metastases, usually to the lungs and skeleton, are common at diagnosis. US and CT frequently show markedly heterogeneous single or multiple liver masses, which may be diagnostic in the proper clinical setting. Angiography shows a characteristic blush and persistence of peripheral enhancement with a central hypovascular area. Treatment consists of surgical resection, which is difficult to achieve owing to the advanced stage of the tumor at the time of diagnosis. Radiation therapy and chemotherapy have not been effective. Most patients die within 6 months of diagnosis.

OTHER PRIMARY MALIGNANT TUMORS OF THE LIVER. Other rare hepatic tumors in the adult liver include squamous cell carcinoma (usually arising in congenital cysts), embryonal sarcoma, fibrosarcoma, leiomyosarcoma, liposarcoma, biliary cystadenocarcinoma, mucoepidermoid carcinoma, malignant rhabdoid tumor, and

carcinosarcomas. These tumors cause symptoms and signs similar to the more common hepatic malignant neoplasms. Diagnosis is usually made by needle biopsy during evaluation or at the time of resection.

METASTATIC TUMORS. Metastatic tumors are the most common malignant neoplasms of the liver in the United States. The most frequent primary tumors to metastasize to the liver include those originating in the gastrointestinal tract (colon, stomach, pancreas, esophagus, extrahepatic cholangiocarcinoma), lung, and breast. Other solid tumors that metastasize to the liver include neuroendocrine tumors, bladder cancer, melanoma, and renal cell carcinoma. The liver is also an extranodal site of involvement for lymphomas and malignant histiocytosis.

Metastatic tumors usually present in the setting of known extrahepatic malignancy, and the diagnosis is often suspected before a liver lesion is found. Metastatic tumors may occasionally present as diffuse involvement and cause rapidly progressive hepatic dysfunction and diagnostic uncertainty. Prognosis is poor once tumor metastases have been found, with a mean survival after diagnosis of 6 months. Selected patients may be surgical candidates for resection of isolated metastases, particularly those from colorectal adenocarcinoma. Patients who have unresectable disease may be offered systemic chemotherapy with the specific protocol depending on the origin of the primary tumor.

Acknowledgment

Thanks to Dr. Miguel R. Arguedas for contributions to the preparation and editing of this work.

Ijzermans JNM, Bac DJ: Recent developments in screening, diagnosis, and surgical treatment of hepatocellular carcinoma. Scand J Gastroenterol 32(Suppl 223):50–54, 1997. *Provides a comprehensive and thorough review of screening strategies for the early detection of hepatocellular carcinoma.*
Kew M: Hepatic tumors and cysts. *In* Feldman M, Scharschmidt BF, Sleisenger MH, (eds): Sleisenger and Fordtran's Gastrointestinal and Liver Disease, 6th ed. Philadelphia, WB Saunders, 1998, pp 1364–1387. *A detailed review of various tumors and cystic lesions of the liver.*
Rubin RA, Mitchell DG: Evaluation of the solid hepatic mass. Med Clin North Am 80:907–926, 1996. *Provides a useful approach to the evaluation of hepatic tumors with emphasis on radiological techniques currently employed.*

---

157 DISEASES OF THE GALLBLADDER AND BILE DUCTS

Z. R. Vlahcevic ■ D. M. Heuman

BILE

The liver is the human body's largest exocrine gland. Its exocrine secretion, bile, provides detergents (bile salts) needed for digestion and absorption of lipids, as well as bicarbonate to neutralize gastric acid. Secretion of bile also has an excretory function because it serves as the major pathway for elimination of many waste products of metabolism as well as exogenous toxins. Bile is formed in bile canaliculi, a network of tubular structures within the hepatocyte plates. The walls of a canaliculus consist of specialized regions of the plasma membranes of two adjacent hepatocytes. The canalicular (biliary) domain of the hepatocyte plasma membrane is separated from the sinusoidal (plasma) domain by tight junctions that allow free passage of water but restrict movement of macromolecules. Bile salts are the most abundant organic solute of hepatic bile (*bile salts* are the ionized species of *bile acids,* and these terms are often used interchangeably by the physiologist) (Fig. 157–1). Bile also contains large amounts of two lipids: phosphatidylcholine (also termed *lecithin*) and unesterified (free) cholesterol. Bilirubin is secreted into bile as monoglucuronides and diglucuronides and is responsible for its yellow color. The total protein content of bile is low (about 1/50 of the plasma protein concentration). A number of biliary proteins appear to stabilize biliary calcium

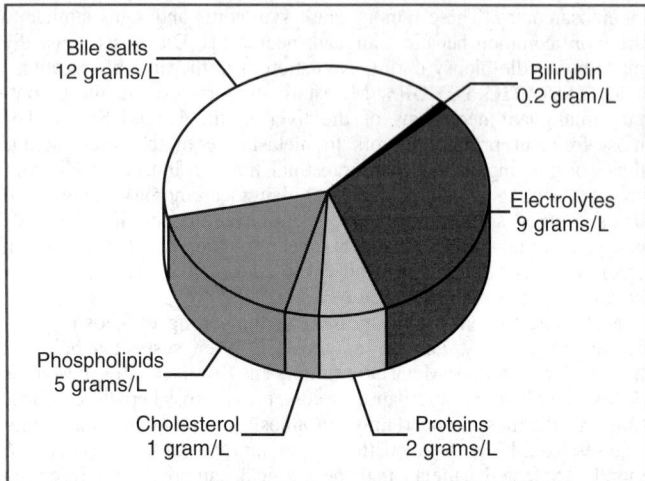

FIGURE 157–1 ■ Solute composition of hepatic bile. Bile salts include principally glycine and taurine conjugates of cholic, chenodeoxycholic, and deoxycholic acids. More than 95% of biliary phospholipid is phosphatidylcholine (lecithin). Cholesterol is present exclusively in its unesterified form. Protein concentration in bile is only 2 to 4% of the plasma protein concentration. Biliary electrolyte composition resembles that of plasma.

salts or lipid aggregates, thus preventing crystal formation. Biliary electrolytes resemble those of plasma (bile is isotonic with plasma) and are responsible for most of the osmotic activity of bile, because bile salts and lipids are present largely in osmotically inactive forms (micelles and vesicles). Under physiologic circumstances, bile flow averages 500 to 1000 mL/day.

Bile salts, the major organic constituents of bile, have a unique

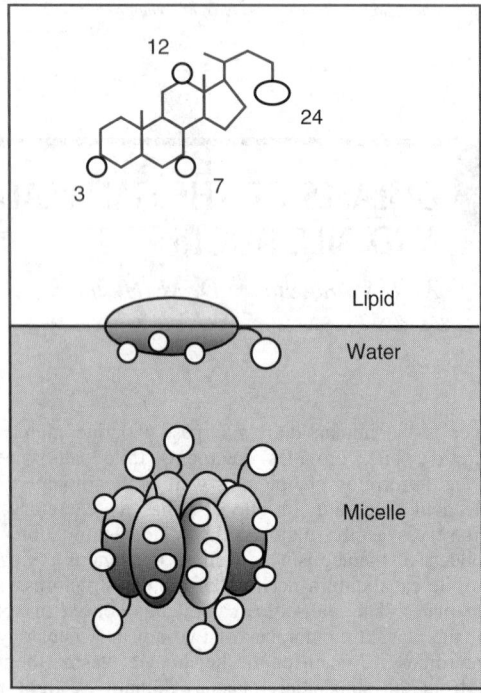

FIGURE 157–2 ■ The molecular structure of a trihydroxy bile salt (cholic acid) is shown in the top figure. The basic sterol nucleus is modified by introduction of polar hydroxyl groups at the 3α, 7α, and 12α positions and by a terminal carboxylic acid moiety at position 24. Because these polar groups are distributed asymmetrically, bile salts are amphiphilic molecules having both lipophilic and hydrophilic surfaces. In aqueous solution at millimolar concentrations, bile salts self-aggregate to form micelles. In bile, bile salt micelles incorporate phospholipid (lecithin) and cholesterol (mixed micelles). In the intestines, bile salts form micelles that incorporate cholesterol, fat-soluble vitamins (A, D, K, and E), and products of lipolysis (monoglycerides and diglycerides, fatty acids).

spectrum of physical and biological properties. Bile salts are biological detergents. Their structure is amphophilic, with both hydrophilic and hydrophobic surfaces (Fig. 157–2). Above a threshold concentration, hydrophobic interaction leads to formation of stable clusters in which the hydrophobic surfaces of the bile salt molecules huddle together, leaving only the hydrophilic surfaces exposed to the aqueous environment. This structure is termed a *micelle*, and the threshold concentration of bile salt at which it forms is termed the *critical micellar concentration*, which is different for different bile salts. Bile salt micelles can incorporate a variety of lipophilic molecules such as cholesterol, phospholipids, and monoglycerides, acting as "carriers" for these lipids in bile and in the intestine. Bile salt secretion represents the major driving force for bile flow and for biliary secretion of cholesterol and lecithin. Finally, bile salt synthesis from cholesterol is a major pathway for elimination of cholesterol from the body: approximately 50% of cholesterol eliminated from the body each day occurs through its degradation to bile salts, and most of the remaining 50% of daily cholesterol elimination occurs through bile salt–induced secretion of free cholesterol into the bile.

The term *primary bile salts* refers to those bile salts that are synthesized in the liver from cholesterol (in humans, *cholic and chenodeoxycholic acids*). Cholesterol's conversion to cholic and chenodeoxycholic acids takes place in the liver through a series of 14 enzymatic reactions in four different organelles (Fig. 157–3). Cholesterol 7α-hydroxylase is the initial and rate-determining enzyme in the main bile salt biosynthetic pathway and is regulated by hydrophobic bile salts in a negative feedback inhibitory manner at the level of gene transcription. This important enzyme is also regulated by cholesterol and certain hormones (glucocorticoids, thyroxine, and glucagon). Before leaving the hepatocyte, bile salts are conjugated (amidated through their carboxyl group) with glycine or taurine, which lowers the pKa and makes them more polar, thereby preventing their absorption from the biliary tree or in the proximal intestine. Alternative pathways of bile acid synthesis have been described.

Bile salts are secreted into bile across the canalicular membrane by active transport. Although the movement of bile salts into the canaliculus is favored by electrochemical forces, it is also driven by adenosine triphosphate (ATP)-dependent active transport and aided by a specific carrier protein, the bile salt export protein, which has recently been identified. The osmotic activity of bile salts and their accompanying cations draws water along with electrolytes through the tight junctions, which are impermeable to bile salts. A small fraction of bile secretion is bile salt independent, driven by secretion of other organic anions such as glutathione and possibly electrolytes. Bile salt secretion draws cholesterol and phospholipid into bile in the form of unilamellar vesicles, which are about 80 nm in diameter and subsequently are dissolved by bile salts to form mixed micelles. The mechanisms by which fluxes of bile salts through hepatocytes mobilize cholesterol and phospholipid and cause their secretion into bile are not well understood.

Canaliculi are surrounded by an actin network and can contract in response to various signals, propelling nascent bile toward larger biliary ductules. Bile ductules are lined by cuboidal epithelium that is both absorptive and secretory. Bile ductular epithelial cells add bicarbonate to bile, stimulated by secretin; biliary bicarbonate contributes to neutralization of gastric acid in the duodenum. The ductules merge into bile ducts, hepatic ducts, and eventually the common hepatic duct. In the interdigestive period, a fraction of bile is diverted to the gallbladder, where it is stored and concentrated. Filling of the relaxed gallbladder is permitted by muscle tone of the sphincter of Oddi in the distal common bile duct, which provides resistance to outflow of bile into the intestine. The gallbladder concentrates bile as much as 10-fold by isotonically reabsorbing Na^+, Cl^-, and HCO_3^- with accompanying water. The gallbladder also secretes mucus and acidifies bile slightly. After food ingestion, gallbladder evacuation is triggered by cholecystokinin, which is released from enterochromaffin cells in the duodenal mucosa in response to the presence of luminal fats and amino acids. Cholecystokinin causes contraction of the gallbladder smooth muscle, which reaches maximum over 10 to 20 minutes, and also simultaneously causes relaxation of the sphincter of Oddi. Between 50 and 90% of the gallbladder contents typically are expelled during normal postprandial gallbladder emptying.

Conjugated bile salts in the proximal intestine play a major role

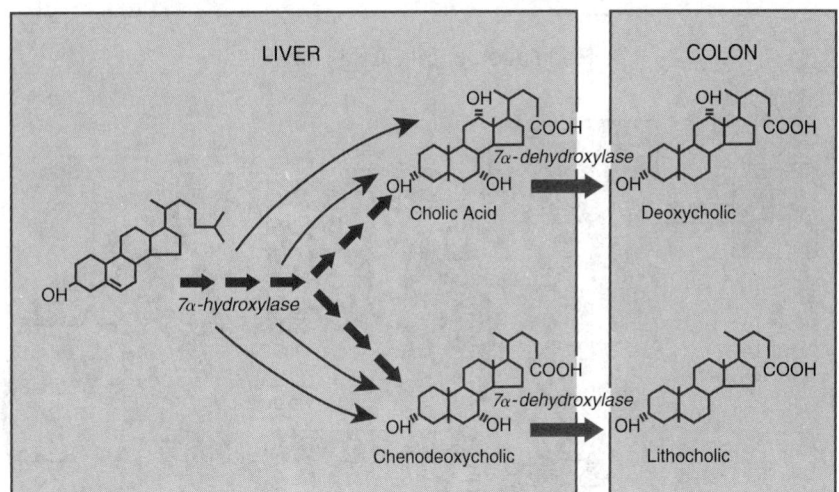

FIGURE 157–3 ■ The primary bile salts of humans, cholic acid and chenodeoxycholic acid, are synthesized from cholesterol exclusively in the liver through a number of intermediary steps. In the colon, anaerobic bacteria deconjugate 7α-dehydroxylate cholic and chenodeoxycholic acid to form the corresponding secondary bile salts, deoxycholic acid and lithocholic acid, respectively. All bile salts are conjugated by the liver with glycine or taurine. In humans, the ratio of glycine to taurine conjugates is 3:1.

in fat digestion. All ingested lipids first undergo emulsification. After emulsification, pancreatic lipase breaks down triglycerides into monoglycerides, diglycerides, and free fatty acids through a process known as lipolysis. In combination with ingested and secreted phospholipids, bile salts form mixed micelles, which have the capacity to solubilize products of lipolysis, cholesterol, and fat-soluble vitamins. The mixed micelles deliver solubilized lipids across the unstirred mucus layer to the apical membranes of enterocytes, where lipid absorption occurs. Reducing the concentration of intestinal bile salts below their critical micellar concentration results in fat maldigestion, a situation that can occur in diseases associated with bile salt wasting (Crohn's disease, ileal resection), in conditions leading to small bowel bacterial overgrowth (Crohn's disease, scleroderma) in which deconjugation of bile salts permits passive reabsorption of free bile salts in the jejunum, and in cholestatic disorders in which delivery of bile salts to the intestine is impaired.

Only a small amount of conjugated bile salt normally is absorbed from the duodenum and jejunum by passive diffusion. Thus, high luminal bile salt concentrations, adequate for micelle formation, normally are maintained throughout those segments of proximal intestine that mediate fat digestion and absorption. In the distal ileum, conjugated bile salts are reabsorbed by an efficient, active, carrier-mediated transport process. A small fraction of bile salt that escapes ileal absorption enters the colon. In the colon, the anaerobic bacteria deconjugate the bile salts and remove the 7-hydroxyl group from cholic or chenodeoxycholic acids to make the secondary bile salts, *deoxycholic and lithocholic acids* (see Fig. 157–3), respectively. Secondary bile salts are strongly lipophilic and can be reabsorbed passively. This pathway salvages about half of the bile salts delivered to the colon. Overall over 95% of the bile salts secreted into the duodenum are recaptured and returned to the liver through the portal blood. Most of the absorption of bile acids takes place in the ileum by an active process mediated by recently cloned carrier proteins called ileal bile acid transporters. Some bile acids are absorbed by passive jejunal or colonic absorption. After absorption, bile acids are bound to albumin or lipoproteins in the portal vein. The liver actively takes up bile salts delivered through the portal vein, clearing 70 to 90% of bile salts from portal blood on a single pass. Hepatic sinusoidal uptake of bile salts is a sodium- and energy-dependent, saturable, carrier-mediated process. The carrier protein, Na^+/cholytaurine cotransporting polypeptide, is responsible for sinusoidal bile salt uptake.

This cycle of biliary secretion followed by intestinal reabsorption and efficient hepatic uptake from the portal blood is termed the *enterohepatic circulation* (Fig. 157–4). The total amount of all bile salts in the enterohepatic circulation ("bile salt pool") averages 2 to 3 g (5–8 mmol). It has been estimated that the entire bile salt pool recirculates six to eight times each day (i.e., two to three times with each meal). Twenty to 30 per cent of the total bile salt pool (roughly 300–600 mg) escapes reabsorption each day and is excreted through the feces. Deoxycholic acid is conjugated by hepato-

cytes and accumulates in the enterohepatic circulation, comprising about 20% of the normal bile salt pool in humans. In contrast, lithocholic acid, which is strongly hydrophobic and cytotoxic, is sulfated by the liver and secreted into the bile, but it is poorly reabsorbed from the intestine. Thus, lithocholic acid does not accumulate in the enterohepatic circulation, and it normally represents less than 3% of the bile salt pool in humans.

Bile salts in the colon induce epithelial cells to initiate net sodium and water secretion; that is, they serve as natural laxatives. This phenomenon may play a role in normal bowel habits; bile salt–binding resins such as cholestyramine or colestipol frequently produce constipation. Bile salt malabsorption is observed in diseases of the ileum or after ileal resection ("bile salt diarrhea"), and administration of bile salt–binding resins relieves bile salt diarrhea in these patients. Massive resection of ileum (> 100 cm) results in bile salt losses that exceed the maximum capacity of the liver to synthesize bile salts, leading to diminution of the bile salt pool, decreased concentrations of intestinal bile salts, fat maldigestion, and steatorrhea.

CHOLESTASIS

Pathophysiology

Cholestasis is the clinical condition that results from impairment of bile secretion. A variety of pathophysiologic mechanisms have been implicated in cholestasis. Functional abnormalities of hepatocytes seen in cholestasis include depressed activity of sinusoidal membrane Na^+,K^+-ATPase, reductions in fluidity of the hepatocyte plasma membrane, decreased basolateral uptake of bile salts and organic anions, altered function of bile salt carrier proteins and microtubules, release of calcium from intracellular stores, and abnormal mitochondrial function with altered cellular redox state and decreased availability of ATP. Canalicular abnormalities may include reduction in microvilli of the canalicular membrane, dilation of the canalicular space, alterations in canalicular membrane fluidity, and disruption of pericanalicular actin microfilaments. Perhaps most important, disruption of tight junctions sealing the canalicular space abolishes both anionic and osmotic gradients necessary for the generation of bile flow and permits back-diffusion of secreted bile components into the plasma. Many of the biochemical abnormalities associated with obstructive cholestasis appear to result from reflux of bile from the canaliculus into the plasma.

Biochemically, cholestasis is characterized by accumulation in plasma of compounds normally secreted into the bile (bilirubin, bile salts) (Table 157–1). Elevated levels of serum bile salts are the most sensitive indicators of cholestasis; this determination is not routinely available and therefore not used widely. Serum cholesterol is commonly increased in cholestasis, reflecting increased cholesterol synthesis and appearance in plasma of lipids normally secreted into bile. The hyperlipidemia of cholestasis is associated with appearance in plasma of lipoprotein X, a discoidal particle

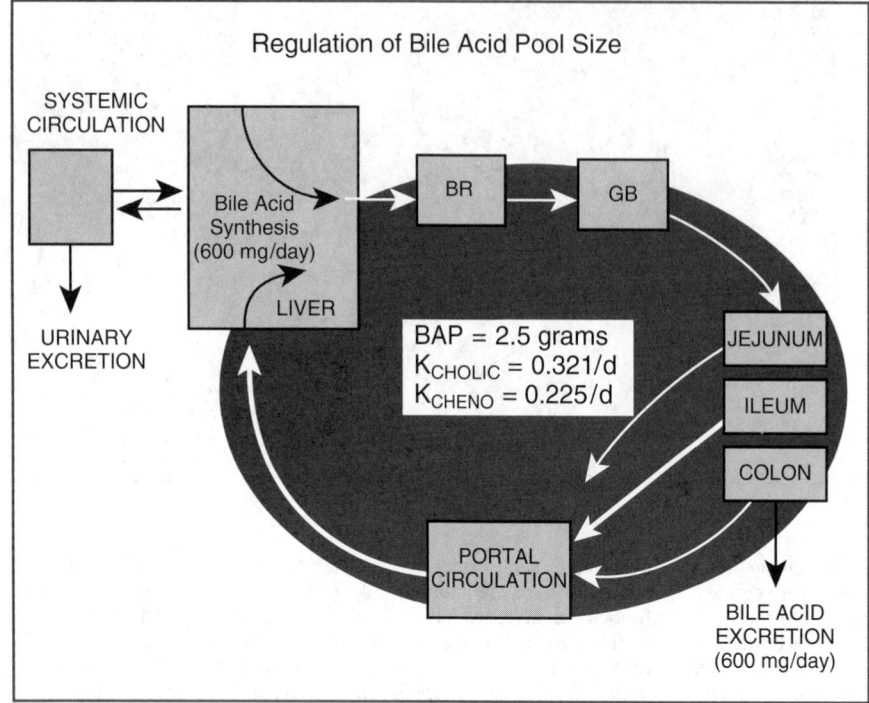

FIGURE 157–4 ■ Enterohepatic circulation of bile salts. Bile salts are secreted by the liver in the biliary radicles and stored in the gallbladder. After meals and the release of cholecystokinin, bile salts are expelled from the gallbladder and into the intestines where they participate actively in the intestinal digestion of fat. Small amounts of bile salts are passively absorbed from the jejunum; they are actively absorbed in the ileum and return to the liver via portal circulation. Following uptake at the sinusoids, bile salts are transferred to the canalicular membrane through the cytosol by binding to bile salt binding proteins and secreted through the canalicular membrane. The total bile acid pool (BAP) circulating in the enterohepatic circulation is 2 to 3 g in normal adults. In steady state, daily bile salt turnover (K) averages 20 to 30% of the bile salt pool.

containing phosphatidylcholine, free cholesterol, albumin, and specific apolipoproteins.

Exclusion of bile from the intestine in severe cholestasis has several consequences. In the absence of bile salts, there is moderate malabsorption of fat and severe malabsorption of cholesterol and fat-soluble vitamins. Cholestasis may be associated with specific vitamin deficiency disorders such as night blindness (vitamin A), osteomalacia (vitamin D), neuropathy (vitamin E), or coagulopathy (vitamin K). Generalized osteoporosis also commonly occurs for unknown reasons. Because bilirubin degradation products are responsible for the normal brown color of stools, pale "acholic" stools are occasionally present in advanced cholestatic disorders. Urobilinogen normally is formed in the colon by bacterial metabolism of bilirubin and is subsequently absorbed and excreted into urine; disappearance of urobilinogen from the urine of a jaundiced patient is indicative of cholestasis.

Certain canalicular membrane enzymes, including alkaline phosphatase, 5' nucleotidase, and γ-glutamyl transpeptidase, also commonly accumulate in plasma of cholestatic patients. These enzymes normally are present on the luminal surface of the canalicular plasma membrane. When canalicular pressure rises (as when flow of bile is obstructed), these enzymes are synthesized in increased amounts, accumulate on the sinusoidal membrane, and are released into the blood. Disproportionately elevated blood levels of these enzymes are useful in establishing the diagnosis of extrahepatic or intrahepatic obstructive cholestasis. Acute obstruction of the common bile duct also can be associated with transient hepatocellular necrosis. For this reason, elevations of serum aminotransferase and lactate dehydrogenase levels may predominate during the early hours after acute biliary obstruction. With time, however, the levels of these enzymes decline, while alkaline phosphatase and other canalicular enzymes rise, producing the typical "cholestatic pattern."

Because of their detergent properties, hydrophobic bile salts retained in cholestasis may contribute to hepatic injury. Bile salt synthesis paradoxically increases in cholestasis, possibly contributing to hepatotoxicity. The liver is not left without defense because it has the capacity to convert hydrophobic bile salts by phase I (cytochrome P-450–mediated hydroxylation) and phase II (sulfation, glucuronidation) pathways to hydrophilic bile acid conjugates, which are eliminated in urine. In high-grade cholestasis, urinary excretion may become the major pathway of bile salt elimination, as compared with the normal situation in which bile acids are eliminated through the feces. Although the role of bile salts in perpetuation of liver injury in cholestasis has not been established with certainty, the administration of hydrophilic bile salts such as ursodeoxycholic acid (UDCA) improves liver function test results, clinical symptoms, and histology.

Patients with advanced cholestasis experience generalized malaise, weakness, easy fatigability, nausea, anorexia, and pruritus. The underlying cause responsible for pruritus in cholestasis is unknown. Although pruritus has been attributed to cutaneous toxicity of retained bile salts, its severity does not correlate with cutaneous bile salt concentrations and treatment with cholestyramine is not invariably helpful in relieving the symptoms. An unknown endogenous opiate receptor agonist is retained in the cholestatic patient and may cause pruritus through direct effects on cutaneous neurons; in recent experimental trials, the severity of pruritus was relieved by administration of opiate antagonists.

Introduction of bacteria into bile above an obstructing lesion can lead rapidly to purulent infection of the biliary tree and liver, termed *ascending cholangitis*. Contributing factors include high biliary pressure and stasis. In the absence of infection, cholestasis may be well tolerated for very long periods of time. Although

Table 157–1 ■ PATHOPHYSIOLOGY OF CHOLESTASIS

Retention of Bile Components in Plasma
Conjugated hyperbilirubinemia with bilirubinuria
Hypercholesterolemia (lipoprotein X) with xanthoma formation
Elevated serum bile salts
Pruritus
Osteoporosis
Exclusuion of Bile Salts From the Intestine
Malabsorption of fat with steatorrhea
Malabsorption of fat-soluble vitamins
    Vitamin A—night blindness
    Vitamin D—osteomalacia
    Vitamin E—neuropathy
    Vitamin K—coagulopathy
Malabsorption of cholesterol
Acholic stools
Osteoporosis
Hepatic Injury
Release of canalicular membrane enzymes into the plasma (alkaline phosphatase, 5'-nucleotidase, α-glutamyltransferase)
Retention of bile salts can contribute to liver injury
Biliary ductular proliferation
Cirrhosis

patients typically do not feel well, hepatic functions unrelated to bile secretion (such as intermediary metabolism, protein synthesis, and toxin degradation) are initially well preserved. If biliary obstruction can be relieved, symptoms and biochemical abnormalities will resolve. However, if allowed to persist, chronic biliary obstruction, regardless of cause, eventually leads to cirrhosis with all its complications. The mechanism by which increased bile secretory pressure leads to cirrhosis has not as yet been established, but it can occur with either extrahepatic or intrahepatic obstruction.

Approach to the Cholestatic Patient

In general, cholestasis may result from conditions affecting large bile ducts (extrahepatic cholestasis) or from disorders of small bile ducts, canaliculi or hepatocytes (intrahepatic cholestasis). The distinction is useful because it has important clinical implications. In extrahepatic cholestasis, bile flow is impaired because of mechanical obstruction of the larger bile ducts due to benign or malignant processes. Increased biliary pressure above the obstruction leads to ductal dilatation. Obstruction of large ducts is usually localized and therefore can be addressed with mechanical measures to effect drainage. In contrast, intrahepatic cholestasis involves either diffuse injury to small bile ducts or metabolic derangements in the bile secretory apparatus at the level of the hepatocyte and canaliculus. Intrahepatic cholestasis is typically not associated with ductal dilatation and is not amenable to mechanical interventions.

Diagnostic evaluation of cholestasis begins with routine blood tests of liver enzymes and liver function to establish the pattern and severity of liver injury. Liver tests typically exhibit a disproportionate elevation of canalicular enzymes such as alkaline phosphatase, 5'-nucleotidase, and γ-glutamyl transpeptidase. Functional abnormalities typically include conjugated hyperbilirubinemia and hypercholesterolemia. Loss of synthetic function manifested by hypoalbuminemia occurs only in patients in whom chronic cholestasis progresses to cirrhosis, but an abnormal prothrombin time may occur relatively early in cholestasis because of malabsorption of vitamin K, which occurs due to decreased concentrations of bile acids in the intestines. Additional blood tests may indicate a specific cause for the cholestasis, such as primary biliary cirrhosis (PBC) (antimitochondrial antibody) (see Chapter 153) or sarcoidosis (see Chapter 81).

Once a cholestatic pattern of liver disease has been established, imaging techniques such as ultrasonography are indicated to determine if there is evidence of large duct obstruction with proximal ductal dilatation. Ultrasonography can also demonstrate the location and nature of the obstructing lesion. This diagnostic modality is a very sensitive and accurate test for detection of gallstones, a common cause of obstructive cholestasis, and also may detect focal mass lesions such as primary or secondary tumors in the liver. Computed tomography (CT) and magnetic resonance imaging (MRI) are more expensive tests that at present offer no advantage over ultrasonography for detection of large duct obstruction. These studies, however, provide additional information about the nature of the obstructing lesion. If cancer is strongly suspected, it may be preferable to image initially with CT or MRI to obtain sectional images of the entire abdomen with high-resolution views of the retroperitoneum and pancreas. The most precise information regarding biliary anatomy is obtained by direct cholangiography (percutaneous transhepatic cholangiography [PTC] or endoscopic retrograde cholangiopancreatography [ERCP]) (Fig. 157–5); these tests may be necessary if non-invasive methods are inconclusive. Very recently, a new non-invasive technique, magnetic resonance cholangiopancreatography (MRCP), was reported to be as useful for diagnosis as ERCP.

If the large bile ducts appear normal with imaging studies, liver biopsy usually is indicated to look for evidence of a parenchymal process. In disorders that diffusely involve the small bile ducts, the pattern of tissue injury on liver biopsy may be diagnostic. Obstruction to bile flow produces a typical histologic pattern that includes retention of bilirubin granules in the hepatic cytoplasm and inspissated "bile plugs" in canaliculi, most prominent in the pericentral zone. Scattered hepatocyte injury, possibly attributable to bile salts, is manifested as feathery degeneration with focal necrosis. Mild edema and polymorphonuclear inflammation of portal tracts may be seen. With prolonged obstruction, the characteristic finding of proliferation of bile ductules is observed. If the duct obstruction is not relieved, an increasing amount of fibrosis occurs around the portal

tracts, accompanied by atrophy of hepatocytes. True cirrhosis with regenerative nodules occurs after months to years of biliary obstruction. The small sample of liver tissue obtained on a percutaneous biopsy is not always representative of the entire liver, and information from a single biopsy must be interpreted with caution.

General principles for therapy of cholestasis include the following:

1. *Specific therapy to cure or control the underlying disorder* usually should be undertaken whenever possible. For example, curative resection is indicated if feasible for an obstructing neoplasm; if clinically indicated, common bile duct exploration will allow cure of gallstones; and repair of biliary strictures may restore normal biliary drainage. Drugs that cause cholestasis should be discontinued. Immune-mediated bile ductular injury may respond to immunosuppressive therapy.

2. *Relief of biliary obstruction* is generally worthwhile for relief of symptoms of cholestasis (pruritus, jaundice), to prevent or relieve ascending cholangitis, and to prevent progression to biliary cirrhosis, even if the underlying disease cannot be cured. Drainage may be achieved by surgical resection or bypass of the obstructed segment, typically by means of a Roux-en-Y choledochojejunostomy. Alternatively, percutaneous and endoscopic approaches may be employed. Strictures may be dilated using balloon catheters passed over guide wires. Malignant biliary obstruction commonly is managed by stenting. In general, the endoscopic retrograde approach is preferable to the percutaneous approach because of the risk of hemorrhage or bile leak with liver puncture.

3. *Palliation of symptoms and supportive measures* are currently the mainstay of treatment for chronic cholestatic disorders such as primary sclerosing cholangitis (PSC) or PBC. Drugs such as rifampin and phenobarbital induce hepatic phase I and phase II drug metabolizing enzymes; therapy with these agents may relieve cholestasis somewhat by enhancing detoxification and elimination of a variety of retained lipophilic compounds, including bile salts. Bile salt–binding resins such as cholestyramine sometimes provide symptomatic relief from pruritus, which may be a serious problem in the more advanced cases. Opiate receptor antagonists such as naloxone may be helpful for treatment of pruritus. Patients with chronic cholestasis and fat maldigestion also require dietary fat restriction, fat-soluble vitamin supplements, and calcium supplements. Complications of cirrhosis should be identified and treated.

   UDCA, the 7β-epimer of chenodeoxycholic acid, is a naturally occurring bile salt in the bear. In contrast to chenodeoxycholic acid, it is a poor detergent because its 7-hydroxyl group projects toward the hydrophobic surface of the molecule, impeding hydrophobic interactions with other lipids. UDCA is intrinsically non-toxic even at supraphysiologic concentrations. It was originally used for dissolution of cholesterol gallstones but was serendipitously found to improve cholestasis and liver injury in a variety of chronic cholestatic liver diseases. It reduces serum bilirubin, transaminase, and alkaline phosphatase levels and can improve clinical symptoms and liver histology. UDCA in various experimental models attenuates toxicity of more hydrophobic bile salts. It also may have direct protective effects on the liver and may alter immunologic function. It is unclear whether UDCA can slow the progression of cholestatic liver disease to biliary cirrhosis.

4. *Hepatic transplantation* (see Chapter 155) can provide a 1-year survival of nearly 90% in certain types of end-stage cholestatic diseases (PBC, PSC, and biliary atresia). Indications for transplantation include intractable symptoms, complications of cirrhosis, or deterioration of prognostic indicators. The healthier the patient at the time of transplantation, the better the outcome; conversely, patients with complications of liver disease frequently die while awaiting transplantation.

DISORDERS ASSOCIATED WITH CHOLESTASIS

Intrahepatic Causes of Cholestasis

Intrahepatic cholestasis may occur because of diffuse obliteration of small bile ducts or because of generalized disorders affecting bile secretion at the level of the hepatocytes or canaliculi. Oblitera-

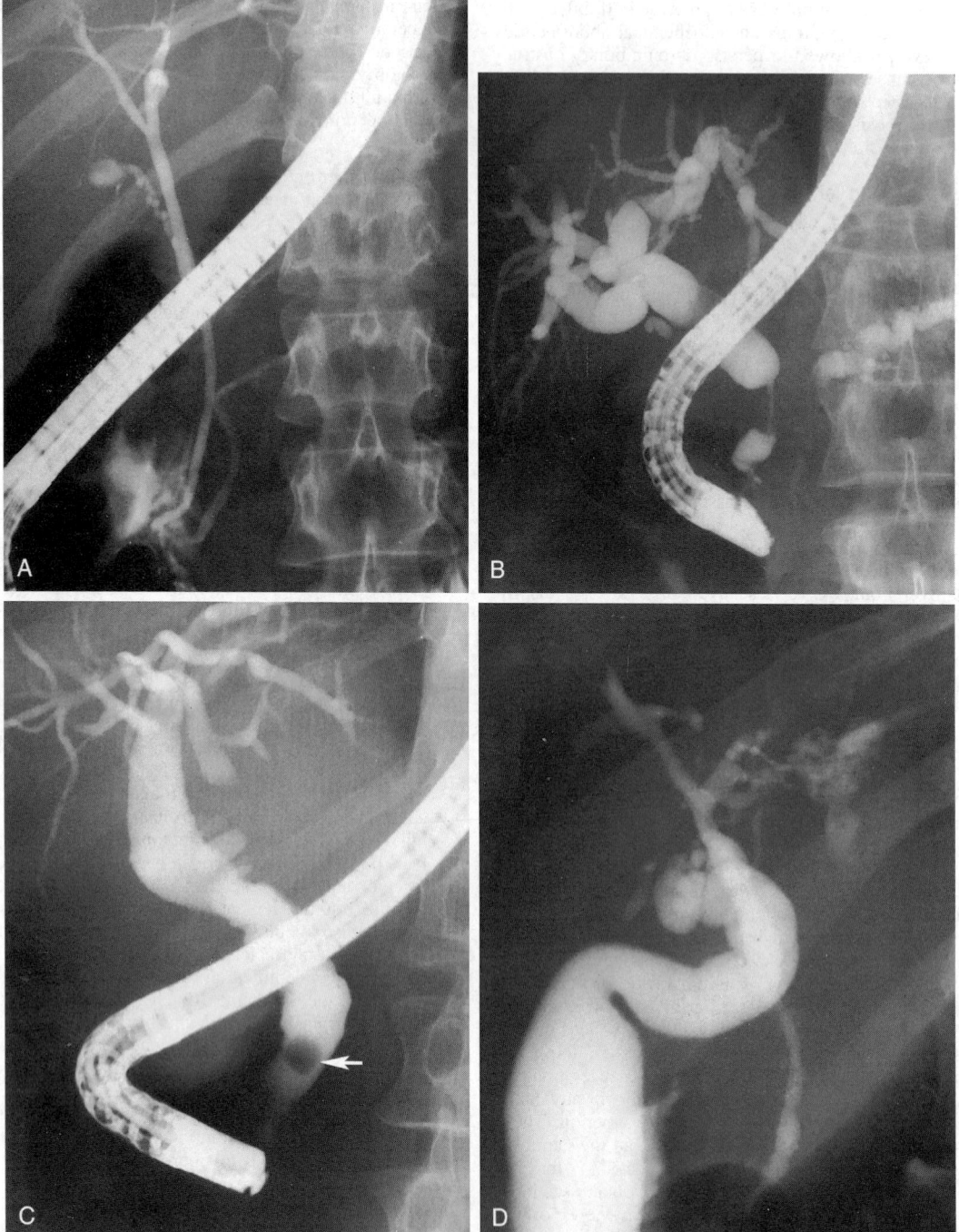

FIGURE 157–5 ■ Cholangiographic appearance of cholestatic disorders. *A,* Normal cholangiogram and pancreatogram. *B,* Pancreatic cancer. The tumor is obstructing the common bile duct and the pancreatic duct, producing proximal dilatation of both (double duct sign). A cannula extending from the endoscope has been passed through the area of obstruction and its tip lies in the proximal common hepatic duct. *C,* Choledocholithiasis. A large cholesterol gallstone in the common bile duct appears as a radiolucent shadow outlined by radiodense contrast material. The common bile duct is dilated. *D,* Primary sclerosing cholangitis. Multiple strictures are present in both the intrahepatic and extrahepatic biliary tree. Intrahepatic ducts are attenuated and reduced in number. Beadlike areas of dilatation can be noted between areas of stricture, but the fibrotic process in the liver prevents generalized dilatation of the proximal biliary ducts. The gallbladder is filled with contrast material and appears normal.

tion of small bile ducts usually leads to chronic progressive cholestasis and biliary cirrhosis. Small duct obliterative disorders, often collectively termed *vanishing bile duct syndromes,* include infiltrating neoplasms (discussed later); granulomatous disorders such as sarcoidosis; and the immune-mediated bile duct destruction of PBC, hepatic allograft rejection, and chronic graft-versus-host disease. Cholestasis of metabolic origin may be seen commonly in severely ill patients and is associated with trauma, surgery, sepsis, and parenteral hyperalimentation. Numerous drugs and estrogen also can produce cholestasis either as a direct effect or as an idiosyncratic reaction (see Chapter 148). Cholestasis of pregnancy appears to reflect sensitivity to the direct cholestatic effects of estrogen.

Non-caseating granulomas are a common and non-specific finding in the liver. In *sarcoidosis* (see Chapter 81), an idiopathic disease characterized by non-caseating granulomas in lung and other tissues, liver involvement is common. Usually these patients are symptom free with mild abnormalities of liver function tests. Granulomas in the portal tracts may produce fibrotic obliteration of small bile ducts. Rarely, bile duct obliteration may be sufficiently severe to produce biliary cirrhosis. Although some experts consider hepatic involvement in sarcoidosis to be an indication for glucocorticoid therapy, glucocorticoids have not been proven to alter the natural history of sarcoidosis involving the liver.

Primary biliary cirrhosis (see Chapter 153) is a progressive cholestatic disorder characterized by autoimmune destruction of small interlobular bile ducts. Injury is thought to occur as a result of cytotoxic T cell–mediated immune attack directed against bile ductular epithelial cells. PBC is primarily a disease of middle-aged women (>10:1 female/male ratio). It may be associated with other autoimmune disorders. A characteristic marker of this disease is antimitochondrial antibody, which is found in 90% of patients with PBC and only rarely in other disorders. PBC generally progresses slowly but relentlessly to cirrhosis and hepatic failure.

Progressive familial intrahepatic cholestasis typically presents as mild to moderate cholestasis in infancy or childhood. Liver biopsy specimens appear generally unremarkable except that bile ductules can be identified in fewer than 50% of portal tracts. The disorder may occur in sporadic or hereditary forms and it may be part of a hereditary condition termed *Alagille's syndrome* or arteriohepatic dysplasia. Severity and prognosis are variable: some patients develop biliary cirrhosis requiring transplantation in childhood, whereas others have an indolent course. A variety of genetic defects in pathways of bile acid synthesis or biliary lipid secretion have been implicated in the pathogenesis of this disorder.

Chronic graft-versus-host disease occurs when T cells from an allogenic source are infused into an immunodeficient patient, most typically at the time of bone marrow transplantation (see Chapter 182). Liver involvement is characterized by mononuclear infiltration of portal tracts with obliteration of small bile ductules, similar to that seen in PBC. Intensive immunosuppression may control the graft-versus-host reaction, and if this fails, UDCA may improve cholestasis; however, the cholestasis often progresses to biliary cirrhosis.

After hepatic transplantation (see Chapter 155), *chronic hepatic allograft rejection* is associated with immunologic injury to biliary ductules and hepatic arterioles. Like PBC and graft-versus-host disease, chronic allograft rejection is associated with T-cell infiltration of the portal tracts and destruction of bile ductules. Arterial intimal injury leading to intimal hyperplasia may compromise hepatic circulation and accelerate the progression of liver injury.

A benign intrahepatic cholestasis of metabolic origin is seen commonly in severely ill patients. Predisposing factors include major trauma or surgery, severe infection, and parenteral hyperalimentation. The mechanism responsible for cholestasis is unknown. Serum bilirubin often is markedly elevated, whereas elevations of the alkaline phosphatase typically are modest, and aminotransferase levels usually are near normal. Liver synthetic function usually is well preserved. Liver biopsy specimens reveal only minimal abnormalities. The etiology of the syndrome is unknown. With elimination of the precipitating factors, cholestasis typically resolves over a few weeks.

Intrahepatic cholestasis of pregnancy is a relatively common disorder that usually appears late during the third trimester of pregnancy, disappears after delivery, and can occur in subsequent pregnancy. In its usual form, the only manifestation is generalized itching (pruritus gravidarum), but more severe cases it may be accompanied by jaundice. It is associated with an increased risk of fetal loss. The pathogenesis is uncertain, but estrogens may cause impaired intracellular transport and/or canalicular excretion of bile salts. There appears to be a familial predisposition to the development of intrahepatic cholestasis of pregnancy.

Drug-induced cholestasis may be a complication of treatment with a number of therapeutic agents (see Chapter 148). Cholestasis induced by estrogens or cyclosporine is not associated with inflammation and is thought to result from metabolic effects at the level of the hepatocyte. Chlorpromazine typically produces an acute febrile illness accompanied by elevation of both aminotransferase and alkaline phosphatase levels; a hypersensitivity mechanism is thought to be responsible. Other common drugs that can produce idiosyncratic cholestatic liver injury include captopril, sulindac, and benoxaprofen. The recognition that drugs frequently can cause intrahepatic cholestasis is important because, in most instances, simple withdrawal of offending agents will result in normalization of liver function tests and clinical symptoms.

Diseases of the Large Bile Ducts and Gallbladder

Primary and Secondary Neoplasms Involving the Bile Ducts

Neoplasms are among the most common and important causes of extrahepatic biliary obstruction. Primary malignancies of the liver, bile ducts, gallbladder, ampulla of Vater, and pancreas in aggregate account for over 50,000 deaths annually in the United States, and patients with these cancers most typically present with jaundice caused by bile duct obstruction. Malignancies classically produce painless obstructive jaundice, but it is more typical for neoplasms involving the liver, bile ducts, or pancreas to cause vague pain in the epigastrium or back; this pain may precede the onset of jaundice. The common bile duct may be obstructed distally by pancreatic cancer or ampullary carcinoma, proximally by hepatocellular carcinoma or gallbladder carcinoma, or anywhere along its length by cholangiocarcinoma. Rare benign neoplasms that may obstruct the common bile duct distally include pancreatic cystadenoma and villous adenoma of the papilla of Vater. Metastatic tumor from any source to lymph nodes in the porta hepatis can also cause extrinsic compression of the proximal common bile duct; this complication is a common cause of cholestasis in patients with cancers of the breast, lung, colon or stomach. Not all cholestasis caused by malignancies is extrahepatic: extensive tumor metastases within the liver parenchyma may produce intrahepatic cholestasis by obstructing smaller intrahepatic ducts. Diffuse infiltration of malignant cells along hepatic sinusoids with consequent cholestasis also may occur, especially in small cell carcinoma of the lung and in lymphoma. Rarely a non-obstructive metabolic cholestasis may occur as a paraneoplastic syndrome complicating extrahepatic malignancies such as lymphoma or renal cell carcinoma (Stauffer's syndrome).

Cholangiocarcinoma is a form of adenocarcinoma that arises from the intrahepatic or extrahepatic biliary epithelium. It occurs somewhat more commonly in males than females. There is a high incidence in the Far East, related to infestation by liver flukes and Oriental cholangiohepatitis. In Western countries there is an increased incidence in patients with PSC or choledochal cysts. Grossly, three patterns of growth are described: polypoid, sclerosing, and infiltrative. Most cancers of the extrahepatic ducts appear as poorly defined gray-white thickenings of the bile duct wall; the lumen is narrowed, often resembling fibrous strictures or sclerosing cholangitis radiographically. Cholangiocarcinomas tend to grow slowly and to infiltrate the wall of the duct and dissect along tissue planes. Perineural invasion and metastasis to regional nodes are common. Tumors at the bifurcation of the common hepatic duct (termed *Klatskin tumors*) commonly invade the liver by direct extension. The usual presentation of cholangiocarcinoma involving the common hepatic or common bile duct is progressive obstructive jaundice. More proximal lesions, which produce localized obstruction of intrahepatic branches of the biliary tree, may cause vague abdominal pain associated with marked elevation of the serum alkaline phosphatase without jaundice. Ultrasonography and CT typically reveal dilated intrahepatic bile ducts with focal narrowing of the biliary tree, sometimes accompanied by a mass. The most useful imaging study is cholangiography, which typically demonstrates segmental narrowing or obstruction. In patients with PSC, diagnosis of cholangiocarcinoma is suggested by rapid worsening of jaundice with a new dominant stricture on cholangiography. Diagnosis may be confirmed by endoscopic brush cytology or needle aspiration, but in some cases the diagnosis can be established only at laparotomy. Only one third of cholangiocarcinomas are resectable for cure at the time of presentation. The 5-year survival after attempted curative resection is about 20%. The best results are obtained with tumors of the distal bile duct and polypoid tumors; absence of lymph node metastases and clear surgical margins also indicate a better prognosis. Radical surgical attempts to cure intrahepatic cholangiocarcinoma by total hepatectomy with hepatic transplantation were disappointing because of a high rate of postoperative recurrence, and this approach has been abandoned by consensus. Response to chemotherapy or radiation is limited, although brachytherapy (intraductal radiation) holds promise as a palliative measure for some patients. Most patients die of local hepatic invasion rather than distant metastases. Overall survival for cholangiocarcinoma is less than 10% at 5 years.

Gallbladder adenocarcinoma is an uncommon malignancy in the United States. Most patients are older than 70 years of age, and women are affected more than men, by a 3:1 ratio. There is a strong association of gallstones with carcinoma of the gallbladder (80–90% of carcinomatous gallbladders have stones), and the risk factors for gallbladder carcinoma by and large are the same as the risk factors for gallstones. In some groups of Native Americans who are genetically predisposed to develop gallstones with very high frequency at relatively young ages, gallbladder adenocarcinoma is 5 to 10 times more common than in the general population. The duration and severity of cholelithiasis appear to correlate with the risk of gallbladder carcinoma. Gallbladder cancer is especially associated with very large gallstones (greater than 3 cm in diameter) or calcification of the chronically inflamed gallbladder wall (porcelain gallbladder), and these findings are therefore considered by many experts to be indications for cholecystectomy even in the asymptomatic patient. However, because the incidence of adenocarcinoma of the gallbladder in patients with cholelithiasis is less than 1 per 1000 patient-years, the prevention of gallbladder cancer currently is not considered a sufficient indication for cholecystectomy in most patients with asymptomatic gallstones. Early symptoms of gallbladder cancer are non-specific and similar to those of cholelithiasis or cholecystitis; later, patients develop persistent pain and *unremitting* jaundice as the tumor invades the liver and bile ducts. Imaging studies such as ultrasonography, CT, and cholangiography can reveal features suggestive of gallbladder cancer, such as thickening or mass of the gallbladder wall or extension of mass to involve the liver, but over 80% of gallbladder cancers are undiagnosed preoperatively. Tumors that are localized to the gallbladder may be cured by cholecystectomy, but these tumors represent fewer than 20% of all patients with gallbladder cancers. Extension to adjacent bile ducts or liver or metastasis to portahepatic lymph nodes or distant organs is common at initial presentation. By the time patients develop jaundice, 85% are unresectable. Chemotherapy and radiation therapy currently are of little benefit. Overall 5-year survival is less than 10%.

New onset of cholestasis over days to weeks in any adult, especially older than age 50, is worrisome for cancer. A palpable, dilated, non-tender gallbladder (Courvoisier's sign) suggests cancer obstructing the common bile duct. Laboratory studies most typically reveal a rapid and progressive increase in serum alkaline phosphatase and bilirubin values. Because cancers are common and may sometimes present as atypical symptoms or laboratory findings, most adults with new onset of abnormal liver tests or jaundice should undergo imaging of the liver and bile ducts to look for masses or ductal dilatation. Ultrasonography is generally the first imaging procedure in a cholestatic patient, but it may be preferable to go directly to CT or MRI if the clinical picture is strongly suggestive of cancer, because these procedures provide more information about the nature and level of the obstructing lesion and the presence of metastases. Further evaluation depends on the initial findings. In patients who appear to be candidates for surgical resection, it may be appropriate to proceed with surgery. The diagnosis of cancer can be established by intraoperative biopsy, and at laparotomy the surgeon can choose between a radical, potentially curative resection, a drainage procedure for palliation of unresectable cancer, or correction of a benign obstructing process. Additional preoperative diagnostic techniques such as cholangiography (see Fig. 157–5B), endoscopic ultrasonography, and angiography may sometimes be helpful in determining resectability and in resolving diagnostic uncertainties. If patients are poor candidates for surgery or have unresectable disease, a diagnosis can be established by CT-guided needle aspiration biopsy of the primary lesion or a metastasis.

When obstructing malignancy is not resectable for cure, relief of cholestasis usually represents a major goal of palliation. Advances in therapeutic radiology and endoscopy over the past decade now permit relief of bile duct obstruction by placement of internal stents without surgery in most patients. Two types of stents are commonly used. Flexible plastic stents ranging in diameter from 7 to 14 French are inexpensive but occlude over a period of months from accumulation of bacterial biofilm and minerals on their inner surface; they must be removed and replaced periodically. Permanently implanted self-expanding metallic mesh stents, introduced in the past few years, provide a much wider lumen (on the order of 1 cm) and occlude less commonly; however they are expensive, and tumors can grow in through the openings in the mesh.

Other Disorders of the Large Bile Ducts

Choledochal cysts are congenital anatomic malformations of the bile duct. Five forms of choledochal cysts are described: type I—fusiform or saccular dilatation of the extrahepatic tree; type II—diverticular common bile duct cyst; type III—choledochocele; type IV—diffuse dilation of common bile duct and hepatic ducts; and type V—intrahepatic ductal dilatation (Caroli's disease). Histologic examination demonstrates a thick-walled structure of very dense connective tissue with smooth muscle fibers. A pericystic inflammatory process or cholangitis frequently accompanies the choledochal cyst. The mechanism of cyst formation is uncertain. If the common bile duct is blocked, patients may present with cholestasis in infancy, resembling patients with biliary atresia. If the common bile duct is patent, patients may remain asymptomatic into adulthood. About half of patients with choledochal cysts present after age 10. In the adult form, the triad of abdominal pain, jaundice, and a palpable mass is the classic presentation. Fever may be present as a result of bile stasis with cholangitis. Complications include primary formation of brown pigment gallstones in the cyst and liver abscesses. Abdominal ultrasonography and CT often demonstrate dilated bile ducts. However, the best method to establish the diagnosis is endoscopic retrograde cholangiopancreatography (ERCP) or MRCP. Once the diagnosis of choledochal cyst is established, the therapy is surgical. Simple cystenterostomy can provide drainage and prevent cholangitis. However, whenever possible, complete surgical excision of the cyst is desirable because there is a high incidence of cholangiocarcinoma in choledochal cysts.

Benign biliary strictures, which are fibrotic narrowings of the large bile ducts, occur as a result of trauma, inflammation, infection, or ischemia. *Surgical injury* to the bile ducts, although uncommon, is a major technical complication of cholecystectomy. Repair of bile duct injuries is technically difficult, and postsurgical strictures are associated with significant chronic morbidity, including biliary cirrhosis. *Chronic pancreatitis* commonly produces fibrotic narrowing of the common bile duct where it passes through the head of the pancreas (see Chapter 141). Although proximal ductal dilatation and alkaline phosphatase elevation are common, significant cholestasis is unusual, and liver failure from biliary cirrhosis is quite uncommon. In patients with chronic pancreatitis who have elevations of serum alkaline phosphatase level or common bile duct dilatation on ultrasound examination, periodic liver biopsy has been recommended to detect progressive hepatic fibrosis. Surgical drainage (choledochojejunostomy) usually is successful in relieving ductal obstruction and halting the progression of biliary cirrhosis in chronic pancreatitis in the few cases in which it is required. Strictures of the bile ducts have been noted after *hepatic irradiation,* possibly secondary to vascular endothelial injury and ischemia. Similarly, strictures have been reported after *chemotherapy* employing intrahepatic arterial infusion of floxuridine or mitomycin C. Surgical drainage is preferred to endoscopic or percutaneous stenting in most patients with benign strictures because of uncertainties regarding long-term patency and late complications of stents.

Liver flukes (see Chapter 432) are trematode parasites that are ingested in food, taken up from the gut, travel through the circulation to the liver, and from there pass into bile. The adult flukes mature in the biliary tree, where they can reside for decades and release eggs into bile. Mild infections usually are asymptomatic; heavier infections may produce fever and eosinophilia initially and later may cause signs and symptoms of biliary obstruction. Chronically, liver flukes may cause ductal fibrosis and strictures. The diagnosis can be established by identifying ova in stool. *Clonorchis sinensis* and *Opisthorchis viverrini* are common in east Asia, where they are acquired through ingestion of raw fish. Praziquantel is the treatment of choice. Fasciola hepatica is found throughout the world. It is acquired from eating wild watercress on which encysted metacercariae have been deposited by snails. The recommended treatment is bithionol.

Liver flukes have been implicated in the pathogenesis of *Oriental cholangiohepatitis,* a chronic inflammatory disorder of the biliary tree associated with bile duct strictures, recurrent episodes of obstructive jaundice and ascending cholangitis, development of brown pigment gallstones in the intrahepatic and extrahepatic bile ducts, and biliary cirrhosis. This disorder is common in east Asia, including China and Japan, and is seen in the United States with some frequency in areas with large Asian immigrant populations. Not all patients have evidence of infection with liver flukes, and other pathogenic factors may be important. The disease is associated with lower socioeconomic class and malnutrition, and its frequency appears to have fallen dramatically in Japan, Hong Kong, and Taiwan since the 1950s. Patients typically are younger than 50 years of age, with males and females affected equally. The usual presentation is an attack of ascending cholangitis associated with fever, right upper quadrant pain, and jaundice. Some attacks respond spontaneously or with antibiotic treatment alone; in others, sepsis may develop and surgical drainage may be required. Attacks may recur at irregular intervals of days to years. Long-term management includes eradication of parasites and elimination of stones and strictures. Intrahepatic stones that cannot be extracted may necessitate resection of hepatic segments. The prognosis varies with the extent of involvement, but death from complications of sepsis and cirrhosis is common.

Cholangiopathy from the acquired immunodeficiency syndrome (AIDS) describes a number of biliary tract abnormalities associated with infection with the human immunodeficiency virus (HIV) (see Chapter 413). Patients with advanced immunodeficiency may develop acalculous cholecystitis, focal distal biliary stenosis at the ampulla of Vater, or multifocal stenoses of the biliary tree resembling PSC. Although the pathogenesis of this complication is not known with certainty, AIDS cholangiopathy is strongly associated with colonization of bile with cryptosporidia or microsporidia. Patients typically complain of right upper quadrant abdominal pain and often have abnormal liver test results, particularly that of alkaline phosphatase. The diagnosis may be suggested when an ultrasound examination of the gallbladder reveals edema of the wall; ERCP demonstrates strictures and delayed emptying and may permit direct sampling of bile for pathogens. No specific therapy is of proven benefit. Cholangiopathy is a late complication of AIDS; although rarely fatal of itself, it portends a poor prognosis.

Biliary atresia is a disorder of infants. Typically, the bile duct is normal at the time of birth; but over the next 6 to 12 weeks, its lumen gradually becomes obliterated and the duct becomes a fibrotic cord. The etiology is unknown. Infants become jaundiced at 4 to 6 weeks of age. Without treatment, over 90% of affected children will die before the age of 1 year from the complications of biliary cirrhosis. If the diagnosis is established promptly, a surgical portoenterostomy (Kasai procedure) can be of benefit. In this procedure, a core of tissue is removed from the hilum of the liver and the ends of the transected bile ducts are allowed to drain into a loop of jejunum. The Kasai procedure improves cholestasis and prolongs survival if performed early in infancy. Even after this procedure, most affected children progress to cirrhosis over the next few years. Biliary atresia is the most common indication for hepatic transplantation in young children.

PSC is a disorder characterized by a patchy obliterative inflammatory fibrosis of the large bile ducts. Chronic inflammation leads to extensive bile duct strictures, cholestasis, and gradual progression to biliary cirrhosis. The etiology of PSC is not known, but both genetic and immunologic abnormalities have been implicated. About 50% of all cases of PSC occur in association with inflammatory bowel disease (see Chapter 135). The frequency of HLA-B8 and HLA-DR3, which are associated with a number of autoimmune diseases, is higher in PSC than in normal subjects. Autoantibodies directed against an epitope present on colonic and biliary epithelial cells have been described in some patients. Unlike other extraintestinal manifestations of ulcerative colitis, PSC shows little correlation with the severity of bowel inflammation and does not remit after colectomy. The definitive diagnostic study for PSC is ERCP (or MRCP), which in classic cases demonstrates multiple areas of irregular stricturing and beadlike dilatations of the intrahepatic and extrahepatic ducts (see Fig. 157–5D). Because the fibrotic process may diffusely involve both intrahepatic and extrahepatic ducts, it is not uncommon for ultrasonography to reveal non-dilated bile ducts. The diagnosis of PSC also may be suggested by liver biopsy showing portal and periportal inflammation with small and large lymphocytes as well as periductular inflammation with epithelial destruction. With the progression of the disease, concentric "onionskin" fibrosis develops around disappearing bile ducts. Liver biopsy staging may be useful to characterize the stage and rate of progression of disease.

Patients with PSC typically present with insidious onset of chronic cholestasis, including jaundice, pruritus, fatigue, and malaise. The disease is often detected in a preclinical stage by routine blood tests revealing marked elevation of the serum alkaline phosphatase level, although in some patients with early disease the alkaline phosphatase value may be normal. About 15% of patients have manifestations suggestive of recurrent bacterial cholangitis,

with episodes of fever, chills, night sweats, right upper quadrant pain, and jaundice. Often the associated inflammatory bowel disease dominates the clinical picture.

There is no specific therapy for sclerosing cholangitis. Corticosteroids, azathioprine, penicillamine, and antibiotics have been proven ineffective. Administration of UDCA often improves liver function tests and sometimes may alleviate symptoms; it has not yet been demonstrated that UDCA retards the progression of the disease. Immunosuppressive therapy with methotrexate and cyclosporine are under study. Antibiotics are indicated for recurrent bacterial cholangitis. Surgical therapy has been directed toward improving biliary drainage. In recent years, endoscopic stenting or balloon dilatation of focal strictures have largely replaced surgery in this disease. Endoscopic drainage in selected cases may improve cholestasis and expedite clearing of biliary infections, but the long-term benefit is generally only marginal. PSC is a common indication for liver transplantation. Several large trials indicate that the mean interval from diagnosis of PSC to death from complications of biliary cirrhosis is 10 to 12 years. In the absence of hepatic transplantation, independent indicators of prognosis include age, serum bilirubin level, histologic stage, and presence of splenomegaly.

Twenty to 30 per cent of patients with advanced PSC may develop secondary cholangiocarcinoma, which is often very difficult to diagnose. Cholangiocarcinoma should be suspected in any patient with this disease who exhibits an abrupt worsening of cholestasis or in whom cholangiography indicates a single dominant stricture. Even with close evaluation and follow-up, cholangiocarcinoma is found incidentally in 10 to 15% of patients with PSC undergoing hepatic transplantation.

Gallstones

Gallstones are concretions that form in the biliary tree, usually in the gallbladder, when certain biliary solutes (cholesterol, calcium) precipitate as solid crystals that subsequently grow and aggregate within the mucin layer lining the gallbladder. The prevalence of gallstones in the U.S. adult population is 10 to 15%, and gallstone disease is responsible for about 10,000 deaths annually. Each year over 500,000 gallbladders are removed at a cost in excess of $6 billion because of gallstone-related disease. In the United States, cholesterol gallstones or cholesterol mixed with calcium bilirubinate account for 80% of stones, whereas the remaining 20% are pigmented or calcium bilirubinate stones.

PATHOGENESIS. The pathophysiology of gallstone formation begins when bile becomes supersaturated with cholesterol or calcium. Next, the solute must nucleate from solution and precipitate as solid crystals (cholesterol or bilirubin). Third, crystals must aggregate and fuse to form stones; this growth and aggregation of crystals occurs in a mucus gel along the wall of the gallbladder. Fourth, gallstone formation may be associated with impaired gallbladder motility, which is thought to be secondary to cholesterol accumulation in the gallbladder muscle, resulting in impaired contractile response to cholecystokinin.

Cholesterol gallstones are yellow-brown and range in size from a few millimeters to 2 to 3 cm. Greater than 50% of their dry weight (often over 90%) consists of crystalline cholesterol monohydrate, but variable amounts of other components, including mucin glycoproteins and calcium bilirubinate, are also present. Cholesterol gallstones can form when the amount of cholesterol secreted into bile exceeds the amount that can be held in stable micellar solution by the concentrations of bile salts and lecithin present. The degree of cholesterol saturation of bile is commonly expressed by a cholesterol saturation index, with index values greater than one indicating supersaturation. In unsaturated bile, newly secreted vesicles containing cholesterol and lecithin are dissolved completely by bile salts as bile is concentrated in the gallbladder. In contrast, as supersaturated bile is concentrated, vesicles fail to dissolve completely and instead fuse to form large, cholesterol-rich multilamellar liquid crystals, from which excess cholesterol may precipitate as plate-like cholesterol monohydrate crystals.

The causes of biliary cholesterol supersaturation generally can be divided into those associated with a primary increase in biliary secretion of cholesterol, by far a more predominant underlying cause, and those associated with deficiency of bile salts. Estrogen causes an increase in absolute rates of biliary cholesterol secretion into bile most likely as a result of up-regulation of low-density lipoprotein receptors and enhanced uptake of cholesterol by the hepatocyte. This fact probably accounts for the two-fold increased risk of cholesterol gallstones in women during their childbearing years and the increased risk of gallstones in multiparous women and women taking oral contraceptives. Progesterone also may play a part in gallstone pathogenesis by impairing gallbladder contractions and by inhibiting an enzyme responsible for esterification of free cholesterol. Obesity is associated with increased biliary cholesterol secretion possibly as a result of an increase in cholesterol synthesis. Some hypocholesterolemic drugs, such as the fibric acid derivatives clofibrate and gemfibrizol, directly stimulate secretion of cholesterol into bile and are associated with increased risk of cholesterol gallstones. Decrease in bile acid pool size may be responsible for increased incidence of cholesterol cholelithiasis in Crohn's disease, in which excessive bile salt losses occur due to ileal resection or diseased ileum. Many non-obese patients with cholelithiasis have a small bile salt pool and lower than normal rates of bile salt synthesis. Bile salt synthesis decreases and biliary cholesterol saturation increases with age, and this trend may account for the progressive increase in prevalence of gallstones with age. Gallstones develop more commonly in first-degree relatives of cholesterol gallstone patients. The high risk of cholesterol gallstones in Native Americans of the southwestern U.S. (greater than 80%) also appears to have a genetic basis. The nature of the genetic predisposition is not well understood, but oversensitive negative feedback regulation of bile salt biosynthesis has been postulated.

Pigment gallstones account for about 20% of U.S. gallstones. The predominant components of these gallstones are calcium salts of organic and inorganic anions, especially bilirubin. Ionized calcium is present in bile at concentrations similar to those of plasma. Unconjugated bilirubin has a low solubility product with calcium, and its presence in bile even in small amounts favors precipitation of calcium bilirubinate. Two subtypes of pigment gallstones have different composition, different pathogenesis, and different risk factors. *Black pigment gallstones* are hard, dense, brittle concretions composed of calcium bilirubinate along with inorganic calcium salts of carbonate and phosphate. The bilirubin in these stones becomes oxidized and polymerized, producing a mixture of altered pigments that absorb light over the entire visible spectrum, thus giving these stones a characteristic jet-black color. The major predisposing factor appears to be an increased heme turnover leading to increased biliary secretion of unconjugated bilirubin, as occurs in hemolytic disorders, hypersplenism (cirrhosis), or disorders associated with ineffective erythropoiesis. *Brown pigment (earthy) gallstones* have a soft, claylike consistency. In addition to calcium bilirubinate, they contain a substantial proportion of calcium soaps of fatty acids. Brown pigment gallstones occur in chronically infected bile in areas of stasis, where bacterial cleavage of phospholipid and conjugated bilirubin releases unconjugated bilirubin and fatty acids. Factors predisposing to this type of stone include biliary strictures, biliary infestation with parasites, Oriental cholangiohepatitis, and choledochal cysts. Most stones forming primarily in the bile ducts are of the brown pigment type.

In addition to bile supersaturation, a variety of other abnormalities contribute to formation of both cholesterol and pigment gallstones (Fig. 157–6). Precipitation of crystals from supersaturated bile requires the formation of an initial solid nidus (nucleation) with subsequent deposition of solute on the surface leading to crystal growth. Many individuals who secrete supersaturated bile have very slow nucleation and do not develop gallstones. Nucleation and growth of cholesterol crystals is much more rapid in bile of gallstone patients than in gallstone-free controls for equal degrees of cholesterol supersaturation. A number of proteins in bile can accelerate or retard the nucleation and growth of crystals, and abnormal levels of these proteins may account for the abnormally rapid crystal appearance in bile of gallstone patients. Nascent cholesterol crystals precipitating from vesicles or mixed micelles are trapped in a mucin gel lining of the gallbladder. Over time these crystals fuse to form macroscopic stones. Mucus secretion is stimulated by prostaglandins; in animal models the prevention of excessive mucin secretion by cyclooxygenase inhibitors can prevent cholesterol gallstone formation. Lastly, many patients with gallstones have defective gallbladder emptying and an abnormally high resid-

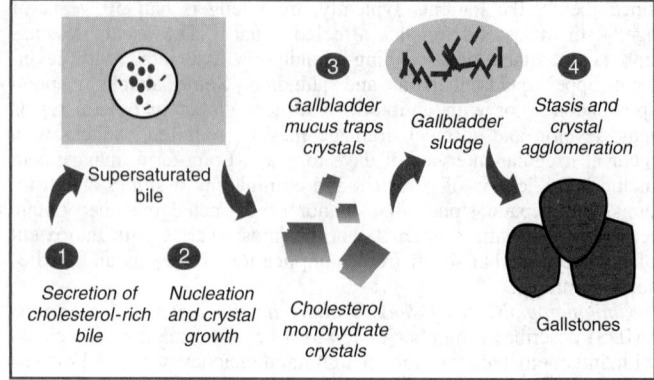

FIGURE 157–6 ■ Pathogenesis of cholesterol gallstones. Canalicular secretion of bile containing excess cholesterol relative to bile salts and phospholipids (supersaturated bile) is necessary but not sufficient. Additional requirements for stone formation are nucleation and growth of crystals, trapping of crystals in a mucin gel, and gallbladder stasis with retention of sludge permitting gradual aggregation and fusion of crystals to form macroscopic stones. Abnormalities in each of these areas have been noted in gallstone patients. In principle, eliminating any of these four steps should prevent gallstone formation.

ual volume after administration of cholecystokinin. Conditions in which gallbladder stasis occurs, such as parenteral alimentation, low-fat weight-reducing diets, and pregnancy are associated with a high rate of rapid gallstone formation.

CLINICAL MANIFESTATIONS. Gallstone disease can be divided conceptually into four stages (Table 157–2). In the first stage ("lithogenic"), no discrete stones have yet formed but the necessary conditions for stone formation (bile supersaturated with cholesterol, rapid nucleation and crystal growth, mucus, and gallbladder stasis) are in place. Identification of patients at high risk for gallstones in this early stage may allow targeted use of preventive therapies. In the second stage, the gallstones have already been formed but are still asymptomatic. Several epidemiologic studies have shown that the majority of gallstones are asymptomatic and may remain so for decades.

Onset of symptoms heralds the third stage of gallstone disease. The typical symptom-complex associated with gallstones is termed *biliary colic.* Biliary colic is thought to result from increased wall tension in the gallbladder and/or bile ducts due to impaction of a stone in the cystic duct or distal common bile duct. It is characterized by continuous severe pain in the epigastrium or right upper quadrant, sometimes radiating to the back or scapula, and typically lasting for more than 30 minutes. The pain is unrelieved by changes in position and often causes the patient to seek emergent medical attention. Biliary colic is frequently associated with nausea and vomiting. Biliary colic is the only pattern of pain that is consistently associated with gallstones; in large prospective studies, the frequency of non-specific symptoms such as vague abdominal discomfort, bloating, and flatulence in individuals with gallstones has been no higher than in the general population. Examination of the abdomen during attacks of biliary colic usually reveals right upper quadrant tenderness but no evidence of peritonitis, and the

Table 157–2 ■ STAGES OF GALLSTONE DISEASE

Lithogenic bile (stage 1)
↓
Asymptomatic gallstones (stage 2)
↓
Symptomatic gallstones (stage 3)
↓
Complications of gallstones (stage 4)
Acute:
  Acute cholecystitis (localized peritonitis, perforation, abscess, sepsis)
  Choledocholithiasis (obstructive jaundice, acute pancreatitis, ascending
    cholangitis)
Chronic:
  Chronic cholecystitis
  Choledochoduodenal fistula with gallstone ileus
  Gallbladder adenocarcinoma

patient is afebrile. Transient elevation of bilirubin, alkaline phosphatase, and aspartate and alanine aminotransferase levels are sometimes noted. In patients who have experienced at least one attack of biliary colic, about two thirds will experience additional attacks of pain during the next 2 years, and biliary colic therefore is commonly an indication for cholecystectomy.

The fourth and most serious stage of gallstone disease is marked by onset of complications. *Acute cholecystitis* (inflammation of the gallbladder) typically presents as acute onset of constant, dull, right upper quadrant pain, fever, shaking chills, nausea, and vomiting. Abdominal pain is often aggravated by coughing or moving; these symptoms are due to localized peritonitis over the area of the gallbladder. A characteristic physical finding is Murphy's sign, defined as tenderness of the gallbladder to palpation during examination of the abdomen. Patients with cholecystitis develop leukocytosis with marked shift to the left, but bilirubin and alkaline phosphatase levels are usually not elevated. In most cases, the cholecystitis develops as a result of impaction of a stone in the neck of the gallbladder. In about 10% of cases, however, no gallstones are present; such *acalculous cholecystitis* may result from impaction of mucus or sludge, from ischemia in vasculitic disorders, or from direct infection of the gallbladder bile. Some cases are sterile, but in the majority bacteria can be cultured from the gallbladder. The usual organisms present are *Escherichia coli* and other enteric gram negatives. If untreated, the gallbladder may become empyematous, develop gangrene, and perforate, leading to peritonitis, subphrenic abscess, and septic shock. Sometimes infection with gas-forming anaerobic organisms may produce emphysematous cholecystitis with air in the gallbladder wall. Acute cholecystitis requires prompt hospitalization. Antibiotic therapy will usually treat the infection and allow for elective surgery. However, acute cholecystitis should be considered a surgical disease requiring a surgical cure as promptly as it can be done safely.

Patients with long-standing gallstone disease frequently develop *chronic cholecystitis*. The evolution of chronic cholecystitis is obscure. It may be the result of repeated bouts of acute cholecystitis in some cases, but many patients cannot relate a history of acute cholecystitis. Often patients note vague, poorly defined, non-specific intermittent epigastric discomfort, but many are asymptomatic. The gallbladder is thickened, fibrotic, and contracted and frequently cannot be seen by oral cholecystography. A chronic inflammatory infiltrate is present, and mucosal pseudodiverticula termed *Rokitansky-Aschoff sinuses* are seen histologically. In long-standing cases, deposition of calcium in the fibrotic gallbladder wall may give an eggshell appearance on a radiograph, termed *porcelain gallbladder*. Chronic cholecystitis, particularly with porcelain gallbladder, is thought to predispose to adenocarcinoma of the gallbladder. In an occasional patient, impaction of a large stone in the cystic duct with persistent obstruction may gradually lead to distention of the gallbladder with clear mucus, a condition termed *gallbladder hydrops (mucocele)*. Calcium salts may become concentrated in the hydropic gallbladder, producing a *limy* or *milk-of-calcium bile*, which may be visible on plain abdominal radiographs.

Rarely in chronic cholecystitis a large gallstone will erode through the wall of the gallbladder or common bile duct into the duodenum, producing a *choledochoenteric fistula*. In the absence of prior biliary surgery, this unusual condition is strongly suggested by the finding of *air in the biliary tree on plain radiographs*. The large stone frequently impacts in the ileum, and patients then present with small bowel obstruction, a phenomenon termed *gallstone ileus*. Fistulization also can occur into other structures adjacent to the gallbladder such as colon, stomach, or abdominal wall.

Gallstones in the common bile duct (choledocholithiasis) may impact at the level of the ampulla of Vater to produce obstructive jaundice and biliary colic (see Fig. 157–5C). Bacterial infection above an obstructing stone in the common bile duct is common and leads to *ascending cholangitis*. Patients with ascending cholangitis typically present with acute onset of high fever and signs of sepsis, right upper quadrant pain and tenderness, and jaundice (Charcot's triad). Leukocytosis with shift to the left, conjugated hyperbilirubinemia, abnormally high alkaline phosphatase, and elevated aminotransferase levels are common. Bacteria often can be cultured from the blood. In severe cases, pus may be present in the biliary tree, and patients may develop multiple hepatic abscesses. The usual pathogens observed in ascending cholangitis are enteric gram-negative bacteria, anaerobes, or occasionally enterococci. Antibiotics are indicated but frequently fail to control sepsis in severe, suppurative cases. Symptoms usually respond rapidly to biliary drainage through surgical, radiographic, or endoscopic means. Endoscopic sphincterotomy with stone extraction and/or temporary stent placement is the least invasive and most rapid way of achieving biliary decompression in most cases of ascending cholangitis.

Attacks of *acute pancreatitis* (see Chapter 141) may be triggered by passage of a gallstone through the ampulla of Vater. The pathogenesis of acute gallstone pancreatitis is not completely understood. It has been speculated that transient obstruction of the pancreatic duct orifice where it joins the common bile duct leads to an increase in pancreatic ductal pressure, which may cause premature activation of proteolytic enzymes within the pancreatic acinar cells. Gallstones are responsible for most cases of pancreatitis in the nonalcoholic. Data suggest that episodes of recurrent acute pancreatitis previously thought to be idiopathic may be caused by small gallstones that are below the limits of detection of the common imaging techniques. A search for cholesterol microcrystals in duodenal bile may be useful in making the diagnosis of *microlithiasis*.

Diagnostic Studies in Gallstone Disease

A variety of diagnostic imaging studies are of value in patients with suspected gallbladder disease (Fig. 157–7). Plain radiographs may reveal calcium-containing (pigment) gallstones, which are usually radiopaque. Occasionally, foci of calcification either in the core or around the rim also can be seen in predominantly cholesterol stones. Air in the biliary tree can be caused by gas-forming organisms or by fistulas between the bowel and biliary tract. Calcification of the gallbladder ("porcelain gallbladder") indicates chronic cholecystitis.

Ultrasonography is a sensitive, specific, non-invasive, and inexpensive test for diagnosis of gallstones. In general, ultrasonography is the only diagnostic procedure needed to make the diagnosis of gallstones in the gallbladder, but it usually will not detect stones in the common bile duct; it may, however, provide clues to the presence of choledocholithiasis, such as dilatation of the major bile ducts. The typical gallstone on ultrasound evaluation appears as an echogenic focus that casts a sound "shadow." Biliary sludge also is diffusely echogenic and located in the dependent gallbladder but lacks acoustic shadowing. In acute cholecystitis, ultrasonography may reveal edema of the gallbladder wall and pericholecystic fluid. The accuracy of ultrasound in diagnosis of gallstones is about 95%. However, ultrasonography does not provide accurate information on the type of gallstone (cholesterol vs. pigmented), number of gallstones, or cystic duct obstruction.

For an oral cholecystogram, patients are given an oral radiocontrast agent, iopanoic acid. The contrast agent is absorbed from the intestine, taken up by the liver, and secreted into the bile. When concentrated by the gallbladder overnight, the contrast agent outlines most of the gallbladder. Radiolucent gallstones appear as negative shadows within the gallbladder. Failure of the gallbladder to visualize generally suggests chronic cholecystitis with loss of gallbladder mucosal function or cystic duct obstruction. Acute and chronic liver disease may also be associated with failure to visualize the gallbladder. The size and type of stones can be estimated with reasonable accuracy by this test. Typical cholesterol gallstones are radiolucent and floating. Because of more extensive information provided by oral cholecystography on the type and size of gallstones and gallbladder visualization, this procedure should be used in evaluating those patients who may be candidates for gallstone dissolution.

Hepatobiliary radionuclide scans employ a variety of iminodiacetic acid (IDA) derivatives (e.g., HIDA, DISIDA, or PIPIDA) to assess the patency of the cystic duct and the common bile duct. These organic anions are administered intravenously, taken up by the liver, and excreted rapidly into bile. Failure of these isotopes to enter the gallbladder or the intestine suggests obstruction of the cystic or common bile ducts, respectively. This test is very useful in the diagnosis of cholecystitis with cystic duct obstruction.

Contrast material may be injected directly into the biliary tree through either a percutaneous, fluoroscopically guided approach (PTC) or a retrograde approach (ERCP). These tests represent the gold standards for examination of the biliary tree and generally will

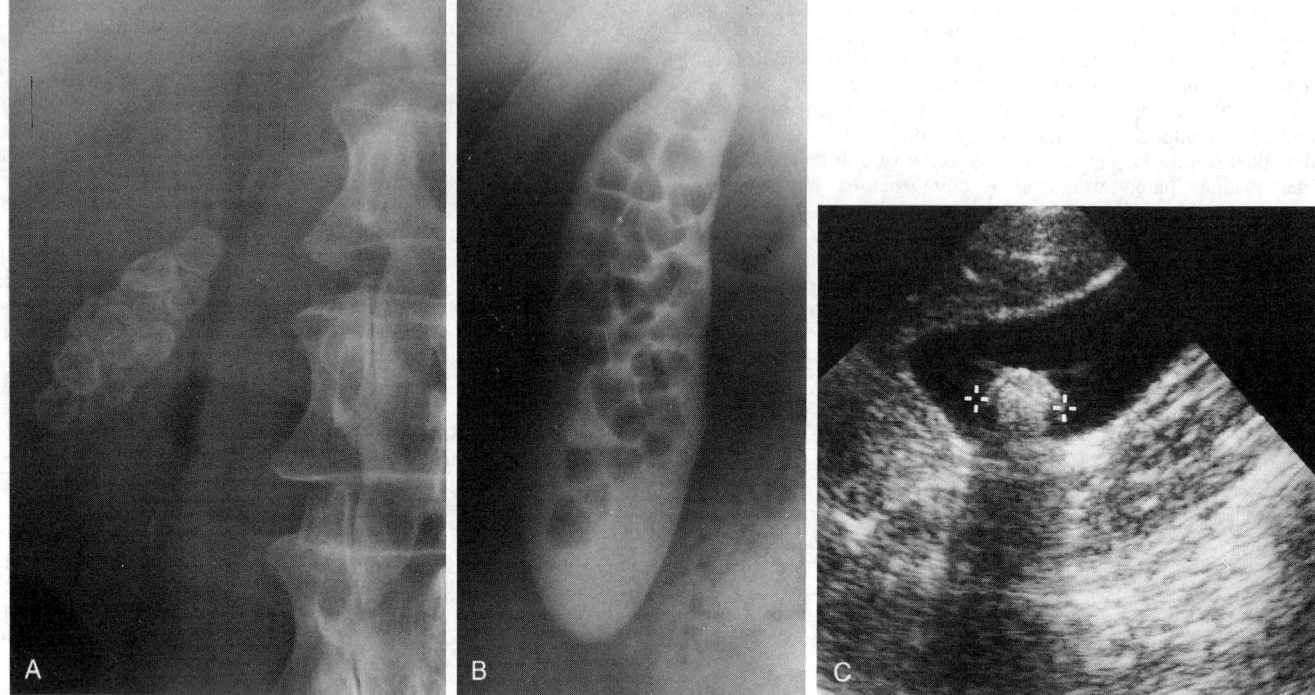

FIGURE 157–7 ■ Images of gallstones. *A,* Plain radiograph reveals calcified pigment gallstones. The more common cholesterol gallstones are not detectable on plain radiographs. *B,* Oral cholecystogram showing contrast material outlining multiple radiolucent cholesterol stones in a normally functioning gallbladder. *C,* Ultrasound examination showing a large gallstone as an echogenic focus that casts a sonic "shadow."

reveal stones or stenosis that are not detectable by other means. In occasional patients in whom gallstones are strongly suspected but all routine studies are negative, microscopic examination of a sample of bile aspirated at ERCP may reveal the presence of calcium bilirubinate or cholesterol crystals.

Therapy for Gallstones

No treatment is usually required for asymptomatic gallstones because of their low propensity to become symptomatic. Longitudinal studies have shown that conversion from asymptomatic to symptomatic stones takes place at the rate of no more than 1 to 2% per year, and risk-benefit analyses indicate that surgery for asymptomatic gallstones generally causes more morbidity than it prevents. Exceptions to this rule may include very large gallstones (>3 cm in diameter) and porcelain gallbladder, both of which have been associated with an increased risk of gallbladder carcinoma. Some experts also would recommend prophylactic cholecystectomy for asymptomatic gallstones in patients with diabetes mellitus or spinal cord injury because gallstone complications such as acute cholecystitis may be more severe and more often life threatening in these groups.

Symptomatic gallstones are cured by cholecystectomy. Surgical removal of the gallbladder is indicated in all instances of acute cholecystitis or in symptomatic patients with non-visualized gallbladder on oral cholecystography. Laparoscopic cholecystectomy is now preferred because of shorter hospitalization time and quicker recovery. Serious bile duct injury, often requiring reconstructive surgery, occurs in about 0.5% of cases but decreases in frequency as the surgeon gains experience with laparoscopic surgery.

Gallstones in the common bile duct may be removed by the surgeon at the time of cholecystectomy. More recently, development of methods for direct choledochoscopy and stone extraction during surgery have reduced the need for common duct exploration (Color Plate 2*D*). Alternatively, stones up to 1.5 cm in diameter can be extracted from the common bile duct by endoscopic methods after endoscopic sphincterotomy. Larger stones can be crushed and extracted in pieces. These techniques are of value when patients are acutely ill with ascending cholangitis or acute pancreatitis or when stones are inadvertently left in the common duct after cholecystectomy.

Ascending cholangitis is treated aggressively with antibiotics and endoscopic sphincterotomy, which removes the obstructed stones and allows for normalization of bile flow. The drainage of infected bile combined with appropriate antibiotic therapy results in quick recovery, after which the patient ordinarily should have an elective cholecystectomy. In patients at high surgical risk, cholecystectomy can be deferred indefinitely after sphincterotomy and stone extraction with only a few per cent per year risk of subsequent gallstone complications.

In addition to surgical therapy, cholesterol gallstones may be treated medically. Oral administration of certain bile salts (chenodeoxycholic acid or UDCA) reduces biliary cholesterol saturation. If the cholesterol saturation index of bile can be brought below 1 with administration of these two bile salts, the gallstone-forming process can be reversed and undersaturated micelles in bile can slowly "leach" cholesterol from the stones. Over a period of time (6 months to 1 year) of continuous therapy, pure cholesterol gallstones will gradually dissolve. Bile salt therapy is most successful in patients with pure cholesterol gallstones and does not work with calcified stones and even mixed stones. Other critical factors for success include small stones, a normally functioning gallbladder, and adequate bile salt dosage. In an ideal group of patients with small, radiolucent, floating stones, 75% dissolution of gallstones within 1 year has been observed. Chenodeoxycholic acid is moderately toxic; it may cause mild to moderate elevations of liver function tests and serum cholesterol. In therapeutic doses, chenodeoxycholic acid is frequently associated with disabling diarrhea. Because of these side effects, the use of chenodeoxycholic acid in patients with gallstones has been abandoned in the United States. UDCA, a 7β-epimer of chenodeoxycholic acid, is a weak detergent and essentially without toxicity; it is equally as efficacious in dissolving gallstones as chenodeoxycholic acid but has practically no side effects. Administration of UDCA is associated with a marked decrease in biliary cholesterol secretion and desaturation of bile with cholesterol; it also appears to stabilize cholesterol-rich lecithin vesicles and liquid crystals in bile. Because oral dissolution therapy is slow and often not successful, it generally is reserved for patients with mildly symptomatic gallstones who are at high risk for surgery or who are otherwise reluctant to undergo cholecystectomy. UDCA is also effective for primary prevention of rapidly forming gallstones in patients with morbid obesity who are experiencing rapid weight loss. Prophylactic administration of UDCA during this period reduces gallstone incidence by more than 80%.

Experimental medical therapies for gallstones include solvent dissolution and extracorporeal shock wave lithotripsy. Cholesterol gallstones can be dissolved rapidly (within hours) when organic solvents such as methyl-tert-butyl ether or ethyl propionate are instilled directly into the gallbladder by percutaneous transhepatic approach. The dissolution rate for non-calcified stones using this modality is close to 100% and the side effects are few. This approach has not gained wide acceptance because of its invasive nature and labor intensity. Extracorporeal shock wave lithotripsy was first introduced with great success for treatment of renal stones and, later, in the mid 1980s, was modified to permit shattering of stones in the gallbladder. Gallstone fragments after lithotripsy are eliminated with bile or can be dissolved with concurrent oral bile salt treatment. This therapy is particularly effective for solitary gallstones. Biliary colic after lithotripsy occurs relatively frequently as a result of elimination of small fragments of pulverized stones; in about 1% of patients, passage of stone fragments causes acute pancreatitis. No gallstone lithotripsy device has been approved for general use in the United States; and with the advent of laproscopic cholecystectomy, this technology has largely been abandoned. A major limitation of all medical treatments of cholesterol gallstones (bile salt dissolution, solvent dissolution, lithotripsy) is gallstone recurrence, which averages about 50% over a period of 5 years. However, only 7.5% of the recurrent stones become symptomatic, and continuous low-dose UDCA administration may prevent or decrease the incidence of stone recurrence.

Other Benign Disorders of the Gallbladder

A number of benign gallbladder wall abnormalities sometimes may mimic cholelithiasis. *Cholesterolosis* of the gallbladder is usually an asymptomatic condition in which cholesterol accumulates within histiocytes in the mucosa of the gallbladder. Aggregates of these lipid-laden macrophages distend and enlarge the mucosal folds. The accumulation of lipid at the tips of these folds is readily visible grossly as yellow streaks or flecks that resemble the seeds of a strawberry, hence the common name "strawberry gallbladder." There is usually no inflammation or calculi. The reason for the accumulation of cholesterol is unknown. Focal aggregation of cholesterol laden macrophages may produce polyps that may be visible on ultrasonography. Other benign gallbladder lesions that may produce polyps of the gallbladder wall include benign *adenomas* and *adenomyomatous hyperplasia*. In general, these lesions are asymptomatic and require no treatment.

Postcholecystectomy Disorders

After cholecystectomy, a small fraction of patients develop mild diarrhea. Increased circulation of the bile salt pool with increased delivery of bile salts to the colon has been implicated in postcholecystectomy diarrhea, and patients with this syndrome often respond well to treatment with cholestyramine. More difficult is the problem of recurrent upper abdominal pain, which is noted in about 5% of patients after cholecystectomy. In some instances, pain may be secondary to retained gallstones in the common bile duct or abscess or other complications of surgery. In the absence of such a specific etiology, biliary type pain after gallbladder removal is termed *post-cholecystectomy syndrome*. This term is a misnomer, since in most cases the pain probably is unrelated to gallstones or cholecystectomy but rather due to an error in the original diagnosis. The prevalence of gallstones is so great that many patients with abdominal pain from other causes are coincidentally found to have gallstones. When these patients undergo cholecystectomy, persistence of symptoms is not surprising. Recurrence of abdominal pain after cholecystectomy should lead the physician to consider other, overlooked causes of pain such as irritable bowel syndrome, peptic ulcer, pancreatitis, and biliary dyskinesia.

Table 157-3 ■ CRITERIA FOR DIAGNOSIS OF BILIARY DYSKINESIA

Right upper quadrant pain associated with transient elevation of alkaline phosphatase, bilirubin, aspartate aminotransferase, and alanine aminotransferase
Diameter of common bile duct >11 mm (ultrasound)
Delayed emptying of common bile duct (>45 min) after endoscopic retrograde cholangiopancreatography or quantitative hepatobiliary scintigraphy
Elevated basal sphincter of Oddi pressure (by manometry)

Biliary Dyskinesia

Biliary dyskinesia refers to a syndrome of repeated attacks of biliary colic resulting from motor dysfunction of the sphincter of Oddi. Bile flow is regulated by the sphincter of Oddi by a combination of phasic contractions superimposed on tonic pressure. The motor activity of the sphincter of Oddi is influenced by hormonal and neural factors. The principal hormone involved in the regulation of sphincter of Oddi and gallbladder contraction is cholecystokinin, which contracts the gallbladder and at the same time relaxes the sphincter of Oddi. After cholecystectomy with loss of the gallbladder reservoir, modest increases normally have been noted in the sphincter of Oddi tone, bile ductal pressure, and common bile ductal diameter. Rarely, patients may develop abnormalities of sphincter of Oddi function, including increased basal tone or increased amplitude and frequency of phasic contraction, which may episodically impede efflux of bile and trigger typical attacks of biliary colic. The association of sphincter of Oddi motor abnormalities with symptoms and signs of functional biliary obstruction is termed *biliary dyskinesia* (Table 157–3). Clinically, biliary dyskinesia produces episodic right upper quadrant abdominal pain mimicking an attack of choledocholithiasis. The diagnosis is suspected when symptoms and laboratory abnormalities suggest intermittent common bile duct obstruction at the level of the ampulla of Vater (elevated alkaline phosphatase, aspartate aminotransferase, and/or bilirubin; dilatation of the common bile duct), but cholangiography reveals no evidence of gallstones. Additional objective signs that support this diagnosis are delayed emptying of the common bile duct at ERCP and abnormal sphincter of Oddi manometry showing an increase in basal pressure to greater than 40 mm Hg. Once the diagnosis is established, endoscopic sphincterotomy is the therapy of choice.

Bates MD, Bucuvalas JC, Alonso MH, Ryckman FC: Biliary atresia: Pathogenesis and treatment. Semin Liver Dis 18:281–293, 1998. *Detailed review of the clinical presentation and therapy of this disorder of 1 per 10,000 live births.*

Czaja AJ: Frequency and nature of the variant syndromes of autoimmune liver disease. Hepatology 28:360–365, 1998. *A clinical review summarizing the similarities and differences among autoimmune hepatitis, primary biliary cirrhosis, and primary sclerosing cholangitis.*

Heuman DM, Moore EW, Vlahcevic ZR: Pathogenesis and dissolution of gallstones. *In* Zakim D, Boyer DT (eds): Hepatology, 3rd ed. Philadelphia, WB Saunders, 1996. *A current review of present gallstone pathogenesis, with particular emphasis on factors involved in pathogenesis of gallstone formation.*

Kaplan MM: The use of methotrexate, colchicine, and other immunomodulatory drugs in the treatment of primary biliary cirrhosis. Semin Liver Dis 17:129–136, 1997. *Review of present modalities of therapy for primary biliary cirrhosis.*

Ko CW, Sekijima JH, Lee SP: Biliary sludge. Ann Intern Med 130:301–311, 1999. *A review of the clinical significance of this ultrasonographic finding.*

Ponsioen CIJ, Tytgat NJ: Primary sclerosing cholangitis: A clinical review. Am J Gastroenterol 93:515–523, 1998. *A detailed review of the natural history of this disease.*

PART XIII

HEMATOLOGIC DISEASES

158 HEMATOPOIESIS AND HEMATOPOIETIC GROWTH FACTORS

Peter Quesenberry

Lymphohematopoiesis is a tightly regulated system in which production of the various blood cell types responds to specific functional demands: red cell production in response to hypoxia, granulocyte/monocyte production in response to infection, lymphocyte production in response to antigen challenge, and platelet production in response to hemorrhage. In this system (or tissue), early multipotent stem cells with extensive proliferative potential, but few differentiated features, reside largely in the bone-encased marrow cavity. These stem cells have the potential, with appropriate inductive signals, to differentiate and give rise to populations of progenitor cells with progressively restricted renewal, proliferative, and lineage potential but with increasing functional characteristics defining a variety of specific lineages (Fig. 158–1). This process eventuates in the cell lineages recognizable by standard Wright-Giemsa stains as erythroid, granulocytic, monocytic, lymphoid, or megakaryocytic. These events occur continuously with a large turnover of differentiated cells, as illustrated by the blood lifespans of human erythrocytes (120 days), platelets (10 days), and granulo-

cytes (9 hours). Lymphocyte (T and B cells) lifespans vary tremendously from hours to years. The production of active blood cell types occurs predominantly in the bone marrow. However, the spleen, lymph nodes, and accessory lymphoid tissues are also ongoing sites of cell production, predominately lymphoid; under stress, myeloid cell production also occurs at these sites. The end cells produced in the marrow are released into the blood stream under various stimuli and circulate in the blood. With the exception of erythrocytes and platelets, they emigrate to the tissues where they have variable lifespans: granulocytes measured in days and monocytes/macrophage/lymphocytes measured in weeks to years.

LYMPHOHEMATOPOIESIS

The classically recognizable differentiated marrow lineages represent the end stages of a carefully orchestrated production system. Progenitors feed into the various blast compartments (myeloblast, proerythroblast, lymphoblast, and megakaryoblast), which, in turn, feed into lineages that show increasingly differentiated characteristics while losing proliferative potency. Myeloblasts become promyelocytes, which then differentiate into myelocytes, the stage at which neutrophilic (Fig 158–2), eosinophilic, and basophilic lineages are distinguished. Erythrocyte and platelet lineages result in anucleate functional cells, whereas B and T lymphocyte lineages give rise to a variety of effector cell populations. This system is an irreversible in-out production system with final demise of end cells in the blood stream (platelets and red cells) or tissues (all others).

The primitive lymphohematopoietic stem cell is the basis for the

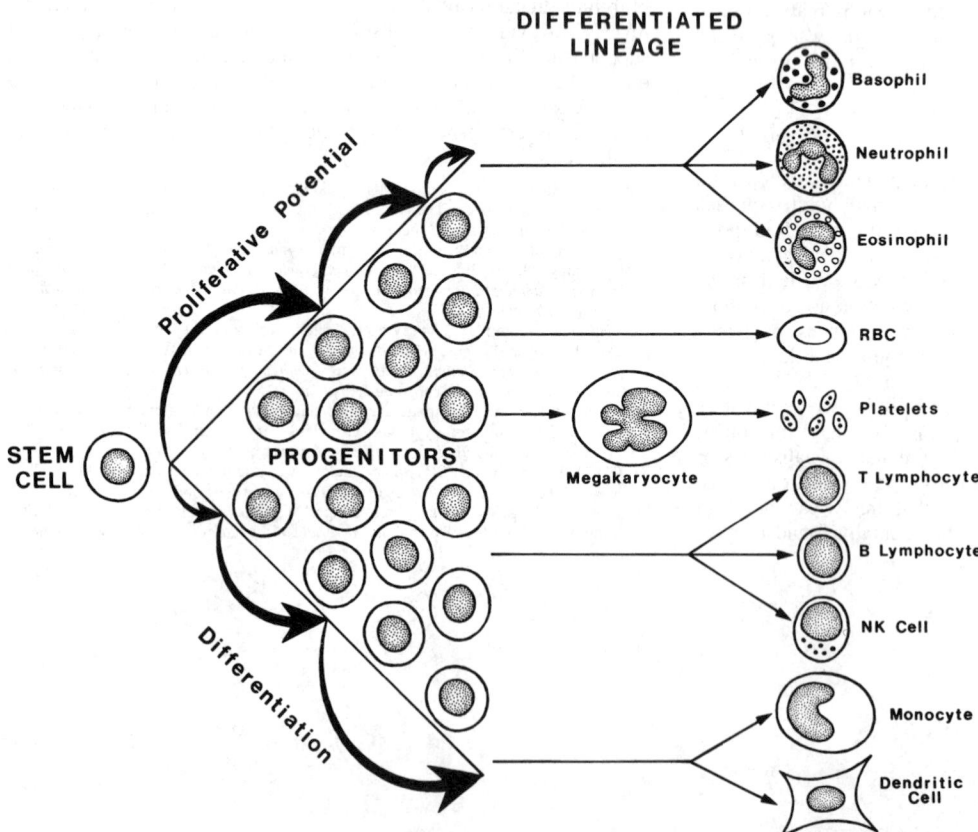

FIGURE 158–1 ■ Hierarchical model of lymphohematopoiesis. RBC-red blood cell; NK cell-natural killer cell.

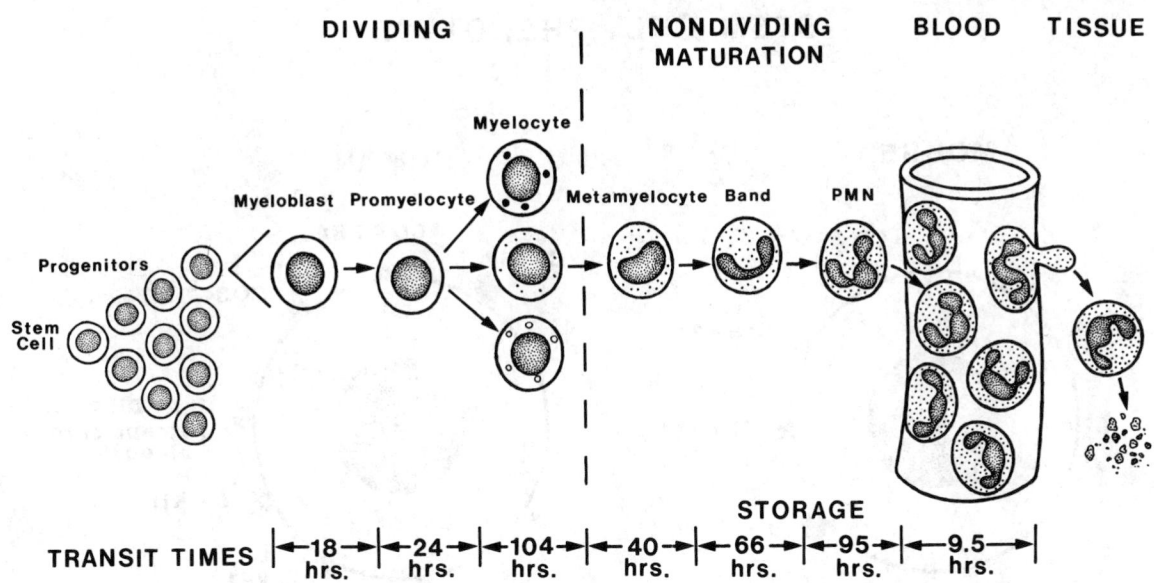

FIGURE 158–2 ■ Neutrophil production system. PMN-polymorphonuclear leukocyte.

ongoing production of lymphohematopoiesis (Table 158–1). The stem cell is defined as a cell with tremendous proliferative potential, the capacity to renew itself on a population basis, and the ability to give rise to large numbers of differentiated progeny eventuating in the end cells just detailed. It immediately gives rise to a wide variety of committed progenitors, ranging from those capable of giving rise to most lineages to progenitors restricted to a single lineage.

STEM CELL ONTOGENY

Early multipotent stem cells are present in the yolk sac and in mesenchymal tissues. These stem cells subsequently traffic predominantly to the liver (and to a lesser extent the kidney), followed by the establishment of marrow as the major site of active hematopoiesis. The earlier in ontogeny stem cells are harvested, the greater their proliferative potential, as illustrated by the proliferative and growth potential of fetal liver and cord blood cells in clinical transplantation.

The hematopoietic cell in both murine and human species has been characterized as to surface proteins and physical, metabolic, and cell cycle characteristics; and these characteristics have been utilized physically to purify stem cells (Fig. 158–3). Early stem cells do not express differentiated lineage markers, but they express certain classes of receptor proteins or other markers; in humans, CD34 and c-*kit* have been proposed as stem cell-specific markers. Studies have indicated that CD34-negative cells (1) have significant stem cell potential but contain no progenitor cells and (2) may give rise to CD34-positive cells. The most primitive stem cells tend to be dormant in G_0 or prolonged G_1 phases and also to show strong

activity of the p170 pump, the multidrug resistance pump that exudes certain chemotherapeutic agents and the dyes rhodamine and Hoechst, from cells. Thus the most primitive stem cells are characterized by very low staining with rhodamine and Hoechst.

LYMPHOHEMATOPOIETIC STEM CELL. The existence of a stem cell, common to all lymphoid and myeloid lineages, was established by studies in mice in which the infusion of a single cytogenetically or retrovirally marked stem cell gave rise to all cell lineages, which then persisted over time. Sustained in vivo engraftment is the gold standard for the true stem cell, although different subpopulations may show different engraftment kinetics, ranging from weeks to over a year in the mouse. The engrafting cell, which is quiescent or dormant, appears to have high p170 pump activity (stains low for rhodamine, a p170-pumped dye). The existence of a similar multipotent stem cell in humans was inferred from studies of marrow and blood cells from patients with chronic myelogenous leukemia, in whom all lineages were marked with the Philadelphia chromosome, and from glucose-6-phosphate dehydrogenase studies of patients with myeloproliferative disorders.

Unfortunately, there is no in vivo engraftment assay in humans, but three in vitro assays appear to measure relatively primitive multilineage cells and have been proposed as true surrogates for the long-term renewal lymphohematopoietic stem cell. The colony-forming unit-blast (an assay in which marrow cells give rise to small colonies of primitive blast cells) with extensive proliferative and differentiative potential may in fact be a good surrogate, but unfortunately few laboratories have mastered this technique, so it is not generally applicable. The high proliferative potential colony-forming cell, an assay in which marrow cells proliferate in the presence of combinations of growth factors to give rise to large (>0.5 mm) colonies in vitro, also appears to be a reasonable surro-

Table 158–1 ■ STEM AND PROGENITOR CELLS

CHARACTERISTIC	STEM CELL	PROGENITOR CELL
Proliferative potential	Tremendous	More limited
Renewal	On a population basis	Probably none
Potential for differentiation	All lymphohematopoietic lineages	Restricted
Differentiated characteristics	Minimal—lineage negative	Progressively increases
Cycle status	Dormant	Cycling
Cytokine responsiveness	Large number of cytokines needed for expression of phenotype	Restricted
Cell of origin	Unknown	Stem cell
Staining with rhodamine and Hoechst dyes (partial measure of p170 pump activity)	Active p170 pump—stains dimly	Less active p170 pump—rhodamine "bright"
Producing long-term hematopoiesis after in vivo transplant	Defines cells	Limited to none
Adheres to marrow stroma	Yes	No or limited

STEM CELL PHENOTYPE

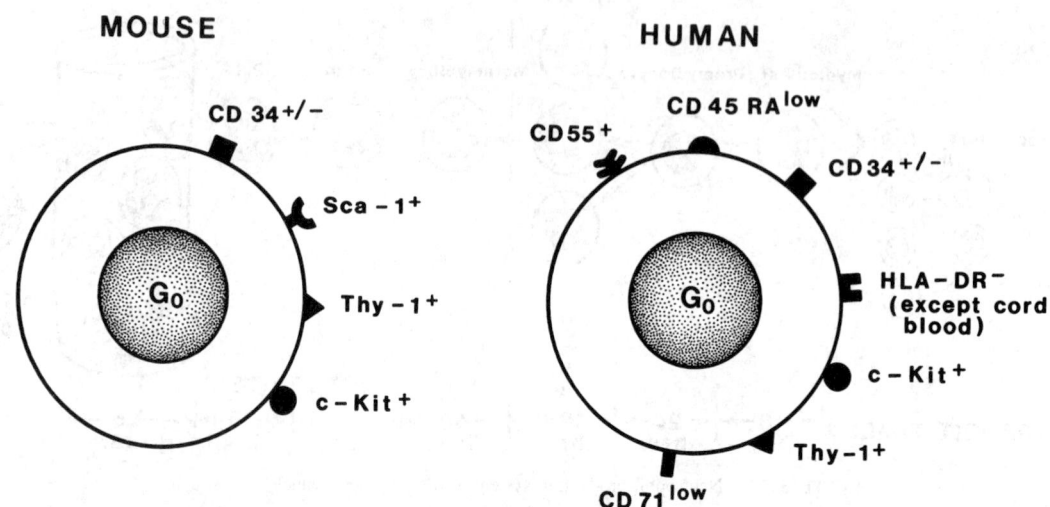

Stains poorly with the supravital dyes rhodamine and Hoechst

Lineage negative

FIGURE 158–3 ■ Characteristics of the lymphohematopoietic stem cell.

gate and probably the best generally available. The stromal-based assays, long-term culture–initiating cell (LTC-IC) and cobblestone-forming assays, are of interest but appear to monitor both primitive and more differentiated cells and are difficult to reproduce. These assays, in which marrow cells grow on an adherent stromal layer, remain interesting research areas without practical applications, although the recently described LTC-IC extended (a 60+ day assay) may come closer to the real stem cell.

Human marrow and cord blood cells have been infused into immunodeficient mice to establish engraftment. Studies with non-obese diabetic–severe combined immunodeficient mice, an immunodeficient animal that will accept human marrow cell engraftment, have been particularly impressive, but the lineages are skewed to lymphoid cells, and engraftment is variable. Thus, this assay has not yet been established as a valid human stem cell assay.

REGULATION AND CYTOKINES. Utilizing both in vitro and in vivo assays, a large number of cytokines have been characterized and shown to affect lymphohematopoiesis. The availability of cloned molecules has provided sufficient quantities of cytokines for in vivo studies and clinical application. Regulation of lymphohematopoiesis is based on a large number of circulating and membrane based cytokines, as well as integrin modulation and antigen presentation to B and T cells. Over 70 cytokines maintain, stimulate, or inhibit various aspects of lymphohematopoiesis (Table 158–2).

Cytokines exert a wide variety of actions on diverse cell types both within and outside specific differentiation lineages, but many

Table 158–2 ■ CHARACTERISTICS OF LYMPHOHEMATOPOIETIC CYTOKINES

Are glycoproteins
Act on cell surface receptors
Initiate complex second messenger and transcriptional and post-transcriptional regulation
May act on stem cell, progenitor cell, and differentiated cells of the same lineage.
May act on multiple different lineages (e.g., erythroid, granulocyte, and lymphoid).
Stimulate or inhibit proliferation, apoptosis, differentiation, or function
Usually act on neoplastic counterpart of normal target cell

have predominant or primary actions, especially when evaluated after in vivo administration (Table 158–3). Erythropoietin (erythroid), macrophage–colony-stimulating factor (M-CSF), and granulocyte-CSF (G-CSF) are examples of cytokines with a relatively high degree of specificity. Most cytokines, however, have multiple actions. Examples include interleukin (IL)-6, which acts on primitive stem cells as well as lymphoid, granulocyte, megakaryocyte, and macrophage lineages, and IL-3, which impacts virtually all lineages. IL-1 induces many other cytokines and illustrates the difficulty in ascertaining primary or secondary effects, especially with the potential for paracrine or autocrine loops.

These cytokines are produced by a large variety of tissues and cell types. Most cells produce multiple cytokines, which can be differentially induced by various stimuli, including other cytokines, such as IL-1. The suggestion that "everything makes everything" is perhaps too drastic, but also not too far off target. The key is in differential production in response to different stimuli, and probably in local production. Monocytes, T lymphocytes, endothelial cells, fibroblasts, and "marrow stromal" cells are important sources of lymphohematopoietic cytokines. Erythropoietin production is an exception to the general rule, because it is largely produced in the kidney in response to hypoxia, although it can also be produced by the liver. Stimuli that induce white blood cell formation are, in general, related to exposure to foreign or noxious agents, whereas platelet production occurs in response to hemorrhage, anemia, and thrombocytopenia.

Perhaps the best way to define the cytokine responsiveness of a particular cell class is to characterize cytokine receptor expression. Each cytokine has its private receptor, but different cytokines may share class-specific signal transducers. Many receptors dimerize on cytokine binding and then activate tyrosine kinase, promoting phosphorylation of intracellular proteins; other receptors do not have intrinsic enzymatic activity but induce protein phosphorylation through associated non–receptor-type tyrosine kinase activities, such as JAK2, Fes, and Lyn. Receptors are expressed in low numbers and do not exceed a few hundred per cell. The multipotent repopulating stem cell possesses receptors for most cytokines, but more mature cells have a more restricted distribution of receptors.

PLATE 5 HEMATOLOGIC DISEASES

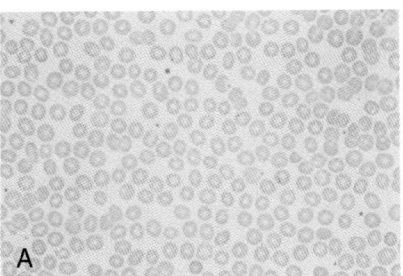

A, Normal peripheral blood smear. The red cells are normocytic (normal size) and normochromic (normal hemoglobin pigment), with central areas of pallor that should occupy less than one half of the diameter of the cells.

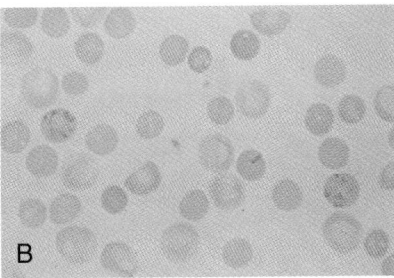

B, Reticulocytes. Special supravital (methylene blue) staining of the blood smear reveals dark purple reticulin, representing residual RNA in immature red cells.

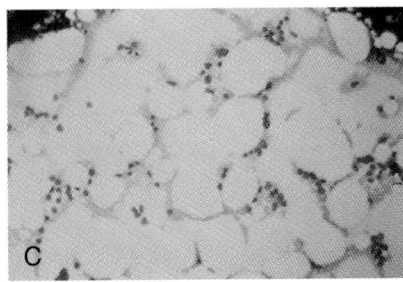

C, Aplastic anemia. Bone marrow biopsy shows a virtually empty marrow.

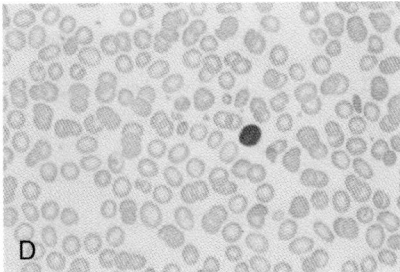

D, Iron deficiency anemia. Many red cells are microcytic (smaller than the nucleus of the normal lymphocyte near the center of the field) and hypochromic (with central areas of pallor that exceed one half of the diameter of the cells).

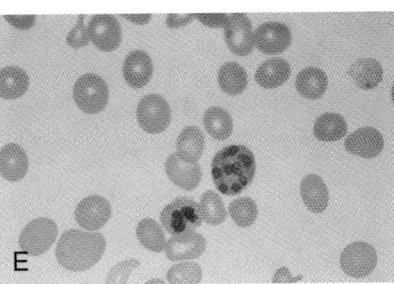

E, Megaloblastic anemia. Peripheral blood with oval macrocytes (large red cells) and marked neutrophil hypersegmentation.

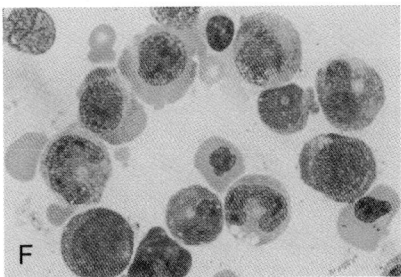

F, Megaloblastic anemia. Bone marrow aspirate shows red cell precursors that are giant megaloblasts, with nuclear-cytoplasmic dissociation (nuclear maturation lagging behind cytoplasmic maturation). Megaloblastic changes in the leukocyte series are demonstrated by the "giant C metamyelocyte."

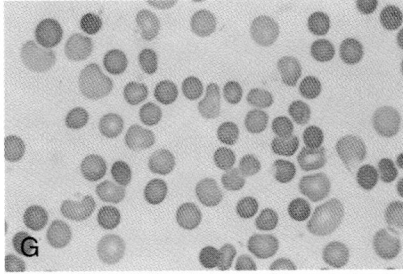

G, Hereditary spherocytosis. Peripheral smear shows a predominance of microspherocytes (small, densely staining red cells with loss of the central areas of pallor) alongside larger, grayish, "polychromatic" cells that probably represent reticulocytes.

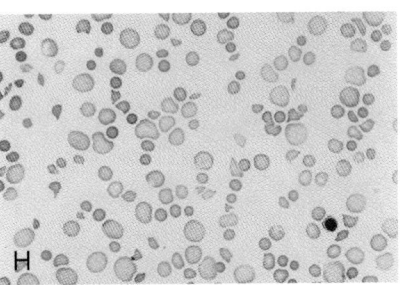

H, Microangiopathic hemolytic anemia. Peripheral smear shows fragmented red cells or "schistocytes" in a variety of shapes and sizes.

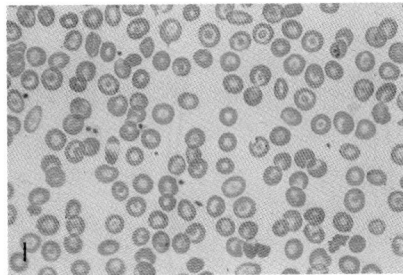

I, Thalassemia minor. Smear shows hypochromic red cells with many target cells.

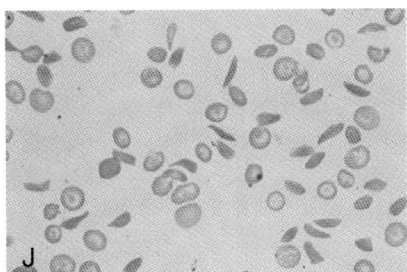

J, Sickle cell anemia. Homozygous SS disease with a predominance of sickled red cells in the peripheral smear.

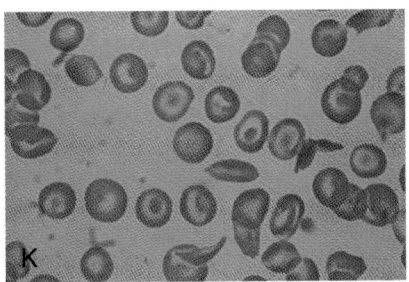

K, Hemoglobin SC disease. Peripheral smear shows frequent target cells interspersed with sickled red cells that are sometimes more plump in appearance than sickle cells in SS disease.

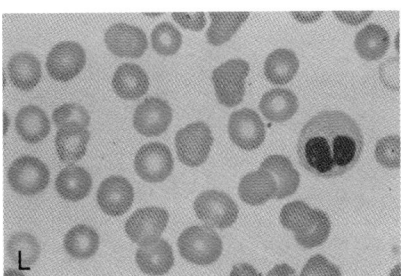

L, Pelger-Huët anomaly. Mature neutrophil with a two-lobed nucleus that has a dumbbell or "pince-nez" appearance. Pseudo-Pelger-Huët anomaly occurs in acquired conditions (e.g., myelodysplasia, myeloproliferative disorders, infections).

PLATE 6   HEMATOLOGIC DISEASES

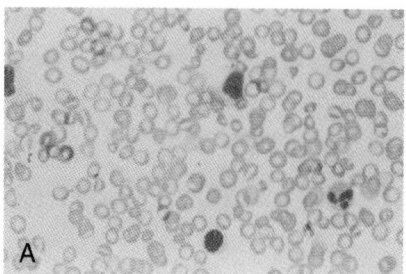

A, Infectious mononucleosis. Peripheral smear shows pleomorphic, atypical (or reactive) lymphocytes.

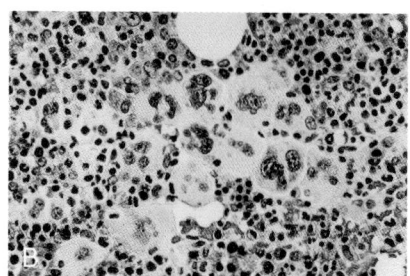

B, Myeloproliferative disorder. Bone marrow shows megakaryocytic clusters seen in essential thrombocythemia and other conditions associated with clonal thrombocytosis.

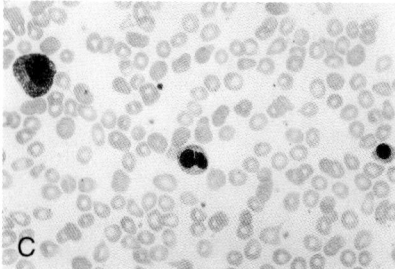

C, Myeloproliferative disorder. A peripheral blood smear in agnogenic myeloid metaplasia showing a leukoerythroblastic picture. The characteristic findings are teardrop-shaped red cells (dacryocytes), nucleated red cells (erythroblasts), and immature granulocyte precursors.

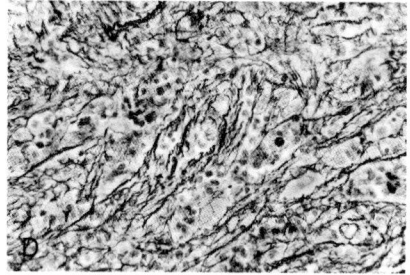

D, Myeloproliferative disorder. A bone marrow biopsy in agnogenic myeloid metaplasia shows reticular fibrosis.

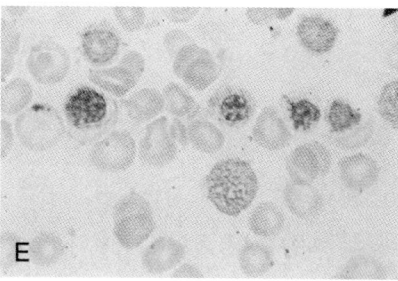

E, Sideroblastic anemia. Prussian blue iron stain of the bone marrow shows ringed sideroblasts, which are nucleated red cell precursors with perinuclear rings of iron-laden mitochondria.

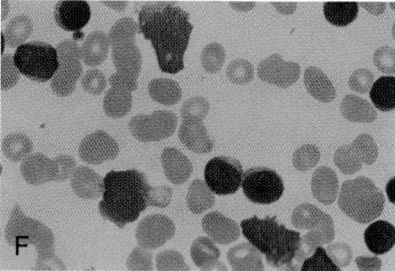

F, Chronic lymphocytic leukemia. Peripheral smear shows that the predominant leukocytes are "normal" mature-appearing lymphocytes, with occasional "smudge" cells.

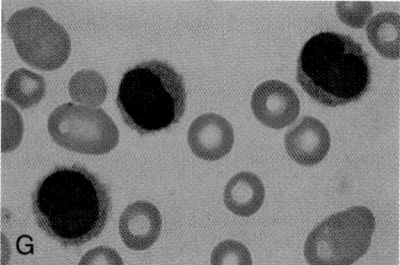

G, Hairy cell leukemia. Peripheral smear shows hairy cells with blue-gray cytoplasm and fine, hairlike projections (resembling ruffles), and oval or slightly indented nuclei with loose chromatin and indistinct nucleoli.

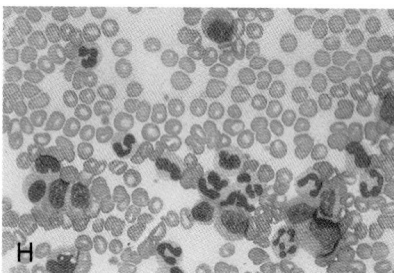

H, Chronic myelogenous leukemia, stable phase. Peripheral smear shows leukocytosis, with representation by the entire spectrum of leukocyte differentiation, ranging from myeloblasts to mature neutrophils.

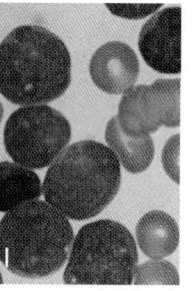

I, Acute leukemia. Left, Acute lymphoblastic leukemia (ALL). Right, Acute myelogenous leukemia (AML). Lymphoblasts in ALL are smaller, with a higher nuclear:cytoplasmic ratio and less distinct nucleoli than myeloblasts in AML. The nucleoli in the myeloblasts are clear and "punched out."

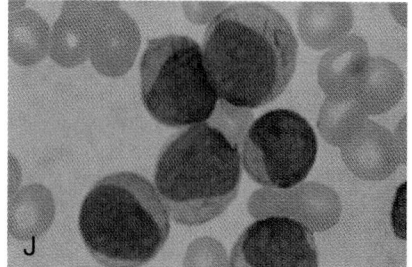

J, Acute non-lymphoblastic leukemia. The myeloblasts in the smear show Auer rods as cytoplasmic inclusions.

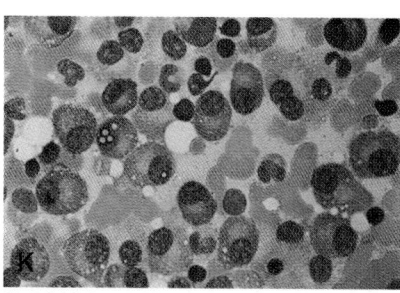

K, Multiple myeloma. Bone marrow aspirate with predominance of plasma cells.

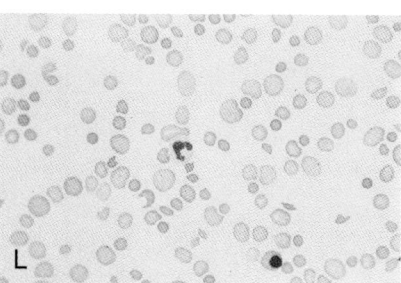

L, Thrombotic thrombocytopenic purpura (TTP). Peripheral smear shows fragmented red cells alongside larger, polychromatophilic cells and a nucleated red cell that reflect hemolysis, as well as a paucity of platelets.

Table 158–3 ■ CYTOKINES ACTIVE ON LYMPHOHEMATOPOIETIC STEM CELLS

CYTOKINE	PRINCIPAL OR HIGHLIGHTED ACTIVITY
Interleukins	
IL-1	Induces production of other cytokines from many cells: co-stimulates early stem cells with other cytokines; modulates immune response.
IL-2	T-cell growth factor; inhibits myelopoiesis and erythropoiesis.
IL-3	Multi-lineage stimulator—myeloid, erythroid, lymphoid, and megakaryocytic; in vivo increases blood monocytes and granulocytes including eosinophils and platelets.
IL-4	Stimulates B cells and dendritic cells and modulates immune response; co-stimulates CFU-GM and CFU-E.
IL-5	Simulates B cells and eosinophils.
IL-6	Stimulates megakaryopoiesis and synergizes with IL-1, IL-2, IL-3, IL-4, GM-CSF, and CSF-1; enhances plasma cell proliferation; role in Castleman's disease and atrial myxoma.
IL-7	Stimulates pre-B cells (with steel factor) and early stem cells.
IL-8	Stimulates production and function of neutrophils; acts as proinflammatory factor.
IL-9	Co-stimulates CFU-GM and CFU-MIX; stimulates BFU-E with erythropoietin; enhances T cell production and, with IL-3, mast cell production.
IL-10	Inhibits cytokine production, modulates immune cells, and stimulates mast cells.
IL-11	Shares most of activities of IL-6; increases neutrophils and platelets in blood in primate model.
IL-12	Increases generation of immunocompetent cells.
IL-13	Enhances steel factor–induced proliferation of Lin− Sca+ murine marrow stem cells; inhibits cytokine production by monocytes; stimulates B cells and activates T cells.
IL-14	B-cell growth factor.
IL-15	Modulates T-cell activity.
IL-16	Acts as immunomodulator.
IL-17	Induces production of other cytokines such as IL-6, IL-8, and G-CSF, and enhances expression of adhesion molecules.
IL-18	Induces GM-CSF and interferon gamma production; inhibits IL-10 production.
Colony-Stimulating Factors, Erythropoietin, and Early Acting Factors	
CSF-1	Enhances production and function of monocytes.
G-CSF	Stimulates granulocyte production and function; co-stimulates early progenitors in synergy with a number of cytokines; stimulates pre-B cells; in vivo stimulates granulocyte production.
GM-CSF	Stimulates GM-CFC and production of monocytes, granulocytes, eosinophils, and basophils; synergizes with IL-4 to produce dendritic cells; co-stimulates many types of progenitors, including early multipotent stem cells.
Erythropoietin	Stimulates erythrocyte production in vitro and in vivo; co-stimulates BFU-E and CFU-MEG and stimulates CFU-E.
FLT-3 ligand	Co-stimulates multipotential stem cells, especially with thrombopoietin and steel factor; stimulates generation of dendritic cells.
Steel factor	Similar to FLT-3; enhances generation of mast cells.
Thrombopoietin, c-mpl ligand	Major regulator of proliferation and differentiation of megakaryocytes; co-stimulates multipotential stem cells in combination with steel factor and IL-11; promotes erythropoiesis in synergy with erythropoietin.
Cytokine Inhibitory Factors and Others	
MIP-1 α	Inhibits early multipotent colony formation but stimulates that of committed precursors.
TGF-β	Suppresses early multipotent progenitors but stimulates later progenitors.
MCAF, platelet factor 4, H-ferritin	Similar to TGF-β
TNF-α	Similar to TGF-β, but a more pronounced effect on BFU-E and CFU-E.
Activin	Enhances IL-3 and erythropoietin stimulated BFU-E and CFU-E; inhibits IL-3 stimulated CFU-GM.
Inhibin	Inhibits CFU-MIX, CFU-GM, and BFU-E.
Interferon- α, β, and γ	Co-inhibits CFU-MIX, CFU-GM, and BFU-E; inhibits production of cytokines; immune modulator.
Prostaglandin E$_2$	Suppresses CFU-M with less or no activity on CFU-GM and CFU-G; enhances BFU-E indirectly through CD8+ lymphocytes.
Glu-Glu-Asp-Asp-Lys (pentapeptide)	Inhibits CFU-S proliferation and CFU-GM.
N-acetyl-Ser-As-Lys-Pro (tetrapeptide)	Inhibits CFU-S and other progenitors entry into cell cycle.
Leukemia inhibitory factor	Inhibits GM-CSF and G-CSF stimulated CFU-GM and CFU-G, respectively.
Insulin-like growth factor II	Stimulates erythroid and granulocyte progenitors.
Hepatocyte growth factor (scatter factor)	Synergistic activity on progenitors.
Basic fibroblast growth factor	Acts in concert with other cytokines on early multipotential and megakaryocyte progenitors.
Platelet-derived growth factor	Stimulates erythroid and granulocyte progenitors.

CFU-GM = colony-forming unit–granulocyte-macrophage; CFU-E = colony-forming unit-erythroid; GM-CSF = granulocyte-macrophage colony-stimulating factor; BFU-E = blast-forming unit-erythroid; G-CSF = granulocyte colony-stimulating factor; GM-CFC = granulocyte-macrophage colony-forming; CFU-MEG = colony-forming unit-megakaryocytes; MIP-1 = macrophage inhibitory protein-1; TGF-β = transforming growth factor-beta; TNF-α = tumor necrosis factor-alpha; CFU-M = colony-forming unit-macrophage; CFU-G = colony-forming unit-granulocyte; CFU-S = colony-forming unit.

Two major receptor families have been described. First, the hematopoietic receptor family includes IL-2, IL-3, IL-4, IL-5, IL-6, IL-7, IL-9, G-CSF, granulocyte-macrophage CSF (GM-CSF), and erythropoietin. The extracellular binding domains of these receptors contain four conserved cysteine residues and a WS-X-WS motif (X is a variable non-conserved amino acid). Some also have an immunoglobulin-like structure. Receptors for GM-CSF, IL-3, and IL-5 each contain specific low-affinity α-chains, but a high-affinity β-chain is shared by all three receptors. The common β-chain plays a role in the competitive binding of these ligands. Second, the tyrosine kinase receptor family includes receptors for FLT3-ligand, steel factor (c-*kit* ligand), CSF-1, and thrombopoietin. These receptors have an immunoglobulin-like structure and 10 conserved cysteines in the extracellular domain, with tyrosine kinase activity in the cytoplasmic domain. Receptors not fitting into these families include those for IL-1 and IL-8.

Signaling through these receptors activates transcription factors that then may direct differentiation toward specific lineages. For example, GATA-1 and FOG promote erythroid and megakaryocyte differentiation, whereas SCL, AML-1, and GATA-2 regulate primitive stem cell differentiation.

Adhesion molecules function both to bind cells or extracellular matrix and as signaling molecules. Steel factor, IL-3, and GM-CSF activate very late antigens 4 and 5 (VLA-4 and VLA-5), which are adhesion molecules expressed on CD34-positive cells. This activation results in promotion of the ability of VLA-4 and VLA-5 to bind fibronectin. Stromal or microenvironmental cells are major regulators of hematopoiesis, both by positioning stem/progenitor

HIERARCHICAL MODEL OF HEMATOPOIESIS

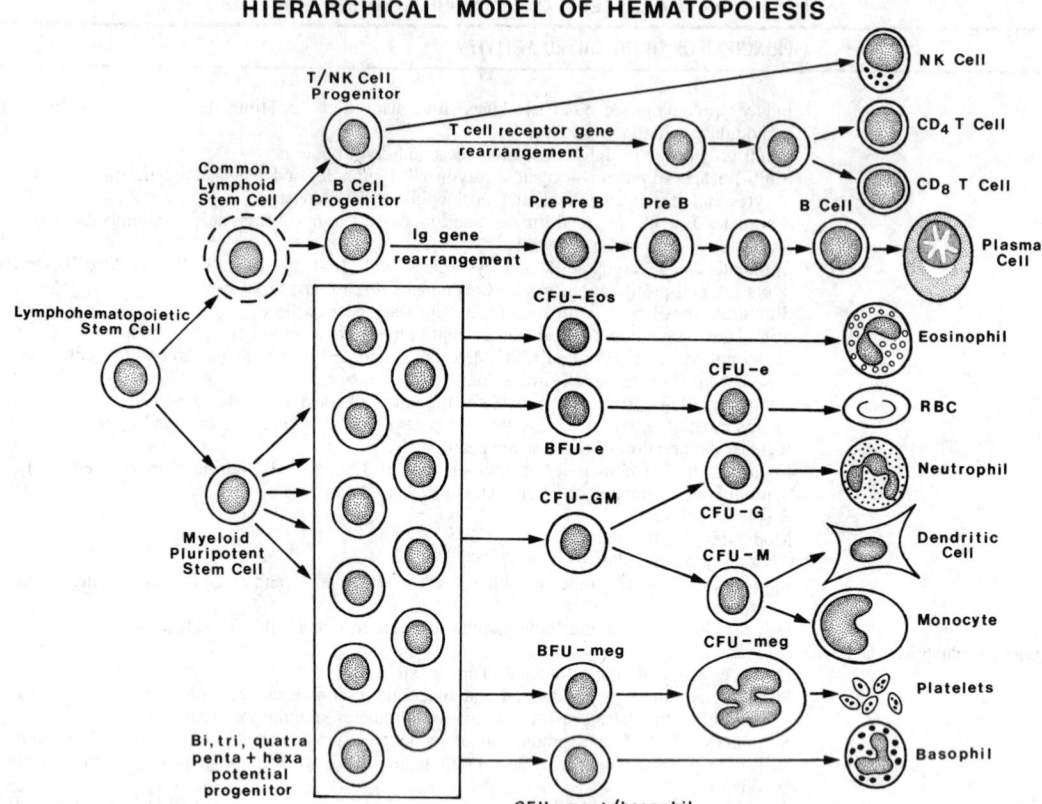

FIGURE 158–4 ■ Hierarchical model of stem cell regulation.

cells and by signaling with secreted and membrane-based cytokines. Homing studies indicate that long-term repopulating lymphohematopoietic stem cells move closely adjacent to osteogenic surfaces; others have suggested that bone cells are major stem cell regulators.

These regulatory influences affect hematopoietic lineages in a variety of ways. An important effect of erythropoietin on erythropoietin progenitors and precursors is to prevent apoptosis and thus maintain the viability of these cells. Cell-cycle transit and the induction of proliferation are major effects of many of the early-acting cytokines, such as steel factor, and all lineages exhibit cytokine-modulated differentiation. Erythropoietin induces erythroid hemoglobulization; G-CSF causes the acquisition of myeloid enzymes in granulocytes; and thrombopoietin induces the expression of platelet-specific proteins. Thus, differentiation is a general feature, although whether this is specifically cytokine-mediated induction from a multipotent cell or simply a manifestation of survival of cells with a genetic probability of differentiation into a specific lineage remains an area of controversy. Regulatory influences also affect the function of many end cells, such as granulocytes, monocytes, T cells, B cells, and dendritic cells. These data, in toto, suggest a hierarchical model of stem cell regulation (Fig. 158–4).

However, there is persuasive evidence that, at least at the more primitive stem cell stages, there may be a cell-cycle component to regulation. Studies have shown that a percentage of daughter cells derived from a single cell from a hematopoietic colony and grown under "permissive" conditions will give rise to totally different lineages. These data suggest that critical commitment decisions are made during one cell-cycle transit. In addition, primitive engrafting stem cells stimulated by cytokine to traverse the cell cycle show dramatic and reversible fluctuations in their ability to engraft and maintain hematopoiesis as they transit the cell cycle. These observations form the basis for the cell-cycle model presented in Figure 158–5.

MOBILIZATION OF STEM/PROGENITOR CELLS. Engraftable, long-term repopulating stem cells and their progenitors are easily mobilized into the peripheral blood by a number of cytokines, including G-CSF, steel factor, FLT-3, IL-11, IL-12, IL-3, IL-8, IL-

7, MIP-1α, and erythropoietin. In addition, previous exposure to cyclophosphamide or other cytotoxic agents also mobilizes stem cells, presumptively through the actions of cytokines. Pretreatment with cyclophosphamide, followed by treatment with steel factor and G-CSF, may be the most potent regimen for mobilizing stem/progenitor cells. In general, mobilized stem/progenitor cells appear to restore hemopoiesis more rapidly than unstimulated marrow, although marrow "primed" with in vivo cytokines may be equivalent to mobilized peripheral blood cells for rapid engraftment. Whether these mobilized stem cells will have the same long-term repopulation capacity as marrow cells remains to be established.

STEM/PROGENITOR CELL EXPANSION. The ability to expand lymphohematopoietic stem cells in vitro has immediate implications for strategies of repetitive transplant, immunotherapy, and gene

CELL CYCLE MODEL OF HEMATOPOIESIS

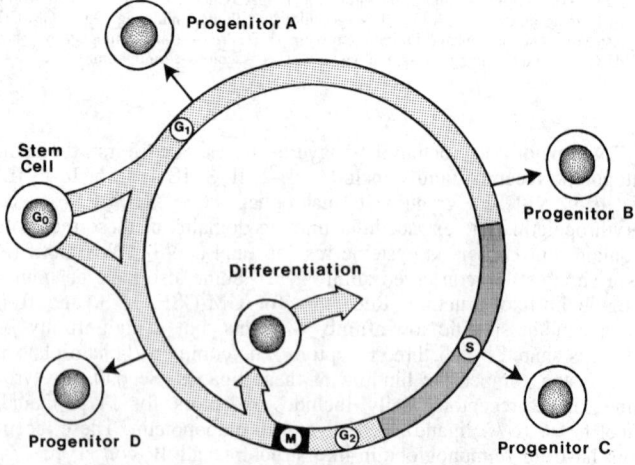

FIGURE 158–5 ■ Cell-cycle–based model of stem cell regulation.

therapy. A large number of studies have established that exposure of marrow cells in liquid culture to a variety of cytokines leads to differentiated and progenitor cell expansion. These cells can also be effective in transplantation, but as yet no study has established expansion of long-term engraftable stem cells, and studies have shown that cytokine stimulation of marrow stem cells can lead to fluctuations in engraftment phenotype that are reversible and correlate with phase of cell cycle; engraftment tends to be lost in the late S/early G_2 phase.

HOMING AND ENGRAFTMENT OF STEM CELLS. Conventional dogma holds that marrow transplant recipients need to be treated with cytotoxic agents, usually irradiation and/or cytotoxic drugs, to open space in the marrow for stem cells to engraft. This turns out to not be the case. Marrow stem cells engraft quantitatively in non-treated hosts, and the final ratio of donor to host cells after transplantation appears to be determined simply by the ratio of donor to host stem cells. Homing to marrow appears complete within 20 hours (probably sooner), and engrafted stem cells rapidly enter cell cycle after intravenous infusion (within 12 hours). They subsequently move to the bone surface, giving rise to both hematopoietic and bone cells. The blood stream clears quickly of stem cells, and there appears to be virtually no primary thymic engraftment, although later secondary engraftment of thymus occurs.

THERAPEUTIC USES OF STEM CELLS AND CYTOKINES

DIAGNOSIS. A number of diseases appear to be stem cell or cytokine diseases. Diseases of deranged or deficient stem cells are usually manifest as cancers or as cell deficiency states (Table 158–4).

THERAPY. Marrow transplantation (see Chapter 182) represents one of the major therapeutic advances of the past 20 years. It has been successfully used to cure marrow deficiency states (largely aplastic anemia), genetic marrow diseases (hemoglobinopathies, enzymopathies), osteopetrosis, and a variety of predominately marrow or lymphoid malignancies. It was initially used to restore deficient cell production (or deficient products from cells) or to restore cell populations after otherwise lethal damage by high-dose radiotherapy/chemotherapy was used to eliminate malignant cell populations; marrow transplantation circumvented the first barrier (killing of marrow stem cells) to dose escalation. More recent studies have indicated that a graft-versus-tumor effect is a major component of the therapeutic efficiency of allogeneic brother/sister transplantation, thus indicating that transplantation may work in part by mediating a cellular immune attack against cancer cells. Marrow cells were the initial source of stem cells for transplantation, but pheresis of peripheral blood stem cells has supplemented marrow in autologous transplantation and is rapidly replacing it in allogeneic transplantation. Fetal liver has been utilized as a source of stem cells, and umbilical cord blood is becoming a major source of cells, especially for unrelated transplantation. Stem cells from these sources are also the most attractive vehicles for a variety of gene therapy approaches, although this is still an evolving area of research.

CYTOKINES IN THERAPY

Interleukin 2 and interferon have been used successfully in therapy for solid tumors and chronic myelogenous leukemia, respectively. The first successful use of a cytokine in the therapy for a cytokine deficiency state was that of erythropoietin to treat the anemia of renal failure. Renal failure represents a true cytokine deficiency state, and thus this is an ideal target for cytokine therapy. Administration of erythropoietin to patients with renal failure corrects or partially corrects the anemia and restores a better state of well-being. Erythropoietin is also used in other settings, where its benefits are less clear (Table 158–5).

Unfortunately, other cytokine deficiency states have been hard to document, and the results of cytokine therapy of other diseases (despite Food and Drug Administration [FDA] approval) are equivocal at best. A major emphasis has been placed on the use of G-CSF and GM-CSF (Table 158–6) for marrow recovery after cytotoxic therapy of cancer. Initial trials escalating the dose of chemotherapy agents in small cell carcinoma indicated that administration of G-CSF enhanced granulocyte recovery and decreased febrile infectious complications. All trials since have been varia-

Table 158–4 ■ STEM CELL DISEASES

DISEASE	MECHANISM
Aplastic anemia	Deficient multipotent stem cell: multiple causes (cell killing or immune)
Neutropenia—Kostmann's, cyclic, and others	Genetic deficiency or regulatory abnormality
Myelodysplastic syndrome	Marrow damage progressing to neoplasm
Acute myelogenous leukemia	Cytogenetic abnormality at stem cell level
Paroxysmal nocturnal hemoglobinuria	Defective glycosylphosphatidylinositol–anchored membrane proteins and mutation in the *PIG-A* gene
Chronic myelogenous leukemia	9:22 translocation moves *abl* oncogene adjacent to *bcr*
Myeloproliferative disorders: polycythemia vera, myelofibrosis, myeloid metaplasia, primary thrombocytosis	Neoplasms of multipotent stem cells

tions on this theme. The critical flaw in these studies is that the dose escalation has not led to better cancer control, and thus the use of G-CSF or GM-CSF has not been of benefit to the underlying problems of these patients. Furthermore, these cytokines may not be cost effective. Although the FDA has approved them for certain indications in cancer, G-CSF and GM-CSF are best treated as interesting experimental therapies at this time. Neither G-CSF nor GM-CSF has proven effective in other conditions such as in active infection; this is not surprising because endogenous levels of G-CSF are already quite high in febrile neutropenic and infected patients.

G-CSF, probably with steel factor or others, has a role in stem cell mobilization and appears effective in certain severe chronic neutropenic states, including Kostmann's neutropenia and cyclic neutropenia. Evolution to leukemia in patients with Kostmann's neutropenia, however, is a real problem. The malignant counterparts of the marrow cells usually retain the cytokine responsiveness of the normal cells, and it is clear that many neoplastic cells will proliferate in response to cytokines. Tumor progression is a risk, but cytokine manipulation of tumor growth, possibly in concert with therapy to kill cycling cells, is an opportunity. G-CSF and

Table 158–5 ■ INDICATIONS FOR THERAPY WITH ERYTHROPOIETIN

DISEASE/CONDITION	THERAPEUTIC EFFICACY
Anemia of renal failure	Improves quality of life and decreases transfusion requirement; there is clinical benefit.
Anemia with human immunodeficiency virus induced by zidovudine with erythropoietin levels < 500/mL	Approved for use in United States but clinical benefit not clear
Chemotherapy-induced anemia	Approved in United States for non-myeloid malignancies. May be of use in selected cases with possible increased quality of life; overall benefit in this setting still unclear
Anemia of inflammation (rheumatoid arthritis and inflammatory bowel disease)	Increases hematocrit without clinical benefit; should not be used
Other conditions under evaluation: perioperative setting; autologous blood collection; anemia of prematurity; anemia of myelodysplasia, lymphoma, or leukemia; anemia with allogeneic transplantation; anemia of pure red cell aplasia; induction of hemoglobin F in sickle cell anemia or thalassemia; and adjuvant for phlebotomy	May be considered in selected individuals but benefit not established (perioperative setting with restrictions has Food and Drug Administration approval)

Table 158–6 ■ G-CSF AND GM-CSF USE IN CLINICAL THERAPY

CONDITION	ESTABLISHED BENEFIT	
	G-CSF	GM-CSF
Chronic neutropenia (cyclic, idiopathic and Kostmann's)	Yes	No
Cancer chemotherapy–induced neutropenia	Uncertain	Uncertain
Stem cell mobilization	Yes	Yes
Active infection	No	No
Other inflammatory conditions	No	No
Drug-induced (not chemotherapy) neutropenia	No	No

GM-CSF stimulate a wide variety of cell types of both hematopoietic and non-hematopoietic origin and, not surprisingly, have a wide variety of side effects, including bone pain; fever and chills; pleural and pulmonary effusions/infiltrates; vasculitis; rashes, including neutrophilic dermatitis (Sweet's syndrome); splenic enlargement, hypersplenism, and, rarely, splenic rupture; and proteinuria.

Recently, agents that stimulate in vivo platelet production have entered clinical trials, and one has been released for clinical use: IL-11 enhances platelet recovery after chemotherapy for cancer. As with G-CSF and GM-CSF, and despite FDA approval, it remains unclear what clinical benefit will accrue from the use of this agent. The ligand for C-mpl or thrombopoietin should also soon be approved for stimulating platelet production. Thus, at present, powerful biologics can increase the red cell, neutrophil, eosinophil, basophil, monocyte, and platelet counts. These are intriguing drugs with great potential, but, with the exceptions of erythropoietin (for the anemia of renal failure) and G-CSF (for chronic neutropenia), their true roles in clinical therapy remain uncertain.

Habibian HK, Peters SO, Hsieh CC, et al: The fluctuating phenotype of the lymphohematopoietic stem cell with cell cycle transit. J Exp Med 188:393–398, 1998. *A focus on stem cell engraftment.*

Kaushansky K: Thrombopoietin: The primary regulator of platelet production. Blood 86:419, 1995. *A review of thrombopoietin.*

Ogawa M: Differentiation and proliferation of hematopoietic stem cells. Blood 81:2844, 1995. *A focus on newer concepts of stem cells.*

Quesenberry PJ: Hemopoietic stem cells, progenitor cells and cytokines. *In* Lichtman M, Kipps T (eds): Williams Textbook of Hematology, 5th ed. New York, McGraw Hill, 1994, p 211. *Review of hemopoiesis.*

159 APPROACH TO THE ANEMIAS

Kenneth S. Zuckerman

DEFINITIONS

Anemia, which is defined as a reduction in the number of circulating erythrocytes, is a common manifestation of primary bone marrow disorders, primary abnormalities of erythrocytes, immunologic disorders, nutritional deficiencies, and a broad spectrum of systemic diseases that secondarily result in anemia. Any condition that can impair the production or increase the rate of destruction or loss of erythrocytes can result in anemia, if the bone marrow is unable to compensate for the rate of loss of red blood cells (RBCs). At least some degree of anemia is detectable in 20 to 40% of hospitalized patients. A considerable amount of information that is useful in determining severity, pathophysiology, and etiology of anemia is provided by electronic, automated blood cell counters (Table 159–1). The hemoglobin (Hgb), measured in grams per deciliter, represents the total amount of hemoglobin in all of the erythrocytes in 100 mL of blood. The hematocrit (Hct) is the percentage of the total blood volume that is composed of erythrocytes. The mean corpuscular or cell volume (MCV) is measured directly on automated cell counters but can be calculated as MCV (μ^3 or fL) = Hct (%) × 10/RBC count (×10^6/μL of whole blood). The mean cell hemoglobin (MCH) is calculated by automated cell counters as MCH (pg) = Hgb (g/dL) × 10/RBC (×10^6/μL). The mean cell hemoglobin concentration (MCHC) is calculated by automated cell counters as MCHC = Hgb (g/dL) × 100/Hct (%). The MCH and MCHC are of limited value because of relatively poor sensitivity for any individual disorders, whereas the MCV is extremely useful in classification and determination of the etiology of anemia. The RBC distribution width (RDW/CV) is a ratio of the width of the RBC size distribution curve at 1 standard deviation from the mean size divided by the MCV. Because this value is a ratio with the MCV as denominator, it tends to magnify any variation in cell size in patients with microcytosis and is relatively insensitive to mild or early macrocytosis. A less frequently used value, the RDW-SD, is the width of the RBC size distribution curve, encompassing 80% of the erythrocytes in the measured population. This latter measurement is particularly sensitive even to small populations of microcytic or macrocytic RBCs. In addition to these standard measurements, automated absolute reticulocyte counts per microliter of blood or evaluations of new methylene blue–stained peripheral blood smears for the percent of positive-staining erythrocytes (reticulocytes) give a measure of the number of newly released (generally 1- to 2-day old) erythrocytes. These newly formed erythrocytes still contain residual ribosomal RNA, which can be recognized easily on supravital staining with new methylene blue. Because the ribosomal RNA is lost from the cell within the first 1 to 2 days in the circulation and erythrocytes in the blood survive an average of about 120 days, reticulocytes comprise about 1% of all erythrocytes in the circulation; a normal, non-anemic adult has 40,000 to 100,000 reticulocytes per microliter of blood. Automated blood cell counters also provide total white blood cell (WBC) count, WBC differential count, and platelet count. All of this information is useful in assessing the mechanism of anemia.

ETIOLOGY AND PATHOGENESIS

Normal Erythropoiesis

The circulating erythrocyte under normal conditions has an average lifespan of approximately 120 days. It is a non-nucleated, non-dividing cell, in which more than 90% of the protein content is the oxygen-carrying molecule, hemoglobin. The erythrocyte's sole responsibility is to deliver oxygen to the tissues of the body. Thus, the primary consequence of anemia is tissue hypoxia. Erythropoiesis is driven by a feedback loop. Oxygen-sensing cells in the area of the juxtaglomerular apparatus of the kidney respond to local tissue hypoxia by increasing production of erythropoietin (EPO), which is the primary regulatory hormone for erythropoiesis. EPO plays little, if any, role in maintaining or producing early hematopoietic precursors or even the earliest detectable erythroid progenitor cells, known as burst forming units-erythroid (BFU-E); however, EPO is absolutely essential for the maturation of BFU-E to late erythroid progenitor cells, known as colony-forming units-erythroid (CFU-E), and to proerythroblasts in the bone marrow. The main mechanism of action of EPO is to prevent apoptosis, also known as programmed cell death, of erythroid precursor cells and to permit their proliferation and subsequent maturation. Once erythroid precursor cells mature to the level of proerythroblasts, further maturation to normoblasts, reticulocytes, and mature erythrocytes no longer requires the presence of EPO. Under normal circumstances, the RBC mass is maintained at a nearly constant level by means of the EPO feedback loop's ability to match new erythrocyte production to the rate of natural senescence and loss of RBCs. Although total absence of EPO in the circulation never or almost never occurs, severe depression of circulating EPO levels results in near cessation of erythrocyte production.

Hypoxia, as sensed in the kidney, results in increased production of EPO, which leads to increased erythrocyte production by the bone marrow. When the local tissue hypoxia is due to a reduction in the number of circulating erythrocytes and amount of hemoglobin and the consequent decreased total-body oxygen-carrying capacity, the increased EPO produced by the kidney stimulates the bone marrow to produce increased numbers of erythrocytes to compensate for the existing deficiency of RBCs. Once an increase in EPO levels in the circulation occurs in response to acute onset of anemia, new proerythroblasts and normoblasts appear in the bone marrow within 2 to 4 days, and new reticulocytes begin to appear

Table 159-1 ■ NORMAL VALUES FOR RED BLOOD CELL MEASUREMENTS

MEASUREMENT	UNITS	NORMAL RANGE (APPROXIMATE)*
Hemoglobin	g/dL	Males: 13.5–17.5 Females: 12.0–16.0
Hematocrit	%	Males: 40–52 Females: 36–48
Red blood cell (RBC) count	× $10^6/\mu L$ of blood	Males: 4.5–6.0 Females: 4.0–5.4
Mean cell volume (MCV)	fL	81–99
Mean cell hemoglobin (MCH)	pg	30–34
Mean cell hemoglobin concentration (MCHC)	g/dL	30–36
Red blood cell size distribution width		
RDW-CV	%	12–14
RDW-SD	%	37–47
Reticulocyte count (absolute number)	No./μL of blood	40,000–100,000
Reticulocyte percentage	% of RBCs	0.5–1.5

*Actual normal ranges for many of these values may vary slightly, depending on such factors as the location and type of equipment used, altitude above sea level, and patient age.

in the peripheral blood within 3 to 7 days. Re-establishment of normal numbers of circulating erythrocytes and normal tissue oxygenation results in reduced production of EPO and then a reduced rate of production of erythrocytes back to the normal basal level that is required to maintain a stable, normal number of erythrocytes in the blood. When hypoxia is caused by decreased ambient oxygen concentration, impaired delivery of oxygen through the lungs and to hemoglobin molecules in erythrocytes, venous to arterial shunting of blood, hemoglobin mutants with increased oxygen affinity and decreased ability to release oxygen in the tissues, or localized renal disease that the renal sensor cannot distinguish from generalized hypoxemia, the increase in EPO results in increased erythropoiesis, erythrocytosis, and secondary polycythemia.

Pathogenesis of Anemias

The basic mechanisms of anemia can be divided into those conditions that result in accelerated destruction or loss of RBCs and those in which the primary abnormality is impaired ability of the bone marrow to produce sufficient numbers of erythrocytes to replace those that are lost. Although this classification makes it easier to understand the pathophysiology of anemia and to determine the proper diagnostic studies to perform, in many patients more than one mechanism may occur simultaneously.

ANEMIAS DUE TO IMPAIRED PRODUCTION OF ERYTHROCYTES BY THE BONE MARROW. If there is a reduced erythrocyte mass due to impaired production of erythroid precursors and mature RBCs by the bone marrow, the number of reticulocytes in the circulating blood and the number of normoblasts in the bone marrow will be lower than would be appropriate in the presence of the existing degree of anemia. A wide variety of conditions can be responsible for impaired erythropoiesis (Table 159–2).

ERYTHROPOIETIN DEFICIENCY. Insufficient production of EPO results in failure of an otherwise normal bone marrow to produce the required number of erythrocytes, despite the production of normal numbers of other hematopoietic cells such as neutrophils and platelets. The prototype for impaired EPO production is renal failure (with particularly severe EPO deficiency after bilateral nephrectomies), in which only very low levels of EPO, generally less than 10% of normal, are produced. The small amount of EPO produced in nephrectomized patients is derived from the liver and is sufficient to generate only a small portion of the required numbers of erythrocytes. Thus, patients with chronic renal failure, and particularly those who have had bilateral nephrectomies, have severe anemia, with Hgb values less than 5 g/dL in the absence of exogenous EPO therapy or RBC transfusions. Rare patients with autoantibodies against EPO have extremely low to undetectable circulating EPO levels and severe anemia, with pure red cell aplasia in the bone marrow. Patients with chronic infectious or inflammatory diseases or cancer can also have anemia that is associated with inappropriately low levels of EPO for their degrees of anemia; in these circumstances, cytokines such as interleukin (IL)-1, IL-6, or tumor necrosis factor (TNF)-α might be responsible, at least in part, for the impaired EPO production.

QUANTITATIVE DEFICIENCY OF HEMATOPOIETIC STEM CELLS AND/OR COMMITTED ERYTHROID PROGENITOR CELLS. A second mechanism of anemia due to reduced production of cells by the bone marrow is deficiency of hematopoietic stem cells and/or committed erythroid progenitor cells. Any condition that is characterized by a deficiency of hematopoietic stem cells and/or committed erythroid precursor cells also will result in anemia. Even if EPO production is appropriately increased for the degree of anemia, anemia will result if the target marrow precursor cells are deficient in number. In almost all such cases, the defect is a more generalized bone marrow abnormality that results in reduced production of all lineages of bone marrow–derived cells, particularly erythrocytes, granulocytes, and platelets. Idiopathic bone marrow failure, commonly known as aplastic anemia, is the prototype of such disorders (see Chapter 160). Bone marrow aplasia or hypoplasia also may occur as a result of toxic substances such as benzene, cancer chemotherapeutic agents, other pharmacologic agents such as chloramphenicol or gold salts, ionizing radiation, or certain viral infections such as Epstein-Barr virus, human immunodeficiency virus (HIV), hepatitis (non-A, non-B, non-C) virus, or dengue virus.

Table 159-2 ■ PATHOPHYSIOLOGIC CLASSIFICATION OF ANEMIAS DUE TO IMPAIRED PRODUCTION OF ERYTHROCYTES BY THE BONE MARROW

Erythropoietin (EPO) deficiency (normocytic anemias)
  Renal insufficiency (worse after bilateral nephrectomies)
  Pure red cell aplasia due to anti-EPO antibodies (extremely rare)
  Anemia of chronic disease (inappropriately low EPO level is a partial contributing factor)
Quantitative deficiency of hematopoietic/erythroid progenitor cells (normocytic anemias)
  Idiopathic bone marrow aplasia/hypoplasia
  Secondary bone marrow aplasia/hypoplasia (drugs, toxins, infections, radiation, malnutrition)
  Myelofibrosis (primary or secondary)
  Bone marrow replacement by neoplastic cells (myelophthisis)
  Myelodysplasia (minority of myelodysplasia patients)
  Paroxysmal nocturnal hemoglobinuria (10–15% of PNH patients)
  Pure red cell aplasia (anti–erythroid precursor cell antibodies, parvovirus B19 infection)
Impaired erythroid precursor cell division and DNA synthesis (macrocytic/megaloblastic anemias)
  Cobalamin (vitamin B_{12}) deficiency
  Folate deficiency
  Myelodysplasia
  Cancer chemotherapeutic drugs and some immunosuppressive and antimicrobial drugs
Impaired heme synthesis in differentiating erythroid cells (microcytic anemias)
  Iron deficiency
  Anemia of chronic disease/inflammation
  Sideroblastic anemias (particularly hereditary forms)
Impaired globin synthesis in differentiating erythroid cells (microcytic anemias)
  Thalassemias

Other conditions such as bone marrow fibrosis (myelofibrosis) or extensive replacement of the bone marrow by neoplastic cells also can result in deficiencies of hematopoietic stem and progenitor cells and/or impaired ability of these cells to proliferate and to differentiate into mature hematopoietic cells. Patients with severe malnutrition, including anorexia nervosa, also may have bone marrow hypoplasia. A minority of patients with myelodysplasia or paroxysmal nocturnal hemoglobinuria also have significant bone marrow hypoplasia. Selective anemia is also seen in pure red cell aplasia; this disorder usually has an immunologic basis, with selective immune-mediated destruction of erythroid progenitor cells and absence or near absence of detectable nucleated erythroid precursors in the bone marrow despite elevated levels of circulating EPO. Viral infection, particularly with parvovirus B19, which selectively infects committed erythroid progenitor cells, also can cause transient or prolonged pure red cell aplasia because of the cytotoxic effect of this virus on the infected erythroid precursor cells.

IMPAIRED ABILITY OF ERYTHROID PROGENITORS TO RESPOND TO ERYTHROPOIETIN. A third general mechanism responsible for reduced erythrocyte production by the bone marrow is impaired responsiveness of erythroid precursors to appropriate circulating EPO concentrations. This category covers a broad range of disorders, including intrinsic erythrocyte abnormalities, exogenous inhibitory effects, and nutritional deficiencies. No mutations or abnormalities of EPO receptors or in EPO-related signal transduction pathways in erythroid precursors have been identified as causes of anemia. There are many potential ways to categorize this large, diverse group of anemias. One method is to divide these conditions pathophysiologically into those in which there is impaired DNA synthesis and cell division and those in which there is impaired synthesis of hemoglobin.

DISORDERS CHARACTERIZED BY IMPAIRED DNA SYNTHESIS: MEGALOBLASTIC ANEMIAS. Impaired DNA synthesis and the resulting impaired cell division by erythroid precursors result in red cell macrocytosis (increased MCV) and variable degrees of anemia (see Chapter 163). These abnormalities may occur whenever there is a significant deficiency of key substrates in the DNA synthetic pathways, as is caused by deficiencies of cobalamin (vitamin B$_{12}$) and folate. Folate deficiency frequently may be due to insufficient dietary intake but also may be due to diffuse intestinal disorders and to drugs that interfere with folate metabolism, such as ethanol, sulfonamides or sulfa-related drugs, trimethoprim, methotrexate, anticonvulsants, and possibly oral contraceptives. Folate deficiency may occur in patients with an increased requirement for folate in such conditions as chronic hemolytic anemias, pregnancy, and in childhood. In addition, severe alcoholics, patients with general malnutrition from any cause, and patients with certain unconventional dietary habits are susceptible to developing folate deficiency. A severely folate-deficient diet will result in clinically significant folate deficiency within about 6 weeks. Cobalamin deficiency almost never occurs because of lack of dietary cobalamin intake; instead, it most often is due to impaired absorption of cobalamin due to lack of intrinsic factor, gastric atrophy, and abnormalities of cobalamin absorption in the terminal ileum. Because of substantial stores and very low daily requirements for cobalamin in normal individuals, deficiency of cobalamin usually takes at least 3 to 5 years to become manifest. In patients with myelodysplasia, one of the mechanisms of anemia and other hematopoietic cell deficiencies can be a moderately severe to severe impairment of DNA synthesis, with development of megaloblastosis and macrocytosis of RBCs. A broad range of cancer chemotherapeutic agents impair DNA synthesis in the short term, and some cause stem cell damage that can result in a long-term adverse effect on DNA synthesis, which may result in mild to moderate anemia or may be manifested only by an increased MCV. In association with the reduced DNA synthesis and delays in or decreased number of cell divisions in megaloblastic anemias, there generally is intramedullary death of hematopoietic precursors, predominantly by apoptosis, and reduced numbers of mature erythrocytes and sometimes granulocytes and platelets released into the blood. This condition of hypercellular bone marrow combined with death of precursors before full maturation xlf hematopoietic cells is called ineffective hematopoiesis, or, in the case of RBCs alone, ineffective erythropoiesis.

IMPAIRED HEMOGLOBIN SYNTHESIS: DISORDERS CHARACTER-

IZED BY DIMINISHED HEME SYNTHESIS. Impaired hemoglobin synthesis occurs with disorders in which there is reduced production of either heme or globin, and, when sufficiently severe, results in microcytic anemias (decreased MCV). The heme synthetic pathway and its defects are described in more detail in other chapters. Most or all of the rare disorders collectively known as hereditary sideroblastic anemias appear to be due to mutations in the coding regions of genes for the erythroid-specific forms of heme synthetic pathway enzymes or erythroid-specific promoters (especially ALA synthase, HMB synthase, and possibly ferrochelatase); the result is reduced heme synthesis in erythroid cells. Iron is required for the final stage of synthesis of heme, and iron deficiency impairs heme synthesis and results in anemia. Although iron-deficiency anemia is associated classically with microcytosis, most patients with mild iron-deficiency anemia actually have normocytic erythrocytes. Over time, iron-deficient patients commonly have a progressive decrease in the MCV within the normal range, and microcytosis occurs generally in the most severe 20 to 30% of cases. In patients with chronic infectious or inflammatory diseases or with cancer, the responsiveness of erythroid precursors to endogenous and exogenous EPO may be impaired. The mechanism for this impaired responsiveness to EPO is unknown, but it is thought to be due to inhibitory cytokines and chemokines. One of the hallmarks of anemia of chronic disease or inflammation is impaired transfer of iron into developing erythroid cells, resulting in a functional iron deficiency in normoblasts even when iron stores in the bone marrow and the rest of the body are adequate. The result is impaired heme synthesis and a mild to moderate normocytic or microcytic anemia. In many of the circumstances in which anemia of chronic disease/inflammation occurs, there also may be concomitant iron deficiency.

IMPAIRED HEMOGLOBIN SYNTHESIS: DISORDERS CHARACTERIZED BY IMPAIRED GLOBIN SYNTHESIS—THALASSEMIAS. Impaired synthesis of α-globin chains in α-thalassemias or β-globin chains in β-thalassemias results in unbalanced synthesis of globin chains and a reduction in the number of hemoglobin α2/β2 hemoglobin tetramers (see Chapter 167). Because of the reduced numbers of hemoglobin tetramer molecules in each cell, thalassemia patients have a microcytic anemia. The unpaired excess β-chains in the erythrocytes of patients with α-thalassemia and unpaired excess α-chains in patients with β-thalassemia tend to aggregate, precipitate, and form insoluble cytoplasmic inclusion bodies that result in oxidative damage to the membranes of developing normoblasts and death of a large proportion of these developing erythroid cells within the marrow, resulting in anemia due to ineffective erythropoiesis. Furthermore, the normoblasts that do survive produce erythrocytes that contain similar inclusions (Heinz bodies), which lead to premature destruction of these cells in the spleen and liver, resulting in a hemolytic component of the anemia. The overall degree of anemia is related to the severity of the defect in globin synthesis, so that patients who have deletion of only one of their four α-globin genes generally have microcytosis but no anemia, those with deletion of two α-globin genes have microcytosis and mild anemia, and those who are heterozygous for β-thalassemia have microcytosis and mild anemia.

INEFFECTIVE ERYTHROPOIESIS. Ineffective erythropoiesis is defined as anemia with increased numbers of erythroid precursor cells in the bone marrow but decreased numbers of mature circulating erythrocytes being released from the bone marrow. Thus, in ineffective erythropoiesis, there are inappropriately low numbers of reticulocytes in the blood. This condition usually is caused by defects that are present in the maturing proerythroblasts and normoblasts in the bone marrow and result in their premature death within the bone marrow. The most common causes of anemia due to ineffective erythropoiesis are myelodysplasia, megaloblastic anemias, and thalassemias.

ANEMIAS DUE TO ACCELERATED DESTRUCTION, CONSUMPTION, OR LOSS OF CIRCULATING ERYTHROCYTES. Any intrinsic defects of erythrocytes or extrinsic conditions that cause erythrocytes to be damaged intravascularly, removed from the circulation prematurely by the spleen or liver, or lost through bleeding result in increased EPO production, increased numbers of maturing erythroid precursors in the bone marrow, and release of increased numbers of newly formed reticulocytes into the blood. Thus, in a patient with a normal bone marrow, accelerated loss of circulating erythrocytes always will be associated with increased erythropoiesis, which can be judged by the presence of an increased reticulocyte count. An increased reticulocyte count implies that there is at least a mildly increased rate of loss or destruction of erythrocytes; if the bone marrow is able to keep up with the increased demand for replacement erythrocytes, the patient will not have a decreased RBC mass. Anemia occurs only if the rate of production of erythrocytes by the bone marrow is unable to compensate completely for the loss or destruction of RBCs. Although chronic hemolysis or blood loss is associated with compensatory increased erythropoiesis (assuming no additional abnormalities of bone marrow, kidney, or required nutrients), signs of compensatory increased erythropoiesis will not appear until several days after acute hemolysis or blood loss.

HEMOLYTIC ANEMIAS DUE TO INTRINSIC RED CELL MEMBRANE DEFECTS. Abnormalities of RBC membrane proteins and lipids lead to deformed erythrocytes, which are prone to be removed prematurely from the circulation, primarily by the filtering functions of the spleen (see Chapter 164). The most common membrane protein abnormalities involve spectrin, ankyrin, band 3 protein, and protein 4.1, and lead to the RBC membranopathies known as hereditary spherocytosis, hereditary elliptocytosis, and hereditary pyropoikilocytosis. In each of these disorders, the decreased deformability of RBCs results in their premature clearance from the blood, primarily in the spleen. Abnormalities of the lipid bilayer of the erythrocyte membrane lead to bizarrely shaped RBCs, which have poor deformability and cytoplasmic projections and also result in an increased rate of destruction of erythrocytes, primarily in the spleen. One abnormality of the lipid bilayer is acanthocytosis or spur cell anemia, which may be caused by hereditary lipoprotein defects such as abetalipoproteinemia, cholesterol metabolism abnormalities that occur in patients with severe liver disease, or the McLeod phenotype of severely deficient Kell blood group antigen on erythrocytes. Stomatocytes or xerocytes result from imbalance in the size of the outer and inner portions of the membrane lipid bilayer and dehydration of erythrocytes; abnormalities of membrane phospholipids or absence of Rh antigens on the surface of RBCs (Rh null phenotype) result in these morphologic abnormalities that may result in mild hemolysis. In paroxysmal nocturnal hemoglobinuria, a defect in a critical membrane-anchoring molecule (glycosylphosphatidylinositol [GPI]), which is responsible for anchoring many cell surface proteins, results in absence of at least three surface proteins that are critical to prevention of complement-mediated cell damage and lysis. The absence or significant reduction in decay accelerating factor (DAF, CD55), membrane inhibitor of reactive lysis (MIRL, CD59), and C8-binding protein result in variably increased susceptibility of these defective cells to lysis by complement.

HEMOLYTIC ANEMIAS DUE TO INTRINSIC RED CELL ENZYMOPATHIES. Red cell enzymopathies (see Chapter 164) that may lead to hemolytic anemia generally fall into two groups. Defects in enzymes in the hexose monophosphate shunt (e.g., glucose-6-phosphate dehydrogenase) or those responsible for maintaining reduced glutathione (e.g., γ-glutamylcysteine synthetase) to prevent oxidative injury to RBCs tend most frequently to be associated with episodic hemolysis during times of physiologic stresses, such as surgery, infections, or oxidants in foods or pharmacologic agents. The oxidant damage causes Heinz body formation. In contrast, deficiencies of enzymes in the Embden-Meyerhof pathway (e.g., pyruvate kinase and glucose phosphate isomerase) or enzymes responsible for supporting nucleotide metabolism (e.g., adenosine deaminase and pyrimidine 5′-nucleotidase) tend to cause chronic hemolytic anemias, presumably as a result of adenosine phosphate deficiency, which leads to impaired homeostasis of water, sodium, potassium, and calcium. Because erythrocytes are unable to synthesize new proteins, older erythrocytes are most likely to have the lowest levels of enzymes that are susceptible to intracellular degradation and thus are the most likely to be removed from the circulation.

HEMOLYTIC ANEMIAS DUE TO HEMOGLOBIN VARIANTS WITH REDUCED SOLUBILITY OR PROTEIN INSTABILITY. More than 100 different structural variants of hemoglobin exhibit either reduced solubility (e.g., hemoglobins S, C, O-Arab, and D-Los Angeles) or a higher susceptibility than normal to oxidation of amino acids within the globin chains (e.g., hemoglobins Zurich, Köln, Hammersmith, and Gun Hill) (see Chapter 168). The less soluble and unstable hemoglobins tend to form abnormal hemoglobin polymers or crystals, to precipitate, and to form cytoplasmic Heinz bodies,

which then become attached to the cell membrane and decrease erythrocyte deformability; the result is membrane damage, followed by sequestration and destruction of erythrocytes in the spleen.

HEMOLYTIC ANEMIAS DUE TO ABNORMALITIES EXTRINSIC TO THE RED CELL. Erythrocytes can be sequestered or destroyed prematurely as a result of other conditions that secondarily cause damage to otherwise normal RBCs. In autoimmune hemolytic anemia, antibodies form against red cell membrane antigens (most commonly Rh-D antigen for so-called warm IgG antibodies and I or i antigen for so-called cold, complement-fixing IgM antibodies) (see Chapter 165). These antibody-coated erythrocytes are recognized by Fc or complement receptors on macrophages in the spleen (especially IgG) or liver (especially C3 complement). IgG-coated red cells usually undergo repeated partial phagocytosis with progressive loss of red cell membrane until the cells that survive and re-enter the circulation are spherocytes, which have decreased deformability and eventually are sequestered and removed permanently from the circulation. A long list of drugs can result in hemolysis by similar mechanisms by causing antierythrocyte antibodies or by causing antidrug antibodies that lead to subsequent immune complex deposition on erythrocytes, which also results in hemolysis by similar mechanisms. Alloimmune hemolysis may result from transfusion of blood with "minor" blood group mismatches into recipients previously sensitized to those antigens by prior transfusions and/or pregnancies. Severe acute intravascular hemolysis (see Chapter 166) can occur from transfusion of ABO incompatible blood and less commonly from transfusion of blood that has Rh or so-called minor blood group antigen mismatches. Microangiopathic hemolysis with fragmented erythrocytes, intravascular release of hemoglobin and other erythrocyte contents, and intravascular and splenic destruction of RBCs occurs in the presence of fibrin deposition in small arterioles, in such conditions as thrombotic thrombocytopenic purpura and disseminated intravascular coagulation, as well as in the presence of diffuse small vessel vasculitis, eclampsia, or malignant hypertension. Prosthetic heart valves or arterial grafts with roughened endothelial surfaces also can cause mechanical fragmentation of erythrocytes. Other causes of mechanical damage to otherwise normal erythrocytes are trauma (e.g., march hemoglobinuria), thermal injury from severe burns, and osmotic lysis due to freshwater drowning or mistaken intravenous infusion of high volumes of hypotonic fluids. Certain infections such as malaria, bartonellosis, and babesiosis can cause direct intravascular destruction of infected erythrocytes, and clostridial sepsis can result in release of toxins that directly damage red cell membrane phospholipids and lyse the cells. Certain snake and spider venoms can cause hemolysis (i.e., cobra venom via phospholipases that destroy the erythrocyte membrane and pit vipers and brown recluse spider venoms via induction of disseminated intravascular coagulation). Finally, a number of drugs and ingested toxins, including nitrofurantoin, phenazopyridine, sulfones, amyl nitrite, naphthalene mothballs, paraquat, and hydrogen peroxide can cause direct oxidative damage to erythrocytes. Several cancer chemotherapeutic agents also probably cause oxidant and/or membrane damage, which can result in anemia within a few days after drug administration.

BLOOD LOSS. Although acute blood loss can result in anemia, it may be much more difficult to document slow, chronic blood loss, in which case the bone marrow almost always is able to compensate until the patient becomes iron deficient. The gastrointestinal tract is a major site of chronic blood loss: malignancies, gastritis, peptic ulcer disease, inflammatory bowel disease, diverticulitis, proctitis, hemorrhoidal bleeding, angiodysplasia, arteriovenous malformations, and hereditary hemorrhagic telangiectasia (Osler-Weber-Rendu syndrome) are among the major causes of chronic or intermittent gastrointestinal blood loss (see Chapter 123). Chronic excessive menstrual blood loss, chronic urinary tract bleeding, and recurrent epistaxis also can lead to iron deficiency and anemia. Because of the substantial consumption of maternal iron by the developing fetus, multiple pregnancies also may contribute to the development of iron deficiency and anemia. Patients with chronic intravascular hemolysis (e.g., paroxysmal nocturnal hemoglobinuria, malaria; or traumatic hemolysis from a prosthetic cardiac valve) lose hemoglobin in the urine and may become iron deficient and anemic. The blood drawn from and lost by a hospitalized patient can also contribute to an otherwise unexplained recent anemia, especially in patients who are unable to mount a reticulocyte response.

DILUTIONAL PSEUDOANEMIA. Certain conditions lead to an expansion of plasma volume, which results in a decreased hemoglobin, hematocrit, and RBC count without any decrease in the patient's total RBC mass. For example, the chronic intravascular volume expansion that occurs in pregnancy can reduce the hemoglobin to a level of as low as about 10 g/dL. Acute volume overload also can cause a dilutional decrease in the concentration of RBCs, which resolves after equilibration and diuresis occur. Certain medications, particularly some cytokines, such as IL-2, IL-11, and granulocyte-macrophage colony-stimulating factor (GM-CSF), also may cause acute dilutional pseudoanemias.

CLINICAL MANIFESTATIONS

There are three main types of clinical manifestations of anemia. In anemia that has developed very rapidly, symptoms related to hypotension may develop as a result of loss of blood volume. In both chronic and acute anemias, tissue and organ hypoxia is a major source of symptoms, although eventually orthostatic and non-orthostatic hypotension and tachycardia may occur due to chronically decreased blood volume. In hemolytic anemias, the products of lysed erythrocytes also may result in separate clinical findings. The specific signs and symptoms of anemia may vary widely from patient to patient with the same degree and tempo of anemia. The major factors that determine the specific response of each individual to anemia include severity of anemia, rapidity of onset of anemia, age of the patient, overall physical condition, and co-morbid events or disorders. Mild anemia often is associated with no clinical symptoms and may be discovered only when a complete blood cell count is done for another reason. The earliest clinical symptoms of mild to modest anemia tend to be a sense of fatigue, generalized weakness, and loss of stamina, followed by tachycardia and exertional dyspnea. In young, healthy patients, these symptoms frequently are not noticed until the hemoglobin level falls to below 7 or 8 g/dL. However, in elderly patients and those with cardiovascular or pulmonary disease, symptoms may occur even with modest degrees of anemia and hemoglobin levels in the range of 9 to 11 g/dL.

Physiologic Compensatory Mechanisms in Anemia

The five main physiologic compensatory responses to anemia vary in prominence depending on rapidity of onset and duration of anemia and the condition of the patient. First, in acute-onset anemia with severe loss of intravascular volume, peripheral vasoconstriction and central vasodilatation preserve blood flow to vital organs. Second, over time and with increasingly severe anemia, systemic small vessel vasodilatation results in increased blood flow to ensure better tissue oxygenation. These vascular compensations result in decreased systemic vascular resistance, increased cardiac output, and tachycardia, which result in a higher rate of delivery of oxygen-bearing erythrocytes to the tissues. Third, RBCs develop an increased level of 2,3-diphosphoglycerate, which interacts with hemoglobin molecules to cause a rightward shift of the hemoglobin oxygen dissociation curve, which in turn enhances the release of oxygen to the tissues at any given partial pressure of oxygen. Fourth, in chronic anemias there is a compensatory increase in plasma volume, which serves to maintain the total blood volume and to enhance tissue perfusion. The fifth compensatory response in otherwise normal individuals is stimulation of EPO production, which in turn stimulates new erythrocyte production. The latter occurs if the stem cells and erythroid precursors are normal, the erythroid precursors are able to respond normally to EPO, and the developing normoblasts are normal.

Clinical Manifestations of Chronic Anemia

Weakness, fatigue, lethargy, decreased stamina, palpitations, dyspnea on exertion, and orthostatic light-headedness are common symptoms in patients with chronic anemia, although the compensatory mechanisms described earlier may prevent these symptoms from being manifested in mild or moderate anemias. Occasional

patients with slowly developing or long-standing anemia may report being asymptomatic even with hemoglobin levels as low as 5 or 6 g/dL, although virtually all such patients notice a distinct improvement in their performance status after correction of anemia. As is true of acute anemias, co-morbid conditions, particularly with impaired blood supply or oxygenation of specific organs, may result in symptoms and signs resulting from organ-specific dysfunction. Thus, anemic patients with prior myocardial dysfunction may have more pronounced edema, dyspnea, orthopnea, tachycardia, fatigue, and loss of stamina. In patients with coronary artery disease, anemia may result in onset or worsening of angina or may even precipitate a myocardial infarction. Anemic patients with significant peripheral arterial disease may develop new or worsening claudication. Anemic patients with cerebrovascular disease may experience more frequent or severe transient ischemic events or strokes. The most prominent general physical examination findings that may occur in patients with significant anemia include pallor of skin and mucosal surfaces, orthostatic hypotension, resting or orthostatic tachycardia, systolic ejection murmur, increased prominence of the cardiac apical impulse, bounding pulses, and wide pulse pressure. The presence of splenomegaly or history of prior splenectomy raises the possibility of a chronic hemolytic anemia. A right upper quadrant surgical scar or history of gallstones and/or cholecystectomy also should raise the possibility of a chronic hemolytic state with formation of bilirubin-containing gallstones. In patients who are anemic without an immediately obvious etiology, careful probing of the patient's past medical history and family history is essential. In particular, it is important to obtain results of previous blood cell counts to determine whether the anemia is of recent to even life-long duration. A careful, in-depth discussion of personal and family history can be very helpful, particularly if positive for anemia, splenectomy, cholecystectomy, gallstones, and/or jaundice at birth or later in life. However, the new mutation rate for congenital/hereditary hemolytic anemias is sufficiently high that a lack of family history should not deter one from the search for such conditions, if the remainder of the clinical picture is compatible with a congenital hemolytic anemia. Mild hereditary and congenital hemolytic anemias sometimes escape detection until patients are elderly or until a second event compromises the ability of the patient's bone marrow to compensate for the chronic, excessive rate of destruction of erythrocytes. In some patients, past treatment may have been inappropriate or ineffective because of inadequate evaluation and incorrect diagnosis.

General Clinical Manifestations of Acute Development of Anemia from Blood Loss or Hemolysis

In a patient with acute severe hemolysis or blood loss, prominent early symptoms include resting or orthostatic hypotension due to a decrease in total blood volume, with subsequent light-headedness or syncope, exertional, orthostatic, and/or resting tachycardia and palpitations, diaphoresis, anxiety, agitation, generalized severe weakness and lethargy, and possibly decreased mental function. All of the physical examination findings described earlier for chronic anemias tend to be more pronounced with anemias of very rapid onset that also are complicated by acute loss of intravascular blood volume. Depending on the severity of the anemia and blood volume depletion, co-morbid conditions, age, and overall patient health, there also may be signs of oxygen deprivation in one or multiple organ systems. Loss of 25 to 35% of the total blood volume in 12 to 24 hours cannot be ameliorated by the normal compensatory mechanisms, and loss of more than 40% of blood volume in 12 hours leads to profound symptoms due more to intravascular volume depletion than to anemia.

Diseases of Other Body Systems that Can Cause or be Associated with Anemia

A broad spectrum of disorders of other organ systems can give rise to anemia. Any chronic infection, chronic inflammatory disease, or malignant disease can result in anemia of chronic disease or inflammation. Patients with lymphoproliferative and rheumatologic diseases may develop autoimmune hemolytic anemia. Any cause of moderate to severe renal insufficiency can cause anemia due to impaired EPO production. Any cause of marked splenomegaly, including myeloproliferative and lymphoproliferative disorders, certain chronic infectious diseases (e.g., malaria, tuberculosis), por-

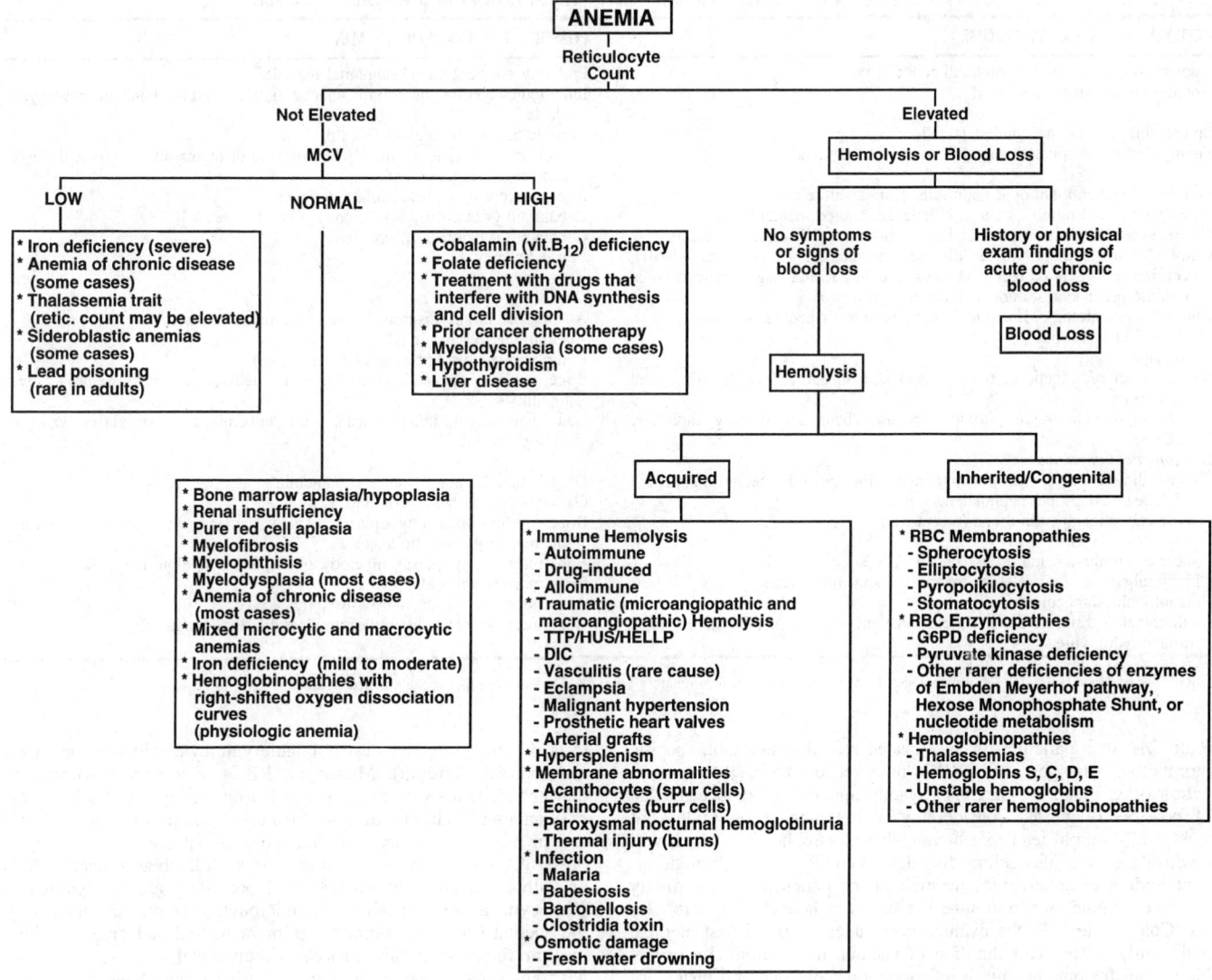

FIGURE 159-1 ■ Algorithm for diagnosis of anemias. TTP = thrombotic thrombocytopenic purpura; HUS = hemolytic-uremic syndrome; HELLP = *h*epatomegaly-*e*levated *l*iver (function tests)-*l*ow *p*latelets; DIC = disseminated intravascular coagulation.

tal vein thrombosis, or portal hypertension may cause excessive red cell sequestration and destruction. Gastritis, peptic ulcer disease, gastrointestinal angiodysplasia, and hereditary hemorrhagic telangiectasia frequently are associated with chronic blood loss that leads to iron deficiency and anemia. Iron deficiency also can be caused by removal or significant dysfunction (e.g., Whipple's disease, Crohn's disease) of the duodenum, which is the major site of iron absorption. Anti–gastric parietal cell antibodies, gastric achlorhydria, prior gastrectomy, intestinal bacterial overgrowth, or dysfunction (e.g., inflammatory bowel disease) or surgical removal of the terminal ileum can result in cobalamin deficiency and anemia. Patients with hypopituitarism or hypothyroidism may have a mild macrocytic anemia. Severe alcoholics may develop folate deficiency from poor dietary intake, iron deficiency from chronic gastric blood loss, or even toxic suppression of the bone marrow, resulting in decreased erythropoiesis. Patients with severe liver disease often have shortened RBC survival due to splenomegaly caused by portal hypertension or due to excess deposition of unesterified cholesterol on erythrocyte membranes and the resulting formation of acanthocytes and schistocytes that are cleared from the blood prematurely. Anemia is a common manifestation of HIV infection and may be multifactorial, including contributions from cytokine-mediated anemia of chronic disease, relative EPO deficiency, malnutrition, myelodysplastic changes in the bone marrow, bone marrow fibrosis and necrosis, immune-mediated hemolysis, and drug (e.g., zidovudine)-induced myelosuppression.

DIAGNOSIS

The initial diagnostic evaluation (Fig. 159–1) of anemia is based on using readily available information, including a careful in-depth evaluation of the patient's past medical history and family history (Table 159–3), physical examination (splenomegaly is the single most important physical finding in the anemic patient), complete blood cell count, reticulocyte count, and microscopic evaluation of the peripheral blood smear (Table 159–4). More specialized laboratory tests are indicated only after these screening studies have been obtained. In the patient with anemia, the first distinction to be made is whether the primary cause of the anemia is failure of the bone marrow to produce sufficient numbers of erythrocytes or accelerated loss or destruction of erythrocytes. A single test, the reticulocyte count, often provides the answer to this question. An elevated absolute reticulocyte count in an anemic patient indicates that the bone marrow is responding to the requirement for new erythrocyte production to replace prematurely destroyed or lost erythrocytes from hemolysis or blood loss. A reticulocyte count that is below normal or in the normal range for non-anemic individuals indicates that the primary cause of the anemia is the inability of the bone marrow to maintain the rate of production of RBCs required to compensate for those lost or destroyed.

Microscopic examination of the morphology of RBCs in a peripheral blood smear is an essential part of the evaluation of both defective production and excessive destruction of RBCs (Color

Table 159-3 ■ USE OF THE PERSONAL AND FAMILY MEDICAL HISTORY IN DIAGNOSIS OF ANEMIAS

HISTORY: SIGNS AND SYMPTOMS	POSSIBLE ETIOLOGY OF ANEMIA
Known normal complete blood cell count in past	Probably not hereditary/congenital disorder
Anemia known since childhood	Inherited/congenital hemolytic anemia or (less likely) bone marrow hypoplasia
Splenectomy, gallstones, and/or jaundice	Chronic hemolytic anemia, liver disease
Family history of splenectomy, gallstones, and/or jaundice	Hereditary hemolytic anemia (RBC enzyme or membrane disorder, thalassemia, or hemoglobinopathy)
Poor or unconventional diet, malnutrition, or severe alcoholism	Bone marrow hypoplasia, folate deficiency
Paresthesias, foot numbness, loss of balance, altered mental status	Cobalamin (vitamin B_{12}) deficiency
Gastrectomy, surgical removal of ileum, chronic malabsorption disorder	Cobalamin (vitamin B_{12}) deficiency
Chronic gastritis, peptic ulcer disease, chronic use of ASA or NSAID, recurrent epistaxis or rectal bleeding, melena, menorrhagia, metrorrhagia, multiple pregnancies, duodenal surgery, gastrectomy	Iron deficiency
Chronic rheumatologic, immunologic, infectious, or neoplastic disease	Anemia of chronic disease, autoimmune hemolytic anemia
Decreased urine output	Anemia due to renal insufficiency
Dark urine	Hemolytic anemia (intravascular hemolysis)
Recent onset of infections, mucosal and skin bleeding, easy bruising, oral ulcerations	Bone marrow aplasia/hypoplasia, acute leukemia, myelodysplasia, myelophthisis
Occupational/environmental toxin exposure (benzene, ionizing radiation, lead)	Bone marrow aplasia/hypoplasia, acute leukemia, myelodysplasia, lead poisoning
Drug/medication exposure:	
Penicillin, cephalosporin, procainamide, quinidine, quinine, sulfonamide	Drug-induced immune hemolytic anemia
Fava beans, dapsone, naphthalene	Oxidant-induced hemolysis (G6PD deficient)
Cancer chemotherapeutic drugs (recent use)	Bone marrow aplasia/hypoplasia, oxidant damage, fluid retention/dilutional anemia, megaloblastic anemia
Cancer chemotherapeutic drugs (past use)	Bone marrow hypoplasia, myelodysplasia, acute myeloid leukemia
Chloramphenicol, gold salts, sulfonamides, anti-inflammatory drugs	Bone marrow aplasia/hypoplasia
Ethanol, chloramphenicol	Acute reversible bone marrow toxicity
Methotrexate, azathioprine, pyrimethamine, trimethoprim, zidovudine, sulfa drugs, hydroxyurea	Bone marrow aplasia/hypoplasia, megaloblastic anemia

RBC = red blood cells; ASA = aspirin; NSAID = non-steroidal anti-inflammatory drug; G6PD = glucose-6-phosphate dehydrogenase.

Plate 5*A*). In a patient with an elevated reticulocyte count, specific morphologic changes in the RBCs observed on microscopic examination often make the diagnosis readily apparent or reduce the list of possible diagnoses considerably. For example, the finding of sickle cells should lead to a hemoglobin electrophoresis, which will confirm the type of sickling disorder (Color Plate 5*J*). A predominant finding of spherocytes means that the patient almost certainly has autoimmune or alloimmune hemolysis or hereditary spherocytosis (Color Plate 5*G*); the evaluation includes a careful past medical and family history (for duration of anemia, medications, history of blood transfusions, anemia in other family members, and history of splenectomy, cholecystectomy, gallstones, and jaundice in the patient and family members), examination of the patient (for splenomegaly, jaundice, or signs of autoimmune disorders), and laboratory studies (including direct and indirect antiglobulin [Coombs]

tests or more sensitive tests of antierythrocyteantibodies and total and indirect bilirubin). Microcytic RBCs in a patient without an elevated reticulocyte count suggest iron deficiency (Color Plate 5*D*), anemia of chronic disease, or thalassemia trait (Color Plate 5*I*) (or, in more severe cases, homozygous β-thalassemia or hemoglobin H disease) as the most likely causes. Sideroblastic anemia with or without myelodysplasia and lead poisoning are rare causes of microcytic anemia in adults. In microcytic anemia, the history of the anemia (including duration; prior menstrual and pregnancy history in females; dietary history; occupational history; history of gastrointestinal, upper respiratory, or urinary tract bleeding; history of chronic infections or autoimmune or chronic inflammatory disorders; response to prior therapy for anemia) and family history of anemia can help greatly to distinguish among these possible causes. A low or low normal RBC count and normal RDW favors anemia

Table 159-4 ■ RED BLOOD CELL MORPHOLOGIC ABNORMALITIES AS CLUES TO THE DIAGNOSIS OF ANEMIAS

RED BLOOD CELL (RBC) MORPHOLOGY	REPRESENTATIVE CAUSES OF ANEMIA
Microcytosis	Iron deficiency, anemia of chronic disease, thalassemia, and (rarely) lead poisoning, vitamin B_6 deficiency, or hereditary sideroblastic anemias
Macrocytosis	Polychromatophilia (reticulocytes), vitamin B_{12} (cobalamin) or folate deficiency, myelodysplasia, use of drugs that inhibit DNA synthesis
Basophilic stippling	Hemolysis, lead poisoning, thalassemia
Target cells	Thalassemia, hemoglobins C, D, E, and S, liver disease, abetalipoproteinemia
Microspherocytes	Autoimmune hemolytic anemia, alloimmune hemolysis, hereditary spherocytosis, some cases of Heinz body hemolytic anemias
Schistocytes and fragmented RBCs	Thrombotic thrombocytopenic purpura, disseminated intravascular coagulation, vasculitis, malignant hypertension, eclampsia, traumatic hemolysis due to prosthetic heart valve or damaged vascular graft, thermal injury (burns), post-splenectomy
Teardrop cells	Myelofibrosis, myelophthisis (bone marrow infiltration by neoplastic cells)
Sickle cells	Hemoglobin SS, SC, or S-β-thalassemia
Acanthocytes (spur cells)	Severe liver disease, malnutrition, McLeod blood group phenotype
Echinocytes (burr cells)	Renal failure, hemolysis due to malnutrition with hypomagnesemia and hypophosphatemia, pyruvate kinase deficiency, common in vitro artifact
Stomatocytes	Alcoholism, hereditary stomatocytosis
"Bite" cells or "blister" cells	Glucose-6-phosphate dehydrogenase deficiency, other oxidant-induced hemolysis, unstable hemoglobins
Howell-Jolly bodies	Post-splenectomy, hyposplenism
Intraerythrocytic parasitic or bacterial inclusions	Malaria (parasites), babesiosis (parasites), bartonellosis (gram-negative coccobacilli)
Agglutinated red blood cells	Cold agglutinin disease, in vitro artifact
Rouleaux formation	Multiple myeloma, monoclonal gammopathy of undetermined significance

Table 159–5 ■ LABORATORY TESTS TO DISTINGUISH IRON DEFICIENCY FROM ANEMIA OF CHRONIC DISEASE (ACD)

MEASUREMENT	UNITS	NORMAL VALUES	IRON DEFICIENCY	ACD	ACD + IRON DEFICIENCY
Serum iron	μg/dL	50–150	↓	Low normal-↓	↓
Serum total iron-binding capacity	μg/dL	250–400	↑	Low normal-↓	Low normal-↓
Transferrin saturation	%	20–50	↓	Normal-↓	Low normal-↓
Serum ferritin	μg/L	20–350	↓	Normal-↑	Normal-↓
Serum soluble transferrin receptor	nM	9–28	↑	Normal	↓
Bone marrow iron stores	0–4+	2–3+	↓	Normal	↓
Iron-containing normoblasts in the bone marrow	%	20–80%	↓		↓

of chronic disease; an elevated RDW in this setting favors iron deficiency; and a high normal or elevated RBC count and normal RDW favors thalassemia. Serum iron, iron-binding capacity, and ferritin levels often can distinguish between anemia of chronic disease and iron-deficiency anemia (Table 159–5); in patients with anemia of chronic disease, an elevated serum soluble transferrin receptor level favors the associated presence of iron deficiency. Determination of marrow iron stores on bone marrow aspiration or biopsy, the gold standard for determining iron stores, rarely is required for this purpose now. However, the diagnosis of myelodysplasia requires microscopic examination of bone marrow cell morphology, and diagnosis of sideroblastic anemia (Color Plate 6*E*) also requires Prussian blue staining (for detection of iron) of normoblasts in the bone marrow (Table 159–6). If there is mild microcytic anemia with significant numbers of target cells, thalassemia trait is the most likely diagnosis. β-Thalassemia heterozygotes who have mild microcytic anemia can be diagnosed with hemoglobin electrophoresis, although more sophisticated tests, including direct sequencing of the β-globin gene, may be needed to determine the specific type of β-thalassemia. α-Thalassemia can be diagnosed definitively only with globin chain synthesis studies, Southern blotting, polymerase chain reaction, or α-globin gene sequencing; however, normal hemoglobin A₂ and F levels in a patient with microcytosis, target cells, and no or mild anemia strongly suggest 1 or 2 gene deletion α-thalassemia trait.

In real life, patients often have multiple potential causes of anemia. A patient with a rheumatologic or lymphoproliferative disease may have anemia of chronic disease but then may have a marked change in the severity of the anemia because of the development of autoimmune hemolysis. A patient with chronic hemolytic anemia such as sickle cell disease, thalassemia, or hereditary spherocytosis may develop folate deficiency or become infected with parvovirus B19, which prevents the bone marrow from continuing to overproduce erythrocytes and leads to a marked increase in the severity of the anemia. If the entire clinical picture cannot be explained by a single cause, the physician must search for secondary factors that may be important contributing components to the patient's anemia.

Berliner N, Duffy TP, Abelson HT: Approach to the adult and child with anemia. *In* Hoffman R, Benz EJ Jr, Shattil SJ, et al (eds): Hematology: Basic Principles and Practice, 2nd ed. New York, Churchill Livingstone, 1995, p 468. *Comprehensive review of the pathophysiology and evaluation of anemias.*

Erslev AJ: Clinical manifestations and classification of erythrocytic disorders. *In* Beutler E, Lichtman MA, Coller BS, Kipps TJ (eds): Williams Hematology, 5th ed. New York, McGraw-Hill, 1995, pp 441–447. *Excellent review of the systemic manifestations of anemia.*

Hillman RS, Ault KA: Hematology in Clinical Practice. New York, McGraw-Hill, 1995. *Excellent summaries of practical approaches to the evaluation and management of anemias.*

Hillman RS, Finch CA: Red Cell Manual, 7th ed. Philadelphia, FA Davis, 1996, pp 3–196. *A definitive text on the production, function, and disorders of erythrocytes.*

Table 159–6 ■ SELECTED LABORATORY STUDIES THAT ARE USEFUL IN THE DIAGNOSIS OF ANEMIAS

IF THIS IS CONSIDERED TO BE A POSSIBLE CAUSE OF A PATIENT'S ANEMIA	THESE ARE POTENTIALLY USEFUL DIAGNOSTIC LABORATORY TESTS
Hypoproliferative Anemias	
Bone marrow aplasia/hypoplasia or myelophthisis	Platelet count, white blood cell count with differential, bone marrow aspirate and biopsy
Myelodysplasia	Bone marrow aspirate and biopsy (including Prussian blue stain of iron), karyotype analysis
Acute leukemia	Bone marrow aspirate and biopsy, flow cytometry, immunohistochemical staining, karyotype analysis
Myelofibrosis	Bone marrow biopsy with stains for collagen (trichrome stain) and reticulin (silver stain)
Iron deficiency	Serum iron, TIBC, ferritin, soluble transferrin receptor (± bone marrow iron stain)
Anemia of chronic disease/inflammation	Serum iron, TIBC, ferritin, soluble transferrin receptor (± bone marrow iron stain)
Folate deficiency	Red blood cell folate level, serum folate level, bone marrow aspirate
Vitamin B₁₂ (cobalamin) deficiency	Serum vitamin B₁₂ level, urine (± serum) methylmalonic acid level, bone marrow aspirate, Schilling tests
Hemolytic Anemias	
General measures of hemolysis (intravascular [T] and extravascular [E])	Reduction in serum haptoglobin (I > E), presence of urine hemoglobin (I) and/or urine hemosiderin (I), increased serum LDH (I > E), and serum unconjugated bilirubin (I > E)
Thalassemias	Hemoglobin electrophoresis, hemoglobin A₂ and hemoglobin F levels, globin DNA analysis (Southern blotting, polymerase chain reaction, sequencing), globin chain synthesis ratios
Sickle cell disorders	Hemoglobin electrophoresis
Autoimmune hemolysis	Direct antiglobulin (Coombs) test, quantitation of red blood cell surface antibodies, cold agglutinin titer
Alloimmune hemolysis	Direct and indirect antiglobulin (Coombs) test with specificity analysis of eluted antibodies
Truamatic (microangiopathic or macroangiopathic) hemolysis	History and physical examination findings of hypertension, pregnancy, prosthetic heart valves or vascular grafts, systemic vasculitis, neurologic changes, fever; schistocytes, anemia, and destructive thrombocytopenia; BUN and creatinine; urinalysis; DIC panel
Hereditary spherocytosis, elliptocytosis, pyropoikilocytosis, and stomatocytosis	Primarily morphologic diagnoses; specific mutations detected by sequencing spectrin, ankyrin, band 3 or protein 4.1 DNA
Red blood cell enzymopathies	G6PD assay (1–2 months after acute hemolysis), Heinz body prep, specific enzyme assays
Unstable hemoglobins	Heat/isopropanol denaturation tests, hemoglobin electrophoresis
Paroxysmal nocturnal hemoglobinuria	Acid hemolysis (Ham) or sucrose hemolysis test, flow cytometry analysis of GPI-anchored cell surface proteins (e.g., CD55, 59)

TIBC = total iron-binding capacity; BUN = blood urea nitrogen; DIC = disseminated intravascular coagulation; G6PD = glucose-6-phosphate dehydrogenase; GPI = glycosylphosphatidylinositol.

160 APLASTIC ANEMIA AND RELATED BONE MARROW FAILURE SYNDROMES

Neal S. Young

Blood cell counts may be low because cells are prematurely removed from the peripheral circulation or are inadequately produced in the bone marrow. Bone marrow failure is often classified by other dominant clinical or morphologic features (e.g., the leukemias) or by specific etiology (e.g., pernicious anemia). The term *bone marrow failure* is vague and inclusive, and it awaits redefinition with more precise understanding of pathophysiologic processes. By default, therefore, the disorders of bone marrow failure are currently defined by their marrow pathology: the fatty bone marrow of aplastic anemia, the disordered hematopoiesis of the myelodysplasias, and the fibrosis of myelofibrosis. Making inferences about disease processes from the appearance of the bone marrow is as misleading as it is inevitable; what is understood must be distinguished from what is conjecture.

APLASTIC ANEMIA

Definition (Table 160–1)

APLASTIC ANEMIA. Aplastic anemia is a disease of the young, with a median age at onset of about 25 years (excluding aplasia secondary to cancer chemotherapy). It is the most common cause of pancytopenia in the adolescent or young adult (Fig. 160–1). The bone marrow usually can be aspirated easily but appears dilute on smear. The biopsy specimen (see Color Plate 5C), often grossly

Table 160–1 ▪ CLASSIFICATION OF APLASTIC ANEMIA AND SINGLE CYTOPENIAS

APLASTIC ANEMIA	CYTOPENIAS
Acquired	**Acquired**
Radiation	*Anemias*
Drugs and chemicals	Pure red cell aplasia (see Table
Regular effects	160–3)
Idiosyncratic reactions	Transient erythroblastopenia of
Viruses	childhood
Epstein-Barr virus (infectious	*Neutropenias*
mononucleosis)	Idiopathic
Hepatitis (non-A non-B non-	Drugs, toxins
C hepatitis)	*Thrombocytopenias*
Human immunodeficiency vi-	Drugs, toxins
rus (AIDS)	**Inherited**
Immune diseases	*Anemias*
Eosinophilic fasciitis	Congenital pure red cell aplasia
Hypoimmunoglobulinemia	*Neutropenias*
Thymoma and thymic carci-	Kostmann's syndrome
noma	Schwachman-Diamond syndrome
Graft-versus-host disease in	Reticular dysgenesis
immunodeficiency	*Thrombocytopenias*
Paroxysmal nocturnal hemoglo-	Thrombocytopenia with absence
binuria	of radii
Pregnancy	Idiopathic amegakaryocytic throm-
Idiopathic—the most frequent	bocytopenia
diagnosis	
Inherited	
Fanconi's anemia	
Dyskeratosis congenita	
Schwachman-Diamond syn-	
drome	
Reticular dysgenesis	
Amegakaryocytic thrombocyto-	
penia	
Familial aplastic anemias	
Preleukemia (e.g., monosomy	
7)	
Non-hematologic syndromes	
(Down, Dubovitz's, Seckel's)	

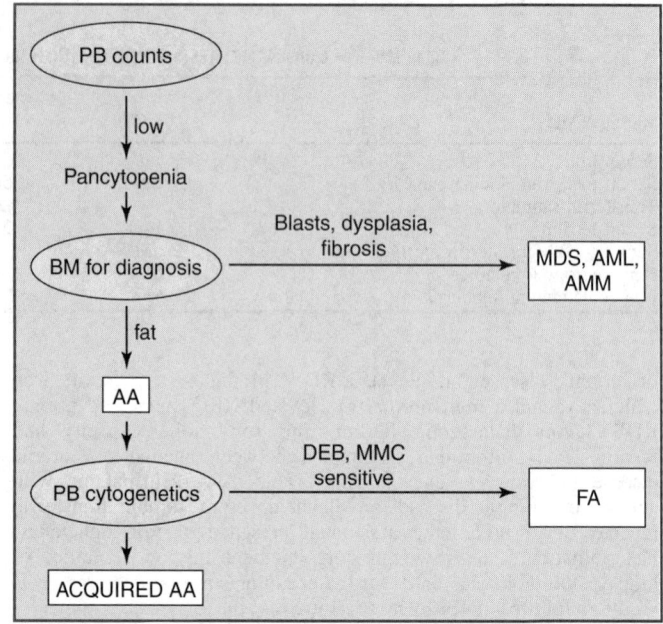

FIGURE 160–1 ▪ Diagnostic decisions in patients who have pancytopenia. PB = peripheral blood; BM = bone marrow; AA = aplastic anemia; MDS = myelodysplastic syndrome; AML = acute myeloid leukemia; AMM = agnogenic myeloid metaplasia; DEB = diepoxybutane; MMC = mitomycin-C; FA = Fanconi's anemia.

pale, shows mainly fat under the microscope; by definition, hematopoietic cells occupy less than 25% of the marrow space and, in the most serious cases, 0 to 5%. Prognosis is determined by the degree of blood cell count depression. The commonly accepted definition for severe disease is two of the following: (1) absolute neutrophil count (percentage of polymorphonuclear and band forms multiplied by the total white blood cell count) of less than 500/mm³; (2) platelets less than 20,000/mm³; and (3) anemia with a reticulocyte count (corrected for hematocrit) less than 1% (or an absolute reticulocyte count less than 40,000/mm³). A subset of very severe aplastic anemia, with the worst prognosis, is defined by more severe neutropenia (absolute neutrophil count less than 200/mm³).

BICYTOPENIA AND SINGLE-LINEAGE FAILURE STATES. Some patients have bone marrow hypocellularity and depression of only two of the three major blood lines; many such cases progress to typical aplastic anemia. Failure of a single lineage also occurs in pure red cell aplasia (rare), megakaryocytic thrombocytopenia (extremely rare), and agranulocytosis (not rare but usually an idiosyncratic drug reaction). These syndromes show the characteristic absence of a single set of recognizable precursor cells in otherwise cellular bone marrow, and in this way they are differentiated from the much more common causes of anemia (e.g., vitamin or iron deficiency and hemolysis) or thrombocytopenia (from peripheral destruction of platelets). The pathophysiology of the more restricted marrow failure states is probably similar to that of general bone marrow failure, but with a more mature target cell.

CONSTITUTIONAL (FANCONI'S) ANEMIA. Fanconi described children with inherited pancytopenia and hypocellular marrows and with associated anomalies of the skeletal and urogenital systems. Fanconi's anemia now is defined by specific chromosomal aberrations in cultured cells after clastogenic stress. Indeed, cytogenetic analysis of families of children with Fanconi's anemia has shown that the majority of patients lack associated anomalies and that the disease can manifest in the third and fourth decades or even later. Congenital pure red cell aplasia (Diamond-Blackfan syndrome) lacks a cytogenetic marker or associated physical abnormalities. Isolated neutropenia or thrombocytopenia occurs in a number of pediatric syndromes.

Etiology

In the majority of patients, aplastic anemia is diagnosed as "idiopathic." There is little to distinguish these cases clinically from those with a presumed cause, such as exposure to a drug or chemical. Even when clinical associations are established, they should not automatically be equated with etiology and pathophysiology.

RADIATION (see Chapter 19). Marrow aplasia is a major acute sequela of radiation exposure. Radiant energy damages DNA; the bone marrow, which is a tissue dependent on active mitosis, is particularly susceptible to its effects. Nuclear accidents and radiation injury can involve not only power plant workers but also employees of hospitals, laboratories, and industry (e.g., food sterilization, metal radiography), as well as persons exposed to stolen, misplaced, or misused radiation sources. The radiation dose can be approximated from the rate and degree of decline in blood cell counts; dosimetry by reconstruction of the exposure can help to estimate the patient's prognosis and also to protect medical personnel from contact with radioactive tissue and excreta. Myelodysplasia and leukemia, but not aplastic anemia, are late effects of irradiation.

CHEMICALS (Table 160–2). Benzene has been clearly linked to bone marrow failure, but the quality of the case reports, many from the early part of the century, usually does not allow accurate discrimination between aplasia and myelodysplasia (benzene exposure also increases the risk of acute leukemia). The occurrence of hematologic abnormalities is roughly correlated with cumulative exposure, but there must also be an important element of susceptibility, because only a minority of even heavily exposed workers develop evidence of myelotoxicity. A history of past employment is important, especially in "open" industries in which benzene is used for a secondary purpose (usually as a solvent) rather than in "closed" industries for chemical production. Benzene-related blood diseases have declined with regulation of industrial exposure, and benzene is not generally available as a household solvent. The benzene content of gasoline increased with the reduction of lead. The association of marrow failure with other organic chemicals is much less well substantiated.

DRUGS. Many of the common cancer chemotherapeutic drugs regularly and predictably suppress the bone marrow. A large and diverse group of other drugs have been linked to idiosyncratic aplastic anemia (see Table 26–5), but some of these associations are based on case reports and are tenuous at best. For example, some incriminated drugs may have been used to treat the first symptoms of bone marrow failure (antibiotics for fever or the preceding viral illness) or may have provoked the first symptom of a pre-existing disease (petechiae produced by non-steroidal anti-inflammatory agents administered to a thrombocytopenic individual). In the context of total drug use, these idiosyncratic reactions, although individually devastating, are very rare events.

Chloramphenicol, the most infamous culprit, reportedly produced aplasia in only about 1 of 60,000 therapeutic courses, and even this number is almost certainly an overestimate. Chloramphenicol also consistently causes dose-related, rather modest marrow depression, mainly reticulocytopenia and altered marrow morphology and iron kinetics. This effect of chloramphenicol use is mechanistically un-

related to and clinically not predictive of the rare, severe reaction, which occurs 1 to 2 months or longer after its routine use. The introduction of chloramphenicol was thought to have produced a notable increase in the number of cases of aplastic anemia, but its diminished use has not been followed by reduced frequency of aplastic anemia. Chloramphenicol remains a popular antibiotic in less-developed countries. Recent epidemiologic studies in Thailand failed to show a relationship between chloramphenicol and aplastic anemia.

Suspected drug reactions account for 15 to 25% of cases of aplastic anemia, whereas most agranulocytosis in adults is drug related. The drugs associated with agranulocytosis are similar, but not identical to, those related to generalized bone marrow failure. Myeloid cells may be uniquely susceptible because of their ability to metabolize drugs, often to toxic intermediate compounds. In contrast to drug-associated aplastic anemia, agranulocytosis should spontaneously resolve with removal of the drug, and the severely neutropenic patient should survive if infection is adequately treated.

INFECTIONS. Hepatitis, which is the most common infection preceding aplastic anemia, accounts for about 5% of cases in Western countries and perhaps twice that proportion in Asia. Typically, severe aplasia occurs in a young man who recovered from a mild bout of hepatitis 1 to 2 months earlier. The hepatitis is non-A, non-B, and non-C by serologic testing. Aplastic anemia can rarely follow infectious mononucleosis; and Epstein-Barr virus, with or without a suggestive preceding history, is found in the marrow of some patients with aplastic anemia. Parvovirus B19 has not convincingly been associated with permanent total bone marrow failure. Moderate marrow depression occurs commonly in the course of many viral and bacterial infections, but the primary disease is usually overt.

IMMUNOLOGIC DISEASE. Fatal aplasia can occur in immunodeficient children who receive unirradiated blood products and in other cases of transfusion-associated graft-versus-host disease. The syndrome eosinophilic fasciitis is associated with aplastic anemia. Pure red cell aplasia is associated with thymoma, and patients with red cell aplasia or pancytopenia may be hypoimmunoglobulinemic.

OTHER ASSOCIATIONS. Aplastic anemia may occur during pregnancy and sometimes resolves with delivery or with spontaneous or induced abortion. Pancytopenia occurs in about one third of patients with paroxysmal nocturnal hemoglobinuria (see Chapter 165), and patients with aplastic anemia may have a positive Ham test, often with hematopoietic recovery; a much larger proportion show evidence of absent cell surface membrane glycophosphoinositol proteins by flow cytometry of granulocytes.

Pathophysiology

TYPES OF INJURY. Most bone marrow failure almost certainly results from damage to the hematopoietic stem cell compartment; little evidence exists of aplastic anemia due to defective stroma or from inadequate production of growth factors. In all patients with aplastic anemia, the numbers of both committed and primitive hematopoietic cells that can be assayed in vitro are markedly diminished, probably to about 1% of normal, by the time of clinical presentation with symptoms. Nevertheless, recovery of peripheral blood cell counts can occur despite low stem cell numbers and does not depend on repopulation of the stem cell compartment.

Although aplastic anemia can result from direct damage to the bone marrow (e.g., due to high doses of physicochemical agents, irradiation, and cytotoxic drugs used to treat cancer), most community-acquired aplastic anemia is caused by immune system attack on the bone marrow and resulting destruction of hematopoietic stem and progenitor cells. The mechanism by which some drugs and chemicals or viruses provoke organ specific autoimmunity in aplastic anemia is unknown, as are the host factors that make only rare individuals susceptible to the idiosyncratic effects of commonly used agents. Specificity of the inciting agent is suggested by the incrimination of a non-A . . . E hepatitis virus in post-hepatitis aplastic anemia (the syndrome is not associated with other known hepatitis viruses [see Chapter 149]) and the involvement of certain types of drugs. On the host side, aplastic anemia has been linked to a few HLA antigens and occurs in association with other autoimmune diseases. Disease is likely the result of a combination

---

Table 160–2 ■ SOME DRUGS AND CHEMICALS ASSOCIATED WITH APLASTIC ANEMIA

Agents That Regularly Produce Marrow Depression as the Major Toxicity in Commonly Employed Doses or Normal Exposures

Cytotoxic drugs used in cancer chemotherapy: alkylating agents, antimetabolites, antimitotics

Some antibiotics

Agents That Frequently But Not Inevitably Produce Marrow Aplasia

Benzene (and benzene-containing chemicals like kerosene, carbon tetrachloride, Stoddard's solvent, chlorophenols)

Agents Probably Associated With Aplastic Anemia But With Relatively Low Probability

Insecticides

Chloramphenicol

Antiprotozoals: quinacrine and chloroquine, mepacrine

Non-steroidal anti-inflammatory drugs (including phenylbutazone, indomethacin, ibuprofen, sulindac, aspirin)

Anticonvulsants (hydantoins, carbamazepine, phenacemide)

Heavy metals (gold, arsenic, bismuth, mercury)

Sulfonamides: some antibiotics, antithyroid drugs (methimazole, methylthiouracil, propylthiouracil), antidiabetes drugs (tolbutamide, chlorpropamide), carbonic anhydrase inhibitors (acetazolamide and methazolamide)

Antihistamines (cimetidine, chlorpheniramine)

D-Penicillamine

Estrogens (in pregnancy and in high doses in animals)

of genetically determined features of the immune response that convert a normal physiologic response to a sustained and abnormal pathologic process.

METABOLIC DRUG INJURY. Most drugs and chemicals, especially if they are polar and have limited water solubility, are metabolized to highly reactive electrophilic intermediates that bind to cellular macromolecules. Excessive generation of such toxic intermediates or failure to detoxify them may be genetically determined and apparent only on drug challenge. The complexity and specificity of the pathways implies multiple susceptible loci. For example, in one case of phenytoin-associated aplastic anemia, a defect in detoxification of that drug's metabolites was detected in the patient after recovery, and cells from the patient's mother were intermediately susceptible; cells from both individuals normally detoxified metabolites generated from drugs closely related to phenytoin.

IMMUNE-MEDIATED INJURY. The recovery of their own marrow function by some patients being prepared for bone marrow transplantation with immunosuppressive horse antilymphocyte globulin first suggested that aplastic anemia might be immune mediated. Blood and bone marrow of patients often suppress normal bone marrow growth in progenitor assays, and removal of T cells from the bone marrow of patients with aplastic anemia can improve colony formation in vitro. Patients with aplastic anemia may have increased numbers of activated cytotoxic lymphocytes (CD8+ cells bearing HLA-DR and interleukin-2 receptors) that overproduce lymphokines (particularly interferon-γ and tumor necrosis factor). The interferon-γ gene is overexpressed in the marrow of most aplastic anemia patients, and lymphocytes containing interferon can be detected by flow cytometric methods in the blood. Both interferon and tumor necrosis factor induce apoptosis in hematopoietic target cells through the Fas pathway; the result is a process of active cell destruction, not simply functional suppression of cell proliferation. The severe and fatal aplastic anemia that accompanies "runt" disease in animals and transfusion-acquired graft-versus-host disease in humans are evidence of the potency of immune cells to ablate bone marrow.

Although immune system abnormalities improve when patients are treated with immunosuppressive therapies, they may not resolve completely even when blood cell counts have improved. The high rate of clinical relapse after discontinuation of immunosuppressive therapy and, conversely, the responsiveness, sometimes dependence, of blood cell counts on cyclosporine administration are further evidence of the pathogenic role of T cells in this disease.

PURE RED CELL APLASIA (Table 160–3). Like aplastic anemia, pure red cell aplasia results from diverse causes. Immune mechanisms have been implicated when pure red cell aplasia is associated with thymoma, systemic lupus erythematosus, and chronic lymphocytic leukemia, but not in failed erythropoiesis secondary to myelodysplasia, myeloproliferative diseases, and distinct cytogenetic abnormalities. Antibodies to red blood cell precursors can be detected in the blood of some patients, but T-cell inhibition is probably the more common mechanism. Cytotoxic lymphocyte activity restricted by histocompatibility locus or specific for cells infected by human T-cell lymphotropic virus (HTLV-I) has been demonstrated in a particularly well-studied case.

Parvovirus B19 represents the best example of the interaction of virus, host hematologic target cell, and immune response. This common virus causes fifth disease, a benign exanthem of childhood, and a polyarthralgia syndrome in adults. In persons with underlying hemolysis, parvovirus infection causes abrupt but temporary worsening of anemia resulting from failed erythropoiesis, a syndrome called transient aplastic crisis. Parvovirus B19 has extreme tropism for human erythroid progenitor cells, owing largely to its employment of red cell P antigen as a cellular receptor. Direct cytotoxicity of the virus causes anemia if demands on erythrocyte production are high. In normal individuals, the temporary cessation of red cell production is not clinically apparent and symptoms are entirely the result of immune complex deposition. In persons unable to mount an adequate antibody response, parvovirus B19 can persist in the bone marrow and cause chronic anemia that resembles pure red cell aplasia. The presence of giant pronormoblasts, the cytopathic sign of the infection, should suggest the diagnosis. Persistent parvovirus infection should be sought in anemic patients with congenital and acquired immunodeficiency syndromes as well as in patients iatrogenically immunosuppressed because it can be effectively treated with immunoglobulin infusions.

Incidence and Epidemiology

The incidence of aplastic anemia is approximately 2 per million in Europe and Israel, but the disease is more frequent in Asia, being 4 per million in Bangkok and higher in rural Thailand. Mortality statistics indicate an equal sex ratio and a preponderance of older persons, but at referral centers the median age is about 25 years. Agranulocytosis has an incidence of 3.4 per million in Europe. Pure red cell aplasia is a very rare disease, with only a few hundred reported cases, and amegakaryocytic thrombocytopenia is rarer still, with only a few dozen cases reported in the literature.

Clinical Description

HISTORY. Bleeding is the most common early symptom of aplastic anemia. Patients commonly report days to weeks of easy bruising, including oozing from the gums, nose bleeds, or heavy menstrual flow; sometimes petechiae will have been noticed. With thrombocytopenia, massive hemorrhage is unusual, but small amounts of bleeding in the central nervous system can result in serious symptoms and signs of intracranial or retinal hemorrhage. In cases of more gradual onset, symptoms of anemia are described: usually lassitude, weakness, shortness of breath, and a pounding sensation in the ears. Infection is unusual as a first symptom in aplastic anemia, in contrast to agranulocytosis, in which pharyngitis, anorectal infection, and frank sepsis may be presenting syndromes. A striking feature of aplastic anemia is the restriction of symptoms to the hematologic system. Patients often feel and look remarkably well despite drastically reduced blood cell counts; systemic complaints and weight loss should point to other causes of pancytopenia. Drug use, chemical exposure, and preceding viral illnesses should be sought with repeated questioning; prompt cessation of drug or chemical exposure is especially important in agranulocytosis, which is usually self-limited.

PHYSICAL EXAMINATION. Petechiae and ecchymoses are frequently present, and there may be retinal hemorrhages. Pelvic and rectal examinations should be performed infrequently and gently to avoid trauma; these examinations may show bleeding from the cervical os and blood in the stool. Pallor of the skin and mucous membranes is also common except in the most acute cases or in those patients who have received transfusions. Infection is uncommon on presentation; however, by the time the patient reaches a referral center, fever and signs of systemic or local infection may well be present. Lymphadenopathy and splenomegaly are very unusual in aplastic anemia. Café-au-lait spots and short stature point to Fanconi's anemia; peculiar nails suggest dyskeratosis congenita.

Diagnosis and Differential Diagnosis

The diagnosis of aplastic anemia is usually straightforward (Table 160–4), based on the combination of pancytopenia with fatty bone marrow. Prompt arrival at the appropriate diagnosis is

---

Table 160–3 ■ CLASSIFICATION OF PURE RED BLOOD CELL APLASIA

Self-limited
Transient erythroblastopenia of childhood
Transient aplastic crisis of hemolysis (parvovirus B19 infection)

Fetal Red Blood Cell Aplasia
Non-immune hydrops fetalis (in utero parvovirus infection)

Hereditary Pure Red Cell Aplasia
Congenital pure red cell aplasia (Diamond-Blackfan syndrome)

Acquired Pure Red Cell Aplasia
Thymoma and malignancy: thymoma, lymphoid malignancies (and more rarely other hematologic diseases), paraneoplastic to solid tumors
Connective tissue disorders with immunologic abnormalities: systemic lupus erythematosus, juvenile rheumatoid arthritis, rheumatoid arthritis, multiple endocrine gland insufficiency
Virus: especially persistent parvovirus B19, more rarely hepatitis, adult T-cell leukemia virus, Epstein-Barr virus
Pregnancy
Drugs: especially phenytoin, azathioprine, chloramphenicol, procainamide, isoniazid
Idiopathic

Table 160-4 ■ DIFFERENTIAL DIAGNOSIS OF PANCYTOPENIA

Pancytopenia With Hypocellular Bone Marrow
Acquired aplastic anemia
Inherited aplastic anemia (Fanconi's anemia)
Some myelodysplasia syndromes
Rare aleukemic leukemia (acute myelogenous leukemia)
Some acute lymphoblastic leukemias in childhood
Some lymphomas of bone marrow
Pancytopenia With Cellular Bone Marrow
Primary Bone Marrow Diseases
Myelodysplasia syndromes
Paroxysmal nocturnal hemoglobinuria
Myelofibrosis
Some aleukemic leukemias
Myelophthisis
Bone marrow lymphoma
Hairy cell leukemia
Secondary to Systemic Diseases
Systemic lupus erythematosus
Hypersplenism
Vitamin B_{12} or folate deficiency
Overwhelming infection
Acquired immunodeficiency syndrome
Alcoholism
Brucellosis
Sarcoidosis
Tuberculosis
Hypocellular Bone Marrow ± Cytopenia
Q fever
Legionnaires' disease
Anorexia nervosa, starvation
Myocobacterial infection

part of the effective management of the patient with aplastic anemia.

BLOOD. The smear typically shows large erythrocytes and a paucity of platelets and granulocytes. Macrocytosis, as determined by automated cell counting, is very common. Lymphocyte numbers may be normal or also reduced. The presence of immature myeloid forms should suggest leukemia or myelodysplasia; nucleated red cells suggest marrow fibrosis or invasion; and abnormal, or large, platelets suggest peripheral destruction, dysplasia, or fibrosis.

BONE MARROW (Fig. 160-1). "Watery" marrow can almost always be obtained, and a "dry tap" occurs in fibrotic or myelophthisic disease. In severe aplasia, the smear of the aspirated specimen shows only residual lymphocytes and stromal cells; in milder cases, the remaining hematopoietic cells can show "megaloblastoid" erythropoiesis. Megakaryocytes are invariably greatly reduced and usually absent. The areas adjacent to the spicule should be searched for myeloblasts, which are not increased in aplastic anemia. Total cellularity is assessed by biopsy (see Color Plate 5C) of a core more than 1 cm in length, which in the most severe cases is virtually 100% fat and in more moderate disease is less than 20% cellular. Nonetheless, the correlation between marrow cellularity and severity is imperfect: some patients with moderate disease according to blood cell counts have empty iliac crest biopsies, and there may be "hot spots" of hematopoiesis in severe cases. In single-lineage failure states, the bone marrow reflects the absence of a specific morphologic subtype, but in both pure red cell aplasia and agranulocytosis, early and mid-mature precursor cells may be present. Granulomas may indicate an infectious cause of the marrow failure.

ANCILLARY STUDIES. Cytogenetic studies of peripheral blood should be performed on younger patients or if there is a suspicious family history or suggestive physical finding. Cytogenetic studies of bone marrow are almost always normal in aplastic anemia and frequently abnormal in myelodysplasia. Testing or abnormal sensitivity of erythrocytes to complement (Ham test) establishes paroxysmal nocturnal hemoglobinuria; flow microfluorometry of granulocytes is much more sensitive for the characteristically underexpressed proteins of this syndrome (see Chapter 165). Serologic studies occasionally show evidence of viral infection, especially antibodies to human immunodeficiency virus or Epstein-Barr virus, but preceding hepatitis is usually indicated by abnormal liver enzymes rather than positive viral serologies. Parvovirus may be detected by DNA hybridization in chronic pure red cell aplasia. Hypoimmunoglobulinemia and thymoma are also associated with pure red blood cell aplasia; a

thymoma should be sought by computed tomography, less because the hematologic disease remits with thymectomy (it often does not) than because a potentially malignant tumor must be removed. If the physical examination of the abdomen is suspicious or unsatisfactory, the size of the spleen should be determined by scanning.

DIFFERENTIAL DIAGNOSIS. Pancytopenia occurs in many diseases, but when secondary blood cell count depression rivals that of severe aplastic anemia, the primary diagnosis is usually obvious from either a history or the physical examination (e.g., the splenomegaly of alcoholic cirrhosis, a history of metastatic cancer or systemic lupus erythematosus, or obvious miliary tuberculosis on the chest radiograph). In practice, the distinction of aplasia from other hematologic diseases, especially hypocellular myelodysplasia, is more difficult.

Treatment (Fig. 160-2)

BONE MARROW TRANSPLANTATION (see Chapter 182). This treatment offers the best therapy for a young patient with a fully histocompatible sibling donor. Survival of patients younger than about 20 years old after bone marrow transplantation is between 65% and 90%. Early consideration of the transplantation option in a child or adolescent can avoid unnecessary transfusions. Transfusions increase the risk of graft rejection, which is already high in patients with aplastic anemia, and graft rejection is a major determinant of successful clinical outcome. Graft-versus-host disease increases progressively with age and occurs in the majority of patients older than 30 years. In older persons, marrow transplantation also carries risks from infections and the effects of the conditioning regimen; as a result, it is usually not recommended for aplastic anemia in patients who are older than 45 to 50. Management of patients in the intermediate range, 20 to 45 years old, depends on their blood counts, especially the neutrophil number, and their general clinical condition. Use of alternative donors, unrelated histocompatible volunteers, or closely but not perfectly matched family members remains experimental; best results have been achieved in selected children employing intensive conditioning regimens, in which survival rates of 50% have been reported.

IMMUNOSUPPRESSION. Most patients with aplastic anemia lack a suitable marrow donor. Antithymocyte globulin (ATG) therapy leads to recovery of autologous bone marrow function in about 50% of patients, usually with independence from transfusion and a leukocyte count adequate to prevent infection. When therapy with ATG fails, about 50% of patients will respond to cyclosporine. For initial therapy for severe aplastic anemia, the combination of ATG and cyclosporine, which is superior to ATG alone, produces hematologic responses in about 70% of cases. Long-term survival rates among respondents are 80 to 90%. Improvement in granulocyte number is generally apparent within 2 months of treatment. In most patients who recover with this treatment, the blood cell counts remain somewhat depressed, the mean corpuscular volume continues to be high, and the bone marrow cellularity returns only very slowly toward normal, if at all. Relapse, meaning the need to treat again, is frequent but does not affect prognosis. Some patients may develop myelodysplasia, paroxysmal nocturnal hemoglobinuria, or acute leukemia years after successful immunosuppressive treatment of their aplastic anemia. Bone marrow examinations should therefore be performed annually or when there is an unfavorable change in blood cell counts, and a Ham test or, preferably, flow cytometry studies should be performed periodically.

ATG can be given intravenously in a regimen of 40 mg/kg/day for 4 days. Anaphylaxis is a rare but occasionally fatal complication of ATG treatment; allergy should be evaluated by a prick test with an undiluted solution and immediate observation of the injected skin. ATG binds to peripheral blood cells, and therefore platelet and granulocyte numbers may fall further during active treatment. Serum sickness often develops about 10 days after initiation of treatment. Most patients receive methylprednisolone (1 mg/kg/day for 2 weeks) to ameliorate the immune consequences of heterologous protein infusion. Cyclosporine is administered orally at an initial dose of 12 mg/kg/day in adults and 15 mg/kg/day in children, with subsequent adjustment according to blood levels obtained every 2 weeks. Nephrotoxicity, hypertension, seizures, and

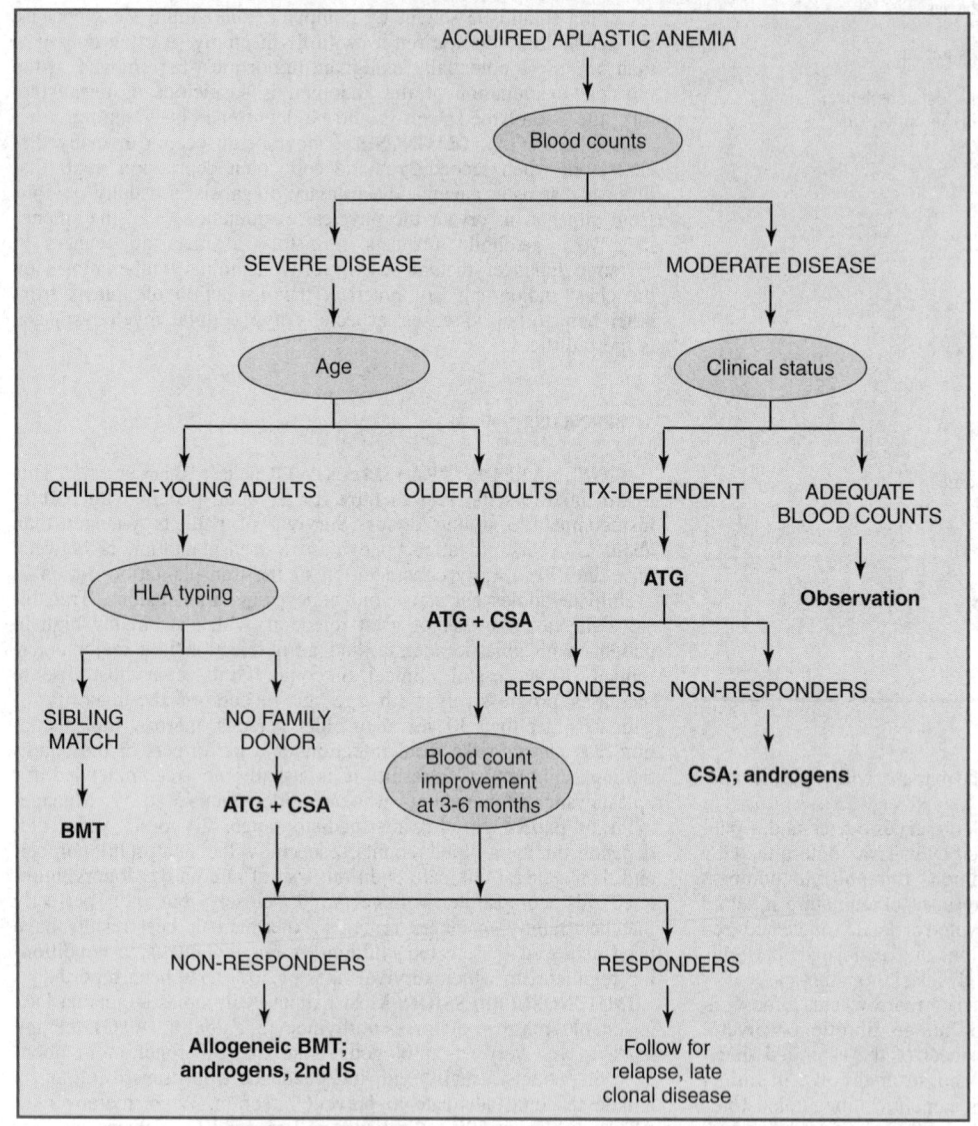

FIGURE 160–2 ■ Therapeutic decisions in patients with aplastic anemia. HLA = human leukocyte antigen; BMT = bone marrow transplantation; ATG = antithymocyte globulin; CSA = cyclosporine; IS = immunosuppression; TX = transfusion.

opportunistic infections (especially *Pneumocystis carinii* pneumonia) are the most serious complications of cyclosporine treatment.

Immunosuppression is also effective in pure red blood cell aplasia and probably in amegakaryocytic thrombocytopenia as well. Immunosuppressive agents include corticosteroids, azathioprine, cyclophosphamide, ATG, or cyclosporine.

OTHER THERAPY. Androgens have not been verified as effective in controlled trials, but occasional patients respond or even demonstrate blood cell count dependence on continued therapy. For patients with moderate disease or for those with severe pancytopenia in whom immunosuppression has failed, a 3-month trial is appropriate: nandrolone decanoate, 5 mg/kg/week given intramuscularly (with firm pressure at the injection site to prevent hemorrhage) or danazol, up to 800 mg/day by mouth.

Cyclophosphamide given intravenously in very high doses, as used for conditioning in marrow transplant (45–50 mg/kg/day for 4 days), also offers effective immunosuppressive therapy and may have the advantage of avoiding the complications of relapse and the evolution of late clonal hematologic disease; because toxicity may be severe, this treatment is best given as part of a research protocol. Hematopoietic growth factors, granulocyte-macrophage and granulocyte colony-stimulating factors (GM-CSF and G-CSF) have not been shown to induce remissions in aplastic anemia, although they may increase the white blood cell count during the period of administration in some patients.

PRINCIPLES OF SUPPORT. Meticulous medical care is required so that the patient can survive to benefit from definitive therapy or,

having experienced treatment failure, can maintain a reasonable quality of life in the presence of pancytopenia. First and most important, infection in the patient with severe neutropenia must be aggressively treated. Parenteral, broad-spectrum antibiotics should be started promptly: monotherapy with a late-generation cephalosporin is a reasonable regimen. Therapy is empirical and must not await results of culture, although specific foci of infection, like oropharyngeal or anorectal abscesses, pneumonia, sinusitis, and typhlitis should be sought on physical examination and with suitable radiographic studies. When indwelling plastic catheters become contaminated, vancomycin is added. Persistent or recrudescent fever implies fungal disease; candidiasis and aspergillosis are common, especially after several courses of antibacterial antibiotics, and a progressive course may be averted by timely initiation of amphotericin. Hand washing, the single most effective method of preventing the spread of infection in the hospital, remains a neglected practice. Non-absorbed antibiotics for gut decontamination may be helpful but are rarely used because of their gastrointestinal side effects. Total reverse isolation is difficult, expensive, psychologically debilitating, inhibitory of nursing and medical attention, and not clearly beneficial in reducing mortality from infections. Now that granulocytes can be efficiently mobilized from normal donors treated with G-CSF, their use in severely neutropenic patients with life-threatening infections will need to be reassessed.

Platelet and erythrocyte levels can be maintained by transfusion. Candidates for bone marrow transplantation should be transfused sparingly and, of course, not with blood products from a family member. Alloimmunization can limit the usefulness of prophylactic platelet transfusions, and single-donor platelets from which leukocytes have been removed by filtration are the best product. There are no direct studies of the value of prophylaxis versus demand platelet transfusions in chronic bone marrow failure. Any rational regimen of prophylaxis requires transfusions once or twice weekly to maintain the platelet count above $10,000/\mu L$ (oozing from the gut, and presumably also from other vascular beds, increases precipitously at values lower than $5000/\mu L$). About one third of patients become refractory to platelet transfusions, sometimes to HLA-matched as well as to random-donor platelets. Inhibitors of fibrinolysis, such as aminocaproic acid, have been reported to be helpful in occasional patients but have not proven beneficial in controlled trials. Menstruation should be suppressed. Aspirin and other non-steroidal inflammatory agents that inhibit platelet function must be avoided.

Red blood cells should be transfused to allow a normal level of activity, usually to a hemoglobin value of 7.0 g/dL (9.0 g/dL if there is underlying cardiac or pulmonary disease). A regimen of 2 units every 2 weeks replaces the normal loss of erythrocytes in a patient without a functioning bone marrow. In chronic anemia, the iron chelator deferoxamine should be considered at about the time the patient receives the 50th transfusion to avoid secondary hemochromatosis.

Prognosis

The natural course of untreated severe aplastic anemia is rapid deterioration and death resulting from infection or hemorrhage; historically, survival in patients with severe disease treated only with transfusions is poor, probably about 20% at 1 year. Fortunately, both transplantation of marrow from a matched sibling donor and intensive immunosuppressive therapies cure or ameliorate aplastic anemia in the great majority of patients. Recent retrospective comparisons from Europe suggest that results from both types of treatment are improving and about equivalent. The physician should inform the patient of the relative values of bone marrow transplantation, which cures the hematologic disease, but at great cost and often with significant morbidity, and immunosuppressive therapy, which is easier but often not completely effective.

Pure red cell aplasia is compatible with long life. Patients with congenital anemias have survived for decades with a combination of transfusions and iron chelation. Probably more than half of patients with acquired red cell aplasia can be cured by immunosuppression.

MYELODYSPLASIA (see Chapter 175)

Myelodysplasia describes a heterogeneous group of hematologic disorders that are defined only broadly by cytopenias associated with dysmorphic or abnormal-appearing bone marrow.

MYELOPHTHISIC ANEMIAS AND MYELOFIBROSIS

Marrow fibrosis is usually accompanied by a characteristic blood smear presentation called leukoerythroblastosis; it can occur as a primary hematologic disease, called myelofibrosis or myeloid metaplasia (see Color Plate 6D), or as a secondary process, called myelophthisis. Myelophthisis represents reaction to invading tumor cells, infectious agents such as mycobacteria or fungi, intracellular lipid deposition in Gaucher's disease, and the granulomas of sarcoidosis (Table 160–5). In secondary fibrosis, the underlying infectious or malignant process is usually obvious. The pancytopenia of human immunodeficiency virus may be associated with moderate marrow fibrosis. Modest degrees of fibrosis can also be a feature of a variety of other hematologic syndromes, especially chronic myelogenous leukemia, poorly differentiated lymphomas, myeloma, and hairy cell leukemia. Marrow fibrosis also occurs in the bony proliferative disease of childhood called osteopetrosis.

The pathophysiology of myelofibrosis has three distinct features: (1) proliferation of fibroblasts in the marrow space; (2) extension of hematopoiesis into the long bones and most peculiarly into extramedullary sites, usually the spleen, liver, and lymph nodes (myeloid metaplasia); and (3) ineffective erythropoiesis. The etiology of fibrosis is unknown but most likely involves dysregulated production of growth factors. Many cell types in the marrow produce growth factors for fibroblasts. Platelet-derived growth factor is one example, and profuse megakaryocytopoiesis and thrombocytosis are often seen early in the course of idiopathic myelofibrosis. Myelofibrosis is remarkable for pancytopenia despite extraordinarily large numbers of circulating hematopoietic progenitor cells. Idiopathic (or agnogenic) myelofibrosis is one of the myeloproliferative syndromes, a category that also includes polycythemia vera, essential thrombocythemia, and chronic myelogenous leukemia (see Chapter 174).

Anderson NS, Appelbaum FR: Myelodysplasia and myeloproliferative syndrome. Curr Opin Hematol 4:261, 1997. *Most current review.*
Young NS, Barrett AJ: The treatment of severe acquired aplastic anemia. Blood 85: 3367, 1995. *Balanced review of transplantation and immunosuppression approaches.*
Young NS, Maciejewski JP: Pathophysiology of acquired aplastic anemia. N Engl J Med 336:1365, 1997. *Stresses immune mechanisms.*

Table 160–5 ■ CAUSES OF MYELOPHTHISIS

Neoplastic Infiltration of the Marrow
Hematologic malignant diseases
Leukemias—acute and chronic
Lymphomas—Hodgkin's and non-Hodgkin's
Plasma cell myeloma
Hairy cell leukemia
Nonhematologic malignant diseases
Carcinomas—especially breast, prostate, lung, stomach
Neuroblastoma
Myelofibrosis
Primary (idiopathic)
Secondary—chronic myeloid leukemia, cancers, vasculitis (lupus, rheumatoid arthritis)
Granulomatous Infections
Tuberculosis
Fungal infections
Metabolic Abnormalities
Lipid storage diseases (e.g., Gaucher's disease)
Osteopetrosis

161 NORMOCHROMIC, NORMOCYTIC ANEMIAS

Thomas P. Duffy

An optimal red blood cell (RBC) mass is maintained within the body via a feedback loop whereby the hormonal stimulus for RBC production, erythropoietin (EPO), is released in response to the hemoglobin needs of the body. EPO is a glycoprotein secreted by renal interstitial cells that respond to the oxidative state of hematin in RBCs perfusing the kidney. As anemia develops, this sensing device within the kidney causes increased EPO secretion, with overdrive of the erythroid component of the marrow. EPO causes amplification of erythroid precursors within the marrow, hastens their differentiation and release from the marrow, and inhibits apoptosis in the erythroid cell line. Under heightened EPO stimulation, normal marrow responds with erythroid hyperplasia and accelerated release of reticulocytes. These reticulocytes can be recognized by supravital staining of their residual polyribosomal reticulated network, which is the marker for these young RBCs in the peripheral blood.

Under normal conditions, the marrow compensates for the 1 to 1.5% of the RBC mass that is lost each day through senescence by replacing it with reticulocytes. When anemia occurs, a physiologic "surge" in reticulocytes should follow if the marrow is capable of responding appropriately to EPO overdrive. This normal response is evidenced by an elevated reticulocyte count, significantly above the normal 1 to 1.5%. If an anemia has its origin within the marrow or is secondary to inadequate EPO stimulation, an appropriate reticulocytosis is not mounted to compensate for the anemia. This reticulocytopenic response indicates that the anemia is due to problems in RBC production within the marrow rather than accelerated RBC loss or destruction in the periphery.

Knowledge of this feedback EPO loop and the reticulocyte count permits a broad dissection of the cause(s) of the anemia (see Chapter 158). Absence of an appropriate reticulocyte response in patients with anemia is the hallmark of hyporegenerative anemias. These conditions have myriad causes that include a lack of marrow precursors (stem cell or pure RBC aplasia), lack of necessary building blocks (iron, vitamin B_{12}, folate), and lack of adequate EPO stimulation, as well as abnormalities in proliferation and differentiation of RBCs (leukemia, myelodysplasias, infiltrative disorders of the marrow). The lesion in hyporegenerative anemias is within the marrow, and bone marrow aspiration and biopsy are the definitive procedures for investigation of such anemias if serum measurements (iron, iron-binding capacity, vitamin B_{12}, folate) do not provide an answer.

The presence of an elevated reticulocyte count has the opposite implications regarding the cause of the anemia (Color Plate 5B). Reticulocytosis indicates the presence of a hyperregenerative anemia in which the marrow is able to respond appropriately to the stimulus of anemia. This lesion has its locus in the periphery, with accelerated loss of RBCs from either premature RBC destruction secondary to hemolysis or excessive loss of blood secondary to bleeding.

Measurement of the mean corpuscular volume (MCV) of RBCs, a value derived from the electronic Coulter counter, can further define anemias with a low reticulocyte count. Anemia with small, or microcytic, RBCs (MCV, <80 fL) is most commonly due to iron deficiency (see Chapter 162). Anemia with large, or macrocytic, cells (MCV, >95 fL) is usually due to abnormalities in nucleic acid metabolism, with vitamin B_{12} or folate deficiency most commonly responsible (see Chapter 163). Anemias with RBCs of normocytic size (MCV, 80 to 95 fL) have numerous causes from faulty production to infiltrative disorders; low EPO states also result in normocytic anemias. The early stages of most anemias are also normochromic/normocytic because of continued presence of the original, normal RBC population manufactured before the new pathologic lesion appeared.

BLOOD LOSS ANEMIA

The hematologic manifestations of bleeding depend on the interval that separates the acute event from measurement of the hematocrit or hemoglobin concentration. Immediately following an acute bleed, the hematocrit is normal because hemodilution has not yet had time to occur and compensate for any reduction in blood volume. Early evidence of acute blood loss may be apparent only in postural changes in blood pressure and pulse rate. After about 24 hours, volume re-expansion corrects this defect by mobilization of extravascular fluid into the intravascular compartment; the result is a fall in hematocrit that parallels the degree of blood loss. After 3 to 5 days, the reticulocyte count rises to compensate for the anemia; this reticulocytosis may lead to confusion with hemolytic anemia— both acute blood loss and hemolytic anemia are normochromic, normocytic anemias with high reticulocyte counts. The MCV may actually be increased in both conditions because reticulocytes are polychromatophilic macrocytes that may elevate the MCV. The two anemias can be distinguished by the byproducts of accelerated RBC breakdown in hemolytic anemias, in which hyperbilirubinemia is frequently, but not always, the marker of hemolysis. Evidence of bleeding is usually clear, but with bleeding into soft tissues or into a body cavity such as the retroperitoneum, resorption of blood may be associated with hyperbilirubinemia; the clinical picture may be confusing until the hematoma extends to the surface as an ecchymosis or a radiographic study identifies retroperitoneal bleeding.

The normochromic, normocytic anemias of both hemolysis and acute post-hemorrhagic states are accompanied by leukocytosis and thrombocytosis; these responses represent cytokine stimulation of all cell lines within the marrow in response to the anemia.

OTHER NORMOCYTIC, NORMOCHROMIC ANEMIAS

ANEMIA OF CHRONIC RENAL INSUFFICIENCY. Chronic renal failure leads to anemia because of the progressive absence of ade-

quate EPO production in the feedback loop for maintenance of erythropoiesis (see Chapter 104). No strict correlation exists between the degree of azotemia and the severity of this anemia, although anemia usually supervenes once the creatinine clearance falls below 35 to 45 mL/minute. Many other factors may also contribute to the development of anemia in renal failure. Bleeding may occur from angiomatous malformations that develop in the gastrointestinal tract in uremia, and the hemostatic platelet defect of renal failure may exaggerate this threat. Significant iron loss also occurs as a byproduct of hemodialysis, and folate stores may be compromised by loss of this dialyzable vitamin. Aluminum toxicity interferes with iron metabolism, and a microcytic anemia may develop in patients whose dialysate baths contain high concentrations of this metal. A microangiopathic process often develops with malignant hypertension, and this same RBC lesion is a hallmark of the hemolytic-uremic syndrome and thrombotic thrombocytopenic purpura.

A modest shortening of RBC survival occurs as a result of a metabolic lesion incurred from uremia. However, this abbreviated RBC survival is only a very minor contribution to anemia in these states because the uncomplicated anemia of renal disease can be reversed with the administration of EPO. EPO is usually administered three times weekly, either subcutaneously or intravenously, following dialysis treatments. Treatment is initiated with EPO doses of 150 U/kg three times weekly and reduced to 50 to 100 U/kg per dose once the desired response has been obtained. Weekly EPO administration is also effective but requires larger amounts (40,000 U) of the recombinant factor. With EPO therapy, the anemia of renal failure has been largely eliminated.

ANEMIA OF LIVER DISEASE. After their release from marrow, RBCs' membranes are remodeled by splenic macrophages, and the lipid constituents of the membrane remain in dynamic equilibrium with plasma lipoproteins. Advanced stages of liver disease are complicated by progressive lipoprotein abnormalities that result in the sequential transformation of normochromic, normocytic RBCs into macrocytes, target cells, echinocytes, and at the final and most severe stage, acanthocytes. Acanthocytes, or spur cells, are converted into spherocytes by the spleen; their lifespan is significantly shortened because the lipid deposition in their membranes interferes with the normal plasticity or deformability of RBCs. In liver disease associated with portal hypertension, hypersplenism may shorten RBC survival even in the absence of any membrane lipid abnormality.

Anemia in liver disease may also have its origin in the several other insults that often accompany hepatic damage. Alcohol, with its effect on folate metabolism, may create a macrocytic, megaloblastic anemia; the same toxin may interfere with heme metabolism and produce a sideroblastic anemia. A metabolic product of alcohol, acetaldehyde is a direct inhibitor of erythropoiesis *in vitro*. Iron deficiency is also not uncommon in liver disease because of blood loss from varices, alcohol-induced gastritis, and the coagulopathy resulting from defective synthesis of coagulation factors. Wilson disease is associated with hemolytic anemia.

ANEMIA OF ENDOCRINE DISORDERS. Dysfunction in hormonal regulation has systemic effects that include the production and survival of RBCs. An anemia, usually normocytic but sometimes macrocytic, accompanies hypothyroidism because of physiologic responses to decreased metabolic needs (see Chapter 239). Menometrorrhagia occurs frequently in hypothyroidism and can lead to iron deficiency anemia. Erythrocytosis may be a feature of Cushing's disease because of androgen overdrive of the marrow; a reduction in RBC mass occurs in Addison's disease, but anemia is not usually evident because of a concomitant reduction in plasma volume caused by mineralocorticoid deficiency. Hypopituitary states are complicated by mild anemias; growth hormone has a growth-stimulating effect on RBCs.

Anemia is not a feature of uncomplicated diabetes mellitus but usually occurs in the course of the disease as renal complications develop. Anemia occurs earlier in diabetic renal disease than in other azotemic states because a poorly documented metabolic lesion shortens RBC survival in uncontrolled diabetes. Severe hemolysis may occur in diabetic ketoacidosis if significant hypophosphatemia appears following insulin treatment.

ANEMIA OF STEM CELL FAILURE. Deficiencies of stem cells, as occurs with aplastic/hypoplastic anemias, cause a normochromic, normocytic (sometimes slightly macrocytic) anemia that is usually part of a pancytopenia with attendant leukopenia and thrombocytopenia (see Chapter 160). Pure red cell aplasia, caused by parvovirus infection of RBC precursors or as a result of humoral or cellular immune mechanisms, may produce a normochromic, normocytic anemia without reticulocytes. Leukemias and lymphomas may replace and inhibit the marrow and cause normochromic, normocytic anemia.

ANEMIA OF CHRONIC DISEASE. Most patients with the anemia of chronic disease have normochromic, normocytic RBC indices. The remainder have a mild hypochromic, microcytic anemia (see Chapter 162).

Bain BJ: Pathogenesis and pathophysiology of anemia in HIV infection. Curr Opin Hematol 6:89–93, 1999. *Review of the multifactorial causes of anemia in HIV infection.*

162   MICROCYTIC AND HYPOCHROMIC ANEMIAS

Thomas P. Duffy

Hemoglobin synthesis for the needs of normal red blood cell (RBC) production requires an adequate supply of iron and intact metabolic pathways for the generation of heme and globin molecules. Any deficiency in this triad of iron, heme, or globin may result in RBCs with a deficient mean corpuscular hemoglobin concentration. Such hemoglobin-deficient RBCs are usually microcytic with a reduced mean corpuscular volume that is attributable to additional divisions in the RBC maturation sequence in bone marrow in the setting of a low hemoglobin concentration. This combination of small and hypochromic RBCs can be detected on examination of the peripheral smear when the process is advanced and can be confirmed by indices generated from measurements of RBC size by electronic Coulter counters. An emerging population of microcytic RBCs at an early stage of iron deficiency anemia can be recognized by studying the red cell distribution width, in which any small cells constitute a peak separate from RBCs of normal size.

Characterization of anemia as hypochromic and microcytic narrows the possible causes of the RBC deficiency to some abnormality in iron, heme, or globin metabolism. Low values for mean corpuscular volume and hemoglobin concentration generated by the electronic counter delimit a small number of possible lesions as the cause of this type of anemia.

IRON DEFICIENCY ANEMIA

DEFINITION. Iron, as the core of the hemoglobin molecule responsible for the oxygen-carrying capabilities of blood, is the most precious element within the body; an efficient system of conservation and recycling of this valuable resource serves to guarantee the amount of iron necessary for daily hemoglobin synthesis. Storage depots of iron (as ferritin and hemosiderin) exist within the reticuloendothelial cells of the liver, spleen, and bone marrow and the parenchymal cells of the liver, and these stores are depleted before any restriction in hemoglobin synthesis occurs. Iron deficiency anemia therefore represents the final temporal development in the chronology of progressive iron deficiency within the body. Because this anemia does not supervene until iron stores are mobilized to maintain an optimal hemoglobin mass, absence of iron stores on examination of the marrow is specific confirmation that iron deficiency is contributing to any anemia that is present.

PREVALENCE. Iron deficiency is the most common cause of anemia throughout the world and one of the most common medical problems that confronts the general physician. Its geographic distribution is determined by dietary deficiencies and intestinal parasitism, especially in Third World countries; hookworm infection has created the same lesion in the American South.

The prevalence of iron deficiency is much higher in women than in men because of the toll of menstruation and pregnancy on the iron stores of women. The expansion of the blood pool that occurs during adolescence also leads to low iron stores that may be further depleted as a result of inadequate dietary intake. The latter factor contributes to the iron deficiency state in many women, even in affluent societies, as they embark on pregnancy.

IRON METABOLISM. Mechanisms exist to ensure that the total-body iron content is maintained within a defined range. In specific contrast with other body constituents, control of iron content is imposed by limiting its entrance into the body rather than by increasing the excretion of any excess. Once iron has entered the plasma after absorption from the gastrointestinal tract or from the breakdown of transfused RBCs, it can be removed only by the withdrawal of blood or by the more laborious process of iron chelation therapy. The normal metabolism of iron is strictly weighted in favor of ensuring adequate iron reserves even at the cost of iron overload, which may result in hemochromatosis with organ damage created by the tissue accumulation of elemental iron.

The major locus of iron within the body is the center of the hemoglobin molecule within RBCs and as part of the myoglobin molecule in muscle; a smaller fraction is a constituent of important tissue-based enzymes. Storage pools of iron in the form of ferritin and hemosiderin are present within the liver, spleen, and bone marrow. These reserves of approximately 1000 mg in males and 500 mg in females are derived from the breakdown of senescent RBCs within the reticuloendothelial system and from any surplus of absorbed iron beyond that needed for hemoglobin synthesis. The disparity in the size of these stores in men and women is attributable to the previously mentioned demands of menstruation and pregnancy in women.

The tiniest compartment of iron within the body is transport iron (7 mg), in which iron travels while linked to the transport protein transferrin. Although transport iron is the smallest compartment, it is kinetically the most active and turns over several times a day as iron is transported to its various destinations within the body. Transferrin picks up iron from the gastrointestinal cells and delivers it primarily to cells engaging in hemoglobin synthesis. Transferrin also picks up iron from the storage depots in the daily recycling of iron stores.

This system of conservation and recycling of iron serves to provide a constant supply of iron for the needs (30 to 35 mg) of daily hemoglobin synthesis. Only a tiny fraction of iron (1 mg) is lost each day via the pathway of sweating and epidermal shedding from the gut and urinary tract; this minuscule amount can easily be replaced from the food in a normal diet. The major source of iron for hemoglobin synthesis is derived from the breakdown of RBCs, which after survival for 90 to 120 days in peripheral blood, undergo phagocytosis by splenic macrophages; the iron released from these senescent RBCs is immediately available for the needs of hemoglobin synthesis, with the excess stored as ferritin and hemosiderin. The vector of iron transport is always in the direction of providing iron to fulfill the body's needs in maintaining an optimal RBC mass.

ABSORPTION. The normal diet in the United States contains approximately 15 to 30 mg of iron each day, with every thousand calories in the diet containing about 6 mg of elemental iron. Iron is present in food as a portion of the heme ring in meats and in a less easily absorbable form as ferric hydroxide complexes in other foods. The acid environment of the stomach and its enzymatic secretions emulsify ingested food and liberate iron for absorption within the small intestine; pancreatic secretions counter this acidic pH and help control excessive absorption of iron.

Iron must be in the reduced or ferrous form to be absorbed. Ingestion of reducing substances such as ascorbate or succinate enhances iron absorption because of their effect on iron valence. Other substances such as phytates in cereals, tannates in tea, antacids, and certain antibiotics (tetracycline) may complex with iron and thereby hinder its absorption. Maximal absorption of iron occurs in the duodenum and upper portions of the jejunum. Malabsorptive states or bypass of these areas by gastrojejunostomy may contribute to iron deficiency.

Iron absorption can be adjusted over a broad range according to the body's needs. In normal health, the body must guard itself against iron overload by absorbing only one tenth of the iron available in the diet. The mechanism whereby such a limitation or "mucosal curtain" is imposed on iron absorption is still not defined; it appears to be regulated by some aspect of dynamic iron turnover because hemolytic anemias, ineffective erythropoiesis, and hypoxemic states all have increased iron turnover and are all associated with increased iron absorption. The mucosal curtain is lowered by imposing a limit on the amount of iron that crosses the gastrointestinal membranes. Whatever iron is not needed by the body is diverted into storage molecules within gastrointestinal mucosal cells; this iron is lost from the body as these cells are exfoliated during the normal cycle of cell turnover. In the presence of iron deficiency, the body can increase its absorption efficiency at least five-fold to compensate easily and rapidly for any deficiency. In iron deficient states, in which iron needs are exaggerated, little iron is diverted to the storage form and the majority of the absorbed iron passes directly through the cells for plasma transport linked to transferrin.

Failure to lower this mucosal curtain properly is thought to be the explanation for iron accumulation in primary hemochromatosis; such patients continue to absorb iron even in the face of total-body iron overload. Increased iron absorption also occurs with pancreatic insufficiency because of absence of the pH alteration contributed by normal pancreatic secretions; absence of this restraint on iron absorption explains in part the iron overload that often occurs in chronic alcoholic states.

TRANSPORT. Transferrin, a glycoprotein with a molecular weight of approximately 80,000, is produced by liver parenchymal cells in inverse proportion to the iron stores within these cells. This matching of transferrin production to iron needs explains in part the elevated transferrin levels or iron-binding capacity that characterizes iron deficiency. Transferrin can bind one or two molecules of ferric iron, a process accompanied by the simultaneous attachment of an equal number of bicarbonate ions; the latter molecules facilitate the uncoupling of iron from the binding protein.

Transferrin binding of iron protects the body against the toxicity of elemental iron and increases the solubility of this molecule within plasma. Transferrin receptors are present on the surface of developing RBCs in direct proportion to their potential for hemoglobin synthesis. Transferrin-bound iron links to these receptors, and the complex enters the RBC by endocytosis; dissociation of the complex occurs following a pH alteration in the vesicle. Iron is released to enter the cycle of heme synthesis, and transferrin leaves the cell to scavenge for other iron molecules. Transferrin is measured in the plasma by quantifying the amount of iron binding sites available, a measurement called the total iron-binding capacity of plasma. Under normal circumstances, total iron-binding capacity is only one third saturated, with the total amount of transferrin within the plasma being approximately 300 mg/dL.

Iron levels vary diurnally, with the highest levels present in the morning; normal iron levels are usually within 60 to 180 mg/dL. A small amount of iron is also present in plasma in the form of the storage molecule ferritin, with the concentration of this molecule generally mirroring the stores of iron within the marrow. Iron also complexes with lactoferrin, which is an iron-binding protein liberated from neutrophilic granules and which is thought to play a role in defense against infection. Lactoferrin rapidly sequesters iron in reticuloendothelial cells, thereby depriving microorganisms of iron, which is an essential growth factor for most microorganisms.

IRON KINETICS. Ferrokinetic measurements using radiolabeled iron-59 can quantify iron absorption, the marrow transit time of iron, and plasma and erythrocyte iron turnover. These studies permit *in vivo* localization of any defect in the uptake, transport, or delivery of iron; such measurements are now primarily investigative tools that are not used in routine clinical situations.

PATHOGENESIS. Conservation and recycling of iron within the body provide an excellent buffer to fulfill the daily needs of iron for hemoglobin synthesis. Iron deficiency anemia occurs only after an extended period of negative iron balance, a period during which the storage pool is exhausted of its reserves. Although this depletion may result from decreased ingestion or absorption of iron, the most common causes of iron deficiency are blood loss from lesions in the gastrointestinal tract or from the demands of menstruation and pregnancy.

DECREASED IRON UPTAKE. To maintain iron balance within the body, the adult male needs to absorb only 1.0 to 1.5 mg of iron each day, whereas an adult female needs to absorb a larger amount (2 to 3 mg) because of the iron losses from menstruation. Each

milliliter of blood contains approximately 0.4 mg of iron, so the monthly menstrual loss of approximately 60 mL creates the need for an additional 20 to 30 mg of iron absorption each month. Pregnancy, with its expansion of the maternal blood pool and additional needs for fetal hemoglobin synthesis, frequently overwhelms an already-marginal iron storage pool and requires supplemental iron as a prophylactic measure against the development of frank anemia.

Because the iron-calorie ratio of the normal U.S. diet is 6 mg iron for every 1000 calories, males usually have no shortage of dietary iron; the restricted diets of some women may not provide a comparable surfeit and may give rise to an iron deficiency state without frank anemia. Diet-related iron deficiency may be aggravated by gastric achlorhydria, with its negative effect on iron absorption, but achlorhydria alone rarely causes iron deficiency anemia.

Gastrojejunostomies and sprue may both result in iron deficiency as a result of loss of the necessary mucosal surface and/or increased intestinal transit time. The anemia seen with gastrojejunal bypass procedures has anastomotic mucosal lesions, with blood loss from these ulcerated sites as the principal cause of iron deficiency.

The modern shift to non–iron-containing cooking utensils has eliminated this rich source of iron from the diet. The popularity of vegetarian diets may also lessen the amount of dietary iron.

A vicious cycle may occur in which patients with iron deficiency acquire an appetite for bizarre foods. This phenomenon, pica, is the only known example of a compulsive appetite or behavior created by the lack of a normal body element. Its victims may ingest clay (geophagia), which in turn may potentiate the problem by chelating iron within the gut, ice (pagophagia), or starch (amylophagia). Iron replacement corrects the problem, which may or may not be accompanied by anemia.

INCREASED IRON LOSS. The most common cause of iron deficiency anemia in both men and women is blood loss; this loss most frequently has its source in gastrointestinal bleeding in the former and menstrual bleeding in the latter. The implication of the discovery of iron deficiency anemia in men and postmenopausal women is the same; the gastrointestinal tract harbors the causal lesion until proved otherwise (see Chapter 123). Even in the absence of occult blood in the stool or a history of melena, it is still imperative to examine the gastrointestinal tract because of its frequent involvement when iron deficiency is present. Iron deficiency may be the initial manifestation of an otherwise occult carcinoma of the gut, with right-sided colon tumors not infrequently having this clinical picture. Multiple other gastrointestinal lesions, such as large hiatal hernias, ulcer disease, inflammatory bowel disease, or angiodysplasias, may all be characterized by iron deficiency.

Ingestion of aspirin and non-steroidal anti-inflammatory agents, often in the treatment of arthritic conditions, may be complicated by gastrointestinal blood loss. Less common causes of excessive iron loss include urinary tract bleeding and renal filtration of hemoglobin released from the breakdown of RBCs; individuals with mechanical heart valves may have traumatic rupture of RBCs as they flow across the artificial surfaces of these valves. Pulmonary sequestration of iron also occurs following some pulmonary hemorrhagic states, with no mechanism available to the body to recapture this closeted iron. The stores of iron may also be depleted by frequent blood donations.

CLINICAL MANIFESTATIONS. Iron deficiency anemia is characterized by a degree of fatigue that may be disproportionate to the apparent severity of the anemia, apparently because of depletion of essential tissue-based iron-containing enzymes with an attendant reduction in energy generation by muscle. Transfusion of RBCs to correct this anemia reverses the symptoms only in part; iron repletion is the definitive treatment for this fatigue.

Iron deficiency has several characteristic clinical manifestations, but all of them are rare relative to the high incidence of this condition. A sore tongue (glossitis), atrophy of the lingual papillae, and erosions at the corners of the mouth (angular stomatitis) are oral manifestations of iron deficiency; atrophy of the gastric mucosa with achlorhydria is a further extension of the same process. An atrophic rhinitis with a foul nasal discharge (ozena) may progress to anosmia in iron-deficient individuals. A greenish hue to the complexion (chlorosis) is an accompaniment of the same deficiency, especially in adolescent girls in Victorian literature. Brittle, fragile fingernails and spooning of the nails (koilonychia) are peripheral clues to the disorder.

Dysphagia, attributable to an esophageal web, occurs most frequently in elderly women with iron deficiency; this lesion, the Plummer-Vinson or Paterson-Kelly syndrome, may later be complicated by the development of esophageal carcinoma. The web may not disappear with iron replacement, and such patients may require dilatation for relief of symptoms.

Splenomegaly has been described as an accompaniment of iron deficiency, although an independent or concomitant thalassemia trait may be the true cause of the enlargement. Pseudotumor cerebri has also been described as a very rare accompaniment of iron deficiency.

LABORATORY FINDINGS. The laboratory findings in full-blown iron deficiency anemia include a reduction in all three parameters (mean corpuscular volume, hemoglobin, hemoglobin concentration) that are generated from the Coulter counter. In contrast, early iron deficiency anemia has normochromic, normocytic indices because the iron-deficient population of RBCs constitutes only a small percentage of the RBC mass. Only when the hematocrit falls below 31 to 32% do the RBC indices become microcytic; a normochromic, normocytic anemia is therefore the earliest form of anemia with iron deficiency.

Coulter counter indices and an elevation of the automated platelet count have generally replaced examination of peripheral blood smears (Color Plate 5D) in the recognition of hypochromia and microcytosis in iron deficiency. Serum iron and transferrin (total iron-binding capacity) levels help confirm the diagnosis of iron deficiency, with a low serum iron and an elevated transferrin level resulting in a transferrin saturation of less than 10 to 15%. Transferrin levels are increased in iron deficiency states because of increased hepatic synthesis of the protein and greater liberation of apotransferrin (the transport protein without iron) from hemoglobin-synthesizing sites. Serum transferrin receptor levels are also increased in iron-deficient states, and their measurement is a possible, but usually unnecessary means of making a diagnosis of iron deficiency. A low iron level is not in itself diagnostic of iron deficiency because many other systemic insults can alter the serum level of iron. Ferritin levels also permit recognition of iron deficiency, with a reduction in this serum protein to less than 10 ng/mL in uncomplicated iron deficiency. The final step in heme synthesis is the incorporation of iron into a protoporphyrin ring; deficient delivery of iron to red cells results in elevated levels of free erythrocyte protoporphyrin as an additional marker of iron-deficient erythropoiesis.

Diagnosis of iron deficiency is usually possible by using the combination of RBC indices and serum measurement of transferrin saturation or ferritin levels. However, because both these levels are altered by perturbations as varied as infection, inflammation, malignancy, and starvation, bone marrow iron stores remain the final arbiter when any uncertainty exists regarding the presence of iron deficiency; the marrow is devoid of macrophage iron, and fewer than 10% of the RBC precursors contain siderotic granules. Absence of iron stores categorically confirms the presence of iron deficiency and serves as the gold standard for making the diagnosis. Serum transferrin receptor levels also help serve to discriminate iron deficiency from the anemias of chronic disease.

TREATMENT. Recognition and treatment of iron deficiency anemia require the identification and reversal, if possible, of its cause; the anemia is a critical sign of an underlying lesion that may be as benign as aspirin ingestion or as threatening as an occult malignancy. Treating the anemia without identifying its cause may mean loss of the only opportunity to discover a malignancy at a potentially curable stage.

Treatment of iron deficiency anemia is made somewhat difficult by the frequent induction of nausea, dyspepsia, constipation, and diarrhea by medicinal iron. These symptoms are usually proportional to the iron content of the prescribed oral iron preparation; the most commonly administered preparation is ferrous sulfate tablets, 300 mg, which contain 60 mg of elemental iron in each tablet. The drug is best absorbed on an empty stomach, but it is frequently prescribed with meals so that it is better tolerated. Most patients tolerate starting with once-daily dosing and escalating to a final dose of three times daily. Persistent intolerance can be addressed by switching to ferrous gluconate, but its lower elemental iron content requires a longer period of iron administration to correct the deficiency state; charting serum ferritin levels permits the ascertainment of adequate replacement with either preparation.

Innumerable iron preparations are marketed, but there is little to recommend these preparations over the cost-effective ferrous sulfate pills. Although ascorbate and succinate enhance the absorption of iron, the addition of these agents to iron preparations is costly and unnecessary in light of the body's efficiency in iron absorption under normal circumstances. Enteric-coated iron tablets may actually be contraindicated because the coating may shield against absorption in the upper portions of the small intestine, where maximal iron absorption takes place. Liquid iron preparations may be better tolerated by some patients and better absorbed in patients with gastrojejunostomies or rapid intestinal transit times; because iron salts can stain the teeth, iron solutions should be ingested through a straw.

At the time that iron therapy is initiated, a baseline reticulocyte count and ferritin level should be obtained. With iron replacement, the symptoms of fatigue and lassitude improve in the first week, but maximal reticulocytosis does not occur for 7 to 10 days. The hemoglobin level does not rise for 2 to 2.5 weeks, and it requires about 2 months of daily iron therapy for the hemoglobin level to return to normal. Measurement of ferritin levels determines when iron stores have been reconstituted and when iron therapy should be discontinued; return of ferritin levels to normal documents that iron stores have been restocked.

In the rare patient who cannot tolerate or cannot absorb iron from the gastrointestinal tract and in individuals who require large iron boluses to compensate for chronic blood loss, parenteral iron is available as an iron-dextran complex; it should be used with restraint because of the threat of acute anaphylaxis and subacute (arthralgias, myalgias, and adenopathy) side effects. This parenteral preparation can be administered intramuscularly or intravenously, with the latter preferred because the total dose can be delivered in a single administration. No more than 2 mL of Imferon, which contains 50 mg iron per milliliter, can be administered at a single intramuscular site; staining of the skin may occur even though the recommended Z-track injection technique is used.

A small test dose (0.25 mL) of the drug should be administered before intramuscular or intravenous injections to determine hypersensitivity to the agent. The dose to be infused for correction of iron deficiency can be calculated according to the following formula:

$$\text{Dose (mL)} = [0.0476 \times \text{wt (kg)} \times (\text{normal Hgb} - \text{observed Hgb})] + (1 \text{ mL}/5 \text{ kg}) \text{ to a maximum of 14 mL to replete iron stores}$$

This total dose can be diluted in normal saline at a 1:20 dilution and infused slowly over several hours while watching for any side effects.

PROGNOSIS. The prognosis in iron deficiency anemia is strictly related to the underlying cause of the anemia. Iron deficiency per se does not usually alter the prognosis because it is easily treated once recognized. The importance of the diagnosis is recognition of the need to identify the underlying cause of the condition and correct this lesion so that the anemia does not recur.

HYPOCHROMIC ANEMIAS NOT CAUSED BY IRON DEFICIENCY

Because characterization of an anemia as hypochromic restricts its cause to some abnormality in iron, heme, or globin metabolism, the elimination of iron deficiency as its cause narrows the choices to these other components of hemoglobin metabolism. Abnormalities in globin chain synthesis, the thalassemias, are a more prominent consideration when hypochromic anemia occurs in the appropriate ethnic groups (see Chapter 167). The sideroblastic anemias are iron-loading anemias caused by abnormalities in heme synthesis; a clue to their presence is nearly total saturation of serum transferrin levels, a striking departure from the findings in iron deficiency. Confirmation of the diagnosis requires bone marrow documentation of ringed sideroblasts, the pathognomonic lesion in this condition.

THE ANEMIA OF CHRONIC DISEASE. Although iron deficiency is the most common anemia in general, anemia of chronic disease is the most common anemia in hospitalized patients. This condition represents a shared hematologic response to systemic insults as varied as infection, inflammation, malignancy, and trauma. The anemia is moderate in degree, with the hematocrit usually in the range of 28 to 32%. The morphology is normochromic/normocytic in 60 to 70% of such patients, with the remainder having a mild hypochromic microcytic anemia. Hypoferremia is characteristic of anemia of chronic disease in the face of marrow iron overload. Confusion of anemia of chronic disease with iron deficiency anemia results from the overlapping of microcytosis and hypoferremia in both disorders. In anemia of chronic disease, the lesion includes deficient delivery of iron to developing RBCs, in addition to other derangements in RBC production.

ETIOLOGY AND PATHOGENESIS. At least three different pathophysiologic mechanisms contribute to anemia of chronic disease, an anemia that develops within a few weeks of the onset of systemic disease and is independent of any marrow involvement or specific hematologic complication of the systemic disease. Accelerated RBC breakdown, abnormalities in iron mobilization and delivery, and cytokine inhibition of erythropoiesis have all been implicated to various degrees. A modest shortening of RBC survival is noted, probably resulting from extravascular sequestration by a stimulated reticuloendothelial system. The degree of hemolysis in anemia of chronic disease is modest, and failure of the host to mount an appropriate reticulocyte response to compensate for the anemia indicates that a hypoproliferative defect rather than hemolysis is the major lesion.

Iron studies reveal low serum iron and transferrin levels in anemia of chronic disease, in contrast to the elevated transferrin levels in iron deficiency. Nevertheless, the transferrin saturation levels in anemia of chronic disease may overlap with those of iron deficiency, further adding to the confusion of these two entities. Anemia of chronic disease is a sideropenic anemia in the face of reticuloendothelial iron overload: both serum ferritin levels and bone marrow iron stores are increased in anemia of chronic disease.

The cause of the hypoferremia in anemia of chronic disease is not strictly defined. The disproportionate incorporation of iron into ferritin in storage depots may explain ferritin elevation as an acute-phase reactant in all the conditions associated with anemia of chronic disease. Another explanation for the hypoferremia in this type of anemia is a form of nutritional deficiency because microorganisms and malignancies require iron for growth and proliferation. In the face of infection and malignancies, normal iron metabolism is subverted to bolster the body's defenses against these assaults; lactoferrin, the product of polymorphonuclear leukocytes, redirects the vector of iron delivery away from RBCs, which lack lactoferrin receptors, to cells of the reticuloendothelial system. Malignancies may themselves alter the vector of iron delivery because many tumors contain siderophores, which are molecules that can effectively extract iron from the surrounding plasma. This closeting of iron explains the fall in serum iron in anemia of chronic disease, although hypoferremia is unlikely to be the primary cause of the anemia. Administration of iron to such patients does not correct the anemia and is not indicated in its management. The hypoferremia is considered an advantage to the body in restraining bacterial or tumor cell growth; the anemia is the cost of the body's defense against invasion.

Elevated ferritin production and lactoferrin linkage are not the only factors causing hypoferremia in patients with anemia of chronic disease; the low serum iron level is now thought to be only part of a more generalized response to infection, malignancy, or inflammation. These systemic threats to the body start a cascade of cytokines initiated by interleukin-1 release from macrophages. Anabolic and catabolic responses result, with an elevation in acute-phase reactants (C-reactive protein, haptoglobin, ceruloplasmin, fibrinogen, ferritin) and a reduction in serum iron and hematocrit levels. Playing an important role in the production of anemia is the liberation of tumor necrosis factor, or cachectin, a product of macrophages and part of the cytokine network. Injection of these substances creates the anorexia, debilitation, and weight loss of chronic disease and also inhibits the growth of erythroid precursor cells; anemia of chronic disease represents "cachexia" of the marrow, a sharing by marrow in the defense of the body against the threat of infection, malignancy, or inflammatory disorders.

CLINICAL MANIFESTATIONS. Anemia of chronic disease is not itself usually a cause of symptoms. The anemia is mild and well tolerated unless it is superimposed on other threatening conditions. The importance of recognizing anemia of chronic disease is in identifying its underlying cause. This type of anemia is not infrequently the initial evidence that otherwise occult disease is present.

DIAGNOSIS. Anemia of chronic disease is a moderate (hematocrit, 28 to 32%), normochromic, normocytic anemia that supervenes during the early course of disorders as diverse as malignancy, infection, inflammation, or trauma. Iron indices usually reveal hypoferremia and a reduced iron-binding capacity. Confusion occurs with iron deficiency anemia because microcytic anemia occurs in 30 to 40% of such cases and transferrin saturation may be reduced to levels seen in iron deficiency. Serum ferritin and serum transferrin receptor levels help distinguish iron deficiency from anemia of chronic disease. Iron deficiency states have elevated serum transferrin receptors relative to a marked lowering of ferritin levels; anemia of chronic disease is characterized by an elevation in ferritin levels, usually greater than 100 ng/mL. When both iron deficiency and anemia of chronic disease are present, as occurs in some patients with rheumatoid arthritis, elevated serum transferrin receptor levels permit recognition of iron deficiency that would otherwise be masked by the alterations in iron/transferrin levels in the anemia of chronic disease. Bone marrow iron stores also distinguish the two because of the presence of marrow iron in anemia of chronic disease; iron deficiency anemia is the only cause of hypochromic, microcytic RBCs in which iron stores are absent from the marrow.

TREATMENT. Anemia of chronic disease is a secondary manifestation of an underlying disorder, and its successful reversal requires recognition and correction of that disorder. Although hypoferremia is present, iron therapy does not correct the anemia and contributes to the usual iron overload in this condition. Blood transfusions are frequently not necessary because the anemia is modest and usually well tolerated. Because anemia of chronic disease results from a cytokine-induced hypoerythropoietin state, the defect can be overridden with erythropoietin administration; however, erythropoietin is commonly not appropriate because anemia of chronic disease is not usually severe.

SIDEROBLASTIC ANEMIAS. Sideroblastic anemias, which are uncommon causes of hypochromic anemia, have their origins in altered production of the heme component of the hemoglobin molecule. The final step in heme synthesis involves the incorporation of iron into the protoporphyrin ring, which is synthesized in and around the mitochondria of developing RBCs. Any defect in the multistep generation of protoporphyrin creates a mismatch between iron delivery and iron incorporation into heme. This mismatch results in iron overloading of the mitochondria because heme, the feedback inhibitor of further RBC iron uptake, is deficient. Cells are designated "ringed" sideroblasts when the iron-laden mitochondria occupy a perinuclear distribution within the developing RBCs; Prussian blue staining of the RBCs within the marrow demonstrates these siderotic granules surrounding the nucleus (Color Plate 6E). The siderotic granules of normal siderocytes are fewer in number and are distributed throughout the cytoplasm of the cell. Mitochondrial accumulation of iron is what distinguishes the sideroblastic anemias.

A clue to the presence of these anemias is the paradoxical finding of hyperferremia and nearly total transferrin saturation in a patient with a hypochromic anemia. The hypochromia has its origin in deficient protoporphyrin ring synthesis, which leads to less hemoglobin in affected cells.

PATHOGENESIS AND CLASSIFICATION. Protoporphyrin ring synthesis is a multistep process that depends on several sequential enzymatic reactions occurring in and around the surface of cell mitochondria. A lesion at any stage in this sequence, whether caused by an enzymatic deficiency or an abnormality in mitochondrial structure or function, may result in faulty protoporphyrin synthesis. These lesions may occur as inherited or acquired defects in the pathway. The inherited forms have both mitochondrial and nuclear genetic mutations as their cause. As with disturbances in other metabolic pathways within the body, drugs and toxins are the major causes of acquired sideroblastic anemia; a less common form of acquired sideroblastic anemia exists as a clonal disorder that is a subgroup of the myelodysplasias.

The primary lesion in sideroblastic anemia results in a mismatch between iron delivery and its incorporation into heme. The unincorporated iron accumulates in the mitochondria and damages these critical organelles. Such iron loading of the mitochondria further contributes to ineffective erythropoiesis. In some patients, cautious phlebotomy may improve the anemia by unloading iron from the mitochondria and correcting this secondary lesion.

The morphologic evidence for the sideroblastic process in peripheral blood is a population of hypochromic RBCs. Transferrin levels are saturated, and ferritin levels are increased, although not usually to the same degree as in hemochromatosis. Rare RBCs containing siderotic granules, or Pappenheimer bodies, may also circulate in the peripheral blood. The diagnosis of sideroblastic anemia is confirmed by the presence of ringed sideroblasts within marrow stained for iron: these forms are nucleated RBCs with a perinuclear collection of iron granules.

ACQUIRED SIDEROBLASTIC ANEMIA. Idiopathic Refractory Sideroblastic Anemia. A hypochromic anemia, frequently with slightly macrocytic (rather than microcytic) indices, develops in elderly individuals as a predominantly erythroid manifestation of a myelodysplastic syndrome (see Chapter 175) The RBC population is often dimorphic, with a varying proportion of hypochromic and normochromic cells; the hypochromic cells have their origin in a clonal population of ringed sideroblasts within the marrow. The cause of the disorder is not known, although its occurrence following chemotherapy suggests that damage to the chromosomal material responsible for normal erythroid development creates this picture.

The lesion is chronic and may remain restricted to the erythroid line with ineffective erythropoiesis in addition to the defect in heme synthesis. The lesion may also evolve into leukemia, but with no firm predictors of whether or when this transition will occur (see Chapter 177). Common antecedents to leukemia transformation are an associated leukopenia, especially when accompanied by leukocyte developmental abnormalities (pseudo–Pelger-Huët anomaly) and alterations in platelet number (Color Plate 5L).

Treatment of the disorder remains experimental. Pharmacologic doses of pyridoxine, a vitamin necessary for the initial step in heme synthesis, usually have no benefit; androgens and erythropoietin are also rarely helpful. The process may be very chronic, with no need for RBC transfusion until late in its course, but prolonged support with RBC transfusions may lead to secondary hemochromatosis and require chelation therapy with deferoxamine.

Sideroblastic anemia may be discovered in the setting of a large variety of medical conditions, including rheumatoid disease, malignancies, and endocrine disorders. The relation to these disorders is probably not causal because treatment or correction of the underlying disorder does not correct the anemia. It is more likely that the medical condition serves to unmask an otherwise undetected anemia.

Sideroblastic Anemia Associated with Drugs or Toxins. Consumption of large amounts of alcohol over a several-week period can induce sideroblastic anemia in the absence of any concomitant vitamin deficiency. The lesion is thought to have its origin in alcohol's interference with pyridoxine metabolism and its essential role as a coenzyme in the δ-aminolevulinic acid synthase step in porphyrin synthesis. Alcohol is also a mitochondrial toxin, and the anemia may be related to damage to mitochondrial function.

In alcoholics with sideroblastic anemia, the marrow lesion persists for 7 to 10 days following the withdrawal of alcohol. Other insults to this metabolic pathway include lead, chloramphenicol, and several antituberculous drugs. All these agents interfere with the initial step in protoporphyrin ring synthesis, with lead also hindering a second site where heme synthetase catalyzes the incorporation of iron into the heme ring in the final step in this pathway.

HEREDITARY SIDEROBLASTIC ANEMIAS. Hereditary sideroblastic anemia is most commonly a moderate to severe hypochromic, normocytic anemia inherited in a sex-linked recessive fashion. A point mutation resulting in an amino acid change near the pyridoxal phosphate binding site of the erythrocytic δ-aminolevulinic acid synthase isoenzyme is the underlying defect in kindreds with this disorder. The anemia does not usually become evident until early adulthood and responds to varying doses of pyridoxine, which are usually much larger than the daily requirements for this vitamin.

Mitochondrial cytopathies may also be responsible for congenital disorders when a sideroblastic anemia is linked to pancreatic, liver,

and kidney dysfunction, as in Pearson's syndrome. These rare syndromes affect infants and are thought to be due to inherited mutations in mitochondrial DNA that result in defective oxidative phosphorylation in the involved organs.

Fitzsimons EJ: The molecular basis of the sideroblastic anemias. Curr Opin Hematol 3: 167, 1996. *A comprehensive review.*

North M, Dallalio G, Donath AS, et al: Serum transferrin receptor levels in patients undergoing evaluation of iron stores: Correlation with other parameters and observed versus predicted results. Clin Lab Haematol 19:93, 1997. *Documents the value of serum transferrin levels.*

Weiss G: Iron and anemia of chronic disease. Kidney Int Suppl 69:S12, 1999. *Reviews role of cytokines and acute-phase reactants.*

Worwood M: The laboratory assessment of iron status—An update. Clin Chim Acta 259:3, 1997. *An excellent review.*

163   MEGALOBLASTIC ANEMIAS
Robert H. Allen

DEFINITION

Megaloblastic anemias are caused by various defects in DNA synthesis that lead to a common set of hematologic abnormalities of bone marrow and peripheral blood. The term *megaloblastic* refers to a morphologic abnormality of cell nuclei that is readily recognizable but difficult to describe. The erythrocytic, granulocytic, and megakaryocytic cell lines are all involved, and pancytopenia may develop. Recognition of megaloblastic anemia is important because two of its most common causes, cobalamin (vitamin B_{12}) deficiency and folate deficiency, are completely corrected with appropriate therapy. Recognition of cobalamin deficiency is of particular importance because it also causes a wide variety of neurologic and psychiatric abnormalities that are preventable or reversible if the diagnosis is made at an early stage.

ETIOLOGY

Etiologic categories of megaloblastic anemia are cobalamin deficiency, folate deficiency, drugs, and miscellaneous causes, including rare enzyme deficiencies and unexplained disorders (Table 163–1). The etiology of cobalamin deficiency can be subdivided into causes of decreased ingestion, impaired absorption, or impaired utilization of the vitamin. Folate deficiency can also be caused by decreased intake, impaired absorption, or impaired utilization or by a number of conditions with an increased requirement for folic acid or an increased loss of folic acid. Drugs causing megaloblastosis can be categorized as those that are purine or pyrimidine antagonists and those that inhibit some other aspect of DNA synthesis. The miscellaneous category includes enzyme defects and some cases of myelodysplastic syndrome and acute leukemia.

It is important to determine the correct etiologic factor in megaloblastic anemia. For example, if a myelodysplastic syndrome is misdiagnosed in a cobalamin-deficient patient, chemotherapy might result in the early death of a patient who could have been completely cured with cobalamin therapy. Similarly, some causes of cobalamin and folate deficiency require therapy for the underlying disease, in addition to replacement therapy with the appropriate vitamin.

INCIDENCE AND PREVALENCE

COBALAMIN DEFICIENCY. The term *pernicious anemia,* often used as a synonym for cobalamin deficiency, should be reserved for conditions in which a gastric mucosal defect results in insufficient intrinsic factor to facilitate the absorption of physiologic amounts of cobalamin. This lack of intrinsic factor, which is by far the most common cause of cobalamin deficiency in the Western hemisphere, occurs in individuals as early as their 20s and can develop in all ethnic groups. Chemically recognized pernicious ane-

Table 163–1 ■ ETIOLOGIC CLASSIFICATION OF THE MEGALOBLASTIC ANEMIAS

CATEGORY	ETIOLOGIC MECHANISMS
I. Cobalamin deficiency	
A. Decreased ingestion	Poor diet, lack of animal products, strict vegetarianism
B. Impaired absorption	1. Failure to release cobalamin from food protein
	Old age
	Gastrectomy (partial)
	2. Intrinsic factor deficiency
	Pernicious anemia
	Gastrectomy (total)
	Destruction of gastric mucosa by caustics
	Congenital abnormal or absence of intrinsic factor molecule
	3. Chronic pancreatic disease
	4. Competitive parasites
	Bacteria in diverticula of bowel, blind loops
	Fish tapeworm infestations (*Diphyllobothrium latum*)
	5. Intrinsic intestinal disease
	Ileal resection, Crohn's disease, radiation ileitis
	Tropical sprue, celiac disease
	Infiltrative intestinal disease (e.g., lymphoma, scleroderma)
	Drug-induced malabsorption
	Congenital selective malabsorption (Imerslund-Graesback syndrome)
C. Impaired utilization	Congenital enzyme deficiencies
	Lack of transcobalamin II
	Nitrous oxide administration
II. Folate deficiency	
A. Decreased ingestion	Poor diet, lack of vegetables
	Alcoholism
	Infancy
B. Impaired absorption	Intestinal short circuits
	Tropical sprue, celiac disease
	Anticonvulsants, sulfasalazine, other drugs
	Congenital malabsorption
C. Impaired utilization	Folic acid antagonists: methotrexate, triamterene, trimethoprim, pyrimethamine, ethanol
	Congenital enzyme deficiencies
D. Increased requirement	Pregnancy, infancy
	Hyperthyroidism
	Chronic hemolytic disease
	Neoplastic disease, exfoliative skin disease
E. Increased loss	Hemodialysis
III. Drugs—metabolic inhibitors	Purine synthesis: methotrexate, 6-mercaptopurine, 6-thioguanine, azathioprine
	Pyrimidine synthesis: methotrexate, 6-azauridine
	Thymidylate synthesis: methotrexate, 5-fluorouracil
	Deoxyribonucleotide synthesis: hydroxyurea, cytosine arabinoside
IV. Miscellaneous	
A. Inborn errors	Lesch-Nyhan syndrome
	Hereditary orotic aciduria
	Others
B. Unexplained disorders	Pyridoxine-responsive megaloblastic anemia
	Thiamine-responsive megaloblastic anemia
	Some cases of myelodysplastic syndrome
	Some cases of acute myelogenous leukemia

mia will develop in about 1.0% of individuals in the United States at some time during their lives. Approximately 10% of the U.S. population older than 70 years have low or low-normal serum cobalamin levels *and* metabolic evidence of cobalamin deficiency (elevated levels of serum methylmalonic acid and homocysteine that fall to normal with cobalamin therapy). The etiology and hematologic and neuropsychiatric significance of these findings are unknown at the present time, although there is increasing evidence of a strong correlation between serum homocysteine levels and all forms of vascular disease.

FOLATE DEFICIENCY, DRUGS, AND OTHER CAUSES. The incidence of folate deficiency and drug-related megaloblastic anemia is less well established. Through its association with alcoholism, folate deficiency is far from a rare condition. The marked increase in the use of chemotherapeutic agents to treat malignant disease and immune disorders suggests that these drugs may now be the most common cause of megaloblastic anemia in the Western hemisphere.

PATHOGENESIS AND PATHOLOGY

MECHANISM OF MEGALOBLASTOSIS. FOLATE DEFICIENCY. Folate functions to transfer one-carbon units, such as methyl, meth-

ylene, and formyl groups, to various substrates in a variety of enzymatic reactions that are intimately related to the synthesis of DNA, RNA, and proteins. In folate deficiency, all forms of folate are reduced within cells, which impairs the growth and maturation of rapidly growing cells such as those in the bone marrow. For example, thymidylate synthase catalyzes the synthesis of thymidine from deoxyuridine and 5,10-methylenetetrahydrofolate. Inhibition of thymidylate synthase leads to increased intracellular concentrations of deoxyuridine triphosphate, which is incorporated into DNA in positions that normally arise from deoxythymidine triphosphate. Attempts to repair this abnormal DNA increase DNA fragmentation, which may play a major role in causing the abnormalities of cell growth and maturation that are present in folate deficiency.

COBALAMIN DEFICIENCY. Cobalamin functions as an essential cofactor for only two enzymes in human cells, methionine synthase and L-methylmalonyl coenzyme A (CoA) mutase (Figs. 163–1 and 163–2). Methionine synthase catalyzes the recycling of homocysteine to methionine; this reaction requires 5-methylcobalamin as a coenzyme (see Fig. 163–1). Methionine, an essential amino acid for protein synthesis, also serves in the form of *S*-adenosylmethionine as the major methyl donor in numerous important enzymatic reactions. In cobalamin deficiency, increasing amounts of intracellular folate are converted to 5-methyltetrahydrofolate in an attempt to prevent intracellular methionine deficiency. The "trapping" of intra-

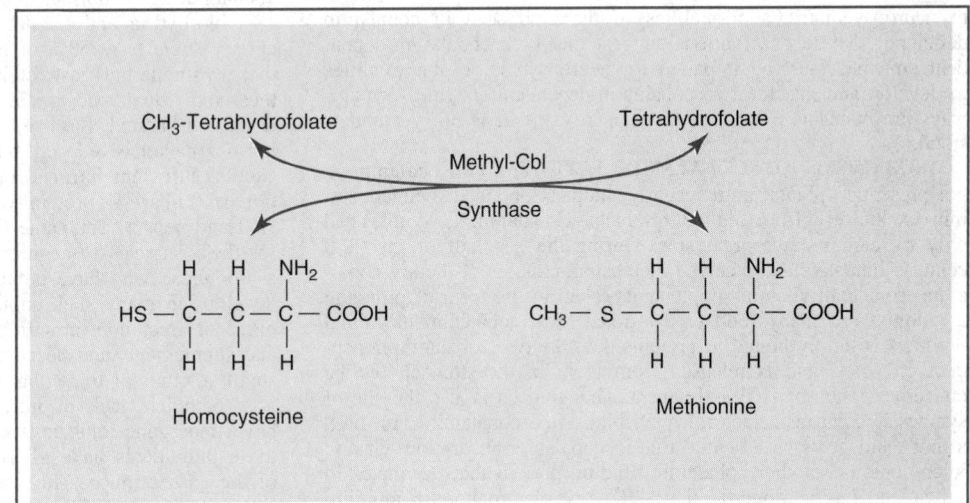

FIGURE 163–1 ■ Reaction catalyzed by methionine synthase that requires methyl-cobalamin (Methyl-Cbl) and transfers the methyl group of 5-methyltetrahydrofolate (CH3-tetrahydrofolate) to homocysteine to form methionine and tetrahydrofolate. Homocysteine accumulates in cobalamin deficiency because of a lack of methyl-cobalamin and in folate deficiency because of a lack of 5-methyltetrahydrofolate.

cellular folate as 5-methyltetrahydrofolate is augmented by the fact that this substance is the major component of plasma folate and is the form that enters cells and must be converted to tetrahydrofolate by methionine synthase before it can enter the folate pool. Thus cobalamin deficiency results in secondary intracellular deficiency of all forms of folate except 5-methyltetrahydrofolate. As a result, the activities of all of the enzymes using folate to transfer one-carbon moieties, including thymidylate synthase, are impaired. This concept of "methylfolate trapping" explains why cobalamin deficiency and folate deficiency produce indistinguishable hematologic abnormalities and why the hematologic abnormalities seen in cobalamin deficiency can be completely reversed by pharmacologic amounts of folic acid. The latter oxidized, non-physiologic form of folate can be directly reduced to tetrahydrofolate without initially being converted to 5-methyltetrahydrofolate. This concept also explains why the hematologic abnormalities caused by folate deficiency respond only slightly, if at all to large amounts of cobalamin.

DRUGS AND OTHER CAUSES. Drugs cause megaloblastic anemia by inhibiting a variety of enzymes involved in DNA synthesis. 5-Fluorouracil (5-FU) inhibits thymidylate synthase directly. The addition of 5-formyltetrahydrofolate (leucovorin) to 5-FU regimens actually increases the inhibition of thymidylate synthase because 5-formyltetrahydrofolate is readily converted to 5,10-methylenetetrahydrofolate, which is involved in the formation of inhibitory ternary complexes between 5,10-methylenetetrahydrofolate, 5-FU, and thymidylate synthase. Why megaloblastic changes occur in some cases of the myelodysplastic syndrome and acute leukemias is un-

known but is probably due to a variety of mutations that alter DNA synthesis.

MECHANISM OF NEUROPSYCHIATRIC ABNORMALITIES IN COBALAMIN DEFICIENCY. A wide variety of neuropsychiatric abnormalities are seen in cobalamin deficiency and appear to be due to an undefined defect involving myelin synthesis. Because these abnormalities are not seen in folate deficiency, it has been tempting to ascribe them to deficient activity of the second cobalamin-dependent enzyme, L-methylmalonyl-CoA mutase, which is unrelated to any folate-dependent enzyme or pathway. This enzyme catalyzes the conversion of L-methylmalonyl-CoA to succinyl-CoA by using adenosylcobalamin as a required coenzyme (see Fig. 163–2). Abnormal odd-carbon and branched-chain fatty acids are formed when the mutase is impaired. The neuropsychiatric abnormalities of cobalamin deficiency are not seen, however, in individuals with genetic defects of the mutase reaction caused either by primary defects in the enzyme itself or by defects in the formation of adenosylcobalamin. Impairment of methionine synthase has also been postulated as the cause of neuropsychiatric abnormalities in view of the importance of methionine and S-adenosylmethionine for the many methylation reactions occurring in the nervous system. As noted, however, the neuropsychiatric abnormalities caused by cobalamin deficiency are not seen in folate deficiency, although methionine synthase appears to be equally impaired in both vitamin deficiencies (based on similar marked elevations in serum homocysteine concentrations). Genetic defects in which the synthesis of both adenosylcobalamin and methylcobalamin is impaired do lead

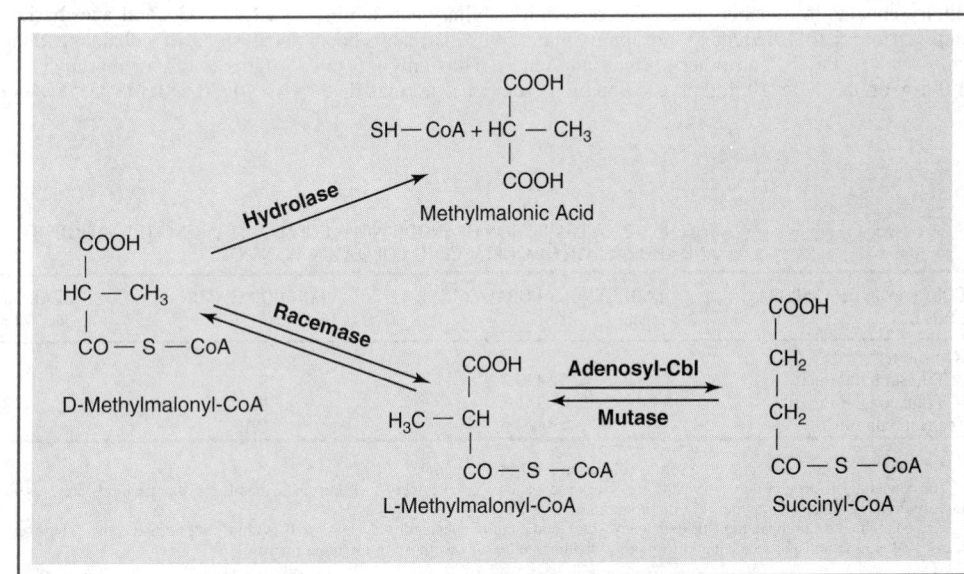

FIGURE 163–2 ■ Reactions involved in the metabolism of D- and L-methylmalonyl coenzyme A(CoA). Methylmalonic acid accumulates in cobalamin deficiency because of a lack of adenosylcobalamin (Adenosyl-Cbl), which leads to an increase in L-methylmalonyl-CoA, which is converted to D-methylmalonyl-CoA and hydrolyzed to methylmalonic acid.

to neuropsychiatric abnormalities of the kind seen in cobalamin deficiency. These observations suggest that both cobalamin-dependent enzymes must be impaired for neuropsychiatric abnormalities to develop and that the two cobalamin-dependent enzymes or pathways are connected or interrelated in a way that is not yet understood.

MECHANISMS OF COBALAMIN DEFICIENCY. Cobalamin is not present in plants; until recently, humans obtained their cobalamin exclusively from animal products. Cobalamin is synthesized only by certain microorganisms. During the last half of the 20th century, humans have received increasing amounts of dietary cobalamin from multivitamin supplements taken in the form of pills and as additives to many food preparations. Most cobalamin in animal products is tightly bound to proteins, i.e., the two cobalamin-dependent enzymes, and is released from them in the stomach by the concerted action of HCl and pepsin. The stomach is also the site of synthesis of intrinsic factor, which binds free cobalamin with high affinity and plays an essential role in cobalamin absorption. Gastric juice contains another cobalamin binding protein that originates in saliva and has a more rapid or "R"-type electrophoretic mobility than does intrinsic factor. R protein binds cobalamin with a higher affinity than does intrinsic factor, particularly at an acid pH.

Thus under normal conditions of gastric acidity, dietary cobalamin enters the duodenum bound to R protein. Additional cobalamin bound to R protein enters the duodenum after secretion into bile by the liver (the only significant route by which cobalamin is lost from the body). Pancreatic proteases partially degrade salivary and biliary R protein–cobalamin complexes in the jejunum; cobalamin is bound to intrinsic factor only after this process occurs. The intrinsic factor–cobalamin complex remains intact until it reaches the distal end of the ileum, where it binds with high affinity to specific receptors located on ileal mucosal cells. Cobalamin then enters these cells and reaches the portal plasma, which contains three cobalamin binding proteins known as transcobalamin I, II, and III (Table 163–2). Although it contains only about 10% of the plasma cobalamin, transcobalamin II is the important transport protein because of its rapid clearance and its ability to deliver cobalamin to all cells within the body. Transcobalamin II–cobalamin is taken up by cells by endocytosis during a process in which the transcobalamin II moiety is degraded and the cobalamin is reduced and eventually converted to its two coenzyme forms, methylcobalamin and adenosylcobalamin. Cobalamin is not stored intracellularly; the entire intracellular vitamin is bound to the aforementioned two enzymes, which are present in greater amounts than is cobalamin.

A large number of acquired and genetic diseases affect the pathway of cobalamin absorption and transport and result in cobalamin deficiency. Strict vegetarians, who ingest neither meat nor other animal products such as milk, cheese, or eggs and who do not ingest multivitamin supplements, become cobalamin deficient on a dietary basis. Ten to 15 years is required for the development of clinical signs of dietary cobalamin deficiency because absorption of biliary cobalamin remains intact. The secretion of biliary cobalamin ranges from 5 to 10 μg/day, and approximately 90% is reabsorbed by strict vegetarians and other normal individuals. Thus only 0.5 to 1.0 μg of the 5 to 10 μg of cobalamin present in a normal diet must be absorbed each day to maintain the total-body content of cobalamin in the normal range of 2000 to 5000 μg.

Achlorhydria and the loss of pepsin secretion are common in elderly subjects (>50% of individuals older than 70 years) and in those with partial gastrectomy. Cobalamin deficiency develops in these individuals because of an inability to liberate cobalamin from its protein-bound form in foods of animal origin. Secretion of intrinsic factor is reduced, but because it is normally formed in vast excess, sufficient intrinsic factor usually remains for the reabsorption of biliary R protein–cobalamin, which is not dependent on HCl and pepsin. The same time span of 10 to 15 years is required for these subjects to acquire clinical signs of cobalamin deficiency as for those who have deficient diets. Cobalamin deficiency never develops in many such subjects, apparently because of the availability of free, non–protein-bound cobalamin in multivitamin pills and supplements and because some natural animal products contain small amounts of free cobalamin.

A complete lack of intrinsic factor occurs in individuals who have undergone total gastrectomy or who have pernicious anemia; these individuals have idiopathic and essentially complete atrophy of the gastric mucosa in association with autoantibodies to parietal cells and intrinsic factor. Only about 3 to 5 years is required for clinical signs of cobalamin deficiency to develop under these circumstances because such individuals demonstrate malabsorption of biliary as well as all forms of dietary cobalamin.

Cobalamin malabsorption occurs commonly in severe pancreatic exocrine insufficiency because of an inability to degrade R protein–cobalamin complexes in the jejunum. Clinically evident cobalamin deficiency rarely occurs, however, probably because oral therapy with pancreatic extract is usually instituted in these patients during the 3 to 5 years necessary for the signs of cobalamin deficiency to develop.

The abnormal presence of high concentrations of bacteria and certain parasites in the small intestine can result in cobalamin malabsorption inasmuch as these organisms can avidly take up and retain cobalamin. Diseases interfering with the integrity of the distal ileal mucosa can also result in cobalamin malabsorption, which occurs invariably after surgical removal of the distal 100 cm of ileum.

A large number of genetic disorders involve the plasma transport of cobalamin, its intracellular conversion to its coenzyme forms, or its utilization by the two cobalamin-dependent enzymes. These disorders usually appear within the first few weeks of life.

The general anesthetic nitrous oxide causes multiple defects in cobalamin utilization, including the following: (1) rapid (within minutes) inhibition of methionine synthase activity with slow (over several days) recovery when nitrous oxide administration is stopped, (2) displacement of cobalamin from methionine synthase, (3) decrease in the level of methylcobalamin, (4) irreversible conversion of cobalamin to inactive and inhibitory cobalamin analogues, (5) gradual (over many weeks) development of cobalamin deficiency, (6) an eventual decrease in L-methylmalonyl-CoA mutase activity, and (7) a further decrease in methionine synthase activity. General anesthesia with nitrous oxide can precipitate clinical signs of cobalamin deficiency in individuals whose cobalamin status is low or marginal.

MECHANISMS OF FOLATE DEFICIENCY. Folate is widely dis-

Table 163–2 ■ DISTRIBUTION OF ENDOGENOUS COBALAMIN AMONG THE VARIOUS TRANSCOBALAMINS AND THEIR RELATIVE IMPORTANCE TO COBALAMIN TRANSPORT*

COBALAMIN TRANSPORT PROTEIN	ENDOGENOUS COBALAMIN (pg/mL)	T½ FOR COBALAMIN CLEARANCE (hr)	COBALAMIN CLEARANCE (pg/mL/24 hr)	SITE OF SPECIFIC UPTAKE
R proteins†				
Transcobalamin I	425–450	240.0	30	None
Transcobalamin III	0–25	0.1	0–4000	Hepatocytes
Transcobalamin II‡	50	0.1	8000	All cells

*In a typical normal subject with a serum cobalamin level of 500 pg/mL.

†In congenital R-protein deficiency, the total serum cobalamin level is very low, but no hematologic abnormalities are present because R proteins do not transport cobalamin to rapidly dividing cells, such as those in the bone marrow.

‡In congenital transcobalamin II deficiency, the total serum cobalamin level is well within the normal range, but severe megaloblastic anemia develops because only transcobalamin II transports cobalamin to rapidly dividing cells, such as those in the bone marrow.

tributed in plants and in products of animal origin; green vegetables are particularly rich sources of folate. Excessive cooking will destroy or remove a high percentage of folate in foods. Folate is either missing or is present only in relatively small amounts (≤800 μg) in non-prescription multivitamin pills and supplements because of the concern that its presence in larger amounts might mask the diagnosis of cobalamin deficiency by correcting the associated hematologic abnormalities without having any beneficial effect on the neuropsychiatric abnormalities. Folates in natural foods are conjugated to chains of polyglutamic acid. Enzymes in the lumen of the small intestine convert the polyglutamate forms of folate to the monoglutamate and diglutamate forms, which are readily absorbed in the proximal portion of the jejunum. Absorption involves both active and passive transport. Most of the folate in plasma is present as 5-methyltetrahydrofolate in the monoglutamate form. The majority is loosely bound to albumin, from which it is readily taken up by the high-affinity folate receptors present on cells throughout the body. Once it enters the cell, 5-methyltetrahydrofolate must be converted to tetrahydrofolate by the cobalamin-dependent enzyme methionine synthase before it can be converted to the polyglutamate form and take part in the other folate-dependent enzymatic reactions. In addition to being secreted into bile and reabsorbed in the small intestine, folates are also degraded and excreted in the urine.

Decreased intake is by far the most common cause of folate deficiency. Normal individuals have approximately 5000 to 20,000 μg of folate in body stores. Because folate is degraded within the body and is excreted in both bile and urine, 50 to 200 μg must be absorbed each day from the average Western diet, which contains about 200 to 500 μg of folate. The amount of dietary folate has increased approximately 100 μg/day in the United States because of the recent mandatory fortification of all grain products that was implemented to reduce the incidence of neural tube defects. Clinical signs of folate deficiency develop after approximately 4 months of decreased intake, as can readily occur in chronic alcoholism.

Absorption of folate is impaired in a variety of diseases affecting the jejunal mucosa, including tropical sprue and celiac disease. Certain drugs such as anticonvulsants and sulfasalazine may impair folate absorption in some individuals. Ethanol and drugs such as triamterene impair the utilization of folate. Certain conditions associated with hypermetabolism or rapid cell growth lead to an increased requirement for folate that often cannot be met by a normal diet; these conditions include hyperthyroidism, pregnancy, chronic hemolysis, and various exfoliative skin diseases. Hemodialysis causes an increased loss of folate from the body.

CLINICAL MANIFESTATIONS OF MEGALOBLASTIC ANEMIA

HEMATOLOGIC MANIFESTATIONS. All causes of megaloblastic anemia produce a common set of hematologic, laboratory, and other abnormalities (Table 163–3). None of the abnormalities are specific for the various diseases that cause megaloblastic anemia, and each may also be present in any combination that may vary greatly from patient to patient. In addition, none of the abnormalities are always seen in conditions that cause megaloblastic anemia, and the absence of any one or more of them cannot be used to exclude any of the diseases that cause megaloblastic anemia in a given patient, including cobalamin or folate deficiency.

Megaloblastic anemia typically develops over many months and may not cause symptoms until the hematocrit falls below 20%. The reticulocyte count is not elevated, in either absolute or relative (percentage) terms, even when the anemia is severe. The mean cell volume is often increased (normal, 80 to 100 fL), with values as high as 140 fL. A review of previous blood counts often reveals a steady increase in mean cell volume over several months or years.

Neutropenia and thrombocytopenia occur less commonly than anemia and are not usually severe. On occasion, however, neutrophil counts of less than 1000 per microliter and platelet counts of less than 50,000 per microliter may be seen. A peripheral blood smear frequently shows neutrophil hypersegmentation (Fig. 163–3 and Color Plate 5E), which may be documented by observing one or more of the following: (1) the presence of at least one neutrophil containing 6 or more lobes, (2) the presence of 5% or more of 5-lobe neutrophils, or (3) an increase above the normal neutrophil lobe average of fewer than 3.4 lobes per neutrophil. Erythrocytes

Table 163–3 ■ HEMATOLOGIC AND OTHER ABNORMALITIES THAT MAY BE DUE TO ANY OF THE VARIOUS CAUSES OF MEGALOBLASTIC ANEMIA*

HEMATOLOGIC	OTHER
Anemia	Glossitis
Reticulocytopenia	Stomatitis
Macrocytosis (increased MCV)	Gastrointestinal symptoms
Neutropenia	Hyperpigmentation
Thrombocytopenia	Infertility
Peripheral blood smear	Orthostatic hypotension
Neutrophil hypersegmentation	Weight loss
Erythrocyte	
Variation in size	
Variation in shape	
Macro-ovalocytes	
Serum	
Elevated lactate dehydrogenase	
Elevated bilirubin	
Elevated iron	
Decreased haptoglobin	
Bone marrow	
Hypercellular	
Megaloblastic morphology	
Giant bands and metamyelocytes	

MCV = mean corpuscular volume.
*These abnormalities may be present in any number or combination in a given patient. Absence of any one or more of them occurs commonly in individual patients with all causes of megaloblastic anemia, including cobalamin deficiency and folate deficiency.

often vary markedly in size and shape, and macro-ovalocytes (large, oval erythrocytes) are frequently present (Fig. 163–4). When the hematocrit is low, nucleated red cells may be seen on the peripheral smear and permit detection of the megaloblastic morphology of the nuclei without the need to perform bone marrow aspiration or biopsy.

Although the reticulocyte count may be normal or low, a number of serum abnormalities often suggest hemolytic anemia: elevated serum levels of lactate dehydrogenase, indirect bilirubin, and iron, as well as decreased levels of haptoglobin. These findings are consistent with the markedly increased red cell production and destruction seen in megaloblastic anemia but confined to the bone marrow and termed intramedullary hemolysis or ineffective erythropoiesis.

The bone marrow is usually hypercellular with an increase in all cellular elements. Megaloblastic morphologic changes are often seen in all cells within the bone marrow but are usually more prominent in the erythroid series. All cells in the erythroid series are larger than their normal counterparts, their cytoplasm appears more mature than their nuclei (nuclear-cytoplasmic asynchrony),

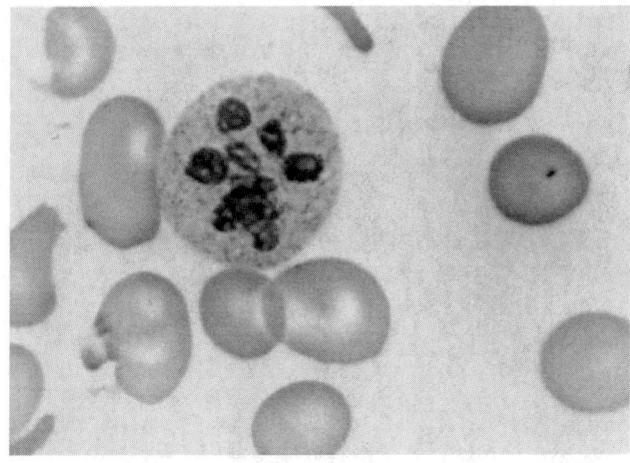

FIGURE 163–3 ■ A hypersegmented neutrophil on a peripheral blood smear from a patient with megaloblastic anemia.

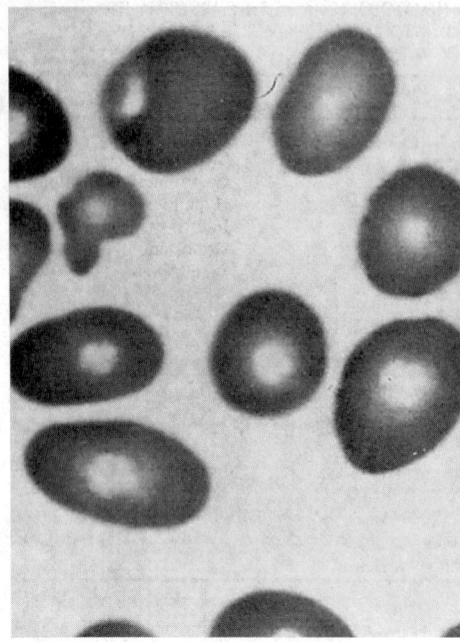
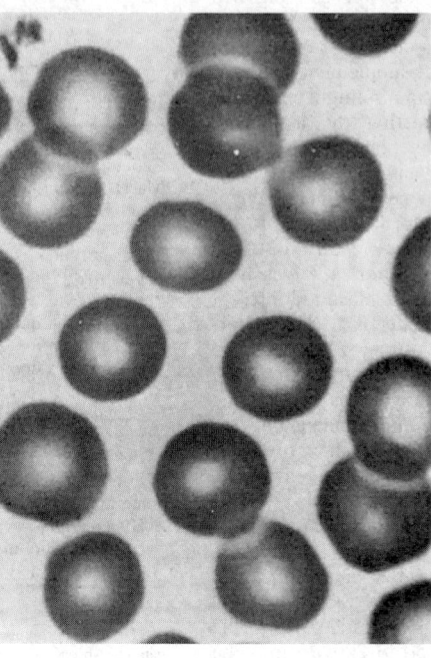

FIGURE 163–4 ■ Peripheral blood smears from a patient with megaloblastic anemia (left) and from a normal subject (right), both at the same magnification. The smear from the patient shows variation in the size and shape of erythrocytes and the presence of macro-ovalocytes.

and the nuclear chromatin has a distinctive open and fine-grained texture (Fig. 163–5 and Color Plate 5F). Similar abnormalities are seen in neutrophil precursors and are usually most striking at the metamyelocyte and band stages, in which "giant metamyelocytes" and "giant bands" are seen. All these features are much more prominent in a Wright-stained smear of bone marrow aspirate than in fixed sections from the bone marrow biopsy. Use of the latter alone can lead to disastrous clinical consequences because even the most experienced hematopathologist can, on the basis of fixed bone marrow sections only, experience difficulty in distinguishing the hypercellularity and abnormal morphology of megaloblastosis from the changes seen in the myelodysplastic syndromes and some cases of acute leukemia. Coexisting iron deficiency may also cause diagnostic problems inasmuch as all of the erythroid megaloblastic changes may be absent, even in Wright-stained smears of aspirated bone marrow. The diagnosis of megaloblastic anemia should never be excluded after bone marrow examination unless bone marrow aspirates have been examined and the presence of bone marrow iron has been established.

Megaloblastic abnormalities may occur in other proliferating body cells, all of which share the underlying defect in DNA synthesis. Such changes have been documented in the epithelial cells of the buccal mucosa, stomach, intestine, and vagina and account for such phenomena as glossitis, stomatitis, and secondary malabsorption. Similar changes may account for the infertility that is sometimes seen.

Few, if any, patients with cobalamin or folate deficiency or other causes of megaloblastic anemia demonstrate all or even most of the classic hematologic or other abnormalities. Even anemia and increased mean cell volume are frequently absent in patients with otherwise severe deficiencies of cobalamin or folate. For example, in a prospective study of 86 consecutive patients with low serum cobalamin levels (<200 pg/mL) *and* one or more objective hematologic and/or neuropsychiatric responses to cobalamin therapy, 44% did not have anemia, 36% had a mean cell volume of 100 fL or less, 86% had a normal white blood cell count, 79% had a normal platelet count, 33% had a normal peripheral smear on routine laboratory study, 43% had normal serum lactate dehydrogenase levels, and 83% had normal serum bilirubin levels.

NEUROPSYCHIATRIC ABNORMALITIES CAUSED BY COBALAMIN DEFICIENCY. Cobalamin deficiency, unlike folate deficiency and other causes of megaloblastic anemia, produces a wide variety of neuropsychiatric abnormalities (Table 163–4). None of these abnormalities are specific for cobalamin deficiency, and any of them may be present alone or in any combination and may vary greatly from patient to patient. None of the abnormalities are always seen in cobalamin deficiency, and the absence of any one or a combination of them does not exclude cobalamin deficiency. The neuropsychiatric abnormalities may occur early or late in the course of cobalamin deficiency and with or without any of the hematologic or other abnormalities listed in Table 163–3. How the deficiency of a single substance, such as cobalamin, can produce a clinical picture with such wide variations in severity and dissociation of various hematologic and neuropsychiatric abnormalities is unknown.

Pathologic studies show loss of myelin with axonal degeneration, most frequently in the dorsal and lateral columns of the spinal cord but also in peripheral and cranial nerves and the cerebral cortex. *Combined systems disease* designates a spinal cord disorder marked by the insidious beginning and gradual progression of demyelination, initially of the dorsal (proprioceptive afferent) and later the lateral (corticospinal efferent) columns. Axonal degeneration affects the same pathways as a late, irreversible change. Demyelinative neuropathy of large peripheral fibers may precede or develop concurrently with the cord changes. Signs and symptoms are usually symmetrical and often include paresthesias in the extremities and impaired vibration and position sense that may progress to an

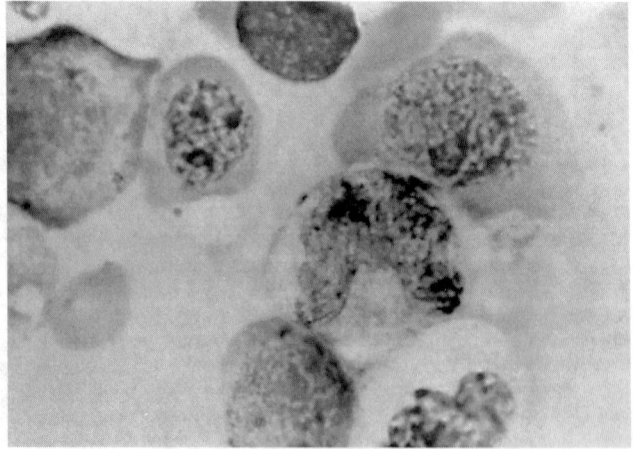

FIGURE 163–5 ■ Erythroid precursors with marked megaloblastic features on a bone marrow smear from a patient with megaloblastic anemia.

Neurologic Abnormalities	Psychiatric Abnormalities
Paresthesia	Depression
Impaired vibration sense	Paranoia
Impaired position sense	Listlessness
Impaired touch or pain perception	Acute confusional state
Ataxia	Hallucinations
Abnormal gait	Delusions
Fatigue	Insomnia
Memory loss	Apprehensiveness
Disorientation	Psychosis
Obtundation	Slow mentation
Decreased reflexes	Paraphrenia
Weakness	Mania
Decreased muscle strength	Panic attacks
Romberg's sign	Personality change
Increased reflexes	Suicide
Spasticity	
Babinski's sign	
Lhermitte's sign	
Urinary or fecal incontinence	
Urinary urgency or nocturia	
Impotence	
Abnormal smell or taste	
Decreased vision or optic atrophy	

*These abnormalities may be present in any number or combination in a given patient. They are seen frequently with *or without* any of the hematologic or other abnormalities listed in Table 163–3.

abnormal gait, spastic ataxia, and quadriparesis. Urinary and fecal incontinence, as well as impotence, may be seen. Cerebral and cranial nerve abnormalities include irritability, memory loss, disorientation, obtundation, and changes in taste and smell; changes in vision can progress to severe optic atrophy and near blindness. Psychiatric abnormalities, which may be prominent and isolated, include depression, hallucinations, agitation, marked personality change, abnormal behavior, and suicide.

The neuropsychiatric abnormalities caused by cobalamin deficiency frequently bear no relationship to the presence or degree of hematologic abnormalities. The severity of neuropsychiatric abnormalities actually bears a striking *inverse correlation* to the degree of anemia. The frequency with which hematologic and neuropsychiatric abnormalities are dissociated is often unappreciated. For example, several clinical studies document that a normal hematocrit, mean cell volume, or both occur in at least 25 to 50% of patients whose neuropsychiatric abnormalities are caused by cobalamin deficiency *and* respond partially or completely to cobalamin therapy. Other hematologic and laboratory abnormalities of the kind

Table 163–5 ■ DIAGNOSTIC APPROACH TO PATIENTS WITH COBALAMIN OR FOLATE DEFICIENCY

I. Initial approach
A. Indications
  1. Any unexplained hematologic or other abnormality of the kind listed in Table 163–3 (cobalamin and folate deficiency)
  2. Any unexplained neuropsychiatric abnormality of the kind listed in Table 163–4 (cobalamin deficiency)
B. Initial tests
  1. Serum cobalamin (normal, 200–900 pg/mL)
  2. Serum folate (normal, 2.5–20 ng/mL)
II. Follow-up
A. Indications
  1. Serum cobalamin <350 pg/mL *or*
  2. Serum folate <5 ng/mL *or*
  3. Clinical condition
    a. Serious unexplained hematologic or neuropsychiatric abnormalities *or*
    b. Very suggestive of cobalamin or folate deficiency
B. Follow-up tests
  1. Serum methylmalonic acid (normal, 70–270 nmol)—elevated in cobalamin deficiency
  2. Serum homocysteine (normal, 5–16 μmol)—elevated in cobalamin and folate deficiency

outlined in Table 163–3 are lacking in a similar or even higher percentage of these patients.

DIAGNOSIS

INDICATIONS. If drugs are excluded as a cause, the differential diagnosis of megaloblastic anemia in adults is usually limited to the important task of distinguishing between cobalamin deficiency and folate deficiency and firmly establishing the presence of one or the other (Table 163–5). Patients should always be evaluated for these two conditions in the presence of any unexplained hematologic or other abnormality of the kind listed in Table 163–3. In addition, patients should always be investigated for cobalamin deficiency in the presence of any unexplained neuropsychiatric abnormality of the kind listed in Table 163–4, regardless of the presence or absence of hematologic abnormalities. The yield may be relatively low because of the non-specific nature of these worrisome abnormalities, but such studies are clearly justified by the fact that all of the hematologic abnormalities caused by cobalamin or folate deficiency are completely corrected by safe and inexpensive therapy with the proper vitamin. In addition, the neuropsychiatric abnormalities caused by cobalamin deficiency are usually partially or completely corrected by cobalamin therapy, and in the small minority of patients who do not improve, cobalamin therapy always prevents subsequent worsening. It is particularly important that the diagnosis of cobalamin deficiency be established with a high degree of certainty because cobalamin therapy must almost always be given for the lifetime of the patient. The distinction between cobalamin deficiency and folate deficiency is also very important because treatment of cobalamin deficiency with folate does not improve the neuropsychiatric abnormalities, although hematologic responses often occur.

SERUM COBALAMIN AND FOLATE. Competitive binding assays for serum cobalamin and serum folate are used as the initial screening tests because they are widely available and relatively inexpensive. Essentially all serum cobalamin assays today use purified intrinsic factor, which neither binds nor measures the serum cobalamin analogues that caused problems with earlier assays.

Normal ranges are defined as the mean ± 2 SD for normal subjects and thus include only 95% of normal individuals. Such normal ranges are approximately 200 to 900 pg/mL for serum cobalamin and approximately 2.5 to 20 ng/mL for serum folate. By definition, 2.5% of normal subjects, or about 6,250,000 persons in the United States, who have no evidence of cobalamin deficiency and who will not benefit in any way from cobalamin therapy, have low serum cobalamin values of less than 200 pg/mL (false-positive readings). This number is much greater than the estimate of approximately 150,000 cobalamin-deficient patients present in the United States at any point in time. The number of false-positive readings will remain large even if cobalamin testing is restricted, as it should be, to individuals with one or more unexplained abnormalities of the kind contained in Tables 163–3 and 163–4. Similar calculations can be made with respect to serum folate values. Serum cobalamin and folate levels therefore cannot be used alone to establish the diagnosis of cobalamin or folate deficiency unequivocally. The problem is compounded by the fact that not all patients with clinically confirmed cobalamin or folate deficiency (defined as those who have objective clinical responses to appropriate therapy) have low values for serum cobalamin or folate. The following distribution of serum cobalamin levels has been noted in clinically confirmed cobalamin-deficient patients: less than 100 pg/mL, approximately 50%; 100 to 200 pg/mL, approximately 40%; 200 to 350 pg/mL, approximately 10%; and higher than 350 pg/mL, approximately 0.1% to 1%. The distribution of serum folate levels in patients with clinically confirmed folate deficiency has been less well studied, but currently available data indicate that only about 75% of such patients have serum folate levels lower than 2.5 mg/mL, with almost all of the remaining 25% falling in the 2.5- to 5.0-ng/mL range.

Perhaps it is not surprising that many patients with clinically confirmed cobalamin or folate deficiency have serum vitamin levels within the normal range. Both vitamins, after all, function within cells and not in plasma. Furthermore, in the case of cobalamin,

Table 163–6 ▪ TYPICAL SERUM FINDINGS IN MEGALOBLASTIC ANEMIA

COMPONENT	NORMAL LEVELS	DEFICIENCY	
		Cobalamin	Folate
Cobalamin	200–900 pg/mL	↓ *	N
Folate	2.5–20 ng/mL	N	↓ *
Methylmalonic acid	70–270 nmol	↑ ↑	N
Homocysteine	5–16 μmol	↑ ↑	↑ ↑

*A significant number of patients with cobalamin deficiency will have serum cobalamin levels in the lower portion of the normal range (see the text). The same is true with respect to folate deficiency and serum folate levels.

serum levels of the vitamin are greatly influenced by levels of plasma binding proteins, which bear no relationship to cellular cobalamin levels. For example, transcobalamin I has no apparent function. Thus assays for serum cobalamin and serum folate are useful as initial screening tests that allow the physician to exclude from consideration almost all patients with serum cobalamin levels of 350 pg/mL or greater and serum folate levels of 5.0 ng/mL or greater. Additional follow-up tests are required for serum cobalamin levels less than 350 pg/mL, serum folate levels less than 5.0 ng/mL, or clinical conditions that are serious or very suggestive of cobalamin or folate deficiency. Examples of such conditions include (1) marked myelodysplasia in a patient who is about to start a regimen of chemotherapy, (2) incapacitating urinary and fecal incontinence of unknown cause in a young patient, (3) pancytopenia with an increased mean cell volume and serum lactate dehydrogenase level, and (4) symmetrical paresthesias in the hands and feet in a patient who also has spastic ataxia and a recent change in personality.

SERUM METHYLMALONIC ACID AND HOMOCYSTEINE. The most useful follow-up tests for diagnosing and distinguishing between cobalamin and folate deficiency are serum levels of methylmalonic acid (normal, 70 to 270 nmol/L) and homocysteine (normal, 5 to 14 nmol/L). For homocysteine, what is actually measured is "total homocysteine," which consists of the sum of homocysteine and homocysteine that is linked via disulfide bond formation in a variety of compounds that include homocystine (homocysteine–homocysteine disulfide), homocysteine-cysteine mixed disulfide, proteins via their cysteine moieties, and peptides such as glutathione via their cysteine moieties. Tests of methylmalonic acid and homocysteine can be performed on serum that remains after cobalamin and folate levels have been determined; these tests are now widely available in the United States through a number of laboratories, including all of the large national reference laboratories. The combined cost of the two tests, which are usually performed together, is similar to the cost of a Schilling test or a bone marrow examination. The serum methylmalonic acid level is elevated in more than 95% of patients with clinically confirmed cobalamin deficiency. Values as high as 2,000,000 nmol/L have been observed, with a median value in the range of 3,500 nmol/L. Serum methylmalonic acid levels are not elevated in folate deficiency. In contrast, serum homocysteine concentrations are elevated in both cobalamin and folate deficiency. Values as high as 500 nmol/L have been observed in cobalamin deficiency, with a median value of 70 nmol/L; values as high as 250 nmol/L have been observed in folate deficiency, with a median value of 50 nmol/L. Except for rare inborn errors of metabolism involving cobalamin- and folate-dependent enzymes or pathways, the only other conditions that also give rise to elevations in serum methylmalonic acid or serum homocysteine are renal failure and intravascular volume depletion. Broad-spectrum antibiotics can lower an elevated serum methylmalonic acid level to normal in patients with cobalamin deficiency by inhibiting the gut microflora, an important source of precursors of methylmalonic acid. Antibiotics do not affect elevated homocysteine levels in these patients, nor do they change any clinical parameters.

Elevated levels of methylmalonic acid and homocysteine resulting from cobalamin deficiency return to normal within 5 to 10 days of starting cobalamin therapy. Elevated levels of homocysteine caused by folate deficiency fall to normal during the same period following folate therapy. Elevations in serum methylmalonic acid and homocysteine secondary to cobalamin deficiency do not respond to pharmacologic doses of folate even in cobalamin-deficient patients, in whom folate causes a marked hematologic improvement (together with no response or a worsening of neuropsychiatric abnormalities). Elevations in homocysteine caused by folate deficiency do not respond to pharmacologic doses of cobalamin. Elevations in methylmalonic acid and homocysteine resulting from renal insufficiency or intravascular volume depletion are not corrected by therapy with either vitamin unless vitamin deficiency coexists. Thus repeat determinations of serum methylmalonic acid and homocysteine levels after a short course of therapy with a single vitamin may provide additional information of diagnostic usefulness.

With few exceptions, patients with serum cobalamin levels lower than 350 pg/mL or serum folate levels less than 5.0 ng/mL do not show objective hematologic or neuropsychiatric responses to cobalamin or folate therapy if their serum levels of methylmalonic acid and homocysteine are normal. Thus the use of serum levels of cobalamin and folate as initial screening tests, together with the use of serum methylmalonic acid and homocysteine determinations as follow-up tests, makes it possible to diagnose cobalamin or folate deficiency and to distinguish between them in the vast majority of patients (see Table 163–5). If in doubt, one can always start empiric therapy, but such therapeutic trials can be difficult to perform (see below) and should be monitored carefully in an attempt to establish a definitive diagnosis. As an alternative, patients can be observed carefully with repeat determinations of methylmalonic acid and homocysteine after 6 months or a year. The usual patterns of serum cobalamin, folate, methylmalonic acid, and homocysteine concentrations in cobalamin and folate deficiency are summarized in Table 163–6.

OTHER TESTS. A number of other tests have been used as diagnostic or follow-up tests in cobalamin deficiency. Serum antibodies to intrinsic factor are present in about 50% of patients with pernicious anemia and are highly specific for that condition. They fail to diagnose about 50% of such cases, however, as well as all cases with other causes of cobalamin deficiency. The standard Schilling test (see Chapter 134 for a complete description of this test) requires a reliable 24-hour urine collection, and because it uses free, i.e., non–protein-bound, cobalamin, it fails to diagnose cobalamin deficiency not only in patients who are strict vegetarians but also, much more commonly, in patients who malabsorb cobalamin from food sources. Both the intrinsic factor antibody test and the Schilling test actually provide information about the etiology of cobalamin deficiency rather than information about the presence or absence of cobalamin deficiency per se. The etiology of cobalamin deficiency (and folate deficiency) should be pursued in unusual patients and those with gastrointestinal symptoms that do not respond to cobalamin therapy because such studies may disclose the presence of a disease that requires additional therapy. It is acceptable practice to institute lifetime cobalamin therapy in individuals with anti–intrinsic factor antibodies or abnormal Schilling tests who lack evidence of current cobalamin deficiency because they will probably become deficient in the future. A normal result with either test should never be used, however, to exclude the diagnosis of cobalamin deficiency or to withhold lifetime therapy.

RESPONSE TO THERAPY. Therapeutic trials with cobalamin or folate must be performed with physiologic levels of either vitamin (1 μg/day for cobalamin and 100 μg/day for folate) inasmuch as larger amounts can give hematologic responses even if the incorrect vitamin is administered. Such trials may require months before responses can be completely evaluated and may be particularly difficult to interpret in patients with neuropsychiatric abnormalities because these complications do not always respond even to large doses of cobalamin, even if cobalamin deficiency is the cause of the abnormalities. Therapeutic trials with pharmacologic doses of folate are potentially dangerous because partial or even complete hematologic responses may be seen in cobalamin-deficient patients while neuropsychiatric abnormalities may progress or develop during folate therapy.

THERAPY

COBALAMIN DEFICIENCY. One option is intramuscular or subcutaneous administration of cyanocobalamin. Because cobalamin is inexpensive and free of any side effects, it is better to give too much than too little. One approach consists of injections of 1000 μg of cyanocobalamin once per week for 8 weeks and then once per month for life. More frequent injections are often used in hospitalized patients or those with marked neuropsychiatric abnormalities, but no evidence of incremental benefit has been demonstrated. Once the weekly injections are completed, the patient or a family member or friend can be taught to give the monthly injections. The absolute requirement of lifetime therapy must be well understood by the patient. Oral therapy with cobalamin in a dose of 10 μg/day can be used with strict vegetarians. In theory, such low-dose therapy could also be used in individuals who malabsorb food cobalamin, but this approach is not recommended because their intrinsic factor production is often precarious and may decrease further over the years. Oral cobalamin therapy in a dose of 1000 to 2000 μg/day has recently been shown to be as effective and possibly superior to the standard parenteral regimen. Both regimens give prompt and equivalent hematologic and neurologic responses, but post-treatment serum cobalamin levels are significantly higher and post-treatment methylmalonic acid levels are significantly lower with the oral regimen. Oral cobalamin, 1000 to 2000 μg/day, is the treatment of choice for most patients.

FOLATE DEFICIENCY. Therapy is usually administered orally in the form of 1-mg tablets of folic acid. Oral therapy is almost always satisfactory, even in the presence of intestinal malabsorption. The usual dose is 1 to 2 mg daily. Therapy limited to several weeks is usually adequate in an alcoholic who begins to eat a normal diet. In patients with chronic conditions such as malabsorption, hemolysis, exfoliative skin diseases, or renal failure requiring hemodialysis, oral folate is continued indefinitely and usually given prophylactically.

COBALAMIN OR FOLATE DEFICIENCY. Red cell transfusions are rarely required because of the well-compensated state of moderately and even severely anemic patients. Such transfusions should be avoided if at all possible because of the associated cost and risk. If a transfusion is required, it should be given very slowly because fluid overload is common and may precipitate lethal congestive heart failure. The only additional therapy is that required for certain underlying causes of cobalamin or folate deficiency, such as antibiotics in bacterial overgrowth or dietary changes in celiac disease.

DRUGS OR OTHER CAUSES. When drugs are responsible for cobalamin or folate deficiency, either administration of them can be stopped or the dosages can be reduced if necessary. In other cases, pyridoxine or thiamine can be tried in pharmacologic doses because occasional patients will respond.

PROGNOSIS

The hematologic abnormalities caused by cobalamin or folate deficiency respond rapidly to therapy with the appropriate vitamin. Reticulocytosis begins by day 5, followed shortly by an increase in the hematocrit, which returns to normal within several months. Neutrophil and platelet counts and other laboratory abnormalities usually return to normal within a week to 10 days. If complete correction of all hematologic abnormalities does not occur, a search should be made for other conditions, such as iron deficiency or hypothyroidism.

The response of the neuropsychiatric abnormalities caused by cobalamin deficiency is less predictable. Cobalamin therapy always prevents such patients from getting worse and most often results in partial or complete correction. Responses may be seen within several days but may take as long as 12 or 18 months. Patients with pernicious anemia have an approximately two-fold increased risk of gastric carcinoma, as well as an increased association with hyperthyroidism, hypothyroidism, and other manifestations of the polyglandular failure syndrome.

Kuzminski AM, Del Giacco EJ, Allen RH, et al. Effective treatment of cobalamin deficiency with oral cobalamin. Blood 92:1191, 1998. *Randomized study showing that oral cobalamin, 2000 μg/day, is at least as effective as parenteral cobalamin, 1000 μg/month.*

Lindenbaum J, Healton EB, Savage DG, et al: Neuropsychiatric disorders caused by cobalamin deficiency in the absence of anemia or macrocytosis. N Engl J Med 318: 1720, 1988. *Detailed description of 42 patients with serious neuropsychiatric abnormalities that responded to cobalamin therapy despite the lack of one or more of the classic hematological abnormalities that are also caused by cobalamin deficiency.*

Stabler SP, Allen RH, Savage DG, et al: Clinical spectrum and diagnosis of cobalamin deficiency. Blood 79:871, 1990. *A total of 145 patients with serum cobalamin levels*

lower than 200 pg/mL were studied before and after cobalamin therapy; 86 had objective clinical responses and 59 did not. The two groups are compared in detail.

Stabler SP, Lindenbaum J, Allen RH: Vitamin B12 deficiency in the elderly: Current dilemmas. Am J Clin Nutr 66:741, 1997. *Extensive review of the high prevalence and potential clinical importance of cobalamin deficiency in the elderly.*

164 HEMOLYTIC ANEMIAS: RED CELL MEMBRANE AND METABOLIC DEFECTS

David E. Golan

NORMAL RED CELL MEMBRANE

Structure

MEMBRANE LIPIDS. The red cell membrane, which was the first biologic membrane to be characterized biochemically, consists of an asymmetrically organized lipid bilayer in which some membrane proteins are embedded and to which other membrane proteins are attached. The lipids consist principally of a mixture of phospholipids and unesterified cholesterol in an approximately 1:1 molar ratio. The cholesterol is randomly distributed between the inner and outer leaflets of the bilayer, but the phospholipids are asymmetrically arranged such that the amino phospholipids (phosphatidylserine and phosphatidylethanolamine) and phosphatidylinositols are localized mainly in the inner leaflet whereas the choline phospholipids (phosphatidylcholine and sphingomyelin) are mainly in the outer leaflet. This phospholipid asymmetry is maintained by the action of a selective amino phospholipid translocase, or "flippase," that uses the energy of adenosine triphosphate (ATP) hydrolysis to translocate phosphatidylserine and phosphatidylethanolamine vectorially from the outer to the inner bilayer leaflet. The action of the translocase is functionally important because exposure of phosphatidylserine and phosphatidylethanolamine at the outer surface of the circulating red cell not only activates the coagulation pathways but also promotes mononuclear phagocyte adhesion, which leads to hemolysis. Red cell membrane lipids appear to exchange freely with those in plasma lipoproteins.

MEMBRANE PROTEINS. Like membrane phospholipids, red cell membrane proteins are asymmetrically arranged to optimize membrane structure and function (Fig. 164–1). The major integral membrane proteins, which penetrate and/or span the lipid bilayer and are commonly decorated with carbohydrate on their extracellular surfaces, include functionally important transport proteins such as band 3 (the anion-exchange protein) and proteins that carry cell-surface antigens such as the glycophorins. The major peripheral membrane proteins, which do not penetrate the lipid bilayer but are instead attached to the intracellular surface of the bilayer by virtue of binding interactions with one or more integral proteins, include structural proteins such as spectrin and actin and some glycolytic enzymes such as glyceraldehyde-3-phosphate dehydrogenase.

The structural proteins are organized into a dense, two-dimensional fibrous meshwork that laminates the inner membrane surface but does not extend into the cytoplasm of the cell. The principal components of this meshwork are spectrin, actin, and protein 4.1. Spectrin is a long, flexible rod-shaped heterodimer consisting of an α- and a β-chain that wrap around one another. These heterodimers associate with one another to form spectrin heterotetramers (and a few higher-order oligomers) at the "head" (self-association) end of the heterodimers and with short filaments of actin at the "tail" end of the heterodimers. The spectrin-actin binding interaction is strengthened by protein 4.1, which binds to both actin and the spectrin β-chain. Because each actin filament can accommodate the binding of about six spectrin heterodimers (this assembly is sometimes called the "junctional complex"), the spectrin–actin–protein

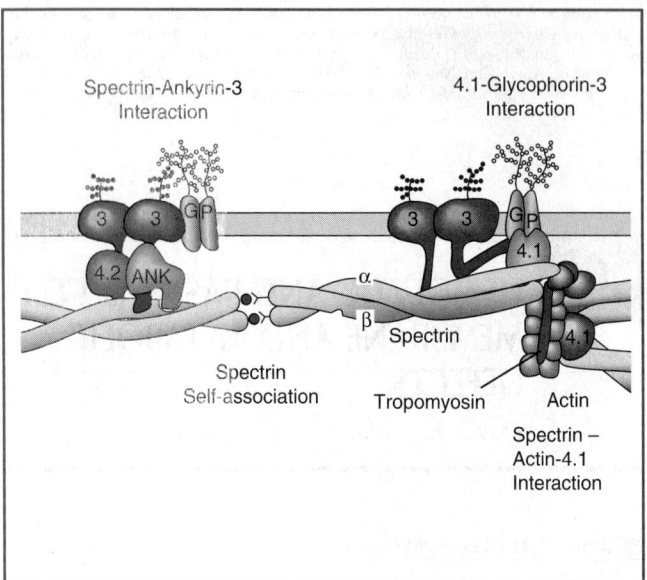

FIGURE 164–1 ■ Molecular binding interactions among the major proteins of the red cell membrane. 3 = band 3; 4.1 = protein 4.1; 4.2 = protein 4.2; ANK = ankyrin; GP = glycophorins.

4.1 complex can extend as a two-dimensional "membrane skeleton" around the entire inner membrane surface.

The membrane skeleton is coupled to the overlying lipid bilayer by the action of several "linking" proteins. The most important linking action is provided by ankyrin, which binds to the spectrin β-chain near the self-association site and to the cytoplasmic domain of the integral protein band 3. Protein 4.2 may play a role in strengthening the spectrin-ankyrin interaction. Other linking mechanisms, the importance of which has recently been demonstrated by the existence of intact (albeit abnormal) red cells in mammalian species that are completely lacking in band 3 protein, include binding interactions between protein 4.1 and glycophorins (especially glycophorin C) and interactions between skeletal proteins (especially spectrin) and inner leaflet membrane lipids.

Function

MEMBRANE STRENGTH AND DEFORMABILITY. The exquisite mechanical coupling between the membrane skeleton and the overlying lipid bilayer confers on the normal red cell its remarkable properties of strength and deformability. Upon release from the bone marrow, mature red cells must withstand the high pressure and shear forces in the heart and large arteries and also traverse the small-diameter microcirculatory vessels for 120 days. The ability of the skeleton-bilayer couple to withstand high shear and to deform readily allows normal red cells to perform these tasks. Abnormal red cells with defective membrane skeletons and/or defective coupling between the skeleton and the overlying bilayer fragment spontaneously in the circulation, which leads to the clinical picture of non-immune hemolytic anemia.

CATION AND VOLUME HOMEOSTASIS. The red cell uses protein pumps and channels in its lipid bilayer membrane to control intracellular concentrations of sodium, potassium, and calcium ions and thereby regulate cell volume. Normal intracellular concentrations of Na^+, K^+, and Ca^{2+} are about 10, 100, and 100 nmol/L, respectively. The physiologically most important pumps include the ATP-dependent Na^+/K^+ exchanger, which uses the energy provided by ATP hydrolysis to pump Na^+ outward against its concentration gradient and K^+ inward against its concentration gradient, and the ATP-dependent Ca^{2+} pump, which pumps Ca^{2+} outward against its concentration gradient. The activities of these pumps counteract the small passive leaks of Na^+, K^+, and Ca^{2+} down their concentration gradients through the relatively impermeable lipid bilayer. Pathologic increases in the passive leak rates of these three cations—or decreases in the activities of these two pumps—can have deleterious effects. A net gain of intracellular cations obligates net water

entry and causes cells to swell, whereas a net loss of intracellular cations dehydrates cells. The free flow of water molecules in both directions across the lipid bilayer is mediated by the aquaporin-1 water channel protein. An increase in intracellular Ca^{2+} concentration can be especially harmful by (1) activating a Ca^{2+}-dependent K^+ channel (the Gardos channel) that mediates K^+ efflux and cell dehydration and (2) at very high concentrations, activating a Ca^{2+}-dependent transglutaminase that cross-links membrane proteins and thereby (among other effects) decreases cell deformability.

CELL SHAPE. The biconcave disk shape of normal red cells is maintained by a balance of forces within the membrane skeleton and between the skeleton and the lipid bilayer. These forces are sufficiently robust to allow normal red cells to deform without fragmenting in the normal circulation. Alterations in membrane skeleton integrity, skeleton-bilayer coupling, intracellular cation and water content, transmembrane protein organization, and hemoglobin denaturation and polymerization can all affect red cell morphology. One major determinant of red cell shape is the ratio between the cell's surface area and volume; decreases and increases in this ratio lead to the formation of sphere-shaped (spherocyte) and cup (stomatocyte) or target-shaped red cells, respectively. Irreversible shape change can also be mediated by permanent deformation of the membrane skeleton; orderly plastic deformation causes the formation of elliptical or oval red cells (elliptocytes or ovalocytes), whereas random membrane injury with denatured hemoglobin precipitation on the skeleton and oxidative cross-linking of proteins leads to the formation of spiculated (echinocyte), irreversibly sickled, and other abnormal red cell forms.

ANION EXCHANGE. The red cell membrane plays an important physiologic role in carbon dioxide (CO_2) transport. CO_2 handling is facilitated by red cell enzyme-mediated conversion of this molecule to bicarbonate in the tissues and back to CO_2 for excretion in the lungs. To increase the HCO_3^- carrying capacity of the blood, some of the HCO_3^- is carried in the plasma. Movement of HCO_3^- in and out of red cells is facilitated by the presence of about 1 million anion-exchange proteins (the band 3 protein) in each red cell membrane. Band 3 mediates the passive bidirectional exchange of HCO_3^- for Cl^-; no energy is required for this process. Band 3 therefore serves at least two important roles in red cell membrane structure and function: coupling the membrane skeleton to the overlying lipid bilayer and mediating anion exchange across the membrane.

INTERACTIONS WITH THE SPLEEN: RED CELL SENESCENCE. Most normal red cells are removed from the circulation by the spleen after a 120-day life span. The fenestrations between splenic cords and sinuses provide mechanical stress as red cells squeeze through these openings, whereas the low-oxygen, low-glucose, low-pH environment of the splenic cords places metabolic stress on the cells. The spleen uses two major mechanisms to sequester and remove aged red cells. First, as red cells become less deformable with age, they are less able to traverse the splenic fenestrations. Second, as red cells age, their membranes are progressively decorated with autoantibodies and/or complement proteins that bind to receptors on mononuclear phagocytes in the spleen; these autoantibodies may be directed against clustered and/or proteolytically altered band 3 at the red cell surface.

RED CELL MEMBRANE DISORDERS

Hereditary Spherocytosis

ETIOLOGY AND INCIDENCE. Hereditary spherocytosis is an inherited hemolytic anemia caused by a defect in one of the proteins that couples the red cell membrane skeleton to the overlying lipid bilayer. These proteins include spectrin (either the α- or the β-chain), ankyrin, band 3, and protein 4.2. Some mutations in these proteins have been identified, and others are the subject of current investigations. Many of the mutations defined to date are unique, thus indicating that no one mutation is common. Autosomal dominant, autosomal recessive, new mutations, and non-classic patterns of inheritance have been observed; approximately 75% of families exhibit the autosomal dominant pattern. The incidence of hereditary spherocytosis is about 1 in 5000 among northern European people, although the disease can occur in any population.

PATHOGENESIS. Molecular defects in spectrin, ankyrin, band 3, and protein 4.2 lead to spectrin deficiency as the "final common pathway" that characterizes all red cells with hereditary spherocytosis. This molecular phenotype results either from a primary deficiency of spectrin or, more commonly, from a deficiency of one of the proteins that allows spectrin to bind with high affinity to the overlying lipid bilayer. Spectrin deficiency appears to cause the spherocytic cellular phenotype by weakening "vertical" interactions between the membrane skeleton and the bilayer and thereby leading to "unsupported" areas of lipid that are spontaneously lost as red cells traverse the circulation. Spherocytic red cells are less able than normal cells to squeeze through the fenestrations between splenic cords and sinuses, and the increased metabolic stress placed on the cells in the environment of the cords leads to further membrane loss. Although some hyperchromic microspherocytes eventually escape back into the peripheral circulation, many of these cells are hemolyzed in the spleen (Fig. 164–2).

The discovery that spectrin deficiency is the *sine qua non* of hereditary spherocytic red cells led some to hypothesize that primary defects in spectrin would be found in most cases of hereditary spherocytosis. Surprisingly, mutations in α-spectrin (autosomal recessive hereditary spherocytosis) and β-spectrin (autosomal dominant hereditary spherocytosis) are each present in only about 10% of patients with hereditary spherocytosis. Instead, mutations in ankyrin (autosomal dominant and recessive hereditary spherocytosis; about 40 to 50% of cases) and band 3 (autosomal dominant hereditary spherocytosis; about 20% of cases) are much more common. Mutations in protein 4.2 (autosomal recessive hereditary spherocytosis) are relatively rare except in Japan, where a number of families have been described. The severity of hemolysis correlates with the cellular spectrin content in spherocytic red cells, providing strong evidence in support of the pathogenetic mechanisms described above.

CLINICAL MANIFESTATIONS: GENERAL. The clinical manifestations of hereditary spherocytosis can vary from a clinically insignificant hemolytic state that is fully compensated by increased marrow erythropoiesis to a life-threatening hemolytic state that is dependent on red cell transfusion. This variation in clinical phenotype is a reflection of the variation in the molecular consequences of the mutations in spectrin, ankyrin, band 3, or protein 4.2, all of which result in weakened interaction between the membrane skeleton and the overlying lipid bilayer. In general, an autosomal recessive inheritance pattern is associated with clinically more severe disease whereas an autosomal dominant pattern is associated with a milder phenotype. Although all cases of hereditary spherocytosis are present from birth, the diagnosis can be made at any age. Clinical manifestations common in hereditary spherocytosis include jaundice and splenomegaly (Table 164–1). Approximately 50% of neonates experience marked jaundice that may require exchange transfusion, and some infants may require periodic red cell transfu-

Table 164–1 ■ HEREDITARY SPHEROCYTOSIS

CLINICAL MANIFESTATIONS	LABORATORY FEATURES
Common Manifestations	
Splenomegaly	Anemia, reticulocytosis, spherocytosis on blood smear
Intermittent jaundice from hemolysis and/or biliary obstruction	Elevated MCHC
	Increased osmotic fragility (especially incubated osmotic fragility) test
Aplastic crises	Negative direct antiglobulin (Coombs') test
Good response to splenectomy	
Rare Manifestations	
Leg ulcers	Decrease in red cell membrane protein(s):
Gout	
Spinal cord dysfunction	Spectrin and/or
Extramedullary hematopoietic tumors of the thorax	Ankyrin and/or
	Band 3 and/or
Cardiomyopathy	Protein 4.2

MCHC = mean corpuscular hemoglobin concentration.

sions to maintain an adequate hematocrit. By several months of age, most patients with hereditary spherocytosis achieve a partially compensated hemolytic state characterized by mild to moderate anemia (hemoglobin, 9 to 11.5 g/dL), intermittent jaundice (exacerbated by viral infection), and splenomegaly. Even in patients with fully compensated hemolysis, states associated with splenic enlargement and/or increased splenic blood flow (such as infectious mononucleosis and, occasionally, intense physical activity) may provoke severe hemolysis and anemia. Previously compensated elderly patients with hereditary spherocytosis may experience more severe anemia with aging because of a decline in compensatory bone marrow activity.

COMPLICATIONS. Common clinical complications of hereditary spherocytosis include occasional crises and the formation of bilirubinate gallstones. Hemolytic crisis appears to be caused by the increased activity of the mononuclear phagocyte (reticuloendothelial) system associated with many infections; such crises are typified by a small decrease in the hematocrit that is not clinically significant. Aplastic crisis is most often associated with parvovirus B19 infection (see Chapter 160); such crises may be clinically severe and require prompt red cell transfusion. Fortunately, infection with parvovirus B19 generally produces lifelong immunity, so most patients are subjected to no more than one such crisis in a lifetime. Megaloblastic crisis is caused by a relative lack of folic

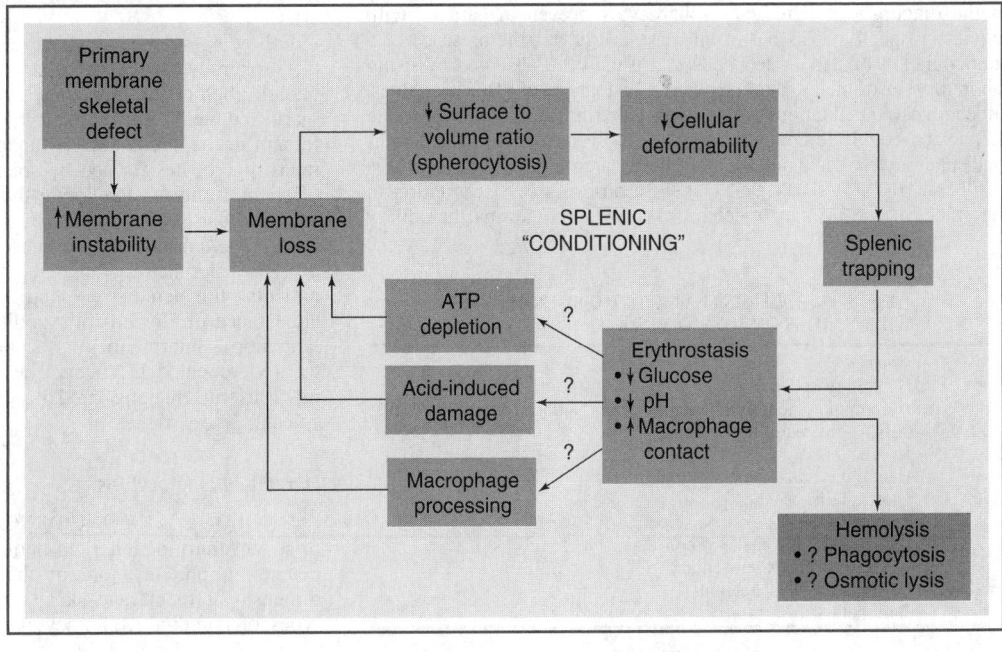

FIGURE 164–2 ■ Model of the pathophysiology of spherocytosis and hemolysis in hereditary spherocytosis.

acid in the diet; because of the increased need for this vitamin during pregnancy, such crises are especially common in pregnant women. The increased generation of bilirubin associated with ongoing hemolysis leads to the formation of bilirubinate gallstones in most untreated teenagers and adults with hereditary spherocytosis. The incidence of this complication increases from about 5% in children 0 to 10 years old, to about 45% in patients aged 11 to 50 years, and to about 65% in older patients. Because a large fraction of bilirubinate gallstones are not radiopaque, abdominal ultrasonography is the most reliable imaging method to detect these stones.

Relatively rare clinical complications of hereditary spherocytosis in adults include gout, rashes, and ulcers of the lower extremities and extramedullary hematopoietic tumors of the thorax. The gout and lower extremity complications usually disappear after splenectomy (see below), but the tumors commonly undergo fatty change after splenectomy and therefore persist on routine chest film. Several families with hereditary spherocytosis and either spinocerebellar degeneration or cardiomyopathy have been described, perhaps suggesting a common genetic basis for these disorders.

DIAGNOSIS. Laboratory features common to all cases of hereditary spherocytosis include an elevated reticulocyte count and the presence of spherocytes on the blood smear (Color Plate 5G). Patients with very mild disease may not be anemic or manifest hyperbilirubinemia, although many patients with hereditary spherocytosis do exhibit mild to moderate anemia and an elevated indirect bilirubin level. The differential diagnosis of spherocytosis includes a number of clinical entities (Table 164–2), but the most common other clinical state characterized by spherocytosis—autoimmune hemolytic anemia—can be readily distinguished from hereditary spherocytosis by the direct antiglobulin (Coombs') test. The laboratory test most commonly used to confirm the presence of spherocytosis is the osmotic fragility test, which measures the ability of red cells to withstand swelling in solutions of decreasing osmotic strength. Because spherocytes have a decreased ratio of surface area to volume, these cells are less able to swell in a hypotonic environment than normal discocytes are. Thus populations of red cells containing a significant proportion of spherocytes exhibit increased osmotic fragility when compared with normal red cell populations. In some cases of mild hereditary spherocytosis, however, neither striking spherocytosis on the blood smear nor an abnormal osmotic fragility test is apparent. The most reliable test in this situation is the incubated osmotic fragility test, in which red cells are metabolically stressed by incubation in the absence of glucose for 24 hours. Whereas normal red cells can withstand this treatment without significant membrane damage, hereditary spherocytic red cells shed bilayer lipids under these conditions and become less able to remain intact in a hypotonic environment. Finally, because hereditary spherocytic red cells tend to be dehydrated, an elevated mean cell hemoglobin concentration (MCHC) can be a helpful clue in the diagnosis of hereditary spherocytosis; even in patients with hereditary spherocytosis but no increase in MCHC, the presence of a subpopulation of dehydrated cells can usually be observed by using laboratory instruments that provide a histogram of MCHC values. Biochemical quantitation of spectrin, ankyrin, band 3, and protein 4.2, which could theoretically yield the most specific test for hereditary spherocytosis, is available only in research laboratories.

TREATMENT AND PROGNOSIS. Because red cell destruction in the spleen is the primary mechanism by which abnormal hereditary

Table 164–2 ■ DISEASES CHARACTERIZED BY PROMINENT SPHEROCYTOSIS ON THE BLOOD SMEAR

Common
Hereditary spherocytosis
Autoimmune hemolytic anemia (warm antibody type)
ABO incompatibility (neonates)
Uncommon to Rare
Hemolytic transfusion reaction
Clostridial sepsis
Severe burn
Spider, bee, and snake venom
Acute red cell oxidant injury
Severe hypophosphatemia
Bartonellosis

spherocytic red cells are prematurely removed from the circulation, splenectomy is highly effective in restoring a normal hematocrit and a near-normal reticulocyte count (1 to 3%) to nearly all patients with hereditary spherocytosis. In patients with the most severe of the disease, a mild anemia may remain after splenectomy; however, this anemia represents a state of compensated hemolysis rather than the transfusion dependence that characterizes such patients pre-splenectomy. In all patients with hereditary spherocytosis, the benefits of splenectomy must be weighed against its risks. The major risks include bacterial sepsis, often caused by pneumococcal, meningococcal, or *Haemophilus influenzae* B bacteria, and mesenteric or portal venous occlusion. The risk of post-splenectomy sepsis is so great in children younger than 3 to 5 years that splenectomy should be avoided in such patients even with the necessity of transfusion dependence. One recent series of 226 adult patients with hereditary spherocytosis estimated the lifetime risk of fulminant post-splenectomy sepsis to be about 2%. After splenectomy, a small but significant increase in the risk of ischemic heart disease has also been reported.

Most hematologists recommend splenectomy for children with severe hereditary spherocytosis, defined as a hemoglobin concentration less than 8 g/dL and a reticulocyte count greater than 10%, and for children with moderate disease (hemoglobin, 8 to 11 g/dL; reticulocyte count, 8 to 10%) if the degree of anemia compromises physical activity. In adults with moderate hereditary spherocytosis, additional indications for splenectomy include a degree of anemia that compromises oxygen delivery to vital organs, the development of extramedullary hematopoietic tumors, and the occurrence of bilirubinate gallstones, which could predispose to cholecystitis and biliary obstruction. Splenectomy is generally deferred in patients with mild hereditary spherocytosis (hemoglobin greater than 11 g/dL; reticulocyte count less than 8%).

Several European groups have recently advocated the use of subtotal splenectomy as a compromise operation that ameliorates most of the extravascular hemolysis associated with splenic function while retaining some immune and phagocytic activity of the normal spleen. In 40 children treated with this operation, the success rate in relieving hemolysis over a 1- to 11-year follow-up period was adequate (although less than that achieved with total splenectomy), and the rate of complications has been low; however, data are currently too limited to recommend this procedure in the general hereditary spherocytosis population.

All patients undergoing splenectomy should receive polyvalent pneumococcal vaccine, preferably several weeks before the operation; children should also receive meningococcal and *H. influenzae* B vaccines. In the first several years after splenectomy, many patients are treated with prophylactic oral penicillin to protect against pneumococcal sepsis, although the emergence of penicillin-resistant pneumococci may force a change in this practice over the coming years. All patients with hereditary spherocytosis should be given 1 mg folate as a daily supplement to prevent megaloblastic crisis.

Following splenectomy, the blood smear in patients with hereditary spherocytosis acquires several characteristic alterations. Howell-Jolly bodies, acanthocytes, target cells, and siderocytes normally mark red cells for removal by the spleen, but such cells now remain in the circulation. Although spherocytes are still present, the microspherocytes formed by splenic conditioning disappear. Failure of splenectomy to ameliorate the degree of hemolysis in hereditary spherocytosis, either immediately after the operation or many years later, is often due to the presence of an accessory spleen. The presence of this structure, which is found in about 15 to 20% of patients with hereditary spherocytosis, can be revealed by the disappearance of Howell-Jolly bodies from the blood smear and/or by laboratory abnormalities associated with hemolysis such as an increased reticulocyte count. The radionuclide liver-spleen scan can be a useful imaging modality when searching for an accessory spleen.

Hereditary Elliptocytosis

ETIOLOGY AND INCIDENCE. Hereditary elliptocytosis comprises a family of inherited hemolytic anemias caused primarily by defects in one or more of the proteins that make up the two-dimensional membrane skeletal network. The four clinical phenotypes of hereditary elliptocytosis appear to be caused by different sets of molecular defects. Mild hereditary elliptocytosis and hereditary pyropoikilocytosis arise most often from α- and/or β-spectrin chain defects that affect the ability of spectrin heterodimers to self-associate, and from protein 4.1 defects that affect the strength of binding in the ternary spectrin–actin–protein 4.1 complex. Spherocytic hereditary elliptocytosis can be caused by defects in the β-chain of spectrin that may affect spectrin-ankyrin binding as well as spectrin self-association; other mutations are the subject of current investigation. In general, mild hereditary elliptocytosis and spherocytic hereditary elliptocytosis are inherited as autosomal dominant traits, and hereditary pyropoikilocytosis is inherited in an autosomal recessive pattern. The incidence of mild hereditary elliptocytosis is about 1 in 2500 among northern Europeans and as common as 1 in 150 in some areas of Africa, although the disease can occur in any population. Hereditary pyropoikilocytosis and spherocytic hereditary elliptocytosis are considerably more rare. Southeast Asian ovalocytosis (SAO) is caused by a specific deletion in band 3 that allows the mutant protein to form linear aggregates in the plane of the lipid bilayer. The incidence of this autosomal dominant disorder is as common as 1 in 3 among some lowland aboriginal populations of Indonesia, Malaysia, Melanesia, and the Philippines, although SAO is rare in other areas of the world.

PATHOGENESIS. In mild hereditary elliptocytosis, a molecular defect near the "head" region of the spectrin heterodimer (i.e., a mutation near the N-terminus of α-spectrin or the C-terminus of β-spectrin) leads to weakening of the "horizontal" interactions that give the red cell membrane skeleton its properties of strength and deformability. Heterozygous deficiency of protein 4.1—or a mutation that prevents formation of the spectrin–actin–protein 4.1 ternary complex at the "tail" region of the spectrin heterodimer—has a similar mechanical effect. In both cases, red cells are released from the bone marrow with a normal discocytic shape, but the membrane skeletons (and consequently, the red cells themselves) undergo plastic deformation to a permanent elliptocytic shape as the cells traverse the microcirculation. Because the "vertical" interactions that couple the membrane skeleton to the overlying lipid bilayer remain intact in these cells, membrane loss does not occur, and the cells may have a relatively normal lifetime in the circulation. Hereditary pyropoikilocytosis, in contrast, results from either a homozygous or a compound heterozygous defect in spectrin (typically, α-spectrin) or protein 4.1. In addition to the defects described above, coinheritance of an α-spectrin mutation with the spectrin α^LELY polymorphism can cause the hereditary pyropoikilocytosis phenotype. In spectrin α^LELY, α-spectrin mRNA splicing is altered such that the resulting protein chains lose the ability to pair with β-spectrin. Because α-spectrin is synthesized in excess of β-spectrin in normal erythropoiesis, the spectrin α^LELY polymorphism is silent by itself. When paired in *trans* with an α-spectrin coding region mutation, however, the polymorphism causes the majority of spectrin heterodimers at the membrane to carry the hereditary elliptocytosis defect, which leads to the much more severe hereditary pyropoikilocytosis phenotype.

In spherocytic hereditary elliptocytosis, the molecular defect in the spectrin β-chain appears to affect both "horizontal" interactions at the spectrin self-association site and "vertical" interactions at the spectrin-ankyrin binding site. This combined defect results in features of both hereditary elliptocytosis (because of the "horizontal" interaction defect) and hereditary spherocytosis (because of the "vertical" interaction defect). The linear aggregates of mutant band 3 protein in SAO red cells are thought to cause extreme rigidification of the membrane by preventing the local expansions and contractions of the membrane skeletal network that are responsible for membrane deformability. Membrane rigidity is likely to be the mechanism by which SAO red cells resist invasion by malaria parasites, which accounts for the high prevalence of this variant in certain areas of Southeast Asia. Interestingly, unlike the non-deformable spherocytes found in hereditary spherocytosis and autoimmune hemolytic anemias, the rigid SAO red cells are not removed prematurely from the circulation. The mechanisms by which SAO cells survive normally in the circulation remain to be elucidated. The SAO mutation must have some deleterious effect on red cell membrane structure and function, however, because the homozygous state appears to be lethal.

CLINICAL MANIFESTATIONS AND DIAGNOSIS. The great majority of individuals with mild hereditary elliptocytosis are hetero-

zygous carriers of a dominantly inherited molecular and cellular defect that is clinically insignificant. These individuals have no anemia, little or no hemolysis (reticulocyte count, 1 to 3%), and no splenomegaly. Diagnosis is based on the presence of prominent elliptocytosis (often greater than 40%) on the blood smear, a normal osmotic fragility test, and a positive family pedigree. Individuals who inherit a mild α-spectrin defect in *trans* with spectrin α^LELY may exhibit mild chronic hemolysis and some fragmented red cells on the blood smear. Mild hereditary elliptocytosis can be associated with significant hemolysis in patients in whom splenic enlargement develops from, for example, viral infection or portal hypertension. Neonates with mild hereditary elliptocytosis often exhibit a syndrome, called transient infantile poikilocytosis, characterized by a moderately severe hemolytic anemia for the initial 6 to 12 months of life. The increased hemolysis in the neonatal and early infant period appears to result from the increase in intracellular 2,3-diphosphoglycerate (2,3-DPG) concentration that is present in fetal red cells. Elevated levels of this normal metabolite weaken the ternary spectrin–actin–protein 4.1 binding interaction and thereby exacerbate the spectrin self-association defect caused by the mild hereditary elliptocytosis mutation. As fetal red cells are lost from the circulation, the intracellular 2,3-DPG concentration falls and the clinical condition spontaneously reverts to that of mild hereditary elliptocytosis.

Hereditary pyropoikilocytosis is a recessively inherited disorder that is clinically manifested by a severe (sometimes life-threatening) hemolytic anemia in which the blood smear contains bizarre poikilocytes and red cell fragments. The mean cell volume is markedly decreased (45 to 75 fL), and because spectrin deficiency and spherocytosis are often secondary consequences of the combined molecular defects, osmotic fragility is increased. The name is derived from the property of hereditary pyropoikilocytosis red cells to fragment at 45 to 46°C rather than the normal 49°C; this abnormal heat sensitivity is most often due to a lowering of the temperature at which the mutant spectrin chains denature. As implied by the name, spherocytic hereditary elliptocytosis has clinical and diagnostic features of both hereditary spherocytosis and mild hereditary elliptocytosis. Patients manifest mild to moderate hemolytic anemia with splenomegaly and intermittent jaundice, the blood smear contains rounded elliptocytes and sometimes spherocytes, and osmotic fragility is increased. In contrast, individuals with the SAO mutation are clinically normal, with little to no anemia or hemolysis; the blood smear shows characteristic rounded elliptocytes that often exhibit a transverse bar dividing the central clear area.

TREATMENT AND PROGNOSIS. Mild hereditary elliptocytosis and SAO are clinically insignificant variants that require no treatment and have no effect on lifespan (other than the beneficial protection against malaria afforded to SAO individuals). Spherocytic hereditary elliptocytosis should be treated like hereditary spherocytosis, with the considerations for and against splenectomy as noted above. Virtually all patients with hereditary pyropoikilocytosis require splenectomy, which ameliorates but does not completely cure the hemolytic anemia. As in treating patients with moderate to severe hereditary spherocytosis, it is important to defer splenectomy until 3 to 5 years of age if possible, especially because of the possibility that a severe poikilocytic anemia in the neonatal and infant period could represent transient infantile poikilocytosis rather than true hereditary pyropoikilocytosis.

Hereditary Defects in Membrane Permeability

HEREDITARY XEROCYTOSIS. The hallmark of this rare autosomal dominant disorder is an alteration in red cell membrane cation permeability that leads to a net loss of intracellular cations and water and to cell dehydration. The molecular defect responsible for this phenotype remains to be elucidated. The dehydrated red cells appear on the blood smear as target cells and/or spiculated acanthocytes, and the increased MCHC leads to relatively non-deformable cells that can be sequestered and removed by the spleen. The differential diagnosis of dehydrated red cells also includes the much more common sickle cell syndromes, hereditary spherocytosis, and hemoglobin C disease.

HEREDITARY STOMATOCYTOSIS. This rare autosomal dominant disorder appears to be due to an inherited defect in Na^+ permeability that leads to a net influx of Na^+ and water and to cell swelling. Several molecular defects are probably responsible for this phenotype because some families with this disorder experience severe hemolytic anemia whereas others have clinically mild disease. The swollen red cells appear on the blood smear to have a "mouth"-like invagination in the membrane and are therefore called stomatocytes. The differential diagnosis of stomatocytosis also includes the much more common acquired effects of acute alcoholism and/or liver disease. Patients with the severe form of hereditary stomatocytosis often respond well to splenectomy.

NORMAL RED CELL METABOLISM

Glycolysis

Normal mature red cells have lost the cellular machinery responsible for oxidative phosphorylation, and the metabolism in these cells is almost entirely anaerobic. The major red cell energy source is glucose, which is metabolized primarily by the glycolytic pathway (also called the Embden-Meyerhof pathway) and secondarily by the pentose phosphate pathway (also called the hexose monophosphate shunt) (Fig. 164–3). The glycolytic pathway converts 90 to 95% of the metabolized glucose in red cells to lactate, in the process generating 2 mol of ATP per mole of glucose consumed. Although this rate of ATP generation is inefficient when compared with that provided in other cells by the tricarboxylic acid cycle, it is sufficient in normal red cells to renew 150 to 200% of the total red cell ATP per hour. ATP is an essential energy source that is used by cation pumps and channels, by protein kinases, and by enzymes that regulate glycolysis, glutathione synthesis, and nucleotide salvage in red cells to maintain homeostasis. Two important metabolic cofactors generated in the glycolytic pathway are reduced nicotinamide adenine dinucleotide (NADH) and 2,3-DPG. NADH is an essential cofactor for the enzyme methemoglobin reductase, which maintains heme iron in the ferrous (Fe^{2+}) state, necessary for the ligation of molecular oxygen by hemoglobin. 2,3-DPG, generated by the Rapoport-Luebering shunt, regulates the affinity of hemoglobin for oxygen and thereby increases oxygen delivery to tissues.

Pentose Phosphate Pathway and Glutathione Metabolism

The pentose phosphate pathway handles 5 to 10% of metabolized glucose in normal red cells, in the process generating 2 mol of reduced nicotinamide adenine dinucleotide phosphate (NADPH) for each mole of glucose metabolized. NADPH is an essential cofactor for the enzyme glutathione reductase, which maintains glutathione in the reduced state necessary for detoxification of toxic oxygen products such as superoxide anion (O_2^-), hydrogen peroxide (H_2O_2), and hydroxyl radical ($OH\cdot$). Normal red cells are continually subjected to these products as a result of intracellular heme oxidation. In addition, certain drugs can markedly enhance oxidant generation by red cells, and many infections can induce oxidant generation by phagocytic cells in the circulation. In the absence of reduced glutathione, toxic oxygen products can damage red cell lipids and proteins and result in hemolysis. Under conditions of oxidative stress, the pentose phosphate pathway can increase in activity to use 50% or more of the available glucose. This increase in activity is stimulated by NADP and inhibited by NADPH, thereby tightly coupling intracellular antioxidant supply and demand.

Glutathione is a tripeptide that is synthesized in relatively high amounts (2-mmol/L steady-state concentration) from the amino acids cysteine, glutamic acid, and glycine by mature red cells. Two enzymes catalyze this synthetic pathway, and two other enzymes couple glutathione metabolism to NADPH oxidation (see Fig. 164–3).

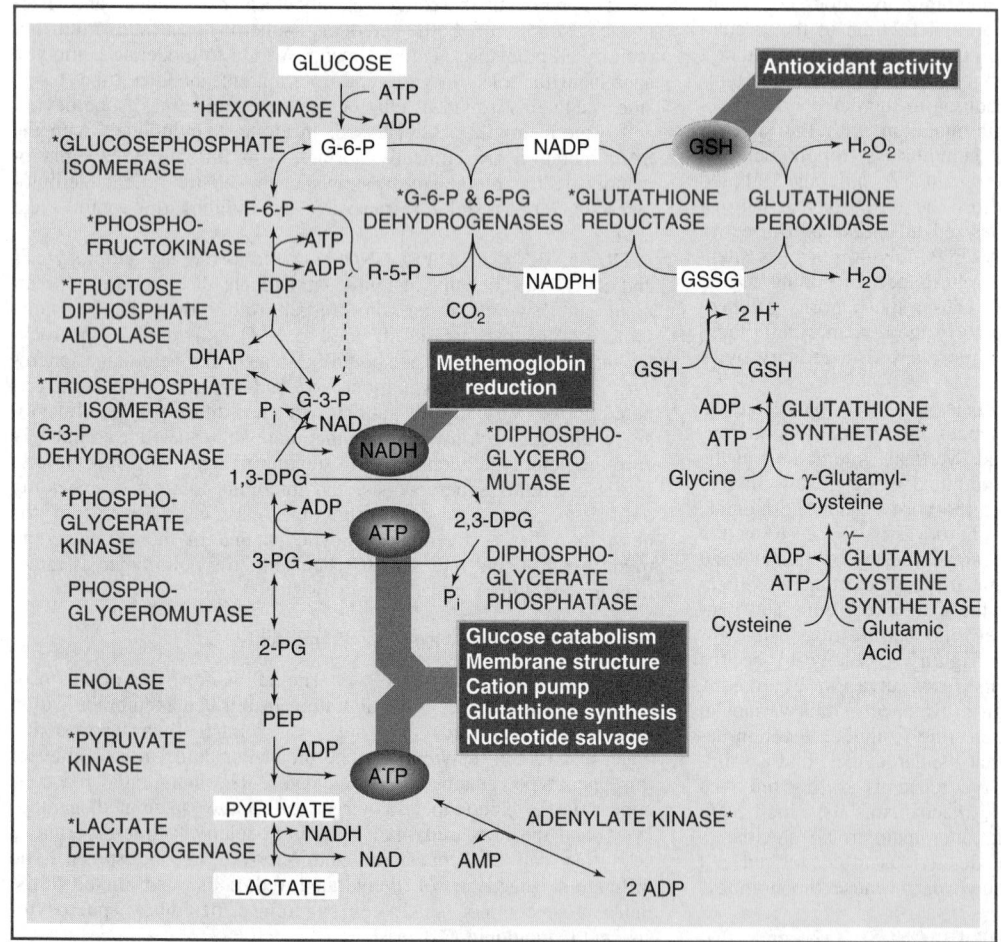

FIGURE 164–3 ■ Biochemical glycolysis, pentose phosphate, and glutathione pathways in human red cell metabolism. Asterisks denote enzymes that have been shown to be deficient in hereditary metabolic defects. ATP = adenosine triphosphate; ADP = adenosine diphosphate; G-6-P = glucose-6-phosphate; NADP = nicotinamide-adenine dinucleotide phosphate; GSH = reduced glutathionine; 6-PG = 6 phosphogluconate; FDP = fructose 1,6-diphosphate; R-5-P = ribose-5-phosphate; NADPH = reduced NADP; GSSG = oxidized glutathionine; DHAP = dihydroxyacetone phosphate; G-3-P = glyceraldehyde-3-phosphate; 1,3-DPG = 1,3-diphosphoglycerate; 3-PG = 3-phosphoglycerate; PEP = phosphoenolpyruvate; AMP = adenosine monophosphate. (From Valentine WN: Hemolytic anemia and inborn errors of metabolism. Blood 54:549, 1979.)

Defects in the Pentose Phosphate Pathway and Glutathione Metabolism

GLUCOSE-6-PHOSPHATE DEHYDROGENASE DEFICIENCY. ETIOLOGY AND INCIDENCE. Glucose-6-phosphate dehydrogenase (G6PD) deficiency, which is by far the most common enzyme defect associated with hereditary hemolytic anemia, affects millions of individuals from all races around the world, and hundreds of G6PD variants have been described. The most common normal variants of the enzyme are called G6PD^B or Gd^B, found in 99% of whites and about 70% of blacks, and Gd^{A+}, found in about 20% of blacks. The most common abnormal variants of the enzyme are called Gd^{A-}, found in about 10% of American blacks and a number of black African populations, and Gd^{Med}, found in Mediterranean (Arabs, Greeks, Italians, Sephardic Jews, and others), Indian, and Southeast Asian populations. Both Gd^{A-} and Gd^{Med} represent mutant enzymes that differ from the respective normal variants by a single amino acid. The prevalence of G6PD deficiency in African black, Mediterranean, Indian, and Southeast Asian populations is thought to derive from the relative protection afforded G6PD heterozygotes against *Plasmodium falciparum* malaria. The electrophoretic mobility of the Gd^B and Gd^{Med} enzymes is identical, and that of the Gd^{A+} and Gd^{A-} isoforms is also identical; however, the overall catalytic activity of the abnormal variants is markedly less than that of the normal variants (see below).

Because the G6PD gene is located on the X chromosome, the inheritance pattern of G6PD deficiency is sex linked. Thus whereas males have either a normal or an abnormal G6PD variant, females can exhibit either homozygous or heterozygous G6PD deficiency. Although relatively rare, homozygous G6PD deficiency in females is phenotypically identical to hemizygous deficiency in males. Even in female heterozygotes, each individual red cell is either normal or abnormal (i.e., there is no intermediate state) because only one X chromosome is active in each somatic cell (according to the Lyon hypothesis). The overall effect of G6PD deficiency in female heterozygotes may be mild, moderate, or severe, depending on the proportion of red cells in which the abnormal G6PD enzyme is expressed.

PATHOGENESIS. The primary metabolic consequence of G6PD deficiency is the diminished ability of the variant enzyme to generate sufficient NADPH to keep up with the requirement for reduced glutathione in a red cell population stressed by oxidizing agents. Depletion of cellular glutathione allows toxic oxygen products to damage red cell macromolecules, including hemoglobin, band 3, spectrin, membrane lipids, and other molecules. Oxidation of the heme iron of hemoglobin generates methemoglobin, which is incapable of ligating molecular oxygen. Oxidative denaturation of the globin chain produces intracellular hemoglobin precipitates called Heinz bodies that localize to the inner surface of the red cell membrane, probably through specific binding interactions between denatured hemoglobin and the cytoplasmic domain of band 3. Heinz bodies cause further oxidative damage to the membrane manifested by clustering of band 3 proteins into large aggregates, which can be recognized by low-affinity autoantibodies and thereby targeted for removal by the mononuclear phagocyte system, and by increasing membrane cation permeability, which is accompanied by changes in cell hydration and deformability. Oxidative cross-linking of spectrin is likely to contribute to the decreased deformability of oxidatively stressed G6PD-deficient red cells, and peroxidation of membrane lipids may be a major contributing factor in the intravascular hemolysis that accompanies acute hemolytic episodes.

Normal and abnormal G6PD variants differ in both the stability and the catalytic activity of the various enzymes. Normal Gd^B and Gd^{A+} enzymes are slowly degraded over the lifetime of a normal red cell in vivo such that intracellular G6PD activity falls to half its original value in about 60 days. This slow decline in enzyme activity over time is clinically inconsequential because even the oldest normal red cells in the circulation retain sufficient G6PD activity to maintain intracellular reduced glutathione levels and to withstand nearly all oxidant stresses (Fig. 164–4). The catalytic activity of the Gd^{A-} variant is mildly reduced when compared with the normal enzyme, but the major defect in Gd^{A-} red cells is the more rapid degradation of Gd^{A-} in comparison with the normal en-

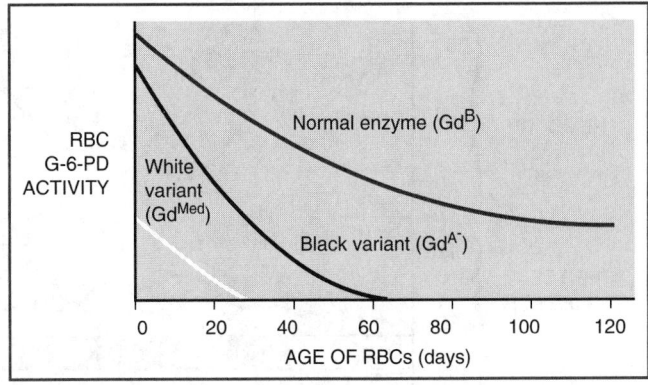

FIGURE 164–4 ■ Decline in red cell glucose-6-phosphate dehydrogenase (G6PD) activity as a function of cell age. Shown are curves for the normal Gd^B enzyme and for the unstable Gd^{A-} and Gd^{Med} variants. Note that although the activity of the normal enzyme declines as red cells age, even the oldest cells have a sufficient level of activity to provide protection against oxidative damage and hemolysis. In contrast, very few Gd^{Med} red cells have sufficient enzyme activity to prevent such damage, whereas a substantial fraction of young Gd^{A-} red cells are so protected. Under oxidative stress, then, nearly all Gd^{Med} cells but only the oldest Gd^{A-} cells are susceptible to hemolysis. Assuming a normally functioning bone marrow, individuals with Gd^{A-} red cells can compensate by increasing the reticulocyte count and thereby populating the red cell pool with younger cells. In this way, G6PD screening assays may be falsely negative in Gd^{A-} males immediately after a hemolytic episode. (Adapted from Lux SE: Hemolytic anemias. Metabolic defects. *In* Beck WS (ed): Hematology, 4th ed. Cambridge, MA, MIT Press, 1985, p 223.)

zyme such that G6PD activity falls to half its original value in only 13 days. Thus young Gd^{A-} red cells are capable of withstanding oxidant stresses, whereas old Gd^{A-} red cells are not. This cellular heterogeneity allows a substantial fraction of Gd^{A-} red cells to survive even severe oxidant stress, and the acute hemolytic episode is therefore self-limited and usually not life threatening. In contrast, both the catalytic activity and the stability of Gd^{Med} are much less than those of either the normal enzymes or Gd^{A-}; this feature renders nearly all Gd^{Med} red cells susceptible to oxidant-induced hemolysis and results in potentially life-threatening acute hemolytic episodes. Chronic ongoing hemolysis is not observed even in Gd^{Med} red cells in vivo, thus suggesting that endogenous oxidant activity must be low in the absence of oxidant stresses such as drugs and infections.

In a Gd^{A-} individual treated with an oxidant drug, the acute hemolytic episode occurs immediately after initiation of drug therapy, as indicated by progressive anemia, hemoglobinuria, and reticulocytosis (Fig. 164–5); during this phase, the older red cells with low G6PD activity are hemolyzing. Despite continuation of the offending drug, however, the hemolysis spontaneously abates, red cell survival improves, and the hematocrit increases; during this phase, the bone marrow is compensating for the acute hemolytic episode by increasing its production of young Gd^{A-} red cells, which have sufficient G6PD activity to withstand the ongoing oxidant stress. Although the individual now appears to be resistant to drug-induced hemolysis, this "resistance" actually results from increased bone marrow erythropoiesis, which compensates for the ongoing hemolysis. The individual's continuing vulnerability to the effects of the drug are unmasked by withdrawing use of the drug for several months to allow the rate of red cell production by the bone marrow to fall to its original value; during this phase, the older red cells are again allowed to survive, and the red cell population is rendered sensitive to drug-induced hemolysis.

CLINICAL MANIFESTATIONS. Except in a few rare cases (see below), the clinical manifestations of G6PD deficiency occur only under conditions of oxidant stress. In the absence of such stress, individuals with the Gd^{A-} and Gd^{Med} variants have a normal blood smear and no hemolysis. In the presence of such stress, individuals with G6PD deficiency manifest hemolysis that can range from a chronic low-level hemolytic state, with a modest (3 to 4 g/dL) de-

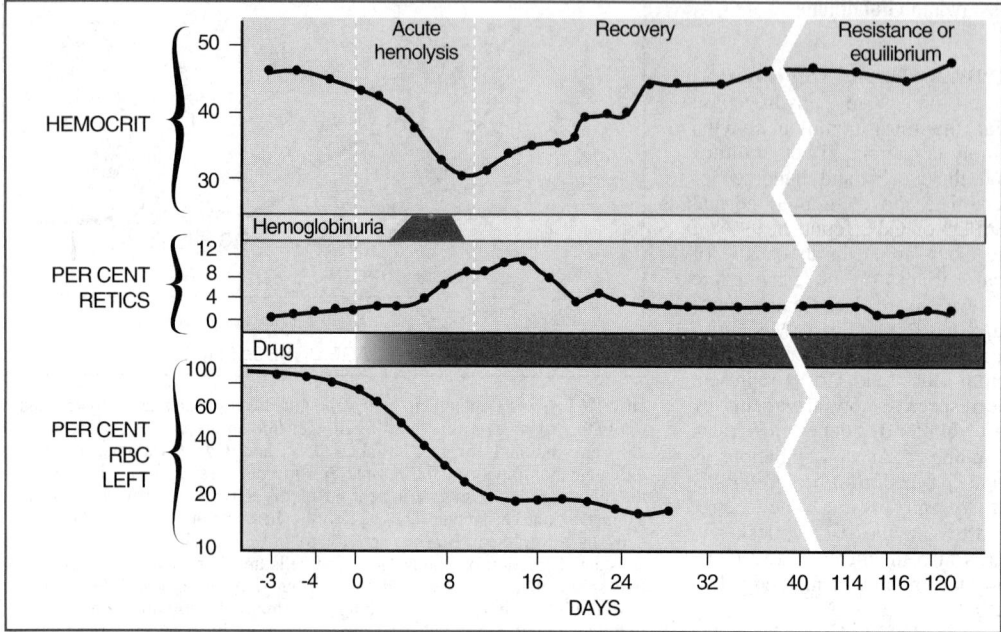

FIGURE 164–5 ■ Time course of primaquine-induced hemolysis in an individual with Gd^A- glucose-6-phosphate dehydrogenase (G6PD) deficiency. Drug was administered from day 0 through day 120. Note that hemolytic anemia, hemoglobinuria, and reticulocytosis develop shortly after starting the drug, but that red cell survival stabilizes and hemolysis abates shortly thereafter because of repopulation of the red cell pool with young cells that have sufficient G6PD activity to protect against oxidative damage and hemolysis. (Modified from Alving AS: Bull World Health Organ 22:621, 1960.)

crease in hemoglobin concentration and a modest increase in the reticulocyte count, to an acute episode of intravascular hemolysis characterized by anemia, hemoglobinemia, hemoglobinuria, hyperbilirubinemia, and jaundice. Severe hemolytic episodes can lead to symptoms of acute anemia such as chest pain, dyspnea, palpitations, dizziness, and headache; to acute abdominal and back pain; and to hemoglobin-induced renal tubular necrosis and renal failure. Changes in the blood smear include the appearance of Heinz bodies (visualized with supravital stains), bite cells (cells with small localized membrane invaginations, probably caused by splenic removal of Heinz bodies at the invagination sites), and blister cells (cells with a hemoglobin-free area adjacent to the membrane) (Table 164–3).

Hemolysis in the setting of G6PD deficiency is most often caused by acute infection, in which oxidant molecules are liberated in large amounts by granulocytes and mononuclear phagocytes. Oxidant drugs represent the other major category of oxidant stress that can lead to acute and/or chronic hemolysis (Table 164–4). Ingestion of fava beans (Italian broad beans) can also cause acute hemolysis in some patients with Gd^Med, probably because of the presence of high levels of oxidant pyrimidine analogues in the beans. Many neonates with G6PD deficiency manifest jaundice at 1 to 4 days of age; although this complication can occasionally require exchange transfusion, it is usually managed successfully with phototherapy. A few rare patients with extremely unstable and/or low-activity G6PD variants have chronic ongoing hemolysis in the absence of oxidant stress.

DIAGNOSIS. The most widely used screening tests for G6PD deficiency rely on a change in NADPH-induced dye decolorization or in methylene blue–mediated methemoglobin reduction to detect a decrease in enzyme activity. These tests suffer from low sensitivity, however, because 30 to 40% of the cells in the sample must be deficient for the abnormal state to be detected and most if not all of the deficient cells may be hemolyzed (especially in Gd^A- individuals) following an acute oxidant stress. More sensitive than these screening tests is the specific enzyme assay, which relies on a direct measurement of NADPH generation; however, even this assay requires that 20 to 30% of the cells be deficient to yield an abnormal result, although careful comparison between the activity of G6PD and that of other age-dependent enzymes in the sample may allow the diagnosis to be made immediately after an acute hemolytic episode. The most sensitive test for G6PD deficiency is the G6PD-tetrazolium cytochemical test, which requires that only 1 to 5% of the cells be deficient to discriminate an abnormal result; this test is capable of not only making the diagnosis after a hemolytic episode but also detecting the enzyme deficiency in female heterozygotes.

TREATMENT AND PROGNOSIS. Because all but a few rare individuals with G6PD deficiency are hematologically normal in the absence of an exogenous oxidant stress, no treatment is required for the deficiency itself. Mild to moderate episodes of acute hemolysis can often be managed by removal of the offending drug or by treatment of the concurrent infection. Severe hemolytic episodes in individuals with Gd^Med and other unstable G6PD variants may require red cell transfusions to alleviate the signs and symptoms of acute anemia, as well as measures designed to protect against the potential renal complications of hemoglobinuria.

DEFECTS IN GLUTATHIONE METABOLISM. Deficiencies in all of the enzymes responsible for glutathione synthesis and metabolism have been described (see Fig. 164–3). Red cells deficient in either γ-glutamylcysteine synthetase or glutathione synthetase, the two enzymes that catalyze glutathione synthesis, have abnormally low levels of glutathione and are sensitive to drug- and infection-induced oxidant hemolysis. Deficiencies of these two enzymes are rare, and the clinical syndromes are similar to G6PD deficiency. Inherited defects in glutathione reductase are also rare; the clinical consequence of this deficiency is uncertain, however, because no case of glutathione reductase–associated hemolysis has been care-

Table 164–3 ■ COMMON FORMS OF GLUCOSE-6-PHOSPHATE DEHYDROGENASE

FEATURE	Gd^A-	Gd^Med
Freqeuncy	Common in African populations	Common in Mediterranean populations
Chronic hemolysis	None	None
Degree of acute hemolysis	Moderate	Severe
Abnormal G6PD activity	Old red cells	All red cells
Hemolysis with		
Drugs	Unusual	Common
Infection	Common	Common
Need for transfusions	Rare	Sometimes

Table 164–4 ■ DRUGS THAT COMMONLY CAUSE HEMOLYSIS IN GLUCOSE-6-PHOSPHATE DEHYDROGENASE DEFICIENCY*

Sulfonamides and Sulfones	*Antimalarials*
Sulfisoxazole (Gantrisin)	**Primaquine§**
Trimethoprim-sulfamethoxazole (Septra)	**Pamaquine****
Salicylazosulfapyridine (Azulfidine, sulfasalazine)	*Anthelmintics*
Sulfanilamide	**β-Naphthol**
Sulfapyridine	**Stibophen**
Sulfadimidine	**Niridazole**
Sulfacetamide (albucid)	*Analgesics‡*
Diaminodiphenylsulfone (dapsone)†	Acetylsalicylic acid (aspirin) (can give moderate doses)
Sulfoxone†	Acetophenetidin (phenacetin)
Glucosulfone sodium (Promin)	*Miscellaneous*
Other Antibacterials	**Probenecid**
Nitrofurans	**Vitamin K analogues** (1 mg menaphthone can be given to infants)
⎯ **Nitrofurantoin (Furadantin)**	**Dimercaprol (BAL)**
⎯ **Nitrofurazone (Furacin)**	Mepacrine (quinacrine HCl)
⎯ **Furazolidone**	**Methylene blue**
Chloramphenicol	**Toluidine blue**
p-Aminosalicylic acid	**Naphthalene (mothballs)†**
Nalidixic acid‡	

*Persons with all forms of G6PD deficiency should avoid the drugs listed in bold print; G6PD-deficient persons of Mediterranean, Middle Eastern, and Asian origin should avoid the drugs listed in bold and plain print.
†These drugs or chemicals may cause hemolysis in normal persons if given in large doses.
‡This drug applies only to individuals with Gd^{A-}.
§Persons with Gd^{A-} may take this drug at reduced dosage (15 mg/day or 45 mg twice weekly) under surveillance.
**Chloroquine may be used under surveillance when required for prophylaxis or treatment of malaria.
‡‡Acetaminophen (paracetamol) is a safe alternative.
Adapted from WHO Working Group: Glucose-6-phosphate dehydrogenase deficiency. Bull World Health Organ 67:601, 1989.

fully documented. Deficiencies in glutathione peroxidase are relatively common, but this disorder appears not to be associated with hemolytic anemia by virtue of the ability of glutathione to reduce hydrogen peroxide by a non-enzymatic as well as an enzymatic route.

Defects in Glycolysis

PYRUVATE KINASE DEFICIENCY. ETIOLOGY AND INCIDENCE. Pyruvate kinase deficiency, which is the most common hereditary defect in the glycolytic pathway, affects hundreds to thousands of individuals worldwide. The disease is inherited in an autosomal recessive pattern; homozygotes manifest clinically significant hemolytic anemia, whereas heterozygote carriers are phenotypically normal.

PATHOGENESIS. Hemolysis in pyruvate kinase deficiency is thought to result from an intracellular deficiency of ATP, which leads to alterations in many of the biochemical pathways responsible for cellular homeostasis (see Fig. 164–3). These inherent biochemical abnormalities are magnified in the stressful environment of the splenic cords. Depending on the level of residual enzyme activity, the degree of hemolysis can range from mild (compensated hemolysis without anemia) to severe (red cell transfusion dependent). One factor that may mitigate the deleterious effects of pyruvate kinase deficiency on ATP generation is the two- to threefold increase in 2,3-DPG that results from the distal block in the glycolytic pathway (see below).

CLINICAL MANIFESTATIONS. Pyruvate kinase deficiency, unlike G6PD deficiency, results in a chronic hemolytic anemia that is not affected by drugs or other oxidant-producing states. Splenomegaly is a common feature of the disorder, probably because the ATP-deficient red cells are not capable of rapidly traversing the splenic fenestrations. The clinical sequelae of hemolytic anemia in pyruvate kinase deficiency are often milder than those seen in other conditions with the same degree of anemia, perhaps because the elevated levels of 2,3-DPG in pyruvate kinase–deficient red cells permit more efficient delivery of oxygen to the tissues for the same concentration of hemoglobin in the blood.

DIAGNOSIS. Pyruvate kinase deficiency is most conveniently diagnosed by spectrophotometric assays of enzyme activity and by measurements of enzyme substrate and product concentrations in the affected red cells. Measurement of red cell ATP content is not a reliable method for determination of pyruvate kinase activity, perhaps because the most severely affected cells with the lowest ATP content are quickly removed from the circulation and because the young reticulocytes that remain in the circulation have a high ATP content. Similarly, the morphology of pyruvate kinase–defi-

cient red cells is often relatively normal in the presence of a functioning spleen.

TREATMENT AND PROGNOSIS. In moderate to severe pyruvate kinase deficiency, splenectomy ameliorates the hemolysis, although the improvement may not be as marked as that seen in diseases such as hereditary spherocytosis. Following splenectomy, a "paradoxical reticulocytosis" (sometimes with a reticulocyte count of 50 to 70%) often occurs despite an improvement in the anemia. This striking finding is thought to be due to improved survival of the pyruvate kinase–deficient reticulocytes, which must depend on mitochondrial oxidative phosphorylation for ATP generation and are therefore susceptible to accelerated splenic "conditioning" (see Fig. 164–2) and extravascular hemolysis in the hypoxic environment of the splenic cords.

OTHER DEFECTS IN GLYCOLYSIS. Although abnormalities in most of the other enzymes in the glycolytic pathway have been described (see Fig. 164–3), the incidence of these deficiencies is so rare that together they affect only 5 to 10% of individuals with pyruvate kinase deficiency. Like pyruvate kinase deficiency, the inheritance pattern of most of these defects is autosomal recessive; the only exception is phosphoglycerate kinase deficiency because the gene coding for this enzyme is located on the X chromosome. The pathogenesis, clinical manifestations, diagnosis, and treatment of these deficiencies are generally similar to those described above for pyruvate kinase deficiency.

Defects in Red Cell Nucleotide Metabolism

Two rare defects in red cell nucleotide metabolism can cause chronic hereditary hemolytic anemia. Pyrimidine-5'-nucleotidase deficiency is inherited in an autosomal recessive pattern. Lack of this enzyme prevents red cell precursor cells from degrading pyrimidine nucleotides to cytidine and uridine, which allows the intracellular accumulation of partially degraded RNA that appears in the mature red cells as basophilic stippling. (This mechanism may also explain the basophilic stippling seen in lead poisoning because the same enzyme is also inhibited by lead.) Although splenomegaly is common in this disorder, splenectomy is of little benefit, thus indicating that the mechanism of hemolysis may be fundamentally different from that involved in the other hereditary anemias discussed in this chapter. Overproduction of adenosine deaminase also causes chronic hemolytic anemia, apparently by depleting the intracellular pool of adenine to the point that ATP synthesis is affected; the molecular mechanism responsible for overexpression of this apparently normal protein remains to be elucidated.

Beutler E: G6PD deficiency. Blood 84:3613, 1994. *Comprehensive review of G6PD molecular variants and clinical aspects of G6PD deficiency. See also periodic* updates of recently described G6PD variants in Blood Cells, Molecules, and Diseases (most recent update by Vulliamy T, Luzzatto L, Hirono A, Beutler E in the Aug 15, 1997 issue).

Gallagher PG, Ferriera JDS: Molecular basis of erythrocyte membrane disorders. Curr Opin Hematol 4:128, 1997. Review of recently described molecular defects in hereditary spherocytosis and hereditary elliptocytosis.

Lux SE, Palek J: Disorders of the red cell membrane. In Handin RI, Lux SE, Stossel TP (eds): Blood: Principles and Practice of Hematology. Philadelphia, JB Lippincott, 1995, pp 1701–1818. Comprehensive review of red cell membrane structure, function, and disorders, especially hereditary spherocytosis and hereditary elliptocytosis. See also periodic updates of recently described membrane protein variants in Blood Cells, Molecules, and Diseases (most recent update by Gallagher PG, Forget BG in the Dec 15, 1998 issue).

Tanaka KR, Paglia DE: Pyruvate kinase and other enzymopathies of the erythrocyte. In Scriver CR, Beaudet AL, Sly WS, Valle D (eds): The Metabolic Bases of Inherited Disease, 7th ed, vol 3. New York, McGraw-Hill, 1995, pp 3485–3511. Comprehensive review of inherited defects in red cell glycolysis, glutathione metabolism, and nucleotide metabolism.

Tchernia G, Bader-Meunier B, Berterottiere P, et al: Effectiveness of partial splenectomy in hereditary spherocytosis. Curr Opin Hematol 4:136, 1997. Suggests that subtotal splenectomy can ameliorate hemolysis in patients with hereditary spherocytosis while preserving phagocytic and immune functions of the spleen. Study of 40 patients monitored for 1 to 11 years each.

165 HEMOLYTIC ANEMIAS: AUTOIMMUNE

Alan D. Schreiber

Immunologic mechanisms play a significant role in the pathophysiology of many disease processes. However, in relatively few disorders is it possible to gain a detailed understanding of the ongoing mechanisms of immune damage in humans. Autoimmune hemolytic anemia is of particular interest in this regard because it is possible to define many of the immunopathologic processes that occur in this disease in molecular and cellular terms. Autoimmune hemolytic anemia represents a group of disorders in which individuals produce antibodies directed toward one or more of their own erythrocyte membrane antigens. This process leads to the destruction of antibody-coated erythrocytes by tissue macrophages.

The most effective way to approach autoimmune hemolytic anemia is to determine which class of antibody is responsible for the hemolysis. In general, two major classes of antierythrocyte antibodies produce hemolysis in humans, IgG and IgM. The pattern of red cell clearance, the site of organ sequestration, the response to therapy, and the prognosis all relate to the class of antierythrocyte antibody involved.

PATHOPHYSIOLOGY OF IMMUNE HEMOLYSIS

IgG-INDUCED IMMUNE HEMOLYTIC ANEMIA. Human erythrocytes are relatively resistant to the lytic action of complement, and their hemolysis, which is mediated by antibody and complement, is primarily extravascular.

Two molecules of IgG antibody need to be in close proximity to one another on the erythrocyte surface for the first component of complement (C1) to bind and initiate activation of the classic complement pathway. With antigens that are widely distributed on the erythrocyte surface, such as the antigens recognized by most antierythrocyte antibodies, many IgG antibody molecules must be deposited on the erythrocyte membrane before two bind sufficiently close to one another to permit complement activation.

IgG-sensitized erythrocytes are removed progressively from the circulation and sequestered predominantly in the spleen. Erythrocyte survival is determined in part by the number of antibody molecules per cell; increasing the number of IgG molecules per cell progressively increases the splenic sequestration of these cells.

In the absence of the third component of complement (C3), the complement activation sequence does not proceed through C3, and erythrocytes do not become coated with C3 in vivo. In this circumstance, IgG-coated erythrocytes are still cleared from the circula-

tion, but not as rapidly as in normal individuals. Complement-independent clearance of IgG-coated erythrocytes is predominately by macrophages in the spleen, and a rather large number of antibody molecules per cell is required.

Although IgG-coated erythrocytes are cleared predominantly in the spleen regardless of whether complement activation occurs, the liver becomes the predominant organ of clearance when very large amounts of IgG are bound to the erythrocytes. In vitro studies have shown that macrophages of the reticuloendothelial system have several classes of surface receptors for the Fc domain of IgG antibodies (Fcγ receptors). These receptors are responsible for the binding and phagocytosis of IgG-coated erythrocytes. One of the Fcγ receptor isoforms is a high-affinity receptor present on macrophages and monocytes, FcγRI. Two low-affinity receptors are also located on macrophages, FcγRIIA and FcγRIIIA. Fcγ receptors are responsible, at least in part, for the clearance of IgG-coated cells. Erythrocytes coated with multiple IgG molecules interact with macrophages with multiple Fcγ receptors; such interaction leads to binding of the erythrocytes to the macrophage surface, which in turn induces phagocytosis.

Macrophages can alter IgG- and/or C3b-coated erythrocytes in a manner that causes the red cells to form microspherocytes. These spherocytes are less able to pass through the splenic cords and sinuses and therefore have decreased survival; their presence in the circulation is an indication of ongoing immune hemolysis. Macrophages also have receptors, designated CR1 and CR2, for the activated third component of complement, which recognize the C3b and iC3b forms of C3b, respectively, and which are capable of binding C3b-coated erythrocytes. The receptors for the various C3 fragments do not recognize native C3; they recognize only fragments of C3 after C3 has undergone activation. Therefore they are capable of efficient function in the presence of normal plasma concentrations of C3. Fcγ receptors and C3b receptors can interact synergistically in their binding of IgG- and C3b-coated cells, and therefore the clearance of erythrocytes coated with IgG and C3b is greater than that of erythrocytes coated with IgG alone.

IgM-INDUCED IMMUNE HEMOLYTIC ANEMIA. Just a single molecule of IgM antibody bound to an erythrocyte membrane can bind C1 and activate the classic complement pathway. Complement is absolutely required for clearance of IgM-coated cells. Erythrocyte survival is proportional to the number of IgM molecules per red cell. IgM-coated cells are cleared rapidly within the liver rather than the spleen.

Macrophages do not have receptors for the Fc domain of IgM antibody, in contrast to their abundant receptors for the Fc domain of IgG antibody. Activation of the complement sequence by IgM results in the deposition of C3b on the erythrocyte surface. Erythrocyte-bound C3b and iC3b can interact with hepatic macrophage C3b and iC3b receptors. This interaction with complement is responsible for the clearance of IgM-coated erythrocytes. Thus IgM-coated erythrocytes require complement for their clearance.

IgM- and C3b-coated erythrocytes are rapidly sequestered within the liver. Subsequently, either they undergo phagocytosis and are destroyed, or they are released from their hepatic macrophage C3b receptor attachment sites back into the circulation, where they then survive normally, even though they still are coated with IgM and C3. This release of IgM- and C3-coated erythrocytes from the macrophage C3 receptor attachment site is not due to elution of the antibody from the surface. Rather, the C3b/iC3b inactivator system, which involves several circulating plasma proteins, including factor I and factor H, causes the release of C3-coated erythrocytes from the macrophage C3b and iC3b receptor attachment sites. These released C3-coated cells have on their surfaces an antigenically altered form of C3 (C3d) that is no longer recognized by macrophage C3b receptors. These C3d-coated erythrocytes then survive normally. Increasing the concentration of IgM per erythrocyte accelerates sequestration by liver macrophages and also decreases the number of erythrocytes released from hepatic macrophage receptor binding sites. Pre-treatment of IgM- and C3-coated erythrocytes with a source of serum C3 inactivator system proteins alters the erythrocyte cell–bound C3 and improves erythrocyte survival.

Thus the two major classes of antibody that cause autoimmune hemolytic anemia, IgG and IgM, differ markedly in their biologic effects. IgG-coated erythrocytes are cleared predominantly in the spleen, whereas IgM-coated erythrocytes are sequestered predominantly within the liver. Splenic macrophage Fc receptors and C3 receptors are responsible for the clearance of IgG-coated cells. IgG-coated erythrocytes do not require complement for their clearance. However, complement accelerates the clearance of IgG-coated erythrocytes in the spleen. Blood flow in the spleen is relatively slow, with close contact between sinusoidal macrophages and circulating red blood cells. This close contact facilitates IgG-mediated splenic macrophage clearance.

The pattern of clearance of IgM-coated erythrocytes is entirely different from that of IgG-coated cells. IgM-coated cells are cleared rapidly by hepatic macrophage C3 receptors. The clearance is entirely complement dependent, and in the absence of complement activation, these cells survive normally. The C3 inactivator system serves as an important control mechanism for the clearance of IgM-coated cells by mediating the release of IgM- and C3-coated cells from their hepatic macrophage C3 receptor attachment sites. Furthermore, exposure of IgM- and C3-coated erythrocytes to C3 inactivator system proteins can attenuate the clearance of these C3-coated cells by hepatic macrophages.

CLINICAL FEATURES

IgG-INDUCED AUTOIMMUNE HEMOLYTIC ANEMIA. Autoimmune hemolytic anemia is most commonly caused by IgG antibodies. The antigen to which the IgG antibody is directed is usually one of the Rh erythrocyte antigens, although often its precise specificity is not easily defined. This antibody usually has its maximal activity at 37° C, and thus this entity has been termed "warm antibody–induced hemolytic anemia."

IgG-induced immune hemolytic anemia can occur without an apparent underlying disease (idiopathic autoimmune hemolytic anemia); however, it can also occur with an underlying immunoproliferative disorder, either malignant or non-malignant, such as chronic lymphocytic leukemia, non-Hodgkin's lymphoma, or systemic lupus erythematosus. In certain patients with immunodeficiency, such as agammaglobulinemia, autoimmune hemolytic anemia can develop as well. Rarely, IgG-induced immune hemolytic anemia has also been observed in patients with an underlying malignant disease that is not an immunoproliferative disorder (Table 165–1). Additionally, bacterial infections such as tuberculosis, viral infections such as cytomegalovirus disease, and chronic inflammatory conditions such as ulcerative colitis have been described as associated conditions. The incidence of idiopathic IgG-induced autoimmune hemolytic anemia varies in different series. Overall, however, approximately half of the patients with IgG-induced immune hemolysis do not have a detectable underlying cause at the time of diagnosis. Regardless of etiology, some patients have immune thrombocytopenia in conjunction with IgG-induced autoimmune hemolytic anemia (Evans' syndrome), and some have immune granulocytopenia as well. It is not clear whether such IgG antibodies directed against blood cells recognize

a common blood cell antigen or represent antibodies with different specificities.

In IgG-induced autoimmune hemolytic anemia, many IgG molecules on the erythrocyte surface are needed to bind and activate a single molecule of C1, the first component of complement, because two IgG molecules in close proximity to each other (a doublet) are required. Once C1 is bound and activated, C4 and C2 activation occurs in a manner similar to that described for IgM antibody (see below), and C3 convertase is formed. C3 cleavage results and C3b is deposited on the erythrocyte surface.

Macrophages within the reticuloendothelial system have receptors not only for C3b but also for the Fc fragment of IgG (Fcγ receptors). These macrophage Fcγ receptors bind IgG-coated erythrocytes and mediate spherocyte formation and phagocytosis. Thus patients who have IgG on the erythrocyte surface in insufficient numbers or distributed in such a way not to allow C1 binding and activation still have a substantial decrease in erythrocyte survival. However, once sufficient IgG is present on the erythrocyte surface so that C1 activation occurs, erythrocyte clearance is further accelerated. In such a circumstance, clearance is due to the macrophage Fcγ receptors and the macrophage C3b receptors. These receptors interact synergistically to induce the binding of erythrocytes coated with IgG and C3b. IgG-coated erythrocytes are cleared progressively from the circulation, primarily in the spleen, and hemolysis is almost always extravascular.

IgM-INDUCED AUTOIMMUNE HEMOLYTIC ANEMIA. In humans, IgM-induced autoimmune hemolytic anemia is caused by an IgM antibody that reacts most efficiently with erythrocytes in the cold; thus this disorder has also been called "cold hemagglutinin disease." The IgM antibody in cold hemagglutinin disease is usually directed against the I antigen or related antigens on the human erythrocyte membrane. As with all IgM antibodies, agglutinating activity is particularly efficient because of the multiple antigen-combining sites on the IgM molecule. The IgM antibody has a particular affinity for its red cell antigen at 0 to 10° C, and the affinity is lower at higher temperatures. Like warm antibody (i.e., IgG-mediated) autoimmune hemolytic anemia, cold hemagglutinin disease can be divided into cases considered primary or idiopathic and those associated with the presence of an underlying disease (secondary).

Chronic cold hemagglutinin disease is due to clonal expansion of lymphocytes in which a monoclonal antibody is produced and recognizes a polysaccharide antigen, termed I or i, on red cells. The most common form of chronic cold hemagglutinin disease, which is the primary or idiopathic form, is usually a disease of older persons, with a peak incidence in the fifties and sixties. Most often this condition initially causes fatigue, anemia, and occasionally jaundice in an elderly individual, but it may be associated with the development of acrocyanosis from sludging of blood in peripheral vessels on exposure to cold or with acute hemolysis. This disease is associated with the presence of a monoclonal IgM antibody, usually exhibiting a high cold agglutinin titer (>1:1000). This IgM antibody binds to erythrocytes avidly in the cold but shows no binding activity at 37° C. In most, but not all patients the antibody is of the κ light-chain type and has specificity for the I antigen present on the erythrocytes of most adults. The I antigenic determinants are closely related to the ABO core antigenic determinants. Although present on the erythrocytes of almost all persons, the antigenic groupings recognized by the antibody develop during childhood and are not present on blood taken from the umbilical vein of the newborn. Thus operationally, specificity is established by the ability of the antibody to agglutinate the blood of almost all adults but an inability to agglutinate the erythrocytes of newborns. Although the monoclonal antibody responsible for development of the cold hemagglutinin syndrome presumably reflects the expansion of a single clone of B cells, the symptom complex associated with multiple myeloma or Waldenström's macroglobulinemia does not develop in these patients. The monoclonal antibody appears to represent a highly restricted clonal response to the I antigen. Although each patient usually has only a single antibody with a single amino acid sequence, the antibodies among patients virtually always differ. Nevertheless, these antibodies tend to share idiotypic determinants consistent with their uniform recognition of the I antigen.

Table 165–1 ■ DISEASES ASSOCIATED WITH AUTOIMMUNE HEMOLYTIC ANEMIA

Infections
Viral infections, especially respiratory infections
Infectious mononucleosis and cytomegalovirus infection
Mycoplasma, especially pneumonia
Tuberculosis
Non-Malignant Disorders
Systemic lupus erythematosus
Rheumatoid arthritis
Thyroid disorders
Ulcerative colitis
Chronic active hepatitis
Immunodeficiency Syndromes
X-linked agammaglobulinemia
Dysgammaglobulinemia
Common variable hypogammaglobulinemia
IgA deficiency
Wiskott-Aldrich syndrome
Malignancies
Non-Hodgkin's lymphoma
Hodgkin's disease
Acute lymphocytic leukemia
Carcinoma
Thymoma
Ovarian cysts and tumors

Secondary cold hemagglutinin disease, or IgM-induced immune hemolytic anemia, is most commonly associated with an underlying *Mycoplasma* infection, particularly *Mycoplasma pneumoniae*, in which antibody with typical anti-I specificity is produced. However, it may also occur with other infections such as infectious mononucleosis, cytomegalovirus, and mumps. With infectious mononucleosis, anti-i (antibody to an antigen related to I, but present on cord blood cells) cold agglutinins are produced, but overt hemolysis is unusual. Under most circumstances with an underlying infection, the cold agglutinin (IgM antibody) is polyclonal, that is, immunochemically heterogeneous.

Cold hemagglutinin disease can also be seen in patients with an underlying immunoproliferative disorder, such as chronic lymphocytic leukemia and non-Hodgkin's lymphoma, or in patients with an underlying connective tissue disease, such as systemic lupus erythematosus. As in idiopathic cold hemagglutinin disease, patients with an underlying malignant immunoproliferative disorder such as one of the non-Hodgkin's lymphomas have a cold agglutinin that is commonly monoclonal or of restricted heterogeneity (oligoclonal). Waldenström's macroglobulinemia (see Chapter 181) is also at times associated with the formation of IgM antibody against red cells. Anti-i, often with λ light chains, may be seen in malignant lymphocytic neoplasias.

The plasma of healthy adults and children contains low levels of antierythrocyte antibodies, that is, low levels of IgM cold agglutinins. Rarely, cold-reacting autoantibodies have been observed with specificity directed against red cell antigens other than I or i, that is, the P and the PR antigens. Also rarely, IgA cold agglutinins have been observed.

The reason for the preferential reaction of cold agglutinin with the human red cell membrane in the cold is not completely understood. Most cold agglutinins have no measurable activity above 30° C. Although it has been postulated that either the antibody or the antigen may undergo a structural change on exposure to cold, most data suggest that the antigen on the erythrocyte surface is altered in the cold.

As in all patients with autoimmune hemolytic anemia, erythrocyte survival is generally proportional to the amount of antibody on the erythrocyte surface. In cold hemagglutinin disease, the extent of hemolysis is a function of the titer of the antibody (cold agglutinin titer), the thermal amplitude of the IgM antibody (the highest temperature at which the antibody is active), and the level of the circulating control proteins of the C3 inactivator system.

In cold hemagglutinin disease, the IgM antibody in the circulation of patients with the disease interacts with the erythrocyte surface, after the cells have circulated to areas below body temperatures, and activates the early steps of the classic complement pathway. Once C1, the first component of complement, is bound to the IgM molecule and activated, it sequentially binds and activates the fourth and second components of complement. The first of these two steps takes place at temperatures as low as 0° C. When the cells return to body temperature, activation proceeds, even though the cold agglutinin antibody can dissociate from the erythrocyte. The C3 convertase (C142) generated cleaves C3 into two antigenic fragments, one of which, C3b (and iC3b), binds to the erythrocyte surface. At this step the IgM effect is considerably amplified, with a single C142 classic pathway C3 convertase capable of cleaving many C3 molecules and depositing many C3b molecules on the erythrocyte surface. In some cases the complement sequence of reactions may be completed with resulting hemolysis, but this event is unusual because of the presence of membrane-bound proteins that restrict complement action. These C3b-coated erythrocytes are recognized by hepatic macrophage complement receptors. The macrophage C3b and iC3b receptors bind, sphere, and may mediate phagocytosis of the C3b-coated erythrocytes. Because no receptors on macrophages are capable of interacting with IgM-coated cells in the absence of complement, IgM-coated red cells have normal survival in the absence of an intact classic complement pathway.

In humans, clearance of IgM-plus-complement–coated cells has been shown to be very rapid and takes place primarily in the liver. However, when large numbers of IgM molecules are present on the erythrocyte surface, sufficient terminal complement components (C5 through C9) are occasionally generated to lyse the erythrocytes in the intravascular space.

Control proteins involved in the C3 inactivator system are particularly important in cold hemagglutinin disease because cell destruction is mediated entirely by C3 and the later complement components. Thus the level of the C3 inactivator proteins in plasma plays an important role in determining hemolysis by regulating the number of active C3 fragments on the cell surface. The C3-coated erythrocytes interacting with C3 inactivator system proteins are degraded to C3dg or C3d. C3dg- or C3d-coated erythrocytes are not bound by macrophage C3 receptors and have normal survival. Thus the presence of C3 (C3dg or C3d)–coated erythrocytes in cold hemagglutinin disease explains the earlier observations of normal erythrocyte survival in patients who still have C3 on their erythrocyte membranes, as detected by the Coombs' antiglobulin test.

The thermal amplitude of the IgM cold agglutinin is important in determining the extent of hemolysis in cold hemagglutinin disease. At a relatively low level of cold agglutinin sensitization, patients with antibodies having higher thermal amplitude (those antibodies that possess activity at temperatures approaching 37° C) may still have considerable hemolysis. Such patients have been described as having a low-titer cold hemagglutinin syndrome with a high–thermal amplitude antibody. The correct diagnosis in such patients is important because they appear to respond to glucocorticoid therapy in a manner different from the usual patient with high-titer cold hemagglutinin disease. Furthermore, some unusual patients have an IgG cold agglutinin. The presence of such an IgG antibody is potentially important inasmuch as it appears to indicate responsiveness to steroids or splenectomy.

GENERAL FEATURES

In large centers, 15 to 30 cases of autoimmune hemolytic anemia are seen yearly, with an annual incidence of approximately 1 case per 75,000 to 80,000 persons in the general population. As with any disease that may require careful serologic study for diagnosis, the level of sophistication and diagnostic capability of the institution influence the reported incidence. There appears to be little genetic predisposition to the development of autoimmune hemolytic anemia except in patients who have a family history of other autoimmune diseases such as autoimmune thrombocytopenia, rheumatoid arthritis, and glomerulonephritis.

Although warm antibody (IgG-induced) immune hemolytic anemia can occur at any age, the peak incidence occurs in the 50-year-old age group. In contrast, idiopathic cold hemagglutinin disease is a disease predominantly of the elderly. Autoimmune hemolytic anemia does not appear to be more prevalent in any particular racial group.

Patients with autoimmune hemolytic anemia vary considerably in their clinical course, which may be either indolent or fulminant. In general, the course of autoimmune hemolytic anemia is more acute in children than it is in adults, often ending in complete resolution of the disease. The fall in hemoglobin may occur over a period of hours to days, with resolution of the disease often within 3 months.

The Donath-Landsteiner cold hemolysin is an unusual IgG antibody with anti-P specificity that was originally noted in cases of congenital or acquired syphilis. The disease it causes is termed "paroxysmal cold hemoglobinuria." Hemolysis in this syndrome most commonly occurs intravascularly, after the antibody has passed through a cell attachment phase in the lower temperatures of the peripheral circulation. The intravascular hemolysis is due to the unusual complement-activating efficiency of this IgG antibody. As its name implies, this antibody is associated with cold hemoglobinuria. This antibody, although uncommon, is most frequently found in children with viral infections. Hemolysis, even though sometimes severe, is usually mild and tends to resolve as the infection clears.

Mortality in the pediatric age group has ranged from 9 to 29%. Death during the acute stage is usually due to severe anemia or hemorrhage from associated thrombocytopenia. Mortality in chronic cases or in adults is higher and usually occurs because of an underlying serious disorder such as Hodgkin's disease or non-Hodgkin's lymphoma or as a complication of therapy. Fatal sepsis has been observed following splenectomy.

Estradiol, in contrast to cortisol, enhances the clearance of IgG-coated erythrocytes by splenic macrophages in a dose-dependent manner. On the other hand, estradiol does not alter the splenic macrophage clearance of heat-altered erythrocytes or the hepatic macrophage clearance of IgM- and C3b-coated erythrocytes. During pregnancy, estrogen concentrations rise to a level similar to that necessary to accelerate the clearance of IgG-coated erythrocytes; as a result, the course of IgG-induced autoimmune hemolytic anemia accelerates.

CLINICAL AND LABORATORY FINDINGS

Many of the symptoms of autoimmune hemolytic anemia, such as weakness, malaise, and light-headedness, are caused by the presence of anemia. Patients who have underlying cardiovascular disease may have significant dyspnea on exertion and peripheral edema, as well as angina pectoris. If the hemolysis is significant, mild jaundice may be noted, particularly in the presence of hepatic dysfunction. In addition, patients with an underlying disease often have the symptoms associated with that disease, for example, fever and weight loss with an underlying malignant disease or joint symptoms secondary to an underlying systemic vasculitis. Physical findings are also generally referable to the underlying disease. For example, in patients with an underlying non-Hodgkin's lymphoma, hepatosplenomegaly and lymphadenopathy are common. Mild splenomegaly may be present in patients with severe autoimmune hemolytic anemia. Massive splenomegaly suggests an underlying disorder such as lymphoma. Other signs that may result from the anemic state include those caused by heart failure (edema, ascites, or pulmonary congestion). Severe jaundice is uncommon.

The common initial symptoms are pallor, jaundice, dark urine, abdominal pain, and fever. Pallor may precede the appearance of jaundice. The clinical status depends on the rapidity of the hemolysis and the severity of the anemia. In mild cases, fatigue may be the only symptom. In severe cases the patient may appear acutely ill or even moribund, with tachycardia, tachypnea, signs of hypoxia, and even cardiovascular collapse. In severe IgM-induced cold hemagglutinin disease, the skin may have a livedo reticularis pattern and the patient may demonstrate acrocyanosis on exposure to cold.

Laboratory data reveal the presence of anemia, reticulocytosis (if bone marrow function is adequate), and a positive result on the direct Coombs' test. Autoantibodies directed against early erythroid precursors are believed to be responsible for the reticulocytopenia in some patients. Examination of the peripheral blood smear may show spherocytes, polychromasia, nucleated red cells, and erythrophagocytosis. Rosetting of red cells around white cells may be visible in a buffy coat preparation. Agglutination of red cells may be evident in cold agglutinin disease. In severe cases, macroagglutination is visible on the microscope slide or in a capillary tube. The white cell count is usually normal or elevated. Autoimmune hemolysis is also associated with thrombocytopenia and/or leukopenia in a small number of patients. Indirect hyperbilirubinemia is common.

The diagnosis of autoimmune hemolytic anemia is most effectively established by directly examining the patient's circulating red cells for the presence of antibody and/or complement components on their surfaces, most easily with a direct Coombs' antiglobulin test. Classically, in this test the patient's red cells are made to interact with a rabbit or goat antihuman serum globulin reagent, and then agglutination of the patient's red cells is assessed. It is also possible to use antibody to human immunoglobulin or complement components as a more specific test reagent. In this case, agglutination induced by anti-IgG (a γ-Coombs' test) indicates the presence of IgG on the surface of the red cells, whereas agglutination with anti-C3 or anti-C4 (a non–γ-Coombs' test) is used to test for the presence of C3 and C4. In IgG-induced hemolytic anemia, IgG or IgG plus complement components is found on the surface of erythrocytes. Therefore, such patients usually have a positive result in the γ-Coombs' test but may have a positive result on the non–γ-Coombs' test as well. In IgM-induced hemolytic anemia (cold hemagglutinin disease), IgG is not found on the red cells, and the IgM cold agglutinin, because of its low affinity for red cell antigens at 37° C, is not found either. In contrast, C3, stably bound at 37° C, is detected on the red cell membrane. Therefore, in cold hemagglutinin disease, usually only a positive result in the non-γ (C3) Coombs' test is observed. Rarely, patients with IgG-induced immune hemolysis have levels of IgG per erythrocyte undetectable

by the standard Coombs' test, which requires the presence of hundreds of molecules of IgG on the erythrocyte surface for the result to be positive. When this phenomenon was originally described, the small amounts of red cell–bound IgG antibody were detected with a complex antiglobulin consumption test. Now, however, a Coombs' test using radiolabeled anti-IgG, which is 10 times more sensitive than the standard Coombs' test, may also be used to detect the antibody.

Thus testing with Coombs' antisera shows several patterns of reactivity. The red cells may be coated with IgG in the presence or absence of detectable complement (warm antibody IgG-mediated autoimmune hemolytic anemia) or with complement protein alone (IgM-induced hemolysis, i.e., cold hemagglutinin disease). Rarely, IgM is detected as well. It is not possible to predict the chronicity or severity of autoimmune hemolytic anemia from the Coombs' testing pattern.

A cold agglutinin titer is also diagnostically helpful. This test is performed by examining the patient's plasma for agglutinating activity directed against normal ABO-compatible erythrocytes containing the I antigen at 0° C. The cold agglutinin titer is the highest dilution of antibody that still agglutinates normal red blood cells in the cold. Most patients with immune hemolysis secondary to cold hemagglutinin disease have cold agglutinin titers greater than 1: 1000.

THERAPY

In many patients with IgG- or IgM-induced immune hemolytic anemia, no therapeutic intervention is necessary because the hemolysis is mild. If an underlying disease is present, control of this disease often brings the hemolytic anemia under control as well. However, if the patient has significant anemia secondary to hemolysis, therapeutic intervention is in order.

GLUCOCORTICOIDS. Patients with IgG antibody–mediated autoimmune hemolytic anemia or immune thrombocytopenic purpura treated with glucocorticoids often respond within days of initiating therapy in dosages equivalent to 1 to 2 mg of prednisone per kilogram of body weight per day. Glucocorticoids are believed to decrease hemolysis in IgG-induced hemolytic anemia by three major mechanisms. First, they decrease production of the abnormal IgG antibody. This effect is common and gradual and can be expected to produce a gradual decrease in the strength of the Coombs' test result and a rise in hemoglobin by 4 to 6 weeks. Second, glucocorticoids are reported to be associated with a fall in the amount of antibody detected by the direct Coombs' test and a rise in the amount detected by the indirect Coombs' test, as though they induce a decrease in antibody affinity; this result is probably an uncommon effect of glucocorticoid therapy. Third, glucocorticoids have been shown in vitro and in vivo to interfere with the macrophage Fcγ receptors responsible for erythrocyte clearance from the circulation. The effect is to improve erythrocyte survival despite the continued presence of IgG on the erythrocyte surface. Thus the Coombs' test in some patients may remain positive in the face of improved erythrocyte survival and a rising hemoglobin concentration. This effect of glucocorticoids may be rapid and could be responsible for the rise in hemoglobin noted to occur in some patients after 1 to 4 days of glucocorticoid therapy. Most patients will respond to glucocorticoid therapy within 2 to 3 weeks. Although 4 to 6 weeks of therapy may be required for a response to be evident, in many of these delayed responders further therapy will be needed.

Approximately 60 to 80% of patients have an initial response to high-dose glucocorticoids. In many patients with acute autoimmune hemolytic anemia and in a small proportion of patients with chronic autoimmune hemolytic anemia, the steroid dosage can be tapered and stopped with the patient remaining in remission. Some patients have control of their hemolytic process with continued low- to medium-dose steroid therapy. Alternate-day therapy may be less effective in autoimmune hemolytic anemia than in some of the inflammatory autoimmune diseases, and patients should be monitored carefully for exacerbation. Great care should be taken in stopping glucocorticoid therapy if the patient continues to demonstrate a positive result on the direct Coombs' test. For patients who are steroid dependent, the initial and long-term side effects of these drugs must be considered (see Chapter 28).

In some patients the presence of a mild hemolytic anemia may be preferable to splenectomy or other treatment options. The initial goal of therapy is to return the patient to normal hematologic values and non-toxic levels of glucocorticoid therapy. However, in some patients, a modified goal of improvement in hemolysis to a clinically asymptomatic state with minimum glucocorticoid side effects is more realistic.

Glucocorticoids are not usually effective in cold hemagglutinin disease, probably because these patients generally have large amounts of IgM antierythrocyte antibody and large numbers of C3 molecules deposited on their red cells. Furthermore, macrophage C3b receptors, in contrast to the case with Fcγ receptors, are less responsive to glucocorticoid therapy. In addition, some of the hemolysis may be intravascular, and glucocorticoids do not inhibit complement-mediated cell lysis. A few patients with a low-titer cold hemagglutinin disease syndrome, in which the antierythrocyte antibody has activity at temperatures approaching 37° C, do respond to steroid therapy. In addition, the few patients described with an IgG cold agglutinin appear to be responsive to both steroids and splenectomy. Patients with cold hemagglutinin disease respond best to the avoidance of cold and control of their underlying disease. Fortunately, in many patients hemolytic anemia is mild.

SPLENECTOMY. The spleen with its resident macrophages is the major site for sequestration of IgG-coated blood cells in humans, as in animals. Splenectomy markedly decreases the sequestration of IgG-sensitized cells. Splenectomy may also lead to a decrease in the production of IgG antierythrocyte antibody because the spleen contains a large B-cell pool. However, as the antibody concentration is increased, splenectomy becomes less effective in preventing the clearance of IgG-coated cells because the liver becomes the dominant organ in erythrocyte clearance.

Splenectomy should be considered in patients who are not responsive to steriods or require more than 10 to 20 mg of prednisone per day or substantial dosages of steroid every other day for maintenance. Each patient requires individual evaluation of underlying diseases, surgical risk, extent of anemia, and steroid intolerance.

The response rate to splenectomy in IgG-mediated disease is approximately 50 to 70%; however, the vast majority of the responses are partial remissions. Probably the patients who are least responsive to splenectomy are those whose erythrocytes are coated with large amounts of IgG. In this circumstance, the liver plays a larger role in clearance. The partial remissions that occur with splenectomy are often quite helpful in that they result in lessening of the hemolytic rate, with a rise in the hemoglobin concentration, and/or allow a reduction in the amount of glucocorticoid needed to control the hemolytic anemia. Because of the increased risk of sepsis, patients should be carefully selected. Patients who are unresponsive to steroids, require moderate to high maintenance doses, or have glucocorticoid intolerance can be considered for splenectomy. ⁵¹Cr-labeled red cell kinetic studies are probably not helpful because the procedure is time consuming, expensive, and not a reliable indicator of response to splenectomy in most cases. Immunization with pneumococcal vaccine should be performed before splenectomy to decrease the likelihood of post-splenectomy pneumococcal infection.

Splenectomy, like glucocorticoid therapy, is usually not effective in patients with cold hemagglutinin disease because IgM-coated erythrocytes are cleared predominately in the liver. An occasional case in which a patient with an apparent IgM-induced hemolytic anemia responded to splenectomy has been reported. This result may be due to decreased production of IgM antibody by the spleen in these few patients or to the presence of an IgG cold agglutinin.

IMMUNOSUPPRESSIVE AGENTS. Several immunosuppressive agents have been used in the treatment of immune hemolytic anemia. The drugs most commonly used include the thiopurines (6-mercaptopurine, azathioprine, and thioguanine) and alkylating agents (cyclophosphamide and chlorambucil). Immunosuppressive agents act by decreasing the production of antibody, and therefore it generally takes at least 4 weeks before any therapeutic result is observed. A reasonable clinical trial consists of 3 to 4 months of

therapy. These drugs are rarely needed in the treatment of childhood autoimmune hemolytic anemia.

Patients are selected for immunosuppressive therapy when a clinically unacceptable degree of hemolytic anemia persists following glucocorticoid therapy and splenectomy. Alternatively, patients may be corticosteroid resistant or intolerant and a poor surgical risk for splenectomy. Clinical benefit has been noted in about 50% of patients. The dosage of drug should be adjusted to maintain the leukocyte count over 4000, the granulocyte count greater than 2000, and the platelet count over 50,000 to 100,000 per microliter. Side effects require that the clinical indications for an immunosuppressive trial be strong and that the patient's exposure to the drug be limited.

Immunosuppressive therapy has been effective in cold hemagglutinin disease. Alkylating agents (cyclophosphamide or chlorambucil) have been used and appear to have a beneficial effect in up to 50 to 60% of patients.

TRANSFUSION THERAPY. The majority of patients with autoimmune hemolytic anemia do not require transfusion therapy because the anemia has developed gradually and physiologic compensation has occurred. However, occasional patients experience acute and/or severe anemia and require transfusions for support until other treatment reduces the hemolysis. Transfusion therapy is complicated by the fact that the blood bank may be unable to find any "compatible" blood because of the presence of an autoantibody directed at a core component of the Rh locus, which is present on the erythrocytes of essentially all potential donors, regardless of Rh subtype. The usual recommendation is for the blood bank to identify the most compatible units of blood of the patient's own major blood group and Rh type and transfuse the patient with these units. With this approach, it is unlikely that the donor blood will have a dramatically shortened red cell survival.

In cold agglutinin disease it is important to pre-warm all intravenous infusions, including whole blood, to 37° C because a decrease in temperature locally in a vein can enhance binding of the IgM antibody to red cells and accelerate the hemolytic process. Furthermore, agglutination of transfused chilled or even room-temperature cells in small peripheral blood vessels can result in severe ischemic changes and vascular compromise.

MISCELLANEOUS THERAPY. Intravenous γ-globulin, which has been used extensively in the treatment of immune thrombocytopenic purpura, may be effective in patients with IgG-induced immune hemolytic anemia, probably by interfering with clearance of the IgG-coated cells. Treatment regimens vary from 400 mg/kg/day for 5 days to 2 g/kg given over 2 days, with additional treatment as needed to maintain the effect. Currently, data are incomplete, but γ-globulin seems less effective in autoimmune hemolytic anemia than in immune thrombocytopenic purpura.

Plasmapheresis or exchange transfusion has been used in patients with severe IgG-induced immune hemolytic anemia but has met with limited success, possibly because more than half of the IgG is extravascular and the plasma contains only small amounts of the antibody (most of the antibody being on the red cell surface). However, plasmapheresis has been effective in IgM-induced hemolytic anemia (cold agglutinin disease) because IgM is a high-molecular-weight molecule that remains predominately within the intravascular space and, at 37° C, most of the IgM is in the plasma fraction. Plasmapheresis is useful only as short-term therapy, but it may be life saving in the rare patient with severe, uncontrollable hemolysis.

Other measures that have been used effectively in some patients with IgG-induced immune hemolysis are vincristine, vinblastine infusions, and hormonal therapy. Because of the limited side effects (limited masculinizing effects and mild weight gain), danazol is an additional agent for use in some patients with IgG-induced immune hemolytic anemia. The results of these agents in IgM-induced hemolysis suggest that such treatment is ineffective. Folic acid should be given to avoid depletion of folate stores from chronic hemolysis caused by either IgG or IgM antibodies.

IMMUNE PANCYTOPENIA

Evans' syndrome refers to autoimmune hemolytic anemia accompanied by thrombocytopenia. It occurs in a small percentage of adults and children with acute autoimmune hemolytic anemia. In an even smaller percentage of patients it is also associated with marked neutropenia. Antibodies directed against red cells, leukocytes, and platelets have been demonstrated in some patients with immune pancytopenia. Suppression of hematopoietic cell maturation by T cells has also been observed. Autoimmune hemolytic anemia in the presence of thrombocytopenia and/or neutropenia is more commonly associated with a chronic or relapsing course. Many patients have associated disorders such as chronic lymphadenopathy or dysgammaglobulinemia. Some patients are hematologically normal between relapses, which may involve depressions in any of the three cell lines. Usually glucocorticoid therapy is effective in controlling the acute episodes and is not needed between relapses. However, some patients have persistent immune cytopenia and require prolonged steroid treatment or more aggressive therapy. Splenectomy may result in improvement, but the risk of infection may be higher in children and adults with pancytopenia than in those with autoimmune hemolytic anemia alone, and relapses are more common.

PAROXYSMAL NOCTURNAL HEMOGLOBINURIA

Paroxysmal nocturnal hemoglobinuria (PNH) is an acquired disorder initially thought to consist of paroxysms of intravascular hemolysis causing nocturnal hemoglobinuria. It is now recognized that chronic intravascular hemolysis is the more frequent clinical finding. PNH is a primary bone marrow disorder that not only affects the red cell lineage but also affects the platelet, leukocyte, and pluripotent hematopoietic stem cell lines. It is believed to be a disorder of stem cells of a clonal nature and can arise from or evolve into other dysplastic bone marrow diseases, including aplastic anemia, sideroblastic anemia, and myelofibrosis. Rarely, PNH may also evolve into acute leukemia. A major clue to the etiology of this disease is provided by the recent finding that patients have a somatic mutation for a protein (phosphatidylinositol glycan class A) important in the pathway that controls formation of the phosphatidylinositol anchor of several membrane proteins, including complement control proteins.

At least 19 proteins are attached to blood cells by a phosphatidylinositol glycan anchor. Three of these proteins protect the cells from complement attack by regulating complement activation on the cell surface. Among the phosphatidylinositol glycan class of proteins are those termed class A, which lack the ability to transfer glucosamine to phosphatidylinositol. The gene responsible for the defect in class A cells and PNH is phosphatidylinositol glycan A (PIG-A). The PIG-A gene is located on the short arm of the X chromosome and consists of six exons coding for a 54-kd protein. The protein is presumed to be an N-acetylglucosamine transferase, and over 100 somatic mutations spread over the entire coding region have been identified. The mutations, mostly deletions or insertions, generally cause a stop codon that results in premature termination of the peptide to yield a truncated protein. These truncated proteins may be either non-functional, partially functional, or unstable. The ultimate result of a non-functional PIG-A gene product can be a PNH III cell, and a partially functional gene product can result in a PNH II cell.

PNH is often a disease of young adults, but it can occur in any age group and in individuals of either sex. Chronic intravascular hemolysis of varying severity is the most common finding. The severity of the hemolysis and the degree of hemoglobinuria depend on the number of circulating abnormal red cells and the degree of expression of the membrane abnormality among these cells. Two to three populations of abnormal red cells, termed PNH type I, II, and III cells, may be present simultaneously and differ in their lytic susceptibility. Patients commonly have iron deficiency anemia as well because of the large amount of iron lost in the urine during intravascular hemolysis via persistent hemoglobinuria and hemosiderinuria. Other frequent clinical complaints include abdominal, back, and musculoskeletal pain. Such pain may be associated with intravascular hemolysis and hemoglobinuria, or it may be ischemic and secondary to the complication of venous thrombosis of major or minor vessels. Thrombosis of the hepatic veins (Budd-Chiari syndrome) and the portal, splenic, mesenteric, cerebral, and other veins may occur and is a common cause of death. Acute intestinal infarction requiring surgical resection has been reported. Thrombotic episodes may require anticoagulant therapy. Platelets and leukocytes also appear to have unusual susceptibility to lysis, and thrombocytopenia, granulocytopenia, or both are common and may be the initial manifestation(s) of the disease. The bone marrow is usually hyperplastic but may be hypocellular, consistent with aplastic anemia. The clinical course is variable and depends on occurrence of the life-threatening complications of progressive bone marrow disease or venous thrombosis. PNH should be considered in everyone with aplastic anemia. In general, patients are not predisposed to the development of infection. At least half the patients live for many years.

PATHOGENESIS. Patients with PNH have an unusual sensitivity of their erythrocytes and often granulocytes and platelets to the lytic action of complement. Activation of complement by either the classic or alternative pathway results in the deposition of larger numbers of C3 molecules on the PNH blood cell surface than on normal cells. The excessive binding of C3 to blood cells in PNH is due to more efficient alternative pathway C3 convertase activity on the cell surface. The surface of a PNH erythrocyte is a better acceptor for C3 than is the surface of a normal cell; the result is greater activation of the terminal complement components C5 to C9, which causes more cell lysis than occurs with normal cells. Furthermore, type II PNH cells are more effectively damaged by the C5b–C9 complex generated on the erythrocyte surface because the C5b–C9 lytic complex penetrates PNH cell membranes more efficiently than normal cell membranes. These patients lack the complement regulatory proteins present on the membranes of all normal blood cells, so their erythrocytes have an increased susceptibility to complement lysis.

Many patients with PNH have several populations of abnormal erythrocytes. The complement lysis sensitivity test, which examines the susceptibility of antibody-sensitized erythrocytes to complement-mediated lysis, can be used to define the various PNH cell populations. PNH type II cells have a moderate increase in susceptibility to complement attack. These erythrocytes appear to have markedly decreased levels of the complement control protein decay-accelerating factor, but they do not have the membrane deficit that leads to sensitivity to attack by the C5b–C9 complex. PNH type III cells are highly susceptible to complement attack. They appear to lack phosphatidylinositol-linked control proteins completely.

DIAGNOSIS. The diagnosis rests on the clinical picture and clinical laboratory measurement of a population of circulating cells with unusual sensitivity to complement-mediated lysis. The diagnosis may be established by the sugar-water test, in which the patient's serum is mixed with 5% dextrose in water and incubated with the patient's cells. In PNH, hemolysis ensues. It has been shown that all individuals have antibody molecules that recognize their own cells under conditions of low ionic strength. These antibodies activate the classic complement pathway. Normal erythrocytes resist lysis, but PNH erythrocytes are susceptible to lytic attack. In Ham's test, the patient's cells are incubated in acidified serum. Under these conditions, the alternative complement pathway is triggered, and lysis of PNH, but not normal cells follows. The Ham test is also positive with some, but not all normal sera from patients with a syndrome of congenital dyserythropoietic anemia (hereditary erythroblastic multinuclearity with positive acidified serum).

THERAPY. A prednisone dose of 15 to 40 mg every other day decreases the rate of hemolysis in some adult patients, but a response is by no means certain. During acute episodes, a higher dose given daily for a short period may help control the hemolysis. In patients with anemia, androgens, including the anabolic steroid danazol, may be effective. Bone marrow transplantation has been successful in some patients, but in general, treatment of PNH has been unsatisfactory.

Patients with PNH may be iron deficient. Acutely, iron replacement may result in increased hemolysis because of the formation and release of a new cohort of sensitive red cells, and hemolysis after iron replacement has been noted. Oral replacement should be used if possible, but parenteral iron therapy may be necessary when iron losses are very large.

DRUG-INDUCED IMMUNE HEMOLYSIS

Drug-induced immune hemolytic anemia may be divided into three primary pathophysiologic entities. The clinical signs and symptoms are identical to those of autoimmune hemolytic anemia. Patients may have chronic hemolytic anemia or, occasionally, catastrophic intravascular hemolysis (quinidine type). Many autoimmune or drug-related hemolytic anemias are accompanied by thrombocytopenia and/or neutropenia as a result of similar pathophysiologic processes. The diagnosis is established primarily by history and *in vitro* assay.

α-METHYLDOPA TYPE. The α-methyldopa type and its derivatives (such as levodopa) produce a clinical syndrome virtually identical to IgG-induced immune hemolytic anemia. This type of drug-induced immune hemolytic anemia is the most common. The mechanisms of IgG antibody formation are poorly understood. This drug stimulates production of IgG warm-reactive antibodies with anti-Rh specificity. A primary mode of action of the drug in this disorder may be an alteration in immunoregulation that allows B lymphocytes that produce Rh antibodies to escape suppression.

It is of interest that antinuclear antibodies develop in 15% of patients receiving α-methyldopa therapy. Many patients, up to 25% exposed to α-methyldopa, have a positive result on the Coombs' test for IgG. Of diagnostic importance is that almost all patients have IgG antierythrocyte antibodies present in their plasma as well. Sufficient IgG coating for hemolysis does not develop in most patients, but patients with the highest amount of erythrocyte-associated IgG appear to have the most significant hemolysis. Overall, significant hemolysis and hemolytic anemia develop in approximately 0.8% of patients 3 to 37 months after the onset of α-methyldopa therapy. The diagnosis can be made by examining patient's red cells and plasma. In vitro, it is not necessary to have the drug present for the patient's plasma to deposit IgG antibody on donor erythrocytes. The Coombs' test result can remain positive in some patients up to 2 years after withdrawal of the drug. A similar syndrome has been reported with mefenamic acid.

HAPTEN TYPE. The hapten type of drug-induced immune hemolysis classically develops in patients exposed to high doses of penicillin. A portion of the penicillin molecule or its active metabolites combines with the erythrocyte surface, acts as a hapten, and induces an antibody response directed against the penicillin-coated erythrocyte membrane. This response usually involves IgG, and complement activation is common. The erythrocytes become coated with IgG and often with C3. This syndrome rarely develops unless patients have received 10 to 20 million U of penicillin per day. The diagnosis can be established by incubating the patient's serum with donor erythrocytes pre-incubated with penicillin. Deposition of IgG antibody will occur only in the presence of penicillin and can be detected with the Coombs' test.

QUINIDINE TYPE. The quinidine type of autoimmune hemolytic anemia usually occurs with quinidine, but it has been reported with quinine, stibophen, chlorpromazine, and sulfonamides. Commonly called an innocent-bystander reaction, it is thought to be due to an antibody directed against quinidine and having a low affinity for the red cell surface. Presumably the drug binds weakly to the cell glycoprotein. The antibody recognizes the complex, and this interaction results in activation of the classic complement pathway and deposition of C3 on the erythrocyte surface. It is believed that the immune complex transiently adheres to the red cell surface, activates complement, and then dissociates. With quinidine it has been shown that an IgM antiquinidine antibody appears to be involved. The diagnosis can be established in vitro by examining deposition of complement on donor erythrocytes by patient serum, which occurs only in the presence of the drug. The Coombs' test is used to detect complement deposition on the erythrocyte surface.

Non-specific coating of the erythrocyte surface has been observed with the cephalosporin antibiotics. Cephalothins become bound to the erythrocyte membrane and cause the red cell to be coated by many plasma proteins. The Coombs' test result is positive. Hemolytic anemia does not occur. Cephalothin, however, can cause hemolytic anemia by acting as a hapten by a mechanism similar to that of penicillin.

In all these drug-induced processes, patients respond to withdrawal of the offending drug. If necessary, a brief course of glucocorticoid therapy can be administered.

McKenzie SE, Schreiber AD: Fcγ receptors in phagocytes. Curr Opin Hematol 5:16, 1998. *A review of Fc receptors.*

Packman CH, Rosenfeld SI, Jenkins DE Jr, et al: Differing susceptibility of two types of paroxysmal nocturnal hemoglobinuria cells to C5b-9. Blood Rev 12:1, 1998. *An update and review of PNH.*

Schreiber AD, Rosse WF, Frank MM: Autoimmune hemolytic anemia. *In* Samter M, Austen KF, Clamens HN, et al (eds): Immunological Diseases, 5th ed. Boston, Little, Brown, 1995. *An in-depth review of autoimmune hemolytic anemia.*

166 HEMOLYTIC ANEMIAS: INTRAVASCULAR

Mark M. Udden

DEFINITIONS

Disorders accompanied by intravascular hemolysis are uncommon, but dramatic causes of anemia. They are marked by destruction of red cells in the circulation, as opposed to extravascular destruction of altered red cells by the reticuloendothelial cells of the spleen, liver, and bone marrow. Recognition and diagnosis of these disorders frequently depend on a careful review of red cell morphology on an ordinary peripheral blood smear. A potent hemolysin or significant mechanical stress is required to dismantle a red cell in the circulation. Subtle red cell abnormalities are more likely to cause extravascular hemolysis in the spleen.

Intravascular hemolysis is the result of a wide range of pathologic conditions (Table 166–1), including small and large vessel lesions, prosthetic circulatory devices, and exertion, as well as chemical and physical agents. Most of these conditions are acquired phenomena extrinsic to the red patient's own red cells. However, some hereditary, intrinsic disorders such as homozygous sickle cell disease and hereditary hydrocytosis and xerocytosis also involve a significant component of intravascular hemolysis. Paroxysmal nocturnal hemoglobinuria is an example of an acquired intrinsic defect, i.e., increased sensitivity to complement, associated with intravascular hemolysis.

CAUSES AND SYNDROMES OF INTRAVASCULAR HEMOLYSIS

MICROANGIOPATHIC HEMOLYTIC ANEMIAS. The combination of small vessel damage and the appearance of fragmented red cells in the peripheral blood defines microangiopathic hemolytic anemia. This syndrome is the end product of a constellation of disorders (Table 166–2) that share endothelial damage as a common feature. Two of the most important microangiopathic hemolytic anemias, thrombotic thrombocytopenic purpura (TTP) (see Chapter 184) and hemolytic-uremic syndrome (HUS) (see Chapter 184), are discussed in detail elsewhere.

The typical findings in autopsy or biopsy tissue are endothelial swelling, hyaline thrombi, and subendothelial deposits of hyaline material. The peripheral blood picture is notable for striking erythrocyte fragmentation. Triangular cells or schistocytes, helmet cells, burr cells, and spherocytes are recognized. Red cell fragmentation in microangiopathic hemolytic anemia has been attributed to interaction of the red cell with fibrin strands in partially thrombosed microvasculature. Red cells are caught on a sharp clothesline of fibrin as they attempt to move past a thrombus. The fibrin strands

Table 166–1 ■ CAUSES OF INTRAVASCULAR HEMOLYSIS

Microangiopathic hemolytic anemia
Valve hemolysis
Exertional hemolysis
Chemical agents
Osmotic lysis
Thermal injury
Infections
Paroxysmal nocturnal hemoglobinuria
Cold agglutinin disease
Venoms

Microangiopathic Hemolytic Anemia
Thrombotic thrombocytopenic purpura
Hemolytic-uremic syndrome
Disseminated intravascular coagulation
Disseminated carcinomatosis
Pregnancy related
    Preeclampsia/eclampsia
    HELLP
    Postpartum hemolytic-uremic syndrome
Glomerulonephritis
Malignant hypertension
Renal cortical necrosis
Allograft rejection
Vasculitis
Diabetic microangiopathy
Hemangiomas
Prosthetic Device and Large Vessel Disorders
Valve hemolysis
Septal patches
Vascular grafts
Arteriovenous fistulas
Circulatory assist devices

HELLP = *h*emolysis, *e*levated *l*iver enzymes, and *l*ow *p*latelet count.

are thought to then scissor the erythrocytes into fragments. Although this phenomenon has been demonstrated in vitro by the fragmentation of red cells after passage through a fibrin clot, there is less evidence that fibrin strands straddle small vessels in microangiopathic lesions in tissue. Another explanation depends on the recently recognized ability of red cells to adhere to cultured endothelial cells under flow conditions. Adhesion events are more frequent when young red cells come into contact with endothelial cells that have been stimulated by cytokines. Adhesion proteins on the red cell interact directly with other adhesive proteins on the endothelial cells or via ligands such as thrombospondin, von Willebrand factor, and fibronectin present in the plasma or in exposed subendothelium. These findings suggest an alternative mechanism for red cell fragmentation in which red cells initially adhere to injured endothelial cells and then fragment as they are sheared away from the endothelium by continued blood flow. Because young red cells are favored in adhesion, reticulocytosis may further accelerate the fragmentation process.

Typical patients have anemia, reticulocytosis, and bizarre erythrocyte morphology—schistocytes, helmet cells, burr cells, and spherocytes (Color Plate 5*H*). The secondary laboratory features of intravascular hemolysis (see below) are present to a varying degree. Renal dysfunction is also common. Thrombocytopenia, prolongation of the prothrombin time (PT) and partial thromboplastin time (PTT), hypofibrinogenemia, and circulating fibrin/fibrinogen degradation products consistent with disseminated intravascular coagulation (DIC) are sometimes found. Because fragmented red cells indicating microangiopathic hemolytic anemia are observed in 10 to 25% of the patients who have DIC, it is clear that the two phenomena are closely associated in some cases; however, DIC is seldom observed in TTP and HUS. Because TTP often responds to plasmapheresis/plasma exchange, it is absolutely critical to review the peripheral blood film personally to identify fragmented red cells in a patient with thrombocytopenia, particularly when the patient has neurologic or renal abnormalities.

The differential diagnosis of microangiopathic hemolytic anemia is largely dependent on an understanding of the patient's clinical situation. Microangiopathic hemolytic anemia is observed in a wide array of multisystem disorders that also affect the kidney, including malignant hypertension, renal cortical necrosis, scleroderma, and vasculitis; it is seen less often with glomerulonephritis and rarely, if ever with acute tubular necrosis. Renal allograft rejection and bone marrow transplantation complicated by fungal infection or graft-versus-host disease have also been associated with microangiopathic hemolytic anemia. It also develops in patients treated with the immunosuppressive agent cyclosporine (less often with tacrolimus). Patients with underlying systemic lupus erythematosus can have a thrombotic microangiopathic syndrome that includes microangiopathic hemolytic anemia, thrombocytopenia, neurologic dysfunction, renal impairment, low complement levels, and antiphospholipid antibodies (see Chapter 289).

Evaluation of a pregnant woman with microangiopathic hemolytic anemia can be particularly difficult inasmuch as TTP, HUS, and eclampsia/preeclampsia share a propensity for proteinuria, thrombocytopenia, and seizures. The HELLP syndrome (*h*emolysis, *e*levated *l*iver function tests, and *l*ow *p*latelet count) should be considered when hepatomegaly, hepatic tenderness, or increased blood transaminases are detected. These patients may suffer hepatic rupture. Microangiopathic hemolytic anemia may also complicate DIC associated with amniotic fluid embolism, premature separation of the placenta, and retained dead fetus. Frequently, delivery will abrogate eclampsia or the HELLP syndrome.

Disseminated carcinomatosis is also a cause of microangiopathic hemolytic anemia. The presence of cancer cells in close proximity to the endothelium or uncovered in tumor vessel walls presents a stimulus for DIC and a trap for erythrocytes. As many as 5% of patients with metastatic cancer will have evidence of microangiopathic hemolytic anemia. The most frequent primary tumor sites are gastric, followed by lung and breast. Mucin-secreting adenomas are also found in association with this form of anemia. Symptoms are related to the anemia and to thrombosis. Intracranial hemorrhage is a frequent complication. In addition to laboratory evidence for intravascular hemolysis and DIC, leukocytosis and a leukoerythroblastic picture are often present. Trousseau's syndrome of cancer associated with thrombophlebitis is also accompanied by any combination of microangiopathic hemolytic anemia, arterial thrombi, marantic endocarditis, and DIC. Cancer-related thrombotic microangiopathic hemolytic anemia may also occur without frank DIC; tumor emboli and fibrin microthrombi are the most common findings at autopsy (see Chapter 193). The outlook for patients with cancer-related microangiopathic hemolytic anemia is poor because the tumors are usually advanced with limited options for effective chemotherapy. The thrombotic complications typically do not respond to warfarin anticoagulation but do improve with heparin. Chemotherapy with mitomycin and other agents has been associated with the development of a HUS-like syndrome months later in the absence of tumor.

Microangiopathic hemolytic anemia also accompanies serious infections, particularly when DIC is present. Purpura fulminans is a striking combination of DIC, protein C deficiency, digital ischemia, and gangrene, as well as symmetrical hemorrhagic bullous skin lesions in fatty areas of the abdomen, thighs, buttocks, and extremities.

Microangiopathic hemolytic anemia has also been described in association with diabetic vasculopathy, ulcerative colitis, Wegener's granulomatosis, Weber-Christian disease, and pulmonary hypertension. It may also develop in infants and adults with giant hemangiomas when associated with DIC—the Kasabach-Merritt syndrome.

VALVE HEMOLYSIS AND RELATED CONDITIONS. Fragmentation hemolysis has been associated with patch repairs of atrial and ventricular defects and after placement of aortic and mitral valves with prosthetic devices. Significant hemolysis is rarely associated with modern valves when they are normally functioning. Evidence of low-grade intravascular hemolysis, including decreased haptoglobin and increased lactate dehydrogenase (LDH), can be detected in most patients with mechanical valves. Patients with multiple mechanical valves or an older valve with a caged ball design are more likely to have hemolysis. Significant hemolysis is more often seen with paravalvular leaks caused by partial valve ring dehiscence or infection. When a paravalvular leak develops, blood flows at high shear rates through a small orifice. Patches placed to close septal wall defects may be the source of hemolysis if they do not support endothelial growth and if flow is turbulent in the area of the patch. Fragmentation has also been observed in patients with artificial hearts, left ventricular assist devices, vascular grafts, traumatic arterial venous fistulas, dialysis catheters, and transjugular portosystemic shunts. Typically, hemolysis associated with cardiac valves, large vessels, or prosthetic devices does not cause thrombocytopenia. Constant intravascular hemolysis and hemoglobinuria will eventually result in iron deficiency. Folate needs are also increased in patients with chronic hemolysis. Patients with significant valve hemolysis do better if iron deficiency is corrected and folate is supplemented. Increased cardiac output accentuates shear stress. Therefore, decreasing cardiac output by correction of anemia with blood transfusions, avoidance of strenuous exercise, and judicious use of afterload reduction or β-blockers may be of benefit. Patients with severe paravalvular leakage may eventually require replacement of the valve.

EXERTIONAL HEMOLYSIS. A little-known consequence of exertion is a mild hemolytic process marked by decreased serum haptoglobin and hemoglobinuria in distance runners, marathon enthusiasts, and triathletes. Destruction of red cells occurs because of repetitive foot strike–induced damage in the small vessels of the feet as they meet hard pavement. March hemoglobinuria was described in soldiers fitted with heavy boots with no cushioning for the feet. The advent of shoes with extensive supportive cushions has reduced the occurrence of foot strike hemolysis. Even so, a "runner's macrocytosis" is still observed and has been attributed to the preferential loss of older and smaller erythrocytes. Reticulocytosis is rarely observed, and other tests for hemolysis are typically uninformative. Lesser degrees of red cell destruction occur with the less traumatic exertion associated with aerobic exercises, rowing, weight lifting, and even swimming. Hemoglobinuria as a result of destruction of erythrocytes by hand trauma also occurs after long sessions playing the conga drum and after enthusiastic karate practices. Hemolysis may be caused by the direct physical trauma to red cells or because the red cells are damaged as they come into contact with damaged endothelium. In occasional patients with known hereditary hemolytic disorders, hemoglobinuria develops with exercise.

The contribution of exertional hemolysis to the mild anemia observed in well-conditioned athletes is uncertain. The plasma volume is expanded as a result of conditioning, and there is evidence of gastrointestinal blood loss following distance running events. The frequent use of non-steroidal anti-inflammatory agents by competitive athletes may also result in gastritis and iron deficiency. Early reports of exertional hemolysis implicated hemoglobinuria as a factor contributing to iron deficiency in athletes. Muscle destruction and myoglobinuria must also be considered in an athlete who overexerts. Better shoes, shorter distances, slower pacing, and running on grass and cinder paths instead of pavement will reduce foot strike hemolysis.

CHEMICAL AND PHYSICAL AGENTS. Intravascular hemolytic anemia and renal failure have been described after intentional ingestion of copper sulfate in suicide attempts and recently in two men after drinking a ceremonial Nigerian "spiritual water." Hemolytic anemia may precede or accompany liver dysfunction in patients with Wilson's disease and may occur when penicillamine treatment is withdrawn. One component of copper toxicity is oxidant damage to the red cell as evidenced by the appearance of Heinz bodies and the greater degree of toxicity for patients who are glucose-6-phosphate dehydrogenase deficient. Other agents that cause oxidant damage to normal red cells include phenazopyridine HCT (Pyridium), dapsone, isobutyl nitrate, amyl nitrite, phenacetin, and potassium and sodium nitrates.

Osmotic lysis of red cells has been reported after near-drowning in fresh water and after exposure of patients to hypotonic fluid during dialysis. Distilled water instilled during prostate surgery has also been associated with osmotic swelling of red cells and hemolysis.

Thermal injury also damages red cells; a brisk intravascular hemolysis accompanied by spherocytosis and unusual red cells with membrane extensions or blebs develops in patients with extensive burns. Less damaged red cells appear to be sequestered in the spleen. In vitro studies show that the principal membrane protein, spectrin, is unstable and unfolds when heated to 49° C. Thermal red cell injury is also recorded with another dialysis misadventure—dialysis with overheated fluid. Hemolysis has also been observed when blood products are excessively warmed before transfusion.

Although infections are associated with microangiopathic hemolytic anemia, a few organisms infect red cells and cause direct destruction in diseases such as malaria, babesiosis, and bartonellosis. Infection with *Clostridium perfringens* occurs in septic abortion, cholecystitis, or biliary duct surgery and also causes significant intravascular hemolysis; phospholipases elaborated by the organism destroy red cell membrane lipids and produce microspherocytosis and intense hemoglobinemia (see Chapter 334). In a few patients, "total hemolysis" was observed a few hours before succumbing to clostridial infection; on the peripheral blood smears of such patients, only white cells and erythrocyte ghosts and membrane remnants were seen. The venom of Indian cobras is hemolytic. Hemolysis can also develop in victims of a brown recluse spider bite.

COMMON CLINICAL FEATURES OF INTRAVASCULAR HEMOLYSIS

Patients may experience symptoms related to anemia or may notice jaundice. Laboratory evaluation depends on adequate assessment of the peripheral blood smear in a patient who has anemia and reticulocytosis. The best direct evidence for intravascular hemolysis includes suggestive red cell morphology (fragmented red cells, spherocytosis) and hemoglobinuria. The indirect fraction of bilirubin is typically increased. Although non-specific, LDH is frequently elevated in patients with intravascular hemolysis and may be a convenient indicator of the patient's progress. In microangiopathic hemolytic anemia associated with malignant hypertension, fragmented red cells will persist in the circulation for weeks after adequate blood pressure control. Decreased haptoglobin is another confirmatory test. Patients with chronic intravascular hemolysis may also have hemosiderinuria. In some patients with chronic hemolysis, tests to determine iron or folate deficiency may be required. Because of the association of microangiopathic hemolytic anemia with DIC, determination of the platelet count, PT, PTT, fibrinogen, and levels of fibrin/fibrinogen degradation products is prudent.

DIFFERENTIAL DIAGNOSIS

A rare cause of hemoglobinuria and intravascular hemolysis is paroxysmal nocturnal hemoglobinuria. Erythrocyte morphology is normal, although patients may be thrombocytopenic and iron deficient. Hemosiderinuria is a sine qua non of this disorder. Cold agglutinin disease and paroxysmal cold hemoglobinuria are causes of intravascular hemolysis and hemoglobinuria (see Chapter 165). When spherocytic morphology predominates, a direct Coombs test should be done to detect autoimmune hemolytic anemia.

Differentiation of myoglobinuria from hemoglobinuria may require specific tests on a urine sample (see Chapter 99). Myoglobin, unlike hemoglobin, is seldom released in enough quantity to color the plasma.

It may be difficult to differentiate intravascular hemolysis from ineffective erythropoiesis associated with megaloblastic anemia (see Chapter 163). In pernicious anemia, for example, fragmentation of the red cells may be striking, even though macro-ovalocytosis and hypersegmentation of granulocytes are usually also prominent. Elevated LDH, low haptoglobin, and increased indirect bilirubin are also observed in pernicious anemia. However, the reticulocyte count is typically low, which makes hemolysis unlikely.

TREATMENT AND PROGNOSIS

Treatment is directed at the underlying disorder. Folate supplementation may be useful and iron replacement may be necessary in a few individuals with valve hemolysis. Because hemolysis is extravascular, splenectomy is seldom beneficial. In some patients, overwhelming hemolysis is catastrophic. Such patients may succumb to shock, DIC, or renal failure. Patients with acute intravascular hemolysis and DIC or acute renal failure may require transfusion support or hemodialysis, respectively. Because thrombosis is a frequent complication of tumor-related microangiopathic hemolytic anemia, anticoagulation with heparin is sometimes offered. The prognosis of patients with intravascular hemolysis depends entirely on the underlying disorder.

Maraj R, Jacobs LE, Ioli A, Kotler MN: Evaluation of hemolysis in patients with prosthetic heart valves. Clin Cardiol 21:387, 1998. *A practical review.*

167 HEMOGLOBINOPATHIES: THE THALASSEMIAS

Griffin P. Rodgers

The *thalassemia syndromes* are a heterogeneous group of inherited anemias characterized by defects in the synthesis of one or more globin chain subunits of the adult hemoglobin tetramer (Hb A). Patients with β-thalassemia have a decrease in β-chain production relative to α-chain production; the converse is the case

Table 167–1 ■ CLINICAL CLASSIFICATION OF THE THALASSEMIAS

CLASSIFICATION	GENOTYPE	CLINICAL SEVERITY*
α Thalassemia Syndromes		
α^+-carrier (silent)	$-\alpha/\alpha\alpha$†	Silent
α-Thalassemia trait	$-\alpha/-\alpha$; $--/\alpha\alpha$	Mild
Hb H disease	$-\alpha/--$	Mild–moderate; hemolytic anemia
Hydrops fetalis	$--/--$	Lethal
Hb Constant Spring genotypes	$\alpha\alpha^{cs}/\alpha\alpha$	Silent–mild
β-Thalassemia Syndromes		
β-Thalassemia minor (trait)	β/β^+‡	Silent
β-Thalassemia intermedia	β/β^0; β^+/β^+; $\beta^+/\beta^0 = \beta^+$	Moderate–severe
	HbE/β^0	
β-Thalassemia major	$\beta^0/\beta^0 = \beta^0$	Severe
Complex β-Thalassemia Syndromes		
Coinherited β-thalassemia†	Various combinations of α- and β-thalassemia syndromes	
Hereditary persistence of fetal hemoglobin	Various point mutations or deletions in or around γ-globin gene	Mild–moderate
γ-Thalassemia	Deletion of one or more γ-genes	
δ-Thalassemia	Deletion of one or more δ-genes	
γ δ β-Thalassemia	Complex deletions of one or more γ-, δ-, β-genes in tandem	

Silent normal or minimally abnormal hematology values; *mild,* hemoglobin level normal or slightly reduced with disproportionate microcytic hypochromic indices; *moderate,* hemolytic anemia, icterus, splenomegaly, although no regular transfusion requirement; *severe,* profound anemia with transfusion dependency, extramedullary hematopoiesis, growth retardation, bone abnormalities, hemosiderosis; *lethal,* death *in utero* from anemic congestive heart failure.

†The α-thalassemia syndromes usually result from deletions in one or more α-genes, indicated by the minus sign, or from mutations in the coding sequence (e.g., α-Constant Spring, α^{cs}).

‡The β-thalassemia syndromes are typically the consequence of mutations that lead to a *decreased* level of normal β-chain production (β^+) or *absence* of β-chain production (β^0). Various combinations of these mutations give rise to syndromes of increasing severity.

in α-thalassemia. The clinical syndromes associated with thalassemia arise from the combined effects of inadequate hemoglobin production and unbalanced accumulation of globin subunits. The former causes hypochromia and microcytosis; the latter leads to ineffective erythropoiesis and hemolytic anemia. Clinical manifestations are diverse and range from asymptomatic hypochromia and microcytosis to profound anemia leading to death in utero or in early childhood if untreated. This clinical heterogeneity reflects the variable severity of the primary biosynthetic defect and coinherited modulating factors, such as accelerated synthesis of fetal hemoglobin subunits, the overall effectiveness of a wide range of cellular and circulatory adaptive factors, and perhaps not yet appreciated environmental factors. These disorders differ from the hemoglobinopathies that result from mutations in the coding sequences of the α- or β-globin genes; such mutations alter protein structure and lead to other disease manifestations (e.g., Hb S in sickle cell disease) (see Chapters 168 and 169). These disorders are not mutually exclusive in that some mutations (e.g., Hb E and Hb Constant

Spring) alter both the structure of a globin chain and the rate at which it is produced. Table 167–1 provides a clinical classification and distinguishing characteristics of specific thalassemia syndromes.

MOLECULAR GENETICS

A number of structural genes encode for the globin polypeptides in maturing human erythroid cells. Normal functional hemoglobin consists of a tetramer of two α-like and two β-like globin polypeptide chains. Two clusters of closely linked genes encode the globin chains. The non-α (β-like) genes reside on chromosome 11 and include the two adult genes δ and β, the two very similar fetal genes (differing by one amino acid, alanine or glycine) $^A\gamma$ and $^G\gamma$, and the single embryonic ε-gene. On chromosome 16 is found the α-like genes, including the duplicated and almost identically functional α-genes ($\alpha_2\alpha_1$), which are present in the fetal and adult stages of erythropoiesis, and the embryonic ζ-gene. A θ-gene

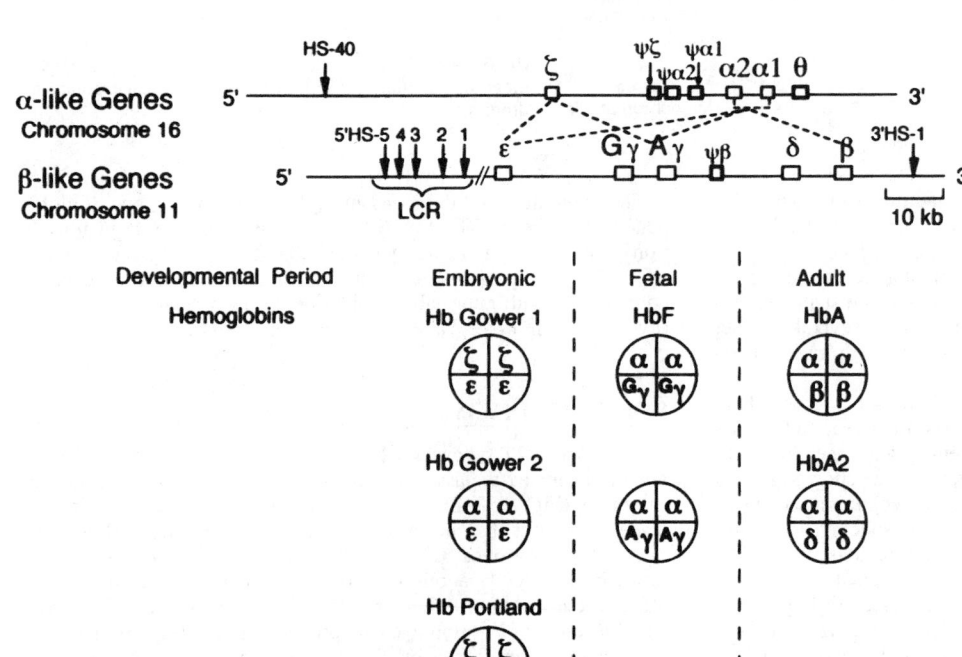

FIGURE 167–1 ■ Organization and expression of the human globin genes. The human globin genes consist of two clusters of closely linked genes on two separate chromosomes encoding the globin chains. The genes are arranged with the same transcriptional orientation arrayed from 5′ to 3′ in the order that they are sequentially expressed during development. The α- and β-globin gene clusters also contain several pseudogenes, indicated by the Ψφ-prefix. Upstream (5′) of these clusters are major transcriptional control elements, HS-40→ (α), LCR→ (β), that are critical for high-level expression in a developmentally specific manner.

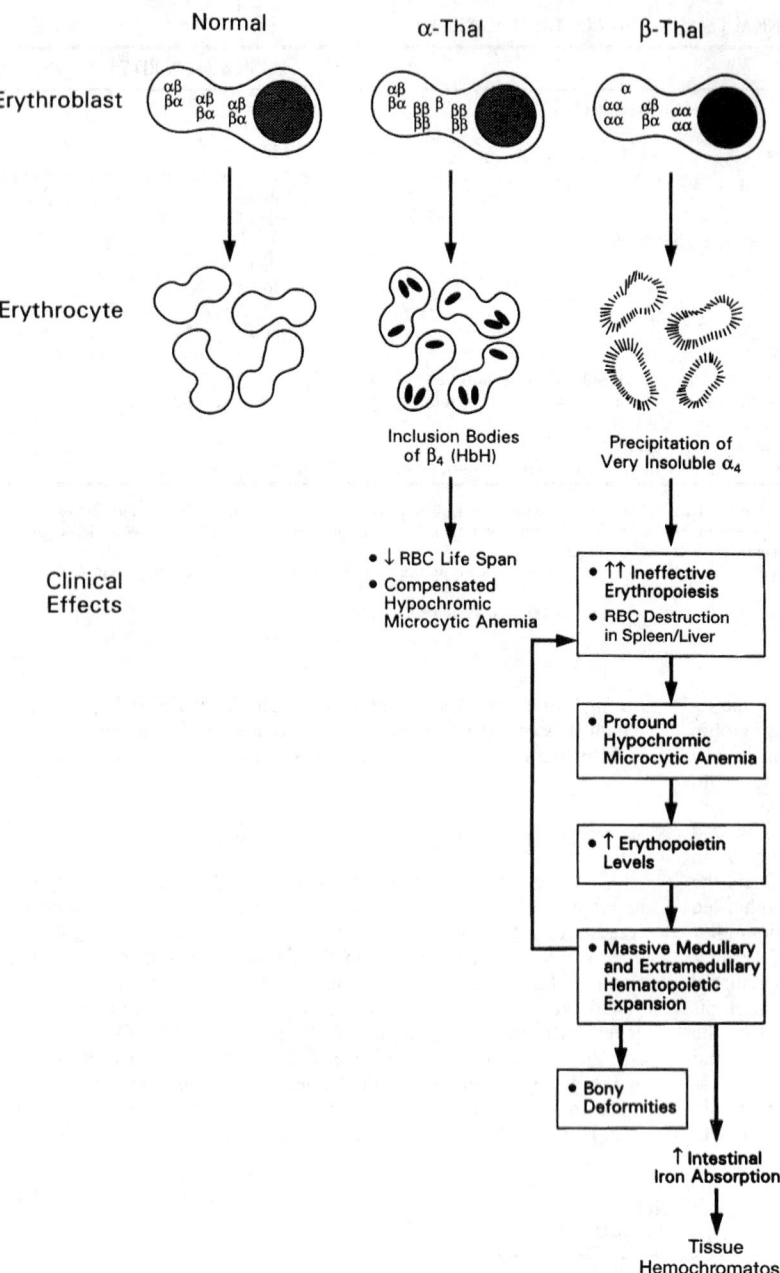

FIGURE 167–2 ■ Schematic representation of the pathophysiology of the clinically significant α- and β-thalassemia syndromes.

downstream from the α_1-gene has now been shown to be a pseudogene incapable of producing normal messenger RNA. High-level tissue and developmentally specific globin gene expression is governed in large part by novel upstream regulatory elements designated HS-40 and LCR for the α- and β-globin clusters, respectively. As the descriptors of these genes imply, several distinct hemoglobin species are present during the transition from intrauterine to adult life (Fig. 167–1).

On a smaller scale, individual α- and β-like globin genes share many general features. Each gene consists of three coding sequences (exons) interrupted by two intervening sequences (introns). As with other eukaryotic genes, globin genes have short segments of 5′ and 3′ untranslated regions, appropriate recognition sequences at the intron/exon junctions to facilitate normal splicing, and polyadenylation sequences in the 3′ untranslated regions. In the 5′ promoter region are three elements critical for normal globin gene expression, including the ATA, CCAAT, and CACCC boxes. Enhancers and silencing elements have also been recognized in these 5′ and 3′ flanking sequences. Mutations (or deletions) in any of these important elements in the promoters, enhancers, or intron-exon junctions lead to a decrease in overall gene transcription.

These mutation or deletions in and around the α- and β-globin genes or in the α-HS-40 or β-LCR may lead to disease manifestations ranging from inconsequential laboratory findings (microcytosis and hypochromia in α- and β-thalassemia trait) to events incompatible with normal intrauterine growth and development (hydrops fetalis) (see Table 167–1 and Fig. 167–2).

MOLECULAR DEFECTS

α-Thalassemia syndromes have been classified by defects resulting in severe (α-thalassemia type 1) and mild (α-thalassemia type 2) forms (Fig. 167–3). This nomenclature is gradually being replaced to reflect the current classification scheme of the β-thalassemias into two groups: α°- and α^+-thalassemia. The α°-thalassemias result in completely abolished production of α-globin chains by the affected chromosome, whereas the α^+-thalassemias are defined by a variable amount of globin chain production resulting from the remaining α-globin genes on the chromosome. The α°-thalassemias usually result from deletion of the α_2- and α_1-globin genes *in cis* (on the same chromosome), the entire cluster together with the

α-Globin Gene		Genotype	Phenotype	# of Functional α-Genes
α2 α1	‡‡	α α/α α	Normal	Normal	4
α2 α1	┿‡	– α/α α	α⁺-thal heterozygote (mild)	Silent carrier α-thal trait	3
α2 α1	|‡	– –/α α	α⁰-thal heterozygote (moderate)	Microcytosis α-thal trait	2
α2 α1	┿┿	– α/– α	α⁺-thal homozygote (moderate)	Microcytosis α-thal trait	2
α2 α1	|┿	– –/– α	α⁰-thal x α⁺-thal (severe)	Hb H disease	1
α2 α1	||	– –/– –	α⁰-thal homozygote (lethal)	Hydrops fetalis with Hb Bart's	0

FIGURE 167-3 ■ The genetic bases of the more common forms of α-thalassemia. The hematologic and clinical severity is directly proportional to the number of deleted α-globin genes, as indicated. (Adapted from Gelehrter TD, Collins FS: Principles of Medical Genetics. Baltimore, Williams & Wilkins, 1990.)

main regulatory sequence (HS40), or the HS40 regulatory element alone. Other less frequent causes of α°-thalassemia include the occurrence of nonsense mutations within a single α-gene *in cis* and deletion of the other α-globin locus.

α^+-Thalassemia usually results from deletion of a single α-gene within the cluster or, less frequently, a thalassemic generating point mutation in either the α_1- or α_2-genes. The point mutation in the 3′ untranslated region (α Constant Spring) is an example of a thalassemic hemoglobinopathy in which a structural variant renders the hemoglobin unstable and thus effectively diminishes the α- to β-globin chain ratio.

In contrast to the α-thalassemia syndromes, the *β-thalassemias* are rarely caused by major structural gene deletions (Fig. 167-4). Deletions that have been described include those in individuals who are heterozygous (with removal of all or a substantial portion of the regulatory elements in the β-LCR), large structural deletions, including the α-δ-β or β-genes (or some subset thereof), or deletions within the critical elements in the β-promoter described previously. The more common cause of β-thalassemia is the so-called non-deletional variant, which affects gene function in many ways, including abnormalities in transcription, RNA processing, or RNA translation of the β-globin gene.

Despite the large number of these mutations—over 200 β-thalassemia alleles have now been characterized—probably only 20 β-thalassemic alleles account for greater than 80% of the β-thalassemia mutations. Transcriptional mutants result from mutations either in the promoter of regulatory elements, generally between position −101 and position −28, or in the 5′ untranslated regions, especially in the region of the canonical CAP site. An example of such a transcriptional mutant is the −28 point mutation, which is common in blacks and Southeast Asians and gives rise to a β^+-phenotype. RNA processing abnormalities, perhaps the most common of all mutations thus characterized, occur near splice junctions next to the consensus splice site (e.g., the IVS 1:5 mutation common in Mediterranean populations, Northern Europeans, and Algerians), in cryptic splice sites in introns (e.g., IVS II:654 producing β°- or β^+-thalassemia in Chinese, Southeast Asians, and Japanese), or in cryptic splice sites in exons (e.g., codon 19 in Southeast Asians). A mutation in codon 26 (GTA → GTG) results in Hb E, prevalent among Southeast Asians, and gives rise to a quantitative reduction in normal β-globin gene mRNA because of activation of a cryptic splice donor site, as well as a qualitative abnormality of the β-globin chain because of substitution of a lysine for the normal glutamic acid (see Chapter 169). The third major category of mutations results in RNA translation abnormalities. These mutations produce a β°-thalassemia phenotype and include abnormalities in the initiation (ATG) codon, the production of nonsense codons (codon 39 in Mediterranean populations), or frame shift mutations such as the codon 41/42 mutations common in Chinese, Southeast Asian, and Asian Indian populations or the codon 71/72 mutations in the Chinese.

PATHOPHYSIOLOGY

Patients with α-thalassemia have a decrease in α-globin chain production relative to β-globin chain, with the formation of β_4 (Hb H) inclusion bodies. Red cells bearing these inclusion bodies are rapidly removed from the circulation by the reticuloendothelial system, thus shortening their survival. The resulting mild anemia is partially compensated by an increase in red cell production.

In contrast, patients with β-thalassemia have a decrease in β-globin chain production relative to α-globin chain production, which leads to an excess of α-globin chains. Although this decrease in β-synthesis is slightly compensated by the γ- and δ-globin chains, the combined β-, δ-, and γ-globin chains are insufficient to match the number of α-globin chains present. Unbound α-globin chains are extremely insoluble and precipitate in red cell precursors and their progeny, a process leading to defective erythroid maturation (ineffective erythropoiesis). The few cells that do emerge into the peripheral circulation are rapidly removed in the spleen and liver. Progressive splenomegaly occurs in an attempt to entrap these abnormal red cells and further exacerbates the anemia by virtue of hemodilution. The resulting profound anemia increases circulating erythropoietin levels and thus causes a massive

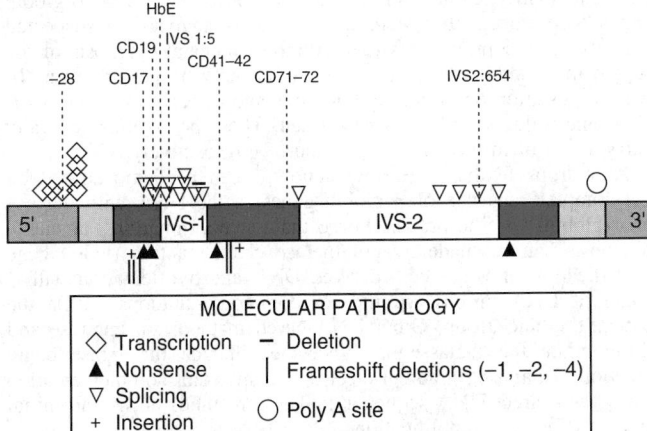

FIGURE 167-4 ■ General structure of the human β-globin gene and the sites (and bases) of some of the more common recessively inherited β-thalassemia mutations. (Adapted from Stamatoyannopoulos G, Neinhuis AW, Leder P, Majerus PW: The Molecular Basis of Blood Disease. Philadelphia, WB Saunders, 1987.)

expansion of medullary and extramedullary hematopoietic tissue. This expansion in turn leads to skeletal abnormalities and various growth and metabolic derangements. Furthermore, the expanded erythroid marrow induces signal(s) (yet uncharacterized) that increase intestinal iron absorption. This process, along with the iatrogenic iron overload (secondary to chronic transfusions), leads to tissue hemochromatosis and its attendant complications.

CLINICAL FEATURES

α-THALASSEMIAS. Deletion of one or both α-globin genes on chromosome 16 is the most common mutation of the human genome. The α-globin gene cluster is a dynamic locus in which tandemly duplicated long blocks of nucleotide sequences promote non-homologous recombination between chromosomes during meiosis. Thus the α-thalassemia syndromes are predominately due to deletions of one or more of the four genes coding for the α-chain, although non-deletional forms have also been described. These disorders have their highest prevalence in blacks (up to 30%), in whom a single α-gene or two α-genes in trans (opposite chromosomes) may be deleted. In contrast, in Southeast Asian populations, where the prevalence may reach up to 40%, more typically two α-genes in cis (on the same chromosome) may be deleted, although single α-gene deletions are also seen (see Fig. 167–3).

The clinical spectrum of the α-thalassemia syndromes is directly related to the number of functioning α-globin genes. Accordingly, deletions of one ($\alpha\alpha/-\alpha$) or two ($-\alpha/-\alpha$, $--/\alpha\alpha$) α-globin genes, which occur very frequently in many parts of the world, are virtually asymptomatic. Correct diagnosis of these genotypes allows for the identification of couples at risk for pregnancies with homozygous fetuses (see below). In addition, proper recognition of these syndromes provides a molecular basis for microcytosis and hypochromia (and possibly mild anemia) and thus averts the injudicious and often extended use of iron supplementation for the erroneous diagnosis of iron deficiency (see Chapter 162). Hb H disease, which is caused by deletions of three genes ($--/-\alpha$), is manifested as a moderately severe anemia with splenomegaly and a hypochromic, microcytic blood film appearance (see Table 167–1). Hb H (β_4) is demonstrable by special staining of the red cell and by hemoglobin electrophoresis. Generally, however, the hemolytic anemia in Hb H disease is partially compensated, with an average hemoglobin value of 8 to 10 g/dL, and therefore chronic transfusion therapy may not be required. However, Hb H is prone to precipitation in red cells during oxidative stress and under conditions of increased temperature, and consequently the hemolytic anemia may be exacerbated in these patients by agents known to induce oxidant injury or by infections. Accordingly, the same drugs that induce hemolysis in glucose-6-phosphate dehydrogenase–deficient patients (see Chapter 164), especially the sulfonamides, should be avoided in susceptible patients with Hb H disease.

In its most severe form, in which all four genes are deleted, α-thalassemia is incompatible with life, and the fetus is stillborn or critically ill with hydrops fetalis. Recent reports indicate that mothers carrying affected fetuses have a high incidence of pregnancy-induced hypertension (up to 75%), seizures, postpartum hemorrhage in 10%, and other peripartum complications. Accordingly, every effort should be made to identify these women (typically Asians or Asian-Americans) during the early course of their pregnancy for appropriate referral.

β-THALASSEMIAS. The β-thalassemia syndromes represent the classic molecular paradigm in which disparate defects in a eukaryotic structural gene can culminate in decreased to absent (β) polypeptide chain production. This diverse group of disorders for the most part is due to single nucleotide changes in or around either or both of the two β-globin genes. Some of the molecular mechanisms accounting for the thalassemic phenotype include nonsense, frame shift, splicing, and polyadenylation mutations, as well as insertions and deletions (see Fig. 167–4). These alterations give rise to significant changes in the level of gene transcription that lead to absent (β°) or markedly diminished (β^+) amounts of β-globin gene mRNA (see Table 167–1). In addition, long deletions lead to more complex forms of β-thalassemia syndromes, such as β-thalassemia or hereditary persistence of fetal hemoglobin. However, such large deletions in the β-globin cluster occur less commonly than in the α-globin cluster.

The condition is ubiquitous, but especially common in Mediterranean, Asian, and African populations (and their American descendants), in whom the high gene frequency has been thought to reflect geographic areas with a high malaria prevalence. Within a given ethnic group, relatively few genotypes account for the majority of the cases, each of which has now been defined by DNA analysis. At a lower level of resolution, the pattern of DNA resolved on gel electrophoresis following restriction enzyme digestion has been used to define certain haplotypes or restriction fragment length polymorphisms. Specific β-globin cluster haplotypes are genetically linked to certain of these thalassemic mutations, and hence haplotype analysis has been used to define mutation prevalence in various populations, as well as to assess population migration.

The clinical spectrum of disease severity in the β-thalassemia syndromes is directly related to the quantitative effect of individual mutations on β-globin synthesis. Whereas β-thalassemia trait is asymptomatic, disease occurs in homozygotes or compound heterozygotes such as β-thalassemia/Hb E (see Table 167–1). In these latter instances, reduced or absent β-globin synthesis results in the accumulation of free α-globin chains that precipitate during early erythroblast development because of their relative insolubility. These inclusions lead to ineffective erythropoiesis in the bone marrow and enhanced peripheral destruction of those erythrocytes that emerge from the bone marrow. The associated pathophysiologic changes resulting from the subsequent anemia include splenomegaly, which may lead to hypersplenism, osteoporosis, and other skeletal and soft tissue changes associated with an expanded bone marrow, and iron overload resulting from a combination of enhanced gastrointestinal iron absorption and red cell transfusions. The liver, heart, pancreas, pituitary, and other endocrine organs serve as the major sites of excessive iron deposition, which ultimately leads to damage and failure of these organs.

LABORATORY DIAGNOSIS

Historically, the diagnosis of β-thalassemia and α-thalassemia has relied heavily on clinical and hematologic features (Color Plate 5I). Very often the patients were referred for the evaluation of anemia and/or microcytosis or in the context of neonatal or population screening. The discovery of low mean corpuscular volume and hemoglobin on automated complete blood counts has increased the number of such referrals. In the presence of normal iron status, increased levels of Hb A_2 (to 4 to 6%) and/or increased Hb F (to 5 to 20%) by quantitative hemoglobin analysis supports the diagnosis. Unfortunately, differentiation between iron deficiency anemia and β- or α-thalassemia trait can be difficult in practice if no reciprocal increases in Hb A_2 levels and/or Hb F are present. Moreover, in the presence of concomitant iron deficiency, Hb A_2 levels in β-thalassemic individuals may fall into the normal range. In these instances, the demonstration of a modified β/α-globin synthetic chain ratio, generally using ^{3}H-leucine to analyze globin chain production in reticulocytes, would be required for a conclusive diagnosis.

In the contemporary era of DNA technology, reference laboratories can swiftly clone and directly sequence the α- or β-globin genes or perform other techniques of DNA analysis on suspected patients. This approach has revolutionized prenatal diagnosis of the severe thalassemia syndromes, which can now be performed at 14 weeks' gestation on amniotic fluid cells and as early as 10 weeks if chorionic villus sampling is performed. These procedures generally carry a risk of miscarriage of 1% and 5%, respectively.

A hydrops fetalis ($--/--$) genotype can be demonstrated by the complete absence of α-globin genes in the DNA with the use of α-globin–specific probes. For β-thalassemia mutations, antenatal diagnosis can be made by polymerase chain reaction (PCR) gene amplification of white cell–derived DNA and hybridization with a panel of DNA probes specific for common mutations within the patient's ethnic group. Other DNA-based methods to diagnose and differentiate the thalassemia syndromes include the ligase chain reaction, denaturing gradient electrophoresis, color complementation assay, and direct DNA sequencing. These methods all use an initial step of PCR gene amplification.

TREATMENT

α-THALASSEMIA. Some deletions of one ($\alpha\alpha/-\alpha$) or two ($-\alpha/-\alpha$, $--/\alpha\alpha$) α-globin genes are asymptomatic, and no therapy is indicated. For Hb H disease (three-gene deletion, $--/-\alpha$), folic acid,

1 mg orally, should be administered daily to compensate for folate loss from accelerated red cell turnover. Splenectomy may be indicated for progressive anemia and is often associated with a mean rise in hemoglobin of 2 to 3 g/dL.

β-THALASSEMIA. Despite a nearly comprehensive understanding of the molecular and cellular pathogenesis of the β-thalassemia syndromes, a widely available curative form of treatment for homozygotes remains elusive. Nonetheless, dramatic improvement in life expectancy and morbidity has been observed over the last two decades, primarily because of aggressive transfusion support and the institution of effective iron chelation therapy in these regularly transfused patients. Thus except for curative allogeneic bone marrow transplantation, therapy is considered symptomatic and supportive. Treatment of compound heterozygotes for Hb S is discussed in Chapter 169.

TRANSFUSION. As treatment of severe β-thalassemia has improved, so has morbidity and median survival. Thus whereas non-transfused patients in the 1920s had a median survival of 2 years, transfusion therapy aimed at maintenance of a hemoglobin concentration of 11 to 13 g/dL (pre-transfusion level, >10 g/dL) has been shown to extend the average survival into the second decade, as well as minimize the bony abnormalities and improve sexual development. Transfusion support is generally initiated once the hemoglobin level drops below 7 g/dL and remains there in the absence of infection, blood loss, etc. To minimize febrile reactions and so as not to prejudice the potential future application of bone marrow transplantation (see below), leukocyte-poor red cells should be administered. An accurate record of the date and amount of blood administered, along with pre- and post-transfusion hemoglobin levels and the occurrence of any transfusion reactions, facilitates optimal therapy. Patients should be tested for the presence of hepatitis B antibodies; those testing negative should be immunized. Splenectomy is usually recommended in children or adolescents (~6 to 7 years of age) when their transfusion requirements exceed 1.5 times normal (e.g., >200 mL/kg/year). Before elective splenectomy, all patients should receive polyvalent pneumococcal vaccine and pediatric patients should also be given *Haemophilus influenzae* and *Neisseria meningitidis* vaccine.

IRON CHELATION. Although intensive transfusion programs have led to markedly improved survival, patients will die of iron overload unless chelation therapy is appropriately instituted and maintained. Currently, this therapy involves subcutaneous deferoxamine, a parenterally administered iron chelator, although a search for an effective oral chelator is currently under way. Many patients can be placed in iron balance by receiving a 12- to 24-hour infusion of deferoxamine 5 or 6 days a week. Chelation therapy should be individualized according to age, risks, compliance history, and other factors. For younger patients who are not yet at risk for the complications of iron overload, 1.5 to 2.0 g/day 5 to 6 days per week should be administered. Individuals aged 13 years or older should receive 2.0 to 2.5 g/day, depending on their ability to tolerate subcutaneous infusions. Patients with high liver iron concentrations (>6000 μg/g dry tissue) or those with evidence of cardiac involvement (i.e., heart failure, arrhythmias) require more intensive intravenous therapy and should be managed at specialized medical centers caring for large numbers of patients requiring chronic transfusion support. Periodic assessment of the effectiveness of chelation therapy should include an estimate of iron burden (e.g., serum iron, total iron binding capacity, ferritin) and an estimate of liver iron concentration by the judicious use of percutaneous liver biopsy or more ideally by validated non-invasive testing. A yearly cardiac evaluation should be performed in an effort to detect clinical evidence of cardiac disease and should include a complete history and physical examination, electrocardiogram, echocardiogram, and chest radiograph. A Holter monitor should be used in any patient who complains of palpitations or who is noted on physical examination to have an irregular heartbeat. Potential iron-induced damage to the endocrine glands should be evaluated by glucose tolerance testing, thyroid function tests, and cortisol determinations. Hormone replacement therapy is dictated by the results of basal and/or provocative endocrine function studies.

Various complications associated with the use of deferoxamine include visual disturbances, tinnitus, and renal dysfunction (azotemia and proteinuria). All of these complications are reversible on discontinuation of treatment with the drug and generally do not recur when the drug is subsequently given at lower doses. For these reasons, annual ophthalmologic and audiologic evaluations are strongly recommended for patients receiving chronic deferoxamine therapy.

STEM CELL TRANSPLANTATION AND EXPERIMENTAL THERAPIES. Allogeneic bone marrow transplantation (see Chapter 182) is increasingly effective for patients with homozygous β-thalassemia. Since the initial report in 1982, over 800 patients have undergone bone marrow transplantation in a single center in Italy, as well as smaller numbers of patients at other institutions. Among good-risk children (defined by good compliance with chelation and the absence of hepatomegaly and portal fibrosis), the 3-year event free survival rate is 95%. Older patients or those exhibiting one or more risk factors have rejection-free survival rates of less than 75%. Thus at the moment, bone marrow transplantation can be recommended as a reasonable option only for selected good-risk pediatric candidates who are fortunate to have an HLA-matched donor.

One alternative form of therapy involves the manipulation of globin gene expression with drugs such as 5-azacytidine, hydroxyurea, erythropoietin, or butyrate analogues. The rationale for such trials is that these agents are known to stimulate fetal hemoglobin synthesis and that γ-globin chain augmentation may compensate for the reduced β-chain synthesis, thereby normalizing the ratio of α- to non-α-chain; the result could be decreased transfusion requirements, decreased extramedullary hematopoiesis, and reduced iron overload. Although some patients have responded to these therapies very impressively, the overall low response rate observed thus far and the requirement for frequent parenteral administration of several of the agents have tempered enthusiasm for this approach. Nonetheless, these initial successes have led investigators to examine the efficacy of related classes of orally administered agents to stimulate Hb F production. It is hoped that these agents, when given alone or in combination, may display increased efficacy in a larger proportion of patients.

Finally, gene therapy has been directed at replacing or compensating for the defective β-globin alleles, especially in view of the comparative ease of obtaining hematopoietic stem cells. Although this approach remains theoretically attractive, its current application is not feasible and will require a convergence of technologic advances in several areas. Improvement in gene transfer methodologies and the ex vivo isolation and expansion of hematopoietic stem cells, as well as other logistic concerns, remain formidable tasks.

Brittenham GM, Griffith P, Nienhuis AW: Desferrioxamine (DFO) use protects against disease and death from transfusional iron overload in thalassemia major. N Engl J Med 331:567, 1994. *Careful study documenting the beneficial effects of aggressive chelation therapy in thalassemia patients with and without established cardiac disease secondary to iron overload.*

Lucarelli G, Galimberti M, Polchi P, et al: Bone marrow transplantation in adult thalassemia. Blood 80:1603, 1992.

Lucarelli G, Galimberti M, Polchi P, et al: Marrow transplantation in patients with thalassemia responsive to iron chelation therapy. N Engl J Med 329:840, 1993. *These two references establish the current protocols, including selection criteria, morbidity, and mortality, in adult and pediatric thalassemia patients undergoing bone marrow transplantation.*

Rodgers GP: Sickle cell disease and thalassemia. *In* Baillieres Clinical Hematology. Philadelphia, WB Saunders, 1998. *Up-to-date summary of the molecular, cellular, and clinical aspects of the congenital disorders of human hemoglobin.*

168 HEMOGLOBINOPATHIES: METHEMOGLOBINEMIAS, POLYCYTHEMIAS, AND UNSTABLE HEMOGLOBINS

Josef T. Prchal ■ *Mary M. Jenkins*

METHEMOGLOBINEMIAS

Methemoglobin Formation

Methemoglobin is the derivative of hemoglobin in which the iron of the heme group is oxidized from the ferrous (Fe^{2+}) to the ferric (Fe^{3+}) state. It is the oxidation state of the iron moiety in hemoglobin that determines its oxygen-carrying capacity. The iron in deoxyhemoglobin is in the ferrous form, which allows oxygen to bind to it easily. In contrast, the ferric hemes of methemoglobin are unable to bind oxygen. In addition, the oxygen affinity of the accompanying ferrous hemes in the hemoglobin tetramer is increased. As a result, the oxygen dissociation curve is left shifted and oxygen delivery is impaired.

Methemoglobin is generated physiologically as a consequence of deoxygenation. During deoxygenation, some oxygen leaves hemoglobin as a superoxide (O_2^-) radical, leaving the iron in a ferric state and creating a steady-state level of methemoglobin. This reaction is referred to as hemoglobin auto-oxidation and occurs spontaneously at a rate of about 3% per day. However, the steady-state blood methemoglobin level is maintained at very low levels ($\leq 1\%$ of total hemoglobin) by endogenous enzymatic hemoglobin reduction mechanisms. Increased levels of methemoglobin above the steady state, termed *methemoglobinemia,* result from either enhanced methemoglobin production or decreased methemoglobin reduction.

Although several potential mechanisms exist to reduce methemoglobin back to hemoglobin, only the reaction catalyzed by the reduced form of nicotinamide-adenine dinucleotide (NADH)-cytochrome b5 reductase (b5R) is physiologically important. Electrons are transferred from NADH (generated by glyceraldehyde 3-phosphate in the glycolytic pathway) to NADH cytochrome b5 reductase, and then to cytochrome b5. In hemoglobin-containing red blood cells, cytochrome b5 transfers electrons directly to methemoglobin to reduce it to hemoglobin. In nucleated cells and reticulocytes, cytochrome b5 transfers electrons to stearyl-CoA desaturase (Fig. 168–1).

A minor alternative pathway of methemoglobin reduction utilizes the reduced form of nicotinamide-adenine dinucleotide phosphate (NADPH), which is generated by glucose-6-phosphate dehydrogenase (G6PD) in the pentose phosphate pathway. Under normal physiologic conditions, electron transfer via NADPH-dependent reductase to methemoglobin is not functionally significant because of the lack of an electron acceptor for this reductase. However, methylene blue, ascorbic acid, or free flavin can all act as exogenous electron acceptors from NADPH reductase in vivo. The NADPH-dependent pathway of methemoglobin reduction is crucial in the treatment of toxic methemoglobinemia. Because the reduction of methemoglobin by methylene blue is dependent on NADPH generated by G6PD, methylene blue may be ineffective in the treatment of methemoglobinemia in individuals with G6PD deficiency. In addition, administration of methylene blue to these patients is potentially dangerous because it may produce hemolysis, presumably due to redox cycling by methylene blue to generate reactive oxygen species.

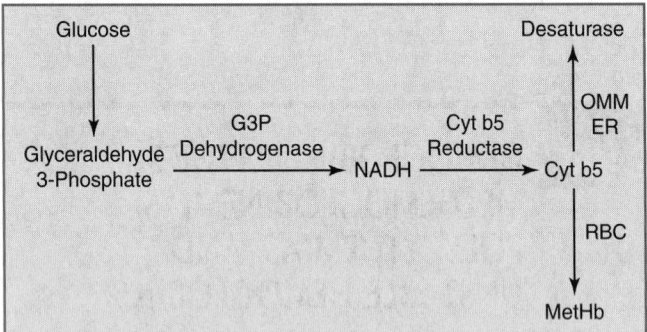

FIGURE 168–1 ■ Pathway of electron transfer. Glucose catabolism through the anaerobic Embden-Meyerhof pathway generates NADH, which serves as a physiologic cofactor for cytochrome b5 reductase. Two electrons are transferred by means of NADH-cytochrome b5 reductase to cytochrome b5. In the red blood cell (RBC), these electrons are then transferred to methemoglobin (MetHb); and in the outer mitochondrial membrane (OMM) and endoplasmic reticulum (ER), these electrons are transferred to stearyl-CoA desaturase.

Table 168–1 ■ MEDICATIONS AND CHEMICALS ASSOCIATED WITH METHEMOGLOBINEMIA

MEDICATIONS	CHEMICALS
Acetaminophen (nitrobenzene derivative)	Acetanilide
	Aniline dyes
Dapsone	Nitric oxide
Flutamide	Nitrites
Metoclopramide	Amyl nitrite
Nitroglycerin	Isobutyl nitrite
Paraquat/monolinuron	Sodium nitrite
Phenacetin	Nitrates (bacterial conversion to nitrites)
Phenazopyridine (pyridium)	Nitrobenzenes/nitrobenzoates
Primaquine	Nitroethane (nail polish remover)
Sulfamethoxazole	Nitrofurans
	4-Amino-biphenyl

Types of Methemoglobinemia

ACQUIRED. The most frequent type of methemoglobinemia is acquired or toxic. It can be induced by certain drugs and other chemicals (Table 168–1). Methemoglobinemia may occur as a result of medication overdoses but may also occur at standard doses, particularly in individuals with partial deficiencies of b5R. Infants are particularly susceptible because their erythrocyte b5R activity is normally 50 to 60% of adult activity. A common clinical scenario leading to symptomatic methemoglobinemia is an infant who receives formula that is diluted with well water that is contaminated with nitrates. In adults, methemoglobinemia usually presents as acute shortness of breath and cyanosis, often mistaken for pulmonary embolism, in a susceptible patient exposed to offending agents. When the evaluation fails to confirm hypoxia, methemoglobinemia should be suspected. Such individuals are often heterozygous for methemoglobin reductase deficiency and will respond rapidly to methylene blue.

CONGENITAL. Hereditary methemoglobinemia was first reported by François, who in 1845 described one of his patients as having long-standing congenital cyanosis without obvious cardiac or pulmonary disease. This subject likely had methemoglobinemia due to cytochrome b5 reductase (b5R) deficiency. These individuals have a decreased ability to reduce the methemoglobin that is formed continuously at physiologic rates because of a deficiency in cytochrome b5 reductase, which, along with NADH, catalyzes the reduction of methemoglobin in normal human erythrocytes. b5R is a constitutively expressed enzyme, a product of a single gene that produces multiple transcripts. The peptide isoforms of this gene have different tissue and subcellular localization. Cytochrome b5 reductase activity decreases slowly during aging of the erythrocytes in the circulation, with a half-life of 240 days.

Of the three types of hereditary methemoglobinemia, two are inherited as autosomal recessives: NADH-cytochrome b5 reductase (b5R) deficiency and cytochrome b5 deficiency. The third type is an autosomal dominant disorder, hemoglobin M (Hb M) disease, in which there is an abnormal globin (Table 168–2).

CYTOCHROME b5 REDUCTASE DEFICIENCY. Type I b5R deficiency. The most common form of congenital methemoglobinemia is due to a deficiency of b5R and is inherited as an autosomal recessive. There are two clinical forms of this disease. The majority of cases of enzymopenic congenital methemoglobinemia are type I, in which the deficiency of b5R is isolated to erythrocytes. Homozygotes or compound heterozygotes have methemoglobin concentrations of 10 to 35% and appear cyanotic but are usually asymptomatic even with levels up to 40%. Symptoms of headache and easy fatigability have been reported by some patients. Life expectancy is not shortened, and pregnancies occur normally. Significant compensatory elevation of hemoglobin concentration (polycythemia, erythrocytosis) is sometimes observed. The cyanosis can be treated effectively with methylene blue or ascorbic acid, both of which facilitate the reduction of methemoglobin through alternative pathways (NADPH-dependent reductase).

There is a worldwide distribution of type I b5R deficiency, but it is endemic in some populations such as the Athabascan Indians, Navajo Indians, and Yakutsk natives of Siberia. However, it re-

Table 168-2 ■ TYPES OF METHEMOGLOBINEMIA

Acquired methemoglobinemia
  Medication/chemicals
  Premature infants and infantile diarrhea
Congenital methemoglobinemia
  Autosomal recessive
    Cytochrome b5 reductase deficiency
    Cytochrome b5 deficiency
  Autosomal dominant
    Hb M disease

mains to be determined if the molecular defect resulting in b5R deficiency is identical in these populations. In other ethnic and racial groups, the defect occurs sporadically.

In contrast to the asymptomatic, chronically methemoglobinemic homozygotes, heterozygous individuals are at risk for developing acute, symptomatic methemoglobinemia after exposure to exogenous methemoglobin-inducing agents. The b5R activity of the erythrocytes of these individuals is approximately 50% of normal. Although this activity level is sufficient to maintain normal methemoglobin levels during normal conditions, oxidant stress can overwhelm the erythrocyte's capacity to reduce methemoglobin. The description of acute toxic methemoglobinemia in U.S. military personnel receiving malarial prophylaxis in Vietnam demonstrated for the first time that heterozygotes for an autosomal recessive disease can, under certain conditions, develop a disease state that is more clinically significant than their asymptomatic homozygous peers.

Type II b5R Deficiency. Ten to 15 per cent of cases of enzymopenic congenital methemoglobinemia are type II, which is caused by a general deficiency of b5R in all cell types. The main symptoms are cyanosis, mental retardation, and severe developmental delay. Life expectancy is significantly shortened. The cyanosis can be effectively treated with methylene blue or ascorbic acid, as in type I b5R deficiency; however, treatment is not indicated except for cosmetic reasons because it has no effect on the neurologic aberrations. Amniotic cells contain an easily measurable b5R activity; thus, prenatal diagnosis of homozygous b5R deficiency is feasible.

Type II b5R deficiency is found sporadically worldwide. Because the b5R enzyme is coded by a single gene, the suggested explanation for the two types of b5R deficiency is that the abnormal gene product is produced at a normal rate but is unstable, and only mature red cells, which cannot synthesize proteins, are affected in the type I deficiency state. By comparison, if the mutations cause structural abnormalities or mutations leading to underproduction of the enzyme, the b5R deficiency is generalized (type II).

CYTOCHROME b5 DEFICIENCY. Deficiency of cytochrome b5 is a rare disorder that also causes congenital methemoglobinemia. Only one well-documented case of cytochrome b5 deficiency has been described compared with over 500 reported cases of b5R deficiency.

HEMOGLOBIN M DISEASE. Five mutations of both α- and β-globin genes have been described as a cause of congenital methemoglobinemia, constituting a phenotype of M hemoglobins or hemoglobin M disease (see Chapter 167). Four of these hemoglobin Ms have a substitution of either a proximal or distal histidine (that binds to the iron atom of heme) by a tyrosine. In contrast to b5R deficiency and cytochrome b5 deficiency that are inherited as autosomal recessive disorders, the methemoglobinemias due to M hemoglobin have autosomal dominant inheritance (see Table 168-2). Affected patients present with cyanosis, which can be viewed as a mainly cosmetic problem that, in contrast to acquired toxic methemoglobinemia and type II b5R deficiency, is otherwise asymptomatic and requires no treatment. Patients inheriting these mutations are generally asymptomatic. Compensatory polycythemia and decreased oxygen affinity, due to an increased 2,3-BPG level, ensure normal oxygen delivery to tissues. Those inheriting α-globin variants are cyanotic at birth, whereas those inheriting β-globin variants have the cyanosis delayed until after fetal hemoglobin is largely replaced by adult hemoglobin at later infancy. Unlike patients inheriting unstable hemoglobins, subjects inheriting stable hemoglobin M mutants have normal red cell morphology.

Not all mutations of α- and β-globin genes leading to hemoglo-

bin M disease are electrophoretically distinguishable; they could be easily missed by routine hemoglobin electrophoresis. More sophisticated laboratory evaluation in a reference or a specialized research laboratory may be needed. Because M hemoglobins (similar to methemoglobin generated from oxidation of a normal hemoglobin molecule) do not participate in oxygen delivery, the decreased tissue oxygenation is generally fully compensated by the increased erythropoiesis that may result in elevated hemoglobin concentration (secondary polycythemia/erythrocytosis).

DIFFERENTIAL DIAGNOSIS. To distinguish the hereditary forms of methemoglobinemia, biochemical analyses and interpretation of family pedigrees are required. Because of its dominant inheritance pattern, cyanosis in successive generations suggests the presence of Hb M disease, whereas normal parents and possibly affected siblings implies the presence of the autosomal recessive cytochrome b5 or b5R deficiencies. Incubation of blood with small amounts of methylene blue will differentially distinguish b5R deficiency from Hb M disease because this treatment will result in the rapid reduction of methemoglobin through alternative pathways in b5R deficiency; by comparison, such reduction will not take place in Hb M disease. To distinguish cytochrome b5 deficiency from b5R deficiency, measurement of the amount of cytochrome b5 and measurement of the level of b5R activity is required.

Diagnosis of Methemoglobinemia

Methemoglobinemia may be clinically suspected by cyanosis, the slate-blue color of the skin, in the presence of a normal partial pressure of arterial oxygen. Other clinical symptoms of methemoglobinemia are generally seen only in acute toxic (acquired) methemoglobinemia and include headache, fatigue, dyspnea, and lethargy. Respiratory depression, altered consciousness, shock, seizures, and death may occur as levels of methemoglobin increase, and oxygen delivery to tissues is impaired. Clinically discernible cyanosis is caused by methemoglobinemia when the absolute level of methemoglobin exceeds 1.5 g/dL (corresponding to 10 to 15% methemoglobin); to discern cyanosis in anemic or polycythemic individuals, the proportion of methemoglobin produced may be higher or lower than 10 to 15%, respectively.

Clinically discernible cyanosis is also associated with sulfhemoglobin when its absolute concentration exceeds 0.5 g/dL. Sulfhemoglobin is an abnormal complex pigment with a different absorption spectrum and is usually produced by methemoglobin degradation in toxic methemoglobinemia. A more commonly encountered clinical situation is cyanosis resulting from desaturated oxyhemoglobin caused by deoxyhemoglobin levels greater than 4 g/dL.

The blood in methemoglobinemia is dark-red or a characteristic "chocolate" color, and the color does not change with the addition of oxygen. Pulse oximetry is inaccurate in monitoring oxygen saturation in the presence of methemoglobinemia. The laboratory diagnosis of methemoglobinemia is based on analysis of its absorption spectra. A fresh specimen should always be tested because methemoglobin levels tend to increase with storage. Methemoglobin has its peak absorbance at 631 nm. The microprocessor-controlled, fixed-wavelength co-oximeter commonly used to assay methemoglobin interprets all readings in the 630-nm range as methemoglobin; false-positive results may occur in the presence of other pigments, including sulfhemoglobin and methylene blue. For a specific diagnosis and accurate quantitation of methemoglobin, a spectrophotometric assay, based on the interaction of methemoglobin with cyanide (CN^-) and ferricyanide and on in vitro generation of cyanomethemoglobin and detection of reaction products by their specific absorption spectra, should be used to confirm methemoglobinemia. Methemoglobin is expressed as a percentage of the total concentration of hemoglobin.

Treatment

Offending agents should be discontinued in the patient with acquired or toxic methemoglobinemia. If the patient is symptomatic, which is often the case in deliberate or accidental overdoses or in toxin ingestion, specific therapy is required. Methylene blue, 1 to 2 mg/kg over 5 minutes, provides an artificial electron acceptor for the reduction of methemoglobin by means of the NADPH-reductase dependent pathway. Response is usually rapid; the dose may be repeated in 1 hour but is frequently unnecessary. Caution should be exercised to avoid overdosage, because large (>7 mg/kg) cumulative doses have been reported to cause dyspnea, chest pain, and hemolysis. Co-oximetry should not be used to follow methemoglobin levels because this method does not distinguish methylene blue from methemoglobin. Before administering methylene blue, populations with a high incidence of G6PD deficiency (e.g., blacks, Mediterraneans, and Southeast Asians) should be screened. Patients with G6PD deficiency should not receive methylene blue but can receive ascorbic acid. For severe cases, hyperbaric oxygen and exchange transfusion have been anecdotally reported to be effective. Treatment of the cyanosis in individuals with type I and II b5R deficiency is indicated for cosmetic reasons only. Treatment options include methylene blue, 100 to 300 mg/day orally, or ascorbic acid, 300 to 1000 mg/day orally in divided doses, although this therapy has been associated with formation of renal calculi. The use of riboflavin (20 to 30 mg/day) has also been reported to be effective. There is currently no therapy for the neurologic disorder associated with type II deficiency. There is also no treatment for methemoglobinemia due to Hb M disease; but, because the patients are asymptomatic, no therapy is warranted.

POLYCYTHEMIA DUE TO MUTANT HEMOGLOBINS AND CONGENITAL RED CELL ENZYME DEFICIENCY

Polycythemias

The polycythemias (also known as erythrocytosis) comprise a group of etiologically diverse disorders characterized by increased red cell mass (see Chapter 174). Absolute polycythemias may be either primary due to an intrinsic defect of hematopoietic progenitors or, more commonly, secondary. Secondary polycythemias are due to stimulation of normal hematopoietic progenitors by extrinsic factors, particularly, erythropoietin. Most of these are due to hypoxia secondary to pulmonary or cardiac disease or high altitude; others are due to autonomous production of erythropoietin. Although most polycythemias are acquired, some are congenital.

FAMILIAL CONGENITAL SECONDARY POLYCYTHEMIAS. MUTANT HEMOGLOBINS WITH INCREASED OXYGEN AFFINITY. Most congenital polycythemias are due to so-called high oxygen affinity hemoglobin mutants. Mutations of both α- and β-globin genes can lead to autosomal dominant polycythemia. More than 50 variants have been described; they are all characterized by an increased oxygen affinity of hemoglobin. The hemoglobin tetramer oscillates between the R (relaxed; fully oxygenated hemoglobin) and T (tense; fully deoxygenated hemoglobin) state of the quaternary protein conformation requiring the cooperative interaction of globin subunits. Mutations affecting the equilibrium between R and T states result in a change of oxygen affinity. Many high-oxygen affinity mutants are located in the α_1/β_2 interface of the hemoglobin tetramer. Some mutations interfere with binding of 2,3-diphosphoglycerate (2,3-DPG) to hemoglobin, whereas others have an amino acid substitution that is located at the C-terminus of one of the globin subunits and that interferes with binding of heme. The functional consequences of the change of oxygen affinity and a decreased P_{50} are a shift in the oxygen saturation curve (Fig. 168–2). The result is decreased delivery of oxygen into the peripheral tissues and compensatory polycythemia. Patients inheriting these mutations are generally asymptomatic because compensatory polycythemia ensures normal oxygen delivery to tissues. It would be expected that those inheriting α-globin variants may have elevated hemoglobin at birth, whereas those inheriting β-globin variants would have detectable abnormalities after fetal hemoglobin ($\alpha_2\gamma_2$) is largely replaced by adult hemoglobin A ($\alpha_2\beta_2$) in later infancy.

2,3-DIPHOSPHOGLYCERATE DEFICIENCY. One rare cause of congenital secondary polycythemia is familial 2,3-DPG deficiency, which results from a deficiency of the red cell enzyme bisphosphoglyceromutase (DPGM). Present in a very high concentration in red blood cells, 2,3-DPG binds hemoglobin, allosterically changing the hemoglobin conformation and modulating its ability to bind oxygen. Thus, a decreased 2,3-DPG level shifts the hemoglobin oxygen dissociation curve to the left (and increases hemoglobin

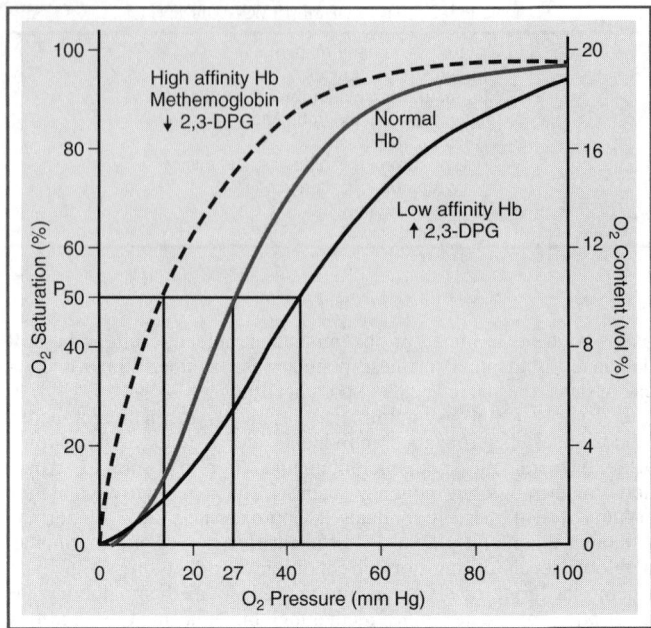

FIGURE 168–2 ■ Hemoglobin oxygen dissociation curve. Left-shifted curve is characteristic of mutant hemoglobins with increased oxygen affinity or decreased 2,3-diphosphoglycerate (2,3-DPG) levels and low P_{50}, whereas the right-shifted curve is characteristic of mutant hemoglobins with decreased oxygen affinity or increased 2,3-DPG levels and increased P_{50}. Normal P_{50} value is 27 mm Hg.

affinity for oxygen). The formation of 2,3-DPG constitutes the Rapoport-Luebering shunt, which is often called an "energy switch" because it bypasses the formation of adenosine triphosphate in the reaction mediated by the glycolytic enzyme phosphoglycerate kinase. A single multifunctional enzyme, DPGM, with both synthase and phosphatase activity, controls this shunt. Deficiency of DPGM leads to a marked decrease in 2,3-DPG levels. The resultant increased hemoglobin oxygen affinity decreases the amount of oxygen released peripherally, leading to a compensatory polycythemia. The deficiency has been reported as either an autosomal dominant or autosomal recessive disease. Thus, some of the heterozygous individuals will not be polycythemic.

Because many of these mutants are electrophoretically silent, the determination of hemoglobin oxygen association kinetics is the best initial screening laboratory test for suspected congenital secondary polycythemia. A decreased P_{50} will likely result from mutant hemoglobin. Unlike patients inheriting unstable hemoglobins, subjects inheriting stable high-oxygen affinity hemoglobin mutants have normal red cell morphology. The definite identification of the mutant globin requires further analytic investigations, such as electrophoretic studies, high-pressure liquid chromatography analysis of hemoglobin and separated globin chains, peptide mapping, and genomic or complementary DNA nucleotide analysis. Once a hemoglobin mutant has been excluded, a biochemical assay of freshly obtained erythrocytes may be used to detect decreased erythrocyte 2,3-DPG. If 2,3-DPG deficiency is found, it should be followed by an assay of DPGM activity. Because inheritance of this defect may, in some families, be autosomal recessive, a family history of this rare deficiency may not be present. As in all rare recessive disorders, consanguinity should be suspected.

CONGENITAL HIGH ERYTHROPOIETIN STATES WITH NORMAL P_{50} AND NORMAL OXYGEN SATURATION. These disorders are poorly understood and probably represent a heterogeneous group. Renal ischemia due to congenital polycystic kidney disorders or renal vascular disease should always be considered. A dysregulation of erythropoietin (EPO) transcription by mutations within the EPO gene locus may account for a subset of the syndrome. Alternatively, abnormalities of genes regulating EPO production, either congenital or acquired, may be involved. Under normal situations, EPO production is stimulated by reduced red cell mass (anemia) or decreased oxygen saturation of red cells (hypoxemia). Both of these states result in tissue hypoxia, which is sensed by a renal oxygen sensor present in the renal peritubular interstitial cells. Hypoxic stimulation of the oxygen sensory pathway results in EPO gene transcription. The only endemic familial polycythemia, congenital polycythemia in Chuvashia, may be an example of a defect in the "oxygen-sensing EPO production pathway." This disorder may affect hundreds or even thousands of individuals and appears to be inherited as an autosomal recessive disorder.

Primary Familial and Congenital Polycythemias. Primary familial and congenital polycythemia (PFCP; also known as familial erythrocytosis) is characterized by elevated red blood cell mass, normal leukocyte and platelet counts, hypersensitivity of erythroid progenitors to EPO in serum containing clonogenic cultures, low serum EPO level, normal oxygen affinity of hemoglobin, absence of progression to leukemia, and typically autosomal dominant inheritance. Mutations in the EPO receptor (EPOR) gene can cause this disease phenotype because of an increased responsiveness of erythroid progenitors to EPO. The result is polycythemia that is thought to be due to the absence of a negative regulatory mechanism in the signal transduction through the EPOR. The lack of down-regulation of the EPOR after ligand binding results in increased proliferation of cells expressing these abnormal receptors. In the majority of PFCP families, however, the PFCP phenotype is not linked to the EPOR gene and the cause of the syndrome remains unclear.

HEMOGLOBIN MUTANTS ASSOCIATED WITH HEMOLYTIC ANEMIA: UNSTABLE HEMOGLOBINS

Unstable Hemoglobins

Approximately 100 different globin mutations have been reported to cause unstable hemoglobins. These mutations interfere with the binding of heme, the secondary structure of hemoglobin, the stabilization of hemoglobin hydrophobic interactions, the tertiary structure that disturbs the hydrophobic interior of hemoglobin, or the quaternary structure of hemoglobin because of deletions of one to five amino acids in one of the globin subunits of hemoglobin.

The hemolysis in this syndrome is inherited as an autosomal dominant phenotype. Most of these patients have enlarged spleens. In some patients, hemolysis is so severe that it may be associated with intravascular hemolysis and hemoglobinuria. Most α-globin mutations that lead to unstable hemoglobins are present at birth. The unstable hemoglobins due to β-globin mutations are noticed after the fetal hemoglobin ($\alpha_2\gamma_2$) is replaced by adult hemoglobin A ($\alpha_2\beta_2$). The β-globin mutants are generally noticed within 6 months of birth. A rare γ-globin mutant has been reported in which the hemolytic anemia was present at birth but disappeared after the fetal hemoglobin was fully replaced by hemoglobin A (hemoglobin F Pool). Because hemoglobin is present at almost saturated concentrations in the red cells, the significant change of its conformation may lead to its decreased solubility and precipitation. Hemoglobin precipitates within red cells are visualized microscopically as Heinz bodies. These rigid particles interfere with the plasticity of red cells and create hindrance in the microcirculation, especially in the spleen, which leads to red cell destruction.

The mechanism of hemoglobin destruction also involves autoxidation of hemoglobin, which leads to release of superoxide radicals and further disturbance of the hemoglobin molecule by its oxidative damage. Fever as well as many oxidant drugs such as sulfonamides lead to exacerbation of hemolysis and acute hemolytic crisis. During infections, oxygen radicals are produced in greater amounts by neutrophils, diffuse into red cells, further accentuate the hemolytic process, and may lead to acute hemolytic crisis.

The diagnosis of hemolysis due to unstable hemoglobin is suspected by demonstration of Heinz bodies in the red cells. These inclusions are specifically visualized by supravital stains, such as methyl violet or brilliant cresyl blue. Hemoglobin electrophoresis is not a reliable way of making a diagnosis because some of these hemoglobin mutants are electrophoretically normal. The definitive diagnosis uses either the isopropanol test or the heat test (incubation of hemolysate at 50° C).

Jaffe E, Hultquist D: Cytochrome b5 reductase deficiency and enzymopenic hereditary methemoglobinemia. *In* Scriver C, Beaudet A, Sly W, Valle D (eds): The Metabolic and Molecular Basis of Inherited Disease, 7th ed. New York, McGraw-Hill, 1995, pp 3399–3415. *A detailed up-to-date reference of the biochemistry of methemoglobinemia and its physiology.*

Jenkins MM, Prchal J: A high frequency polymorphism of NADH-cytochrome b5 reductase in African-Americans. Hum Genet 99:248, 1997. *First description of high-frequency polymorphism, which appears to be specific for African-Americans.*

Prchal JF, Prchal JT: Molecular basis for polycythemia. Cur Opin Hematol 6:100, 1999. *An updated review.*

Prchal JT, Gregg X: Red cell enzymopathies. *In* Hoffman R: Hematology, 3rd ed. Philadelphia, WB Saunders, 1999. *A detailed up-to-date description of enzyme disorders leading to methemoglobinemias, hemolytic anemias, and polycythemic disorders, with references to mid-1998.*

169 SICKLE CELL ANEMIA AND ASSOCIATED HEMOGLOBINOPATHIES

Stephen H. Embury

Sickle cell disease is an inherited multisystem disorder caused by the abnormal properties of red blood cells containing mutant sickle cell hemoglobin (HbS). Chronic hemolytic anemia, recurrent painful episodes, and acute and chronic organ dysfunction are the cardinal features of this disease. Traditional understandings of sickle cell disease attribute all disease features to a causative cascade: an A→T nucleotide substitution in the sixth codon of the β-globin gene, a β-globin Val→Glu substitution on the surface of the HbS tetramer; the abnormal solubility and polymerization of HbS when deoxygenated; the impaired deformability and sickling of polymer-containing erythrocytes; and the occlusion of the microvasculature by poorly deformable red cells. The fundamental importance of these sequential events notwithstanding, a comprehensive understanding of sickle cell pathophysiologic features requires inclusion of numerous polymerization-independent mechanisms (Figure 169–1).

The different sickle cell syndromes that result from distinct inheritance patterns of the sickle cell gene (β^S gene) are divided into sickle cell disease and sickle cell trait. The former is associated with chronic anemia and recurrent pain. The latter is largely asymptomatic. Common varieties of sickle cell disease are inherited as homozygosity for the β^S gene, called *sickle cell anemia* (Hb SS), or as compound heterozygosity of the β^S gene with another mutant β-globin gene—sickle cell-β^0 thalassemia (HbS-β^0 thal), sickle cell-Hb C disease (Hb SC disease), and sickle cell-β^+ thalassemia (HbS-β^+ thal). Sickle cell trait is inherited as simple heterozygosity for the β^S gene (Hb AS).

Clinical management of these disorders is accomplished most effectively by comprehensive approaches that predict, prevent, or treat specific disease manifestations.

HISTORICAL BACKGROUND

Sickle cell disease had been recognized as a clinical entity in Africa well before the seminal account by Dr. James Herrick in 1910. That report contained the initial description of the sickle-shaped erythrocytes (Figure 169–2; Color Plate 5*J*), and the first suggestion of a linkage between these abnormal cells and the recurrent pain and anemia of their Granadian patient. An important insight into the pathobiologic characteristics of these abnormal cells derived from the 1927 report by Hahn and Gillespie of deoxygenation-induced red cell deformation or "sickling."

The role of the hemoglobin within sickle cells as the cause of these cellular changes was first suggested by the 1940 discovery that deoxygenation caused changes in the optical birefringence of sickle erythrocytes. This finding led to the discovery by Pauling, Itano, Singer, and Wells in 1949 of the abnormal electrophoretic mobility of sickle cell hemoglobin (HbS). The critical importance of HbS to cell sickling was established in 1950 by Harris and by Perutz and Mitchison, who reported independently the reversible, deoxygenation-induced gelation of HbS solutions. In 1957, Ingram reported the substitution of valine for glutamic acid as the sixth

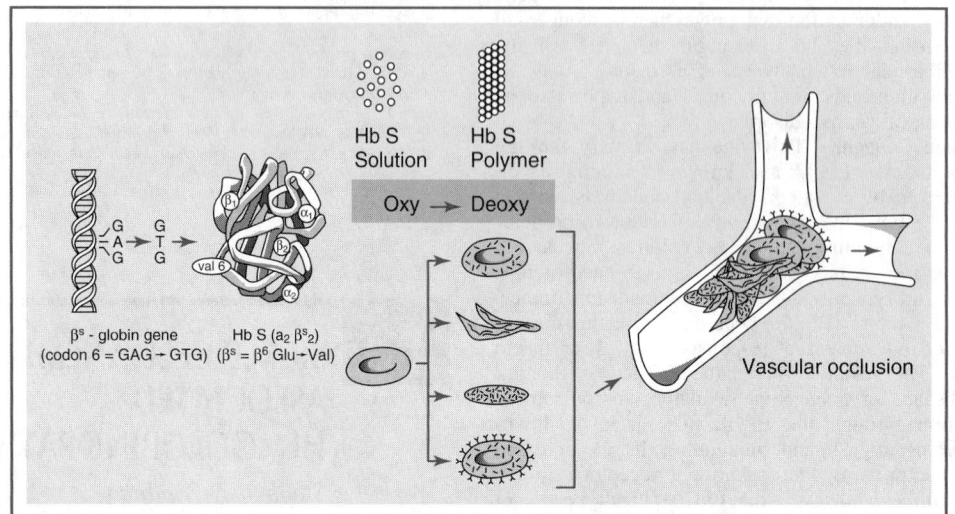

FIGURE 169–1 ■ A schematic view of the pathophysiologic characteristics of sickle cell disease. The double-stranded DNA molecule on the left represents a β-globin gene in which a GAG→GTG substitution in the sixth codon has created the sickle cell gene. The product of this gene is the β^S-globin variant, in which valine is substituted for glutamic acid as the sixth amino acid. The mutant hemoglobin tetramer $\alpha_2\beta^S_2$ is HbS, which loses solubility and polymerizes when deprived of oxygen. Upon deoxygenation, most sickle cells accumulate polymer and lose deformability; some cells sickle; a fraction of cells become dehydrated, irreversibly sickled, and poorly deformable; and a few cells accrue cytoadherence molecules on their surface. Dehydrated and highly adherent cells also may be generated by polymerization-independent processes. Vaso-occlusion, shown on the right, is initiated by adherent cells sticking to the vascular endothelium, thereby creating a nidus that traps rigid cells and facilitates polymerization.

amino acid of β-globin, which unified the abnormalities of electrophoretic mobility and solubility of the mutant HbS.

GENETICS, EVOLUTION, AND MALARIA

Consideration of the high frequency of both normal and sickle cell alleles in given populations led Allison to the concept of genetic polymorphism: The stable frequency of the sickle cell gene in areas of hyperendemic falciparum malaria was the result of balanced gene exclusion from early death of homozygotes and gene selection from protection of heterozygotes against death by malaria. Mechanisms for this "heterozygous advantage" are effected at a stage of the symbiotic parasite-erythrocyte relationship after initial parasitization. As a result of these influences, the worldwide distribution of sickle cell anemia mirrors the "malaria belt." In the United States more than 90% of patients are black.

Near the β-globin gene on chromosome 11 are a series of restriction fragment length polymorphisms (RFLPs), combinations of which define ethnogeographic-specific β-globin haplotypes. The association of the sickle cell gene with five different haplotypes demonstrates the multiple occurrence of the sickle cell mutation among peoples of Senegal, Benin, Bantu, Cameroon, and Arab-Indian origins. There is no evidence to suggest that these haplotypes have provided selective evolutionary pressures on the β^S gene. The effect of glucose-6-phosphate dehydrogenase (G6PD) deficiency, another common African polymorphism, on the sickle cell gene remains controversial, but there is no apparent higher frequency of the mutant G6PD gene, greater hemolysis, or more frequent pain among males with coexistent sickle cell disease and G6PD deficiency.

PREVALENCE. The prevalence of sickle cell trait is 8 to 10% among black newborns in the U. S. and as high as 25 to 30% in western Africa. Calculations based on the frequency among black American of the β^S (0.045), Hb C (β^C) (0.015), and β-thalassemia (0.004) genes indicate that in the United States there are 4000 to 5000 pregnancies at risk for sickle cell disease each year. It is estimated that there are approximately 50,000 to 60,000 patients with sickle cell disease living in the United States. In Africa 120,000 babies with sickle cell disease are born each year.

PATHOPHYSIOLOGIC CHARACTERISTICS

Deoxygenation-induced polymerization of HbS, sickling of erythrocytes, and increased viscosity of blood are the sine qua non of sickle cell disease. Despite this absolute requirement for HbS polymerization, the pathophysiologic characteristics of sickle cell disease require additional consideration.

HbS POLYMER. Although oxygenated HbS and Hb A are equally soluble, the solubility of deoxygenated HbS is severely reduced. The insolubility of deoxy-HbS is related to the presence of valine rather than glutamic acid as the sixth amino acid of β^S globin and to the resultant increased surface hydrophobicity of HbS molecules. The intermolecular bonding of deoxy-HbS generates polymer filaments, which associate into bundles that can be discerned by electron microscopy. One of the two β^S valines forms a lateral contact with the β^{85} phenylalanine and β^{88} leucine within a hydrophobic pocket of an adjacent HbS tetramer. Additional intermolecular bonds form axial and lateral contacts within double filaments and lateral contacts between double filaments. Differences in the surface hydrophobicities of HbS and Hb F are responsible for the inhibitory effect of Hb F on HbS polymerization.

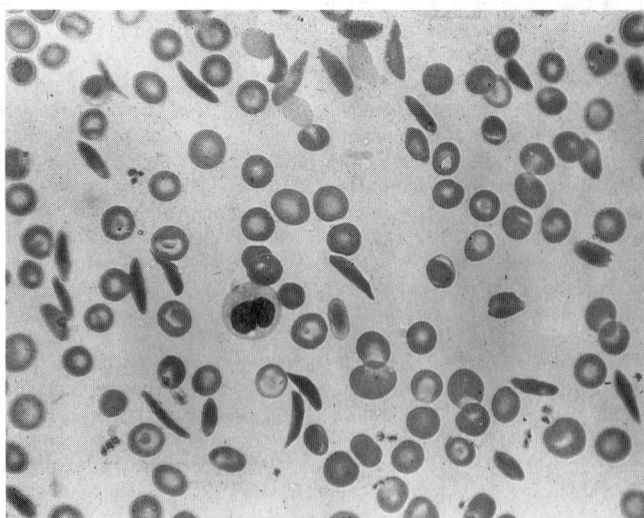

FIGURE 169–2 ■ A peripheral blood smear showing the "peculiar elongated forms of the red corpuscles" originally reported by Herrick (1910).

POLYMERIZATION. The solubility of deoxy-HbS is 17 g/dL, far less than the usual 34-g/dL concentration of hemoglobin within sickle erythrocytes. Deoxygenation promotes rapid supersaturation, aggregation, and polymerization, with the progression from nuclear aggregation to polymer formation having a delay time inversely related to the 30th power of the deoxy-HbS concentration. Resultant polymer fibers provide additional nuclei for further polymer formation. Kinetic interpretations of polymerization hold that because delay times usually exceed capillary transit times, cells usually do not accumulate significant amounts of polymer until they are in a large vein where they cannot elicit vaso-occlusion; local vascular perturbations that cause unusual delays in the transit time are important to this version of sickle cell pathophysiologic mechanisms. Individual thermodynamic parameters for each cell dictate the amount of polymer that will accumulate with each capillary transit, thereby affording a different version of pathophysiologic processes.

INHERITED INFLUENCES ON POLYMERIZATION. The switch from γ- to β-globin production begins in the fetus and results in replacement of fetal hemoglobin (Hb F) by adult HbS. The retardant effect of Hb F on HbS polymerization and cellular sickling masks the expression of sickle cell disease until approximately 6 months of age, when HbS levels increase to about 75%. Preservation of high Hb F levels into adulthood similarly mitigates the course of sickle cell disease: That is, sickle cell–hereditary persistence of fetal hemoglobin (HbS-HPFH) and sickle cell-β-thalassemia both have higher Hb F levels and milder clinical courses than sickle cell anemia. Polymerization is also influenced by elevated levels of Hb A_2 in sickle cell-β^0- and -β^+-thalassemia and by Hb A levels of 5 to 30% in sickle cell-β^+-thalassemia. Hb F inhibits polymerization 100 to 10,000 times more actively than Hb A does. This difference is accounted for by the exclusion of both Hb F and $\alpha_2\beta^S$ γ hybrid tetramers from polymer compared with the exclusion of Hb A and inclusion of $\alpha_2\beta^A$ γ hybrid tetramers. Another influence retarding polymerization in sickle cell-β-thalassemia is the lower intraerythrocytic HbS concentration. Hematologic values for sickle cell anemia, the sickle cell-β-thalassemias, and HbS-HPFH are shown in Table 169–1.

α-Thalassemia also reduces the mean corpuscular hemoglobin concentration (MCHC) and influences certain aspects of sickle cell disease. The silent carrier of α-thalassemia syndrome (genotype $-\alpha/\alpha\alpha$) exists in about 30% of black Americans and α-thalassemia trait (genotype $-\alpha/-\alpha$) in 2%. The lower intraerythrocytic concentrations of HbS associated with either the $-\alpha/\alpha\alpha$ or the $-\alpha/-\alpha$ genotype modulate, after 7 years of age, the hematologic, pathophysiologic, and clinical manifestations of disease, particularly the severity of anemia. Average hemoglobin levels associated with different α-globingeno types in adults are 7.9 g/dL for $\alpha\alpha/\alpha\alpha$, 8.7 g/dL for $-\alpha/\alpha\alpha$, and 9.0 g/dL for $-\alpha/-\alpha$.

CELLULAR SICKLING. Deoxygenation of sickle cell suspensions results in generation of deoxy-HbS polymer, alteration of cellular morphologic characteristics, and increased viscosity of the cell suspension. Accrual of polymer is prompt and precedes changes in cell morphologic properties during deoxygenation. Polymer is lost before cells regain normal shape during re-oxygenation. Polymer alignment and the number of intracellular polymer domains that influence the rheologic properties of sickle cells are affected by both deoxygenation rate and shear stress. During slow deoxygenation, classic crescent-shaped cells with a single domain of highly aligned polymer arise by homogeneous nucleation from a single nucleus; with faster deoxygenation, holly leaf–shaped cells with a greater number of less well-aligned domains are generated by heterogeneous nucleation from a few nuclei; and with very rapid deoxygenation, granular cells with multiple poorly aligned domains

are derived by heterogeneous nucleation from many nuclei. Shear stress during polymerization creates more nucleation sites, shortens the delay time, and increases cell viscosity; shear applied after polymerization has begun breaks the polymer and diminishes viscosity.

IRREVERSIBLY SICKLED CELLS. Those cells that do not unsickle when re-oxygenated, the "irreversibly sickled cells" (ISCs), are the least deformable sickle cells and have the shortest circulatory survival. Their rheologic impairment is related more to the effects of severe cellular dehydration on intraerythrocytic HbS concentration, cytoplasmic viscosity, and polymerization tendency than to rigidly deformed skeletal proteins. ISCs had been assumed to be old cells damaged by repeated cycles of sickling and unsickling until Bertles and Milner found reticulocytes having very low Hb F content among the ISCs. Lacking the protective effects of Hb F against polymerization and sickling, these young red cells are predestined to rapid dehydration.

Sickled forms seen on the peripheral blood smear are ISCs. Their number does not change with complications of disease (such as the acute painful episode), is generally constant in individual patients, and correlates mainly with the degree of anemia. ISCs exist in all sickle cell disease genotypes but not in sickle cell trait.

CATION HOMEOSTASIS AND CELL DEHYDRATION. During their brief survival in the circulation, sickle cells become dehydrated, some achieving MCHC over 50 g/dL, which greatly enhances polymerization. The sodium-potassium pump, in attempting to restore the perturbations in cation homeostasis caused by deoxygenation-induced passive cation leaks, depletes cells of monovalent cations as a result of its fixed stoichiometry of three sodium ions pumped out for every two potassium ions pumped in. A more important cause of cell dehydration involves the interdependent actions of calcium-dependent potassium loss (Gardos pathway) and potassium chloride cotransport on a population of calcium-sensitive reticulocytes. Gardos-mediated potassium efflux lowers the intracellular pH, thereby activating the volume-regulatory K-Cl cotransport activity, which further depletes cells of potassium and water.

Specific clinical complications demonstrate the importance of cell dehydration. First, the hematuria and diminished concentrating ability of subjects with sickle cell trait demonstrate that even Hb AS cells sickle and occlude vessels when dehydrated in the 1300-mOsm environment of the renal medulla. Second, the clinical manifestations of Hb SC disease demonstrate that even heterozygous amounts of HbS can cause clinical morbidity when the HbS is sufficiently concentrated within the cell. That is, the cellular dehydration effected by HbC–induced potassium-chloride cotransport increases intraerythrocytic HbS concentration and polymerization to a degree that individuals with Hb SC disease, in contrast to those having sickle cell trait, experience anemia and pain. Third, the interaction of α thalassemia and sickle cell anemia is more important for broadening pathophysiologic interpretations than for recapitulating the polymerization principle. The less severe anemia associated with coexistent α thalassemia is related to better cell hydration, lower MCHC, fewer dense cells and ISCs, and greater deformability of α-thalassemic sickle cells—all consistent with a retardant effect on polymerization. Yet, coexistent α thalassemia is associated with more severe vaso-occlusion—more frequent pain and osteonecrosis and a higher mortality rate after the age of 20 years. These conflicting influences of α thalassemia demonstrate the need for a pathophysiologic understanding that includes polymerization-independent mechanisms. Therapeutic strategies that improve cellular hydration include inhibiting the Gardos phenomenon with

Table 169–1 ■ HEMATOLOGIC VARIABLES ASSOCIATED WITH SICKLE CELL ANEMIA, THE SICKLE CELL-β-THALASSEMIA SYNDROMES, AND SICKLE CELL-HPFH

GENOTYPE	Hb	%Hb A	%Hb F	%Hb A_2	MCV	% RETICULOCYTE
Hb SS	7.8	0	4.6	2.9	85.9	10.2
Hb S-β^0-thalassemia	8.9	0	5.9	5.0	69.3	7.2
Hb S-β^+-thalassemia	8.4–11.6	3–25	5.1–6.8	4.7–4.9	64–73	1.3–9.7
Hb S-HPFH	14.6	0	25.8	2.0	81.7	2.4

Hb SS = homozygosity for the β^s gene: sickle cell anemia; Hb S-β^0-thalassemia = compound heterozygosity of the β^s gene with another mutant β-globin gene: sickle cell = β^0 thalassemia; Hb S-β^+-thalassemia = sickle cell-β^+ thalassemia; Hb S-HPFH = sickle cell-hereditary persistence of fetal hemoglobin.

cetiedil citrate or clotrimazole and blocking K-Cl cotransport with Mg²⁺ salts.

OXIDATIVE DAMAGE. In addition to having abnormal electrophoretic and solubility properties, HbS is unstable. Its oxidation results in increased generation of methemoglobin, heme, and oxidative radicals. Resultant oxidative stresses affect red cell metabolism, membrane lipids, membrane proteins, and HbS itself. Decreased reduced nicotinamide-adenine dinucleotide (NADH) redox potential, hexomonophosphate shunt activity, and reduced glutathione (GSH) content contribute significantly to sickle cell pathobiologic processes. Hemichrome aggregates on the cytoplasmic portion of band 3 initiate membrane coclustering of band 3 molecules, assembly of immunoglobulin G (IgG) and complement on their extracellular domains, and sickle cell adherence to macrophages and endothelial cells. Oxidative radicals oxidize spectrin, ankyrin, band 3, and band 4.1; disrupt membrane skeletons; and impair spectrin assembly in sickle cell membranes. Oxidative damage to membrane lipids causes their reduced lateral mobility in cell membranes and the loss of phosphatidylinositol-anchored complement-regulatory proteins of the membrane, such as DAF and MIRL.

SICKLE CELL ADHERENCE. The notion that vaso-occlusion is initiated by the adherence of sickle erythrocytes to vascular endothelium is derived from the close correlation of clinical severity with the adhesivity of sickle cells for endothelial cells and from ex vivo flow studies showing that vaso-occlusion is initiated by adherence of sickle cell reticulocytes to vascular endothelium and propagated by trapping of poorly deformable ISCs (Figure 169–3). Adherence of sickle erythrocytes to endothelial cells is mediated by numerous receptors and ligands.

THE IMPORTANCE OF NEUTROPHILS (POLYMORPHONUCLEAR NEUTROPHIL LEUKOCYTES). In HbSS there is a direct relationship of the leukocyte count with mortality rate, hemorrhagic stroke, and acute chest syndrome, and the clinical response to hydroxyurea correlates with reduction in polymorphonuclear neutrophil leukocyte (PMN) count. The mechanisms by which PMNs influence vaso-occlusion may involve their poor deformability, their increased adherence to endothelium and frequent up-regulation of CD64 during pain crisis, their activation by sickle erythrocytes, and their important role in the ischemia/reperfusion process, which resembles the characterisitc blood flow in sickle cell disease.

COAGULATION ABNORMALITIES. The continuous perturbation and activation of the hemostatic system disease suggest that a steady state of normal vascular flow in sickle cell may be illusory. There is evidence for ongoing platelet activation, which is increased during acute vaso-occlusive episodes. The activation of coagulation in sickle cell disease is demonstrated by evidence of increased thrombin generation, such as elevated levels of thrombin-antithrombin III complexes, prothrombin activation fragment 1.2, and fibrinopeptide A. One source of hemostatic activation unique to sickle cell disease is the phosphatidylserine contained in the outer membrane leaflet of ISC and of deoxygenated, reversibly sickled cells. Phosphatidylserine is capable of activating the coagulation system, as are phosphatidylserine-rich vesicles exovesiculated from sickle erythrocyte membranes during sickling, activated endothelial cells, and activated monocytes. Another hemostatic activator is the tissue factor expressed by circulating endothelial cells that have been dislodged from their vascular moorings in the course of vascular perturbations in this disease.

PATHOPHYSIOLOGIC MECHANISMS OF VASO-OCCLUSION. Although polymerization of deoxy-HbS and sickling of erythrocytes provide the basis of sickle cell disease, a critical assessment of their role in vaso-occlusion illustrates the need for a more comprehensive view of pathophysiologic processes. Evidence for the importance of polymerization is provided by the detrimental influence of high intraerythrocytic HbS concentration in Hb SC disease, the protective effect of large amounts of Hb F in all cells in HbS-HPFH, and the induction of vaso-occlusive complications by known precipitants of polymerization. However, there are sufficient exceptions to this model so that polymerization may be regarded as necessary but not sufficient for vaso-occlusion. Sickle cells become deoxygenated more frequently than once a minute, demonstrating that "sickling" is a constant, unrelenting process rather than an occasional cataclysmic one. The chronic activation of several processes involved in vaso-occlusion hints that there is probably no

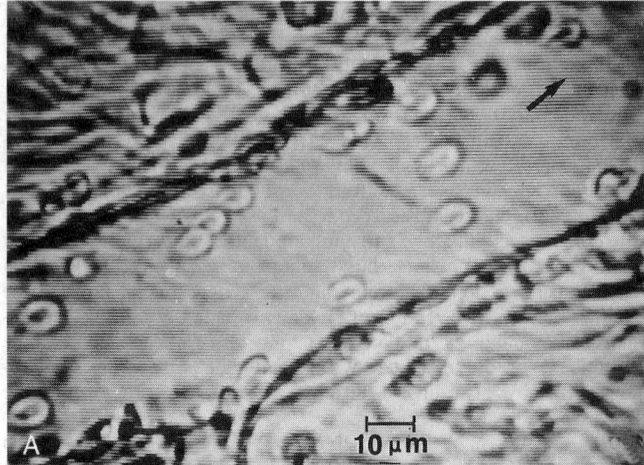
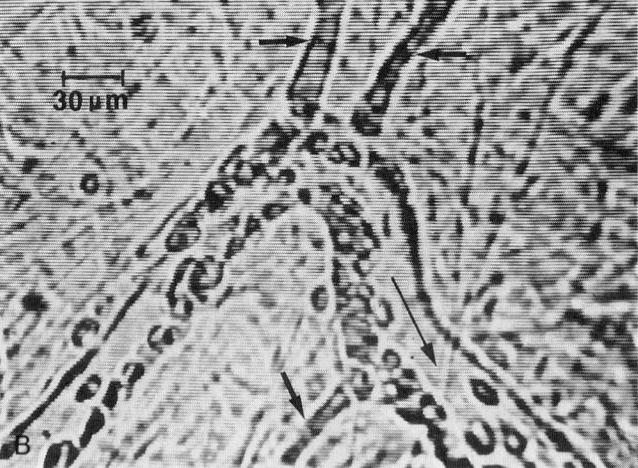

FIGURE 169–3 ■ Adhesion of sickle erythrocytes in venules. *A,* Adherent discocytic sickle cells tethered to the endothelial wall of a venule and aligned in the direction of the flow (*arrow*). *B,* Increased adherence of sickle cells at venule or bending and at junctions of smaller-diameter postcapillary venules. The post-capillary vessels (*small arrows*) are totally blocked. Large arrow indicates flow direction. (From Kaul DK, et al: Microvascular sites and characteristics of sickle cell adhesion to vascular endothelium in shear flow conditions: Pathophysiologic implications. Proc Natl Acad Sci USA 86:3356, 1989, with permission.)

normal "steady-state" blood flow in sickle cell disease. Despite the considerable effect of a high MCHC on polymerization, there is no greater frequency of pain in patients with a high ISC number. Furthermore, ex vivo studies show that vaso-occlusion is initiated by cells with low MCHC adhering to vascular endothelium (Figure 169–3), not by the polymerization-prone ISC. Although polymerization tendencies provide a first approximation of sickle cell disease severity, transient changes in vascular flow are best understood in terms of a broader group of pathophysiologic processes.

MECHANISMS OF HEMOLYSIS. Hemolysis of sickle cells is both extravascular and intravascular. The former is due to the effects of unstable HbS and recurrent sickling on causing oxidative damage to cell membranes. Binding of oxidatively denatured HbS to the cytosolic portion of band 3 induces adherence of IgG and complement to extracellular band 3, thereby promoting cell recognition by macrophages. Also, the very rigid ISCs that are generated by recurrent sickling and by sickling-independent cell dehydration are trapped extravascularly, accounting for their short circulatory survival and correlation with the severity of anemia. Elevated free plasma hemoglobin levels suggest that one third of sickle cell hemolysis is intravascular. One mechanism relates to sickling-induced exovesiculation of vesicles enriched in phosphatidylinositol-anchored membrane proteins, which depletes cells of complement-regulatory proteins and leaves them susceptible to complement-mediated lysis. A second mechanism involves the mechanical fragility of cells, which accounts for accelerated hemolysis during exercise.

IMMUNE DEFICIT. The propensity of children with sickle cell disease to *Streptococcus pneumoniae* infection relates to their impaired splenic function and diminished serum opsonizing activity. The function of the spleen is deficient even before its eventual autoinfarction, but prior to the second decade function is restorable by transfusion. The greater the rate of hemolysis, the earlier the age at which splenic function is lost: sickle cell anemia > Hb SC disease > sickle cell-β^+-thalassemia. The decreased titer of antibody against *S. pneumoniae* antigens following splenectomy in individuals without sickle cell disease suggests that splenic hypofunction may mediate opsonic deficiency in sickle cell disease.

CLINICAL MANIFESTATIONS

Clinical manifestations of sickle cell disease vary greatly between and among the disease genotypes. Even within the most severe genotype, sickle cell anemia, asymptomatic patients may be detected incidentally whereas others are disabled by disease complications. The typical patient is anemic but asymptomatic except during painful episodes. Most organ systems are subject to vaso-occlusion, resulting in the characteristic acute and chronic multisystem failure. Important clinical features less directly related to vaso-occlusion are growth retardation, psychosocial problems, and susceptibility to infection. Therapeutic interventions are directed to specific complications.

LIFE EXPECTANCY. The current mean survival is 42 years for men and 48 years for women with sickle cell anemia. This improved life expectancy compared with that of earlier eras is mainly the result of better general medical care, such as prophylactic penicillin therapy for preventing *S. pneumoniae* bacteremia in children.

CHRONIC ANEMIA. Sickle cells are destroyed randomly with a mean lifespan of 17 days. The degree of anemia is most severe in sickle cell anemia and HbS-β^0-thalassemia, milder in HbS-β^+-thalassemia and Hb SC disease, and, among patients with sickle cell anemia, less severe in those who have coexistent α-thalassemia. In addition to hemolysis, inappropriately low erythropoietin levels contribute to the anemia.

EXACERBATIONS OF ANEMIA. The reasonably constant level of hemolytic anemia may be exacerbated by several different causes, most commonly aplastic crises. Aplastic crises are transient arrests of erythropoiesis characterized by abrupt falls in hemoglobin levels, reticulocyte number, and red cell precursors in the marrow. Anemia becomes severe as hemolysis continues in the absence of red cell production, but these episodes typically last only a few days. Although general mechanisms that impair erythropoiesis in inflammation occur in all types of infection, parvovirus B19 specifically invades proliferating erythroid progenitors, accounting for its importance in sickle cell disease. Parvovirus B19 accounts for approximately two thirds of aplastic crises in children with sickle cell disease, but the high frequency of protective antibodies in adults makes parvovirus a less frequent cause in this age group. Bone marrow necrosis, with attendant fever, bone pain, reticulocytopenia, and leukoerythroblastic response, is another cause of aplastic crisis; it is sometimes associated with parvovirus infection. High oxygen tensions during oxygen inhalation suppress erythropoietin production promptly and, within 2 days, impair red cell production. Red cell transfusion is the main treatment for aplastic crises. When transfusion is necessitated by cardiorespiratory symptoms, a single transfusion usually suffices, as reticulocytosis soon resumes spontaneously. Transfusion sometimes may be avoided by enforcing bed rest and avoiding unnecessary oxygen therapy.

Acute splenic sequestration is characterized by acute exacerbation of anemia, persistent reticulocytosis, a tender enlarging spleen, and sometimes hypovolemia. Patients whose spleen has not undergone fibrosis are at risk—young patients with sickle cell anemia and adults with Hb SC disease or sickle cell-β^+-thalassemia. Thirty percent of children experience splenic sequestration, and 15% of the attacks are fatal. Transfusion is given to restore blood volume and red cell mass. Splenic sequestration recurs in half the cases, so splenectomy is recommended after the acute event. Acute sequestration also may occur in the liver.

Hyperhemolytic crisis is characterized by sudden exacerbation of anemia and increased reticulocytosis and bilirubin level. Apparent hyperhemolytic crises are usually occult splenic sequestration or aplastic crises detected during the resolving reticulocytosis. Actual hyperhemolysis may occur with coexistent glucose-6-phosphate dehydrogenase (G6PD) deficiency.

Chronic worsening of anemia may be related to incipient renal insufficiency or lack of folic acid or iron. Inadequate erythropoietin (EPO) production in renal failure limits compensation for hemolysis. This complication has been treated by using hydroxyurea and/or recombinant human EPO. Chronic hemolysis consumes folic acid stores, potentially resulting in megaloblastic crises. The combination of nutritional deficiency and urinary iron losses may result in iron deficiency. This diagnosis may be obscured by the elevated serum iron levels associated with hemolysis and often depends upon finding low serum ferritin or elevated serum transferrin levels.

THE ACUTE PAINFUL EPISODE. The acute painful episode of sickle cell disease was originally called "sickle cell crisis." Acute pain is often the first symptom of disease, is the most frequent complication after the newborn period, and is the most common reason why patients seek medical attention. Although there is a general association between vaso-occlusive severity and genotype, tremendous variability exists within genotypes and in the same patient over time. One third of patients with sickle cell anemia rarely have pain, one third are hospitalized for pain two to six times per year, and one third have more than six pain-related hospitalizations per year; 5% of patients account for one third of emergency department visits. The frequency of pain is highest in the third and fourth decades, and after the second decade frequent pain is associated with increased mortality rates. Factors associated with more frequent pain are high hemoglobin levels, α-thalassemia, low Hb F levels, and sleep apnea. The frequency of pain is decreased during chronic transfusion therapy.

Painful episodes are caused by vaso-occlusion and may be precipitated by cold, dehydration, infection, stress, menses, or alcohol consumption, but the cause of most episodes is indeterminate. Pain affects any area of the body, most commonly the back, chest, extremities, and abdomen. Severity varies from trifling to agonizing, and the duration is usually a few days. Frequent pain may cause despair, depression, and apathy, which predispose the patient to an existence that revolves around pain—a chronic debilitating pain syndrome.

Half of painful episodes are associated with objective clinical signs—fever, swelling, tenderness, tachypnea, hypertension, nausea, and vomiting. Potential laboratory indicators are a decline in the dense fraction of sickle cells and also an increase in overall red cell deformability and in levels of acute phase reactants, serum lactic dehydrogenase (LDH), interleukin 1, tumor necrosis factor, and serum viscosity. Clinical application of these tests requires baseline data with which to compare acute variations.

PSYCHOSOCIAL ISSUES. Particular challenges to psychosocial adjustment are recurrent pain and the response to it, limitation of activity due to pain, misinterpretation of the meaning of pain, and depression leading to learned helplessness. Some patients become addicted to narcotics, but addiction is uncommon and most often the result of social influences rather than appropriate analgesia therapy. Signs of good adjustment are active coping strategies and support from the family and the extended family unit. Interventional approaches emphasize recognizing and reinforcing individual strengths, confronting pathologic behavior, and establishing coping skills such as re-interpreting pain, diverting attention from pain, and utilizing support systems. Attention to psychosocial welfare is critical to the health and integration into society of patients with sickle cell disease.

GROWTH AND DEVELOPMENT. Growth retardation affects weight more than height and has no clear gender difference. By adulthood normal height is achieved, but weight remains abnormally low. More severe growth delay is noted in children with sickle cell anemia and sickle cell-β^0-thalassemia than in those with Hb SC disease. Skeletal maturation is also delayed. Retarded sexual maturation is greater in sickle cell anemia and sickle cell-β^0-thalassemia than in Hb SC disease or sickle cell-β^+-thalassemia; it is associated with elevated gonadotropin levels for the stage of sexual development and in girls with delayed menarche. Retarded sexual maturation in males can be the result of primary hypogonadism, hypopituitarism, or hypothalamic insufficiency. Impaired development may be the effect of hemolysis on increased protein turnover and basal metabolic rate and can be reversed after splenectomy. In severely delayed growth and development, hormonal therapy should be tailored to the specific deficiency.

INFECTIONS. Infectious complications of sickle cell disease are a major cause of morbidity and mortality (Table 169–2). *S. pneumoniae,* the most common cause of bacteremia in children with sickle cell disease, may be accompanied by aplastic crisis, disseminated intravascular coagulation (DIC), and a 20 to 50% mortality rate. The second most common cause of bacteremia, *Haemophilus Influenzae* type b, affects older children, is less fulminant, but also may be fatal. Results of pneumococcal vaccination had been disappointing, but newer vaccines in which *S. pneumoniae* carbohydrates are conjugated to diphtheria or tetanus toxins offer promise. Vaccination and regular re-immunization are now recommended. *H. influenzae* type b vaccination, prophylactic penicillin, and the long-acting, broad-spectrum antibiotic ceftriaxone have greatly impacted childhood bacteremia. Prophylactic penicillin beginning in infancy has reduced the incidence of *S. pneumoniae* bacteremia in newborns by 84%, and its use is recommended through the age of 5 years. Penicillin-resistant microorganisms have emerged, and local patterns of resistance vary. The efficacy of ceftriaxone for *S. pneumoniae* and *H. influenzae* infection has led to increased outpatient therapy in children with fever. However, patients with a history of previous *S. pneumoniae* bacteremia should not be treated as outpatients, and vancomycin should be used in areas in which antibiotic resistance is frequent. Urinary tract infections and bacteremia in older patients are more likely due to *Escherichia coli* and other gram-negative organisms.

Meningitis in sickle cell anemia is primarily a problem of infants and young children, and *S. pneumoniae* is the most frequent cause. Because meningitis occurs commonly in association with bacteremia, rapid administration of antibiotics for bacteremia has resulted in a much lower incidence of meningitis. *H influenzae* type b is a less common cause of meningitis.

Bacterial pneumonia is one cause of the acute chest syndrome. Patients with any combination of dyspnea, cough, chest pain, fever, tachypnea, or leukocytosis should be evaluated by chest radiograph, arterial blood gas measurement, blood and sputum culture, cold agglutinins, and serologic study for *Mycoplasma pneumoniae, Chlamydia pneumoniae,* and *Legionella* spp. *Mycoplasma pneumoniae* and *Chlamydia pneumoniae* account for approximately 20% of cases of acute chest syndrome. *S. pneumoniae* and *H. influenzae* type b are less common causes.

Osteomyelitis occurs more commonly in sickle cell disease, probably as a result of infection of infarcted bone. Among sickle cell patients, osteomyelitis is commonly caused by *Salmonella* species. *S. aureus* accounts for < 25% of cases. Infection is often at multiple sites in long bones. Diagnosis is made by culture of blood or infected bone. Articular infection is less common and often due to *S. pneumoniae.*

NEUROLOGIC COMPLICATION. Neurologic complications occur in 25% of patients with sickle cell disease, and common events are transient ischemic attacks (TIA), cerebral infarction, cerebral hemorrhage, seizures, and unexplained coma. Cerebrovascular accident (CVA) may occur spontaneously or intercurrently with complications, such as pneumonia, aplastic crises, painful episodes, or dehydration. Patients at higher risk for CVA are those with more severe anemia, higher reticulocyte counts, lower Hb F levels, higher white blood cell (WBC) counts, sleep apnea, and sickle cell anemia rather than Hb SC disease or sickle cell-β-thalassemia. Cerebral thrombosis accounts for 70 to 80% of CVAs and is due to large vessel obstruction rather than the microvascular occlusion commonly associated with sickle cell disease. Thrombotic CVAs may be heralded by focal seizures or TIA, are fatal in approximately 20% of cases, recur within 3 years in nearly 70%, and frequently cause motor and cognitive impairment.

Many patients with sickle cell disease develop collateral vessels that appear as puffs of smoke (*moyamoya* in Japanese) on angiography. These friable pseudomoyamoyas are vulnerable to both thrombosis and hemorrhage. Improved treatment of this complication has been achieved with surgical extracranial-intracranial shunting. Coma is more frequently associated with hemorrhage than with thrombosis, and the combination of coma and seizures without hemiparesis is strongly suggestive of hemorrhage. Although the mortality rate with hemorrhage is 50%, the morbidity rate of survivors is low. The favorable neurosurgical outcome in subarachnoid hemorrhage from ruptured aneurysm justifies aggressive diagnosis, transfusion, vasodilatory therapy, and surgery.

Patients presenting with symptoms and signs of CVA should be evaluated immediately by computed tomographic (CT) scanning or magnetic resonance imaging (MRI) to distinguish among TIA, cerebral thrombosis, and hemorrhage. In hemorrhage, angiography is indicated but is performed only after a partial exchange transfusion to prevent complications associated with injected contrast material. In thrombosis, prompt partial exchange transfusion is indicated, and chronic transfusion to maintain the HbS level below 30% is initiated to prevent recurrent thrombosis and promote resolution. Transfusion therapy provides the current best means of preventing recurrence. Transfusion may be required indefinitely for those with persistent flow abnormalities after 5 years of transfusion and for those in whom thrombosis recurs soon after discontinuing chronic transfusion.

MRI and transcranial Doppler (TCD) flow studies are useful in detecting subclinical cerebral infarction. Neurodevelopmental abnormalities have been found to result from silent cerebral infarcts. The ability to predict the occurrence of strokes by detecting arterial stenosis with TCD and to prevent the occurrence of such strokes with chronic transfusion has led to the recommendation that TCD be used for routine screening and that transfusion be instituted upon detection of arterial stenosis.

PULMONARY COMPLICATIONS. The "acute chest syndrome" consists of dyspnea, chest pain, fever, tachypnea, leukocytosis, and pulmonary infiltrate indicated on chest radiograph. It affects approximately 30% of patients with sickle cell disease and may be life-threatening. The usual causes are vaso-occlusion, infection, and pulmonary fat embolus from infarcted marrow. Microbial pathogens are more commonly isolated in children, in whom the mortality rate is one fourth that in adults. Pre-morbid events in the 2 weeks

Table 169–2 ■ ORGAN RELATED INFECTION IN SICKLE CELL DISEASE

PRIMARY SITES OF INFECTION	MOST COMMON PATHOGENS	OTHER PATHOGENS	PATHOPHYSIOLOGY	PREVENTION	MANAGEMENT
Septicemia	*S. pneumoniae*	*H. influenzae* type b, *E. coli, Salmonella* sp.	Defective splenic function; deficiency of opsonic antibody	Vaccines*, prophylactic penicillin	Empiric intravenous antibiotics for fever
Meningitis	*S. pneumoniae*		Same as for septicemia		
Osteomyelitis and septic arthritis	*Salmonella* sp. *S. pneumoniae*	*E. coli* *Proteus* sp., *S. aureus*	Ischemic or infarcted tissue	—	Surgical drainage; prolonged course of intravenous antibiotics
Pneumonia	*Mycoplasma pneumoniae* Respiratory viruses	*Chlamydia pneumoniae, S. pneumoniae*	Concomitant infection and intrapulmonary vaso-occlusion leading to infarction and/or sequestration	Vaccines*	See Pulmonary and Therapy sections for management of acute chest syndrome

*Against *S. pneumoniae* and *H. influenzae* type b.
Reprinted with permission from Buchanan GR: Infections. *In* Mohandas SH, Steinberg MH (eds): Sickle Cell Disease; Basic Principles and Clinical Practice. New York, Raven Press, 1994, pp 567–587.

preceding the acute chest syndrome are likely to be febrile events in children and acute painful events in adults. Often, when common pathogens are not detected on culture, one of the "atypical" agents, *Mycoplasma, Chlamydia,* or *Legionella,* is responsible, and its presence suggests a specific therapeutic response. Pulmonary fat embolism has a severe clinical course and can be diagnosed by a positive stain finding for fat in sputum macrophages. When patients have a progressive course associated with severely decreased arterial oxygen tension, intensive care may be required. When arterial oxygen tension cannot be maintained above 70 mm Hg using inhaled oxygen, partial exchange transfusion is indicated. Extracorporeal membrane oxygenation may be required for severe cases.

Evaluation of chronic pulmonary status in patients with sickle cell anemia may reveal restrictive lung disease, hypoxemia, and pulmonary hypertension, singly or in combination, often preceded by a history of acute chest syndrome. Causes unrelated to prior acute episodes may relate to chronic vascular insufficiency. Blood gas and pulmonary function measurements should be obtained as baseline data. Airway hyperreactivity and sleep apnea are more common in sickle cell disease and are treatable causes of morbidity.

HEPATOBILIARY COMPLICATIONS. Pigmented gallstones develop as a result of the chronic hemolysis of sickle cell disease and eventually will occur in at least 70% of patients. Because of the advent of laparoscopic cholecystectomy, surgery for asymptomatic gallstones has become a feasible approach for preventing subsequent confusion of gallbladder pain with acute painful episodes.

Chronic hepatomegaly and liver dysfunction caused by trapping of sickle cells, transfusion-acquired infection, and iron overload are associated with centrilobular parenchymal atrophy, accumulation of bile pigment, periportal fibrosis, hemosiderosis, and cirrhosis. In acute hepatic events, the combination of hemolysis, hepatic dysfunction, and renal tubular defects often results in dramatically high serum bilirubin levels, sometimes exceeding 100 mg/dL. Acute hepatic complications may result from viral hepatitis, benign cholestasis (which causes severe hyperbilirubinemia but not fever, pain, or mortality), and ischemic "hepatic crisis" (which causes severe hyperbilirubinemia, fever, pain, abnormal liver function test, findings, and hepatic failure). Hepatitis C occurs with high frequency. Autoimmune liver disease has been treated successfully in sickle cell disease with immune suppression. Liver transplantation has been used successfully for hepatic failure.

OBSTETRIC AND GYNECOLOGIC ISSUES. The major reproductive concern in patients with sickle cell disease is pregnancy. Fetal complications of pregnancy relate to impaired placental blood flow and include spontaneous abortion, intrauterine growth retardation, low birth weight, pre-eclampsia, and death. Maternal complications include increased rates of painful episodes and infections, severe anemia, and death. Prophylactic transfusions do not improve fetal outcome, and their routine application is not recommended. Oral contraceptives containing low-dose estrogen are a safe and recommended method of birth control. Barrier methods and injections of medroxyprogesterone every 3 months may also be useful.

RENAL COMPLICATIONS. Renal complications result from medullary, distal tubular, proximal tubular, and glomerular abnormalities. Occlusion of the vasa recta compromises blood flow to the medulla, causing impaired urinary concentrating ability, papillary infarction, hematuria, incomplete renal tubular acidosis, and abnormal potassium clearance. Isosthenuria is reversible with red cell transfusions up to the age of 8 years. Sickle cell trait is a common cause of hematuria among black Americans. Patients with sickle cell disease or trait who have hematuria should be evaluated by ultrasonography or magnetic resonance imaging to exclude life-threatening causes. Therapeutic options include standard hydration, alkalization of the urine, and diuresis. In unresponsive cases, ε-aminocaproic acid, vasopressin, intravenous distilled water, and nephrectomy have been used. Proximal tubular dysfunction may result in hyperuricemia and is aggravated by chronic use of analgesics.

Glomerular abnormalities result from vaso-occlusion, hyperperfusion, immune complex nephropathy, and parvovirus B19 infection. Hypertension, proteinuria, hyperkalemia, and worsening anemia may herald chronic renal insufficiency, the average age of onset of which is 23 years in sickle cell anemia and 50 years in Hb SC disease. Angiotensin-converting enzyme inhibitors diminish hyperperfusion and proteinuria but do not increase glomerular filtration

rate. Renal transplantation is effective therapy for end-stage renal disease.

PRIAPISM. Priapism, an unwanted painful erection, has been reported to affect from 6.4 to 42% of males with sickle cell disease and strikes most commonly between the ages of 5 to 13 years and 21 to 29 years. Its onset can be acute, recurrent, chronic, or "stuttering." In the priapism of sickle cell disease, the corpora cavernosa are usually engorged and the glans penis and corpus spongiosum are spared. In a minority of patients there is tricorporal priapism, which can be diagnosed by using nuclear scanning of the penis. Priapism, particularly tricorporal priapism, may eventuate in impotence.

Recurrent priapism can be prevented by oral self-administration of the α-adrenergic agent etilefrine and by its intracavernous injection for episodes lasting over an hour. Recurrences may be prevented also by the administration of diethylstilbestrol.

More traditional therapy can be monitored by intercavernous pressure measurements. If there is no response to 12 hours of intravenous hydration and analgesia, partial exchange transfusion is employed. If there is still no resolution within 12 hours, corporal aspiration with saline solution and α-adrenergic agents is used. If there is no response within the next 12 hours, a fistula is created surgically between the glans penis and the corpora cavernosa by inserting a large-bore needle through the glans (the Winter procedure). In 45% of patients who experience priapism, some degree of impotence develops.

OCULAR COMPLICATIONS. Ophthalmologic features include tortuosity of conjunctival vessels, anterior chamber ischemia, retinal artery occlusion, angioid streaks, proliferative retinopathy, and retinal detachment and hemorrhage. The earlier onset and greater frequency of proliferative retinopathy in Hb SC disease and sickle cell-β^+-thalassemia than in sickle cell anemia and sickle cell-β^0-thalassemia suggest that retinal vessels are particularly vulnerable to occlusion by more viscous blood, rather than to the rigidity of individual sickle cells. Annual retinal examination is part of routine health care maintenance. The retinopathy is often seen best by using fluorescein angiography. Peripheral sickle retinopathy may require therapy with laser photocoagulation.

BONE COMPLICATIONS. Osteonecrosis may cause compression of vertebrae, shortening of cuboidal bones of the hands and feet, and acute "aseptic or avascular necrosis." The painful bone infarction of the "hand-foot syndrome" is often the first symptom of sickle cell disease in children. Nuclear medicine scintigraphy and magnetic resonance imaging are sensitive means of detecting bone infarcts. Bone marrow infarction may be distinguished from osteomyelitis by using triple scans that specifically identify osteoclasts, bone marrow macrophages, and inflammatory cells, but cultures taken directly from the affected tissue should be obtained before starting antibiotic therapy for osteomyelitis.

Osteonecrosis is most sensitively detected by magnetic resonance imaging. Necrosis of femoral heads commonly progresses to joint destruction, which may be prevented or delayed by core decompression surgery to relieve increased intraosseous pressure. In advanced disease, major reconstructive therapy can be attempted to prevent permanently limited joint mobility. Among the sickle cell syndromes, osteonecrosis occurs most frequently in sickle cell anemia with coexistent α-thalassemia.

Arthritic pain, swelling, and effusion may be the result of periarticular infarction or gouty arthritis. Non-steroidal anti-inflammatory agents are useful therapies.

Bone marrow infarction may cause reticulocytopenia, exacerbation of anemia, a leukoerythroblastic appearance, and sometimes pancytopenia. It may also cause pulmonary fat embolism, which has a severe clinical course. This constellation of events may be caused by parvovirus B 19 infection.

DERMATOLOGIC COMPLICATIONS. Leg ulcers begin spontaneously or result from trauma, arise near the medial or lateral malleolus, and frequently occur bilaterally. They may become infected and cause systemic infection, osteomyelitis, or tetanus. They rarely occur before the age of 10 years and are less frequent in those who have coexistent α-thalassemia. Males have a three-fold greater incidence. Ulcers are resistant to healing and recur in well over half the cases. Treatment requires weeks for healing. Initial therapy is intended to remove non-viable, superficial tissue using wet to dry dressings or adhesive hydrocolloid dressings (Duo-Derm). After débridement, zinc oxide–impregnated Dane-paste bandages (Unna's boots) are applied. Bed rest, elastic stockings, and leg elevation control edema and facilitate healing.

The myofascial syndrome consists of soft tissue swelling and subcutaneous edema, which may cause a "peau d'orange" appearance. These lesions may be large or only a few centimeters in diameter, are probably the result of dermal or subdermal vaso-occlusion, and are treated symptomatically.

CARDIAC COMPLICATIONS. Although there is no cardiomyopathy specific for sickle cell disease, management of sickle cell patients requires consideration of the cardiac status. The chronic anemia of sickle cell disease is compensated by increased cardiac output, stroke and chamber volumes, and heart size, beginning in childhood. Despite diminished exercise capacity and progressive loss of cardiac reserve, overt heart failure is uncommon in sickle cell patients unless they are stressed with volume overload, exacerbations of anemia, or hypertension. Myocardial infarction occurs in the absence of coronary disease; in one autopsy series, evidence of such events was found in 10% of patients, perhaps as a result of increased oxygen demand exceeding limited oxygen carrying capacity or as a result of microcirculatory impairment. Septal hypoperfusion affecting the atrioventricular (AV) node and bundle of His has been observed to cause second-degree AV block during a painful episode, and it has been suggested that cardiac autonomic dysfunction may account for the increased rate of sudden death observed in sickle cell disease.

VARIANT SICKLE CELL SYNDROMES

In addition to homozygous sickle cell anemia, sickle cell syndromes result from simple heterozygous inheritance of the sickle cell gene (i.e., sickle cell trait) and from its compound heterozygous inheritance with other mutant β-globin genes (e.g., Hb SC disease, sickle cell-β-thalassemia).

SICKLE CELL TRAIT. The approximate prevalence of sickle cell trait is 9% among black Americans and 25 to 30% in regions of western Africa. Those heterozygous for the sickle cell gene number approximately 2.5 million in the United States and 30 million worldwide. Sickle cell trait is a benign carrier condition with no hematologic manifestations. Sickle forms (ISCs) are not seen on the peripheral blood smear. The fractional partition of Hb A and HbS is usually 60:40 as a result of a greater post-translational affinity of α-chains for β^A than for β^S chains. Coinherited α-thalassemia reduces the availability of α chains, thereby enhancing this preferential affinity and decreasing the percentages of HbS according to the number of α-globin genes deleted (i.e., 40, 35, 29, and 21%, HbS, respectively, for the genotypes $\alpha\alpha/\alpha\alpha$, $-\alpha/\alpha\alpha$, $-\alpha/-\alpha$, and $--/-\alpha$).

Few clinical complications are associated with sickle cell trait. Splenic infarction at high altitude affects whites with sickle cell trait more frequently than those of African ancestry. Sickle cell trait is a common cause of hematuria among black Americans. The impaired urinary concentrating ability is directly related to the intraerythrocytic concentration of HbS, inversely related to the presence of α-thalassemia, and reversed by transfusion up to age 8 years. There is no increased incidence of anesthetic complications. The 30-fold greater frequency of unexplained sudden death in military recruits during basic training appears to be the result of exercise-induced vaso-occlusion and rhabdomyolysis.

Despite its known complications, the rare clinical events do not justify regarding sickle cell trait as anything but a benign carrier condition. Newborn screening programs identify infants with sickle cell trait whose parents require genetic counseling. Parents must understand that their child has a benign hereditary condition, not a disease, but that there may a risk for a subsequent child to be born with sickle cell disease.

Certain individuals appear to have sickle cell trait but are symptomatic. In these the diagnosis must be verified. Rare hemoglobins other than S may polymerize and account for reports of symptomatic "sickle cell trait," i.e., heterozygous HbS[Antilles] and Hb Quebec-CHORI.

Hb SC DISEASE. The frequency of the Hb C gene ($\alpha_2\beta_2^{6Glu\rightarrow Lys}$) among black Americans is approximately one fourth that of the β^S gene, resulting in a prevalence for Hb SC disease that is one fourth that of sickle cell anemia. Although oxy-Hb C forms intraerythrocytic crystals, Hb C does not participate in deoxy-HbS polymerization. The fundamental contribution of Hb C to sickle erythrocyte pathobiologic mechanisms is the sustained potassium-chloride cotransport that induces cellular desiccation, thereby raising intraerythrocytic HbS concentrations to levels that support polymerization, sickling, and clinical symptoms.

As a result of a longer circulatory survival of Hb SC red cells (i.e., 27 days compared with 17 days for Hb SS red cells) the degree of anemia and reticulocytosis is frequently milder. Target cells predominate on the peripheral smear (Color Plate 5K). ISCs, folded (pita bread) cells, "billiard ball" cells, and crystal-containing cells also are found. The clinical heterogeneity within the Hb SC genotype notwithstanding, the clinical course is generally milder than that of sickle cell anemia. Compared with sickle cell anemia, the frequency of painful episodes is approximately half, the life expectancy is 20 years longer, the persistence of splenic function is extended, and the incidence of fatal bacterial infection is lower. There is a higher incidence of proliferative sickle retinopathy in Hb SC disease, but the reported higher incidence of osteonecrosis has been challenged.

Hemoglobin C was the second hemoglobin variant discovered. The β^c gene arose almost exclusively in the area of Ghana and Burkina Faso in Africa and is associated with different β-globin haplotypes than is the β^s gene. The β^c mutation affects the same codon as HbS, the sixth codon of the β-globin gene, but the GAG→AAG substitution results in lysine instead of glutamic acid as the sixth amino acid. Hemoglobin C tetramers are poorly soluble when oxygenated and form intraerythrocytic oxy-Hb C crystals. The interaction of Hb C with negatively charged erythrocyte membrane proteins causes sustained potassium-chloride cotransport, loss of erythrocyte potassium and water, and cell dehydration with attendant elevation of the MCHC.

Simple heterozygosity for Hb C (Hb AC) is not associated with anemia, hemolysis, or splenomegaly. Target cells are present on the peripheral smear, but spherocytes, Hb C crystals, and thin red cells folded over upon themselves, "pita bread cells," are lacking. On electrophoresis there are about 50 to 60% Hb A and 40 to 50% Hb C.

Homozygosity for Hb C (Hb CC) results in mild to moderate hemolytic anemia, with hematocrit values ranging from 25 to 37% and moderate reticulocytosis. Splenomegaly is usual, gallstones are common, and aplastic crisis may occur. The MCHC is elevated to approximately 38 g/dL. Prominent spherocytes, target cells, a few Hb C crystals, and "pita bread cells" are observed on the peripheral smear.

Compound heterozygosity for Hb C and β-thalassemia results in moderately severe hemolytic anemia with microcytosis, hypochromia, and target cells. Hb C-β^0-thalassemia is characterized by more severe hemolytic anemia and splenomegaly than Hb C-β^+-thalassemia. Both are associated with a risk for gallstones and aplastic crisis. Although both Hb C-β^0-thalassemia and Hb CC are predominantly characterized by Hb C on electrophoresis, the former is distinguishable by its lower mean corpuscular volume (MCV) (55–70 versus 72 fL), lower mean corpuscular hemoglobin (MCH)(18–21 versus 27 pg), and higher Hb F level (3–10 versus <3%). Hb C-β^+-thalassemia is characterized by the electrophoretic finding of 65 to 80% Hb C, 20 to 30%. Hb A, and 2 to 5% Hb F.

SICKLE CELL-β-THALASSEMIA. The frequency of β-thalassemia genes among black Americans is one tenth that of the β^S gene, resulting in a prevalence for compound heterozygous sickle cell-β-thalassemia that is one tenth that of sickle cell anemia. Sickle cell-β-thalassemia comprises sickle cell-β^+-thalassemia and sickle cell-β^0-thalassemia, which have, respectively, reduced amounts of or no Hb A present. The percentage of Hb A present in sickle cell-β^+-thalassemia varies from 3 to 25%, according to the degree to which specific thalassemia mutations impair β-globin gene expression. Eighty percent of black American β-thalassemia is due to the mild -88 (C→T) and -29 (A→G) promoter region mutations, which generate relatively large amounts of Hb A.

Sickle cell-β-thalassemia red cells are hypochromic and microcytic. ISCs present on the peripheral blood smear are more numerous in sickle cell-β^0-thalassemia than in sickle cell-β^+-thalassemia. The hematologic severity is a function of the amount of Hb A inherited. The clinical nature of sickle cell-β^+-thalassemia is also more benign than that of sickle cell-β^0-thalassemia, as reflected by its three-fold higher rate of incidental diagnosis, later age of presentation, three-fold less frequent leg ulcers, half as frequent acute chest syndrome, lower frequency of priapism and aplastic crisis, and less severe retardation of growth and development. Splenomegaly occurs in approximately one third of both groups. Proliferative retinopathy is more frequent in sickle cell-β^{+}-thalassemia, consistent with the notion that those sickle cell syndromes associated with higher hematocrits have more frequent ocular complications.

SICKLE CELL ANEMIA WITH COEXISTENT α-THALASSEMIA. The α-globin gene deletion responsible for α-thalassemia among black Americans has a frequency of 0.16 in this population—nearly one in three are silent carriers of α-thalassemia (genotype $-\alpha/\alpha\alpha$), and 2% have α-thalassemia trait due to homozygous α-thalassemia 2 (genotype $-\alpha/-\alpha$). This high frequency, combined with the powerful effect of HbS concentration on polymerization, originally suggested that the lower MCHC of thalassemia would influence a large number of patients with sickle cell anemia. This notion was substantiated by the finding of milder anemia in sickle cell anemia associated with the deletion of either one (genotype $-\alpha/\alpha\alpha$) or two (genotype $-\alpha/-\alpha$) α-globin genes.

In addition to less rapid hemolysis and milder anemia, α-thalassemia is associated with fewer reticulocytes and ISCs. Coinherited α-thalassemia results in a decreased incidence of leg ulcers but an *increased* incidence of osteonecrosis, frequency of acute painful episodes, incidence of CVA, and mortality rate after the age of 20 years. The conflicting clinical correlates of α-thalassemia demonstrate the vagaries of trying to predict clinical severity by using formulas of polymerization tendencies.

SICKLE CELL-$\delta\beta^{0}$-THALASSEMIA. The $\delta\beta$-thalassemia locus is one of several large deletions of the δ- and β-globin genes. It allows the switch from fetal to adult hemoglobin production, which in this case is an attempted switch in expression from γ-globin genes to genes that are not present. Sickle cell-$\delta\beta^{0}$-thalassemia is an uncommon compound heterozygous condition in which HbS, F, and A$_2$ exist. The 15 to 25% Hb F is distributed heterocellularly. Anemia is mild, and clinical complications are infrequent.

SICKLE CELL-HEREDITARY PERSISTENCE OF FETAL HEMOGLOBIN. Classic hereditary persistence of fetal hemoglobin (HPFH) results from one of several large deletions of the δ- and β-globin genes that retard the switch from the production of Hb F to adult hemoglobin. Non-deletional types of HPFH are due to one of many nucleotide substitutions that up-regulate the expression of the γ-globin gene. The clinical expressions of deletional and non-deletional HPFH differ in that heterozygosity for the former results in 15 to 35% Hb F, distributed in all red cells (pancellularly), and for the latter in 1 to 5% Hb F distributed unevenly in the red cell population (heterocellularly). Certain mild varieties of HPFH do not express high Hb F levels in simple heterozygosity but do with erythropoietic stress, such as compound heterozygosity with the β^{S} gene. The gene frequency of deletional HPFH among black Americans is 0.0005, resulting in an incidence of sickle cell-deletional HPFH that is 1/100 that of sickle cell anemia. Individuals with the pancellular distribution of 25% Hb F associated with sickle cell-deletional HPFH are neither anemic nor afflicted with vaso-occlusive manifestations, providing evidence that Hb F inhibits HbS polymerization. Hemoglobin electrophoresis reveals only HbS, F, and A$_2$, which is distinguished from sickle cell anemia, sickle cell-β^{0}-thalassemia, and sickle cell-$\delta\beta^{0}$-thalassemia by the pancellular distribution of 15 to 35% Hb F and Hb A$_2$ levels <2.5%.

SICKLE-CELL-Hb LEPORE DISEASE. Hb Lepore, which is a crossover fusion product of the δ- and β-globin genes, has the same electrophoretic mobility as HbS. Thalassemic expression of the Hb Lepore gene results in only 12% Hb Lepore in simple heterozygotes. Compound heterozygous HbS-Hb Lepore is similar to sickle cell anemia or sickle cell-β^{0}-thalassemia on electrophoresis, but the anemia is less severe. The combination of predominantly HbS with microcytosis resembles sickle cell-β-thalassemia, but low to low-normal Hb A$_2$ levels due to crossover incapacitation of one δ-globin gene suggest HbS-Hb Lepore. The peripheral smear reveals microcytosis, hypochromia, and ISC. Vaso-occlusive complications and splenomegaly occur.

SICKLE CELL-Hb D DISEASE. Hb SD disease was first reported as an unusual case of sickle cell anemia, because Hb D^{Punjab} or Hb D$^{Los\ Angeles}$ ($\alpha_2\beta_2^{\ 121Glu \rightarrow Gln}$) has an alkaline electrophoretic mobility similar to that of HbS. Hb D is distinguishable from HbS by acid electrophoresis or isoelectric focusing. The peripheral smear shows marked anisocytosis and poikilocytosis, target cells, and ISCs.

There is moderately severe hemolytic anemia, and the clinical manifestations are similar to those of sickle cell disease.

SICKLE CELL-Hb O ARAB DISEASE. Hb O^{Arab} ($\alpha_2\beta_2^{\ 121Glu \rightarrow Lys}$) was first described in an Israeli Arab family, but its distribution is widespread. On alkaline electrophoresis, Hb S-O^{Arab} disease resembles Hb SC disease, but either acid electrophoresis or isoelectric focusing distinguishes the Hb O^{Arab} from Hb C. There is moderately severe hemolytic anemia, and anisocytosis, poikilocytosis, and ISCs are found on the peripheral smear.

SICKLE CELL-Hb E DISEASE AND OTHER Hb E SYNDROMES. Hb E ($\alpha_2\beta_2^{\ 26Glu \rightarrow Lys}$) is a β-thalassemic hemoglobinopathy found predominantly among Southeast Asians. Hb E has an electrophoretic mobility similar to that of Hb A$_2$, C, and O Arab under alkaline conditions, but it can be distinguished by acid electrophoresis or isoelectric focusing. The codon 26 GAG$\rightarrow$AAG mutation activates a cryptic splice site in the first intron, which decreases expression of the β^{E} gene. Hb E constitutes 30% of the hemoglobin in Hb SE disease, and there is mild microcytosis. Despite reports that Hb SE disease (compound heterozygosity for Hb S and E) causes only mild hemolysis without vaso-occlusive complications or abnormalities of red cell morphologic characteristics, there is sufficient experience to the contrary to indicate that Hb SE disease should be included among the sickle cell diseases.

Hemoglobin E is classified as a thalassemic hemoglobinopathy because of its having features both of quantitatively reduced production and of structural aberrance. It was the fourth mutant hemoglobin reported. The β^{E} gene has arisen mostly in Southeast Asia and exists in β-globin haplotypes that differ from those of β^{S} and β^{C}. The mutation is a GAG$\rightarrow$AAG substitution in the 26th codon of the β-globin gene and results in the production of the structural variant $\beta^{E(26Val \rightarrow Lys)}$. The thalassemic quality of this variant is due to the nucleotide substitution's activation of a cryptic splice site, which results in the abnormal splicing of β^{E} mRNA transcripts and the quantitatively diminished production mature β^{E} mRNA, β^{E} globin, and Hb E. Hemoglobin E tetramers are slightly unstable, but the instability contributes little to the clinical picture of the Hb E syndromes. The inheritance of the β^{E} gene results in several syndromes that are of particular importance among individuals of Southeast Asian background.

Simple heterozygosity for Hb E (Hb AE) is not associated with anemia, hemolysis, or splenomegaly but usually is associated with mild microcytosis (average MCV ~ 74 fL) and target cells on the peripheral smear. The imbalanced proportions of Hb E (27%) and Hb A (73%) on electrophoretic analysis are largely the result of the thalassemic synthesis of β^{E}-globin and Hb E, although a difference in the electrostatic affinities of β^{E} and of β^{A} chains for α-globin also influences this distribution. The lower proportion of Hb E provides a clue for distinguishing carriers of Hb E and C, which co-migrate on standard alkaline electrophoresis.

In homozygous Hb E (Hb EE) there is no or mild anemia. Microcytosis is more pronounced than in Hb AE (average MCV ~ 67 fL) and there are more target cells on the peripheral smear.

The most significant clinical syndrome associated with Hb E is the compound heterozygous condition Hb E-β-thalassemia. Because of the thalassemic nature of both the β^{E} and β^{Thal} alleles, the clinical severity of this condition usually resembles that of homozygous β-thalassemia major. The high frequencies of these two genes in Southeast Asia make this combination the most common cause of thalassemia major. By far the most frequent β-thalassemia alleles in this population completely abolish β-globin production by causing premature termination of translation due to a frameshift deletion (codon 41/42 - TTCT), premature termination of translation due to a non-sense mutation (codon 17 A$\rightarrow$T), or defective splicing of mRNA transcripts (C $\rightarrow$ T substitution at nucleotide 654 of the second intervening sequence). Because of the absence of β^{A}-globin synthesis in Hb E-β^{0}-thalassemia, no Hb A is detected on hemoglobin electrophoresis. Mostly Hb E and variably elevated levels of Hb F are observed. The Hb A$_2$ present is not distinguishable from Hb E on routine laboratory testing. This condition is associated with severe transfusion-requiring hemolytic anemia (average Hb = 6.4 g/dL), reticulocytosis, and severe microcytosis. The remarkably abnormal peripheral smear is notable for microcytosis, hypochromia, target cells, poikilocytosis, anisocytosis, nucleated red cells, and a variable degree of basophilic stippling. Clinical features include splenomegaly, icterus, growth retardation, skeletal changes, iron overload, endocrine deficiency, susceptibility to infection, hypersplenism, aplastic crises, folic acid deficiency, and extramedullary bone marrow tumors. Hb E-β^+-thalassemia is far less prevalent than Hb E-β^0 thalassemia. The most common β^0 thalassemia allele in Southeast Asians is a -28 A→G substitution that attenuates transcription promoter function. Hb A is present in proportions twice that encountered in Hb AS or AC as a result of the thalassemic production of Hb E. This may result in diagnostic difficulty, but Hb E-β^+-thalassemia is readily distinguishable from Hb AE by its greater clinical severity. The hematologic and clinical manifestations are similar to but milder than those of Hb E-β^0-thalassemia. The average Hb level is 8.2 g/dL.

A great number of genetically and clinically complex Hb E syndromes result from the coinheritance of α-thalassemia genes, which are also highly prevalent in Southeast Asia. The diagnostic challenge presented by these combinations underscores the importance of DNA-based diagnosis for accurate diagnosis and counseling.

DIAGNOSIS

Methods of diagnosing sickle cell syndromes and goals of diagnostic programs vary with developmental stage and emerging clinical manifestations. In fetal and newborn periods, the predominance of Hb F confounds characterization of the adult hemoglobins that are present. As HbS increases and Hb F declines in infancy, clinical manifestations of sickle cell anemia evolve—ISCs appear on the peripheral smear at 3 months of age, and by 4 months of age hemolytic anemia presents. General diagnostic methods include those that separate hemoglobin species having different amino acid compositions (i.e., hemoglobin electrophoresis, thin-layer isoelectric focusing), solubility testing, and review of the peripheral blood smear.

OLDER CHILDREN AND ADULTS. The purpose of diagnosis is to identify those with the disease or trait who need treatment or counseling. Hb S, G, and D have the same electrophoretic mobility on cellulose acetate electrophoresis at pH 8.4, which is the standard method of separating HbS from other variants. However, HbS has a different mobility than Hb D and G using citrate agar electrophoresis at pH 6.2. The solubility test (Sickledex) also distinguishes HbS, which is not soluble, from Hb D and G, which are. Thin-layer isoelectric focusing separates Hb S, D, and G but also requires confirmatory solubility testing. The "sickle cell prep" using metabisulfite or dithionite is currently of historical interest only.

In sickle cell anemia and sickle cell-β^0-thalassemia, HbS constitutes nearly all the hemoglobin present. Useful indicators of sickle cell-β^0-thalassemia are microcytosis or a parent lacking HbS. Sickle cell-β^+-thalassemia and sickle cell trait both have Hb A and HbS. Sickle cell trait has neither anemia nor microcytosis; it has a Hb A fraction that exceeds 50%. Sickle cell-β^+-thalassemia has anemia, microcytosis, and a Hb A fraction between only 5 and 25%. Solubility tests yield positive findings in both sickle cell-β^+-thalassemia and sickle cell trait, but sickled forms (ISCs) occur on the peripheral smear only in sickle cell-β^+-thalassemia, not in sickle cell trait. In Hb SC disease nearly equal amounts of Hb S and C are present.

NEWBORN SCREENING. Incentive for early identification of infants with sickle cell disease derives from the tremendous reduction in mortality rate effected by the use of prophylactic penicillin and comprehensive medical care in the first 5 years of life. Universal newborn screening of all ethnic backgrounds is recommended. Tests used in newborn screening must distinguish Hb F, S, A, and C. Patterns of hemoglobins detected are listed, according to convention, in descending order according to their quantities. In this developmental period, sickle cell anemia has predominantly Hb F with small amounts of HbS and no Hb A (FS pattern), which is also seen in sickle cell-β^0-thalassemia, sickle cell-HPFH, and sickle cell-Hb D or sickle cell-Hb G (i.e., Hb D and G have the same electrophoretic mobility as HbS). Family studies, DNA-based testing, or repeat hemoglobin analysis at age 3 to 4 months can be used to establish difficult diagnoses.

Sickle cell trait and sickle cell-β^+-thalassemia have Hb F, Hb A, and HbS. In the former, quantities of Hb A exceed those of HbS

(FAS pattern). In the latter, quantities of HbS exceed those of Hb A (FSA pattern). When it is not possible to distinguish FAS and FSA patterns in newborns, DNA-based testing or repeat hemoglobin testing at age 3 to 6 months is required.

PRENATAL DIAGNOSIS. The limited efficacy of current treatments for sickle cell disease emphasizes the importance of prenatal diagnosis. The development of DNA-based testing methods led to the use of amniocentesis for fetal DNA for testing in the second trimester. The polymerase chain reaction (PCR) method of amplifying β-globin DNA sequences in vitro allowed testing of minute quantities of DNA and motivated the development of a host of new methods for detecting the sickle cell gene, including restriction analysis (Figure 169-4), allele-specific hybridization, and reverse dot blotting. PCR-based diagnosis for Hb SC disease is also possible by using specific molecular methods for detecting the Hb C gene. The diagnosis of sickle cell-β thalassemia can be made using

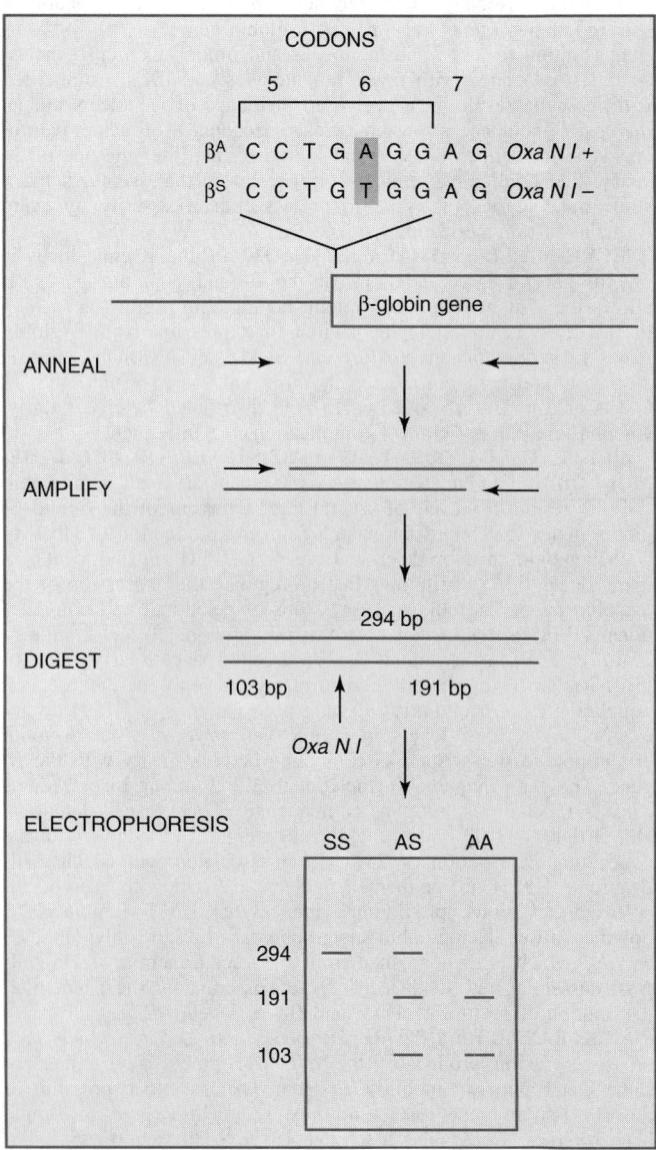

FIGURE 169-4 ■ PCR-based restriction analysis for the sickle cell gene. The target β-globin DNA containing the sixth codon, which is mutated in the sickle cell gene, is flanked by the two annealed PCR primers so that this codon is included in the PCR amplification product. The CCTNAGG cleavage site for the restriction enzyme OxaN I found in normal β-globin DNA is abolished by the GAG→GTG sickle cell mutation. The electrophoretic gel shows the OxaN I digestion products of PCR amplified DNA with the sizes in base pairs shown at the left. The genotypes of the DNA samples tested are shown above the gel. The fragments from normal β-globin DNA (AA) show complete OxaN I cleavage; from sickle cell trait DNA (AS) shows partial cleavage; and from sickle cell anemia, (SS) shows no cleavage; PCR-polymerase chain reaction. (Figure adapted with permission of YW Kan.)

reverse dot blot methodology to screen the many American β-thalassemia mutations and the HbS and Hb C mutations in a single hybridization reaction. Currently, fetal DNA samples are obtained by chorionic villus sampling at 8 to 10 weeks gestation.

OTHER LABORATORY TESTING. The hemolytic anemia of sickle cell disease is associated with mildly to moderately reduced hematocrit, hemoglobin, and red cell levels; reticulocytosis of approximately 3 to 15%; unconjugated hyperbilirubinemia; elevated LDH levels; and low haptoglobin levels. The peripheral blood smear reveals polychromasia related to reticulocytosis and Howell-Jolly bodies indicative of hyposplenia. Sickle cells are normochromic, except with coexistent thalassemia or iron deficiency. Hb F levels are slightly to moderately elevated, with average values of 5 to 6%. White blood cell (WBC) and platelet counts tend to be elevated in sickle cell anemia but not in Hb SC disease or sickle cell-β⁺-thalassemia. Serum bilirubin levels reflect the greater hemolytic rate in sickle cell anemia compared with that in Hb SC disease and sickle cell-β⁺-thalassemia.

THERAPY

HEALTH CARE MAINTENANCE. Routine clinical visits are important for patients with sickle cell disease to establish baseline clinical and laboratory findings for comparison at times of clinical exacerbations, relationships with health care professionals, and red cell phenotypes and individualized blood bank files. Counseling regarding the disease, genetic characteristics and psychosocial issues are best accomplished during routine visits. Folic acid, 1 mg/day orally, is administered. Non-invasive surveillance of cerebral blood flow using transcranial Doppler assessment is a useful predictor of CVA and should be performed regularly to identify those in whom chronic transfusion should be initiated to prevent this outcome. Retinal evaluation is begun at school age and continued routinely. Sexually active women receive routine pelvic exams. Oral contraception with low-dose estrogen can be administered safely. Immunization using conjugated vaccines for *S. pneumoniae* and *H. influenzae* type b should be employed. Re-immunization for *S. pneumoniae* is recommended every 6 to 8 years.

INFECTIONS. Outpatient ceftriaxone is recommended for children with fevers >38.5° C unless they appear toxic, have temperature > 40° C, are not receiving prophylactic penicillin, have previously documented *S. pneumoniae* bacteremia, or live in areas where antibiotic-resistant *S. pneumoniae* has evolved. In these situations, hospitalization is recommended with cultures of blood and cerebrospinal fluid and use of antibiotics likely to be effective against local strains of *S. pneumoniae*. Treatment of meningitis should cover *S. pneumoniae* and *H. influenzae* type b and be continued for at least 2 weeks.

Antibiotic therapy for the acute chest syndrome should provide coverage for *S. pneumoniae, H. influenzae* type b, *Mycoplasma pneumoniae,* and *Chlamydia pneumoniae.* Cefuroxime and erythromycin combinations are recommended.

The diagnosis of osteomyelitis is confirmed by culture of blood or infected bone, after which parenteral antibiotics that cover *Salmonella* spp. and *S. aureus* are administered. Antibiotic therapy is tailored by using culture and sensitivity results and continued for 2 to 6 weeks. Surgical drainage or sequestrectomy may be required.

TRANSFUSION THERAPY. Patients with sickle cell disease have similar requirements for transfusion to other patients—oxygen carrying capacity and blood volume replacement (e.g., aplastic crisis, splenic sequestration). They also have indications unique to their disease—protection from imminent danger (e.g., acute chest syndrome, septicemia, metabolic acidosis) and improved rheologic properties of blood (e.g., prevention of recurrent CVA, priapism, pre-operatively). The routine acute painful crisis is not an indication for transfusion. Transfusion complications are alloimmunization, iron overload, and transmission of viral illness. Antibodies against the Rh (E, C), Kell (K), Duffy (Fya, Fyb), and Kidd (Jk) antigens present the greatest problem in transfusion of these patients. Transfusing extended-matched, phenotypically compatible blood has been documented to diminish alloimmunization rates.

As sickle cell patients live longer and are transfused more, iron overload becomes a greater problem. Deferoxamine chelation should be considered for those with elevated total body iron level, i.e., serum ferritin levels that exceed 2000 ng/mL. This therapy is inconvenient, uncomfortable, and expensive. The anticipated availability of oral chelating agents will be a tremendous asset for the management of these patients. Transmission of human immunodeficiency virus (HIV), hepatitis B and C, and human T-lymphotropic virus 1 (HTLV-1) has diminished with improved screening, and it is anticipated that the use of leukocyte-depleted red cell transfusion will reduce this hazard further.

Preoperative transfusion is recommended for patients with sickle cell anemia. Both simple transfusion to reduce HbS to <60% and raise the hemoglobin level to 10 g/dL and aggressive partial exchange transfusion to reduce HbS to <30% will reduce the incidence of perioperative acute chest syndrome; simple transfusion is equally efficacious and is associated with fewer complications. Partial exchange transfusion may be advantageous in Hb SC disease, in which the higher hemoglobin levels may not accommodate simple transfusion.

Simple transfusion is used to restore oxygen carrying capacity or blood volume. Partial exchange transfusions are used for acute emergencies and chronic transfusion programs, in the latter case because of their beneficial impact on blood viscosity and body iron burden. For average size adults, it is anticipated that each unit of red cells will increase the hemoglobin level approximately 1 g/dL. Partial exchange transfusion in adults is accomplished by phlebotomizing 500 mL, infusing 300 mL normal saline solution, phlebotomizing another 500 mL, and infusing 4 to 5 units packed red cells.

PAIN MANAGEMENT. Acute painful episodes are the most common cause of sickle cell patients' seeking medical care. The physician must exclude causes other than vaso-occlusion, maintain optimal hydration by oral or intravenous fluid administration, and use analgesics aggressively, but cautiously. Neither red cell transfusion nor oxygen administration is indicated in treating the routine acute painful episode, although oxygen inhalation is recommended for those who are hypoxemic. Health care providers should be familiar with the pharmacologic characteristics of analgesia (Table 169–3) and must overcome fears of narcotic addiction to treat pain optimally and to prevent prolonging the duration of pain, which promotes a "drug-seeking" ("pain-relieving"?) behavior pattern.

Optimal treatment of patients in pain is in a familiar setting that avoids the hectic environment of the emergency department. The treatment of severe pain may require hospitalization, intravenous fluid administration, and narcotics. Intravenous morphine is recommended for prompt pain relief, and patient-controlled analgesia is an excellent means of subsequent ("rescue") pain control. Patients with sickle cell disease metabolize narcotics more rapidly than normal and may respond poorly to conventional doses of analgesia. Comprehensive approaches to the biopsychosocial experience of pain includes psychosocial support systems, local anesthetics, epidural anesthetics, combinations of nonsteroidal anti-inflammatory agents and narcotics, and antidepressive drugs. The potent nonsteroidal anti-inflammatory drug ketorolac (Toradol) can be given by injection or orally, provides analgesia superior to that of parenteral meperidine especially for bone pain, and prevents respiratory depression. Tramadol is an orally administered, centrally acting analgesic that binds to the μ-opioid receptor, causes minimal respiratory depression, and has a low potential for abuse or addiction. The chronic sickle cell pain syndrome is rare; its therapy may require approaches similar to that used for the management of terminal cancer pain, i.e., long-acting morphine and fentanyl patches.

HYDROXYUREA. The unrelenting search for a pharmacologic agent capable of inducing Hb F production led to the momentous discovery and characterization of hydroxyurea. In a large multicenter study, the capacity of this ribonucleotide reductase inhibitor to suppress hematopoiesis was documented by significant reductions in leukocyte, PMN, and reticulocyte counts. Its ability to induce beneficial effects was confirmed by significant reductions in dense sickle cell counts and increased levels of hemoglobin, hematocrit, MCV, Hb F, F cells, and F reticulocytes. Salient clinical changes were a lower rate of acute painful episodes, longer interval to first and second acute painful episodes, decrease in episodes of acute chest syndrome, and diminished number of subjects and units transfused. No short-term toxicity was observed. At the time of this writing there is no convincing evidence for a leukemogenic effect in patients who lack a preexistent potential for leukemia.

Table 169–3 ■ RECOMMENDED DOSE AND INTERVAL OF ANALGESICS NECESSARY TO OBTAIN ADEQUATE PAIN CONTROL IN SICKLE CELL DISEASE

	DOSE/RATE	COMMENTS
Severe/Moderate Pain		
1. Morphine	**Parenteral:** 0.1–0.15 mg/kg/dose every 3–4 hr. Recommended maximum single dose 10 mg **P.O.:** 0.3–0.6 mg/kg/dose every 4 hr.	Drug of choice for pain; lower doses in the elderly, infants, and those with liver failure or impaired ventilation.
2. Meperidine (Demerol)	**Parenteral:** 0.75–1.5 mg/kg/dose every 2–4 hr; recommended maximum dose 100 mg **P.O.:** 1.5 mg/kg/dose every 4 hr	Increased incidence of seizures, total daily dose not to exceed 1200 mg, avoid in patients who have renal or neurologic disease or receiving monoamine oxidase inhibitors; weak analgesic effect
3. Hydromorphone	**Parenteral:** 0.01–0.02 mg/kg/dose every 3–4 hr	
4. Oxycodone	**P.O.:** 0.04–0.06 mg/kg/dose every 4 hr; recommended maximum dose 0.15 mg/kg every 4 hr	
5. Ketorolac	**Intramuscular:** Adults: 30- or 60-mg initial dose, followed by 15 to 30 mg every 6–8 hr Children: 1 mg/kg load, followed by 0.5 mg/kg every 6 hr	Equal efficacy to 6 mg morphine sulfate; helps narcotic-sparing effect, not to exceed 5 days, maximum 150 mg first day, 120 mg maximum subsequent days, may cause GI irritation
6. Butorphanol	**Parenteral:** Adults: 2 mg every 3–4 hr	Agonist-antagonist, can precipitate withdrawal if given to patients being treated with agonists
Mile Pain		
1. Codeine	**P.O.:** 0.5–1 mg/kg/dose every 4 hr Maximum dose 60 mg	Mild to moderate pain not relieved by aspirin or acetaminophen; can cause nausea and vomiting
2. Aspirin	**P.O.:** Adults: 0.3–0.6 g/dose every 4–6 hr, children: 10 mg/kg/dose every 4 hr	Often given with a narcotic to enhance analgesia; can cause gastric irritation; avoid in febrile children
3. Acetaminophen	**P.O.:** Adults: 0.3–0.6 g every 4 hr; children: 10 mg/kg/dose	Often given with a narcotic to enhance analgesia
4. Ibuprofen	**P.O.:** Adults: 300–400 mg/dose every 4 hr; children: 5–10 mg/kg/dose every 6–8 hr	Can cause gastric irritation
5. Naproxen	**P.O.:** Adults: 500 mg/dose initially, then 250 every 8–12 hr; children: 10 mg/kg/day (5 mg/kg every 12 hr)	Long duration of action; can cause gastric irritation
6. Indomethacin	**P.O.:** Adults: 25–50 mg/dose every 8 hr; children: 1–3 mg/kg/day given 3–4 times	Contraindicated in psychiatric, neurologic, renal diseases; high incidence of gastric irritation; useful in gout

GI = gastrointestinal. Adapted from Charache S, Lubin B, Reid C, et al: Management and Therapy of Sickle Cell Disease, 3rd ed. Bethesda, MD, NIH publication #95–2117, 1995, pp. 1–114.

The mechanism of action of hydroxyurea is unknown. Although the original interest in this agent was generated by its potential for up-regulating Hb F production, there is evidence for therapeutic responses independent of changes in Hb F levels, for improved erythrocyte hydration and deformability, and for decreased sickle cell–endothelial cell adherence, which may be due to decreased $\alpha_4\beta_1$ and CD36 molecules on sickle cells. The therapeutic benefit of hydroxyurea may also be related to its lowering of the PMN count. General guidelines recommend administration of hydroxyurea to patients who consider themselves impaired by painful episodes, who are willing to comply with frequent monitoring for myelosuppression, and who will adopt a program that may improve their quality of life.

NEW THERAPEUTIC MODALITIES

Membrane-active agents that improve sickle cell hydration have shown therapeutic promise. Oral administration of agents that inhibit the cellular dehydration caused by the Gardos and potassium-chloride cotransport pathways, such as the imidazole compound clotrimazole, which inhibits the Gardos pathway, or Mg supplements that inhibit potassium-chloride co-transport, have been shown to improve the pathobiologic features of sickle erythrocytes and may have application for treating sickle cell disease in the future. Cetiedil, despite its ability to preserve sickle cell hydration, had limited therapeutic benefit in a controlled clinical trial. Membrane-active compounds, such as pentoxifylline, generally are not efficacious.

Artificial surfactant (Pluronic F-68, RheothRx, or poloxamer 188) improves rheologic properties of sickle erythrocytes and inhibits their adherence to the vascular endothelium. This agent, given by intravenous infusion, may reduce narcotic requirements, shorten the duration of pain, and gain a therapeutic role for acute painful episodes. Vasodilating agents that improve membrane deformability have not been found effective.

Nitric oxide (NO) has several biologic effects, including increasing the oxygen affinity of sickle erythrocytes and decreasing vascular tone, which may contribute to the potential utility of inhaled NO for the treatment of acute chest syndrome and painful episodes. Its endogenous level in the blood varies inversely with vaso-occlusive severity.

Both warfarin and minidose heparin have been suggested to have beneficial effects in sickle cell disease. Methylprednisolone has been reported to provide pain relief, albeit with a high rebound pain rate after its discontinuation.

The ability of butyric acid compounds to delay the switch from fetal to adult hemoglobin production has not been matched by clinical efficacy. Although arginine butyrate induces increase in numbers of Hb F–containing reticulocytes, there has been no consistent improvement in levels of Hb F or hemolysis to justify its reported risks. New orally absorbable butyrate formulations are being evaluated. Valproic acid may stimulate Hb F production and have therapeutic potential in selected patients with sickle cell disease.

Bone marrow transplantation (BMT) (Chapter 182) has been used successfully for sickle cell anemia. One major challenge with this approach is identification of appropriate recipients. Another pertains to the decision whether to await serious complications before employing BMT, which may result in disability prior to definitive therapy, or to subject those with mild disease to what may be unnecessary risk. In the United States, the practice has been closer to the former. The initial results with BMT revealed an unacceptable rate of neurologic complications, which has been redressed by aggressive maintenance of hemoglobin levels, platelet counts, and normal blood pressure. Comparing the cost of $150,000 to $200,000 for uncomplicated BMT in the United States with up to $112,000 annually for conventional care of a patient on long-term transfusion and chelation suggests that BMT may be more cost-effective. Another major hurdle pertains to the availability of suitable donors, which is further complicated in sickle cell disease: the usual one compatible donor per three siblings ratio is lessened further by the presence of sickle cell disease in the family. Broadening the ethnic composition of the registry donor pool, using partially matched donors, and correcting the sickle cell gene in autologous marrow erythroid precursors may improve the outcome with BMT. Of particular interest is the development of cord blood stem cells for transplantation, an approach that may obviate the occurrence of graft-versus-host disease and allow crossing of the human leukocyte antigen (HLA) barrier with partially matched donor sources.

Recent advances in gene therapy technology provide promise for the future of sickle cell disease. Gene transfer can be accomplished efficiently by using a variety of non-viral or replicative defective or non-virulent viral vectors. A high level of expression has been attained by including locus control region regulatory sequences in the vector and by inserting the normal gene into its native environment by using homologous recombination, which also knocks out the mutant gene by inserting the normal sequence. Transfer of the normal gene into self-replicating stem cells allows sustained expression of the corrected gene. The practicality of these approaches and safety of gene therapy remain to be established.

Adams RJ, McKie VC, Hsu L, et al: Prevention of a first stroke by transfusions in children with sickle cell anemia and abnormal results on transcranial Doppler ultrasonography. N Engl J Med 339:5, 1998. *A breakthrough study that defined the state of the art approach to diagnosing subclinical cerebrovascular disease and preventing stroke.*

Charache S, Barton FB, Moore RD, et al: Hydroxyurea and sickle cell anemia: Clinical utility of a myelosuppressive "switching" agent: The Multicenter Study of Hydroxyurea in Sickle Cell Anemia. Medicine (Baltimore) 75:300, 1996. *A thorough data analysis, discussion, and review of the hydroxyurea experience.*

Fucharoen S, Winichagoon P: Hemoglobinopathies in southeast Asia: Molecular biology and clinical medicine. Hemoglobin 21:299, 1997. *An up-to-date account of these globally important conditions with an emphasis on molecular biology.*

Steinberg MH: Management of sickle cell disease. N Engl J Med 340:1021, 1999. *Recent review emphasizing new therapeutic approach to sickle cell disease.*

Vichinsky E, Styles L: Pulmonary complications. Hematol/Oncol Clin North Am 10: 1275, 1996. *A thoughtful treatment of this major cause of morbidity and mortality.*

Walters MC, Patience M, Leisenring W, et al: Barriers to bone marrow transplantation for sickle cell anemia. Biol Blood Marrow Transplant 2:100–104, 1996. *A comprehensive discussion of this important therapeutic modality.*

170 BLOOD TRANSFUSION

Jay E. Menitove

Red blood cells (or packed cells) are prepared by separating red cells from the plasma contained in whole blood. The approximately 325-mL red cell concentrate includes 100 mL of an additive solution that contains nutrients for maintaining cell viability at 1° to 6° C during the 42-day storage interval. The hematocrit is approximately 55%.

Blood donors undergo a multilayer screening approach designed to interdict those at risk for transmitting retroviruses and hepatitis. Laboratory testing is performed to detect hepatitis B surface antigen (HBsAg); antibodies against human immunodeficiency virus (HIV) types 1 and 2, hepatitis C, hepatitis B core antigen, and human T-lymphotropic virus (HTLV) types I and II; syphilis; alanine aminotransferase; and, if indicated, antibodies against cytomegalovirus (CMV). Because donations may occur during the window period between infectivity and serodetection, transmission of infectious agents cannot be eliminated. This consideration and other adverse consequences of transfusion should be part of the decision-making process for ensuring that anticipated benefits outweigh potential transfusion risks.

INDICATIONS FOR WHOLE BLOOD TRANSFUSION

Whole blood is indicated when there are concomitant deficits of oxygen-carrying capacity, blood volume, and coagulation factors. Whole blood contains red cells and plasma. Factors V and VIII, present in plasma, are labile and decrease during ex vivo blood storage. For patients with acute blood loss, crystalloid or colloid solutions should be used to restore intravascular volume until hemorrhage leads to impaired oxygen delivery. At that point, red cell transfusion should be done. If there is continued blood loss, whole blood is an appropriate choice for additional red cell support and coagulation factor replacement (other than Factors V and VIII).

INDICATIONS FOR TRANSFUSION OF RED BLOOD CELLS

Red cell transfusions are used to alleviate signs and symptoms attributable to diminished oxygen-carrying capacity in patients unable to tolerate anemia pending the effect of iron, folic acid, vita-min B_{12}, exogenous erythropoietin, or other specific therapeutic interventions to increase hemoglobin/hematocrit levels. Signs and symptoms attributable to anemia include fatigue, syncope, dyspnea on exertion, decreased exercise capacity, decreased mental acuity, tachycardia, angina, postural hypotension, or transient ischemic attack. In general, transfusions should be avoided in asymptomatic patients regardless of the hemoglobin/hematocrit. If symptoms do occur, transfusions should be administered on a case-by-case and unit-by-unit basis (Fig. 170–1).

Compensatory mechanisms for augmenting oxygen delivery to tissues allow patients to tolerate modest degrees of anemia. These mechanisms include increasing cardiac output by raising stroke volume or heart rate; redistributing blood to areas requiring more oxygen; enhancing oxygen extraction by tissues; increasing coronary artery blood flow, ventilatory volume, and respiratory rates; and augmenting oxygen unloading as a result of elevated 2,3-diphosphoglycerate (2,3-DPG) levels.

In the absence of cardiopulmonary dysfunction or ischemic co-morbidities, otherwise healthy patients usually do not have signs or symptoms of anemia at rest when the hemoglobin concentration is greater than 7 to 8 g/dL. Dyspnea on exertion occurs at this level. Weakness occurs at a hemoglobin of 6 g/dL, dyspnea at rest occurs when the hemoglobin concentration falls to 3 g/dL, and the risk of heart failure is significant when the hemoglobin is less than 2.5 g/dL.

When transfusions are prescribed for patients with chronic anemia, the therapeutic goals are to avoid inadequate tissue oxygenation and heart failure. The strategy for transfusion support involves an assessment of symptoms caused by or aggravated by anemia; a determination of whether these symptoms resolve with transfusion; the minimal hemoglobin concentration at which patients function satisfactorily; and consideration of life-style factors, coexisting medical disorders, the duration of anemia, and the overall prognosis. Other factors influencing the need for transfusion include the patient's activity level and fitness, the likelihood of ongoing blood loss, the rapidity of onset of anemia, physiologic adaptations, cardiopulmonary function, and history of ischemic co-morbidities. Currently, factors other than hemoglobin or hematocrit levels comprise the major criteria for ordering transfusions, although most transfusions are given at hemoglobin concentrations of 7 to 9 g/dL.

With chronic anemia, symptomatic patients receive 2 to 3 units of blood at 2- to 3-week intervals. One unit of red cells raises the hemoglobin/hematocrit by approximately 1 g/dL (or a hematocrit increase of 3%).

Acute anemia is tolerated less well than chronic anemia. In patients with acute anemia, transfusion is indicated to alleviate signs or symptoms of anemia caused by blood loss after correction of volume deficits with either crystalloid or colloid solutions.

LEUKOCYTE-REDUCED RED BLOOD CELLS. White blood cells contained in red cell transfusions cause febrile, non-hemolytic transfusion reactions, alloimmunization to human leukocyte antigen (HLA) and other non–red cell alloantigens, and immunomodulatory effects of blood transfusion such as the possibly increased rate of postoperative infections in transfused versus non-transfused surgical patients. In addition, white blood cells provide a reservoir for infectious agents, including CMV and HTLV I/II. During storage, leukocytes produce various cytokines, including interleukin (IL)-1, IL-6, and IL-8 and tumor necrosis factor-α (TNF-α), that relate etiologically to some febrile transfusion reactions.

Red cells and whole blood contain approximately 10^9 white blood cells per unit. Experimental and observational data indicate that reduction of white cell levels to less than 2×10^8 per unit alleviates recurrent febrile, non-hemolytic transfusion reactions; and levels less than 5×10^6 reduce the incidence of alloimmunization against HLA antigens and decrease transmission of CMV. Currently, leukocyte reduction filters routinely reduce white cell content below 5×10^6 per unit.

To date, there is no consensus about whether all patients or only certain patients, such as those receiving outpatient or perioperative transfusions, are most likely to benefit from leukocyte reduction. Other issues under consideration include venue and whether to remove leukocytes before or after storage. Filtration may be performed in the laboratory setting to reduce variation or through leukocyte reduction filters at the bedside to provide a pragmatic

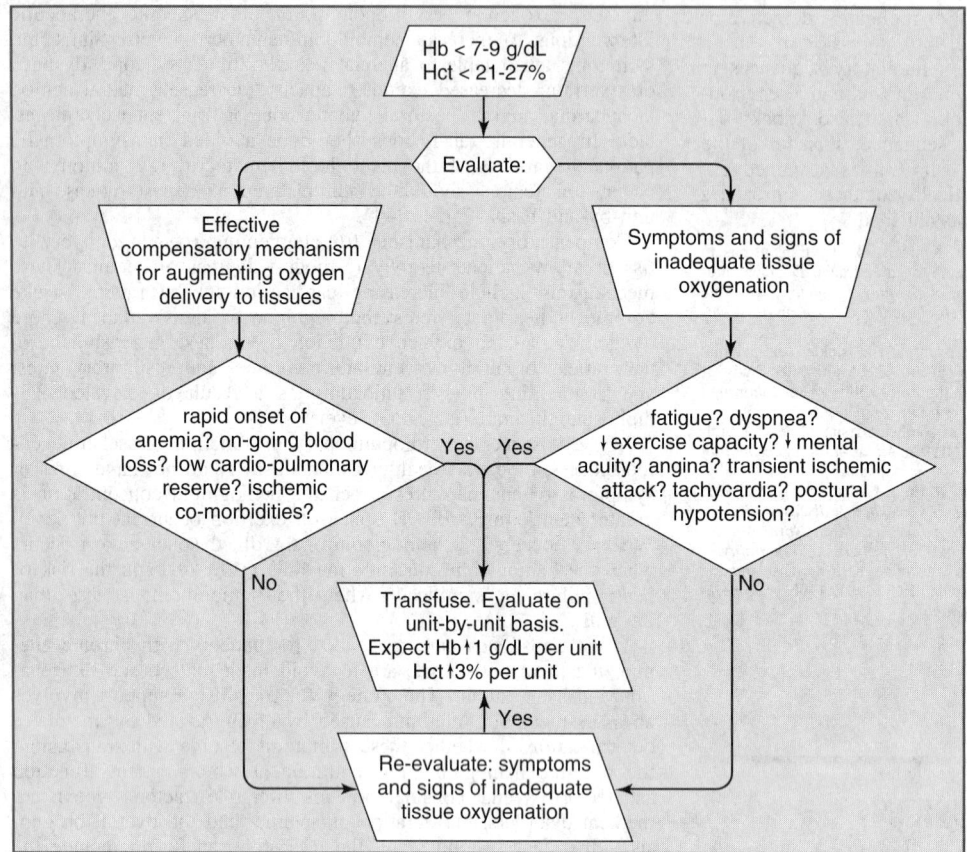

FIGURE 170–1 ■ An approach to deciding when to transfuse patients with anemia and/or blood loss.

approach. Concerns about cytokine accumulation favor removal of white cells within a few days of collection rather than waiting until infusion.

WASHED RED BLOOD CELLS. Washed red cells are prepared by adding saline to blood cells, subjecting the container to centrifugation to separate the red cells and diluted plasma, decanting the plasma/saline mixture, and resuspending the red cells in saline. Washing removes plasma proteins, including IgA.

RED BLOOD CELLS STORED IN THE FROZEN STATE. The cryoprotective agent glycerol is added to red cells before storing the cells in the frozen state for up to 10 years. When needed for transfusion, the red cells are thawed and washed to remove the glycerol. Frozen red cells are used primarily for maintaining repositories of red cell units with uncommon phenotypes needed for patients with alloantibodies against commonly occurring antigens.

IRRADIATED RED BLOOD CELLS. Irradiated components are used to prevent graft-versus-host disease (GvHD) by eliminating the proliferative capacity of T lymphocytes. The midplane of the blood container should receive 25 Gy. Patients at risk for GvHD include bone marrow, peripheral blood progenitor cell, or umbilical cord blood transplant recipients; patients with congenital immunodeficiency syndromes; infants weighing less than 1000 g at birth; fetuses receiving intrauterine transfusions; neonates who receive intrauterine transfusions; patients with Hodgkin's disease, non-Hodgkin's lymphoma, and hematologic and solid tumor malignancies profoundly immunosuppressed by chemotherapy; recipients of transfusions from blood relatives; and recipients of HLA-selected components.

AUTOLOGOUS TRANSFUSION

Autologous transfusion involves collection and reinfusion of a patient's own blood to reduce allogeneic blood exposure. Blood donation may be performed as frequently as every 3 days—but at least 72 hours—before a scheduled surgical procedure. The hemoglobin concentration should be more than 11 g/dL before each donation. Oral iron supplementation is given. Collections should begin as soon as possible before the scheduled surgery, noting the

maximal 42-day shelf life of routinely stored red cells. Autologous donations should be restricted to those likely to need a transfusion because only 50% of autologous units are returned to the donor and, in general, autologous units are not placed into the general blood supply. Perioperative blood salvage and acute normovolemic hemodilution are other alternatives to autologous transfusion.

DIRECTED DONATION

A directed donation refers to blood provided by a donor (usually a family member or friend) selected by the patient. Available data do not support the contention that blood from directed donors is "safer" than general blood supply.

TRANSFUSION PRACTICE

Clinicians are responsible for obtaining informed consent and discussing alternatives to allogeneic transfusion with their patients. Optimally, consent for elective situations should be obtained in time to permit consideration of autologous or directed donations. Physicians are responsible for documenting and reporting suspected adverse transfusion reactions to the hospital transfusion service. The transfusion service must report to the U.S. Food and Drug Administration any reactions associated with fatalities. Required reporting of accidents or errors, such as those involving incorrect identification of samples used in compatibility testing, is under consideration.

IMMUNOHEMATOLOGY

BLOOD GROUPS. The antigenicity of the various red cell blood groups serves as the basis for serologic reactions and compatibility testing. The various blood groups are assigned to 23 systems, nine collections, and several low-incidence and high-incidence antigen series on a genetic basis. The blood group systems include ABO, Rh, MNS, Kell, Duffy, Kidd, and others. These antigens are controlled at a single gene locus, or by two or more closely linked homologous genes. Collections include Cost, Ii, Er, and others and consist of serologically, biochemically, or genetically related antigens that do not fulfill the criteria for systems. The low-incidence antigens refer to those occurring in less than 1% of the population and high-incidence antigens to those occurring in more than 90% of the population. Low-incidence antigens include Batty and Christiansen; examples of high-incidence antigens include Vel, Sd^a, and JMH.

An oligosaccharide structure, formed by glycosyltransferases, gives rise to A and B antigens. The A phenotype is the result of N-acetylgalactosaminyl transferase activity, and the B phenotype arises from galactosyl transferase. Other oligosaccharide structure antigens function as receptors (e.g., the P antigen serves as the receptor for parvovirus B19 and the Le^b antigen is the epithelial receptor for *Helicobacter pylori*). Fetal red cells, those produced under hematopoietic stress, and red cells from patients with congenital dyserythropoietic anemia type II express the i antigen, whereas normal adults express I.

Protein-based antigens include Rh, Gerbich, Diego, Wright, Duffy, and other antigens. The Rh blood group antigens are expressed by a complex of two polypeptide chains, each with a molecular weight of 32 to 34 kd. The *RHD* and *RHCE* genes each consist of 10 exons. RHD codes for the D antigen, which confers Rh positivity, and RHCE codes for C, c, E, and e. Several strategies are used for performing DNA-based Rh typing for prenatal testing and investigation of Rh polymorphisms. Gerbich antigens reside on glycophorins C and D. These minor erythrocyte membrane proteins are the major protein ligands of cytoskeletal protein band 4.1. Specific variants or the lack of glycophorins C and D are associated with partial band 4.1 deficiency and elliptocytosis (see Chapter 164). Erythrocyte band 3, or anion exchanges protein AEI, carries the Diego blood group antigens and Wright a and b amino acid polymorphisms. Mutations of band 3 protein have been implicated in Southeast Asian ovalocytosis, hereditary spherocytosis, congenital acanthocytosis, and an inherited form of renal tubular acidosis. The Duffy blood group antigens reside on a protein receptor for chemokines IL-8 and RANTES. Lack of Duffy a and b antigen expression confers resistance to *Plasmodium vivax* and *P. knowlesi* infection. Phosphatidylinositol-linked proteins include Cromer, Cartwright, Dombrock, JMH, and Emm blood groups.

The clinical importance of a particular blood group depends on its frequency in the population, the immunogenicity of the antigen, and whether alloantibodies directed against it are IgG or IgM or activate complement. IgM anti-A and anti-B are "naturally occurring" antibodies; that is, they are present in the absence of previous transfusion or pregnancy. Intravascular hemolysis may result if these antibodies are present at high titer and incompatible blood is infused. Approximately 80% of Rh-negative persons exposed to Rh-positive blood form anti-Rh antibodies. Anti-Rh antibodies, usually IgG, are implicated in hemolytic reactions and cross the placenta to cause hemolytic disease of the newborn.

A, B, and D are potent immunogens. Kell (K), c, and E are less immunogenic but are stronger antigenically than Fy^a and Jk^a. As a result of differences in antigenicity and frequency, anti-K, anti-D, anti-E, anti-Fy^a, anti-Jk^a, and other antibodies against Rh antigens comprise the majority of alloantibodies detected by hospital transfusion services. Generally, 1% of hospitalized patients have red cell alloantibodies, compared with 10 to 30% of multitransfused patients.

COMPATIBILITY TESTING. Compatibility testing involves determination of the donor's and recipient's ABO groups and Rh types and the presence of unexpected antibodies (i.e., antibodies other than anti-A and anti-B) in the recipient's serum. A system must be in place to ensure accurate identification of the recipient, all blood samples, a review of previous records, and resolution of any discrepancies. If the recipient serum does not have unexpected antibodies, a "type and screen" procedure is acceptable in lieu of a major crossmatch. When blood is needed, the patient's serum is reacted with donor red cells and centrifuged briefly (immediate spin crossmatch). If agglutination or hemolysis does not occur, ABO compatibility is assumed and the blood is released for transfusion.

If unexpected antibodies are present, blood that does not contain the corresponding antigen is selected. Currently, this selection process involves testing donor blood with human- or animal-derived polyclonal and laboratory-derived monoclonal antibodies with

known specificity against blood group antigens. Subsequently, a major crossmatch is performed with donor red cells, patient sera, and antiglobulin reagents.

Computerized crossmatching is gaining acceptance because of reported cost savings and the trend toward centralized crossmatch services. The serologic evaluation is limited to testing a current recipient sample for ABO, Rh, and unexpected antibodies. The computer crossmatch requires the system to contain logic to detect discrepancies between donor and recipient ABO and Rh results and to ensure that ABO compatible blood is selected.

Recipients of whole blood must receive blood from a donor with the same ABO group because infusion of plasma with anti-A and/or anti-B present may cause destruction of recipient red cells. For example, group O whole blood must be given only to group O patients, and group AB patients must receive only group AB whole blood. Because the amount of plasma is reduced in red cells (packed cells), recipients of this component may be compatible rather than identical to the donor; that is, group O (universal donor) red cells may be given to group A, B, or AB patients, and group AB patients (universal recipients) may receive group O, A, or B red cells. Rh-negative patients should receive Rh-negative whole blood or red cells. Rh-positive recipients may receive either Rh-positive or Rh-negative blood.

If a patient's physician is concerned that a delay in transfusion will unduly jeopardize the patient, blood is issued without pretransfusion testing provided the physician documents the urgent need for transfusion. If the ABO type of the recipient is not known, group O red cells should be provided. If the ABO group was determined by the transfusion service, ABO group-compatible red cells may be given. Whole blood must be ABO group identical.

ADVERSE EVENTS ASSOCIATED WITH TRANSFUSION (Table 170–1)

ACUTE REACTIONS. Acute reactions caused by transfusion occur within minutes or hours after infusing red cells or components. Because of significant overlap in the presenting signs and symptoms, a laboratory investigation is required for making a definite diagnosis (Table 170–2).

Table 170–1 ■ **FREQUENCY OF ADVERSE REACTIONS TO BLOOD TRANSFUSION**

	RISK PER UNIT INFUSED
Acute	
Hemolytic transfusion reactions	1:25,000
Fatal hemolytic transfusion reaction	1:600,000
Febrile non-hemolytic transfusion reactions	1:200
Transfusion-related acute lung injury	1:5,000–10,000
Allergic reactions (urticaria)	1:30–100
Anaphylactic reactions	1:150,000
Hypervolemia	Infrequent
Bacterial transmission	
Platelets	1:2,000–12,000
Red blood cells	1:500,000
Delayed	
"Hemolytic" transfusion reactions	
Serologic	1:300–1,600
Hemolytic	1:1,500–8,000
Graft-versus-host disease	Infrequent
Iron overload	Following 60–210 units
Post-transfusion purpura	Infrequent
Transfusion-Transmitted Infections	
Hepatitis A	Infrequent
B	1:63,000–1:233,000
C	~1:120,000
D	Infrequent
Retroviral infection	
HIV 1–2	~1:676,000
HTLV-I/II	~1:640,000
Cytomegalovirus	Varies according to patient's status
Malaria	1:4 million
Chagas' disease	Infrequent
Syphilis	No recent cases
Creutzfeldt-Jakob disease	No cases reported

Table 170-2 ■ SIGNS AND SYMPTOMS OF ACUTE ADVERSE REACTIONS TO BLOOD TRANSFUSION

REACTION	FEVER	CHILLS/ RIGORS	NAUSEA/ VOMITING	CHEST DISCOMFORT/ PAIN	FACIAL FLUSHING	WHEEZING/ DYSPNEA	BACK/ LUMBAR PAIN	DISCOMFORT AT INFUSION SITE	HYPOTENSION	BLEEDING/ DIC	HEMOGLOBINURIA	HIVES/ PRURITUS
Acute hemolytic	X	X	X	X	X	X	X	X	X	X	X	X
Febrile non-hemolytic	X	X		X	X							
Non-immune hemolysis											X	
Acute lung injury	X			X		X			X			
Allergic												X
Massive transfusion complications	X	X	X							X		
Anaphylaxis	X	X	X	X	X	X	X	X	X			X
Passive cytokine infusion												
Hypervolemia						X						
Bacterial sepsis	X	X	X				X	X	X			
Air embolus				X		X						

DIC = Disseminated intravascular coagulation.

ACUTE HEMOLYTIC TRANSFUSION REACTIONS. The majority of these reactions result from a clerical error occurring at the time of sample collection, in the laboratory, or in administering the transfusion. The major sequelae are shock, disseminated intravascular coagulation (DIC), or acute renal failure. The initiating event, infusion of immunologically incompatible blood, leads to complement activation and release of red cell stroma, antibody-antigen complexes, and hemoglobin into the circulation. Shock and DIC result from inflammatory response mediators. Renal failure occurs as a result of ischemia associated with shock and DIC and also of direct toxicity from hemoglobin and nitric oxide antagonism. In vitro models of IgM-mediated red cell incompatibility demonstrate that TNF-α release peaks 2 hours after adding group A red cells to group O whole blood. Subsequently, IL-8 and monocyte chemoattractant protein-1 concentrations increase. Monocyte activation in the absence of lymphocyte activation has been observed. TNF release is associated with fever, hypotension, and capillary leak. In contrast, in vitro studies involving IgG-mediated hemolysis demonstrate markedly diminished TNF responses. This finding in IgG-mediated hemolysis may, in part, account for its other clinical differences from IgM-mediated hemolysis, including opsonization without complement activation and extravascular rather than intravascular sites of red cell destruction.

The majority of acute hemolytic reactions involve ABO incompatibility (Table 170–3); the mortality rate is 5 to 10%. If antibodies coat red cells but complement is not fully activated, the opsonized red cells are removed by tissue macrophages. Antibodies directed against Rh, Kell, and Duffy antigens usually cause extravascular rather than intravascular hemolysis.

Fever is the most frequent sign of a hemolytic reaction. Nausea, vomiting, and chest pain occur less often. Wheezing and dyspnea, back pain, restlessness, and discomfort at the infusion site may occur. Additional clinical findings include hemoglobinuria, intravascular coagulation abnormalities, hemolysis, renal failure, and hypotension.

FEBRILE NON-HEMOLYTIC TRANSFUSION REACTIONS. These reactions occur in patients with cytotoxic or agglutinating antibodies against donor lymphocytes, granulocytes, or platelets previously stimulated by alloantigen exposure through transfusion or pregnancy. Alternatively, febrile reactions occur as a result of passive infusion of cytokines IL-1, IL-6, IL-8, and TNF, produced during storage by leukocytes contained in the blood.

Within an hour after beginning a transfusion, the diastolic blood pressure increases and headache, chills or frank rigors, or fever with at least a 1° C or 2° F temperature elevation occurs. Fewer than 15% of patients suffer a recurrence when transfused subsequently. When a reaction is suspected, the infusion must be stopped immediately, and a laboratory investigation must be initi-

ated to determine whether hemolysis occurred. The diagnosis of a febrile, non-hemolytic transfusion reaction is made by excluding evidence of hemolysis such as hemoglobinemia, hemoglobinuria, or a positive direct antiglobulin test result. Treatment involves antipyretics and other supportive measures. Patients suffering recurrent reactions should receive leukocyte-reduced blood components.

TRANSFUSION-RELATED ACUTE LUNG INJURY. This clinical disorder occurs within 4 hours of transfusion and consists of severe dyspnea, cyanosis, cough, blood-tinged sputum, hypoxemia, fever, and hypotension. Radiographic evaluation shows diffuse, patchy infiltrates. Auscultatory findings include crackles and rales. Decreased pulmonary compliance with normal cardiac function, resembling non-cardiogenic pulmonary edema, has been described in this syndrome. Rapid intervention with respiratory support and mechanical ventilation is required. Recovery usually ensues within 48 hours.

The pathogenesis presumably involves passive infusion of HLA antibodies, anti-HLA-DR, or granulocyte antibodies from donor blood. Recently this hypothesis has been challenged by a suggestion that affected patients have predisposing clinical conditions such as recent surgery, active inflammation, or infection combined with a second event that leads to neutrophil priming and adherence to endothelial cells.

ALLERGIC REACTIONS. Urticarial eruptions and pruritus are caused by an interaction between donor plasma proteins and recipient IgE antibody. The reactions are usually mild and respond to antihistamines. The transfusion may be continued after hives subside.

Anaphylactic reactions develop in some IgA-deficient patients (approximately 1 per 500 to 1000 persons) who have IgE anti-IgA antibodies against IgA contained in donor plasma. Facial flushing, generalized urticaria, laryngeal or facial edema with bronchospasm, hypotension, vomiting, or diarrhea occurs. Treatment with intravenous epinephrine may be indicated. If subsequent red cell transfusions are required, the components should be washed to remove IgA.

HYPERVOLEMIA. Patients with impaired myocardial reserve are at risk of hypervolemia and heart failure. With the exception of acute blood loss situations, infusion rates should be 2 to 4 mL/kg/hour but reduced to 1 mL/kg/hour in patients known to be at risk for hypervolemia.

BACTERIAL SEPSIS. Septic transfusion reactions result from contamination of blood by skin flora or low level bacteremia at the time of phlebotomy. Bacteria proliferate during storage. For example, *Yersinia enterocolitica* grows preferentially at cold temperatures in iron-rich environments. After infusion of only 50 to 70 mL

Table 170–3 ■ CLINICALLY SIGNIFICANT RED CELL ANTIGENS/ANTIBODIES

	FREQUENCY %		ASSOCIATED WITH ACUTE HEMOLYTIC REACTIONS		
BLOOD GROUPS	Whites	Blacks	Intravascular	Extravascular	Delayed
ABO					
A	41	27	X		
B	10	20	X		
O	45	49			
AB	4	4			
Rh					
D	85	92		X	X
C	70	27		X	X
c	80	96		X	X
E	30	22		X	X
e	97	98		X	X
Kell					
K	9	3		X	X
k	99.8	99.9		X	X
Duffy					
Fyᵃ	66	11	Rare	X	X
Fyᵇ	83	23	Very rare	X	X
Kidd					
Jkᵃ	77	92	X	X	X
Jkᵇ	74	46	X	X	X
Ss					
S	55	31	Some	X	X
s	89	94	Rare	X	X

of blood, patients develop chills, frank rigors, or vomiting. Subsequently, fever with temperature elevation of 1° to 3.5° F or 1° to 2° C, hypotension, shock, and DIC may occur within 90 minutes of transfusion. The profound symptoms are related to endotoxin produced by gram-negative organisms. Less dramatic clinical presentations occur when gram-positive organisms are involved. *Yersinia* causes the majority of septic red cell reactions, but other organisms such as *Pseudomonas putida* and *P. fluorescence* can contaminate red cell transfusions. When a septic reaction is suspected, the infusion must be stopped immediately, followed by supportive care and broad-spectrum antibiotic coverage. A microbacteriologic examination, including a Gram stain or similar assessment and culture of non-infused blood, should be performed. Visualization of bacteria supports the diagnosis, but sepsis can occur despite a negative Gram stain.

DELAYED REACTIONS. Delayed or non-immediate adverse consequences of blood transfusion occur days to years after the transfusion.

DELAYED HEMOLYTIC TRANSFUSION REACTIONS. Three to 8 days (range, 3 to 21 days) after transfusion, some patients have anamnestic or newly formed antibodies that were not present or not detected at the time of pretransfusion testing. The direct antiglobulin test is positive, but fewer than 20% of patients develop clinical evidence of hemolysis. Specific therapy is rarely needed. Anti-E, anti-Jk[a], anti-K, anti-c, anti-C, anti-Fy[a], and anti-S are commonly associated with these reactions. Surprisingly, a positive direct antiglobulin test persists in many of these patients for months after the sensitized red cells are expected to have been removed. Laboratory evaluation suggests that some patients have autoantibodies in addition to alloantibodies. In multitransfused patients with sickle cell anemia and pain crises, evidence suggests bystander hemolysis in which autologous red cells as well as allogeneic, antigen-positive transfused red cells are destroyed; the mechanism(s) of action is under investigation.

GRAFT-VERSUS-HOST DISEASE. Transfused lymphocytes engraft, recognize, and react against the host (recipient). The pathogenesis involves transfer of immunocompetent T lymphocytes from donors who partially share HLA phenotypes with the patient. Severely immunocompromised patients are at greatest risk, but GvHD has been reported in immunologically normal patients. Transfusion-associated GvHD occurs 4 to 30 days after infusion. In contrast to marrow transplantation-associated GvHD, the marrow is affected, resulting in pancytopenia, infection, and hemorrhage. The mortality rate is approximately 90% in patients with these complications. Hence, prevention is a primary goal and is accomplished by subjecting blood and components to 25 to 30 Gy gamma irradiation.

IRON OVERLOAD. Endocrine, cardiac, and liver dysfunctions occur in adults who receive 60 to 210 (mean, 120) units of blood. Each unit of blood contains approximately 250 mg of iron. Iron chelation therapy or possibly exchange transfusion reduces iron stores or iron accumulation.

POST-TRANSFUSION PURPURA. This infrequently occurring syndrome is manifested by profound thrombocytopenia 5 to 9 days after transfusion. The exact cause is uncertain. Primary therapy involves intravenous gamma globulin infusion; plasma exchange is an alternative.

IMMUNOMODULATORY EFFECTS OF TRANSFUSION. Several reports implicate blood transfusion as a cause of immunosuppression. Some studies report a higher incidence of postoperative infection in transfused than in non-transfused patients. Although the data are conflicting, it appears that the use of leukocyte-reduced blood components reduces this putative immunomodulatory effect. Available evidence provides less support for concluding that patients with malignancies given transfusions in the perioperative period have a greater recurrence rate and lower survival rate than non-transfused patients.

TRANSFUSION-TRANSMITTED DISEASES. These complications are among the most feared consequences of transfusion. Significant improvements in donor screening and laboratory testing procedures lessen the risk.

HEPATITIS. Transfusion-transmitted hepatitis A infection occurs infrequently because few donations are made during the asymptomatic viremic phase. Hepatitis B transmission by transfusion results from donations given by hepatitis B surface antigen and hepatitis B core antibody negative donors who have circulating hepatitis B virus DNA. Currently, the risk of transfusion-associated hepatitis B per unit varies between 1 per 63,000 and 1 per 233,000 units. The risk of hepatitis C infection after transfusion relates to the 70- to 82-day "window period" between infection and detection of hepatitis C antibodies. Infectivity occurs during this interval with the resultant risk of hepatitis C infection per unit of approximately 1 per 103,000 to 121,000 units. Use of nucleic acid amplification assays should decrease the current risk.

RETROVIRAL INFECTIONS. The initial reports of hemophilic patients with the acquired immunodeficiency syndrome (AIDS) appeared in 1982. By December 1997, there were 4922 hemophilic and other patients with coagulation factor deficiencies who had acquired AIDS, and 8575 AIDS cases occurred in recipients of blood transfusions. Almost all of these infections occurred before introduction of HIV antibody testing in the spring of 1985. Currently, the mean "window period" between HIV infection and detection by HIV-1 or HIV-2 antibody or HIV-1 p24 antigen testing is 16 days, with a residual risk per unit of 1 in 670,000.

HUMAN T-LYMPHOTROPIC VIRUSES. HTLV-I is associated with adult T-cell leukemia/lymphoma and with HTLV-I associated myelopathy/tropical spastic paraparesis. HTLV-II infected persons appear to have an increased risk of bacterial, mycobacterial, and fungal infections. These viruses reside intracellularly in leukocytes and, therefore, transfusion transmission is linked to cellular components (i.e., transmission does not occur through plasma or cryoprecipitate transfusions). The interval between exposure and antibody detection is approximately 51 days; the risk per unit is 1 in 640,000.

CYTOMEGALOVIRUS. This latent virus, present in polymorphonuclear leukocytes and lymphocytes, rarely causes symptomatic illness in immunocompetent patients. In contrast, CMV-seronegative patients who receive allogeneic bone marrow transplants from CMV-seronegative donors and infants weighing less than 1200 g born to seronegative mothers have significant morbidity and mortality if they become infected with CMV as a result of transfusion. Others at high risk of transfusion-transmitted CMV infection include the fetus of a CMV-seronegative pregnant woman, CMV-seronegative AIDS patients, and possibly CMV-seronegative transplant recipients of solid organs from CMV-seronegative donors or CMV-seronegative candidates for bone marrow transplantation. Transfusion transmission is reduced by selecting blood components from CMV antibody–negative donors or by removing leukocytes through filtration with appropriate leukocyte reduction filters. This intracellular virus is not transmitted by non-cellular components.

MALARIA. Transfusion-induced malaria occurs in approximately 1 per 4 million recipients. The incubation period after transfusion ranges from 7 to 50 days (average, 20 days). The risk of this complication is reduced by not accepting blood donations from persons who have traveled to or emigrated from endemic areas.

CHAGAS' DISEASE. *Trypanosoma cruzi,* transmitted by transfusion, may cause fulminant illness in immunocompromised patients. Less severe disease may occur in immunocompetent patients. Preliminary studies in the United States, involving follow-up of recipients of donations made by persons with environmental or serologic evidence of *T. cruzi* exposure, do not show evidence of *T. cruzi* transmission. Further evaluation is required to determine the risk of transmitting this agent by transfusion.

PARVOVIRUS. In children, parvovirus B19 causes a viral exanthem known as fifth disease. In some patients with sickle-cell anemia, thalassemia, entities associated with enhanced red cell production, HIV-infected patients, solid organ transplant recipients, and children with malignancies, the virus can cause acute aplastic or hypoplastic anemia. Transmission by transfusion occurs, but symptomatic sequelae are infrequent. Immune globulin infusion reverses aplasia in some patients.

CREUTZFELDT-JAKOB DISEASE (CJD). Transmission of this disease by blood or plasma derivatives has not been reported. However, cases have been linked to iatrogenic events such as exposure to contaminated human pituitary-derived growth hormone and dura mater transplants. Animal model experiments suggest transmission requires the presence of B lymphocytes. In response to the threat of transmission, plasma derivatives, albumin, and coagulation factor concentrates are withdrawn if any of the donors subsequently develop CJD. Physicians caring for recipients of previous red cell or other blood component transfusions from donors developing CJD or at risk for CJD are notified so they can decide whether to inform patients who receive such blood components.

OTHER INFECTIOUS AGENTS. Other infectious agents that are transmitted infrequently by blood transfusion include *Babesia, Bartonella,* Epstein-Barr virus, and *Toxoplasma.* No cases of transfusion-associated syphilis have been reported recently. Human herpesvirus 8, a virus linked to Kaposi's sarcoma, has been shown to be transmitted to virus-negative mononuclear cells in vitro; however, Kaposi's sarcoma occurs infrequently among HIV-infected transfusion recipients and hemophilic patients, suggesting the risk is remote.

SUMMARY

Red blood cell transfusions increase oxygen-carrying capacity. Transfusion of 1 unit of red cells increases the hemoglobin concentration by 1 g/dL and the hematocrit by 3%. The decision to transfuse red cells rests with a careful clinical assessment of the effectiveness of compensatory mechanisms for maintaining tissue oxygen delivery. A pre-set hemoglobin/hematocrit level should not be the sole reason for ordering transfusions. Patients without pulmonary, cardiac, cerebrovascular, or peripheral vascular disease tolerate a hemoglobin concentration of about 8 g/dL (range, 7 to 10 g/dL) without symptoms other than decreased capacity for activity. Patients with impairment of critical organs or tissues may require transfusion at higher hemoglobin/hematocrit levels. To avoid complications associated with transfusion, the physician must evaluate the patient's age, adaptation to anemia, cardiopulmonary status, ischemic co-morbidities, and prognosis, as well as the expected response to alternative therapy, such as replacement of vitamin deficiencies or the use of recombinant erythropoietin. When prescribed, transfusions should be given on a unit-by-unit and case-by-case basis.

Aubuchon JP, Birkmeyer JD, Busch MP: Safety of the blood supply in the United States: Opportunities and controversies. Ann Intern Med 127:904, 1997. *The authors provide an assessment of the blood supply and offer comments about potential failure improvements.*

Cummings JP: UHC Clinical Practice Advancement Center. Technical Assessment: Red Blood Cell Transfusion Guidelines. 1997. *This compendium analyzes the multiple transfusion guidelines prepared by professional organizations and academic medical centers and makes recommendations.*

Expert Working Group: Guidelines for red blood cell and plasma transfusion for adults and children. Can Med Assoc J 156:S1, 1997. *These guidelines contain an excellent review and analysis of issues relating to transfusion decision making and include a discussion of transfusion risks.*

Goodenough LT, Brecher ME, Kanter MH, et al: Transfusion medicine–blood transfusion. N Engl J Med 340:438–447; 525–533, 1999. *An excellent two-part summary of risks and benefits of blood transfusion.*

Telen MJ: Erythrocyte blood group antigens: Polymorphisms of functionally important molecules. Semin Hematol 33:302, 1996. *The biochemical and molecular bases of erythrocyte blood group antigens provide explanations for biological roles of red cell antigenic structures.*

171 DISORDERS OF PHAGOCYTE FUNCTION

Laurence A. Boxer

Neutrophils and mononuclear phagocytes are essential components of the host defense system. Both cell types are made in the bone marrow, and both accomplish most of their purpose by protecting and maintaining the organism's internal biologic environment. Mononuclear phagocytes are versatile cells whose functions include the consumption and destruction of invading pathogens, elimination of debris from the blood stream and sites of tissue damage, remodeling of normal tissue, release of immune regulators, and presentation of antigens to lymphocytes. Neutrophils remain dedicated primarily to the destruction of invading microbes. To appreciate deranged function of phagocytes, the normal physiology of the phagocytes must be considered.

THE NEUTROPHIL

ORIGIN. Like other cells in the circulation, neutrophils originate from pluripotential stem cells in the bone marrow. Depending on environmental influences, pluripotential stem cells may give rise to the committed progenitors of blood cells. Partial purification of human pluripotential stem cells has been accomplished by using an antibody to the cell-surface antigen CD34, which marks cells that are used in human stem cell transplantation. These pluripotential stem cells give rise to more mature stem cells that are committed to either lymphoid or myeloid development. Myelopoiesis begins with about 10^6 stem cells in the bone marrow; these cells undergo both self-renewal and differentiation to produce all the individual types of blood cells. The individual types of blood cells arise from the ability of their precursors to express lineage-specific growth factor receptors. These single-lineage progenitors proliferate and differentiate into their respective precursors in response to the growth factors that bind to their unique receptors. The proliferation, differentiation, and survival of immature hematopoietic progenitor cells are governed by a family of glycoproteins termed the hematopoietic growth factors (see Chapter 158). The mechanism that determines whether a stem cell simply self-renews or differentiates is probably governed by the different signaling pathways used between cell-surface receptors and the cell nucleus, but the precise pathway for each cytokine remains poorly defined. Cell proliferation and differentiation are also influenced by interleukins and the local hematopoietic microenvironment, which is defined by extracellular matrix proteins and their stromal elements. Colony-stimulating factors are rarely lineage specific and usually influence multiple steps in hemolymphopoiesis, often in synergy with as many as four or five other factors. As cells mature, they lose receptors for most cytokines, especially those that influence early cell development such as stem cell factor. However, once the cells have matured, they express receptors for chemokines, which help direct the cells to sites of inflammation.

NEUTROPHIL MATURATION AND KINETICS. Based on kinetic studies, four cellular compartments containing myeloid cells are generally recognized: (1) the marrow mitotic compartment; (2) the marrow post-mitotic and storage compartment; (3) the vascular compartment, which in the case of neutrophils is divided into a circulating pool and a marginating pool; and (4) the tissue compartments. During infection, tissue macrophages can engage the invading microbes, release cytokines such as interleukin-1 (IL-1) and tumor necrosis factor (TNF) that activate stromal cells, and activate T lymphocytes to produce additional growth factors. Early progenitor cells in the marrow are then stimulated to proliferate and differentiate. This step markedly shortens the time of maturation of myeloid precursors through the post-mitotic pool. Increased numbers of neutrophils are then released from the marrow storage compartment into the circulation. These same neutrophils are then primed by either granulocyte or granulocyte-macrophage colony-stimulating factor for enhanced bactericidal activities.

STRUCTURE. The neutrophil is a terminally differentiated, nondividing cell that is well equipped for removing microorganisms. The cell is packed with granules whose contents kill and degrade target microorganisms. The granules are primarily of three types. *Azurophil granules* contain proteases and other hydrolytic enzymes, defensins, other microbicidal peptides, and myeloperoxidase, a Cl⁻-oxidizing enzyme. *Specific granules* contain, among other things, apolactoferrin, collagenase, and an as yet unidentified enzyme that releases C5a from complement component C5. The membranes of the granules contain receptors for chemoattractants, extracellular matrix proteins, and cytochrome b_{558}. *Gelatinase granules* contain gelatinase, and the membranes bear the CD11/18 receptor essential to cell adhesiveness. In addition to granules are vesicles that bear membranes containing the CD11/18 receptor, cytochrome b_{558}, and CR1, a receptor for the complement component C3b. The nucleus is a vestigial structure that can no longer replicate its DNA. The plasma membrane contains some of the neutrophil's killing equipment, sensors that locate the microorganisms to which the neutrophil responds, such as chemokines, chemotactic factors, and adhesion molecules. The cytoskeleton of the neutrophil is a complex system of microfilaments and microtubules and is responsible for the orderly movement of this highly motile cell.

FUNCTION. Chemotactic factors generated by the interaction of plasma proteins with antigens, pathogens, chemokines released by activated T cells attract neutrophils from the blood to sites of infection. Diffusion of these factors creates a chemical gradient that directs the migration of neutrophils toward the source of the chemotactic factor (Fig. 171–1). Plasma, in addition to elaborating chemoattractants, provides antibodies and complement that coat microorganisms in a process called opsonization, which is derived from the Greek word for "providing victuals." Neutrophils ingest the opsonized microorganisms by surrounding them with moving pseudopodia that fuse to enclose the microbe within a vesicle called the phagosome. The cytoplasmic granules of the neutrophil fuse with the phagosome and discharge their contents through the membrane, a process called degranulation. The neutrophil reduces molecular oxygen enzymatically to generate "activated" metabolites such as superoxide (O_2^-) and hydrogen peroxide (H_2O_2), which join with material discharged into the phagosome from the granules to destroy the ingested microbes. Granule contents and oxygen metabolites under certain circumstances may leak from the activated neutrophil into extracellular fluid, where they can injure surrounding tissue and engender tissue inflammation.

ADHESION. Because neutrophils move by crawling, they must adhere to surfaces to migrate through the tissues to an inflammatory site. A likely sequence of events leading to neutrophil activation during the acute inflammatory response in vivo is becoming better understood. Activated neutrophils enter post-capillary venules adjacent to inflammatory foci and develop low avidity, adhesive interactions with inflamed endothelium via specific classes of adhesion molecules that include L-selectin, E-selectin (ELAM-1), and P-selectin (GMP-140) (Fig. 171–2). Endothelial cells inducibly express selectins following exposure to inflammatory cytokines (TNF and IL-1). Specific oligosaccharide molecules expressed on the neutrophil membrane glycolipids and glycoproteins serve as counterreceptors for E-selectin and P-selectin (sialyl-Lewis X and Lewis X, respectively). In conjunction with neutrophil membrane L-selectin, which recognizes oligosaccharide molecules expressed by endothelial cells, the selectins promote low-affinity neutrophil-endothelial binding under flow conditions termed neutrophil "rolling." Neutrophil rolling is a prerequisite for higher-affinity interactions with the inflamed endothelium. Subsequent to neutrophil rolling, high-affinity interactions are induced by a separate class of adhesion molecules (e.g., intracellular adhesion molecule type 1 [ICAM-1]) whose functional affinity is increased by high and prolonged local concentrations of TNF and IL-1. ICAM-1 serves as a recognition receptor for the neutrophil β_2-integrin counterreceptors CD11/CD18. This latter agent's relative affinity for ICAM-1 is increased by neutrophil exposure to activating stimuli including platelet activating factor expressed by the inflamed endothelium, as well as by soluble chemotactic stimuli (formyl bacterial peptides, C5a, IL-8 and leukotriene B₄) (see Fig. 171–2). During neutrophil activation, a reciprocal relationship between the expression of L-selectin and

β_2-integrin on the plasma membrane leads to a release of L-selectin, followed by a dramatic increase in the number and affinity of surface CD11/CD18 receptors. Once the neutrophils adhere through their β_2-integrin receptors to the endothelium, subsequent transendothelial migration by neutrophils occurs in response to local gradients of chemotactic factors.

CHEMOTAXIS. The neutrophil finds its target through a chemical sensor that detects substances known as *chemotactic factors*. These factors are continuously released at sites where microorganisms have invaded tissue, thereby establishing a concentration gradient. Circulating neutrophils recognize this gradient and travel toward its source by migrating between endothelial cells and penetrating the subendothelial basement membrane. Once outside the capillaries, they continue their directed migration, eventually reaching the microorganism-invaded site in which the chemotactic factors originated.

INGESTION. Contact between the neutrophil and the microorganism sets the stage for ingestion. This step proceeds as the neutrophil recognizes opsonins on the surface of the invading microorganisms and attaches to them (see Fig. 171–1). The opsonins themselves consist of antibodies belonging to the IgG subclass and the complement components C3b and C3bi (an important stable opsonin formed by the cleavage of C3b by C3b inactivator). The actual binding takes place between opsonic antibodies and the Fc receptors FcR11 and FcR111, plus the C3b and C3bi receptors on the surface membrane of the neutrophils. As the opsonic target attaches to the neutrophil surface, ingestion begins. The neutrophilic membrane and the region of the attached complement particle invaginate into the cell. Once fully internalized, the invagination closes at its neck to form an internal *phagocytic vesicle* that is lined with the neutrophil plasma membrane and kills the ingested organisms. (see Fig. 171–1).

BACTERICIDAL KILLING. Killing involves two separate actions on the part of neutrophils: degranulation and activation of the respiratory burst. Degranulation refers to a calcium-dependent process by which the granule membranes fuse with the plasma membrane and release the granule contents into either a phagocytic vesicle (see Fig. 171–1) or the external environment. Azurophil granules degranulate almost exclusively into the phagocytic vesicles, so their microbicidal proteins destroy the ingested microorganisms; myeloperoxidase reacts with H_2O_2 and a halide to produce hypochlorous acid (HOCl). Specific granules degranulate into both the phagocytic vesicles and the external environment to destroy their ingested microorganisms.

The respiratory burst refers to a metabolic event that produces potent microbicidal oxidants through partial reduction of oxygen. The burst is activated by the same stimuli that provoke degranulation of the specific granules—namely, primary contact with ingestible particles and exposure to chemotactic factors. These stimuli initiate the translocation of 47- and 67-kd cytosolic proteins along with a small-molecular-weight G protein to the membrane containing cytochrome b₅₅₈. This step initiates the reduction of oxygen to O_2^- at the expense of the reduced form of nicotinamide adenine

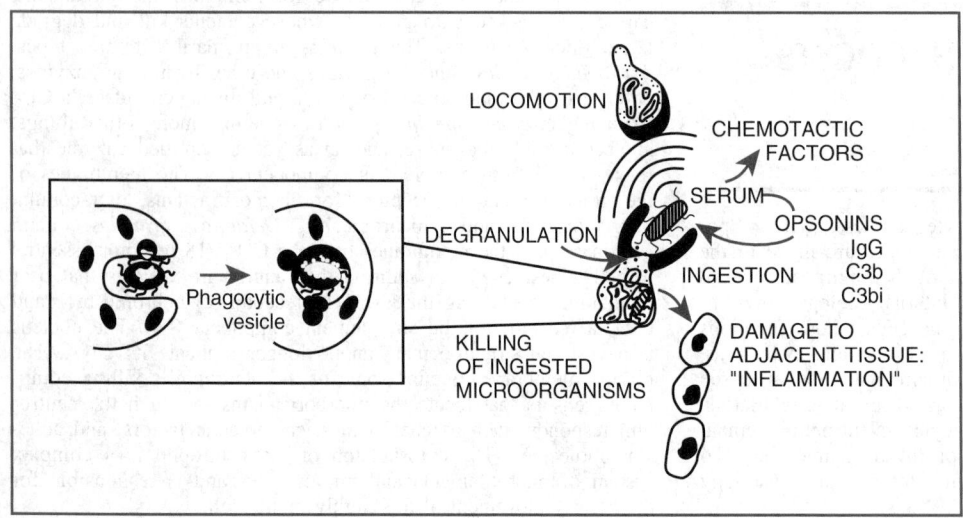

FIGURE 171–1 ■ Functional activities of the neutrophil. The neutrophil is shown in a polarized shape responding to chemotactic factors. Subsequently opsonins, either IgG and/or C3b or C3bi, coat the bacteria for subsequent ingestion by neutrophils. (The insert shows degranulation into a phagocytic vesicle. Granules migrate toward the phagocytic vesicle and eventually fuse with it. After fusion, the contents of the granule are released into the vesicle, and the granule membrane becomes incorporated into the vesicle wall.) Bacterial killing occurs following activation of the respiratory burst. Granule contents and oxygen metabolites (under certain circumstances before closure of the phagosome occurs) may leak from the activated neutrophil into the extracellular fluid and cause inflammatory damage to adjacent tissue.

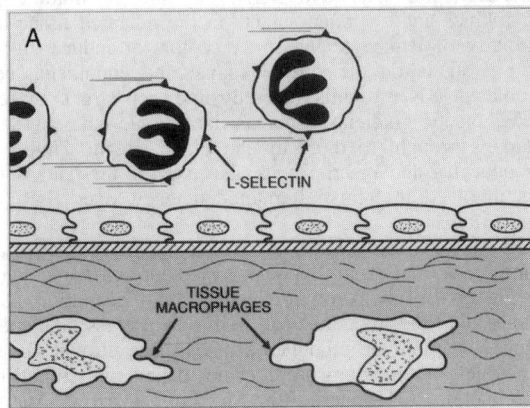
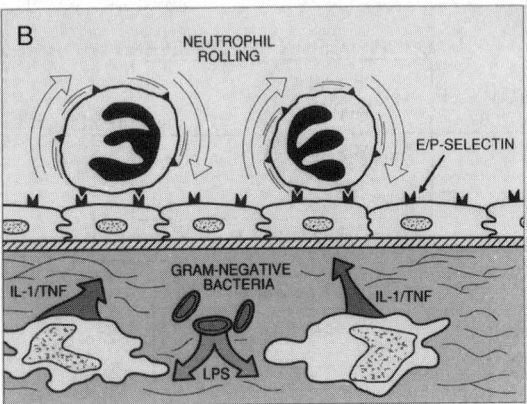
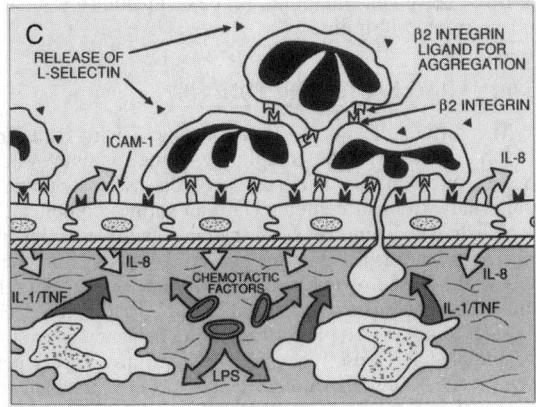
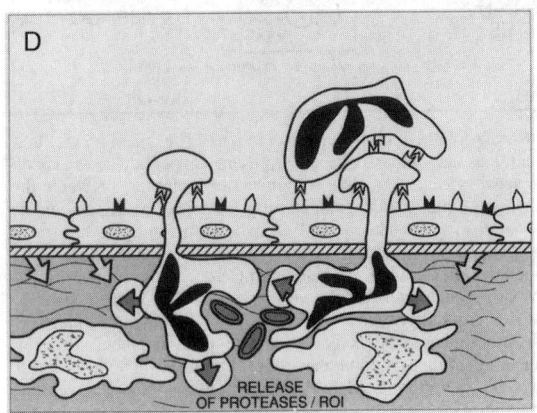

FIGURE 171–2 ■ The neutrophil-mediated inflammatory response (see the text for details). *A,* Unstimulated neutrophils (expressing L-selectin) entering a post-capillary venule. *B,* Invasion of gram-negative bacteria stimulates low-avidity neutrophil rolling. *C,* Leukocyte spreading and the start of transendothelial migration. *D,* Neutrophils invade through the vascular basement membrane with the release of proteases and reactive oxidative intermediates (ROI). IL-1 = interleukin=1; TNF = tumor necrosis factor; LPS = lipopolysaccharide; ICAM = intracellular adhesion molecule. (Redrawn from Smolen JE, Boxer LA: Functions of neutrophils. *In* Williams WJ, Beutler E, Erslev AJ, et al (eds): Hematology, 5th ed. New York, McGraw-Hill, 1994, p 779.)

dinucleotide phosphate (NADPH). Most of the O_2^- reacts with itself to yield H_2O_2, and NADPH is regenerated concurrently by the way of the hexose monophosphate shunt. A portion of the H_2O_2 oxidizes Cl^- to the highly microbicidal HOCl, a reaction catalyzed by myeloperoxidase. Another portion of the H_2O_2 is converted to the reactive hydroxyl radical ($\cdot OH$) in an iron-catalyzed reaction with O_2^-. These and related oxidants attack and kill ingested microorganisms by oxidizing their cellular constituents.

MONONUCLEAR PHAGOCYTES

ORIGIN AND STRUCTURE. The first recognizable monocyte precursor is the monoblast. The next stage is the promonocyte, a somewhat larger cell with cytoplasmic granules and an indented nucleus containing freely divided chromatin. Finally, the fully developed monocyte appears. Larger than the neutrophil and with a large horseshoe-shaped nucleus containing disperse chromatin, the mature monocyte has a cytoplasm filled with granules whose content includes hydrolytic enzymes and other proteins necessary for the cell's activities. The transition from monoblast to mature circulating monocyte requires about 5 days.

Unlike neutrophils, monocytes have a limited capacity to divide, and they undergo considerable further differentiation. After circulating in the blood stream, they enter the tissues where they differentiate into mature macrophages that live for weeks to months. Topologic factors seem to influence their final differentiation and endow each type with particular metabolic and structural features. Those in the liver, for example, become the Kupffer cells, spidery phagocytes that bridge the sinusoids separating adjacent plates of hepatocytes. Those in the lungs become large ellipsoidal alveolar macrophages.

Macrophages are important components of the inflammatory reactions elicited by microorganisms and foreign bodies. Some of the macrophages that appear at a site of inflammation are recruited from the surrounding tissue, whereas others are derived from monocytes that have migrated from the blood stream. Once at the inflamed site, macrophages can be stimulated by opsonized particles. Monocytes and macrophages share the receptors described for neutrophils and, in addition, express other receptors. The contact between a suitable particle and its receptor on the surface of the macrophage elicits the transient production of compounds that include reactive oxygen species, nitric oxide, and arachidonate metabolites. Besides phagocytosable particles, many soluble substances can activate macrophages to release a number of mediators or affect their own signal transduction. Some activators, e.g., interferon-γ (IFN-γ), also confer the ability to kill tumor cells and inactivate specific pathogens.

FUNCTIONS. Despite their functional specialization, macrophages have at least three major functions in common: presentation of antigens, phagocytosis, and immunomodulation.

ANTIGEN PRESENTATION. Activation of mononuclear phagocytes by IFN-γ is one of a series of mutually potentiating interactions between these cells and lymphocytes that take place at sites of inflammation (Fig. 171–3). Both T and B lymphocytes participate in these interactions.

PHAGOCYTOSIS. Mononuclear phagocytes ingest material for two purposes: to eliminate waste and debris (scavenging) and to kill invading pathogens. In their role as general scavengers, mononuclear phagocytes dispose of effete cells, a process exemplified by splenic phagocytes disposing of aged red cells or by macrophagic destruction of cells that have not undergone programmed cell death (apoptosis). Similarly, phagocytes remove foreign material from the

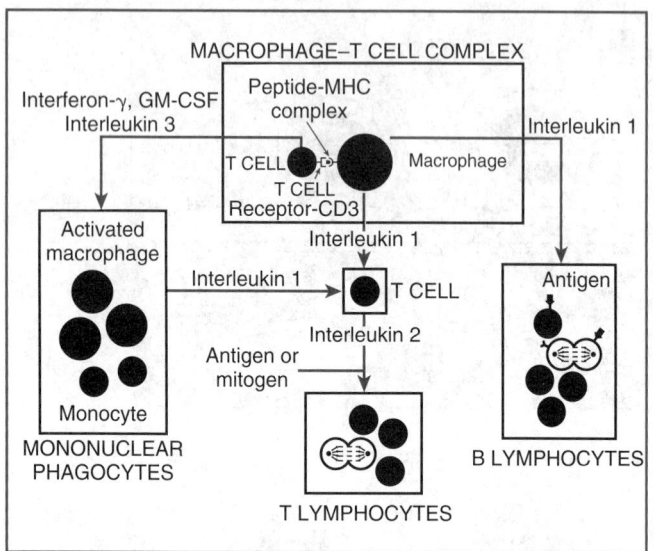

FIGURE 171–3 ■ Macrophage-lymphocyte interactions. The macrophage, acting in its capacity as an "accessory cell," presents a peptide to a T cell equipped with specific receptors that recognize the complex between the peptide and a class II major histocompatibility complex (MHC) molecule on the macrophage surface. The T cell to which the antigen has been presented undergoes activation and begins to secrete lymphokines. The lymphokines include interferon-γ, granulocyte-macrophage colony-stimulating factor (GM-CSF), and interleukin-3 (IL-3); they cause macrophages to accumulate and undergo activation at the site of the initial macrophage–T cell interaction. Macrophages so activated secrete IL-1, a potent mediator capable, among other things, of inducing the proliferation of both B and T cells. B cells are directly stimulated by IL-1 to proliferate and differentiate into antibody-secreting plasma cells. T cells, however, proliferate under the influence of a mediator known as IL-2 (T-cell growth factors), itself a T-cell product. IL-1 promotes the proliferation of T cells indirectly by inducing them to secrete IL-2.

blood stream and clean up debris at sites of infection or tissue damage.

A dense network of resident macrophages lying chiefly in the liver and spleen remove material from the blood stream. Bacterial products such as lipopolysaccharide that enter the blood stream from the large intestine are removed principally by the Kupffer cells of the liver during the process of gastrointestinal venous drainage. Similarly, macrophages recruited to the damaged area dispose of dead cells and tissue fragments at sites of infection or injury. Activated macrophages also secrete neutral proteases that break down damaged connective tissue and fibrin mesh to clear the way for the reconstitution of injured tissues.

Mononuclear phagocytes also eliminate from the circulation denatured proteins, protein fragments, and activated clotting factors. Some proteins are eliminated through pinocytosis, a process in which the detritus is taken into the cell by an invagination of the cell membrane that buds off and enters the cytoplasm as a pinocytotic vesicle. Other proteins are eliminated by receptor-mediated endocytosis. For instance, the lipids of arthrosclerotic lesions are derived from lipoproteins that have been taken into the macrophage by receptor-mediated endocytosis. On occasion, monocytes will ingest oxidized lipoproteins, which transform them into foam cells and contribute to the generation of arthrosclerotic plaque.

KILLING. Mononuclear phagocytes can kill invading microorganisms. Like neutrophils, monocytes can adhere to endothelial cells by multiple adhesion molecules, including the selectins and β_2-integrins. Monocytes differ importantly from neutrophils in that they express significant levels of β_1 (VLA) integrin receptors, including VLA-4, which binds to VCAM-1 on activated endothelial cells. Neutrophils are initially the predominant leukocytes at sites of acute inflammation, with the peak of immigration generally occurring in the first several hours. Subsequently, mononuclear phagocytes derived from blood monocytes become the most abun-

dant cell type. These differences in the kinetics of immigration and accumulation can be explained by the elaboration of particular cytokines and chemoattractants in the inflamed tissue that alter the affinity of leukocyte integrin receptors or induce up-regulation or down-regulation of both leukocyte and endothelial cell adhesion molecules. Neutrophils generally find their targets by responding to chemotactic gradients, whereas fixed tissue macrophages have their targets brought to them by the blood stream. Unlike neutrophils, monocytes and macrophages also express the CD4 antigen, which is involved in human immunodeficiency virus (HIV) uptake and infection.

IMMUNOMODULATION. Activated monocytes also release IL-1 and IL-6, TNF, and INF-α/β—cytokines that are involved in the regulation of hematolymphopoiesis and activation of endothelial cells and the mononuclear cells themselves. Another important source of immune modulation takes place through the role of chemokines. Chemokines are considered potential stimuli of leukocyte production and release from the bone marrow. Additionally, the chemokines MIP-1α, MIP-1β, and RANTES, produced by CD8+ T cells, are potent inhibitors of HIV infection by monocyte/macrophage-trophic-1 strains.

EVALUATING NEUTROPHIL FUNCTION

The differential diagnosis for a patient with recurrent infections is formidable given the complexity of the immune system. Similarities in the clinical manifestation of diseases, including the neutrophil, antibody, and complement, can further complicate attempts to establish the diagnosis. Most patients with recurrent infections do not have an identifiable phagocyte defect or immune deficiency. Given the low probability of identifying a discrete immune defect, clinicians are faced with the difficult question of deciding which patients merit a complete evaluation. In general, evaluation should be initiated for those who have had within a 1-year period at least one of the following clinical features: (1) more than two systemic bacterial infections, (e.g., sepsis, meningitis, osteomyelitis); (2) three serious respiratory infections (e.g., pneumonia, sinusitis) or three bacterial infections (e.g., cellulitis, draining otitis media, lymphadenitis); (3) the presence of an infection at an unusual site (e.g., hepatic or brain abscess); (4) infections with unusual pathogens (e.g., *Aspergillus* pneumonia, disseminated candidiasis, or infection with *Serratia marcescens, Nocardia* spp., and *Berkoldaria cepacia*); and (5) infections of unusual severity.

Neutrophils have a particularly important role in protecting the skin, the mucous membranes, and the lining of the respiratory and gastrointestinal tracts. As such, they form the initial line of defense against microbial invasion. During the critical 2- to 4-hour period following invasion by microbial organisms, neutrophils must arrive at the site of invasion if infection is to be contained. Patients whose neutrophils have defects in adhesion or cell motility generally suffer cutaneous abscesses with common pathogens such as *Staphylococcus aureus* or have mucous membrane lesions caused by microbes such as *Candida albicans*. A profound defect in adhesion and chemotaxis is often reflected by a paucity of neutrophils at the site of inflammation. Disorders of phagocyte microbicidal activity, especially as observed in chronic granulomatous disease (CGD), are also associated with cutaneous abscesses and pulmonary infections.

Once the decision is reached that a phagocyte evaluation is warranted, a thorough clinical history, physical examination, and laboratory testing (Fig. 171–4) should provide the diagnosis and help formulate an appropriate therapeutic plan. Despite the rarity of the inherited disorders, the understanding gleaned from evaluating their molecular mechanisms has contributed immensely to our knowledge of normal neutrophil function.

ACQUIRED DISORDERS. Neutrophils may exhibit decreased adhesiveness and chemotaxis following exposure to a variety of drugs, the most common being corticosteroids and epinephrine (Table 171–1). Clinically, the diminished adhesiveness induced by these drugs is manifested by a dramatic rise in the total neutrophil count in the blood as cells from the marginating pool are quickly released into the circulating pool. Although the mechanism by which corticosteroids alters adherence remains unknown, epinephrine exerts its effects indirectly by causing endothelial cells to release cyclic adenosine monophosphate, which impairs the ability of neutrophils to adhere to endothelium. In contrast, the adhesive-

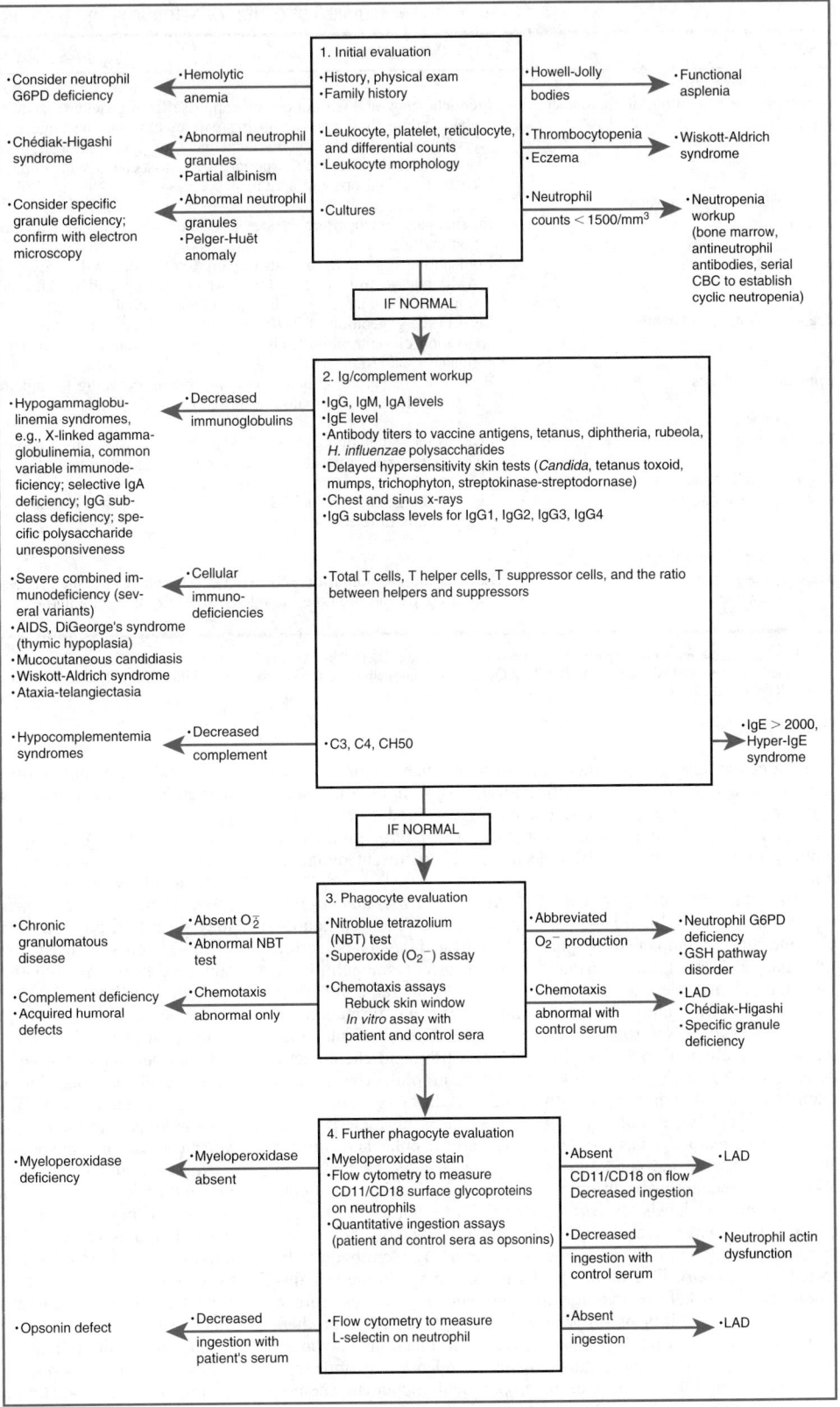

FIGURE 171–4 ■ Algorithm for the evaluation of patients with recurrent infections. CBC = complete blood count; Ig = immunoglobulin; G6PD = glucose-6-phosphate dehydrogenase; LAD = leukocyte adhesion deficiency. (Modified from Curnutte JT: Chronic granulomatous disease: Clinical and genetic aspects. Ann Intern Med 109:138, 1988.)

ness of neutrophils can be dramatically enhanced in a variety of clinical conditions that generate biologically active complement fragments (e.g., C5a), cytokines (e.g., TNF and IL-1), and chemokines (e.g., IL-8). Disorders associated with gram-negative bacterial sepsis, severe thermal injury, pancreatitis, trauma, and exposure of neutrophils to artificial membrane surfaces during hemodialysis and cardiopulmonary bypass can all be associated with activation of neutrophils and, in extreme cases, lead to adult respiratory distress syndrome. In these various conditions, generation of C5a and cytokines promotes enhanced neutrophil adhesiveness, possibly because of enhanced expression of β_2-integrins. Under these conditions, neutrophils undergo increased aggregation with each other and become trapped within the capillary beds of the lungs. It is believed that the aggregated neutrophils then generate toxic oxygen radicals and release proteases that damage structural proteins such as collagen and elastin.

Table 171–1 ■ ACQUIRED DISORDERS OF NEUTROPHIL DYSFUNCTION

DISORDER	ETIOLOGY	CLINICAL CONSEQUENCE
Disorders of Chemotaxis		
Defects in the generation of chemotactic signals	IgG deficiency and C3 deficiency can arise from genetic or acquired abnormalities, e.g., protein-losing enteropathy and systemic lupus erythematosus, respectively. Deficiency of IgG can lead to reduced opsonic activity. C3 deficiency is associated with impaired chemotaxis and opsonic activity	Recurrent pyogenic infections
Direct Inhibition of Neutrophil Mobility		
Drugs	Ethanol and glucocorticoids are associated with impaired locomotion and ingestion	Possible cause of infection
	Epinephrine is associated with impaired adherence following cyclic AMP release from endothelium, which in turn shifts neutrophils from the marginating pool to the circulating pool	Neutrophilia
Trauma, burns, pancreatitis	Lead to the generation of TNF and C5a, which activate neutrophils Activation of neutrophils leads to impaired locomotion secondary to enhanced adhesion to substrates	Tissue damage and, in severe situations, adult respiratory distress syndrome
Immune complexes	Bind to Fc receptors on neutrophils in disorders leading to impaired chemotaxis, e.g., rheumatoid arthritis, lupus erythematosus	Recurrent infection
Adhesion Abnormalities		
Trauma, burns, pancreatitis	Lead to the generation of TNF, IL-1, C5a, and IL-8, which activate neutrophils and promote enhanced adhesion to substrates	Enhanced accumulation of neutrophils at inflammatory sites
Degranulation Abnormalities		
Trauma, burns, pancreatitis	Lead to the generation of TNF, IL-1, C5a, and IL-8, which activate neutrophils to release proteases	Tissue damage and, in severe situations, adult respiratory distress syndrome
Defects of Microbicidal Activity		
Trauma, burns, pancreatitis	Lead to the generation of TNF, IL-1, C5a, and IL-8, which activate neutrophils and promote the release of H_2O_2 and chloramines	Tissue damage and, in severe situations, adult respiratory distress syndrome

AMP = adenosine monophosphate; TNF = tumor necrosis factor; IL-1 = interleukin-1.
Modified from Boxer LA: Neutrophil disorders: Qualitative abnormalities of the neutrophil. *In* Williams WJ, Beutler E, Erslev AJ, Lichtman MA (eds): Hematology, 5th ed. New York, McGraw-Hill, 1994, p 828.

Immune complexes are found in disorders such as rheumatoid arthritis and systemic lupus erythematosus, as well as after bone marrow transplantation. Immune complexes can bind to Fc receptors on neutrophils and impair their motility. In turn, diminished motility of neutrophils may be associated with recurrent pyogenic infections.

INHERITED DISORDERS. CHEMOTAXIS. *The hyperimmunoglobulin E syndrome* (Table 171–2) is characterized by reduced neutrophil motility accompanied by markedly elevated levels of serum IgE that lead to chronic dermatitis and recurrent sinopulmonary infections. Skin infections in these patients remarkable for their absence of surrounding erythema and subsequent formation of "cold abscesses." Neutrophils and monocytes from patients with this syndrome exhibit a variable, but at times profound chemotactic defect that appears to be extrinsic to the neutrophil. The clinical manifestations of hyperimmunoglobulin E syndrome can begin as early as 1 to 8 weeks of age. This syndrome is characterized by chronic eczematoid rashes, which are typically papular and pruritic and often involve the face and extensor surface of the arms and legs. Most frequently the offending pathogen is *S. aureus*. Patients have serum IgE levels exceeding 2500 IU/mL, but unlike atopic patients who may have similarly elevated IgE levels, those with hyperimmunoglobulin E syndrome have serum IgE antibodies directed to *S. aureus*. The molecular basis for the syndrome remains unknown. Some believe that the immunologic basis arises from a deficiency in the ability of suppressor T cells to inhibit IgE production. Alternatively, a predisposition to bacterial infections may arise from production of a chemotactic inhibitor released by mononuclear cells that inhibits normal neutrophil and monocyte chemotaxis. Preliminary studies indicate that some patients improve clinically following the administration of INF-γ (50 μg/m² given three times per week subcutaneously).

FAMILIAL MEDITERRANEAN FEVER. *Familial Mediterranean fever* is an inherited, recurrent inflammatory diseases prevalent among people of the Near East—Arabs, Turks, Armenians, and Sephardic Jews. It is transmitted as an autosomal recessive trait (see Table 171–2). The disease is characterized by acute self-limited attacks of fever often accompanied by pleuritis, peritonitis, arthritis, pericarditis, inflammation of the tunica vaginalis of the testes, and erythematous skin lesions. The first attacks may begin in infancy, although more commonly they begin in childhood or adolescence. Most patients have the first attack by 20 years of age.

Etiology. The gene responsible for familial Mediterranean fever is located on chromosome 16. It encodes for a 781–amino acid protein called pyrin. Homology searches indicate that pyrin is a new member of the *RetRo* gene family and suggests that pyrin itself may be a transcription factor presumably regulating the expression of target genes, at least some of which are probably involved in the suppression of inflammation. The gene is expressed in neutrophils but not lymphocytes or monocytes. Pyrin has been designated as the gene for familial Mediterranean fever because missense mutations have been identified in exon 10 in most of the affected patients but not in normal subjects. These mutations have not been found in all patients, thus indicating that other mutations are likely to be discovered.

Pathology. The pathologic findings in familial Mediterranean fever are those of non-specific acute inflammation. Neutrophilic infiltration predominates, and exudates develop in the peritoneal, pleural, and/or joint spaces at the time of acute attacks. In about 25% of affected patients, a form of renal amyloidosis develops in which the amyloid is derived from a normal serum protein called serum amyloid A (amyloidosis of the AA type). Amyloidosis usually progresses over a period of years to renal failure, and almost all causes of death in familial Mediterranean fever can be attributed to this complication.

Clinical Manifestations. The duration and frequency of attacks vary considerably even in the same patient. Acute attacks frequently last 24 to 48 hours and recur once or twice per month. In some patients, attacks may recur as frequently as several times a week or as infrequently as once a year, and symptoms may persist for as long as a week during individual episodes. Some patients experience spontaneous remission that persists for years, followed by recurrence of frequent attacks. Peritonitis secondary to familial Mediterranean fever may resemble an acute abdomen, thereby leading to potential uncertainties about the clinical management of acute abdominal episodes.

Pleuritic pain occurs during attacks in 75% of patients. Symptoms of pleuritis may sometimes precede abdominal pain, and a few patients experience pleuritic attacks without abdominal symp-

Table 171–2 ■ INHERITED DISORDERS OF NEUTROPHIL DYSFUNCTION

DISORDER	ETIOLOGY	CLINICAL CONSEQUENCE
Disorders of Chemotaxis		
Hyperimmunoglobulin E syndrome	Autosomal dominant; variable expression of a soluble inhibitor from mononuclear cells affecting neutrophil chemotaxis; high levels of antistaphylococcal IgE leads to impaired IgG opsonization of *Staphylococcus aureus*	Recurrent skin and sinopulmonary infections
Familial Mediterranean fever (FMF)	Autosomal recessive; the gene responsible for FMF is located on chromosome 16 and encodes for a protein called "pyrin." Pyrin may modify neutrophil activation	Recurrent fevers, peritonitis, pleuritis, arthritis, and amyloidosis
Adhesion Abnormalities		
Leukocyte adhesion deficiency	Autosomal recessive; absence of CD11/CD18 surface adhesive glycoprotein (β_2-integrins) on leukocyte membranes arising from failure to express CD18 mRNA leads to decreased binding of C3bi to neutrophils and impaired adhesion of neutrophils to ICAM-1	Neutrophilia; recurrent bacterial infections associated with a lack of pus formation
Leukocyte adhesion deficiency type 2	Autosomal recessive (?); absence of neutrophil sialyl-Lewis X leading to decreased adhesion to inflamed endothelium	Neutrophilia; recurrent bacterial infections associated with a lack of pus formation
Degranulation Abnormalities		
Chédiak-Higashi syndrome	Autosomal recessive; disordered coalescence of lysosomal granules leading to decreased neutrophil chemotaxis; degranulation, and bactericidal activity. Responsible gene found at 1q42-q45. The encoded protein has structural features homologous to a vacuolar sorting protein	Neutropenia; recurrent pyogenic infections, propensity for the development of marked hepatosplenomegaly in the accelerated phase
Defects of Microbicidal Activity		
Chronic granulomatous disease	X-linked and autosomal recessive; failure to express functional gp91phox in the phagocyte membrane in X-linked CGD; failure to express functional protein in the phagocyte membrane in p22phox (autosomal recessive). Other autosomal recessive CGD arises from failure to express protein p47phox or p67phox. The absence of either gp91phox, p47phox, or p67phox leads to failure to activate the neutrophil respiratory burst and failure to kill catalse-positive microbes	Recurrent pyogenic infections with catalase-positive microorganisms
G6PD deficiency	Autosomal recessive; <5% of normal activity of G6PD leads to failure to activate NADPH-dependent oxidase	Infections with catalase-positive microorganisms
Myeloperoxidase deficiency	Autosomal recessive. Failure to process modified precursor protein arising from a missense mutation. The lack of myeloperoxidase leads to delay in microbial killing	None

ICAM = intracellular adhesion molecule; CGD = chronic granulomatous disease; phox = phagocytic oxidase; p = protein of a given molecular weight; G6PD = glucose-6-phosphate dehydrogenase; NADPH = reduced form of nicotinamide adenine dinucleotide phosphate.
Modified from Boxer LA: Neutrophil disorders: Qualitative abnormalities of the neutrophil. *In* Williams WJ, Beutler E, Erslev AJ, Lichtman MA (eds): Hematology, 5th ed. New York, McGraw-Hill, 1994, p 828.

toms. Mild arthralgia is a common feature of febrile attacks; monarticular or oligoarticular arthritis may occur. Arthritis usually affects the large joints, the knee in particular, and effusions are common.

As many as one third of patients experience transient erysipelas-like skin lesions that typically appear on the lower part of the leg, ankle, or dorsum of the foot. These painful erythematous areas of swelling usually subside within 24 to 48 hours.

Laboratory findings in familial Mediterranean fever are non-specific. During acute attacks, prominent leukocytosis (up to 30,000/mm^3) is present, and the erythrocyte sedimentation rate is increased. Between attacks the leukocyte count is normal.

Diagnosis. The diagnosis of familial Mediterranean fever is based primarily on clinical findings and the history. In individuals of appropriate ethnic background with typical recurrent, self-limited attacks, diagnosis is not difficult; in such individuals, delay in recognizing the disease usually occurs because the diagnosis is not considered.

Treatment. Colchicine treatment is effective in familial Mediterranean fever and may prevent the development of amyloidosis. Prophylactic colchicine, 0.6 mg orally two or three times per day, prevents or substantially reduces acute attacks of familial Mediterranean fever in 75 to 90% of patients. Some patients can abort attacks with intermittent doses of colchicine beginning at the onset of attacks (0.6 mg orally every hour for 4 hours, then every 2 hours for 4 hours, and then every 12 hours for 2 days). In general, patients who benefit from intermittent colchicine therapy are those who experience a recognizable prodrome before fever and clear-cut acute symptoms develop.

Prognosis. The prognosis for normal longevity for patients with familial Mediterranean fever is excellent, and given the efficacy of

colchicine, most patients can be maintained almost entirely symptom free. Once amyloidosis appears, it is associated with the nephrotic syndrome or uremia. The likelihood of eventual death from renal failure remains substantial unless the patient receives a renal transplant.

ADHESION ABNORMALITIES. Leukocyte adhesion deficiency (LAD) is a rare autosomal recessive disorder of leukocyte function. LAD-1 affects about 1 in 10^6 individuals; it is characterized by recurrent bacterial and fungal infections, as well as a depressed inflammatory response despite striking blood neutrophilia.

Etiology. Individuals with LAD-1 have mutations of the gene on chromosome 21q22.3 encoding CD18, the 95-kd β_2-integrin subunit. Normal neutrophils express three heterodimeric adhesion molecules known as LFA-1 (CD 11a/CD18), Mac-1 (CD11b/CD18, also known as CR3 or C3bi receptor), and p150,95 (CD11c/CD18). These three transmembrane adhesion molecules are composed of unique α-subunits, all of which are encoded on chromosome 16, and they share a common β_2-subunit. In patients with LAD-1, expression of the β_2-subunit can be either absent or diminished, or alternatively, mutations in the CD18 gene affect the structure of the synthesized CD18 peptide and lead to abnormal post-translational processing and loss of function. The lack of a β-chain prevents active $\alpha\beta$-dimers from forming. Diminished or absent surface expression of these proteins accounts for the failure of patients' neutrophils to migrate to specific sites of inflammation. The impaired function of their neutrophils arises from the inability to adhere firmly to inflamed endothelial surfaces and to undergo transendothelial migration, a function dependent on β_2-integrin binding to endothelial ICAM-1.

Clinical Manifestations. LAD-1 is characterized by recurrent soft tissue infections, delayed wound healing, and severe impaired pus formation despite a striking blood neutrophilia. The onset of clinical manifestations begins in the newborn period and is usually characterized by delayed separation of the umbilical cord, with patients often not surviving beyond the toddler age. Patients with moderate disease can survive into adulthood. Patients with severe LAD involvement (i.e., total lack of CD11/CD18 on membranes) suffer from recurrent and gangrenous soft tissue infections of subcutaneous tissues or mucous membranes. Patients with moderate involvement have fewer and less severe infections. The diagnosis is most readily made by flow cytometric measurement of surface CD11/CD18 in stimulated and unstimulated neutrophils by using monoclonal antibodies directed against CD11/CD18. Assessment of neutrophil monocyte adherence, aggregation, chemotaxis, and C3bi-mediated phagocytosis will generally demonstrate striking abnormalities that directly correspond to the molecular deficiency.

In contrast to LAD-1 patients, two patients have been described with neutrophilia, recurrent bacterial infections, and an inability to form pus. Both patients had the Bombay blood phenotype, short-limbed dwarfism, and mental retardation. Functionally, their neutrophils were unable to adhere to cytokine-activated endothelial cells expressing E-selectin. The neutrophils expressed normal levels of CD11/CD18 integrins but were deficient in the carbohydrate moiety of sialyl-Lewis X, which renders the cells unable to adhere to E-selectin on activated endothelial cells. Neutrophils from these two patients are unable to tether to inflamed venules for subsequent activation and spreading on the endothelium and thereby undergo subsequent transendothelial migration. This disorder is recognized as LAD-2.

Treatment. Treatment of LAD-1 is largely supportive. Patients with a history of recurrent infections can take prophylactic trimethoprim-sulfamethoxazole. Marrow transplantation from HLA-compatible siblings or parental donors has resulted in engraftment and restoration of neutrophil function and remains the treatment of choice in patients with the severe phenotype of LAD-1. Although gene replacement therapy is not yet available, LAD-1 is an ideal candidate for this approach because the clinical history and mild forms of LAD-1 support the notion that even a low level of neutrophil function will attenuate the severity of the disease.

DEGRANULATION ABNORMALITIES. *Chédiak-Higashi syndrome* (see Table 171–2) is a rare autosomal recessive disease in which neutrophils, monocytes, and lymphocytes contain giant cytoplasmic granules. About 200 cases have been reported. The disorder is characterized by generalized cellular dysfunction involving increased fusion of cytoplasmic granules. Affected patients with this disorder are usually recognized in infancy, and only a few patients may survive into early adulthood.

Pathogenesis. The gene for Chédiak-Higashi syndrome has been cloned. The gene is located on chromosome 1q42-q44 and has structural features homologous to a vacuolar sorting protein termed VPS15 in yeast. It is believed that the Chédiak-Higashi protein may be associated with vesicle transport and mediate protein-protein interactions.

Almost all cells of patients with Chédiak-Higashi syndrome show some aspect of oversized and dysmorphic lysosomes, storage granules, or related vesicular structures. For example, the melanosomes or melanocytes are oversized, and compromised dispersion of melanosomes in keratinocytes and hair follicles leads to pigmentary dilution involving the hair, skin, and ocular fundi. This same abnormality in melanocytes leads to the macroscopic impression of hair that is lighter than expected from parental coloration and to the partial ocular albinism associated with light sensitivity. Patients with this syndrome exhibit an increased susceptibility to infection that can be explained in part by the presence of giant neutrophil granules. The granules alter cell motility by compromising neutrophils' ability to traverse the narrow passages between endothelial cells.

Clinical Manifestations. Features of the disease include neutropenia arising from ineffective myelopoiesis, a platelet defect associated with a mild bleeding disorder, natural killer cell abnormalities, and peripheral neuropathies. The most serious clinical problem, however, is caused by abnormalities in neutrophil chemotaxis, degranulation, and bactericidal activity. Patients with Chédiak-Higashi syndrome are at any time in life subject to the accelerated phase of the disorder, which is characterized by polyclonal T-cell prolifera-

tion in the liver, spleen, and bone marrow. Typically, hepatosplenomegaly and high fever develop in the absence of bacterial sepsis. Pancytopenia becomes pronounced and often leads to hemorrhage and further increased susceptibility to infection. Onset of the accelerated phase may be related to the inability of these patients to contain and control the Epstein-Barr virus and leads to features in common with viral-mediated hemophagocytic syndrome.

Diagnosis. The diagnosis is made by demonstrating giant granules in neutrophils and eosinophils. Diagnosis of the accelerated phase depends on finding the characteristic infiltrate of T cells in a biopsy sample of involved tissue. Occasionally, giant granules may be observed in acute myelogenous leukemia.

Treatment. Management of the early stage of Chédiak-Higashi syndrome amounts to the management of infectious complications. Prophylactic antibiotics (trimethoprim-sulfamethoxazole) should be given, and infections should be treated vigorously with appropriate antibiotic therapy. Ascorbic acid (20 mg/kg/day) has corrected the microbicidal defect in some patients with Chédiak-Higashi syndrome. Treatment of the accelerated phase is unsatisfactory; splenectomy and chemotherapy are ineffective. Bone marrow transplantation remains the treatment of choice during progression to the accelerated phase.

DEFECTS OF MICROBICIDAL ACTIVITY—CHRONIC GRANULOMATOUS DISEASE. CGD (see Table 171–2) is a genetic disorder affecting 4 to 5 per million humans. Neutrophils and monocytes from affected individuals ingest but do not kill catalase-positive microorganisms because of their inability to generate antimicrobial oxygen metabolites. CGD is caused by genetic defects affecting one X-linked and three autosomal recessive chromosomes encoding the components of NADPH oxidase.

Pathogenesis. The inability of phagocytes to generate superoxide anion (O_2^-) is caused by the absence of one of the components of the NADPH oxidase system (Fig. 171–5). Approximately two thirds of affected patients lack the membrane-bound component of the oxidase cytochrome b_{558}. The gene for the heavy chain of this protein, which is a heterodimeric protein, is located on the X

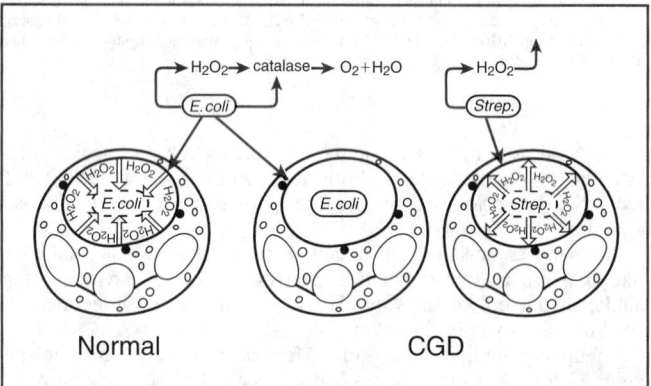

FIGURE 171–5 ■ Pathogenesis of chronic granulomatous disease (CGD). The manner in which the metabolic deficiency of neutrophils in patients with CGD predisposes the host to infection is shown schematically. Normal neutrophils stimulate hydrogen peroxide production in the phagosome containing ingested *Escherichia coli*. Myeloperoxidase is delivered to the phagosome by degranulation, as indicated by the closed circles. In this setting, hydrogen peroxide acts as a substrate for myeloperoxidase to oxidize halide to hypochlorous acid in chloramines that kill the microbes. The quantity of hydrogen peroxide produced by a normal neutrophil is sufficient to exceed the capacity of catalase, a hydrogen peroxide–catabolizing enzyme of many aerobic microorganisms, including most gram-negative enteric bacteria, *Staphylococcus aureus*, *Candida albicans*, and *Aspergillus* spp. When organisms such as *E. coli* gain entry into neutrophils from patients with CGD, they are not exposed to hydrogen peroxide because the neutrophils do not produce it and the hydrogen peroxide generated by microorganisms themselves is destroyed by their own catalase. When CGD-involved neutrophils ingest streptococci or pneumococci, these organisms, which lack catalase, generate enough hydrogen peroxide to result in a microbicidal effect. As indicated in the middle drawing, catalase-positive microbes such as *E. coli* can survive within the phagosomes of CGD-affected neutrophils. (From Boxer LA: Neutrophil disorders: Qualitative abnormalities of the neutrophil. *In* Williams WJ, Beutler E, Erslev AJ, et al (eds): Hematology, 5th ed. New York, McGraw-Hill, 1994, p 828.)

chromosome. Not surprisingly, family histories of patients with the X-linked variety of CGD often include male maternal relatives who died of infection at a young age. Most all other patients with CGD lack one of two identified cytosolic factors, either a 47-kd protein or 67-kd protein. Rarely, patients may lack the genes responsible for expression of the light chain of cytochrome b_{558}. These latter three deficiencies are inherited in an autosomal recessive pattern.

Clinical Manifestations. Although the clinical picture is variable, several clinical features suggest the diagnosis of CGD. Any patient with recurrent lymphadenitis should be considered to have CGD. Additionally, bacterial hepatic abscesses, osteomyelitis at multiple sites or in the small bones of the hands and feet, and a family history of recurrent infections or unusual catalase-positive microbial infections all suggest the disorder. The onset of clinical signs and symptoms may occur from early infancy to young adulthood. The severity and frequency of infections vary widely. The most common offending organism is *S. aureus,* although any catalase-positive microorganism may be involved. Infection with *S. marcescens, Pseudomonas* species, *Aspergillus* species, or *C. albicans* occurs frequently. Pneumonias, lymphadenitis, and skin infections remain the most commonly encountered infections. Often the infections are characterized by microabscesses and granuloma formation. Patients may suffer from the sequelae of chronic infection, including anemia of chronic disease, lymphadenopathy, hepatosplenomegaly, chronic purulent dermatitis, restrictive lung disease, gingivitis, hydronephrosis, and gastrointestinal narrowing.

Diagnosis. The diagnosis is usually suggested with use of the nitroblue tetrazolium (NBT) test, in which the yellow, water-soluble tetrazolium dye is reduced to a blue and insoluble formazan pigment by O_2^- generated from activated normal phagocytes. Phagocytes from patients with CGD fail to reduce NBT because they cannot produce O_2^-. Because carriers of X-linked CGD are mosaics, only a fraction of their neutrophils are able to generate O_2^-; the NBT test stains only that fraction and leaves the rest of the cells unstained. The NBT test is rapidly being replaced by the more accurate flow cytometry test using dihydrorhodamine-123 fluorescence. This test detects oxidant production because it increases fluorescence when oxidized by H_2O_2. Leukocytes from patients with CGD have normal glucose-6-phosphate dehydrogenase (G6PD) activity. A few individuals with apparent CGD, however, have neutrophils that lack almost all G6PD activity. Erythrocytes from these patients also lack G6PD and are subject to chronic hemolysis. In cases of severe neutrophil G6PD deficiency, an attenuated respiratory burst progressively decreases because of the depletion of intracellular NADPH, the primary substrate for the respiratory burst oxidase. G6PD deficiency and CGD can be distinguished from each other by the presence of hemolysis in G6PD deficiency.

Treatment. Management of CGD consists of long-term antibiotic prophylaxis (trimethoprim-sulfamethoxazole, 5 mg trimethoprim per kilogram per day), long-term IFN-γ (50 μg/m² body surface given three times per week), vigorous treatment of acute infections with antibiotics in adequate doses, and surgery, if indicated. Families of patients with CGD should be investigated to ascertain the mode of disease transmission. Genetic counseling should be offered.

MYELOPEROXIDASE DEFICIENCY. Deficiency of myeloperoxidase (see Table 171–2), an autosomal recessive disorder, is the most common inherited disorder of neutrophil function, with an incidence of 1 in 4000 individuals. Individuals with this trait do not have an increased rate of infection or clinical manifestations of disease. Mutations in the myeloperoxidase gene causing this defect have been defined and provide insight into the post-translational processing of this azurophil granule protein. Myeloperoxidase deficiency is caused by a missense mutation in the myeloperoxidase gene that leads to a myeloperoxidase precursor that does not incorporate heme. Partial or complete myeloperoxidase deficiency leads to diminished production of HOCl and HOCl-derived chloramines. Lack of HOCl in the phagosome causes a delay in the microbicidal activity of neutrophils early after the ingestion of microorganisms. Eventually, however, effective killing of bacteria occurs. Myeloperoxidase-deficient neutrophils accumulate more hydrogen peroxide than do normal neutrophils, which improves the bactericidal activity of affected neutrophils. Clinically, myeloperoxidase deficiency is almost completely silent. The most frequent problem is an increase in *Candida* infections in occasional patients with coincident diabetes mellitus. The diagnosis is made from a peroxidase stain of the blood film. In myeloperoxidase deficiency, peroxidase activity is missing from neutrophils and monocytes but is present in the eosinophils. Treatment is unnecessary for myeloperoxidase deficiency.

Dinauer MC: The phagocyte system and disorders of granulopoiesis and granulocyte function. *In* Nathan DG, Orkin SH (eds): Hematology of Infancy and Childhood, 5th ed. Philadelphia, WB Saunders, 1997. *This chapter discusses at length neutrophil, monocyte, and eosinophil disorders, both qualitative and quantitative.*
Malech HL, Nauseef WM: Primary inherited defects in neutrophil function: Etiology and treatment. Semin Hematol 34:279, 1997. *This chapter is the most recent update on the inherited defects of neutrophils with a strong emphasis on the molecular abnormalities underlying these disorders.*

172 LEUKOPENIA AND LEUKOCYTOSIS

Grover C. Bagby, Jr.

The normal peripheral blood white cell count ranges from 5.0 to 10.0×10^9/L, and a low total white blood count (less than 4.5×10^9/L) is known as leukopenia. When leukopenia is discovered, the single most important first step is to determine which type of white blood cell is lower than normal. Circulating leukocytes consist of heterogeneous cell types (neutrophils, monocytes, basophils, eosinophils, B lymphocytes, T lymphocytes, and natural killer cells), each of which serves a unique purpose and each of which represents a different fractional component of the total body leukocyte population. Taking this leukocyte heterogeneity into account, patients may be severely neutropenic or lymphocytopenic despite having total white blood counts that fall within the normal range. Consequently, in a number of clinical settings (e.g., patients with recurrent infections) differential white blood cell counts are important even in the absence of leukopenia.

NEUTROPENIA

DEFINITION. Neutropenia exists when the peripheral *neutrophil* count is less than 2.0×10^9/L. Because the normal range in blacks and Yemenite Jews is somewhat lower, neutropenia in these populations is defined as counts less than 1.5×10^9/L. The role of the neutrophil in phagocytic defense of the host is generally met if the neutrophil count is above 1.0×10^9/L. If the neutrophil count drops further, particularly below 0.5×10^9/L, the incidence of serious, recurrent, and difficult-to-treat infections rises markedly.

PATHOPHYSIOLOGIC CONSIDERATIONS. The multiple pathophysiologic types of neutropenia are best described in the context of normal neutrophil kinetics. Such a description also simplifies initial diagnostic and therapeutic approaches to patients with neutropenia. Neutrophils arise from a pool of marrow precursor cells through serial divisions and synchronous maturation steps (Fig. 172–1). The rate of neutrophil production is astonishingly high, more than 10^{11} cells/day. In the bone marrow, neutrophil precursors that retain replicative potential (myeloblasts, promyelocytes, and myelocytes) comprise the mitotic pool. Later differentiation stage cells (metamyelocytes, bands, and segmented neutrophils) do not replicate and therefore form a non-mitotic precursor pool. An additional pool of fully developed neutrophils form a neutrophil storage pool, a population of cells held in reserve ready for release when needed to combat microbial invaders.

Released after a few days in the bone marrow, neutrophils circulate freely for only a matter of hours before crawling into the extravascular space looking for things to engulf and kill. Half of the neutrophils in the peripheral blood are "marginated" along the endothelium and are, therefore, not measured in the white blood cell count. Accordingly, the true intravascular neutrophil number, consisting of the circulating and the marginated pools, is ordinarily twice that measured by the neutrophil count. Taking these kinetic considerations into account, a simple pathophysiologic classification

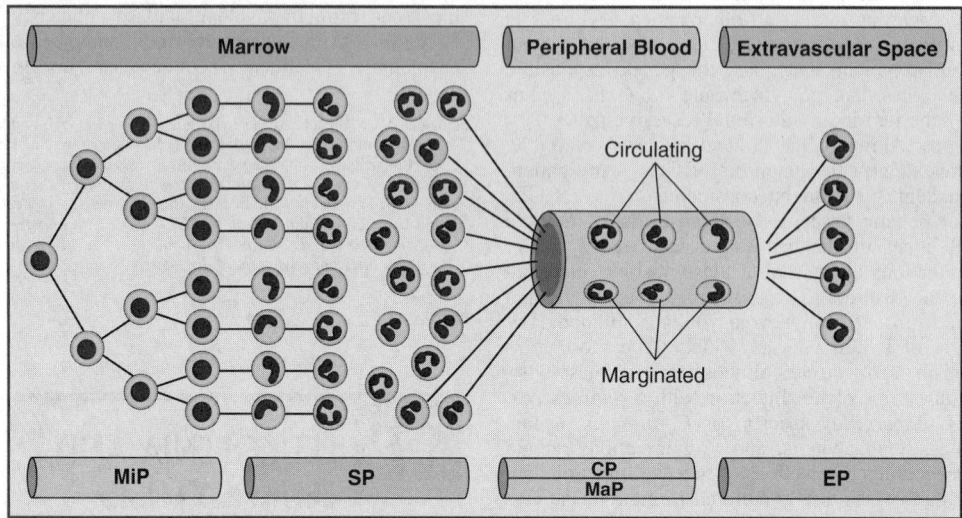

FIGURE 172-1 ■ Production and distribution of neutrophils involve three generic compartments: the marrow, peripheral blood, and extravascular space. Unlike red cells, phagocytes of all kinds are destined to function primarily in the extravascular space. The critical issue for clinicians to consider, therefore, is whether the delivery of phagocytes to this space is adequate. Stem cells, committed progenitor cells, and morphologically recognizable bone marrow precursor cells proliferate and mature; they differentiate under the influence of a variety of humoral regulatory factors that govern the production of neutrophils (granulocyte colony-stimulating factor [G-CSF]), monocytes (macrophage colony-stimulating factor [M-CSF]), and eosinophils (interleukin [IL]-5). These replicative responses occur in the "mitotic pool" (MiP). Once more differentiated cells reach the intermediate maturation stage known as the metamyelocyte, they stop proliferating but continue differentiating to bands and segmented neutrophils. These cells, although capable of leaving the marrow when needed (e.g., in the setting of an acute bacterial infection), spend, in the steady state, about 5 days in the marrow in the "storage pool" (SP). The neutrophils then enter the blood stream. Half of these circulating cells adhere to endothelial cells and compose the "marginated pool" (MaP). The non-marginated cells make up the "circulating pool" (CP). After their very brief sojourn in the peripheral blood, the neutrophils invade the extravascular compartments of most organs, where they are used as defenders or garbage disposal devices (a process that involves both destruction of the offending organism and self-destruction), or they die within 1 to 2 days.

of neutropenia can be derived from the three-compartment model: (1) the marrow compartment, (2) the peripheral blood compartment, (3) the extravascular compartment, or (4) combinations of the above (Fig. 172–2).

ABNORMALITIES IN THE MARROW COMPARTMENT. Bone marrow defects (failure to produce and release neutrophils at a normal rate) account for the majority of neutropenias in clinical practice. Failure of the marrow compartment can occur as a result of direct injury, in which case the marrow usually contains fewer than normal hematopoietic cells, or from maturation defects of hematopoietic cells, principally characterized by normal or increased numbers of morphologically abnormal hematopoietic cells. In either case, neutropenia of this type frequently occurs along with abnormalities in the number of platelets and red cells.

Marrow injury can occur as a consequence of a variety of diseases, but drug-induced injury is most common (Table 172–1). Antineoplastic and immunosuppressive agents are generally designed to inflict injury on a proliferative population of cells (e.g., neoplastic cells); myelosuppressive toxicity is the rule but is generally predictable because its intensity varies directly with the dose. Drugs that usually are not myelosuppressive and well tolerated in the majority of patients can sometimes induce either marrow injury or peripheral neutrophil destruction. These drug-induced reactions can result from direct drug-mediated cytotoxicity or from an immune mechanism in which (1) neutrophils are destroyed in extramedullary sites as a result of antineutrophil antibodies (e.g., the penicillins) or (2) the marrow compartment is injured (e.g., procainamide, chloramphenicol, dapsone, tocainide).

Radiation (see Chapter 19) may result in acute self-limited bone marrow injury and chronic marrow failure. Chronic radiation-induced injury can also result in the later development of myelodysplasia and non-lymphocytic leukemia, both of which may present with neutropenia. Benzene toxicity can also result in acute or chronic neutropenia and, like radiation-induced marrow failure, is associated with a high risk of acute non-lymphocytic leukemia.

Immune-mediated bone marrow failure can be mediated by autoantibodies or by T lymphocytes that inhibit the growth of bone marrow precursor cells. Apart from those with acquired aplastic

anemia (often immunologically mediated), most patients with immune-mediated leukopenia have concurrent rheumatic or autoimmune diseases; these diseases are especially likely if the neutropenia is the only defect in patients with normal red cell and platelet counts. Infection of the marrow per se is unusual and most often does not result in neutropenia; some exceptions include mycobacterial infection (especially those caused by *Mycobacterium tuberculosis* and *M. kansasii*) and certain viral infections.

Bone marrow invasion by abnormal cells can result in neutropenia. Carcinoma of the lung, breast, prostate, and stomach as well as malignant hematopoietic disorders can occupy enough of the medullary space to cause global marrow failure. Similarly, in certain of the myeloproliferative diseases and leukemias, bone marrow fibroblasts can proliferate significantly in the marrow and contribute to bone marrow failure (see Fig. 172–2).

Maturation arrest can result in functional bone marrow failure even though the bone marrow is full of granulocyte precursors. In the bone marrows of patients with folate or vitamin B$_{12}$ deficiency, for example, numerous, morphologically abnormal granulocyte precursors fail to mature normally and therefore suffer a high rate of intramedullary death because of the effects of the vitamin deficiency state on nuclear replication (see Chapter 163). The marrow is hypercellular but is packed with peculiar cells exhibiting dyssynchronous nuclear and cytoplasmic maturation (e.g., primitive nuclei and very differentiated cytoplasm [the hallmark of megaloblastic change]). Hematopoietic activity in the primitive cell population is intensely active, but the proliferative activity is ineffective at delivering terminally differentiated cells into the blood stream—the process is known as "ineffective hematopoiesis." Certain congenital neutropenias also represent maturation abnormalities, as do the acute non-lymphocytic leukemias, myelodysplastic syndromes, and paroxysmal nocturnal hemoglobinuria.

ABNORMALITIES IN THE PERIPHERAL BLOOD COMPARTMENT. Perturbations of the peripheral blood compartment result from shifts in the circulating pool (see Figs. 172–1 and 172–2). In pseudoneutropenia, neutrophil production and utilization are normal, but the size of the marginated pool is increased and the circulating pool is decreased. Because these marginated cells, while

Marrow

ABNORMALITIES IN THE BONE MARROW
COMPARTMENT

1. Bone Marrow Injury
   A. Drugs
      Cytotoxic and noncytotoxic agents
   B. Radiation
   C. Chemicals
      Benzene, DDT, dinitrophenol, arsenic,
      bismuth, nitrous oxide
   D. Certain congenital and hereditary
      neutropenias
   E. Immunologically mediated (largely seen
      in patients with rheumatic disorders)
      Cytotoxic T cell-mediated (T)
      Antibody-mediated (Ab)
      Mechanisms that require both T and Ab
   F. Infection
      Viral (hepatitis, parvovirus, AIDS)
      Bacterial (*M. tuberculosis, M. kansasii*)
   G. Bone marrow replacement (infiltrative
      diseases)
      Malignancies (lung, breast, prostate,
      stomach, lymphomas, and lymphoid leukemias)
      Fibrosis
      Agnogenic myeloid metaplasia
      Long-standing polycythemia vera
      Chronic myelogenous leukemia
      Radiation injury
      Injury from chronic cytotoxic drug therapy
      Acute megakaryocytic leukemia

2. Maturation Defects
   A. Acquired
      Folic acid deficiency
      Vitamin B_{12} deficiency
   B. Neoplastic and other clonal disorders
      Congenital neutropenias
      Acute nonlymphocytic leukemia
      Myelodysplastic syndromes
      Paroxysmal nocturnal hemoglobinuria

Peripheral Blood

ABNORMALITIES IN THE PERIPHERAL
BLOOD COMPARTMENT

1. Shift of neutrophils from the
   circulating to the marginated
   pool (known as pseudoneutropenia)
   A. Hereditary or constitutional
      benign pseudoneutropenia
   B. Acquired
      Acute: Severe bacterial
      infection, frequently
      associated with endotoxemia
      Chronic: Protein-calorie
      malnutrition, malaria
2. Intravascular sequestration
   A. In lung (complement-mediated
      leukoagglutination)
   B. In spleen (hypersplenism)

Extravascular

ABNORMALITIES IN THE
EXTRAVASCULAR COMPARTMENT

1. Increased utilization
   A. Severe bacterial, fungal, viral, or
      rickettsial infection
   B. Anaphylaxis

FIGURE 172–2 ■ The causes of neutropenia have been arranged according to the compartment with which the pathophysiologically relevant mechanism is linked. The approach to the neutropenic patient should begin by determining which of the three major compartments is likely the critical pathophysiologic point. The approach to the neutropenic patient whose neutrophil production is reduced is entirely different than that taken for neutropenic patients whose production is normal and whose rate of delivery to the extravascular compartment is normal or appropriately increased in the context of an acute infection.

hidden from the counting machine, maintain their capacity to migrate to sites of infection, patients with pseudoneutropenia are not at increased risk of infection unless a neutrophil function abnormality coexists. Acquired pseudoneutropenia often occurs as an acute or subacute response to systemic infections; it is generally associated with acute changes in other compartments (Fig. 172–3) and resolves when the infection is appropriately treated or spontaneously abates.

DEMANDS OF THE EXTRAVASCULAR COMPARTMENT. Neutrophils and their precursors respond to a number of environmental cues in a highly regulated fashion. The most frequent of these cues evolve in response to infections. The responses of neutrophils to infection are governed by a variety of hematopoietic growth factors, adhesion molecules, and interleukins, including two granulopoietic factors, granulocyte-macrophage colony stimulating factor (GM-CSF) and granulocyte colony stimulating factor (G-CSF), and an important chemokine, interleukin (IL)-8. These factors, along with IL-1 and tumor necrosis factor-α (TNF-α), which are cytokines that induce synthesis and release of granulopoietic factors, account for (1) a prompt increase in the rate of production of neutrophils in the mitotic compartment, a response mediated by a complex network of cellular and humoral regulatory interactions, (2) early release of neutrophils from the marrow storage pool to the peripheral blood pool, (3) an increase in the rate of neutrophil egress from the

peripheral blood pool to the invaded tissue or tissues, and (4) increased phagocytic and bactericidal activity of the neutrophils. Rarely, increased demand for neutrophils in the extravascular compartment can lead to transient neutropenia, especially in patients with severe acute infections (see Fig. 172–3). In such cases, the immediate demand for neutrophils in the zone of infection calls forth such a substantial release response that the marrow storage pool is used up before it can be restored by increased proliferative activity of granulocyte progenitor cells. Therefore, for a brief period (sometimes up to 5 to 6 days), the infected tissue serves as a sink for neutrophils. Ultimately, under even these conditions, the neutrophil count generally rises well above normal within a few days because the bone marrow is highly effective in responding to infectious events, so that the demand for neutrophils almost never exceeds the capacity of the mitotic pool to supply them. In contrast, neutrophil consumption in patients with autoimmune neutropenia and hypersplenism can outstrip marrow production.

CLINICAL MANIFESTATIONS. Neutropenia can occur as a manifestation of a wide variety of systemic diseases (see Fig. 172–2), the manifestations of which may dominate the clinical picture. Many neutropenic patients remain asymptomatic, most often those whose neutrophil count exceeds 1.0×10^9/L or those whose neutropenia is acute and/or of brief duration. When symptoms do occur, they generally result from recurrent, often severe, bacterial

Table 172-1 ■ DRUGS THAT CAUSE NEUTROPENIA

Antiarrhythmics
  Tocainide, procainamide, propranolol, quinidine
Antibiotics
  Chloramphenicol, penicillins, sulfonamides, p-aminosalicylic acid (PAS), rifampin, vancomycin, isoniazid, nitrofurantoin
Antimalarials
  Dapsone, quinine, pyrimethamine
Anticonvulsants
  Phenytoin, mephenytoin, trimethadione, ethosuximide, carbamazepine
Hypoglycemic agents
  Tolbutamide, chlorpropamide
Antihistamines
  Cimetidine, brompheniramine, tripelennamine
Antihypertensives
  Methyldopa, captopril
Anti-inflammatory agents
  Aminopyrine, phenylbutazone, gold salts, ibuprofen, indomethacin
Antithyroid agents
  Propylthiouracil, methimazole, thiouracil
Diuretics
  Acetazolamide, hydrochlorothiazide, chlorthalidone
Phenothiazines
  Chlorpromazine, promazine, prochlorperazine
Immunosuppressive agents
  Antimetabolites
Cytotoxic agents
  Alkylating agents, antimetabolites, anthracyclines, *Vinca* alkaloids, cisplatin, hydroxyurea, dactinomycin
Other agents
  Recombinant interferons, allopurinol, ethanol, levamisole, penicillamine, zidovudine, streptokinase, carbamazepine

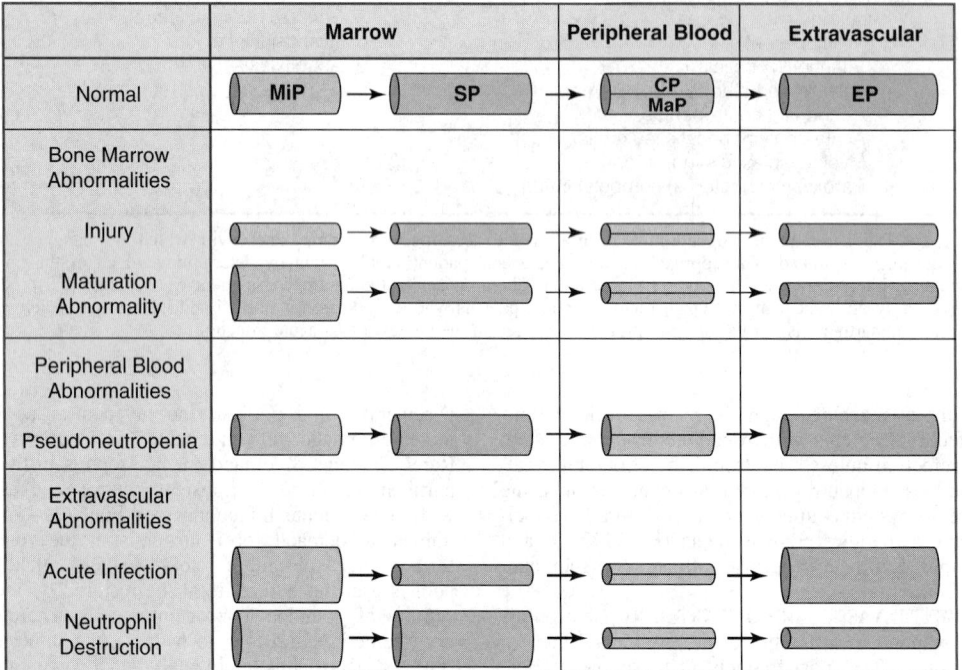

FIGURE 172-3 ■ Pathophysiologic mechanisms of neutropenia. The size of a given compartment is represented by the size of the corresponding cylindrical pool. The relative number of cells leaving one compartment and headed for the next (highly variable from case to case) is represented by the size of the arrow between those compartments. Flow between compartments is unidirectional. MiP = mitotic pool; SP = storage pool; CP = circulating pool; MaP = marginated pool; EP = extravascular pool. Notice that in every case the circulating neutrophil pool is small, but the size of the other pools is variable. In marrow injury, there is a global decline in the size of all pools. A maturation abnormality (e.g., folic acid or vitamin B_{12} deficiency), however, is characterized by an increase in the number of precursor cells that do not mature, resulting in an absolute decrease in mature neutrophils in the marrow, blood, and tissues. Pseudoneutropenia is characterized by a movement of circulating neutrophils to the marginated pool, but, because delivery of the cells to the extravascular space is usually normal, such patients are not at increased risk of infections. In patients who have acute infections, the demand for neutrophils in the infected extravascular site can result in a transient loss of storage pool neutrophils before the hypercellular (but as yet immature) mitotic compartments can renew the storage pool. This kind of neutropenia is very transient and occurs most often in overwhelming infections, although certain organisms (e.g., *Salmonella typhosa*) seem to induce this kind of response more than others. Finally, excessive destruction of neutrophils can result in neutropenia.

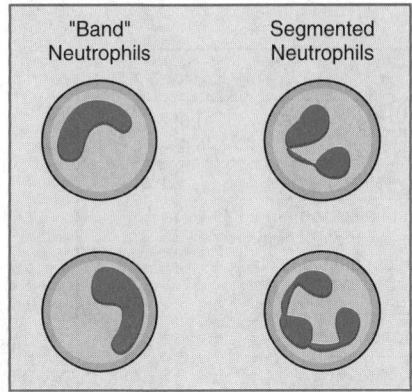

FIGURE 172-4 ■ The nuclear lobes in a segmented form are separated by fine filaments absent in the band. Band neutrophils are "younger" forms than segmented neutrophils. In time, bands residing in the bone marrow will undergo segmentation. Normally, band neutrophils account for less than 4% of total circulating neutrophils. Band percentages greater than 6 to 7% suggest that the storage pool is releasing granulocytes early under the influence of increased levels of granulopoietic factors and suggests that neutrophils are being consumed in the periphery. Alternatively, if neutropenia is the result of bone marrow failure, the bone marrow may be in the midst of an early recovery.

infections because of the pivotal importance of the neutrophil in the defense of the host against microorganisms (see Chapter 171).

This risk of bacterial infection increases slightly as the peripheral neutrophil count falls below 1.0×10^9/L but is substantially increased at levels below 0.5×10^9/L. The degree to which monocytosis compensates for neutropenia may modify the risk. Some patients with severe congenital neutropenia have such substantial compensatory monocytosis that their clinical course is very mild. Because of the capacity of the extra monocytes to "cover" for neutrophil deficiencies, such rare patients have few bacterial infections.

Lungs, genitourinary system, gut, oropharynx, and skin are the most frequent sources of infection in neutropenic patients. The infecting organisms are the "usual suspects" for the given anatomic site with the caveat that, for patients who have recurrent infections and require prolonged and recurrent antibacterial therapy, unusual (often hospital-acquired) organisms can colonize and subsequently cause infection. Consequently, the antibiotic history of infected neutropenic patients is important to obtain. It is absolutely essential to recognize that the usual signs and symptoms of infection are often diminished or absent in patients with neutropenia because the cell that mediates much of the inflammatory responses to infection is absent. Thus, neutropenic patients with severe bilateral bacterial pneumonia can present, initially, with minimal infiltrates demonstrable on chest radiograph (sometimes no infiltrates at all until about 3 or 4 days of full-blown symptoms) and can have benign-looking, non-purulent sputum; patients with pyelonephritis may not exhibit pyuria; patients with bacterial pharyngitis may not have purulence in the oropharynx; and patients with severe bacterial infection of the skin may present only with some mild erythroderma rather than furunculosis. In the neutropenic patient, infections that in an otherwise normal individual might have been well localized become quickly disseminated. Therefore, not only is the infected neutropenic patient a diagnostic problem but, in addition, because any given infection is more likely to be widespread at the time of diagnosis, these patients are often gravely ill at the time they initially present to their caregivers.

DIAGNOSIS. The diagnostic evaluation of neutropenia is influenced by its severity and the clinical setting in which it occurs. The assessment of patients with neutrophil counts of less than 0.5 to 1.0×10^9/L must proceed briskly. The patient with fever, sepsis, or both in whom neutropenia is discovered for the first time presents a particularly difficult problem. In such patients it is impossible to determine immediately whether the neutropenia antedated sepsis, a situation with both prognostic and therapeutic implications, or whether the neutropenia is merely a short-lived response to the infection itself (see Fig. 172-3). Examination of the peripheral blood smear and differential white blood cell count can be

helpful in such cases. An increase in the fraction of circulating band neutrophil forms to levels above 20% suggests that marrow granulopoietic activity is responding appropriately (Fig. 172-4). Although the clinical context is more important to consider than this single data point, colloquially known as "bandemia," it is, nonetheless, a data point more compatible with the notion that the bone marrow of the patient is in the midst of recovering from injury or that the neutropenia is derived from a transient shift to the marginated pool or to the extravascular compartment.

The diagnostic evaluation of neutropenia must first address the question of the severity and then whether the patient has fever, sepsis, or both. The patient with sepsis and severe neutropenia should be treated promptly with intravenous antibiotics after obtaining appropriate cultures but *without waiting for the results of those cultures.* Once these important initial questions are answered, the remainder of the diagnostic evaluation can proceed (Fig. 172-5): (1) identifying any potential drugs and toxins to which the patient might have been exposed (see Table 172-1); (2) determining, if possible, the chronicity of the neutropenia (e.g., ask whether there is evidence that the patient ever had a normal white blood cell count and when); (3) ascertaining whether there have been recurrent infections; (4) identifying any underlying systemic disease that might be causative; and (5) examining the blood counts and blood morphology and bone marrow (marrow examination is virtually always warranted unless a diagnosis is clear based on simple blood tests, e.g., serum folate, homocysteine, methylmalonate, or vitamin B_{12} levels) to determine the most likely pathophysiologic explanation. In some cases, specialized bone marrow studies (e.g., progenitor cell colony assays before and after removing T lymphocytes from the sample) are warranted even with a clear diagnosis. Felty's syndrome, for example, a well-recognized syndrome of neutropenia in patients with rheumatoid arthritis, is caused by one of two pathophysiologic mechanisms. One is mediated by antineutrophil antibodies, the other by T lymphocyte–mediated bone marrow failure. Each mechanism has different therapeutic implications.

After the severity of the neutropenia is determined, careful examination of the peripheral blood counts and blood smear is in order (Fig. 172-5). Patients with selective neutropenia are approached differently than those with additional deficiencies of platelets and red cells, although drugs or toxins may be involved in either category. Potentially offending drugs should obviously be discontinued if such a maneuver is possible based on the nature of the disease for which the agent was prescribed and the availability of alternative drugs. Patients with selective neutropenia but with no drug or toxin exposure, no history of recurrent sepsis, and no underlying chronic inflammatory or autoimmune disease may have stable and benign neutropenia; this category includes some cases of familial and congenital neutropenia and pseudoneutropenia. Any patient with selective neutropenia with a history of sepsis and all patients with known toxin exposure should have a bone marrow examination to assess (1) the cellularity of each compartment (storage and mitotic pools), (2) the distribution of differentiation stages found in each pool, and (3) whether any morphologic abnormality (e.g., acute leukemia or myelodysplasia) exists in the hematopoietic cells.

In patients with pancytopenia or bicytopenia, bone marrow examination, which must include not only aspiration but also biopsy, is almost always indicated. The only arguable exception to this rule would include patients with unambiguous evidence of vitamin B_{12} or folate deficiency (see Chapter 163).

TREATMENT. Rational treatment of the neutropenic patient follows accurate diagnosis and involves treatment of the underlying disease or discontinuation of suspected toxins or drugs. The nature of the specific therapy naturally depends on the pathophysiology of the neutropenia in a given patient. The abiding rule of "treatment-after-diagnosis" does not hold for the infected neutropenic patient. As mentioned earlier, blood and fluids from these patients should be quickly cultured, and then empirical antibiotic therapy must be started promptly, without waiting for the results of the cultures to be reported.

TREATMENTS SPECIFICALLY DESIGNED TO INCREASE THE NEUTROPHIL COUNT. Immunosuppressive therapy, including glucocorticoids or azathioprine, almost always elicits a favorable response in patients with marrow failure mediated by cytotoxic T lymphocytes.

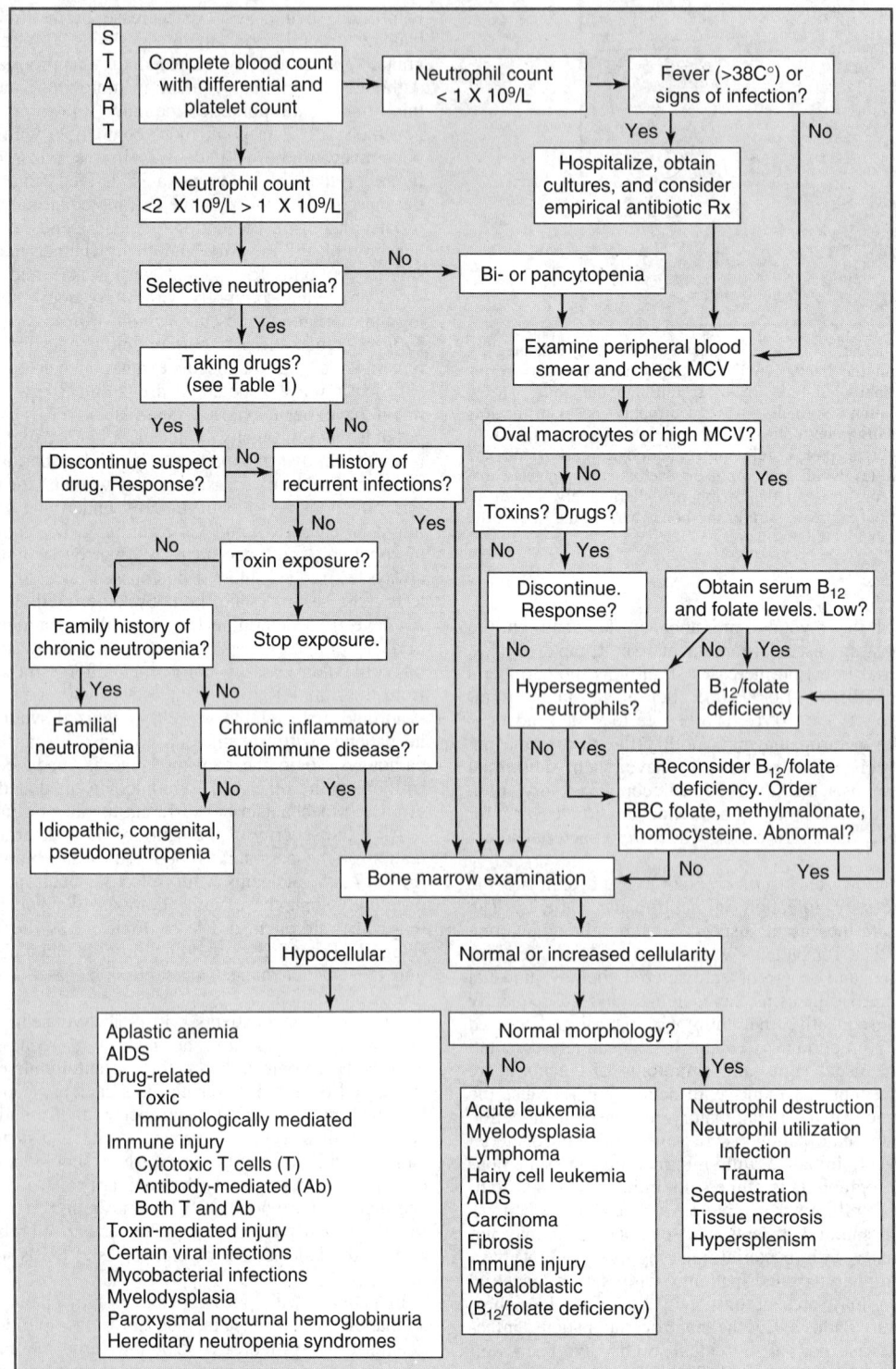

FIGURE 172–5 ■ A practical algorithm for the evaluation of patients with neutropenia. The fundamental diagnostic principle is that for patients with severe neutropenia or for those with bicytopenia or pancytopenia, bone marrow examination will likely be necessary unless the following diagnoses are made: (1) a nutritional (folate or vitamin B_{12}) deficiency or (2) drug or toxin-induced neutropenia in a patient whose neutropenia resolves after discontinuation of the offending agent.

In vitro clonogenic cultures of bone marrow cells in severely neutropenic patients can aid in the identification of patients likely to respond to such therapy. Some responses to immunosuppressive therapy have also occurred in patients whose neutropenia resulted from antineutrophil antibodies. Splenectomy is rarely helpful in the management of neutropenic patients, even those with Felty's syndrome; it is now reserved for patients with unambiguous hypersplenism in whom bone marrow function is normal.

RECOMBINANT HUMAN GRANULOPOIETIC FACTORS. GM-CSF and G-CSF, both of which are approved by the U.S. Food and

Drug Administration, are capable of increasing the neutrophil count in selected neutropenic patients. In normal volunteers, GM-CSF and G-CSF reliably induce neutrophilic leukocytosis; GM-CSF also induces the appearance of eosinophils and monocytes. As a general rule, patients with drug-induced neutropenia (e.g., after cancer chemotherapy) recover more rapidly if they receive either GM-CSF or G-CSF. However, other than the settings of (1) bone marrow transplantation, (2) the management of selected patients with congenital neutropenia, (3) induction of stem cell mobilization from marrow to peripheral blood in preparation for transplantation, and

Abnormalities of Lymphocyte Production
Protein–calorie malnutrition
Radiation
Immunosuppressive therapeutic agents
    Glucocorticosteroids
    Cyclosporine
Congenital immunodeficiency states
    Wiskott-Aldrich syndrome
    Nezelof's syndrome
    Adenosine deaminase deficiency
Viral infections
Hodgkin's disease
Multiple myeloma
Widespread granulomatous infection (mycobacterial, fungal)
Cytotoxic chemotherapy
    Direct dose-related effects (e.g., fludarabine)
    Long-term effects (e.g., cyclophosphamide)
Idiosyncratic drug reactions (e.g., quinine)

Alterations in Lymphocyte Traffic
Acute bacterial/fungal infection
Surgery
Trauma
Hemorrhage
Glucocorticosteroid therapy
Viral infection
Widespread granulomatous infection
Hodgkin's disease

Lymphocyte Destruction or Loss
Viral infection (e.g., human immunodeficiency virus)
Antibody-mediated lymphocyte destruction
Protein-losing enteropathy
Chronic right ventricular failure
Thoracic duct drainage or rupture
Extracorporeal circulation

(4) a combination with erythropoietin for selected patients with myelodysplastic syndromes, the role of these agents in clinical practice is still unclear. Granulopoietic factor therapy is in widespread use to support bone marrow recovery in cancer patients after cytotoxic therapy. However, large clinical studies indicate that while G-CSF hastens neutrophil recovery, it does not reduce the rate of hospitalization for febrile episodes, prolong survival, reduce culture-positive infections, or reduce the costs of supportive care, whether given pre-emptively or to treat neutropenic fever. In summary, in selected cases, the use of G-CSF or GM-CSF treatment is of substantial value and no doubt saves lives. However, considering the attendant costs of growth factor therapy, the routine use of G-CSF or GM-CSF to *prevent infection in neutropenic cancer patients* cannot be encouraged outside the setting of well-designed controlled clinical trials. For non-transplant patients not participating in such studies, it seems most rational to use these granulopoietic factors in those undergoing cytotoxic chemotherapy only if dose intensity of the chemotherapeutic agents has a demonstrated

impact on overall survival (e.g., Hodgkin's disease, germ cell neoplasms) *and* one of following three criteria apply: (1) the patient has developed, in prior rounds of therapy, serious potentially life-threatening complications of neutropenia (e.g., documented bacterial infection), (2) the potential for prolonged myelosuppression is high (e.g., patients seropositive for human immunodeficiency virus [HIV]-1), or (3) the patient has persistent neutropenia between cycles.

BONE MARROW TRANSPLANTATION. In severe aplastic anemia, the role of bone marrow transplantation is well established (see Chapter 182). Other marrow failure states (e.g., myelodysplastic syndromes and congenital neutropenias) may also respond to transplantation. Before transplantation is seriously considered, the duration and severity of the neutropenia must be assessed; marrow failure must be established as the primary cause, and immunologically mediated marrow failure should probably be excluded. If the patient has an identical twin, transplantation might be attempted with fewer constraints, but allogeneic transplantation should always be reserved for individuals with severe and symptomatic neutropenia caused by marrow failure.

TREATMENT OF THE INFECTED NEUTROPENIC PATIENT. Each patient with neutropenia should understand the function of neutrophils, the consequences of neutrophil deficiency, and the importance of communicating with his or her physician the moment signs and symptoms of infection occur. If a neutropenic patient is afebrile and there is no sign of sepsis, the diagnostic work-up of the neutropenia should take place in the outpatient setting to avoid unnecessary exposure to nosocomial organisms. Patients with severe neutropenia and fever, however, generally should be hospitalized. Cultures of urine, blood, and other relevant sites should be obtained, but broad-spectrum antibiotics should be given without waiting for the results of these cultures. One of three responses will be seen:

1. A causative organism will be identified, in which case the spectrum of antimicrobial agents can be promptly and appropriately narrowed.
2. A candidate organism will not be found, but the patient still improves with empirical therapy. In this situation, a full course of broad-spectrum antibiotics should be given. Moreover, after a full course of parental antibiotics, some of which may be given on an outpatient basis, another 7 to 14 days of oral antibiotics should be considered, especially in patients with invasive infections associated with necrosis, slow responses to initial antibiotic therapy, or recurrent infections in the same anatomic site.
3. No organism is found, and the clinical picture has not changed for the better after 3 days of empirical treatment. This unsettling situation occurs with some regularity in practice, and the approach at this point depends on the seriousness of the infection. For a patient who has localized disease and who is not critically ill, it is sometimes helpful for empiric therapy to be discontinued and for repeat cultures to be obtained. If the patient is

Table 172–3 ■ CAUSES OF LEUKOERYTHROBLASTOSIS

Normal Bone Marrow
Severe acute hemolytic anemia
Acute infection in hyposplenic patients

Abnormal Bone Marrow
Marrow infiltration
    Metastatic malignancy (e.g., carcinoma of lung, breast, prostate, or stomach)
    Hematologic malignancies
        Acute leukemia
        Multiple myeloma
        Chronic myeloproliferative diseases (e.g., myeloid metaplasia or chronic myelogenous leukemia)
        Lymphoma
    Granulomatous diseases
        Mycobacterial infection
        Fungal diseases
Other Disorders
    Osteopetrosis
    Gaucher's disease
    Amyloidosis
    Paget's disease of bone
    Severe tissue hypoxia
    Multiple fractures

critically ill, however, antibiotics should be discontinued only if other antibiotics are substituted. Among those antibiotics to consider under these circumstances is amphotericin B. Amphotericin B definitely should be added to the therapeutic regimen in certain clinical settings (i.e., for patients with acute leukemia, diabetes, dysphagia and/or esophagitis, endophthalmitis, or defective cell-mediated immunity [including those receiving immunosuppressive therapy] and for those who have received prolonged treatment with broad-spectrum antibacterial agents in the recent past).

DEFICIENCIES OF OTHER CIRCULATING PHAGOCYTES

Monocytopenia, eosinopenia, and basophilopenia are seen in most of the bone marrow failure states associated with neutropenia. Isolated monocytopenia, however, is very unusual. In view of the heterogeneous and critical roles played by the monocyte-macrophage in normal physiology, complete failure of monocyte production for a period of more than 9 to 10 months (the estimated lifespan of tissue macrophages) is probably incompatible with life.

Eosinopenia and basophilopenia are more common than monocytopenia in clinical practice and most often represent redistributional mechanisms resulting from stress, including acute infections, widespread neoplasms, and severe injury (e.g., burns). A variety of humoral factors, including glucocorticoids, prostaglandins, and epinephrine, are released in such settings and are known to induce eosinopenia. In fact, because of the reliable reduction of peripheral eosinophils during infectious events, *if a patient with bacterial infection does not have eosinopenia,* one should consider that adrenocortical insufficiency or a primary myeloproliferative syndrome may coexist.

LYMPHOCYTOPENIA

Lymphocyte production and traffic are difficult to assess because (1) both T and B lymphocytes replicate in heterogeneous anatomic sites, including the lymph nodes, spleen, tonsils, and bone marrow; and (2) lymphocytes are capable of leaving and then later re-

entering a given compartment. Given these variables, it is surprising that the lymphocyte counts in the peripheral blood are so tightly regulated; normal counts range from 2 to 4×10^9/L; approximately 20% are B lymphocytes, and 70% are T lymphocytes. Lymphocytopenia is defined as a peripheral blood lymphocyte count below 1.5×10^9/L, but severe lymphocytopenia is considered to be less than 0.7×10^9/L.

ETIOLOGY AND PATHOGENESIS. Lymphocytopenia can result from three types of abnormalities: (1) lymphocyte production, (2) lymphocyte traffic, and (3) lymphocyte loss and destruction (Table 172–2).

REDUCED PRODUCTION OF LYMPHOCYTES. The most common cause of reduced lymphocyte production in the world is protein-calorie malnutrition. The immunologic paresis resulting from malnutrition contributes substantially to the high incidence of infection in malnourished populations. Radiation and immunosuppressive agents, including alkylating agents and antithymocyte globulin, can induce lymphocytopenia by injuring the progenitor pool and inhibiting replication of more well-differentiated cells. A variety of congenital lymphocytopenic immunodeficiency states exist, some of which result in selective deficiencies of B lymphocytes, some of T cells, and some of combined deficiencies of both T cells and B cells. The mechanisms by which production and maturation of B and T lymphocytes are impaired in these patients are heterogeneous; many remain ill defined, although in many cases inactivating mutations of receptors for lymphopoietic factors are the cause. Even in the absence of lymphocytopenia, immunodeficiency states can clearly exist because of abnormal lymphocyte function or selective deficiency of a component of the circulating lymphocyte population.

Certain viruses are capable of inducing lymphocytopenia; some of these agents infect lymphoid cells and cause their destruction. Such viruses include measles, polio, varicella zoster, and HIV. HIV does not frequently cause lymphocytopenia, but it infects the helper (CD4+) subset of T lymphocytes and destroys them, a process that results in a marked decline in the absolute numbers of helper (CD4+) T cells in the peripheral circulation. Patients with untreated Hodgkin's disease occasionally have lymphocytopenia, especially during the late stages of the disease and with the least favorable histologic subtypes (see Chapter 180).

ALTERATIONS IN LYMPHOCYTIC TRAFFIC. Redistribution of lym-

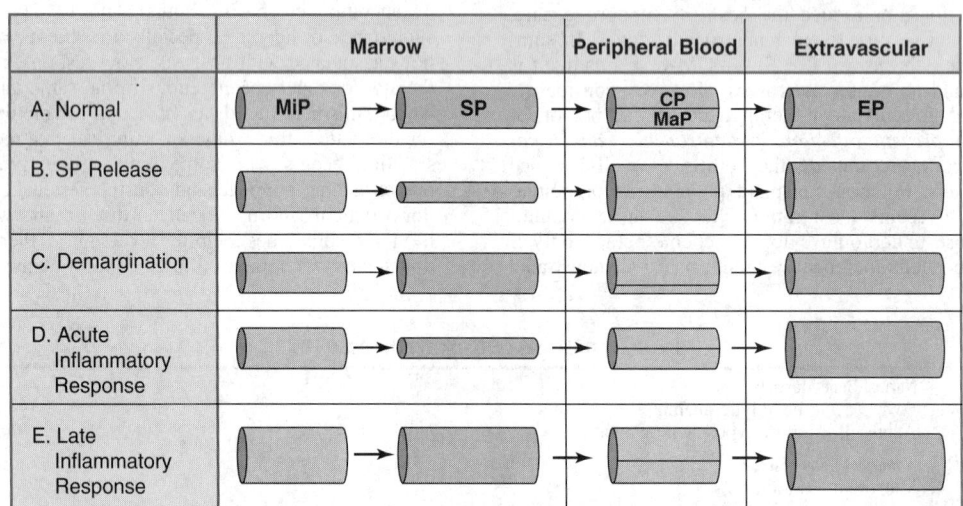

	Marrow		Peripheral Blood	Extravascular
A. Normal	MiP →	SP →	CP / MaP →	EP
B. SP Release				
C. Demargination				
D. Acute Inflammatory Response				
E. Late Inflammatory Response				

FIGURE 172–6 ■ Pathophysiologic mechanisms of neutrophilia. *A,* In this figure, the size of a given compartment is represented by the relative size of the cylinder shaped "pool." The number of cells leaving any pool for the next one is represented by the size of the arrows between the pools. MiP = the mitotic pool of neutrophil precursor cells; SP = the neutrophil storage pool; CP = the circulating granulocyte pool; MaP = the marginated pool; EP = the extravascular pool. Notice that in every case the circulating neutrophil pool is large (necessarily true for patients with neutrophilic leukocytosis), but the size of the other pools is variable. *B,* A variety of stresses, such as infection, can result in the release of storage pool granulocytes, probably mediated through the actions of glucocorticosteroids or the granulopoietic factors G-CSF and GM-CSF. *C,* The circulating granulocyte pool can also increase in size because of a shift of neutrophils from the marginated to the circulating pool. The demargination response can be regularly elicited by the administration of epinephrine or glucocorticosteroids. This is a response that also occurs in infections, but generally not without other dynamic alterations of other pools. *D,* In most bacterial infections and other inflammatory processes, the demand for neutrophils in the infected extravascular site results in the simultaneous release of storage pool neutrophils and demargination. *E,* Later in the inflammatory response, after the hematopoietic growth factors released in response to the inflammatory stimulus (see Fig. 172–8) have induced a few days of proliferation in the mitotic pool, the content of neutrophils in all pools increases and delivery to the tissues is maximized.

phocyte traffic is common and most frequently represents transient responses to a variety of stressful events, including bacterial infections, surgery, trauma, and hemorrhage. These responses are likely mediated by high levels of endogenous glucocorticoids that induce rapid declines in circulating levels of B and T lymphocytes. In hospitalized patients with lymphocytopenia, glucocorticosteroid therapy is the third most common cause, after acute bacterial or fungal infections and surgery. The lymphocytopenic response to this type of steroid results from a self-limited shift of lymphocytes away from the peripheral blood compartment. Lymphocyte values generally return to normal within 24 to 48 hours. For this reason, the transient declines induced by endogenous steroid production are not associated with functional immunologic deficiency. Certain viruses can also bind to lymphocyte populations and cause their departure from the blood compartment into other sites.

More persistent lymphocytopenia has been described in patients with widespread granulomatous disease, a phenomenon that is likely multifactorial, deriving from both inhibition of production and alterations of traffic. Patients with these disorders are often difficult to treat. In daily practice, establishing a cause-and-effect relationship between the infection and lymphocytopenia can be difficult when one considers that the reverse might just as easily be true; consider, for example, the frequency of mycobacterial infection in patients with the acquired immunodeficiency syndrome.

INCREASED DESTRUCTION OF LYMPHOCYTES. Viral infections or antilymphocyte antibodies, especially in patients with underlying autoimmune or rheumatic diseases, increase lymphocyte destruction. Losses of viable lymphocytes can also occur because of structural defects in sites of high-density lymphocyte traffic (e.g., through thoracic duct fistulas). In such patients, both T cells and B cells decline in the peripheral blood. Loss of lymphocytes from intestinal lymphatics can occur in protein-losing enteropathies, severe heart failure, or primary diseases of the gut or intestinal lymphatics (see Table 172–2).

CLINICAL MANIFESTATIONS AND DIAGNOSIS. There are no specific clinical manifestations of lymphocytopenia per se. Whether the patient exhibits signs of immunologic deficiency depends on the pathophysiology of the disorder, the duration of the disease, the type of lymphocytes affected most significantly, the intactness of nodal tissues, and the degree to which cellular or humoral immunity is functionally perturbed. Accordingly, unless the clinical setting is clearly one in which transient lymphocytopenia is likely, the approach to diagnosis should involve comprehensive assessment of the integrity of the immune apparatus. Specifically, the subsets of lymphocytes remaining in the circulating blood should be quantified, including B cells, helper-inducer T cells (CD4+), and cytotoxic-suppressor T cells (CD8+). In addition, quantitative immunoglobulin levels should be measured in the serum and a series of skin tests should be performed to detect deficiencies of cell-mediated immunity.

TREATMENT. Because lymphocytopenia ordinarily represents a response to an underlying disease, primary attention must be paid to establishing the nature of that disease and instituting therapy for it. Patients whose lymphocytopenia is accompanied by hypogam-

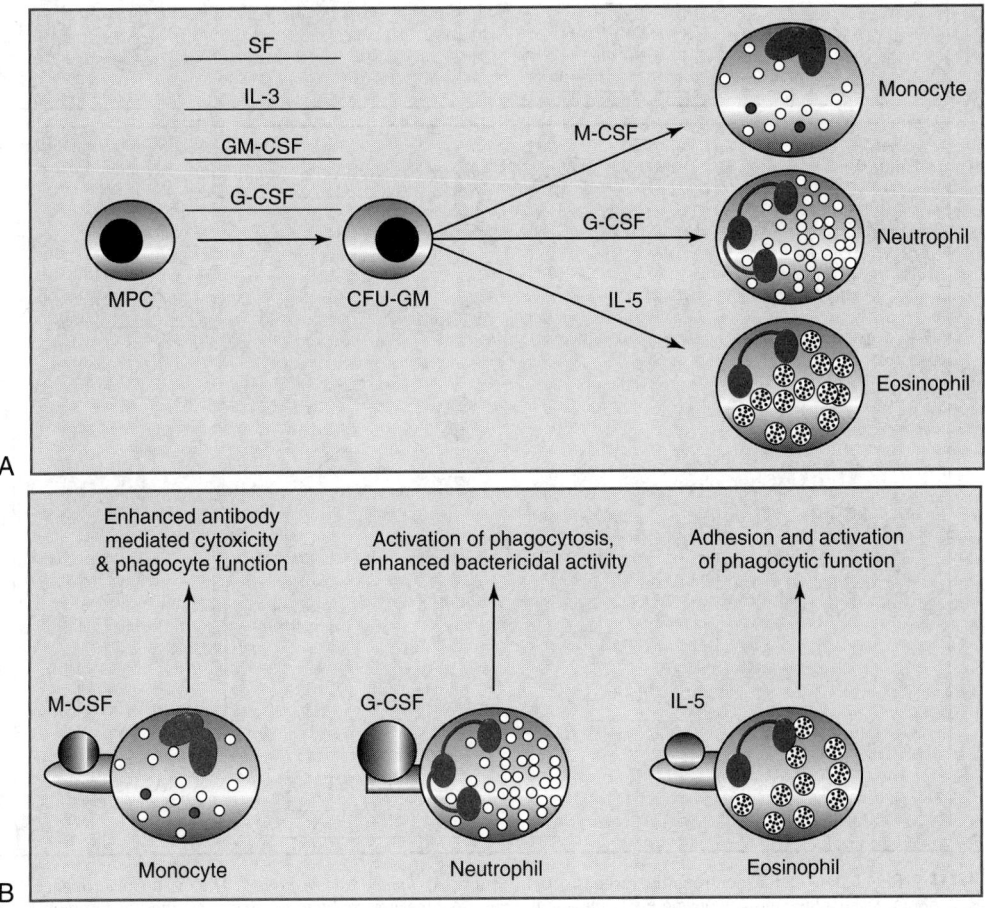

FIGURE 172–7 ■ Cytokine control of phagocyte production and activation. *A,* Steel factor (SF, also known as stem cell factor), interleukin-3 (IL-3), granulocyte macrophage colony-stimulating factor (GM-CSF), and granulocyte colony-. stimulating factor (G-CSF) can each influence the growth and differentiation of multilineage progenitor cells (MPC) to the committed granulocyte macrophage progenitor cell (CFU-GM), but they work best in synergy with each other. Specific factors govern the production of specific phagocytes, each serving as a survival factor for that lineage. M-CSF is a survival factor for monocytes and their precursors, G-CSF for neutrophil precursors, and IL-5 for eosinophil precursors. *B,* Factors that serve as growth and differentiation factors for a specific lineage also act as activation factors for the terminally differentiated forms of the same lineage. The horizontal projections from the cell borders are meant to represent receptor molecules while the spherical shapes represent the ligands. M-CSF activates the function of monocytes and macrophages, G-CSF activates neutrophils, and IL-5 activates eosinophil function.

maglobulinemia may benefit significantly from administration of intravenous immunoglobulin, which often reduces the incidence of infectious events. The treatment of severe deficiencies of cell-mediated immunity remains experimental. Responses have been described with transplantation of allogeneic bone marrow, fetal liver, or thymic epithelial cells. Recent progress has been made in the therapy for adenosine deaminase deficiency, which is a cause of severe combined immunodeficiency, using adenosine deaminase conjugated to polyethylene glycol. Some syndromes may also respond in the future to gene therapy.

LEUKOCYTOSIS AND LEUKEMOID REACTIONS

Circulating leukocytes consist of neutrophils, monocytes, eosinophils, basophils, and lymphocytes (T cells, B cells, and natural

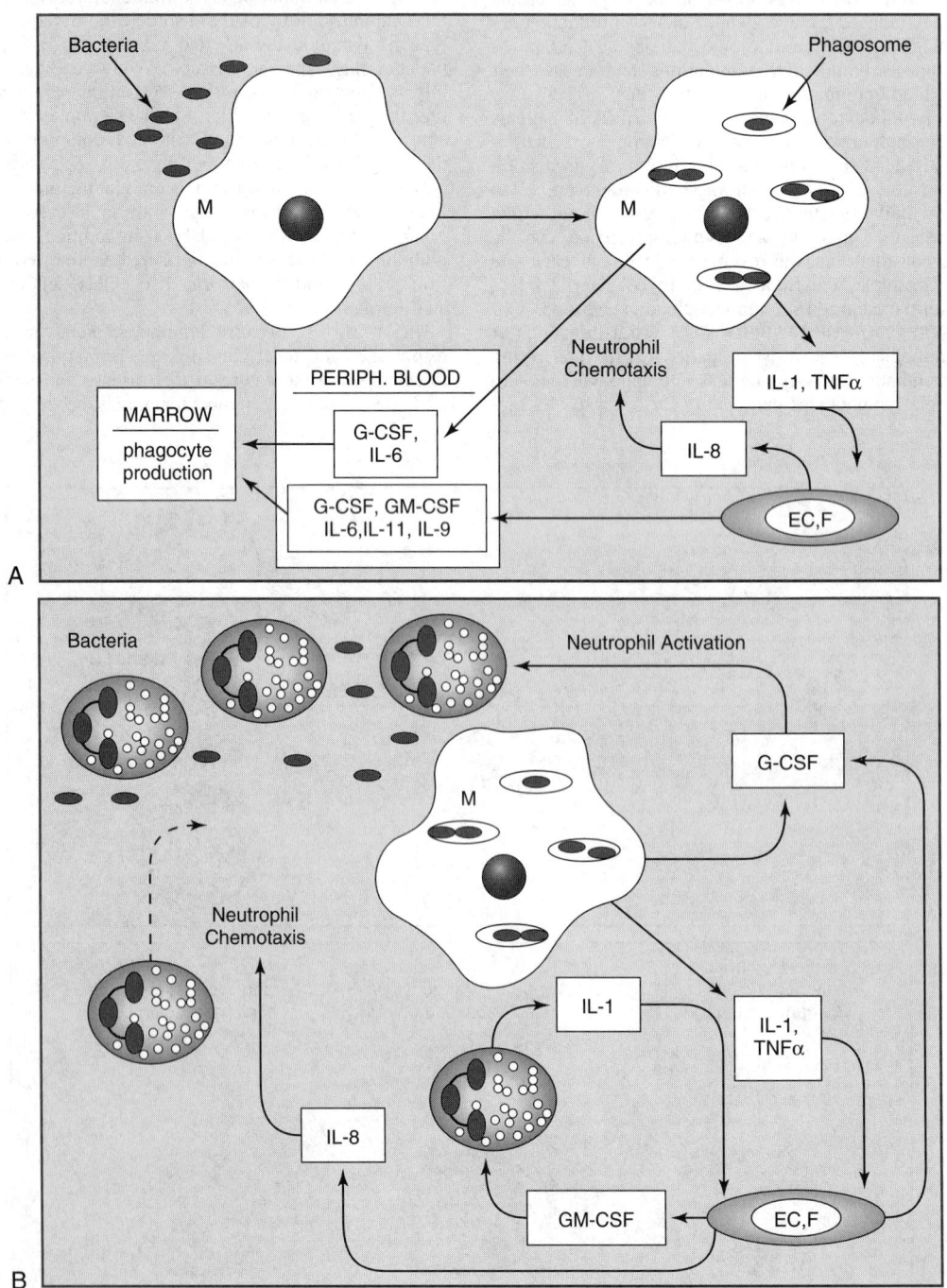

FIGURE 172–8 ■ Regulation of the neutrophilic response to infection. *A, Immediate response:* The tissue macrophage (M) is the first line of defense and plays more than merely a phagocytic role. As the macrophage engages and ingests offending organisms, it releases hematopoietic growth factors (G-CSF and IL-6) into the peripheral blood ("periph. blood") that ultimately stimulate the production of neutrophils by the bone marrow progenitor cell pool. Activated macrophages also release the master switch cytokines TNF-α and IL-1, both of which induce secretory responses in neighboring stroma cells (shown as endothelial cells [EC] and fibroblasts [F]). Stromal cells also release a wide variety of factors that call forth a neutrophil chemotactic response (e.g., IL-8) and also induce neutrophil production (G-CSF, GM-CSF, IL-6, IL-11, and IL-9). *B, Early response:* Within hours, neutrophils move to the invasion site. Neutrophils move out of the circulating blood into the site of infection under the influence of IL-8, a potent neutrophil chemotactic factor. They also come under the influence of G-CSF that activates their phagocytic and bactericidal capacity. Finally, neutrophils, too, can play a secretory role, augmenting release of additional cytokines. Specifically, under the influence of GM-CSF, neutrophils release IL-1 that, in turn, induces more IL-8 and G-CSF production. This secretory capacity of neutrophils is a classic cytokine amplification mechanism.

killer cells). Any one or all of these cell types can increase to abnormal levels in peripheral blood in response to various stimuli. Each type of leukocyte is produced in the bone marrow (and in the case of lymphocytes, in lymph nodes, spleen, and thymus as well) in response to specific growth factors, and in the case of some lymphocytes, in response to antigenic stimuli. The term *leukocytosis* is used to describe a total leukocyte count above $11.0 \times 10^9/L$; it is a common and diagnostically important finding in clinical practice. Once leukocytosis is discovered, it is first essential to examine the differential white blood cell count so that one can determine which of the white cell types is increased. The terms *neutrophilia* (neutrophilic leukocytosis), monocytosis, lymphocytosis, eosinophilia, and basophilia suggest specific sets of diagnostic considerations.

Leukocytosis is a common finding in acutely ill patients. When the leukocyte count exceeds 25 to $30 \times 10^9/L$, it is sometimes termed a *leukemoid reaction*. Leukemoid reactions generally reflect the response of healthy bone marrow to cytokines released by auxiliary cells (lymphocytes, macrophages, and stromal cells) exposed to infection or trauma. Leukemoid reactions are not synonymous with *leukoerythroblastosis*, which indicates the presence of immature white cells and nucleated red cells in the peripheral blood irrespective of the total leukocyte count. Leukoerythroblastosis is less common than leukemoid reactions but often, especially in the adult patient, reflects serious marrow dysfunction (Table 172–3). Consequently, the finding of leukoerythroblastosis represents a clear indication to perform bone marrow aspiration and biopsy, unless the clinical setting is specifically an acute severe hemolytic anemia, sepsis in a patient with hyposplenism, or acute massive trauma with multiple fractures.

NEUTROPHILIA

PATHOPHYSIOLOGY. The number of neutrophil precursors in the marrow mitotic pool (MiP) (Fig. 172–6) is largely influenced by the hematopoietic growth factors, the most neutrophil lineage specific of which is the granulopoietic factor G-CSF. G-CSF not only functions to stimulate the growth and differentiation of granu-locyte progenitor cells but also functionally activates neutrophils, enhancing their capacity to kill ingested organisms. The same holds true for macrophage colony-stimulating factor (M-CSF; the growth factor for mononuclear phagocytes) and IL-5 (the growth factor for eosinophils) (Fig. 172–7).

The marrow storage pool is sufficient to provide the periphery with neutrophils for about 5 days in the steady state, even if it were unsupported by the MiP. Neutrophils are released from the storage pool into the circulating pool in response to a variety of physiologic stresses, including endogenous glucocorticoids (see Fig. 172–6B). Normally, peripheral neutrophils are equally divided between the circulating pool and the marginated pool. Neutrophilia can therefore result from a shift of neutrophils from the marginated to the circulating pool—"demargination" (see Fig. 172–6C). This response is rapid and can be induced by injections of epinephrine and glucocorticosteroids. In patients with acute inflammatory illnesses, storage pool release and demargination usually occur together (see Fig. 172–6D).

Neutrophilic leukocytosis is the most common type of leukocytosis in clinical practice. It evolves in response to the release of factors that govern the production and traffic of this cell type, including G-CSF and the factors that augment the mitotic activity of G-CSF, including IL-3 and Steel factor (SF) (see Fig. 172–2). These factors are produced by a complex network of auxiliary cells in the bone marrow, including mononuclear phagocytes, microvascular endothelial cells, fibroblasts, and lymphocytes. These growth factor producing cells respond to acute inflammatory events by augmenting production of the critically important colony-stimulating factors (CSFs) (Fig. 172–7). The CSFs stimulate replication of granulopoietic progenitor cells, which leads to expansion of the neutrophil storage pool and subsequent neutrophilia (see Fig. 172–6E). In response to the infection and the induced cytokines and adhesion molecules, the transit time of neutrophils in the mitotic and post-mitotic pools in the bone marrow are shorter than in the uninfected state, and immature neutrophils (bands and metamyelocytes) are released from the storage pool. This new high level of production persists until the inflammatory process resolves.

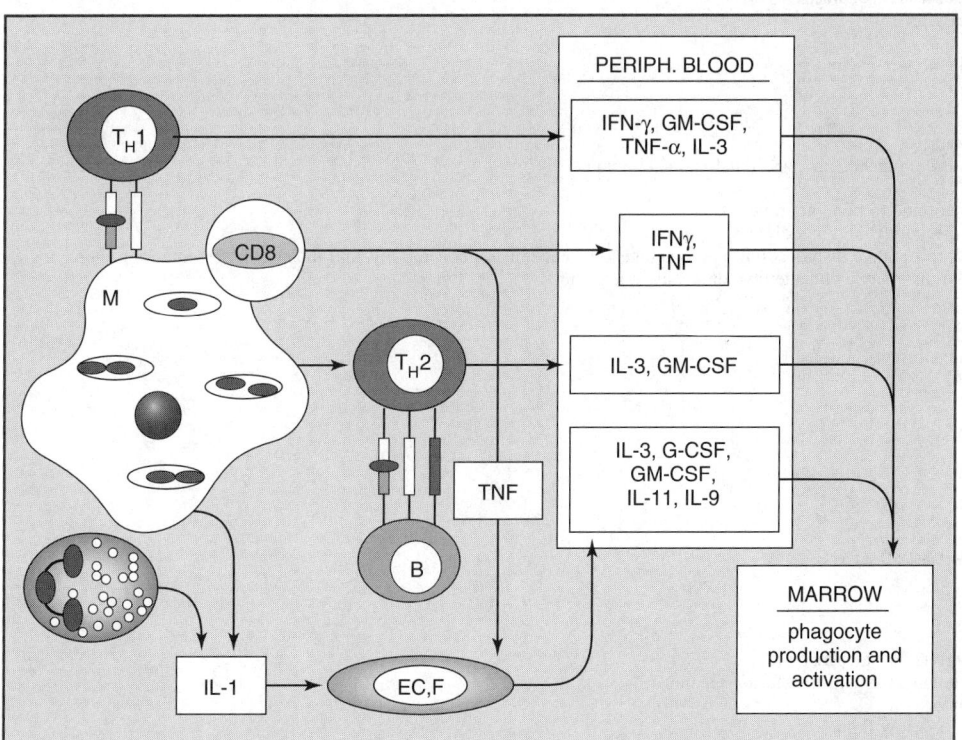

FIGURE 172–8 ■ *Continued. C, Fully established inflammatory response:* Macrophages and neutrophils at the invasion site continue to produce IL-1, but macrophages also begin to present antigen (bacterial in this case) to T lymphocytes, which themselves release a wide variety of factors that have a direct impact on the production and activation of neutrophils. At this point, the granulopoietic response is in full swing and the proliferation of CFU-GM is at its peak. In summary, when a tissue is infected, the need for new neutrophils is answered by a highly complex and interdependent intercellular network of interleukins, chemotactic factors, and hematopoietic growth factors, some of which are shown here. Macrophages, stromal cells, lymphocytes, and even neutrophils amplify the initial inductive signals that begin at the site of invasion in macrophages.

CAUSES. Neutrophilia (neutrophil counts greater than 7.5×10^9/L), a common finding in clinical practice, usually reflects the inflammatory response to acute or subacute infections (Fig. 172–8; Table 172–4). Neutrophilia is a finding that should first trigger a diagnostic search for its cause. Such searches usually involve a careful history and physical examination and just a few inexpensive laboratory tests (the nature of which depends on the findings on physical examination) because in most cases the cause will become apparent and usually proves to be an active infectious process.

When neutrophilia occurs in the absence of evidence of acute inflammation or illness, three explanations should be considered: (1) chemical effects, including agents such as glucocorticoids, lithium chloride, or epinephrine; (2) malignant tumors, in which cancer cells may inappropriately express certain of the CSF genes, thereby increasing CSF blood levels; and (3) chronic myeloproliferative disorders, including chronic myelogenous leukemia, agnogenic myeloid metaplasia, essential thrombocytosis, and polycythemia vera.

DIAGNOSIS. The diagnostic approach to patients with neutrophilia (Fig. 172–9) leads quickly to the performance of bone marrow aspiration and biopsy for patients with leukoerythroblastosis. In patients without leukoerythroblastosis, neutrophilic leukocytosis generally results from acute toxic, inflammatory, or traumatic stresses, and it is usually best to observe the course of neutrophilia to determine its degree of linkage with the underlying disease. If the underlying disease resolves and the neutrophilia does not, other, less common explanations must be pursued.

NEUTROPHIL MORPHOLOGY. Neutrophil morphology can lead to early diagnosis. Toxic granulation of neutrophils, the presence of Döhle bodies, and the presence of vacuoles in the neutrophil cytoplasm suggest that overt or subclinical inflammation, toxin exposure, trauma, or neoplasia exist. Because glucocorticoids induce prompt eosinopenia and basophilopenia, these cells are almost universally absent in the blood of the acutely injured or infected patient. Thus, their presence should indicate that (1) the acutely ill patient may have concomitant adrenocortical insufficiency, (2) the neutrophilia derives from the inappropriate production of GM-CSF (e.g., by malignant cells), or (3) the neutrophilia is one manifestation of a hematopoietic neoplasm (a chronic myeloproliferative disorder, myelodysplastic syndrome, lymphoma, or acute nonlymphocytic leukemias associated with eosinophilia).

LEUKOCYTE ALKALINE PHOSPHATASE. Leukocyte alkaline phosphatase (LAP) is an enzyme found in neutrophils. When neutrophilia represents a reaction to an acute illness, the LAP levels usually increase substantially. In chronic myelogenous leukemia (CML), however, the LAP score is markedly decreased. A low LAP level in a patient with neutrophilia should therefore lead to a diagnostic evaluation designed to exclude CML (Table 172–5, see Fig. 172–8).

DIFFERENTIAL DIAGNOSIS OF NEUTROPHILIC LEUKEMOID REACTIONS. Neutrophilic leukemoid reactions generally occur in patients who are obviously systemically ill. When the neutrophil count exceeds 80×10^9/L or when the mildness of the systemic illness seems discordant with the extremely high level of neutrophils in the peripheral blood, the diagnosis most often considered is CML or chronic myelomonocytic leukemia (CMML). A number of additional features distinguish leukemoid reactions from CML and

---

Table 172–4 ■ COMMON CAUSES OF NEUTROPHILIC LEUKOCYTOSIS

Infections
Bacteria
Viruses
Fungi
Parasites
Rickettsia

Rheumatic and Autoimmune Disorders
Rheumatoid arthritis
Vasculitis
Autoimmune hemolytic anemia
Colitis
Gout

Neoplastic Disorders
Pancreatic, gastric, bronchogenic, and renal cell carcinoma
Melanoma
Any cancer metastatic to bone marrow
Lymphoma, especially Hodgkin's disease
Chronic myeloproliferative disorders (chronic myelogenous leukemia, agnogenic myeloid metaplasia, essential thrombocytosis, polycythemia vera)
Myelodysplastic disorders and acute myelomonocytic leukemia

Chemicals
Mercury poisoning
Venoms (reptiles, insects, jellyfish)
Ethylene glycol
Histamine

Trauma
Thermal injury
Hypothermia
Crush injury
Electrical injury

Endocrine and Metabolic Disorders
Ketoacidosis
Lactic acidosis
Thyrotoxicosis

Hematologic Disorders (Non-neoplastic)
Acute hemolytic anemias and transfusion reactions
Postsplenectomy
Recovery from marrow failure

Other Disorders
Tissue necrosis
Pregnancy
Eclampsia
Exfoliative dermatitis
Hypoxia
Drugs: corticosteroids, lithium, epinephrine, granulocyte colony-stimulating factor, granulocyte-macrophage colony-stimulating factor

CMML (see Table 172–5). The diagnostic tests for CML are those designed to identify the classic balanced chromosomal rearrangement (a chromosome 9;22 translocation) either morphologically (cytogenetic analysis) or by molecular methods (identification of the bcr/abl DNA, mRNA, or protein).

MONOCYTOSIS

Monocytosis is defined as absolute peripheral blood monocyte counts greater than 0.80×10^9/L in children and greater than 0.50×10^9/L in adults. Monocytes present processed antigens to lymphocytes, mediate cellular cytotoxicity, release procoagulants, participate in bone remodeling and wound repair, dispose of damaged cells, and regulate immune and hematopoietic responses by producing IL-1, TNF-α, G-CSF, IL-6, and certain interferons. The most specific growth/survival factor for mononuclear phagocytes is M-CSF (known as CSF-1 in the mouse) (see Fig. 172–8) produced by stromal cells, including endothelial cells and fibroblasts. M-CSF knockout mice have monocytopenia and macrophage deficiency, but GM-CSF knockout mice do not.

The mononuclear phagocyte is more sluggish than the neutrophil in moving toward and killing bacteria but is as effective, if not more so, in killing obligate intracellular parasites such as fungi, yeasts, and viruses. In addition, the mononuclear phagocyte participates substantially in all types of granulomatous inflammation. Accordingly, monocytosis is often seen in patients with tuberculosis, syphilis, fungal infections, ulcerative and granulomatous colitis, and sarcoidosis (Table 172–6). Mild monocytosis is common in patients with Hodgkin's disease and a variety of cancers. High levels of monocytes in the blood are most often seen in patients with hematopoietic malignancies, including acute and chronic myelomonocytic leukemia, acute monocytic leukemia, and chronic myelogenous leukemia of the juvenile type.

EOSINOPHILIA

Eosinophilic leukocytosis (eosinophilia) exists when the eosinophil count in the peripheral blood exceeds 0.4×10^9/L (see Chapter 173). Eosinophils are produced by progenitor cells in the marrow largely under the influence of IL-5, a protein that also stimulates

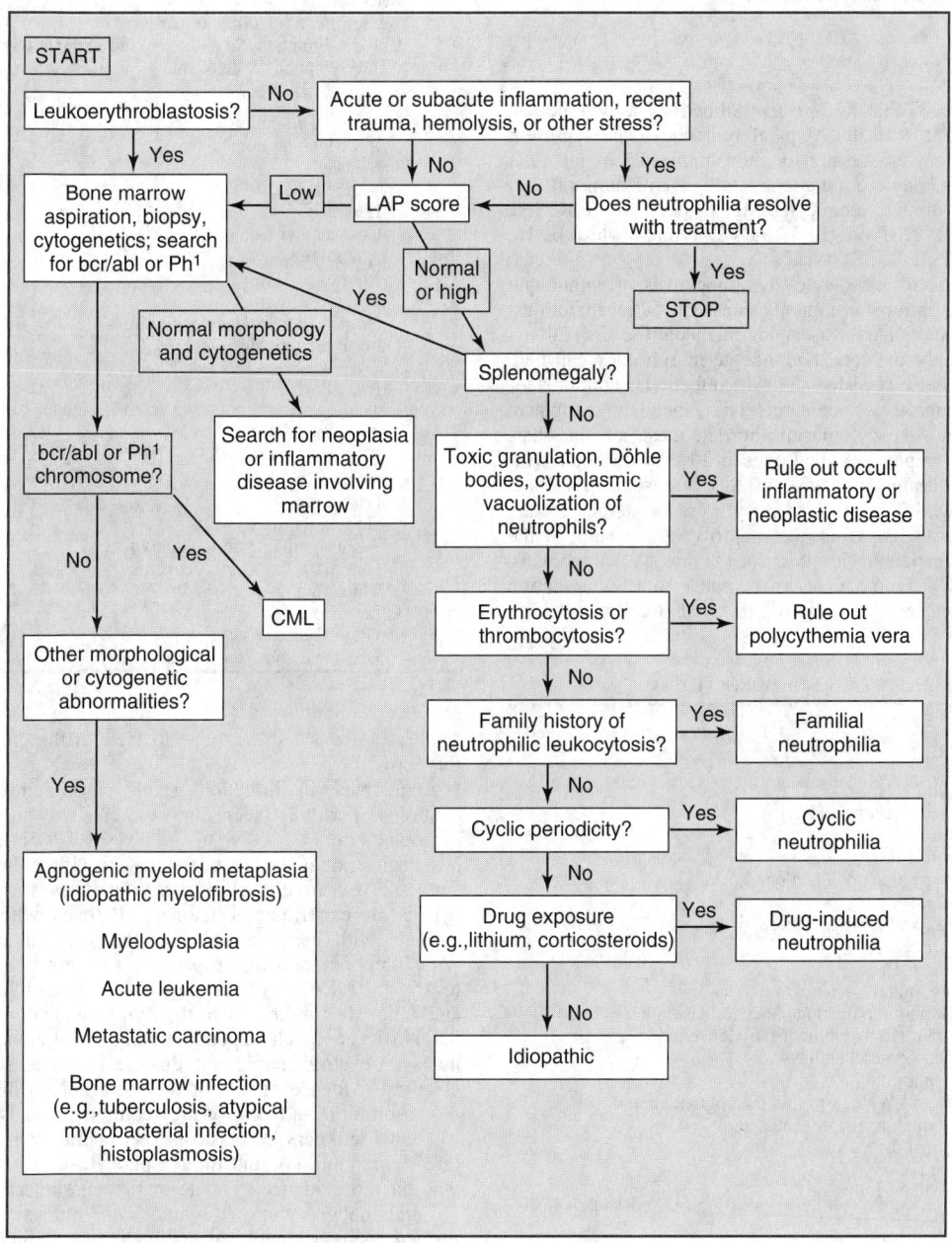

FIGURE 172–9 ■ Evaluation of patients with neutrophilic leukocytosis. LAP = leukocyte alkaline phosphatase; Ph¹ = Philadelphia chromosome; bcr/abl = the translocation of the c-abl gene from chromosome 9 to the bcr gene on chromosome 22q; CML = chronic myelogenous leukemia.

Table 172–5 ■ DISTINCTIONS BETWEEN NEUTROPHILIC LEUKEMOID REACTIONS AND CHRONIC MYELOGENOUS LEUKEMIA (CML)

FINDING/RESULT	LEUKEMOID REACTION	CML
Presence of fever or other manifestations of acute or subacute inflammation	Usual*	Infrequent†
Splenomegaly	Rare	Frequent
Natural course of neutrophilia	Resolution linked with abatement of underlying disease	Progressive slow increase over time
Peripheral blood basophilia	Rare‡	Common
LAP score	High	Low§
Philadelphia chromosome	Absent	Frequent (~85%)
bcr/abl translocation	Absent	Frequent (>90%)

*Exceptions include patients with leukemoid reactions associated with certain cancers.
†Patients with CML can also develop infections. The time to evaluate this possibility is when the inflammatory process resolves and the neutrophilia does not.
‡Patients with acute allergic reactions and patients with parasitic diseases are exceptions to this rule.
§LAP scores can be normal in some CML patients, particularly after splenectomy.

the growth and differentiation of B lymphocytes. Eosinophils not only function as phagocytes but also play an extraordinarily important role in modulating the potentially toxic effects of mast cell degranulation in hypersensitivity reactions.

LYMPHOCYTOSIS

Lymphocytosis (see Table 172–7) is defined as a lymphocyte count in excess of 5.0×10^9/L. Atypical lymphocytosis is present when atypical lymphocytes account for more than 20% of the total peripheral blood lymphocyte population. A number of humoral factors induce growth of T lymphocytes (IL-2, IL-3, IL-7, IL-15), natural killer cells (IL-2, IL-12, IL-1), and B lymphocytes (IL-10, IL-6, IL-5, IL-4, IL-7, IL-13, IL-14, IL-15).

DIAGNOSIS. Mild to moderate lymphocytosis (lymphocyte counts $<12 \times 10^9$/L) is most commonly caused by viral infections, including infectious mononucleosis and viral hepatitis. Careful examination of the peripheral blood lymphocyte morphology can help distinguish between these two disorders. In infectious mononucleosis, many of the lymphocytes are large, with abundant cytoplasm and a "ballerina skirt"-like cytoplasmic border; these are the characteristic "atypical" lymphocytes that exceed 20% of the total lymphocyte population during the course of this disease (Color Plate 6A). Interestingly, while the B lymphocyte is the target of the causative Epstein-Barr (EB) virus, the majority of the cells in the peripheral blood of patients with this disease are T lymphocytes. This proliferation of T lymphocytes in response to EBV infection of B cells plays a role in eradicating the infected B-cell population.

Table 172–7 ■ CAUSES OF LYMPHOCYTOSIS

High ($>15 \times 10^9$/L)
Infectious mononucleosis
Pertussis
Acute infectious lymphocytosis
Chronic lymphocytic leukemia and variants thereof
Acute lymphocytic leukemia

Moderate ($<15 \times 10^9$/L)
Many viral infections
  Infectious mononucleosis
  Measles
  Varicella
  Hepatitis
  Coxsackievirus
  Adenovirus
  Mumps
  Cytomegalovirus
  Human immunodeficiency virus-1 (acute lymphadenopathy)
Other infectious diseases
  Toxoplasmosis
  Brucellosis
  Tuberculosis
  Typhoid fever
  Syphilis (secondary)
Neoplastic disorders
  Carcinoma
  Hodgkin's disease
  Acute lymphocytic leukemia (early)
  Chronic lymphocytic leukemia
  Thymoma
Other disorders
  Graves' diseases
  Drug reactions (e.g., tetracycline)

Table 172–6 ■ CAUSES OF MONOCYTOSIS

Infections
  Tuberculosis
  Brucellosis
  Endocarditis
  Typhoid and paratyphoid
  Syphilis
  Fungal infections
  Recovery from acute infections
  Protozoal infections
  Viral (e.g., varicella) infections
Neoplastic diseases
  Hodgkin's disease
  Carcinoma (many varieties)
  Acute and chronic myelomonocytic leukemia
  Juvenile chronic myelomonocytic leukemia
  Acute monocytic leukemia
  Myelodysplasia
  Myeloma and Waldenström's macroglobulinemia
  Chronic lymphocytic leukemia (rare)
Gastrointestinal disorders
  Ulcerative colitis
  Granulomatous colitis
  Cirrhosis
Sarcoidosis
Drug reactions
Recovery from marrow suppression
Congenital neutropenia

This response is a critical one in view of the oncogenic potential of this virus.

Acute bacterial infections rarely cause lymphocytosis. One exception is pertussis (seen almost exclusively in children), in which profound lymphocytosis (up to 60×10^9/L) is sometimes seen. It has been known for 30 years that specific soluble factors derived from the causative organism, *Bordetella pertussis,* induce lymphocytosis in experimental animals. Perhaps with the exception of patients with early chronic lymphocytic leukemia, most patients with lymphocytosis and especially substantial lymphocytosis (>12 to 15×10^9/L) have overt signs of an underlying illness involving anatomic sites other than the lymphohematopoietic system. The diagnostic approach depends simply on establishing a tissue diagnosis to exclude malignant disease in patients who do not have clear-cut evidence of one of the more benign disorders. Bone marrow aspiration and biopsy are required when lymphocytosis coexists with leukoerythroblastosis, peripheral lymphocytes are immature (lymphoblasts), and the lymphocytosis is persistent in a patient who has no evidence of acute or subacute infection.

Immunophenotyping ("lymphocyte markers") should be performed using monoclonal antibodies to definitive integral membrane proteins. Not only will such studies provide evidence for or against dominance of one lymphocyte type and differentiation stage, but also analyses of immunoglobulin light chain types can determine whether B lymphocytes in the circulation are all members of a single (therefore, likely neoplastic) clone.

Blay JY, Chauvin F, LeCesne A, et al: Early lymphopenia after cytotoxic chemotherapy as a risk factor for febrile neutropenia. J Clin Oncol 14:636–643, 1996. *This article suggests that assessment of lymphocyte counts in neutropenic chemotherapy patients can predict the risk of neutropenic fever.*

Castelino DJ, McNair P, Kay TW: Lymphocytopenia in a hospital population—what does it signify? Aust NZ J Med 27:170–174, 1997. *A retrospective review of clinical records of patients with lymphocyte counts less than $0.6 \times 10^9/L$ reveals that the two most common clinical settings were the postoperative period or bacterial/fungal sepsis, followed by corticosteroid treatment and malignancy.*

Greenberg PL: The role of hemopoietic growth factors in the treatment of myelodysplastic syndromes. Int J Pediatr Hematol Oncol 4:231, 1997. *Review of the role of G-CSF and erythropoietin therapy in selected patients with myelodysplasia, including the synergistic activity of erythropoietin combined with G-CSF in these disorders.*

Hartmann LC, Tschetter LK, Habermann TM, et al: Granulocyte colony-stimulating factor in severe chemotherapy-induced afebrile neutropenia. N Engl J Med 336: 1776, 1997; and Pui CH, Boyett JM, Hughes WT, et al: Human granulocyte colony-stimulating factor after induction chemotherapy in children with acute lymphoblastic leukemia. N Engl J Med 336:1781, 1997. *These two articles demonstrate that shortening the duration of neutropenia in patients who receive G-CSF after receiving cytotoxic chemotherapy does not necessarily reduce the number of infectious complications.*

Lieschke GJ: CSF-deficient mice—what have they taught us? Ciba Found Symp 204: 60–74, 1997. *This concise review demonstrates the power of this genetic methodology. These models have also helped us understand exactly which cytokines are in control during the inflammatory response.*

Moses AV, Nelson J, Bagby GC: The influence of HIV-1 on hematopoiesis. Blood 91: 1479, 1998. *This literature review presents an overview of regenerative bone marrow failure in the light of recent evidence that progenitors and stem cells are rarely infected by HIV-1 but bone marrow and lymph node stromal cells are often infected and malfunction as a result of it.*

Nichols CR, Fox EP, Roth BJ, et al: Incidence of neutropenic fever in patients treated with standard-dose combination chemotherapy for small-cell lung cancer and the cost impact of treatment with granulocyte colony-stimulating factor. J Clin Oncol 12:1245–1250, 1994. *Pre-emptive therapy with G-CSF is best considered for clinical situations in which maintaining very high doses of cytotoxic agents results in clear clinical benefit (increased survival, increase in response rates).*

173 EOSINOPHILIC SYNDROMES

Peter F. Weller

Eosinophilia, often with heightened production of eosinophils as well as increased blood and tissue eosinophil accumulation, is associated with distinctive disease processes that include helminthic parasitic infections, allergic diseases, and a diversity of diseases of often ill-defined etiology (see Chapters 270 and 420). In comparison with other leukocytes, eosinophils are distinguished by their morphology, constituents, products, and associations with specific diseases.

Eosinophils are produced in the bone marrow. The cytokine interleukin-5 specifically promotes the development and terminal differentiation of eosinophils and is principally responsible for increases in eosinophilopoiesis. Normally, eosinophils are primarily tissue-dwelling cells; the greatest numbers of eosinophils are found in tissues with a mucosal epithelial interface with the environment, including the respiratory, gastrointestinal, and lower genitourinary tracts. The lifespan of eosinophils is longer than that of neutrophils, and eosinophils may survive for weeks within tissues. Eosinophils, similarly sized to neutrophils but with usually bilobed nuclei, are morphologically characterized by their cytoplasmic granules. Specific granules, the most numerous of several types of cytoplasmic granules, have unique, ultrastructurally distinct crystalloid cores and contain eosinophil-specific cationic proteins. These cationic granule proteins, which bind acidic dyes such as eosin, are responsible both for the tinctorial properties of eosinophils and for many of the functional properties of eosinophils. The four eosinophil cationic proteins are major basic protein, eosinophil peroxidase, eosinophil cationic protein, and eosinophil-derived neurotoxin. Another predominant eosinophil constituent that is not derived from specific granules is the protein, a lysophospholipase, that forms bipyramidal Charcot-Leyden crystals, often found in sputum, feces, and tissues as a hallmark of eosinophil-related diseases. In addition to their content of pre-formed granule proteins, eosinophils also elaborate newly synthesized lipid mediators, including the 5-lipoxygenase pathway–derived eicosanoid leukotriene C_2 and platelet activating factor. Eosinophils are also the source of many cytokines.

Eosinophils are equipped to serve several immunologic functions. Like neutrophils, eosinophils can serve as end-stage effector cells, but eosinophils have specialized roles in host defense and act primarily against multicellular parasites that cannot be eradicated by phagocytosis. Although eosinophils are capable of phagocytosing and killing bacteria and other small microbes, eosinophils do not have a major role in vivo in host defense against such microbial pathogens and cannot constitute an effective defense against bacterial infections in situations in which neutrophil function is deficient. Rather, eosinophils function in host defense against large, nonphagocytosable organisms, most notably the multicellular, helminthic parasites. Eosinophils can invoke several mechanisms, including their cytotoxic cationic granule proteins, for antiparasitic host defense.

Pertinent to the eosinophil's involvement in allergic diseases, including asthma, is the capacity of eosinophils to elaborate specific lipid mediators, including leukotriene C_4 and platelet activating factor, which can contract airway smooth muscle, promote mucus secretion, alter vascular permeability, and elicit eosinophil and neutrophil infiltration. Some of the mechanisms beneficial in eosinophils' role in host defense can prove detrimental to the host. Released eosinophil cationic proteins are toxic to host cells, and the dysfunction and damage elicited by eosinophil granule proteins may contribute to the pathogenesis of diseases in which heightened numbers of eosinophils are found within involved tissues. The effector functions of mature eosinophils, whether they are mediated by release of pre-formed granule proteins or by the synthesis of new lipid mediators, can be stimulated by cytokines, including interleukin-5 and granulocyte-macrophage colony-stimulating factor. Additional immunologic functions, based on the eosinophil's capabilities to interact with lymphocytes and other cells, are beginning to be defined and may further contribute to the understanding of eosinophil participation in normal mucosal immune responses and in eosinophil-related diseases.

Blood eosinophil numbers do not always reflect the extent of eosinophil involvement in affected tissues in various diseases. Eosinophils usually number less than $450/\mu L$ in the blood; the count has a mild diurnal variation, being higher in the early morning and falling as endogenous glucocorticosteroid levels rise. Eosinopenia occurs with corticosteroid administration and is also frequent with active bacterial and viral infections. In patients with eosinophilia of various etiologies, circulating blood eosinophils can exhibit morphologic and functional changes consequent to their activation. In some, but not necessarily all patients with sustained blood eosinophilia, organ damage can develop, especially cardiac, as found in the idiopathic hypereosinophilic syndrome. Undoubtedly, the development of such complications of sustained eosinophilia reflects not just heightened numbers of eosinophils but also some activating events, as yet ill defined, that promote eosinophil-mediated tissue damage. Patients with sustained eosinophilia should be monitored for evidence of cardiac disease (see below).

DISEASES ASSOCIATED WITH EOSINOPHILIA (Table 173–1)

PARASITIC DISEASES. Eosinophilia is not elicited by infections with single-celled protozoan parasites (with the exception of the intestinal coccidian parasite *Isospora belli* [see Chapter 429]), but rather by the multicellular helminthic parasites. The level of eosinophilia tends to parallel the magnitude and extent of tissue invasion, especially by larvae. Eosinophilia may be absent in established infections that are well contained within tissues or solely intraluminal in the gastrointestinal tract (e.g., *Ascaris*, tapeworms). Even with severe helminthic diseases such as disseminated strongyloidiasis (see Chapter 433), superimposed bacterial infections can suppress eosinophilia. In evaluating a patient with unexplained eosinophilia, geographic and dietary histories are germane in indicating potential exposure to helminthic parasites. Stool examinations for diagnostic ova and larvae should be performed, and for evaluation of *Strongyloides* infection, an enzyme-linked immunosorbent assay for antigens should be performed. In addition, for a number of the helminthic parasites that cause eosinophilia, diagnostic para-

Table 173–1 ■ DISEASES ASSOCIATED WITH EOSINOPHILIA

"Allergic" Diseases
Atopic and related diseases
Medication-related eosinophilias
Infectious Diseases
Parasitic infections, mostly with helminths
Specific fungal infections: allergic bronchopulmonary aspergillosis, coccidi-
 oidomycosis (acute and sometimes disseminated)
Other infections—infrequent, including HIV-1 and HTLV-1
Hematologic and Neoplastic Disorders
Hypereosinophilic syndrome
Leukemia
Lymphomas, including nodular sclerosing Hodgkin's disease
Tumor associated
Mastocytosis
Diseases with Specific Organ Involvement
Skin and subcutaneous diseases, including urticaria, bullous pemphigoid,
 eosinophilic cellulitis (Well's syndrome), episodic angioedema with eo-
 sinophilia
Pulmonary diseases, including acute or chronic eosinophilic pneumonia,
 allergic bronchopulmonary aspergillosis
Gastrointestinal diseases, including eosinophilic gastroenteritis
Neurologic diseases (e.g., eosinophilic meningitis)
Rheumatologic diseases, especially Churg-Strauss vasculitis; also eosino-
 philic fasciitis
Cardiac diseases (e.g., endomyocardial fibrosis)
Renal diseases, including drug-induced interstitial nephritis, eosinophilic
 cystitis, dialysis
Immunologic Reactions
Specific immune deficiency diseases: hyper-IgE syndrome, Omenn's syn-
 drome
Transplant rejection: lung, kidney, liver
Endocrine
Hypoadrenalism: Addison's disease, adrenal hemorrhage
Other
Atheroembolic disease
Irritation of serosal surfaces, including peritoneal dialysis
Inherited

site stages are never present in feces. Hence negative stool examinations do not necessarily exclude a helminthic etiology for eosinophilia, and examination of blood or appropriate tissue biopsy
material, as guided by the clinical findings and exposure history,
may be needed to diagnose specific tissue or blood-dwelling infections, including trichinosis, filarial infections, and in children, visceral larva migrans.

OTHER INFECTIOUS DISEASES. The characteristic response in
acute bacterial and viral infections is eosinopenia, although in the
convalescent phase of these diseases eosinophil numbers return to
normal and at times to above normal, as seen with scarlet fever.
Two fungal diseases may be associated with eosinophilia: aspergillosis (see Chapter 401), but only in the form of allergic bronchopulmonary aspergillosis and not as invasive disease; and coccidioidomycosis (see Chapter 395), following primary infection,
especially in conjunction with erythema nodosum and at times with
progressive disseminated disease. On occasion, eosinophilia may be
present in chronic tuberculosis (see Chapter 358).

ALLERGIC DISEASES. Allergic rhinitis and asthma (see Chapters 74 and 274) are commonly associated with eosinophilia. Hypersensitivity drug reactions can elicit eosinophilia without accompanying manifestations such as drug fever or organ dysfunction.
When organ dysfunction develops, cessation of drug administration is
necessary. Drug-induced interstitial nephritis (see Chapter 107) may
be accompanied by blood eosinophilia and eosinophils in the urine.

MYELOPROLIFERATIVE AND NEOPLASTIC DISEASES. Idiopathic hypereosinophilic syndrome is a myeloproliferative disease
characterized by sustained overproduction of eosinophils. The three
diagnostic criteria for this disorder are (1) eosinophilia in excess of
$1500/\mu L$ persisting for longer than 6 months; (2) lack of an identifiable parasitic, allergic, or other etiology for eosinophilia; and (3)
signs and symptoms of organ involvement. Not all patients with
prolonged eosinophilia develop organ involvement, and many have
benign courses. Moreover, the above diagnostic criteria are sufficiently broad potentially to include eosinophilic disorders of other
etiologies, currently unrecognized, that may have more favorable
courses. The presence of angioedema is a good prognostic

sign in hypereosinophilic patients, and this finding may be related
to the more recent identification of a distinct clinical syndrome of
recurrent episodic angioedema with eosinophilia, not complicated
by the development of hypereosinophilic cardiac disease.

The clinical signs and symptoms of hypereosinophilic syndrome
can be heterogeneous because of the diversity of potential organ
involvement. One of the most serious and more frequent complications in this disorder is cardiac disease secondary to endomyocardial thrombosis and fibrosis. Mitral and tricuspid regurgitation may
result from progressive fibrotic damage to the chordae tendineae,
and heart failure can develop from valvular incompetence and endomyocardial fibrosis. Cardiac involvement in hypereosinophilic
syndrome, which may require surgical valve replacement, has developed in association with eosinophilias of other recognized etiologies, occasionally including parasitic infections. A pathologically
similar disease, Löffler's endocarditis and endomyocardial fibrosis,
has been noted in tropical regions, where it is possible that antecedent parasite-elicited eosinophilias were responsible for the development of this cardiac disease. Echocardiography can facilitate detection and monitoring of these changes. Neurologic involvement
can take three forms: embolic disease originating from the heart,
diffuse encephalopathy, and peripheral neuropathy, especially
mononeuritis multiplex. Other organ systems that can be involved
include the skin, liver, spleen, gastrointestinal tract, and lungs. For
patients with prominent organ involvement, mortality without therapy is about 75% after 3 years. Therapy is aimed at suppressing
eosinophilia and is initiated with corticosteroids, to which about
one third of patients will respond. In those unresponsive to corticosteroids, hydroxyurea and interferon-α have also proved beneficial.

Eosinophilic leukemia is distinctly uncommon. Eosinophilia may
accompany chronic myelogenous leukemia (see Chapter 176), often
with basophilia, and some subtypes of acute myelogenous leukemia
(see Chapter 177), but it is uncommon with acute lymphoblastic
leukemia (see Chapter 177). In a minority of patients with Hodgkin's disease (see Chapter 180), blood eosinophils are elevated,
occasionally to high levels. Increases in marrow and lymph node
eosinophilia are more common. A small proportion of patients with
carcinomas, especially of mucin-producing epithelial cell origin,
have associated blood eosinophilia. Eosinophilia develops in some
patients with mastocytosis.

CUTANEOUS DISEASES. In addition to the neoplastic involvement of skin, a number of cutaneous diseases can be associated
with increased blood eosinophils, including scabies (see Chapter
435), bullous pemphigoid (see Chapter 522), and two diseases
associated with pregnancy: herpes gestationis and the syndrome of
pruritic urticarial papules and plaques of pregnancy. In episodic
angioedema with eosinophilia (see Chapter 273), recurrences are
marked by blood eosinophilia and prominent angioedema, at times
with significant weight gain from fluid retention, and less frequently by fever. This entity is responsive to corticosteroids.

PULMONARY EOSINOPHILIAS. Blood eosinophilia can infrequently accompany pleural fluid eosinophilia, which is a non-specific response seen with various disorders, including trauma and
even repeated thoracenteses.

GASTROINTESTINAL DISEASES. Eosinophilic gastroenteritis
(see Chapter 136) is often associated with blood eosinophilia. Eosinophils are often present in the lesions of ulcerative colitis, and
increased blood eosinophilia is occasionally found in both ulcerative colitis and Crohn's disease.

IMMUNE DISEASES. Of the various forms of vasculitis (see
Chapter 292), only two are commonly associated with eosinophilia:
hypersensitivity vasculitis and allergic granulomatous angiitis, or
the Churg-Strauss syndrome, in which asthma, eosinophilia, and
pulmonary and neurologic involvement are frequent. Although eosinophilia may uncommonly accompany rheumatoid arthritis (see
Chapter 286), any associated eosinophilia is more commonly due to
medications used to treat the disease. Cholesterol embolization (see
Chapter 112) is at times associated with eosinophilia and hypocomplementemia, thus suggesting a secondary immunologic component.
Some primary immunodeficiency syndromes are associated with
eosinophilia, including the hyper-IgE syndrome and Omenn's syndrome. Eosinophilic fasciitis is commonly associated with blood
eosinophilia.

OTHER DISEASES. Irritation of serosal surfaces can be associated with eosinophilia, and related diseases can include Dressler's
syndrome; eosinophilic pleural effusions; peritoneal and, at times,

blood eosinophilia developing during chronic peritoneal dialysis; and perhaps the eosinophilia that follows abdominal irradiation. Two notable, apparently toxic diseases, the eosinophilia-myalgia syndrome caused by contaminated L-tryptophan (see Chapter 510) and the earlier toxic oil syndrome in Spain, were prominently associated with eosinophilia. Loss of normal adrenoglucocorticosteroid production in Addison's disease (see Chapter 240), adrenal hemorrhage, or hypopituitarism can cause blood eosinophilia.

Lim K, Weller PF: Eosinophilia and eosinophil-related disorders. *In* Adkinson NF Jr, Busse WW, Ellis EF, et al. (eds): Allergy: Principles and Practice, 5th ed. Mosby, St Louis, 1998, pp 783–798. *Provides a comprehensive review of clinical conditions associated with eosinophilia.*

Weller PF, Bubley GJ: The idiopathic hypereosinophilic syndrome. Blood 83:2759, 1994. *Reviews the manifestations, differential diagnosis, and management of idiopathic hypereosinophilic syndrome.*

174 MYELOPROLIFERATIVE DISEASES

Ayalew Tefferi ■ Murray N. Silverstein

Blood cells are, in general, specified as being either lymphoid or myeloid (granulocytes, monocytes, erythrocytes, and platelets). Accordingly, hematologic malignancies are organized into lymphoproliferative or myeloproliferative disorders. Each of these disorders is operationally classified as being acute or chronic, depending on the proportion of immature precursor cells (blasts) in the bone marrow. In the myeloid lineage, the presence of more than 30% blasts in the bone marrow defines acute myeloid leukemia. A myeloid disorder that is not acute myeloid leukemia is referred to as either a myelodysplastic syndrome or a chronic myeloproliferative disease based, respectively, on the presence or absence of trilineage morphologic dysplasia, primarily involving the red blood cell series. The chronic myeloproliferative diseases include chronic myelogenous leukemia (CML), essential thrombocythemia, polycythemia vera, and agnogenic myeloid metaplasia. Occasionally, a chronic myeloid disorder is not classifiable as either myelodysplastic syndrome or chronic myeloproliferative disease. Examples are atypical CML and chronic neutrophilic leukemia.

As a group, the chronic myeloproliferative diseases are interrelated in that the clonal process originates at the myeloid progenitor cell level and may, secondarily, cause marrow fibrosis or undergo leukemic transformation. Among the chronic myeloproliferative diseases, only CML has been biologically characterized by the presence of a reciprocal genetic translocation between chromosomes 9 and 22. A similar consistent genetic abnormality has not been associated with the other chronic myeloproliferative diseases, and specific diagnosis is based on the presence or absence of certain clinical and laboratory characteristics. An increased red blood cell mass is required for the diagnosis of polycythemia vera. Similarly, the presence of substantial bone marrow fibrosis not associated with CML or polycythemia vera is the hallmark of agnogenic myeloid metaplasia. The diagnosis of essential thrombocythemia is one of exclusion, representing clonal thrombocytosis that is not classifiable as agnogenic myeloid metaplasia, polycythemia vera, myelodysplastic syndrome, or CML.

ESSENTIAL THROMBOCYTHEMIA

Epidemiology

Many retrospective studies of essential thrombocythemia suggest an incidence rate of 1.5 per 100,000 and a median age at diagnosis of 60 years. Because of referral bias, the epidemiologic information derived from these studies may not be generalizable to the population at large. Accordingly, a higher incidence rate (2.5 per 100,000) and median age at diagnosis (72 years) were noted in a population-based study from Olmsted County, Minnesota. Essential thrombocythemia has been described in children, and approximately 20% of patients are younger than 40 years. Females are overrepresented (1.6:1) in most studies, but the age-adjusted incidence rates may not be significantly different. Long-term use of dark hair dyes,

living in a tuff house, and working as an electrician have all been implicated as possible environmental risk factors.

Pathogenesis

Essential thrombocythemia is a clonal process arising from the multipotent hematopoietic progenitor cell, manifested by spontaneous colony formation in vitro. However, recent clonality studies using refined methods of X-linked DNA analysis have demonstrated both monoclonal and polyclonal hematopoiesis, supporting the contention that it is pathogenetically heterogeneous. Similar studies have also shown variable lineage involvements among affected cases, suggesting clonal origination at different hierarchical levels. Regardless, the preferential expansion of megakaryocytes and platelets remains unexplained.

A megakaryocyte growth factor gene has recently been cloned, and its protein, called thrombopoietin, has been shown to promote proliferation and maturation of megakaryocytes. Exogenous administration of thrombopoietin increases platelet production in humans. A point mutation in the thrombopoietin gene has been associated with hereditary essential thrombocythemia, but similar genetic lesions of thrombopoietin or its receptor (*c-mpl*) have not been found in nonconsanguineous essential thrombocythemia. Furthermore, the demonstration of reduced platelet *c-mpl* expression makes it unlikely that thrombopoiesis in essential thrombocythemia is growth factor–dependent. Instead, the low levels of *c-mpl* expression may explain the above-normal thrombopoietin levels.

Despite the description of numerous platelet function abnormalities in patients with essential thrombocythemia, a correlation of these defects with thrombotic or hemorrhagic risk has not been possible. Furthermore, the mechanisms of vasomotor symptoms, bleeding, and thrombosis are poorly understood. Clonal platelets in essential thrombocythemia may mediate small-vessel endothelial inflammation or occlusion, resulting in erythromelalgia and other functional symptoms. Similar to the situation with *c-mpl*, α-adrenergic and prostaglandin D_2-receptors are markedly reduced in platelets of patients with essential thrombocythemia. Acquired type II von Willebrand's disease is occasionally associated with markedly increased platelet counts and may involve abnormal platelet adsorption of the von Willebrand factor multimers.

Diagnosis

Before making a diagnosis of essential thrombocythemia, reactive thrombocytosis should first be excluded (Table 174–1). A persistent increase of the platelet count not associated with iron deficiency, splenectomy, surgery, an infectious or inflammatory condition, or metastatic cancer strongly suggests clonal thrombocytosis (Fig. 174–1). When a potential cause for reactive thrombocytosis is not clinically identifiable, laboratory evaluation of serum ferritin, the peripheral blood smear, and C-reactive protein may be helpful in the diagnostic process. A low serum ferritin value is diagnostic of iron deficiency. The peripheral blood smear reveals red blood cell Howell-Jolly bodies after splenectomy. C-reactive protein levels should be normal in uncomplicated essential throm-

Table 174–1 ■ CAUSES OF REACTIVE THROMBOCYTOSIS

ACUTE CONDITIONS
Acute bleeding
Postsurgical period
Acute hemolysis
Infections
Tissue damage (acute pancreatitis, myocardial infarction, trauma, burns)
Coronary artery bypass grafting
Rebound recovery from chemotherapy or immune thrombocytopenia
CHRONIC CONDITIONS
Iron-deficiency anemia
Surgical or functional asplenia
Metastatic cancer, lymphoma
Inflammation (rheumatoid arthritis, vasculitis, allergies)
Renal failure, nephrotic syndrome

From Tefferi A, Silverstein MN: Chronic myeloproliferative disorders. *In* Wachter RM, Hollander H, Goldman L (eds): Hospital Medicine. Baltimore, Williams & Wilkins, in press.

Note: Mayo Foundation retains copyright to Mayo copyrighted illustrations. Mayo Foundation is "author" for purposes of copyright ownership under the "work made for hire" provision of the copyright law.

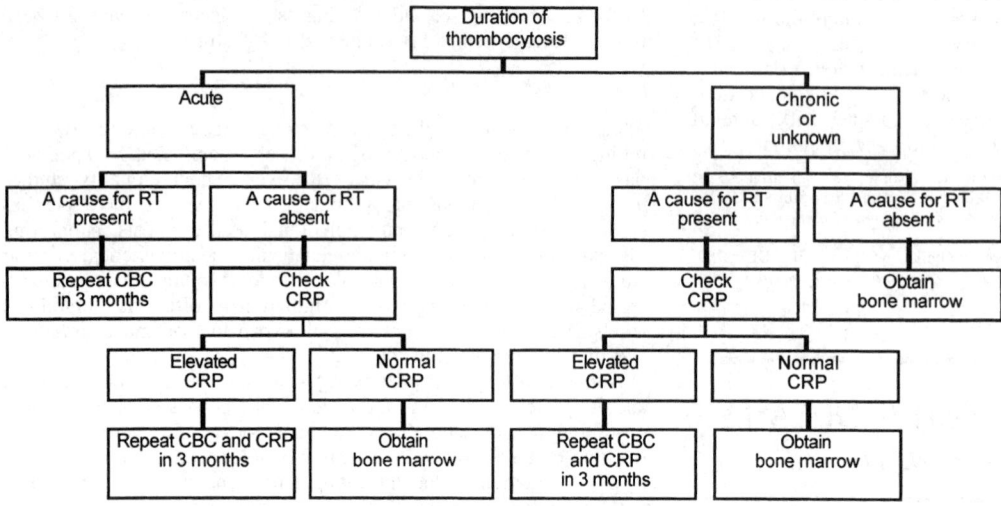

FIGURE 174–1. ■ A diagnostic approach to the asymptomatic patient with thrombocytosis. CBC = complete blood cell count; CRP = C-reactive protein; RT = reactive thrombocytosis.

bocythemia and increased in most cases of reactive thrombocytosis (Fig. 174–2). Serum thrombopoietin levels are increased in both reactive and primary thrombocytosis and are not diagnostically helpful.

If the clinical and laboratory evaluation is unrevealing for reactive thrombocytosis, bone marrow examination is needed. A bone marrow examination is also recommended, regardless of the possibility of reactive thrombocytosis, if clinical findings (splenomegaly, persistent leukocytosis or erythrocytosis, generalized pruritus, unusual thrombosis, erythromelalgia) consistent with chronic myeloproliferative disease accompany the thrombocytosis. The bone marrow in essential thrombocythemia commonly shows atypical megakaryocytes and megakaryocytic clusters (Color Plate 6B). In addition, some cases may show evidence of bone marrow fibrosis by a reticulin stain. Cytogenetic abnormalities are detected in approximately 6% of patients with essential thrombocythemia.

Once clonal thrombocytosis is suspected, a peripheral smear and a bone marrow examination with cytogenetic studies are recommended to distinguish essential thrombocythemia from the other chronic myeloid disorders. An increased red blood cell mass indicates polycythemia vera. The demonstration of t(9;22) or the *bcr-abl* rearrangement on DNA analysis is consistent with the diagnosis of CML, even if the patient presents with isolated thrombocytosis. Substantial bone marrow fibrosis is characteristic of agnogenic my-

eloid metaplasia. The presence of dyserythropoiesis suggests a diagnosis of myelodysplastic syndrome. These distinctions are important because the prognoses of the other chronic myeloid disorders are not as favorable as that of essential thrombocythemia, and treatment may be different.

Clinical Features and Prognosis

Life expectancy in essential thrombocythemia is near normal, and the risk of leukemic conversion or post-thrombocythemic myelofibrosis is less than 5%. However, the clinical course is complicated by frequent vasomotor and thrombohemorrhagic events. Vasomotor symptoms (headache, erythromelalgia, acroparesthesia, visual symptoms) may occur in more than one-third of patients and are usually controlled by the use of acetylsalicylic acid. Erythromelalgia refers to a burning pain and erythema of the extremities. Associated leukocytosis and palpable splenomegaly occur in approximately one-third and one-quarter of patients, respectively.

Compared with a control population, patients with essential thrombocythemia have a significantly increased risk for thrombosis (1% versus 7% per patient-year). The thrombotic risk is highest for patients older than 60 years (15% per patient-year) and for those with a prior history of thrombosis (31% per patient-year). Interestingly, the degree of thrombocytosis or platelet function abnormalities has not been correlated with thrombotic risk. Therefore, currently defined risk factors in essential thrombocythemia are a history of thrombosis and age older than 60 years.

Bleeding complications, in the absence of antiplatelet therapy, are infrequent and usually nonconsequential. In one large study, only 5% of the patients had a bleeding history at diagnosis, and an additional 5% had hemorrhages in a 5-year follow-up. In contrast, thrombotic events were noted in 15% of the patients at diagnosis and in 11% during follow-up. A fatal outcome was associated more with thrombosis than with hemorrhage.

Treatment

Treatment is aimed at alleviating vasomotor symptoms and reducing thrombotic and bleeding complications without increasing the intrinsically low risk of leukemic transformation. The use of low-dose acetylsalicylic acid (81 mg daily) is effective for controlling vasomotor symptoms. Occasionally, a platelet-lowering agent may be required for stubborn cases. In the absence of vasomotor symptoms, the avoidance of nonsteroidal anti-inflammatory agents is often adequate to prevent catastrophic hemorrhage.

The use of platelet-lowering agents is primarily for prevention of thrombosis, which is uncommon (3%) in young patients (age less than 60 years) who do not have a history of thrombosis; therefore, these patients may not require therapy. These drugs are also discouraged in women of childbearing age because of an increased risk of first-trimester spontaneous abortion (45%), which is neither predictable nor influenced by specific therapy. After the first trimes-

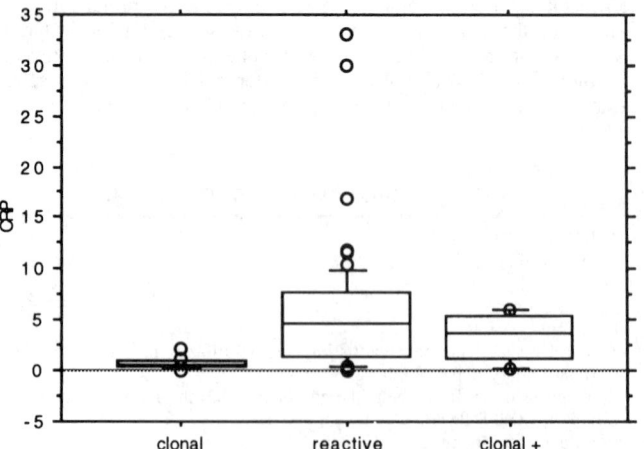

FIGURE 174–2. ■ Plasma C-reactive protein values in 20 patients with clonal thrombocytosis (clonal), 64 patients with reactive thrombocytosis (reactive), and 7 patients with clonal thrombocytosis who also had conditions associated with reactive thrombocytosis (clonal +). (From Tefferi A, Ho TC, Ahmann GJ, et al: Plasma interleukin-6 and C-reactive protein levels in reactive versus clonal thrombocytosis. Am J Med 97:374, 1994. By permission of Excerpta Medica.)

ter, complications are rare, and drugs or platelet apheresis during delivery may not be needed. In high-risk patients (prior history of thrombosis or age older than 60 years), hydroxyurea significantly reduces thrombotic events compared with no treatment (3.6% versus 24%) and is reasonable, starting at 500 mg orally twice a day.

Concern regarding the potential leukemogenicity of hydroxyurea has led to the exploration of alternative therapeutic agents in essential thrombocythemia. Anagrelide is an oral imidazoquinazolin derivative that has recently been approved by the Food and Drug Administration as a platelet-lowering agent in essential thrombocythemia; it lowers platelet counts by interfering with the maturation of megakaryocytes. The starting dose is 0.5 mg orally three times a day. Side effects occur in one-third of patients and include headache, fluid retention, dizziness, palpitations, tachycardia, diarrhea and, rarely, heart failure. The response rate is more than 90%, and response occurs at a median of 3 weeks. Anagrelide does not affect the leukocyte count or the hemoglobin level. Interferon-α lowers platelet counts by suppressing progenitor cell proliferation and therefore causes a concomitant decrease in leukocytes. In essential thrombocythemia, interferon-α controls thrombocytosis, splenomegaly, and disease-associated symptoms in approximately 80% of patients. Starting doses are 3 to 5 million units subcutaneously daily, and the average response time is 12 weeks. Side effects include a transient influenza-like syndrome associated with fever and chills, myalgias, headache, and arthralgias. Chronic side effects include fatigue, nausea, anorexia, weight loss, diarrhea, increase in liver aminotransferase levels, altered mental status, and depression. However, neither anagrelide nor interferon-α has been tested in randomized trials.

The issue of drug leukemogenicity in essential thrombocythemia has not been settled. Acute leukemia has been reported in the presence or absence of antecedent chemotherapy, and there is no controlled study demonstrating an increased incidence of leukemia in association with drug use. The leukemogenic potential of hydroxyurea in essential thrombocythemia, if any, is very small and does not prohibit its use in patients older than 60 years. In younger patients with a history of thrombosis, anagrelide is a reasonable alternative if there is a concern about the leukemogenicity of hydroxyurea, and interferon-α is preferred for women of childbearing age who require treatment. Regardless of the particular platelet-lowering agent used, the platelet count should be kept less than 400,000/μL when treatment is indicated.

POLYCYTHEMIA VERA

Epidemiology

Reported population incidence rates for polycythemia vera have ranged from 0.5 to 3.5 per 100,000, and evidence suggests a higher incidence in Jews. In a population-based study from Olmsted County, Minnesota, the incidence rates did not increase with time, and the average was about 2.3 per 100,000. In general, the median age at diagnosis is approximately 60 years and, unlike essential thrombocythemia, polycythemia vera has a male preponderance (1.6:1) that is more pronounced when adjusted for age (2.2:1). Polycythemia vera is rarely described in children, and congenital and secondary causes of erythrocytosis must be excluded before the diagnosis is established in children. An excess number of cases of polycythemia vera have been reported among participants of a nuclear weapons test.

Pathogenesis

More than 20 years have elapsed since the original glucose-6-phosphate dehydrogenase isoenzyme studies suggested the clonal nature of polycythemia vera. Recent X-linked DNA studies have confirmed these observations, including multilineage involvement by the clonal process. Accordingly, monoclonal proliferations of all myeloid cells, including erythrocytes, platelets, granulocytes, and monocytes, have been demonstrated in polycythemia vera. Molecular lesions responsible for the predominantly erythroid clonal expansion have not been defined. Recent studies have focused on genes regulating the production and expression of the erythroid growth factor erythropoietin (EPO) and its receptor (EPO-R). So far, EPO-R genes have been shown to be intact in polycythemia vera, whereas point mutations have been demonstrated in some patients with familial erythrocytosis.

In view of the clonal nature of the disease, serum EPO levels are often suppressed in patients with polycythemia vera. Similarly, unlike in normal individuals, erythroid progenitor cells from patients with polycythemia vera can produce in vitro erythroid colonies without the addition of EPO to the culture medium. Some progenitor cells appear to be totally EPO-independent, whereas others are hypersensitive to very low concentrations of EPO. This growth factor hypersensitivity in patients with polycythemia vera is also seen with myeloid growth factors and insulin-like growth factor-1, suggesting a defective signal transduction pathway common to both EPO and other growth factors.

Quantitative and qualitative abnormalities of red cells and platelets have been implicated in the pathogenesis of thrombosis and bleeding in polycythemia vera. Hematocrit levels of more than 45% have been associated with an increased incidence of clinical thrombosis and decreased cerebral blood flow. The coexisting clonal abnormalities of platelets may play a major role during microvascular occlusions. The increased whole blood viscosity associated with increased hematocrit levels and the promotion of increased interactions between platelets and the endothelium due to in vivo flow dynamics are believed to contribute to the development of thrombosis in polycythemia vera. A therapeutic reduction in hematocrit levels and platelet counts decreases but does not abolish the risk of thrombosis in polycythemia vera. The mechanisms behind this residual risk are currently unknown.

Diagnosis

Ideally, the diagnosis of polycythemia vera requires the demonstration of an increased red cell mass, exclusion of secondary erythrocytosis, and some evidence of a chronic myeloproliferative disease. Approximately 30 years ago, the Polycythemia Vera Study Group developed a set of criteria to ensure uniform accrual of patients with polycythemia vera to treatment protocols (Table 174–2). Inadvertently, these criteria have since been used to diagnose polycythemia vera. The subsequent demonstration of early cases of polycythemia vera that do not fulfill the diagnostic criteria and inaccuracies inherent in measurements of red blood cell mass have necessitated a revision in diagnostic criteria. The process has been facilitated by the current availability of reliable serum EPO (sEPO) assays and culture methods to grow endogenous erythroid colonies.

The first step in evaluating erythrocytosis is to determine whether it is acquired (Fig. 174–3) or congenital. A working diagnosis of polycythemia vera is made when the sEPO level is lower than normal, and further laboratory investigations are undertaken to confirm the diagnosis. The diagnosis is seriously considered when the low sEPO level is associated with any one of the following: a hematocrit level of more than 60% (53% in women), splenomegaly, persistent leukocytosis, persistent thrombocytosis, microcytosis, unusual thrombotic history, post-bath pruritus, erythromelalgia, bone marrow panhyperplasia with atypical megakaryocytes, bone marrow reticulin fibrosis, clonal cytogenetic abnormalities, or in vitro formation of endogenous erythroid colonies. If none of these factors

Table 174–2 ■ POLYCYTHEMIA VERA STUDY GROUP DIAGNOSTIC CRITERIA FOR POLYCYTHEMIA VERA*

MAJOR CRITERIA
1. Increased red cell mass
   Males, $\geq$36 mL/kg
   Females, $\geq$32 mL/kg
2. Normal arterial oxygen saturation $\geq$92%
3. Splenomegaly

MINOR CRITERIA
1. Platelets >400,000/μL
2. Leukocytes >12,000/μL
3. Leukocyte alkaline phosphatase >100
   or
   Vitamin B$_{12}$ >900 pg/mL
   or
   Unbound B$_{12}$ binding capacity >2200 pg/mL

*Diagnosis of polycythemia vera requires the presence of all three major criteria or the presence of the first two major criteria and any two minor criteria.
Modified from Berlin NI: Diagnosis and classification of the polycythemias. Semin Hematol 12:339, 1975. By permission of Grune & Stratton.

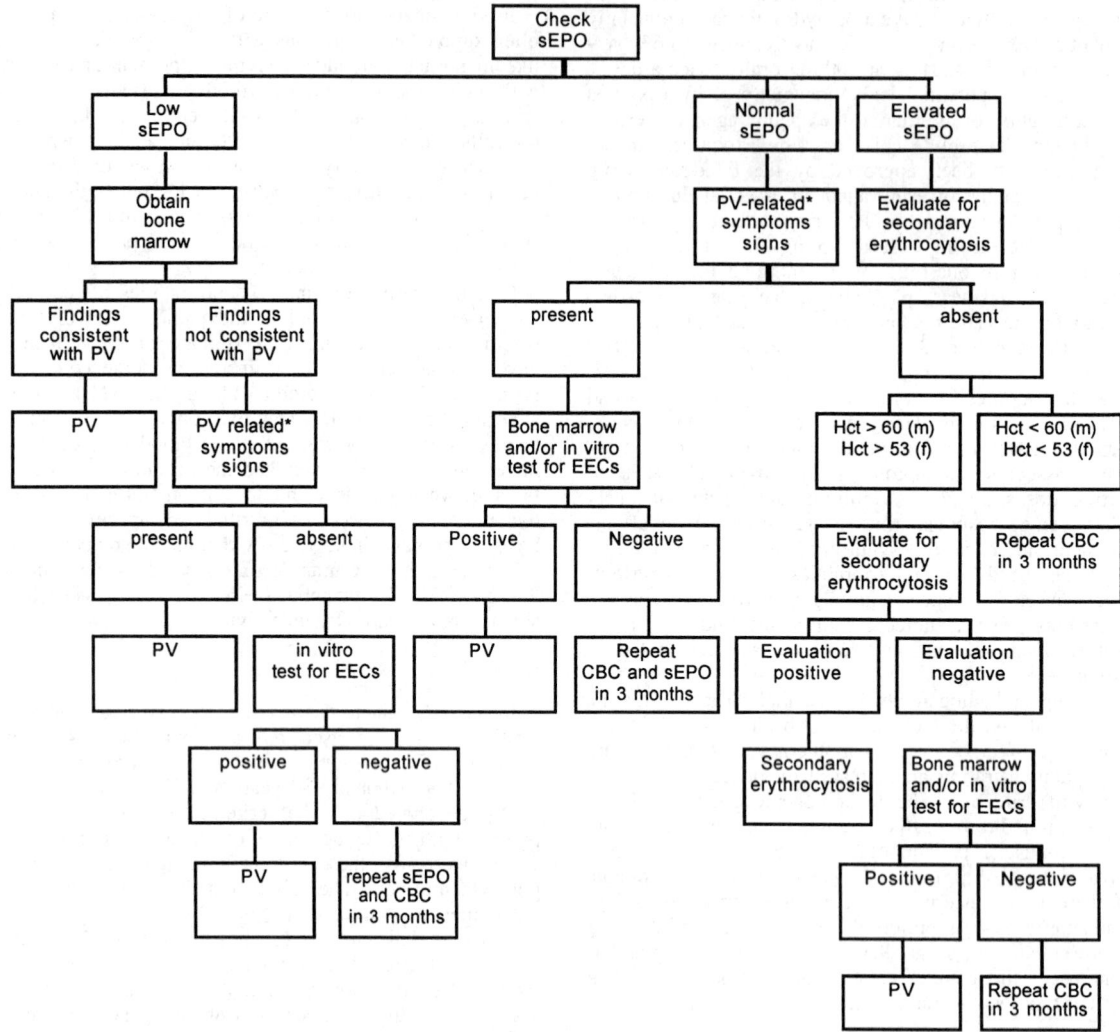

FIGURE 174–3. ■ A diagnostic approach to acquired erythrocytosis. CBC = complete blood cell count; EEC = endogenous (spontaneous) erythroid colonies; f = female; Hct = hematocrit; m = male; PV = polycythemia vera; sEPO = serum erythropoietin level. *PV-related symptoms and signs include unusual thrombosis, generalized pruritus, splenomegaly, persistent leukocytosis or thrombocytosis, and erythromelalgia.

are present, then the sEPO level and complete blood cell count should be determined again in 3 months.

A normal sEPO level does not exclude the possibility of polycythemia vera, and in the presence of any polycythemia vera–related features (unusual thrombosis, erythromelalgia, post-bath pruritus, splenomegaly, persistent leukocytosis or thrombocytosis, microcytosis) a bone marrow examination or an in vitro test for endogenous (spontaneous) erythroid colonies is appropriate. In the absence of polycythemia vera–related features, further investigation depends on the hematocrit level. If the value is less than 60% (53% in women), then observation with a repeat test of the hematocrit level in 3 months is recommended. "Apparent erythrocytosis" (a seemingly high hematocrit level not associated with increased red blood cell mass) has been associated with dehydration, use of diuretics, tobacco use, and hypertension. If a normal EPO level is associated with a hematocrit value of more than 60% (53% in women), then evaluation for secondary erythrocytosis is appropriate, followed, if negative, by bone marrow examination or in vitro testing for endogenous erythroid colony formation.

The bone marrow examination in polycythemia vera typically shows panhyperplasia and atypical megakaryocytes with or without associated bone marrow fibrosis. The rate of cytogenetic abnormalities is approximately 12% in untreated cases and 40% in treated cases. The most frequent abnormalities include trisomy 8, trisomy 9, and deletion of the long arm of chromosome 20 (20q-).

Erythrocytosis associated with an increased sEPO level is very unlikely to represent polycythemia vera and, instead, a working diagnosis of congenital or acquired secondary erythrocytosis is made (Table 174–3). Levels of sEPO may be normal in certain types of secondary erythrocytosis, both congenital and acquired. Acquired secondary erythrocytosis is associated with either an "appropriate EPO production" in response to tissue hypoxia or an "oxygen-independent EPO production" by tumors.

A congenital erythrocytosis is suspected in the presence of disease onset at an early age and a family history of erythrocytosis. Laboratory investigation begins with the determination of the oxygen pressure at 50% hemoglobin saturation (P_{50}). A low P_{50} suggests either a high-oxygen-affinity hemoglobinopathy (autosomal-dominant) or familial 2,3-diphosphoglycerate deficiency (autosomal-recessive). In both of these disorders, sEPO levels are usually low. A normal P_{50} in congenital erythrocytosis is consistent with either autosomal-dominant (benign) familial erythrocytosis or autosomal-recessive familial erythrocytosis. Benign familial erythrocytosis is associated with a low or normal sEPO level and erythroid progenitor EPO hypersensitivity. EPO-R mutations have been recognized in some patients with the benign form. Recessive familial erythrocytosis is the most frequent form of familial erythrocytosis and is prevalent in Russia.

Clinical Features and Prognosis

At presentation, patients are either asymptomatic or manifest symptoms and signs related to hyperviscosity and tumor burden, including headaches, dizziness, visual symptoms, paresthesias, fa-

Table 174-3 ■ CAUSES OF SECONDARY ERYTHROCYTOSIS

CONGENITAL
Low P_{50}*
High-oxygen-affinity hemoglobinopathy
2,3-Diphosphoglycerate deficiency
Normal P_{50}*
Autosomal-dominant (benign) familial erythrocytosis
Autosomal-recessive familial erythrocytosis
ACQUIRED
Appropriate erythropoietin response
   Chronic lung disease
   Arteriovenous or intracardiac shunts
   High-altitude habitat
   Chronic carbon monoxide exposure (smoking)
Pathologic erythropoietin production
   Tumors (liver, kidney, cerebellum)
   Uterine fibroids
   Postrenal transplant
   Benign renal disorders (e.g., polycystic kidneys)

*Oxygen pressure at 50% hemoglobin saturation.
From Tefferi A, Silverstein MN: Chronic myeloproliferative disorders. *In* Wachter RM, Hollander H, Goldman L (eds): Hospital Medicine. Baltimore, Williams & Wilkins, in press.

tigue, abdominal discomfort, weight loss, and night sweats. Generalized pruritus (exacerbated by contact with water) is a poorly understood, frequent disease manifestation. Clinical examination may reveal plethora (facial erythema), retinal vein distention, and palpable splenomegaly. More than one-half of patients have associated leukocytosis or thrombocytosis. Microcytosis is frequent and indicates iron deficiency from phlebotomy or occult gastrointestinal blood loss. Nonspecific additional laboratory abnormalities include increases of leukocyte alkaline phosphatase score, serum B_{12}, and uric acid.

The primary morbid conditions associated with polycythemia vera are thrombosis and bleeding, which are direct consequences of not only increased red blood cell mass but also of other unidentified disease-related conditions. The thrombotic events include cerebrovascular accident, transient ischemic attack, retinal vein thrombosis, central retinal artery occlusion, myocardial infarction, angina, pulmonary embolism, hepatic and portal vein thrombosis, deep vein thrombosis, and peripheral arterial occlusion. Bleeding occurs usually in the gastrointestinal tract. In addition, patients may experience vasomotor disturbances (headache, dizziness, acral dysesthesia, erythromelalgia, visual symptoms). Furthermore, polycythemia vera is associated with a delayed risk of transformation into acute leukemia and myelofibrosis, the latter sometimes referred to as "spent phase."

Despite these complications, median survival in young patients exceeds 15 years. In one of the largest studies ever conducted in patients with polycythemia vera, thrombosis was found in 19% of 1213 patients followed for a median of 5.3 years. Risk of thrombosis correlated with advanced age (more than 4% per year for patients older than 60 years versus 1.8% per year for those younger than 40 years) and a history of thrombosis. These and other risk factors for thrombosis (treatment with phlebotomy alone, phlebotomy requirement more than six times per year) were previously identified during the original studies of the Polycythemia Vera Study Group.

Treatment

Introduced in the first decade of the 20th century, phlebotomy (venesection) remains the cornerstone of therapy. With the current use of phlebotomy alone as initial therapy, the estimated median survival is between 12.5 and 13.5 years. To date, no other form of initial therapy has been shown to result in better survival, and overall survival in a large randomized trial conducted by the Polycythemia Vera Study Group was actually lower when chlorambucil or radioactive phosphorus was used with phlebotomy as initial therapy because of excess late fatalities from both hematologic and nonhematologic malignancies. Although secondary malignancies contribute to late fatalities, the most frequent cause of death in the study was thrombosis (29.2%). In the first 3 years of therapy, patients randomized to the phlebotomy-alone arm had significantly

more thrombotic events. Subsequent studies showed that the use of acetylsalicylic acid (300 mg three times daily) and dipyridamole (75 mg three times daily) in addition to phlebotomy did not reduce the risk of early thrombosis but instead significantly increased the incidence of gastrointestinal hemorrhage. By comparison, the same Polycythemia Vera Study Group reported that the 9.8% rate of thrombotic events in the first 7 years in hydroxyuria-treated patients was significantly less than the 33% rate in a historical control group treated with phlebotomy alone. After a median follow-up period of 8.6 years, acute leukemia developed in 5.9% of the hydroxyurea-treated patients who remained "on-study." Therefore, hydroxyurea reduced early thrombosis without either compromising survival or significantly increasing the rates of acute leukemia or post-polycythemic myelofibrosis. Other prospective studies, however, have reported variable results regarding the leukemogenic potential of hydroxyurea, and the issue remains unsettled.

New drugs, including interferon-α and anagrelide, lack intrinsic mutagenicity. Interferon-α (3 million units subcutaneously three times a week) controls erythrocytosis, thrombocytosis, splenomegaly, and pruritus in most patients with polycythemia vera. Anagrelide (0.5 mg orally four times a day) effectively lowers platelet counts in patients with polycythemia vera. Both of these new drugs are more expensive and toxic than hydroxyurea, and their role in the overall management of patients with polycythemia vera has not been defined. Recent studies have shown effective suppression of platelet thromboxane A_2 production with low-dose acetylsalicylic acid (40 mg) and have revived interest in its use to prevent thrombotic complications in polycythemia vera.

Based on currently available information, all patients should undergo phlebotomy with the goal of keeping the hematocrit values less than 45% in men and 42% in women. Approximately 500 mL of blood may be removed daily (in symptomatic patients) or weekly (in asymptomatic patients) until the target hematocrit level is reached. Thereafter, the frequency is adjusted to maintain the required hematocrit level at all times. No additional therapy may be required in patients who are at low risk for thrombosis (age less than 60 years, no history of thrombosis). In patients at high risk for thrombosis, hydroxyurea (starting dose 500 mg orally twice a day) is recommended as a supplement to phlebotomy.

For patients who do not tolerate hydroxyurea because of either side effects or neutropenia, interferon-α is a reasonable alternative. Interferon-α may also be considered an alternative to hydroxyurea in women of childbearing age and in young patients (age less than 50 years) in whom many years of therapy with hydroxyurea are anticipated. Radioactive phosphorus (2.3 mCi/m^2) may be considered if life expectancy is less than 10 years or compliance is an issue. In the absence of a history of thrombosis, it is unclear whether drug supplement to phlebotomy benefits young patients with cardiovascular risk factors or thrombocytosis. Low-dose acetylsalicylic acid (81 mg daily) is effective for alleviating vasomotor symptoms and is recommended if there are other treatment indications; whether it is safe and effective for preventing early thrombosis associated with polycythemia vera is being evaluated in a randomized study.

AGNOGENIC MYELOID METAPLASIA AND MYELOFIBROSIS

Epidemiology

Agnogenic myeloid metaplasia has the lowest incidence rate among the chronic myeloproliferative diseases. In a recent population-based study from Olmsted County, only 21 cases were identified over 20 years, and the incidence rate was 1.3 per 100,000. Reported population incidence rates were 0.5 per 100,000 from Western Australia and 0.7 per 100,000 from Northern Israel. The incidence rates were significantly higher in the older age groups, and the median age at diagnosis ranged from 60 to 70 years. Approximately 10% of the patients are younger than 50 years, and the disease has rarely been reported in children. The sex distributions vary among different studies, but they show a slight male preponderance. An excess of myelofibrosis has been reported among patients exposed to thorium dioxide, among survivors of the atomic bomb explosion at Hiroshima, and among workers at petroleum manufacturing plants.

Table 174–4 ■ CAUSES OF BONE MARROW FIBROSIS

MYELOID DISORDERS	NONHEMATOLOGIC DISORDERS
Chronic myeloproliferative diseases	Metastatic cancer
Agnogenic myeloid metaplasia	Connective tissue disease
Polycythemia vera	Systemic lupus erythematosus
Chronic myelogenous leukemia	Progressive systemic sclerosis
Essential thrombocythemia	Infections
Myelodysplastic syndrome	Human immunodeficiency virus disease
Acute myelofibrosis	Disseminated mycobacterial or fungal infections
Acute megakaryoblastic leukemia	Vitamin D deficiency rickets
Acute myeloid leukemia	Renal osteodystrophy
Mast cell disease	Parathyroid disease
Malignant histiocytosis	Paget's disease
LYMPHOID DISORDERS	Gray platelet syndrome
Hodgkin's disease	Osteopetrosis
Non-Hodgkin's lymphoma	
Hairy cell leukemia	
Multiple myeloma	
Acute lymphocytic leukemia	

From Tefferi A, Silverstein MN: Chronic myeloproliferative disorders. *In* Wachter RM, Hollander H, Goldman L (eds): Hospital Medicine. Baltimore, Williams & Wilkins, in press.

Pathogenesis

Several pathogenetic mechanisms work together to bring about the ineffective hematopoiesis, bone marrow fibrosis, and extramedullary hematopoiesis associated with agnogenic myeloid metaplasia. The aboriginal process is the generation of clonal megakaryocytes as part of a multilineage myeloproliferation. Studies based on analyses of glucose-6-phosphate dehydrogenase isoenzyme patterns, cytogenetics, N-*ras* mutations, and X-linked DNA analyses have all supported the multipotent hematopoietic progenitor cell origin of the clonal process in agnogenic myeloid metaplasia. In contrast, the collagen-secreting fibroblasts are polyclonal and are secondarily affected by megakaryocyte-derived growth factors. The primary growth factor implicated in the pathogenesis of bone marrow fibrosis is transforming growth factor (TGF)-β. TGF-β is a potent stimulator of collagen biosynthesis by fibroblasts. Other growth factors that may collaborate with TGF-β include platelet-derived growth factor, epidermal growth factor, and basic fibroblast growth factor. Similarly, it has been suggested that vascular endothelial growth factors may be involved in the pathogenesis of extramedullary hematopoiesis and thrombosis associated with agnogenic myeloid metaplasia. Recent experiments involving the injection of high doses of thrombopoietin (TPO) or promoting endogenous TPO excess by retrovirally transferring the TPO gene have been associated with induction of both increased levels of TGF-β and bone marrow fibrosis in mice, supporting the important role of megakaryocytes in bone marrow fibrosis.

Diagnosis and Clinical Presentation

The peripheral blood smear provides the first clue to the diagnosis by revealing a leukoerythroblastic blood picture (the presence of nucleated red blood cells, immature granulocytes, and teardrop-shaped red blood cells) (Color Plate 6C). The diagnosis is confirmed by a bone marrow biopsy. Collagenous fibers are appreciated in sections of marrow stained with hematoxylin-eosin, and a "reticulin" stain with silver impregnation provides additional detail (Color Plate 6D). However, bone marrow fibrosis is not specific to agnogenic myeloid metaplasia and can accompany any of the other chronic myeloproliferative diseases and myelodysplastic syndromes. In addition, other hematologic and nonhematologic diseases may be associated with reactive bone marrow fibrosis (Table 174–4). Therefore, a careful clinical and bone marrow morphologic evaluation and cytogenetic studies are strongly recommended before making the diagnosis of agnogenic myeloid metaplasia. Cytogenetic abnormalities, including del(13q) and del(20q), occur in approximately one-third of patients at diagnosis.

Approximately one-fifth of patients may present with asymptomatic splenomegaly. Of the remaining, about half present with mild to moderate anemia and the other half with severe anemia and marked splenomegaly (Fig. 174–4). Constitutional symptoms (weight loss, fever, sweats) prevail during the advanced stages of the disease, and a few patients may manifest bleeding or thrombotic complications. Laboratory features at diagnosis include a hemoglobin level less than 10 g/dL in 45% of patients, leukocyte value of more than 30,000/μL in 11%, and thrombocytopenia in 26%. A few patients have mild prolongations of the prothrombin and partial thromboplastin times along with decreased levels of factors V and VIII. These abnormalities may or may not be accompanied by laboratory features of low-grade disseminated intravascular coagulation.

Clinical Course and Prognosis

The median survival in agnogenic myeloid metaplasia may be as long as 8 years or as short as 1 year depending on the absence or presence of unfavorable clinical characteristics, including anemia, thrombocytopenia, left-shifted leukocytosis, and cytogenetic abnormalities. Causes of death include heart failure, infection, and leukemic transformation, the latter occurring in approximately 10% of patients. Most patients experience progressive anemia requiring frequent red blood cell transfusions and massive hepatosplenomegaly associated with the hypercatabolic symptoms of profound fatigue, weight loss, night sweats, and low-grade fever. In addition, some patients may develop extramedullary hematopoiesis in the spinal cord, the pleural and peritoneal cavities, and other organs. Disease progression into a clinical picture identical to agnogenic myeloid metaplasia occurs in approximately 9% of patients with polycythemia vera and less than 2% of those with essential thrombocythemia. Treatment of patients with post-polycythemic or post-thrombocythemic myelofibrosis is similar to that of patients with agnogenic myeloid metaplasia.

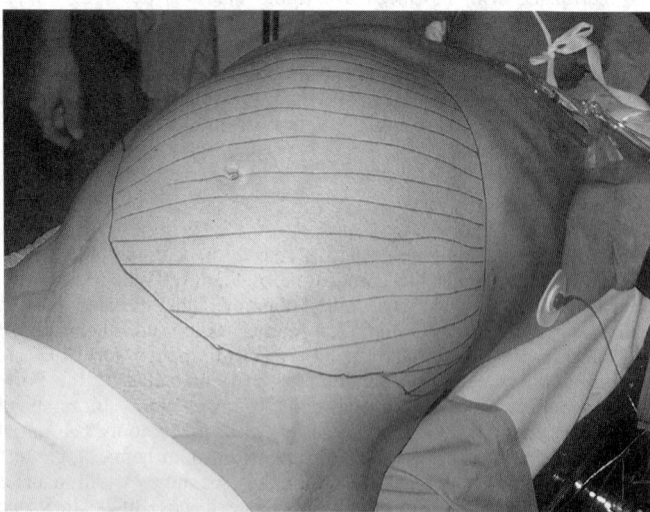

FIGURE 174–4. ■ Marked splenomegaly in a patient with agnogenic myeloid metaplasia.

Except for allogeneic bone marrow transplantation (see Chapter 182), current therapy is not curative, does not prevent leukemic transformation, and may not prolong life. Therefore, treatment efforts have been largely palliative and mostly directed at improving anemia and alleviating symptomatic organomegaly. In the very few patients who are appropriate candidates for allogeneic transplantation, the procedure is potentially curative in one-third.

As initial treatment of anemia, a combination of an androgen preparation (fluoxymesterone, 10 mg orally twice a day) and a corticosteroid (prednisone, 30 mg orally) is used. Approximately one-third of patients respond to this combination. After 1 month of therapy, fluoxymesterone treatment is continued in responding patients, whereas the corticosteroid is tapered. For steroid-dependent patients and for those who do not respond to fluoxymesterone, danazol (400 mg orally twice a day) may be useful in approximately 20% of patients. All patients treated with androgens should have periodic monitoring of liver function, and male patients should be screened for prostate cancer before initiating therapy. In addition, the virilizing side effects should be emphasized to female patients.

In patients who do not respond to androgen therapy, a therapeutic trial of EPO (10,000 units subcutaneously three times a week) may benefit the occasional patient with an endogenous EPO level of less than 100 mU/mL. Patients in whom both androgen and EPO therapy fail may experience an improvement in their anemia after splenectomy. Despite these treatment options, periodic red blood cell transfusion remains the major supportive therapy. Secondary hemosiderosis from chronic blood transfusion may result in heart failure and liver injury. Deferoxamine (2 g by daily continuous 12-hour subcutaneous injection) may prevent complications of iron overload.

Splenectomy is considered for patients with symptomatic splenomegaly (mechanical discomfort, refractory thrombocytopenia, hypercatabolic symptoms, portal hypertension). Laboratory evidence of disseminated intravascular coagulation before splenectomy may increase the risk of perioperative bleeding, and it is recommended that the procedure be postponed until the abnormalities are corrected. At experienced centers, the mortality rate associated with the procedure should be less than 10%. Postsurgical complications include intra-abdominal bleeding, subphrenic abscess, sepsis, large vessel thrombosis, extreme thrombocytosis, and accelerated hepatomegaly. The thrombocytosis and hepatomegaly may be transiently controlled with hydroxyurea (starting dose 500 mg orally three times daily) or 2-chlorodeoxyadenosine.

After splenectomy, almost all patients experience improvement in hypercatabolic symptoms and portal hypertension. In addition, approximately one-half of patients with refractory anemia or thrombocytopenia may benefit from splenectomy. In poor surgical candidates, the alternative to splenectomy is splenic irradiation (200 to 300 cGy delivered in 10 to 15 daily fractions), which usually provides a transient (3 to 6 months) benefit. Fatal myelosuppression after splenic irradiation is not infrequent. Radiation therapy is most useful in the management of extramedullary hematopoiesis.

Cortelazzo S, Finazzi G, Ruggeri M, et al: Hydroxyurea for patients with essential thrombocythemia and a high risk of thrombosis. N Engl J Med 332:1132, 1995. *Randomized study in patients with essential thrombocythemia, proving the benefit of hydroxyurea in high-risk patients.*

Dupriez B, Morel P, Demory JL, et al: Prognostic factors in agnogenic myeloid metaplasia: A report on 195 cases with a new scoring system. Blood 88:1013, 1996. *Prognostic guidelines in patients with agnogenic myeloid metaplasia.*

Gruppo Italiano Studio Policitemia: Polycythemia vera: The natural history of 1213 patients followed for 20 years. Ann Intern Med 123:656, 1995. *The largest study of patients with polycythemia vera, it contains information on the incidence and outcome of thrombotic and bleeding events.*

Harrison CN, Gale RE, Machin SJ, et al: A large proportion of patients with a diagnosis of essential thrombocythemia do not have a clonal disorder and may be at lower risk of thrombotic complications. Blood 93:417, 1999. *A study showing pathogenetic heterogeneity of essential thrombocythemias with both monoclonal and polyclonal hematopoiesis.*

Schafer AI: The primary and secondary hypercoagulable states. *In* Schafer AI (ed): Molecular Mechanisms of Hypercoagulable States. Austin, TX, Landes Bioscience, 1997, pp 1–48. *An authoritative and comprehensive review of mechanisms of thrombosis and hemorrhage.*

Sterkers Y, Preudhomme C, Laï J-L, et al: Acute myeloid leukemia and myelodysplastic syndromes following essential thrombocythemia treated with hydroxyurea: High proportion of cases with 17p deletion. Blood 91:616, 1998. *Discusses the leukemogenic effect of hydroxyurea in patients with essential thrombocythemia.*

Tefferi A, Elliott MA, Solberg LA Jr, Silverstein MN: New drugs in essential thrombocythemia and polycythemia vera. Blood Reviews 11:1, 1997. *Summarizes therapeutic options in essential thrombocythemia and polycythemia vera and discusses their mechanism of action.*

175 MYELODYSPLASTIC SYNDROME

D. Gary Gilliland

DEFINITION. Myelodysplastic syndrome (MDS) refers to a heterogeneous group of acquired bone marrow disorders characterized by dysplastic growth of hematopoietic progenitors, a hypercellular bone marrow with peripheral cytopenia, and propensity to progress to acute myelogenous leukemia (AML).

ETIOLOGY. Although there are rare kindreds in which there is an inherited predisposition to develop MDS, the vast majority of cases are sporadic. In most instances the etiology of de novo MDS is unknown, although exposure to chemical solvents, including benzene, and to pesticides have been identified as risk factors. De novo MDS occurs only rarely in young patients, but therapy-related MDS and acute myelogenous leukemia (t-MDS/AML) is increasingly recognized as a potentially fatal complication of chemotherapy and/or radiation therapy for other malignancies.

INCIDENCE AND EPIDEMIOLOGY. De novo MDS is rare, occurring at a frequency of approximately 1 per 100,000 per year in the general population. However, the incidence increases dramatically with age, with an incidence of 25 to 50 per 100,000 per year in populations older than the age of 60. In this age group, the incidence approximates other common hematologic malignancies, such as chronic lymphocytic leukemia and multiple myeloma. It is likely that, as demographics in developed countries shift in favor of older patient populations, the prevalence of MDS will increase. Similarly, it is anticipated that the incidence of t-MDS/AML will increase in younger patient populations as more intensive therapeutic regimens are employed in the treatment of solid tumors. With advances in technology that include the use of stem cell support and hematopoietic growth factors, the dose intensity and duration for treatment of cancer have increased dramatically. To the extent that these therapeutic maneuvers are successful in eradicating the underlying disease, the incidence of t-MDS/AML is likely to increase.

The treatment of Hodgkin's disease and non-Hodgkin's lymphoma (NHL) is an example of the problem. Autologous bone marrow transplantation (BMT) has proven to be a significant advance in the treatment of Hodgkin's disease and NHL, with cure rates approaching 40 to 50% in patient subgroups in whom the expected survival had been lower than 20%. The counterpoint to the success of intensive therapy has been an increased risk of t-MDS/AML in this population. Because autologous BMT is a relatively new procedure and follow-up is not sufficiently long, the exact incidence of secondary t-MDS/AML in this population is not known. However, reported actuarial incidences of t-MDS/AML in patients undergoing autologous BMT for Hodgkin's disease and NHL range from 4 to 18%. That is, in some centers as many as one in five patients cured of their underlying lymphoma will develop the life-threatening complication of t-MDS/AML. It is not clear whether t-MDS after autologous BMT is due to pretransplant chemotherapy and radiation therapy or due to damaged hematopoietic progenitors that survive the transplant conditioning regimen. However, the problem of t-MDS/AML is likely to increase with increasing intensity of therapy for solid tumors.

PATHOGENESIS. CLONALITY. MDS is a clonal disorder with an acquired somatic mutation that affects an early hematopoietic progenitor and gives rise to clonally derived neutrophils, red cells, and platelets. There is no convincing evidence for clonal involvement of B and T cells. Evidence that MDS is a clonal disorder includes the presence of clonal cytogenetic abnormalities, as described later, and analysis using X-inactivation–based clonality assays.

CYTOGENETIC ABNORMALITIES. Identification of mutant genes in MDS has been difficult, in part because MDS is characterized by loss of genetic material, in contrast to the balanced reciprocal chromosomal translocations typical of de novo AML. Consistent loss of genetic material has led to the hypothesis that MDS is caused by homozygous loss of genes with tumor suppressor activity. The most common cytogenetic abnormalities in MDS are deletions of the long arm of chromosome 5 and/or 7. 5q− is present in approximately 15% of de novo MDS and 50% of t-MDS, and abnormalities of 5q and/or 7 are present in 70% of t-MDS. Although there has been significant progress in identifying the critically deleted regions on chromosome 5 and 7, the gene(s) responsible for the pathogenesis of MDS associated with 5q− or 7q− have not yet been isolated.

There has been more success in cloning rare but recurring chromosomal translocations associated with MDS. For example, the *MLL (HRX)* gene localized to chromosome 11q23 has been implicated in the pathogenesis of de novo AML. It has been shown that t-MDS/AML patients with 11q23 abnormalities also have involvement of the *MLL* gene and that rearrangements of *MLL* in t-MDS/AML correlate with use of topoisomerase inhibitors (e.g., epipodophyllotoxins). Furthermore, the t(11;16)(q23;p13) is exclusively associated with t-MDS/AML and results in fusion of *MLL* to the transcriptional co-activator *CBP* (CREB binding protein).

The t(3;21)(q22;q22) translocation, which is associated with some cases of t-MDS/AML as well as with chronic myelogenous leukemia (CML) in blast crisis, has also been cloned. The consequence of the translocation in t-MDS/AML is fusion of *AML1* with one of several fusion partners on chromosome 3, including *EAP*, *EVI1*, and *MDS1*. *AML1* is also involved in the t(8;21) translocation in de novo AML and contains a highly conserved DNA binding domain that regulates expression of myeloid specific genes, including myeloperoxidase and neutrophil elastase. It has been suggested that the t(3;21) and t(8;21) fusions disrupt *AML1* function and thereby inhibit early myeloid differentiation.

t(5;12)(q33;p13) is a rare recurring translocation associated with the chronic myelomonocytic leukemia subtype of MDS (see Classification). The consequence of the translocation is fusion of the tyrosine kinase domain of the platelet-derived growth factor-β receptor (PDGFRβ) to a member of the ETS family of transcription factors, TEL. Fusion of TEL to PDGFRβ constitutively activates the tyrosine kinase domain of PDGFRβ, leading to abnormal myeloid proliferation.

POINT MUTATIONS. Activating mutations, which confer transforming potential to the *RAS* gene family, occur in 5 to 10% of MDS patients. Mutations are rare in *p53,* in the macrophage colony stimulating receptor gene *(M-CSFR),* and in the neurofibromatosis gene *NF1,* which acts in the *RAS* signal transduction pathway.

CELL CULTURE ANALYSIS. Hematopoietic progenitors from MDS patients grow poorly in culture, although poor growth can be partially overcome by addition of exogenous growth factors such as granulocyte-macrophage colony-stimulating factor (GM-CSF). There are functional defects in neutrophils (decreased phagocytosis, chemotaxis, microbicidal activity), red cells (ringed sideroblasts with defective iron processing, qualitative defects in red cell glycolytic enzymes), and platelets (defects in aggregation and morphology). Most patients have normal T- and B-cell numbers and normal levels of immunoglobulins and hence are not particularly prone to opportunistic infections unless treated with immunosuppressive agents.

CLINICAL MANIFESTATIONS. The clinical presentation of MDS is frequently referable to cytopenia in one or more hematopoietic cell lineages, with neutropenia occurring in 24 to 39% of patients, anemia in 45 to 93%, and thrombocytopenia in 28 to 45% in various series. In the geriatric population, patients may present with symptoms related to co-morbid illnesses. For example, a patient with coronary artery disease may present with mild anemia associated with an increase in the frequency and duration of angina. Other common presenting symptoms include easy bruisability, epistaxis or petechiae, and signs and symptoms of infection. Because infection may itself suppress myelopoiesis, any patient with a mild cytopenia in the setting of infection should have follow-up blood cell counts to determine if the cytopenia persists after the infection has resolved. This evaluation is particularly important because MDS confers not only a quantitative defect in the production of myeloid lineage cells but also a qualitative defect in function of those cells. Therefore, a patient with a mild leukopenia may have MDS and be highly susceptible to bacterial infections due to abnormal neutrophil function. Patients with MDS usually have normal number and function of T and B cells and rarely present with evidence of opportunistic infections. Infections due to opportunistic pathogens are usually seen only in MDS patients who have been

heavily treated with antibacterial antibiotics for extended periods of time or who have received marrow suppressive therapy for MDS.

The clinical course of MDS is characterized by inexorably progressive pancytopenia. Although the rate of decline of peripheral blood cell counts is highly variable and may affect one hematopoietic lineage more than another, there is rarely if ever clinically significant improvement in blood cell counts during the course of MDS. The clinical problems encountered during the course of MDS depend in part on co-morbid illness and the extent to which each of the hematopoietic lineages is involved. For example, although it is relatively easy to provide red cell transfusion therapy for patients with isolated macrocytic anemia as the primary manifestation of MDS, anemia may be a significant and life-threatening problem in an elderly MDS patient with coexistent severe coronary artery disease. Similarly, an elderly MDS patient with diabetes may encounter little difficulty with anemia or thrombocytopenia but may have recurrent life-threatening infections requiring frequent hospitalization from persistent neutropenia in the setting of diabetes. Because de novo MDS occurs most commonly in the elderly, about 30% of patients will die of underlying medical conditions unrelated to MDS. About 40% of patients die of complications of marrow failure, such as infection or bleeding, and about 30% die of transformation to acute leukemia and attendant complications.

DIAGNOSIS AND CLASSIFICATION OF MDS. Examination of the peripheral blood smear is often helpful in establishing the diagnosis of MDS. Granulocytes are poorly granulated and may be hyposegmented and display the Pelger-Huët anomaly (Color Plate 5L). Red cells are usually hypochromic with polychromasia. Other abnormalities in red cell morphology can include teardrop-shaped cells, especially in the subset of MDS patients with bone marrow fibrosis, as well as red cell fragments and nucleated cells. Mild macrocytosis is a hallmark of MDS, with mean corpuscular volume (MCV) in the 100 to 110 range. MCVs outside this range make a diagnosis of MDS less likely. Platelets may be large, and megakaryocyte fragments may be present.

A bone marrow aspirate and biopsy are required to provide a definitive diagnosis. Evidence of dysmyelopoiesis can include abnormal granules, such as large primary granules or decreased numbers of granules, the presence of bizarre nuclear forms in myeloid lineage cells, the Pelger-Huët anomaly, and Auer rods. Signs of dyserythropoiesis may include multinuclear forms, nuclear fragments, megaloblastic changes, nuclear:cytoplasmic dyssynchrony, and ringed sideroblasts. Finally, dysplasia affecting megakaryocyte lineage cells can include bizarre nuclear figures, decreased ploidy, separated nuclei (so-called pawn ball nuclei), and micro-megakaryocytes. The percentage of myeloblasts may be increased and is used as part of the classification of MDS described later. The bone marrow cellularity is usually normal or increased, which is a paradox because most patients present with peripheral blood cytopenia.

Characteristic cytogenetic abnormalities are another helpful clue in the diagnosis of MDS, although normal cytogenetics do not exclude the diagnosis. Most cytogenetic abnormalities in MDS are characterized by loss of genetic material through deletions. Nonrandom chromosomal abnormalities associated with MDS include 5q−, which occurs in approximately 15% of de novo MDS and 50% of secondary MDS, monosomy 7, trisomy 8, 21q−, 17q−, and 20q−. As many as 80% of patients have detectable chromosomal abnormalities.

A diagnosis of MDS requires the exclusion of other disorders that may cause peripheral cytopenias (Table 175–1). The evaluation of a patient with unexplained cytopenia should always include exclusion of congenital disorders associated with cytopenia, exclusion of vitamin deficiencies, and, in particular, the possibility that drugs may be contributory. Whenever possible, patients should be taken off any medications that can cause cytopenia for at least 6 to 8 weeks. A careful physical examination for evidence of hypersplenism should be part of the evaluation of cytopenia, with attention to various potential underlying causes, such as myelofibrosis, hepatic cirrhosis, and other hematologic disorders (e.g., hairy cell leukemia or primary splenic lymphoma). Alcoholic patients may present with a combination of vitamin deficiency, alcoholic myelosuppression, and hypersplenism that may resemble MDS. Some physicians will incorporate testing for autoimmune diseases, such as antinuclear antibody tests, in the evaluation of cytopenia, although it is rare that cytopenia is the only presenting finding for autoimmune disorders. In addition, there is an association between

Table 175–1 ■ DIFFERENTIAL DIAGNOSIS OF MDS

Congenital disorders
  Hereditary sideroblastic anemia
  Fanconi's anemia
  Diamond-Blackfan syndrome
  Kostmann's syndrome
  Shwachman syndrome
  Down syndrome
Vitamin deficiency
  B$_{12}$, folate, or iron deficiency
Drug toxicity
  Marrow suppression from oral or parenteral medications
  Toxins
  Chemotherapy and/or radiation therapy
  Alcohol
Anemia of chronic disease
  Renal failure
  Chronic infection, including tuberculosis
  Rheumatologic disorders
Viral marrow suppression
  Including Epstein-Barr virus, parvovirus B19, human immunodeficiency
    virus, and others
Marrow infiltration
  Acute and chronic leukemias
  Metastatic solid tumor infiltration
Paroxysmal nocturnal hemoglobinuria
Hypersplenism

---

autoimmune disease and MDS, such that a prior diagnosis of inflammatory bowel disease or arthralgias does not exclude the possibility that a patient may have MDS.

When the initial physical examination, laboratory evaluation, and removal of potentially causative drugs fail to disclose a cause for a cytopenia, bone marrow aspiration and biopsy with cytogenetic analysis should be performed to address the possibility that the patient may have MDS. The bone marrow examination will determine whether the patient has MDS and exclude other potential causes of cytopenia, including aplastic anemia, leukemia, and marrow infiltration by malignant cells.

MDS patients are divided into subgroups based on the French-American-British (FAB) classification scheme. The designations delineate subgroups of MDS based on the presence or absence of ringed sideroblasts and the percentages of blood and bone marrow blasts. Patients with refractory anemia (RA) have less than 5% marrow blasts and less than 1% blasts in the peripheral blood. Refractory anemia with ringed sideroblasts (RARS) meets the same criteria for blasts as RA but contains a high percentage of ringed sideroblasts in marrow. Refractory anemia with excess blasts (RAEB) has between 5 and 20% bone marrow blasts and less than 5% circulating blasts, whereas in refractory anemia with excess blasts in transition (RAEB-T) the patients have 20 to 30% marrow blasts and may have more than 5% peripheral blasts. Chronic myelomonocytic leukemia (CMML) is a distinct subgroup of MDS characterized by dysplastic monocytosis that shares features with myeloproliferative syndromes, and some have argued that it may be better characterized as a myeloproliferative disorder. Patients are approximately equally distributed among FAB subtypes at the time of diagnosis. Survival and probability of leukemic transformation can be estimated only approximately based on the FAB subtype, and the FAB classification system does not consider the generally poor prognosis of t-MDS patients. The International Prognostic Scoring System (IPSS), described later in the chapter, provides more reliable estimates of survival and likelihood of progression to AML.

TREATMENT. No treatment has been shown to prolong survival of MDS patients except for allogeneic BMT in suitable candidates (see Chapter 182). Supportive care remains the mainstay of therapy, including transfusion of red cells with chelation therapy to prevent iron overload, prevention and treatment of infection, and transfusion of platelets for clinically significant bleeding.

Numerous agents have been tested for efficacy in MDS, including pyridoxine, vitamins, androgens, corticosteroids, differentiating agents, and chemotherapy. The rationale for the use of pyridoxine, a cofactor in heme biosynthesis, is the potential for improvement in ineffective erythropoiesis. Pyridoxine is non-toxic and is usually given for 3 months in patients with anemia from MDS; responses are rare. There is no clear role for corticosteroids, androgens, or other vitamins in the therapy of MDS, although there are anecdotal reports of response. Drugs that promote differentiation of hematopoietic progenitors, such as low-dose cytarabine, low-dose etoposide, retinoic acid derivatives including all-trans retinoic acid, vitamin D$_3$ derivatives, interferon, and hexamethylene bisacetamide, have been tested extensively in MDS. Despite anecdotal reports of responses to each, clinical trials do not support their general use. 5-Azacytidine, which interferes with DNA methylation, has shown some promise in clinical trials but is not known to prolong survival.

Thus far, there is no known survival benefit from administration of any hematopoietic growth factors, either alone or in combination. In 15 separate trials of erythropoietin (EPO) involving 308 MDS patients, there has been an overall response rate of approximately 20%, generally in patients with serum EPO levels less than 500 mU/mL. Most trials used high doses of EPO, which may not be cost effective when compared with transfusion therapy. However, it may be reasonable to consider a trial of EPO in MDS patients in the range of 150 to 300 U/kg three times per week by subcutaneous injection, especially in patients with low serum EPO levels relative to their degree of anemia. Several phase II trials have suggested that G-CSF augments the response to EPO. Interleukin (IL)-3, GM-CSF + erythropoietin, IL-3 + erythropoietin, and IL-3 + GM-CSF are not effective.

CONVENTIONAL CHEMOTHERAPY. In trials conducted in the 1980s, remission rates for MDS or secondary AML (evolving from MDS) ranged from 18 to 44% with standard anti-leukemia regimens; treatment-related deaths occurred in as many as half of patients. It has been reported that treatment with FLAG (fludarabine 30 mg/m^2, and ara-C [cytarabine], 2 g/m^2, daily for 5 days, coupled with granulocyte colony-stimulating factor [G-CSF] therapy beginning the day before chemotherapy and continuing until complete remission) results in complete response rates comparable to those for induction chemotherapy for de novo AML. However, duration of remission and median survival were short in these studies, and it is not yet clear whether intensive chemotherapy prolongs survival. Newer chemotherapeutic agents are being investigated, but intensive chemotherapy, with or without growth factor support, can be recommended only under the auspices of a clinical trial.

STEM CELL TRANSPLANTATION (see Chapter 182). Related or unrelated donor BMT remains the only known cure for MDS and should be considered the treatment of choice for patients who meet age and donor criteria. Disease-free survivals of up to 15 years may be seen, and the age at which allogeneic BMT can be considered has been liberalized for related donor BMT up to the age of 65. Thus, approximately one half of patients with de novo MDS may be candidates for allogeneic BMT. Although most centers place an upper age limit of 55 years for unrelated donor BMT, this therapeutic modality may also be an option for the smaller group of de novo MDS patients younger than the age of 55 and for many

Table 175–2 ■ INTERNATIONAL PROGNOSTIC SCORING SYSTEM

PROGNOSTIC VARIABLE	SCORE VALUE				
	0	0.5	1.0	1.5	2.0
Bone marrow blasts (%)	<5	5–10	—	11–21	21–30
Karyotype*	Good	Intermediate	Poor		
Cytopenias†	0 or 1	2 or 3			

Karyotype scores:*
Good: normal - Y, del(5q), del(20q)
Poor: complex (greater than or equal to 3), any abnormality of chromosome 7
Intermediate: any other cytogenetic abnormality
  Cytopenias:†
Hemoglobin less than 10 g/dL
Absolute neutrophil count less than 1,500/μL
Platelet count less than 100,000/μL
  Score for each of the three variables are summed for an overall score. Overall scores for risk groups are low: 0; intermediate-1: 0.5–1.0; Intermediate-2: 1.5–2.0; and high: ≥2.5.
  From Greenberg P, Cox C, LeBeau MM, et al: International scoring system for evaluating prognosis in myelodysplastic syndromes. Blood 89:2079, 1997.

of the therapy-related MDS patients. In most cases, MDS patients proceed to BMT without prior chemotherapy, although patients with greater than 15% bone marrow blasts are more likely to relapse. In one analysis of 70 patients with refractory anemia transplanted between 1981 and 1993, young age and short disease duration before transplant were favorable prognostic indicators.

The largest series of 93 MDS patients undergoing BMT included 65 patients with HLA-compatible sibling donors and 28 with other family members or unrelated donors. At 4 years, overall disease-free survival was 41%, relapse rate was 28%, and non-relapse mortality was 43%. Comparable results have been obtained in four other large trials. Overall there was a 42% disease-free survival at 4 years, which is considerably better than would be predicted based on FAB subtype analysis. However, in an elderly patient population, the risk of BMT is likely to be significantly higher than for trials reported to date, in which the upper age limit for BMT

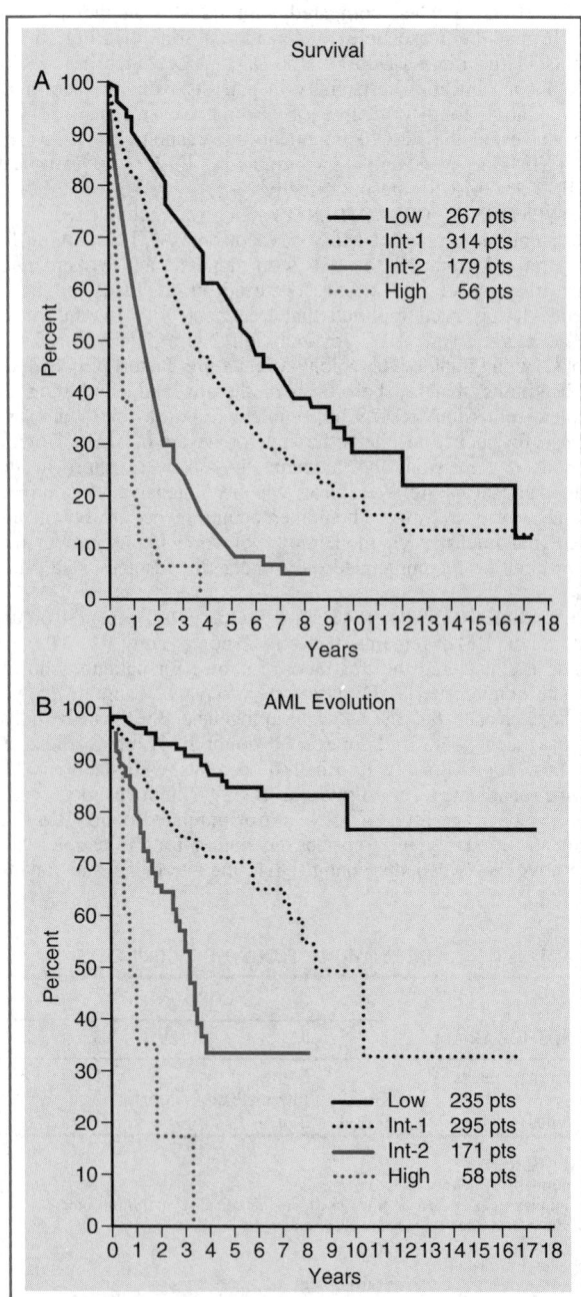

FIGURE 175-1 ■ International MDS risk classification by IPSS for survival and evolution to acute myelogenous leukemia. (From Greenberg P, Cox C, LeBeau MM, et al: International Scoring System for Evaluating Prognosis in Myelodysplastic Syndromes. Blood 89:2079, 1997.)

ranged between 50 and 55. BMT should therefore still be considered an investigational approach in the majority of de novo MDS patients who are over the age of 55. Analysis of unrelated donor BMT data has suggested that unrelated donor transplant is approximately comparable to allogeneic BMT from an HLA-identical sibling, with 2-year disease-free survival, relapse, and non-relapse mortality rates of 38%, 28%, and 48%, respectively.

PROGNOSIS. An International Prognostic Scoring System has been developed to provide risk classification for overall survival and progression to AML (Table 175–2). Points are assigned for blast percentage, karyotype, and the presence of cytopenias; the resulting overall score correlates well with overall survival and likelihood of progression to AML (Fig. 175–1). The IPSS may prove useful to identify high-risk patients who are most likely to benefit from intensive therapy with curative intent, such as BMT, or from more "conservative" treatment with investigational chemotherapy protocols.

Anderson JE, Anasetti C, Appelbaum FR, et al: Unrelated donor bone marrow transplantation for myelodysplasia (MDS0 and MDS-related acute myeloid leukemia). Br J Haematol 93:59, 1996.

Anderson JE, Appelbaum FR, Fisher LD, et al: Allogeneic bone marrow transplantation for 93 patients with myelodysplastic syndrome. Blood 82:677, 1993. *These two papers summarize the largest single institution experience with stem cell transplantation for MDS.*

Greenberg P, Cox C, LeBeau MM, et al: International Scoring System for Evaluating Prognosis in Myelodysplastic Syndromes. Blood 89:2079, 1997. *The new IPSS for risk classification of MDS patients for overall survival and likelihood of progression to AML.*

Kouides PA, Bennett JM: Advances in the therapy of the myelodysplastic syndromes. Cancer Treat Res 99:335, 1999. *Discussion of potential efficacy of differentiation-induction/antiapoptotic agents in myelodysplastic syndromes, and current therapeutic strategies based on risk stratification, degree of cytopenia, and age.*

176 THE CHRONIC LEUKEMIAS

Michael J. Keating

CHRONIC MYELOGENOUS LEUKEMIA (CHRONIC MYELOID LEUKEMIA, CHRONIC MYELOCYTIC LEUKEMIA, CHRONIC GRANULOCYTIC LEUKEMIA)

DEFINITION. Chronic myelogenous leukemia (CML) is a disease characterized by overproduction of cells of the granulocytic, especially the neutrophilic, series and occasionally the monocytic series, leading to marked splenomegaly and very high white blood cell (WBC) counts. Basophilia and thrombocytosis are common. A characteristic cytogenetic abnormality, the Philadelphia (Ph¹) chromosome, is present in the bone marrow cells in more than 95% of cases. The granulocytes usually appear relatively normal, although those of many patients exhibit dysplastic changes, including Pelger-Huët anomalies. Neutrophil functions, such as phagocytosis and bactericidal activity, are largely preserved. Before effective treatment was available, patients survived, on the average, approximately 2 years after diagnosis.

ETIOLOGY. Usually no etiologic agent can be incriminated in CML. Exposure to ionizing radiation increases the risk of subsequent CML. Survivors of the atomic bomb explosions in Japan in 1945 have had an increased incidence of CML, with a peak occurring 5 to 12 years after exposure and seeming to be dose related. The relative risk has been falling since that time but is still above the expected rate for Japan. Radiation treatment of ankylosing spondylitis and cervical cancer has increased the incidence of CML. No increase in the risk of CML has been demonstrated in individuals working in the nuclear industry. Radiologists working without adequate protection before 1940 were more likely to develop myeloid leukemia, but no such association has been found in recent studies. Benzene exposure increases the risk of acute myelogenous leukemia (AML) but not of CML. Patients with CML have an increased frequency of the Cw3 and Cw4 human leukocyte antigens (HLAs). CML is not a frequent secondary leukemia following the treatment of other cancers with radiation and/or alkylating agents.

INCIDENCE. CML constitutes one fifth of all cases of leukemia in the United States. It is diagnosed in 1 or 2 persons per 100,000 per year and has a slight male preponderance. This incidence has not changed significantly in the past few decades. The incidence of CML increases with age; the median age at diagnosis is 45 to 50 years. Ph¹-positive CML is uncommon in children and adolescents. Patients older than 60 years have a poorer prognosis. No familial association of CML has been noted.

MOLECULAR PATHOGENESIS. The striking feature in CML is the presence of the Ph¹ chromosome in the bone marrow cells of more than 90% of patients with typical CML. The Ph¹ chromosome results from a balanced translocation of material between the long arms of chromosomes 9 and 22. As more chromosomal material is lost from chromosome 22 than is gained from chromosome 9, the Ph¹ chromosome is a shortened chromosome 22 containing approximately 60% of its normal complement of DNA. The break, which occurs at band q34 of the long arm of chromosome 9, allows translocation of the cellular oncogene *C-ABL* to a position on chromosome 22 called the breakpoint cluster region (*bcr*). The breakpoint in the *bcr* varies from patient to patient but is identical in all cells of any one patient. *C-ABL* is a homologue of *V-ABL*, the Abelson virus that causes leukemia in mice. The apposition of these two genetic sequences produces a new hybrid gene (*BCR/ABL*), which codes for a novel protein of molecular weight 210,000 kd (P210). The P210 protein, a tyrosine kinase, may play a role in triggering the uncontrolled proliferation of CML cells. The Ph¹ chromosome occurs in erythroid, myeloid, monocytic, and megakaryocytic cells, less commonly in B lymphocytes, rarely in T lymphocytes, but not in marrow fibroblasts. This extensive cellular distribution places the abnormality in CML close to the pluripotent stem cell. Studies of glucose-6-phosphate dehydrogenase (G6PD) isoenzymes support the finding of multilineage monoclonal proliferation, because a single isoenzyme is present in the aforementioned cells in some patients with CML. Insertion of a retrovirus encoding P210 (*BCR/ABL*) into cells of mice has led to the development of a disease closely resembling CML in some of these animals, giving credence to the hypothesis that the *BCR/ABL* hybrid gene is sufficient to cause CML. *C-sis,* the homologue of the simian sarcoma virus, is also translocated from chromosome 22 to chromosome 9 in CML but is distant from the breakpoint and not expressed in benign-phase CML. *C-sis* codes for a protein identical to platelet-derived growth factor (PDGF).

The fusion *BCR/ABL* gene and the P210 protein can be found in many cases of typical CML in which no cytogenetic abnormality occurs or in which changes other than typical t(9;22)(q34;q11) are identified. These patients have a survival rate and a response to therapy that are similar to those in Ph¹-positive patients. Patients with atypical CML who are Ph¹ and *BCR/ABL* negative have a different natural history than do patients who are either Ph¹ positive or Ph¹ negative with *BCR/ABL* positivity. They resemble more closely patients with myelodysplastic syndrome (MDS). Thus, three groups of patients with CML can be identified: (1) positive for Ph¹ and *BCR/ABL*, (2) Ph¹ negative but *BCR/ABL* positive, and (3) negative for Ph¹ and *BCR/ABL* (Table 176–1).

Although 100% of the metaphases on cytogenetic analysis usually show the presence of the Ph¹ chromosome, some normal stem cells must remain. Normal diploid cells emerge on long-term bone marrow culture and after treatment with interferon, high-dose chemotherapy, and autologous bone marrow transplantation.

SYMPTOMS AND SIGNS. CML is increasingly being diagnosed in asymptomatic patients owing to the use of hematologic studies in routine physical examinations or in evaluations of other illnesses. In these patients the WBC count may be relatively low at the time of diagnosis. The WBC count correlates well with tumor mass as defined by spleen size. Patients with higher WBC counts

and larger spleens have more symptoms. The symptoms of CML, which usually are nonspecific, are caused by anemia, spleen size, or an increased basal metabolic rate, but most patients are asymptomatic or only mildly symptomatic. Fatigue, weight loss, malaise, easy satiety, and a sense of left upper quadrant fullness are the major symptoms of CML. Rarely, bleeding (associated with a low platelet count and/or platelet dysfunction) or thrombosis (associated with thrombocytosis and/or marked leukocytosis) occurs. The serum uric acid level is commonly elevated at diagnosis, and acute gouty arthritis may follow treatment. An elevated blood histamine level (related to the basophil cell mass) can cause upper gastrointestinal ulceration and bleeding. Neutrophil function is usually normal or only modestly impaired, and neutrophil numbers are markedly increased; infections are therefore uncommon at the time of diagnosis. Headaches, bone pain, arthralgias, pain from splenic infarction, and fever are uncommon in the early stages of CML but become more common as the disease progresses. Priapism is occasionally noted, usually in patients with marked leukocytosis or thrombocytosis. Leukostatic symptoms, such as dyspnea, drowsiness, loss of coordination, or confusion, which are due to sludging in the pulmonary or cerebral vessels, are uncommon in the benign (chronic) phase of CML despite WBC counts that may exceed 400,000/μL. These symptoms appear more frequently in later stages of the disease (i.e., in the accelerated or blast crisis phases, in which more immature cells predominate). All symptoms subside as the WBC count falls and the splenomegaly decreases as a result of effective treatment.

Splenomegaly, by far the most consistent physical sign in CML, occurs in more than 60% of cases. The spleen may extend to the pelvic brim and across the midline of the abdomen. Hepatomegaly is less common and is usually minor (1 to 3 cm below the right costal margin). Lymphadenopathy is very uncommon, as is infiltration of skin and other tissues. If present, these findings suggest Ph¹-negative CML or accelerated phase or blastic crisis of CML.

NATURAL HISTORY. More than 90% of patients present with CML in the benign (chronic) phase, in which the disease behaves in a predictable fashion, with the symptoms, abnormal physical signs, and abnormal blood findings returning to normal after treatment. This satisfactory response is transient; all patients eventually develop a variety of changes in the behavior of the disease. Most frequently there is a "blast crisis," a clinical picture resembling that of acute leukemia. Rarely, patients initially present in blast crisis. This change can be abrupt, but more frequently it is preceded by a period of progressively greater difficulty in maintaining the WBC count at a level of less than 20,000/μL and of other manifestations, such as increasing splenomegaly, hepatomegaly, and infiltration of nodes, skin, bones, or other tissues; the appearance of blast cells or basophils in the peripheral blood; development of anemia and/or thrombocytopenia; or fever, malaise, and weight loss. These features, termed the *accelerated phase* of CML, demand re-evaluation of the bone marrow, which, in the accelerated phase, often shows dysplastic changes in the myeloid and other cell lineages and may show an increase in the percentage of blast cells (5–29%) and an increase in basophils. Aspiration of bone marrow may be difficult, especially in patients who have developed myelofibrosis subsequent to the CML. Chromosomal abnormalities in addition to the Ph¹ chromosome occur in both the accelerated and the blastic phases of CML. Blast crisis is diagnosed when 30% or more blast cells are present in the bone marrow and/or peripheral blood.

When the accelerated phase or blast crisis is suspected (more than 10% blasts in bone marrow), the patient should be further observed in 2 to 4 weeks, because the percentage of blasts in the

Table 176–1 ■ CLASSIFICATION OF CHRONIC MYELOGENOUS LEUKEMIA (CML)

DISEASE	Ph¹ PRESENT	BCR/ABL REARRANGEMENT	PROGNOSIS (SURVIVAL)
Classic CML	Yes	Yes	Median 5–7 yr
bcr+, Ph¹−	No	Most	Median 5–7 yr
CMML/CMoL/*bcr*− CML	No	No	Median 18–24 mo

bcr = breakpoint cluster region; *BCR/ABL* = a hybrid gene (see text); CMML = chronic myelomonocytic leukemia; CMoL = chronic monocytic leukemia; Ph¹ = Philadelphia chromosome.

blood and bone marrow can increase transiently after the treatment of CML is discontinued, especially if the patient had been treated with hydroxyurea or interferon. It is important to be cautious in classifying patients as having blast crisis or accelerated phase because of the adverse prognostic implications (Fig. 176–1). Criteria for accelerated phase are the following: an increase in blast cells (>15%) or basophils (>20%) in the blood or bone marrow, thrombocytopenia (<100,000/μL), serious anemia (hemoglobin [Hb] <7 g/dL); documented extramedullary leukemia, or development of clonal evolution (new chromosomal changes in addition to the Ph[1] chromosome). The risk of developing accelerated phase or blast crisis in CML is relatively low in the first 2 years after diagnosis (~10% per year) but then increases and remains constant (15 to 20% per year) thereafter unless therapy such as interferon or bone marrow transplantation (BMT) is used.

LABORATORY FINDINGS. All patients with untreated CML have an elevated WBC count, ranging from 10,000/μL to more than 1 million/μL. The predominant cells are of the neutrophil series, with a left shift extending to blast cells. In addition, eosinophils and basophils are commonly increased in number. Monocytes may be slightly increased in some cases that overlap with chronic myelomonocytic leukemia (CMML) (see Chapter 175). The bone marrow is hypercellular with marked myeloid hyperplasia and sometimes shows evidence of increased reticulin or collagen fibrosis. The myeloid:erythroid ratio is 15:1 to 20:1. About 15% of patients have 5% or more blast cells in the peripheral blood or bone marrow at diagnosis. T cells (both T helper and T suppressor), but not B cells, are increased in number in CML. A hemoglobin of less than 11 g/dL is present in one third of patients. The red cells are usually normochromic and normocytic, but nucleated red cells are present in the blood of one fourth of the patients at diagnosis. Autoimmune hemolytic anemia and thrombocytopenia (<100,000/μL) are rare in CML, but thrombocytosis (>450,000/μL) occurs in almost half of the patients.

Biochemical abnormalities in CML include a leukocyte alkaline phosphatase (LAP) score that is markedly decreased in the neutrophils of 90% or more of patients and is zero in 5 to 10% of cases. A low LAP score also occurs in some patients with agnogenic myeloid metaplasia, which is sometimes difficult to differentiate from CML. The serum levels of transcobalamins I and III, cobalamin-binding glycoproteins produced by neutrophils, are elevated in accord with the increased neutrophils. This elevation leads to extremely high serum cobalamin values (e.g., vitamin B$_{12}$ levels > 10 times normal). Serum levels of lactate dehydrogenase, uric acid, and lysozyme are often increased. The lysozyme levels are modestly increased in CML compared with CMML, in which the levels in blood and urine are often markedly increased. Kinetic studies show an increased neutrophil production rate related to a markedly expanded myeloid mass. The number of colony-forming cells in the blood in CML is increased, but the number in the bone marrow is in the normal range. Defective feedback control of WBC production is common in CML; some patients demonstrate a cyclic oscillation of the WBC count. The labeling index of myeloblasts in

CML is lower than in normal bone marrow, and the generation time is prolonged, confirming the concept that CML is an accumulative rather than a proliferative disease: neutrophils in CML survive slightly longer in the intravascular circulation than do normal granulocytes.

DIAGNOSIS. The diagnosis of typical CML is not difficult. The presence of unexplained myeloid leukocytosis (Color Plate 6H) with splenomegaly should lead to a LAP test on the peripheral blood neutrophils (usually zero or a low value) and bone marrow examination with a cytogenetic analysis. Marrow myeloid hyperplasia and hypercellularity further suggest the diagnosis. The standard diagnostic test remains the cytogenetic analysis; the presence of the Ph[1] chromosome in this clinical setting establishes the diagnosis. When the Ph[1] chromosome is not found in a patient with suspected CML, molecular evidence for the presence of the hybrid BCR/ABL gene should be sought, because 40 to 50% of Ph[1]-negative patients with CML have BCR/ABL rearrangement. The Ph[1] chromosome is usually present in 100% of metaphases, ordinarily as the sole abnormality. Ten to 15 percent of patients at initial presentation have an additional chromosomal change, such as loss of the Y chromosome, trisomy 8, an additional loss of material from 22q, or an atypical translocation. Many patients who have atypical complex chromosomal changes, which may or may not involve chromosome 9 or chromosome 22 morphologically, demonstrate evidence of the hybrid BCR/ABL gene when molecular techniques are used.

CML must be differentiated from leukemoid reactions, which usually produce WBC counts lower than 50,000/μL, toxic granulation vacuolation, Döhle bodies in the granulocytes, absence of basophilia, a normal or increased LAP level, and a clinical history and physical examination suggesting the origin of the leukemoid reaction. Corticosteroids can rarely cause extreme neutrophilia together with the left shift, but this response is self-limited and short in duration and thus seldom a cause of diagnostic difficulty.

CML may be more difficult to differentiate from other myelodysplastic or myeloproliferative syndromes (see Chapters 174 and 175). Patients having agnogenic myeloid metaplasia with or without myelofibrosis have splenomegaly and often have neutrophilia and thrombocytosis. Polycythemia rubra vera with associated iron deficiency, which causes a normal hemoglobin level and hematocrit value, can manifest with an elevated neutrophil and platelet count. Such patients usually have a normal or increased LAP score, a WBC count less than 25,000/μL, and no Ph[1] chromosome.

The greatest diagnostic difficulty lies with patients who have splenomegaly and leukocytosis but who do not have the Ph[1] chromosome. Many of these patients have the usual blood and marrow findings of Ph[1]-positive CML, and the BCR/ABL hybrid gene can be demonstrated despite a normal or atypical cytogenetic pattern. Patients who are Ph[1] negative and BCR/ABL negative are considered to have Ph[1]-negative CML or CMML (see Table 176–1). The cytogenetic findings in patients with CMML are normal or involve an additional chromosome 8 or findings other than the Ph[1] chromosome. Patients with CMML have ras mutations in 50 to 60% of cases. Rarely, patients have myeloid hyperplasia, which involves almost exclusively the neutrophil, eosinophil, or basophilic cell lineage. These patients are described as having chronic neutrophilic, eosinophilic, or basophilic leukemia and do not have evidence of the Ph[1] chromosome or BCR/ABL gene. Isolated megakaryocytic hyperplasia can give rise to a syndrome called idiopathic thrombocythemia with marked thrombocytosis and splenomegaly. These conditions are considered to fall under the general category of myeloproliferative disorders and have a better prognosis than does CML. Some patients who present with clinical characteristics of essential thrombocythemia (with marked thrombocytosis but without marked leukocytosis) actually have CML, with a Ph[1] chromosome and/or the BCR/ABL rearrangement (see Chapter 174).

EVOLUTION OF CML. Death occurs rarely during the chronic phase of CML, but over time the clinical behavior of the disease changes. One third of patients abruptly develop an acute transformation (blast crisis of CML); the other two thirds respond progressively less well in the control of the WBC count and spleen size with conventional agents such as busulfan and hydroxyurea. This loss of control (accelerated phase) is often associated with an increased proportion of blasts, promyelocytes, and basophils in the peripheral blood and bone marrow and is often accompanied by anemia and thrombocytopenia. Some patients develop bone marrow failure in which anemia and thrombocytopenia are accompanied by increasing evidence of dysplastic changes in the marrow and mye-

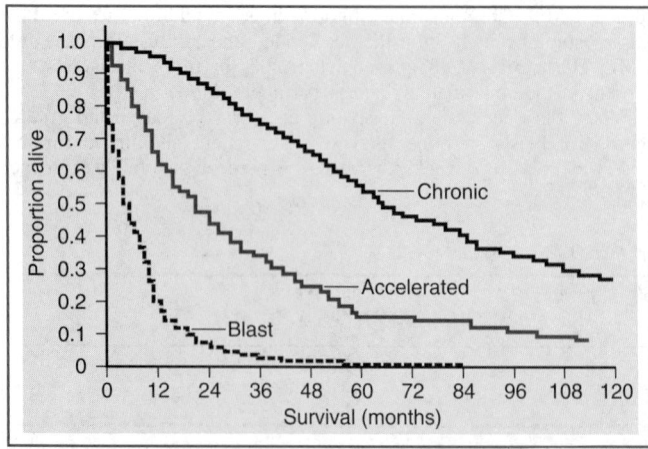

FIGURE 176–1 ■ Survival of M. D. Anderson Cancer Center patients with chronic myelogenous leukemia by phase of disease, 1970–1997.

lofibrosis. The median survival after developing a blast crisis of CML is only 3 months (see Fig. 176–1). The survival after development of the accelerated phase of CML is 12 to 18 months if the blood and bone marrow contain more than 30% blasts plus promyelocytes or more than 20% basophils or if the platelet count falls to less than 100,000/μL. Most patients with blast crisis or accelerated phase have additional chromosomal abnormalities (clonal evolution), such as duplication of the Ph[1] chromosome, trisomy of chromosome number 8, or development of an isochromosome number 17. Clonal evolution usually presages the accelerated phase or blast crisis of CML. The blast cells in blast crisis are usually myeloblasts, but less commonly erythroid, monocytoid, or megakaryoblastic transformations occur. In one fourth of cases, the blast cells are lymphoid, as demonstrated by cytochemical stains (terminal deoxynucleotidyl transferase), immunophenotyping, and immunoglobulin heavy-chain rearrangement studies. In 10% of cases, the blast cells are completely undifferentiated. Some patients with acute leukemia and the Ph[1] chromosome abnormality presumably have had blast crises that occurred before the diagnosis of CML was made. These cases have the P210 protein and 8.5-kb fusion messenger RNA. Patients with acute lymphoblastic leukemia (ALL) with a Ph[1] chromosome usually have a P190 protein or a 7.0-kb fusion messenger RNA probably restricted to the lymphoid cells. Extramedullary blast crisis of CML can occur in the spleen, lymph nodes, skin, meninges, bone, and other sites. This initial extramedullary transformation is usually shortly followed by evidence of marrow involvement.

CMML and Ph[1]-negative and *BCR/ABL*-negative CML appear to overlap clinically in some instances, and their clinical behavior, progress, and response to therapy resemble those of the myelodysplastic syndromes more than Ph[1]-positive CML (see Chapter 175). A male preponderance is noted, splenomegaly is common (60 to 70%), and the WBC count, while elevated, is usually in the 25,000 to 100,000/μL range. Anemia and thrombocytopenia are more common than in Ph[1]-positive CML, and eosinophilia and basophilia are less common. The median survival is 18 to 24 months, with patients dying of infection, bleeding, or transformation to acute leukemia.

TREATMENT. Immediate treatment of CML is not necessary unless the WBC count exceeds 200,000/μL or there is evidence of leukostasis (priapism, venous thrombosis, confusion, or dyspnea) or unless painful splenomegaly suggests splenic infarction. Hyperuricemia is common at the diagnosis of CML and should be treated with allopurinol, 300 mg/day, and adequate hydration while the WBC count is higher than 25,000/μL to prevent renal dysfunction. Acute gouty arthritis is rare.

PALLIATIVE TREATMENT. CML had been treated traditionally with oral busulfan or hydroxyurea, which, if used prudently, gives smooth, sustained control of the WBC count, platelet count, and spleen size. Both agents have a high level of acceptance by the patient, and both control the manifestations of the disease in 90% of cases when first used; over time, however, they produce progressively shorter and less complete reductions in the WBC count and spleen size. Leukapheresis can also be used on a short-term basis to decrease the leukocyte or platelet counts rapidly.

Hydroxyurea is the preferred oral agent and is given at dosages of 1 to 4 g/day, again according to the WBC count and body size. The WBC count falls in similar fashion to that induced by busulfan, but severe marrow hypoplasia is rare. The dosage of hydroxyurea is decreased as the leukocyte count decreases and can be discontinued when the WBC count is 5000 to 10,000/μL. Some physicians prefer to treat patients with intermittent courses, whereas others maintain patients on 0.5 to 2 g/day. The drug can be given as a single dose or fractionated throughout the day. Although close monitoring of the blood cell count is necessary initially with hydroxyurea, the pattern of response is usually predictable with repeated courses. Side effects are uncommon, although rash, mucositis, skin ulcers, and diarrhea can occur.

Busulfan should rarely be used because of its adverse reaction profile and because the survival of patients treated with hydroxyurea is superior to that of those treated with busulfan. Busulfan exposure before allogeneic transplant is also an adverse factor for survival.

CYTOGENETICALLY DIRECTED THERAPY. Busulfan and conventional-dose hydroxyurea rarely eliminate the Ph[1] chromosome from marrow cells. A return to a normal chromosomal pattern is a reasonable therapeutic goal; patients who achieve a normal karyo-

type survive longer than those who do not. Three therapeutic initiatives have been developed based on this concept: the use of interferons, intensive chemotherapy, and BMT.

Interferon. Both human leukocyte interferon and recombinant interferon-α (r-IFNα) can produce hematologic and cytogenetic remissions in CML. Complete hematologic remissions are obtained in 75 to 80% of patients treated with r-IFNα, and 30 to 40% of the patients have complete or major suppression in the Ph[1] chromosome. Interferon-γ does not have a significant therapeutic effect. Return of normal metaphases after the use of r-IFNα is associated with a longer survival than is seen in patients without a cytogenetic response. The dosage of r-IFNα is 2 to 5 million units/m²/day, administered subcutaneously. The response rate is higher with higher doses. The most common acute side effects (musculoskeletal discomfort, fever, and chills) subside in most patients but are often replaced by symptoms of fatigue, depression, lethargy, inattention, loss of weight, lack of libido, and mild alopecia. These toxicities are more common in patients older than 60 years of age. Reactions at the injection site occur in approximately 5% of patients. Hypothyroidism, thrombocytopenia, anemia, arthritis, nephrotic syndrome, and seizures can occur. Loss of disease control, together with lack of side effects, may signal the development of neutralizing antibodies to interferon. Studies suggest that a combination of cytarabine and interferon results in superior survival to interferon alone.

Aggressive Chemotherapy. Regimens commonly employed for the treatment of AML have been used in an attempt to suppress the Ph[1] chromosome. In more than 50% of the treated patients, the percentage of Ph[1]-positive metaphases is greatly reduced, and about one third become transiently diploid for 2 to 12 months. Research protocols use chemotherapy induction therapy followed by r-IFNα.

Allogeneic Bone Marrow Transplantation. BMT (see Chapter 182) has been performed in patients with benign-phase CML. The risk of early death due to complications of BMT (20–35%) is balanced against the observation that 50 to 60% of patients will be in hematologic or cytogenetic remission 5 to 10 years afterward. Favorable factors for survival are age younger than 30 years, BMT within 1 year of diagnosis, and absence of severe graft-versus-host disease (GVHD). Long-term survival rates after BMT for accelerated and blast phases of CML are only 10 to 15%. In one series, syngeneic (identical twin) BMT provided 75% rate of persistent complete hematologic and cytogenetic remission; the possibility exists that many of these patients will be cured. Conversely, results with autologous BMT and peripheral blood stem cell support after ablative chemotherapy and radiation therapy have been disappointing. Because only one third of all patients have a matched related donor, matched unrelated donor transplants are being investigated, with promising results but substantial early morbidity (≈50%).

TREATMENT OF ACCELERATED CML AND BLAST CRISIS OF CML. Loss of control of CML with agents such as busulfan, hydroxyurea, or interferon is a feature of the development of the accelerated

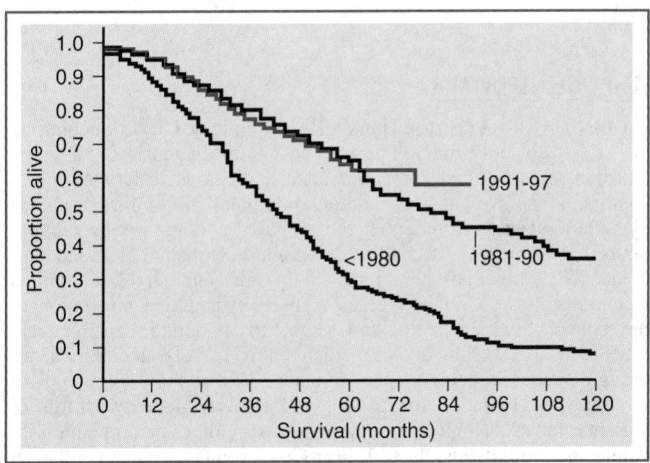

FIGURE 176–2 ■ Survival of M. D. Anderson Cancer Center patients with chronic (benign) phase chronic myelogenous leukemia by year of diagnosis, 1970–1997.

Table 176-2 ■ ADVERSE PROGNOSTIC FACTORS IN CHRONIC MYELOGENOUS LEUKEMIA

Older age
Large spleen size
Large liver
Increase or decrease in platelet count
High white blood cell count
Basophilia
Clonal evolution

From Kantarjian HM, Keating MJ, Smith TL, et al: Proposal for a simple synthesis prognostic staging system in chronic myelogenous leukemia. Am J Med 88:1, 1990.

phase of CML. Many of these patients develop additional cytogenetic abnormalities (clonal evolution) and increasing dysplasia, a left shift (5 to 29% blast cells), eosinophilia, and basophilia in the marrow. Change of therapy from busulfan to hydroxyurea or vice versa is successful for a short time (3 to 6 months) in a few patients. Splenectomy occasionally corrects the thrombocytopenia. If the proportion of blast cells in bone marrow exceeds 30%, the patient is considered to be in blast crisis (acute transformation of CML). The blast crisis, or refractory accelerated phase of CML, is usually treated with regimens designed for the treatment of acute leukemia. Treatment of myeloid, undifferentiated, or mixed-lineage blast crisis is usually unsatisfactory, with only 25 to 30% of patients achieving complete remission. Patients with a lymphoid blast crisis phenotype have a better chance (50 to 65%) of achieving complete remission on regimens using vincristine, corticosteroids, cyclophosphamide, asparaginase, and/or anthracyclines. The Ph[1] chromosome usually persists, and the duration of response is usually short (2 to 6 months), with no prospect of cure. Only 10 to 15% of patients with blast crisis survive for more than 1 year (see Fig. 176–1). Allogeneic BMT should be offered to patients with blast crisis (with active disease or after remission is obtained) if a suitable donor is available, because few of these patients have survived more than 5 years. The mortality rate and relapse rate after allogeneic BMT for CML blast crisis are much higher than for CML in the benign (chronic) phase.

PROGNOSIS. The median survival in Ph[1]-positive CML was 3 to 4 years for patients treated in the 1970s, with a range of 1 to 20 years (Fig. 176–2). The median survival at one institution for patients in whom the diagnosis was made after 1980 is greater than 5 years. The risk of death is 5 to 8% per year for the first 24 months and increases to 15 to 20% per year for the next 2 years and 25% per year thereafter. No patients are projected to be cured with palliative busulfan or hydroxyurea. Treatment with interferon, aggressive chemotherapy, or allogeneic BMT contributes to the improved survival of patients. Large spleen, increased liver size, elevated platelet counts, high marrow and blood blast and basophil percentages, advanced age, and clonal evolution are consistent adverse prognostic factors (Table 176–2) and have been combined into a simple staging system. This system identifies a high-risk group (30–40%) of patients with a median survival of only 2 years.

HAIRY CELL LEUKEMIA

CLINICAL FEATURES. Hairy cell leukemia (HCL) is uncommon (1–2% of all leukemias). The median age at diagnosis is 50 years, and there is a 4:1 male preponderance. Patients have fatigue due to anemia, fever, weight loss, and/or abdominal discomfort produced by splenomegaly. Sometimes the disease is diagnosed when patients have infection secondary to granulocytopenia or monocytopenia. The only consistent physical findings are slight to marked splenomegaly (75–80% of cases) caused by massive infiltration of the spleen by hairy cells and slight to moderate hepatomegaly (33% of cases). Clinical lymphadenopathy is very uncommon, although retroperitoneal lymphadenopathy is noted on computed tomography (CT) in 20 to 25% of cases. More than two thirds of patients have anemia (hemoglobin < 10 g/dL), neutropenia (absolute neutrophil count < 1500/μL), thrombocytopenia (platelet count <100,000/μL), and monocytopenia (absolute monocyte count <100/μL). The total WBC count is usually lower than 4000/μL at

diagnosis, but marked thrombocytopenia is rare. The cytopenias are due to a combination of bone marrow production failure caused by leukemic infiltration and of hypersplenism. Marrow failure may be due in part to inhibitory factors (e.g., tumor necrosis factor) produced by the leukemic infiltrate, because the pancytopenia is often much more marked than would be anticipated from the degree of leukemic infiltration. During the course of the illness, patients often experience repeated infections and, more rarely, a systemic vasculitis resembling polyarteritis nodosa. Patients also rarely have osteolytic bone lesions, usually affecting the upper femora. Although gram-positive or gram-negative infections occur as expected with neutropenia, patients with HCL have a predilection to develop tuberculosis, atypical mycobacterial infections, or fungal infections, perhaps related to the severe monocytopenia that is characteristic of this disorder. Pneumonia and septicemia are common causes of death in HCL.

DIAGNOSIS. In conjunction with the described clinical features, examination of the blood often suggests the diagnosis of HCL. In addition to the cytopenias described earlier, the peripheral blood film usually demonstrates relative or absolute lymphocytosis, composed of cells with cytoplasmic projections, giving rise to the name hairy cell leukemia (see Color Plate 6G). The cytoplasmic projections are best seen using phase contrast or electron microscopy. The hairy cells are 10 to 15 mm in diameter with pale blue cytoplasm and a nucleus with a loose chromatin structure and one or two indistinct nucleoli. Bone marrow aspiration is usually inadequate owing to increased reticulin, collagen, and fibrin deposition; bone marrow biopsy is usually necessary. The biopsy demonstrates increased cellularity with a diffuse or occasionally patchy infiltrate with hairy cells. The infiltrate is loose and spongy, with pale-staining cytoplasm surrounding bland, monotonous round or ovoid nuclei.

Hairy cells exhibit a strong acid phosphatase (isoenzyme 5) cytochemical reaction in 95% of cases, a reaction that is resistant to the inhibitory effect of tartaric acid (TRAP). Other lymphoproliferative diseases are rarely TRAP positive. Electron microscopy exquisitely demonstrates the microvillar projections. Often, ribosomal-lamellar complexes can be identified; these are characteristic, but not diagnostic, of HCL. The peroxidase stain is negative, and lysozyme activity is absent in hairy cells, differentiating the cells from monocytes.

The cell of origin of HCL is the B lymphocyte, as documented by the demonstration of heavy- and light-chain immunoglobulin gene rearrangements. Hairy cells express CD19 and CD20, FMC7, and CD22, but not CD21 or CD5. Cell-surface immunoglobulins can be immunoglobulin G (IgG) or immunoglobulin A (IgA), which are rare in chronic lymphocytic leukemia (CLL). The cells demonstrate a κ or λ light-chain phenotype excess. The cells are CD25 (TAC or low-affinity interleukin-2 [IL-2] receptor) positive and anti-HC2 positive, and they are positive for an early plasma cell antigen PCA-1 but not a late plasma cell antigen PC1. These findings suggest that hairy cells are late B lymphocytes or early plasma cells. High levels of soluble IL-2 receptors (> five times normal) are present in the sera of almost all patients with HCL, with extremely high levels being noted in many cases. Some cases of HCL have a 14q+ cytogenetic abnormality with a breakpoint at 14q32 (the locus of the Ig heavy chain gene). Hairy cells have a low proliferative index, with fewer than 1% being in the S phase of the cell cycle. Immune dysfunction is wide ranging in HCL. Monocytopenia is universal; B and T lymphocytes are decreased in number; the CD4/CD8 ratio is often inverted; and skin test reactivity to recall antigens is impaired, as is antibody-dependent cellular cytotoxicity. Humoral immunity is relatively preserved with normal immunoglobulin levels. Patients with HCL may have markedly impaired production of INF-α.

DIFFERENTIAL DIAGNOSIS. The differential diagnosis is most difficult between HCL and patients with lymphoma or CLL who have predominant splenomegaly and minimal lymphadenopathy. Some patients with a myelodysplastic or myeloproliferative syndrome have marked splenomegaly and pancytopenia with only a few atypical cells. Patients with other diseases, such as systemic lupus erythematosus and other autoimmune diseases, infiltrative splenomegaly, or tuberculosis, may have splenomegaly and cytopenia, but these diagnoses can usually be made by history, physical examination, and appropriate blood and bone marrow tests. Splenomegaly, cytopenia, and inaspirable marrow in a male should create a very high index of suspicion for HCL.

Other pathologic conditions to be differentiated from HCL by special tests are HCL variant, splenic lymphoma with villous lymphocytes, B-cell and T-cell prolymphocytic leukemia, and CLL with splenomegaly and no lymphadenopathy. Splenectomy and lymph node biopsy are sometimes necessary to establish the diagnosis in difficult cases. Cases of HCL variant manifest with higher WBC counts, are TRAP negative, have prominent nucleoli, and are only occasionally positive for antibodies against CD25. HCL variant responds poorly to interferon or deoxycoformycin, which are very effective agents in the management of typical HCL.

TREATMENT. A small proportion (<5%) of patients with HCL do not require therapy. These patients have mild cytopenias, are not transfusion dependent, have no history of infections, and have a low level of marrow infiltration by hairy cells.

Splenectomy was often used in the past as the first treatment of most patients with complications from HCL; it temporarily improves blood cell counts in two thirds of patients, usually within 1 to 4 weeks, but does not decrease the infiltration of hairy cells in the marrow or reduce the incidence of infections. Splenectomy is now recommended mainly for patients with splenic infarcts or massive splenomegaly.

Human leukocyte interferon (HuIFN) or r-IFNα rapidly improves (1 to 3 months) granulocyte, platelet, and hemoglobin levels; reduces spleen size; and consistently decreases marrow infiltration. Peripheral blood cell counts return to normal in 80% of cases, and these patients achieve complete remission (no hairy cells in the marrow) or partial remission (> 50% reduction in marrow HCL infiltration). Most patients achieve partial remission by 6 months and complete remission by 12 to 18 months. Lack of response or loss of an initial response may result from the development of neutralizing antibodies to r-IFNα, especially if the antibody titer is high. When treatment is discontinued, most cases relapse within 1 to 2 years but can respond to re-treatment.

Pentostatin, an adenosine deaminase inhibitor, produces complete remissions in 50 to 60% of patients and partial remissions in 40%. The response to treatment is more rapid than for interferon, occurring within 2 to 4 months after the initiation of therapy. Pentostatin is active in patients previously treated with interferon. Responses appear to be more durable than those seen in interferon-treated patients. Toxicity includes nausea and vomiting, infection, renal and hepatic dysfunction, conjunctivitis, and photosensitivity.

2-Chlorodeoxyadenosine (2-CDA), an adenosine analogue that is resistant to deamination by adenosine deaminase, produces complete remissions in more than 90% of HCL patients with a single course of 0.1 mg/kg/day for 7 days by continuous intravenous infusion. Patients for whom previous splenectomy or interferon therapy had failed usually respond to 2-CDA; patients resistant to pentostatin can also respond to 2-CDA. Remissions are very durable, and the few patients who experience relapse can attain second remissions after re-treatment with 2-CDA. The drug is very well tolerated, with a low infection rate. Despite long-lasting suppression of CD4+ lymphocyte counts from 2-CDA, there does not appear to be an increase in late opportunistic infections or second malignancies. The low doses and brief exposure to 2-CDA that are required to treat HCL, and the durability of 2-CDA–induced responses, strongly suggest that this drug may become established as the first therapy of choice in HCL.

Chemotherapy for HCL with alkylating agents, corticosteroids, androgens, and anthracyclines is not effective. Granulocyte colony-stimulating factor (G-CSF) has been reported to correct the granulocytopenia in HCL.

PROGNOSIS. The median survival of patients with HCL before interferon therapy was 2 to 3 years. A return to normal leukocyte counts in HCL diminishes the risk of infection and is certain to improve the survival of patients with HCL. More than 90% of patients treated with interferon, 2-CDA, or pentostatin are projected to be alive at 5 years.

CHRONIC LYMPHOCYTIC LEUKEMIA

CLL is a neoplasm characterized by accumulation of monoclonal lymphocytes, usually of B-cell immunophenotype (> 95% of cases) and more rarely of T-cell immunophenotype. The cells accumulate in the bone marrow, lymph nodes, liver, spleen, and occasionally other organs. CLL is the most common leukemia (one third of all cases) in the Western world and is twice as common as CML. The disease occurs rarely in those younger than 30; most patients with CLL are older than 60 years of age. CLL increases in incidence exponentially with age; by age 80 the incidence rate is 20 cases per 100,000 persons per year. The male:female ratio is approximately 2:1. Asians in Japan and China have an incidence of CLL only 10% of that in the United States and other Western countries. Intermediate incidence rates exist for persons of Hispanic origin.

ETIOLOGY. The cause of CLL is unknown. Ionizing radiation and viruses have not been associated with CLL. Familial clustering in CLL is more common than in other leukemias; first-degree relatives of patients have a twofold to fourfold higher risk and develop CLL at a younger age than does the general population. Farmers have a higher incidence of CLL than do those in other occupations, raising the question of the possible etiologic role of herbicides or pesticides. No definite leukemogenic role of chemicals, including benzene, has been established for CLL.

PATHOGENESIS. Leukemia cells in CLL are usually remarkably homogeneous. The cells express low-intensity monoclonal surface immunoglobulin (SmIg, usually immunoglobulin M [IgM] ± immunoglobulin D [IgD]) of a single κ or λ light chain phenotype. A number of patients with CLL have SmIg molecules that cross react with IgM rheumatoid factor paraprotein. CLL cells are early B cells and have lost terminal deoxynucleotidyl transferase activity. The CLL cells express the pan–B cell antigens CD19, CD20, and CD24 in almost all cases and CD23 and CD21 (which includes the receptor for the Epstein-Barr virus and the C3D component of complement) and CD23 in more than 75% of cases. The C3B complement component receptor is expressed in fewer than 20% of cases. Almost all cells exhibit Ia antigen, receptors for the Fc fragment of IgG, and spontaneously form rosettes with mouse erythrocytes. In 95% of cases, the CLL cells co-express pan–B cell antigens and CD5 (Leu 1, T1, and T101), a pan–T cell antigen. Other T-cell antigens and common acute lymphocytic leukemia antigen (CALLA) (CD10) are absent. CD25 (TAC, IL-2 receptor) antigen is positive in more than 20% of cells in 20% of cases. Monoclonality of the B cells is demonstrated by marked preponderance of κ or λ light chains, by evidence of immunoglobulin gene rearrangement, by the presence of monoclonal serum Ig peaks in some cases, and by G6PD isoenzyme studies.

CLL is an accumulative rather than a proliferative disease, because the CLL cells have a low proliferative index. Patients with higher WBC counts and more advanced stages have higher proliferative indices and shorter survivals. Most of the CLL cells in the blood and bone marrow are in the G0 phase of the cell cycle, with only a small proportion of larger cells in the marrow and lymph nodes being in the other phases. The CLL cells have a longer lifespan in the blood than do normal B cells and have impaired egress from the blood. The CLL B cells have impaired responses to B-cell mitogens and to B-cell growth factors. The cells appear to be blocked in differentiation, with a high content of cytoplasmic IgM but a low surface IgM. Although most of the cells do not secrete immunoglobulins, in about 5% of cases a paraprotein of the same type as that on the surface of the CLL cells is present in the plasma or urine. The stimulatory effect of the CLL cells is low or absent in allogeneic or autologous mixed lymphocyte cultures. The CLL cells can be stimulated to differentiate into cells resembling hairy cells or plasma cells under the influence of phorbol esters, B-cell mitogens, or growth factors.

T-cell function is invariably abnormal in CLL. T cells are increased in number in the blood, bone marrow, and lymph nodes of patients with CLL; but they are polyclonal, and T-cell receptor gene rearrangement is rare. The CD4/CD8 (T-helper/T-suppressor) ratio is often close to unity or is inverted owing to a relatively greater increase in the CD8-positive cells. The T cells have a blunted response to T-cell mitogens in unseparated blood and decreased delayed hypersensitivity reactions to recall antigens. The T-cell defects worsen as the disease progresses to a more advanced stage. Purified T cells have a normal response to T-cell mitogens.

CLINICAL FEATURES. Most patients with CLL are asymptomatic, and the disease is diagnosed when absolute lymphocytosis is noted in the peripheral blood (Color Plate 6*F*) during evaluation for other illnesses or when the patient undergoes a routine physical examination. Symptoms such as fatigue, lethargy, loss of appetite, weight loss, or reduced exercise tolerance are non-specific. These features are occasionally greater than can be explained by the degree of anemia or extent of tumor burden. Many patients have enlarged lymph nodes (usually cervical) noted by themselves or others. Fever, night sweats, and documented infections are uncommon initial symptoms (<5%) but become more prominent as the disease progresses. Sinopulmonary infections occur during the early phase of the disease; but as the disease progresses, the frequency of neutropenia, T-cell deficiency, and hypogammaglobulinemia increases, resulting in gram-negative bacterial, fungal, and viral infections. Herpes zoster, herpes simplex, and cytomegalovirus infections usually occur later in the disease.

The major physical findings relate to infiltration of the reticuloendothelial system. Lymphadenopathy with discrete, rubbery, mobile lymph nodes is present in two thirds of patients at diagnosis. Later, as the lymph nodes enlarge, they become matted. Enlargement of the liver or spleen is less common at diagnosis (approximately 10% and 40% of cases, respectively). Less commonly, and usually late in the disease, clinically significant infiltration of skin, eyelids, heart, lungs, pleura, or gastrointestinal tract may occur, suggesting MALT or mantle cell leukemia. Organ failure due to infiltration with CLL is uncommon, with pulmonary symptoms being most likely to cause clinical problems. Infiltration of the central nervous system in CLL is rare, and central nervous system symptoms are more likely to be due to opportunistic infections, such as cryptococcosis or listeriosis. The extent of involvement varies from only a single node or node group to enlargement of virtually all nodes. Later in the disease, massive adenopathy may develop and cause luminal obstruction, such as obstructive jaundice, obstructive uropathy, dysphagia, or partial bowel obstruction. Unilateral or bilateral leg edema can occur, owing to obstruction of the lymphatic and/or venous systems. Pleural effusions and ascites can also develop and are associated with a poor prognosis.

DIAGNOSTIC FEATURES. CLL is characterized by absolute lymphocytosis in the peripheral blood—a minimal level of more than 5000/μL, but more usually in the range of 40,000 to 150,000/μL. Extreme leukocytosis approaching $1 \times 10^6/\mu$L occurs late in the disease, and hyperviscosity symptoms can occur if the WBC count is higher than 500,000/μL. If the lymphocyte count is 5,000 to 15,000/μL, supportive evidence for clonality (κ or λ light chain excess or immunoglobulin gene rearrangement) should be present before the diagnosis is made. Most physicians also document lymphocytosis in the bone marrow (>30% lymphocytes) and perform a bone marrow biopsy. Anemia (hemoglobin <11 g/dL) is present in 15 to 20% of patients at diagnosis and thrombocytopenia (platelet count <100,000/μL) in 10%. Both bone marrow replacement and hypersplenism contribute to the anemia and thrombocytopenia in most cases. The anemia is usually normochromic and normocytic, and the reticulocyte count is normal unless the patient has autoimmune hemolytic anemia, which usually results from the development of a warm-reacting IgG antibody. The diagnosis of autoim-

mune hemolytic anemia, which occurs in the course of 8 to 10% of cases, is confirmed by a positive direct Coombs' test, reticulocytosis, and an elevated unconjugated serum bilirubin level (see Chapter 165). In such patients, reactive erythroid hyperplasia as a response to the hemolysis may be masked in the bone marrow by the marked lymphocytic infiltration. Cold agglutinin hemolysis occurs rarely in CLL. Autoimmune thrombocytopenia (immune thrombocytopenic purpura [ITP]) can be diagnosed in some cases with a positive test for platelet antibodies (see Chapter 184). The antibodies causing the red cell and platelet destruction are not produced by the CLL cells, and the mechanism for the autoimmune diseases is not known. Pure red cell aplasia associated with T-suppressor cell activity is an additional reported cause of anemia in CLL.

The lymphocytes in CLL are indistinguishable on light or electron microscopy from normal small B lymphocytes. On bone marrow aspiration, the proportion of lymphocytes is greater than 30% and may extend up to 100% in patients with newly diagnosed CLL. The remainder of the cells are normal myeloid and erythroid cells. Four patterns of lymphocyte infiltration on bone marrow biopsy occur and have prognostic value in CLL: (1) nodular (15%), (2) interstitial (30%), (3) mixed nodular and interstitial (30%), and (4) diffuse (35%). Most early-stage cases have patterns 1, 2, or 3; diffuse histology is most common in advanced-stage disease and becomes more prominent as the disease evolves. A diffuse histologic pattern confers a poor prognosis regardless of the stage of disease. Hypogammaglobulinemia is common in CLL and predisposes to infections, especially with encapsulated microorganisms. Low levels of IgG, IgA, or IgM occur in 25% of newly diagnosed patients, are more common in advanced stages, and increase in frequency to 50 to 70% as the disease progresses.

Non-random cytogenetic abnormalities in CLL include trisomy 12 (40%), 14q+ abnormalities (25%), and abnormalities in the long arm of chromosomes 6, 11, and 13. Single abnormalities are more common in early and recently diagnosed cases, and additional changes develop with time (clonal evolution). The site of the breakpoint on chromosome 14 (q32) is close to the site of the Ig heavy-chain gene. Recent molecular studies suggest that deletion of genetic material from chromosome 13 or 14 occurs in two thirds of the cases.

STAGING SYSTEMS. Two major staging systems are used. The Rai staging system (1975) defines five stages and is most frequently used in the United States, whereas the Binet system (1981) defines three stages and is most frequently used in Europe (Table 176–3). Both systems have the advantage of simplicity, low cost, and reproducibility and have been prospectively validated (Figs. 176–3 and 176–4). Within the stages, outcome is variable; other prognostic factors, such as the bone marrow histologic pattern, provide additional prognostic information. Patients with anemia and thrombocytopenia (Rai stages III and IV, Binet C) have, on the average, a poor prognosis; patients with lymphocytosis alone (Rai 0, some Binet A patients) have an excellent prognosis. The prognosis of the other patients is heterogeneous and, as might be expected, is worse in patients with a greater tumor burden. Rai stage II patients who have splenomegaly without lymphadenopathy (pure splenic form) have a better prognosis than do other stage II patients. Although useful in the design and analysis of clinical trials,

Table 176–3 ■ RAI AND BINET STAGING SYSTEMS IN CHRONIC LYMPHOCYTIC LEUKEMIA

	LYMPHOCYTOSIS	LYMPHADENOPATHY	HEPATOMEGALY OR SPLENOMEGALY	HEMOGLOBIN (g/dL)	PLATELETS × 10³/µL
Rai Stage					
0	+	−	−	≥11	≥100
I	+	+	−	≥11	≥100
II	+	±	+	≥11	≥100
III	+	±	±	<11	≥100
IV	+	±	±	Any	<100
Binet Stage					
A	+	±	± (<3 Lymphatic groups* positive)	≥10	≥100
B	+	±	± (≥3 Lymphatic groups* positive)	≥10	≥100
C	+	±	±	<10 and/or	<100

*(1) Cervical, axillary, and inguinal nodes; (2) liver; and (3) spleen; each group is considered one group whether unilateral or bilateral.

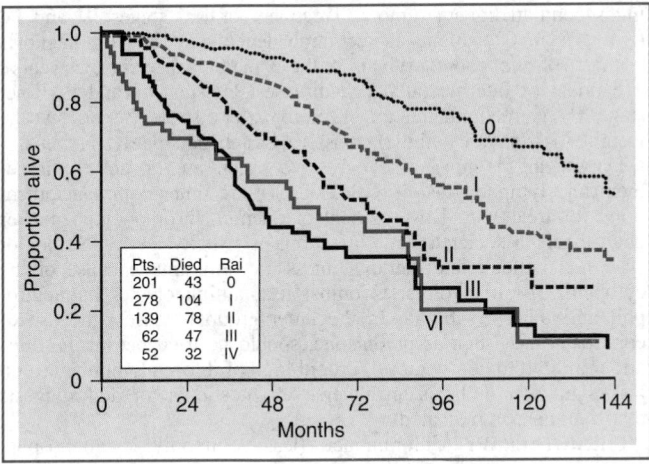

FIGURE 176–3 ■ Survival of untreated patients with chronic lymphocytic leukemia by Rai stage.

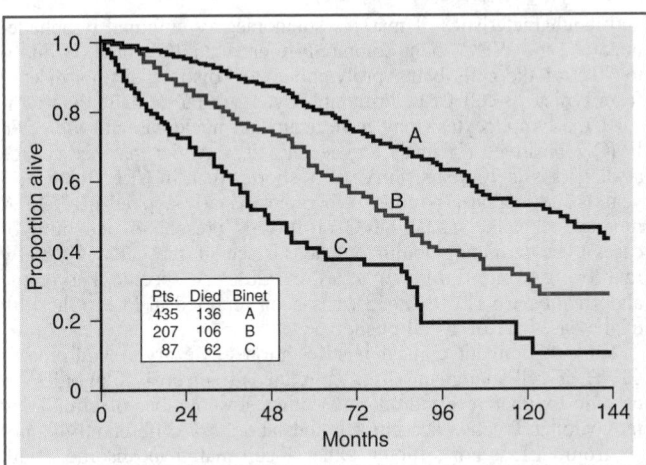

FIGURE 176–4 ■ Survival of untreated patients with chronic lymphocytic leukemia by Binet stage.

the staging systems are not particularly useful for individual patients because of the heterogeneity of outcome. A group of patients with a lymphocyte count of less than 30,000/μL, hemoglobin higher than 11 g/dL, platelet count higher than 100,000/μL, fewer than three involved node areas, and lymphocyte doubling time of greater than 12 months has been described as having "smoldering" CLL, with a survival equal to that of an age- and sex-matched population. Studies suggest that serum levels of β_2-microglobulin and soluble CD23 are more strongly predictive for prognosis than stage.

Patients tend to progress through stages, with many patients developing more sites of involvement with time and eventually experiencing marrow failure, but anemia and thrombocytopenia can develop abruptly even without antibody-mediated destruction or increasing tumor burden.

DIFFERENTIAL DIAGNOSIS. Many diseases can cause lymphocytosis: pertussis, infectious lymphocytosis, cytomegalovirus and Epstein-Barr virus mononucleosis, tuberculosis, toxoplasmosis, chronic inflammatory disorders, and autoimmune syndromes. Although these conditions may superficially resemble CLL, their clinical pictures seldom are confused with that of B-cell CLL. Many of these patients are younger, have fever or other acute symptoms, or exhibit other clinical features, such as rash and joint symptoms, that are uncommon in CLL. The lymphocytosis (usually <15,000/μL) is not sustained. If doubt persists, immunophenotype studies distinguish the monoclonal lymphocytosis in CLL from the polyclonal B cell proliferation in the other disorders.

The more difficult differential diagnosis is from other lymphoproliferative disorders, such as prolymphocytic leukemia (PLL), splenic lymphoma with villous lymphocytes (SLVL), HCL, the leukemic phase of mantle cell lymphoma, Waldenström's macroglobulinemia, and T-cell CLL. Whereas certain clinical features are

more common in some of these disorders (e.g., marked splenomegaly with minimal or no lymphadenopathy in prolymphocytic leukemia, splenic lymphoma, and HCL versus extensive lymphadenopathy with or without splenomegaly in CLL), none of these differential features is specific. The differential diagnosis therefore depends largely on histopathologic and, more specifically, immunophenotypic features (Table 176–4).

Small lymphocytic lymphoma (SLL) shares histopathologic and immunophenotypic features with CLL, differing only in lacking absolute monoclonal lymphocytosis in the peripheral blood (see Chapter 179). The bone marrow in SLL may or may not have more than 30% lymphocytes. LFA-1 adhesion protein is much more commonly expressed on SLL cells than CLL cells. Occasionally, other lymphomas, such as follicular small cleaved cell lymphoma (FSCCL) and mantle cell lymphoma, manifest in a leukemic phase. These cells are often cleaved on light microscopy, have bright staining for SmIg, and are commonly FMC-7 and CD 10 positive. Lymph node biopsy should be performed to identify these cases with greater precision. The presence of lymphoma cells in the blood in SLL and FSCCL is more common later in the disease. FSCLL can usually be identified by the presence of the translocation t(14;18) on cytogenetic analysis and consequent *bcl*-2 rearrangement, both of which are rare in CLL. The WBC count in Waldenström's macroglobulinemia at diagnosis is usually much lower than in CLL (< 10,000/μL), and many patients are leukopenic. The cells have a plasmacytoid appearance, CD38 and PCA-1 positivity, and more SmIg and cytoplasmic Ig. A monoclonal IgM plasma peak is present in almost all cases of Waldenström's macroglobulinemia, is common in splenic lymphoma, but is rare in CLL.

PLL is an uncommon disease (10% of the incidence of CLL);

Table 176–4 ■ DIFFERENTIAL DIAGNOSIS OF INDOLENT LYMPHOPROLIFERATIVE DISORDERS

DISEASE	LYMPHADENOPATHY (%)	SPLENOMEGALY (%)	CELL OF ORIGIN (B/T)	POSITIVE MARKERS*			
				SmIg	CD5	CD19,20 (%)	Other Positives
Chronic lymphocytic leukemia (CLL)	75	50	B (20:1)	Weak	>90%	≥90	Mouse red blood cell (RBC) receptors
Prolymphocytic leukemia (PLL)	33	95	B (4:1)	Bright	T cell PLL	75	FMC-7
Hairy cell leukemia	<10	80	B (T rare)	Bright	—	>90	CD25, CD11C
Lymphoma (leukemic phase)	90	90	B (T rare)	Bright	Some	>90	CD10
Splenic lymphoma with villous lymphocytes	10	80	B	Bright	20%	>90	FMC-7, CD22
Waldenström's macroglobulinemia	33	33	All B	Weak	Some	Many	CD38, PCA-1
Large granular lymphocytosis	10	10	All T	Absent	—	—	CD2, CD3, CD8

*CD5—pan T cell, B CLL
  CD19—early pan B cell
  CD20—pan B cell
  FMC-7—PLL and hairy cell
  CD2—pan T cell
  CD3—pan mature T cell

CD8—T cell (suppressor-cytotoxic)
CD10—early B cell
CD11C—hairy cell, activated T cell, NK cell
CD38—activated B cell, thymocyte, plasma cell
PCA-1—plasma cell
CD25—low-affinity interleukin-2 (IL-2) receptor

and its characteristics of massive splenomegaly, minimal lymphade-nopathy, and WBC count commonly more than 100,00/μL, with 10 to 90% of the cells being prolymphocytes, distinguish this disease from typical B-cell CLL. Prolymphocytes are larger cells than typical CLL lymphocytes; they have a distinct nucleolus and are often FMC-7 positive. The male:female ratio is 4:1, and the median age at diagnosis is 70 years. Survival is shorter than in CLL (median, 3 years), and response is poor to therapies usually applied in CLL. A monoclonal spike, usually IgG or IgA, is present in one third of cases. The immunoglobulin on the surface of the cells is usually IgG or IgA, not IgM ± IgD, as in CLL. A specific karyotypic abnormality, t(6;12) (q15;q13), has been reported in PLL. One fifth of the cases are of T-cell phenotype.

The predominant clinical manifestation in Sézary's syndrome (a CD4+ T-cell malignant disorder related to mycosis fungoides) is chronic exfoliative erythroderma with a low number of circulating monoclonal T cells. The clinical and laboratory differential diagnosis from CLL is not difficult. Other T-cell malignant disorders with peripheral blood involvement are adult T-cell leukemia-lymphoma and large granular lymphocytosis (LGL), also referred to as "large granular lymphoproliferative disorder," "T-cell lymphocytosis with neutropenia," or "T-gamma lymphocytosis syndrome." Adult T-cell leukemia-lymphoma is associated with a retrovirus (human T-cell leukemia-lymphoma virus [HTLV-I]) and is common in Japan and the Caribbean. It is frequently manifested by lytic bone lesions and hypercalcemia. In T-LGL the absolute lymphocyte count is usually low (<5000/μL), with a CD2+, CD3+, CD8+ and CD16+(T-suppressor) phenotype (T-gamma cells). These patients often have splenomegaly, neutropenia, and rheumatoid arthritis–like symptoms and serology. Some, called NK-LGL, have a natural killer phenotype (CD16−) and have no molecular evidence of T-cell receptor rearrangement. The lymphocytes have abundant cytoplasm with azurophilic granules. In most patients, a benign course is noted, although repeated infections can occur.

PROGNOSTIC FACTORS. In addition to the impact of tumor burden and marrow function on prognosis, as reflected in the Rai and Binet staging systems, other adverse factors include a diffuse pattern of lymphocytic infiltration observed on bone marrow biopsy; an abnormal karyotype (e.g., trisomy 12 or multiple chromosomal abnormalities); advanced age; male sex; elevated serum levels of thymidine kinase, β_2-microglobulin, uric acid, alkaline phosphatase, or lactate dehydrogenase; rapid lymphocyte doubling time; and an increased proportion of large or atypical lymphocytes in the peripheral blood. A poor response to therapy is an adverse factor in all phases of the disease. As the disease progresses, a worsening of stage and the development of prolymphocytic leukemia (10% of cases), large cell lymphoma, or myelomatous or acute lymphocytic leukemia (rare) are grave prognostic features. Multiple chromosomal abnormalities identify patients at risk of developing a large cell lymphomatous transformation (Richter's syndrome), which occurs in 5 to 10% of CLL patients as a terminal event. Richter's syndrome should be suspected whenever a single lymph node area or the spleen begins to enlarge in CLL or when unexplained clinical deterioration occurs. The transformation does not always share immunophenotypic or cytogenetic features with the original CLL clone and may be a coincidental second tumor. Response to therapy in Richter's transformation is not as satisfactory as for de novo large cell lymphoma.

A high incidence of second malignant tumors (10–20% of patients) either precedes or follows the diagnosis of CLL, with the roles of therapy versus impaired immune surveillance as causative factors being unclear. Skin cancer, including melanoma, colorectal and lung cancers, and sarcomas are common in patients with CLL. Hypogammaglobulinemia may have an adverse impact on survival. Patients who develop repeated infections fare less well than other patients.

TREATMENT. The major therapeutic questions for CLL are when to treat and which therapeutic agent or agents to use.

WHEN TO TREAT. Patients with CLL are usually elderly, and the prognosis of the disease is variable (with some early-stage cases being stable for 5 to 20 years). It is traditional, therefore, to delay treatment of early-stage CLL (Rai 0, Binet A) until the disease progresses. Early treatment with alkylating agents does not prolong survival and may be associated with a heightened risk of developing second malignant tumors. Treatment of Rai stages III and IV (Binet stage C) patients is recommended at the time of diagnosis because of the poor survival of these patients (median, 3 years). Treatment of intermediate-stage disease (Rai stages I and II, Binet stage B) is recommended if symptomatic disease (fever, sweats, weight loss, severe fatigue), massive lymphadenopathy, or hepatosplenomegaly is present. Progressive organ and/or node enlargement and lymphocytosis (>100,000/μL) are other common indications for treatment. Development of anemia, thrombocytopenia, or neutropenia associated with infections is usually an indication for systemic antileukemic therapy unless an autoimmune cause of the cytopenia (positive direct Coombs' test, antiplatelet or antineutrophil antibodies) is found. In the latter group of cases, the use of corticosteroids, such as prednisone, should be tried before the initiation of cytotoxic therapy. A doubling of blood lymphocytes in less than 12 months is an adverse prognostic factor and suggests that treatment is indicated.

CHEMOTHERAPY. Chlorambucil (less commonly, cyclophosphamide) is traditionally the first chemotherapeutic agent used. Corticosteroids are often used concurrently, but with no clearly demonstrated advantage in therapeutic response or survival. Chlorambucil regimens vary widely. In the chronic low-dosage daily regimen, 0.1 to 0.2 mg/kg/day of chlorambucil is continued for 3 to 6 weeks until the desired effect is obtained or until thrombocytopenia or neutropenia develops. The dosage is then adjusted for maintenance and is continued for 6 to 12 months. For intermittent high-dosage (pulse) schedules, chlorambucil (0.5 to 2 mg/kg) is given over 1 to 4 days every 4 weeks or at half dosage every 2 weeks. No dosage schedule for chlorambucil has been established as being superior. If prednisone is given concurrently with chlorambucil, the dosage is 60 to 100 mg/day in the pulse schedule. Continuous prednisone is not recommended in this elderly population but can be given at a dosage of 40 to 60 mg/day for 4 weeks initially, tapering to 10 to 20 mg/day when combined with chlorambucil in the continuous-therapy schedule. Myelosuppression is the most common toxicity with chlorambucil, although occasionally rash, nausea, or pulmonary toxicity occurs. After therapy, the condition of many patients remains stable for months to years before disease progression indicates the need for further treatment. The end points for response to therapy have not been well defined, because treatment is usually strictly palliative. Most physicians try to achieve the disappearance of lymphadenopathy and splenomegaly and the return to a normal WBC count but rarely normal bone marrow (Table 176–5).

Fludarabine monophosphate and 2-CDA, both adenosine analogues, and pentostatin (deoxycoformycin), an adenosine deaminase inhibitor, have exhibited striking therapeutic efficacy in CLL. Fludarabine monophosphate (25 mg/m²/day for 5 days every 4 weeks) leads to complete remission in 30% of untreated patients and 10% of those previously treated with alkylating agents. The dose-limiting toxicity is myelosuppression. The course of therapy may be complicated by infections with organisms usually associated with immunodeficiency syndromes involving T lymphocytes (e.g., those caused by *Pneumocystis carinii,* herpesviruses). Fludarabine has been shown to have a higher complete remission rate and longer time to disease progression than chlorambucil or combination chemotherapy with the CAP regimen (see later). 2-CDA delivers similar results with a lower complete remission rate and more myelosuppression. Deoxycoformycin has not been as widely studied in CLL.

The COP regimen (cyclophosphamide, 100 to 300 mg/m²/day given orally on days 1 through 5; vincristine [Oncovin], 2 mg given intravenously on day 1; and prednisone, 100 mg administered orally on days 1 through 5) does not have any advantage over chlorambucil. Regimens using cyclophosphamide, doxorubicin (Adriamycin), and prednisone with vincristine (CHOP) or without vincristine (CAP) have produced response rates of 50 to 70% in previously untreated patients with Binet stage C disease and are well tolerated in CLL despite the advanced age of most patients.

Corticosteroids, usually prednisone (60 to 100 mg/day), are indicated as treatment for Coombs-positive autoimmune hemolytic anemia and for some cases of immune-mediated thrombocytopenia (ITP) in CLL. If there is no response in 3 to 4 weeks, the treatment has failed, and the dose should then be tapered over 1 to 2 weeks. If a response is obtained, the dose is usually reduced by 25% each

Table 176–5 ■ DEFINITION OF REMISSION IN CLL: COMPARISON OF THE INTERNATIONAL WORKSHOP IN CLL (IWCLL) AND THE NATIONAL CANCER INSTITUTE WORKING GROUP (NCI–WG) CRITERIA

CRITERIA	COMPLETE REMISSION		PARTIAL REMISSION	
	IWCLL	NCI–WG	IWCLL	NCI–WG
Physical examination				
Nodes	None	None	Shift to a lower Binet stage, e.g., C → A or B, B → A	≥50% decrease
Liver/spleen	Not palpable	Not palpable		≥50% decrease
Symptoms	None	None		N/A
Peripheral blood				
Neutrophils	≥1500/μL	≥1500/μL		≥1500/μL or ≥50% ↑ from baseline
Platelets	>100,000/μL	>100,000/μL		100,000/μL or ≥50% ↑ from baseline
Hemoglobin	Not specified	>11 g/dL		>11 g/dL or >50% ↑ from baseline
Lymphocytes	<4000/μL	≤4000/μL		>50% decrease
Bone marrow	Normal aspirate and biopsy*			N/A
Lymphocytes		<30%		N/A

*Nodules or focal aggregates of lymphocytes are compatible with complete remission.

week over 4 weeks. Patients in whom corticosteroids fail often respond well to splenectomy and sometimes to intravenous therapy with high doses of immunoglobulin or cyclosporin. Autoimmune hemolytic anemia and immune-mediated thrombocytopenia do not correlate closely with the activity of CLL.

RADIATION THERAPY. In CLL, radiation therapy is usually restricted to external irradiation of localized nodal masses or an enlarged spleen that has been refractory to chemotherapy. Repeated leukapheresis and extracorporeal irradiation of blood can decrease the tumor burden in CLL and occasionally increase hemoglobin and platelet levels but are not practical for long periods.

OTHER THERAPY. Intravenous immunoglobulin (400 mg/kg every 3 to 4 weeks) significantly decreases the incidence of infections of minor to moderate severity in CLL patients with hypogammaglobulinemia, but the cost of this therapy is substantial. Although ineffective in patients with advanced-stage CLL, INF-α may significantly decrease the lymphocyte count in 50 to 70% of early-stage cases as well as increase the absolute granulocyte count, improve the serum immunoglobulin level, and improve T-helper/T-suppressor ratios. Early studies of monoclonal antibodies directed against CLL cells have not as yet resulted in consistent benefit to patients. The efficacy of autologous and allogenic transplantations is being studied in CLL.

PROGNOSIS IN CLL. The median survival of patients with CLL is 4 to 5 years after initiation of treatment (see Figs. 176–3 and 176–4). As expected, patients with early-stage cases (Rai 0 to II) survive significantly longer, a median of 7 to 8 years. No current treatment strategy has demonstrated a survival advantage over conventional therapy with chlorambucil.

CLL tends to develop in elderly patients; death often occurs, therefore, from other intercurrent illnesses of this age group. Younger patients (< 60 years of age) almost all die as a result of CLL or one of its complications, especially infections. Gram-positive organisms usually cause non-fatal infections early in CLL, but most deaths due to infection are associated with gram-negative bacterial or fungal infections. Infection with other opportunistic organisms, such as *Mycobacterium tuberculosis,* herpesvirus, and *Pneumocystis carinii,* may also be fatal.

Cortes JE, Talpaz M, Kantarjian H: Chronic myelogenous leukemia: A review. Am J Med 100:555, 1996. *Comprehensive review with emphasis on therapeutic options.*

DiGiuseppe JA, Borowitz MJ: Clinical utility of flow cytometry in the chronic lymphoid leukemias. Semin Oncol 25:6, 1998. *Review of immunophenotypic analysis in the diagnosis of CLL.*

Hallek M, Kuhn-Hallek I, Emmerich B: Prognostic factors in CLL. Leukemia 11 (Suppl 2):S4, 1997. *Discussion of the heterogeneity of clinical course of CLL.*

Reed JD: Molecular biology of CLL. Semin Oncol 25:11, 1998. *Review emphasizing the molecular biology of CLL, with particular focus on cytogenetic abnormalities and the role of programmed cell death.*

Sawyers CL: Chronic myeloid leukemia. N Engl J Med 340:1330, 1999. *Concise up-to-date review of the molecular pathophysiology, mechanism of leukemogenesis, and treatment options, including novel strategies, for CML.*

177 THE ACUTE LEUKEMIAS

Frederick R. Appelbaum

DEFINITION

Normal hematopoiesis requires tightly regulated proliferation and differentiation of pluripotent hematopoietic stem cells that become mature peripheral blood cells. Acute leukemia is the result of a malignant event or events occurring in an early hematopoietic precursor. Instead of proliferating and differentiating normally, the affected cell gives rise to progeny that fail to differentiate and instead continue to proliferate in an uncontrolled fashion. As a result, immature myeloid cells (in acute myelogenous leukemia [AML]) or lymphoid cells (in acute lymphocytic leukemia [ALL]), often called blasts, rapidly accumulate and progressively replace the bone marrow; diminished production of normal red cells, white cells, and platelets ensues. This loss of normal marrow function in turn gives rise to the common clinical complications of leukemia: anemia, infection, and bleeding. With time, the leukemic blasts pour out into the blood stream and eventually occupy the lymph nodes, spleen, and other vital organs. If untreated, acute leukemia is rapidly fatal; most patients die within several months of diagnosis. With appropriate therapy, the natural history of acute leukemia can be markedly altered, and many patients can be cured.

ETIOLOGY

In most cases acute leukemia develops for no known reason, but sometimes a possible cause can be identified.

RADIATION. Ionizing radiation is leukemogenic. ALL, AML, and chronic myelogenous leukemia (CML) are all increased in incidence in patients given radiation therapy for ankylosing spondylitis and in survivors of the atomic bomb blasts at Hiroshima and Nagasaki. The magnitude of the risk depends on the dose of radiation, its distribution in time, and the age of the individual. Greater risk results from higher-dose radiation delivered over shorter periods to younger patients. In areas of high natural background radiation (often from radon), chromosomal aberrations have been reported to be more frequent, but an increase in acute leukemia has not been consistently found. Recently, concern has been raised about the possible leukemogenic effects of extremely low-frequency non-ionizing electromagnetic fields emitted by electrical installations. If such an effect exists at all, the magnitude of the effect is small.

ONCOGENIC VIRUSES. The search for a viral cause of leukemia has been intensely pursued, but none has been found, except for two rare leukemias associated with retroviruses. Human T-cell lymphotropic virus type I (HTLV-I), an enveloped, single-stranded RNA virus, is considered the causative agent of adult T-cell leukemia. This distinct form of leukemia is found within geographic clusters in southwestern Japan, the Caribbean basin, and Africa. The virus can be spread vertically from mother to fetus or horizontally by sexual contact or through blood products. Although previously rare in the United States, HTLV-I seropositivity has been found with increasing frequency among patients undergoing frequent transfusions and among intravenous drug users. Screening of blood products for antibodies to HTLV-I is now routine practice in blood banks in the United States. A second human retrovirus, termed HTLV-II and genetically distinct from HTLV-I, has been isolated from several patients with a syndrome resembling hairy cell leukemia. The etiologic link between HTLV-II and malignancy is uncertain.

GENETICS AND CONGENITAL FACTORS. If leukemia develops before 10 years of age in a patient with an identical twin, the unaffected twin has a one in five chance of leukemia subsequently developing. In occasional families, an identical form of leukemia has developed in multiple members. Several autosomal recessive disorders associated with chromosomal instability are prone to terminate in acute leukemia, including Bloom syndrome, Fanconi's anemia, and ataxia-telangiectasia. Other congenital disorders associated with an increased incidence of leukemia are Down syndrome and infantile X-linked agammaglobulinemia.

CHEMICALS AND DRUGS. Heavy occupational exposure to benzene and benzene-containing compounds such as kerosene and carbon tetrachloride may lead to marrow damage, which can take the form of aplastic anemia, myelodysplasia, or AML. A link between leukemia and tobacco use has recently been reported.

Prior exposure to alkylating agents such as melphalan and the nitrosoureas is associated with an increased risk of AML. These so-called secondary leukemias are often manifested as a myelodysplastic syndrome, frequently have abnormalities of chromosomes 5, 7, and 8, but have no distinct morphologic features; they typically develop 4 to 6 years after alkylating agent exposure, and their incidence may be increased with greater intensity and duration of drug exposure. Prolonged exposure to epipodophyllotoxins (teniposide or etoposide) has also been identified as a risk factor for the development of AML. The secondary leukemias associated with epipodophyllotoxin exposure tend to have a shorter latency period (1 to 2 years), lack a myelodysplastic phase, have a monocytic morphology, and involve abnormalities of the long arm of chromosome 11 (band q23). Recently, an association between the development of acute promyelocytic leukemia (APL) and prior treatment for psoriasis with bimolane, a dioxopiperazine derivative, has been reported.

INCIDENCE

The annual new case incidence of all leukemias is 8 to 10 per 100,000. This rate has remained static over the past three decades. The relative incidences for the four categories of leukemia are as follows: ALL, 11%; chronic lymphocytic leukemia, 29%; AML, 46%; and CML, 14%. The leukemias account for about 3% of all cancers in the United States. The impact of leukemia is heightened because of the young age of some patients. For example, ALL is the most common cancer and the second leading cause of death in children younger than 15 years. ALL has a maximal incidence between 2 and 10 years of age, with a second, more gradual rise in frequency later in life. The incidence of AML gradually increases with age, without an early peak. Approximately half of AML cases occur in patients younger than 50 years.

PATHOPHYSIOLOGY

The precise molecular event or events that cause leukemic transformation are unknown; the end result, however, is relentless proliferation of immature hematopoietic cells that have lost their capacity to differentiate normally. The development of leukemia may be a multistep process, as demonstrated by the fact that in many cases acute leukemia develops in patients with a pre-existing myelodysplastic disorder. The disease is monoclonal, i.e., the final leukemic event occurs in a single cell. The level of differentiation at which malignancy becomes evident is variable. In some cases of AML it appears that malignancy occurs in a very undifferentiated cell, similar to the normal hematopoietic stem cell, in that red cell, platelet, and myeloid precursors are all products of the malignant clone. In other cases of AML, the malignant event may occur in a more differentiated cell; granulocyte and monocyte precursors develop from the malignant cell, whereas red cell and platelet precursors do not. In almost all cases of ALL, the myeloid lineage is not malignant, which suggests that in ALL the malignant event occurs in a cell that is at least partially differentiated. Although the majority of leukemic cells are relatively undifferentiated, some mature circulating cells may be products of the malignant clone.

As the malignant clone expands, it does so at the expense of normal hematopoiesis. The mechanism of normal marrow suppression in leukemia is complex; in many patients with hypercellular marrow, the pancytopenia is probably the result, at least in part, of physical replacement of normal marrow precursors by leukemic cells. In some patients with acute leukemia, however, a pancytopenia with hypocellular marrow develops, thus suggesting that marrow failure is not simply due to physical replacement of the marrow space but may also be due to substances released by the malignant cells.

CLASSIFICATION

The acute leukemias can be classified in a variety of ways, including morphology, cytochemistry, cell-surface markers, cytoplasmic markers, cytogenetics, and oncogene expression (Table 177–1). The most important distinction is between AML and ALL because these two diseases differ considerably in their clinical behavior, prognosis, and response to therapy. The various subgroups of AML and ALL also have some important differences.

MORPHOLOGY. Leukemic cells in AML are typically 12 to 20 mm in diameter, with discrete nuclear chromatin, multiple nucleoli, and cytoplasm that usually contains azurophilic granules. Auer rods, which are slender, fusiform cytoplasmic inclusions that stain red with Wright-Giemsa stain, are virtually pathognomonic of AML. The French-American-British (FAB) collaborative group has subdivided AML into eight subtypes based on morphology and histochemistry: M0, M1, M2, and M3 reflect increasing degrees of differentiation of myeloid leukemic cells; M4 and M5 leukemias have features of the monocytic lineage; M6 has features of the erythroid cell lineage; and M7 is acute megakaryocytic leukemia.

The leukemic cells in ALL tend to be smaller than AML blasts and relatively devoid of granules. ALL can be divided, by FAB criteria, into L1, L2, and L3 subgroups. L1 blasts are uniform in size, with homogeneous nuclear chromatin, indistinct nucleoli, and scanty cytoplasm with few, if any granules. L2 blasts are larger and more variable in size and may have nucleoli. L3 blasts are quite distinct, with prominent nucleoli and deeply basophilic cytoplasm with vacuoles.

CELL-SURFACE MARKERS. Monoclonal antibodies reactive with cell-surface antigens have been used to classify acute leukemias. Antibodies that react with antigens found on normal immature myeloid cells, including CD13, CD14, CD33, and CD34, also react with blast cells from most patients with AML. Exceptions are the M6 and M7 variants, which have antigens restricted to the red cell and platelet lineage, respectively. Myeloid leukemia blasts also express HLA-DR antigens but usually lack T-cell, B-cell, and other lymphoid antigens. In 10 to 20% of patients, however, AML blasts will express antigens usually restricted to B- or T-cell lineage. Expression of lymphoid antigens by AML cells does not change either the natural history or the therapeutic response of these leukemias.

ALL can be divided into several forms based on cell-surface antigen expression. Approximately 60% of cases of ALL express the common ALL antigen (CALLA) on the cell surface. CALLA (CD10) is a glycoprotein also found on occasional normal early lymphocytes and other non-hematopoietic tissues. Cases of CALLA-positive ALL are thought to represent an early pre–B-cell differentiation state. About 20% of cases of CALLA-positive ALL

Table 177–1 ■ CLASSIFICATION OF ACCUTE LEUKEMIAS

| SUBTYPE | MORPHOLOGY | HISTOCHEMISTRY | | | MONOCLONAL REACTIVITY | CYTOGENETIC ABNORMALITIES |
		Myeloperoxidase	Non-specific Esterase	PAS		
M0, Acute undifferentiated leukemia	Uniform, very undifferentiated	−	−	−		Various
M1, Acute myeloid leukemia with minimal differentiation	Very undifferentiated, few azurophilic granules	+/−	+/−	−		Various
M2, acute myeloid leukemia with differentiation	Granulated blasts predominate; Auer rods may be seen	+++	+/−	+	For subtypes M0–M5b, approximately 90% of cases will react with at least one of the following antimyeloid antibodies: anti-CD13 anti-CD14 anti-CD33 anti-CD34	Various, including t(8;21)
M3, acute promyelocytic leukemia	Hypergranular promyelocytes	+++	+	+		t(15:17)
M4, acute myelomonocytic leukemia	Both monoblasts and myeloblasts are present	++	+++	++		Various, including inv/del(16)
M4E	Like M4 but with eosinophils					
M5, acute monocytic leukemia	Monoblasts predominate					
M5a	Type a, >80% monoblasts;	+/−	+++	++		Various, including abnormalities of 11q23
M5b	type b, >20% promonocytes					
M6, acute erythroleukemia	Erythroblasts and megaloblastic red cell precursors seen	−		++	Antiglycopherin, antispectrin	Various
M7, Acute megakaryocytic leukemia	Undifferentiated blasts	−	+/−	+	CD41, 61	Various
L1, Acute lymphoid leukemia, childhood variant	Small, uniform blasts, nucleoli indistinct	−	−	+++	65% react with anti-CD10 (anti-CALLA); 20% react with anti-CD5, 3, or 2 (anti–T cell)	Various including t(9;22), t(4;11), and t(1;9)
L2, Acute lymphoid leukemia, adult variant	Larger, more irregular nucleoli present		−	++		
L3, Burkitt-like acute lymphoid leukemia	Large with strongly basophilic cytoplasm and vacuoles	−	−	−	Anti–surface immunoglobulin, anti-CD19, anti-CD20	t(8:14)

PAS = periodic acid–Schiff.

have intracytoplasmic immunoglobulin and are termed pre–B-cell ALL. B-cell ALL is signified by the presence of immunoglobulin on the cell surface and accounts for fewer than 5% of cases of ALL. About 20% of cases of ALL are of the T-cell phenotype and express antigens found on normal early T cells such as CD5, CD3, or CD2. Approximately 15% of cases of ALL fail to express CALLA, B-, or T-cell markers and are termed null cell ALL. In about 25% of patients with ALL, the leukemic cells also express myeloid antigens. The presence of such antigens defines a group of patients who historically have had a somewhat worse prognosis; even with current, more aggressive regimens, however, outcomes seem to be similar.

CYTOGENETICS AND MOLECULAR BIOLOGY. In most cases of acute leukemia, an abnormality in chromosome number or structure is found. These abnormalities are clonal, essentially involving all of the malignant cells in a given patient, are acquired and not found in the normal cells of the patient, and are referred to as "non-random" because specific abnormalities are found in multiple cases of AML and are associated with distinct morphologic or clinical subtypes of the disease. These abnormalities may be simply the gain or loss of whole chromosomes, but more often they include chromosomal translocations, deletions, or inversions. When patients with acute leukemia and a chromosomal abnormality are treated and enter into complete remission, the chromosomal abnormality disappears; when relapse occurs, the abnormality reappears.

In AML, the most frequent changes are a gain of chromosome 8 or loss of part or all of chromosome 7 or 5. These abnormalities are each seen in anywhere from 7 to 12% of cases and are not associated with a particular morphologic subtype of AML. They are, however, more frequently seen in patients with secondary leukemia and are associated with an unfavorable prognosis. Whether these abnormalities cause leukemia or occur secondarily is uncertain, but the presence of tumor suppressor genes on chromosomes 5 and 7 could explain the association. Two other chromosomal abnormalities seen in AML, inv(16) and t(18;21), interfere with DNA transcription, which is normally regulated by a protein complex that includes core building factors (CBF) α and β. The t(8;21) results in an abnormal CBF α-subunit (AML1/ETO), whereas

inv(16) results in an abnormal CBF β-subunit (CBFβ/MYH11). Both of these "core binding factor" AMLs are characterized by a high complete response rate and relatively favorable long-term survival. The two differ in that t(8;21) is normally associated with FAB M2 whereas inv(16) is associated with a unique morphologic subtype, M4 with abnormal eosinophils. A third translocation seen in AML, t(15;17), involves two genes, PML and RARα (a gene encoding the α-retinoic acid receptor) and is invariably associated with APL, the M3 subtype of AML. Leukemia develops in transgenic mice containing the PML/RARα fusion gene after a variably long latency period. A final group of translocations involve the MLL gene located at chromosome band 11q23. MLL is among the most promiscuous oncogene partners in oncology, with over 30 fusions partners identified. MLL gene rearrangements account for as many as 85% of all secondary leukemias arising from exposure to epipodophyllotoxins or topoisomerase II inhibitors. In addition to the chromosomal gains, losses, and translocations, occasional cases of AML are associated with point mutations in n-ras or c-fms.

The most common cytogenetic abnormality seen in adults with ALL is the Philadelphia (Ph) chromosome [t(9;22)], a translocation that results in fusion of the bcr gene on chromosome 22 to the abl tyrosine kinase gene on chromosome 9. This translocation appears to result in the constitutive activation of abl, but the precise mechanism by which this activity is linked to the development of leukemia is unclear. The bcr/abl fusion is associated with both ALL and CML, with a minor difference in the breakpoint of bcr distinguishing the two. A slightly smaller 190-kd protein is generally found in ALL, whereas a larger 21-kd protein is characteristic of CML. The t(9;22) abnormality is seen in approximately 20% of adult ALL cases and 5% of childhood cases and is associated with a poor prognosis. The most common translocation seen in childhood ALL is t(12;21), which involves the genes TEL and AML1. Like the AML-associated translocation t(8;21) and inv(16), t(12;21) is thought to result in abnormal DNA transcription by interfering with the normal function of CBF. The t(12;21) is difficult to diagnose by routine cytogenetics, but by molecular studies it has been shown to account for 25% of childhood ALL and 4% of adult ALL. Other abnormalities sometimes seen in B-cell ALL include t(8;14) and t(8;22), which result in translocation of the *myc* gene on chromosome 8 and immunoglobulin enhancer response genes on chromosomes 14 or 22, and abnormalities involving 11q23. T-cell ALLs are frequently associated with abnormalities of chromosomes 7 or 14 at the sites of T-cell receptor enhancer genes on these chromosomes. The leukemia cells in about 20% of patients with ALL have a propensity to gain chromosomes, sometimes reaching an average of 50 to 60 chromosomes per cell. Patients with such hyperdiploid leukemias tend to respond well to chemotherapy.

CLINICAL MANIFESTATIONS

The signs and symptoms of acute leukemia result from decreased normal marrow function and invasion of normal organs by leukemic blasts. Anemia is present at diagnosis in most patients and causes fatigue, pallor, and headache and, in predisposed patients, angina or heart failure. Thrombocytopenia is usually present, and approximately one third of patients have clinically evident bleeding at diagnosis, usually in the form of petechiae, ecchymoses, bleeding gums, epistaxis, or hemorrhage. Most patients with acute leukemia are significantly granulocytopenic at diagnosis. As a result, approximately one third of patients with AML and slightly fewer patients with ALL have significant or life-threatening infections when initially seen, most of which are bacterial in origin.

In addition to suppressing normal marrow function, leukemic cells can infiltrate normal organs. In general, ALL tends to infiltrate normal organs more often than AML does. Enlargement of lymph nodes, liver, and spleen is common at diagnosis. Bone pain, thought to result from leukemic infiltration of the periosteum or expansion of the medullary cavity, is a common complaint, particularly in children with ALL, in many of whom the original diagnosis was juvenile rheumatoid arthritis. Leukemic cells sometimes infiltrate the skin and result in a raised, non-pruritic rash, a condition termed "leukemia cutis." Leukemic cells may infiltrate the leptomeninges and cause leukemic meningitis. Signs of leukemic meningitis are headache and nausea. As the disease progresses, central nervous system (CNS) palsies and seizures may develop. Although fewer than 5% of patients have CNS involvement at diagnosis, the CNS is a frequent site of relapse, particularly with ALL; because of the so-called blood-brain barrier, the CNS requires special therapy. Testicular involvement is also seen in ALL and the testicles are a frequent site of relapse. In AML, collections of leukemic blast cells, often referred to as chloromas or myeloblastomas, can occur in virtually any soft tissue and appear as rubbery, fast-growing masses.

Certain clinical manifestations are unique to specific subtypes of leukemia. Patients with APL (M3) commonly have subclinical or clinically evident disseminated intravascular coagulation (DIC) (see Chapter 183) caused by tissue thromboplastins that are present in the leukemic cells and released as these cells die. Acute monocytic or myelomonocytic leukemias are the forms of AML most likely to have extramedullary involvement. M6 leukemia often has a long prodromal phase. Patients with T-cell ALL frequently have mediastinal masses.

LABORATORY MANIFESTATIONS

Abnormalities in peripheral blood counts are usually the initial laboratory evidence of acute leukemia. Anemia is present in most patients. Most are also at least mildly thrombocytopenic, and up to one quarter have severe thrombocytopenia (platelets, <20,000/μL). Although most patients are granulocytopenic at diagnosis, the total peripheral white cell count is more variable; approximately 25% of patients have very high white cell counts (>50,000/μL), approximately 50% have white cell counts between 5000 and 50,000, and about 25% have a low white cell count (<5000/μL). In most cases, blasts are present in the peripheral blood, although in some patients the percentage of blasts may be quite low or blasts may be absent.

The diagnosis of acute leukemia is generally established by marrow aspiration and biopsy, usually from the posterior iliac crest. Marrow aspirates and biopsy specimens are generally hypercellular and contain 30 to 100% blast cells, which largely replace the normal marrow (Color Plates 6*I* and 6*J*). Occasionally, in addition

to the blast cell infiltrate, other findings are present, including marrow fibrosis (especially with M7 AML) or bone marrow necrosis.

The prothrombin and partial thromboplastin times are sometimes elevated. In APL, reduced fibrinogen and evidence of DIC are also often seen. Other laboratory abnormalities frequently present are hyperuricemia, especially in ALL, and increased serum lactate dehydrogenase. In cases of high cell turnover and cell death, such as ALL-L3, evidence of tumor lysis syndrome may be noted at diagnosis, including hypocalcemia, hyperkalemia, hyperphosphatemia, hyperuricemia, and renal insufficiency. This syndrome, which is more commonly seen shortly after therapy is begun, can be rapidly fatal if untreated.

DIFFERENTIAL DIAGNOSIS

The diagnosis of acute leukemia is usually straightforward but can occasionally be more difficult. Both leukemia and aplastic anemia can be manifested by peripheral pancytopenia, but the finding of hypoplastic marrow without blasts usually distinguishes aplastic anemia. Occasionally a patient may have hypocellular marrow and a clonal cytogenetic abnormality, which establishes the diagnosis of myelodysplasia or hypocellular leukemia. A number of processes other than leukemia can lead to the appearance of immature cells in the peripheral blood. Although other small round cell neoplasms can infiltrate the marrow and sometimes mimic leukemia, immunologic markers are effective in differentiating the two. Leukemoid reactions to infections such as tuberculosis can result in the outpouring of large numbers of young myeloid cells, but virtually never does the proportion of blasts in marrow or peripheral blood reach 30% in a leukemoid reaction (see Chapter 172). Infectious mononucleosis and other viral illnesses can sometimes resemble ALL, particularly when large numbers of atypical lymphocytes are present in the peripheral blood and when the disease is accompanied by immune thrombocytopenia or hemolytic anemia.

TREATMENT

With the development of effective programs of combination chemotherapy and advances in marrow transplantation, many patients with acute leukemia can be cured. These therapeutic measures are complex and are therefore best carried out at centers with appropriate support services and experience in treating leukemia. Because leukemia is a rapidly progressive disease, specific antileukemic therapy should be started as soon after diagnosis as possible, usually within 48 hours. Before therapy is started, hemorrhage and infection should be brought under control, if possible. To prevent uric acid nephropathy, patients should be hydrated and given allopurinol, 100 to 200 mg orally three times per day. The diagnosis of leukemia usually comes as a profound psychological shock to the patient and family. Therefore, in addition to stabilizing the patient hematologically and metabolically, it is worthwhile having at least one formalized conference in which the patient and the family are advised about the meaning of the diagnosis of leukemia and the consequences of therapy before treatment is initiated.

Management of Emergencies

Patients sometimes have treatable emergencies that require immediate attention before specific antileukemic therapy is begun. Severe bleeding usually results from thrombocytopenia, which can be reversed with platelet transfusions. Once thrombocytopenic bleeding is stopped, continued prophylactic transfusions of platelets may be warranted to maintain the platelet count above 20,000/μL. Occasionally, patients also have evidence of DIC, usually associated with the diagnosis of M3 AML. If active bleeding is due to DIC, low doses of heparin (50 U/kg) given intravenously every 6 hours can often be of benefit. Platelets and fresh-frozen plasma (or cryoprecipitate) should be transfused to maintain platelets over 50,000/μL and fibrinogen levels above 100 mg/dL until the DIC abates. Whether heparin should be given prophylactically to patients with laboratory evidence of DIC but no active bleeding is an often debated, but unsettled question. Patients with fever and granulocytopenia should have blood cultures; while awaiting culture results, infection should be assumed and broad-spectrum antibiotics begun empirically. It is preferable to bring an infection under control before starting initial chemotherapy if the patient has an adequate granulocyte count. However, patients often have infection but essentially no granulocytes; in this situation, delaying chemotherapy is unlikely to be of benefit. Patients with very high blast counts (>150,000/μL) may have symptoms attributable to the effect of masses of these immature cells on blood flow. The leukostasis may evolve into vascular injury and local hemorrhage. If this situation occurs in the CNS, the outcome may be fatal. Leukapheresis, immediate whole-brain irradiation (600 cGy in one dose), and administration of hydroxyurea (3 g/m^2 given orally for 2 or 3 days) can usually prevent this complication. Patients with very high white cell counts may also have uremia and anuria secondary to greatly increased serum uric acid levels, with subsequent intratubular crystallization. Rehydration, urine alkalinization with acetazolamide (500 mg/day), and prevention of uric acid production with allopurinol may lead to improved renal function. If patients do not respond and remain uremic, dialysis should be begun before the institution of chemotherapy.

Treatment of ALL

After the patient's condition has been stabilized, antileukemic therapy should be started as soon as possible. Initial therapy for ALL can be divided into three phases: remission induction, post-remission therapy, and CNS prophylaxis.

REMISSION INDUCTION. The initial goal of treatment is to induce complete remission, which is usually defined as the reduction of leukemic blasts to undetectable levels and restoration of normal marrow function. A number of different chemotherapeutic combinations can be used to induce remission; all include vincristine and prednisone, and most add L-asparaginase and/or daunorubicin, administered over a period of 3 to 4 weeks. With such regimens, complete remission is achieved in 90% of children and 75% of adults. Because vincristine, prednisone, and L-asparaginase are relatively non-toxic to normal marrow precursors, the disease often enters complete remission after a relatively brief period of myelosuppression. Failure to achieve complete remission is usually due either to resistance of the leukemic cells to the drugs used or to progressive infection. These two complications occur with approximately equal frequency.

POST-REMISSION CHEMOTHERAPY. If no further therapy is given after induction of complete remission, virtually all cases relapse, most within several months. This fact demonstrates the need for further post-remission therapy. Chemotherapy after complete remission can be given in a variety of combinations, dosages, and schedules. The term consolidation chemotherapy generally refers to short courses of further chemotherapy given at doses similar to those used for initial induction and thus requiring rehospitalization. Attempts are usually made to select different drugs for consolidation than were used to induce the initial remission. In the case of ALL, such drugs include high-dose methotrexate, cyclophosphamide, and cytarabine, among others. Maintenance involves the administration of low-dose chemotherapy on a daily or weekly outpatient basis for long periods. The most commonly used maintenance regimens in ALL are daily 6-mercaptopurine and weekly or biweekly methotrexate. The optimal duration of maintenance chemotherapy is unknown, but maintenance is usually given for 2 to 3 years. Optimal chemotherapy for ALL requires both consolidation and maintenance chemotherapy.

CENTRAL NERVOUS SYSTEM PROPHYLAXIS. Most chemotherapeutic agents, when given intravenously or orally, do not penetrate the CNS well, thus making it a common site of relapse unless specific measures are taken. Effective regimens for CNS prophylaxis include the use of intrathecal methotrexate alone, intrathecal methotrexate combined with 2400 cGy to the cranium, or 2400 cGy to the craniospinal axis.

PROGNOSIS AFTER INITIAL CHEMOTHERAPY. A number of factors are predictive of outcome in ALL, the most consistent of which are age, white cell count at diagnosis, and cytogenetics. With currently available treatment regimens, 50 to 70% of children and 25 to 45% of adults who initially achieve complete remission maintain complete remission for more than 5 years, and thus these patients are probably cured of their disease. In both children and adults, a low white cell count at diagnosis predicts a favorable outcome, whereas a high white cell count at diagnosis does the reverse. Patients with Ph-positive leukemia, t(4;11), or t(1;19) have

a poor prognosis, as do patients with the L3 mature B-cell variant of ALL characterized by t(8;14). Accordingly, these patients are more often treated with marrow transplantation while in first remission.

TREATMENT OF RELAPSED ALL. Most relapses occur within 2 years of diagnosis, and most occur in the marrow. Occasionally, relapse may initially be found in an extramedullary site such as the CNS or testes. Extramedullary relapse is usually followed shortly by systemic (marrow) relapse and should thus be considered part of a systemic recurrence. With the use of chemotherapeutic regimens similar to those used for initial induction, 50 to 70% of patients achieve at least short-lived second remissions. A small percentage of patients in whom the initial remission was longer than 2 years may be cured with salvage chemotherapy. If the CNS or testes are the initial site of the relapse, specific therapy to that site is also required, along with systemic retreatment. Because the prognosis of relapsed leukemia treated with chemotherapy is so poor, marrow transplantation is now generally recommended in this setting.

MARROW TRANSPLANTATION. The use of high-dose chemoradiotherapy followed by marrow transplantation (see Chapter 182) from an HLA-identical sibling can cure 20 to 40% of patients with ALL who fail to achieve an initial remission or who have a relapse after an initial complete remission. The major limitations of transplantation are graft-versus-host disease, interstitial pneumonia, and disease recurrence. If an HLA-identical sibling is not available, alternative sources are marrow from a partially matched family member, marrow from an HLA-matched unrelated donor, or autologous marrow that has been removed during remission, treated in vitro to remove contaminating tumor cells, and then subsequently stored. The outcome of transplantation of either autologous marrow or alternative sources of marrow has not been as favorable as that using matched allogeneic family member donors.

Treatment of AML

REMISSION INDUCTION. Treatment with a combination of an anthracycline (daunomycin or idarubicin) and cytarabine leads to complete remission in 60 to 80% of patients with AML. Profound myelosuppression always follows when these agents are used at doses capable of achieving complete remission. Failure to achieve complete remission is usually due either to drug resistance or to fatal complications of myelosuppression.

POST-REMISSION THERAPY. Intensive consolidation chemotherapy with repeated courses of daunomycin and cytarabine at conventional doses, high-dose cytarabine, or other agents prolongs the average remission duration and improves the chances for long-term disease-free survival. The best results reported to date with chemotherapy have generally used repeated cycles of high-dose cytarabine. Unlike the situation in ALL, low-dose maintenance therapy is of limited benefit after intensive consolidation treatment. In AML, leukemic recurrence occurs less often in the CNS, being seen in only approximately 10% of cases, most commonly in patients with the M4 or M5 variants. There is no evidence that CNS prophylaxis improves overall disease-free survival in AML.

PROGNOSIS AFTER INITIAL CHEMOTHERAPY. Among patients in whom complete remission is achieved, 20 to 40% remain alive in continuous complete remission for more than 5 years, thus suggesting probable cure. As with ALL, younger patients and those with a low white cell count at diagnosis have a more favorable outcome. Patients whose disease is characterized by certain chromosomal abnormalities, particularly t(8;21), t(15;17), and inv(16), do somewhat better, whereas those with 5q−, −7, 11q23, inv(3) or t(6;9) do worse. Patients who have a pre-leukemic phase before their condition evolves into acute leukemia and those whose leukemia is secondary to prior exposure to alkylating agents or radiation respond poorly to chemotherapy. Expression of the multidrug resistance gene 1 (MDR1) is also associated with a worse outcome.

TREATMENT OF RECURRENT AML. Patients whose AML recurs after initial chemotherapy can achieve second remission in about 50% of cases following retreatment with daunomycin-cytarabine or high-dose cytarabine. Unfortunately, these remissions tend to be short lived, and few patients in whom relapse occurs after first-line chemotherapy are cured by salvage chemotherapy.

TREATMENT OF ACUTE PROMYELOCYTIC LEUKEMIA. Recent studies demonstrate that complete remissions can be induced in at least 80% of patients with APL by using all-*trans*-retinoic acid (ATRA). Patients treated with ATRA usually have their coagulation disorders corrected within several days, but up to 2 or 3 months of therapy may be required to achieve complete remission. ATRA works by inducing differentiation of leukemic cells. A unique toxicity of ATRA in the treatment of APL is the development of hyperleukocytosis accompanied by respiratory distress and pulmonary infiltrates. The syndrome responds to temporary discontinuation of ATRA and the addition of corticosteroids. If patients are treated for APL with ATRA alone, disease inevitably recurs, which suggests that ATRA should be combined with or followed by other therapy. A recently completed large randomized trial found that the best results in APL can be achieved if ATRA is combined with an anthracycline-containing induction regimen and if ATRA is added during maintenance.

BONE MARROW TRANSPLANTATION. For patients with AML in whom an initial remission cannot be achieved or for patients who have a relapse after chemotherapy, marrow transplantation (see Chapter 182) from an HLA-identical sibling offers the best chance for cure. If carried out when patients have end-stage disease, approximately 15% of patients can be saved. If the procedure is applied earlier, the outcome with marrow transplantation improves: approximately 30% of patients who undergo transplantation at first relapse or second remission are cured, and 50 to 60% of patients are cured if transplantation is performed in the first remission. Several studies have prospectively compared the outcome of allogeneic marrow transplantation with that of chemotherapy in patients with AML in first remission. The trend in all of these studies has been in favor of transplantation, although not all studies have shown a statistically significant difference. Currently, transplantation is the treatment of choice for patients with AML who have suffered an initial relapse, and it should be strongly considered for most patients while in first remission. The major limitations to allogeneic transplantation are graft-versus-host disease, interstitial pneumonia, and disease recurrence. Because the incidence of graft-versus-host disease increases with age, most centers limit transplantation to patients of 55 years old or younger. Autologous transplantation offers an alternative for patients without matched siblings to serve as donors. In recently completed randomized trials, the use of autologous marrow transplantation after consolidation chemotherapy significantly prolonged the duration of disease-free survival and overall survival for patients with AML in first remission.

Supportive Care

Treatment of acute leukemia, especially AML, is accompanied by a number of complications, the two most serious and frequent being infection and bleeding. During the granulocytopenic period following induction and consolidation chemotherapy, most patients become febrile, and in approximately 50% of cases a bacterial infection can be documented. The most commonly isolated organisms vary somewhat from medical center to medical center, but generally, gram-positive organisms such as *Staphylococcus epidermidis* and gram-negative enteric organisms such as *Pseudomonas aeruginosa, Escherichia coli,* and *Klebsiella/Aerobacter* are the most commonly isolated bacteria. Even if no cause for fever is found, bacterial infection should be assumed, and in general, all patients with fever and neutropenia should begin receiving broad-spectrum antibiotics. Commonly used antibiotic combinations include a cephalosporin and a semisynthetic penicillin or a semisynthetic penicillin and an aminoglycoside. Once begun, antibiotic use should be continued until patients recover their granulocyte count, even if they become afebrile first. If documented bacterial infection persists despite appropriate antibiotics, the physician should consider removing indwelling catheters and giving granulocyte transfusions. It may be possible to reduce the incidence of bacterial infection through the use of selective gastrointestinal decontamination with, for example, ciprofloxacin or a combination of trimethoprim-sulfamethoxazole plus colistin. The use of protective environments can also reduce the incidence of infection, but this approach is costly and has not been shown to influence overall survival.

Frequently, patients taking broad-spectrum antibiotics become afebrile for a time, only to have a second fever develop. Such patients should be carefully reassessed with a high index of suspicion for fungal infection. Granulocytopenic patients who remain febrile for more than a week while taking broad-spectrum antibiotics should be treated empirically with amphotericin for presumed fungal infection. The prophylactic use of fluconazole can reduce the incidence of invasive candidal infections but does not change overall survival.

In addition to being granulocytopenic, patients undergoing induction chemotherapy for leukemia have deficient cellular and humoral immunity, at least temporarily, and thus are subject to infections common in other immunodeficiency states, including *Pneumocystis carinii* infection and a variety of viral infections. *P. carinii* infection can be prevented by prophylactic use of trimethoprim-sulfamethoxazole. Cytomegalovirus (CMV) infection can be prevented in a CMV-seronegative patient by the sole use of CMV-seronegative blood products. Herpes simplex can often complicate existing mucositis and can be treated successfully with acyclovir. Acyclovir is also useful for the treatment of disseminated varicella-zoster virus infection.

Myeloid growth factors (granulocyte or granulocyte-macrophage colony-stimulating factor), if given shortly after the completion of chemotherapy, shorten the period of severe myelosuppression by, on average, approximately 4 days. In most studies this accelerated recovery has resulted in fewer days with fever and less use of antibiotics, but it has not improved the complete response rate or altered survival.

The platelet count that signals a need for platelet transfusion has been the subject of recent debate. Traditionally, platelet transfusions from random donors were used to maintain platelet counts above 20,000/μL, but more recently it has been demonstrated that lowering this threshold to 10,000/μL is safe in patients with no active bleeding. In 30 to 50% of cases, patients eventually become alloimmunized and require the use of HLA-matched platelets. Occasionally, cells (presumably T cells) within the blood product can engraft in an immunosuppressed leukemic patient and cause a graft-versus-host reaction. Transfusion-induced graft-versus-host disease is manifested as a rash, low-grade fever, elevated values in liver function tests, and falling blood counts. This syndrome can be prevented by irradiating all blood products with at least 1500 cGy before transfusion.

Burnett AK, Goldstone AH, Stevens RM, et al, for the UK Medical Research Council Adult and Children's Leukaemia Working Parties: Randomised comparison of addition of autologous bone-marrow transplantation to intensive chemotherapy for acute myeloid leukaemia in first remission: Results of MRC AML 10 trial. Lancet 351: 700, 1998. *A large randomized trial that demonstrated the benefits of autologous marrow transplantation in first remission for adults with AML.*

Cline MJ: The molecular basis of leukemia. N Engl J Med 330:328, 1994. *An outstanding review of the various categories of genetic abnormalities associated with leukemia, including the types of genes involved, the molecular alterations seen, and the presumed functional changes that result.*

Tallman, MS, Anderson, JW, Schiffer, CA, et al: A prospective randomized study of all-*trans*-retinoic acid induction and maintenance therapy for patient with acute promyelocytic leukemia. N Engl J Med 337:1021, 1997. *Report of a large randomized trial demonstrating the efficacy of ATRA for both induction and maintenance therapy in APL.*

Zittoun RA, Mandelli F, Willemze R, et al: Autologous or allogeneic bone marrow transplantation compared with intensive chemotherapy in acute myelogenous leukemia. N Engl J Med 332:217, 1995. *A large prospective trial in adult AML comparing three forms of post-remission therapy, allogeneic marrow transplantation, autologous marrow transplantation, and intensive chemotherapy.*

178 APPROACH TO THE PATIENT WITH LYMPHADENOPATHY AND SPLENOMEGALY

James O. Armitage

LYMPHADENOPATHY

PHYSIOLOGY AND ANATOMY. Lymph nodes are found throughout the body along the course of lymphatics, strategically located to allow filtering of lymphatic fluid and interdiction of microorganisms and abnormal proteins. Lymphatic fluid enters the node in afferent lymphatic vessels that empty into the subcapsular sinus. The fluid then transverses the node to exit in a single efferent lymphatic vessel. In doing so, the lymph and its contents are exposed to immunologically active cells throughout the node. Lymph nodes are populated predominantly by macrophages, dendritic cells, B lymphocytes, and T lymphocytes. B lymphocytes are located primarily in the follicles and perifollicular areas, whereas T lymphocytes are found primarily in the interfollicular or paracortical areas of the lymph node. These cells function together to provide antigen processing, antigen presentation, antigen recognition, and proliferation of effector B and T lymphocytes as part of the normal immune response to microorganisms or foreign proteins.

Because the normal immune response leads to proliferation and expansion of one or more of the cellular components of lymph nodes, it also often leads to significant lymph node enlargement. In young children, who are continuously undergoing exposure to new antigens, palpable lymphadenopathy is the rule. In fact, the absence of palpable lymphadenopathy would be considered abnormal. In adults, lymph nodes larger than 1 to 2 cm in diameter are generally considered abnormal. However, lymph nodes 1 to 2 cm in diameter in the groin are sufficiently frequent to often be considered "normal."

Lymphoid proliferation is a normal response to exposure to foreign antigens. The location of the enlarged lymph nodes will often reflect the site of invasion. For example, cervical lymphadenopathy would be typical in a patient with pharyngitis. Generalized immune proliferation and lymphadenopathy can occur with a systemic disorder of the immune system, disseminated infection, or disseminated neoplasia. Malignancies of the immune system might be manifested as localized or disseminated lymphadenopathy.

DIFFERENTIAL DIAGNOSIS. The differential diagnosis of lymphadenopathy (Table 178–1) is vast, with the underlying causes responsible for either proliferation of immunologically active cells or infiltration of the lymph node by foreign cells or substances. In practice, the cause of enlarged lymph nodes is often not certain even in retrospect; in these cases, unrecognized infectious processes are generally blamed.

Infections by bacteria, mycobacteria, fungi, chlamydiae, parasites, and viruses are the major causes of lymph node enlargement. Lymph nodes in the drainage area of essentially all pyogenic infections can enlarge. In certain infections such as bubonic plague caused by *Yersinia pestis,* dramatic regional lymph node enlargement with fluctuant lymph nodes (i.e., bubos) can be a hallmark of the disease (see Chapter 348). Other bacterial infections have lymph node enlargement as a prominent feature (e.g., cat-scratch disease) and can mimic lymphoproliferative disorders (see Chapter 357). In some parts of the world, cervical lymphadenopathy is a sufficiently frequent manifestation of tuberculosis to lead to the institution of antituberculosis therapy rather than biopsy. Disseminated lymphadenopathy can be seen in infections by a variety of

Table 178–2 ■ MOST FREQUENT CAUSES OF LYMPHADENOPATHY IN ADULTS IN AMERICA

Unexplained
Infection
  In drainage area of infection (e.g., cervical adenopathy with pharyngitis)
  Disseminated (e.g., mononucleosis, HIV infection)
Immune disorders (e.g., rheumatoid arthritis)
Neoplasms
  Immune system malignancies (e.g., leukemia and lymphomas)
  Metastatic carcinoma or sarcoma

organisms such as *Toxoplasma,* Epstein-Barr virus (i.e., infectious mononucleosis), cytomegalovirus, and human immunodeficiency virus (HIV).

A variety of non-malignant disorders of the immune system can lead to localized or disseminated lymphadenopathy (see Chapter 282). Autoimmune diseases such as rheumatoid arthritis and systemic lupus erythematosus often have accompanying lymphadenopathy, which can pose a diagnostic challenge because of the increased incidence of lymphoma in patients with these disorders. In the lymphadenopathy that occurs as a reaction to drugs such as phenytoin, lymph node biopsy findings can sometimes be confused with those of lymphoma. Benign proliferative diseases of the immune system that can also be confused with lymphoma include Castleman's disease (angiofollicular lymph node hyperplasia) sinus histiocytosis with massive lymphadenopathy, and disorders seen more frequently in Asia such as Kawasaki syndrome and Kimura's disease.

All of the cells in the immune system can become malignant. Several of these malignancies are usually manifested as lymphadenopathy, and it can be seen in all. Lymphadenopathy as the initial manifestation is the rule for Hodgkin's disease and non-Hodgkin's lymphoma and is common in Waldenström's macroglobulinemia and B-cell chronic lymphocytic leukemia, but it is only occasionally seen in the myeloid leukemias (see Chapters 176, 177, and 179 to 181). Malignancies of all organ systems can metastasize to the lymph nodes and cause lymphadenopathy, which is usually seen in the drainage area of the primary tumor, e.g., axillary lymph nodes in patients with breast cancer, hilar lymph nodes in patients with lung cancer, and cervical lymph nodes in patients with head and neck cancer. However, widespread lymphadenopathy can also be seen with many solid tumors.

Other disorders that can have lymphadenopathy as an initial finding include storage diseases such as Gaucher's disease, endocrinopathies such as hyperthyroidism, sarcoidosis, and dermatopathic lymphadenitis. Amyloidosis can cause lymphadenopathy in patients with multiple myeloma, hereditary amyloidosis, or amyloidosis associated with chronic inflammatory states.

In patients actually seen in practices in the United States with lymphadenopathy, diagnoses will not be determined in a high proportion of patients (Table 178–2). In these cases the lymphadenopathy will usually be blamed on infection. When the lymphadenopathy is in the drainage site of a known infection (e.g., cervical lymphadenopathy in a patient with pharyngitis) or the patient has a known infection associated with lymphadenopathy (e.g., infectious mononucleosis), this infectious assumption is usually correct. Alternatively, if a patient has an immunologic disorder that is known to cause lymphadenopathy, such as rheumatoid arthritis, this disorder is usually an acceptable explanation; however, progressive lymphadenopathy in such patients should trigger a biopsy because these patients are at a increased risk for lymphoma. Localized, progressive lymphadenopathy, particularly when associated with fever, sweats, or weight loss, requires biopsy to exclude lymphoma.

LYMPH NODE EVALUATION. Evaluation of a patient with lymphadenopathy includes a careful history, a thorough physical examination, laboratory tests, and sometimes imaging studies to determine the extent and character of the lymphadenopathy (Table 178–3). The age of the patient and any associated systemic symptoms might be important hints in the evaluation. Cervical lymphadenopathy in a child would be much less worrisome than equally prominent lymphadenopathy in a 60-year-old. The occurrence of fever, sweats, or weight loss raises the possibility of a malignancy of the immune system. The explanation for the lymphadenopathy

Table 178–1 ■ CAUSES OF LYMPHADENOPATHY

Infection
  Bacterial (e.g., all pyogenic bacteria, cat-scratch disease, syphilis, tularemia)
  Mycobacterial (e.g., tuberculosis, leprosy)
  Fungal (e.g., histoplasmosis, coccidioidomycosis)
  Chlamydial (e.g., lymphogranuloma venereum)
  Parasitic (e.g., toxoplasmosis, trypanosomiasis, filariasis)
  Viral (e.g., Epstein-Barr virus, cytomegalovirus, rubella, hepatitis, HIV)
Benign disorders of the immune system (e.g., rheumatoid arthritis, systemic lupus erythematosus, serum sickness, drug reactions such as to phenytoin, Castleman's disease, sinus histiocytosis with massive lymphadenopathy, Langerhans' cell histiocytosis, Kawasaki syndrome, Kimura's disease)
Malignant disorders of the immune system (e.g., chronic and acute myeloid and lymphoid leukemia, non-Hodgkin's lymphoma, Hodgkin's disease, angioimmunoblastic-like T-cell lymphoma, Waldenström's macroglobulinemia, multiple myeloma with amyloidosis, malignant histiocytosis)
Other malignancies (e.g., breast carcinoma, lung carcinoma, melanoma, head and neck cancer, gastrointestinal malignancies, germ cell tumors, Kaposi's sarcoma)
Storage diseases (e.g., Gaucher's disease, Niemann-Pick disease)
Endocrinopathies (e.g., hyperthyroidism, adrenal insufficiency, thyroiditis)
Miscellaneous (e.g., sarcoidosis, amyloidosis, dermatopathic lymphadenitis)

Table 178–3 ■ FACTORS TO CONSIDER IN THE DIAGNOSIS OF LYMPHADENOPATHY

Associated systemic symptoms
Patient age
History of infection, trauma, medications, travel experience, previous malignancy, etc.
Location: cervical, supraclavicular, epitrochlear, axillary, intrathoracic (hilar versus mediastinal), intra-abdominal (retroperitoneal versus mesenteric versus other), iliac, inguinal, femoral
Localized versus disseminated
Tenderness/inflammation
Size
Consistency

might become apparent by identification of a site of infection, a particular medication, a travel history, or a previous malignancy.

Physical examination allows the identification of localized versus widespread lymphadenopathy. The particular sites of involvement can be important hints to the diagnosis inasmuch as infections and carcinomas are likely to cause lymphadenopathy in the lymphatic drainage of the site of the disorder. In general, lymph nodes that are tender are more likely to be due to an infectious process, whereas painless adenopathy raises the concern of malignancy. Lymph node consistency can also aid in the diagnosis: typically, lymph nodes containing metastatic carcinoma are rock hard, lymph nodes containing lymphoma are firm and rubbery, and lymph nodes enlarged in response to an infectious process are soft.

The larger the lymph node, the more likely a serious underlying cause exists, and lymph nodes greater than 3 to 4 cm in diameter in an adult are very concerning. Physical examination to assess lymph node size is only marginally accurate and reproducible; although it is by far the most widely used method, more precise methods are available with various imaging techniques.

Imaging studies using routine radiographs or computed tomography (CT), ultrasonography, lymphangiography, magnetic resonance imaging (MRI), and gallium scans provide the only methods to assess the extent of lymphadenopathy in the chest and abdomen (Table 178–4). Chest radiographs provide the most economical and easiest method to assess mediastinal and hilar lymphadenopathy but are not as accurate as CT of the chest. Although the technique is no longer widely available today, lymphangiography provides an extremely accurate assessment of the lower abdominal lymph nodes and, because of retained contrast material, allows repeat examinations and assessment of the response to therapy. CT and ultrasound provide the most useful ways to assess abdominal and retroperitoneal lymphadenopathy. In most patients, CT is probably the most accurate approach, but ultrasound has the advantage of being less expensive and not requiring radiation exposure. MRI and gallium scanning are not first-line studies for the assessment of lymphadenopathy. Gallium scans are frequently positive in patients with Hodgkin's disease and aggressive non-Hodgkin's lymphomas and can assess the presence of active lymphoma in patients with lymphadenopathy and a proven diagnosis; they are especially useful for re-evaluating patients after therapy because the lymph nodes do not always regress to normal size after therapy, particularly in the mediastinum and retroperitoneum.

Lymph node aspiration or biopsy is often necessary for an accurate diagnosis of the cause of the lymphadenopathy. Fine-needle

Table 178–4 ■ METHODS OF LYMPH NODE EVALUATION

Physical examination
Imaging
   Chest radiography
   Lymphangiography
   Ultrasonography
   Computed tomography
   Magnetic resonance imaging
   Gallium scanning
   Positron emission tomography
Sampling
   Needle aspiration
   Cutting needle biopsy
   Excisional biopsy

Table 178–5 ■ AN APPROACH TO THE PATIENT WITH LYMPHADENOPATHY

1. Does the patient have a known illness that causes lymphadenopathy? Treat and monitor for resolution.
2. Is there an obvious infection to explain the lymphadenopathy (e.g., infectious mononucleosis)? Treat and monitor for resolution.
3. Are the nodes very large and/or very firm and thus suggestive of malignancy? Perform a biopsy.
4. Is the patient very concerned about malignancy and unable to be reassured that malignancy is unlikely? Perform a biopsy.
5. If none of the preceding are true, perform a complete blood count and if it is unrevealing, monitor for a pre-determined period (usually 2 to 6 weeks). If the nodes do not regress or if they increase in size, perform a biopsy.

aspiration is currently popular and is often an accurate way to diagnose infection or carcinoma involving a lymph node. Although lymphomas can sometimes be diagnosed with this approach, it is inappropriate as an initial diagnostic maneuver for lymphoma. Cutting needle biopsies will occasionally provide sufficient material for an unequivocal diagnosis and subtyping of the lymphoma. However, in general, excisional biopsy, which is most likely to provide the pathologist with adequate material to perform histologic, immunologic, and genetic studies, is the most appropriate approach.

AN APPROACH TO THE PATIENT WITH LYMPHADENOPATHY. Patients with lymphadenopathy (Table 178–5) come to medical attention in several ways. Perhaps the most common is a patient who has felt a lymph node in the neck, axilla, or groin and then seeks a physician's opinion. Lymphadenopathy might also come to medical attention as an unexpected finding on routine physical examination or as part of the evaluation of another complaint. Finally, patients might be found to have unexpected lymphadenopathy on imaging studies of the chest or abdomen.

The approach to a patient complaining of newly discovered lymphadenopathy in the neck, axilla, or groin will depend on the size, consistency, and number of enlarged lymph nodes and the patient's general health. In general, very large or very firm lymph nodes in the presence of systemic symptoms such as unexplained fever, sweats, or weight loss should lead to a lymph node biopsy. Patients who have lymph nodes in the drainage area of a previously treated malignancy (e.g., neck nodes in a patient with a history of head and neck cancer) might be best approached by lymph node aspiration. Carcinoma can often be diagnosed in this manner, although it is a poor approach for the diagnosis of lymphoid malignancies. For cervical lymph nodes, excisional biopsy should be delayed in a patient who has head and neck cancer as a diagnostic consideration. These patients should initially undergo careful ear, nose, and throat examinations to avoid performing a biopsy that complicates the patient's subsequent therapy.

For the most common situation, in which a lymph node is soft, not larger than 2 to 3 cm and the patient has no obvious systemic illness, observation for a brief period is usually the best approach. Performance of a complete blood count and examination of a peripheral smear can be helpful in recognizing a systemic illness (e.g., infectious mononucleosis) (Color Plate 6A). These patients are often also given antibiotics. If the lymph node does not regress over the course of a few weeks or if it grows in size, a biopsy should be performed.

Part of the care of such patients involves the art of medicine and responsiveness to the patient's particular needs. For example, a biopsy might be done more quickly in a patient who is very anxious about malignancy or who needs a definitive diagnosis expeditiously.

SPLENOMEGALY

PHYSIOLOGY AND ANATOMY. The spleen is the largest lymphatic organ in the body and is sometimes approached clinically as though it were a very large lymph node. However, although it also participates in the primary immune response to invading microorganisms and foreign proteins, the spleen has many other functions. It functions as a filter for the blood and is responsible for removing from the circulation senescent red cells, as well as blood cells and other cells coated with immunoglobulins. Blood enters the spleen, filters through the splenic cords, and is exposed to the immunologically active cells in the spleen.

The splenic red pulp occupies more than half the volume of the spleen and is the site where senescent red cells are identified and destroyed and red cell inclusions are removed by a process known as pitting. In the absence of splenic function, inclusions known as Howell-Jolly bodies are seen in circulating red blood cells. The presence of Howell-Jolly bodies in the peripheral blood indicates that the patient has had a splenectomy or has a process that has rendered the spleen non-functional.

The white pulp of the spleen contains macrophages, B lymphocytes, and T lymphocytes, participates in the recognition of microorganisms and foreign proteins, and is involved in the primary immune response. Absence of this splenic function makes individuals particularly sensitive to certain infections, including sepsis with encapsulated organisms such as *Streptococcus pneumoniae*.

CAUSES OF SPLENOMEGALY. As with lymphadenopathy, the conditions associated with splenomegaly are extremely numerous (Table 178–6). A wide variety of infections can lead to splenomegaly (see Chapter 310). Certain bacterial infections such as endocarditis, brucellosis, and typhoid fever have splenomegaly as a frequent manifestation. Disseminated tuberculosis is often associated with splenomegaly, and splenomegaly can also be seen in disseminated histoplasmosis and toxoplasmosis. Splenomegaly is an almost constant accompaniment of malaria. Rickettsial disorders such as Rocky Mountain spotted fever are frequently associated with splenomegaly. A wide variety of viral infections usually cause splenomegaly, including infectious mononucleosis associated with Epstein-Barr virus and viral hepatitis. Splenomegaly can accompany HIV infection.

Splenomegaly is also seen in a variety of benign disorders of the immune system (see Chapter 282), including rheumatoid arthritis, where some patients will have Felty's syndrome and accompanying granulocytopenia. Splenomegaly is frequently seen in systemic lupus erythematosus, certain drug reactions, and serum sickness.

Malignancies of the immune system and non-immune organs can also lead to splenomegaly. Splenomegaly is usually seen in patients with chronic myeloid leukemia and is frequent in chronic lymphoid leukemia. It is often seen in patients with acute myeloid or lymphoid leukemia, non-Hodgkin's lymphoma, Hodgkin's disease, and Waldenström's macroglobulinemia. The condition previously known as angioimmunoblastic lymphadenopathy, which is now known usually to represent a T-cell lymphoma, often has splenomegaly as one manifestation. Metastasis of carcinomas and sarcomas to the spleen is unusual except for malignant melanoma; even in melanoma, however, palpable splenomegaly is an unusual finding.

Splenomegaly can develop from increased pressure in the splenic circulation, especially in portal hypertension caused by a variety of hepatic disorders, including alcoholic cirrhosis. However, it also can be due to splenic or portal vein thrombosis.

Hematologic disorders that can lead to palpable splenomegaly include autoimmune hemolytic anemia, hereditary spherocytosis,

Table 178–6 ■ CAUSES OF SPLENOMEGALY

Infection
  Bacterial (e.g., endocarditis, brucellosis, syphilis, typhoid, pyogenic abscess)
  Mycobacterial (e.g., tuberculosis)
  Fungal (e.g., histoplasmosis, toxoplasmosis)
  Parasitic (e.g., malaria, leishmaniasis)
  Rickettsial (e.g., Rocky Mountain spotted fever)
  Viral (e.g., Epstein-Barr virus, cytomegalovirus, HIV, hepatitis)
Benign disorders of the immune system (e.g., rheumatoid arthritis with Felty's syndrome, systemic lupus erythematosus, drug reactions such as to phenytoin, Langerhans' cell histiocytosis, serum sickness)
Malignant disorders of the immune system (e.g., acute or chronic myeloid or lymphoid leukemia, non-Hodgkin's lymphoma, Hodgkin's disease, Waldenström's macroglobulinemia, angioimmunoblastic-like T-cell lymphoma, malignant histiocytosis)
Other malignancies (e.g., melanoma, sarcoma)
Congestive splenomegaly (e.g., portal hypertension secondary to liver disease, splenic or portal vein thrombosis)
Hematologic disorders (e.g., autoimmune hemolytic anemia, hereditary spherocytosis, thalassemia major, hemoglobinopathies, elliptocytosis, megaloblastic anemia, extramedullary hematopoiesis)
Storage diseases (e.g., Gaucher's disease)
Endocrinopathies (e.g., hyperthyroidism)
Miscellaneous (e.g., sarcoidosis, amyloidosis, tropical splenomegaly, cysts)

Table 178–7 ■ METHODS FOR EVALUATION OF THE SPLEEN

Physical examination
Imaging
  Ultrasonography
  Computed tomography
  Liver-spleen scanning
  Gallium scanning
  Positron emission tomography
Biopsy
  Needle aspiration
  Splenectomy
    Laparotomy (total or partial splenectomy)
    Laparoscopy

and a number of other anemias. In idiopathic myelofibrosis, the spleen is frequently a site of extramedullary hematopoiesis.

A variety of less common conditions can lead to splenomegaly. The storage disorder Gaucher's disease is usually manifested as splenomegaly. Splenomegaly can be seen in endocrinopathies such as hyperthyroidism. Sarcoidosis and amyloidosis can be manifested as splenomegaly. Tropical splenomegaly is a term used to describe the palpable spleens found in patients who live in tropical areas and might have numerous causes.

EVALUATION OF SPLENIC SIZE AND FUNCTION. The ability to perform an accurate physical examination and determine the presence of an enlarged spleen (Table 178–7) is an important skill, but it is not easily learned. Physical examination of the spleen can be performed with the patient supine or in the right lateral decubitus position. Inspection, percussion, auscultation, and palpation can all be important in accurate assessment. It is rare to have a spleen so large that it is visible and can be seen to move with respiration. However, in such patients it is possible to miss the splenomegaly by failing to start palpation sufficiently low to find the edge. Occasionally, percussion of the left upper quadrant will help identify an area of dullness that moves with respiration and can lead to identification of splenomegaly. Splenic size is usually recorded as the number of centimeters that the spleen descends below the left costal margin in the midclavicular line on inspiration. Although auscultation is not usually a regular part of splenic examination, the existence of a splenic rub on inspiration can lead to the diagnosis of splenic infarct. The left kidney is sometimes confused with the spleen on physical examination, but failure to move with respiration in the way typical for the spleen will usually allow easy distinction.

Laboratory studies are frequently valuable in assessing splenic function. Patients with an absent spleen or non-functional spleen will have Howell-Jolly bodies seen in circulating red cells. Splenic hyperfunction (i.e., a condition often referred to as hypersplenism) is associated with cytopenias: the spleen is the normal reservoir for a significant proportion of platelets, and this reservoir function can lead to thrombocytopenia in patients with splenomegaly. Patients with autoimmune hemolytic anemia usually have palpable splenomegaly, but patients with idiopathic (immune) thrombocytopenic purpura usually do not.

The spleen can be imaged with ultrasound, CT, traditional radionuclide scans, and positron emission tomography. Ultrasonography can provide accurate determination of splenic size and is easy to repeat. CT will frequently give a better view of the consistency of the spleen and can identify splenic tumors or abscesses that would otherwise be missed. Radionuclide scans such as gallium scans can identify active lymphoma or infections. The technetium liver-spleen scan can be important in identifying liver disease as the cause of splenomegaly; in patients with cryptogenic cirrhosis, a technetium liver-spleen scan that shows higher activity in the spleen than the liver might be the initial hint of liver disease.

Because of the spleen's location and its propensity to bleed, needle aspiration or cutting needle biopsy of the spleen is rarely performed. In general, a splenic "biopsy" involves splenectomy, which can be performed at laparotomy or with laparoscopy. However, a splenectomy done via laparoscopy leads to maceration of the organ and reduces the diagnostic information. In very young children, in whom splenectomy causes a high risk for serious infections such as pneumococcal septicemia, partial splenectomy can

Table 178–8 ■ AN APPROACH TO THE PATIENT WITH SPLENOMEGALY

1. Does the patient have a known illness that causes splenomegaly (e.g., infectious mononucleosis)? Treat and monitor for resolution.
2. Search for an occult infection (e.g., infectious endocarditis), hematologic disorder (e.g., hereditary spherocytosis), occult liver disease (e.g., cryptogenic cirrhosis), autoimmune disease (e.g., systemic lupus erythematosus), or storage disease (e.g., Gaucher's disease). If found, manage appropriately.
3. If systemic symptoms are present and suggest malignancy and/or focal replacement of the spleen is seen on imaging studies and no other site is available for biopsy, splenectomy is indicated.
4. If none of the above are true, monitor closely and repeat studies until the splenomegaly resolves or a diagnosis becomes apparent.

sometimes be performed. Patients who undergo splenectomy at the time of splenic trauma and rupture can have seeding of splenic cells to other sites in the abdomen. Some patients will have additional small or accessory spleens. Persistent, functional splenic tissue can be the explanation for recurrent immune thrombocytopenia after splenectomy and might be recognized by the absence of Howell-Jolly bodies in circulating red blood cells.

AN APPROACH TO THE PATIENT WITH SPLENOMEGALY. Patients with splenomegaly might come to medical attention for a variety of reasons (Table 178–8). Patients might complain of left upper quadrant pain or fullness or of early satiety. Rarely, splenomegaly can initially present with the catastrophic symptoms of splenic rupture. Some patients will be found to have splenomegaly as a result of evaluation for unexplained cytopenias. Splenomegaly can be discovered incidentally on physical examination. In recent years, splenomegaly has been frequently discovered on imaging studies of the abdomen performed for other purposes.

The presence of a palpable spleen on physical examination is almost always abnormal. The one exception to this rule is a palpable spleen tip in a slender, young woman. In general, the presence of a palpable spleen should be considered a serious finding and an explanation should be sought. It is less clear that the same rules would apply to borderline splenomegaly discovered incidentally on routine imaging studies.

The approach to a patient with an enlarged spleen should focus initially on excluding a systemic illness that could explain the splenomegaly. The presence of infectious mononucleosis, leukemia or lymphoma, rheumatoid arthritis, sarcoidosis, cirrhosis of the liver, malaria, or a host of other illnesses would be accepted as a reasonable explanation for the splenomegaly. The systemic condition should be treated and then the spleen re-evaluated. If the systemic illness can be treated successfully, the spleen should regress to normal size over time.

Patients with no obvious explanation for an enlarged spleen present a difficult diagnostic problem. Careful follow-up of these patients will sometimes reveal occult liver disease or an autoimmune process that initially defied diagnosis. Concerns about malignancy, particularly in patients with systemic symptoms such as fever, sweats, or weight loss or in patients in whom imaging studies show a focal abnormality, are sometimes indications for splenectomy. However, in the absence of such findings, it is generally preferable to monitor patients closely with repeated attempts to establish the diagnosis by approaches other than splenectomy. It is particularly important to avoid splenectomy in a patient with occult liver disease and portal hypertension.

Armitage JO: The spleen. *In* Walker HK, Hlal WD, Hurst JW (eds): Clinical Methods: The History, Physician and Laboratory Examinations. Butterworths, 1990, pp 715–717.
Barkun AN, Camus M, Green L, et al: The bedside assessment of splenic enlargement. Am J Med 91:512, 1991.
Castell DO: The spleen percussion sign: A useful diagnostic technique. Ann Intern Med 67:1265, 1967.
These articles present the methods and pitfalls of the clinical evaluation of splenic enlargement.
McIntyre OR, Ebaugh FG Jr: Palpable spleens in college freshmen. Ann Intern Med 66:301, 1967. *A classic manuscript showing that normal spleens can sometimes be palpated in slender young women.*
Pangalis GA, Vassalikopoulos TP, Boussiotis VA, Fessas P: Clinical approach to lymphadenopathy. Semin Oncol 20:570, 1993.
Skolnik PR, Mark EJ: Case Records of the Massachusetts General Hospital: A 37-year-old man with fever and diffuse lymphadenopathy. N Engl J Med 340:545–554, 1999. *An excellent case discussion.*
Williamson HA Jr: Lymphadenopathy in a family practice: A descriptive study of 240 cases. J Fam Pract 20:449, 1985.
These articles present the problems in lymph node evaluation and the diagnoses actually made in routine clinical practice.

179 NON-HODGKIN'S LYMPHOMAS

Margaret A. Shipp ■ *Nancy L. Harris*

EPIDEMIOLOGY

The non-Hodgkin's lymphomas (NHLs) include over 20 discrete entities (Table 179–1) with characteristic morphologic, immunophenotypic, genetic, and clinical features. These lymphoid neoplasms are the 6th most common cause of cancer-related deaths in the United States. Over 53,000 patients were diagnosed with NHLs in 1997, and slightly less than half of these patients are expected to die of their diseases. In the past 15 years the incidence of NHLs has increased 50%, partly as a result of the increased numbers of young men in whom NHLs are developing in association with acquired immune deficiency syndrome (AIDS). However, the incidence of NHLs has also increased in older patients without additional apparent predisposing factors.

Although NHLs occur in all parts of the world, certain entities occur more frequently in specific geographic locations. For example, Burkitt's lymphoma occurs more frequently in tropical Africa, and adult T-cell leukemia-lymphoma is more common in southwest Japan and the Caribbean basin.

ETIOLOGY

The etiology of most NHLs remains unknown. However, certain congenital and acquired immunodeficiency states, autoimmune disorders, infectious agents, and physical and chemical agents have been associated with an increased risk for NHLs.

IMMUNE DEFICIENCY. In the congenital and acquired immunodeficiencies, long-standing immune dysregulation and ongoing,

Table 179–1 ■ WORLD HEALTH ORGANIZATION CLASSIFICATION OF NEOPLASTIC DISEASES OF THE HEMATOPOIETIC AND LYMPHOID TISSUES: LYMPHOID NEOPLASMS

B-Cell Neoplasms
Precursor B-cell lymphoblastic leukemia/lymphoma*
Mature B-cell neoplasms
  B-cell chronic lymphocytic leukemia/small lymphocytic lymphoma
  B-cell prolymphocytic leukemia
  Lymphoplasmacytic lymphoma
  Splenic marginal zone B-cell lymphoma
  Hairy cell leukemia
  Extranodal marginal zone B-cell lymphoma of the mucosa-associated lymphoid tissue type
  Mantle cell lymphoma
  Follicular lymphoma
  Nodal marginal zone lymphoma with or without monocytoid B cells
  Diffuse large B-cell lymphoma
  Burkitt's lymphoma
  Plasmacytoma
  Plasma cell myeloma
T-Cell Neoplasms
Precursor T-cell lymphoblastic lymphoma/leukemia
Mature T-cell and NK cell neoplasms
  T-cell prolymphocytic leukemia
  T-cell large granular lymphocytic leukemia
  NK cell leukemia
  Extranodal NK/T-cell lymphoma, nasal and nasal type
  Mycosis fungoides/Sézary syndrome
  Primary cutaneous anaplastic large cell lymphoma
  Subcutaneous panniculitis-like T-cell lymphoma
  Enteropathy-type intestinal T-cell lymphoma
  Hepatosplenic γ/δ T-cell lymphoma
  Angioimmunoblastic T-cell lymphoma
  Peripheral T-cell lymphoma (unspecified)
  Anaplastic large cell lymphoma, primary systemic type
  Adult T-cell lymphoma/leukemia (HTLVI+)

NK = natural killer; HTLV = human T-cell leukemia virus.
*The most common B- and T-cell malignancies are in bold.
Modified from Jaffe E, Bernard C, Harris N, et al: Proposed World Health Organization classification of neoplastic diseases of hematopoietic and lymphoid tissues. Am J Surg Pathol 21:114, 1997.

chronic antigenic stimulation increase the likelihood of developing a secondary NHL. Congenital disorders such as ataxia-telangiectasia, Wiscott-Aldridge syndrome, common variable immunodeficiency, severe combined immunodeficiency, and X-linked lymphoproliferative syndrome have all been associated with an increased incidence of aggressive B-cell malignancies (see Chapter 272). Acquired immunodeficiencies resulting from immunosuppressive therapies or infectious agents also increase the incidence of NHLs. For example, patients who receive immunosuppressive therapy following solid organ transplantation have an approximately 25 to 50-fold higher relative risk of developing a secondary lymphoid malignancy. The spectrum of post-transplant lymphoproliferative disorders ranges from polyclonal B-cell hyperplasia to monoclonal diffuse large B-cell lymphomas with extranodal and central nervous system (CNS) involvement. Patients with long-standing human immunodeficiency virus (HIV) infection are also estimated to have a 100-fold increased risk of the development of NHLs (see Chapter 416).

AUTOIMMUNE DISORDERS. Autoimmune disorders such as Hashimoto's thyroiditis and Sjögren's syndrome promote the development of mucosa-associated lymphoid tissue (MALT) and increase the risk of subsequent B-cell malignancies. Non-tropical sprue also increases the incidence of enteropathy-associated T-cell lymphoma. The association of rheumatoid arthritis and systemic lupus erythematosus with NHLs is less certain because patients with these disorders often receive additional chronic immunosuppressive therapy.

INFECTIOUS AGENTS (OTHER THAN HIV). HELICOBACTER PYLORI. *H. pylori* infection of the stomach results in chronic gastritis and the development of MALT and associated primary gastric lymphomas (see Chapter 125). The link between *H. pylori* infection and primary gastric MALT lymphomas has prompted the development of treatment strategies based on eradicating the *H. pylori* infection (see Treatment).

EPSTEIN-BARR VIRUS. The Epstein-Barr virus (EBV), which infects and immortalizes B lymphocytes in vitro, is implicated in the pathogenesis of African Burkitt's lymphoma and B-cell malignancies in immunocompromised patients. In residents of the African malarial belt and in patients with congenital and acquired immunodeficiencies, B-cell lymphomas may result from impaired immunosurveillance of EBV-infected cells.

HUMAN T-CELL LEUKEMIA VIRUS. The human T-cell leukemia virus (HTLV) is a type C retrovirus that was originally isolated from patients with adult T-cell lymphoma/leukemias in the United States and Japan. HTLV-I is endemic in several regions, including the southernmost islands of Japan and certain areas of the Caribbean basin. HTLV-I–associated T-cell disorders range from a smoldering disease with normal lymphocyte counts and no lymphadenopathy to chronic lymphocytoses, lymphomas, and acute leukemias.

KAPOSI'S SARCOMA–ASSOCIATED HERPESVIRUS. The Kaposi's sarcoma–associated herpesvirus (KSHV) was initially identified in AIDS-related Kaposi's sarcoma lesions and subsequently in HIV-associated lymphoid malignancies (see Chapter 522). KSHV-associated lymphomas are body cavity–based diseases characterized by lymphomatous pleural, pericardial, or peritoneal effusions.

CHEMICAL AND PHYSICAL AGENTS. Certain chemical and physical agents have also been associated with an increased risk of NHL. An increased incidence of NHL is also noted in the survivors of nuclear explosions or reactor accidents and in patients with other tumors that have been treated with certain chemotherapies and/or radiation.

MORPHOLOGIC, IMMUNOPHENOTYPIC, AND CLINICAL FEATURES

PRINCIPLES OF LYMPHOMA CLASSIFICATION. Over the years the NHLs have been classified in a variety of ways. Earlier schemes such as the Rappaport classification were based solely on morphology. Specific entities were classified according to pattern (nodular or diffuse), cytologic subtype, and degree of differentiation. Thereafter, the Luke-Collins and the Kiel classifications attempted to correlate specific lymphoid neoplasms with their normal counterparts in the immune system. Subsequently, an international collaborative group compared these major pathologic classifications and developed a common NHL classification, the Working Formulation. In the Working Formulation, lymphoma subtypes were identified on the basis of morphology and natural history; specific entities were given alphabetical letters (A to J) and grouped into low-, intermediate-, and high-grade categories (Table 179–2).

Recent advances in immunophenotypic, genetic, and morphologic characterization of the NHLs are reflected in the recently proposed "Revised European-American Classification of Lymphoid Neoplasms." This classification and the subsequent World Health Organization (WHO) classification include newly identified entities such as mantle cell, MALT, and anaplastic large cell lymphoma. These entities are divided into disorders of bone marrow–derived B- or T-cell precursors and diseases of peripheral "mature" circulating or nodal B or T cells (see Table 179–1). The most common lymphoid malignancies included in the WHO classification are compared with those recognized by the Working Formulation in Table 179–2. The salient morphologic, immunophenotypic, genetic, and clinical features of these most common B- and T-cell NHLs are discussed below.

B-CELL CHRONIC LYMPHOCYTIC LEUKEMIA/SMALL LYMPHOCYTIC LYMPHOMA (WORKING FORMULATION: SMALL LYMPHOCYTIC, CONSISTENT WITH CHRONIC LYMPHOCYTIC LEUKEMIA). MORPHOLOGY. B-cell chronic lymphocytic leukemia (B-CLL) and small lymphocytic lymphoma (B-SLL) are composed of small lymphocytes with condensed chromatin; these cells are only slightly larger than normal lymphocytes.

IMMUNOPHENOTYPE, GENETIC FEATURES, AND POSTULATED NORMAL COUNTERPART. The tumor cells of B-CLL/SLLs express faint surface immunoglobulin M (sIgM), B-cell–associated antigens (CD19, CD20, CD79a), CD5, and CD23 (Table 179–3). CD23 is particularly useful in distinguishing B-CLL/SLL from mantle cell lymphoma, which lacks CD23. Most cases of B-CLL/SLL are

---

Table 179–2 ■ COMPARISON OF THE WORKING FORMULATION AND THE WORLD HEALTH ORGANIZATION CLASSIFICATION OF LYMPHOID NEOPLASMS

	WHO CLASSIFICATION	
WORKING FORMULATION	**B-Cell Neoplasms**	**T-Cell Neoplasms**
Low Grade		
A. Small lymphocytic consistent with CLL	B-cell CLL/SLL	
B. Follicular, predominantly small cleaved cell	Follicular lymphoma, grade I	
C. Follicular, mixed small cleaved and large cell	Follicular lymphoma, grade II	
Intermediate Grade		
D. Follicular, large cell	Follicular lymphoma, grade III	
E. Diffuse, small cleaved cell	Mantle cell lymphoma	
F. Diffuse, mixed small and large cell	Large B-cell lymphoma (rich in T cells)	Peripheral T cell, unspecified
G. Diffuse, large cell	Diffuse large B-cell lymphoma	Peripheral T cell, unspecified
High Grade		
H. Large cell immunoblastic	Diffuse large B-cell lymphoma	Peripheral T cell, unspecified
I. Lymphoblastic	Precursor B lymphoblastic	Precursor T lymphoblastic
J. Small non-cleaved cell	Burkitt's lymphoma	
Burkitt's		
Non-Burkitt's		

CLL = chronic lymphocytic leukemia; SLL = small lymphocytic lymphoma.

Table 179–3 ■ IMMUNOPHENOTYPIC AND GENETIC FEATURES OF NON-HODGKIN'S LYMPHOMAS

NEOPLASM	IMMUNOPHENOTYPE*								GENETIC ABNORMALITY
	sIg; cIg	CD5	CD10	CD23	CD43	Pan-T (CD2, CD3)	Cyclin D₁		
B-cell CLL/SLL	+; −/+	+	−	+	+	−	−/+		Trisomy 12 (30%)
MALT lymphoma	+; +/−	−	−	−/+	−/+	−	−		Trisomy 3
Follicular lymphoma	+; −	−	+/−	−/+	−	−	−		t(14;18) (bcl-2)
Mantle cell lymphoma	+; −	+	−	−	+	−	+		t(11;14) (bcl-1)

	Ig	CD19	CD20	CD3	CD5	CD7	CD10	TdT	
Diffuse large B-cell lymphoma	+/−	+	+	−	−/+	−	−/+	−	t(14;18) (bcl-2) t(8;14) (myc), 3q (bcl-6)
ALCL	−	−	−	+/−	+/−	NA	−	−	t(2;5) (NPM/ALK)
PTCL	−	−	−	+/−	+/−	+/−	−	−	
Burkitt's	+	+	+	−	−	−	+	−	t(8;14), t(2;8), t(8;22), (myc), EVB −/+
T-LBL	−	−	−	+/−	+/−	+	−/+	+	Multiple
ATL/L	−	−	−	+	+	−/+	−	−	HTLV-I+

sIg = surface immunoglobulin; cIg = cytoplasmic immunoglobulin; CLL = chronic lymphocytic leukemia; SLL = small lymphocytic lymphoma; MALT = mucosa-associated lymphoid tissue; TdT = terminal deoxynucleotidyl transferase; ALCL = anaplastic large cell lymphoma; PTCL = peripheral T-cell lymphoma; EBV = Epstein-Barr virus; T-LBL = T-lymphoblastic lymphoma/leukemia; ATL/L = adult T-cell lymphoma/leukemia; HTLV = human T-cell lymphoma/leukemia virus.
*+ = >90% positive; +/− = >50% positive; −/+ = <50% positive; − = <10% positive.
Modified from Shipp MA, Harris NL, Mauch PM: The non-Hodgkin's lymphomas. In DeVita VT, Hellman S, Rosenberg SA (eds): Cancer: Principles & Practice of Oncology. Philadelphia, JB Lippincott, 1997, pp 2165–2220.

thought to correspond to recirculating CD5+, CD23+ naive B cells, which are found in the peripheral blood, primary follicle, and follicle mantle zone (Fig. 179–1). Trisomy 12 is reported in one third of B-CLL/SLLs, and 13q is seen in up to 25% of these disorders; t(11;14) bcl-1 rearrangements have also been described.

CLINICAL FEATURES. In the United States and Europe, over 90% of B-CLL/SLLs are manifested as chronic lymphoid leukemias; fewer than 5% of these disorders are manifested as lymphomas without a significant leukemic component. Patients with B-CLL/SLL are typically older adults with bone marrow and peripheral blood involvement at diagnosis; generalized lymphadenopathy, hepatosplenomegaly, and extranodal infiltrates may occur. Although the extent of the disease at diagnosis is the best predictor of survival, chromosomal abnormalities and immunophenotype may also have prognostic significance. Patients with B-CLL/SLL often have hypogammaglobulinemia and associated infectious complications and autoimmune phenomena such as hemolytic anemia or thrombocytopenia. Approximately 5% of B-CLL/SLLs undergo transformation to an aggressive lymphoma (Richter's syndrome), which is often fatal.

EXTRANODAL MARGINAL ZONE B-CELL LYMPHOMA (LOW-GRADE B-CELL MALT LYMPHOMA) (WORKING FORMULATION: NOT SPECIFICALLY LISTED). MORPHOLOGY. Extranodal marginal zone B-cell (MALT) lymphoma is characterized by an infiltrate of small lymphocytes, marginal zone and monocytoid B cells, and plasma cells. These extranodal marginal zone B cells infiltrate epithelial tissue and form characteristic lymphoepithelial lesions.

IMMUNOPHENOTYPE, GENETIC FEATURES, AND POSTULATED NORMAL COUNTERPART. MALT lymphomas typically express sIg and B-cell–associated antigens (CD19, CD20, CD22, CD79a) but lack CD5 and CD10. Immunophenotyping studies are useful to exclude CD5+ B-CLL/SLL or mantle cell lymphoma and CD10+ follicular lymphomas. The postulated normal counterpart is a post–germinal center memory B cell with the capacity to differentiate into marginal zone, monocytoid, and plasma cells (see Fig. 179–1).

CLINICAL FEATURES. The majority of low-grade gastric lymphomas and almost 50% of all gastric lymphoid neoplasms are MALT lymphomas. Forty per cent of orbital lymphomas and the majority of indolent pulmonary, thyroid, and salivary gland B-cell malignancies are also MALT lymphomas. Many patients with MALT lymphoma have a history of Helicobacter gastritis or an autoimmune disease such as Sjögren's syndrome or Hashimoto's thyroiditis. In these settings, chronic infection or autoimmune disease generates MALT, which is the substrate for lymphoma development. Recent studies suggest that therapy directed at the antigen (H. pylori in gastric lymphoma) may eliminate early lesions (see Treatment).

Like many other indolent B-cell neoplasms, marginal zone B-cell (MALT) lymphoma may transform into more aggressive, diffuse large B-cell lymphomas.

FOLLICULAR LYMPHOMA (WORKING FORMULATION: FOLLICULAR, SMALL CLEAVED, MIXED, OR LARGE CELL). MORPHOLOGY. Follicular lymphomas are composed of mixtures of small cleaved and large non-cleaved follicle center cells. Because follicular lymphomas have a continuous gradation in their numbers of large cells, the terms follicular lymphoma, grade I, grade II, and grade III, are preferred to the older Working Formulation terms follicular small cell, mixed cell, and large cell lymphoma (see Table 179–2).

IMMUNOPHENOTYPE, GENETICS, AND POSTULATED NORMAL COUNTERPART. Follicular lymphomas are usually sIg+ and express pan-B-cell–associated antigens; approximately 60% of tumors are CD10+ and the majority are CD5−, CD23−/+, and CD43− (see Table 179–3). The postulated normal counterparts are small cleaved and large non-cleaved follicular center cells from the germinal center (see Fig. 179–1). The t(14;18) translocation is present in 95% of grade I and II follicular lymphomas and a smaller proportion of grade III follicular lymphomas. The t(14;18) translocation results in expression of the bcl-2 "antiapoptosis" gene, which is normally switched off in germinal center cells.

CLINICAL FEATURES. Over 75 to 80% of indolent B-cell lymphomas are follicular lymphomas. These lymphomas are primarily diseases of older adults, who often have widespread nodal disease, as well as splenic and bone marrow involvement. Although the clinical course is usually indolent, follicular lymphomas are not curable with currently available standard therapy. With sufficient follow-up, up to 40% of follicular lymphomas undergo transformation to diffuse large B-cell lymphomas. Transformation is generally regarded as an ominous event associated with refractoriness to therapy. De novo follicular large cell (grade III) lymphomas are often treated similarly to diffuse large B-cell lymphomas (see Treatment).

MANTLE CELL LYMPHOMA (WORKING FORMULATION: NOT SPECIFIED, OFTEN PREVIOUSLY DIAGNOSED AS DIFFUSE SMALL CLEAVED CELL). MORPHOLOGY. Most cases of mantle cell lymphoma are composed exclusively of small to medium-sized lymphoid cells with slightly irregular or "cleaved" nuclei. The category mantle cell lymphoma comprises most of the cases that were previously classified as diffuse small cleaved cell lymphoma in the Working Formulation.

IMMUNOPHENOTYPE, GENETIC FEATURES, AND POSTULATED NORMAL COUNTERPART. Mantle cell lymphomas express bright sIgM and IgD and B-cell associated antigens; although tumor cells express CD5, they lack CD23 (see Table 179–3). In contrast to follicular lymphoma, mantle cell lymphoma is usually CD10− and CD43+. In the majority of mantle cell lymphomas, the t(11;14)

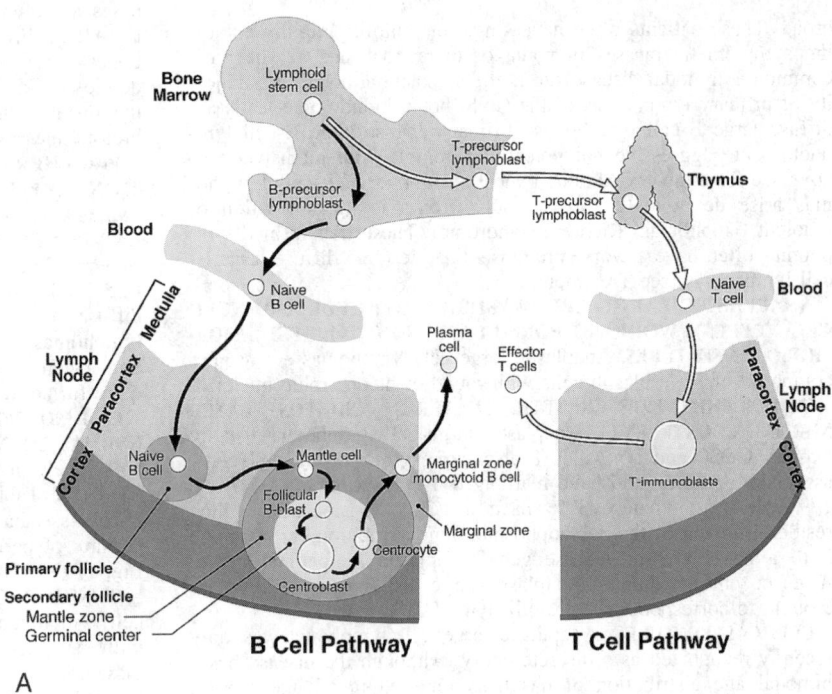

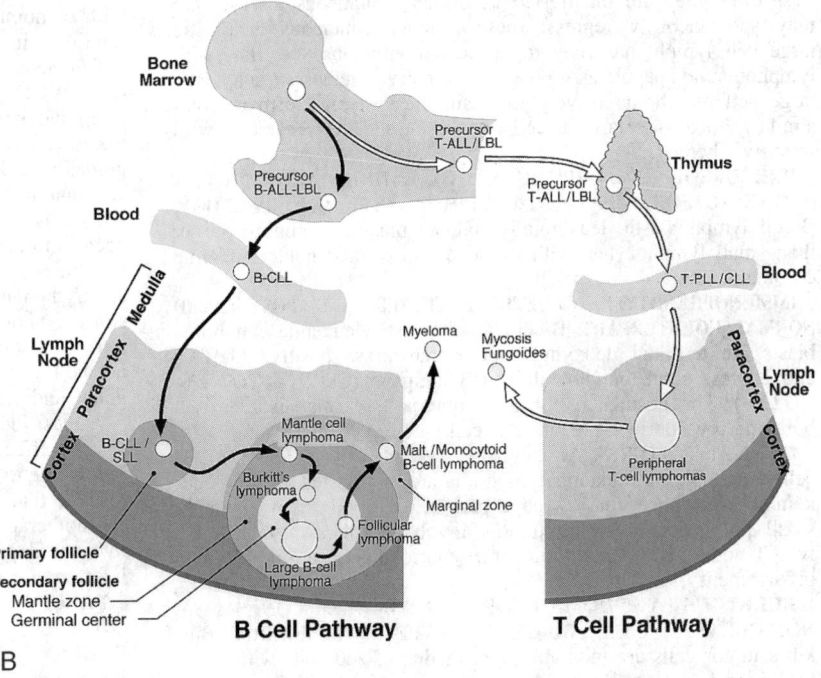

FIGURE 179–1 ■ Postulated normal counterparts of currently recognized B- and T-cell malignancies. *A,* Schema of normal B- and T-cell differentiation. Bone marrow–derived lymphoid stem cells differentiate into committed B-cell precursors or T-cell precursors that undergo further maturation in the thymus. Thereafter, these B- and T-cell precursors mature into naive B or T cells that circulate to lymph nodes. After antigen exposure, normal B blasts proliferate and undergo further differentiation in the germinal center of the secondary follicle. The germinal center is surrounded by a mantle zone and marginal zone. Antigen-specific B cells generated in the germinal center leave the follicle and reappear in the marginal zone. Thereafter, immunoglobulin-producing plasma cells accumulate in the lymph node medulla and subsequently exit to the periphery. Antigen-dependent T-cell proliferation occurs in the lymph node paracortex. After antigen exposure, mature T cells become immunoblasts and, subsequently, antigen-specific effector T cells that exit to the periphery. The postulated normal counterparts of many currently recognized T- and B-cell neoplasms are shown. *B,* T- and B-cell malignancies derived from the postulated normal counterparts shown in *A.*

translocation results in overexpression of PRAD1 (cyclin D_1). For this reason, immunoperoxidase staining for cyclin D_1 is useful in distinguishing mantle cell lymphoma from other indolent B-cell lymphomas. The postulated normal counterpart of mantle cell lymphoma is a naive B cell of follicle, mantle, or germinal center origin that is distinct from both the recirculating B cell of B-CLL/SLL and the later small cleaved and large non-cleaved germinal center cells of follicular lymphomas (see Fig. 179–1A and B).

CLINICAL FEATURES. Mantle cell lymphoma is typically a tumor of older adults with a marked male preponderance. Patients usually have widespread disease involving the lymph nodes, spleen, Waldeyer's ring, and extranodal sites, including bone marrow, blood, and the gastrointestinal tract (lymphomatous polyposis). The course is moderately aggressive, with a median survival of 3 to 5 years.

DIFFUSE LARGE B-CELL LYMPHOMA (WORKING FORMULATION: DIFFUSE LARGE CELL, LARGE CELL IMMUNOBLASTIC, OCCASIONALLY DIFFUSE MIXED SMALL AND LARGE CELL). MORPHOLOGY. Diffuse large B-cell lymphomas are composed of large cells that resemble centroblasts or immunoblasts. Occasional tumors may be rich in small T lymphocytes or histiocytes.

IMMUNOPHENOTYPE, GENETIC FEATURES, AND POSTULATED NORMAL COUNTERPART. Diffuse large B-cell lymphomas often (but not always) express sIg and one or more B-cell–associated antigens (CD19, 20, CD22, CD79a) (see Table 179–3); these tumors may also coexpress CD10. The *bcl*-2 gene is rearranged in about 30% of diffuse large B-cell lymphomas; c-*myc* is occasionally rearranged, and the *bcl*-6 gene is rearranged in 20 to 40% of cases (see Table 179–3). The postulated normal counterpart of diffuse large B-cell lymphomas is a germinal center or post-germinal center proliferating B cell (see Fig. 179–1).

CLINICAL FEATURES. Over 30% of adult NHLs are diffuse large B-cell lymphomas. Although the median age of patients with diffuse large B-cell lymphoma is in the sixth decade, the range is broad. These patients often have single or multiple, rapidly enlarging symptomatic masses in nodal or extranodal site(s). The most common extranodal disease site is the stomach, although the majority of primary lymphomas of the CNS, bone, kidney, and testis are diffuse large B-cell lymphomas. Primary diffuse large B-cell lymphomas are aggressive but potentially curable with intensive therapy (see Treatment). Although most diffuse large B-cell lymphomas arise de novo, a subset results from the transformation of indolent lymphomas (Richter's syndrome). These transformed lymphomas often have a worse prognosis than de novo diffuse large B-cell lymphomas (see Treatment).

ANAPLASTIC LARGE CELL LYMPHOMA (T-CELL AND NULL CELL TYPES) (WORKING FORMULATION: NOT LISTED). MORPHOLOGIC FEATURES. Anaplastic large cell lymphomas are usually composed of large blastic cells with round or pleomorphic nuclei.

IMMUNOPHENOTYPE, GENETIC FEATURES, AND POSTULATED NORMAL COUNTERPART. Anaplastic large cell lymphomas usually express CD30 and EMA; 60% also express one or more T-cell–associated antigens and have rearranged T-cell receptors (see Table 179–3). Approximately 30% have a t(2;5) translocation, which results in fusion of the nucleophosmin gene (*NPM*) on chromosome 5 to a novel tyrosine kinase gene (anaplastic lymphoma kinase, *ALK*) on chromosome 2. Anaplastic large cell lymphoma cells are thought to correspond to extrafollicular CD30+ blasts.

CLINICAL FEATURES. Anaplastic large cell lymphoma was only recently recognized as a discrete entity. Although the disease has a bimodal age distribution, it has been reported in all age groups. Most anaplastic large cell lymphomas are manifested as systemic diseases involving the lymph nodes and/or extranodal disease sites. Less often they are manifested as primary cutaneous disease that may spontaneously regress; these primary cutaneous anaplastic large cell lymphomas may represent a continuous spectrum with lymphomatoid papulosis. Whereas primary cutaneous anaplastic large cell lymphoma is very indolent, the systemic form behaves similarly to diffuse large B-cell lymphoma and may be cured with intensive therapy.

PRECURSOR B-LYMPHOBLASTIC LEUKEMIA/LYMPHOMA (WORKING FORMULATION: LYMPHOBLASTIC). MORPHOLOGY. B-cell lymphoblastic leukemia/lymphoma blasts are slightly larger than small lymphocytes, with round or convoluted nuclei and fine chromatin.

IMMUNOPHENOTYPE, GENETIC FEATURES, AND POSTULATED NORMAL COUNTERPART. B-cell lymphoblastic leukemia/lymphoma blasts are terminal deoxynucleotidyl transferase positive (TdT+) and express some but not all pan-B antigens (CD19+, CD79a+, CD22+). The postulated normal counterpart of this disorder is a bone marrow–derived precursor B cell (see Fig. 179–1A and B).

CLINICAL FEATURES. Although the vast majority of cases of B-cell lymphoblastic leukemia/lymphoma are manifested as acute leukemias with bone marrow and peripheral blood involvement, a small proportion are solid tumors involving the skin, bone, and lymph nodes, with or without bone marrow and peripheral blood involvement.

BURKITT'S LYMPHOMA (WORKING FORMULATION: SMALL NON-CLEAVED CELL, BURKITT'S TYPE). MORPHOLOGY. Burkitt's tumor cells are monomorphic, medium-sized cells with round nuclei and basophilic cytoplasm. The characteristic "starry-sky" pattern is imparted by infiltrating benign macrophages that have ingested apoptotic tumor cells. In some cases the larger tumor cells resemble those seen in diffuse large B-cell lymphoma; such borderline cases are often called "non-Burkitt's" or "Burkitt's-like" lymphomas.

IMMUNOPHENOTYPE, GENETIC FEATURES, AND POSTULATED NORMAL COUNTERPART. Burkitt's lymphomas express sIgM, B-cell–associated antigens, and CD10; these tumors lack CD5 and CD23 (see Table 179–3). Most Burkitt's lymphomas have a translocation of c-*myc* from chromosome 8 to either the immunoglobulin heavy chain region on chromosome 14 [t(8;14)] or one of the light chain loci on chromosome 2 [t(2;8)] or 22 [t(8;22)]. African Burkitt's lymphomas frequently contain EBV genomes; 25 to 40% of AIDS-associated Burkitt's lymphomas also contain EBV. The postulated normal counterpart of Burkitt's lymphoma may be a B-cell blast of early germinal center origin (see Fig. 179–1A and B).

CLINICAL FEATURES. Burkitt's lymphoma is most common in

children (30% of non-African pediatric lymphomas). Rare adult cases are often associated with immunodeficiency syndromes such as AIDS. In African (endemic) cases, the jaw and other facial bones are often involved. The majority of non-African (non-endemic) Burkitt's lymphomas occur in the abdomen, often involving the distal ileum, cecum, and/or mesentery; ovaries, kidneys, and breasts may also be involved.

PERIPHERAL T-CELL LYMPHOMAS (WORKING FORMULATION: DIFFUSE SMALL CLEAVED CELL, DIFFUSE MIXED SMALL AND LARGE CELL, DIFFUSE LARGE CELL, AND LARGE CELL IMMUNOBLASTIC). MORPHOLOGIC FEATURES. Peripheral T-cell lymphomas typically contain a mixture of small and large cells and include entities that were previously identified as diffuse mixed small and large cell or large cell immunoblastic lymphomas in the Working Formulation. The category of peripheral T-cell lymphoma contains a number of rare diseases that require further definition.

IMMUNOPHENOTYPE, GENETIC FEATURES, AND POSTULATED NORMAL COUNTERPART. Peripheral T-cell lymphomas express variable levels of T-cell–associated antigens such as CD3, CD2, and CD5 (see Table 179–3); CD4 is expressed more often than CD8. B-cell–associated antigens are absent. The postulated normal counterparts of peripheral T-cell lymphomas are peripheral T cells (see Fig. 179–1A and B).

CLINICAL FEATURES. Recent studies suggest that peripheral T-cell lymphomas represent fewer than 10% of all NHLs. Patients with peripheral T-cell lymphoma are usually initially seen with disseminated disease and occasional eosinophilia, pruritus, or hemophagocytic syndromes; lymph nodes, skin or subcutis, liver, spleen, and other viscera may be involved. Although the clinical course is usually aggressive, these diseases are potentially curable with combination chemotherapy. However, relapses are more common than in diffuse large B-cell lymphomas (see Treatment).

Cutaneous T-cell lymphomas are related T-cell neoplasms of mature CD4+ cells that home to the skin and T-cell zone of lymphoid structures but do not characteristically involve the bone marrow. The previously described clinical entities of mycosis fungoides and Sézary syndrome are now recognized as different clinical manifestations of cutaneous T-cell lymphomas (Color Plate 13F). They are most common in adults aged 40 to 60 years and occur more frequently in males and blacks. The classic mycosis fungoides manifestation of cutaneous T-cell lymphoma begins with an erythematous macular eruption in sun-shielded areas; these lesions eventually become more palpable and subsequently develop into frank tumors that extend beneath the dermis. Thereafter, cutaneous T-cell lymphoma nodules may disseminate to involve distant nodal and visceral sites. In cutaneous T-cell lymphoma, prognostic variables include the type of skin lesion(s), percentage of skin surface affected, and the presence or absence of nodal and visceral involvement and circulating tumor cells. Patients with early-stage disease that is localized to the skin may be cured with topical chemotherapy (carmustine or nitrogen mustard), systemically administered psoralens that are activated in the skin with ultraviolet light, and/or superficial radiation therapy.

PRECURSOR T-LYMPHOBLASTIC LYMPHOMA/LEUKEMIA (WORKING FORMULATION: LYMPHOBLASTIC, OR NOT OTHERWISE SPECIFIED). MORPHOLOGY. T-cell lymphoblastic lymphomas/leukemias are morphologically identical to precursor B-cell lymphoblastic lymphomas/leukemias. Immunophenotyping studies are necessary to distinguish precursor B- and T-cell malignancies.

IMMUNOPHENOTYPE, GENETIC FEATURES, AND POSTULATED NORMAL COUNTERPART. The majority of T-cell lymphoblastic lymphomas/leukemias are CD7+ and CD3+; cytoplasmic CD3 is usually present even when surface antigen is absent. Expression of other T-cell–associated antigens (CD2, CD5) is variable (see Table 179–3). Tumors are typically TdT+ and often CD4 and CD8 double positive or double negative; occasional cases express natural killer antigens (CD16, CD57). The postulated T-cell lymphoblastic lymphoma/leukemia counterparts are precursor T-cells (see Fig. 179–1A and B).

CLINICAL FEATURES. Although most patients with T-cell lymphoblastic lymphoma/leukemia are adolescents or young adult males, older adults may be affected. These patients typically have mediastinal (thymic) masses and/or peripheral lymphadenopathy; CNS involvement is common. Untreated T-cell lymphoblastic lymphoma/leukemia is rapidly fatal, frequently terminating in acute leukemia.

ADULT T-CELL LYMPHOMA/LEUKEMIA (WORKING FORMULATION: DIFFUSE SMALL CLEAVED CELL, DIFFUSE MIXED SMALL AND LARGE CELL, DIFFUSE LARGE CELL, AND LARGE CELL IMMUNOBLASTIC). MORPHOLOGY. Adult T-cell lymphoma/leukemia histology is variable, with a mixture of small and large atypical cells.

IMMUNOPHENOTYPE, GENETIC FEATURES, AND POSTULATED NORMAL COUNTERPART. Adult T-cell lymphoma/leukemia cells express T-cell–associated antigens (CD2, CD3, CD5) but usually lack CD7 (see Table 179–3). Although most tumors are CD4+, CD25+, rare CD8+ cases have been reported. In adult T-cell lymphoma/leukemia, T-cell receptor genes are clonally rearranged, and the HTLV-I genome is clonally integrated. The postulated normal counterparts of adult T-cell lymphoma/leukemia are peripheral CD4+ T cells in various stages of transformation.

CLINICAL FEATURES. Patients with adult T-cell lymphoma/leukemia are usually adults with detectable HTLV-I antibodies. Adult T-cell lymphoma/leukemia is most common in Japan, although an endemic focus is located in the Caribbean and additional sporadic cases can be found in the United States. Patients with "acute" adult T-cell lymphoma/leukemia have a high white blood cell count, hepatosplenomegaly, hypercalcemia, and lytic bone lesions; survival is often only a few months. A less common lymphomatous form of adult T-cell lymphoma/leukemia is characterized by isolated lymphadenopathy or extranodal tumors without leukemic involvement. A chronic form of adult T-cell lymphoma/leukemia with less marked lymphocytosis and no hypercalcemia or hepatosplenomegaly has a slightly longer survival. Rare smoldering cases have been described with mild (clonal) lymphocytosis and a very indolent course.

STAGING SYSTEMS

Ann Arbor Classification

Patients with NHL are currently staged with the Ann Arbor classification, which was originally developed for Hodgkin's disease. The Ann Arbor staging system is based on the number of sites of involvement, the presence of disease above or below the diaphragm, the existence of systemic symptoms, and the presence of extranodal disease (Table 179–4).

CLINICAL PROGNOSTIC FACTORS. Because the patterns of disease spread in Hodgkin's disease and NHLs are somewhat different, it is not surprising that the Ann Arbor classification is less accurate in identifying prognostic subgroups of NHL. For this reason, investigators have used additional clinical prognostic factors and associated classification schema to reflect the behavior of NHLs more accurately. A widely accepted prognostic factor model for patients with aggressive NHLs has been developed using the following clinical features: age, serum lactate dehydrogenase, performance status, stage, and number of extranodal disease sites. These features were incorporated into a model, the International Prognostic Index (IPI), that identified groups of patients with different risks for death (Table 179–5). Because the relative risk associated with each of the clinical features was comparable, an individual patient's relative risk for death was determined by adding the number of adverse prognostic factors present at diagnosis. Four risk groups of patients (low risk, low-intermediate, high-inter-

mediate, or high risk) were subsequently identified. Because younger and older patients had significantly different outcomes and patients 60 years or younger were more likely to be candidates for intensive experimental regimens, an age-adjusted model for patients 60 years or younger (age-adjusted IPI) was also developed. Although the IPI was specifically developed to predict outcome in patients with aggressive NHLs, the model is also highly predictive in patients with other subtypes of lymphoma. For example, the IPI predicts survival in a variety of indolent lymphomas and additional newly identified lymphoid neoplasms.

RECOMMENDED STAGING PROCEDURES. It is not possible to recommend a uniform approach to the evaluation of all NHLs because specific lymphoid neoplasms have unique natural histories and patterns of manifestation. Common staging procedures are listed below; additional specific information is available in recently developed national treatment guidelines.

HISTORY AND PHYSICAL EXAMINATION. The initial history should include the duration and rate of lymph node enlargement; the presence or absence of fever, night sweats, and/or unexplained weight loss (B symptoms); and the presence or absence of symptoms such as bone pain or gastrointestinal discomfort that might indicate extranodal involvement. The physical examination should be directed toward node-bearing areas and sites of common extranodal involvement. The site and size of all abnormal lymph nodes should be recorded. Because hepatosplenomegaly frequently correlates with tumor involvement in the NHLs, the size of the liver and spleen should also be noted.

The physical examination and subsequent special studies are dictated in part by the specific lymphoid neoplasm and the sites of disease at initial evaluation. For example, patients with pre-auricular lymph node enlargement often have disease that is in Waldeyer's ring and can be identified only with indirect laryngoscopy. Waldeyer's ring involvement can also be associated with gastrointestinal involvement and should prompt contrast studies of the gastrointestinal tract in patients who appear to have localized disease. Because patients with lymphoma of the skin often have multiple cutaneous lesions that may be remote from one another, the skin should be inspected carefully and suspicious lesions biopsied. Patients with lymphoma of the paranasal sinuses or orbit have a high risk of CNS involvement; for this reason, radiographic studies of the CNS and analysis of cerebrospinal fluid are appropriate in such patients.

LABORATORY STUDIES. Blood analysis may provide additional site-specific and prognostic information. An elevated creatinine level may indicate renal insufficiency resulting from obstruction caused by retroperitoneal disease. Elevation of liver enzymes, bilirubin, and alkaline phosphatase may be signs of liver involvement and/or bone involvement. Serum lactate dehydrogenase and β_2-microglobulin levels are indirect measurements of tumor burden.

RADIOGRAPHIC STAGING. Plain films and Computed Tomography. Chest radiographs can be used to identify hilar or mediastinal adenopathy, pleural or pericardial effusions, or parenchymal involvement. In patients with abnormal chest radiographs, thoracic computed tomographic (CT) scans provide important additional information regarding the extent of disease. CT scanning is also useful for monitoring the response to treatment of mediastinal, pericardial, and hilar disease. Abdominal-pelvic CT scans are recommended for evaluating mesenteric and retroperitoneal disease and measuring the dimensions of involved nodal areas. Renal and bulky splenic and hepatic disease can also be identified on abdominal-pelvic CT scans.

Magnetic Resonance Imaging. Magnetic resonance imaging may be most valuable in evaluation of the brain and spinal cord and detection of occult bone marrow involvement.

Nuclear Medicine Studies. Gallium-67 scans are positive in nearly all aggressive lymphomas and in approximately 50% of indolent lymphomas at diagnosis. In gallium-avid lymphomas, properly performed gallium-67 scans can identify initial sites of disease, reflect response to therapy, and detect early recurrence. Gallium scans complement CT scans in determining response to treatment.

Invasive Procedures. *Bone Marrow Biopsies.* Unilateral bone marrow biopsies should be performed as part of the initial staging evaluation and also as part of the follow-up of patients whose marrow is positive at diagnosis. Specific lymphoid neoplasms tend

---

Table 179–4 ■ ANN ARBOR STAGING SYSTEM

Stage I	Involvement of a single lymph node region (I) or a single extralymphatic organ or site (IE)
Stage II	Involvement of two or more lymph node regions on the same side of the diaphragm (II) or localized involvement of an extralymphatic organ or site (IIE)
Stage III	Involvement of lymph node regions on both sides of the diaphragm (III) or localized involvement of an extralymphatic organ or site (IIIE), the spleen (IIIS), or both (IIISE)
Stage IV	Diffuse or disseminated involvement of one or more extralymphatic organs with or without associated lymph node involvement

Identification of the presence or absence of symptoms should be noted with each stage designation. A = asymptomatic; B = fever, sweats, or weight loss greater than 10% of body weight.

Table 179–5 ■ THE INTERNATIONAL PROGNOSTIC INDEX FOR NON-HODGKIN'S LYMPHOMA

RISK GROUP (PATIENTS OF ALL AGES)	RISK FACTORS*	DISTRIBUTION OF CASES, %	COMPLETE RESPONSE RATE (%)	5-YEAR SURVIVAL RATE (%)
Low	0.1	35	87	73
Low-intermediate	2	27	67	51
High-intermediate	3	22	55	43
High	4.5	16	44	26

*Age ($\leq$60 versus >60); serum lactate dehydrogenase (normal versus >1 × normal); performance status (0 or 1 versus 2 to 4); stage (I or II versus III or IV); and extranodal involvement ($\leq$1 site versus >1 site).

Modified from Shipp M, Harrington DP, Anderson J, et al: International non-Hodgkin's lymphoma prognostic factors project: A predictive model for aggressive non-Hodgkin's lymphoma. N Engl J Med 329:987, 1993.

to have identifiable patterns of bone marrow involvement. For example, follicular lymphoma involves the paratrabecular spaces, whereas aggressive lymphomas have widespread bone marrow involvement.

MOLECULAR ANALYSIS OF MINIMAL RESIDUAL DISEASE. Clonal rearrangements of immunoglobulin or T-cell receptor genes and specific chromosomal translocations can be considered molecular signatures of specific lymphoid neoplasms. With the advent of polymerase chain reaction (PCR) technology, it is now possible to identify specific immunoglobulin gene rearrangements or chromosomal translocations with a sensitivity of 1 in 10^5 cells and to assess the significance of minimal residual disease in a variety of lymphoid neoplasms. Although early studies failed to correlate PCR positivity with risk of relapse, more recent analyses suggest that these techniques may be useful. It is still too early to recommend changes in staging or treatment based on molecular analysis of minimal residual disease; however, these techniques are likely to affect treatment strategies in the future.

TREATMENT OF NON-HODGKIN'S LYMPHOMAS

THERAPEUTIC OPTIONS. Therapeutic approaches to the NHLs are based on the specific lymphoid neoplasm, the stage of disease, and the prognosis and physiologic status of the patient. Treatment options for indolent diseases such as B-CLL/SLL and follicular lymphoma include no therapy with careful follow-up, radiation therapy alone, single-agent chemotherapy, mild combination chemotherapy, aggressive combination chemotherapy, and treatment with newer experimental agents. Virtually all patients with aggressive entities such as the diffuse large B-cell and peripheral T-cell lymphomas require combination chemotherapy with or without additional radiation therapy. Patients with highly aggressive lymphomas such as precursor B-cell or T-cell lymphoblastic lymphoma/leukemia and Burkitt's lymphoma require specialized leukemia-like regimens with CNS prophylaxis. Current approaches to the most common NHLs are discussed below and presented in more detail in recently developed national treatment guidelines.

B-CELL SMALL LYMPHOCYTIC LYMPHOMA/CHRONIC LYMPHOCYTIC LEUKEMIA. Therapeutic approaches to these entities are discussed in Chapter 176.

EXTRANODAL MARGINAL ZONE B-CELL LYMPHOMA (MALT). Indolent extranodal MALT lymphomas such as those of the gastrointestinal tract, salivary glands, breast, thyroid, orbit, conjunctiva, and lung tend to remain localized for long periods. For this reason, local treatment (surgery or local/regional irradiation) is often very effective. Chemotherapy is less commonly used in MALT lymphomas and is primarily administered to patients with advanced-stage disease.

GASTRIC MALT LYMPHOMA. Because chronic *H. pylori* infection leads to the development of gastric MALT and subsequent gastric MALT lymphoma, patients with localized gastric MALT lymphomas and documented *H. pylori* infection are frequently treated with antibiotic therapy alone (see Chapters 125 and 138). Tumor regression and *H. pylori* eradication have been documented. In patients with bulky gastric MALT lymphomas, the data on antibiotic therapy are more limited and less encouraging.

FOLLICULAR LYMPHOMA, GRADES 1 AND 2 (FOLLICULAR SMALL CELL AND MIXED CELL LYMPHOMAS). TREATMENT

OF LOCALIZED-STAGE (STAGE I–II) DISEASE. Only 15% of patients with follicular lymphoma are initially seen with stage I or II disease. A number of studies have demonstrated the efficacy of directed radiation therapy in this setting.

TREATMENT OF ADVANCED-STAGE (III–IV) DISEASE. The majority of patients with follicular lymphoma have advanced-stage disease. However, the optimal treatment strategy for advanced-stage patients remains to be determined. Patients can be treated conservatively with an approach that includes no initial treatment, followed by palliative single-agent (e.g., chlorambucil) or combination chemotherapy (e.g., cyclophosphamide, vincristine, and prednisone) or involved-field radiotherapy as needed. Alternatively, patients may be treated aggressively with initial combination chemotherapy (e.g., cyclophosphamide, doxorubicin, vincristine, and prednisone [CHOP] or fludarabine-containing regimens) and/or radiation therapy. This dichotomy exists because there is still no evidence that immediate aggressive therapy is more effective than symptom-based conservative therapy in terms of overall survival.

The majority of patients who are initially managed without treatment require chemotherapy or radiation therapy within 2 to 4 years of diagnosis. Furthermore, many patients with symptomatic disease will require treatment at diagnosis. Therapeutic alternatives for advanced-stage follicular lymphoma include single-agent chemotherapy (e.g., chlorambucil), radiation therapy, combination chemotherapy (e.g., CHOP or fludarabine-containing regimens), combined modality therapy, or the use of new agents alone or in combination with chemotherapy. Although these approaches are frequently associated with clinically meaningful responses, the responses are not durable and last a median of only 2 years. Despite the lack of durable complete remissions, median survival in advanced-stage follicular lymphoma is over 7 years.

FOLLICULAR LYMPHOMA, GRADE 3 (FOLLICULAR LARGE CELL LYMPHOMA). Grade 3 (large cell) follicular lymphomas make up fewer than 10% of all follicular lymphomas. The current approach to treatment of this disease is similar to that for diffuse large B-cell lymphoma (see below).

NEW AGENTS AND APPROACHES TO THE TREATMENT OF FOLLICULAR LYMPHOMAS. The lack of curative therapy and the continuous pattern of relapse in advanced-stage follicular lymphomas have prompted a search for new active agents. The nucleoside analogues 2'-deoxycoformycin (pentostatin), 2-chlorodeoxyadenosine, and fludarabine all have activity in follicular lymphomas. Interferon-α also appears to prolong remission in patients who receive this cytokine in association with conventional combination chemotherapy. Monoclonal antibodies directed against B-cell surface antigens have also been used to treat follicular lymphomas that are resistant to conventional therapy. For example, a chimeric antibody consisting of human IgG-κ constant regions and murine anti-CD20 variable regions has been approved for the treatment of relapsed follicular lymphoma. Monoclonal antibodies directed against B-cell surface antigens have also been linked to radioisotopes, including iodine-131 and yttrium-90, and are being used in ongoing studies. High-dose chemotherapy with or without total-body irradiation, followed by autologous bone marrow transplantation, has also been used as consolidation therapy for patients with recurrent follicular lymphoma and high-risk newly diagnosed follicular lymphoma.

MANTLE CELL LYMPHOMA. Mantle cell lymphoma shares some of the least favorable clinical characteristics of both the indolent and the aggressive lymphomas. Like other indolent lymphomas, mantle cell lymphoma has a pattern of continued relapse despite combination chemotherapy (e.g., cyclophosphamide, vincristine, and prednisone or CHOP). However, the natural history of mantle cell lymphoma is more aggressive than that of other indolent lymphomas. The uniquely unfavorable natural history of mantle cell lymphoma suggests that innovative approaches to this disease are needed.

DIFFUSE LARGE B-CELL ANAPLASTIC AND PERIPHERAL T-CELL LYMPHOMA. INDUCTION THERAPY. To date, induction therapy for patients with these aggressive lymphomas has been similar and based on the presence of localized versus advanced-stage disease. Patients with localized disease are commonly treated with anthracycline-containing combination chemotherapy (e.g., CHOP). However, recent studies suggest that it may be possible to reduce the number of cycles of chemotherapy administered to early-stage patients who receive additional directed radiation therapy.

Anthracycline-containing combination chemotherapy is also the treatment of choice for advanced-stage diffuse large B-cell anaplastic or peripheral T-cell lymphoma. The initial successes with the "first-generation" CHOP regimen stimulated subsequent studies of additional "second- and third-generation" regimens such as methotrexate, bleomycin, doxorubicin, cyclophosphamide, vincristine, dexamethasone, and leucovorin; methotrexate, doxorubicin, cyclophosphamide, vincristine, prednisone, bleomycin, and leucovorin; and prednisone, doxorubicin, cyclophosphamide, etoposide, cytarabine, bleomycin, vincristine, methotrexate, and leucovorin. However, recent randomized trials indicate that CHOP is as effective as these second- and third-generation regimens in unselected patients with aggressive lymphomas. Nevertheless, CHOP cures fewer than about 40% of patients with aggressive lymphoma, which underscores the need to develop more effective treatment strategies.

Consensus is emerging that patients with these aggressive lymphomas who fall into either the high-intermediate– or high-risk categories of the IPI may be appropriate candidates for experimental therapy. This conclusion is particularly true for younger patients, who are more likely to tolerate intensive experimental approaches to their disease. To date, treatment strategies for such patients have been based on increasing the doses of chemotherapy with or without additional radiation therapy and hematopoietic stem cell support.

THERAPY FOR RELAPSED DISEASE. Numerous salvage regimens have been used in patients who relapse after standard induction therapy. These regimens typically incorporate drugs that were not used in the first-line induction therapy such as cisplatin, etoposide, cytarabine, and ifosfamide. In general, 20 to 35% of relapsed complete responders achieve a second (short-lived) complete remission with standard salvage chemotherapy. In contrast, a subset of patients with relapsed aggressive lymphoma achieve durable remissions when treated with high-dose chemotherapy and autologous stem cell support.

BURKITT'S AND BURKITT'S-LIKE LYMPHOMAS. Although Burkitt's and Burkitt's-like variant lymphomas differ in morphology, molecular genetics, and clinical features, these diseases are currently treated in the same way. Most treatment regimens for adult Burkitt's lymphoma are based on pediatric protocols, which include brief high-dose combination chemotherapy and CNS prophylaxis with or without cranial irradiation.

LYMPHOBLASTIC LYMPHOMAS. Lymphoblastic lymphomas are treated similarly to acute lymphoblastic leukemias (see Chapter 177).

HIV-ASSOCIATED LYMPHOMAS. By definition, HIV-associated lymphoma conveys a poor prognosis. The median survival for patients with HIV-related lymphoma is less than 12 months, and fewer than 10% of patients survive beyond 2 years. However, aggressive treatment with CHOP or other similar regimens may significantly improve survival in patients who have CD4+ lymphocyte counts greater than 200/mm³ and lymphoma as their initial AIDS-defining condition. Nevertheless, HIV-infected patients have underlying immunodeficiencies and associated infections that make them less able to tolerate aggressive chemotherapeutic regimens.

The Non-Hodgkin's Lymphoma Classification Project: A clinical evaluation of the International Lymphoma Study Group classification of non-Hodgkin's lymphoma. Blood 89:3909, 1997. *This study characterizes the frequency and natural history of currently recognized lymphoid neoplasms.*

Harris N, Jaffe E, Stein H, et al: A revised European-American classification of lymphoid neoplasms: A proposal from the International Lymphoma Study Group. Blood 84:1361, 1994. *The REAL classification includes additional immunophenotypic, genetic, and morphologic data and identifies several additional discrete entities.*

Jaffe E, Berard C, Harris N, et al: Proposed World Health Organization classification of neoplastic diseases of hematopoietic and lymphoid tissues. Am J Surg Pathol 21:114, 1997. *The proposed WHO classification updates the information included in the Revised European-American Lymphoma classification.*

Magrath I, Adde M, Shad A, et al: Adults and children with small non–cleaved-cell lymphoma have a similar excellent outcome when treated with the same chemotherapy regimen. J Clin Oncol 14:925, 1996. *The study describes one of the most effective current regimens for Burkitt's lymphoma.*

Miller TP, Dahlberg S, Cassady JR, et al: Chemotherapy alone compared with chemotherapy plus radiotherapy for localized intermediate- and high-grade non-Hodgkin's lymphoma. N Engl J Med 339:21, 1998. *The superiority of combined modality therapy in localized aggressive lymphomas is demonstrated in this randomized trial.*

Philip T, Guglielmi C, Hagenbeek A, et al: Autologous bone marrow transplantation as compared with salvage chemotherapy in relapses of chemotherapy-sensitive non-Hodgkin's lymphoma. N Engl J Med 333:1540, 1995. *This phase III study demonstrates that autologous bone marrow transplantation improves disease-free and overall survival in chemotherapy-sensitive relapsed aggressive NHL.*

Shipp M, Ambinder R, Appelbaum F, et al: NCCN preliminary non-Hodgkin's lymphoma practice guidelines. Oncology 11:281, 1997. *The National Cancer Center Network treatment guidelines for the most common NHLs are included in this review.*

Shipp MA, Abeloff MD, Antman KH, et al: International consensus conference on high-dose therapy with hematopoietic stem cell transplantation in aggressive non-Hodgkin's lymphomas: report of the jury. J Clin Oncol 17:423–429, 1999. *Updated recommendations.*

Wilson LD, Kacinski BM, Edelson RL, Heard PW: Cutaneous T cell lymphomas. *In* DeVita VT, Hellman S, Rosenberg SA (eds): Cancer: Principles & Practices of Oncology. Philadelphia, JB Lippincott, 1997, p 2220. *This review describes the natural history and varied clinical features of cutaneous T-cell lymphomas and summarizes current approaches to the treatment of these diseases.*

180 HODGKIN'S DISEASE

Carol S. Portlock ■ Joachim Yahalom

Hodgkin's disease, a distinct malignant disorder of the lymphatic system that primarily affects the lymph nodes, serves as a paradigm of the successful evolution of modern oncologic concepts. The management of Hodgkin's disease provides a multidisciplinary challenge, from an accurate diagnosis to a comprehensive staging evaluation and appropriate treatment recommendation. Particularly important is the collaboration between the medical and radiation oncologist because treatments often involve combined chemotherapy/radiation strategies, and single-modality alternatives may affect future treatment options if relapse occurs. These complexities make the disease best treated by experienced multidisciplinary teams working in major medical centers.

EPIDEMIOLOGY AND ETIOLOGY. In the United States, approximately 7500 new cases of Hodgkin's disease are diagnosed annually. In contrast to the increasing incidence of non-Hodgkin's lymphoma, the annual incidence of Hodgkin's disease has remained stable over the past several decades. In developed Western countries, the age-specific incidence of the disease is bimodal, with its greatest peak in the third decade of life and a second, smaller peak after age 50. The second peak is probably an artifact of histologic misclassification because recent studies have shown that many of the older-age cases originally diagnosed as Hodgkin's disease turned out to be non-Hodgkin's lymphomas. The age-specific incidence differs markedly in different countries. In Japan, where the overall incidence is low, no early peak exists. In some developing countries, the peak shifts into childhood. Hodgkin's disease is more common in males (ratio of 1.3:1.0) and less common in African Americans. Genetic factors appear to affect disease expression. Same-sex siblings have a 10 times greater risk of the disorder; monozygotic twin siblings' risk is 99 times higher than that of dizygotic twins if one affected twin has Hodgkin's disease. Parent-child combinations have been more common than spouse pairing incidences, which possibly could reflect the influence of an infectious or environmental agent during childhood or early adolescence. Persons who grow up with few siblings or in single-family houses and persons who had early birth order and fewer playmates show a higher risk of Hodgkin's disease. The incidence of clinical infectious mononucleosis is also associated with these factors; indeed, infectious mononucleosis becomes clinically detectable only after early childhood. Some believe that a viral infection at a certain age and host circumstances may induce a malignant transformation. For a short period, it was thought that Hodgkin's disease might be contagious because of reports of clustering, but that concern has been effectively dispelled.

There have been no conclusive studies regarding the possible increased frequency of Hodgkin's disease in patients with human immunodeficiency virus (HIV) infection. However, Hodgkin's disease in HIV-positive patients is associated with advanced stage and poor therapeutic outcome.

In the past, because of the high incidence of tuberculosis in Hodgkin's disease, *Mycobacterium tuberculosis* was suspected to be the causative organism. More recently, the Epstein-Barr virus (EBV) has been implicated in epidemiologic and serologic studies. A small increase in incidence of Hodgkin's disease has been detected among patients with a history of infectious mononucleosis. More importantly, perhaps, the proportion of patients with Hodgkin's disease who possess high titers of antibody against the viral-capsid antigen of EBV was found to be larger than expected. Furthermore, enhanced activation of EBV was shown to precede the development of Hodgkin's disease. A variety of techniques have demonstrated that 50% or more of Hodgkin's biopsy specimens contain the EBV genome, that the EBV nucleic acid is localized to the Reed-Sternberg cell and its variants, and that the infected cells are monoclonal. These data suggest that EBV alone or with other carcinogens may contribute directly to the pathogenesis of Hodgkin's disease. Alternatively, it is possible that EBV is only a marker of a more fundamental disruption of the immune system of the host. Hodgkin's disease may represent a final common response to diverse pathologic processes such as viral infection, environmental or occupational exposures (e.g., woodworking), and a genetically determined host response.

PATHOLOGY. The diagnosis of Hodgkin's disease requires expert hematopathologic interpretation of a properly processed lymph node specimen. The Reed-Sternberg (R-S) cell is the diagnostic tumor cell that must be identified within the appropriate cellular milieu of lymphocytes, eosinophils, and histiocytes. Hodgkin's disease is unique pathologically because the tumor cells compose a minority of the cell population, whereas normal inflammatory cells are the major cell component. As a result, it sometimes may be difficult to identify the diagnostic R-S cells. Also, other lymphoproliferations may have cells that resemble R-S cells. The R-S cell is characterized by its large size and classic binucleated structure with large eosinophilic nucleoli. R-S variants may have single nuclei, so-called popcorn cells and lacunar cells. The cellular origin of the R-S cell is uncertain. However, recent information supports the notion that R-S cells are of B-cell origin. It has characteristics of both a macrophage and a lymphocyte, including the ability to phagocytose. Genetically, the cell is hyperdiploid without recurring karyotypic abnormalities. Two antigenic markers are thought to provide diagnostic information: CD-30 or Ber-H2 and CD-15 or Leu M-1. These markers reside on the R-S cells or their variants and not on the background inflammatory cells.

Hodgkin's disease has four histologic subtypes. Each is based on the number and appearance of R-S cells as well as the background milieu. Lymphocyte-predominant Hodgkin's disease (LPHD) is a rare form of Hodgkin's disease in which few R-S cells may be identified. The cellular background consists primarily of lymphocytes in a diffuse or sometimes nodular pattern, which may be mistaken for a low-grade non-Hodgkin's lymphoma. Unlike other histologic types of Hodgkin's disease, the lymphocytic infiltrate in LPHD is of B-cell polyclonal origin. This finding has led investigators to propose that LPHD is a non-Hodgkin's lymphoma unrelated to the other three histologic types of Hodgkin's disease. LPHD is more often clinically localized, usually effectively treated with radiation alone, and may have late relapses (clinical features reminiscent of low-grade lymphoma).

Nodular sclerosing Hodgkin's disease (NSHD) is the most common subtype and typically affects young females with early-stage supradiaphragmatic presentations. The number of R-S cells is greater than in LPHD, and they may sometimes be found in clusters. The distinguishing feature is the presence of broad birefringent bands of collagen that divide the cellular process into macroscopic nodules. The tumors contain large numbers of T lymphocytes, eosinophils, neutrophils, and histiocytes. The so-called lacunar cell R-S variants often appear in the "cellular phase" of NSHD. Sclerosis is not a diagnostic feature limited to Hodgkin's disease; it may occur in non-Hodgkin's lymphomas as well, particularly those involving the mediastinum or retroperitoneum. The most difficult differential diagnosis pathologically is between NSHD and Ki-1 (CD-30) diffuse large cell lymphoma (anaplastic large cell lymphoma). Both entities may include sclerosis, large binucleated giant cells, and a T-cell lymphocytic infiltrate. Ki-1 lymphoma (see Chapter 179) is a non-Hodgkin's lymphoma in which both the large and small cells are malignant. In such lymphomas, R-S–like cells are found that are CD30 or Ber H-2 positive but CD15 or Leu M-1 negative. Accurate pathologic diagnosis is critical because the two diseases often affect the same young female population and present as large mediastinal masses, but treatment and prognosis may be decidedly different.

Mixed-cellularity Hodgkin's disease (MCHD) is the second most common histologic type. It is diagnosed more often in males, usually presents as generalized lymphadenopathy or as disease in extranodal sites, and produces associated systemic symptoms. R-S cells are frequently identified and bands of collagen are absent, although a fine reticular fibrosis may exist. The cellular background includes lymphocytes, eosinophils, neutrophils, and histiocytes.

Lymphocyte-depletion Hodgkin's disease (LDHD) is a rare disorder, particularly so because antigen marker studies have demonstrated that in the past many such cases were misdiagnosed and would now be classified as non-Hodgkin's lymphomas. R-S cells are numerous and may be pleomorphic, the cellular background is sparse, and diffuse fibrosis and necrosis may be present. This is the histologic subtype that may be associated with HIV infection and is most commonly diagnosed in elderly persons and in underdeveloped countries. By the time of diagnosis, affected patients usually have advanced-stage disease, extranodal involvement, an aggressive clinical course, and poor prognosis.

As a general rule, findings in extranodal tissues should not be used to diagnose Hodgkin's disease unless R-S cells are conclusively identified. Extranodal sites may contain non-caseating granulomas that are neither diagnostic of Hodgkin's nor indicators of active disease. Rather, granulomas appear to be a non-specific finding in Hodgkin's disease and may denote a favorable prognosis.

DIFFERENTIAL DIAGNOSIS. Hodgkin's disease is a lymph node–based malignancy and uniquely consists of lymphadenopathy in predictable clinical locations. More than 80% of patients present with lymphadenopathy above the diaphragm, often involving the anterior mediastinum; less than 10 to 20% present with lymphadenopathy limited to regions below the diaphragm. Therefore, the differential diagnosis is usually not that of generalized lymphadenopathy but, more commonly, that of regional lymphadenopathy in selected sites.

MEDIASTINAL PRESENTATIONS. Hodgkin's disease frequently affects the anterior mediastinum, and this may be the only site of involvement. In this location, the differential diagnosis is limited to neoplasms (Hodgkin's disease, aggressive non-Hodgkin's lymphomas, germ cell tumors, thymoma), infections (tuberculosis), and sarcoidosis. Hodgkin's disease is remarkably silent when it involves the mediastinal structures. Masses may reach a large size before patients complain of symptoms such as cough, wheeze, chest discomfort, or tightness. Unlike aggressive non-Hodgkin's lymphomas or other neoplasms, Hodgkin's disease rarely causes superior vena cava obstruction, phrenic nerve involvement with diaphragmatic paralysis, or laryngeal nerve compression and hoarseness. A common complaint of patients with large mediastinal masses due to Hodgkin's disease compressing the trachea is a cough or shortness of breath that intensifies when lying supine but is relieved by sitting upright.

REGIONAL LYMPH NODE PRESENTATIONS. Cervical, supraclavicular, axillary, or, uncommonly, inguinal lymphadenopathy may be the initial complaint. Lymph nodes that are unlikely to be involved with Hodgkin's disease at diagnosis include those in Waldeyer's tonsillar ring, as well as at preauricular, occipital, epitrochlear, posterior mediastinal, mesenteric, and popliteal sites. Involvement, if any, of these areas is more likely to occur in non-Hodgkin's lymphomas. In addition, retroperitoneal lymphadenopathy rarely oc-

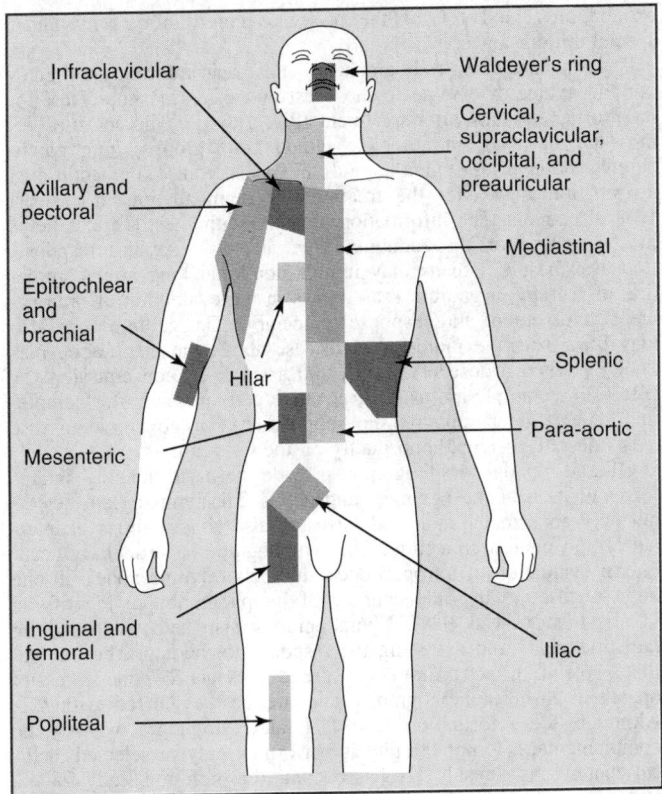

FIGURE 180–1 ■ Anatomic definition of lymph node regions for staging of Hodgkin's disease. (From Kaplan HS, Rosenberg SA: The treatment of Hodgkin's disease. Med Clin North Am 50:1591, 1966.)

curs as the only site of Hodgkin's disease but rather is accompanied by other supradiaphragmatic presentations and/or inguinal adenopathy. Many conditions can cause regional lymphadenopathy, including infections with reactive lymphadenopathy (particularly frequent in the cervical and inguinal distributions); neoplasms (such as primary head and neck, lung or thyroid, breast, rectum), and autoimmune disorders. It is important to keep in mind that patients with lymphoma may develop superimposed regional reactive lymphadenopathy that may improve partially with a course of antibiotics. When residual lymphadenopathy persists, however, it deserves further investigation.

GENERALIZED LYMPH NODE PRESENTATIONS. Disseminated lymphadenopathy is infrequent in Hodgkin's disease. When present, it is usually associated with systemic symptoms and often extranodal involvement as well. This presentation is sufficiently uncommon that one must consider other causes of widespread lymphadenopathy: infections (viral, bacterial, fungal, mycobacterial), autoimmune disorders, HIV-associated lymphadenopathy, and non-Hodgkin's lymphomas.

EXTRANODAL INVOLVEMENT. Hodgkin's disease may affect extranodal tissues by direct invasion (contiguity), the so-called E-lesion, or by hematogenous dissemination, that is, stage IV disease. Isolated extranodal presentations (e.g., cutaneous nodules or gastric involvement) without nodal involvement usually denote a non-Hodgkin's lymphoma except when associated with HIV disease. When extranodal involvement is suspected, one must also consider the possibility that the patient has an infection concurrent with regional Hodgkin's disease. Examples include patients who have bulky mediastinal involvement that produces tracheal or bronchial compression and an obstructive pneumonia as well.

Sites of extranodal involvement that suggest a diagnosis other than Hodgkin's disease include meninges, parenchymal brain involvement, nasal sinuses, lung lesions without mediastinal adenopathy, gastrointestinal tract invasion, ascites or mesenteric nodal disease, and genitourinary structures (kidney, bladder, testis, or ovary). All these areas are more commonly affected by a non-Hodgkin's lymphoma, other neoplasms, or infectious processes.

SYSTEMIC MANIFESTATIONS OF HODGKIN'S DISEASE. Occasionally, patients come to attention because of systemic complaints or findings. These findings include chronic pruritus, which may be intense and produce destructive excoriation; systemic "B" symptoms of fever, night sweats, or weight loss; lymph node pain with alcohol consumption; an abnormal blood profile, such as leukocytosis with neutrophilia, eosinophilia, or thrombocytosis; or rarely hypercalcemia, nephrotic syndrome, or pancytopenia with a fibrotic bone marrow and splenomegaly.

STAGING. The next step after the diagnosis of Hodgkin's disease is the staging process, that is, the classification of the tumor according to its extent. Precise definition of the extent of nodal and extranodal involvement with Hodgkin's disease is made according to a standard staging classification system and is critical for selection of the proper treatment. Detailed documentation of the extent of disease also provides the baseline for evaluating the response to therapy and for monitoring potential relapse. Accurate delineation of disease sites is mandatory for the design of radiation therapy fields. The use of a standard staging system also allows comparison of the results of therapeutic interventions in different clinical trials.

The Ann Arbor staging classification has been the basis for treatment decisions for Hodgkin's disease patients since 1971. It was originally designed to distinguish patients who would benefit from extended-field radiation therapy from those who would require systemic chemotherapy. The staging system is an anatomic one and describes the sites of tumor in relation to the diaphragm (Fig. 180–1). The Ann Arbor staging classification was revised at a meeting in Cotswolds, England, to recognize the importance of tumor bulk (Table 180–1).

The assignment of stage is based on the number of sites of involvement, whether lymph nodes are involved on both sides of the diaphragm, whether this involvement is bulky (particularly in the mediastinum), whether there is contiguous extranodal involvement (E sites) or disseminated extranodal disease, and, additionally, whether typical systemic symptoms (B symptoms) are present (Table 180–2). In defining a patient's stage, it is important to note how the information was obtained to reflect remaining uncertainties: clinical staging (CS) refers to information that has been obtained by initial biopsy, history and physical examination, and radiographic studies only; a pathologic stage (PS) is determined by more extensive surgical assessment of potentially involved sites, such as by surgical staging laparotomy and splenectomy.

HISTORY AND PHYSICAL EXAMINATION. The history should give special attention to the presence or absence of disease-associated symptoms, which may occur in up to one third of patients and include fever, night sweats, weight loss (B symptoms), pruritus, and, less commonly, pain in involved regions after ingestion of alcohol. In each anatomic stage, the presence of B symptoms is an adverse prognostic indicator that may affect the treatment choice. Unexplained fever is defined as recurrent temperatures above 38° C during the previous month, night sweats are considered present if

Table 180–1 ■ THE COTSWOLDS STAGING CLASSIFICATION FOR HODGKIN'S DISEASE

Stage I	Involvement of a single lymph node region or a lymphoid structure (e.g., spleen, thymus, Waldeyer's ring)
Stage II	Involvement of two or more lymph node regions on the same side of the diaphragm (i.e., the mediastinum is a single site, hilar lymph nodes are lateralized). The number of anatomic sites should be indicated by a subscript (e.g., II₂).
Stage III	Involvement of lymph node regions or structures on both sides of the diaphragm: III₁: With or without involvement of splenic, hilar, celiac, or portal nodes III₂: With involvement of para-aortic, iliac, or mesenteric nodes
Stage IV	Involvement of extranodal site(s) beyond that designed E

Designations applicable to any disease stage
A: No symptoms
B: Fever, drenching sweats, weight loss
X: Bulky disease:
  >1/3 the width of the mediastinum
  >10 cm maximal dimension of nodal mass
E: Involvement of a single extranodal site, contiguous or proximal to a known nodal site
CS: Clinical stage
PS: Pathologic stage

Table 180–2 ■ RECOMMENDED PROCEDURES IN STAGING HODGKIN'S DISEASE

1. Adequate surgical biopsy reviewed by an experienced pathologist
2. History and physical examination with particular attention to the presence and duration of B symptoms (see Table 180–1) and pruritus
3. *Imaging studies*
   Plain chest radiograph
   CT of thorax
   CT of abdomen and pelvis
   Gallium scan
4. *Hematologic studies*
   Complete blood cell count
   Erythrocyte sedimentation rate
   Bone marrow biopsy
5. *Biochemical studies*
   Liver function tests
   Renal function tests
   Lactate dehydrogenase, albumin, calcium
6. *Under special circumstances*
   Bipedal lymphography
   Magnetic resonance imaging
   Technetium bone scan
   Percutaneous or laparoscopic liver biopsy
   Staging laparotomy

they are drenching and recurrent, and unexplained weight loss is significant only if at least 10% of body weight is lost within the preceding 6 months. Although pruritus is no longer considered a B symptom, the presence of generalized itching is considered by many to be an adverse prognostic symptom. Certain combinations of B symptoms have been found to be more prognostically significant than others. For example, the combination of fever and weight loss has a more adverse prognosis than night sweats alone. B symptoms probably reflect the end-product manifestation of cytokines produced by the tumor cells.

The physical examination should carefully determine the location and size of all palpable lymph nodes. An inspection of Waldeyer's ring, detection of splenomegaly or hepatomegaly, and evaluation of the cardiac and respiratory status are important.

LABORATORY STUDIES. The initial laboratory studies should include a complete blood cell count with white cell differential and platelet count, an erythrocyte sedimentation rate (ESR), tests for liver and renal function, and assays for serum alkaline phosphatase and lactate dehydrogenase.

Mild to moderate anemia with normal indices of the type often found in patients with other malignancies or chronic disease may accompany Hodgkin's disease and does not necessarily indicate bone marrow involvement or hypersplenism. A moderate to marked leukemoid reaction and thrombocytosis are common, particularly in symptomatic patients, and usually disappear with treatment. Mild eosinophilia frequently exists, especially in patients with pruritus. Patients with advanced stage disease and those with HIV-related Hodgkin's disease may show absolute lymphopenia (<1000 cells/mm^3), which usually denotes a poor prognosis.

The ESR may provide helpful prognostic information. At some centers, treatment programs for patients with early-stage disease are influenced by the degree of ESR elevation. Changes in the ESR after therapy also may correlate with response and relapse. Other acute-phase reactants, such as serum copper, have been proposed as reliable non-specific markers of disease activity but have shown no advantage over ESR.

Abnormalities of liver function studies should prompt further evaluation of that organ, with imaging and possible biopsy. An elevated alkaline phosphatase value may be a non-specific marker, but it also may indicate bone involvement that should be appropriately evaluated by a radionuclide bone scan and directed skeletal radiographs. An appreciably elevated LDH has been associated with a poor prognosis in some studies.

IMAGING STUDIES. Radiologic studies should include a chest radiograph and computed tomography (CT) of the chest, abdomen, and pelvis with intravenous contrast medium enhancement. In most patients, a bipedal lymphogram and a gallium radionuclide scan provide important information and are highly recommended. Radionuclide bone scan, magnetic resonance imaging (MRI) of the chest

or abdomen, and CT of the neck are contributory only under special circumstances.

The standard chest radiograph provides basic information regarding the extent of disease in the chest and offers a simple test for monitoring patients after treatment (Fig. 180–2). Thoracic CT details the status of intrathoracic lymph node groups, lung parenchyma, pericardium, pleura, and the chest wall. This additional information may alter the treatment recommendation in at least 10% of patients. The information obtained with chest CT also helps in the design of the radiation field and in assessing response. Because chest CT scans may remain abnormal long after completion of therapy, a gallium scan assists in the evaluation of pretreatment involvement and response to therapy. The gallium scan also may be a sensitive indicator of disease above the diaphragm, particularly when a dose of 10 mCi and a single-photon emission CT (SPECT) technique are used. A negative gallium scan after completion of treatment supports the supposition that no active disease exists despite residual abnormality on the CT scan.

CT and bipedal lymphography provide the basic imaging studies for evaluation of the abdomen and pelvis. The lymphogram detects not only abnormal lymph node size but also abnormalities of internal lymph node architecture. The lymphogram is particularly accurate in evaluation of retroperitoneal and pelvic lymph nodes. In one large series, the overall accuracy of lymphography in identifying involved nodes was 92%. Lymphography also helps in designing radiation fields and assessing the response to therapy. The internal iliac, splenic hilar, porta hepatis, and mesenteric nodes are not opacified during lymphography and are best evaluated with CT. Although the information from CT and lymphography may be complementary, lymphography is performed only in selected medical centers. As a result, CT has become the preferred study for the abdomen and pelvis in most institutions.

The current use of MRI is under study. MRI of the chest may help to differentiate residual fibrosis from active disease and to assess chest wall and pericardial invasion. So far MRI has been found to be of little advantage over CT in evaluating abdominal involvement. Radionuclide bone scans are appropriate for investigating the nature of bone pain or an elevated serum alkaline phosphatase. MRI may be a sensitive indicator of bone or bone marrow involvement.

BONE MARROW BIOPSY. Bone marrow involvement is relatively uncommon, but because of the impact of a positive biopsy on further staging and treatment, unilateral iliac crest bone marrow biopsy should be part of the staging process. Because the disease involves the marrow non-homogeneously, single biopsies are not always adequate, and bilateral biopsies may be warranted in evaluating extent of disease in patients with widespread nodal disease or B symptoms.

STAGING LAPAROTOMY. Staging laparotomy is the most definitive method for detecting occult infradiaphragmatic Hodgkin's disease. A major problem with all imaging techniques for Hodgkin's disease is their inability to identify splenic involvement. In about one third of patients with normal-size spleens, Hodgkin's disease is found in the resected organ. Conversely, approximately half of patients found to have clinical or radiologic enlargement of the spleen do not have pathologic involvement of the removed organ. Staging laparotomy includes splenectomy and sampling of the splenic hilar, porta hepatis, para-aortic, and iliac nodes (with special attention given to areas that look suspicious on imaging studies). The procedure also samples the liver with a wedge and needle biopsy under direct vision and obtains open iliac crest bone marrow biopsy, if not performed previously. Areas of biopsy are marked with a clip, and an abdominal radiograph during or after laparotomy assists in verifying the removal of suspicious nodes shown by lymphography.

The complications of staging laparotomy include the non-specific risks of general anesthesia and abdominal surgery. Reviews of laparotomy series report the risk of major postoperative complications to be 3 to 7%. Surgical mortality is rare (<1%) and is zero in many large series. Because of occasional severe bacterial infections occurring after splenectomy, pneumococcal vaccine should be administered before staging laparotomy.

Laparotomy is not a routine staging procedure and should be considered only if the additional information may alter the choice of treatment. Thus, it is relevant only for patients who are potential candidates for radiation therapy alone. Although staging laparotomy

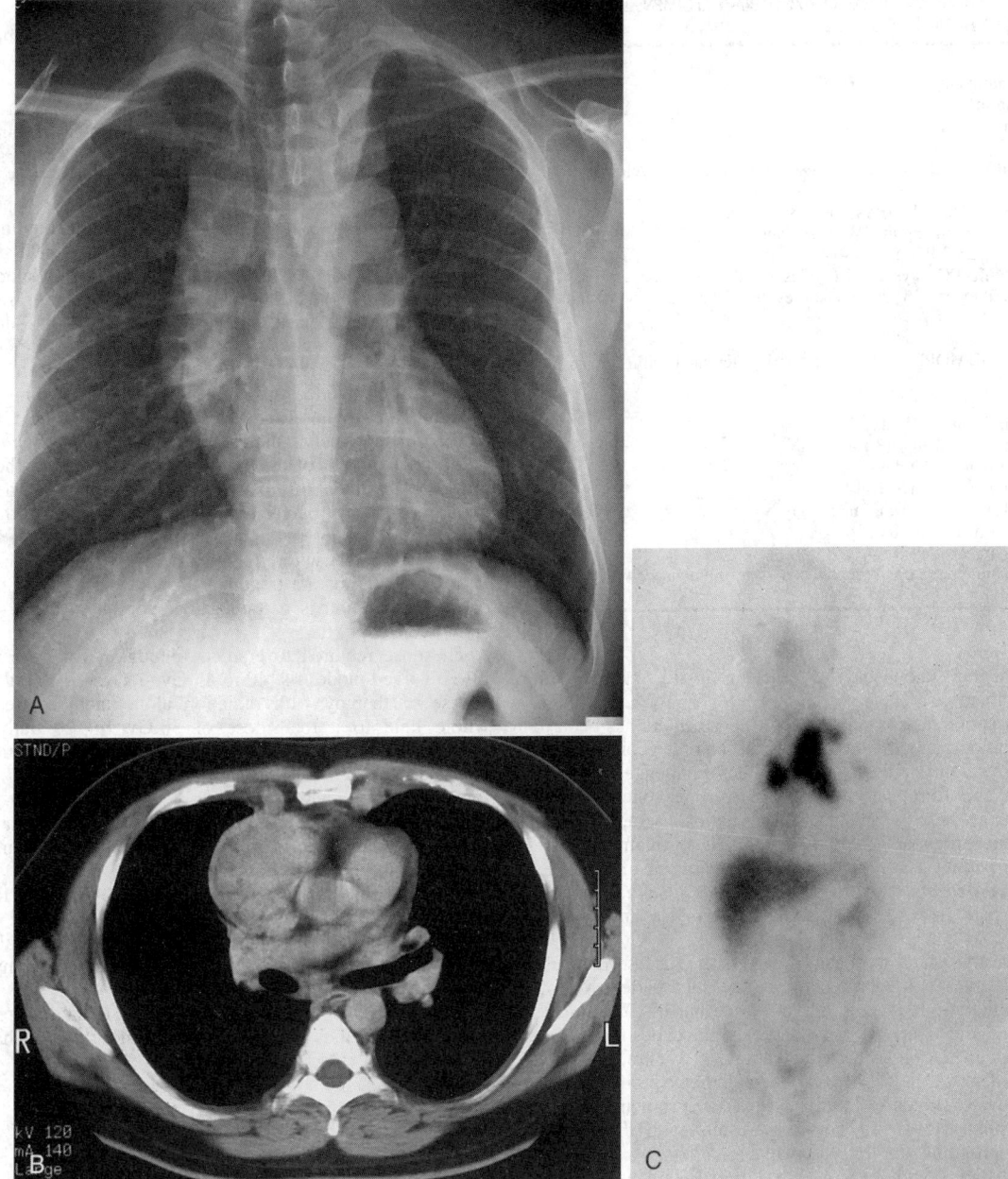

FIGURE 180-2 ■ Bulky Hodgkin's disease as seen on chest radiograph (*A*), CT scan of the chest (*B*), and gallium scan (*C*).

remains the most precise way to determine the presence and extent of infradiaphragmatic Hodgkin's disease, it is currently used less frequently than in the past because clinical prognostic factors allow adequate selection of patients for radiation therapy alone and because randomized studies have not demonstrated an advantage for performing a staging laparotomy. Moreover, combined modality therapy in many treatment plans has replaced radiation therapy alone, further limiting the need for precise surgical staging.

TREATMENT. Over the past three decades, advances in radiation therapy and the development of effective combination chemotherapy have resulted in the cure of more than 75% of all newly diagnosed patients with Hodgkin's disease. All patients, regardless of stage, can and should be treated with curative intent.

The stage of the disease is the most important determinant of treatment options and outcome, so precise definition of the extent of nodal and extranodal involvement during staging is critical to select the proper treatment strategy. Hodgkin's disease is very sensitive to radiation and to many chemotherapy drugs; in most stages, more than one option provides effective treatment. Because most patients are expected to have a normal life expectancy, new treat-

ment programs must pay particular attention to minimizing future toxicity. Any changes must be undertaken without compromising the excellent cure rates obtained by well-established therapies.

Effective treatment of Hodgkin's disease is complex, requiring the expertise of a multidisciplinary team consisting of a pathologist, diagnostic radiologist, and medical and radiation oncologists during staging of the disease and subsequent treatment. Because radiation plays an important role in the treatment, the use of a modern, high-quality radiation therapy facility staffed with an experienced team yields the best treatment results.

EARLY-STAGE DISEASE. The curative treatment of early-stage Hodgkin's disease was established in the 1960s and 1970s using radiation alone, and this single modality remains the gold standard for the management of most patients with early-stage disease. In patients who were pathologically (laparotomy) staged and treated with primary irradiation alone, several large series reported a 15- to 20-year survival of nearly 90% and a relapse-free survival rate of 75 to 80%. Most relapses (75%) occur within the first 3 years after completing therapy; late relapses are uncommon. It is important to note that more than half of the patients who experience relapse

Table 180–3 ■ COMBINATION CHEMOTHERAPY REGIMENS IN
ADVANCED HODGKIN'S DISEASE

ABVD
Doxorubicin (Adriamycin), 25 mg/m² IV
Bleomycin, 10 mg/m² IV
Vinblastine (Velban), 6 mg/m² IV
DTIC, 375 mg/m² IV
ABVD is repeated every 2 weeks; two treatments equal one cycle.
MOPP
Nitrogen mustard, 6 mg/m² IV days 1 and 8
Vincristine (Oncovin), 1.4 mg/m² IV days 1 and 8
Procarbazine, 100 mg/m² PO days 1–14
Prednisone, 40 mg/m² PO days 1–14 (cycles 1 and 4 only)
MOPP is repeated every 28 days; each cycle is one 28-day course of
  therapy.
MOPP-ABVD
One 28-day cycle of MOPP with prednisone is alternated with one 28-day
  cycle of ABVD
MOPP-ABV hybrid
Nitrogen mustard, 6 mg/m² IV day 1
Vincristine (Oncovin), 1.4 mg/m² IV day 1
Procarbazine, 100 mg/m² PO days 1–8
Prednisone, 40 mg/m² PO days 1–14
Doxorubicin (Adriamycin), 35 mg/m² IV day 8
Bleomycin, 10 mg/m² IV day 8
Vinblastine, 6 mg/m² IV day 8
Pneumocystis carinii pneumonia prophylaxis is recommended with the hy-
  brid regimen.

after radiation therapy alone have disease that is still curable with
standard chemotherapy.

The standard approach in many United States centers has been to
insist on a pathologic staging of the disease before recommending
radiation therapy alone. This notion has been challenged by data
from Canadian and European studies that show excellent overall
survival results in patients selected for radiation therapy on the
basis of clinical prognostic factors alone. Thus, treatment with
radiation alone can be safely offered to clinically staged patients
with favorable prognostic factors. With a clinical staging policy,
however, more patients receive chemotherapy, either as initial or as
salvage therapy.

An alternative treatment approach to early-stage disease is to use
both radiation therapy and chemotherapy in selected patients. Combined-modality therapy reduces the relapse rate but in most studies
does not change the overall survival rate while exposing all patients to the added toxicity of chemotherapy. New strategies that
combine less intensive and less toxic chemotherapy regimens with
radiation therapy to clinically involved sites have shown excellent
preliminary results. However, long-term results with these combined-modality programs are not yet available.

Early-stage patients with bulky mediastinal disease and significant B symptoms or clinically staged patients at high risk for
subdiaphragmatic involvement (e.g., mixed cellularity or lymphocyte-depletion histology, age > 40) attain better relapse-free survival rates with combined-modality therapy including chemotherapy
(Table 180–3) than with radiation therapy alone.

Two prospective randomized studies compared the efficacy of
MOPP chemotherapy alone with radiation therapy alone in early-
stage patients. Whereas a study from the National Cancer Institute
(NCI) showed equivalent results for the two modalities, other analyses found a significantly lower survival rate among patients
treated with MOPP than among those treated with standard radiation therapy. Although other drug combinations such as ABVD
may be more effective and less toxic than MOPP, they have not
been tested without radiation in early-stage Hodgkin's disease and
should not be used alone outside a controlled clinical trial.

RADIATION THERAPY. The cure of early-stage Hodgkin's disease
with radiation alone became possible only after the recognition that
all involved sites, as well as adjacent nodal areas, need to be
treated with tumoricidal doses. Proper irradiation technique requires
the use of linear accelerators that produce 6- to 10-MV photons.
This degree of energy permits the exposure of large volumes to an
adequate and homogeneous radiation dose with a modest degree of
skin sparing. Treatment planning should be performed on a dedicated radiation CT-based simulator that duplicates the features of

the treatment unit. The plan itself is based on detailed imaging
information that has been obtained during the staging process and
during the simulation. The radiation field is shaped to conform to
the patient's anatomy and tumor configuration. Routine field verification (port films) is essential for controlling the proper delivery of
treatment.

Successful therapy with radiation alone requires treatment of all
clinically involved lymph nodes and all nodal and extranodal
regions at risk for subclinical involvement. Certain standard large
radiation therapy fields (Fig. 180–3) have been designed for the
treatment of Hodgkin's disease. The fields are shaped to include
multiple adjacent lymph node sites while accounting for normal
tissue tolerance and the technical constraints of field size.

The mantle radiation field covers the lymph node areas above the
diaphragm, including the submandibular, cervical, supraclavicular,
infraclavicular, axillary, mediastinal, and hilar nodal areas. The
para-aortic field includes the para-aortic lymph nodes from the
diaphragm to the aortic bifurcation and the spleen or the splenic
pedicle (after splenectomy). The pelvic field encompasses the iliac,
inguinal, and femoral nodes. The inverted-Y field combines the
para-aortic and pelvic fields. The term *total lymphoid irradiation*
refers to treatment of all three fields. Subtotal lymphoid irradiation
indicates treatment of the mantle and para-aortic fields only. To
avoid excessive toxicity, the radiation fields are treated sequentially, the total dose is fractionated, and the radiated volumes are
carefully tailored with individualized divergent blocks. When patients require separate treatment to adjacent regions, the calculation
of field separation is particularly important to avoid overlap at the
spinal cord.

The dose required to eradicate Hodgkin's disease in demonstrably involved nodes is 40 to 45 Gy (1 Gy = 100 rad). A standard
course of therapy with radiation alone includes treatment of the
whole field to a total dose of 36 Gy (in 20 daily fractions of
1.8 Gy each, over a period of 4 weeks), with additional radiation
restricted to the clinically apparent disease sites of 4 to 9 Gy. A
lower dose of radiation, in the range of 24 to 36 Gy, is used when
radiation is administered as adjuvant or consolidation treatment
after chemotherapy. In such programs, the radiation port may be
limited to the clinically involved sites.

SIDE EFFECTS AND COMPLICATIONS OF RADIATION THERAPY.
Early Effects. These effects depend on the radiated volume, dose
administered, and technique employed. They are also influenced
by the extent and type of prior chemotherapy, if any, and by the
patient's age.

The acute side effects of mantle field radiation are usually mild
and transient: they may include mouth dryness, change in taste,

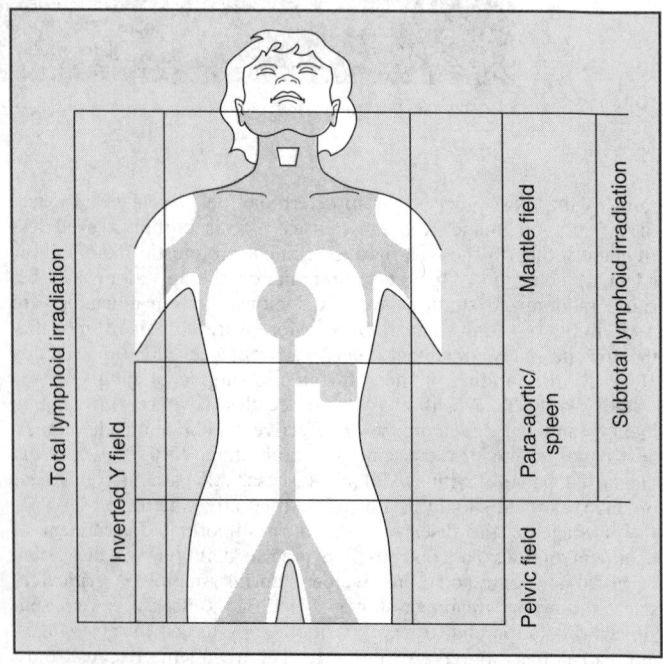

FIGURE 180–3 ■ Standard radiation fields for Hodgkin's disease.

pharyngitis, nausea, dry cough, dermatitis, and fatigue. These side effects are managed symptomatically and subside gradually soon after the completion of radiation therapy. The main potential side effects of subdiaphragmatic radiation are loss of appetite, nausea, and increase in bowel movements. These reactions are usually mild and can be minimized with standard antiemetic medications. Irradiation of more than one field, particularly after chemotherapy, can cause myelosuppression, and treatment delays may be required during therapy.

Six weeks to 3 months after completion of mantle therapy, approximately 15% of patients may develop Lhermitte's sign: patients note an electric shock sensation radiating down the backs of both legs when the head is flexed. Lhermitte's sign may be secondary to transient demyelinization of the cervical spinal cord; it resolves spontaneously after a few months and is not associated with late or permanent cord damage. During the same period, radiation pneumonitis and/or acute pericarditis may occur in less than 5% of patients, more often in those who had extensive mediastinal disease. Both inflammatory processes have become rare with modern radiation techniques. Patients with Hodgkin's disease, regardless of treatment type, have a propensity to develop herpes zoster infection within 2 years after the onset of therapy. Usually the infection is confined to a single dermatome and is self-limited. If the cutaneous eruption is identified promptly, treatment with systemic acyclovir limits the duration and intensity of the infection.

Late Effects. Mantle field radiation therapy can induce subclinical hypothyroidism, detected by elevation of the level of thyroid-stimulating hormone, in about one third of patients. Thyroid replacement with L-thyroxine is recommended, even for asymptomatic patients, to prevent the development of overt hypothyroidism and to decrease the risk of developing benign thyroid nodules. Radiation of the pelvic field may have deleterious effects on fertility; in most patients this effect can be avoided by appropriate gonadal shielding. In females, the ovaries can be moved (oophoropexy) into a shielded area laterally or inferomedially near the uterine cervix. Irradiation of the mantle and para-aortic fields alone does not increase the risk of sterility.

Hodgkin's disease patients who were cured with radiation therapy and/or chemotherapy have an increased risk of developing secondary solid tumors and non-Hodgkin's lymphoma 10 or more years after treatment. Unlike MOPP and similar chemotherapy combinations, radiation therapy for Hodgkin's disease is not leukemogenic. The most frequent solid tumors reported after radiation therapy or chemotherapy for Hodgkin's disease are lung cancer, breast cancer, stomach cancer, and melanoma. Patients who smoke should be strongly encouraged to stop because the increase in lung cancer after irradiation or chemotherapy has been detected mostly in smokers. The increase in breast cancer risk is inversely related to the age at Hodgkin's disease treatment; in women irradiated after the age of 30 years, no increase in the risk of breast cancer has been found. Breast cancer is curable in its early stages, and early detection significantly improves survival. Breast examination should be part of the routine follow-up program for women cured of Hodgkin's disease, and routine mammography should begin about 7 years after treatment of Hodgkin's disease.

An increase in the risk of coronary artery disease has been reported for patients who have received mediastinal irradiation. To reduce this hazard, patients should be monitored and advised to avoid other established coronary disease risk factors such as smoking, hyperlipidemia, hypertension, and poor dietary and exercise habits. In children, high-dose radiation affects bone and muscle growth and may result in deformities. Current programs for pediatric Hodgkin's disease are chemotherapy based, and radiation therapy is limited to low doses.

ADVANCED-STAGE DISEASE. The mainstay of treatment in advanced Hodgkin's disease (stages IIIB and IV) is combination chemotherapy. Before embarking on a therapeutic regimen, it is important to document carefully the diagnosis, clinical or pathologic stage, and possible medical contraindications to systemic therapy. The possible side effects of the treatment plan should be outlined given the reasonable expectation of a curative outcome.

In selecting a combination chemotherapy regimen, it is important to evaluate the relative effectiveness, as well as potential acute and long-term side effects. Several combination chemotherapy regimens have been developed since their introduction in the 1960s and

1970s, but few studies have prospectively compared their efficacy. The most frequently used drug programs are MOPP, ABVD, MOPP-ABVD, and MOPP-ABV hybrid (see Table 180–3). MOPP and ABVD are considered non-cross-resistant drug regimens; alternating and hybrid regimens have been developed to take advantage of this characteristic. In prospective, randomized studies, ABVD chemotherapy has been found to be at least as effective as MOPP and MOPP-ABVD; likewise, MOPP-ABV hybrid has been shown to be equivalent to MOPP-ABVD; and ABVD has been found equivalent to MOPP-ABV hybrid. Thus, ABVD is now considered the preferred drug combination in Hodgkin's disease treatment because it is at least equally effective and avoids exposure to the toxic drugs in MOPP or MOPP-containing regimens. In prospective comparisons, MOPP-containing regimens have had significantly greater risks of infection and late development of secondary myelodysplasia, leukemia, and solid tumors. Results of combination chemotherapy reveal a complete response rate of approximately 80%, a disease-free survival of complete responders of 50 to 60%, and an overall survival of 40 to 50%. Adverse prognostic factors include the presence of systemic symptoms, tumor bulk, multiple extranodal sites, age older than 40 years, and male gender.

To increase the cure rate of advanced Hodgkin's disease, the most important strategy is to administer the planned drug regimen according to the dose and schedule of the empirically developed schema. Retrospective analyses have demonstrated that the relative dose intensity (amount of drug per unit time) of the drug regimen correlates with treatment outcome. Another approach, which is to add regional irradiation as a consolidative local therapy after chemotherapy induction, is routinely recommended when patients have bulky disease presentations (masses >10 cm) and often applied when residual masses remain after chemotherapy. Routine use of widefield consolidative radiation, either low dose or full dose, without these specific indications remains controversial, although retrospective studies and some prospective trials support this approach. Investigative strategies to increase the cure rate further include the use of intensive short-course combination chemotherapy with involved-field irradiation (e.g., BEACOPP or Stanford V) and consolidative autologous stem cell transplantation in first clinical remission, but these approaches have not yet proven to be superior to the standard drug regimens.

When administering chemotherapy, the physician must pay attention to the rate of disease regression, remaining particularly alert to the rare situation in which response is sluggish (<50% tumor reduction in the first three cycles) or completely absent. In this setting, pathologic diagnosis must be seriously questioned (e.g., the disease may be a non-Hodgkin's lymphoma) or it may be that the patient has primary refractory disease requiring a change in chemotherapy. In most patients, response is rapid, although a residual mass often persists at the completion of four to six cycles of chemotherapy. It is generally recommended to continue treatment for at least two cycles beyond a clinical complete remission. Response is measured by physical examination, chest radiography, CT (when appropriate), and gallium scanning. If the response remains equivocal at the end of a chemotherapy regimen, it may be appropriate to evaluate the treatment effect with biopsy, particularly if there is residual gallium avidity.

TOXICITIES OF COMBINATION CHEMOTHERAPY. ABVD is a well-tolerated drug regimen whose major consistent toxicities include modest hair loss, fatigue, and myelosuppression (particularly neutropenia). Side effects in some patients include nausea and vomiting, not completely controlled even with the routine use of ondansetron; pulmonary toxicity (which must be monitored closely with measures of diffusion capacity and for which bleomycin must be discontinued as soon as symptoms or a significant decrease in diffusion capacity is identified); vinblastine-associated peripheral or autonomic neuropathy; and symptomatic phlebitis. Rarely, patients may develop doxorubicin-induced cardiomyopathy or extravasation necrosis at injection sites.

In cancer centers, MOPP is used much less frequently than ABVD because it is considered an equivalent or less effective drug program and has several less acceptable side effects, including greater myelosuppression (particularly thrombocytopenia) and susceptibility to infection; permanent infertility in most males and many older females; greater autonomic and peripheral neuropathy with vincristine; and, most importantly, the possible late toxicity of secondary myelodysplasia or acute myeloid leukemia is approximately 5% at 10 years. MOPP-ABV hybrid uses half the number of MOPP treatments and thereby reduces some of these risks. Nevertheless, permanent infertility and secondary blood dyscrasias are still a concern. Secondary myelodysplasia or leukemia has been reported rarely after ABVD. However, an increased incidence of secondary solid tumors and non-Hodgkin's lymphoma has been detected in patients treated for Hodgkin's disease with any form of chemotherapy alone or with combined-modality therapy.

ABVD causes a transient azoospermia but not permanent infertility in men and only temporarily disrupts menstrual function in most women. Older women, however, may suffer permanent menopause or infertility. Because preservation of fertility is an important consideration in this young, potentially curable patient group, sperm banking should be recommended before chemotherapy. Many men have low sperm counts before any treatment as a result of chronic illness. After ABVD or pelvic radiation, counts generally recover within 1 to 2 years.

RELAPSED HODGKIN'S DISEASE. Hodgkin's disease may be cured even if the initial treatment fails. The choice of salvage approach depends on the history of prior treatments, considering the relapse sites as well as the patient's age and general medical condition.

For patients who relapse after radiation therapy, combination chemotherapy such as ABVD is the treatment of choice. If the relapse is regional and outside the prior radiation field, involved- or extended-field irradiation may be added. The salvage rate in this group is excellent (10-year relapse-free survival of 50 to 60%). The most important prognostic factor after relapse in a patient who has received radiation therapy is the extent of disease at the time of relapse, emphasizing the importance of careful follow-up.

Standard-dose chemotherapy seldom salvages patients who fail to attain a complete response with chemotherapy or who relapse early after completion of combination chemotherapy (or combined modality therapy). High-dose chemotherapy accompanied by autologous stem cell transplantation (HD-ASCT) has become the preferred choice in this situation (see Chapter 182). A randomized study demonstrated the advantage of HD-ASCT over standard-dose salvage in refractory and relapsed patients. Results of transplantation are best in patients who have chemoresponsive disease at relapse, few prior therapies, and good performance status and who lack bulky disease or bone/bone marrow involvement. Favorable patients have a curative potential of 50 to 80% in most series. By contrast, only 10 to 30% of poor-risk patients remit. Less than 5% of patients die of transplant complication. Carefully selected patients with a late first relapse (>2 years after completion of standard-dose chemotherapy) may be salvaged with a second standard-dose combination chemotherapy, with or without involved-field irradiation.

HD-ASCT is a cumbersome, toxic, and expensive process, making it important to identify proper candidates accurately. All should have histologic proof of active Hodgkin's disease at relapse because residual masses are common and may not represent active tumor. Consolidation HD-ASCT is not recommended in first remission. At relapse, there is no standard reinduction chemotherapy, and it may include drugs used at initial therapy or new agents. The most commonly used HD-ASCT conditioning regimen is CBV (cyclophosphamide, BCNU [carmustine], and VP 16 [etoposide]). Other combinations also have demonstrated efficacy, and some programs also incorporate standard involved-field or intensive large-field radiation therapy. The autologous stem cell product may be provided from the patient's own bone marrow and/or peripheral blood with hematopoietic growth factor support.

SPECIAL CIRCUMSTANCES. Pregnancy may complicate the management of initial or relapsed Hodgkin's disease. When the pregnancy is first diagnosed, it is important to stage the patient clinically by history and physical examination; posteroanterior chest radiograph; ultrasonography; MRI of the chest, abdomen, and pelvis (as indicated); and bone marrow biopsy. Before recommending medical management, it must be kept in mind that Hodgkin's disease is often an indolent tumor and may be clinically silent or asymptomatic for many months. For that reason, it may be possible to monitor a patient and defer treatment during the pregnancy. If treatment is indicated, options include involved-field radiation with

shielding of the pregnant uterus, single-agent chemotherapy such as vinblastine, or even combination chemotherapy with ABVD. Treatment selection depends on disease sites at risk, age and size of the developing fetus, tumor bulk, the patient's symptoms, and predicted delivery date. Very rarely it may be necessary to consider therapeutic abortion if the diagnosis of advanced and/or symptomatic Hodgkin's disease is made early in the pregnancy.

HIV-associated Hodgkin's disease is much less frequent than non-Hodgkin's lymphoma; the most important consideration is to establish an accurate diagnosis (see Chapter 416). Clinical staging often reveals more advanced disease than in non-HIV patients, and extranodal involvement is more frequent. It is important to distinguish between Hodgkin's disease and infectious causes of apparent extranodal involvement (such as pulmonary nodules) before determining a final treatment plan. Staging laparotomy is generally not justified in HIV-affected patients. Primary radiation, based on clinical stage, with or without adjuvant chemotherapy is appropriate for early-stage presentations; chemotherapy alone, with or without consolidative radiation, is given in advanced disease. ABVD is a suitable combination regimen but may need to be modified to avoid bleomycin pulmonary toxicity. *Pneumocystis carinii* pneumonia prophylaxis should be instituted routinely. HIV antiviral therapy may be administered during chemotherapy as indicated and tolerated. Whenever possible, these patients should be approached with curative intent. Primary Hodgkin's disease regimens are not so immunosuppressive as to be contraindicated except in unusual circumstances.

TREATMENT RECOMMENDATIONS. After an accurate histologic diagnosis and staging, the following general guidelines may be used in recommending therapy. For clinical stage I and IIA good-risk patients with a low likelihood of abdominal involvement, primary irradiation without staging laparotomy is appropriate. Combined-modality therapy (ABVD plus extended field radiation) is a less acceptable alternative because it exposes patients to the toxicities of both modalities in a low-risk setting.

For clinical stage I and IIA or B, moderate-risk (see earlier) patients in whom the risk for abdominal involvement is greater than 10%, primary irradiation remains an appropriate therapy but requires staging laparotomy to confirm pathologic stage I or II disease. A frequently used alternative is combined modality therapy (ABVD plus involved-field or extended-field radiation), thus obviating the need for laparotomy. For all patients with clinical stage IIIA disease, combined modality therapy or ABVD alone are the acceptable options. Primary irradiation is not indicated in such patients, even when staging laparotomy reveals III₁A disease.

Table 180–4 ■ RECOMMENDED FOLLOW-UP IN TREATED HODGKIN'S DISEASE

1. **End of therapy**
   Repeat all studies initially positive for baseline values. If suspicious, consider biopsy.
2. **0 to 3 years after therapy**
   Visits: Every 3 to 4 months
   Imaging: Chest radiography each visit, unless CT of chest obtained
      CT of chest every 6 months × 2, then yearly
      CT of abdomen and pelvis yearly
   Laboratory: With each visit: Complete blood cell count, platelets, erythrocyte sedimentation rate
            Liver and renal function tests
            Lactate dehydrogenase
      Every 6 months: Thyroid-stimulating hormone
3. **3 to 5 years after therapy**
   Visits: Every 6 months
   Imaging: Chest radiography each visit, unless CT of chest obtained
      CT of chest, abdomen, pelvis yearly
   Laboratory: As in 2
4. **More than 5 years after therapy**
   Visits: Yearly
   Imaging: Chest radiography; CT only as indicated
   Laboratory: As in 2
5. **Other considerations, as indicated**
   Mammography
   Lipid profile
   Pulmonary function studies
   Echocardiography
   Hormone replacement if menopausal

For the bulky early-stage presentations, clinical stage IX or IIX disease, combined-modality therapy is essential. The choice of combination chemotherapy regimen is discussed earlier; usually this is ABVD. After successful induction of complete clinical remission, consolidative radiation should be administered. For advanced-stage disease (IIIB and IV), combination chemotherapy alone (ABVD) or combined with involved- or extended-field radiation is recommended.

Follow-up studies for successfully treated patients are listed in Table 180–4.

Connors JM, Klimo P, Adams G, et al: Treatment of advanced Hodgkin's disease with chemotherapy—comparison of MOPP/ABV hybrid regimen with alternating courses of MOPP and ABVD: A report from the National Cancer Institute of Canada clinical trials group. J Clin Oncol 15:1638, 1997. *A prospective randomized trial demonstrating the value of doxorubicin-containing regimens.*

Hancock SL, Hoppe RT: Long-term complications of treatment and causes of mortality after Hodgkin's disease. Semin Radiat Oncol 6:225, 1996. *An outstanding review of long-term complications and their management.*

Loeffler M, Brosteanu O, Hasenclever D, et al: Meta-analysis of chemotherapy versus combined modality treatment trials in Hodgkin's disease. J Clin Oncol 16:818, 1998. *A meta-analysis of 1740 patients evaluating the role of chemotherapy with or without irradiation.*

Mauch P: What is the role for adjuvant radiation therapy in advanced Hodgkin's disease? J Clin Oncol 16:815, 1998. *Companion editorial to previous article discussing the merits of the meta-analysis.*

Nautiyal J, Weichselbaum RR, Vijayakumar S: Radiation therapy techniques in the treatment of Hodgkin's disease. Semin Radiat Oncol 6:131, 1996. *An excellent review of radiation therapy for Hodgkin's disease.*

Yahalom J: Management of relapsed and refractory Hodgkin's disease. Semin Radiat Oncol 6:210, 1996. *This review of relapse/refractory management discusses in detail autologous stem cell transplantation and the role of radiation therapy in salvage strategies.*

181　PLASMA CELL DISORDERS

Robert A. Kyle

The plasma cell disorders are a group of neoplastic or potentially neoplastic diseases associated with proliferation of a single clone of immunoglobulin-secreting plasma cells derived from the B-cell series of immunocytes. This group of disorders has been referred to as monoclonal gammopathies, immunoglobulinopathies, paraproteinemias, and dysproteinemias.

The plasma cell disorders are characterized by the secretion of electrophoretically and immunologically homogeneous (monoclonal) proteins. Each monoclonal protein (M-protein, myeloma protein, or paraprotein) consists of two heavy (H) polypeptide chains of the same class and subclass and two light (L) polypeptide chains of the same type (see Fig. 270–2). The heavy polypeptide chains are designated by Greek letters: γ in immunoglobulin G (IgG), α in immunoglobulin A (IgA), μ in immunoglobulin M (IgM), δ in immunoglobulin D (IgD), and ϵ in immunoglobulin E (IgE). The subclasses of IgG are IgG1, IgG2, IgG3, and IgG4. There are two subclasses of IgA—IgA1 and IgA2. No subclasses of IgM, IgD, or IgE have been recognized. The light-chain types are kappa (κ) and lambda (λ). Both heavy chains and light chains have "constant" and "variable" regions with respect to amino acid sequence. Class specificity of each immunoglobulin is defined by a series of antigenic determinants on the constant regions of the heavy chains (γ, α, μ, δ, and ϵ) and the two major classes of light chains (κ and λ). The amino acid sequence in the variable regions of the immunoglobulin molecule corresponds to the active antigen-combining site of the antibody, whereas the constant regions convey other biologic properties (see Chapter 270).

RECOGNITION OF MONOCLONAL PROTEINS

High-resolution agarose gel electrophoresis is preferred for the detection of monoclonal proteins (M-proteins). Immunofixation should be used to confirm the presence of an M-protein and to distinguish the immunoglobulin class and its light-chain type.

Note: Mayo Foundation retains copyright to Mayo copyrighted illustrations. Mayo Foundation is "author" for purposes of copyright ownership under the "work made for hire" provision of the copyright law.

Analysis of Serum

Serum protein electrophoresis should be done when multiple myeloma or Waldenström's macroglobulinemia is suspected because of unexplained weakness or fatigue, anemia, back pain, osteoporosis, osteolytic lesions or spontaneous fracture, elevation of the erythrocyte sedimentation rate, hypercalcemia, Bence Jones proteinuria, renal insufficiency, immunoglobulin deficiency, or recurrent infections. It should also be considered in adults with sensorimotor peripheral neuropathy, carpal tunnel syndrome, refractory heart failure, nephrotic syndrome, orthostatic hypotension, or malabsorption, because a spike or localized band is strongly suggestive of primary systemic amyloidosis (AL).

An M-protein is usually seen as a narrow peak (like a church spire) in the densitometer tracing or as a dense, discrete band on agarose gel (Fig. 181–1). Although the immunoglobulins (IgG, IgA, IgM, IgD, and IgE) compose the gamma component, they are also found in the β-γ or β region, and IgG may actually extend to the α_2-globulin area. Consequently, an IgG M-protein may range from the slow gamma (cathode) to the α_2-globulin region. In contrast, an excess of polyclonal immunoglobulins (having one or more heavy-chain types and both κ and λ light chains) produces a broad-based peak or broad band. It is usually limited to the γ region (Fig. 181–2). It is important to differentiate between an M-protein and a polyclonal increase because the former is associated with a malignant process or a potentially neoplastic condition, whereas a polyclonal increase in immunoglobulins is associated with a reactive or inflammatory process. In 3% of sera with a monoclonal peak, there is an additional M-protein of a different immunoglobulin class. This condition is designated as a biclonal (double) gammopathy.

The presence of an M-protein is most suggestive of monoclonal gammopathy of undetermined significance (MGUS), multiple myeloma, primary amyloidosis, Waldenström's macroglobulinemia, or other lymphoproliferative disease (Table 181–1). Rarely, other conditions may also simulate the presence of an M-protein in the serum (e.g., free hemoglobin-haptoglobin complexes resulting from hemolysis, large amounts of transferrin in patients with iron-deficiency anemia, or the presence of fibrinogen). On the other hand, an M-protein may appear as a rather broad band on agarose gel or as a broad peak in the densitometer tracing, owing to the complexing of an M-protein with other plasma components or aggregates of IgG, polymers of IgA, or dimers of IgM.

An M-protein can be present when the total protein concentra-

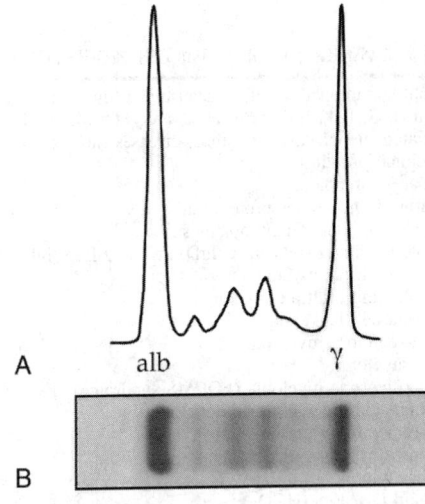

FIGURE 181–1 ■ *A,* Monoclonal pattern of serum protein as traced by densitometer after electrophoresis on agarose gel: tall, narrow-based peak of γ mobility. *B,* Monoclonal pattern from electrophoresis of serum on agarose gel (anode on left): dense, localized band representing monoclonal protein of γ mobility. (From Kyle RA, Katzmann JA: Immunochemical characterization of immunoglobulins. *In* Rose NR, Conway de Macario E, Folds JD, et al [eds]: Manual of Clinical Laboratory Immunology, 5th ed. Washington, DC, ASM Press, 1997, p 156, with permission of the American Society for Microbiology.)

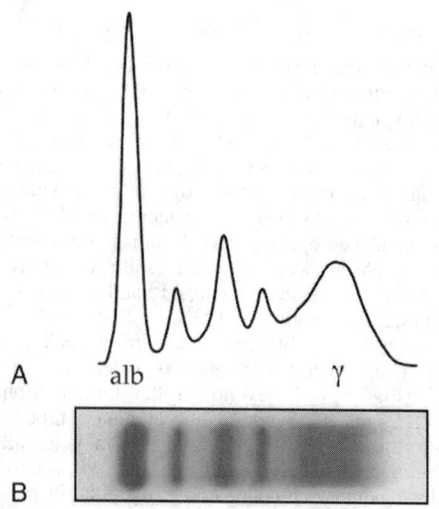

FIGURE 181–2 ■ *A*, Polyclonal pattern from densitometer tracing of agarose gel: broad-based peak of γ mobility. *B*, Polyclonal pattern from electrophoresis of agarose gel (anode on left). Band at right is broad and extends throughout the γ area. (From Kyle RA, Katzmann JA: Immunochemical characterization of immunoglobulins. *In* Rose NR, Conway de Macario E, Folds JD, et al [eds]: Manual of Clinical Laboratory Immunology, 5th ed. Washington, DC, ASM Press, 1997, p 156, with permission of the American Society for Microbiology.)

tion, β- and γ-globulin levels, and quantitative immunoglobulin values are all within normal limits. A small M-protein may be concealed in the normal β or γ areas and may be overlooked. In addition, the presence of a monoclonal light chain (Bence Jones proteinemia) is rarely seen in the agarose gel. In the heavy chain diseases, the M-component is usually not apparent.

Immunofixation, a useful technique for identifying an M-protein, should be performed when a peak or band is seen on protein electrophoresis or when multiple myeloma or related disorders are suspected despite a normal protein electrophoresis. Immunofixation is especially useful when one is searching for a small M-protein in primary amyloidosis, solitary plasmacytoma, or extramedullary plasmacytoma, or after successful treatment of multiple myeloma or macroglobulinemia.

Table 181–1 ■ **CLASSIFICATION OF PLASMA CELL PROLIFERATIVE DISORDERS**

I. Monoclonal Gammopathies of Undetermined Significance (MGUS)
   A. Benign (IgG, IgA, IgD, IgM, and, rarely, free light chains)
   B. Associated neoplasms or other diseases not known to produce monoclonal proteins
   C. Biclonal gammopathies
   D. Idiopathic Bence Jones proteinuria
II. Malignant Monoclonal Gammopathies
   A. Multiple myeloma (IgG, IgA, IgD, IgE, and free light chains)
      1. Overt multiple myeloma
      2. Smoldering multiple myeloma
      3. Plasma cell leukemia
      4. Non-secretory myeloma
      5. IgD myeloma
      6. Osteosclerotic myeloma (POEMS syndrome)
      7. Solitary plasmacytoma of bone
      8. Extramedullary plasmacytoma
   B. Waldenström's macroglobulinemia
      1. Other lymphoproliferative diseases
III. Heavy-Chain Diseases (HCDs)
   A. γ HCD
   B. α HCD
   C. μ HCD
IV. Cryoglobulinemia
V. Primary Amyloidosis (AL)

From Kyle RA: Classification and diagnosis of monoclonal gammopathies. *In* Rose NR, Friedman H, Fahey JL (eds): Manual of Clinical Laboratory Immunology, 3rd ed. Washington, DC, American Society for Microbiology, 1986, p 152.

Quantitation of Immunoglobulins

This procedure is more useful than immunofixation for the detection of hypogammaglobulinemia. Rate nephelometry is the preferred method.

Serum Viscometry

Serum viscometry should be measured when the IgM monoclonal level is more than 4 g/dL, when the IgA or IgG value is more than 5 g/dL, or when the patient has oronasal bleeding, blurred vision, or other symptoms suggestive of a hyperviscosity syndrome.

Analysis of Urine

Dipstick tests are used in many laboratories to screen for protein, but unfortunately they are often insensitive to Bence Jones protein. Consequently, sulfosalicylic acid or Exton's reagent is best for the detection of protein.

Screening tests for Bence Jones proteins (monoclonal light chain in the urine) that use their unique thermal properties are not recommended because of their serious shortcomings. Immunofixation of an adequately concentrated 24-hour urine specimen reliably detects Bence Jones protein. An M-protein appears as a dense, localized band on the agarose gel or a tall, narrow, homogeneous peak in the densitometer tracing, and its amount can be calculated on the basis of the size of the spike and the amount of total protein in the 24-hour specimen. It is not uncommon to have a negative reaction for protein and no obvious spike on electrophoresis and yet for immunofixation of a concentrated urine specimen to show a monoclonal light chain. Immunofixation should also be done on the urine of every adult older than age 40 who develops a nephrotic syndrome of unknown cause. The presence of a monoclonal light chain in nephrotic urine is strongly suggestive of primary amyloidosis or light chain deposition disease.

MONOCLONAL GAMMOPATHY OF UNDETERMINED SIGNIFICANCE

The term *monoclonal gammopathy of undetermined significance* (benign monoclonal gammopathy) denotes the presence of an M-protein in persons without evidence of multiple myeloma, macroglobulinemia, amyloidosis, or other related diseases. The term *benign monoclonal gammopathy* is misleading because at diagnosis it is not known whether the process producing an M-protein will remain stable and benign or will develop into symptomatic multiple myeloma, macroglobulinemia, amyloidosis, or a related disorder. MGUS is characterized by a serum M-protein concentration less than 3 g/dL; fewer than 5% plasma cells in the bone marrow; no or only small amounts of M-protein in the urine; absence of lytic bone lesions, anemia, hypercalcemia, and renal insufficiency; and, most important, the stability of the amount of the M-protein and the failure of other abnormalities to develop.

Incidence

More than 50% of patients with a serum M-protein will have an initial clinical diagnosis of MGUS (Fig. 181–3). The prevalence of MGUS is 1% of patients older than 50 years and 3% of those older than 70 years. Because of this high prevalence, it is crucial to determine whether the M-protein will remain benign or will evolve to multiple myeloma, amyloidosis, macroglobulinemia, or another lymphoproliferative disease.

Prognosis

In one series of 241 patients followed long-term after a diagnosis of benign monoclonal gammopathy (i.e., patients in whom multiple myeloma, macroglobulinemia, amyloidosis, lymphoma, or related diseases were excluded), the median age of the patients was 64 years at the time when the M-protein was recognized. Of note was that about 75% of the patients had other conditions that brought them to medical attention but that were seemingly unrelated to the monoclonal gammopathy. In these patients, the M-protein level ranged from 0.3 to 3.2 g/dL (median, 1.7 g/dL) and consisted of IgG (73%), IgA (11%), and IgM (14%) or was biclonal (2%). An M-protein was found in the urine in only 9 patients, and bone marrow plasma cells ranged from 1 to 10% (median, 3.0%). Anemia,

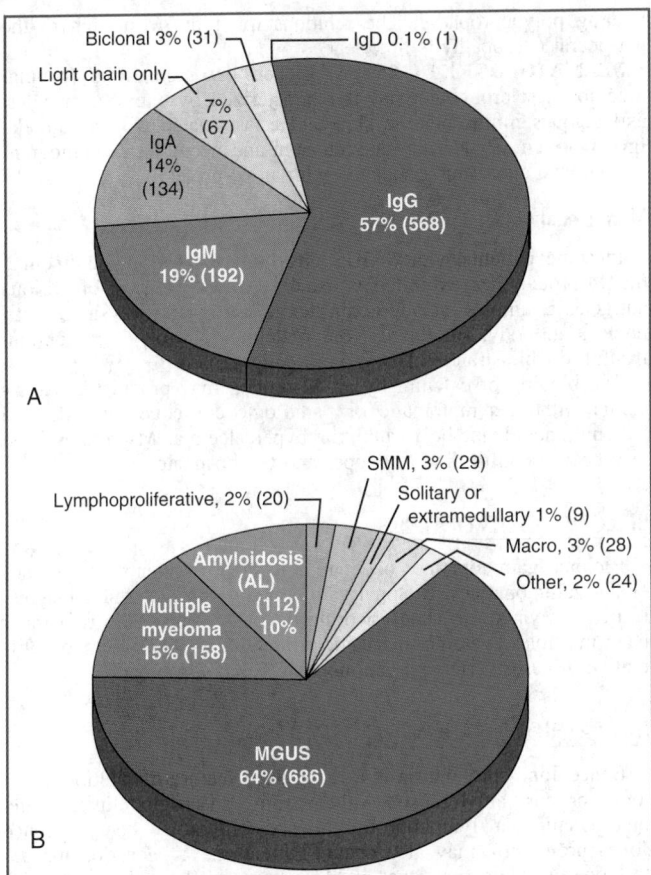

A

B

FIGURE 181-3 ■ A, Distribution of serum monoclonal proteins in 993 patients seen at the Mayo Clinic during 1996. B, Diagnoses in 1066 cases of monoclonal gammopathy seen at the Mayo Clinic during 1996. CLL = chronic lymphocytic leu-kemia; Macro = macroglobulinemia; MGUS = monoclonal gammopathy of undetermined significance; SMM = smoldering multiple myeloma. (From Kyle RA: Multiple myeloma, macroglobulinemia, and the monoclonal gammopathies. *In* Duffy T [ed]: Current Practice of Medicine, 2nd ed. Philadelphia, Current Science, in press, with permission of the publisher.)

leukopenia, leukocytosis, thrombocytopenia, renal insufficiency, and hypercalcemia, when present, were unrelated to the M-protein.

At follow-up, 24 to 38 years later, the 241 patients could be divided into four groups. Approximately one tenth of the patients have remained stable and could be classified as having benign monoclonal gammopathy, although they must continue to be observed because serious disease may still develop. No initial laboratory measurements or clinical factors were predictive of which patients would remain in this stable or benign group. In 11% of the patients, the M-protein level increased to more than 3 g/dL, but they did not develop symptomatic multiple myeloma, macroglobulinemia, or related disorders; their condition remained clinically "benign," although with an M-protein level that causes concern. More than half of the patients died of seemingly unrelated causes without developing multiple myeloma, macroglobulinemia, or related disorders. Approximately one fourth of the patients (26%) developed multiple myeloma (18%), macroglobulinemia (3%), amyloidosis (3%), or related disorders (2%), with an actuarial rate of 16% at 10 years, 33% at 20 years, and 40% at 25 years (Fig. 181–4). The interval from the time of recognition of the M-protein to the diagnosis of serious disease ranged from 2 to 29 years (median, 10 years). In seven patients, multiple myeloma was diagnosed more than 20 years after detection of the serum M-protein.

Differentiation of MGUS from Multiple Myeloma and Macroglobulinemia

Differentiation of the patient with benign monoclonal gammopathy from one in whom multiple myeloma, macroglobulinemia, or a related disorder eventually develops is very difficult when the M-protein is first recognized. The size of the M-protein is of some help—levels greater than 3 g/dL usually indicate overt multiple myeloma or macroglobulinemia, but some exceptions, such as smoldering multiple myeloma (SMM), exist. Levels of the immunoglobulin classes other than the M-protein (i.e., the normal polyclonal or background immunoglobulins) are almost always reduced in multiple myeloma or Waldenström's macroglobulinemia, but a reduction may also occur in benign monoclonal gammopathy. The association of a monoclonal light chain (Bence Jones proteinuria) with a serum monoclonal gammopathy suggests multiple myeloma or macroglobulinemia, but many patients with small amounts of monoclonal light chain in the urine have stable M-protein levels in the serum for many years. The presence of more than 10% plasma cells in the bone marrow suggests multiple myeloma, but some patients with more plasma cells have remained stable for long periods. The presence of osteolytic lesions strongly suggests multiple myeloma, but metastatic carcinoma may produce lytic lesions

FIGURE 181-4 ■ Incidence of multiple myeloma, macroglobulinemia, amyloidosis, or lymphoproliferative disease after recognition of monoclonal protein. (From Kyle RA: Multiple myeloma, macroglobulinemia, and the monoclonal gammopathies. *In* Duffy T [ed]: Current Practice of Medicine, 2nd ed. Philadelphia, Current Science, in press, with permission of the publisher.)

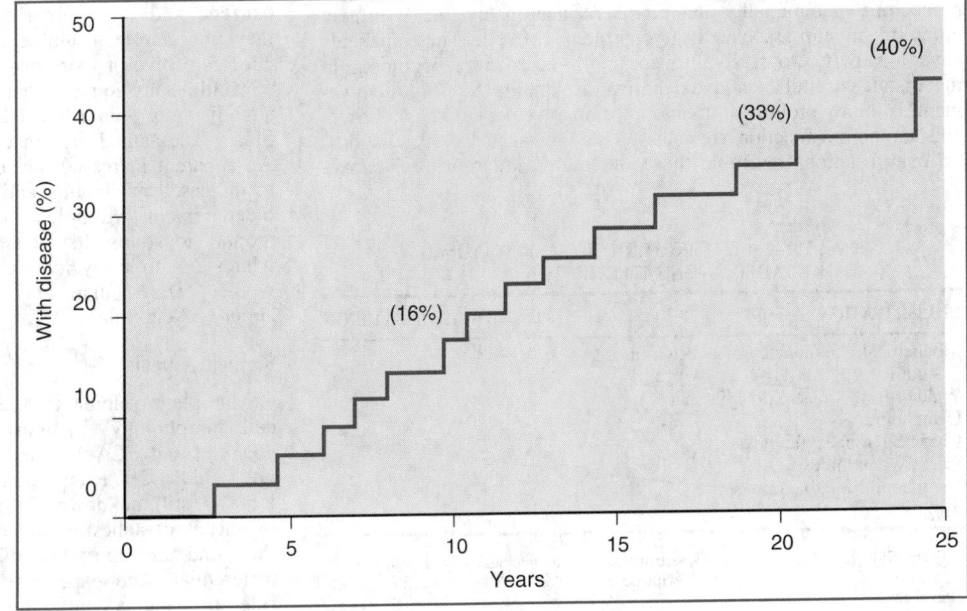

as well as plasmacytosis and may be associated with an unrelated monoclonal gammopathy.

Certain procedures show promise in differentiating the patient with MGUS or SMM from the patient with multiple myeloma. The plasma cell labeling index measures the synthesis of DNA; when elevated, it is good evidence that the patient has multiple myeloma or will soon have symptomatic disease. The presence of circulating plasma cells in the peripheral blood usually indicates active multiple myeloma.

However, no single technique reliably differentiates a patient with a benign monoclonal gammopathy from one who will subsequently have symptomatic multiple myeloma or other malignant disease. The M-protein level in the serum and urine should be serially measured, together with periodic re-evaluation of clinical and other laboratory features, to determine whether multiple myeloma or another related disorder is present. In general, if the serum M-protein is less than 2.0 g/dL, electrophoresis should be repeated at 6 months; if it is stable, it should be checked annually. If the serum M-protein is 2.0 g/dL or more without evidence of myeloma or related disorders, electrophoresis should be repeated in 3 months; if it is stable, the test should be repeated annually. If an M-protein is present in the urine, the patient should be followed more closely by repeating serum and urine protein levels at 6-month intervals rather than annually.

Association of Monoclonal Gammopathies with Other Diseases

Monoclonal gammopathy frequently exists without other abnormalities. However, certain diseases are associated with it more often than expected by chance.

LYMPHOPROLIFERATIVE DISORDERS. An M-protein is found in 3 to 4% of patients with a diffuse lymphoproliferative process but in fewer than 1% of those with a nodular lymphoma. IgM monoclonal gammopathies are more common than IgG or IgA in lymphoproliferative diseases.

In a large series of patients in whom a serum IgM monoclonal gammopathy was identified, more than half were originally considered to have MGUS (Table 181–2). During follow-up, 17% of patients with MGUS of the IgM class developed a malignant lymphoid disease, most frequently Waldenström's macroglobulinemia.

LEUKEMIA. M-proteins occur in the sera of some patients with chronic lymphocytic leukemia but with no recognizable effect on the clinical course. M-proteins have also been recognized in hairy cell, adult T cell, chronic myelogenous, acute promyelocytic, and acute myelomonocytic leukemias, but without a documented increased prevalence over that in the normal population. M-proteins may also be found after liver, bone marrow, or kidney transplantation.

NEUROLOGIC DISORDERS. Approximately 5% of patients with sensorimotor peripheral neuropathy of unknown cause have an associated monoclonal gammopathy. In half of those with an IgM monoclonal gammopathy and peripheral neuropathy, the M-protein binds to myelin-associated glycoprotein (MAG). These patients have a slowly progressive sensorimotor neuropathy beginning in the distal extremities and extending proximally. Sensory involvement is more prominent than motor involvement. Cranial nerves and autonomic function are intact. The clinical and electrodiagnostic manifestations resemble those of chronic inflammatory demyelinating polyneuropathy. The relationship of the M-protein to the peripheral neuropathy is not clear.

DERMATOLOGIC DISEASES. Lichen myxedematosus (papular mucinosis, scleromyxedema) is characterized by papules, macules, and plaques infiltrating the skin and is associated with a cathodal IgG λ protein. Pyoderma gangrenosum and necrobiotic xanthogranuloma have also been associated with an M-protein.

Monoclonal Gammopathies with Antibody Activity

In some patients with MGUS, myeloma, or macroglobulinemia, the M-protein has exhibited unusual specificity to one of various antigens. Examples include actin, dextran, anti–streptolysin O, antinuclear antibody, riboflavin, von Willebrand factor, thyroglobulin, insulin, double-stranded DNA, and apolipoprotein.

The binding of calcium by an M-protein may produce hypercalcemia without symptomatic or pathologic consequences. Affected patients should not be treated for hypercalcemia. M-proteins have also been found to bind to copper and to phosphate.

BICLONAL GAMMOPATHIES

Biclonal gammopathies occur in 2 to 3% of patients with monoclonal gammopathies. Biclonal gammopathy of undetermined significance accounts for about two thirds of patients. The remainder have multiple myeloma, macroglobulinemia, or other lymphoproliferative diseases. Triclonal gammopathies may also occur.

IDIOPATHIC BENCE JONES PROTEINURIA

Bence Jones proteinuria is a recognized feature of multiple myeloma, primary amyloidosis, Waldenström's macroglobulinemia, and other malignant lymphoproliferative disorders. A benign Bence Jones proteinuria may also occur. Patients have been documented to have a stable serum level of M-protein and Bence Jones proteinuria for more than 15 years without developing multiple myeloma or related disorders.

MULTIPLE MYELOMA

Multiple myeloma (myelomatosis, plasma cell myeloma, or Kahler's disease) is characterized by the neoplastic proliferation of a single clone of plasma cells engaged in the production of a monoclonal immunoglobulin. This clone of plasma cells proliferates in the bone marrow and frequently invades the adjacent bone, producing extensive skeletal destruction that results in bone pain and fractures. Anemia, hypercalcemia, and renal insufficiency are other important features.

Etiology and Epidemiology

The cause of multiple myeloma is unclear. Exposure to radiation, benzene and other organic solvents, herbicides, and insecticides may play a role. Multiple myeloma has been reported in familial clusters of two or more first-degree relatives and in identical twins.

Multiple myeloma accounts for 1% of all malignant disease and slightly more than 10% of hematologic malignancies in the United States. The annual incidence of multiple myeloma is 4 per 100,000. An apparent increased incidence in recent years is probably related to increased availability and use of medical facilities, especially in older persons. Multiple myeloma occurs in all races and all geographic locations. Its incidence in blacks is almost twice that in whites. Multiple myeloma is slightly more common in men than in women. The median age of patients at the time of diagnosis is about 65 years; only 2% of patients are younger than 40.

Biologic Aspects

Multiple myeloma is a B-cell malignancy with mature plasma cell morphology. In most cases, the plasma cells are CIg+, CD38+, and PCA-1+, and only a minority express CD10, HLA-DR, and CD20. However, the nature of clonogenic cells in myeloma is still unknown. Circulating clonogenic pre-myeloma cells, by means of adhesion molecules, may home to the marrow, where they find an appropriate microenvironment (cytokine network) to differentiate and expand further. T cells may play an important role. In patients with multiple myeloma, CD4 T cells are often

Table 181–2 ■ CLASSIFICATION OF IgM MONOCLONAL GAMMOPATHIES AMONG 430 PATIENTS

CLASSIFICATION	PERCENTAGE OF PATIENTS
Monoclonal gammopathy of undetermined significance	56
Waldenström's macroglobulinemia	17
Lymphoma	7
Chronic lymphocytic leukemia	5
Primary amyloidosis (AL)	1
Lymphoproliferative disease	14
Total	100

From Kyle RA, Garton JP: The spectrum of IgM monoclonal gammopathy in 430 cases. Mayo Clin Proc 62:719, 1987, with permission of the Mayo Foundation, Rochester, MN.

reduced. Interleukin-6 (IL-6) is an important growth factor for myeloma cells. Elevated levels of IL-6 have been found in patients with progressive myeloma, in contrast to those with MGUS.

Increased expression of c-*myc*, H-*ras*, and *bcl*-2 has been found in myeloma. *Ras* mutations as well as point mutations of the tumor suppressor gene *p53* have been seen. Thus, c-*myc*, H-*ras*, and *p53* genes may be involved in the pathogenesis of myeloma.

Cytogenetic Abnormalities

Flow cytometry studies have shown aneuploidy in about 80% of patients, hyperdiploidy in 70%, and hypodiploidy in the remaining 10%. Fluorescence in situ hybridization (FISH) using chromosome-specific probes reveals chromosome abnormalities in over 80% of patients with multiple myeloma. Structural changes of chromosomes 1, 11, and 14, monosomies and trisomies, and translocations have been detected, but no specific abnormality has been demonstrated.

Clinical Manifestations

SYMPTOMS (Table 181–3). Bone pain, particularly in the back or chest and less often in the extremities, is present at the time of diagnosis in more than two thirds of patients. The pain is usually induced by movement and does not occur at night except with change of position. The patient's height may be reduced by several inches because of vertebral collapse. Weakness and fatigue are common and often are associated with anemia. Fever is rare and, when present, is usually from an infection. The major symptoms may result from an acute infection, renal insufficiency, hypercalcemia, or amyloidosis.

PHYSICAL FINDINGS. Pallor is the most frequent physical finding. The liver is palpable in about 20% of patients and the spleen in 5%. Occasionally, extramedullary plasmacytomas may appear.

Laboratory Findings

A normocytic, normochromic anemia is present initially in two thirds of patients but eventually occurs in nearly every patient with multiple myeloma. The serum protein electrophoretic pattern shows a peak or localized band in 80% of patients, hypogammaglobulinemia in almost 10%, and no apparent abnormality in the remainder. IgG M-protein is found in 53%, IgA in 20%, light chain only (Bence Jones proteinemia) in 17%, IgD in 2%, and biclonal gammopathy in 1%, and 7% have no serum M-protein at diagnosis.

Immunofixation of the urine reveals an M-protein in approximately 75% of patients. The κ/λ ratio is 2:1. Ninety-eight per cent of patients with multiple myeloma have an M-protein in the serum or urine at the time of diagnosis.

In the bone marrow of patients with multiple myeloma, plasma cells usually account for 10% or more of all nucleated cells, but they may range from less than 5% to almost 100% (Fig. 181–5; Color Plate 6*J*). Bone marrow involvement may be focal rather than diffuse, requiring repeated bone marrow examinations for diagnosis. Identification of a monoclonal immunoglobulin in the cytoplasm of plasma cells by immunoperoxidase staining is helpful for differentiating monoclonal plasma cell proliferation in multiple myeloma from reactive plasmacytosis due to connective tissue disease, metastatic carcinoma, liver disease, and infections. The immunoperoxidase technique is also useful in recognizing neoplastic plasma cells that have atypical features.

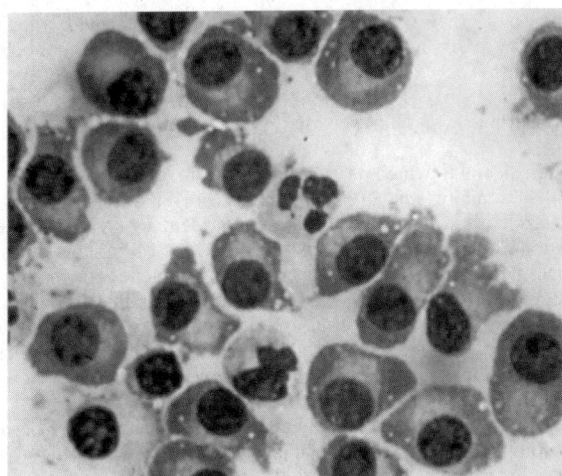

FIGURE 181–5 ■ Bone marrow aspirate containing increased numbers of abnormal plasma cells.

Radiologic Findings

Conventional radiographs reveal abnormalities consisting of punched-out lytic lesions (Fig. 181–6), osteoporosis, or fractures in 75% of patients. The vertebrae, skull, thoracic cage, pelvis, and proximal humeri and femora are the most frequent sites of involvement. Technetium-99m bone scanning is inferior to conventional radiography and should not be used. Computed tomography (CT) or magnetic resonance imaging (MRI) is helpful in patients who have skeletal pain but no abnormality on radiographs.

Diagnostic Criteria

Minimal criteria for the diagnosis of multiple myeloma are a bone marrow containing more than 10% plasma cells or a plasmacytoma plus at least one of the following: (1) M-protein in the serum (usually greater than 3 g/dL), (2) M-protein in the urine, and (3) lytic bone lesions. These findings must not be from metastatic carcinoma, connective tissue diseases, chronic infection, or lymphoma. Patients with multiple myeloma must be differentiated from those with MGUS and smoldering multiple myeloma.

Organ Involvement

RENAL. Bence Jones proteinuria detected by immunofixation is present in 75%. The serum creatinine value is increased initially in almost half of patients and is 2 mg/dL or more in one fourth.

The two major causes of renal insufficiency are "myeloma kidney" and hypercalcemia. Myeloma kidney is characterized by the

---

Table 181–3 ■ CLINICAL MANIFESTATIONS OF MULTIPLE MYELOMA

Skeletal involvement: pain, reduced height, pathologic fractures, hypercalcemia
Anemia: due mainly to decreased erythropoiesis; produces weakness and fatigue
Renal insufficiency: mainly due to "myeloma kidney" from light chains or hypercalcemia; rarely from amyloidosis
Recurrent infections: respiratory and urinary tract infections or septicemia due to gram-positive or gram-negative organisms
Bleeding diathesis: from thrombocytopenia or coating of platelets with M-protein
Amyloidosis: develops in 10 to 15%
Extramedullary plasmacytomas: occur late in the disease
Cryoglobulinemia type I: rarely symptomatic

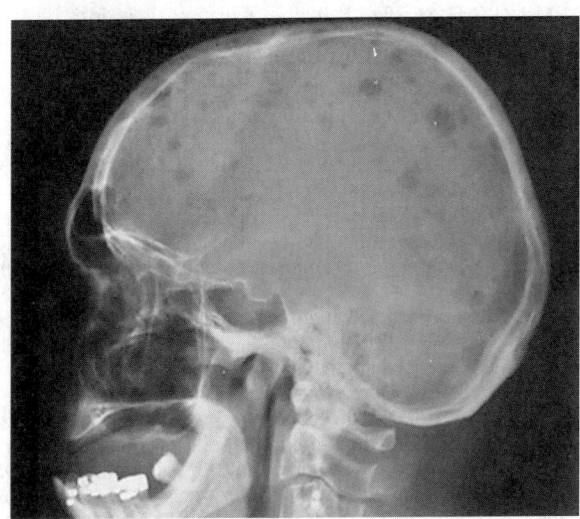

FIGURE 181–6 ■ Skull roentgenogram showing multiple lytic lesions.

presence of large waxy laminated casts in the distal and collecting tubules. The casts are composed mainly of precipitated monoclonal light chains. The extent of cast formation correlates directly with the amount of free urinary light chain and with the severity of renal insufficiency. With dehydration, acute renal failure may occur.

Hypercalcemia, which is present in 15 to 20% of patients initially, is a major and treatable cause of renal insufficiency. It results from destruction of bone. Hyperuricemia may contribute to renal failure. Amyloidosis occurs in 10 to 15% of patients and may produce nephrotic syndrome or renal insufficiency or both. Acquired Fanconi's syndrome, characterized by proximal tubular dysfunction, results in glycosuria, phosphaturia, and aminoaciduria. Deposition of monoclonal light chains in the renal glomerulus (light-chain deposition disease) may produce renal insufficiency and the nephrotic syndrome.

NEUROLOGIC. Radiculopathy, the single most frequent neurologic complication, is usually in the thoracic or lumbosacral area and results from compression of the nerve by the vertebral lesion or by the collapsed bone itself. Compression of the spinal cord occurs in up to 10% of patients. Peripheral neuropathy is uncommon in multiple myeloma and, when present, is usually caused by amyloidosis. Rarely, myeloma cells diffusely infiltrate the meninges. Intracranial plasmacytomas almost always represent extensions of myelomatous lesions of the skull.

Other Systemic Involvement

Hepatomegaly from plasma cell infiltration is uncommon. Ascites is rare. Plasmacytomas of the ribs are common and present either as expanding bone lesions or as soft tissue masses. The incidence of infections is increased in multiple myeloma. *Streptococcus pneumoniae* and *Staphylococcus aureus* organisms have been the most frequent pathogens, but gram-negative organisms now account for more than half of all infections. Propensity to infection results from impairment of antibody response, deficiency of normal immunoglobulins, and neutropenia. Bleeding from coating of the platelets by the M-protein may occur. Occasionally, a tendency to thrombosis is present.

Treatment

Not all patients who fulfill the minimal criteria for the diagnosis of multiple myeloma should be treated. Patients with MGUS or SMM should not be treated. The patient's symptoms, physical findings, and all laboratory data must be considered. An increasing level of the M-protein in the serum or urine suggests that therapy will be needed in the near future. Indications for therapy include the development of significant anemia, hypercalcemia, or renal insufficiency; the occurrence of lytic bone lesions; and the finding of extramedullary plasmacytomas. If there is doubt in the physician's mind, it is usually better to withhold therapy and to re-evaluate the patient in 2 or 3 months.

RADIATION THERAPY. Palliative radiation in a dose of 20 to 30 Gy should be limited to patients who have multiple myeloma with disabling pain and a well-defined focal process that has not responded to chemotherapy. Analgesics in combination with chemotherapy usually can control the pain.

AUTOLOGOUS STEM CELL TRANSPLANTATION. If the patient is younger than 70 years, the physician should discuss the possibility of autologous peripheral blood stem cell transplantation (see Chapter 182), ideally as part of a prospective study. Peripheral blood stem cells are preferable to bone marrow transplantation because engraftment is more rapid and there is less contamination of the infused cells with tumor cells. Most investigators prefer vincristine, doxorubicin (Adriamycin), and dexamethasone, the VAD regimen, as the initial therapy because these drugs do not damage hematopoietic stem cells. The patient is treated initially with VAD or a similar program for 3 to 4 months to reduce the number of tumor cells in the bone marrow and peripheral blood. The patient is then given high-dose cyclophosphamide followed by granulocyte colony-stimulating factor, and the peripheral stem cells are collected. One can proceed with the transplantation, in which the patient is given high-dose melphalan and total-body irradiation or a similar preparative regimen followed by infusion of the periph-

eral blood stem cells. The alternative is to treat the patient with alkylating agents until a plateau state is reached and then maintain the patient with α_2-interferon or no therapy until early relapse. At that point, the patient is given high-dose melphalan and total-body irradiation, and the previously collected peripheral blood stem cells are infused.

In a randomized prospective study comparing autologous bone marrow transplantation with conventional chemotherapy, the median survival was longer with transplantation than with chemotherapy. In a study of 496 patients enrolled in a non-randomized transplant program, complete response was obtained in 36% of patients, and the transplant-related mortality rate was 7%. The median duration of survival from the time of the first transplantation was 41 months.

Autologous peripheral stem cell or bone marrow transplantation is applicable for up to 50% of patients with multiple myeloma. However, two major problems exist: (1) the multiple myeloma is not eradicated even with large doses of chemotherapy and total-body irradiation, and (2) infused peripheral blood stem cells or bone marrow cells are usually contaminated by myeloma cells or their precursors and may contribute to relapse.

The complete remission rate is higher with high-dose chemotherapy, but the duration of response is relatively short, ranging from 1 to 3 years. Few, if any, patients are cured. Autologous transplantation should not be performed if the patient has received long-term chemotherapy and has refractory multiple myeloma. Purging of tumor cells or collection of CD34+ cells is of potential value. However, delayed engraftment may occur with stem cell selection because stem cells may be lost during collection.

ALLOGENEIC BONE MARROW TRANSPLANTATION. Ninety to 95 per cent of patients with multiple myeloma cannot have an allogeneic bone marrow transplantation because of their age, lack of an HLA-matched sibling donor, and inadequate renal, pulmonary, or cardiac function. Allogeneic transplantation has the advantage that the graft does not contain tumor cells, and it can produce a graft-versus-myeloma effect. Unfortunately, the mortality rate from the procedure is approximately 25% within the first 3 months and approaches 40% overall. Although complete response occurs in 40% of patients, most will relapse; and in long-term follow-up there is no apparent survival plateau. The use of T cell–depleted peripheral blood stem cells decreases the incidence of graft-versus-host disease and reduces transplant-related mortality. Donor lymphocyte infusions have produced significant benefit in up to one half of patients after allogeneic transplantation.

CHEMOTHERAPY. Chemotherapy is the preferred initial treatment for overt, symptomatic multiple myeloma in patients older than 70 years or in younger patients in whom transplantation is not feasible. The oral administration of melphalan and prednisone produces objective response in 50 to 60% of patients. Melphalan can be given daily in a dosage of 0.15 mg/kg for 7 days (8–10 mg/day), with 20 mg of prednisone three times daily for the same 7 days. The melphalan must be given while the patient is fasting, because food reduces absorption. Leukocyte and platelet levels should be determined every 3 weeks after beginning each cycle of therapy, and the melphalan and prednisone treatment should be repeated every 6 weeks. The dosage of melphalan must be adjusted until mid-cycle cytopenia occurs. Unless the disease progresses rapidly, at least three courses of melphalan and prednisone should be given before therapy is discontinued. Because the natural course of multiple myeloma is to progress, alleviation of pain and stabilization of disease usually indicate some therapeutic benefit. An objective improvement may not be achieved for 6 to 12 months or longer in some patients. Because of the obvious shortcomings of melphalan and prednisone, various combinations of therapeutic agents have been tried. Generally, objective responses are higher, but no differences in survival have been reported in most studies.

Chemotherapy should be continued for at least 1 year or until the patient is in a plateau state. At that point, interferon-α_2 may be given; it prolongs the duration of the plateau state but does not generally produce significant survival benefit. If relapse occurs while in the plateau state, the initial chemotherapeutic regimen should be reinstituted. Most patients will respond, but the duration and quality of response are usually inferior to those of the initial response.

Refractory Multiple Myeloma

Almost all patients with multiple myeloma will eventually relapse. The highest response rates for patients resistant to alkylating agents have been with the VAD regimen. Dexamethasone is administered in a dosage of 40 mg/day on days 1–4, 9–12, and 17–20. The cycles are repeated every 28 days. Dexamethasone is usually given only on days 1–4 in even-numbered cycles because of toxicity. Most of the VAD activity is from the corticosteroid effects of dexamethasone. Methylprednisolone, 2 g three times weekly intravenously for a minimum of 4 weeks, is helpful for patients with pancytopenia and may have fewer side effects than from dexamethasone. If there is a response, methylprednisolone is reduced to once or twice weekly.

VBAP (vincristine, carmustine [BCNU], and doxorubicin [Adriamycin]) on day 1 and prednisone daily for 5 days every 3 to 4 weeks benefits 30% of patients. It is well tolerated. If the patient's leukocyte and platelet levels are satisfactory, cyclophosphamide, 600 mg/m²/day intravenously for 4 days (days 1–4), plus prednisone, 50 mg twice a day for the same 4-day period, followed by granulocyte colony-stimulating factor, has been helpful in patients with refractory advanced disease. The use of interferon as a single agent for these patients has been disappointing.

The reversal of resistance to chemotherapeutic agents is an important area of research. The use of verapamil or quinine to reverse the resistance to doxorubicin has been disappointing. PSC-833, an analogue of cyclosporin A, is being investigated in an effort to reduce multidrug resistance to *Vinca* alkaloids and anthracyclines.

Management of Complications

HYPERCALCEMIA. Hypercalcemia, present in 15 to 20% of patients at diagnosis, should be suspected in the presence of anorexia, nausea, vomiting, polyuria, polydipsia, increased constipation, weakness, confusion, or stupor. If hypercalcemia is untreated, renal insufficiency may develop. Hydration, preferably with isotonic saline plus prednisone (25 mg four times per day), relieves the hypercalcemia in most cases. The dosage of prednisone must be reduced and its use discontinued as soon as possible. If these measures fail, bisphosphonates such as pamidronate disodium or etidronate disodium are beneficial. Patients with myeloma should be encouraged to be as active as possible because prolonged bed rest contributes to hypercalcemia.

RENAL INSUFFICIENCY. This complication occurs in half of patients with multiple myeloma and may develop insidiously or rapidly (acute renal failure). Hydration and prednisone are necessary if there is accompanying hypercalcemia. Furosemide is helpful for maintaining a high urine flow rate (100 mL/hr). Hemodialysis is necessary in the event of symptomatic azotemia. Plasmapheresis may be helpful for regaining renal function, but patients with severe myeloma cast formation or other irreversible changes are unlikely to benefit from plasmapheresis. Allopurinol is necessary if hyperuricemia is present. Renal transplantation for myeloma kidney has been followed by prolonged survival. Maintenance of a high urine output (3 L/day) is important for preventing renal failure in patients with Bence Jones proteinuria.

INFECTION. Prompt, appropriate therapy for bacterial infections is necessary. Prophylactic penicillin often benefits patients with recurrent gram-positive infections. Intravenously administered γ-globulin is helpful but expensive. Pneumococcal and influenza immunizations should be given to all patients.

SKELETAL LESIONS. Patients should be encouraged to be as active as possible but to avoid trauma. Fixation of fractures or impending fractures of long bones with an intramedullary rod and methyl methacrylate has produced good results. Patients in a prospective study receiving 90 mg of pamidronate every 4 weeks had fewer skeletal complications and improved quality of life; this medication is recommended for myeloma patients with skeletal involvement.

MISCELLANEOUS COMPLICATIONS. Symptomatic hyperviscosity should be treated with plasmapheresis. Hyperviscosity is usually manifested by oronasal bleeding, blurred vision, or heart failure. Serum viscosity levels do not correlate well with the symptoms or clinical findings. Plasmapheresis promptly relieves the symptoms and should be done regardless of the viscosity level, if the patient is symptomatic. Anemia during the plateau state often responds to erythropoietin.

Spinal cord compression from an extramedullary plasmacytoma should be suspected in patients with severe back pain, the development of weakness or paresthesias of the lower extremities, or bladder or bowel dysfunction. MRI, CT, or myelography must be done immediately. Dexamethasone and radiation therapy are usually helpful. If the neurologic deficit increases, surgical decompression is necessary.

Prognosis

Multiple myeloma has a progressive course, and the median survival is approximately 3 years. The bone marrow plasma cell labeling index and β₂-microglobulin level are the most important prognostic factors in previously untreated multiple myeloma. Cytogenetics contribute important and independent prognostic information: partial or complete deletion of chromosome 13, chromosome 11q abnormalities, and the presence of any translocation are predictors of a poor outcome. The level of C-reactive protein correlates with the serum IL-6 level and is a useful prognostic factor. An increased lactase dehydrogenase level is a predictor of poor prognosis. Advanced age, plasmablastic morphology, circulating myeloma cells in the peripheral blood, increased myeloma colony growth, and increased levels of IL-6 are all associated with more aggressive disease. Patients who respond rapidly to chemotherapy and who have an increased plasma cell labeling index have a shorter remission and survival. Twenty to 30 per cent of patients survive 5 or more years, but fewer than 5% survive longer than 10 years. In some patients, an acute or aggressive terminal phase is characterized by rapid tumor growth, pancytopenia, soft tissue subcutaneous masses, decreased M-protein levels, and fever; the survival in this subset is usually only a few months.

VARIANT FORMS OF MULTIPLE MYELOMA (See Table 181–1)

Smoldering Multiple Myeloma

The diagnosis of SMM depends on the presence of an M-protein level of more than 3 g/dL in the serum and more than 10% plasma cells in the bone marrow, but no anemia, renal insufficiency, or skeletal lesions. Often, a small amount of M-protein is found in the urine and the concentration of normal immunoglobulins in the serum is decreased. The plasma cell labeling index is low. Biologically, patients with SMM have a benign monoclonal gammopathy (MGUS), but it is difficult to accept that diagnosis initially when the M-protein level is greater than 3 g/dL and the bone marrow contains more than 10% plasma cells. These patients must be observed over time because symptomatic multiple myeloma develops in many of them. However, SMM should be recognized because patients must not be treated unless progression occurs.

Plasma Cell Leukemia

Patients with plasma cell leukemia have greater than 20% plasma cells in the peripheral blood and an absolute plasma cell count of at least 2000/μL. Plasma cell leukemia is classified as primary when it is diagnosed in the leukemic phase (60%) or as secondary when there is leukemic transformation of a previously recognized multiple myeloma (40%). Patients with primary plasma cell leukemia are younger and have a greater incidence of hepatosplenomegaly and lymphadenopathy, a higher platelet count, fewer bone lesions, a smaller serum M-protein component, and a longer survival (median, 6.8 vs. 1.3 months) than patients with secondary plasma cell leukemia. Treatment of plasma cell leukemia is unsatisfactory, but partial responses occur with melphalan and prednisone or with a combination of alkylating agents. Autologous stem cell transplantation after myeloablative therapy is beneficial for some patients. Secondary plasma cell leukemia rarely responds to chemotherapy because the patients have already received chemotherapy and are resistant.

Non-Secretory Myeloma

Patients with non-secretory myeloma have no M-protein in either the serum or the urine and account for only 1 to 2% of those with myeloma. For certainty of diagnosis, an M-protein must be identified in the plasma cells by immunoperoxidase or immunofluorescence methods. More than a dozen patients in whom no M-protein could be found within the myeloma cell have been described. Response to therapy and survival rate of patients with non-secretory myeloma are similar to those in patients with a serum or urinary M-component, but renal involvement is less.

IgD Myeloma

The M-protein is smaller than in IgG and IgA myelomas, and Bence Jones proteinuria of the λ-type is more common. Amyloidosis and extramedullary plasmacytomas are more frequent with IgD myeloma. Survival is generally believed to be shorter than with other myeloma types, but IgD myeloma is often not diagnosed until later in its course.

Osteosclerotic Myeloma (POEMS Syndrome)

This syndrome is characterized by *p*olyneuropathy, *o*rganomegaly, *e*ndocrinopathy, *M*-protein, and *s*kin changes (POEMS). The major clinical features are a chronic inflammatory-demyelinating polyneuropathy with predominantly motor disability and sclerotic skeletal lesions. Except for the presence of papilledema, the cranial nerves are not involved. The autonomic nervous system is intact. Hepatomegaly occurs in almost one half of patients, but splenomegaly and lymphadenopathy occur in a minority. Hyperpigmentation and hypertrichosis are usually evident. Gynecomastia and atrophic testes as well as clubbing of the fingers and toes may be seen. In contrast to multiple myeloma, the hemoglobin level is usually normal or elevated and thrombocytosis is common. The bone marrow usually contains fewer than 5% plasma cells, and hypercalcemia and renal insufficiency rarely occur. Most patients have a λ protein. Evidence of Castleman's disease may be found. Diagnosis is confirmed by the identification of monoclonal plasma cells obtained at biopsy of an osteosclerotic lesion.

If the lesions are in a limited area, radiation therapy will produce substantial improvement of the neuropathy in more than half of the patients. If the patient has widespread osteosclerotic lesions, chemotherapy with melphalan and prednisone may be helpful.

Solitary Plasmacytoma (Solitary Myeloma) of Bone

Diagnosis of this disease is based on histologic evidence of a tumor consisting of monoclonal plasma cells identical to those seen in multiple myeloma. In addition, complete skeletal radiographs must show no other lesions of myeloma, the bone marrow aspirate must contain no evidence of multiple myeloma, immunofixation of the serum and concentrated urine should show no M-protein. Exceptions to the last-mentioned criterion occur, but therapy for the solitary lesion usually results in the disappearance of the M-protein. Almost 50% of patients with solitary plasmacytoma are alive at 10 years, and disease-free survival at 10 years ranges from 15 to 25%. Treatment consists of radiation in the range of 40 to 50 Gy. There is no evidence that chemotherapy affects the incidence of conversion to multiple myeloma. Progression usually occurs within 3 to 4 years, but the most uncertain criterion for diagnosis is the duration of observation necessary before deciding that the disease will not become generalized.

Extramedullary Plasmacytoma

Extramedullary plasmacytoma is a plasma cell tumor that arises outside the bone marrow. The tumor is found in the upper respiratory tract in approximately 80% of cases, especially in the nasal cavity and sinuses, nasopharynx, and larynx. Extramedullary plasmacytomas may also occur in the gastrointestinal tract, central nervous system, urinary bladder, thyroid, breast, testes, parotid gland, or lymph nodes. The diagnosis is based on the finding of a plasma cell tumor in an extramedullary site and the absence of multiple myeloma on bone marrow examination, radiography, and appropriate studies of blood and urine. Treatment consists of tumoricidal irradiation. The plasmacytoma may occur locally, metastasize to regional nodes, or, rarely, develop into multiple myeloma.

WALDENSTRÖM'S MACROGLOBULINEMIA (PRIMARY MACROGLOBULINEMIA)

Macroglobulinemia is the result of an uncontrolled proliferation of lymphocytes and plasma cells in which a large IgM M-protein is produced. The cause is unknown, but it occurs more frequently in certain families. The median age of patients at the time of diagnosis is about 65 years, and about 60% are male.

Clinical Presentations

Weakness, fatigue, and bleeding (especially oozing from the oronasal area) are common presenting symptoms. Blurred or impaired vision, dyspnea, loss of weight, neurologic symptoms, recurrent infections, and heart failure may occur. In contrast to multiple myeloma, lytic bone lesions, renal insufficiency, and amyloidosis are rare. Physical findings include pallor, hepatosplenomegaly, and lymphadenopathy. Retinal hemorrhages, exudates, and venous congestion with vascular segmentation ("sausage" formation) may occur. Sensorimotor peripheral neuropathy is common. Pulmonary involvement is manifested by diffuse pulmonary infiltrates and isolated masses. Pleural effusion may occur. Diarrhea and steatorrhea are uncommon.

Laboratory Evaluation

Almost all patients have moderate to severe normocytic, normochromic anemia. Coombs-positive hemolytic anemia is uncommon. The serum cholesterol value is often low. The serum electrophoretic pattern is characterized by a tall, narrow peak or dense band and is usually of λ mobility. Seventy-five per cent of the IgM proteins have a κ light chain. Low-molecular-weight IgM (7S) is present and may account for a significant part of the elevated IgM level. A monoclonal light chain is present in the urine of 80% of patients. The amount of urinary protein is usually modest.

The bone marrow aspirate is often hypocellular, but the biopsy is hypercellular and extensively infiltrated with lymphoid cells and plasma cells. The number of mast cells is frequently increased. Rouleaux formation is prominent, and the sedimentation rate is markedly increased unless gelation of the plasma occurs. About 10% of macroglobulins have cryoproperties.

Diagnosis

The combination of typical symptoms and physical findings, the presence of a large IgM M-protein (usually greater than 3 g/dL), and lymphoid–plasma cell infiltration of the bone marrow provide the diagnosis. Multiple myeloma, chronic lymphocytic leukemia, and MGUS of the IgM type must be excluded.

Treatment

Patients should not be treated unless they have anemia; constitutional symptoms such as weakness, fatigue, night sweats, or weight loss; hyperviscosity; or significant hepatosplenomegaly or lymphadenopathy. Chlorambucil (Leukeran) is usually given orally in a dosage of 6 to 8 mg/day and is reduced when the leukocyte or platelet value decreases. Patients should be treated until the disease has reached a plateau state; the treatment can be discontinued and the patients observed closely. Chemotherapy should be reinstituted when the disease relapses. Combinations of alkylating agents, such as the M2 protocol (vincristine, BCNU, melphalan, cyclophosphamide, and prednisone), may be beneficial. α₂-Interferon may be of some use. Eighty per cent of previously untreated patients have been reported to respond to fludarabine or 2-chlorodeoxyadenosine. Autologous stem cell transplants have been performed in some cases, but series results have not been published.

Transfusions of packed red blood cells should be given for symptomatic anemia. Spuriously low hemoglobin and hematocrit levels may occur because of the increased plasma volume from the large amount of M-protein. Consequently, transfusions should not be given solely on the basis of the hemoglobin or hematocrit value. Symptomatic hyperviscosity should be treated with plasmapheresis. The median survival in macroglobulinemia is 5 years.

HYPERVISCOSITY SYNDROME

Chronic nasal bleeding and oozing from the gums are frequent, but postsurgical or gastrointestinal bleeding also may occur. Retinal hemorrhages are common, and papilledema may be seen. The patient occasionally complains of blurring or a loss of vision. Dizziness, headache, vertigo, nystagmus, decreased heating, ataxia, paresthesias, diplopia, somnolence, and coma may occur. Hyperviscosity can precipitate or aggravate heart failure. Most patients have symptoms when the relative viscosity is greater than 4 centipoises (cP), but the relationship between serum viscosity and clinical manifestations is not precise. Patients with symptomatic hyperviscosity should be treated with plasmapheresis. Plasma exchange of 3 to 4 L should be performed daily until the patient is asymptomatic. The plasma should be replaced with albumin rather than plasma.

HEAVY CHAIN DISEASES

The heavy chain diseases (HCDs) are characterized by the presence of an M-protein consisting of a portion of the immunoglobulin heavy chain in the serum or urine or both. These heavy chains are devoid of light chains and represent a lymphoplasma cell proliferative process. There are three major types: γ-HCD, α-HCD, and μ-HCD.

γ-HCD

The abnormal protein consists of γ chain with significant deletions of amino acids, including the C_{H1} domain of the constant region. The median age of patients is approximately 60 years, although the condition has been noted in persons younger than 20. Patients with γ-HCD often present with a lymphoma-like illness, but the clinical findings are diverse and range from an aggressive lymphoproliferative process to an asymptomatic state. Hepatosplenomegaly and lymphadenopathy occur in about 60% of patients. Anemia is found in about 80% initially and in nearly all eventually. A few patients have had a Coombs-positive hemolytic anemia. The electrophoretic pattern often shows a broad-based band more suggestive of a polyclonal increase than an M-protein. The urinary protein value ranges from a trace to 20 g/day, but it is usually less than 1 g/24 hours.

Increased numbers of lymphocytes, plasma cells, or plasmacytoid lymphocytes are seen in the bone marrow and lymph nodes. The histologic pattern varies, usually including generalized or localized lymphoma or myeloma, but in some cases there is no evidence of a lymphoplasmacytic proliferative process.

Treatment is indicated only for symptomatic patients. Many different drugs have been used, but the results have been inconsistent and generally disappointing. Therapy with cyclophosphamide, vincristine, and prednisone is a reasonable choice. If there is no response to this regimen, doxorubicin should be added. The prognosis of γ-HCD is variable and ranges from a rapidly progressive downhill course of a few weeks' duration to the asymptomatic presence of a stable monoclonal heavy chain in the serum or urine.

α-HCD

This most common HCD occurs in patients from the Mediterranean region or Middle East, usually in the second or third decade of life. About 60% are men. Most commonly, the gastrointestinal tract is involved, resulting in severe malabsorption with diarrhea, steatorrhea, and loss of weight. Plasma cell infiltration of the jejunal mucosa is the most frequent pathologic feature. Immunoproliferative small intestinal disease is restricted to patients with small intestinal lesions who have the same pathologic features as those of α-HCD, but these patients do not synthesize α heavy chains.

The serum protein electrophoretic pattern is normal in half the cases, and in the remainder an unimpressive broad band may appear in the α_2 or β regions. The diagnosis depends on the recognition of a monoclonal α heavy chain. The amount of α heavy chain in the urine is small, and Bence Jones proteinuria has never been reported.

Most often, α-HCD is progressive and fatal, but it may respond to melphalan or to cyclophosphamide and prednisone. Antibiotics such as tetracyclines may also produce a remission.

μ-HCD

This disease is characterized by the demonstration of a monoclonal μ-chain fragment in the serum. The patient may present with chronic lymphocytic leukemia or lymphoma, but it is likely that the clinical spectrum will broaden when more cases are recognized.

The serum protein electrophoretic pattern is usually normal except for hypogammaglobulinemia. Bence Jones proteinuria has been found in two thirds of cases. An increase in lymphocytes, plasma cells, and lymphoplasmacytoid cells is seen in the bone marrow.

Vacuolization of the plasma cells is common and should suggest the possibility of HCD. The course of μ-HCD is variable, and survival ranges from a few months to many years. Treatment with corticosteroids and alkylating agents has produced some benefit.

CRYOGLOBULINEMIA

Cryoglobulins are proteins that precipitate when cooled and dissolve when heated. They are designated as idiopathic or essential when they are not associated with any recognizable disease. Cryoglobulins are classified into three types: type I (monoclonal), type II (mixed), and type III (polyclonal).

Type I (monoclonal) cryoglobulinemia is most commonly of the IgM or IgG class, but IgA and Bence Jones cryoglobulins have been reported. Most patients, even with large amounts of type I cryoglobulin, are completely asymptomatic from this source. Others with monoclonal cryoglobulins in the range of 1 to 2 g/dL may have pain, purpura, Raynaud's phenomenon, cyanosis, and even ulceration and sloughing of skin and subcutaneous tissue on exposure to the cold because their cryoglobulins precipitate at relatively high temperatures. Type I cryoglobulins are associated with macroglobulinemia, multiple myeloma, or MGUS.

Type II (mixed) cryoglobulinemia typically consists of an IgM M-protein and polyclonal IgG, although monoclonal IgG or monoclonal IgA may also be seen with polyclonal IgM. Serum protein electrophoresis usually shows a normal pattern or a diffuse, polyclonal hypergammaglobulinemic pattern. The quantity of mixed cryoglobulin is usually less than 0.2 g/dL. Vasculitis, glomerulonephritis, lymphoproliferative disease, and chronic infectious processes are common. Purpura and polyarthralgias are frequently seen. Involvement of the joints is symmetric, but joint deformities rarely develop. Raynaud's phenomenon, necrosis of the skin, and neurologic involvement may be present. In almost 80% of renal biopsy specimens, glomerular damage can be identified. Nephrotic syndrome may result, but severe renal insufficiency is uncommon. Hepatic dysfunction and serologic evidence of infection with hepatitis C virus are common.

Early administration of corticosteroids is the most frequent therapy. α_2-Interferon has been of benefit, but relapse is common after cessation of therapy. Cyclophosphamide, chlorambucil, or azathioprine should be used if there is no response. Plasmapheresis has been effective in some instances.

Type III (polyclonal) cryoglobulinemia is not associated with a monoclonal component. Type III cryoglobulins are found in many patients with infections or inflammatory diseases and are of no clinical significance.

PRIMARY AMYLOIDOSIS (AL)

Amyloid, stained with Congo red, produces an apple-green birefringence under polarized light. It is a fibrous protein that consists of rigid, linear, non-branching, aggregated fibrils of 7.5 to 10 nm width and of indefinite length. The type of amyloid cannot be differentiated by organ distribution or by electron microscopy. The amyloid fibrils in AL consist of the variable portion of a monoclonal light chain or, in some instances, the intact light chain (Table 181–4). The light-chain class is more frequently λ than κ (2:1), with a predominance of the λ_{VI} subclass. Patients with AL may have aberrant de novo synthesis or abnormal proteolytic processing of light chains. Rarely, the fibril consists of a monoclonal heavy chain. Amyloid P-component (AP) is a glycoprotein found in all types of amyloid, but its function is unknown. The catabolism, or breakdown, of amyloid fibrils is an important but poorly understood factor in pathogenesis.

Clinical Features

The median age at diagnosis is 64 years, and only 1% of patients are younger than 40. Two thirds are male. Weakness or fatigue and loss of weight are the most frequent symptoms. Dyspnea, pedal edema, paresthesias, light-headedness, and syncope are frequently seen in patients with heart failure or peripheral neuropathy. Hoarseness or change of voice as well as jaw claudication may occur.

The liver is palpable in one fourth of patients, but splenomegaly

Table 181-4 ■ CLINICAL CLASSIFICATION OF AMYLOIDOSIS

AMYLOID TYPE	CLASSIFICATION	MAJOR PROTEIN COMPONENT
AL	Primary	κ or λ light chain
AA	Secondary	Protein A
AL	Localized	κ or λ light chain
ATTR	Familial	
	Neurologic	Transthyretin mutant (prealbumin)
	Cardiopathic	Transthyretin mutant (prealbumin)
	Nephropathic	
	Familial Mediterranean fever	Protein A
	Senile systemic amyloidosis	Normal transthyretin (prealbumin)
$A\beta_2M$	Long-term dialysis	β_2-Microglobulin

occurs in only 5%. Macroglossia is present in 10%. Purpura often involves the neck, face, and eyes. Ankle edema is common.

Almost one third of patients have nephrotic syndrome. Carpal tunnel syndrome, heart failure, peripheral neuropathy, and orthostatic hypotension are other major presenting syndromes (Fig. 181–7). The presence of one of these syndromes and an M-protein in the serum or urine is a strong indication of amyloidosis, for which appropriate biopsy specimens must be taken for diagnosis.

Laboratory Findings

Anemia is not a prominent feature, but, when present, it is usually due to renal insufficiency, multiple myeloma, or gastrointestinal bleeding. Thrombocytosis occurs in 10% of patients. Proteinuria is present initially in 80% and renal insufficiency in almost 50% of patients. Elevation of the serum alkaline phosphatase value is not uncommon. Hyperbilirubinemia is infrequent, but, when present, it is an ominous sign. Hypoalbuminemia and elevation of the cholesterol and triglyceride values are common with the nephrotic syndrome. The Factor X level is decreased in more than 10% of patients but is rarely the cause of bleeding. The prothrombin time is increased in about 15% of patients, and the thrombin time is prolonged in 60%.

A localized band or spike in the serum protein electrophoretic pattern is found in about half of patients, but it is modest in size (median, 1.4 g/dL). Hypogammaglobulinemia is present in about 20%.

Immunofixation reveals an M-protein in the serum and in the urine of more than 70% of patients. An M-protein is found in the serum or urine in almost 90% of patients at diagnosis.

Bone marrow plasma cells are usually only modestly increased, with a median value of 7%. Less than one fifth of patients have more than 20% plasma cells in the marrow. Radiographs of the bones are normal unless the patient has multiple myeloma.

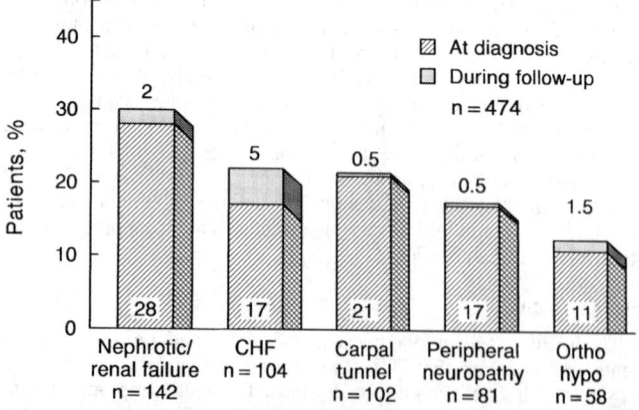

FIGURE 181-7 ■ Syndromes seen at diagnosis and during follow-up of patients with primary amyloidosis. Some patients had more than two syndromes at presentation. CHF = congestive heart failure; Ortho hypo = orthostatic hypotension. (From Kyle RA, Gertz MA: Primary systemic amyloidosis: Clinical and laboratory features in 474 cases. Semin Hematol 32:45, 1995.)

Organ System Involvement

CARDIAC AND CIRCULATORY. Heart failure is present in approximately 20% of patients at diagnosis and develops during the course of the disease in an additional 10%. The electrocardiogram frequently shows either low voltage in the limb leads or features consistent with an anteroseptal infarction (loss of anterior forces), but there is no evidence of myocardial infarction at autopsy. Atrial fibrillation, atrial or junctional tachycardia, ventricular premature complexes, and heart block are common electrocardiographic features.

Echocardiography is valuable for evaluation of amyloid heart disease. Increased thickness of the ventricular wall and septum correlates with an increased prevalence of heart failure (see Chapter 64). Early cardiac amyloidosis is characterized by abnormal relaxation, whereas advanced involvement is characterized by restrictive hemodynamics. Intermittent claudication of the lower extremities, the upper extremities, or the jaw may be a prominent feature. Orthostatic hypotension occurs in about 15%.

OTHER ORGANS. Nephrotic syndrome is present in more than one fourth of patients at the time of diagnosis. The degree of proteinuria does not correlate well with the extent of amyloid deposition in the kidney. Gross hematuria is rare. Other organ involvement includes the lungs and gastrointestinal tract, but it is asymptomatic in most instances. Sensorimotor peripheral neuropathy characterized by dysesthetic numbness involving the lower extremities occurs in one sixth of patients. Autonomic dysfunction may be a prominent feature and is usually manifested by orthostatic hypotension, diarrhea, or impotence. Amyloidosis can involve the periarticular structures and produce the shoulder pad syndrome. Rarely, osteolytic lesions from amyloid may occur. Pseudohypertrophy of skeletal muscles from amyloid deposition may be impressive. Petechiae, ecchymoses, papules, plaques, nodules, tumors, bullous lesions, thickening of the skin, and dystrophy of the nails may occur.

The diagnosis of amyloidosis depends on histologic proof. The initial diagnostic procedure should be abdominal fat aspiration, which is positive in 80% of patients. A bone marrow aspiration and biopsy should be done to determine the degree of plasmacytosis, and results are positive for amyloid in more than one half of patients. The abdominal fat or bone marrow biopsy results are positive in 90%. If subcutaneous fat and bone marrow biopsies are negative, a rectal biopsy should be done, or tissue should be obtained from a suspected organ.

Specific antisera are helpful for identifying the type of systemic amyloidosis. Antiserum to AP reacts with all amyloid types and is useful in demonstrating the presence of amyloid.

Prognosis

Currently, the median survival of patients with AL amyloidosis is 13 months. Survival varies greatly, depending on the associated syndrome; it is 4 months after the onset of heart failure. Patients with only peripheral neuropathy have a median survival of 2 years.

Treatment

Therapy of AL amyloidosis is not satisfactory. In a prospective study of treatment with melphalan and prednisone compared with colchicine, no significant difference in survival was noted (25 and 18 months, respectively). When the survival of patients who received only one regimen was analyzed, or when survival was determined from the time of entry into the study to the time of death or progression of disease, significant differences favoring melphalan and prednisone therapy were evident.

In a randomized trial, patients with AL received melphalan and prednisone, colchicine, or a combination of the three. Survival of those receiving the two melphalan/prednisone–containing regimens was superior to that of those with the colchicine schedule.

Substantial clinical improvement has been observed with the administration of 4'-iodo-4'-deoxyrubicin (I-DOX) in patients with primary amyloidosis. This agent appears to bind to amyloid fibrils and thus to contribute to the resolution of amyloid deposits. Encouraging results have been reported with high-dose intravenous melphalan (200 mg/m$_2$) followed by autologous peripheral stem cell rescue. However, because of the short-term follow-up, the impact of this approach is still unknown.

The nephrotic syndrome should be managed with salt restriction and diuretic agents as needed. If symptomatic azotemia develops, chronic renal dialysis is necessary. Salt restriction and the judicious use of diuretic drugs are helpful for heart failure. Digitalis must be avoided or used with great care because patients are unusually sensitive to the drug, and heart block and arrhythmias are common. Elastic stockings or leotards may be of benefit in patients with orthostatic hypotension; fludrocortisone may also be useful, but it leads to retention of fluids.

Agnello V: The etiology and pathophysiology of mixed cryoglobulinemia secondary to hepatitis C virus infection. Springer Semin Immunopathol 19:111, 1997. *This is a review of mixed cryoglobulinemia associated with hepatitis C virus infection.*

Attal M, Harousseau J-L: Standard therapy versus autologous transplantation in multiple myeloma. Hematol Oncol Clin North Am 11:133, 1997. *This is an update of the first prospective study comparing autologous transplantation and chemotherapy for multiple myeloma.*

Bataille R, Harousseau J-L: Multiple myeloma. N Engl J Med 336:1657, 1997. *This article reviews the highlights of the biology of multiple myeloma.*

Berenson JR, Lichtenstein A, Porter L, et al, for the Myeloma Aredia Study Group: Long-term pamidronate treatment of advanced multiple myeloma reduces skeletal events. J Clin Oncol 16:593, 1998. *This prospective study indicates that pamidronate reduces the number of skeletal complications and improves the quality of life in patients with myeloma.*

Dimopoulos MA, Alexanian R: Waldenström's macroglobulinemia. Blood 83:1452, 1994. *This review covers features of the disease, complications, and therapy.*

Falk RH, Comenzo RL, Skinner M: The systemic amyloidoses. N Engl J Med 337:898, 1997. *This is an excellent review of amyloidoses.*

Frassica DA, Frassica FJ, Schray MF, et al: Solitary plasmacytoma of bone: Mayo Clinic experience. Int J Radiat Oncol Biol Phys 16:43, 1989. *In 46 cases of solitary plasmacytoma of bone, the presence of an M-protein did not significantly alter the survival or duration of disease-free survival.*

Gertz MA, Kyle RA: Hyperviscosity syndromes. J Intensive Care Med 10:128, 1995. *Comprehensively reviews the pathophysiology, clinical features, and treatment of hyperviscosity.*

Gillmore JD, Hawkins PN, Pepys MB: Amyloidosis: A review of recent diagnostic and therapeutic developments. Br J Haematol 99:245, 1997. *This is an extensive review of amyloidosis.*

Jagannath S, Tricot G, Barlogie B: Autotransplants in multiple myeloma: Pushing the envelope. Hematol Oncol Clin North Am 11:363, 1997. *This is an extensive and detailed report of autologous transplants in multiple myeloma.*

Kyle RA: "Benign" monoclonal gammopathy—after 20 to 35 years of follow-up. Mayo Clin Proc 68:26, 1993. *Of 241 patients with MGUS, 24% developed multiple myeloma, macroglobulinemia, amyloidosis, or related disorders.*

Kyle RA, Gertz MA: Primary systemic amyloidosis: Clinical and laboratory features in 474 cases. Semin Hematol 32:45, 1995. *A review of the clinical and laboratory data on 474 primary amyloidosis patients seen at one institution from 1981–1992 within 30 days of diagnosis.*

Kyle RA, Gertz MA, Greipp PR, et al: A trial of three regimens for primary amyloidosis: Colchicine alone, melphalan and prednisone, and melphalan, prednisone, and colchicine. N Engl J Med 336:1202, 1997. *This is a prospective study demonstrating that melphalan-prednisone was superior to colchicine in 220 patients with primary amyloidosis.*

Schey S: Osteosclerotic myeloma and "POEMS" syndrome. Blood Rev 10:75, 1996. *This is a well-written review of the POEMS syndrome (osteosclerotic myeloma).*

Susnerwala SS, Shanks, JH, Banerjee SS, et al: Extramedullary plasmacytoma of the head and neck region: Clinicopathological correlation in 25 cases. Br J Cancer 75:921, 1997. *Only 2 of the 25 patients with extramedullary plasmacytomas had development of multiple myeloma.*

182 STEM CELL TRANSPLANTATION

Malcolm K. Brenner

Hematopoietic stem cell transplantation derives its feasibility from the biologic properties of these cells. Even in small numbers ($<10^6$/kg), infused hematopoietic stem cells can completely and permanently repopulate a host with every marrow-derived lineage, including erythrocytes, myelocytes, monocytes, platelets, and T and B lymphocytes. Consequently, stem cell transplantation can treat defects arising in any of these lineages, and it can also be used to rescue patients from marrow aplasia arising from primary marrow disease or from the intensive cytotoxic chemotherapy that is used to treat malignancy. More recently, stem cell transplantation has been used to equip patients with genetically modified cells intended to combat several different inherited or acquired disorders and may also be valuable for mesenchymal cell disorders such as osteogenesis imperfecta (Table 182–1). The two types of stem cell transplantation are autologous, in which the patient is the cell donor, and allogeneic, in which the stem cells are derived from a separate individual.

ALLOGENEIC TRANSPLANTATION

Identification of HLA antigens, the human major histocompatibility complex, paved the way for transplantation of stem cells be-

Table 182–1 ■ CONDITIONS FOR WHICH ALLOGENEIC BONE MARROW TRANSPLANTATION MAY BE UNDERTAKEN

Malignancy	Defective Hematopoiesis
Acute myeloid leukemia	Aplastic anemia
Acute lymphoid leukemia	Fanconi's anemia
Chronic myeloid leukemia	Sickle cell disease
Chronic lymphoic leukemia	Thalassemia
Myelodysplasia	Granulocyte disorders
Hodgkin's disease	Kostmann's syndrome
Non-Hodgkin's lymphoma	Chronic granulomatous disease
Multiple myeloma	Chédiak-Higashi syndrome
	Adhesion molecule deficiencies
Immunodeficiency	Platelet disorders
Severe combined immunodeficiency	Glanzmann's thrombasthenia
	Bernard-Soulier syndrome
Wiscott-Aldrich syndrome	Metabolic storage diseases
Adenosine deaminase deficiency	Osteopetrosis
X-linked lymphoproliferative syndrome	Congenital hemophagocytic syndrome
Cartilage-hair hypoplasia	

tween individuals. Initially, only sibling donors with an identical HLA genotype could safely be used. More recently, the development of international computer-linked panels consisting of millions of tissue-typed donors has made it possible to perform transplants between unrelated, but phenotypically HLA-matched individuals. It is also possible to perform transplants between close relatives who are only partially matched at HLA loci. The morbidity of allogeneic stem cell transplantation increases as major and minor histocompatibility differences between the donor and patient increase. This increased morbidity largely results from alloreactivity, the recognition of self/non-self by donor and patient T lymphocytes. Alloreactivity causes graft-versus-host disease (GVHD), in which donor alloreactivity dominates, or graft rejection, in which the recipient immune system gains the upper hand. The success of allogeneic transplantation depends on balanced modulation of alloreactivity to allow engraftment without the production of GVHD.

AUTOLOGOUS TRANSPLANTATION

One of the fundamental concepts of medical oncology is that intensification of therapy will increase the cure rate of chemosensitive/radiosensitive tumors. Dose intensification is limited by damage to normal organs, among the most sensitive of which is the bone marrow. One way of overcoming this limitation is to harvest and freeze hematopoietic stem cells from patients who have received conventional levels of therapy. This material is then infused to produce hematologic rescue following doses of chemotherapy/radiotherapy that would otherwise be lethal from marrow ablation. Because autologous transplants are not alloreactive, the procedure has a lower treatment-related morbidity and mortality than seen with allografting. However, the lack of an alloreactive "graft-versus-tumor" effect may explain why autografting generally has a higher risk of tumor relapse than allografting does. Relapse may also be associated with contamination of the graft with tumorigenic cells if these cells survive the conventional levels of chemotherapy that were given before stem cell harvest. Efforts to remove these cells by treating marrow with physical, pharmaceutical, or immunologic techniques are of uncertain benefit and may retard engraftment.

Autografting is currently in wide clinical practice as treatment of a variety of hematologic and solid malignancies, including lymphoma and breast cancer. Unfortunately, there has been a disappointing lack of randomized studies to confirm that the approach genuinely increases patient survival in comparison to conventional chemotherapy/radiotherapy. The few completed randomized studies have produced mixed results. Some (for example, in patients with advanced Hodgkin's lymphoma and myeloma) show an advantage for autologous transplants; others (for example, in children with acute myeloid leukemia) show limited benefit. Hence the usefulness of autologous transplantation in many malignant diseases remains uncertain.

More recently, autologous transplantation has been used as a means of introducing genetically modified cells to treat inherited or acquired disorders of hematopoietic cells. This approach is of great promise but is limited by the inefficiency of current gene transfer technologies. The value of autologous transplantation as treatment of severe autoimmune disorders is also under investigation. This approach is based on animal models in which it has been shown that "resetting" the immune system in this way may produce a long-term cure.

CHOICE BETWEEN AUTOGRAFT AND ALLOGRAFT. For most non-malignant indications, allogeneic stem cell transplantation is the only current option. In malignant disease, either autografts or allografts are feasible. Here the choice will be influenced primarily by the results of comparative studies in each disease and by variables that affect outcome, including the patient's age and fitness, the availability of donors, previous treatment, and current status.

SOURCES OF HEMATOPOIETIC STEM CELLS

Originally, hematopoietic stem cells for transplantation were always obtained from bone marrow. Under general anesthetic, marrow is removed though needle punctures made in the iliac crest. Sufficient marrow is removed to ensure engraftment ($>1 \times 10^8$ nucleated cells per kilogram for autografting or $>2 \times 10^8$ nucleated cells per kilogram for allografting); in adults, this number of cells usually translates to a volume between 0.5 and 1 L. Serious complications of this procedure are rare, although bruising and pain at aspiration sites are common. Infrequent but serious sequelae include the complications of anesthesia, as well as infection or cardiorespiratory instability.

PERIPHERAL BLOOD. Peripheral blood stem cell (PBSC) harvest has become a preferred alternative to marrow harvesting for most autologous transplants and is increasing in popularity for allografts. This approach has been made feasible by the ability to mobilize stem cells (identified by the CD34 phenotypic marker) from the marrow into the peripheral blood. PBSCs are collected by apheresis after patients are treated with chemotherapy and/or granulocyte or granulocyte-macrophage colony-stimulating factor (G- or GM-CSF). A typical regimen is to inject G-CSF, 5 μg/kg for 5 to 8 days, and collect peripheral blood mononuclear cells on days 4 and/or 5, when the numbers of CD34-positive cells are usually at their peak. Once a minimum of 2×10^6 CD34+ cells per kilogram has been collected, the product may be cryopreserved and reinfused following ablative chemotherapy.

PBSCs have a number of advantages over marrow-derived stem cells. No general anesthetic or hospital stay is required, and the procedure can be performed by technical rather than medical staff. More importantly, time to engraftment, particularly of platelets, is reduced (often by a week or more), probably because PBSCs contain greater numbers of more mature progenitor cells than marrow does. These characteristics not only reduce both the costs of the procedure and the accompanying morbidity but may also increase overall patient survival after autologous transplantation. However, some patients—especially those who have received extensive prior chemotherapy—may fail to mobilize and may then require marrow harvest in addition. The increased numbers of T lymphocytes present in PBSCs as compared with marrow may also increase the risk of chronic GVHD if this source is used for allogeneic transplantation.

PLACENTAL BLOOD. Patients with diseases that would benefit from allogeneic transplantation but who lack sibling donors may receive stem cell grafts from HLA-matched unrelated donors located through international registries of tissue-typed donors. However, locating and counseling prospective donors, performing phenotypic and molecular tissue typing, and harvesting the marrow require an average of 120 days, a delay that may doom a seriously ill patient. Moreover, patients from many minority groups simply may not have a suitable donor. Interest has therefore increased in transplanting the stem cells present in placental blood. After birth, the 50 to 150 mL of fetal blood remaining in the placenta is aspirated, tissue-typed, and sent to the placental blood bank, which then stores the graft itself rather than just the prospective donor's tissue type. Hence placental blood transplantation is available as soon as typing is confirmed. Moreover, T lymphocytes in placental blood appear to be less alloreactive than T cells from adults and hence less likely to produce GVHD; a greater degree of HLA disparity may therefore be acceptable. It should also be possible to

store blood from ethnically diverse groups. At present, the results of placental blood transplantation appear relatively comparable to results using more conventional sources of stem cells in children and small adults. Because volumes of placental blood are small, however, they may be insufficient for engraftment in large adults, and outcomes in some diseases such as aplastic anemia and chronic myelocytic anemia appear to be less good.

STEM CELL TRANSPLANT PROCEDURE AND ASSOCIATED COMPLICATIONS

Before transplantation occurs, patients are treated with a preparative regimen of chemoradiotherapy. The intensity of this treatment regimen depends on the type of donor and on the underlying condition, but for hematologic malignancy it typically consists of a combination of high doses of one or more cytotoxic drugs such as cyclophosphamide ($\sim$200 mg/m^2) with total-body irradiation ($\sim$1400 cGy) given in several fractions. Patients may also receive immunosuppressive antibodies such as antithymocyte globulin. This preparative regimen fills a number of functions. In allograft recipients, it ablates host hematopoiesis and lymphopoiesis to allow engraftment. In patients with malignant disease, the treatment also reduces or obliterates residual tumor.

Preparative regimens produce a number of potentially lethal adverse effects. The two most common severe problems are hepatic veno-occlusive disease and hemorrhagic cystitis. Veno-occlusive disease of the liver can occur in a third or more of allograft recipients. It results from treatment-mediated damage to hepatic venous endothelium and is characterized by weight gain, hepatomegaly, and hyperbilirubinemia, often with ascites and refractory thrombocytopenia. Contributory factors include pre-transplant liver dysfunction, the intensity of previous chemotherapy, the type of transplant, and the method of GVHD prophylaxis. Distinction from other causes of hepatic dysfunction such as GVHD, drug toxicity, or sepsis may be difficult. Although ultrasound may show dilated portal veins or reversal of flow, it is not definitive, and liver biopsy is hazardous in these patients. When biopsy is considered essential to define the source of liver dysfunction, a transvenous approach is preferable. If veno-occlusive disease progresses, renal insufficiency and cardiopulmonary failure may ensue. In up to 20% of affected patients, death results from multiorgan failure. In the absence of a clear understanding of pathogenesis, prevention and treatment have been based on reported perturbations in clotting mechanisms and hepatic microcirculation. Heparin, tissue plasminogen activator, and prostaglandin E_1 have all been used with uncertain benefit. Supportive measures to maintain fluid and electrolyte balance, if necessary by hemodialysis, are the mainstays of treatment.

Hemorrhagic cystitis occurs in 5 to 50% of patients following treatment with preparatory regimens containing high-dose cyclophosphamide and has been attributed to the presence of activated drug metabolites in the uroepithelium. Its incidence is affected by factors such as prior alkylating therapy and radiotherapy to the bladder. Hemorrhagic cystitis usually develops in the initial few weeks after transplantation, but it may occur even during the preparatory regimen or be delayed for several months. Its severity ranges from asymptomatic microscopic hematuria to massive hemorrhage from the entire uroepithelium, with hemodynamic instability, incapacitating bladder spasm, and urinary outflow obstruction. The differential diagnosis includes infectious causes of hemorrhagic cystitis, of which adenovirus infection is now the most common. The complication itself is treated symptomatically. Limited hemorrhage is treated by ensuring a brisk urine output (>60 mL/kg/day) to reduce clot formation and by maintaining platelet counts above 50,000/mm^3. More severe manifestations require irrigation through an indwelling urinary catheter, along with analgesia and antispasmodics. Refractory severe hematuria requires cystoscopy and instillation of aluminum hydroxide, silver nitrate, or formalin and may also necessitate the placement of ureteric stents, nephrostomy, or even cystectomy. Hemorrhagic cystitis usually resolves, but it may leave the patient with a scarred and dysfunctional urinary tract.

Gastrointestinal mucositis with painful oral ulceration, dysphagia, vomiting, and diarrhea occurs almost universally, and it may be exacerbated by GVHD regimens that contain methotrexate. Patients require good oral and perianal hygiene and adequate analgesia until the condition resolves in 10 to 21 days. Most patients also require intravenous hyperalimentation to maintain adequate nutrient intake.

Pneumonitis and acute carditis represent less than 2% of the regimen-related toxicity and usually occur in patients who have received extensive prior treatment. The mortality is high. Other pulmonary problems such as capillary leak syndrome and pulmonary alveolar hemorrhage occur with greater frequency but have a lower mortality. Treatment is symptomatic.

To avoid these major complications, recent efforts have attempted sub-ablative or "mini" transplants using lower doses of cytotoxic drugs and radiation together with immunosuppressive agents. The donor immune system is then able to engraft, to achieve the final hematopoietic ablation, and to allow the donor hematopoietic system to follow.

CELL INFUSION. Once the preparative regimen is completed, fresh stem cell products are infused by the usual procedures for blood product infusion, but without in-line filters. Most patients tolerate infusion well, although care must be taken to avoid volume overload, particularly when peripheral stem cells are used. Cryopreserved products are usually thawed at the bedside immediately before infusion. The dimethyl sulfoxide used as a cryoprotectant may cause nausea and cardiovascular instability; because the agent is a mercaptan, which is excreted through the lungs, it causes a garlic-like odor for 24 to 72 hours. Recipients of cryopreserved products should be well hydrated because red cell degradation products can precipitate acute renal failure.

COMPLICATIONS AFTER TRANSPLANTATION

Complications post-transplantation are due either to hematopoietic and immune system aplasia or to alloreactivity. Because preparative regimens destroy the recipient's own immune and hematopoietic system, recovery is dependent on engraftment and proliferation of the infused stem cells. This process is lengthy, and post-transplant immunodeficiency is associated with a high incidence of infection and considerable morbidity and mortality. The degree of risk is greater in allogeneic than autologous transplantation and is also increased by the presence of GVHD. To reduce this risk, a variety of precautions are taken. Rigorous hand washing before entering patients' rooms is probably the most important single preventive measure, but most units also isolate patients in positive-pressure rooms in which particulate matter is reduced by air filtration with high-efficiency particulate air filters or laminar flow. A variety of prophylactic antibiotic and antifungal regimens have been used in addition to these physical methods of protection, but to date no consensus has been reached on their value.

In the initial post-transplantation period when patients are neutropenic, the primary risk is bacterial and fungal infection. The problem is exacerbated by mucositis from the preparative regimen, and both gram-positive and gram-negative bacteria may produce overwhelming infections. Fungal disease, most commonly with *Aspergillus* or *Candida* species, also occurs at this time. Temperatures higher than 38° C will develop in more than 65% of patients during the period of neutropenia, a sign that is always assumed to indicate sepsis. Treatment with broad-spectrum antibiotics is critical, and many different regimens have been designed to offer broad and effective coverage. Amphotericin is added when cultures are negative but fever persists. Parenteral antibiotics are continued until myeloid engraftment is stable and the patient is afebrile; amphotericin may be required for several weeks longer if fungal lesions are documented.

Intravenous administration of the granulocyte growth factors G-CSF or GM-CSF from the time of marrow infusion or at the time of initial engraftment accelerates the recovery of neutrophils, particularly after autologous transplantation. However, these cytokines have little impact on the period of absolute neutropenia when patients are most vulnerable to infection, nor can they reduce the period of thrombocytopenia. Overall, the use of growth factors after transplantation may abbreviate the hospital stay if discharge is triggered by the point at which patients reach a specific neutrophil count. It has been much harder to demonstrate that these agents substantially reduce patient morbidity or mortality, and their cost-effectiveness is controversial.

The risk of bacterial infection (Table 182–2) decreases after neutrophil recovery, but because the immune system is much slower to recover, recipients of allografts remain at risk of infection with viruses and other opportunistic pathogens for some months. Many post-transplant infections result from reactivation of latent

Table 182–2 ■ INFECTIOUS COMPLICATIONS OF TRANSPLANTATION

PATHOGEN	SUGGESTED TREATMENT
Pre-engraftment	
Fever of unknown origin	Broad-spectrum antibiotics, usually in combination, e.g., oxacillin and a cephalosporin
Gram-positive bacteria	Vancomycin
Gram-negative bacteria	Aminoglycoside or cephalosporin
Fungi	Amphotericin B
Herpes simplex virus	Acyclovir
Respiratory syncytial virus	Inhaled ribavirin
Post-engraftment	
Cytomegalovirus	Ganciclovir/IVIG
Epstein-Barr virus	? Interferon-α, ? anti–B-cell antibodies, ? donor T cells
Varicella zoster	Acyclovir
Pneumocystis	Co-trimoxazole or pentamidine
Adenovirus	? IV ribavirin
Fungi	Amphotericin B
Encapsulated bacteria	Penicillin/erythromycin
Hepatitis C	Interferon-α, lamivudine

IVIG = intravenous immunoglobulin.

herpesviruses, including cytomegalovirus (CMV), Epstein-Barr virus (EBV), herpes simplex, and herpes zoster. Until recently, CMV was the cause of death in 10 to 20% of allograft recipients, usually from reactivation of host or donor virus but occasionally secondary to primary infection from blood products. CMV reactivation can cause disease affecting the lungs, liver, marrow, and gut. CMV disease occurs in fewer than 3% of autograft recipients, but CMV pneumonitis (the most severe manifestation), which has been fatal in 80 to 90% of cases, will develop in about half of allograft recipients who have evidence of CMV reactivation/infection (see Chapter 386). Two developments have reduced the magnitude of this problem. Primary infections in CMV-negative recipients of CMV-negative stem cells can be reduced to almost zero if they receive leukocyte-filtered blood or blood products from CMV-negative donors. For CMV-positive donor/recipients, prophylaxis with ganciclovir (10 mg/kg intravenously for 5 days weekly) and immunoglobulin (0.4 g/kg intravenously weekly) has proved highly effective. Treatment of established disease requires these same agents in therapeutic doses (ganciclovir, 10 mg/kg daily, or foscarnet, 180 mg/kg daily, and immunoglobulin, 0.5 g/kg for 3 days weekly).

EBV infection has become more problematic with the wider use of matched unrelated donor grafts, particularly if these transplants are also depleted of T lymphocytes to prevent GVHD (see below). EBV reactivation in these immunocompromised patients may be associated with uncontrolled lymphoproliferation and the development of frank immunoblastic lymphoma in 3 to 25% of recipients. Treatment has been difficult: withdrawal of immunosuppression may be insufficient to restore immunocompetence, and antiviral agents such as interferon-α or acyclovir have been of limited value. At present, the most effective way of preventing or treating the complication is to infuse donor T lymphocytes, preferably in the form of EBV-specific T-cell lines.

Herpes simplex may become reactivated in the first 2 to 3 months post-transplant. Herpes zoster reactivation may occur at a later date, and one third of allograft recipients will have an episode of shingles in the first year post-transplant. Acyclovir (1400 mg/m² in divided doses daily for 10 to 14 days) is usually effective therapy for this complication.

Many other viral infections, including respiratory syncytial virus, parainfluenza, and adenovirus, may cause significant morbidity and mortality after transplantation, particularly when they produce pneumonitis. No therapies have been established for these viruses, which are treated with supportive care. Hepatitis B and C may cause severe liver disease, either from reactivation in seropositive patients or following transmission by blood products. Liver biopsy is usually required to differentiate viral hepatitis from other causes of abnormal liver function after transplantation. Interferon-α has proved beneficial in patients with hepatitis B, and some data support the use of lamivudine for hepatitis C.

Complications caused by alloreactivity are manifested as rejection (host dominant) or GVHD (donor dominant). The risk of rejection increases with increasing donor/recipient disparity, being least in syngeneic grafts between twins and greatest between mismatched unrelated donors. Rejection is also increased by graft manipulations intended to reduce the incidence of GVHD (such as T-lymphocyte depletion) and by alloimmunization of recipients from the prior administration of blood products. Rejection occurs in up to 20% of the most at-risk group. The complication may be manifested as primary failure to engraft (defined as failure to attain a count of >500 × 10⁶ neutrophils per liter for 3 consecutive days) or failure to maintain this count once achieved. Previous efforts to treat rejection by the administration of hematopoietic growth factors or by reconditioning of the patient and retransplantation have worked poorly, so the complication had been associated with a high mortality. More promising results have been reported following a combination of immunosuppressive antibody therapy with infusion of donor PBSCs.

GVHD occurs when the donor's CD4+ and CD8+ T lymphocytes recognize major or minor histocompatibility antigens on host tissues. Like rejection, the risks increase with greater donor-recipient genetic disparity, and the risk is also greater in male recipients of female (multiparous) donor stem cells. The major targets for attack are the skin, gut, and liver. GVHD of the skin is manifested as erythema that initially affects the face, hands, and feet and then progresses to diffuse erythema with bullae and desquamation. In the gut, the complication is characterized by watery diarrhea that may progressively increase in volume and become bloody. The diarrhea is associated with abdominal distention and cramps. In the liver, the disease is typically manifested by hyperbilirubinemia and an elevated alkaline phosphatase concentration. Aminotransferase levels may remain almost normal even in liver GVHD. The diagnosis is confirmed by histologic examination of clinically affected tissue. GVHD is graded from I to IV according to severity. Following conventional matched sibling transplants, GVHD greater than grade II develops in 30 to 50% of recipients, and 10 to 15% died of the disease or associated complications. Mortality is substantially higher when the donor and recipient are HLA mismatched or unrelated. Fortunately, a number of recent advances in GVHD prophylaxis have helped reduce this toll. The combination of cyclosporine begun on day −1 (either a fixed dose of 5 mg/kg or targeted dosing to achieve plasma concentrations of 250 to 350 μg/L) with methotrexate (e.g., 10 mg/m² on days 0, 3, 7, and 11) after transplantation has proved very effective. As a substitute for cyclosporine, the fungal-derived immunosuppressive tacrolimus has recently been used with apparent success. T-lymphocyte depletion of the donor graft by means of monoclonal antibodies, erythrocyte rosetting, or elutriation is an even more effective means of preventing GVHD. Complete prevention of GVHD by removal of all T cells may not be of unalloyed benefit inasmuch as antihost reactivity has a potentially important role to play. The residual host hematopoietic and immune system cells that have survived the preparative regimen are important targets of the incoming donor T lymphocytes. Destruction of these host cells appears essential to ensure complete host engraftment and may also represent a major component of the antitumor effect of allogenic transplantation. This activity, termed the graft-versus-leukemia effect, has been especially well documented in chronic myeloid leukemias. Hence the most effective methods of GVHD prevention are often associated with the highest risk of rejection and relapse. Once GVHD has occurred, intravenous methylprednisolone in doses between 1 and 10 mg/kg/day is given. If the condition worsens or persists, additional immunosuppressive agents are given, including antithymocyte globulin and monoclonal anti–T-cell antibodies. However, severe steroid-resistant GVHD continues to carry a poor prognosis, with a 60 to 90% death rate. Patients with severe GVHD die of either end-organ failure or the immunosuppression that accompanies the condition and its treatment.

The acute form of GVHD may be followed by chronic GVHD, although this complication may arise *de novo* after day 40. Any organ may be affected and manifestations are protean, so chronic GVHD is graded by the extent and sites of organ involvement. Chronic diffuse GVHD is often manifested as a systemic sclerosis-like syndrome affecting the skin, eyes, gut, liver, and lungs. Although skin involvement limited to the more superficial layers may be successfully treated with psoralens and ultraviolet light, disseminated and progressive chronic GVHD is very disabling. Treatment with immunosuppressive drugs, including prednisolone, cyclosporine, mycophenolic acid, azathioprine, and thalidomide, are often of only modest benefit, and the condition has a high mortality from end-organ failure and infection.

Although recurrence of malignant disease is not strictly a complication of transplantation, it remains a major cause of treatment failure. Relapse is more common after autologous transplantation because of the lack of a graft-versus-malignancy effect and perhaps also because the stem cell graft may be contaminated with malignant cells. Although disease relapse may be treated by further doses of chemotherapy and even by additional transplantation, these approaches are rarely curative and have high treatment-associated mortality. An alternative approach after allografting is to use the graft-versus-leukemia effect by infusing donor T cells; alloreactive T lymphocytes may then eradicate resurgent host hematopoietic malignancy. Although this approach is associated with a risk of inducing severe GVHD and even marrow aplasia (if host hematopoiesis has come to predominate), it can produce remission in up to 70% of patients with relapsed chronic myeloid leukemia. In combination with chemotherapy, the approach induces prolonged remission in 20% or more of patients with acute myeloid leukemia, and it may also be effective in patients with relapsed myeloma. To date, only anecdotal success has been reported in acute lymphocytic leukemia or lymphoma.

LONG-TERM COMPLICATIONS

Most late effects of bone marrow transplantation are related either to chronic GVHD or to the toxicity of chemotherapy and radiotherapy conditioning regimens. Post-transplant hemolytic-uremic syndrome (also called radiation nephritis) is seen primarily in patients who have received extensive previous chemotherapy. It generally occurs about 6 months post-transplant, and clinical findings include renal insufficiency, hematuria, and anemia with evidence of microangiopathic hemolysis. In most recipients, the syndrome is self-limited and resolves with no specific therapy. Occasionally the course is progressive and renal failure develops. Hemorrhagic cystitis may also occur or recur as a late complication.

The major causes of pulmonary complications during the later post-transplant period are infection and regimen-related toxicity. Bacterial, fungal, and viral infections occurring at this time are usually associated with continuing immune deficiency from chronic GVHD. Less commonly, chronic obstructive lung disease, usually directly associated with chronic GVHD, develops in long-term survivors. The pathologic abnormality is obliteration of the bronchioles. The syndrome responds poorly to therapy with steroids, tends to progress, and has a poor prognosis. Independent of GVHD, a restrictive defect caused by interstitial fibrosis develops in many patients, although this complication is usually asymptomatic and detected only on pulmonary function tests.

The risk of endocrine dysfunction is greater in patients who receive total-body irradiation, and abnormal thyroid function test results will develop in about 50% of such patients. In most cases the abnormality is subclinical, with elevated thyroid-stimulating hormone levels and increased response to thyroid-releasing hormone, but about 10% will eventually require replacement therapy. Growth hormone deficiency may also occur, especially in pediatric patients who have received prior cranial irradiation. In women who receive a transplant post-puberty with total-body irradiation as part of the conditioning regimen, ovarian failure is evidenced by increased levels of follicle-stimulating hormone and luteinizing hormone in the presence of low estrogen. Even conditioning regimens that use chemotherapy alone produce ovarian failure, but some of these patients may recover, and a small number of pregnancies have been reported. Ovarian hormone replacement is generally used in premenopausal women to prevent menopausal symptoms. In men who receive transplants after puberty, testosterone levels remain normal but spermatogenesis rarely recovers.

Cataracts occur in about 20% of patients who have received fractionated total-body irradiation and in almost 80% of patients who have received single-dosage regimens. Steroid therapy is another risk factor for this complication. Cataracts begin to develop between 5 and 10 years post-transplant and respond well to excision. Aseptic osteonecrosis occurs in 10 to 20% of long-term transplant survivors; it primarily involves the hip joints and is exacerbated by steroid therapy for GVHD or by ovarian failure in females. Several studies have shown a higher incidence of a second malignancy in transplant recipients, particularly in those who received radiation as part of their conditioning. In one series of 2246 patients, the relative risk was 6.7 times that observed in the general population adjusted for age. Both lymphoid and myeloid acute leukemias are increased, and the most common post-transplant solid tumors are melanoma and glioblastoma.

OUTCOME

Despite the daunting list of short- and long-term complications, the safety of stem cell transplantation has improved substantially over the past decade. This effect can most readily be seen in patients receiving unrelated donor allografts for hematopoietic malignancies. In the past, these patients had a mortality that was more than 50% higher than that of recipients of grafts from HLA-identical sibling donors treated for the same disease at an equivalent stage of development. As a result of advances in tissue typing, GVHD prophylaxis, and antiviral prophylaxis, the survival rates of these two groups of patients are now nearly identical; a residual excess of procedure-related mortality in the unrelated donor recipients is offset by a lower relapse risk, presumably because of increased graft-versus-leukemia effects. Disease-free survival rates approaching or exceeding 90% can now be expected for individuals with aplastic anemia, chronic myeloid leukemia in the first chronic phase, or thalassemia without liver damage. Conversely, survival rates for patients with advanced malignancy remain low; the combination of both severe regimen-related toxicities in these heavily pre-treated patients and a high relapse rate means that only 5 to 30% may survive 5 years.

FUTURE TRENDS

In allografting, the safety and effectiveness of preparative regimens should continue to improve. The trend has been toward a reduction in the intensity of the preparative regimen, with a correspondingly increased reliance on the ability of the donor immune system to eradicate host hematopoietic and malignant cells. A combination of this approach with the introduction of monoclonal antibodies (coupled to radionuclides or toxins) that specifically target the hematopoietic system without damaging other host organs should reduce the incidence and severity of complications associated with current preparative regimens. "Graft engineering," in which the component cells in a graft are separated and functionally modified, will probably be of increasing importance. These modifications are intended to produce a graft that lacks the capacity to induce GVHD but retains activity against pathogens and residual malignancy. The availability of improved growth factors with activity on stem cells and on all hematopoietic lineages should enable rapid ex vivo and/or in vivo expansion of the donor hematopoietic cells, thereby accelerating engraftment and minimizing the consequence of marrow aplasia. Finally, it is likely that hematopoietic stem cells will increasingly be used as vehicles for gene transfer to allow autologous transplantation to be curative for a number of inherited and acquired disorders currently amenable only to allogeneic therapies.

Armitage JO: Bone marrow transplantation. N Engl J Med 330:827, 1994. *An excellent overview of the indications for marrow transplantation.*

Blazar BR, Korngold R, Vallera DA: Advances in graft-versus-host disease (GvHD) prevention. Immunol Rev 157:79, 1997. *Reviews the biology and treatment of this complication.*

Brenner MK: Gene transfer to hematopoietic cells: N Engl J Med 335:337, 1996. *Summarizes the potential and the problems of hematopoietic stem cell gene therapy.*

Gerson SL: Mesenchymal stem cells: No longer second class marrow citizens. Nature Med 5:262, 1999. *A description of mesenchymal cells in marrow and their possible applications after transplantation.*

Giralt S, Estey E, Ibitar M, et al: Engraftment of allogeneic hematopoietic progenitor cells with purine analog-containing chemotherapy harnessing graft versus leukemia without myeloablative chemotherapy. Blood 89:4531, 1997. *How the immune system can help eradicate leukemia in the absence of ablative conditioning.*

Hansen JA, Petersdorf E, Martin PJ, et al: Hematopoietic stem cell transplants from unrelated donors. Immunol Rev 157:141, 1997. *A review of unrelated donor transplants.*

Kolb HJ, Poetscher C: Late effects after allogeneic bone marrow transplantation. Curr Opin Hematol 4:401, 1997. *A good discussion of the longer-term problems of the procedure and how they affect quality of life.*

Rubinstein P, Carrier C, Scaradavou A, et al: Outcomes among 562 recipients of placental blood transplants from unrelated donors. N Engl J Med 339:1565, 1998. *A large-scale multicenter account of the use of cord blood transplantation, mainly in patients with malignant disease.*

183 APPROACH TO THE PATIENT WITH BLEEDING AND THROMBOSIS

Andrew I. Schafer

MECHANISMS OF HEMOSTASIS AND THROMBOSIS

The intimal surface of the vasculature throughout the circulatory tree is lined by a monolayer of endothelial cells. These cells constitutively express anticoagulant properties that promote blood fluidity under normal circumstances. At a site of vascular injury, however, endothelial cells are either "activated," and are thereby converted from an antithrombotic to a prothrombotic state, or become detached to expose circulating blood to thrombogenic constituents of the subendothelial vessel wall. These processes result in the rapid formation of a hemostatic plug that consists of platelets and fibrin. Activation of platelets and formation of fibrin occur essentially simultaneously and interdependently to effect hemostasis. Subsequently, vessel wall repair is accomplished by thrombolysis and recanalization of the occluded site.

In the presence of intact endothelium, platelets are repelled from the vessel wall and circulate passively. Prostacyclin and nitric oxide are among the potent, locally active platelet inhibitors (and vasodilators) that are elaborated by normal endothelial cells to promote blood fluidity. At a site of vascular damage, these antiplatelet substances are lost, and platelets adhere to the de-endothelialized intimal surface. Platelet "adhesion" (platelet–vessel wall interaction) is mediated by von Willebrand factor, which anchors the platelets to the vessel wall by binding to its platelet receptors localized in membrane glycoprotein Ib (GPIb). Adherent platelets then undergo the "release reaction," during which they discharge constituents of their storage granules, including adenosine diphosphate (ADP), and synthesize thromboxane A_2 (TXA_2) from arachidonic acid by means of the aspirin-inhibitable cyclooxygenase reaction. ADP, TXA_2, and other components of the release reaction then act in concert to recruit and activate additional platelets from the circulation to the site of vascular injury. These activated platelets expose binding sites for fibrinogen by forming the surface membrane glycoprotein IIb-IIIa (GPIIb-IIIa) complex. In the process of platelet "aggregation" (platelet-platelet interactions), fibrinogen (or von Willebrand factor under conditions of high shear stress) mediates the formation of an occlusive platelet plug.

The fibrin, which anchors the hemostatic platelet plug, is formed from soluble plasma fibrinogen by the action of the potent protease enzyme thrombin (Fig. 183–1). The fibrin mesh is then stabilized by covalent crosslinking mediated by Factor XIII. Thrombin is formed from its inactive (zymogen) plasma precursor, prothrombin, by the action of activated Factor X (Xa) and its cofactor, Factor Va. This sequence of reactions has been classically referred to as the "common pathway" of coagulation. Factor X can be activated, in turn, by either the tissue factor ("extrinsic") pathway or the contact activation ("intrinsic") pathway of coagulation. The former is initiated by the complex of tissue factor and Factor VIIa. The latter involves a series (or cascade) of zymogen-protease reactions that are initiated by contact activation of Factor XII to XIIa. High-molecular-weight kininogen and prekallikrein are two other plasma protein components of the contact activation system that leads to the generation of Factor XIIa. Factor XIIa then converts Factor XI to XIa, followed by Factor XIa–mediated activation of Factor IX to IXa. Factor IXa then serves as the enzyme to convert Factor X to Xa, a reaction that requires Factor VIIIa as a cofactor.

In the interpretation of screening in vitro laboratory tests of coagulation, it is still convenient to separate the "extrinsic" and "intrinsic" pathways of coagulation that converge as alternative

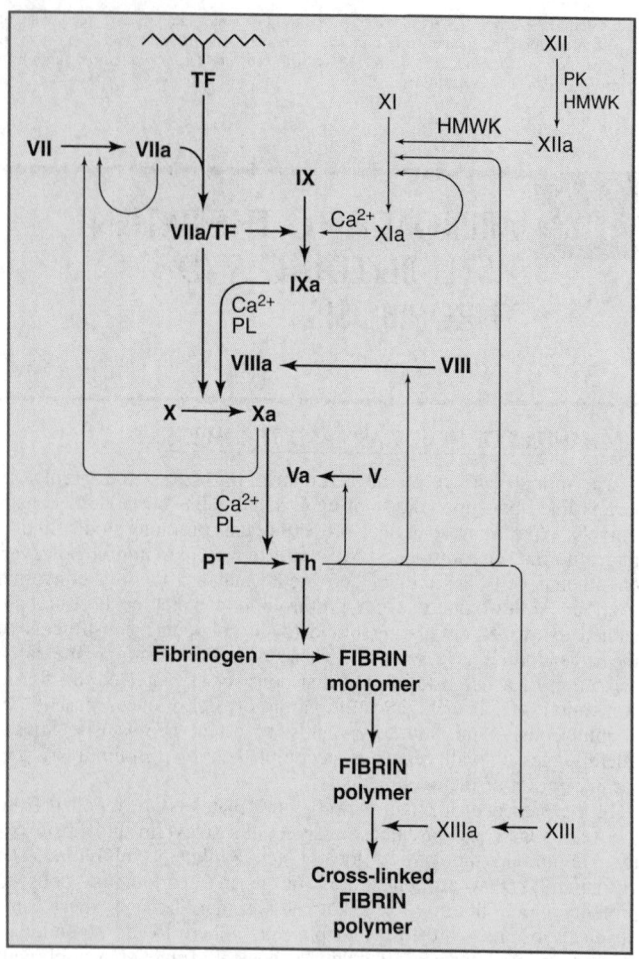

FIGURE 183–1 ■ The coagulation cascade. This scheme emphasizes recent understanding of (1) the importance of the tissue factor pathway in initiating clotting in vivo; (2) the interactions between pathways; and (3) the pivotal role of thrombin in sustaining the cascade by feedback activation of coagulation factors. HMWK = high-molecular-weight kininogen; PK = prekallikrein; PL = phospholipid; PT = prothrombin; TF = tissue factor; Th = thrombin. (From Schafer AI: Coagulation cascade: An overview. In Loscalzo J, Schafer AI [eds]: Thrombosis and Hemorrhage. Cambridge, MA, Blackwell Scientific Publications, 1994, pp 3–12.)

prekallikrein, Factor XII) has cast doubt on the physiologic importance of the intrinsic pathway in hemostasis.

Just as intact, normal endothelium promotes blood fluidity by inhibiting platelet activation, it likewise plays a critical role in naturally anticoagulating blood by preventing fibrin accumulation. Among the physiologic antithrombotic systems that produce this effect are (1) antithrombin III; (2) protein C and protein S; (3) tissue factor pathway inhibitor (TFPI); and (4) the fibrinolytic system. Antithrombin is the major protease inhibitor of the coagulation system: it inactivates thrombin, as well as other activated coagulation factors. Heparin functions as an anticoagulant by binding to antithrombin and thereby greatly accelerating its ability to inhibit the coagulation proteases. Heparin and heparin sulfate proteoglycans are naturally present on endothelial cells, so antithrombin inactivation of thrombin and other coagulation proteases most likely occurs physiologically on vascular surfaces rather than in fluid phase plasma. Activated protein C, with its cofactor, protein S, functions as a natural anticoagulant by destroying Factors Va and VIIIa, two essential cofactors of the coagulation cascade. Thrombin itself is the activator of protein C, and this reaction again occurs rapidly only on the surfaces of intact vascular endothelial cells where thrombin binds to the glycosaminoglycan thrombomodulin. Thus, in the presence of normal vessel wall intima, small amounts of thrombin that are generated in the circulation bind to endothelial cell thrombomodulin, thereby not only removing it from the circulation but also activating anticoagulant protein C, which inhibits its further production. TFPI is another plasma protease inhibitor that quenches tissue factor–induced coagulation. Although inherited deficiencies of antithrombin, protein C or protein S are associated with a lifelong thrombotic tendency (hypercoagulable state), TFPI deficiency has not yet been related to clinical problems. Finally, what little fibrin can be produced, despite these potent physiologic antithrombotic mechanisms, is rapidly digested by the endogenous fibrinolytic system, in which endothelium-derived tissue plasminogen activator (t-PA) converts the plasma zymogen, plasminogen, to the active fibrinolytic protease, plasmin.

Thrombus formation occurs wherever vascular damage causes loss of the natural endothelium-dependent antiplatelet and anticoagulant mechanisms or in disorders in which one or more of these protective systems is deficient. Thrombi are composed of platelets and fibrin, although their relative contributions vary with the site of thrombosis: the former tend to predominate in the high-shear arterial circulation, whereas the latter predominate in the venous system. Regardless of the site of thrombus formation, platelet activation and fibrin production occur simultaneously and in an interdependent manner: thrombin generation occurs most efficiently on the surfaces of activated platelets, whereas thrombin itself is a potent stimulus for further platelet activation.

EVALUATION OF THE PATIENT WITH A POSSIBLE BLEEDING DISORDER

There are three general clinical settings in which patients may be required to undergo evaluation for a possible bleeding disorder. First, patients may present with a history or physical signs of bleeding that provoke suspicion of a systemic coagulopathy. Sec-

mechanisms to activate Factor X, leading to the "common" pathway that culminates in fibrin formation. However, it is now understood that this is an inaccurate oversimplification of the situation in vivo. For example, Factor IX (an intrinsic factor) can be activated by Factor VII (an extrinsic factor). Furthermore, the absence of any clinical bleeding problems in patients with inherited deficiencies of the contact activation factors (high-molecular-weight kininogen,

Table 183–1 ■ CHARACTERISTIC PATTERNS OF BLEEDING IN SYSTEMIC DISORDERS OF HEMOSTASIS

TYPE OF DISORDER	SITES OF BLEEDING				ONSET OF BLEEDING	CLINICAL EXAMPLES
	General	Skin	Mucous Membranes	Others		
Platelet-vascular disorders	Superficial surfaces	Petechiae, ecchymoses	Common: oral, nasal, gastrointestinal, genitourinary	Rare	Spontaneous or immediately after trauma	Thrombocytopenia, functional platelet disorder, vascular fragility Disseminated intravascular coagulation, liver disease
Coagulation factor deficiency	Deep tissues	Hematomas	Rare	Common: joint, muscle, retroperitoneal	Delayed after trauma	Inherited coagulation factor deficiency, acquired inhibitor, anticoagulation Disseminated intravascular coagulation, liver disease

ond, asymptomatic patients may be incidentally discovered to have laboratory abnormalities that suggest a bleeding disorder. Third, patients may be asked to undergo routine testing for bleeding risk before surgery or an invasive procedure.

A thorough history is of paramount importance in all three of these settings. Not only should the patient be asked about spontaneous bleeding episodes in the past, but the response to specific hemostatic challenges should also be recorded. A bleeding tendency may be suspected if a patient has experienced excessive hemorrhage after previous surgery or trauma, including commonly encountered events, such as circumcision, tonsillectomy, labor and delivery, menses, dental procedures, vaccinations, and injections. Conversely, the history of normal blood clotting after such challenges in the recent past is at least as important to note because it may provide a better test of systemic hemostasis than any laboratory measurement could provide.

Evaluation of the Patient With a History of Bleeding

In a patient with a history of excessive or unexplained bleeding, the initial problem is to determine whether the cause is a systemic coagulopathy or an anatomic or mechanical problem. This situation is most frequently encountered in postoperative patients with excessive bleeding. A history of prior bleeding suggests a coagulopathy, as does the finding of bleeding from multiple sites. However, even diffuse bleeding may arise from anatomic rather than hemostatic abnormalities (e.g., recurrent mucosal hemorrhage in patients with hereditary hemorrhagic telangiectasia). Conversely, a single episode of bleeding from an isolated site may be the initial manifestation of a systemic coagulopathy.

The history must also include a survey of coexisting systemic diseases and drug ingestion that may affect hemostasis. For example, renal failure and the myeloproliferative disorders are associated with impaired platelet–vessel wall interactions and qualitative platelet abnormalities, connective tissue disease and lymphomas are associated with thrombocytopenia, and liver disease causes a complex coagulopathy. Aspirin and other non-steroidal anti-inflammatory drugs cause platelet dysfunction: these drugs are often contained in over-the-counter preparations that patients may neglect to report without specific questioning. Other drugs, such as antibiotics, also may be associated with a bleeding tendency by causing abnormal platelet function or thrombocytopenia. Finally, it is important to elicit a family history of bleeding problems. Whereas a positive history provides a clue to a possible inherited coagulopathy, a negative history does not exclude a familial etiology; for example, up to 20% of patients with classic hemophilia have a completely negative family history of bleeding.

Patterns of clinical bleeding, as revealed by the history and physical examination, may be characteristic of certain types of coagulopathy (Table 183–1). In general, patients with thrombocytopenia or qualitative platelet and vascular disorders present with bleeding from superficial sites in the skin and mucus membranes; these may involve petechiae, which are pinpoint cutaneous hemorrhages that appear particularly over dependent extremities (characteristic of severe thrombocytopenia), ecchymoses (common bruises), purpura, gastrointestinal and genitourinary tract bleeding, epistaxis, and hemoptysis. In these disorders, bleeding from these sites tends to occur spontaneously or immediately after trauma. In contrast, patients with inherited or acquired coagulation factor deficiencies, such as hemophilia or therapeutic anticoagulation, tend to bleed from deeper tissue sites (e.g., hemarthroses, deep hematomas, retroperitoneal hemorrhage) and in a delayed manner after trauma.

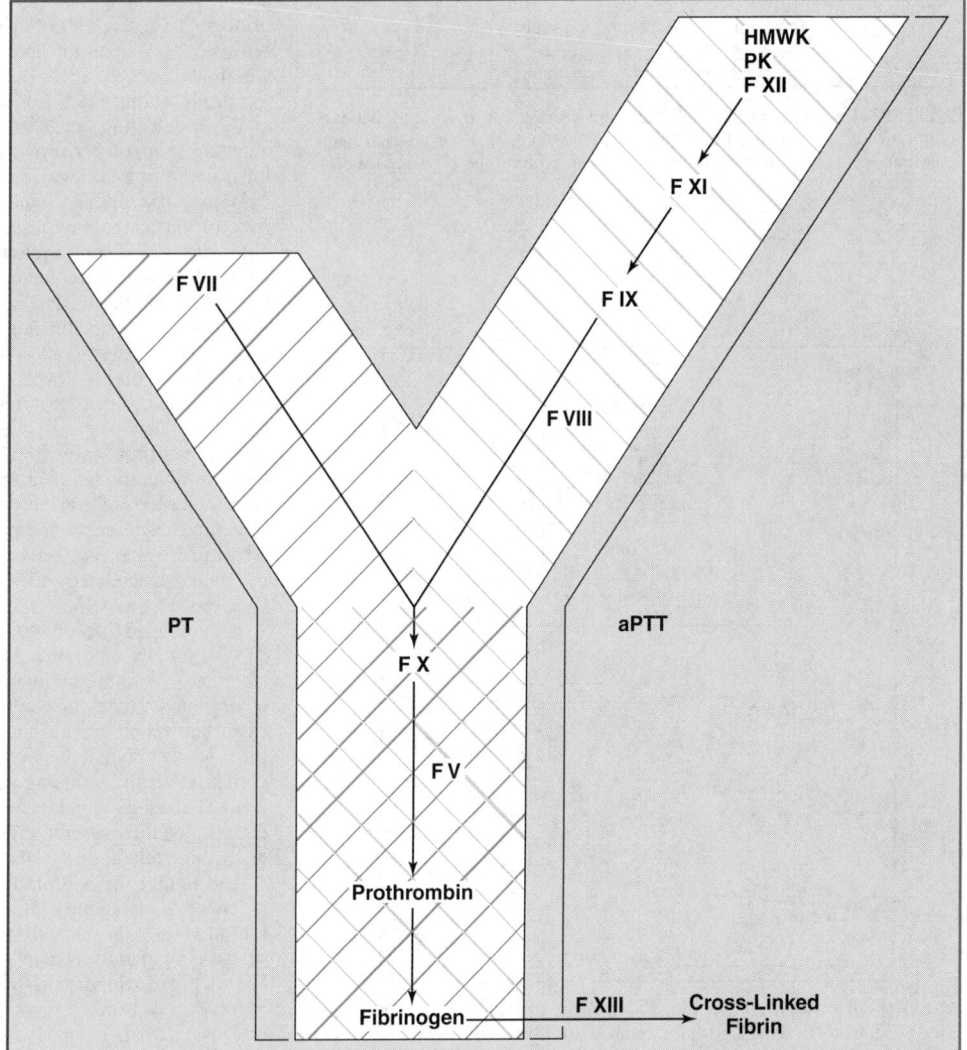

FIGURE 183–2 ■ Classic coagulation cascade, in which the prothrombin time (PT) measures the integrity of the extrinsic and common pathways, while the activated partial thromboplastin time (aPTT) measures the integrity of the intrinsic and common pathways. Note that Factor (F) XIII deficiency is not detected by the PT or aPTT. HMWK = high-molecular-weight kininogen; PK = prekallikrein.

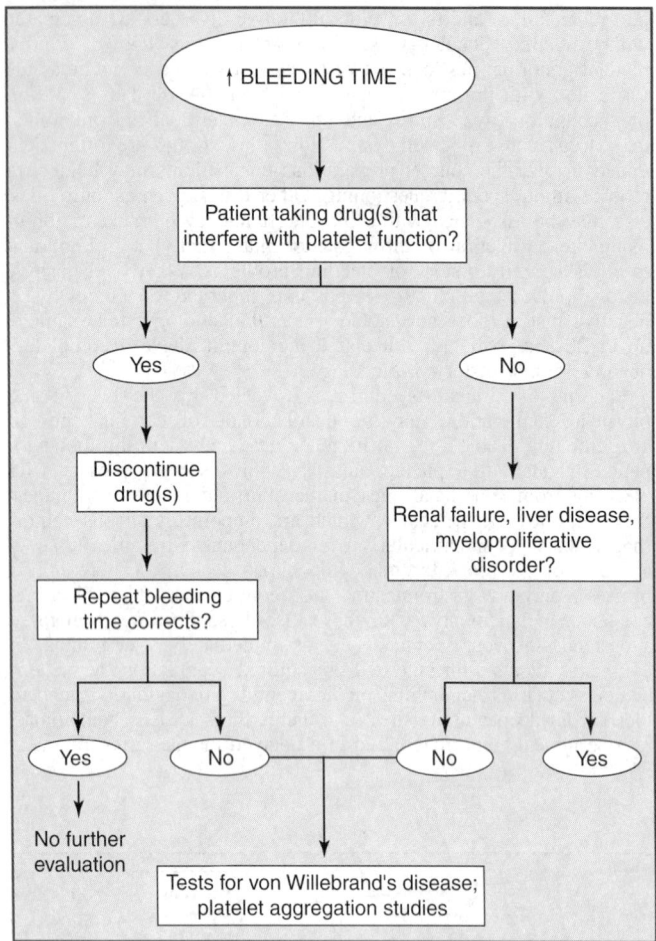

FIGURE 183-3 ■ An algorithm for diagnostic decisions in evaluating patients with a prolonged bleeding time. The scheme assumes that the platelet count is normal, because thrombocytopenia itself can prolong the bleeding time.

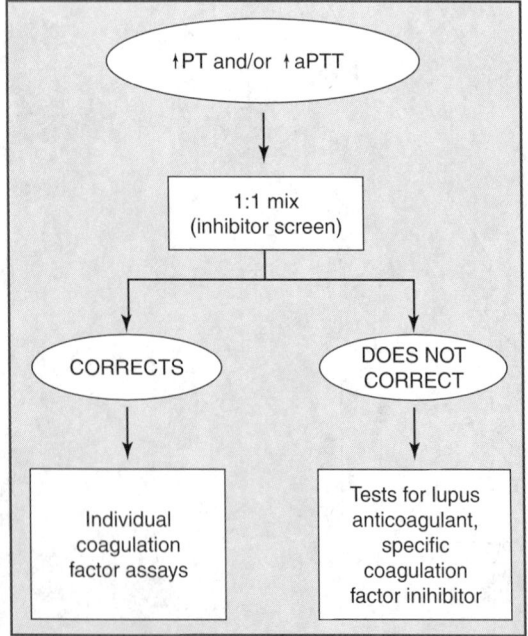

FIGURE 183-4 ■ Approach to evaluating patients with prolonged prothrombin time (PT) and/or activated partial thromboplastin time (aPTT).

Four simple, rapid screening tests are generally used in the initial evaluation of patients with a suspected coagulopathy: (1) platelet count, (2) bleeding time, (3) prothrombin time (PT), and (4) activated partial thromboplastin time (aPTT). It is also from one or more of these tests that asymptomatic individuals may be incidentally found to have abnormalities that suggest a bleeding disorder and prompt further evaluation.

Thrombocytopenia, routinely reported by electronic particle counting, should be verified by examination of the peripheral smear. "Pseudothrombocytopenia," a laboratory artifact of ex vivo platelet clumping, may be caused by the EDTA anticoagulant used in tubes for blood cell counts, other anticoagulants, or cold agglutinins acting at room temperature; it should be suspected whenever a very low platelet count is reported in a patient who does not exhibit any clinical bleeding, and it has no known pathologic correlates. Pseudothrombocytopenia is indicated by the finding of platelet clumps on the peripheral smear, and the diagnosis is supported by the finding of simultaneously normal platelet counts in blood samples obtained by fingerstick, in tubes containing other anticoagulants, or when the tube of blood is maintained at 37° C before platelet counting. Examination of the blood smear in patients with real thrombocytopenia can also reveal clues to the cause, such as fragmented red cells in thrombotic thrombocytopenic purpura.

The bleeding time is the most widely used clinical screening test for disorders of platelet–vessel wall interactions. It measures the time to cessation of bleeding after a standardized incision over the volar aspect of the forearm, now most commonly performed by disposable automated devices. The bleeding time is prolonged in (1) thrombocytopenia, (2) qualitative platelet abnormalities, (3) defects in platelet–vessel wall interactions (e.g., von Willebrand's disease), or (4) primary vascular disorders. The bleeding time usually is not prolonged in patients with coagulation factor deficiencies. However, the test is prone to problems of reproducibility, sensitivity, and specificity.

The PT measures the integrity of the extrinsic and common pathways of coagulation (Factors VII, X, V, prothrombin, and fibrinogen) (Fig. 183-2). The aPTT measures the integrity of the intrinsic and common pathways of coagulation (high-molecular-weight kininogen; prekallikrein; Factors XII, XI, IX, VIII, X, and V; prothrombin; and fibrinogen). The sensitivity of the PT and aPTT in detecting coagulation factor deficiencies may vary with the reagents used to perform these tests, and therefore each laboratory must determine its own reference standards.

With a few notable exceptions, as follows, normal results for all four of the screening tests of hemostasis essentially exclude any clinically significant systemic coagulopathy. Patients with Factor XIII deficiency may have a serious bleeding diathesis but have normal screening tests; specific tests for Factor XIII deficiency should be performed when this disease is suspected. The PT and aPTT detect only more severe deficiencies of coagulation factors, generally involving levels of less than 30% of normal; therefore, specific factor levels should be determined if a mild coagulation factor deficiency is suspected. Patients with von Willebrand's disease sometimes have normal bleeding times and usually do not have sufficiently reduced levels of Factor VIII to affect the aPTT. Rare disorders of fibrinolysis may also be associated with normal screening tests, necessitating more specialized tests when indicated. Abnormalities in the screening tests of hemostasis may be pursued by more specialized tests to establish a specific diagnosis (see Chapters 184 to 187).

A prolonged bleeding time in the absence of thrombocytopenia should initially be approached by determining if the patient is taking any drugs that might interfere with platelet function (e.g., aspirin, other non-steroidal anti-inflammatory drugs) or has coexisting diseases that might explain the finding (e.g., renal failure) (Fig. 183-3). If these conditions are not found, or if the bleeding time fails to correct after discontinuing any potential offending drugs, further specialized testing may include platelet aggregation studies to identify specific qualitative abnormalities of platelet function and specific assays to exclude one of the types of von Willebrand's disease.

The finding of a prolonged PT and/or aPTT indicates that there is either a deficiency of one or more coagulation factors or an inhibitor, usually an antibody, directed at one or more components of the coagulation system (Fig. 183-4). These two possibilities can be readily distinguished by performing an inhibitor screen, which involves a 1:1 mix of patient and normal plasma. The premise of the test is that, even if a patient's plasma is completely deficient

Table 183–2 ▪ CLINICAL CHARACTERISTICS OF PATIENTS
WITH INHERITED HYPERCOAGULABLE STATES

Venous thromboembolism (>90% of cases)
  Deep vein thrombosis of lower limbs (common)
  Pulmonary embolism (common)
  Superficial thrombophlebitis
  Mesenteric vein thrombosis (rare but characteristic)
  Cerebral vein thrombosis (rare but characteristic)
Frequent family history of thrombosis*
First thrombosis usually at young age (<40 yr)*
Frequent recurrences*
Neonatal purpura fulminans (homozygous protein C and protein S deficiency)

*All these features are less evident in patients with activated protein C resistance, who appear to be less severely affected clinically.
  From De Stefano V, Finazzi G, Manucci PM: Inherited thrombophilia: Pathogenesis, clinical syndromes, and management. Blood 87:3531–3544, 1996.

(0% level) in a certain factor, mixing it 1:1 with normal plasma (100% level) should bring the concentration of the factor to 50% of the mixture, which, as noted earlier, is sufficient to correct the prolonged PT and/or aPTT; then, individual coagulation factor levels should be assayed for a specific deficiency state. If the 1:1 mix fails to correct the prolonged PT and/or aPTT, an inhibitor is likely to be present in the patient's plasma and to be interfering with coagulation in both patient and normal plasma; then specific assays should be performed to determine if there is a true inhibitor against a coagulation factor (e.g., Factor VIII antibody) or if the inhibitor is a lupus anticoagulant.

Evaluation of the Asymptomatic Patient With Abnormal Coagulation Tests

In asymptomatic individuals who are incidentally discovered to have abnormalities in screening laboratory tests of hemostasis, the first critical question is whether the findings are clinically relevant. For example, patients with inherited deficiencies of one of the contact activation coagulation factors (Factor XII, high-molecular-weight kininogen, prekallikrein) characteristically have a markedly prolonged aPTT, yet they clearly do not have a clinical bleeding tendency. Likewise, patients with lupus anticoagulants typically have prolongations of the aPTT, and sometimes also the PT; yet they more often have thrombotic rather than bleeding complications. In patients with heparin-induced thrombocytopenia, a marked decrease in the platelet count is sometimes associated with arterial and venous thrombosis. It is, therefore, critically important to view the clinical setting, history, physical examination, and screening laboratory tests as complementary facets of the approach to patients with suspected coagulopathies.

Evaluation of the Preoperative Patient

The platelet count, bleeding time, PT, and aPTT have become widely ingrained in surgical practice as components of a coagulation panel to screen patients for bleeding risk before elective surgery. However, increasing evidence from many studies now indicates that such routine screening of all preoperative patients is not only uninformative but may even be counterproductive when follow-up testing causes unnecessary expense and delays in the surgery. Preoperative bleeding time, PT, and aPTT do not predict surgical bleeding risk in patients who are not found to be at increased risk on clinical grounds, so a thorough clinical assessment should serve as the guide to the need for obtaining these preoperative screening tests. Laboratory testing, and possibly further specialized tests of coagulation, is clearly indicated in patients whose bleeding histories are suspicious for a hemostatic abnormality. Preoperative screening tests of coagulation are probably also warranted in patients in whom adequate clinical assessment is impossible, as well as in those who are to undergo procedures in which even minimal postoperative hemorrhage could be hazardous.

EVALUATION OF THE PATIENT WITH A POSSIBLE HYPERCOAGULABLE STATE

Many, and possibly most, patients with venous thromboembolism have an inherited basis for hypercoagulability (see Chapter 187). Most patients with inherited hypercoagulable states (or thrombophilia) present with their initial episode of venous thromboembolism in early adulthood, but thrombotic manifestations may begin at any time from early childhood to old age. Patients typically have deep vein thrombosis of the lower extremities or pulmonary embolism, but other unusual sites of venous thrombosis may be involved. Arterial thrombosis is distinctly unusual in patients with inherited hypercoagulable states, with the exception of hyperhomocysteinemia. Arterial thrombosis that occurs prematurely or in the absence of apparent risk factors should trigger a different line of investigation, including possible evaluation for vasculitis, myeloproliferative disorders, antiphospholipid syndrome, and other acquired disorders, as well as potential sources of systemic embolization.

The primary or hereditary hypercoagulable states (see Table 187–1) result from specific mutations, mostly in genes encoding a plasma protein that serves as a physiologic anticoagulant. The hereditary form of heterozygous hyperhomocysteinemia, which often presents in adulthood with venous or arterial thrombosis, is caused by discrete mutations in the enzymes that mediate homocysteine metabolism. In contrast, the secondary or acquired hypercoagulable states (see Fig. 187–1) represent a heterogeneous group of disorders that predispose to thrombosis by complex mechanisms. Venous thrombosis is often precipitated by the combination of a hypercoagulable phenotype and an acquired prothrombotic, hypercoagulable state, such as pregnancy, immobilization, or the postoperative state. Certain clinical characteristics suggest the presence of an inherited hypercoagulable state (Table 183–2). Patients with recurrent thrombosis should be tested for these disorders and, in most cases, committed to lifelong prophylactic anticoagulation. It is not clear at this time whether or not it is essential to order these tests after a single episode of venous thromboembolism. Even when patients are not maintained on chronic anticoagulation, those with diagnosed primary hypercoagulable states should receive prophylactic anticoagulation during situations that pose a high risk for thrombosis, such as the peripartum period. There is no simple screening test(s) for primary hypercoagulable states, and the timing of obtaining these tests is critical to avoid erroneous diagnoses. Acute thrombosis itself can cause transient decreases in the levels of antithrombin, protein C, and protein S. Heparin therapy can cause a decrease in plasma antithrombin activity. Warfarin therapy lowers the functional levels of protein C and protein S. Therefore, inherited deficiency states can be spuriously diagnosed under these conditions.

Patients who present with venous thromboembolism probably have an increased risk of harboring an occult malignancy. This association is further increased in those who have recurrent and idiopathic thrombosis. Evaluation for occult malignancy in these patients need not be exhaustive, however, and can be limited to a thorough history, physical examination, a routine complete blood cell count and chemistries, test of fecal occult blood, urinalysis, mammogram (in women) and chest radiograph; further testing should then be guided only by any abnormalities found in this initial evaluation.

In addition to classic deep vein thrombosis and pulmonary embolism, certain characteristic types of thrombosis may provide important clues to the etiology and trigger specific evaluation. Migratory, superficial thrombophlebitis (Trousseau's syndrome), or non-bacterial thrombotic endocarditis suggest the presence of an occult malignancy. Hepatic vein thrombosis (Budd-Chiari syndrome) or portal vein thrombosis might be indicative of a myeloproliferative disorder or paroxysmal nocturnal hemoglobinuria. Warfarin-induced skin necrosis strongly suggests an underlying protein C or protein S deficiency. Recurrent, spontaneous miscarriages are associated with the antiphospholipid syndrome.

Clemetson KJ: Primary haemostasis: sticky fingers cement the relationship. Curr Biol 9:R110, 1999. *Current concepts of the basic mechanisms of platelet aggregation and hemostatic plug formation.*
De Stefano V, Finazzi G, Mannucci PM: Inherited thrombophilia: Pathogenesis, clinical syndromes, and management. Blood 87:3531, 1996. *Comprehensive review of the major primary hypercoagulable states currently recognized.*

184 HEMORRHAGIC DISORDERS: ABNORMALITIES OF PLATELET AND VASCULAR FUNCTION

Marc Shuman

The normal sequence of events leading to clotting is initiated by trauma to the vessel, which constricts reflexively to reduce blood flow. Platelets adhere to the subendothelial matrix in the injured vessel, and platelet aggregation and thrombus formation begin simultaneously (see Chapter 183). A variety of drugs can interfere with different aspects of hemostasis (Table 184–1), and therefore a medication history is particularly important.

PATHOLOGIC HEMOSTASIS. Thrombus formation is similar to normal hemostasis except that abnormalities in activation, inhibition, or fibrinolysis result in pathologic clots. Derangements may occur in (1) the vessel wall, e.g., atherosclerosis; (2) platelets, e.g., myeloproliferative disorders; and (3) regulation of the coagulation system, e.g., antithrombin III deficiency, Factor V Leiden, etc. Anatomic and/or biochemical alterations of the vascular intima are by far the most frequent causes of pathologic thrombosis. A variety of pathologic alterations of the vessel wall modify endothelial function in a prothrombotic fashion. At one extreme, the endothelial lining may be physically disrupted with exposure of circulating blood to extracellular matrix and tissue factor. Also, several substances may induce intact endothelium to promote thrombosis. Thus interleukin-1 (IL-1), tumor necrosis factor, and endotoxin increase both endothelial plasminogen activator inhibitor type 1, inhibitor of fibrinolysis, and endothelial tissue factor. Moreover, endothelial cells express receptors for several of the coagulation factors, including Factors Va, IXa, and Xa, so that once coagulation is initiated, it can be amplified on the endothelial cell surface. It is not difficult to imagine how rupture of an atherosclerotic plaque results in pathologic initiation of clotting that terminates in vascular occlusion. Thrombosis is an important event in atherosclerotic vascular disease: (1) platelet thrombi are found in the coronary circulation in fatal myocardial infarction, and (2) fibrinolytic therapy can restore blood flow early in coronary occlusion.

BLOOD PLATELETS

FORMATION AND KINETICS. Platelets are disk-shaped cells 2 to 4 mm in diameter normally found in the peripheral blood (150,000 to 300,000 per microliter). In Wright-stained blood smears, they are identified by their blue-gray cytoplasm and red (lysosomal) granules and by lack of a nucleus.

Platelets are formed in the bone marrow from giant polyploid cells called megakaryocytes. Megakaryocytes mature by a series of nuclear replications within a common cytoplasm (endomitosis) that lead to four- to six-lobed nuclei, as well as by elaboration of specific granules in the cytoplasm. Following maturation, the megakaryocyte cytoplasm becomes demarcated into platelet subunits, and the platelets are released into the circulation through the marrow sinusoids. A hematopoietic growth factor specific for megakaryocytes, thrombopoietin, has been identified. Various forms of the recombinant protein are currently being tested in clinical trials. The expectation is that it will be approved for the treatment of patients with thrombocytopenia caused by inadequate production of platelets. IL-11 also stimulates platelet production. IL-11 has been approved for use in patients with thrombocytopenia secondary to treatment of malignancy with high-dose chemotherapy.

Ordinarily, each megakaryocyte produces 1000 to 3000 platelets. Normally, 3 to 10 megakaryocytes are seen in bone marrow smears under low-power magnification, but none appear in peripheral blood. Platelets circulate for 9 to 10 days. Approximately one third reside in a splenic pool, which exchanges freely with the circulating pool. In diseases associated with platelet antibodies, the spleen is frequently the site of destruction. In addition, in disorders causing secondary splenic enlargement, thrombocytopenia may result from splenic sequestration (see Chapter 178). Conversely, follow-

Table 184–1 ■ DRUGS THAT MAY ALTER HEMOSTASIS

Drugs Reported to Cause Thrombocytopenia
 Immune mechanism proposed*

Quinine/quinidine	Ranitidine
Sulfa compounds	Cimetidine
Ampicillin	Danazol
Penicillin	Procainamide
Thiazide diuretics	Carbamazepine
Furosemide	Acetaminophen
Chlorthalidone	Phenylbutazone
Phenytoin	*p*-Aminosalicylate
α-Methyldopa	Rifampin
Heparin	Acetazolamide
Digitalis derivatives	Anazolene
Aspirin	Arsenicals
Valproic acid	

 Non-immune mechanisms
  (Hemolytic-uremic syndrome/thrombotic thrombocytopenic purpura)
  Ticlopidine
  Mitomycin
  Cisplatin
  Cyclosporine
 Mechanism undefined
  Gold compounds
  Indomethacin
Drugs That Alter Platelet Function
 Primary antiplatelet agents

Aspirin	Sulfinpyrazone
Dextran	Ticlopidine
Dipyridamole	

 Drugs in which inhibition of platelet function is associated with prolongation of the bleeding time
  Non-steroidal anti-inflammatory agents
  β-Lactam antibiotics
  ε-Aminocaproic acid (>24 g/day)
  Heparin
  Plasminogen activators (streptokinase, urokinase, tissue plasminogen activator)
Drugs That Affect Coagulation Factors
 Induction of antibodies inhibiting function
  Lupus anticoagulant†‡
   Phenothiazines
   Procainamide
  Factor VIII antibodies
   Penicillin
  Factor V antibodies
   Aminoglycosides
  Factor XIII antibodies
   Isoniazid
  Inhibitors of synthesis of vitamin K–dependent clotting factors (Factors II, VII, IX, X; proteins C and S)
   Coumarin compounds
   Moxalactam
  Inhibitor of fibrinogen synthesis
   L-Asparaginase‡

*The list is limited to drugs for which there are multiple reports and in vitro or in vivo evidence of antiplatelet antibodies.
†Does not cause bleeding.
‡May cause thrombosis.

ing splenectomy, the platelet count may increase transiently to 10^6 per microliter.

An estimate of platelet number in the peripheral blood film (normal, increased, decreased) is useful in detecting patients with abnormally low platelet counts. Normally, 3 to 10 platelets per high-power (oil immersion) field appear on peripheral smears. Platelets are counted directly by an automated particle counter.

PLATELET FUNCTION. Platelets contain three types of secretory granules: lysosomes, α-granules, and dense bodies (electron-dense organelles) (Fig. 184–1). α-Granules contain platelet-specific proteins: platelet factor 4, β-thromboglobulin, and several growth factors, including platelet-derived growth factor, platelet-derived endothelial cell growth factor, and transforming growth factor β. α-Granules also contain several hemostatic proteins, including fibrinogen, Factor V, and von Willebrand factor, which is synthesized by megakaryocytes. Dense bodies (δ-granules) contain adenosine triphosphate, adenose diphosphate (ADP), Ca^{2+}, and serotonin.

In addition to release of potent vasoconstrictors from intracellular

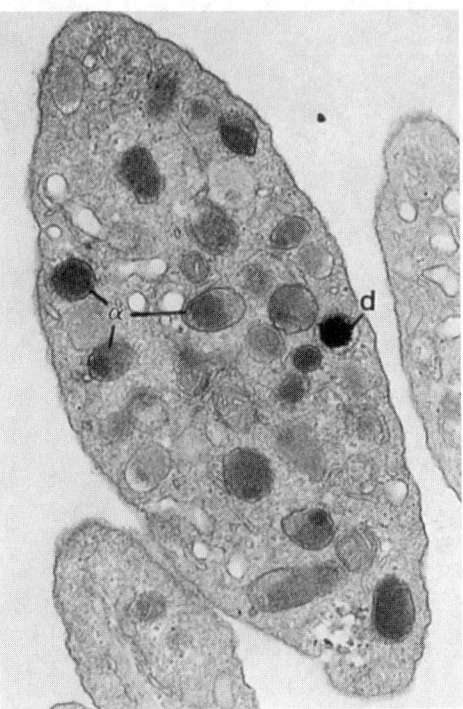

FIGURE 184–1 ■ Electron micrograph of an unstimulated platelet. α = α-granule; d = dense body (×24,000). (Courtesy of Dr. Dorothy Bainton, University of California, San Francisco.)

granules in response to a variety of substances and aggregation to form a plug at the site of vessel injury, platelets provide a surface for the activation of soluble coagulation factors (Fig. 184–2). Activated platelets expose specific receptors that bind Factor Xa and Va and in this way increase their local concentration, thus accelerating prothrombin activation. Factor X is also activated by Factors IXa and VIII (antihemophilic factor) on the platelet surface.

Platelets contain a membrane phospholipase C that, upon stimulation by activating agents, hydrolyzes endogenous phosphatidylinositol to form a diglyceride. The diglyceride, in turn, is converted to arachidonic acid by a diglyceride lipase. Arachidonic acid is a substrate for prostaglandin synthetase (cyclooxygenase), a reaction inhibited by aspirin and non-steroidal anti-inflammatory drugs, and is subsequently converted to prostaglandins. The prostaglandin endoperoxide PGG_2 is required for ADP-induced aggregation and release; both PGG_2 and thromboxane A_2 are potent platelet-aggregating agents.

PLATELET FUNCTION TESTS. BLEEDING TIME. (See Chapter 183.) The bleeding time is prolonged when the platelet count falls below 90,000 per microliter or when a functional platelet abnormality exists. Von Willebrand disease prolongs the bleeding time not as a result of a platelet defect but rather because of the lack of a plasma factor important for normal platelet function. Although imperfect, the bleeding time is the only test of platelet function that correlates with susceptibility to bleeding. Even though patients with a prolonged bleeding time may be at risk for increased bleeding with surgery, not all have abnormal bleeding.

PLATELET AGGREGOMETRY. The response of platelets to a variety of aggregating agents can be quantitated in platelet-rich plasma or whole blood. The aggregometer measures temporal, semiquantitative, and qualitative parameters of in vitro aggregation. This technique is of greatest value in diagnosing congenital qualitative platelet disorders.

ABNORMALITIES IN PLATELET COUNT

Thrombocytopenia

Low platelet counts (thrombocytopenia) (Fig. 184–3) can be caused by disturbances in production, distribution, or destruction. The consequences are entirely hemostatic. With normally functioning platelets, the following is expected: when the platelet count is 100,000 per microliter or greater, patients have no abnormal bleeding even with major surgery; with a platelet count of 50,000 to 100,000 per microliter, patients may bleed longer than normal with severe trauma; with a platelet count of 20,000 to 50,000 per microliter, bleeding occurs with minor trauma, but spontaneous bleeding is unusual; with a platelet count less than 20,000 per microliter, patients may have spontaneous bleeding; and when the platelet count is less than 10,000 per microliter, patients are at high risk for severe bleeding.

Decreased Production of Platelets

Hypoplasia of hematopoietic stem cells may cause thrombocytopenia (Table 184–2). Examination of the bone marrow reveals decreased numbers of megakaryocytes and either an overall decrease in cellularity or infiltration by abnormal cells.

Decreased production of platelets may also be due to abnormal maturation of megakaryocytes. Deficiency of either vitamin B_{12} or folate can cause thrombocytopenia owing to ineffective thrombocytopoiesis (see Chapter 163). Similarly, abnormal platelet production is common in hematopoietic dysplasias (see Chapter 175). In both disorders, megakaryocytes are usually increased. In hematopoietic dysplasia, megakaryocytes may be abnormal in appearance, such as micromegakaryocytes occasionally with a single-lobed nucleus.

Increased Peripheral Destruction of Platelets (see Table 184–2)

IMMUNE DISORDERS. Three types of immunologic reactions cause premature destruction of platelets: (1) development of autoantibodies against platelet-membrane antigens, (2) binding of immune complexes to platelet Fc receptors, and (3) lysis of platelets because of fixation of complement on their surface.

IDIOPATHIC THROMBOCYTOPENIC PURPURA. Idiopathic thrombocytopenic purpura (ITP) is an autoimmune bleeding disorder characterized by the development of antibodies to one's own platelets, which are then destroyed by phagocytosis in the spleen and, to a lesser extent, the liver. The spleen is the principal reticuloendothelial site of platelet destruction, as well as the major site of synthesis of antibody production in ITP. Childhood ITP is usually acute and follows recovery from a viral infection. The incidence is equal in boys and girls. In adults, the onset is usually more gradual, without a preceding illness and with a chronic course. In a small percentage of adult cases, the disease has an acute onset. Ninety per cent of adults with ITP are younger than 40 years, and the ratio of women to men is 3 to 4:1. Some patients' sera contain antibodies against platelet glycoproteins IIb and IIIa. Petechiae, ecchymoses, and epistaxis develop in this patients. Menorrhagia may develop in women. The incidence of death, reported in older series to be about 5%, is likely to be significantly lower now. Adverse risk factors are severe thrombocytopenia (platelet count, <15,000), advanced age, and concomitant bleeding diatheses. Cerebral bleeding occurs in approximately 1% of cases.

The diagnosis of ITP depends on the exclusion of underlying systemic disorders that result in increased peripheral destruction or decreased production of platelets. On physical examination, the spleen is not enlarged, although it may be in childhood ITP as a consequence of viral infection. In ITP the hemoglobin is normal unless the patient has significant bleeding. Peripheral blood smears reveal normochromic, normocytic red blood cells. Similarly, the leukocyte count and differential are normal, although these values may reflect a preceding viral illness in children. The value of assays for detecting antiplatelet antibodies on the platelet surface is unclear; most of the tests do not distinguish between autoantibodies and immune complexes that bind to the platelet Fc receptor. Furthermore, the assays do not differentiate between specific antiplatelet antibodies and non-specifically adsorbed IgG. In most cases of ITP the diagnosis is clear-cut, thus making it unnecessary to confirm the presence of antiplatelet antibodies. In complex cases, the antibody test may be helpful. The level of platelet-associated IgG does not correlate with the severity of thrombocytopenia. In over 90% of cases of chronic ITP, the antibody is IgG.

If the general clinical evaluation and blood tests do not identify a systemic cause of thrombocytopenia, the bone marrow should be examined. In ITP the marrow is normal, although megakaryocytes may be increased in number.

In children, ITP is self-limited. Approximately 70% recover within 4 to 6 weeks. In adults, indications for treatment depend on the severity of bleeding and the degree of thrombocytopenia.

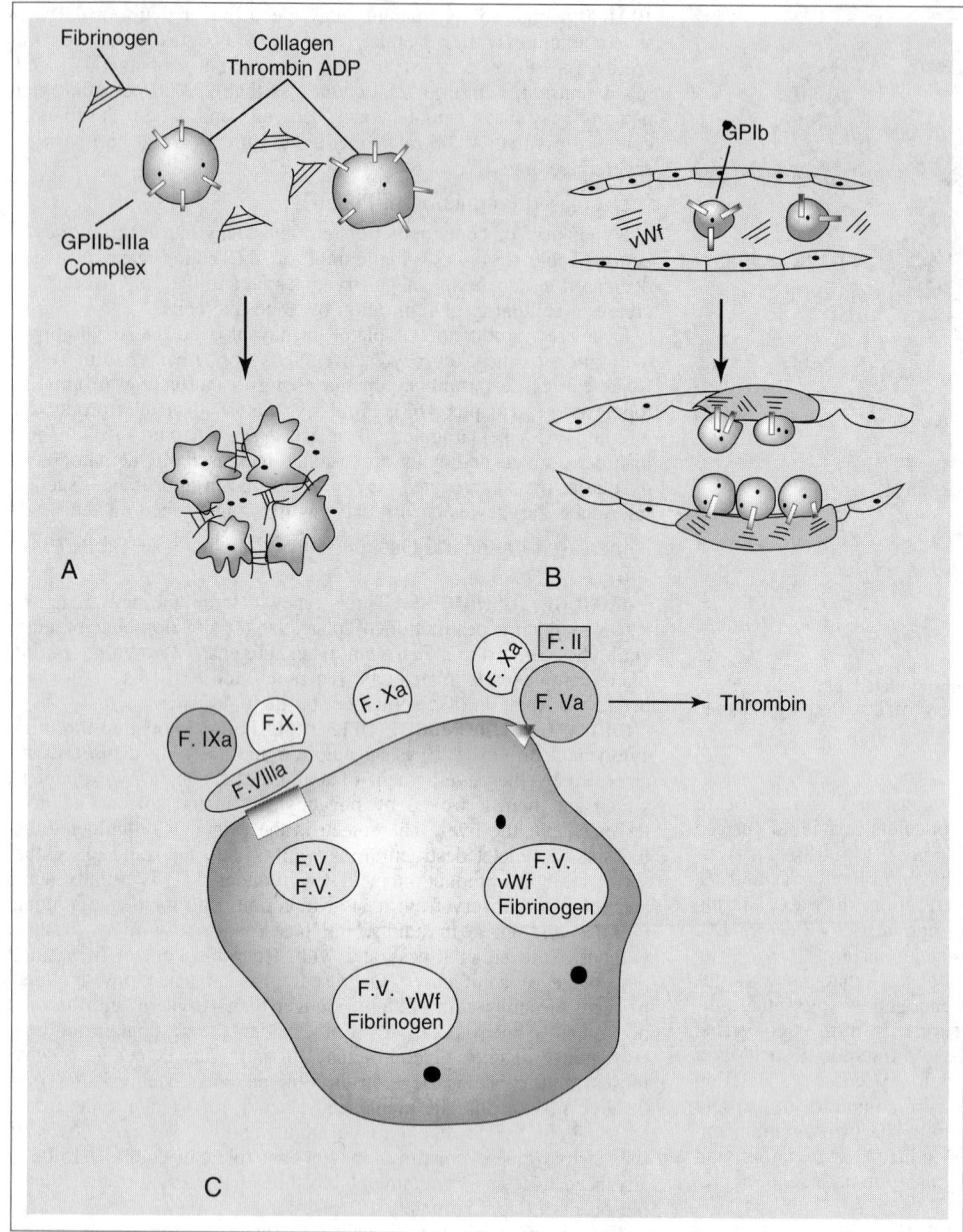

FIGURE 184–2 ■ Platelet aggregation, adhesion, and enhancement of coagulation. *A,* Platelet aggregation. Activation of platelets by several physiologic stimuli results in fibrinogen binding to specific receptors, GPIIb-IIIa. Binding of fibrinogen is followed by platelet aggregation. *B,* Platelet adhesion. Injury to the vascular endothelium results in exposure of extracellular matrix. Under high shear, von Willebrand factor (vWf) binds to the platelet receptor GPIb. The platelet-vWf complex then binds to the subendothelium. *C,* Amplification of thrombin formation by platelets. Coagulation Factors IXa, VIIIa, and X form a Ca^{2+}-dependent trimolecular complex on the platelet surface. Activation of Factor X is amplified several hundred thousand–fold. Coagulation Factors Xa, Va, and prothrombin form a Ca^{2+}-dependent trimolecular complex on platelets. Thrombin formation is amplified several hundred thousand–fold.

Asymptomatic patients with platelet counts greater than 40,000 per microliter can be observed with periodic evaluation to determine the natural fluctuations of their disease. Patients with platelet counts less than 20,000 per microliter are usually symptomatic and require treatment. Patients with platelet counts over 30,000 per microliter who have bleeding may have an acquired platelet function abnormality caused by the antibody. Initially, bleeding associated with ITP is treated with prednisone at a dose of 1 to 2 mg/kg/day. Prednisone inhibits macrophage ingestion of antibody-coated platelets, in addition to suppressing antibody synthesis. Prednisone has also been shown to have a stabilizing effect on small blood vessels in thrombocytopenic animals. In 80 to 90% of patients, the platelet count rises to hemostatic levels within 2 to 3 weeks. Failure to respond to steroids is indicated by a platelet count lower than 50,000 per microliter after 4 weeks of treatment or a subnormal platelet count after 6 weeks. Once the platelet count has reached its apex and is stable, the steroid dose should be tapered slowly. When the dose of prednisone is tapered, however, most patients (>90%) exhibit a relapse of thrombocytopenia. Thus the primary benefit of prednisone is in the acute management of bleeding.

Another effective approach to managing patients who are actively bleeding or for whom major surgery is necessary is the use of intravenous γ-globulin. Intravenous immune globulin (IVIG) concentrates raise the platelet count within 3 to 5 days in most patients and is the most rapidly active agent. Unfortunately, the therapeutic effect is usually transient because the platelet count falls to baseline levels over the next month. In rare instances, repeated infusions of IVIG have led to sustained remissions after discontinuation of therapy. It is proposed that IVIG works by blocking Fc receptors on macrophages, thereby inhibiting phagocytosis. The dosage is 1 g/kg/day on 2 successive days. In 80% of patients, subsequent platelet counts rise above 50,000 per microliter. A less expensive alternative is RhoGAM, anti-Rh antibody. The principle is the same as that in IVIG, reticuloendothelial blockade.

Owing to the lack of a sustained remission in most patients with severe thrombocytopenia treated with steroids or IVIG, a more definitive approach is necessary. Splenectomy improves the platelet count in 70% of patients with ITP and induces sustained remission in approximately 60%, but no test can reliably predict which patients will respond. The platelet count rises, usually within a few days or at most 1 to 2 weeks after splenectomy.

A variety of other therapies can induce partial or complete remissions in chronic ITP when splenectomy has failed. Danazol, 200 mg three times per day, induces a remission in approximately

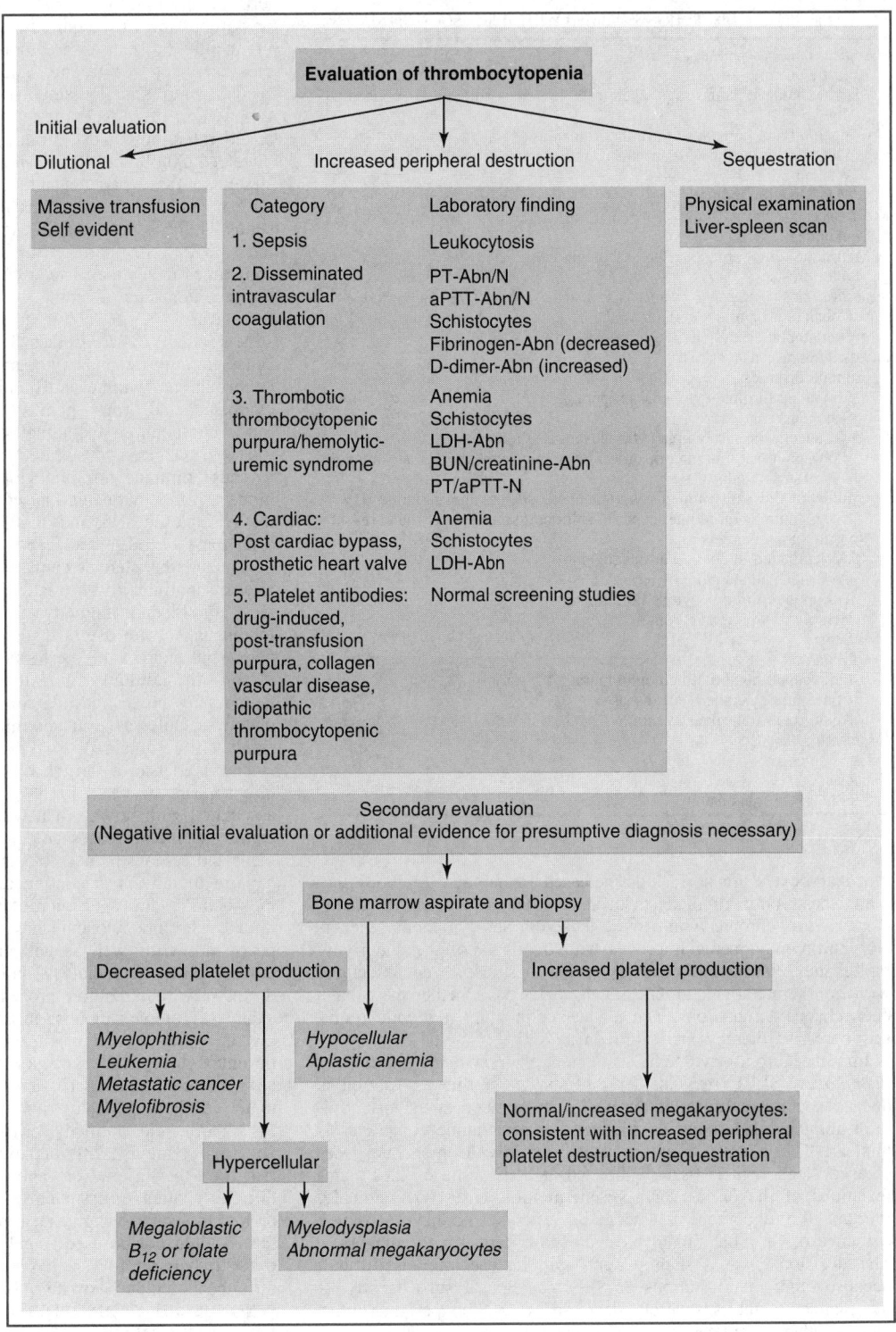

FIGURE 184–3 ■ Evaluation of thrombocytopenia. Abn = abnormal; N = normal; PT = prothrombin time; aPTT = activated partial thromboplastin time; LDH = lactate dehydrogenase; BUN = blood urea nitrogen.

40% of cases of chronic ITP. Response is delayed and takes 4 to 6 weeks. The mechanism remains unknown. Intravenous vincristine and vinblastine also raise the platelet count in ITP, usually within 1 to 2 weeks. Responses are transient and remissions are not sustained.

Immunosuppressive agents—cyclophosphamide and azathioprine—improve the platelet count in 20 to 30% of cases of chronic ITP. The potential benefit of these drugs must be weighed against the risks of toxicity. In one small series, 60% of patients with refractory ITP had complete remissions with combination chemotherapy. Pulsed, high-dose dexamethasone has also been reported to be effective therapy in patients with refractory ITP.

Management of ITP in pregnancy is complicated by the addi-

tional risk to the fetus of thrombocytopenia secondary to maternal antibodies. Intraventricular hemorrhage, gastrointestinal bleeding, and death have been reported in newborns. Whether the mother had ITP before pregnancy is critical. When ITP initially develops in women during pregnancy, the risk of serious bleeding in the newborn is negligible. Conversely, neonates born to women with a history of ITP preceding pregnancy have a 20% risk of severe thrombocytopenia. In addition to treating the underlying ITP, cesarean delivery is recommended to decrease the risk of intracranial bleeding in these newborns.

PLATELET ANTIBODIES ASSOCIATED WITH SYSTEMIC DISORDERS. Antibodies directed against platelets and causing thrombocytopenia occur in several types of disorders in which bone marrow

Table 184–2 ■ DISORDERS ASSOCIATED WITH THROMBOCYTOPENIA

Hypoplasia of Hematopoietic Stem Cells
  Aplastic anemia
  Marrow damage from drugs, chemicals, ionizing radiation, alcohol, infection
  Congenital and hereditary thrombocytopenias
    Thrombocytopenia with absent radii syndrome
    Wiskott-Aldrich syndrome
    May-Hegglin anomaly
Replacement of Normal Marrow
  Leukemias
  Metastatic tumor (prostate, breast, lymphoma)
  Myelofibrosis
Ineffective Thrombocytopoiesis (Normal or Increased Numbers of Megakaryocytes)
    Cobalamin or folate deficiency
    Hematopoietic dysplastic syndromes
Increased Destruction of Platelets
  Immune disorders
    Idiopathic thrombocytopenic purpura
    Secondary causes
      Cancer: chronic lymphocytic leukemia, lymphoma
      Systemic autoimmune disorders: systemic lupus erythematosus, polyarteritis nodosa
    Infectious diseases: infectious mononucleosis, cytomegalovirus, HIV
    Drugs: quinine/quinidine, heparin, sulfa compounds (see Table 184–1)
  Non-immune disorders
    Disseminated intravascular coagulation
    Cavernous hemangioma
    Thrombotic thrombocytopenic purpura
    Hemolytic-uremic syndrome
    Sepsis
    Malaria
    Paroxysmal nocturnal hemoglobinuria
    Congenital cyanotic heart disease
    Acute renal transplant rejection
Disorders of Distribution
  Hypersplenism
Dilutional
  Secondary to transfusion

megakaryocytes are normal or increased in number. Antibody-mediated destruction of platelets occurs in *lymphoproliferative disorders* such as chronic lymphocytic leukemia and lymphoma. Generally, thrombocytopenia improves with treatment of the underlying malignancy. Immune thrombocytopenia has also been associated with non-hematologic tumors, but it is unclear whether these have been chance associations. The platelet count improves with immunosuppressive therapy such as prednisone.

Immune thrombocytopenia is common in *systemic lupus erythematosus* (SLE) (see Chapter 289). Whether this association is due to specific antiplatelet antibodies, to antibodies against common antigens also found on platelets, or to immune complexes is unclear. The platelet count is usually mildly to moderately decreased. Treatment is usually directed at SLE because other manifestations of the disease are present in most cases. Occasionally, immune thrombocytopenia occurs in patients who have serologic evidence of SLE but fail to meet all the criteria for the diagnosis. The decision to treat such patients with splenectomy is difficult because other manifestations of SLE may appear subsequently. If the platelet count is severely decreased (<30,000 per microliter) and no other complications of SLE exist, splenectomy is a reasonable choice. If the platelet count is moderately decreased (230,000 to 40,000 per microliter) and major bleeding problems are absent, careful observation may be the best course. Monthly intravenous cyclophosphamide, 0.75 to 1.0 g/m² body surface area, normalizes platelet counts within 2 to 18 weeks in patients with SLE who are also taking prednisone. Such therapy allows a substantial reduction in steroid dosage.

Thrombocytopenia associated with antiplatelet antibodies has been reported in patients with *viral* illnesses, including infectious mononucleosis, human immunodeficiency virus (HIV) infection, and cytomegalovirus (CMV) infection. In the case of infectious mononucleosis and CMV infection, thrombocytopenia is usually self-limiting, with recovery in 3 to 4 weeks. For patients with severe thrombocytopenia, a short course of glucocorticoids may be

indicated. The nature of the immune reaction has not been characterized. In HIV-infected patients, thrombocytopenia is frequent with or without the full acquired immune deficiency syndrome (AIDS). Frequently the causes are multifactorial: (1) infection causing increased platelet destruction and/or inhibition of platelet production secondary to granulomatous replacement of the bone marrow, (2) suppression of hematopoiesis by drugs used to treat AIDS or associated infections, and (3) immune destruction of the patient's own platelets. Antibodies associated with platelets have been demonstrated in these patients, although the cause is unclear. Treatment with prednisone is hazardous because of the immunocompromised status of these patients. Splenectomy has the disadvantage of further compromising the immune system. Zidovudine treatment sometimes raises the platelet count in mild to moderate thrombocytopenia. For acute bleeding, IVIG raises the platelet count within a few days.

More than 50 *drugs* (see Table 184–1) have been reported to cause immune thrombocytopenia, but infrequently with conclusive confirmation. Quinine and quinidine often cause immune thrombocytopenia, and drug-dependent antibodies have been demonstrated. Sulfa compounds, including sulfisoxazole, sulfonamide, sulfamethoxypyridazine, and sulfamethazine, have also been demonstrated to cause immune thrombocytopenia. Multiple reports describe immune thrombocytopenia caused by hydrochlorothiazide, phenytoin, methyldopa, heparin, and digitalis derivatives. In most instances the drug must be present to cause antibody binding and thrombocytopenia, and the platelet count returns to normal within a few days after discontinuation of treatment. Glucocorticoids do not accelerate recovery. Platelet antibody tests with and without the putative offending agent are useful in determining the cause of thrombocytopenia but cannot be performed until the drug clears from the plasma. In addition, a drug metabolite rather than the parent compound may be responsible for antibody formation and binding to platelets. Unless the metabolite is specifically tested, a negative result will be obtained.

The incidence of thrombocytopenia associated with *heparin therapy* appears to be 3 to 5%, with a higher percentage of cases associated with bovine than with porcine preparations. The platelet count usually decreases gradually after the first few days of treatment and seldom induces bleeding. The count corrects rapidly after heparin therapy is discontinued. Nevertheless, if the platelet count falls below 50,000 per microliter, heparin therapy should be discontinued. Thrombocytopenia has been reported with the usual therapeutic doses, as well as with the very low doses used for procedures such as hemodialysis and "flushing" of vascular catheters or during revascularization procedures. The antibody appears to be against a complex of heparin and platelet factor 4, a glycosaminoglycan α-granule component with high affinity for heparin. Immune thrombocytopenia also occurs with low-molecular-weight heparins as well (e.g., enoxaparin and dalteparin [Fragmin]). In approximately 50% of patients with immune thrombocytopenia secondary to heparin, the antibody cross-reacts with low-molecular-weight heparins. Patients with heparin-induced thrombocytopenia are at risk for either arterial or venous thrombosis and pose an extremely difficult challenge inasmuch as treatment with either unfractionated or low-molecular-weight heparin is contraindicated. Moreover, warfarin should not be used acutely as the sole anticoagulant. Alternatives to heparin for acute anticoagulation of patients with active thrombosis include new thrombin inhibitors or heparinoids.

NON-IMMUNE DISORDERS ASSOCIATED WITH INCREASED CONSUMPTION OF PLATELETS. DISSEMINATED INTRAVASCULAR COAGULATION. (See Chapter 186). In this syndrome, pathologically activated coagulation results in thrombin formation and the subsequent removal of platelets from the circulation.

THROMBOTIC THROMBOCYTOPENIC PURPURA. A rare disease of unknown etiology, thrombotic thrombocytopenic purpura (TTP) is characterized by severe thrombocytopenia, microangiopathic hemolytic anemia (>96% of patients), and neurologic abnormalities (>92% of patients). Fever and renal involvement—proteinuria, hematuria, azotemia, and casts—are present in 98 and 88% of patients, respectively. Renal abnormalities are usually mild; the creatinine rarely exceeds 3.0 mg/dL. Azotemia usually reverses as remission occurs, in contrast to the hemolytic-uremic syndrome (HUS) (see below). In the involved organs, arterioles and capillaries become occluded by a hyaline material consisting principally

Table 184-3 ■ DIFFERENTIAL DIAGNOSIS OF ANEMIA AND THROMBOCYTOPENIA

DIAGNOSTIC STUDY	AUTOIMMUNE DISORDERS (EVANS' SYNDROME/ COLLAGEN-VASCULAR DISEASE)	DISSEMINATED INTRAVASCULAR COAGULATION	THROMBOTIC THROMBOCYTOPENIC PURPURA/HEMOLYTIC-UREMIC SYNDROME
Peripheral blood smear	Microspherocytes	Schistocytes (+)	Schistocytes (+++)
Reticulocyte count	Increased (+++)	N/increased (+)	Increased (+++)
Coombs' test	Positive	Negative	Negative
Coagulation tests	N	Abn (+++)	N/Abn (+)

N = normal; Abn = abnormal.

of platelet thrombi plus fibrin deposits in the vessel wall. Virtually any organ may be involved. Symptoms frequently wax and wane, presumably because of platelet aggregation and disaggregation. Thus patients may have evanescent headache, aphasia, or stupor one moment and be alert the next.

TTP must be considered when thrombocytopenia and anemia occur acutely with microangiopathic changes of red blood cells on the peripheral blood smear and the absence of evidence of other disorders (Tables 184–3 and 184–4; Color Plate 6L). Although findings in disseminated intravascular coagulation are similar, patients with TTP have minimal changes in coagulation tests. Evans' syndrome, which is autoimmune hemolytic anemia and thrombocytopenia, is characterized by a positive Coombs' test and by microspherocytes rather than schistocytes on peripheral smear. Rarely, TTP has been reported to complicate SLE. More commonly, patients with SLE have immune thrombocytopenia and anemia of chronic disease or immune hemolytic anemia (see Chapter 289). TTP has also been reported in association with oral contraceptives and pregnancy. In most cases the diagnosis of TTP is straightforward. When the diagnosis is uncertain, gum, skin, or bone marrow biopsy may be helpful, with positive results reported in 40 to 60% of cases. It is critical to establish the diagnosis and begin treatment rapidly inasmuch as delay can result in severe morbidity or mortality. Most untreated patients die within 3 months. Large-volume plasmapheresis, approximately two plasma volumes with replacement infusion of normal plasma, is the treatment of choice for TTP and cures approximately 70% of patients. The best indication of a successful response is a rise in the platelet count. Plasmapheresis/infusion should be continued until the platelet count becomes normal and stable. Normalization of anemia and neurologic abnormalities usually follows. Approximately 10% of patients have a chronic, relapsing form of TTP. The plasma of patients with chronic TTP in remission contains abnormally large multimers of von Willebrand factor.

HEMOLYTIC-UREMIC SYNDROME. Primarily a disorder of infants and young children, HUS rarely occurs in adults. Like TTP, HUS produces a microangiopathic hemolytic anemia, but thrombocytopenia is mild to moderate and neurologic abnormalities are absent. Unlike TTP, acute renal failure is a prominent feature in HUS, frequently necessitating hemodialysis. Severe hypertension is also a prominent feature. Children typically have gastrointestinal signs and

TABLE 184-4 ■ DISORDERS ASSOCIATED WITH THROMBOCYTOPENIA AND MICROANGIOPATHIC ANEMIA

Thrombotic thrombocytopenic purpura
Hemolytic-uremic syndrome
Disseminated intravascular coagulation
Malignant hypertension
Eclampsia
Vasculitis
   Systemic lupus erythematosus
   Polyarteritis nodosa
Cavernous hemangioma
   (Kasabach-Merritt syndrome)
Disseminated carcinoma
Renal allograft rejection
Prosthetic heart valves
Malignant angioendotheliomatosis

symptoms—abdominal pain and diarrhea. HUS may occur in women who are in the postpartum period or are taking oral contraceptives. HUS has also been reported in cancer patients receiving mitomycin or cisplatin chemotherapy.

SEPSIS. Gram-negative (more commonly than gram-positive) sepsis causes accelerated platelet destruction, presumably a result of binding of bacterial immune complexes to the platelet. Severe thrombocytopenia may follow.

Disorders of Distribution of Platelets

With splenic enlargement, platelet pooling increases (e.g., Gaucher's disease, congestive splenomegaly, lymphoma) and may cause thrombocytopenia (see Chapter 178). Platelet counts lower than 30,000 to 50,000 per microliter are unusual.

Dilutional Thrombocytopenia

When packed erythrocytes or non-fresh whole blood is transfused to replace blood loss, thrombocytopenia may ensue. Approximately 35 to 40% of platelets remain after replacement of one blood volume; microvascular bleeding secondary to thrombocytopenia occurs rarely after the replacement of one to two volumes. Platelets should be transfused only if thrombocytopenia and bleeding are present.

Thrombocytosis

Elevation of the platelet count above the normal range reflects increased production, either reactive or the result of a myeloproliferative disorder. Most thrombocytosis occurs secondary to an underlying disorder unassociated with complications. When caused by a primary disorder of hematopoiesis, however, thrombocytosis can cause serious bleeding and/or thrombotic complications, which makes it important to determine its cause.

ESSENTIAL THROMBOCYTHEMIA. Essential thrombocythemia (see Chapter 174) and other myeloproliferative diseases such as agnogenic myeloid metaplasia and polycythemia vera are also associated with an elevated platelet count. The count may be elevated in chronic myelogenous leukemia but rarely results in complications.

REACTIVE THROMBOCYTOSIS. Elevated platelet counts occur secondarily in a number of unrelated disorders (counts higher than 10^6 per microliter are unusual): iron deficiency anemia; hemorrhage; splenectomy (see Chapter 178); inflammatory disorders, particularly inflammatory bowel disease; neoplasms (e.g., lung, gastrointestinal); and leukemoid reaction (see Chapter 172).

No convincing evidence exists that reactive thrombocytosis increases the risk of thrombosis. Therefore it should not be treated. With successful treatment of the primary disease, the count returns to normal.

ABNORMALITIES IN PLATELET FUNCTION

Acquired Disorders of Platelet Function

DRUGS THAT INHIBIT PLATELET FUNCTION. (See Table 184–1.) Non-steroidal anti-inflammatory agents inhibit platelet function by blocking platelet synthesis of prostaglandins. Aspirin (acetylsalicylic acid) irreversibly acetylates prostaglandin synthetase (cyclooxygenase) and, as a result, impairs platelet function for its lifespan. One aspirin tablet (300 mg) is sufficient to cause this effect. Fortunately, in normal people this dose does not result in excessive bleeding, but in patients with von Willebrand disease or those with severe coagulation factor deficiency (Factor VIII or IX), serious bleeding can result. For this reason, aspirin is contraindicated in these disorders.

High doses of *β-lactam antibiotics* such as penicillin and related compounds induce an abnormality in platelet function that persists for 2 to 3 days after treatment with the drug is discontinued. The mechanism is unclear. The bleeding time is prolonged, and patients may have increased bleeding.

RENAL FAILURE. Platelets function abnormally in patients with renal failure. The uremic metabolites responsible for this dysfunction are uncertain. Guanidinosuccinic acid and phenolic compounds that accumulate in uremia may inhibit platelet aggregation. Abnormal platelet adhesion and activation may occur in uremia as well as thrombocytopenia. The latter is usually mild and may be due to the underlying cause of the renal disease.

Uremic bleeding is usually mucocutaneous and reflects abnormal platelet and/or vascular hemostatic functions. The bleeding time is commonly prolonged, but other causes of prolongation must be excluded (e.g., medication, congenital platelet disorders, and von Willebrand disease). Low hematocrits (<24%) prolong the bleeding time in uremia. Transfusion of packed red blood cells or recombinant erythropoietin to elevate the hematocrit above 26% shortens the bleeding time and corrects abnormal platelet aggregation in hemodialysis patients. Although the mechanism for improved hemostasis is uncertain, it may be due in part to increased platelet radial movement and interaction with the endothelium. Tests of coagulation are normal.

When a uremic patient bleeds, a structural lesion or other hemostatic abnormalities must be suspected; platelet abnormalities are seldom the cause. When the hemostatic defect of renal failure is believed to be a significant contributing factor in bleeding, either peritoneal dialysis or hemodialysis can usually reverse the hemostatic defect. If the bleeding time remains prolonged and the patient is bleeding, low-dose estrogens, 1-deamino-8-D-arginine vasopressin (DDAVP), or cryoprecipitate can be tried. All three raise the plasma levels of Factor VIII (antihemophilic factor/von Willebrand factor), but their efficacies have not been firmly established. Platelet transfusion usually has no benefit.

HEPATIC FAILURE. (See Chapter 154.) Platelet function is sometimes abnormal in liver disease, but why this is so and the extent to which it contributes to bleeding are unclear. The bleeding time may be prolonged in moderately severe liver disease when the platelet count is greater than 90,000 per microliter. DDAVP has been reported to improve the bleeding time in these circumstances. More commonly in hepatic failure, a bleeding diathesis is due to deficiencies in coagulation factors.

PARAPROTEINEMIAS. (See Chapter 181.) Abnormal platelet function occurs in a subset of patients with multiple myeloma or Waldenström's macroglobulinemia. The bleeding time is usually prolonged, and bleeding can be moderately severe. If the level of the paraprotein is lowered by plasmapheresis and/or chemotherapy, the bleeding time and bleeding improve, thus suggesting a direct effect of the paraprotein on platelet function. Paraproteins may impair platelet function by inhibiting platelet-fibrinogen interaction.

ACQUIRED STORAGE POOL DISEASE. Mild platelet function abnormalities may develop from loss of storage granules. Some of the disorders in which this finding has been reported include cardiopulmonary bypass surgery, hairy cell leukemia, and conditions with antiplatelet autoantibodies. Platelet dysfunction following bypass surgery is transient and not of clinical importance beyond the initial 24 hours after surgery.

MYELOPROLIFERATIVE DISORDERS. Patients with essential thrombocythemia and, less commonly, agnogenic myeloid metaplasia and polycythemia vera may have abnormalities of platelet function. In essential thrombocythemia, abnormalities usually occur at platelet counts greater than 10^6 per microliter and may lead to abnormal bleeding, thrombosis, or both. Although the functional abnormalities are not specific, a prolonged bleeding time indicates that the patient is at risk for bleeding. Treatment of bleeding patients with thrombocytosis should be directed at lowering the platelet count as rapidly as possible.

Hereditary Disorders of Platelet Function

The bleeding history is similar among these rare diseases. Patients provide a lifelong history of easy bruising, epistaxis, and prolonged oozing after venipuncture, dental extractions, and other challenges to hemostasis.

GLANZMANN'S THROMBASTHENIA. This autosomal recessive bleeding disorder is characterized by a prolonged bleeding time and platelets that fail to aggregate normally when stimulated with ADP, epinephrine, collagen, or thrombin. In Glanzmann's thrombocytopenia, two membrane glycoproteins (GPIIb, GPIIIa) that normally serve as the receptor for fibrinogen in activated platelets are markedly deficient (see Fig. 184–2). Fibrinogen binding to platelets is required for platelet aggregation. The diagnosis is confirmed by demonstrating a deficiency of platelet GPIIb-IIIa. The platelet count is always normal.

BERNARD-SOULIER SYNDROME. This autosomal recessive disorder is caused by deficiency of a platelet membrane glycoprotein complex, GPIb-IX. As a result, "giant" platelets appear in the peripheral blood smear. Frequently, the platelet count is mildly decreased. In laboratory studies, platelets aggregate normally in response to ADP, collagen, or epinephrine but fail to aggregate in response to ristocetin. Physiologically, platelets fail to adhere normally to subendothelial connective tissue because of defective binding of von Willebrand factor.

STORAGE POOL DISEASE. In this autosomal dominant disorder, platelet storage granules are decreased in number and/or content, presumably because of abnormal granule formation in megakaryocytes. The bleeding diathesis is mild and affects mostly women. With the deficiency in dense granules, platelets aggregate abnormally because of inadequate secretion of ADP. Dense-granule storage pool disease is also associated with several other congenital disorders, including oculocutaneous albinism in both the Hermansky-Pudlak and Chédiak-Higashi syndromes, the Wiskott-Aldrich syndrome, and a syndrome that includes thrombocytopenia and absent radii. Patients may also be deficient in α-granules, either in combination with denser-granule deficiency or independently. The gray platelet syndrome refers to the latter situation, in which the absence of granule staining confers a gray color to the platelets. Mild thrombocytopenia may also be present.

VON WILLEBRAND DISEASE. This disease, the most common congenital bleeding disorder that also affects platelet function, is discussed in Chapter 185.

PLATELET TRANSFUSIONS

INDICATIONS. When serious bleeding complicates thrombocytopenia, platelet transfusions are effective only when the cause is decreased production. Thrombocytopenia caused by increased peripheral destruction or sequestration is usually refractory to platelet transfusion. Bleeding caused by qualitative platelet disorders ordinarily responds to platelet transfusions except when secondary to uremia or hepatic failure or when an offending drug remains in the circulation.

For patients with congenital platelet disorders, platelet transfusion must be given judiciously because repeated transfusions stimulate alloantibodies. Eventually it may become impossible to raise the platelet count through transfusion. Accordingly, platelet transfusions should be reserved for serious bleeding or in preparation for surgery on patients with moderately severe platelet defects.

Platelet transfusions are indicated for patients who are bleeding actively and have either a platelet count lower than 50,000 per microliter or a qualitative platelet abnormality as manifested by a prolonged bleeding time. Platelet transfusions may also be indicated prophylactically before surgery or other invasive procedures. Before surgery, platelet counts should be greater than 50,000 per microliter in most cases and greater than 90,000 per microliter for procedures such as neurosurgery or ophthalmologic surgery in which any abnormal bleeding may cause excessive morbidity. For invasive procedures such as kidney or liver biopsies, a platelet count over 50,000 per microliter is probably sufficient, assuming normal platelet function.

CHRONIC THROMBOCYTOPENIA. In the absence of active bleeding, recommendations are based on the cause of the thrombocytopenia. When thrombocytopenia is due to decreased production, the platelet count should be maintained at 10,000 to 20,000 per microliter. When accelerated destruction of platelets exists, transfusion is seldom effective. Patients with ITP frequently tolerate low platelet counts with little bleeding because of the excellent function of the younger platelets available in the circulation.

DOSAGE. For patients who require platelet transfusions chronically, platelets should be obtained from a single donor for each transfusion (generally 6 to 7 U) to reduce the risk of formation of multiple alloantibodies (see below). In a 70-kg patient, 1 U of platelets usually raises the platelet count by approximately 10,000 per microliter. The count should be repeated 10 to 60 minutes after transfusion to assess the compatibility of the transfused platelets and to determine whether the desired count has been achieved. In actively bleeding patients, the platelet count should be maintained above 50,000 per microliter.

ALLOANTIBODIES AGAINST PLATELETS. In approximately 50 to 60% of patients who become refractory to random donor platelets, anti-HLA antibodies appear to be responsible. The other presumed antigens have not yet been identified. In one rare form of alloimmunization, antibodies develop against the PL antigen, an epitope on platelet glycoprotein IIIa. The difference between PL^{AI} positive and negative (PL^{A2}) is a single amino acid. Of the normal population, 98% have PL^{AI}-positive platelets.

When PL^{AI}-negative patients are transfused with PL^{AI}-positive blood, they produce anti-PL^{AI} antibodies and post-transfusion purpura may develop. Previous immunization is necessary, either by transfusion or by pregnancy. Why this syndrome is rare and selectively high in women despite the frequency of PL^{AI} negativity in the population is unknown. These patients not only rapidly clear transfused platelets from their circulation but also destroy their own platelets and become thrombocytopenic usually 5 to 10 days after transfusion. If patients with antibodies against the PL^{AI} antigen become severely thrombocytopenic, treatment with plasmapheresis or exchange transfusion is necessary because bleeding from thrombocytopenia can be life-threatening.

NEONATAL ALLOIMMUNE THROMBOCYTOPENIA. Thrombocytopenia caused by maternal alloantibodies against fetal platelet antigens occurs in approximately 1 in 2000 to 4000 fetuses. Affected infants may have intracranial hemorrhage (estimated at between 10 and 30%); in families with an affected infant, the risk of recurrence is at least 75%. PL^{AI} antibodies have been identified in most cases as being responsible for thrombocytopenia. Affected infants are treated by transfusion with washed maternal platelets. Women with a prior history of an affected infant should give birth by cesarean section. Also, IVIG given to pregnant mothers with a prior affected infant raises fetal platelet counts and reduces the rate of intracranial hemorrhage.

VASCULAR DISORDERS (TABLE 184–5)

Normal vascular function is necessary for effective hemostasis (see Fig. 184–1). Alteration in the integrity or structure of blood vessels can lead to a bleeding diathesis, the symptoms and signs of which are indistinguishable from those of a platelet disorder.

Table 184–5 ■ VASCULAR DISORDERS ASSOCIATED WITH BLEEDING

Congenital
Hereditary hemorrhagic telangiectasia
Cavernous hemangioma
Connective tissue disorders
    Ehlers-Danlos syndrome
    Osteogenesis imperfecta
    Pseudoxanthoma elasticum
Acquired Disorders Affecting Vascular Hemostatic Function
Scurvy
Immunoglobulin disorders
    Cryoglobulinemia
    Benign hyperglobulinemia
    Waldenström's macroglobulinemia
    Multiple myeloma
    Henoch-Schönlein purpura
Glucocorticoid excess
    Cushing's syndrome
    Glucocorticoid therapy

Congenital Vascular Disorders Associated with Bleeding

HEREDITARY HEMORRHAGIC TELANGIECTASIA (RENDU-OSLER-WEBER DISEASE). This disorder, the most common genetic cause of vascular bleeding, is inherited as an autosomal dominant trait. Its most frequent symptom is spontaneous epistaxis. More than half of these patients have epistaxis by 20 years of age and 90% by age 45. Telangiectasia occurs most frequently on the face in two thirds of patients, on the mouth in half, and on the cheeks, tongue, nose, and lower lip in approximately one third. In about 40%, the hands and wrists are also involved. Beyond this cutaneous or mucosal involvement, the organ system affected most often is the gastrointestinal tract (15%). Death from intestinal bleeding occurs in 12 to 15% of patients with symptomatic gastrointestinal involvement. The liver, lungs, central nervous system, and urinary tract are involved in decreasing order of frequency. Pulmonary arteriovenous fistulas, present in approximately 5% of patients, are manifested by cyanosis, dyspnea, clubbing, and thoracic murmurs. Hemoptysis is unusual. Surgical resection is successful in managing this complication in most instances. Coil embolization of these fistulas has also been used successfully. Stroke may occur with central nervous system involvement, a complication that tends to affect younger patients (mean age, 33 years). Careful inspection of the nose and mouth usually reveals the diagnosis. In other cases, endoscopy or angiography may be necessary. Pathologic examination of involved tissue demonstrates dilated capillaries with loss of subendothelial structures.

Tests of platelet function and bleeding time are normal. Although no therapy is consistently effective, based on a few case reports and one small series of patients, conjugated estrogen-progestin therapy appears to be efficacious in decreasing the number of bleeding episodes. Generally, the prognosis is relatively good.

CAVERNOUS HEMANGIOMA (KASABACH-MERRITT SYNDROME). Congenital subcutaneous and visceral hemangiomas may be associated with thrombocytopenia and bleeding in infants and children. Bleeding occurs at the site of the lesions or systemically secondary to thrombocytopenia. Platelets are activated within the hemangioma and subsequently removed from the circulation. In addition, mild disseminated intravascular coagulation may occur with consumption of fibrinogen. Thrombocytopenia is more severe than the coagulation abnormalities. Spontaneous regression of hemangiomas may occur over a period of years. In cases in which thrombocytopenia is severe and tumors are few, surgery and/or radiation therapy may be effective. Intentional thrombosis of hemangiomas by the administration of inhibitors of fibrinolysis, with or without cryoprecipitate, has been successful in managing thrombocytopenia in a few cases. Also, interferon-α has been observed to cause significant regression of hemangiomas.

DISORDERS OF CONNECTIVE TISSUE. Genetic abnormalities in structural glycoproteins such as collagen can result in vascular fragility caused by weakening of the vessel wall. Bleeding may be limited to increased bruising or may be manifested as internal hemorrhaging. Ehlers-Danlos syndrome (see Chapter 216), osteogenesis imperfecta (see Chapter 217), and pseudoxanthoma elasticum (see Chapter 218), are examples of inherited disorders of connective tissue that may be associated with a bleeding diathesis on this basis.

Acquired Disorders of Blood Vessels Causing Bleeding

SCURVY. Severe vitamin C deficiency results in defective collagen formation in small blood vessels. Bleeding may occur in any tissue but is prominent in the lower extremities and is perifollicular in distribution. Other sites where bleeding is common include the gums, the subperiosteum in children, and muscle.

PURPURA ASSOCIATED WITH IMMUNOGLOBULIN DISORDERS. CRYOGLOBULINEMIA. (See Chapter 181.) Patients with any of the three types of cryoglobulinemia have purpura as a complication of their disease. In type I, bleeding may be due to obstruction of blood flow in the microcirculation at cold temperatures by cryoprecipitates, with subsequent increased vascular fragility. In type II and type III cryoglobulinemia, bleeding may be due to leukocytoclastic vasculitis associated with the immune complexes. Purpura occurs most commonly in the distal ends of the extremities.

BENIGN HYPERGLOBULINEMIA (WALDENSTRÖM'S PURPURA). In this syndrome, patients have polyclonal hyperglobulinemia associated with purpura of the lower extremities. Leukocytoclastic involvement of the vessel wall may account for the increased vascular fragility and bleeding. Commonly, the onset of purpura is preceded by a stinging sensation in areas of involvement. Although generally no evidence of systemic vasculitis is seen, the disorder may evolve into Sjögren's syndrome or SLE.

AMYLOIDOSIS. Amyloid deposition in the skin and subcutaneous tissue alters the normal structural support for small blood vessels and thereby results in increased vascular fragility. Purpura can occur at any site; for unclear reasons, periorbital hemorrhage is a characteristic finding.

WALDENSTRÖM'S MACROGLOBULINEMIA AND MULTIPLE MYELOMA. (See Chapter 181.) Abnormalities in platelet function may occur with M proteins, as noted above. An additional contributing factor is hyperviscosity when it complicates these diseases. Slowing of blood flow and increased hydrostatic pressure may increase vascular fragility and lead to purpura.

HENOCH-SCHÖNLEIN PURPURA. Symmetrical purpura and arthralgias of the lower extremities, abdominal pain, and melena characterize this childhood disorder. Rarely, adults are affected. Patients may give a history of a recent infectious illness. The disease has an acute onset with a maculopapular rash evolving into palpable purpura. Other complications include glomerulonephritis and hypertension (both of which are self-limiting) and intussusception. Involved tissues, including the skin, demonstrate vasculitis with IgA and complement deposition.

Henoch-Schönlein purpura usually remits spontaneously over a period of 1 to 2 months, although the course is often punctuated by flaring of symptoms and signs. Symptomatic improvement is obtained with glucocorticoids.

Miscellaneous Disorders

CUSHING'S SYNDROME. Cushing's disease or chronic administration of glucocorticoids results in increased bruising, particularly in the extremities. Abnormal bleeding probably results from alterations in the structure of the perivascular matrix, with loss of normal elasticity.

AUTOERYTHROCYTE SENSITIZATION (GARDNER-DIAMOND SYNDROME). This bizarre syndrome is characterized by the development of purpura at any site on the body, preceded by pain and burning. It occurs almost exclusively in women. Usually, affected women have a history of severe stress and emotional problems. Tests for abnormalities in hemostasis are all normal.

The diagnostic test is the development of large ecchymoses within 24 to 48 hours at the site of subcutaneous injection of a small amount (~0.1 mL) of the patient's own blood or erythrocytes. Injection should be at sites inaccessible to the patient, and a concurrent control injection should be administered. The primary differential diagnosis is factitious purpura.

PURPURA SIMPLEX. Purpura simplex denotes easy bruising, commonly observed in young children and middle-aged women and primarily affecting the lower extremities. Laboratory evaluation, including the bleeding time, is normal, and no evidence of vascular abnormalities is present. Affected women do not experience excessive bleeding with surgery, nor do they suffer from internal bleeding.

Louwes H, Lathor OAZ, Vellenga E, deWolf JTLM: Platelet kinetic studies in patients with idiopathic thrombocytopenic purpura, Am J Med 106:430, 1999. *Study suggesting that most patients with ITP have reduced platelet survival but some have decreased production.*

McMillan R: Therapy for adults with refractory chronic immune thrombocytopenic purpura. Ann Intern Med 126:307, 1997. *Reviews experience with therapeutic options in ITP as well as experimental approaches.*

Ravandi-Kashani F, Schafer AI: Microvascular disturbances, thrombosis, and bleeding in thrombocythemia: Current concepts and perspectives. Semin Thromb Hemost 23:479, 1997. *Review of the pathophysiology of thrombocytosis and its complications in myeloproliferative disorders.*

Rebulla P, Finazzi G, Marangoni F, et al: A multicenter randomized study of the threshold for prophylactic platelet transfusions in adults with acute myeloid leukemia. Gruppo Italiano Malattie Ematologiche Maligne dell'Adulto. N Engl J Med 337:1870, 1997. *Establishes guidelines for platelet transfusion in hypoproliferative thrombocytopenia.*

Sarode R, Gottschall JL, Aster RH, et al: Thrombotic thrombocytopenic purpura: Early and late responders. Am J Hematol 54:102, 1997. *Comprehensive examination of therapeutic efficacy of plasmapheresis.*

185 COAGULATION FACTOR DEFICIENCIES

Craig M. Kessler

Severe coagulation deficiencies, or coagulopathies, are typically characterized by the development of excessive bleeding precipitated by trivial incidental or surgical trauma. Frequently, these conditions produce life- and limb-threatening complications. Moderate and mild coagulopathies may remain clinically silent until they are detected serendipitously on routine laboratory screening assays for global coagulation, e.g., the prothrombin time (PT) or activated partial thromboplastin time (aPTT), or when these assays are ordered to evaluate the etiology of abnormal bleeding or easy bruisability. Much of the morbidity of coagulopathies can be minimized or avoided altogether by advanced awareness and prophylactic replacement of the deficient clotting factor protein(s). In contrast to the lifelong clinical manifestations of hereditary/congenital coagulopathies, acquired deficiencies usually occur in previously asymptomatic individuals, may not be suspected immediately on examination, and may remit spontaneously or after eradication of an inciting disease state or withdrawal of treatment with an offending medication. Interestingly, acquired coagulation disorders are often associated with more severe bleeding than the congenital forms. Coagulopathies predominantly result from quantitative defects in biosynthesis of the coagulation factor protein(s), but qualitative defects can also result in bleeding.

HEREDITARY COAGULATION DEFICIENCIES

THE HEMOPHILIAS. The first written documentation for the existence of a sex-linked hereditary coagulation disorder dates back to a fifth century description in the Talmud and was eventually termed *hemophilia* ("love of bleeding") in the 19th century German medical literature. The pathogenesis of this hemorrhagic process was not elucidated completely until 1952, when a mixture of plasma from two hemophilic individuals with similar clinical and hereditary pictures corrected their respective prolonged clotting assays. This incident eventually resulted in the recognition of hemophilia A, caused by a deficiency of clotting protein Factor VIII (antihemophilic factor), and hemophilia B, caused by a deficiency of Factor IX (antihemophilic Factor B, plasma thromboplastin component, or Christmas factor, named after an individual with the disease). A deficiency of either of these two intrinsic coagulation pathway components results in inefficient and inadequate generation of thrombin, which cannot be circumvented or supplemented by a normal extrinsic pathway because of the strong modulatory effects of tissue factor pathway inhibitor.

EPIDEMIOLOGY. The sex-linked recessive disorders of hemophilia A and B are estimated to occur in approximately 1 per 5000 and 1 per 30,000 male births, respectively. The significantly increased incidence of hemophilia A may be due to the greater amount of DNA "at risk" for mutation in the Factor VIII gene (186,000 base pairs) as compared with the Factor IX gene (34,000 base pairs). Hemophilia A and B are observed throughout all races and ethnic groups. About 20,000 individuals have hemophilia in the United States, with a peak prevalence in the second or third decade of life. Suspected or confirmed pregnant carriers have not always opted to undergo prenatal testing or terminate their pregnancies if an affected fetus is detected, and a substantial number (up to 30%) of hemophiliacs result from unanticipated new spontaneous mutations.

GENETICS. As sex-linked recessive diseases, the genes for Factor VIII and IX are located on the long arm of the X chromosome. Males with a defective allele on their single X chromosome will not transmit this gene to their sons, but all of their daughters will be obligate carriers. In turn, female carriers will transmit the coagulation disorder to half of their sons, whereas half of their daughters become carriers. Female carriers can manifest hemophilia-like symptoms when the alleles on the X chromosome are unequally inactivated (lyonization); the defective hemophilic allele is expressed in preference to the normal allele, and a phenotypic hemophiliac is produced. Female hemophilia can arise as the result of mating between a hemophilic male and a female carrier (homozygous for the defective Factor VIII or IX gene) or in carrier females who have the 45 XO karyotype (Turner's syndrome) (hemizygous for the defective hemophilia gene). Evaluation of hemophilia in a female should address the aforementioned processes, as well as von Willebrand's disease (vWD) and its variants, e.g., type 2 Normandy, and exclude the rare, but reported situation of a normal male karyotype associated with testicular feminization.

No single mutation is responsible for the hemophilias, and many missense and nonsense point mutations, deletions, and inversions have been described. Up to 50% of all severe hemophilia A is due to a unique inversion involving intron 22 (the largest of the Factor VIII introns) and homologous DNA outside the gene. The encoded proteins resulting from these mutations are defective and do not express any Factor VIII activity. Mild and moderate hemophilia A is commonly associated with point mutations and deletions. In contrast, Factor IX mutations are more diverse, and severe hemophilia B is more likely caused by large deletions. Hemophilia B may also result from mutations altering the γ-glutamyl residues of the Factor IX protein, which normally become carboxylated through a vitamin K–dependent process and then assemble on a phospholipid surface for eventual activation. Mutated clotting factor genes responsible for the hemophilias may code for the production of defective non-functional proteins that circulate in the plasma and can be detected by immunoassays. Designated cross-reacting material, these proteins have no clinical relevance except that individuals without cross-reacting material may be more susceptible to alloantibody inhibitor formation.

CARRIER DETECTION AND PRENATAL DIAGNOSIS. Carrier detection is particularly useful for women who are related to males with hemophilia and who anticipate becoming pregnant. Coagulation laboratory diagnosis of the carrier state or prenatal involvement is based on measurement of Factor IX activity or Factor VIII activity in comparison to von Willebrand factor antigen (vWF:Ag). This phenotypic approach is 90% accurate but cannot be applied easily to fetal blood specimens or amniotic fluid. Genotypic analysis via restriction fragment length polymorphisms is more accurate if the specific gene defect is known and genetic material is available from the propositus and the carrier. Polymerase chain reaction amplification of DNA and denaturing gradient gel electrophoresis analysis are useful for detection of the intron 22 inversion associated with half of the cases of severe hemophilia A.

CLINICAL FEATURES. The clinical pictures of hemophilia A and B are indistinguishable from each other, with their clinical severity corresponding inversely to the circulating levels of plasma coagulant Factor VIII or IX activity. Thus individuals with less than 1% of normal Factor VIII or IX activity have severe disease characterized by frequent spontaneous bleeding events in joints (hemarthrosis) and soft tissues and by profuse hemorrhage with trauma or surgery. Spontaneous bleeds are uncommon with mild deficiencies of greater than 5% of normal activity; however, excessive bleeding can still occur with trauma or surgery. A moderate clinical course is associated with Factor VIII or IX levels between 1 and 5%. Approximately 60% of all cases of hemophilia A are clinically severe, whereas only 20 to 45% of cases of hemophilia B are severe.

Severe hemophilia is typically suspected and diagnosed during infancy in the absence of a family history. Although the trauma of uncomplicated childbirth (vaginal or cesarean section) rarely produces intracranial hemorrhage, prolonged labor, forceps delivery, and the use of vacuum extraction are major risk factors. Circumcision within days of birth is accompanied by excessive bleeding in fewer than half of severely affected boys. The first spontaneous hemarthrosis usually occurs in severely affected hemophiliacs between 12 and 18 months of age, when ambulation begins, and in moderately affected individuals at about 2 to 5 years of age. The knees are the most prominent sites of spontaneous bleeds, followed by the elbows, ankles, shoulders, and hips; wrists are less commonly involved.

Acute hemarthroses originate from the subsynovial venous plexus underlying the joint capsule and produce a tingling or burning sensation, followed by the onset of intense pain and swelling. On physical examination the joint is swollen, hot, and tender to palpation, with erythema of the overlying skin. Joint mobility is compromised by pain and stiffness, and the joint is usually maintained in a flexed position. Replacement of the deficient clotting factor to normal hemostatic levels rapidly reverses the pain. Swelling and joint immobility improve as the intra-articular hematoma resolves. Intra-articular needle aspiration of fresh bleeding is not recommended because of the risk of introducing infection. Short courses of oral corticosteroids may be helpful in reducing the acute joint symptoms in children but are rarely used in adults.

Recurrent or untreated bleeds result in chronic synovial hypertrophy and eventually damage the underlying cartilage, with subsequent subchondral bone cyst formation, bony erosion, and flexion contractures. Abnormal mechanical forces from weight bearing can produce subluxation, misalignment, loss of mobility, and permanent deformities of the lower extremities. These changes are accompanied by chronic pain, swelling, and arthritis. Radiographic and clinical examination of chronic hemarthroses often underestimates the extent of bone and joint damage; serial ultrasonography and magnetic resonance imaging (MRI) are the most sensitive and specific monitoring and diagnostic techniques.

The pain that accompanies acute hemarthroses responds to immediate analgesic relief, temporary immobilization, and restraint from weight bearing, as well as clotting factor replacement. Narcotic analgesics such as codeine or synthetic derivatives of codeine should be prescribed alone or combined with acetaminophen. Although these medications do not possess significant anti-inflammatory activity, they are preferable to non-steroidal anti-inflammatory drugs or aspirin, which may exacerbate bleeding complications through their anti–platelet aggregatory effects. Similar analgesia can be used for the chronic arthritic symptoms produced by recurrent hemarthroses; however, psychological and physical addiction is more likely to occur. Alternative approaches to pain control include acupuncture, transdermal nerve stimulation, and hypnosis, which may reduce narcotic consumption but may also mask joint pain so that proper immobilization and timely replacement therapy are delayed or ignored, with eventual worsening of the joint damage. Strategies intended to prevent end-stage joint destruction should be initiated at an early age. Synovectomy via open surgery or arthroscopy removes the inflamed tissue and should result in substantially decreased pain and recurrent bleeding. Non-surgical synovectomy ("synoviorthesis"), which involves the intra-articular administration of a radioisotope, is particularly useful in high-risk patients or those with alloantibody inhibitors against Factor VIII or IX. Neither of these procedures reverses joint damage, but both may delay its progression. Non–weight-bearing exercises such as swimming and isometrics are important to periarticular muscle development and maintenance of joint stability for ambulation. Intractable pain and severe joint destruction secondary to repeated hemorrhage require prosthetic replacement. Chronic ankle pain responds best to open surgical or arthroscopic fixation and fusion (arthrodesis).

The ultimate strategy to minimize or eliminate progressive joint destruction by recurrent hemarthroses is predicated on the concept of primary prophylaxis—the planned administration of clotting factor concentrates two (for Factor IX products) or three (for Factor VIII replacement) times weekly at doses to maintain trough clotting factor activity levels above 1 to 2% of normal. These regimens prevent the development of joint deformities and the need for orthopedic surgery, significantly reduce the frequency of spontaneous bleeds, and translate into increased productivity and improved performance status. Although the short-term costs of clotting factor replacement are greater with primary prophylaxis versus traditional "on-demand" therapy for each acute bleeding event, the substantial long-term benefits derived from primary prophylaxis actually reduce the overall cost of hemophilia care. Primary prophylaxis is facilitated by the implantation of a permanent indwelling central catheter for venous access.

Intramuscular hematomas account for about 30% of the bleeding events in individuals with hemophilia and are rarely life threatening. They are usually precipitated by physical or iatrogenic trauma, i.e., following intramuscular injection of vaccines or medications, and can compromise sensory and/or motor function and arterial circulation when they entrap and compress vital structures in closed fascial compartments. Retroperitoneal hematomas may be clinically confused with appendicitis or hip bleeds. Unless these bleeding episodes are treated immediately and aggressively, permanent anatomic deformities such as flexion contractures and pseudotumors (expanding hematomas that erode and destroy adjacent skeletal structures) will occur. Bleeding from mucous membranes, a frequent and troublesome complication in hemophilia, is due to the degradation of fibrin clots by proteolytic enzymes contained in the secretions. Bleeding involving the tongue or the retropharyngeal space can rapidly produce life-threatening compromise of the airways. Gastrointestinal hemorrhage in hemophiliacs typically originates from anatomic lesions proximal to the ligament of Treitz and can be exacerbated by esophageal varices secondary to cirrhosis and portal hypertension and by the use of non-steroidal anti-inflammatory drugs for the treatment of hemarthroses. Ninety per cent of hemophiliacs will experience at least one episode of gross hematuria or hemospermia. Spontaneous bleeding in the genitourinary tract secondary to hemophilia is a diagnosis of exclusion after renal stones and infection are ruled out. Ureteral blood clots produce renal colic, which may be worsened by the use of antifibrinolytic agents.

Intracranial bleeds are the second most common cause of death in hemophiliacs after acquired immune deficiency syndrome (AIDS). They occur in 10% of patients, are usually induced by trauma, and are fatal in 30%. The risk of development of an intracranial hemorrhage is approximately 2.0% per year. Neuromuscular defects, seizure disorders, and intellectual deficits may ensue.

TREATMENT. Reversal and prevention of acute bleeding events in hemophilia A and B are based on replacement of the missing or deficient clotting factor protein to restore adequate hemostasis. Severely affected adolescents or adults consume an average of 50,000 to 80,000 IU of Factor VIII or IX concentrate yearly at a cost ranging between $20,000 and $100,000, depending primarily on the choice of replacement product, e.g., recombinant or plasma derived. Data indicate that the morbidity, mortality, and overall cost of care for individuals with hemophilia are significantly reduced if patients are managed and treated by comprehensive hemophilia centers, where the multispecialty expertise, specialized coagulation laboratory, and diagnostic capabilities exist to coordinate and monitor specific patient needs.

Replacement guidelines (see Table 185–2) are intended to achieve plasma levels of Factor VIII and IX activity of 25 to 30% for minor spontaneous or traumatic bleeds, e.g., hemarthroses, persistent hematuria; at least 50% clotting factor activity for the treatment or prevention of severe bleeds, e.g., major dental surgery, maintenance replacement therapy following major surgery or trauma; and 80 to 100% activity for any life- or limb-threatening hemorrhagic event, major surgery, trauma, etc. Following major trauma or if visceral or intracranial bleeding is suspected, replacement therapy adequate to achieve 100% clotting factor activity should be administered before initiating diagnostic procedures. Although replacement dosing is often empirical, for each unit of Factor VIII administered per kilogram of body weight, plasma Factor VIII activity will increase about 2% (0.02 U/mL), and for each unit of Factor IX administered per kilogram of body weight, Factor IX activity will increase about 1% (0.01 U/mL). The initial dose of Factor IX diffuses into the extravascular space and binds to endothelial cell surfaces to a much greater degree than Factor VIII does. Thus a 70-kg individual with severe hemophilia A or B (Factor VIII or IX activity less than 1% of normal) who requires replacement to 100% activity for major surgery should initially receive 3500 U Factor VIII or 7000 U Factor IX concentrate, respectively. The circulating kinetics of Factors VIII and IX require subsequent dosing every 8 to 12 hours and every 18 to 24 hours, respectively, individualized according to the peak recovery increment within 15 to 30 minutes after bolus infusion and according to trough activity levels. The frequency of repeat dosing is also determined by the rapidity of pain relief, recovery of joint function, and resolution of active bleeding. Replacement is usually maintained for up to 10 to 14 days after major surgery to allow for proper wound healing. Bolus dosing typically results in wide fluctuations in clotting factor activity levels and requires frequent laboratory monitoring to avoid suboptimal troughs. Continuous infusion regimens consisting of 1 to 2 U Factor VIII or IX concentrate per kilogram per hour following a bolus dose maintain a plateau level without the necessity for frequent laboratory testing and reduce total concentrate consumption 30 to 75% in surgical settings.

Thrombogenicity is a major complication of repeated administration of high doses of prothrombin complex concentrates in hemophilia B over short time intervals. Disseminated intravascular coagulation, deep venous thromboses, acute cerebrovascular accidents, and acute myocardial infarctions have been associated with these products but can be avoided by the use of high-purity Factor IX concentrates, which lack activated vitamin K–dependent clotting factors.

Although cryoprecipitate (the precipitate remaining after fresh-frozen plasma [FFP] is thawed at −4° C) is a rich source of Factor VIII and FFP contains both Factors VIII and IX, they are not the replacement products of choice for hemophilia A and B because of their potential to transmit blood-borne pathogens. Plasma-derived clotting factor concentrates (Table 185–1) are manufactured from the plasma donations of over 10,000 individual donors and are then subjected to various types of viral inactivation techniques. Unfortunately, only lipid-enveloped viruses are susceptible to these procedures, which increases the risk that these products can transmit viruses such as parvovirus B19 and hepatitis A and increases the theoretic concern that new viruses and/or prions could contaminate these products in the future. Most manufacturers in the United States are screening donated plasma pools for hepatitis A, B, and C virus, human immunodeficiency virus (HIV), and parvovirus B19 by polymerase chain reaction to enhance the viral safety of the final product. Recombinant Factor VIII and IX concentrates (see Table 185–1) are also available. However, most are stabilized in human albumin and produced by genetically transformed murine cell lines in fetal calf serum, which introduces similar theoretic risks of potential transmission of prions or murine viruses. All concentrates available in the United States, whether plasma derived or recombinant, are equally efficacious and are considered extremely safe; no concentrate has been implicated in the transmission of prions thus far.

As obligate recipients of clotting factor replacement, virtually all hemophiliacs treated before 1985, when techniques for elimination of lipid-enveloped viruses were introduced, have been exposed to hepatitis C virus, often with multiple genotypes (see Chapter 149). Seropositivity to hepatitis G, caused by another lipid-enveloped virus, has been observed in 15 to 25% of hemophiliacs; like hepatitis C virus, it is believed to be susceptible to current viral attenuation procedures. Hepatitis B virus, also lipid enveloped, is a rare problem for hemophiliacs now because vaccination at an early age is the standard of care; however, approximately 5% of those exposed before 1985 are chronic carriers of hepatitis B surface antigen. Hepatitis A virus is not lipid coated and has been transmitted to a small but significant number of patients through solvent detergent–treated Factor VIII and IX concentrates; hepatitis A vaccination should now eliminate this risk. Parvovirus B19 seroprevalence approaches 80% in hemophiliacs; although the long-term clinical consequences are unclear, transmission symbolizes the vulnerability of hemophiliacs to blood-borne pathogens that escape viral attenuation processes.

Ancillary treatment strategies for hemophilias include the use of antifibrinolytic agents, e.g., ε-aminocaproic acid or tranexamic acid, to minimize mucous membrane bleeding and the application of fibrin glues to bleeding sites. Desmopressin (DDAVP) is useful in patients with mild hemophilia A inasmuch as an adequate incremental rise in Factor VIII activity can circumvent the use of clotting factor concentrates. Repeated administration of DDAVP (intravenously or by intranasal spray) can be complicated by tachyphylaxis, hyponatremic seizures, and angina.

PROGNOSIS. The life expectancy of severe hemophiliacs approached 62 years by the mid 1980s with the introduction of clotting factor concentrates; however, HIV has tripled the death rate and is currently responsible for over 55% of all hemophilia deaths. In contrast, the lifetime risk of intracranial hemorrhage is 2 to 8%. Over 75% of adults with hemophilia A and 46% of those with hemophilia B are HIV positive. Otherwise, life expectancy is related to the severity of hemophilia, with the mortality rate of severely affected patients being four to six times greater than that of patients with mild deficiencies. The mortality of patients with inhibitors is significantly greater than that of non-inhibitor patients. Defects in normal growth and development are also exaggerated in HIV-infected boys, with increased cortical atrophy on MRI (15% in HIV-positive versus 6.5% in HIV-negative boys) and delayed growth velocity in adolescence. IQ does not appear to be affected by either HIV or hemophilia.

ALLOANTIBODY AND AUTOANTIBODY INHIBITORS TO FACTORS VIII AND IX. Alloantibody inhibitors arise predominantly in individuals with severe congenital deficiencies of Factors VIII or IX and are suspected when replacement therapy does not provide the usual immediate relief in bleeding symptoms. These IgG antibodies (usually IgG4 subclass) completely neutralize clotting factor activity; no or reduced increments in Factor VIII or IX levels are observed following the administration of bolus doses of concentrate. These inhibitors are time and temperature dependent. The strength of the inhibitor is quantitated in Bethesda units (BU); 1 BU is arbitrarily defined as the amount of inhibitor that neutralizes 50% of the specific clotting factor activity in normal plasma. Patients with high-titer inhibitor, or "high responders," have greater than 5 BU, and an anamnestic antibody enhancement usually develops 5 to 7 days following subsequent exposure to the antigenic clotting factor protein. Low-titer inhibitor patients, i.e., less than 5 BU, are "low responders" and do not manifest anamnesis. Low-titer inhibitor patients can easily be overwhelmed by large amounts of human Factor VIII or IX concentrate, usually three to four times the usual dose. Treatment of patients with high-titer inhibitor against Factor VIII or IX is complicated by the observation that no single approach is uniformly successful. For intermittent bleeds and on-demand regimens, Factor IX complex concentrates of the standard inactivated or activated varieties (see Table 185–1) can be used at an empirical dose of 75 U/kg every 12 to 18 hours. Approximately 48 to 64% of bleeding events will respond favorably. These products contain activated vitamin K–dependent clotting factors that "bypass" the intrinsic pathway inhibitor. As a result, their use is limited by potential thrombogenicity, and the aPTT and clotting factor assays are useless monitors of adequate hemostasis. Alternatively, for patients with inhibitor titers less than 50 BU against

human Factor VIII, porcine Factor VIII concentrate can be administered at a dose between 50 and 100 U/kg with an 80% excellent or good response rate. Cross-reactivity Factor VIII assays should be performed before use to exclude the possibility that the antihuman Factor VIII antibodies will neutralize the effectiveness of the porcine Factor VIII. Factor VIII activity can be measured after its administration and provides objective laboratory evidence of hemostasis. This product is non-thrombogenic, but anamnestic immune responses can result in increased antibody titers against both porcine and human Factor VIII. Recombinant Factor VIIa appears to be an additional new and effective therapy in patients with high-titer Factor VIII and IX inhibitors.

Immune tolerance induction regimens have emerged as a useful adjunctive therapy to eradicate alloantibody inhibitors. Consisting of daily administration of Factor VIII or IX concentrates to inhibitor patients, this regimen is essentially a desensitization process with up to a 68% success rate. Young age, low-titer inhibitor, and immediate initiation following detection of the inhibitor increase the likelihood of success. Once tolerance has been achieved, maintenance prophylaxis with factor concentrate administered two to three times weekly (20 U/kg) is necessary.

Alloantibodies are usually detected in childhood after a median of 9 to 12 days of exposure to clotting factor. These inhibitors occur with an increased incidence in sibships, are more common in those with large, multidomain Factor VIII and Factor IX gene deletions, and manifest a racial predilection. The incidence of Factor VIII alloantibodies is 24 to 52%, with an increased frequency in blacks and perhaps Hispanics. Factor IX alloantibodies are observed with a 1.5 to 3.0% incidence and predominate in Scandina-

Table 185–1 ■ CLOTTING FACTOR CONCENTRATES FOR HEMOPHILIA A AND B AVAILABLE IN THE UNITED STATES

VIRUCIDAL TECHNIQUE	TYPE/NAME OF PRODUCT (MANUFACTURER)	SPECIFIC ACTIVITY (U/mg protein discounting albumin)
	Ultrapure Recombinant Factor VIII	
Immunoaffinity chromatography	Recombinate (Baxter), Bioclate (Baxter, distributed by Centeon); both synthesized in Chinese hamster ovary cell lines	>3000
	KOGENATE (Bayer), Helixate (Bayer, distributed by Centeon); both synthesized in baby hamster kidney cell lines	>3000
	Ultrapure Plasma-Derived Factor VIII	
Immunoaffinity chromatography and pasteurization (60° C, 10 hr)	Monoclate P (Centeon)	>3000
Immunoaffinity chromatography, solvent detergent (TNBP/Triton X-100), and terminal heating (25° C, >10 hr)	Hemofil M (Baxter), Monarc M (Baxter, distributed by the American Red Cross, which also provides the donor plasma)	>3000
	Intermediate-Purity and High-Purity Plasma-Derived Factor VIII	
Affinity chromatography, solvent detergent (TNBP/polysorbate 80), and terminal heating (80° C, 72 hr)	Alphanate (Alpha Therapeutics)	~8–30 (>400 when corrected for von Willebrand factor protein content)
Solvent detergent (TNBP/polysorbate 80)	Koāte-HP (Bayer)	~9–22
Pasteurization (60° C, 10 hr)	Humate-P (Centeon-Pharma)	~1–2
	Ultrapure Recombinant Factor IX	
Affinity chromatography and ultrafiltration (Chinese hamster ovary cell lines maintained in fetal calf serum–free medium)	BeneFix (Genetics Institute)	>200 (albumin free)
	Very Highly Purified Plasma-Derived Factor IX	
Dual-affinity chromatography, solvent detergent (TNBP/polysorbate 80), and nanofiltration	AlphaNine SD (Alpha Therapeutics)	>200
Immunoaffinity chromatography, solvent detergent (sodium thiocyanate), and ultrafiltration	Mononine (Centeon)	>160 (albumin free)
	Low-Purity Plasma-Derived Factor IX Complex Concentrates	
Solvent detergent (TNBP/polysorbate 80)	Profilnine SD (Alpha Therapeutics)	~4.5
Vapor heat (10 hr 60° C, 1190 mbar pressure plus 1 hr, 80° C, 1375 mbar)	Bebulin VH (Immuno, distributed by Baxter)	~2
	Activated Plasma-Derived Factor IX Complex Concentrates (Reserved Primarily for Inhibitor Patients)	
Dry heat (68 °C, 144 hr)	Autoplex T (Baxter, distributed by NABI)	~5
Vapor heat (10 hr, 60° C, 1190 mbar plus 1 hr, 80° C, 1375 mbar)	Feiba VH (Immuno, distributed by Baxter)	~0.8

vians. Factor IX inhibitor patients appear to be susceptible to anaphylaxis and the development of nephrotic syndrome with subsequent exposure to sources of Factor IX.

Autoantibody inhibitors occur spontaneously in individuals with previously normal hemostasis (non-hemophiliacs). Although approximately 50% have no obvious underlying etiology, the remainder are associated with autoimmune diseases, lymphoproliferative disorders, idiosyncratic drug associations, and pregnancy. Patients typically have massive hemorrhagic events, usually much more severe than those produced by alloantibodies; the laboratory expression of autoantibodies is similar to that of alloantibodies except that clotting factor activity is not completely neutralized. Residual clotting factor activities between 3 and 20% of normal are frequently observed in autoantibody patients. The same principles of replacement therapy for alloantibodies also apply to these inhibitors. Porcine Factor VIII concentrate is particularly useful in acquired hemophilia A because very little cross-reactivity usually occurs even with extremely high titers of antihuman Factor VIII antibodies. Immunosuppressive therapy with steroids and cytotoxic agents is a necessary component of the overall treatment to suppress the inhibitor. High-dose intravenous γ-globulin may be a useful adjunctive therapy. Immune tolerance induction is rarely successful in eradicating autoantibody inhibitors and is not usually attempted. For hemorrhagic catastrophes related to either alloantibodies or autoantibodies, extracorporeal plasmapheresis over a staphylococcal protein A column may remove enough of the IgG to allow for replacement therapy with enough factor concentrates to achieve hemostasis.

VON WILLEBRAND DISEASE. In 1926 Erik von Willebrand described an autosomal dominantly inherited hemorrhagic disease affecting both sexes that was subsequently recognized as a deficiency in vWF. It has emerged as the most common bleeding disorder, with a prevalence of 1 to 3% of the population without any ethnic predominance. Homozygous patients are rare and are the result of a recessive mutant gene.

Normal vWF is a large multimeric glycoprotein with monomeric subunits of 220,000 daltons. Its total molecular weight may reach 20 million daltons, with its platelet agglutination properties mediated predominantly by the highest-molecular-weight multimers. The phenotypic classification of vWD recognizes three major types of the disease based on their multimeric structure and function of the vWF protein (Table 185–3). Type 1 vWD accounts for up to 75 to 80% of patients and is inherited predominantly via an autosomal dominant mode; a qualitative defect is present in which the vWF structure is normal but vWF antigen and activity are concurrently reduced. Type 2 vWD includes approximately 20% of vWD patients, is inherited in either a dominant or recessive pattern, and is characterized by qualitative and quantitative abnormalities in the vWF protein. Further subclassification is based on multimeric structure and responses in the ristocetin-induced platelet aggregation assay. Up to 30 variants have been described, each with unique aberrations in vWF multimer structure. Type 2A is the most common variant, with loss of the largest and intermediate-sized multimers, and type 2B lacks the only the largest vWF multimers. The multimeric patterns in type 2A may result from defective synthesis of the vWF protein or increased susceptibility of vWF to proteolysis in vivo. In type 2B, the highest-molecular-weight multimers of vWF are adsorbed preferentially and with abnormally high affinity to the glycoprotein Ib receptor binding site on the platelet membrane surface. Alternatively, a structural defect in the glycoprotein Ib platelet receptor binding site for vWF can produce a multimeric pattern similar to that of type 2B by virtue of its preferential adsorption of the highest-molecular-weight multimers from normal vWF in the circulation. This latter variant is designated platelet-

Table 185–2 ■ COAGULATION PROTEINS AND REPLACEMENT THERAPY

COAGULATION PROTEIN DEFICIENCY	INHERITANCE PATTERN	PREVALENCE	MINIMUM HEMOSTATIC LEVEL	REPLACEMENT SOURCES
Factor I (fibrinogen)			100 mg/dL	Cryoprecipitate/fresh-frozen plasma, viral-treated Factor VIII concentrates (intermediate purity)
Afibrinogenemia	Autosomal recessive	Rare (<300 families)		
Dysfibrinogenemia	Autosomal dominant or recessive	Rare (>300 variants)		
Factor II (prothrombin)	Autosomal dominant or recessive	Rare (~25 kindreds)	30% of normal	Fresh-frozen plasma, Factor IX complex concentrates
Factor V (labile factor)	Autosomal recessive	1 per million births	25% of normal	Fresh-frozen plasma
Factor VII	Autosomal recessive	1 per 500,000 births	25% of normal	Fresh-frozen plasma, Factor IX complex concentrates, or recombinant Factor VIIa
Factor VIII (antihemophilic factor)	X-linked recessive	1 per 5,000 male births	80–100% for surgery/life-threatening bleeds, 50% for serious bleeds, 25–30% for minor bleeds	Factor VIII concentrates (see Table 185–1)
Von Willebrand disease Type 1 and 2 variants	Usually autosomal dominant	1% prevalence	>50% vWF antigen and ristocetin cofactor activity	DDAVP for mild to moderate vWD (except 2B. Variable response to 2A); cryoprecipitate and fresh-frozen plasma (not preferred except in emergencies); Factor VIII concentrates, viral attenuated, intermediate purity (preferred for vWD unresponsive to DDAVP and for Type 3) (see Table 185–1)
Type 3	Autosomal recessive	1 per million births		
Factor IX (Christmas factor)	X-linked recessive	1 per 30,000 male births	25–50% of normal, depending on extent of bleeding and surgery	Factor IX concentrates; fresh-frozen plasma is not preferred except in dire emergencies (see Table 185–1)
Factor X (Stuart-Prower factor)	Autosomal recessive	1 per 500,000 births	10–25% of normal	Fresh-frozen plasma or Factor IX complex concentrates
Factor XI (hemophilia C)	Autosomal dominant: severe type is recessive	~4% Ashkenazi Jews; 1 per million general population	20–40% of normal	Fresh-frozen plasma or Factor XI concentrate
Factor XII (Hageman factor), prekallikrein, high-molecular-weight kininogen	Autosomal recessive	Not available	No treatment necessary	
Factor XIII (fibrin stabilizing factor)	Autosomal recessive	1 per 3 million births	5% of normal	Fresh-frozen plasma, cryoprecipitate, or viral-attenuated Factor XIII concentrate

vWF = von Willebrand factor; DDAVP = desmopressin

Table 185–3 ■ PATTERNS OF VON WILLEBRAND DISEASE

TYPE	VWF:Ag/vWF:RCoF	RIPA	RIPA–LOW DOSE	MULTIMERIC PATTERN
1 (classic)	↓ / ↓	± ↓	Absent	Uniform ↓ in all multimers
2 (Variant)				
2A	↓ / ↓ ↓ ↓	↓ ↓	Absent	↓ in large and intermediate multimers
2B	± ↓ / ± ↓	Normal	Increased	↓ in large multimers
2N (Normandy)	Normal/normal	Normal	↓	Normal
Platelet type	± ↓ / ± ↓	± ↓	Increased	↓ in large multimers
3 (Homozygote or compound heterozygote)	Absent/absent	Absent	Absent	Absent

vWF:Ag = von Willebrand factor antigen; vWF:RCoF = Willebrand factor ristocetin cofactor activity; RIPA = ristocetin-induced platelet aggregation.

type pseudo-vWD. Type 2N (Normandy) is an unusual variant that resembles hemophilia A, although it is inherited in an autosomal dominant pattern. The defective vWF protein is normal from functional and multimeric perspectives but lacks an intact binding site for Factor VIII. Thus unbound Factor VIII is cleared from the circulation with a very rapid half-life. Finally, type 3 vWD, an exceedingly rare variant that occurs in 1 per 1 million individuals, is characterized by nearly complete absence of circulating vWF.

Most patients with vWD have mild disease that may go undiagnosed until trauma or surgery. Symptomatic individuals manifest easy bruisability and mucosal surface bleeding, including epistaxis and gastrointestinal hemorrhage. Menorrhagia affects 50 to 75% of women and may be the initial symptom. These symptoms are consistent with platelet-based defects and reflect the critical role of vWF protein in mediating platelet-platelet and platelet–subendothelial matrix interactions in the process of vascular plug formation and primary hemostasis. The use of aspirin or non-steroidal anti-inflammatory drugs with anti–platelet aggregation effects may exacerbate the symptoms. Deep subcutaneous and intramuscular bleeds, hemarthroses, and intracranial hemorrhage are unusual in vWD, except in the rare type 3 variant. The Factor VIII deficiency is due to the absence of vWF protein, which normally complexes with Factor VIII, delivers it to sites of ongoing coagulation, and prevents its clearance from the circulation.

Physical examination usually reveals non-specific evidence of easy bruising and bleeding. The bleeding time is variably prolonged in patients with vWD and may be influenced by the thrombocytopenia associated with vWD type 2B. The aPTT is also variably increased because of concurrent Factor VIII deficiency; however, a normal aPTT does not exclude the diagnosis of vWD. The vWF activity assay or ristocetin cofactor activity (vWF:RCoF) is the most specific test for vWF function but may be only slightly decreased in mild vWD. The vWF:Ag assay measures the immunologic expression of vWF and is usually performed via electroimmunoassay or enzyme-linked immunosorbent assay. It is slightly reduced in mild vWD and its variants and virtually absent in type 3. Because these assays are sensitive to the molecular mass of vWF, vWF:RCof activity is discordantly low as a result of a low-normal or slightly reduced vWF:Ag level in the type 2 variants of vWD. Furthermore, vWF:RCoF and vWF:Ag are acute phase reactants and are increased by exercise, stress, pregnancy, oral contraceptives, and liver disease and decreased with hypothyroidism and in the presence of blood group O. vWD subtypes can be analyzed by in vitro platelet aggregation assays in which the patient's platelet-rich plasma is activated by the addition of standard and low concentrations of ristocetin or cryoprecipitate. Types 1 and 3 vWF will show mild or marked hyporesponsiveness, respectively, to the standard concentration of ristocetin, whereas type 2B and the rare platelet-type pseudo-vWD will hyperaggregate with half-standard concentrations of ristocetin. Platelet-type pseudo-vWD can be differentiated from type 2B by observing spontaneous platelet agglutination following the addition of cryoprecipitate. With type 2B vWD, the defect responsible for the high-affinity vWF-platelet interaction is present in the vWF protein, whereas in the platelet type the defect resides in the platelet glycoprotein Ib/IX complex.

Gene-based assays are the most specific for diagnosing vWF variants via restriction enzyme mapping of the vWF gene. Type 3 vWF has large deletions whereas the others are caused by variable point mutation defects. Type 2N has defects in the functional domain coding for vWF binding to Factor VIII.

TREATMENT. The goals of therapy for vWD consist of correcting the deficiencies in vWF protein activity to above 50% of normal and Factor VIII activity to levels appropriate for the clinical situation. Although cryoprecipitate is licensed by the FDA for prophylaxis or treatment of vWD-related bleeding complications, the lack of viral safety relegates its use exclusively to emergency circumstances when no other options are readily available. Replacement therapy with viral-attenuated, intermediate- or high-purity Factor VIII concentrates containing high-molecular-weight multimers of vWF, e.g., Humate-P or Alphanate, is preferred and should be reserved for patients with type 1 and 2A variants who are unresponsive to DDAVP and for patients with type 2B and type 3 disease. These products are also indicated for the 2N variant and provide a source of normal vWF to complex with the normal intrinsic Factor VIII. Dosing of Factor VIII concentrates for vWD is calculated according to Factor VIII activity increments, assuming that these materials have a 1:1 relationship between Factor VIII and vWF content. On-demand and continuous infusion regimens have been used successfully. An ultrahigh-purity plasma-derived vWF concentrate is available for clinical research protocols; however, this product will have little value for type 3 individuals, who require simultaneous sources of Factor VIII. All these plasma-derived concentrates may precipitate thrombotic complications or exacerbate the thrombocytopenia in platelet-type pseudo-vWD. These individuals should receive transfusions with normal platelets that possess glycoprotein Ib/IX complexes with normal vWF affinity. Otherwise, DDAVP (0.3 μg/kg in 50 mL normal saline infused over a 20-minute period or intranasally at 150 μg per nostril for adults) is the recommended treatment and eliminates potential exposure to blood-borne pathogens.

The adjunctive use of antifibrinolytic agents such as ε-aminocaproic acid is useful following DDAVP therapy for bleeds. These agents should not be used for renal bleeds or menorrhagia.

The following important caveats for vWD treatment should be considered: (1) A prolonged bleeding time does not need to be normalized to achieve adequate hemostasis following replacement therapy. Correction of vWF and Factor VIII activity will suffice and correlates closely with the clinical risk of bleeding. (2) DDAVP administration should be avoided in most individuals with type 2B variant vWD. Their thrombocytopenia may worsen inasmuch as DDAVP induces the release of abnormal vWF into the circulation with additional in vivo platelet agglutination/aggregation. (3) Individuals with variant type 2N may not manifest a sustained response to DDAVP because the vWF released cannot complex with the simultaneously released Factor VIII and prevent its clearance from the circulation. (4) Individuals who respond adequately to intravenously administered DDAVP may not respond adequately to the intranasal DDAVP preparation. Ideally, patients should be tested for their responses *before* needing it for surgery, etc. (5) Pregnant women with type 2B variant vWD may experience an exacerbation of their thrombocytopenia as pregnancy progresses. Levels of the abnormal vWF increase as estrogen levels increase. (6) Free water intake, whether intravenous or by mouth, should be severely restricted for 4 to 6 hours after DDAVP administration to minimize the risk of hyponatremia and seizures. (7) vWD is clinically associated with Osler-Weber-Rendu syndrome (hereditary hemorrhagic telangiectasia), so gastrointestinal bleeding may occur. (8) Replacement therapy in type 3 vWD may occasionally precipitate the formation of alloantibody inhibitors that neutralize vWF activity.

Acquired vWD is a rare condition and usually occurs as a complication of autoimmune, myeloproliferative, or lymphoproliferative disorders. The acquired vWD associated with neuroblastoma is secondary to proteolysis of vWF by tumor-secreted hyaluronidase. Abnormal vWF multimeric composition is a hallmark of these syndromes. Treatment is similar to that for congenital vWD, but responses are unpredictable.

FACTOR XI DEFICIENCY (HEMOPHILIA C). Factor XI deficiency occurs at a prevalence of 1 per million in the general population and 1 per 500 births in Ashkenazi Jewish families. Factor XI is the only component of the contact phase system of coagulation (Factor XII, pre-kallikrein, and high-molecular-weight kininogen) that is associated with excessive bleeding complications when a deficient state exists. Factor XI deficiency is diagnosed in the laboratory by a prolonged aPTT, normal PT, and decreased Factor XI activity ascertained in a specific quantitative clotting assay (normal range, 60 to 130%). The clinical bleeding tendencies in Factor XI deficiency are less severe than those seen with severe hemophilia A or B and are not necessarily correlated with the extent of the deficiency. Most individuals with Factor XI levels less than 20% of normal activity experience excessive bleeding following trauma or surgery; however, a small number will not bleed. In contrast, bleeding has been observed in approximately 35 to 50% of mildly affected patients with Factor XI levels between 20 and 50%. Spontaneous hemorrhagic episodes, hemarthroses, and intramuscular and intracerebral bleeds are very unusual; traumatic and surgical bleeds typically involve the mucous membranes. Patients undergoing tonsillectomies, prostatectomies, and dental extractions are at highest risk for bleeding unless replacement therapy is administered. Women may experience significant menorrhagia.

GENETICS. Factor XI deficiency is an autosomal disorder that can be inherited in both recessive and dominant patterns. The Factor XI gene is located on chromosome 4. In Ashkenazi Jewish individuals, two predominant gene mutations occur with equal frequency and are designated type II (a stop codon in exon 5) and type III (a single base defect in exon 9). The most severe clinical disease is observed in homozygous type II patients, who usually have less than 1% Factor XI activity. Homozygous type III individuals also manifest severe symptoms, typically less severe than those in individuals with type II, and have slightly higher Factor XI levels of about 10 to 20%. Compound heterozygotes, type II/III, make up the bulk of Factor XI–deficient patients and are clinically mild, with Factor XI levels between 30 and 50%. Genotypic identification of affected patients is determined practically by Factor XI levels rather than by defining their specific gene defect.

TREATMENT. Although Factor XI activity in plasma may not correlate with the severity of clinical bleeding, individuals with severe deficiencies, i.e., less than 20% of normal, are at particular risk of bleeding from surgery and trauma. Replacement therapy for prophylaxis and treatment of acute bleeding events should increase Factor XI levels to at least 40%. FFP is the traditional replacement product of choice because of its rapid effects; however, this approach is associated with potential transmission of blood-borne viruses because FFP is not viral attenuated. In older adults, the volume of FFP required to raise Factor XI activity to adequate hemostatic levels may precipitate heart failure. An emerging alternative to FFP is solvent detergent–treated frozen plasma (currently awaiting FDA approval), which is as efficacious as FFP with substantially decreased risks of viral transmission.

Recently, clinical studies have evaluated a high heat–treated (80° C) viral-attenuated high-purity Factor XI concentrate available on a compassionate basis (Bio Products Laboratory, Elstree, United Kingdom). Although very effective clinically, its usefulness has been compromised somewhat by it potential thrombogenicity manifested by the onset of occasional fatal disseminated coagulation, myocardial infarction, and acute cerebrovascular accident. These complications have usually occurred postoperatively in older individuals with pre-existing hypercoagulable conditions such as malignancy. Factor XI concentrate should be avoided or administered judiciously with careful patient selection. Replacement dosing lev-

els should never exceed 70% Factor XI activity. Repeat dosing with FFP or Factor XI concentrate should account for the very long 60- to 80-hour biologic half-life of Factor XI in vivo.

The decision to treat heterozygotes with Factor XI at levels greater than 20% is somewhat empiric and should be based on the individual's prior history of bleeding after trauma or surgery. Alternatively, the family medical history of previous bleeding complications can be considered. For symptomatic patients, the preoperative or post-trauma use of FFP and pooled plasma products can be minimized or avoided by administering DDAVP, 0.3 μg/kg intravenously. Because hemorrhagic complications originate most commonly from mucosal membrane surfaces, antifibrinolytic agents such as ϵ-aminocaproic acid or tranexamic acid are frequently helpful as adjunctive therapy.

The poor correlation between Factor XI levels and bleeding risk has prompted a search for concurrent defects in coagulation and platelet function. Preliminary data suggest that individuals with absent platelet Factor XI content are at risk. In addition, a significant association is seen between an increased bleeding tendency in patients with mild Factor XI deficiency and coincident mild vWD.

CONTACT ACTIVATION FACTORS. Although Factor XI is important for activating Factor IX in the intrinsic pathway generation of thrombin, it is only one of the four components of the contact phase of coagulation. Deficiencies in any of the other three factors (Factor XII, pre-kallikrein, and high-molecular-weight kininogen) will produce in vitro laboratory abnormalities but no clinical bleeding and therefore require no replacement therapy. Deficiencies of each of these contact factors prolong the aPTT, which may normalize after prolonged incubation of the patient's plasma at 37° C with a negatively charged activator of the aPTT assay, e.g., kaolin or celite. Specific assays are also available to quantitate each of the contact factors.

Counterintuitively, 8 to 10% of individuals with severe Factor XII deficiency (<1% activity) have experienced premature venous thromboembolic events, occasionally fatal in nature. This finding has led to speculation that Factor XII deficiency may lead to hypercoagulability through defective participation of the contact phase proteins in the activation of fibrinolysis.

FACTOR XIII (FIBRIN-STABILIZING FACTOR) DEFICIENCY. Factor XIII is a transglutaminase that is activated by thrombin and subsequently cross-links fibrin to protect it from lysis by plasmin. It is also involved in wound healing and tissue repair and appears to be critical for maintaining a viable pregnancy. Homozygous severe deficiency states are rare and inherited in an autosomal recessive manner with a prevalence of 1 per 3 million births. Consanguinity is common. Typically, patients are first seen shortly after birth with persistent bleeding around the umbilical stump. Intracranial bleeding events, usually precipitated by minimal trauma, occur commonly enough in infants to justify initiating a primary prophylaxis regimen of replacement therapy. Delayed bleeding after surgery and trauma is the hallmark of the disease; however, easy bruisability, poor wound healing with defective scar formation and dehiscence, and hemarthroses are characteristic. Spontaneous abortions are increased in severely affected women. The diagnosis is usually suspected on clinical grounds inasmuch as Factor XIII deficiency is not detected by the conventional screening coagulation assays, e.g., the aPTT or the PT. Most laboratories use a rapid screening assay that assesses the ability of a fibrin clot to remain intact with incubation in 5 mol/L urea or 1% monochloroacetic acid. With Factor XIII levels less than 1% of normal, the clot dissolves within 2 to 3 hours.

Replacement therapy for prophylaxis or treatment of acute bleeds can be accomplished by administering cryoprecipitate, FFP, or preferably, plasma-derived Factor XIII concentrate (pasteurized for viral safety and available in the United States via compassionate IND through Centeon Pharma, King of Prussia, PA). Clinical studies are in progress to evaluate a placentally derived product. Normal hemostasis is achieved with a Factor XIII level of only 5% of normal. The circulating half-life of Factor XIII is up to 10 days, so prophylaxis replacement can be scheduled every 3 to 4 weeks. Acquired alloantibody inhibitors can develop in severely affected individuals. Autoantibodies also occur, usually in association with systemic lupus erythematosus.

DYSFIBRINOGENEMIA AND AFIBRINOGENEMIA. Approximately 300 abnormal fibrinogens have been described; however, very few cause symptoms.

very few cause symptoms. Abnormalities are usually detected incidentally when routine coagulation screening assays reveal decreased fibrinogen concentrations and prolonged thrombin clotting times. On further evaluation, discordance between functional and immunologic fibrinogen levels (>50 mg/dL more antigenic than functional) is observed; plasma-based clotting times with substitution of snake venom for thrombin, e.g., reptilase and ancrod, are variably prolonged. Abnormal fibrinogens are rare autosomally inherited proteins. Their characterization has provided valuable structure-function information and better understanding of wound healing and fibrinolysis.

Over 50% of the dysfibrinogenemias are asymptomatic, 25% are associated with a mild hemorrhagic tendency (commonly caused by defective release of fibrinopeptide A), and 20% predispose individuals to thrombophilia (usually caused by impaired fibrinolysis). Concurrent bleeding and thrombosis may also occur. The prevalence of dysfibrinogenemia in patients with a history of thromboembolic episodes approaches 0.8%, typically occurring in late adolescence and early adulthood. Females experience a high incidence of pregnancy-related complications such as spontaneous abortions and postpartum thromboembolic events. Thrombin and reptilase times are not helpful in predicting whether an abnormal fibrinogen will be prothrombotic, prohemorrhagic, or asymptomatic, but clinical history, fibrinopeptide release studies, and fibrin polymerization studies may be useful. Clinically insignificant dysfibrinogenemias may be acquired in association with hepatocellular carcinoma.

In contrast to the hepatic synthesis of a qualitatively abnormal protein in dysfibrinogenemia, congenital afibrinogenemia, an autosomal recessive disorder, represents the markedly deficient production of a normal protein. Severe life-threatening hemorrhagic complications can occur at any site, beginning at birth with umbilical bleeding. Intracranial hemorrhage is a frequent cause of death. Poor wound healing is characteristic. All coagulation-based assays dependent on detection of a fibrin clot end point are markedly prolonged. Afibrinogenemia is usually detectable by either specific functional or immunologic assays. Platelet dysfunction may accompany afibrinogenemia and exacerbate bleeding.

Deficiencies of fibrinogen may be corrected by the administration of fresh-frozen plasma (FFP) or cryoprecipitate; however, viral safety remains an issue. Intermediate-purity Factor VIII concentrates from FFP that have been viral attenuated and treated with solvent detergent (when licensed by the FDA) are preferable alternatives. The replacement goal is 100 mg/dL fibrinogen. With a circulating biologic half-life of at least 96 hours, treatment every 3 to 4 days is adequate. Primary prophylaxis regimens may be useful in afibrinogenemia; on-demand or prophylactic replacement for trauma or surgery is recommended for prohemorrhagic dysfibrinogenemias. Individuals with thrombophilic manifestations should receive anticoagulation indefinitely.

FACTOR V (PROACCELERIN, LABILE FACTOR) DEFICIENCY. Factor V is a component of the prothrombinase complex that assembles Factors Va and Xa on the phospholipid membrane of the platelet for prothrombin (Factor II) activation to thrombin. Deficiency of Factor V is a very uncommon autosomal recessive disorder (1 per 1 million births). The severity of the plasma Factor V reduction correlates less well with the risk of clinical bleeding than does the platelet Factor V content in the α-granule. This observation illustrates the critical role of the platelet in promoting adequate hemostasis at bleeding sites and explains why transfusions of normal platelets may be preferred over FFP for the treatment of hemorrhagic episodes secondary to congenital or acquired Factor V deficiency. Thus hemostasis can be maintained without correcting plasma Factor V activity (>25% of normal). The Factor V Leiden protein, which is responsible for resistance to activated protein C and thrombophilia, does not affect Factor V coagulant activity (see Chapter 187).

Combined deficiencies of Factors V and VIII occur as an autosomal recessive disorder with a prevalence of 1 per 100,000 births in Jews of Sephardic origin. The severity of bleeding is determined by the levels of these factors, usually ranging from 5 to 30% of normal. Replacement therapy should be aimed at normalizing both clotting protein activities. Factors V and VIII are structurally homologous proteins.

Acquired Factor V deficiency has been described in individuals exposed to bovine Factor V, which contaminates the thrombin preparations used topically to control bleeding during cardiovascular surgery. This abnormality probably represents the development of antibovine Factor V antibodies that cross-react with the human Factor V protein. Profuse bleeding accompanies this complication.

DEFICIENCIES OF VITAMIN K–DEPENDENT COAGULATION FACTORS II, VII, AND X. Congenital deficiencies of Factors II, VII, and X are rare autosomally inherited disorders. Heterozygotes (with factor levels ~20% of normal) are typically asymptomatic except in the immediate newborn period, when physiologic vitamin K deficiency exacerbates the underlying clotting factor deficiency. Homozygotes with clotting factor levels less than 10% of normal manifest variable symptoms. As with other coagulopathies, these deficiencies are usually suspected after the onset of neonatal umbilical stump bleeding. Thereafter, unless replacement or prophylactic therapy is provided, such patients are subject to mucosal bleeding from epistaxis, menorrhagia, and dental extractions; to hemarthroses and intramuscular hematomas; and to post-surgical/trauma bleeding.

In the coagulation laboratory, Factor VII deficiency is associated with a prolonged PT and normal aPTT. This pattern localizes the deficiency to the extrinsic pathway. In contrast, deficiencies of Factors II and X prolong both the PT and aPTT, with the defects localized to the common pathway of coagulation. A Russell's viper venom–based clotting assay can differentiate between these two deficiencies because as a direct activator of Factor X, the Russell's viper venom assay will be prolonged with Factor X but not Factor II deficiency. Mixing patient plasma with normal plasma will demonstrate correction of these assays; specific clotting assays using plasma deficient in the coagulation protein to be studied confirm the diagnosis.

Replacement therapy is indicated for acute symptomatic bleeds and for prophylaxis for surgery. In addition to FFP, which has the potential to transmit blood-borne viruses, Factor IX complex concentrates can be administered to achieve hemostatic levels of any of these vitamin K–dependent factors (>25 to 30% of normal).

Additional issues that should be considered when a deficiency of these or other coagulation factors is confirmed include the following:

1. Acquired severe deficiency of Factor X, often accompanied by deficiencies of other vitamin K–dependent factors, occasionally occurs in individuals with systemic amyloidosis. Because amyloid fibrils in the reticuloendothelial system bind both endogenous and exogenous sources of Factor X, replacement therapy with FFP or Factor IX complex concentrates, even in large quantities, may not always be sufficient. Splenectomy may ameliorate or reverse the bleeding complications.
2. Acquired Factor IX deficiency has been associated with Gaucher's disease because Factor IX binds to glucocerebroside (see Chapter 208).
3. Factor IX deficiency may accompany Noonan's syndrome, an autosomal dominant disease complex characterized by congenital heart disease, abnormal facies, and excessive bleeding or bruising.
4. The genetic Factor II variant resulting from a G to A mutation at nucleoside 20210 is associated with elevated prothrombin levels and an increased risk of venous and arterial thrombosis (see Chapter 187). The PT and aPTT are not affected.
5. Bleeding complications caused by acquired IgG autoantibodies directed against any coagulation factor protein may be rapidly but temporarily reversed by extracorporeal immunoadsorption over a Sepharose-bound polyclonal antihuman IgG or staphylococcal A column with concomitant replacement therapy and initiation of immunosuppression.
6. Acquired Factor VII deficiency has been associated with Dubin-Johnson and Gilbert syndromes.

LUPUS ANTICOAGULANTS

The lupus anticoagulant may be discovered incidentally when routine coagulation assays reveal prolongations in the PT and/or the aPTT, when young women experience recurrent spontaneous miscarriages and/or pregnancy-related thromboembolic events, when young women and elderly men are detected with cerebral arterial thromboses, when patients are affected by systemic lupus erythematosus (20 to 40%) or other autoimmune diseases or lymphoproliferative malignancies, and when patients have been receiving long-term therapy with psychotropic medications, e.g., chlorpromazine. Lupus anticoagulant can also occur with the active opportunistic infections and malignancies associated with AIDS.

The lupus anticoagulant is an IgG or IgM antiphospholipid antibody directed against the phospholipids that function as templates for activation of the prothrombinase complex in vivo and in coagulation assays in vitro. Anticardiolipin antibodies, which are a subset of the antiphospholipid antibody family, can be purified with cardiolipin liposomes and demonstrate anticoagulant activity similar to that of lupus anticoagulants. Recent data suggest, however, that anticardiolipin antibody and lupus anticoagulant may represent separate types of antibodies with different specificities and binding kinetics to phospholipid. Occasionally, individuals may have discordant test results for lupus anticoagulant and the anticardiolipin and antiphospholipid antibodies, particularly during an acute thrombotic event. For practical purposes, one or a combination of these antibodies can be associated with thrombotic complications. These antibodies are diagnosed when mixing studies of patient and normal plasma reveal immediate inhibition of the aPTT or PT at baseline with no additional prolongation after a 2-hour incubation (in contrast to Factor VIII autoantibody). Confirmatory assays include the dilute Russell's viper venom time, tissue thromboplastin time, and platelet neutralization assay. The lupus anticoagulant precipitates bleeding complications in the presence of prothrombin (Factor II) deficiency, probably because of clearance of complexes from the circulation, and when the lupus anticoagulant targets platelet membranes and produces quantitative and/or qualitative platelet abnormalities. The pathologic mechanism for thrombotic complications is not clear; however, lupus anticoagulant may activate platelets and/or inhibit prostacyclin synthesis by endothelial cells or interfere with thrombomodulin function. β_2-Glycoprotein 1, a serum protein that mediates binding of anticardiolipin antibodies to phospholipid, may be critical to the development of thrombotic complications. β_2-Glycoprotein 1 functions as a natural anticoagulant and appears to inhibit thrombin generation. Induction of antiphospholipid antibodies may be stimulated by the exposure of new epitopes that form after β_2-glycoprotein 1 binds to phospholipid/cardiolipin. It has been shown in vitro that these antibodies can cross-react with β_2-glycoprotein 1 and neutralize its anticoagulant capacity and may therefore promote the development of thrombotic complications.

The approach to the management of lupus anticoagulant or antiphospholipid antibody varies according to the severity of symptoms and the clinical circumstances. Although daily low-dose aspirin (81 mg) and/or corticosteroids had been considered an important cornerstone in the prevention of spontaneous miscarriage secondary to lupus anticoagulant or antiphospholipid antibody, a recent large randomized trial found this combination to be ineffective in promoting live births. When a miscarriage has been associated with lupus anticoagulant or antiphospholipid antibody, the preponderance of evidence indicates that more aggressive anticoagulation with full-dose or minidose unfractionated heparin regimens alone or in combination with low-dose aspirin should be used to reduce subsequent fetal losses and to protect the mother who has experienced a previous thrombotic event. Clinical trials with low-molecular-weight heparin (LMWH) preparations and immunosuppressive agents such as intravenous γ-globulin are in progress.

Non-pregnant individuals with thrombotic manifestations of lupus anticoagulant or antiphospholipid antibody have up to a 50% risk of experiencing recurrent events over a 5-year period. Typically, recurrent hypercoagulable episodes occur in a pattern consistent with the initial findings; i.e., venous recurrence follows an initial deep venous thrombosis. Conventional oral anticoagulation to maintain the International Normalized Ratio (INR) between 2.0 and 3.0 does not effectively prevent recurrent events; therefore, a more aggressive regimen intended to achieve an INR of 3.0 to 3.5 is recommended.

The non-virilizing androgen preparations danazol and stanazol may be helpful in raising depressed Factor II levels into the hemostatic range. Asymptomatic individuals may benefit from prophylactic aspirin therapy, which has a favorable risk-to-benefit profile.

COAGULOPATHIES SECONDARY TO ANTICOAGULATION

The most common acquired clinical coagulopathies are secondary to anticoagulation with warfarin and other coumarin analogues and to heparin. Vitamin K–dependent clotting Factors II, VII, IX, and X are functionally defective after warfarin because post-translational carboxylation of their γ-glutamyl residues cannot be accomplished (see Chapter 186). The risks for bleeding increase proportionally with the intensity of anticoagulation and rising INRs. Warfarin effects can be exaggerated by potentiating medications, excessive ethanol use, and simultaneous dietary vitamin K deficiency. Bleeding may be severe or occult and may unmask the presence of pathologic lesions such as carcinomas. For acute and profuse bleeding events caused by warfarin, vitamin K_1, 1 to 5 mg, should be administered subcutaneously or intravenously in conjunction with FFP (10 to 20 mL/kg) or small amounts of Factor IX complex concentrates (20 to 50 U/kg). Bleeding due to over-anticoagulation with warfarin has also been reversed successfully and efficiently by infusions of recombinant Factor VIIa concentrate. For minor bleeding or a markedly increased INR without bleeding, warfarin should be withheld for 1 to 2 days and vitamin K_1 administered at 1 to 2 mg subcutaneously or intravenously. This approach allows for easy reinitiation of warfarin with appropriate dose adjustment. Warfarin effects on the PT can be reversed in vitro by mixing patient plasma with normal plasma. Although the PT is the first coagulation screening parameter that is prolonged after warfarin therapy, this prolongation simply reflects decreased Factor VII activity. Protein C activity has a circulating half-life that parallels that of Factor VII. Thus in early anticoagulation, a potential paradoxical thrombogenic state is produced despite an increased PT. Simultaneous heparin therapy with a 5-day overlap with warfarin will minimize these risks.

Heparin anticoagulation can also induce life-threatening hemorrhagic complications. The aPTT and thrombin times will be prolonged even with minimal amounts of heparin in the circulation or contaminating indwelling catheters from which blood specimens are obtained. The reptilase time can be used to distinguish heparin from other causes of thrombin time prolongation, e.g., fibrin degradation products, or abnormal fibrinogens. The PT may be prolonged in the presence of large concentrations of heparin. Heparin functions as a circulating inhibitor, so mixing studies of patient plasma with normal plasma will not result in correction of the aPTT. LMWH preparations will not affect the aPTT but may affect the thrombin time, depending on the thrombin concentration used in the assay (see Chapter 188). The anticoagulant properties of LMWHs can be monitored by the anti–Factor Xa assay. Acute and profuse bleeding episodes secondary to heparin can be reversed by administering protamine sulfate (1 mg/100 U of residual heparin). Overdosing with protamine sulfate can produce its own coagulopathy. Otherwise, the circulating half-life of standard heparin is short enough (2 to 4 hours) to allow the anticoagulant state to dissipate on its own. The half-life of LMWH is longer, but bleeding is uncommon. The anticoagulation effects of LMWH may be reversed with protamine sulfate, although the response may be marginal and unpredictable.

Bolton-Maggs PHB: Factor XI deficiency. Baillieres Clin Haematol 9:355, 1996. *A comprehensive discussion of genetic aspects and treatment.*

Brettler DB: Inhibitors of factor VIII and IX. Haemophilia 1(Suppl. 1):35, 1995. *A good review of the detection and treatment of this significant complication.*

Cohen AJ, Kessler CM: Treatment of inherited coagulation disorders. Am J Med 99: 675, 1995. *A review of preferred products for replacement therapy for all congenital coagulopathies.*

Cohen AJ, Kessler CM: Acquired inhibitors. Baillieres Clin Haematol 9:331, 1996. *Basic concepts in the diagnosis and treatment of acquired inhibitors to coagulation proteins.*

Di Bona E, Schiavoni M, Castaman G, et al: Acquired haemophilia: Experience of two Italian centres with 17 new cases. Haemophilia 3:183, 1997.

Lee CA (ed): Haemophilia. Baillieres Clin Haematol 9:1, 1996. *This volume contains a comprehensive review of all aspects of hemophilia A and B, including descriptions of molecular diagnostics, new therapeutic modalities, prospects for successful gene therapy, and complications and treatment of alloantibody inhibitors.*

Martinez J: Congenital dysfibrinogenemia. Curr Opin Hematol 4:357, 1997. *An excellent overview of the structure-function relationships of abnormal fibrinogens and their clinical features.*

Perry DJ: Factor X and its deficiency states. Haemophilia 3:159, 1997. *An excellent summary of a rare condition with application for all vitamin K–dependent clotting factor protein deficiencies.*

Sadler JE: A revised classification of von Willebrand disease. Thromb Haemost 71: 520, 1994. *A good reference for interpretation of clinical and laboratory data.*

HEMORRHAGIC DISORDERS: MIXED ABNORMALITIES

Andrew I. Schafer

DISSEMINATED INTRAVASCULAR COAGULATION

Disseminated intravascular coagulation (DIC), also referred to as consumptive coagulopathy or defibrination, is caused by a wide variety of serious disorders (Table 186–1). In most patients, the underlying process dominates the clinical picture, but in some cases (e.g., occult malignancy, envenomation), DIC may be the initial manifestation of the disorder.

PATHOPHYSIOLOGY. DIC is primarily a thrombotic process, even though its clinical manifestation may be widespread hemorrhage in acute, fulminant cases. The basic pathophysiology (Fig. 186–1), irrespective of etiology, is entry into the circulation of procoagulant substances that trigger systemic activation of the coagulation system and platelets and thereby lead to the disseminated deposition of fibrin-platelet thrombi. In most cases, the procoagulant stimulus is tissue factor, a lipoprotein that is not normally exposed to blood. In DIC, tissue factor gains access to blood by tissue injury, its elaboration by malignant cells, or its expression on the surfaces of monocytes and endothelial cells by inflammatory mediators. Tissue factor then triggers generation of the coagulation protease thrombin, which induces fibrin formation and platelet activation. In some specific cases of DIC, procoagulants other than tissue factor (e.g., a cysteine protease or mucin in certain malignancies) and proteases other than thrombin (e.g., trypsin in pancreatitis, exogenous proteins in envenomation) provide the procoagulant stimulus.

In acute, uncompensated DIC, coagulation factors are consumed at a rate in excess of the capacity of the liver to synthesize them, and platelets are consumed in excess of the capacity of bone marrow megakaryocytes to release them. The resulting laboratory manifestations are a prolonged prothrombin time (PT) and activated partial thromboplastin time (aPTT), as well as thrombocytopenia. Increased fibrin formation in DIC stimulates the compensatory process of secondary fibrinolysis in which plasminogen activators generate plasmin to digest fibrin (and fibrinogen) into fibrin(ogen)

Table 186–1 ■ MAJOR CAUSES OF DISSEMINATED INTRAVASCULAR COAGULATION

Infections
  Gram-negative bacterial sepsis
  Other bacteria, fungi, viruses, Rocky Mountain spotted fever, malaria
Obstetric complications
  Amniotic fluid embolism
  Retained dead fetus
  Abruptio placentae
  Toxemia
  Septic abortion
Malignancies
  Pancreatic carcinoma
  Adenocarcinomas
  Acute promyelocytic leukemia
  Other neoplasms
Liver failure
Acute pancreatitis
Envenomation
Transfusion reactions
Respiratory distress syndrome
Trauma, shock
  Brain injury
  Crush injury
  Burns
  Hypothermia/hyperthermia
  Fat embolism
  Hypoxia, ischemia
  Surgery
Vascular disorders
  Giant hemangioma (Kasabach-Merritt syndrome)
  Vascular tumors

degradation products (FDPs). FDPs are potent circulating anticoagulants that further contribute to the bleeding manifestations of DIC. Intravascular fibrin deposition can cause fragmentation of red cells and thereby lead to the appearance of schistocytes in blood smears; however, frank hemolytic anemia is unusual in DIC. Microvascular thrombosis in DIC can also cause tissue necrosis and end-organ damage.

ETIOLOGY. DIC always has an underlying etiology, which must generally be identified and eliminated for successful treatment of the coagulopathy. Infection is the most common cause of DIC. The syndrome is particularly associated with gram-negative sepsis, although it can be triggered by a wide variety of bacterial, fungal, viral, rickettsial, and protozoal microorganisms. The placenta and uterine contents are rich sources of tissue factor and other procoagulants that are normally excluded from the maternal circulation; a spectrum of clinical manifestations of DIC may therefore accompany obstetric complications, especially in the third trimester. These syndromes range from acute, fulminant, and often fatal DIC in amniotic fluid embolism to chronic or subacute DIC with a retained dead fetus. Other obstetric problems associated with DIC include abruptio placentae, toxemia, and septic abortion. Chronic forms of DIC accompany a variety of malignancies, particularly pancreatic cancer and mucin-secreting adenocarcinomas of the gastrointestinal tract, in which thrombotic manifestations predominate (see Chapter 197), and acute promyelocytic leukemia, in which acute exacerbation of chronic DIC can be precipitated by cytotoxic chemotherapy. It is not known whether liver failure can actually cause DIC or whether its coexistence merely exacerbates intravascular coagulation because of impaired clearance of activated clotting factors, plasmin, and FDPs. Snake venom contains a variety of substances that can affect coagulation and endothelial permeability. Bites from rattlesnakes and other vipers can induce profound DIC by introducing these exogenous toxins, as well as by endogenous tissue factor released by tissue necrosis. The likelihood and degree of DIC caused by trauma, surgery, and shock are related to the extent of tissue damage and the organs involved; the brain is a particularly rich source of tissue factor, so traumatic brain injury can precipitate acute DIC. Aortic aneurysms, giant hemangiomas, and other vascular malformations can cause subclinical or clinical DIC that is initiated locally in the abnormal vasculature but can "spill" into the systemic circulation.

CLINICAL MANIFESTATIONS. The clinical manifestations of DIC are determined by the nature, intensity, and duration of the underlying stimulus. The coexistence of liver disease enhances DIC of any etiology. Low-grade DIC is often asymptomatic and diagnosed only by laboratory abnormalities. Thrombotic complications of DIC occur most often with chronic underlying diseases, as exemplified by Trousseau's syndrome in cancer (see Chapter 197). Gangrene of the digits or extremities, hemorrhagic necrosis of the skin, or purpura fulminans may also be manifestations of DIC. Bleeding is the most common clinical finding in acute, uncompensated DIC. Bleeding can be limited to sites of intervention or anatomic abnormalities, but it tends to be generalized in more severe cases, including widespread ecchymoses and diffuse oozing from mucosal surfaces and orifices.

DIAGNOSIS. The laboratory diagnosis of severe, acute DIC is not usually difficult. Consumption and inhibition of the function of clotting factors cause prolongation of the PT, aPTT, and thrombin time. Consumption of platelets causes thrombocytopenia. Secondary fibrinolysis generates increased titers of FDPs, which can be measured by latex agglutination or D-dimer assays. Some schistocytes may be seen in the peripheral blood smear, but this finding is neither sensitive nor specific for DIC. Chronic or compensated forms of DIC are more difficult to diagnose, with highly variable patterns of abnormalities in "DIC screen" coagulation tests. Increased FDPs and prolonged PT are generally more sensitive measures than are abnormalities of the aPTT and platelet count. Overcompensated synthesis of consumed clotting factors and platelets in some chronic forms of DIC may actually cause shortening of the PT and aPTT and/or thrombocytosis, even while elevated levels of FDPs indicate secondary fibrinolysis in such cases.

The most difficult differential diagnosis of DIC occurs in patients who have coexisting liver disease. The coagulopathy of liver failure is often indistinguishable from that of DIC, partly because ad-

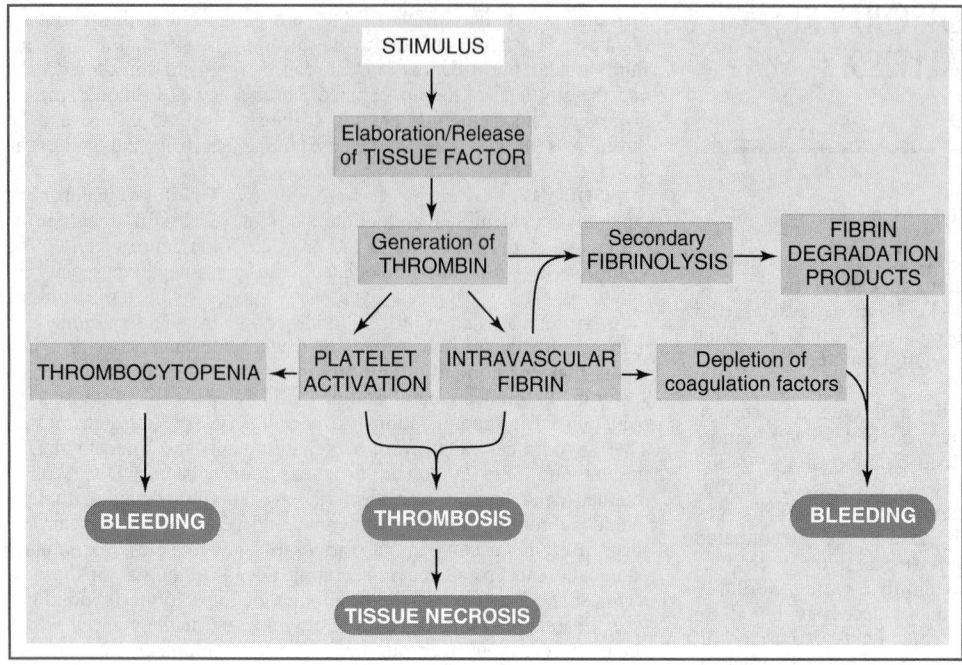

FIGURE 186–1 ■ Pathophysiology of bleeding, thrombosis, and ischemic manifestations in disseminated intravascular coagulation.

vanced hepatic dysfunction is necessarily accompanied by a state of DIC. In liver failure, the combination of decreased synthesis of clotting factors, impaired clearance of activated clotting factors, secondary fibrinolysis, and thrombocytopenia from portal hypertension and hypersplenism may make the coagulopathy practically impossible to differentiate from DIC. In thrombotic microangiopathies, including thrombotic thrombocytopenic purpura and hemolytic-uremic syndrome, platelet consumption and thrombocytopenia are not accompanied by activation of clotting factors or secondary fibrinolysis; hence the PT, aPTT, thrombin time, and FDPs are generally normal in these disorders. Furthermore, schistocytes, often with frank hemolysis, are much more prominent in the peripheral smear in thrombotic thrombocytopenic purpura and hemolytic-uremic syndrome than in DIC.

"Primary fibrinolysis" is disputed as a distinct entity. However, some patients with a serious clinical bleeding diathesis have laboratory evidence of predominantly fibrinolysis, including very high levels of FDPs (D-dimers) and severe hypofibrinogenemia, with relatively little consumption of coagulation factors and normal or near-normal platelet counts. These unusual findings, which approximate those expected with fibrinolytic therapy, are occasionally encountered, particularly in patients with prostate cancer.

TREATMENT. Successful treatment of DIC (Table 186–2) requires that the underlying cause be identified and eliminated. All other therapies, including hemodynamic support, coagulation factor and platelet replacement, and pharmacologic inhibitors of coagulation and fibrinolysis, are only temporizing measures. In many patients with asymptomatic, self-limited DIC who have only laboratory manifestations of the coagulopathy, no treatment may be necessary. In patients with DIC who are actively bleeding or who are at high risk of bleeding, the blood component treatments of choice are transfusions of platelets to improve the thrombocytopenia and fresh-frozen plasma to replace all consumed coagulation factors and thereby correct the prolonged PT and aPTT. The theoretic concern that these blood products may "fuel the fire" and exacerbate the DIC has not been supported by clinical experience. In some patients who have particularly profound hypofibrinogenemia, the additional transfusion of cryoprecipitate, a plasma concentrate that is enriched in fibrinogen, may also be useful. Although not of proven efficacy in human forms of DIC, the infusion of antithrombin III concentrate may be considered as an adjunctive measure in selected cases.

The use of pharmacologic inhibitors of coagulation and fibrinolysis in DIC is controversial. Heparin is of theoretic benefit because it blocks thrombin activity and thereby quenches intravascular coagulation and the resultant secondary fibrinolysis. However, in practice, heparin might exacerbate the bleeding tendency in acute DIC. Heparin is therefore usually reserved for special forms of DIC, including those manifested by thrombosis or acrocyanosis and those that accompany cancer, vascular malformations, retained dead fetus, and possibly acute promyelocytic leukemia. Antifibrinolytic agents, including ε-aminocaproic acid and tranexamic acid, are generally contraindicated in DIC. By blocking the secondary fibrinolytic response to DIC, these drugs will cause unopposed fibrin deposition and may therefore precipitate thrombosis. However, antifibrinolytic agents may be effective in decreasing life-threatening bleeding in DIC, particularly in extreme cases in which aggressive blood component replacement fails to control the hemorrhage; the simultaneous infusion of low doses of heparin may reduce the risk of thrombosis in such situations.

LIVER FAILURE

Bleeding complications in patients with advanced liver disease can be very severe and even fatal and directly account for about 20% of the deaths associated with hepatic failure. The extent of the bleeding tendency depends on the severity and type of liver disease involved. About one third of deaths in patients undergoing liver transplantation are attributable to perioperative hemorrhage.

PATHOPHYSIOLOGY. The pathophysiology of bleeding in liver failure is complex and multifactorial. Anatomic abnormalities are frequently the major cause of gastrointestinal bleeding in patients with liver disease. These changes usually result from portal hyper-

Table 186–2 ■ TREATMENT OF DISSEMINATED INTRAVASCULAR COAGULATION

Identify and eliminate the underlying cause
No treatment if mild, asymptomatic, and self-limited
Hemodynamic support, as indicated, in severe cases
Blood component therapy
  Indications: Active bleeding or high risk of bleeding
    Fresh-frozen plasma
    Platelets
    In some cases, consider cryoprecipitate, antithrombin III
Drug therapy
  Indications: Heparin for DIC manifested by thrombosis or acrocyanosis;
    antifibrinolytic agents generally contraindicated except with life-threatening bleeding and failure of blood component therapy
    Heparin
    Antifibrinolytic agents (generally contraindicated)

tension. Upper gastrointestinal bleeding can be caused by esophageal varices or hemorrhagic gastritis (congestive gastropathy), whereas lower gastrointestinal bleeding, although seldom life-threatening, can be due to hemorrhoids.

The complexity of the systemic coagulopathy of liver failure is not surprising inasmuch as the liver is the principal organ site for the synthesis of coagulation and fibrinolytic factors and their protein inhibitors (Table 186–3). Hepatocytes produce all of the clotting factors except von Willebrand factor, and advanced parenchymal liver disease therefore results in impaired synthesis of these proteins. When superimposed on this quantitative synthetic defect, liver disease can also produce impairment in vitamin K–dependent γ-carboxylation of the procoagulant Factors II, VII, IX, and X, as well as the anticoagulant factors protein C and protein S because of either an intrinsic enzymatic abnormality or vitamin K malabsorption and deficiency in cholestatic forms of liver disease. In addition to a quantitative deficiency of fibrinogen, functional abnormalities of this protein, termed dysfibrinogenemias, are frequently found in various forms of liver disease, particularly in hepatomas. Most forms of advanced liver disease are accompanied by some degree of DIC caused by impaired synthesis of inhibitors of blood coagulation and defective hepatocellular clearance of activated coagulation factors. DIC is an especially important potential complication of LeVeen shunts used for the treatment of intractable ascites because this procedure introduces procoagulant-rich ascitic fluid into the systemic circulation. In many such cases, shunt ligation is required to terminate the DIC. DIC and bleeding risk are exacerbated by the enhanced fibrinolytic activity of liver disease that is caused by increased levels of tissue plasminogen activator accompanied by decreased synthesis of inhibitors of both plasminogen activator and plasmin.

Quantitative and qualitative abnormalities of platelets also contribute to the bleeding diathesis of liver failure. Congestive splenomegaly secondary to portal hypertension causes increased pooling of platelets in the spleen (hypersplenism). The resultant thrombocytopenia, the degree of which generally correlates with spleen size, rarely causes a reduction in the platelet count below 50,000/mm^3. In alcoholic patients, suppression of bone marrow thrombopoiesis by the acute toxic effects of alcohol or folate deficiency may contribute to the thrombocytopenia. Qualitative platelet abnormalities have also been described in patients with liver disease.

Liver transplantation poses special problems to the coagulation system. During the anhepatic stage of surgery, which lasts about 2 hours, the complete cessation of synthesis of coagulation factors causes further prolongations in the PT and aPTT. Release of tissue plasminogen activator from the newly grafted liver then leads to increased fibrinolysis and transient exacerbation of bleeding risk in the postoperative period.

CLINICAL MANIFESTATIONS. The most common hemorrhagic complication of liver disease is gastrointestinal bleeding, which is usually caused by anatomic abnormalities and exacerbated by the systemic coagulopathy of liver failure. Bleeding from other mucosal sites, extensive ecchymoses, or more serious hemorrhage into the retroperitoneum or central nervous system generally indicates more significant derangements of the coagulation system.

DIAGNOSIS. Routine coagulation tests are usually sufficient to diagnose the coagulopathy of liver failure. Although both the PT and aPTT are often prolonged in advanced liver disease, the former tends to be a more sensitive assay early in the course; in fact, a disproportionate prolongation of the aPTT should raise suspicion of a coexisting coagulation abnormality, such as a lupus anticoagulant or clotting factor inhibitor. The prolonged PT is also a useful prognostic indicator of poor outcome in patients with cirrhosis,

acute acetaminophen hepatotoxicity, and acute viral hepatitis; in the latter, it is a better index of prognosis than the serum albumin or transaminases. A disproportionate prolongation of the thrombin time should suggest the presence of dysfibrinogenemia. Hypersplenism, possibly associated with nutritional folate deficiency or the acute toxic effects of alcohol on bone marrow, often causes mild to moderate thrombocytopenia in patients with liver disease; however, consideration should be given to other coexisting causes of thrombocytopenia if the platelet count is much below 50,000/mm^3.

The coagulopathy of liver failure is sometimes indistinguishable from that of DIC, in part because some degree of DIC is a necessary accompaniment of advanced liver disease. However, in general, patients with DIC have more marked decreases in levels of Factor VIII and increases in titers of FDPs, particularly D-dimers, than do those with liver failure.

TREATMENT. Therapy for the coagulopathy of liver disease may be directed at preventing the hemorrhagic complications of invasive procedures or treating active bleeding. Bleeding risks of surgical procedures in patients with liver failure are poorly defined. However, it is usually recommended that attempts be made to correct PT prolongations of over 3 seconds and platelet counts below 70,000/mm^3 before surgical interventions, including percutaneous liver biopsy. The most effective treatment is blood component therapy with fresh-frozen plasma (which contains all of the coagulation factors) and platelet transfusions. Some patients require large volumes of fresh-frozen plasma (15 to 20 mL/kg) to lower the prolonged PT; rarely, plasmapheresis with plasma exchange is required to avoid fluid overload in such situations. Because of the short half-lives of some clotting factors, fresh-frozen plasma may have to be administered as frequently as every 8 to 12 hours to maintain acceptable coagulation test parameters. In some patients, especially those with cholestasis, parenteral administration of vitamin K can at least partially reverse the coagulation abnormalities; however, in patients with advanced hepatocellular failure, vitamin K is largely ineffective. Prothrombin complex concentrates are relatively contraindicated in liver failure, as in DIC, because of the risk of thrombotic complications. Platelet transfusions are not as effective as in thrombocytopenias caused by decreased platelet production. Because of immediate pooling of transfused platelets in the enlarged spleens of patients with hypersplenism, a higher than calculated dose of platelet concentrates is usually required to raise the circulating platelet counts significantly. Desmopressin (DDAVP), which can shorten the bleeding time of patients with cirrhosis, may be used as ancillary therapy.

VITAMIN K DEFICIENCY

Vitamin K is required for γ-carboxylation of glutamic acid residues of the procoagulant Factors II (prothrombin), VII, IX, and X and the anticoagulant factors protein C and protein S. This posttranslational modification normally renders these proteins functionally active in coagulation. Severe vitamin K deficiency can lead to a hemorrhagic diathesis that is characterized by prolongations of the PT and sometimes also the aPTT. The PT is more sensitive than the aPTT in detecting vitamin K deficiency states because Factor VII, the only one of the vitamin K–dependent factors that is in the extrinsic pathway of coagulation, is the most labile of these proteins.

The two major sources of vitamin K are dietary intake and synthesis by the bacterial flora of the intestine. Therefore, in the absence of malabsorption, nutritional deficiency alone rarely causes clinically significant vitamin K deficiency. However, such a condition can arise when eradication of gut flora is combined with inadequate dietary intake. This situation typically occurs in critically ill patients in intensive care units who have no oral intake and are receiving broad-spectrum antibiotics for prolonged periods. Vitamin K deficiency can also develop in patients receiving total parenteral nutrition unless the infusions are supplemented with vitamin K.

Vitamin K is absorbed predominantly in the ileum and requires the presence of bile salts. Therefore, clinically significant vitamin K deficiency occurs with malabsorption of fat-soluble vitamins secondary to obstructive jaundice or with malabsorption caused by intrinsic small bowel diseases, including celiac sprue, short-bowel

Table 186–3 ■ COAGULATION ABNORMALITIES IN LIVER DISEASE

Abnormalities of Coagulation
Decreased synthesis of coagulation factors
Impaired vitamin K–dependent γ-carboxylation
Dysfibrinogenemia
Disseminated intravascular coagulation
Increased fibrinolytic activity
Abnormalities of platelets
Thrombocytopenia (hypersplenism)
Abnormal platelet function

syndrome, and inflammatory bowel disease. Finally, warfarin acts as an anticoagulant by competitive antagonism of vitamin K.

Correction of vitamin K deficiency, when clinically significant, can be achieved with oral supplementation, unless malabsorption is present. In the latter case, parenteral vitamin K (10 mg subcutaneously daily) should be administered. Emergency treatment of bleeding caused by vitamin K deficiency is transfusion of fresh-frozen plasma.

Carey MJ, Rodgers GM: Disseminated intravascular coagulation: Clinical and laboratory aspects. Am J Hematol 59:65, 1998. *Review of concepts of diagnosis and treatment of DIC, including discussion of novel approaches.*

Furie B, Bouchard BA, Furie BC: Vitamin K dependent biosynthesis of gamma-carboxyglutamic acid. Blood 93:1798, 1999. *Comprehensive review of basic mechanisms of vitamin K metabolism.*

Staudinger T, Locker GJ, Frass M: Management of acquired coagulation disorders in emergency and intensive-care medicine. Semin Thromb Hemost 22:93, 1996. *Emphasis on a practical clinical approach to the treatment of bleeding problems in DIC and liver failure.*

187 THROMBOTIC DISORDERS: HYPERCOAGULABLE STATES

Andrew I. Schafer

The "hypercoagulable states" encompass a group of inherited or acquired disorders that cause a pathologic thrombotic tendency or risk of thrombosis. These conditions are also known as "pre-thrombotic" states. A hereditary tendency to thrombosis, irrespective of its cause, is sometimes referred to as "thrombophilia."

The primary hypercoagulable states (see Chapter 183) are caused by quantitative or qualitative abnormalities of specific coagulation proteins that lead to a prothrombotic state. Most of these disorders involve inherited mutations in one of the physiologic antithrombotic factors (see Chapter 183). Particularly when combined with other prothrombotic mutations (multigene interactions), these primary hypercoagulable states are associated with a lifelong predisposition to thrombosis. The trigger for a discrete, clinical thrombotic event is often the development of one of the acquired, secondary hypercoagulable states superimposed on an inherited state of hypercoagulability. The secondary hypercoagulable states, a diverse group of mostly acquired conditions (Fig. 187–1), cause a thrombotic tendency by complex and often multifactorial mechanisms.

PRIMARY HYPERCOAGULABLE STATES

MOLECULAR MECHANISMS AND FREQUENCY. ANTITHROMBIN III DEFICIENCY. Inherited quantitative or qualitative deficiency of antithrombin III leads to increased fibrin accumulation and a lifelong propensity to thrombosis (see Chapter 183). Antithrombin is the major physiologic inhibitor of thrombin and other activated coagulation factors, and its deficiency leads to unregulated protease activity and fibrin formation. Two basic phenotypes of inherited antithrombin deficiency are recognized. Patients with type I antithrombin deficiency have proportionately reduced plasma levels of antigenic and functional antithrombin that result from a quantitative deficiency of the normal protein. Impaired synthesis, defective secretion, or instability of antithrombin in type I antithrombin-deficient individuals is caused by major gene deletions, single nucleotide changes, or short insertions or deletions in the antithrombin gene. Patients with type II antithrombin deficiency have normal or nearly normal plasma antigen accompanied by low activity levels, thus indicating a functionally defective molecule. Type II antithrombin deficiency is further subdivided into subtypes in which abnormalities affect the reactive protease inhibitory activity, the heparin binding site, or both. Type II deficiency is usually caused by specific point mutations leading to single amino acid substitu-

tions that produce a dysfunctional protein. Over 80 different mutations causing type I or type II antithrombin deficiency have been recognized to date.

The pattern of inheritance of antithrombin deficiency is autosomal dominant. Most affected individuals are heterozygotes whose antithrombin levels are typically about 40 to 60% of normal but may have the full clinical manifestations of hypercoagulability. Rare homozygous antithrombin-deficient patients usually have type II deficiency with reduced heparin affinity, a variant that is associated with a low risk of thrombosis in its heterozygous form.

The frequency of asymptomatic heterozygous antithrombin deficiency in the general population may be as high as 1 in 350. Most of these individuals have clinically silent mutations and will never have thrombotic manifestations. The frequency of symptomatic antithrombin deficiency in the general population has been estimated to be between 1:2000 and 1:5000. Among all patients seen with venous thromboembolism, antithrombin deficiency is detected in only about 1%, but it is found in about 2.5% of selected patients with recurrent thrombosis and/or thrombosis at a younger age (<45 years).

PROTEIN C DEFICIENCY. Protein C deficiency leads to unregulated fibrin generation because of impaired inactivation of Factors VIIIa and Va, two essential cofactors in the coagulation cascade. As with antithrombin deficiency, two general forms of protein C deficiency are recognized: type I, with proportionate decreases in protein C antigen and activity, and type II, in which qualitative defects in protein C are associated with disproportionately reduced protein C relative to antigen. More than 160 mutations are known to cause protein C deficiency. In type I, frameshift, nonsense, or missense mutations cause premature termination of protein synthesis or loss of protein stability. In type II, different mutations can cause abnormalities in protein C activation or function.

The mode of inheritance of protein C deficiency is autosomal dominant. As in antithrombin deficiency, most affected individuals are heterozygotes. The prevalence of protein C deficiency in the general population is 1:200 to 1:300 when an antigenic assay is used and 1:500 when a functional assay with confirmatory DNA analysis is used. Protein C deficiency is found in 3 to 4% of patients with venous thromboembolism.

PROTEIN S DEFICIENCY. Protein S is the principal cofactor of activated protein C (APC), and therefore its deficiency mimics that of protein C in causing loss of regulation of fibrin generation by impaired inactivation of Factors VIIIa and Va. Unlike protein C, protein S circulates in plasma partly in complex with C4b binding protein; only free protein S, which normally constitutes about 35 to 40% of total protein S, can function as a cofactor of APC. As in antithrombin and protein C deficiencies, both quantitative (type I) and qualitative (type II) forms of inherited protein S deficiency are known. In addition, type III protein S deficiency is characterized by normal plasma levels of total protein S but low levels of free protein S.

Relatively few specific mutations of the protein S gene have been described to date, most involving frameshift, nonsense, or missense point mutations. The prevalence of protein S deficiency in the general population is unknown. However, its frequency among patients evaluated for venous thromboembolism (2 to 3%) is comparable to that of protein C deficiency.

ACTIVATED PROTEIN C RESISTANCE. Inherited APC resistance causing thrombophilia was originally detected by the finding that the activated partial thromboplastin times (aPTTs) of the plasma of affected individuals could not be appropriately prolonged by the addition of exogenous APC in vitro. It was subsequently recognized that the great majority of subjects with functional APC resistance have a single, specific point mutation in the Factor V gene. This mutation, termed "Factor V Leiden," replaces guanine with adenine at nucleotide 1691 (G1691A), which leads to the amino acid substitution of Arg504 by Gln and thereby renders Factor Va incapable of being inactivated by APC. Heterozygosity for the autosomally transmitted Factor V Leiden increases the risk of thrombosis by a factor of 5 to 10, whereas homozygosity increases the risk by a factor of 50 to 100.

The Factor V Leiden mutation is remarkably frequent (3 to 7%) in healthy white populations but appears to be far less prevalent or even non-existent in certain black and Asian populations. In various studies, APC resistance was found in a wide range (10 to 64%) of patients with venous thromboembolism.

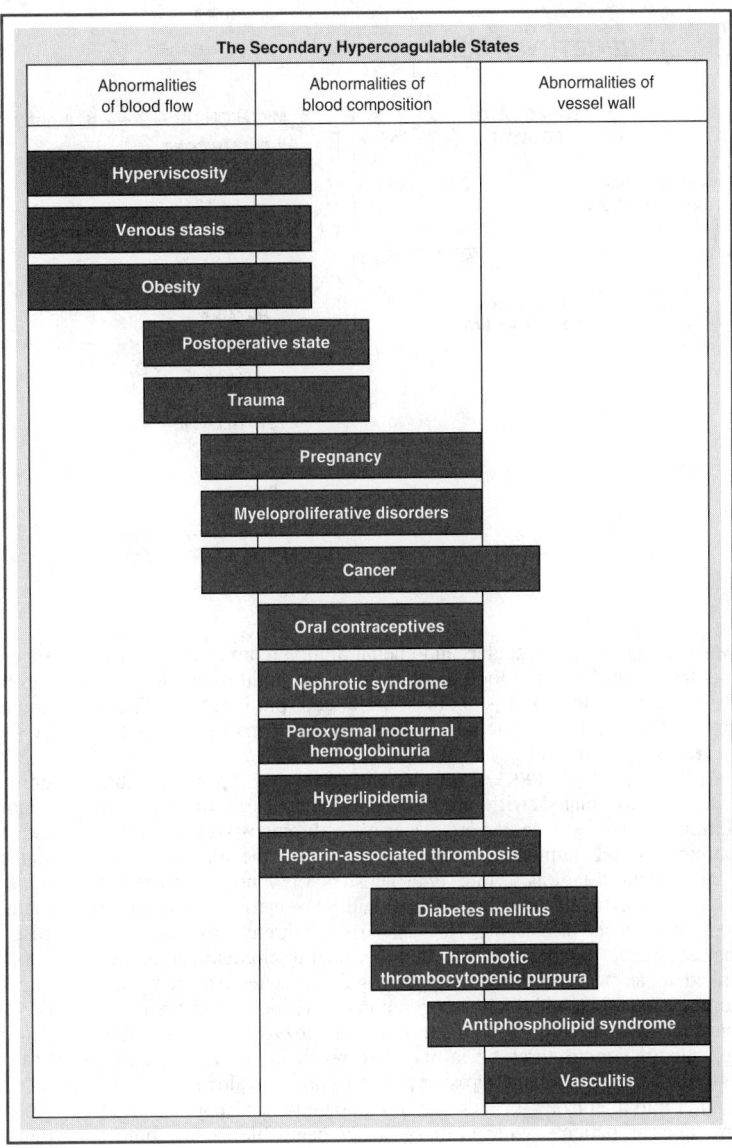

The Secondary Hypercoagulable States

Abnormalities of blood flow	Abnormalities of blood composition	Abnormalities of vessel wall
Hyperviscosity		
Venous stasis		
Obesity		
Postoperative state		
Trauma		
Pregnancy		
Myeloproliferative disorders		
Cancer		
Oral contraceptives		
Nephrotic syndrome		
Paroxysmal nocturnal hemoglobinuria		
Hyperlipidemia		
Heparin-associated thrombosis		
Diabetes mellitus		
Thrombotic thrombocytopenic purpura		
Antiphospholipid syndrome		
Vasculitis		

FIGURE 187–1 ■ The secondary hypercoagulable states. The pathophysiologic basis of thrombotic risk in these diverse disorders is complex and multifactorial. Predominant mechanisms of thrombosis for the different secondary hypercoagulable states shown are based on Virchow's triad of thrombogenesis: abnormalities in blood flow, abnormalities in blood composition, abnormalities of the vessel wall. (Modified from Schafer AI: The primary and secondary hypercoagulable states. *In* Schafer AI (ed): Molecular Mechanisms of Hypercoagulable States. New York, Chapman & Hall, 1997, p 16.)

PROTHROMBIN GENE MUTATION. The substitution of G for A at nucleotide 20210 of the prothrombin gene has been associated with elevated plasma levels of prothrombin and an increased risk of venous thrombosis. The allele frequency for the prothrombin gene mutation is 1.2% in a Dutch population, which makes it second only to Factor V Leiden as a genetic risk factor for venous thrombosis, at least in certain white populations. This prothrombin gene mutation is found in 6 to 18% of patients with venous thromboembolism.

OTHER PRIMARY HYPERCOAGULABLE STATES. A number of other inherited abnormalities of specific physiologic antithrombotic systems may be associated with a thrombotic tendency. However, most of these conditions are limited to case reports or family studies, their molecular genetic bases are less well defined, and their prevalence rates are unknown but are probably much lower than those of the disorders described above. The other primary hypercoagulable states include heparin cofactor II deficiency, dysfunctional thrombomodulin, and a number of fibrinolytic disorders that lead to impaired fibrin degradation, including hypoplasminogenemia, dysplasminogenemia, plasminogen activator deficiency, and certain dysfibrinogenemias that cause a thrombotic rather than a bleeding diathesis.

HYPERHOMOCYSTEINEMIA. Hyperhomocysteinemia is due to elevated blood levels of homocysteine, a sulfhydryl amino acid derived from methionine; when blood levels are sufficiently increased, particularly in homozygous children, homocystinuria develops. Homocysteine can be metabolized by either of two remethylation pathways (catalyzed by methionine synthase, which requires folate and cobalamin, or by betaine-homocysteine methyltransferase); alternatively, homocysteine is converted to cystathionine in a transsulfuration pathway catalyzed by cystathionine β-synthase, with pyridoxine used as a cofactor (Fig. 187–2). Inherited hyperhomocysteinemia is most commonly caused by deficiency of cystathionine β-synthase, whereas a minority of cases are caused by hereditary defects in the remethylation pathways.

Homozygous deficiency states that lead to severe hyperhomocysteinemia cause premature arterial atherosclerotic disease and venous thromboembolism, as well as mental retardation, neurologic defects, lens ectopy, and skeletal abnormalities. However, adults with heterozygous deficiency states, with resultant mild to moderate hyperhomocysteinemia, may have only venous or arterial thrombotic manifestations. The frequency of heterozygous cystathionine β-synthase deficiency in the general population is 0.3 to 1.4%. The allele frequencies of the remethylation pathway defects appear to be lower. Acquired causes of hyperhomocysteinemia in adults most commonly involve nutritional deficiencies of the cofactors required for homocysteine metabolism, including pyridoxine, cobalamin, and folate.

Acquired as well as inherited hyperhomocysteinemia is a likely risk factor for arterial and venous thrombosis. The mechanism of homocysteine-induced thrombosis and atherogenesis involves complex and probably multifactorial effects on the vessel wall. Homo-

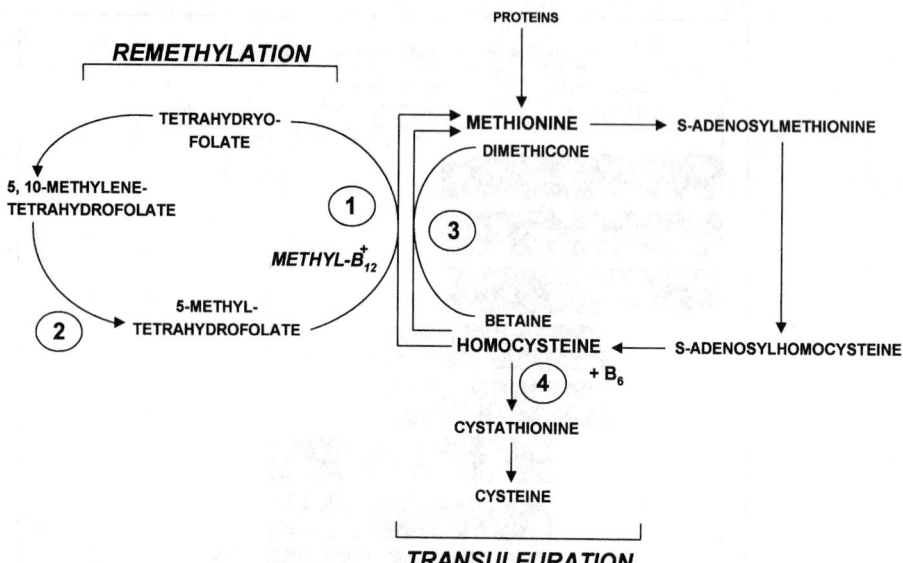

FIGURE 187-2 ■ Intracellular metabolism of homocysteine occurs through remethylation to methionine or transsulfuration to cysteine. Numbered circles indicate the principal enzymes involved: (1) methionine synthase; (2) 5,10-methylenetetrahydrofolate reductase; (3) betaine-homocysteine methyltransferase; (4) cystathionine β-synthase. (Modified from De Stefano V, Finazzi G, Mannucci PM: Inherited thrombophilia: Pathogenesis, clinical syndromes, and management. Blood 87:3531, 1996.)

cysteine can cause vascular endothelial injury, conversion of the endothelial surface of blood vessels from an antithrombotic to a prothrombotic one, and smooth muscle cell proliferation. These toxic effects of homocysteine on the vessel wall may be mediated by free oxygen radicals.

CLINICAL MANIFESTATIONS. The primary hypercoagulable states are associated with predominantly venous thromboembolic complications (see Chapter 69). Deep vein thrombosis of the lower extremities and pulmonary embolism are by far the most frequent clinical manifestations. More unusual sites of venous thrombosis include superficial thrombophlebitis and mesenteric and cerebral vein thrombosis (see Table 183–2). Arterial thrombosis involving the coronary, cerebrovascular, and peripheral circulations is not linked to any of the primary hypercoagulable states except hyperhomocysteinemia, although some reports have described their occurrence with protein S deficiency and homozygous antithrombin deficiency. Venous thrombosis may also result in arterial occlusion by paradoxical embolism across a patent foramen ovale.

The initial episode of venous thromboembolism may occur at any age in patients with primary hypercoagulable states, but it typically occurs in early adulthood. The risk of recurrence is increased in these patients, and positive family histories of thrombosis can frequently be elicited. The risk of thrombosis varies among the individual primary hypercoagulable states and is relatively lower in patients with APC resistance; it is markedly increased with the coexistence of other prothrombotic mutations. Rare patients with homozygous deficiency states tend to have more severe thrombotic complications. A peculiar manifestation of homozygous protein C or protein S deficiency is neonatal purpura fulminans. This serious and sometimes fatal syndrome is caused by widespread thrombosis of small cutaneous and subcutaneous vessels that leads to ischemic necrosis. Fatal purpura fulminans associated with a bleeding diathesis has also been described in a patient with an acquired IgG inhibitor of protein C. Warfarin-induced skin necrosis may infrequently complicate the initiation of oral anticoagulant therapy in patients with heterozygous protein C or protein S deficiency. Because both of these proteins are vitamin K dependent for normal function, their plasma levels in patients with inherited deficiency states may drop to nearly zero within a few days of starting therapy with warfarin, a vitamin K antagonist, and lead to a transient prothrombotic imbalance and skin necrosis caused by dermal vascular thrombosis. Nevertheless, oral anticoagulation clearly provides effective long-term antithrombotic prophylaxis in these patients.

In most patients with primary hypercoagulable states, discrete clinical thrombotic complications appear to be precipitated by acquired prothrombotic events (e.g., pregnancy, use of oral contraceptives, surgery, trauma, immobilization), many of which are the secondary hypercoagulable states discussed below. In particular, thrombosis complicates pregnancy, especially in the puerperium, in about 30 to 45% of women with antithrombin deficiency, 10 to 20% with protein C or protein S deficiency, and almost 30% with APC resistance, unless prophylactic anticoagulation is administered during this period. The clinical manifestations and circumstances of venous thromboembolism in hyperhomocysteinemia are essentially indistinguishable from those of the other primary hypercoagulable states. However, in contrast to the other disorders, hyperhomocysteinemia is also an independent risk factor for arterial thrombosis, including myocardial infarction, stroke, and peripheral arterial disease.

DIAGNOSIS. Laboratory diagnosis (see Chapter 183) of the primary hypercoagulable states requires testing for each of the disorders individually because no general screening test is available to determine whether a patient may have such a condition. At this time, functional, immunologic, or DNA-based assays are available to test for antithrombin deficiency, protein C deficiency, protein S deficiency, APC resistance (Factor V Leiden), the prothrombin gene mutation, and hyperhomocysteinemia.

The scope and timing of laboratory testing for primary hypercoagulable states should be individualized. For example, an otherwise healthy, younger patient who has suffered a single episode of deep vein thrombosis or pulmonary embolism should probably be evaluated for each of the major primary hypercoagulable states, particularly if high-risk characteristics are present (see Table 183–2). Conversely, a patient with a terminal metastatic malignancy and recurrent or refractory thrombosis does not require such testing if its results will not alter the treatment strategy. Individuals with arterial thrombosis should generally not be tested for any of these disorders except hyperhomocysteinemia because other primary hypercoagulable states (Table 187–1) are not clearly associated with an increased risk of arterial thrombosis.

In general, testing for these disorders is not recommended immediately after a major thrombotic event. Active thrombosis may transiently consume and deplete some of the proteins in plasma and lead to the erroneous diagnosis of inherited antithrombin, protein C, or protein S deficiency. In addition to acute thrombosis, pregnancy, estrogen use, liver disease, and disseminated intravascular coagulation (DIC) may cause acquired deficiencies of antithrombin, protein C, and/or protein S. Anticoagulation may also interfere with some of the tests for primary hypercoagulable states. Heparin treatment can cause a decline in antithrombin levels to the deficiency range even in individuals who do not have underlying antithrombin deficiency. In contrast, warfarin can elevate antithrombin levels into the normal range in patients who do have an inherited deficiency state. Warfarin therapy also reduces the functional levels and, less prominently, the immunologic levels of protein C

Table 187-1 ■ THE PRIMARY HYPERCOAGULABLE STATES

Antithrombin (III)/Heparin Disorders
Antithrombin deficiency
Heparin cofactor II deficiency
Protein C/Protein S Disorders
Protein C deficiency
Protein S deficiency
Activated protein C resistance
   Factor V Leiden
Thrombomodulin dysfunction
Prothrombin Gene Mutation
Fibrinolytic Disorders
Hypoplasminogenemia
Dysplasminogenemia
Plasminogen activator deficiency
Dysfibrinogenemia
Hyperhomocysteinemia
Cystathionine β-synthase deficiency
Remethylation pathway defects
Acquired hyperhomocysteinemia
   Pyridoxine, cobalamin, folate deficiency

Table 187-2 ■ LONG-TERM MANAGEMENT OF PATIENTS WITH PRIMARY HYPERCOAGULABLE STATES

RISK CLASSIFICATION	MANAGEMENT
High risk	Indefinite anticoagulation or lifelong chronic anticoagulation
2 or more spontaneous thromboses	
1 spontaneous life-threatening thrombosis	
1 spontaneous thrombosis at an unusual site (e.g., mesenteric, cerebral venous)	
1 spontaneous thrombosis in the presence of more than a single hypercoagulable state	
Moderate risk	Vigorous prophylaxis during high-risk situations
1 thrombosis with an acquired prothrombotic stimulus	
Asymptomatic	

Modified from Bauer K: Approach to thrombosis. *In* Loscalzo J, Schafer AI (eds): Thrombosis and Hemorrhage, 2nd ed. Baltimore, Williams & Wilkins, 1998, pp 477–490.

and protein S, potentially leading to misdiagnosis of inherited deficiency. Therefore, all these tests are optimally performed in clinically stable patients at least 2 weeks after completing oral anticoagulation following a thrombotic episode. When testing is indicated in patients in whom interruption of prophylactic oral anticoagulation is considered too risky, protein C and protein S levels can be determined after warfarin therapy has been discontinued under heparin coverage for at least 2 weeks. Testing of first-degree family members can also confirm an inherited deficiency state.

Functional assays are the best screening tests for antithrombin, protein C, and protein S deficiencies because these assays will detect both quantitative and qualitative defects; antigenic (immunologic) assays detect only quantitative deficiencies of these proteins. However, functional coagulation assays for protein C and protein S may yield spuriously low values if APC resistance is present. APC resistance can be diagnosed by either of the newer, high-sensitivity and high-specificity coagulation assays or by DNA analysis of peripheral blood mononuclear cells for the Factor V Leiden mutation. Hyperhomocysteinemia is currently diagnosed by measurement of total plasma homocysteine after an overnight fast. Discrimination of affected individuals from normal subjects can be improved if the fasting plasma homocysteine level increment is measured following ingestion of a standardized oral methionine load.

TREATMENT. The initial treatment of acute venous thrombosis or pulmonary embolism in patients with primary hypercoagulable states is not different from that in those without genetic defects (see Chapter 84). As in patients without known thrombophilia, thrombolytic therapy should be considered following massive venous thrombosis or pulmonary embolism. Acute management is initiated with at least 5 days of unfractionated or low-molecular-weight heparin. Oral anticoagulation with warfarin can be started on the first day of heparin use and continued for at least 3 months, with regulation of the dose to maintain an International Normalized Ratio (INR) of the prothrombin time between 2.0 and 3.0.

Recommendations for long-term management are compromised at this point by the lack of data from rigorously controlled clinical trials (Table 187-2). Continuing oral anticoagulant prophylaxis beyond the initial 6 months following an acute episode of venous thromboembolism must be weighed against continued exposure of the individual patient to the significant risk of bleeding complications. Patients with primary hypercoagulable states who have suffered two or more thrombotic events should receive lifelong prophylactic anticoagulation with warfarin. In fact, indefinite or lifelong anticoagulation is probably indicated for individuals with recurrent thrombosis even in the absence of identifiable primary hypercoagulable states.

The decision to continue prophylactic oral anticoagulation beyond the initial period following the initial episode of thrombosis is more difficult. Recent data indicate that the risk of recurrent thrombosis up to 8 years after an initial episode in patients heterozygous for Factor V Leiden is significantly greater than in genetically unaffected individuals. However, these findings should not be ex-

trapolated to other inherited primary hypercoagulable states. Furthermore, despite the increased risk of thrombosis recurrence over several years in individuals with Factor V Leiden and the clear efficacy of prophylactic warfarin therapy, it is not yet clear whether the protection afforded by oral anticoagulation outweighs the risk of serious bleeding complications associated with it. Following a single episode of thrombosis, patients with inherited hypercoagulable states should probably receive indefinite or lifelong anticoagulation if their initial episodes were life threatening or occurred in unusual sites (e.g., mesenteric, cerebral venous thrombosis) or if they have more than one prothrombotic genetic abnormality. In the absence of these characteristics, particularly if the initial episode was precipitated by a transient acquired prothrombotic situation (e.g., pregnancy, postoperative state, immobilization), it is reasonable at this time to discontinue warfarin therapy after 6 months and administer subsequent prophylactic anticoagulation only during high-risk periods.

Asymptomatic individuals with known thrombophilia who have not had previous thrombotic complications do not require prophylactic anticoagulation except during periods of high risk for thrombosis. Because about half of the first-degree relatives of a patient with a primary hypercoagulable state should be affected, such individuals should be counseled about the implications of making a diagnosis.

The management of pregnancy in women with primary hypercoagulable states requires special consideration because of the high risk of thrombosis, particularly in the puerperium. Women with thrombophilia who have had previous thrombosis—and probably also asymptomatic women with thrombophilia—should receive prophylactic anticoagulation throughout pregnancy and for 4 to 6 weeks postpartum, a particularly high-risk period. Heparin is presently the anticoagulant of choice because of the risk of embryopathy in the first trimester and bleeding late in pregnancy with the use of warfarin. The options are adjusted-dose unfractionated heparin given by subcutaneous injection every 8 or 12 hours, with doses adjusted to maintain a mid-interval aPTT of 1.5 times the control INR, or fixed-dose, low-molecular-weight heparin.

Because warfarin-induced skin necrosis is a very rare problem, screening of all patients for inherited protein C or protein S deficiency, conditions that are known to predispose to this complication, is not indicated before starting warfarin therapy. Most cases can be avoided by not initiating warfarin therapy with high loading doses and by concomitant coverage with heparin. When the complication does occur, as manifested by painful red and subsequently dark, necrotic skin lesions within a few days of starting warfarin, warfarin therapy must be immediately discontinued, vitamin K administered, and heparin started. The use of fresh-frozen plasma or purified protein C concentrate to rapidly normalize protein C levels can improve results. Despite this rare complication, warfarin is an effective, long-term prophylactic anticoagulant in patients with inherited protein C or protein S deficiency.

Antithrombin III concentrate purified from normal human plasma may be a useful adjunct to anticoagulation in "heparin-resistant" patients, who represent unusual cases of type II antithrombin deficiency, and in antithrombin-deficient patients with recurrent thrombosis despite adequate anticoagulation. Antithrombin concentrate infusion can also be considered in some perioperative or obstetric settings in which anticoagulation poses an unacceptable bleeding risk. Purified protein C concentrate has been used to initiate warfarin therapy in severe protein C deficiency and in the initial treatment of neonatal purpura fulminans.

It is not clear at this time whether comparable guidelines for anticoagulation are applicable to patients with hyperhomocysteinemia and venous thrombosis. Vitamin supplementation with folate, pyridoxine, and cobalamin can normalize elevated blood levels of homocysteine, but it is not known whether such treatment reduces the risk of thrombosis. Until such information becomes available, the safety and low cost of supplementation make this treatment advisable for patients with hyperhomocysteinemia associated with thrombosis. The recommended daily doses are 1 mg folate, 100 mg pyridoxine, and 0.4 mg cobalamin.

SECONDARY HYPERCOAGULABLE STATES

The secondary hypercoagulable states (see Fig. 187–1) are diverse, mostly acquired disorders that predispose patients to thrombosis by complex, multifactorial pathophysiologic mechanisms. Many of these conditions also represent the acquired precipitating stimuli for clinical thrombotic events in individuals with a genetic predisposition (primary hypercoagulable states). Although each disorder causes thrombosis primarily through abnormalities in blood flow (rheology), blood composition (coagulation factors and platelet function), or the vessel wall, multiple overlapping mechanisms are operative in many of them.

MALIGNANCY. Certain malignant tissues may stimulate thrombosis directly by elaborating procoagulant substances that initiate a systemic process of chronic DIC. For example, the leukocytes of patients with acute promyelocytic leukemia produce tissue factor–like procoagulant activity. Tumor-associated monocytes may also be activated to express surface tissue factor, thereby indirectly activating the coagulation system and inducing chronic DIC. The thrombotic tendency of patients with cancer may also be related to mechanical factors such as immobility or a bulky tumor mass compressing vessels, as well as to co-morbid conditions such as liver dysfunction secondary to metastases, sepsis, surgery, and the prothrombotic effects of certain antineoplastic agents.

The incidence of thrombotic complications in cancer patients depends in part on the type of malignancy. Hypercoagulability appears to be most prominent in patients with pancreatic cancer, adenocarcinomas of the gastrointestinal tract or lung, and ovarian cancers. The presence of underlying malignancy compounds the independent risk of thrombosis in the postoperative state. Although thrombosis most commonly occurs in patients with established malignancy, it can also antedate the diagnosis by months or even years (see Chapters 69 and 197).

The most common thrombotic manifestations in patients with neoplasms are deep vein thrombosis and pulmonary embolism, but more unusual and distinctive thrombotic complications are also found. Trousseau's syndrome, characterized by migratory superficial thrombophlebitis of the upper or lower extremities, is strongly linked to cancer. Non-bacterial thrombotic endocarditis involves fibrin-platelet vegetations on heart valves, which produce clinical manifestations by systemic embolization (see Chapter 197). As many as 75% of cases of non-bacterial thrombotic endocarditis have underlying malignancies at autopsy. Because the valve vegetations are often too small to be detected by auscultation of murmurs or by echocardiography, the diagnosis should be suspected in individuals with systemic embolic signs, including acute stroke syndromes. Both Trousseau's syndrome and non-bacterial thrombotic endocarditis are highly associated with adenocarcinomas and laboratory evidence of DIC (see Chapter 197). The occurrence of either syndrome in patients without known cancer demands a more vigorous search for occult malignancy than in those with deep vein thrombosis or pulmonary embolism. Thrombotic microangiopathy,

characterized by hemolysis with red cell fragmentation, thrombocytopenia, and microvascular thrombosis with involvement of target organs, occurs in about 5% of patients with metastatic carcinomas, most commonly with gastric, lung, and breast primary sites.

Treatment of acute venous thromboembolism in cancer patients should be initiated as in other patients, but subsequent prophylactic anticoagulation probably should be continued while active malignancy is present. Many cancer patients are difficult to anticoagulate and may be resistant to warfarin prophylaxis. Anticoagulation also can be complicated by bleeding into tumors. In some cases, only continuous heparin infusion, delivered by pump, is effective in suppressing the thrombotic process.

MYELOPROLIFERATIVE DISORDERS AND PAROXYSMAL NOCTURNAL HEMOGLOBINURIA. Thrombosis and, apparently paradoxically, bleeding are major causes of morbidity and mortality in the myeloproliferative disorders, a group of bone marrow hematopoietic stem cell disorders that include polycythemia vera, essential thrombocythemia, chronic myelogenous leukemia, myelofibrosis and myeloid metaplasia (see Chapter 174), and in the related stem cell disorder, paroxysmal nocturnal hemoglobinuria. In uncontrolled polycythemia vera, increased whole blood viscosity contributes to the thrombotic tendency. Thrombocytosis, abnormal platelet function, and other less well understood factors are also probably involved in the hemostatic defect of the myeloproliferative disorders and paroxysmal nocturnal hemoglobinuria.

In addition to deep vein thrombosis and pulmonary embolism, some distinctive thrombotic manifestations are seen. Hepatic vein thrombosis (Budd-Chiari syndrome), as well as portal and other intra-abdominal venous thrombosis, is associated with myeloproliferative disorders and paroxysmal nocturnal hemoglobinuria and may be the initial manifestations of the disease. Myeloproliferative disorders, particularly essential thrombocythemia, may cause erythromelalgia, a syndrome of microvascular thrombosis that is manifested by intense pain accompanied by warmth, duskiness, and mottled erythema, sometimes resembling livedo reticularis, in a patchy distribution in the extremities, most prominently in the feet; digital microvascular ischemia progressing to vascular insufficiency and gangrene may ensue. A wide spectrum of neurologic manifestations may be caused by cerebrovascular ischemia, especially in essential thrombocythemia. As in the antiphospholipid antibody syndrome, pregnancy in patients with myeloproliferative disorders may be complicated by recurrent spontaneous abortions, fetal growth retardation, and premature deliveries, probably secondary to placental insufficiency caused by thrombosis and infarctions.

Treatment of venous thromboembolism in the myeloproliferative disorders and paroxysmal nocturnal hemoglobinuria should be initiated as in patients without these hematologic disorders. In patients with thrombosis associated with polycythemia vera, the hematocrit should be maintained in the normal range with phlebotomies and/or chemotherapy; in those with essential thrombocythemia, cytoreduction of the elevated platelet count should be achieved with chemotherapy. Long-term prophylaxis of recurrent thrombosis in these patients may also be achieved with antiplatelet (aspirin) therapy, but caution should be exercised because of the increased risk of bleeding complications.

ANTIPHOSPHOLIPID ANTIBODY SYNDROME. The antiphospholipid antibody syndrome is characterized by both venous and arterial thrombosis, recurrent spontaneous abortions (which may also be due to thrombosis), thrombocytopenia, and a variety of neuropsychiatric manifestations. The syndrome is associated with a heterogeneous group of autoantibodies that bind to anionic phospholipid-protein complexes, the critical protein cofactor of which is probably α_2-glycoprotein I. Patients with this syndrome have any combination of positive tests to detect plasma antiphospholipid-protein antibodies: anticardiolipin antibodies, lupus anticoagulants, and/or biologic false-positive VDRL. Although animal models have now begun to demonstrate a pathogenetic relationship, it has not yet been conclusively proved that these antibodies are the cause of the hypercoagulable state rather than just epiphenomena. Even though the antiphospholipid-protein antibodies may cause activation of platelets and the coagulation system, their predominant prothrombotic effects are probably directly on the vessel wall.

About two thirds of thrombotic events in these patients are venous, typically deep vein thrombosis or pulmonary embolism, and one third are arterial. Cerebrovascular events are the most common arterial thrombotic complications and are manifested as stroke, transient ischemic attacks, multi-infarct dementia, or retinal artery occlusion. Peripheral and intra-abdominal vascular occlusion is encountered more rarely. Echocardiographic studies have revealed that about one third of these patients have non-bacterial heart valve vegetations (Libman-Sacks endocarditis). The most prominent obstetric complications of the antiphospholipid antibody syndrome are recurrent, spontaneous abortions and fetal growth retardation, which are probably due to thrombosis of placental vessels. Thrombotic complications are largely limited to patients with "primary" antiphospholipid antibody syndrome or those in whom the antibodies are associated with collagen-vascular disease, not with drugs or infections.

Acute management of thrombosis in these patients is essentially the same as that in other individuals. Monitoring of heparin anticoagulation is difficult in patients who have a lupus anticoagulant because they already have a prolonged aPTT at baseline; the use of low-molecular-weight heparin, which does not require monitoring, can circumvent this problem. Warfarin is effective in preventing recurrent thrombosis but usually requires prolonged therapy with intermediate- to high-intensity doses to achieve an INR greater than 2.6, with a target INR of 3.0. No established treatment of women with antiphospholipid antibody syndrome has been shown to prevent recurrent fetal loss. Treatment during pregnancy with prednisone and aspirin is not effective in promoting live birth and may actually increase the risk of prematurity.

PREGNANCY AND ORAL CONTRACEPTIVES. The pathophysiology of hypercoagulability associated with pregnancy involves a progressive state of DIC throughout the course of pregnancy. Activation of the coagulation system is initiated locally in the uteroplacental circulation, where the placenta is the source of increased thrombin generation. Platelet activation and increased platelet turnover also occur during normal pregnancy, and about 8% of healthy women at term have mild thrombocytopenia. Simultaneously, the fibrinolytic system is progressively blunted throughout pregnancy because of the action of placental plasminogen activator inhibitor type 2. The net effect of these coagulation changes is to produce a state of hypercoagulability that makes pregnant women vulnerable to thrombosis, particularly in the puerperium. These systemic alterations are compounded by prothrombotic mechanical and rheologic factors in pregnancy, including venous stasis in the legs caused by the gravid uterus, pelvic vein injury during labor, and the trauma of cesarian section. Oral contraceptives induce systemic coagulation changes that are similar to those found in pregnancy.

Deep vein thrombosis and pulmonary embolism are the most common thrombotic complications of pregnancy and oral contraceptive use. Coexisting primary hypercoagulable states represent a major additive risk factor. Increasing age, increasing parity, cesarean delivery, prolonged bed rest or immobilization, obesity, and previous thromboembolism are additional prothrombotic risk factors in pregnant women. Most thrombotic events associated with pregnancy occur in the peripartum period, especially after delivery.

POSTOPERATIVE STATE AND TRAUMA. Postoperative thrombosis is caused by a combination of local mechanical factors, including decreased venous blood flow in the lower extremities, and systemic changes in coagulation. Activation of the coagulation system is most likely initiated by the release of tissue factor from injured tissue and is accompanied by decreased plasma levels of physiologic anticoagulants and, particularly in orthopedic surgery, an antifibrinolytic response.

The level of risk of postoperative thrombosis depends largely on the type of surgery performed. It is probably compounded by coexisting risk factors such as an underlying inherited primary hypercoagulable state or malignancy, as well as by advanced age and prolonged procedures. Postoperative deep vein thrombosis and pulmonary embolism, the most common thrombotic complications, are often asymptomatic but detectable by non-invasive studies. The incidence of deep vein thrombosis following general surgical procedures is about 20 to 25%, with almost 2% of such patients having clinically significant pulmonary embolism. The risk of deep vein thrombosis after hip surgery and knee reconstruction ranges from 45 to 70% without prophylaxis, and clinically significant pulmonary embolism occurs in as many as 20% of patients undergoing hip surgery. Postoperative thrombosis risk following urologic and

gynecologic surgery more closely approximates that found after general surgery. Although the process of thrombosis usually begins intraoperatively or within a few days of surgery, the risk of this complication can be protracted beyond the time of discharge from the hospital, particularly in hip replacement patients.

Venous thromboembolism is also one of the most common causes of morbidity and mortality in survivors of major trauma, and asymptomatic deep vein thrombosis of the lower extremities has been detected by venography in over 50% of hospitalized trauma patients. The risk of venous thrombosis after trauma is increased by advanced age, need for surgery or transfusions, and the presence of lower extremity fractures or spinal cord injury. The striking but highly variable incidence of venous thromboembolism after surgery or trauma has led to risk stratification and recommendations for prophylactic anticoagulation.

Bauer K: Approach to thrombosis. *In* Loscalzo J, Schafer AI (eds): Thrombosis and Hemorrhage, 2nd ed. Williams & Wilkins, Baltimore, 1998, pp 477–490. *Clinical approach to patients with suspected hypercoagulable state, with an emphasis on evaluation of inherited disorders.*

De Stefano V, Fanizzi G, Mannucci PM: Inherited thrombophilia: Pathogenesis, clinical syndromes, and management. Blood 87:3531, 1996. *Comprehensive review with practical guidelines to diagnostic methods.*

Schafer AI: The primary and secondary hypercoagulable states. *In* Schafer AI (ed): Molecular Mechanisms of Hypercoagulable States. New York, Chapman & Hall, 1997, p 16. *Detailed overview of inherited and acquired thrombotic disorders. Other chapters in the book provide more encyclopedic reviews of individual hypercoagulable states.*

Schafer AI: Venous thrombosis as a chronic disease. N Engl J Med 340:955, 1999. *Editorial commenting on recent finding that secondary prevention of venous thromboembolism requires more prolonged oral anticoagulation.*

188 ANTITHROMBOTIC THERAPY

Laurence A. Harker

Antithrombotic therapies involve the use of thrombolytic agents, antiplatelet drugs, and anticoagulants. Selection of appropriate antithrombotic therapy depends on the location, size, and flow characteristics of the thrombosed vasculature; the risk of propagation, embolization, and recurrence; and the relative antithrombotic benefits and hemorrhagic risk. The clinical presumption of vaso-occlusive thrombosis (see Chapter 67) or thromboembolism (see Chapter 84) generally requires objective confirmation. Complementary mechanical measures for restoring peripheral arterial patency include balloon catheter thrombectomy or surgical embolectomy (see Chapter 84). Transcutaneous deployment of caval filters may be useful in preventing pulmonary thromboembolism when immediate anticoagulant therapies are not possible or are contraindicated (see Chapter 69). Coronary thrombosis may be treated by catheter-based techniques in conjunction with antithrombotic therapy (see Chapter 60).

Kearon C, Julian JA, Newman TE, Ginsberg JS: Non-invasive diagnosis of deep venous thrombosis. Ann Intern Med 128:663, 1998. *This objective evaluation of diagnostic methods contributes appropriate strategies for non-invasive assessment.*

Verstraete M, Fuster V, Topol EJ (eds): Cardiovascular Thrombosis, 2nd ed. Philadelphia, Lippincott-Raven, 1998. *This volume is an excellent up-to-date review of antithrombotic therapy.*

THROMBOLYTIC THERAPY

Fibrinolytic therapy is useful in the treatment of patients with acute arterial and venous thrombo-occlusive events. Early intravenous thrombolytic therapy is convincingly beneficial in patients with acute myocardial infarction (MI), acute arterial thromboembolic occlusion, severe deep venous thrombosis (DVT), and threatening pulmonary embolism (PE). Overall, the clinical benefits, as well as the bleeding risks, are equivalent for the four approved thrombolytic agents: streptokinase, recombinant tissue plasminogen activator (t-PA), urokinase plasminogen activator, and anisoylated plasminogen-streptokinase activator complex (anistreplase).

Acute Arterial Thrombo-occlusive Events

ACUTE CORONARY THROMBOSIS. In patients with acute MI, extensive data from controlled clinical trials have clearly established that intravenous thrombolytic therapy salvages ischemic myocardium when given within the initial 6 hours and probably within the initial 12 hours after symptoms develop by recanalizing approximately 75% of the occluded coronary arteries. Although t-PA appears to re-establish flow more quickly than does streptokinase or anistreplase, this early advantage is lost within the initial 24 hours except when front-loaded t-PA regimens are used (see Chapter 60).

Thrombolytic agents convert plasminogen to plasmin (Table 188–1). Newer derivatives or alternative fibrinolytic agents evaluated in controlled clinical trials have not shown superiority over established thrombolytic agents.

Residual thrombus remaining after successful thrombolytic reperfusion is highly thrombogenic and initiates rethrombosis. Consequently, adjunctive antiplatelet or anticoagulant therapy improves patency rates in patients with acute MI treated with thrombolytic therapy. The Second International Study of Infarct Survival Collaborative Group demonstrated improved mortality in patients with acute MI who were receiving adjuvant aspirin (160 mg). Abciximab, a potent antiplatelet $\alpha_{IIb}\beta_3$-integrin fibrinogen receptor antibody antagonist, produces additional improvement in outcomes when used as an adjunctive to thrombolysis (see below). Clinical trial data also suggest that direct antithrombins (bivalirudin or hirudin) improve reperfusion patency and outcomes after thrombolytic therapy. Adjuvant heparin is beneficial for patients with acute MI who are receiving t-PA, as shown by the GUSTO trials, but evidence supporting heparin's use with other thrombolytic agents is less compelling. Current guidelines recommend adjuvant heparin for acute MI patients receiving other thrombolytic agents who are at high risk for systemic emboli. Adjuvant regimens achieving optimum benefit with acceptable hemorrhagic risk have not yet been adequately established. Newer data suggest a possible role for the combination of low-dose thrombolytic therapy combined with urgent percutaneous transluminal coronary angioplasty for acute MI (see Chapter 60).

SYSTEMIC THROMBOEMBOLIC OCCLUSIVE EVENTS. Fibrinolytic therapy is an alternative to mechanical or surgical intervention for treating arterial thrombo-occlusive disease (see Chapter 67). Although opinions vary, fibrinolytic therapy is generally used initially, with surgical intervention reserved for resistant occlusive thrombi. Catheter delivery of thrombolytic agents directly into the occluding thrombus usually recanalizes occluded arteries. However, bleeding complications occur with either local or systemic forms of therapy. Most bleeding occurs at sites of diagnostic or interventional arteriotomy. No controlled trials have directly compared outcomes after different thrombolytic agents or mechanical/surgical interventions in peripheral arterial thrombo-occlusive disease.

Venous Thrombosis and Pulmonary Embolism

DEEP VENOUS THROMBOSIS. (See Chapter 69.) Fibrinolytic agents are indicated in the treatment of massive DVT. The theoretic advantages of managing proximal vein thrombosis with thrombolytic agents include preservation of valvular structures in the deep veins to prevent the post-phlebitic syndrome and lysis of thrombi more rapidly and completely than occurs by endogenous fibrinolysis. Despite the lack of adequately controlled clinical trials, many recommend fibrinolytic therapy for DVT if a massive thrombus is present.

ACUTE PULMONARY EMBOLISM. (See Chapter 84.) Thrombolytic therapy is more effective than heparin anticoagulation in the removal of acute PE, as measured by angiography, perfusion lung scans, or hemodynamic assessments. No differences in these outcomes have been documented for streptokinase, urokinase plasminogen activator, or t-PA. However, the early flow benefits of thrombolytic therapy disappear within 1 week, and no improvement in mortality or short-term morbidity has been shown in controlled clinical trials. Unfortunately, thrombolytic therapy in patients with PE substantially increases bleeding complications.

Complications of Thrombolytic Therapy

Because severe bleeding is the principal limiting complication of thrombolytic therapy, medical thrombolysis is contraindicated in patients with recent surgery or trauma, malignant disease, recent stroke, active peptic ulcer disease, recent liver or renal biopsy, and recent arterial puncture. The frequency of clinical bleeding complications, including intracranial bleeding, which occurs in 0.3 to 1.0% of patients with acute MI, is comparable for all thrombolytic drugs. Concomitant use of other antithrombotic therapies appears to aggravate bleeding.

ISIS-3 Collaborative Group: ISIS-3: A randomised comparison of streptokinase vs tissue plasminogen activator vs anistreplase and of aspirin plus heparin vs aspirin alone among 41,299 cases of suspected acute myocardial infarction. Lancet 339:753, 1992. *This study randomizing patients with acute MI demonstrated that 35-day*

Table 188–1 ■ THROMBOLYTIC AGENTS

FEATURE	SK	APSAC (ANISTREPLASE)	u-PA	t-PA
Structure	47-kd bacterial non-enzymatic trypsin-like protein	SK complexed with *p*-anisoylated plasminogen	54-kd human 2-chain serine protease	68-kd human single-chain fibrin-dependent serine protease
Mode of action	SK forms complex with plasminogen, which converts plasminogen to plasmin	Anistreplase forms complex with plasminogen and generates plasmin gradually as active-center *p*-anisoylated groups hydrolyze	u-PA directly cleaves plasminogen to form plasmin	t-PA forms complex with fibrin, which converts plasminogen to plasmin
Removal from plasma (T_{50})	30 min	100 min	15 min	5 min
Advantages/disadvantages	Relatively inexpensive, produces systemic fibrinogenolysis, immunogenic	Prolonged disappearance from plasma permits easy bolus administration, produces systemic fibrinogenolysis, immunogenic	Produces systemic fibrinogenolysis, not immunogenic	More rapid lysis, less systemic fibrinogenolysis, not immunogenic, expensive
Dose regimen				
AMI (within 6–12 hr)	1.5 million U IV over 60 min	30 U IV bolus	Not adequately validated	100 mg IV infusion over 90 min with heparin
DVT/PE	250,000 U IV bolus and 100,000 U/hr for 24 hr with heparin	Not adequately validated	4400 U/kg IV bolus and 4400 U/kg/hr for 24 hr with heparin	1–2 mg/kg per 24 hr for 2–4 d
Complications	Abnormal bleeding, allergic reactions	Abnormal bleeding, allergic reactions	Abnormal bleeding	Abnormal bleeding

SK = streptokinase; APSAC = anisoylated plasmin-streptokinase activator complex; u-PA = urokinase plasminogen activator; t-PA = tissue plasminogen activator; AMI = acute myocardial infarction; DVT/PE = deep vein thrombosis/pulmonary embolism.

mortality was equivalent for patients receiving initial therapy with three different thrombolytic agents.

The GUSTO Investigators: An international randomized trial comparing four thrombolytic strategies for acute myocardial infarction. N Engl J Med 329:673, 1993. *This study of 41,021 patients compared the relative efficacy of different thrombolytic agents with intravenous heparin as adjunctive therapy. The results suggest that t-PA plus intravenous heparin is of greater benefit than streptokinase plus heparin or streptokinase and t-PA with heparin.*

The International Study Group: In-hospital mortality and clinical course of 20,891 patients with suspected AMI randomized between alteplase and SK with or without heparin. Lancet 336:71, 1990. *This study combined 8401 patients; no differences in mortality were found between patients treated with streptokinase and those treated with t-PA.*

ANTIPLATELET THERAPY

Coronary and cerebral atherosclerotic vascular diseases give rise to heart attacks and strokes by inducing thrombotic occlusion at sites of plaque stenosis and rupture. These thrombotic processes are platelet dependent and thrombin mediated but largely unresponsive to heparin or warfarin anticoagulation (Fig. 188–1).

The benefits of antiplatelet therapy in this setting have been convincingly shown by the Antiplatelet Trialists' Collaboration. This meta-analysis, which included more than 200 randomized trials involving more than 100,000 patients, confirmed that aspirin reduces the relative risk of acute MI, ischemic stroke, and vascular death by about 25% in patients with symptomatic atherosclerotic disease, including males and females, diabetics and non-diabetics, and old and young. Oral aspirin (75 to 325 mg/day) produces its antithrombotic effects by irreversibly blocking platelet cyclooxygenase and, consequently, thromboxane A_2–dependent platelet recruitment (see Chapter 29).

The Antiplatelet Trialists' Collaboration also concluded that ticlopidine (250 mg twice daily) reduced stroke, acute MI, and vascular death approximately 10% more effectively than aspirin did. Clopidogrel (75 mg daily), a ticlopidine-like drug, also reduces the combined risk of ischemic stroke, MI, or vascular death approximately 10% more effectively than aspirin does, as shown in a randomized, blinded trial of clopidogrel versus aspirin in more than 19,000 patients with symptomatic atherosclerotic vascular disease. Clopidogrel has none of the troublesome adverse effects plaguing ticlopidine and is at least as safe as moderate-dose aspirin (325 mg/day). After oral absorption and hepatic modification, clopidogrel irreversibly inactivates platelet adenosine diphosphate (ADP) receptors in a dose-dependent manner. Whereas several days of 75 mg/day clopidogrel is needed to interrupt ADP-induced platelet activation fully, administering an initial dose that is several-fold higher achieves immediate inactivation of platelet ADP receptors.

Because aspirin and clopidogrel inactivate separate pathways of platelet recruitment, combined aspirin and clopidogrel are predicted to produce additive antithrombotic effects. This postulate is strongly supported by pre-clinical findings, as well as by the enhanced antithrombotic effects produced by aspirin and ticlopidine in patients undergoing endovascular stenting. Clinical trials are presently evaluating the potential usefulness of combined aspirin and clopidogrel.

Striking antithrombotic effects are produced by antagonists of platelet $\alpha_{IIb}\beta_3$-integrin fibrinogen receptors by interrupting the final common pathway mediating platelet participation in thrombus formation. Because these agents also impair platelet hemostatic function, their use is generally reserved for transient interruption of high-risk thrombosis. Three fibrinogen receptor antagonists are presently available for parenteral use: abciximab (humanized monoclonal antibody), eptifibatide (synthetic cyclic peptide), and tirofiban (synthetic antagonist).

Atherosclerotic Vascular Disorders.

Aspirin, clopidogrel, or ticlopidine decrease the risk of thrombo-occlusion and thromboembolism for all major vascular distributions, irrespective of the anatomic site producing symptoms (Table 188–2).

CEREBROVASCULAR DISEASE. (See Chapters 469 and 470) Treatment of patients with transient ischemic attacks (TIAs) or mild strokes with aspirin, ticlopidine, or clopidogrel reduces the risk of subsequent stroke, MI, or vascular death. Although aspirin therapy is associated with a small increase in hemorrhagic stroke, the overall reduction in all strokes far outweighs that complication. In patients with prior thromboembolic stroke, ticlopidine reduced the risk of stroke, MI, and vascular death by 30% in the Canadian-American Ticlopidine Study. When compared with aspirin, ticlopidine reduced the risk of stroke and death by 12% in the Ticlopidine-Aspirin Stroke Study, whereas clopidogrel decreased the relative risk of ischemic stroke by 7 to 8% in the CAPRIE (Clopidogrel versus Aspirin in Patients at Risk of Ischaemic Events) Study. The effect of dipyridamole in stroke patients remains controversial. Although dipyridamole has recently been reported to enhance the effects of aspirin, this outcome is inconsistent with previous controlled trials reporting that aspirin alone produces equivalent outcomes to the combination of aspirin and dipyridamole and that dipyridamole alone fails to prevent subsequent stroke when compared with placebo.

CORONARY ARTERY DISEASE. (See Chapters 59 and 60) In patients with prior MI, aspirin reduces the risk of stroke, MI, and vascular death by about 25%. Clopidogrel (or ticlopidine) is more effective than aspirin in reducing the risk of stroke, MI, and vascular death in patients with prior MI by about 10% (CAPRIE Study and Antiplatelet Trialists' Collaboration). Aspirin is also beneficial in acute MI in that it reduces the risk of subsequent vascular events by 29%. Several large independent studies have established that aspirin decreases the risk of MI or cardiac death by about 50% in patients with unstable angina. Although there is much less experience in acute ischemic coronary syndromes, the available evidence suggests that clopidogrel or ticlopidine may exhibit similar effects.

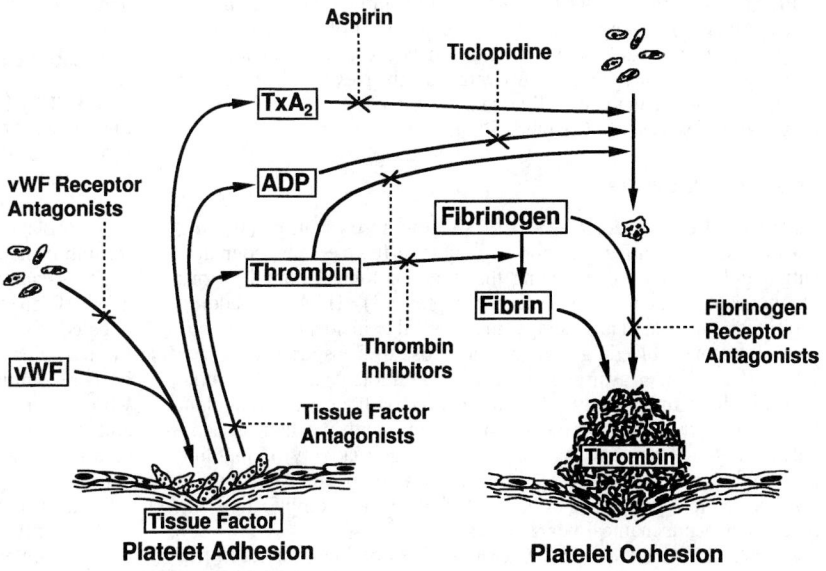

FIGURE 188–1 ■ *Antiplatelet strategies for vascular thrombogenesis.* At sites of denuding arterial damage, platelets attach, undergo activation, and recruit ambient platelets by three independent pathways: platelet production of thromboxane A_2 (TxA_2), which is inhibited by aspirin; platelet secretion of granular adenosine diphosphate (ADP), which is blocked by the platelet ADP receptor antagonists ticlopidine and clopidogrel; and thrombin, which involves tissue factor (TF) initiation and sequential activation of coagulation serine proteases. Free and fibrin-bound thrombin is inactivated by direct thrombin inhibitors such as hirudin, bivalirudin, or argatroban. Platelet-platelet cohesion proceeds by adhesive proteins binding functional platelet $\alpha_{IIb}\beta_3$-integrin fibrinogen receptors that are expressed by activated platelets, and cohesion is interrupted by $\alpha_{IIb}\beta_3$-integrin fibrinogen receptor antagonists, including abciximab, eptifibatide, or tirofiban.

Table 188–2 ■ COMPARISON OF ANTIPLATELET AGENTS

FEATURE	ASPIRIN	THIENOPYRIDINES (CLOPIDOGREL AND TICLOPIDINE)	$\alpha_{IIb}\beta_3$ ANTAGONISTS
Mode of action	Irreversible acetylation of platelet cyclooxygenase within minutes of oral dose	Irreversible inactivation of platelet ADP receptors after oral dosing	Dose-dependent competitive inhibition of adhesive protein bridging between activated platelets
Oral dose	75–325 mg daily	Clopidogrel, 75 mg daily; ticlopidine, 250 mg twice daily	Variable oral dosing (generally at least twice daily)
Clinical indications	Symptomatic atherosclerotic vascular disease	Systemic atherosclerotic vascular disease (particularly aspirin failures)	Risk of thrombosis after interventional procedures, acute coronary syndromes, ?thrombolysis for MI, ?endovascular stents
Usefulness	Risk reduced by 25% for symptomatic disease and 44% for vascular procedures	More effective than aspirin by about 10%	Highly effective in preventing platelet-dependent thrombosis
Complications	Gastrointestinal bleeding increased with surgery, allergic reactions	At least as safe as aspirin (ticlopidine produces diarrhea and neutropenia)	Hemostatic impairment comparable to antithrombotic benefits

ADP = adenosine diphosphate; MI = myocardial infarction.

Other more potent parenteral agents that inhibit platelet $\alpha_{IIb}\beta_3$-integrin fibrinogen receptors and have been approved for the treatment of acute ischemic coronary syndromes include abciximab, eptifibatide, and tirofiban. These agents effectively block platelet recruitment into the thrombus, regardless of the inducing mechanism (see Fig. 188–1). Because effective antithrombotic doses of these agents concurrently inhibit platelet hemostasis, abnormal bleeding may complicate their use, particularly in association with invasive procedures.

CORONARY ARTERY BYPASS GRAFTS. (See Chapter 62) Aspirin (160 to 325 mg) improves the patency of aortocoronary saphenous vein and internal mammary artery bypass grafts by approximately 40%. To maintain graft patency without increasing surgical bleeding, patients undergoing saphenous vein or internal mammary artery aortocoronary grafting should receive aspirin (325 mg/day) within hours after completing the procedure and continue aspirin therapy for 1 year. Although optimum regimens involving clopidogrel, ticlopidine, or platelet $\alpha_{IIb}\beta_3$-integrin fibrinogen receptor antagonists have not been established, these agonists may also produce beneficial effects.

PERIPHERAL VASCULAR DISEASE. (See Chapter 67) Aspirin improves patency after vascular angioplasty and grafting. Clopidogrel (or ticlopidine) is more effective than aspirin in reducing fatal and non-fatal cardiovascular events in patients with peripheral vascular disease (CAPRIE Study and Antiplatelet Trialists' Collaboration). Ticlopidine decreases the risk of stroke, MI, or vascular death by 20% in patients with atherosclerotic peripheral arterial disease (Swedish Ticlopidine Multicentre Study).

PRIMARY PREVENTION. Aspirin significantly decreased the incidence of MI in a large primary prevention trial of men older than 40 years, but the study was discontinued because continuation was unlikely to show a reduction in overall death. Nevertheless, aspirin is often recommended in individuals whose principal risk is coronary artery disease (see Chapters 59 and 60).

Cardiovascular Devices

MECHANICAL HEART VALVES. Low-dose aspirin (100 mg daily) and oral anticoagulation are more effective than coumarin anticoagulants alone in reducing the thromboembolic complications of mechanical heart valves (see Chapter 63). However, adding aspirin to anticoagulant therapy increases the incidence of serious gastrointestinal bleeding when the dose of aspirin exceeeds 100 mg/day. When aspirin fails or is contraindicated, dipyridamole (100 mg four times daily) in combination with oral anticoagulant therapy is currently recommended in patients with mechanical heart valves in the aortic and mitral positions. Alternatively, ticlopidine (or clopidogrel) may also be used in addition to oral anticoagulation to reduce thromboembolic occlusive events complicating the placement of mechanical heart valves.

PROSTHETIC VASCULAR GRAFTS. The combination of aspirin and ticlopidine (or clopidogrel) reduces vascular occlusive events in patients with peripheral vascular disease who are undergoing grafting procedures and in hemodialysis patients receiving arteriovenous access grafts. However, these therapies fail to decrease the formation of stenotic anastomotic vascular lesion formation, which is the principal underlying cause of graft failure.

ENDOVASCULAR STENTS. Combining aspirin and ticlopidine (or presumably aspirin and clopidogrel) therapy for several weeks following the deployment of coronary artery endovascular stents substantially decreases stent thrombotic vascular occlusion when compared with aspirin alone (see Chapter 61). These results support the concept that concurrent inhibition of the thromboxane A_2 and ADP pathways of platelet recruitment produce additive antiplatelet benefits and justify formal testing of this possibility.

HIGH-RISK ANGIOPLASTY. Thrombo-occlusive events complicate coronary angioplasty in high-risk patients despite treatment with aspirin and heparin (See Chapters 61). Resistance to aspirin is explained by the dominance of thrombin, as opposed to thromboxane A_2 in mediating the thrombogenic process initiated by mechanical vascular injury. Resistance to heparin is attributable to the inaccessibility of bound thrombin to inhibition by the heparin-antithrombin complex, together with the local heparin-inhibiting effects of proteins secreted by activated platelets (platelet factor 4).

Powerful antiplatelet therapy interrupting resistant vascular thrombosis targets platelet $\alpha_{IIb}\beta_3$-integrin fibrinogen receptors (see Table 188–2). By blocking this final common pathway regulating platelet recruitment, the participation of platelets in thrombus formation is abolished. However, these agents also impair platelet hemostatic function.

Pharmacologic Agents

ASPIRIN. (See Chapter 29) Oral aspirin potently and irreversibly inactivates cyclooxygenase in all circulating platelets, thereby interrupting thromboxane A_2 generation. Platelet hemostasis is minimally impaired. Aspirin at 1 mg/kg is as effective as higher doses in the majority of patients at risk. Because just 10% non–aspirin-treated platelets in the circulation are sufficient to generate full thromboxane A_2–dependent platelet aggregation in the blood of aspirin-treated patients, aspirin should be given every day to inhibit newly formed platelets. The ideal dose of aspirin continues to be debated. Some patients may need 325 mg aspirin daily because of limited bioavailability. Larger doses of aspirin (~1 g/day) have been recommended for stroke-prone patients by some neurologists, who reason that dose-response data are inadequate in stroke trials and platelet aggregation results suggest the possibility of resistance to aspirin inhibition. However, because the gastrointestinal complications of aspirin are dose dependent, most practitioners prescribe daily aspirin at a dose of 75 to 325 mg.

TICLOPIDINE. Ticlopidine has no inhibitory effect on ADP-induced platelet aggregation when added in vitro. After oral absorption and hepatic modification, ticlopidine produces cumulative irreversible inactivation of platelet ADP receptors, with 7 to 8 days of 250 mg twice daily required to fully inhibit ADP-induced platelet aggregation. Ticlopidine is more effective than aspirin in patients at risk for vascular events and maybe preferred in patients with TIAs, prior stroke, unstable angina, recent MI, and peripheral arterial disease. Ticlopidine in combination with aspirin is currently used in patients undergoing coronary artery stenting. Unfortunately, ticlopidine has several limiting adverse effects, including neutropenia (in 1%), diarrhea (in 10%), skin rash, and rare, but devastating thrombotic thrombocytopenic purpura.

CLOPIDOGREL. Clopidogrel, a thienopyridine closely related to ticlopidine, requires hepatic modification after oral dosing to inhibit ADP-induced platelet aggregation. Clopidogrel irreversibly inactivates platelet ADP receptors in a dose-dependent manner. Several days of cumulative receptor inactivation is required to produce maximal inhibition of ADP-induced platelet aggregation when administering the recommended chronic oral dose of 75 mg/day. However, increasing the initial dose several-fold produces immediate receptor inactivation. Experimental studies confirm that combining clopidogrel and aspirin produces additive antithrombotic effects with minimal inhibition of platelet hemostatic function.

PLATELET FIBRINOGEN RECEPTOR ANTAGONISTS. Three parenteral platelet $\alpha_{IIb}\beta_3$-integrin fibrinogen receptor antagonists provide effective antithrombotic therapy for high-risk angioplasty, ischemic coronary syndromes, and adjuncts to thrombolytic therapy in acute MI. These agents include abciximab, eptifibatide, and tirofiban. Orally active small molecule antagonists to platelet $\alpha_{IIb}\beta_3$-integrin fibrinogen receptor are being developed for chronic therapy. This therapeutic strategy has several unresolved issues, including requirements for the drug to have an appropriate pharmacokinetic profile ensuring once-daily use, acceptable antithrombotic efficacy versus hemostatic risk, competitive cost, and occasional adverse effects such as thrombocytopenia.

Antiplatelet Trialists' Collaboration: Collaborative overview of randomised trials of antiplatelet therapy. I. Prevention of death, myocardial infarction, and stroke by prolonged antiplatelet therapy in various categories of patients. BMJ 308:81, 1994. *Initial report from this important analysis evaluating antiplatelet therapy in patients with symptomatic atherosclerosis.*

Antiplatelet Trialists' Collaboration: Collaborative overview of randomised trials of antiplatelet therapy II. Maintenance of vascular graft or arterial patency by antiplatelet therapy. BMJ 308:159, 1994. This *large-scale meta-analyses showed that aspirin reduces vascular occlusive events in about one fourth of patients with symptomatic vascular disease and in patients undergoing vascular procedures.*

CAPRIE Steering Committee: A randomised, blinded, trial of clopidogrel versus aspirin in patients at risk of ischaemic events (CAPRIE). Lancet 348:1329, 1996. *This report of the largest blinded controlled trial in patients with symptomatic atherosclerotic vascular disease provides convincing evidence for the efficacy and safety of clopidogrel therapy.*

Chesebro JH, Badimon JJ: Platelet glycoprotein IIb/IIIa receptor blockade in unstable coronary disease. N Engl J Med 338:1539, 1998. *Summary of small molecule antagonist of $\alpha_{IIb}\beta_3$-integrin fibrinogen receptor.*

IMPACT-II Investigators: Randomised placebo-controlled trial of effect of eptifibatide on complications of percutaneous coronary intervention: IMPACT-II (Integrilin to Minimise Platelet Aggregation and Coronary Thrombosis-II). Lancet 349:1422, 1997. *This report demonstrates that peptide antagonists of platelet fibrinogen receptors decrease the thrombotic risk of angioplasty.*

ANTICOAGULANT THERAPY

Low-molecular-weight heparin (LMWH) given subcutaneously (1 mg/kg every 12 hours) effectively substitutes for dose-adjusted unfractionated heparin for all indications. Because LMWH requires no monitoring and has a longer elimination time, it is suited for out-of-hospital management of acute DVT. LMWHs are expected to displace standard heparin as they become more cost competitive. Monitored oral anticoagulation using coumarin drugs, usually warfarin, is indicated for long-term out-of-hospital prophylaxis of DVT, PE, and systemic thromboembolism.

Anticoagulant Therapy for Venous Thrombosis and Thromboembolism (see Chapters 69 and 84)

ACUTE DVT AND PE. (See Table 188–3.) Immediate treatment with LMWH or heparin benefits patients with DVT or PE by markedly reducing mortality from recurrent PE and preventing extension or embolization of DVT. LMWH may be started as acute treatment in outpatients (Table 188–4). Warfarin (0.1 mg/kg/day but not exceeding 10 mg) is begun after initiating the heparin infusion, while monitoring the response with the International Normalized Ratio (INR) (see Table 188–3). Because the risk of recurrence remains elevated for months, uncomplicated DVT requires at least 3 months of warfarin therapy, and at least 6 months of treatment is generally recommended for major or complicated DVT. Patients with recurrent DVT or a continuing risk factor such as deficiencies in antithrombin III (AT-III), protein C, or protein S, resistance to activated protein C, or malignancy should be treated indefinitely with oral anticoagulants, although emerging data may moderate these recommendations in the future.

PROPHYLAXIS OF SURGICAL DVT AND PE. No specific prophylaxis is required for low-risk general surgery patients younger than 40 years or those undergoing minor operations with no clinical risk factors other than early ambulation postoperatively.

Moderate-risk general surgery patients who are older than 40 years and undergoing major surgery without additional risk factors should be treated prophylactically with low-dose heparin (5000 U subcutaneously every 12 hours). Low-dose subcutaneous heparin begun before surgery and continuing until the patient is ambulatory reduces the incidence of venous thrombosis by two thirds and PE by half. Patients older than 40 years who are undergoing major surgery and have additional risk factors should receive low-dose subcutaneous heparin (5000 U every 8 hours) or LMWH every 12 hours.

Patients undergoing hip surgery should receive prophylaxis with LMWH, adjusted-dose heparin (to prolong the activated partial thromboplastin time [aPTT] in the upper half of the normal range), or moderate-dose warfarin (to maintain the INR at 2.0 to 3.0). Recent controlled clinical trials demonstrate that subcutaneous hirudin (15 mg twice daily) reduces thromboembolic complications after orthopedic surgery more effectively than heparin or LMWH does. Approval for this indication is pending. Patients undergoing intracranial neurosurgical procedures or urologic surgery should not generally receive anticoagulants but should be treated with intermittent pneumatic compression only; the availability of LMWH may change this recommendation.

PROPHYLAXIS OF MEDICAL DVT AND PE. Low-dose heparin is recommended for the prophylaxis of DVT and PE in medical patients at prolonged bed rest, such as patients with acute MI or heart failure. Full-dose anticoagulation is also effective. Similarly, prophylaxis should be provided for patients with ischemic stroke and lower-extremity paralysis in the form of low-dose heparin or LMWH.

DVT AND PE DURING PREGNANCY. Pregnant patients with a history of previous venous thromboembolic disease are at increased risk for DVT and PE; these patients should be given low-dose subcutaneous heparin (5000 U twice daily) throughout their pregnancy. Women who have DVT during pregnancy should receive

Table 188–3 ■ ANTICOAGULANT THERAPY FOR DEEP VENOUS THROMBOSIS AND PULMONARY EMBOLISM

Initiate Therapy with Heparin
Administer LMWH at doses indicated for "Acute Treatment" in Table 188–4; no aPTT monitoring required

  Alternative 1: Administer intravenous heparin and adjust based according to aPTT results (see Table 69–5)

  Alternative 2: Administer heparin subcutaneously every 12 hr beginning with an initial dose of 18,000 U. Check aPTT after 4 hr and adjust subsequent doses to prolong a aPTT to 1.5–2.5 times control; monitor and maintain range for 5–7 days

Maintenance Anticoagulation
Oral anticoagulants
1. Give warfarin, 5–10 mg, during first hospital day
2. Check PT daily
3. Adjust dose to prolong PT to INR of 2–3 (1.3–1.5 times control with most rabbit brain thromboplastins)
4. Discontinue heparin after minimum of 5 d when PT reaches desired range
5. Continue warfarin as outpatient for at least 3–6 mo

Heparin
Heparin subcutaneously every 12 hr in a dose to prolong the mid-interval aPTT to 1.5 times control

LMWH = low-molecular-weight heparin; aPTT = activated partial thromboplastin time; PT = prothrombin time; INR = International Normalized Ratio.

Table 188–4 ■ ANTICOAGULANT PROFILES, MOLECULAR WEIGHTS, PLASMA HALF-LIVES, AND RECOMMENDED DOSES OF COMMERCIAL LOW-MOLECULAR-WEIGHT HEPARINS

AGENT	Anti-Xa–TO–Anti-IIa RATIO	MOLECULAR WEIGHT	PLASMA HALF-LIFE (min)	RECOMMENDED DOSE (INTERNATIONAL ANTI-Xa UNITS)		
				General Surgery Prophylaxis	Orthopedic Surgery Prophylaxis	Acute Treatment
Enoxaparin	2.7:1	4500	129–180	2000 U s.c. daily	4000 U s.c. daily or 3000 U s.c. BID	7000 U s.c. BID*
Dalteparin	2.0:1	5000	119–139	2500 U s.c. daily	2500 U s.c. BID or 5000 U s.c. daily	8400 U s.c. BID*
Nadroparin	3.2:1	4500	132–162	7500 U/IC s.c. daily†		31,500 U/IC daily†
Tinzaparin (Innohep)	1.9:1	4500	111	3500 U s.c. daily	50 U/kg s.c. daily	12,250 daily*
Ardeparin	2.0:1	6000	200		50 U/kg s.c. BID	
Danaparoid‡	20:1	6500	1100		750 U s.c. BID	1250 U s.c. BID

*Weight-adjusted dose; stated dose for 70-kg patient.
†U/IC = Institute Choay units; 3 ICU = 1 IU.
‡Danaparoid sodium is a heparinoid.

full-dose intravenous heparin by continuous infusion for 5 to 7 days or subcutaneous LMWH twice daily, followed by twice-daily adjusted-dose subcutaneous heparin until term. If pregnancy is planned while the patient is receiving long-term anticoagulant prophylaxis, subcutaneous heparin anticoagulation should be substituted for the warfarin before pregnancy begins. Although no validating randomized studies have been carried out, pregnant patients with mechanical heart valves or atrial fibrillation and documented systemic embolization are often treated with twice-daily LMWH or adjusted-dose subcutaneous heparin from the time pregnancy is diagnosed until delivery.

Prevention of Systemic Thromboembolism

ATRIAL FIBRILLATION AND VALVULAR HEART DISEASE. (See Chapters 51 and 63.) Long-term warfarin therapy sufficient to maintain the INR at 2.0 to 3.0 should be given to patients with atrial fibrillation and valvular heart disease, except patients younger than 60 years who have no associated cardiovascular disease. Long-term warfarin therapy (INR of 2.0 to 3.0) is also recommended for patients with rheumatic mitral valvular disease and normal sinus rhythm if the left atrial diameter is larger than 5.5 cm.

Long-term antithrombotic therapy is not indicated in patients with aortic valve disease in the absence of associated mitral valve disease or atrial fibrillation. Additionally, antithrombotic therapy is not indicated in patients with mitral valve prolapse who have not experienced systemic embolism, unexplained TIAs, or atrial fibrillation. Warfarin therapy (INR of 2.0 to 3.0) before elective cardioversion of atrial fibrillation is guided by the presence or absence of left atrial clot by transesophageal echocardiography and the duration of the arrhythmia (see Chapter 51).

MECHANICAL HEART VALVES. All patients with mechanical heart valves should be treated with long-term warfarin at a dose sufficient to maintain the INR at 2.5 to 3.5 (see Chapter 63). If systemic embolization occurs despite warfarin, daily aspirin (100 mg/day) should be added and the INR maintained at 2.5 to 3.5. Dipyridamole (400 mg/day) with warfarin may also be beneficial. Although clopidogrel (or ticlopidine) would presumably produce similar protection, no formal confirmation has been reported. Antiplatelet agents alone, without warfarin, do not offer sufficient protection against systemic embolism.

Patients with bioprosthetic mitral valves should be treated for the first 3 months after valve insertion with warfarin to maintain an INR of 2.0 to 3.0. Patients with bioprosthetic valves who have atrial fibrillation, exhibit left atrial thrombus at the time of surgery, have a history of systemic embolism, or show evidence of a left atrial thrombus at surgery should also be treated with long-term warfarin therapy (INR of 2.0 to 3.0). Patients with bioprosthetic valves and sinus rhythm or valves in the aortic position may benefit from long-term aspirin therapy (325 mg/day) without anticoagulants.

ACUTE MI. (See Chapter 60.) Patients with anterior Q wave acute MI are at increased risk of systemic embolism and should receive full-dose heparin therapy by continuous infusion or twice-daily subcutaneous injections of LMWH, followed by warfarin therapy to maintain an INR of 2.0 to 3.0 for 1 to 3 months. Patients with acute MI who have an increased risk of systemic embolism because of atrial fibrillation, a history of previous pulmonary or systemic embolism, or heart failure are also appropriate for heparin or LMWH therapy followed by warfarin therapy to prolong the prothrombin time (PT) to an INR of 2.0 to 3.0 for at least 3 months. Although long-term anticoagulation therapy is not generally recommended for patients with acute MI, long-term warfarin therapy is recommended for those with risk factors for pulmonary or systemic embolism, such as atrial fibrillation, previous systemic embolism, venous thromboembolism, or severe heart failure.

Pharmacologic Agents

STANDARD HEPARIN. Because standard (unfractionated) heparin must be given parenterally, with regular monitoring of its anticoagulant effects and frequent adjustment of dosage, its use is largely limited to in-hospital settings. Heparin is indicated for prevention of DVT and PE, early treatment of unstable angina, chronic prevention of DVT and PE during pregnancy, treatment of resistant thrombotic processes, and transient anticoagulation when using cardiovascular devices and procedures. Tests of intrinsic clotting such as the aPTT have intermediate sensitivity to heparin, i.e., clotting times are doubled by therapeutic heparin levels (0.2 to 0.3 IU/mL). Because the PT is only slightly prolonged by relatively high heparin concentrations, it is a reliable means of assessing the status of oral anticoagulation during therapeutic heparin infusions.

Standard heparin may be administered intravenously by bolus injection, continuous infusion, or subcutaneous injection. Continuous infusion is associated with fewer bleeding complications than intermittent bolus injection is and provides excellent protection against recurrent venous disease. The half-life of therapeutic heparin following bolus intravenous administration averages about 60 to 90 minutes, depending on the dose and the patient; the response to heparin varies considerably among different individuals and even in the same individual at different times during the course of therapy because heparin binds to a number of other basic proteins in plasma that compete with AT-III, including fibronectin, vitronectin, von Willebrand factor, histidine-rich glycoprotein, and platelet factor 4. Variable binding of standard heparin to these proteins contributes to standard heparin's reduced bioavailability at low concentrations, variability in anticoagulant response after fixed dosing, and resistance to therapy. Thus the anticoagulant response to heparin is not linear but increases disproportionately in intensity and duration with increasing doses.

When given by continuous infusion, standard heparin requires accurate administration and should be given in a separate intravenous line. The initial loading dose is 75 IU/kg body weight by intravenous bolus injection, followed by infusion at 10 to 25 IU/kg/hour, depending on the patient and the clinical situation. The aPTT should be maintained at about 1.5 to 2 times baseline (heparin levels, 0.2 to 4 IU/mL). Appropriate therapeutic aPTTs are 50 to 80 seconds. The aPTT should be adjusted by changing the infusion rate. After each adjustment, the aPTT should be checked after 4 hours to assess effects of the dose change; monitoring should be performed daily.

Plasma heparin levels are unexpectedly low after subcutaneous administration because entry of heparin into the intravascular space from the subcutaneous deposits is delayed, thereby enhancing rapid saturable clearance by binding to endothelium and macrophages. This effect seriously complicates initial therapy with subcutaneous heparin for DVT management by delaying the time required to attain full antithrombotic heparin levels.

LOW-MOLECULAR-WEIGHT HEPARIN. LMWHs are effective and safe for preventing and treating venous thromboembolism and are now approved for this purpose. LMWHs are fragments of commercial-grade standard heparin produced by either chemical or enzymatic depolymerization and are approximately one third the size of standard heparin (see Table 188–4). Like standard heparin they are heterogeneous in size, but average 4000 to 5000 daltons. Depolymerization of standard heparin changes its anticoagulant profile, bioavailability, pharmacokinetics, and effects on platelet function and experimental bleeding. LMWHs produce their principal anticoagulant effect via pentasaccharide-dependent binding to AT-III. Whereas approximately one third of unfractionated heparin fragments exhibit these binding domains, a lower proportion of LMWH molecules bind plasma AT-III. Although a minimum chain length of 18 saccharides (including the pentasaccharide sequence) is required for ternary complex formation with thrombin, inactivation of Factor Xa by AT-III depends only on the pentasaccharide. The various commercial LMWHs have anti–Factor Xa-to-antithrombin ratios varying between 4:1 and 2:1, as compared with the 1:1 ratio for standard heparin.

Because LMWHs bind much less avidly to heparin-binding plasma proteins and endothelium than standard heparin does, LMWHs exhibit superior bioavailability, longer rates of elimination, and more predictable anticoagulant responses. When compared on a gravimetric basis in experimental models of venous thrombosis, LMWHs are less effective than heparin as antithrombotic agents but produce much less bleeding than standard heparin does in models measuring blood loss from a standardized injury, perhaps related to attenuated effects on platelet function and vascular permeability.

In patients, LMWHs also exhibit greater bioavailability, a longer plasma half-life, and a more predictable anticoagulant response than standard heparin does, which allows LMWHs to be administered subcutaneously twice daily without laboratory monitoring. LMWHs also produce less bleeding than standard heparin does for an equivalent antithrombotic effect, thereby permitting patients to be treated with higher anticoagulant doses of LMWHs without compromising patient safety. This latter potential advantage of LMWHs has been demonstrated in patients undergoing hip surgery who are at high risk of thrombosis.

COUMARIN-TYPE ANTICOAGULATION. Oral coumarin-type anticoagulation is indicated for preventing chronic out-of-hospital venous thrombosis, PE, and systemic embolism in patients at increased risk.

The PT is the most common laboratory test for monitoring oral anticoagulant therapy because it is sensitive to alterations in prothrombin and Factors X and VII, three of the vitamin K–dependent coagulation factors that are inhibited by coumarin-type oral anticoagulants, including warfarin. The pharmacologic response of warfarin depends on the net effect on the activity levels of these factors because they have different half-lives; for example, a reduction in Factor VII, which has a 6-hour half-life, prolongs the PT within 24 hours after large doses of warfarin before significant changes occur in the other factors. It is therefore common practice to begin warfarin therapy at 5 to 10 mg for each of the initial 2 days and then adjust the dose, usually downward, based on results of the daily PT until it equilibrates in the therapeutic range.

A properly standardized PT is used for monitoring warfarin therapy. The observed PT ratio obtained with the local thromboplastin is converted into an INR, which is calculated as follows: INR = observed ratio^c, where C is the constant that represents the international sensitivity index (ISI). The INR is therefore the PT ratio that reflects the result that would have been obtained if the reference thromboplastin had been used to perform the test. For practical purposes, it is sufficient to know that the primary human brain reference thromboplastin, which is very responsive to the anticoagulant effects of warfarin, has an ISI of 1.0 and that the ISI value increases as the thromboplastin exhibits less responsiveness. Clinical trials have provided good evidence that a targeted INR range of 2.0 to 3.0 is effective in treating venous thrombosis after an initial course of heparin and in preventing venous thrombosis and systemic embolism.

Because drug interactions significantly affect the dose of warfarin needed to maintain optimal therapy, great care is required to maintain therapeutic INR control in patients receiving other medications, particularly drugs used for changing symptoms. The introduction of any new medication prompts an assessment of its effects on the INR.

Complications of Anticoagulant Therapy.

The major risk of anticoagulant therapy is bleeding secondary to excessive anticoagulation, the patient's underlying clinical disorder, or the concurrent use of high-dose aspirin. Patients treated with standard doses of either heparin or warfarin have a 2 to 4% per year frequency of bleeding episodes requiring transfusion. The risk of a fatal hemorrhage is about 0.2% per year for patients taking oral anticoagulants. The risk of major bleeding is increased in patients older than 65 years; in patients with a history of stroke, gastrointestinal bleeding, atrial fibrillation, and co-morbid conditions such as uremia and anemia; and with infrequent monitoring. The most common minor episodes involve urinary, gastrointestinal, and vaginal bleeding. In general, any new or painful symptom in a patient receiving anticoagulants should be considered a manifestation of a potential bleeding complication until proved otherwise.

The risk of clinically important bleeding is minimized by maintaining the INR at 2.0 to 3.0. Bleeding episodes occurring within this therapeutic range are frequently due to focal pathologic lesions such as an occult neoplasm unmasked by the therapy, especially in the gastrointestinal or genitourinary tract. Full evaluation is warranted.

Reversal of heparin is achieved by protamine sulfate, a basic nuclear histone containing one third of its residue as arginine. Protamine binds heparin more tightly than any plasma protein, including AT-III. It is routinely given after heparinization during cardiopulmonary bypass surgery in amounts approximately equal to the total administered heparin. The protamine may dissociate or metabolize more rapidly than heparin, thereby accounting for the occasional open heart surgical patient who exhibits "rebound" heparinization after surgery.

Heparin-associated thrombocytopenia occurs in about 1 to 3% of treated patients (see Chapters 183 and 184). Thus it is prudent to check the platelet count before heparin is given and on the fifth day after initiating heparin therapy or with any bleeding episode. Thrombocytopenia may be induced by heparin derived from bovine or porcine sources, administered either intravenously or subcutaneously, or as LMWH derivatives (although LMWH is associated with one tenth the frequency of inducing heparin-associated thrombocytopenia). Two main clinical types are recognized: the more common modest thrombocytopenia of early onset, possibly caused by the platelet proaggregating effect of some contaminating fraction of heparin itself, and the less common severe delayed-onset thrombocytopenia caused by heparin-dependent immune destruction. Occasionally, patients with severe thrombocytopenia also experience threatening thromboembolic events attributable to platelet activation mediated by heparin-induced antibodies. The laboratory diagnosis of heparin-induced thrombocytopenia may be confirmed by demonstrating platelet activation by heparin-induced antibodies in the patient's plasma. In patients with severe thrombocytopenia, heparin therapy should be stopped and an alternative direct antithrombin used, such as hirudin, bivalirudin, or argatroban. Alopecia and osteoporosis also complicate heparin therapy after prolonged use of full-dose heparin for several months.

Management of bleeding in patients receiving warfarin depends on the seriousness of the bleeding episode. If the INR is outside the therapeutic range but less than 6.0, the patient is not bleeding, and no invasive procedures are planned, several doses of warfarin are omitted and the drug is recommended at a lower dose. If the

INR is between 6.0 and 10.0 and the patient is not bleeding or more rapid reversal is needed to prepare for some invasive procedure, the intravenous injection of 1 mg vitamin K_1 often restores the INR to the therapeutic range within 24 hours. If the INR is between 10.0 and 20.0, an intravenous dose of 5 mg vitamin K_1 is recommended, with repeat dosing indicated if the INR remains prolonged at 12 to 24 hours. For more rapid reversal in patients with an INR greater than 20.0, 10 mg intravenous vitamin K_1 should be given and the INR checked every 6 hours. Vitamin K_1 may need to be repeated every 12 hours and supplemented with fresh-frozen plasma transfusion or factor concentrate, depending on the urgency of the situation. With serious bleeding, replacement with factor concentrates of vitamin K–dependent clotting factors is indicated in addition to supplemental intravenous vitamin K_1 (10 mg repeated every 12 hours until the INR is corrected). If the patient requires antithrombotic protection after administration of high-dose vitamin K, heparin should be used until the patient again becomes responsive to warfarin.

During the first trimester of pregnancy, warfarin therapy is associated with a fetal skeletal embryopathy. Women receiving warfarin should be advised against pregnancy because of this risk. If pregnancy develops, full-dose subcutaneous heparin should be substituted for warfarin. Poisoning with warfarin has occurred in children ingesting coumarin-type rat poisons. Rarely, areas of skin necrosis are seen, particularly after large loading doses of warfarin; these lesions are associated with thrombi in the microcirculation. In a proportion of these patients, early depletion of protein C and protein S by warfarin in the absence of heparin coverage may explain this thrombotic complication. Consequently, warfarin therapy is generally initiated under the cover of heparin or LMWH anticoagulation.

Hirsh J, Granger CB: Unfractionated and low molecular weight heparin. *In* Verstraete M, Fuster V, Topol EJ (eds): Cardiovascular Thrombosis: Thrombocardiology and Thromboneurology, 2nd ed. Philadelphia, Lippincott-Raven 1998, pp 189–219. *Reviews heparin and low-molecular-weight heparin mechanisms of action and current therapeutic use.*

Kakkar VV, Marder VJ: Low molecular weight heparins and antithrombotic therapy. Sem Hematol 34(Suppl. 4):1, 1997. *Recent review of low-molecular-weight heparin usage.*

Turpie AG, Gent M, Laupacis A, et al: A comparison of aspirin with placebo in patients treated with warfarin after heart-valve replacement. N Engl J Med 329:524, 1993. *Combining aspirin with warfarin reduces thromboembolic events more effectively than warfarin alone, without significantly increasing bleeding complications in patients with mechanical valves.*

Vorchheimer DA, Badimon JJ, Fuster V: Platelet glycoprotein IIb/IIIa receptor antagonists in cardiovascular disease. JAMA 281:1407, 1999. *A comprehensive review.*

PART XIV

ONCOLOGY

189 INTRODUCTION

Joseph V. Simone

BACKGROUND

DEFINITIONS, INCIDENCE, AND MORTALITY. Cancer describes a class of diseases characterized by the uncontrolled growth of aberrant cells. Cancers kill by the destructive invasion of normal organs through direct extension and spread to distant sites through the blood, lymph, or serosal surfaces. The abnormal clinical behavior of cancer cells is often mirrored by biologic aberrations such as genetic mutations, chromosomal translocations, expression of fetal or other discordant ontologic characteristics, and the inappropriate secretion of hormones or enzymes. All cancers invade or metastasize, but each specific type has unique biologic and clinical features that must be appreciated for proper diagnosis, treatment, and study.

About 1.2 million new cases of invasive cancer are diagnosed each year in the United States, and about 500,000 people die annually of the disease. Cancer is the second most deadly disease and is expected to surpass heart disease early in the 21st century to top that nefarious list (see Chapter 193). Over the past half century, the frequency of most cancers has been stable, but some dramatic changes have taken place. Steady declines in stomach and uterine cancer have occurred, the latter undoubtedly due to routine cytologic screening for cervical cancer. The cause of the decline in stomach cancer is unclear but may in part relate to increased use of antibiotics and their effect on chronic *Helicobacter pylori* infection. The most striking change has been the increases in lung cancer in both men and women, undoubtedly related to smoking. Other cancers with increasing mortality, particularly in the elderly, include melanoma, non-Hodgkin's lymphoma, and brain tumors. There have been speculations but little firm evidence to explain these changes. The overall mortality, particularly for those younger than age 65, has declined, primarily due to more effective therapy for cancers of fetal and hematopoietic origin that occur in the younger population.

ETIOLOGY AND PREVENTION. A broad array of agents can cause or directly contribute to a sequence of events or sensitize cells in such a way that cancer develops (see Chapter 190). The final common pathway in virtually every instance is a cellular genetic mutation that converts a well-behaved cellular citizen of the body into a destructive renegade that is unresponsive to the ordinary checks and balances of a normal community of cells. Promoters (oncogenes) and suppressors (like the retinoblastoma or *p53* gene) play a central role in many cases (see Chapter 191). Chemicals such as benzene and nitrosamines, physical agents such as gamma and ultraviolet radiation, and biologic agents such as the Epstein-Barr and hepatitis viruses contribute to carcinogenesis under certain circumstances. Evidence exists to link dietary factors to carcinogenesis; although not as clear as one would like, the evidence is strong enough to recommend diets low in fat and high in fiber. A sensible diet is based on grains, vegetables, and fruits, with smaller than the current average proportions of fat. Inherited susceptibilities are becoming more evident and probably play a key role in a significant number of cancers of the breast and colon. Down syndrome and the Li-Fraumeni syndrome are well-known harbingers of a substantial risk for developing cancer.

The single most important carcinogen in the United States and Europe is tobacco (see Chapter 13), because it causes or contributes to the development of about one third of all cancers: primarily lung, esophageal, head and neck, and bladder. Less well appreciated is the contribution tobacco may make to causing breast, colon, and gastric cancer. Tobacco-related cancer is also important because it is preventable by the obvious, inexpensive, and 100% effective means of abstention. Although the total number of smokers in the United States has declined, women smoke more than ever, adolescents continue to view smoking as socially chic, and the number of smokers in Asia and developing countries is growing at an alarming rate.

EARLY DETECTION OF CANCER. When prevention of cancer is not possible because effective means are lacking, early detection is the next best strategy to reduce cancer mortality. As a general rule, the smaller and more confined the tumor, the more likely therapy will result in permanent cure. This approach has been most successful for directly accessible tumors that have an early malignant or premalignant state. Examples include Papanicolaou smears and surgical conization for cancer of the uterine cervix, physical removal of early skin cancer, and colonoscopic removal of colorectal polyps. Physical examination and indirect methods, such as

Table 189–1 ■ SUMMARY OF AMERICAN CANCER SOCIETY RECOMMENDATIONS FOR THE EARLY DETECTION OF CANCER IN ASYMPTOMATIC PEOPLE

	POPULATION		
TEST OR PROCEDURE	**Sex**	**Age**	**Frequency**
Sigmoidoscopy, preferably flexible	M & F	50 and over	Every 3–5 years
Fecal occult blood test	M & F	50 and over	Every year
Digital rectal examination	M & F	40 and over	Every year
Prostate examination*	M	50 and over	Every year
Papanicolaou test	F		All women who are or who have been sexually active, or have reached age 18, should have an annual Papanicolaou test and pelvic examination. After a woman has had three or more consecutive satisfactory normal annual examinations and Papanicolaou tests, screening may be performed less frequently at the discretion of her physician.
Pelvic examination	F	18–40	Every 1–3 years with Papanicolaou test
		Over 40	Every year
Endometrial tissue sample	F	At menopause, if at high risk†	At menopause and thereafter at the discretion of the physician
Breast self-examination	F	20 and over	Every month
Breast clinical examination	F	20–40	Every 3 years
		Over 40	Every year
Mammography‡	F	40–49	Every 1–2 years
		50 and over	Every year
Health counseling and cancer checkups§	M & F	Over 20	Every 3 years
	M & F	Over 40	Every year

*Annual digital rectal examination and prostate-specific antigen should be performed on men 50 years and older. If either is abnormal, further evaluation should be considered.

†History of infertility, obesity, failure to ovulate, abnormal uterine bleeding, or unopposed estrogen or tamoxifen therapy.

‡Screening mammography should begin by age 40.

§To include examination for cancers of the thyroid, testes, prostate, ovaries, lymph nodes, oral region, and skin.

From Cancer Facts and Figures—1998. Atlanta, American Cancer Society, 1998.

screening mammography for breast cancer and prostate-specific antigen blood tests for prostate cancer, can also be effective at detecting small malignant or premalignant tumors. However, it is not clear that all in situ breast and prostate cancers will become invasive and fatal, so there is some risk of overtreatment, particularly for prostate cancer.

The American Cancer Society (ACS) has recommended a series of cancer screening procedures for asymptomatic individuals (Table 189–1). Not all experts agree on the frequency or age ranges for employing such procedures, but the ACS recommendations are a well-considered and useful guide that, at the very least, indicates the cancers most amenable to clinically useful early detection by conventional techniques. An even more exciting development in this effort has been the emergence of genetic screening and counseling of families at high risk for developing cancer. Individuals at risk are identified largely by analysis of family pedigrees, and the increasing availability of the revolutionary tools of molecular biology can identify specific genetic mutations (see Chapter 191). It is certain that many such genes will be identified, focusing the cancer screening and early detection efforts more efficiently and productively on high-risk populations (see Chapter 190).

CANCER TUMOR GROWTH. Although it is impossible to know the specific details of early in vivo tumor growth and the efficiency of tumor cell renewal of human cancer, clinical and laboratory observations have provided a reasonable conceptual framework. This framework should be used with caution, however, because it is certain that the intrinsic factors that control tumor growth and propagation are far more complex, episodic, and heterogeneous than currently known, even within a single tumor mass. Furthermore, the stromal environment and neovascularization of tumors have become more central to our understanding of this process than heretofore. Nonetheless, the following description can be a useful reference point.

A tumor reaches the size of clinical detectability when it contains about 10^9 cells, weighing about 1 g and occupying a volume of about 1 mL. A three-log increase to 10^{12} cells, 1 kg, and 1000 mL is often lethal. Below 10^9 cells, the tumor is usually undetectable, but it has already undergone at least 30 doublings, and only 10 further doublings will produce the 1 kg of tumor. This exercise illustrates how much has already occurred, with all the opportunities for the cancer to undergo advantageous mutation and metastasis, before clinical detection. Once the tumor has grown into the clinically evident range, it tends to grow progressively slower with increasing size. This deceleration of growth probably occurs because the tumor outgrows its blood supply, reaches anatomic boundaries, and responds to yet undiscovered feedback regulation from other members of the now larger and more heterogeneous mass of tumor cells. Thus, cancers probably grow much like bacteria after inoculation into a favorable medium. The phases of bacterial growth describe a sigmoid curve (Fig. 189–1): an early lag phase of inapparent or slow growth followed by exponential growth. Growth then slows when new cell production and cell death are nearly equal, with the latter phase in culture due to crowding and inadequate nutrients. Of course, in bacteria as well as cancers, the specific growth characteristics differ among types as well as within types that have developed subpopulations of mutant clones.

Most chemotherapy acts by damaging DNA, so it tends to be most effective in rapidly growing tumors such as acute leukemia, lymphomas, and testicular cancers. Also, after gross surgical removal, residual cancer cells may grow more rapidly and be more sensitive to subsequent ("adjuvant") chemotherapy. The sensitivity or resistance to chemotherapy or irradiation, however, probably has as much or more to do with the specific biochemical and metabolic features of the cancer cell as with its growth characteristics (see Chapter 198).

MANAGEMENT OF THE PATIENT WITH CANCER

Oncology has been transformed over the past 40 years. From a diverse set of orphan diseases usually managed by surgeons alone and viewed with despair by most physicians, it has become a complex and exciting discipline that draws its strength from the essential partnership of specialists in medicine, surgery, pediatrics, pathology, radiation oncology, diagnostic imaging, psychiatry, and others. This remarkable evolution can be credited to therapeutic successes and biologic advances that could not be imagined in the early 1950s. Oncology has pointed the way to an understanding of the biologic variability of cancer and the success that is possible with a coordinated multimodal approach to therapy.

GOALS. Any physician who seriously and expertly assumes responsibility for the management of patients with cancer should have three sets of goals: therapeutic, human, and scientific. The initial therapeutic goal is to cure patients and return them to a normal place in society. This goal, which should be attempted in virtually all cancers, even when the likelihood of cure is small, requires an attitude of reasonable hope and determination as well as a willingness to attempt difficult, dangerous, and sometimes daring approaches to fundamentally resistant diseases. If, after a reasonable attempt, permanent cure is not possible, the physician must not abandon the patient but rather should aim for a secondary goal—a long, qualitatively satisfactory remission. If and when this second goal is no longer possible, the tertiary level of therapeutic intent is to obtain a remission of any kind and duration; however, at this stage and later, one is less willing to expose the patient to the possibility of serious side effects or long hospitalization. When the possibility of remission of any type becomes remote, the fourth goal is to control the disease and symptoms by the judicious use of palliative therapeutic measures. The objective in this final stage is terminal comfort care, which is always difficult because it requires the admission that specific therapy is no longer of any value. Instead of blood transfusions, antibiotics, or chemotherapeutic agents, the physician must use pain medications, sedation, psychosocial support, and other comfort measures with the thought of returning the patient to the home or another appropriate setting and to the support of family.

The human goals in oncology are inextricably linked with the therapeutic and scientific goals. Physicians, nurses, and other health care providers must be sensitive to the particular needs of the patient and family and understand the social environment from which they came and to which they must return. The physician must help patients maintain their dignity, understand their weaknesses, and refuse to allow any frustration, animosity, or excessive friendship to develop and threaten good judgment and the best interests of the patient.

The use of scientific methods in oncology is only in its adolescence, and definitive treatment has been established for only a small proportion of the circumstances and types of cancers that can arise. Systematic protocol studies yield useful information about a new drug, a novel regimen, or a biologic feature. Presentation and

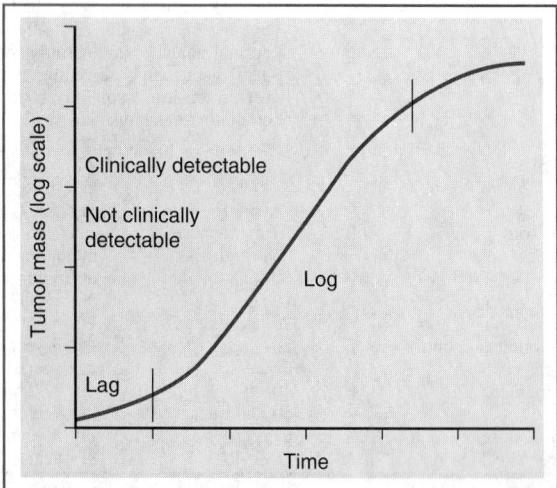

FIGURE 189–1 ■ A schematic representation of the phases of growth of a cancer. After a period of inapparency (lag phase), growth tends to be logarithmic, followed by deceleration due to inadequate nutrients, competitive inhibition among cells, or a lack of neovascularization. (This growth resembles the growth curve of bacteria inoculated into a favorable medium.) The tumor has gone through many doublings before it becomes clinically apparent.

criticism of each other's efforts in a collegial and scientific manner are essential to advancing the knowledge about a particular treatment. Physicians who manage a small number of patients per year cannot possibly have the background and support necessary to treat these complex diseases adequately. This task is best left to specialists who participate in active scientific programs and have the resources to deliver optimal clinical care. It is also important to understand the limitations of science; at times, the best option is no specific anticancer treatment at all.

DIAGNOSTIC PRINCIPLES. The first diagnostic principle is that adequate tissue must be obtained from the tumor to establish the specific diagnosis and subtype of cancer. The rare exceptions are instances in which a biopsy might be life threatening and the anatomic location is virtually pathognomonic of a specific histology; two notable examples are brain tumors and anterior mediastinal tumors that compress the trachea and blood vessels. In the latter situation, often due to a lymphoma, corticosteroids may reduce the tumor size and relieve symptoms before a biopsy is attempted. More often, an adequate sample must be obtained before therapy is started unless complete surgical excision is definitively diagnostic and therapeutic. Because management of each type and subtype of cancer is often distinctive, every effort must be made to obtain appropriate samples, even if therapy is delayed for a short time. A specific diagnosis is seldom a problem in the leukemias because bone marrow aspiration usually affords a ready answer; solid tumors may present greater difficulty. Cancer diagnosis also requires an understanding of paraneoplastic syndromes (see Chapter 195), endocrine (see Chapter 194) and cutaneous manifestations of cancer (see Chapter 196), and oncologic emergencies (see Chapter 199).

A second diagnostic principle is to establish the extent of the disease. In the leukemias, this goal can be accomplished readily by physical examination, routine laboratory tests, chest roentgenography, and examination of cerebrospinal fluid. With solid tumors, determination of the extent of the disease, that is, the *stage* of the tumor, often involves major surgery and an extensive examination that includes diagnostic imaging. A coordinated approach involving the surgeon and pathologist is crucial to determine the extent of tumor invasion; without this approach, one may lack essential information for planning treatment and for judging its success. Failure to detect a tumor that has extended to regional lymph nodes can lead to undertreatment and a false impression that the local treatment, whether surgery or radiation therapy, was adequate. Generic staging systems (Table 189–2) can be supplemented by detailed and specific staging systems that have been developed for most cancers to recognize peculiar pathogenetic features, modes of spread, and potential curability. In addition, modern oncology demands an extensive biologic classification of leukemias and solid tumors, often requiring sophisticated scientific approaches not available a few years ago: monoclonal antibodies to determine the phenotype of lymphomas and leukemias; light and electron microscopy with special stains to determine the presence of glycogen, enzymes, or other substances that help to classify solid tumors; chromosomal analysis and modern molecular probes that identify unique characteristics of a disease; and responsible oncogenes, suppressor genes, and familial genes (see Chapter 191).

Table 189–2 ■ SIMPLIFIED GENERIC CANCER STAGING SYSTEM

Stage 1	Localized. Usually confined to the organ of origin. Usually curable with locally effective measures such as surgery or irradiation.
Stage 2	Regional. Extends beyond organ of origin but remains nearby, in lymph nodes, for example. Often curable by local measures alone or in combination (surgery ± irradiation) or by a local modality with chemotherapy.
Stage 3	Extensive. Has extended beyond regional site of origin, crossing several tissue planes or extending more distantly via lymphatics or blood. Also may be confined to an organ or region, but be unresectable because of anatomic extent or location. This stage is used rather than stage 2 or stage 4 depending on the usefulness of local and systemic treatment modalities and the likelihood of cure for that specific cancer.
Stage 4	Widely disseminated. Often involves the bone marrow or multiple distant organs. Rarely curable with current armamentarium.

THERAPEUTIC PRINCIPLES. The first step in treatment is to know the patient. All pertinent information—medical, developmental, and social—must be sought before treatment is planned. The second step is to know the tumor: its usual behavior, usual rate of growth, mode of spread, whether it is local or systemic, and any features that may provide prognostic or therapeutic leads. Third, the physician must know the available therapies: not only the therapeutic modalities such as chemotherapy, radiation therapy, and surgery, but also the skills and limitations of colleagues. Finally, the physician must know his or her own skills, experience, objectivity, and limitations. All these factors shape decisions concerning the patient. Caring for patients with cancer is not easy; the physician must be prepared for disappointment as well as success.

Clarity of intent—whether curative, palliative, or supportive—will avoid confusion of approach and method. Treatment protocols, either research or "standard of care" regimens, are important tools that allow strategies to be planned before immediate decisions become necessary. Protocols are also more likely to provide useful conclusions from a study or experience, because a scientific question or a uniform approach has been formulated and data have been collected in a systematic manner. A protocol is, however, only a road map. The planned therapy may require adjustment if complications develop after treatment has begun. Although many of these adjustments can be anticipated and specified in the protocol, not every circumstance can be foreseen. A protocol also is intended to provide practical information that will lead to improved treatment of subsequent patients.

THERAPEUTIC MODALITIES. There are four principal therapeutic modalities for cancer. *Surgery* is the oldest and most definitive when the tumor is localized under the most favorable anatomic circumstances. For example, for a small tumor localized in the breast, the interior of one kidney, or the peripheral edge of the liver, surgery is usually definitive, curative, and leaves no undue side effects. For many solid tumors, however, surgery alone is inadequate because of local or distant spread. Surgery is also crucial in establishing the extent of a tumor. Considerable surgical skill and experience are required to approach a tumor that may or may not be resectable, achieve tumor-free margins, and obtain the necessary tissue without causing further dissemination.

Radiation therapy is most useful for localized tumors that cannot be resected at all or without serious morbidity and for tumors, such as Hodgkin's disease, that tend to spread to predictable contiguous sites. Therefore, a port of radiation can be enlarged beyond the known extent of the tumor and be quite effective. Radiation therapy is also sometimes useful before surgery to reduce tumor size or after surgery to reduce the risk of recurrence. For some cancers, radiation therapy may also be used in combination with chemotherapy. Unfortunately, radiation therapy can have serious side effects (see Chapter 19), especially in children who are growing and developing. The dosage of radiation therapy is based on an estimate of the dose absorbed by tumor, measured in units called centigrays (cGy) or grays (Gy), where 100 cGy = 1 Gy.

Chemotherapy was the first systemic treatment for any cancer. It most often consists of a combination of drugs, which is almost always more effective than the sequential use of single agents. Because tumors develop subpopulations of cells that differ in their sensitivity to antineoplastic drugs, combinations of agents destroy more cells more rapidly, thereby reducing the frequency of emergence of resistant clones. The mechanisms of action differ widely among common chemotherapeutic agents, although DNA damage is the common final pathway. Toxicity also differs among agents; myelosuppression and gastrointestinal disorders are the most common disturbances. Although toxicity is a concern, for many cancers the best therapeutic results depend on the intensity of the dosage; that is, effective agents given at higher doses over a shorter period are more efficacious than less intensive regimens. The physician must straddle the fine line between too much and too little. Chemotherapy is used (1) as a definitive treatment, as in leukemia and some lymphomas; (2) as a principal form of treatment, as in testicular cancer and Ewing's sarcoma; or (3) as an adjuvant to another modality, such as amputation for osteosarcoma or surgical resection for breast or bowel cancer.

Biologic therapy for cancer includes, in addition to bone marrow transplantation, biologic response modifiers such as lymphokines or monoclonal antibodies and agents such as retinoic acid that may cause tumor cells to undergo differentiation and become harmless. These approaches, although still under development, show promise for the future.

The success of cancer therapy often depends on the skillful combination of two or more treatment modalities necessitating close cooperation of medical specialists. Failure to coordinate the effort may lead to the use of modalities in a useless or harmful sequence with an ineffective result.

Supportive care encompasses skilled general medical care; it includes management of infectious, metabolic, and cardiopulmonary disorders that frequently occur in patients undergoing aggressive treatment or surgical procedures. The judicious use of blood products is an essential part of supportive care, and infectious complications in the immunosuppressed patient must be anticipated. Because infections account for a large proportion of hospitalizations and deaths in patients with cancer, modern cancer therapy requires appropriate support from specialists in infectious diseases. In addition, loss of appetite is common among cancer patients, and special effort is required to maintain adequate nutrition. Dietitians with cancer care experience can be extremely helpful in prescribing palatable diets with high nutritional value.

After specific anticancer therapy, patients may require rehabilitation therapy. Common examples include physical therapy after amputation or bed confinement, speech therapy after head and neck surgery, and psychosocial therapy for depression or familial disruption. Patients require emotional support, adequate pain control, and a supportive environment. Care of terminally ill cancer patients is difficult: acute care hospitals often are not staffed to provide such care. Hospice and home care are often the best choices, provided continuing physician and nursing attention is available.

MEASURES OF SUCCESS. The measures of success in the treatment of patients with cancer are relatively simple, although not always precise. The first is survival without recurrence of tumor. Unfortunately, some malignancies recur many years after apparently successful control. An operative definition of cure, therefore, differs for each cancer. A patient who remains tumor free for 2 years after completing therapy is probably cured if the tumor was neuroblastoma, lung cancer, acute myeloid leukemia, or Burkitt's lymphoma. A much longer period would be needed to assume a cure for breast cancer, Ewing's sarcoma, Hodgkin's disease, or acute lymphoblastic leukemia of childhood.

The second measure of success is resumption of a normal life pattern without sequelae from the disease or its treatment. The number of cancer survivors is, happily, increasing rapidly. However, these patients require long-term follow-up for reasons other than cancer recurrence. In addition to the physical, social, and emotional rehabilitation that might be needed, patients may suffer a variety of late effects. A second malignancy may emerge because of a genetic predisposition, a side effect of irradiation or chemotherapy, or both. The growing and developing tissues of children are especially sensitive to therapeutic late effects. Neuropsychological disorders may emerge in children given brain irradiation and chemotherapy for brain tumors or acute leukemia. Radiation therapy and chemotherapy can also cause sterility, hypothyroidism, and cardiopulmonary dysfunction, as well as other functional disorders that may appear a few years or decades after therapy. Patients and their family physicians should be made aware of such possibilities and encouraged to be diligent.

PATIENT-FAMILY-PHYSICIAN RELATIONSHIP. Patients with cancer and their families face an extremely difficult time. They need a physician who is hopeful, truthful, compassionate, understanding, accessible, informative, and knowledgeable. Although cancer patients understand that several physicians and other professionals will be involved in their care, they prefer and need one physician who can assume ultimate responsibility for their myriad needs.

Patients should be told of plans and procedures in language that is understandable and appropriate. Some idea of the nature of cancer can be provided by analogy. For example, one may compare leukemia to the overgrowth of a farmer's field (bone marrow) by weeds (leukemia cells) that prevent the growth and export of crops (normal blood cells). Because the weeds cannot be removed manu-

ally from the marrow, chemicals are used to destroy the weeds and allow the crops to grow.

Physicians and family often mistakenly believe that the patient is concerned only with the possibility of death. In fact, patients are often equally or more concerned with the immediate implications of disease, for example, separation from family, pain, disfigurement, lengthy hospitalization, financial ruin, or missed time at work or school. Sensitive caregivers will understand and try to address these issues. Some patients and families become very knowledgeable about the disease and may know as much as or more than physicians about certain details; this knowledge should be viewed as an asset that can aid the physician in management. Physicians, nurses, and other caregivers may become emotionally attached to a patient or the family; this attachment need not be avoided if the necessary professional relationship and sound medical judgment are sustained. The physician must realize that, above all, the patient and family want an expert physician, not a pal or buddy.

When the cancer becomes resistant to therapy and death is imminent, the patient and family need support more than ever to help them through the last days. The family must understand that no known effective therapy remains and that the goal of management must change from destroying cancer cells to providing comfort. Once this decision is made, chemotherapy, transfusions, antibiotics, blood cell counts, and other laboratory tests are no longer necessary. The patient should be hospitalized only if proper supportive care or pain medication cannot be given at home. For pain that cannot be controlled by oral analgesics, parenteral morphine is the drug of choice and is most effective when given by continuous intravenous infusions, which can be self-regulated (see Chapter 27). The inadequate control of cancer pain in the United States is a national scandal. The demonstrably unwarranted fear of narcotic addiction, the rigid adherence to timed dosages irrespective of need, and the lack of knowledge and human insensitivity of doctors and nurses are widespread and indefensible. There is no reason for any cancer patient to suffer severe unremitting pain, a consequence of cancer more feared than death by most patients.

Terminally ill patients themselves seldom ask the physician whether they are going to die, probably because they already know or suspect the truth and do not want to confront the physician with an uncomfortable question. Should the question be asked, however, the patient probably knows the answer already; to deny the truth is worse than useless. Although guidelines can be provided for the caring of patients during this difficult period, the medical staff must adopt an approach that is suitable to the particular patient and circumstances. Most of all, the patient needs palpable demonstration that the medical staff is readily available and willing to listen, to comfort, to provide any possible service, and simply to be there. Even patients who are at home should not be abandoned; telephone communication can provide welcome support to the family. Both hospice care and home visits by nurses can be a godsend to patients and their families.

Li FP: Cancer control in susceptible groups. J Clin Oncol 17:719, 1999. *Review of genetic screening.*

190 CANCER PREVENTION

Gilbert S. Omenn

Cancers are estimated to have claimed an estimated 560,000 lives in the United States during 1998, one fourth of all deaths; approximately 1.2 million people were estimated to have newly diagnosed cancer (not including 1 million squamous or basal cell skin cancers). Fear of cancer, suffering from cancer and its treatment, and the limited benefit of therapy for most common cancers combine to make prevention an increasingly high priority in clinical medicine and public health.

The leading cancer killer by far in both men and women is lung cancer, followed by cancer of the prostate, colon and rectum, and pancreas in men and cancer of the breast, colon and rectum, ovary, and pancreas in women (Fig 190–1). Nine screening-accessible cancers (breast, colon, rectum, cervix, prostate, testis, tongue,

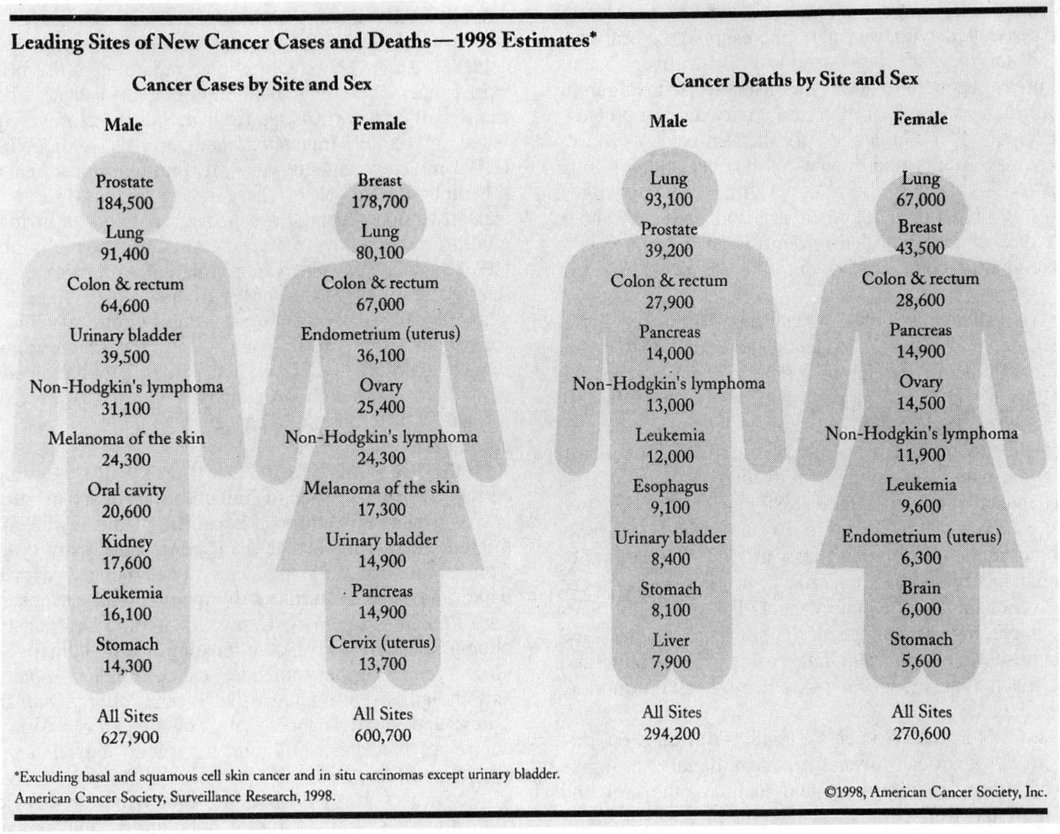

Leading Sites of New Cancer Cases and Deaths—1998 Estimates*

FIGURE 190–1 ■ Leading sites of cancer incidence and death—1998 estimates. (From Cancer Facts and Figures—1998. Atlanta, American Cancer Society, 1998.)

mouth, skin) are targets for early diagnosis. Currently, no effective screening tests are available for pancreatic and pulmonary cancers.

The primary modalities for cancer prevention (Table 190–1) require changes in behavior, especially smoking, alcohol, diet, and physical activity. Reduction of exposures to carcinogenic agents from all environmental sources is a complementary approach. Meanwhile, hormonal, nutritional, and pharmacologic interventions and genetic screening, counseling, and treatments for those with testable inherited predispositions are under intensive investigation. New animal models and genetic markers of high risk for colon and breast cancer offer promising means of screening and testing agents and risk factor modifications on a scientifically sound basis.

SMOKING CESSATION AND SMOKING PREVENTION. (See Chapter 13.) Diseases related to cigarette smoking represent a 20th century epidemic and are rapidly spreading globally. Smoking is the primary cause of cancer of the lungs, larynx, oral cavity, and esophagus (approximately 10 to 20 times the risk in non-smokers) and contributes to leukemia and to cancer of the pancreas, bladder, kidney, stomach, and cervix (about 2 times increased risk). Smoking acts synergistically with chemical and radiation carcinogens in the lung and with alcohol in the esophagus and oral cavity. Former smokers, after a lag of up to 4 years, show a progressively lower relative risk than continuing smokers do, and the rate of increase is comparable to the slowly rising rate among never-smokers as they age. However, unlike the risk of coronary heart disease, the absolute risk of lung cancer in former smokers probably never declines to the level of non-smokers. Low-tar, low-nicotine, and filtered cigarettes have had little or no protective effect because the smokers of these products tend to inhale more deeply and more frequently. Smokeless tobacco and snuff dipping have also been successfully promoted to children and adolescents in recent years. Leukoplakia, a white patch involving the oral mucosa epithelium, is a telltale pre-malignant lesion found in up to half of tobacco chewers, with a 5% risk of epidermoid carcinoma. Finally, environmental tobacco smoke, or second-hand smoke, has been declared a definite human carcinogen by the Environmental Protection Agency; 6000 cases of lung cancer per year are attributed to environmental tobacco smoke by the National Research Council.

A huge literature attests to the difficulty of helping smokers quit and remain abstinent. About 5% quit by themselves for at least a 6-month period each year. Physicians play a key role in urging smokers to quit and in guiding them to self-help materials, classes, or pharmacologic aids to try to avoid relapse. Work site, family, and community reinforcement is essential; increased taxes (prices) on tobacco products also reduce smoking. Prevention of smoking, especially in young people, minorities, and women, can be enhanced by organized community and school programs, as well as regulatory actions and physician advice.

MODERATION OF ALCOHOL INTAKE. (See Chapter 16.) The National Cancer Institute Dietary Guidelines recommend that con-

Table 190–1 ■ PROPORTIONS OF CANCER DEATHS ATTRIBUTED TO VARIOUS PREVENTABLE FACTORS

FACTOR OR CLASS OF FACTOR	BEST ESTIMATE	RANGE OF ESTIMATES
Tobacco	30	25–40
Alcohol	3	2–4
Diet	35	10–70
Food Additives*	<1	−5–2
Reproductive/sexual behavior	7	1–13
Occupation	4	2–8
General pollution	2	1–5
Industrial products	<1	<1–2
Medical procedures	1	0.5–3
Geophysical factors†	3	2–4
Infections	10?	1–?

*Minus indicates potential benefits from antioxidants and other additives.
†Ultraviolet and cosmic radiation included; perhaps 1% and truly avoidable.
From Doll R, Peto R: The causes of cancer: Quantitative estimates of avoidable risks of cancer in the United States today. J Natl Cancer Inst 66:1193, 1981. These conclusions and estimates were updated and reaffirmed in a special supplement to Cancer Causes & Control 7 (Suppl. 1), 1996, edited by Colditz et al.

sumption of alcoholic beverages, if any, be moderate. Alcohol intake is highly associated with cancer of the esophagus, oral cavity, pharynx, and larynx and, less strikingly, with liver, rectal, pancreatic, and breast cancer. It acts synergistically with cigarette smoking and poor diet, especially in the oral cavity and esophagus.

DIET. (See Chapter 11.) Guidelines for healthy diets strongly recommend decreases in fat and increases in fiber intake, most easily described as "five-a-day" portions of fruit and vegetables. Such advice aims at preventing colon, breast, and prostate cancer, as well as heart disease and bowel disorders. High calcium intake may be protective against colon cancer, but data are inconclusive at present.

The typical U.S. diet has 39% of calories from fat, about 150 g/day. Experimental studies in rodents show that dietary fat may exert tumor-enhancing or tumor-promoting effects on the breast directly through changes in cell membranes or indirectly through neuroendocrine systems. In the colon, fat may influence bile acids, sterol substrates, and fecal microflora. International, migrant, and time-trend data indicate that a reduction in dietary fat to 20% of caloric intake might reduce breast cancer risk by two thirds, but most case-control (retrospective) and cohort (prospective) epidemiologic studies have found less striking correlations or none at all. Similar inconsistencies underlie positive associations of fat intake with colorectal and prostate cancer. Fat intake involves many variables, including percentage of calories, grams per day, saturated versus unsaturated fats and fatty acids, overweight, and duration of diet. Each type of cancer possesses other confounding or interacting risk factors.

A feasibility study for the Women's Health Trial showed that women aged 45 to 69 years can lower their mean dietary fat intake to below 25% of energy requirements and maintain the diet and good health for 2 years. Reduction in dietary fat intake is a major component of the Women's Health Initiative, a massive trial aimed at reducing breast cancer, heart disease, and osteoporosis in postmenopausal women by means of hormone replacement therapy, calcium and vitamin D, five-a-day diet change, and exercise.

INCREASE IN DIETARY FIBER. The highest rates of colon cancer occur in Western countries, which are associated with a high intake of refined carbohydrates as compared with the naturally occurring, fiber-rich foods common in African and Asian countries, where colon cancer rates are low. Among Western countries, low colon cancer rates and a mean intake of 31 g of fiber per day in Finland contrast with high colon cancer rates in Denmark and New York and 17 g of fiber per day despite similar fat intake. "Fiber," defined by plant origin and resistance to digestion by human enzymes, is highly heterogeneous, thus making measurement difficult. Soluble fiber (gum, mucilage, pectin, and hemicellulose) delays gastric emptying, slows glucose absorption, and lowers serum cholesterol levels, with lesser effects on bulk and transit time. Insoluble fiber increases fecal bulk and decreases intestinal transit time; cellulose and hemicellulose are prominent in cereals and grains, lignin in berry fruits, and pectin in citrus fruits and apples. Although a number of epidemiologic studies suggested a link between higher dietary fiber intake and colorectal cancer, a recent large study found no association.

INCREASED PHYSICAL ACTIVITY. Overcoming sedentary or inactive lifestyles benefits the cardiovascular, respiratory, muscular, cognitive, and metabolic systems. Increased physical activity seems to offer significant protection against colon cancer. Physical activity differences may be influential in cross-national and cross-cultural studies and should be carefully monitored in chemoprevention studies.

REDUCTION IN ENVIRONMENTAL AND OCCUPATIONAL EXPOSURE TO CARCINOGENIC CHEMICALS, PHYSICAL AGENTS, AND INFECTIOUS AGENTS. Asbestos fibers, inorganic arsenic compounds, bis-chloromethyl ether, chromium compounds, mustard gas, nickel dust, and polycyclic aromatic hydrocarbons from coal and gasoline combustion are lung carcinogens; vinyl chloride causes a distinctive angiosarcoma of the liver; some pesticides are associated with the development of non-Hodgkin's lymphoma; aromatic amine dyestuffs can cause bladder cancer; leather production

and isopropyl alcohol manufacturing are associated with nasal cancer; and benzene can cause acute myelogenous leukemia. Tobacco smoke is the most prevalent chemical carcinogen, probably followed by charbroiled meat and fish.

PHYSICAL AGENTS. Ultraviolet radiation is the primary cause of skin cancer, including melanoma and lip cancer. The risk of squamous cell cancers arising from actinic keratoses is greatly exacerbated in organ transplant and human immunodeficiency virus (HIV)-infected patients who are immunosuppressed after infection; preemptive removal of these pre-cancerous lesions and fastidious sun protection are required in such patients. Ionizing radiation (including radiotherapy) increases rates at essentially all exposed sites (see Chapter 19). The Environmental Protection Agency estimates that as many as 21,000 cases of lung cancer (see Chapter 85) per year may be attributed to α-particle–emitting radon gas in homes, for which simple testing and venting procedures are available to reduce exposure and risk. Non-ionizing radiation and electromagnetic fields, although previously suspected of increasing leukemia (of any type) and brain cancer, seem not to raise risks based on current data in aggregate.

INFECTIOUS AGENTS (SEE CHAPTER 193.) Certain cancers are causally related to specific infections: Primary hepatocellular cancer is associated with chronic hepatitis B and C infections, with distinctive mutations in the *p53* gene, and with synergistic effects from aflatoxins; cervical cancer is associated with certain human papillomaviruses; Burkitt's lymphoma and nasopharyngeal cancer with Epstein-Barr virus; Kaposi's sarcoma and non-Hodgkin's lymphoma with HIV-1; T-cell leukemia with human T-cell leukemia virus type I; urinary bladder cancer (*Schistosoma haematobium*) and cholangiocarcinoma of the liver (*Clonorchis sinensis*) with parasites; and gastric cancer with *Helicobacter pylori*. Environmental control of parasites, antibiotic treatment of *Helicobacter*, interferon treatment of hepatitis, and/or vaccines to protect against exposure to the viruses and *Helicobacter* should be effective cancer prevention strategies. For example, population-wide neonatal immunization against hepatitis B virus is expected to eliminate the scourge of primary liver cancer in Taiwan.

PHARMACEUTICAL AGENTS. Alkylating agents can cause leukemias; androgens and anabolic steroids, liver cancer; chlornaphazine, bladder cancer; estrogens (possibly also "environmental estrogens"), cancer of the vagina and cervix (diethylstilbestrol), endometrium (postmenopausal estrogens), or liver and cervix (steroid contraceptives); azathioprine and cyclosporine immunosuppressants, non-Hodgkin's lymphoma and skin cancer; and phenacetin-containing analgesics, renal pelvic tumors. Careful indications for use and surveillance are essential.

CHEMOPREVENTION. Population trials of chemopreventive agents are under way worldwide. Many candidate agents are natural products, food constituents, or pharmaceuticals already approved for other indications. Various agents block activation of procarcinogens, enhance detoxification of carcinogens, block the carcinogenic action, or make the cells less responsive to carcinogenic effects. Carotenoids and retinoids have been prime candidates based on observational epidemiologic work and animal and cell culture findings suggesting protective effects through antioxidant, tumor suppressor, or immunomodulatory actions. 13-*cis*-Retinoic acid may be effective in prevention of recurrences of head and neck cancer. 4-Hydroxyretinamide and 9-*cis*-retinoic acid are prime candidates for prevention of breast cancer. Antioxidants (vitamins E and C and selenium), isoflavones, phytosterols in soybeans, polyphenols in green tea, and many other inhibitors of cellular proliferation or tumor promotion are being investigated in animal models and in phase I and phase II human studies. For example, calcium supplementation, aspirin, and other non-steroidal anti-inflammatory agents can reduce colonic cell proliferation in humans; selective inhibitors of cyclooxygenase 2 are particularly promising for preventing colon cancer.

The largest studies of the past 15 years involved β-carotene alone (22,000 male physicians), β-carotene plus vitamin E (29,000 male smokers in Finland), β-carotene plus vitamin A (14,000 male and female U.S. smokers and 4000 asbestos-exposed workers), and β-carotene plus vitamin E and aspirin (40,000 female health professionals). The Alpha-Tocopherol/Beta-Carotene study in Finland found no benefit from vitamin E or from β-carotene; instead, the men receiving β-carotene, 20 mg/day, had an 18% higher rate of lung cancer and 8% higher overall mortality. In 1996, confirmatory results of no benefit from β-carotene were noted in the Physicians Health Study, and confirmation of adverse effects (28% higher lung cancer incidence and 17% higher mortality) was provided by the Beta-Carotene and Retinol Efficacy Trial (CARET). CARET and the Finland trial also found excess cardiovascular mortality; even though β-carotene is carried in the low-density lipoprotein (LDL) particles in blood, it fails to protect against LDL oxidation in vivo. As a result, β-carotene was removed from cereals and many vitamin supplements, and subsequent laboratory studies noted that specific epoxides and ketones of β-carotene increase the formation of B[a]P-DNA adducts in rat microsomes. These adverse effects of β-carotene have also stimulated a search for other chemopreventive constituents of fruit and vegetables, of which the many candidates include folic acid and calcium D-glucarate.

CHEMOPREVENTION WITH HORMONES. In the United States, cancer of hormone-responsive tissues accounts for 20% of the newly diagnosed cancers in men and more than 40% in women. Thus chemoprevention with "antihormones" represents a promising approach. Although the early sequential oral contraceptives increased endometrial cancer risk, modern estrogen-progesterone combinations are potent chemopreventive agents. Women with 6 or more years of oral contraceptive use have less than one sixth the risk of endometrial cancer when compared with never-users, and the effect lasts at least 15 years after discontinuation of the oral contraceptives. Combination oral contraceptives also suppress gonadotropin levels and ovulation, thereby decreasing the risk for epithelial ovarian cancer by about 40%, independent of parity. The breast responds differently: progesterone increases the rate of cell division beyond that induced by estrogen, so there is a potential increase in breast cancer.

In premenopausal women, a strategy for gaining the benefits of oral contraceptives while reducing breast cancer (and cardiovascular) risk involves the use of luteinizing hormone–releasing hormone (LHRH) antagonists to create a "reversible bilateral oophorectomy," combined with low-dose estrogen to overcome the hypoestrogenic effects and with a quarterly progestogen. Antiestrogenic agents such as tamoxifen reduce the incidence of new primary cancers in the other breast of breast cancer survivors. In a subsequent double-blind, randomized, multiple–end point trial in 13,000 women, tamoxifen halved the rates of invasive and noninvasive breast cancer and fractures, so the trial was halted after 5 years, 2 years ahead of schedule; however, endometrial cancer rates and venous/pulmonary thromboses were significantly increased among those receiving tamoxifen. Among candidate agents, the 2-arylbenzothiophene raloxifene is a target-site selective estrogen receptor modulator that has estrogen agonist effects on bone and serum lipids but estrogen antagonist effects on the breast and uterus. Preliminary findings from randomized double-blind trials in 12,000 postmenopausal women with osteoporosis to reduce the risk of fractures within the first 2 years indicate that raloxifene reduces the incidence of breast and endometrial cancer, with the difference in breast tumors being due to fewer that are positive for estrogen or progesterone receptors.

Diethylstilbestrol and LHRH agonists are therapeutically effective against metastatic prostate cancer by reducing testosterone-mediated maintenance of prostate tissue. Finasteride, a testosterone 5α-reductase inhibitor, is being tested in 18,000 men for primary prevention of prostate cancer.

GENETIC SCREENING. Molecular studies of cancer have revealed numerous oncogenes, tumor suppressor genes, and other genes affecting cell division, cell cycle, and cell proliferation (see Chapter 191). The host of potential molecular targets for cancer prevention include those identified in inherited cancer syndromes, such as retinoblastoma and polyposis coli, and those identified in molecular analyses of sporadic cancers.

American Cancer Society: Cancer Facts and Figures—1998. Atlanta, American Cancer Society, 1998. *Excellent annual update on cancer statistics and advances.*

Fuchs CS, Giovannucci EL, Colditz GA: Dietary fiber and the risk of colorectal cancer and adenoma in women. N Engl J Med 340:169, 1999. *A study of nearly 90,000 women showing no association of dietary fiber with colorectal cancer.*

Omenn GS, Goodman GE, Thornquist MD, et al: Effects of a combination of beta-carotene and vitamin A on lung cancer and cardiovascular disease. N Engl J Med 334:1150, 1996. *Confirmation of lack of benefit and strong evidence of adverse effects of the intervention. Long-term follow-up continuing.*

ONCOGENES AND SUPPRESSOR GENES: GENETIC CONTROL OF CANCER

Edison T. Liu

THE ONCOGENE THEORY AND HUMAN CANCERS

Oncogenes encode proteins that, when activated, induce cancer; by contrast, tumor suppressor genes cause cancer when their function is blocked. The observation that mutant chicken and mouse oncogenes not only are associated with but also are causal in human cancers provided the first concrete evidence that human and animal cancers follow the same genetic rules and led to a new cancer model that stressed the importance of mutations in resident genes (also called proto-oncogenes) rather than the introduction of foreign genes. The concept that genes involved in cancer are the same as those controlling normal cellular processes further generalized the malignant process as a part of normal biology. The primacy of genes in defining cellular phenotype would predict that the mutational profile of a cancer cell may presage clinical outcome, or at least explain cancer cell behavior. Indeed, this prediction has become reality.

THE MANY ROADS TO CANCER: ABERRATIONS OF SIGNALING PATHWAYS

Viral oncogenes were the first evidence that endogenous genes can directly cause cancer. Normal cellular genes (proto-oncogenes, designated by the "c" prefix) are "captured" or transduced by the retrovirus and mutated through the error-prone replicative process of the retroviral life cycle. The result is a viral oncogene (v-*onc*) that is often structurally distinct from its normal cellular counterpart and is functionally arrested in a biochemically activated form. Extensions of these early investigations revealed that the oncogene precursors, the proto-oncogenes, act as biochemical switches in cellular command and control processes, specifically relaying signals from the outside of the cell to the nucleus. The progressive and controlled transfer of extracellular signals is bypassed when one of the relay members is rendered constitutively activated, resulting in a characteristic of a cancer cell: unmanaged growth.

Nature has provided ample evidence for oncogenic mutations in members of signaling pathways. The receptor tyrosine kinase epidermal growth factor receptor (EGFR, mutated or overexpressed in brain and epithelial cancers, homologous retroviral oncogene = v-*erbB*), when stimulated with one of its ligands, tumor growth factor-α (TGF-α; found to be overexpressed in some human cancers), interacts with *ras* (retroviral homologue = v-H-*ras*, or v-K-*ras*, mutated in 10–20% of all human cancers) through bridging proteins. *Ras*, in turn, is controlled by guanosine triphosphatase–activating proteins (GAPs, oncogenic homologue = *NF1*, the gene involved in neurofibromatosis) and transmits signals through activation of *raf* (retroviral homologue, v-*raf*). Stimulation of the *ras/raf* pathway leads to augmented expression of the nuclear proteins *jun*, *fos*, and *myc* (retroviral homologues = v-*jun*, v-*fos*, v-*myc*; *myc* is mutated and rearranged in lymphoid malignancies and amplified in breast cancers), some of which are proteins that induce the expression of other genes (called transcription factors). Thus, every relay node in this signal transduction pathway is a potential site for oncogenic conversion. The complexity of the transformation process is further augmented by the existence of multiple parallel signaling pathways that are promiscuous in their selection of biochemical partners. For example, the receptor tyrosine kinase HER-2 forms dimers either with itself or with related receptor tyrosine kinases, such as EGFR, HER-3, and HER-4; *ras* can be regulated by either *ras*-GAP or *NF1;* and stimulation of the *ras* pathway activates a number of mitogen-activated protein kinases (MAPKs).

THE WRONG PLACE AT THE WRONG TIME. In human cancers, mutations in proto-oncogenes lead to altered function. However, another avenue to cancer is the inappropriate expression of structurally normal proteins. Several transcription factors fall into this category: *myc, tal-1/SCL, lyl-1, Ttg-1,* and *Ttg-2.* These oncoproteins are structurally identical to their normal forms but are either expressed inappropriately in the cell cycle or in inappropriate tissues. *myc* is ubiquitously expressed in cells and plays a role in cell division and differentiation. Activation of *myc* due to the t(8; 14)(q24;q32) seen in Burkitt's lymphomas and B-cell acute lymphoblastic leukemias (ALLs) deregulates *myc* expression such that the exquisite control of *myc* transcription is lost. In lymphoid tissues, the result is expansion of the pre–B-cell compartment in *myc*-containing transgenic mice and ultimately to the emergence of a monoclonal lymphoid malignancy. By contrast, the other members on this list (*tal-1/SCL, lyl-1, Ttg-1,* and *Ttg-2*) are linked to T-cell ALL. In this group, oncogenic potential is activated by expression in an inappropriate cell type: *tal-1* is normally expressed in erythroid and myeloid precursors and not T cells; *lyl-1* is expressed only in myeloid and B-lymphoid cells; and *Ttg-2* transcripts are found in liver, spleen, and kidney but not in activated T cells. The exception is *Ttg-1,* which is mainly a neural associated transcription factor that is expressed at low levels in normal T cells; however, in T-cell leukemias with the t(11;14) translocation, *Ttg-1* RNA levels are extraordinarily high. In each case, the inappropriate expression of a transcription factor serves as a molecular switch to induce a malignancy.

THE MANY ROADS TO CANCER: RELEASE OF SUPPRESSION

Whereas proto-oncogenes are identified by a gain of function after mutational damage, another class of cancer genes—tumor suppressor genes—contribute to malignancy by a loss of function. To this end, well-known tumor suppressor genes such as the retinoblastoma gene (*Rb-1*) and *p53* can act as "brakes" to cellular proliferation, and each appears to function through distinct pathways. *Rb-1* negatively regulates an important transcription factor, E2F, and the deletion of the *Rb* gene (as seen in congenital retinoblastoma) or sequestration of its protein product (as seen in the presence of the adenovirus E1A protein, or the human papilloma viral protein, E7) releases the suppression of E2F. *p53* enhances the expression of *p21/CIP1*, which is a potent suppressor of cell cycle regulatory kinases (CDKs). Activation of these CDKs is necessary for progression through the cell cycle, and CDK inhibitors block this process. The loss of *p53* and the associated loss of *p21/CIP1* expression control result in unmanaged progression through the cell cycle.

That both *Rb* and *p53* are involved in the genesis of cancer is supported by the identification of germline mutations in patients with cancer predisposition syndromes such as congenital retinoblastoma (*Rb*) and the Li-Fraumeni multicancer syndrome (*p53*). As is the case with transforming oncogenes, the presence of a single abnormal tumor suppressor allele is insufficient for cancer to form; lesions at other genetic loci are necessary. For example, both *Rb* and *p53* may need to be inactivated for some primary cells to be rendered immortal, one of the first steps in transformation. The DNA tumor virus, human papillomavirus (HPV), which is etiologic in cervical, anal, and penile carcinomas, has engineered itself to inhibit both of these critical proteins by binding with the HPV viral proteins E6 and E7. Through this mechanism, HPV biochemically achieves the same outcome that carcinogens accomplish by inactivating genetic mutations. In colon cancers, mutations in *p53* frequently accompany several other genetic lesions, including those involved in cytoskeletal organization (*APC* gene of familial adenomatous polyposis), signal transduction (*ras*), and cellular adhesion (*DCC* gene in colon cancers) for an invasive cancer to emerge.

By using the definition of a tumor suppressor gene as any gene whose loss of function contributes to cancer progression, functional categories of molecules involved in maintaining cellular "contain-

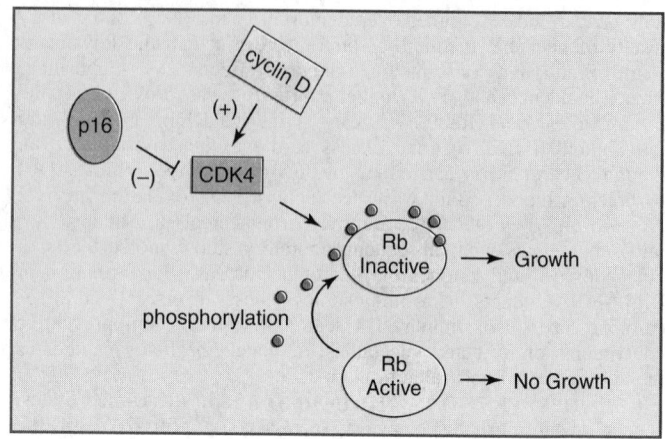

FIGURE 191–1 ■ The interaction between p16, cyclin D, the cyclin-dependent kinases (CDKs), and *Rb.*

ment" can be devised. One category of suppressor genes includes the inhibitors of the CDKs. CDKs are kinases that control progression through the cell cycle. They, in turn, are controlled by protein activators (called cyclins) and inhibitors (called CDK inhibitors). The loss of expression of CDK inhibitors such as *p16, p27,* and *p57* has been associated with a wide range of cancers, including lung, head and neck, breast, pancreas, and melanoma. In malignant melanoma, the loss of both *p16* alleles identified in most primary tumors led to the finding that inactivating germline mutations in *p16* segregate with familial melanomas and with some familial pancreatic cancer syndromes. Therefore, CDK inhibitors such as *p16* maintain the normal cellular phenotype by regulating cell proliferation, and abrogation of inhibitor function leads to cancer. The story of *p16* reiterates the importance of viewing cancer genetics in the context of signaling relays. *Rb* acts to inhibit cell proliferation. Biochemically, *Rb* function is inhibited by CDK4 phosphorylation. Cyclin D is a necessary activator of CDK4, and *p16* blocks CDK4-dependent *Rb* phosphorylation. Inactivating mutations in *Rb* and in *p16,* activation of CDK4 through mutation, and amplification or overexpression of cyclin D have all been implicated in human cancers. Thus, *Rb,* CDK4, cyclin D, and *p16* are components of a signaling "relay station" that regulates traverse through the G₁ portion of the cell cycle. Abnormalities in any of these components lead to the same outcome—cancer (Fig. 191–1).

THE MANY ROADS TO CANCER: BLOCK IN CELL DEATH

The accumulation of cancer cells can be accomplished by a decrease in cell death as well as by an increase in cellular proliferation. Current evidence suggests that the abrogation of programmed cell death (apoptosis) may be an important concomitant to neoplastic transformation. Certain cellular events, such as cytokine signaling (e.g., tumor necrosis factor, interleukin-3 withdrawal) or DNA damage, can trigger a cascade of events culminating in activation of intracellular proteases. These events result in the regulated cleavage of cellular constituents, including proteins and DNA, and ultimately to cell death. The cell exerts exquisite control of this process using redundant systems to induce or to block apoptosis, and some of these control switches are involved in cancer induction and in the response to cancer treatment.

The clearest example of an oncogene modulating the apoptotic process is *bcl-2,* found to be the important oncogene in patients with the t(14q;18q) translocation frequently detected in follicular lymphomas. *bcl-2* blocks apoptosis when overexpressed or inappropriately expressed, and, in lymphomas, perturbations in *bcl-2* may be among the earliest oncogene abnormalities acting to prolong the lifespan of cells that are prone to accumulate genetic mutations. In experimental lymphomas, *bcl-2* does not cause cancer directly but allows the cell to survive to undergo subsequent mutations involving rearrangements at other oncogenes, such as the c-*myc,* that result in accelerated progression of the lymphoma. This *bcl-2/myc* interaction underscores another principle of oncogene action: more than one cancer gene must be perturbed for a malignancy to arise.

Other bcl-2–related proteins have recently been identified, all capable of physically interacting with each other as homodimers or heterodimers: bcl-X$_L$, like bcl-2, is antiapoptotic; however, overexpression of bax, bak, bcl-X$_S$, and BAD actually induces apoptosis. Thus, the ratio of antiapoptotic:proapoptotic factors of related structure determine the cell's "set point" that triggers apoptosis. Significantly, this set point is associated with responsiveness to irradiation and chemotherapy.

More recently, growth factor receptors and other surface signaling molecules have been directly linked with the control of apoptosis. Many receptor kinase systems such as platelet-derived growth factor receptor (PDGFR) and met recruit and activate the phosphatidylinositol 3-kinase (PI 3-kinase). PI 3-kinase is now known to activate the Akt protein kinase, which supports cell survival through its phosphorylation and inactivation of BAD, a bcl-2–related protein that promotes cell death. Therefore, augmented Akt function induced by certain ligand receptor interactions is predicted to have a significant antiapoptotic effect. It is not clear why certain tumors directly alter bcl-2 to modulate apoptotic potential whereas others primarily use alternative pathways to accomplish the same ends. Nevertheless, the underlying principle is that normal cells have self-policing mechanisms that activate suicide programs: when the mutational load of a cell exceeds a critical level, self-destruct processes are activated. Cancer, however, may result when genetically aberrant cells are not cleared but rather permitted to proliferate, thus accumulating mutations in important cancer genes.

A second principle that has emerged is that many of the common oncogenes known to transform cells paradoxically also have proapoptotic functions. For example, myc is capable of transforming rat fibroblasts; however, in situations of cellular stress, such as serum starvation or when coupled with exposure to certain chemotherapeutic agents, myc triggers cell death in the same cells. Activated ras oncogenes, which are potent transforming genes in immortalized cell lines, also induce apoptosis under similar stress conditions. However, when myc and ras are co-introduced into primary murine fibroblasts, unequivocal transformation occurs. When the biochemical components necessary for apoptosis were investigated for myc, it was found that bcl-2 overexpression or specific activation of insulin-like growth factor receptor (IGFR) by IGF-1 can block myc-induced apoptosis. Taken together, it now appears that oncogenes can induce both growth and death, and that modulation of cooperating pathways (e.g., bcl-2, ras, and IGFR) can tip the balance toward transformation. These observations raise the intriguing possibility that transformation is not an inevitable outcome of oncogene activation and that biochemical manipulation of pro-apoptotic signals can result in clearing mutant cells before they convert to cancers or can augment therapeutic responses.

THE MANY ROADS TO CANCER: ABNORMALITIES IN GENETIC STABILITY

A characteristic of a cancer cell is its inherent ability to undergo and to sustain genetic mutations. Normal cells have the ability not only to identify and repair DNA damage but also to prevent the propagation of mutation-laden daughter cells by suicide mechanisms such as apoptosis. Although defects in DNA repair, found in rare disorders such as xeroderma pigmentosum and ataxia-telangiectasia, are associated with cancer risk, only recently has an abnormality in a repair process been linked to a common human cancer. Hereditary non-polyposis colon cancer (HNPCC) is an inherited syndrome characterized by increased risk for colon cancer without associated polyposis. In addition, these individuals also harbor a heightened risk for endometrial cancer. It was found that affected individuals show signs of a defect in the repair of DNA mismatches: additions or reductions in the number of dinucleotide repeats (called microsatellite instability) were clonally detected in their tumors. Although DNA mutations are commonly seen in cancer cells, this type of abnormality is a signature for a specific kind of repair defect previously studied mainly in bacteria and in yeast. When incorrectly paired nucleotides occur within a DNA duplex, either through misincorporations, nucleotide damage, or genetic recombination, cells use a mismatch repair (MMR) system to identify and to excise the mismatch. This recognition is mediated by the mammalian protein products of the MSH2, MSH3, MSH6, MLH1,

PMS1, and PMS2 genes. HNPCC patients primarily have mutations in MSH2 and MLH1, although mutations in the others are also found in a small proportion of HNPCC patients. That lesions in the MMR genes lead to cancer has been confirmed in mice genetically engineered to have deleted the MSH2, MLH1, PMS1, and PMS2 homologues. These animals have a high potential of developing hematopoietic malignancies and intestinal adenocarcinomas and adenomas. The clinical consequence of this molecular defect in humans is the emergence of colon cancers that differ from the sporadic variety and are characterized by fewer ras and p53 mutations, as well as less allelic losses. Moreover, colon cancer in HNPCC patients appears to have a better prognosis than its sporadic counterparts.

ONCOGENES AS POINTS OF ORIGIN: MOLECULAR PATHWAYS DEFINE A CANCER

Certain oncogenes are closely associated with specific malignancies, suggesting that they may be causative for that disease. Chronic myelogenous leukemia (CML) is characterized by a genetic rearrangement juxtaposing the beginning of the bcr gene on chromosome 22 with the abl proto-oncogene on chromosome 9 (see Chapter 176). The resultant bcr-abl hybrid protein activates the tyrosine kinase activity of abl and, in animal models, has been shown to be the direct cause of the CML phenotype. Intriguingly, 10 to 25% of de novo ALL also harbor the same t(9;22) translocation, but the rearrangement occurs at a slightly different genetic location to generate a distinctly smaller hybrid bcr-abl oncoprotein with increased biochemical activity. Thus, not only does the bcr-abl induce a specific hematologic disease, CML, but minor alterations of the same aberrant protein result in a different clinical picture, ALL. Another example of specific oncogene-cancer associations is the t(15;17) translocation found exclusively in acute promyelocytic leukemia (APL); it causes the aberrant fusion of the retinoic acid receptor alpha (RARA) with another transcription factor, PML. This abnormal protein is seen in no other cancers. Lastly, rearrangements of the bcl-2 locus and translocations involving the myc proto-oncogene are found solely in lymphomas.

In solid tumors, genetic perturbations of the ret oncogene have been identified only in cancers, and germline mutations in this receptor tyrosine kinase give rise to the heritable multiple endocrine neoplasia syndrome. Germline APC mutations give rise predominantly to colorectal cancers, and constitutive BRCA1 and BRCA2 mutations result mainly in breast and ovarian cancers. The near exclusivity of the involvement of some of these genes with the induction of specific cancers suggests a potential "gatekeeper" function for these genes. Although the exact mechanism is unclear, such putative gatekeeper genes are responsible for the maintenance of the non-cancerous phenotype in restricted tissue types.

Less exclusive oncogene-cancer associations occur more frequently and are also helpful in mapping pathways of cancer progression. Overexpression or amplification of the HER-2 gene is seen in 20 to 30% of invasive breast cancers and is correlated with a worse outcome. The concordance observed in the HER-2 status between carcinomas in situ, invasive carcinomas, and their metastases from individual patients suggests that perturbations at the HER-2 locus occur early in breast tumorigenesis and mark a distinct progression pathway for the tumor. Similar findings have been observed in other cancers: p53 mutations are found only in cervical carcinomas not induced by oncogenic papillomaviruses. Ras mutations are detected in 20% of de novo acute myelogenous leukemia but are very rare in CML (in either chronic or blast phase) or in APL. The initiation by one gene may not only define a particular molecular progression pathway but may also predict some tumor characteristics as well. Bcr-abl–positive ALLs are associated with earlier relapse and may account for the poorer prognosis in adult ALL (in which the bcr-abl rearrangement is seen in 25–40% of patients) as compared with childhood ALL (in which only 5% are bcr-abl positive). HER-2 overexpression or amplification is found frequently in ductal breast carcinomas but rarely in lobular carcinomas. N-myc amplification remains one of the most potent predictors of poorer survival in childhood neuroblastomas. Thus, oncogene mutations can be used not only in cancer diagnostics but also as useful markers of prognosis.

CONVERGENCE OF PATHWAYS: TOWARD A UNIFYING EXPLANATION OF CANCER

The many oncogenes involved in malignancies highlight the complexity of the cancer process. However, the dissection of the biochemical pathways used by these oncogenes is uncovering interactions that may begin to unify empirical observations of human tumor biology. One example is found in ras. Ras activity is down-regulated by GAP, and oncogenic ras is resistant to the effects of GAP, suggesting that mutations abrogating GAP's negative effects on ras might promote cancer. Although abnormalities in ras-GAP have not been found, the gene associated with congenital neurofibromatosis, NF1, is structurally a GTPase-activating protein that functionally interacts with ras. Mutations in NF1, seen in neurofibromatosis, block its ability to down-regulate ras activity. This biochemical interaction between ras and NF1 is manifested clinically in an unusual form of leukemia. Mutations in ras are a common genetic abnormality in adult acute myelogenous leukemia (AML), and epidemiologic and molecular data support a role for ras in the induction of myeloid leukemias. Interestingly, children with neurofibromatosis have a higher rate of developing a rare myeloproliferative syndrome that often progresses to AML. The biochemical pathway, therefore, predicts the clinical convergence.

How the molecular pathways explain some manifestations of a disease also can be found in the example of von Hippel-Lindau disease (VHL). Von Hippel-Lindau disease is a heritable disorder characterized by renal cell carcinomas, retinal and cerebellar hemangioblastomas, pancreatic cysts, pheochromocytomas, and endolymphatic sac tumors. Linkage analysis led to the identification of the VHL gene as causative in the syndrome, and as the important gene within the 3p deletions seen in the majority of sporadic renal cell cancers. Many of the VHL tumors, notably the renal cell carcinomas and the retinal and cerebellar hemangioblastomas, are highly vascular tumors. This finding is particularly pertinent because the VHL protein product is now thought to be involved in the post-transcriptional regulation of cellular mRNA, particularly those produced in response to hypoxic stress: the presence of an intact VHL protein reduces the stability of RNA transcripts for the gene encoding the angiogenic factor, vascular endothelial growth factor (VEGF), and erythropoietin (EPO). Mutations in the VHL gene seen in both hereditary and sporadic renal cell carcinoma frequently result in higher levels of VEGF and EPO. These higher levels explain, to a great extent, the highly vascular nature of renal cell carcinomas and the generation of vascular tumors such as hemangioblastomas in individuals with the von Hippel-Lindau syndrome (due to the VEGF), and the association of elevated red cell mass in patients with renal cell carcinoma (due to the EPO).

FRUIT FLIES AND HUMAN CANCER. One aspect of biology and medicine that has become apparent is how seemingly unrelated fields and biological systems are uncovering common truths through the study of related genes. The underlying principle is that any biochemical switch can be usurped to control oncogene processes. This is evident in the observation that many oncogenes function as genetic switches in the development of diverse systems such as *Drosophila melanogaster* (fruit fly).

As is the case for all oncogenes, their non-oncogenic counterparts, the proto-oncogenes, act as switches for normal cellular functions. In the fruit fly, body segmentation during embryogenesis is controlled by the regulated expression of a series of related genes called homeobox (HOM) genes. Abnormalities in one such molecular "switch" are found in the homeotic mutation called antennapedia, which induces a condition in which legs develop where antennae are normally found. The human homologues are called HOX genes, and 22 of the 39 human HOX genes are expressed in different subpopulations of hematopoietic progenitor cells, functioning as signals for hematopoietic differentiation. As might be predicted, abnormalities in some of these HOX genes are associated with human leukemias: for example, the HOXA9-NUP98 fusion

transcript is generated in the t(7;11) translocation, and the HOX11 gene is activated in the t(10q;14q) translocation. Intriguingly, the genes that interact or control HOM expression in *Drosophila* are also specifically and frequently implicated in human leukemia. The translocated genes involved in t(8;21)(q22;q22) of AML-M2 include AML1, which is related to the *Drosophila* pair rule gene, *runt,* which acts temporally and spatially to regulate the expression of specific patterns of the HOM genes. The normal AML1 binds to a protein partner called CBFβ to exert its physiologic function. Remarkably, CBFβ is also involved in leukemias with eosinophilia harboring the inv(16) translocation that generates the fusion protein CBFβ-MYHII. Similarly, rearrangements involving the t(4q21; 11q23) translocation observed in both AML and ALL create fusion oncogenes mutating the ALL1/MLL gene (residing on 11q23). ALL1/MLL is homologous to another *Drosophila* gene, *trithorax,* that maintains the cell-type specific expression patterns of the HOM genes. Once expressed, HOM proteins interact with the extradenticle (exd) protein to exert its physiologic effects. In the related human situation, the mammalian counterpart to exd, PBX1, is rearranged to form the E2A-PBX1 fusion oncoprotein seen in pre–B-cell leukemias. Thus, at every node of signaling control, perturbations induce aberrations of differentiation and growth.

ONCOGENES AND CANCER TREATMENT

A goal of oncogene research has been the potential targeting of oncogenes as specific therapies for cancer. This goal is now in reach because of a better understanding of their biochemistry and the growing awareness that activating some oncogenes may render cancer cells more sensitive to chemotherapy. One of the most mature forms of antioncogene therapeutics is in the use of all-trans-retinoic acid in the treatment of APL (see Chapter 177). APL is characterized by the t(15;17) translocation that generates a fusion protein between PML and RARA. The PML-RARA fusion results in aberrant signaling leading to an arrest in differentiation that appears to be corrected by interaction with the retinoic acid ligand. All-trans-retinoic acid is an effective treatment for APL and, in conjunction with standard induction chemotherapy, results in a high rate of complete remission.

Because activation of ras appears to be involved in a wide variety of cancers, ras has become an attractive target for gene-directed therapeutics. The transforming activity of ras requires that the oncoprotein be bound to the cell membrane through fatty acid modification at a four amino acid motif: CAAX (representing the sequence: cysteine–aliphatic amino acid–aliphatic amino acid–any amino acid). Synthetic CAAX peptides effectively block ras transformation in vitro, but the excitement is in the fact that the growth of cancer cells not transformed by mutant ras can also be inhibited by these CAAX peptides. The requirement, however, is that the activated pathway uses ras as an intermediary. Therefore, cells transformed by membrane-bound tyrosine kinases such as src, HER-2, and the EGFR are predicted to be inhibited by anti-ras approaches. More direct inhibition of oncogenic tyrosine kinases (such as EGFR, JAK, PDGFR, and SRC) is also being developed using small molecules that disrupt the normal function of the enzymatic site.

Aside from being targets, oncogenes can function as markers of cancer behavior that help in defining optimal therapy. For example, the presence of either the t(8;21) or the inv(16) translocations in AMLs (resulting in abnormalities in the AML1 and the CBFβ transcription factors, respectively) portend for a good response to standard leukemic chemotherapy. The presence of 11q23 abnormalities with mutations in the ALL1 gene or of a bcr-abl rearrangement are markers of inherent resistance to standard treatment and may require transplantation. Recently, the stimulation of HER-2 and EGFR by antibodies against their respective extracellular domains has been found to augment sensitivity to alkylating agents, possibly by inhibiting DNA repair. In clinical trials, the adverse effects of HER-2 overexpression and amplification on the survival of women with node-positive breast cancer potentially can be reversed by dose-intensive adjuvant therapy. Thus, the presence of poor prognostic factors may not necessarily mean irreversibly unfavorable outcomes; instead, the profile of oncogene abnormalities in a particular tumor may be used to choose optimal therapy.

MOLECULAR ONCOLOGY AND PUBLIC HEALTH

In the past, oncogene sciences have centered on understanding molecular mechanisms and applications to clinical care. Recent advances have placed oncogenes more prominently in public health and, in the process, have moved the field into the realm of cancer prevention. This fusion of disciplines has been necessitated by the identification of a growing number of cancer susceptibility genes and by the finding that oncogene mutations in some cases may represent "signatures" of carcinogen exposure. Data emerging from molecular epidemiologic investigations have identified predictable mutations in the *p53* gene associated with aflatoxin exposure in hepatocellular carcinoma and with ultraviolet light exposure in skin cancers. Cancer susceptibility genes for colon cancer (*APC, MSH2, MLH1*), for breast cancer (*BRCA1* and *BRCA2*), for retinoblastoma (*Rb*), for the Li-Fraumeni syndrome (*p53*), for the von Hippel-Lindau syndrome (*VHL*), for the multiple endocrine neoplasia syndrome (*RET*), and for neurofibromatosis (*NF1*) have already been cloned and can be used for direct screening of cancer susceptibility (Table 191–1). The availability of these genetic tests raises some interesting and, simultaneously, troubling questions: Who should be tested, and how young? What are the environmental factors modifying the genetic risk? Do all mutations in the susceptibility gene give the same cancer phenotype? What kind of screening or surveillance is optimal? What is the best timing for surgical prophylaxis? Is surgical prophylaxis efficacious? What safeguards to privacy can we provide our patients?

An example of the complexities is seen in the emerging management of *BRCA1* and the *BRCA2* carriers. Mutations in these two genes account for many, but clearly not all, of the familial breast or breast and ovarian cancer syndromes. Once testing programs were initiated, difficult and sometimes troublesome questions emerged. First, in the absence of a functional assay, it was not clear what constituted a mutation that changed protein activity as compared with what constituted a simple polymorphism that has no functional impact. Unforeseen, often adverse, psychological effects were noted in patients who were tested regardless of the outcome of the genetic test; moreover, relationships within families can change once test results are disclosed. Even when firm linkages could be made between a truncation mutation and cancer susceptibility, the therapeutic options remain limited: mammography before the age of 40 has no proven benefit in reducing breast cancer mortality, there are no validated screening measures for ovarian cancer, and no definitive study has shown a reduction in mortality using prophylactic mastectomy or oophorectomy. As the genetic tests for carrier status become more available, concerns about confidentiality and insurability severely restrict their clinical application.

LESSONS LEARNED AND FUTURE CHALLENGES

Our understanding of cancer genes has dramatically altered the conceptual landscape of basic biology. The implications for clinical cancer care are just beginning to be understood but will undoubt-

edly be equally profound. The promise of oncogene research is for more precise and effective therapy and for more rational prevention measures. The challenge in the future, however, will be to extend this process to the public health arena.

Fearon ER: Human cancer syndromes: Clues to the origin and nature of cancer. Science 278:1043, 1997.

Levine AJ: p53, the cellular gatekeeper for growth and division. Cell 88:323, 1997.
These references provide a general background on oncogenes and their role in human cancers.

Look AT: Oncogenic transcription factors in the human acute leukemias. Science 278: 1059, 1997.

Gibbs JB, Oliff A, Kohl NE: Farnesyltransferase inhibitors: *Ras* research yields a potential cancer therapeutic. Cell 77:175, 1994.
These references address the issue of oncogenes and cancer treatment.

Reed JC: Bcl-2 family proteins: Strategies for overcoming chemoresistance in cancer. Adv Pharmacol 41:501, 1997.

Reed JC: Mechanism of apoptosis avoidance of cancer. Curr Opin Oncol 11:68, 1999.
Emphasizes the importance of natural apoptotic mechanisms.

192 TUMOR MARKERS
Dennis L. Cooper

Since the first report of the use of serum carcinoembryonic antigen (CEA) levels in colon cancer, an increasing number of serum tumor markers have been validated for the purpose of assessing prognosis and response to therapy. Tumor markers also may substantially precede other evidence of disease progression or recurrence. In the latter situations, the ultimate utility of serum tumor markers is often compromised by a lack of effective therapy. Nevertheless, some tumor markers now have proven clinical value for diagnosis and treatment (Table 192–1).

COLORECTAL CARCINOMA

SCREENING. Although an increase in the serum level of CEA was initially thought to be indicative of colorectal cancer, it is now appreciated that abnormal CEA levels are observed in a variety of adenocarcinomas (lung, breast, pancreas, and stomach) as well as medullary cancer of the thyroid and some squamous cell cancers of the head and neck. In addition, serum CEA is often not increased in early-stage colon cancer and may be modestly increased in smokers and in association with a variety of benign conditions, including bronchitis, diverticulitis, peptic ulcer disease, fibrocystic breast disease, and a number of liver disorders. In view of the lack of sensitivity (percentage of patients with disease who have abnormal test) or specificity (percentage of patients without disease who have normal test results) for colorectal cancer, CEA is not an effective screening test.

PROGNOSIS. Preoperative increases in CEA appear to provide prognostic information independent of Dukes' stage. Thus, in one large study, a preoperative CEA above 2.5 ng/mL was associated with 1.62-fold increased risk of recurrence in patients with disease that had not apparently penetrated through the bowel wall. The risk of recurrence increased to 3.25-fold if the CEA was greater than 10 ng/mL. In patients who developed recurrent disease, the time to recurrence was also shorter in patients with higher preoperative CEA levels. Nevertheless, from a practical point of view, a high preoperative CEA is, at present, of limited value because there are no data to suggest that a different or more intensive therapy will lead to a better outcome. However, if knowledge of an increased CEA will change the surgical approach or if the CEA level plays a role in decisions about adjuvant therapy, then its use is recommended.

MONITORING DISEASE RESPONSE. In patients undergoing therapy for metastatic colorectal cancer, a decline in CEA generally indicates a favorable response. In such patients, the CEA can be substituted for more costly imaging procedures. Conversely, a rising CEA suggests disease progression, although the latter should be

Table 191–1 ■ SOME GENES INVOLVED IN CANCER SUSCEPTIBILITY

DISORDER	GENE
Familial retinoblastoma	*Rb*
Li-Fraumeni syndrome	*p53*
Familial breast and ovarian cancer	*BRCA1*
Familial breast cancer	*BRCA2*
Cowden's disease	*PTEN*
Familial adenomatous polyposis	*APC*
Hereditary non-polyposis colorectal cancer (HNPCC)	*MSH2, MLH1, PMS1, PMS2*
von Hippel-Lindau syndrome	*VHL*
Familial papillary renal cell carcinoma	*MET*
Nevoid basal cell carcinoma	*PTCH*
Familial melanoma	*p16*
MEN1	*MEN1*
MEN2	*RET*
Neurofibromatosis	*NF1* and *NF2*
Ataxia-telangiectasia	*ATM*
Wilms' tumor	*WT-1*

Table 192-1 ■ USE OF SERUM TUMOR MARKERS FOR SCREENING, PROGNOSIS, MONITORING RESPONSE TO THERAPY, AND DETECTING RECURRENCE

TUMOR	MARKER(s)	UTILITY OF MARKERS			
		Screening	Prognosis	Monitoring	Recurrence
Colorectal	CEA	No	Yes	Yes	Yes
Ovary	CA-125	No	No	Yes	Yes
Testicle	hCG, AFP	No	In some studies	Yes	Yes
Prostate	PSA	Yes?	Yes	Yes	Yes
Breast	CA15-3, CEA	No	No	Yes	Yes
Non-Hodgkin's lymphoma	LDH	No	Yes	No	Yes
Myeloma	β_2-M	No	Yes	Yes	Yes
Hepatoma	AFP	Yes, in high-risk patient*	No	Yes	Yes

CEA = carcinoembryonic antigen; hCG = human chorionic gonadotropin; AFP = α-fetoprotein; PSA = prostate-specific antigen; LDH = lactate dehydrogenase; β_2-M = β_2-microglobulin.

*Screening studies have been useful in Asian patients with evidence of previous hepatitis infection. Controlled trials are lacking. In the United States and Europe, patients with cirrhosis are often followed with AFP and ultrasound without definitive data from clinical trials.

confirmed radiographically before changing to an alternative treatment. The CEA is most useful when serial tests are followed over several months. Because therapy may acutely cause an increase in CEA as a manifestation of tumor response, measurements should be obtained just before a course of therapy rather than soon after treatment.

A RISING CEA AND SURGICAL RE-EXPLORATION. A small percentage of patients with local-regional recurrence or single liver metastases can be cured with second resections. In fact, although "second-look" resections are now more commonly thought of in association with ovarian cancer, the procedure was first described in patients with colon cancer. Because an increase in the CEA may precede other evidence of recurrence by several months, monitoring the CEA every 3 to 6 months during the first 2 years after surgery has become "standard practice" in many centers. Unfortunately, the available evidence suggests that only a small percentage of patients are helped by this strategy. In a controversial retrospective study in which the CEA was measured at the investigators' discretion, curative second resections were no more common in the group that had an increase in the CEA than in a group of patients who were monitored but did not have an increase in the CEA or in a third group of patients who did not have CEA measurements performed. Moreover, an abnormal CEA level alone without other evidence of disease recurrence proved to be of limited value: no disease was found in 8 of 29 patients with an isolated abnormal CEA, and curative resections could be performed in just 4 of the other 21 patients, only 1 of whom remained alive and free of disease at the end of the study period. These data suggest that CEA testing is of limited value in the follow-up of patients with colorectal cancer.

OVARIAN CANCER

SCREENING. Analogous to the use of CEA in colon cancer, the serum CA 125 is neither sensitive nor specific for the diagnosis of ovarian cancer. CA 125 may be normal in up to 50% of patients with stage I (limited to one ovary) disease and may be increased in patients with other types of adenocarcinomas. In addition, abnormal CA 125 levels are not limited to patients with malignant disease; increased levels have been seen in patients with endometriosis, pelvic inflammatory disease, benign ovarian cysts, the first trimester of pregnancy, menstruation, and liver disease. Because of the limited specificity of CA 125 and the low prevalence of ovarian cancer, it is predicted that less than 5% of women with an abnormal CA 125 would be found to have ovarian cancer at exploratory laparotomy. Even if CA 125 screening is limited to women with pelvic tumors, the positive predictive value (the percentage of patients with an abnormal CA 125 who have ovarian cancer) depends on the age of the woman. Thus, because benign conditions associated with an increased CA 125 are more common in premenopausal women, only 15 to 36% of premenopausal women with a pelvic mass will be found to have ovarian cancer. On the other hand, in women older than age 50, 80 to 90% of women with a pelvic mass and an increased CA 125 will be found to have ovarian cancer. If

the CA 125 is greater than 65 U/mL, 93% of such patients will be found to have ovarian cancer. Patients in the latter category are most appropriately referred to a gynecologic oncologist who can perform a definitive procedure at the initial laparotomy.

Importantly, although a high CA 125 in a postmenopausal woman with a pelvic mass is highly suggestive of ovarian cancer, a normal CA 125 does not exclude ovarian cancer. In one study of women with pelvic masses and ovarian cancer, 18 to 28% did not have an abnormal CA 125.

MONITORING RESPONSE TO THERAPY. Monitoring the level of CA 125 has proved invaluable for observing patients with ovarian cancer. Particularly in patients with disease that has been optimally debulked surgically, the CA 125 level may be the most sensitive indicator of the response to treatment. In addition, monitoring of the CA 125 is less expensive than serial computed tomography. Studies have shown that a 50 to 75% reduction in the CA 125 level is consistent with a more than 50% shrinkage of tumor. Moreover, the rate of fall of CA 125 also provides prognostic information. In one study, if the CA 125 was less than 10 U/mL after three cycles of therapy, the median survival was 60 months; however, if it was greater than 100 U/mL, the median survival was 7 months.

Nevertheless, the CA 125 has limited sensitivity for the detection of microscopic disease. Thus, approximately two thirds or more of patients with advanced ovarian cancer and an abnormal CA 125 will respond to therapy, and in a substantial number of patients the CA 125 will return to normal. However, even in the latter group of patients, only about 50% of patients have a pathologic complete remission at the time of surgical re-exploration and approximately 50% of the patients with a pathologic complete remission will eventually relapse. These results suggest that a significant volume of disease is required to produce an abnormal CA 125, a finding that also can be inferred by the poor sensitivity of CA 125 in patients with early ovarian cancer.

Failure of CA 125 to return to normal after chemotherapy is indicative of drug-resistant disease, and an increase (>15%) in the CA 125 may be the first sign of disease progression or recurrence. However, as is the case with the use of other tumor markers, changes in treatment should not be considered on the basis of one measurement. Particularly given the increasing number of second-line treatments available for ovarian cancer and the better outlook for patients with low-volume disease, it seems likely that early detection of disease progression by CA 125 monitoring may be advantageous; however, this assumption has not yet been confirmed in clinical trials.

BREAST CANCER

SCREENING. At present there is no evidence that the most commonly used tumor markers, CA 15-3 or CEA, have any role in screening patients for breast cancer. They are not usually abnormal in early-stage disease, nor are they specific for breast cancer.

MONITORING RESPONSE TO THERAPY. As in the use of tumor markers for monitoring patients with colon and ovarian cancer, a rising level of CA 15-3 or CEA in patients with breast cancer is often the first sign of disease progression. Analogous to ovarian cancer, tumor markers play an even more important role in monitoring response to therapy in patients with disease that cannot be followed well by physical examination or with radiographic studies. For example, in patients with disease limited to bone, the bone scan may lag behind improvements in tumor marker levels by many months. Similarly, in patients with abdominal carcinomatosis, tumor marker measurements may substitute for more costly computed tomographies.

An important caveat to the use of tumor markers in patients on hormonal therapy is that some patients will have a "flare" (worsening clinical disease and increase in tumor markers) weeks to months after beginning hormonal therapy. Because these patients predictably go on to have excellent responses, such patients should not have therapy changed prematurely.

PROSTATE CANCER

SCREENING. In large cohorts of asymptomatic men, screening with prostate-specific antigen (PSA) consistently detects approximately a third more cancers than digital rectal examination. Nevertheless, because a variable number of cancers have been found by digital rectal examination alone, both tests are recommended by proponents of screening. However, the routine use of the PSA for the detection of organ-confined prostate carcinoma remains controversial. If a cutoff of 4.0 ng/mL is used to separate normal from abnormal, then 38 to 48% of patients with organ-confined cancer will be missed because they fall within the normal range. Conversely, a great number of patients who do not have prostate cancer will be subjected to biopsies, thus increasing the cost of health care without any benefit. Because the PSA normally increases with age, using an age-adjusted PSA rather than the usual cutoff of 4.0 ng/mL may increase the sensitivity (percentage of patients with cancer who have an abnormal test) of screening in younger patients and improve specificity (percentage of patients without cancer who have a normal value) in older patients. Thus, a PSA of 3.8 ng/mL is inappropriately high for a 52-year old and requires further investigation. Conversely, a PSA of 4.2 ng/mL is probably normal in a 72-year old and, in the absence of an abnormal digital rectal examination, should not result in more extensive evaluation. Unfortunately, there are important limitations of the age-adjusted PSA because the range may be slightly different in white, black, and Asian men. In addition, tolerating higher values in older men will decrease the sensitivity of PSA screening in the population at greatest risk for cancer.

Recently, it has been observed that there are different forms of circulating PSA and that PSA produced by prostate carcinoma tends to be bound by plasma proteins whereas PSA produced by normal cells is more likely to be free in plasma. Thus, a high normal (2.5–4.0 ng/mL) or marginally increased (4.0–10.0) PSA is of more concern if the percent free PSA is relatively low. Conversely, a high percent free PSA might be able to eliminate the need for blind biopsies in patients with marginally increased PSA values. For example, in one study, a percent free PSA of less than or equal to 19 detected 90% of organ-confined cancers when the PSA was between 3.0 and 4.0 ng/mL. Conversely, when the total PSA was between 4.0 and 10.0 ng/mL, using a slightly higher percent free PSA was able to maintain the sensitivity of prostate cancer detection to between 90 and 95% and, at the same time, decrease the number of biopsies by 13 to 31%. The use of free percent PSA is undergoing testing in larger cohorts.

DECISIONS REGARDING INITIAL THERAPY. Nearly 50% of prostate cancers resected with curative intent are not confined to the prostate at the time of surgery. Recently, based on preoperative data from a large cohort of patients, the PSA, Gleason grade, and clinical TNM stage have been combined to construct nomograms to indicate the chance of finding tumor extending outside the prostate gland (see Chapter 118). These data can theoretically be used to counsel patients before attempted definitive therapy with the anticipated result that fewer patients would opt for surgery in the face of a high chance of extra-organ tumor extension. Nevertheless, the most appropriate therapy for patients with early-stage prostate can-

cer by clinical criteria but with a high likelihood of extra-organ extension has not been defined.

ASSESSMENT OF THE ADEQUACY OF DEFINITIVE THERAPY. Because PSA is organ specific, patients with completely resected prostate cancer should have undetectable levels of PSA. Thus, patients with measurable levels of PSA 6 to 8 weeks after surgery generally have persistent disease. Similarly, the re-emergence of detectable PSA after surgery is indicative of recurrent prostate cancer. Although some investigators have suggested that pelvic radiation is indicated in patients with late (>1 year after surgery) detection of PSA, at present there are not enough data to support this practice. Nevertheless, given the increasing number of radical prostatectomies being done, the appropriate management of persistently detectable PSA levels or late increases in PSA are an important area of clinical research.

After potentially curative radiation, local or systemic spread of cancer is likely if the PSA does not drop below 1.0 ng/mL. However, similar to the situation after surgery, a consensus on appropriate salvage treatment has not been reached.

MONITORING THE RESPONSE OF HORMONAL ABLATION THERAPY. Androgen ablation therapy is the most effective treatment for patients with metastatic prostate cancer. Although it is now clear that androgen ablation can reduce PSA independent of any antitumor effect, PSA remains an excellent tumor marker in patients receiving androgen ablation treatment. This finding is particularly important because patients with metastatic prostate cancer generally do not have easily measurable disease. Several studies also show that the rate and depth of fall of PSA after androgen ablation correlate with the duration of response. It is rare for patients to have progression of disease in the absence of an increasing PSA.

TESTICULAR CANCER

SCREENING. Human chorionic gonadotropin (hCG) and α-fetoprotein (AFP) have no value in screening because they are detected in fewer than 20% of patients with stage I tumors.

DIAGNOSIS. Although 15% of seminomatous germ cell tumors are associated with an increased hCG, high levels of hCG are often associated with a non-seminomatous tumor component; an increased level of AFP is diagnostic of the presence of non-seminomatous tumor. The importance of this distinction is that non-seminomatous germ cell tumors (NSGCT) are treated with chemotherapy, whereas non-bulky seminomas confined to the abdomen are treated with radiation. In patients with midline tumors (pineal, mediastinal, and retroperitoneum regions), markedly elevated germ cell markers are diagnostic of a testicular or extragonadal germ cell tumor and do not require biopsy for diagnosis. However, low-level elevation of hCG may be seen in patients with lung, breast, gastrointestinal, and ovarian tumors and, as a result, is not diagnostic of a germ-cell tumor.

MONITORING RESPONSE TO THERAPY. Because either hCG or AFP is increased in 89% of patients with NSGCT, they are useful in monitoring response after chemotherapy or for detecting recurrence after the completion of treatment. Generally, during chemotherapy, the hCG should fall by at least 1 log after each treatment, and the AFP should fall by 50% approximately every 7 days. However, in view of the exquisite sensitivity of germ cell tumors to therapy, it is not unusual for patients to have a temporary rise in tumor markers early after chemotherapy, presumably owing to tumor cell necrosis, before a subsequent fall. If the tumor markers do not return to normal after chemotherapy, residual disease is almost invariably present. In patients with very high tumor markers at diagnosis, the tumor markers may not return to normal until 1 or 2 months after therapy is completed. However, nearly one third of patients with normal markers and residual masses will have residual disease. Thus, in patients with NSGCT with residual retroperitoneal or pulmonary masses and negative markers, surgical resection is advised.

HEPATOMA USING AFP

SCREENING. For a screening test to be effective, the disease in question must be relatively common, and efforts to detect early-stage disease must be focused in high-risk patients. Thus, screening with AFP and liver ultrasound have been relatively successful and cost-effective in Asian countries where hepatoma is common and high-risk patients can be identified by hepatitis B and C serology tests (see Chapter 150). In contrast, studies in Europe, where the prevalence of hepatoma is much lower and the majority of screened patients have cirrhosis unrelated to hepatitis infection, have not been particularly successful in detecting small and potentially resectable tumors. It has been suggested but not proved that more aggressive screening (AFP testing and ultrasonography every 3 to 6 months) as done in Japan will be more successful. Importantly, because of the lower prevalence of hepatoma and more expensive testing in the United States, it has been estimated that the cost of detecting one hepatoma is as high as $270,000 compared with $8,000 in Japan. Nevertheless, despite the absence of confirmatory data, many hepatologists perform surveillance testing with AFP and/or liver ultrasonography in all patients with end-stage liver disease. Increases in AFP are particularly difficult to interpret in patients with chronic hepatitis B; in one study, only 6 of 44 patients with increases in AFP had hepatocellular carcinoma.

MULTIPLE MYELOMA

PROGNOSIS. Multiple myeloma is a malignant lymphoproliferative disorder that is inevitably fatal in a period ranging from a few months to several years (see Chapter 181). Because of the extreme variability in the aggressiveness of disease even in patients who have the same clinical stage, it is helpful to identify patients with more aggressive disease who might benefit from experimental treatment, including bone marrow transplantation. Although a number of clinical and laboratory tests have been used to predict prognosis, at present the β_2-microglobulin (β_2-M) level is the most important (and generally available) prognostic factor in multiple myeloma. In a large cooperative group study, patients with a β_2-M level less than 6 μg/mL had a median survival of 36 months compared with a median survival of 23 months in patients with a β_2-M greater than 6 μg/mL. If serum albumin also was considered, patients could be divided into three prognostic groups. The median survival of younger patients (<60 years) with a serum albumin level greater than 3.0 and a β_2-M less than 6 μg/mL was projected at greater than 48 months, whereas older patients with both a low serum albumin level and a high β_2-M value had an average survival of just over 1 year.

MONITORING. After treatment, the β_2-M level generally parallels the decline in serum monoclonal protein, but persistently elevated levels of β_2-M may occasionally identify patients with brief responses. In patients with light chain disease or non-secretory myeloma, who do not have a measurable serum monoclonal protein, the β_2-M can be used to follow the response to treatment.

NON-HODGKIN'S LYMPHOMA

PROGNOSIS. In view of data showing that second- and third-generation chemotherapy regimens are generally no better than earlier regimens (see Chapter 179), current treatment studies in younger (<age 60) patients with aggressive non-Hodgkin's lymphoma (NHL) have focused on identifying patients with high-risk disease so they can be given myeloablative doses of chemotherapy as part of their initial treatment. One randomized study showed that this approach was superior to standard treatment. Therefore, in view of the potential morbidity, mortality, and expense of high-dose therapy, it has become increasingly important to identify patients who are unlikely to be cured with conventional chemotherapy. One of the most important prognostic factors is the serum lactate dehydrogenase level (LDH). High pretreatment serum LDH levels have been consistently shown to be an adverse risk factor, presumably because they reflect the growth rate and tumor burden. Patients with a high LDH and either advanced stage disease or a poor performance status have less than a 50% chance of durable remission with standard therapy.

MONITORING THE RESPONSE TO TREATMENT. In contrast to the value of the pre-treatment LDH, values obtained during therapy

may be difficult to interpret. In one study, the LDH increased as much as twofold to fourfold during therapy and remained elevated for up to 1 month after the conclusion of treatment. In addition, the LDH value may increase in patients treated with hematopoietic colony-stimulating factors, presumably due to increased progenitor cell turnover in the bone marrow.

TUMORS OF UNKNOWN ORIGIN

Five to 10 percent of patients who present with cancer have tumors with an unknown primary site (see Chapter 200). Although squamous cell histology limits the site of origin to the head and neck, lung, skin, or cervix, it is more common for patients to have adenocarcinoma or a poorly differentiated tumor. In view of the lack of specificity of tumor markers for a specific tissue and the lack of effective therapy for most adenocarcinomas, tumor markers are not generally helpful in predicting the site of origin for recommending therapy. One important exception is prostate cancer where a high serum PSA should result in an examination of the tumor tissue for expression of PSA. Levels of AFP and hCG may also be helpful in selected circumstances (see Chapter 118).

Clinical practice guidelines for the use of tumor markers in breast and colorectal cancer. J Clin Oncol 14:2843–2877, 1996. *Utility of CA 15-3 and CEA levels to document treatment failure in the absence of clinically-detectable disease.*

Collier J, Sherman M: Screening for hepatocellular carcinoma. Hepatology 27:273–278, 1998. *Levels of α-fetoprotein are useful but not diagnostic.*

Partin AW, Kattan MW, Subong ENP, et al: Combination of prostate-specific antigen, clinical stage, and Gleason score to predict pathological stage of localized prostate cancer. JAMA 277:1445, 1997. *A multifactorial approach to staging prostate cancer.*

193 THE EPIDEMIOLOGY OF CANCER
William J. Blot

DESCRIPTIVE PATTERNS

THE GEOGRAPHY OF CANCER. Cancer affects all the world's populations, with nearly a fourfold difference between areas with the highest and lowest age-adjusted rates for all cancers combined. For certain cancers, the difference exceeds 100-fold (Table 193–1). One of the most distinctive geographic patterns is seen for esophageal cancer, with pockets of exceptionally high mortality in areas of north central China, the Caspian littoral of Iran, and South Africa. In Linxian, China, for as yet unknown reasons, esophageal/gastric cardia cancer is the most common cause of death, causing over one third of all fatalities among adults. Clustering of elevated esophageal cancer rates also has been observed in parts of Europe and the United States, primarily due to heavy alcohol intake.

Geographic variation for other tumors is also noteworthy. Rates of oral cancer are highest in India and parts of south central Asia. Within the United States, elevated oral cancer mortality among females is found in the southern states, especially in rural areas. In both instances, the cause is the same, namely, high use of smokeless tobacco. In southeastern China, nasopharyngeal cancer is the most common malignancy; it is also a leading cancer among Alaskan Aleuts and Eskimos and occurs more frequently among Chinese than white or black Americans. The primary cause of nasopharyngeal cancer in southern China appears to be consumption of salted fish, especially during weaning and early childhood. The importance of early life events is also suggested by the up to threefold higher rates of nasopharyngeal cancer among Chinese-Americans born and raised in China than among those born and raised in the United States. Similar migrant effects are seen for stomach cancer: Japanese-Americans born in Japan, where rates of stomach cancer are among the highest in the world, have a twofold to threefold higher incidence of this cancer than Japanese-Americans born in the United States, who still have more than double the incidence of stomach cancer of white Americans. Such differences in rates imply the influence of environmental factors.

Table 193-1 ■ INTERNATIONAL VARIATION IN AGE-ADJUSTED INCIDENCE RATES FOR SELECTED CANCERS

CANCER SITE	HIGH-RATE AREAS*	RATE†	BASELINE RATE‡
Oral cavity	France, India	35–45	1–2
Nasopharynx	China, Hong Kong	30	<1
Esophagus	China, Iran	100+	1–2
Stomach	Japan	80–90	5
Colon/rectum	U.S. Japan, New Zealand	50–60	6
Liver	China, Japan, Thailand	40–90	1
Pancreas	U.S. blacks	15	1
Larynx	Brazil, Italy, Spain	15–20	2
Lung	U.S. blacks, New Zealand Maori	110–120	6
Skin melanoma	Australia	30	<1
Breast	U.S.	100	20
Uterine cervix	Brazil, Paraguay, Peru, Colombia, India	40–50	4
Ovary	Norway, Iceland, Switzerland	15	4
Prostate	U.S. blacks	120+	2
Bladder	U.S. whites, Italy, Spain	25–35	2
Thyroid	Pacific Islands	25	<1
Non-Hodgkin's lymphoma	Switzerland, U.S., Canada	10–15	1
Hodgkin's disease	Ireland, Italy	4	<1
Multiple myeloma	U.S. blacks	10	<1
Leukemia	Canada	12	2–3

*Country in which high-rate areas occur is listed. The high rates do not necessarily persist throughout the country.

†Approximate age-adjusted (world standard) incidence rate per year 100,000 population among males (except for breast, cervix, and ovarian cancers). Data collection periods vary by area but typically center around the mid-1980s.

‡Approximate age-adjusted incidence rate in typical low-rate areas.

The most common cancers in Western countries, those of the lung, large bowel, and breast, also vary geographically. Within the United States, the highest rates of lung cancer are now found in southern rural counties, where lung cancer mortality in the 1980s surpassed that in northern cities, reversing a long-standing pattern. These shifts follow changes in cigarette smoking, now more prevalent in the South than elsewhere in the United States. In addition, certain southern port and coastal areas have had excess lung cancer rates among males as a legacy of occupational exposures to asbestos in shipyards during World War II, when shipbuilding was the largest manufacturing industry in the United States. In contrast, for colon and breast cancer, higher rates occur in the Northeast and lower rates in the South, but the differentials are not large.

U.S. CANCER RATES AND TRENDS. It is estimated that in 1998 about 1.25 million Americans will develop and nearly 600,000 will die of cancer (Fig. 190–1). Cancer, excluding basal and squamous cell skin cancers, is newly diagnosed annually in about 500 of every 100,000 males and 350 of every 100,000 females. The leading cancers among men are those of the prostate, lung, and colon/rectum, whereas among women the top three are breast, colon/rectum, and lung. If mortality rather than incidence data are considered, the order shifts. Among males, lung cancer is by far the leading age-adjusted cause of cancer death (73.2 deaths per year per 100,000), followed by prostate (26.5 per 100,000) and colon/rectum (22.4 per 100,000) cancer. Among females, age-adjusted death rates of lung cancer (32.8 per 100,000) now exceed rates for breast (26.4 per 100,000) and colon/rectum (16.3 per 100,000) cancer.

For nearly all cancers, the incidence rates are higher among men than women, the exceptions being gallbladder and thyroid cancers. For some cancers, explanations for the male excess are evident (e.g., higher tobacco and alcohol intake account for most of the higher rates of oral, esophageal, laryngeal, and lung cancer among males), but for others (e.g., stomach cancer, leukemia) the reasons are enigmatic.

Rates of most cancers, particularly those deriving from epithelial tissue, rise steadily with advancing age, often exponentially. Some cancers show a bimodal age distribution. Leukemia and nervous system tumors display an early childhood (age <5 years) peak, then rates decline before rising again in late middle age. Testis cancer occurs primarily between the ages of 20 and 40, whereas Hodgkin's disease incidence is highest at ages 20 to 30, declines somewhat, then rises again after age 50.

Racial differences in cancer occurrence are sometimes marked. Total cancer incidence during 1990 to 1994 was higher among black than white males by 26%, whereas rates were higher among white than black females by 3%. The black/white differences among males were particularly pronounced for esophageal, stomach, pancreas, and lung cancer and for multiple myeloma, with age-adjusted incidence from 50% to 160% higher among blacks than whites.

Mortality rates of several cancers have changed over the past decades (Fig. 193–1). Most notable has been the rise in lung cancer. Lung tumors were rarely diagnosed before the early 1900s, but incidence and mortality began a steady rise in the 1920s that has continued until recently. The epidemic increase in lung cancer, almost entirely attributable to cigarette smoking, has now ended among males. Whereas rates among males peaked in the late 1980s and are now declining, the leveling off and subsequent decrease in lung cancer rates among females will not take place until after the year 2000. Rates of stomach and cervical cancers, the leading tumors early in this century, have declined, the former for reasons not yet fully understood, the latter, at least in part, due to cytologic screening for cervical pathology. The decreases in these tumors are beginning to end, however, and rates of gastric cardia cancer are now rising.

Although not shown in Figure 193–1, there has been nearly a doubling in incidence of melanoma and a 50% rise in non-Hodgkin's lymphomas among whites since the early 1970s. In addition, among blacks the excess in lung, oral, laryngeal, and esophageal cancer has been increasing. For esophageal cancer, however, striking differences exist by cell type: rates of adenocarcinomas of the esophagus have been rising, especially among whites, and account for most esophageal cancers among white men, whereas squamous cell carcinomas of the esophagus predominate among black men. Reasons for the growing racial disparity are not entirely evident, although higher prevalences of cigarette smoking, heavy alcohol consumption, and nutritional disadvantages are suspected.

In the United States, a sharp rise in the incidence of prostate cancer occurred in the late 1980s, owing mainly to the increased detection of early tumors because of expanded screening with prostate-specific antigen testing. The result was a far higher incidence for prostate cancer than for any other malignancy (Fig. 190–1). The rise abated by the mid-1990s, most likely because the cancers that ordinarily would have been detected then had already been diagnosed by the earlier screening.

THE CAUSES OF CANCER

Cancer is believed to be largely preventable. The causes of most cancers of the oral cavity and pharynx, esophagus, liver, larynx,

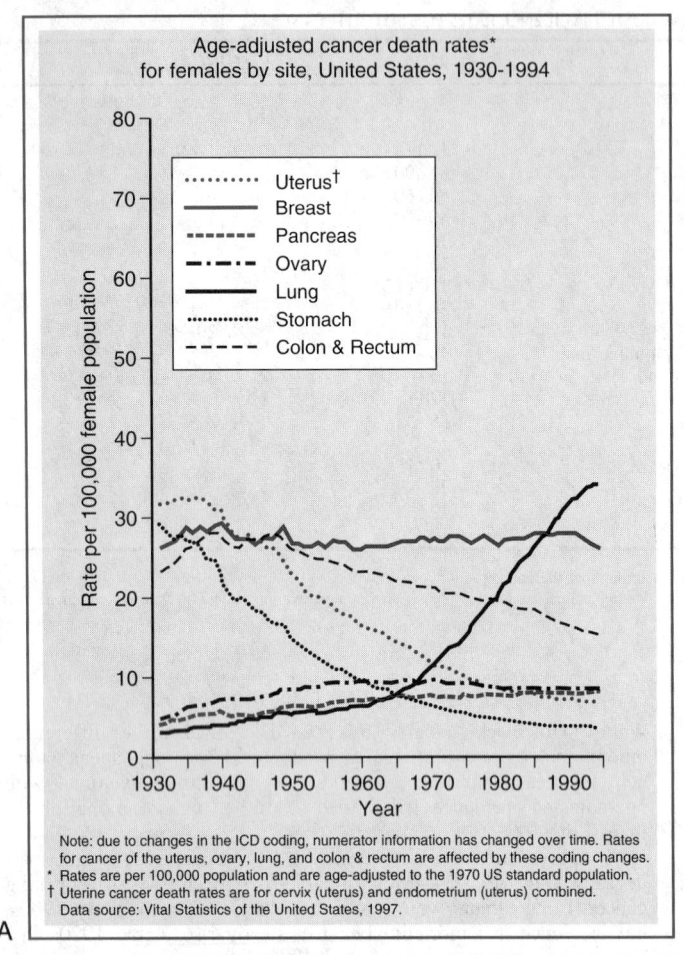

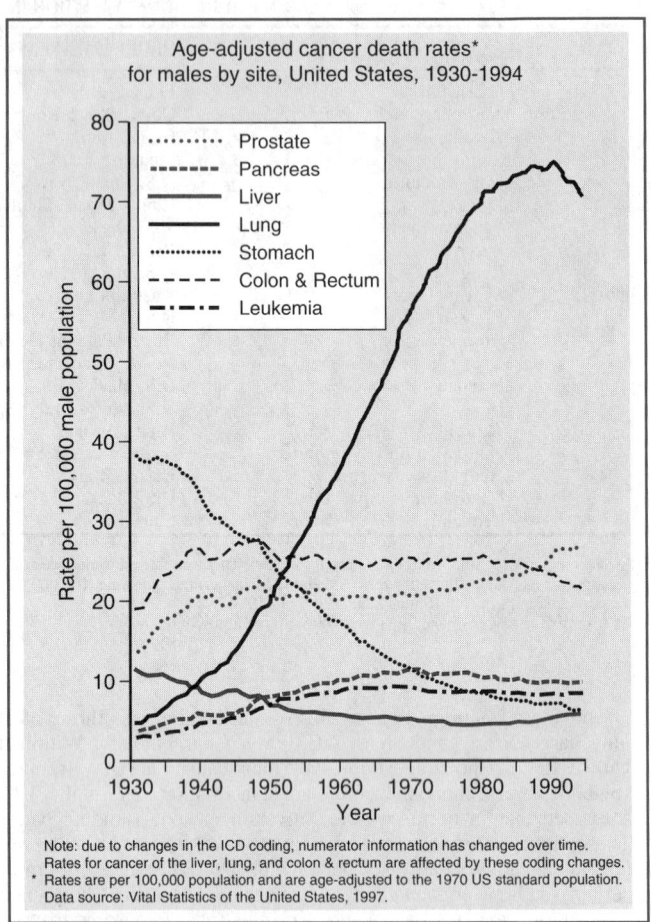

FIGURE 193-1 ■ *A* and *B,* Trends during 1930–1994 in age-adjusted mortality rates for selected cancers in the United States. (Adapted from Landis SH, et al: Cancer statistics, 1998. CA Cancer J Clin 48:6, 1998.)

lung, and uterine cervix are now known. Risk factors also have been identified for other cancers, but the search continues to clarify the factors that account for the bulk of malignancies in the United States and around the world. Most current information on risk factors for cancer has come from case-control studies assessing various characteristics and exposures of patients with individual cancers and from cohort studies determining rates of cancer among groups exposed to particular agents suspected of carcinogenic potential. The leads for these epidemiologic investigations often have arisen from descriptive studies of cancer rates and statistics and from alert clinical observations.

The striking variation in cancer rates within and between countries, the differing rates among migrants from one place to another, and the often marked trends over time suggest that environmental factors (using the term *environmental factors* in its broadest sense to encompass all exogenous, non-genetic exposures) induce most cancers, perhaps through interaction with host susceptibility traits.

TOBACCO (SEE CHAPTERS 13 AND 190). Cigarette smoking is the dominant cause of the leading cancer (i.e., lung cancer) in the United States and many other Western nations. The association was first suspected by clinical observations that new lung cancer patients were often smokers and then confirmed in the 1950s by case-control and cohort studies in the United States and Great Britain. In the years since the first U.S. Surgeon General's report on smoking in 1964, additional evidence has documented that risks of lung cancer rise in proportion to both duration of smoking and amount smoked per day, with risks of lung cancer more than 20 times greater among long-term heavy smokers than among non-smokers. Lifelong filter smokers have experienced a somewhat lesser risk than lifelong non-filter smokers, but the greatest protection comes from smoking cessation. Risks 10 years after quitting are typically only one third or less those of continuing cigarette smokers. Smoking affects all major types of lung cancer, but squamous and small

cell carcinomas more so than adenocarcinomas. Cigarette smoking also is a principal cause of cancers of the oral cavity and pharynx, esophagus, larynx, and renal pelvis; is a major contributor to cancers of the pancreas, bladder, and kidney; and is implicated to a moderate degree in cancers of the stomach and uterine cervix. Smokeless tobacco is the predominant cause of buccal mucosa cancers in some populations. In total, tobacco use is thought to account for nearly one third of all cancers in the United States and thus is the largest single preventable cause of cancer.

Although the effects of smoking are far greater for smokers themselves, the consensus of evidence from over 30 worldwide epidemiologic studies since the early 1980s indicates that long-term exposure to environmental tobacco smoke also increases the risk of lung cancer among non-smokers. The excess risk of lung cancer among non-smoking women married to smokers has averaged about 30%. Because of tobacco's harmful effects, efforts to induce smokers to quit and to encourage non-smokers, particularly adolescents, not to start smoking must be continued. Smoking prevalence among adult men in the United States has declined from a peak of nearly 60% in the 1950s to nearly 25% today. Further reductions are attainable and critical to the nation's public health.

ALCOHOL (SEE CHAPTERS 16 AND 190). Alcohol combines with tobacco to cause cancers of the oral cavity and pharynx, esophagus, and larynx. Alcoholic beverages also have been implicated in the etiology of liver, rectal, and breast cancers, although the latter associations may not be conclusive. A large case-control study involving more than 1100 oral and pharyngeal cancer patients in the United States found that cancer risk increased progressively with increasing intake of alcoholic beverages among non-smokers as well as smokers. Smoking and drinking multiplied each other's effects so that the risk of oral cancer was increased over 35-fold among two-pack-a-day smokers who consumed more than four alcoholic drinks per day compared with abstainers of both products.

Similar tobacco-alcohol interactions have been observed for esophageal and laryngeal cancer. Although not carcinogenic in animal models, ethanol seems likely to be the etiologic agent in humans, because all types of alcoholic beverages (beer, wine, dark and light spirits) have been linked with increased risk in epidemiologic studies.

OCCUPATIONAL HAZARDS. Occupational exposures have long been recognized as causes of cancer, beginning with the observation in the 1700s of scrotal cancer among chimney sweeps in London. Today, at least 20 substances in the workplace have been associated with increased cancer risk (Table 193–2). About one half have been implicated in lung cancer, occasionally in an interactive manner with cigarette smoking. Asbestos exposure has accounted for the largest number of occupational cancers, although its impact is diminishing because of curtailments in asbestos exposure instituted more than 2 decades ago. Increased rates of lung cancer and mesothelioma have been found among asbestos miners and millers; factory workers handling asbestos, textile, and other products; shipyard, railroad, and construction workers; and employees working in other industries that manufacture or use this material. Rates of lung cancer and mesothelioma vary, however, according to intensity and type of asbestos exposure, with the majority of asbestos-related tumors due to high levels of exposure to amphibole fibers.

Radon and its daughter products (see Chapters 19 and 190), another group of potent carcinogens, exist in high levels in underground mines throughout much of the world. Over 20-fold increases of lung cancer have been reported in some groups of radon-exposed miners, most of whom are also smokers, with the excesses most pronounced for small cell anaplastic carcinomas. Several chemicals, including inorganic arsenic, benzene, β-naphthylamine and other aromatic amines, bischloromethylether, mustard gas, certain nickel compounds, and polycyclic hydrocarbons also have induced cancer in exposed workers. All except arsenic are carcinogenic also in animals, with the carcinogen often (but not always) inducing similar tumors in the animals as in humans. Some reviews have included beryllium and cadmium compounds, as well as 2,3,7,8-tetrachlorodibenzo-para-dioxin, on the list of known occupational carcinogens, but the epidemiologic evidence for these agents is still equivocal.

Among all cancers, those of the urinary bladder and nasal cavity and sinuses have the highest proportion related to occupational exposures. It has been estimated that among American men, up to 25% of all bladder cancers are occupationally related. In a Swedish nationwide survey of all nasal adenocarcinomas over a recent 19-year period, nearly 25% occurred among furniture makers, possibly as a result of wood dust exposures. Wood dust exposures, however, have not been related to as exceptionally high a risk of nasal cancer in North America as they have in Europe. The percentages of other tumors due to occupational exposures are lower, and for all cancers combined it is generally thought that fewer than 5% have been induced by workplace exposures.

ENVIRONMENTAL POLLUTION. Carcinogens have in some instances been identified in the air we breathe and the water we drink. Quantifying the effects of air and water pollution has been extremely difficult, however, because of uncertainty over the amount and characteristics of exposures actually received by individuals. Before the discovery of the carcinogenic effects of cigarette smoking, air pollution, primarily from combustion products, was thought to be involved in the rise in lung cancer in the United States and other countries. It is now believed that the degree of air pollution found in most urban areas contributes to less than 10% of cases of this cancer. The percentage rises in some areas of the world, including parts of China, where excessive rates of lung cancer affect non-smokers living in chimneyless houses and in homes heavily polluted by coal-burning heating systems. Increased risks of lung cancer also have been found among residents living near copper smelters suspected of emitting inorganic arsenic into the air. Mesotheliomas have been diagnosed among women married to asbestos workers, presumably from handling clothing or otherwise being exposed to fibers brought home by their husbands. Concern has arisen over possible health risks from much lower levels of asbestos exposure that may occur in homes, schools, and other public places, but few such environmentally induced cancer cases seem likely. Pollutants in drinking water also have aroused concern. Rates of bladder cancer have correlated with levels of halogenated compounds in municipal water supplies; some of these agents have shown carcinogenicity in animal studies. Laboratory tests also indicate an increased risk of osteogenic sarcomas after high levels of exposure to fluoride in exposed animals, but epidemiologic investigations have found few or no unexpected changes in cancer rates after fluoridation of water supplies.

MEDICINAL AGENTS. Among chemicals considered to be causally associated with cancer in humans, nearly one half are medications (Table 193–3), including drugs used in cancer treatment. The occurrence of second primary cancers in 5 to 10% or more of patients who have received chemotherapy suggests that risks as well as benefits of such agents must be carefully assessed, particularly for patients whose long-term prognosis is otherwise highly favorable. Exogenous estrogens have been implicated in cancer risk. Diethylstilbestrol taken during pregnancy has resulted in vaginal adenocarcinomas in offspring exposed in utero. Conjugated estrogens given to menopausal women in the 1970s induced a rising rate of endometrial cancer, and rates dropped abruptly when the drug was discontinued. The link to breast cancer is less clear, although aggregate data suggest an increased risk among women receiving long-term postmenopausal estrogen replacement therapy. Extended use of oral contraceptives before a first pregnancy also has been reported to increase subsequent risk of breast cancer, but the widespread introduction of oral contraceptives in the 1960s has not significantly influenced national rates of breast cancer in the United States. Combined (estrogen plus progestogen) oral contraceptives have been associated with a reduced risk of endometrial and ovarian cancer.

Immunosuppressive agents sharply increase the risk of cancer; for example, renal transplant recipients have over a 30-fold in-

Table 193–2 ▪ **OCCUPATIONAL EXPOSURES RECOGNIZED AS HUMAN CARCINOGENS**

EXPOSURE	SITE OF CANCER
4-Aminobiphenyl	Bladder
Arsenic	Lung, skin
Asbestos	Lung, pleura, peritoneum
Benzene	Leukemia
Benzidine	Bladder
β-Naphthylamine	Bladder
Bischloromethylether	Lung
Chromium (hexavalent) compounds	Lung
Coal tars and pitches	Lung, skin
Mineral oils	Skin
Mustard gas	Pharynx, lung
Nickel compounds	Lung, nasal sinuses
Radon	Lung
Soot, tars, and oils (polycyclic hydrocarbons)	Lung, skin
Strong inorganic acid mists containing sulfuric acid	Lung
Talc containing asbestiform fibers	Lung
Vinyl chloride	Liver
Wood dusts (furniture)	Nasal sinuses

Table 193-3 ■ MEDICINAL AGENTS RECOGNIZED AS HUMAN CARCINOGENS

DRUG	SITE OF CANCER
Azathioprine	Lymphoma, skin, soft tissue sarcoma
Chlornaphazine	Bladder
Cyclosporine	Lymphoma
1,4-Butanediol dimethanesulfonate (Myleran)	Leukemia
Combined chemotherapy for lymphoma, including MOPP*	Leukemia
Chlorambucil	Leukemia
Cyclophosphamide	Leukemia, bladder
Estrogens—conjugated	Endometrium
Estrogens—synthetic (diethylstilbestrol)	Vagina, cervix
Estrogens—steroid contraceptives	Benign liver tumors
Melphalan	Leukemia
Methoxsalen with ultraviolet A therapy (PUVA)	Skin
Phenacetin-containing analgesics	Renal pelvis
Tamoxifen	Uterus
Thiotepa	Leukemia
Treosulfan	Leukemia

*MOPP = nitrogen mustard, vincristine, procarbazine (Oncovin) and prednisone.

creased risk of subsequent lymphomas. The excess risk begins within months of starting immunosuppressive therapy, the fastest onset of any environmentally induced cancer.

RADIATION (SEE CHAPTER 19). Follow-up of survivors of the atomic bombs of Hiroshima and Nagasaki and of groups of patients receiving radiation therapy for ankylosing spondylitis, cancer, and certain other conditions demonstrates that ionizing radiation can induce cancer in humans as it does in lower animals. Leukemia is the initial carcinogenic consequence, occurring most frequently 5 to 10 years after exposure, with increased risks of a variety of solid tumors, particularly breast, thyroid, and lung cancers, following thereafter. Significantly increased risks of breast cancer have been detected among atomic bomb survivors at doses somewhat below 0.5 Gy, and head and neck tumors have followed less than 0.1 Gy of scalp irradiation for tinea capitis in Israeli children. The findings suggest the need for prudence in the use of medical irradiation. Improvements in radiologic equipment, however, have resulted in lower radiation doses. Thus, for example, risks associated with mammography are now believed to be low enough to justify routine periodic screening for breast cancer among U.S. women aged 50 and older, and the American Cancer Society recommends beginning at age 40.

Ultraviolet radiation from sun exposure is the dominant cause of basal and squamous cell carcinoma and melanoma of the skin. The key to prevention is reduced solar exposure, even though there is uncertainty regarding variations in effect according to extent and timing of exposure. For melanoma, intermittent heavy sun exposures, particularly during childhood and adolescence, may carry the greatest risk.

DIET AND NUTRITION (SEE CHAPTERS 11 AND 190). Strong evidence indicates that diet and nutrition can influence cancer risk. Clearest are the inverse associations between risk of certain epithelial cancers, particularly oral, esophageal, stomach, and lung cancers, and intake of fresh fruits and vegetables. Risk of these cancers among persons in the highest quartile of consumption is lower, sometimes by more than one half, than among those in the lowest quartile of intake. The ingredients responsible for the protective effects in humans remain to be clarified. Epidemiologic studies have shown that carotenoids, but not animal sources of vitamin A (retinols), link fairly consistently to reduced cancer risk, but vitamins C and E, which can inhibit the formation of carcinogenic N-nitroso compounds in vivo, folate, and other possibly protective nutrients also have been identified. In a randomized clinical trial in an area of China characterized by chronic nutrient deficiencies, daily supplementation with a combination of β-carotene, vitamin E, and selenium reduced cancer mortality. Selenium supplementation also was associated with reduced risk of several cancers in a smaller randomized trial in the United States. No similar benefit, however, was observed in trials of cigarette smokers in Finland taking supplements of β-carotene or vitamin E, of American physicians taking β-carotene, or of American smokers and asbestos workers taking β-carotene plus retinol. Indeed, the Finnish and American smokers trials showed small but significant increases in

lung cancer among those supplemented with β-carotene. This unexpected result cautions against supplementation with high levels of β-carotene among smokers and indicates that the link between diet and cancer is more complex than originally believed.

Recent studies in China and Italy suggest that garlic, onions, and other allium vegetables may reduce the risk of stomach cancer. Compounds in allium vegetables exhibit strong anticancer effects in experimental animals. Animal studies also show protection against cancer by polyphenols and other compounds in tea and certain other foods. Several epidemiologic studies have shown lower risk of some cancers in tea drinkers, but the evidence is mixed. Some food products may also contain substances that may increase cancer risk; for example, some food contaminants, including aflatoxins sometimes found in moldy peanuts or grains, are strong animal carcinogens. Rates of liver cancer tend to be high in parts of Asia and Africa where aflatoxin contamination is common, but information on the effect of these substances in humans is scanty.

Dietary fat, particularly saturated fat, and calories have been implicated in the risk of colon and other cancers, although the etiologic nature of the associations is still not well established. The relationship between dietary fiber and the risk of colon cancer is unclear. Despite these uncertainties, it has been estimated that a high percentage of colorectal cancers have a dietary etiology. Diet and breast cancer have been linked, in part because of the much higher rates of these cancers in Western nations with high-fat, low-fiber diets, but the evidence is inconsistent. In total, some estimates suggest that one third or more of all cancers may be related to dietary and nutritional practices.

INFECTIOUS AGENTS. Several viral agents have been associated with human cancer, particularly cancers of the liver in endemic areas and of the uterine cervix worldwide. Hepatitis B virus (HBV) is the primary cause of hepatocellular carcinoma in China and other areas where infections are prevalent. Prospective follow-up studies show large increases in risk, with nearly all liver cancers arising among persons with prediagnosis HBV surface antigen positivity. The epidemiologic patterns of cervical cancer (with risks elevated among those with multiple sexual partners and/or early age at coitus) have long suggested a venereal component to etiology. Only recently have laboratory techniques enabled detection of human papillomavirus (HPV) as a likely etiologic agent in a high percentage of cases. Herpes simplex virus type 2 has been associated with cervical cancer, but its independent or interactive role with HPV remains to be clarified. The Epstein-Barr virus has been implicated in both nasopharyngeal cancer and Burkitt's lymphoma, whereas certain human retroviruses have been associated with adult T-cell leukemias in Japan and the Caribbean. The human immunodeficiency virus, the cause of AIDS, is associated not only with Kaposi's sarcomas but also with clearly increased risk of lymphoma among survivors of AIDS. Infection with Schistosoma haematobium has been implicated in increased risk of bladder cancer in parts of Africa, and infection with the liver fluke (Opisthorchis viverrini) has been linked to liver cancers, predominantly cholangiosarcomas, in Thailand. Recently, sufficient data have accumulated to declare that infection with *Helicobacter pylori* increases risk of gastric cancer, including gastric lymphomas. *Helicobacter pylori* thus becomes the first bacterial agent to be recognized as a cause of human cancer.

GENETIC SUSCEPTIBILITY. A history of cancer in the family often increases cancer risk. The increases for common cancers such as those of the lung, colon, and breast are typically on the order of twofold to threefold. Shared environmental factors may contribute to the familial clustering, but strong associations among subgroups with early age at onset of cancer or bilateral presentation of breast cancer indicate a genetic predisposition. The most marked genetic effects are seen for skin cancer, with tumors rarely appearing in persons inheriting darkly pigmented skin. A few cancers show mendelian inheritance patterns, including retinoblastomas and melanomas arising from familial dysplastic nevi. In addition, certain hereditary precancerous syndromes have been linked to increased cancer risk: neurofibromatosis and other phacomatoses (associated with nervous system cancer), xeroderma pigmentosum and albinism (skin cancer), ataxia-telangiectasia and certain other immunodeficiency syndromes (lymphoma, leukemia, and other cancers), Bloom's syndrome (lymphoma, leukemia, and other cancers), and Fanconi's anemia (leukemia).

Investigations of families with unusually large numbers of members with the same or different cancers have provided insight into genetic patterns. In larger epidemiologic studies, increasing attention is being paid to systematic evaluations of genetic factors as reliable markers of host susceptibility become available. The search for indicators of individual susceptibility to specific carcinogenic exposures has intensified in hopes of identifying persons at high risk of cancer who could then be counseled to avoid exposure and be examined for early detection of cancer. The process of establishing relevant markers is complex, and promising leads sometimes fail to materialize. Nevertheless, the rapid expansion of research on susceptibility factors should prove highly fruitful in understanding the mechanisms of carcinogenesis as well as delineating groups and individuals at high risk for targeted interventions.

International Agency for Research on Cancer: Overall Evaluations of Carcinogenicity: An updating of IARC Monographs Volumes 1 to 42. Monographs on the Evaluation of Carcinogenic Risks to Humans. Supplement 7. Lyon, World Health Organization, 1987; and Volumes 43 to 69, 1987 to 1998. *A systematic review of epidemiologic and experimental evidence regarding carcinogenicity of over 150 substances.*

Landis SH, Murray T, Bolden S, Wingo PA: Cancer statistics, 1999. CA Cancer J Clin 49:8 1999. *The most recent compilation of cancer frequency, incidence, mortality, and survival data for the United States.*

Ries LA, Kosary CL, Hankey BF, et al (eds): Cancer Statistics Review 1973–1994. Bethesda, MD, US Department of Health and Human Services, NIH publication No. 97-2789, 1997. *Cancer incidence, mortality, and survival rates in the United States.*

Schottenfeld D, Fraumeni JF Jr (eds): Cancer Epidemiology and Prevention, 2nd ed. Oxford, Oxford University Press, 1996. *A comprehensive review of cancer epidemiology, with individual chapters assessing cancers and causative agents, as well as basic concepts in cancer etiology and control.*

194 ENDOCRINE MANIFESTATIONS OF TUMORS: "ECTOPIC" HORMONE PRODUCTION

Robert F. Gagel

It is now commonly accepted that genetic abnormalities cause disordered cell growth that leads to the transformation of the phenotype. A corollary of this fundamental tenet is that changes in a handful of important cellular genes can result in altered expression of other genes, leading to the production of cellular proteins not normally expressed in the differentiated cell type. Among the more interesting and clinically relevant types of abnormal protein are those associated with "ectopic" hormone syndromes, a small but clinically important group of disorders.

There are several patterns of "ectopic" hormone production. The most common is the production of small polypeptide hormones by tumors derived from a specific class of neuroendocrine cells. These neuroendocrine cells are widely dispersed throughout the lung, gastrointestinal tract, pancreas, thyroid gland, adrenal medulla, breast, prostate, and skin; they share several common cytologic and biochemical characteristics (amine precursor uptake and decarboxylation [APUD]), are derived from the neural crest, and normally produce both biogenic amines and small polypeptide hormones. The list of hormones produced by tumors derived from members of this group of neuroendocrine cells includes corticotropin (ACTH), calcitonin (CT), vasoactive intestinal peptide (VIP), growth hormone–releasing hormone (GHRH), corticotropin-releasing hormone (CRH), somatostatin (SRIH), and other small peptides. A second group of tumors, generally derived from squamous epithelium, produce parathyroid hormone–related protein (PTHrp) and vasopressin.

Current evidence suggests aberrant hormone production is due to reversion to an earlier state of differentiation and an earlier developmental pattern of transcription factor expression. Expression of human acheate-scute homologue (hASH), a helix-loop-helix transcription factor, is necessary for differentiation of pulmonary neuroendocrine cells, the cell type involved in small cell carcinoma of the lung (SCCL). This factor is not expressed normally in the differentiated cell type, but it is expressed at high levels in SCCL. Recent studies have shown that a negative regulator of hASH, hairy enhancer of split-1 (HES-1), is expressed at low levels in SCCL and that overexpression of this gene in SCCL and other neuroendocrine carcinoma cell lines returns the cell to a more differentiated phenotype. These results suggest that a perturbation in a normal differentiation factor is involved not only in the development of the transformed phenotype, but also in the aberrant expression of several small polypeptide hormones.

In a second common hormonal syndrome, hypercalcemia caused by ectopic production of PTHrp, activation of the *ras*-MAP kinase signaling pathway, through mutation, appears to be responsible for PTHrp production by squamous epithelium. For example, normal fibroblasts can be stimulated to overexpress PTHrp by combined expression of an activated *ras* gene and a mutated tumor suppressor gene, *p53*. In this example, a combinatorial effect of common genetic changes in human cancer apparently results in abnormal expression of this hypercalcemic peptide.

CLINICAL SYNDROMES

The clinical syndromes associated with "ectopic" hormone production are important because they are often difficult diagnostic dilemmas, they are a major cause of morbidity and death in cancer patients, and their therapy can be challenging. Management of these clinical syndromes is often difficult because of the necessity to treat both the cancer and the syndrome caused by excessive hormone production.

HUMORAL HYPERCALCEMIA OF MALIGNANCY

Hypercalcemia is one of the most common hormonal syndromes associated with cancer and one of the most difficult to manage. Hypercalcemia is the final common manifestation for several different pathophysiologic processes, so each patient must be approached in an organized manner to facilitate correct diagnosis and treatment. Measurement of an intact serum parathyroid hormone (iPTH) provides a useful starting point (Figure 194–1). An elevated parathyroid hormone level in the context of hypercalcemia should prompt further evaluation for parathyroid disease (Chapter 264). However, in the majority of cancer patients with hypercalcemia, the iPTH value will be suppressed, indicating that the malignancy is generating the hypercalcemia. Several different clinical syndromes have been elucidated.

Parathyroid Hormone–Related Protein

Parathyroid hormone–related protein (PTHrp) is normally involved in chondrocytic and dermatologic differentiation. Eight of the first 16 amino acids of PTHrp are homologous with PTH, and both peptides exert their various effects through interaction with the osteoblast PTH receptor. Activation of the PTH receptor increases

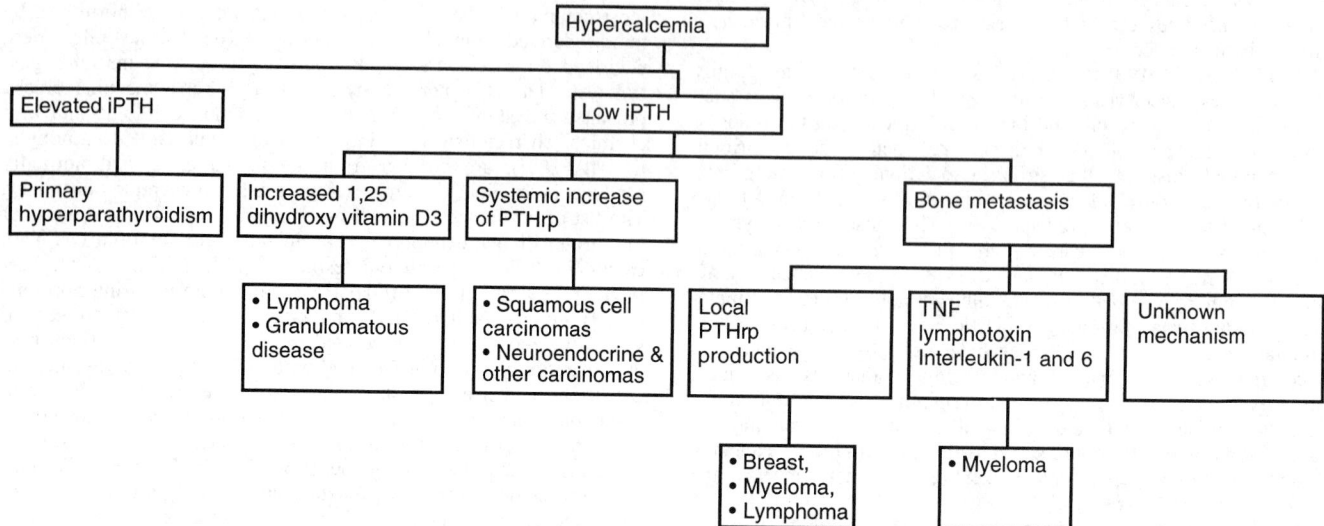

FIGURE 194–1 ■ A strategy for the evaluation of hypercalcemia in the context of malignancy based on measurement of intact parathyroid hormone (iPTH).

the expression of an osteoblast-specific cell surface protein, osteo-protegrin ligand (OPGL) or RANK ligand (RANKL). Cell-to-cell communication of OPGL or RANKL with the RANK receptor on the undifferentiated osteoclast causes increased osteoclast differenti-ation, bone resorption, and hypercalcemia. Ectopic production of PTHrp by a wide variety of tumors is one of the most common causes of hypercalcemia associated with malignancy. The clinical syndrome is nearly identical to that observed with hyperparathy-roidism and includes increased osteoclast-mediated bone resorption as well as an increase in renal tubular calcium resorption and a decrease in phosphorus resorption. The only significant clinical difference between PTHrp and PTH-mediated hypercalcemia is the finding of increased serum calcitriol (1,25-dihydroxycholecalciferol) levels in hyperparathyroidism and low or normal values in PTHrp-mediated hypercalcemia, presumably because of the effects of can-cer on the 1-α-hydroxylase. PTHrp production is most commonly associated with squamous cell carcinomas, although production has been observed in other types of tumors including breast, neuroen-docrine, renal, melanoma, and prostate tumors.

Increased Production of Calcitriol

Increased production of calcitriol occurs in a high percentage of patients with lymphoma. There is compelling evidence for in-creased expression of 1-α-hydroxylase by lymphomatous tissue. Other granulomatous conditions such as sarcoid, berylliosis, and tuberculous or fungal infections may also cause this clinical syn-drome. Other clinical features in this group of patients include a suppressed iPTH level (Figure 194–1), an increased or normal serum phosphorus level, hypercalciuria, and no evidence of bone metastasis. An elevated serum calcitriol concentration is found in approximately one half of hypercalcemic cancer patients.

Bone Metastasis

Bone metastasis should always be considered in the differential diagnosis of hypercalcemia in the cancer patient. Bone metastases are frequently associated with local production of cytokines, PTHrp, or other substances that cause increased bone resorption. Indeed, the distinctions between humoral hypercalcemia of malig-nancy and localized osteolysis have become blurred because of evidence that tumors such as breast carcinoma or myeloma cause localized osteolysis by local production and secretion of PTHrp. In breast carcinoma, there is considerable evidence supporting a local regulatory loop between transforming growth factor β (TGF-β) and PTHrp production. TGF-β is a normal component of bone matrix. Local PTHrp production by breast carcinoma cells can stimulate osteoclastic bone resorption and TGF-β release, which in turn stim-ulate greater PTHrp production, thereby accelerating the osteolytic process. Other activators of bone resorption, including tumor necro-sis factor, lymphotoxin, interleukin 1 (IL-1), and IL-6, can be

produced by other tumors that metastasize to (renal cell carcinoma) or reside in (myeloma) bone.

Therapy

Management of hypercalcemia should focus initially on reversing dehydration and increasing urine calcium excretion by infusion of normal saline solution at rates of 100 to 300 mL/hour, depending upon cardiac status. A patient with a serum calcium concentration >13 mg% (3.25 mM/L), altered mental status, or renal dysfunction should also be treated with bisphosphonate (intravenous [IV] pami-dronate 60–90 mg/4 hours), glucocorticoids (40–60 mg/day predni-sone or methyl prednisolone), gallium nitrate (200 mg/M²/day, in-fused for 7 days), or salmon calcitonin (100–200 units, IV or subcutaneously [SQ] every 6 to 12 hours) alone or in combination. PTHrp-mediated or localized osteolysis is most responsive to bis-phosphonates or gallium nitrate; vitamin D–mediated hypercal-cemia is most responsive to glucocorticoid therapy (Chapter 264).

Long-term management is focused on therapy of the underlying malignancy. The average survival in a patient with PTHrp-mediated hypercalcemia is less than 3 months, in part related to the underly-ing malignancy. Long-term therapy of PTHrp-mediated hypercal-cemia, like that associated with parathyroid carcinoma, is difficult: patients tend to become less responsive to the effects of bisphos-phonate or salmon calcitonin therapy over time and may experience renal toxicity from gallium nitrate therapy when it is used for extended periods.

ECTOPIC ACTH SECRETION

Inappropriate secretion of ACTH is a rare but important cause of morbidity and mortality in cancer patients. It can be caused by two different mechanisms: expression of the pro-opiomelanocortin (POMC) gene by a tumor or ectopic expression of CRH. In cell types that express the POMC gene, post-translational processing of this gene product can proceed down one of several mutually exclu-sive pathways resulting in expression of β-lipotropin, γ-lipotropin, and β-endorphin, or big melanocyte–stimulating hormone and ACTH. Although POMC expression by malignant tumors is rela-tively common, the enzymes necessary to cleave ACTH from the precursor are found less frequently outside the pituitary gland. ACTH production occurs in a broad spectrum of tumors, but it is most commonly associated with SCCL or more classic neuroendo-crine tumors such as pulmonary carcinoid, medullary thyroid carci-noma, islet cell adenomas or carcinomas, pheochromocytoma, and occasional neural tumors such as ganglioneuroma. Ectopic ACTH production causes adrenal cortical hyperplasia and excessive corti-sol production.

Ectopic production of CRH causes a clinical syndrome character-ized by pituitary corticotrope hyperplasia and laboratory results that

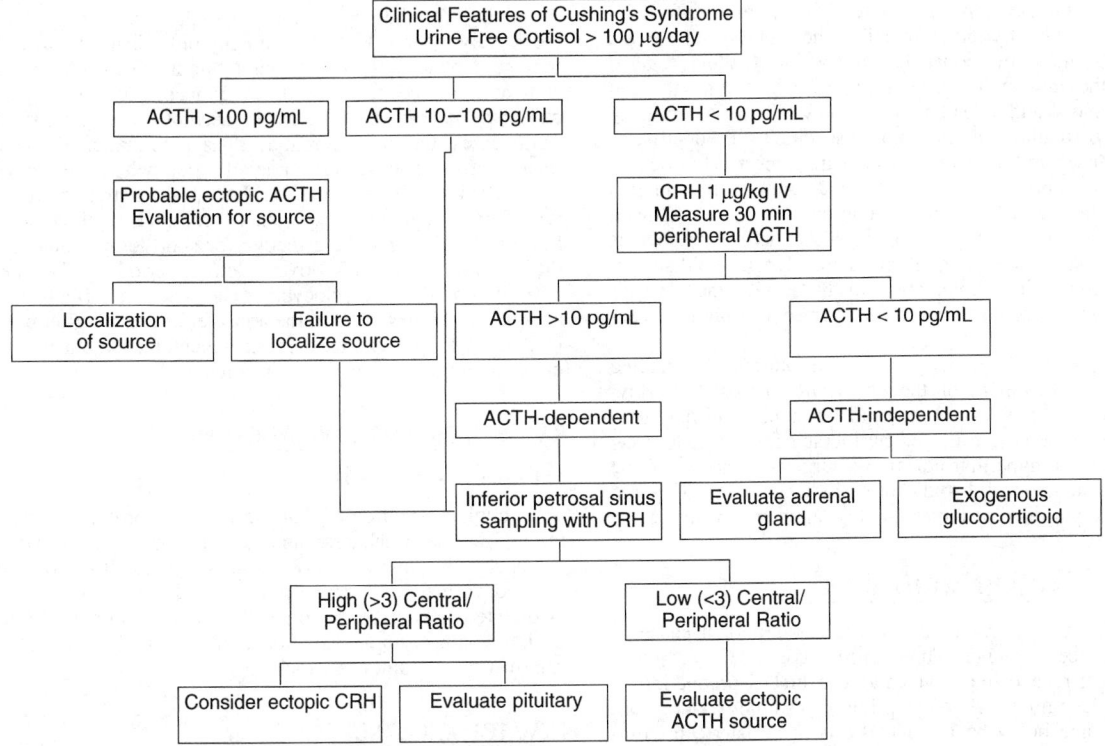

FIGURE 194–2 ■ An evaluation strategy for a patient with Cushing's syndrome and suspected ectopic ACTH production. In patients with a plasma ACTH concentration >100 pg/mL, ectopic ACTH concentration should be considered, although some patients with pituitary Cushing's disease may have values in this range. In patients with a plasma ACTH concentration between 10 and 100 pg/mL, inferior petrosal sinus sampling (IPSS) for ACTH should be performed after peripheral CRH injection (Chapter 240) to separate a pituitary (high central/peripheral ACTH ratio) from an ectopic ACTH (low central/peripheral ACTH ratio) source. In patients with a low basal peripheral ACTH value (<10 pg/mL), a low-dose CRH test (1 μg/kg) should be performed, followed by IPPS in individuals whose plasma ACTH concentration rises to >10 pg/mL. ACTH = corticotropin; CRH = corticotropin-releasing hormone.

mimic those of pituitary Cushing's disease (Figure 194–2). Diagnosis requires a high index of suspicion, combined with either measurement of CRH in the blood or identification of a neoplasm outside the pituitary. Some neoplasms produce both ACTH and CRH. Tumors reported to produce CRH include medullary thyroid carcinoma, paragangliomas, prostate cancer, and islet cell neoplasms.

Hypercorticism associated with ectopic ACTH syndrome may present with classic features of Cushing's syndrome such as easy bruisability, centripetal obesity, muscle wasting, hypertension, diabetes, and metabolic alkalosis. In other patients, particularly those with rapidly growing SCCL, the clinical picture may be dominated by profound hypokalemic metabolic alkalosis and hypertension without the other clinical findings of Cushing's syndrome.

Several different approaches have evolved for evaluation of Cushing's syndrome (Chapter 240). One approach (Figure 194–2) is based on the plasma ACTH measurement in a patient with clinical and laboratory features of Cushing's syndrome. The finding of a marked elevation of the plasma ACTH concentration (> 100 pg/mL) should prompt a search for an ectopic source of ACTH. In a patient with a plasma ACTH value greater than 10 pg/mL but less than 100 pg/mL, a more detailed evaluation is appropriate. The differentiation between a pituitary and an ectopic source may require stimulation of ACTH secretion by CRH combined with measurement of ACTH in blood from the pituitary venous drainage (inferior petrosal sinus sampling). Lack of an increase in the inferior petrosal sinus ACTH concentration (more than three times the peripheral ACTH) following peripheral CRH stimulation should prompt a search for an ectopic source. In patients who have an increased (more than three times the peripheral level) inferior petrosal sinus ACTH following CRH, a pituitary source is likely. Ectopic CRH can yield confusing results and may not be diagnosed unless the clinician considers the possibility and measures a plasma CRH or looks for an ectopic source.

Other approaches have also been applied to the diagnosis of ectopic ACTH syndrome. For example, ACTH production from an ectopic source is not generally suppressed by high-dose dexamethasone. In a patient with an ACTH >10 pg/mL, administration of a single 8-mg oral dose of dexamethasone at 11:00 P.M. followed by measurement of serum cortisol level at 8:00 A.M. can differentiate between a pituitary and an ectopic source. The serum cortisol level in pituitary Cushing's syndrome will generally be suppressed 50% after dexamethasone, whereas levels in ectopic ACTH generally are not suppressed. However, false-positive or false-negative results occur with each of these testing procedures, making the differential diagnosis of Cushing's syndrome among the most challenging in medicine.

Hypercortisolism associated with ectopic ACTH can be managed by removal of the ACTH- or CRH-producing tumor or by inhibition of cortisol synthesis with metyrapone (1 to 4g/day orally), aminoglutethimide (250 mg orally [PO] four times/day with upward titration), or ketoconazole (200–400 mg twice a day orally). Replacement glucocorticoid therapy is needed to prevent adrenal insufficiency. If surgical removal of an ACTH- or CRH-producing tumor is not possible and inhibition of cortisol synthesis is inadequate, bilateral adrenalectomy (with replacement glucocorticoid therapy) may be required. In patients with a rapidly progressive SCCL and ectopic ACTH syndrome, the oncologic imperative to initiate immediate cytotoxic therapy must be counterbalanced by the desire to normalize cell-mediated immunity by normalizing cortisol secretion, hypokalemia, and metabolic alkalosis. Cytotoxic chemotherapy generally should be delayed, if possible, until the serum cortisol level is normalized, because of the high rate of infection in neutropenic patients with hypercortisolism.

HUMAN CHORIONIC GONADOTHROPIN PRODUCTION

Two different genes encode the α- and β-subunits of human chorionic gonadotropin (hCG). The α-subunit is common to all of the pituitary glycoprotein hormones (luteinizing hormone, follicle-stimulating hormone, thyroid-stimulating hormone, and hCG), whereas each of these hormones has a specific β-subunit gene. Production of the α-subunit occurs in a variety of pituitary and non-pituitary tumors and does not cause any discernible clinical syndrome. The β-subunit confers biologic specificity. Production of intact hCG occurs commonly in trophoblastic tumors (choriocarcinomas, testicular embryonal carcinomas, and seminomas) and less commonly in other tumors such as lung and pancreas. Clinical syndromes associated with production of hCG include precocious puberty, gynecomastia, and hyperthyroidism. Hyperthyroidism results from the low-affinity interaction of hCG with the thyroid-stimulating hormone receptor when hCG is present at high concentrations.

Therapy for precocious puberty and gynecomastia is directed toward removal or treatment of the underlying tumor. Hyperthyroidism is treated by inhibition of thyroid hormone synthesis, usually by thionamide therapy, followed by therapy for the underlying tumor. Treatment of hyperthyroidism by surgical removal of the thyroid gland or ablation with radioactive iodine is rarely required since the hyperthyroidism resolves rapidly after treatment of the underlying tumor.

HYPOGLYCEMIA ASSOCIATED WITH CANCER

Tumor-associated hypoglycemia is a rare but important cause of morbidity for cancer patients. Three different clinical syndromes cause most cancer-related hypoglycemia. The first is production of insulin by an islet tumor. Although primary insulinomas are rare, dedifferentiation and bulky hepatic metastasis of an islet cell carcinoma may be associated with excessive insulin production (Chapter 243). A second cause of hypoglycemia, insufficient gluconeogenesis to maintain the plasma glucose concentration in the fasting state, is caused by near-complete replacement of the liver by metastatic tumor. A third cause of hypoglycemia is increased concentrations of insulin-like growth factor II (IGF-II), a ligand that interacts with the insulin receptor in large abdominal tumors, most commonly fibrosarcomas, hemangiopericytomas, or hepatomas. This increase appears to be due to the failure to form normal IGF binding protein 3 (IGFBP-3) and the acid labile subunit (ALS) complex that normally binds IGF-II; the result is an increase in free IGF-II concentrations.

In all three types of hypoglycemia, the patient is at greatest risk for symptoms during periods of fasting, most commonly during sleeping hours. Therapy should focus on surgical excision, where possible, or antineoplastic therapy directed at the tumor. Initial therapy of hypoglycemia is focused on frequent meals, and patients may occasionally be maintained symptom-free if awakened for one or more snacks during sleeping hours. If there is progression of the tumor or the patient's caloric intake is inadequate, additional measures may be required. In patients in whom hepatic replacement by tumor is evident, a continuous infusion of 20% dextrose through a central line may be required, especially during sleeping hours. In patients with insulin-producing or large retroperitoneal tumors, glucagon infusion (0.5–2 mg/hour) stimulates hepatic gluconeogenesis and prevents hypoglycemia, although in rare patients the rash associated with glucagonoma may develop. A glucose response to a single injection of glucagon (1 mg) should be documented before initiating therapy. In patients with large retroperitoneal tumors, treatment with growth hormone (3–6 μg/kg SQ) or glucocorticoids (20–40 mg/day) may reverse hypoglycemia possibly by facilitating IGFBP-3/ALS complex formation, thereby reducing free serum IGF-II levels. Growth hormone doses as high as 2600 μg/day have been administered in this condition, although long-term treatment with this dose may cause acromegalic side effects. Somatostatin analogues (octreotide or lanreotide) are generally not effective for normalizing the plasma glucose level in patients with islet cell tumors; diazoxide (3–8 mg/kg/day in two or three divided doses) may be effective, but problems with fluid retention frequently preclude its long-term use.

SYNDROME OF INAPPROPRIATE ANTIDIURETIC HORMONE

Ectopic production of vasopressin by head and neck tumors (3%), SCCL (15%), and other lung carcinomas (1%) causes a clinical syndrome characterized by hyponatremia, hypo-osmolality, excessive urine sodium excretion, an inappropriately high urine osmolality for the low serum osmolality, and normal function of the kidneys, adrenal glands, and thyroid (Chapter 238). Other malignant neoplasms (primary brain tumors, hematologic neoplasms, skin tumors, and gastrointestinal, gynecologic, breast, and prostate cancers, and sarcomas) are rare causes of this clinical syndrome. In most cases the hyponatremia is asymptomatic, although altered mental status and seizures may develop when the serum sodium concentration falls below 120 mEq/L; hyponatremic women of the reproductive age may experience profound cerebral degeneration. Fluid restriction may be effective for short-term management but is difficult to maintain over long periods. Treatment with 150–300 mg/day demeclocycline can block the effects of vasopressin on the kidney and is the most effective long-term therapy in patients with cancer. Vasopressin receptor antagonists are in clinical trials but are not currently available.

RARE ECTOPIC HORMONE SYNDROMES

Oncogenic Osteomalacia

A clinical syndrome characterized by profound hypophosphatemia, muscle weakness, and osteomalacia can be produced by mesenchymal tumors (osteoblastomas, giant cell osteosarcomas, hemangiocytomas, and rarely prostate and lung carcinoma). Therapy is directed toward correction of hypophosphatemia with either oral or intravenous supplementation and vitamin D treatment. Surgical removal of the tumor is curative.

HEMATOLOGIC SYNDROMES

The kidney is the primary site of erythropoietin production, and, therefore, the relatively common erythropoietin production by benign or malignant renal tumors is not an "ectopic" hormone syndrome. Production of erythropoietin by cerebellar hemangioblastoma, uterine fibroids, pheochromocytomas, and ovarian and hepatic tumors is generally considered "ectopic." Patients with excessive erythropoietin production may or may not have polycythemia. Other ectopic syndromes, less well defined, include production of thrombopoietin, leukopoietin, or colony-stimulating factor by some tumors. These conditions are treated by removal of the tumor or by appropriate chemotherapy.

HYPERTENSION

Renal (Wilms' tumor, renal cell carcinoma, or hemangiopericytoma), lung (SCCL, adenocarcinoma), hepatic, pancreatic, and ovarian carcinomas may produce renin. The clinical presentation in these patients can include hypertension, hypokalemia, and evidence of increased aldosterone production. Therapy with spironolactone (Aldactone) or angiotensin-converting enzyme inhibitors may be effective.

GROWTH HORMONE AND PROLACTIN PRODUCTION

Rare examples of growth hormone (GH) production have been identified in lung and gastric adenocarcinoma. Ectopic production of GHRH has been documented for islet cell tumors, bronchogenic carcinoids, and SCCL. Increased prolactin production is a rare phenomenon associated with lung and renal carcinoma; it produces galactorrhea and amenorrhea in women and produces hypogonadism and gynecomastia in men.

Berenson JR: Bisphosphonates in the treatment of malignant bone disease. Annu Rev Med 50:237, 1999. *Review of the use of bisphosphonates in reducing skeletal complications in patients with bone metastases.*

Hoff AO, Vassilopoulou-Sellin R: The role of glucagon administration in the diagnosis and treatment of patients with tumor hypoglycemia. Cancer 82:1595, 1998. *Excellent review of clinical management of hypoglycemia associated with cancer and the use of a glucagon stimulation test to determine response to glucagon infusion.*

Miller M: Inappropriate antidiuretic hormone secretion. Curr Ther Endocrinol Metab 6: 206, 1997. *Current review of status of diagnosis and management of SIADH.*

Mundy GR, Guise TA: Hypercalcemia of malignancy. Am J Med 103:134, 1997. *An overview of several mechanisms of hypercalcemia.*

Winquist EW, Laskey J, Crump M, et al: Ketoconazole in the management of paraneoplastic Cushing's syndrome secondary to ectopic adrenocorticotropin production. J Clin Oncol 13:157, 1995. *Approach to medical management of ectopic ACTH syndrome.*

NONMETASTATIC EFFECTS OF
CANCER: THE NERVOUS SYSTEM

Jerome B. Posner

When nervous system dysfunction develops in patients with cancer, metastasis is usually the cause, but cancer also can exert deleterious effects on the nervous system by mechanisms other than metastasis. Recognition of these non-metastatic neurologic complications can prevent inappropriate and perhaps harmful therapy directed at a non-existent metastasis. Sometimes the nervous system symptoms precede discovery of the cancer and can, if correctly interpreted, lead the physician to the diagnosis of an otherwise occult neoplasm.

An almost bewildering variety of neurologic disorders have been ascribed to the effects of systemic cancer (Table 195–1). Most patients with nervous system dysfunction not caused by metastases are eventually found to be suffering from infection, vascular or metabolic disorders, or neurotoxicity secondary to chemotherapy. However, two other types of nervous system damage related to cancer are paraneoplastic syndromes (Table 195–2) and radiation injury.

Paraneoplastic syndromes, also called "remote effects of cancer on the nervous system," refer to neurologic dysfunction caused by cancer but not ascribable to such well-defined secondary effects of cancer as infection, coagulation abnormalities, nutritional and metabolic disorders, or side effects of therapy (see Table 195–1). Similar clinical disorders occur in the absence of cancer, and thus in any given patient, the cancer must be identified to document that the neurologic disorder is paraneoplastic. If patients with mild peripheral neuropathy or myopathy possibly associated with cachexia are excluded, remote effects of cancer affect fewer than 1% of patients with cancer. Lung cancer accounts for more than 50% of cases; the incidence is greatest in patients with ovarian cancer, small cell lung cancer, and Hodgkin's disease. Because of its rarity, the diagnosis of paraneoplastic syndrome should never be accepted until a thorough evaluation has excluded metastatic or other non-metastatic causes of neurologic dysfunction. In particular, infiltration of nerve roots by tumor in the leptomeninges may mimic paraneoplastic peripheral neuropathy. An exception exists when the serum of a patient suspected to be suffering from a paraneoplastic syndrome is found to contain an antibody reacting with both the cancer and the nervous system (onconeuronal antigen).

Increasing evidence suggests that the etiology of most or all remote effects is autoimmune. Patients with Lambert-Eaton myasthenic syndrome (see below) harbor an IgG antibody that reacts with P/Q voltage-gated calcium channels on the pre-synaptic neuromuscular junction. Complexing of these channels by the antibody prevents normal release of acetylcholine, which in turn causes the clinical symptoms of the disorder. About two thirds of patients with Lambert-Eaton myasthenic syndrome have small cell lung

Table 195–1 ■ NON-METASTATIC EFFECTS OF CANCER ON THE NERVOUS SYSTEM

Paraneoplastic syndromes or remote effects of cancer (see Table 195–2)
Side effects of therapy
  Chemotherapy
  Radiation therapy (see Table 195–3)
Metabolic and nutritional abnormalities
  Destruction of vital organs (e.g., liver)
  Elaboration of hormonal substances by tumor (e.g., carcinoid)
  Competition between tumor and brain for essential substrates (e.g., glucose)
  Malnutrition
Infections (usually associated with lymphomas)
  Parasites (e.g., toxoplasmosis)
  Fungi (e.g., cryptococcosis, aspergillosis, mucormycosis)
  Bacteria (e.g., *Listeria monocytogenes*)
  Viruses (e.g., herpes zoster)
Vascular disease
  Intracranial hemorrhage
  Cerebral infarction

Table 195–2 ■ PARANEOPLASTIC SYNDROMES OF THE NERVOUS SYSTEM

Brain and Cranial Nerves
Limbic encephalitis*
Brain stem encephalitis
Cerebellar degeneration*
Opsoclonus-myoclonus*
Paraneoplastic visual syndromes
  Cancer-associated retinopathy*
  Optic neuritis
Spinal Cord
Necrotizing myelopathy
Myelitis
Motor neuron syndrome
Subacute motor neuronopathy
Dorsal Root Ganglia
Paraneoplastic sensory neuronopathy
Peripheral Nerves
Autonomic neuropathy
Acute sensorimotor neuropathy
  Polyradiculoneuropathy (Guillain-Barré syndrome)
  Brachial neuritis
Chronic sensorimotor neuropathy
  Sensorimotor neuropathies associated with plasma cell dyscrasias
Vasculitic neuropathy
Neuromyotonia
Neuromuscular Junction and Muscle
Lambert-Eaton myasthenic syndrome*
Myasthenia gravis
Polymyositis/dermatomyositis
Acute necrotizing myopathy
Cachectic myopathy
Carcinoid myopathy*
Myotonia
Multiple Levels of Involvement or Uncertain Site
Encephalomyelitis†
Stiff-person syndrome
Carcinomatous neuromyopathy*

*In some groups of patients (e.g., children with opsoclonus, postmenopausal women with cerebellar dysfunction), the neurologic disorder is associated with a tumor in more than 50% of instances.
†Can include cerebellar symptoms, autonomic dysfunction, and sensory neuronopathy.

cancer cells that also express the P/Q calcium channel protein. Removal of anti–calcium channel IgG from the serum of a patient with Lambert-Eaton myasthenic syndrome ameliorates the neuromuscular symptoms, and injection of that IgG into experimental animals reproduces the neurologic disorder. High titers of antibodies against other onconeuronal antigens are found in several other paraneoplastic syndromes, thus suggesting a mechanism similar to that in Lambert-Eaton syndrome.

PARANEOPLASTIC SYNDROMES

Paraneoplastic syndromes are usually classified by the anatomic site of neurologic disability (see Table 195–2). However, it is common for more than one anatomic site to be involved, e.g., dementia and myelopathy or limbic encephalitis and sensory neuronopathy. Sometimes, two different syndromes develop together, e.g., Lambert-Eaton myasthenic syndrome and cerebellar degeneration.

Brain

CEREBRUM. Loss of recent memory (limbic encephalitis) and affective alterations, either anxiety or depression, are the usual findings. Seizures are prominent in some patients; others have a fluctuating confusional state. When other abnormal neurologic signs are present, they usually point to the brain stem, cerebellum, or peripheral nerves (encephalomyelitis). Cerebrospinal fluid (CSF) usually contains 10 to 40 lymphocytes per cubic milliliter, with a slight elevation in protein concentration. Magnetic resonance imaging (MRI) is usually normal, but in some patients abnormalities can be found in the medial temporal areas. Limbic encephalitis can be associated with anti-Hu antibodies in some patients with small cell lung cancer, and anti-TC antibodies in some patients with testicular cancer.

Pathologically, two main groups of cerebrum involvement can be differentiated. In some patients, no significant pathologic changes are found in the cerebrum despite clinical dementia. Other patients demonstrate widespread cerebral neuronal loss, gliosis, and perivascular collections of lymphocytes, particularly in the medial temporal lobes (limbic encephalitis) or the thalamus. In patients who have anti-Hu antibodies in blood and CSF, the same antibodies can also be identified in the brain. The differential diagnosis includes brain or leptomeningeal metastases; fungal, parasitic, or viral infections (including multifocal leukoencephalopathy); metabolic encephalopathy; and nutritional deficits (e.g., thiamine deficiency leading to the memory loss and brain stem dysfunction of Wernicke-Korsakoff syndrome). These other disorders are usually readily identified by appropriate imaging studies, CSF examination, and other laboratory tests. The rapid onset of dementia in middle age accompanied by cerebellar, brain stem, or peripheral nerve dysfunction but no other focal cerebral signs suggests paraneoplastic dementia as a remote effect of cancer. Paraneoplastic dementia may be confused with Creutzfeldt-Jakob disease, but other degenerative dementias such as Alzheimer's disease are usually slower in onset and have a more protracted course. No specific treatment is available for paraneoplastic dementias, but they occasionally improve spontaneously with successful treatment of the cancer.

CEREBELLUM. Cerebellar symptoms usually evolve over weeks, with bilateral and symmetrical ataxia of gait and the arms and legs. Severe dysarthria is usually present; vertigo and diplopia are common, but nystagmus may be absent. Some patients have neurologic signs pointing to disease outside the cerebellum (e.g., extensor plantar responses, diminished or exaggerated tendon reflexes, dementia). Early in the disorder, CSF pleocytosis is present, and an elevated CSF IgG content is common. In about half of patients, the neurologic findings precede discovery of the cancer, but the clinical picture is so characteristic that cancer should be suspected. Cerebellar atrophy may be seen on MRI. In a subset of patients with gynecologic cancers (ovarian, uterine, fallopian tube, breast), an antibody (anti-Yo) reacting with cerebellar Purkinje cells and with the underlying tumor allows a definitive diagnosis to be made before the tumor is discovered. Other antibodies associated with paraneoplastic cerebellar degeneration include anti-Tr (Hodgkin's disease), anti-Hu (small cell lung cancer), and anti-Ma (several different cancers).

Pathologic changes consist of loss of cerebellar Purkinje cells with or without lymphocytic cuffing of blood vessels in the deep nuclei. Cerebellar dysfunction is also caused by cerebellar or leptomeningeal metastases and by Listeria meningitis or progressive multifocal leukoencephalopathy. These disorders can easily be identified by MRI and CSF examination. In alcohol-nutritional cerebellar degeneration, truncal and lower extremity ataxia is prominent, but nystagmus, dysarthria, and upper extremity ataxia are mild or absent. Sporadic or familial cerebellar degenerative disorders are much slower in onset. Cerebellar dysfunction associated with viral infections (varicella, infectious mononucleosis) or with chemotherapy (5-fluorouracil, cytosine arabinoside) may mimic paraneoplastic cerebellar degeneration. Paraneoplastic cerebellar degeneration usually runs a subacute course and then stabilizes or occasionally improves with successful treatment of the tumor.

Cranial Nerves

Two rare but striking paraneoplastic syndromes affect the eyes. Carcinoma-associated retinopathy is characterized by rapid onset of blindness caused by retinal degeneration, usually of photoreceptors, and is associated with antibodies that recognize the retinal antigen recoverin. Optic neuritis, which does not differ clinically in any way from the idiopathic disorder, has also been described in some patients with underlying neoplasms. Opsoclonus (saccadic conjugate involuntary movement of the eyes), also called "saccadomania," is often a paraneoplastic disorder. About 50% of infants and children with opsoclonus have underlying neuroblastoma. In adults, about 20% of patients with opsoclonus probably have an underlying cancer, usually gynecologic or lung cancer, that is sometimes associated with the anti-Ri antibody. Except when this autoantibody is present, paraneoplastic opsoclonus cannot be clinically distinguished from opsoclonus caused by metabolic or structural abnormalities of the brain stem or cerebellum.

Spinal Cord

Several distinct myelopathies complicate cancer. Subacute motor neuronopathy affects anterior horn cells, usually in patients with Hodgkin's disease or other lymphomas. The course is subacute, with progressive painless asymmetrical lower motor neuron weakness of the legs and arms. Some patients complain of sensory symptoms, but sensory loss is mild or absent despite profound weakness. Examination may also demonstrate extensor plantar (Babinski) reflexes, indicating that corticospinal tracts are also involved. The major pathologic finding is degeneration of anterior horn cells. Sometimes the anterior horns and ventral nerve roots are inflamed, in addition to demyelination in the white matter of the spinal cord. The clinical course is different from most remote effects of cancer in that some patients improve spontaneously, independently of the course of the underlying lymphoma. The etiology is unknown, but a similar disorder in mice with lymphomas appears to be caused by a retrovirus. Typical amyotrophic lateral sclerosis is rarely paraneoplastic, but primary lateral sclerosis, which is a variant of motor neuron disease that affects only the corticospinal tracts and hence causes weakness and spasticity, may complicate breast cancer.

In subacute necrotic myelopathy, both gray and white matter are affected equally. Clinically, rapidly ascending sensory and motor loss is present, usually to the mid-thoracic levels; the patient becomes paraplegic and incontinent within hours or days. The neurologic symptoms often precede discovery of the neoplasm, and the illness is clinically and pathologically indistinguishable from idiopathic subacute necrotic myelopathy. Because epidural or intramedullary spinal metastases and arteriovenous spinal cord anomalies may present similar clinical signs, an MRI scan is essential.

The stiff-person syndrome is characterized by rigidity and spasms of muscles associated with antiamphiphysin antibodies and breast cancer. Most "stiff persons" do not have cancer, but they produce antibodies against glutamic acid decarboxylase that cause both diabetes and the neurologic disorder.

Peripheral Nerves and Dorsal Root Ganglia

Four clinical peripheral nerve disorders occur in association with cancer. Characteristic of carcinoma is subacute sensory neuronopathy marked by loss of sensation with relative preservation of motor power. The illness usually precedes appearance of the carcinoma and progresses over a few months, and the patient is left with moderate or severe disability. CSF pleocytosis and increased IgG content are common. Pathologically, destruction of posterior root ganglia with perivascular lymphocytic cuffing and wallerian degeneration of sensory nerves is noted. Many patients also have encephalomyelitis with inflammatory and degenerative changes in the brain and spinal cord. The disorder, when associated with small cell carcinoma, is characterized by anti-Hu antibodies.

More common than sensory neuronopathy is a distal sensorimotor polyneuropathy characterized by motor weakness, sensory loss, and absence of distal reflexes in the extremities. The illness is pathologically characterized by either segmental demyelination or axonal degeneration (or both) of sensory and motor peripheral nerves. Pathologically and clinically, the sensorimotor neuropathy is indistinguishable from polyneuropathies not associated with cancer. Indeed, some have suggested that late or terminal polyneuropathy may be due to nutritional deprivation associated with cancer. Its etiology, however, is not clear, and it does not respond to treatment with vitamins or other nutritional supplements.

A polyneuritis clinically and pathologically indistinguishable from acute post-infectious polyneuropathy (Guillain-Barré syndrome) also complicates cancers, particularly Hodgkin's disease. A few patients with neuropathy limited to the autonomic nervous system have been reported.

Neuromuscular Junction and Muscles

NEUROMUSCULAR JUNCTION. Myasthenia gravis is associated with thymomas but not usually with other systemic tumors. The Lambert-Eaton myasthenic syndrome is characterized by weakness and fatigability of proximal muscles, particularly of the pelvic girdle and thighs. The cranial nerves and respiratory muscles are usually spared. Patients often complain of dryness of the mouth, impotence, pain in the thighs, and peripheral paresthesias. Proximal muscles are weak, but strength increases over several seconds of sustained contraction. Deep tendon reflexes are diminished or absent. The diagnosis is made by electromyographic studies in which repeated nerve stimulation at rates above 10 per second causes a progressive *increase* in the size of the muscle action potential (the opposite of myasthenia gravis). About two thirds of patients with this syndrome either have cancer or will develop cancer, usually small cell carcinoma of the lung. Most patients harbor P/Q-type voltage-gated calcium channel antibodies in their serum, an excellent diagnostic test. Plasmapheresis and immunosuppressant drugs usually relieve the symptoms, as may successful treatment of the neoplasm. The illness responds poorly to anticholinesterase drugs but does respond to 3,4-diaminopyridine in doses up to 100 mg/day.

MUSCLE. Typical *dermatomyositis* or *polymyositis* may occur as a remote effect of cancer (see Chapter 296). Fewer than 10% of patients with this disorder have cancer, but the figure is higher in older patients. The clinical picture of polymyositis associated with cancer (i.e., subacute development of weakness, particularly weakness involving the proximal muscles and sometimes the bulbar muscles) is indistinguishable from dermatomyositis or polymyositis not associated with cancer. Pathologically, it is possible to differentiate two groups: one with the typical inflammatory lesions of polymyositis and one with little inflammation but severe muscle necrosis. The latter group may suffer an explosive clinical course. These patients respond less well to corticosteroid therapy than do those with dermatomyositis unaccompanied by cancer, although substantial improvement with steroid treatment sometimes occurs. Intravenous immunoglobulin may help.

Some patients with cancer complain of *weakness* and *fatigability* that seem worse than can be accounted for by their cancer alone. Cachexia and weight loss alone do not usually cause measurable muscle weakness. The weakness is usually proximal and produces particular difficulty climbing stairs or getting out of low chairs. Ankle reflexes may be diminished or absent. Further neurologic evaluation does not yield findings diagnostic of one of the remote effects of cancer described above. Brain and colleagues have labeled this entity "neuromyopathy" because its exact anatomic locus is unclear, but others have suggested that it is a non-specific accompaniment of cachexia and systemic illness. Specific (type II) muscle fiber atrophy develops early in patients with systemic cancer. The cause and treatment of the weakness are unknown.

NERVOUS SYSTEM INJURY FROM THERAPEUTIC RADIATION

Adverse effects of ionizing radiation on the nervous system (Table 195-3) are related to the total dose of radiation, the size of each fraction, the total duration over which the dose is received, and the volume of nervous system tissue irradiated. Other factors such as underlying nervous system disease (e.g., brain tumor, cerebral edema), previous surgery, concomitant use of chemotherapeutic agents, and individual susceptibility make it impossible to define precisely a safe dose of radiation therapy for a given individual. However, guidelines generally allow the radiation therapist to calculate safe nervous system doses. Adverse effects may involve any portion of the central or peripheral nervous system and may occur acutely or be delayed weeks to years following irradiation.

CLINICAL MANIFESTATIONS. *Acute encephalopathy* may follow large radiation doses to the brains of patients with increased intracranial pressure, particularly in the absence of corticosteroid prophylaxis. Immediately following treatment, headache, nausea,

vomiting, somnolence, fever, and occasionally worsening of neurologic signs develop in susceptible patients; rarely, the syndrome culminates in cerebral herniation and death. Acute encephalopathy usually follows the initial radiation fraction and becomes progressively less severe with each ensuing fraction. This disorder is believed to result from increased intracranial pressure or brain edema from radiation-induced alteration of the blood-brain barrier. It responds to corticosteroids.

Early delayed reactions appear 6 to 16 weeks after therapy and persist for days to months. A transient, diffuse encephalopathy commonly follows prophylactic irradiation of the brain for leukemia in children and for small cell lung cancer in adults. The disorder is characterized by somnolence, often associated with headache, nausea, vomiting, and sometimes fever. Whole-brain irradiation for brain tumor sometimes causes lethargy and worsening of focal neurologic signs suggestive of progression of the brain tumor. MRI scans may also suggest worsening. Both disorders usually respond to steroids but resolve spontaneously even if untreated. Rarely, a brain stem disorder characterized by diplopia, ataxia, dysarthria, and dysphagia and associated with foci of demyelination resembling acute multiple sclerosis follows irradiation to the brain stem.

Early delayed myelopathy follows radiation therapy to the neck or upper part of the thorax and is characterized by Lhermitte's sign (an electric shock–like sensation radiating into various parts of the body when the neck is flexed). The symptoms resolve spontaneously. Early delayed radiation syndromes are believed to result from demyelination, possibly caused by radiation-induced damage to oligodendroglia.

Late delayed radiation injury appears months to years after radiation therapy and may affect any part of the nervous system. In the brain, two clinical syndromes of late delayed radiation injury may occur. The first follows whole-brain irradiation either prophylactically or, in some patients, for primary and metastatic brain tumors. The disorder is characterized either by dementia alone or by dementia with gait abnormalities and incontinence. Cerebral atrophy may occur alone or with diffuse white matter hyperintensity on MRI scans. Ventricular shunting may improve symptoms in some patients. The second disorder, radionecrosis, affects patients who receive either focal brain irradiation during therapy for extracranial neoplasms or irradiation for intracranial neoplasms. Neurologic signs suggest a tumor and include headache, focal or generalized seizures, and hemiparesis. MRI reveals a hypointense mass, sometimes with contrast enhancement. Neuropathologic features include coagulative necrosis of white matter, telangiectasia, fibrinoid necrosis of blood vessels with thrombus formation, glial proliferation, and bizarre multinucleated astrocytes. The clinical and imaging findings cannot be distinguished from those of brain tumor, and the diagnosis can be made only by biopsy. Positron emission tomography with radiolabeled glucose usually shows decreased metabolism in areas of radiation damage, whereas most malignant tumors show increased metabolism. Corticosteroids sometimes ameliorate the symptoms. Improvement in symptoms may be sustained even after corticosteroid withdrawal; however, if symptoms recur, the treatment of radionecrosis, if focal, is surgical removal.

Late delayed myelopathy is characterized by progressive paralysis, sensory changes, and sometimes pain. A Brown-Séquard syndrome (weakness and loss of proprioception in the extremities of

Table 195-3 ■ RADIATION INJURY TO THE NERVOUS SYSTEM

TIME AFTER RADIATION THERAPY	ORGAN AFFECTED	CLINICAL FINDINGS
Primary injury		
Immediate (minutes to hours)	Brain	Acute encephalopathy
Early delayed (6–16 wk)	Brain	Somnolence, focal signs
	Spinal cord	Lhermitte's sign
Late delayed (months to years)	Brain	Dementia, focal signs
	Spinal cord	Transverse myelopathy
	Peripheral nerves	Paralysis, sensory loss
Secondary injury (years)	Several	Brain, cranial and/or peripheral nerve sheath tumor
	Arteries (atherosclerosis)	Cerebral infarction
	Small vessel telangiectasia	Cerebral or spinal hemorrhage
	Endocrine organs	Metabolic encephalopathy

one side accompanied by loss of pain and temperature sensation on the other) is often present at onset. Patients occasionally respond transiently to steroids, and the disorder may stop progressing; generally, however, patients become paraplegic or quadriplegic. Pathologic changes include necrosis of the spinal cord. *Late delayed neuropathy* may affect any cranial or peripheral nerve. Common disorders are blindness from optic neuropathy and paralysis of an upper extremity from brachial plexopathy after therapy for lung or breast cancer. The pathogenesis is probably fibrosis and ischemia of the plexus. No treatment is available.

Radiation-induced tumors, including meningiomas, sarcomas, or less commonly, gliomas, may appear years to decades after cranial irradiation and may follow low-dose irradiation. Malignant or atypical nerve sheath tumors may follow irradiation of the brachial, cervical, and lumbar plexuses. The central nervous system may also be damaged when radiation alters extraneural structures. Radiation therapy accelerates atherosclerosis, and cerebral infarction associated with carotid artery occlusion in the neck may occur many years after neck irradiation. Endocrine (pituitary, thyroid, parathyroid) dysfunction from radiation may be associated with neurologic signs. Hypothyroidism is often manifested as a neurologic disorder, and hyperthyroidism or hyperparathyroidism from radiation may also cause an encephalopathy.

Keime-Guibert F, Napolitano M, Delattre JY: Neurological complications of radiotherapy and chemotherapy. J Neurol 245(11): 695, 1998. *A comprehensive review.*
Nathanson L, Hall TC: Paraneoplastic syndromes. Semin Oncol 24:265, 1997. *An entire issue devoted to paraneoplastic syndromes, including those involving the nervous system.*
Peterson K, Rottenberg DA: Radiation damage to the brain. *In* Vecht CJ (ed): Handbook of Clinical Neurology, vol 67. Amsterdam, Elsevier, 1997, pp 325–352. *Comprehensive review of nervous system radiation changes.*
Posner JB: Neurologic Complications of Cancer. Philadelphia, FA Davis, 1995. *Comprehensive chapters on radiation damage to the central and peripheral nervous systems (Chapter 13) and paraneoplastic syndromes (Chapter 15).*

196 NONMETASTATIC EFFECTS OF CANCER: THE SKIN

Frank Parker

Cutaneous changes associated with internal malignant conditions are diverse. Some of these skin alterations are clear indicators of underlying malignant disease. Others, less specific, arise in either the presence or absence of malignancy, but occur with sufficient frequency to arouse suspicion and require a search for underlying carcinomas or lymphomas. These various skin findings may precede signs of the internal malignancy; they are therefore of crucial importance in early identification and cure of internal neoplasms.

Skin manifestations of internal malignancy can be classified into two groups: (1) those in which malignant cells are found in the skin on biopsy (specific skin lesions) and (2) those in which malignant cells cannot be identified in a skin biopsy (non-specific skin lesions). The specific lesions are diagnostic of the internal neoplasm, whereas non-specific skin alterations may or may not be associated with a neoplasm. Some non-specific skin changes are clear indicators of underlying tumor. Others merely alert the physician to the possibility of serious internal problems.

SPECIFIC SKIN LESIONS ASSOCIATED WITH INTERNAL MALIGNANT DISEASE

Carcinomas, leukemias, lymphomas, plasma cell dyscrasias, and sarcoma can affect the skin specifically in clinically identifiable patterns. A skin biopsy of the lesions is diagnostic because the tissue of origin of the primary underlying neoplasm can be identified.

NON-SPECIFIC SKIN LESIONS ASSOCIATED WITH INTERNAL MALIGNANT DISEASE

Malignant cells are not seen in the skin in a wide variety of cutaneous associations of internal malignancy (Table 196–1). The pathogenesis of these disparate skin reactions is obscure. Often the only evidence that malignancy and cutaneous changes are related is the observation that following removal of the tumor, the skin change subsides or resolves and may subsequently become exacerbated if the neoplasm recurs. Skin manifestations may coincide with, antedate, or follow the clinical diagnosis of internal malignant disease.

Although non-specific skin reactions are suggestive of underlying malignancy, they are more frequently seen with non-malignant conditions. When these skin changes are observed, therefore, an internal neoplasm is only one of several possibilities in the differential diagnosis.

Non-specific skin manifestations can be considered under two major categories: (1) skin changes common to many skin diseases, including internal malignancies, and (2) syndromes and entities commonly associated with internal neoplasia.

Skin Changes Common to Many Skin Conditions, Including Internal Malignancy

Pruritus, or itching, unassociated with skin changes except for secondary lesions such as excoriations or prurigo-like papules, may be an important clue to various internal malignant and pre-malignant diseases, especially lymphomatous conditions. Hodgkin's disease, lymphocytic leukemia, polycythemia vera (in which pruritus often occurs or intensifies after exposure to heat), myeloid metaplasia, carcinoid, and less commonly, carcinomas cause itching. In Hodgkin's disease, itching is usually continuous and may be localized to the feet and lower part of the body, only later to become centralized. Up to 30% of patients with Hodgkin's disease may itch. Pruritus occurring with carcinoma is generally not as severe or intolerable as it is with lymphomas. Carcinomas of the gastrointestinal tract, lung, ovary, and prostate may also be associated with itching that may precede recognition of the cancer by a year.

Table 196–1 ■ NON-SPECIFIC SKIN LESIONS ASSOCIATED WITH INTERNAL MALIGNANCIES

Skin Lesions Common to Many Skin Conditions, Including Internal Malignancy
Pruritus
Erythroderma
Figurate erythemas
Urticarial-like lesions
Herpes zoster
Paraneoplastic pemphigus
Syndromes and Entities Commonly Associated with Internal Malignancy
Non-genetic syndromes
  High incidence of association with internal malignancy
    Paget's disease
    Stewart-Treves syndrome
    Acanthosis nigricans
    Dermatomyositis
    Leser-Trélat syndrome
    Bazex's syndrome
    Pulmonary osteoarthropathy
    Carcinoid syndrome
    Lymphomatoid papulosis
  Low incidence of association with malignancy
    Sweet's syndrome
    Amyloid
    Urticaria pigmentosa and mastocytosis syndrome
    Bowen's disease
Genetic syndromes
  High incidence of association with malignancy
    Torres' syndrome
    Gardner's syndrome
    Cowden syndrome
    Multiple endocrine neoplasia IIB
    Ataxia-telangiectasia
  Low incidence of association with malignancy
    Neurofibroma
    Peutz-Jeghers syndrome
    Basal cell carcinoma nevus syndrome
    Bloom's syndrome

Although dry skin (xerosis) is the most common cause of pruritus (especially in the elderly as a result of winter weather and excessive bathing), other systemic causes in addition to malignant disease include drug reactions, cholestatic liver disease, uremia, diabetes, thyroid disease, and emotional problems.

Erythroderma, or exfoliative dermatitis, is a cutaneous reaction with redness, edema, scaling, and lichenification. In 10% of cases it is associated with malignancy, especially lymphomas, leukemia, and mycosis fungoides. In clinical practice the usual cause of erythroderma is either a drug reaction or a generalized exacerbation of a pre-existing dermatosis such as atopic eczema, psoriasis, or contact dermatitis. When it is due to malignant disease, erythroderma is most pathognomonic of Hodgkin's disease, less frequently seen with lymphocytic leukemia, and rarely associated with underlying solid tumor (stomach, liver, lung, prostate, thyroid). Erythroderma may be the first sign of Hodgkin's disease or leukemia. It is to be stressed that skin biopsies in these instances do not reveal lymphomatous or leukemic infiltrates, although the patients appear clinically identical to those with Sézary syndrome (in which skin biopsies display diagnostic cutaneous T-cell lymphoma with Sézary cells). Lymphadenopathy and hepatosplenomegaly are more important clues to the underlying lymphoma or leukemia. Erythroderma and itching improve or resolve with treatment and remission of the lymphoma or leukemia.

Figurate erythemas are red, persistent, gyrate, serpiginous, and annular bands with a fine trailing scale that take on a pattern of wood grain; they have been given descriptive names such as erythema gyratum repens and erythema annulare centrifugum. The lesions, which persist and expand over large areas of the skin, have been associated with breast, stomach, bladder, prostate, cervix, tongue, and uterine cancer. Dramatic to moderate improvement occurs when the cancer is successfully treated.

Urticarial-like lesions, or flesh-colored to red pruritic papules, nodules, and wheal-like plaques, at times accompany leukemia and are called leukemids. They may precede the development of leukemia by many months, and biopsy of the lesions does not show malignant cells. Treatment and control of the leukemic process often result in resolution of the skin lesions.

Herpes zoster occurs with considerable frequency, especially with lymphomas (Hodgkin's disease), chronic lymphocytic leukemia, and a variety of neoplasms that are being managed with chemotherapy. Zoster and carcinoma, primarily breast cancer, are also linked. The painful, unilateral, grouped, clear, and often hemorrhagic umbilicated vesicles develop in a dermatomal distribution. About 1 week after the initial dermatomal outbreak, widespread vesicles on a red base ("dew drops on a rose petal"—as seen in varicella) can disseminate widely throughout the body, especially in patients who are immunosuppressed because of an underlying malignancy or chemotherapy. As a result, patients with destructive varicella lesions, disseminated disease, and a prolonged course need to be investigated for underlying neoplasia.

Paraneoplastic pemphigus is a recently recognized condition with persistent, painful erosions of the oropharynx, vermilion border of the lips, and conjunctivae, as well as cutaneous pemphigus-like superficial intraepidermal bullae and non-healing erosions. Target lesions suggestive of erythema multiforme are seen on the extremities. Biopsy shows lesions identical to pemphigus vulgaris: suprabasilar intraepidermal acantholysis and IgG deposition on the surface of the epidermal cells on direct immunofluorescence. Patients have circulating autoantibodies that not only react against the tumor tissue but also cross-react with similar antigens found in the epidermal cell junction of normal skin. Underlying neoplasms related to this syndrome are most commonly T-cell and B-cell lymphomas, benign and malignant thymomas, chronic lymphatic leukemia, sarcomas, and Waldenström's macroglobulinemia.

A number of miscellaneous dermatoses have been associated with internal malignancies, but it is not entirely clear whether these associations are real or fortuitous. Table 196–2 lists some of these associations.

Syndromes and Entities Involving the Skin and Internal Malignancies

A number of unique cutaneous syndromes are associated with internal neoplasms with sufficient frequency to alert the clinician to look for these tumors when they are potentially curable. Some

Table 196–2 ■ **DERMATOSES ASSOCIATED WITH INTERNAL MALIGNANT DISEASE**

DERMATOSES	ASSOCIATED NEOPLASM
Bullous lesions: pemphigus, pemphigoid, dermatitis herpetiformis	Rectal, breast, larynx, lymphoma
Tylosis: palmar hyperkeratoses	Esophagus
Acquired ichthyosis	Gastrointestinal leiomyosarcoma, lymphoma, multiple myeloma
Acquired hypertrichosis lanuginosa (malignant down)	Breast, uterine, pancreatic, lung, gastrointestinal cancers and lymphomas
Generalized hyperpigmentation	ACTH-secreting tumors—pancreas, ovary, colon, breast, thyroid
Gynecomastia	Bronchogenic carcinoma, hepatoma
Cutaneous-systemic angiitis	Lymphomas, leukemia, colon, breast, lung, prostate cancers

ACTH = adrenocorticotropic hormone.

syndromes are non-genetic and others are genetic in origin. Certain skin lesions have a high prevalence of associated neoplasia, whereas in others the prevalence is low.

Non-Genetic Syndromes and Entities with Skin Changes Associated with Internal Malignancy

CUTANEOUS LESIONS ASSOCIATED WITH A HIGH PREVALENCE OF INTERNAL MALIGNANCY. *Paget's disease* of the breast is characterized by erythematous scaling or weeping, sharply marginated, eczematous patches on the nipple extending to the areola. A breast mass may not be palpable or may not even be found with mammography, but in virtually every case an underlying cancer is found. The lesion mimics eczema, which improves with topical therapy; any eczematous lesion on the nipple that does not respond to topical steroids should undergo biopsy, which shows diagnostic pathologic changes. Paget's disease can also be found in the anogenital area (extramammary Paget's disease). In this disorder, eczematous, pruritic, crusted, lichenified, well-demarcated patches may involve the lower part of the abdomen, inguinal regions, genitalia, or perianal area. The color of the lesions varies from red to whitish gray. Patients are usually older than 50 years, and an underlying carcinoma of the rectum, prostate, urethra, other parts of the genitourinary tract, or apocrine glands is found in up to 50%. The most common sites of metastasis, when present, are regional inguinal and pelvic lymph nodes, bone, liver, lung, brain, and bladder. Biopsy samples taken from patients with mammary and extramammary Paget's disease show the same diagnostic features, namely, large, round cells with clear cytoplasm in the epidermis (Paget's cells).

Stewart-Treves syndrome is the occasional occurrence of a lymphangiosarcoma as a complication of chronic lymphedema of the arm after radical mastectomy for carcinoma of the breast. Angiomatous, livid, or dusky red blobs and nodules may evolve 2 to 20 years following the onset of postoperative lymphedema. Angiosarcoma has also developed in congenital lymphedema, as well as in lymphedema of the legs following surgery for cervical cancer.

Acanthosis nigricans (see color Plate 14*A*) is characterized by soft, velvety, verrucous, brown hyperpigmentation with skin tags in the body folds, especially those of the neck, axilla, and groin. When it occurs in patients older than 40 years, it is often a sign of an underlying malignant tumor, usually adenocarcinoma (most often of the stomach, gastrointestinal tract, and uterus; less commonly of the ovary, prostate, breast, and lung; and rarely lymphoma). Acanthosis nigricans involving the tongue and oral mucosa is highly suggestive of an underlying neoplasm. In 80% of cases, the cancer is abdominal; in 60% of cases, the cancer is found in the stomach. Special concern must be given to non-obese adults in whom pigmented verrucous areas have recently developed in the body folds; in 80 to 90%, an underlying gastric cancer is present. Of patients with acanthosis and malignancy, the skin abnormalities precede the appearance of the neoplasm in 20% of cases. The skin findings often regress following successful antitumor therapy and reappear with recurrence of the tumor, which suggests that the underlying tumor secretes an unidentified substance that is responsible for the verrucoid skin lesions. Acanthosis nigricans is more commonly found in individuals younger than 40 years, in whom it is not usually associated with malignancy but rather with obesity, a familial occurrence, or a variety of endocrinopathies (Cushing's disease, acromegaly, polycystic ovaries, hypothyroidism, hyperthyroidism, and insulin-resistant diabetes).

Dermatomyositis (see Color Plate 14*B*) is recognized by proximal muscle pain and weakness and a characteristic dermatitis that includes a heliotrope rash (edematous, violaceous, telangiectatic discoloration of the eyelids) along with a violaceous, erythematous, telangiectatic scaling rash on the cheeks, forehead, V of the neck, elbows, and knees. Gottron's papules, slightly elevated, red to violaceous plaques over the knuckles, are also an important finding. In individuals older than 40 years, the prevalence of internal carcinoma, primarily breast and lung tumors, is increased (see Chapter 296). Not uncommonly, the dermatomyositis resolves on removal of the carcinoma, but it may recur if the tumor reappears. In some instances, the dermatomyositis precedes the cancer by several years. Neoplasm should be especially suspected if the dermatomyositis does not respond to conventional therapy, if the patient has a history of previous malignant disease, or if atypical symptoms of dermatomyositis are present.

The Leser-Trélat sign, or the sudden or eruptive appearance or increase in size of multiple seborrheic keratoses, occurs with underlying cancer in the elderly. This sign has been the subject of controversy because seborrheic keratoses are common in the elderly, as are cancers, so their simultaneous occurrence may not have any relationship. Nevertheless, several case reports have described new and enlarging keratoses in association with cancer of the lung, adenocarcinoma of the bowel, mycosis fungoides, and Sézary syndrome; in some of these patients, the keratoses regressed when the malignant tumor was treated.

Lymphomatoid papulosis is an uncommon condition of cutaneous lymphoid infiltration clinically characterized by involuting and recurring purplish red papules, plaques, and nodules. In 10 to 20% of patients the condition develops or evolves into a cutaneous T-cell lymphoma or Hodgkin's disease. Based on histologic features, lymphomatoid papulosis has been divided in two types: type A lesions contain large anaplastic tumor cells, whereas type B lesions have cerebriform mononuclear cells and epidermotropism indistinguishable from the changes seen in mycosis fungoides. In some patients, both histologic types are seen even within the same lesions. The lesions may wax and wane, and lymphoma does not develop in most patients. Unfortunately, no single clinical or pathologic feature distinguishes lymphomatoid papulosis from lymphoma. At onset, however, the presence of skin lesions larger than 3 cm in diameter, persistence without spontaneous regression, lymphadenopathy, and systemic symptoms (fever, weight loss) are suggestive of lymphoma. Later in the disease course, multiple, rapidly growing lesions that fail to regress spontaneously or become resistant to therapy (such as psoralen plus ultraviolet A or low-dose methotrexate) usually signal transformation to lymphoma.

Necrolytic migratory erythema associated with α-cell tumors of the pancreas and elevated glucagon levels evolves as enlarging erythematous patches with central, superficial blister formation progressing to central crusting and healing. Annular lesions result, with exudative, erosive areas most pronounced in the perineum, groin, and perioral areas. The legs, feet, and hands may be involved, and painful glossitis, angular cheilitis, anemia, weight loss, and diarrhea are often seen. The rash and glossitis resolve rapidly after the tumor is removed.

Bazex's syndrome, or acrokeratosis paraneoplastica, is a unique marker of carcinomas of the upper respiratory tract, especially squamous cell carcinomas of the oral, pharyngeal, laryngeal, esophageal, and bronchial tissues, primarily in males. When the tumor is asymptomatic, red to violaceous, scaling, eczematous, and psoriasiform patches are found over the nose, fingers, toes, and margins of the ear helices. The nail folds are red, scaling, and tender, with grooving of the nails and onycholysis. Later, the acral lesions become more extensive and spread from the digits to the palms and soles, which in turn become red and scaling and form a honeycomb-like thickening. The fingers and toes become violaceous and bulbous. In a still later stage, if the tumor has not been treated, new scaling lesions resembling psoriasis spread over the face,

trunk, knees, arms, and scalp, with extensive nail dystrophy. In the majority of cases, cutaneous lesions improve significantly if the underlying neoplasm is successfully treated.

Clubbing of the fingers is a significant sign of underlying bronchogenic carcinoma, mesothelioma, metastatic carcinoma to the thorax (from the colon, larynx, breast, or ovary), and occasionally, Hodgkin's disease. *Hypertrophic pulmonary osteoarthropathy* is new bone formation along the shafts of the long bones of the extremities and digits. Joints of the ankles, knees, wrists, and hands are swollen and painful. In some patients, cutaneous thickening of the legs and forearms produces enlargement of the limbs; facial features may become coarse with deep facial furrows simulating acromegaly, and deep confluent skin wrinkles evolve over the forehead and scalp, a condition termed *pachydermoperiostosis.*

Carcinoid (see Chapter 245), a malignant tumor of the chromaffin cells of the gastrointestinal tract and bronchus, may be associated with intermittent scarlet to red flushing of the head, neck, and upper part of the trunk. Eventually, the erythema becomes permanent, and telangiectasis and tortuous veins evolve in the flushed areas.

CUTANEOUS LESIONS ASSOCIATED WITH A LOW PREVALENCE OF MALIGNANCY. *Amyloid deposits* may occur in the skin without obvious cause (cutaneous amyloidosis) as part of an inherited syndrome or secondary to plasma cell dyscrasias—either primary systemic amyloidoses or multiple myeloma (see Chapter 297) In plasma cell dyscrasias, unique, shiny, translucent, waxy, firm, purpuric papules and plaques occur around the mucocutaneous junctions of the eyes, nose, and mouth. Occasionally, infiltrated papules are not apparent, and only purpuric lesions evolve around the eyes (raccoon eyes). Macroglossia is also common.

Urticaria pigmentosa consists of red-brown macules and papules on the trunk and extremities caused by the accumulation of mast cells in the dermis. Light stroking of the skin lesion causes urtication with edema and a red flare as a result of release of histamine from the mast cells infiltrating the skin (Darier's sign). Rarely, the skin lesions are found in association with systemic mastocytosis (mast cell infiltrates of the bone, liver, spleen, and lymph nodes—see Chapter 280) or, even less commonly, with mast cell leukemia or myeloproliferative disorders.

Bowen's disease of the skin consists of multiple, superficial squamous cell cancers over the non–sun-exposed areas of the body, particularly in individuals with a history of chronic exposure to arsenicals (drinking well water, exposure to insecticides or industrial arsenicals). Bowen's lesions appear as discreet, scaling, red, flat to elevated patches that mimic eczematous or psoriatic patches. The skin lesions should be removed to prevent progression to invasive squamous cell carcinoma and the possibility of metastasis. The relation of these lesions to internal malignancy is controversial, but cancers of the larynx, lung, esophagus, liver, and bladder should be considered.

Sweet's syndrome may be the harbinger of underlying myelogenous or lymphoblastic leukemia, hairy cell leukemia, lymphoma, and solid carcinoma (breast, stomach, lung, colon) in 25% of cases. The unique syndrome consists of painful, raised erythematous plaques with sterile vesicles or pustules studding the surface of the face, trunk, and extremities. Fever occurs in 80% of cases and is often accompanied by arthritis, leukocytosis, and an elevated sedimentation rate; however, no obvious underlying infection is apparent. Skin biopsy shows the same band-like infiltration with neutrophils in the upper dermis in patients with or without internal malignancy.

Genetic Syndromes Associated with Internal Malignant Disease

CUTANEOUS LESIONS ASSOCIATED WITH A HIGH PREVALENCE OF INTERNAL MALIGNANCY. *Gardner's syndrome* consists of multiple epidermal and sebaceous cysts of the face and scalp, fibrous tissue tumors of the skin (desmoid tumors, fibromas, and fibrosarcomas), osteoma of the membranous bones of the face and head, and polyps of the gastrointestinal tract. Adenocarcinomas of the bowel develop in most patients by the seventh decade.

Cowden's disease, a condition characterized by numerous hamartomas of the skin, mucous membranes, and internal organs, is associated with malignant neoplasms of the breast and thyroid in a high percentage of patients. The hamartomas occur on the skin as warty keratotic papules and nodules on the central part of the face (trichilemmomas) and on the hands and arms. Papular cobblestone lesions may appear on the gingiva, palate, tongue, nose, and larynx. Multiple lipomas and cavernous hemangiomas occur in half of the cases.

Torre's syndrome, another autosomal dominant condition, consists of multiple sebaceous gland tumors, sebaceous adenomas, sebaceous hyperplasia, and basal cell cancers with sebaceous differentiation. The skin lesions appear as yellow to red papules and nodules. Gastrointestinal and genitourinary carcinomas arise up to 30 years after the cutaneous lesions. In the majority of cases, the colon and rectum are the sites of internal malignancy, but other associated cancers are found in the esophagus, stomach, duodenum, ovary, kidney, bladder, prostate, testes, and ampulla of Vater.

Multiple endocrine neoplasia type IIB (see Chapter 244) consists of medullary carcinoma of the thyroid and pheochromocytoma in association with a marfanoid habitus and multiple whitish to pink papular mucosal neuromas studding the lips, tip of the tongue, buccal mucosa, gingivae, palate, and pharynx. Neuromas also develop on the conjunctivae and corneas; thickened corneal nerves may be found by slit-lamp examination.

Ataxia-telangiectasia, an autosomal recessive disorder associated with lymphomas, is recognized by telangiectases over the ears, eyelids, nose, butterfly area of the face, and conjunctivae in association with profound immunologic deficiency and sinopulmonary infections. Hodgkin's disease, non-Hodgkin's lymphoma, or leukemia develops in 10% of patients, with other neoplasms such as ovarian dysgerminomas, gliomas, medulloblastomas, and gastric adenocarcinomas occurring less frequently.

Persons with *Wiskott-Aldrich syndrome* also display a propensity to lymphomas (79%) or leukemias (13%) by the age of 10 years, probably related to the immunologic abnormalities of both the humoral and cell-mediated systems found in this condition. The skin changes are similar to atopic dermatitis.

CUTANEOUS LESIONS ASSOCIATED WITH A LOW PREVALENCE OF INTERNAL MALIGNANCY. Some autosomal dominantly inherited conditions are associated with internal malignancy, but the relationship is not frequently found. Thus patients with *neurofibromatosis* (see Chapter 522), who have café au lait spots, axillary freckles, and multiple neurofibromas, are prone to the development of pheochromocytomas (10% of the patients by the age of 60 years), acoustic neuromas, and neurofibrosarcomas.

Patients with *Peutz-Jeghers syndrome* have numerous brown-black macules on the lips, perioral regions, hands, and feet in association with hamartomatous polyps of the small bowel, stomach, and less commonly, the colon (see Chapter 139). Malignancy can occasionally develop in the polyps, pancreas, ovary, and testes.

Nevoid basal cell carcinoma syndrome can be associated with medulloblastomas and fibrosarcoma of the jaw, in addition to multiple basal cell skin cancers. *Bloom's syndrome* (telangiectatic redness of the skin in photoexposed areas and stunted growth) and *Chédiak-Higashi* syndrome (light coloration of the skin and hair) are autosomal recessive conditions associated with a propensity for leukemias and lymphomas.

Anhatt AJ: Paraneoplastic pemphigus. *In* Janes WD (ed): Advances in Dermatology, vol 12. St. Louis, CV Mosby, 1998, pp 77–96. *Excellent review and new information on a newly recognized condition.*
Braverman IM (ed): Skin Signs of Systemic Disease, 3rd ed. Philadelphia, WB Saunders, 1998. *A remarkably comprehensive review of all skin signs of systemic disease, including those related to underlying malignancies; extensive bibliography and referencing.*

197 NONMETASTATIC EFFECTS OF CANCER: OTHER SYSTEMS

Marc S. Ernstoff
Kenneth R. Meehan

In contrast to the direct effects that both primary and metastatic foci of malignancies may have on the body, paraneoplastic syn-

Table 197–1 ■ PARANEOPLASTIC SYNDROMES

Endocrine	See Chapter 194
Neurologic	See Chapter 195
Dermatologic and arthritic	See Chapter 196
Renal	Glomerular abnormalities, miscellaneous: amyloidosis, myeloma, kidney. See Chapter 106
Hematologic	Erythrocytosis, thrombocytosis, leukemoid reaction, anemia (chronic disease, aplastic anemia, microangiopathic hemolytic anemia), granulocytopenia, thrombocytopenia
Coagulation	Disseminated intravascular coagulation, superficial venous thromboembolism, marantic endocarditis, thrombotic microangiopathy
Miscellaneous	Hepatopathy, cancer-related cachexia, pulmonary osteoarthropathy

dromes (Table 197–1), which constitute signs and symptoms resulting from distant effects of the tumor on various body systems, can affect a variety of organ systems in addition to the endocrine system (see Chapter 194), the nervous system (see Chapter 195), and the skin (see Chapter 196). These indirect effects can be due to the tumor's production and release of growth factors, biologically active hormones, immune mechanisms (antigen-antibody reactions), or other unidentified substances. Many paraneoplastic syndromes are due to excessive production of hormones resulting in signs or symptoms indistinguishable from primary endocrine diseases. Successful treatment of the underlying malignancy is associated with dramatic improvement in the paraneoplastic syndrome.

The general approach to paraneoplastic syndromes requires careful diagnosis and therapy (Table 197–2). Diagnosing the presence of a paraneoplastic syndrome is critical because these syndromes generally parallel the course of the underlying malignancy. In some cases, signs and symptoms may precede the diagnosis of cancer or signal the recurrence of a prior malignancy. Paraneoplastic syndromes may cause signs and symptoms that can be confused with direct effects of the primary tumor or metastases, infection, toxicity of therapy, or co-morbid illnesses. Thus it is important that a correct diagnosis be made to permit the institution of appropriate cancer-directed treatment and symptomatic therapy. Most of these syndromes occur rarely (<15% of patients); however, if cachexia or anemia is included, the majority of cancer patients will demonstrate one or more of these findings.

CANCER-RELATED CACHEXIA

CLINICAL FEATURES. The clinical syndrome of cancer cachexia includes weight loss, anorexia, muscle atrophy, immune dysregulation (resulting in anergy), and sometimes organ atrophy as noted on post-mortem examination. These manifestations are related to the presence of the malignancy and may abate once treatment is initiated. These signs are often discovered before the diagnosis of cancer, which should prompt the physician to evaluate for an underlying malignancy. No correlation is seen between the presence or severity of these signs and the type of malignancy, the amount of disease, or sites of disease.

Table 197–2 ■ EVALUATION OF A PATIENT FOR PARANEOPLASTIC SYNDROMES

List and make a full description of the signs and symptoms.
Consider the pathophysiology of the signs and symptoms.
Create a differential diagnosis.
Perform appropriate clinical and laboratory tests to confirm the diagnosis.
If no underlying pathophysiology explains the signs and symptoms, consider paraneoplastic syndromes.
If signs and symptoms are consistent with a known paraneoplastic syndrome, undertake a search for an unknown primary cancer or recurrence or progression of a known primary tumor.
Perform appropriate clinical and laboratory tests, if available, to confirm a paraneoplastic syndrome.
Consider treatment of cancer and/or appropriate palliative treatment for paraneoplastic symptoms when possible.

PATHOPHYSIOLOGY. The etiologies of cancer-related cachexia are multifactorial and may be the result of cytokine release by the tumor, side effects of anticancer therapy (treatment-related nausea, vomiting), or an inability to eat or digest food because of physical abnormalities (gastrointestinal obstruction) or emotional difficulties (depression). Tumor necrosis factor α (TNF-α), also known as cachectin, is postulated to be the major cytokine released from macrophages that mediates this syndrome. Other potential cytokines include interleukin-1 (IL-1), IL-6, and interferon-γ (IFN-γ). The production and release of these cytokines cause an overall catabolic state. The resulting effects include increased protein turnover, increased rate of lipolysis, and inhibition of enzymes that promote the uptake of glucose into muscle and the liver. Simultaneously, endogenous glucose production is increased from hepatic gluconeogenesis.

DIAGNOSIS. The non-specific complaints and the absence of specific laboratory tests make the diagnosis difficult. The signs and symptoms in the appropriate clinical setting should prompt the physician to evaluate for a possible paraneoplastic etiology. It is important to note that a correlation is not always found between the TNF-α level and the clinical syndrome, and the resulting cachexia may be out of proportion to the size or extent of the underlying malignancy.

TREATMENT. Therapy is directed at the underlying malignancy, with supplemental alimentation when appropriate (e.g., surgical candidates or patients with a significant likelihood of response to treatment). Parenteral nutrition or nutritious supplements may be offered but are not often helpful because of the global systemic effects of this syndrome. High doses (400 to 800 mg/day of the liquid formulation) of the progestational hormone megestrol acetate can improve appetite in a significant percentage of cancer patients. Corticosteroids can also be considered.

CANCER-ASSOCIATED IMMUNOLOGIC DYSFUNCTION

CLINICAL FEATURES. Although not commonly thought of as a paraneoplastic syndrome, the impaired immune suppression observed in cancer patients is associated with tumor-associated immunosuppressive factors. Because of this immune dysregulation, actively treated cancer patients or patients with a history of a malignancy are at increased risk for the development of infections.

PATHOPHYSIOLOGY. Impaired cell-mediated immunity, as detected by the delayed-type hypersensitivity reaction, can be identified in patients with lymphoid and non-lymphoid malignancies, including patients with isolated brain tumors. Some of this impairment may be due to cytotoxic therapy, but a number of studies have documented this problem in patients with newly diagnosed cancer. In addition, despite eradication of the tumor, the immune defects may persist.

Immune abnormalities include a decrease in the number of T lymphocytes (with no effect on B-cell numbers) and impaired proliferative responses of lymphocytes. Some evidence suggests that cancer patients may generate suppressor T lymphocytes, further hindering the immune response, while simultaneously suppressing the cytotoxic activity of natural killer cells, lymphokine-activated killer cells, and cytotoxic T lymphocytes. Fas ligand has been identified in the serum of patients with cancer and may play a role in immunosuppression by down-regulating the toxicity of cytotoxic T lymphocytes. In general, humoral immunity often remains intact.

PARANEOPLASTIC HEMATOLOGIC DISORDERS

Paraneoplastic hematologic disorders can be quite diverse and include clotting or bleeding abnormalities, erythrocytosis, leukemoid reaction, and thrombocytosis.

ANEMIA OF MALIGNANCY. Anemia is seen in patients with cancer and may be secondary to chronic disease, red cell aplasia, bone marrow invasion, blood loss, chemotherapy, radiation therapy, nutritional deficiencies, or autoimmune or microangiopathic hemolysis. It is critical to determine whether the anemia is due to direct effects of the tumor or its treatment or whether it is secondary to a paraneoplastic syndrome. Pure red cell aplasia is most frequently associated with thymoma. Immune hemolytic anemia may be due to warm antibody–mediated hemolytic anemia (with 20% of cases observed in lymphoproliferative malignancies), cold agglutinin disease (as observed in the lymphomas), or hemolysis resulting from procoagulant substances released by mucin-producing adenocarcinomas such as ovarian or gastrointestinal malignancies. Chemotherapy may directly affect the marrow or, in the case of cisplatin, cause a reduction in endogenous erythropoietin production. Treatment of chemotherapy-induced anemia with recombinant erythropoietin is successful in 30 to 40% of cases.

The cause of the hypoproliferative anemia of malignancy is unknown. Postulated mechanisms include a shortened red blood cell lifespan, suppressed or hypoproliferative bone marrow, or impaired iron utilization by the hematopoietic system. A novel protein called anemia-inducing substance alters osmotic resistance in red blood cells and may therefore shorten red blood cell survival. A hypoproliferative bone marrow may be due to the reduced levels of erythropoietin found in many cancer patients, although a reduced erythropoietin level does not always correlate with the degree of bone marrow hypoproliferation. In vitro studies show that various cytokines produced by tumors, especially IL-1 and TNF-α, inhibit mRNA synthesis of erythropoietin. As a result, erythropoietin secretion and production are inhibited, and hematopoietic cells in the bone marrow have a decreased response to erythropoietin. Finally, IL-1 and TNF-α, as well as IFN-γ, IL-6, and transforming growth factor β, have been implicated in the hindrance of iron metabolism.

COAGULATION ABNORMALITIES. CLINICAL FEATURES. The interaction of components of the coagulation cascade and tumor cells is intricate and complex and could result in thrombotic or hemorrhagic tendencies. Systemic activation of coagulation may result in disseminated intravascular coagulation, superficial venous thromboembolism (Trousseau's syndrome), marantic endocarditis, or thrombotic microangiopathy. Although abnormal coagulation parameters are frequently observed in patients with cancer, the relationship to clotting or bleeding abnormalities is often unrelated and the significance unknown. Malignancies prominently associated with coagulation abnormalities include adenocarcinomas (particularly mucin-secreting carcinomas) and acute promyelocytic leukemia.

PATHOPHYSIOLOGY. Tumor cells may release procoagulant materials such as tissue factor–like substances that activate Factor X, the sialic acid portion of secreted mucin, or "thromboplastin-like" substances. Tumor procoagulants include tissue factor and cancer procoagulant. Tissue factor can serve as a cofactor to Factor VIIa for the activation of Factor X, whereas cancer procoagulant directly activates Factor X without a need for Factor VII. Tumor cells can release adenosine diphosphate, which activates platelets and thereby results in adhesion and aggregation and also stimulates monocyte/macrophage release of cytokines, especially TNF-α, that will act as procoagulants. Tumor cells can also secrete cytokines, including IL-1 and TNF-α, that induce normal endothelial cells to express tissue factor, as well as stimulate TNF-α production by monocytes. The end result is the formation of a clot while stimulating platelet–tumor cell interaction.

DIAGNOSIS. Although controversy exists concerning the relationship of an occult malignancy and thrombosis, about 10% of patients with a new thrombotic event will subsequently be found to have cancer. Signs or symptoms suggestive of underlying malignancy and the presence of migratory or recurrent thrombophlebitis should precipitate a search for an occult malignancy, especially in patients with recurrent or migratory venous thrombosis affecting unusual sites such as subclavian veins or the veins of the upper extremities, axilla, or neck. The evaluation should include a careful history, physical examination, and routine laboratory tests (including blood counts, serum chemistries, urinalysis, chest radiograph, mammogram, stool for occult blood), in addition to aggressive pursuit of any abnormalities revealed by this screening evaluation. It is important to exclude inherited clotting disorders, such as Factor V Leiden abnormalities or deficiencies of protein C, protein S, and antithrombin III, dysfibrinogenemia, and plasminogen deficiency, which may appear in young patients (i.e., aged 20 to 40 years) and can result in recurrent thrombosis in unusual locations (see Chapter 187).

TREATMENT. Anticoagulant therapy should be initiated in a cancer patient cautiously and only after careful consideration because such patients may have an increased tendency for hemorrhage from a tumor invading blood vessels or the presence of central nervous system metastasis. Other causes of coagulation abnormalities need to be excluded, including sepsis, hemolytic-uremic syndrome, acidosis, or hypoxemia. The most effective therapy is treatment of the underlying disease. Generally, the coagulation abnormalities will be corrected if the underlying tumor responds to cytotoxic therapy. Acute symptomatic relief can sometimes be achieved with heparin, occasionally in combination with fresh-frozen plasma to provide clotting factors and cryoprecipitate (to maintain a plasma fibrinogen level of 150 to 200 mg/dL). Chronic therapy may include warfarin or low-molecular-weight heparin as an outpatient, although the long-term prognosis is dependent on the primary tumor's response to cytotoxic therapy. Experience with the use of aspirin and dipyridamole has been minimal.

PARANEOPLASTIC LEUKEMOID REACTION. Leukemoid reactions are defined as a peripheral white blood cell count of greater than 20,000 cells/mm³ without evidence of infection or leukemia. The white blood cell count is generally shifted to the left, with mature neutrophils representing the majority of cells. These high white cell counts are asymptomatic. Paraneoplastic leukemoid reaction can occur in patients with solid tumors or hematologic malignancies and can be associated with fever; it should be differentiated from leukoerythroblastosis secondary to malignant involvement of the bone marrow. Granulocyte-colony stimulating factor production has been observed in a number of malignancies (malignant fibrous histiocytoma, nasopharyngeal carcinoma, transitional cell carcinoma of the urinary bladder) and is probably the cause of paraneoplastic leukemoid reaction. Other colony-stimulating factors that may contribute include granulocyte-macrophage, macrophage, and IL-3. Clinically, the diagnosis of paraneoplastic leukemoid reaction is made by exclusion of a primary hematologic malignancy such as chronic myelogenous leukemia (see Chapter 176), which is associated with splenomegaly, basophilia, and a left shift of the white blood cells with an increase in all early myeloid progenitors. Treatment of paraneoplastic leukemoid reaction involves therapy directed at the underlying malignancy.

CANCER-ASSOCIATED ERYTHROCYTOSIS. (See Chapter 174) The liver and kidney normally produce erythropoietin. As a result, malignancies involving these organs may result in erythrocytosis. Cancer-associated erythrocytosis is most frequently seen in malignant and benign conditions of the kidney (renal cell carcinoma, Wilms' tumor, cystic kidney, and hydronephrosis) or the liver (hepatoma). Cerebellar hemangioblastoma is another etiology. Pheochromocytomas, uterine fibroids, sarcomas, and aldosterone-secreting tumors are also associated with cancer-associated erythrocytosis. This paraneoplastic syndrome is associated with increased levels of endogenous erythropoietin in 50% or fewer of patients; in some cases, cancer-associated erythrocytosis may be secondary to the overproduction of androgens, prostaglandins, and other, yet unidentified substances. Treatment of the underlying tumor will result in beneficial effects on the cancer-associated erythrocytosis.

CANCER-ASSOCIATED THROMBOCYTOSIS. (See Chapter 174) A true paraneoplastic cancer-associated thrombocytosis is seen in patients with Hodgkin's disease, non-Hodgkin's lymphoma, leukemias, and other solid malignancies and may be related to the overproduction of thrombopoietin(s). This condition must be differentiated from a primary hematologic disorder such as a myeloproliferative disorder (chronic myelogenous leukemia or primary thrombocythemia) or a secondary cause (chronic inflammation, severe iron deficiency, acute bleeding, or post-splenectomy status). Treatment of the malignancy will generally result in a decrease in the platelet count. Despite the elevated platelet count, secondary thrombocytosis is not generally associated with clinical evidence of thrombotic or bleeding disorders.

RENAL PARANEOPLASTIC SYNDROMES

Nephrotic syndrome in the setting of malignancy can be due to direct kidney involvement by the cancer, renal vein thrombosis, or a paraneoplastic syndrome. Paraneoplastic nephrotic syndrome usually improves dramatically when the underlying malignancy is successfully treated. Paraneoplastic nephrotic syndrome is most commonly seen in association with Hodgkin's disease and is usually characterized by lipoid nephrosis (minimal glomerular nephrosis),

which may be caused by deficient T-lymphocyte function. Other glomerular lesions, which occur in approximately 20% of cases of paraneoplastic nephrotic syndrome, include membranous glomerulopathy, focal sclerosis, and membranoproliferative glomerulonephritis and may be associated with non-Hodgkin's lymphoma, colon cancer, bronchogenic carcinoma, and prostate cancer. Deposition of tumor-associated antigen-antibody complexes can cause membranous glomerulonephritis.

MISCELLANEOUS PARANEOPLASTIC SYNDROMES

PARANEOPLASTIC HEPATOPATHY. Paraneoplastic hepatopathy, also known as Stauffer's syndrome, is characterized by hepatic dysfunction, fever, and weight loss and is most commonly seen in non-metastatic renal cell carcinoma. The cause of Stauffer's syndrome is uncertain but probably involves an autoimmune process directed at hepatic cells or substances released by the tumor that result in elevated liver enzymes and hepatic dysfunction.

Patients often have fever and weight loss, in addition to hepatomegaly, elevated aminotransferase levels, and poor liver synthesizing ability (indicated by an elevated prothrombin time). Hematologic abnormalities such as thrombocytosis may also exist. A liver biopsy may reveal Kupffer cell hyperplasia with fairly nonspecific inflammatory changes.

In the presence of non-metastatic hypernephroma, treatment directed at the primary lesion generally results in resolution of the syndrome. Surgical resection of the primary tumor has also been reported to reverse the liver abnormalities. If signs or symptoms persist, an evaluation for metastatic disease should be initiated.

PULMONARY OSTEOARTHROPATHY. Pulmonary osteoarthropathy consists of symmetrical clubbing of the nails, active synovitis, and periosteal inflammation of the long bones (often manifested as "arthritis" of the elbows, wrists, knees, or ankles). Pulmonary osteoarthropathy can precede the diagnosis of cancer by months; it is generally observed with lung carcinoma (non–small cell lung histology) but has also been described with metastatic lung lesions, non-pulmonary malignancies, and a number of non-malignant conditions.

PATHOPHYSIOLOGY. The development of pulmonary osteoarthropathy may be based on two components: a neurogenic vascular component and a humorally mediated osteogenic element. The bilateral nature of the disease suggests a cytokine-mediated component. Vagotomy will partially reverse some symptoms, thus supporting the neurogenic vascular etiology. Other possible etiologies include an immune-mediated response or release of growth factor(s) by the tumor.

The classic triad of clubbing, synovitis, and periostitis may appear at different times in the clinical course. Although the joints of the lower extremities may be painful, red, and swollen, physical examination may reveal that the "arthritis" is discomfort caused by pain in the adjacent long bone, especially the distal ends of the radius/ulna and tibia/fibula. Plain radiographs may reveal the periosteal elevations. Bone scans appear to be more sensitive than plain radiographs and may confirm the diagnosis. Pulmonary osteoarthropathy can be differentiated from metastatic bone disease or rheumatoid arthritis by the symmetrical bilateral findings and the absence of rheumatoid factor.

The presence of pulmonary osteoarthropathy does not alter the patient's prognosis. Because pulmonary osteoarthropathy is not life threatening, treatment is often palliative. Arthritic symptoms may be treated with aspirin and/or non-steroidal anti-inflammatory drugs. Vagotomy often results in analgesia within days to weeks. Atropine may also be helpful. Surgery of the primary malignancy may improve the articular complaints, sometimes within hours. Chemotherapy or radiotherapy may provide a gradual beneficial effect.

Dalmau JO, Posner JB. Paraneoplastic syndromes. Arch Neurol 56:405, 1999. *Review of recent advances in the pathophysiology of paraneoplastic nervous system disorders.*

Maesaka JK, Mittal SK, Fishbones S: Paraneoplastic syndromes of the kidney. Semin Oncol 24:373, 1997. *A comprehensive review.*

Walther MM, Johnson B, Culley D, et al: Serum interleukin-6 levels in metastatic renal cell carcinoma before treatment with interleukin-2 correlates with paraneoplastic syndromes but not patient survival. J Urol 159:178, 1998.

198 PRINCIPLES OF CANCER THERAPY

Joseph R. Bertino ■ *Sydney E. Salmon*

The development of effective anticancer drugs has progressively integrated medical management with surgery and radiation therapy in the multimodal treatment of cancer. The development of new cytotoxic and endocrine agents and the introduction of biologic therapy based on recombinant synthesis of interferons and cytokines have expanded medical management, as has the treatment of the complications of cancer. The physician also must be familiar with palliative aspects of cancer care, including management of pain (see Chapter 27) and treatment of life-threatening complications (see Chapter 199).

Although current systemic therapy can cure few forms of metastatic cancer, it is now increasingly effective as a component of multimodal management of apparently localized cancers known to have a high frequency of occult micrometastatic spread. This approach is predicated on the availability of specific systemic agents with antitumor activity in advanced cancers of the same histopathology. Not all patients are candidates for attempts at cancer therapy because of limitations in available drugs or co-morbidity from other medical problems. To a significant extent, cancer is a disease of the elderly, and treatment for many types of cancer in patients older than the age of 65 remains difficult because of the reduced host tolerance to the toxicities of many cancer chemotherapeutic agents. Patients and families must be fully informed about the nature of planned treatment, whether curative or palliative in intent. Inasmuch as prognosis for individual patients is currently based on statistical estimates, the physician must evaluate each patient individually in relation to relevant prognostic factors in attempting to develop a treatment plan.

DEVELOPMENT OF A TREATMENT PLAN

The major clinical features of cancer to be considered in developing a treatment plan include (1) specific histologic diagnosis of the neoplasm, (2) tumor burden and extent of specific organ involvement (stage), and (3) biologic characteristics and other prognostic factors relevant to the specific type of cancer.

DIAGNOSIS. Accurate histologic diagnosis and staging critically influence treatment selection. Increasingly, immunohistochemical analysis helps in subtyping lymphomas and distinguishing among various morphologically "undifferentiated" neoplasms (see Chapter 200). Tumors of diverse histogenesis can have markedly different prognosis and treatment. Electron microscopy sometimes can help by identifying specific morphologic features such as melanosomes (in melanoma) or desmosomes (in carcinomas) that permit more specific classification. Other distinctive biologic markers include immunohistochemistry (e.g., overexpression of cyclin D in mantle cell lymphoma), hormone receptor expression, serum or urinary tumor markers (e.g., β-human chorionic gonadotropin, α-fetoprotein, carcinoembryonic antigen, CA-125, myeloma proteins, urinary 5-hydroxyindole acetic acid), karyotype, or molecular analysis. Increasingly, molecular biologic methods for DNA analysis are also playing a role in diagnosis by identifying characteristic gene rearrangements (e.g., Southern blots), gene deletions, or oncogene expression. Cellular proto-oncogene amplification and expression have been linked to the pathogenesis of various neoplasms (see Chapter 191). Recently identified genes regulate the cell cycle and provide "checkpoints" when damage to DNA occurs. Determination of the status of the products of the *p53* and retinoblastoma genes is becoming increasingly important in assessing tumor biology and prognosis, because tumors with mutant or null *p53* and lacking a functional retinoblastoma protein may have a poor prognosis.

In the leukemias and lymphomas, such information can prove important for selecting appropriate treatment approaches. For example, the approach to treatment of T-cell or B-cell lymphomas dif-

fers as a function of cell lineage, which often cannot be identified with standard histologic approaches. Specialized studies can in some instances provide evidence for a treatable or curable form of cancer that might otherwise go unrecognized.

STAGING. Assessment of the body burden and spread of cancer by clinical means (staging) is important in developing the treatment plan. Most staging systems assess the size of the primary tumor and define regional lymph node involvement as well as the presence or absence of distant metastatic disease. It is important to distinguish between clinical and pathologic staging and to recognize that pathologic staging employing surgical biopsy is generally more accurate. Increasingly, staging can be accomplished by using non-invasive imaging procedures such as chest radiography and magnetic resonance imaging (MRI) or computed tomography (CT). In the diagnostic evaluation of specific forms of cancer, such as breast or prostate cancer, bone scans can be useful to evaluate advanced disease but have minimal use in early localized disease unless the patient has skeletal symptoms. For multiple myeloma, bone scans are of less use than skeletal radiographs. The temptation to use a variety of redundant and expensive tests such as CT, MRI, and ultrasonography to examine the same site should be avoided. It is important to focus on the benefit-to-risk ratio of invasive procedures such as staging laparotomy. The patient's age, performance status, concomitant medical problems, and histologic diagnosis all must be considered; then the procedure should be performed only if it may influence the treatment plan. For patients who present with life-threatening local complications of cancer (e.g., spinal cord compression, upper airway obstruction, the superior vena cava syndrome, or obstructive jaundice) (see Chapter 199), it is usually necessary first to treat the local complication. Even in these cases, a pathologic diagnosis should be established if at all possible before treatment is started.

OVERALL ASSESSMENT. Once diagnosis and staging have been performed, the information must be integrated into an optimal treatment plan. For patients with apparently localized cancers, multidisciplinary input is important, because a combined-modality approach may be indicated. The biologic characteristics of the specific cancer must be considered. For many tumor types, histopathologic features such as grade of tumor cell differentiation are important, with a less differentiated or undifferentiated phenotype indicating a more aggressive neoplasm. For some sites, other biologic factors are of greater value than histologic grade. For example, in breast cancer, the presence or absence of estrogen or progesterone receptors and the DNA-index and ploidy status as determined by flow cytometry provide useful information in developing a treatment plan. Some patients with a minimal tumor burden (e.g., stage I) of currently incurable B-cell neoplasms (e.g., chronic lymphocytic leukemia [CLL] and multiple myeloma) are best watched expectantly rather than treated. By contrast, almost all patients with diffuse large cell (intermediate- or high-grade) lymphoma should be treated aggressively with curative intent, irrespective of stage, unless they are very elderly and have other major medical problems.

In any given patient, it is important to decide whether curative therapy is available or not, and, if so, whether the patient's age and overall medical condition permit a curative approach. If cure is not an option, one must consider whether palliation with prolongation of survival (and relief of symptoms) can be achieved. For old and infirm patients, a palliative approach may be preferable, particularly if there is significant morbidity associated with the treatment approach under consideration. On the other hand, some forms of cancer therapy are very effective and well tolerated even with advanced age (e.g., use of tamoxifen in adjuvant therapy of postmenopausal breast cancer or of chlorambucil for chronic lymphocytic leukemia). For many tumor types, it is important to examine results of recent prospective clinical trials relevant to the patient's diagnosis and clinical setting and, if possible, to enter patients in clinical trials.

THERAPEUTIC MODALITIES

Three primary therapeutic approaches dominate the treatment of cancer: surgery, radiation therapy, and medical therapy. A fourth modality, biologic therapy (cytokines, antibodies, vaccines), is beginning to add another dimension to treatment programs.

Surgery

Cancer surgery is most useful to establish a tissue diagnosis, to excise the primary tumor with clear surgical margins free of tumor, and to determine the extent of cancer with staging procedures. Surgery is a simple and safe means to remove solid tumors when the tumor is confined to a specific anatomic site of origin. However, in the case of some solid tumors, most patients already have metastatic disease at the time of presentation. In evaluating major surgery for an individual patient, it is important to assess the operative risk-to-benefit ratio for the procedure in the context of the patient's general health status, the extent of the tumor, and the likelihood that it can be completely removed. Additionally, the technical complexity of the surgical procedure, the type of anesthesia needed, and the experience of the personnel must also be considered.

With advances in both radiation and chemotherapy, the need for radical surgery has diminished. However, it remains a major primary approach to curative cancer therapy. For testicular cancer, even in the presence of limited metastatic disease, regional lymphadenectomy after radical orchiectomy can be curative and eliminate the need for chemotherapy in some patients who have metastases only to retroperitoneal lymph nodes. For many other sites, surgical resection of regional lymph nodes is performed for diagnostic rather than therapeutic purposes. For example, in breast cancer, the presence or absence of axillary lymph node involvement is the single most important factor in evaluating the likelihood of distant recurrence, and this information is currently not obtainable by non-surgical means. Similarly, surgical staging of nodal involvement in colorectal cancer plays an important role in deciding whether adjuvant systemic chemotherapy is indicated.

Initial cancer therapy often requires a multimodal approach to maximize the chance of cure while simultaneously reducing the extent of surgery required. Multimodal approaches require close communication among the involved physicians before surgery. Early communication is improved by obtaining histopathologic diagnosis by needle biopsy or local excision of the primary cancer before more extensive therapy. Two examples are of note in this regard: (1) the management of osteogenic sarcoma with limb salvage surgery, irradiation, and adjuvant chemotherapy and (2) the management of early breast cancer with lumpectomy, axillary staging followed by primary irradiation, and adjuvant systemic administration of cytotoxic or endocrine agents. In both instances, the combined approach yields a better cosmetic and functional outcome. Screening mammography can establish a diagnosis of breast cancer when the tumor is less extensive and when likelihood of cure is greater. Improved plastic surgical techniques have also made breast reconstruction possible for women who either require or prefer mastectomy rather than lumpectomy followed by radiation therapy.

In addition to its use in diagnosis, staging, and primary therapy, cancer surgery also plays an important role in the management of some patients with more extensive cancer. In ovarian cancer, when the gynecologic oncologist "debulks" peritoneal and omental spread and leaves the patient with minimal residual disease, patients become better candidates for systemic chemotherapy and have a better survival. Additionally, early resection of pulmonary metastases of soft tissue sarcomas or of solitary brain metastases in melanoma, colon, or breast cancer may provide marked palliation and improved survival, albeit with only occasional cures.

Radiation Therapy

Radiation therapy has made major strides in instrumentation, physics, radiobiology, treatment planning, and applications to curative and palliative cancer therapy. In general, the term *radiation* refers to ionizing radiation that is either electromagnetic or particulate (e.g., x-rays). Compared with surgery, radiation therapy has distinct advantages in the locoregional treatment of cancer. Radiation causes less acute morbidity and can be curative for some specific sites while preserving organ or tissue structure and function. An example is the use of radiation for the curative treatment of early-stage laryngeal cancer wherein vocal function can be preserved.

The basic unit of ionizing irradiation is the gray (Gy), which has superseded the rad (1 Gy = 100 rads = 100 cGy) (see Chapter 19).

By interaction with molecular oxygen, radiation induces the formation of superoxide, hydrogen peroxide, or hydroxyl radicals that damage or break cellular DNA, the critical target for radiation-induced cell death. Both single- and double-strand breaks of the DNA helix can be induced, with the latter constituting lethal damage. Single-strand breaks, if not repaired by the cell, can also result in cell death. High linear energy transfer (LET) radiation can induce direct damage to the molecular structure of DNA.

Radiation has limitations in the treatment of bulky tumors. Large tumors frequently have poorly perfused, hypoxic zones in which radiation often fails to induce needed reactive intermediaries. Various forms of irradiation are used for different therapeutic objectives. For example, electron-beam irradiation deposits most of its energy in the skin and soft tissues and can be useful for superficial therapy of skin neoplasms such as mycosis fungoides. Low-energy (kilovoltage) x-rays expend most of their effects on the overlying tissues above a deep-seated tumor and therefore cause considerable normal tissue damage. By contrast, higher-energy x-rays (megavoltage) or x-irradiation from a cobalt-60 source spare the skin, deposit their energy at greater depth, and provide a better approach to treating deep-seated neoplasms. Use of radioactive implants also can be useful in some settings (e.g., cervical cancer, prostate cancer). The use of multiple irradiation fields reduces the dose to normal tissue while increasing the dose to the tumor. The use of fractionated doses causes less cumulative damage to normal tissues than to the tumor, because the normal tissues are often able to repair sublethal damage more quickly. Additionally, as a tumor shrinks with therapy, its oxygenation can improve and render it more radiosensitive. The selection of treatment is based on the relative radiosensitivity of the tumor and of the normal organs and tissues within the radiation field (Table 198–1).

The combined use of multiple fields, fractionated irradiation, and megavoltage radiation equipment is optimized by treatment individualized to the patient's tumor. Although the major uses of radiation therapy involve local irradiation of sites of tumor involvement, total-body irradiation or total lymphoid irradiation is a valuable part of a preparative regimen for allogeneic or autologous bone marrow transplantation for leukemia or lymphoma (see Chapter 182).

Radiation therapy has important palliative applications. One of these is for bone pain due to metastatic involvement of the skeleton. Irradiation can also cause sufficient cytoreduction of tumor in bone to permit healing of osteolytic lesions and thereby prevent pathologic fractures of weight-bearing bones. Other examples include tumor shrinkage to relieve postobstructive infection in lung cancer and to suppress bronchial or gastric bleeding secondary to cancer.

Although modern radiation therapy with megavoltage equipment has proved to be extremely useful, even higher energy radiation approaches are currently in development. These include the use of higher LET sources of irradiation (e.g., neutrons, charged particles, heavy ions), which may also provide selective advantages for specific tumor sites and reduce the need for oxygenation of tumor tissue. Additionally, several classes of compounds are under study as radiosensitizers to enhance the cytotoxic effects of radiation on tumor cells. One class is the halopyrimidines, including bromodeoxyuridine, fluorouracil, and fluorodeoxyuridine, which sensitize

Table 198–1 ■ TOLERANCE OF NORMAL TISSUES TO IRRADIATION

TISSUE	TOXIC EFFECT	LIMITING DOSE (Gy)*
Bone marrow	Aplasia	2.5
Lung	Pneumonitis, fibrosis	15.0
Kidney	Nephrosclerosis	20.0
Liver	Hepatitis	25.0
Spinal cord	Infarction, necrosis	45.0
Intestine	Ulceration, fibrosis	45.0
Heart	Pericarditis, myocarditis	45.0
Brain	Infarction, necrosis	50.0
Skin	Dermatitis, sclerosis	55.0

*Radiation in 2.0-Gy fractions to the whole organ for 5 days weekly produces a 5% incidence of the listed toxicities at the limiting doses listed.

DNA to strand breakage by radiation. Other chemotherapeutic agents, including gemcitabine and taxol, are also under investigation as radiosensitizing agents. Several sulfhydryl compounds (e.g., amifostine) are also under investigation as potential radioprotective agents.

Although the term *radiation* normally refers to ionizing irradiation, several other forms of radiation are also used in cancer treatment. These include hyperthermia and photodynamic therapy, both of which are still undergoing development. Some tumors show thermal sensitivity to temperatures in the range of 41° to 43° C and may be more sensitive than surrounding normal tissues. Hyperthermia appears to work best on bulky tumors with poor blood supply in which the tumor cells are in an acidic environment. A variety of approaches can induce local or regional hyperthermia (e.g., ultrasonography, microwaves, regional perfusion) and may enhance the effects of ionizing irradiation or chemotherapy on local tumors.

Photodynamic therapy (PDT) involves the preliminary systemic administration of a photosensitizing compound such as a hematoporphyrin derivative (e.g., dihematoporphyrin ether, Photofrin II). Such hematoporphyrins are concentrated in the vicinity of local tumors and can be activated with local exposure to visible red light (usually 630 nm), with a resulting preferential toxicity to cancer cells. The intense light used for PDT can be delivered by means of a fiberoptic probe, which can be used for various internal sites as well as on the skin. The mechanism of action of PDT is poorly understood but may involve vascular damage or a direct toxic effect on tumor cells. Side effects of photodynamic therapy include hypersensitivity to light (skin and eyes). Locally, PDT induces transient sunburn and hyperpigmentation as well as local tumor necrosis. Tumor sites amenable to PDT include skin recurrences of breast cancer (e.g., chest wall) and malignant lesions in the endobronchus, peritoneal cavity, and bladder. Photodynamic therapy has not been approved by the U.S. Food and Drug Administration (FDA) and remains investigational.

Medical Therapy

Curative therapy has been developed for a series of relatively uncommon disseminated neoplasms, and useful palliative therapy has been developed for some common forms of cancer (Table 198–2). With rare exceptions, effective therapy has used combinations of anticancer drugs. Increasingly, anticancer drugs are used in concert with surgery and/or irradiation.

Ideally, anticancer drugs should eradicate cancer without harming normal tissues; however, this goal has not been achieved, and most useful drugs have significant side effects. The introduction of anticancer drugs for clinical use has largely been predicted from ani-

Table 198–2 ■ **RESPONSIVENESS OF CANCER TO CHEMOTHERAPY**

Cure (>30%) of Advanced Disease
Choriocarcinoma
Acute lymphocytic leukemia (childhood)
Malignant lymphoma (Hodgkin's disease, diffuse high-grade or intermediate-grade non-Hodgkin's lymphoma)
Hairy cell leukemia
Testicular cancer
Childhood solid tumors (embryonal rhabdomyosarcoma, Ewing's sarcoma, Wilms' tumor)
Acute myelocytic leukemia
Acute lymphocytic leukemia (adult)
Promyelocytic leukemia
Significant Palliation, Some Cures of Advanced Disease (5–30%)
Ovarian cancer
Bladder cancer
Small cell lung cancer
Gastric cancer
Palliation, Probably Increases Survival
Breast cancer
Multiple myeloma
Head and neck cancer
Adjuvant Treatment Leading to Increased Cure
Breast cancer
Colon cancer
Osteogenic sarcoma
Early-stage large cell lymphoma

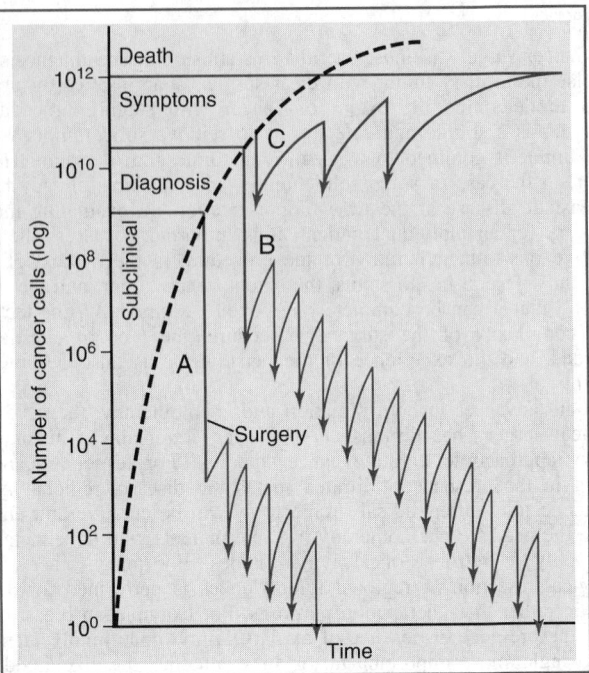

FIGURE 198–1 ■ The relationship of tumor growth and tumor burden to treatment strategies and outcome with systemic chemotherapy. Human tumors grow in accord with the Gompertz curve (dashed line), with a decreasing doubling time as tumor burden increases. Treatment interventions relate to tumor type and extent of disease. A, Surgery followed by pulse courses of adjuvant chemotherapy. B, Systemic chemotherapy for stage III Hodgkin's disease. C, Palliative chemotherapy for advanced non–small cell cancer. In A, combined modality has curative potential with the addition of chemotherapy after surgery. Cure is also possible in B with prolonged administration of combination chemotherapy. In C, the patient's tumor burden is too great and the potency of the drugs for this specific form of cancer is inadequate because of development of drug resistance. (Modified from Salmon SE, Sartorelli AC: Cancer chemotherapy. *In* Katzung BG [ed]: Basic and Clinical Pharmacology, 4th ed. Norwalk, CT, Appleton & Lange, 1989, p 685.)

mal tumor models. Perhaps because the initial murine models were for acute leukemia, many of the developed drugs are general antiproliferative agents. Accordingly, they are more effective against rapidly proliferating tumors than against some of the more slowly growing solid tumors and are more toxic to rapidly growing tumors than to normal host tissues. Nevertheless, such generally antiproliferative agents can have important toxic side effects on normal tissues that divide rapidly, such as bone marrow, gastrointestinal mucosa, and skin.

CELL KINETICS AND RESPONSE TO CHEMOTHERAPY. A number of related factors, including total tumor burden, cell kinetics, and intrinsic sensitivity, influence the response to anticancer drugs. In both animal models and human tumors, growth occurs in accord with gompertzian kinetics. Initially, growth occurs rapidly, and most tumor cells traverse the complete cell cycle. As the tumor burden grows larger, the rate of tumor cell doubling progressively slows (Fig. 198–1), and the fraction of cells traversing the cell cycle decreases as more and more cells remain "hung up" in a G_0 phase. Whereas the population doubling time may be in the range of 1 to 2 days at the subclinical phase (with less than 1 g of tumor), by the time the tumor burden has reached 1 kg or more, the tumor cell population doubling time may be 3 to 6 months. A significant problem in the treatment of high tumor burden metastatic solid tumors is that the tumor exhibits a significant degree of heterogeneity; subpopulations of cells exhibit differing biologic, kinetic, antigenic, and drug-sensitivity profiles.

Several important features related to cell kinetics and tumor burden are important with respect to drug dose, scheduling, and response to chemotherapy. Anticancer drugs can be classified as either cell cycle specific (CCS) or cell cycle non-specific (CCNS) (Table 198–3). CCNS agents have greater effects on cycling than on non-cycling cells but nonetheless can exert anticancer effects on non-cycling cells, whereas CCS agents do not. Endocrine agents

Table 198-3 ■ RELATIONSHIP OF TUMOR CELL CYCLE TO ACTIVITY OF MAJOR CLASSES OF CYTOTOXIC ANTICANCER DRUGS

CELL CYCLE–SPECIFIC (CCS) AGENTS	CELL CYCLE–NON-SPECIFIC (CCNS) AGENTS
Antimetabolites (cytarabine, fluorouracil, methotrexate, mercaptopurine, hydroxyurea)	Alkylating agents (busulfan, cyclophosphamide, mechlorethamine, melphalan, thiotepa, chlorambucil)
Anthracyclines (doxorubicin, daunorubicin)	Antibiotics (dactinomycin, mitomycin)
Bleomycin	Platinum compounds (cisplatin, carboplatin)
Camptothecins (irinotecan, topotecan)	Nitrosoureas (BCNU, CCNU)
Plant alkaloids (vincristine, vinblastine, etoposide, taxol)	Dacarbazine
	L-Asparaginase

are also in a sense cycle active, because they block the transition of tumor cells from G_1 to the S phase of the cell cycle. However, certain endocrine agents (e.g., tamoxifen, progestins) are considered to suppress growth rather than kill tumor cells. Endocrine agents are therefore often given for many years, whereas cytotoxic agents are usually given over a time course measured in months.

An important concept in cancer chemotherapy is that cellular killing with cytotoxic agents follows first-order kinetics, with a given dose of drug killing only a fraction of the tumor cells. This "fractional kill hypothesis" is particularly relevant to CCNS agents and predicts that the greater the dose of drug administered, the greater the "log kill" of tumor cells that will occur.

The concept of combination chemotherapy was developed to take advantage of the fact that many anticancer agents have differing mechanisms of action and side effects. This concept was based on the hypothesis that giving drugs with differing mechanisms of action may achieve synergistic antitumor effects while simultaneously retarding the rate of development of drug resistance. Additionally, by careful selection of drugs in a combination to include those with known single-agent activity against the tumor and different normal tissue toxicities, the side effects would be "spread" across different tissues and organs. The validity of this concept has been borne out clinically. Optimal results for most tumor types sensitive to chemotherapy have been achieved with drug combinations, often employing CCNS and CCS agents possessing different mechanisms of action. For example, cisplatin has demonstrated clear-cut synergy with etoposide in testicular cancer and small cell lung cancer and with fluorouracil in both head and neck and esophageal cancer. The major potential toxicity for cisplatin is nephrotoxicity, whereas myelosuppression is the major side effect for both etoposide and fluorouracil.

New drugs entering clinical trials are normally first tested in patients with a large tumor burden of metastatic cancer who have relapsed from known effective chemotherapy regimens. Although this approach is ethically most acceptable, it nonetheless represents a significant obstacle to new drug development, because these patients have a lower probability of response to a new drug than those with a lower tumor burden or those who have not been previously treated. The presence of the blood-brain barrier has been a major obstacle to the development of chemotherapy for primary or metastatic tumors in the brain. At present, brain tumors are treated chiefly with surgery and radiation therapy.

DRUG RESISTANCE. For many of the drug-responsive tumor types (see Table 198–2), major cytoreduction occurs with initial chemotherapy. Some months to years thereafter, however, tumor regrowth occurs and continues even though the same drugs are reinstituted. This observation usually reflects the acquisition of drug resistance by the tumor to the specific drugs. Most drug resistance is considered to result from the high spontaneous mutation rate of cancer cells, which leads to the development of heterogeneous subpopulations, some of which exhibit resistance to various drugs. Perhaps the most important form of resistance is multidrug resistance (MDR), mediated by a cell membrane glycoprotein (the P-glycoprotein), which is thought to function as an energy-dependent efflux pump that actively extrudes a variety of cytotoxic agents from the cell (Fig. 198–2).

Drugs pumped out of the cancer cell by the P-glycoprotein include natural products such as plant alkaloids (vincas, podophyllotoxins, taxol), antibiotics (dactinomycin, doxorubicin, daunorubicin), and some synthetic agents (e.g., mitoxantrone). The P-glycoprotein is normally expressed in tissues such as the gut and the kidney, perhaps to deal with toxic products in the environment.

Cancer cells with mutations to "switch on" the expression of the gene responsible for encoding the P-glycoprotein show resistance to a wide variety of useful anticancer drugs. Techniques such as immunohistochemistry, Western blots, and Northern blots can be used to detect the presence of P-glycoprotein in tumor tissues. Clinical studies suggest that patients whose tumors express P-glycoprotein have a poor prognosis. Culture studies performed on biopsy specimens in vitro have documented that P-glycoprotein–positive tumors usually exhibit resistance to doxorubicin. Tumor types such as sarcoma, neuroblastoma, malignant lymphoma, and myeloma are usually P-glycoprotein negative at the time of diagnosis but are frequently positive for P-glycoprotein when the patient relapses from chemotherapy. A series of non-cytotoxic drugs has been identified to reverse drug resistance mediated by P-glycoprotein (e.g., verapamil, cyclosporine). In drug-resistant patients with malignant lymphoma and multiple myeloma, high doses of verapamil given simultaneously with vincristine and doxorubicin can reverse resistance to these agents, with some patients regaining remission. Although verapamil is not an ideal chemosensitizer (because of its cardiovascular side effects), other potential chemosensitizers are now being tested in an effort to identify more effective and less toxic chemosensitizers. In the long run, such chemosensitizers may find their major use to prevent development of MDR expression. Other mechanisms of multidrug resistance include an increase in proteins called MRP and LRP, and mutations in topoisomerase II, which is the target for the anthracycline drugs and for etoposide.

Drug-specific resistance mechanisms also occur (Table 198–4). For example, intrinsic or natural resistance of patients with acute

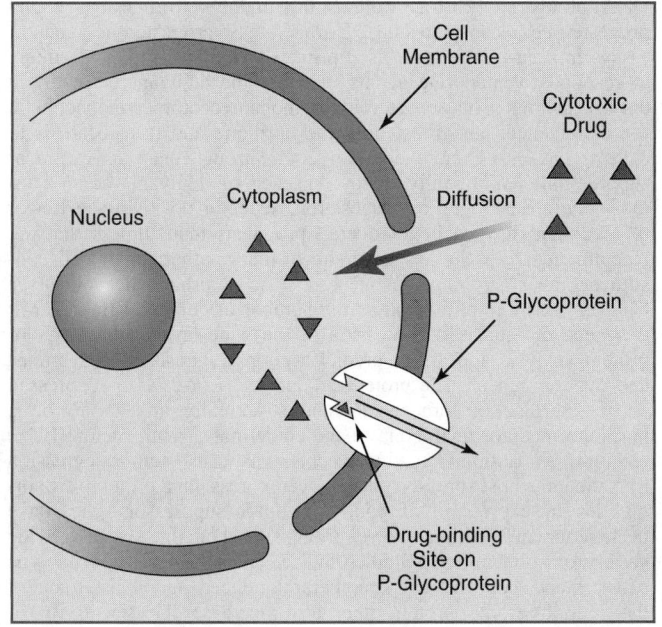

FIGURE 198-2 ■ Model of cancer cell expressing P-glycoprotein. This transmembrane protein is believed to function as an energy-dependent efflux pump or drug transporter. It has acceptor sites to which various natural product anticancer drugs bind, after which they are pumped out of the cell. Chemosensitizers such as verapamil also bind to the drug acceptor sites on P-glycoprotein and can competitively inhibit its function.

Table 198–4 ■ SOME MECHANISMS OF RESISTANCE TO CHEMOTHERAPY DRUGS

DRUG	MECHANISMS OF RESISTANCE
Methotrexate	Impaired transport or amplification of dihydrofolate reductase
Cytarabine	Decreased deoxycytidine kinase or increase in cytidine deaminase
5-Fluorouracil	Increase in thymidylate synthase
Cisplatin	Decreased uptake
	Increase in repair enzymes
Taxol, *Vinca* alkaloids	MDR expression
	Mutations in tubulin (decreased binding)
Doxorubicin	MDR expression
	Decrease or alterations in topoisomerase II
Irinotecan, topotecan	Decrease in topoisomerase I

myelogenous leukemia to methotrexate is attributed to lack of retention of this drug by leukemic blasts. These cells form low levels of methotrexate polyglutamates, the drug species that are retained by cells. In contrast, acute lymphocytic leukemia blasts (pre-B, not T cells) convert methotrexate to its polyglutamates efficiently and are sensitive to treatment with this drug. Acquired resistance, fortunately now noted in the minority of patients with this disease treated with combination chemotherapy, has been found to be associated with impaired uptake due to abnormalities in the reduced folate carrier transport protein, or to low-level amplification of the dihydrofolate reductase gene, whose product is the target for methotrexate.

PREDICTIVE TESTING IN VITRO. Many approaches have been developed to assess the probability of relapse after primary therapy or response to a given type or class of endocrine or cytotoxic agents. The "S-phase" fraction of the tumor cell population undergoing DNA synthesis as well as DNA ploidy can be determined by flow cytometry. For several tumor types, patients with a high percentage of tumor cells in DNA synthesis and/or hyperdiploidy have a high likelihood of relapsing early after local primary cancer therapy. Taken with other prognostic characteristics, such flow cytometry assays may aid in identifying patients who should receive adjuvant chemotherapy. This approach is currently being applied to patients with stage I breast cancer in an effort to decide which patients are at higher risk for recurrence.

Diagnostic laboratories can provide the results of S-phase and DNA ploidy analysis as well as the findings from estrogen and progesterone receptor testing. Estrogen and progesterone receptor assays in breast cancer are used primarily to identify patients likely to respond to endocrine agents in either the adjuvant or recurrent disease setting. The sex steroid hormone receptors are located in the cell nucleus and must bind the hormone and translocate it to cellular DNA to exert endocrine action through gene activation or suppression. Additionally, in the absence of adjuvant therapy, tumors that are estrogen or progesterone receptor positive take longer to recur and have a better overall prognosis than tumors that are receptor negative. Studies have shown that another tumor cell constituent, the *HER-2/neu* oncogene, can be of prognostic value (see Chapter 258). Amplification of the number of copies of the *HER-2/neu* gene or increased expression of the gene product by RNA or protein analysis appears to predict a poor prognosis in both breast and ovarian cancer. The protein product of *HER-2/neu* is expressed on the surface of tumor cells and structurally appears to be a hormone receptor analogous to the epidermal growth factor (EGF) receptor. An antibody to this receptor can cause tumor regression in patients whose breast cancers overexpress this protein. Abnormalities in expression of *p53*, the tumor suppressor gene, have been associated with a worse prognosis when present in a wide variety of solid tumors. Studies indicate that the lack of wild type *p53* protects cells from chemotherapy-induced apoptosis. Lack of the retinoblastoma protein may also decrease the sensitivity of tumor cells to antimetabolites. Thus, measurement of abnormalities of these tumor suppressor genes in tumors may be an additional prognostic factor in treatment outcome.

Chemosensitivity assays appear to predict drug resistance but are somewhat less accurate for predicting which drugs will be useful for an individual patient. Another type of testing for drug resistance that is now being applied to fresh frozen (and in some instances to fixed) tissues is immunohistochemical testing for P-glycoprotein expression.

Knowledge of the mechanism of action of certain drugs has been used to predict sensitivity to these agents. For example, fresh sarcoma cells in short-term mixture have been shown to be useful for evaluating potential anticancer effects of various folate analogues as measured by inhibitors of thymidylate synthesis in a whole-cell assay. In addition, the low levels of thymidylate synthase mRNA expression in tumors has also correlated well with response to fluorouracil treatment among patients with gastric or colon cancer, and studies are in progress to determine if this assay may be used to select patients for treatment with this drug.

PHARMACOKINETIC CONSIDERATIONS. Although intrinsic drug sensitivity appears to be the most critical determinant of response to chemotherapy, pharmacokinetic factors related to the route of administration, bioavailability, metabolism, and elimination are probably of greater importance in cancer therapy. Many cytotoxic agents have a steep dose-response curve and a resulting narrow therapeutic index. Thus, at too low an available dose level within the tumor, no response is seen. On the other hand, at higher doses, host toxicity supervenes and is usually dose limiting. Because of the steep dose-response relationship, doses of most cytotoxic agents are calculated in relation to body surface area, a more accurate approach than dose calculations based on body weight. Patients usually prefer the oral route of drug administration, but marked variations in bioavailability among oral formulations plus inconsistent patient compliance tend to limit such an approach. For example, with the alkylating agent melphalan, more than a 10-fold variation in plasma levels has been documented after standard dosing. Unfortunately, plasma assays are not routinely available for most anticancer drugs, and the only semiquantitative indicator of bioavailability of cytotoxic agents is the occurrence of myelosuppression after drug administration. For patients presenting with hypercalcemia or other complications of myeloma, oral melphalan therefore seems undesirable, because such patients need to achieve effective plasma levels immediately. Similar difficulties are faced with oral administration of fluorouracil, methotrexate, and 6-mercaptopurine. Bioavailability is adequate after oral administration of agents such as tamoxifen and cyclophosphamide.

The intravenous route of drug administration is preferable for most cytotoxic anticancer drugs, because it ensures adequate plasma levels while minimizing compliance problems. For some agents, continuous intravenous drug administration for 4 days or longer provides better results and less toxicity than do bolus or short-duration infusions because tumor response for many agents can be related to the "area under the plasma disappearance curve (AUC)" for the drug, whereas toxicity generally relates more directly to peak plasma concentrations than to the AUC. With the advent of vascular access devices such as subcutaneous ports, external catheters, and infusion pumps, outpatient continuous infusion chemotherapy can now be used for stable drugs such as fluorinated pyrimidines, anthracyclines, and *Vinca* alkaloids. Subcutaneous administration can be used effectively with drugs such as cytarabine, interferon-α, and erythropoietin. Subcutaneous dosing provides more sustained plasma levels than can be obtained with intravenous administration. Depot intramuscular formulations are available for a variety of endocrine agents used in treatment of breast or prostate cancer.

Regional administration of chemotherapy can be effective for several tumor sites. For metastatic colon cancer limited to the liver, hepatic artery catheterization for arterial infusion of 5-fluorodeoxyuridine or 5-fluorouracil can be used effectively by connection of the catheter to an external pump or to an implantable perfusion pump. In either instance, arterial infusions are often administered for 14 days, followed by a similar rest period. A relatively high objective response rate of metastatic colon cancer in the liver can be obtained by this means, but this route is ineffective for metastases outside the liver. Hepatic artery chemotherapy is expensive and associated with complications, including arterial thrombosis, biliary sclerosis, and chemical hepatitis. Nonetheless, it can induce sustained remissions for a year or more in selected patients. Regional infusion or isolated perfusion has been used with melanomas and sarcomas of the lower extremity. With melanoma metastases of the lower extremity, melphalan or cisplatin has been administered in this fashion with or without regional hyperthermia.

Intraperitoneal drug administration has also gained increasing popularity and appears to show particular promise for patients with peritoneal carcinomatosis, where it can induce remissions of established metastatic disease. In ovarian cancer, intraperitoneal chemotherapy is being studied as a follow-up to cytoreductive surgery. Diffusion of intraperitoneally administered drugs is limited to a few millimeters of tumor tissue. Accordingly, intraperitoneal chemotherapy is seldom warranted in patients with bulky tumor masses. For optimal distribution, the drug is usually diluted in 2 L of parenteral fluid for injection. Preferred drugs for intraperitoneal administration are those that tend to be limited largely to the peritoneal cavity, have good properties for tumor penetration, and produce little or no local toxicity. Mitoxantrone, fluorodeoxyuridine, and cisplatin have these favorable characteristics and can be quite useful. With each of these drugs, the intraperitoneal concentration can be 1000-fold higher than measured in the systemic circulation. Other agents sometimes used in intraperitoneal administration include thiotepa, fluorouracil, and methotrexate. Intraperitoneal drug administration can be performed at repeated intervals with relative ease if a surgically implanted Tenkoff catheter is connected to a subcutaneous port. Mild to moderate chemical peritonitis and the development of peritoneal adhesions are common complications of intraperitoneal chemotherapy and limit repeated use. Intracavitary drug administration with instillation of a biologic agent such as bacille Calmette-Guérin (BCG) or interferon or a variety of cytotoxic agents (e.g., thiotepa, doxorubicin, mitomycin, cisplatin) is used to treat superficial bladder cancer.

The intrathecal route can be used to deliver therapy to the meninges. Methotrexate, cytarabine, and thiotepa can be given by this route to prevent meningeal leukemia and treat central nervous system leukemia or lymphoma or meningeal carcinomatosis. Intrathecal methotrexate has been used effectively for acute lymphoblastic leukemia as an adjuvant to initial systemic chemotherapy and has reduced the frequency of central nervous system relapse in patients in complete peripheral remission.

EVALUATION OF RESPONSE. Objective measurement of tumor shrinkage with medical or radiation therapy has prognostic importance. Reduction of symptoms alone does not indicate a response. Cure or significant prolongation of survival occurs in patients who achieve complete response (disappearance of all evidence of cancer). Whenever possible, confirmation of response should be obtained pathologically through the use of restaging procedures. Many patients achieve only a partial response, defined as a reduction of tumor burden by 50% or greater. Patients achieving partial responses generally have palliation of symptoms and usually have a prolonged period without tumor growth. Modest improvements in survival accompany some partial responses.

Tumor markers in the blood or urine can be useful in monitoring response to therapy (see Chapter 192). Patients with testicular germ cell tumors and gestational choriocarcinoma cannot be considered potentially cured unless the titer of marker substance falls below the limit of detection. Tumor marker studies are also useful in judging responses in ovarian cancer, prostatic carcinoma, colon cancer, multiple myeloma, neuroblastoma, and the carcinoid syndrome.

Response to adjuvant chemotherapy cannot be evaluated by these methods, because insufficient tumor usually remains to employ physical or imaging studies or tumor markers. However, in the neoadjuvant setting in which chemotherapy is used before local surgery, the response to chemotherapy provides an "in vivo sensitivity test" to determine whether the employed agents can provide effective therapy after surgery.

CYTOTOXIC ANTICANCER DRUGS. Safe and effective cytotoxic cancer chemotherapy requires considerable understanding of the pharmacology and toxicology of these drugs. Drug doses are cited for single-agent chemotherapy; when drugs are used in combinations (Table 198–5), lower doses may be required for some agents. Therefore, it is wise to use effective and well-established combination protocols with known side-effect profiles rather than to improvise combinations. The development of new combinations of standard drugs is best done in the research setting.

ALKYLATING AGENTS. The major clinically useful alkylating agents (Table 198–6) kill cells by binding to and cross-linking DNA through a bis(chloroethyl)amine, ethyleneimine, or nitrosourea moiety. Although these agents likely kill cells by alkylating DNA (primarily at the N7 position of guanine), they also react chemically with nucleophilic molecules (e.g., sulfhydryl, amino, hydroxyl, and phosphate groups). Alkylating agents differ in the severity of early and late side effects. The major acute side effects are gastrointestinal (nausea and vomiting) and hematologic (myelosuppression). Most alkylating agents cause local skin and subcutaneous tissue necrosis when infiltrated into the skin.

All alkylating agents can potentially induce ovarian or testicular failure as well as acute leukemia. Agents such as melphalan and chlorambucil appear to be more leukemogenic than cyclophosphamide, whereas busulfan and the nitrosoureas cause more persistent damage to hematopoietic stem cells and more prolonged myelosuppression.

Cyclophosphamide and Ifosfamide. Cyclophosphamide (Cytoxan) is the most widely used alkylating agent and is effective in the treatment of both hematologic malignancies and solid tumors. It does not have significant vesicant effects, because it is a prodrug that requires bioactivation in the liver. Metabolism of cyclophosphamide by cytochrome P-450 produces the active metabolite phosphoramide mustard plus acrolein. Cyclophosphamide is available in both intravenous and oral formulations and is well absorbed by the oral route. A commonly used single-agent dosage schedule for intravenous cyclophosphamide is 1.0 g/m^2 every 3 weeks. Cyclophosphamide produces a less severe pattern of myelosuppressive toxicity than other alkylating agents; it can cause severe neutropenia but usually of relatively short duration, and thrombocytopenia is less severe than with other alkylators. Other toxicities of cyclophosphamide include alopecia and immunosuppression. When high doses are used (e.g., for bone marrow transplantation), cyclophosphamide can also cause myocardial necrosis or the syndrome of inappropriate secretion of antidiuretic hormone. Although cyclophosphamide can cause acute non-lymphocytic leukemia and pulmonary fibrosis, these toxicities are more common with other alkylating agents. Both cyclophosphamide and a related analogue, ifosfamide (Ifex), can cause hemorrhagic cystitis. Bladder toxicity can be blocked by administration of the uroprotective agent mesna (Mesnex), which is concentrated in the urine and inactivates the toxic metabolite acrolein. Mesna is particularly valuable with ifosfamide, which otherwise routinely causes bladder toxicity. Ifosfamide causes somewhat less hematologic toxicity than other alkylating agents and at present is used mostly for second-line therapy (e.g.,

Table 198–5 ■ COMMON COMBINATION CHEMOTHERAPY REGIMENS

ABBREVIATION	DRUGS EMPLOYED	INDICATION
MOPP	Nitrogen mustard (Mustargen), vincristine (Oncovin), prednisone, procarbazine	Hodgkin's disease
ABVD	Doxorubicin (Adriamycin), bleomycin, vinblastine, dacarbazine	Hodgkin's disease
CHOP	Cyclophosphamide, hydroxydaunomycin (doxorubicin), vincristine (Oncovin), prednisone	Non-Hodgkin's lymphomas
CMF	Cyclophosphamide, methotrexate, 5-fluorouracil	Breast cancer
CAF	Cyclophosphamide, doxorubicin (Adriamycin), 5-fluorouracil	Breast cancer
M-VAC	Methotrexate, vinblastine, doxorubicin (Adriamycin), cisplatin	Bladder cancer
PVB	cisplatin, vinblastine, bleomycin	Testicular cancer
VAD	Vincristine, doxorubicin (Adriamycin), dexamethasone	Multiple myeloma

Table 198–6 ■ ALKYLATING ANTICANCER DRUGS

DRUG	MAJOR INDICATIONS
Nitrogen mustard	Hodgkin's disease
Melphalan	Multiple myeloma
Chlorambucil	Chronic lymphocytic leukemia
Busulfan	Chronic myelocytic leukemia
Cyclophosphamide	Lymphoma, breast cancer, bladder cancer
Ifosfamide	Soft tissue sarcoma, lymphoma
Nitrosoureas (carmustine, lomustine)	Brain tumors, lymphoma
Procarbazine	Hodgkin's disease
Dacarbazine	Melanoma, Hodgkin's disease
Cisplatin, carboplatin	Testicular, ovarian cancer, head and neck, lung cancer

for therapy for testicular cancer, lymphoma, or metastatic sarcomas).

Chlorambucil. Chlorambucil (Leukeran) has antitumor activity similar to that of cyclophosphamide and is also well absorbed after oral administration. It is used primarily in the treatment of chronic lymphocytic leukemia, low-grade lymphomas, macroglobulinemia, and polycythemia vera. Chlorambucil does not cause hemorrhagic cystitis or alopecia, and its gastrointestinal side effects are mild. However, it is myelosuppressive. Acute non-lymphocytic leukemia has been reported in patients treated with chlorambucil for polycythemia vera or other disorders.

Melphalan. Melphalan (Alkeran) is L-phenylalanine mustard and gains access to cells through an amino acid transport system. Melphalan is commonly given orally in a dosage of 10 mg/m^2/day for 4 days every 3 to 4 weeks. Some patients do not absorb the drug; generally, the only clue, other than drug levels, is the absence of myelosuppression. If myelosuppression does not occur, melphalan dosage should be increased in subsequent courses until moderate myelosuppression is induced. Melphalan is commonly used in the treatment of multiple myeloma and ovarian cancer and occasionally for other tumor types. The drug induces acute non-lymphocytic leukemia in some patients treated for myeloma or ovarian cancer.

Busulfan. Busulfan (Myleran) is a methane-sulfonate–based alkylating agent that has specificity for myeloid neoplasms and appears to have less antitumor activity in other forms of cancer. It is available only for oral administration and is used primarily for treatment of chronic myeloid leukemia (CML) or as part of marrow ablative regimens followed by stem cell transplantation. Busulfan can produce protracted myelosuppression, and hematologic recovery should be complete before the next course is administered. Busulfan can also cause pulmonary fibrosis, hyperpigmentation, weakness, and wasting. Adrenal function remains normal.

Nitrosoureas. Carmustine (BCNU) and lomustine (CCNU) are rapidly biotransformed through non-enzymatic hydrolysis to release intermediates with alkylating and carbamoylating activities. Carmustine is available for intravenous use, and lomustine is given orally. The major toxicity of nitrosoureas at standard dosage levels is on hematopoietic stem cells; delayed, prolonged myelosuppression can result. At high doses (e.g., in preparative regimens for bone marrow transplantation), nitrosoureas can induce a chemical hepatitis or pneumonitis. Prolonged use with total doses greater than 1500 mg/m^2 can also result in pulmonary fibrosis or renal failure. Because of their high lipid solubility and ability to cross the blood-brain barrier, the nitrosoureas have some activity against primary brain tumors. The nitrosoureas also are useful in the management of Hodgkin's disease and multiple myeloma and as part of combined-modality therapy for cancers of the anal canal.

Platinum Compounds. Cisplatin and carboplatin are platinum-coordination compounds with broad-spectrum antitumor activity and synergistic interactions with a variety of other cytotoxic agents, including alkylating agents, antimetabolites, and natural products. Although their mechanism of action is not completely understood, they act similarly to alkylating agents in terms of their ability to bind to the N7 position of guanine and crosslink DNA. However, cross-linking with adenine and cytosine also occurs, as does binding to RNA and protein.

Cisplatin and carboplatin differ in their toxicity profiles. Both drugs are administered intravenously. Cisplatin is commonly given in a dose of 100 mg/m^2 every 3 weeks, whereas the dose of carboplatin is in the range of 450 mg/m^2 at similar intervals, although larger doses may be tolerated. After intravenous infusion, the major acute toxicity for both cisplatin and carboplatin is nausea and vomiting, which is worse with cisplatin. Satisfactory suppression of the gastrointestinal side effects of platinum compounds requires potent antiemetic agents, often in combination. Large cumulative doses of cisplatin also cause renal toxicity, which can be largely prevented if the patient is well hydrated with simultaneous saline infusions and diuretics. Large cumulative doses can also cause a progressive neuropathy. Myelosuppression is minimal with cisplatin but is dose limiting with carboplatin. Although carboplatin is less toxic than cisplatin, its efficacy is equivalent for some, but not all, tumors. The lack of myelosuppression favors cisplatin for use in some drug combinations with myelosuppressive agents. A new platinum analogue, oxaloplatin, may have activity against colon cancer comparable with that of fluorouracil.

ANTIMETABOLITES. The antimetabolites (Table 198–7) are structural analogues of normal biochemical compounds, most of which are involved in DNA or RNA synthesis and generally function as CCS agents. Antimetabolites are classed in relation to their mechanisms of action.

Pyrimidine Antagonists. *Cytarabine (Cytosine Arabinoside, Cytosar-U, Ara-C).* Cytarabine is an S-phase–specific agent that is particularly useful in acute non-lymphocytic leukemia and, to a lesser extent, in other hematologic malignancies. Its active form, ara-CTP, competitively inhibits DNA polymerase, blocking DNA synthesis. Ara-C also blocks chain elongation and ligation of fragments into newly synthesized DNA. Ara-C is given intravenously and crosses the blood-brain barrier. It is administered either by continuous infusion or in bolus doses by the intravenous or subcutaneous route for 5 to 7 days. In an alternative schedule that exceeds the manufacturer's recommended maximum, high-dose ara-C is administered in doses of 1 to 3 g every 12 hours for 3 to 5 days and yields higher response rates. The duration of intracellular retention of ara-CTP appears to predict ara-C antileukemic effects, with best results in patients who have the longest ara-CTP retention times. Both standard and high-dose ara-C can produce severe myelosuppression. With the high-dose regimen, chemical conjunctivitis is common and can be ameliorated with corticosteroid ophthalmic drops. With rare exception, complete remissions can be achieved in acute leukemia only if ara-C is administered with sufficient intensity to drive the bone marrow to severe hypocellularity and destroy the leukemic blast population. Thereafter, the marrow is repopulated by residual normal progenitors that were suppressed by the leukemia. Ara-C is generally used in combination with daunorubicin in the treatment of acute non-lymphocytic leukemia but also acts synergistically with other drugs, including cisplatin. Cytarabine can also be given intrathecally in doses of 75 to 100 mg as treatment for leukemic or carcinomatous meningitis.

Gemcitabine. Gemcitabine (Gemzar), is a novel nucleoside analogue with structural similarities to cytarabine. Both drugs are metabolized by cytidine deaminase and require intracellular phos-

Table 198–7 ■ ANTIMETABOLITE ANTICANCER DRUGS

DRUG	MAJOR INDICATIONS
Folic acid antagonists (methotrexate)	Acute lymphocytic leukemia, choriocarcinoma, breast cancer, bladder cancer, head and neck cancer, lymphoma
5-fluorouracil	Gastrointestinal cancer, breast cancer, cancer of the head and neck
5-fluorodeoxyuridine	Regional therapy (intra-arterial or intraperitoneal) for colon cancer metastasis
Cytarabine	Acute leukemia
Gemcitabine	Cancer of the pancreas
6-Mercaptopurine, 6-thioguanine	Acute leukemia
Fludarabine	Chronic lymphocytic leukemia, low-grade lymphoma
2-Chlorodeoxyadenosine	Hairy cell leukemia, low-grade lymphoma
Deoxycoformycin	Hairy cell leukemia, T-cell lymphoma
Hydroxyurea	Chronic myelocytic leukemia

phorylation for activation. The drug is approved for use in the treatment of patients with advanced pancreatic carcinoma. Gemcitabine significantly improves disease related symptoms in approximately 25% of patients, and a modest increase in survival was demonstrated in patients with pancreatic carcinoma when compared with treatment with 5-fluorouracil. The drug is well tolerated; reversible myelosuppression is the dose-limiting toxicity. The drug is administered intravenously over 30 minutes, weekly for 3 weeks followed by 1 week of rest.

Fluorouracil and Floxuridine. Fluorouracil (5-FU) is an important anticancer agent used to treat a variety of solid tumors, including cancers of the head and neck, esophagus, breast, and colon. It acts synergistically with a variety of agents, including platinum compounds and radiation therapy. Studies indicate that "pulse" or bolus injections of 5-FU are cytotoxic mainly as a result of incorporation into RNA, whereas continuous infusions of this drug (2 or more days) kill cells by inhibiting DNA synthesis and producing "thymine-less death." 5-FU is usually given intravenously by bolus or infusion schedules but can also be used in intra-arterial, intracavitary, and topical therapy. An optimal schedule for 5-FU administration is a 5-day continuous infusion at a dose rate of 1.0 g/m^2/day. This schedule causes some gastrointestinal toxicity but only a mild degree of myelosuppression. Full doses of cisplatin can be administered additionally, providing an active treatment program in the neoadjuvant chemotherapy of head and neck and esophageal cancer. 5-FU administered on a weekly intravenous bolus schedule produces greater hematologic toxicity and mucositis than lower total doses. Less common toxicities observed with 5-FU include a neurologic syndrome associated with ataxia, chemical conjunctivitis, and a syndrome including chest pain and cardiac enzyme elevation consistent with myocardial ischemia. The bioavailability of 5-FU after oral administration is erratic, and the drug is metabolized mostly during its first pass through the liver.

Both the gastrointestinal toxicity and the antitumor activity of 5-FU can be enhanced by administration of leucovorin, which increases the binding of fluorodeoxyuridine phosphate to thymidylate synthase. This combination appears to increase the antitumor activity of 5-FU in breast and colon cancer. Interferon-α and levamisole also appear to enhance 5-FU activity in colorectal cancer. Levamisole potentiation has been observed only in the adjuvant setting. Recent studies showed that 6 months of treatment with 5-FU and leucovorin in the adjuvant setting is the regimen of choice for patients with colorectal cancer. Both 5-FU and floxuridine (5-FUDR) can be given by hepatic artery infusion to treat patients with colorectal carcinoma with metastases confined to the liver. With the use of a surgically placed vascular access catheter, outpatient hepatic artery infusions can be administered using either an internal or a portable external pump. A limitation is that either 5-FU or 5-FUDR can induce a chemical hepatitis and biliary sclerosis with jaundice. Hepatic dysfunction can be most readily detected by obtaining liver chemistries on day 14 when 5-FU is to be discontinued. Studies indicate that the response rate and duration of remission are increased by the addition of leucovorin (folinic acid) or dexamethasone to 5-FUDR.

Purine Antagonists. *6-Mercaptopurine and 6-Thioguanine.* In contrast to 6-mercaptopurine (6-MP), some 6-thioguanine (6-TG) metabolites are incorporated into both DNA and RNA. 6-TG has some uses in acute non-lymphocytic leukemia in combination with cytarabine, whereas 6-MP is used primarily in acute lymphoblastic leukemia, particularly in childhood. Absorption of 6-MP is variable, but plasma monitoring can identify poor absorbers who have a high likelihood of developing recurrent leukemia, presumably because of inadequate bioavailability of 6-MP. The 6-MP analogue azathioprine is a useful immunosuppressive agent. Because both 6-MP and azathioprine are catabolized by xanthine oxidase, patients must have their thiopurine doses reduced to 25% of their standard doses if they are also receiving the xanthine oxidase inhibitor allopurinol. 6-TG is not catabolized by xanthine oxidase, and dose correction is not required for allopurinol.

Fludarabine. Fludarabine (Fludara, 5-fluoroadenosine monophosphate) is an analogue of adenine that inhibits DNA polymerase and ribonucleotide reductase. Fludarabine is the single most active agent available in the treatment of chronic lymphocytic leukemia and also exhibits some antitumor activity in other indolent lymphomas and macroglobulinemia. Fludarabine is often given intravenously in a dose of 25 mg/m^2/day over 30 minutes for 5 days

every 4 weeks. The major toxicity is myelosuppression. Higher doses administered in early trials in patients with acute non-lymphocytic leukemia occasionally produced cortical blindness. In the lower-dosage schedule used in chronic lymphocytic leukemia and other lymphoid neoplasms, side effects are usually mild and reversible.

Additional purine antagonists include deoxycoformycin (DCF) and 2-chlorodeoxyadenosine (2-CDA). Both DCF and 2-CDA are extremely active agents in the treatment of hairy cell leukemia and can produce prolonged remissions after a single course of treatment. Both agents also exhibit some antitumor activity in other low-grade lymphoid neoplasms (e.g., CLL and low-grade lymphomas).

Folic Acid Antagonists. Methotrexate (MTX) is a structural analogue of folic acid and is currently the only FDA-approved member of this group. Clinical trials of new antifolates are targeting not only dihydrofolate reductase (e.g., trimetrexate) but also other folate-requiring enzymes such as thymidylate synthase (e.g., raltitrexed). MTX can be administered orally, intramuscularly, or intravenously and is useful primarily as a component of chemotherapy combinations for various types of cancer, including acute lymphoblastic leukemia, small cell lung cancer, bladder cancer, head and neck cancer, and breast cancer. When used in high dosage with leucovorin rescue, it exerts antitumor activity in osteogenic sarcoma. Intracellular formation of polyglutamated forms of MTX is important to the action of MTX, because the polyglutamated forms have equivalent ability to inhibit dihydrofolate reductase action but have a longer intracellular retention time than MTX. The polyglutamates also inhibit other folate-dependent enzymes, including thymidylate synthase. Given satisfactory renal function and adequate hydration, MTX is excreted unchanged mainly in the urine within 12 hours of administration.

Major toxicities of MTX are to rapidly dividing tissues, including the bone marrow, gastrointestinal mucosa, and, to a lesser extent, skin. At high dosages or in patients with impaired renal function, MTX also can induce renal toxicity. Chronic extended use of MTX (e.g., for maintenance treatment of patients with acute lymphocytic leukemia or long-term treatment of patients with psoriasis), occasionally leads to liver fibrosis and cirrhosis. The toxic effects on the rapidly dividing tissues can be circumvented by administering the reduced folate leucovorin (folinic acid) within 36 hours after MTX administration. Leucovorin rescue also can be used when MTX is intentionally administered in higher than manufacturer's recommended maximum dose (e.g., 1500 mg/m^2 or more). When high-dose MTX is administered, leucovorin must be administered 24 to 36 hours after MTX in dosages of 15 to 50 mg/m^2 every 6 hours for 48 hours, with the duration of rescue contingent on the serum MTX level. Increased leucovorin dosage and longer periods of rescue are needed in patients with impaired renal function. The high-dose MTX/leucovorin rescue regimen therefore requires good renal function.

NATURAL PRODUCT ANTICANCER DRUGS. The two main classes of natural antitumor products are plant alkaloids and antibiotics (Table 198–8). Resistance to the natural products, with the exception of bleomycin, can be mediated by the P-glycoprotein multidrug resistance mechanism.

PLANT ALKALOIDS. Vincristine and Vinblastine. The *Vinca* alkaloids were isolated from the common periwinkle (*Vinca rosacea*). The major Vinca alkaloids in clinical use, vincristine (Oncovin) and vinblastine (Velban), precipitate tubulin and disrupt cellular microtubules. Whereas the primary toxicity of vinblastine is hematopoietic, vincristine's major toxicity affects peripheral nerves, resulting in sensorimotor and autonomic neuropathies. Common symptoms are paresthesias ("pins and needles sensation") in the digits and progressive muscular weakness with areflexia, particularly in the lower extremities. Footdrop can develop, as can occasional cranial, bladder, or bowel neuropathies. The neurotoxicity subsides slowly after the drug is discontinued, with improvement requiring months, especially if motor function is impaired. The lack of bone marrow toxicity of vincristine has made it useful for combination chemotherapy regimens. The *Vinca* alkaloids have vesicant effects and can be administered only intravenously. Both provide antitumor activity in leukemias and lymphomas as well as in selected solid tumors, including small cell lung cancer and breast cancer. Vincristine is used in various drug combinations, in-

Table 198-8 ■ NATURAL PRODUCT ANTICANCER DRUGS

DRUGS	MAJOR INDICATIONS
Plant Alkaloids	
Vincristine	Lymphoid malignancies
Vinblastine	Hodgkin's disease, testicular cancer
Vinorelbine	Small cell lung cancer
Podophyllotoxins	
Etoposide (VP-16)	Small cell lung cancer, lymphoma
Teniposide (VM-26)	Acute lymphocytic leukemia
Paclitaxel (Taxol)	Ovarian cancer, breast cancer
CPT-11	Colon cancer
Antibiotics	
Anthracyclines	
Doxorubicin	Lymphoma, breast cancer, sarcomas
Daunorubicin	Acute leukemia
Idarubicin	Acute leukemia
Mitoxantrone (synthetic)	Acute leukemia, lymphoma
Mitomycin	Gastrointestinal malignancies
Dactinomycin	Choriocarcinoma, Wilms' tumor, Ewing's sarcoma, rhabdomyosarcoma
Bleomycin	Lymphoma, head and neck cancer
Miscellaneous Agents	
Hexamethylmelamine	Ovarian cancer
Asparaginase	Acute lymphocytic leukemia

cluding MOPP, CHOP, MACOP-B, and M-BACOD for the treatment of lymphomas (see Chapter 179), and VMCP and VAD in the treatment of multiple myeloma (see Chapter 181). Vinblastine's greatest use has been in its incorporation into the PVB regimen for the treatment of non–seminomatous testicular cancers (see Chapter 247), and in the ABVD regimen to treat Hodgkin's disease (see Chapter 180). Vinblastine is also used in combination with cisplatin in non–small cell lung cancer and with mitomycin in metastatic breast cancer.

Vinorelbine. Vinorelbine (Navelbine) is a semisynthetic *Vinca* alkaloid approved for use in the treatment of non–small cell lung cancer. Its spectrum of antitumor activity and its mechanism of action are similar to those of vinblastine and vincristine. In humans, its limiting toxicity, like that of vinblastine is hematologic, and its spectrum of activity and use in combinations is under investigation.

PODOPHYLLOTOXINS. Etoposide. Etoposide (VP-16, VePesid), a semisynthetic glucoside, is produced from extracts of the root of the mayapple or mandrake (*Podophyllum peltatum*). A closely related analogue, teniposide (VM-26), has not been approved in the United States by the FDA. Mechanistically, podophyllotoxins are thought to act as inhibitors of nuclear topoisomerase II, leading to DNA strand breaks. Additional effects include inhibition of nucleoside transport and mitochondrial electron transport. Etoposide is highly lipid soluble and water insoluble and requires a special formulation for intravenous administration. An oral formulation is also available. Good tissue distribution is achieved in all sites other than the brain. A commonly used schedule administers etoposide intravenously for 3 days at a dosage of 150 to 200 mg/m²/day. Etoposide is excreted primarily in the urine and to a lesser extent in the bile. Its dosage should be reduced by half in patients with impaired renal function. The main side effect is myelosuppression, although gastrointestinal toxicity and alopecia also can occur. Etoposide is used primarily to treat metastatic testicular cancer in combination with cisplatin and bleomycin. The combination substitutes etoposide for vinblastine, yielding a less toxic but equally effective regimen. Etoposide also exerts potent effects against small cell lung cancer, lymphomas, and monocytic leukemia.

Paclitaxel. The taxoids are an important new class of anticancer agents that appear to stabilize tubulin as their major mechanism of action. Paclitaxel (Taxol) has been approved for use in the United States for the treatment of breast cancer and ovarian cancer and is also widely used for other epithelial tumors (head and neck, esophagus, non–small cell lung cancer) in combination therapy regimens. For example, the combination of cisplatin and paclitaxel is now first line treatment with a 10 to 20% cure rate for patients with ovarian cancer, where it improves survival compared with cisplatin

and cyclophosphamide. The drug may cause hypersensitivity reactions (e.g., hypotension, dyspnea, bronchospasm and urticaria). Typically, premedications are administered before paclitaxel administration to prevent these reactions: dexamethasone, 20 mg orally or intravenously, 12 and 6 hours before treatment; diphenhydramine, 50 mg, 30 minutes before treatment; and an H₂ antagonist (e.g., cimetidine), 300 mg, intravenously, 30 minutes before treatment. Other toxicities include neutropenia, which is dose limiting, myalgias, and peripheral neuropathy, the latter which generally occurs only after multiple courses at conventional doses (135 to 250 mg/m² over 24 hours). Other dosage schedules (3-hour, 96-hour) are under investigation.

Docetaxel. Docetaxel (Taxotere) is a semisynthetic analogue of paclitaxel and has been approved for use in the treatment of locally advanced or metastatic breast cancer that has progressed during anthracycline-based therapy. This drug also has anticancer activity in patients with non–small cell lung cancer. The recommended dose is 60 to 100 mg/m² intravenously every 3 weeks.

ANTITUMOR ANTIBIOTICS. Doxorubicin, Daunorubicin, and Idarubicin. These anthracycline antibiotics were isolated from a variant of *Streptomyces peucetius* and are extremely useful in cancer chemotherapy. Daunorubicin (daunomycin) was the first agent in this class and is active in the treatment of acute leukemia. Its congener, doxorubicin (Adriamycin), has a broader spectrum of antitumor activity, including both hematologic malignancies and a variety of solid tumors such as carcinoma of the breast and thyroid, lymphoma, and myeloma, as well as osteogenic and soft tissue sarcomas. Daunorubicin is frequently used in combination with cytarabine in the treatment of acute myelocytic leukemia, whereas doxorubicin is incorporated into regimens for solid tumors along with cyclophosphamide, fluorouracil, etoposide, vincristine, or cisplatin. Mechanistically, the anthracyclines intercalate with high affinity into DNA and inhibit the action of topoisomerase II, resulting in DNA strand breaks. Anthracycline cardiac toxicity may also be related in part to the generation of free radicals. Both doxorubicin and daunorubicin must be administered intravenously by either bolus injection or prolonged infusion. Extravasation can lead to severe tissue injury. Immediate topical application of 1.5 mL of 99% dimethylsulfoxide (DMSO) has been reported to prevent subsequent ulceration. For prolonged anthracycline infusions, use of a vascular access catheter is advisable. Ulceration and necrosis after anthracycline extravasation usually require surgical débridement of the damaged tissues plus skin grafting.

The most common acute toxicities of the anthracyclines include alopecia, nausea, vomiting, mucositis, and myelosuppression. A dose-dependent, delayed, and potentially irreversible cardiomyopathy with reduced cardiac contractility can develop in patients who receive large cumulative doses of doxorubicin or daunorubicin (see Chapter 64). Acute cardiac arrhythmias are uncommon.

Periodic monitoring for cardiac effects of anthracyclines is normally initiated when a patient has received a total doxorubicin dose of 350 to 400 mg/m². Endomyocardial biopsy can also be used. Cardiac toxicity is uncommon with cumulative bolus doses of doxorubicin of less than 550 mg/m², above which the incidence rises progressively. Elderly patients and others with risk factors for cardiac disease (e.g., hypertension) are at somewhat higher risk for anthracycline cardiomyopathy. Anthracyclines are not recommended for patients who have major pre-existing heart disease. When doxorubicin is administered by continuous infusion (e.g., for 4 to 5 days), there is less cardiotoxicity, and a significantly larger cumulative dose in the range of 1000 mg/m² can usually be administered. However, regular cardiac monitoring is required, and doxorubicin should be discontinued if the left ventricular ejection fraction falls by 15 percentage points and to below 50%. Idarubicin is another anthracycline recently approved for use in the treatment of acute myelocytic leukemia. In controlled studies, idarubicin in combination with cytarabine induced higher remission rates than daunorubicin and cytarabine.

An agent that protects the heart from anthracycline toxicity, dexrazoxane, has been approved for use by the FDA for patients who are treated with cumulative doses of doxorubicin greater than 300 mg/m². Liposomal preparations of doxorubicin are also being evaluated as potentially less cardiotoxic formulations. Toxicities associated with dexrazoxane are pain at the injection site and modest neutropenia and thrombocytopenia. The possibility that dexrazoxane may have an adverse effect on tumor response led to the FDA recommendation that treatment with this drug should be initiated only when the cumulative dose of 300 mg/m² of doxorubicin was reached.

Bleomycin. Bleomycin (Blenoxane) comprises 11 closely related glycopeptide moieties produced by *Streptomyces verticillus*. The major components are bleomycins A2 and B2. Bleomycin action involves its binding to DNA and generation of superoxide and other reactive oxygen species, including hydroxyl radicals. DNA fragmentation appears to result from the oxidation of a DNA-bleomycin-Fe²⁺ complex. Bleomycin's antitumor activity is schedule dependent, acting primarily at the G₂ phase of the cell cycle. It can be administered by subcutaneous, intramuscular, and intravenous routes. Its major uses are in combination therapy to treat carcinoma of the testis and squamous cell carcinomas of the head and neck, cervix, skin, penis, and rectum. It is also used in combination regimens for treatment of lymphomas (ABVD).

Bleomycin has minimal myelosuppressive effects and is useful in combination with drugs that cause leukopenia. Acute toxicities include anaphylactoid reactions and fever associated with hypotension and dehydration. Patients who have not received bleomycin previously should receive a test dose (e.g., 1 to 2 mg) to discover such adverse reactions. Individual therapeutic doses of bleomycin are usually in the range of 5 to 10 units/m².

The most serious chronic reaction to bleomycin is pulmonary fibrosis related to the cumulative dose of drug and manifested by cough, dyspnea, and bilateral basilar infiltrates on chest radiography. It is possible to screen for earlier pulmonary abnormalities such as a decline in the diffusion capacity, which is usually detectable at total doses of bleomycin above 250 units. If the pulmonary diffusion capacity falls abnormally, bleomycin should be discontinued. The incidence of pulmonary fibrosis rises at total doses above 450 units and is higher in patients with pre-existing pulmonary disease, after lung irradiation, and in the elderly. This toxicity may be irreversible, although corticosteroids may be of some use. Other reactions to bleomycin include skin toxicity with blistering, desquamation, hyperkeratosis of the palms, and hyperpigmentation of creases.

Mitomycin. Mitomycin (Mutamycin, Mitocin-C, Mitomycin C) is isolated from *Streptomyces caespitosus*. Its structure includes quinone, carbamate, and aziridine groups, which may contribute to its antitumor activity. Mitomycin functions as a CCNS alkylating agent after it has been activated in various tissues by the cytochrome P-450 system. Thereafter, it can alkylate DNA to form intrastrand and interstrand crosslinks resulting in cell death. Mitomycin has "bioreductive" properties, with increased cytotoxic effects on poorly oxygenated tumor cells in solid tumors, and has been used in combination with irradiation to treat patients with cancer of the head and neck. Mitomycin's clinical spectrum of antitumor activity includes breast, lung, gastrointestinal, genitourinary, and gynecologic cancers. Mitomycin has been incorporated into a variety of cytotoxic drug combinations for systemic administration, often as second-line therapy for patients who relapse from initial chemotherapy. It is usually administered intravenously but can be used for intravesical therapy of superficial bladder cancer. Its normal intravenous dosage range is 10 to 15 mg/m².

The major toxicity of mitomycin is delayed myelosuppression, usually appearing 4 to 6 weeks after injection. Mitomycin has a cumulative effect on bone marrow stem cells, which can lead to protracted marrow hypoplasia for 3 to 6 months after discontinuing the drug. Nausea, vomiting, and anorexia often occur at the time of administration but can usually be managed effectively with antiemetic agents. Occasionally, mitomycin can induce interstitial pneumonitis, nephrotoxicity, or hemolytic-uremic syndrome.

Dactinomycin. Dactinomycin (Actinomycin D, Cosmegen) was the first effective antitumor antibiotic isolated from *Streptomyces*. It binds to the DNA helix by intercalation between adjacent guanine-cytosine base pairs; it inhibits DNA-dependent RNA synthesis and leads to cessation of most protein synthesis in sensitive cells. The drug is administered intravenously, and its major toxicity is myelosuppression, usually appearing 7 to 10 days after injection. Dactinomycin also causes significant gastrointestinal toxicity with abdominal cramps and diarrhea as well as mucositis. The drug also can cause a radiation "recall" reaction in which cutaneous erythema redevelops at a site of prior irradiation. The principal use of dactinomycin is in pediatric oncology in combination chemotherapy for the treatment of Wilms' tumor, Ewing's sarcoma, and embryonal

rhabdomyosarcoma. It has some utility in adults in third-line therapy of germ cell tumors of the testis or ovary, gestational choriocarcinoma, and soft tissue sarcomas.

TOPOISOMERASE 1 INHIBITORS. This class of drugs binds to topoisomerase I. Two inhibitors of this enzyme have now been approved for clinical use: irinotecan and topotecan.

Irinotecan. Irinotecan (CPT-11, Camptosar) is a prodrug that is rapidly hydrolyzed in vivo to SN-38, a potent inhibitor of topoisomerase I. It has been approved for use in the treatment of patients with colorectal cancer. The dose schedule used most commonly is a single infusion (200 mg/m²) every 3 weeks, although other dose schedules are being explored. The principal dose-limiting toxicities are non-hematologic, in particular diarrhea. Diarrhea may be seen within the first 24 hours of treatment, or later, occurring 4 to 8 days after treatment. Aggressive treatment with loperamide or octreotide at the first sign of diarrhea has allowed patients to tolerate this drug. Severe neutropenia may also occur with CPT-11. Current studies are evaluating combinations of this drug with fluorouracil or raltitrexed (Tomudex), an investigational drug that targets the enzyme thymidylate synthase.

Topotecan. Topotecan (Hycamtin) is approved for use in previously treated patients with ovarian cancer. Its mechanism of action is similar to that of irinotecan, namely, inhibition of topoisomerase I. Topotecan also has activity in other tumors, including hematologic malignancies, small cell lung cancer, neuroblastoma, and rhabdomyosarcoma. The recommended dose is 1.5 mg/m²/day infused intravenously over 30 minutes for 5 consecutive days, every 3 weeks. The dose limiting and most common toxicity is myelosuppression, especially neutropenia.

MISCELLANEOUS ANTICANCER AGENTS. PROCARBAZINE. Procarbazine (Matulane) is an orally administered methylhydrazine derivative that has antitumor activity in Hodgkin's disease (as part of MOPP combination chemotherapy) and in non-Hodgkin's lymphomas, lung cancer, and brain tumors. Procarbazine is usually given in a dose of 100 mg/m²/day for 10 to 14 days in each chemotherapy cycle. Procarbazine is activated metabolically to produce a methyldiazonium ion that binds to nucleic acids, proteins, and phospholipids to inhibit macromolecular synthesis. Its mechanism of cytotoxicity is thought to involve DNA strand scission, possibly through generation of H₂O₂. Procarbazine's principal toxicities are nausea, vomiting, and myelosuppression. One of procarbazine's metabolites is a monoamine oxidase (MAO) inhibitor that can cause toxicity when the patient is taking other MAO inhibitors. Patients taking procarbazine may develop hypertension if they ingest tyramine-rich foods such as ripe cheese, wine, and bananas. Disulfiram-like reactions are also seen, with sweating and headache after alcohol ingestion. Other infrequent reactions include hemolytic anemia and pulmonary reactions. Procarbazine is also known to be leukemogenic, carcinogenic, and mutagenic and is considered to play a significant role in the development of late leukemias and other second malignancies in patients with Hodgkin's disease. Procarbazine also produces azoospermia and anovulation. Because alternative combinations lacking procarbazine can be used in the treatment of Hodgkin's disease (e.g., ABVD), the benefits versus risks of using this agent must be carefully considered.

DACARBAZINE. Dacarbazine (DTIC, dimethylimidazole carboxamide) is activated by oxidative *N*-demethylation. A methyl carbonium ion metabolite is thought to be the cytotoxic intermediate with alkylating activity. Dacarbazine is administered intravenously either in a single-day infusion schedule of 750 mg/m² or in fractionated bolus doses over 5 days or more. DTIC causes severe nausea and vomiting, and potent antiemetic agents are required. Myelosuppression is relatively mild. Dacarbazine is used in combination chemotherapy for Hodgkin's disease (ABVD), for soft tissue sarcomas in combination with doxorubicin and other agents, and in single-agent chemotherapy for metastatic melanoma.

HEXAMETHYLMELAMINE (HMM). This agent is available only in an oral formulation because of its sparing solubility. Oral bioavailability of HMM is quite variable, however, and nausea and vomiting can be dose limiting. The gastrointestinal distress increases with daily use, limiting the length of treatment courses (at doses of up to 12 mg/kg/day) to 2 to 3 weeks. Mild myelosuppression occurs. Additionally, HMM can induce both central and peripheral neurotoxicities, including altered mood, hallucinations, and peripheral neuropathy. HMM is thought to act as an alkylating agent, possibly through the enzymatic hydroxylation of its demethyl metabolites to cytotoxic methylol compounds. HMM exhibits antitumor activity in alkylating agent-resistant ovarian cancer and, to a lesser extent, in several other neoplasms (lung, breast cancer, lymphomas).

HYDROXYUREA. Hydroxyurea (Hydrea, HU) acts as an inhibitor of ribonucleotide reductase, resulting in intracellular depletion of deoxynucleoside triphosphates and inhibition of DNA synthesis. It is available for clinical use in oral formulation. HU's major toxicity is to the bone marrow, and it causes transient dose-related myelo-suppression. At high dosage, a megaloblastic anemia can develop, which is non-responsive to vitamin B_{12} or folic acid. Gastrointestinal side effects of nausea and vomiting are also common with high-dose therapy. HU is used primarily to treat chronic myeloid leukemia and polycythemia vera, but it also has some use in head and neck cancer and metastatic melanoma and as a radiosensitizer.

MITOXANTRONE. Mitoxantrone (Novantrone) is an anthracenedi-one with a structure that appears analogous to that of the anthra-cyclines. It has been approved by the FDA as a second-line agent for treatment of acute leukemia in relapse but is also useful in the treatment of breast cancer and lymphoma. Mitoxantrone binds to DNA and causes strand breaks and inhibits DNA and RNA synthesis. In terms of cellular response by tumor cells, there is not complete cross-reactivity between mitoxantrone and the anthracyclines. Mitoxantrone dosage for acute leukemia is higher than for solid tumors. Comparative studies in patients with advanced breast cancer suggest that it is less active and less toxic than doxorubicin. Its major acute toxicity is myelosuppression. Gastrointestinal side effects, including nausea, vomiting, and mucositis as well as alopecia, are less severe than with the anthracyclines. Mitoxantrone can cause some cardiac toxicities, usually manifest by development of arrhythmia at the time of injection, and can exacerbate pre-existing anthracycline-induced cardiomyopathy. It can be used intraperitoneally in patients with ovarian cancer, because most of the drug remains in the peritoneal cavity. This approach reduces systemic toxicity, but it can induce chemical peritonitis and adhesions.

ASPARAGINASE. L-Asparaginase (Crasnitin, Elspar) is a bacterial enzyme isolated from *Escherichia coli* or *Erwinia carotovora*. Its major use is to treat lymphoblastic leukemias and some lymphomas with a deficiency in asparagine synthetase and cellular dependence on exogenous asparagine. L-Asparagine is a non-essential amino acid, and most normal cells can synthesize their required asparagine. Therapeutically, L-asparaginase depletes the plasma of asparagine by converting it to aspartic acid and ammonia. Most patients develop fever and chills as well as nausea and vomiting after administration, but these symptoms can usually be reduced or prevented by premedication with antiemetics and anti-inflammatory agents. Asparaginase toxicity can produce abnormal liver function tests (aspartate aminotransferase T, alkaline phosphatase, and bilirubin) as well as hypoalbuminemia and reductions in plasma levels of clotting factors and insulin. Other occasional toxicities include pancreatitis and central nervous system abnormalities, which can lead to confusion or coma. Repeated use of asparaginase leads to the development of antibodies that can inhibit its activity and accelerate its clearance as well as induce hypersensitivity reactions. Patients developing hypersensitivity after asparaginase administration may exhibit hypotension, laryngeal edema, bronchospasm, and urticaria. Switching to an asparaginase derived from a different bacterial species can bypass neutralizing antibodies in hypersensitive patients. The lack of myelosuppressive or gastrointestinal toxicity has facilitated incorporation of L-asparaginase into drug combinations for the treatment of acute lymphocytic leukemia (ALL). A useful combination in ALL is methotrexate, followed 24 hours later by L-asparaginase.

MANAGEMENT OF TOXICITY

Most cytotoxic drugs are also toxic for host cells, and treatment schedules must take this into account.

DOSE ADJUSTMENTS FOR BONE MARROW TOXICITY. Doses of myelosuppressive agents often must be adjusted downward to avoid serious or life-threatening side effects such as granulocytopenic fever and thrombocytopenic bleeding. For most drugs, empir-ical schedules have been developed for drug administration with single agents or combinations of myelosuppressive drugs normally given every 3 to 4 weeks. The interval between treatments provides time for hematopoietic recovery of normal myeloid progenitors in the bone marrow and avoids cumulative myelosuppression. It is essential to check the patient's white blood cell count, differential, and platelet count immediately before each course of myelosuppressive chemotherapy. During the first few cycles of chemotherapy, and at intervals thereafter, it is useful to check counts between treatment courses, particularly to determine the nadir of absolute granulocyte count (AGC). Falls of AGC below $1000/\mu L$ increase the risk of infection; AGCs below $500/\mu L$ represent a potentially fatal risk. Because hematopoietic recovery can occur rapidly after the nadir, the AGC immediately before the next course can be normal even though the nadir count may have been very low. For some drug combinations with low but brief AGC nadirs, prophylactic antibiotic agents (e.g., ciprofloxacin, sulfamethoxazole-trimethoprim) that will bracket the AGC nadir can protect against infection secondary to neutropenia. In general, if the AGC immediately before the next course of chemotherapy is less than $2000/\mu L$, the dose of myelosuppressive drugs should be reduced by 50%. With an AGC of less than $1500/\mu L$, doses should be reduced by 75%. If less than $1000/\mu L$, the drug should be withheld until hematologic recovery occurs. An additional approach to problems of myelosuppression involves the use of bone marrow growth factors, as discussed below under Biologic Agents.

DOSE ADJUSTMENTS FOR IMPAIRED HEPATIC OR RENAL FUNCTION. It is important to make downward dosage adjustments for specific drugs when altered hepatic or renal function plays a major role in drug metabolism. The metabolism of doxorubicin depends on good hepatobiliary function. Patients with a serum bilirubin value of greater than 3.0 mg/dL should have their doxorubicin dose reduced by at least 50% until drug tolerance is established.

Cisplatin, methotrexate, etoposide, hydroxyurea, and bleomycin all are cleared predominantly through renal excretion. Doses of these agents should be decreased approximately in proportion to the decline in renal function as determined by creatinine clearance and reflected by the serum creatinine value.

ENDOCRINE AGENTS

Cancer cells often exhibit susceptibility to hormonal control mechanisms that regulate growth of the normal organ or tissue from which the neoplasm arose. Endocrine therapy (Table 198–9) appears generally to work through cytostatic rather than cytotoxic mechanisms and usually requires long-term suppression. Endocrine therapy includes the use of both hormones and "antihormones," which are either antagonists or partial agonists for a given endocrine mechanism. Inasmuch as the effects of hormones are receptor mediated, evaluation of receptors capable of binding hormones has played an important role in assessing both tumor types and individual patients for possible endocrine therapy.

STEROID HORMONES AND ANTIHORMONES. Cancers arising from endocrine organs and the immune system are susceptible to the effects of steroid hormones, steroid hormone antagonists, and hormone deprivation. The sex steroids and their antagonists represent major agents for the treatment of common cancers arising from the breast, prostate gland, and uterus. The role of endocrine ablation procedures (hypophysectomy, adrenalectomy, oophorectomy, orchiectomy) has diminished as systemic agents have been identified to replace surgical procedures. Nonetheless, oophorectomy and orchiectomy are still useful in the treatment of endocrine-sensitive cancers of the breast and prostate, respectively.

ESTROGENS AND ANTIESTROGENS. Pharmacologic doses of estrogen have therapeutic effects in cancers of the prostate and the breast. Orchiectomy is equally efficacious and lacks feminizing side effects. No evidence suggests an additive effect of the two.

The antiestrogen tamoxifen (Nolvadex) improves survival of postmenopausal women with estrogen and/or progesterone receptor-positive breast cancer in both the adjuvant and metastatic settings. Recent but still controversial studies also suggest that tamoxifen may be a useful adjuvant for hormone receptor–negative cancers in postmenopausal women. A recent breast cancer prevention

Table 198–9 ■ HORMONALLY ACTIVE AGENTS IN CANCER TREATMENT

REPRESENTATIVE AGENTS	DOSE (ORAL UNLESS SPECIFIED)	TOXICITY (A = ACUTE; D = DELAYED)	USES
Glucocorticoids			
Prednisone	20–100 mg/d or 50 mg qod (single dose)	A: Fluid retention, hyperglycemia, euphoria, depression, hypokalemia	Leukemia Lymphoma
Dexamethasone	4–16 mg/d or 40 mg/d for 4-day pulses every 2–4 weeks	D: Osteoporosis, immunosuppression, gastrointestinal ulcers, cushingoid appearance, cataracts	Myeloma Breast cancer Brain metastases
Estrogen			
Diethylstilbestrol	5 mg tid (breast); 1–3 mg qd (prostate)	A: Nausea, vomiting, fluid retention, hypercalcemia (flare reaction with bone metastases), uterine bleeding	Breast cancer Prostate cancer
		D: Feminization, accelerated coronary artery disease	
Antiestrogen			
Tamoxifen	20 mg qd	A: Occasional nausea, fluid retention, hot flashes	Breast cancer
		D: Retinal degeneration	
Toremifene			Breast cancer
Aromatase Inhibitor			
Aminoglutethimide (plus hydrocortisone 20 mg bid)	250 mg bid (breast); 250 mg qid (prostate)	A: Dizziness D: Rash (transient)	Breast cancer Prostate cancer
Anastrozole	1 mg/d	A: Nausea, vomiting	
Progestins			
Megestrol acetate	40 mg qid	A: Increased appetite (megestrol), fluid retention	Breast cancer
Hydroxyprogesterone	1 g IM biw	D: Weight gain, thromboembolism	
Androgens			
Fluoxymesterone	10–20 mg qd	A: Cholestatic jaundice (with oral drug)	Breast cancer
Testosterone	600 mg IM q4–6 wk	D: Virilization	
Antiandrogen			
Flutamide	250 mg tid	D: Gynecomastia	Prostate cancer
Gonadotropin-releasing hormone agonists (depot formulations)			
Leuprolide acetate	7.5 mg SQ monthly	A: Transient flare of symptoms	Prostate cancer
Goserelin acetate	3.6 mg SQ monthly		Breast cancer (?)

trial involving more than 1300 women at high risk for breast cancer showed that women taking tamoxifen had a lower incidence of disease than those taking a placebo. Raloxifene, also an estrogen antagonist, has been shown to reduce breast cancer risk without increasing the incidence of uterine cancer, which is a concern with tamoxifen prophylaxis. In general, cytotoxic chemotherapy rather than endocrine therapy is recommended for women with hormone-receptor–negative breast cancer. Tamoxifen is available only in 10-mg tablets for oral administration, with a manufacturer's recommended dose of 10 mg twice daily. The schedule lacks a good scientific rationale because, with chronic therapy, tamoxifen and its active metabolite dihydroxytamoxifen achieve a steady state with a large deep tissue reservoir. Accordingly, use of a single dose of 20 mg should be an acceptable alternative schedule with fewer problems with compliance. Serious or life-threatening toxicities of tamoxifen (thromboembolic disease, retinitis) are rare. Common side effects include hot flashes and weight gain, sometimes due to fluid retention. Mild nausea also may occur. In premenopausal women with hormone receptor–positive neoplasms and overt metastatic disease, both oophorectomy and antiestrogen therapy can be useful. However, cytotoxic chemotherapy remains the treatment of choice, because it appears to have curative potential. The role of ovarian ablation or antiestrogen therapy added to chemotherapy in the adjuvant setting remains to be defined. Tamoxifen has been reported as occasionally having palliative effects in other neoplasms such as ovarian or endometrial cancer. Toremiphene, an estrogen antagonist, has also been approved for the treatment of breast cancer. It appears to have similar response rates to tamoxifen in the treatment of this disease.

ANDROGENS AND ANTIANDROGENS. Androgen therapy is contraindicated in prostate cancer because it stimulates growth. Virilizing androgens such as testosterone propionate, fluoxymesterone (Halotestin), and testosterone enanthate (Delatestryl) have all been used beneficially in the treatment of metastatic breast cancer with hormone receptor–positive disease. However, androgen therapy has largely been replaced with antiestrogen therapy because the antiestrogen does not cause hirsutism, deepening of the voice, or changes in libido. Additionally, the oral halogenated androgens (e.g., fluoxymesterone) also can cause cholestatic jaundice. The antiandrogen flutamide (Eulexin) is a useful agent in the treatment of prostate cancer in combination with one of the gonadotropin-releasing hormone agonists (leuprolide, goserelin), and these combinations function as a "medical orchiectomy."

PROGESTINS. Progestins are useful in palliative management of metastatic breast or endometrial cancer and can cause tumor regression in endocrine-sensitive disease. No evidence suggests their utility in the adjuvant setting in either of these neoplasms. Occasional patients with prostate cancer also appear to benefit from progestational therapy. The most commonly used progestins include megestrol acetate (Megace), medroxyprogesterone (Provera), and hydroxyprogesterone caproate (Delalutin). Megestrol acetate is useful for second-line endocrine therapy for patients with metastatic breast cancer who initially respond to tamoxifen. In patients who experience disturbing side effects from tamoxifen (e.g., severe hot flashes), megestrol acetate may represent a reasonable alternative. In addition to its antitumor effects, megestrol acetate improves appetite in some patients with cancer-induced cachexia.

GLUCOCORTICOIDS. Adrenal steroid hormones of the glucocorticoid class (e.g., prednisone, methylprednisolone, dexamethasone) are useful in treating lymphoid malignancies and may also potentiate the effects of cytotoxic agents in these tumor types as well as in breast cancer and perhaps other neoplasms. The glucocorticoids play an important role in treating complications of cancer (hypercalcemia, cerebral edema). Glucocorticoids are lympholytic and non-myelosuppressive and have been incorporated into combination chemotherapy for acute and chronic lympholytic leukemia, malignant lymphoma, and multiple myeloma. Glucocorticoids appear to induce cell death in some lymphoid malignancies by apoptosis.

AROMATASE INHIBITORS. AMINOGLUTETHIMIDE (CYTADREN). Aminoglutethimide inhibits the first step in adrenal steroid synthesis. Additionally, and probably more importantly, aminoglutethimide also inhibits the extra-adrenal conversion of the adrenal androgen androstenedione to estrone by the enzyme aromatase. Aromatase is found in body fat and some other tissues and explains the presence of the weak estrogen estrone in the plasma of postmenopausal women. Aminoglutethimide is useful in the palliative treatment of recurrent breast cancer in hormone receptor–positive patients. Used in combination with hydrocortisone, it suppresses endogenous steroid hormone synthesis (including androstenedione) as well as ACTH production and slows the catabolism of aminoglutethimide. Aminoglutethimide is commonly administered in a dose of 250 mg twice daily along with 20 mg of hydrocortisone. Somewhat higher doses have been employed for second-line endocrine therapy for metastatic prostate cancer. Patients receiving aminoglutethimide and hydrocortisone should be cautioned against abrupt cessation of therapy to avoid symptoms of adrenal insufficiency.

ANASTROZOLE. Anastrozole (Arimidex) is a selective non-steroidal aromatase inhibitor. Unlike aminoglutethimide, which is neither a selective nor a powerful aromatase inhibitor, anastrozole is the first orally administered aromatase inhibitor approved by the FDA for the treatment of postmenopausal women with advanced breast cancer. The drug has an excellent toxicity profile, and only a small percentage of patients who receive a 1-mg/day dose experience nausea, asthenia, headache, or hot flashes.

GONADOTROPIN-RELEASING HORMONE (GnRH, LHRH) AGONISTS. Several synthetic analogues of natural GnRH (LHRH) are now clinically available. Both leuprolide acetate (Lupron) and goserelin acetate (Zoladex) are available in long-acting parenteral-depot formulations. These analogues function more potently than natural GnRH agonists and also have an unusual effect on the pituitary, consisting of initial stimulation followed by long-term inhibition of the release of follicle-stimulating hormone and leuteinizing hormone. This initial increase in gonadotropins can cause a transient increase in symptoms in patients with bone metastases. The inhibition of release of the gonadotropin reduces testicular androgen synthesis in men and ovarian estrogen production in women. Accordingly, GnRH offers an alternative to surgical orchiectomy in patients with prostate cancer and avoids the gynecomastia, nausea, vomiting, edema, and thromboembolic disease that estrogens may induce. The effectiveness of GnRH agonists is enhanced by administration in combination with an antiandrogen (flutamide), and the combination has been reported to be more effective than a GnRH agonist alone in patients with stage D metastatic prostate cancer. Impotence results from this form of "medical orchiectomy," as it does from surgical orchiectomy, but the effects of medical therapy are potentially reversible if treatment is discontinued. Medical orchiectomy is more expensive but acceptable to patients who decline surgical orchiectomy. GnRH agonists now show promise in combination with antiestrogens as endocrine therapy for premenopausal women with hormone receptor–positive breast cancer. The GnRH agonists are abortifacients in animals and should not be given to women who are or may become pregnant.

BIOLOGIC THERAPY

A new form of cancer therapy, still in its evolution, is the use of recombinant cytokines, vaccine growth factors, and monoclonal antibodies for the treatment of cancer (Table 198–10). The term *biologic therapy* describes this heterogeneous group of agents that either are normal mammalian mediators or achieve antitumor effects through endogenous host defense mechanisms. The biologic agents have also been termed *biologic response modifiers*. Both the cellular and humoral limbs of immunity can be exploited in cancer therapy. The cellular defenses include several classes of cytotoxic lymphocytes (natural killer cells), lymphokine-activated killer (LAK) cells, tumor infiltrating lymphoma, and cytotoxic T lymphocytes, as well as antibody-dependent cytotoxic cells. The non-specific cells of the reticuloendothelial system, including activated macrophages, also may be important. Humoral agents with antitumor activities include cytokines such as interferons and interleukins as well as specific antibodies. Most of these humoral agents interact with specific immune effector cells in a coordinated and synergistic fashion. The general availability of cytokines and growth

Table 198–10 ■ BIOLOGIC THERAPY OF CANCER: APPROACHES AND AGENTS

APPROACH	AGENTS
Active immunotherapy	
Non-specific	Adjuvants: BCG, levamisole
	Cytokines: Interferons, interleukin-2
Specific	Tumor cell vaccines
Passive serotherapy	
Antibodies	Polyclonal or monoclonal antibodies (alone or conjugated with drugs, radionuclides, or toxins)
Adoptive cellular therapy	Lymphokine-activated killer cells
	Tumor-infiltrating lymphocytes
Immunomodulators	Levamisole, thymic hormones
Bone marrow growth factors	G-CSF, GM-CSF, M-CSF, interleukin-3, erythropoietin
Growth factor antagonists	Suramin
	Antibodies to growth factor receptors (e.g., epidermal growth factor, HER-2/neu, interleukin-2 receptors)
Antiangiogenesis agents	Endostatin
	Angiostatin

G-CSF, GM-CSF, and M-CSF = granulocyte, granulocyte-macrophage, and macrophage colony-stimulating factors.

factors has been facilitated by the development of recombinant DNA technology. Antibodies are highly specific and generally interact directly with their tumor targets when they are targeted against cell-surface constituents. Some humoral agents, including the tumor necrosis factors-α and -β, have demonstrated potent local antitumor properties in preclinical models but have yet to be shown to be clinically useful.

Vaccines based on specific bacterial agents or extracts from bacteria can non-specifically activate the host immune system. By using BCG, this approach has been applied successfully to intravesical therapy of in situ cancer of the urinary bladder. Specific cancer-associated antigen vaccines are under active investigation.

INTERFERONS. The interferons (IFNs) are a family of antiviral proteins that differ in their cellular origin and polypeptide structure as well as in their clinical applications. The three major molecular species are IFN-α, -β, and -γ. IFN-α and -β mediate their action by binding to the same cell surface receptor, whereas a second cell-surface receptor mediates the action of IFN-γ. IFN-α is the major species for use in the treatment of hematologic malignancies and solid tumors. Whether IFN-β or -γ will have sufficient advantage over IFN-α in any specific cancer indication to gain regulatory approval is uncertain.

INTERFERON-α. Recombinant IFN-α (IFN-α_2, Intron-A, Roferon-A), a polypeptide cytokine with antiviral properties, is useful for single-agent treatment of selected hematologic malignancies and solid tumors. The precise mechanism of action of IFN is still poorly understood, but it is known to activate the transcription of a number of cellular genes. Additionally, IFN inhibits the synthesis of a number of proteins in sensitive tumor target cells, including ornithine decarboxylase, a rate-limiting enzyme in polyamine metabolism. Although IFN-α also has antiviral and immunoregulatory properties that alter the biologic function of many cell types involved in humoral and cellular immunity, it is unclear whether these functions influence its antitumor properties above and beyond its direct receptor-mediated effects on sensitive tumor cells. The antitumor properties of IFN-α also appear to be schedule dependent with a cytostatic mode of action. Most remissions induced by IFN are only partial.

IFN-α can be administered parenterally by intravenous, intramuscular, subcutaneous, and intracavitary routes. Its preferred route is by subcutaneous administration, which provides the longest duration of action. The dosage schedules are quite variable, with higher dosages required for some tumor types. Hairy cell leukemia is the tumor most sensitive to IFN-α. Usual dosages are in the range of 3 million IU administered subcutaneously three times weekly. At these low levels, IFN usually causes only mild side effects such as fever and chills with the first few doses. For Kaposi's sarcoma, far more aggressive and toxic IFN schedules are required and can cause anorexia, weight loss, failure in concentration, and profound weakness. High-dose IFN can also induce occasional cardiac arrhythmias, nausea, vomiting, leukopenia, myalgias, proteinuria, and hepatic dysfunction. Elderly patients appear to develop more marked side effects at all dosage schedules.

IFN-α is also useful in the treatment of chronic myeloid leukemia, multiple myeloma, some of the low-grade non-Hodgkin's lymphomas, and in some patients with metastatic melanoma or renal cell carcinoma. In melanoma, the use of high doses of IFN-α in an adjuvant mode has been shown to decrease the relapse rate. In myeloma, IFN-α appears to lengthen remissions induced by chemotherapy. Patients receiving recombinant IFN-α for hairy cell leukemia, CML, or renal cancer have developed neutralizing antibodies to the recombinant product when the disease progresses again after an IFN-induced remission. A limited number of patients with neutralizing antibodies have been successfully re-treated by switching to non-recombinant IFN-α. IFN-α has been incorporated into combination therapy with various cytotoxic and endocrine agents. At present, use of IFN-α in combination with 5-FU is being explored in combination with *cis*-retinoic acid to treat renal and cervical cancers. Although the clinical indications for IFN therapy continue to grow gradually, it has lacked the type of broad-spectrum anticancer effects that were initially envisioned.

INTERLEUKIN-2. Interleukin-2 (IL-2, Proleukin) is an immunomodulatory cytokine that acts on T-cell progenitors to produce LAK cells. Recombinant IL-2 has been approved for therapeutic use in renal cancer. Direct intravenous infusion induces LAK cells in the patient. Additionally, leukapheresis can obtain circulating lymphocytes that can then be exposed to IL-2 in tissue culture to activate lymphoid progenitors into LAK cells, which are then reinfused into the patient. There is now general agreement that either IL-2 or IL-2/LAK can induce tumor regression in 10 to 20% of patients with renal carcinoma or melanoma.

Whereas the infusion of LAK cells causes relatively few side effects, IL-2 induces considerable toxicity. Patients receiving high-dose IL-2 must be in an intensive-care unit with close management of blood pressure, fluids, and electrolytes. The high-dose regimens are suitable only for younger patients without other significant disease or impairment of cardiac, pulmonary, hepatic, or renal function. Common side effects of high-dose IL-2/LAK are probably due to lymphoid infiltrates in major organs and an induced capillary leak syndrome. Shortly after initiation of high-dose IL-2 therapy, tachycardia develops, and a significant drop in arterial blood pressure occurs. As IL-2 administration continues, compensatory fluid retention occurs in association with weight gain, oliguria, and azotemia. Vasopressors are often needed. Even at lower doses that can be used in a conventional hospital or outpatient setting (e.g., 3 million IU/m^2/day by intravenous infusion for 2 weeks), hypotension and fluid retention are not uncommon.

Pulmonary metastases appear to be somewhat more sensitive to IL-2 or IL-2/LAK therapy than are other tumors. With the adoptive immunotherapy approach using IL-2/LAK, a small percentage of patients who had undergone prior removal of the primary tumor achieved complete remission, with all evidence of metastatic disease disappearing for prolonged periods of time. Some controversy nonetheless remains as to whether the use of high-dose IL-2/LAK has any advantage over administration of IL-2 alone at a lower and better-tolerated dosage level.

LEVAMISOLE. Levamisole (Ergamisole) is an anthelmintic agent possessing immunopotentiating properties. It has been reported to enhance various tests of cell-mediated immunity in patients with Hodgkin's disease but has not been shown to have a therapeutic effect. When combined with 5-FU, however, levamisole has been reported to enhance adjuvant chemotherapy of patients with Dukes' C colon cancer, although this regimen has been largely supplanted by treatment with 5-FU and leucovorin. In patients with overt metastatic colon cancer, the combination of 5-FU and levamisole does not appear to be any more useful than 5-FU alone.

ANTITUMOR ANTIBODY THERAPY

RITUXIMAB. Rituximab (Rituxan) is a genetically engineered chimeric murine/human monoclonal antibody directed against the CD-20 antigen found on the surface of normal and malignant B-lymphocytes. It is the first antibody approved for therapeutic use in humans. Approximately 50% of patients with relapsed or refractory low-grade lymphoma treated with 375 mg/m^2 of this agent given as an IV infusion weekly for four doses had a partial or complete remission lasting 10 to 12 months. Current studies are exploring the use of this antibody together with chemotherapy and/or irradia-

tion. Use of this antibody to deliver radioactivity to lymphoma tumor sites is also under investigation. Infusion-related side effects consisting of fever, chills, and rigors occur in the majority of patients during the first infusion. Subsequent infusions are associated with fewer side effects.

TRASTUZUMAB (HERCEPTIN). This genetically engineered monoclonal antibody is directed against cells overexpressing the HER-2 protein, a transmembrane glycoprotein. Approximately 30% of breast cancers overexpress this protein. The response rate to the antibody alone in this group of patients is low (about 15%); however, in combination with taxol or doxorubicin, augmented response rates have been reported, leading to the approval of this antibody for clinical use by the FDA. An unexpected side effect of this treatment has been an increased incidence of cardiac toxicity when this antibody is used in combination with doxorubicin or taxol.

GROWTH FACTOR ANTAGONISTS. The use of antagonists to polypeptide growth factors is an extension of neuroendocrine therapy but represents a form of biologic therapy as well. One growth factor antagonist that has been recognized to have anticancer properties is suramin, which has been used since the 1920s for the treatment of African sleeping sickness. Suramin is a polysulfonated napthylurea that binds tightly to heparin-binding growth factors such as fibroblast growth factor (FGF), platelet-derived growth factor (PDGF), and insulin-like growth factor (IGF-1). Exclusion of growth factors from their receptors can result in "programmed cell death." Suramin actively treats prostate cancer, presumably by blocking the action of FGF and other growth factors. Suramin also inhibits the function of a variety of enzymes and other proteins, so its precise mechanism of antitumor action remains to be defined. Suramin's multiple actions also account for a broad range of toxicities, which can be severe or irreversible. One of these is adrenal insufficiency, which requires long-term adrenal steroid replacement. Frequent plasma monitoring of suramin concentrations is essential, because there is the potential for serious neuropathy when suramin concentrations exceed 300 mg/mL. Suramin represents the first member of a new class of investigational agents for cancer therapy. Another approach to growth factor receptor blockade involves use of monoclonal antibodies to epidermal growth factor (EGF) receptor and the IL-2 receptor.

BONE MARROW GROWTH FACTORS (See Chapter 158). A new approach to supportive care for bone marrow failure associated with cancer and for maintaining adequate hematopoietic function between courses of myelosuppressive chemotherapy is to administer bone marrow growth factors to stimulate an increased rate of production of myeloid progenitors (Table 198–11). The bone marrow growth factors are glycoproteins that function in an overlapping and hierarchic manner on bone marrow progenitors and not only result in cell proliferation but also activate differentiation and cell trafficking. The major factors also potently stimulate the proliferation of myeloid precursors. Several of these recombinant proteins, including granulocyte colony stimulating factor (G-CSF), granulocyte-macrophage colony stimulating factor (GM-CSF), and erythropoietin (Epogen, EPO), are widely used in cancer treatment. IL-3, macrophage colony-stimulating factor (M-CSF), and thrombopoietin are at an earlier stage of development, and their role in supportive care is currently uncertain. Clinical trials using subcutaneously administered G-CSF or GM-CSF have shown that either can shorten the duration of granulocytopenia, the frequency of

Table 198–11 ■ **RECOMBINANT BONE MARROW GROWTH FACTORS OF POTENTIAL IMPORTANCE IN SUPPORTIVE CARE OF CANCER PATIENTS**

GROWTH FACTOR	EFFECTS
G-CSF	Stimulates granulocyte production
GM-CSF	Stimulates granulocyte, macrophage, and eosinophil production
M-CSF	Stimulates macrophage production and activation
Interleukin-3	Stimulates granulocyte, macrophage, and platelet production
Erythropoietin	Stimulates production of red blood cells
Interleukin-11	Stimulates platelet production
Thrombopoietin	Stimulates platelet production

G-CSF, GM-CSF, M-CSF = granulocyte, granulocyte-macrophage, and macrophage colony-stimulating factors.

infectious complications, and the duration of hospitalization after chemotherapy combinations that normally require inpatient administration. With bone marrow transplantation, in which high-dose chemotherapy and/or total body radiation is used, both myelosuppressive and nonmyelosuppressive side effects can be diminished with the use of G-CSF or GM-CSF. Preliminary evidence suggests that IL-3 (multi-CSF) can stimulate platelet and red blood cell as well as granulocyte production.

In preclinical studies, IL-3 also appears to act synergistically with GM-CSF to produce more complete and rapid recovery of circulating granulocytes and platelets. The major toxicities of the growth factors that stimulate white blood cell production include fever, myalgias, and occasional rashes. Pericarditis has been reported with high-dose GM-CSF or G-CSF. Recombinant EPO is already in general clinical use for the anemia of renal failure. Preliminary studies also suggest that when used in pharmacologic doses, EPO can restore normal red blood cell counts in some patients with multiple myeloma and perhaps in some other hematologic malignancies as well. EPO also has promise for reducing the degree of anemia induced by cytotoxic chemotherapy.

DIFFERENTIATION THERAPY. All-*trans*-retinoic acid is the first effective differentiation agent introduced into routine clinical care. It causes a high percentage of complete remissions in patients with acute promyelocytic leukemia. Retinoids are also under investigation as chemotherapeutic and chemopreventive agents.

ANTIANGIOGENESIS TREATMENTS. An attractive target for anticancer drug development is the neovasculature elicited by growth of tumors. Natural substances derived from precursor proteins (e.g., endostatin, a 20 kd-terminal fragment of collagen, and angiostatin, a 38-kd internal fragment of plasminogen), show encouraging antitumor effects in animal models. These studies have also stimulated a search for natural products as well as new synthetic agents with the goal of generating small molecule inhibitors of tumor cell vasculature. This approach may provide relatively non-toxic treatment of tumor cell growth because tumor-derived endothelial cells proliferate rapidly but normal endothelial cells usually do not replicate.

Chabner BA, Longo DL: Cancer Chemotherapy: Principles & Practice, 2nd ed. Philadelphia, JB Lippincott, 1996. *An excellent reference on cancer chemotherapy, including a detailed discussion of the pharmacology of anticancer drugs.*

DeVita VT, Hellman S, Rosenberg SA: Cancer: Principles and Practice of Oncology, 5th ed. Philadelphia, JB Lippincott, 1997. *A standard reference.*

Holland JF, Frei E III, Bast RC Jr, et al: Cancer Medicine, 4th ed. Philadelphia, Lea & Febiger, 1997. *A comprehensive textbook covering clinical, diagnostic, and therapeutic approaches for all major forms of cancer. Major modalities of treatment as well as drug combination schedules are delineated in detail in relation to relevant tumor types.*

199 ONCOLOGIC EMERGENCIES

Stephen M. Hahn

The clinical course of patients with cancer is characterized by the development of complications from either the underlying malignancy or from therapy. To avoid significant morbidity and mortality, the clinician must be aware of the signs and symptoms of these complications and perform a rapid evaluation followed by the appropriate institution of treatment. Several types of cancer are now routinely cured; and for others, treatment brings an increase in the patient's quality of life and survival time. Therefore, the early recognition and treatment of oncologic emergencies has an important role in the medical management of cancer patients.

FEVER AND NEUTROPENIA. One of the most common oncologic emergencies is fever (a single temperature of 38.5° C [101.3° F] or three temperatures of 38° C [100.4° F] within a 24-hour period) and neutropenia (absolute neutrophil count less than 1000/mm³). Neutropenic cancer patients have an increased risk of systemic infection and may rapidly develop sepsis (see Chapter 96). Emergent empiric antibiotic therapy is crucial.

The risk of infection increases once the neutrophil count drops below 1000/mm³. Disruptions of other host defenses will also predispose to infection. Paramount among these is breakdown of the gastrointestinal barrier with mucositis. Additional factors include indwelling catheters, invasive procedures, and abnormal cellular and humoral immunity.

The febrile, neutropenic patient usually presents with few signs or symptoms other than fever. Localized infection may be present but not clinically apparent. The absence of an adequate number of leukocytes may make the detection of an active infection difficult. A careful history and physical examination must be performed, focusing on common sites of infection. The oral cavity should be inspected for evidence of mucositis and lesions suggestive of anaerobic, viral (especially *Herpes simplex*), and fungal (especially *Candida* species) infection. Examination of soft tissue and skin, especially at catheter sites, may show early cellulitis or septic phlebitis. A perirectal abscess should be excluded by careful palpation of the anorectal area for induration, fluctuance, or tenderness.

Before initiation of antibiotic therapy, cultures should be performed on all patients and sent routinely for isolation of bacteria and fungi. Blood cultures must be obtained both from the port of an indwelling central catheter and from peripheral veins. If an indwelling catheter is suspected to be the source of infection, removal of the catheter is not always required but must be considered. If the catheter is removed, the tip should be sent for Gram stain and culture. Sputum examination by Gram stain and culture are usually not helpful but are obtained if sputum is produced. Gram stain as well as bacterial, fungal, and viral cultures should be ordered for all oral, skin, and soft tissue lesions. Biopsies of cutaneous lesions may be especially helpful in the diagnosis of systemic viral and fungal infections and can be safely performed in the neutropenic patient. A chest radiograph, urinalysis with microscopy and culture, and evaluation of ascites and pleural fluid should be performed. Although meningitis is not typically encountered in febrile neutropenic cancer patients, a lumbar puncture should be performed when suggestive clinical signs or symptoms exist.

Use of indwelling urinary tract catheters and unnecessary intravenous catheters is to be avoided. Strict hand washing by all hospital personnel is required. Aggressive prophylactic or therapeutic mouth care (suggested regimen: nystatin suspension, diphenhydramine [Benadryl]/antacid/lidocaine mixture, and 5% sodium bicarbonate solution, alternating each every 2 hours, administered as swish and spit) will provide relief of symptoms and may improve the patient's course.

Once evaluated and hospitalized, the patient should be started without delay on broad-spectrum antibiotics that include coverage for *Pseudomonas* species and other gram-negative organisms. Recently there has been a shift toward gram-positive organisms as the cause of infection in the neutropenic patient. Therefore, antibiotic regimens with broad coverage are required. Many antibiotic regimens have been evaluated in prospective studies, and there is no clearly superior regimen. Emerging antimicrobial resistance at an individual institution may dictate the antibiotics administered to the neutropenic patient. Suggested regimens are (1) monotherapy with a third- or fourth-generation cephalosporin (cefepime, 2 g every 12 hours, or ceftazidime, 1 to 2 g every 8 hours intravenously), (2) a semisynthetic penicillin (piperacillin, 3 to 4 g every 4 hours intravenously) plus an aminoglycoside (gentamicin or tobramycin, 2 mg/kg loading dose followed by one to three divided doses daily depending on renal function), or monotherapy with imipenem (50 mg/kg divided every 6 hours intravenously). If a specific organism is suspected, appropriate antibiotics should be added to the initial regimen. For example, if infection of an indwelling catheter is likely, additional gram-positive coverage with vancomycin (500 mg every 6 hours intravenously) should be added to cover infection with *Staphylococcus aureus* and *Staphylococcus epidermidis*. For patients with mucositis, periodontal infections, or perianal infections, anaerobic coverage with either metronidazole (15 mg/kg loading dose intravenously and 7.5 mg/kg intravenously every 6 hours) or clindamycin (300 mg intravenously every 6 hours) should be started while awaiting culture results. Antifungal agents such as fluconazole should be given to patients who present with suspected oral thrush or esophagitis, but these agents do not replace amphotericin B in the treatment of documented or suspected invasive fungal infections. Fluconazole prophylaxis to prevent invasive mycotic infections is of unknown benefit and is not routinely recommended at this time.

If fever persists after the initiation of antibiotics, cultures and diagnostic studies should be repeated and the spectrum of antibiotic coverage should be broadened. Patients with prolonged neutropenia who are receiving broad-spectrum antibiotics are at high risk for fungal infection, and early institution of antifungal therapy may be life saving. If the patient remains febrile for 5 to 7 days, empiric antifungal therapy should be started with amphotericin B (0.25 to 1.0 mg/kg/day intravenously). If neutropenic patients remain febrile despite broad-spectrum therapy, diagnostic possibilities include a second bacterial isolate, superinfection with gram-positive organisms, abscess, anaerobic infection, *Clostridium difficile* enteritis, atypical organisms, fungi, viruses, and drug fever.

An infection is identified in approximately 40% of patients with fever and neutropenia. If a causative organism or a specific infection is discovered, specific therapy should be initiated; however, broad-spectrum antibiotics should not be discontinued, because there is a significant chance of developing infection with a second isolate when antibiotic therapy is narrowed. Patients with documented infections require treatment for a full, usually 2-week, course of antibiotic therapy. If the patient is afebrile and no specific infection has been identified, antibiotics may be discontinued when the absolute neutrophil count exceeds 1000/mm³. Antibiotics should be continued until the neutropenia resolves in the patient who remains neutropenic despite becoming afebrile because otherwise clinical deterioration or recurrent fever will develop in a significant proportion of these patients.

The treatment of febrile neutropenic patients who are at low risk for infectious complications has not been completely defined; the oral antibiotic combination of ciprofloxacin and amoxicillin-clavulanic acid is under active investigation. Until prospective, randomized trials define the proper treatment for low-risk patients, the administration of broad-spectrum intravenous antibiotics should be considered standard. In general, the patient should remain hospitalized and receive intravenous antibiotics until the neutropenia resolves. However, there is a trend toward early discharge with outpatient oral or intravenous antibiotics in low-risk patients.

The introduction of the recombinant hematopoietic cytokines granulocyte colony-stimulating factor (G-CSF) and granulocyte-macrophage colony-stimulating factor (GM-CSF) has improved the treatment of neutropenia in cancer patients. G-CSF has been studied more extensively and may have a lower toxicity profile. These cytokines are administered prophylactically (24 hours after the last dose of cytotoxic chemotherapy) or therapeutically (when the patient develops fever and/or neutropenia). The prophylactic use of cytokines reduces the duration of neutropenia, decreases the frequency of febrile neutropenia, and in some studies reduces the use of antibiotics and the number of hospital days. It should be noted, however, that a survival benefit has not been demonstrated from the use of G-CSF. G-CSF prophylaxis is often recommended for patients who are treated with chemotherapy regimens that result in a high frequency of febrile neutropenia, patients with poor bone marrow reserve, and possibly in those who have experienced febrile neutropenia with a previous cycle of chemotherapy. The routine use of prophylactic G-CSF is not recommended.

The therapeutic use of cytokines is theoretically attractive, but randomized clinical trials have not demonstrated a clinically significant benefit. Therefore, the use of G-CSF in addition to broad-spectrum antibiotics during an episode of febrile neutropenia is not routinely recommended. Clinical judgment with regard to the severity of the patient's illness and the expected duration of neutropenia will ultimately determine whether therapeutic administration of cytokines is indicated. G-CSF is administered initially as a subcutaneous injection (5 μg/kg). Higher doses (10 μg/kg) may be necessary in some patients. The drug is well tolerated by most patients, although bone pain, fever, allergic reactions, and lethargy have been reported.

At one time, white blood cell transfusions were believed to benefit patients with gram-negative infection and prolonged neutropenia. Such transfusions are not now recommended because their benefit is questionable and the risks, such as alloimmunization, pulmonary toxicity, and infections are significant.

SPINAL CORD COMPRESSION. Back or neck pain can be a harbinger of spinal cord compression; and in the cancer patient (most commonly, lung cancer, breast cancer, lymphoma, and prostate cancer), this symptom merits immediate, careful evaluation. The pain of intraspinal lesions is worsened by straining, sneezing, coughing, movement, and recumbency. Complaints may precede the diagnosis by days to months, but once neurologic signs exist, progression is usually rapid. Typically, midline back pain progresses to radicular pain followed by weakness, sensory loss, paralysis and/or loss of sphincter control at or below the level of the lesion. Early recogni-

tion is important, because ambulatory ability and maintenance of bowel and bladder control at the time when therapy is begun correlates highly with the ultimate functional outcome. Less than 15% of patients with paraplegia or loss of sphincter tone due to metastatic or primary spinal cancer regain function. The location of such lesions correlates with the volume and number of vertebral bodies (thoracic > lumbar > cervical).

The physical examination determines the pace of evaluation and treatment (Fig. 199–1). Patients who show signs of spinal cord compression require immediate treatment with dexamethasone (10 mg intravenously plus 4–6 mg every 6 hours) followed by emergent evaluation. About 60% to 80% of patients with spinal cord compression will have plain film spine radiographs showing erosion or loss of pedicles, partial or complete collapse of vertebral bodies, or a paraspinous mass. Therefore, the patient with no neurologic findings but with plain film evidence of spine metastases should be evaluated emergently. Patients with no neurologic findings and no plain film abnormalities usually may be expeditiously evaluated as outpatients; the exception is patients with lymphoma, who more frequently may have epidural tumor without plain film abnormalities. The evaluation of patients with neurologic abnormalities should proceed directly to magnetic resonance imaging (MRI) with gadolinium enhancement. MRI will delineate intramedullary, extramedullary, intradural, and extradural lesions as well as encroachment on the cord through the spinal foramina. Although MRI of the suspected site of compression is usually performed emergently, a screening MRI of the entire spine is preferable because malignancies (especially lung, breast, and prostate) often produce multiple noncontiguous bone metastases that should be included in any planned radiation therapy. Metrizamide myelography, previously considered the diagnostic test of choice in spinal cord compression, should be considered in patients who cannot tolerate an MRI or in whom an MRI is contraindicated. If, after a lumbar injection, a myelographic block is identified, a C1–2 puncture should be performed to visualize the extent of the block, as well as to define other rostral lesions (15%); computed tomography (CT) focused on the spinal block, can then be performed to delineate the lesion further.

Although treatment should be individualized, palliative radiation therapy is the treatment of choice for patients who have slowly evolving neurologic symptoms, incomplete block, cauda equina involvement, or widely metastatic disease. A commonly used radiation regimen is 3000 cGy (30 Gy) delivered in 10 fractions of 300 cGy per fraction. Corticosteroid doses can be reduced judiciously as radiation therapy proceeds. Surgery is recommended for spinal cord compression in the non-terminal patient if a tissue diagnosis is needed; for rapidly developing neurologic signs; if neurologic dys-

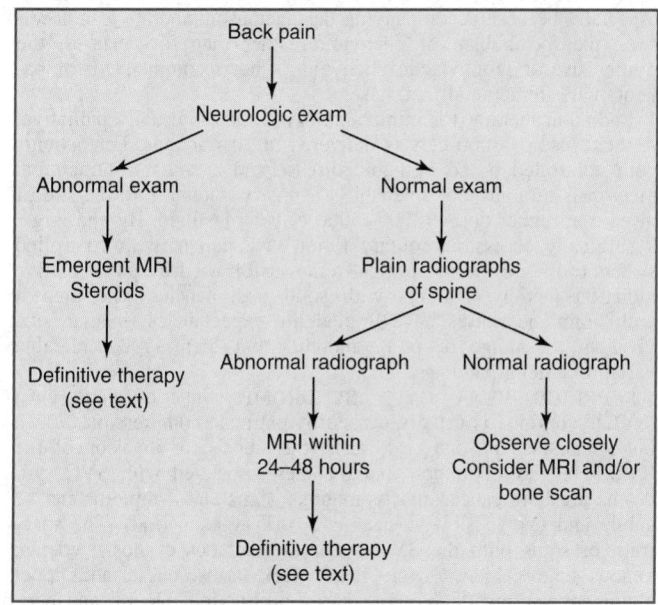

FIGURE 199–1 ■ Flow diagram for evaluation of spinal cord compression in the cancer patient.

function progresses despite radiation treatment; if there is recurrent spinal cord compression in an area of previous radiation therapy; or if there is spinal instability resulting from vertebral body collapse or bony protrusion into the spinal cord. Simple laminectomy is not usually effective and may lead to spinal instability. The surgical procedure is dictated by tumor location and surgical experience and expertise. If surgery is used, radiation therapy should be administered postoperatively. For chemosensitive malignancies, chemotherapy may be considered in addition to irradiation or surgery. For the majority of patients with solid tumors, spinal cord compression can be palliated, but curative therapy is not available (exceptions are patients with lymphoma or testicular cancer). The patient's prognosis is related to the tempo of the underlying cancer, the presence of other metastases, and other medical problems.

INTRACRANIAL METASTASES. Headache, altered mental status, seizures, or a focal neurologic examination in cancer patients may signal intracranial metastases (most commonly melanoma and cancers of the lung and breast). Brain metastases are amenable to treatment but are fatal if left untreated. The differential diagnosis in a cancer patient includes iatrogenic causes (chemotherapy agents, narcotic analgesics, hypnotics, and antiemetics), metabolic disorders (hypercalcemia, hyponatremia, hypoglycemia, hyperviscosity, hepatic encephalopathy), paraneoplastic syndromes (subacute cerebral degeneration, dementia, limbic encephalitis, optic neuritis, progressive multifocal leukoencephalopathy), strokes (coagulation abnormalities, Trousseau's syndrome), sepsis, and intracranial metastases. A careful history and physical examination and laboratory evaluation are critical and should guide decisions for further evaluation. In acutely ill cancer patients, cranial CT with contrast medium enhancement should be performed to define the presence and characteristics of the intracerebral lesion. MRI is more sensitive in defining metastatic lesions and differentiating between vascular and malignant lesions and should be considered as an alternative to CT or if there is a need to clarify CT findings. If no mass lesion is demonstrable, leptomeningeal carcinomatosis should be considered as the cause of neurologic signs and symptoms and sought by examination of cerebrospinal fluid.

Patients who are deteriorating neurologically or who show signs of impending intracerebral herniation should be intubated and hyperventilated to maintain the PCO_2 between 25 and 30 mm Hg. Mannitol, up to 1.5 g/kg, should be administered immediately and repeated every 6 hours. If signs of increased intracranial pressure exist with or without impending herniation, intravenous dexamethasone (16 mg every 6 hours) should be administered to lessen cerebral edema. Status epilepticus requires immediate-acting drugs, such as benzodiazepines, and close attention to respiratory status. Seizures, other than status epilepticus, caused by intracranial metastasis are managed by phenytoin (oral loading dose 1 g in divided doses followed by 300 mg/day). Drug levels should be monitored, especially because accompanying dexamethasone therapy can accelerate the metabolism of phenytoin. Other than for seizures, the routine use of prophylactic phenytoin is not recommended for patients with intracranial metastases.

Radiation therapy for intracranial metastasis is usually palliative. A total dose of 3000 cGy is delivered in 10 fractions. For patients with controlled or no systemic disease and a solitary intracranial metastasis in a site not amenable to surgery, radiation to the site of disease at higher doses (4000–5000 cGy) is justified. By and large, a surgically accessible solitary lesion in a patient with controlled systemic disease merits surgical removal followed by postoperative radiation therapy. Patients with solid malignancies who present with brain metastases have limited life expectancies (median survival in the range of 6–12 months), but there is considerable variation among patients.

SUPERIOR VENA CAVA SYNDROME. Superior vena cava (SVC) syndrome is usually caused by extrinsic compression (90%), but it can also be due to fibrosis, thrombosis, or invasion of the SVC. The most common malignancies associated with SVC syndrome are lung cancer and lymphoma. Signs and symptoms can be subtle and evolve slowly (over a 2- to 5-week period). The spectrum of signs with the SVC syndrome includes cyanosis; edema; venous engorgement of the head, neck, arms, chest, and upper abdomen; varying degrees of airway obstruction; pleural and pericardial effusions; and tracheal edema. Non-pitting edema of the neck (Stokes' collar) can also be found. Symptoms, which fre-

quently worsen when the patient lies down or leans forward, may include fullness or stuffiness in the ears or nose, visual disturbances, facial swelling, shortness of breath, cough, chest pain, voice changes (hoarseness), dysphagia, headache, stupor, seizures, and syncope. Back pain may herald simultaneous spinal cord compression by a contiguously extending tumor. Upper extremity venography complements either CT or MRI in defining the level of SVC obstruction.

In the past, malignancy-associated SVC syndrome was considered an oncologic emergency that merited immediate radiation therapy to avoid death from respiratory arrest or intracranial hemorrhage. Immediate therapy is indicated for impending airway obstruction (stridor) or increased intracranial pressure (stupor, seizure), particularly in a thrombocytopenic patient. However, given the vast array of benign causes of SVC syndrome and the frequency of chemosensitive malignancies such as small cell lung cancer and lymphomas, its cause should be determined while the patient is closely observed and managed symptomatically. Sputum cytology, bone marrow, lymph node biopsy, thoracentesis, bronchoscopy, and thoracotomy may confirm the diagnosis.

Once a neoplastic cause of SVC syndrome has been established, appropriate treatment should be initiated. In most cases, radiation therapy remains the primary treatment, commonly using doses of 150 to 300 cGy per fraction to a total dose of 3000 to 5000 cGy. About 85% of patients improve within 3 weeks, but symptoms usually recur. If small cell lung cancer, testicular cancer, or lymphoma causes SVC obstruction, chemotherapy should be delivered through a lower extremity vein. Corticosteroids may improve cerebral or laryngeal edema.

The increasing use of subclavian catheters to deliver chemotherapy has increased the frequency of SVC thromboses. Low-dose warfarin (1 to 2 mg/day) may prevent such thromboses. Localized fibrinolytic therapy should be considered for patients with catheter-associated thrombosis who have recently developed SVC syndrome if there is not a high risk of bleeding. After successful fibrinolysis, heparinization and subsequent warfarin therapy should be instituted to prevent recurrent SVC syndrome and to maintain the indwelling catheter. The prognosis of the patient with SVC is related to the underlying malignancy. Patients with lymphomas and Hodgkin's disase may be cured with appropriate therapy.

CARDIAC TAMPONADE (SEE CHAPTER 65). Cardiac tamponade in a cancer patient may have a non-cancerous cause, may be the first manifestation of malignancy, or may signify disease progression. Prompt diagnosis is necessary because tamponade is life threatening, but successful treatment improves survival. Tamponade may be caused by primary tumors of the pericardium (mesothelioma, sarcoma, and teratoma) or, more frequently, by metastatic disease from breast, lung, leukemia, lymphoma, melanoma, and epidemic or non-epidemic Kaposi's sarcoma. When fluid pressure within the pericardial sac approaches right atrial and ventricular diastolic pressure, cardiac tamponade occurs. As intrapericardial pressure increases, heart rate, myocardial contractility, and systemic resistance increases. If intrapericardial pressure increases rapidly, between 150 to 250 mL of fluid (normal volume <50 mL) may cause tamponade; if fluid accumulates slowly, however, more than 1 L may be accommodated without producing decompensation. Symptoms are non-specific and include shortness of breath, chest pain, cough, hoarseness, nausea, abdominal pain, hiccoughs, and anxiety. The chest radiograph may show an enlarged globular (water bottle) heart and possibly pleural effusions. Two-dimensional echocardiography (see Chapters 43 and 65) is the non-invasive, preferred diagnostic study that provides both anatomic and physiologic information (Fig. 199–2).

Pericardiocentesis is lifesaving: it provides fluid for diagnosis; and with insertion of a pigtail catheter, it permits measurement of the rate of fluid reaccumulation and the instillation of drugs for sclerosis. Fluid can be serous, serosanguinous, or frankly hemorrhagic. If fluid is hemorrhagic, a hematocrit lower than systemic and the absence of clot weigh against the fluid resulting from puncture of the myocardium. Fluid should be sent for cultures and cytology. Once a malignancy has been established and intrapericardial pressures are reduced, there are several treatments available. Radiation therapy up to 40 Gy is highly successful (approaching 100%) in treating effusion caused by leukemias or lymphomas; however, radiation is not the preferred course of treatment for these patients because of the potential cardiac toxicity, and systemic chemotherapy is often preferred. The most common surgical ap-

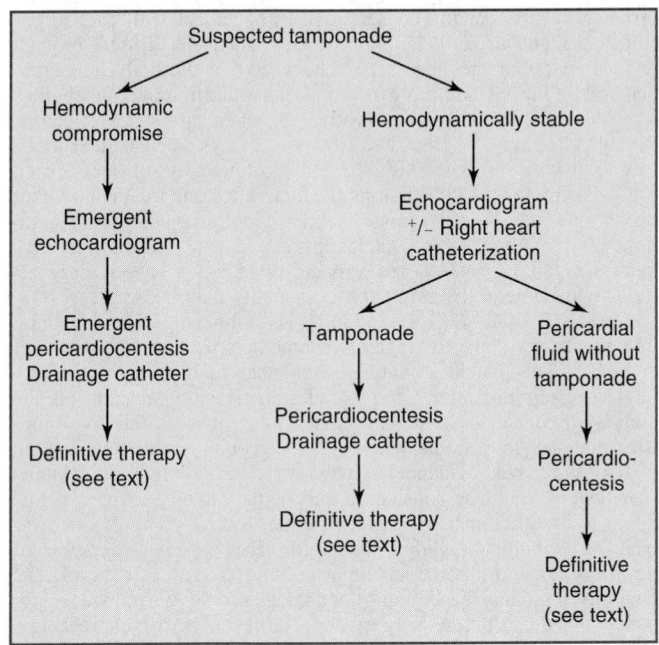

FIGURE 199-2 ■ Flow diagram for evaluation of cardiac tamponade in the cancer patient.

proach to a malignant pericardial effusion is a subxiphoid pericardial window; the window can also be performed with a thoracoscopic approach if a larger pericardial biopsy is needed for diagnosis or if the chest cavity requires evaluation. However, patients with malignant pericardial tamponade (especially those with solid tumors) often have such a poor prognosis that surgical approaches are not pursued. After placement of a pigtail catheter, sclerosis of the pericardial space may be considered with various chemotherapeutic agents, radioisotopes, or doxycycline. Doxycycline is highly effective in sclerosing the pericardial space and eliminating fluid recurrence, but patients should be monitored during and immediately after sclerosis because many develop transient fevers, arrhythmias, or chest pain after treatment.

HEMOPTYSIS. The most common causes (bronchitis, tuberculosis, fungal infections, lung abscess, bronchiectasis, and bronchial adenoma) of hemoptysis are not neoplastic; however, malignancies, especially of bronchogenic origin, are most common among older patients. Hemoptysis associated with respiratory compromise, major hemoptysis ($\geq$ 200 mL in 24 hours) or massive hemoptysis ($\geq$ 1000 mL in 24 hours) should be considered an emergency.

Minor hemoptysis often presages major hemoptysis. The tempo of the bleeding should dictate the pace and aggressiveness of the intervention. Patients with massive hemoptysis should be admitted to an intensive-care unit. The first intervention is to place the patient on his or her side with the bleeding lung down. Correction of coagulopathy and thrombocytopenia, repletion of blood volume, and determination of the site and cause of bleeding are undertaken simultaneously. Flexible bronchoscopy allows for better visualization and is the diagnostic procedure of choice to determine the site and cause of bleeding and to provide direct therapeutic intervention. However, if vigorous suctioning is needed, a rigid bronchoscope should be used. Endobronchial tamponade using an 8-French Fogarty catheter is a temporizing procedure. In terms of definitive therapy, surgical resection should be considered if the patient can tolerate the procedure and if the site can be localized. Bronchial artery angiography and embolization is another alternative therapy. For non-massive bleeding, radiation therapy can be delivered to sites of hemoptysis and is effective in up to 80% of patients. Another treatment option for non-emergent situations is neodymium:yttrium-aluminum-garnet (Nd:YAG) laser–induced coagulation.

AIRWAY OBSTRUCTION. Airway obstruction by an intrinsic or extrinsic malignancy is an emergency, and management depends on the tempo of narrowing, its location, previous treatment, and the type of tumor (most commonly lung cancer). Corticosteroids should be given to lessen edema and, in the case of lymphomas, to begin treatment. Obstruction at or above the larynx and high tracheal region should first be relieved by tracheostomy with subsequent radiation therapy or surgery performed in a non-emergency setting.

More distal obstructions can be treated with surgery, the placement of an expandable stent, and/or radiation therapy (external and/or brachytherapy). A stent placed under fluoroscopic guidance has become a preferred method of palliation. The Nd:YAG laser has been useful in treating high-grade, incomplete, centrally obstructing airway lesions; the technique is quick and safe and provides immediate relief. Restrictions to its use include lobar or segmental level lesions, extraluminal compression, total luminal obstruction, upper lobe lesions, and the presence of a tracheoesophageal fistula. The use of visible light lasers and fiberoptics with photosensitizers (photodynamic therapy [PDT]) also may relieve obstructed airway lesions; lesions that totally obstruct may be completely removed. Furthermore, PDT can be repeated. Repeat bronchoscopy 2 to 3 days after endobronchial PDT should be performed to remove necrotic tissue and evaluate the status of treatment.

HYPERCALCEMIA (See Chapter 264). Hypercalcemia occurs in approximately 10% of all cancer patients. Lung, particularly squamous cell, and breast cancers account for 40 to 60% of all cases. Bone metastases frequently accompany hypercalcemia.

Malignancy-associated hypercalcemia is often caused by tumors that secrete a parathyroid-related protein that causes increased osteoclastic activity and results in increased bone and renal tubular calcium reabsorption (see Chapter 194). Likewise, osteolytic metastases can act directly on bone to cause calcium resorption or can secrete factors that result in bone resorption or activation of osteoclasts. Approximately 45% of calcium is ionized (non–protein bound), and total calcium levels must be corrected for changes in serum albumin concentration. Most laboratories now report ionized calcium levels.

In patients with symptomatic hypercalcemia, laboratory values usually show an elevated serum calcium, commonly above 12 mg/dL. The clinical manifestations may be non-specific and depend in part on the general metabolic condition and associated illnesses of the patient, as well as on the degree and rapidity of calcium elevation. Symptoms include polyuria, nocturia, polydipsia, anorexia, nausea, vomiting, abdominal pain, constipation, fatigue, lethargy, confusion, psychosis, agitation, stupor, obtundation, and coma. The electrocardiogram may show a narrowed QT interval.

For patients who are symptomatic or have serum calcium levels above 13 mg/dL, treatment should be immediate and aggressive. Because of the reversible defects of renal tubular absorption and subsequent fluid loss coupled with decreased oral intake, the patient is invariably volume depleted. Volume repletion with normal saline at a rate of 200 to 300 mL/hour will result in calciuresis. Once rehydration is accomplished, urinary output should be maintained at 100 to 200 mL/hour. Saline-induced calciuresis can be augmented by furosemide. Electrolytes, including magnesium, should be checked frequently and, when necessary, repleted. Once the patient is initially stabilized, the optimal treatment becomes therapy for the underlying malignancy. Steroids can be effective in reducing hypercalcemia in multiple myeloma, lymphoma, and occasionally breast cancer.

For the chronic management of hypercalcemia, several agents are available. The bisphosphonates, the most commonly used agents, bind to hydroxyapatite crystals and inhibit their dissolution. These drugs should be administered only after the patient has been hydrated and adequate urine output has been established. Two bisphosphonates, etidronate and pamidronate, are now available and are the treatments of choice for malignancy-associated hypercalcemia in the United States. Pamidronate is administered in a single dose of 60 to 90 mg by slow intravenous infusion over 24 hours. Etidronate is initially given intravenously (7.5 mg/kg/day) for 3 days followed by oral etidronate 20 mg/kg/day for 30 days if a response is observed to the intravenous drug. The bisphosphonates will reduce serum calcium levels to the normal range in at least 60% of patients. These compounds are very well tolerated, although a transient temperature elevation may be observed 24 to 48 hours after administration. Caution should be exercised if administration is planned for patients with renal insufficiency. Gallium nitrate, usually administered as a continuous IV infusion (100–200 mg/m^2/day) for up to 5 days, is also available for the treatment of hypercalcemia; toxicities include nephrotoxicity and acute optic neuritis. Calcitonin (4 IU/kg every 12 hours increased to 8 IU/kg every 8–12 hours) can lower the serum calcium by 2 to 3 mg/dL within a few hours. The effects of natriuresis and calcitonin are short lived. Intravenous plicamycin (previously known as mithramycin) (10 to 25 μg/kg over a period of 4–6 hours) may be given every 48 hours for up to three doses. The response to plicamycin may last up to 3 weeks. After the initial course, plicamycin may be administered up to twice weekly to maintain normocalcemia. The use of plicamycin to treat hypercalcemia has declined because of concern over toxicities that include hypotension, hepatic and renal dysfunction, and bone marrow suppression, especially thrombocytopenia. Patients being treated with any of these agents should be observed closely for the development of hypocalcemia.

TUMOR LYSIS SYNDROME. Tumor lysis syndrome is a metabolic emergency that can be anticipated and prevented. Rapid tumor lysis is usually encountered after initiation of chemotherapy for rapidly proliferating malignancies such as high-grade lymphomas or acute leukemias. Rarely, it has been reported to occur in solid tumors. The syndrome can occur within 48 hours after arterial embolization of large tumors within the liver. Tumor lysis syndrome causes rapid and severe metabolic changes, including hyperkalemia, hyperuricemia, hyperphosphatemia, and hypocalcemia. Hyperuricemia or hyperphosphatemia can cause renal failure secondary to uric acid or calcium phosphate crystallization in the tubules. Hypocalcemia caused by precipitation of calcium phosphate and lowered calcitriol levels can result in neuromuscular irritability, tetany, and obtundation. Hyperkalemia can be sufficiently severe to cause cardiac arrhythmias and sudden death.

Treatment begins with identification of the patient at risk and prevention of the metabolic and end-organ changes. If a patient is likely to develop rapid tumor lysis associated with chemotherapy, hospital admission and initiation of measures to circumvent the syndrome are necessary. Volume status should be assessed and electrolytes, blood urea nitrogen, creatinine, uric acid, phosphorus, and calcium serum levels should be obtained before beginning chemotherapy. If possible, intravenous hydration should begin before the administration of chemotherapy. If patients present with evidence of tumor lysis syndrome before chemotherapy, every effort should be made to correct the metabolic abnormalities before starting the drugs. It is not always possible to postpone chemotherapy, however, and in such a setting, hemodialysis may be necessary. Hyperkalemia must be treated aggressively (see Chapter 102). To avoid uric acid precipitation in the renal tubules, the urine should be alkalinized with 0.25 normal sodium chloride containing two ampules (100 mEq) of sodium bicarbonate; additional bicarbonate is titrated to maintain urine pH between 7.0 and 8.0, and acetazolamide (250 mg by mouth once or twice daily) may be administered in the first several days to hasten urine alkalinization. Urinary output between 100 to 200 mL/hour should be maintained; loop diuretics (furosemide) may be necessary to maintain urine flow. Allopurinol should be administered before chemotherapy (500 mg/m^2 by mouth on day one and 300 mg on subsequent days) because it decreases uric acid production by inhibiting xanthine oxidase. It should be noted that calcium phosphate crystal formation theoretically can be increased by alkalinization of the urine (pH >8). However, practical considerations would dictate that excretion of uric acid is of primary importance and high volume urinary output, even when alkaline, will dilute calcium phosphate in the urine and lessen the danger of phosphate crystalluria. Hypocalcemia will occasionally require therapy with intravenous calcium. Rarely, calcitriol replacement will be necessary to obviate persistent hypocalcemia caused by low calcitriol levels. Hemodialysis should be initiated when volume status, urinary output, acid-base status, and electrolyte changes signal its necessity.

HEMORRHAGIC CYSTITIS. Patients who have received or are receiving cyclophosphamide or ifosfamide may develop a life-threatening urologic emergency, hemorrhagic cystitis, caused by metabolites (chlorethylazeridine, chloroacetic acid, and acrolein) of either chemotherapy agent. Because metabolites are excreted by the kidneys, high concentrations can accumulate in the bladder. The bladder grossly appears hyperemic and edematous with areas of punctate hemorrhage; mucosal erosions and sloughing are common. The best management entails prevention by maintaining a high urinary output to decrease the concentration of metabolites in the bladder and by correcting any coagulation defect. Systemic use of sodium 2-mercaptoethanesulfonate (mesna) prevents mucosal irritation by detoxifying the metabolites within the bladder. Once hem-

orrhagic cystitis occurs, conservative management with care to ensure excellent urinary output is often adequate. Blood product replacement may be necessary. The use of a urethral catheter to perform saline lavage, remove blood clots, and remove metabolites may be considered. If conservative management is not effective, the bladder may be irrigated by N-acetylcysteine. If that fails, irrigation with 1.0% to 2.0% formalin solution by an experienced urologist frequently (85%) stops bleeding after one treatment. Other agents that may be efficacious include the intravesicular administration of 1% alum or prostaglandins E$_2$ and F$_2$. If conservative measures fail to control hemorrhage, diversion of hypogastric arteries with ureteral diversion and cystectomy may be necessary.

HEMATOLOGIC EMERGENCIES. Thrombocytopenia is common in patients who are undergoing chemotherapy (see Chapters 183 and 184). The platelet count threshold that should trigger the prophylactic administration of a platelet transfusion depends on the clinical circumstances. At many institutions, it is routine to administer platelets to patients whose platelet count is below 15,000 to 20,000/mm^3, but evidence suggests that a prophylactic platelet transfusion should be considered only if the platelet count is below 5,000 to 10,000/mm^3). However, uremia, fever, or any evidence of bleeding should raise this threshold. The expected duration of thrombocytopenia is also an important consideration. If the platelet count is less than 50,000/mm^3, platelets should be transfused for active bleeding, before surgery, or before an invasive procedure. When the patient is symptomatic from an associated anemia or has a hemoglobin value less than 8.0 g/dL, red blood cells should also be administered. Thrombopoietin, a stimulator of platelet production, appears to speed the recovery of the platelet count in patients with chemotherapy-induced thrombocytopenia.

Leukostasis may result when the white blood cell count exceeds 100,000/mm^3, most often in chronic myelogenous leukemia or acute myelogenous leukemia. An oncologic emergency is not defined by the degree of leukocytosis but rather by the symptoms associated with elevated white blood cell count. The ensuing clinical dysfunction results from the lack of deformability of white blood cell blasts, with subsequent plugging of small vessels. The leukostasis syndrome affects the central nervous system, causing stupor, dizziness, visual problems, ataxia, coma, intracranial hemorrhage, and sudden death. It also affects the lungs, producing pulmonary infiltrates and hypoxia that can progress to pulmonary failure with a clinical picture similar to the adult respiratory distress syndrome. Because extreme leukocytosis results in hyperviscosity, diuresis and volume depletion should be avoided. The primary goal of treatment is to reduce the white blood cell count by leukopheresis (decrease white blood count by 20 to 60% over 3 to 4 hours), followed by immediate effective therapy of the underlying leukemia. Because of the potential of leukemic cell lysis, measures should be instituted to prevent the tumor lysis syndrome.

Chanock SJ, Pizzo PA: Fever in the neutropenic host. Infect Dis Clin North Am 10: 777, 1996. *A practical review of the approach to the patient with fever and neutropenia including the use of colony-stimulating factors.*

Loblaw DA, Laperriere NJ: Emergency treatment of malignant extradural spinal cord compression: An evidence-based guideline. J Clin Oncol 16:1613, 1998. *A comprehensive review of the literature for malignant spinal cord compression including general treatment guidelines.*

Markman M: Diagnosis and management of superior vena cava syndrome. Cleve Clin J Med 66:59, 1999. *A review of the malignant and benign causes of SVC syndrome with an emphasis on the practical aspects of management and treatment.*

Mundy GR, Guise TA: Hypercalcemia of malignancy. Am J Med 103:134, 1997. *A scholarly, well-referenced review of the pathophysiology, natural history, and treatment of malignancy-associated hypercalcemia.*

200 APPROACH TO THE PATIENT WITH METASTATIC CANCER, PRIMARY SITE UNKNOWN

Daniel C. Ihde

DEFINITION. Cancers may first become manifest with visceral or nodal metastases without an obvious primary lesion. Patients presenting in this fashion are said to have metastatic cancer, primary site unknown (MCPSU). Other terms used to denote this clinical entity include cancer (or carcinoma) of unknown primary site and metastases of unknown origin. There is no consensus regarding the extent of clinical evaluation required before the conclusion is reached that the site of origin of the primary tumor cannot be found; as a result, there is considerable heterogeneity in the frequency with which MCPSU is ultimately diagnosed and in the clinical features of patients deemed to have this syndrome. Most authorities agree that complete history and physical examination, blood cell counts, a chemistry screening panel, tests for occult blood in urine and stool, mammography in women, and routine histologic evaluation of the diagnostic pathologic specimen should be performed. Other major sources of heterogeneity include the differing degrees of certainty that individual pathologists require to make a more specific diagnosis, the differing numbers and types of pathologic studies employed before the diagnosis of MCPSU is made, and the extent of imaging studies ordered by clinicians in patients exhibiting this syndrome.

ETIOLOGY. The syndrome of MCPSU by definition results from an occult primary cancer that produces clinically documented metastases. The etiology of this process varies markedly depending on the organ of origin of the malignancy. In a minority of patients, the primary site is not apparent even at autopsy. In a large series of 302 patients with MCPSU who eventually had a postmortem examination, the primary tumor site was eventually identified in 27% of individuals during life and an additional 57% at autopsy; in a residual 16% of cases, even autopsy could not discover the primary neoplasm. When autopsy is not performed, the fraction of cases in which the origin of cancer is not discovered is as high as 70 to 80%.

INCIDENCE. Because there is no standard definition of the MCPSU syndrome, its incidence can only crudely be estimated. Various authors suggest that from 2 to 12% of all cancer patients present in this fashion, with the higher estimates usually based on series from tertiary care centers. Because 1,229,000 individuals in the United States will be diagnosed with cancer in 1998, approximately 86,000 of them (the median of 2–12%) will have MCPSU.

PATHOGENESIS AND PATHOLOGY. The primary pathogenesis of the MCPSU syndrome is the sequence of events that produced the occult primary cancer and its metastases. These events differ greatly, depending on the primary neoplasm. Why the primary cancer is not discovered by routine diagnostic evaluation is a question of major interest. The most common explanation is that the primary tumor is simply too small to be detected by physical examination and imaging studies. Other possibilities include prior surgical excision of the primary lesion, as can occasionally be established in malignant melanoma presenting as an MCPSU; hemorrhagic infarction with resulting necrosis and scarring, as is thought to occur in some testicular choriocarcinomas; and spontaneous regression, which occurs rarely in renal cancers and melanomas and may be mediated by immunologic mechanisms.

Because pathologic confirmation of a malignant neoplasm must be obtained and a search for the primary cancer by routine evaluation must be unrewarding before a tentative diagnosis of MCPSU is made, careful scrutiny of the pathologic specimen assumes critical importance. Discussion between clinician and pathologist should always occur and may sometimes reveal that available pathologic material is inadequate for a more specific diagnosis because of the suboptimal amount of tissue or a poorly processed specimen. This situation occurs with pathologically undifferentiated neoplasms or when the diagnosis of malignancy rests solely on cytologic material obtained by fine-needle aspiration, which sometimes provides little information on tissue architecture and may be insufficient for detailed immunohistochemical or electron microscopic studies that sometimes elucidate the primary site of malignancy. When the pathologist believes examination of additional tissue could lead to a more definitive diagnosis, careful communication is essential to ensure that a repeat biopsy will yield sufficient, properly processed material.

Once an adequate pathologic specimen is available, routine light microscopic examination will reveal adenocarcinoma in approximately 40% of MCPSU patients, undifferentiated carcinoma or malignant neoplasm in 40%, squamous carcinoma in 10%, and, in fewer than 5% each, melanoma, neuroblastoma, neuroendocrine tumor, or other cancers. The pathologist must determine that the presumed metastasis is not the primary tumor. Carcinoma occurring

in a setting of epithelial dysplasia suggests a primary neoplasm, whereas certain types of cells not normally present at the biopsy site, such as epithelial acinar structures in lymph nodes, confirm that the tumor is metastatic. Light microscopic examination can sometimes reveal structural features that suggest the origin of the cancer. For example, papillary adenocarcinoma most often arises in the thyroid, ovary, or lung; and signet ring carcinoma arises in the gastrointestinal tract. Rosetting malignant cells are characteristic of neuroblastoma, and psammoma bodies, of thyroid or ovarian carcinoma.

More specialized studies, particularly immunohistochemical techniques (Table 200–1), may be useful in diagnosing undifferentiated carcinomas or malignant neoplasms, which usually prove to be poorly differentiated squamous or adenocarcinoma, lymphoma, amelanotic melanoma, germ cell carcinoma, or undifferentiated sarcoma, and may identify the organ in which some carcinomas arise. However, the clinical behavior and response to therapy of these malignancies, particularly of undifferentiated neoplasms diagnosed exclusively by immunohistochemical means, may not be identical to corresponding neoplasms diagnosed routinely by light microscopy.

Although not used as often as immunohistochemistry, electron microscopic examination of certain tissue specimens may sometimes be useful, particularly in undifferentiated neoplasms. Ultrastructural demonstration of microvilli is characteristic of adenocarcinoma, desmosomes of squamous carcinoma, premelanosomes or melanosomes of malignant melanoma, and cytoplasmic dense-core granules of neuroendocrine carcinomas such as small cell lung cancer.

CLINICAL MANIFESTATIONS. The first clinical manifestation and site of initial pathologic diagnosis of cancer in patients with MCPSU most often occurs in the lung or pleural space, liver, bone, or lymph nodes. Less frequent presentations include cancer in the peritoneum or pelvis, brain, epidural space, and skin. The distribution of metastases is clearly different in patients with MCPSU as compared with tumors that have an obvious primary site. For example, bone metastases are uncommon in typical cases of pancreatic cancer but are frequent in pancreatic cancer presenting as MCPSU. Liver and lung metastases are uncommon in typical prostatic cancer but occur much more frequently in prostatic cancer with a clinically undetected primary site.

The most common ultimately detected primary sites of cancer in MCPSU patients arise in the pancreas, lung, colon, and hepatobiliary organs. In MCPSU cases presenting above the diaphragm, the lung is the most common primary cancer that is eventually discovered. For infradiaphragmatic presentations, the pancreas is the most frequent primary site.

The distribution of eventually proven sites of cancer origin in patients with MCPSU is also somewhat different from the frequency of various malignancies in the general cancer population. Germ cell, adrenal, hepatobiliary, pancreatic, and renal cancers are relatively overrepresented among patients with the MCPSU syndrome, whereas malignancies of the breast, endometrium, cervix, lung, and prostate are relatively underrepresented because these latter tumors are more readily diagnosed by simple means such as physical examination and chest radiography.

STAGING EVALUATION. Staging of the extent of tumor dissemination is somewhat atypical in patients with MCPSU because the presence of metastatic cancer has already been documented. Attempting to discover the primary malignancy is most often a futile

Table 200–1 ■ IMMUNOHISTOCHEMICAL TECHNIQUES IN CANCER DIAGNOSIS

ANTIBODY REACTIVITY	LIKELY DIAGNOSIS
Leukocyte common antigen	Lymphoma
S-100 antigen	Melanoma, sarcoma
Epithelial membrane antigen	Carcinoma
Cytokeratin	Carcinoma
Prostate-specific antigen	Prostate cancer
Thyroglobulin	Thyroid cancer
Human chorionic gonadotropin	Germ cell tumor
α-Fetoprotein	Germ cell tumor, hepatoma
Gross cystic disease protein	Breast cancer

exercise because the great majority of these patients will prove to have advanced carcinoma refractory to therapy. Furthermore, performing extensive testing to identify the site of the tumor's origin can sometimes occupy a considerable fraction of the patient's usually short remaining life span.

Discovery of the primary tumor will, however, be beneficial to a small minority of patients. Tumor confined to a single peripheral lymph node region may potentially be eradicated with surgery and/or radiation, making identification and control of the primary cancer in the area drained by affected lymph nodes a potentially curative procedure. A pertinent example is occult primary squamous carcinoma of the head and neck region presenting in cervical lymph nodes. Second, documenting that effective systemic treatment is available for the primary tumor (e.g., breast cancer) strongly supports a trial of such therapy. Finally, location of a primary tumor that is producing or is about to produce disabling symptoms may permit institution of specific palliative therapy.

Identification of additional asymptomatic visceral metastatic sites of tumor is of no value in a patient with known visceral metastases. However, in patients whose MCPSU arises in a single peripheral lymph node region, discovery of visceral or distant nodal metastases may prevent unnecessarily radical local or regional therapy.

There is virtually a universal agreement that radiographic barium studies of the upper gastrointestinal tract and colon and intravenous pyelography are of no value in the absence of symptoms or signs suggestive of an occult primary cancer in the region being imaged, because false-positive studies occur more frequently than do true-positive results. Computed tomographic (CT) scans of the abdomen and chest have a higher yield, but in most cases they will detect only a poorly treatable malignancy, such as pancreatic or non–small cell lung cancer. In all patients with MCPSU, any imaging studies that are suggested by the evaluation of the pathologic specimen and that might support the diagnosis of a treatable malignancy (e.g., prostatic ultrasonography in an adenocarcinoma reacting with antibodies to prostate-specific antigen or an abdominal CT scan to detect retroperitoneal lymphoma in an undifferentiated neoplasm reacting with leukocyte common antigen) should be performed. Imaging studies are often appropriate to evaluate symptoms because detection of a symptomatic metastatic tumor requiring palliative therapy (e.g., intestinal bypass for bowel obstruction) may be initiated.

Serum biochemical studies that may help to diagnose a treatable neoplasm (e.g., human chorionic gonadotropin and/or α-fetoprotein in germ cell carcinoma and prostate-specific antigen in prostatic cancer) should be obtained in the appropriate clinical and pathologic setting. However, only markedly elevated levels of these biomarkers are specific for germ cell (or hepatocellular cancer in the case of α-fetoprotein), because benign conditions, such as liver disease and prostatic hypertrophy, can yield false-positive results. Moderate elevations do, however, support further evaluation for the specific treatable neoplasm in question. Estrogen receptors can be performed on an appropriately prepared tumor biopsy, but only markedly elevated values strongly support the diagnosis of hormonally responsive breast or endometrial cancer, because many types of carcinoma can exhibit modestly elevated receptor protein levels.

The remainder of the staging evaluation in patients with MCPSU should be closely tailored to the specific clinical presentation. It is most useful to segregate patients into two groups, those with known tumor confined to lymph nodes and those with tumor in visceral site(s), with or without nodal involvement.

MCPSU CONFINED TO LYMPH NODES. Malignant melanoma and lymphoma can present as isolated lymphadenopathy in any node-bearing region. If neither is excluded by pathologic evaluation, a primary cutaneous melanoma (and any previously excised skin lesions) should be re-reviewed and other sites of adenopathy should be sought.

In patients with middle and upper cervical adenopathy in whom biopsy reveals squamous or poorly differentiated carcinoma, complete endoscopic examination with blind biopsies and CT scan to identify areas of submucosal thickening may disclose a primary cancer of the upper aerodigestive tract. Patients with supraclavicular adenopathy more often prove to have an adenocarcinoma that is likely to originate in the lung, breast, or (principally in the left fossa) the gastrointestinal tract.

Adenocarcinoma presenting as isolated axillary adenopathy most likely originates in the breast in the female, with lung cancer another possibility in both sexes. Careful breast examination and mammography should always be performed in this setting. Even if there is no evidence of a mammary tumor after this evaluation, axillary dissection and either breast irradiation or surgery is often recommended. With pathologic diagnoses other than adenocarcinoma, lung and skin of the upper extremity should be considered as primary sites. Isolated inguinal adenopathy may be either squamous or adenocarcinoma; the primary cancer often originates in genitalia, skin of the lower extremities, and anorectal structures, all of which should be carefully examined.

MCPSU IN VISCERAL SITES. Approximately 85% of MCPSU patients will present with visceral metastases; no effective systemic therapy is available for the great majority. The clinician should focus on identifying neoplasms for which effective systemic therapy exists, specifically chemotherapy-responsive breast and ovarian cancer, pulmonary and extrapulmonary small cell carcinoma, germ cell carcinoma, and lymphoma; hormonally responsive prostatic, breast, and endometrial carcinoma; and papillary carcinoma of the thyroid, which responds to administration of radioactive iodine. Unfortunately, no more than 10% of MCPSU patients with visceral metastases will be shown to have one of these diagnoses.

In women, pelvic examination should be performed and mammography obtained if pathologic evaluation does not exclude breast cancer. Any suspicion of gynecologic neoplasm should lead to abdominal and pelvic CT or pelvic ultrasonography. Some women who present with malignant ascites revealing adenocarcinoma on cytologic examination and no evidence of metastases outside the peritoneal cavity have tumors with clinical behavior similar to ovarian carcinoma. They are candidates for exploratory laparotomy and should generally be treated as if they had ovarian cancer. In men, prostatic examination and ultrasonography should be performed, and blind prostatic biopsy may be appropriate if suspicion of cancer is high. A previously overlooked subareolar breast mass should be sought. The thyroid gland should be carefully examined for masses in both sexes.

TREATMENT. MCPSU CONFINED TO LYMPH NODES. In patients who, after the staging outlined earlier, have all known tumor confined to a single lymph node region the disease should be approached aggressively, because a fraction of these patients will attain 5-year survival and even cure. Patients with melanoma should undergo radical lymphadenectomy; the expectation is a 5-year survival of 15 to 35%, depending on the number and volume of nodal metastases, an outcome similar to stage III melanoma managed with excision of the skin primary and radical lymphadenectomy. If malignant lymphoma is the suspected diagnosis, combination chemotherapy appropriate for these diseases should be administered, followed by radiation therapy to the initial area of involvement.

Squamous and undifferentiated carcinoma in the middle to upper cervical nodes is often managed with radical neck dissection and irradiation, although irradiation alone may be sufficient for low-volume disease. The radiation field usually includes the nasopharynx, oropharynx, and laryngopharynx in order to treat the most likely sites where the primary tumor originated. Five-year survival of 25 to 40% can be anticipated, depending on tumor volume. The outlook for patients with adenocarcinoma in supraclavicular node metastases is much more problematic, with only occasional 5-year survivors.

Isolated axillary adenopathy in women with biopsy-proven adenocarcinoma is usually treated as if it were breast cancer. Axillary node dissection and modified radical mastectomy are often advocated in this setting and yield 5-year survival rates of 30 to 70%, results at least as good as in overt stage II breast cancer. Only half of modified radical mastectomy specimens will reveal a primary tumor. More recently, similar survival rates have been reported in patients treated with axillary node dissection in conjunction with breast irradiation. Because a fraction of these patients clearly have breast cancer, systemic adjuvant therapy appropriate for stage II breast cancer, either chemotherapy, tamoxifen, or both modalities, should be administered.

Men and women with squamous or undifferentiated carcinoma confined to axillary nodes should be considered for node dissection, because about 20% of such patients so treated will live 5 or more years after surgery. Although physical examination usually reveals the primary cancer in patients with inguinal nodes, surgical extirpation or irradiation alone yields 5-year survival of approximately 25% in cases without a documented primary site.

In younger men with predominant midline nodal presentations and minimal visceral tumor, historical evidence of rapid tumor growth, or response to previous chemotherapy, the still incompletely characterized syndrome of "poorly differentiated carcinoma of unknown primary site" should be considered. This syndrome, although not yet well defined, is of importance because a fraction of patients with some or all of the above characteristics obtain complete remissions, sometimes durable, with cisplatin-based chemotherapy programs similar to those employed in men with testicular cancer. Originally, these cases were thought to represent germ cell carcinomas in which a definitive pathologic diagnosis could not be rendered. Recent retrospective reviews indicate that fewer than 5% of patients have initially unrecognized germ cell tumors. The pathogenesis of this syndrome remains obscure, and until clinical trials using strict eligibility criteria for patient entry and adherence to a uniform therapeutic regimen are completed, the fraction of patients who benefit from therapy will remain uncertain.

MCPSU IN VISCERAL SITES. Palliative or supportive care is usually the major focus of management in MCPSU patients with visceral metastases, because most have widely disseminated cancer for which no effective systemic treatment is available. However, palliative irradiation, for example of bone metastases, is often effective in ameliorating associated pain. In rare instances, such as intestinal obstruction by tumor, surgical resection of symptomatic metastases may be indicated. Chemotherapy and, in some instances, hormonal therapy or radioactive iodine are the only maneuvers that address the problem of distant metastatic disease, but success is expected in few patients.

In women with isolated malignant ascites, laparotomy with maximum feasible resection of tumor masses, provided they are confined to the peritoneal cavity, is often appropriate. Whether or not a primary ovarian tumor is identified, one study reports a relatively indolent course in these patients, with some complete responses to chemotherapy regimens utilized in ovarian cancer.

Whenever detailed review of the pathologic material or the staging evaluation raises reasonable suspicion of a primary cancer that might be expected to respond to systemic treatment, a trial of appropriate therapy may be initiated, provided a favorable risk-benefit ratio is thought to exist in the individual patient. For the remaining patients with visceral MCPSU, there is no evidence that any treatment improves survival. Close observation with palliation of symptoms as they arise is an appropriate management strategy. For fully ambulatory patients who understand the limitation of chemotherapy but still desire it, investigational therapies or empirical chemotherapy regimens, for which responses have occasionally been reported, may be tried.

PROGNOSIS. The prognosis of the great majority of patients with MCPSU is poor. In several large series of patients accrued in single institutions, median survival is 5 to 6 months and 5-year survival is 3 to 7%. The most important prognostic features, as in most cancers, are ambulatory status, sites and volume of tumor involvement, and degree of weight loss. Five-year survival is reported to be 25 to 50% for patients whose tumor is confined to peripheral lymph nodes and less than 3% for all other patients.

Abbruzzese JL, Abbruzzese MC, Hess HR, et al: Unknown primary carcinoma: Natural history and prognostic factors in 657 consecutive patients. J Clin Oncol 12:1272, 1994. *A large institutional series of consecutive MCPSU patients emphasizing detailed information on prognostic factors.*

Daugaard G: Tumour review: Unknown primary tumours. Cancer Treat Rev 20:119, 1994. *Work-up should concentrate on identifying the occasional tumor responsive to treatment.*

Lembersky BC, Thomas LC: Metastases of unknown primary site. Med Clin North Am 80:153, 1996. *Effective therapy does not exist for most patients with metastases of unknown primary site, but modern pathologic techniques provide better diagnostic precision and can identify some patients with better prognosis.*

PART XV

METABOLIC DISEASES

201 APPROACH TO THE PATIENT WITH METABOLIC DISEASE

Louis J. Elsas II

In this chapter we approach the principles of screening, diagnosing, and treating inherited metabolic diseases, many of which are detailed in subsequent chapters. In Chapter 32, inborn errors of metabolism are defined in terms of the function and location of proteins and the pathophysiologic consequences to the human organism when they are impaired. Here we invoke a genetic approach through the use of predictive genetic testing to identify and prevent irreversible damage from an inborn error of metabolism. The goal is to diagnose the disorder and intervene to prevent damage by a return to metabolic homeostasis before the disease is irreversible. Genetic screening of symptomatic and pre-symptomatic individuals is used to accomplish this objective. Once the disorder is diagnosed, if its pathophysiology is understood, intervention can restore metabolic homeostasis and prevent progressive disease.

Genetic screening is a process by which a small population of individuals at high risk for a genetic disorder are selected from a much larger group. From this smaller population, a diagnosis, preferably pre-symptomatic, is made. Screening is performed in at least five categories of heritable risk, age, or reproductive condition.

Non-selected screening of a pre-symptomatic population is performed to identify homozygous affected individuals and to prevent death, mental retardation, and other irreversible clinical manifestations. Certain principles are used to determine which diseases would be ethically, legally, and socially acceptable for such a universal public health activity (Table 201–1). At present, universal screening is limited to newborns because of this population's accessibility, the rapidity of progression, and the lifelong burden of disease processes. Disorders currently being screened for in various combinations include phenylketonuria, maple syrup urine disease, galactosemia, homocystinuria, tyrosinemia, sickle cell disease, congenital adrenal hyperplasia, biotinidase deficiency, hypothyroidism, and cystic fibrosis.

Selective screening of symptomatic newborns, children, and adults is performed to identify inherited disorders that may be preventable or ameliorated, not only in the patient but in extended family members at risk as well. The objectives of diagnosis are to provide treatment; determine the genetic component of the disorder; provide genetic counseling, including heterozygote detection and prenatal diagnosis, to patients, parents, and relatives; provide new information about the disorder's pathophysiology; and develop prevalence data. The laboratory diagnostic methods used in selective screening are different from those used in non-selective mass

screening, and clinical judgment is the primary criterion for a given patient's entry into this type of genetic screening. The preventive aspects of genetic screening of a symptomatic patient are important, particularly in disorders in which the onset of irreversible manifestations requires time for full expression. Given a specific diagnosis, genetic counseling may alter reproductive or life-planning behavior. Examples of heritable disorders amenable to selective screening are various cancers (breast, colon, medullary thyroid), peroxisomal disorders, Wilson's disease, cystinuria, familial hypercholesterolemia, early-onset heart disease associated with hyperlipidemia or hyperhomocystinuria, cirrhosis, organic acidemias, mucopolysaccharidosis and other lysosomal disorders, cystinosis, Duchenne's muscular dystrophy, disorders of mitochondrial function, and disorders of connective tissue.

Selective and non-selective genetic screening in pregnant women is achieved by fetal sonography, chorionic villus biopsy, or amniocentesis coupled with biochemical, chromosomal, or molecular analyses of cultured fetal cells. Maternal blood is commonly screened for α-fetoprotein, chorionic gonadotropin, and estradiol to detect the fetal disorders Down syndrome and spina bifida. If maternal blood concentrations of α-fetoprotein, chorionic gonadotropin, or estriol vary above or below the mean values of normal at a specific age of gestation, further fetal studies by sonography and amniocentesis are indicated. Considerable research is in progress to isolate fetal cells from maternal blood to avoid the invasion of the amniotic cavity currently required for prenatal screening.

Screening selected populations at risk for environmental hazards is generally applied to the adult population. Pharmacogenetic disorders fall into this category and include screening plasma pseudocholinesterase concentrations preoperatively to detect *pseudocholinesterase deficiency* and prevent death from succinyldicholine and determining α_1-antitrypsin genotypes in individuals exposed to dust to prevent occupation-related, early-onset emphysema from α_1-antitrypsin deficiency. Screening for the HLA-H mutations causing hemochromatosis may prevent cirrhosis from iron overload.

Screening for asymptomatic heterozygotes in a "high-risk" population is another preventive approach to inborn errors of metabolism. The objective is to detect reproductive couples who carry high-burden recessive genes and provide genetic counseling and reproductive alternatives in high-risk matings. An example is screening for *Tay-Sachs disease* carriers in the Ashkenazi Jewish population (see Chapter 31) and for cystic fibrosis carriers in white couples planning pregnancy. Screening for heterozygotes requires consideration and fulfillment of ethical issues, including patient autonomy, beneficience to the patient, and confidentiality to prevent discrimination by insurers and employers and stigmatization by society.

TREATMENT OF INHERITED DISEASE

Because the metabolic diseases considered in this section have in common that they are inherited and caused by genes of large effect, a general approach to their treatment is appropriate. These approaches are outlined in Table 201–2. The level at which therapy is rendered depends on the level of understanding of the pathophysiologic mechanisms producing disease and the interventional methods available. Genetic counseling is used for all inherited diseases, even those whose mechanisms are not yet understood and for which no clear beneficial treatment is available.

Genetic counseling is a unique and fundamental aspect of management in inherited metabolic diseases. Patients and relatives usually ask the following questions: Why did this disease occur? Will this disease happen to me or my other children? Can it be cured or

---

Table 201–1 ■ **PRINCIPLES FOR NON-SELECTIVE GENETIC SCREENING**

The disorder should produce a high burden to the affected individual yet be preventable.

Methods for screening, retrieval, diagnosis, and management must be practical and available to the target population as a whole.

The inheritance and pathogenesis of the disease should be understood and genetic counseling available.

The benefit-to-cost ratio of the program should be greater than 1.

Patients' rights should be protected (voluntariness, informed consent, confidentiality).

Sensitivity and specificity should be high for the methods used.

Genetic Counseling: Prospective Therapy
Diagnosis, risk assessment, informational transfer, support for resource allocation
Reproductive alternatives: Contraception, abstinence, artificial insemination, in vitro fertilization, risk taking with or without prenatal monitoring
Environmental Engineering
Avoiding the offending agent
Supplemental physical, speech, developmental therapy
Nutritional management
    Limit toxic precursor
    Provide deficient product
    Detoxify through alternative metabolic route
    Provide feedback inhibitor
    Provide supraphysiologic amounts of vitamin precursor
    Induce protein (enzyme) production
    Chemoprevention
Protein and Enzyme Replacement
Infuse protected pure enzyme
Provide clotting factors and peptide hormones
Transplantation (prospective)
    Organ transplant
    Bone marrow transplant
Genetic Engineering
Somatic gene therapy
    Random insertion
    Homologous recombination (site specific)
Germ line therapy

---

prevented? Genetic counseling tries to answer these questions through processes involving several elements (see Chapter 37). One cannot overemphasize the importance of an accurate clinical and genetic diagnosis and the availability of a genetic discriminant for other family members before entering into formal genetic counseling.

Surgical intervention may be a useful adjunct for treating heritable disorders. For example, stabilizing hypoplastic cervical vertebrae may prevent quadriparesis or death in a variety of *chondrodysplasias* and *mucopolysaccharidoses* accompanied by hypoplasia of the odontoid process. In Marfan syndrome, careful monitoring of aortic root diameter with surgical removal of the aorta and prosthesis may prevent a lethal aortic dissection. Similarly, evaluation of polyps and early colectomy may prevent disseminated adenocarcinoma in families with the autosomal dominant forms of *familial polyposis coli.* Molecular diagnoses of mutations in the *APL* gene help identify at-risk family members. Preventing heritable cancer by early surgical excision is therapeutic for *medullary thyroid carcinoma, Wilms' tumors,* and neurofibromas of *von Recklinghausen's disease.* Other examples of the benefit of preventive surgery for inborn errors include splenectomy for hemolytic anemias associated with spherocytosis and pyloroplasty in pyloric stenosis.

Environmental engineering is the most commonly used approach to preventing disease in patients affected by inherited metabolic disease. The environment (nutritional intake, exposure to toxins, sun, stress, climatic variation, and drug therapy) may produce a disease state in individuals who have inherited single genes or polygenic susceptibility to the environmental stress. Many inborn errors of metabolism detected by newborn screening identify infants susceptible to the stress of lactose or protein in human or cow's milk. Restriction and replacement of lactose with sucrose will save the lives of infants with galactosemia. Pharmacogenetic disorders exemplify the simple treatment of *avoidance* once the genetic susceptibility is identified. Health can then be viewed as a continual adaptation between the individual and the environment. Environmental engineering is a form of genetic therapy in which individual genetic susceptibility is identified and the environment is altered to provide optimal health for that individual's unique genetic constitution. The frequency of diseases caused by genetic susceptibility to the environment varies from rare to 100%. *Scurvy* develops in all humans unless ascorbate is provided in the diet because we are all unable to convert glucuronic acid to glucuronolactone and ascorbate. Humans and primates lost this anabolic pathway during evolution. By contrast, humans readily synthesize tetrahydrobiopterin, a cofactor in many hydroxylase reactions, including phenylalanine hydroxylase. In some rare diseases (about 1 in 500,000) of increased blood phenylalanine and severe neurodegeneration, biopterin is not synthesized. Biopterin replacement may

treat defects in biosynthesis and exemplifies a group of metabolic disorders known as *vitamin dependency disorders.*

Nutritional management and chemoprevention involve correction of the metabolic imbalance and return of the patient to homeostasis through diet manipulation and drug therapy. Many of the diseases listed in this section are amenable to this approach and use the pathophysiologic mechanisms listed in Table 201-2. For example, in disorders of the urea cycle, protein intake is limited to reduce ammonia accumulation. Arginine is supplemented to provide deficient product of the blocked reaction, and alternative pathways are induced for nitrogen excretion. The latter therapy is made possible by a ubiquitous enzyme, *N*-glycine-acylase, that forms adducts with benzoic acid and glycine to produce hippuric acid, which is excreted, thus ridding the body of one nitrogen molecule. Orotic aciduria is caused by mutations in the bifunctional enzyme orotate phosphoribosyl transferase-orotidine-5′-monophosphate decarboxylase. The disease process, which includes severe anemia and immune deficiency, is caused by a deficient end product, uridine, and is treated by replacing 100 to 200 mg/kg/day of uridine (orally). Feedback inhibition of pituitary adrenocorticotropic hormone production is important in treating congenital adrenal hypertrophy with replacement doses of hydrocortisone to prevent virilization from testosterone overproduction. Glucose decreases overproduction of the precursors δ-aminolevulinic acid and porphobilinogen in acute intermittent porphyria caused by porphobilinogen deaminase deficiency. Using supraphysiologic amounts of a specific vitamin is important if it is the precursor of a coenzyme required for holoenzyme function. Many vitamin-dependent metabolic disorders are known and include pyridoxine (vitamin B_6)-dependent homocystinuria and vitamin C–dependent Ehlers-Danlos syndrome type VI. In vitamin B_6–dependent homocystinuria, mutant cystathionine synthase is stabilized to biologic degradation when saturated with pyridoxal phosphate. Others include vitamin B_{12}-dependent methylmalonic aciduria, thiamine-dependent maple syrup urine disease, and biotin-dependent multiple carboxylase deficiency. Some blocked metabolic reactions can be augmented by inducing transcription of their gene. For example, phenobarbital and several other drugs induce hepatic uridine diphosphate glucuronyl transferase gene expression and reduce the accumulation of unconjugated bilirubin in Gilbert's syndrome. On the horizon is chemoprevention of common diseases such as breast cancer. Trials with estrogen receptor inhibitors in pre-symptomatic, high-risk members of families with breast and ovarian cancer are promising. Similar trials to prevent colorectal cancer by preventing polyps in at-risk offspring of patients are also promising.

If the specific protein or enzyme has been purified and engineered to function in its specified organ or subcellular organelle, it can be used to treat an inherited metabolic disease. One good example is glucocerebrosidase, which has been purified in large quantities from placenta and from recombinant mammalian cells. The secreted enzyme is biochemically engineered to contain the mannose recognition site for cellular uptake into lysosomal compartments. It has been used successfully to prevent and reverse the hypersplenism, pancytopenia, and bone disease of *type 1 Gaucher's disease* (see Chapter 208). Many proteins are now made through recombinant techniques to treat metabolic disease and bypass the risks of acquired immune deficiency syndrome and hepatitis attendant on using human-derived biologicals. These agents include *glucocerebrosidase,* Factor VIII for *hemophilia type A,* and growth hormone for *growth hormone deficiency.* Several other engineered proteins used to treat inherited metabolic disease include 1-deamino-8-D-arginine vasopressin to treat *X-linked recessive diabetes insipidus* and recombinant α_1-antitrypsin made stable by inactivating methionine 385 in the treatment of α_1-*antitrypsin deficiency.* Some enzymes such as adenosine deaminase have been modified with polyethylene glycol to reduce immunogenicity and prolong their biologic half-life in blood. It is used to treat *severe combined immunodeficiency.* Chemoprevention is being developed for heritable disorders such as cancer. For *BRCA1* mutation carriers, anti–estrogen receptor medications such as tamoxifen may become an alternative preventive therapy to mastectomy and oophorectomy.

For metabolic disorders that are lethal and have no other available therapy, organ transplantation may be life saving. Transplantation with histocompatible organs is clinically available because of advances in immunology that not only allow for better tissue typing but also enable chronic immunosuppression with such drugs as cyclosporine, azathioprine, and prednisone to prevent rejection.

Several principles are required for successful treatment of an inherited metabolic disorder by organ transplantation: (1) The normal enzyme, protein, or function must be provided by the transplanted organ. (2) Usually the affected organ must be removed. (3) The host must be immunologically tolerant to the gene product being introduced in addition to the transplanted organ itself. These principles are particularly relevant when displacement bone marrow transplantation is used. In the latter, normal donor stem cells differentiate and provide their enzymes to the recipient's reticuloendothelial system. Diseases associated with accumulation of products in the central nervous system are not yet ameliorated by bone marrow transplantation, although accumulation in bone, liver, and spleen is reduced. One group of metabolic diseases uses stem cell bone marrow transplantation to prevent leukemia caused by inherited syndromes that are associated with defective DNA repair, such as *Fanconi's anemia, Bloom's syndrome,* and *ataxia-telangiectasia.* Liver or kidney transplantation can reverse growth and develop-

mental delay in type I glycogen storage disease, cystinosis, acute intermittent porphyria, type I tyrosinemia, Fabry's disease, oxalosis, and non-neuronotrophic lysosomal storage diseases. Lung transplantation has been successful in cystic fibrosis and α_1-antitrypsin deficiency, and prophylactic aortic transplantation has prevented aortic dissection in Marfan syndrome.

In the past decade somatic cell gene therapy to treat patients afflicted with genetic disease has entered the arena of clinical research. Numerous laboratories throughout the world are actively designing strategies by which exogenous DNA can be incorporated into the genomic DNA of specific organs to provide a missing gene function. It is not overly optimistic to assume that some form of *somatic gene therapy* for a number of inherited metabolic diseases will become routinely available (see Chapter 33).

Elsas LJ: Newborn screening. *In* Rudolph AM (ed): Pediatrics, 20th ed. New York, Appleton-Century-Crofts, 1996, pp 282–291. *Approaches to genetic screening.*

Elsas LJ, Acosta PB: Nutrition support of inherited metabolic diseases. *In* Shils ME, Olson JA, Shike M (eds): Modern Nutrition in Health and Disease, 9th ed. Philadelphia, Lea & Febiger, 1998. *Complete discussion of how to manage metabolic disease by diet.*

NIH Consensus Statement: Genetic testing for cystic fibrosis. NIH Consens Statement 15(4):1, 1997. *A summary of issues both medical and ethical pertaining to genetic screening of asymptomatic adults.*

■ DISORDERS OF CARBOHYDRATE METABOLISM

202 GALACTOSEMIA

Robert K. Naviaux ■ *William L. Nyhan*

Galactosemia is an inborn error of carbohydrate metabolism in which the activity of galactose 1-phosphate uridyltransferase is deficient (Fig. 202–1). Patients are unable to metabolize galactose, a component of the disaccharide lactose, whose source in the diet is milk or milk products. Two other disorders, galactokinase deficiency and uridine diphosphate (UDP) epimerase deficiency, also represent abnormalities in this pathway and lead to excretion of galactose in the urine (Table 202–1). The treatment of each of these disorders is elimination of galactose from the diet.

ETIOLOGY. Classic galactosemia and the other disorders of ga-

lactose metabolism are all transmitted by autosomal recessive genes. The gene for uridyl transferase is located on chromosome 9p13. The gene has been cloned and a number of mutations identified (Table 202–2). The most common missense mutation in galactosemia (G) is a change in the codon for glutamine at position 188 to arginine in exon 6. More than 60% of white patients are homozygous or heterozygous for this mutation. Another common abnormal uridyl transferase enzyme, the Duarte variant (D), results from an A-to-G mutation in exon 10 that changes asparagine 314 to aspartic acid. Heterozygous carriers for the galactosemia (G) variant display transferase activity about half that of normal individuals. Homozygotes for the Duarte (D) variant also have about 50% of normal activity, but heterozygotes for this variant have about 75% of normal activity. Study of parents or assessment of the mutation will distinguish individuals with the Duarte variant from G heterozygotes. This distinction can also be made electrophoretically.

PREVALENCE. In central Europe the prevalence of galactosemia

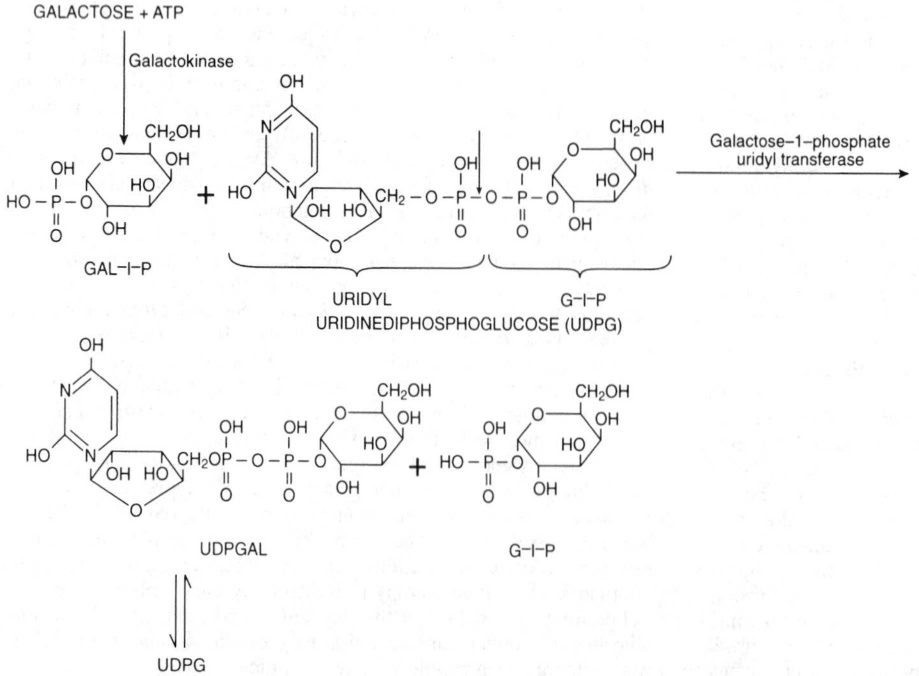

FIGURE 202–1 ■ Galactose 1-phosphate uridyltransferase, the site of the enzyme defect in patients with classic galactosemia. Shown also are the galactokinase and the epimerase reactions.

Table 202-1 ■ DISORDERS OF GALACTOSE METABOLISM

DEFECTIVE ENZYME	METABOLIC PATTERN	CLINICAL MANIFESTATIONS
Galactose 1-phosphate uridyltransferase	Galactose 1-phosphate Galactose	Classic galactosemia
Galactokinase	Galactose	Cataracts; pseudotumor cerebri
UDPglucose 4-epimerase	Galactose 1-phosphate UDPgalactose	May be asymptomatic; may have the classic galactosemic phenotype

UDP = uridine diphosphate.

(GG) is 1 in 55,000; data from neonatal screening programs in California and Massachusetts yielded figures of 1 in 86,000 and 1 in 62,000. Prevalence of the GD compound has ranged from 1 in 3000 to 1 in 38,000. Infants with the GD phenotype have transferase activity 10 to 25% that of control erythrocytes. In general, this activity is sufficient and treatment is not required.

Galactokinase deficiency is quite rare, with a prevalence of 1 in 500,000 to 1 in 1 million births. Epimerase deficiency is even rarer. The benign type has mainly been described in Swiss and Japanese populations. Two patients have been detected with symptomatic epimerase deficiency.

PATHOGENESIS. Three distinct enzymes catalyze the conversion of galactose to glucose. They also create the activated UDPgalactose needed for glycoprotein and glycolipid synthesis (see Fig. 202-1). In normal individuals, administered galactose disappears rapidly from the blood and leads to an increase in the concentration of glucose.

The defective enzyme in galactosemia is galactose 1-phosphate uridyltransferase. In individuals with the classic (G) variant, this activity is virtually completely absent. The immediate consequence of defective activity is the accumulation of galactose 1-phosphate. Ingested galactose is found in the blood and excreted in the urine. When concentrations of galactose are increased, alternative pathways are called into play. In one of these pathways galactose is reduced at carbon 1 to form galactitol, a sugar alcohol. In another, galactose is oxidized to galactonic acid. Both of these metabolites are found in tissues and are excreted in considerable amounts in the urine.

The pathogenesis of many of the acute clinical manifestations of classic galactosemia has been related to the accumulation of galactose 1-phosphate in tissues. Among the best evidence for this pathogenesis are the observations that therapeutic measures that result in a reduction in intracellular concentrations of galactose 1-phosphate lead to prevention or disappearance of the acute symptoms. At the same time, it should be recognized that although this association is clinically useful, the mechanism of pituitary, hepatic, renal, and cerebral damage is unknown. It is clear that these complications do not occur in galactokinase deficiency. Therefore, it is clear that they are not due to galactose itself. Cataracts are, on the

other hand, found in patients with galactokinase deficiency, as well as uridyl transferase deficiency. Cataracts appear to result from the accumulation of galactitol in the lens, where it causes osmotic swelling, precipitation of protein, and disruption of fibers. Osmotic swelling resulting from galactitol also appears to be the mechanism of production of acute cerebral edema. Pseudotumor cerebri occurs in patients with galactokinase deficiency, as well as in those with uridyl transferase activity. The galactitol theory of the genesis of cataracts is strengthened by the prevention of cataracts in galactose-treated rats by sorbinil, an aldose reductase inhibitor that prevents the formation of galactitol.

The pathogenesis of the late-appearing manifestations in the ovary, in speech development, and in the brain are not clear. One theory is that of autointoxication, in which galactose 1-phosphate is formed from UDPgalactose, which is made from uridine diphosphoglucose via the epimerase reaction and thus from dietary glucose in the absence of dietary galactose. Another is a deficiency of intracellular UDPgalactose. Epimerase maintains a steady-state ratio of uridine diphosphoglucose (UDP glucose) to UDPgalactose of 3:1, which might be required for the synthesis of cerebral galactolipids. Low levels of UDPgalactose in erythrocytes have been reported in some patients with galactosemia. Abnormally low galactosylation of fibroblast glycoproteins has also been observed.

CLINICAL MANIFESTATIONS. Vomiting and jaundice usually develop in infants with galactosemia within days of the initiation of feedings containing milk. Vomiting may be so severe that pyloric stenosis is diagnosed and surgery performed. The infant feeds poorly and fails to thrive. Hepatomegaly is a regular finding, and the hepatic damage is progressive to typical Laënnec's cirrhosis. Edema, ascites, hypoprothrombinemia, and bleeding may be present, and splenomegaly develops with increased portal pressure. In the presence of continued milk feedings, this clinical picture rapidly leads to death. Granulocyte function may be impaired by galactose or its metabolites. Infants may have sepsis, most commonly caused by Escherichia coli. Fulminant septicemia may cause an early demise or complications such as osteomyelitis, meningitis, and gangrene. Cataracts are characteristic features. They may occur in very young infants. Pseudotumor cerebri in patients with galactosemia may be recognized by bulging of the anterior fontanelle or

Table 202-2 ■ MUTATIONS* ASSOCIATED WITH GALACTOSEMIA

CODON AND AMINO ACID SUBSTITUTION	NUCLEOTIDE CHANGE	PHENOTYPE	PREVALENCE IN CLASSIC GALACTOSEMIA		
			White	Hispanic	Black
Q188R	CAG → CGG	G	62%	58%	12%
S135L	TCG → TTG	G	0%		48%
V44M	GTG → ATG	G			
M142K	ATG → AAG	G			
R148W	CGG → TGG	G			
L195P	CTG → CCG	G			
R231H	CGT → CAT	G			
H319Q	CAC → CAA	G			
R333W	CGG → TGG	G			
N314D	AAC → GAC	Duarte†			

*In the gene for galactose 1-phosphate uridyltransferase (GALT).
†Found in 5.9% of non-galactosemic controls.

by computed tomography or magnetic resonance imaging (MRI), which reveals cerebral edema. The renal abnormality in galactosemia is a renal Fanconi syndrome, in which renal tubular glycosuria, generalized aminoaciduria, proteinuria, and systemic hyperchloremic acidosis are present. Some patients have polyuria.

In most patients with galactokinase deficiency, lenticular cataracts are the only clinical manifestation. A few infants have been reported with pseudotumor cerebri. Most patients with epimerase deficiency are asymptomatic. A very few have had a clinical picture identical to that of classic galactosemia.

LONG-TERM COMPLICATIONS OF GALACTOSEMIA. Although dietary therapy for galactosemia has effectively eliminated the acute toxicity syndrome of classic galactosemia, long-term complications have become evident as significant problems, even under ideal conditions of management and patient compliance.

Ovarian failure in female patients may be manifested as either primary or secondary amenorrhea with hypergonadotropic hypogonadism (primary ovarian failure, resistant ovary syndrome, premature menopause). This complication in seen in 75 to 96% of female patients before the age of 30. The incidence of ovarian failure is unrelated to the patient's age at diagnosis or the level of dietary control in sibling pairs. The mechanism of this ovarian failure remains enigmatic. Impaired oocyte maturation and accelerated atresia have both been reported. One patient had normal ovaries at laparoscopy at 7 years of age and streak ovaries 10 years later, thus suggesting a time-dependent effect. Pregnancies have occurred in female patients with classic galactosemia, although they are very rare. In one patient who successfully gave birth, ovarian failure later developed. The male gonad is not affected.

The second major later complication of classic galactosemia is delayed speech and language. Most children with galactosemia have delayed language development associated with a verbal dyspraxia that is often overcome with time. This complication also appears to be unrelated to the time of diagnosis or the level of compliance as assessed by erythrocyte levels of galactose 1-phosphate.

Mental retardation is the most important long-term consequence of the disease. It is most severe in patients in whom diagnosis and treatment occurred late. Prior to the advent of neonatal screening, 11 of 85 patients had IQ levels below 70. An average IQ of 84 was seen in 32 highly compliant patients and an IQ of 77 in 22 poorly compliant patients.

Early information on the development of patients in whom galactosemia was diagnosed early and who were compliant with therapy was optimistic. By 1972, data from the largest experience in the United States suggested that such patients had normal levels of IQ, and it appeared that the earlier diagnosis, the higher the IQ. However, more recent experience has led to a much more pessimistic prognosis. The results of a retrospective questionnaire survey of 298 patients from the United States and Europe on whom IQ data were available indicated that 45% of those at least 6 years old were developmentally delayed. This survey provided the first evidence of a definite decline in IQ with age; furthermore, the decline in females was significantly greater than that in males. A more recent retrospective study of 134 galactosemic patients in Germany also provided evidence of a decline in IQ with age in that 4 of 34 patients younger than 6 years had IQs less than 85 whereas 10 of 18 between 7 and 12 years of age and 20 of 24 older than 12 years had such levels. A best-fit regression line suggested a mean loss in cognitive performance of 2 IQ points per year (40 points in 20 years). Of course, most of these patients, especially the older ones, antedated nationwide neonatal screening in Germany, and in the earlier international study 270 patients had clinical symptoms before diagnosis and treatment. Data were not specifically set out in either study for patients in whom the diagnosis was made while pre-symptomatic and who were managed carefully. Nevertheless, decline with age in the earlier study was even shown in individuals tested at different ages. In addition, patients in both studies had evidence of microcephaly and specific neurologic manifestations such as progressive ataxia and tremor.

MRI of the brain has revealed a substantial number of patients with cerebral atrophy. White matter abnormalities occurred in 95%

(52 of 55) older than 1 year. In addition, many patients, even those with normal IQs, have had problems with behavior and school performance.

DIAGNOSIS. The ideal approach to the diagnosis of galactosemia is through routine neonatal screening for the activity of galactose 1-phosphate uridyltransferase in dried blood on filter paper. A positive screening test is confirmed by quantification of activity in freshly obtained erythrocytes in the fluorometric assay for reduced nicotinamide-adenine dinucleotide phosphate formed along with glucose 6-phosphate from the glucose 1-phosphate product. In classic galactosemia the activity approximates zero. Variants with greater activity than this can be elucidated by electrophoresis or by mutational analysis.

In populations in which neonatal screening for galactosemia is not available, the disease is usually initially recognized after the development of symptoms by means of a test for the presence of reducing substance in the urine. It is important to emphasize that testing of the urine with glucose oxidase (Clinistix, Tes-Tape) will not detect galactose, which is a strong argument for continued use of the older methods for urinary sugar (Benedict's or Fehling's test; Clinitest). Galactosuria is also dependent on the dietary intake of lactose. A patient who is admitted to the hospital acutely ill and treated with parenteral fluid therapy may have a negative urine test because galactose has been absent from the diet for 24 to 48 hours. Characterization of the reducing substance found in a urine sample can be done in a number of ways, including paper chromatography, but sugar in an infant's urine that is positive for reducing substance and negative for glucose oxidase is galactose until proved otherwise. Confirmation is by assay of the enzyme.

Galactokinase deficiency is usually detected by assay of the urine for reducing substance in an infant or child with cataracts. The diagnosis is confirmed by assay of the enzyme in erythrocytes or cultured fibroblasts.

Epimerase deficiency is suspected in a patient with signs of galactosemia and normal transferase activity. The diagnosis is confirmed by assay of the erythrocyte activity of the epimerase.

TREATMENT. Treatment of galactosemia is exclusion of galactose from the diet, which involves the elimination of milk and its products. The mainstay of the diet for an infant is the substitution of casein hydrolysate for milk formulas. Soybean preparations may also be used. Some fruits and vegetables such as watermelons and tomatoes are avoided. Education of parents and children as they grow older on the galactose content of foods is important. Lists of foods are available that are useful in management.

Determination of the galactose 1-phosphate content of erythrocytes is useful in monitoring adherence to the diet. An acceptable level has been set at 150 μmol/L (4 mg/dL).

PROGNOSIS. Abundant experience with early treatment supports the concept that effective treatment instituted in the initial weeks of life can prevent all of the acute clinical manifestations of the disease. At the other end of the scale, mental retardation, once established, is irreversible, and if the diagnosis is delayed, some damage to the brain is inevitable. Abnormalities of visual perception, behavior problems, or convulsions may be present. Cataracts are reversible if treatment is started within the initial 3 months of life. Hepatic and renal manifestations of the disease are reversible.

Late manifestations such as ovarian failure, white matter abnormalities, and problems with speech development are not prevented by exemplary treatment. These complications will require new insight into pathogenesis for effective prevention.

PREVENTION. Prenatal diagnosis can be accomplished by assay of uridyl transferase in chorionic villus sampling or in cultured amniocytes or by quantification of galactitol in amniotic fluid by gas chromatography–mass spectrometry.

Elsas LJ, Langley S, Paulk EM, et al: A molecular approach to galactosemia. Eur Int Pediatr 154(Suppl. 2):21, 1995. *Mutational analysis of the human uridyl tranferase gene in the most common clinical phenotypes elucidates the frequency of mutations by demonstrating the high incidence of the arginine substitution for glutamine at position 188 (Q188R) in classic galactosemia and N314D in the Duarte variant.*

Nyhan WL, Ozand PT: Galactosemia. *In* Atlas of Metabolic Disease. London, Chapman & Hall, 1998, pp 322–329. *An illustrated treatment of the clinical, molecular, and therapeutic aspects of the disease.*

Segal S, Berry G: Disorders of galactose metabolism. *In* Scriver CH, Beaudet AL, Sly WS, et al (eds): The Metabolic and Molecular Bases of Inherited Disease, 7th ed. New York, McGraw-Hill, 1995. *A monograph providing the molecular bases of all aspects of galactose metabolism, galactosemia, and the pathophysiology of galactose intoxication.*

203 GLYCOGEN STORAGE DISEASES

Harry L. Greene

Glycogen is the storage form of glucose and is present in varying amounts in virtually all cells, although the liver is the primary organ for storage and subsequent release of glucose into the circulation. Glycogen is synthesized from glucose and glucose hydrolyzed and released from glycogen; this highly regulated process helps maintain normal blood glucose concentrations during fasting. At least eight enzymes involved in glycogen synthesis and the hydrolysis to glucose are utilized in this control.

Glycogen storage diseases are characterized by an abnormal tissue concentration (> 70 mg/g of liver or > 15 mg/g of muscle) and/or an abnormal structure of the glycogen molecule. During the past four decades, patients who have deficient activity in virtually every enzyme important in the normal synthesis or degradation of glycogen have been identified. More recently, identification of the genetic mutations have led to more specific molecular classifications. Clinical expression of the disease can usually be traced to either the liver or the muscle.

HEPATIC FORMS OF GLYCOGENESIS

The various hepatic enzymatic deficiencies are expressed primarily as hypoglycemia and hepatomegaly, and three defects (branching enzyme, glycogen synthetase, and debranching enzyme) result in the accumulation of abnormally structured glycogen and may cause progressive hepatic cirrhosis and associated splenomegaly. Conversely, the accumulation of normally structured glycogen, as seen with deficiency of phosphorylase, phosphorylase b kinase, acid α-glucosidase, or glucose-6-phosphatase, is usually not associated with hepatic fibrosis and splenomegaly. Figure 203–1 summarizes the general location of enzymatic defects resulting in the hepatic forms of glycogenesis. With the exception of lysosomal acid glucosidase deficiency, hypoglycemia is a common presenting feature. Clinical and biochemical expressions of the various types of glyco-gen storage diseases are summarized in Table 203–1, and the more commonly diagnosed types are discussed below.

GLUCOSE-6-PHOSPHATASE DEFICIENCY (TYPE I GLYCOGEN STORAGE DISEASE, GSD-I). The incidence of GSD-I is 1:100,000 to 1:300,000 live births and has been subcategorized into types a, b, or c, with type a the most common; but all types have similar clinical features. As noted in Figure 203–1, all other enzymatic defects directly affect the formation or degradation of glycogen, with the exception of glucose-6-phosphatase. Similarly, the clinical expression of this defect is distinctly different from that of the other forms of glycogenosis. For example, fasting-induced hypoglycemia may be extreme, and associated with lactic acidosis, hyperlipidemia, and hyperuricemia. The mechanism for the striking abnormalities in lipid and purine metabolism results primarily from overproduction of substrate in response to a decline in blood glucose, as indicated in Figure 203–1. The documented reversal of these abnormalities by treatment that maintains the blood glucose level between 80 and 90 mg/dL supports this postulate. Therapeutic intervention aimed at maintenance of blood glucose concentrations within these physiologic ranges has resulted in favorable development of many patients with delivery of unaffected offspring.

Late Complications. As more patients have survived and developed into active, functioning adults, two subsequent, unexpected complications have become apparent: (1) single or multiple hepatic adenomas, developing between ages 16 and 22, and (2) progressive glomerulosclerosis with renal failure. Because adenomas may become malignant, annual monitoring by ultrasonography is recommended. Any rapidly expanding lesion should be considered potentially malignant and should undergo surgical biopsy because serum α-fetoprotein measurements have been an unreliable marker for malignant transformation. There has been some indication that the adenomas could be prevented or reduced in younger children by more stringent dietary control; however, this hypothesis has not been substantiated in older individuals.

The development of progressive glomerulosclerosis, proteinuria, hypertension, and renal failure has been a recent observation and usually occurs in older patients (> 18 years) who are less well managed and exhibit recurrent hypoglycemic episodes, chronic hypertriglyceridemia, and lactic acidosis. The mechanism(s) causing the renal lesion is not defined, although some improvement in proteinuria has been seen after better glucose control and use of angiotensin-converting enzyme inhibitors.

Identification of several gene mutations in patients with GSD-I has led to a better understanding of the variability in clinical expression of the disease.

DEBRANCHING ENZYME DEFICIENCY (TYPE III GLYCOGEN STORAGE DISEASE). GSD-III has an incidence of about 1:100,000 live births. This disease most often affects only the liver but may affect muscle as well, although a single variant in North African Jews show both liver and muscle involvement with a prevalence of 1:5,400. Elevated serum creatine kinase concentrations indicate muscle involvement, but these concentrations may not become elevated until later childhood or adolescence. Hypoglycemia with fasting is less severe (usually 40 to 50 mg/dL) than in patients with GSD-I, although hepatic enlargement may be substantially greater. Serum aspartate aminotransferase and alanine aminotransaminase concentrations are commonly above 500 units/mL. Correspondingly, hepatic fibrosis of varying degrees is usually present during childhood and may be progressive. Adult patients may present with "cryptogenic cirrhosis."

Treating patients with GSD-III has not been advocated because the natural course of the disease has been thought to be benign. However, because growth retardation and cirrhosis may be serious complications, several patients have been treated with frequent feedings and raw cornstarch to maintain blood glucose levels between 75 and 100 mg/dL. Treated patients often show a significant reduction in serum transaminase levels and improvements in growth, and they may demonstrate improved muscle strength, although serum creatine kinase activities remain elevated. Identification of specific gene mutations should provide better prognostic predictions.

Clinical and laboratory features of the other, less common forms of hepatic glycogenesis are presented in Table 203–1.

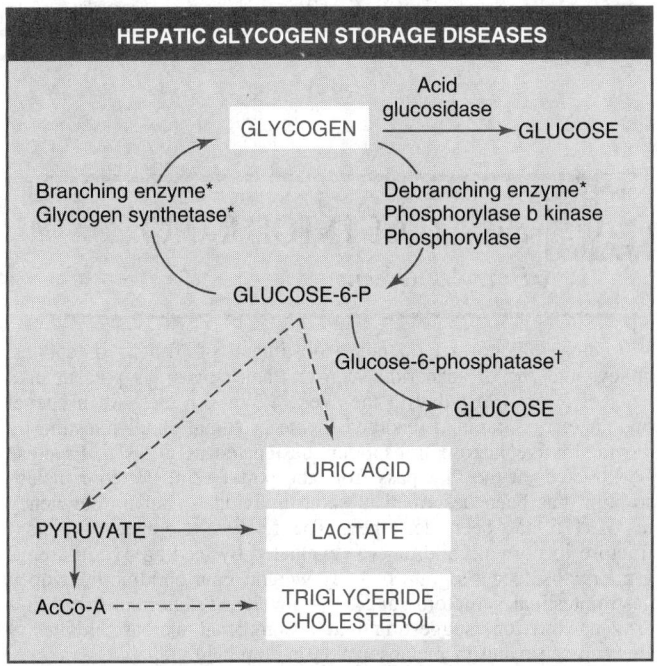

FIGURE 203–1 ■ Mechanism for abnormalities in lipid, purine, and carbohydrate metabolism in type I (glucose-6-phosphatase deficiency) glycogen storage disease. * = associated with hepatic cirrhosis. † = associated with elevated serum uric acid, lactate, and lipid levels and with hepatic adenoma.

Table 203–1 ▪ CLASSIFICATION OF GLYCOGEN STORAGE DISEASES

TYPE	ENZYME AFFECTED	PRIMARY ORGAN INVOLVED	MANIFESTATIONS
O	Glycogen synthetase	Liver	Hypoglycemia, hyperketonia, FFT, early death
Ia	Glucose-6-phosphatase	Liver	Enlarged liver and kidney growth failure, fasting hypoglycemia, acidosis, thrombocyte dysfunction
Ib	Microsomal membrane G-6-P translocase	Liver	As in Ia; in addition, recurrent neutropenia, bacterial infections
Ic	Microsomal membrane P-transporter	Liver	As in Ia
II	Lysosomal acid glucosidase	Skeletal and cardiac muscle	*Infantile form:* early-onset, progressive muscle hypotonia, cardiac failure, death before 2 years *Juvenile form:* late-onset myopathy and variable cardiac involvement *Adult form:* limb-girdle muscular dystrophy-like feature
III	Amylo-1,6-glucosidase (debrancher enzyme)	Liver, skeletal muscle, heart	Fasting hypoglycemia, hepatomegaly in infancy; some have myopathic features, rarely clinical cardiac features
IV	Amylo-1,4-1,6-transglucosidase (brancher enzyme)	Liver, muscle	Hepatosplenomegaly, cirrhosis; may have late-onset myopathy
V	Muscle phosphorylase	Skeletal muscle	Exercise-induced muscular pain, cramps, and progressive weakness, sometimes with myoglobinuria; symptoms usually begin during adolescence or early adulthood
VI	Liver phosphorylase	Liver	Hepatomegaly, mild hypoglycemia, good prognosis
VII	Phosphofructokinase	Muscle, red blood cells	As in V; in addition, mild hemolytic anemia
Formerly VIb, VIII, or IX	Phosphorylase b kinase	Liver, leukocytes, (?) muscle	As in VI; X-linked inheritance
X	Cyclic AMP-dependent kinase	Liver, muscle	Hepatomegaly, mild hypoglycemia

MUSCULAR FORMS OF GLYCOGEN STORAGE

ACID α-GLUCOSIDASE DEFICIENCY (POMPE'S DISEASE, TYPE II GLYCOGEN STORAGE DISEASE). In this condition, virtually all tissues have an increased glycogen content. However, presenting clinical manifestations of the illness are cardiac enlargement, myocardial failure, and generalized muscle hypotonia without muscle wasting. The classic infantile form manifests during the first months of life, and few infants survive past the first year. The juvenile variant presents in later infancy or early childhood and progresses more slowly, with death in the second or third decade. The adult type manifests as a slowly developing adult-onset myopathy. In each case, the diagnosis is dependent on finding deficient activity of acid α-1,4-glucosidase in muscle specimens or cultured fibroblasts. More recently, diagnosis is possible by identification of genetic mutations. No treatment, including bone marrow transplantation and systemic enzyme infusion, has proved to be of long-term benefit to these patients. The finding of chimerization in other tissues after liver transplant in two patients with GSD-IV may offer some encouragement for future treatment for GSD-II.

MYOPHOSPHORYLASE DEFICIENCY (TYPE V GSD, MCARDLE'S DISEASE). Most of these patients are asymptomatic during early childhood and escape diagnosis until the second or third decade of life. A history of muscle pain and cramps after exercise, signs of myoglobinuria, and painful cramping on an ischemic exercise test are characteristic. The diagnosis is suggested by an elevation in serum muscle creatine kinase isoenzyme activity and by failure to elevate the serum lactate level with exercise. The diagnosis is established by documenting elevated muscle glycogen in the sarcolemmal regions and reduced muscle phosphorylase activity. Glucose or fructose ingestion before exercise is said to reduce the symptoms.

MUSCLE PHOSPHOFRUCTOKINASE DEFICIENCY (MUSCLE PHOSPHOGLYCERATE MUTASE DEFICIENCY, LACTATE DEHYDROGENASE [LDH-M] SUBUNIT DEFICIENCY, TYPE VII GSD). These muscle glycogenoses are rare and clinically similar to myophosphorylase deficiency. Patients with phosphofructokinase deficiency may also show a mild hemolytic anemia. Diagnosis depends on muscle enzyme analysis or identification of the genetic mutations. Treatment is aimed at avoiding strenuous exercise.

DIAGNOSIS AND PRENATAL DIAGNOSIS OF GLYCOGEN STORAGE DISEASE

Diagnostic enzyme or genetic analysis of fibroblasts or hepatic or muscle tissue for most types of glycogen storage diseases can usually be performed at Duke Medical Center, Division of Genetics (Dr Y. T. Chen).

Dimauro S, Tsujino S, Shanske S, et al: Biochemistry and molecular genetics of human glycogenoses: An overview. Muscle Nerve 3:S10, 1995. *This extensively referenced article provides information on the molecular and biochemical aspects of the glycogen storage diseases.*

Ding JH, deBarsy T, Brown B, et al: Immunoblot analyses of glycogen debranching enzyme in different subtypes of glycogen storage disease type III. J Pediatr 116:95, 1990. *Provides newer insights into the molecular basis of type III glycogenoses.*

Ghishan FK, Greene HL: Inborn errors of metabolism that lead to permanent liver injury. *In* Zakim D, Boyer TD (eds): Hepatology: A Textbook of Liver Disease, 3rd ed. Philadelphia, WB Saunders, 1996. *An extensively referenced review that focuses on the altered metabolism, treatment, and outcome of the hepatic forms of glycogenesis.*

Ke-Jian L, Shelly LL, Chi-Jiunn P, et al: Mutations in the glucose-6-phosphatase gene that cause glycogen storage disease type 1a. Science 262:580, 1993. *First identification of the molecular basis of this disease.*

Parker PH, Ballew M, Greene HL: Nutritional management of glycogen storage disease. Annu Rev Nutr 13:83, 1993. *Combines the biochemical abnormalities of the glycogenoses and associated research findings with a practical guide to dietary management of children and adults.*

204 FRUCTOSE INTOLERANCE

Harry L. Greene

Fructose, a normal dietary constituent of fruits, vegetables, honey, and the disaccharide sucrose (table sugar), is present at a level of 50 to 100 g/day in the average Western diet. At this level of intake, it is rapidly absorbed in the proximal small intestine by the facilitative hexose transporter, designated as GLUT5. Fructose is extracted on the first pass from the portal vein. Fructose malabsorption has been described in some individuals, but no deficiency in GLUT5 has been described. The relative tolerance of dietary fructose in normal children was evaluated by feeding 31 children 2 g of fructose per kilogram of body weight. Four children developed gastrointestinal symptoms and 71% developed abnormal breath hydrogen excretion, suggesting that a significant increase in dietary fructose can result in malabsorption in some individuals.

Initial metabolism of fructose primarily involves three enzymes: fructokinase, aldolase B, and triokinase (Fig. 204–1), although hexokinase phosphorylates some of the fructose. Five enzymatic defects involving fructose metabolism have been identified: (1) fructokinase deficiency, (2) aldolase A deficiency, (3) aldolase B

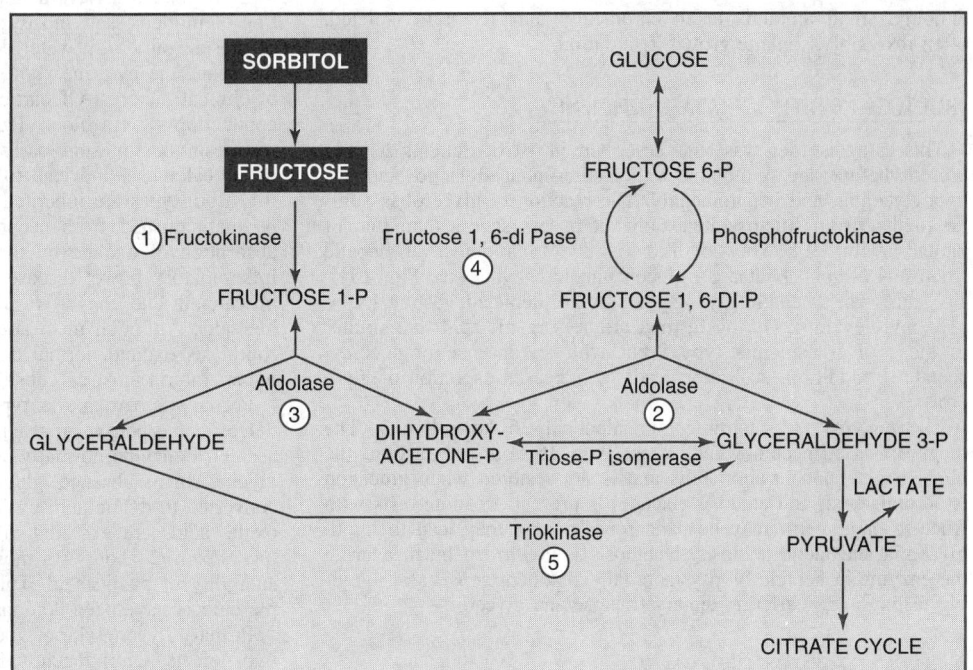

FIGURE 204–1 ■ The major pathway for fructose metabolism in the liver, showing the five defects discussed in the text. Aldolase deficiency consists primarily of defects in aldolase B (3). Aldolase A deficiency (2) is extremely rare and is expressed primarily during embryogenesis.

deficiency, (4) fructose-1,6-diphosphatase deficiency, and (5) D-glycerate kinase deficiency. The enzymatic defects in fructose metabolism are illustrated in Figure 204–1 and are discussed below.

FRUCTOKINASE DEFICIENCY

Fructokinase deficiency (essential fructosuria) is a rare (about 1:130,000 live births), asymptomatic, autosomal-recessive condition caused by deficient activity of fructokinase, the first enzyme in fructose utilization. Because no pathologic condition results from this defect, the primary concern relates to the fact that fructose is a reducing sugar. Thus, a positive reaction with urinary Clinitest tablets may result in the erroneous suggestion of diabetes unless glucose oxidase is determined with a dipstick.

ALDOLASE DEFICIENCY

Three aldolases (A, B, and C) are responsible for the conversion of fructose-1,6-diphosphate into glyceraldehyde-3-phosphate and dihydroxyacetone phosphate. Embryonic tissue produces aldolase A; adult liver, kidney, and intestine express aldolase B; and nervous tissue expresses aldolase C. Although all three aldolases are tetramers of identical 40-kd subunits, each is coded for different genes on different chromosomes: aldolase A on chromosome 16,16q22-q24, aldolase B on chromosome 9,9q13-q32, and aldolase C on chromosome 17,17 cen-q 21.

ALDOLASE A DEFICIENCY. Aldolase A deficiency may be detrimental because of its pivotal role in glycolysis. This is apparently of special relevance to the developing embryo, which expresses only aldolase A. Only a few patients with this deficit have been described, and not all symptoms are expressed to the same degree. Potential symptoms include mental retardation, short stature, hemolytic anemia, and abnormal facial appearance. Because aldolase B becomes normal at birth as aldolase A declines, newborns with hereditary fructose intolerance (HFI) do not show fructosuria, explaining why neonates with HFI are unaffected *in utero.*

ALDOLASE B DEFICIENCY (HEREDITARY FRUCTOSE INTOLERANCE). Aldolase B deficiency (prevalence about 1:23,000 live births) is a potentially life-threatening autosomal-recessive disorder than can be effectively treated by eliminating dietary fructose. This disorder is due to deficiency of fructose-1-phosphate aldolase (aldolase B). Aldolase B is normally present in large amounts in the liver, intestine, and renal cortex; thus, excessive fructose intake by patients with HFI adversely affects each of these organs. Recent expression of the C134R mutation showed partial activity of the

enzyme, explaining why gluconeogenesis/glycolysis is maintained in patients with HFI.

Symptoms become manifested only when patients ingest fructose or sorbitol-containing foods. Because lactose is the carbohydrate source in mammalian milk, infants do not develop symptoms until the introduction of dietary fruits or other fructose-containing foods or medication (e.g., fruits, fruit juices, medicinal syrups, sucrose-containing infant formulas, or sorbitol-sweeteners). The primary presentation is vomiting and other features of hypoglycemia within 20 to 30 minutes after fructose ingestion. These acute manifestations may not be apparent after lower chronic intakes, for example with fructose-containing infant formulas or sorbitol-containing gum. In these instances, failure to thrive, hepatomegaly, and cirrhosis may represent the dominant presenting features. Concomitant laboratory findings include an acute decrease in serum glucose and phosphate concentrations and an elevated uric acid concentration. With continued exposure to fructose, hyperbilirubinemia, lactic acidosis, hepatosplenomegaly, and liver failure develop in conjunction with renal tubular dysfunction (bicarbonaturia, aminoaciduria, phosphaturia). At this stage, fatty infiltration of liver, cellular necrosis, and mild bile duct proliferation with fibrosis occur. If exposure to fructose continues, progressive fibrosis, cirrhosis, and death from liver failure follow. The brain may also show diminished neurons.

The diagnosis is suggested by the presence of urinary reducing sugar detectable by Clinitest tablets and not by urinary dipstick, which measures glucose oxidase. Because similar clinical features may be present with galactosemia or tyrosinemia, diagnosis can be confirmed by genetic screen. An intravenous fructose tolerance test (0.2 to 0.3 g/kg in adults or 3 g/m^2 in children) after restriction of dietary fructose for several weeks has been used to confirm the illness, but this procedure may cause hypoglycemia and is no longer recommended.

At present, 21 mutations of HFI have been reported; 15 are single base substitutions, resulting in nine amino acid replacements, four nonsense codons, and two putative splicing defects. Two large deletions, two four-base deletions, a single-base deletion, and a seven-base deletion/one-base insertion have been found. Regions of the enzyme where mutations have been observed recurrently are encoded by exons 5 and 9. The three most common mutations are found in these exons, making screening methods more feasible.

In spite of recurrent bouts of hypoglycemia and substantial liver disease, restriction of dietary fructose usually results in almost complete recovery during a 3- to 5-week period, and affected adults have normal intelligence. Older children and adults are protected from large dietary intakes of fructose by an aversion to sweets, although small amounts taken chronically may result in isolated, often reversible, somatic growth retardation.

FRUCTOSE-1,6-DIPHOSPHATASE DEFICIENCY

This rare disorder was first described in 1970. Patients usually present before age 6 months with fasting-induced lactic acidosis, hypoglycemia, and hepatomegaly. The reaction to glycerol is similar to that from fructose ingestion but is less severe than that of patients with HFI. The condition is due to a defect of hepatic fructose-1,6-diphosphatase, a gluconeogenic enzyme (see Fig. 204–1). Thus, when hepatic glycogen stores are depleted, fasting hypoglycemia develops. During fasting, urinary organic acids are similar to those of tyrosinemia type I but with an absence of succinyl acetate. In addition, starvation leads to increased excretion of glycerol.

The enzyme is a tetramer for identical 36 kd subunits. The diagnosis is suspected when, after 12 to 16 hours of fasting, the blood sugar concentration falls and is not restored when glucagon is administered, and acidosis (lactate) is present. Loading tests with fructose or glycerol may be dangerous because they lead to hypoglycemia and lactic acidosis. Diagnosis is confirmed by measuring the enzyme in hepatic biopsy material. Treatment consists of avoiding fasting and restricting dietary fructose and glycerol.

D-GLYCERATE KINASE DEFICIENCY
(D-GLYCERIC ACIDURIA)

This is a rare, clinically variable disorder resulting in either no symptoms, or metabolic acidosis and failure to thrive, and profound psychomotor retardation and seizures. The variable phenotypic expression has not been fully explained on the basis of the enzymatic defect, but all patients who show a substantial increase in D-glycerate excretion after fructose ingestion should avoid dietary fructose.

Cox TM: Iatrogenic deaths in hereditary fructose intolerance. Arch Dis Child 69:413, 1993. *This paper illustrates the need to restrict intravenous sorbitol as well as fructose in patients with HFI.*
Hommes FA: Inborn errors of fructose metabolism. Am J Clin Nutr 58(Suppl):788, 1993. *A recent correlation between the genotype and phenotype of five common defects in fructose metabolism.*
Tolan DR: Molecular basis of hereditary fructose intolerance: Mutations and polymorphisms in the human aldolase B gene. Hum Mutat 6:210, 1995. *An extensively referenced review that focuses on the new advances in genetic methods for identification and screening methods of HFI.*

205 PRIMARY HYPEROXALURIA

Richard E. Hillman

Primary hyperoxaluria refers to two different peroxisomal enzyme deficiencies that are characterized by massive synthesis and urinary excretion of oxalic acid. Until recently, primary hyperoxaluria was considered a very rare disease. However, the ready availability of oxalate assays in the past few years has led to the description of milder cases, mostly type II, which are either asymptomatic or present only with water deprivation. Oxalate is also deposited in the heart, the eye, the skin, and other organs, leading to a variety of clinical pictures. Of particular interest, oxalate has led to cardiac conduction system block. Particularly in type I disease, the clinical manifestations present early in childhood with nephrolithiasis or nephrocalcinosis and lead to renal failure within the first decade of life. Both types are inherited as autosomal recessive traits and must be distinguished from secondary hyperoxalurias due to increased absorption of oxalate by the gut. These secondary causes include inflammatory bowel disease and fat malabsorption, which may tie up calcium and convert insoluble calcium oxalate to more absorbable salts. Although most adult patients with calcium oxalate nephrolithiasis excrete normal amounts of oxalate, it is now clear that hyperoxaluria must be considered in the differential diagnosis.

Primary hyperoxaluria type I (glycolic aciduria) is caused by a defect in the peroxisomal enzyme alanine:glyoxylate aminotransferase. This enzyme normally converts glycolic acid to the amino acid glycine. In its absence, glycolic acid leaves the peroxisome and is converted to oxalic acid by lactic dehydrogenase. Both glycolic and oxalic acids are excreted in large amounts, usually more than 60 mg/1.73 m²/24 hours. In most cases, this concentration exceeds the solubility of oxalic acid. This enzyme has been cloned, and multiple defects have been demonstrated.

Primary hyperoxaluria type II (glyceric aciduria) is due to one of two defects. Until recently it was believed that the defect was in the enzyme D-glyceric dehydrogenase. This enzyme leads to the accumulation of hydroxypyruvic acid, which is reduced in the cytoplasm to L-glyceric acid. It had been unclear why this defect caused hyperoxaluria. Recently, it was suggested that this enzyme may be the same as glyoxalate reductase, which leads to accumulation of glyoxalate and production of oxalate by lactate dehydrogenase. Type II is a much milder disease in most cases than type I. Asymptomatic cases or cases with only a single attack of oxaluria have been reported. Two patients in recent cases developed symptoms only after experiencing severe water deprivation (one while sailing and one while running in hot weather).

Some patients with type I disease respond to large doses of pyridoxine (20 to 200 mg/day). This vitamin is the cofactor for the enzyme. It appears to act by stabilizing the remaining activity and is effective only in patients with some enzyme, in general the milder cases. Dilute urine should be maintained by high fluid intake, and some reports suggest that diuretics may help. Attempts to form more soluble salts of oxalate, particularly with magnesium orthophosphate and citrate, have met with some success. The only "cure" for this disease has been a combined renal and liver transplant. Renal transplants alone have failed, owing to the accumulation of oxalate produced in the liver. Therapeutic outcomes in type II patients are very variable. Pyridoxine has no effect. Other measures that maintain a dilute urine seem to be enough in the milder cases.

Danpure CJ, Purdue PE: Primary hyperoxaluria. *In* Scriver CR, Beaudet AL, Sly WS, et al (eds): The Metabolic Basis of Inherited Disease, 7th ed. New York, McGraw-Hill, 1995, p 2385. *A general review of the biochemistry of primary oxalosis and related secondary disorders.*
Danpure CJ, Purdue PE, Fryer P, et al: Enzymological and mutational analysis of a complex primary hyperoxaluria type I phenotype. Am J Hum Genet 53:417, 1993. *The latest data on type I enzyme deficiencies, including variability.*

DISORDERS OF LIPID METABOLISM

206 THE HYPERLIPOPROTEINEMIAS

Joseph L. Witztum ■ *Daniel Steinberg*

Hyperlipidemia, abnormal elevation of plasma cholesterol and/or triglyceride levels, is one of the most common clinical problems that confront the physician in daily practice. Much attention has been focused on these disorders because there is a strong association of hyperlipidemia—especially hypercholesterolemia—with development of atherosclerosis, and of hypertriglyceridemia with pancreatitis. Hyperlipidemia may occur because of a primary genetic disorder or as a result of environmental influences secondary to other medical conditions, or any combination of these factors. Because lipids are transported in plasma as components of lipoprotein complexes, understanding lipoprotein physiology is necessary for informed diagnosis and therapeutic planning.

Table 206-1 ■ APOLIPOPROTEIN CHARACTERISTICS

APOPROTEIN	LIPOPROTEINS	FUNCTION
Apo B-100	VLDL, IDL, LDL	Secretion of VLDL from liver. Structural protein of VLDL, IDL, and LDL. Ligand for the LDL receptor
Apo B-48	Chylomicrons, remnants	Secretion of chylomicrons from intestine
Apo E	Chylomicrons, VLDL, IDL, HDL	Ligand for binding of IDL and remnants to LDL receptor and LRP
Apo A-I	HDL, chylomicrons	Structural protein of HDL Activator of LCAT
Apo A-II	HDL, chylomicrons	Unknown
Apo C-II	Chylomicrons, VLDL, IDL, HDL	Activator of LPL
Apo C-III	Chylomicrons, VLDL, IDL, HDL	Inhibitor of LPL activity

PHYSIOLOGY OF LIPOPROTEIN TRANSPORT

Lipoproteins are complex macromolecules that transport nonpolar lipids through the aqueous environment of plasma. The more nonpolar lipids—triglycerides and cholesteryl esters—are carried almost exclusively in the central core of the spherical lipoprotein particles. The more polar lipids (such as phospholipids and free cholesterol), together with amphipathic apolipoproteins, form a surface monolayer that serves to "solubilize" the particles and allows them to remain in stable solution in the aqueous plasma.

Each lipoprotein particle contains on its surface one or more apolipoproteins that have a variety of functional and structural roles. Some apolipoproteins provide structural stability to the lipoprotein, serve as ligands for cellular lipoprotein receptors that help determine the metabolic fate of individual particles, and act as cofactors for plasma enzymes involved in plasma lipid and lipoprotein metabolism. Other apolipoproteins play several roles; for example, apolipoprotein B (apo B) is the major structural apolipoprotein of the triglyceride-rich lipoproteins secreted by the liver (very low-density lipoproteins [VLDL]), but it also serves as the ligand for binding of low-density lipoproteins (LDL) (formed from VLDL) to cellular LDL receptors. Table 206-1 lists major apoproteins, lipoproteins on which they reside, and known or postulated functions.

The most widely used classification of lipoproteins is based on their different densities, which determine their behavior during preparative equilibrium ultracentrifugation. The fact that lipoprotein particles exist as relatively discrete species when separated this way led to the currently used density classification system outlined in Table 206-2. A second classification system originally proposed many years ago assigns priority to the apoprotein content of the lipoproteins. For example, in the high-density lipoprotein (HDL) density class there are lipoprotein particles that contain mainly apo A-I and others that contain both apo A-I and apo A-II; these are designated LpA-I and LpA-I, A-II, respectively. Current research suggests that it is primarily LpA-I that confers the anti-atherogenic properties of HDL. Thus, in the future, full evaluation may include this type of analysis, but for now more research is needed to determine its clinical value.

An older classification system of the lipoproteins, based on their electrophoretic patterns (lipoprotein pattern typing), while important historically for the development of our understanding of lipid transport disorders, is not used commonly today. However, for the sake of completeness, the electrophoretic mobility of each lipoprotein class is also given in Table 206-2.

SYNTHESIS AND TRANSPORT OF ENDOGENOUS LIPIDS. The endogenous lipid transport system can be divided into two major classes: the apo B-100 lipoprotein system (VLDL, IDL [intermediate-density lipoproteins], and LDL) and the apo A-I lipoprotein system (HDL).

METABOLISM OF VERY LOW-DENSITY LIPOPROTEINS. Between meals, free fatty acids are mobilized from the adipose tissue and serve as a major source for hepatic triglyceride synthesis. Lipogenesis, the synthesis of fatty acids de novo from carbohydrate or protein, also can occur in the liver. Fatty acids can either enter mitochondria (where β-oxidation occurs) or they can undergo esterification to form triglycerides in the cytosol. Control of triglyceride synthesis is a complex process that appears to be regulated in part by changes in insulin and glucagon that occur with feeding. Glucagon enhances fatty acid oxidation, whereas insulin prevents it. In addition, insulin may induce lipogenic enzymes in the liver. Triglycerides, together with cholesterol synthesized de novo in the liver or delivered to the liver by chylomicron remnants, are packaged together with apo B and phospholipids and form a nascent VLDL (Fig. 206-1).

The details of the packaging process are still being worked out, but it is known that a microsomal triglyceride transfer protein (MTP) is essential for normal VLDL assembly and secretion from the hepatocyte. When mutations in MTP occur, the newly synthesized apo B is not lipidated within the lumen of the endoplasmic reticulum (ER), and as a result the apo B is degraded, leading to abetalipoproteinemia, even though the apo B gene is normal. This results in a serious clinical syndrome in which patients lack any apo B–containing lipoproteins in their plasma.

Plasma VLDL also contain other apolipoproteins, including the C apoproteins and apo E. Apo B is found as a full-length protein termed apo B-100 (or apo B), which is made by the liver, or as a shortened form termed apo B-48, which is made in humans only by the intestine. Apo B is an obligatory component for nascent VLDL assembly and secretion from the hepatocyte; other apoproteins are added to VLDL after their entry into plasma. The size of the VLDL particle released depends on the availability of triglycerides in the liver. Very large triglyceride-rich VLDL are secreted when excess hepatic triglyceride synthesis is occurring, as in obesity, non–insulin dependent diabetes, and excess alcohol consumption. In contrast, small VLDL are secreted when availability of triglyceride, but not cholesterol, is decreased. Each VLDL particle contains one molecule of apo B, yet under ordinary circumstances the rate of apo B synthesis is not rate limiting for VLDL secretion. Although enhanced triglyceride synthesis can lead to enhanced triglyceride output, the *number* of VLDL particles released is not necessarily increased. Instead, *larger* individual VLDL particles containing more triglyceride are released. Understanding the processes regulating VLDL assembly and release by the hepatocytes is necessary to understand the etiology of clinically important disorders, such as familial combined hyperlipidemia or hyperapobetalipoproteinemia, which are characterized by increased rates of secretion of VLDL particles from the liver. Other lipoprotein disorders (familial hypertriglyceridemia) are caused by hepatic secretion of a normal number of VLDL particles but ones that are enriched with triglycerides. The half-life of VLDL in plasma is about 1 hour or less.

The primary function of lipoprotein particles is to transport lipids from one site to another. Triglyceride-rich lipoproteins serve to transport endogenously synthesized triglyceride to adipose tissue

Table 206-2 ■ CHARACTERISTICS OF MAJOR LIPOPROTEIN CLASSES

LIPOPROTEIN CLASS	DENSITY (g/mL)	DIAMETER (nm)	MAJOR LIPID	ELECTROPHORETIC MOBILITY
Chylomicron and remnants	<<1.006	500–80	Dietary triglycerides	Remains at origin
VLDL	<1.006	80–30	Endogenous triglycerides	Pre-β
IDL	1.006–1.019	35–25	Cholesteryl esters, triglycerides	Slow pre-β
LDL	1.019–1.063	25–18	Cholesteryl esters	β
HDL	1.063–1.210	5–12	Cholesteryl esters, phospholipids	α
Lp(a)	1.055–1.085	30	Cholesteryl esters	Slow pre-β

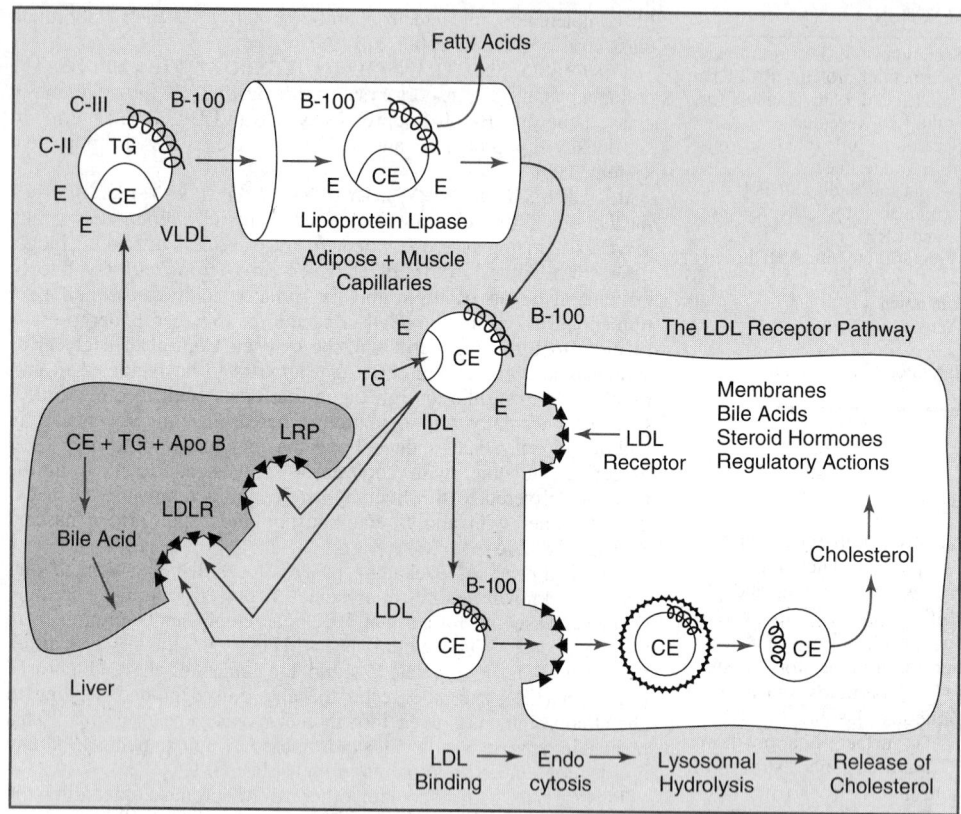

FIGURE 206–1 ■ Simplified scheme of metabolism of apo B–containing lipoproteins. In the liver, triglyceride (TG), cholesteryl esters (CE), and apolipoprotein B-100 (B-100) are packaged and released into plasma as very low-density lipoproteins (VLDL). In capillary beds, lipoprotein lipase hydrolyzes TG to release free fatty acids. The TG-depleted particle is termed an intermediate-density lipoprotein (IDL). The particle is further metabolized to CE-rich low-density lipoprotein (LDL). A major fraction of IDL particles is removed from plasma by hepatic receptors, both by LDL receptors (LDLR) and LDL receptor–related protein (LRP). A portion of IDL is converted to LDL, which is then removed from plasma by LDLR on liver and peripheral cells. Uptake of LDL through the LDLR pathway leads to regulation of cholesterol synthesis and LDLR synthesis as explained in text. (Modified from Witztum JL: Current approaches to drug therapy for the hypercholesterolemic patient. Circulation 80: 1101, 1989. By permission of the American Heart Association, Inc.)

for storage in the fed state or to muscle for utilization in the fasting state. The enzyme that catalyzes peripheral triglyceride uptake is lipoprotein lipase (LPL). This enzyme is synthesized in adipose tissue and skeletal muscle cells, secreted, and transported across the capillary endothelial cell, where it binds to glycoproteins on the endothelial luminal surface. When VLDL binds to LPL, the LPL is activated by apo C-II present on the surface of the VLDL particle. This leads to triglyceride hydrolysis and release of fatty acids, which are then transported into the fat (or muscle) cell where they are re-esterified with glycerol and stored as intracellular triglyceride. The vast majority of triglyceride in adipose tissue is acquired by this mechanism because essentially no lipogenesis occurs de novo from glucose in human adipose tissue. The activity of LPL in adipose tissue is increased in the fed state, effectively providing for triglyceride storage. Insulin is required to maintain adequate LPL levels in adipose tissue. It appears to do so by maintaining synthesis and release, but it does not acutely affect changes in LPL levels. This is in contrast to "hormone-sensitive lipase" (HSL), an enzyme that hydrolyzes intracellular triglycerides, releasing fatty acids to plasma for uptake by the liver. HSL is acutely inhibited by insulin, whereas glucagon increases its activity. Thus, after a meal, high insulin levels serve to promote storage of fatty acids in the adipocyte as triglyceride, whereas in the fasting state hydrolysis is promoted, providing fatty acids for uptake by muscle and liver.

As noted earlier, the action of LPL requires the cofactor, apo C-II. Shortly after VLDL enters into plasma, apo C-II is transferred to VLDL from a reservoir on circulating HDL. After hydrolysis of triglyceride in VLDL, the apo C-II is released and presumably picked up again by HDL. The importance of apo C-II is demonstrated by individuals with genetic deficiency of C-II, which leads to impaired LPL activity and massive hypertriglyceridemia. Other apolipoproteins, such as C-III, are also transferred between VLDL and HDL. In vitro, apo C-III can inhibit LPL-mediated hydrolysis, but its physiologic role in vivo is still unclear. Evidence from studies with transgenic mice supports the idea that increased plasma levels of apo C-III cause hypertriglyceridemia, directly or indirectly, by inhibiting LPL-mediated hydrolysis.

Hydrolysis of triglycerides in VLDL profoundly alters the structure of the VLDL with collapse of the core. The excess surface components, including cholesterol, phospholipids, and the non–apo

B apoproteins, are transferred to HDL. The triglyceride-depleted VLDL, with its associated loss of other lipids and apoproteins, now becomes an IDL, cholesterol-enriched and containing only apo B and apo E. Under normal conditions this particle is rapidly removed from plasma by the liver through a complex interaction with several hepatic receptors, including the LDL receptor, which recognizes apo B and apo E, and with another receptor, termed the *remnant receptor,* which is specific for apo E. This latter receptor is thought to be the LDL-receptor–related protein (LRP). Whereas the majority of IDL particles are normally removed from plasma by this process in other species, in humans a significant fraction is converted into LDL. By the time the cholesterol-rich LDL has been formed, most of the triglyceride has been removed and apo B is now the sole apoprotein remaining from the original VLDL particle. Under normal circumstances, most of the cholesterol found in plasma is present in the form of LDL particles, and only minute amounts of IDL are present.

Apo E, which acts as a ligand for both the LDL receptor and the LRP, appears to be crucial for both the direct removal of IDL and conversion of IDL particles to LDL particles. Patients who either lack apo E or are homozygous for apo E isoforms (E2) that bind less efficiently to these receptors may have excess plasma accumulation of IDL particles (and chylomicron remnants) and are both hypercholesterolemic and hypertriglyceridemic, a condition known as dysbetalipoproteinemia.

METABOLISM OF LDL. Each LDL particle is derived from VLDL via IDL and contains one copy of apo B. All other apolipoproteins have now been removed, together with much of the phospholipid and triglyceride and some of the cholesterol. Although only a small percentage of VLDL particles ultimately end up as LDL particles, the bulk of plasma cholesterol is accounted for by LDL particles because of the relatively slow rate of clearance of LDL from plasma (half-life of 2 to 3 days). Because LDL particles contain only apo B, their efficient clearance can occur only by way of the LDL receptor pathway. In normal humans, approximately 75% of LDL particles are cleared by the LDL receptor pathway and approximately two thirds of LDL particles are removed by the liver. Nobel Prize winners Brown and Goldstein elucidated the LDL receptor pathway, one of the major achievements of modern medical science. The rate of LDL removal through this pathway is the primary determinant of LDL levels. The LDL receptor, which binds apo B with high affinity and leads to internalization of the LDL particle is found on virtually every mammalian cell. As shown in the right side of Figure 206–1, the LDL particle binds to the receptor on the surface of the cell, and subsequently the receptor and the bound LDL particle are internalized. LDL is then delivered to the lysosome, but the receptor recycles to the surface of the cell. Within the lysosome, the protein component, apo B, is degraded to amino acids or oligopeptides. The cholesteryl ester is hydrolyzed to free cholesterol, which can now leave the lysosome and is used by the cell for a variety of cellular processes, including new cell membrane synthesis, hormone synthesis (in adrenal, ovarian, or testicular cells), bile acid production (in hepatocytes), or for re-esterification to be stored as a cholesteryl-ester droplet. In addition, when sufficient cholesterol has been accumulated, down-regulation of the LDL receptors is accomplished, as well as inhibition of the cell's own cholesterol synthetic pathway. Thus, this efficient regulatory pathway provides a cell with sufficient cholesterol for its physiologic needs, but it prevents the overaccumulation of cholesterol, which could be toxic. In particular, regulation of the *hepatic* LDL receptor pathway is a dominant mechanism for regulating plasma LDL levels in humans, and the ability to manipulate this pathway by therapeutic agents forms the basis of most of our current techniques to lower LDL levels.

It should also be appreciated that apo B–containing lipoproteins may be removed by the liver by inefficient, low-affinity pathways as well. For example, in subjects with homozygous familial hypercholesterolemia, who have no functional LDL receptors, the fractional clearance of LDL is drastically reduced, but a new steady state is reached because of the nonspecific pathways for LDL removal. However, greatly elevated LDL levels occur, creating a very high risk for premature atherosclerosis. A scavenger pathway involving the macrophage system may also remove LDL particles by non–LDL receptor pathways, and in the artery wall this may play an important role in the genesis of the atherosclerotic lesion.

SYNTHESIS AND TRANSPORT OF EXOGENOUS (DIETARY) LIPIDS. After a triglyceride-rich meal, triglycerides and cholesterol are absorbed into the mucosal cells of the small intestine as free fatty acids and free cholesterol. There they are re-esterified to triglyceride and cholesteryl esters and incorporated into the core of a nascent lipoprotein, the chylomicron. The surface coat of the chylomicron is composed of phospholipid and apo A-I, A-II, and A-IV. Apo B-48 is a crucial component of chylomicrons and is a product of the same gene that codes for the intact, full-length apo B-100. Apo B-48 is so named because it is identical to the first 48% (the amino terminal portion) of apo B-100. In humans, the intact, full-length apo B-100 is made only in the liver, whereas apo B-48 is made only in the intestine. Apo B-48 is transcribed from the apo B-100 gene, but the mRNA is first edited by a cytosine-to-uracil change creating a stop-codon. The domain of intact apo B-100 that binds to the LDL receptor is contained in the carboxyterminal end. Because apo B-48 lacks this domain it is unable to bind to LDL receptors. Thus, once the chylomicron has been secreted by the intestine, apo B-48 functions primarily as a structural component.

Triglycerides constitute more than 90% by weight of the chylomicron particle, and consequently the density of this lipoprotein is the lowest of any in plasma. When plasma is left overnight in the refrigerator, if chylomicrons are present, they will float to the top and appear as a layer of "cream" on top, which is the basis for the chylomicron test. In normal individuals, this test is always negative after an 8- to 12-hour fast, because chylomicrons have a short half-life in plasma. The presence of a positive chylomicron test in a 12-hour fasting sample is abnormal and indicative of marked delay in chylomicron clearance.

Chylomicrons are delivered to the plasma via the thoracic duct (Fig. 206–2). While in the lymph and after entering plasma, chylomicrons acquire apo C-II, C-III, and apo E by transfer. After having acquired sufficient apo C-II, which is absolutely required for LPL activity, the chylomicron can interact with LPL in a manner analogous to that of VLDL particles. After sufficient triglyceride hydrolysis has occurred, the remaining chylomicron particle, now termed a *remnant,* has a markedly reduced core volume and its excess surface components, including apoproteins such as C-II, C-III, and some of the apo E, are transferred to HDL particles as described for the VLDL particles. The remnant particle is still

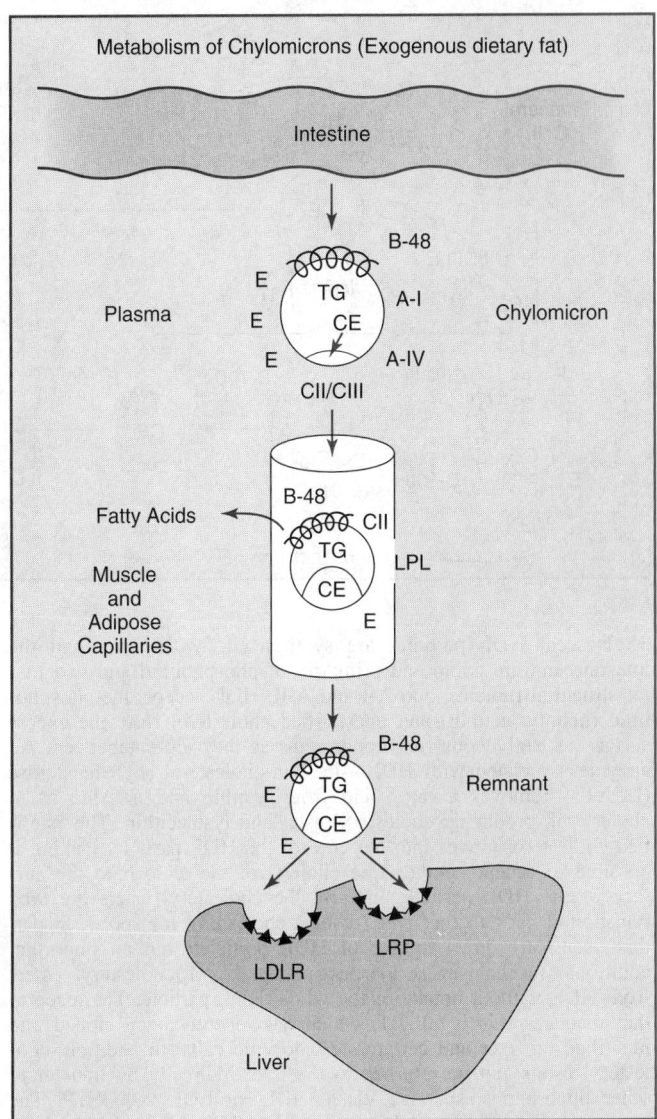

FIGURE 206–2 ■ Metabolism of chylomicrons (exogenous dietary fat). In the intestine, triglyceride (TG) and small amounts of cholesteryl esters (CE) are packaged with apo B-48, apo A-I, and apo A-IV and released into lymph. The chylomicron particle acquires apo E and apo C-II/C-III in lymph and plasma. In capillary beds, TG is hydrolyzed by lipoprotein lipase (LPL). The remnant particle is then removed primarily by liver, mediated by binding to LRP and LDLR as well as to surface proteoglycans. Chylomicron remnants are not a source of LDL.

relatively cholesteryl-ester-rich. In part, this cholesterol comes from dietary sources, but a significant amount is also transferred into the particle from HDL particles mediated by cholesterol ester transfer protein (CETP). In addition, because it is still a relatively large particle, it contains many copies of apo E on its surface, and it is believed that this represents the ligand that leads to rapid interaction with remnant receptors in the liver and efficient removal from the circulation. The exact pathway for uptake of chylomicron remnants by the liver is still being investigated but probably includes the LRP, the LDL receptor itself, as well as cell-surface glycosaminoglycans that can also bind apo E. Apo E is central to the process of remnant removal, just as it is for IDL uptake. Individuals who either lack apo E or synthesize only apo E isoforms that bind poorly to receptors can accumulate chylomicron remnants in plasma.

HDL-CONTAINING LIPOPROTEINS. When chylomicrons and VLDL particles are hydrolyzed by LPL to release fatty acids for peripheral use, their surface coat of unesterified cholesterol, phospholipid, and various apoproteins forms excess surface material that must be disposed of. HDL plays a principal role in this by acting as an acceptor or "sink" for this excess surface material (Fig. 206–

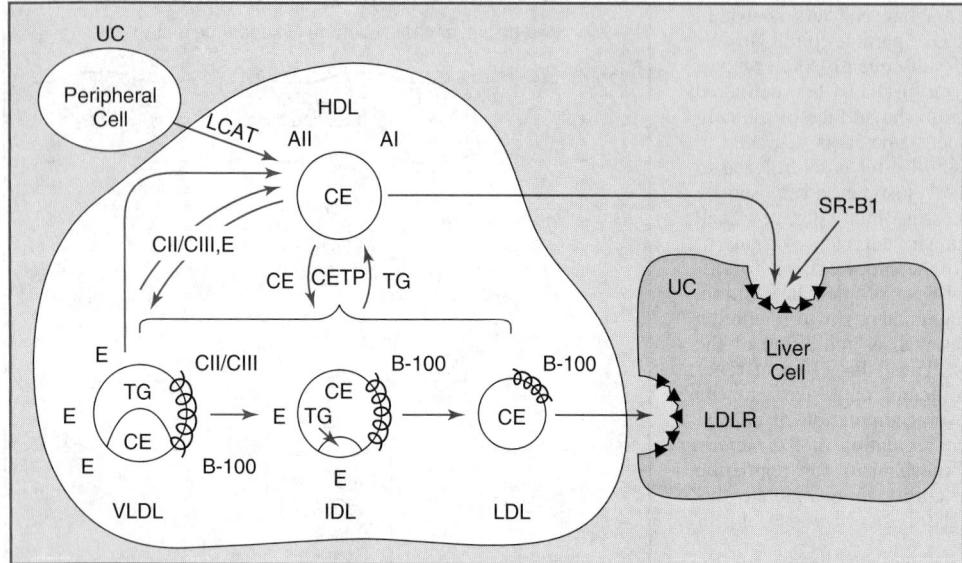

FIGURE 206–3 ■ Interactions of high-density lipoproteins (HDL) and apo B–containing lipoproteins. HDL has particles containing apo A-I and particles containing apo A-I, A-II. Nascent HDL, made primarily by liver and intestine, accepts unesterified cholesterol (UC) from VLDL and from membranes of cells. The enzyme lecithin-cholesterol-acyltransferase (LCAT), which is associated with HDL, esterifies the cholesterol to form cholesteryl esters (CE), which then form the core of the HDL. The enzyme cholesterol ester transfer protein (CETP) transfers CE from HDL into apo B–containing lipoproteins in exchange for TG. HDL also serves as a "sink" for apoproteins C-II/C-III and E, which shuttle back and forth from the HDL to VLDL and IDL. HDL also returns CE to the liver by binding to SR-B1, leading to selective delivery of CE into liver cells.

3). Nascent HDL particles are synthesized by the liver and the intestine and are composed primarily of phospholipid and two major structural proteins, apo A-I and A-II. HDL accepts the phospholipid (mainly lecithin) and unesterified cholesterol from the excess surface of triglyceride-rich lipoproteins as they are catabolized. An enzyme associated with HDL—lecithin-cholesterol acyl transferase (LCAT)—removes a fatty acid from lecithin and transfers it to cholesterol, producing cholesteryl ester and lysolecithin. The esterified cholesterol moves into the core of the HDL particle, making it possible to accept another free cholesterol molecule onto the surface of the HDL particle. In turn, the cholesteryl esters are then transported back to the liver (reverse cholesterol transport). In part this occurs by direct uptake of HDL particles, but an important additional mechanism is a selective uptake of cholesteryl esters from HDL without uptake of the whole HDL particle. The receptor that mediates this is SR-B1, which has recently been cloned and identified on liver and certain steroidogenic cells, In addition, cholesteryl esters can be returned to the liver indirectly by transfer to other lipoproteins, such as VLDL, IDL, or LDL via CETP. The uptake of these cholesteryl-ester–enriched lipoproteins by the liver results in net removal from plasma of cholesteryl esters. This HDL/LCAT/CETP system plays a pivotal role in removing excess cellular cholesterol, facilitating its transfer back to the liver for excretion. The removal of excess cholesterol from arterial wall cells by such a mechanism could play a crucial role in minimizing cholesterol accumulation in the artery wall and thus inhibiting atherogenesis (see Chapter 58). Thus, HDL may be viewed as playing a vital role in transporting excess cholesterol from extrahepatic tissues back to the liver where it is excreted in the bile. In addition to their role in reverse cholesterol transport, HDL may also serve as the reservoir for apoproteins such as C-II, C-III, and E as they shuttle back and forth from triglyceride-rich lipoproteins while being catabolized.

BILE ACID PRODUCTION (SEE CHAPTER 146). Nearly all cells of the body have the capacity to synthesize cholesterol de novo, but none has the ability to degrade it completely. However, hepatocytes have the capacity to convert cholesterol into bile acids, which can then be secreted into the bile along with free cholesterol and phospholipids. Nearly 95% of secreted bile acids are reabsorbed in the distal ileum and enter the enterohepatic circulation; that is, they are taken up by the liver and recycled. Cholesterol delivered to the liver in the form of chylomicrons or other lipoproteins could be recycled and secreted as VLDL or converted to bile acids for secretion into the bile.

DISORDERS OF LIPOPROTEIN METABOLISM

Disorders of lipoprotein metabolism can lead to hypercholesterolemia or hypertriglyceridemia or both. Although these disorders appear to be common in the general population, the molecular events responsible for them are only currently being elucidated. For purposes of organization the hyperlipoproteinemias are grouped into disorders leading primarily to hypercholesterolemia (due to elevations of LDL levels) or to hypertriglyceridemia (due to elevations of VLDL or chylomicrons) or to combined elevations of both triglycerides and cholesterol. Several monogenic disorders have been defined that lead to each type of hyperlipidemia, but for many cases the etiology is likely to be polygenic. These disorders affect plasma lipoprotein levels by overproduction of lipoproteins and/or decreased clearance.

Hyperlipoproteinemia Resulting Primarily in Hypercholesterolemia

FAMILIAL HYPERCHOLESTEROLEMIA AND FAMILIAL DEFECTIVE APOLIPOPROTEIN B. Familial hypercholesterolemia (FH) is a common autosomal dominant disorder due to absence of or defective LDL receptors resulting in decreased capacity to remove plasma LDL. Familial defective apolipoprotein B is an autosomal dominant disorder in which the ligand binding region of apo B is defective, also leading to delayed plasma LDL clearance. In both disorders LDL-cholesterol levels are strikingly increased, frequently associated with characteristic xanthomas in the Achilles tendons, the patellar tendons, the extensor tendons of the hands, and by the presence of xanthelasma. It is frequently associated with early coronary artery disease (CAD). In heterozygous FH, estimated to be present in 1 in 500 individuals, there is one abnormal allele for the LDL receptor. The abnormal allele may produce no receptors or produce abnormal LDL receptors that are largely nonfunctional. In the heterozygote, a 50% decrease exists in hepatic LDL receptor number, a corresponding decrease in LDL catabolism, and an approximately twofold to threefold increase in plasma LDL levels. In the rare homozygous FH patient (only 1 in 1 million people) almost no functional LDL receptors are found, and plasma LDL levels may be increased 6-fold to 10-fold. In this situation, LDL can be removed from plasma only by low-affinity pathways. In familial defective apolipoprotein B, the ligand-binding domain of apo B is defective because of a missense mutation at amino acid 3500. This mutation leads to impaired binding of the LDL to the LDL receptor and clinical consequences similar to those seen in FH. It is likely that other mutations in apo B affecting its ability to bind to the LDL receptor also occur.

These disorders are characterized by greatly elevated concentrations of LDL cholesterol. If untreated, patients with FH have premature CAD, as well as other clinical manifestations of atherosclerosis (see Chapter 58). Peripheral vascular disease and cerebral vascular disease are also increased, although not as much as CAD. Tendon xanthomas are seen only in FH and in patients with familial defective apo B. Bilateral, irregular, firm and nodular thickenings in the Achilles tendons or extensor tendons of the hands or knees are usually present and can be so large as to interfere with normal functions, such as wearing shoes. Xanthelasma typically occurs in this setting, and corneal arcus is frequently seen as well, although this latter entity occurs in other lipoprotein disorders and can be found in elderly, normolipidemic patients as well.

Plasma cholesterol levels in heterozygous FH exceed the upper 1% of levels seen in the general population and are generally in the range of 300 to 500 mg/dL. In rare patients, homozygous for FH, plasma cholesterol levels can exceed 800 to 1000 mg/dL. Triglyceride levels are usually normal, but in 10% of subjects may be mildly elevated. Patients with defective remnant removal or with marked chylomicronemia may also have markedly elevated cholesterol levels, but they will have very high triglyceride levels as well. In addition, their plasma will appear turbid or creamy, in contrast to plasma in FH patients, which is always clear.

Because myocardial infarction can occur in men with heterozygous FH when they are in their early 40s, these subjects deserve vigorous therapy to lower LDL levels and to decrease other risk factors as well. Women with FH also have an accelerated risk for CAD, although the absolute risk is less than that of men and the CAD occurs at a later age. For both men and women the risk of atherosclerosis is greatly accelerated by the presence of other risk factors such as smoking, hypertension, diabetes, low HDL-cholesterol levels, and high Lp(a) levels. A diet low in saturated fat and cholesterol should be initiated in all affected individuals with this disorder, although frequently only modest reductions in LDL levels occur. Effective therapy can be achieved using HMG-CoA reductase inhibitors, a class of compounds termed *statins,* as first-line therapy because they effectively lower LDL-cholesterol levels by 20 to 45% and infrequently have side effects. When these statins are combined with a bile acid–binding resin, decreases of LDL levels by 50 to 60% or greater can frequently be achieved. In some individuals, triple therapy with a statin, a bile acid–binding resin, and niacin may be necessary to normalize LDL levels. Unfortunately, subjects homozygous for FH will usually not respond to these measures, which work in large part by increasing the LDL receptor activity. For such individuals, heroic measures are required, such as repeated plasmapheresis or a more specialized procedure, termed *LDL apheresis,* in which apo B–containing lipoproteins are removed from blood as it passes extracorporeally through a column that binds apo B. In selected individuals, liver transplantation has been used. In the future it is hoped that gene therapy may lead to correction of the primary genetic defect.

POLYGENIC HYPERCHOLESTEROLEMIA. Irrespective of one's definition of hypercholesterolemia, it is clear that a large number of individuals in the general population have elevated LDL-cholesterol levels (see Table 206–4). If one uses the conventional definition that the top 5% of the general population have hypercholesterolemia, then on average only 1 of 25 of such hypercholesterolemic individuals will have FH, and only 2 will have familial combined hyperlipidemia (described later). The large majority have hypercholesterolemia due to a complex interaction of multiple genetic factors and environmental factors, that is, polygenic hypercholesterolemia. The cause of the hypercholesterolemia is unknown, but it is likely, due to the convergence of several subtle alterations that affect regulation of LDL levels. Differences may exist in dietary responsiveness to cholesterol and saturated fat, differences in regulation of cholesterol and/or bile acid biosynthesis, and/or differences in regulation of LDL receptor activity and in the secretion and intravascular catabolism of apo B–containing lipoproteins.

FAMILIAL HYPERALPHALIPOPROTEINEMIA. Occasionally, patients are seen who have mildly elevated total cholesterol levels due to elevated HDL-cholesterol. They usually have normal levels of LDL and VLDL. In these individuals the elevated HDL-cholesterol level is genetic, and in some families it is inherited as an autosomal dominant trait. In other families the etiology appears to be polygenic. High HDL levels can also be seen with chronic alcoholism, in response to estrogen administration, and after exposure to chlorinated hydrocarbon pesticides. In some families a genetic deficiency of CETP is associated with strikingly elevated HDL-cholesterol levels, especially in Japanese populations. Individuals with hyperalphalipoproteinemia do not have any unusual clinical features, and they have been reported to have slightly increased longevity because of a decreased incidence of CAD.

Hyperlipoproteinemias Resulting Primarily in Hypertriglyceridemia

LIPOPROTEIN LIPASE DEFICIENCY AND APO C-II DEFICIENCY. LPL deficiency is a rare autosomal recessive trait that is

characterized by the absence of active LPL in all tissues, leading to massive hypertriglyceridemia from birth and the clinical consequences of eruptive xanthoma and episodes of pancreatitis. This same clinical syndrome may also occur with deficiency of apo C-II, an obligatory activator of LPL, although clinical manifestations tend to occur later in life.

In infants and young children with LPL deficiency, the hypertriglyceridemia results primarily from chylomicron accumulation, whereas impairment of VLDL triglyceride removal becomes more important in later life. Homozygosity for LPL deficiency or for apo C-II deficiency is necessary for this disorder to occur. Heterozygosity for LPL deficiency may lead to moderate hypertriglyceridemia and may be one factor in the etiology of familial combined hyperlipidemia. Infants with homozygous LPL deficiency have massive hypertriglyceridemia and grossly lipemic serum. They frequently fail to thrive and have severe abdominal pain and pancreatitis as a consequence of their marked hyperchylomicronemia. Eruptive xanthomas can occur on the extensor surfaces, notably on the elbows, knees, back, and buttocks, but can occur elsewhere, and when seen are pathognomonic for chylomicronemia. Hepatomegaly is frequent, as is splenomegaly, which occurs because of the accumulation of lipid-laden foam cells. LPL activity can be measured by assaying plasma after injection of heparin, which releases LPL into plasma. Apo C-II levels can be assayed by immunoassay. The clinical manifestations will rapidly disappear with elimination of fat from the diet, which leads to elimination of the chylomicronemia. With effective fat restriction, plasma triglyceride levels can usually be maintained between 500 and 800 mg/dL or lower; and at this level, episodes of eruptive xanthoma, abdominal pain, and pancreatitis can usually be avoided. Substances that increase endogenous VLDL output, such as alcohol and glucocorticoids, must be avoided. With effective attention to diet, individuals can grow and easily reach adulthood without difficulty. There is no indication that any increased risk for atherosclerosis exists in this disorder.

FAMILIAL HYPERTRIGLYCERIDEMIA. Individuals with this condition have marked hypertriglyceridemia, normal to low LDL levels, and marked decreases in HDL-cholesterol levels. When studied in detail, the number of VLDL particles is relatively normal, but they are triglyceride enriched. LPL-related triglyceride removal and remnant removal appears to be normal. HDL particle number is also relatively normal, but the triglyceride content in the HDL, which is normally very low, is considerably increased at the expense of cholesterol. The underlying defect in this disorder is postulated to be enhanced hepatic triglyceride synthesis. This disorder has been defined as an autosomal dominant trait that is quite common. There is some controversy about the association of this disorder with CAD. These patients are usually detected only because of routine lipid screening, or occasionally as a result of complications of marked hypertriglyceridemia. They do not have xanthomas unless there is chylomicronemia. Affected individuals usually have hypertriglyceridemia in adulthood, and they appear to be unusually sensitive to factors that are known to be associated with hypertriglyceridemia, such as diabetes, obesity, excess alcohol consumption, or use of estrogen, diuretics, glucocorticoids, or β-adrenergic blockers, which can greatly exaggerate the degree of hypertriglyceridemia and even precipitate the chylomicronemia syndrome. Although the reasoning is somewhat circular, most experts would not treat individuals with isolated hypertriglyceridemia, (e.g., triglyceride levels of 250 to 500 mg/dL), if they come from families without evidence of increased atherosclerosis.

Hyperlipoproteinemias Resulting in Mixed or Combined Hyperlipidemia

DYSBETALIPOPROTEINEMIA. Dysbetalipoproteinemia, also known as broad-beta or type III hyperlipoproteinemia, is a condition in which there is abnormal accumulation of cholesterol-rich IDL-type particles, commonly termed β-VLDL. This disorder is due to interaction of (1) an autosomal recessive defect in apo E that leads to abnormal remnant catabolism and (2) an independent aggravating environmental factor (e.g., obesity, diabetes, pregnancy) or genetic factor (FCH) leading to overproduction of apo B–containing lipoproteins. The combination of these two factors leads to accumulation of IDL-like particles (resulting from impaired VLDL catabolism) and remnants (resulting from impaired chylomicron metabolism) that lead to xanthomas, peripheral vascular disease, and CAD.

There are three major alleles for apo E, differing from each other by a single amino acid substitution at one or two sites. These are named E_2, E_3, and E_4. An individual can be homozygous for any of these alleles, or heterozygous for any combination. The apo E encoded by the E_2 allele has sharply reduced ability to bind to lipoprotein receptors. Individuals homozygous for this allele (i.e., E_2/E_2 homozygotes), who compose about 2% of the population, have a relative defect in IDL and remnant catabolism. This can lead to relative accumulation in plasma of cholesteryl-ester–rich IDL and chylomicron remnant particles (β-VLDL) and corresponding decrease in LDL levels because of defective conversion of VLDL to LDL (see Fig. 206–1). Yet, in the absence of aggravating factors, total plasma cholesterol levels are actually low in such individuals and triglyceride levels are normal. However, in an estimated 1 in 100 individuals with E_2/E_2 homozygosity, there is also an associated condition leading to overproduction of VLDL. This combination results in the absolute accumulation of β-VLDL particles, which are atherogenic when present in excess. This is expressed as marked hypertriglyceridemia and hypercholesterolemia. Normally, VLDL particles have "pre-β" mobility on agarose gel electrophoresis, but the VLDL remnants in dysbetalipoproteinemia are much closer to LDL in composition and therefore have "β" mobility ("β-VLDL"). Hence, the designation *dysbetalipoproteinemia*. Because individuals who are homozygous for the E_2 allele will have low levels of such qualitatively abnormal VLDL present in plasma even when total lipids are normal (or even low), some experts use the term dysbetalipoproteinemia to refer to the condition of homozygosity for E_2, whereas the term type III hyperlipoproteinemia or broad-beta syndrome is reserved for those individuals with associated hyperlipidemia. The type III hyperlipoproteinemia phenotype can also be caused by total absence of apo E, which has been observed in rare families.

When overproduction of VLDL occurs, or when there is delayed clearance, marked hyperlipidemia appears, and this disorder may present as premature clinical atherosclerosis with peripheral vascular disease and/or CAD. The presence of hypothyroidism has been noted frequently in individuals with clinical symptoms. These patients frequently have highly characteristic planar xanthomas in the creases of the palms as well as tuberous or tuberoeruptive xanthomas on the elbows or knees that are virtually diagnostic for this disorder. Occasionally these manifestations can be seen with obstructive liver disease. Although the apo E abnormality is present from birth, it is unusual to see hyperlipidemia in a male younger than age 30 and in a female before menopause. The presence of hypertriglyceridemia accompanied by unusual degrees of hypercholesterolemia when associated with palmar or tuberous xanthomas is highly suggestive of this disorder. Liver disease and hypothyroidism need to be excluded. Electrophoresis of a VLDL fraction of plasma will reveal particles of β mobility, rather than the typical pre-β mobility. The E_2 isoforms can be identified by isoelectric focusing in specialty laboratories, and genotyping is also available. The concentration of LDL is typically low even in hyperlipidemic patients, and a normal or elevated LDL level should make one consider an alternative diagnosis. HDL levels are normal or slightly decreased, depending on the degree of hypertriglyceridemia.

In many E_2/E_2 adults with clinical manifestations of hyperlipidemia, there is associated obesity, and weight reduction is of primary importance. In postmenopausal women, low-dose estrogen replacement frequently normalizes the abnormal lipoprotein profile and corrects the hyperlipidemia. All patients should be checked for mild degrees of hypothyroidism using sensitive thyroid-stimulating hormone (TSH) assays; if hypothyroidism is present, treatment may frequently completely normalize the lipoprotein profile. Gemfibrozil is frequently effective in decreasing lipid levels in these individuals; high-dose nicotinic acid may also be useful. Use of an HMG-CoA reductase inhibitor has been found to be quite successful in reducing the hypercholesterolemia and, when combined with low-dose gemfibrozil, has frequently normalized triglyceride levels in severe cases.

FAMILIAL COMBINED HYPERLIPIDEMIA. Among patients with myocardial infarction, a significant number have an apparently dominantly inherited pattern of hyperlipoproteinemia that is ex-

pressed by a variable lipoprotein phenotype. Thus, individuals may have increased VLDL or LDL levels or both. Some first-degree relatives have elevated VLDL levels, some have elevated LDL, and some have both. This entity appears to be monogenic and inherited in an autosomal dominant manner and has been termed familial combined hyperlipidemia (FCH) or familial multiple lipoprotein-type hyperlipidemia. The lipoprotein phenotype is not stable over time. A person can have VLDL elevations noted on one visit but marked increases in LDL, or both VLDL, and LDL, at another visit. Although there remains much uncertainty about classification of this disorder, all clinicians seeing patients with premature CAD recognize the frequency of this pattern. A characteristic of this disorder is increased accumulation of small LDL particles, which are cholesterol depleted. Thus, patients may have a relatively normal "LDL cholesterol" level, yet the number of LDL particles is increased and therefore the LDL–apo B level is increased. Some investigators have termed this condition familial hyper*apo*betalipoproteinemia. Most evidence suggests that the underlying defect is increased hepatic secretion of VLDL. The VLDL appear to be smaller than normal, with less triglyceride per particle. Undoubtedly this disorder represents several different genetic traits interacting with the basic defect–overproduction of VLDL. For example, overproduction of VLDL may become manifested primarily as elevations in VLDL levels if a relative or absolute defect in VLDL catabolism occurs in addition, as for example, with relative deficiency in LPL activity. Recently, a number of cases of heterozygous LPL deficiency have been found in association with this phenotype. Conversely, in the face of appropriate VLDL and IDL catabolism, LDL may accumulate because of the increased rate of generation of LDL and/or functional disturbances in LDL catabolic mechanisms. These individuals also typically have low levels of HDL with decreases in both HDL-cholesterol and apo A-I.

This phenotype is associated with a clinical constellation that includes mild abdominal obesity, insulin resistance, mild hypertension, elevated VLDL levels, the presence of an excess number of small dense LDL, and decreased HDL. This syndrome has been referred to as the insulin-resistance syndrome or syndrome X (see Chapter 242). This disorder is more typically seen in men and is associated with a strikingly high rate of premature CAD. The effect of other risk factors appears to be greatly exaggerated in these individuals, and a history of smoking is frequently found in those with early CAD. Patients do not have any characteristic xanthomas, and the diagnosis is made by a characteristic family history that is unusually positive for early CAD, by documentation of the variable lipoprotein phenotype, and, if possible, by lipoprotein phenotyping of first-degree relatives. Women may also be affected by this phenotype, although the clinical manifestations of CAD appear to be expressed later in life. Because this disorder is associated with a high risk of premature CAD, vigorous efforts should be made to lower lipoprotein levels of affected individuals. Nicotinic acid may be quite efficacious in some individuals in lowering VLDL and raising HDL levels. Other regimens include the use of an HMG-CoA reductase inhibitor alone or in combination with niacin or fibrates, such as gemfibrozil, although use of these combinations poses a small but increased risk of myositis (see later). The use of gemfibrozil alone to lower VLDL levels will often be highly effective but is almost always associated with significant rises in LDL.

OTHER FORMS OF HYPERTRIGLYCERIDEMIA. Mild hypertriglyceridemia is one of the most commonly encountered hyperlipidemias. Although many patients with hypertriglyceridemia will fit into one of the categories noted earlier, there are many other patients with triglyceride levels of 400 to 2000 mg/dL who do not seem to fall into any of those categories. They may have a family history of hypertriglyceridemia and/or quite commonly have one of the secondary forms of hypertriglyceridemia, such as that due to excess alcohol use or diabetes mellitus. Frequently, treating the underlying cause will ameliorate the hypertriglyceridemia, but often a milder form remains, probably indicative of an underlying as yet undefined genetic defect.

ACQUIRED DISORDERS OF LIPOPROTEIN METABOLISM

Many medical conditions are associated with mild or even severe hyperlipidemia in the absence of underlying genetic hyperlipoproteinemia. With underlying genetic hyperlipidemia, acquired disor-

Hypercholesterolemia
Nephrotic syndrome
Hypothyroidism
Dysgammaglobulinemia
Acute intermittent porphyria
Obstructive liver disease
Combined Hyperlipidemia
Nephrotic syndrome
Hypothyroidism
Glucocorticoid excess/Cushing's disease
Diuretics
Uncontrolled diabetes
Hypertriglyceridemia
Diabetes mellitus
Uremia
Sepsis
Obesity
Systemic lupus erythematosus
Dysgammaglobulinemia
Glycogen storage disease, type I
Lipodystrophy
Drugs
　Alcohol
　Estrogens
　β-Adrenergic blocking agents
　Isotretinoin (13-*cis*-retinoic acid)

ders can lead to greatly exaggerated effects on lipoprotein levels. Table 206–3 lists disorders commonly associated with changes in lipoprotein levels.

DIABETES MELLITUS (SEE CHAPTER 242). Persons with untreated insulin-dependent diabetes, as well as uncontrolled non-insulin-dependent diabetes, frequently have hypertriglyceridemia, low HDL levels, and associated small dense LDL particles. These individuals appear to have low adipose tissue or muscle LPL activity that leads to relative impairment in VLDL clearance. Although LDL levels are not absolutely elevated in these individuals as a rule, for the degree of hypertriglyceridemia, the LDL levels are higher than expected. In part, this may be due to non-enzymatic glycosylation of the LDL particle caused by hyperglycemia as well as by down-regulation of LDL receptors because of insulin lack.

CHRONIC UREMIA AND DIALYSIS (SEE CHAPTER 105). Many individuals with chronic uremia have elevated VLDL levels with associated hypertriglyceridemia and low HDL-cholesterol levels. This condition persists even after initiation of maintenance hemodialysis or peritoneal dialysis. These lipoprotein abnormalities are related to defects in LPL-mediated triglyceride removal and/or associated overproduction.

ALCOHOL AND OTHER DRUGS. Among the many associated factors that cause mild degrees of hypertriglyceridemia, alcohol consumption is probably the most common; it increases triglyceride levels in most individuals. This occurs because both fatty acid synthesis and VLDL output are stimulated, and LPL activity is inhibited. In individuals with normal baseline VLDL levels this is not usually a problem, but in those in whom there is excess VLDL secretion or some other additional basis for impairment in VLDL clearance, marked hypertriglyceridemia ensues with alcohol use. Diuretic agents and β-adrenergic blocking agents are also frequently associated with mild increases in triglyceride levels in patients with no underlying abnormality in lipoprotein metabolism but with quite marked increases in those with underlying hypertriglyceridemia. In individuals with genetic hypertriglyceridemia or FCH, estrogen use may also lead to marked increases in VLDL levels. Hypertriglyceridemia occurs in 25% of people given isotretinoin (13-*cis*-retinoic acid) for cystic acne.

HYPOTHYROIDISM (SEE CHAPTER 239). Thyroid hormone is crucial in many steps of lipoprotein metabolism. LDL receptor activity is particularly sensitive to thyroxine levels, and in hypothyroidism LDL levels are elevated because of down-regulation of LDL receptor number. In addition, LPL activity is low, leading to elevated VLDL levels and even, rarely, chylomicronemia, especially in subjects with dysbetalipoproteinemia.

NEPHROTIC SYNDROME (SEE CHAPTER 106). With massive proteinuria and with hypoalbuminemia, a compensatory increase occurs in overall hepatic protein synthesis, and in particular there is

marked increase in VLDL output. An associated defect in VLDL catabolism is also seen, in part due to depressed LPL activity.

HYPERLIPOPROTEINEMIA AND ATHEROSCLEROSIS

The etiology of atherosclerosis is multifactorial; a more general discussion of its pathogenesis can be found in Chapter 58. However, the cause-and-effect relationship between hypercholesterolemia and atherosclerosis has been proved in a large number of animal model studies and by large randomized, double-blind clinical intervention trials. Reducing plasma LDL-cholesterol levels sharply reduces the risk of subsequent clinical CAD in both patients with pre-existing CAD and in patients free of CAD at the beginning of the study. In studies extending over 5 to 7 years, morbidity and mortality from new coronary events have been reduced by as much as 30 to 40%. A statistically significant decrease in *total* mortality was also seen in two large studies, the Scandinavian Simvastatin Survival Study and the West of Scotland Coronary Prevention Study. Angiographic studies have documented that intensive cholesterol-lowering regimens slow progression of coronary lesions: in some cases there has even been significant regression of lesions. Plasma triglyceride levels also correlate very significantly with risk of CAD, but the interpretation of this correlation is less clear, because elevation of triglyceride levels is frequently associated with other factors that may be more immediately relevant to the increase in CAD risk.

CHYLOMICRONS AND VLDL. Almost no evidence exists that chylomicrons are proatherogenic, and they are probably too large to penetrate into the artery. VLDL may also be too large, but CAD risk correlates with hypertriglyceridemia almost as well as it does with hypercholesterolemia in the fasting state and most of the triglycerides in plasma are carried in VLDL. This correlation may be explained by the frequent association of hypertriglyceridemia with obesity, low HDL levels, small, dense LDL, and diabetes mellitus. More likely is the possibility that the catabolic products of VLDL, the IDL, are atherogenic. Indeed, in hyperlipidemic patients with dysbetalipoproteinemia, the lipoprotein that accumulates is a type of IDL—so-called β-VLDL. Such patients are at increased risk of atherosclerosis and its complications. Moreover, the lipoprotein class that accumulates in experimental animals fed a high-fat, high-cholesterol diet is predominantly the same sort of β-VLDL.

LDL. There is no doubt about the atherogenicity of LDL. Patients with FH have strikingly premature atherosclerosis. However, in addition to greatly increased LDL levels, they also have some increase in IDL levels. Yet patients with a mutation of apo B that reduces its affinity for the LDL receptor accumulate *only* LDL, and their risk of premature CAD at any given plasma cholesterol level appears to be just as great as that of patients with LDL receptor deficiency. Increasing evidence suggests that oxidative modification of LDL within the artery is important, if not obligatory, for mediating the atherogenicity of LDL. Much evidence has been obtained that oxidized LDL is formed in the artery wall. Products of oxidized LDL may contribute to atherogenesis by many mechanisms, including attracting monocytes to the lesion and facilitating their conversion into macrophages. In turn, macrophages express scavenger receptors that take up oxidized LDL, leading to foam cells and the fatty streak lesion. In addition, products of oxidized LDL are toxic, producing endothelial damage and initiation of thrombosis. Treatment with antioxidants has been shown to slow the progress of atherosclerosis in several animal models, but similar data are not yet available in humans.

HDL. A wealth of epidemiologic evidence establishes that high plasma HDL levels are associated with a lower risk of CAD. Until recently it was not certain whether the protective effect of a high HDL level was referable to a direct effect of the HDL or whether it represented a "marker" for some other factor. Studies in transgenic mice have now shown that increasing HDL reduces the susceptibility of these mice to atherosclerosis. It is widely believed that HDL protects against atherosclerosis by facilitating reverse cholesterol transport, that is, the ability of HDL to accept excess cholesterol from tissues and return it to the liver either directly or via other lipoproteins, but this has not been explicitly proved.

Lp(a). An increased risk for CAD has been found in many populations in association with increased levels of Lp(a), in particular when elevated LDL levels are also present. However. Lp(a) appears to be an independent risk factor. Lp(a) is an LDL particle to which an additional large protein, termed apo (a), is attached via a disulfide bond. There are many different allelic forms of apo (a) protein, varying widely in molecular size and determined in large part by genetic factors. Apo (a) has high homology to plasminogen but lacks the catalytically active site. Speculation has centered on the possibility that it interferes with plasminogen binding to its receptors and thus inhibits plasmin formation and thrombolysis. Alternatively, Lp(a) may have increased binding to the extracellular matrix of the artery, leading to greater deposition of the associated LDL. To date, no therapy has been found to effectively lower elevated Lp(a) levels, although niacin may lower it modestly.

PRACTICAL MANAGEMENT OF HYPERLIPIDEMIA

TREATMENT OF HYPERCHOLESTEROLEMIA. Irrespective of the cause of elevated LDL levels, patients are usually managed similarly. In almost all cases, lowering LDL levels is achieved first by dietary intervention and then, if necessary, by adding drug therapy. Because the LDL receptor plays such an important role in regulating plasma LDL levels, therapy is aimed at achieving maximal expression of hepatic LDL receptor activity. Dietary cholesterol and saturated fat both lead to suppression of hepatic LDL receptor activity, and therefore reduction of these dietary components leads to up-regulation of hepatic LDL receptors and lowered plasma cholesterol levels. Individuals heterozygous for FH are more restricted in their response, and generally even stringent diets lower their LDL levels by no more than 5 to 10% below baseline levels. However, all individuals should be instructed in these diets, because some are unusually responsive.

Regulation of hepatic LDL receptor activity also appears to underlie mechanisms by which many commonly used hyperlipidemic drugs affect plasma cholesterol levels. As shown in Figure 206–4, the hepatocyte is the primary site of cholesterol synthesis. The cholesterol made by this cell is either excreted into plasma in the form of VLDL or is converted into bile acids, which are released into the intestine in response to meals. Normally, more than 95% of bile acids are reabsorbed and transported to the liver through the enterohepatic circulation and recycled through the liver up to six to seven times per day. Bile acid–binding resins work by binding bile acids in the intestine and promoting their subsequent loss in the stool. This prevents reabsorption and results in depletion of hepatic bile acid pools. In response, the hepatocyte actually increases cholesterol (and triglyceride) synthesis, as well as compensatory bile acid synthesis to replete the depleted bile acid pool. Despite this enhanced cholesterol synthesis, it is not sufficient to compensate for depletion of some crucial intracellular sterol pool, and the

hepatocyte responds by also increasing LDL receptor expression. In turn, this directly removes LDL particles (or their precursors) from circulation. In this way, a non-systemic agent leads to enhanced removal of plasma LDL particles and lowered plasma cholesterol levels. Very likely the soluble dietary fibers, such as oat bran, also lower plasma cholesterol by binding bile acids in a similar manner. For many individuals, this degree of plasma cholesterol lowering is sufficient. However, in others the enhanced cholesterol (and triglyceride) synthesis leads to enhanced VLDL synthesis and release, and in effect, negates in part the cholesterol-lowering effect. In fact, many patients develop a transient or even permanent increase of plasma triglycerides (VLDL) in response to bile sequestrant therapy, even as LDL levels are lowered. This enhanced production of VLDL leads to generation of more LDL, which offsets in part the enhanced LDL removal, leading to suboptimal lowering of LDL levels. For this reason, a second agent, in combination with a bile sequestrant, is frequently used and leads to synergistic lowering of LDL levels. For example, nicotinic acid, which effectively inhibits release of lipoproteins from the liver, is quite effective when combined with a bile acid–binding resin. Even more effective is the use of an HMG-CoA reductase inhibitor. This class of drugs, which have been termed *statins,* directly inhibits cholesterol biosynthesis and as a result not only inhibits the production of new lipoproteins but also, by apparently depleting still further specific hepatic sterol pools, leads to maximal expression of hepatic LDL receptor activity (see Fig. 206–4). Because of their ease of administration and relatively low incidence of side effects, they are widely used as the primary therapy to lower elevated LDL levels. This effect is greatly enhanced when used in combination with a bile acid–binding resin and can lower LDL levels by more than 50%. If these two drugs are combined with nicotinic acid as a third agent, LDL levels can be lowered by as much as 70% or more.

WHOM TO TREAT. The definition of hypercholesterolemia has been undergoing marked changes in recent years because it has become clear that "ideal" or "optimal" cholesterol levels are quite different from "normal" levels, which have been arbitrarily defined as values below the 90th or 95th percentile of the bell-shaped curve of the general population. The expert panel of the National Cholesterol Education Program (NCEP) has recommended specific desirable blood cholesterol levels for the population as a whole (Table 206–4). Many experts have argued that any plasma cholesterol level above 160 to 180 mg/dL is above *ideal* values, such as those found in the Japanese, for example, who have a low inci-

Table 206–4 ■ **BLOOD CHOLESTEROL LEVELS**

(mg/dL)	DESIRABLE	BORDERLINE	HIGH
Total blood cholesterol	<200	200–239 (borderline high)	>240
LDL	<130	130–159	>160

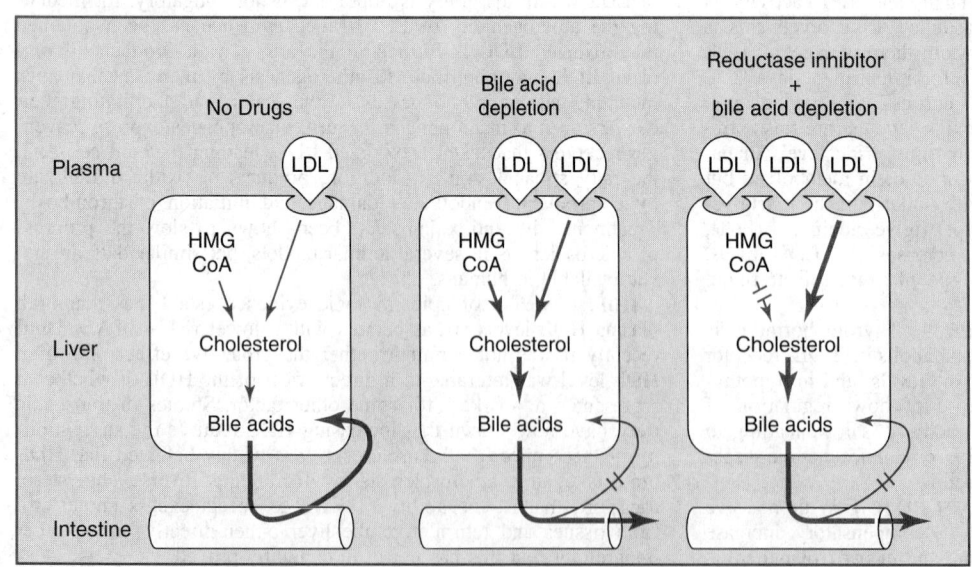

FIGURE 206–4 ■ Mechanisms by which a bile acid–binding resin and an HMG CoA-reductase inhibitor lower plasma LDL levels. (From Brown MS, Goldstein JL: A receptor-mediated pathway for cholesterol homeostasis. Science 232:34, 1986. Copyright 1986 by the American Association for the Advancement of Science.)

dence of CAD. Unfortunately the vast majority of people in the United States have plasma cholesterol levels that are far above this ideal. For this reason, there is an intensive ongoing effort to educate the general public as to appropriate dietary guidelines to lower plasma cholesterol levels.

It should be appreciated that these cutoff points are appropriate for the population as a whole, but assessment of appropriate cholesterol levels for any given patient must take into account the presence of other risk factors. Although many individuals with very high plasma cholesterol levels clearly are at increased risk for CAD (see Chapter 59), most patients who develop CAD actually have total and LDL cholesterol levels that would place them in the borderline or, not infrequently, even below the borderline category. Thus, individuals with hypertension, smoking history, obesity, or diabetes are clearly at increased risk at any given plasma cholesterol level. Individuals with low HDL levels (i.e., <35 mg/dL) are also at significantly increased risk. A strong family history of heart disease is highly predictive of those individuals who are at increased risk. Finally, for patients who have existing CAD and, in particular, for those who have already undergone coronary artery bypass graft or other types of intervention, the cholesterol levels listed in Table 206–4 are probably still too high. Achievement of ideal plasma cholesterol levels (i.e., 160 mg/dL) is probably more appropriate. Studies in experimental animals and data from clinical trials show that the greater the reduction in plasma cholesterol levels, the greater the clinical benefit achieved.

The NCEP has devised a protocol for screening and management of blood cholesterol in the general population. It is recommended that plasma total cholesterol levels should be measured in all adults older than age 20 at least once every 5 years. HDL-cholesterol should be measured at the same time whenever possible. These measurements may be made in the non-fasting state. In individuals free of CAD, total cholesterol levels are classified into desirable, borderline, and high levels. It should be appreciated that the cutoff point that defines high blood cholesterol, 240 mg/dL, is a value that represents the top 20th percentile of the U.S. adult population and corresponds to a value at which risk for CHD rises more steeply. Similarly, an HDL-cholesterol level less than 35 mg/dL is defined as low and represents an independent risk factor. For individuals with desirable blood cholesterol levels (<200 mg/dL) the level of HDL-cholesterol determines the appropriate follow-up. Those with HDL-cholesterol levels greater than 35 mg/dL are advised about dietary modification, physical activity, and other risk-reduction activities and to have repeat determinations of total cholesterol and HDL-cholesterol levels in 5 years. Those with HDL-cholesterol levels less than 35 mg/dL and/or those who have two or more risk factors should have a formal lipoprotein analysis in the fasting state. Among those potentially at risk are men who are older than age 45 years and women who are older than age 55 years or who are prematurely (post)menopausal and who are not taking estrogen. Other risk factors include a positive family history of premature CAD, history of smoking, hypertension, diabetes, obesity, and, as mentioned, an HDL-cholesterol level below 35 mg/dL. The lipoprotein analysis includes measurement of fasting levels of total cholesterol, total triglyceride, and HDL cholesterol. From these values, LDL cholesterol is calculated as follows:

LDL-cholesterol = Total cholesterol − HDL-cholesterol
− (triglycerides/5).

Further classification is based on LDL values: LDL-cholesterol levels less than 130 mg/dL are defined as desirable; those 130 to 159 mg/dL as borderline high-risk; and those greater than 160 mg/dL as high-risk LDL-cholesterol levels. Patients with desirable LDL-cholesterol levels can be provided education about general dietary habits and risk factor modification. Patients with borderline elevated levels and with fewer than two risk factors can similarly be given dietary instruction with re-evaluation annually. Patients with borderline LDL elevations and two or more risk factors should undergo thorough evaluation, receive dietary therapy, and be considered for drug therapy if they fail to respond. Finally, individuals with high-risk LDL-cholesterol levels, greater than 160 mg/dL, should have a thorough evaluation to rule out any secondary causes and the presence of a familial lipoprotein disorder and then should begin dietary therapy. Presently the American Heart Association step I or step II diets, which restrict dietary saturated fat and cholesterol, should be prescribed to all individuals with greater than desirable cholesterol levels. This diet is safe for a wide spectrum of individuals, from those as young as age 2 years to the elderly, and usually works best when followed by the whole family.

The NCEP guidelines suggest that all patients with existing CAD have a formal lipoprotein analysis. If LDL-cholesterol levels are less than 100 mg/dL, patients should receive individual instruction on diet and risk-factor reduction. If LDL-cholesterol levels are more than 100 mg/dL, patients should be instructed on an appropriate diet and be considered for drug therapy. Patients with diabetes should also be considered in this category as well. The therapeutic goal for treatment of hypercholesterolemia is listed in Table 206–5. The decision to initiate drug therapy for elevated LDL-cholesterol levels should be considered in most patients only after the individual has been on a diet for 3 to 6 months. In general, a young or middle-aged adult who has been on such a diet, yet continues to have LDL-cholesterol levels greater than 190 mg/dL is a candidate for drug therapy even in the absence of other risk factors. Individuals with existing CAD or those who have high LDL cholesterol levels of 160 to 190 mg/dL and other risk factors are also candidates for drug therapy, including an HMG-CoA reductase inhibitor, bile acid–binding resins, and nicotinic acid. In patients with existing CAD, diet and drug therapy may be initiated simultaneously.

The statin class of drugs, which are used most frequently as primary therapy, lower LDL levels by 25 to 45%. Combinations of a statin and a bile acid–binding resin are also highly efficacious, and LDL lowering of more than 50% can frequently be achieved. They have now been in use for more than 15 years with practically no serious side effects. A myositis-like picture has been rarely associated with their use, particularly when combined with nicotinic acid, gemfibrozil, or, rarely, with erythromycin and certain antifungal agents. This appears as muscle pain and is associated with increases in muscle creatine kinase. Rarely, frank rhabdomyolysis has occurred. This side effect has been seen particularly in transplant patients treated with cyclosporine. Abnormalities in liver function tests occur occasionally, but frequently when this occurs there is associated excess alcohol use. Creatine kinase levels should be measured before the start of statin therapy to obtain baseline levels, at bimonthly intervals during initial use of therapy, and semiannually after that.

TREATMENT OF MILD HYPERTRIGLYCERIDEMIA. The NCEP guidelines do not directly address the issue of hypertriglyceridemia. As noted earlier, the link between triglycerides and CAD is complex and may be explained by associations between high triglyceride and low HDL levels and atherogenic forms of LDL. Patients with milder degrees of hypertriglyceridemia should be treated initially with non-pharmacologic therapy. This should in-

Table 206–5 ▪ THERAPEUTIC GOAL FOR TREATMENT OF HYPERCHOLESTEROLEMIA

THERAPEUTIC GOAL LDL CHOLESTEROL (mg/dL)	PATIENT CATEGORIES
<130	Moderate risk for CAD
	Patients with no family history of CAD and no other CAD risk factors
	Young adults with familial hypercholesterolemia
	Adults with familial hypercholesterolemia and no other risk factors
<100	High risk for CAD
	With family history of CAD or two or more CAD risk factors
	Adult familial hypercholesterolemia patients with family history of CAD or one or more risk factors
	Individual with existing CAD
	Individual after CABG
	Individual with low HDL cholesterol and family history of CAD

LDL = low-density lipoprotein; HDL = high-density lipoprotein; CAD = coronary artery disease; CABG = coronary artery bypass graft surgery.

clude weight reduction in overweight patients, increased physical activity, and low-fat diets. Alcohol should be restricted. Gemfibrozil lowers VLDL levels, but frequently there is an associated rise in LDL levels. Niacin has been used to both decrease VLDL and increase HDL. Many experts now use a statin as initial therapy for treating patients with familial combined hyperlipidemia. VLDL levels are lowered, HDL levels increase, and there is no increase in LDL levels. In some patients a combination of a statin and niacin is used, and in others the combined use of gemfibrozil and a statin has been useful, but these combinations may increase slightly the risk of myositis.

RECOGNITION AND TREATMENT OF MARKED HYPERTRIGLYCERIDEMIA: THE CHYLOMICRONEMIA SYNDROME. Marked chylomicronemia with plasma triglyceride levels more than 1000 mg/dL is associated with a combination of signs and symptoms that has been termed the *chylomicronemia syndrome.* Prompt and effective therapy is indicated to prevent severe medical complications, including pancreatitis. This syndrome occurs whenever there is excess accumulation of chylomicrons. Rarely this occurs as a result of homozygous LPL deficiency, or apo C-II deficiency. More commonly this may be due to a combination of an inherited defect in a factor involved in triglyceride clearance (e.g., heterozygosity for LPL deficiency) and an acquired exacerbating problem (see Table 206–3). Uncontrolled diabetic ketoacidosis is a common cause.

Plasma triglyceride levels may become exceedingly high, with values well in excess of 20,000 mg/dL. For reasons that are not understood the clinical signs and symptoms do not necessarily correlate with the level of hypertriglyceridemia, and patients who have triglyceride levels as high as 20,000 mg/dL can be asymptomatic, whereas other individuals with triglyceride levels of 3000 mg/dL or lower may have abdominal pain and/or pancreatitis. Lipemia retinalis can often be observed, and eruptive xanthomas are also frequently seen. Patients may complain of paresthesias of the extremities, particularly on the dorsum of the hands and feet, and frequently have an erythematous flush on the face and chest. With marked hyperchylomicronemia, impairment of recent memory has been noted. Patients also may complain of symmetric arthralgia, although physical findings or joint involvement is not found. In diabetics, this syndrome may be associated with marked insulin resistance, marked hyperglycemia, and frequently diabetic ketoacidosis. Because of the marked hyperchylomicronemia, an increased proportion of the total blood volume is occupied by fat, and many routine laboratory tests will be invalid because fat is sampled as well as the water space. For example, hyponatremia is frequently seen in samples from hyperchylomicronemic subjects, but this is a "pseudo hyponatremia" that occurs because of inclusion of lipid in the aliquot of blood sampled, and lipid does not contain sodium. Simple removal of chylomicrons from plasma by a brief centrifugation step before laboratory tests can eliminate such artifacts. Frequently a false-negative test for amylase occurs in lipemic plasma, apparently due to an inhibitor of amylase activity.

The diagnosis is made by the presence of chylomicrons in fasting plasma, which will always appear milky. Plasma will usually appear turbid when plasma triglycerides are greater than 350 mg/dL, because of the excess accumulation of VLDL, and will appear grossly lipemic when triglycerides are greater than 1000 mg/dL. With extreme degrees of hypertriglyceridemia the whole blood takes on the appearance of cream of tomato soup, and plasma allowed to sit in a refrigerator overnight will develop a thick layer of chylomicrons on top. Because the major cause of hyperchylomicronemia is accumulation of dietary-induced fat, the treatment is absolute elimination of fat from the diet until triglyceride levels have fallen to a safe level. With associated pancreatitis, patients usually receive nothing orally; and in this setting plasma triglyceride levels will usually fall by 50% every 2 to 3 days. When refeeding begins, fat (of all kinds) must be totally avoided initially and then replaced very gradually.

RARE DISORDERS OF LIPOPROTEIN METABOLISM

There are a number of inherited disorders of lipoprotein metabolism that are rare but that have taught us a great deal about lipoprotein function. Patients with *hypobetalipoproteinemia* have mutations in one or both apo B alleles that lead to truncated apo B proteins. Because of defective synthesis and/or enhanced intravascular catabolism, there are markedly reduced levels of apo B-containing lipoproteins in plasma. Heterozygotes may have LDL-cholesterol levels less than or equal to 50 mg/dL, and rare compound heterozygotes may have LDL-cholesterol levels less than or equal to 5 mg/dL. Usually these patients are asymptomatic and long lived. Patients with the rare autosomal recessive disorder of *abetalipoproteinemia* have total inability to release apo B-48 from intestinal cells or apo B-100 from liver. As noted earlier, they have a normal apo B gene, but lack MTP, which is required for assembly of lipoproteins. Because they cannot make chylomicrons, they malabsorb fat and fat-soluble vitamins. They manifest ataxia, neuropathy, and retinitis pigmentosa and are responsive to high doses of vitamin E. Patients with *Tangier disease* have virtually no HDL in plasma, apparently because of abnormally rapid removal of HDL from plasma. This leads to generation of abnormal chylomicron remnants, which are stored as cholesteryl esters in phagocytotic cells. Patients typically have enlarged, orange tonsils and develop corneal opacities and polyneuropathy. Premature atherosclerosis does not seem to occur. No therapy is indicated.

Patients with mutations in *cholesterol ester transfer protein* have also recently been described, particularly in Japanese populations, and this is associated with cholesteryl ester enrichment of HDL and greatly elevated HDL-cholesterol values, frequently more than 100 mg/dL. Although not proven, it is generally believed that this mutation is associated with protection from CAD. In contrast, in patients with deficiency of *lecithin cholesterol acyltransferase,* unesterified cholesterol accumulates in plasma and tissues, and patients may develop premature CAD. In addition, they have corneal opacities, hemolytic anemia, and early renal failure. Therapy consists of renal transplantation and fat-restricted diets. Two rare disorders leading to accumulation of abnormal sterols have also been described. Patients with *cerebrotendinous xanthomatosis* have defective bile acid synthesis with associated oversynthesis and accumulation of cholestanol and cholesterol in brain, tendons, and other tissues. They can have neurologic symptoms (including cerebellar ataxia and dementia), tendon xanthomas, atherosclerosis, and cataracts. Finally, patients may have large tendon xanthomas due to abnormal accumulation of plant sterols, chiefly β-sitosterol. Normally, plant sterols are not absorbed, but in patients with *sitosterolemia* there is unexplained intestinal absorption and accumulation of β-sitosterol in plasma and tendons. Treatment consists of diets low in plant sterols and cholesterol and the use of cholestyramine to promote gastrointestinal loss.

Breslow J: Familial disorders of high-density lipoprotein metabolism. *In* Scriver CR, Baudet AL, Sly WS, Valle D (eds): The Metabolic and Molecular Basis of Inherited Disease. New York, McGraw-Hill, 1995, p 2031. *Comprehensive overview of HDL metabolism.*

Brown MS, Goldstein JL: A receptor-mediated pathway for cholesterol homeostasis, Science 232:34, 1986. *Classic citation describing the LDL receptor pathway—this was the lecture delivered on the occasion of receipt of the Nobel Prize.*

Brunzell JD: Familial lipoprotein lipase deficiency and other causes of the chylomicronemia syndrome. *In* Scriver CR, Baudet AL, Sly WS, Valle D (eds): The Metabolic and Molecular Basis of Inherited Disease. New York, McGraw-Hill, 1995, p 1913. *Comprehensive description of disorders leading to accumulation of chylomicrons.*

Goldstein JL, Hobbs HH, Brown MS: Familial hypercholesterolemia. *In* Scriver CR, Baudet AL, Sly WS, Valle D (eds): The Metabolic and Molecular Basis of Inherited Disease. New York, McGraw Hill, 1995, p 1981. *Comprehensive description of pathogenesis and clinical description of this important cause of hypercholesterolemia.*

Havel RJ, Kane JP: Introduction: Structure and metabolism of plasma lipoproteins. *In* Scriver CR, Baudet AL, Sly WS, Valle D (eds): The Metabolic and Molecular Basis of Inherited Disease. New York. McGraw-Hill, 1995, p 1841. *Excellent overview of lipoprotein metabolism.*

Kane JP, Havel RJ: Disorders of the biogenesis and secretion of lipoproteins containing the B-apolipoproteins. *In* Scriver CR, Baudet AL, Sly WS, Valle D (eds): The Metabolic and Molecular Basis of Inherited Disease. New York. McGraw-Hill, 1995, p 1853. *Comprehensive and current concepts of metabolism of apo B-containing lipoproteins.*

Mahley RW, Rall SC: Type III hyperlipoproteinemia (dysbetalipoproteinemia): The role of apolipoprotein E in normal and abnormal lipoprotein metabolism. *In* Scriver CR, Baudet AL, Sly WS, Valle D (eds): The Metabolic and Molecular Basis of Inherited Disease. New York, McGraw-Hill, 1995, p 1953. *Most comprehensive and up-to-date discussion of role of apo E in lipoprotein metabolism.*

Steinberg D, Olefsky JM: Hypercholesterolemia and Atherosclerosis: Pathogenesis and Prevention. New York, Churchill Livingstone, 1987. *Easy-to-read book covering both basic research and clinical aspects of lipoprotein metabolism and their relationship to atherosclerosis.*

207 DISORDERS OF PURINE AND PYRIMIDINE METABOLISM

Beverly S. Mitchell
■ Michael S. Hershfield

PURINE ENZYME DEFICIENCIES AND DISORDERS OF IMMUNE FUNCTION

ADENOSINE DEAMINASE DEFICIENCY. Adenosine deaminase (ADA) deficiency in its usual severe form causes the syndrome of severe combined immunodeficiency disease (SCID) with absence of both T- and B-lymphocyte function. Less complete ADA deficiency is associated with T-cell dysfunction and more variable loss of B-cell function. It is now recognized that ADA deficiency can result in slowly progressive immune dysfunction in adolescents or adults. ADA deficiency accounts for approximately 14% of all cases of SCID and for one third to one half of those with autosomal recessive inheritance. Several hundred families with ADA deficiency have been identified to date. The frequency of ADA deficiency has been estimated at 1 in 200,000 to 1 in a million births.

ETIOLOGY AND PATHOGENESIS. The gene for ADA is located on chromosome 20q. Over 40 single base changes have been identified within the coding region, as well as several deletions and splicing mutations leading to loss of enzymatic activity. The great majority of affected individuals are heteroallelic for two different molecular defects. A so-called partial deficiency of ADA activity resulting from mutations that cause a less severe loss of enzymatic activity in the absence of clinical manifestations has been identified in population screening programs.

ADA catalyzes the irreversible deamination of adenosine to inosine and that of 2'-deoxyadenosine to 2'-deoxyinosine (Fig. 207–1). In the absence of ADA activity, plasma levels of both adenosine and 2'-deoxyadenosine are increased to the range of 0.5 to 10 μmol/L; high levels of 2'-deoxyadenosine, but not adenosine, are excreted in the urine. The pathogenesis of this disorder and its selectivity for cells of the immune system have been the subject of considerable interest. The major pathogenic mechanism appears to involve the preferential phosphorylation of 2'-deoxyadenosine and subsequent accumulation of 2'-deoxyadenosine tri-

phosphate (2'-deoxyATP) in developing thymocytes, with resultant cytotoxicity and thymocyte depletion. The possible metabolic sequelae of 2'-deoxyATP pool expansion are several. This metabolite inhibits the enzyme ribonucleotide reductase, thus inhibiting DNA replication. 2'-DeoxyATP has also been demonstrated to activate a caspase proteolytic cascade that directly results in apoptosis and to accumulate in a subpopulation of thymocytes that express low levels of the antiapoptotic protein Bcl-2. Finally, accumulation of 2'-deoxy-ATP is associated with the induction of single-strand breaks in DNA and activation of a DNA repair pathway that consumes both nicotinamide adenine dinucleotide and ATP. Other pathogenic mechanisms that may play a role in the selective lymphocytotoxicity include inhibition of the enzyme *S*-adenosylhomocysteine hydrolase by 2'-deoxyadenosine, which results in a decrease in transmethylation reactions mediated by *S*-adenosylmethionine, and a direct toxic effect of adenosine on lymphocytes mediated by adenosine receptors.

CLINICAL MANIFESTATIONS. ADA deficiency is most frequently diagnosed in children with signs of immunodeficiency manifested as lymphopenia, failure to thrive, and recurrent infections with both ordinary pathogens and opportunistic organisms. *Pneumocystis carinii* infections and candidiasis are commonly observed, as well as cytomegalovirus, varicella, and other viral pneumonias and infections. Vaccination with live organisms may be fatal, and an increased incidence of B-cell lymphomas has been reported. Although the diagnosis has most commonly been made in very young children, less severe forms of ADA deficiency are increasingly being recognized in adults with lymphopenia and chronic infections. Recurring respiratory infections may lead to pulmonary insufficiency in older individuals. Physical findings are unremarkable with the exception of an absence of lymph nodes and tonsillar tissue and the presence in some affected infants of very prominent costochondral junctions. Neurologic abnormalities have been reported in occasional cases, as have autoimmune abnormalities such as hypothyroidism, hemolytic anemia, and immune thrombocytopenic purpura. Chest radiographs reveal the absence of a thymus, and peripheral blood examination usually demonstrates an absolute lymphopenia of less than 500/μL with a marked reduction in mature T cells and a more variable decrease in B cells associated with hypogammaglobulinemia and lack of specific antibody response to immunization. In vitro tests of lymphocyte function, including proliferative responses to mitogens and antigen, are abnormal.

DIAGNOSIS. The disorder should be looked for in individuals with recurrent infections associated with unexplained lymphopenia. The diagnosis is made by measuring ADA activity in the hemolysates of untransfused patients. Determining the degree of elevation of 2'-deoxyATP and inhibition of *S*-adenosylhomocysteine hydrolase activity in erythrocytes may help gauge the severity of ADA deficiency. In kindreds in which mutations in the ADA gene have been identified because of a previously affected sibling, the diagnosis can be made at the molecular level by amplifying specific regions of the gene by polymerase chain reaction and DNA sequencing or restriction enzyme digestion. Pre-natal diagnosis can be accomplished by assay of ADA activity in cultured amniotic or chorionic villi cells, as well as by DNA analysis when the mutations are known.

TREATMENT. Specific antibiotic treatment for infections is essential. In addition, patients should receive prophylaxis for *P. carinii* and fungal infections and should not receive live virus vaccines or unirradiated blood products. Most patients are also treated with intravenous immunoglobulin. Once the diagnosis is established, the patient is a candidate for either bone marrow transplantation from an HLA-identical or HLA-haploidentical donor or enzyme replacement therapy with polyethylene glycol (PEG)-conjugated bovine ADA. The long-term survival rate for engraftment of 2nd siblings (who are less ill at diagnosis) with HLA-identical transplants is greater than 90%, and marrow transplantation remains the treatment of choice if a donor is available. Haploidentical transplants with T-cell–depleted marrow have been less successful, with the probability of long-term survival rates ranging from 28 to 67%. Enzyme replacement with PEG-conjugated ADA (PEG-ADA), which maintains high levels of ADA activity in plasma, is uniformly effective in correcting the metabolic abnormalities caused by ADA defi-

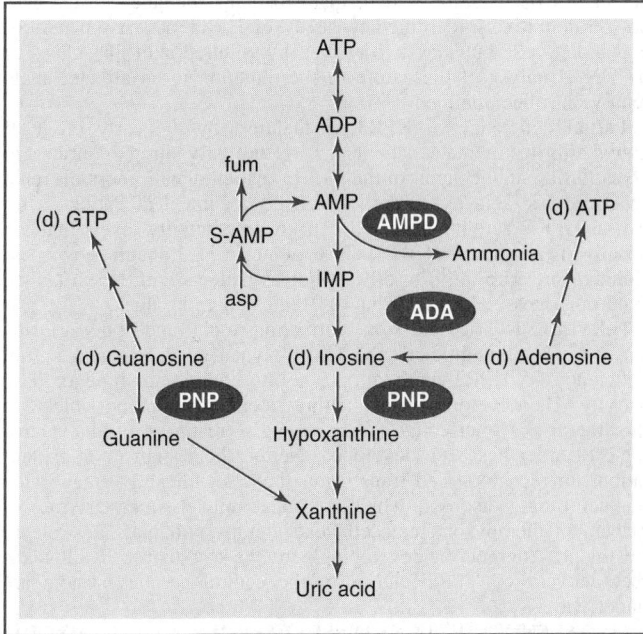

FIGURE 207–1 ■ Schema of purine metabolism demonstrating metabolic reactions catalyzed by adenosine deaminase (ADA), purine nucleoside phosphorylase (PNP), and adenosine monophosphate (AMP) deaminase (AMPD). ATP = adenosine triphosphate; asp = aspartate; fum = fumarate.

ciency. Improving lymphocyte counts and function and restoration of the thymus have occurred within weeks to a few months of intramuscular treatment with PEG-ADA given once or twice weekly. Although lymphocyte counts do not return to normal, the majority of patients have a major reduction in infectious episodes and have resumed growth and normal activities. Experimental somatic cell gene therapy has been used in 10 patients treated concomitantly with PEG-ADA. The majority of these patients were treated recurrently with autologous T cells that had been transfected with a retroviral vector containing the ADA cDNA, whereas 3 received transfected CD34+ umbilical cord stem cells. Although the vector was found in 1 to 10% of T cells at 3 years in the latter group of patients, a finding consistent with a positive selection for lymphocytes expressing ADA, all patients continued to receive PEG-ADA. The future success of the gene therapy approach will depend on the development of improved vectors that enable higher transduction efficiencies.

PURINE NUCLEOSIDE PHOSPHORYLASE DEFICIENCY. Purine nucleoside phosphorylase (PNP) catalyzes the reversible phosphorolysis of the nucleosides inosine and 2'-deoxyinosine to the base hypoxanthine and guanosine and 2'-deoxyguanosine to guanine (see Fig. 207–1). Deficiency of PNP has been reported in approximately 50 individuals, whereas specific mutations in the PNP gene located on chromosome 14q have been identified in 8. Lack of PNP activity is associated primarily with T-cell depletion and cellular immune dysfunction, although either B-cell dysfunction or B-cell hyperactivity associated with autoimmune disorders also occurs in about one third of patients. Neurologic abnormalities, including spasticity, ataxia, behavioral abnormalities, and hypertonia or hypotonia, have been observed in over 50% of affected individuals. Patients are generally seen in childhood with recurrent infections associated with markedly reduced T-lymphocyte counts and are found to lack a thymus gland on chest radiography. Absence or a marked reduction in PNP activity in erythrocytes is diagnostic. Supportive laboratory tests consist of a marked decrease in uric acid because of the inability to convert PNP substrates to hypoxanthine and guanine. Serum and urinary levels of all four nucleoside substrates of PNP are increased. The metabolite of 2'-deoxyguanosine, 2'-deoxyguanosine triphosphate, is found in erythrocytes and is believed to be causally associated with the T-cell depletion because it accumulates in T-cell precursors and results in inhibition of DNA synthesis. Treating this disorder with either red cell transfusions or infusions of deoxycytidine aimed at restoring DNA replication has not resulted in any consistent therapeutic response. Only 2 of 8 patients have had long-term engraftment following bone marrow transplantation. PEG-conjugated PNP and gene therapy remain developmental, and the small number of affected patients makes clinical research on this disorder difficult.

LESCH-NYHAN SYNDROME. The Lesch-Nyhan syndrome is an X-linked disorder caused by the absence or severe deficiency of the enzyme hypoxanthine phosphoribosyltransferase (HPRT). It is manifested as a devastating neurologic disorder consisting of compulsive self-mutilation, choreoathetosis, spasticity, and often mental retardation. The syndrome occurs at a frequency of 1 in 100,000 births and is associated with a marked overproduction of purines resulting in hyperuricemia and gout (see Chapter 299). Partial deficiency of the enzyme also causes hyperuricemia, but without severe neurologic deficits, and accounts for fewer than 1% of patients with gout.

ETIOLOGY AND PATHOGENESIS. The molecular basis of HPRT deficiency has been studied in detail, and a large number of point mutations, splicing defects, and deletions have been identified. HPRT catalyzes the reaction whereby the purine bases hypoxanthine and guanine are condensed with ribose-5-PO_4 derived from phosphoribosylpyrophosphate to form the corresponding nucleotides inosine and guanosine monophosphate, thus salvaging the purine bases for nucleotide metabolism. In the absence of HPRT activity, hypoxanthine and guanine can only be catabolized through xanthine to uric acid, which causes hyperuricemia and markedly increased uric aciduria. In addition, an increase in the intracellular concentration of phosphoribosylpyrophosphate and reduced formation of inosine and guanine monophosphate lead to a marked increase in the overall rate of de novo synthesis of purine nucleotides, further increasing the generation of uric acid. The clinical sequelae of

hyperuricemia and increased uric acid excretion are the juvenile onset of uric acid stone formation and gouty arthritis. The pathogenesis of the neurologic defects is not completely understood but could involve guanine nucleotide deficiency as a result of decreased guanine salvage in neurons that depend on the salvage pathway for purine nucleotide synthesis. Positron emission tomography has demonstrated a selective decrease in dopamine transporters of 50 to 70% in the caudate and putamen. Although anatomic studies of the brains of affected individuals have not revealed any structural lesions, imaging studies have revealed a significant reduction in caudate volume.

CLINICAL MANIFESTATIONS. The Lesch-Nyhan syndrome is manifested in affected males during the 1st year of life by an initial delay in motor development, followed by extrapyramidal signs leading to choreoathetosis and, at approximately age 1, by pyramidal tract involvement with hyperreflexia, clonus, and scissoring of the legs. Compulsive self-destructive behavior appears sometime between early childhood and adolescence and is a behavior pattern unique to this disorder. Affected individuals will bite their fingers, lips, and buccal mucosa; this behavior necessitates restraints and in some cases edentulation. Repeated attempts at self-injury, such as placing extremities in dangerous areas and self-inflicted head trauma, are common. Mental and growth retardation also occur in the majority of cases. Uric acid crystalluria may be noted as orange crystals in the diaper during the first weeks of life and, if untreated, may lead to nephrolithiasis, obstructive uropathy, and azotemia. Hyperuricemia is usually present and may attain levels of 18 mg/dL. Gout may develop later in the course of the disease, but generally not before puberty. Death usually occurs in the 2nd or 3rd decade from infection or renal failure.

Uric acid crystalluria and renal calculi develop in childhood in patients with partial deficiency of HPRT, and gouty arthritis often occurs before age 20. Neurologic manifestations, including mental retardation, mild spastic quadriplegia, dysarthria, cerebellar ataxia, and seizures, are noted in 20% of patients, but self-mutilation does not develop. Patients with partial HPRT deficiency may seek medical attention after passing a renal calculus or following an attack of gouty arthritis. Life expectancy is normal.

DIAGNOSIS. The clinical diagnosis of Lesch-Nyhan syndrome is strongly suggested by the self-mutilation and characteristic choreoathetosis; mental retardation of other origins is very rarely accompanied by self-injury, especially in the presence of intact sensation. The presence of hyperuricemia supports the diagnosis. The definitive diagnosis is made by demonstrating a lack of HPRT enzymatic activity in red cells or other tissues. The molecular defect has been established in many patients. Female carriers cannot be definitively identified by assay of HPRT activity in peripheral blood cells but may be detected by cultured skin fibroblasts or by DNA analysis if the nature of the mutation in an affected male relative has been defined.

Partial deficiency of HPRT is manifest by the early onset of gouty arthritis in male patients or by the early onset of uric acid crystalluria and/or nephrolithiasis. In patients with normal renal function, uric acid overexcretion can be documented. Patients with partial HPRT activity have red cell enzyme activity levels that are usually in the range of 0.2 to 5% of normal, although they occasionally range up to 30 to 50%, whereas patients with Lesch-Nyhan syndrome have values less than 0.01% of control values.

TREATMENT. Uric acid stone formation, tophi, and gouty arthritis can be controlled in both the Lesch-Nyhan syndrome and partial deficiency of HPRT with allopurinol to inhibit xanthine oxidase activity. The development of xanthine stones remains possible with this therapy. No effective pharmacologic treatment of the neurologic disorder has been developed. Neither bone marrow transplantation nor red blood cell transfusions have significantly ameliorated the neurologic disorder, which makes it unlikely that enzyme replacement therapy or stem cell gene therapy will play any role in treatment. Attempts at developing viral vectors that will allow direct delivery of HPRT cDNA to the central nervous system are under way.

MYOADENYLATE DEAMINASE DEFICIENCY AND MYOPATHY. Myoadenylate deaminase is the muscle-specific isoenzyme of adenosine monophosphate deaminase (AMPD). It catalyzes the deamination of adenosine monophosphate to inosine monophosphate and is the product of one (AMPD1) of three distinct genes encoding AMPD isoenzymes. This enzyme activity is an integral part of the purine nucleotide cycle that in subsequent steps regenerates adenosine monophosphate from inosine monophosphate, with the production of fumarate (see Fig. 207–1), and appears to play a major role in energy production in skeletal tissue. Deficiency of AMPD1 has been documented in 2% of all muscle biopsies submitted for histologic examination. Inherited deficiency of myoadenylate deaminase is associated with exercise-related cramps and myalgias. An acquired deficiency of AMPD1 is associated with a number of primary muscle disorders.

ETIOLOGY AND PATHOGENESIS. The *AMPD1* gene is located on chromosome 1 and is expressed predominantly in skeletal muscle, whereas *AMPD2* and *AMPD3* are expressed in other tissues. Normal expression of *AMPD1* is associated with an alternatively spliced 12–base pair 2nd exon of the gene, so 0.6 to 2% of the mRNA in human skeletal muscle lacks exon 2 and encodes a protein of four fewer amino acids. A single nonsense mutation within this 2nd exon has been identified at frequencies ranging from 0.13 to 0.19 in the general population and is associated in its homozygous form with a marked reduction in AMPD1 protein. To date, no other mutations have been identified as causing this enzyme deficiency state. Acquired AMPD1 deficiency is associated with decreased AMPD1 mRNA levels that may be due to a regulatory defect in gene expression in a variety of muscle disorders.

AMPD1 protein has been shown to bind to myosin heavy chain in skeletal muscle. During contraction, the activity of AMPD1 increases markedly. Operation of the next two steps in the purine nucleotide cycle regenerates adenosine monophosphate and produces fumarate, an intermediate in the citric acid cycle, as a by-product. Patients deficient in AMPD1 do not generate inosine monophosphate, NH$_3$, or fumarate in skeletal muscle during exercise.

CLINICAL MANIFESTATIONS. Fatigue, cramps, or myalgias may develop in individuals with the inherited form of AMPD deficiency following vigorous exercise; myoglobinuria has been reported occasionally. The majority of these patients are initially seen between childhood and early adulthood, and the disorder has been documented in over 200 individuals. With the high frequency of the nonsense mutation in the general population, it is apparent that a large number of homozygous mutant individuals must exist who do not have clinical symptoms severe enough to warrant medical evaluation. It has been postulated that the low level of normal alternative splicing that eliminates the exon containing the nonsense codon results in the production of a protein product with some enzymatic activity in many homozygous individuals. Deficiency of AMPD1 is also found in a number of other muscle diseases, including neurogenic disorders, divergent myopathies, and collagen-vascular disorders. The clinical symptoms of these individuals are dictated by the primary muscle disease. Whether the clinical heterogeneity of this disorder relates to expression of the spliced variant of the enzyme and/or to expression of other AMPDs in muscle tissue or indeed whether the enzyme deficiency state is causally associated with symptoms is under investigation.

DIAGNOSIS. Individuals with AMPD1 deficiency do not produce NH$_3$ on ischemic exercise of the forearm and may have an elevated creatine phosphokinase concentration in 50% of cases. Histochemical stains and determination of enzyme activity demonstrate an absence of AMPD1 enzyme in muscle biopsy tissue. The genetic abnormality may be detected by an altered restriction enzyme digestion site in genomic DNA.

TREATMENT. No treatment has been demonstrated to be highly effective. Oral ribose administered in an attempt to enhance the synthesis of purine nucleotides has met with variable subjective improvement.

2,8-DIHYDROXYADENINE RENAL STONES. Deficiency of the enzyme adenine phosphoribosyltransferase (APRT) leads to an accumulation of its substrate adenine, which in turn is oxidized, although inefficiently, by xanthine oxidase to 2,8-dihydroxyadenine. Because of the insolubility of this product, patients with the autosomal recessive form of this disorder are predisposed to radiolucent renal calculi composed of 2,8-dihydroxyadenine. Renal stones may develop within the 1st months of life or occur as late as the 5th decade, although stones never develop in many APRT-deficient individuals. The diagnosis may be made by analyzing the stones with ultraviolet, infrared, or mass spectrometry or x-ray crystallography. Definitive diagnosis requires demonstrating the absence of APRT activity in erythrocyte lysates. No other biochemical or clinical abnormalities have been reported in individuals homozygous

for this enzyme deficiency; heterozygous individuals have no clinical abnormalities. Mutations at the APRT locus are particularly common in individuals of Japanese ancestry, and investigation of the molecular basis of this defect reveals a single base mutation at codon 136 in 68% of the defective alleles, with two other mutations accounting for 28% of the defects. Analysis of both germline and somatic cell mutations in non-Japanese subjects has revealed clustering of the mutations at the intron 4 splice donor site and at codon 87. Thus the molecular basis of this disorder appears to result from relatively few mutations. Therapy for individuals with 2,8-dihydroxyadenine calculi consists of restricting dietary purines, high fluid intake, and treatment with allopurinol to prevent the oxidation of adenine by xanthine oxidase.

XANTHINURIA. Classic xanthinuria results from deficiency of the enzyme xanthine oxidase. As a consequence, the xanthine and hypoxanthine produced by the catabolism of purines cannot be oxidized to uric acid, and therefore serum urate and urinary uric acid excretion values are very low. Serum oxypurine (xanthine and hypoxanthine) concentrations and urinary oxypurine excretion are increased. This disorder has been identified in over 60 individuals, with radiolucent renal calculi composed of xanthine developing in approximately one third. Crystalline deposits of xanthine and hypoxanthine in muscle have been described in a few individuals with muscle cramps following exercise and may also be associated with polyarthritis. The diagnosis is strongly suggested by the presence of low serum and urinary uric acid levels in conjunction with elevated serum and urinary oxypurine concentrations. Deficiency of xanthine oxidase activity can be confirmed by direct enzymatic assay. Therapy for xanthine calculi consists primarily of increasing fluid intake.

A combination of xanthine oxidase deficiency and sulfite oxidase deficiency may also result in xanthinuria and has been attributed to an absence of the molybdenum cofactor for catalytic activity required for both enzymes to be active. The few reported patients with this disorder have been seen in infancy with a severe neurologic disorder characterized by seizures, nystagmus, enophthalmos, ocular lens dislocation, and Brushfield spots characteristic of sulfite oxidase deficiency.

DISORDERS OF PYRIMIDINE METABOLISM

Hereditary orotic aciduria is a rare genetic disorder of pyrimidine metabolism characterized by megaloblastic anemia, leukopenia, retarded growth and development, and high levels of urinary orotic acid excretion, frequently associated with crystal or stone formation. The disorder is inherited as an autosomal recessive defect and results from deficient activity of the bifunctional enzyme uridine monophosphate synthase, which in two steps catalyzes the conversion of orotic acid to uridine monophosphate. This enzyme is therefore essential for the *de novo* synthesis of pyrimidine nucleotides. The gene encoding this enzyme has been localized to the long arm of chromosome 3, and point mutations in the cDNA encoding the enzyme that result in loss of its activity and manifestation of the clinical syndrome have been described. Administering uridine (2 to 4 g/day) has been demonstrated to ameliorate the clinical sequelae of this enzymatic defect through direct phosphorylation to uridine monophosphate.

Pyrimidine 5′-nucleotidase deficiency is an autosomal recessive disorder that results in hereditary hemolytic anemia associated with prominent basophilic stippling of red blood cells. Erthrocytes contain high levels of cytidine and uridine monophosphates, which are substrates for the enzyme, as well as a number of pyrimidine conjugates, including cytidine diphosphate–choline, cytidine diphosphate–ethanolamine, and uridine diphosphate–glucose. Hemolysis is believed to result in part from increased oxidative stress because of inhibition of the pentose phosphate shunt pathway. Acquired pyrimidine 5′-nucleotidase deficiency is found in association with lead toxicity and is also associated with the induction of basophilic stippling from undegraded ribosomal nucleoprotein. Diagnosis of the hereditary disorder is made by measuring erythrocyte pyrimidine 5′-nucleotidase enzymatic activity or by demonstrating elevated pyrimidine nucleotides by ultraviolet absorption spectra in red cell lysates.

Dihydropyrimidine dehydrogenase deficiency is a rare autosomal recessive disorder characterized by deficiency of the enzymatic activity responsible for degrading the pyrimidine bases uracil and thymidine. High levels of these metabolites are found in the urine and may be detected when screening for organic aciduria. Although no clinical symptoms have been associated with this defect, administering fluoropyrimidines (5-fluorouracil, 5-fluorodeoxyuridine) to enzyme-deficient patients with malignancy can result in severe and prolonged drug-related toxicity.

Hershfield MS, Mitchell BS: Immunodeficiency diseases caused by adenosine deaminase deficiency and purine nucleoside phosphorylase deficiency. *In* Scriver CR, Beaudet AL, Sly WS, et al (eds): The Metabolic and Molecular Basis of Inherited Disease, 8th ed. New York, McGraw-Hill, 1999, in press. *Highly detailed discussion of the clinical, metabolic, and molecular aspects of ADA and PNP deficiency states.*
Nyhan WL, Wong DF: New approaches to understanding Lesch-Nyhan disease. N Engl J Med 334:1602, 1996. *Review of metabolic abnormalities in the central nervous system, including studies documenting abnormalities in dopaminergic function.*
Sabina RL, Holmes EW: Myoadenylate deaminase deficiency. *In* Scriver CR, Beaudet AL, Sly WS, et al (eds): The Metabolic and Molecular Basis of Inherited Disease, 8th ed. New York, McGraw-Hill, 1999, in press. *In-depth description of the clinical and biochemical abnormalities associated with myoadenylate deficiency states.*

208 LYSOSOMAL STORAGE DISEASES

Margaret M. McGovern ■ Robert J. Desnick

The lysosomal storage diseases are a family of more than 30 disorders resulting from different defects in lysosomal function. Although most of these disorders are caused by deficiency of a specific hydrolytic enzyme, others are due to impaired receptors or deficiencies of crucial cofactors or protective proteins. Prevalent among these disorders are Fabry's disease, Gaucher's disease, and Niemann-Pick disease, i.e., lipid storage diseases that result from mutations in specific genes that encode lipid-degrading enzymes. The respective enzymatic defects lead to the storage in lysosomes of specipic lipids and their metabolites. All three of these disorders have later-onset forms that can begin in adult life. In addition, Gaucher's disease and Niemann-Pick disease have severe, fatal infantile forms that are described briefly.

FABRY'S DISEASE

DEFINITION. Fabry's disease is an X-linked inborn error of glycosphingolipid metabolism characterized by angiokeratomas (telangiectatic skin lesions), hypohidrosis, corneal and lenticular opacities, acroparesthesias, and vascular disease of the kidney, heart, and/or brain. The disease has an estimated incidence of 1 in 40,000 males.

ETIOLOGY AND PATHOGENESIS. Fabry's disease is an X-linked recessive trait that is manifested in affected hemizygous males. Atypical hemizygous males with residual α-galactosidase A activity may be asymptomatic or have late-onset, mild disease manifestations primarily limited to the heart. Heterozygous females are usually asymptomatic or exhibit mild manifestations. The disease results from the deficient activity of a lysosomal hydrolase (Table 208–1). The course of the disease is more severe in affected males with blood group B or AB because the blood group B substance also accumulates inasmuch as it is normally degraded by α-galactosidase A. The molecular basis of Fabry's disease has been identified for a number of patients (Table 208–2).

PATHOLOGY. Fabry's disease is characterized by marked deposition of globotriaosylceramide and related glycosphingolipids with terminal α-galactosyl moieties primarily in the plasma and in the lysosomes of endothelial, perithelial, and smooth muscle cells of blood vessels. These glycosphingolipid deposits are also prominent in epithelial cells of the cornea, in glomeruli and tubules of the kidney, in muscle fibers of the heart, and in ganglion cells of the dorsal roots and autonomic nervous system. The skin lesions are telangiectases. Capillaries, venules, and arterioles show pathologic lipid storage, and the capillaries of the dermal papillae just below the epidermis are markedly dilated. The larger lesions are usually located in the upper dermis, where they may produce elevation, flattening, or hypertrophy of the epithelium along with keratosis—hence the term angiokeratoma. Ultrastructurally, the glycosphingolipid inclusions in lysosomes have a concentrically arranged lamellar or myelin-like structure.

CLINICAL MANIFESTATIONS. Angiokeratomas usually occur in childhood, which may lead to early diagnosis. They increase in size and number with age and range from barely visible to several millimeters in diameter. The lesions are punctate, dark red to blue-black, and flat or slightly raised. They do not blanch with pressure, and the larger ones may show slight hyperkeratosis. Characteristically the lesions are most dense between the umbilicus and knees, in the "bathing trunk area," but may occur anywhere, including the oral mucosa. The hips, thighs, buttocks, umbilicus, lower part of the abdomen, scrotum, and glans penis are common sites, and a tendency toward bilateral symmetry is noted. Variants without skin lesions have been described. Sweating is usually decreased or absent. Corneal opacities and characteristic lenticular lesions, observed in slit-lamp examination, are present in affected males as well as in about 70% of asymptomatic heterozygotes. Conjunctival and retinal vascular tortuosity is common and results from systemic vascular involvement.

Pain is the most debilitating symptom in childhood and adolescence. Fabry crises, lasting from minutes to several days, consist of agonizing, burning pain in the hands and feet and proximal parts of the extremities and are usually associated with exercise, fatigue, and/or fever. These painful acroparesthesias usually become less frequent in the 3rd and 4th decades of life, although in some men they may become more frequent and severe. Attacks of abdominal or flank pain may simulate appendicitis or renal colic.

With increasing age, the major morbid symptoms result from progressive involvement of the vascular system. Early in the course

Table 208–1 ■ BIOCHEMICAL AND PHENOTYPIC CHARACTERISTICS OF LYSOSOMAL STORAGE DISEASES

DISEASE	DEFICIENCY	ACCUMULATION	ACCUMULATION SITE	RESULTANT COMPLICATIONS
Fabry's	α-Galactosidase A	Primarily globotriaosylceramide	Lysosomes of vascular endothelial and smooth muscle cells	Ischemia, infarction
Gaucher's				
Type 1	Acid β-glucosidase	Primarily glucosylceramide	Macrophage-monocyte system	Infiltration of bone marrow, progressive hepatosplenomegaly, skeletal complications
Type 2	Acid β-glucosidase	Primarily glucosylceramide	Macrophage-monocyte system, CNS	Infiltration of bone marrow, progressive hepatosplenomegaly, skeletal complications, neurodegeneration
Type 3	Acid β-glucosidase	Primarily glucosylceramide	Macrophage-monocyte system, CNS	Progressive neurodegeneration
Niemann-Pick				
Type A	Acid sphingomyelinase	Sphingomyelin	Monocyte-macrophage system, CNS	Hepatosplenomegaly, progressive neurodegeneration
Type B	Acid sphingomyelinase	Sphingomyelin	Monocyte-macrophage system	Progressive hepatosplenomegaly, infiltrative lung disease

Table 208–2 ▪ MOLECULAR GENETICS OF FABRY'S, GAUCHER'S, AND NIEMANN-PICK DISEASES

DISEASE	CHROMOSOME ASSIGNMENT	MOLECULAR CHARACTERISTICS	COMMENTS
Fabry's	Xq22	cDNA, entire genomic sequences, >50 mutant alleles known	Many mutations responsible for disease, including amino acid substitutions, gene rearrangements, mRNA splicing defects
Gaucher's	1q21	cDNA, functional and pseudogenomic sequences, >35 mutant alleles known	4 mutations (N370S, L444P, 84insG, IVS2^{+1}) account for 90–95% of mutant alleles in Ashkenazi Jewish patients
Niemann-Pick			
Types A and B	11p15.1 to p15.4	cDNA, entire genomic sequence, >30 mutant alleles known	3 mutations account for >90% of mutant alleles in Ashkenazi Jewish patients with type A disease
Type C	18	—	Specific gene and nature of the cholesterol defect unknown

cDNA = complementary DNA; mRNA = messenger RNA.

of the disease, casts, red cells, and lipid inclusions with characteristic birefringent "Maltese crosses" appear in the urinary sediment. Proteinuria, isothenuria, and gradual deterioration in renal function and the development of azotemia occur in the 2nd to 4th decades. Cardiovascular findings may include hypertension, left ventricular hypertrophy, anginal chest pain, myocardial ischemia or infarction, and congestive heart failure. Mitral insufficiency is the most common valvular lesion. Abnormal electrocardiographic and echocardiographic findings are common. Cerebrovascular manifestations result primarily from multifocal small vessel involvement. Other features may include obstructive airway disease that increases with age, lymphedema of the legs without hypoproteinemia, episodic diarrhea, osteoporosis, retarded growth, and delayed puberty. Death most often results from uremia or vascular disease of the heart or brain. Before the advent of hemodialysis and renal transplantation, the mean age at death for affected men was 41 years. Atypical male variants with residual α-galactosidase A activity who are asymptomatic or mildly affected have been described, and more recently, several patients with late-onset isolated cardiac or cardiopulmonary disease have been reported. These patients do not have the early classic manifestations. These "cardiac variants" have cardiomegaly, usually involving the left ventricular wall and interventricular septum, and electrocardiographic abnormalities consistent with cardiomyopathy. Others have had hypertrophic cardiomyopathy and/or myocardial infarction.

DIAGNOSIS. The diagnosis in classically affected males is most readily made from a history of painful acroparesthesias, hypohidrosis, the presence of characteristic skin lesions, and observation of the characteristic corneal opacities and lenticular lesions. The disorder is often misdiagnosed as rheumatic fever, erythromelalgia, or neurosis. The skin lesions must be differentiated from benign angiokeratomas of the scrotum (Fordyce's disease) or from angiokeratoma circumscriptum. Angiokeratomas identical to those of Fabry's disease have been reported in fucosidosis, aspartylglycosaminuria, late-onset GM$_1$ gangliosidosis, galactosialidosis, α-N-acetylgalactosaminidase deficiency, and sialidosis. Diagnosis of the mild cardiac variants should be considered in individuals with left ventricular hypertrophy and/or cardiomyopathy. The diagnosis of classic and variant cases is confirmed biochemically by markedly decreased α-galactosidase A activity in plasma, isolated leukocytes, or cultured fibroblasts or lymphoblasts.

Heterozygous females may have corneal opacities, isolated skin lesions, and intermediate activities of α-galactosidase A in plasma or cell sources. Rare female heterozygotes may have manifestations as severe as those in affected males. However, in asymptomatic at-risk females in families affected by Fabry's disease, optimal diagnosis should be by direct analysis of the family's specific mutation. Prenatal detection of affected males can be accomplished by demonstrating deficient α-galactosidase A activity or by detecting the family's specific gene mutation in chorionic villi obtained in the 1st trimester of pregnancy or in cultured amniocytes obtained by amniocentesis in the 2nd trimester.

TREATMENT. Phenytoin and carbamazepine have been shown to decrease the frequency and severity of the chronic acroparesthesias and the periodic crises of excruciating pain. Otherwise, treatment of the disease complications is supportive and non-specific: Renal

transplantation and long-term hemodialysis have become life-saving procedures. Replacement therapy using partially purified human enzyme has proved to be biochemically effective in pilot trials. The recent availability of cDNA encoding human α-galactosidase A has permitted the expression of sufficient quantities of recombinantly produced, active enzyme for further trials of enzyme replacement therapy, which have recently been initiated.

Desnick RJ, Ioannou YA, Eng CM: Fabry disease: α-Galactosidase deficiency and Schindler disease: α-N-acetylgalactosaminidase deficiency. *In* Scriver CR, Beaudet AL, Sly WS, Valle D (eds): The Metabolic and Molecular Bases of Inherited Disease, 7th ed. New York, McGraw-Hill, 1995. *Definitive chapter describing the clinical, pathologic, biochemical, and molecular manifestations of Fabry's disease with more than 400 references.*

Eng CM, Desnick RJ: Molecular basis of Fabry disease: Mutations and polymorphisms in the human α-galactosidase A gene. Hum Mutat 3:103, 1994. *Description of mutations in classic and variant cases.*

GAUCHER'S DISEASE

DEFINITION. Gaucher's disease is a lipid storage disease characterized by the deposition of glucocerebroside in cells of the macrophage-monocyte system. Three clinical subtypes are delineated by the absence or presence and progression of neurologic involvement: type 1, or the adult, non-neuronopathic form; type 2, the infantile or acute neuronopathic form; and type 3, the juvenile or Norrbotten form. All three subtypes are inherited as autosomal recessive traits. Type 1 disease is the most common lysosomal storage disease and the most prevalent genetic disorder among Ashkenazi Jewish individuals, with an incidence of about 1 in 1000 and a carrier frequency of about 1 in 16 to 18.

ETIOLOGY AND PATHOGENESIS. All three subtypes of Gaucher's disease result from deficient activity of a lysosomal hydrolase (see Table 208–1). The molecular basis of Gaucher's disease has been identified for 90 to 95% of Ashkenazi Jewish patients (see Table 208–2). Genotype/phenotype correlations have been noted for the different subtypes and may provide the molecular basis for the remarkable clinical variation in type 1 Gaucher's disease. Presumably, the amount of residual enzymatic activity determines disease subtype and severity. For example, type 1 patients homozygous for the milder *N370S* mutation tend to have a later onset and milder course than do patients with one *N370S* allele and another mutant allele. However, the wide variability in clinical finding among patients with Gaucher's disease cannot be fully explained by the underlying acid β-glucosidase mutations. The lesions causing the severe type 2 (infantile) disease express little if any enzymatic activity in vitro.

PATHOLOGY. The pathologic hallmark is the presence of the Gaucher cell in the macrophage-monocyte system, particularly in the bone marrow. These cells, which are 20 to 100 μm in diameter, have a characteristic wrinkled-paper appearance resulting from intracytoplasmic substrate deposition. These cells stain strongly positive with periodic acid–Schiff, and their presence in bone marrow and/or other tissues suggests the diagnosis (Fig. 208–1). The accumulated glycolipid glucosylceramide is derived primarily from the phagocytosis and degradation of senescent leukocytes and to a lesser extent from erythrocyte membranes. Glycolipid storage results in organomegaly and pulmonary infiltration. Neuronal cell

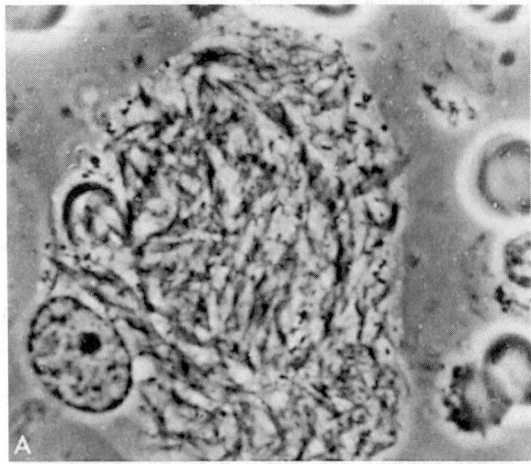

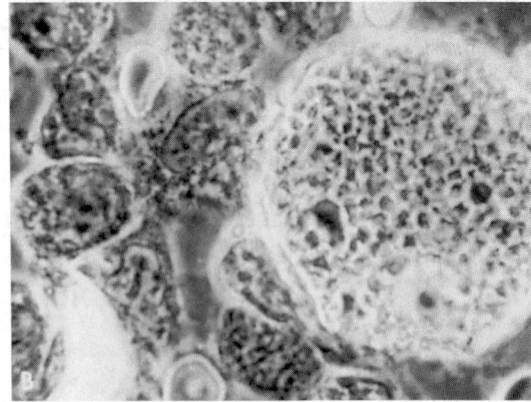

FIGURE 208–1 ■ Typical Gaucher cell *(A)* and a foam cell seen in Niemann-Pick disease *(B)*. Both are viewed under phase microscopy with unstained smears of aspirated bone marrow. Magnification can be estimated from adjacent red cells.

loss in patients with type 2 and 3 disease is presumably caused by accumulation of the cytotoxic glycolipid glucosphingosine in the brain as a result of the severe deficiency of acid β-glucosidase activity. Glucosylceramide accumulation in the bone marrow, liver, spleen, lungs, and kidney leads to pancytopenia, massive hepatosplenomegaly, diffuse infiltrative pulmonary disease, and nephropathy or glomerulonephritis. The progressive infiltration of Gaucher cells in the bone marrow causes thinning of the cortex, pathologic fractures, bone pain, bony infarcts, and osteopenia. Central nervous system involvement occurs only in patients with type 2 and 3 disease.

CLINICAL MANIFESTATIONS. A broad spectrum of clinical expression is seen in patients with type 1 disease, in part because of a combination of different mutant alleles. The onset of clinical manifestations occurs from early childhood to late adulthood, with most seen by adolescence. At examination, patients may have easy bruisability because of thrombocytopenia, chronic fatigue secondary to anemia, hepatomegaly with or without elevated liver function test results, splenomegaly, and bone pain or pathologic fractures. Occasional patients have pulmonary involvement. Patients whose disease is diagnosed in the first 5 years of life are frequently non-Jewish and typically have a more malignant disease course. Patients with milder disease are discovered later in life during evaluations for hematologic or skeletal problems or are found to have splenomegaly on routine examination. In symptomatic patients, splenomegaly is progressive and can become massive. Clinically apparent bone involvement, which occurs in more than 20% of patients, can be manifested as bone pain or pathologic fractures. Most patients have radiologic evidence of skeletal involvement, including an Erlenmeyer flask deformity of the distal end of the femur, which is an early skeletal change. In patients with symptomatic bone disease, lytic lesions can develop in the long bones, ribs, and pelvis, and osteosclerosis may be evident at an early age.

Bone crises with severe pain and swelling can occur. Bleeding secondary to thrombocytopenia may be manifested as epistaxis and bruising and is frequently overlooked until other symptoms become apparent. Children with massive splenomegaly are short of stature because of the energy expenditure required by the enlarged organ.

Type 2 disease, which is rare and pan-ethnic in distribution, is characterized by a rapid neurodegenerative course with extensive visceral involvement and death within the first 2 years of life. The disease occurs in infancy and is associated with increased tone, strabismus, and organomegaly. Failure to thrive and stridor from laryngospasm are typical. The progressive psychomotor degeneration leads to death, usually secondary to respiratory compromise.

Type 3 disease is noted in infancy or childhood. In addition to the organomegaly and bone involvement, neurologic involvement is present. A high frequency of type 3 disease is noted in Sweden (1 in 50,000) and has been traced to a common founder in the 17th century. Type 3 has been further classified as type 3a and 3b based on the extent of neurologic involvement and whether progressive myotonia and dementia (type 3a) or isolated supranuclear gaze palsy (type 3b) is present.

DIAGNOSIS. Gaucher's disease should be considered in the differential diagnosis of patients with unexplained organomegaly, easy bruisability, and/or bone pain. Bone marrow examination usually reveals the presence of Gaucher cells; however, all suspected diagnoses should be confirmed by demonstrating deficient acid β-glucosidase activity in isolated leukocytes or cultured fibroblasts. For possible genotype/phenotype correlations, the specific acid β-glucosidase mutation may be determined, particularly in Ashkenazi Jewish patients. Carrier identification can be achieved by enzymatic assay confirmed with DNA testing in most Jewish families. Testing should be offered to all family members, but it should be kept in mind that heterogeneity even among members of the same kindred can be so great that cases may be diagnosed in asymptomatic affected individuals during such testing. Prenatal diagnosis is possible by determining enzymatic activity or specific mutations in chorionic villi or cultured amniotic fluid cells.

TREATMENT. In the past, management of patients with type 1 disease was primarily symptomatic and included blood transfusions for anemia, partial or total splenectomy for severe mechanical cardiopulmonary compromise or hypersplenism, analgesics for bone pain, and orthopedic procedures for joint replacement. A small number of patients have also undergone bone marrow transplantation, which if successful is curative. However, a matched donor is required, and significant morbidity and mortality are associated with the procedure. No effective treatment is known for the neurologic involvement in type 2 and 3 disease. More recently the safety and efficacy of enzyme replacement with purified placental or recombinant acid β-glucosidase have been demonstrated in type 1 disease. Clinical trials have demonstrated that most extraskeletal symptoms are reversed by initial debulking doses of enzyme (30 to 60 IU/kg) administered by intravenous infusion every other week. The effectiveness of enzyme replacement in reversing and preventing bone manifestations is still under study; however, early data indicate that it may be efficacious. However, it has been demonstrated that enzyme replacement is effective in normalizing linear growth in affected children. Efforts are also under way to develop gene therapy for type 1 disease.

Beutler E, Grabowski G: Gaucher disease. *In* Scriver CR, Beaudet AL, Sly WS, Valle D (eds): The Metabolic and Molecular Bases of Inherited Disease, 7th ed. New York, McGraw-Hill, 1995. *Comprehensive review of the clinical, biochemical, and molecular features of Gaucher's disease.*

Pastores GM, Sibille AR, Grabowski GA: Enzyme therapy in Gaucher disease type 1: Dosage efficacy and adverse events in 33 patients treated for 6 to 24 months. Blood 82:408, 1991. *Description of the initial experience with enzyme replacement therapy.*

NIEMANN-PICK DISEASE

DEFINITION. The four major subtypes of Niemann-Pick disease are characterized by an accumulation of sphingomyelin and cholesterol in the lysosomes of cells of the macrophage-monocyte system. Type A disease is a fatal disorder of infancy, whereas type B disease is a non-neuronopathic form in which most affected individuals live into adulthood and suffer primarily from hepatic and pulmonary involvement. Types C and D are neurodegenerative disorders with onset in early or late childhood. All four subtypes are inherited as autosomal recessive traits and display variable clinical features.

ETIOLOGY AND PATHOGENESIS. Types A and B Niemann-Pick disease result from deficient activity of a lysosomal hydrolase (see Table 208–1). In types C and D, the genetic defect(s) involve the defective transport of cholesterol from the lysosome to the cytosol. The gene encoding the defect in type C disease has been localized (see Table 208–2), but the specific gene and nature of the cholesterol transport defect remain unknown.

PATHOLOGY. The pathologic hallmark in types A and B Niemann-Pick disease is the histochemically characteristic lipid-laden foam cell, often referred to as the Niemann-Pick cell. These cells, which can be readily distinguished from Gaucher cells by their histologic and histochemical characteristics, are not pathognomonic for Niemann-Pick disease because histologically similar cells are found in patients with Wolman's disease, cholesterol ester storage disease, and lipoprotein lipase deficiency and in some patients with GM_1 gangliosidosis type 2. Sphingomyelin is the major lipid that accumulates in the cells and tissues of patients with types A and B Niemann-Pick disease. In most normal tissues, sphingomyelin constitutes 5 to 20% of the total cellular phospholipid content; however, in patients with types A and B, sphingomyelin levels may be elevated up to 50-fold and thus constitute about 70% of the total phospholipid fraction. Lysosomal sphingomyelin accumulation in the brain, liver, kidney, and lungs has been documented in organs from patients with types A and B Niemann-Pick disease; they contain about the same amount of sphingomyelin, with the notable exception that patients with type B Niemann-Pick disease have little or no lipid storage in their central nervous system. In general, patients with type A disease have less than 5% of normal acid sphingomyelinase activity when determined in cultured fibroblasts and/or lymphocytes, whereas cells from type B patients typically have 10 to 20% of normal activity that presumably prevents the development of neurologic symptoms.

CLINICAL MANIFESTATIONS. The clinical features and course of type A Niemann-Pick disease are relatively uniform and are characterized by normal appearance at birth, although the newborn period is sometimes complicated by prolonged jaundice. Hepatosplenomegaly, moderate lymphadenopathy, and psychomotor retardation are evident by 6 months of life and are followed by rapid neurodegeneration. The loss of motor function and deterioration in intellectual capabilities are progressive. In later stages, spasticity and rigidity are evident, with affected infants experiencing complete loss of contact with their environment.

In contrast to the predictable natural history of the A phenotype, the clinical features and course in patients with type B disease are variable. Most cases are diagnosed in infancy or childhood, when enlargement of the liver and/or spleen is detected during routine physical examination. At diagnosis, type B patients also have evidence of mild pulmonary involvement, usually detected as a diffuse reticular or finely nodular infiltration on chest radiography. In most patients, hepatosplenomegaly is particularly prominent in childhood, but with increasing linear growth the abdominal protuberance decreases and becomes less conspicuous. In mildly affected patients the splenomegaly may not be noted until adulthood, and disease manifestations may be minimal. In most patients with type B disease, decreased pulmonary diffusion secondary to alveolar infiltration becomes evident in childhood and progresses with age. Severely affected individuals may experience significant pulmonary compromise by age 15 to 20. Such patients have low PO_2 values and dyspnea on exertion. Life-threatening bronchopneumonia may occur and cor pulmonale has been described. Severely affected patients may also have liver involvement leading to life-threatening cirrhosis, portal hypertension, and ascites. Clinically significant pancytopenia from secondary hypersplenism may necessitate partial or total splenectomy. However, removal of the spleen can lead to significant worsening of the pulmonary involvement. Typically, patients with type B disease do not have neurologic involvement and are intellectually intact.

Patients with type C disease often have prolonged neonatal jaundice, appear normal for 1 to 2 years, and then experience a slowly progressive and variable neurodegenerative course. Their hepatosplenomegaly is less severe than in patients with type A or B disease, and they may survive into adulthood. Neurologic symptoms develop in patients with type D Niemann-Pick disease later in childhood, and these patients have a slower neurodegenerative course than do patients with type C. Most patients with type D disease share a common ancestry traceable to the Acadians from Yarmouth County, Nova Scotia. It appears that these patients also have an abnormality in cholesterol metabolism and that the defect may be allelic with that causing type C disease.

DIAGNOSIS. Type A disease is diagnosed in the patient's first year of life by failure to thrive, organomegaly, and severe psychomotor retardation. In type B Niemann-Pick disease, splenomegaly is usually noted early in childhood; however, in very mild cases, the enlargement may be subtle and detection may be delayed until adolescence or adulthood. The presence of the characteristic Niemann-Pick cells in the bone marrow supports the diagnosis. However, patients with types C and D disease also have extensive infiltration of these cells in the bone marrow. Thus all suspected cases should be evaluated enzymatically to confirm the clinical diagnosis by measuring the sphingomyelinase activity level in peripheral leukocytes, cultured fibroblasts, and/or lymphoblasts. Patients with types A and B disease will have markedly decreased levels of enzymatic activity (1 to 10% of normal), whereas patients with types C and D disease may have slightly decreased sphingomyelinase activity (50 to 75% of normal) and patients with Gaucher's disease and other storage disorders characterized by hepatosplenomegaly and/or neurologic involvement will have normal or near-normal levels. Types C and D disease can be biochemically documented by demonstrating the cholesterol transport defect in cultured fibroblasts. The enzymatic identification of type A carriers and of type B carriers is problematic. However, in families in which the specific molecular lesion has been identified, family members can be accurately tested for heterozygote status by DNA analysis. Heterozygote identification for types C and D disease is unavailable. Prenatal diagnosis of types A and B disease may be reliably made by measuring acid sphingomyelinase activity in cultured amniocytes or chorionic villi. In families in which the specific molecular lesions are known, prenatal diagnosis can be made by DNA analysis of fetal cells.

TREATMENT. At present, no specific treatment is available for any of the Niemann-Pick disease subtypes. Orthotopic liver transplantation in an infant with type A disease and amniotic cell transplantation in several patients with type B disease have been attempted with little or no success. Bone marrow transplantation in a type B patient was successful in reducing the spleen and liver volumes, the sphingomyelin content of the liver, the number of Niemann-Pick cells in the marrow, and radiologically detected infiltration of the lungs. However, no long-term information is available because this patient died 3 months after transplantation. To date, lung transplantation has not been performed in any severely compromised patient with type B disease. Future prospects for treatment of type B disease include enzyme replacement and gene therapy. Treatment of types A, C, and D disease is presently precluded by the severe neurologic involvement.

Schuchman EH, Desnick RJ: Types A and B Niemann-Pick disease. *In* Scriver CR, Beaudet AL, Sly WS, Valle D (eds): The Metabolic and Molecular Bases of Inherited Disease, 7th ed. New York, McGraw-Hill, 1995. *The most up-to-date description of the clinical, metabolic, and molecular nature of Niemann-Pick disease types A and B.*

INBORN ERRORS OF AMINO ACID METABOLISM

209 THE HYPERPHENYLALANINEMIAS AND ALKAPTONURIA

Charles R. Scriver

THE HYPERPHENYLALANINEMIAS

DEFINITIONS. A widely accepted medical model of disease attributes manifestations (signs and symptoms) to a deviant underlying process (pathogenesis) that has its origins in both proximate and ultimate causes. According to this model, phenylketonuria (MIM 261600),* the best known form of hyperphenylalaninemia (HPA), is no longer a disease, although it continues to be a risk factor, because its principal manifestations (mental retardation, pigment dilution, mousy odor, neurotransmitter deficiency) occur only in rare cases escaping early diagnosis and treatment. This satisfactory turn of events came about because pathogenesis from hyperphenylalaninemia (the risk factor) is offset by treatment (low phenylalanine diet). Genetic forms of hyperphenylalaninemia are described here; they are all autosomal recessive disorders. About 0.01% of live births are affected. Physicians for adult-age patients must be aware of maternal hyperphenylalaninemia and its consequences for the fetus (see later).

PHENYLALANINE METABOLISM. Phenylalanine is an essential amino acid. The normal concentration in plasma is less than 125 μmol/L (0.125 mM) (1 μmol = 165 μg). Metabolic utilization is largely controlled by a hydroxylation reaction (Fig. 209–1A) and impaired hydroxylation is the chief explanation for hyperphenylalaninemia. The reaction requires the apoenzyme phenylalanine hydroxylase (a monooxygenase), molecular oxygen, and tetrahydrobiopterin cofactor; the last-named is consumed in stoichiometric amounts to form tyrosine, the reaction product. The catalytic property of phenylalanine hydroxylase requires both moment-to-moment regeneration of tetrahydrobiopterin from 4α-carbinolamine and dihydrobiopterin, consecutive byproducts of the hydroxylating reaction, and long-term renewal of the tetrahydrobiopterin pool by synthesis from precursors. The former is achieved by the enzymes 4α-carbinolamine dehydratase and dihydropteridine reductase, the latter by a synthesis pathway in which several enzymes act in sequence. Accordingly, there are several ways to impair phenylalanine hydroxylation. Failure to recognize the biologic heterogeneity of hyperphenylalaninemia may lead to erroneous counseling and the wrong treatment; all of its forms require special management of women during the reproductive years.

DISORDERS OF PHENYLALANINE HYDROXYLASE INTEGRITY. The phenylalanine hydroxylase enzyme is multimeric and homopolymeric. The polypeptide is encoded by a gene (symbol, *PAH*) on chromosome 12, region q24.1, which is expressed only in liver in humans. *PAH* mutations are "severe" and cause phenylketonuria (with plasma phenylalanine values > 1 mM on a normal diet) or "mild" and cause non-phenylketonuric hyperphenylalaninemia (values < 1 mM but > 0.125 mM). Phenylketonuria is typically associated with mental retardation in the untreated patient; the other form is not. The incidence and relative frequencies of the two forms (together about 1 per 10,000 births) vary widely among population.

The hydroxylation reaction accounts for about three fourths of the moment-by-moment metabolic outflow of phenylalanine; incor-

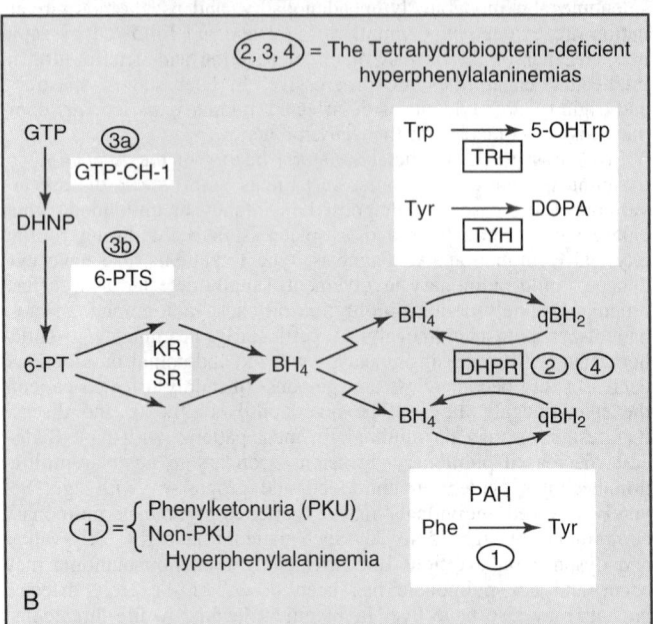

FIGURE 209–1 ■ *A*, Intake of phenylalanine (an essential amino acid supplied only by diet) and its disposal by hydroxylation (1) (representing three fourths of normal runout), transamination (2), decarboxylation (3), and incorporation into proteins (4) (representing a fourth of runout). *B*, Interrelations between phenylalanine hydroxylase (PAH), dihydropteridine reductase (DHPR), and the tetrahydrobiopterin (BH$_4$) biosynthesis pathway serving aromatic amino acid hydroxylation reactions. Mutations at the relevant chromosomal loci impair the hydroxylation reactions with effects on PAH activity only (1); DHPR activity (2); GTP-cyclohydrolase 1 (GTP-CH-1) activity (3a); 6-pyruvoyltetrahydropterin synthase activity (6-PTS) (3b); and 4α-carbinolamine dehydratase (4). Disorders 2, 3a, 3b, and 4 can impair function of three hydroxylases: PAH, tyrosine hydroxylase (TYH), and tryptophan hydroxylase (TRH). GTP = guanosine triphosphate; DHNP = dihydroneopterin triphosphate; 6-PT = 6-pyruvoyltetrahydropterin; KR = 2′-ketotetrahydropterin reductase; SR = sepiapterin reductase; qBH$_2$ = quinonoid dihydrobiopterin.

---

*MIM: (Online) Mendelian Inheritance in Man (catalogues of Mendelian traits); the URL is http://www.ncbi.nlm.nih.gov/OMIM

poration into protein is the other important route (see Fig. 209–1A). If there is deficient hydroxylating activity, and dietary intake is not curtailed, free phenylalanine accumulates in body fluids. Overflow into the alternative pathways generates excessive amounts of metabolites derived from phenylalanine, such as the pyruvic (causing "phenylketonuria"), lactic, and acetic acid derivatives. Overburden of phenylalanine impairs brain development in ways still not fully understood.

Phenylketonuria was first described as a clinical entity in 1934 by Asbjørn Følling, who surmised that the disorder was autosomal recessive and an "inborn error of metabolism." In the following three decades, phenylketonuria was seen as a paradigm for the biochemical basis of mental disease, of disease that could be prevented by deliberately restoring normal metabolism, and of chemical individuality that could be used as the basis for a screening test and early diagnosis. Newborn screening for hyperphenylalaninemia is now one of the most widely applied "genetic" tests. The incidence of the risk factor has not changed, but the frequency of the associated disease is now trivial in screened populations. The practical issues for non-specialist physicians are interpretation of a positive screening test result, referral of the patient for reliable treatment, and monitoring for maternal hyperphenylalaninemia (all discussed later).

TETRAHYDROBIOPTERIN-DEFICIENT FORMS OF HYPERPHENYLALANINEMIA. Not every case of persistent hyperphenylalaninemia is explained by a primary hydroxylase deficiency. Tetrahydrobiopterin insufficiency impairs function of three hydroxylases (for phenylalanine, tryptophan, and tyrosine) and synthesis of their products, notably 5-hydroxytryptophan (the precursor of serotonin) and L-dopa (the precursor of catecholamines) (see Fig. 209–1B). The products function as neurotransmitters in the brain, and a deficiency of them gives rise to central nervous system disease (including retarded psychomotor development, basal ganglion dysfunction, and unstable body temperature). Regeneration of tetrahydrobiopterin is necessary to maintain catalytic function of the three hydroxylases. Deficient activity of quininoid dihydropteridine reductase (gene symbol *QDPR* on chromosome 4, region p15.31) or of 4α-carbinolamine dehydratase (gene symbol *DCOH*, chromosome 10q22) impairs recycling of dihydrobiopterin. Deficient activity of quanosine triphosphate cyclohydrolase I (gene symbol *GCH1*, chromosome 14q21–q22.2) or 6-pyruvoyl tetrahydropterin synthase (gene symbol *PTS*, chromosome 11q22.3–q23.3) impairs synthesis of tetrahydrobiopterin.

SCREENING AND DIAGNOSIS. Screening newborns for hyperphenylalaninemia is public policy. Capillary blood collected on filter paper from heel puncture is analyzed by the bacterial inhibition (Guthrie) assay, fluorimetric analysis, or other quantitative methods. Blood phenylalanine values greater than 2 mg/dL (125 μM) on the first day of life or thereafter are considered abnormal and require further investigation; false-negative results do occur, some for biologic reasons. Urine screening for "phenylketones" is not reliable. The HPA phenotype test is still the most efficient; DNA-based tests will detect over 400 mutations in the *PAH* gene and dozens in the genes controlling tetrahydrobiopterin homeostasis, but none is common to every case of HPA.

Every infant with persistent hyperphenylalaninemia is investigated to rule out disorders of tetrahydrobiopterin homeostasis. Urine pterin metabolites or blood cofactor levels are measured under special conditions; there are distinctive urine profiles as well as low blood levels in the disorders of tetrahydrobiopterin homeostasis. The tests are done at established centers and require experienced interpretation. Direct measures of phenylalanine hydroxylase and 4α-carbinolamine hydratase require liver biopsy and are not necessary. Deficiency of dihydropteridine reductase can be confirmed in blood spots, fibroblasts, and amniocytes; of cyclohydrolase in phytohemagglutinin-stimulated leukocytes; and of synthase in erythrocytes.

After excluding disorders of tetrahydrobiopterin metabolism, hyperphenylalaninemia is classified as follows. About one half of cases with primary phenylalanine hydroxylase deficiency have *phenylketonuria,* a generic term for severe hyperphenylalaninemia (>1 mM), low phenylalanine tolerance (<500 mg/day; normal tolerance > 1000 mg/day), and high risk of mental retardation in the absence of treatment. The remainder have non-phenylketonuric hyperphenylalaninemia with lower blood phenylalanine values (<1

mM), higher tolerance for dietary phenylalanine (>500 mg/day), and much lower risk for mental retardation if not treated. There is a correlation between level of hepatic hydroxylase activity and clinical form; in broad terms, activity is less than 1% of normal in phenylketonuria and more than 1% of normal in non-phenylketonuric hyperphenylalaninemia.

DNA analysis, which is increasingly available, identifies mutations, and interprets phenotypes by mutation analysis, is beginning to have clinical relevance. Prenatal diagnosis by analysis of DNA (for linked markers or mutations) in chorionic villus samples or amniocytes is now feasible for (>85%) couples at risk; these tissues do not express the enzyme. Mutation databases exist for phenylketonuria (http://www.mcgill.ca/pahdb) and for disorders of tetrahydrobiopterin homeostasis (http://www.unizh.ch/~blau/bh4.htmL).

TREATMENT. The mainstay of treatment for primary phenylalanine hydroxylase deficiency is dietary restriction of the amino acid. There are several semisynthetic diet products ("orphan foods") for this purpose. Phenylketonuric patients can tolerate only 250 to 500 mg of phenylalanine per day (normal intake >1000 mg) to maintain the blood phenylalanine level well below 1 mM. Intake, blood levels of phenylalanine, and growth rate are monitored at frequent intervals to avoid undertreatment or overtreatment. Treatment into adult life is now recommended to maintain normal neuropsychologic function. Well-treated patients have normal or near-normal intellectual development.

The tetrahydrobiopterin-deficient forms require continuous replacement therapy of cofactor alone or in combination with neurotransmitter precursors. Whether postnatal treatment of these disorders is fully effective remains to be seen.

MATERNAL HYPERPHENYLALANINEMIA. *This problem is relevant to all practitioners who counsel women about pregnancy.* Intrauterine hyperphenylalaninemia places the fetus at risk of microcephaly, mental retardation, and organ malformations (notably cardiac). Accordingly, all females with hyperphenylalaninemia should be identified, followed (registries are appearing for this purpose, e.g., Metabolic Information Network, email: mizesg@ix,netcom.com), counseled about risk when they attain reproductive age, and treated with diet to maintain near-normal blood phenylalanine levels before conception and throughout the pregnancy.

GENETICS. Mutant alleles (at all relevant loci) are recessive. Their aggregate frequency in the population is about 0.01, meaning that 2% of the population is heterozygous. Observed explanations for the high allelic frequency of this "rare" phenotype include founder effect and genetic drift in some populations and mutability at the *PAH* locus.

ALKAPTONURIA

DEFINITION. Alkaptonuria (MIM 203500) is an autosomal recessive disorder in which homogentisic acid oxidase activity is missing. Homogentisic acid produced during the metabolism of phenylalanine and tyrosine accumulates and is excreted in the urine. It causes pigmentation of cartilage and other connective tissue (ochronosis) and in later years a degenerative arthritis of the spine and the larger peripheral joints. The disease has historical significance, for it was chiefly on the basis of his study of families with alkaptonuria that Sir Archibald Garrod developed the concept of the "inborn error of metabolism." The alkaptonuria gene (symbol *AKU*), encoding homogentisic acid oxidase, has been mapped to human chromosome 3q21–q23, cloned, and characterized; and mutations have been identified—a major advance in the alkaptonuria saga.

INCIDENCE AND PREVALENCE. The trait is rare (< 1 per 250,000 births), but cases are still being reported (now > 600), including one in a 3500-year-old Egyptian mummy.

PATHOGENESIS. The activity of homogentisic acid oxidase in the normal adult human liver is sufficient to metabolize over 1600 g of homogentisic acid per day. Normally, no homogentisic acid can be detected in plasma or urine. In alkaptonuric individuals there is no detectable activity of this enzyme in liver, kidney, or prostrate where it is normally abundant. Plasma levels of homogentisic acid rise to about 3 mg/dL, and the urinary excretion ranges from 4 to 8 g/day. Mammalian tissue also contains an enzyme called homogentisic acid polyphenoloxidase that catalyzes the oxidation of homogentisic acid to an ochronotic pigment, but pigment can also be produced non-enzymatically in the presence of oxygen and alkali, as, for example, in urine. The homogentisic acid polymer has a high affinity for cartilage and connective tissue macromolecules. The stained tissue is fragile and eventually may break down, leading to degenerative intervertebral disk or joint disease. Homogentisic acid may also have a direct effect on collagen synthesis through inhibition of lysyl hydroxylase.

PATHOLOGY. In the adult alkaptonuric patient, costal, laryngeal, and tracheal cartilages are densely pigmented, sometimes appearing coal-black. Pigmentation is also present throughout the body in fibrous tissue, fibrocartilage, tendons, ligaments, epidermis, endocardium, and intima of larger vessels in various organs including kidney, lung, and prostrate.

CLINICAL MANIFESTATIONS. Homogentisic acid is present in urine from birth. Urine is colorless when passed but darkens when alkaline or after long exposure to air. Generally, the earliest physical sign is a slight pigmentation of the sclerae or the ears, beginning at age 20 to 30 years. The cartilage of the ears may be slate blue or gray and feel irregular and thickened. Sometimes dusky discolorations of underlying tendons can be seen through the skin over the hands. Pigment in perspiration stains clothing in the axillary and genital regions. The arthritis causes limitation of motion of the hips, knee joints, or shoulders; and there may be periods of acute inflammation. Limitation of motion and ankylosis in the lumbosacral region is a late finding. In addition, alkaptonuric patients appear to have a high incidence of cardiovascular disease; at least one degenerated pigmented aortic valve has been replaced with a prosthesis. Other complications include ruptured intervertebral disks, prostatitis, and renal stones.

RADIOGRAPHIC CHANGES. Almost pathognomonic, the changes affect vertebral bodies of the lumbar spine, which show degeneration of the intervertebral disks, narrowing of the space, dense calcification of remaining disk material, and variable fusion of vertebral bodies, but little osteophyte formation and minimal calcification of intervertebral ligaments. The degenerative changes of ochronotic arthritis are most severe in the hip, shoulder, and knee; and there may be calcific deposits in the tendons. The sacroiliac joints and smaller joints of the extremities usually show little or no abnormality. Ear cartilage may be calcified.

DIAGNOSIS AND DIFFERENTIAL DIAGNOSIS. The diagnosis is suggested by urine discoloration and presence of non-glucose reducing substance, pigmentation of sclerae or cartilage, arthritic episodes, and typical radiographic changes of the lumbar spine. Homogentisic acid in urine can be identified by chromatographic or enzymatic assays.

The ochronotic changes of skin and cartilage, in the past, have been confused with an effect of prolonged use of quinacrine (Atabrine) or of carbolic acid dressings for chronic cutaneous ulcers. The arthritis must be differentiated from rheumatoid arthritis, osteoarthritis, and gout.

TREATMENT. A low protein diet for life would be prudent. Dietary restriction of phenylalanine and tyrosine of the degree necessary to reduce homogentisic aciduria is impractical and potentially deleterious. Pharmacologic doses of ascorbic acid, early and continuously, might reduce polymerization and pigmentation because ascorbic acid inhibits the polyphenol oxidase. It does not alter the primary metabolic defect. NTBC (2-(2-nitro-4-trifluoromethylbenzoyl)-1,3-cyclohexanedione), the potent inhibitor of p-hydroxyphenylpyruvic acid oxidase, would prevent excess formation of homogentisic acid by blocking the pathway prior to the mutant step.

Fernandez-Cañón JM, Granadino B, Beltran-Valero de Bernabe D, et al: The molecular basis of alkaptonuria. Nat Genet 14:19, 1997. *A modern classic describing cloning of the HGO (AKU) gene and proof that it is the AKU locus harboring mutations causing alkaptonuria; companion papers (Genomics 43:115, 1979; Am J Hum Genet 62:776, 1998) document HGO gene structure and multiple AKU mutations.*

La Du BN: Alkaptonuria. *In* Scriver CR, Beaudet AL, Sly WS, Valle D (eds): The Metabolic and Molecular Bases of Inherited Disease, 7th ed. New York, McGraw-Hill, 1995, p 1371. *A detailed discussion of the history, clinical features, and biochemical derangements of alkaptonuria and ochronosis.*

Levy HL: Maternal phenylketonuria. Prog Clin Biol 281:227, 1988. *A good discussion of an important problem (maternal hyperphenylalaninemia).*

Scriver CR, Kaufman S, Eisensmith RC, Woo SLC: The hyperphenylalaninemias. *In*

Scriver CR, Beaudet AL, Sly WS, et al (eds): The Metabolic and Molecular Bases of Inherited Disease, 7th ed. New York, McGraw-Hill, 1995, p 1015. *A reference covering most issues concerning the hyperphenylalaninemias; also see URL websites for mutation data: http://www.mcgill.ca/pahdb; http://www.unizh.ch/~blau/bh4.htmL.*

210 THE HYPERPROLINEMIAS AND HYDROXYPROLINEMIA

James M. Phang

There are three autosomal recessive genetic disorders in the degradative pathways for proline and hydroxyproline. Although these rare disorders are generally benign, the resulting metabolic abnormalities, at least for one of the disorders, are associated with neurologic manifestations in childhood.

The α-nitrogen of the imino acids proline and hydroxyproline is incorporated within a pyrrolidine ring. This feature confers structural and functional properties to proteins. Because of the ring structure, the metabolism of proline, including biosynthesis from glutamate and ornithine and degradation back to glutamate, is catalyzed by a specific set of enzymes. Both synthetic and degradative pathways share Δ^1-pyrroline-5-carboxylate as an intermediate. The cycling of proline may mediate the transfer of reducing-oxidizing potential that may be important under certain conditions. Studies suggest that proline oxidation is increased during apoptosis. Preformed hydroxyproline is not incorporated into proteins. Instead, hydroxyproline is formed from peptide-linked proline primarily in collagen.

HYPERPROLINEMIAS. The two genetic disorders in proline metabolism are characterized by hyperprolinemia and iminoglycinuria, but they are due to different enzyme deficiencies; type II hyperprolinemia can be diagnosed directly. This disorder is due to a deficiency of Δ^1-pyrroline-5-carboxylate dehydrogenase, which catalyzes the second step in the degradative pathway for proline (Fig. 210–1); the deficiency in enzyme activity can be determined in extracts of circulating leukocytes or cultured fibroblasts. Hyperprolinemia in type II is more marked than in type I, but the distin-

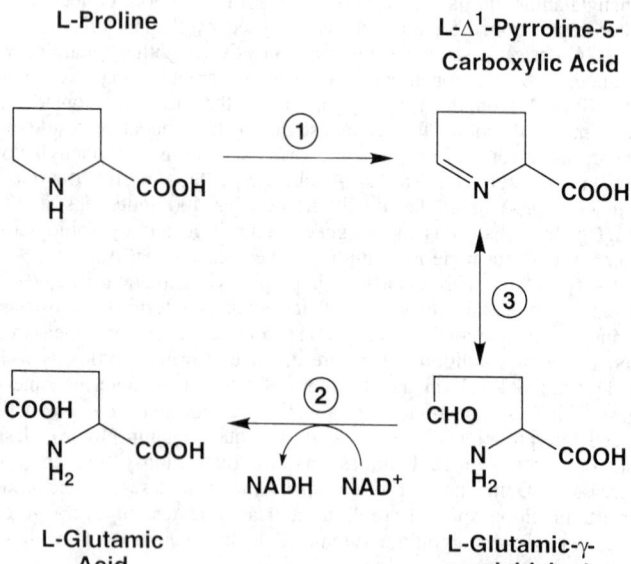

FIGURE 210–1 ■ Schematic of the degradative pathway for proline. Reaction 1 is catalyzed by proline oxidase (EC number unassigned); reaction 2 is catalyzed by Δ^1-pyrroline-5-carboxylic acid dehydrogenase (EC 1.5.1.12); and reaction 3 is spontaneous. Type I hyperprolinemia is due to blockade at reaction 1 (deficiency of proline oxidase), and type II hyperprolinemia is due to blockade at reaction 2 (deficiency of Δ^1-pyrroline-5-carboxylic acid dehydrogenase).

guishing feature of type II is the accumulation of Δ^1-pyrroline-5-carboxylate in plasma and its excretion in urine. The hyperprolinemia in type I is due to a deficiency of the first enzyme in the pathway, proline oxidase. Although plasma proline is generally lower than in type II, the diagnosis of type I is one of exclusion, that is, hyperprolinemia unaccompanied by Δ^1-pyrroline-5-carboxylate in urine or plasma.

Clinical manifestations have been described with the hyperprolinemias, but the association may be due to chance because, in most cases, hyperprolinemia was identified fortuitously in patients presenting with clinical abnormalities (biased ascertainment). This is true especially for type I hyperprolinemia in which renal disease and mental retardation found in some pedigrees were shown to segregate independently of hyperprolinemia. For type II hyperprolinemia, however, clinical associations untainted by biased ascertainment have been identified. Screening a large pedigree in Ireland identified 14 new cases confirmed by elevated plasma Δ^1-pyrroline-5-carboxylate levels and undetectable enzyme activity in leukocytes. Nine of these 14 new subjects had a history of recurrent childhood febrile seizures requiring hospitalization and treatment with anticonvulsants. Thus, the association of type II hyperprolinemia with a predisposition to seizures appears convincing. Adults in this pedigree were fertile and otherwise normal. Although the mechanism for this association remains unclear, the identification of a high-affinity proline transporter in rat brain suggests that proline or its metabolites may have a neuromodulatory function.

HYDROXYPROLINEMIA. Hydroxyprolinemia with hydroxyprolinuria, but without hyperprolinemia or prolinuria, has been described in members of several families. Although the degradation of hydroxyproline parallels that of proline, the pathway enzymes are distinct except the second degradation step is catalyzed by a common enzyme that dehydrogenates both Δ^1-pyrroline-5-carboxylate (see earlier) and 3-OH-Δ^1-pyrroline-5-carboxylate. The first step in the degradation, however, is catalyzed by distinct oxidases. The absence of urinary Δ^1-pyrroline-5-carboxylate or its hydroxylated congener leads to the conclusion that this autosomal recessive disorder is due to a deficiency of hydroxyproline oxidase. In this disorder there are no clinical manifestations related to abnormalities in collagen metabolism or central nervous system function and therapy is not indicated.

Flynn MP, Martin MC, Moore PT, et al: Type II hyperprolinaemia in a pedigree of Irish travellers (nomads). Arch Dis Child 64:1699–1707, 1989. *Documents the association of type II hyperprolinemia with seizures.*

Fremeau RT Jr, Caron MG, Blakely RD: Molecular cloning and expression of a high affinity L-proline transporter expressed in putative glutamatergic pathways of rat brain. Neuron 8:915–926, 1992. *First report of high affinity transporters in the central nervous system.*

Phang JM, Yeh GC, Scriver CR: Disorders of proline and hydroxyproline metabolism. *In* Scriver CR, Beaudet AL, Sly WS, Valle D (eds): The Metabolic and Molecular Basis of Inherited Disease, 7th ed. New York, McGraw-Hill, 1995, pp 1125–1146. *Review of proline metabolism.*

Polyak K, Xia Y, Zweier JL, et al: A model for p53-induced apoptosis. Nature 389:300–395, 1997. *Report of proline oxidase induction with apoptosis.*

211 DISEASES OF THE UREA CYCLE

Stephen D. Cederbaum

Ammonia is a highly toxic metabolic product, which, when present at levels no more than two times the upper limits of normal (10 to 25 μM), may cause symptoms. The urea cycle is a five-step metabolic pathway in which two ammonia molecules and one bicarbonate molecule are converted to the relatively easily excreted and non-toxic urea. It is the only major pathway to remove waste nitrogen derived from ingested protein or from normal or augmented protein turnover in the body. The urea cycle occurs predominantly or possibly exclusively in the liver.

In children, the vast majority of cases of hyperammonemia are the result of inborn errors of metabolism, primarily of the urea cycle. In adults, a larger proportion of cases are due to liver failure and less frequently to toxic ingestion. Nevertheless, with the wider availability of blood ammonia tests, the increased recognition of urea cycle disorders, and more successful treatment modalities, the inherited disorders of ammonia metabolism are being recognized with greater frequency in adolescents and adults with acute or intermittent organic brain syndrome. Hyperammonemia appears to be better tolerated in infants and young children, in part because the cranium is more compliant. Ammonia levels that leave minimal residual damage in infants may be deadly in adults. Ammonia itself appears to be the metabolite toxic to the central nervous system; however, there is some speculation that the accumulation of glutamine, a compound in equilibrium with ammonia, may be involved as well. The primary toxic effect appears to be the uptake of fluid into astrocytes, causing cerebral edema. Death is caused acutely by herniation of the brain through the foramen magnum with consequent cerebral ischemia, but survivors may have various degrees of brain damage.

The urea cycle is shown in Figure 211–1. The five enzymes generally associated with it are carbamoylphosphate synthetase 1 (CPS-1) and ornithine transcarbamoylase (OTC), both found in the mitochondrion, and argininosuccinate synthetase (ASAS), argininosuccinate lyase (ASAL), and arginase 1 (ARG-1) found in the cytoplasm. *N*-Acetylglutamate synthetase catalyzes the synthesis of *N*-acetylglutamate, which activates CPS-1 and modulates urea cycle function, and the ornithine transporter recycles ornithine to the mitochondrion. Deficiency of these latter enzymes has been associated with symptomatic hyperammonia, the former only in infants.

The normal urea cycle can increase its ureagenic capacity greatly in response to ammonia challenge. The genes for all five enzymes have been cloned and are available for defining mutations, prenatal diagnosis, and population studies.

Disorders of the urea cycle are estimated to occur in 1 in 25,000 births. It is probable that 2 to 4% of the population is heterozygous for a urea cycle defect, although only women who are carriers of ornithine transcarbamoylase deficiency are known to be prone to disease. It is unclear whether patients receiving intensive chemotherapy for leukemia, in whom hyperammonemia occurs rarely, or patients receiving valproate anticonvulsant therapy, in whom it occurs more mildly, are heterozygotes for one or another of these enzyme deficiencies.

Complete deficiency of any of the first four enzymes in the cycle usually leads to severe hyperammonemia in the first 2 to 4 days of life. The patients have irritability, lethargy, and poor feeding that progress rapidly to stupor, seizures, coma, respirator dependence, and death. The plasma ammonia level often exceeds 1000 μM, and urea levels are extremely low. Episodic hyperammonemia occurs in association with periods of endogenous protein catabolism and severely affects patients, such as those with severe OTC deficiency; they almost certainly die or suffer severe neurologic impairment during one of these episodes. Patients with partial deficiency of urea cycle enzymes or those who avoid hyperammonemia in the neonatal period may present at any time later in life, from infancy to adulthood. Older patients have irritability, vomiting, and disorientation, which may progress (as in the infants) to stupor, seizures, coma, and death. These episodes are often precipitated by severe infection, excessive protein intake, parturition, or rarely menstruation, or they may have no apparent cause.

Some general genetic characteristics of defects in the urea cycle are presented in Table 211–1.

ENZYME DEFICIENCIES

DEFICIENCY OF CARBAMOYL PHOSPHATE SYNTHETASE. CPS-1, the first enzyme in the urea cycle, constitutes up to 25% of the mitochondrial matrix protein in liver, and ordinarily all of the carbamyl phosphate synthesized from ammonium and bicarbonate by CPS-1 is used to produce urea. Orotic acid and pyrimidine are products of carbamoylphosphate as well, which is synthesized by a second, independently regulated cytoplasmic enzyme. Patients with both the neonatal and later-onset forms have been described. Diagnosis may be inferred from hyperammonemia, low to absent levels of citrulline in the plasma amino acid profile, and normal or elevated bicarbonate levels. During acute hyperammonemia there is

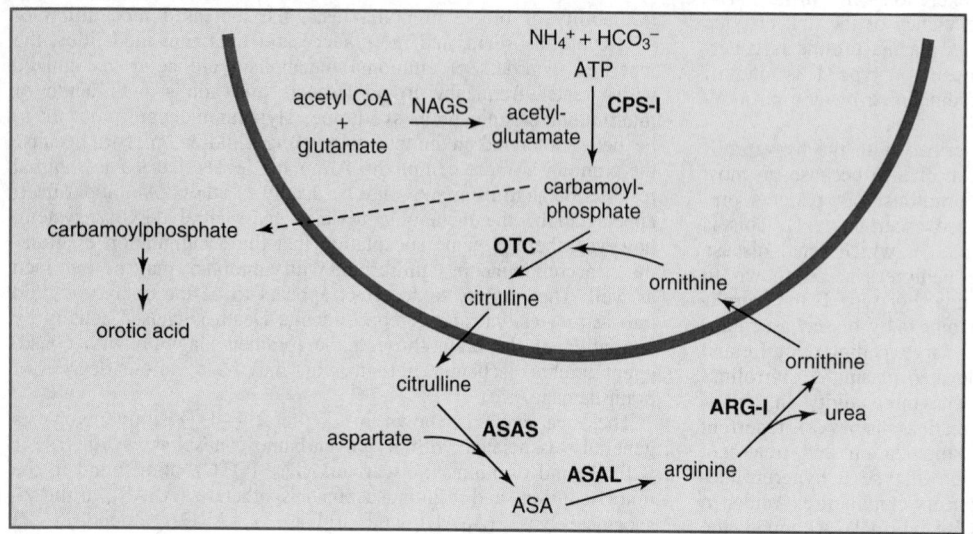

FIGURE 211–1 ■ Abbreviated pathway for the urea cycle. NAGS = *N*-acetylglutamate synthetase; CPS-1 = carbamoyl-phosphate synthetase 1; OTC = ornithine transcarbamoylase; ASAS = argininosuccinate synthetase; ASAL = agininosuccinate lyase; ARG-1 = arginase 1. Enzymes within the bold line function within the mitochondrial matrix.

usually a generalized hyperaminoacidemia with particular prominence of glutamine. Liver transplantation alone offers definitive treatment. Restricting dietary protein, supplementing essential amino acids and citrulline, hospitalizing for "catabolic crises," hemodialysis or peritoneal dialysis, and administering phenylacetate (or phenylbutyrate) and benzoate to divert ammonia to phenylacetylglutamine and benzoylglycine (hippurate) are used to control symptoms and treat crises (Fig. 211–2). Patients with this and other urea cycle defects are prone to develop severe hyperammonemia with valproate anticonvulsant therapy.

DEFICIENCY OF ORNITHINE TRANSCARBAMOYLASE. This mitochondrial enzyme catalyzes the reaction of carbamyl phosphate with ornithine to form citrulline, which is then transported out of the mitochondrion for further metabolism. The acute form of this X-linked enzyme deficiency usually occurs in males. Uncommonly a newborn female may be severely affected, thought to be due to non-random, X-chromosome inactivation. Female carriers of this co-dominant trait usually escape obvious symptoms, but those who have them usually present later in life or at parturition with hyperammonemic crises, some of which may be severe enough to be fatal. A number of males with partial enzyme deficiency may present later as well. Patients with this "later-onset" form of the disease may suffer from severe and otherwise inexplicable protein intolerance. The amino and organic acid profiles resemble those of CPS-1 deficiency. OTC deficiency is distinguished by extraordinarily high levels of orotic acid in the urine, formed when the excess carbamoyl phosphate accumulating in the mitochondrion leaks into the cytoplasm and is channelled into the pyrimidine biosynthetic pathway (see Fig. 211–1). Orotic acid levels may be normal when ammonia has been controlled. Because of this typical clinical biochemical picture, liver biopsy to confirm enzymes is less frequently undertaken than in CPS-1 deficiency. An allopurinol challenge may be necessary to detect carrier females, a test with less than 100% accuracy. The treatment is identical to that described for CPS-1 deficiency.

DEFICIENCY OF ARGININOSUCCINATE SYNTHETASE (CITRULLINEMIA). This cytoplasmic enzyme condenses the citrulline synthesized by OTC with aspartate to form argininosuccinate in a reaction that introduces the second ammonia nitrogen for excretion as urea. ASAS deficiency leads to hyperammonemia, greatly increased blood citrulline levels, and excretion of excessive amounts of citrulline and orotic acid in the urine. Here, too, neonatal, later-onset, or symptomless deficiency of the enzyme has been reported. Genetic heterogeneity at the ASAS locus has been demonstrated by residual enzyme activity or by study of the gene and its messenger RNA.

Treatment is similar to that for CPS-1 and OTC deficiencies except that arginine is supplemented instead of citrulline. Citrulline excretion is more complete than that of ammonia, and managing this condition is somewhat easier than managing hyperammonemia.

DEFICIENCY OF ARGININOSUCCINATE LYASE (ARGININOSUCCINIC ACIDURIA). ASA is cleaved into two smaller product molecules, arginine and fumarate, in a reaction catalyzed by ASA lyase. This enzyme deficiency results in massive accumulation and excretion of ASA. Variable onset or lack of symptoms characterizes this enzyme deficiency as well. ASA is actively secreted by the renal tubules, and its synthesis can be stimulated by stoichiometric amounts of arginine as a source of ornithine to drive the urea cycle. By this means, ammonia levels are rapidly reduced and can be controlled more reliably than in any other urea cycle disorder.

DEFICIENCY OF ARGINASE 1 (HYPERARGININEMIA). Arginase, the final enzyme in the urea cycle, catalyzes the hydrolysis of arginine to urea and ornithine, the latter returned to the mitochondrion to participate in another cycle of ammonia detoxification (see Fig. 211–1). Clinical symptoms of hyperargininemia, the rarest of the urea cycle defects, are of later onset, are more gradual and relentless in progression, and are less frequently or seriously punctuated by apparent episodes of acute hyperammonemia and organic brain syndrome. Rather typically, normal patients begin to develop gait abnormalities and spasticity at age 2 to 3, and cortical and pyramidal tract dysfunction progresses slowly. More than 80% of the reported patients are still alive, some at age 30 or older. The diagnosis is often suspected when arginine levels are found to be elevated in blood or urine. Excess arginine excretion in urine along with secondary cystinuria pattern is more variable and less reliable

Table 211–1 ■ GENETIC CHARACTERISTICS OF DISORDERS OF THE UREA CYCLE

ENZYME DEFECT	INHERITANCE PATTERN	HETEROZYGOTE DETECTION	HETEROZYGOTE SYMPTOMS	PRENATAL DIAGNOSIS*
Carbamoyl phosphate synthetase	AR	No†	No	Yes
Ornithine transcarbamoylase	X-linked	Yes, in most instances*	Yes	Yes
Argininosuccinate synthetase	AR	No†	No	Yes
Argininosuccinate lyase	AR	Yes	No	Yes
Arginase 1	AR	Yes	No	Yes

*With varying degrees of ease.

†Heterozygotes for all disorders can be detected, if the specific base change in the gene has been ascertained. This is not practical at this time outside the research laboratory.

AR = Autosomal recessive.

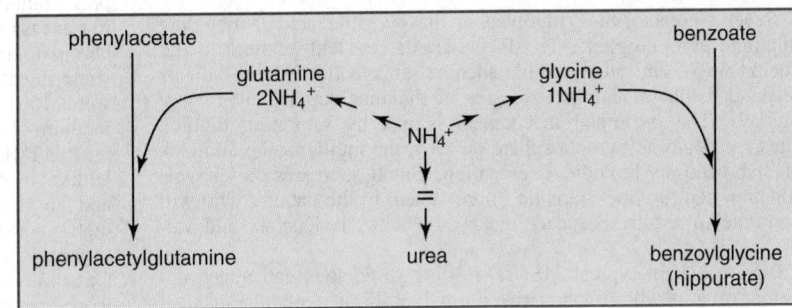

FIGURE 211–2 ■ Mechanisms of ammonia diversion from the urea cycle with administration of sodium phenylacetate and sodium benzoate.

as a screening method. Hyperammonemia is usually seen only during acute catabolic episodes.

Although most patients have been moderately to severely retarded at detection, treatment by limiting protein and diverting ammonia reverses many of the most severe manifestations of the disease, and presymptomatic treatment has allowed two patients to reach the age of 20 or older without apparent clinical manifestations.

FUTURE TREATMENT

Urea cycle defects, originally considered a pediatric problem, are moving into the realm of internal medicine. Internists must cast aside the lactulose used for hyperammonemia of liver failure and gastrointestinal bleeding in favor of diversion therapy and hemodialysis. Soon liver replacement, the artificial liver, and gene therapy will be more widely used. As breakthroughs in gene technology allow us to dissect the pathobiology of the acute catabolic process, efforts to control this process rather than control its consequences will become increasingly important.

Brusilow SW, Horwich AL: Urea cycle enzymes. *In* Scriver CR, Beaudet AL, Sly WS, Valle D (eds): The Metabolic and Molecular Bases of Inherited Disease, 7th ed. New York, McGraw-Hill, 1995. *The definitive clinical and molecular discussion of these inborn errors.*
Elsas III LJ, Acosta PB: Nutritional support of inherited metabolic diseases. *In* Shils ME, Olson JA, Shike M (eds): Modern Nutrition in Health and Disease, 9th ed. Malvern, PA, Lea & Febiger, 1998, 1003–1056. *A practical guide to the nutritional aspects of treating this and other metabolic disorders.*
Leonard JV: Urea cycle disorders. *In* Fernandes J, Saudubray J-M, Van Den Bergh G (eds): Inborn Metabolic Diseases. New York, Springer-Verlag, 1995, p 167. *A practical clinical chapter on urea cycle disorders reflecting a transatlantic perspective.*

212 BRANCHED-CHAIN AMINOACIDURIAS

Louis J. Elsas II

MAPLE SYRUP URINE DISEASE (MSUD). Maple syrup urine disease, also called *branched-chain* α-ketoaciduria, derives its name from the burnt-sugar smell of affected infants. MSUD is caused by impaired branched-chain α-ketoacid dehydrogenase, which catalyzes decarboxylation of the α-ketoacid derivatives of all three of the branched-chain amino acids: leucine, isoleucine, and valine. They are essential amino acids that share branching, aliphatic chains. Isovaleric acidemia affects the next step but only for products of leucine catabolism. Leucine is transaminated to α-ketoisocoproate, which is decarboxylated to isovaleric acid. Isovaleric acidemia is caused by defects in isovaleryl coenzyme A (CoA) dehydrogenase. Both disorders conform to autosomal recessive patterns of inheritance. The affected homozygote for maple syrup urine disease exhibits impaired activity in the branched-chain α-ketoacid dehydrogenase (BCKD) multienzyme complex. This enzyme catalyzes oxidative decarboxylation and transacylation of α-ketoisocoproate, α-keto-β-methylvalerate, and α-ketoisovalerate, which are derived from deamination of leucine, isoleucine, and valine, respectively. The blocked reaction is

$$\text{Branched-chain} - \overset{\displaystyle O}{\overset{\|}{C}} - \text{COOH} + \text{CoASH} + \text{NAD}^+$$

$$\downarrow \text{TP} \sim \text{P}$$

$$\text{Branched-chain} - \overset{\displaystyle O}{\overset{\|}{C}} - \text{CoA} + \text{CO}_2 + \text{NADH} + \text{H}^+$$

If impaired, branched-chain α-ketoacids and amino acids accumulate throughout the body and produce neurotoxicity mechanisms, which include competitive inhibition by branched-chain α-ketoacids of mitochondrial oxidative phosphorylation in the brain.

The disease is caused by mutations in one of six genes, which code for the six different proteins that make up the branched-chain α-ketoacid dehydrogenase multienzyme complex. A wide range of mutations is defined, along with the severity of impaired enzyme and consequent clinical manifestations (Table 212–1).

These mitochondrial proteins are encoded in the nuclear genome. Once translated in the cytosol, they are guided to the mitochondria by their intrinsic amino terminal leader sequences and chaperone proteins. They then transmigrate through outer and inner mitochondria membranes and assemble in the mitochondrial matrix. The six proteins are (1) E1α, and (2) E1β, which produce the dimeric branched-chain α-ketoacid decarboxylase; (3) a branched-chain dihydrolipoamide acyltransferase (E2); (4) lipoamide oxidoreductase (E3); (5) E1 α-kinase; and (6) E1 α-phosphatase.

Table 212–1 ■ GENES, PROTEINS, AND MUTATIONS IN THE HUMAN BRANCHED-CHAIN α-KETOACID DEHYDROGENASE COMPLEX

NAME (FUNCTION)	CHROMOSOME LOCUS	GENE SIZE (kb)	MATURE PROTEIN (kd)	MUTATION
E1α (decarboxylase)	19q13.1–q13.2	55	47	Y393N (Mennonite missense mutation)
E1β (stabilizes decarboxylase)	6p21–p22	100	37	11bp deletion (frameshift with premature STOP)
E2 (acyltransferase)	1p31	68	52	E163STOP
				F215C (exonic and intronic insertions, deletions, and transitions)
E3 (dehydrogenase)	**7q31**	**20**	55	Affects other substrate-specific dehydrogenases (α-ketoglutarate and pyruvate)
E1α kinase (inactivates)	?	?	43	?
E1α phosphatase (activates)	?	?	?	?

Several cofactors are involved in the overall reaction, including thiamine pyrophosphate, TP~P, lipoamide covalently bound to E2, coenzyme A, and nicotinamide adenine dinucleotide. Many patients respond to pharmacologic excesses of thiamine supplement (8 mg/kg/day). The presumed mechanism is that by saturating binding sites for thiamine pyrophosphate on E1α, the multienzyme complex is stabilized to biologic degradation. Small increases in enzyme function can provide dramatic improvement to the patient, who will continue to require reduced intake of leucine, isoleucine, and valine.

DIAGNOSIS. In typical MSUD, feeding difficulties and apnea develop in a newborn who was normal at birth. Convulsions and decorticate rigidity may develop, and before newborn screening affected infants died or were severely damaged. With newborn screening, retrieval, diagnosis, and diet intervention before age 2 weeks, these children not only survive but have reached adulthood.

In surveyed populations the frequency of MSUD varies from 1 in 760 (in Mennonites) to an average U.S. figure of 1 in 200,000 newborns. Atypical cases with less severe clinical manifestations may be missed in newborn screening and appear with intermittent ataxia in later childhood or early adulthood. The diagnosis should be suspected clinically when a patient has intermittent symptoms related to protein ingestion and sweet smell to the earwax. A positive dinitrophenylhydrazine reaction is seen in affected patients' urine, and the diagnosis is confirmed by the abnormal excesses of branched-chain amino acids and keto acids in blood and urine. The enzyme defect is demonstrable in leukocytes and fibroblasts, and prenatal monitoring has been accomplished both biochemically and through DNA analysis of specific mutations when known.

TREATMENT. Treatment is aimed at limiting intake of branched-chain amino acids to prevent accumulation of neurotoxic branched-chain α-ketoacids and at maintaining an anabolic state through non-protein caloric intake. Branched-chain amino acids are essential and must be ingested in quantities sufficient to allow new protein synthesis and normal growth but below levels that result in accumulation of toxic precursors in the blocked reaction. Commercial formulas are necessary to accomplish this goal. In infancy and early childhood, anabolism is encouraged by providing excess calories and maintaining branched-chain amino acid–restricted protein intake at the recommended daily allowance. Treatment is monitored clinically in terms of growth and development and biochemically through analysis of plasma amino acid and urine organic acid concentrations. Because leucine residues are more frequent than isoleucine and valine in natural proteins, care must be taken not to overrestrict isoleucine and valine while attempting to lower blood concentrations of leucine by restricting natural dietary protein. Thiamine supplements allow increased natural protein intake in thiamine-responsive patients. Chronic acidosis may deplete carnitine, which should also be monitored in blood and supplemented if deficient.

ISOVALERIC ACIDEMIA. Isovaleryl CoA is the product formed from BCKD action on α-ketoisocaproate (leucine's derivative). Isovaleryl CoA is then converted to β-methylcrotonyl CoA by isovaleryl CoA dehydrogenase.

When isovaleryl dehydrogenase is impaired, isovaleric acid accumulates in blood and urine and produces a foul odor similar to that of rancid cheese or sweaty feet. Symptoms are severe in the first week of life and consist of vomiting, acidosis, hypoglycemia, tremors, coma, and death. Leukopenia, anemia, thrombocytopenia, and hyperammonemia may occur during acute attacks. Emergency therapy consists of eliminating dietary leucine and supplementing with intravenous, oral, and colonic infusion of glycine (300 mg/kg/day) to provide an alternate excretory pathway for the non-toxic adduct, isovaleryl glycine. Carnitine (100 mg/kg/day) may provide nontoxic adducts of isovaleryl carnitine. Both adducts are excreted in the urine. Emergency therapy also requires producing anabolism by using excess calories from carbohydrates, fat, and non-leucine-containing protein. As patients mature, they have less frequent attacks and are developmentally normal. "Attacks" are caused by excess leucine ingestion, starvation, infections, or other causes of catabolism. Chronic intermittent forms of this disorder have not been differentiated from acute infantile forms at the biochemical or molecular level of enzyme or gene analysis and may result from epigenetic phenomena.

DIAGNOSIS. The diagnosis is suspected as a result of the clinical presentation and associated odor and is established by demonstrating excess isovaleric acid and its adducts in the urine by gas-liquid chromatography. The gene has been cloned and sequenced and some mutations have been defined. The gene is located on chromosome 15q13 and the coding sequence has homology to short- and medium-chain acyldehydrogenase.

TREATMENT. Chronic therapy includes reduced intake of leucine. Unlike in MSUD, normally valine and isoleucine are catabolized and are required as essential nutrients in normal amounts in the diet. Supplements of glycine (90 to 100 mg/kg/day) and carnitine (10 mg/kg/day) are used as part of chronic dietary management. Outcome is excellent in both infantile and later-onset forms of isovaleric acidemia diseases if the acute, irreversible effects of the neonatal disease are prevented.

Danner DJ, Elsas LJ: Disorders of branched chain amino and keto acid metabolism. *In* Scriver CR, Beaudet A, Sly W, Valle D (eds): The Metabolic and Molecular Bases of Inherited Disease, 7th ed. New York, McGraw-Hill Book Co., 1995. *Sophisticated discussion of clinical, biochemical, and pathophysiologic characteristics of these diseases (268 references).*
Elsas LJ, Acosta PB: Nutrition support of inherited metabolic disease. *In* Shils ME, Olson JE, Shike M (eds): Modern Nutrition in Health and Disease, 9th ed. Malvern, PA, Lea & Febiger, 1998. *A complete approach to dietary therapy of these diseases.*

213 HOMOCYSTINURIA

Bruce A. Barshop

DEFINITIONS. Homocysteine is a non-protein amino acid and an intermediate in methionine metabolism that arises when methionine (through S-adenosylmethionine) acts as a donor in methylation reactions (Fig. 213–1). The fate of homocysteine is either remethylation to methionine or transulfuration (through cystathionine) of serine to cysteine. Homocystinuria results from defective disposal of homocysteine because of a defect in either transulfuration or remethylation. The classic finding of the disulfide homocystine in urine gives this class of disorders its common name. The free sulfhydryl form, homocysteine, is present in lower amounts in blood; total homocyst(e)ine is the term used to described the mix of sulfhydryl and disulfide. The defining finding in blood is hyperhomocyst(e)inemia, which is distributed about 10% as free homocysteine and 90% as protein-bound and soluble disulfides (homocystine, cysteine-SS-homocysteine, etc.).

ETIOLOGY. The classic form of homocystinuria is cystathionine β-synthase deficiency, which results in decreased transulfuration and hypermethioninemic hyperhomocyst(e)inemia. Homocystinuria may also result from defective remethylation, as in a deficiency of methylenetetrahydrofolate reductase, or from a disorder of the delivery, generation, or utilization of the methylcobalamin cofactor of methionine synthase. Defects of remethylation give rise to hyperhomocyst(e)inemia with normal or low methionine. All these disorders are inherited in an autosomal recessive manner (Table 213–1).

INCIDENCE AND PREVALENCE. Minimum estimates of the incidence of cystathionine β-synthase deficiency by newborn screening programs have ranged from 1:300,000 to 1:60,000 live births, varying with the population and method. Estimates of its incidence in Europe have been in the range of 1:40,000, which corresponds to a carrier (heterozygote) frequency of about 1%. The incidence of severe homocysteine remethylation defects appears to be less than 1:500,000. On the other hand, partial remethylation deficiencies seem to have a much greater incidence, which may be clinically relevant in predisposing individuals to thrombotic disorders; evidence of deficiency has been reported in 15 to 30% of some series of patients presenting with vaso-occlusive disease.

PATHOGENESIS AND MECHANISMS. Homocysteine has effects on vascular endothelium, platelets, and coagulation factors that predispose to thrombosis. Modification of connective tissue proteins may cause the skeletal and ocular manifestations associated with homocystinuria. These effects are particularly likely in relation to fibrillin, which is a component of the matrix of periosteum and perichondrium, the major component of the zonular fibers of the

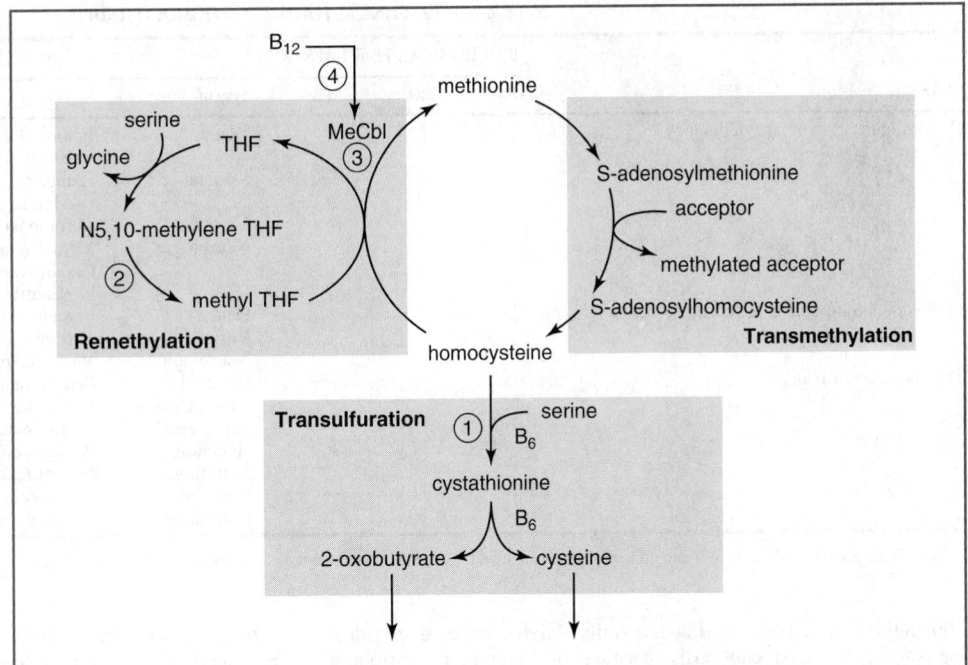

FIGURE 213–1 ■ Pathways of homocysteine metabolism. The systems of transmethylation, remethylation, and transulfuration are marked. Steps discussed are numbered: (1) cystathionine β-synthase; (2) methylenetetrahydrofolate reductase; (3) methionine synthase and methyltransferase reductase; (4) systems of cobalamin absorption, distribution, and reduction. THF = tetrahydrofolate; MeCbl = methylcobalamin; B_{12} = cyanocobalamin/hydroxocobalamin; B_6 = pyridoxine.

ocular lens, and a protein singularly rich in cysteine. Fibrillin structure may be affected either by cysteine limitation or by homocysteinylation; the result is features of homocystinuria that are also associated with fibrillin mutations (Marfan syndrome). The neurologic effects of homocysteine may be due predominantly to agonism of the N-methyl-D-aspartate receptor by homocysteic acid, although cerebral vascular effects may contribute as well.

CLINICAL MANIFESTATIONS. Cystathionine β-synthase deficiency is pleiotropic, with effects in the eye, skeleton, and central nervous and vascular systems (Table 213–2). Eye and skeletal system changes resemble those in Marfan syndrome. Non-traumatic dislocation of the ocular lens can be an initial finding. Some abnormality of the skeletal system develops in almost all untreated patients. Between one third and three fourths of untreated patients have mild or moderate mental retardation, and cerebrovascular thrombosis may play a role in the neurologic picture. Affected patients have a lifelong danger of thromboembolic phenomena, which are the major cause of mortality in untreated disease. Arterial and venous occlusion, in small or large vessels, may occur at any time in life, including infancy. Treatment with pyridoxine, the cofactor of the enzyme, may be effective in nearly half of these patients, particularly those with relatively high residual activity and spared amounts of immunologically detectable enzyme. Blood total homocyst(e)ine concentrations may be intermediately elevated in heterozygotes, particularly after a methionine load, and heterozygotes are at some increased risk for vaso-occlusive events. Although increased vascular complications have not been formally demonstrated in outcome studies of obligate heterozygotes, a considerable number of studies show a highly disproportionate fraction of patients with various vaso-occlusive complications who manifest either total blood homocyst(e)ine concentrations or fibroblast cystathionine β-synthase activities that fall in the range observed for heterozygotes.

Methylenetetrahydrofolate reductase deficiency has been described in a limited number of patients, with a spectrum of manifestations including neurologic symptoms, thromboses, and lens dislocation, but without conspicuous skeletal changes. Partial deficiencies and thermolabile variants have been observed in otherwise normal subjects who have premature vaso-occlusive disorders. Polymorphisms are also found in the methylenetetrahydrofolate reductase gene in association with spinal closure defects, a class of disease that has been known to be influenced by folate. Cobalamin metabolic disorders generally occur in early childhood and are characterized by neurologic symptoms, megaloblastic anemia, and in some cases, methylmalonic acidemia.

DIAGNOSIS. Qualitative detection using sodium nitroprusside led to the recognition of homocystinuria early in the history of biochemical genetics, but it is neither specific nor sensitive. Assay of plasma amino acids by routine methods may not reveal homocysteine because of the high degree of protein binding. Because of lower protein concentrations, routine amino acid analysis of urine is more successful, hence the common name homocystinuria. The preferred diagnostic method is total homocyst(e)ine, which is measured in plasma treated with a reducing agent to release bound homocysteine before deproteinization. Plasma amino acids will indicate a transulfuration or remethylation defect, depending on the presence or absence of hypermethioninemia (see Table 213–2). The clinical diagnosis of remethylation defects is facilitated by detection of urine methylmalonate and blood B_{12} and folate. The normal range of total homocyst(e)ine in blood extends up to around 15 μmol/L and may be more than 50% higher 2 to 4 hours after an oral methionine load. A standard methionine load (100 mg/kg) may identify individuals with partial defects, which could increase the susceptibility to vascular disease.

TREATMENT. Cystathionine β-synthase deficiency is responsive to the cofactor pyridoxine in about 50% of cases. Doses of 100 to

Table 213–1 ■ GENETIC DEFECTS ASSOCIATED WITH HOMOCYSTINURIA

FUNCTIONAL DEFECT	COMMON NAME	ENZYME DEFECT	CHROMOSOME LOCUS
Transulfuration	"Classic" homocystinuria	Cystathionine β-synthase	22q22.3
Remethylation	Folate-dependent homocystinuria	Methylenetetrahydrofolate reductase	1p36.3
	Cbl G	Methionine synthase (methyltransferase)	5p15.2-p15.3
	Cbl E	Methyltransferase reductase	1q43
Cobalamin transport	TC-II	Transcobalamin II	22q11-q13.1
	Cbl F	Lysosomal B_{12} translocase	—
Cobalamin reductase	Cbl C, Cbl D	Unknown	—

Table 213–2 ■ CLINICAL FEATURES OF HOMOCYSTINURIA

| CLASS | BIOCHEMICAL FEATURES | | | CLINICAL FEATURES | |
	Hcys	met	MMA	System	Signs
Cystathionine β-synthase deficiency	↑	↑	−	Ocular	Ectopia lentis, myopia, glaucoma, optic atrophy, retinal detachment
				Skeletal	Elongated and thinned bones, arachnodactyly, genu valgum, pectus malformation, scoliosis
				Vascular	Thromboembolic events (arterial or venous)
				Neurologic	Mental retardation often in untreated cases
					Cerebrovascular thromboses, seizures
					Psychiatric disorders, personality disorder
Methylenetetrahydrofolate reductase deficiency	↑	↓	−	Ocular	Ectopia lentis
				Vascular	Thromboses
				Neurologic	Variable–psychiatric to severe neurologic
Transcobalamin II deficiency	−/↑	−/↓	+/−	Hematologic	Pancytopenia, macrocytosis
				Pansystemic	MMA, ketoacidosis, stomatitis
Cbl F	−/↑	?	+/−	Pansystemic	MMA, macrocytosis, stomatitis
Cbl C, Cbl D	−/↑	−/↓	+	Hematologic	Pancytopenia
				Neurologic	Mental retardation
Cbl E, Cbl G	↑	−/↓	−	Vascular	Vaso-occlusive phenomena
				Neurologic	Spasticity, dystonia

Hcys = homocyst(e)inemia/homocystinuria; met = plasma methionine; MMA = methylmalonic acidemia; Cbl = cobalamin.

500 mg/day have been used successfully. Higher doses of pyridoxine should be used cautiously because of the risk of peripheral neuropathy. Responsiveness is documented by the elimination of free homocysteine in blood and urine as pyridoxine is added, but measurement of total homocyst(e)ine demonstrates that the effect is generally far less than complete. Betaine (*N,N,N*-trimethylglycine) has recently become available commercially, and it is effective in reducing homocysteine through an alternative remethylation step. Betaine is generally given at 6 g/day in divided doses, but considerably higher doses have been used. It is particularly important in pyridoxine-unresponsive cases but may also be used as an adjunct in responsive patients. In the absence of vitamin responsiveness, special diets are adopted to restrict methionine and supplement cysteine. Folic acid may be effective in remethylation defects, and it is also generally used as a supplement (10 to 20 mg/day) in all forms of homocystinuria. Vitamin B$_{12}$ preparations may be life saving in disorders of cobalamin metabolism, although its effectiveness in the most common forms of cobalamin C or D defects is generally far from complete. Initial doses are usually 1000 μg/day, and hydroxocobalamin may be more effective than cyanocobalamin. It is prudent to adopt measures to decrease thrombosis, such as using low-dose aspirin or dipyridamole and avoiding smoking and birth control pills. Nitrous oxide may also be relatively contraindicated inasmuch as it can inhibit methionine synthase. Surgery poses serious risks but can be performed safely as long as attention is paid to hydration and coagulation status.

PROGNOSIS. In cystathionine β-synthase deficiency, pyridoxine responsiveness generally correlates with higher residual activity, and the prognosis is significantly better than that for unresponsive cases, with or without treatment. Skeletal, ocular, vascular, and neurologic risks are all reduced with successful treatment. Without early institution of treatment, the median IQ in a large outcome study was 57 for unresponsive and 78 for responsive patients. With early treatment, pyridoxine-unresponsive patients have nearly normal median IQ. With treatment in responsive patients, the prognosis for intellectual development is very good, but significant increases in total homocyst(e)ine generally still persist and some increased risk of vascular complications probably does remain.

Kraus JP: Molecular basis of phenotype expression in homocystinuria. J Inherit Metab Dis 17:383, 1994. *Discussion of the early mutational analysis in cystathionine synthase, with interesting correlations.*
Mudd SH, Levy HL, Skovby F: Disorders of transulfuration. *In* Scriver CR, Beaudet AL, Sly WS, Valle D (eds): The Metabolic and Molecular Bases of Inherited Disease, vol 1. New York, McGraw-Hill, 1995, pp 1279–1327. *A definitive review with extensive references; although a new edition is awaited, this reference is invaluable.*
Nygard O, Vollset SE, Refsum H, et al: Total plasma homocysteine and cardiovascular risk profile: The Hordaland study. JAMA 274:1526, 1995. *A large population study regarding homocysteine in association with cardiovascular risk factors, with references to other studies treating it as an independent risk factor.*
Rozen R: Genetic predisposition to hyperhomocysteinemia: Deficiency of methylenetetrahydrofolate reductase (MTHFR). Thromb Haemost 78:523, 1997. *A review of methylenetetrahydrofolate reductase in homocystinuria and multifactorial disease.*

■ INHERITED DISORDERS OF CONNECTIVE TISSUE

214 THE MUCOPOLYSACCHARIDOSES

Hans C. Andersson ■ *Emmanuel Shapira*

The mucopolysaccharidoses (MPSs) are a heterogeneous group of inherited lysosomal storage disorders. The common feature of these disorders is intracellular storage and urinary excretion of glycosaminoglycans (GAGs), previously termed acidic mucopolysaccharides. GAGs result from the proteolytic cleavage of large macromolecules—the proteoglycans. They are highly glycosylated and sulfated molecules that are normally degraded in a stepwise manner in the lysosome by specific enzymes that either cleave terminal sulfate or glycosyl groups or acetylate the GAG to facilitate further degradation. MPSs result from deficient activity of one of these lysosomal enzymes. This deficiency arrests further degradation of GAGs and leads to their storage in various tissues. Such storage causes progressive disruption of cellular function and leads to physical deformation of various tissues.

The group of MPS disorders demonstrates two principles of

Table 214–1 ■ THE MUCOPOLYSACCHARIDOSES

MPS TYPE	EPONYM	ENZYME DEFICIENCY	URINARY GAG	CLINICAL FEATURES
I				
I-H	Hurler	α-L-Iduronidase	DS HS	Onset <2 yr, early corneal clouding and organomegaly, coarse facies, MR; later onset of cardiorespiratory failure
I-S	Scheie	α-L-Iduronidase	DS	Later onset (>5 yr), similar to I-H but with normal intellect, milder skeletal involvement, and slower progression
II	Hunter	Iduronate sulfatase	DS HS	Onset <4 yr, early skeletal involvement, organomegaly, but no corneal clouding; X-linked inheritance, MR usually severe; mild form with normal intelligence and slower progression
III	Sanfilippo			Same for all types (A–D)
IIIA		Heparan-N-sulfatase	HS	Onset >2 yr, rapidly progressive neurologic/intellectual regression; late mild visceral and skeletal involvement
IIIB		α-N-acetylglucosaminidase		
IIIC		N-acetyl-CoA: α-glucosaminide acetyltransferase		
IIID		N-acetylglucosamine-6-sulfatase		
IV	Morquio			
IVA		N-acetyl-galactosamine-6-sulfatase	KS	Onset <4 yr, mainly skeletal involvement, rapidly progressive kyphoscoliosis, short stature, odontoid hypoplasia, late corneal clouding, normal intellect
IVB		β-Galactosidase	KS	Same as IVA but MR may develop
VI	Maroteaux-Lamy	Arylsulfatase B	DS	Onset <4 yr, phenotype as in MPS I-H, but with normal intellect; rare adult form with slower progression
VII	Sly	β-Glucuronidase	HS DS ChS	Variable age of onset, MR, and skeletal involvement; some patients have hydrops fetalis

MPS = mucopolysaccharide; GAG = glycosaminoglycan; DS = dermatan sulfate; HS = heparan sulfate; MR = mental retardation; KS = keratan sulfate; ChS = chondroitin sulfate.

human genetics—heterogeneity and variability. Heterogeneity refers to the observation that mutations in different enzymes located at different loci can lead to clinically indistinguishable phenotypes. This phenomenon is exemplified by the four types of MPS III (Sanfilippo). Within each type of MPS, considerable clinical variability exists regarding the age of onset, the rate of progression, and the extent to which various organs are involved. Typically, these disorders are manifested within a spectrum of severity from early, severe childhood forms to milder, late childhood or adolescent forms. This clinical variability can sometimes be explained by the biochemical and molecular observation of particular mutations with varying degrees of residual enzyme activity. Many of the genes coding for enzymes involved in the MPS diseases have been cloned, thus making possible mutation analysis in individual patients. The more severely affected patients have a mutation resulting in the complete absence of detectable enzyme protein in their tissues, whereas mildly affected patients have point mutations leading to an amino acid substitution with detectable enzyme protein but markedly decreased residual activity. Other factors in addition to the specific gene mutation may also be involved in modifying the patient's clinical characteristics.

CLINICAL FEATURES. Most patients with MPS diseases appear normal at birth, with pathologic findings gradually developing in the first 2 years of life. The various MPSs share multiple organ system involvement, organomegaly, dysostosis multiplex, and facial coarsening. Dysostosis multiplex refers to the collective bony abnormalities, including a thickened calvarium, J-shaped sella, anterior vertebral hypoplasia leading to kyphoscoliosis, impaired long bone growth with irregular metaphyses, poorly formed pelvis, and oar-shaped ribs that invariably lead to short stature. MPS I, II, III, and VII are usually also characterized by central nervous system (CNS) storage, and consequently result in progressive mental retardation. MPS IV (Morquio) spares the CNS but has unusually severe skeletal abnormalities, including odontoid hypoplasia that may become life-threatening. In many of the MPSs, sensorineural and conductive hearing loss and vision defects (corneal and retinal) may also contribute to poor intellectual development. Cardiac disease from GAG stored in valve leaflets, endocardium, myocardium, and coronary arteries is a common feature in middle childhood and often the cause of death.

The MPSs are inherited as autosomal recessive disorders, with the exception of MPS II, which has an X-linked mode of inheritance. The incidence of each of the various MPSs is relatively rare, in the range of 1 in 40,000 to 1 in 100,000 live births. Table 214–1 summarizes some of the distinguishing clinical and biochemical features of the MPSs.

DIAGNOSIS. Whenever the diagnosis of MPS is suspected, a urine-screening test for GAGs should be performed. The most commonly used screening test is the toluidine blue spot test; it is relatively sensitive but has a significant false-positive rate because of reactivity with chondroitin sulfate, which is a normal finding in the urine. In some patients with MPS III and IV, the spot test can be falsely negative. In patients with a positive spot test and those suspected of being falsely negative, the various GAGs in the urine should be identified by either thin-layer chromatography or electrophoresis. Based on the clinical findings and the pattern of urinary GAGs, the diagnosis should be established by demonstration of the specific enzyme deficiency in leukocytes, fibroblasts, or other tissues (see Table 214–1). Mutation analysis is available for most MPS disorders, and a genotype-phenotype correlation has been established for some mutations.

MANAGEMENT AND TREATMENT. SUPPORTIVE CARE. In managing families with an MPS-affected member, proper counseling is one of the most important and difficult tasks (see Chapter 37). Basic explanation of the pathophysiology of the disease, while emphasizing that nothing that the parents did or did not do led to the disorder, can alleviate the guilt and anger that parents of children with newly diagnosed MPS experience. The risk for other unaffected family members should be provided, including the option of prenatal diagnosis in future pregnancies in all family members with an increased risk for having affected offspring.

Treatment of patients with MPS is mainly symptomatic because treatments of the primary defect are few and variably effective. Supportive treatment should be aimed at the following complications:

1. Orthopedic: Because of the generalized and progressive nature of the skeletal involvement, a conservative orthopedic approach is most appropriate, with minimization of surgical treatment. Surgical intervention is critical in patients with spinal cord com-

pression and atlantoaxial instability. Orthopedic shoes and ankle braces can be used to maintain mobility in the early stages of the disease. In some patients, elongating the Achilles tendon may be helpful. Surgery is advised for carpal tunnel syndrome when progressive median nerve compression is documented.

2. Cardiorespiratory: Early alveolar involvement is relatively common in some of the MPSs. Small airway obstruction by accumulated storage material, thickened mucosal secretions, hypertrophy of the tonsils/adenoids, and the associated macroglossia contribute to the respiratory problems. Sleep apnea should be considered and treated in the early stages of the disease, whereas tracheostomy might be considered in very advanced stages of the disorder. Managing a tracheostomy can be difficult because of tenacious secretions. Cardiac insufficiency may be palliated by medical therapy, but valvular dysfunction is more difficult to correct, especially because these are very high-risk anesthesia patients.

3. Hernias: Inguinal and umbilical hernias are relatively common and often require surgical correction.

4. Neurologic: Only the relatively rare complication of hydrocephalus can be treated by ventriculoperitoneal shunting. Anticipatory diagnostic studies should attempt to ascertain patients at risk for atlantoaxial dislocation.

5. Anesthesia: Patients with MPS should be considered at high risk whenever general anesthesia is contemplated because of the associated respiratory complications, temporomandibular ankylosis, and atlantoaxial instability. General anesthesia should be restricted to mandatory surgical procedures that cannot be performed under local anesthesia.

6. Dental care: Dental care is a relatively common problem in MPSs because of the decreased mouth opening, gingival hypertrophy, and poor dental hygiene in patients with mental retardation. Awareness of the need for continuous dental care should be maintained.

ENZYME AND GENE THERAPY. Attempts to treat patients with MPS types I and II by high-volume plasma transfusions were made nearly 25 years ago. The amount of enzyme that could be provided with the maximal plasma transfusion led to some decreased urinary excretion of GAGs but no meaningful phenotypic improvement. Attempts to purify large quantities of enzymes from human tissues (placental) or by genetic engineering are currently under way in several laboratories. Thus far, the amount of purified enzyme required for clinical trials is not available for MPS therapy. The additional problem of targeting enzyme to the affected tissue, especially the brain, must still be overcome.

Enzyme replacement by bone marrow transplantation has been attempted in a limited number of patients. Some of the patients with MPS VI who have received a bone marrow transplant had significant clinical improvement with complete or nearly complete arrest of the progressive disorder. The recent national collaborative study of bone marrow transplantation in patients with MPS I suggests an improved developmental outcome when compared with untransplanted patients, especially when transplantation is conducted before 2 years of age. Bone marrow transplantation did not prevent the severe skeletal deformities in MPS IV or the severe neurologic regression in patients with MPS III. The clinical indications for bone marrow transplantation in patients with MPS I-H and MPS II have not been established because of a lack of consistent improvement in the neurologic sequelae. Because transplantation can only arrest the progression but not reverse the symptoms, attempts were made to provide this treatment to patients in the early stages of the disease. It is not clear whether the few patients who appeared to benefit from bone marrow transplantation had mutations with residual activity and therefore had better outcomes. The correlation of genotype with phenotype that is becoming available might enable a conclusive answer to this question.

Gene therapy (see Chapter 33) for MPSs by providing the normal gene carried by one vector or another to the affected tissue remains a desirable goal for the future. Major hurdles that need to be overcome include choosing the vector, establishing stable incorporation of the normal gene, and targeting the gene to the affected tissue.

Gieselmann V: Lysosomal storage diseases. Biochem Biophys Acta 1270:1, 1995. *An excellent review of the molecular understanding of lysosomal enzymes and their mutations, with an emphasis on genotype-phenotype correlation.*

Neufeld EF, Muenzer J: The mucopolysaccharide storage diseases. *In* Scriver CR, Beaudet AL, Sly WS, Valle D (eds): The Metabolic and Molecular Bases of Inherited Disease, 7th ed. New York, McGraw-Hill, 1995. *The most comprehensive review of MPSs available in the definitive reference text for metabolic diseases. This discussion of basic science and clinical issues related to lysosomal storage diseases offers a biochemical understanding of these diseases.*

Peters C, Shapiro EG, Anderson J, et al: 1. Hurler syndrome: II. Outcome of HLA-genotypically identical sibling and HLA-haploidentical related donor bone marrow transplantation in fifty-four children. The Storage Disease Collaborative Study Group. Blood 91:2601, 1998. *This study suggests that bone marrow transplantation may slow the neurologic progression and offer prolonged survival of MPS I-H patients if performed early and with HLA genotypically identical siblings or HLA-haploidentical related donors.*

Shapiro SG, Lockman LA, Balthazor M, Krivit W: Neuropsychological outcomes of several storage diseases with and without bone marrow transplantation. J Inherit Metab Dis 18:413, 1995. *This paper reviews the intellectual outcomes after bone marrow transplantation in a number of lysosomal storage diseases and fails to provide convincing proof of the treatment's efficacy.*

Whitley CB: The mucopolysaccharidoses. *In* Beighton P (ed): McKusick's Heritable Disorders of Connective Tissue, 5th ed. St Louis, Mosby–Year Book, 1993. *An extremely readable clinical summary of MPSs with many illustrative graphs and clinical photographs. Gives the non-geneticist a concise overview of the MPSs.*

215 MARFAN SYNDROME

Reed Edwin Pyeritz

DEFINITION. Marfan syndrome is characterized by autosomal dominant inheritance; pleiotropic features in multiple tissues and organs, including the ocular, skeletal, muscular, cardiovascular, and pulmonary systems and skin; and a defect in the extracellular microfibril.

ETIOLOGY AND PATHOGENESIS. The cause of Marfan syndrome was defined in 1991 when mutations were discovered in the gene encoding fibrillin-1, the principal component of the extracellular microfibril. This gene, *FBN1*, spans over 200 kb of chromosome 15 and consists of 65 exons specifying a 365-kd glycoprotein. Over 200 different mutations have been described in persons with Marfan syndrome, with very few recurrences in unrelated individuals. Fibrillin monomers polymerize and combine with incompletely characterized other proteins to form microfibrils. Microfibrils exist in the extracellular matrices of most tissues and perform various functions. In the eye, microfibrils are the zonules that attach the lens to the ciliary bodies. In skin, microfibrils are arrayed perpendicular to the epidermal-dermal junction and seemingly have a structural role. Deeper in the dermis, in the media of arteries, and in the lung, microfibrils combine with tropoelastin to form elastic fibers. The pathogenesis of Marfan syndrome stems from the diverse functions normally played by the microfibrils, many of which are unclear. Although subluxation of the ocular lens is directly attributable to defective microfibrils, how these structures are involved in controlling bone growth is unknown. The predisposition to aortic root dilatation and aortic dissection undoubtedly stems from the defective elastic fibers, but the intermediate steps are still the subject of much experimental work.

PREVALENCE. Marfan syndrome is one end of a spectrum of heritable disorders of connective tissue, and the line of demarcation among these other disorders is arbitrary. Thus, prevalence is something of an artificial concept. However, estimates of classic Marfan syndrome in all populations range from 1 per 3000 to 10,000. No racial or ethnic group seems predisposed. About one fourth of newly diagnosed individuals represent the first case in the family; the cause is a new mutation in the egg or the sperm that participated in that conception. A paternal age effect, which is typical of many autosomal dominant disorders, strongly suggests that most new mutations occur in spermatocytes.

PATHOLOGY. In the eye, the globe tends to be elongated and the cornea flattened. The lens subluxation, which is present in only about 50% of patients, is typically superior. The lenticular cataract is nuclear and otherwise unremarkable. The elastic fibers of the skin and the aortic media show varying degrees of fragmentation and disarray. Immunohistopathologic analysis with a primary antibody against fibrillin shows decreased presence of fibrillin associated with the elastic fibers. However, this assay is neither sensitive nor specific enough to be used as a diagnostic test.

Aortic dilatation usually involves only the sinuses of Valsalva and the proximal ascending aorta. The histopathology used to be called *cystic medial necrosis,* but this term is imprecise because there are no cysts (just pools of proteoglycan) and little, if any, necrosis. *Medial degeneration* is a better term, but in any event, the histopathology is not specific for Marfan syndrome. The mitral apparatus shows the same myxomatous alterations found in idiopathic mitral valve prolapse; some patients have considerable redundancy in the mitral leaflets and dilatation of the annulus, whereas a small percentage develop marked calcification of the mitral annulus. Dissection typically occurs after the root has dilated and begins just above the coronary ostia. The dissection may be confined to the ascending aorta, but it usually progresses along the entire course and past the bifurcation. Occlusion of a coronary ostium accounts for some sudden death in persons with acute ascending dissection. Retrograde dissection produces pericardial tamponade, the most common cause of sudden death. About 15% of dissections begin in the proximal descending thoracic aorta (type B).

CLINICAL MANIFESTATIONS. All of the manifestations show considerable variability, even among relatives. Patients are generally taller than their genes and environment would otherwise predict, but few are exceptionally tall. The stature is disproportionate, with arms and legs particularly long. The ribs also overgrow, and push the sternum in (pectus excavatum) or out (pectus carinatum). Joint laxity is common, especially of the elbows, wrists, and digits; however, congenital contractures of the elbows and digits also occur. Ligamentous laxity also contributes to the predisposition to scoliosis and to flat feet (pes planus). The palate tends to be narrow and high, and the teeth are crowded and maloccluded. Skeletal muscle development is poor in many persons, which contributes to the asthenic habitus. Lens dislocation can be present at birth or appear at any time during growth of the eye. Myopia is the most common ocular sign and can be severe. Strabismus and astigmatism are also common. If the ocular problems are not detected in early childhood, amblyopia becomes a permanent problem. Glaucoma and cataract are much more common than in the young and middle-aged adult without Marfan syndrome. The lung is subject to spontaneous pneumothorax from rupture of apical blebs (5%). The dura stretches in the lumbosacral region, producing a capacious thecal sac (dural ectasia) and occasionally anterior meningoceles, which can cause radicular pain and neuropathy and have occasionally been misdiagnosed as ovarian cysts.

The life-threatening complications are mainly cardiovascular. The aortic root may be enlarged at birth and typically dilates progressively throughout life. This process is painless and, in the absence of appropriate imaging, goes unrecognized until the symptoms of aortic regurgitation or aortic dissection appear. When the aorta is substantially dilated, the risk of dissection during pregnancy and the peripartum is high. Mitral valve prolapse occurs in most persons with Marfan syndrome and shows the same characteristics as in the general population, although the tendency to progress is higher in individuals with Marfan syndrome. Severe mitral regurgitation is the most common indication for cardiac surgery in children with Marfan syndrome.

DIFFERENTIAL DIAGNOSIS. Marfan syndrome is one end of a continuum of connective tissue disorders that includes some variants of Ehlers-Danlos syndrome, mitral valve prolapse syndrome and the MASS phenotype, familial aortic dissection, familial aortic aneurysm, familial ectopia lentis, congenital contractural arachnodactyly, and the Stickler syndrome. The diagnostic criteria are based on the clinical features and rely heavily on major criteria that are uncommon in the general population, such as ectopia lentis, aortic dissection, and dural ectasia. Testing of fibrillin-1 or *FBN1* for mutations is of limited benefit, because defects in this gene have also been found in patients with many of the related conditions one is attempting to exclude. The exceptions include studying relatives of someone with Marfan syndrome in whom an *FBN1* mutation has been found and linkage analysis using markers in and around *FBN1* in families large and cooperative enough for such studies. Homocystinuria due to deficiency of cystathionine β-synthase has a similar skeletal and ocular phenotype in some respects but is also accompanied by mental retardation and a risk of occlusive vascular disease; analysis of plasma homocysteine excludes this diagnosis.

TREATMENT AND CARE. The key to effective management is early diagnosis. This is much more easily achieved when a family history of Marfan syndrome heightens awareness and suspicion. Unfortunately, in some patients the syndrome is not detected until a major complication occurs. Diagnosis of the first case in any family should prompt evaluation of close relatives.

Early evaluation by an ophthalmologist familiar with Marfan syndrome is key to preventing amblyopia. With improved ocular surgery, lens removal for valid indications is much less risky. Little can be done to affect growth, although young girls predicted to become exceptionally tall can be taken through puberty early by administering estrogen and progesterone and thereby reduce their adult height. Scoliosis screening should begin in early childhood and bracing instituted. Curves greater than about 40 degrees require surgical stabilization. Severe pectus excavatum can be surgically repaired to improve respiratory mechanics and to present the cardiovascular surgeon with improved access to the heart and aorta.

One key to managing the cardiovascular features is echocardiography. By this tool, the size of the aortic root can be followed, cardiac and valvular function quantified, and the effects of therapy gauged. The most effective therapy is early administration of a β-adrenergic blocking agent. The intent is to reduce both inotropy and chronotropy to reduce hemodynamic stress on the aorta and delay or prevent dilatation and dissection. When the aortic root reaches 50 to 55 mm in the adult, strong consideration to prophylactic aortic replacement should be given. The long-term responses to this approach have been gratifying, with life expectancy having risen over the past three decades from the mid-40s to the late 60s.

Dietz HC, Pyeritz RE: Mutations in the human gene for fibrillin-1 (*FBN1*) in the Marfan syndrome and related disorders. Hum Mol Genet 4:1799–1809, 1995. *A review of the first 100 mutations in fibrillin-1 associated with Marfan syndrome and disorders often considered in the differential diagnosis.*
Gott VL, Greene PS, Alejo DE, Cameron DE, Naftel DC, Miller DC, Gillinov AM, Laschinger JC, Pyeritz RE: Surgery for ascending aortic disease in Marfan patients: A multicenter study. N Engl J Med 1999;340:in press. *Long-term outcomes of 676 patients undergoing aortic surgery; confirms the highly positive outlook for patients having prophylactic repair.*
Pyeritz RE: Marfan syndrome and other disorders of fibrillin. *In* Rimoin DL, Connor JM, Pyeritz RE (eds): Principles and Practice of Medical Genetics, 3rd ed. New York, Churchill Livingstone, 1997, pp 1027–1066. *A review of the clinical, pathologic, and molecular aspects of this group of related disorders.*
Shores J, Berger KR, Murphy EA, Pyeritz RE: Chronic β-adrenergic blockade protects the aorta in the Marfan syndrome: A prospective, randomized trial of propranolol. N Engl J Med 330:1335–1341, 1994. *The first randomized trial concluding that medication can reduce the risk of dissection and delay aortic dilatation.*

216 EHLERS-DANLOS SYNDROMES

Reed Edwin Pyeritz

DEFINITION. The Ehlers-Danlos syndromes (EDSs) are clinically variable and genetically heterogeneous. Diagnoses are still largely based on the bedside examination, and the classification scheme and diagnostic criteria have been revised recently. The unifying themes among the disorders are fragility of tissues, joint hypermobility, and skin hyperextensibility.

ETIOLOGY AND PATHOGENESIS. Defects in collagen in the extracellular matrices of various tissues underlie all forms of EDS that have been elucidated thus far. The specific genetic mutations occur in any of a number of genes, with the effect of altering the structure, synthesis, post-translational modifications, or stability of the collagens involved. The known molecular defects are listed in Table 216–1.

PREVALENCE. No accurate data exist, but an incidence of about 1 in 5000 births is a reasonable estimate of how many individuals will qualify for one of the EDS diagnoses. Each of the types represents something of a clinical spectrum, with the mild end merging with what might be considered normal variation. Hence just as the diagnostic criteria are arbitrary, so will any determina-

Table 216-1 ■ EHLERS-DANLOS SYNDROMES

TYPE	FORMER NAME	CLINICAL FEATURES*	INHERITANCE	OMIM†	MOLECULAR DEFECT
Classic	EDS I & II	Joint hypermobility; skin hyperextensibility; atrophic scars; smooth, velvety skin; subcutaneous spheroids	AD	130000 130010	Structure of type V collagen ?COL5A1, COL5A2
Hypermobility	EDS III	Joint hypermobility; some skin hyperextensibility, with or without smooth and velvety texture	AD	130020	?
Vascular	EDS IV	Thin skin; easy bruising; pinched nose; acrogeria; rupture of large- and medium-caliber arteries, uterus, and large bowel	AD	130050 (225350) (225360)	Deficient type III collagen COL3A1
Kyphoscoliotic	EDS VI	Joint hypermobility; congenital, progressive scoliosis; scleral fragility with globe rupture; tissue fragility, aortic dilatation, MVP	AR	225400	
Arthrochalasia	EDS VII A & B	Joint hypermobility, severe, with subluxations; congenital hip dislocation; skin hyperextensibility; tissue fragility	AD	130060	No cleavage of N-terminus of type I procollagen due to mutations in COL1A1 or COL1A2
Dermatosparaxis	EDS VII C	Severe skin fragility; decreased skin elasticity; easy bruising; hernias; premature rupture of fetal membranes	AR	225410	No cleavage of N-terminus of type I procollagen due to deficiency of peptidase
Unclassified types	EDS V	Classic features	XL	305200	?
	EDS VIII	Classic features and periodontal disease	AD	130080	?
	EDS X	Mild classic features, MVP	?	225310	?
	EDS XI	Joint instability	AD	147900	?
	EDS IX	Classic features; occiptial horns	XL	309400	Allelic to Menkes syndrome

EDS = Ehlers-Danlos syndrome; AD = autosomal dominant; AR = autosomal recessive; MVP = mitral valve prolapse; XL = X-linked.
*Listed in order of diagnostic importance.
†Entries in Online Mendelian Inheritance in Man (http://www.ncbi.nlm.nih.gov/OMIM).

tion of prevalence based on phenotypic criteria. The extent to which normal variation in joint hypermobility, skin elasticity, and tissue fragility represents genetic variation at loci that encode collagen or other extracellular matrix genes is in need of considerable research.

PATHOLOGY. Little of routine pathologic evaluation distinguishes among the various types of EDS or even distinguishes individual types from normal. Thickness of the dermis is decreased in some forms, especially the vascular type, and the walls of arteries are also reduced in thickness in this type. By electron microscopy, the classic, hypermobile, and kyphoscoliotic types have abnormal collagen fibers, especially when viewed in cross section (variable and often increased fiber diameter with an irregular outline). In the vascular type, some patients have dilated endoplasmic reticulum consistent with aberrant secretion of type III collagen molecules.

CLINICAL MANIFESTATIONS. The major and minor features of each type are detailed in Table 216-1. Infants with the classic type are often born prematurely by 4 to 8 weeks because of rupture of fetal membranes. Diagnosing the vascular and kyphoscoliotic types is important because of their cardiovascular features. The vascular type, previously termed EDS IV, is characterized by a troublesome tendency to suffer spontaneous rupture of large arteries and hollow organs, especially the colon and uterus. Because these events carry considerable morbidity, life expectancy is reduced, on average, by more than half. Women with this form of EDS are especially vulnerable during pregnancy. In the kyphoscoliotic type, aortic root dilatation and aortic regurgitation can develop. Patients with most forms of EDS are prone to the development of mitral valve prolapse, and progression to mitral regurgitation occurs more often than in the common form of mitral valve prolapse.

DIFFERENTIAL DIAGNOSIS. By carefully adhering to the clinical features shown in Table 216-1 and judicious use of laboratory tests, the various defined types of EDS can be differentiated. A number of specific non-EDS syndromes need to be excluded. Infants with the kyphoscoliotic type of EDS share some features with severe Marfan syndrome. Patients with the Larsen syndrome may resemble those with the arthrochalasis type of EDS. The skin redundancy and loss of elasticity of the dermatosparaxis type of EDS is reminiscent of autosomal dominant cutis laxa, which is not associated with easy bruising or tissue fragility.

The most difficult decision is whether a person warrants any diagnosis of EDS. Patients who have only joint hypermobility without skin changes should not be labeled with EDS; a diagnosis of familial joint hypermobility might be more appropriate. Familial joint instability involves a predisposition to dislocations of major joints that is rare in most types of EDS except for arthrochalasis.

TREATMENT AND CARE. Management of most skin and joint problems should be conservative and preventive. Sutures need to be placed with careful attention to approximating the margins and avoiding tension; removable sutures should be left in place for twice the usual time. Most joint hypermobility and pain in EDS does not require surgical treatment. Benefit is often derived from physical therapy designed to strengthen the muscles that need to provide support for the loose ligaments. All patients should receive genetic counseling about the mode of inheritance and their risk of having children affected with EDS. The possibility of prenatal diagnosis exists for all of the types with defined molecular or biochemical defects.

The vascular type requires particular surgical care; the ruptured arteries are difficult to repair because of the pronounced vascular fragility. Rupture of the bowel is a surgical emergency. Because the risk of vascular rupture is especially high during pregnancy in women with the vascular form, this condition is one in which women should be advised to avoid pregnancy. Patients should be advised to avoid contact sports and to treat aggressively blood pressure elevations. Genetic screening holds the potential for relieving relatives at risk by discovering that they do not have a defect in type III collagen.

The kyphoscoliotic type may improve with large doses of ascorbic acid (1 to 4 g/day) because vitamin C is a cofactor for the enzyme that is deficient. No other metabolic or genetic therapy is yet effective in other forms of EDS.

Beighton P, De Paepe A, Steinmann B, et al: Ehlers-Danlos syndromes: Revised nosology, Villefranche, 1997. Am J Med Genet 77:31, 1998. *Major revision of the classification scheme and diagnostic criteria.*

Byers PH: The Ehlers-Danlos syndromes. *In* Rimoin DL, Connor JM, Pyeritz RE (eds): Principles and Practice of Medical Genetics, 3rd ed. New York, Churchill Livingstone, 1997, p 1067. *A review of the clinical and biochemical features of EDS.*

Steinmann B, Royce PS, Superti-Furga A: The Ehlers-Danlos syndrome. *In* Royce PM, Steinmann B (eds): Connective Tissue and Its Heritable Disorders: Molecular, Genetic, and Medical Aspects. New York, Wiley-Liss, 1993, p 351. *An excellent review chapter based on the old classification scheme for EDS.*

217 OSTEOGENESIS IMPERFECTA SYNDROMES

Reed Edwin Pyeritz

DEFINITION. The heterogeneous group of disorders known as osteogenesis imperfecta includes, at one end of the severity spectrum, a type lethal prenatally or in the neonatal period and, at the other, such mild features that distinguishing those affected from the general population is difficult. The unifying feature is hereditary osteopenia (insufficient bone), with primary defects in the protein matrix in bone and other tissues. The clinical syndromes all involve osteoporosis with liability to fracture.

ETIOLOGY AND PATHOGENESIS. Patients in whom mutations have been found all have defects of one sort or another in the two genes that encode the procollagen chains of type I collagen, *COL1A1* and *COL1A2*. Type I collagen is composed of two $\alpha 1$(I) and one $\alpha 2$(I) procollagen chains; the mature fiber requires considerable post-translational modification that only occurs appropriately if the three procollagen chains have intertwined to form a triple helix that is both perfect and completed at the right speed (see also Chapter 283). Thus a mutation that affects formation of the triple helix, such as substitution of one of the mandatory glycine residues that occurs at every 3rd position, will also have adverse effects on modifications that render the molecule capable of forming effective mature fibers. As a result, a single nucleotide change ("point mutation") may have profound effects on the extracellular matrix and produce a severe condition. Alternatively and at first glance paradoxically, a mutation that eliminates an entire allele, or at least production of any product capable of intertwining with normal procollagen chains, will have a much milder effect on the matrix and the severity of osteogenesis imperfecta. Examples of the most common classes of mutations are shown in Table 217–1. Hundreds of mutations have been described.

PREVALENCE. No careful epidemiologic study has been performed, and the milder forms of type I osteogenesis imperfecta merge with the phenotypes found in the general population. A crude estimate of its overall prevalence is 1 per 10,000. The neonatal lethal form (type II), which is nearly always due to a new mutation in a parental gamete, has an incidence of about 1 in 50,000.

PATHOLOGY. Other than the gross pathology associated with the clinical manifestations, the most characteristic pathology is a primary reduction in bone matrix with secondary undermineralization.

CLINICAL MANIFESTATIONS. The major phenotypic features of osteogenesis imperfecta are shown in Table 217–1. The most severe type is II, followed in decreasing order by III, IV, and I. In type II, infants are either stillborn or succumb soon after birth on account of pulmonary failure secondary to the small thorax, which is usually compromised further by myriad rib fractures. A few infants have experienced survival for at least a few years but require enormous attention to their medical needs.

Type III may be confused with type II at birth, but survival alone helps make the distinction. Bony deformity is pronounced and not necessarily due to fractures. Mobility is impaired, and most patients require a wheelchair at an early age. Stature may be severely compromised. Because of progressive vertebral column deformity and rib fractures, restrictive lung disease is a common problem as patients age; many die of pulmonary complications. Basilar impression causing compression of the brain stem and the craniocervical junction can produce central sleep apnea, headache, and upper motor neuron signs.

Patients with type IV osteogenesis imperfecta generally have reduced stature, some bony deformity, and abnormal teeth that are opalescent and wear easily (dentinogenesis imperfecta). As in type I osteogenesis imperfecta, the tendency to fracture is highest in childhood and lessens with adolescence. A distinguishing characteristic of type IV is a normal scleral hue.

Type I osteogenesis imperfecta is probably the most common form and is associated with a bluish or blue-gray scleral hue. People with type I osteogenesis imperfecta who also have dentinogenesis imperfecta tend to have more severe skeletal problems. The risk of fracture diminishes during adulthood but re-emerges as a major concern for women after menopause. Hearing impairment in all forms of osteogenesis imperfecta is common and age related, being rare before adolescence. The deficits are of a mixed or predominantly conductive form.

DIFFERENTIAL DIAGNOSIS. The range of diagnostic possibilities in a person with multiple fractures is largely dependent on the age. In infancy, the genetic conditions hypophosphatasia, severe osteochondrodysplasias (such as achondrogenesis and forms of spondyloepiphyseal dysplasia), and Menkes syndrome need to be excluded when a diagnosis of type II or III osteogenesis imperfecta is considered. The radiologic features eventually become entirely diagnostic, but often the neonatologist has to arrive at a definitive answer in short order. Analysis of serum alkaline phosphatase and copper can be helpful. In childhood, the most common situation leading to a consideration of a mild form of osteogenesis imperfecta is child abuse. Here, the pattern of fracture is usually distinct, and bone mineralization should be normal if the child is the object of non-accidental or even repeated accidental trauma. Abnormal scleral hue, dentinogenesis imperfecta, and wormian bones (microfractures along the cranial sutures) all support the diagnosis of osteogenesis imperfecta. In older children, the disorder idiopathic juvenile osteoporosis should be considered in any patient seen initially with repeated fractures. Occasionally, studies of skin fibroblasts are needed to document whether a defect in type I collagen (which would be characteristic of osteogenesis imperfecta) is

Table 217–1 ■ OSTEOGENESIS IMPERFECTA

TYPE	CLINICAL FEATURES	INHERITANCE	OMIM*	BASIC DEFECTS
I	Fractures variable in number; little deformity; stature normal or nearly so; blue sclerae; hearing loss common but not always present; DI uncommon	AD	166200	Typically, one nonfunctional *COL1A1* allele
II	Lethal *in utero* or shortly after birth; many fractures at birth involving ribs (may appear "beaded") and other long bones; little mineralization of calvarium; pulmonary hypertension	AD	166210	*COL1A1* or *COL1A2*: typically substitution of glycyl residues; occasionally deletions of a portion of the triple-helical domain
		AR	259400	Deletion in *COL1A2* plus a nonfunctional allele
III	Fractures common, but long bones progressively deform starting *in utero*; stature markedly reduced; sclerae often blue, but become lighter with age; DI and hearing loss common	AD	259420	One single–amino acid substitution
		AR (rare)	259440	Two mutations in *COL1A1* and/or *COL1A2* (rarely)
IV	Fractures common; stature usually reduced; bone deformity common, but rarely severe; scleral hue normal to grayish; hearing loss variable; DI common	AD	166220	Point mutations in *COL1A1* or *COL1A2*
		AD	166240	Exon skipping mutations in *COL1A2*

DI = dentinogenesis imperfecta; AD = autosomal dominant; AR = autosomal recessive.
*Entry in Online Mendelian Inheritance in Man (http://www.ncbi.nlm.nih.gov/OMIM).

present. A number of osteochondrodysplasias are associated with short stature, skeletal deformity, and a tendency to fracture. However, both pyknodysostosis and osteopetrosis are associated with sclerotic bones rather than osteoporotic ones. In adulthood, early-onset osteoporosis may be confused with osteogenesis imperfecta. Indeed, mutations in type I collagen also cause familial osteoporosis, and the skeletal phenotypes merge; patients with true osteogenesis imperfecta may have scleral, hearing, or dental abnormalities and a positive family history.

TREATMENT AND CARE. Management of the skeletal complications largely depends on orthopedic, physical, and occupational therapy approaches. Although no medical treatment has yet been proved to improve the quality of the bone, studies of growth hormone and bisphosphonates are under way. The long-term goal is to maintain function and independence as an individual. These goals can be advanced in some by judicious use of intramedullary rods in the long bones of the legs; if mobility and especially ambulation can be maintained, the demineralization associated with inactivity can be avoided.

Unaffected parents of a child with osteogenesis imperfecta and all affected individuals should have genetic counseling. For the parents of a child with type II osteogenesis imperfecta, the possibility of germinal mosaicism (which has been well documented in this condition) should not be overlooked. If one parent has a "new" mutation in one of the type I procollagen genes and multiple gonadal cells carries this mutation, the risk of recurrence in future children is not negligible. If the mutation in the affected child can be defined, the risk of recurrence can be quantified (through molecular analysis of sperm) if the mutation arose in the father.

Glorieux FH, Bishop NJ, Plotkin H, et al: Cyclic administration of pamidronate in children with severe osteogenesis imperfecta. N Engl J Med 339:947–952, 1998. *In a preliminary study, children with type III OI had improved bone density and growth when treated with a bisphosphonate compound that inhibits bone resorption.*

Horowitz EM, Prockop DJ, Marini JC, et al: Bone marrow transplantation to correct the mesenchymal defect of children with osteogenesis imperfecta. Nat Med 5:309–313, 1999. *Mesenchymal stem cells in allogenic bone marrow populated the marrow of children with type III OI in sufficient quantity to increase bone density and reduce the rate of fracture.*

Sillence DO: Disorders of bone density, volume, and mineralization. *In* Rimoin DL, Connor JM, Pyeritz RE (eds): Principles and Practice of Medical Genetics, 3rd ed. New York, Churchill Livingstone, 1997, p 2817. *A review of the clinical, pathologic, and molecular aspects of a diverse group of related disorders, including osteogenesis imperfecta.*

218 PSEUDOXANTHOMA ELASTICUM

Reed Edwin Pyeritz

DEFINITION. Pseudoxanthoma elasticum is a heritable disorder of connective tissue with pleiotropic manifestations wherever elastic fibers are found, but primarily in the skin, eye, and vasculature. Life expectancy is reduced on average because of a predisposition to myocardial infarction and gastrointestinal hemorrhage.

ETIOLOGY AND PATHOGENESIS. At least two forms exist, autosomal recessive (the more common) and autosomal dominant. A gene for both forms has been mapped to human chromosome 16, but its identity is not yet known. Because of the prominent histopathologic feature of calcification of elastic tissue, speculation about pathogenesis has focused on tropoelastin (the gene for which has been excluded), components of the microfibril, and factors important in calcium homeostasis. However, it remains unclear whether the calcification is a primary or secondary phenomenon.

PREVALENCE. The exact frequency of pseudoxanthoma elasticum is unknown, but it is probably underdiagnosed. Rough approximations suggest a prevalence of 1 in 25,000 to 100,000. Males and females are equally frequently affected, although women are more likely to seek medical attention out of concern for the skin changes.

PATHOLOGY. The hallmark of pseudoxanthoma elasticum—and

an important diagnostic clue—is the histopathologic finding of hyperproliferated elastic fibers in the mid-dermis; these fibers become fragmented, clumped, and calcified. An arteriolar sclerosis develops in the media of muscular arteries and arterioles; the lumen may become progressively and concentrically narrowed. Alternatively, microaneurysms can form. Thickening of the endocardium, especially atrial endocardium, develops in some patients. In the eye, Bruch's membrane becomes calcified and fragmented.

CLINICAL MANIFESTATIONS. Because of the pleiotropic nature of pseudoxanthoma elasticum, the diagnosis is initially suspected by any of a variety of clinicians, especially dermatologists, ophthalmologists, cardiologists, and gastroenterologists. The condition gains its name from the dermatologic feature of yellowish papules that appear at areas of flexural stress, especially the neck, groin, popliteal and cubital fossae, and periumbilical regions and on the buccal mucosa. The appearance of affected skin has been likened to that of a "plucked chicken." Over time, affected areas coalesce and become thickened.

Changes in the eye begin as a generalized, subtle mottled pattern in the retina ("peau d'orange") and progress to the characteristic angioid streaks. The latter changes are not specific for pseudoxanthoma elasticum and can be seen in diabetes mellitus, sickle cell disease, and a variety of other conditions. Streaks represent breaks in Bruch's membrane, an elastic lamina that lies between the retinal vasculature and the choroid. Spontaneous hemorrhages, especially those involving the macula, lead to progressive visual loss.

Involvement of arteries of various caliber produces problems because of occlusion and hemorrhage. The lifetime risk of serious gastrointestinal hemorrhage from any site, but especially the stomach, is about 10%. Hypertension is relatively common, in part because of involvement of the renal vasculature. Progressive occlusion of peripheral arteries leads to absence of pulses; acral ischemia is rare because of the development of collaterals. The risk for stroke, myocardial infarction, abdominal angina, and intermittent claudication is increased independent of other risk factors.

DIFFERENTIAL DIAGNOSIS. An acquired form of pseudoxanthoma elasticum has been reported and is also of unclear etiology. This form is difficult to differentiate from a sporadic case potentially caused by a new mutation or heterozygous parents, but it tends to affect only the skin. As suggested by the name, the cutaneous features of pseudoxanthoma elasticum need to be differentiated from true xanthoma resulting from a disorder of lipid metabolism. The dermatologic manifestations need to be differentiated from Miescher's elastoma, elastic tissue nevi (Buschke-Ollendorff syndrome), and solar elastosis.

TREATMENT AND CARE. No cure for or means of preventing pseudoxanthoma elasticum is known. Based on one report of an association between calcium intake in early life and later severity of pseudoxanthoma elasticum, restriction of dietary calcium, primarily dairy products, may have a role. However, no clinical trials have been performed. In many instances, careful attention to the ocular features by a retinal specialist experienced in pseudoxanthoma elasticum can delay but not prevent loss of vision. The risk of gastrointestinal hemorrhage suggests that patients should avoid gastric irritants such as aspirin, non-steroidal anti-inflammatory drugs, and excessive alcohol. Stool should be checked regularly for occult blood, and angiography may be necessary to detect the source of bleeding. All standard risk factors for atherosclerosis should be managed aggressively. Complaints of chest pain should prompt a rigorous investigation for coronary artery disease. Angioplasty has not been reported to be effective, and the coronary lesions tend to be diffuse. Coronary artery bypass has been performed, but long-term results have not been reported. It may be theoretically advantageous to use vein grafts rather than the internal mammary artery for bypass. The excessive wrinkling and pseudoxanthoma in exposed areas can be ameliorated by plastic surgery.

Lebwohl M, Nelder K, Pope FM, et al: Classification of pseudoxanthoma elasticum: Report of a consensus conference. J Am Acad Dermatol 30:103, 1994. *A group of experienced clinicians proposed a classification scheme.*

Pope FM: Pseudoxanthoma elasticum. *In* Rimoin DL, Connor JM, Pyeritz RE (eds): Principles and Practice of Medical Genetics, 3rd ed. New York, Churchill Livingstone, 1997, p 1083. *A comprehensive review of all aspects of pseudoxanthoma elasticum by an experienced clinician.*

Struk B, Nelder KH, Rao VS, et al: Mapping of both autosomal recessive and dominant variants of pseudoxanthoma elasticum to chromosome 16p13.1. Hum Mol Genet 6:1823, 1997. *The first report of localizing the gene for pseudoxanthoma elasticum by linkage analysis.*

▪ DISORDERS OF PORPHYRINS AND METALS

219 THE PORPHYRIAS

Karl E. Anderson

Porphyrias are due to deficiencies of specific enzymes of the heme biosynthetic pathway and, when clinically expressed, are associated with striking accumulations of heme pathway intermediates. Most porphyrias are inherited, but other factors are important in determining their severity. These conditions are more prevalent and more often manifested in adults than are most metabolic diseases and are likely to be encountered by physicians in many disciplines. The three most common porphyrias differ considerably from each other and are managed very differently.

THE HEME BIOSYNTHETIC PATHWAY AND THE PORPHYRIAS

The genes for all eight enzymes of this important pathway (Fig. 219–1) have been cloned and characterized at the molecular level and their chromosomal locations identified (Table 219–1). Mutations of the erythroid-specific form of δ-aminolevulinic acid (ALA) synthase, the first enzyme, are found in X-linked sideroblastic anemia. Mutations in genes for the other seven enzymes are found in the porphyrias. (Standard abbreviations for these diseases are shown in Table 219–1). These diseases are all heterogeneous at the molecular level. Therefore, different mutations commonly occur in unrelated families with any given type of porphyria.

Heme is synthesized in the largest amounts in bone marrow and liver, where it is used primarily to make hemoglobin and cytochrome P-450 enzymes, respectively. Hepatic heme biosynthesis is regulated primarily by ALA synthase, which is rate limiting and under sensitive feedback control by the cellular free heme content. Hepatic ALA synthase is induced by many of the same drugs and steroids that induce P-450 enzymes. Additional pathway enzymes and cellular uptake of iron are important in regulating heme synthesis in erythroid cells.

Most heme pathway intermediates (see Fig. 219–1) are conserved and excreted only in small amounts. ALA and porphobilinogen (PBG) are normally excreted in much larger amounts than porphyrins. Porphyrinogens (hexahydroporphyrins) undergo autooxidation outside cells and are excreted primarily as porphyrins. ALA, PBG, and porphyrinogens are colorless and non-fluorescent. Porphyrins are reddish and fluoresce when exposed to long-wave ultraviolet light. ALA, PBG, uroporphyrin, and heptacarboxyl, hexacarboxyl, and pentacarboxyl porphyrins are excreted mostly in urine, coproporphyrin (a tetracarboxyl porphyrin) in urine and bile, and harderoporphyrin (a tricarboxyl porphyrin) and protoporphyrin (a dicarboxyl porphyrin) in bile and feces.

CLASSIFICATION

Two major types of clinical manifestations are characteristic of porphyrias. *Neurologic effects* occur in porphyrias characterized by accumulation of the porphyrin precursors ALA and PBG. These "acute porphyrias" share many clinical features and are similarly managed. *Cutaneous photosensitivity* occurs in types of porphyria in which porphyrins accumulate. Porphyrins are activated by long-wave ultraviolet light and generate oxygen radicals that damage the skin. Several of the "cutaneous porphyrias" are associated with similar skin lesions but differ considerably in terms of treatment and prognosis. The cutaneous features of erythropoietic protopor-

phyria (EPP) are distinct. Traditionally, porphyrias have also been divided into erythropoietic and hepatic types. Now that these disorders are well characterized, they are best classified in terms of their specific enzyme deficiencies.

It is important to appreciate that the three most common types of porphyria that are likely to be encountered periodically by any physician differ markedly from each other with regard to major clinical manifestations, exacerbating factors, tests important for diagnosis, and effective therapies (Table 219–2). Because their features are so distinct, a feature learned about one of these porphyrias will not apply to the others. On the other hand, two of these conditions are prototypic: They share some important features with the other less common porphyrias, which should be evident from the brief descriptions of each of the porphyrias that follow.

δ-AMINOLEVULINIC ACID DEHYDRATASE–DEFICIENT PORPHYRIA. In this very rare autosomal recessive disorder, ALA dehydratase is markedly reduced (1 to 2% of normal). Symptoms resemble those of acute intermittent porphyria (AIP) but may begin in childhood. Hemolysis is sometimes present. Urinary ALA and coproporphyrin III and erythrocyte zinc protoporphyrin are increased. In this and other disorders in which ALA accumulates, coproporphyrin III may originate from excess ALA by metabolism to coproporphyrin III in tissues other than the tissue of origin of the excess ALA.

Several other conditions are associated with ALA dehydratase deficiency and increased ALA. Lead poisoning and hereditary tyrosinemia can cause symptoms (abdominal pain, ileus, and motor neuropathy) that are strikingly similar to those of the acute porphyrias. Lead concentrates in erythroid cells. Deficient erythrocyte ALA dehydratase in lead poisoning can be restored to normal in vitro with dithiothreitol. Erythrocyte protoporphyrin and urinary coproporphyrin are increased. In hereditary tyrosinemia, a deficiency of fumarylacetoacetase leads to the accumulation of succinylacetone (2,3-dioxoheptanoic acid). This structural analogue of ALA is a potent inhibitor of ALA dehydratase. Other heavy metals or styrene exposure can also inhibit ALA dehydratase.

ACUTE INTERMITTENT PORPHYRIA. AIP is an autosomal dominant disorder that results from an approximately 50% deficiency of PBG deaminase. The enzyme is deficient in all individuals who inherit the mutant gene and remains fairly constant over time. The majority of subjects with PBG deaminase deficiency remain asymptomatic.

PREVALENCE. AIP occurs in all races. Its prevalence in most countries has not been precisely estimated but may be most common (perhaps 5 per 100,000) in northern European populations.

ETIOLOGY AND PATHOGENESIS. More than 100 different mutations of the PBG deaminase gene have been identified in unrelated AIP lineages. Two isoenzymes of PBG deaminase are known, an erythroid-specific and a non-erythroid or "housekeeping" form. Both are transcribed by alternative mRNA splicing from the same gene, which contains 15 exons. The erythroid-specific isoenzyme is encoded by exons 2 to 15; the erythroid promoter, which functions only in erythroid cells, is found immediately upstream from exon 2. The non-erythroid enzyme is encoded by exons 1 and 3 to 15; the non-erythroid promoter is immediately upstream from exon 1. PBG deaminase is decreased in all tissues of most patients with AIP. However, if the mutation is in or near exon 1, only the non-erythroid isoenzyme is deficient. Therefore, in individuals with this type of mutation, enzyme activity is deficient in non-erythroid tissues but is normal in erythrocytes. Homozygous AIP is extremely rare.

Most individuals with clinically latent AIP have normal levels of ALA and PBG and apparently normal hepatic cytochrome P-450

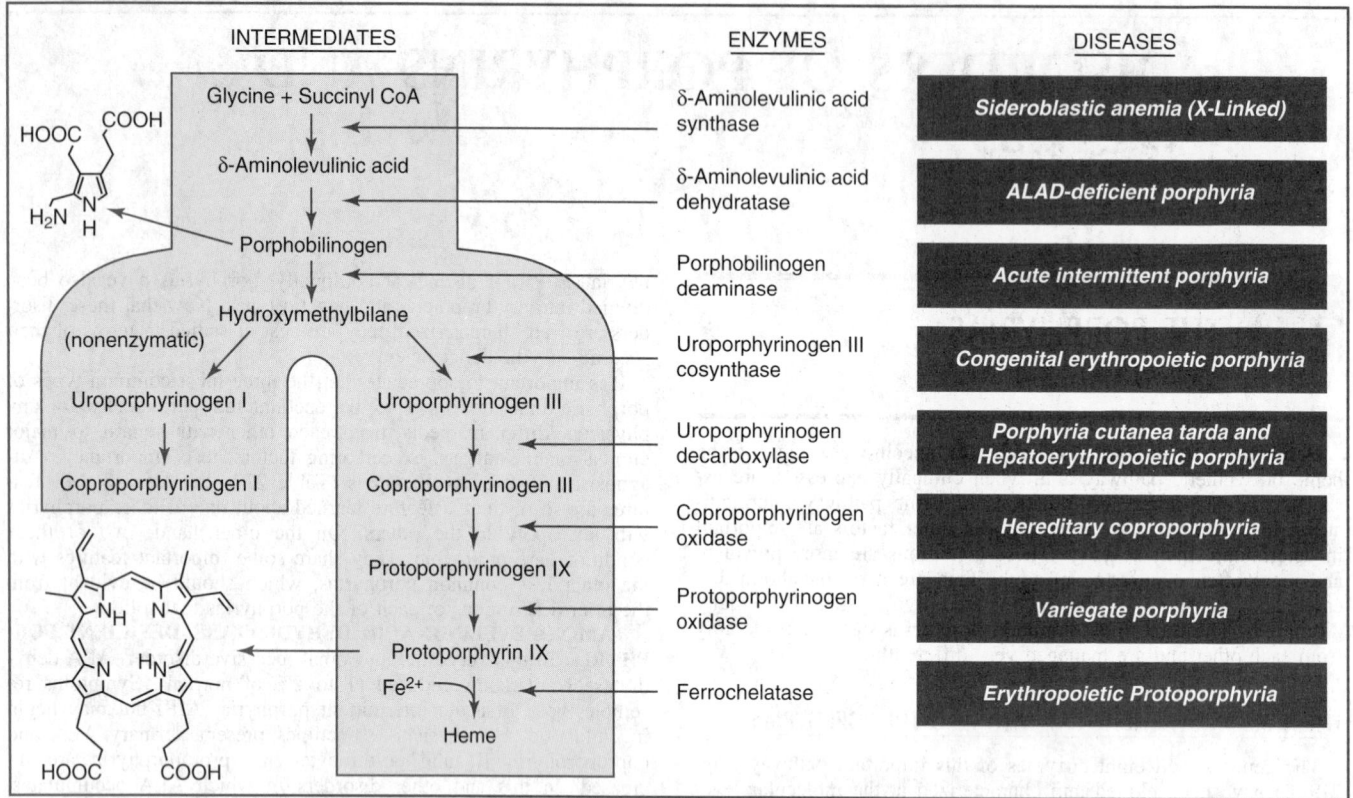

| INTERMEDIATES | ENZYMES | DISEASES |

FIGURE 219-1 ■ Intermediates and enzymes of the heme biosynthetic pathway and the major diseases of porphyrin metabolism that have been associated with deficiencies of specific enzymes. The initial and last three enzymes (in red) are mitochondrial and the other four (in black) are cytosolic. Heme is synthesized from glycine and succinyl coenzyme A (CoA). Intermediates in the pathway include δ-aminolevulinic acid (an amino acid), porphobilinogen (a pyrrole), and hydroxymethylbilane (a linear tetrapyrrole). Uroporphyrinogen III cosynthase catalyzes the closure of hydroxymethylbilane, with inversion of one of the pyrroles, to form a porphyrin macrocycle, uroporphyrinogen III. (Non-enzymatic closure occurs without inversion of this pyrrole to form uroporphyrinogen I, which is not metabolized beyond coproporphyrinogen I.) The next two enzymes result in decarboxylation of six of the eight side chains of uroporphyrinogen III, with sequential formation of hepta-, hexa-, and pentacarboxyl porphyrinogens, coproporphyrinogen III, tricarboxyl porphyrinogen, and protoporphyrinogen IX. The final two enzymes catalyze the oxidation of protoporphyrinogen IX to protoporphyrin IX and the insertion of ferrous iron into the porphyrin macrocycle to form heme (iron protoporphyrin IX). With the exception of protoporphyrin IX, all porphyrin intermediates are in their reduced forms (hexahydroporphyrins or porphyrinogens). Chemical structures of two intermediates are shown.

content, which indicates that the partial deficiency of PBG deaminase does not of itself greatly impair hepatic heme synthesis or induce ALA synthase. However, when the demand for hepatic heme is increased by drugs, hormones, or nutritional factors, the deficient enzyme can become limiting for heme synthesis. Induction of hepatic ALA synthase is then accentuated and ALA and PBG accumulate in the liver and increase in plasma and urine. Excess porphyrins originate non-enzymatically from PBG or enzymatically from ALA transported to tissues other than the liver.

Most drugs that are harmful in AIP induce hepatic ALA synthase and cytochrome P-450 enzymes. Sulfonamide antibiotics are not inducers and may inhibit PBG deaminase. Reduced caloric and carbohydrate intake enhances the induction of ALA synthase in animals and in AIP can increase ALA and PBG and precipitate symptoms. Administration of carbohydrate can reduce hepatic ALA synthase and P-450 enzymes.

The mechanism of neural damage in AIP is unknown. Porphyrias and related disorders associated with increased ALA have similar neurologic manifestations. ALA is structurally analogous to γ-aminobutyric acid (GABA) and can interact with GABA receptors. However, ALA and other products of the heme pathway have not been convincingly shown to be neurotoxic. The suggestion that heme deficiency may occur in nervous tissue in these disorders is also unproved.

CLINICAL MANIFESTATIONS. Symptoms rarely occur before puberty and seldom if ever recur throughout adult life. Characteristically, attacks last for several days or longer, often require hospitalization, and are followed by complete recovery. Abdominal pain is the most common symptom, is usually steady and poorly localized,

but may be cramping. Tachycardia, hypertension, restlessness, fine tremors, and excess sweating may be due to sympathetic overactivity. Other manifestations include nausea and vomiting; constipation; pain in the limbs, head, neck, or chest; muscle weakness; and sensory loss. Ileus with distention and decreased bowel sounds is common. However, increased bowel sounds and diarrhea may be seen. Because the abdominal symptoms are neurologic rather than inflammatory, tenderness, fever, and leukocytosis are generally absent or mild. Dysuria and bladder dysfunction may occur. Recurrent attacks tend to be similar in a given patient.

Peripheral neuropathy in AIP is primarily motor, results from axonal degeneration, and does not develop in all patients with acute attacks, even when abdominal symptoms are severe. Rarely, neuropathy develops apart from abdominal symptoms. Weakness most commonly begins in proximal muscles (often requiring a careful examination to detect) and more often in the arms than the legs. It can be asymmetric and focal. Tendon reflexes may be little affected or hyperactive in the early stages but are usually decreased or absent with advanced neuropathy. Cranial and sensory nerves can be affected. Progression to respiratory and bulbar paralysis and death seldom occurs unless the porphyria is not recognized, the use of harmful drugs is not discontinued, and appropriate treatment is not instituted. Sudden death, presumably from cardiac arrhythmia, may also occur.

The central nervous system can be involved. Anxiety, insomnia, depression, disorientation, hallucinations, and paranoia, which can be especially severe during acute attacks, may suggest a primary mental disorder or hysteria. Seizures may occur as an acute neurologic manifestation of AIP, as a result of hyponatremia, or second-

Table 219–1 ∎ ENZYMES OF THE HEME BIOSYNTHETIC PATHWAY AND CLASSIFICATION AND INHERITANCE OF DISEASES ASSOCIATED WITH THEIR DEFICIENCIES*

ENZYME	CHROMOSOMAL LOCATION	DISEASE	INHERITANCE	CLASSIFICATIONS OF PORPHYRIAS			
				Hepatic	Erythropoietic	Acute	Cutaneous
ALA synthase							
Erythroid	Xp11.21	Sideroblastic anemia	X-linked recessive				
Non-erythroid	3p21	None known					
ALA dehydratase	9q34	δ-Aminolevulinic acid dehydratase–deficient porphyria (ADP)	Autosomal recessive	?X		X	
Porphobilinogen deaminase†	11q24.1 —> q24.2	Acute intermittent porphyria (AIP)	Autosomal dominant	X		X	
Uroporphyrinogen III co-synthase	10q25.2 —> q26.3	Congenital erythropoietic porphyria (CEP)	Autosomal recessive		X		X
Uroporphyrinogen decarboxylase	1p34	Porphyria cutanea tarda‡ (PCT)	Autosomal dominant	X			X
		Hepatoerythropoietic porphyria (HEP)	Autosomal recessive	X	X		X
Coproporphyrinogen oxidase	3q12	Hereditary coproporphyria (HCP)	Autosomal dominant	X		X	X
Protoporphyrinogen oxidase	1q22 or 23	Variegate porphyria (VP)	Autosomal dominant	X		X	X
Ferrochelatase	18q21.3 or 22	Erythropoietic protoporphyria (EPP)	Autosomal dominant		X		X

*The most precise classification is according to the specific enzyme deficiencies. Other classifications based on the major tissue site of overproduction of heme pathway intermediates (hepatic versus erythropoietic) or the type of major symptoms (acute neurovisceral versus cutaneous) are useful but not precise or mutually exclusive.
†This enzyme is also known as hydroxymethylbilane synthase and formerly as uroporphyrinogen I synthase.
‡Inherited deficiency of uroporphyrinogen decarboxylase is partially responsible for the familial (type II) form.

ary to causes unrelated to porphyria. Hyponatremia may be due to hypothalamic involvement and inappropriate antidiuretic hormone secretion; vomiting, diarrhea, and poor intake; or excess renal sodium loss.

After several days, an attack may resolve quite rapidly, with abdominal pain disappearing within a few hours and paresis within a few days. Attacks during the luteal phase of the menstrual cycle usually resolve with the onset of menses. Even advanced neuropathy is potentially reversible. Pain, depression, and other symptoms are sometimes chronic.

Chronic hepatic abnormalities are common in AIP, and affected patients have an increased risk of hepatocellular carcinoma (apparently not associated with hepatitis B or C). AIP may predispose to chronic hypertension and be associated with impaired renal function. The mechanisms of these associations are unknown.

PRECIPITATING FACTORS. Recognition of precipitating factors is important in management. Endogenous steroid hormones are probably most important. AIP is characterized by rarity of symptoms and excess ALA and PBG before puberty, more frequent clinical expression in women, premenstrual attacks in some women, and exacerbations after the administration of sex steroid preparations. Some patients manifest increased proportions of 5β-hydroxysteroid metabolites, which are potent inducers of hepatic ALA synthase. Recurrent cyclic attacks are troublesome in some women and occur when progesterone levels are highest. Progesterone and its metabolites are potent inducers of ALA synthase, whereas estrogens are

not. Pregnancy is usually well tolerated despite high progesterone levels. Some women are more prone to attacks during pregnancy, possibly partly because of hyperemesis gravidarum and reduced caloric intake.

Drugs remain important as causes of AIP attacks. Published information is insufficient to allow most drugs to be classified as definitely harmful or safe. The major drugs known to be harmful or safe in the acute porphyrias are listed in Table 219–3. Barbiturates and sulfonamides are the most notorious. Benzodiazepines are much less hazardous. Some drugs may exacerbate porphyria cutanea tarda (PCT) but not acute porphyrias (see below). Advice can be sought from a center with experience in porphyria with regard to the use of drugs.

Reduced caloric intake, usually instituted in an effort to lose weight, is a common cause of attacks. Attacks are also provoked by intercurrent infections, major surgery, and other conditions. Cigarette smoke contains chemicals that can induce hepatic heme synthesis and may predispose to attacks. Attacks are almost always due to two or more factors acting in an additive fashion. Probably for this reason, (1) drugs may produce attacks in adults but are rarely reported to do so in children with PBG deaminase deficiency, (2) anticonvulsants do not produce attacks in some PBG deaminase–deficient subjects, and (3) barbiturate anesthetics more frequently exacerbate porphyria if symptoms are present before anesthetic exposure.

DIAGNOSIS AND DIFFERENTIAL DIAGNOSIS. AIP and other acute

Table 219–2 ∎ THREE MOST COMMON HUMAN PORPHYRIAS AND MAJOR DIFFERENTIATING FEATURES

DISORDER	INITIAL SYMPTOMS	EXACERBATING FACTORS	MOST IMPORTANT SCREENING TESTS	TREATMENT
Acute intermittent porphyria	Neurovisceral (acute)	Drugs (mostly P-450 inducers), progesterone, dietary restriction	Urinary porphobilinogen	Heme, glucose
Porphyria cutanea tarda	Blistering skin lesions (chronic)	Iron, alcohol, estrogens, hepatitis C virus, halogenated hydrocarbons	Plasma (or urine) porphyrins	Phlebotomy, low-dose chloroquine
Erythropoietic protoporphyria	Painful skin and swelling (mostly acute)		Plasma (or erythrocyte) porphyrins	β-Carotene

Table 219–3 ■ DRUGS CONSIDERED UNSAFE AND SAFE IN ACUTE INTERMITTENT AND VARIEGATE PORPHYRIA AND HEREDITARY COPROPORPHYRIA

UNSAFE	SAFE
Barbiturates*	Narcotic analgesics
Sulfonamide antibiotics*	Aspirin
Meprobamate* (also mebutamate*, tybuta-	Acetaminophen
mate*)	Phenothiazines
Carisoprodol*	Penicillin and derivatives
Glutethimide*	Streptomycin
Methyprylon	Glucocorticoids
Ethchlorvynol*	Bromides
Phenytoin*	Gabapentin
Mephenytoin	Insulin
Succinimides (ethosuximide, methsuximide)	Atropine
Carbamazepine*	Cimetidine
Clonazepam	Ranitidine*†
Primidone*	Erythropoietin*†
Valproic acid*	? Estrogens*‡
Pyrazolones (aminopyrine, antipyrine)	
Griseofulvin*	
Ergots	
Metoclopramide*	
Rifampin*	
Pyrazinamide*	
Diclofenac and possibly other NSAIDs*	
Progesterone and synthetic progestins*	
Danazol*	
Alcohol	

NSAIDs = non-steroidal anti-inflammatory drugs.

*Porphyria is listed as a contraindication, warning, precaution, or adverse effect in U.S. labeling for these drugs. For drugs listed here as unsafe, absence of such cautionary statements in U.S. labeling does not imply lower risk.

†Although porphyria is listed as a precaution in U.S. labeling, these drugs are regarded as safe by other sources.

‡There is little evidence that estrogens alone are harmful in acute porphyrias. They have been implicated as harmful mostly from experience with estrogen-progestin combinations and because they can exacerbate porphyria cutanea tarda.

porphyrias are uncommon, their symptoms are non-specific, and physical findings are minimal. Therefore, a high index of suspicion is necessary for diagnosis. The diagnosis is established by demonstrating a marked increase in urinary PBG by quantitative assay (see the later discussion of laboratory methods). During an acute attack, PBG excretion is generally in the range of 50 to 200 mg/day (reference range, 0 to 4 mg/day), and ALA excretion is 20 to 100 mg/day (reference range, 0 to 7 mg/day). Such increases virtually ensure a diagnosis of AIP, variegate porphyria (VP), or hereditary coproporphyria (HCP). ALA and PBG excretion generally decreases with clinical improvement. Such decreases are particularly dramatic (but transient) after heme therapy. After an attack it is distinctly unusual for ALA and PBG to decrease to persistently normal levels, except after prolonged periods of latency. In HCP and VP, urinary ALA and PBG may be less increased and decrease to normal levels more readily than in AIP. Fecal porphyrins are usually normal or minimally increased, which distinguishes AIP from HCP and VP. Urinary uroporphyrin and coproporphyrin and erythrocyte protoporphyrin may be increased, but these findings are not specific.

Decreased PBG deaminase (most conveniently measured in erythrocytes) confirms a diagnosis of AIP. However, as already noted, some mutations of the PBG deaminase gene only reduce the non-erythroid enzyme. Furthermore, erythrocyte PBG deaminase has a wide normal range (up to three-fold) that somewhat overlaps the AIP range and is increased by inapparent concurrent conditions that stimulate erythropoiesis. The enzyme is not reduced in HCP and VP, which are also important to consider when acute porphyria is suspected. For these reasons, measurement of erythrocyte PBG deaminase is not useful in acutely ill patients. On the other hand, its measurement is highly useful for analysis of pedigrees of known AIP patients, if it is established that the propositus has a low value. In screening family members, urinary PBG should also be measured. Diagnosis of AIP in utero is possible but seldom indicated in view of the favorable outlook for most PBG deaminase–deficient subjects.

No single laboratory test fully excludes AIP, HCP, and VP. However, a normal result of a quantitative test for urinary PBG virtually excludes AIP and is strong evidence against HCP and VP as a cause of the current symptoms. Attempting to provoke increases in ALA and PBG for diagnostic purposes by glycine loading or administration of phenobarbital may be dangerous and is not definitive.

TREATMENT. Acute attacks usually require hospitalization for the treatment of severe pain, nausea, and vomiting and for the administration of intravenous glucose and heme. Hospitalization also facilitates observation for neurologic complications, electrolyte imbalances, and nutritional status, as well as investigation of precipitating factors. Symptomatic therapy includes narcotic analgesics, which are usually required for abdominal pain, and small to moderate doses of a phenothiazine for nausea, vomiting, anxiety, and restlessness. Chloral hydrate can be used for insomnia. Diazepam in low doses is probably safe if a minor tranquilizer is required. Bladder distention may require catheterization. After recovery, continued treatment with a phenothiazine is seldom indicated.

Heme therapy and carbohydrate loading are specific therapies because they repress hepatic ALA synthase and overproduction of ALA and PBG. Heme therapy is most effective in this regard and should be initiated early, but only after the diagnosis of a porphyric attack is confirmed by a marked increase in urinary PBG. Diagnosis is more difficult after heme therapy, which can at least transiently normalize ALA and PBG.

The standard regimen for heme therapy is 3–4 mg heme per kilogram body weight infused intravenously once daily for 4 days. A longer course of treatment is seldom necessary if treatment is started early. Efficacy is reduced and recovery less rapid when treatment is delayed and neuronal damage is more advanced. It is not effective for chronic symptoms of AIP. A lyophilized hematin (hydroxyheme) preparation is available in the United States. The manufacturer recommends reconstitution with sterile water. However, the product is unstable and degradation products adhere to endothelial cells, platelets, and coagulation factors and cause a transient anticoagulant effect and phlebitis at the site of infusion. Reconstitution with human albumin enhances the stability of hematin and prevents these side effects. Heme arginate, which is available in Europe and South Africa, is much more stable than hematin and also does not have these side effects. It is an investigational drug in the United States.

Carbohydrate loading may suffice for mild attacks and can be given orally as sucrose, glucose polymers, or carbohydrate-rich foods. If oral intake is poorly tolerated or is contraindicated by distention and ileus, intravenous administration of glucose (at least 300 g daily) is usually indicated. A central venous line facilitates more complete parenteral nutrition support and avoids excess fluid volumes. Parenteral nutrition support may be indicated in some patients who require heme therapy.

Treatment of seizures is problematic because almost all antiseizure drugs can exacerbate AIP. Bromides, gabapentin, and probably vigabatrin can be given safely. β-Adrenergic blocking agents may control tachycardia and hypertension in acute attacks of porphyria, but they may be hazardous in patients with hypovolemia, in whom increased catecholamine secretion may be an important compensatory mechanism. Numerous other therapies have been tried in this disease but have not been consistently useful.

PROGNOSIS. In the past 20 years, attacks of porphyria have rarely been fatal. If acute attacks are treated appropriately, inciting factors are removed, and precautions are taken to prevent further attacks, the outlook for patients with AIP is usually excellent. Recurrent attacks of porphyria occur in some patients and can be disabling, but they do not occur throughout adult life. Occasionally, chronic pain and other symptoms develop, but they may improve in the long term. Chronic symptoms and depression increase the risk of suicide and thus require careful management.

Symptoms never develop in the great majority of relatives with PBG deaminase deficiency, especially if they have normal urinary porphyrin precursors. Although such individuals are less sensitive to inducing drugs, etc., than are patients with prior porphyric symptoms, they should follow the same precautions as patients with AIP. Latent AIP should never be construed as a health risk that limits the availability of health insurance.

PREVENTION. Some specific measures are helpful in preventing clinical expression of AIP. (1) Family members should be screened to detect latent cases. (2) Harmful drugs should be avoided. (3) "Crash diets" for weight reduction and even brief periods of starvation (e.g., during postoperative periods or intercurrent illnesses) should be avoided. Diet regimens for obesity should provide for gradual weight loss during periods of clinical remission of porphyria. (4) Gonadotropin-releasing hormone analogues (for women with frequent cyclic attacks) or periodic heme infusions can prevent attacks. Oophorectomy is not an acceptable option for preventing cyclic attacks. Because suicide is a risk in AIP, a preventive approach is appropriate, especially in patients with chronic symptoms and depression.

CONGENITAL ERYTHROPOIETIC PORPHYRIA. Congenital erythropoietic porphyria (CEP) is an autosomal recessive disorder that is due to a deficiency of uroporphyrinogen III cosynthase. Fewer than 200 cases have been reported. CEP occurs in several animal species (including all fox squirrels).

ETIOLOGY AND PATHOGENESIS. Many different mutations of the uroporphyrinogen III cosynthase gene have been identified in CEP. Most patients have unrelated parents and have inherited a different mutation from each parent. The severity of the disease is variable and relates to the degree of enzyme deficiency caused by the particular mutations. There is considerable accumulation of hydroxymethylbilane (the substrate of the deficient enzyme), which is converted non-enzymatically to uroporphyrinogen I. Uroporphyrin I and other porphyrins accumulate in bone marrow erythroid cells that are actively synthesizing hemoglobin and lead to intramedullary and intravascular hemolysis. Even in the most severe cases some residual cosynthase activity is noted, and heme production is actually increased in response to hemolysis. Excretion of type III porphyrin isomers is also increased. Splenomegaly can contribute to anemia and cause leukopenia and thrombocytopenia. Sunlight, other sources of ultraviolet light, and minor trauma to friable skin are other determinants of clinical expression. Drugs, steroids, and nutrition have little influence.

CLINICAL MANIFESTATIONS. Clinical expression is variable. In most cases, reddish urine and severe cutaneous photosensitivity are noted in early infancy. In a few very severe cases, CEP has been manifested as non-immune hydrops and intrauterine transfusions were administered. If CEP was not recognized, marked photosensitivity developed when phototherapy was initiated for neonatal jaundice. In some milder cases, symptoms begin in adult life. Cutaneous features resemble those in PCT but are usually more severe. Lesions on sun-exposed skin include bullae and vesicles, which are prone to rupture and become infected, hypopigmented or hyperpigmented areas, and hypertrichosis. Loss of digits and facial features and corneal scarring can be severe. Porphyrins are deposited in the teeth (producing a reddish brown color termed "erythrodontia") and in bone. Bone demineralization can be substantial. No neurologic manifestations are known, but hemolysis and splenomegaly are almost always present. Life expectancy is often shortened by infections or hematologic complications.

DIAGNOSIS AND DIFFERENTIAL DIAGNOSIS. In CEP, porphyrin excretion and porphyrin levels in red cells and plasma are generally much greater than in other forms of porphyria. Porphyrins in urine are primarily uroporphyrin and coproporphyrin, and in feces porphyrins mostly consist of coproporphyrin. ALA and PBG are normal. In most cases, uroporphyrin I predominates in erythrocytes. A predominance of protoporphyrin in red cells has been described in some cases and is characteristic of bovine CEP. CEP is readily distinguished from EPP clinically but may resemble HEP and homozygous cases of AIP, VP, and HCP.

TREATMENT. Protection of the skin from sunlight and minor trauma and prompt treatment of secondary bacterial infections help prevent scarring and mutilation. Improvement may occur after splenectomy. Oral charcoal may be helpful by increasing fecal excretion of porphyrins. Blood transfusions sufficient to suppress erythropoiesis and bone marrow transplantation may be the most effective current therapies but entail significant risks. Gene therapy may eventually be possible.

PREVENTION. In affected families, heterozygotes with intermediate deficiencies of the cosynthase can be detected, and CEP can be diagnosed in utero. Therefore, options are available for preventing genetic transmission.

PORPHYRIA CUTANEA TARDA. PCT is the most common and readily treated form of porphyria and is caused by a deficiency of uroporphyrinogen decarboxylase in the liver. It is most common in men but has become more frequent in women in association with alcohol and estrogen use.

ETIOLOGY AND PATHOGENESIS. Both acquired and inherited factors can play causative roles in PCT. Individual cases can be classified as "sporadic" (type I) or "familial" (type II). The majority of cases are type I, in which uroporphyrinogen decarboxylase mutations are not found and the enzyme is deficient in the liver but not in erythrocytes and other tissues. The amount of hepatic uroporphyrinogen decarboxylase protein, as measured immunochemically, is normal, thus suggesting that an acquired process has inactivated the enzyme. With treatment and remission of the disease, enzyme activity gradually increases to normal. Familial (type II) PCT is distinguished from type I by an inherited, approximately 50% deficiency of the decarboxylase in all tissues, including erythrocytes. This deficiency is an autosomal dominant trait and can result from a number of different mutations of the uroporphyrinogen decarboxylase gene. Apparently, type II PCT is not manifested clinically until the product of the normal allele is inactivated in the liver, as in type I PCT. A type III PCT has been described in which the enzyme is deficient in the liver but not in other tissues and more than one family member is affected. Types I to III are clinically similar and often difficult to distinguish, and they respond to the same therapies.

Examples of *toxic porphyria* have resembled PCT. Most notably, an extensive outbreak of porphyria occurred in eastern Turkey in 1955–1958 after seed wheat containing the fungicide hexachlorobenzene was used for food. Dichlorophenols, trichlorophenols, and 2,3,7,8-tetrachlorodibenzo-*p*-dioxin (TCDD, dioxin) have been implicated in smaller outbreaks and single cases in humans. When administered to animals, these chemicals decrease uroporphyrinogen decarboxylase (only in the liver) and induce a pattern of excess porphyrins resembling PCT. A history of exposure to such chemicals is seldom found in sporadic (type I) PCT.

A notable feature of PCT is massive accumulation of porphyrins in the liver, which may develop over many months. This accumulation precedes the appearance of excess porphyrins in plasma and urine. Hepatic ALA synthase may be little increased because the amount of excess porphyrins produced in PCT is small relative to the rate of hepatic heme formation. By contrast, during attacks of the acute porphyrias, much larger amounts of intermediates are excreted (as porphyrin precursors) and ALA synthase is substantially induced. Worsening of PCT by factors (other than alcohol) that induce heme synthesis is seldom reported.

The pattern of porphyrins that accumulate in PCT is complex and characteristic. The enzyme-catalyzed decarboxylation of uroporphyrinogen occurs in four sequential steps. Therefore, when the enzyme is markedly deficient, uroporphyrin and the heptacarboxyl, hexacarboxyl, and pentacarboxyl porphyrins (type I and III isomers and porphyrins derived from the corresponding porphyrinogens) accumulate. In addition, pentacarboxyl porphyrinogen can be metabolized by coproporphyrinogen oxidase to a series of tetracarboxyl porphyrins termed isocoproporphyrins. These substances are excreted primarily in bile and feces and are diagnostic of uroporphyrinogen decarboxylase deficiency.

Multiple factors may contribute to the inactivation of hepatic uroporphyrinogen decarboxylase. (1) A normal or increased amount of hepatic iron seems essential in this disease. Patients with PCT are homozygous or heterozygous for the *HFE* gene mutation, which is associated with genetic hemochromatosis more commonly than expected by chance. Ferrous iron may directly inhibit uroporphyrinogen decarboxylase. Iron may catalyze the formation of free radicals that damage the enzyme protein or oxidize its porphyrinogen substrates to porphyrins. (2) Cytochrome P-450 enzymes may also be involved in the oxidation of porphyrinogen substrates. (3) Alcohol intake may promote iron absorption, stimulate hepatic heme and porphyrin synthesis, or generate free radicals that damage the decarboxylase. (4) Levels of antioxidant vitamins (C and E) may be decreased. (5) Estrogens but apparently not other steroids can exacerbate PCT, perhaps by an unknown oxidative mechanism. (6) The strong association with chronic hepatitis C virus infection suggests that the hepatocellular damage induced by this virus, which appears to be accentuated by iron, can involve specific cellular proteins, including uroporphyrinogen decarboxylase. Drugs may worsen PCT; those so indicated in U.S. labeling are several non-steroidal anti-inflammatory drugs, sulfonylureas, and busulfan.

CLINICAL MANIFESTATIONS. Most patients with PCT have a history of moderate or heavy alcohol intake. The disease may develop in men treated with estrogens for prostate cancer and in women taking oral contraceptives or replacement estrogens. Cutaneous photosensitivity is the major clinical feature. Vesicles and bullae develop on the face, dorsum of the hands and feet, forearms, and legs. Sun-exposed skin becomes friable, and minor trauma may precede the formation of bullae or cause denudation of the skin. Small white plaques ("milia") may precede or follow vesicle formation. Involved skin tends to heal slowly. Hypertrichosis and hyperpigmentation sometimes occur even in the absence of vesicles. Thickening, scarring, and calcification of affected skin ("pseudoscleroderma") may be striking. Neurologic effects are not observed.

Liver histopathology is not usually diagnostic of alcoholic liver disease. Cirrhosis and hepatocellular carcinomas are most common in older patients and at autopsy. In some locations as many as 80% of patients with PCT are chronically infected with hepatitis C virus. This strong association may explain much of the chronic liver damage and many of the hepatocellular carcinomas that have been observed in patients with PCT. However, liver damage occurs in PCT in the absence of hepatitis C. Liver iron may be increased and *HFE* mutations present. The disease is also associated with systemic lupus erythematosus and acquired immune deficiency syndrome.

PCT sometimes occurs in patients with advanced renal disease. Skin lesions may be more severe and plasma porphyrin levels much higher in this setting because urinary excretion of porphyrins is not possible and they are poorly dialyzed.

Very rarely, hepatic tumors themselves contain and presumably produce excess porphyrins. Some of these cases have resembled PCT.

DIAGNOSIS AND DIFFERENTIAL DIAGNOSIS. Skin lesions in PCT, VP, and HCP are indistinguishable clinically and histologically. It is important to differentiate these conditions by laboratory testing before starting therapy. A predominance of uroporphyrin and heptacarboxyl porphyrin in urine and increased isocoproporphyrin in feces is diagnostic of PCT. In PCT, urinary ALA may be slightly increased, whereas PBG is normal. Total fecal porphyrins are usually less increased in PCT than in other types of porphyria with photosensitivity. Plasma porphyrins are virtually always increased in patients with skin lesions from any type of porphyria; the fluorescence spectrum of plasma can distinguish VP and EPP from PCT (see below).

TREATMENT. A course of phlebotomies is the preferred treatment and almost always produces a remission. Patients are also advised to discontinue the use of alcohol, estrogens, iron supplements, or other contributing factors. Because iron stores in PCT are seldom markedly increased and may be normal, removal of only 5 to 6 U of blood at 1- to 2-week intervals is usually sufficient. Many more phlebotomies may be needed in patients who also have hemochromatosis. Plasma (or serum) ferritin and porphyrin levels should be monitored (Fig. 219–2). Deferoxamine, an iron chelator, may be effective but is much less efficient.

A course of low-dose chloroquine, 125 mg twice weekly, or hydroxychloroquine, 100 mg twice weekly for several months, is usually effective when repeated phlebotomies are contraindicated. The mechanism of their effects in PCT has not been established. One hypothesis is that chloroquine forms complexes with porphyrins and promotes their removal from the liver. If usual doses of these drugs are given to patients with PCT, marked increases in photosensitivity and porphyrin levels in plasma and urine are seen and may be accompanied by nausea, malaise, fever, and hepatocellular damage. Although these adverse effects are generally transient and are followed by complete remission, it is prudent to avoid them by using a low-dose regimen.

Therapy is more difficult when PCT occurs with advanced renal disease because phlebotomy is usually contraindicated by anemia (usually because of erythropoietin deficiency). Recent studies indicate that genetic recombinant erythropoietin can mobilize excess iron, support phlebotomy, and lead to remission of PCT in these patients.

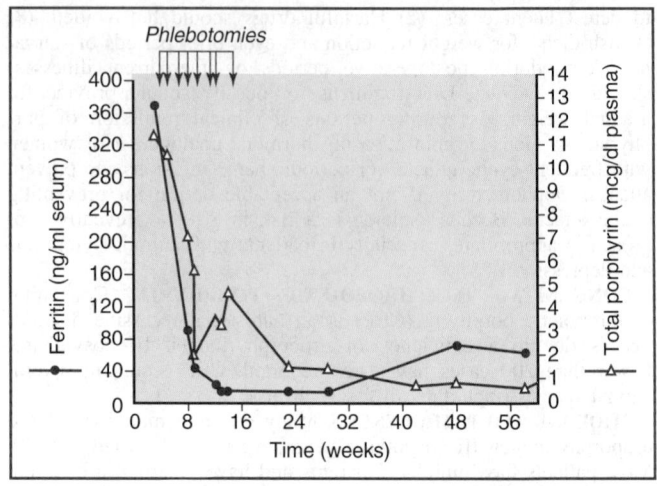

FIGURE 219–2 ■ Treatment of porphyria cutanea tarda by repeated phlebotomy. The patient was a 37-year-old woman with a history of excess alcohol intake and chronic hepatitis C. Each arrow indicates removal of 450 mL of whole blood. Phlebotomies are stopped when serum ferritin is near the lower limit of normal. Further iron depletion is of no additional benefit and may cause anemia and associated symptoms. Plasma porphyrins become normal and the appearance of new skin lesions ceases within several months. After remission, ferritin can return to normal without recurrence, in most cases. In some cases, relapses occur and respond to another course of phlebotomies. (Modified from Anderson KE: The porphyrias. *In* Zakim D, Boyer T (eds): Hepatology. Philadelphia, WB Saunders, 1996, pp 417–463.)

HEPATOERYTHROPOIETIC PORPHYRIA. This rare autosomal recessive disease is clinically similar to CEP but is distinguished by excess isocoproporphyrin in feces and urine and decreased uroporphyrinogen decarboxylase activity in erythrocytes (and other tissues). Mild cases may resemble PCT. Mutations in the uroporphyrinogen decarboxylase gene are found in this disease and are associated with some residual enzyme activity. Increased erythrocyte protoporphyrin probably reflects an earlier accumulation of uroporphyrinogen in erythroblasts, which after completion of hemoglobin synthesis is metabolized to protoporphyrin. A similar explanation can account for increased erythrocyte protoporphyrin in other homozygous forms of porphyria.

HEREDITARY COPROPORPHYRIA AND VARIEGATE PORPHYRIA. These autosomal dominant acute hepatic porphyrias are clinically similar to AIP but are much less common in most countries. Unlike AIP, these disorders can cause cutaneous photosensitivity. VP is quite prevalent in South Africa, where most cases have been traced to a couple who immigrated from Holland in the late 1600s.

ETIOLOGY AND PATHOGENESIS. HCP and VP are due to approximately 50% deficiencies of coproporphyrinogen oxidase and protoporphyrinogen oxidase, respectively. Many different mutations in the genes for these enzymes have been described. A specific mutation of the protoporphyrinogen oxidase gene is common in South Africa. ALA and PBG are increased during acute attacks, although the degree and duration of increases are less than in AIP. Increases in ALA and PBG occur when hepatic ALA synthase is induced by factors such as endogenous steroids, drugs, and nutritional alterations and because PBG deaminase activity is almost as low as ALA synthase activity even in normal liver. Coproporphyrinogen III may accumulate in VP because of a functional association between coproporphyrinogen oxidase and the deficient protoporphyrinogen oxidase in mitochondria. Furthermore, coproporphyrinogen is more readily lost from the liver than are other porphyrinogens, and its loss increases further when heme synthesis is stimulated. The excess porphyrinogens are auto-oxidized to the corresponding porphyrins. In one form of HCP termed *harderoporphyria*, a structurally altered coproporphyrinogen oxidase with reduced substrate affinity results in the accumulation of harderoporphyrin (tricarboxyl porphyrinogen) as well as coproporphyrin. A few homozygous cases of HCP and VP have been described.

CLINICAL MANIFESTATIONS. Drugs, steroids, and nutritional factors that are detrimental in AIP provoke exacerbations of HCP and VP. Neurologic manifestations are identical to those in AIP. Skin manifestations are similar to those of PCT and may occur apart from the neurovisceral symptoms. Impaired biliary excretion by concurrent liver diseases or drugs such as contraceptive steroids can cause porphyrin retention and worsen photosensitivity.

DIAGNOSIS AND DIFFERENTIAL DIAGNOSIS. Urinary ALA and PBG are commonly increased during acute attacks. With resolution of symptoms, ALA and PBG normalize more readily than in AIP. Increases in urinary porphyrins are more persistent. A marked, isolated increase in fecal coproporphyrin (especially isomer III) is distinctive for HCP. Fecal coproporphyrin and protoporphyrin are about equally increased in VP. The fluorescence spectrum of plasma porphyrins (at neutral pH) is characteristic and very useful for rapidly distinguishing VP from the other porphyrias. This test is probably the most sensitive porphyrin measurement for detecting VP, including latent cases, at least in adults.

TREATMENT AND PROGNOSIS. Acute attacks of VP are treated as in AIP. Phlebotomies and chloroquine are not effective. The striking decreases in attacks and deaths from VP in South Africa have been attributed to identification of latent cases, avoidance of harmful drugs, and better treatment during acute attacks. Measures that protect the skin from sunlight are helpful for photosensitivity. Cholestyramine may decrease the photosensitivity occurring with liver dysfunction.

ERYTHROPOIETIC PROTOPORPHYRIA. EPP was not clearly described until 1961, perhaps because it seldom causes blistering of the skin and urine porphyrins are not increased. Now recognized as the third most common porphyria, EPP is due to a deficiency of ferrochelatase, with increased protoporphyrin in erythrocytes, plasma, bile, and feces.

ETIOLOGY AND PATHOGENESIS. Many different mutations in the ferrochelatase gene have been identified in various EPP families. Most of these mutant alleles express little or no ferrochelatase. The pattern of inheritance often appears to be autosomal dominant, but some obligate carriers have little or no increase in red cell protoporphyrin. Co-inheritance of a common ferrochelatase allele that expresses low levels of enzyme may explain an incompletely dominant trait, at least in some families.

Ferrochelatase is deficient in all tissues in clinically expressed EPP but becomes rate limiting for protoporphyrin metabolism primarily in bone marrow reticulocytes, which are the primary source of the excess protoporphyrin. Circulating erythrocytes and the liver contribute smaller amounts. Protoporphyrin is increased in plasma and is excreted in bile and feces. Protoporphyrin in erythrocytes in patients with EPP is not complexed with zinc and, when compared with zinc protoporphyrin (found in lead poisoning, iron deficiency, and homozygous forms of porphyria), diffuses more readily into plasma. Zinc protoporphyrin dissociates less readily from hemoglobin binding sites and persists in the red cell as long as it circulates. Disposition of the excess protoporphyrin in EPP depends on hepatic uptake, biliary excretion, and the degree of enterohepatic circulation. These processes are impaired by liver damage.

CLINICAL MANIFESTATIONS. Cutaneous manifestations usually begin in childhood and are distinctly different from those of other porphyrias. Burning, itching, erythema, and swelling can occur within minutes of sun exposure. Diffuse edema of sun-exposed areas may resemble angioneurotic edema. Other characteristic skin changes include lichenification, leathery pseudovesicles, labial grooving, and nail changes. Scarring is rarely severe or deforming. Vesicles, pigment changes, friability, and hirsutism are unusual. No fluorescence of the teeth and (except with severe hepatic failure) no neuropathic manifestations are present. Drugs that exacerbate hepatic porphyrias are not known to worsen EPP, although they are generally avoided as a precaution.

Hemolysis is uncommon or very mild in uncomplicated cases. Erythropoiesis and iron metabolism are generally normal. Mild anemia with hypochromia and microcytosis is noted in some cases and is unexplained. Gallstones containing protoporphyrin may develop in patients with EPP.

Liver function is usually normal in EPP. In a minority of patients with EPP, liver disease with protoporphyrin deposition can develop and progress rapidly to death from liver failure. Liver complications may be more likely to develop in individuals who have inherited certain ferrochelatase mutations. Excess protoporphyrin itself may have cholestatic effects and damage hepatocytes. Intercurrent factors such as viral hepatitis, alcohol, iron deficiency, fasting, and oral contraceptive steroids have played a role in some

patients. Marked photosensitivity with blistering and motor neuropathy have occurred in some patients with EPP and liver failure.

DIAGNOSIS AND DIFFERENTIAL DIAGNOSIS. Protoporphyrin is increased in bone marrow, erythrocytes, plasma, bile, and the feces of patients with EPP. Urinary porphyrins and porphyrin precursors are normal. Hepatic complications of EPP are often preceded by increasing levels of erythrocyte and plasma protoporphyrin, abnormal liver function tests, marked deposition of protoporphyrin in liver cells and bile canaliculi, and increased photosensitivity.

TREATMENT AND PROGNOSIS. β-Carotene (Lumitene, Tishcon) was developed primarily for treating EPP. Its clinical benefits have been substantiated in large series of patients. No side effects other than a mild and dose-related skin discoloration because of carotenemia have been noted. Its mechanism of action may involve quenching of singlet oxygen or free radicals. Cholestyramine may reduce protoporphyrin levels by interrupting its enterohepatic circulation. Iron deficiency, caloric restriction, and drugs or hormone preparations that impair hepatic excretory function should be avoided.

Hepatic complications may resolve spontaneously if a reversible cause of liver dysfunction such as viral hepatitis or alcohol is contributing. Transfusions or heme therapy may suppress erythroid and hepatic protoporphyrin production. Splenectomy, correction of iron deficiency, and cholestyramine or activated charcoal may be beneficial. Liver transplantation is sometimes required. Operating room lights have produced severe skin and peritoneal burns in some patients.

DUAL PORPHYRIA. Dual porphyria refers to patients with porphyria and deficiencies of more than one enzyme of the heme biosynthetic pathway. Examples include double heterozygotes with both VP and familial PCT, deficiencies of both PBG deaminase and uroporphyrinogen decarboxylase (with symptoms of AIP, PCT, or both), and deficiencies of both coproporphyrinogen oxidase and uroporphyrinogen III cosynthase.

LABORATORY DIAGNOSIS OF PORPHYRIAS

Appropriate laboratory testing for these disorders is both specific and sensitive. An array of tests for porphyria are available, but some are subject to overuse and misinterpretation. Porphyrias can be readily detected and misdiagnoses avoided by relying primarily on a few first-line tests. The preferred approach for screening, as outlined in Table 219–4, is to rely on measurement of *urinary porphyrin precursors (ALA and PBG) and total porphyrins* for patients with neurovisceral symptoms and a fluorometric measurement of *plasma total porphyrins* when it is suspected that skin photosensitivity might be due to porphyria.

In acutely ill patients, it is important to identify or exclude acute porphyria promptly. Urinary PBG (and ALA) is virtually always markedly increased during acute attacks of AIP. ALA and PBG may be less increased in HCP and VP, but urinary total porphyrins are consistently markedly increased in symptomatic patients. Normal levels of ALA, PBG, and total porphyrins effectively exclude all acute porphyrias as potential causes of the current symptoms. Because increases are so striking during an attack, quantitation on a random urine sample is highly informative. Assays for PBG use Ehrlich's aldehyde (*p*-dimethylaminobenzaldehyde), which forms reddish purple chromogens with PBG, urobilinogen, and other substances in urine. Qualitative methods (e.g., the Watson-Schwartz and Hoesch tests) are still widely used to screen for increased PBG. They are subject to misinterpretation and false-positive reports, do not quantitate PBG, and are less sensitive and only slightly more rapid than quantitative methods, which separate PBG from interfering substances by ion exchange chromatography. If a qualitative test for PBG is used for screening, positive samples should be retested by a quantitative method.

Total plasma porphyrins are virtually always increased in patients with active skin lesions from porphyrias. Normal plasma porphyrin levels exclude porphyria as a cause of cutaneous symptoms, especially if the measurement is carried out by a simple and direct fluorometric method. Plasma porphyrins in VP are mostly covalently bound to plasma porphyrins and may not be detected by other methods.

More extensive testing is required if an initial screening test for

Table 219-4 ■ FIRST-LINE LABORATORY TESTS FOR SCREENING FOR PORPHYRIAS AND SECOND-LINE TESTS FOR FURTHER EVALUATION WHEN INITIAL TESTING IS POSITIVE

	SYMPTOMS SUGGESTING PORPHYRIA	
TESTING	Acute Neurovisceral Symptoms	Cutaneous Photosensitivity
First line	Urinary ALA, PBG, and total porphyrins (quantitative, random urine)	Total plasma porphyrins*
Second line	Urinary ALA, PBG, and total porphyrins† (quantitative, 24-hr urine)	Erythrocyte porphyrins
	Total fecal porphyrins†	Urinary ALA, PBG, and total porphyrins† (quantitative, 24-hr urine)
	Erythrocyte PBG deaminase	Total fecal porphyrins†
	Total plasma porphyrins*	

ALA = δ-aminolevulinic acid; PBG = porphobilinogen.
*The preferred method is by direct fluorescent spectrophotometry.
†Urinary and fecal porphyrins are fractionated only if the total is increased.

porphyria provides a positive result; such testing may also be necessary initially if subclinical porphyria is suspected. Interpretation of urine, fecal, and erythrocyte porphyrin levels is often problematic for the following reasons. (1) These measurements do not individually detect all cutaneous porphyrias. (2) Urine and erythrocyte porphyrins can be increased in many conditions other than porphyria, whereas an increased plasma porphyrin concentration is much more specific for porphyria. (3) Fecal porphyrin determinations are semiquantitative and subject to interference by diet and other factors.

Laboratory testing of relatives is not usually appropriate until test results have firmly established a diagnosis of porphyria in the propositus. Results of testing the propositus guide the choice of tests for relatives. Cytosolic heme biosynthetic pathway enzymes (ALA dehydratase, PBG deaminase, uroporphyrinogen III cosynthase, and uroporphyrinogen decarboxylase) can be measured in erythrocytes. These assays are not recommended for the initial screening of patients with symptoms suggestive of porphyria. The other heme pathway enzymes are mitochondrial and are not reliably measured in erythrocytes. Demonstrating a specific mutation in a family greatly facilitates the detection of relatives who carry the same mutation. Consultation with a physician and a laboratory experienced in testing for porphyrias is helpful in these situations.

Laboratory data that were the basis for an original diagnosis of porphyria should remain available for future reference. Incorrect diagnoses of porphyria are not uncommon in patients with symptoms from other diseases. Not very much evidence supports recent suggestions that porphyria is common in disorders such as multiple chemical sensitivity syndrome.

Anderson KE: The porphyrias. In Zakim D, Boyer T (eds): Hepatology. Philadelphia, WB Saunders, 1996, pp 417–463. One of several recent and detailed reviews on the genetic, biochemical, and clinical aspects of the porphyrias.
Mustajoki P, Nordmann Y: Early administration of heme arginate for acute porphyric attacks. Arch Intern Med 153:2004, 1993. A large series of patients treated with intravenous heme, with an emphasis on the importance of early treatment.
Roberts AG, Whatley SD, Morgan RR, et al: Increased frequency of haemochromatosis Cys282Tyr mutation in sporadic porphyria cutanea tarda. Lancet 349:321, 1997. Homozygotes for this mutation may be seen late in life with PCT rather than hemochromatosis.
Schmid R (ed): The porphyrias. Semin Liver Dis 18:1, 1998. A collection of reviews emphasizing recent progress in the cellular and molecular biology of these diseases.

220 WILSON DISEASE

William A. Gahl

DEFINITION. Wilson disease (hepatolenticular degeneration) is a rare, potentially fatal disorder of copper toxicity characterized by progressive liver disease, neurologic deterioration, or both.

ETIOLOGY. The Wilson disease gene, *ATP7B*, is located on chromosome 13q14.3 and codes for a copper-transporting P-type adenosinetriphosphatase (ATPase). *ATP7B* has 60% identity with *MNK*, the gene involved in Menkes' disease, a neurologic disorder of copper enzyme deficiency. Both genes code for a transporter that has six copper-binding motifs, an adenosine triphosphate–binding domain, an aspartyl kinase domain, a phosphatase domain, and eight membrane-spanning regions. *ATP7B* has 21 exons and is expressed primarily in the liver and kidney, with a shorter, alternatively spliced form in the brain. The full-length gene product has been localized to the trans-Golgi, whereas the truncated product is found in the cell cytoplasm. By late 1997, at least 27 distinct mutations in 20 different exons had been reported; the most common, His1069Gln, was present in one third of patients of European ancestry with Wilson disease. Correlations between genotype and phenotype are weak.

PREVALENCE. An autosomal recessive disorder, Wilson disease occurs throughout the world; the prevalence in the United States approximates 1 in 40,000.

PATHOGENESIS. In normal adults, the intestines absorb 1 to 5 mg of copper each day; net balance is achieved by the regulated biliary excretion of copper in a non-resorbable form. Urinary excretion is minimal in the absence of copper overload or excessive wasting of certain amino acids to which copper binds. In Wilson disease, biliary excretion of copper is reduced to approximately 20% of normal, and copper progressively accumulates in the liver. Increased hepatic copper damages the liver and overflows to other tissues. These complications occur at extremely variable rates that are influenced by allelic differences, other genes, dietary copper intake, and viral infections. Acute, substantial liver damage, for any reason, releases copper for uptake by the brain, cornea, kidney, muscle, bones, and joints.

Ceruloplasmin is an α₂-globulin glycoprotein that carries over 80% of the copper present in human plasma. It has amine oxidase activity, by which the holoenzyme can be assayed, and may play a role in copper transport from the liver to other tissues. Soon after delivery from the intestine to the liver, copper is incorporated into ceruloplasmin. This process appears to be impaired in Wilson disease; 95% of patients have reduced ceruloplasmin levels despite having normal amounts of other copper enzymes.

The dual defects of reduced ceruloplasmin levels and impaired biliary copper excretion can be explained by a copper-transporting ATPase located in the Golgi that fails to incorporate copper into proteins destined for secretion. Presumably, one of these proteins is ceruloplasmin secreted into the circulation and another is a non-resorbable copper-binding protein (perhaps ceruloplasmin) secreted into the bile. Alternatively, the protein(s) may incorporate copper but fail to leave the hepatocyte. Animal models of Wilson disease such as the Long-Evans cinnamon rat and the toxic milk mouse may help elucidate the precise metabolic defect in Wilson disease.

PATHOLOGY. The liver in patients with Wilson disease shows non-specific changes, including piecemeal necrosis and lymphocytosis progressing to fibrosis and cirrhosis, usually micronodular. Copper staining with rhodanine can be patchy and variable. In the brain, the basal ganglia can be atrophic, and the cerebrum may also show involvement. Descemet's membrane in the cornea contains granular deposits of copper.

CLINICAL MANIFESTATIONS. In general, one third of patients with Wilson disease have liver disease, one third have neurologic impairment, and one third have both. Because copper initially accumulates in the liver, patients with hepatic symptoms are younger, as a rule, than those with extrahepatic symptoms. The liver damage associated with Wilson disease frequently resembles viral hepatitis and appears between 8 and 16 years of age with jaundice, anorexia, malaise, and increased serum liver enzymes. It sometimes follows a waxing and waning course, and portal hypertension is common. Hepatic coma and death may occur precipitously without the benefit of a diagnosis. Cirrhosis eventually develops in all untreated patients.

Neurologic symptoms of Wilson disease occur rarely before adolescence but commonly in early adulthood. They include dysarthrias and loss of fine motor coordination, abnormal tone, dystonic posturing, unsteady gait, and uncontrolled, involuntary movements including chorea and wing-beating proximal tremors. Psychiatric, intellectual, emotional, and behavioral disturbances often occur, and decreased school performance can be an initial sign. Organic dementia is usually present in neurologically involved patients. Seizures are rare. A pseudobulbar palsy may develop at any time and can be fatal.

Copper overflow to the cornea results in Kayser-Fleischer rings, characteristic yellow-brown deposits at the limbus of the cornea, especially apparent at the upper and lower poles. Early in the disease, slit-lamp examination is required to see the rings, but they are easily visible in later stages. Kayser-Fleischer rings are present in nearly all patients with neurologic symptoms, in most patients with liver disease (including children), and in some asymptomatic but affected siblings of confirmed patients. However, some patients with Wilson disease plus hepatic disease do not have Kayser-Fleischer rings, and the rings do occur in patients without Wilson disease but with severe liver disease and copper overload.

As a heavy metal, copper is toxic to the kidney tubules. Hence Wilson disease is one of the known causes of renal tubular Fanconi syndrome and may involve glucosuria, aminoaciduria, poor growth, electrolyte wasting (with acidosis), phosphaturia (with occasional hypophosphatemic rickets), or hypercalciuria (with renal stone formation). Other complications of Wilson disease include acute hemolysis caused by rapid hepatic copper release as a result of infarction or viral infection. Copper can also settle in bones and joints and cause osteomalacia, osteoporosis, osteophytes, lax ligaments, and arthritis. The pancreas, heart, and parathyroid glands may be damaged by copper accumulation, and sunflower cataracts occur in a few patients.

Heterozygotes for Wilson disease are clinically normal.

DIAGNOSIS. The diagnosis of Wilson disease involves the classic triad of clinical, biochemical, and molecular findings. Clinically, Wilson disease must be the primary consideration in children and young adults with chronic liver disease or any unusual hepatitis and should be part of the differential diagnosis in adolescents and adults with characteristic neurologic manifestations. Routine studies such as serum liver enzymes and urine glucose and electrolyte measurements, slit-lamp examination of the corneas, electroencephalograms, and computed tomography and magnetic resonance imaging of the brain may show abnormalities, but suspicion of Wilson disease should lead to more specific biochemical tests.

In Wilson disease, serum ceruloplasmin is below normal (200 to 400 mg/L) in over 80% of patients, but this acute phase reactant rises with inflammation and pregnancy. In the serum, total copper is reduced (normal, 11 to 24 μmol/L). Elevated *non-ceruloplasmin* copper binds to amino acids in the circulation, and urinary copper excretion is 2.5- to 20-fold elevated (normal, approximately 40 μg/day). A 5-mg liver biopsy specimen will give copper values of 200 to 3000 μg/g dry weight (normal, 20 to 50); the preferred method of assay is graphite furnace atomic absorption spectrometry or neutron activation; copper staining of a liver specimen should not be relied upon. Every liver biopsy should be assayed for copper regardless of the putative diagnosis.

Evaluation of tests for Wilson disease requires caution. Copper measurements can be spuriously high if the tubes for blood collection or the containers for liver biopsy are contaminated. Laboratory consistency between ceruloplasmin and serum copper levels can be checked by multiplying the ceruloplasmin (milligrams per liter) by 3, which equals its contribution to serum copper in micrograms per liter. Some young patients with Wilson disease have normal ceruloplasmin, and liver copper can be elevated above 300 μg/g dry weight in severe liver disease not caused by Wilson disease. In equivocal cases, injection of copper isotope (^{64}Cu) can make the diagnosis. In this test, isotope appears progressively in the circulation 4 to 48 hours after injection because of its incorporation into ceruloplasmin; patients with Wilson disease show no such rise in circulating isotope.

The many different mutations causing Wilson disease militate against an easy molecular diagnosis. A specific mutation can be sought in at-risk relatives of a patient with molecularly diagnosed Wilson disease, and this approach is relevant to prenatal diagnosis as well. Full siblings of a patient in whom Wilson disease is diagnosed carry a 25% risk of having the disorder and should undergo biochemical or molecular testing for Wilson disease and prophylactic treatment if the disease is diagnosed.

TREATMENT. The era of efficacious therapy for Wilson disease began in 1956 with Walshe's use of penicillamine, a free thiol that chelates copper for urinary excretion. Adult doses of D-penicillamine are 1 g/day in two to four doses away from meals, although up to 3 g daily has been given; children receive 0.5 to 1 g/day. The dose is titrated every 1 or 2 months so that urinary copper losses are 2 mg/day in the first year or two of therapy and 1 mg/day thereafter. Pyridoxine (25 mg daily) is often given at the same time. Penicillamine therapy takes weeks to relieve the neurologic symptoms and months to improve liver function. In fact, mobilization of hepatic copper by D-penicillamine may exacerbate the neurologic symptoms in the first days of treatment, sometimes irreversibly. Patients with severe hepatic dysfunction engage in a race between liver regeneration and continued cell damage from copper release. This process can last 3 to 6 months, and sometimes only hemofiltration, peritoneal dialysis, or plasmapheresis can remove copper and provide time enough for the liver to recover. Hemodialysis is ineffective.

In 10 to 30% of patients, D-penicillamine has significant but reversible side effects, including skin rashes, neutropenia and thrombocytopenia, nephrotic syndrome, arthritis, and connective tissue laxity. These problems disappear with cessation of therapy and may not recur on resumption of treatment if 40 mg of prednisone is given before restarting the D-penicillamine. The occurrence of aplastic anemia precludes future use, and elastosis perforans may be irreversible. A penicillamine embryopathy consisting of connective tissue abnormalities has been reported in patients treated for cystinuria and rheumatoid arthritis, but over 50 pregnancies in patients with Wilson disease treated with D-penicillamine have yielded normal infants. Interruption of decoppering therapy during pregnancy is not recommended.

The adverse effects of D-penicillamine have prompted use of the chelators trientine (triethylenetetramine dihydrochloride, 400 to 800 mg three times daily) and ammonium tetrathiomolybdate. Trientine but has no serious reported side effects. Tetrathiomolybdate is an extremely potent copper chelator suitable for acute copper reduction in neurologically affected patients or if rapid copper loss is required to win the race for liver regeneration. It is not generally recommended for long-term use and has not been approved by the Food and Drug Administration.

Oral zinc acetate (100 to 150 mg/day in three to four doses away from meals) induces gastrointestinal cell synthesis of the copper-binding protein metallothionein; subsequent sloughing of the mucosal cells rids the body of copper. Increased hepatic metallothionein synthesis also means that liver copper is complexed and rendered non-toxic; liver histologic status improves. Other advantages to zinc are its low toxicity and the fact that in treated patients, urinary copper accurately reflects the hepatic copper load. However, experience with long-term zinc treatment is less than with D-penicillamine therapy, and zinc is relatively slow in its decoppering activity.

For irreversible liver disease, orthotopic liver transplantation has proved curative in over 50 patients with Wilson disease; the survival rate for the procedure approximates 70%. Dietary copper restriction can be helpful and consists of avoiding shellfish and liver. Neurologic symptoms may be improved by L-dopa.

PROGNOSIS. Therapy for Wilson disease can prevent further neurologic and hepatic damage and reverse most if not all the symptoms and signs, including the Kayser-Fleischer rings. However, if long-term chelating therapy is stopped, irreversible and often fatal liver damage will occur within 1 to 2 years.

Brewer GJ, Yuzbasiyan-Gurkan V: Wilson disease. Medicine (Baltimore) 71:139, 1992. *A practical review antedating elucidation of the Wilson disease gene and emphasizing zinc therapy.*

Cuthbert JA: Wilson's disease: A new gene and an animal model for an old disease. J Invest Med 43:323, 1995. *This easy read summarizes all aspects of the disorder without giving excruciating detail.*

Danks DM: Disorders of copper transport. *In* Scriver CR, Beaudet AL, Sly WS, Valle

D (eds): The Metabolic and Molecular Bases of Inherited Disease, 7th ed. New York, McGraw-Hill, 1995, pp 2211–2235. *This chapter, like the bible it resides in, has a strong biochemical and genetic bent; look for the 8th edition to include molecular studies.*

221 IRON OVERLOAD (HEMOCHROMATOSIS)

Virgil F. Fairbanks ■ *David J. Brandhagen*

DEFINITION

Hemochromatosis is a state of iron overload that results in parenchymal tissue damage. In persons of European descent, the disorder is most often *hereditary (primary) hemochromatosis. Secondary hemochromatosis* occurs in a variety of chronic anemias caused by ineffective erythropoiesis, as in thalassemia major, or as the result of multiple transfusions or one of the less frequent conditions listed in Table 221–1.

PREVALENCE, GENETICS, AND CAUSE

Hereditary hemochromatosis, transmitted by an autosomal recessive trait, is the most common single-gene disorder of people of northern European origin, particularly among those whose forebears inhabited the littoral of the North Sea or North Atlantic. Approximately 3 to 5 persons/1000 are homozygous for the disease in the United States, Canada, France (particularly in Brittany), Iceland, the British Isles, the Netherlands, Germany, Denmark, Sweden, Norway, Australia, New Zealand, and South Africa. Approximately 10 to 15% of the white population of these countries are heterozygous for the major hemochromatosis gene. The hemochromatosis gene is less frequent in eastern and southern Europe, and of low frequency in North Africa and the Middle East. Black Americans have a lower prevalence of homozygous hemochromatosis, but it is thought to be about 0.3 to 0.5/1000. Hemochromatosis is rare in Asians. The paradoxical occurrence of hemochromatosis in successive generations of some kindreds is best explained by homozygotes marrying heterozygotes. This occurs in approximately 10% of hemochromatosis kindreds because of the high heterozygote frequency in whites.

The hemochromatosis gene is in linkage disequilibrium with the human leukocyte antigen A (HLA-A) and HLA-B genes. Seventy percent of persons with hemochromatosis have HLA-A3 antigens, compared with 28% in the general population. They also possess increased frequencies of HLA-B7 and -B14 antigens. In the course of numerous generations, the effect of normal meiotic recombination should have rendered the HLA allele frequencies in hemochro-

Table 221–1 ■ DISORDERS ASSOCIATED WITH IRON OVERLOAD

Hereditary hemochromatosis
Chronic anemias
  Thalassemia major
  Sideroblastic anemia
    Hereditary sideroblastic anemia
    Refractory anemia with ringed sideroblasts
  Congenital dyserythropoietic anemia
Exogenous iron overload
  Transfusion-dependent anemia
  Chronic oral iron ingestion (in absence of iron deficiency)
African (Bantu) hemochromatosis
Porphyria cutanea tarda
Portacaval shunt
Juvenile hemochromatosis
Neonatal hemochromatosis
Congenital atransferrinemia

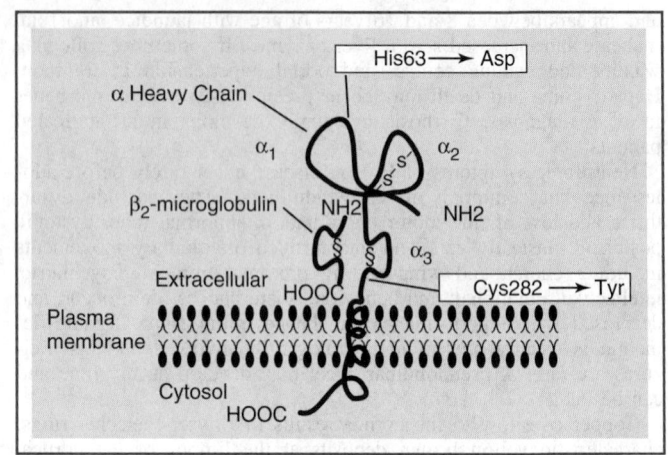

FIGURE 221–1 ■ The structure of the HFE protein as postulated from the nucleotide sequence. See text for explanation. (From Feder KM, Gnirke A, Thomas W, et al: A novel MHC class 1–like gene is mutated in patients with hereditary haemochromatosis. Nature Genetics 13:399–408, 1996, with permission.)

matosis similar to those in the general population. The most likely explanation for the high frequencies of certain HLA alleles is that the mutation is relatively recent, although it occurred and became widely prevalent before Europeans colonized North America, Australia, New Zealand, and South Africa.

The gene that is responsible for hemochromatosis is located 4 million nucleotide base pairs (4 Mb) telomeric to the major histocompatibility complex (MHC) on the short arm of chromosome 6. The corresponding HFE protein contains 343 amino acids (Figure 221–1). It is similar to MHC class I molecules, including a signal sequence, a peptide-binding region, an immunoglobulin-like domain, a transmembrane region, and a small cytoplasmic portion. The extracellular portion of the molecule, as in other MHC class I proteins, has three domains, designated $\alpha1$, $\alpha2$, and $\alpha3$. Each of these contains several β-pleated sheets. The $\alpha3$ domain is closely associated with β_2-microglobulin, which is encoded by a gene on chromosome 15. The HFE protein is expressed in nearly all cell lines that have been tested. Its normal function appears to be the control of iron uptake by cells through its interaction with transferrin receptor. Two mutations of the *HFE* gene have been described that are responsible for 90% of the cases of hereditary hemochromatosis in people of northern European origin. The more important of these is a guanine to adenine (G → A) mutation at codon 845 (therefore designated 845A) that causes a substitution of tyrosine (Y) for cysteine (C) at position 282 in the HFE protein (therefore designated C282Y). Among whites of North America and northern Europe, Australia, New Zealand, and South Africa, 10 to 15% are heterozygous for the 845A (C282Y) mutation, and 83% of cases of hereditary hemochromatosis are homozygous for this mutation. Another mutation at codon 187, of cytosine to guanine, or C → G (therefore designated 187G), causes the substitution histidine (H) to aspartic acid (D) at amino acid position 63 in the HFE protein (therefore designated H63D). Among North Americans and Europeans, approximately 2 out of every 7 are heterozygous for this 187G (H63D) mutation, and 1 out of every 12 is homozygous. Heterozygotes for either *HFE* mutation alone have negligible risk of hemochromatosis. Compound heterozygotes, who have both mutations, have increased risk of hemochromatosis and constitute approximately 5% of cases of this disease in North America and Europe. Those who are homozygous for the 187G mutation are at slightly increased risk for hemochromatosis. Even for those who are homozygous for 845A (C282Y), the more severe mutation, the exact level of risk is still uncertain and is the subject of current investigations. Furthermore, 10% or more of patients with clinically severe hereditary hemochromatosis do not appear to have either mutation; other mutations still to be identified presumably are responsible. This fact limits the value of DNA tests for diagnostic purposes.

Normal adult males must absorb approximately 1 mg/day of iron from the intestinal tract in order to balance iron loss. Normal women, during the reproductive years, must absorb approximately 2 mg/day of iron, the greater need reflecting menstrual iron loss.

Persons homozygous for hereditary hemochromatosis absorb from their intestinal tracts only a few milligrams of iron each day in excess of need, and the excess accumulates particularly in the liver but also in other critical organs. Clinical manifestations usually appear after the fourth decade but may appear even before age 20, when there has been a total iron accumulation of 15 to 40 g. Not all homozygotes experience overt disease, however, because the development of clinical manifestations is influenced by age, sex, iron content of the diet, alcohol, and other unknown factors. For example, women regularly lose iron during menses and childbirth, and this iron loss delays the onset of tissue damage. Thus, despite an equal frequency of homozygosity, women express the disease much less frequently than males. Ethanol abuse and hepatitis accelerate the development of liver and pancreatic disease in hereditary hemochromatosis. Alcohol abuse characterizes as many as one third of patients with hemochromatosis. The frequency of serum antibodies to hepatitis C is higher in hemochromatosis patients than in the normal population; that observation suggests a contributory role of this virus.

METABOLIC AND TISSUE EFFECTS

Iron accumulates over decades, as ferritin and hemosiderin, in nearly all cells of the body. Tissue damage that leads to morbidity occurs in the liver, thyroid, hypothalamus, heart, pancreas, gonads, and joints. This leads to cirrhosis of the liver, hypothyroidism, hypothalamic hypogonadotropic hypogonadism, cardiomyopathy, diabetes mellitus, arthralgias, and deforming arthritis. There is pigment deposition in skin, principally melanin. Cardiac deposition of ferritin and hemosiderin causes cardiac arrhythmias and impaired contractility of cardiac muscle.

The liver is a target organ because iron that is absorbed from the intestinal tract enters the portal circulation and passes through the liver before it enters any other organ. Quantities of iron that exceed the binding capacity of transferrin are deposited in the liver. In hereditary hemochromatosis, excess iron is deposited initially as hemosiderin granules in hepatocytes, in a periportal pattern; i.e., the heaviest deposition is at the periphery of the lobule. There is also marked deposition of hemosiderin in the epithelial cells of the biliary canaliculi. As iron overloading progresses, some hemosiderin deposits in Kupffer cells. Signs of hepatocellular injury are also first apparent and most pronounced in the periphery of the lobule. These changes consist of cytoplasmic ballooning and fatty change. As the disease progresses, filaments of fibrous tissue begin to traverse the lobules. As fibrosis develops, it is predominantly periportal. The other changes of severe cirrhosis follow. Similar histologic changes occur in the pancreas, heart, and other organs.

In secondary hemochromatosis, as in that which may follow numerous transfusions for chronic anemia, hemosiderin deposition is initially more marked in Kupffer cells. Ultimately, however, the histologic pattern becomes indistinguishable from that of hereditary hemochromatosis. Furthermore, other histologic changes may be indistinguishable between late-stage hemochromatosis and alcoholic cirrhosis, except for the marked hemosiderosis in the former.

CLINICAL MANIFESTATIONS

Most people with hemochromatosis are asymptomatic. All homozygotes are at risk, however, for development of severe dysfunction of the heart, liver, pancreas, pituitary, gonads, or joints, as well as for fatal peritonitis or sepsis.

Clinical manifestations are more common in males older than 20, and in post-menopausal women. Rare cases may involve adolescent children and young women. Table 221–2 lists the potential symptoms, signs, and abnormal laboratory findings of hemochromatosis. The most common symptoms are fatigue that may be overwhelming, arthralgias, abdominal discomfort, impotence, amenorrhea, and palpitations. Cardiac arrhythmia is a common presenting sign and may be either atrial or ventricular. Suntan-like hyperpigmentation of the skin can affect both exposed and non-exposed areas as well as scars. In advanced cases, the skin may be slate gray. Hepatosplenomegaly, ascites, pleural effusion, and arthritis can be a late development. The arthritis may affect any joint but most commonly involves the second and third metacarpophalangeal joints, knees, and hips. The affected joints may be deformed with or without inflammatory signs. Signs of hypothyroidism and testicular atrophy often appear along with loss of hair on body and extremities. Mild abdominal pain is common. Infrequently, there may be an abrupt onset of abdominal pain followed by prostration, shock, and death.

Hemochromatosis, because of its associated asthenia, cardiac, hypogonadal, or multiple-organ abnormality, may cause patients initially to seek the attention of general physicians, cardiologists, pediatricians, urologists, endocrinologists, neurologists, or psychiatrists. Therefore, its features should be understood by all physicians because concentrating on a particular organ system—like one of "the Six Blind Men of Hindustan"—may preclude early diagnosis and preventive treatment, which critically influence prognosis.

LABORATORY ABNORMALITIES AND DIAGNOSIS

The most useful laboratory test to ascertain hemochromatosis is measuring serum iron concentration, total iron binding capacity, and transferrin saturation. These should be done together. The transferrin saturation, as a percentage, is calculated from 100 times serum iron concentration divided by total iron binding capacity. Characteristically, the transferrin saturation is >60% and may approach 100% in hemochromatosis, whereas normally it is 20 to 50%. Other conditions may also elevate serum iron concentration and transferrin saturation, particularly the recent ingestion of medicinal iron or iron-fortified vitamin preparations, or oral contraceptives (Table 221–3). Therefore, if the transferrin saturation is elevated, the test should be repeated after eliminating such confounding variables. If it is still elevated, serum ferritin assay should be performed. When there is marked iron overload, as in advanced hemochromatosis, the serum ferritin concentration commonly exceeds 500 μg/L and may be >5000 μg/L. Each 1 μg/L of serum ferritin concentration is roughly equivalent to 120 μg of iron stores/kg of body weight (with 95% confidence limits of about

Table 221–2 ■ CLINICAL AND LABORATORY MANIFESTATIONS OF HEMOCHROMATOSIS

SYMPTOMS	SIGNS	ABNORMAL LABORATORY FINDINGS
None (common)	Alopecia	Increased serum iron concentration
Fatigue	Hyperpigmentation	Serum transferrin saturation >60%
Weakness	Tender, swollen joints	Increased serum ALT or AST transaminase level
Arthralgia	Cardiac arrhythmia	Increased blood glucose level
Abdominal pain	Cardiomegaly	Abnormal glucose tolerance
Impotence	Hepatomegaly	Low serum testosterone level
Amenorrhea	Splenomegaly	Low serum estrogen and progesterone levels
Dyspnea	Pleural effusion	Low FSH and LH levels
Abdominal swelling	Ascites	Low serum T_4, high TSH level
Weight loss	"Spider" telangiectases	Azoospermia
	Signs of hypothyroidism	Thrombocytopenia
	Testicular atrophy	Macrocytosis
		Electrocardiographic abnormalities
		Echocardiographic abnormalities
		Roentgenographic and imaging abnormalities

ALT = alanine aminotransferase; AST = aspartate aminotransferase. FSH = follicle-stimulating hormone; LH = Luteinizing hormone; T_4 = thyroxine; TSH = thyrotropin.

Table 221–3 ■ PHENOMENA KNOWN TO AFFECT SERUM IRON CONCENTRATION, TOTAL IRON-BINDING CAPACITY, AND TRANSFERRIN SATURATION

PHENOMENON	EFFECT
Menstrual cycle	Pre-menstrually, elevated values (SI increased by 10–30%); at menstruation, low values (SI decreased by 10–30%)
Pregnancy	May elevate SI through increased progesterone; may lower SI through Fe deficiency
Ingestion of iron (including iron-fortified vitamins)	High values (SI may rise by 300+ μg/dL and transferrin saturation to 75%)
Iron contamination of tube (Vacutainer) or other glassware (phenomenon may be rare, sporadic, very difficult to prove)	High values (SI 200–300 μg/dL, transferrin saturation of 75–100%)
Iron dextran injection	Very high values (SI may be >500 μg/dL, transferrin saturation 100%, probably from circulating iron dextran; effect may persist for several weeks)
Hepatitis (including steatohepatitis)	Very high values (SI may exceed 1000 μg/dL through hyperferritinemia from hepatocyte injury)
Acute inflammation (respiratory infection, abscess, immunization, myocardial infarction	Low or normal SI; normal or low Tsat
Chronic inflammation or malignancy	Low or normal SI; normal or low Tsat
Iron deficiency	Low or normal SI; increased TIBC; low or normal Tsat
Iron overload (hemochromatosis)	High SI, high Tsat

Abbreviations: SI = serum iron; TIBC = total iron-binding capacity; Tsat = transferrin saturation (percentage).

±30%). A 70-kg person with a serum ferritin concentration of 3000 μg/g has approximately 17 to 33 g of storage iron in ferritin and hemosiderin. This contrasts with the normal iron stores of about 0.5 to 0.8 g in adult males or about 0 to 0.3 g in adult women. However, since serum ferritin is an acute-phase reactant, elevated values may result from chronic disease, such as inflammation (as in rheumatoid arthritis), or from malignancies. Liver injury from hepatitis or alcohol abuse also elevates both the serum iron and the serum ferritin concentrations. High values of serum ferritin may be observed in Gaucher's disease and in a rare familial disorder associated with congenital cataracts (the hyperferritinemia-cataract syndrome), without concomitant excess iron accumulation in the liver or other organs. Therefore, elevated values of serum ferritin concentration must be interpreted in the context of the presence or absence of these other conditions.

Among other frequent abnormal laboratory findings are elevated blood glucose concentration, abnormal glucose tolerance test results, elevated serum aspartate aminotransferase (AST) or alanine aminotransferase (ALT) activity, low serum thyroxine level, elevated serum thyroid stimulating hormone level, low serum values for pituitary gonadotropins, and thrombocytopenia (reflecting liver disease). Hemoglobin concentration, hematocrit, erythrocyte count, erythrocyte indices, and leukocyte count and differential are usually normal, although chronic liver disease may be reflected in macrocytosis. Bone marrow examination with iron stain variably shows increase in hemosiderin, hence is not reliable for diagnosis of iron overload.

Roentgenographic examinations of affected joints show soft tissue swelling, narrowing of joint spaces, irregular articular surfaces, osteoporosis, and subcapsular cysts. There may be chondrocalcinosis or calcification of periarticular ligaments. Synovial fluid often contains calcium pyrophosphate and apatite crystals. Distinction from either degenerative arthritis or rheumatoid arthritis may be difficult.

Electrocardiography may reveal atrial or ventricular arrhythmia, low QRS amplitude, and repolarization abnormalities of ST segment and T waves. Echocardiography and cinecardiography may show dilated, or, less commonly restrictive, cardiomyopathy. There may be radiographic evidence of pulmonary vascular congestion or pleural effusion.

Traditionally, diagnosis has required liver biopsy. This also permits evaluation of the severity of liver injury and thus the prognosis. In addition to hematoxylin and eosin stain, the biopsy specimen should be examined for iron by Perls' stain. In the absence of iron overload, the stainable iron is 0 to 1+. In heterozygotes or those with alcoholic cirrhosis it is 1 to 2+; in those with homozygous hemochromatosis it is 3 to 4+. These semiquantitative estimates from iron stain correlate with quantitative measurements of hepatic iron concentration. The hepatic iron concentration can be measured in the liver biopsy specimen. Normal hepatic iron concentrations are <40 (males) and <33 (females) μmol/g of tissue (dry weight). In alcoholic cirrhosis, and in heterozygotes for hemochromatosis, the hepatic iron concentration is <100 μmol/g of tissue. In homozygous hemochromatosis, the hepatic iron concentration usually exceeds 200 μmol/g of tissue. A useful index is obtained by dividing the hepatic iron concentration in micromoles per gram (μmol/g) by the patient's age in years. This *hepatic iron index* is usually >1.9 in homozygous hemochromatosis.

DNA testing for the hemochromatosis mutations of the *HFE* gene may be useful for confirmation of the diagnosis or for testing of other family members. This may replace the need for liver biopsy in patients who are less than 40 years of age, who have no laboratory evidence of liver disease, and whose serum ferritin concentration is <1000 μg/L. As a screening method, however, it would miss too many cases of hemochromatosis: 10% in some populations and a much higher proportion of cases in other populations.

Imaging methods, such as computed tomography or magnetic resonance imaging, have led to the correct diagnosis of hemochromatosis in many instances. However, compared with conventional laboratory methods, imaging procedures are too expensive to be used in screening for hemochromatosis.

HLA typing is of little value for diagnosis of hemochromatosis. Of persons whose leukocytes have the HLA-A3 antigen, only about 1 in 90 will be found to have hemochromatosis. Such persons are more likely to be normal or to have alcoholic cirrhosis than hereditary hemochromatosis. As a screening test, HLA typing would yield unacceptably high frequencies of both false-positive and false-negative results. Therefore, this quite expensive test has no place in screening for hemochromatosis. It may be used, however, to help identify affected siblings of a person known to be affected. When so used, it does not matter what the HLA type is: Within a sibship, those whose HLA genotype is identical with that of a sibling who is proved to be affected are also presumed to have homozygous hemochromatosis.

Physicians must examine other members of a sibship for hemochromatosis, since within any hemochromatosis sibship, on average 25% of sibs will be homozygous for hemochromatosis. Measuring transferrin saturation and serum ferritin concentration is sufficient to identify other affected sibs. The DNA test for the *HFE* gene mutation may also be used for this purpose when the index case, in any kindred, is known to be homozygous for the 845A (C282Y) mutation.

TREATMENT

The treatment of hemochromatosis is by repeated phlebotomy. This is the most efficient, least inconvenient, and least expensive way to remove excess iron from the body. There is no place for chelating therapy or dietary manipulation in treating hereditary hemochromatosis. Since iron stores may be 25 to 40 g of iron, and each half liter of blood removed contains approximately 200 mg of iron, phlebotomies can be sustained at the rate of one to two times/week for 1 to 3 years or longer before the iron stores become depleted. Patients should be advised that they may need to have 50 to 100 or more phlebotomies before their iron stores are reduced to normal. This is usually done at the rate of one to two phlebotomies per week until the venous hemoglobin concentration or hematocrit begins to decline and does not return to normal (Figure 221–2). Then, serum ferritin assay determines whether additional phlebotomies are required. The objective is to lower the serum ferritin concentration to <20 μg/L before reducing the rate of phlebotomy.

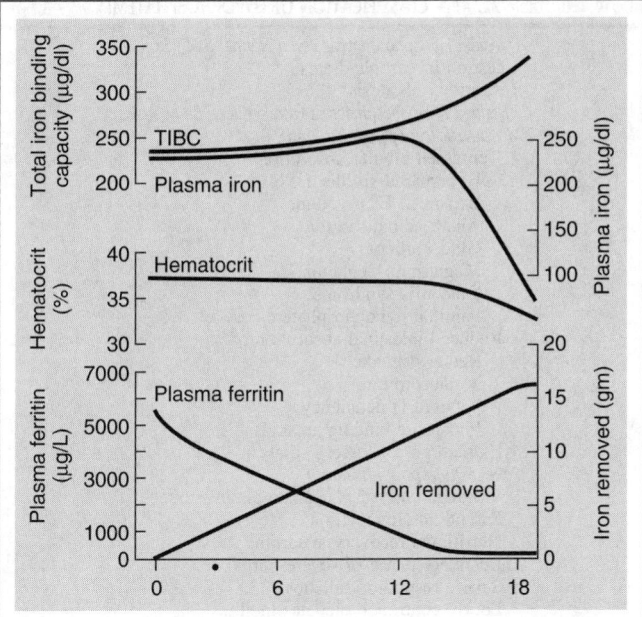

FIGURE 221–2 ■ Serial changes in the hematocrit, serum (plasma) iron concentration, total iron-binding capacity, and serum (plasma) transferrin concentration in a patient with hereditary hemochromatosis during phlebotomy therapy. (N.B. Although shown as plasma iron and ferritin in the illustration, serum specimens are used for these assays, since EDTA-anticoagulated specimens do not have measurable plasma iron by most commonly used methods). EDTA = ethylenediaminetetraacetic acid. (From Bothwell TH, Carlton RW, Cook JD, et al: Idiopathic haemochromatosis. *In* Iron Metabolism in Man. Oxford, Blackwell Scientific, 1979.)

After that, most patients require four to six phlebotomies annually to keep the serum ferritin concentration in the normal range. Since the transferrin saturation is often high irrespective of the state of iron stores, the measurement of serum iron, total iron-binding capacity (TIBC), and transferrin saturation is less reliable for determining when additional phlebotomies are needed.

People with hemochromatosis should abstain from handling or eating uncooked shellfish or marine fish, since they are susceptible to fatal septicemia from the marine bacterium *Vibrio vulnificus*. No other dietary restrictions should be imposed. However, complete abstinence from use of alcohol must be observed.

In addition to these measures directed toward removing iron from the body, treating cardiac dysfunction may require cardiac glycosides or diuretics, diabetes may require insulin, hypothyroidism requires thyroid replacement, impotence may be relieved with androgens, and painful joints may require salicylates or nonsteroidal anti-inflammatory agents. in advanced cases, liver transplantation may be required. Early diagnosis and vigorous treatment should prevent the need for these drastic and costly measures that have high morbidity rate and uncertain outcomes.

PROGNOSIS

Historically, the median survival was about 2 years from diagnosis. A greatly improved prognosis results from early diagnosis and treatment. When the diagnosis precedes onset of signs and symptoms, and in the absence of hepatic cirrhosis or diabetes, survival is the same as for the age- and-sex-matched cohort of the general population. When cirrhosis or diabetes is already present at the time of diagnosis, the outlook is poorer. Cirrhosis rarely disappears as a result of phlebotomy therapy. Patients may die of hepatic or cardiac failure or may exsanguinate from ruptured esophageal varices. They are at risk of death from infections, such as peritonitis. Patients with cirrhosis have a 30% probability of development of hepatocellular carcinoma, even after iron stores are depleted by phlebotomy. Diabetes is not improved by removing iron, but it may not progress as rapidly. Arthritis is not improved by iron removal and, unfortunately, may first appear after adequate removal of excess iron. However, cardiac dysfunction is often substantially improved. Impotence requires continued androgen therapy. Azosper-

mia is not alleviated. Amenorrhea may rarely be alleviated. Osteoporosis that follows premature menopause requires estrogen therapy. The risk of sudden death from sepsis or peritonitis is diminished.

It is tragic whenever this easily diagnosed and easily treated disorder is permitted to evolve unrecognized and untreated. Patients for whom the diagnosis is not made in a timely manner may experience cirrhosis or severe cardiac dysfunction or both. Fewer than 100 such patients, who could not otherwise be salvaged, have had liver or heart transplantation or both. Such procedures may be warranted, although extremely costly (>$250,000) and attended by long-term morbidity even when successful. The long-term survival rate of patients who have had transplantation for cirrhosis due to hemochromatosis is poorer than for those with alcoholic cirrhosis, although half have survived as long as 5 years after liver transplantation. Every far-advanced case of hemochromatosis poses the dilemma whether procedures so costly, attended by a high morbidity rate and uncertain outcome, can be justified. This dilemma may prove even more troublesome in an era of cost containment.

Balan V, Baldus WP, Fairbanks VF, et al: Screening for hemochromatosis: A cost-effectiveness study based on 12,258 patients. Gastroenterology 107:453–459, 1994. *This study extensively analyzed all the considerations and costs that attend screening for hemochromatosis, follow-up tests, and examinations. A reasonable estimate of the cost of screening, and the potential for salvaging years of life, is approximately $2,000 per year of life saved per person who is homozygous for hereditary hemochromatosis (an extremely favorable cost-benefit relationship). Indeed, the cost-benefit ratio for hemochromatosis screening is much more favorable than is the cost-benefit ratio for such widely accepted screening procedures as those for breast cancer, colon cancer, cancer of the uterine cervix, and neonatal screening for congenital hypothyroidism, phenylketonuria, or galactosemia.*

Beutler E, Gelbart T, West C, et al: Mutation analysis in hereditary hemochromatosis. Blood Cells Mol Dis 23(2):187–194, 1996. *This article was the first to confirm the HFE gene mutations responsible for hemochromatosis (see also Feder et al).*

Fairbanks VF, Brandhagen DJ, Thibodeau SN, et al: H63D is an haemochromatosis-associated allele. GUT 43(3), 441, 1998. *This letter reviewed all the published data concerning the association of hemochromatosis with mutations of the HFE gene.*

Fargion S, Mandelli C, Piperno A, et al: Survival and prognostic factors in 212 Italian patients with genetic hemochromatosis. Hepatology 15:655–1078, 1992. *Patients adequately treated by phlebotomy before development of cirrhosis had normal survival rate; for cirrhotic patients, median survival was 8 years.*

Feder KM, Gnirke A, Thomas W, et al: A novel MHC class 1–like gene is mutated in patients with hereditary haemochromatosis. Nature Genetics 13:399–408, 1996. *A fundamental breakthrough in the genetics of hemochromatosis was the identification of both the 845A (C282Y) and the 187C (H63D) mutations and their frequencies in hemochromatosis patients. The article also described the putative structure of the HFE protein in terms of nucleotide sequence (see Figure 221–1).*

Mendlein J, Cogswell ME, McDonnell SM, et al (eds): Iron overload, public health and genetics. Ann Intern Med 129 (Suppl.):920–996, 1998. *A set of 11 articles that address the issues of public health and screening for hemochromatosis.*

Summers KM, Halliday JW, Powell LW: Identification of homozygous hemochromatosis subjects by measurement of hepatic iron index. Hepatology 12:20–25, 1990. *The hepatic iron index, obtained by dividing hepatic iron concentration, in micromoles per gram (μmol/g) by patient's age, provides the best criterion for identifying homozygotes with iron overload.*

Witte DL, Crosby WH, Edwards CQ, et al: Practice parameter for hereditary hemochromatosis. Clin Chim Acta 245:139–200, 1996. *This article, by a College of American Pathologists Hemochromatosis Task Force, is an extensive compilation of published observations concerning the prevalence, diagnosis, and management of hereditary hemochromatosis.*

222 PHOSPHORUS DEFICIENCY AND HYPOPHOSPHATEMIA

Wadi N. Suki

Phosphorus is an integral constituent of all body tissues. It is a component of hydroxyapatite, the main crystalline structure of bone, and a component of the phospholipids in all cell membranes. It is a constituent of nucleotides and furnishes the backbone of DNA. It is also a component of the second messengers cyclic adenosine monophosphate (cAMP) and cyclic guanosine monophosphate. Enzymes are activated following phosphorylation by kinases. As a component of 2,3-diphosphoglycerate, phosphorus facilitates the release of oxygen to tissues from oxyhemoglobin. In adenosine triphosphate (ATP) and creatine phosphate, it serves as an energy store, and when excreted in the urine, it serves as an important buffer to facilitate the excretion of urinary acid. When all the functions of phosphate are considered, it becomes evident why severe deficiency of this anion can lead to disordered function of a large number of systems.

NORMAL PHOSPHORUS METABOLISM. More than 700 g (22 mol) of phosphorus is present in an average-sized adult: 80% of the total phosphorus is present in bone; 10% is present in skeletal muscle. In muscle cells and in other cells, phosphate in the form of phospholipids, phosphoproteins, and phosphosugars represents the major intracellular anion and is present in a concentration of approximately 100 mmol/L of cell water.

In the extracellular fluid, phosphorus is present in a concentration of 4.0 to 7.0 mg/dL in children and 2.7 to 4.5 mg/dL in adults. Phosphate in blood is mostly free (only 10% is protein bound) and is present in two ionic forms, dibasic (HPO_4^{2-}) and monobasic ($H_2PO_4^-$), the relative amounts of which vary with the blood pH, being present in a ratio of 4:1 at pH 7.4. Therefore, the phosphate concentration in blood should be considered in terms of millimoles (0.9 to 1.5 mmol/L in adults and 1.4 to 2.2 mmol/L in children) rather than milliequivalents (which would vary with blood pH).

Depending on the composition of the diet, the average adult in the United States consumes 800 to 1500 mg of phosphorus daily, derived primarily from dairy products and meat. Most of the ingested phosphorus is absorbed, and except in growing children, most is excreted in the urine. Urinary excretion depends on glomerular filtration and tubular reabsorption, with only 12% of the filtered load being excreted in the urine. Intestinal absorption of phosphate is augmented by the active metabolites of vitamin D, whereas renal tubular absorption is inhibited by parathyroid hormone acting through its second messenger cAMP.

HYPOPHOSPHATEMIA. Moderate or severe hypophosphatemia is seen in approximately 2% of hospitalized patients.

ETIOLOGY. Hypophosphatemia may result from a shift of phosphorus into cells, in which case body phosphorus stores are normal. On the other hand, hypophosphatemia may be associated with depleted total body stores resulting from poor dietary intake, reduced gastrointestinal absorption, or increased renal losses (Table 222–1).

Hypophosphatemia may be sustained or may be transient. Transient hypophosphatemia is seen after the ingestion of carbohydrates and is caused by the phosphorylation of sugars before they enter the body cells, or it is seen in respiratory alkalosis, wherein alkalinization of the cytosol activates intracellular glycolysis and increases the formation of phosphorylated sugars.

MODERATE HYPOPHOSPHATEMIA. Carbohydrate administration and respiratory alkalosis cause moderate hypophosphatemia (serum phosphorus, 1 to 2.5 mg/dL). Other disorders that also result in moderate hypophosphatemia may be classified into those that increase renal losses of phosphate, decrease intestinal absorption of phosphate, or increase extracorporeal loss of phosphate such as in hemodialysis against a phosphate-free dialysate. Renal losses of phosphate are increased when tubular absorption is depressed, as seen in hyperparathyroidism (see Chapter 264), expansion of the extracellular fluid volume, administration of alkali or glucocorticoids, hypomagnesemia and magnesium depletion, and renal tubular defects such as Fanconi's syndrome (see Chapter 109) or familial hypophosphatemic rickets (see Chapter 263).

Reduced intestinal absorption may be caused by drastically reduced intake, malabsorption, vitamin D deficiency, and the use of phosphate-binding antacids. Moderate hypophosphatemia causes only osteomalacia.

SEVERE HYPOPHOSPHATEMIA. Severe hypophosphatemia (serum phosphorus, <1 mg/dL) causes serious systemic manifestations that demand prompt attention and correction. The most common causes of this disorder are prolonged use of phosphate-binding antacids, hyperalimentation, nutritional recovery syndrome and recovery from severe burns, severe respiratory alkalosis, poorly controlled diabetes mellitus, and alcoholism and alcohol withdrawal syndrome. Phosphate-binding compounds such as aluminum and magnesium oxides bind phosphate in the intestinal lumen and impair its absorption. Excessive use of these compounds by patients with peptic ulcer disease or by patients with chronic renal failure who are treated with these compounds to prevent the development of

Table 222–1 ■ CLASSIFICATION OF HYPOPHOSPHATEMIA

Transient Hypophosphatemia with Normal Body Stores
Ingestion of carbohydrates
Respiratory alkalosis
Sustained Hypophosphatemia with Reduced Body Stores
  Moderate hypophosphatemia
    Depressed tubular absorption
      Hyperparathyroidism
      Expanded ECF volume
      Alkali administration
      Glucocorticoids
      Magnesium depletion
      Fanconi's syndrome
      Familial hypophosphatemic rickets
    Reduced intestinal absorption
      Reduced intake
      Malabsorption
      Vitamin D deficiency
      Phosphate-binding antacids
    Extracorporeal losses—dialysis
  Severe hypophosphatemia
    Prolonged use of phosphate-binding antacids
    Parenteral alimentation
    Nutritional recovery syndrome
    Recovery phase of severe burns
    Severe respiratory alkalosis
    Poorly controlled diabetes mellitus
    Alcoholism and alcohol withdrawal

ECF = extracellular fluid.

hyperphosphatemia results in phosphate depletion. Enteral and parenteral alimentation, if not supplemented with phosphate, can also result in phosphate depletion. Phosphate excretion in the urine is increased by administering glucose and amino acids. Furthermore, glucose and amino acids entering into cells and their incorporation into intracellular compounds consume phosphate and deplete body

Table 222–2 ■ MANIFESTATIONS OF HYPOPHOSPHATEMIA

SYMPTOMS AND SIGNS	COMMENTS
Central Nervous System	
Symptoms and signs of metabolic encephalopathy	Irritability, malaise, ataxia, seizures, coma
Neuromuscular	
Generalized muscle weakness or paralysis	Ventilatory insufficiency, respiratory failure
Rhabdomyolysis	Increased creatine kinase, large-muscle tenderness; may mask underlying hypophosphatemia
Cardiac muscle dysfunction	Congestive cardiomyopathy
Hematologic	
Altered red cell function	Depleted 2,3-DPG shifts oxyhemoglobin dissociation curve to the left and impairs tissue oxygen delivery. Depleted ATP increases intracellular calcium, thereby causing hemolysis
Impaired leukocyte function	Impaired leukotaxis, phagocytosis, and bactericidal activity; susceptibility to infection
Impaired platelet aggregation	Bleeding tendency from lips and oral mucosa
Bone	
Bone resorption, osteomalacia, increased 1α-hydroxylation of vitamin D	Increased calcium absorption, mild increase in serum calcium, depressed PTH secretion, marked renal hypercalciuria
Renal	
Impaired tubular function	Increased urine calcium and magnesium, renal glucosuria, decreased ammoniagenesis, metabolic acidosis
Liver	
Transient hyperbilirubinemia	
Metabolism	
Hypoglycemia	

2,3-DPG = 2,3-diphosphoglycerate; ATP = adenosine triphosphate; PTH = parathyroid hormone.

Table 222–3 ■ MANAGEMENT OF HYPOPHOSPHATEMIA

STATUS	TREATMENT	DOSE
Normal Body Phosphorus Stores		
Transient hydrophosphatemia	Treat underlying disorder	No phosphate replacement
Reduced Body Phosphorus Stores		
Moderate hypophosphatemia	Minimize urinary losses, reduce sodium diuresis, enhance gastrointestinal absorption, discontinue phosphate binders	
	If patient capable of oral intake:	
	High-phosphate foods	e.g., skimmed cow's milk (contains 1 mg P/mL)
	Oral supplements:	
	Sodium salt	Phospho-Soda, 750 mg P/5 mL
	Potassium salt (potassium not contraindicated/desirable)	Neutra-Phos, 250 mg P/capsule with 7 mEq of K; Neutra-Phos K, 250 mg P/capsule with 14 mEq of K; K Phos, 150 mg P/tablet with 3.65 mEq K; or K-Phos Neutral, 250 mg P with 2 mEq K
Severe hypophosphatemia		
Patient incapable of oral/enteral intake or with organ manifestations of P depletion	Parenteral P	P 2.5–5 mg/kg body weight (0.08–0.16 mmol/kg) infused over 6 hr repeated every 6 hr until serum P is 2.0–2.5 mg/dL
Hypocalcemic patient, renal failure		Lower dose than above

stores. Overzealous refeeding of severely malnourished subjects may also result in multiple deficiencies, including thiamine, potassium, and phosphate. Providing these nutritional components generally obviates the severe disorder once encountered in this setting. In the case of severely burned subjects, healing results in reabsorption of the edema fluid and consequent diuresis, which may be responsible for substantial renal phosphate loss. Furthermore, as new tissue is rebuilt, phosphate is taken up by the newly formed cells, thus aggravating the depletion of body phosphate stores. Unlike metabolic alkalosis, which may result in a modest drop in serum phosphorus, prolonged vigorous hyperventilation and respiratory alkalosis can result in profound hypophosphatemia. Urinary phosphate excretion in respiratory alkalosis is extremely low, whereas phosphate excretion in metabolic alkalosis is increased. In poorly controlled diabetes mellitus, the glucosuria and resulting osmotic diuresis increase urinary phosphate loss. Acetoacetate and β-hydroxybutyrate also increase urinary phosphate loss. Finally, the acidosis per se also increases urinary phosphate loss. However, serum phosphorus is not generally depressed when poorly controlled diabetics are initially evaluated, probably because phosphate shifts to the extracellular compartment from the intracellular space. Only after starting therapy with insulin and intravenous fluids does the hypophosphatemia become manifested.

In alcoholics, hypophosphatemia and phosphate depletion are caused by multiple factors: the phosphaturic effects of ethanol and magnesium depletion, poor dietary intake, and ketoacidosis. Other contributing factors can be vomiting, diarrhea, and the use of phosphate-binding antacids.

MANIFESTATIONS. Severe hypophosphatemia alters cell membrane composition and function, depletes intracellular phosphorylated compounds such as ATP and 2,3-diphosphoglycerate, and increases intracellular calcium (Table 222–2). This constellation of disorders results in disturbed function of multiple body systems.

MANAGEMENT. When total body phosphorus stores are normal, phosphate supplementation is unnecessary (Table 222–3). When body phosphate stores are reduced, urinary losses need to be minimized, gastrointestinal absorption needs to be enhanced, and phosphate supplements may be necessary. To replete body phosphorus stores, 1000 to 2000 mg of phosphorus may need to be supplemented daily for up to 2 weeks. Whenever phosphate replacement is given, serum calcium, magnesium, phosphorus, and electrolytes should be monitored closely. The complications of administering phosphate include diarrhea (after oral administration), hypocalcemia, metastatic calcification, hypotension, hyperkalemia and/or hypernatremia, and metabolic acidosis.

Crook M, Swaminathan R: Disorders of plasma phosphate and indications for its measurement. Ann Clin Biochem 33:376, 1996. *A well-referenced review of the clinical disorders of phosphate and their pathophysiology, manifestations, and treatment.*

223 DISORDERS OF MAGNESIUM METABOLISM

Allen C. Alfrey

Magnesium is the second most common intracellular cation, with only three other cations—potassium, calcium, and sodium—occurring with greater abundance in the body. It plays a crucial role in storing and using energy inasmuch as all enzymatic reactions involving adenosine triphosphate frequently require magnesium. Because magnesium is also an essential element for plants in that it is a constituent of chlorophyll, it is present in virtually all food sources. Despite this wide distribution, the average dietary intake of magnesium is about 25 mEq/day, which only marginally meets the recommended daily requirements for this element. Fractional absorption of magnesium varies from 80% on a magnesium-restricted diet to less than 10% when large oral loads of magnesium are consumed. Renal magnesium reabsorption occurs in multiple nephron segments, and a tubular maximum (TM_{Mg}) may be described for the whole kidney. Normal tubular reabsorption for magnesium is very close to the TM_{Mg}. Therefore, small changes in serum magnesium levels are accompanied by rather rapid increases or decreases in urinary magnesium excretion. This intrinsic TM_{Mg} phenomenon, which is not directly controlled hormonally, allows the kidney to be the major determinant of plasma magnesium levels.

MAGNESIUM DEPLETION. The prevalence of hypomagnesemia in a general hospital setting has been estimated to range from 6.9 to 12% and is as high as 20% in patients in an intensive care unit. Clinical findings of severe hypomagnesemia are mainly confined to the neuromuscular system and consist of muscle fasciculations and tremors, positive Chvostek and Trousseau signs, overt tetany, weakness, anorexia, apathy, and rarely seizures. However, cardiac arrhythmias and increased sensitivity to digoxin may also occur. The biochemical findings of symptomatic hypomagnesemia are serum magnesium levels usually less than 1 mEq/L in association with hypokalemia and hypocalcemia.

MECHANISMS. Magnesium depletion can result from either gastrointestinal or renal causes (Table 223–1). When serum magnesium falls only slightly and if the kidneys respond normally, urinary magnesium excretion falls to less than 12 mg (1 mEq) per day. Therefore, urine magnesium is low if magnesium depletion results from gastrointestinal causes; however, urinary magnesium excretion is in the normal range (120 to 160 mg/day) if depletion results from a renal leak.

Table 223–1 ■ CAUSES OF HYPOMAGNESEMIA

Gastrointestinal	Steatorrheic states
	Severe diarrhea
	Familial magnesium malabsorption
	Protein-calorie malnutrition
Renal	Gitelman's syndrome
Intrinsic	Bartter's syndrome
	Renal transplantation
	Post-obstructive uropathy diuresis
	Therapeutic agents (drugs)
Extrinsic	Volume expansion
	Hypercalciuria
	Diabetic ketoacidosis
	Diuretics
Miscellaneous	Alcoholism
	Thyrotoxicosis
	Burns
	Post-parathyroidectomy
	Lactation

Magnesium depletion has been found in 35% of patients with steatorrheic states. The fecal magnesium content correlates with the amount of stool fat, which suggests that magnesium malabsorption is a result of magnesium forming an insoluble complex with fat in the gastrointestinal tract. Any severe diarrheal state such as ulcerative colitis, amebic colitis, and intestinal resection can also deplete magnesium. Another gastrointestinal cause of magnesium depletion is an isolated defect in magnesium absorption that usually occurs in infants. Magnesium depletion can rarely result from poor intake as found in protein-calorie malnutrition and patients receiving total parenteral nutrition without magnesium supplementation.

Renal magnesium wasting (see Table 223–1) can result from an intrinsic disorder of the renal tubule or from extrinsic or reversible factors. The major intrinsic causes of renal magnesium wasting are Bartter's syndrome, Gitelman's syndrome, post-obstructive diuresis, renal transplantation, and a number of therapeutic agents. Bartter's syndrome tends to occur more commonly in infants and is usually associated with only mild asymptomatic hypomagnesemia. In contrast, Gitelman's syndrome occurs in older children and adults and is frequently accompanied by severe symptomatic hypomagnesemia, hypocalcemia, and hypocalciuria. Gitelman's syndrome has recently been shown to be an autosomal recessive disease resulting from mutations in the gene encoding the renal thiazide-sensitive Na-Cl cotransporter in the distal convoluted tubule. Drugs that most commonly cause magnesium depletion are aminoglycosides, cyclosporine, pentamidine, foscarnet, and cis-diamminedichloroplatinum (cisplatin). Cisplatin commonly causes renal magnesium wasting that can persist for months after use of the drug has been discontinued. A number of extrinsic or intrarenal factors, including virtually all diuretics, volume expansion, diabetic ketoacidosis, and hypercalciuria, can cause mild to moderate renal magnesium wasting. Several miscellaneous causes of hypomagnesemia are also possible, including alcoholism, thyrotoxicosis, pancreatitis, lactation, parathyroidectomy, and burns. Alcoholism is the most important. Magnesium depletion in this condition results from a number of causes, including poor dietary intake and somewhat enhanced renal excretion of this cation. Hypomagnesemia, which correlates with the severity of the hyperthyroid state, is a result of redistribution rather than deficiency of this element. Hypomagnesemia can also be caused by redistribution following parathyroidectomy, which results from magnesium being incorporated into bone, along with calcium salts, during the rapid healing that follows parathyroid surgery.

EFFECT OF MAGNESIUM ON CALCIUM METABOLISM. Magnesium depletion is the most common cause of hypocalcemia in the general hospital population. Parathyroid hormone (PTH) levels have been shown to be either low or inappropriately normal when the patient has hypomagnesemia-induced hypocalcemia. This problem is one of release rather than synthesis of PTH in that PTH levels rapidly increase within minutes of giving magnesium replacement. Besides affecting PTH secretion, with more severe magnesium depletion, bone resistance to PTH is also encountered, as manifested by lack of a calcemic response.

INTERRELATIONSHIP BETWEEN MAGNESIUM AND POTASSIUM. Approximately 40% of hypomagnesemic patients have coexisting hypokalemia. In muscle and myocardium, when either intracellular magnesium or potassium falls, a corresponding decrease in the other cation takes place. Conversely, primary potassium depletion is characterized by intracellular muscle magnesium depletion without hypomagnesemia. The interrelationship between intracellular potassium and magnesium is further demonstrated by the fact that repletion of potassium frequently cannot be accomplished without concomitantly administering magnesium. The term "refractory potassium repletion states" has been used to describe this condition. Intracellular depletion of magnesium has been suggested as being responsible for causing a variety of cardiovascular alterations, including increased sensitivity to digitalis toxicity and cardiac arrhythmias such as premature ventricular contractions and torsades de pointes. However, it is unclear whether these cardiovascular alterations are a direct result of magnesium depletion or a consequence of the associated intracellular potassium depletion.

DIAGNOSIS AND MANAGEMENT OF MAGNESIUM DEPLETION. Magnesium depletion is usually readily diagnosed by measuring the serum magnesium level. Mild asymptomatic magnesium depletion requires no treatment if the patient is able to eat a normal diet. Patients with symptomatic hypomagnesemia usually require parenteral magnesium replacement. As a rule, the magnesium deficit can be roughly calculated by assuming that the space of distribution is the extracellular volume. Because half the administered magnesium is excreted in urine, replacement is approximately twice the calculated deficit. Although an occasional patient may require intravenous replacement, the intramuscular route is safer and the preferred method of administering magnesium. Suggested regimens of magnesium replacement for hypomagnesemic states are given in Table 223–2. It has been suggested that intravenous magnesium be routinely given to patients with acute myocardial infraction to replace depleted intracellular magnesium, partially based on the finding of reduced muscle magnesium and potassium levels, especially in patients receiving diuretics. This approach has been suggested to enhance tissue potassium repletion, decrease death rates, and reduce the number of episodes of arrhythmias in this patient population. The evidence is good that magnesium replacement can enhance intracellular potassium replacement and under certain conditions is necessary for potassium repletion. However, a recent large controlled trial involving 58,050 patients (ISIS-4) failed to show any benefit of intravenous magnesium therapy in patients with acute myocardial infarction.

HYPERMAGNESEMIA. Mild hypermagnesemia is seen in patients with hypothyroidism, adrenal insufficiency, and advanced renal failure. The majority of cases of symptomatic hypermagnesemia have resulted from administering large oral loads of magnesium in the form of laxatives or antacids to patients with advanced renal insufficiency. In patients with normal renal function, life-threatening hypermagnesemia has been described in only a few unusual circumstances. Several fatalities in children have resulted from accidentally ingesting Epsom salts (magnesium sulfate). Normal subjects receiving 800 to 1600 mEq of magnesium sulfate per rectum have been found to have serum magnesium levels of 6 to 16 mEq/L. Administering hypertonic magnesium solutions poses an additional risk of producing magnesium intoxication in patients with normal renal function. With hypertonic magnesium solutions, i.e.,

Table 223–2 ■ MANAGEMENT OF HYPOMAGNESEMIA

Severe hypomagnesemia (serum Mg, <1 mEq/L)
  IM replacement: 4 mL of 50% magnesium sulfate heptahydrate ($MgSO_4 \cdot 7H_2O$, 16 mEq Mg (196 mg) IM every 4 hr for the 1st 24 hr. Subsequent replacement as required for persistent hypomagnesemia should be 2 mL of 50% $MgSO_4 \cdot 7H_2O$ IM every 6 hr
  IV replacement: Initially 12 mL of 50% $MgSO_4 \cdot 7H_2O$ (49 mEq Mg) in 1000-mL solution of 5% dextrose infused over 3 hr with 2 additional L containing 12 mL of 50% $MgSO_4 \cdot 7H_2O$ administered over the remainder of the 1st 24-hr period. Over the next 3 to 4 d, 49 mEq Mg/day may be given IV
Symptomatic hypomagnesemia (tetany or seizures): 4 mL (16.3 mEq Mg) of a 50% $MgSO_4 \cdot 7H_2O$ solution diluted to 100 mL and infused over a 10-min period
Chronic oral replacement therapy (steatorrheic states and renal magnesium wasting): Magnesium oxide (550 mg Mg/g), 250 to 500 mg four times daily as tolerated without diarrhea developing

50% MgSO$_4$, fluid moves from the extracellular space into the gastrointestinal tract. This shift decreases the effective blood volume and reduces renal perfusion, which compromises the ability to excrete the magnesium absorbed from the large gastrointestinal load. This combination of increased absorption and decreased ability to excrete magnesium can cause life-threatening hypermagnesemia.

SYMPTOMS. Usually no symptoms are noted until serum magnesium is greater than 4 mEq/L, at which time deep tendon reflexes may be slightly depressed. When serum magnesium increases to 10 to 15 mEq/L, deep tendon reflexes are absent and a flaccid quadriplegia may also develop. Other symptoms include lethargy, nausea, dilated pupils, respiratory depression, hypotension, bradycardia, and rarely, complete heart block and cardiac arrest.

TREATMENT OF ACUTE HYPERMAGNESEMIA. Severe hypermagnesemia requires emergency management because patients can die of respiratory failure or cardiac arrest. Calcium is a direct antagonist to magnesium, and as little as 5 to 10 mEq of calcium administered intravenously can readily reverse these potentially lethal complications. This step should be followed by methods to reduce the serum magnesium concentration. In patients with reasonable renal function, the combination of furosemide and 0.5 N saline to replace urine volume and maintain diuresis can augment magnesium excretion. The most effective way of reducing plasma magnesium levels is hemodialysis with a magnesium-free dialysate.

al-Ghamdi SM, Cameron EC, Sutton RA: Magnesium deficiency: Pathophysiologic and clinical overview. Am J Kidney Dis 24:737, 1994. *A recent review that is well referenced.*

ISIS-4: A randomised factorial trial assessing early oral captopril, oral mononitrate and intravenous magnesium sulphate in 58,050 patients with suspected acute myocardial infarction. ISIS-4 (Fourth International Study of Infarct Survival) Collaboration Group. Lancet 345:669, 1995. *A well-controlled study documenting the lack of protective effect of intravenous magnesium in acute myocardial infarction.*

Millane TA, Ward DE, Camm AJ: Electrophysiology, pacing and arrhythmia. Clin Cardiol 15:103, 1992. *An excellent, well-referenced review on the interrelationship between magnesium and potassium and cardiac arrhythmias.*

Simon DB, Nelson-Williams C, Bia MJ, et al: Gitelman's variant of Bartter's syndrome, inherited hypokalemic alkalosis is caused by mutations in the thiazide-sensitive Na-Cl cotransporter. Nat Genet 12:24, 1996. *A comparison of Bartter's and Gitelman's syndromes documenting evidence for a mutation of the thiazide-sensitive Na-Cl transporter in Gitelman's syndrome.*

Whang R, Whang DD, Ryan MP: Refractory potassium repletion. A consequence of magnesium deficiency. Arch Intern Med 152:40, 1992. *Emphasizes the need for combined replacement with potassium and magnesium in certain conditions.*

PART XVI

NUTRITIONAL DISEASES

224 NUTRITION'S INTERFACE WITH HEALTH AND DISEASE

Douglas C. Heimburger

OLD AND NEW PARADIGMS

Nutrition science has been characterized by two major phases in the 20th century. During the first phase, nutrition scientists discovered, characterized, and synthesized the various vitamins and described their deficiency syndromes in detail. The dietary requirements for these nutrients were determined and have been periodically updated by the National Academy of Sciences as the *Recommended Dietary Allowances* (Table 224–1). These allowances are estimated with a margin of error designed to prevent classic deficiencies in practically all persons and do not represent minimum requirements. For nutrients for which too little information exists to estimate recommended intakes, the academy has published *Estimated Safe and Adequate Daily Dietary Intakes* (Table 224–2).

The second phase of modern nutrition science has focused on the relationship of diet and nutritional status to the diseases that plague western societies, such as coronary heart disease (CHD), cancer, and the other leading causes of death. Particularly during the last decade, this focus has led to expansion of the perspectives of nutrition scientists and the evolution of a new paradigm for understanding nutrition, which is contrasted with the older paradigm in Table 224–3. It is likely that this development will produce exciting changes in the way that nutrition and health are understood during the next decade.

NUTRITION'S INFLUENCE ON MORTALITY AND MORBIDITY

The causal connections between diet and chronic disease are difficult to tease out of the complex network of other risk factors, including social and behavioral variables, so a wide variety of studies must be relied on to establish these connections with reasonable certainty. The first links between diet and disease are often derived from epidemiologic studies, but such studies are unable to infer causal relationships and may be confounded by variables that have not been examined. Epidemiologic studies are also challenged by the difficulty of accurately assessing the diets of free-living individuals. Animal and in vitro studies can overcome some of these drawbacks but may be confounded by experimental conditions that differ from those encountered by humans. A large number of prospective, randomized human intervention trials have been undertaken to test the effects of dietary change on the risk for disease. However, even these trials will not always be conclusive because of pitfalls associated with selecting study populations and isolating individual dietary factors.

Nevertheless, taken together, epidemiologic, animal, in vitro, and intervention studies are proving that human dietary habits contribute importantly to the pathogenesis of most of the major causes of death in developed countries. The 10 leading causes of death in the United States are listed in Table 224–4 and includes several other morbid conditions that have well-established dietary links.

Nutritional influences on the most common cause of death in the United States, CHD, have been the subject of a great deal of productive research. The overall U.S. mortality rate from CHD peaked in the 1960s and, in a trend that surprised medical science, has declined steadily ever since. Although the causes of the decline are not firmly established, it is apparent that changes in lifestyle, including diet, are probably more responsible than is high-tech care of patients with established CHD. Elevated plasma low-density lipoprotein cholesterol (LDL-C) levels are a major risk factor for CHD and peripheral atherosclerosis and correlate strongly with dietary saturated fat intake and less strongly with cholesterol intake. Intake of both of these substances in the United States is derived largely from foods of animal origin such as meats, dairy products, and eggs. Attempts to produce less atherogenic substitutes for some of these foods have not always proved beneficial. For instance, hydrogenation of vegetable oils to create margarine and shortening results in the formation of *trans* fatty acids, which affect serum cholesterol levels in a manner similar to the saturated fatty acids found in butter and lard. LDL-C levels can be lowered modestly by increasing the intake of soluble fiber from legumes, fruits, and vegetables. LDL must be oxidized before it induces injury to arterial wall epithelial cells: adequate dietary levels of the antioxidant vitamins C and E and β-carotene have been shown to inhibit LDL oxidation.

Epidemiologic evidence suggests that fish consumption may reduce CHD risk; perhaps through the action of ω-3 fatty acids. Evidence also indicates that moderate consumption of alcohol, especially wine, is associated with decreased risk for CHD, possibly through increasing high-density lipoprotein cholesterol levels or preventing oxidation of LDL. Circulating levels of the amino acid homocysteine, which are asymptomatically elevated in 20 to 25% of Americans, have been strongly correlated with risk for CHD. Homocysteine levels can be reduced by increasing the intake of folic acid (mainly from legumes and vegetables) and decreasing the intake of methionine (principally from animal protein). A conservative estimate suggests that moderate dietary modification by the U.S. population consisting mainly of replacing saturated fats with complex carbohydrates, fiber, monounsaturated fats, and fish should lead to a 10% reduction in serum cholesterol levels and a 20% reduction in CHD mortality in comparison to 1987 levels.

Nutrients, non-nutritive dietary constituents, and nutritional status can influence the risk for cancer in a variety of ways. Nutrition interacts with each step of carcinogenesis (carcinogen activation and tumor initiation, promotion, and progression). Humans are exposed to countless potential carcinogens, but to many anticarcinogens as well, each day through dietary and other means. Excess caloric intake may favor the generation of free radicals and reduce the body's ability to detoxify carcinogens. By contrast, antioxidant nutrients scavenge free radicals and other (pre)carcinogens and thereby inhibit their activation and/or their ability to initiate mutations. Folic acid may improve a cell's ability to preserve, repair, and methylate its DNA, either preventing or reversing the tendency to mutation. Obesity, excess dietary fat intake, and excess alcohol appear to promote tumor growth.

Much evidence indicates that the number one cancer killer, lung cancer, is strongly influenced by diet. Although the most important causal factor is cigarette smoking, consumption of fruits and vegetables is inversely associated with lung cancer risk in both smokers and non-smokers. It is probable that many nutrients in fruits and vegetables, such as β-carotene and folic acid, as well as non-nutritive components, are partly responsible for the protective effects. Moreover, in view of the disappointing results of randomized trials of supplementation with β-carotene, antioxidant supplements should not be relied on to reduce disease risk. It is noteworthy that plasma levels of antioxidant nutrients (β-carotene and vitamins C

Table 224–1 ■ FOOD AND NUTRITION BOARD, NATIONAL ACADEMY OF SCIENCES—NATIONAL RESEARCH COUNCIL RECOMMENDED DIETARY ALLOWANCES,* REVISED 1989

CATEGORY	AGE (yr) OR CONDITION	WEIGHT† kg	WEIGHT† lb	HEIGHT† cm	HEIGHT† in	PROTEIN (g)	FAT-SOLUBLE VITAMINS Vitamin A (µg RE)‡	Vitamin D (µg)§	Vitamin E (mg α-TE)**	Vitamin K (µg)	WATER-SOLUBLE VITAMINS Vitamin C (mg)	Thiamine (mg)	Riboflavin (mg)	Niacin (mg NE)††	Vitamin B₆ (mg)	Folate (µg)	Vitamin B₁₂ (µg)	MINERALS Calcium (mg)	Phosphorus (mg)	Magnesium (mg)	Iron (mg)	Zinc (mg)	Iodine (µg)	Selenium (µg)
Infants	0.0–0.5	6	13	60	24	13	375	7.5	3	5	30	0.3	0.4	5	0.3	25	0.3	400	300	40	6	5	40	10
	0.5–1.0	9	20	71	28	14	375	10	4	10	35	0.4	0.5	6	0.6	35	0.5	600	500	60	10	5	50	15
Children	1–3	13	29	90	35	16	400	10	6	15	40	0.7	0.8	9	1.0	50	0.7	800	800	80	10	10	70	20
	4–7	20	44	112	44	24	500	10	7	20	45	0.9	1.1	12	1.1	75	1.0	800	800	120	10	10	90	20
	7–10	28	62	132	52	28	700	10	7	30	45	1.0	1.2	13	1.4	100	1.4	800	800	170	10	10	120	30
Males	11–14	45	99	157	62	45	1,000	10	10	45	50	1.3	1.5	17	1.7	150	2.0	1,200	1,200	270	12	15	150	40
	15–18	66	145	176	69	59	1,000	10	10	65	60	1.5	1.8	20	2.0	200	2.0	1,200	1,200	400	12	15	150	50
	19–24	72	160	177	70	58	1,000	10	10	70	60	1.5	1.7	19	2.0	200	2.0	1,200	1,200	350	10	15	150	70
	25–50	79	174	176	70	63	1,000	5	10	80	60	1.5	1.7	19	2.0	200	2.0	800	800	350	10	15	150	70
	51+	77	170	173	68	63	1,000	5	10	80	60	1.2	1.4	15	2.0	200	2.0	800	800	350	10	15	150	70
Females	11–14	46	101	157	62	46	800	10	8	45	50	1.1	1.3	15	1.4	150	2.0	1,200	1,200	280	15	12	150	45
	15–18	55	120	163	64	44	800	10	8	55	60	1.1	1.3	15	1.5	180	2.0	1,200	1,200	300	15	12	150	50
	19–24	58	128	164	65	46	800	10	8	60	60	1.1	1.3	15	1.6	180	2.0	1,200	1,200	280	15	12	150	55
	25–50	63	138	163	64	50	800	5	8	65	60	1.1	1.3	15	1.6	180	2.0	800	800	280	15	12	150	55
	51+	65	143	160	63	50	800	5	8	65	60	1.0	1.2	13	1.6	180	2.0	800	800	280	10	12	150	55
Pregnant						60	800	10	10	65	70	1.5	1.6	17	2.2	400	2.2	1,200	1,200	320	30	15	175	65
Lactating	1st 6 months					65	1,300	10	12	65	95	1.6	1.8	20	2.1	280	2.6	1,200	1,200	355	15	19	200	75
	2nd 6 months					62	1,200	10	11	65	90	1.6	1.7	20	2.1	260	2.6	1,200	1,200	340	15	16	200	75

*The allowances, expressed as average daily intakes over time, are intended to provide for individual variations, among most normal persons as they live in the United States under usual environmental stresses. Diets should be based on a variety of common foods to provide other nutrients for which human requirements have been less well defined. These allowances have been designed for the maintenance of good nutrition of practically all healthy people in the United States.
†Weights and heights of reference adults are actual medians for the designated age, as reported by NHANES II (National Health and Nutrition Examination Survey II). Use of these figures does not imply that the height-to-weight ratios are ideal.
‡Retinol equivalents. 1 retinol equivalent = 1 µg retinol or 6 µg β-carotene.
§As cholecalciferol. 10 µg cholecalciferol = 400 IU vitamin D.
**Tocopherol equivalents. 1 mg D-α-tocopherol = 1 α-TE.
††One niacin equivalent (NE) is equal to 1 mg of niacin or 60 mg of dietary tryptophan.

Table 224–2 ■ ESTIMATED SAFE AND ADEQUATE DAILY DIETARY INTAKES OF SELECTED VITAMINS AND MINERALS*

| CATEGORY | AGE (yr) | VITAMINS | | TRACE ELEMENTS† | | | | |
		Biotin (μg)	Pantothenic Acid (mg)	Copper (mg)	Manganese (mg)	Fluoride (mg)	Chromium (μg)	Molybdenum (μg)
Infants	0–0.5	10	2	0.4–0.6	0.3–0.6	0.1–0.5	10–40	15–30
	0.5–1	15	3	0.6–0.7	0.6–1.0	0.2–1.0	20–60	20–40
Children and adolescents	1–3	20	3	0.7–1.0	1.0–1.5	0.5–1.5	20–80	25–50
	4–6	25	3–4	1.0–1.5	1.5–2.0	1.0–2.5	30–120	30–75
	7–10	30	4–5	1.0–2.0	2.0–3.0	1.5–2.5	50–200	50–150
	11+	30–100	4–7	1.5–2.5	2.0–5.0	1.5–2.5	50–200	75–250
Adults		30–100	4–7	1.5–3.0	2.0–5.0	1.5–4.0	50–200	75–250

*Because less information on which to base allowances is available, these figures are not given in Table 224–1 and are provided here in the form of ranges of recommended intakes.

†Because the toxic levels for many trace elements may be only several times the usual intake, the upper levels for the trace elements given in this table should not be habitually exceeded.

From the National Research Council: Recommended Dietary Allowances, 10th ed. Washington, DC, National Academy Press, 1989.

Table 224–3 ■ OLD AND NEW PARADIGMS IN NUTRITION

OLD PARADIGM	NEW PARADIGM
Major nutritional problems are classic deficiency syndromes	Major nutritional problems are chronic diseases
Micronutrients (vitamins, minerals, trace elements) function primarily as cofactors in biochemical reactions	Micronutrients also function as antioxidants, regulators of genes and cell-cell communications, hormones, and pharmacologic agents
Nutrient needs (Recommended Dietary Allowances) determined by amounts required to prevent classic deficiency syndromes	Nutrient needs (not yet distilled into consensus recommendations) determined by amounts required to provide optimal function and health and prevent chronic disease; amounts are affected by individual's genetic makeup and environmental exposures
Micronutrient deficiencies are global, affecting the whole body	Micronutrient deficiencies may be localized and affect the functions of specific tissues
General effects of nutrients	Specific effects of nutrient subtypes, e.g., individual fatty acids, amino acids, and particular forms of micronutrients
All benefits of food are derived from nutrients; many can be obtained from supplements	Many non-nutritive components of foods, e.g., fiber, pigments, protease inhibitors, flavonoids, and others, have important effects; even if some become available through supplements, many undetected ones may exist in foods

Table 224–4 ■ DIETARY INFLUENCES ON MAJOR CAUSES OF DEATH AND MORBIDITY IN THE UNITED STATES

	POSSIBLE BENEFICIAL INFLUENCES	POSSIBLE DELETERIOUS INFLUENCES
Cause of Death		
Coronary heart disease	Complex carbohydrates, particular fatty acids (e.g., monounsaturated, polyunsaturated, and ω-3 fatty acids from fish), soluble fiber, antioxidants (vitamins E, C; β-carotene, selenium), folic acid, moderate alcohol	Saturated fat, cholesterol; excess calories, sodium, animal protein; abdominal distribution of body fat
Cancer	Fruits and vegetables (for β-carotene, vitamins A, C, D, E, folic acid, calcium, selenium, phytochemicals), fiber	Excess calories, fat, alcohol, red meat, salt- and nitrite-preserved meats, possibly grilled meats; abdominal distribution of body fat
Stroke	Potassium, calcium ω-3 fatty acids	Sodium, alcohol (as with hypertension)
Accidents		Alcohol
Diabetes mellitus	Fiber	Excess calories, fat, alcohol; abdominal distribution of body fat
Suicide		Alcohol
Chronic liver disease		Alcohol
Atherosclerosis (peripheral)	Particular fatty acids (e.g., monounsaturated and ω-3 fatty acids), soluble fiber, antioxidant vitamins	Saturated fat, cholesterol
Cause of Morbidity		
Obesity		Excess calories and fat
Hypertension	Potassium, calcium, ω-3 fatty acids, fruits and vegetables	Sodium, alcohol, excess calories, and saturated and total fat; abdominal distribution of body fat
Osteoporosis	Calcium, vitamin D	Sodium, phosphorus, protein
Diverticular disease, constipation		Fiber
Neural tube defects	Folic acid	

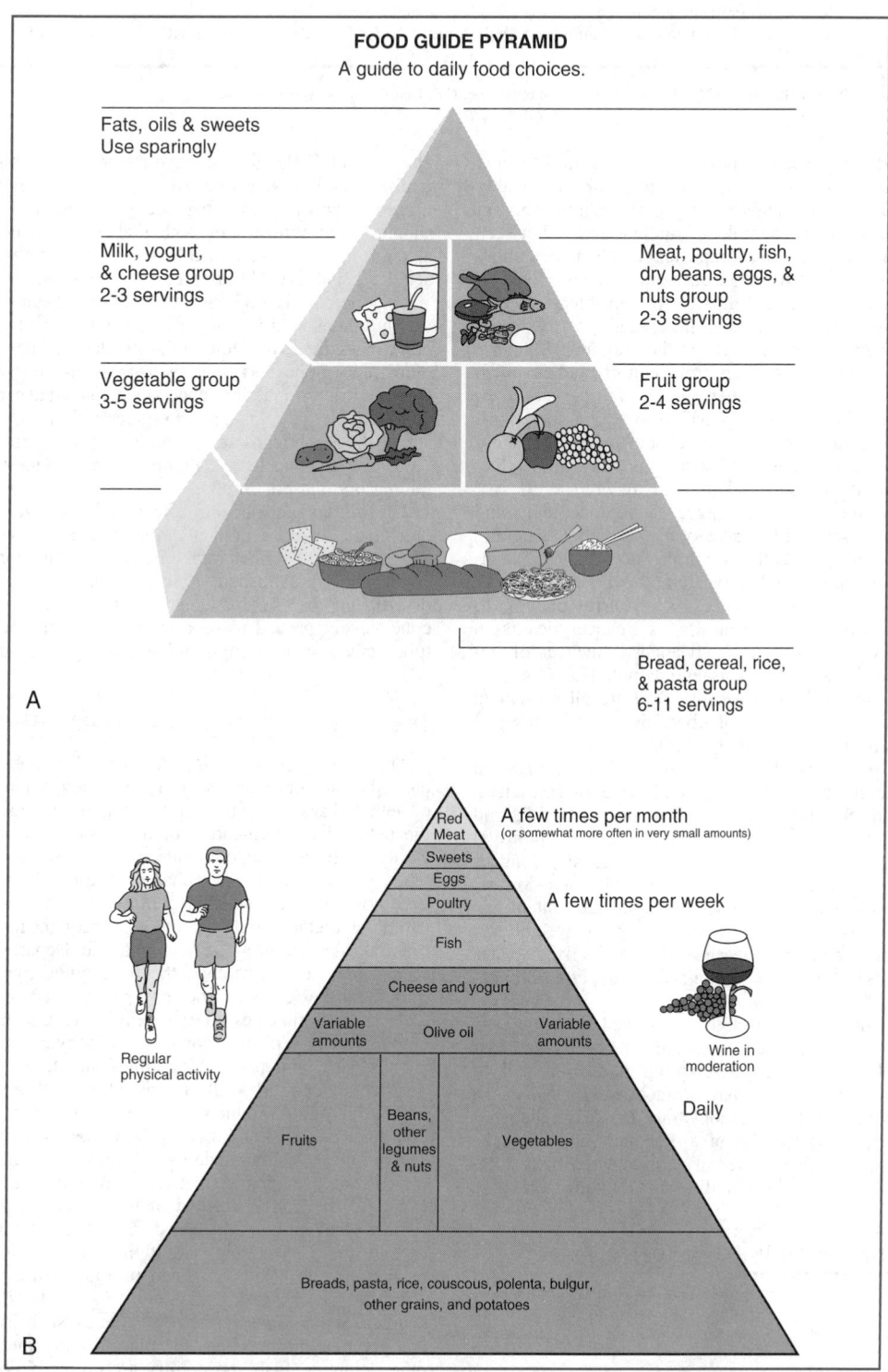

FIGURE 224–1 ■ *A.* U.S. Department of Agriculture/Department of Health and Human Services Food Guide Pyramid. *B.* Traditional healthy Mediterranean diet pyramid. (*A.* From USDA/DDHS. *B.* Copyright 1994. Oldways Preservation & Exchange Trust and The President and Fellows of Harvard College. Used by permission.)

Table 224–5 ■ DEFINITIONS OF TERMS USED ON FOOD LABELS

Low fat	≤3 g per serving
Low saturated fat	≤1 g per serving, ≤15% of calories
Low calorie	≤40 calories per serving
High	≥20% of the desired daily value per serving
Light	Half the fat or one third the calories of the regular product
Reduced	≤75% of the content of the regular product
Free	None or insignificant amount (e.g., <1 g fat or <$\frac{1}{2}$ g sugar per serving)
Healthy	Low total and saturated fat, sodium, and cholesterol; ≥10% of the daily value for vitamin A, vitamin C, iron, calcium, protein, or fiber

From U.S. Department of Health and Human Services, Food and Drug Administration, U.S. Department of Agriculture.

and E) and folic acid are lower in smokers than non-smokers and intermediate in persons passively exposed to smoke. Probably caused by oxidants in cigarette smoke and poorer dietary habits in smokers, this difference is an example of an interaction between nutritional factors and environmental exposure that explains more of the variation in cancer incidence than does either factor alone.

The 2nd largest cause of cancer deaths in women, breast cancer, is positively associated with dietary fat intake and obesity, especially when the latter predominantly affects the abdomen. Because of the inconsistencies between ecologic and cohort studies noted earlier, however, it is unclear whether dietary fat per se, total calorie intake, or other factors are responsible for the associations. Epidemiologic evidence suggests that alcohol intake may also be a risk factor for this disease. Colorectal cancer is the 2nd leading cause of cancer mortality in men and the 3rd in women. Its risk correlates positively with dietary fat intake in both ecologic and cohort studies and inversely with intake of dietary fiber, calcium, and folic acid. Other malignant diseases for which dietary fat intake appears to increase risk include prostate and ovarian cancer.

The interaction of all these influences is powerful enough to indicate that diet contributes to about 35% of cancer deaths in Western countries. Even though the independent influences of potentially protective nutrients such as carotenoids, vitamins C and E, folic acid, and fiber are not known because they are all present in vegetables and fruits, the evidence that liberal intake of fruits and vegetables reduces cancer risk is overwhelming.

Hypertension is a major risk factor for stroke, CHD, congestive heart failure, peripheral vascular disease, and renal disease. It is often associated with obesity, especially abdominal obesity, and weight reduction in obese hypertensives usually leads to improvement in blood pressure. Sodium restriction also usually reduces blood pressure levels. A diet rich in fruits, vegetables, and low-fat dairy products and with reduced saturated and total fat content can also decrease blood pressure levels, even when body weight and sodium intake are held constant. Because alcohol intake elevates blood pressure, its use should be minimized in hypertensive patients.

Type II diabetes mellitus is strongly associated with obesity. This relationship is especially true for abdominal obesity and less so for peripheral obesity. Sugar consumption does not lead to diabetes except to the extent that it may promote weight gain. Past recommendations to restrict total carbohydrate intake in diabetics have been abandoned, so 55 to 60% of a diabetic's energy intake should come from carbohydrate, preferably unrefined carbohydrates that include fiber. Because higher-fat diets tend to promote both

obesity and CHD, for which diabetics are at high risk, dietary fat intake should be kept low. Alcohol can cause hypoglycemia, hyperglycemia, and increased triglyceride levels in diabetics, and its use should be minimized. In both diabetics and non-diabetics, excess alcohol intake is responsible for many deaths, particularly from accidents and liver disease, and is a factor in some suicidal deaths.

Osteoporosis is influenced by several dietary factors. Inadequate calcium intake during adolescence may result in suboptimal peak bone mass in early adulthood, and during later life it may lead to more rapid bone loss, thereby increasing the risk for osteoporosis. Other nutrients that influence bone mass have received much less attention. Sodium, phosphorus, and protein, all of which are consumed by Americans in greater quantities than required, may promote excess bone loss. Vitamin D and magnesium assist in maintaining optimal bone mass.

The causes and health effects of obesity, the most prevalent nutritional disorder in the United States, are reviewed in Chapter 228. Low dietary fiber intake causes constipation, and although not conclusively established, it is thought to be a cause of intestinal diverticular disease. Inadequate maternal folic acid intake has been conclusively proved to be a major risk factor for congenital neural tube defects such as spina bifida and myelomeningocele.

TRANSLATING EVIDENCE INTO DIETARY CHANGE

Thus strong evidence has surfaced that dietary habits can influence the incidence and severity of many potentially incapacitating or lethal diseases in the United States. No justification exists for the belief that modification of the "usual" American diet is unnecessary or futile. The only questions are whether it is feasible and what is required to effect change. Various health agencies and the U.S. government have used public education, particularly the publication of dietary goals, as their primary means. The U.S. Department of Agriculture (USDA) and the Department of Health and Human Services developed the food guide pyramid to replace the traditional basic four food groups in educating the public (Fig. 224–1A). It indicates that a healthy diet should be founded on ample servings of the complex carbohydrates present in breads, cereals, rice, and pasta. Vegetables and fruits should be a prominent component as well. Foods of animal origin, such as meat, eggs, and dairy products, should form a less central part of the diet, and fats, oils, and sweets should be used sparingly.

Even these recommendations do not typify an ideal diet based on the available evidence; instead, they reflect a consensus on what can be realistically expected of the American public. A potentially more "ideal" pyramid, based on observations of low rates of chronic disease and high adult life expectancies in the Mediterranean region in 1960, has been promulgated by the Department of Nutrition at Harvard University (Fig. 224–1B). In this pyramid, sources of monounsaturated fatty acids such as olive oil and nuts are given a more prominent place in the diet, as are beans and other legumes. Fish and poultry are preferable over red meat. Moderate consumption of wine (normally with meals) is recommended as optional, unless it would put the individual or others at risk.

Beginning in May 1994, the U.S. Food and Drug Administration and USDA initiated a major public education effort by requiring substantial changes in the listing of nutrient contents and health claims on food labels. Issues that were previously left to the discretion of food manufacturers, such as the serving sizes and the particular nutrients listed, are now stipulated. Labels must delineate

Table 224–6 ■ PERMISSIBLE HEALTH CLAIMS FOR FOOD LABELS

Calcium	May lower risk for osteoporosis
Fat	May increase risk for cancer
Saturated fat and cholesterol	Increase risk for coronary heart disease
Fiber-containing grain products, fruits, and vegetables	May reduce risk for coronary heart disease and cancer
Sodium	May increase risk for high blood pressure
Fruits and vegetables	May reduce risk for cancer
Folic acid supplementation	Reduces risk for neural tube defects

From U.S. Department of Health and Human Services, Food and Drug Administration, U.S. Department of Agriculture.

total calories, percentage of calories from fat, and amounts of total fat, saturated fat, cholesterol, sodium, total carbohydrates, dietary fiber, sugars, protein, vitamins A and C, calcium, and iron. Labels must also indicate how a food's content of these nutrients conform to recommended intakes based on a reference 2000-calorie diet. Definitions for "low," "high," "light," "reduced," "free," and "healthy" have been standardized (Table 224–5). Furthermore, only the particular health claims listed in Table 224–6 are permitted on food labels. As further evidence accumulates on the relationships between diet and disease, the approved claims will undoubtedly be revised.

For more details on the rationale for and methods of implementing the recommended dietary changes, please see Chapter 225. Physicians can importantly influence their patients' health by encouraging them to optimize their dietary habits and providing them with instructional materials and assistance from dietitians to help them make needed changes.

National Academy of Sciences: Diet and Health: Washington, DC, 1989. *Comprehensive and easily readable analysis of the scientific evidence on the role of diet in the etiology and prevention of chronic disease in the United States; prepared by a committee of experts.*

Shils, ME, Olson JA, Shike M, Ross, AC (eds): Modern Nutrition in Health and Disease, 9th ed. Baltimore, Williams & Wilkins, 1999. *Comprehensive and detailed source for information on all aspects of human nutrition.*

USDA: Dietary Guidelines for Americans. Washington, DC, USDA, 1995. *A concise and practical summary of the recommended dietary habits to promote health and prevent disease. Available at www.nal.usda.gov/fric/dga/dguide95.html.*

World Cancer Research Fund/American Institute for Cancer Research: Food, Nutrition, and the Prevention of Cancer: A Global Perspective. Washington, DC, WCRF/AICR, 1997.

225 NUTRITIONAL ASSESSMENT

Bruce R. Bistrian

Nutritional assessment in clinical medicine has three primary goals: to identify the presence and type of malnutrition, to define health-threatening obesity, and to devise suitable diets as prophylaxis against disease later in life. The focus of this chapter is on the diagnosis of protein-energy malnutrition because of its wide prevalence and major impact on disease outcome. Other deficiency diseases are of much less relevance in that most occur in conjunction with protein-energy malnutrition or with specific disease states, such as thiamine deficiency with alcoholic liver disease or fat-soluble vitamin deficiency with malabsorptive states. The classic deficiency diseases, either primary or secondary, are considered elsewhere in this volume. The widespread availability of parenteral and enteral therapeutic measures over the past decade that can provide adequate feeding regimens for virtually any disease condition makes a rudimentary knowledge of the pathophysiology of protein-energy malnutrition and its nutritional assessment essential for all primary care practitioners (see Chapter 224).

CLINICAL NUTRITIONAL ASSESSMENT. Clinical assessment of protein nutritional status is based principally on the clinical history, simple anthropometry, and measurement of the levels of several secretory proteins. Although detailed dietary assessment can at times be helpful, in most circumstances physicians can safely limit their diet questions to whether patients have been following a prescribed diet and how much alcohol they drink. In ambulatory patients the ability to maintain usual and adequate weight generally indicates that serious micronutrient deficiency is probably not due to dietary inadequacy. Isolated vitamin deficiencies in the absence of weight loss or symptoms are rare, except perhaps for folate and vitamin B_{12}. Although nutritional anemias do exist, the role of dietary deficiency in folic acid– or vitamin B_{12}–related anemias is minimal in the absence of underlying disease or weight loss. Only iron deficiency is a reasonable cause as a dietary anemia. By contrast, full dietary assessment and diet prescriptions are likely to help conditions such as fat malabsorption accompanied by weight loss, cramps, or diarrhea. Such evaluations are most effectively carried out by dietitians. Thus detailed nutritional assessment of protein-energy malnutrition with secondary assessment of vitamin

and mineral deficiencies is usually needed only when protein-energy malnutrition or a specific disorder known to interfere with nutrient metabolism coexists, such as celiac disease, pernicious anemia, or nutrient-drug interactions. Even then, the assessment should emphasize the likely deficiencies. For fat malabsorption, one should check levels of the fat-soluble vitamins A, D, E, and K, as well as important divalent and trivalent cations (Ca^{2+}, Zn^{2+}, Mg^{2+}, Fe^{3+}). When ileal resection has occurred, serum B_{12} levels should be measured. Weight loss resulting from short-gut syndrome should prompt assessment of the fat-soluble vitamins, folic acid, vitamin B_{12}, calcium, magnesium, zinc, and iron. Measurements of body water status (blood urea nitrogen, creatinine, serum sodium) and acid-base balance (CO_2 combining power, chloride, potassium, urine, and arterial pH) should be obtained if the diarrhea is profuse.

Clinically obvious marasmus and hypoalbuminemic malnutrition affect 25 to 50% of patients hospitalized for acute care. Many of these patients can benefit from nutritional support and require a thorough clinical nutritional assessment, including a dietary history, physical examination, and laboratory tests that serve to confirm clinical impressions. The history should list information about the timing and amount of weight loss, medical illnesses, medications, gastrointestinal symptoms (abdominal pain, diarrhea, dysphagia), diet habits (eating fewer than two meals per day, alcohol consumption, dental status), social habits (eats alone, needs assistance in self-care), economic status (enough money for food), and mental status, particularly the presence of depressive symptoms. A special focus should be reserved for the elderly, in whom protein-energy malnutrition secondary to these last factors is more common.

Three factors principally determine the timing and appropriateness of nutritional support, (1) the presence and severity of protein-energy malnutrition, defined primarily by weight loss and serum albumin; (2) the presence and severity of the systemic inflammatory response, also defined by serum albumin but in addition including fever, leukocytosis, and increased band forms; and (3) the actual or expected duration of inadequate nutritional intake. Well-nourished individuals have a 7- to 10-day reserve of energy and protein to withstand a moderate systemic inflammatory response without adverse nutritional consequences. Greater degrees of systemic inflammatory response or pre-existing protein-energy malnutrition dramatically shorten the period that semistarvation, defined as consuming less than 50% of the energy and protein needs, can be tolerated.

WEIGHT LOSS. A recent unintended weight loss of 10 lb or more than 5% of usual weight should prompt efforts to diagnose the underlying disorder or social circumstance. Weight loss alone does not distinguish the composition of tissue loss, which can range from 25 to 30% lean tissue in semistarvation to 50% lean tissue loss following starvation plus injury. Therefore, unintentional weight loss of more than 10 lb indicates a need for thorough nutritional assessment. Weight loss in excess of 10% of usual weight should be considered to represent protein-energy malnutrition that will impair physiologic function, particularly muscle strength and endurance. Weight loss in excess of 20% should be considered severe protein-energy malnutrition that will substantially impair most organ systems. If major elective surgery is planned, such individuals would benefit from adequate feeding preoperatively. If palliative or curative radiotherapy or systemic chemotherapy is planned, adequate feeding during therapy with the use of supplemental formulas, tube feeding, or parenteral nutrition (in that order) is indicated. However, if the weight loss represents end-stage systemic illness (e.g., cancer, end-stage liver disease, acquired immune deficiency syndrome) for which no primary therapy is planned or effective, invasive nutritional support is rarely indicated.

PHYSICAL EXAMINATION. Although the patient's external appearance and a check of the skin, eyes, mouth, hair, and nails often provide a clue to the presence of nutritional abnormalities (Table 225–1), the physical findings of deficiency syndromes of vitamins, essential fatty acids, and trace metals are relatively insensitive and non-specific. With respect to protein-energy malnutrition, only the marasmic form of semistarvation is evident at examination. Loss of subcutaneous fat and skeletal muscle is manifested by sunken temples, thin extremities, wasting of the muscles of the hand, and rarely edema. Although kwashiorkor in children is characterized by severe edema and a potbelly appearance from hepatomegaly and

Table 225–1 ■ CLINICAL SIGNS AND SYMPTOMS OF NUTRITIONAL INADEQUACY IN ADULT PATIENTS

	CLINICAL SIGN OR SYMPTOM	NUTRIENT
General	Wasted, skinny	Calorie
	Loss of appetite	Protein-energy, zinc
Skin	Psoriasiform rash, eczematous scaling	Zinc, vitamin A, EFA
	Pallor	Folate, iron, vitamin B_{12}, copper
	Follicular hyperkeratosis	Vitamin A, vitamin C
	Perifollicular petechiae	Vitamin C
	Flaking dermatitis	Protein-energy, niacin, riboflavin, zinc
	Bruising	Vitamin C, vitamin K
	Pigmentation changes	Niacin, protein-energy
	Scrotal dermatosis	Riboflavin
	Thickening and dryness of skin	Linoleic acid
Head	Temporal muscle wasting	Protein-energy
Hair	Sparse and thin, dyspigmentation	Protein
	Easy to pull out	Protein
	Corkscrew hairs	Vitamin C
Eyes	History of night blindness (also impaired visual recovery after glare)	Vitamin A, zinc
	Photophobia, blurring, conjunctival inflammation	Riboflavin, vitamin A
	Corneal vascularization	Riboflavin
	Xerosis, Bitot spots, keratomalacia	Vitamin A
Mouth	Glossitis	Riboflavin, niacin, folic acid, vitamin B_{12}, pyridoxine
	Bleeding gums	Vitamin C, riboflavin
	Cheilosis	Riboflavin, pyridoxine, niacin
	Angular stomatitis	Riboflavin, pyridoxine, niacin
	Hypogeusia	Zinc
	Tongue fissuring	Niacin
	Tongue atrophy	Riboflavin, niacin, iron
	Nasolabial seborrhea	Pyridoxine
Neck	Goiter	Iodine
	Parotid enlargement	Protein
Thorax	Thoracic rosary	Vitamin D
Abdomen	Diarrhea	Niacin, folate, vitamin B_{12}
	Distention	Protein-energy
	Hepatomegaly	Protein-energy
Extremities	Edema	Protein, thiamine
	Softening of bone	Vitamin D, calcium, phosphorus
	Bone tenderness	Vitamin D
	Bone ache, joint pain	Vitamin C
	Muscle wasting and weakness	Protein, calorie, vitamin D, selenium, sodium chloride
	Muscle tenderness, muscle pain	Thiamine
Nails	Spooning	Iron
	Transverse lines	Protein
Neurologic	Tetany	Calcium, magnesium
	Paresthesias	Thiamine, vitamin B_{12}
	Loss of reflexes, wristdrop, footdrop	Thiamine
	Loss of vibratory and position sense	Vitamin B_{12}
	Ataxia	Vitamin B_{12}
	Dementia, disorientation	Niacin
Blood	Anemia	Vitamin B_{12}, folate iron, pyridoxine
	Hemolysis	Phosphorus, vitamin E

EFA = essential fatty acids.
Modified from Russell RM: Nutritional assessment. *In* Wyngaarden JB, Smith LH Jr, Bennett JC: Cecil Textbook of Medicine, 19th ed. Philadelphia, 1992, WB Saunders, pp 1151–1155.

ascites, one rarely encounters these clinical signs in hypoalbuminemic malnutrition.

The most useful element in the physical examination is body weight, which is expressed as a relative value to evaluate the patient in relation to the healthy population. Weight and height are easily obtained, and standards for comparison have been established (Table 225-2). Although newer standards are available, they reflect the increasing prevalence of obesity in the U.S. population. Use of the 1959 standards allows the same tables to be used to diagnose significant protein-energy malnutrition (less than 85% of desirable weight, which approximates the 5th percentile) and significant obesity, defined as obesity predisposing to excessive mortality risk (greater than 130% of desirable weight). Although severe protein-energy malnutrition will often occur at levels greater than 85% of desirable weight, this condition will generally be detected by percent weight loss or upper arm anthropometry. Height can be measured in a reclining patient with a tape measure, and in certain situations the patient history may be relied upon. The major confounding variable that limits the value of weight and height as an index of protein-energy malnutrition is the tendency for water retention with disease, and thus weight gain may not reflect an increase in lean body mass or protein content. Fluid retention is particularly a problem with hypoalbuminemic malnutrition because of the effects of aldosterone, antidiuretic hormone, and insulin stimulated by the stress response to cause sodium and fluid retention. Fluid retention, however, is not common in patients first seen at the physician's office or initially at the hospital, except in those with diseases such as cardiac failure, end-stage liver disease, and severe renal disease.

The body mass index (BMI), which is the weight in kilograms divided by the height in meters squared, has recently gained favor as a nutritional measure because of two valuable attributes. The measure is relatively independent of height, and the same standards apply to males and females. Normal nutrition is defined as a BMI of 18 to 25, with significant obesity defined as a BMI greater than 28. Evidence from less developed countries suggests that the BMI is better correlated with outcome than are weight and height.

UPPER ARM ANTHROPOMETRY. Approximately 50% of body fat is subcutaneous. The use of skinfold calipers to define the triceps skinfold is the most practical technique to estimate body fat. Standards for skinfold measurements are available from the National Health and Nutrition Examination Survey I and II and were

Table 225-2 ■ DESIRABLE WEIGHT IN POUNDS IN RELATION TO HEIGHT FOR ADULT MEN AND WOMEN 25 YEARS OR OLDER*

MEN, MEDIUM FRAME				WOMEN, MEDIUM FRAME			
Height		Weight (lb)		Height		Weight (lb)	
ft	in.	Range	Midpoint	ft	in.	Range	Midpoint
				4	8	93–104	98.5
				4	9	95–107	101
				4	10	98–110	104
				4	11	101–113	107
				5	0	104–116	110
5	1	113–124	118.5	5	1	107–119	113
5	2	116–128	122	5	2	110–123	116.5
5	3	119–131	125	5	3	113–127	120
5	4	122–134	128	5	4	117–132	124.5
5	5	125–138	131.5	5	5	121–136	128.5
5	6	129–142	135.5	5	6	125–140	132.5
5	7	133–147	140	5	7	129–144	136.5
5	8	137–151	144	5	8	133–148	140.5
5	9	141–155	148	5	9	137–152	144.5
5	10	145–160	153	5	10	141–156	148.5
5	11	149–165	157				
6	0	153–170	161.5				
6	1	157–175	166				
6	2	162–180	171				
6	3	167–185	176				

*Corrected to nude weights and heights by assuming 1-inch heel for men, 2-inch heel for women, and indoor clothing weight of 5 and 3 lbs for men and women, respectively.
Adapted from the Metropolitan Life Insurance Company Statistical Bulletin 4:1, 1959.

derived from a probability sample of the U.S. population. Generally, less than the 5th percentile is used to define abnormality (Table 225-3). The principal value of the triceps skinfold (TSF) is to determine the arm muscle circumference (AMC) or arm muscle area.

$$AMC (cm) = arm\ circumference - (\pi)(TSF\ [mm])/10$$

The arm muscle circumference is a specific measure of protein-energy malnutrition if the 5th or 10th percentile is chosen as the cutoff point, and it is particularly valuable in edematous states or in amputees, in whom weights are inaccurate or insensitive. The triceps skinfold and arm muscle circumference measurements are most useful in initial defining of marasmic-type malnutrition or the mixed disorder. Nearly all dietitians are skilled in upper arm anthropometry.

SERUM PROTEINS. Despite many concerns, the serum albumin level remains the traditional standard for nutritional assessment by virtue of its extensive history and its continued use to separate the two principal forms of protein-energy malnutrition. Hypoalbuminemia is a strong predictor of risk for morbidity and mortality in both hospitalized and ambulatory patients. In almost all cases, except perhaps for hereditary analbuminemia, excessive loss secondary to nephrosis, and occasionally, protein-losing enteropathy, hypoalbuminemia identifies the systemic inflammatory response and thus the presence of an illness with the accompanying effects of anorexia and depression of immune function. Given a half-life for albumin of 18 to 20 days and the fractional replacement rate of about 10% per day, the return of serum albumin to normal takes about 2 weeks of feeding when the stress response remits. Levels of other proteins such as transferrin, pre-albumin, and retinol-binding protein with respective half-lives of 7 days, 2 days, and ½ day also fall acutely with injury and respond more quickly when stress remits. However, serum transferrin also varies with iron status, and pre-albumin and retinol-binding protein vary with dietary carbohydrate and renal function. As a result, these proteins do not identify the presence and severity of the stress response any better than albumin does.

NUTRITIONAL THERAPY AND ITS ASSESSMENT. The same indices that are used in the baseline nutritional assessment can be used to assess response to therapy, provided that certain points are kept in mind. In a stressed, hospitalized patient receiving nutritional support, day-to-day weight changes generally reflect shifts in fluid balance rather than energy balance. In an ambulatory setting, weight increases or decreases are most likely to reflect changes in protein nutritional status and body fat because the underlying illness is usually less severe. Even the most sensitive research methods for assessing changes in lean body mass, however, do not offer major improvements in diagnosis in the more seriously ill. Techniques that measure total body water such as isotope dilution and underwater weighing, from which lean tissue is extrapolated, fail to account for the distortion in hydration of lean tissue with illness. Surrogate measures of total body protein to estimate lean tissues such as total body potassium measurement do not adjust for differing potassium/nitrogen ratios with disease. A newer method, multifrequency body impedance, does show promise as a simple, accurate, non-invasive method that may allow distinction between intracellular and extracellular water, with the former used to estimate lean tissue.

In an unstressed patient with marasmus, appropriate protein and calorie intake should cause a positive nitrogen balance of 2 to 6 day (60 to 180 g lean tissue) and slow weight gain, depending

Table 225-3 ■ 5TH, 10TH, AND 50TH PERCENTILE FOR TRICEPS SKINFOLD (TSF) AND MID UPPER ARM MUSCLE CIRCUMFERENCE (MUAMC) OF AMERICAN MEN AND WOMEN FROM THE NHANES I SURVEY

Age Group	MUAMC (cm)			TSF (mm)		
	Percentile			Percentile		
	5th	10th	50th	5th	10th	50th
Male						
18–24	23.8	24.8	27.9	4.5	6.0	11.0
18–24	23.5	24.4	27.2	4.0	5.0	9.5
25–34	24.2	25.3	28.0	4.5	5.5	12.0
35–44	25.0	25.6	28.7	5.0	6.0	12.0
45–54	26.0	26.9	28.1	5.0	6.0	11.0
55–64	22.8	26.4	27.9	5.0	6.0	11.0
65–74	22.5	23.7	26.9	4.5	5.5	11.0
Female						
18–24	13.4	19.0	21.8	11.0	13.0	22.0
18–24	17.7	18.5	20.6	9.4	11.0	18.0
25–34	18.3	18.9	21.4	10.5	12.0	21.0
35–44	18.5	19.2	22.0	12.0	14.0	23.0
45–54	18.8	19.5	22.2	13.0	15.0	25.0
55–64	18.6	19.5	22.6	11.0	14.0	25.0
65–74	18.6	19.5	22.5	11.5	14.0	23.0

NHANES = National Health and Nutritional Examination Survey I.
From Bishop CW, Bowen PE, Ritchey SJ: Norms for nutritional assessment of American adults by upper arm anthropometry. Am J Clin Nutr 34:2530, 1981.

the positive energy balance. For instance, a 300-kcal excess of intake over expenditure would provide approximately 120 g of lean tissue (100 kcal equivalent) plus 200 kcal (22 g) as fat for a total of around 140 g, or about ⅓ lb of weight per day. Weight gains in excess of this figure probably reflect sodium and water retention from the insulin stimulated by dietary carbohydrate. Such overhydration can be improved by reducing salt and limiting fluid intake. In patients with hypoalbuminemic malnutrition who are no longer stressed, a similar nutritional regimen will lead to a comparable gain of tissue, but weight change may vary as edema becomes mobilized, with normalization in serum albumin in 2 to 4 weeks and transferrin pre-albumin and transferrin more quickly. In stressed patients with hypoalbuminemic malnutrition, appropriate nutritional support will often not restore lean tissue but will improve other important functions such as wound healing and immune competence. Both the systemic inflammatory response and the limited activity level reduce the efficiency of skeletal muscle repletion, which represents 30% of body weight and 75% of actively metabolizing lean tissue. Functional testing of muscle strength and endurance such as hand dynamometry may prove useful as a means of assessment in the future. Similarly, any reduction in other physiologic functions or impairment in performing the usual activities of daily living will accentuate the protein-energy malnutrition.

Although caloric expenditure can now be reliably and easily measured with portable indirect calorimeters, estimated energy expenditure is sufficient in most clinical situations. The three components of total energy expenditure are basal energy expenditure (about 55 to 65% of total energy expenditure), thermal effect of feeding (about 10% of total energy expenditure), and activity energy expenditure (the remainder). An energy intake of 30 to 35 kcal/kg of body weight will maintain most sedentary ambulatory patients, with adjustments upward or downward in 200- to 300-kcal increments as prompted by biweekly changes in weight. Although young, severely burned, or traumatized patients may require 35 to 40 kcal/kg in the acute phase to meet total energy expenditure, most postoperative patients who require invasive nutritional support for mechanical or infectious complications need no more than 30 kcal/kg because of their older age and reduced activity and energy expenditure. Overfeeding should be avoided in such patients.

Daley BJ, Bistrian BR: Nutritional assessment. *In* Zaloga G (ed): Nutrition in Critical Care. St Louis, CV Mosby, 1993, pp 9–33. *Discusses etiologic factors in the development of protein-caloric malnutrition and nutritional assessment methods.*

Hill G: Body composition research: Implications for the practice of clinical nutrition. JPEN J Parenter Enteral Nutr 16:197, 1992. *Superb presentation of clinical nutritional assessment in critically ill patients.*

Stack JA, Babineau TJ, Bistrian BR: Assessment of nutritional status in clinical practice. Gastroenterologist 4(Suppl. 1):8, 1996. *Discusses in detail the use of nutritional assessment tools.*

226 PROTEIN-ENERGY MALNUTRITION

Samuel Klein

Normal nutritional status represents a healthy relationship between nutrient intake and nutrient requirements. An imbalance between intake and requirements can over time lead to malnutrition manifested by alterations in intermediary metabolism, organ function, and body composition. The term *protein-energy malnutrition* has been used to describe macronutrient deficiency syndromes, which include kwashiorkor, marasmus, and nutritional dwarfism in children and wasting associated with illness or injury in children and adults.

Primary protein-energy malnutrition is caused by lack of access adequate nutrient intake and usually affects children and elderly persons. The functional and structural abnormalities associated with primary protein-energy malnutrition are often reversible with nutri-

tional therapy. However, prolonged primary protein-energy malnutrition can cause irreversible changes in organ function and growth.

Secondary protein-energy malnutrition is caused by illnesses that alter appetite, digestion, absorption, or nutrient metabolism and can be divided into three general, but often overlapping categories: (1) diseases that affect gastrointestinal tract function, (2) wasting disorders, and (3) critical illness. Gastrointestinal disease can cause protein-energy malnutrition by pre-mucosal (maldigestion), mucosal (malabsorption), or post-mucosal (lymphatic obstruction) defects (Table 226–1). The nutritional status of patients with protein-energy malnutrition caused by gastrointestinal tract dysfunction can often be restored to normal if adequate nutritional support can be provided by dietary manipulations, enteral tube feeding, or parenteral nutrition. Wasting disorders such as cancer, acquired immune deficiency syndrome, and rheumatologic diseases are characterized by involuntary loss of body weight and muscle mass in the setting of a chronic illness. These patients often experience wasting because of (1) inadequate nutrient intake related to anorexia and possibly gastrointestinal tract dysfunction and (2) metabolic abnormalities caused by alterations in regulatory hormones and cytokines. The alterations in metabolism are responsible for the greater loss of muscle tissue observed in these patients than in those with pure starvation or semistarvation. Restoration of muscle mass is unlikely with nutrition support unless the underlying inflammatory disease is corrected. Weight gain that occurs after nutrition support is initiated is usually caused by increases in fat mass and body water without significant increases in lean tissue. Patients with critical illness exhibit marked metabolic alterations manifested by increases in energy expenditure, endogenous glucose production, lipolytic rates, and protein breakdown. Therefore, protein and energy requirements are increased in critically ill patients. However, providing aggressive nutrition support may ameliorate but does not prevent net lean tissue losses without correction of the underlying illness or injury.

PROTEIN-ENERGY MALNUTRITION IN CHILDREN

Undernutrition in children differs from that in adults because it affects growth and development. Much of our understanding of undernutrition in children comes from observations and studies in underdeveloped nations, where poverty, inadequate food supply, and unsanitary conditions lead to a high prevalence of protein-energy malnutrition. The Waterlow classification of malnutrition takes into account the fact that children grow and undernutrition affects their growth. Therefore, nutritional status can be assessed by comparing a child's weight for height (wasting) and height for age (stunting) with normal standards (Table 226–2). The characteristics of the three major clinical syndromes of protein-energy malnutrition in children are outlined in Table 226–3. Although these three syndromes are classified separately, they may coexist in the same patient.

MARASMUS. Weight loss and marked depletion of subcutaneous fat and muscle mass are the characteristic features in children with marasmus. Loss of fat and muscle make ribs, joints, and facial bones prominent. The skin is thin and loose and lies in folds.

KWASHIORKOR. The word "kwashiorkor" comes from the Ga language of West Africa and can be translated as "disease of the displaced child" because it was commonly seen after weaning. The presence of peripheral edema distinguishes children with kwashiorkor from those with marasmus and nutritional dwarfism (Fig. 226–1). Children with kwashiorkor also have typical skin and hair changes (see the sections on hair and skin changes below). The abdomen is protuberant because of weakened abdominal muscles, intestinal distention, and hepatomegaly, but ascites is never present. In fact, the presence of ascites should prompt the clinician to search for liver disease or peritonitis. Children with kwashiorkor are typically lethargic and apathetic when left alone but become quite irritable when picked up or held. Kwashiorkor is not caused by a relative deficiency in protein intake as has previously been believed; in fact, protein and energy intake is similar in children with kwashiorkor and those with marasmus. Kwashiorkor is related to the physiologic stress of an infection that induces a deleterious metabolic cascade in an already malnourished child. Therefore kwashiorkor is an acute illness when compared with chronic undernutrition, although some of the features of marasmus and kwashior-

Table 226-1 ■ CLASSIFICATION OF MALDIGESTIVE AND MALABSORPTIVE DISORDERS

PRIMARY ABNORMALITY	PATHOPHYSIOLOGY	REPRESENTATIVE DISORDERS
Pre-mucosal defect	Pancreatic insufficiency	Chronic pancreatitis
		Cystic fibrosis
	Bacterial overgrowth	Pancreatic duct obstruction
		Motility diseases
		Blind loop syndromes
		Small intestine diverticula
Mucosal defect	Rapid gastric emptying and intestinal transit	Post–gastric surgery syndrome
	Inadequate bowel syndrome	Intestinal resection
		Gluten-sensitive enteropathy
		Immunoproliferative small bowel disease
		Radiation enteritis
		Intestinal ischemia
		AIDS enteropathy
Post-mucosal defect	Lymphatic obstruction	Congenital intestinal lymphangiectasia
		Milroy's disease
		Secondary intestinal lymphangiectasia
		Retroperitoneal carcinoma
		Lymphoma
		Retroperitoneal fibrosis
		Chronic pancreatitis
		Tuberculosis
		Sarcoidosis
		Crohn's disease
		Whipple's disease
		Constrictive pericarditis
		Chronic congestive heart failure

kor overlap. Kwashiorkor is characterized by leaky cell membranes that permit the movement of potassium and other intracellular ions to the extracellular space. The increased osmotic load in the interstitium causes water movement and edema. These changes occur despite increased "sodium pump" (Na⁺, K⁺-adenosinetriphosphatase [Na⁺, K⁺-ATPase]) activity, which also contrasts with a slowing down of the sodium pump in pure undernutrition.

NUTRITIONAL DWARFISM. Children with failure to thrive may have normal weight for height but short stature and delayed sexual development. Providing appropriate feeding can stimulate catch-up growth and sexual maturation.

PROTEIN-ENERGY MALNUTRITION IN ADULTS

The diagnosis of protein-energy malnutrition is different in adults than children because adults are no longer growing in height. Therefore, undernutrition in adults causes wasting rather than stunting and can be assessed by determining body mass index, defined as the patient's weight (in kilograms) divided by height (in meters squared) (Table 226–4). In addition, although kwashiorkor and marasmus can occur in adults, most studies of adult protein-energy malnutrition have evaluated hospitalized patients who had secondary protein-energy malnutrition and coexisting illness or injury. The current methods that are used clinically to evaluate protein-energy malnutrition in hospitalized adult patients shifts nutritional assessment from a diagnostic to a prognostic instrument in an attempt to identify patients who can benefit from nutritional therapy. Therefore, common nutritional assessment parameters are affected by non-nutritional factors, which makes it difficult to separate the influence of the disease itself from the contribution of inadequate nutrient intake. At present, no "gold standard" exists for determining protein-energy malnutrition in ill patients. The most commonly used methods include a careful history, physical examination, and selected laboratory tests (see Chapter 225).

METABOLIC RESPONSE TO STARVATION

The adaptive response to starvation involves specific metabolic alterations that enhance the chance for survival by increasing the use of body fat as a fuel, sparing the use of glucose, minimizing body nitrogen losses, and decreasing energy expenditure. A marked shift in fuel use occurs during the first day of starvation. By 24 hours of fasting, the use of glucose as a fuel has decreased; only 15% of liver glycogen stores remain, and the rates of hepatic glucose production and whole-body glucose oxidation have decreased. Conversely, endogenous fat stores become the body's major fuel, and the rates of adipose tissue lipolysis, hepatic ketone body production, and fat oxidation are increased. After 3 days of fasting, the rate of glucose production is reduced by half and the rate of lipolysis is more than double the values found at 12 hours of fasting. The increase in fatty acid delivery to the liver, in conjunction with an increase in the ratio of plasma glucagon to insulin, enhances hepatic ketone body production. By 7 days of fasting, plasma ketone body concentrations have increased 75-fold and ketone bodies provide 70% of the brain's energy needs. In contrast to fatty acids, ketone bodies can cross the blood-brain barrier and provide a water-soluble fuel derived from water-insoluble adipose tissue triglycerides. The use of ketone bodies by the brain greatly diminishes glucose requirements and thus spares the need for muscle protein degradation to provide glucose precursors. Furthermore, thyroid hormone inactivation and plasma ketones inhibit muscle protein breakdown and prevent rapid protein losses. If post-absorptive protein breakdown rates were to continue throughout starvation, a potentially lethal amount of muscle protein would

Table 226-2 ■ WATERLOW CLASSIFICATION OF PROTEIN-ENERGY MALNUTRITION IN CHILDREN

FEATURE	NORMAL	MILD	MODERATE	SEVERE
Weight for height (wasting)				
Percentage of median NCHS standard	90–110	80–89	70–79	<70
Standard deviation from the NCHS median	+Z to −Z	−1.1 Z to −2 Z	−2.1 Z to −3 Z	<−3 Z
Height for age (stunting)				
Percentage of median NCHS standard	95–105	90–94	85–89	<85
Standard deviation from the NCHS median	+Z to −Z	−1.1 Z to −2 Z	−2.1 Z to −3 Z	<−3 Z

NCHS = National Center for Health Statistics.

Table 227–3 ■ FEATURES OF PROTEIN-ENERGY MALNUTRITION SYNDROMES IN CHILDREN

FEATURE	KWASHIORKOR	MARASMUS	NUTRITIONAL DWARFISM
Weight for age (% of expected)	60–80	<60	<60
Weight for height	Normal or decreased	Markedly decreased	Normal
Edema	Present	Absent	Absent
Mood	Irritable when picked up Apathetic when alone	Alert	Alert
Appetite	Poor	Good	Good

be catabolized in less than 3 weeks. As fasting continues, the kidney becomes an important site for glucose production; glutamine, released from muscle, is converted to glucose in the kidney and accounts for almost half of the total glucose production. The resting metabolic rate decreases by approximately 15% at 7 days.

Adaptation is maximal during more prolonged starvation (>14 days of fasting). At this time, adipose tissue provides more than 90% of the daily energy requirements. Total glucose production has decreased to ~75 g/day and provides fuel for glycolytic tissues (40 g/day) and the brain (35 g/day). Muscle protein breakdown has decreased to less than 30 g/day, which causes a marked decrease in urea nitrogen production and excretion. The diminished urea load to the kidneys decreases urine volume to 200 mL/day, thereby minimizing fluid requirements. Resting energy expenditure is decreased by approximately 25%.

UNDERNUTRITION-INDUCED ALTERATIONS IN TISSUE MASS AND FUNCTION

BODY COMPOSITION. All body tissue masses are affected by undernutrition, but fat mass and muscle mass are the most affected. In lean adults, these two tissues account for almost two thirds of body weight. Therefore, the loss of weight that occurs in malnourished patients is principally due to loss of muscle and fat mass. Body adipose tissue can be almost completely depleted and up to half of muscle mass can be consumed before death from starvation occurs.

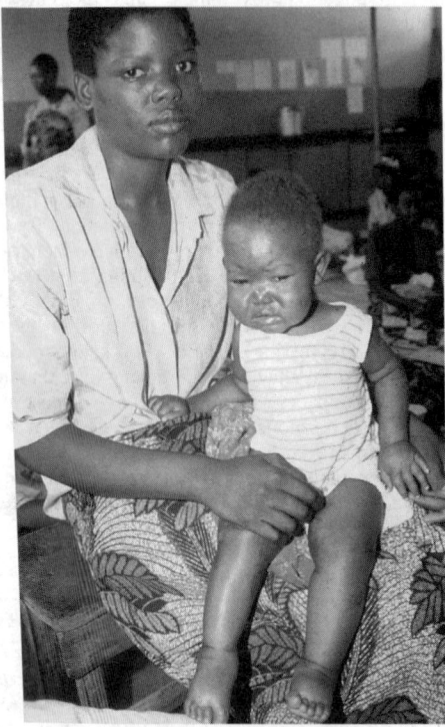

URE 226–1 ■ Mother with a child suffering from kwashiorkor in Blan-
, Malawi. The child manifests some of the classic features of kwashior-
including leg edema, reddish blond hair discoloration, and irritability.
ograph courtesy of Mark Manary, M.D.)

BODY WATER. Many patients who are malnourished have intravascular volume depletion because of inadequate water and sodium intake. However, the percentage of body weight that is composed of water may be increased. Decreased plasma proteins, "leaky" capillaries, "leaky" cells, and increased interstitial ion content may cause intravascular volume depletion and expansion of the interstitial space. Therefore, malnourished patients may have diminished intravascular volume in the face of whole-body fluid overload.

SKIN. The skin is a large organ that regenerates rapidly; a basal cell of the dermis reaches the cornified layer and dies in 10 to 14 days. Frequently, undernutrition causes the skin to be dry, thin, and wrinkled with atrophy of the basal layers of the epidermis and hyperkeratosis. Severe malnutrition may cause considerable depletion of skin protein and collagen. Patients with kwashiorkor experience sequential skin changes in different locations. Hyperpigmentation occurs first, followed by cracking and stripping of superficial layers, thereby leaving behind hypopigmented, thin, and atrophic epidermis that is friable and easily macerated.

HAIR. Scalp hair becomes thin and sparse and is easily pulled out. In contrast, the eyelashes become long and luxuriant and children may have excessive lanugo hair. Children with kwashiorkor experience hypopigmentation with reddish brown, gray, or blond discoloration. Adults may lose axillary and pubic hair.

GASTROINTESTINAL TRACT. Starvation and malnutrition cause structural and functional deterioration of the intestinal tract, pancreas, and liver. The total mass and protein content of the intestinal mucosa and pancreas are markedly reduced. Mucosal epithelial cell proliferation rates decrease and intestinal mucosa becomes atrophic with flattened villi. Synthesis of mucosal and pancreatic digestive enzyme is reduced. Intestinal transport and absorption of free amino acids are impaired, whereas hydrolysis and absorption of peptides are maintained. Gastric and biliary secretions are diminished. The abdomen may become protuberant because of hypomotility and gas distention. Hepatomegaly is common in severe malnutrition because of excessive fat accumulation caused by decreased very-low-density lipoprotein synthesis and triglyceride export. Decreased synthesis of most hepatic proteins is noted.

HEART. Chronic undernutrition affects cardiac mass and function. Cardiac muscle mass decreases and is accompanied by fragmentation of myofibrils. Bradycardia (the heart rate can decrease to less than 40 beats per minute) and decreased stroke volume can cause a marked decrease in cardiac output and low blood pressure. For example, a hypocaloric diet in normal volunteers that caused a 24% decrease in body weight was associated with a 38% decrease in the cardiac index.

LUNGS. Respiratory muscle function is altered by malnutrition, as evidenced by a decrease in vital capacity, tidal volume, and minute ventilation.

KIDNEYS. Renal mass and function are relatively well preserved during undernutrition, provided that adequate water is consumed to

Table 226–4 ■ CLASSIFICATION OF PROTEIN-ENERGY MALNUTRITION IN ADULTS

BODY MASS INDEX (kg/m²)	NUTRITIONAL STATUS
≥18.5	Normal
17.0–18.4	Mildly malnourished
16.0–16.9	Moderately malnourished
<16.0	Severely malnourished

prevent a severe decrease in renal perfusion and acute renal failure. However, when malnutrition is severe, decreases are seen in kidney weight, glomerular filtration rate, and the ability to excrete acid, excrete sodium, and concentrate urine. Mild proteinuria may also occur.

BONE MARROW. Severe undernutrition suppresses bone marrow red blood cell and white blood cell production and leads to anemia, leukopenia, and lymphocytopenia.

MUSCLE. Muscle function is impaired by malnutrition because of both a loss of muscle mass and impaired metabolism. Decreased "sodium pump" activity causes an increase in intracellular sodium and a decrease in intracellular potassium, which affects myocyte electrical potential and thereby contributes to fatigue.

BRAIN. The weight and protein content of the brain remain relatively stable even during long-term starvation. Therefore, the integrity of the brain is preserved at the expense of other organs and tissues.

IMMUNE SYSTEM. Severe undernutrition causes atrophy of all lymphoid tissues, including the thymus, tonsils, and lymph nodes. Cell-mediated immunity is diminished more than antibody production. Alterations in cell-mediated immunity cause impaired delayed cutaneous hypersensitivity and anergy. The ability to kill bacteria is diminished because of decreased complement and impaired neutrophil function. Gastrointestinal IgA secretion is also decreased. Malnourished patients are at increased risk for opportunistic infections and should be considered immunocompromised.

ENDOCRINE SYSTEM. Decreased plasma insulin concentrations and glucose intolerance are common in severe malnutrition. Growth hormone is usually increased, with the increase being much greater in the kwashiorkor type than the marasmic type of protein-energy malnutrition. Serum thyroxine levels are low and the conversion of thyroxine to triiodothyronine is decreased with increased conversion to reverse triiodothyronine. The plasma cortisol concentration is usually greater than normal.

ENERGY METABOLISM. Starvation and undernutrition decrease basal energy expenditure because of diminished organ size and function, increased conversion of active thyroid hormone to its inactive form, decreased sodium pump activity, decreased protein turnover, decreased body core temperature, absence of shivering and non-shivering thermogenesis, and suppression of sympathetic nervous system activity. Energy is also conserved by the onset of fatigue, which causes a decrease in physical activity.

DEATH FROM STARVATION

At the terminal phase of starvation, body fat mass, skeletal muscle mass, and the size of most organs are markedly decreased. During this final phase of starvation, body fat stores are nearly depleted, energy derived from body fat decreases, and muscle protein catabolism is accelerated. The mechanism(s) responsible for death from starvation in humans is not well understood, but many patients ultimately succumb to infection. It has been suggested that humans are subject to lethal levels of body weight loss (loss of 40% of body weight), protein depletion (loss of 30 to 50% of body protein), fat depletion (loss of 70 to 95% of body fat stores), or body size (body mass index of 13 kg/m^2 for men and 11 kg/m^2 for women). The duration of survival depends on the amount of available endogenous fuel and the amount of lean tissue. Data from Irish Republican Army hunger strikers demonstrate that death occurs in lean men after approximately 2 months of starvation when more than 35% (~25 kg) of body weight is lost. Obese persons can survive much longer periods of starvation because of their increased fat stores and lean tissue mass. The longest reported fast is that of a severely obese (207 kg) man, who safely lost 61% (126 kg) of his initial weight after completing a 382-day fast in which he ingested only acaloric fluids, vitamins, and minerals.

CLINICAL MANAGEMENT OF SEVERELY MALNOURISHED PATIENTS

INITIAL EVALUATION. A careful clinical examination is needed to identify life-threatening complications of protein-energy malnutrition that require immediate treatment. The presence of fluid, plasma glucose, electrolyte, and acid-base abnormalities should be determined. A search for infections (e.g., obtaining a white blood cell count, urinalysis and urine culture, blood cultures, and chest

radiograph) should be considered even in the absence of physical findings because many patients are not able to mount a normal inflammatory response. The evaluation must also include a careful analysis of the possible route for nutrition support and whether the gastrointestinal tract can be used or parenteral nutrition will be needed for refeeding.

INITIAL SUPPORTIVE CARE. Judicious resuscitation with fluids and electrolytes may be necessary before beginning feeding, along with frequent evaluation to prevent congestive heart failure from excessive fluid. Vitamin supplementation should be given routinely. Severely malnourished patients are poikilothermic, so warm ambient temperature and warming blankets may be necessary to slowly raise the core temperature. However, if warming blankets are being used, patients must be carefully monitored to avoid hyperthermia.

REFEEDING. The goal of feeding severely malnourished patients can be divided into three phases: (1) prevention of further deterioration and correction of life-threatening abnormalities, (2) restoration of normal organ function and metabolism, and finally (3) repletion of deficient nutrient stores. Oral or enteral tube feedings are preferred over parenteral feeding because of fewer serious complications and enhanced gastrointestinal tract recovery. Feedings should be given in small amounts at frequent intervals to prevent overwhelming of the body's limited capacity for nutrient processing and to prevent hypoglycemia, which can occur during brief non-feeding intervals. Therefore, the patient should receive small amounts of oral feeds frequently (every 1 to 4 hours), enteral tube feeding by continuous drip, or parenteral nutrition by continuous infusion. Sodium intake should be limited during early refeeding, but liberal amounts of phosphorus, potassium, and magnesium should be given to patients who have normal renal function. Daily monitoring of body weight, fluid intake, urine output, and plasma glucose and electrolyte values is critical during the first few days of refeeding so that nutritional therapy can be appropriately adjusted when necessary. Appetite has usually improved during the second phase. Protein and energy intake should be marginally above the estimated requirements to provide for adequate maintenance and repair. Additional protein and energy should be provided during phase 3 for repletion and synthesis of new tissue.

REFEEDING COMPLICATIONS. Refeeding can be harmful and even cause death because of impaired organ function and depleted nutrient stores from previous starvation. The adverse consequences caused by initiating feeding too aggressively are known as the "refeeding syndrome" and usually occur within the first 5 days. Refeeding syndrome complications include fluid overload, electrolyte imbalances, glucose intolerance, cardiac arrhythmias, and diarrhea.

FLUID OVERLOAD. Severely malnourished patients are at increased risk for fluid retention and congestive heart failure after nutritional therapy because of compromised cardiac and renal function. The ability to excrete sodium is impaired, so even normal amounts of dietary sodium intake can be excessive. In addition, carbohydrates increase the concentration of circulating insulin, which stimulates sodium and water reabsorption by the renal tubule. The presence of heart failure requires discontinuation of feeding until the cardiac status is stabilized.

MINERAL DEPLETION. Carbohydrate refeeding stimulates insulin release and intracellular uptake of phosphate, which is used for protein synthesis and glucose metabolism. Therefore, plasma phosphorus concentrations can sometimes fall precipitously to below 1 mg/dL after initiating nutritional therapy if adequate phosphate is not given. Severe hypophosphatemia, which is associated with muscle weakness, paresthesias, seizures, coma, cardiopulmonary decompensation, and death, has occurred in severely malnourished patients after receiving enteral or parenteral nutritional therapy.

Decreased body cell mass and decreased Na$^+$, K$^+$-ATPase activity or leaky cell membranes in a malnourished patient lead to depletion of the major intracellular cations potassium and magnesium. Nonetheless, serum potassium and magnesium concentrations may remain normal or nearly normal during starvation because of their release from tissue and bone stores. During refeeding, increases in protein synthesis, body cell mass, and glycogen stores require generous intake of potassium and magnesium. In addition, hyperinsulinemia during refeeding increases cellular uptake of p tassium and can cause a rapid decline in extracellular concentrations.

GLUCOSE INTOLERANCE. Malnourished patients are predisposed to hypoglycemia because of decreased hepatic glucose production. However, starvation and malnutrition impair insulin's ability to suppress endogenous glucose production and stimulate glucose uptake and oxidation. Therefore, providing enteral or parenteral carbohydrate can cause hyperglycemia, glucosuria, dehydration, and hyperosmolar coma. Furthermore, because of the importance of thiamine in glucose metabolism, carbohydrate refeeding in patients who are thiamine deficient can precipitate Wernicke's encephalopathy.

CARDIAC ARRHYTHMIAS. Sudden death from ventricular arrhythmias can occur during the first week of refeeding in severely malnourished patients and has been reported in conjunction with severe hypophosphatemia. A prolonged QT interval may contribute to the rhythm disturbances.

GASTROINTESTINAL DYSFUNCTION. Alterations in gastrointestinal tract function limit the ability of the gastrointestinal tract to digest and absorb food. Mild diarrhea after initiating oral/enteral feeding usually resolves and is not clinically important if fluid and electrolyte homeostasis can be maintained. However, in some severely malnourished patients, oral feeding is associated with severe diarrhea and death. Therefore, aggressive fluid and electrolyte replacement and a search for enteric pathogens should be considered in patients with prolonged or severe diarrhea.

Golden MHN: Severe malnutrition. *In* Weatherall DJ, Ledington JGG, Warrell DA (eds): Oxford Textbook of Medicine, 3rd ed. New York, Oxford University Press, 1996, pp 1278–1296. *Excellent review of the pathophysiology, clinical findings, and management of malnutrition in children.*

Klein S, Jeejeebhoy KN: The malnourished patient: Nutritional assessment and management. *In* Feldman M, Scharschmidt BF, Sleisenger M (eds): Gastrointestinal Disease, 6th ed. Philadelphia, WB Saunders, 1997, pp 235–253. *Reviews nutritional assessment and management of severely malnourished adult patients and basic principles of nutritional metabolism.*

Waterlow JC: Protein-Energy Malnutrition. London, Edward Arnold, 1992. *Comprehensive book that carefully discusses all major aspects of protein-energy malnutrition in children in underdeveloped countries.*

227 THE EATING DISORDERS
Delia Smith

DEFINITION

The eating disorders are a group of psychiatric disorders characterized by aberrant eating patterns and disturbed attitudes about the importance of body weight and shape, specifically, the evaluation of self-worth based on weight. The most well known and well characterized of the eating disorders are anorexia nervosa and bulimia nervosa. The hallmark of anorexia nervosa is the pursuit of thinness in the presence of severe emaciation. The defining features of bulimia nervosa are a cycle of binge eating followed by inappropriate compensatory behavior to avoid weight gain (e.g., self-induced vomiting, misuse of laxatives or diuretics, fasting, excessive exercise) and undue concern about body weight.

ETIOLOGY

ANOREXIA NERVOSA. Although anorexia nervosa has long been recognized and well described, the etiology of the disorder is not well understood. Societal influences promoting an unrealistically thin body size and a cultural environment that associates slimness with happiness and success have been implicated in the development of anorexia nervosa.

Genetic vulnerabilities also appear to play a role in the development of anorexia nervosa. Concordance rates for anorexia nervosa higher in monozygotic than dizygotic twins. Furthermore, the prevalence of anorexia nervosa, as well as mood disorders, is higher in first-degree relatives of affected individuals than in the general population, thus suggesting genetic aggregation. Although the indications are strong for genetic influences on the development of anorexia nervosa, the relative contributions of genetics and environmental influences remain unclear.

Neuroendocrine abnormalities have been studied extensively in anorexia nervosa, and questions remain about which aspects of the observed hypothalamic dysfunction are primary and which are secondary to the starvation state. Some patients experience amenorrhea before weight loss and some continue to have abnormal neuroendocrine function after weight restoration.

BULIMIA NERVOSA. As with anorexia nervosa, a sociocultural emphasis on pursuit of an unrealistically thin body weight and unobtainable body shape has been suggested as a causative factor in the etiology of bulimia nervosa. Over the previous decades, culturally desirable body shapes have become thinner and more unobtainable for the average woman, in parallel with increases in bulimia nervosa rates. Dieting to lose weight is nearly epidemic in some cultures, and peer pressure to maintain a low body weight is strong. Dieting has been shown to predispose young girls to bulimia nervosa, and a history of obesity, as well as significant fluctuations in weight, has been observed among women in whom the disorder develops. However, being discontented with body size or weight is not uncommon among women in general, and dieting is endemic in our society. Therefore, sociocultural factors alone cannot account for the development of bulimia nervosa in a specific individual.

The aggregation of bulimia nervosa in families suggests a genetic vulnerability. Twin studies indicate that approximately 50% of the variability in the development of bulimia nervosa can be attributed to genetic factors. Depression, anxiety disorders, and substance abuse (particularly alcoholism) have also been shown to be more common in the families of patients with bulimia nervosa than in the general population. Thus a vulnerability to psychiatric disorders in general and eating disorders in particular may be transmitted genetically. However, the influence of environmental and individual factors remains substantial.

EPIDEMIOLOGY

ANOREXIA NERVOSA. Anorexia nervosa is relatively rare, with lifetime prevalence rates of 0.5% among women and few cases noted in men. The age of onset is bimodal, with peaks around 14 and 18 years of age. The natural course of anorexia nervosa appears to have high mortality rates, with long-term studies reporting 10 to 20% mortality, although recent reports have noted higher survival rates. The disorder appears to be more common among women in higher socioeconomic groups and among whites; furthermore, anorexia nervosa is overrepresented in professions that emphasize low body weight, such as fashion models, ballet dancers, and gymnasts.

BULIMIA NERVOSA. Bulimia nervosa is more common than anorexia nervosa and in general has a more optimistic prognosis. Approximately 1 to 2% of women and 0.1% of men will meet the diagnostic criteria for bulimia nervosa sometime in their life. The average age at onset is around 20 years. Although patients with bulimia nervosa from higher socioeconomic groups seek treatment more often than lower income patients do, population-based studies indicate that rates of the disorder are similar. The disorder is more prevalent among whites, but an increasing number of patients in other groups have been described in recent years.

CLINICAL MANIFESTATIONS

ANOREXIA NERVOSA. Apart from the severe emaciation and amenorrhea central to the disorder, anorexia nervosa has no consistent pathologic or physiologic characteristics. The majority of medical complications seen are sequelae of the starvation state and usually remit with appropriate nutritional remediation. Signs commonly noted on physical examination include hypotension, dry skin or lanugo (downy fine hair), and bradycardia.

ENDOCRINE ABNORMALITIES. Perturbations in endocrine function are invariably present (see also Chapters 235, 237, and 250).

Amenorrhea and hypofunction of the hypothalamic-pituitary axis (reduced luteinizing and follicle-stimulating hormone) develop in females. Secondary amenorrhea is most common, although primary amenorrhea may occur. Amenorrhea may precede weight loss in some patients and may persist after weight restoration. Estrogen metabolism can also be disturbed (low plasma and urinary estrogen levels that rebound with weight gain) and may be associated with irreversible osteopenia and pathologic fractures. Male anorectics have diminished testosterone levels and loss of libido, as well as infertility. Pre-pubertal patients may have arrested sexual maturation and diminished overall physical growth. Abnormalities in thyroid function tests are common. Low triiodothyronine levels are found consistently, accompanied by normal or low thyroxine levels, and probably reflect adaptations to starvation. Thyroid abnormalities usually reverse with weight restoration, and exogenous thyroid replacement therapy is not indicated.

CARDIOVASCULAR ABNORMALITIES. Disturbed cardiovascular function is common and reflects adaptation to starvation. Orthostatic hypotension is frequently observed. Electrocardiograms often reveal bradycardia, ST segment depression, or T wave morphology changes. Arrhythmias (tachycardia, sinus arrest with ectopic atrial rhythm, nodal escape beats, or junctional rhythms) can develop, even in the absence of electrolyte disturbance. The use of emetics such as syrup of ipecac can cause myopathy, including cardiomyopathy. Sudden death from cardiac failure is a risk but uncommon.

FLUID AND ELECTROLYTE DISTURBANCE/RENAL COMPLICATIONS. Dehydration is a common complication, particularly with protracted purging (self-induced vomiting, laxative or diuretic abuse). Hypokalemic, hypochloremic alkalosis is the most frequently occurring electrolyte abnormality. Elevated blood urea nitrogen is often found, although serum creatinine is usually normal. Chronic hypokalemia can cause proteinuria and renal damage; therefore, renal function should be evaluated in all severely emaciated patients.

PSYCHIATRIC FEATURES. In addition to pathologic attitudes about eating and weight that are pathognomonic, patients with anorexia nervosa may display psychiatric features secondary to severe malnutrition, including irritability, mood lability, social withdrawal, anxiety, depression, concentration impairment, food preoccupation, obsessive-compulsive symptoms regarding foods, or bizarre food preferences. These features usually diminish after nutritional replenishment. However, a minority of patients can have co-morbid psychiatric disorders (particularly major depression and, in a small number of patients, obsessive-compulsive disorder) that are not secondary to starvation and warrant specific assessment and treatment.

GASTROINTESTINAL COMPLICATIONS. Patients may suffer from gastrointestinal motility problems. Abdominal pain, bloating, and postprandial distress are very common, as is constipation. These complaints can be troublesome for patients who need to eat more to gain weight. Acute gastric dilation and rupture are possible with overaggressive refeeding or large binge episodes.

BULIMIA NERVOSA. The majority of the medical complications associated with bulimia nervosa reflect the binge eating and purgative behavior (self-induced vomiting, laxative and diuretic abuse). No specific signs and symptoms are associated with bulimia nervosa. Patients frequently complain of constipation, bloating and abdominal pain, and lethargy and impaired concentration. Menstrual irregularities are common. Dehydration may be evident, particularly in patients who purge excessively or restrict fluid intake. Erosion of dental enamel and excessive caries are present in some patients. Physical examination seldom reveals the nature of the problem; therefore, a comprehensive history that includes assessment of psychological and behavioral aspects of the disorder is critical.

Serious medical complications can be associated with chronic vomiting or laxative or diuretic abuse. Electrolyte disturbances (metabolic alkalosis, hypochloremia, hypokalemia), elevated serum amylase, gastric and esophageal irritation, and large bowel abnormalities from laxative abuse are the more common physical complications.

DIAGNOSIS

ANOREXIA NERVOSA. The essential features of anorexia nervosa are an intense fear of weight gain or becoming fat in spite of

---

Table 227–1 ■ DSM-IV DIAGNOSTIC CRITERIA FOR ANOREXIA NERVOSA

A. Refusal to maintain body weight at or above a minimally normal weight for age and height (e.g., weight loss leading to maintenance of body weight less than 85% of that expected or failure to make expected weight gain during period of growth resulting in body weight less than 85% of that expected).
B. Intense fear of gaining weight or becoming fat even though underweight.
C. Disturbance in the way in which one's body weight or shape is experienced, undue influence of body weight or shape on self-evaluation, or denial of the seriousness of the current low body weight.
D. In post-menarchal females, amenorrhea, i.e., the absence of at least three consecutive menstrual cycles. (A woman is considered to have amenorrhea if her periods occur following only hormone, e.g., estrogen, administration.)

Specify type:

Restricting type: During the current episode of anorexia nervosa, the person has not regularly engaged in binge-eating or purging behavior (i.e., self-induced vomiting or the misuse of laxatives, diuretics, or enemas).

Binge-eating/purging type: During the current episode of anorexia nervosa, the person has regularly engaged in binge-eating or purging behavior (i.e., self-induced vomiting or the misuse of laxatives, diuretics, or enemas).

Used by permission from the American Psychiatric Association Diagnostic Manual of Mental Disorders (DSM-IV), 4th ed, Washington, DC, American Psychiatric Association, 1994.

---

significantly low body weight (Table 227–1). Two types of anorexia nervosa can be differentiated: restricting, in which weight loss occurs primarily through dieting, fasting, or excessive exercise, and binge-purge, in which the patient engages in binge eating and/or purging. About half of patients with anorexia nervosa are the restricting type and occasionally some individuals will alternate over time between the restricting and binge-purge types. The diagnostic challenge with anorexia nervosa is to distinguish it from other causes of malnutrition or starvation. The attitudinal and behavioral features of individuals with anorexia nervosa are therefore vital in making the differential diagnosis. Evaluation of fears of fatness or pursuit of thinness despite significant underweight and undue influence of body weight on self-evaluation is crucial; however, accurate assessment can be challenging because patients often deny the extent of their problems. Thus it is important to probe about weight preoccupations, the potential response to weight regain, and underlying schemas of self-evaluation, in addition to the medical complications associated with low body weight.

BULIMIA NERVOSA. The defining characteristics of bulimia nervosa are the recurrent episodes of binge eating and inappropriate compensatory behavior to avoid weight gain (Table 227–2). An excessive concern about weight and self-evaluation based on weight are also typical of the disorder. Two types of bulimia nervosa have been identified and are distinguished by the methods used to compensate for excessive calorie intake during binge episodes. Those with the purging type engage in self-induced vomiting or laxative or diuretic abuse, whereas individuals with the nonpurging type use other methods (e.g., severe caloric restriction, excessive exercise). The purging type is the more common type, and self-induced vomiting is the most common method of purging.

During binge episodes, large amounts of food are consumed, usually in secret. Loss of control over eating (i.e., unable to stop once started eating) is a defining feature of the binge episode. This loss of control may take the form of frenzied, rapid eating of available food or planned binges for which the patient acquires specific foods in advance for periods when secretive eating can occur. Some patients report dissociative experiences during the binge episode when they "tune out" and are unaware of what or how much they are eating.

Patients with bulimia nervosa are typically of average weight, although both overweight and underweight bulimia nervosa patients exist. Bulimia nervosa is frequently accompanied by depressive symptoms, and patients often meet the diagnostic criteria for major depressive disorder. Depressive symptoms typically remit with su

Table 227–2 ■ DSM-IV DIAGNOSTIC CRITERIA FOR BULIMIA NERVOSA

A. Recurrent episodes of binge eating. An episode of binge eating is characterized by both of the following:
  1. Eating, in a discrete period (e.g., within any 2-hr period), an amount of food that is definitely larger than most people would eat during a similar period and under similar circumstances.
  2. A sense of lack of control over eating during the episodes (e.g., a feeling that one cannot stop eating or control what or how much one is eating).
B. Recurrent inappropriate compensatory behavior to prevent weight gain such as self-induced vomiting; misuse of laxatives, diuretics, enemas, or other medication; fasting; or excessive exercise.
C. The binge-eating and inappropriate compensatory behaviors both occur, on average, at least twice a week for 3 months.
D. Self-evaluation is unduly influenced by body shape and weight.
E. The disturbance does not occur exclusively during episodes of anorexia nervosa.
Specify type:
  Purging type: During the current episode of bulimia nervosa, the person has regularly engaged in self-induced vomiting or the misuse of laxatives, diuretics, or enemas.
  Non-purging type: During the current episode of bulimia nervosa, the person has used other inappropriate compensatory behaviors, such as fasting or excessive exercise, but has not regularly engaged in self-induced vomiting or the misuse of laxatives, diuretics, or enemas.

Used by permission from the American Psychiatric Association Diagnostic Manual of Mental Disorders (DSM-IV), 4th ed. Washington, DC, American Psychiatric Association, 1994.

cessful treatment of the bulimia nervosa and can be viewed as secondary. However, in a minority of cases, concomitant mood disorders precede the bulimia nervosa or fail to improve with adequate treatment and require specific attention. Concurrent substance abuse may occur and often requires assessment and treatment before addressing the bulimia nervosa.

TREATMENT

The long-term treatment goal for both disorders is to ameliorate the psychological and behavioral patterns that promote and maintain aberrant eating habits and the attitudinal disturbances. A second goal is to address the medical complications that accompany these behavioral and psychological patterns, particularly for anorexia nervosa, where weight restoration is a primary emphasis in the initial treatment.

ANOREXIA NERVOSA. Anorexia nervosa requires a comprehensive, multidisciplinary approach to treatment that integrates medical management, individual psychotherapy, and family therapy. Currently, the best results have been shown with weight restoration accompanied by family therapy for patients with adolescent-onset anorexia nervosa and individual therapy for patients with onset after 18 years of age. Inpatient treatment is often required.

NUTRITIONAL REHABILITATION. Weight restoration is a primary initial goal of treatment of a seriously underweight patient. Weight regain programs incorporating behavioral modification strategies appear to be the most effective. Clear goals are outlined (e.g., daily calorie intake, weekly weight gain, abstinence from purging), and patients are rewarded for achieving them by praise and privileges (e.g., time out of bed, time off the unit, visitors, opportunity to exercise). The goal for weight restoration is usually no more that 1 to 2 kg/week, with the ultimate target weight determined individually for each patient. An individually specific healthy weight (i.e., one at which normal reproductive function resumes and bone demineralization ceases) is selected. Weight at discharge in relation to goal weight must also be individually determined, depending on the likelihood of sustained weight regain.

Weight restoration can be accomplished with nutritional hyperalimentation. Daily calorie intake will depend on the patient's degree of underweight, and methods of refeeding will depend on the condition and approbation of the patient. Oral supplementation can be helpful for patients with moderate malnutrition. Nasogastric tube feeding should not be used routinely; however, this route may be

more palatable for refeeding severely malnourished patients. Those who do not tolerate feeding tubes may require parenteral supplementation. However, this form of feeding should be used only in life-threatening situations and with recognition of the significant dangers associated with parenteral supplementation in this patient population (e.g., severe edema and possible cardiac failure). It is generally recommended that forced nutritional hyperalimentation or supplementation continue only until the patient is out of medical danger. At that time, even if not yet at a healthy body weight, the patient should resume total calorie intake from food. This approach facilitates re-establishment of normal eating patterns and allows hunger and satiety sensations to begin to normalize, both of which are important treatment goals.

PSYCHOTHERAPY. A first step for psychotherapy is to engage the patient as a motivated and willing partner in the process and establish a trusting therapeutic relationship. The long-term goals are to address the fear of fatness, which is central to the disorder, as well as ameliorate self-concept inadequacies, perfectionistic tendencies, disturbed social relationships, and separation or autonomy concerns. Family therapy is particularly effective with younger patients, whereas individual psychotherapy appears most helpful for older patients. Cognitive behavioral treatments have shown promise.

MEDICATION. Although a range of pharmacotherapies for anorexia nervosa have been examined, no pharmacologic agent has demonstrated effectiveness. However, patients with persistent depression may require antidepressant treatment, which should be undertaken with care because malnourished patients with anorexia nervosa may be particularly prone to side effects, especially hypotension and arrhythmia.

BULIMIA NERVOSA. Cognitive behavioral treatment is generally regarded as the treatment of choice for bulimia nervosa. The rationale underlying a cognitive behavioral approach is that dysfunctional beliefs about the importance of weight and shape are primary factors in the development and maintenance of the disorder. Treatment focuses on modifying these cognitions. Behavioral strategies are used to interrupt the cycle of dieting, binge eating, and purging and to gradually resume regular eating habits, as well as expand the range of foods that can be eaten without loss of control. Self-monitoring helps patients identify antecedents that trigger binge eating and purging and the consequences that reinforce the behavior. Cognitive strategies to identify and challenge dysfunctional beliefs are used, specifically, strategies to target rigid and perfectionistic attitudes about dieting and self-evaluation. Problem-solving skills and relapse prevention techniques are also provided. Cognitive behavioral treatment is usually offered on an outpatient basis over the course of 16 to 20 sessions. Inpatient treatment is indicated only when a patient's health or safety is of concern (e.g., suicide or medical risk). A longer course of treatment is required for more complicated cases (e.g., patients with concomitant personality disorder). Most patients improve following cognitive behavioral therapy, with reductions of approximately 80% in the frequency of both binge episodes and purging. Over half of treated patients are abstinent from both bingeing and purging after treatment and remain so at 1-year post-treatment. Preliminary studies indicate that interpersonal psychotherapy can also be effective in treating bulimia nervosa.

MEDICATIONS. Antidepressant medication has a role in the treatment of bulimia nervosa. When experienced cognitive-behavioral therapists are not available, tricyclic and monoamine oxidase inhibitor antidepressants have been shown to be effective in reducing binge eating and purging. Antidepressants are effective even among patients who do not have major depression, and doses similar to those used for mood disorders are recommended. However, relapse may occur when the use of these medications is discontinued.

Fairburn CG, Wilson GT (eds): Binge Eating: Nature, Assessment and Treatment. New York, Guilford Press, 1993. *Practical manual that includes the state-of-the-art clinical interview for diagnosis and a session-by-session outline for cognitive-behavioral treatment.*
Garner DM, Garfinkel PE (eds): Handbook of Treatment for Eating Disorders. New York, Guilford Press, 1997. *Comprehensive reviews of issues in the diagnosis and treatment of eating disorders that address a range of psychotherapeutic approaches, as well as pharmacologic management.*
Smith DE, Marcus MD, Eldredge KL: Binge eating syndromes: A review of assessment and treatment with an emphasis on clinical application. Behav Ther 25:635, 1994. *Review of the literature on the diagnosis, etiology, and treatment of binge-eating syndromes, with special attention to issues relevant to clinicians treating patients who binge-eat.*

228 OBESITY

F. Xavier Pi-Sunyer

Obesity is a frustrating condition for patient and physician alike. Its underlying cause is rarely clear, and its treatment is fraught with difficulty and failure. Management of obesity therefore requires much understanding and persistence.

About 97 million adult Americans (55% of those aged 20 to 75 years) are overweight or obese. The percentage of adult men who are overweight or obese (59.4%) is somewhat greater than that of women (50.7%).

DEFINITION

Visual inspection of a patient can give a subjective but fairly accurate estimate of the degree of obesity. More objective measures are height-weight tables, weight-related indices, and other anthropometric measurements.

The three most commonly used indices are (1) tables of average weights by height and age; (2) tables of desirable weights for height associated with lowest mortalities in insured populations; and (3) indices derived from height and weight, of which the body mass index is the most useful.

TABLES OF AVERAGE WEIGHTS. National Health and Nutrition Examination Surveys (NHANES) are periodically conducted on a representative United States population and then compiled in percentile tables as weights for height for gender. These cross-sectional data can be used for defining obesity, with a commonly made arbitrary decision that a weight above the 85th percentile for a young adult population is "overweight" for everyone. This comparison to a reference population makes no statement as to health risk involved at any weight level. A problem is finding an appropriate reference population, particularly for minorities.

IDEAL WEIGHT TABLES. The Metropolitan Life Insurance Company Tables of Heights and Weights indicate the weight at which longevity is greatest, based on those insured. The 1983 tables were derived from the pooled data of 25 insurance companies in the United States and Canada, including about 4.2 million policies issued between 1950 and 1971. People with major diseases were screened out. The tables show weights based on lowest mortality for men and women from ages 25 to 59 years by height and body frame.

The Metropolitan tables have been criticized as being inaccurate because (1) insured subjects do not represent a random sample of the population; (2) insured subjects are screened for illness and so are healthier than average; (3) no actual body frame measurements were taken when data were gathered so that the division into three frame categories (small, medium, and large) was a post hoc manipulation of the data; (4) about 20% of the subjects used in the tables reported their heights and weights but were not actually measured (the bias being that women tend to underreport their weight and men to overreport their height); (5) the tables do not distinguish between obesity and overweight.

BODY MASS INDEX. A third way to classify overweight is by computing the body mass index (BMI):

$$BMI = kg/(height\ in\ meters)^2$$
$$or\ BMI = lb/(height\ in\ inches)^2 \times 703.1$$

This simple measurement correlates well with other estimates of fatness, although some very muscular or very short individuals may be classified as obese when they are not. It is also a somewhat more accurate index of fatness for males than for females.

The mean BMI (weighted for the height distribution of the U.S. population) taken from the midpoint of the medium frame of the 1983 Metropolitan tables is 22.4 kg/m² for men and 22.5 kg/m² for women. Patients can be divided for degree of overweight and obesity as shown in Table 228–1. Health risks increase as BMI increases above 25.

Aging is a fattening process, so that a young and old person of comparable body weight are not comparably obese (Fig. 228–1).

Table 228–1 ■ CLASSIFICATION OF OVERWEIGHT AND OBESITY BY BODY MASS INDEX (BMI)

	OBESITY	BMI (kg/m²)
Underweight		<18.5
Normal		18.5–24.9
Overweight		25.0–20.0
Obesity	I	30.0–34.9
	II	35.0–39.9
Extreme obesity	III	≥40

This has led to controversy concerning whether it is the total weight of an individual that should stay constant from 25 years to 70 years or the fat-free mass, that is, the working cellular mass of the body plus the skeleton. The average weight data from the U.S. population show a gradually increasing weight with age, more pronounced and sustained for women than for men (Fig. 228–2).

Whereas many studies suggest that an increase from one's weight at 25 years old may increase mortality, a number have suggested that for the lowest mortality, the pattern of body weight should be leanness in the 20s followed by a very moderate weight gain as one gets older. The minimal mortality points in relation to BMI for each age-gender grouping have been calculated. The regression lines, computed separately for men and women, are presented in Figure 228–3. Clearly, age strongly affects the BMI associated with the lowest mortality. Also, the regression lines for men and women are nearly the same. The "best" BMI gradually increases with age in both genders, with no consistent difference between men and women. As a result, a single set of weight goal tables (Table 228–2) can be constructed that are applicable for both men and women. The goals, which are somewhat more liberal for certain age groups than are the Metropolitan tables, are given by decade of age, with generally higher allowable weights as persons get older. Until the issue is further clarified, these goals seem

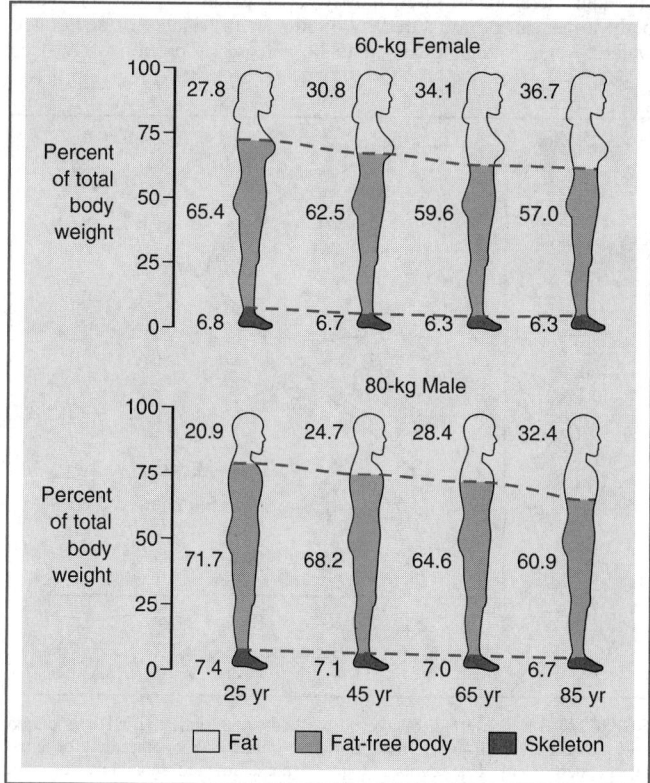

FIGURE 228–1 ■ Body composition change with aging of representative normal adults. (Adapted from Moore FD, Olesen KH, McMurrey JE, et al: The Body Cell Mass and Its Supporting Environment. Philadelphia, WB Saunders, 1963.)

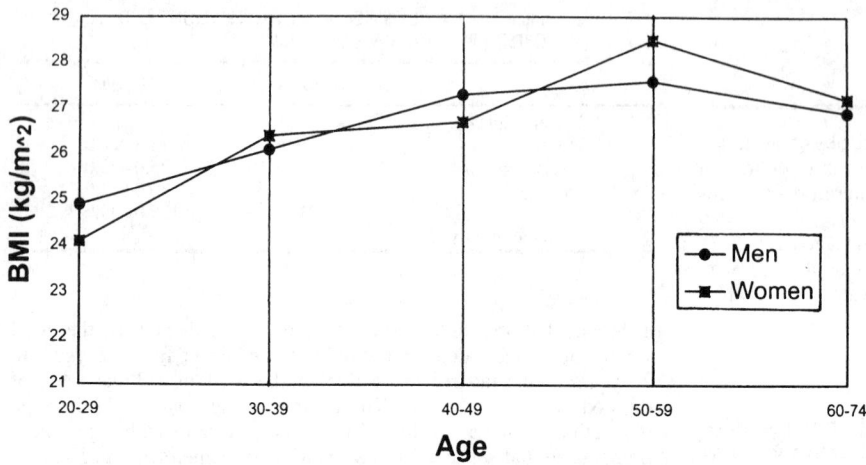

FIGURE 228-2 ■ Weight change with aging for men and women. (Adapted from National Center for Health Statistics: JAMA 272:208, 1994.)

to be reasonable for a physician to utilize in counseling patients in preventive medicine. Two caveats must be added. First, these tables have been derived from and are applicable primarily to white men and women in the United States. Second, the tables have been derived from populations without known risk factors. Patients with significant risk factors such as coronary artery disease, hypertension, and diabetes mellitus are better counseled on stricter tables, such as the Metropolitan Life Tables of 1983 (see Chapter 225).

OTHER METHODS. Over half of the fat in the body is deposited under the skin. Its thickness can be measured at various sites using standard skin calipers. It is not difficult to become adept in the use of the calipers, and a running record of a patient's estimated body fat can be easily kept. The most useful and accurate tables are based on the measurement of four skinfold thicknesses—biceps, triceps, subscapular, and suprailiac. (For such tables, see the *British Journal of Nutrition* 2:77, 1974.)

Other methods of defining obesity are more difficult and expensive and therefore are used mostly for research purposes: (1) Total body water can be measured by dilution with tritiated or deuterated water. Water is then assumed to be a fixed proportion of fat-free mass (FFM = water mass/0.73), and FFM is subtracted from total body weight to obtain total body fat. (2) Body density can be measured by underwater weighing (with accurate correction for lung and abdominal air) and the amount of fat-free mass and body fat can be calculated. (3) The amount of body potassium can be estimated by measuring the amount of its naturally radioactive isotope ^{40}K in a whole-body counter. From this figure the lean body mass can be calculated as LBM = total K^+ (mmol)/68.1. Total body fat can be calculated as total weight minus LBM.

ETIOLOGY

Very little is known about the etiology of obesity. There are probably many different causes, and some may even coexist in one individual. Obviously excess lipid deposition occurs because energy intake exceeds energy expenditure. An obese individual may have increased intake, decreased expenditure, or both.

GENETICS VS. ENVIRONMENT. Recent twin and adoption studies indicate that human fatness is under strong genetic influence. From 25 to 35% of the variance in skinfold thickness, body mass index, and relative weight has been attributed to genetic factors. Obesity is a polygenic disease, and its genetic determinants are complex and not yet well described. The genes involved may affect food intake and/or energy expenditure, increasing one and decreas-

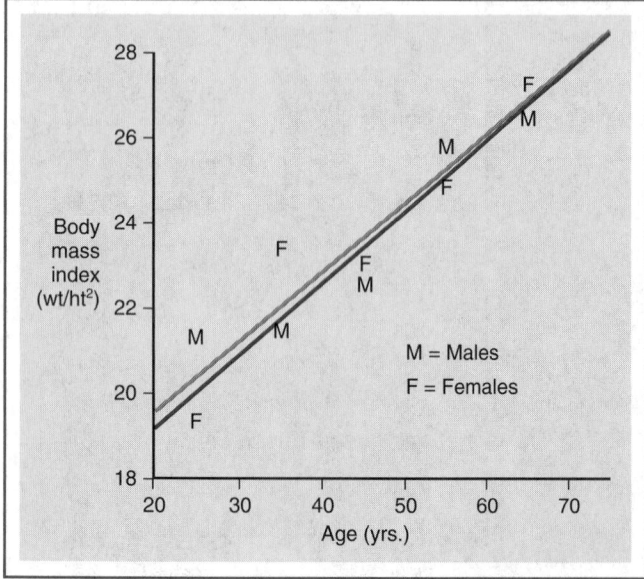

FIGURE 228-3 ■ The effect of age on the body mass index (BMI) associated with lowest mortality. Minimal mortality points were computed for each age-gender group. The regression lines were computed separately for men (dark line) and women (light line). Note that a strong effect of age on the BMI is associated with lowest mortality and that the regression lines for men and women are nearly identical. (From The Build Study, 1979. Adapted by Andres R: *In* Andres R, Bierman EL, Hazzard WR, Blass JP [eds]: Principles of Geriatric Medicine. Copyright © 1990 by McGraw-Hill. Used by permission of McGraw-Hill Book Company.)

Table 228-2 ■ AGE-SPECIFIC WEIGHT-FOR-HEIGHT TABLES (GERONTOLOGY RESEARCH CENTER)

HEIGHT (FT-IN)	WEIGHT RANGE (LB) FOR MEN AND WOMEN BY AGE†				
	25 yr	35 yr	45 yr	55 yr	65 yr
4–10	84–111	92–119	99–127	107–135	115–142
4–11	87–115	95–123	103–131	111–139	119–147
5–0	90–119	98–127	106–135	114–143	123–152
5–1	93–123	101–131	110–140	118–148	127–157
5–2	96–127	105–136	113–144	122–153	131–163
5–3	99–131	108–140	117–149	126–158	135–168
5–4	102–135	112–145	121–154	130–163	140–173
5–5	106–140	115–149	125–159	134–168	144–179
5–6	109–144	119–154	129–164	138–174	148–184
5–7	112–148	122–159	133–169	143–179	153–190
5–8	116–153	126–163	137–174	147–184	158–196
5–9	119–157	130–168	141–179	151–190	162–201
5–10	122–162	134–173	145–184	156–195	167–207
5–11	126–167	137–178	149–190	160–201	172–213
6–0	129–171	141–183	153–195	165–207	177–219
6–1	133–176	145–188	157–200	169–213	182–225
6–2	137–181	149–194	162–206	174–219	187–232
6–3	141–186	153–199	166–212	179–225	192–238
6–4	144–191	157–205	171–218	184–231	197–244

*Values in this table are for height without shoes and weight without clothes. To convert inches to centimeters, multiply by 2.54; to convert pounds to kilograms, multiply by 0.455.

†Data from Andres R: Baltimore, Gerontology Research Center, National Institute of Aging.

ing the other. The studies that have shown this degree of variance describe the genetic influences found in persons living under particular environmental conditions, namely those of Western society. Because the environment in which heritable characteristics are expressed affects the expression, these variance ranges may not apply to all societies. Not only is there a strong genetic component to fatness, but there is also a similarly strong genetic component to regional fat distribution. Thus, a person's genotype is an important determinant of how adaptation to excess energy intake occurs. Environment is also clearly important. This has been well-described in populations that have changed environment from a less "developed" to a more "developed" Western one. The interrelation of genetics to particular environments needs to be further investigated. The combination of the increased availability of low-cost, very palatable, high-energy-density food and a great decrease in physical activity has caused waist girth and weight to rise dramatically.

A number of rare genetic diseases are associated with obesity, and appear to be inherited as autosomal recessive disorders: the Prader-Willi syndrome, the Laurence-Moon-Biedl syndrome, the Alström syndrome, the Cohen syndrome, the Carpenter syndrome, and Blount's disease. The reader is referred to textbooks on genetic disorders for further descriptions of these entities.

THE REGULATION OF BODY WEIGHT

The regulation of body weight comprises a complex homeostatic system that results in a balance between energy intake and energy expenditure. The hypothalamus is the central coordinating area for this system. It has been known for many years that lesions in differing hypothalamic areas can result in either hyperphagia or hypophagia with resulting obesity or cachexia. A number of discrete molecules are involved in neurotransmission in the hypothalamus, some producing satiety and others hunger. Among the former are cholecystokinin, insulin, corticotropin-releasing hormone, bombesin, urocortin, and glucagon-like peptide-1; among the latter are neuropeptide Y, peptide YY, MCH (melanocortin-concentrating hormone), and galanin. The classical neurotransmitters serotonin, norepinephrine, and dopamine are also involved in decreasing hunger and/or increasing satiety.

In an effort to try to clarify this system further, molecular geneticists have turned to animal models of obesity that occur as a result of single-gene mutations. Table 228–3 shows a group of such mouse and rat models. The ob/ob mouse is hyperphagic and hypometabolic and very obese. The ob/ob gene has been identified by positional cloning and has been found to produce a messenger RNA (mRNA) that encodes a protein, which has been named leptin. Leptin is produced only in adipose cells and has been found to vary in plasma according to weight and fat mass, increasing with fat gain and decreasing with fat loss. There are also acute drops in the plasma level of leptin with a decrease in food intake. Thus, leptin plasma levels rise with increased food intake and increased fatness and fall with decreased intake and decreased fatness. The gene mutation in the ob/ob mouse leads to synthesis of a truncated leptin or to defective leptin production.

Leptin has been found to have many actions, but the two primary ones are inhibition of food intake and an enhancement of energy expenditure. Because of this, when first discovered, leptin was thought to be the long-sought substance that acted as a body mass sensor for the homeostatic control of body weight (Fig. 228–4). However, it has been found that obese persons accurately increase their leptin levels as they gain weight (Fig. 228–5). Also,

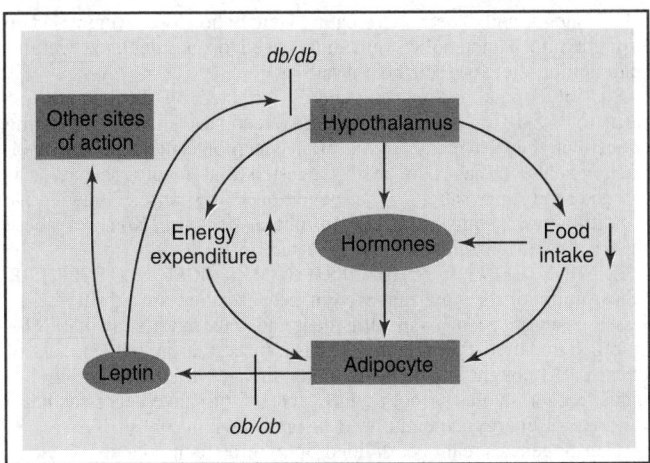

FIGURE 228–4 ▪ Secretion of leptin by adipocytes sends a signal back to the central nervous system about the amount of stored energy, thereby regulating body weight via a feedback mechanism. This system is defective in *ob/ob* mice due to lack of circulating leptin, and in *db/db* mice due to defective leptin receptors, both resulting in obesity.

the human leptin receptor has been cloned and has been found to be normal in most obese persons. Although a handful of very obese persons have been identified as having a leptin gene mutation, this is a very rare condition and is not the cause of obesity in the great majority of people who develop this problem. So if leptin biology is defective in obese persons, it must be due to poor transport of leptin into the central nervous system or to a postreceptor defect in the transmission of the signal to hypothalamic effectors.

ENERGY INTAKE. Hyperphagia is the striking cause of obesity in a number of animal models (both genetic and brain-lesioned). The cause of human obesity is much less straightforward. Obesity has been regarded as an eating disorder for centuries, but the presumed abnormality has been difficult to document. Measuring food intake in a free-living environment is subject to large errors. Most studies have suggested that obese persons do overeat (at least in their weight-gaining phases). Many reports describe individuals

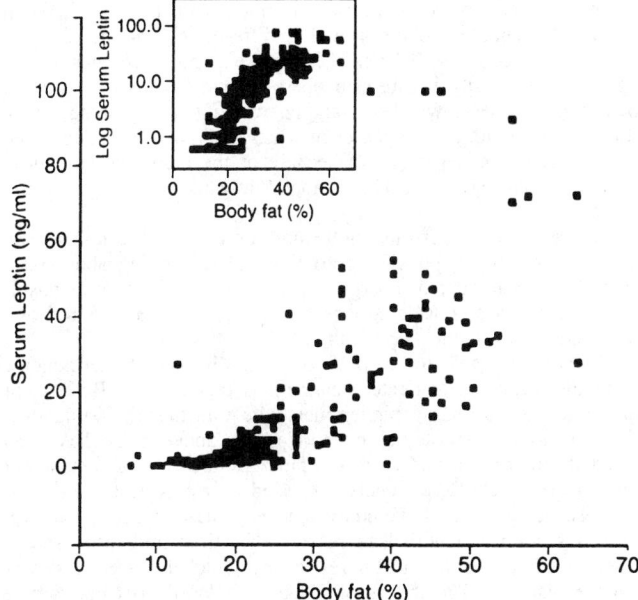

FIGURE 228–5 ▪ The relationship between percent body fat and serum leptin concentrations in 139 obese and 236 lean subjects. (Reprinted with permission from Considine RV, Sinha MK, Heiman ML, et al: Serum immunoreactive-leptin concentrations in normal-weight and obese humans. N Engl J Med 334:292–295. © 1996, Massachusetts Medical Society. All rights reserved.)

Table 228–3 ▪ GENETIC MODELS OF OBESITY IN MICE AND RATS

SINGLE GENE MUTATIONS	GENE PRODUCT
Mice	
ob/ob	OB protein
db/db	(leptin)
fat/fat	OB-R receptor
tub/tub	Carboxypeptidase E
agouti	TUB protein
	AGOUTI protein
Rats	
fa/fa or Zucker (rat equivalent of *db/db*)	OB-R receptor
LA/N *f/f* (corpulent)	OB-R receptor

who categorically deny overeating but who lose weight when brought into a metabolic ward and placed on a calculated weight-maintaining diet for their height and age.

Possibly obese persons are unduly attracted by the hedonic aspects of food, or they have impaired feedback signals registering satiety, or they have insensitive brain receptor centers for the feedback signals. It has also been suggested that feeding behavior is learned and that satiety is a conditioned response. Maladaptive conditioning is said to occur in obese persons. None of these theories has been scientifically validated.

ENERGY EXPENDITURE. RESTING METABOLIC EXPENDITURE. Obese individuals may gain weight because they are "thrifty": i.e., less ingested nutrient is spent as heat and thus more is available for storage. Impaired thermogenesis exists in certain animal models of obesity. Although it has been more difficult to document in humans, recent studies in both adults and infants have reported that a low rate of energy expenditure may predispose to obesity.

Thermogenesis can be divided into three components—resting metabolic rate (RMR), thermic effect of food (TEF), and thermic effect of exercise or activity (TEE).

RMR is the energy expended in the postabsorptive state to drive basic life-supporting processes under thermoneutral conditions. RMR, expressed as total amount of energy spent per unit time, is higher in obese persons than in lean ones. RMR can be well correlated with total weight but can be better correlated with lean body mass (LBM). This explains why men have higher RMRs than women and why RMRs decrease with age.

Obese individuals have a greater LBM than those who are lean because they require an extra amount of sustaining cell mass to maintain the extra fat. When RMR is expressed as kilocalories per kilogram of LBM, obese persons have values equivalent to those of lean. It is only when RMR is expressed as kilocalories per kilogram of body weight that they have values below those who are lean. This is because per unit of weight they have a relatively lower amount of metabolizing cell mass and a larger amount of stored fat, which is relatively inert in energy utilization. In terms of basal or resting energetics, therefore, the obese, once they are obese, do not have impaired RMRs and are not more "efficient" than lean persons.

The RMR varies as much as ±15% from individual to individual, even when matched for age, gender, and surface area. If a difference in metabolic rate between individuals can be as great as this, it is clear that at a given caloric intake one individual may gain weight and another may lose it. Energy balance depends on matching intake to expenditure. It is not surprising that different individuals maintain weight on widely differing caloric intakes.

EXPENDITURE IN ACTIVITY. The obese expend more energy during physical activity because an obese person is moving a greater load through space, whether walking, running, or climbing stairs. This is true, although less so, even when body weight is supported as in cycle ergometer exercise, because of the higher cost of moving the larger leg mass. Thus, more kilowatts of energy are expended.

Studies of obese persons show most of them to be less active, both in engaging in physical activities and in moving about once engaged. The amount of energy expended over 24 hours in physical activity varies considerably from individual to individual, however, and it is difficult to generalize.

EXPENDITURE AFTER FOOD. Food is an important thermogenic stimulant because it generates heat as it is metabolized. Because of this, a fed person has a higher metabolic rate than a fasting one. This elevation of postcibal metabolic rate above basal has been called the thermic effect of food (TEF). With a mixed diet, about 10% of the metabolizable energy ingested is lost as heat.

Obese persons may have equivalent or somewhat depressed TEF responses compared with lean persons. The impaired response appears to be related to insulin resistance, which leads to a slower glucose disposal. The thermogenic defect relating to carbohydrate disposal is found in obese patients who are insulin resistant and not found in those who are equivalently obese but insulin sensitive. However, even insulin-resistant obese persons with a decreased TEF have a total energy expenditure greater than do lean persons for the 3- to 4-hour period after the meal, because the slight decrease in TEF is less than the inherent elevation in their RMR.

In summary, although hypometabolism may predispose to obesity in some cases, RMR is higher once obesity is present. Thermogenic responses to ordinary stimuli (food, stress, cold) are small per se, and differences between lean and obese persons are small to nonexistent. The net result is that 24-hour energy expenditure in the typical obese person is greater than that of the typical sedentary lean person.

EXPENDITURE AFTER OVERFEEDING. Small rodents can waste rather than store much of excess ingested calories. This is mediated through the sympathetic nervous system, which activates a protein named thermogenin, or uncoupling protein (UCP1), which is present in brown adipose tissue (BAT), a tissue that is specialized to generate heat. Thermogenin bypasses the usual biochemical pathway for adenosine triphosphate (ATP) synthesis and allows energy production to occur "uncoupled" from the usual respiration process. A deficient ability to burn off excess calories has been documented in a number of genetically obese rodents. Although humans do not have an adequate amount of brown fat to mount a similar excess of heat production, this may occur through other newly discovered uncoupling proteins, UCP2 and UCP3.

In lean humans, significant overfeeding (of the order of 2000 extra calories per day) for about 10 days or more may lead to energy wastage. In the few studies of overfeeding done in obese volunteers, no evidence of similar energy wastage was found, but few long-term studies are available.

Do obese people lack a protective mechanism, i.e., heat dissipation, that lean people possess if they overeat? There is not much convincing experimental evidence to date, although it is a tempting hypothesis that needs to be further investigated.

PATHOPHYSIOLOGY

FAT CELLS. Fat cells (adipocytes) form a reservoir of energy that expands or contracts according to the energy balance of the organism. Fat cells develop from precursor preadipocytes, which are indistinguishable from fibroblasts, to accommodate excess nutrient calories. Individual adipocytes gradually increase in volume to about 1 μg of mass, at which point little further enlargement seems to be possible. With continuing positive energy balance, new adipocytes form from precursor cells and the total cell number increases. Adipocytes can increase in number in an unlimited fashion, so that fat mass can reach huge dimensions through fat cell hyperplasia.

Once fat cells are formed, it is difficult to de-differentiate them. This has been termed the "ratchet effect," because a ratchet turns in only one direction. Even though weight may be lost, fat cell numbers remain fixed. As a result, fat cell size reverts toward normal and with sustained weight loss may actually go below normal.

What the stimulus is for the differentiation of preadipocytes into adipocytes is unclear, but there are a series of steps that are dependent on certain transcription factors, including peroxisome proliferator-activator receptor γ (PPARγ) nuclear peptides. Once differentiated, adipocytes are active secretors of a number of peptides into the circulation. In addition to leptin, these include adipsin, tumor necrosis factor α (TNFα), angiotensinogen, and lipoprotein lipase (LPL). TNFα may be involved in the production of insulin resistance in obesity. Adipose tissue LPL may be involved. LPL acts to break down triglyceride to glycerophosphate and free fatty acids (FFA). Whereas LPL activity seems to rise with weight loss and is thought to be important in the accelerated weight regain of many patients, it seems to drop after the maintenance of weight loss for a time, suggesting that its elevation in the obese patient may be secondary rather than primary.

REGIONAL DISTRIBUTION OF ADIPOSE TISSUE. Fat mass is distributed differently in men and women. The android, or male, pattern is characterized by fat distributed predominantly around the waist and on the upper body, whereas the gynecoid, or female, pattern shows fat predominantly in the lower body, that is, lower abdomen, buttocks, hips, and thighs. Central or upper body fat has a significantly worse prognosis for morbidity and mortality than does lower body fat. Some evidence suggests that the intra-abdominal or visceral component of fat rather than the subcutaneous abdominal component is responsible, but this is still controversial. The regional distribution can be measured in a variety of ways. The easiest, most common, and very useful way is by measuring body circumference at the waist. A value of greater than 35 inches in women and greater than 40 inches in men can be considered abnormally high (see Table 228–2).

Fat cells from the upper body seem to be functionally different from fat cells in the lower body. They are more sensitive to catecholamines and insulin. It is likely that the greater lipolytic and lipogenic potential of the upper body cells is related to an underlying difference in sex-hormone response of the two tissues. Thus, testosterone and estrogen influences may be important and may act differently on upper and lower body fat cells.

Abdominal or android fatness carries a greater risk for hypertension, cardiovascular disease, hyperinsulinemia, diabetes mellitus, gallbladder disease, stroke, and cancer of the breast and endometrium. It also carries a greater risk of overall mortality. Because more men than women have the android distribution, they are more at risk for most of these conditions. Also, women who deposit their excess fat in a more android manner have a greater risk than women whose fat distribution is more gynoid. Upper body fat deposition tends to occur primarily by hypertrophy of the existing cells, whereas lower body fat deposition is by differentiation of new fat cells, i.e., hyperplasia. Reducing a normal number of enlarged fat cells to normal size is easier than reducing large numbers of the smaller cells in the lower body hyperplastic depot to normal or below normal size. This may explain the weight loss difficulties of many women with lower body obesity.

Thus, three components of body fat are associated with health risk: percent body fat, subcutaneous truncal or abdominal fat, and intra-abdominal fat. While partly correlated with each other, they do show independence of expression.

CLINICAL MANIFESTATIONS

INSULIN RESISTANCE. Obesity induces an insulin-resistant state in man, one that is associated with both basal and stimulated hyperinsulinemia. As mentioned, this may be partly mediated by an increased secretion of TNFα from adipocytes. This results from a change in β-cell insulin release rather than in the threshold to glucose stimulation. The enlarged fat cell is less sensitive to the antilipolytic and lipogenic actions of insulin. Although a decreased number of insulin receptors contributes to the insulin resistance, the resistance is generally much greater than would be predicted from the magnitude of this decrease. A "postreceptor" defect therefore occurs as well. This defect in glucose utilization occurs also in other insulin-sensitive tissues, particularly muscle. The liver is also less responsive to insulin. As the insulin resistance becomes more profound, glucose uptake in peripheral tissues is impaired and hepatic glucose output increases.

DIABETES MELLITUS. In a certain number of obese individuals, type 2 diabetes mellitus occurs (see Chapter 242). The prevalence of diabetes is approximately three times higher in overweight than in non-overweight persons. In the United States about 85% of patients with type 2 diabetes are obese. Clinically manifest diabetes develops only with the appropriate genetic legacy, but obesity, by enhancing insulin resistance, increases the demand on the pancreatic islets and tends to unmask and exacerbate an underlying genetic propensity.

HYPERTENSION. The prevalence of hypertension (blood pressure greater than 140/90 mm Hg) is approximately three times higher for the obese than for the nonobese. In the Framingham Study, high blood pressure developed 10 times more often in persons who were 20% or more overweight than in those of normal weight.

The mechanism by which obesity contributes to high blood pressure is not clear. Hyperinsulinemia leading to increased tubular reabsorption of sodium may be a factor; increased sympathetic tone may be another; and increased activity of the angiotensin system may be a third. Whatever the mechanism, weight loss from dieting leads to a fall in arterial pressure, even when salt intake is not restricted.

CARDIOVASCULAR DISEASE. Obesity has been shown to be an independent risk factor for coronary artery disease in both men and women. In obesity, increased blood volume, stroke volume, left ventricular end-diastolic volume, and filling pressure result in a high cardiac output. This can lead to predominantly left ventricular hypertrophy and dilatation. Hypertension also contributes to left ventricular hypertrophy. Thus, obese hypertensive patients are at greater risk for congestive heart failure and sudden death.

BLOOD LIPIDS. Obese people seem to have an adverse pattern of plasma lipoproteins. This is manifested particularly by a low concentration of high-density-lipoprotein (HDL) cholesterol. LDL cholesterol may be elevated. Hypertriglyceridemia is more prevalent in obese persons, possibly because the insulin resistance and hyperinsulinemia of obesity lead to increased hepatic production of triglycerides. Levels of LDL cholesterol may be elevated, but they are often normal; however, LDL lipoprotein particles are smaller, denser, and more atherogenic. The lipid abnormalities generally improve with weight loss, but if a true genetic lipoprotein disorder coexists, more intensive therapy specific for the lipoprotein abnormality may be required (see Chapter 206).

RESPIRATORY PROBLEMS. Severe obesity can lead to chronic hypoxia with cyanosis and hypercapnia. Associated with this are an increased demand for ventilation, an increased breathing workload, respiratory muscle inefficiency, and decreased functional reserve capacity and expiratory reserve volume. Peripheral lung units can close, resulting in a ventilation-perfusion mismatch.

The end-stage associated with severe obesity is the pickwickian syndrome, in which hypoventilation is so marked that hypoxia leads to long periods of somnolence. In these patients, pulmonary hypertension occurs and cardiac failure may supervene.

SLEEP APNEA. Sleep apnea is common in severely obese patients (see Chapter 87). The relationship between obesity and sleep apnea is unclear because the most obese individuals are not necessarily the most severely affected. Apnea can be obstructive or central in nature; both forms are more prevalent in obese persons. The upper airways may be obstructed by the large local accumulation of fat tissue, often in combination with micrognathia and enlarged tonsils and adenoids. The obstruction leads to hypoventilation and hypoxia, which trigger apneic episodes that then worsen the hypoxia and hypercapnia. Affected patients benefit from weight loss and sometimes from surgical removal of some of the obstructive tissue. Central apnea is characterized by a cessation of ventilatory drive from brain centers, so that diaphragmatic excursions stop for periods of 10 to 30 seconds. The reason obese persons are prone to this condition is unknown. Pharmacotherapy sometimes helps. Daytime somnolence is common in obese patients with apnea, partly from hypoxia and partly from the continual disturbance of sleep at night, because they tend to awaken after each apneic episode.

VENOUS CIRCULATORY DISEASE. Severely obese individuals often have varicose veins and venous stasis. Congestive heart failure may add to dependent edema, with the further complications of trophic changes of the skin and an increased propensity for thrombophlebitis and thromboembolism. Pulmonary embolism is much more common in the obese than in those of normal weight (see Chapter 84).

CANCER. Endometrial cancer is two to three times more common in obese than in lean women. Risk of breast cancer increases with increasing BMI in postmenopausal women. It has been speculated that this increased risk is due to the stimulatory effect of increased levels of estrogen in the postmenopausal period. Obese women also have a higher incidence of cancer of the gallbladder and of the biliary system. Obese men have a higher mortality from cancer of the colon, rectum, and prostate for reasons that are unknown.

GASTROINTESTINAL DISEASE. Cholesterol gallstones are more prevalent in obesity. The pathogenetic sequence is presumed to be that of greater cholesterol production in the increased body fat depots, greater biliary excretion of cholesterol, and a resulting supersaturation of the cholesterol in bile. The gallstones can lead to cholecystitis (see Chapter 157) and the need for cholecystectomy. The obese carry a greater risk for complications and mortality from such abdominal surgery.

Many obese patients have fatty livers with modest abnormalities of liver function tests, but hepatic diseases in general are not more common in obese than in lean persons.

ARTHRITIS. As the severity of obesity increases, joint symptoms related to osteoarthritis become common. Excess stress is particularly placed on joints of the lower extremities and the lower back, but particularly in the knees.

Body weight and serum uric acid level often correlate. With obesity, urate clearance is decreased and urate production increased. Because hypertension and diabetes mellitus also correlate with elevated uric acid levels, the relationship between hyperuricemia and obesity is multifactorial.

SKIN. Skin problems are common in obesity, particularly intertrigo in redundant folds of skin. Fungal and yeast infections of the skin are common. Acanthosis nigricans occurs in a minority of morbidly obese patients. These patients can manifest a syndrome that includes severe insulin resistance.

PSYCHOLOGICAL MANIFESTATIONS

The psychological toll of severe obesity is large. Poor self-image and impaired social relationships are common. Obese individuals are often discriminated against in educational and professional settings, engendering anxiety, anger, and self-doubt. There is no evidence, however, of any particular neurotic or psychotic character in obese individuals. The depression and anxiety seem to be situational rather than endogenous; they usually improve if the obesity can be ameliorated.

MORTALITY

Obesity is associated with increased mortality. The effect of obesity on cardiovascular mortality generally occurs through linkage with other risk factors such as hypertension, diabetes, and dyslipidemia. Obesity, however, also makes an independent contribution to mortality. In the Framingham Study, for every 10% rise in relative weight, systolic blood pressure rose 6.5 mm Hg, plasma cholesterol 12 mg/dL, and fasting blood glucose 2 mg/dL. The causes of increased mortality for those 20% or more overweight include coronary heart disease, stroke, diabetes, digestive diseases, and cancer (Table 228-4). The risk of mortality is higher for those with upper body obesity than those with lower body obesity. A number of prospective studies have now described this, particularly as it relates to cardiovascular disease risk.

OBESITY AND THE ENDOCRINE SYSTEM

Although obesity has often been described as an "endocrine" disease, <1% of obese patients have any measurable endocrine dysfunction. Hypothalamic, pituitary, thyroid, adrenal, ovarian, and possibly pancreatic endocrine syndromes have been related to obesity.

HYPOTHALAMIC DISEASE. In this type of obesity, the appetite systems or tracts located in the hypothalamus are affected. Bilateral damage in the ventromedial hypothalamus produces hyperphagic obesity in the rat; conversely, bilateral damage in the extreme lateral portion of the hypothalamus causes aphagia. Rather than a single balance of a "feeding center" and a "satiety center," however, it is now clear that diffuse excitatory and inhibitory neuronal systems controlling feeding course through the limbic system and the whole brain. Following trauma, inflammation, or a tumor (particularly craniopharyngioma) involving the hypothalamus, a few patients develop hyperphagic obesity, most of them after surgery

Table 228-4 ■ PATTERN OF EXCESS MORTALITY VARIATION WITH EXCESS WEIGHT (MEN AGES 15 TO 34 YEARS AT ENTRY)

WEIGHT RELATIVE TO AVERAGE WEIGHT (%)	MORTALITY RATIO
105–115	110
115–125	127
125–135	134
135–145	141
145–155	211
155–165	227

Adapted from Society of Actuaries and Association of Life Insurance Medical Directors of America: *Build Study 1979.* Chicago, Society of Actuaries, March 1980, p 82.

for hypothalamic tumors. The diagnosis is usually based on history, physical findings, and brain imaging studies.

PITUITARY AND ADRENAL DYSFUNCTION. Cushing's disease is the most common form of pituitary dysfunction leading to obesity (see Chapter 237). ACTH is excessively produced, which leads to excess production of cortisol by the adrenal cortex. Cushing's syndrome can also have a variety of other causes, including exogenous glucocorticoids, primary disorders of the adrenal, and paraneoplastic syndromes of excess ACTH production. The hypercortisolism causes adipocytes located primarily at the center of the body to expand, whereas those at the extremities do so much less. With this central obesity comes hypertension and diabetes.

THYROID DISEASE. Obesity is often ascribed to "hypometabolism" caused by underactivity of the thyroid gland, but this is in fact seldom true. Severe hypothyroidism can lead to some increased fat, but most of the excess weight is actually edema, which is lost with the institution of thyroid hormone replacement.

POLYCYSTIC OVARIAN SYNDROME. Mild hirsutism, irregular menses or amenorrhea, and obesity have been linked in the polycystic ovarian syndrome (PCOS). In this disorder the ovaries have atretic follicles, the patient is anovulatory, and menstrual disturbance (long-term amenorrhea to oligomenorrhea) is the rule. The ovaries overproduce androgens. Although hirsutism is common, virilization is not. Obesity and PCOS often coexist. Their relationship is not clear, but hyperinsulinemia has been implicated in the development of PCOS.

ENDOCRINE CONSEQUENCES OF OBESITY. One of the pathophysiologic consequences of obesity may be certain endocrine abnormalities. The sex-hormone abnormalities associated with obesity are different in males and females. Whereas mildly obese men have no detectable abnormalities, severely obese men have mild hypogonadotropic hypogonadism, with less than two thirds the normal mean plasma levels of total testosterone, free testosterone, and folicle-stimulating hormone. Gonadotropic hormones are suppressed by elevated plasma estrogens derived from increased aromatization of adrenal steroids in the excessive body fat. Obesity may be associated with increased metabolic clearance rates of testosterone, caused partly by decreased sex hormone-binding globulin (SHBG). Spermatogenesis, libido, and potency, however, are generally normal.

Estrogens are not elevated in obese premenopausal women, probably because the amount of estrone conversion by the adipose tissue is small in comparison with regular ovarian estradiol production. Estrogens are elevated, however, in postmenopausal obese women, most likely owing to increased peripheral conversion of the prehormone androstenedione to estrone. This may be a partial explanation as to why there is less osteoporosis in obese women.

There are differences in the androgen-estrogen environment in persons with upper (UBO) and lower (LBO) body obesity. This is more clearly defined in women. Women with UBO have higher androgen production rates and higher concentrations of testosterone and estradiol levels than those with LBO. They also have decreased levels of SHBG, so that free testosterone concentrations are higher. Women with LBO have increased estrone from peripheral aromatization of circulating androgens.

In obesity, insulin resistance develops and hyperinsulinemia results. Whether impaired glucose tolerance or frank diabetes ensues depends on the degree of insulin resistance and the underlying genetic make-up of the individual, but both are common. Triiodothyronine (T_3) may be elevated to high normal in conditions of high caloric intake with adequate carbohydrate, while thyroxine levels and TSH levels are normal. Slightly low blood cortisol levels may be present in obesity, probably because of enhanced turnover rates of cortisol. The circadian rhythm of cortisol secretion is usually normal in obesity. Urinary free cortisol levels are generally normal if related to the lean body mass or urinary creatinine. Also, obese patients usually suppress normally with dexamethasone (see Chapter 237). Leptin has been found to inhibit the hypothalamic-pituitary-adrenal axis in rodents. It is possible that, if obese humans have peptin resistance, subtle adrenal disinhibition may occur.

Pseudotumor cerebri (benign intracranial hypertension) occurs most commonly in obese young women. No intracranial pathology has been found, although headache, blurred vision, and papilledema occur. Why obesity affects so many of these patients is unclear.

Hypothalamic control of prolactin and growth hormone is often defective in obesity, with poor responses to insulin hypoglycemia.

These abnormalities generally revert to normal with weight loss, but not always. Whether these pituitary abnormalities reflect altered hypothalamic control due to obesity or abet the obesity in some way is unclear.

TREATMENT

Obesity is very difficult to treat, because the primary emphasis must be on active patient self-control rather than on passive drug therapy. The responsibility of the physician is to be as supportive and helpful as possible. The three approaches to weight control are diet, exercise, and drugs.

DIET. A truly motivated individual must stay on a diet for a long time, initially for weight loss and then for weight maintenance. Crash diets for a few days or weeks are ineffective. Because of the long-term requirement, a diet must be tailored to a person's tastes and habits.

The diet must be nutritionally adequate. It is not possible to calculate a diet under 1100 calories that contains adequate amounts of vitamins and minerals. If the diet is lower in calories than this, vitamin and mineral supplements are necessary. The goal of weight loss is to lose as much fat while losing as little lean body mass as possible. A mixed, balanced diet is a sensible approach to long-term weight reduction. A diet that contains at least 0.8 to 1.2 g of protein per kilogram of desirable body weight will minimize nitrogen losses. The protein should be of high quality, so that essential amino acids can be utilized to maintain lean body mass.

A useful strategy to induce and maintain weight reduction is to educate the obese patient with regard to the caloric content of foods. Particularly important is to emphasize the high caloric density of some foods, especially those high in fat and sugar. The fat content of the diet should drop below 30% of total calories. This will help to lower the caloric content of the diet. Foods high in fiber should be used liberally because of their low caloric density. Refined sugars should be reduced because these provide calories without any useful vitamins or minerals.

VERY-LOW-CALORIE DIETS. Very-low-calorie diets (VLCD) severely limit daily intake to 300 to 700 calories. Some diets are strictly limited to protein and have been called protein-supplemented modified fasts (PSMF). Others allow both protein and carbohydrate. The concept of protein-supplemented fasting arose because the regimen improves nitrogen balance over fasting programs. There is little evidence, however, that at equicaloric levels protein alone is better than protein with carbohydrate. The extra weight lost early in the diet when protein alone is given is that of water. With this water diuresis there is electrolyte loss as well. The calories can be given either in liquid formula form or as natural foods. High-quality protein must be given. Adequate supplements of vitamins and minerals must also be taken. These very severe diets have been given for extensive periods of time, but it is unwise to allow them to last longer than 16 weeks. The heavier the patient, the safer the diet seems to be. The lighter the patient, the more LBM is lost per unit of weight loss, so that more caution, more liberal calories, and a shorter time period of dieting should be followed. These diets, especially those relying on liquid formulas have been popular because of their relative ease and because, since they are so hypocaloric, the weight loss is more rapid. However, they can have serious side effects.

Side effects of these severe diets include orthostatic hypotension (secondary to both sodium loss and impaired norepinephrine secretion), fatigue, cold intolerance, dry skin, hair loss, and menstrual irregularities. Cholelithiasis, cholecystitis, and rarely pancreatitis can occur. Unfortunately, most individuals rapidly regain weight after being on these crash programs, perhaps in large measure because the very low caloric content and the liquid form of the diet do not educate the patient to make the adjustments in lifestyle and eating behavior necessary to subsequently maintain the weight loss.

EXERCISE. Obese persons tend to be inactive; it is therefore important to increase activity and thus overall energy expenditure. Patients should be taught the approximate number of calories being expended over basal level in individual activities. Most are surprised at how much exercise it takes to expend just a few calories (Table 228–5).

Moderate exercise only transiently increases the metabolic rate. The calories expended are the calories of work done. In the obese,

Table 228–5 ▪ APPROXIMATE ENERGY EXPENDITURE IN SELECTED ACTIVITIES FOR PEOPLE OF DIFFERENT WEIGHTS (CALORIES PER 30 MINUTES)*

ACTIVITY	WEIGHT (LB)					
	110	130	150	170	190	210
Aerobic dancing						
"Walking pace"	99	114	132	150	168	156
"Jogging pace"	159	186	213	243	270	300
"Running pace"	204	240	276	315	351	387
Basketball	207	243	282	318	357	396
Canoeing—leisure	66	78	90	102	114	126
Canoeing—racing	156	183	210	237	267	294
Carpentry	78	93	105	120	135	147
Cycling—5.5 mph	96	114	132	147	165	183
Cycling—9.4 mph	150	177	204	231	258	285
Dancing—ballroom	78	90	105	117	132	144
Dancing—disco	156	183	210	237	267	294
Gardening	150	177	204	231	258	285
Golf	129	150	174	195	219	243
Judo	294	345	399	450	504	558
Lying or sitting down	33	39	45	51	57	63
Mopping floor	96	105	120	138	153	171
Running						
11.5 minutes per mile	204	240	276	315	351	387
9 minutes per mile	291	342	393	447	498	552
7 minutes per mile	366	417	468	522	573	624
5.5 minutes per mile	435	513	591	669	747	828
Skiing, cross-country	216	252	291	330	369	408
Standing quietly	39	45	51	57	66	72
Swimming						
Backstroke	255	300	345	390	435	486
Crawl	192	228	261	297	330	366
Table tennis	102	120	138	156	174	195
Tennis	165	192	222	252	282	312
Walking						
3 mph	102	114	126	138	153	165
4 mph	120	141	162	186	207	228

*Adapted from Gutin B: The High Energy Factor. New York, Random House, 1983. Copyright © 1983 by Bernard Gutin and Gail Kessler. Reprinted by permission of Random House, Inc.

moderate exercise does not actually lower food intake, but intake does not increase to keep pace with the extra expenditure, as it does in lean persons. This is helpful in inducing and particularly in maintaining weight loss.

BEHAVIOR MODIFICATION. Psychoanalysis and psychotherapy have not been very helpful in weight control. An extended change in eating behavior requires a great change in lifestyle, however, so behavior modification programs have proliferated. Behavior therapy is a fundamental departure from the traditional "dietary" training of the past, in which a list of foods, the allowable quantities, and specific menus were supplied. In behavior modification the patient is first made aware of what and how much he or she eats as a background for changing that behavior. Many persons eat quite unconsciously, with little thought of how much they eat and with little or no knowledge of its caloric content. In the education process, careful food intake diaries are kept. Patients record not only what and how much was eaten, but where, with whom, how, their feelings, and their degree of hunger. These diaries are analyzed, and nutrient densities of foods are discussed. New modes of eating are suggested, including not eating between meals, eating always at table, eating only three times per day, watching the portions of food eaten, not doing other activities while eating, and eating slowly with concentration. Behavior modification also strives at stimulus control, cognitive re-structuring, and environmental management. The aim is to break learned associations between environmental cues and food intake. Particular situations that trigger eating are avoided or controlled. Behavior change also includes increasing physical activity. Behavior modification therapy is usually done in groups, with continued dialogue between the trained group leader (psychologist, nutritionist, physician), the other group members, and the patient.

DRUG THERAPY. Drugs in weight control have been used in the past as short-term adjunctive therapy to diet and exercise. Over the long term the use of drugs has been disappointing, owing to small effects on weight loss or adverse side effects. In general, drugs affect appetite modestly. Anorectic drugs act centrally through brain catecholamine, dopamine, or serotonin pathways. For example, the derivatives of amphetamine seem to produce anorexia through stimulating the central hypothalamic neurochemical pathways in which norepinephrine and/or dopamine are the principal neutransmitters.

Amphetamine-like drugs not only decrease appetite; they also elevate mood and increase arousal, probably mediated through making norepinephrine and dopamine more abundant at synapses. This is true of phendimetrazine, phentermine, phenylpropanolamine, and diethylpropion. Mazindol probably works by blocking norepinephrine uptake. It therefore appears that increasing the activity of norepinephrine, dopamine, and/or serotonin at certain central nervous system sites can lead to anorexia and weight loss.

All of the drugs mentioned have a greater effect on appetite control than do placebos. Problems arise, however, from abuse potential and side effects. Amphetamine has clearly addictive properties and is no longer used for appetite suppression. Benzphetamine and phendimetrazine may have disturbing side effects, such as sleep disturbances, agitation, and psychosis, and are scheduled substances. Irritability and insomnia have been reported with diethylpropion, mazindol, and phentermine. Contraindications include severe hypertension, coronary artery disease, glaucoma, and a history of drug abuse. The use of fenfluramine and dexfenfluramine has been terminated after many patients developed heart valve lesions.

These drugs should only be prescribed for short periods of time, in an effort to help patients over difficult weight "plateaus" or crisis periods. They have not been tested for effectiveness or adverse effects for long-term periods.

Because obesity is a chronic condition and sustained treatment often fails, the chronic use of drugs has been suggested. Two drugs have been tested long-term: sibutramine (Meridia) and Xenical (Orbistat). Sibutramine has been tested in a large number of subjects for 1 year, with acceptable risk to benefit ratio. It is uniquely both a serotonin and norepinephrine reuptake inhibitor. Potential side effects are blood pressure and heart rate elevation, and these must be monitored. Xenical has been tested for 2 years and is now approved for use in much of the world, though not in the United States. It inhibits fat absorption in the intestine by blocking pancreatic lipase. As a result, about 30% of ingested fat is passed in the stool. Side effects are gastrointestinal, e.g., looser and more frequent stools and steatorrhea. These drugs, in comparison to placebo, lower weight, on average, an additional 4 to 5% in long-term trials, which is a modest effect. However, some patients lose more than this, and evidence now indicates that with a loss of weight of 10 to 15% below baseline, a large effect on risk factors can occur.

GOALS. Very often patients, and sometimes physicians, have unrealistic goals of what can be accomplished. One pound of fat is equivalent to 4000 kcal. With a deficit of 400 kcal/day, losing 1 lb takes 10 days. The more accurate the knowledge of daily energy expenditure and energy intake, the closer a physician can predict the rate of weight loss. This may prevent unrealistic goals and disappointment by both patient and therapist. The initial goal for weight loss should be modest, with an effort made to lose 10 to 15% of weight rather than to strive for an "ideal" or "normal" weight. With even this amount of loss, detectable improvement can occur in co-morbid conditions. Only if such weight loss can be maintained for a period of months should a further effort be attempted.

SURGERY. Patients who have severe obesity (greater than 100% over desirable weight), have tried weight control programs without success, and often have complications such as sleep apnea, heart failure, phlebitis, and arthritis have a life expectancy that is much lower than normal. These patients may be candidates for surgery because nonoperative management rarely leads to permanent weight reduction.

Surgery for obesity should be considered experimental, as there is no one accepted procedure, and all carry significant risks and complications. Because of the severe side effects of previously done intestinal surgery, gastric surgical procedures have become popular. A small fundic pouch or reservoir is created so that individuals are severely limited in the amount of food that they can eat. The distal stoma created for the pouch has variably been designed to empty into the rest of the stomach or into a loop of jejunum, with the rest of the stomach and duodenum becoming a blind loop. Alternatively, in vertical-banded gastroplasty, as opposed to horizontal banding, only a small tubular reservoir remains for food entering from the esophagus. Side effects include gastric distress, vomiting, and electrolyte disturbances. Also, some patients do not lose much weight, because many eat "around" the small reservoir with frequent servings of liquid or semisolid foods. A mean weight loss of two thirds of excess weight has been reported, but failure is not uncommon. Dilatation of the gastric pouch, stomal dilation, stomal obstruction, and gastric dehiscence can occur as complications.

Surgery may be advisable in some patients. Because life-long follow-up and vitamin and mineral supplementation are necessary, a responsible and cooperative patient and an experienced surgeon are a requisite duo.

WEIGHT REGAIN The most difficult problem in the treatment of obesity is the maintenance of a reduced body weight.

A person who is modestly overweight with enlarged adipocytes but little proliferation of extra adipocytes can more easily maintain weight loss. The adipocyte hyperplasia of greater obesity is likely to create a much greater problem in maintenance of weight loss. The degree of filling of adipocytes is very likely a regulated factor in energy balance, with leptin playing a role. Obese persons with adipocyte hyperplasia begin to decrease the mass of each adipocyte as they lose weight. If the adipocyte mass drops below a normal lower level of about $0.5 \mu g$ per cell, individuals seem to have greater difficulty in maintaining weight reduction. Adipocyte mass is regulated with a feedback effect on energy intake and energy expenditure, so that the reduced obese experience strong food intake cues that they have trouble resisting and lower their metabolic rate.

Lipogenic enzyme activities increase when a hypocaloric diet is liberalized as a patient goes from a weight-loss to a weight-maintenance period. This is consequent to an increase in caloric intake rather than being primarily caused by the reduction in weight. Reduced obese individuals have been reported to require about 25% fewer calories per square meter of surface area to maintain their body weight than do either normal persons or obese individuals who have not dieted and lost weight. This is because, as obese persons reduce, the energy expended in general activity decreases owing to the smaller mass they carry. Their RMR is appropriate to the new lean body mass, but their thermic effect of activity drops unless they can greatly increase their activity pattern over the previous one. Therefore, exercise is very important in the weight maintenance phase.

PREVENTION The propensity toward obesity is partially inherited, but a large component is also environmental. Obesity leads to an increased morbidity and mortality from a number of diseases, especially for those who are younger than 45 years. Being overweight in early adult life is more dangerous than it is at older ages.

It is incumbent on physicians to make their patients aware of these risks and try to keep patients at a BMI of ≥25 (see Fig. 228–1). This is particularly true for those patients who already have, or have a family history of, the diseases that are precipitated and abetted by obesity.

Campfield LA, Smith FJ, Burn P: The OB protein (leptin) pathway: A link between adipose tissue mass and central networks. Horm Metab Res 28:619–632, 1996.
Pi-Sunyer FX: Medical hazards of obesity. Ann Intern Med 119:655–660, 1993.
Pi-Sunyer FX: Short-term medical benefits and adverse effects of weight loss. Ann Intern Med. 119:722–726, 1993.

229 ENTERAL NUTRITION

John L. Rombeau

Enteral nutrition is the provision of liquid formula diets into the gastrointestinal (GI) tract. When compared with total parenteral nutrition (TPN), enteral nutrition measurably increases intestinal mucosal growth and function and is less costly. Because of these acknowledged benefits, enteral nutrition is being used with increasing frequency in medical patients. It is therefore incumbent on physicians to be familiar with the rationale, indications, administration, and prevention of complications of enteral nutrition.

RATIONALE FOR PROVISION Of ENTERAL NUTRIENTS

EFFECTS ON INTESTINAL GROWTH AND FUNCTION. The most important stimulus for gut growth and function is the presence of nutrients within the GI tract. Enteral nutrients mediate such effects both directly and indirectly. The presence of nutrients within the intestinal lumen directly increases epithelial proliferation and enhances mucosal cell renewal. In the absence of luminal stimuli or intestinal nutrients, the small and large bowels atrophy, not only in the absorptive cells and brush border enzymes but also in the mucus-secreting cells and the gut-associated lymphoid tissue. These entities are important protective components of the intestinal barrier against bacteria, endotoxins, and other antigenic macromolecules and may provide a rationale for using small volumes (e.g., 10 mL/hour) of continuous enteral feeding in critically ill patients even if they cannot tolerate larger volumes and must be fed parenterally as well.

Enteral nutrients mediate many of their indirect enterotropic effects by stimulating gut hormones such as gastrin, neurotensin, bombesin, and enteroglucagon. Gastrin exerts trophic effects on the stomach, duodenum, and possibly the colon. Enteral nutrients given to animal models increase the production of additional enterotropic hormones such as glucagon-like peptide 2. Furthermore, because of reduced manufacturing costs of its nutrient components, enteral feeding is less costly than TPN and may be more cost-effective than hand-feeding disabled or debilitated patients.

INDICATIONS

General indications for enteral nutrition include the following: (1) the presence of protein-energy malnutrition (see Chapter 226), (2) a GI tract that can safely tolerate enteral formulas, and (3) anticipated inadequate oral intake for at least 7 days. Safe usage of the GI tract is possible in the absence of obstruction, severe intractable diarrhea, or massive bleeding. The anticipated duration of inadequate oral intake is based solely on the clinical judgment of the primary physician. Table 229–1 indicates examples of specific medical indications for enteral nutrition. Figure 229–1 gives an algorithm for determining the method of feeding.

DIETARY FORMULAS

Commercial enteral formulas have proliferated rapidly. Table 229–2 outlines the nutrient composition of some of these agents, including polymeric balanced diets, modified formulas, and modular supplements.

POLYMERIC BALANCED FORMULAS. Polymeric formulas are "complete" balanced, isotonic diets containing 100% of the Recommended Daily Allowance for substrates, vitamins, and minerals when prescribed in the recommended amounts. These formulas are palatable and are the first choice for oral supplementation or tube feeding when digestion and absorption are reasonably normal. The nitrogen source consists of an intact or partially hydrolyzed natural protein (e.g., soy, egg, lactalbumin) that requires the patient's ability to digest protein, in addition to carbohydrate and fat. The caloric density of these formulas is usually 1 kcal/mL but can be as high as 1.5 to 2 kcal/mL. Calorie-dense formulas are reasonable choices for patients who have unusually high caloric requirements,

Table 229–1 ■ INDICATIONS FOR THE USE OF ENTERAL NUTRITION IN ADULT MEDICAL PATIENTS

Protein-energy malnutrition with anticipated significantly decreased oral intake for at least 7 d
Anticipated significantly decreased oral intake for 10 d
Severe dysphagia
Massive small bowel resection (used in combination with total parenteral nutrition)
Low-output (<500 mL/day) enterocutaneous fistula

can tolerate only limited feeding volumes, or require fluid restriction. Most importantly, polymeric balanced formulas are less expensive than the other formulas. Their major disadvantage is a fixed nutrient composition.

MODIFIED FORMULAS. Conventional modified diets are also "complete" diets. Composed primarily of pre-digested or "elemental" nutrients, they require minimal digestion and are almost completely absorbed. Although the protein source can be crystalline amino acids, some pancreatic function is required to digest carbohydrates (oligosaccharides and disaccharides) and fats (up to 30% of which are provided as medium-chain triglycerides). In addition, absorption of glucose, sodium, amino acids, fat, vitamins, and trace elements requires intact mucosal transport systems.

Unlike the polymeric balanced diets, modified diets are hyperosmolar, unpalatable, and relatively expensive, costing between 3 and 10 times as much per calorie as polymeric balanced formulas. They may produce osmotic diarrhea if administered too rapidly and require flavoring supplements for oral use. Modified diets may be indicated in conditions of digestive or absorptive insufficiency, in which polymeric diets are not well tolerated. Examples of such limiting conditions include chronic pancreatitis, short-bowel syndrome, and prolonged ileus.

DISEASE-SPECIFIC FORMULAS. Certain modified formulas are designed for patients with specific nutritional needs. Formulas that contain only essential amino acids as the protein source are designed for patients with renal failure. Formulas that have a protein source high in branched-chain amino acids and low in aromatic amino acids have been formulated for patients with hepatic encephalopathy, severe trauma, and sepsis. Formulas that are high in fat content (~55% of calories) and low in carbohydrate content (~28% of calories) have been recommended for patients with respiratory insufficiency because their oxidation produces less carbon dioxide. The high fat content of these formulas may produce diarrhea in critically ill patients. Recently, diets supplemented with fish oils, arginine, and nucleotides have been developed to allegedly enhance the immune response of critically ill and postoperative patients. These diets are very expensive. Well-controlled and properly designed clinical trials are needed before recommending their use. Little objective evidence justifies the use of any of these expensive, disease-specific formulas; their use should be restricted to patients with specific nutrient needs who cannot tolerate polymeric and conventional modified diets.

MODULAR SUPPLEMENTS. Modular supplements, which consist of single or multiple nutrients, can be added to existing "fixed-ratio" diets without affecting the quality or quantity of other nutrients. They are designed for patients for whom standard fixed-ratio formulas are suboptimal. Commercially available modules include carbohydrate, fat, protein, mineral, electrolyte, and vitamin formulations.

ENTERAL NUTRITION ADMINISTRATION

ACCESS. Selection of the access site for delivery of enteral nutrients is based on the anticipated duration of forced feeding and the potential risk of aspiration. Ideally, enteral nutrition is given by the oral route to alert patients with intact gag reflexes who require nutritional supplementation only with meals. For patients who cannot tolerate oral nutrition, other access techniques include nasogastric tube, nasoenteric tube, and tube enterostomy.

Nasogastric or nasoenteric tubes are ideal for patients who require short-term (less than 4 weeks) enteral nutrition. To use these access routes safely, patients must have intact gag reflexes and competent lower esophageal sphincters. Ideal candidates are those with poor oral intake such as occurs with cancer of the head and neck and the lung. The stomach is the preferred site of delivery, but the nasoenteric tube should be advanced into the jejunum in patients with gastroparesis and a high risk of aspiration.

Permanent access through tube enterostomies is the preferred route of delivery for long-term enteral nutrition (more than 4 weeks). Tube enterostomies are inserted either endoscopically, laparoscopically, or operatively into the pharynx, stomach, and jejunum.

The percutaneous endoscopic approach is the preferred method

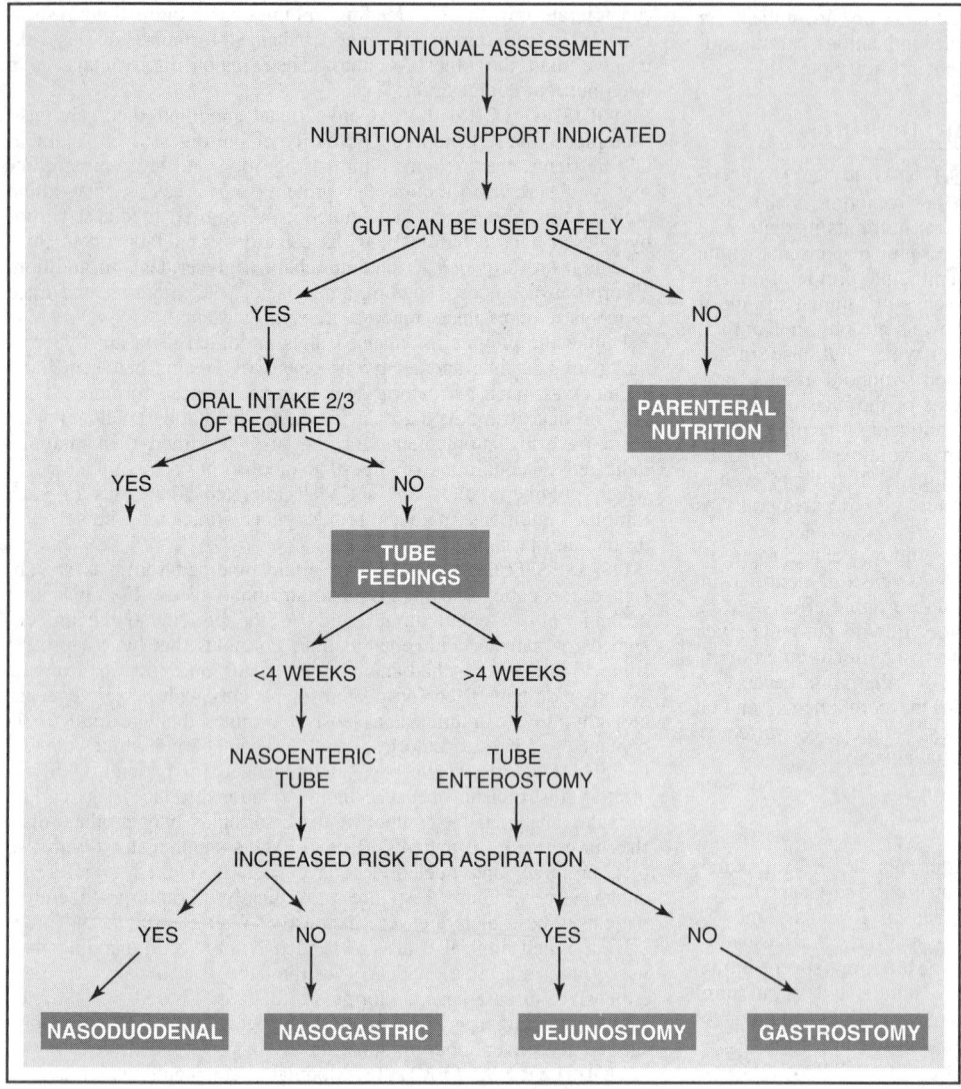

FIGURE 229–1 ■ Decision approach for the type and route of nutritional support.

for gastrostomy placement. It has the advantage of decreased procedure time, local anesthesia, absence of an incision, and avoidance of ileus. The speed, simplicity, low cost, and low complication rate of percutaneous endoscopic gastrostomy have resulted in its replacement of surgical gastrostomy in most hospitals. Surgical gastrostomy for feeding is indicated for patients unable to tolerate percutaneous endoscopic gastrostomy or for individuals undergoing concomitant GI surgery.

Jejunostomy is indicated for patients who need long-term enteral nutrition and have chronic aspiration, gastric outlet obstruction, or stomach or duodenal cancer or for patients who have had a gastrectomy.

DELIVERY. Formulas are delivered intermittently or continuously. Intermittent feeding is preferred for delivery into the stomach because it is more physiologic and "frees" the patient from the feeding equipment. Feedings of polymeric diets in a volume of 240 to 400 mL every 4 hours are well tolerated. The disadvantages of intermittent feedings consist of an initial requirement for nursing supervision, such as monitoring for gastric residuals, and a higher risk of aspiration if delayed gastric emptying is present. Slow administration of small volumes into the stomach (25 to 40 mL/hour) is well tolerated and avoids the abdominal discomfort often caused by the increased rate and volume of intermittent feedings.

Continuous feeding, administered by infusion pump over a period of 18 to 24 hours, requires less nursing supervision and results in smaller residual volumes and a lower risk of aspiration than does intermittent feeding. When feeding into the duodenum or jejunum, continuous feeding is required to avoid distention of the bowel, fluid and electrolyte shifts, and diarrhea, all of which can

occur with intermittent feeding. Feedings into the small bowel usually consist of isotonic polymeric solutions, initially at a rate of 30 mL/hour. The rate is increased approximately 25 mL/hour/day until the desired volume is achieved to meet the patient's nutrient requirements. Infusions should be initiated at very low rates (10 mL/hour) in critically ill patients. Disadvantages of continuous feeding include the expense of the volumetric infusion pump and the limitation it places on ambulatory patients.

MONITORING. Patients receiving enteral feedings require the same careful monitoring as do those who receive parenteral nutrition. This need for monitoring is especially true in critically ill patients. Routine monitoring is best accomplished by following a protocol that ensures complete and detailed surveillance to reduce the possibility of error in formula choice and nutrient administration and to assess progress toward nutritional goals (Table 229–3).

Special attention must be paid to GI tolerance to the formula. The patient's condition should be evaluated daily for diarrhea, constipation, nausea, cramping, vomiting, and abdominal distention. Clinical evidence of abdominal distention is a contraindication to enteral feeding. One must give close attention to the patient's metabolic status and fluid and electrolyte balance. In many instances, potential complications can be avoided by simple maneuvers such as changing the infusion rate, caloric density, or formulation.

Periodic nutritional assessment is required to evaluate the adequacy of the nutritional support. Nitrogen balance, body weight change, and serum protein status should be monitored and the nutrient prescription amended when indicated. Because of frequent disruptions in feeding attempts, it is not uncommon for hospitalized

Table 229–2 ■ COMMONLY USED ADULT COMMERCIAL ENTERAL FEEDING FORMULAS*

CATEGORY	1.0 kcal/mL	1.2 kcal/mL	1.5 kcal/mL	2.0 kcal/mL
Polymeric Balanced				
≤16% protein	Ensure, Resource, Isocal, Osmolite, Nutren 1.0		Nutren 1.5, Ensure Plus, Resource Plus, Boost Plus, Comply	Nutren 2.0, Deliver, Magnacal
17–20% protein	Osmolite HN, Isocal HN, Ensure HN, Ultracal, Jevity		Ensure Plus HN	TwoCal HN
≥20% protein	Sustacal, Replete, Promote, Protain XL (22%), Isosource VHN (25%)		TraumaCal	
Modified–Conventional				
≤16% protein	Peptamen, Reabilan, Vivonex Plus, Criticare HN			
17–20% protein	Vital HN, Reabilan HN, AlitraQ			
Peptide based	Peptamen (16%), Reabilan (12.5%), Criticare HN (14%), Peptamen VMP (25%), Reabilan HN (17.5%), AlitraQ (21%), Vital HN (16%), SandaSource Peptical (20%)		Crucial (25%)	
Elemental	Tolerex (8%), Vivonex T.E.N. (15%), Vivonex Plus (18%)			
Modified—Disease Specific (% protein)†				
Critical care	Immun-Aid (32%), Impact (22%), Impact/Fiber (22%)	Perative (20%)		
Glucose intolerance	Glytrol (18%), Choice dM (17%), Glucerna (16.7%), Diabeta Source (20%)			
Hepatic	Travasorb Hepatic (11%), Hepatic-Aid (15%)	Hepatic-Aid II (15%)	Nutrihep (11%)	
Malabsorption			Lipisorb (17%)	
Renal			Travasorb Renal (7%)	Renal Cal (6–9%), Amin-Aid (4%)
Pulmonary			NutriVent (18%), Respalor (20%), Pulmocare (16.7%)	
Modular Supplements				
Protein	Casec, ProMod,			
Carbohydrate	Moducal, Polycose,			
Fat	Microlipid, MCT oil			

*This table includes only a partial listing of commercial products.

†Manufacturers market these products as disease specific. The author's use of this designation is intended neither to endorse the manufacturers' claims of special efficacy in the diseases specified nor to deny that some of the polymeric-balanced or modified-conventional formulas might be appropriate or even superior in these conditions.

patients to receive as little as 70% of the enteral calories ordered on a daily basis. These considerations may make it necessary to increase the infusion rate or to supplement infusions with parenteral feeding until satisfactory enteral intake is achieved.

Table 229–3 ■ STANDARD ORDER FORM FOR PATIENTS RECEIVING ENTERAL NUTRITION

Obtain an abdominal radiograph to confirm tube location before feeding.

Elevate the head of the bed 30 degrees when feeding into the stomach.

Record the name, volume, and strength of the formula and the duration and rate (mL/hr) of feeding.

Check the gastric residual every 4 hr in patients receiving gastric feedings. Withhold feedings for 4 hr if the residual is greater than 150 mL. Notify the physician if two consecutive measurements detect excessive residual.

Weigh the patient on Monday, Wednesday, and Friday.

Record input and output daily. Every 8 hr, chart the volume of formula administered separately from water or other oral intake.

Change administration tubing daily.

Irrigate the feeding tube with 20 mL of water at the completion of each intermittent feeding, when the tube is disconnected, after delivery of crushed medications, or if feeding is stopped for any reason.

When the patient is ingesting oral nutrients, request calorie counts daily upon request.

Obtain a complete blood count with red blood cell indices, SMA 12, serum iron, serum magnesium albumin, transferrin, and pre-albumin every Monday.

Obtain an SMA 6 every Thursday.

Collect urine for 24 hr starting at 8 A.M., and analyze for urea nitrogen and creatinine upon request.

Hold feedings for nausea, vomiting, distension. Call a house officer.

COMPLICATIONS

Clinically significant complications of enteral feeding, although few, should be promptly recognized and treated aggressively. As noted, a standardized monitoring protocol helps prevent and detect possible problems. Complications of enteral feeding are grouped into four major categories: gastrointestinal, metabolic, infectious, and mechanical.

GASTROINTESTINAL. Diarrhea, defined as stool weight (or volume) of more than 200 g (or milliliters) per 24 hours, the most common complication of enteral nutrition, occurs in 10 to 20% of patients. Its possible causes are listed in Table 229–4. Tube feeding–related factors that have been suggested to predispose to diarrhea but not documented by controlled studies include formula hyperosmolality, lactose in the presence of relative lactase deficiency, and bacterial contamination of the enteral products and delivery systems. Although contamination is not a frequent cause of diarrhea, formula containers and administration tubing should be changed daily to avoid this complication. High-fat formulas may cause diarrhea, when patients suffer from fat malabsorption (as with pancreatic exocrine insufficiency, biliary obstruction, ileectomy, or ileitis). Enterally administered medications, including antibiotics, hyperosmolar drug solutions such as sorbitol-containing elixirs, and magnesium-containing antacids, can cause diarrhea. Many elixir medications contain substantial amounts (up to 65%) of sorbitol, although the agent is listed in alphabetic order in the drug information insert only as an "inactive" ingredient. For this reason, all elixir medications must be considered potential causes of diarrhea in tube-fed patients, and it is often prudent to discontinue them or change them to tablet or intravenous forms to determine their responsibility.

Table 229-4 ■ CAUSES OF DIARRHEA IN TUBE-FED PATIENTS

Common Causes Unrelated to Tube Feeding
Elixir medications containing sorbitol
Magnesium-containing antacids
Antibiotic-induced sterile gut
Pseudomembranous colitis
Possible Causes Related to Tube Feeding
Inadequate fiber to form stool bulk
High fat content of formula (in the presence of fat malaborption syndrome)
Bacterial contamination of enteral products and delivery systems (causal
 association with diarrhea not documented)
Rapid advancement in rate (after the GI tract is unused for prolonged
 periods)
Unlikely Causes Related to Tube Feeding
Formula hyperosmolality (proven not to be a cause for diarrhea)
Lactose (absent from nearly all enteral feeding formulas)

Treatment of diarrhea is directed at the underlying cause; however, several therapeutic options are available when no cause is clearly identifiable. Decreasing the feeding flow rate may alleviate diarrhea by allowing time for intestinal mucosal adaptation to occur when the GI tract has not been used for extended periods (i.e., in starvation and TPN-induced intestinal atrophy). The flow rate is then slowly increased over several days. Parenteral feeding may be necessary to meet full nutrient requirements during this interval. Non-specific treatment with antidiarrheal agents can also be tried cautiously. Supplementation of formulas with fiber may help solidify the stool and slow transit time in patients not receiving broad-spectrum antibiotics. The fiber contained in some commercial formulas (usually soy polysaccharide) has not been shown to reduce the incidence of diarrhea.

METABOLIC. Metabolic complications include abnormalities in fluid and electrolyte balance, hyperglycemia, trace element deficiencies, vitamin K deficiency, and abnormalities in protein tolerance.

Overhydration occurs in 20 to 25% of patients receiving enteral nutrition. Cardiac failure and renal insufficiency aggravate the problem and complicate its management. Slowing of the infusion rate or substitution of a 1.5- to 2-kcal/mL formula usually provides adequate treatment, and diuretics are rarely necessary for acute control. Although uncommon, hypertonic dehydration also can occur in patients fed calorie-dense formulas, especially when they cannot communicate their thirst.

Hyperglycemia occurs in 10 to 30% of tube-fed patients. High-calorie enteral diets may unmask adult-onset diabetes mellitus. Hyperglycemia is corrected by decreasing the formula flow rate, administering insulin, or implementing both of these measures. Because hyperglycemia can cause osmotic diuresis, the patient's fluid status must be carefully monitored.

Abnormalities of most electrolytes and trace elements have been reported. Routine screening of many of these substances permits early detection before clinical manifestations are apparent. Such screening is especially important in patients with renal, cardiac, or hepatic insufficiency.

INFECTIOUS. The most common infectious complication of enteral nutrition is aspiration pneumonia, which is potentially fatal. Its incidence varies from 1 to 44%, depending on how it is defined. Aspiration can occur subtly, without witnessed episodes of vomiting, and it should be suspected with new onset of tachycardia, tachypnea, fever, hypoxemia, or chest radiographic changes. Patients fed nasogastrically appear to have a higher likelihood of aspiration than do patients fed by gastrostomy or jejunostomy. Those with an endotracheal tube or a tracheostomy have an especially high risk. Feeding beyond the duodenum probably lowers the incidence of aspiration, although no conclusive evidence supports this premise.

Preventive measures include elevating the head of the bed to 30 degrees, periodic measuring of gastric residuals, and inflating endotracheal tube cuffs. Correct techniques to insert the soft feeding tubes and careful observation of the tube's position may prevent potentially lethal bronchopleural complications. A chest radiograph should be obtained before initiating feeding in every patient with a newly inserted nasogastric or nasoenteric tube if gastric contents cannot be withdrawn through the tube. Methods for detecting the

"silent" aspiration of enteral formulas in intubated patients include checking tracheal aspirates for the presence of glucose with the use of oxidant reagent strips or placing methylene blue dye in the formula as a potential marker in tracheal aspirates.

MECHANICAL. Mechanical complications associated with enteral nutrition generally relate to the tube itself or to its anatomic position. Nasoenteric tubes can cause nasopharyngeal erosions and discomfort, sinusitis, otitis media, gagging, esophagitis, esophageal reflux, tracheoesophageal fistulas, and rupture of esophageal varices. Feeding tubes can become knotted or clogged. Gastrostomy or jejunostomy tubes can cause mechanical obstruction of the pylorus or small bowel. Additional complications of percutaneous tubes include leakage around the tube, dislodgment to an intraperitoneal position, and occlusion, especially of small-bore needle-catheter jejunostomies.

Guenther PA, Settle RG, Perlmutter S, et al. Tube feeding–related diarrhea in acutely ill patients. JPEN J Parenter Enteral Nutr 15:277, 1991. *Review of the causes and potential treatments for diarrhea in patients receiving enteral nutrition.*
Moore FA, Feliciano DV, Andrassy RJ, et al. Early enteral feeding, compared with parenteral, reduces postoperative septic complications: The results of a metaanalysis. Ann Surg 216:172, 1992. *Review of published clinical trials of enteral nutrition versus TPN. Significant increases in infectious complications were noted in patients receiving TPN.*
Rombeau JL, Rolandelli RH (eds): Clinical Nutrition: Enteral and Tube Feeding. 3rd ed. Philadelphia, WB Saunders, 1997. *Detailed and extensively illustrated text includes scientific principles and practical clinical aspects of enteral nutrition.*
The Veterans Affairs Total Parenteral Nutrition Cooperative Study Group: Perioperative total parenteral nutrition in surgical patients. N Engl J Med 325:525, 1991. *Largest published prospective, controlled clinical trial of TPN. Significant increases in infectious complications were noted in patients receiving TPN.*

230 PARENTERAL NUTRITION

M. Molly McMahon

It was first appreciated in 1968 that patients could receive all of their nutritional requirements intravenously. This advance was a landmark in the field of nutrition and clinical medicine. Although parenteral nutrition can be essential or even life saving, its substantial cost and potential for complications necessitate judicious use.

DEFINITION. The term *parenteral nutrition* should be used in place of intravenous hyperalimentation, a term coined at a time when provision of an excess of calories was believed to be beneficial. Parenteral nutrition provides amino acids (nitrogen), dextrose (carbohydrate), fat, electrolytes, minerals, trace elements, vitamins, and water by central vein (central parenteral nutrition) or by peripheral vein (peripheral parenteral nutrition). The enteral route should always be selected for the provision of nutrition in malnourished patients with a functional gastrointestinal tract because the bowel atrophies when nutrients are provided exclusively by vein. In addition, when compared with parenteral nutrition, tube feeding is less expensive and associated with fewer metabolic complications and does not require a central venous catheter for feeding.

PARENTERAL NUTRITION CONTENT

PROTEIN. Nitrogen is required for protein synthesis and is thus an essential component of parenteral nutrition. All currently manufactured parenteral nutrition solutions use crystalline amino acids as the source of nitrogen. Each gram of protein provides 4.0 kcal. Protein solutions are available with or without added electrolytes and minerals. For a well-nourished healthy subject without stress, the recommended dietary allowance of protein is 0.8 g/kg/day, provided that total caloric intake is adequate. Although protein is a metabolic fuel, its structural functions are as important as its fuel functions. At steady state, protein oxidation equals protein intake. Therefore, caloric requirements should be estimated as total calories rather than as non-protein calories.

Protein breakdown and synthesis are dynamic processes. During severe illness, protein catabolism exceeds protein synthesis, and a net loss of body protein results. Body protein stores are minimal, and net protein loss results in a loss of tissue function. The increase in proteolysis is primarily caused by the actions of hormones and cytokines, with additional protein losses occurring in specific disease states. Diminished protein synthesis results from bed rest and decreased food intake. In general, hospitalized patients with normal renal and hepatic function should receive 1.0 to 1.5 g of protein per kilogram of body weight per day, with stressed patients requiring the higher amount. For the majority of patients, provision of greater amounts of protein does not provide benefit, and the excess protein results in ureagenesis. For obese patients (weight greater than 120% of ideal weight), it may be appropriate to provide 1.5 g of protein per kilogram of estimated ideal weight, although data to support this recommendation are limited. The administration of nutrition support to critically ill, immobilized patients can decrease but not prevent the loss of body protein.

Modified amino acid solutions have been formulated for use in specific disease states. For example, the use of branched-chain enriched amino acid solutions (providing up to 50% of amino acids as leucine, isoleucine, and valine) has been suggested for patients with hepatic encephalopathy. These patients have decreased plasma levels of branched-chain amino acids and increased levels of aromatic amino acids. Branched-chain amino acids are uniquely oxidized in skeletal muscle and adipose tissue rather than the liver. Several studies indicate that patients prone to encephalopathy can tolerate more protein being given as branched-chain enriched solutions than as the standard solution. However, the clinical effectiveness of formulas with high levels of branched-chain amino acids is controversial inasmuch as few prospective randomized trials have compared this treatment with standard therapy. Once the encephalopathy has resolved, the less costly standard amino acid solution should be used. Patients with liver disease but no encephalopathy can tolerate the less costly standard amino acid solutions. Limited data support the use of branched-chain amino acid solutions for patients with renal failure or severe stress.

Another example of a modified amino acid formulation is a more concentrated (15%) amino acid base solution. Use of this product enables higher caloric and protein supplementation in less volume to patients with excess total body water and salt. The disadvantages of this product are similar to those of branched-chain solutions: its expense and the lack of prospective, randomized trials confirming its efficacy. Parenteral nutrition supplementation with the amino acid glutamine is undergoing investigation. Currently, glutamine is not present in commercially available parenteral nutrition solutions in the United States because it has a shorter shelf life than the more commonly used amino acids and has been considered a nonessential amino acid. During critical illness, however, glutamine appears to be an essential amino acid for the intestinal tract. For patients undergoing bone marrow transplantation, the use of glutamine-supplemented parenteral nutrition (as compared with the standard amino acid solution) has been shown to improve clinical outcome with fewer infections and shortened hospital stay. Additional prospective randomized trials of these modified formulas are needed.

CARBOHYDRATE. Parenteral carbohydrate provided in the form of dextrose is a vital source of fuel and has important nitrogen-sparing effects. Solutions of dextrose in concentrations of 10 to 70% are mixed with the appropriate quantity of amino acids to obtain the desired solution. Each gram of hydrated dextrose monohydrate provides 3.4 kcal. The minimum daily glucose requirement is the amount necessary to meet brain glucose needs (100 to 150 g) because body carbohydrate stores are limited. Providing calories as glucose stimulates insulin secretion, reduces muscle protein breakdown, and decreases hepatic glucose release, thus decreasing the need for skeletal muscle to provide amino acid precursors for gluconeogenesis. Glucose oxidation is also stimulated, thus sparing the oxidation of amino acids.

INTRAVENOUS FAT EMULSION. Fat emulsions provide an intravenous source of fat calories and the essential linoleic and linolenic fatty acids. Currently, intravenous fat emulsions consist of 10% (1.1 kcal/mL) or 20% (2.0 kcal/mL) solutions. The emulsions contain long-chain fatty acids (derived from safflower and/or soybean oil), egg yolk phospholipids as emulsifying agents, and glycerin to make the solution isotonic with plasma. Intravenous fat is calorically dense (9 kcal/g), isotonic, and protein sparing and can prevent essential fatty acid deficiency. In addition, provision of a portion of calories as fat allows lower rates of dextrose infusion, which results in less hyperglycemia and hyperinsulinemia and a

lower incidence of abnormalities in liver function tests. The fat can be administered intravenously either by piggyback infusion or as a three-in-one admixture of fat, dextrose, and protein in one container. The fat emulsion is hydrolyzed by lipoprotein lipase to free fatty acids and glycerol. When fatty acids are oxidized for fuel, the respiratory quotient and therefore carbon dioxide production rates are lower than those observed if carbohydrate or protein is oxidized; this feature may be advantageous in certain clinical situations such as severe pulmonary disease.

Adverse effects, including hypoxemia, hepatic dysfunction, and impaired immune function from fat uptake by the reticuloendothelial system, have been reported with intravenous fat administration. At very high infusion rates, enzymatic removal systems for free fatty acids become saturated and hypertriglyceridemia can result. However, all of these effects have been demonstrated at the higher infusion rates achieved during 8- to 12-hour infusions rather than during 24-hour infusions. No data suggest that the continuous infusion of intravenous fat emulsion at recommended rates to normolipidemic patients results in any adverse effects. Thus continuous fat infusion is preferable to intermittent fat infusion. If the plasma triglyceride concentration exceeds 400 mg/dL, the intravenous fat emulsion infusion rate should be reduced or the infusion discontinued. Although the optimal percentage of calories that should be infused as fat is unclear, provision of 20 to 30% of total calories as fat is generally recommended for stressed patients receiving parenteral nutrition.

The role of fat extends beyond that of energy substrate alone inasmuch as substitution of different fat sources has been reported to beneficially modify the patient's response to illness. Active investigation is under way to determine the optimal type (e.g., medium-chain triglycerides, short-chain triglycerides, structured triglycerides, ω-3 fatty acids) and quantity of fat to be provided in parenteral nutrition solutions.

ELECTROLYTES, MINERALS, TRACE ELEMENTS, AND MULTIVITAMINS. The electrolytes and minerals required for health are sodium, potassium, chloride, calcium, phosphorus, magnesium, and sulfur. The electrolytes are supplied as salts, e.g., sodium chloride, potassium chloride, calcium gluconate, potassium phosphate, and magnesium sulfate, and provide maintenance intake for most adult patients. Most sodium and potassium cations are added to the parenteral nutrition solution as chloride or acetate salts after the phosphate requirement is met. Acetate is further metabolized by the liver to bicarbonate to provide an alkaline buffer.

Trace elements are commercially available as combination products or as single-item injections; 1 mL of a multiple trace element injection contains zinc, copper, manganese, and chromium in amounts that are suggested for medically stable adult patients (Table 230–1). This amount may be adjusted as needed for individual patients. Because iron, iodine, and selenium are not always added to parenteral nutrition solutions, monitoring of levels and supplementation of these trace elements may be required for patients receiving longer-term administration of parenteral nutrition.

The composition of intravenous multivitamin products has been established in accordance with the guidelines of the American Medical Association Nutrition Advisory Group. One adult multivitamin formulation and one pediatric multivitamin formulation are currently available commercially. The adult formulation provides the daily maintenance for three fat-soluble and nine water-soluble vitamins (Table 230–2). For patients requiring short-term nutrition, vitamin K is often not routinely added to parenteral nutrition solutions. Accordingly, the prothrombin time (International Normalized Ratio) should be monitored to determine whether vitamin K supplementation is needed. The daily multivitamin dose may be increased for patients with suspected or documented vitamin deficien-

Table 230–1 ■ STANDARD ADULT TRACE ELEMENT INJECTION

TRACE ELEMENT	AMOUNT PER DOSE PER DAY
Zinc	4 mg
Copper	0.8 mg
Manganese	0.4 mg
Chromium	8 μg
Selenium	48 μg

Table 230-2 ■ STANDARD ADULT MULTIVITAMIN INJECTION

VITAMIN	AMOUNT PER DOSE PER DAY
A (retinol)	3300 IU
D (ergocalciferol)	200 IU
E (dl-α-tocopheryl acetate)	10 IU
C (ascorbic acid)	100 mg
B₁ (thiamin)	3 mg
B₂ (riboflavin)	3.6 mg
B₆ (pyridoxine)	4 mg
B₁₂ (cyanocobalamin)	5 μg
Folic acid	400 μg
Niacin	40 mg
Pantothenic acid	15 mg
Biotin	60 μg

cies. Serious consequences can result from providing less than the standard replacement amounts of vitamins. During the recent nation-wide shortages of intravenous multivitamin preparations, several patients receiving thiamin-deficient parenteral nutrition died with refractory lactic acidosis, clinical courses suggestive of beriberi, and brain lesions diagnostic of acute thiamin deficiency.

INDICATIONS FOR NUTRITIONAL SUPPORT

MALNUTRITION. Protein catabolism (with eventual depletion of body protein leading to protein-calorie malnutrition) can be a consequence of starvation, severe illness, or a combination of the two. Malnutrition is difficult to define and thus inevitably arbitrary. The need for nutritional support in malnutrition is a reflection of the timing and extent of recent (previous 3- to 6-month interval) unintentional weight loss, the presence or absence of clinical markers of stress, and the anticipated time that the patient will be unable to meet nutritional requirements orally. Studies that have demonstrated a beneficial influence of nutritional support on clinical outcome have provided nutrition for a minimum of 1 week. Currently, no evidence suggests that nutrition support of briefer duration is beneficial. Additional research is needed to develop clinical markers for malnutrition and identify patients who will benefit from nutrition support.

DELIVERY OF PARENTERAL NUTRITION

INDICATIONS. Once it has been determined that nutrition support should be initiated, the route of nutrient delivery should be selected. Parenteral nutrition should be used whenever nutrition support is indicated in a patient with a non-functioning gastrointestinal tract. As examples, parenteral nutrition should be considered in malnourished patients with persistent distal bowel obstruction, serious gastrointestinal motility disorders combined with intolerance of tube feeding, short-bowel syndrome with insufficient intestinal adaptation to maintain nutritional status via the enteral route, and severe pancreatitis, as well as in patients in whom a feeding tube cannot be placed in the desired location. Although it is difficult to establish absolute criteria for the use of parenteral nutrition, the American Society for Parenteral and Enteral Nutrition has published guidelines for the general use of parenteral nutrition, as well as recommendations for its use in selected disease states. Once the decision has been made that parenteral nutrition is required, the clinician is faced with the challenge of selecting peripheral parenteral nutrition or central parenteral nutrition as the preferred form of nutrition.

PERIPHERAL VERSUS CENTRAL PARENTERAL NUTRITION: INDICATIONS, ADVANTAGES, AND LIMITATIONS. With the lower caloric and protein requirements that can be provided by this form of nutrition, peripheral parenteral nutrition may be considered in medically stable patients who require short-term (e.g., 7 to 10 days) parenteral nutrition. It is not possible to peripherally administer the high-osmolarity solutions used for central parenteral nutrition because of phlebitis. For this reason, the osmolarity of peripheral parenteral nutrition solutions should not exceed 1000 mOsm/L. The addition of isotonic lipid to dextrose and amino acids may enhance vein tolerance to peripheral parenteral nutrition solutions.

Peripheral parenteral nutrition avoids the use of central vein catheterization. However, there are limitations to the use of peripheral parenteral nutrition. The cost of the solution is similar to that of central parenteral nutrition solutions. Furthermore, critically ill patients will not tolerate the high volume rates required to meet nutrition needs. Central parenteral nutrition is necessary to provide adequate nutrition to patients who are moderately or severely stressed or who are anticipated to require longer use of parenteral support.

VASCULAR ACCESS. Selection of the site for catheter insertion should be individualized for each patient. Cannulation of a high-flow central vessel permits infusion of hyperosmolar nutrient solutions that are not tolerated by smaller low-flow peripheral veins. In general, the preferred site of central catheter insertion is the subclavian vein both for patient comfort and for ease of management. Central vein cannulation for parenteral nutrition should never be considered an emergency procedure. Coagulation studies should be checked before catheterization, and patients should be adequately hydrated. Sterile technique during catheter insertion is mandatory. Whereas placement of double- or triple-lumen catheters is appropriate in patients who require multiple infusions or hemodynamic monitoring in addition to parenteral nutrition, medically stable patients should receive nutrition via a single-lumen catheter. Before initiation of central parenteral nutrition, a chest radiograph should be obtained to confirm catheter tip location in the distal end of the superior vena cava.

A peripherally inserted central catheter for parenteral nutrition may be used effectively in selected adult patients. These radiopaque catheters, inserted in the basilic or cephalic vein via the antecubital fossa and advanced to the distal end of the superior vena cava for infusion of central parenteral nutrition, provide reliable venous access for medically stable patients requiring from 1 week to as long as 6 months of central parenteral nutrition. Early reports noted a high incidence of phlebitis with peripherally inserted central catheter use, but more recent studies report more favorable results. The use of peripherally inserted central catheters eliminates many of the risks associated with central venous catheter insertion.

ESTIMATION OF DAILY CALORIC REQUIREMENTS. The daily caloric requirement of patients can be estimated by use of a formula such as the Harris-Benedict equation or measured by indirect calorimetry (Table 230-3). For many years it was believed that patients requiring nutritional support had elevated caloric requirements, especially when stressed by surgery, trauma, or sepsis. Over the last decade, however, numerous studies have shown that the majority of hospitalized patients have surprisingly normal energy expenditure, usually between 100 and 120% of predicted caloric expenditure. As mentioned earlier, data about how to feed obese patients are limited. Some groups advocate provision of basal caloric requirements based on the obese weight, whereas other groups base the requirement on an adjusted weight.

Overfeeding of sick patients can result in serious sequelae. Excess calories can increase oxygen consumption, carbon dioxide production, minute ventilation, and the work of breathing, which can

Table 230-3 ■ GUIDELINES FOR ESTIMATING DAILY CALORIC, PROTEIN, AND FAT REQUIREMENTS OF HOSPITALIZED PATIENTS*

Calories†	Basal Harris-Benedict to Harris-Benedict plus 20%
Protein‡	1.0–1.5 g/kg body weight
Fat	20–30% of total calories during 24-hr infusion

Harris-Benedict equation:

Females: $65.5 + (9.6 \times \text{weight, kg}) + (1.8 \times \text{height, cm}) - (4.7 \times \text{age, yr})$

Males: $66.5 + (13.8 \times \text{weight, kg}) + (5.0 \times \text{height, cm}) - (6.8 \times \text{age, yr})$

*An indirect calorimetric measurement of daily caloric needs may be helpful in the following group of patients: severely stressed patients (e.g., following closed head injury, multiple trauma, severe burn), volume-overloaded patients in whom the "dry weight" estimate is uncertain, nutritionally supported patients in whom weaning from mechanical ventilation is difficult, or patients receiving home parenteral nutrition.

†If patient weight is 120% or more of ideal body weight, the basal Harris-Benedict estimate of caloric needs (based on current weight or adjusted weight) and 1.5 g of protein per kilogram (based on estimated ideal weight) may be adequate. Ideal body weight can be estimated by the following method: females, 45.4 kg for 1.5 m and 2.3 kg per additional 2.5 cm; males, 48.1 kg for 1.5 m and 2.7 kg per additional 2.5 cm.

‡Assumes normal or nearly-normal hepatic and renal function.

Modified from McMahon M, Farnell M, Murray M: Nutritional support of critically ill patients. Mayo Clin Proc 69:911, 1993.

fatigue patients with impaired lung function. Overfeeding can also cause hyperglycemia, which may adversely affect fluid balance and immune function. A growing body of clinical evidence links hyperglycemia to nosocomial infection in stressed hospitalized patients. Finally, excessive calories can cause abnormal liver test results.

To design a specific parenteral nutrition program, the clinician should first determine the appropriate volume for the individual patient, then estimate the caloric requirement, and finally estimate the protein and fat requirements. The remaining caloric requirements are provided as carbohydrate (Table 230–4).

MONITORING PARENTERAL NUTRITION. After initiation of parenteral nutrition, the patient's vital signs and laboratory values must be carefully monitored. The source of fever should always be investigated in a patient with a central venous catheter. Hemodynamic data, fluid balance, and creatinine, urea, and sodium should be reviewed to help determine the appropriate parenteral nutrition volume. Daily weight should be interpreted in light of the fluid balance; weight increases exceeding 0.25 kg over a 24-hour period usually reflect fluid gain.

Before initiation of parenteral nutrition, patients should have a recent glucose, sodium, potassium, creatinine, urea, aspartate aminotransferase, calcium, phosphorus, and albumin level determined. For patients with pancreatitis or poorly controlled diabetes mellitus or those receiving medications formulated in fat emulsion (e.g., propofol), a triglyceride level should be checked before initiation of fat emulsion. For patients with known hypertriglyceridemia, a triglyceride level should be checked before and during intravenous fat emulsion administration. Plasma magnesium, zinc, and copper levels should be measured in patients with impaired absorption or increased gastrointestinal (zinc, copper) or renal (magnesium) output. The calcium, magnesium, and zinc values should be interpreted with knowledge of the albumin level because they are albumin bound. In addition, plasma levels do not reflect tissue stores. The extent and frequency of biochemical monitoring following initiation of parenteral nutrition should be individualized; at a minimum, plasma glucose, electrolytes, and phosphorus levels should be checked until stable. During short-term hospitalization, a serum

---

Table 230–4 ■ **DESIGN OF PARENTERAL NUTRITION PROGRAMS: EXAMPLES**

Non-obese patient weighing 60 kg; assume basal Harris-Benedict equation estimate of daily caloric requirements of 1250 kcal/day

A. Patient characteristics:
  1. Euvolemic, normal urine output, and no unusual gastrointestinal losses; therefore, appropriate initial estimate of daily fluid requirement is 30 mL/kg body weight
  2. Moderately stressed with normal renal and hepatic function; therefore, appropriate to provide 1.2 g protein per kg body weight
  3. Non-obese; therefore, appropriate to provide Harris-Benedict estimate plus 20% for calories, i.e., 1250 plus 20% = 1500 kcal
B. Program design:
  1. Fluid requirement: 30 mL times body weight; 30 times 60 = 1800 mL
  2. Caloric requirement: Harris-Benedict estimate plus 20%; 1250 plus 250 = 1500 kcal
  3. Protein requirement for moderately stressed patient: 1.2 g/kg body weight; 60 times 1.2 = ~70 g protein. 70 g protein times 4 kcal/g protein = 280 kcal
  4. Fat requirement: 30% of total calories; 30% times 1500 kcal = 450 kcal
  5. Carbohydrate requirement: caloric requirement minus the sum of protein and fat calories; 1500 minus (280 plus 450 kcal) = 770 kcal. 770 kcal carbohydrate divided by kcal/g carbohydrate (3.4) = ~225 g carbohydrate
  6. Therefore, consider the following PN formula: 1.5 L amino acids, 5%, dextrose, 15%, plus 250 mL of 20% fat emulsion, which provides 1750 mL, 1565 kcal, 75 g protein, 225 g carbohydrate, and 500 fat calories. Note that amino acids, 5%, equals 50 g protein per liter.
  7. If institution uses 3-in-1 admixture compounding (amino acids plus dextrose plus fat in one container and stock solutions of amino acids, 10%, dextrose, 70%, and lipid, 20%), a comparable PN program would be 1.5 L amino acids, 5%, dextrose, 15%, fat, 3.5%
C. Similar patient characteristics except patients volume-expanded:
  1. Consider the following fluid-restricted PN formula: 1 L of amino acids, 7%, dextrose, 20%, plus 250 mL 20% fat emulsion which provides 1250 mL, 1460 calories, 70 g protein, 200 g carbohydrate, and 500 fat calories

PN = parenteral nutrition.

---

glucose goal range of 100 to 200 mg/dL is appropriate. If glucose values exceed 180 to 200 mg/dL, regular insulin may be added to the parenteral nutrition admixture. Initiation of a subcutaneous regular insulin algorithm is often necessary. If glycemic control cannot be achieved with parenteral nutrition supplementation of insulin and the regular insulin algorithm, a separate insulin infusion should be considered.

Parenteral nutrition should not constitute the sole treatment of acute abnormalities in volume or electrolyte disturbances, but it is an effective vehicle to replace chronic losses. Knowledge of the volume of gastrointestinal and renal losses allows an estimation of electrolyte and mineral losses and appropriate parenteral nutrition supplementation. A daily review of the medication profile is essential to anticipate and manage metabolic status (e.g., amphotericin: hypokalemia, hypomagnesemia, renal tubular acidosis; corticosteroids: hyperglycemia, hypokalemia; insulin: hypokalemia, hypophosphatemia, hypomagnesemia; diuretics: hypokalemia, hypomagnesemia, metabolic alkalosis; propofol: this anesthetic agent is in a 10% fat emulsion, and its administration may temporarily eliminate or decrease the requirement for additional fat). The acetate and chloride content of the parenteral nutrition admixture should be adjusted for acid-base disturbances. Acetate and chloride balance is best assessed by reviewing the blood gas (arterial or venous) and electrolyte results and by the volume of gastrointestinal or renal losses. For example, the parenteral nutrition acetate content may be increased and the chloride content decreased in metabolic acidosis; the converse is true for metabolic alkalosis. Although the extent of the daily examination must be individualized, the catheter site, heart, and lungs should always be examined and the possible development of peripheral edema assessed. Use of a patient monitoring record that combines information about the composition of the parenteral nutrition solution with biochemical data facilitates prompt recognition of metabolic abnormalities. The daily goal is to determine whether the parenteral nutrition program (volume or composition) needs modification in light of the patient's current condition. Once the gastrointestinal tract regains function, the enteral route should always be used for nutrition.

VOLUME-RESTRICTED PARENTERAL NUTRITION. Patients with excess total body water and salt following major surgery or illness are often those most in need of nutrition support. The ability to concentrate medications, intravenous infusions, and central parenteral nutrition solutions may allow earlier and more adequate nutrition support. By using concentrated commercial solutions of 10% amino acids and 70% dextrose, 1 L can, for example, provide 70 g protein and 200 g dextrose (960 total calories) (see Table 230–4). Fat should be added when a larger volume can be tolerated. To further restrict volume, the parenteral nutrition admixture may be used as a vehicle for drugs with a stable dose requirement, provided that therapeutic efficacy has been documented for continuous drug infusion. Medications commonly added to the parenteral nutrition admixture include histamine receptor antagonists and regular insulin.

COMPLICATIONS

The complications associated with parenteral nutrition can be categorized into catheter related (mechanical, infectious, and thrombotic), metabolic, and gastrointestinal. Studies have demonstrated that the use of organized interdisciplinary nutrition support teams reduces complications.

Pneumothorax, the most common mechanical complication, is most often related to improper central vein cannulation technique. Anatomic factors (such as cachexia, barrel chest deformity, kyphosis, and morbid obesity) can increase the risk even with satisfactory technique. An important predictor of complications associated with central catheter insertion is the physician's experience in catheter insertion.

Catheter malposition is generally not serious if recognized early. Misdirection most often involves a subclavian catheter traveling up the ipsilateral internal jugular vein. The catheter can usually be repositioned by either the catheter guidewire technique or fluoroscopic manipulation. Other uncommon complications related to catheter placement are air embolism, subclavian or internal carotid artery puncture, hemothorax, hemomediastinum, catheter embolism, thoracic duct injury, and brachial plexus injury.

Bacteremia and fungemia are serious complications, and the catheter should always be evaluated as a potential source of infection. Most catheter-related septicemias begin with focal infections of the catheter wound; organisms from the patient's own cutaneous flora invade the intracutaneous tract when the catheter is inserted and thereafter. Hub contamination may also cause catheter-related septicemia. In addition, hematogenous seeding of the fibrin sheath on the catheter tip can occur during an episode of bacteremia or fungemia. Sterile technique and the use of effective antiseptics during catheter insertion are the most important measures to prevent catheter sepsis.

The two types of infection that occur most often are catheter infection and catheter-related septicemia. Quantitative cultures of the external surface of the catheter differentiate infection from contamination more reliably than the broth culture method does. Infection is diagnosed when culture of the catheter grows more than 15 colony-forming units. Catheter-related septicemia is diagnosed by semiquantitative catheter cultures and blood cultures that are positive for the same species. The most common organisms that cause catheter-related sepsis are coagulase-negative staphylococci, *Staphylococcus aureus,* and yeast. In selected circumstances (unexplained fever or leukocytosis), replacement of the catheter by guidewire exchange technique is appropriate. Catheters should always be removed immediately if patients appear septic. Blood (peripheral and central) and catheter cultures should always be performed; if applicable, the catheter site should also be cultured. New types of catheters and cuffs are being developed to reduce the risk of device-related infection.

Although subclinical venous thrombosis commonly occurs in patients receiving central parenteral nutrition, clinically significant thrombosis is uncommon during short-term nutrition use. The incidence of thrombosis, however, is greater in patients receiving long-term parenteral nutrition. The diagnosis should always be considered when swelling develops in the arm and neck ipsilateral to the catheter and swollen veins develop in the neck. The use of very low doses of heparin (5000 to 6000 U in parenteral nutrition per day) or warfarin (approximately 1 mg/day) can reduce the incidence of central vein thrombosis without causing adverse hemorrhagic effects and should be considered for patients requiring long-term parenteral nutrition.

Serious metabolic disturbances can result from providing parenteral calories in excess of needs, the exclusive use of dextrose as the caloric source, or an excess or deficiency of nutrients. Serious and life-threatening complications of sudden refeeding, coined the refeeding syndrome, have been recognized since the advent of parenteral nutrition therapy. The refeeding risk increases when chronically malnourished patients are too rapidly refed. The acute increase in plasma insulin concentration caused by feeding can lead to severe hypokalemia, hypomagnesemia, and hypophosphatemia if replacement is inadequate. Hyperinsulinemia promotes the passage of potassium from the extracellular space into the intracellular space and results in hypokalemia. Glucose- and insulin-stimulated glycolysis enhances cellular uptake and the use of phosphorus for the phosphorylation of glycolytic intermediates and for adenosine triphosphate synthesis. Hyperinsulinemia can also increase tissue uptake of magnesium with subsequent hypomagnesemia. The adverse sequelae resulting from hypokalemia, hypophosphatemia, and hypomagnesemia are discussed in Chapters 102.3, 222, and 223. In addition, acute hyperinsulinemia promotes renal tubular reabsorption of sodium, which can expand the extracellular fluid and provoke cardiac decompensation in extremely malnourished patients with decreased left ventricular mass. Patients receiving long-term parenteral nutrition are at increased risk for metabolic bone disease.

Hepatic abnormalities, the most common gastrointestinal complication associated with parenteral nutrition, may be caused by the therapy itself or by the patient's underlying disease or medications. In adults, parenteral nutrition–related hepatic abnormalities are common and are generally benign and temporary. Some patients requiring long-term parenteral nutrition, however, have persisting abnormalities in liver function tests associated with fibrotic and/or cholestatic damage. Complications may be biochemical (elevation of serum aminotransferase, alkaline phosphatase, or bilirubin) or

histologic (steatosis, portal triaditis). Transaminase elevations generally occur early in therapy (1 to 2 weeks after initiation of parenteral nutrition) and often resolve without change in the program. Bilirubin and alkaline phosphatase elevations usually appear slightly later (2 to 3 weeks into therapy). Although the etiology of parenteral nutrition–related hepatic abnormalities has not been clearly elucidated, many factors have been proposed, including the parenteral nutrition solution (excessive dextrose or total calories or fat-free parenteral nutrition), nutritional deficiencies (carnitine, taurine, essential fatty acid deficiency), and cholestasis. Biliary complications associated with parenteral nutrition include acalculous cholecystitis, gallbladder sludge, and cholelithiasis. Sludge, the most common of these complications, occurs when the gastrointestinal tract is not used. Abnormal liver function test results should not automatically lead to stopping or altering the parenteral nutrition solution inasmuch as abnormal liver function results may not represent true liver dysfunction. Other causes of abnormal hepatic function, such as extrahepatic obstruction, medications, or infection, should be excluded. The nutrition program should be reviewed to be certain that the caloric intake is not excessive and that a mixed-fuel system (i.e., dextrose, protein, and fat) is being infused.

Parenteral nutrition is an essential form of nutrition for malnourished patients with non-functioning gastrointestinal tracts. An understanding of the indications for use, appreciation of the significant cost and potential complications, and the ability to design a nutrition program and monitoring plan are important to effective use of this therapy. Future prospective randomized trials are needed to establish outcome data in appropriate patient groups. Evidence is accumulating that the use of alternative fuel sources may beneficially modify the body's response to illness; this concept is stimulating research that may expand the role of nutritional support.

ASPEN: Guidelines for the use of parenteral and enteral nutrition in adult and pediatric patients. JPEN J Parenter Enteral Nutr 17(Suppl.):1, 1993. *Position statement providing concise guidelines (and recent references) for the use of parenteral nutrition.*

Klein S, Kinney J, Jeejeebhoy K, et al: Nutrition support in clinical practice. Review of published data and recommendations for future research directions. Am J Clin Nutr 66:683, 1997. *Summarizes the current literature evaluating the clinical use of nutrition support.*

McMahon M, Farnell MB, Murray MJ: Nutritional support of critically ill patients. Mayo Clin Proc 68:911, 1993. *Review of the pathophysiology of malnutrition and the principles of nutrition assessment, nutrition program design, and monitoring of hospitalized patients receiving nutrition support.*

231 CONSEQUENCES OF ALTERED MICRONUTRIENT STATUS

Joel B. Mason

Micronutrients are a highly diverse array of dietary components necessary to sustain health. The physiologic roles of micronutrients are as varied as their composition: Some are used in enzymes as either coenzymes or prosthetic groups, others are used as biochemical substrates or hormones, and in some instances, the functions are not well defined. Under normal circumstances, the average daily dietary intake for each micronutrient required to sustain normal physiologic operations is measured in milligrams or smaller quantities. This quantification distinguishes micronutrients from macronutrients, the latter category encompassing carbohydrates, fats, and proteins, as well as the macrominerals calcium, magnesium, and phosphorus.

For homeostasis to proceed properly, most dietary nutrients must be ingested in quantities that are neither too small nor too great. Disorders may arise when this "physiologic window" is either not met or exceeded. The size of the window varies for each micronutrient and should be kept in mind, particularly in present-day circumstances when the administration of large quantities of certain micronutrients is being increasingly explored for possible therapeutic implications. Many factors determine the dietary requirement for a particular micronutrient, only one of which is the amount needed to sustain those physiologic functions for which it is used (Table

Physiologic Factors
1. *Bioavailability:* the proportion of an ingested micronutrient that can be assimilated and used for physiologic purposes
2. Quantity required to fulfill physiologic roles
3. Extent to which the body can reuse the micronutrient
4. Distribution of nutrient in the body: storage compartments, etc.
5. Influence of gender
6. Stage of life cycle: intrauterine development, childhood, adulthood, elder adulthood, pregnancy, lactation

Pathophysiologic and Pharmacologic Factors
1. Inborn errors of metabolism that variously affect assimilation, utilization, or excretion of micronutrients
2. Acquired disease states that alter the amounts required to sustain homeostasis (e.g., malabsorption, maldigestion, states that increase utilization)
3. Lifestyle habits, e.g., smoking, ethanol consumption
4. Drugs: may alter bioavailability and/or utilization

231–1). The *U.S. Recommended Daily Allowances* (RDAs) provide dietary guidelines that indicate how much of each nutrient is "adequate to meet the known nutrient needs of practically all healthy persons"; the RDAs are listed in Table 224–1). Adequate intake, which is the amount necessary to prevent a deficiency state, is not necessarily synonymous with optimal intake, an issue this chapter discusses in more detail.

SALIENT FEATURES OF VITAMINS AND TRACE ELEMENTS: TRADITIONAL PERSPECTIVES

VITAMINS. Vitamins have long been categorized as either fat soluble (A, D, E, K) or water soluble (all the others) (Table 231–2). Such differentiation remains a physiologically meaningful manner of categorization. None of the fat-soluble vitamins appear to serve as a coenzyme. Their absorption is primarily through a micellar route, and pathophysiologic conditions associated with fat malabsorption are frequently associated with selective deficiencies of the fat-soluble vitamins. In contrast, most water-soluble vitamins function as coenzymes. Furthermore, the water-soluble vitamins are not absorbed through the lipophilic phase in the intestine.

TRACE ELEMENTS. Fifteen trace elements have been identified as essential for health in animal studies: iron, zinc, copper, chromium, selenium, iodine, fluorine, manganese, molybdenum, cobalt, nickel, tin, silicon, vanadium, and arsenic. Nevertheless, only for the first 10 of these elements is there compelling evidence of essentialness in humans (Table 231–3). Cobalt seems to be essential solely as a component of vitamin B_{12}; an isolated deficiency state has never been described. Deficiency syndromes for several of the other essential trace elements were not recognized until recently because of their exceedingly small requirements and their ubiquitous nature in foodstuffs. Only under exceptional circumstances, such as long-term dependence on total parenteral nutrition (TPN) that lacked the elements (a situation that has since been corrected), have some of the deficiency syndromes been observed.

The biochemical functions of trace elements have not been as well characterized as those for the vitamins, but most of their functions appear to be as components of prosthetic groups or as cofactors for a number of enzymes. Determination of essential trace element status is problematic except for iron, selenium, and iodine. The vanishingly low concentrations of these elements in body fluids and tissues, the fact that blood levels frequently do not correlate well with levels in the target tissues, and the fact that functional tests cannot be devised until biochemical functions are better understood preclude an accurate and convenient laboratory method of assessment for most of the trace elements.

CONDITIONS THAT INCREASE THE REQUIRED DIETARY INTAKE FOR VITAMINS AND MINERALS

Many physiologic, pathophysiologic, and pharmacologic factors increase the dietary requirements for micronutrients (see Table 231–1), and these factors, when compounded, enhance the risk of development of a deficiency state.

PHYSIOLOGIC FACTORS. Stages of the life cycle have an important impact on the requirements of certain nutrients. Phases of rapid growth and development, such as in utero development, infancy, adolescence, and pregnancy, are associated with remarkable increases in the utilization of certain micronutrients on a per-kilogram basis. Requirements for most micronutrients increase in pregnancy; those for iron and folate are particularly increased because of the rapid proliferation of placental and fetal tissue. Periods of lactation are similarly associated with remarkable increases in requirements. A lactating woman experiences disproportionately large increases in her requirements for zinc and vitamins A, E, and C, in addition to the needs for pregnancy, to meet the metabolic demands incurred by milk production.

Infancy carries with it particular vulnerabilities to specific micronutrient inadequacies: Healthy infants in the United States are typically supplemented with vitamin K at birth and with iron and vitamin D during the course of the first year because of their particular susceptibility to deficiencies of these nutrients.

The ability to maintain adequate iron status from menarche through menopause is compromised in women by the additional losses incurred by menstruation, pregnancy, and lactation. As a result, the highest rate of iron deficiency affects women of childbearing age.

Specific dietary recommendations for the elderly have not yet been formally adopted, but such recommendations will inevitably appear because aging also affects the requirements for certain micronutrients. Vitamin B_{12} status, for instance, declines significantly with aging because of the high prevalence of atrophic gastritis and its associated impairment in protein-bound B_{12} absorption. The average decline is big enough to put a measurable proportion of the elderly population at risk of clinically important B_{12} deficiency and thus warrants an increase in B_{12} intake in this age group. Elderly persons, particularly those institutionalized for a long time, are also susceptible to vitamin D deficiency; increased intake is therefore indicated. The causes include diminished cutaneous synthesis of vitamin D by senile skin and decreased sun exposure, as well as smaller dietary intake in many instances.

PATHOPHYSIOLOGIC AND PHARMACOLOGIC FACTORS. Intestinal malabsorptive and maldigestive states predispose to multiple micronutrient deficiencies. Both fat-soluble and water-soluble micronutrients are absorbed predominantly in the proximal portion of the small intestine, the only exception being vitamin B_{12}. Diffuse mucosal diseases that affect the proximal portion of the gastrointestinal tract are therefore very likely to result in deficiencies. Even in the absence of mucosal disease of the proximal part of the small intestine, however, extensive ileal disease, small bowel bacterial overgrowth, and chronic cholestasis can each interfere with maintenance of adequate intraluminal conjugated bile acid concentrations and thereby impair absorption of fat-soluble vitamins. Maldigestion is usually the result of chronic pancreatitis. Untreated, it frequently causes malabsorption and deficiencies of fat-soluble vitamins. Vitamin B_{12} malabsorption can often be demonstrated in this setting and is a result of inadequate R-protein digestion, but clinical B_{12} deficiency is rarely reported in patients with pancreatitis.

A myriad of rare inborn errors of metabolism that impair an individual's ability to assimilate, use, or retain a particular vitamin or mineral have been described. Such defects are usually partial and can often be overcome, at least in part, by administering doses of the nutrient that are several degrees of magnitude greater than usually required. Suspicion for such defects should be entertained if (1) a known defect exists in the family, (2) a deficiency syndrome arises at birth or during infancy, and (3) the deficiency syndrome is present despite adequate dietary intake and the absence of any disease that would impair the ability to assimilate the nutrient.

The long-term administration of many drugs may adversely affect micronutrient status and may either induce an overt deficiency syndrome or predispose to one. The manner in which drug-nutrient interactions occur varies; some of the more common mechanisms are outlined in Table 231–4. Some drugs exert their therapeutic effects by specifically inhibiting the actions of a micronutrient. Examples include coumarin, which inhibits γ-carboxylation reactions mediated by vitamin K, and methotrexate, which binds tightly to dihydrofolate reductase, thereby inhibiting folate metabolism.

Tobacco smoking alters the metabolism of several micronutrients, including folate, β-carotene, and vitamins C and E. In large surveys, diminished plasma levels of folate and ascorbic acid have been observed in long-time smokers. Smoking is also associated with diminished levels of folate in cells of the oral mucosa, diminished ascorbic acid levels in leukocytes, and decreased concentrations of vitamin E in lung alveolar fluid.

NEW FRONTIERS IN MARGINAL DEFICIENCY STATES

REDEFINING THE CONCEPT OF NUTRIENT DEFICIENCY. An important evolution in the understanding of micronutrient requirements has occurred over the past century: As nutritional science has expanded its appreciation for additional physiologic functions

of micronutrients, an ever-increasing need to redefine the concept of deficiency has ensued. The original means by which the necessary intake of these nutrients was defined was typically based on a disease entity that occurred as a result of flagrant deficiency of the nutrient, the so-called classic deficiency syndrome. In retrospect, this concept was naive because it is now evident that most, if not all micronutrients serve important functions in a wide variety of distinct biochemical systems. As the science of nutrition has come to appreciate this diversity in function, new deficiency syndromes are being defined.

Nevertheless, redefinition of micronutrient deficiencies and re-

Table 231-2 ■ VITAMINS AND THEIR FUNCTIONS

FAT-SOLUBLE VITAMINS

	Biochemistry and Physiology	Deficiency	Toxicity	Assessment of Status
Vitamin A	A subset of the retinoid compounds with biologic activity qualitatively similar to that of retinol. Carotenoids are structurally related to retinoids. Some carotenoids, most notably β-carotene, are metabolized into compounds with vitamin A activity and are considered to be provitamin A compounds. Vitamin A is an integral component of rhodopsin and iodopsin, light-sensitive proteins in retinal rod and cone cells.	Follicular hyperkeratosis and night blindness are early indicators. Conjunctival xerosis, degeneration of the cornea (*keratomalacia*), and dedifferentiation of rapidly proliferating epithelia indicate more severe deficiency. *Bitot spots* (focal areas of the conjunctiva or cornea with a foamy appearance) are an indication of xerosis. Blindness, due to corneal destruction and retinal dysfunction, ensues if left uncorrected. Increased susceptibility to infection also a consequence.	In adults, >500,000 IU may cause *acute* toxicity: intracranial hypertension, skin exfoliation, and hepatocellular necrosis. *Chronic* toxicity may occur with habitual daily intake of >25,000 IU: alopecia, ataxia, dermatitis, pseudotumor cerebri, hepatocellular necrosis, and hyperlipidemia. Daily ingestion of >15,000 IU during early pregnancy can be teratogenic. Excessive intake of most carotenoids causes a benign, yellowish discoloration of the skin. Large doses of canthaxanthin, a carotenoid, can induce retinopathy.	Retinol concentrations in plasma as well as vitamin A concentrations in milk and tears are reasonably accurate measures. Toxicity best assessed by elevated levels of retinyl esters in plasma. Quantitative measures of dark adaptation for night vision and electroretinograms are useful functional tests.
Vitamin D	A group of sterol compounds whose parent structure is cholecalciferol (vitamin D_3). Cholecalciferol is formed in the skin from 7-dehydrocholesterol by exposure to UV-B radiation. A plant sterol, ergocalciferol, can be similarly converted into vitamin D_2 and has similar vitamin D activity. Maintains intracellular and extracellular concentrations of calcium and phosphate by enhancing intestinal absorption of the two ions and, in conjunction with parathormone, promoting their mobilization from bone mineral.	Deficiency results in *rickets* in childhood and *osteomalacia* in adults. Expansion of the epiphyseal growth plates and replacement of normal bone with unmineralized bone matrix are the cardinal features. Deformity of bone and pathologic fractures occur. Serum concentrations of calcium and phosphate may decline.	Excess amounts result in abnormally high serum concentrations of calcium and phosphate; metastatic calcifications, renal damage, and altered mentation may ensue.	The serum concentration of the major circulating metabolite, 25-hydroxyvitamin D, indicates systemic status, except in chronic renal failure, in which the impairment in renal 1-hydroxylation results in disassociation of the monohydroxy- and dihydroxyvitamin concentrations. Measuring the serum concentration of 1,25-dihydroxyvitamin D is then necessary.
Vitamin E	A group of at least 8 naturally occurring compounds that share a spectrum of biologic activities. Some are tocopherols and some are tocotrienols. The most biologically active of the vitameric forms is α-tocopherol. Acts as an antioxidant and free radical scavenger in lipophilic environments, most notably in cell membranes. Acts in conjunction with other antioxidants such as selenium.	Deficiency due to dietary inadequacy rare in developed countries. Usually affects premature infants, individuals with fat malabsorption, and persons with abetalipoproteinemia. RBC fragility can produce hemolytic anemia. Neuronal degeneration produces peripheral neuropathies, ophthalmoplegia, and destruction of posterior columns of the spinal cord. Neurologic disease frequently irreversible if deficiency is not corrected early enough. May contribute to hemolytic anemia and retrolental fibroplasia in premature infants.	Depressed levels of vitamin K–dependent procoagulants and potentiation of oral anticoagulants have been reported, as has impaired leukocyte function. Doses of ≥50 IU/d may slightly increase the incidence of hemorrhagic stroke.	Plasma or serum concentration of α-tocopherol is most commonly used. Additional accuracy is obtained by expressing this value per mg of total plasma lipid. The RBC peroxide hemolysis test is not entirely specific, but is a useful functional measure of antioxidant potential of cell membranes.
Vitamin K	A family of naphthoquinone compounds with similar biologic activity. Phylloquinone (vitamin K_1) is derived from plants; a variety of menaquinones (vitamin K_2) are derived from bacterial sources. Serves as an essential cofactor in the post-translational α- or γ- carboxylation of glutamic acid residues in many proteins. These proteins include several circulating procoagulants and anticoagulants, as well as proteins in the bone matrix and renal epithelium.	Deficiency syndrome uncommon except in (1) breast-fed newborns, in whom it may cause "hemorrhagic disease of the newborn"; (2) adults with fat malabsorption or who are taking drugs that interfere with vitamin K metabolism (e.g., coumarin, phenytoin, broad-spectrum antibiotics); and (3) individuals taking large doses of vitamin E and anticoagulant drugs. Excessive hemorrhage is the usual manifestation.	Rapid intravenous infusion of K_1 has been associated with dyspnea, flushing, and cardiovascular collapse, probably related to dispersing agents in the solution. Supplementation may interfere with coumarin-based anticoagulation. Pregnant women taking large amounts of the provitamin menadione may deliver infants with hemolytic anemia, hyperbilirubinemia, and kernicterus.	The prothrombin time is typically used as a measure of functional vitamin K status; it is neither sensitive nor specific for vitamin K deficiency. Determination of undercarboxylated prothrombin or PIVKA II (proteins induced in vitamin K absence or antagonism) in plasma is more accurate but less widely available.

Table 231-2 ■ VITAMINS AND THEIR FUNCTIONS *Continued*

FAT-SOLUBLE VITAMINS

	Biochemistry and Physiology	Deficiency	Toxicity	Assessment of Status
Thiamine (vitamin B$_1$)	A water-soluble compound containing substituted pyrimidine and thiazole rings and a hydroxyethyl side chain. The coenzyme form is thiamine pyrophosphate (TPP). Serves as a coenzyme in many α-keto-acid decarboxylation and transketolation reactions. Inadequate thiamine availability leads to impairment of the above reactions and consequently to inadequate ATP synthesis and abnormal carbohydrate metabolism. May have an additional role in neuronal conduction independent of above-mentioned actions.	Classic deficiency syndrome ("beriberi") described in Asian populations consuming a polished rice diet. Alcoholism and chronic renal dialysis are also common precipitants. High carbohydrate intake increases need for B$_1$. Deficiency produces various combinations of peripheral neuropathy are cardiovascular and cerebral dysfunction. Cardiovascular involvement ("wet beriberi") includes congestive heart failure and low peripheral vascular resistance. See Chapter 48 for neurologic changes. Deficiency syndrome responds to parenteral thiamine, but is at least partially irreversible after a certain stage.	Excess intake is largely excreted in the urine although parenteral doses >400 mg/d are reported to cause lethargy, ataxia, and reduced tone of the gastrointestinal tract.	The most effective measure of B$_1$ status is the erythrocyte transketolase activity coefficient, which measures enzyme activity before and after addition of exogenous TPP: RBCs from a deficient individual express a substantial increase in enzyme activity with addition of TPP. Thiamine concentrations in the blood or urine are also used.
Riboflavin (vitamin B$_2$)	A compound consisting of a substituted isoalloxazine ring with a ribitol side chain. Serves as a coenzyme for diverse biochemical reactions. The primary coenzymatic forms are flavin mononucleotide and flavin adenine dinucleotide. Riboflavin holoenzymes participate in oxidation-reduction reactions in myriad metabolic pathways.	Deficiency is usually found in conjunction with deficiencies of other B vitamins. Isolated deficiency of riboflavin produces hyperemia and edema of nasopharyngeal mucosa, cheilosis, angular stomatitis, glossitis, seborrheic dermatitis, and a normochromic, normocytic anemia.	Toxicity not reported in humans.	The most common assessment is determining the activity coefficient of glutathione reductase in RBCs (the test is invalid for individuals with glucose-6-phosphate dehydrogenase deficiency). Measurements of blood and urine concentrations are less desirable methods.
Niacin (vitamin B$_3$)	Refers to nicotinic acid and the corresponding amide nicotinamide. The active coenzymatic forms are composed of nicotinamide affixed to adenine dinucelotide to form NAD or NADP. Over 200 apoenzymes use these coenzymes as electron acceptors or hydrogen donors. The essential amino acid tryptophan is used as a precursor of niacin; 60 mg of dietary tryptophan yields approximately 1 mg of niacin. Dietary requirements depend partly on the tryptophan content of diet.	*Pellagra* is the classic deficiency syndrome and often affects populations where corn is the major source of energy. Still endemic in parts of China, Africa, and India. Diarrhea, dementia (or symptoms of anxiety or insomnia), and the pigmented dermatitis that develops in sun-exposed areas are typical. Glossitis, stomatitis, vaginitis, vertigo, and burning dysesthesias are early signs. Seen also in carcinoid syndrome, which diverts tryoptophan to other synthetic pathways.	Human toxicity known largely through studies examining hypolipidemic effects. Includes vasomotor phenomenon (flushing), hyperglycemia, parenchymal liver damage, and hyperuricemia.	Assessment is problematic: Blood levels of vitamin not reliable. Measurements of urinary excretion of the niacin metabolites *N*-methylnicotinamide and 2-pyridone are thought to be the most effective means of assessment at present.
Vitamin B$_6$	Refers to several derivatives of pyridine, including pyridoxine, pyridoxal, and pyridoxamine. The co enzymatic forms are pyridoxal-5-phosphate (PLP) and pyridoxamine-5-phosphate. As a coenzyme, B$_6$ is involved in many transamination reactions (and thereby in gluconeogenesis), in the synthesis of niacin from tryptophan, and in the synthesis of several neurotransmitters, and δ-aminolevulinic acid (and therefore in heme synthesis).	Deficiency usually seen in conjunction with other water-soluble vitamin deficiencies. Stomatitis, angular cheilosis, glossitis, irritability, depression, and confusion occur in moderate to severe depletion; normochromic, normocytic anemia has been reported in severe deficiency. Abnormal EEGs and, in infants, convulsions have been observed. Some sideroblastic anemias respond to B$_6$ administration. Isoniazid, cycloserine, penicillamine, ethanol, and theophylline can inhibit B$_6$ metabolism.	Chronic use with doses exceeding 200 mg/d (in adults) may cause peripheral neuropathies and photosensitivity.	Many laboratory methods of assessment exist. Plasma or erythrocyte PLP levels are most common. Urinary excretion of xanthurenic acid after an oral tryptophan load or activity indices of RBC alanine or aspartic acid transaminases (ALT and AST, respectively) all functional measures of B$_6$-independent enzyme activity.
Folate	A group of over 35 related pterin compounds. The fully oxidized form, folic acid, is not found in nature but is the pharmacologic form of the vitamin. All folate functions relate to their ability to transfer one-carbon groups. The step is essential in the de novo synthesis of nucleotides and in the metabolism of several amino acids and is an integral component for regeneration of the "universal" methyl donor *S*-adenosylmethionine. Inhibition of bacterial and cancer cell folate metabolism is the basis for the sulfonamide antibiotics and chemotherapeutic agents such as methotrexate and 5-fluorouracil.	Women of childbearing age are the most likely individuals to have a deficiency. The "classic" deficiency syndrome is megaloblastic anemia. The hematopoietic cells in the bone marrow develop megaloblastic features reflecting ineffective DNA synthesis. The peripheral blood smear demonstrates macro-ovalocytes and polymorphonuclear leukocytes with an average of more than 3.5 nuclear lobes. Megaloblastic changes in the oral and gastrointestinal epithelia often occur and produce glossitis and diarrhea, respectively. Sulfasalazine and phenytoin inhibit absorption and predispose to deficiency.	Dose >400 μg/d may partially correct the anemia of B$_{12}$ deficiency and mask (and perhaps exacerbate) the associated neuropathy. Doses >400 μg are also reported to lower the seizure threshold in individuals prone to seizures. Rarely, parenteral administration is reported to cause allergic phenomena, but the allergy symptoms are probably due to dispersion agents.	Serum folate measures short-term folate balance, whereas RBC folate better reflects tissue status. Serum homocysteine rises early in deficiency but is non-specific because B$_{12}$, deficiency or renal insufficiency also may cause elevations.

Table continued on following page

Table 231–2 ■ VITAMINS AND THEIR FUNCTIONS *Continued*

FAT-SOLUBLE VITAMINS

	Biochemistry and Physiology	Deficiency	Toxicity	Assessment of Status
Vitamin C (ascorbic and dehydroascorbic acid)	Ascorbic acid readily oxidizes to dehydroascorbic acid. Because the latter can be reduced in vivo, it possesses vitamin C activity. Total vitamin C is therefore measured as the sum of ascorbic and dehydroascorbic acid concentrations. Because of its reductant properties, it serves primarily as a biologic antioxidant and free radical scavenger in aqueous environments. The biosynthesis of collagen, carnitine, bile acids, and norepinephrine, as well as proper functioning of the hepatic mixed-function oxygenase system, all depends on these properties. Vitamin C in foodstuffs increases the intestinal absorption of non-heme iron.	Overt deficiency is uncommonly observed in developed countries. The classic deficiency syndrome is *scurvy,* characterized by fatigue, depression, and widespread abnormalities in connective tissue such as inflamed gingivae, petechiae, perifollicular hemorrhage, impaired wound healing, coiled hair, hyperkeratosis, and bleeding into body cavities. In infants, defects in ossification and bone growth may occur. Tobacco smoking lowers plasma and leukocyte vitamin C levels.	Quantities exceeding 500 mg/d (in adults) sometimes cause nausea and diarrhea. Acidification of the urine with supplementation and the potential for enhanced oxalate synthesis have raised concerns regarding nephrolithiasis, but this has yet to be demonstrated. Supplementation may interfere with laboratory tests based on redox potential (e.g., fecal occult blood testing, serum cholesterol and glucose). Withdrawal from chronic ingestion of high doses of vitamin C supplements should occur gradually over a month because accommodation does occur and thus raises a concern of "rebound scurvy."	Plasma ascorbic acid concentrations reflect recent dietary intake, whereas leukocyte levels more closely reflect tissue stores. Women's plasma levels are approximately 20% higher than men's for any given dietary intake.
Vitamin B$_{12}$	A group of closely related cobalamin compounds composed of a corrin ring (with a cobalt atom in its center) connected to a ribonucleotide via an aminopropanol bridge. Microorganisms are the ultimate source of all naturally occurring B$_{12}$. The two active coenzyme forms are deoxyadenosylcobalamin and methylcobalamin. Both are needed for the synthesis of succinyl CoA, which is essential in lipid and carbohydrate metabolism, as well as the synthesis of methionine. The latter reaction is essential for amino acid metablism, for purine and pyrimidine synthesis, for many methylation reactions, and for the intracellular retention of folates.	Dietary inadequacy rarely causes deficiency except in strict vegetarians. Most deficiencies reflect loss of intestinal absorption, which may result from pernicious anemia, pancreatic insufficiency, atrophic gastritis, small bowel bacterial overgrowth, or ileal disease. Megaloblastic anemia and megaloblastic changes in other epithelia (see Folate) are the result of sustained depletion. Details of the hematologic (see Chapter 158) and neurologic (see Chapter 501) complications are described elsewhere. Hematologic and neurologic complication may occur independently.	A few allergic reactions to crystalline B$_{12}$ preparations have been reported but are probably due to impurities, not the vitamin.	Serum or plasma concentrations are generally accurate. Subtle deficiency with neurologic complications, as described in the text, can best be confirmed by measuring the concentration of serum methylmalonic acid, which is a sensitive indicator of cellular deficiency.
Biotin	A bi-cyclic compound consisting of a uredio ring fused to a substituted tetrahydrothiophene tring. Most dietary biotin is linked to lysine, a compound called biotinyl lysine, or biocytin. The lysine must be hydrolyzed by an intestinal enzyme called biotinidase before intestinal absorption occurs. Acts primarily as a coenzyme for several carboxylases; each holoenzyme catalyzes an ATP-dependent CO$_2$ transfer. The carboxylases are critical enzymes in carbohydrate and lipid metabolism.	Isolated deficiency is rare. Deficiency in humans has been produced experimentally, by prolonged diets lacking the vitamin, and by ingestion of large quantities of raw egg white, which contains avidin, a protein that binds biotin with extremely high affinity. Alterations in mental status, myalgias, hyperesthesias, and anorexia occur. Later a seborrheic dermatitis and alopecia develop. Biotin deficiency is usually accompanied by lactic acidosis and organic aciduria.	Toxicity has not been reported in humans with doses as high as 60 mg/d in children.	Plasma and urine concentrations of biotin are diminished in the deficient state. Elevated urine concentrations of methyl citrate, 3-methylcrotonylglycine, and 3-hydroxyisovalerate are observed in deficiency.
Pantothenic acid	Consists of pantoic acid linked to β-alanine through an amide bond. Pantothenate serves as an essential precursor of CoA. CoA is essential for the synthesis and β-oxidation of fatty acids and the synthesis of cholesterol, steroid hormones, vitamins A and D, and other isoprenoid derivatives. CoA is also involved in the synthesis of several amino acids and δ-aminolevulinic acid, a precursor for the corrin ring of vitamin B$_{12}$ and the porphyrin ring of heme and the cytochromes. CoA is also necessary for the acetylation and fatty acid acylation of a variety of proteins.	Usually seen in conjunction with other water-soluble vitamin deficiencies. Experimental, isolated deficiency in humans produces fatigue, abdominal pain and vomiting, insomnia, and paresthesias of the extremities.	Doses exceeding 10 g/d may induce diarrhea.	Whole blood and urine concentrations of pantothenate are indicators of status; serum levels are not accurate.

examination of recommended daily intakes have proved difficult for several reasons. In some instances there continues to be less than definitive evidence for the role of a particular micronutrient in a new function that has been proposed. Furthermore, even if a novel biochemical or physiologic role is well demonstrated for a nutrient, an appropriate question is whether optimization of such function translates into optimization of health. For example, providing supplemental vitamin E to elderly individuals who are vitamin E replete enhances T-lymphocyte responsiveness to mitogens. Nevertheless, it is unclear whether this approach diminishes infection rates among the elderly. Another difficult problem pertains to the use of micronutrients in supraphysiologic quantities, i.e., intakes that greatly exceed all conventional concepts of what is necessary for health. When taken in large quantities, some micronutrients affect physiologic functions beneficially (e.g., gram quantities of niacin to reduce low-density lipoprotein [LDL] cholesterol). Such physiologic effects are not observed at more conventional levels of intake and are therefore usually considered to be "pharmacologic" effects of the nutrient. Nevertheless, if the dietary requirement of a nutrient is strictly defined as the minimal dose necessary for the mainte-

Table 231–3 ■ NUTRITIONAL TRACE ELEMENTS AND THEIR CLINICAL IMPLICATIONS

TRACE ELEMENTS

	Biochemistry and Physiology	Deficiency	Toxicity	Assessment of Status
Chromium	Dietary chromium consists of both inorganic and organic forms. Its primary function in humans is to potentiate insulin action, which it accomplishes as a circulating dinicotinoglutathione complex called glucose tolerance factor. It thereby has an impact on carbohydrate, fat, and protein metabolism.	Deficiency in humans described only in long-term TPN patients receiving insufficient chromium. Hyperglycemia or impaired glucose tolerance is uniformly observed. Elevated plasma free fatty acid concentration, neuropathy, encephalopathy, and abnormalities in nitrogen metabolism are also reported. Whether supplemental chromium may improve glucose tolerance in mildly glucose-intolerant but otherwise healthy individuals remains controversial.	Toxicity after oral ingestion is uncommon and seems confined to gastric irritation. Airborne exposure may cause contact dermatitis, eczema, skin ulcers, and bronchogenic carcinoma.	Plasma or serum concentrations of chromium are crude indicators of chromium status; they appear to be meaningful when their value is markedly above or below the normal range.
Copper	Copper is absorbed by a specific intestinal transport mechanism. It is carried to the liver, where it is bound to ceruloplasmin, which circulates systematically and delivers copper to target tissues in the body. Excretion of copper is largely through bile into feces. Absorptive and excretory processes vary with the levels of dietary copper and thereby provide a means of copper homeostasis. Copper serves as a component of many enzymes, including amine oxidases, ferroxidases, cytochrome-*c* oxidase, dopamine *β*-hydroxylase, superoxide dismutase, and tyrosinase.	Dietary deficiency is rare; it has been observed in premature and low-birthweight infants fed exclusively a cow's milk diet and in individuals receiving long-term TPN lacking copper. Clinical manifestations include depigmentation of skin and hair, neurologic disturbances, leukopenia, hypochromic microcytic anemia, and skeletal abnormalities. The anemia arises from impaired utilization of iron and is therefore a conditioned form of iron deficiency anemia. The deficiency syndrome, except for the anemia and leukopenia, is also observed in Menke's disease, a rare inherited condition associated with impaired copper utilization.	Acute copper toxicity has been described after excessive oral intake and with absorption of copper salts applied to burned skin. Milder manifestations include nausea, vomiting, epigastric pain, and diarrhea; coma and hepatic necrosis may ensue in severe cases. Toxicity may be seen with doses as low as 70 μg/kg/d. Chronic toxicity is also described. Wilson disease is a rare, inherited disease associated with abnormally low ceruloplasmin levels and accumulation of copper in the liver and brain, eventually leading to damage to these two organs (see Chapter 120).	Practical methods for detecting marginal deficiency are not available. Marked deficiency is reliably detected by diminished serum copper and ceruloplasmin concentrations, as well as by low erythrocyte superoxide dismutase activity.
Fluorine	Known more commonly by its ionic form, fluoride. It is incorporated into the crystalline structure of bone, thereby altering its physical characteristics.	Intake of <0.1 mg/d in infants and <0.5 in children is associated with an increased incidence of dental caries. Optimal intake in adults is between 1.5 and 4 mg/d.	Acute ingestion of >30 mg/kg body weight fluoride is likely to cause death. Excessive chronic intake (>0.1 mg/kg/d) leads to mottling of the teeth (dental fluorosis), calcification of tendons and ligaments, and exostoses and may increase the brittleness of bones.	Estimates of intake or clinical assessment are used because no good laboratory test exists.
Iodine	Readily absorbed from the diet, concentrated in the thyroid, and integrated into the thyroid hormones thyroxine and triiodothyronine. The hormones circulate largely bound to thyroxine-binding globulin. They modulate resting energy expenditure and, in the developing human, growth and development.	In the absence of supplementation, populations relying primarily on food from soil with a low iodine content have endemic iodine deficiency. Maternal iodine deficiency leads to fetal deficiency, which produces spontaneous abortions, stillbirths, hypothyroidism, cretinism, and dwarfism. Permanent cognitive deficits may also be induced by iodine deficiency during infancy and childhood. In the adult, compensatory hypertrophy of the thyroid (goiter) occurs along with varying degrees of hypothyroidism.	Large doses (>2 mg/d in adults) may induce hypothyroidism by blocking thyroid hormone synthesis. Supplementation with >100 μg/day to an individual who was formerly deficient occasionally induces hyperthyroidism.	Iodine status of a population can be estimated by the prevalence of goiter. Urinary excretion of iodine is an effective laboratory means of assessment. The thyroid-stimulating hormone level in the blood is an indirect and therefore not entirely specific means of assessment.

Table continued on following page

Table 231–3 ■ NUTRITIONAL TRACE ELEMENTS AND THEIR CLINICAL IMPLICATIONS *Continued*

TRACE ELEMENTS

	Biochemistry and Physiology	Deficiency	Toxicity	Assessment of Status
Iron	Participates in redox reactions in a number of metalloproteins such as hemoglobin, myoglobin, and the cytochrome enzymes. Primary storage form is ferritin. Intestinal absorption is 15–20% for "heme" iron and 1–8% for the iron contained in vegetables. Absorption of the latter form is enhanced by the ascorbic acid in foodstuffs; by poultry, fish, or beef; and by an iron-deficient state; it is decreased by phytate and tannins.	The most common micronutrient deficiency in the world. Women of childbearing age constitute the highest-risk group because of menstrual blood loss, pregnancy, and lactation. The classic deficiency syndrome is hypochromic, microcytic anemia. Glossitis and koilonychia (spoon nails) are also observed. Easy fatigability often develops as an early symptom. In children, mild deficiency insufficient to cause anemia is associated with behavioral disturbances and poor school performance.	Iron overload occurs when habitual dietary intake is extremely high, intestinal absorption is excessive, or repeated parenteral administration occurs. Excessive iron stores usually accumulate in reticuloendothelial tissues and cause little damage (hemosiderosis). If overload continues, iron eventually begins to accumulate in tissues such as the liver, pancreas, heart, and synovium; the result is hemochromatosis (see Chapter 221). Hereditary hemochromatosis arises as a result of homozygosity of a common recessive trait. Excessive intestinal absorption of iron is observed in homozygotes.	Negative iron balance initially leads to depletion of iron stores in the bone marrow and an associated decrease in serum ferritin. As the severity of deficiency proceeds, serum iron (SI) decreases and total iron-binding capacity (TIBC) increases. An iron saturation (SI/TIBC) <16% suggests iron deficiency (see Chapter 221).
Manganese	A component of several metalloenzymes. Most manganese is in mitochondria, where it is a component of manganese superoxide dismutase.	Manganese deficiency in the human has not been conclusively demonstrated. It is said to cause hypocholesterolemia, weight loss, hair and nail changes, dermatitis, and impaired synthesis of vitamin K–dependent proteins.	Toxicity by oral ingestion unknown in humans. Toxic inhalation causes hallucinations, other alterations in mentation, and extrapyramidal movement disorders.	Until the deficiency syndrome is better defined, an appropriate measure of status will be difficult to develop.
Molybdenum	A cofactor in several enzymes, most prominently xanthine oxidase and sulfite oxidase.	A probable case of human deficiency is described as being secondary to parenteral administration of sulfite and resulted in hyperoxypurinemia, hypouricemia, and low sulfate excretion.	Toxicity not well described in the human, although it may interfere with copper metabolism at high doses.	Laboratory means of assessment not meaningful until deficiency syndrome is better defined.
Selenium	Selenium is a component of several enzymes, most notably glutathione peroxidase. This enzyme appears to prevent oxidative and free radical damage to various cell structures. Evidence suggests that the antioxidant protection conveyed by selenium operates in conjunction with vitamin E because deficiency of one seems to enhance damage induced by a deficiency of the other. Selenium also participates in the enzymatic conversion of thyroxine to its more active metabolite triiodothyronine.	Deficiency is rare in North America except in individuals receiving long-term TPN lacking selenium. Such individuals have myalgias and/or cardiomyopathies. Populations in some regions of the world, most notably some parts of China, have marginal intake of selenium. In these regions, *Keshan disease,* a condition characterized by cardiomyopathy, is endemic. The disease can be prevented (but not treated) by selenium supplementation.	Toxicity is associated with nausea, diarrhea, alterations in mental status, peripheral neuropathy, and loss of hair and nails; such symptoms were observed in adults who inadvertently consumed between 27 and 2400 mg.	Erythrocyte glutathione peroxidase activity and plasma, or whole blood, selenium concentrations are moderately accurate indicators of status.
Zinc	Intestinal absorption occurs by a specific process that is enhanced by pregnancy and corticosteroids and diminished by coingestion of phytates, phosphates, iron, copper, lead, or calcium. Diminished intake of zinc leads to increased efficiency of absorption and decreased fecal excretion, thus providing a means of zinc homeostasis. Zinc is a component of over 100 enzymes, among which are DNA polymerase, RNA polymerase, and tRNA synthetase.	Mild deficiency causes growth retardation in children. More severe deficiency is associated with growth arrest, teratogenicity, hypogonadism and infertility, dysgeusia, poor wound healing, diarrhea, a dermatitis on the extremities and around orifices, glossitis, alopecia, corneal clouding, loss of dark adaptation, and behavioral changes. Impaired cellular immunity is observed. Excessive loss of gastrointestinal secretions through chronic diarrhea, fistulas, etc., may precipitate deficiency. *Acrodermatitis enteropathica* is a rare, recessively inherited disease in which intestinal absorption of zinc is impaired.	Acute zinc toxicity can usually be induced by ingestion of >200 mg of zinc in a single day (in adults). It is manifested by epigastric pain, nausea, vomiting, and diarrhea. Hyperpnea, diaphoresis, and weakness may follow inhalation of zinc fumes. Copper and zinc compete for intestinal absorption. Chronic ingestion of >150 mg/d has been reported to cause gastric erosions, low HDL cholesterol levels, and impaired cellular immunity and may lead to copper deficiency.	No accurate indicators of zinc status are available for routine clinical use. Plasma, erythrocyte, and hair zinc concentrations are frequently misleading. Acute illness, in particular, is known to diminish plasma zinc levels, in part by inducing a shift of zinc out of the plasma compartment and into the liver. Functional tests that determine dark adaptation, taste acuity, and rate of wound healing lack specificity.

nance of optimal health, as has been suggested, supraphysiologic doses may have to be considered the dietary requirement in such instances. Thus determination of "optimal" nutrient intake depends considerably on which physiologic effect is sought. Furthermore, if only a segment of the population will benefit from supraphysiologic quantities of a nutrient, should dietary guidelines for the entirety be established according to this effect?

Determining an adequate level of intake implies the existence of

Table 231–4 ■ EXAMPLES OF DRUG-MEDIATED EFFECTS ON MICRONUTRIENT STATUS

DRUG(s)	NUTRIENT	MECHANISM OF INTERACTION
Dextroamphetamine, fenfluramine, levodopa	Potentially all micronutrients	Induce anorexia
Cholestyramine	Vitamin D, folate	Adsorbs nutrient, decreases absorption
Omeprazole	Vitamin B$_{12}$	Induces modest bacterial overgrowth; decreases gastric acid, thereby impairing absorption
Sulfasalazine, methotrexate	Folate	Impair absorption and/or inhibit folate-dependent enzymes
Isoniazid	Pyridoxine	Impairs utilization of B$_6$
Non-steroidal anti-inflammatory agents	Iron	Gastrointestinal blood loss
Penicillamine	Zinc	Increases renal excretion

a means of measuring nutrient status. In seeking such indices, the diversity of function often makes it difficult to decide the most germane measurement. Tobacco smoking, for example, appears to diminish vitamin E levels in alveolar fluid but not in serum. The concepts of "localized" nutrient deficiencies and tissue-specific requirements add a level of complexity to the determination of nutrient status.

The following examples illustrate how advances in nutritional science are prompting the redefinition of micronutrient requirements.

FOLATE. Guidelines regarding the necessary intake of folate were based, until recently, on the prevention of megaloblastic anemia. Measurements of serum and erythrocyte folate concentrations have been the most common means of assessing status; maintaining such levels within accepted normative ranges provides good assurance that folate status is adequate to prevent anemia.

It has become increasingly evident, however, that low folate levels that are insufficiently severe to cause anemia may still disturb normal biochemical and physiologic homeostasis. This is evidenced in part by an increase in serum homocysteine, an amino acid that is normally metabolized by a folate-dependent pathway. Some nutritional surveys have observed elevated serum homocysteine levels in individuals whose habitual intake of folate is at or just above the U.S. RDA (see Table 224–1), as well as in those whose serum folate levels are marginally above the conventional thresholds of deficiency. This elevation reflects less than optimal disposal of homocysteine and is now believed to probably be an independent risk factor for the development of occlusive vascular disease. Vitamins B$_6$ and B$_{12}$ are also important components of the biochemical pathways by which the body disposes of homocysteine, although their responsibility for hyperhomocysteinemia in the population is less evident.

Ingestion of folate in quantities considerably above the present recommended allowances appears to have other health benefits. Women taking folate supplements at the time of conception have a significantly lower risk of delivering a baby with a neural tube defect than do women who do not take folate supplements but whose dietary intake or serum folate levels fall within conventionally accepted ranges. This observation alone prompted the U.S. government to begin supplementation of folic acid in flour and other uncooked cereal grains starting in 1998. A more controversial observation is the inverse relationship that exists between the ingestion of folate and the incidence of neoplasia of the uterine cervix, the colorectum, and the bronchopulmonary tree; this inverse relationship is observed even when folate status (or dietary intake) falls within the range of conventionally accepted norms.

These observations suggest that ingestion of folate in quantities above what is presently regarded as adequate may contribute to the optimization of health. Substantial increases in the suggested intake of any micronutrient must be tempered, however, by the consideration of toxicity: With folate, toxicity is primarily related to its ability to mask B$_{12}$ deficiency when taken in doses exceeding 400 μg/day.

ANTIOXIDANT AND FREE RADICAL–SCAVENGING VITAMINS/PROVITAMINS. Vitamins A, C, and E, as well as many of the carote-

noids, are effective antioxidants. In addition, vitamins C and E and some of the carotenoids can scavenge free radicals when taken in adequate quantities. Such properties have long been appreciated, but it is only recently that oxidation and free radical damage have been thought to play important roles in common degenerative illnesses such as atherosclerosis, cancer, cataracts, retinal degeneration, and neurodegenerative disorders.

LDL can undergo oxidation in vivo, and growing evidence indicates that LDL thus transformed is particularly atherogenic. Prevention of LDL oxidation, at least in animal models, retards the process of atherogenesis. Supplementation in human subjects with several-fold the RDA of vitamin E, and perhaps some of the other antioxidant micronutrients, is an effective means of preventing LDL oxidation. Such intervention, however, remains unproved as a way to confer beneficial effects on human atherogenesis. Although some evidence suggests that large doses of β-carotene and vitamin E may protect against the recurrence of coronary heart disease, no clear consensus of such an effect has been reached in the several intervention trials that have been performed.

Many epidemiologic studies indicate that the occurrence of cancer of the oral cavity, lung, esophagus, stomach, and perhaps colorectum is inversely related to the dietary intake of fresh vegetables and fruit. Careful dissection of dietary data suggests that β-carotene and vitamin E are the most protective components of these foodstuffs. High doses of vitamin A and some of its synthetic analogues (e.g., 13-cis-retinoic acid) can effectively reduce the recurrence of head and neck cancers, although hepatic toxicity is sometimes a limiting factor. Similarly, when taken in large doses, these agents, as well as β-carotene and vitamin E, have been shown to promote the regression of oral leukoplakia, a pre-malignant lesion. Daily supplementation with one to three times the U.S. RDA of β-carotene, selenium, and vitamin E has been found to reduce the incidence of gastric adenocarcinoma in a disease-prevalent region of China. Contrarily, two large intervention trials that used considerably larger doses of β-carotene have shown an increase in lung cancer in smokers with daily supplementation of the carotenoid. Further investigation is necessary to more precisely define those circumstances under which antioxidant nutrients can prevent cancer.

Epidemiologic associations also suggest an inverse relationship between lens cataracts, macular degeneration, and the intake of vitamins C and E, and selected carotenoids. Considerable experimental evidence indicates that photo-oxidation, as well as other oxidative processes, contribute to both of these common degenerative conditions of the eye. In animal models, the development of cataract has been retarded by supraphysiologic supplementation with vitamin C or E. Furthermore, individuals who ingest vitamin

Table 231–5 ■ NEWLY IDENTIFIED ROLES FOR VITAMINS

VITAMIN OR PROVITAMIN	CLASSIC ROLE(S)	NEW ROLE(S)
β-Carotene	Provitamin A	Antioxidant, free radical scavenger, cell-cell gap junction modulation
Niacin	NAD/NADP coenzyme	Reduction in LDL cholesterol and elevation in HDL cholesterol
Folate	Hematopoietic factor	Diminishes homocysteinemia, incidence of neural tube defects
Vitamin A	Transduction of visual input in retina	Induction and maintenance of epithelial differentiation, maintenance of cell-mediated immunity, morphogenetic signal in embryogenesis
Vitamin D	Regulator of calcium, phosphate metabolism	Modulates epithelial proliferation and promotes differentiation
Vitamin B$_6$	Coenzyme for transamination	Modulation of steroid activity
Vitamin C	Hydroxylation coenzyme	Antioxidant

NAD = nicotinamide adenine dinucleotide; NADP = nicotinamine-adenine dinucleotide phosphate; LDL = low-density lipoprotein; HDL = high-density lipoprotein.

C in excess of the U.S. RDA have a lower incidence of cataract than to those ingesting the RDA, thus suggesting a preventive role for larger than conventionally recommended doses of these nutrients. Nevertheless, insufficient prospective data exist at the present time to conclude that antioxidants specifically prevent cataracts and macular degeneration.

VITAMIN B$_{12}$ AND NEUROPSYCHIATRIC DISEASE Plasma B$_{12}$ concentrations are considered to be an accurate indication of B$_{12}$ status. The normal range for a healthy population has typically been considered 150 to 900 pg/mL: values above 150 or 200 pg/mL were believed to exclude B$_{12}$ deficiency as a cause of neurologic or psychiatric syndromes. Some observations, however, suggest that in 7 to 10% of individuals who have plasma B$_{12}$ values between 150 and 400 pg/mL, neuropsychiatric complications of B$_{12}$ deficiency may develop in the absence of megaloblastic anemia. Such persons can be identified by an elevated level of methylmalonic acid in the blood that decreases to normal after parenteral B$_{12}$ administration.

An elevation in serum methylmalonic acid is both a sensitive and specific indication of cellular B$_{12}$ deficiency. Awareness of this phenomenon is particularly important because it is now clear that atrophic gastritis, an asymptomatic condition that affects approximately 30% of the elderly population, frequently produces a modest decrease in B$_{12}$ absorption.

Table 231–5 lists several examples of biochemical functions of vitamins that have only recently been identified. As nutritional science proceeds with defining the clinical significance of each of these new roles and determines what quantities of each vitamin are necessary to optimize such functions, redefinition of the desirable range of vitamin status may well occur.

Sauberlich H, Machlin L (eds): Beyond Deficiency: New Views on the Function and Health Effects of Vitamins. Ann N Y Acad Sci 1992, vol 669. *Excellent collection of discussions pertaining to new perspectives on functions of vitamins and how these perspectives have an impact on the definition of deficiency.*
Shils M, Olsen J, Shike M, Ross AC: Modern Nutrition in Health and Disease, 9th ed. Baltimore, Williams & Wilkins, 1998. *Comprehensive, up-to-date reviews of the biochemistry, physiology, and nutrition of each micronutrient.*

PART XVII

ENDOCRINE DISEASES

232 PRINCIPLES OF ENDOCRINOLOGY

Gordon N. Gill

Communication is essential for all life processes. Accurate sensing of the environment and appropriate coordinated responses depend on the nervous and endocrine systems, which are tightly interwoven. Nervous system functions are mediated by hormones, and the endocrine system is centrally controlled by the nervous system. Communication between cells is necessary for development from a single fertilized egg to a mature adult, for an orderly reproductive cycle, and for homeostatic adjustments to a constantly changing environment. Hormones, distinct chemical messengers, transmit information from one cell to another to coordinate homeostatic adaptations, growth, development, and reproduction. *Hormones,* a word derived from Greek meaning "excite" or "set in motion," bind with high affinity and specificity to receptors, which are allosteric proteins. Receptor proteins have two essential functional characteristics: (1) a recognition site, which binds hormones with high specificity and affinity, and (2) an activity site, which transduces the information received into a biochemical message. Allosteric receptor proteins adopt various conformational states; binding of the hormone ligand results in the active conformation. The initial event in hormone action is thus a bimolecular reaction dependent on the concentration of hormone, the concentration of receptor, and the affinity of receptor for hormone.

$$[\text{Hormone}] + [\text{Receptor}] \underset{\text{Inactive}}{\overset{k_1}{\underset{k_{-1}}{\longleftrightarrow}}} [\text{Hormone-Receptor}]_{\text{Active}}$$

Factors that control the concentration of both hormone and receptor determine biologic responses of cells, of organs, and of the whole organism.

Classic endocrinology dealt with the glands that produce hormones and the concentration of hormone to which cells expressing receptors are exposed. Biosynthesis, secretion, transport of hormone to target cells, and metabolic inactivation determine the effective hormone concentration. Diseases of endocrine glands that impair hormone production result in deficiency states, whereas diseases that cause excessive production result in hormone excess states. Expression of receptor is equally important in forming the active hormone-receptor complex. Genetic and acquired diseases that impair receptors result in deficiency states even though hormone concentrations are compensatorily increased. Increased receptor expression results in an excess state, an event that occurs with growth factor receptors in malignant transformation.

Hormones are produced not only by the glands of internal secretion but by a variety of cells throughout the body. Neurohormones, produced in the hypothalamus, are also produced in cells throughout the nervous system to modulate neuronal function. Gastrointestinal hormones are produced within the nervous system. Hormones that regulate production and maturation of cells of the hematopoietic and immune systems are made in cells of these lineages and in endothelial and mesenchymal cells. Growth-promoting and growth-inhibiting hormones (growth factors and growth inhibitors) are produced by macrophages and mesenchymal cells. Many of these signaling molecules do not travel long distances through the blood to reach target cells as do classic hormones (endocrine) but act on target cells in the vicinity of the producer cell (paracrine) or even on the producer cell itself (autocrine). During development, cell surface hormones may act on the cell surface receptor of a neighbor cell as a cell-cell communication system. Regardless of signaling distance, the same principles of hormone-receptor interactions operate.

HOW HORMONES WORK

Two classes of hormones operate via two types of receptors (Fig. 232–1). Peptide hormones are synthesized as parts of larger protein molecules and processed as secretory proteins. They act via receptors located in the cell membrane with the recognition/binding site exposed on the cell surface and the activity domain facing the inside of the cell. Activated cell surface receptors use a variety of strategies to transduce signal information, often activating second messengers, which amplify and distribute the molecular information. Many peptide hormones ultimately signal via regulation of protein phosphorylation. In this most common process through which proteins are covalently modified, a phosphate group is donated to the protein by adenosine triphosphate. This allows peptide hormones to change rapidly the conformation and thus the function of existing cell enzymes. It also allows somewhat slower changes in gene transcription to regulate the concentration of enzyme proteins. Biogenic amines function like peptide hormones.

Steroid hormones are synthesized from precursor cholesterol. Thyroid hormone, retinoic acid (vitamin A), and vitamin D are synthesized through separate pathways but act through the same family of receptors and mechanisms as do steroid hormones. This group of hormones acts via structurally related receptors that bind to DNA recognition sites to regulate transcription of target genes.

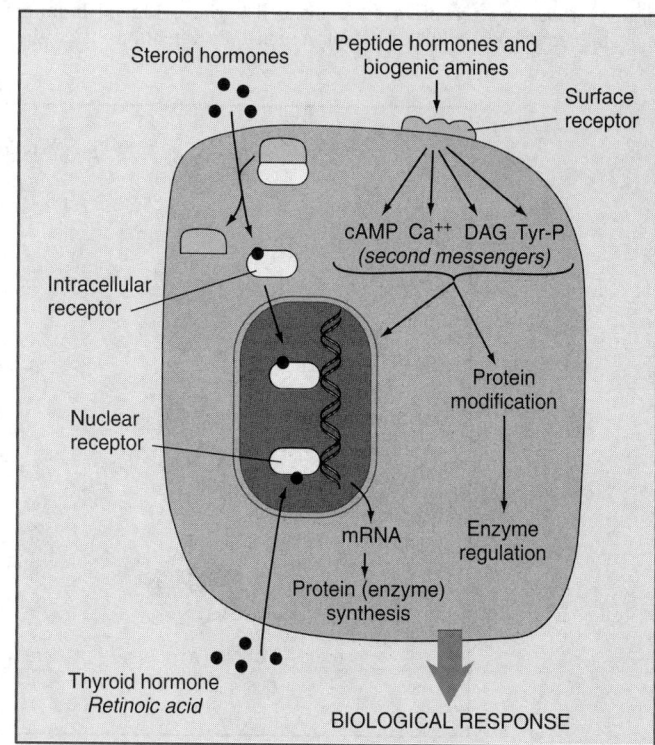

FIGURE 232–1 ■ Mechanisms by which peptide and steroid hormones signal.

They change the concentration of cell proteins, primarily enzymes, and thus the metabolic activity underlying the physiologic response.

Peptide Hormones Act Via Cell Surface Receptors

HORMONE BINDING AND SIGNAL TRANSDUCTION. Peptide hormone receptors have one of three general structures (Fig. 232–2): (1) a seven-membrane spanning structure in which the recognition site is formed by exterior sequences between membrane-spanning helices and the activity site is formed by interhelical regions inside the cell; (2) a single membrane-spanning helical structure separating the recognition domain from the cytoplasmic domain, which contains an intrinsic enzyme activity; and (3) a single membrane-spanning helix that separates the recognition domain from an intracellular domain that couples to second messenger systems, as do the seven-membrane spanning receptors. The protein coupled may be an intracellular tyrosine kinase or other enzyme.

Hormone ligands and receptors bind with high affinities (equilibrium dissociation constants $[K_D]$ of nanomolar to picomolar), thus providing the specificity necessary for cells to decode the information provided by the low concentration of hormone present among the many other circulating and extracellular proteins. The conformational change resulting from peptide hormone binding activates receptors to signal from the cell surface. Removal of receptors from the cell surface results in down-regulation and attenuation of the response. Binding affinities and dose-response curves for the initial event in cell signaling are the same. Biologic responses consequent to these initial events occur through a series of amplifications, each with its own affinity. The result is a dose-response curve for biologic activities that is more sensitive than that for binding and activation of the initial response. Full biologic responses may thus occur at a low concentration of hormone, resulting in occupancy of only 10% or less of receptors. This provides high sensitivity to small changes in hormone concentration. It also provides significant reserve. Hormone-induced down-regulation may remove 90% of receptors from the cell surface. This renders the cell refractory to the initial hormone concentration, but if the need is great enough, hormone concentrations can increase 10-fold and fully activate the residual 10% of receptors to give full biologic responses. Such a response system provides high initial sensitivity, buffering via down-regulation against excessive hormone responses, but reserve that can operate when the signal strength is strong enough.

Receptors are mobile in the plane of the membrane. Ligand binding not only transduces signals but also induces down-regulation by removing receptors from the cell surface. Ligand binding may induce sequestration of receptors and their retention inside the cell via interactions with cell proteins, as occurs with rhodopsin and adrenergic receptors. Ligand binding may induce endocytosis through clathrin-coated pits with ultimate degradation by lysosomal enzymes, as occurs with insulin and epidermal growth factor receptors. The concentration of cell surface receptors is regulated by interaction with hormone ligand and by other signals that regulate its synthesis and affinity. The concentration of receptors determines the cells' responsiveness. Antagonists occupy receptors but in general do not induce desensitization. When antagonists are removed, receptor concentrations are high and cells are very responsive to hormone exposure. Effects on receptor concentration are seen clinically as up-regulation (e.g., as excessive adrenergic responses when β blockers are rapidly withdrawn) and as down-regulation (e.g., insulin resistance in type II diabetes). Regulation of receptor synthesis is an important mechanism by which one hormone regulates responsiveness to another to coordinate biologic effects.

A class of cell surface receptors serves a nutrient delivery rather than an informational function. These molecules include the low density lipoprotein (LDL) receptor, the transferrin receptor, and the asialoglycoprotein receptor. LDL and transferrin receptors, which are clustered in coated pits, internalize, deliver LDL (cholesterol) and iron to the cell interior, and then recycle to the cell surface. Such receptors do not down-regulate but undergo repeated rounds of recycling to provide the cell with essential nutrients.

INTRACELLULAR SECOND MESSENGERS. CYCLIC AMP AND CYCLIC GMP. The concept of second messengers was established by Earl Sutherland, who discovered cyclic adenosine monophosphate (AMP), an intracellular allosteric effector that mediates the action of many peptide hormones. Hormone receptors are coupled to catalytic adenylate cyclase through guanosine nucleotide binding (G) proteins, the β-adrenergic receptor being a paradigm for this signaling pathway (Fig. 232–3). This receptor belongs to the seven-membrane spanning class. On ligand binding, the receptor interacts with a G protein trimer consisting of α, β, and γ subunits. Because G proteins bind guanosine diphosphate (GDP) with higher affinity than guanosine triphosphate (GTP), guanine nucleotide exchange is triggered by proteins that facilitate exchange of GTP for GDP; activity is reversed by hydrolysis of GTP to GDP. Binding of hormones to receptors that operate through the cyclic AMP second messenger system results in a conformational change causing receptors to bind to G proteins. Ligand-activated receptors facilitate exchange of GTP for GDP so that the activated $G_\alpha s$ (stimulating α GTP-binding subunit) dissociates from the β and γ subunits. The [ligand·hormone receptor]·[$G_\alpha S·GTP$] complex activates adenylate cyclase to catalyze formation of cyclic AMP from adenosine triphosphate (ATP). Each hormone ligand induces formation of multiple cyclic AMP molecules through this mechanism.

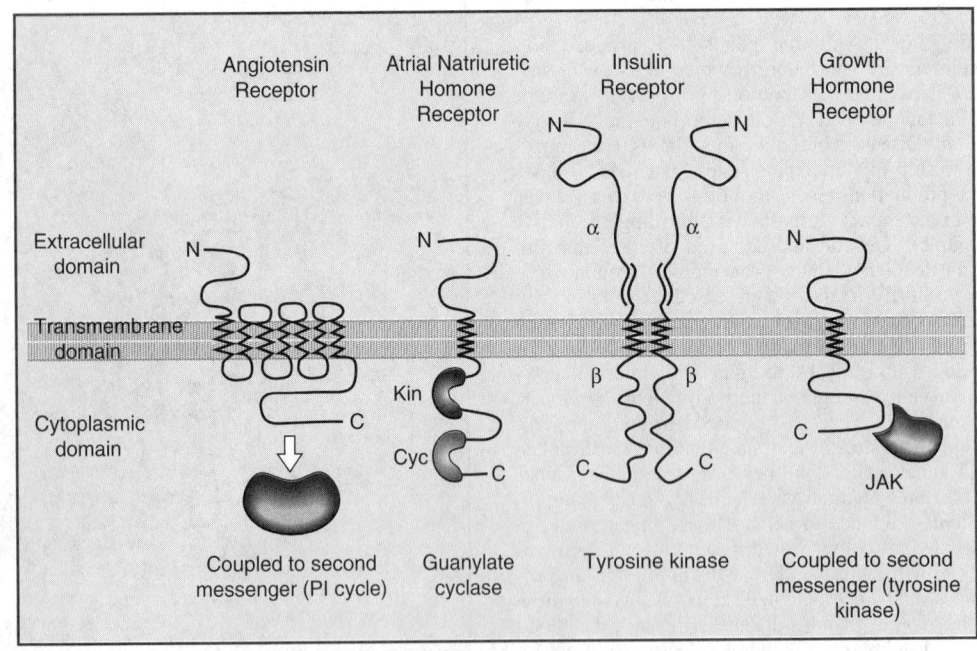

FIGURE 232–2 ■ Structures of peptide hormone receptors.

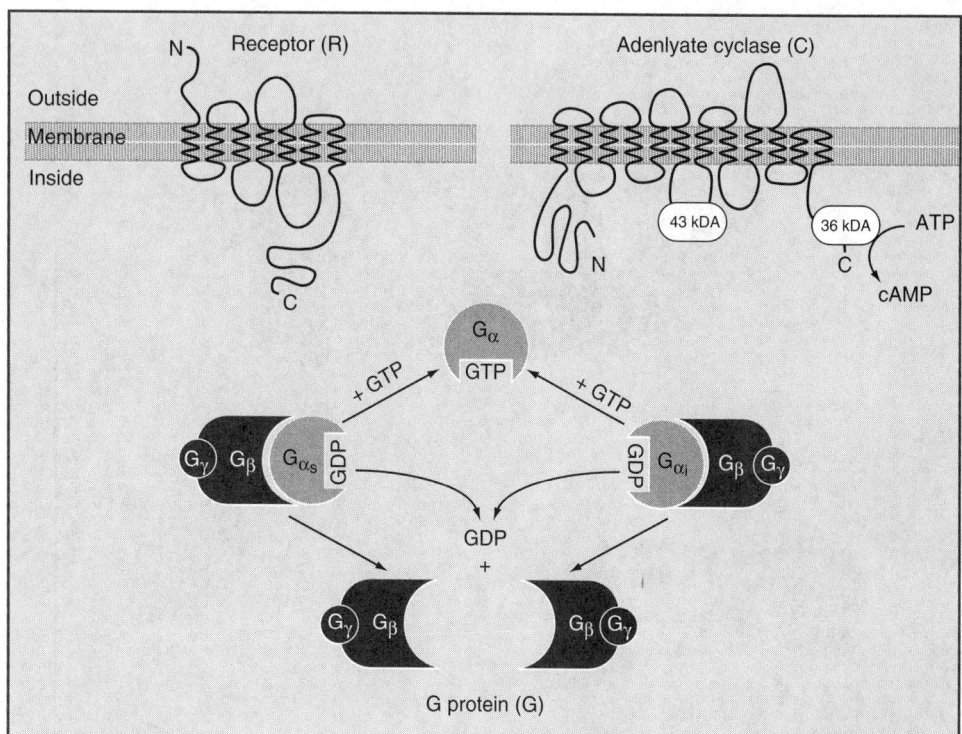

FIGURE 232-3 ■ Hormone-regulated adenylate cyclase.

Inhibitory G proteins operate in a similar manner to decrease cyclic AMP formation. In both cases, ligand-activated receptors act to exchange GTP for GDP, analogous to proteins that catalyze this process to regulate protein synthesis.

Adenylate cyclase is a large complex molecule with a 12-membrane spanning structure. The two large cytoplasmic domains have internal sequence similarities and are related to sequences in guanylate cyclase. Eight adenylate cyclases have been identified, and their channel-like structure suggests that they may function as transporters in addition to catalyzing formation of cyclic AMP.

Activation of adenylate cyclase is buffered and terminated by several mechanisms: (1) Hormone dissociates from receptor. Binding of $G_{\alpha} \cdot$ GTP to the receptor decreases affinity for hormone about one order of magnitude to facilitate this dissociation. (2) Receptors desensitize and are removed from the cell surface by a process involving phosphorylation and interaction with cell proteins termed *arrestins*. If hormone exposure is short, receptors are dephosphorylated and reappear on the cell surface; if exposure is prolonged, receptors are degraded and resensitization requires new receptor synthesis. (3) Most importantly, G_{α} proteins possess intrinsic GTPase activity so that GTP is hydrolyzed to GDP and, on GDP binding, G_{α} is inactivated and reassociates with the β/γ subunits.

There are many consequences when this mechanism of signal transduction is perturbed. Mutations in seven-membrane spanning receptors may inactivate so that signaling is defective; some mutations, such as those observed in thyroid-stimulating hormone (TSH) receptors in hyperfunctioning thyroid nodules, may activate so that receptors signal in the absence of hormone. Continuous exposure to hormone results in desensitization or tachyphylaxis. Deficiency of G protein, which occurs in certain forms of pseudohypoparathyroidism, results in insensitivity to hormone. Cholera toxin, which activates ADP ribosylation of $G_{\alpha}s$, inhibits GTPase activity and interferes with reversibility so that profound and prolonged elevations in cyclic AMP occur. Mutations in G_{α} proteins that are predicted to impair GTPase activity have been described in endocrine tumors.

Cyclic AMP, an intracellular allosteric effector, binds to the regulatory subunit of cyclic AMP–dependent protein kinase. A-kinase is a tetrameric protein consisting of two regulatory and two catalytic subunits. Binding of cyclic AMP dissociates the inhibitory regulatory subunits as a dimer from the two catalytic subunits. The latter then catalyze the transfer of the γ phosphate of ATP to serine and threonine residues in proteins. This covalent modification by

phosphorylation causes an allosteric conformational change in the substrate protein that results in a change in its activity. The hormonal signal is transduced into an alteration in enzyme activity and thus in cell function. Phosphorylation of cytoplasmic proteins results in alterations such as glycolysis; the activated catalytic kinase subunit also migrates to the nucleus to phosphorylate and activate transcription factors such as the cyclic AMP response element binding protein (CREB).

Cyclic AMP actions are reversed by hydrolysis of cyclic AMP by phosphodiesterase to $5'$ AMP, and protein phosphorylation is reversed by the action of phosphatases. Phosphodiesterases are regulated and are a frequent target of inhibitor drugs such as methylxanthines, which prolong cyclic AMP action by blocking its degradation. Phosphatases are regulated by phosphatase-inhibitor proteins, which are fine tuned by phosphorylation of these molecules.

A conceptually similar but structurally distinct system provides signal transduction through the second messenger cyclic guanosine monophosphate (GMP). Two forms of guanylate cyclase catalyze formation of cyclic GMP from GTP. The best-characterized mammalian enzyme is the receptor for atrial natriuretic hormone (ANH). The binding site for ANH is located on the extracellular portion of its receptor separated by a single membrane-spanning domain from the cytoplasmic guanylate cyclase (see Fig. 232–2). In contrast to adenylate cyclase, receptor and catalytic activities reside in the same molecule. Activity is regulated primarily by ligand binding but also depends on phosphorylation of the enzyme, with dephosphorylation causing desensitization. A cytoplasmic form of guanylate cyclase contains a heme moiety and is activated by nitrous oxide and free radicals.

Cyclic GMP acts by binding to the regulatory domain of cyclic GMP-dependent protein kinase. G-kinase, a dimeric enzyme that is evolutionarily related to A-kinase, is allosterically activated on cyclic GMP binding. Like A-kinase, it catalyzes protein phosphorylation to alter enzyme function and physiologic responses. Reactions are terminated by cyclic GMP phosphodiesterase and protein phosphatases. Cyclic GMP phosphodiesterase is activated by binding of calcium·calmodulin, a mechanism providing biochemical communication between two signaling systems.

CALCIUM AND DIACYLGLYCEROL. Hormone receptors that activate the phosphatidylinositol (PI) cycle transmit information to the interior of the cell by two second messengers: calcium (Ca^{2+}) and

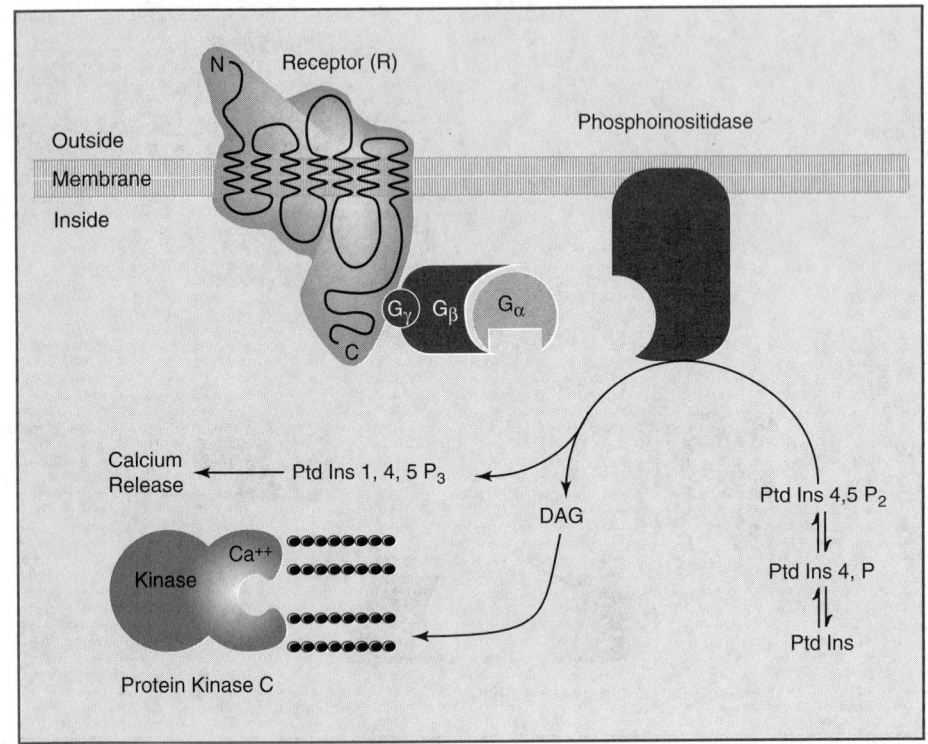

Outside
Membrane
Inside

Receptor (R)

Phosphoinositidase

Calcium
Release ← Ptd Ins 1, 4, 5 P$_3$ ←

DAG

Ptd Ins 4,5 P$_2$

Ptd Ins 4, P

Ptd Ins

Kinase

Ca^{++}

Protein Kinase C

FIGURE 232–4 ■ The phosphatidylinositol signaling pathway.

diacylglycerol (DAG) (Fig. 232–4). The cycle of PI metabolism consists of synthesis of this phospholipid, its breakdown, and its resynthesis. PI is composed of a three-carbon glycerol backbone with long-chain fatty acids esterified at carbons 1 and 2 and an inositol ring esterified via a phosphoester bond at carbon 3. Distinct kinase enzymes catalyze phosphorylation of the inositol ring at positions 3, 4, and 5. Quantitatively, the principal phosphorylations occur sequentially at positions 4 and then 5. The principal function of activated hormone receptors is to stimulate phosphoinositidase (phospholipase C), which releases the phosphorylated inositol to generate inositol trisphosphate (IP$_3$, inositol 1,4,5 P$_3$) and DAG (the glycerol backbone with fatty acids attached at carbons 1 and 2). IP$_3$ increases the concentration of cytoplasmic [Ca^{2+}]. It mobilizes stored intracellular Ca^{2+} by binding to specific receptors on intracellular membranes and by facilitating opening of calcium channels. The concentration of basal cytoplasmic Ca^{2+} is at least 1000-fold less than that in storage sites and outside the cell. The release from intracellular stores or entry of Ca^{2+} into the cell rapidly increases cytoplasmic [Ca^{2+}].

Ca^{2+} plays a regulatory role in muscle contraction, in neuromuscular transmission, and in hormone signaling. Ca^{2+} binds to calmodulin and alters its conformation, causing the Ca^{2+}·calmodulin complex to bind to a variety of enzymes to regulate their activities. Ca^{2+}·calmodulin regulates protein kinases, including myosin light chain kinase involved in smooth muscle contraction, phosphorylase kinase involved in breakdown of glycogen, and calmodulin-dependent protein kinase important in synaptic transmission. Ca^{2+}·calmodulin regulates cyclic nucleotide phosphodiesterase and adenylate and guanylate cyclases to influence cyclic AMP and cyclic GMP concentrations, and it is involved in microtubule assembly and disassembly. Ca^{2+}·calmodulin is thus able to bind to a variety of other proteins and to alter their activity in response to information provided by the cytoplasmic Ca^{2+} concentration.

DAG acts as a second messenger by binding to protein kinase C to activate this important regulatory enzyme. Protein kinase C also requires Ca^{2+} for activation, so both second messengers of this pathway cooperate to increase the activity of this enzyme. Tumor promoters, such as active phorbol esters, are DAG analogues and act via protein kinase C.

The components of this second messenger system are diverse and complex. There are multiple isoenzyme forms of protein kinase

C and of phosphoinositidase. Although one isoenzyme form of phosphoinositidase is activated via receptor-coupled G proteins, another is activated by binding to receptor tyrosine kinases and undergoing tyrosine phosphorylation. Additional kinases phosphorylate alternate positions on the inositol ring; PI 3-kinase is activated by certain tyrosine kinases to yield unique PI metabolites with functions distinct from Ca^{2+} mobilization. Ptd Ins, which is phosphorylated at the 4, 5 position, functions in recognizing PH domains to localize and activate kinases and other proteins, and Ptd Ins 3 (P) binds to FYVE domains in proteins. Sphingosine, a component of glycosphingolipid metabolism, inhibits protein kinase C, which provides dual regulation of this protein. Specific phosphatases remove the phosphate groups from the inositol ring to terminate its activity; lithium blocks the activity of one of these phosphatases to enhance accumulation of the biologically active inositol phosphates. Like other information pathways, this one is diffused to generate coordinated cellular responses and is buffered and ultimately turned off when the signal strength decreases.

PROTEIN TYROSINE KINASES. A group of peptide hormone receptors contains intrinsic protein tyrosine kinase activity. Ligand binding to the extracellular domain results in an allosteric change that is transmitted across the single membrane-spanning segment to activate the cytoplasmic kinase domain (see Fig. 232–2). In a second structural motif a transmembrane receptor is coupled to a distinct cytoplasmic tyrosine kinase subunit. The growth hormone receptor and JAK2 belong to this second class.

Within the cell the great majority of protein-bound phosphate is attached to serine and threonine residues, with only a small fraction being attached to tyrosine. Numerous kinases, however, covalently modify tyrosine residues in proteins as a central regulatory function in cell proliferation, developmental processes, and differentiated function. The extracellular ligand-binding domains of receptors of this class contain cysteine-rich regions that create the binding sites either as monomers (epidermal growth factor [EGF] receptor) or as dimers (insulin receptor) or contain immunoglobulin-like structures (platelet-derived growth factor [PDGF] and fibroblast growth factor [FGF] receptors). The cytoplasmic protein tyrosine kinase domains are highly homologous, containing ATP and substrate-binding sites, but different receptors recognize distinct substrates to give specific biologic responses. For example, insulin stimulates glucose uptake whereas EGF stimulates cell proliferation. The tyrosine kinases contain variable domains on both sides of the tyrosine kinase core as well as inserts within the kinase domain, which provide regulatory sites that modulate ligand-activated tyrosine kinase activity.

Information received by a cell surface tyrosine kinase receptor is transmitted through a signal transduction pathway that begins with direct physical coupling of two proteins and proceeds through the GTP-binding protein *ras* (Fig. 232–5). In response to ligand binding, receptor tyrosine kinases either self-phosphorylate or phosphorylate a linker substrate. Proteins that contain a 100-amino acid domain homologous to a region in *src*, SH2, bind tightly to these sites of tyrosine phosphorylation. The growth factor receptor binding protein 2 (Grb2) is a molecular coupler containing an SH2 domain that plugs into a tyrosine phosphorylation site. Shc is another molecule coupler frequently used. Grb2 also contains two SH3 domains that act as a receptacle for proline-rich domains of the guanine nucleotide exchange protein SOS. These high-affinity protein-to-protein interactions bring SOS to the cell membrane, where *ras* is present in its inactive GDP-bound form. Activated GTP-bound *ras* then couples to a serine/threonine protein kinase cascade involving first *raf*-1, then MEK and MAP (mitogen-activated protein) kinases. Information is thus relayed, expanded, and diffused to ultimately control gene expression and cell division. Operative mechanisms for this, as for other hormone-signaling pathways, include ligand or protein-protein interactions, activated GTP-bound G proteins, and protein phosphorylation. Receptor tyrosine kinases also couple to additional signaling pathways via SH2 domains in other proteins and via tyrosine phosphorylation of these proteins including phospholipase C-γ, transcription control proteins termed *signal transducers, and activators of transcription* (STAT) and PI 3-kinase.

Increased tyrosine kinase activity is reversed by four principal mechanisms: (1) ligand-induced endocytosis and down-regulation of surface receptors, (2) tyrosine phosphatases, which specifically remove phosphate from tyrosine residues, (3) reversal of the kinase reaction to transfer the phosphate from tyrosine residues in protein to adenosine diphosphate (ADP), and (4) hydrolysis of *ras*-bound GTP to GDP.

Regulation and reversibility of ligand-activated tyrosine kinases are important. Mutations involving these proteins occur frequently in cells transformed from normal to cancerous patterns of growth. These mutations may bypass regulatory features so that the kinases are constitutively active. The kinases may be overexpressed, most frequently owing to gene amplification but also owing to enhanced

transcription, or the ligand may be constitutively expressed to activate receptors continuously. Mutant *ras* proteins may be constitutively active owing to decreased GTPase activity or to a defect in a protein that stimulates the GTPase activity of *ras*. Any of these changes converts a normal regulatory protein into an oncoprotein, one capable of causing neoplastic transformation.

Steroid Hormones Act Via Nuclear Receptors

THE SUPERFAMILY OF STEROID HORMONE RECEPTORS. All steroid hormone receptors share structural similarities indicative of a common ancestral molecule. The most conserved structural feature is the DNA-binding domain that contains zinc "fingers." The diagnostic spacing of cysteine residues creates a structure coordinated to a Zn^{2+} atom and a helix that binds to the major groove of DNA. Because the energy of protein-DNA interaction depends on the area of contact, most proteins bind DNA as complexes. Steroid hormone receptors of the glucocorticoid receptor subfamily bind to DNA as homodimers; receptors of the thyroid hormone receptor subfamily may bind as homodimers but more commonly bind as heterodimers with a common partner, the retinoid X receptor (RXR) (Fig. 232–6).

The DNA recognition element consists of two half-sites of six base pairs, each half binding one monomer surface of the dimeric receptor protein. The half-sites are arranged as direct, inverted, or everted repeats. Receptors of the glucocorticoid receptor subfamily most often bind to palindromic sites, whereas receptors of the thyroid hormone receptor subfamily most often bind to sites made up of directly repeated DNA sequences. Small variations in the DNA-binding domain and in the DNA recognition element provide specificity for hormone action. One important determinant for receptor binding and activity is the spacing between the two half-sites for dimeric receptor binding. The spacing rules for DNA recognition elements that are arranged as direct repeats (DR) indicate that a spacing of 1 (DR + 1) directs RXR homodimer binding and 9-*cis*-retinoic acid responses, DR + 3 directs vitamin D receptor·RXR binding and vitamin D responses, DR + 4 directs thyroid hormone receptor·RXR binding and thyroid hormone responses, and DR + 5 directs retinoic acid receptor·RXR binding and all-*trans*-retinoic acid responses. RXR binds to the upstream half and the hormone-specific receptor binds to the downstream

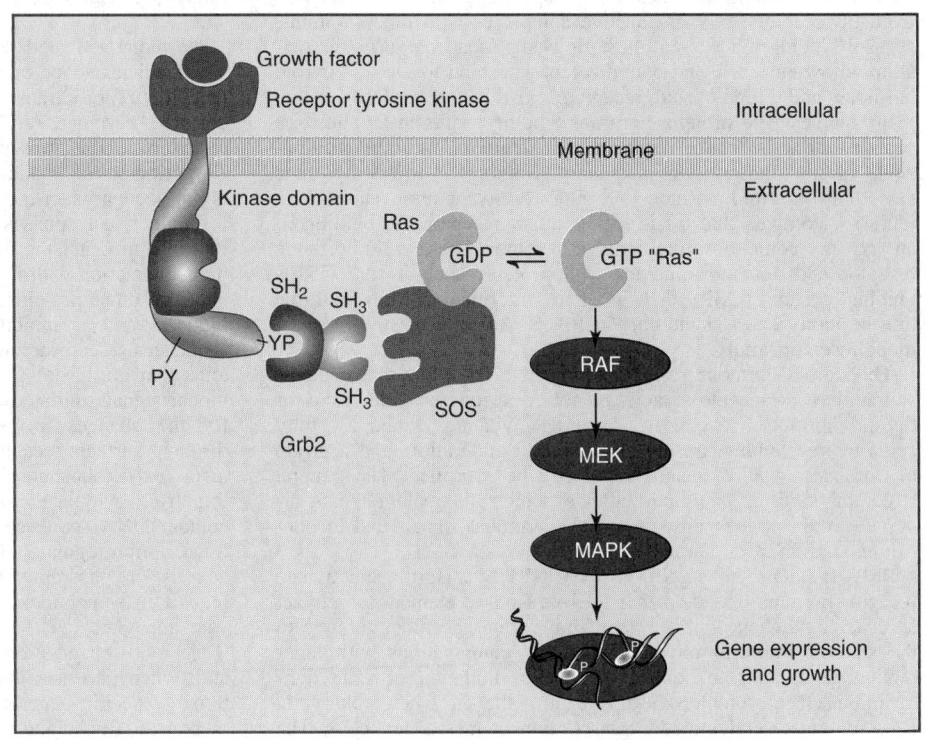

FIGURE 232–5 ■ Information transfer through a receptor tyrosine kinase pathway. Sites of receptor tyrosine self-phosphorylation, Y-P, are recognized by the SH2 domain of the linker Grb2, which brings the guanine nucleotide exchange factor SOS to the membrane where *ras* is located. Activated GTP-bound *ras* initiates signaling by contacting *raf*, a serine threonine kinase, to initiate a cascade of kinase activations.

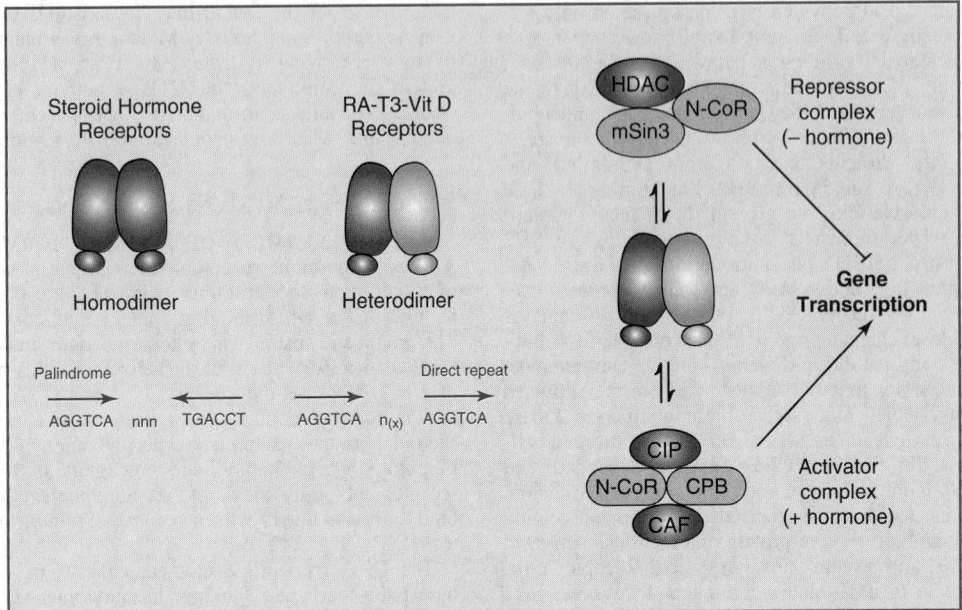

FIGURE 232–6 ■ How steroid hormone receptors work. *Left,* Glucocorticoid receptor family members bind as homodimers to palindromic DNA sites. Thyroid hormone receptor family members bind primarily as heterodimers with retinoid X receptor to direct repeat DNA sites separated by varying numbers of base pairs. *Right,* As a result of hormone binding, repressor complexes dissociate and activator complexes bind to nuclear receptors. Repressor complexes contain histone deacetylase (HDAC) and activator complexes contain histone acetylase (CAF).

half of these DNA response elements to mediate hormone-dependent changes in transcription. Spacing between half-sites is crucial for binding homodimeric receptors of the glucocorticoid receptor class, but the sequence of the half-site provides an essential discriminant. Specificity is quantitative, not absolute. For example, progesterone receptors bind to glucocorticoid response elements, and retinoic acid receptors bind to thyroid hormone receptor DNA response elements. Specificity is sufficient for generating hormone-specific responses but may permit overlapping functions as in lig-and-activated progesterone receptor induction of glucocorticoid-regulated genes.

Hormone binding activates the biologic function of the receptor. Cortisol receptors exist in inactive complexes with other proteins; cortisol binding induces an allosteric change that facilitates dissociation, allowing the ligand-bound receptor to bind to DNA. Thyroid hormone and retinoic acid receptors exist bound to DNA rather than complexed to protein; hormone binding results in an allosteric change that activates the receptor, so it interacts with other components of the transcription machinery. Binding of triiodothyronine (T_3) to the thyroid hormone receptor results in dissociation of a repressor complex that binds to the empty receptor and binding of an activator complex to the liganded receptor. The thyroid hormone receptor and activator interact with proteins such as the CREB binding protein (CBP) that integrate information from multiple transcription factors, including CREB, STAT, and the thyroid hormone receptor family.

The steroid hormone receptor family is a large one that includes subfamilies of receptors: at least four for retinoic acid, two for thyroid hormone, several for $1,25(OH)_2$ vitamin D and for fatty acids or metabolites causing perixosome proliferation, and a group of "orphans" whose ligands remain to be identified. The general structural motif is an important one, which, in evolution, has diverged to specify responses to many hormonal signals and to control expression of numerous genes.

REGULATION OF GENE TRANSCRIPTION. Hormone-activated receptor proteins bound to their DNA response element targets act as *cis*-active enhancers. They act from various positions relative to the start of transcription and in various combinations with other regulatory proteins to control the rate of initiation of gene transcription. Gene promoters lie upstream of the site where eukaryotic RNA polymerase II initiates transcription of messenger RNA. The best-characterized promoter contains a TATA box that binds a protein, transcription factor II-D (TF II-D), which directs accurate transcription by RNA polymerase II about 30 base pairs downstream. Seven proteins (TATA-associated factors [TAFs]) associate with TF II-D in a specific complex that provides a molecular surface for interaction with the transcription-regulatory proteins, which are bound elsewhere to DNA. Other promoter motifs include a basal initiator and GC-rich regions in which multiple transcription start sites exist. Gene expression is induced by increasing the rate of transcription. Mechanisms involved in enhancing rates of initiation of transcription include summing of multiple weak protein·protein interactions and acetylating histones to change their interaction with DNA at the transcription start site.

Hormone-activated receptors can also repress transcription. Negative feedback loops operate through this process. Activated cortisol receptors repress transcription of the gene encoding the adrenocorticotropic hormone (ACTH) precursor; activated thyroid hormone receptors inhibit transcription of both α- and β-TSH subunit genes. The principle of ligand-activated receptors binding to specific DNA target sequences in the regulated gene is the same as that required for inductive responses. The receptor may inhibit transcription by multiple mechanisms, including deacetylating histones, to increase their interaction with DNA.

Many other proteins regulate initiation of transcription, both as inducers and as inhibitors. These bind to DNA through specific sequences, as do steroid receptors, or they may interact with proteins that do. These proteins may be modified in response to hormonal signals initiated at the cell surface. Such alterations account for the changes in gene transcription due to hormones acting through surface receptors. Two general and cooperative mechanisms exist: phosphorylation and translocation of transcription factors from cytoplasm to nucleus. Genes regulated by cyclic AMP contain DNA sequences that specify binding of a specific nuclear transcription regulator (CREB). CREB, which undergoes changes in activity on phosphorylation, is a required final mediator of gene induction by peptide hormones that act at the cell surface to activate adenylate cyclase and cyclic AMP-dependent protein kinase. STAT and related proteins are phosphorylated on tyrosine residues and, when phosphorylated, enter the nucleus to activate transcription of specific genes. This chain of effects alters transcription of messenger RNAs and cell protein concentrations to dictate changes in cell function and organ physiology.

SYNTHESIS AND DELIVERY OF PEPTIDE HORMONES. Peptide hormones are small secretory proteins; their biosynthesis and secretion occur via the same processes as other non-hormonal secretory proteins. In general, peptide hormones are synthesized as part of larger precursor proteins that contain additional information. The precursor protein is cleaved, covalently modified, and folded into the form that will be ultimately secreted.

The precursor structure may have a variety of functions. Precursors for antidiuretic hormone (ADH) and oxytocin contain specific neurophysins that serve as carriers of the peptides from the site of synthesis in the hypothalamus to storage granules in axon terminals in the posterior pituitary. The ACTH precursor, pro-opiomelanocortin, contains information for several peptides that may be coordinately involved in stress responses. Structures in the precursor protein may serve to fold the peptide correctly. The connecting peptide in the insulin precursor between the β and the α subunits facilitates folding for formation of mature insulin with correctly formed disulfide bonds between and within the two chains. The connecting peptide is then excised and removed from mature α-β insulin.

Within the endoplasmic reticulum and Golgi apparatus, glycosylation of TSH, luteinizing hormone (LH), follicle-stimulating hormone (FSH), and human chorionic gonadotropin (hCG) occurs. Secretory granules containing highly concentrated hormone accumulate in the unstimulated cell. During secretion, the membrane of the secretory granule fuses with the plasma membrane and stored hormone is discharged into the circulation, a process termed *exocytosis*. Rapid release of hormone in response to stimuli reflects discharge of secretory granules, whereas prolonged secretion reflects release of newly synthesized hormone.

Peptide hormones may also be derived from precursors with receptor-like structures or from circulating forms. EGF and transforming growth factor-α (TGF-α) are made as a part of the surface domain of a transmembrane protein with a receptor-like structure. These are released by proteolysis, although they may act on adjacent cells without processing to provide cell-to-cell communication. Renin, an enzyme released from juxtaglomerular cells, acts on angiotensinogen secreted from liver. Active angiotensin is synthesized by progressive proteolysis of a precursor outside of cells: renin to yield angiotensin I and angiotensin-converting enzyme to yield angiotensin II.

Secreted peptide hormones have a short half-life of 3 to 7 minutes in the circulation. Glycoprotein hormones have longer half-lives of 1 to 4 hours. The short circulating half-life and peptide degradation by gastric acid and intestinal enzymes have precluded oral use of this class of hormones. Several attempts to prolong half-lives have met with partial success: Complexing with Zn^{2+} and protamine creates a slowly absorbed and longer-acting form of injectable insulin; removing the amino group from the N terminal amino acid and substituting a D-arginine creates a longer-acting ADH, which can be absorbed from nasal mucous membranes. At present, direct use of peptide hormones is limited to injectable forms. Prolonged action results in receptor desensitization, so recapitulation of normal cyclic secretion typical of endogenous production presents a second difficulty. Use of gonadotropin releasing hormone (GnRH) must be both by the parenteral route and pulsatile to induce ovulation and successful pregnancy.

SYNTHESIS AND TRANSPORT OF STEROID HORMONES. Steroid hormones are derived from cholesterol provided by de novo cellular synthesis from acetate or by uptake of circulating cholesterol made in the liver and delivered to cells by means of LDL particles. Synthesized steroid hormones are not stored, so secretory rates directly reflect production rates. In adrenal and gonadal tissues the rate-limiting step for increased steroid hormone biosynthesis is transfer of substrate cholesterol to the side chain cleavage enzyme located in the inner mitochondrial membrane. Cleavage of the side chain of cholesterol is catalyzed by a cytochrome P-450 enzyme that resembles other steroid hydroxylases. These enzymes progressively modify the cholesterol nucleus by the sequential addition of hydroxyl groups to specific sites. The rate-limiting step is stimulated in target cells by ACTH, LH, and FSH to result in rapid increases in steroid hormone biosynthesis. The trophic stimulatory hormones also maintain the structure of the target glands and induce each of the enzymes involved in hormone biosynthesis. With

hypophysectomy or feedback inhibition of pituitary hormone production, the entire steroid biosynthetic pathway decreases and the adrenal, ovary, and testis atrophy. Addition of trophic hormones induces enzymes and regrowth of target glands. Induction of biosynthetic enzymes appears directly mediated through second messenger pathways, primarily cyclic AMP, but growth requires coordinate provision of growth factors because cyclic AMP, in general, inhibits growth.

The pattern of biosynthetic enzymes expressed during cell differentiation determines which steroid hormone is produced and is the basis of the differentiated function of the adrenal and gonads. The fascicularis zone of the adrenal cortex expresses cytochrome P-450 enzymes that catalyze hydroxylations at carbons 21, 17, and 11. They also express 3β-hydroxysteroid dehydrogenase, $\Delta^{4,5}$ isomerase, which forms cortisol. The zona glomerulosa of the adrenal cortex makes aldosterone through a similar series of reactions, but the pathway lacks 17α-hydroxylase and contains an activity that acts at carbon 18. The testis lacks 21- and 11β-hydroxylases, so reactants flow to testosterone. Ovarian synthesis of estradiol requires cooperation between adjacent theca interna and granulosa cells. Granulosa cells express aromatase, the enzyme that catalyzes placement of three double bonds in the A ring of estrogens but cannot provide precursor androstenedione, which is synthesized in the theca interna cell located adjacent to the granulosa cell. Granulosa cells efficiently convert precursor androstenedione provided by the theca interna to estrone and estradiol.

The active form of vitamin D, 1, 25 $(OH)_2$ vitamin D, is also made from cholesterol, but the biosynthetic enzymes are located in three separate organs: skin, liver, and kidney. Vitamin D_3 is formed from 7-dehydrocholesterol by ultraviolet irradiation of skin. Vitamin D_3 is then hydroxylated at carbon 25 in the liver to yield 25(OH) vitamin D. This is converted by 1α-hydroxylase to 1, 25 $(OH)_2$ vitamin D in proximal tubule cells of the kidney. In this unique endocrine system, the major site for regulation is the final 1α-hydroxylation in renal proximal tubule cells, a step controlled by parathyroid hormone (PTH) and phosphate.

In contrast to peptide hormones, steroid hormones have longer circulating half-lives and may be active when administered orally. After secretion into the circulation, steroid hormones are bound to transport glycoproteins made in the liver. The transport proteins, which have a binding but not an activity site, provide a reservoir of hormone, protected from metabolism and renal clearance, that can be released to cells. Three transport proteins have been characterized: CBG, which binds cortisol and progesterone, sex steroid hormone–binding globulin (SHBG), which binds testosterone with greater affinity than estradiol, and vitamin D–binding protein, which binds precursor 25 (OH) vitamin D with greater affinity than 1, 25 $(OH)_2$ vitamin D. Thyroid-binding globulin (TBG) binds L-thyroxine (T_4) to provide its uniquely long half-life of 7 days. Estrogens induce and androgens inhibit synthesis of these transport proteins. Albumin provides a large carrier system that weakly binds hormones.

Free steroid hormone, which is in equilibrium with that bound to transport protein, enters cells to bind intracellular receptors and generate biologic responses. The free fraction is also the active one in feedback regulation, so it is the concentration of free hormone that is altered in homeostatic responses. The free fraction is very small compared with the bound fraction, but total hormone concentrations from both fractions are measured in most clinical assays. Conditions such as pregnancy, which alter binding protein concentrations, alter total measured hormone but not the biologically relevant free hormone concentration. In special clinical situations, measurement of binding protein concentration and of free hormone may be required for accurate assessment.

Steroid hormones are metabolized principally in the liver to inactive water-soluble metabolites. Cortisol is inactivated by reduction of the double bond in the A ring and conjugation to glucuronide or sulfate at carbon 3 to make it water soluble for renal excretion. However, not all peripheral metabolic alterations are inactivating. 5α-Reductase converts testosterone to 5α-dihydrotestosterone, which is the biologically active species in male reproductive tract and skin. Androstenedione produced in the ovary and the adrenal gland can be converted to testosterone in peripheral tissues. Significant quantities of estradiol are produced by conversion of circulating precursors.

Like their hormonal ligands, receptor synthesis is highly regulated to control cellular responses and sensitivity to hormones. Receptor synthesis is increased in response to environmental or developmental need or is repressed in negative feedback loops and during stages of development. Receptor concentration is as important as hormone concentration in determining cell responses. Regulation of receptor synthesis is therefore central to providing coordinated and appropriate endocrine responses.

INTEGRATION OF ENDOCRINE RESPONSES

FEEDBACK LOOPS. Multiple hormones cooperate to coordinate development, reproduction, and homeostasis. When a hormone has elicited an appropriate response, the signal must be terminated. In addition to the buffering that occurs in target cells, feedback control is the principal mechanism through which this occurs (Fig. 232–7). Feedback loops are especially important for communication between organs that are spatially separated. The hormonal products of peripheral endocrine glands such as thyroid, adrenal cortex, ovary, and testis exert negative feedback control over the synthesis and secretion of the stimulatory pituitary hormone. Feedback, which occurs at the level of the pituitary cell and in the hypothalamus, operates by control of several essential steps. The neurohormone thyrotropin-releasing hormone (TRH) stimulates thyrotropes of the anterior pituitary to synthesize and secrete TSH, which, in turn, increases synthesis and secretion of thyroid hormone. Increased production of thyroid hormone induces appropriate metabolic responses in target organs; it also inhibits production of TSH to return the system to baseline. The prohormone T_4 is con-

verted in the pituitary thyrotrope to active T_3, and T_3 binds to nuclear T_3 receptors to inhibit transcription of both α and β-TSH subunit genes. T_3-bound receptors also decrease synthesis of TRH receptors, rendering cells less responsive to stimulatory TRH. In addition, T_3 inhibits hypothalamic production of TRH. Conversely, when thyroid hormone concentrations are low, feedback inhibition is relieved and TRH stimulates increased production of TSH, which increases production of T_4 and thus re-establishes homeostasis. Feedback principles provide an exquisitely sensitive system for making appropriate changes and then returning to the homeostatic set point.

Feedback operates not only through steroid and thyroid hormones but also through peptides and ions. Pituitary FSH production is feedback regulated by the ovarian steroid hormone estrogen and by the ovarian peptide hormone inhibin. PTH regulates serum Ca^{2+} concentrations; with hypocalcemia, PTH increases and re-establishes normocalcemia. The increase in serum $[Ca^{2+}]$ feedback inhibits PTH synthesis and secretion to re-establish serum PTH concentrations appropriate to normocalcemia. With mutations in the $[Ca^{2+}]$ receptor on parathyroid cell membranes, feedback sensing is impaired and excessive PTH is made.

RECRUITMENT OF COORDINATE RESPONSES. Physiologic responses result from many different cell types and organs acting in concert. The necessary coordination is provided both by a hormone acting at multiple sites and by each hormone eliciting multiple responses, which sum to give the overall effect. Integrated responses require that one hormone regulate the synthesis or action of another; the nervous system is integrated into the overall response. Paradigms of such coordinated responses include stress, fasting, and reproduction.

A major stress, such as trauma with pain and hypovolemia, initiates a central nervous system response that includes synthesis and secretion of corticotropin-releasing hormone (CRH) and ADH.

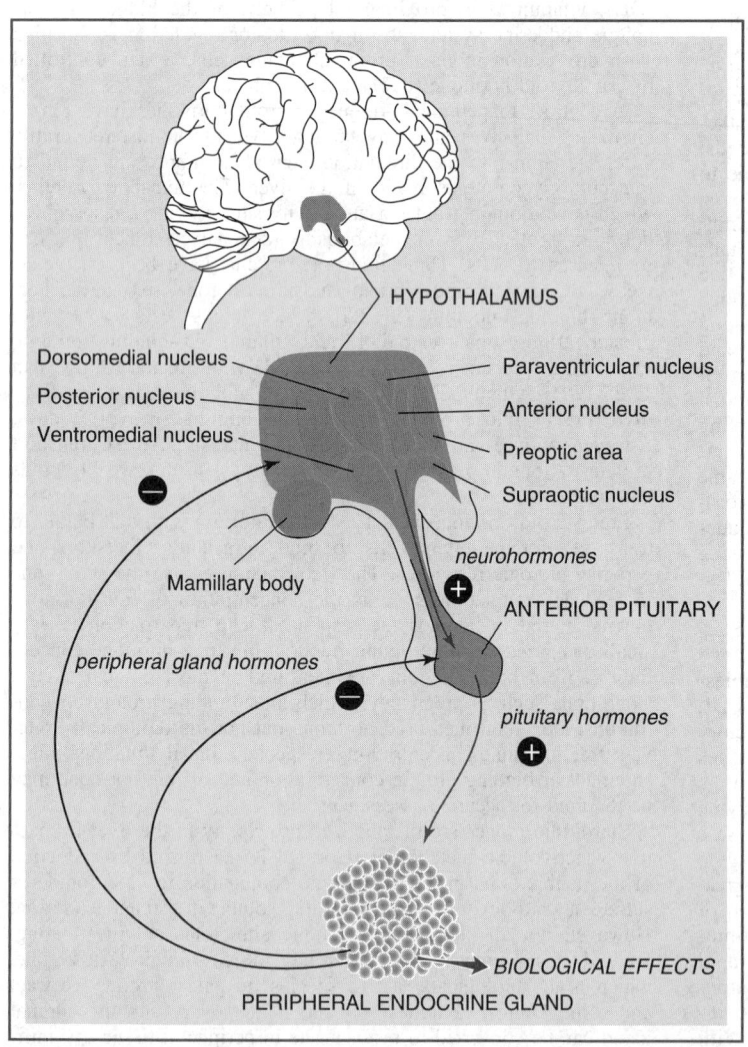

FIGURE 232–7 ■ Forward regulation and negative feedback.

CRH is the major stimulus to increase pituitary secretion of ACTH, which increases adrenal cortisol production. Cortisol maintains not only blood glucose but also vascular responsiveness to epinephrine and norepinephrine. It limits excessive inflammatory responses to prevent further volume loss and tissue damage. CRH acts, in the central nervous system, to stimulate the peripheral sympathetic nervous system. Increased sympathetic nervous system activity mediates adaptive cardiovascular responses, including increased blood pressure and pulse rate. It also induces appropriate behavioral responses. ADH increases permeability of the collecting duct of the distal nephron to conserve water and intravascular volume. It facilitates CRH-stimulated ACTH secretion. With hypovolemia the renin-angiotensin-aldosterone system is also activated to enhance vasoconstriction and to conserve sodium and intravascular volume. These responses of the hypothalamus, pituitary, and adrenal cortex together facilitate survival from stresses.

With fasting, blood glucose concentrations are maintained for 12 to 24 hours by glucagon- and epinephrine-mediated release of glucose from glycogen stores. With more prolonged fasting, cortisol-stimulated gluconeogenesis is the major mechanism that sustains blood glucose. Insulin secretion is suppressed. Metabolic demands are decreased by inhibition of 5'-deiodinase to decrease conversion of T_4 to active T_3 in peripheral tissues. Growth-promoting hormones, such as insulin-like growth factor I, are also suppressed under conditions of substrate lack. With starvation, gonadotropin secretion decreases and reproductive capacity is diminished.

Female reproductive cycles result from coordinated signaling by hypothalamic, pituitary, and ovarian hormones. Pulsatile secretion of GnRH stimulates pituitary production of LH and FSH. During the follicular phase of the menstrual cycle these peptide hormones regulate ovarian secretion of estrogen and direct maturation of follicles, one of which increases 1000-fold in diameter and becomes dominant for ovulation. FSH induces LH receptors in ovarian granulosa cells, and both LH and FSH induce aromatase as part of the mechanism that enhances estrogen production. LH and FSH increase during the follicular phase and, with follicle development, estrogen secretion rises. Positive feedback effects of estrogen result in the mid-cycle surge of LH and FSH, which induces ovulation. The remaining granulosa and theca cells reorganize to form the corpus luteum, which produces progesterone as well as estrogen. Concentrations of these hormones negatively inhibit FSH and LH production and induce additional uterine changes necessary for implantation. Ovarian inhibin also inhibits FSH production. If fertilization and implantation occur, the corpus luteum is regulated by hCG until placental steroidogenesis is established. If fertilization does not occur, negative feedback of estrogen and progesterone inhibits LH and FSH, and the luteal phase of the menstrual cycle ends after about 10 days when the corpus luteum, now deprived of trophic stimulation, decreases estrogen and progesterone production. Menstruation occurs and, in the absence of negative feedback, FSH and LH again rise to initiate a subsequent reproductive cycle.

CYCLES AND RHYTHMS. Nervous system rhythms are evident within feedback loops and coordinate hormonal responses. Several pituitary hormones are secreted with a frequency of 15 to 60 minutes, owing to pulsatile secretion of hypothalamic hormones. Longer rhythms are superimposed on these pulses. Pulsatile secretion of peptide hormones maximizes target cell responses by preventing excessive receptor down-regulation. ACTH and, consequently, cortisol exhibit a diurnal rhythm, with early morning secretion exceeding evening secretion at least twofold. Growth hormone is entrained to deep sleep, with maximal daily production occurring coincident with electroencephalographically defined slow wave sleep. Cycles also occur at different stages of development. At puberty, nocturnal increases in gonadotropins occur, a rhythm much less pronounced in adult life. Measured hormone levels must be interpreted relative to these rhythms and cycles, as well as to stages of the menstrual cycle when assaying reproductive hormones.

ASSESSMENT OF ENDOCRINE FUNCTION

QUANTITATION OF CIRCULATING HORMONES AND METABOLIC PRODUCTS. Endocrine function is assessed by accurately measuring the concentration of hormones present in blood. Even though circulating concentrations are low (nanomolar to micromolar

for steroid hormones and thyroxine and picomolar to nanomolar for peptide hormones), precise assays based on competitive protein binding are widely available. Improved sensitivity and accuracy of hormone measurements reduce the need to perform more complex stimulation and suppression tests. Even with sensitive and precise assays of hormone concentration, clinical assessment is essential. Measured values must be interpreted in relation to clinical signs and symptoms. It is also extremely helpful to measure both arms of a feedback loop. Most hormone concentrations exhibit a gaussian distribution of normal values, so an individual measurement at either end of the normal range may be normal or abnormal for that individual. Coincident measurement of TSH and T_4, LH and testosterone, ACTH and cortisol, and PTH and Ca^{2+} gives greater information than either combination alone. A T_4 value at the lower end of the normal range with an elevated TSH concentration indicates thyroid gland failure, whereas the same T_4 value with a normal TSH value likely indicates a euthyroid state. An elevated cortisol with suppressed ACTH indicates autonomous production of cortisol by an adrenal tumor. Cycles and rhythms of hormone secretion must also be considered. Evening cortisol concentrations are half or less of peak morning values. Coincident measurement of ACTH clarifies whether a low cortisol represents diurnal rhythm or adrenal insufficiency; an elevated ACTH level when the cortisol level is low suggests adrenal insufficiency. Measurement of gonadotropins, estradiol, and progesterone must be related to normal values for follicular and luteal phases of the menstrual cycle.

Steroid and thyroid hormones are bound to carrier proteins. In pregnancy, in which estrogen increases hepatic production of carrier proteins, total cortisol and T_4 values are elevated but ACTH and TSH values are normal. On occasion, it is necessary to measure the free, active hormone concentration. Because the free fraction is very small relative to the total amount, careful separation of bound from free fractions without the use of organic solvents is necessary, and very sensitive detection systems are required. Assays for free T_4 and for ionized Ca^{2+} are available for specialized clinical circumstances. One can assess the amount of binding globulin directly or can indirectly measure unoccupied binding sites (T_3 resin uptake test).

Measurement of urinary excretion of some hormones provides an integrated value for daily production rates. Measurement of urinary free cortisol is particularly useful because cortisol-binding globulin, which binds 1 cortisol molecule per molecule of protein, is approximately saturated at the peak morning cortisol concentration. Free unbound cortisol that exceeds binding capacity is filtered at the glomerulus, so an elevated 24-hour urine free cortisol determination provides an accurate assessment in cortisol excess syndromes.

Measurement of metabolic effects is an essential component of endocrine evaluation. Insulin function is assessed by measuring plasma and urine glucose concentrations, PTH by measuring serum Ca^{2+}, aldosterone by measuring serum K^+, and ADH by measuring serum and urine osmolalities.

STIMULATION AND SUPPRESSION TESTS. Measurement of both arms of a feedback loop provides sufficient laboratory information in most endocrine deficiency or excess states. Additional diagnostic information can be gained, however, by perturbing the feedback system through administration of hormones. For stimulation tests, a hormone is administered and the ability of the target gland to respond is assessed by measuring its product. This provides an estimate of the ability of the target gland to synthesize hormone, of its trophic maintenance, and of its exposure to feedback inhibition. Baseline measurements are made before hormone administration and at the established normal time of peak target gland response. Ranges of normal responses have been established for comparison. Examples include TRH stimulation tests, in which levels of pituitary-produced TSH are measured. In hypopituitarism, serum TSH fails to rise in response to a standard intravenous injection of TRH. In primary hypothyroidism, in which feedback inhibition by thyroid hormone is small, TSH rises excessively, whereas in hyperthyroidism, excessive feedback inhibition results in minimal or no increases in TSH. For ACTH stimulation tests, $ACTH_{1-24}$ is administered as an intravenous injection to assess the ability of the adrenal cortex to produce cortisol. A low baseline cortisol level that fails to rise indicates adrenal insufficiency. Interpretation requires integration of clinical information because failure to respond to ACTH may also occur when the adrenal cortex has been suppressed, owing to treatment with synthetic glucocorticoids. A variation of stimulation tests involves interruption of the feedback loop by metabolic inhibitors of hormone biosynthesis. Metyrapone, an inhibitor of 11β-hydroxylase, decreases serum cortisol, relieving feedback suppression of ACTH production. The resulting increase in ACTH can be measured directly; or ACTH-stimulated 11-desoxycortisol, the precursor of cortisol, can be measured as an indicator of increased ACTH. The metyrapone test provides an assessment of pituitary corticotrope function and reserve. Stimulation tests are most useful in suspected endocrine deficiency states.

Suppression tests, which measure the ability of administered hormone to provide feedback inhibition, are most useful in evaluating hormone excesses. Dexamethasone, a potent synthetic glucocorticoid, is administered to inhibit ACTH production. Because dexamethasone is not detected in cortisol assays, more easily measured cortisol rather than ACTH can be used as an endpoint. In Cushing's syndrome, the source of cortisol excess can be deduced using dexamethasone suppression. Pituitary tumors that produce excess ACTH frequently retain susceptibility to feedback inhibition. These tumors are resistant to doses of dexamethasone that suppress normal corticotrope ACTH production but are inhibited by higher doses of dexamethasone. In contrast, adrenal gland tumors and tumors that ectopically produce ACTH are resistant to even high doses of dexamethasone.

ANATOMIC ASSESSMENT. Imaging of endocrine glands is important, especially when considering surgical therapy. The high sensitivity and precision of computed tomography and nuclear magnetic resonance imaging allow detection of even small endocrine tumors such as pituitary, parathyroid, and adrenal adenomas. Ultrasonographic techniques are also useful for imaging the thyroid gland, ovaries, testes, and pancreas. Radionuclide imaging may also be useful. Radioactive isotopes of iodine (^{123}I, ^{131}I) or compounds that are concentrated by the thyroid gland similar to iodine, such as ^{99}Tc, are used to determine anatomy and imply function of the thyroid gland.

Measurement of hormone concentrations in venous effluent of glands may be useful in specialized circumstances to localize the source of abnormal production. Measurement of ACTH in petrosal sinus blood may be useful in localizing pituitary tumors, of PTH in neck and chest veins in localizing unusually located parathyroid adenomas, and of insulin in mesenteric venous drainage in localizing pancreatic insulinomas.

Cytologic and immunocytochemical techniques are important. Fine-needle aspiration of thyroid nodules with cytologic examinations analogous to those used in Papanicolaou smears has become the procedure of choice to distinguish benign and malignant thyroid nodules. Staining of surgical tissues with antihormone antibodies provides proof of hormone production and a guide to future therapy.

Receptors are not routinely measured but can be quantitated using immunologic techniques. Recombinant DNA technologies can be used to define inherited defects in receptors. When oncogenes are identified in specific endocrine neoplasms, these can be measured and mutations identified using DNA hybridization techniques. Autoimmune endocrine diseases can be documented by quantitating antibodies directed against specific organs (thyroid-stimulating immunoglobulin, anti-islet cell antibodies, antiadrenal antibodies).

ABERRATIONS IN DISEASE

DEFICIENCY STATES. The most prevalent endocrine disorders result from hormone deficiencies. A variety of disease states impair or destroy endocrine glands: defects in organ development, genetic defects in biosynthetic enzymes, immune-mediated destruction, neoplasia, infections, hemorrhage, nutritional deficits, and vascular insufficiency. Endocrine gland failure may be acute, with rapid development of symptoms or chronic with slower development of symptoms but more pronounced physical changes. Defects in a gland such as the thyroid may result in a multisystem disorder due to failure to produce a single hormone, whereas defects in the hypothalamus or pituitary may result in a multisystem disorder, including thyroid deficiency, due to failure to produce many hor-

mones. Multiple endocrine gland deficiencies may also result from autoimmune-mediated mechanisms in the polyglandular autoimmune deficiency syndromes. Because hormones participate in coordinated responses, secondary changes in other endocrine responses often result from deficiency of a single hormone.

Deficiency states also result from defects in hormone receptors and in signaling mechanisms. Defects may be inherited or acquired. Genetic abnormalities in androgen receptors result in unresponsiveness to androgens and an XY male with a female phenotype; defects in vitamin D receptors result in vitamin D-resistant rickets; defects in thyroid hormone receptors result in the resistance to thyroid hormone of Refetoff's syndrome; defects in growth hormone receptors result in ateliotic dwarfism of Laron's syndrome. Acquired receptor defects most often result from immunologic mechanisms where antibodies bind to receptors, blocking ligand access.

Post-receptor defects may occur. A defect in $G_{\alpha}s$ results in pseudohypoparathyroidism, in which unresponsiveness to PTH occurs. Such patients fail to respond normally to other hormones whose receptors couple to adenylate cyclase (TSH, glucagon, LH). Type II diabetes mellitus, which is inherited, is characterized by insulin resistance. The molecular defect has not yet been characterized, but understanding this pathophysiology underlies therapeutic approaches directed at reducing resistance to and augmenting secretion of insulin. Because receptor and post-receptor defects are characterized by hormone resistance, feedback does not occur; and producer glands enlarge and circulating hormone concentrations are high despite clinical evidence for deficiency.

EXCESS STATES. Excessive production of hormone and clinical evidence of such excess implies failure of normal feedback mechanisms. This occurs most commonly with neoplasia and with autoimmunity, in which antireceptor antibodies act as hormone agonists. Tumors of endocrine glands characteristically produce excessive amounts of the hormone made by the cell of origin but are no longer subject to normal feedback controls. Some tumors, such as pituitary adenomas that produce ACTH, retain feedback but require higher concentrations of cortisol to suppress ACTH. Prolactinomas retain dopamine suppression, and both their function and growth can be inhibited by dopamine agonists. Tumors arising in peripheral endocrine glands that are under pituitary trophic hormone regulation are autonomous because they are not normally subject to negative feedback. More undifferentiated tumors may also be insensitive to feedback regulation.

Hormones may be produced in excess by tumors arising from cells that do not normally produce the hormone. Ectopic production of peptide hormones is common in a variety of neoplasms, and symptoms due to the hormone excess may contribute significantly to morbidity. Because steroid hormones are made via a multienzyme pathway, excesses of these hormones occur only with tumors arising in the producer gland or with excessive production of the trophic peptide hormone. Cortisol excess may result from adrenocortical tumors or from excessive stimulation by ACTH produced by pituitary or ectopic neoplasms.

The most prevalent disease due to agonistic antibodies is Graves' disease, in which antibodies are produced that activate the TSH receptor. Because many hormones are available as therapeutic agents, some patients take excessive amounts and present with an endocrine excess syndrome.

GENETIC DETERMINANTS OF DISEASE. Many endocrine diseases result from genetic mutations. Genetic defects in biosynthetic enzymes may result in deficiency states: Hypothyroidism may result from thyroid peroxidase or deiodinase enzyme defects; adrenal insufficiency may result from 21-hydroxylase deficiency or a defect in other steroid biosynthetic enzymes; a form of male hypogonadism may result from 5α-reductase deficiency. Receptor defects are thought to be uncommon, but methods to define these have only recently become available. Type II diabetes, the most common endocrine abnormality, is inherited, but its molecular basis is not yet known. Autoimmune endocrine disease also has a genetic basis involving an inherited defect in immune surveillance. Multiple endocrine neoplasia syndromes are due to activating mutations in the *ret* tyrosine kinase receptor so that cell growth and function are constitutively stimulated without ligand.

Methods using nucleic acid probes can be used to make precise diagnoses in disease states and to provide predictive information before overt disease develops. Because genetic defects are present in all DNA, peripheral blood cells or skin fibroblasts provide a ready source of material for assay. Acquired mutations can be assessed by assay of material obtained by biopsy.

Darnell JE Jr: Stats and gene regulation. Science 277:1630, 1997. *Summary of a major pathway through which information is transferred from the cell surface to the nucleus.*
Glass CK, Rose DW, Rosenfeld MG: Nuclear receptor coactivators. Curr Opin Cell Biol 9:222, 1997. *Concise review of mechanisms by which hormone binding switches nuclear receptors from repressors to activators of gene transcription.*
Marks F (ed): Protein phosphorylation. Weinheim, Germany, VCH, 1996. *Contains chapters on various protein kinases, their structure, function, and postulated role in biologic processes.*
Pawson AJ (ed): Protein modules in signal transduction. *In* Current Topics in Microbiology and Immunology. Berlin, Springer-Verlag, 1998. *A single small volume that contains reviews of many of the modules that direct protein . protein interactions that are essential to signal transduction.*

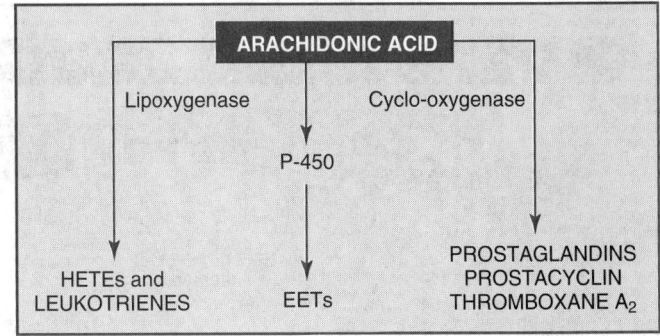

FIGURE 233–1 ■ Major pathways of metabolism of arachidonic acid. HETEs = hydroxyeicosatetraenoic acids; EETs = epoxy-eicosatrienoic acids.

233 PROSTAGLANDINS AND RELATED COMPOUNDS*

Perry V. Halushka

Prostaglandins, thromboxanes, leukotrienes, C_{20}-hydroxy-fatty acids, and lipoxins belong to a large family of oxygenated fatty acids collectively named eicosanoids because they are metabolites of polyunsaturated eicosanoic (C_{20}) acids. With the exception of seminal fluid, the eicosanoids are not stored in tissues or cells, but rather are rapidly synthesized from precursor fatty acids. Of the three fatty acid precursors for the eicosanoids, arachidonic acid, which is derived from dietary sources, is the predominant one. It is transported in plasma in both esterified and non-esterified forms primarily bound to lipoproteins and albumin, respectively. Esterified arachidonic acid in low-density lipoproteins is taken up by cells by a process dependent on the low-density lipoprotein receptor. The fatty acids are stored in the sn-2 position of phospholipids and compartmentalized in the cell membranes, which is important for the availability of their release.

Arachidonate release may occur via several mechanisms and is the rate-limiting step in formation of the eicosanoids. Cleavage of arachidonic acid from either phosphatidylcholine or phosphatidylethanolamine occurs after cytosolic phospholipase A_2 is translocated to the membrane. Phosphorylation by mitogen-activated kinase and protein kinase C permits its calcium-dependent translocation to the cell membrane. Other phospholipases and triglyceride lipases may also participate in arachidonate release. Phosphatidylinositol may be hydrolyzed by a phosphatidylinositol-specific phospholipase C to yield diacylglycerol and inositol phosphate. Diacylglycerol is then further hydrolyzed to yield free arachidonic acid and other fatty acids. Subsequent oxygenation by either fatty acid cyclooxygenases, lipoxygenases, or cytochrome P-450 give rise to biologically active compounds (Fig. 233–1).

The profile of enzymatic products that are formed is highly cell specific. Because of their diverse biologic properties and rapid metabolism to inactive products, the eicosanoids have been implicated as local mediators or modulators of receptor-dependent events in a range of physiologic processes and diverse human diseases, including bronchial asthma, inflammatory processes, and renal, vascular, and coronary artery diseases. Arachidonic acid itself and its metabolites may also function as intracellular second messengers, particularly in the modulation of ion channels, ras activity, and perhaps gene expression.

THE CYCLOOXYGENASE PATHWAY

The initial oxygenation of arachidonic acid that ultimately leads to the formation of thromboxane A_2 (TxA_2), prostacyclin (PGI_2), prostaglandin E_2 (PGE_2), $PGF_{2\alpha}$, and PGD_2 is catalyzed by the enzyme fatty acid cyclooxygenase (Fig. 233–2). The product of

*Revised and updated from the chapter by G.A. Fitzgerald in the 20th edition of the *Cecil Textbook of Medicine.*

cyclooxygenase is an unstable endoperoxide, PGG. A second oxygen molecule introduced at C_{15} results in formation of the 15-hydroperoxyendoperoxide PGH and liberates a free radical. Two *COX* (cyclooxygenase) genes have been identified. A constitutive form *(COX-1)* is expressed ubiquitously and is inducible in certain constrained circumstances (e.g., by certain cytokines in bone marrow–derived mast cells or by male sex hormones in the ram seminal vesicle). Expression of *COX-2* is induced by cytokines, endotoxin, tumor promoters, growth factors, and gonadotropins. Its induced expression occurs in macrophages, monocytes, synoviocytes, ovarian follicles, colonic adenomas and cancer cells, vascular smooth muscle cells, and amnion. Consequently, it is presumed to be the cyclooxygenase of predominant importance in the generation of prostaglandins in inflammation and, possibly, cancer, mitogenesis, and induction of parturition.

Arachidonic acid contains four double bonds ($D^{5,8,11,14}$); however, after metabolism by fatty acid cyclooxygenase (see Fig. 233–2), only two double bonds remain. This phenomenon is denoted by the subscript 2, as in TxA_2 and PGE_2. Analogous metabolism of other fatty acid substrates gives rise to monoenoic or trienoic prostaglandins and thromboxanes. For example, metabolites of eicosatrienoic acid ($C_{20:3}$ n-6)(di-homo-γ-linolenic acid), which is found in oil of evening primrose, contain only one (D^{13}) double bond. Eicosapentaenoic acid ($C_{20:5}$ n-3), which is prevalent in certain fish and aquatic mammals, is transformed by cyclooxygenase to metabolites with three ($D^{5,13,17}$) double bonds, such as PGI_3 and TxA_3. Structurally, prostaglandins possess a cyclopentane ring and differ only in their substituent groups and their positions, which confers the letter designation.

THROMBOXANE A_2. TxA_2 is the predominant cyclooxygenase product formed by platelets and human monocytes. It stimulates platelet aggregation and secretion and is mitogenic for and constricts vascular and bronchial smooth muscle. These biologic properties are shared by the prostaglandin endoperoxides. A single gene encodes a human thromboxane receptor, which is a member of the G protein–coupled receptor superfamily. Two carboxyl terminal tail splice variants have been described, and they differ in their preferential linkage to G proteins and in aspects of their desensitization. Expression of the receptors is transcriptionally regulated by certain growth factors and male sex steroids. A mutation in the first intracellular loop of the thromboxane receptor has been linked to a bleeding disorder characterized by a selective defect in the signal transduction and aggregation of platelets induced by thromboxane agonists.

PROSTACYCLIN. PGI_2, the predominant cyclooxygenase product of arachidonic acid formed by vascular endothelium and subendothelium, both inhibits the aggregation of platelets and causes disaggregation. PGI_2 inhibits the adherence of platelets and neutrophils to foreign surfaces and damaged endothelium and dilates both bronchial and vascular smooth muscle. A PGI_2 receptor exhibits 30 to 40% homology with other eicosanoid receptors. Deletion of this receptor in mice results in decreased pain perception and inflammation and increased thrombotic responses, thus supporting a role for PGI_2 in these processes. Another potentially important property of PGI_2 is modulation of cholesterol efflux from arterial walls. Nan-

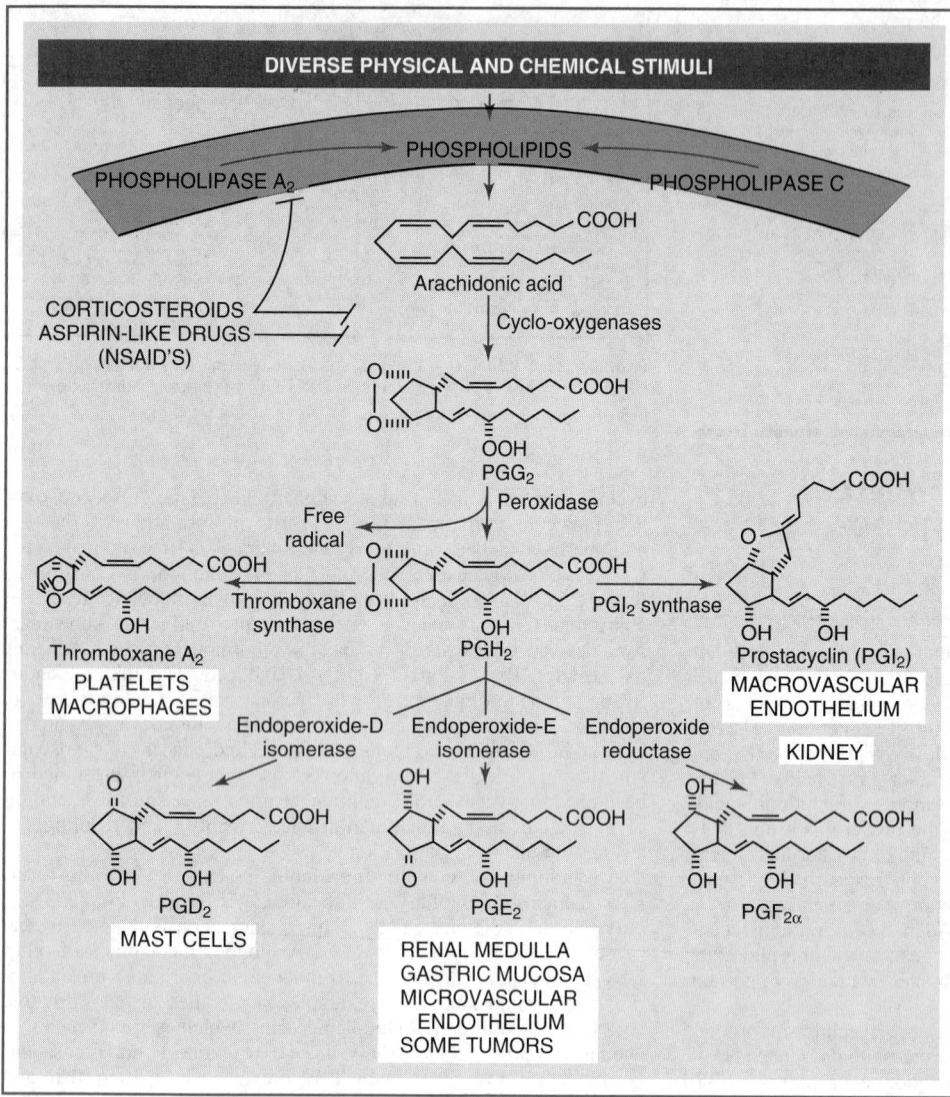

FIGURE 233–2 ■ Metabolism of arachidonic acid by fatty acid cyclooxygenase. The major tissues of origin of the eicosanoids are shown. PGG$_2$ = prostaglandin G$_2$.

omolar quantities of PGI$_2$ stimulate the activity of both the lysosomal and cytoplasmic cholesterol ester hydrolases but have no effect on the microsomal acyl coenzyme A cholesterol acyltransferase, which re-esterifies free cholesterol. Both PGI and TxA synthase are cytochrome P-450 enzymes.

PGI$_2$ biosynthesis is increased in several human diseases in which evidence of platelet activation is present, including severe peripheral arterial disease and unstable coronary artery disease, thus implying a homeostatic role for this eicosanoid.

PROSTAGLANDIN D$_2$. PGD$_2$, the principal cyclooxygenase product of the mast cell, is released, together with histamine and other mediators, by IgE and other stimuli. Infusion of PGD$_2$ in humans results in nasal stuffiness, systemic hypotension, and flushing. PGD$_2$ is increased in bronchoalveolar lavage fluid following antigen challenge in atopic individuals, which suggests that it contributes to bronchospasm in allergic asthma. PGD$_2$ is a minor product of platelet cyclooxygenase. Both PGD$_2$ and its $9\alpha,11\beta$-PGF metabolite inhibit platelet aggregation by stimulating adenylate cyclase. In experimental animals, central administration of PGD$_2$ induces sleep, an event that is countered by infusion of PGE$_2$. Two forms of PGD synthase exist—one in brain and the other in blood cells. The former is highly expressed in the leptomeninges and choroid plexus, where it may increase PGD levels in cerebrospinal fluid (CSF). Elevated CSF levels of PGD have been reported in patients with African sleeping sickness.

PROSTAGLANDIN E$_2$. The formation of PGE$_2$ from PGH$_2$ is catalyzed by PGE$_2$ isomerase, which is present in the renal medulla, gastric mucosa, platelets, and other tissues. PGE$_2$ rather than PGI$_2$

may be the predominant prostaglandin formed by microvascular endothelium. In the kidney, PGE$_2$ acts both as a vasodilator and as an inhibitor of tubular sodium reabsorption. Together with PGI$_2$, it helps maintain renal blood flow during activation of the renin-angiotensin and sympathoadrenal systems and in patients with mild renal insufficiency. Four PGE receptor genes (*EP1*, *EP2*, *EP3*, and *EP4*) yield tissue-specific carboxyl terminal splice variants that couple with differing preference to discrete effector pathways.

Other biologic properties of PGE$_2$ include relaxation of bronchial smooth muscle, contraction of gravid uterine smooth muscle (19-hydroxylated E prostaglandins are the major arachidonic acid products in human semen), and modulation of lymphocyte function. PGE$_2$ modulates neurotransmission via pre-synaptic receptors on adrenergic neurons.

PROSTAGLANDIN F$_{2\alpha}$. PGF$_{2\alpha}$, formed from PGH$_2$ by the action of endoperoxide reductase, contracts bronchial and uterine smooth muscle and vasoconstricts uterine vessels and veins. Although increases in PGF$_{2\alpha}$ metabolites have been described during dysmenorrhea and allergen-evoked bronchospasm, a unique site for formation of this prostaglandin and its role in pathophysiology remain to be determined. It does play an important role in parturition.

PROSTAGLANDIN J$_2$. PGJ$_2$ is a non-enzymatically formed dehydration product of PGD$_2$. $^\Delta$12-PGJ$_2$ has been found to inhibit tumor cell growth via induction of apoptosis and suppression of the c-*myc* gene and to modulate macrophage function. It appears that these effects result from stimulation of the peroxisome proliferator–activated receptor γ, but the significance of these pharmacologic effects is uncertain.

CYCLOOXYGENASE INHIBITORS. Non-steroidal anti-inflammatory drugs (NSAIDs) prevent the formation of prostaglandins by inhibiting fatty acid cyclooxygenases. This group of drugs includes aspirin, indomethacin, and all other NSAIDs. Acetaminophen is a considerably less potent inhibitor than the other compounds, except perhaps in the brain. It has considerably greater potency in inhibiting COX-1 than COX-2, which may account for its lack of anti-inflammatory effects. Aspirin differs from other NSAIDs in that it acetylates a serine residue in the active site of COX-1 and irreversibly inhibits the enzyme. This property accounts for the long-lived effects of aspirin on platelet COX-1. Whereas other cells have the capacity for de novo protein synthesis, the anucleate platelet does not; thus inhibition of TxA$_2$ formation by aspirin persists for the lifetime of the platelet. In contrast, the effects of aspirin on eicosanoid formation by other cells (e.g., PGI$_2$ biosynthesis by vascular endothelium) that express both COX-1 and COX-2 are not so prolonged owing to their capacity to generate new enzymes. The irreversible actions of aspirin on platelet cyclooxygenase also account for the cumulative inhibition of platelet TxA$_2$ formation by the repeated administration of low doses of aspirin (20 to 40 mg/day; an adult aspirin tablet contains 325 mg). This phenomenon results in partial inhibition of platelet cyclooxygenase after single-dose administration. Even though low doses of aspirin depress PGI$_2$ formation, the effect is more pronounced on platelet TxA$_2$ biosynthesis during long-term therapy. The serine target for aspirin acetylation is conserved in COX-2, and aspirin is a non-selective inhibitor of the two enzymes. However, coincident with prostaglandin inhibition, aspirin acetylation of COX-2 but not COX-1 results in increased formation of 15-R-hydroxyeicosatetraenoic acid.

THE LIPOXYGENASE PATHWAY

Arachidonic acid is also subject to lipoxygenation reactions (Fig. 233–3). In neutrophils, insertion of an oxygen molecule adjacent to one of the double bonds yields the hydroperoxy derivative 5-hydroperoxyeicosatetraenoic acid (5-HPETE). This byproduct can undergo further metabolism to either a 5-hydroxyeicosatetraenoic acid (5-HETE) or to an unstable 5,6-epoxide intermediate, leukotriene A$_4$ (LTA$_4$). This metabolite can be hydrolyzed to 5,12-dihydroxyeicosatetraenoic acids (5,12-DiHETE), one of which is LTB$_4$. The subscript 4 refers to the number of double bonds. The site of the initial lipoxygenation reaction tends to vary with the cell type. Thus 12-HETE is formed predominantly in platelets, 5-HETE by polymorphonuclear leukocytes, and 5-HETE, 11-HETE, and 15-HETE by endothelial cells.

The 5-lipoxygenase of human neutrophils, a cytosolic enzyme, is translocated to the membrane for metabolism of arachidonic acid. It requires the 5-lipoxygenase activating protein (FLAP) for full activation. Analogous activating proteins do not appear necessary for the expression of 12- and 15-lipoxygenase activity. Two distinct 12-lipoxygenases are recognized. One, in porcine leukocytes and brain and in human tracheal cells, is closely related to 15-lipoxygenase, whereas the human platelet 12-lipoxygenase is a distinct gene product. Platelet 12-lipoxygenase is translocated from the cytosol to the membrane in a calcium-dependent manner, and 12-HETE inhibits the mobilization of a glycoprotein IIb-IIIa complex that is analogous to the receptor for adhesive macromolecules, such as fibrinogen, in activated platelets. Formation of 15-HETE is increased in atherosclerotic blood vessels, and in situ hybridization studies suggest that expression of the enzyme is increased and colocalized with oxidized low-density lipoproteins in human atherosclerotic plaque.

LTA$_4$ is conjugated enzymatically with glutathione to yield LTC$_4$. This compound is metabolized to LTD$_4$ and LTE$_4$ by successive elimination of a γ-glutamyl residue and glycine. The cysteinyl-containing leukotrienes are powerful bronchoconstrictors and vasoconstrictors, dilate microvessels, increase vascular permeability, potentiate the effects of histamine on bronchial smooth muscle, and stimulate mucus secretion. LTC$_4$ causes pulmonary bronchoconstriction, an effect that is partially blocked by cyclooxygenase inhibitors, which implies that this effect may be mediated via the release of a bronchoconstrictor prostaglandin such as TxA$_2$. LTC$_4$ may cooperate with luteinizing hormone–releasing hormone in the control of luteinizing hormone release by cells of the anterior pituitary.

LTB$_4$ stimulates adhesion, migration, aggregation, enzyme release, and generation of superoxide by polymorphonuclear leukocytes. These biologic properties indicate a role for lipoxygenase products in both inflammation and antigen-evoked bronchoconstriction. LTB$_4$ levels are significantly increased in the synovial fluid of patients with gout and may be one of the chemotactic stimuli for the infiltration of polymorphonuclear leukocytes.

DiHETEs can be formed via transcellular metabolism. Examples include 12,20-DiHETE formed by a mixed suspension of platelets

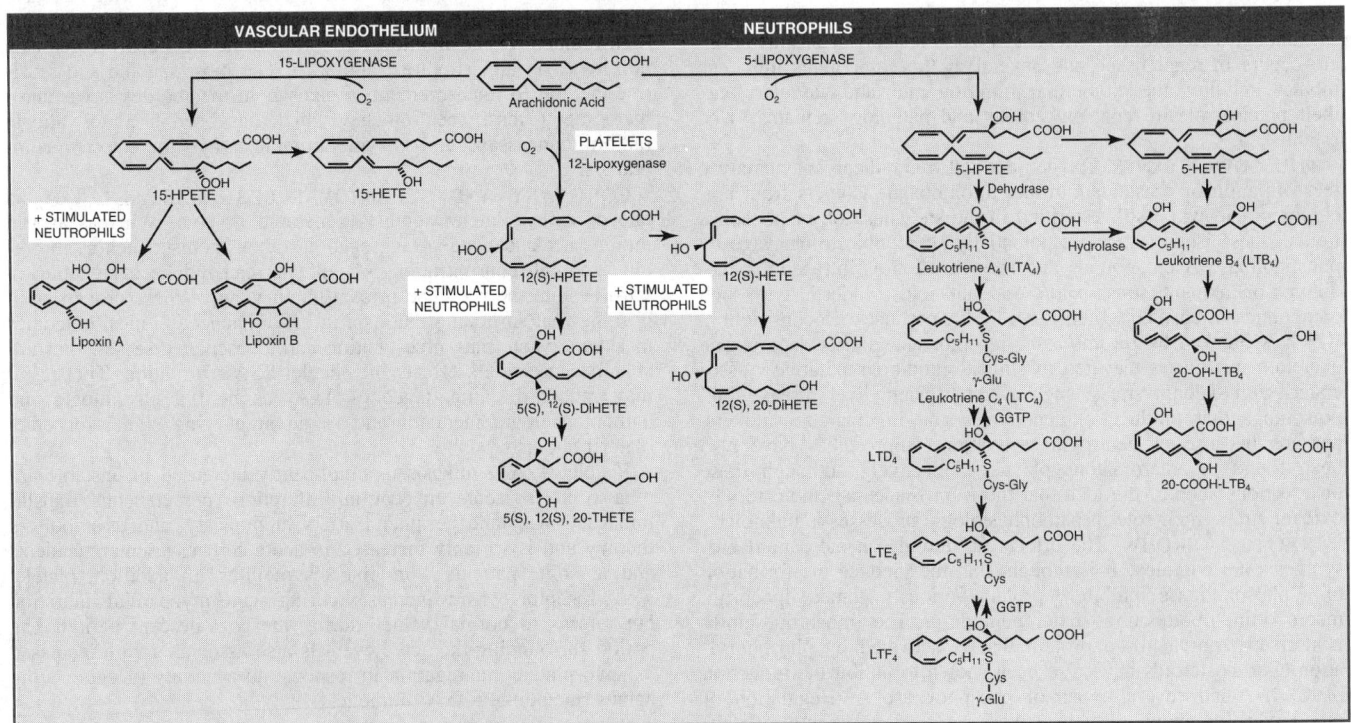

FIGURE 233–3 ■ Metabolism of arachidonic acid by lipoxygenase enzymes. HPETE = hydroperoxyeicosatetraenoic acid; HETE = hydroxyeicosatetraenoic acid; GGTP = γ-glutamyltranspeptidase.

and polymorphonuclear leukocytes. Leukocytes can use erythrocyte LTA_4 to generate LTB_4, and endothelial cells can use platelet-derived PGH_2 to generate PGI_2.

Stimulated human leukocytes can convert 15-HPETE to lipoxins containing a characteristic tetraenoic structure (see Fig. 233–3). The two major products are identified as lipoxin A and B. Lipoxin A is a potent stimulus to superoxide generation by neutrophils and contracts pulmonary tissue. Both lipoxin A and B inhibit natural killer cell cytotoxicity by a mechanism distinct from that of PGE_2, which decreases the binding between target and effector cells. Another series of compounds with potent biologic properties in vitro are the hepoxilins, which are formed by an intramolecular rearrangement of 12-HETE. Glutathione conjugates of hepoxilin A_3 cause hyperpolarization of rat brain neurons at nanomolar concentrations.

THE EPOXYGENASE PATHWAY

In addition to metabolism by cyclooxygenase and lipoxygenase enzymes, arachidonic acid is subject to ω and ω-1 oxidation by cytochrome P-450 enzymes located in microsomes. A specific cytochrome P-450 enzyme with high affinity for arachidonic acid catalyzes the formation of 19-OH- and 19-oxo-eicosatetraenoic acid (by ω-1 oxidation) and 20-OH-eicosatetraenoic and eicosatetraene-1,20-dioic acids (by ω oxidation). In addition, a series of epoxides, e.g., 14(15)-epoxy-, 11(12)-epoxy-, 8(9)-epoxy-, and 5(6)-epoxy-eicosatrienoic acids (EETs), can be formed by this enzyme from arachidonic acid. These compounds can be further transformed to vicinyl diols by epoxide hydrolases. One such compound, 11,12-dihydroxyeicosatrienoic acid, inhibits the Na^+, K^+-adenosinetriphosphatase enzyme in vascular smooth muscle. 5(6)-EET inhibits sodium absorption and potassium secretion by the rabbit cortical collecting duct, and synthetic 5(6)-EET stimulates the release of luteinizing hormone and somatostatin by pituitary cells in culture. Interestingly, 8,9-EET and 14,15-EET stereospecifically inhibit human platelet cyclooxygenase. By contrast, all EETs studied inhibit platelet aggregation in vitro by a non-specific mechanism independent of an effect on thromboxane formation. EETs weakly inhibit monocyte and platelet adherence to endothelial cells. Urinary excretion of the vicinyl diols of the EETs (DiHETs) is increased in normal pregnancy, and further increments, particularly of 14(15)-DiHET, are observed in patients with pregnancy-induced hypertension. 5(6)-EET biosynthesis is increased in syndromes of salt and water retention.

Although cytochrome P-450–catalyzed metabolism of arachidonate occurs in renal tissue and several of the compounds influence tubular ion flux, the glomerular filtration rate, and vascular tone, their precise role in renal physiology and pathology remains to be established.

THE ISOPROSTANES. Oxygen-derived free radicals may catalyze the formation of prostaglandin and thromboxane isomers from arachidonic acid while still esterified in the sn-2 position of phospholipids. These isoprostanes are potentially susceptible to cleavage by phospholipase A compounds and may function as intracellular mediators of oxidant stress and/or as autacoids. Indeed, two such compounds, 8-epi-$PGF_{2\alpha}$ and 8-epi-PGE_2, produce vasoconstriction, which is blocked by thromboxane receptor antagonists. Isoprostane excretion in urine is elevated in clinical conditions putatively associated with oxidant stress, such as reperfusion, liver disease, and poisonings that produce oxidant stress and in cigarette smokers, perhaps because of neutrophil activation. Isoprostanes have also been found in atheromatous plaque. Collectively, although these observations support the idea that the isoprostanes are indicators of oxidant stress, their role in pathophysiologic processes is unknown.

CORTICOSTEROIDS. The effects of steroids on eicosanoid biosynthesis are complex. It is thought that they induce the formation of a phospholipase inhibitory protein variously named lipocortin, macrocortin, lipomodulin, and renomodulin. The lipocortin family is derived from a 40-kd protein that is activated by phosphorylation. Corticosteroids have also been shown to inhibit the induction of COX-2 and several types of phospholipase A. Regulation of other inducible enzymes such as nitric oxide synthase is also probably of relevance to the anti-inflammatory properties of these compounds.

DIETARY SUBSTRATE MODIFICATION. Mortality from coronary heart disease seems to be lower in populations that consume large quantities of ω-3 fatty acids, such as eicosapentaenoic acid, derived from aquatic mammals or salt and cold water fish. One hypothesis is that a shift toward the formation of TxA_3 (which is less biologically active than TxA_2) and PGI_3 (which is a platelet inhibitory, vasodilator compound like PGI_2) may favorably influence platelet–vessel wall interactions. Although fish oil supplementation of the Western diet has only modest effects on platelet function, it has caused regression of atherosclerosis in several animal models. It has also been shown to decrease triglycerides and has variable effects on cholesterol. However, efforts to modify the rate of restenosis after coronary angioplasty by fish oil supplementation have been unsuccessful. Attempts to relate dietary fish intake to cardiovascular morbidity and mortality have provided conflicting results.

Supplementation of the diet with ω-3 fatty acids lowers blood pressure in patients with mild essential hypertension. This effect is not obviously related to altered eicosanoid formation.

Fish oil supplementation in animal models of inflammation, particularly renal disease and cyclosporine-induced nephropathy, have produced modest positive effects. It has been hypothesized that marine oils might modulate inflammatory or immune diseases by altering the profile of lipoxygenase or cyclooxygenase product formation.

HUMAN DISEASES INVOLVING EICOSANOIDS

The evidence implicating arachidonate metabolites in human diseases is derived from measurements of their biosynthesis and from the effects of drugs that prevent their formation or antagonize their actions. Because of the evanescent nature of the primary compounds, estimates of in vivo synthesis have largely been based on measurement of long-lived but biologically inactive metabolites. Quantitative assays for the major urinary metabolites of the primary prostaglandins PGD_2, PGE_2, PGI_2, and TxA_2 have been useful in identifying potential targets for drugs designed to modulate their actions. Similar methodology is now available to explore lipoxygenase and epoxygenase product formation in vivo. The capacity of tissues to generate arachidonic acid metabolites greatly exceeds the actual production rates in vivo. Thus artifacts related to sample collection (for example, platelet activation ex vivo during blood sampling, catheter-induced vascular trauma, or formation of free radical–catalyzed derivatives during sample storage) can seriously confound attempts to measure these compounds in the bloodstream. Measurement of metabolite excretion in urine has been favored as a non-invasive, albeit indirect approach. The most specific and sensitive method for measurement of eicosanoid metabolites is gas chromatography–mass spectrometry, which has been used to validate radioimmunoassays and enzyme immunoassays for selected compounds.

CORONARY AND CEREBROVASCULAR DISEASES. TxA_2 is one of many platelet agonists generated in vivo. Whereas aspirin inhibits TxA_2-dependent aggregation, other agonists such as thrombin and high concentrations of collagen can induce aggregation in vitro despite the presence of aspirin. In view of these properties, it is somewhat surprising that aspirin has influenced clinical outcomes in a variety of trials investigating cardiovascular diseases, presumably because of its effects on platelet TxA_2 formation. This result may reflect the importance of TxA_2 as both a physiologic and pathophysiologic mediator and as an amplifying signal for other platelet agonists.

Platelet TxA_2 synthesis is significantly increased in unstable angina pectoris, acute myocardial infarction, percutaneous transluminal coronary and peripheral artery angioplasty, and thrombolysis therapy and is variably increased in acute cerebrovascular accidents and in some patients with diabetes mellitus. In addition, platelet TxA_2 receptor density increases during acute myocardial infarction but returns to normal values during the convalescent period. The period surrounding the acute event is also associated with increased ex vivo platelet aggregation in response to a variety of aggregating agents, including a TxA_2 mimetic.

Aspirin significantly reduces the incidence of stroke in patients suffering transient ischemic attacks or with non-valvular atrial fibrillation. It also reduces the incidence of thrombotic occlusion following coronary artery bypass grafting and the incidence of myocardial infarction and death in patients with unstable angina pectoris. Aspirin reduces the risk of a combined end point of myocardial infarction, stroke, and vascular death by about 25%. The most convincing evidence that aspirin reduces mortality in patients who have suffered an acute myocardial infarction is provided by the ISIS-2 study of more than 17,000 patients. The reduction in mortality achieved by aspirin and the thrombolytic agent streptokinase was comparable and additive. Importantly, aspirin did not increase the incidence of stroke when combined with streptokinase.

Clear-cut evidence of the benefit of aspirin has been obtained in smaller trials of patients with unstable angina. This benefit may reflect the early initiation of aspirin therapy and the more prominent role of thrombosis in determining outcome in these patients. Angioscopic and angiographic evidence of thrombosis is present in unstable angina, and phasic increases in TxA_2 formation coincide with episodes of cardiac ischemia. By contrast, the alteration in TxA_2 formation after myocardial infarction is transient, and there is little evidence of sustained platelet activation in patients with chronic stable angina. Controlled trials have, however, established that aspirin reduces the incidence of myocardial infarction and death in patients with chronic stable angina. Presumably, they are at greater risk for platelet-dependent coronary events, such as unstable angina or myocardial infarction, than their peers without coronary disease. Nonetheless, they represent a population more dilute with respect to susceptibility to the benefits of aspirin than patients with unstable angina or myocardial infarction.

Exploration of the potential benefits of aspirin in the primary prevention of cardiovascular disease requires larger studies than those reported to date. Aspirin (325 mg every other day) has been shown to reduce the incidence of myocardial infarction, but not death, in healthy U.S. physicians but not in the British physicians study (500 mg/day). A trend toward increased hemorrhagic stroke in the aspirin group in the U.S. physicians study did not attain statistical significance. Although aspirin has been used in combination with dipyridamole in many of these studies, there is little evidence that this latter drug contributes to the antithrombotic efficacy of aspirin or has any significant efficacy of its own in humans. The lowest dose of aspirin that has been shown to be effective in unstable angina has been 75 mg/day. The American Diabetes Association has recently made the recommendation that aspirin should also be given to patients with diabetes mellitus as prophylaxis against cardiovascular disease.

DUCTUS ARTERIOSUS OF THE NEWBORN. Closure of a persistent ductus arteriosus can be achieved with a single oral dose of indomethacin in the neonatal period in approximately 80% of infants, which implies that a cyclooxygenase metabolite contributes to ductal patency, most likely PGE_2. In fact, infusion of PGE_1 has been used to maintain a patent ductus, the fetal circulation, and reasonable oxygenation in infants with right heart lesions and cyanosis until corrective or palliative surgery is performed.

PRIMARY PULMONARY HYPERTENSION. Intravenous infusions of PGI_2 for prolonged periods (over 1 year) have been found to significantly decrease pulmonary vascular resistance and improve symptoms. In one study it was more effective than adenosine.

SEPSIS. Human septic shock has been associated with increased plasma and urinary metabolite levels of PGE_2, 6-keto-$PGF_{1\alpha}$, and TxB_2. Experimental models of sepsis and endotoxic shock have also demonstrated increased levels of the eicosanoids, and NSAIDs have been shown to improve morbidity and mortality. In a small clinical trial, ibuprofen was found to decrease urinary metabolite excretion and had positive effects on some clinical parameters but no effect on renal function. In a large multicenter controlled clinical trial, ibuprofen decreased PGI_2 and thromboxane synthesis, fever, tachycardia, oxygen consumption, and lactic acidosis but did not prevent the development of shock or the acute respiratory distress syndrome and had no significant effect on final outcome.

ASTHMA. TxA_2 and leukotriene biosynthesis is increased coincident with the bronchoconstrictor response to inhaled allergen. However, studies with aspirin and thromboxane antagonists suggest that TxA_2 does not play a major pathophysiologic role. In contrast, 5-lipoxygenase inhibitors and LTD_4 receptor antagonists have been found to be beneficial in the chronic treatment of asthma (see Chapter 74). These compounds decrease basal bronchial tone and improve forced expiratory volume in 1 second in asthmatic subjects but have no effect in normal subjects. They decrease the use of β-adrenoreceptor agonists and may also decrease the use of corticosteroids. A minority of asthmatics, perhaps 10%, exhibit bronchoconstriction and hypersensitivity reactions to aspirin. This phenomenon appears to indicate a role for prostaglandins, TxA_2, or leukotrienes inasmuch as these attacks are provoked by a range of structurally distinct inhibitors of cyclooxygenase but rarely by salicylate, which resembles aspirin but is at best a weak inhibitor of cyclooxygenase. Drug-induced reactions in such patients may be quite severe and often feature profuse rhinorrhea and flushing in addition to bronchospasm. Whether such attacks are mediated by differential inhibition of bronchoconstrictor versus bronchodilator prostaglandins or by a shunting of the arachidonate substrate toward lipoxygenation and the formation of bronchoconstrictor leukotrienes is uncertain. However, the latter is more likely because LTD_4 receptor antagonists can reduce aspirin-induced bronchoconstriction.

Aspirin may also trigger a hypersensitivity response in which alterations in blood pressure, flushing, tachycardia, and diarrhea predominate over bronchospasm. Some of these patients have systemic mastocytosis.

ADULT RESPIRATORY DISTRESS SYNDROME. Adult respiratory distress syndrome (ARDS) is associated with significant increases in urinary and bronchoalveolar lavage fluid levels of leukotrienes. Experimental models of lung injury also demonstrate a significant increase in leukotriene formation, and treatment with either 5-lipoxygenase inhibitors or sulfidopeptide leukotriene inhibitors significantly decreases the severity of the injury. Whether these drugs will have a significant impact on ARDS remains to be determined.

THE GASTROINTESTINAL TRACT. PGE_2 is the predominant COX-1 product of arachidonic acid formed in the gastric mucosa. It stimulates bicarbonate and mucus secretion, decreases acid secretion, and may regulate gastric blood flow, which most likely plays a role in limiting the effects of diverse physical and chemical insults to the gastric mucosa. This "cytoprotective" property is shared by PGI_2. The dose-related gastrointestinal side effects of NSAIDs are thought to reflect increased susceptibility to local injury (e.g., H^+ back-diffusion) because of inhibition of these prostaglandins. To reduce the incidence of NSAID-induced ulcers, the 15-methyl-PGE_1 analogue (misoprostol) is added as a protective adjunct. Recent studies, however, have shown that omeprazole is better than ranitidine but equivalent to misoprostol for the healing of NSAID-induced ulcers. Omeprazole was more effective than either misoprostol or ranitidine for prophylaxis against recurrence. COX-1 but not COX-2 appears to be expressed in the normal gastrointestinal tract. Thus recently developed, highly selective COX-2 inhibitors may provide anti-inflammatory and analgesic effects devoid of gastrointestinal side effects.

The watery diarrhea associated with multiple endocrine neoplasia often responds to treatment with cyclooxygenase inhibitors. Excessive formation of LTB_4 has been demonstrated in colonic mucosa and rectal dialysates obtained from patients with inflammatory bowel disease, but the significance of this finding is uncertain because a trial of a 5-lipoxygenase inhibitor in these patients failed to produce significant improvements.

COLON CANCER. Recent epidemiologic data have suggested that aspirin intake is inversely associated with the incidence of colorectal cancer. Treatment with sulindac, a non-selective cyclooxygenase inhibitor, decreased or caused regression of polyp formation in patients with familial polyposis coli. Increased expression of COX-2 is noted in polyps and in colonic cancers, as well as increased prostaglandin formation. Increasing the expression of COX-2 in intestinal cell lines is associated with increased expression of metalloproteinases and decreased apoptosis, effects consistent with increasing the metastatic potential of cancer cells. In a mouse model of familial adenomatous polyposis, selective inhibition or selective knockout of COX-2 resulted in a significant decrease in polyp formation. The clinical potential of cyclooxygenase inhibitors and, in particular, selective COX-2 inhibitors in these disorders remains to be explored.

RENIN RELEASE AND RENAL FUNCTION. Although sympathoadrenal activity is a major regulator of renin release, it appears to occur via a cyclooxygenase metabolite of arachidonic acid. PGI_2 is the most potent of the prostaglandins as a renin secretagogue. Sodium depletion in rats has been found to result in an increased expression of COX-2 in the macula densa. Inhibition of cyclooxygenase by NSAIDs may thus lead to a decrease in renin release.

Although metabolites of arachidonic acid contribute little to the regulation of renal blood flow under physiologic circumstances, it appears that preservation of renal blood flow becomes increasingly dependent on the generation of vasodilator prostaglandins in patients with increased renal vasoconstrictor tone, chronic glomerulonephritis, the nephritis of systemic lupus erythematosus, congestive heart failure, or combined hepatic and renal dysfunction. Physiologic stress has been shown to induce spatially selective expression of COX-2 in the central nervous system, and this mechanism may also operate in the renal vasculature. Administration of NSAIDs or high doses of aspirin to these patients may lead to a significant decline in renal function or even reversible renal failure.

The kidney possesses the capacity to generate TxA_2, particularly in response to inflammatory stimuli. Renal biosynthesis of TxA_2 is increased in some patients with active nephritis in association with systemic lupus erythematosus. Although infusion of a TxA_2 receptor antagonist improved indices of renal function in such patients, it is not known whether long-term use of TxA_2 receptor antagonists will modify the progression of renal disease. Increased TxA_2 biosynthesis by the kidney has been demonstrated in animal models in response to ureteric obstruction, renal vein thrombosis, and the development of hypertension following partial renal ablation and diabetes mellitus and coincident with the development of cyclosporine-induced nephrotoxicity. Increased TxA_2 formation during renal allograft rejection has been reported. Misoprostol has been used as an adjunct to cyclosporine in renal transplantation and has been found to delay renal allograft rejection in humans. Although the mechanism for this beneficial effect is uncertain, it may be due to both the immunosuppressive and vasodilator effects of misoprostol.

PGE_2 is the major product formed from arachidonic acid in the renal medulla, where it inhibits sodium reabsorption in the distal tubule. PGE receptor subtypes are spatially segregated within the kidney and may thus subserve different roles in renal function. The sodium retention caused by the administration of NSAIDs persists only for a day or two, after which a new steady-state sodium balance is achieved despite continued treatment. The use of NSAIDs in patients with hypertension may result in the loss of blood pressure control in patients previously well controlled with medicines.

Vasopressin increases renal PGE_2 synthesis, which in turn modulates its effects on the distal nephron. Indomethacin augments the effects of vasopressin and diminishes the excessive water elimination in nephrogenic and lithium-induced diabetes insipidus. Interestingly, embryonic stem cell disruption of the COX-2 gene results in marked polydipsia and polyuria in surviving animals.

BARTTER'S SYNDROME. Bartter's syndrome (see Chapter 109), a congenital abnormality of the kidney, is associated with increased plasma renin activity, hyperaldosteronism, profound hypokalemia, and resistance to the vasoconstrictor effects of angiotensin II. Urinary excretion of PGE_2 is markedly increased in these patients, and treatment with indomethacin and other NSAIDs decreases PGE_2 synthesis, restores the sensitivity to angiotensin II, and partially corrects the hypokalemia.

PARTURITION. Biosynthesis of prostaglandins increases during pregnancy, particularly during labor, and may reflect induction of COX-2, which is regulated by gonadotropic hormones. Both PGE_2 and $PGF_{2\alpha}$ are potent stimulants of myometrial contraction. High concentrations of $PGF_{2\alpha}$ and thromboxane receptor mRNA are found in myometrium. Recently, a $PGF_{2\alpha}$ receptor knockout mouse was bred and the homozygous females were unable to undergo spontaneous or oxytocin-induced parturition because of failure of the luteolysis normally induced by $PGF_{2\alpha}$.

Misoprostol has been used in conjunction with either RU 486 (mifepristone) or methotrexate for the premature termination of pregnancy, with a very high success rate. An analogue of $PGF_{2\alpha}$ has been used instead of hypertonic saline to induce abortion, as well as postpartum to decrease uterine bleeding. Cyclooxygenase inhibitors are currently being evaluated for the treatment of premature labor. A potential hazard of this approach is premature closure

of the ductus arteriosus, although the incidence of this complication is unknown.

PREGNANCY-INDUCED HYPERTENSION. During pregnancy, prostaglandin and thromboxane formation is significantly increased. Biosynthesis of PGI_2 is increased markedly from as early as the first trimester. This increment is less pronounced in patients with pregnancy-induced hypertension. Indeed, diminished PGI_2 biosynthesis is apparent before the rise in blood pressure. TxA_2 biosynthesis is also increased, thus indicating that platelet activation may be present in normal pregnancy and is further increased in patients with severe pregnancy-induced hypertension. Platelet TxA_2 receptor density is also increased in women with pregnancy-induced hypertension and is highest in the most severely affected patients. TxA_2 is a potent vasoconstrictor in the placental bed and may contribute to the depressed placental blood flow that is a hallmark of this disorder. Multicenter trials have been performed to determine whether low-dose aspirin will reduce the incidence of pregnancy-induced hypertension in women at risk for the disease. Studies have yielded equivocal results, with the larger trials failing to show any benefit of aspirin over placebo.

ERECTILE DYSFUNCTION. Because of its vasodilator properties, PGE_1 has been used to treat erectile dysfunction in men. It can be delivered either as an injection (alprostadil [Caverject]) into the corpus cavernosum or via a urethral suppository (alprostadil [MUSE]). It is effective in men with neurogenic, vasculogenic, and psychogenic causes, with the latter two groups appearing to require lower doses.

MASTOCYTOSIS. Systemic mastocytosis is associated with excessive mast cell production of PGD_2 and its major metabolite $9\alpha,11\beta$-PGF_2. Many of the life-threatening symptoms, particularly the bronchospasm, can be relieved by treatment with aspirin in combination with H_1- and H_2-receptor antagonists.

HYPERCALCEMIA OF CANCER. In a minority of patients with solid tumors, PGE_2 production by the tumor causes hypercalcemia via stimulation of osteoclast activity (see Chapter 264). In such cases, suppression of PGE_2 biosynthesis with indomethacin lowers the level of serum calcium. In patients with elevated parathyroid hormone levels or when metastases to bone occur, indomethacin is not effective.

FEVER AND INFLAMMATION. Cyclooxygenase inhibitors (NSAIDs) share antipyretic, analgesic, and anti-inflammatory actions. Acetaminophen differs from the other compounds in being an efficient antipyretic despite weak anti-inflammatory properties in the periphery. In animal experiments it has been demonstrated that CSF levels of PGE_2 increase in response to pyrogenic stimuli and that concomitant with the administration of acetaminophen, PGE_2 levels decrease and core body temperature decreases back to normal. Administration of PGE_2 into the anterior hypothalamus can result in an increase in core body temperature in animals.

Vasodilator prostaglandins seem to act in concert with other mediators to augment the inflammatory response. Among these may be the leukotrienes, which enhance capillary permeability and function as chemoattractants and leukocyte activators.

Morrow JD, Hill KE, Burk RF, et al: A series of prostaglandin F_2–like compounds are produced in vivo in humans by a non-cyclooxygenase, free radical–catalyzed mechanism. Proc Natl Acad Sci USA 87:9383, 1990. *The first description of isoprostanes in human plasma and urine.*

Murata T, Ushikubi F, Matsuoka T, et al: Altered pain perception and inflammatory response in mice lacking prostacyclin receptor. Nature 388:678, 1997. *The first definitive study demonstrating a role for PGI_2 in inflammation, pain perception, and thrombosis.*

Patrono C: Aspirin as an antiplatelet drug. N Engl J Med 330:1287, 1994. *A comprehensive review of the prototypic prostaglandin inhibitor.*

234 NATRIURETIC HORMONES

Garner T. Haupert, Jr.

For more than two decades, considerable interest has focused on endogenous factors that play a role in the regulation of water and electrolyte balance. Isolation and cloning of the cardiac-derived atrial natriuretic peptide (ANP) have led to rapid definition of its biosynthesis, storage, release response, and action.

Two structurally related peptides, brain natriuretic peptide (BNP) and C-type natriuretic peptide (CNP), have subsequently been isolated, sequenced, and cloned. Detailed information on the physiologic effects of these peptides is available. Some of the uncertainties about their importance in physiology and pathophysiology have recently been addressed in genetic manipulation studies. So far, routine clinical application has not been achieved. A second compound (or compounds), classically called natriuretic hormone, has finally been characterized as a glycosylated steroid derivative distinct in structure and mechanism from ANP. Its physiology, pathophysiology, and therapeutic potential now await the availability of chemically synthetic material permitting direct testing.

NATRIURETIC HORMONE

Experimental observations led to the concept of the existence of an endogenous regulator of mammalian Na^+, K^+-adenosinetriphosphatase (Na^+, K^+-ATPase) (the Na^+ pump) more than 30 years ago. At that time, intravascular expansion with saline in dogs produced a brisk natriuresis with no change in renal perfusion pressure, glomerular filtration rate (GFR), or mineralocorticoid activity. The natriuretic effects of extracellular fluid volume expansion in one animal also occurred in a second animal cross-circulated with the blood of the first. The presumption was that the natriuresis was due to a circulating substance that exerted its effects directly on the renal tubular Na^+ reabsorptive process without affecting renal hemodynamics. Further experiments confirmed that active extracts from plasma, urine, and tissue sources that were natriuretic in vivo had a direct effect on transepithelial sodium transport. These substances have digitalis-like characteristics. The digoxin radioimmunoassay has been used to detect digitalis-like immunoactivity in the urine and plasma of sodium-loaded normal human subjects and in uremic and hypertensive subjects. Discovery of digitalis-like structure(s) in mammalian tissues and the existence of isoforms of Na^+, K^+-ATPase with differing affinities for cardiac glycosides suggests that the mammalian sodium pump is endogenously regulated by this compound. Whether natriuretic hormone and the digitalis-like endogenous Na^+, K^+-ATPase inhibitor are the same molecule remains to be proved.

BIOLOGIC ACTIVITIES. The biologic effects that have been claimed for the putative natriuretic hormone include (1) natriuresis in vivo, (2) inhibition of active sodium transport in vitro, (3) Na^+, K^+-ATPase inhibition, (4) positive cardiac inotropism, and (5) increased vascular reactivity.

BIOCHEMICAL CHARACTERIZATION. Recently, the chemical structure of the endogenous Na^+, K^+-ATPase inhibitor from the hypothalamus was chemically characterized as an isomer of the plant-derived cardiac glycoside ouabain. This mammalian molecule inhibits active sodium transport in renal tubular cells and has positive inotropic and vasoconstrictive properties consistent with the natriuretic hormone hypertension hypothesis. A compound with identical physicochemical properties has been extracted from human plasma. Although less characterized biologically than the hypothalamic compound, a substance with structural similarity to the amphibian-derived bufodienolides was extracted from human cataractous lenses, and a compound indistinguishable by nuclear magnetic resonance analysis from plant-derived ouabain itself has been recovered from bovine adrenal glands, which raises the possibility that more than one digitalis-like compound may be present in mammals, including humans.

SITE OF ORIGIN. The site of origin of natriuretic hormone also remains uncertain, but the brain has been favored because the natriuretic effects of extracellular fluid volume expansion appear to depend on an intact central nervous system. The hypothalamus is an enriched source of an endogenous inhibitor of Na^+, K^+-ATPase, if not the site of its production.

An ouabain-like compound has been isolated from human cerebrospinal fluid, and other evidence suggests that the adrenal gland may be a source. It is also possible that multiple tissues can produce natriuretic hormone, which could act locally as a paracrine hormone. Preliminary results using adrenal tissue suggest that biosynthetic pathways exist for natriuretic hormone, starting with known steroid precursors.

NATRIURETIC HORMONE AND THE PATHOPHYSIOLOGY OF ESSENTIAL HYPERTENSION. Natriuretic hormone may play a role in normal volume regulation and in the pathophysiology of hypertension and secondary edema states. Natriuretic hormone may have an extrarenal action leading to enhanced vascular reactivity. The hypothesis proposed is that hereditary forms of hypertension have a persistent tendency toward renal retention of sodium, possibly because of the increased Na^+-K^+ cotransport or Na^+-H^+ exchange in the proximal tubule that occurs as a manifestation of a generalized genetic defect in Na^+-Na^+ (Na^+-Li^+) countertransport. This defect exists in the erythrocytes of some patients with essential hypertension and in their first-degree normotensive relatives. Recent studies in the Milan strain of the genetically hypertensive rat (MHS), which has been shown to have abnormally high levels of the hypothalamic Na^+, K^+-ATPase inhibitor in the midbrain and blood, indicate that genetic polymorphism affecting the cytoskeletal protein adducin leads to enhanced Na^+, K^+-ATPase activity in the MHS renal tubule with resulting enhanced Na^+ reabsorption. The renal sodium retention leads to a transient increase in extracellular fluid volume, which serves as a stimulus for the release of a Na^+, K^+-ATPase inhibitor. The sodium pump inhibitor acts on the renal tubule to promote sodium excretion, thus restoring extracellular fluid volume to normal levels. It has similar inhibitory effects on Na^+, K^+-ATPase in vascular smooth muscle cells or on adrenergic nerve endings at the neuromuscular junction and results in a tonic increase in vascular tone, increased total peripheral resistance, and hypertension. The same genetic polymorphism for adducin has been found in a subset of human essential hypertensive patients. It is assumed that Na^+, K^+-ATPase inhibition in vascular smooth muscle results in an increase in cytosolic free calcium concentration, which must occur to produce the arterial vasoconstriction. How this occurs is unsettled. One hypothesis is that altered Na^+-Ca^{2+} exchange resulting from partial sodium pump inhibition may account for an increase in the intracellular free Ca^{2+} concentration. Currently this remains attractive but unproved. Alternatively, enhanced norepinephrine activity caused by Na^+ pump inhibition in adrenergic neurons, either in the central nervous system or peripherally, can be responsible for altered renal sodium reabsorption and vasoconstriction. Consistent with this mechanism is the observation that intrathecal administration of high NaCl, plant ouabain, and mammalian-derived ouabain-like factor stimulates renal sympathetic nerves, increased peripheral resistance, and hypertension in normal rats. In general, the developing body of physiologic information involving the endogenous Na^+, K^+-ATPase inhibitor has shifted to its cardiovascular effects. However, the existence of renal tubular Na^+, K^+-ATPase isoforms or genetic polymorphisms with high affinity for the inhibitor could produce Na^+ reabsorption regulation and natriuresis consistent with the original hypothesis that the endogenous Na^+ pump inhibitor and natriuretic hormone are one and the same.

NATRIURETIC PEPTIDE

ANP is a peptide hormone secreted primarily by the cardiac atria and produces natriuresis, diuresis, smooth muscle relaxation, and inhibition of renin and aldosterone secretion. Its major sites of action include the cardiovascular, renal, and endocrine systems. Although the exact mechanisms triggering the release of ANP are not clear, stretching of the atria appears to be the principal stimulus.

It has been known for several decades that membrane-bound secretory granules exist in the cardiac atria. In 1981 in a pioneering report, DeBold and colleagues observed that bolus injection of crude extracts of rat atria, but not ventricles, produced a rapid, massive, and short-lasting diuresis and natriuresis and a modest kaliuresis. This observation suggested the existence of a natriuretic hormone in the atrial granules. Subsequently, this unique hormonal system has been thoroughly studied. The amino acid sequence of the active circulating peptide and its pre-hormone forms has been defined together with their gene structure, target tissue receptors, and signal transduction pathways. Close on the heels of ANP came the isolation and structural characterization of related peptides, first BNP and then CNP. BNP is found mainly in the cardiac ventricle, has biologic effects similar to ANP, and is increased in the circulation in cardiopathologic states such as congestive heart failure (CHF). CNP probably does not circulate normally, is found mainly in the brain and vascular endothelium, has little intrinsic natriuretic activity, and may play a local (paracrine) role in vasodepression and vascular remodeling (antimitogenesis). All three natriuretic peptides show structural similarity, are derived from the C-terminal ends of their precursors, and interact with specific receptors.

STRUCTURE, BIOSYNTHESIS, AND SECRETION. The atrium first produces a pre-pro-ANP (151 amino acids), the final 126 amino acids of which represent pro-ANP. Pro-ANP, the principal storage form of the hormone in the atrial granules, is the immediate precursor of the biologically active 28–amino acid ANP, the predominant circulatory peptide. Pro-BNP and the 32–amino acid active form also circulate. All natriuretic peptides have a 17–amino acid ring with a cysteine-cysteine disulfide cross-link that is essential for activity.

The human gene for pre-pro-ANP is located on the short arm of chromosome 1. Transcription of the gene for pre-pro-ANP proceeds at a high rate in the cardiac atria and is estimated to involve 1% of all mRNA in atrial cardiocytes. Expression of the gene for ANP is transcriptionally regulated by dexamethasone and thyroid hormone. ANP is also expressed at very low levels in other tissues such as the brain, anterior pituitary, adrenal medulla, lung, kidney, thyroid, and submandibular gland. Pro-ANP is cleaved by a specific atrial protease, probably at the time of exocytotic fusion of atrial granules with the plasma membrane and possibly even soon after secretion from the myocyte; consequently, ANP is the predominant form entering the coronary sinus blood.

STIMULI FOR RELEASE. Atrial stretch, measured as atrial transmural pressure, is the principal stimulus for ANP secretion into the circulation. Atrial pressure is also correlated with the release of ANP. During infusion of isotonic saline in humans, plasma ANP increases in parallel with the increase in right atrial pressure. This increase results from rapid conversion of pro-ANP to ANP and/or release of ANP. With cardiovascular or pulmonary disease, a significant correlation exists between circulating ANP levels and right and left atrial pressures. BNP secretion is stimulated by increased ventricular wall tension. CNP production may be stimulated by cytokines acting on vascular endothelium and by ANP and BNP directly. ANP synthesis within brain tissue may be stimulated by systemic volume, catecholamines, cyclic adenosine monophosphate, and endothelin. Factors regulating brain production of BNP and CNP are unknown.

Mineralocorticoids, as well as glucocorticoids administered in high doses, increase mRNA encoding for pre-pro-ANP and circulating ANP levels and thus result in an increase in ANP production and release. In addition, adrenalectomized rats do not respond to increased atrial pressure with increased atrial and circulating ANP levels in the absence of glucocorticoid or mineralocorticoid replacement. Thus these hormones may play a permissive role in the volume response mediating ANP release, as well as induction of ANP secretion directly.

NATRIURETIC PEPTIDE RECEPTORS. Natriuretic peptide receptors (NPRs) are localized on the cell surface of target tissues, including most notably the adrenal, the kidney, and the vasculature. They are also found, to a lesser extent, in the central nervous system, hepatocytes, colonic smooth muscle, and lung. In the kidney, ANP binding sites are most prevalent in large vessels, glomeruli, and the renal medulla. In the adrenal, ANP binding is limited primarily to the zona glomerulosa.

Molecular cloning has defined three NPRs. The first is the NPR-C clearance receptor, which is not coupled to cyclic guanosine monophosphate (cGMP) production, the signal transduction pathway involved in natriuretic peptide action. Clearance receptors do not mediate any known physiologic effect. The receptors for ANP in the kidney and vascular smooth muscle are predominantly clearance receptors. Their abundance accounts for the short half-life of circulatory ANP (2 to 4 minutes in humans). It seems probable that the atrial peptide system has a novel receptor-mediated sequestration and clearance mechanism that is responsible, at least in part, for maintaining plasma levels of the hormone. In humans, ANP clearance is also mediated by a tissue endopeptidase (EC 24.11) found in multiple tissues, including vascular endothelium, that

opens the ring inactivating the hormone. The other ANP receptors are two structurally similar plasma membrane receptors, NPR-A and NPR-B, the biologically active receptor forms. Binding of natriuretic peptide to the extracellular domain of NPR-A or NPR-B activates the cytoplasmic domain of the receptor, which is a guanylate cyclase responsible for generation of the second messenger cGMP. NPRs bind the three natriuretic peptides differentially, with NPR-A having greater affinity for ANP than for BNP and much greater affinity for ANP than for CNP; and NPR-B having much greater affinity for CNP than for ANP and greater affinity for CNP than for BNP.

CELLULAR ACTION. The most apparent action of ANP is to increase the intracellular cGMP concentration. ANP is a unique peptide hormone in its use of cGMP as a second messenger, which mediates most of the physiologic actions of the hormone. ANP also influences intracellular calcium homeostasis, which may be responsible for some of its biologic effects.

The physiologic responses to ANP include (1) relaxation of vascular and other smooth muscle, (2) increase in the GFR and inhibition of tubular water and sodium transport in the kidney, and (3) inhibition of hormone secretion (Fig. 234–1).

KIDNEY ACTION. The kidney is the primary target organ for ANP. ANP causes natriuresis and diuresis by a concerted action at several nephron segments. The primary sites of action of ANP are the glomerulus, the renal vasculature, and the inner medullary collecting duct, although other nephron segments may be involved in the response to ANP. In pharmacologic doses, ANP can increase the GFR by raising the glomerular hydraulic pressure gradient from the capillary lumen to Bowman's space through differential effects on afferent and efferent arteriole tone. By relaxing glomerular mesangial cells, ANP also increases the glomerular ultrafiltration coefficient Kf. The combined effects result in increased filtration pressure and thus an increased filtration fraction, with a higher load of salt and water being delivered to the tubules for excretion.

The increased quantity of sodium filtered is not completely reabsorbed. An increased amount of sodium is delivered to the distal tubule and collecting duct, where ANP reduces sodium reabsorption and vasopressin-induced water reabsorption and thus causes a profound natriuresis. In addition, redistribution of blood flow from the cortex to inner medulla, which dilutes the papillary interstitium, results in an increase in sodium and water excretion.

At *physiologic* doses an increase in GFR is not observed, and the natriuretic effects are due mainly to inhibited Na⁺ transport in the inner medullary collecting duct. A slightly elongated (four amino acid residues) form of ANP called urodilatin is produced in the kidney and may be responsible for paracrine regulation of sodium and water excretion by acting on sodium transport in the inner medullary collecting duct.

CARDIOVASCULAR ACTION. ANP directly relaxes arterial vascular smooth muscle through the action of its second messenger cGMP. This ANP-induced vasorelaxation occurs independent of the presence of endothelium. ANP at pharmacologic concentrations reduces mean arterial pressure in humans by reducing peripheral vascular resistance and decreasing intravascular volume. This activity is followed by a decrease in cardiac output attributed to (1) a shift of volume from the intravascular to the extravascular space caused by elevated capillary hydraulic conductivity and resulting transcapillary flow and (2) pre-load reduction from relaxation of venous smooth muscle leading to an augmentation of venous capacitance and a reduction in venous return. Hemoconcentration secondary to decreased plasma volume may occur in humans in response to ANP.

ENDOCRINE ACTION. ANP modulates renin-angiotensin-aldosterone secretion. Administration of ANP causes a prompt decline in circulatory renin and aldosterone levels. ANP blocks both basal and agonist-stimulated (angiotensin II, adrenocorticotropic hormone, K⁺) secretion of aldosterone in isolated adrenal zona glomerulosa cells. Direct inhibition of steroidogenesis has been shown. In addition, ANP decreases the biosynthesis and release of vasopressin, which may potentiate a decrease in vascular tone and augment diuresis and natriuresis.

COMPARATIVE EFFECTS OF NATRIURETIC PEPTIDES. Most information on the biologic actions of natriuretic peptides is derived from studies of ANP. Considerably less is known about the effects and significance of BNP and CNP. In general, in normal humans the actions and potency of BNP appear to parallel those of

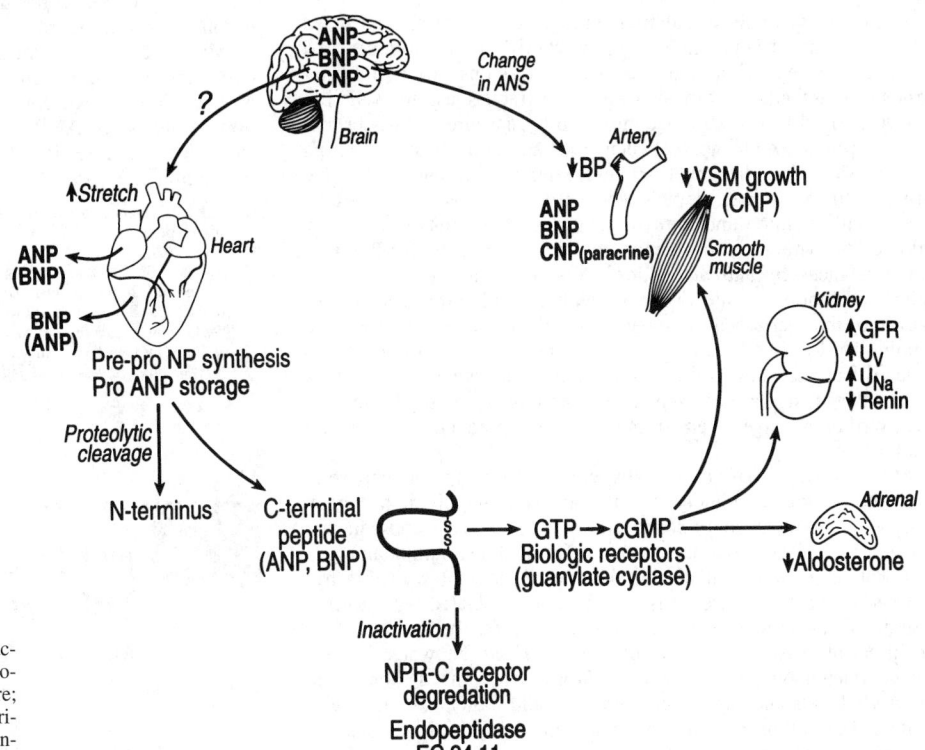

FIGURE 234–1 ■ Major target organs and actions of natriuretic peptides. ANS = autonomic nervous system; BP = blood pressure; GFR = glomerular filtration rate; U_v = urinary volume; cGMP = cyclic guanosine monophosphate; GTP = guanosine triphosphate.

ANP. Physiologic effects appear to be additive, not synergistic. In animal studies, CNP has been shown to suppress aldosterone production, perhaps through stimulation of ANP and BNP, but it does not have the hemodynamic and vascular permeability actions of the latter. In rats, chronic infusion of CNP suppresses restenosis in injured arteries, thus suggesting a possible role for vascular remodeling.

SIGNIFICANCE OF ATRIAL NATRIURETIC PEPTIDE IN BODY FLUID HOMEOSTASIS

Despite the wealth of information on the physiologic actions of ANP, its relevance to blood pressure and fluid volume homeostasis has remained controversial. The primary reason for this controversy lies in a lack of correlation between ANP levels and natriuresis experimentally in humans, the presence of postprandial natriuresis with salt feeding where ANP levels are not elevated, and only modest natriuresis with ANP infusions to produce levels in the physiologic range.

Classically, the physiologic effects of a substance can be better elucidated by nullifying its effects through blockers or inhibitors. In the case of ANP, both antagonists to cGMP production and antibodies to ANP itself have been studied, with conflicting results. To this point, none of the studies with antagonists or antibodies has answered the question of ANP's role in volume homeostasis and blood pressure control under normal physiologic conditions.

Perhaps more promise lies in gene-targeting studies. In this approach, gene knockout animals (mice) can be produced in which hybrid animals are normal other than for the specific gene mutated or deleted. Alternatively, transgenic mice can be created in which an extra copy of a gene is added to the genome. Early results are available in mice with both techniques. Transgenic mice with endogenous 10-fold elevations of ANP or BNP are found to have markedly lower arterial blood pressure and increased plasma cGMP levels. In knockout experiments, mice that are homozygous for a disrupted pro-ANP gene had blood pressure significantly higher than that in the wild type and heterozygous mutants, and plasma volume was increased. The homozygote mutants also had cardiomegaly and higher blood pressure in response to intermediate dietary salt than did wild-type and heterozygotes. These early studies support the notion that the gene for ANP has a definite effect on

blood pressure and intravascular volume and that ANP modulates the blood pressure response to dietary salt, at least in mice.

ROLE OF ATRIAL NATRIURETIC PEPTIDE IN PATHOPHYSIOLOGY

Diseases of Disordered Volume Regulation (Edematous States)

The common edematous disorders clinically typified by CHF, decompensated cirrhosis of the liver, and nephrotic syndrome represent pathophysiologic states in which renal Na⁺ reabsorption is avid despite excess total body Na⁺ and extracellular fluid volume accumulation. Antinatriuretic forces are generated by peritubular physical factors and enhanced activity of the renin-angiotensin system, catecholamines, and vasopressin on renal Na⁺ and water reabsorption. If ANP plays a central role in homeostatic renal regulation of volume, the edematous disorders can be viewed as failure of the endogenous ANP system to combat these antinatriuretic forces and brings into question whether pharmacologic treatments with ANP can reverse the pathophysiology.

CONGESTIVE HEART FAILURE. CHF is associated with increased atrial pressure and elevated ANP levels. Despite high circulating ANP, however, these patients retain salt and water. CHF is associated with a decreased response of the kidney to ANP, which could result from receptor down-regulation because of high plasma ANP concentrations. The direct correlation between the severity of the heart failure and plasma ANP has allowed the use of ANP levels to serve as a marker for CHF in adults and children, including those with congenital heart disease. The natriuresis and diuresis associated with pharmacologic dose infusions of ANP in normal subjects does not occur in patients with heart failure. Early studies with BNP were believed to show more promise as an intravenous therapy for CHF, but a recent study of long-term infusion to achieve a circulating dose equivalent to that found in severe CHF failed to show any increase in cardiac output, urinary volume, or urinary Na⁺ excretion, although favorable hemodynamic changes (systemic arterial pressure, pulmonary artery mean and capillary wedge pressure, and systemic vascular resistance) did occur.

CIRRHOSIS. Progressive cirrhosis of the liver is accompanied by renal sodium and water retention along with the development of ascites and edema. ANP levels may be normal or moderately elevated. Expansion of the intravascular volume by infusion of ascitic fluid into the systemic circulation through a LeVeen shunt caused an increase in plasma ANP, urinary cGMP, urine volume, and urine Na+ concentration. This result argues against the notion that cirrhosis is associated with an acquired refractoriness to ANP because increased levels were accompanied by natriuresis. It is probable that a complex balance between ANP and antinatriuretic factors is responsible for the renal sodium retention in early and late cirrhosis. In the former, hepatic venous outflow obstruction results in renal salt retention and intravascular volume expansion (overflow hypothesis), which in turn leads to an elevation in ANP levels counterbalanced by antinatriuretic factors such that the net effect is ascites formation. In late cirrhosis, with loss of intravascular volume into the peritoneal compartment (underfill hypothesis), the stimulus for ANP secretion is reduced and ANP plasma levels no longer offset the antinatriuretic processes. Unfortunately, efforts to induce natriuresis by intravenous infusion of ANP in decompensated cirrhotics have been stymied by the production of severe hypotension.

NEPHROTIC SYNDROME. Why edema forms in the nephrotic syndrome is not completely understood. Traditionally it has been suggested that renal sodium and water retention is a consequence of the lower plasma oncotic pressure from hypoalbuminemia and the resultant reduction in plasma volume. Consistent with this hypothesis, nephrotic syndrome is found to be associated with normal or diminished circulatory levels of ANP that can be stimulated to rise after intravascular volume expansion. Head-out water immersion conducted on patients with nephrotic syndrome demonstrated that ANP levels increased but renal salt and water excretion was blunted. There thus appears to be an impaired renal response to ANP in the nephrotic syndrome.

ESSENTIAL HYPERTENSION. The wide range of plasma ANP concentrations found in patients with essential hypertension suggests that the contribution of ANP may vary in the heterogeneous population of patients with this disease. This finding precludes the use of ANP levels to differentiate among the various causes of hypertension. However, as noted above, detection of genetic polymorphisms in the ANP gene family in humans could help define that segment of the hypertensive population with salt sensitivity.

RENAL DISEASE. Progressive renal disease is frequently associated with plasma volume expansion and elevated ANP levels. Two observations suggest that ANP may be involved in the adaptive increased fractional excretion of sodium by preserved nephrons in chronic renal failure. Infusion of ANP in such patients increases the GFR and fractional Na+ excretion, and infusion of ANP antiserum leads to decreased fractional excretion of Na+ without affecting the GFR or renal plasma flow. In patients undergoing regular dialysis, ANP levels can be used as an indicator of volume status. Decreased levels correlate with the amount of weight lost by fluid removal in dialysis patients. Plasma ANP levels remaining resistant to dialysis treatment may be a poor prognostic sign. Preliminary data that intravenous ANP alters the course of oliguric acute renal failure in human patients has not been confirmed in subsequent clinical trials.

THERAPEUTIC POTENTIAL

The hoped-for use of ANP and then BNP as pharmaceutical interventions to treat fluid and electrolyte disturbances has largely not materialized. As noted above, use of these peptides to treat edematous disorders complicating CHF, cirrhosis, and nephrotic syndrome has been disappointing because the renal response to infusions is either ineffective or blunted. An additional problem is that the depleted intravascular volume in cirrhosis and nephrotic syndrome and diminished effective circulating plasma volume in CHF make these patients particularly susceptible to the hypotensive actions of natriuretic peptide infusions. Although ineffective as natriuretic and diuretic agents in CHF, favorable hemodynamic changes are produced. Another disadvantage is that as peptides, natriuretic peptides must be administered intravenously. However, new understanding of the metabolism of natriuretic peptides and appreciation of the important role of C receptors suggest alternative approaches to augment endogenous levels of natriuretic peptides by blocking the degrading mechanisms. Thus the use of endopeptidase

inhibitors, with or without C-receptor blockers such as C-ANP$_{4-23}$, may hold promise in the treatment of CHF or hypertension. Recognition of antiproliferative effects, particularly of CNP, raises the possibility that long-term use of metabolic blockers might be effective against vascular smooth muscle hypertrophy and endothelial proliferation. As we enter the era of gene therapy, direct introduction of genes for ANP or CNP into affected vessels provides new technology to take advantage of natriuretic peptide's antiproliferative actions.

Goetz KL: Evidence that atriopeptin is not a physiological regulator of sodium excretion. Hypertension 15:9, 1990. *Debate on the role that ANP plays in body fluid homeostasis.*

Haupert GT: Structure and biological activity of the Na+-K+-ATPase inhibitor isolated from bovine hypothalamus: Difference from ouabain. *In* Bamberg E, Schoner W (eds): The Sodium Pump. New York, Steinkopff Darmstadt Springer, 1994, pp 732–742. *Review of current knowledge of the hypothalamic ouabain-like factor.*

Levin ER, Gardner DG, Samson WK: Natriuretic peptides. N Engl J Med 339:321, 1998. *Succinct review of the field with a detailed bibliography.*

235 NEUROENDOCRINOLOGY AND THE NEUROENDOCRINE SYSTEM

Mark E. Molitch

NEUROENDOCRINE REGULATION

Neuroendocrinology refers to the general area of endocrinology in which the nervous system interacts with the endocrine system to link aspects of cognitive and non-cognitive neural activity with metabolic and hormonal homeostatic activity. Neural cells that can secrete hormones, i.e., *neurosecretory* cells, serve as the final common pathway linking the brain with the endocrine system. The *neurohypophysial* neurons originate from the paraventricular and supraoptic nuclei, traverse the hypothalamic-pituitary stalk, and release vasopressin and oxytocin from nerve endings in the posterior pituitary. The *hypophysiotropic* neurons, localized in specific hypothalamic nuclei, project their axons to the median eminence to secrete their peptide and bioamine releasing and inhibiting hormones into the proximal end of the hypothalamic-pituitary portal vessels (Fig. 235–1). Neurons from other nuclei within the hypothalamus and other parts of the brain influence pituitary hormone secretion by interacting with these specific neurons. The median eminence receives its blood supply from the superior hypophysial artery, which arborizes into a rich capillary bed. The capillary loops extend into the median eminence and coalesce to form the long portal veins that traverse the pituitary stalk and end in the pituitary. The capillary walls are "fenestrated" and allow entry of the peptides secreted by the axon terminals. At the pituitary end of the stalk the portal vessels again branch to form an extensive capillary plexus.

The neuroendocrine system operates through a series of feedback loops that control pituitary and target organ hormone levels precisely. Target organ hormones can feed back at both the hypothalamic and pituitary levels to complete the loop, and efferent controller factors from the hypothalamus may include both stimulatory and inhibitory substances. The feedback loops can be perturbed and result in temporary or prolonged alterations of set points by such factors as length of day (circadian periodicity), stress, nutritional status, and systemic illness. The suprachiasmatic nuclei, located just above the optic chiasm, are important in regulating circadian rhythms of the body.

HYPOPHYSIOTROPIC HORMONES

Regulation of pituitary hormones by the hypophysiotropic hormones is quite complex, in part because of the multiplicity of substances present in the hypothalamus that can affect pituitary hormone secretion and in part because of the redundancy and overlapping nature of the feedback loops alluded to above. In

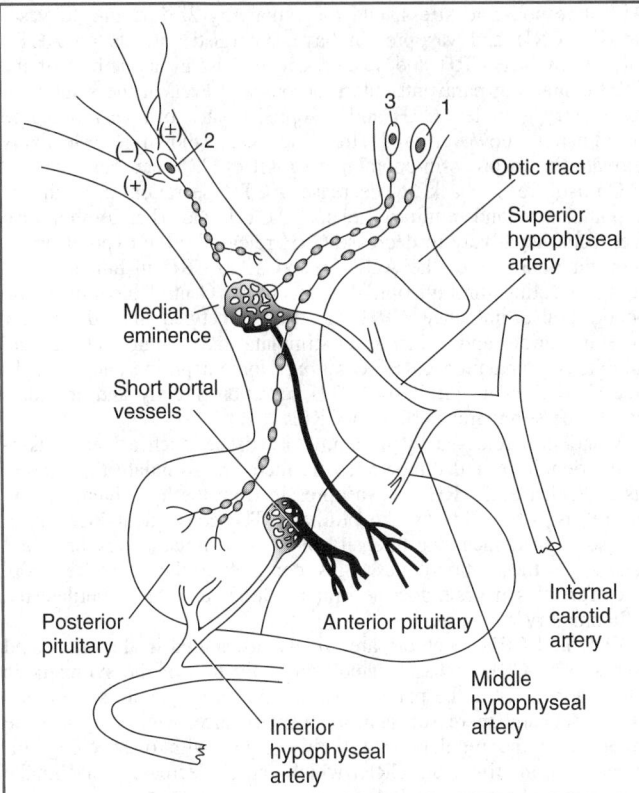

FIGURE 235-1 ■ Neuroendocrine organization of the hypothalamus and pituitary gland. The posterior pituitary is fed by the inferior hypophyseal artery and the hypothalamus by the superior hypophyseal artery, both branches of the internal carotid artery. A small portion of the anterior pituitary also receives arterial blood from the middle hypophyseal artery. Most of the blood supply to the anterior pituitary is venous by way of the long portal vessels, which connect the portal capillary beds in the median eminence to the venous sinusoids in the anterior pituitary. Hypophysiotropic neuron 3 in the parvocellular division of the paraventricular nucleus and neuron 2 in the arcuate nucleus are shown to terminate in the median eminence on portal capillaries. These neurons of the tuberoinfundibular system secrete hypothalamic releasing and inhibiting hormones into the portal veins for conveyance to the anterior pituitary gland. Neuron 2 is innervated by monoaminergic neurons. Note that the multiple inputs to such neurons, using neuron 2 as an example, can be (a) stimulatory, (b) inhibitory, or (c) neuromodulatory, in which another neuron may affect neurotransmitter release. Neuron 1 represents a peptidergic neuron originating in the magnocellular division of the paraventricular nucleus or supraoptic nucleus and projects directly to the posterior pituitary by way of the hypothalamic-neurohypophyseal tract. (Courtesy of Ronald M. Lechan, M.D., and modified from Lechan RM: Neuroendocrinology of pituitary hormone regulation. Endocrinol Metab Clinic North Am 16:475, 1987, with permission.)

addition, some hypophysiotropic hormones exert effects on more than one pituitary hormone (Fig. 235-2). Some of the hypophysiotropic hormones are also found elsewhere in the body, particularly the gastrointestinal tract and placenta, where they may have significant physiologic functions. All of the hypophysiotropic hormones are also present in extrahypothalamic brain tissue and function as neurotransmitters. Several hormones can occur in the same hypothalamic nucleus. In each instance, the action of the hypophysiotropic hormone is mediated first by binding to specific receptors and then by alteration of intracellular transduction mechanisms.

THYROTROPIN-RELEASING HORMONE. Thyrotropin-releasing hormone (TRH) is a tripeptide whose secretion is stimulated by norepinephrine and dopamine but is inhibited by serotonin. The primary neuroendocrine functions of TRH are to stimulate the synthesis and release of thyroid-stimulating hormone (TSH) and prolactin. It has been estimated that a single molecule of TRH, through its TSH-releasing effect, induces the release of more than 100,000 molecules of thyroxine from the thyroid. In hypothyroidism, the increased TRH synthesis and binding to the pituitary result in increased basal and TRH-stimulated TSH and prolactin levels. Correction of the hypothyroidism with thyroid hormones decreases the elevated TSH and prolactin levels. Conversely, in hyperthyroid-

ism, basal and TRH-stimulated TSH levels are markedly suppressed; basal prolactin levels are not low, but the prolactin response to TRH is markedly blunted and returns to normal with correction of the hyperthyroidism. The feedback effects of thyroid hormones, therefore, although occurring primarily at the pituitary, also occur at the hypothalamus.

Although TRH is the major regulator of TSH synthesis and secretion, the role of TRH as a physiologic prolactin releasing factor (PRF) remains questionable. TRH can also stimulate growth hormone (GH) secretion in patients with acromegaly, as well as in several states associated with decreased insulin-like growth factor type I (IGF-I) feedback on GH secretion, such as cirrhosis, renal insufficiency, anorexia nervosa, poorly controlled type I diabetes mellitus, and malnutrition. Such responses are also seen in patients with depression and schizophrenia, which may be associated with disordered central bioaminergic regulation. TRH can also stimulate follicle-stimulating hormone (FSH) secretion in some patients with gonadotroph adenomas, but not in normal individuals. Obviously, somatotroph and gonadotroph cells must have TRH receptors, but "activation" of such receptors, which may involve alteration of intracellular transduction mechanisms, occurs only in special circumstances.

GONADOTROPIN-RELEASING HORMONE. Gonadotropin-releasing hormone (GnRH) is a 10–amino acid peptide. Embryologic studies suggest that GnRH neurons originally develop in the epithelium of the medial part of the olfactory placode. During fetal development, these cells migrate across the cribriform plate, enter the forebrain with the nervus terminalis and vomeronasal nerves, travel medial to the olfactory bulbs, and eventually enter the septal–pre-optic region of the hypothalamus. This demonstration of the origin of GnRH-producing neurons from olfactory epithelium is of clinical interest with respect to the entity of Kallmann's syndrome, in which GnRH deficiency is associated with anosmia secondary to agenesis of the olfactory bulbs. At least one form of Kallmann's syndrome has now been found to be due to a gene defect resulting in loss of function of a protein that facilitates the embryologic migration of these GnRH-producing neurons. GnRH secretion is stimulated by dopamine and norepinephrine and inhibited by serotonin.

The primary function of GnRH is to stimulate the secretion of luteinizing hormone (LH) and FSH. Although early studies suggested the presence of separate LH and FSH releasing factors, only one GnRH has been identified and the differential secretion of LH and FSH is due to variations in sensitivity of the feedback effects of steroid and peptide hormones and variations in sensitivity to GnRH. GnRH pulsatile secretion also directly up-regulates its own receptors, i.e., it causes an increase in GnRH receptor number. In contrast, continuous administration of GnRH is associated with a "down-regulation" of gonadotropin synthesis and secretion as a result of decreased receptor numbers, as well as post-receptor mechanisms.

In women, positive and negative steroid hormone feedback regulation of the hypothalamic-pituitary-gonadal axis occurs at both the pituitary and hypothalamic levels, the hypothalamic effects being

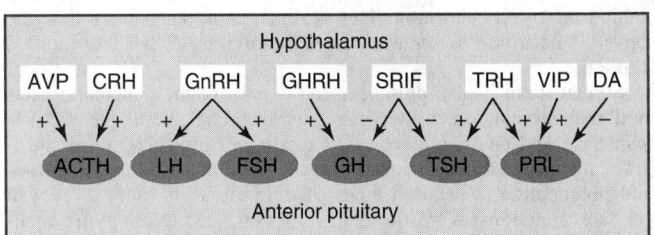

FIGURE 235-2 ■ Interrelationships between hypothalamic and pituitary hormones. Plus signs indicate stimulatory effects and minus signs indicate inhibitory effects. AVP = arginine vasopressin; CRH = corticotropin-releasing hormone; GnRH = gonadotropin-releasing hormone; GHRH = growth hormone–releasing hormone; SRIF = somatotropin release–inhibiting factor [somatostatin]; TRH = thyrotropin-releasing hormone; VIP = vasoactive intestinal polypeptide; DA = dopamine; ACTH = adrenocorticotropic hormone; LH = luteinizing hormone; FSH = follicle-stimulating hormone; TSH = thyroid-stimulating hormone; PRL = prolactin.

alteration of GnRH pulse amplitude and frequency and the pituitary effects being modulation of the gonadotropin response to GnRH. In the follicular phase of the menstrual cycle, estrogen feeds back negatively on gonadotropin secretion. At mid-cycle, estrogen feedback becomes positive and rising estrogen levels from the developing follicle stimulate the ovulatory surge of LH and FSH. Following ovulation, the feedback again becomes negative, and the estrogen and progesterone produced by the corpus luteum result in decreasing levels of LH and FSH. In males, testosterone decreases GnRH pulsatile secretion with a resultant decrease in gonadotropin pulse amplitude and frequency, as well as a decreased gonadotropin response to exogenous GnRH.

The negative-feedback effects of inhibin, a peptide produced by testicular Sertoli cells and ovarian granulosa cells, are predominantly on FSH at the pituitary. Inhibin causes a dose-related decrease in the sensitivity of gonadotrophs to GnRH, but a hypothalamic site of action may also be present. The related ovarian protein activin stimulates basal and GnRH-stimulated FSH synthesis and release from the pituitary. Another gonadal peptide, follistatin, also inhibits the oophorectomy- and GnRH-induced rise in FSH selectively, primarily by binding to activin. These ovarian peptides are also found in the pituitary and may therefore have additional local effects on gonadotropin secretion.

The hormone levels and feedback loops mentioned are primarily those of mature adults. In children, gonadotropin and gonadal steroid levels are very low. At puberty, negative feedback of steroid hormones decreases and gonadotropin and steroid levels gradually rise. During this pubertal development, variation in negative and positive estrogen feedback develops in females and eventually precipitates the changes resulting in the ovulatory menstrual cycle. At menopause, ovarian estrogen and inhibin production cease, gonadotropin levels rise markedly, and the symptoms associated with estrogen deficiency develop. In men, aging sometimes produces a decrease in testosterone production with a modest rise in gonadotropins, but no clinical syndrome similar to menopause affects men.

GnRH itself has been administered in pulsatile fashion to individuals with hypogonadotropic hypogonadism secondary to GnRH deficiency with great success, i.e., restoration of normal sexual function and fertility. Long-acting GnRH agonists have been used to down-regulate GnRH receptors and gonadotropin secretion in a variety of conditions, including precocious puberty, prostate cancer, breast cancer, uterine fibroids, and endometriosis. Direct GnRH antagonists that competitively compete for the GnRH receptor are being explored for similar conditions.

SOMATOSTATIN. Somatostatin (also known as somatotropin release–inhibiting factor) is a tetradecapeptide; a 28–amino acid precursor also has GH inhibitory properties. Somatostatin blocks the rise in GH that occurs with all stimuli in a dose-dependent fashion. The interaction of somatostatin and growth hormone–releasing hormone (GHRH) on GH secretion is complex. GH secretory episodes are associated with increased GHRH secretion, often accompanied by low somatostatin levels; the basal or trough GH levels are associated with low GHRH levels and more elevated somatostatin levels. Somatostatin also inhibits basal and stimulated TSH secretion. However, dose-response studies using somatostatin infusions in humans have shown that GH is about 10-fold more sensitive to inhibition by somatostatin than is TSH, thus suggesting that the physiologic role of somatostatin in inhibiting TSH secretion is limited.

Somatostatin is also present in the D cells of the pancreatic islets and the gut mucosa, as well as the myenteric neural plexus. Via paracrine and endocrine actions it suppresses the secretion of insulin, glucagon, cholecystokinin, gastrin, secretin, vasoactive intestinal polypeptide (VIP), and other gastrointestinal hormones, as well as such functions as gastric acid secretion, gastric emptying, gallbladder contraction, and splanchnic blood flow. Recently, analogues of somatostatin have been developed for the treatment of acromegaly, carcinoid tumors, VIP-secreting tumors, TSH-secreting pituitary tumors, islet cell tumors, and diarrhea of a number of causes.

CORTICOTROPIN-RELEASING HORMONE. Corticotropin-releasing hormone (CRH) releases adrenocorticotropic hormone (ACTH), β-endorphin, β-lipotropin, melanocyte-stimulating hormone (MSH), and other peptides generated from pro-opiomelanocortin (POMC) in equimolar amounts. CRH mediates 75% of the

ACTH response to stress, and the remaining 25% is due to vasopressin. CRH and vasopressin have synergistic effects on ACTH release. In fact, CRH and vasopressin coexist in about half of the CRH-containing paraventricular neurons and even in the same neurosecretory granules. CRH and vasopressin are not always released coordinately, however, and stress has been shown to selectively activate the vasopressin-containing subset of CRH neurons.

Cortisol feeds back to decrease ACTH secretion at both the hypothalamic and pituitary levels. ACTH and β-endorphin also feed back negatively to decrease CRH release by the hypothalamus. Morphine suppresses the ACTH response to CRH in humans, presumably acting through opioid μ-receptors. Central bioamines and peptides also influence CRH secretion. Acetylcholine, dopamine, norepinephrine, and epinephrine stimulate and γ-aminobutyric acid inhibits hypothalamic CRH secretion. Norepinephrine and epinephrine also stimulate pituitary ACTH secretion directly and are additive to the stimulatory effect of CRH.

Monokines released by inflammatory tissue, such as interleukin-1, interleukin-6, and tumor necrosis factor α, stimulate the synthesis and release of CRH and vasopressin from the hypothalamus and the release of ACTH by the pituitary. The consequent increase in cortisol then reduces the intensity of the inflammatory response and release of these monokines, thus completing the feedback loop. Therefore this neuroendocrine-immune loop serves to modulate the inflammatory response.

CRH and CRH receptors are widely distributed in the brain, and increases in CRH are associated with activation of the sympathetic and suppression of the parasympathetic nervous system, stimulation of arousal, and increased learning performance. CRH may also be involved in the regulation of body weight; with overfeeding, increased leptin stimulates CRH, which causes decreased food intake and increased energy expenditure.

Biosynthetic human CRH has recently become available for clinical use. Its major utility is in the differential diagnosis of Cushing's disease versus ectopic ACTH syndrome, with the finding that patients with Cushing's disease respond with greater than a 35% increment whereas those with ectopic ACTH secretion have a lesser response. If the results are equivocal, CRH testing during bilateral inferior petrosal sinus sampling for ACTH often provides additional discriminatory information.

GROWTH HORMONE–RELEASING HORMONE. GHRH dose-dependently stimulates GH secretion, and in some individuals GHRH is capable of eliciting a small increase in prolactin as well. With repetitive administration every 3 hours, GHRH can cause the release of sufficient GH in children with GHRH deficiency to result in an increase in IGF-I levels and an acceleration of growth. Both IGF-I and GH itself feed back negatively on GH secretion, with the negative feedback mediated by both a decrease in GHRH and an increase in somatostatin. This feedback effect of IGF-I is clinically relevant, as documented by the high circulating GH levels that occur in IGF-I–deficient states such as renal insufficiency and cirrhosis. In children with mutations of the GH receptor resulting in their not being responsive to GH (GH insensitivity syndrome, also known as Laron-type dwarfism), IGF-I levels are very low and GH levels are correspondingly elevated. α_2-Adrenergic receptors and serotonin activate GHRH and GH secretion, but γ-aminobutyric acid is inhibitory to GHRH secretion.

A recently described, separate GH-stimulating system for GH secretion involves a distinct receptor that interacts with a six–amino acid GH-releasing peptide (GHRP), although the physiologic ligand for this receptor has still not been identified. Receptors for GHRP are present in the pituitary and hypothalamus of humans, and GHRP and orally active non-peptide mimetics of GHRP are capable of releasing GH. Such substances may have potential diagnostically and therapeutically in the future.

PROLACTIN INHIBITORY FACTOR. The inhibitory component of hypothalamic regulation of prolactin secretion predominates over the stimulatory component. Dopamine is the predominant physiologic prolactin inhibitory factor, and the concentration of dopamine found in pituitary stalk blood is sufficient to decrease prolactin levels. It is likely that in most physiologic circumstances that cause a rise in prolactin, such as lactation, a simultaneous fall in dopamine occurs along with a rise in a PRF such as VIP. Blockade of endogenous dopamine receptors by a variety of drugs, such as the neuroleptics, causes a rise in prolactin. Lesions that interrupt the basal hypothalamic neuronal pathways carrying dopamine to the median eminence or that interrupt portal blood flow result in decreased dopamine reaching the pituitary and hyperprolactinemia.

PROLACTIN RELEASING FACTOR. A number of hypothalamic peptides other than TRH have also been shown to have PRF activity. VIP stimulates prolactin synthesis and release at concentrations found in hypothalamic-pituitary portal blood. Within the VIP precursor is another similarly sized peptide known as peptide histidine methionine, which also has PRF activity. Complicating the role of VIP as a PRF is the finding that VIP is actually synthesized by anterior pituitary tissue. The precise roles of VIP versus peptide histidine methionine and hypothalamic VIP versus pituitary VIP are still not clear.

ENDOGENOUS OPIOID PEPTIDES. In the mid-1970s, discovery of the opiate receptors and the fact that some of the endogenous opioid peptide ligands for these receptors were present within POMC, the precursor to ACTH, prompted widespread speculation about the importance of this system in neuroendocrine regulation, as well as the interaction of neuroendocrinology, mental illness, and opiate addiction. Most data now suggest, however, at most a modest role for endogenous opioid peptides in neuroendocrine regulation.

The endogenous opioid peptides have a common five–amino acid sequence at their amino termini (Tyr-Gly-Gly-Phe-Met [or Leu]) that is important for their binding to endogenous opioid receptors and bioactivity. Three major opioid peptide receptors and three major groups of opioid peptides (Fig. 235–3) are recognized, but the correspondence is not one for one. The μ-receptor mediates most of the endocrine effects and analgesia, morphine is its prototypic agonist, and naloxone is its prototypic antagonist. The primary peptide ligand for the μ-receptor is β-endorphin, which is derived from POMC, although β-endorphin also binds to the δ-receptor and the enkephalins can also bind to the μ-receptor. The δ-receptor mediates behavioral, analgesic, and some endocrine effects and has as its primary peptide ligands met- and leu-enkephalins, which are derived from proenkephalin A. It is much less well blocked by naloxone than is the μ-receptor. The κ-receptor mediates sedation and ataxia and binds primarily dynorphin and the neoendorphins, which are derived from proenkephalin B (prodynorphin). The importance of other opioid receptors, σ and ε, is not clear.

POMC is a 31,000-dalton precursor peptide that harbors within it ACTH, β-lipotropin, and β-endorphin; the last substance corresponds to the C-terminal 31 amino acids of β-lipotropin. POMC undergoes tissue-specific post-translational processing, i.e., in the anterior pituitary the major cleavage products are β-lipotropin and ACTH, with a significant proportion of β-lipotropin being further processed to β-endorphin, but in the pituitary intermediate lobe, the major products are α-MSH, corticotropin-like intermediate peptide, β-endorphin, and γ-lipotropin. Brain POMC, however, is processed primarily to β-endorphin, γ-lipotropin, and ACTH, with most of the ACTH being further processed to corticotropin-like intermediate peptide and α-MSH. All neuronal perikarya containing POMC-derived peptides are located in the arcuate nucleus, from which β-endorphin– and α-MSH–containing fibers project to the median eminence; ventromedial, dorsomedial, paraventricular, and periventricular nuclei of the hypothalamus; amygdala; pre-optic area; periaqueductal gray matter; reticular formation; stria terminalis; locus caeruleus; striatum; and hippocampus. The projection to the median eminence results in significant quantities of β-endorphin being found in portal blood. POMC-derived peptides are also found in the placenta, thyroid C cells, pancreas, testes, ovaries, adrenal medulla, gastric antrum, and macrophages. Anterior pituitary β-endorphin is secreted with ACTH after CRH and vasopressin stimulation (see above), but the only factors known to decrease hypothalamic β-endorphin are dopamine and estradiol.

The pentapeptide enkephalins are derived from the 28-kd precursor proenkephalin A, which contains six copies of the met-enkephalin sequence and one copy of the leu-enkephalin sequence. Other extended cleavage products with biologic activity may also exist, and the ratio of met- to leu-enkephalin ranges between 5:1 and 10:1 in various places in the brain, possibly representing evidence of differences in tissue-specific cleavage and/or degradation. Neuronal perikarya containing the enkephalins are widely distributed throughout the brain, as are fiber networks. Most enkephalinergic neurons are short and have the characteristics of interneurons. Rich enkephalinergic neural fiber networks can be found in the globus pallidus, amygdala, and midbrain, with specific areas of innervation including the origin of the central noradrenergic system, the locus

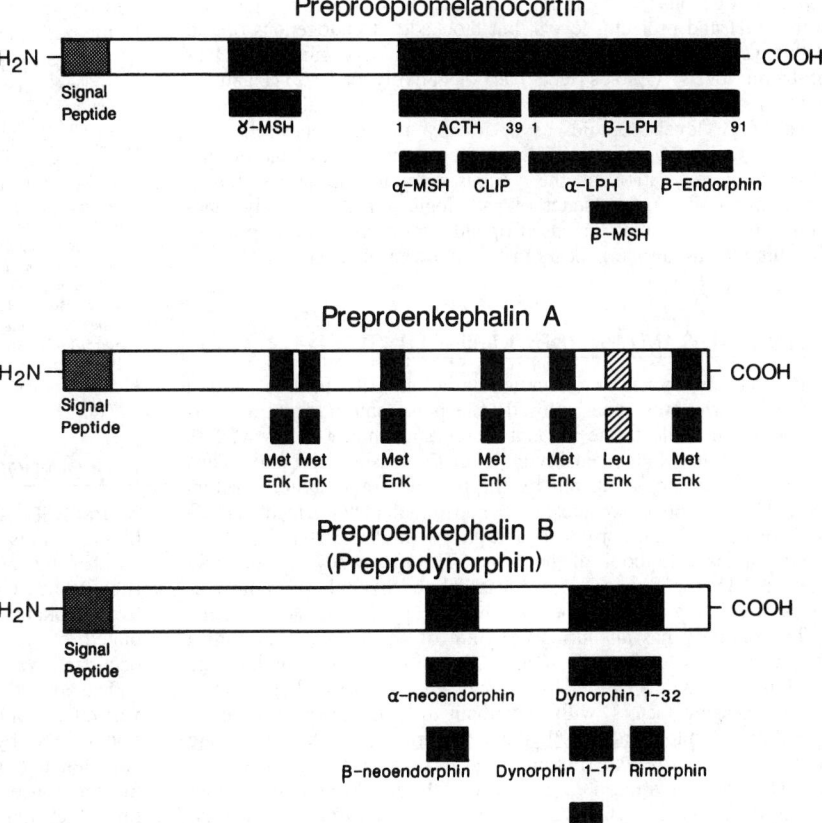

FIGURE 235–3 ■ Structures of the precursors of the endogenous opioid peptides. Pre-pro-opiomelanocortin (POMC) generates several peptides, including β-lipotropin (β-LPH), β-endorphin, adrenocorticotropic hormone (ACTH), α-melanocyte-stimulating hormone (α-MSH), β-MSH, γ-MSH, and corticotropin-like intermediate lobe peptide (CLIP). Pre-proenkephalin A generates six copies of methionine enkephalin (met-enk) and one copy of leucine-enkephalin (leu-enk). Pre-proenkephalin B (pre-prodynorphin) generates α- and β-neoendorphins; dynorphins 108, 1-7, and 1-32; and rimorphin.

caeruleus, the origin of the central serotoninergic system, the raphe nuclei, and the origin of the striatal dopaminergic system, the substantia nigra. Enkephalinergic neurons in the magnocellular portion of the paraventricular and supraoptic nuclei project to the posterior pituitary. Within the pituitary, enkephalins have been detected primarily in the posterior pituitary. Enkephalins have also been found in the adrenal medulla, gut, heart, lung, sympathetic ganglia, vagus, and retina.

Dynorphin is a 17–amino acid peptide derived from a 28-kd precursor called proenkephalin B or prodynorphin. Shorter peptides termed α- and β-neoendorphin, which have 10 and 9 amino acids, respectively, have also been isolated. These peptides react almost exclusively with the κ-receptor. Dynorphin-containing cells also project from the magnocellular neurons of the paraventricular nucleus to the posterior pituitary. Other tissues containing dynorphin include the gut, lungs, and adrenal medulla.

The three main opioid receptors μ, δ, and κ have all been cloned and found to be members of the G protein–coupled, seven-transmembrane class of receptors; they have 61% sequence identity at the amino acid level. The δ-receptors are located predominantly in the thalamus, hippocampus, periaqueductal gray matter, and neocortex, and the receptors are located primarily in the amygdala, nucleus accumbens, and hypothalamus. Dynorphin receptors have been localized to the cerebral cortex, the thalamus, and the caudate nucleus. The anterior pituitary itself is poor in opioid receptors but the hypothalamus is quite rich, and it has been suggested that the effects of opioid peptides on anterior pituitary hormone secretion are produced via modulation of hypothalamic bioamines and hypophysiotropic factors.

The specific functions of the various opioid peptides and the opioid receptors are still not completely understood, although evidence links them to a number of body functions, including stress, mental illness, narcotic tolerance and dependence, eating, drinking, gastrointestinal function, learning, memory, reward, cardiovascular responses, respiration, thermoregulation, seizures, brain electrical activity, locomotor activity, pregnancy, and neuroimmune activity. More specific functions regarding neuroendocrine regulation have been documented, however. In general, endogenous opioids have an inhibitory influence on gonadotropin secretion through action on GnRH secretion, probably by inhibition of noradrenergic neuronal input. Exogenous β-endorphin and enkephalin analogues increase serum GH and prolactin levels, but blockade of endogenous opioid pathways with naloxone does not alter basal or stimulated GH or prolactin levels. Opioids feed back negatively on ACTH and β-endorphin secretion, and naloxone can increase basal and stimulated ACTH levels. Opioids have virtually no effect on TSH secretion. Overall, the effects of the endogenous opioids on normal physiologic regulation of the various pituitary hormones appear quite minimal. In some states of pathologic gonadotropin dysfunction it is possible that increased opioid peptidergic tone is present, but this increased tone appears to be somewhat inconsistent.

CNS RHYTHMS AND NEUROENDOCRINE FUNCTION

Pituitary hormones are secreted in a pulsatile fashion with a number of rhythms superimposed. The pulse amplitude of a pituitary hormone reflects the amount of releasing hormone, as well as factors that may alter sensitivity to that releasing hormone. Thus the amplitude can be altered by the presence of inhibitory factors (e.g., GHRH versus somatostatin), nutritional factors, feedback effects of target organ hormones, and prior stimulation that depletes a readily releasable pool of hormone. The frequency is generally governed by the frequency of release of the hypophysiotropic factor, which is regulated by the hypothalamic pulse generator system.

The pituitary has an intrinsic rhythm of small amplitude with a frequency of every 2 to 10 minutes. Superimposed on this intrinsic rhythm is a rhythm caused by the pulsatile release of hypophysiotropic releasing factors, with or without the withdrawal of a corresponding inhibitory factor. Rhythms that are shorter than a day are referred to as *ultradian* rhythms. The next layer of rhythmicity is the *circadian* rhythm, i.e., rhythms with approximately 24-hour periodicity. These rhythms are usually synchronized with the 24-hour period by a periodic environmental cue such as the dark-light

cycle. The suprachiasmatic nucleus functions as a circadian pacemaker and receives light-induced electrical impulses from the retina via the retinohypothalamic tract, finally transmitting those impulses to the pineal gland, where they are converted to hormonal signals. Signals for a rhythm with a periodicity longer than 24 hours, i.e., an *infradian* rhythm, include the gravitational influence of the moon, which gives rise to the menstrual cycle.

A number of factors may influence circadian and infradian rhythms. One of the most important is the sleep-wake cycle. GH, TSH, prolactin, ACTH, and pubertal LH secretion are all entrained more to the sleep-wake cycle than the dark-light cycle. Each has an increase and maximal level that occur following sleep onset. The profound diurnal variation in cortisol and ACTH is often used as an index of "normality" of the system. Loss of this diurnal rhythm occurs with disordered regulation by CRH, which may be due to endogenous depression or excessive alcohol intake, as well as autonomous secretion of ACTH in Cushing's disease. Loss of the diurnal rhythm of cortisol has been used as a diagnostic test for Cushing's syndrome.

Interesting changes occur in gonadotropin secretion as a child passes through puberty into adulthood. Early in puberty the amplitude of the pulses increases during sleep at night, especially for LH, but in adulthood this nocturnal rise is lost. In patients with anorexia nervosa, the pattern of gonadotropin secretion often reverts to this pubertal pattern, only to lose this pattern again with weight gain. This phenomenon suggests that body composition may in some way affect regulation of the pulsatile secretion of gonadotropins. In fact, the percentage of body composition that is fat has been proposed as being important in the timing of the onset of puberty. Recent studies implicate leptin as the signal indicating this change in body composition.

Endocrine rhythms appear to reflect a rather primitive organizing influence that helps an animal adapt to the environment. Circadian synchronization with the light-dark cycle and sleep and infradian synchronization with seasonal changes are present very early phylogenetically. However, because humans are able to alter the light-dark cycles, they are less tied to environmental changes. This adaptation has led to new, modern problems with these rhythms such as jet lag, which involves rapid resynchronization of the rhythms with several-hour time zone displacements. Because not all rhythms resynchronize at the same rates, some of the disorientation and other symptoms associated with jet lag may be due to abnormal phase relationships of various body rhythms to each other and to the dark-light cycle.

Akil H, Meng F, Devine DP, Watson SJ: Molecular and neuroanatomical properties of the endogenous opioid system: Implications for treatment of opiate addiction. Semin Neurosci 9:70, 1997. *A review of the endogenous opioid peptides and their receptors and implications for new directions in drug abuse research.*

Chrousos GP: The hypothalamic-pituitary-adrenal axis and immune mediated inflammation. N Engl J Med 332:1351, 1995. *Review of the various interactions between the hypothalamic-pituitary-adrenal axis, stress, and the immune system, including possible therapeutic consequences.*

Vale W, Vaughan J, Perrin M: Corticotropin-releasing factor (CRF) family of ligands and their receptors. Endocrinologist 7(Suppl.):3, 1997. *An authoritative, brief review of CRF by the laboratory that initially characterized this substance.*

Van Cauter E: Diurnal and ultradian rhythms in human endocrine function: A minireview. Horm Res 34:45, 1990. *This article reviews the physiology and clinical relevance of the rhythms characterizing hormone secretion.*

Woodruff TK, Mather JP: Inhibin, activin and the female reproductive axis. Annu Rev Physiol 57:219, 1995. *Inhibin, activin, and follistatin are discussed along with a critical review of past misinformation that may have occurred because of assay problems.*

NEUROENDOCRINE DISEASE

DISEASES OF THE HYPOTHALAMUS. Diseases may affect the hypothalamus by being localized to the hypothalamus, by being part of more generalized central nervous system (CNS) disease such as neurosarcoidosis, or by indirect means such as causing hydrocephalus (Table 235–1). Furthermore, hormonal changes mediated by functional alterations in hypothalamic regulation may occur in a variety of psychiatric disorders or systemic illnesses.

The axons projecting to the median eminence that contain the various hypophysiotropic factors are concentrated in the basal portion of the hypothalamus. Thus lesions located within this final common pathway might be expected to cause significant decreases in secretion of some or all of the pituitary hormones except prolactin, which may increase because of the elimination of tonic inhibition by dopamine. Diabetes insipidus may also occur. Other func-

Neonates

Intraventricular hemorrhage
Meningitis: bacterial
Tumors: glioma, hemangioma
Trauma
Hydrocephalus, hydranencephaly, kernicterus

1 Month–2 Years

Tumors: glioma, especially optic glioma, histiocytosis X, hemangiomas
Hydrocephalus, meningitis
"Familial" disorders: Laurence-Moon-Bardet-Biedl, Prader-Labhart-Willi

2–10 Years

Tumors: craniopharyngioma, glioma, dysgerminoma, hamartoma, histiocyto-
  sis X, leukemia, ganglioneuroma, ependymoma, medulloblastoma
Meningitis: bacterial, tuberculous
Encephalitis: viral and demyelinating, various viral encephalitides and exan-
  thematous demyelinating encephalitides, disseminated encephalomyelitis
"Familial" disorders: diabetes insipidus, etc.
Damage from nasopharyngeal radiation therapy

10–25 Years

Tumors: craniopharyngioma, pituitary tumors, glioma, hamartoma, dysger-
  minoma, histiocytosis X, leukemia, dermoid, lipoma, neuroblastoma
Trauma
Subarachnoid hemorrhage, vascular aneurysm, arteriovenous malformation
Inflammatory diseases: meningitis, encephalitis, sarcoidosis, tuberculosis
Disease associated with midline brain defects: agenesis of corpus callosum
Chronic hydrocephalus or increased intracranial pressure

25–50 Years

Nutritional: Wernicke's disease
Tumors: glioma, lymphoma, meningioma, craniopharyngioma, pituitary tu-
  mors, angioma, plasmacytoma, colloid cysts, ependymoma, sarcoma, his-
  tiocytosis X
Inflammatory sarcoidosis, tuberculosis, viral encephalitis
Subarachnoid hemorrhage, vascular aneurysms, arteriovenous malformation
Damage from pituitary radiation therapy

50 Years and Older

Nutritional: Wernicke's disease
Tumors: sarcoma, glioblastoma, lymphoma, meningioma, colloid cysts,
  ependymoma, pituitary tumors
Vascular: infarct, subarachnoid hemorrhage, pituitary apoplexy
Infectious: encephalitis, sarcoidosis, meningitis

Adapted from Plum F, Van Uitert R: Non-endocrine diseases of the hypothalamus. *In* Reichlin S, Baldessarini RJ, Martin JB (eds): The Hypothalamus. New York, Raven Press, 1978, p 415.

tions of the hypothalamus are more diffusely located, such as the regulation of temperature, food intake, and blood pressure.

Symptoms resulting from hypothalamic dysfunction are related to the size of the lesion and consequently to the area of the hypothalamus involved, as well as the rapidity of the increase in lesion size. Slowly growing lesions tend to cause problems of hormone dysregulation rather than dramatic symptoms. Large, slowly growing lesions can cause more acute problems, however, when a slight increment in growth eliminates the remaining vestiges of vasopressin or ACTH secretion or completely occludes the aqueduct of Sylvius and precipitates hydrocephalus.

The best way of discerning lesions affecting the hypothalamus is by magnetic resonance imaging (MRI) with gadolinium enhancement, although computed tomographic (CT) scanning with intravenous contrast is also quite good. Formal visual field testing may discern impingement of the optic nerves and chiasm by hypothalamic lesions, including the suprasellar extension of pituitary tumors. Detailed testing of hypothalamic-pituitary function may reveal evidence of functional hypothalamic disruption with great sensitivity.

CONGENITAL EMBRYOPATHIC DISORDERS. The most common embryopathic disorders to affect the hypothalamus are the midline cleft syndromes, which cause varying degrees of defects of midline structures, especially the optic and olfactory tracts, the septum pellucidum, the corpus callosum, the anterior commissure, the hypothalamus, and the pituitary. The clinical features of patients with midline cleft defects varies in severity from cyclopia to cleft lip and from isolated hypothalamic hormone defects to panhypopituitarism. The combination of absent septum pellucidum associated with optic nerve hypoplasia is referred to as *septo-optic dysplasia*

and is associated with abnormalities of hypothalamic and other diencephalic structures. Some patients with septo-optic dysplasia and hypothalamic hypopituitarism have sexual precocity, presumably caused by a lack of inhibitory influences from other parts of the hypothalamus and intact GnRH-producing structures. Children with very mild midline cleft defects consisting of just cleft lip, cleft palate, or both have been found to have a markedly increased risk of having GH and other pituitary hormone deficiencies. Recent MRI studies of patients with "idiopathic" GH deficiency show absence of the infundibulum in nearly 50%.

Kallmann's syndrome is a condition characterized by anosmia or hyposmia and hypogonadotropic hypogonadism. The diagnosis is made by finding anosmia and low gonadotropin levels, and MRI will show absence or hypoplasia of the olfactory bulbs. The X-linked form of Kallmann's syndrome is due to a gene defect (*KAL*) resulting in loss of function of a protein that facilitates the embryologic migration of GnRH-producing neurons from the olfactory placode to the hypothalamus and the olfactory nerves to the olfactory bulbs. The pituitary is usually intact in this condition, and treatment with pulsatile GnRH therapy or gonadotropins results in spermatogenesis and normal gonadal function. In some patients, other neurologic abnormalities may be present, including cerebellar ataxia, nerve deafness, color blindness, cleft lip and palate, mental retardation, and disordered thirst.

TUMORS. The most common tumors affecting the hypothalamus are *pituitary adenomas* that have significant suprasellar extension. These tumors can cause varying degrees of hypopituitarism, diabetes insipidus, and hyperprolactinemia either by compressing the normal pituitary or, more commonly, by affecting the pituitary stalk and mediobasal hypothalamus. Evidence that hypopituitarism is caused by pituitary compression includes a low serum prolactin level and a lack of TSH response to TRH; pituitary function in such cases usually does not improve after treatment. In patients with normal or elevated prolactin levels, pituitary function often returns following therapy.

Craniopharyngiomas are the next most common tumors affecting the hypothalamus. Microscopically, craniopharyngiomas consist of cysts alternating with stratified squamous epithelium. The cyst fluid is usually thick and dark and the material is often calcified. They arise from remnants of Rathke's pouch. A closely related, less common lesion is a *Rathke cleft cyst,* which develops from the space between the anterior and rudimentary intermediate lobes. Rathke's cleft cysts are lined with cuboidal as opposed to squamous epithelium, and the cyst fluid is usually a white, mucoid fluid. Craniopharyngiomas may be difficult to remove in their entirety, and postoperative radiation reduces recurrences. Rathke's cleft cysts less commonly recur. Craniopharyngiomas most commonly arise during childhood, but they may also occur in adults and even the elderly. These tumors come to attention because of mass effects, including headache, vomiting, visual disturbance, seizures, hypopituitarism, and polyuria. Some patients have galactorrhea, amenorrhea, and hyperprolactinemia, features suggestive of a prolactinoma. Careful endocrine testing reveals varying degrees of hypopituitarism in 50 to 75% and modest hyperprolactinemia in 25 to 50%. Surgical extirpation of craniopharyngiomas commonly causes a worsening of pituitary function, often resulting in complete panhypopituitarism and diabetes insipidus because of stalk section. Irradiation may also be helpful, especially in children.

Suprasellar dysgerminomas arise from primitive germ cells that have migrated to the CNS during fetal life and are structurally identical to germ cell tumors of the gonads. They most commonly occur in children, in whom they cause decreased growth because of hypopituitarism, as well as diabetes insipidus and visual problems. Hyperprolactinemia occurs in more than 50%, and 10% have precocious puberty from the production of chorionic gonadotropin by the tumor. As opposed to craniopharyngiomas, these tumors are very radiosensitive and radiation therapy is the preferred treatment.

A hypothalamic *hamartoma* is a nodule of growth of hypothalamic neurons attached by a pedicle to the hypothalamus between the tuber cinereum and the mamillary bodies and extending into the basal cistern. Asymptomatic hamartomas may be present in up to 20% of random autopsies; rarely, these lesions may enlarge and disrupt hypothalamic function because of compression of adjacent tissue. A variant of hamartoma consisting of similar tissue present within the anterior pituitary but without a neural attachment to the hypothalamus is called a choristoma or gangliocytoma. These neuronal tumors are of particular endocrine interest because they can produce hypophysiotropic hormones. A number of cases associated with precocious puberty have been reported in which the hamartomas produced GnRH. Successful treatment has been reported with surgery and with the administration of a long-acting GnRH analogue, which suppresses gonadotropin secretion but does not affect the tumor itself. Medical therapy with the GnRH analogue may be the best choice because surgery can be non-curative or even fatal, if the hamartoma does not cause other problems from mass effects. Some gangliocytomas have been reported that produce GHRH and acromegaly or CRH and Cushing's syndrome.

Other tumors and space-occupying lesions occurring in the suprasellar area include arachnoid cysts, meningiomas, gliomas, astrocytomas, chordomas, infundibulomas, cholesteatomas, neurofibromas, lipomas, and metastatic cancer (particularly breast and lung). Any such lesion may be manifested by varying degrees of hypopituitarism, diabetes insipidus, and hyperprolactinemia, and surgical therapy often worsens the hormonal deficit.

INFLAMMATORY DISORDERS. CNS involvement in *sarcoidosis* occurs in 1 to 5% of patients, as determined on clinical grounds, and in up to 16% of cases at autopsy. Isolated CNS sarcoidosis is quite uncommon, however. When sarcoidosis does involve the CNS, the hypothalamus is involved in 10 to 20%. Sarcoid granulomas can involve the hypothalamus, stalk, or pituitary and may be infiltrative or occur as a mass lesion. Rarely, sarcoid granulomas can be manifested as an expanding intrasellar mass mimicking a pituitary tumor. The most common endocrine findings are varying degrees of hypopituitarism, diabetes insipidus, and hyperprolactinemia. Obesity secondary to hypothalamic involvement by sarcoidosis has also been reported. In patients with isolated CNS sarcoidosis, the diagnosis may be extremely difficult. Examination of cerebrospinal fluid usually shows elevated protein levels, low glucose levels, pleocytosis, and variable elevations of angiotensin-converting enzyme. However, biopsy is often necessary. Although corticosteroid therapy has been reported to at least partially reverse the thirst disorders, anterior pituitary hormone deficits usually do not respond.

Langerhans cell histiocytosis or eosinophilic granulomatous infiltration of the hypothalamus may cause diabetes insipidus, varying degrees of hypopituitarism, and hyperprolactinemia. It is the most common cause of diabetes insipidus in children. Usually this infiltration will appear as a thickening of the pituitary stalk, but it may also appear as a mass lesion of the hypothalamus or the pituitary. Osteolytic lesions may be present in the jaw or mastoid, so radiographs of the jaw are a worthwhile part of the diagnostic evaluation of an unknown suprasellar mass or diabetes insipidus for this reason. Therapy consists of local surgery, focal irradiation, or chemotherapy with alkylating agents and high-dose corticosteroids.

VASCULAR DISEASE. An enlarging aneurysm may be manifested as a mass lesion of the hypothalamic-pituitary area and may cause hypopituitarism and visual field defects. Obviously, the distinction must be made before surgery. Tumors and aneurysms may also coexist, and careful radiologic evaluation with MRI is necessary to discern such association. Hypothalamic disease caused by vascular infarction is extremely rare.

TRAUMA. Head trauma can cause defects ranging from isolated ACTH deficiency to panhypopituitarism with diabetes insipidus. Within the first 72 hours of trauma, GH, LH, ACTH, TSH, and prolactin levels may actually be elevated in blood, perhaps because of acute release. These levels subsequently fall and either patients return to normal or hypopituitarism develops. In patients dying of head injury, anterior pituitary infarction has been found in 16% of cases, posterior pituitary hemorrhage in 34%, and hypothalamic hemorrhage or infarction in 42% of cases. The paraventricular and supraoptic nuclei and median eminence are particularly involved with microhemorrhages, hence the high frequency of panhypopituitarism with diabetes insipidus. With frontal injuries the brain travels backward but the pituitary cannot move; consequently, the pituitary stalk becomes avulsed, with interruption of the portal vessels. Most patients with head injury are hyperprolactinemic, which clinically confirms that the hypothalamus and/or stalk is the primary site of injury.

IRRADIATION. Whole-brain irradiation for intracranial neoplasms frequently results in hypothalamic dysfunction, as evidenced by endocrine abnormalities and behavioral changes. The most common endocrine abnormality is hyperprolactinemia, but hypopituitarism can also occur. When the radiotherapy is targeted to the hypothalamic area, as in patients with tumors in that area or nasopharyngeal carcinomas, hypopituitarism occurs even more frequently. The frequencies of loss of pituitary function are so high that all patients who have had their pituitary and hypothalamic areas irradiated must be monitored closely for the purpose of detecting these deficits when they occur.

EFFECTS OF HYPOTHALAMIC DISEASE ON PITUITARY FUNCTION. Hypothalamic disease can cause both pituitary hyperfunction and hypofunction in varying degrees of severity. Although severe disease can cause absolute deficiencies of the various hormones, milder disease may cause a subtle alteration in feedback loops and timing such that, for example, the integration of signals necessary for menstrual cycling is lost, with subsequent "hypothalamic" amenorrhea. Furthermore, the hypothalamic defects may be interrelated. The rather common finding of hyperprolactinemia occurring with hypothalamic dysfunction causes a hypogonadotropic hypogonadism that is reversible when the elevated prolactin levels are brought down to normal. In many cases no structural lesion can be found on MRI, and a functional defect caused by altered neurotransmitter regulation is invoked.

GROWTH HORMONE. Loss of normal GH secretion is the most common hormonal defect occurring with structural hypothalamic disease. Congenital idiopathic GH deficiency is a heterogeneous disorder consisting of hypothalamic and pituitary defects. The diagnosis is usually made between 1 and 3 years of age because of impaired growth. Between 5 and 30% of subjects with idiopathic GH deficiency have an affected relative, and thus their defect is thought to have a genetic basis. One autosomal dominant form of complete GH deficiency has been found to be associated with deletion of the gene for GH. About three quarters of cases have a normal GH response to exogenous GH, which implies that the defect is probably disordered hypothalamic regulation. Defects in the gene for GHRH have not been found, but a rare form of GH deficiency has been found to be caused by a mutation in the GHRH receptor. As noted above, nearly half of children with idiopathic GH deficiency have midline cleft defects, and MRI scans should be performed routinely as part of the evaluation.

A reversible form of idiopathic GH deficiency caused by inadequate parental care and affection is referred to as the emotional deprivation syndrome or psychosocial dwarfism. Restoration of a proper social environment for such a child results in prompt normalization of GH secretion and growth. It has been hypothesized that the disordered GH regulation is due to psychogenic alteration of the neurotransmitter balance necessary for normal GHRH and somatostatin secretion. Other systemic illnesses such as inflammatory bowel disease, often occult, may also cause decreased GH secretion and growth; treatment of the systemic illness will correct the growth abnormality. Treatment of children and adults with GH deficiency is discussed in Chapter 237.

GONADOTROPINS. Hypothalamic Hypogonadism. The primary defect in this group of disorders is thought to involve the secretion of GnRH, with resultant impairment in pituitary gonadotropin secretion and gonadal function. The disorders causing these conditions may be primary, i.e., congenital defects, or acquired. Depending on the time of onset, they are manifested as either delayed puberty, interruption of pubertal progression, or loss of adult gonadal function. The lesions causing these disorders may cause loss of other hormones or may be isolated to GnRH. Loss of gonadotropin secretion as the result of hypothalamic structural damage is the second most common defect after GH deficiency. However, a substantial portion of these defects are due to hyperprolactinemia and are reversible with correction of the hyperprolactinemia. In some cases the defect is idiopathic. Defects in the gene for GnRH have not been found, but a rare familial form has been found to be due to a mutation in the GnRH receptor.

Lesions occurring pre-pubertally result in the failure of onset of puberty or in incomplete progression of puberty if the defect is partial. If the disorder is limited to GnRH and the gonadotropins, prior growth and development will be normal. However, the growth spurt occurring at puberty will be lost. Undescended testes are present in 50% of patients with GnRH deficiency, probably secondary to the absence of gonadotropins during fetal development. The most common congenital lesion causing pre-pubertal GnRH deficiency is Kallmann's syndrome, which affects 50% of males and 37% of females seen with isolated gonadotropin deficiency. In patients with idiopathic GnRH deficiency, the gene for GnRH appears to be normal. However, indirect measures of functional GnRH secretion show that disorders of pulse amplitude and/or frequency may be present. When hyperprolactinemia occurs before puberty, it can prevent the onset of puberty and must always be looked for in this setting.

The ideal therapy for patients with GnRH deficiency is replacement of GnRH via subcutaneous administration every 2 hours with a portable pump. This treatment causes a rapid rise in LH and FSH responses to GnRH, a rise in testosterone to normal, and the development of normal spermatogenesis. Similar approaches in women result in ovulatory cycles in 80%. The success of such therapy confirms the original hypothesis of a primary defect of GnRH secretion. In men, comparable results can be obtained with exogenous gonadotropins given three times per week. Replacement with testosterone alone causes adequate androgenization but does not result in an increase in testicular size or in spermatogenesis.

Loss of formerly normal GnRH secretion in adults may be due to structural hypothalamic damage such as a tumor, a functional change unassociated with a detectable lesion, or hyperprolactinemia. Structural disease must be excluded in such patients by CT or MRI. Most but not all cases of functional hypogonadotropic hypogonadism occur in women, the most common causes being weight loss, excessive exercise, psychogenic stress, or systemic illness. In some the exercise results in a loss of body fat not detected with total body weight measures, and it is unclear whether the hypogonadism is directly due to the loss of body fat or the exercise per se. Studies of pulsatile gonadotropin secretion in such patients reveal absent pulses. Usually the gonadotropin response to injected GnRH is normal. Regain of weight and stopping of the exercise result in resumption of normal gonadal function. Hyperprolactinemia occurring post-pubertally can also decrease GnRH and the pulsatile secretion of LH and FSH and thereby result in anovulation with oligomenorrhea/amenorrhea in women and impotence and infertility in men.

Therapy should be directed at the underlying process, if possible. Efforts at weight gain and restricting exercise should be made when appropriate. Two goals in the treatment of idiopathic, functional hypogonadotropic amenorrhea are (1) restoration of a normal estrogen status to promote well-being and to prevent osteoporosis and (2) facilitation of ovulation for fertility. The former can generally be achieved with cyclic estrogen and progesterone, whereas the latter may require clomiphene or GnRH or gonadotropin therapy.

Hypothalamic Hypergonadism (Precocious Puberty). Precocious puberty is defined as the onset of puberty before the ages of 8 in girls and 9 in boys. "Pseudo"-precocious puberty is that resulting from peripheral (gonadal or adrenal) causes. Central, "true," or GnRH-dependent precocious puberty is characterized by hormonal changes similar to those that occur at the time of normal puberty,

i.e., an increase in the pulsatile release of LH, an increase in the gonadotropin response to GnRH, and an increase in gonadal steroid secretion. GnRH-dependent precocious puberty therefore represents premature activation of this GnRH pulse generator by a variety of lesions, or it may also be idiopathic. Fewer than one quarter of cases of central precocious puberty occur in boys, but they tend to have more serious underlying disease. In boys with central, GnRH-dependent precocious puberty, hypothalamic hamartomas account for 38% of cases, other CNS lesions represent 31%, familial disease accounts for 23%, and idiopathic disease accounts for only 8%. The picture is quite different in girls, however: hypothalamic hamartomas account for only 15% of cases, other CNS lesions represent 14%, the McCune-Albright syndrome (polyostotic fibrous dysplasia) accounts for 6%, and fully 65% are idiopathic. Dysgerminomas in the suprasellar or pineal region can produce chorionic gonadotropin, which acts like LH in its stimulation of gonadal function. Usually such tumors cause increased sex steroid formation but fail to cause ovulation.

Therapy for central GnRH-dependent precocious puberty consists of surgical removal of the tumor or medical therapy with a long-acting GnRH analogue. The latter can suppress gonadotropin and sex steroid hormone levels and cause a stabilization or even regression of secondary sex characteristics and a slowing of growth and bone maturation in most cases. When therapy is discontinued at the normal time of puberty, sex steroid levels increase, secondary sexual characteristics again develop, growth increases, and regular menses develop spontaneously. For patients who do not respond to GnRH analogues, treatment with medroxyprogesterone acetate or testolactone, an aromatase inhibitor, is indicated.

PROLACTIN. Hypothalamic Hyperprolactinemia. Structural or infiltrative lesions of the hypothalamus, such as those discussed above, can decrease the amount of dopamine reaching the lactotrophs and thus cause modest hyperprolactinemia. Prolactin elevations resulting from such lesions rarely exceed 150 ng/mL and are usually less than 100 ng/mL. Similar elevations are also seen in patients with the empty-sella syndrome. Because their therapy is quite different, it is very important to differentiate non-secreting pituitary adenomas with extensive suprasellar extension causing prolactin elevations in this range from prolactin-secreting adenomas, which when of such a large size usually cause prolactin elevations 5 to 50 times higher. A number of medications can cause hyperprolactinemia primarily by interfering with central catecholamine, dopamine in particular (Table 235–2).

Therapy is generally directed at the underlying cause. The hyperprolactinemia itself may impair gonadal function, so efforts may also be made to lower prolactin levels with bromocriptine or other dopamine agonists. Prolactin levels usually fall quite readily in such patients. Restoration of gonadal function is not automatic, however, because the primary hypothalamic lesion may also directly impair release of GnRH. In that circumstance both bromocriptine and sex steroid replacement may be necessary. When administration of psychotropic medications that cause the

Table 235–2 ■ **ETIOLOGIES OF HYPERPROLACTINEMIA**

Pituitary Disease	*Neurogenic*	*Medications*
Prolactinomas	Chest wall lesions	Phenothiazines
Acromegaly	Spinal cord lesions	Haloperidol
Empty-sella syndrome	Breast stimulation	Monoamine oxidase inhibitors
Lymphocytic hypophysitis		Tricyclic antidepressants
Cushing's disease	*Other*	Reserpine
Pituitary stalk section	Pregnancy	Methyldopa
	Hypothyroidism	Metoclopramide
Hypothalamic Disease	Chronic renal failure	Amoxapine
Craniopharyngiomas	Cirrhosis	Cocaine
Meningiomas	Pseudocyesis	Verapamil
Dysgerminomas	Adrenal insufficiency	Fluoxetine
Non-secreting pituitary adenomas		
Other tumors	*Idiopathic*	
Sarcoidosis		
Eosinophilic granuloma		
Neuraxis irradiation		
Vascular		

Modified from Molitch ME: Diagnosis and treatment of prolactinomas. Adv Intern Med 44:117, 1999.

hyperprolactinemia cannot be stopped, dopamine agonists may be used but might exacerbate the psychosis. In such cases and others in which fertility is not an issue, treatment with cyclic estrogen/progestin replacement can be carried out safely.

Idiopathic Hyperprolactinemia. Idiopathic hyperprolactinemia is a diagnosis of exclusion. Prolactin levels in this condition are usually less than 100 ng/mL. In such cases, small pituitary or hypothalamic tumors could exist that are beyond the resolution of current imaging techniques, but when such patients are monitored for many years, it is very uncommon for tumors to later be visualized. Idiopathic hyperprolactinemia can cause amenorrhea, galactorrhea, impotence, infertility, and loss of libido, just as occurs with hyperprolactinemia of other causes, so the idiopathic hyperprolactinemia may need to be treated. Premature osteoporosis related to the estrogen deficiency may also occur. The only possible treatment is bromocriptine or another dopamine agonist, and these agents are successful in more than 90% of cases. Alternatively, cyclic estrogen/progesterone replacement may be given, but fertility will not be restored.

THYROID-STIMULATING HORMONE. *Hypothalamic hypothyroidism*, also referred to as tertiary hypothyroidism, is due to a central lesion that impairs the secretion of TRH, usually along with the loss of other hormones. It occurs considerably less commonly than hypothalamic GH and gonadotropin deficiency. Defects in the gene for TRH have not been detected, but a case has been reported of a TRH receptor mutation causing hypothyroidism. TSH levels in this syndrome are generally normal or even slightly elevated, and the response to TRH is delayed, peaking at 60 to 120 minutes rather than at 20 to 30 minutes. TSH in these patients is biologically less active than normal and binds to the TSH receptor less well because of altered glycosylation as a result of the TRH deficiency. Treatment is with L-thyroxine.

ADRENOCORTICOTROPIC HORMONE. *Hypothalamic ACTH deficiency* caused by hypothalamic lesions is uncommon. It may occur with the loss of other hormones but may also appear as an isolated deficiency. In the absence of CNS lesions or a history of trauma, most cases of isolated ACTH deficiency appear to be a pituitary autoimmune disorder. However, in patients with hypothalamic disease as the etiology, basal ACTH levels are low and the ACTH response to injected CRH may be prolonged and exaggerated, much as is the TSH response to TRH. The best test remains a comparison of ACTH responses to hypoglycemia, which is clearly mediated by the hypothalamus, and to CRH. The ACTH response is low in response to hypoglycemia but increased and delayed in response to CRH in most patients with hypothalamic CRH deficiency. Treatment is with glucocorticoids, and mineralocorticoids are not needed.

VASOPRESSIN. Diabetes insipidus can develop as a result of destructive lesions in the supraoptic and paraventricular nuclei or in the mediobasal hypothalamus in the path of the neural fibers containing vasopressin (see Chapter 102.1) that are passing on to the posterior pituitary. Irritative lesions can trigger the release of vasopressin in an unregulated fashion and thereby result in the syndrome of inappropriate antidiuretic hormone (vasopressin) secretion.

EFFECTS OF HYPOTHALAMIC DISEASE ON OTHER NEUROMETABOLIC FUNCTIONS. A number of functions that affect the internal milieu, in addition to anterior and posterior pituitary function, are regulated, at least in part, by the hypothalamus and include temperature control, behavior, consciousness, memory, sleep, food intake, and carbohydrate metabolism.

ALTERATIONS IN FOOD INTAKE. Body weight is kept relatively constant in non-obese individuals through the integration of a number of factors relating to the intake of nutrients and the output of energy; these functions are also affected by hormonal, environmental, and genetic factors. As with the regulation of hormone secretion, regulation of food intake can be conceptually regarded as an adjustment of food intake and energy expenditure around "set points" that may be different for body weight, total body fat, and lean body mass. The primary regulatory system involves production of the hormone leptin by adipocytes, which binds to hypothalamic leptin receptors and feeds back negatively on food intake and energy expenditure, but a number of other peptides are involved as well (see Chapter 228). A number of areas of the hypothalamus are involved in the regulation of energy balance.

Hypothalamic Obesity. Destruction of the mediobasal hypothalamus will sometimes inhibit satiety and may result in hyperphagia and hypothalamic obesity. The hyperphagia is due to destruction of noradrenergic fibers originating in the paraventricular nucleus and passing through the mediobasal hypothalamus. Because of their location, such lesions also usually produce hypopituitarism and diabetes insipidus. In a number of rare syndromes with obesity as a major characteristic, a hypothalamic etiology has been postulated. Prader-Willi is the most common of these syndromes and occurs in 1 in 25,000 births. It is characterized by hypotonia, obesity, short stature, mental deficiency, hypogonadism, and small hands and feet. About half have a chromosome 15 deletion. In the few cases studied at autopsy, no discernible hypothalamic lesions were detected. In the other syndromes (Laurence-Moon-Biedl-Bardet, Altrom-Hallgren), no specific hypothalamic lesions have been found.

Hypothalamic Anorexia. Lesions of the lateral hypothalamus, which destroy nigrostriatal dopaminergic fibers that pass through this area, produce hypophagia along with an increase in peripheral norepinephrine turnover and metabolic rate. This syndrome is very rare, probably owing to the requirement of bilateral lesions. The hormonal changes that occur in anorexia nervosa appear to all be secondary to the weight loss, and no evidence for a primary hypothalamic disorder in this syndrome has been found.

HYPERGLYCEMIA. Hypothalamic activation as part of the generalized response to stress can cause release of GH, prolactin, and ACTH, which serve as counterregulatory hormones with respect to insulin. These hormones promote lipolysis, gluconeogenesis, and insulin resistance, thereby resulting in glucose elevation. Of more importance in the acute response to stress, this hypothalamic response results in sympathetic activation with release of catecholamines that inhibit insulin secretion and stimulate glycogenolysis. In rare circumstances of acute hypothalamic injury from trauma, stroke, or infection, severe hyperglycemia can occur that is similar to the hyperglycemia seen in animals when the floor of the 4th ventricle is pricked with a needle, a phenomenon referred to as "piqûre" diabetes by Claude Bernard.

TEMPERATURE REGULATION. The anterior hypothalamus and preoptic area contain temperature-sensitive neurons that respond to internal temperature changes by initiating certain thermoregulatory responses necessary to restore a constant temperature. Measures that dissipate heat include cutaneous vasodilation, sweating, panting, and behavioral changes that result in attempts to alter the environment. Measures that increase body heat include increasing metabolic heat production, shivering, cutaneous vasoconstriction, and similar behavioral changes. In humans, much of the increase in metabolic heat production occurs via sympathetic activation. The thermosensitive neurons are affected by endogenous pyrogens and drugs that alter thermoregulation, as well as input from thermoreceptors in the skin and spinal cord.

Rare patients have been reported with anterior hypothalamic lesions that caused sustained hypothermia from failure of heat generation by shivering and vasoconstriction but who had intact heat dissipation or resetting of the temperature set point lower. Paroxysmal hypothermia lasting for minutes to days from the sudden onset of sweating, vasodilation, and a fall in core temperature has been reported in a number of patients in association with demonstrated lesions such as tumors and agenesis of the corpus callosum. Some of these patients had evidence of other hypothalamic dysfunction, including diabetes insipidus, hypogonadism, and precocious puberty.

Fever as a manifestation of hypothalamic disease is uncommon but has been reported in association with trauma or bleeding into the region of the anterior hypothalamus. Such fevers rarely persist more than 2 weeks. Paroxysmal hyperthermia secondary to hypothalamic dysfunction also occurs. Some cases of paroxysmal hypothermia and hyperthermia respond to anticonvulsant medications, which suggests that the neuronal discharge effecting the temperature changes are seizure-like.

Poikilothermy results from an inability to dissipate or generate heat to keep the body temperature constant in the face of varying ambient temperatures. This condition results from bilateral lesions in the posterior hypothalamus and rostral mesencephalon, which are the areas responsible for the final integration of thermoregulatory neural efferents. Patients with this condition do not feel discomfort with temperature changes and are unaware of having a problem. Depending on the ambient temperature, they may experience life-threatening hypothermia or hyperthermia. Poikilothermy is normally present in infants and frequently occurs in elderly individuals.

Constine LS, Woolf PD, Cann D, et al: Hypothalamic-pituitary dysfunction after radiation for brain tumors. N Engl J Med 328:87, 1993. *In this series of 32 patients, over two thirds had some hormonal dysfunction 2 to 13 years following cranial irradiation. Studies like this point out the need for endocrine evaluation of all patients undergoing cranial irradiation.*

DeRoux N, Young J, Misrahi M, et al: A family with hypogonadotropic hypogonadism and mutations in the gonadotropin-releasing hormone receptor. N Engl J Med 337: 1597, 1997. *This case report is illustrative of the new molecular approaches to diagnosis, i.e., being able to document the precise mutation in the GnRH receptor causing hypogonadotropic hypogonadism.*

Freda PU, Wardlaw SL, Post KD: Unusual causes of sellar/parasellar masses in a large surgical series. J Clin Endocrinol Metab 81:3455, 1996. *This series of patients illustrates the types of parasellar lesions that can be found clinically.*

Molitch ME: Diagnosis and treatment of prolactinomas. Adv Intern Med, 44:117, 1999. *This review covers current knowledge of the regulation of prolactin secretion, various causes of hyperprolactinemia, and the therapeutic options available.*

Mukherjee JJ, Islam N, Kaltsas G, et al: Clinical, radiological and pathological features of patients with Rathke's cleft cysts: Tumors that may recur. J Clin Endocrinol Metab 82:2357, 1997. *Rathke's cleft cysts may recur at rates greater than previously thought, as indicated in this series.*

Puchner MJA, Lüdecke DK, Saeger W, et al: Gangliocytomas of the sellar region—A review. Exp Clin Endocrinol 103:129, 1995. *This review explores all aspects of these rare but fascinating lesions.*

Quinton R, Duke VM, de Zoysa PA, Bouloux P-MG: The neurobiology of Kallmann's syndrome. Hum Reprod 11:121, 1996. *This short review discusses the pathophysiology and genetics of Kallmann's syndrome, as well as its clinical features.*

Triulzi F, Scotti G, di Natale B, et al: Evidence of a congenital midline brain anomaly in pituitary dwarfs: A magnetic resonance imaging study in 101 patients. Pediatrics 93:409, 1994. *In this series of children with idiopathic GH deficiency, a high proportion were found to have structural abnormalities of the pituitary stalk, thus making these anomalies of midline embryologic development. As imaging techniques improve, more and more "idiopathic" disorders may be found to have structural etiologies.*

236 THE PINEAL GLAND

Alfred J. Lewy

The mammalian pineal gland is located in the "center" of the brain (above the quadrigeminal plate, just behind the posterior commissure), but it is actually outside the blood-brain barrier. Postganglionic neurons from the superior cervical ganglia release norepinephrine which stimulates β_1-adrenergic receptors on the pinealocytes (Fig. 236–1). Such stimulation results in the synthesis and release of melatonin, the principal putative hormone of the pineal gland, into the cerebrospinal fluid and venous circulation. The (paired) suprachiasmatic nuclei are the source of an approximately 24-hour rhythm in melatonin production that persists in conditions of constant darkness or blindness. Photic input, conveyed to the suprachiasmatic nuclei via the retinohypothalamic tracts, synchronizes (entrains) the suprachiasmatic nuclei and their output circadian rhythms to the 24-hour light/dark cycle. Between the suprachiasmatic nuclei and the cell bodies of the pre-ganglionic sympathetic neurons in the spinal cord are synapses in the paraventricular nuclei.

Melatonin production by the human pineal gland is decreased by β-blockers and α_2-agonists and is increased by certain tricyclic antidepressants that block reuptake of norepinephrine. Melatonin production is also increased by extreme physical exercise, norepinephrine, and psoralen. In general, diet and activity have no effect. Increased melatonin in manic states and decreased melatonin in depression probably occur but most likely represent epiphenomena following changes in adrenergic activity.

FUNCTION OF MELATONIN

The function of melatonin in humans remains elusive. In some fish and reptiles, melatonin coalesces melanin-containing melanosomes and in this way causes blanching, but this effect has been lost in most animals. Melatonin may possibly have this effect on the mammalian retinal pigmented epithelium. The association of pineal tumors with disorders of puberty is most likely explained by compression of the hypothalamus inasmuch as no melatonin-secreting tumor has yet been found. Furthermore, it now appears that the

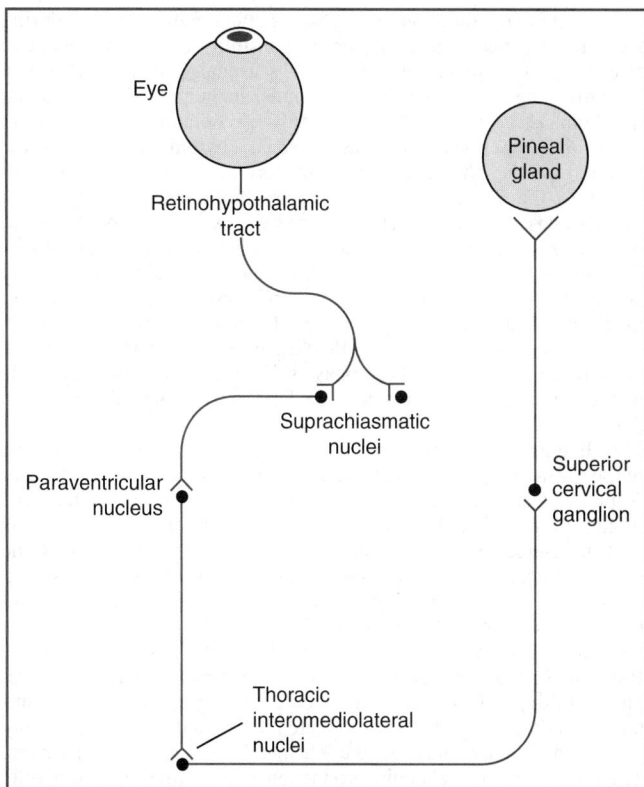

FIGURE 236–1 ■ Schematic diagram depicting neuroanatomic regulation of the timing of mammalian melatonin production (see the text). (Adapted by permission of the publisher from "Biochemistry and regulation of mammalian melatonin production" by AJ Lewy, in The Pineal Gland, edited by RM Relkin, pp 77–128. Copyright 1983 by Elsevier Science Publishing Co., Inc.)

main effect of melatonin on the reproductive system lies in its ability to communicate the time of the year to animals that are seasonal breeders. In such animals it can have either antigonadal or progonadal activity, depending on whether the species is a spring or fall breeder respectively. The reproductive and endocrine effects of exogenous melatonin administration, not to mention endogenous melatonin secretion, have not been well documented in humans, with the possible exception that melatonin at certain doses can increase prolactin levels in humans.

CHRONOBIOLOGY OF MELATONIN

Melatonin is produced only during nighttime darkness in both diurnal and nocturnal animals, with an approximately 12-hour "on" phase and a 12-hour "off" phase. Many blind people with complete absence of light perception have free-running endogenous circadian rhythms. When these individuals' melatonin rhythms are out of phase with their sleep/wake cycles (which have remained more or less synchronized to clock time), they are prone to nocturnal insomnia and daytime sleepiness. A pattern of insomnia that recurs every few weeks is almost pathognomonic for free-running circadian rhythms in totally blind individuals.

Although darkness does not induce melatonin production, in sighted people exposure to sufficiently bright light during the night immediately suppresses melatonin production. Two models have been proposed to explain how the nightly melatonin profile is shaped. In the *two-pacemaker model*, it is hypothesized that separate endogenous pacemakers control the onset and offset of melatonin production, cued primarily to dusk and dawn, respectively. In the *"clock-gate" model*, the suppressant effect of light (unique to melatonin) participates in shortening the duration of nighttime melatonin production during long photoperiods. Both models attempt to explain the shorter duration of melatonin secretion during the briefer summer nights than during the longer winter nights.

The changing duration of nighttime melatonin secretion during the calendar year seems to be responsible for the reproductive effects of the light/dark cycle in seasonal breeders. Seasonal rhythms have not been well documented in humans, but it is clear that humans have most, if not all of the circadian rhythms found in other higher animals. Whereas seasonal rhythms respond to the duration of the photoperiod or scotoperiod, circadian rhythms respond to the 24-hour light/dark cycle. In animals, the light/dark cycle's phase-shifting effects on circadian rhythms can be described by a phase response curve (PRC). This phenomenon appears to be the case in humans as well. The PRC can be explained as follows: delay responses (shifts to a later time) result when exposure to light occurs during the 1st part of the night; advance responses (shifts to an earlier time) result when exposure occurs during the latter part of the night. These phase shifts are greatest in magnitude in the middle of the night and are least during the middle of the day.

Although the suppressant effect of light is unique to melatonin, phase shifting by light affects the endogenous circadian pacemaker (suprachiasmatic nuclei) and all of its driven rhythms. In fact, the timing of the circadian rhythms of the suprachiasmatic nuclei is best measured by the circulating levels of melatonin. In some species, injections of exogenous melatonin are capable of causing phase shifts and/or entrainment. In lizards, a PRC for melatonin has been described that is about 12 hours out of phase with the PRC for light; that is, the melatonin PRC resembles a dark-pulse PRC. In humans, exogenous melatonin appears to have circadian phase-shifting effects that can be described by a PRC that resembles a dark-pulse PRC. Thus melatonin—which is produced only during the night—may be the chemical messenger of darkness. Therefore, human melatonin production may normally have a role, however small, in entrainment of the circadian rhythms of the suprachiasmatic nuclei. Not being seasonal breeders, perhaps humans have retained the suppressant effect of light in order to use endogenous melatonin to more effectively augment the entrainment and phase-shifting effects of the light/dark cycle. The melatonin PRC may also provide the rationale for precise scheduling of exogenous melatonin administration for therapeutic purposes, such as to treat chronobiologic sleep and mood disorders and to facilitate adaptation to shift work and air travel.

PINEAL TUMORS

The three main types of tumors that usually arise in the pineal gland are (1) pineoblastomas or pineocytomas, the term used depending on the degree of differentiation of this tumor of the pineal parenchyma; (2) germ cell tumors, including germinomas and embryonal carcinomas; and (3) glial tumors. Symptomatic enlargement of the pineal gland due to cysts has also been reported, but these conditions are almost always asymptomatic. Destruction of pineal tissue can reduce or even ablate melatonin production, but pineocytomas have rarely been associated with increased circulating levels of melatonin. Melatonin production decreases with age, but this decrease does not seem to be related to pineal calcification. By occluding the cerebral aqueduct, pineal tumors can produce symptoms associated with increased intracranial pressure, sometimes necessitating a shunt. Through pressure on the quadrigeminal plate, pineal tumors can produce Parinaud's syndrome, which includes paresis of upward conjugate gaze. Some germinomas and embryonal carcinomas secrete human chorionic gonadotropin, which has been implicated in cases of delayed onset of puberty. Treatment modalities include surgical extirpation, radiation, and chemotherapy, depending on tumor type and location and the absence or degree of metastases.

Lewy AJ, Bauer VK, Ahmed S, et al: The human phase response curve (PRC) to melatonin is about 12 hours out of phase with the PRC to light. Chronobiol Int 15: 71, 1998.

Lewy AJ, Cutler NL, Sack RL: The endogenous melatonin profile as a marker for circadian phase position. J Biol Rhythms (in press), 1999.

Lewy AJ, Wehr TA, Goodwin FK, et al: Light suppresses melatonin secretion in humans. Science 210:1267, 1980.

Neuwelt EA (ed.): Diagnosis and Treatment of Pineal Region Tumors. Baltimore, Williams & Wilkins, 1984.

237 ANTERIOR PITUITARY

Mark E. Molitch

ANATOMY AND EMBRYOLOGY

The pituitary is a relatively small gland that is located in the sella turcica at the base of the brain. It has a bilobed shape and weighs about 0.6 g (range, 0.4–0.9 g), being somewhat larger in women than in men. The pituitary is divided into anterior and posterior lobes, with the anterior lobe comprising about 80% of the gland. The posterior pituitary or neurohypophysis consists of the pituitary stalk as well as the posterior lobe (see Chapter 238). Superiorly, the pituitary is covered by the diaphragma sella, a reflection of the dura mater that forms the roof of the sella and is attached to the clinoid processes. The diaphragma sella has a central opening that is penetrated by the pituitary stalk and its blood vessels. Importantly, the optic chiasm, formed by the decussation of the optic nerves, is positioned directly above the pituitary gland and below the third ventricle. The exact position of the chiasm is variable, affecting the pattern of visual field changes experienced by patients with pituitary tumors that expand into the suprasellar region. The lateral boundaries of the sella are formed by the cavernous sinuses, which contain the internal carotid artery and cranial nerves III, IV, V_1, V_2, and VI.

The blood supply to the pituitary gland is derived from the superior and inferior hypophyseal arteries, branches of the internal carotid arteries. Specialized vascular structures, referred to as gomitoli, are located in the median eminence of the hypothalamus and consist of short terminal arterioles that drain into portal veins that course down the pituitary stalk to join the sinusoidal capillaries of the anterior lobe. Hypothalamic hormones enter fenestrations in the perigomitolar capillaries to flow from the hypothalamus to the anterior pituitary. Venous drainage from the anterior lobe enters the posterior pituitary capillary bed before draining into the cavernous sinuses. The cavernous sinuses are interconnected by means of channels that encircle the pituitary, and they drain into the petrosal sinuses. The petrosal sinuses can be catheterized for hormone sampling in the diagnosis of adrenocorticotropic hormone (ACTH)-secreting pituitary tumors.

The six major pituitary cell types include somatotrophs (growth hormone [GH] producing), lactotrophs (prolactin [PRL] producing), corticotrophs (ACTH producing), thyrotrophs (thyroid-stimulating hormone [TSH] producing), gonadotrophs (follicle-stimulating hormone [FSH] and luteinizing [LH] producing), and folliculostellate cells that do not produce the classic pituitary hormones but may have paracrine functions. The biochemical characteristics of the major anterior pituitary hormones are summarized in Table 237–1.

The pituitary is formed early in embryonic life from the fusion of Rathke's pouch (which gives rise to the anterior pituitary) and a portion of the ventral diencephalon (which gives rise to the posterior pituitary). Rathke's pouch is an ectodermal evagination in the roof of the primitive oropharynx. However, there is some evidence that the anterior pituitary may develop from a more rostral neuroectoderm fold rather than this ectodermal tissue. The ontogeny of hormone production during anterior pituitary development has been characterized in detail. The pituitary anlage expresses the glycoprotein hormone α gene even as the progenitor cells are arising from Rathke's pouch. Subsequently, pro-opiomelanocortin (POMC)-producing cells can be seen in the hypothalamus and in the pituitary. An evanescent group of TSH-producing cells appear, but then fade away, to be followed later by a distinct population of TSH cells in a different location in the pituitary. After gonadotrophs develop, GH- and PRL-producing cells appear and later form distinct populations of somatotrophs and lactotrophs. The transcription factor Pit-1, a member of the Pou-Homeodomain family, is produced in somatotrophs, lactotrophs, and thyrotrophs. Mutations in Pit-1 prevent the development of these cells and cause deficiencies of GH, PRL, and TSH. This lineage relationship probably accounts for the observation that some GH-producing tumors also secrete PRL and about one third of TSH-producing tumors co-secrete GH.

Table 237-1 ■ FEATURES OF THE MAJOR ANTERIOR PITUITARY HORMONES*

HORMONE	AMINO ACIDS	MW (kd)	SERUM HALF-LIFE (min)	CELL TYPE	TARGET GLAND
Growth hormone (GH)	191	22	20	Somatotroph	Multiple
Prolactin (PRL)	198	23	20	Lactotroph	Breast
Adrenocorticotropic hormone (ACTH)	39	4.5	8	Corticotroph	Adrenal
Thyroid-stimulating hormone (TSH)	α-subunit, 92	14	50	Thyrotroph	Thyroid
	β-subunit, 118	17			
Luteinizing hormone (LH)	α-subunit, 92	14	50	Gonadotroph	Gonad
	β-subunit, 121	18			
Follicle-stimulating hormone (FSH)	α-subunit, 92	14	220	Gonadotroph	Gonad
	β-subunit, 111	18			

*The amino acid lengths are based on the cloned complementary DNAs and differ in some cases from the lengths of the sequenced proteins, perhaps because of proteolysis. The indicated molecular weights (MW) include the contributions of the carbohydrates in the case of the glycoprotein hormones (TSH, LH, FSH). The serum half-lives assume single compartment monoexponential decay.

Anterior pituitary hormone production is largely established by the ninth week of gestation, and the anatomic and biosynthetic mechanisms that comprise an active hypothalamic-pituitary system appear to be functional by 12 to 17 weeks of gestation. In anencephaly, all anterior pituitary cell types, with the exception of corticotrophs, are capable of hormone synthesis and secretion, indicating that the embryonic pituitary develops relatively normally in the absence of hypothalamic stimulation.

Somatotrophs, which constitute 40 to 50%, and lactotrophs, which make up 15 to 25%, of anterior pituitary cells, are located predominantly in the lateral aspects of the anterior pituitary. Corticotrophs constitute 10 to 20% of anterior pituitary cells and are located mainly in the central region of the anterior pituitary. Gonadotrophs, which account for about 10% of pituitary cells, produce both FSH and LH, although a small fraction of gonadotrophs appear to selectively secrete only one of the hormones. Only 5% of pituitary cells are thyrotrophs. The folliculostellate cells have long irregular processes that extend between the hormone-producing cells. They do not contain secretory granules but have been shown to produce growth factors such as basic fibroblast growth factor, vascular endothelial growth factor, and follistatin, among others.

Asa SL, Kovacs K, Melmed S: The hypothalamic-pituitary axis. In Melmed S (ed): The Pituitary. Cambridge, MA, Blackwell Science, 1995, pp 3–44. A definitive summary of pituitary anatomy, normal histology, and pathology.

Voss JW, Rosenfeld MG: Anterior pituitary development: Short tales from dwarf mice. Cell 70:527–30, 1992. A review of a remarkable series of studies that define pituitary cell lineages.

RADIOLOGY OF THE PITUITARY

Radiologic imaging of the pituitary gland primarily involves computed tomography (CT) and magnetic resonance imaging (MRI). CT scans are performed using high-resolution (1.5 mm), contrast medium–enhanced procedures with direct coronal sections. Although CT provides excellent resolution, problems include artifacts from metallic objects and dental fillings, and some patients have difficulty assuming the position required for coronal sections. Pituitary adenomas are hypodense on both unenhanced and contrast medium–enhanced CT scans.

Overall, MRI is the technique of choice for evaluating the sellar region. MRI provides multiplanar imaging and excellent resolution of the pituitary and surrounding cerebrospinal fluid and vascular and central nervous system structures. There is less radiation exposure with MRI than with CT, allowing repeated imaging as required for evaluation and follow-up. However, bone structures are not well defined by MRI. The normal anterior pituitary appears isointense with brain white matter, whereas the posterior pituitary exhibits high signal intensity. The optic chiasm can be readily identified superior to the pituitary gland because it is surrounded by hypodense structures. MRI detects pituitary microadenomas in nearly all patients with surgically proven tumors. Pituitary adenomas typically appear hypointense on T1-weighted images and show less enhancement with gadolinium than surrounding normal tissue. Focal hypodense areas are also seen in about a fourth of normal individuals, which may correspond to cysts or small adenomas that have been described in autopsy series, emphasizing the importance

of endocrine evaluation in making the diagnosis of pituitary tumors.

Freda PU, Post KD: Differential diagnosis of sellar masses. Endocrinol Metab Clin North Am 28:81–117, 1999. A brief review of the differential diagnosis of sellar masses.

Molitch ME: Pituitary incidentalomas. Endocrinol Metab Clin North Am 26:725–740, 1997. A brief discussion of how to approach the patient with an incidentally found abnormality in the sella on CT or MRI.

Naidioh MJ, Russell EJ: Current approaches to imaging of the sellar region and pituitary. Endocrinol Metab Clin North Am 28:45–79, 1999. A review of the radiologic features of pituitary adenomas, craniopharyngiomas, meningiomas and other masses commonly seen in the sellar area.

REGULATION OF THE PITUITARY AXIS

The concept of positive and negative feedback control represents a fundamental tenet of endocrinology. The pituitary gland integrates the influences of an array of positive and negative signals to modulate hormone secretion within a narrow range (Table 237–2). The major hypothalamic-pituitary-target gland axes include the thyrotropin (TRH)-TSH-thyroid hormone axis; corticotropin-releasing hormone (CRH)-ACTH-cortisol axis; gonadotropin-releasing hormone (GnRH)-LH/FSH-gonads axis; and GH-releasing hormone (GHRH)-GH-insulin-like growth factor (IGF)-1 axis. PRL is the only major pituitary hormone that is not subject to feedback inhibition by hormones produced in target tissues. However, it is controlled by positive and negative input from the hypothalamus.

The principles of feedback regulation are well illustrated by the hypothalamic-pituitary-thyroid axis (see Fig. 239–1). Hypothalamic TRH stimulates TSH secretion from the pituitary. TSH increases thyroid hormone secretion, which in turn suppresses hypothalamic TRH as well as pituitary TSH. A typical regulatory loop therefore has both positive (TRH, TSH) and negative (thyroxine [T_4], triiodothyronine [T_3]) components, allowing a high degree of control of hormone levels. In this case, the pituitary gland integrates positive TRH signals and the negative effects of thyroid hormone. The concept of feedback regulation is important not only for understanding pituitary physiology but also because it provides the basis for analyzing pituitary gland function using stimulation and suppression tests.

The feedback regulatory systems just described are superimposed on hormonal rhythms that are used for adaptation to the environ-

Table 237-2 ■ FACTORS THAT REGULATE PITUITARY HORMONE SECRETION

HORMONE	RELEASING FACTORS	INHIBITING FACTORS
GH	GHRH	Somatostatin, IGF-1
PRL	TRH, VIP, E_2	Dopamine
ACTH	CRH, vasopressin	Cortisol
TSH	TRH	T_4, T_3, somatostatin, dopamine
LH	GnRH	E_2, testosterone
FSH	GnRH, activin	Inhibin, E_2, testosterone

GHRH = Growth hormone–releasing hormone; IGF-1 = insulin-like growth factor-1 (formerly called somatomedin C); TRH = thyrotropin-releasing hormone; VIP = vasoactive intestinal peptide; E_2 = estradiol; CRH = corticotropin-releasing hormone; T_4 = thyroxine; T_3 = triiodothyronine. The gonadal steroids E_2 and testosterone exert much of their inhibitory effects on gonadotropin secretion at the hypothalamic level.

ment. Seasonal changes, the daily occurrence of the light-dark cycles, and stress are but a few of many environmental events that have major impacts on the secretion of pituitary hormones. Some hormonal pathways, such as ACTH, GH, and PRL secretion, are entrained to the sleep-wake cycle, causing characteristic peaks of ACTH and cortisol production in the early morning with a nadir in the late afternoon and evening. The early pubertal surges of LH occur at night and usually in association with sleep. The menstrual cycle provides an example of a pituitary rhythm that occurs on a much longer time scale (approximately 28 days). The pattern of the menstrual cycle is coupled to cycles of follicular development in the ovary. As follicular development progresses, levels of gonadal steroids and inhibin feed back on the hypothalamus and pituitary to modulate LH and FSH secretion.

Because many hormones are released in a pulsatile manner and in a rhythmic fashion, it is important to be aware of these characteristics of secretion when attempting to relate serum measurements to normal values. Although it is possible to characterize pulsatile patterns of hormone secretion using frequent blood sampling (every 10 minutes) over several hours, this is not practical in a clinical setting. Alternative approaches include stimulation and suppression tests or the use of "integrated" measurements of hormone production such as 24-hour urine free cortisol as an index of ACTH secretion or IGF-1 as a biologic marker of GH action.

Van Cauter E: Diurnal and ultradian rhythms in human endocrine function: A mini-review. Horm Res 34:45, 1990. *This article reviews the physiology and clinical relevance of the rhythms characterizing hormone secretion.*

HYPOPITUITARISM

Hypopituitarism implies diminished production of one or more anterior pituitary hormones. Although the recognition of complete or panhypopituitarism is usually straightforward, the detection of partial or selective hormone deficiencies is more challenging. Pituitary hormone deficiencies can be caused by loss of hypothalamic stimulation (tertiary hormone deficiency) or by direct loss of pituitary function (secondary hormone deficiency). The distinction between hypothalamic and pituitary causes of hypopituitarism is important for establishing the correct diagnosis and for applying and interpreting the relevant diagnostic endocrine tests. With improved procedures for testing the hypothalamic-pituitary axis, it is apparent that hypothalamic causes of hypopituitarism are more common than previously appreciated (see Chapter 235). When hypopituitarism is accompanied by diabetes insipidus or hyperprolactinemia, one should particularly consider hypothalamic causes of pituitary dysfunction.

CAUSES OF HYPOPITUITARISM. A variety of congenital and acquired causes of hypopituitarism have been described (Table 237–3). Sporadic and familial forms of panhypopituitarism occur, but the underlying genetic or developmental defects have not been elucidated. Congenital combined deficiencies of GH, PRL, and TSH are caused by mutations in the gene encoding Pit-1, a pituitary-specific transcription factor that is involved in the development of somatotroph, lactotroph, and thyrotroph cell lineages. Different types of Pit-1 mutations are inherited in an autosomal dominant or recessive pattern. Gene mutations have been found at several steps leading to pituitary hormone secretion, including mutations in the hypophysiotropic releasing factor receptors for GnRH, GHRH, and TRH; mutations in the pituitary hormone structural genes for GH, ACTH, and the α subunits of FSH, TSH, and LH; and mutations in the pituitary hormone receptors for GH, ACTH, TSH, and LH. Best studied are mutations of the GH gene, and these have proved to be heterogeneous. Some include large deletions of the GH gene that are inherited in an autosomal recessive manner and involve genetic recombination between related DNA sequences in the duplicated GH gene cluster. Point mutations have also been described in the GH gene, and some of these can be inherited in an autosomal dominant manner, apparently because the mutant hormone impairs GH biosynthesis and normal function of the somatotroph cell. Mutations of the other types described earlier generally cause autosomal recessive forms of selective hormone deficiencies. The congenital embryopathic disorders causing hypopituitarism are discussed in Chapter 235.

Neoplastic lesions, particularly pituitary adenomas, are the most

Table 237–3 ■ CAUSES OF HYPOPITUITARISM

Genetic Defects
  Hypophysiotropic hormone gene defects
  Hypophysiotropic hormone receptor gene defects
    GHRH receptor defect
    GnRH receptor defect
    TRH receptor defect
  Pituitary hormone gene defects
    Gonadotropins: LH β- and FHS β-subunit gene defects
    Growth hormone: defects in GH gene
    Thyrotropin: defects in TSH β-subunit
    Multiple hormone (GH, PRL, TSH) defects: due to mutation in Pit-1 gene and Propl gene
  Pituitary hormone receptor genetic defects
    Growth hormone receptor defects: GH insensitivity syndrome (Laron-type dwarfism)
    ACTH receptor defects: congenital insensitivity to ACTH
    LH receptor defects
    TSH receptor defects
Congenital Embryopathic Defects
  Anencephaly
  Midline cleft defects: septo-optic dysplasia, basal encephalocele, cleft lip and palate
  Pituitary aplasia
  Kallmann's syndrome (GnRH defect with anosmia)
Acquired Defects
  Tumors: pituitary adenomas, craniopharyngiomas, dysgerminomas, meningiomas, gliomas, metastatic tumors, hamartomas, Rathke's cleft cysts
  Irradiation
  Trauma: surgery, external blunt trauma
  Empty sella syndrome
  Vascular
    Pituitary apoplexy
    Sheehan's syndrome
    Internal carotid aneurysm
    Vasculitis
  Inflammatory/infiltrative diseases
    Sarcoidosis
    Langerhans' cell histiocytosis (histiocytosis X, eosinophilic granuloma)
    Tuberculosis, syphilis
    Meningitis
    Lymphocytic hypophysitis, infundibulohypophysitis
  Metabolic
    Hemochromatosis
    Amyloidosis
    Critical illness
    Malnutrition
    Anorexia nervosa
    Psychosocial deprivation
  Idiopathic

GHRH = Growth hormone releasing hormone; GnRH = gonadotropin-releasing hormone; TRH = thyrotropin-releasing hormone; LH = luteinizing hormone; FSH = follicle-stimulating hormone; GH = growth hormone; TSH = thyroid-stimulating hormone; PRL = prolactin; ACTH = adrenocorticotropic hormone.

common cause of acquired hypopituitarism. Pituitary adenomas cause hypopituitarism in several different ways. In some cases there is direct destruction or compression of the normal pituitary. Compression of the pituitary stalk can impair blood supply to the pituitary as well as decrease input from hypothalamic hormones. Hemorrhage into tumors can lead to pituitary infarction. When tested carefully, most patients with macroadenomas have partial deficiencies of one or more pituitary hormones, most often involving GH and gonadotropins. A mild degree of hyperprolactinemia is characteristic of disorders that cause stalk compression, and hyperprolactinemia further impairs gonadotropin secretion. A variety of other neoplasms that occur near the sella, such as craniopharyngiomas, can also cause hypopituitarism (see Table 237–3).

Radiation causes hypopituitarism primarily because of its effects on hypothalamic function, although high-dose radiation (e.g., proton beam) can also cause direct pituitary damage. The sellar region is subjected to radiation in the treatment of pituitary adenomas, craniopharyngiomas, clivus chordomas, optic gliomas, meningiomas, dysgerminomas, and neoplasms of the oropharynx. Importantly, the effects of radiation can be delayed as much as several years, and patients at high risk should be evaluated at about yearly intervals for radiation-induced hypopituitarism. Although GH and gonadotropin deficiencies develop first in most patients, ACTH or

TSH deficiencies occasionally occur first, emphasizing the need to evaluate each of the major axes.

Empty sella syndrome can occur as a primary or as an acquired condition. It is caused by defects in the diaphragma sella that allow herniation of the arachnoid membrane into the hypophyseal fossa. In long-standing cases, sellar enlargement occurs, probably because of persistent transmission of intracranial pressure. With appropriate imaging studies, the pituitary gland can be seen as a flattened rim of tissue along the floor of the sella. Primary empty sella occurs most commonly in women and may be associated with features of benign intracranial hypertension. Pituitary function in patients with primary empty sella syndrome is usually normal, although 15% have mild hyperprolactinemia, probably because of stretching of the pituitary stalk. Acquired forms may occur as a result of surgery, radiation, or pituitary infarction (usually of an adenoma).

Pituitary apoplexy is usually caused by hemorrhage into a tumor with associated infarction. In the absence of a tumor, predispositions to apoplexy include trauma, pregnancy, anticoagulation, sickle cell anemia, and diabetes mellitus. Pituitary infarction in the peripartum period is referred to as Sheehan's syndrome and is usually associated with significant obstetric hemorrhage and hypovolemia. Although Sheehan's syndrome may present acutely with vascular collapse, it more commonly has a subacute presentation consisting of postpartum inability to lactate, amenorrhea, and symptoms of adrenal insufficiency. Sheehan's syndrome is now infrequent, owing to improvements in obstetric care.

Infiltrative diseases such as sarcoidosis, histiocytosis, and tuberculosis usually cause hypopituitarism by infiltrating the hypothalamus and stalk rather than the pituitary and are discussed in Chapter 235. In lymphocytic hypophysitis, there is massive infiltration of the pituitary by lymphocytes and plasma cells with destruction of the parenchyma and it is believed to have an autoimmune basis. The lesion that develops is usually large, and patients present with either symptoms or signs of hypopituitarism or those of a mass lesion (i.e., visual field defects and/or headaches). Some patients may have mild hyperprolactinemia and diabetes insipidus. Almost all cases have been reported in women, and most present during or after pregnancy. Because of the presentation as a mass lesion during pregnancy, such lesions may be confused with prolactinomas, but the mild PRL elevation points to a non-secretory lesion rather than a prolactinoma. MRI cannot differentiate pituitary adenoma from hypophysitis. Diagnosis is usually made by biopsy, but the lesion may be suspected clinically if the lesion presents during or just after pregnancy. Careful pituitary function testing is mandatory, because many of the patients in the reported cases went undiagnosed and died of adrenocortical insufficiency. Although the prognosis is not clear, a number of cases have resolved spontaneously. An entity with similar histologic findings involving the stalk and posterior pituitary, referred to as infundibuloneurohypophysitis, can cause diabetes insipidus. The causes and interrelationships between these entities remain unknown.

The pituitary may undergo damage because of iron deposition in

Table 237-4 ■ **TESTS OF PITUITARY INSUFFICIENCY**

HORMONE	TEST	INTERPRETATION
Growth hormone (GH)	*Insulin tolerance test:* Regular insulin (0.05–0.15 U/kg) is given IV and blood is drawn at −30, 0, 30, 45, 60, and 90 min for measurement of glucose and GH.	If hypoglycemia occurs (glucose < 40 mg/dL), GH should increase to >7 mg/L.
	L-Dopa test: 10 mg/kg PO with GH measurements at 0, 30, 60, and 120 min.	Normal response is GH > 7 mg/L
	L-Arginine test: 0.5 g/kg (max. 30 g) IV over 30 min with GH measurements at 0, 30, 60, and 120 min.	Normal response is GH > 7 mg/L
Prolactin (PRL)	*TRH test:* 200–500 μg IV with measurements of TSH and PRL at 0, 20, and 60 min.	Normal prolactin is >2 mg/L and >200% increase after TRH.
ACTH	*Insulin tolerance test:* Regular insulin (0.05–0.15 U/kg) is given IV and blood is drawn at −30, 0, 30, 45, 60, and 90 min for measurement of glucose and cortisol.	If hypoglycemia occurs (glucose < 40 mg/dL), cortisol should increase by >7 mg/dL or to >20 μg/dL.
	CRH test: 1 μg/kg ovine CRH IV at 8 AM with blood samples drawn at 0, 15, 30, 60, 90, 120 min for measurement of ACTH and cortisol.	In most normals, the basal ACTH increases twofold to fourfold and reaches a peak (20–100 pg/mL). ACTH responses may be delayed in cases of hypothalamic dysfunction. Cortisol levels usually reach 20–25 μg/dL.
	Metyrapone test: Metyrapone (30 mg/kg–max. 2 g) at midnight with measurements of plasma 11-deoxycortisol and cortisol at 8 AM. ACTH can also be measured. A 3-day test is also available. Basal cortisol should be > 5–6 μg/dL before test.	A normal response is 11-deoxycortisol > 7.5 μg/dL or ACTH > 75 pg/mL. Plasma cortisol should fall below 4 μg/dL to ensure an adequate response.
	ACTH stimulation test: ACTH 1-24 (Cosyntropin), 0.25 mg IM or IV. Cortisol and aldosterone are measured at 0, 30, and 60 min. A 3-day ACTH stimulation test consists of 0.25 mg ACTH 1-24 given IV over 8 hr each day.	A normal response is cortisol > 18 μg/dL and aldosterone response of >4 ng/dL above baseline. In suspected hypothalamic-pituitary deficiency, 3-day ACTH test should result in 17-hydroxysteroids of >25 mg/24 hr.
TSH	*Basal thyroid function tests:* free T₄, free T₃, TSH.	Low free thyroid hormone levels in the setting of TSH levels that are not appropriately increased.
	TRH test: 200–500 μg IV with measurements of TSH at 0, 20, and 60 min.	TSH should increase by more than 5 mU/L unless thyroid hormone levels are increased. Peak may be delayed if hypothyroidism due to hypothalamic disease.
LH, FSH	*Basal levels of LH, FSH, testosterone, estrogen*	Basal LH and FSH should be increased in postmenopausal women. Low testosterone levels in conjunction with low or low-normal LH and FSH are consistent with gonadotropin deficiency.
	GnRH test: GnRH (100 μg) IV with measurements of serum LH and FSH at 0, 30, and 60 min.	In most normal persons, LH should increase by 10 IU/L and FSH by 2 IU/L. Normal responses are variable, and repeated stimulation may be required.
	Clomiphene test: Clomiphene citrate (100 mg) is given orally for 5 days. Serum LH and FSH are measured on days 0, 5, 7, 10, and 13.	A 50% increase should occur in LH and FSH, usually by day 5.
Multiple hormones	*Combined anterior pituitary test:* GHRH (1 μg/kg), CRH (1 μg/kg), GnRH (100 μg), TRH (200 μg) are given sequentially IV. Blood samples are drawn at 30, 15, 30, 60, 90, and 120 min for measurements of GH, ACTH, LH, FSH, and TSH.	Combined or individual releasing hormone responses must be evaluated in the context of basal hormone values and may not be diagnostic (see text).

TRH = Thyrotropin-releasing hormone; TSH = thyroid-stimulating hormone; ACTH = adrenocorticotropic hormone; T₄ = thyroxines; T₃ = triiodothyronine; LH = luteinizing hormone; FSH = follicle-stimulating hormone; GnRH = gonadotropin-releasing hormone; GHRH = growth hormone–releasing hormone; CRH = corticotropin-releasing hormone.

Table 37–5 ■ HORMONAL REPLACEMENT THERAPY IN HYPOPITUITARISM*

PITUITARY AXIS	HORMONAL REPLACEMENTS
Growth hormone (GH)	In children, GH (0.05 mg/kg) SC daily. In adults, GH (0.025 mg/kg) SC daily.
Prolactin	None
ACTH–cortisol	Prednisone (5 mg PO qAM; 2.5 mg PO qPM) or hydrocortisone (20 mg PO qAM; 10 mg PO qPM). Dose adjusted on clinical basis.
Thyroid-stimulating hormone–thyroid	L-Thyroxine (0.075–0.15 mg) PO qd
Gonadotropins–gonads	Pulsatile GnRH (via pump) can be used for GnRH-deficient subjects, or FSH and LH (or hCG) can be used to induce ovulation in women. hCG alone, or FSH and LH, can be used to induce spermatogenesis in men.
	In men, testosterone enanthate (100–300 mg) IM q1–3 weeks or testosterone cyclopentylpropionate (100–300 mg) IM q1–3 weeks. Testosterone transdermal patches can also be used on the scrotum (4–6 mg qd) and other areas of the skin (5 mg qd).
	In women, conjugated estrogens (0.625–1.25 mg) or mestranol (35 mg) PO days 1–25 each month cycled with medroxyprogesterone acetate (5–10 mg) PO qd days 15–25 each month. Low-dose contraceptive pills may also be used. Estrogen-containing transdermal patches are also available.
Posterior pituitary	Desmopressin, 0.05–0.2 mL (5–20 μg) intranasally once or twice daily, or tablets (0.1–0.4 mg every 8–12 hr) or 0.5 mL (2 μg) SC.

*Replacement therapy is dictated by the types of hormone deficiencies and by the clinical circumstances. In each case, the recommended preparations and doses are representative, but need to be adjusted for individual patients. Other hormonal preparations are also available.

GnRH = Gonadotropin-releasing hormone; FSH = follicle-stimulating hormone; LH = luteinizing hormone; hCG = human chorionic gonadotropin.

patients with hemochromatosis and amyloid fibrils in patients with systemic amyloidosis. Functional, reversible hypopituitarism of varying degrees occurs in patients with severe systemic illness, severe psychosocial and emotional deprivation, and severe weight loss, and particularly in those with anorexia nervosa.

DIAGNOSIS AND TREATMENT. The diagnosis of hypopituitarism rests on the stimulation tests that are summarized in Table 237–4. The therapy for hypopituitarism depends on the nature and severity of the hormone deficiencies as well as on the desired clinical endpoints. The goal is to replace hormones in a physiologic manner, with efforts to avoid the consequences of overreplacement. In patients with acquired forms of hypopituitarism (e.g., pituitary tumors, radiation treatment), it is not uncommon to encounter a mixture of partial hormone deficiencies. It is generally prudent to provide hormone replacement if partial deficiency is suspected because patients may experience symptoms over a number of years before an unequivocal diagnosis of hormone deficiency is made. Examples of hormonal replacement paradigms are provided in Table 237–5. Even when conventional hormone replacement (adrenal, thyroid, gonadal) is carried out appropriately, there is an approximately twofold excess risk of death reported in patients with hypopituitarism. Although untreated GH deficiency has been hypothesized to be the cause of this excess risk, this has not been proven.

Bates AS, Van't Hoff W, Jones PJ, et al: The effect of hypopituitarism on life expectancy. J Clin Endocrinol Metab 81:1169–1172, 1996. *This paper is one of several that documents the excess risk of death in patients with hypopituitarism.*

MacCagnan P, Macedo CLD, Kayath MJ, et al: Conservative management of pituitary apoplexy: A prospective study. J Clin Endocrinol Metab 80:2190–2197, 1996. *An excellent description of the clinical manifestations of pituitary apoplexy with discussion about therapeutic concerns.*

Meling TR, Nylen ES: Growth hormone deficiency in adults: A review. Am J Med Sci 311:153–166, 1996. *A review of the clinical features of GH deficiency in adults.*

Pellegrini-Bouiller I, Belicar P, Barler A, et al: A new mutation of the gene encoding the transcription factor Pit-1 is responsible for combined pituitary hormone deficiency. J Clin Endocrinol Metab 81:2790–2796, 1996. *One of several reports of Pit-1 mutations in humans.*

Vance ML: Hypopituitarism. N Engl J Med 330:1651–1662, 1994. *A review of causes, diagnosis, and management of hypopituitarism.*

PITUITARY TUMORS

CLASSIFICATION. Pituitary tumors are classified according to the hormones that they produce and their size: microadenomas, less than 10 mm in diameter; macroadenomas, more than 10 mm in diameter; and macroadenomas with extrasellar extension. In general, the levels of hormones produced by the tumors parallel the size of the tumors, although exceptions occur. The approximate prevalence of the different types of pituitary adenomas, based on surgical data, is summarized in Table 237–6. Immunohistochemical studies, using antibodies specific for each of the major pituitary hormones, have been used to define tumor phenotype. Electron microscopy can provide additional ultrastructural information but is not employed routinely. Pituitary adenomas are very rarely malignant but can be locally invasive.

THEORIES OF PITUITARY TUMORIGENESIS. A long-standing controversy exists concerning the clonality of pituitary tumors. Monoclonal tumors arise from a single progenitor cell, presumably because of a somatic mutation to create an oncogene or to inactivate a tumor suppressor gene. Polyclonal tumors, on the other hand, reflect hyperplasia caused by exogenous stimulation of a group of cells by a growth factor or hypothalamic releasing hormone. By using recombinant DNA techniques to track X-chromosome inactivation as an index of cell lineage, it has been shown that the vast majority of pituitary tumors are monoclonal. This finding does not exclude a role for hormonal stimulation as a predisposing factor for somatic mutations, and the hormonal environment may also affect the rate of tumor growth (e.g., Nelson's syndrome).

Supporting the concept that somatic mutations lead to pituitary tumorigenesis, a subset (35–40%) of somatotroph adenomas have mutations in two different amino acids (Arg201 and Glu227) that result in activation of the Gsα-subunit. Either mutation prevents hydrolysis of guanosine triphosphate, causing the Gsα-subunit to stimulate adenylyl cyclase in a constitutive manner. The elevated

Table 237–6 ■ PREVALENCE OF DIFFERENT TYPES OF PITUITARY ADENOMAS

TYPE OF PITUITARY ADENOMA	DISORDER	HORMONE PRODUCED	PREVALENCE (%)*
Somatotroph	Acromegaly/gigantism	Growth hormone	10–15
Lactotroph (prolactinoma)	Hypogonadism, galactorrhea	Prolactin	25–40
Corticotroph	Cushing's disease	ACTH	10–15
Gonadotroph	Mass effects, hypopituitarism	FSH and LH	10–15
Thyrotroph	Hyperthyroidism	TSH	<3
Nonfunctioning/null cell	Mass effects, hypopituitarism	None	10–25

*The prevalence rates represent ranges described in several different large series. Mixed tumors (e.g., growth hormone and prolactin) and plurihormonal adenomas are not shown. Rates vary depending on methods used to establish the diagnosis. Prolactinomas were underestimated in most recent pathologic series because they are largely managed medically. Most glycoprotein hormone–producing pituitary tumors were classified as non-functioning adenomas until the application of immunohistochemical studies.

ACTH = Adrenocorticotropic hormone; FSH = follicle-stimulating hormone; LH = luteinizing hormone; TSH = thyroid-stimulating hormone.

intracellular cyclic adenosine monophosphate (AMP) levels lead to increased cell growth as well as GH production. Mutations in other oncogenes, such as *ras*, *Rb*, and *p53* are uncommon in pituitary tumors. Thus, the nature of the somatic defects in most pituitary tumors remains unknown.

Two types of inherited predispositions to pituitary tumors are recognized. Patients with McCune-Albright syndrome occasionally develop pituitary adenomas as well as characteristic abnormalities in other tissues, particularly the ovary, bone, and thyroid. Interestingly, the McCune-Albright syndrome is also caused by mutations in the Gsα-subunit. However, the somatic mutations in McCune-Albright occur early during development, rather than only in the pituitary gland, so that multiple tissues are affected. In multiple endocrine neoplasia type 1 (MEN-1), the predisposition to pituitary tumors is inherited in an autosomal dominant manner and occurs in conjunction with tumors of the parathyroid and pancreas. The MEN-1 gene has been localized on the long arm of chromosome 11 (11q13). Individuals with MEN-1 are thought to inherit one mutant allele with tumorigenesis occurring after a "second hit" mutates or deletes the normal MEN-1 gene. Deletions of portions of chromosome 11 have also been described in sporadic pituitary tumors. Deletions of other chromosomal regions (loss of heterozygosity) suggest that several different tumor suppressor genes may play a role in the development of pituitary tumors.

Burgess JR, Shepherd JJ, Parameswaran V, et al: Spectrum of pituitary disease in multiple endocrine neoplasia Type 1 (MEN 1): Clinical, biochemical, and radiological features of pituitary disease in a large MEN 1 kindred. J Clin Endocrinol Metab 81:2642–2646, 1996. *This paper outlines the types of pituitary lesions that may be seen in a large kindred with MEN 1.*

Clayton RN, Boggild M, Bates AS, et al: Tumour suppressor genes in the pathogenesis of human pituitary tumours. Horm Res 47:185–193, 1997. *The types of tumor suppressor gene mutations that may be etiologic in pituitary tumors are reviewed.*

MASS EFFECTS OF PITUITARY ADENOMAS. Many of the clinical manifestations of pituitary adenomas are related to the hypersecretion of hormones. However, the mass effects of the enlarging tumor can also lead to specific signs and symptoms. Particularly in the case of non-functioning tumors or in those that produce gonadotropins, the primary clinical manifestations are related to effects of the tumor on surrounding structures.

Headaches are common in patients with macroadenomas and appear to be caused by expansion of the diaphragma sella or by invasion of bone. Headaches may be retro-orbital or referred to the top of the skull, but the location is variable. The sudden onset of severe headache associated with nausea, vomiting, and altered consciousness can also be caused by infarction of a pituitary adenoma. In severe cases, pituitary apoplexy can occur, requiring glucocorticoid treatment and possible surgical decompression.

The effects of pituitary tumors on the visual fields are well explained by the relationship of the optic chiasm to the sella turcica. Expansion of macroadenomas into the suprasellar region exerts pressure on the optic chiasm, usually in the central region where nerves emanating from the inferior and medial part of the retina (superior and temporal visual fields) cross. Consequently, bitemporal hemianopsia is the most common visual field abnormality associated with pituitary adenomas. However, the exact pattern of visual field loss is variable and is affected by the location and flexibility of the chiasm as well as the direction and extent of tumor growth. Large tumors may grow asymmetrically and invade the cavernous sinus or surround an optic nerve, leading to other patterns of visual field changes or loss of visual acuity. The size and direction and degree of extrasellar extension are best evaluated with MRI with gadolinium infusion. If the tumor abuts the chiasm on MRI, then formal visual field testing should be performed by an ophthalmologist. Even long-standing visual field changes may be reversible by surgical or medical decompression.

The normal pituitary is often compressed into a thin rim of tissue by large pituitary adenomas. Hypopituitarism probably results more from compression of the hypothalamic-pituitary stalk than from direct replacement or pressure on the normal pituitary. GH deficiency and hypogonadotropic hypogonadism are particularly common. Slightly elevated PRL levels (generally < 100 ng/mL) occur in cases of stalk compression because of diminished inhibition by dopamine. It is important not to mistake such tumors for prolactinomas because they will not decrease in size in response to medical therapy with bromocriptine. Preoperative hypopituitarism caused by a large pituitary mass is reversible in up to half of patients after surgical decompression. Diabetes insipidus (vasopres-sin deficiency) is rarely caused by pituitary tumors and should raise the suspicion of a craniopharyngioma or other disorders that are likely to cause hypothalamic dysfunction.

Arafah BM, Nekl KE, Rold RS, et al: Dynamics of prolactin secretion in patients with hypopituitarism and pituitary macroadenomas. J Clin Endocrinol Metab 80:3507–3512, 1995. *This study of a large number of patients with macroadenomas illustrates how pituitary tumors can cause hypopituitarism and hyperprolactinemia by compression of the pituitary stalk.*

THERAPY FOR PITUITARY ADENOMAS. Surgical Treatment. Except for prolactinomas, surgery is the primary mode of therapy for most pituitary tumors that warrant intervention. Indications for surgery include reduction in hormone levels and decompression to relieve mass effects or to prevent further tumor expansion. Currently, the transsphenoidal route is used almost exclusively for decompression or extirpation of pituitary tumors. Because of substantially greater morbidity, subfrontal craniotomy is reserved for patients with tumors that require extensive exploration of the suprasellar region and surrounding structures, including invasion into the third ventricle. The transsphenoidal approach usually involves a sublabial incision allowing ready access to the sphenoidal sinus that leads to the floor of the sella. After entering the sella, the tumor is identified and resected in fragments under microscopy. Decompression of the sellar contents can allow tumor in the suprasellar region to drop into the surgical field to allow further resection. In experienced hands, transsphenoidal surgery is effective and complications are uncommon (<5% complication rate) but include cerebrospinal fluid leak, hemorrhage, optic nerve injury, hypopituitarism, and sinusitis. Transient diabetes insipidus occurs in about 5% of patients after surgery but rarely persists long-term. Mortality rates are less than 1%.

Surgical cure rates are largely a function of the size and location of the pituitary mass. When stringent hormonal criteria are used to assess surgical success rates, less than 30% of macroadenomas are cured by transsphenoidal surgery, although considerable improvements in hormone levels or mass effects can be achieved. On the other hand, hormone hypersecretion by microadenomas can be corrected completely in up to 80 to 90% of patients, although the cure rates vary considerably at different institutions.

Radiation Therapy. Irradiation has been used as a primary mode of treatment of pituitary adenomas and as adjunctive therapy after surgery or in combination with medical therapy. Radiation is typically administered over 5 weeks at a dose of 45 Gy using cobalt-60 or a linear accelerator. Proton-beam therapy has also been used and delivers very high doses of radiation within a localized region, but it is limited to intrasellar lesions and is not widely available. More recently, a radiation therapy technique referred to as "gamma knife" technique or radiosurgery has been employed for many patients with pituitary tumors. With this technique approximately the same dosage of radiation is administered as a single dose through over 100 ports using a computerized matching of irradiation to tumor geometry. Because response rates are slow (several years) and complete remission is rarely achieved for all of these types of irradiation, primary radiation therapy is generally reserved for patients who cannot or choose not to undergo surgery. Radiation therapy is more commonly used as adjunctive therapy after incomplete transsphenoidal resection. The decision regarding adjunctive radiotherapy involves a number of issues, including hormone levels, amount and location of residual tumor, rate of tumor growth, and degree of invasiveness. Because the time to recurrence for most non-functioning macroadenomas is 5 to 10 years and not all recur, it is often reasonable to follow patients with imaging techniques, reserving irradiation for those with evidence of recurrence. Complications of irradiation are dose related but can also be idiosyncratic. Partial or complete hypopituitarism occurs in 50 to 70% of patients and is primarily due to hypothalamic injury. Second tumors occur in the radiation field in about 2% of patients over a 20-year period. Less common complications include optic nerve damage, brain necrosis, vascular damage, and cognitive dysfunction.

Medical Therapy. The emergence of medical therapies for pituitary tumors has dramatically impacted patient management. Dopamine agonists, which include bromocriptine, pergolide, and cabergoline, have a primary role in the management of prolactinomas. They induce a rapid fall in PRL levels and, importantly, decrease tumor size. Dopamine agonists are also used in the management of acromegaly, although the GH responses and effects on tumor size are generally much less pronounced than in prolactinomas. Somatostatin analogues, such as octreotide, act to suppress the secretion of a number of hormones, including GH and TSH. Octreotide has been used to treat acromegaly and TSH-producing tumors. Long-acting GnRH agonists and antagonists have been studied in gonadotropin-producing tumors. Unlike the situation in normal individuals, the long-acting agonists do not cause desensitization and suppression of gonadotropins in most pituitary tumors. GnRH antagonists are more effective, reducing FSH in the majority of patients examined, but these agents have little effect on tumor growth. Medical therapy for Cushing's disease is primarily directed toward inhibition of steroid biosynthesis. These drugs include ketoconazole, metyrapone, aminoglutethimide, and mitotane. Because of substantial side effects and because patients with Cushing's disease tend to escape from the cortisol-suppressing effects of these drugs by producing more ACTH, medical therapy is used primarily as an adjunctive treatment or to reduce cortisol levels preoperatively.

Hansen LJ, Molitch ME: Is irradiation indicated postoperatively for patients with clinically nonfunctioning pituitary adenomas? Endocrinologist 8:71–78, 1998. *A review of the issues surrounding postoperative irradiation of pituitary adenomas.*

Jackson IMD, Noren G: Role of gamma knife in the management of pituitary tumors. Endocrinol Metab Clin North Am, 28:133–142, 1999. *A thorough review of the new technique of "gamma knife" radiotherapy in the treatment of pituitary adenomas.*

Laws EW Jr, Thapar K: Pituitary surgery. Endocrinol Metab Clin North Am 28:119–131, 1999. *The surgical treatment of pituitary adenomas is reviewed here.*

Tsang RW, Brierley JD, Panzarella T, et al: Role of radiation therapy in clinical hormonally-active pituitary adenomas. Radiother Oncol 41:45–53, 1996. *Data are presented on a large series of patients undergoing radiation therapy for various types of pituitary tumors.*

GROWTH HORMONE

The pituitary gland contains large amounts of stored GH (5–10 mg), a 191-amino acid, single-chain protein that contains two intramolecular disulfide bonds (see Table 237–1). The GH gene is located on chromosome 17 and is part of a five-member gene cluster. In addition to the normal GH gene, the gene cluster includes a GH variant gene that is expressed in the placenta, two placental lactogen (hPL) genes that are also referred to as chorionic somatomammotropin (hCS), and an hPL pseudogene that is not expressed. Highly repetitive sequences within the gene cluster appear to account for the propensity for recombination and deletions of the GH gene, causing one form of GH deficiency.

The predominant circulating form of GH is a 22-kd protein. However, a splicing variant creates a 20-kd form that constitutes 10 to 15% of circulating GH and is biologically active. GH also forms high-molecular-weight oligomers and is complexed in the circulation to two different binding proteins. The high-affinity binding protein has been identified as a circulating form of the extracellular domain of the GH receptor. In addition to greatly reducing the clearance of GH, this binding protein may also modulate GH action.

GH production is controlled by a complex interplay of hypothalamic stimulatory and inhibitory peptides, neurotransmitters, growth factors, sex steroids, and nutritional conditions. The most important regulators of GH are the hypothalamic hormones: GHRH, which is stimulatory, and somatostatin, which is inhibitory. GH increases the production of IGF-1 (also known as somatomedin C), which, in turn, inhibits GH production. GHRH acts by a G-protein coupled receptor that is structurally related to receptors in the vasoactive intestinal peptide (VIP), glucagon, and secretin family. GHRH stimulates cyclic AMP, activates phospholipase C, and causes an increase in intracellular calcium. GHRH causes somatotroph proliferation as well as increases GH biosynthesis and secretion. The Gsα-subunit, which is coupled to the GHRH receptor, is one of the targets for activating mutations that lead to somatotroph adenomas. Somatostatin binds to receptors that inhibit adenylate cyclase and thereby lower cyclic AMP levels. As a result, GHRH and somatostatin act antagonistically at the level of signal transduction. When both hormones are added concomitantly, somatostatin appears to act dominantly and GH secretion is inhibited.

IGF-1 also inhibits GH secretion, and it acts at both the pituitary and hypothalamic levels. In addition to reflecting GH action (primarily at the liver), serum IGF-1 is also sensitive to nutritional and metabolic changes. In starvation and anorexia nervosa, IGF-1 levels are low, resulting in increased levels of GH. In obesity, GH levels are low and GHRH responses are blunted. Stress, exercise, and a variety of neurogenic stimuli also increase GH secretion. Estrogens stimulate GH secretion, but their effects are less pronounced than for PRL.

Large bursts of GH secretion characteristically occur at night in association with slow-wave sleep. GH levels tend to be greatest during puberty and decline gradually in adulthood. The amplitude of GH pulses is greater in women than in men, likely reflecting the effects of estrogens. Spontaneous GH pulses can reach 50 ng/mL and are cleared rapidly with a half-life of about 20 minutes. Consequently, random GH levels can be very low or high. In addition, GH responses to GHRH are highly variable even within an individual, probably reflecting variations in endogenous somatostatin tone.

GH acts through a single transmembrane receptor that is structurally related to PRL and cytokine receptors (e.g., erythropoietin and colony-stimulating factors). This group of receptors associates with adaptor tyrosine kinases, one of which is referred to as Janus-associated kinase 2 (JAK2). After GH stimulation, JAK2 is phosphorylated and initiates a signaling cascade. The GH molecule has two distinguishable receptor binding domains that allow it to contact two separate receptor molecules to induce receptor dimerization. Mutations in the GH receptor cause GH resistance and severe growth retardation, a condition referred to as the GH insensitivity syndrome (Laron-type dwarfism). GH levels are elevated and IGF-1 levels are low, reflecting the inability of the mutant receptor to transduce the GH signal.

Many of the growth and metabolic effects of GH are transmitted indirectly through the actions of IGF-1. GH stimulates IGF-1 production in most tissues, where it then exerts autocrine or paracrine effects. Circulating IGF-1 is derived predominantly from the liver and is a useful marker of GH action because it has a longer half-life and integrates the effects of GH pulses. Although IGF-1 levels are used in the diagnosis of acromegaly and to assess the integrity of the GH axis, factors other than GH (e.g., malnutrition) can alter IGF-1 levels. IGF-1 acts through widely distributed receptors that are structurally related to insulin receptors. In addition to its growth-promoting and anabolic effects, IGF-1 also stimulates mitogenesis in many tissues. The bioactivity of IGF-1 is itself modulated by six IGF binding proteins (IGFBPs). These IGFBPs can inhibit or enhance IGF actions and may even function as independent cell regulators. IGFBP-3 is the major IGFBP in plasma; it is regulated by GH, and its levels generally parallel those of IGF-1 itself, both reflecting GH bioactivity.

GH has its major effects on linear growth but also influences a variety of metabolic pathways. Some of these effects are mediated by GH directly, whereas others are conferred by IGF-1. Although the relative roles of GH and IGF-1 are debated, their actions are cooperative in many cases. The effects of GH on linear growth appear to be mediated largely by IGF-1, which has been used to stimulate growth in patients with GH insensitivity syndrome. Linear growth in the fetus and neonate is not GH dependent, as illustrated by the fact that GH-deficient infants have normal birth lengths although intrauterine IGF-1 and IGF-2 may be important for fetal growth independent of GH. In contrast, normal postnatal linear growth requires GH, as illustrated by the clinical manifestations of GH deficiency. GH and IGF-1 act together to markedly accelerate linear growth, particularly at the time of puberty when sex steroids enhance GH and IGF-1 levels.

GH also induces lipolysis and stimulates anabolic activity, including amino acid uptake and protein synthesis. As a result, it reduces body fat, increases lean body mass, and leads to positive nitrogen balance. These properties of GH are most strikingly seen in GH-deficient children who have undergone replacement. GH opposes many of the actions of insulin and can be considered diabetogenic. In diabetic individuals, nocturnal GH secretion accounts in large part for the dawn phenomenon, in which there is a decrease in glucose utilization, causing a tendency toward hyperglycemia.

GROWTH HORMONE DEFICIENCY. Causes of GH deficiency include hypothalamic/pituitary disorders, GHRH receptor mutations, GH gene mutations, combined pituitary hormone deficiencies, GH receptor mutations, IGF-1 receptor mutations, radiation, and psychosocial deprivation (see also Chapter 235). The clinical manifestations of GH deficiency depend on the time of onset and the severity of hormone deficiency. Children with complete GH deficiency have slow linear growth rates (~ 3 cm/yr), and they rapidly fall below normal on standardized growth charts. GH-deficient children have normal skeletal proportions, and many have a pudgy, youthful appearance because of decreased lipolysis. Particularly in the setting of cortisol deficiency, there is a predisposition to hypoglycemia.

Basal GH does not provide a reliable measure of GH reserve, whereas low IGF-1 and low IGFBP-3 levels are consistent with GH deficiency. GH deficiency is most frequently assessed using insulin-induced hypoglycemia, which activates central nervous system pathways leading to stimulation of both GH and ACTH secretion (see Table 237–4). The insulin tolerance test requires careful monitoring for symptoms of severe hypoglycemia, such as confusion or depressed consciousness. This test should be avoided in patients with seizure disorders or coronary artery disease. Insulin doses (0.1–0.15 U/kg) may need to be decreased if glucocorticoid deficiency is suspected or increased in conditions of insulin resistance (e.g., obesity). Alternatives to the insulin tolerance test for evaluation of GH include stimulation by L-dopa or arginine. Stimulation tests with GHRH have not been well standardized and appear to show substantial variation even within an individual, perhaps because of changing somatostatin tone.

In children with well-documented GH deficiency, GH replacement is effective and it is essential to increase final adult height. In a typical regimen, recombinant GH (0.05 mg/kg) is given daily as subcutaneous injections. The efficacy of GH treatment depends on when it is initiated as well as replacement of other hormone deficiencies, if they co-exist. In the setting of multiple hormone deficiencies, replacement of thyroid hormone and cortisol is necessary for effective GH action. On the other hand, sex steroids (estrogen in particular) lead to epiphyseal closure and limit linear growth. Consequently, GH is more effective before puberty; if exogenous sex steroids are given, low doses should be used. GH has also been shown to increase the final height of girls with Turner's syndrome (chromosomal XO state), and this use has been approved by the U.S. Food and Drug Administration (FDA).

Although the potential role of GH replacement in adults is debated, it has been approved by the FDA for the treatment of adults with organic causes of GH deficiency. Short-term studies show that it can increase lean body mass, decrease fat mass, and improve the sense of well-being in adults with documented GH deficiency, but safety data for long-term GH administration are meager and data documenting clinically significant increased muscle strength and endurance are lacking. Whether GH treatment in adults will affect the increased mortality associated with hypopituitarism remains to be seen. Adverse effects occur at lower doses in adults compared with children, and a dose of 0.025 mg/kg/day has been recommended. Although GH therapy has also been approved by the FDA for the treatment of wasting due to the acquired immunodeficiency syndrome and it has been used short term to reduce acute catabolism, such as burns and sepsis, long-term clinical benefits have not yet been shown conclusively and potential adverse effects exist so that such use should be considered experimental.

GROWTH HORMONE EXCESS: ACROMEGALY AND GIGANTISM. Etiology and Pathogenesis. GH-producing pituitary tumors involve the neoplastic proliferation of somatotroph cells and account for 10 to 15% of pituitary tumors (see Table 237–6). GH-producing tumors are frequently mixed tumors that secrete more than one hormone. PRL is produced in about 40% of somatotroph adenomas, and some patients may present because of symptoms due to the hyperprolactinemia (i.e., amenorrhea and/or galactorrhea). A subset of these tumors are categorized morphologically as mammosomatotroph adenomas. GH-producing tumors can also co-secrete glycoprotein hormones, most frequently the common α-subunit (10–30%) or, rarely, TSH.

Considerable progress has been made concerning the cause of GH-producing pituitary tumors. Ectopic production of GHRH (usually carcinoid or pancreatic islets) is a well-documented but rare (<1%) cause of acromegaly that can result in somatotroph hyperplasia. Gsα-subunit mutations occur in 35 to 40% of somatotroph adenomas. Molecular defects in the remaining 60 to 65% of somatotroph adenomas need to be identified.

Clinical Features. GH-secreting tumors cause acromegaly in adults and gigantism in children in whom GH excess occurs before epiph-

yseal closure. The annual incidence of acromegaly has been estimated at about 3 per million. It affects men and women with equal frequency and is most often recognized when patients are in their 30s or 40s, usually after a decade of GH excess. The clinical features of acromegaly are summarized in Table 237–7. The most striking features of acromegaly usually involve the face, hands, and feet. The diagnosis is often suspected because of changes in facial appearance that include enlargement of the lower jaw (prognathism), the nose and lips, and sinuses (causing frontal bossing) (Fig. 237–1). Oral cavity changes including malocclusion, increased spacing between the teeth, and enlargement of the tongue may lead to recognition of the disorder by dentists. A hollow, resonant voice is caused by changes in the vocal cords and the soft tissues of the hypopharynx. Sleep apnea may occur in patients with soft tissue obstruction of the pharynx but may also occur because of a central disorder. Few acromegalic patients wear rings because they have long since outgrown them, and they usually have a history of progressive increase in shoe size and width. In addition to bony enlargement, there is a marked increase in the soft tissue of the hands and feet. A moist, doughy, enveloping handshake is characteristic of acromegaly. Heel pad thickness (which can be assessed radiographically) correlates well with IGF-1 levels and other clinical features of the disease. Arthritis (hands, feet, hips, knees) is common (75%) and is caused by cartilage and synovial overgrowth. Some degree of carpal tunnel syndrome is seen in about half of patients. Skin changes include increased skinfolds, particularly over the brow and forehead. The skin is usually oily, owing to increased sebaceous activity and sweating. Skin tags are common, and their presence correlates with the presence of colonic polyps. Galactorrhea may be seen in women, and reproductive dysfunction occurs in both women and men when PRL levels are elevated. Headaches, visual field defects, and other neurologic symptoms depend on the location and extent of tumor growth.

Acromegaly causes as much as a twofold to threefold increase in mortality. Most of the increased mortality can be attributed to cardiovascular and cerebrovascular diseases and may be related in part to the increased prevalence of hypertension (25–35%) and diabetes mellitus (10–25%) in acromegaly. There is evidence for cardiac hypertrophy in the majority of acromegalics, and symptomatic heart disease, consisting of coronary ischemia and/or congestive heart failure, occurs in 15 to 20% of patients. Sleep apnea may predispose patients to cardiac dysrhythmias. There is an increased risk of premalignant polyps and colon cancer in acromegaly, and screening with colonoscopy is generally recommended in men, particularly those older than the age of 50 and with skin tags. The disfigurement, metabolic complications, and increased mortality associated with acromegaly emphasize the importance of early diagnosis and implementation of appropriate therapy to lower the GH levels into the normal range.

Diagnosis. Because GH is secreted in a pulsatile manner, and because the amplitude of normal GH pulses can be large (>50 ng/mL), random GH levels are not very useful in making the diagnosis of acromegaly. IGF-1 levels provide an integrated index of GH production and provide a better screening test for acromegaly. IGF-

Table 237–7 ■ CLINICAL FEATURES OF ACROMEGALY

CLINICAL FEATURES	NO. OF SUBJECTS*	YEARS OR FREQUENCY*
Age at diagnosis	885	42 yr
Delay to diagnosis	680	8.7 yr
Gender (% male)	1331	48%
Acral/facial changes	595	98%
Oligo/amenorrhea (females)	366	72%
Hyperhidrosis	751	64%
Headaches	825	55%
Paresthesias/carpal tunnel	725	40%
Impotence (males)	355	36%
Hypertension	630	28%
Goiter	705	21%
Visual field defects	993	19%

*From Molitch ME: Clinical manifestations of acromegaly. Endocrinol Metab Clin North Am 21:597, 1992.

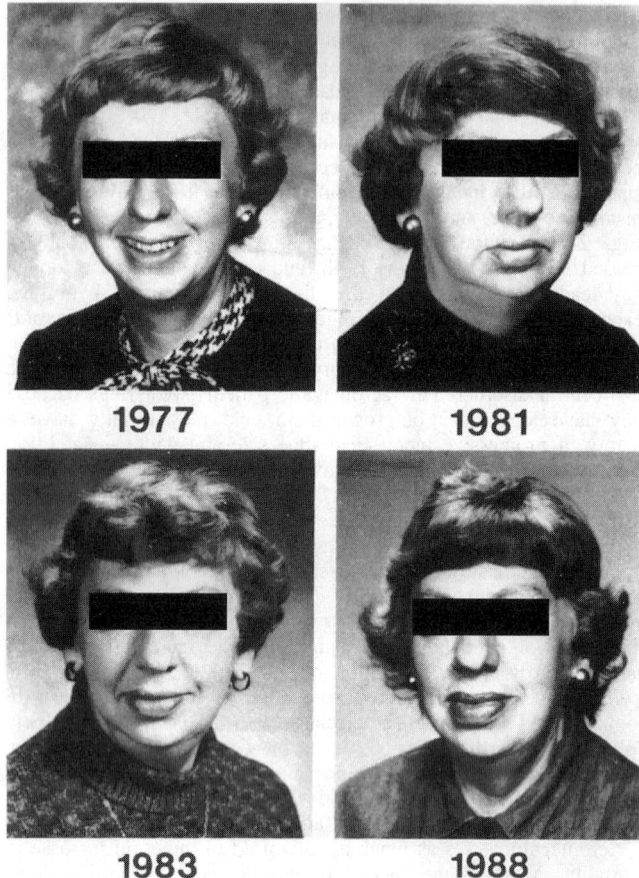

FIGURE 237–1 ■ Clinical features of acromegaly. Serial photographs of a 64-year-old woman with acromegaly. Over an 11-year period there is a progressive coarsening of facial features, including enlargement of the nose and lips and development of prognathism. She also experienced hypertension, arthropathy, and enlargement of the hands (not shown). (From Molitch ME: Clinical manifestations of acromegaly. Endocrinol Metab Clin North Am 21:597–614, 1992.)

1 levels are normally elevated during puberty and pregnancy and decrease with age so that normal ranges must be age adjusted. IGF-1 levels correlate well with 24-hour GH production rates and with disease activity. The most reliable test for acromegaly is the glucose tolerance test (Table 237–8). In acromegaly, increased glucose levels fail to suppress GH levels to below 2 ng/mL and may even cause a paradoxical increase in GH. More than half of patients with acromegaly exhibit a paradoxical stimulation of GH in response to TRH. Co-secretion of PRL should be evaluated, and the common α-subunit of the glycoprotein hormones may provide an additional marker of tumor activity. After the diagnosis of acromegaly is made, radiologic studies, preferably using MRI, should be used to evaluate the extent of tumor growth. Unlike in Cushing's disease and prolactinomas, the majority of patients with acromegaly have macroadenomas. In the absence of an apparent pituitary tumor, the possibility of ectopic GHRH secretion causing somatotroph cell hyperplasia should be considered.

Therapy. The goals of therapy in acromegaly are to reverse or prevent tumor mass effects and to reduce the long-term morbidity and mortality that result from excess GH production. Correction of the disorder prevents further physical disfigurement and can result in substantial resolution of soft tissue changes and improvements in metabolic derangements. Although reductions in GH levels are associated with improvements in symptoms, the ultimate goal is to achieve normal GH and IGF-1 levels and to prevent tumor recurrence without incurring hypopituitarism.

Transsphenoidal surgery results in GH levels below 5 ng/mL in about 60% of patients with microadenomas. Not all of these patients are cured of their tumor when assessed by more stringent criteria, such as GH suppression below 2 ng/mL during an oral glucose tolerance test or a normal IGF-1 level. Patients with mac-

roadenomas are less often cured by surgery (<30%) but usually have reductions in GH levels.

Medical therapies for acromegaly include dopamine agonists, such as bromocriptine, and somatostatin analogues, such as octreotide. Responsiveness to both of these agents depends on the presence and density of receptors on tumor cells. Although bromocriptine can reduce GH and IGF-1 levels in many patients, normal levels are achieved in only 10 to 20% and high doses (up to 30 mg/day) may be needed. Octreotide reduces GH and IGF-1 levels in almost all patients, with normal levels of IGF-1 being achieved in over half. Octreotide reduces tumor size modestly in about half. Octreotide is useful as adjunctive therapy in patients who are not cured by surgery and/or radiation. Although octreotide has a much longer half-life than somatostatin, it must be given in doses of 100 to 200 μg, every 6 to 8 hours by subcutaneous injection to maintain GH suppression; some patients benefit from continuous subcutaneous infusion using a pump. Longer-acting preparations of octreotide and other somatostatin analogues that can be given by intramuscular injection every 2 to 4 weeks have now become available. Side effects of octreotide include diarrhea and increased risk of cholelithiasis, although cholecystitis and need for cholecystectomy are rare. Because of ease of use and lower cost, bromocriptine is usually tried before octreotide but, because of relative efficacies, most patients end up on octreotide as adjunctive therapy. In addition, some patients experience additive beneficial effects from combining the two medications while keeping the dose of each drug low enough to avoid adverse effects.

Radiation is not recommended as primary therapy for acromegaly because of the long length of time (5–10 years) required for reductions in GH levels and the high incidence of hypopituitarism and other complications discussed earlier. Adjunctive radiation therapy may be required for patients with macroadenomas when GH levels or mass effects persist after transsphenoidal surgery and medical therapy. Recent data suggest that gamma knife radiotherapy may be the most efficacious form of radiotherapy for acromegaly.

Carroll PV, Christ ER, Bengtsson BÅ, et al: Growth hormone deficiency in adulthood and the effects of growth hormone replacement: A review. J Clin Endocrinol Metab 83:382–395, 1998. *A comprehensive review of the benefits and risk of GH treatment in adults.*

Hoffman DM, O'Sullivan AJ, Baxter RC, Ho KK: Diagnosis of growth-hormone deficiency in adults. Lancet 343:1064–1068, 1994. *Data from a large series of patients documenting the best ways of diagnosing GH deficiency in adults.*

Newman CB, Melmed S, Snyder PJ, et al: Safety and efficacy of long-term octreotide therapy of acromegaly: Results of a multicenter trial in 103 patients. J Clin Endocrinol Metab 80:2768–2775, 1996. *Results from the largest study of octreotide use in acromegaly, documenting the benefits and risks of such use.*

PROLACTIN

PRL and GH appear to be derived from a common ancestral gene, accounting for the similarities in their present-day structures and some overlap in their functional properties. The PRL gene is located on chromosome 6 and encodes a 198-amino acid protein (23 kd) that is produced in the lactotroph cells. PRL contains three intramolecular disulfide bonds, and high molecular variants are reported that may represent dimers or protein aggregates. Although the larger molecular weight forms of PRL react in radioimmunoassays, they have diminished biologic potency. Estrogen stimulates lactotroph proliferation, and their number is consequently greater in females than in males, and during pregnancy (approximately 70% of pituitary cells).

PRL secretion is controlled by tonic inhibition by dopamine, which acts through D_2-type receptors on lactotrophs. PRL biosynthesis and secretion are stimulated by the hypothalamic peptides TRH and VIP. Hypothyroidism causes increased TRH output and increased sensitivity of the lactotrophs to TRH and can result in hyperprolactinemia. VIP, which acts through receptors that increase cyclic AMP, may be responsible, along with a decrease in dopamine, for PRL increases associated with suckling. VIP is also found in the pituitary, where it may act as an autocrine or paracrine regulator of PRL secretion. On balance, dopamine inhibition is the dominant influence for PRL secretion so that PRL is the one pituitary hormone that increases after pituitary stalk section. A variety of pharmacologic agents can stimulate PRL secretion, in many cases by impairing dopamine secretion or action (see Table 237–2).

PRL secretion is pulsatile and increases with sleep, stress, chest

Table 237–8 ■ SELECTED TESTS OF EXCESS PITUITARY FUNCTION

HORMONE	TEST	INTERPRETATION
Growth hormone (GH)	*Basal IGF-1*	Elevated IGF-1 levels are consistent with acromegaly when interpreted in the context of age and nutritional status.
	Oral glucose suppression test: After 75-g glucose load, GH is measured at -30, 0, 30, 60, 90, 120 min.	GH should be suppressed to <2 μg/L in normals. GH may paradoxically increase in acromegaly.
	TRH test: TRH (200 μg) is given IV with serum GH measurements at 0, 20, 60 min.	GH is not stimulated by TRH in most normals. A GH increase of 10 μg/L or greater than 50% of baseline is consistent with acromegaly, but it can also occur in other disorders. The test is most useful for evaluating surgical cure.
Prolactin	*Basal prolactin levels*	Elevated prolactin (>200 μg/L) is consistent with a prolactinoma. When prolactin levels are between 20–200 μg/L, other causes of hyperprolactinemia should be considered.
ACTH	*Measurement of 24-hr urine free cortisol*	Elevated urine free cortisol level is suggestive of Cushing's syndrome, but it has several other causes as well.
	Overnight dexamethasone suppression test: Dexamethasone (1 mg) PO at midnight followed by 8 AM plasma cortisol.	In normal persons AM cortisol should be suppressed to <5 μg/dL. Normal dexamethasone suppression excludes Cushing's syndrome. Several other disorders can cause failure to suppress normally.
	Low-dose dexamethasone suppression test: Dexamethasone (0.5 mg) q6h for eight doses with basal and end of treatment measurements that may include 24-hr urine collections for free cortisol or 17-hydroxysteroids and AM plasma cortisol and ACTH.	17-Hydroxysteroids should be suppressed to <4 mg/24 hr; urine free cortisol should be <20 μg/24 hr; serum cortisol should be suppressed to <6 μg/dL. Failure to suppress cortisol production is consistent with the diagnosis of Cushing's syndrome.
	High-dose dexamethasone suppression test. Dexamethasone (2 mg) q6h for eight doses with basal and end of treatment measurements that may include 24-hr urine collections for free cortisol or 17-hydroxysteroids and AM plasma cortisol and ACTH.	The high dose test is intended to distinguish Cushing's disease (pituitary adenoma), ectopic ACTH production, and adrenal adenoma. The 50% suppression of 17-hydroxy steroids or 90% suppression of urine free cortisol production is suggestive of Cushing's disease. Less than 50% suppression suggests ectopic ACTH or adrenal adenoma. Low ACTH levels are consistent with adrenal adenoma.
	CRH test: Ovine CRH (1 μg/kg) is administered IV and ACTH and cortisol are drawn at -15, 0, 15, 30, 60, 90, and 120 min.	In Cushing's disease, there is usually a 50% increase in ACTH and a 20% increase in cortisol. Adrenal adenoma is associated with suppressed ACTH. Ectopic ACTH is associated with high basal ACTH and cortisol levels that are not affected by CRH.
	Petrosal sinus ACTH sampling: The inferior petrosal sinus is catheterized, ideally bilaterally, and plasma ACTH is compared with simultaneous peripheral samples. The sampling can be done in conjunction with CRH stimulation.	In Cushing's disease, the ratio of ACTH in the petrosal sinus/periphery is at least 2. In ectopic ACTH, the ratio of petrosal sinus/peripheral level is <1.5.
TSH	*Basal thyroid function tests*	An inappropriate normal or elevated TSH in the setting of increased free thyroid hormone levels is consistent with a TSH-producing tumor or other causes of inappropriate TSH secretion.
	Free α-subunit level	Elevated free α-subunit levels associated with inappropriately elevated TSH are suggestive of a TSH-producing tumor.
FSH, LH	*Basal FSH, LH, testosterone*	Increased LH and testosterone levels in males are consistent with LH-secreting tumors. Elevated FSH and low-normal testosterone is suggestive of an FSH-producing tumor if primary gonadal failure is not present. In females, assessment of excess hormone secretion is difficult because of changes during the menstrual cycle and at menopause.
	TRH test: TRH (200 μg) is given IV with measurements of serum FSH, LH, FSHβ, and LHβ subunits at 0, 20, 60 min.	Stimulation of LH, FSH, or their free β-subunits is suggestive of a gonadotropin-producing adenoma.

IGF = Insulin-like growth factor; TRH = thyrotropin-releasing hormone; ACTH = adrenocorticotropic hormone; CRH = corticotropin-releasing hormone; TSH = thyroid-stimulating hormone; FSH = follicle-stimulating hormone; LH = luteinizing hormone.

wall stimulation, and pregnancy. PRL levels are usually less than 15 to 20 ng/mL in women and 10 to 15 ng/mL in men. The primary function of PRL is to induce and sustain lactation. However, PRL binds to specific receptors that are located in several tissues, including breast, gonads, lymphoid cells, and liver. There are several different forms of PRL receptors, which, like the GH receptor, are members of a cytokine family of receptors. During pregnancy, PRL levels increase, and, in conjunction with other hormones (estrogens, progesterone, thyroid hormone, cortisol, and insulin) breast epithelium is stimulated to proliferate and milk synthesis is induced. High levels of estrogen and progesterone inhibit lactation during pregnancy. The rapid decline in these steroids in the postpartum period permits lactation to occur. Neural pathways leading to the secretion of oxytocin provide the "let-down" reflex that induces lactation in response to suckling. Early in the postpartum period, PRL secretion is stimulated by suckling, but this response becomes damped with time as the frequency of suckling episodes decreases. PRL also suppress gonadotropins, probably by a direct action on GnRH-secreting neurons. As a result, breast-feeding can suppress ovulation. The role of PRL in other tissues is not well understood. High levels of PRL are present in amniotic fluid and it is produced in the decidual layer of the placenta.

PROLACTIN DEFICIENCY. PRL deficiency is rare and occurs primarily in the setting of combined hormone deficiencies. PRL levels at or below the limits of detection of radioimmunoassays and an absent rise of PRL after TRH stimulation are consistent with the diagnosis. The only recognized consequence of PRL deficiency is the absence of postpartum lactation. No effects on breast development or other tissues have been described in PRL deficiency.

HYPERPROLACTINEMIA. Etiology and Pathogenesis. Hyperprolactinemia can occur as a consequence of pharmacologic alterations in the pathways that control PRL secretion or of physiologic or metabolic effects on PRL production and clearance or as a neoplastic condition (see Table 237–2). Prolactinomas are neoplastic growths of lactotroph cells and are the most common type of pituitary adenoma (25 to 40%). Theories concerning the causes of prolactinomas have centered around hormonal stimuli that influence lactotroph growth and PRL secretion. Estrogen is a potent stimulus for lactotroph proliferation. In rats, chronic estrogen exposure induces lactotroph hyperplasia and prolactinomas, but there is no clear association between estrogens (e.g., oral contraceptive use) and the incidence of prolactinomas in humans. It is possible that estrogen may rarely stimulate the growth of pre-existing prolactinomas and the very high estrogen levels present during pregnancy may cause about 15% of large prolactinomas to increase in size during pregnancy. Diminished dopamine tone results in increased PRL but has not been shown to cause prolactinomas. PRL secretory dynamics are generally restored to normal on resection of prolactinomas, suggesting that an underlying hypothalamic abnormality is not present. Analyses of tumor DNA from a relatively small number of prolactinomas are consistent with a monoclonal origin, but molecular defects in prolactinomas have not been readily identified. Mutations in *ras* and other oncogenes have been found in sporadic case reports but are not found in most prolactinomas.

Microprolactinomas constitute the great majority of tumors in premenopausal women. In contrast, macroadenomas are more commonly seen in men and postmenopausal women. The predominance of smaller tumors in premenopausal women may be accounted for by a bias of ascertainment because elevated PRL levels in this group lead to clinical manifestations (amenorrhea, galactorrhea, or infertility). It is likely that subclinical prolactinomas exist in men and many older women, because about 10% of individuals have PRL-positive microadenomas in autopsy series.

Clinical Features. Hyperprolactinemia causes galactorrhea and oligo/amenorrhea in premenopausal women. Estrogen facilitates PRL-induced galactorrhea, explaining why it is less common in postmenopausal women or in women with prolonged hypogonadism. Amenorrhea is primarily a consequence of PRL suppression of GnRH, although PRL may also have inhibitory effects at the level of the pituitary and the gonad. Amenorrhea is associated with infertility, and PRL levels should be a routine part of the hormonal evaluation of infertility. Estrogen deficiency can cause decreased libido, vaginal dryness, and dyspareunia. Long-standing estrogen deficiency also leads to osteopenia in some women. A subset of patients have hirsutism and can exhibit elevations of adrenal androgens. Oral contraceptives may mask PRL-induced oligo/amenorrhea that becomes apparent on their discontinuation. In postmenopausal women, prolactinomas are often identified because of mass effects rather than because of their hormonal effects.

In men, hyperprolactinemia causes hypogonadism with suppressed LH and FSH levels and low testosterone levels. Hypogonadism causes diminished libido, impotence, infertility, and rarely gynecomastia or galactorrhea. Diminished libido may also reflect suppression of GnRH because testosterone replacement is not as effective as suppression of hyperprolactinemia. Hyperprolactinemia is found in up to 5% of men being evaluated for sexual dysfunction.

Diagnosis. There are four primary categories of causes of hyperprolactinemia that must be distinguished if the correct therapy is to be instituted: (1) physiologic/metabolic hyperprolactinemia; (2) pharmacologic hyperprolactinemia; (3) hypothalamic or pituitary stalk compression; and (4) prolactinoma (see Table 237–2). With the exception of pregnancy and renal failure, physiologic causes of increased PRL result in minor elevations in PRL (usually less than 50 ng/mL), which may not be present on repeat testing. Primary hypothyroidism should be excluded as a cause of mild hyperprolactinemia. A careful drug history should be obtained in all patients with hyperprolactinemia because of the large number of agents that can stimulate PRL secretion. Psychotropic medications, in particular, can increase PRL either by reducing dopamine production or by blocking its action. In most cases, the degree of hyperprolactinemia caused by drugs is less than 100 ng/mL. A variety of suprasellar and parasellar mass lesions cause hyperprolactinemia (generally between 20–100 ng/mL) because of compression of the hypothalamus or pituitary stalk. Unless there is very good evidence for physiologic or drug-induced hyperprolactinemia, even patients with mild hyperprolactinemia should be evaluated with CT or MRI to distinguish among idiopathic hyperprolactinemia, microprolactinomas, and other large mass lesions that cause stalk compression, resulting in decreased dopamine reaching the lactotrophs. When no pituitary lesions are seen by radiographic studies and physiologic and pharmacologic causes of hyperprolactinemia cannot be identified, the diagnosis of idiopathic hyperprolactinemia is made. Idiopathic hyperprolactinemia may represent microprolactinomas too

small to be detected accurately by current imaging techniques or altered hypothalamic regulation of PRL secretion. Whether such patients should be treated depends on the clinical effects of hyperprolactinemia. When followed for several years, few of these patients develop large tumors, only 10 to 15% show MRI evidence of microadenomas, and in one third of cases the hyperprolactinemia resolves.

Therapy. The natural history of prolactinomas has been evaluated in several series. Although large prolactinomas clearly must evolve from smaller lesions, it is uncommon (approximately 7%) for microprolactinomas to progress to macroadenomas. When patients with microadenomas are observed over 3 to 5 years but not treated, PRL levels decrease in 20 to 30% and increase in less than 10% of patients. Decreased PRL may occur because of spontaneous tumor infarction. Because of the slow rate of growth, it is reasonable to monitor patients with microprolactinomas without treatment unless the hyperprolactinemia is causing symptoms that warrant therapy.

When hyperprolactinemia causes hypogonadism, osteopenia, or infertility, a dopamine agonist such as bromocriptine or cabergoline is the therapy of choice. Dopamine agonists normalize PRL levels and correct amenorrhea-galactorrhea in 80 to 90% of patients. Bromocriptine is usually started as a half tablet (1.25 mg) given at bedtime with a snack to avoid side effects (nausea, dizziness, somnolence, and nasal stuffiness). After adaptation to the drug, the dose can be increased gradually over several weeks. A typical final dose is 2.5 mg, two or three times a day with meals, but up to 20 mg/day may be required. The lowest effective dose should be used after achieving adequate suppression of PRL levels. Dopamine agonists may cause a considerable reduction in tumor size in patients with macroprolactinomas, about 40% having a more than 50% reduction in tumor size, about 25% having a 25 to 50% reduction in tumor size, and the remainder having little or no response. Visual field defects are a very sensitive index of tumor size, and improvements can be seen in about 90% of patients. Thus, it is reasonable to use bromocriptine as first-line therapy even in patients with visual field defects as long as visual acuity is not threatened by rapid progression or recent tumor hemorrhage. Ten to 20 per cent of patients can maintain normal PRL levels after stopping treatment, and 70 to 80% with marked tumor size reduction may not experience tumor re-expansion with stopping therapy. In patients with very large tumors who have excellent tumor size reduction, stopping therapy must be done very cautiously, if at all. Cabergoline is a new dopamine agonist that is even more effective and has less adverse side effects than bromocriptine and has the additional advantage in only having to be taken once or twice weekly. In some cases, prolactinomas appear to be resistant to a dopamine agonist, but it is important to ensure compliance and to be certain that the underlying lesion is a prolactinoma and not some other cause of hyperprolactinemia. In these cases, an alternative dopamine agonist may be successful. Alternatively, transsphenoidal surgery may be used. Although initial remission rates (70 to 80%) for transsphenoidal surgery of microprolactinomas are good, there is long-term recurrence in about 20% of patients. For macroprolactinomas, the initial remission rates are closer to 30%, with a similar recurrence rate. Radiation therapy is reserved for those patients with macroadenomas not responding to either medical or surgical treatment.

Bromocriptine therapy for infertility, or when there is a possibility of pregnancy, deserves special consideration. Bromocriptine can induce ovulation in 80 to 90% of patients with hyperprolactinemia. Although bromocriptine has not been associated with congenital malformations or complications during pregnancy, most physicians and patients prefer to avoid its use during pregnancy if possible. A form of barrier contraception is usually recommended until two to three regular menstrual cycles have occurred. Subsequently, pregnancy can be confirmed if a menstrual period is missed, allowing discontinuation of bromocriptine with exposure of the fetus to the drug for only 3 to 5 weeks. At present, the safety data for pregnancy outcome are much more limited for cabergoline; therefore, bromocriptine is the preferred drug when fertility is desired. Less than 2% of patients with microadenomas, but 15% of patients with macroadenomas develop symptoms of tumor enlargement (headaches, visual field defects) during pregnancy. If symptoms develop, an MRI and formal visual field testing should be performed. If there is evidence of visual field compromise or tumor growth, bromocriptine therapy should be restarted to shrink the tumor. PRL levels are not very useful because they are normally increased in pregnancy and PRL production by an enlarging tumor may not increase substantially. Because problems of tumor growth occur most often in patients with macroadenomas, consideration should be given to the option of transsphenoidal decompression before pregnancy in women with large tumors, as long as fertility can be preserved.

Colao A, DeSarno A, Landi ML, et al: Long-term and low-dose treatment with cabergoline induces macroprolactinoma shrinkage. J Clin Endocrinol Metab 82: 3574–3579, 1997. *A recent study documenting the efficacy of cabergoline in the shrinkage of PRL-secreting macroadenomas.*

Jeffcoate WJ, Pound N, Sturrock NDC, Lambourne J: Long-term follow-up of patients with hyperprolactinaemia. Clin Endocrinol 45:299–303, 1996. *Presented here are long-term follow-up studies of patients treated with dopamine agonists as well as those not receiving any treatment.*

Molitch ME: Diagnosis and treatment of prolactinomas. Adv Intern Med 44:117, 1999. *A concise review of the diagnosis and treatment of prolactinomas.*

Molitch ME, Thorner MO, Wilson C: Therapeutic controversy: Management of prolactinomas. J Clin Endocrinol Metab 82:996–1000, 1997. *A discussion of the advantages and disadvantages of medical versus surgical treatment for prolactinomas.*

ACTH

STRUCTURE. ACTH is a 39-amino acid peptide that is derived from a precursor polypeptide POMC (241 amino acids), which encodes several peptides, including an amino-terminal peptide, joining peptide, ACTH, and β-lipotropin (β-LPH) (see also Chapter 235). The functional roles of the POMC-encoded peptides other than ACTH have not been fully defined. β-LPH, in addition to ACTH, may stimulate melanocytes and contribute to hyperpigmentation in conditions of POMC stimulation. β-LPH can be processed further to yield γ-lipotropin and β-endorphin. The biologically active portion of ACTH resides within the first 18 of its 39 amino acids. However, because a synthetic peptide (cosyntropin) that includes the first 24 amino acids has a longer half-life, it is used clinically to assess adrenocortical function. The half-life of ACTH is relatively short (<10 minutes), and pulses of ACTH secretion are discrete. Levels of precursor peptides, such as β-LPH, do not always parallel those of ACTH because of their slower clearance rates. β-LPH, but not ACTH, is also elevated in renal failure. In cases with neoplastic ectopic production of ACTH, the levels of precursor peptides or their processed products may be elevated. The POMC gene can also be expressed from alternate transcription start sites, giving rise to aberrant POMC transcripts in ectopic tumors.

The primary effect of ACTH is to stimulate the adrenal gland to produce cortisol. It also stimulates secretion of adrenal androgens and mineralocorticoids, although production of mineralocorticoids is controlled primarily through non–ACTH-dependent mechanisms (see Chapter 240). Consequently, mineralocorticoid function is preserved in ACTH deficiency, in contrast to primary adrenal insufficiency, which is characterized by loss of glucocorticoid and mineralocorticoid function.

ACTH binds to a high-affinity receptor that is a member of the seven transmembrane class of receptors that are coupled to G proteins. ACTH acts as a trophic hormone as well as causing the immediate secretion of cortisol and other adrenal steroids. Long-term stimulation by ACTH causes adrenal hyperplasia and enlargement. On the other hand, ACTH deficiency leads to adrenal atrophy, and several days of ACTH stimulation are required before steroid synthesis returns to normal.

The secretion of ACTH is regulated by the hypothalamic-pituitary-adrenal axis. Hypothalamic CRH is the most important stimulator of ACTH secretion. CRH is a 41-amino acid peptide that is produced in the paraventricular nucleus of the hypothalamus and in other sites in the nervous system and peripheral tissues (see Chapter 235). The CRH receptor is structurally related to the calcitonin/VIP/GHRH subfamily of seven membrane spanning, G protein-coupled receptors. CRH stimulates cyclic AMP production and increases POMC gene transcription as well as ACTH secretion. Chronic stimulation by CRH also causes corticotroph cell hyperplasia, which can be seen in cases of ectopic CRH production.

Arginine vasopressin (AVP) weakly stimulates ACTH when given alone, but it acts synergistically when administered with CRH and functions as a physiologic stimulus to ACTH secretion along with CRH. About half of the CRH-containing paraventricular neurons also contain AVP. CRH and vasopressin are not always released coordinately, however, and stress has been shown to selectively activate the vasopressin-containing subset of CRH neurons.

Several other hypothalamic factors (angiotensin II, VIP, gastrin-releasing peptide, catecholamines) also enhance ACTH secretion, either by stimulating CRH or by acting at the level of the pituitary gland. ACTH secretion is inhibited by glucocorticoids, which act at both the hypothalamic and pituitary levels. Cortisol inhibits POMC gene transcription by binding to glucocorticoid receptors that interact with negative glucocorticoid response elements in the POMC promoter. Cortisol also inhibits ACTH secretion, and it blunts the ACTH response to CRH. Consequently, ACTH responses to CRH stimulation tests are dependent on ambient concentrations of cortisol and are most robust at night when cortisol levels are low. Cortisol inhibits CRH production and may also act at higher CNS levels. After prolonged glucocorticoid suppression of the hypothalamic-pituitary-adrenal axis, the amount of endogenous CRH secretion appears to be rate limiting and can require several months to recover.

Plasma ACTH is secreted in discrete pulses (10–80 pg/mL) that occur about once an hour. Because of the marked variation in ACTH levels, random measurements are of little value, and most clinical tests are therefore based on levels of cortisol or its metabolites, which tend to integrate the effects of ACTH. ACTH secretion exhibits a marked diurnal rhythm, being greatest at night several hours after the initiation of sleep. ACTH in turn induces a diurnal pattern of cortisol secretion. Cortisol levels are greatest in the early morning and reach a nadir in the late afternoon and evening. Patients with Cushing's disease lose or exhibit a blunted diurnal rhythm of ACTH secretion. ACTH secretion can be stimulated by a variety of different forms of stress, including psychologic stimuli such as fright, anticipation of athletic competition, or surgery. Depression is associated with activation of the hypothalamic-pituitary-adrenal axis and impairs dexamethasone suppressibility. Hypoglycemia induces ACTH secretion through a central mechanism. The resulting increase in cortisol secretion represents one of several counterregulatory mechanisms that increase glucose production. Insulin-induced hypoglycemia provides a mechanism for testing the integrity of the hypothalamic-pituitary-adrenal axis (see Table 237–4). Serious trauma and infection activate an array of cytokines that stimulate CRH and ACTH secretion. Because cortisol levels are often increased up to 10-fold in these circumstances, similar adjustments in cortisol replacement doses may be required in seriously ill patients with adrenal insufficiency.

ACTH DEFICIENCY: SECONDARY HYPOCORTISOLISM. Secondary hypocortisolism causes symptoms of glucocorticoid deficiency including nausea, vomiting, weakness, fatigue, fever, and hypotension. In addition to reduced levels of cortisol, abnormal laboratory tests can include hyponatremia, hypoglycemia, and eosinophilia. Depending on its cause, the severity of cortisol deficiency in secondary adrenal insufficiency is often not as marked as in primary adrenal insufficiency. In addition, mineralocorticoid function is preserved in secondary adrenal deficiency. Consequently, the clinical manifestations of volume depletion are less pronounced and hyperkalemia is not a feature of ACTH deficiency. Because ACTH levels are low in secondary adrenal insufficiency, hyperpigmentation is not seen as in primary adrenal insufficiency. In women, reduced adrenal androgens can decrease libido and cause loss of axillary and pubic hair.

The most common cause of ACTH deficiency is treatment with exogenous glucocorticoids, which causes suppression of the hypothalamic-pituitary-adrenal axis. Sudden withdrawal of glucocorticoids or an increased requirement induced by the superimposition of severe illness can elicit symptoms of glucocorticoid deficiency. Congenital forms of ACTH deficiency are rare. When it is present, ACTH deficiency usually occurs in combination with the loss of other pituitary hormones, although acquired, isolated ACTH deficiency does occur.

ACTH reserve is most often evaluated using CRH or the insulin tolerance test. Caution should be exercised before inducing hypoglycemia in patients with suspected adrenal insufficiency. Insulin-induced hypoglycemia stimulates central responses to neuroglycopenia and mimics some but not all stresses that activate ACTH secretion. CRH testing (ovine CRH 1 μg/kg IV) may be useful for distinguishing hypothalamic and pituitary causes of ACTH deficiency, because it will still induce an ACTH response in most patients with hypothalamic dysfunction and blunted responses to hypoglycemia. The metyrapone test provides an alternative to the insulin tolerance test. By blocking the 11-hydroxylation step, metyrapone inhibits cortisol production, resulting in stimulation of ACTH secretion and an increase in precursor adrenal steroids (e.g., 11-deoxycortisol). Patients should be monitored closely for evidence of adrenal insufficiency, and metyrapone should only be used in patients with at least some evidence of adrenocortical function. ACTH stimulation tests using ACTH$_{1-24}$ (cosyntropin) can accurately evaluate primary adrenocortical insufficiency but do not accurately assess secondary adrenal insufficiency.

ACTH deficiency is treated by replacement with glucocorticoids. Doses need to be individualized and are based largely on clinical criteria in which symptoms of glucocorticoid deficiency are balanced against features of glucocorticoid excess. Patients should wear MedicAlert tags and be instructed in the warning signs of cortisol deficiency, including nausea, vomiting, abdominal pain, low-grade fever, fatigue, and postural dizziness. Stress doses of steroids should be used during times of illness. Mineralocorticoid replacement is not required in patients with ACTH deficiency.

CUSHING'S DISEASE. Etiology and Pathogenesis. Cushing's *disease* results from a pituitary adenoma that causes excess production of ACTH (see also Chapter 240). It is to be distinguished from a variety of other causes of Cushing's *syndrome* (glucocorticoid excess), which include adrenal causes of cortisol excess, ectopic production of ACTH and CRH, and physiologic states that result in overproduction of cortisol. Cushing's disease accounts for 60 to 70% of cases of Cushing's syndrome. Ten to 15 per cent of pituitary tumors secrete ACTH. For unknown reasons, Cushing's disease occurs about eight times more often in women than in men.

The cause of Cushing's disease has been the subject of a longstanding controversy. The observation that CRH stimulates corticotroph hyperplasia and that some patients with Cushing's disease have corticotroph hyperplasia when the pituitary is subjected to pathologic evaluation support the idea of a hypothalamic cause of Cushing's disease. This concept has been used to explain the occasional recurrence of Cushing's disease after apparent cure following transsphenoidal surgery. On the other hand, most ACTH-producing pituitary neoplasms, like other pituitary tumors, are monoclonal. A primary defect in corticotroph cells is also supported by several clinical observations. First, most patients who undergo successful removal of a corticotroph adenoma exhibit suppression of the hypothalamic-pituitary-adrenal axis after surgery, suggesting that CRH is low rather than high. Second, many patients with Cushing's disease respond to exogenous CRH, suggesting that endogenous CRH levels are not high. On balance, the great majority of cases of Cushing's disease likely arise from a primary defect at the level of the pituitary, with rare cases possibly being caused by hypothalamic dysregulation. In addition, there are rare cases of corticotroph hyperplasia causing Cushing's syndrome that are secondary to CRH production by either adjacent CRH-producing intrasellar gangliocytomas or ectopic CRH-producing cancers.

In contrast to other pituitary tumors, the great majority (80–90%) of ACTH-secreting tumors are microadenomas at the time of diagnosis. The clinical features of cortisol excess may allow detection of corticotroph adenomas before they have grown to a larger size. High levels of cortisol may also restrain tumor growth. ACTH-secreting macroadenomas tend to be locally invasive.

Clinical Features. The clinical features of Cushing's disease are caused by the effects of excess glucocorticoids and by the hypersecretion of ACTH and other POMC peptide products. The severity of the features of Cushing's disease varies greatly and appears to reflect not only the level of free cortisol but also the duration of the disease and perhaps the sensitivity to glucocorticoid action. In florid cases of Cushing's disease (Fig. 237–2), the constellation of symptoms and physical features is readily recognized. However, early in the disease or in mild cases, it can be extremely challenging to distinguish the clinical features of Cushing's disease from similar traits that are seen in the normal population. Clinical suspicion is of paramount importance because it establishes the first screening test before embarking on laboratory studies. On the other hand, one must be discriminating and not formally evaluate everyone with obesity, hypertension, and glucose intolerance. Of the many features listed in Table 237–9, some are relatively specific for Cushing's disease. For example, the centripetal distribution of fat with the characteristic "buffalo hump," "moon facies," and deposition in supraclavicular area, with minimal fat in the extremities, is much more specific than generalized obesity. Striae that are wide (>1 cm) and purple reflect steroid-induced thinning of the dermis and can be distinguished from the more common "stretch marks." Numerous spontaneous ecchymoses also occur because of thinning of the skin and capillary fragility. Proximal muscle weakness represents another manifestation of glucocorticoid excess. Osteopenia and hypokalemia, when present, provide objective evidence consistent with ACTH excess. Hypokalemia results from the effects of ACTH on mineralocorticoid production but also from the ability of high levels of cortisol to saturate 11β-dehydrogenase, an enzyme in the kidney that inactivates cortisol. As a result, cortisol can "spill over" and act on mineralocorticoid receptors in the distal tubule. The hyperpigmentation associated with Cushing's disease is not as

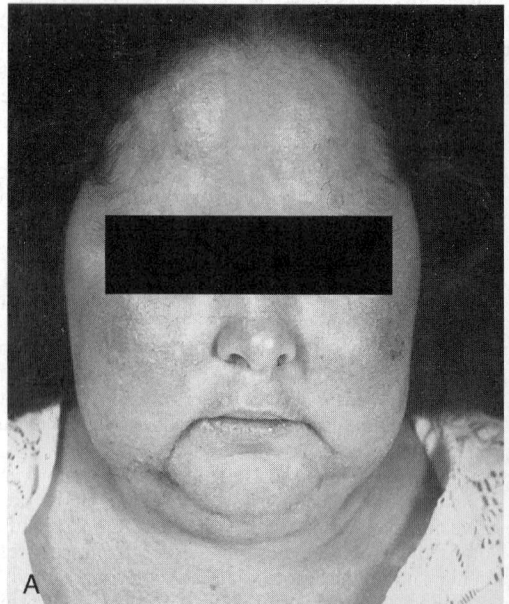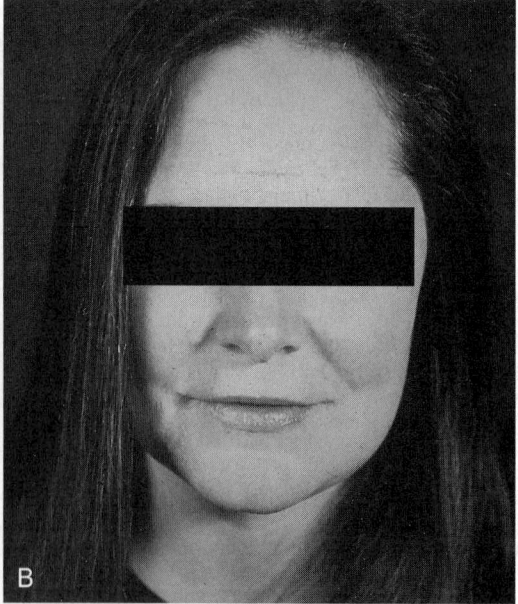

FIGURE 237–2 ▪ Clinical features of Cushing's disease. A 25-year-old woman presented with severe Cushing's disease. *A*, Facial features of Cushing's syndrome including plethora, moon facies, and hirsutism are evident. *B*, Dramatic resolution of the manifestations of cortisol excess after successful transsphenoidal surgery. (Photographs courtesy of Dr. Beverly M. K. Biller.)

General
Obesity (centripetal distribution)
"Moon facies" and mild proptosis
Increased supraclavicular fat and "buffalo hump"
Hypertension

Skin
Hyperpigmentation
Facial plethora
Hirsutism
Violaceous striae and thin skin
Capillary fragility and easy bruising
Acne
Edema

Musculoskeletal
Muscle weakness (proximal)
Osteoporosis and back pain

Reproductive
Decreased libido
Oligoamenorrhea

Neuropsychiatric
Depression
Irritability and emotional lability
Psychosis

Metabolic
Hypokalemia and alkalosis
Hypercalciuria and renal stones
Glucose intolerance or diabetes mellitus
Impaired wound healing
Impaired resistance to infection
Granulocytosis and lymphopenia

Tumor Mass Effects
Headache
Visual field loss
Hypopituitarism

striking as one encounters with Addison's disease or in ectopic ACTH syndrome; but in association with other findings, it should raise the suspicion of Cushing's disease and help to distinguish it from adrenal causes of hypercortisolemia. Hirsutism and acne are caused by the increased production of adrenal androgens and are more prominent in Cushing's disease than in adrenal adenomas, in which glucocorticoids tend to be the predominant product. Oligo/amenorrhea probably has several causes, including androgen effects on the reproductive axis and glucocorticoid inhibition of GnRH, which may also account for diminished libido. Hypertension and glucose intolerance are caused by glucocorticoid excess. Immune suppression, opportunistic infections, and impaired wound healing can lead to considerable morbidity. Neuropsychiatric symptoms, including depression, can be prominent effects of Cushing's disease. Suicide occurs with increased frequency in persons who receive no treatment for Cushing's disease.

Diagnosis. The screening tests and differential diagnosis of Cushing's syndrome represent one of the greatest diagnostic challenges in endocrinology (see Chapter 240) In most cases, the complete evaluation of Cushing's syndrome can take place in the outpatient setting. The first step is to determine whether a patient truly has cortisol excess. After confirmation of Cushing's syndrome, one must distinguish among (1) adrenal causes of cortisol excess; (2) pituitary causes of ACTH excess (Cushing's disease); (3) ectopic sources of ACTH; and (4) ectopic CRH (Table 237–10).

In screening for hypercortisolism, random cortisol levels are not useful because of diurnal variation of the hormone. The overnight dexamethasone test is the most widely used screening test (see

Table 237–8). A normal dexamethasone test essentially excludes Cushing's syndrome. It should be noted, however, that abnormal overnight dexamethasone suppression can be seen in up to 30% of hospitalized patients and in many patients with depression or during alcohol withdrawal. An elevated 24-hour urine free cortisol value provides an alternative, or additional screening test for hypercortisolism. Often, two sequential specimens are collected because of day-to-day variations in hormone production. The sensitivity and specificity of urinary free cortisol measurements are greater than those of the overnight dexamethasone suppression test, particularly in hospitalized patients.

After demonstrating that cortisol excess is present, the next step is to determine the source of excess ACTH or cortisol. The classic approach is to perform a low-dose, followed by a high-dose, dexamethasone suppression test (see Tables 237–8 and 237–10). The low-dose dexamethasone test excludes or confirms the presence of Cushing's syndrome. On the second day of the test, normal individuals suppress plasma cortisol to less than 5 μg/dL and reduce the 17-hydroxysteroids to less than 2.5 mg/24 hr or urinary free cortisol to less than 20 μg/24 hr. All forms of Cushing's syndrome fail to suppress according to these criteria.

The high-dose dexamethasone test is one of several means to distinguish ACTH-independent and ACTH-dependent causes of Cushing's syndrome and to discriminate between pituitary and ectopic causes of ACTH-dependent Cushing's (see Table 237–10). Because adrenal sources of cortisol excess are autonomous and ACTH independent, plasma and urinary cortisol levels are not affected by dexamethasone suppression, even at high doses. In addition, plasma ACTH levels are low in adrenal causes of Cushing's syndrome because the hypothalamic-pituitary axis is suppressed. Pituitary and ectopic causes of Cushing's disease are both ACTH dependent but respond differently to high-dose dexamethasone. Pituitary adenomas have an altered set point for glucocorticoid inhibition but retain a partial ability to respond to high-dose dexamethasone. The exact criteria for dexamethasone suppression in the high-dose test are debated. In most cases of ACTH-producing pituitary adenomas, 17-hydroxysteroids are suppressed to less than 50% of baseline and urinary free cortisol is suppressed below 90% of baseline during the high-dose dexamethasone test.

The ectopic ACTH syndrome should be suspected in patients with known malignancies, particularly small cell carcinoma of the lung, bronchial, thymic, or gastrointestinal carcinoids, islet cell tumors, medullary carcinoma of the thyroid, and others. Plasma ACTH levels are often very high (>200 pg/mL) and can be associated with hyperpigmentation. Clinical features of Cushing's syndrome may be altered by the rapid onset of extreme hypercortisolemia coincident with elements of tumor cachexia. Pronounced weakness, fluid retention, glucose intolerance, hypokalemia, and poor skin integrity are often seen.

Ectopic ACTH syndrome is readily recognized in its classic form. However, a subset of tumors, particularly carcinoids, exhibit dexamethasone suppression that is similar to that seen with pituitary adenomas. When suspected, carcinoids can sometimes be detected by CT or MRI, but many are too small to be seen even with these techniques. Because of these exceptions to the high dose dexamethasone test, a variety of procedures have been devised in an attempt to further distinguish ectopic and pituitary dependent sources of ACTH. The metyrapone test takes advantage of the fact that inhibition of 11β-hydroxylase blocks cortisol production. As a result, negative feedback is reduced and pituitary dependent sources

Table 237–10 ■ TESTS USED IN THE DIFFERENTIAL DIAGNOSIS OF CUSHING'S SYNDROME

ETIOLOGY	OVERNIGHT DEXAMETHASONE SUPPRESSION TEST	PLASMA ACTH	LOW-DOSE DEXAMETHASONE	HIGH-DOSE DEXAMETHASONE	CORTICOTROPIN-RELEASING HORMONE STIMULATION OF ACTH	PETROSAL/PERIPHERAL ACTH RATIO
Normal	Suppression	Normal	Suppression		Normal	
Pituitary	No suppression	Normal or High	No suppression	Suppression	Normal or increased	>2
Ectopic	No suppression	High or normal	No suppression	No suppression	No response	<1.5
Adrenal	No suppression	Low	No suppression	No suppression	No response	

Classic responses are indicated. Certain cases of ectopic adrenocorticotropic hormone (ACTH) production are suppressed by high-dose dexamethasone or are stimulated by corticotropin-releasing hormone. In these cases, petrosal sinus sampling is the most reliable method for distinguishing pituitary and etopic sources of ACTH.

of ACTH typically exhibit an increase in ACTH that stimulates the production of precursor adrenal steroids (e.g., 11-deoxycortisol) (see Table 237–4). Although most ectopic causes of ACTH exhibit a blunted response to the decreased cortisol levels, the subset of ectopic tumors that respond atypically to dexamethasone are most likely to give a positive response in the metyrapone test.

In recent years, inferior petrosal sinus sampling has been used to distinguish pituitary and ectopic sources of ACTH when the source of ACTH is not obvious based on the clinical circumstances, biochemical evaluation, and imaging studies. This test requires an experienced radiologist for safe and effective catheterization of the petrosal sinuses (which drain the pituitary venous effluent). Blood samples are taken simultaneously from the left and right petrosal sinuses and from the periphery. In the case of ACTH-producing pituitary adenomas, there is a gradient in ACTH levels between the central and peripheral blood specimens. Administration of CRH stimulates ACTH and tends to enhance the gradient. A gradient of 2:1 (central:peripheral) on either the left or the right is consistent with a pituitary source of ACTH. When clinical and biochemical studies suggest the presence of a pituitary adenoma, pituitary imaging should be performed using CT or MRI. Most ACTH-secreting pituitary adenomas are small and scans are normal in more than half of patients.

Therapy. The efficacy of transsphenoidal surgery for Cushing's disease is greatly aided by making the correct diagnosis preoperatively. In experienced hands, surgical cures of ACTH-producing microadenomas occur in 75 to 90% of patients undergoing a first operation. As in other pituitary tumors, complete remissions with macroadenomas are much less common. In the event of surgical remission or cure, postoperative hypocortisolism is to be expected because of suppression of the hypothalamic-pituitary axis. After coverage for steroid withdrawal in the postoperative period, cortisol replacement should gradually be decreased to allow recovery of the hypothalamic-pituitary-adrenal axis.

If transsphenoidal surgery is unsuccessful, reoperation may be indicated and can result in remission in up to 50% of patients. If transsphenoidal surgery cannot be performed or has failed, alternative forms of therapy should be used to prevent the long-term consequences of hypercortisolism. Pituitary irradiation is usually the second line of treatment for Cushing's disease. It is more efficacious in children and in younger patients, but even in older adults remissions can be achieved in 50 to 60% within 2 years. To prevent the continued ravages of hypercortisolism during this period, however, concomitant medical therapy is usually given. Bilateral adrenalectomy represents another alternative for patients with severe hypercortisolism after transsphenoidal surgery. It rapidly and effectively lowers cortisol levels but is associated with relatively high morbidity and mortality (as high as 5%) because of the associated metabolic and immune system alterations caused by hypercortisolism. After adrenalectomy, patients must be maintained on glucocorticoids and mineralocorticoids and are at risk for the development of Nelson's syndrome.

Medical therapy for Cushing's disease has its primary role in preparation for surgery or for control of hypercortisolism during the interval when radiation therapy is taking effect. Because most pituitary adenomas are responsive to changes in cortisol levels, they have a tendency to "escape" from adrenal blockade caused by some therapies by producing higher levels of ACTH. The antifungal agent ketoconazole is highly effective in decreasing glucocorticoid biosynthesis and also inhibits ACTH secretion so that it has become the medical therapy of choice. Alternative medications include metyrapone, aminoglutethimide, and mitotane.

NELSON'S SYNDROME. Nelson's syndrome was initially described as the appearance of a pituitary adenoma after bilateral adrenalectomy. In addition to an enlarging pituitary mass, the syndrome is characterized by very high ACTH levels and hyperpigmentation. It is caused by a pre-existing ACTH-producing tumor that grows in the absence of feedback inhibition by high levels of glucocorticoids. The incidence of clinically significant Nelson's syndrome after adrenalectomy for Cushing's disease varies from 10 to 50% in different series. Patients with Cushing's disease who have undergone adrenalectomy should be followed with imaging studies and plasma ACTH levels because tumors that cause Nelson's syndrome can be very aggressive. When there is evidence of

mass effects or rapid growth, transsphenoidal surgery should be performed. Postoperative irradiation may provide additional benefit, although it appears to be less efficacious than in other ACTH-producing adenomas.

Estrada J, Boronat M, Mielgo M, et al: The long-term outcome of pituitary irradiation after unsuccessful transsphenoidal surgery in Cushing's disease. N Engl J Med 336: 172–177, 1996. *This report of a large series of patients documents the rather surprising rapid benefit of irradiation after unsuccessful transsphenoidal surgery.*
Findling JW: Differential diagnosis of Cushing's syndrome. Endocrinologist. 7:17s–23s, 1997. *A brief review of the various tests used to evaluate patients with Cushing's syndrome with an emphasis on CRH testing and inferior petrosal sinus sampling.*
Orme SM, Peacey SR, Barth JH, Belchetz PE: Comparison of tests of stress-released cortisol secretion in pituitary disease. Clin Endocrinol 45:135–140, 1996. *This report stresses the need to perform insulin tolerance tests rather than ACTH$_{1-24}$ stimulation tests in the assessment of the hypothalamic-pituitary-adrenal axis in patients with pituitary disease.*

GONADOTROPINS (FOLLICLE-STIMULATING HORMONE AND LUTEINIZING HORMONE)

The pituitary glycoprotein hormones include FSH, LH, and TSH. Chorionic gonadotropin, which is structurally very similar to LH, is made in the placenta. Each of the glycoprotein hormones has a specific β-subunit that forms a non-covalent dimer with the common α-subunit. The α- and individual β-subunits are encoded by separate genes. The β-subunit genes are evolutionarily related and share a common gene structure as well as having nucleotide and amino acid sequence homology. Similarities in the structures of the β-subunits account for their ability to form non-covalent dimers with the common α-subunit. The α- and β-subunits each undergo glycosylation, which is important for correct hormone folding, intracellular transport, and secretion. Glycosylation is also required for biologic activity, presumably because of effects on the tertiary structure of the hormones.

The half-life of LH (approximately 50 minutes) is shorter than that of FSH (approximately 220 minutes), accounting for the more rapid secretory dynamics of LH, even though both hormones are secreted together. Differences in FSH and LH sequences between the conserved cysteines provide distinct "determinant loops" that allow the hormones to bind to specific receptors. Receptor contacts are made by both the α- and β-subunits. The receptors for FSH and LH are also structurally related and are members of the G-protein coupled seven transmembrane family. After binding to their receptors, LH and FSH stimulate cyclic AMP production, phosphatidylinositol turnover, and mobilization of calcium.

The gonadotropins are involved in sexual differentiation, sex steroid production, and gametogenesis. The regulation and physiologic roles of gonadotropins are quite different in males and females. In males, receptors for FSH are located on Sertoli cells and seminiferous tubules, whereas LH receptors are located on Leydig cells in the testis. LH stimulates androgen production by the Leydig cells. FSH is involved primarily in sperm maturation in the seminiferous tubules. Thus, FSH and LH act together to induce spermatogenesis (see Chapter 247).

In females, ovarian FSH receptors are located on granulosa cells where they induce enzymes involved in estrogen biosynthesis. LH receptors are located predominantly on thecal cells in the ovary and stimulate the production of ovarian androgens and steroid precursors that are transported to granulosa cells for aromatization to estrogens. The pattern of FSH and LH secretion during the menstrual cycle results in follicular recruitment and maturation (largely FSH-mediated), followed by ovulation (largely LH-mediated) and steroid production by the corpus luteum.

Gonadotropin secretion is regulated primarily by the hypothalamic decapeptide GnRH. The receptor for GnRH is a member of the G-protein–coupled seven transmembrane family of receptors. GnRH stimulates an immediate release of intracellular calcium followed by a second phase of extracellular calcium influx. GnRH also activates phosphatidylinositol turnover, resulting in production of diacylglycerol and inositol triphosphate, which act together to stimulate the protein kinase C pathway. The gonadotroph cell is exquisitely sensitive to the pattern of GnRH stimulation. Continuous, rather than pulsatile exposure to GnRH causes gonadotroph desensitization and suppression of LH and FSH. Gonadotroph sensitivity to GnRH is modulated by sex steroids and probably other hypothalamic peptides, such as neuropeptide Y. Increased GnRH secretion in combination with a higher density of GnRH receptors and rising estradiol concentrations accounts in part for the dramatic release of gonadotropins that induces ovulation.

The hypothalamic-pituitary-gonadal axis is activated during fetal development. However, during the first 2 years of life, LH and FSH levels fall and remain suppressed until puberty. The physiologic basis for gonadotropin suppression during early childhood is not well understood but involves tonic inhibition of the GnRH pulse generator by the central nervous system as the pituitary gland is still responsive to exogenous GnRH. Most theories hold that the onset of puberty reflects disinhibition of the pulse generator. Puberty occurs between ages 8 and 13 in girls and between ages 9 and 14 in boys. In the peripubertal period, sleep-associated bursts of LH secretion can first be detected at night. Subsequently, there is a gradual increase in LH pulse frequency and amplitude, such that LH pulses are detected during the day and night.

In women, the pattern of GnRH pulse frequency varies across the menstrual cycle (see Part XVIII). The combination of GnRH stimulation, in conjunction with ovarian feedback regulation, results in a complex orchestration of positive and negative hormonal signals that converge at the gonadotroph to regulate LH and FSH secretion. The typical 28-day menstrual cycle is divided into follicular and luteal phases that are separated by ovulation on day 14. Unlike chronic exposure to low concentrations of estrogens, which exert negative feedback regulation and inhibit GnRH, the increasing concentration of estrogen before the LH surge exerts positive feedback regulation that results in increased GnRH pulse frequency. Increased GnRH, in combination with increased gonadotroph sensitivity to GnRH, results in the LH/FSH surge. During the luteal phase, the gonadotropin pulse frequency is reduced. In addition to feedback regulation by steroids, ovarian peptides such as inhibin also play a role in control of the reproductive axis. Inhibin causes selective suppression of FSH, without affecting LH secretion. A homodimer of inhibin β-subunits, referred to as activin, has opposite actions and selectively stimulates FSH. Circulating inhibin provides one of the negative feedback inputs that leads to FSH suppression as the follicle develops.

The perimenopause is characterized by a gradual cessation of ovarian function. After several years of menstrual cycles that are sometimes anovulatory or irregular, menses cease, thereby defining the menopause. Although there is considerable variation, menopause usually occurs at about age 50. At this point, ovarian follicles have been depleted, and the production of sex steroids changes such that there is minimal production of estrogen and progesterone, but ovarian androgens continue to be made at lesser levels, primarily by stromal cells. The chronic decline in estrogen and progesterone causes loss of feedback inhibition and a marked increase in LH and FSH levels.

In males, the regulation of the hypothalamic-pituitary-gonadal axis is relatively constant. After early puberty, LH and FSH pulses occur about once an hour during the night and day. It is notable that there is considerable variation in LH pulse frequency among normal individuals. Because each pulse of LH stimulates testosterone secretion, one also observes pulses of testosterone after LH, although these pulses are muted somewhat by the presence of serum binding proteins that delay clearance. Nevertheless, testosterone levels can drop below the "normal" range in individuals with slow LH pulse frequencies. Testosterone inhibits the hypothalamic-pituitary axis, although its actions are mediated, in part, by aromatization to estrogens, as has been shown in rare patients who are unable to convert testosterone to estrogen because of a deficiency of aromatase. Much of the inhibition by gonadal steroids occurs at the hypothalamic level, but there is also evidence for weak inhibition of the gonadotroph at the level of the pituitary gland. In contrast to women, there is no abrupt change in hormone levels analogous to the menopause. There is, however, a gradual decline in testosterone levels associated with an increase in LH and FSH with aging.

HYPOGONADOTROPIC HYPOGONADISM. Clinical features of hypogonadotropic hypogonadism in women are primarily due to estrogen deficiency and include breast atrophy, vaginal dryness, and diminished libido. Hot flashes are uncommon, in contrast to postmenopausal estrogen deficiency. In premenopausal women, normal menstrual cycles provide evidence for an intact hypothalamic-pituitary-gonadal axis. LH and FSH levels should be increased in postmenopausal women. Hypogonadism in men causes decreased libido and sexual function. In men, low testosterone without elevation of

LH and FSH is consistent with impaired hypothalamic-pituitary reserve. GnRH stimulation can distinguish hypothalamic and pituitary deficiency but may require multiple injections to prime the pituitary, if GnRH deficiency is of long standing.

In premenopausal women, preparations of estrogen and progestins should be used for hormonal replacement and to allow cyclical growth of the endometrium. Pulsatile GnRH (for GnRH-deficient subjects) or gonadotropins can be given to induce ovulation and fertility when desired. Testosterone can be replaced in men using intramuscular injections that are given at 2- to 4-week intervals. Doses and the intervals between injections should be adjusted on an individual basis using libido and testosterone levels before the next injection as a guide. Oral preparations of androgens should be avoided because of hepatotoxicity. Transdermal preparations are also available, but there is less experience with their long-term acceptance and efficacy. Induction of spermatogenesis requires pulsatile GnRH (for GnRH-deficient subjects) or injections of gonadotropins.

A congenital form of hypogonadotropic hypogonadism is caused by deficiency of GnRH, which in turn, causes deficiencies of LH and FSH. When associated with anosmia (absent sense of smell), the condition is referred to as Kallmann's syndrome (see Chapter 235). Pulsatile GnRH has been used to induce puberty and fertility in both males and females with Kallmann's syndrome.

Secondary hypogonadotropic hypogonadism is relatively common. In most cases it is reversible and is caused by weight loss, anorexia nervosa, stress, heavy exercise, or severe illness. Reversible forms of secondary hypogonadotropic hypogonadism are caused by GnRH deficiency and are more common in women than men. The condition is ideally treated by correcting the underlying cause. Many women have a discrete threshold for weight or exercise level that will cause loss of menstrual periods. When it is not possible to correct the underlying abnormality, hormonal replacement can be used in women for protection against osteopenia and to cycle the endometrium.

A variety of pathologic conditions can cause secondary hypogonadotropic hypogonadism, often in association with deficiencies of other pituitary hormones (see Table 237–3). These include hypothalamic lesions or central nervous system irradiation. Pituitary tumors can suppress gonadotropins because of stalk compression and disruption of pulsatile GnRH input as well as by direct destruction of normal pituitary tissue. Hyperprolactinemia can suppress GnRH and lead to reduced gonadotropin levels. In contrast to the aforementioned causes of hypogonadotropic hypogonadism, which result from GnRH deficiency, primary deficiencies of LH and FSH are uncommon. An acquired form of isolated gonadotroph deficiency is rarely encountered and may have an autoimmune basis. Mutations in the LHβ or FSHβ genes have been described in case reports and cause selective loss of individual gonadotropins. Inactivating mutations in the GnRH receptor and the LH receptor causing hypogonadotropic hypogonadism have also been reported.

FSH- AND LH-PRODUCING TUMORS. Etiology and Pathogenesis. Although most early series suggested that gonadotropin-producing adenomas were relatively uncommon, recent studies using sensitive techniques to characterize tumor phenotype show a prevalence (10–15%) that is similar to that of corticotroph or somatotroph adenomas (see Table 237–6). The majority (70–80%) of pituitary tumors classified previously as non-functioning adenomas can be shown to produce low levels of intact glycoprotein hormones or their uncombined α- or β-subunits. Biosynthetic defects in the tumor cells account for relatively inefficient hormone secretion as well as the propensity to produce uncombined subunits. FSH is produced more commonly than LH. Elevated levels of free α-subunits are noted more often than free β-subunits.

Clinical Features. Gonadotropin-producing tumors are somewhat more common in men than women and increase in prevalence with age. FSH- and LH-producing tumors do not usually cause a characteristic hormone excess syndrome. The tumors are typically large macroadenomas and present as clinically non-functioning tumors with symptoms and signs related to local mass effects. Visual field loss due to suprasellar extension and compression of the optic chiasm is found in more than 70% of patients. Many of these tumors are detected incidentally by CT and MRI that are performed for unrelated indications. Symptoms of hypopituitarism, including hypogonadism with loss of libido, are also common. Men with predominantly FSH-secreting tumors may present with testicular enlargement from hypertrophy of the seminiferous tubules but also can paradoxically present with hypogonadal features that are related to low levels of testosterone. These patients must be distinguished from those with primary hypogonadism who have testicular dysfunction. Tumors that primarily secrete LH are rare but can cause increased testosterone levels. Premenopausal women with gonadotropin-producing tumors may experience menstrual irregularity or secondary hypogonadism. Postmenopausal women often show reduced gonadotropin levels because the mass effects of the gonadotropin-producing tumors cause stalk compression, impairing GnRH stimulation of gonadotropins from both normal and pituitary tumor cells.

Diagnosis. Because of the absence of a clinical syndrome in most patients, the preoperative diagnosis of gonadotropin-producing pituitary tumors has relied on imaging studies and laboratory tests. Unfortunately, the laboratory diagnosis of gonadotropin-producing tumors is less than satisfactory. First, the tumors synthesize gonadotropins inefficiently and hormone levels are usually not markedly elevated. Second, because the secretion of gonadotropins is pulsatile, random LH and FSH values are difficult to interpret. Furthermore, gonadotropin levels vary widely and are normally elevated in postmenopausal women. GnRH stimulation tests also do not clearly distinguish gonadotropin-producing tumors from normal subjects and suppression tests have not proven useful. However, paradoxical responses to TRH have helped to identify gonadotropin-secreting tumors. In contrast to its effect on normal persons, TRH stimulates secretion of intact gonadotropins or the uncombined FSHβ- and LHβ-subunits in most patients with gonadotropin tumors. Once identified, the uncombined α- or β-subunits can serve as tumor markers and can be useful for monitoring responses to therapy.

Men with proven gonadotropin-producing tumors typically have high-normal or elevated FSH levels but low levels of testosterone. Moderately elevated PRL levels are common and are caused by tumor mass effects. It is important to distinguish this group from patients with true prolactinomas. As noted earlier, many women, including those in the postmenopausal group have paradoxically low gonadotropin levels. Thus, the absence of elevated gonadotropins does not exclude the diagnosis of a gonadotropin-producing tumor.

The postoperative diagnosis of gonadotropin-producing tumors can be made based on immunohistochemical analyses or using more sophisticated studies of gonadotropin gene expression. These types of analyses confirm that the great majority of clinically nonfunctioning tumors are composed of gonadotropin-producing cell types.

Treatment. Because the major symptoms of the gonadotropin-producing tumors are due to extrasellar extension and local mass effects, the main aim of treatment is reduction in the size of the tumor. Complete or partial reversal of visual field defects and hypopituitarism can be accomplished by surgery, unless these have been of long standing. However, transsphenoidal surgery is rarely curative of this group of macroadenomas. Patients with significant residual tumor may benefit from radiation therapy, although there are no large series in which patients have been randomly allocated to treatment groups. Because most tumors are slow growing, one approach when no tumor is visible postoperatively by MRI is to monitor tumor recurrence using visual fields and CT or MRI. If tumor markers, such as free α- or β-subunit levels are available, they can be used alone, or in conjunction with TRH testing, to monitor tumor function. When follow-up studies show tumor regrowth, repeat surgery and/or radiation therapy are indicated.

There has been great interest in medical therapies that might be useful as adjuncts to surgery or even as primary therapies in patients not requiring immediate decompression. The success of bromocriptine and somatostatin analogues in treating hormone oversecretion and tumor mass in prolactinomas and acromegaly have not been seen in most patients with gonadotropin-producing tumors, although exceptions have been described in selected patients. The efficacy of long-acting GnRH agonists or antagonists, which suppress LH and FSH in normal individuals has also been examined. The GnRH agonists stimulate gonadotropin secretion from tumors, without apparent desensitization, and have not been

useful. GnRH antagonists have been shown to suppress FSH levels in small series of patients, but these agents have not been found to reduce tumor size.

Nachtigall LB, Boepple PA, Pralong FP, Crowley WF Jr: Adult-onset idiopathic hypogonadotropic hypogonadism—a treatable form of male infertility. N Engl J Med 336:410–415, 1996. *In this series of men with acquired, idiopathic hypogonadotropic hypogonadism, fertility could be induced with pulsatile GnRH secretion.*
Young WF, Scheithauer BW, Kovacs KT, et al: Gonadotroph adenoma of the pituitary gland: A clinicopathologic analysis of 100 cases. Mayo Clin Proc 71:649–656, 1996. *The clinical, hormonal, and pathologic characteristics of a large number of cases is summarized in this report.*

THYROID-STIMULATING HORMONE

Like the other glycoprotein hormones, TSH is a heterodimer composed of the common α-subunit and the unique TSH β-subunit. Both subunits are glycosylated, and the composition of carbohydrates is thought to alter the biologic activity of the hormone. TSH is produced in thyrotroph cells that account for about 5% of pituitary cell types. TSH is measured by highly sensitive immunoradiometric assays that use antisera directed toward the TSHβ-subunit. Normal levels of TSH range from 0.4 to 4.0 μU/mL. The detection limit for current TSH assays is less than 0.01 μU/mL, allowing measurement of suppressed TSH levels in hyperthyroidism.

TSH controls thyroid hormone (T_4 and T_3) synthesis and secretion from the thyroid gland. TSH receptors are members of the G-protein–coupled seven transmembrane family and are structurally related to LH and FSH receptors. TSH stimulates cyclic AMP production and acts as a trophic hormone as well as stimulating hormone biosynthesis in the thyroid. TSH secretion from the pituitary gland is regulated by the hypothalamic-pituitary-thyroid axis. Hypothalamic TRH is a tripeptide that stimulates TSH synthesis and secretion. TRH, acting through its G-protein–coupled receptor elicits phosphatidylinositol turnover and induces release of intracellular calcium followed by an influx of extracellular calcium. TSH secretion appears to be modulated by alterations in calcium flux, whereas biosynthesis may be controlled by activation of other pathways, such as protein kinase C. A variety of other hypothalamic hormones including somatostatin and dopamine can inhibit TSH secretion, but their roles in normal physiology have not been clearly elucidated.

Thyroid hormones have an inhibitory effect on the production of TRH and TSH and comprise a powerful negative feedback loop in the hypothalamic-pituitary-thyroid axis. The direct effects of thyroid hormone at the level of the pituitary gland are well illustrated by TSH responses to TRH stimulation tests. In hypothyroidism, TSH responses to exogenous TRH are exaggerated. In hyperthyroidism, TSH responses to TRH are blunted or flat, indicating that the inhibitory effects of thyroid hormone override the stimulatory effects of TRH. Thyroid hormones act via nuclear receptors that function at the transcriptional level to suppress expression of the TRH gene as well as the α- and β-subunit genes of TSH. In hypothyroidism, expression of the α and TSHβ genes is stimulated and hormone production is markedly enhanced.

TSH secretion is pulsatile, but the amplitude of the pulses is relatively small and does not create the difficulties in measurement of TSH that are encountered with measurements of other pituitary hormones. TSH levels are elevated in infants in the immediate postpartum period. Thereafter, thyroid function tests remain remarkably constant throughout life. There is a diurnal rhythm of TSH secretion with a small increase at night. Because of the integrated nature of the hypothalamic-pituitary-thyroid axis, thyroid function tests are best interpreted when concentrations of TSH, free T_4, and free T_3 levels are known. Except in conditions of secondary hypothyroidism or TSH-secreting pituitary tumors (see later), TSH levels provide an excellent screening test for thyroid dysfunction. In primary hypothyroidism, TSH levels are elevated as TSH increases logarithmically in response to falling thyroid hormone levels (see Chapter 239). In hyperthyroidism, TSH is suppressed to levels below or near the detection limits of most sensitive assays.

CENTRAL HYPOTHYROIDISM. Central forms of hypothyroidism include secondary hypothyroidism, which is caused by TSH deficiency, and tertiary hypothyroidism, which is caused by TRH deficiency. Three different types of congenital TSH deficiency are caused by genetic mutations. One type involves mutations in the TSHβ gene in which several different types of mutations have been described. A second involves mutations in Pit-1, which causes combined deficiencies of GH, PRL, and TSH (see earlier). A third involves a mutation in the gene for TRH. Acquired, central forms of hypothyroidism are often associated with other pituitary hormone deficiencies and usually there is no goiter because of low TSH levels. Suspicion of central hypothyroidism should prompt measurements of T_4, T_3, and TSH as well as other pituitary hormones. When TSH deficiency is documented, thyroid hormone is replaced using daily doses of L-thyroxine (0.05–0.15 mg/day). Because TSH cannot be used as an endpoint, one monitors serum levels of free T_4 and T_3.

Tests for TSH deficiency are best performed by analyzing free T_4 levels in combination with TSH. Low free T_4 without elevated TSH is consistent with central hypothyroidism. Free T_4 measurements should be used rather than total T_4 to avoid confusion caused by thyroxine-binding globulin (TBG) deficiency (which is suggested by high T_3 resin uptake tests). In some patients with hypothalamic disease, the TSH level is partially elevated in the presence of low free T_4, but the bioactivity of the TSH is reduced. Central forms of hypothyroidism must be distinguished from patients with the sick-euthyroid condition (see Chapter 239). Laboratory tests in the sick-euthyroid syndrome progress through several phases but can include prolonged periods when both TSH and free thyroid hormone levels are low. It can be very difficult in these patients to unequivocally exclude central hypothyroidism. In addition to the clinical setting in which thyroid function tests are measured, the presence of normal thyroid function tests before the illness and the absence of known hypothalamic or pituitary disease make true central hypothyroidism unlikely. Increased levels of reverse T_3 are suggestive of sick-euthyroidism and free T_4 and T_3 may be in the normal or low normal range in sick-euthyroid patients.

TSH-SECRETING TUMORS. Etiology and Pathogenesis. TSH-secreting tumors are rare and account for between 1% and 3% of pituitary tumors. Like gonadotropin-producing tumors, a subset of tumors classified as clinically non-functioning tumors can be shown to produce TSH, often at subclinical levels. However, because TSH overproduction can cause hyperthyroidism, TSH-secreting tumors are more readily detected than FSH- and LH-producing tumors. As many as 30% of TSH-producing tumors are plurihormonal. GH and PRL are co-secreted most often, perhaps reflecting a common cellular lineage for thyrotrophs, somatotrophs, and lactotrophs. Long-standing severe hypothyroidism can cause thyrotroph hyperplasia and pituitary enlargement. However, these hyperplastic masses regress on thyroid hormone replacement. Most true TSH-producing tumors are relatively autonomous and respond weakly, if at all, to TRH stimulation or thyroid hormone suppression.

Clinical Features. TSH-secreting tumors are usually macroadenomas by the time a diagnosis has been made. Consequently, many patients exhibit mass effects of the tumor as well as hyperthyroidism. However, now that measurement of TSH is being used as the initial assessment for hyperthyroidism, smaller tumors are being seen more commonly than previously. The clinical features of TSH-secreting tumors resemble those of Graves' disease except that features of autoimmunity such as ophthalmopathy are absent. Circulating levels of T_4 and T_3 range widely but can be elevated as much as twofold to threefold. Diffuse goiter is present in the majority of patients with TSH-producing tumors, and the 24-hour uptake of radioiodine is elevated.

Diagnosis. Because feedback inhibition of TSH is impaired in TSH-producing tumors, TSH levels are inappropriately elevated in the presence of high levels of T_4 and T_3. TSH levels produced by tumors range from the low normal range to as high as 500 μU/mL, but most levels are minimally elevated. By using ultrasensitive TSH assays, it is now possible to detect non-suppressed TSH levels without the need for TRH testing. Free α-subunit measurements can be very helpful in confirming the diagnosis of a TSH-secreting tumor. Most TSH-producing tumors (> 80%) secrete excess free α-subunit. Thus, the diagnosis of a TSH-secreting tumor can usually be made by demonstrating that a hyperthyroid patient has a detectable serum TSH associated with excess secretion of the free α-subunit. The finding of a mass lesion on CT or MRI confirms the diagnosis. Several other causes of inappropriate TSH secretion should be considered, including resistance to thyroid hormone and familial dysalbuminemic hyperthyroxinemia and other disorders that alter serum thyroid hormone binding proteins.

Treatment. The goals of therapy are to treat the underlying TSH-secreting tumor and to correct the hyperthyroidism. Transsphenoidal surgery alone is rarely curative because of the large size of most tumors, but it can alleviate mass effects and lower TSH levels. As in other large pituitary tumors, adjunctive irradiation may be required to control tumor growth. Somatostatin analogues (e.g., octreotide) have been used as adjunctive medical therapy and decrease TSH and α-subunit levels in about 80% patients with TSH-secreting tumors, but consistent effects on tumor growth have not been demonstrated. Hyperthyroidism caused by TSH-secreting tumors can also be treated using antithyroid drugs or radioiodine.

Chanson P, Weintraub BD, Harris AG: Octreotide therapy for thyroid-stimulating hormone–secreting pituitary adenomas: A follow-up of 52 patients. Ann Intern Med 119:236–240, 1993. *The literature of patients with these tumors is summarized, and their responses to octreotide are detailed.*

Collu R, Tang J, Castagne J, et al: A novel mechanism for isolated central hypothyroidism: Inactivating mutations in the thyrotropin-releasing hormone receptor gene. J Clin Endocrinol Metab 82:1361–1365, 1997. *A mutation in the TRH receptor acts like a mutation in the TSH gene, causing mild hypothyroidism with a mild elevation in TSH that is biologically less active than normal.*

NULL CELL PITUITARY TUMORS. Null cell adenomas, or clinically non-functioning tumors, are variably defined depending on the criteria used to analyze tumor cell phenotype. As noted earlier, the majority of clinically non-functioning adenomas can be shown to produce low levels of the free α-subunit, free β-subunits of FSH and LH, and intact FSH and LH when analyzed by immunocytochemistry or for messenger RNA expression. A smaller fraction can be shown to produce low levels of other pituitary hormones, particularly ACTH or GH, that escaped detection based on routine endocrine testing. Even with detailed analyses of hormone production, a subset (10–20%) of non-functioning adenomas do not appear to produce one of the major pituitary hormones.

The clinical features and management of null cell tumors are similar to those for gonadotropin-producing tumors. The major signs and symptoms result from tumor mass effects that cause visual field defects, headache and other neurologic symptoms, and hypopituitarism. Transsphenoidal surgery is the primary mode of treatment, with a goal of debulking the tumor to relieve mass effects. Because there are no serum tumor markers, patients must be followed by CT or MRI in conjunction with visual field tests.

Warnet A, Harris AG, Renard E, et al, and the French Multicenter Octreotide Study Group: A prospective multicenter trial of octreotide in 24 patients with visual defects caused by nonfunctioning and gonadotropin-secreting pituitary adenomas. Neurosurgery 41:786–797, 1997. *A large series of patients with these clinically non-functioning adenomas and their responses to octreotide.*

---

238 POSTERIOR PITUITARY

Alan G. Robinson

ANATOMY AND HORMONE SYNTHESIS. The hormones of the posterior pituitary, vasopressin and oxytocin, are synthesized in specialized neurons in the hypothalamus, the magnocellular neurons. These neurons are specific for each hormone and are noted for their large size. In the hypothalamus the magnocellular neurons are clustered in the paired paraventricular nuclei and the paired supraoptic nuclei (Fig. 238–1). Vasopressin and oxytocin are also synthesized in parvicellular (small cell) neurons of the paraventricular nuclei, and vasopressin (but not oxytocin) is synthesized in the suprachiasmatic nucleus. Transcription of vasopressin and oxytocin mRNA and translation of vasopressin and oxytocin prohormone occur entirely in the cell bodies of the hormone-specific neurons. The preprohormones are cleaved from the signal peptide in the endoplasmic reticulum, and the prohormones propressophysin and pro-oxyphysin are packaged with processing enzymes into neurosecretory granules. In the magnocellular neurons the neurosecretory granules are transported out of the perikaryon via microtubules down the long axons that form the supraopticohypophysial tract to terminate in axon terminals in the posterior pituitary. During transport the processing enzymes cleave propressophysin to vasopressin (8 amino acids), vasopressin-neurophysin (95 amino acids), and

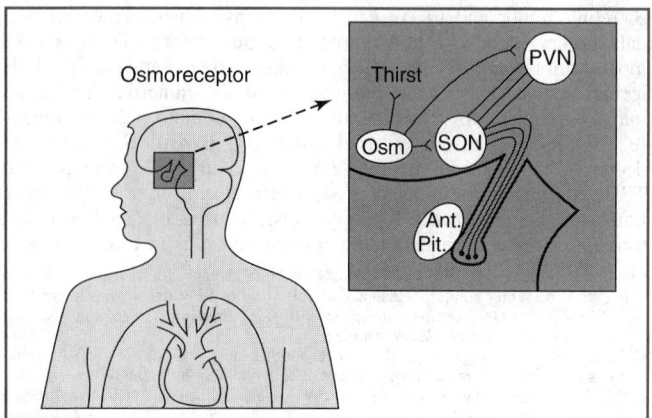

FIGURE 238–1 ■ Sagittal view of the head demonstrating the position of the neurohypophysis. The magnocellular neurons are clustered in two paraventricular nuclei (PVN) and two supraoptic nuclei (SON). Only one nucleus of each pair is illustrated. The supraoptic nuclei are located lateral to the edge of the optic chiasm, whereas the paraventricular nuclei are central in the wall of the 3rd ventricle. The osmostat and thirst center are located in the hypothalamus anterior to the third ventricle. The axons of the four nuclei combine to form the supraopticohypophyseal tract as they course through the pituitary stalk to their storage terminals in the posterior pituitary. (From Buonocore CM, Robinson AG: Diagnosis and management of diabetes insipidus during medical emergencies. Endocrinol Metab Clin North Am 22:411, 1993.)

vasopressin glycopeptide (39 amino acids). Pro-oxyphysin is similarly cleaved to oxytocin and oxytocin-neurophysin, but not glycopeptide. Within the neurosecretory granules, neurophysins form neurophysin-hormone complexes that stabilize the hormones. Crystallography demonstrates that tetramers of neurophysin form specific binding sites for five molecules of hormone. Stimulatory (e.g., cholinergic and angiotensin) neurotransmitter terminals and inhibitory (e.g., γ-aminobutyric acid, noradrenergic, atrial natriuretic peptide [ANP]) neurotransmitter terminals control the release of vasopressin by the activity of contacts on the cell body. Physiologic release of vasopressin or oxytocin into the general circulation is at the level of the posterior pituitary, where in response to an action potential, intracellular calcium is increased to cause the neurosecretory granules to fuse with the axon membrane and release (via exocytosis into the pericapillary space) the entire contents of the granule. Once released, the hormone has no further association with its respective neurophysin, and each of the peptide products can be independently detected in the general circulation. Factors that stimulate the release of vasopressin also stimulate synthesis; however, whereas release is instantaneous, synthesis requires a longer time. This difference may explain the physiologic advantage of the large store of hormone in the posterior pituitary. In most species, sufficient hormone is stored in the posterior pituitary to support maximum antidiuresis for several days and to maintain baseline levels of antidiuresis for weeks without the synthesis of new hormone.

The axons of the parvicellular neurons of the paraventricular nuclei terminate in the median eminence of the basal hypothalamus, where similar to other hypothalamic releasing factors the hormones are secreted into the portal capillary system and where vasopressin serves as one of the regulators of secretion of adrenocorticotropic hormone (ACTH). Yet other axons secrete hormone into the cerebrospinal fluid of the third ventricle; however, the function of this secretion is unknown.

SECRETION. VASOPRESSIN AND REGULATION OF OSMOLALITY.

The primary physiologic action of vasopressin is its function as a water-retaining hormone. The central sensing system (osmostat) for control of release of vasopressin is anatomically discreet, located in a small area of the hypothalamus just anterior to the 3rd ventricle (see Fig. 238–1). The osmostat controls release of vasopressin to cause water retention and also stimulates thirst to cause water repletion. Osmotic regulation of vasopressin release and osmotic regulation of thirst are usually tightly coupled, but experimental lesions and some pathologic situations in humans demonstrate that the regulation can be independent. The primary extracellular osmo-

lyte to which the osmoreceptor responds is sodium. Glucose and urea under normal physiologic conditions readily traverse neuron membranes and do not affect the release of vasopressin. Although osmolality in normal subjects is between 275 and 295 mOsm/kg of water, for each person extracellular fluid osmolality is maintained in a narrow range. An increase in plasma osmolality as little as 1% will stimulate the osmoreceptors to cause release of vasopressin. Basal levels of vasopressin are 0.5 to 2 pg/mL, which will maintain urine osmolality above plasma osmolality and urine volume at less than 2 L/day. Increases in plasma osmolality cause a linear increase in plasma vasopressin and a linear increase in urine osmolality as illustrated in Figure 238–2. At a plasma osmolality of about 294 mOsm/kg of water, urine osmolality is maximally concentrated at about 1200 mOsm/kg. Thus the entire physiologic range of urine osmolality is accomplished by changes in plasma vasopressin of 0.5 to 5 pg/mL.

To maintain fluid balance, water must not just be conserved but consumed as well to replace obligate insensible water loss and obligate urine output. In animals, drinking behavior increases linearly with increases in osmolality, similar to the release of vasopressin. In humans, thirst has been less well studied than vasopressin secretion, but it is thought that thirst is not stimulated until a somewhat higher osmolality than the threshold for release of vasopressin. Most humans in a normal day get sufficient water from the catabolism of food or from fluids taken daily that marked thirst is seldom sensed.

Vasopressin acts on V_2, or antidiuretic, receptors in the kidney to cause water retention by stimulating cyclic adenosine monophosphate production in the luminal cell membranes of the collecting duct. Activation of V_2 receptors initiates the movement of aquaporin-2 water channels from the cytoplasm to the apical membrane of the cells. These channels specifically allow the free movement

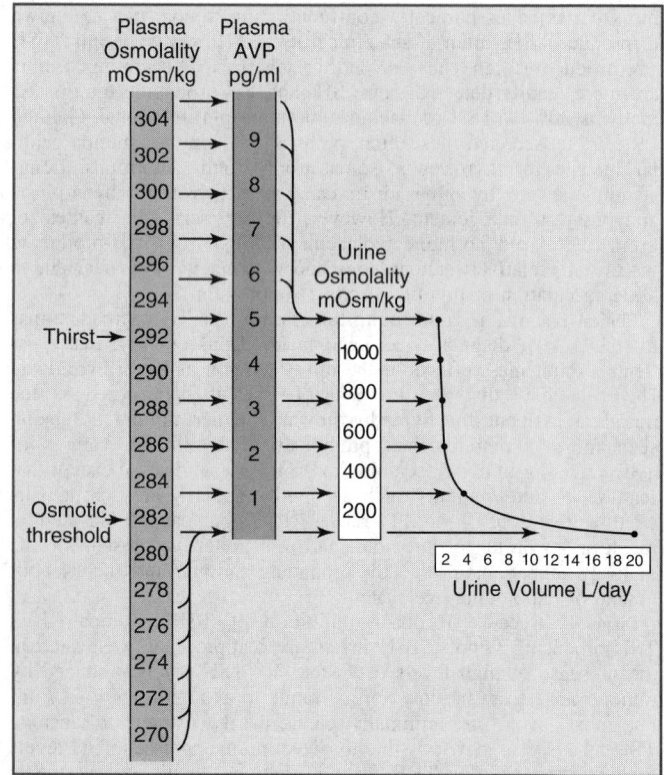

FIGURE 238–2 ■ Idealized schematic of the normal physiologic relationships among plasma osmolality, plasma vasopressin, urine osmolality, and urine volume. The entire physiologic range of urine osmolality occurs with 0.5 to 5 pg/mL of vasopressin. Increases in plasma osmolality above approximately 294 mOsm/kg of water result in increases in plasma vasopressin, but no further concentration of urine, which is limited by the concentration in the renal inner medulla. Decreases in plasma osmolality below approximately 282 cause no further decrease in vasopressin or increase in urine volume. Note that urine volume is plotted as a horizontal scale to emphasize the geometric relationship between urine volume and urine osmolality. (Adapted from Robinson AG: Disorders of antidiuretic hormone secretion. Clin Endocrinol Metab 14:55, 1985.)

of water into the cell. Water exits the cell through the basolateral membrane via aquaporin-3 and aquaporin-4 water channels, which are constitutively present. In the absence of vasopressin, the aquaporin-2 channels rapidly move out of the apical membrane. In addition to this "shuttling" of aquaporin-2 channels, vasopressin also acts via V_2 receptors to regulate the synthesis of aquaporin-2, i.e., increased vasopressin stimulates aquaporin-2 synthesis and the absence of vasopressin suppresses aquaporin-2 synthesis. The hypertonic medullary interstitium determines the maximum concentration of the final urine, which is isotonic with the inner medulla of the kidney (see Chapter 101). Whereas the increase in urine osmolality is linear with increases in plasma vasopressin, the changes in urine volume are geometric. This difference is illustrated in Figure 238–2. Urine volume is maintained at less than 4 L/day until plasma vasopressin is nearly absent; when maximum urine osmolality decreases to less than 50 mOsm/kg, urine volume increases rapidly to 18 to 20 L/day.

VASOPRESSIN AND PRESSURE AND VOLUME REGULATION. In contrast to the osmoregulatory system, volume regulation is anatomically diffuse. High-pressure (baro) receptors are located in the aorta and carotid sinus, and low-pressure volume receptors are located in the left atrium. Stimuli for pressure and volume receptors pass via the glossopharyngeal (9th) and vagal (10th) cranial nerves to the brain stem and through the nucleus tractus solitarii to finally converge on the magnocellular neurons, where the predominant action is inhibitory. Decreases in blood pressure or vascular volume stimulate vasopressin release, whereas maneuvers that increase volume or left atrial pressure (e.g., negative-pressure breathing) decrease the secretion of vasopressin. The release of vasopressin in response to changes in volume or pressure is less sensitive than release in response to osmoreceptors, and a 10 to 15% reduction in blood volume or pressure is needed to stimulate the release of vasopressin. However, once vasopressin is stimulated, the increase in response to baroreceptors is logarithmic, and the levels of vasopressin achieved are markedly above those achieved by osmotic stimulation. Other non-osmotic stimuli such as nausea and intestinal traction probably act through similar neural pathways to release vasopressin. The effector of the pressor component is the V_1 receptor located on vascular smooth muscle. For V_1 receptors the mechanism of action of vasopressin is to increase intracellular calcium rather than stimulate adenylate cyclase. In intact animals the pressor activity of vasopressin is weak because of compensatory vasodilatory systems that tend to modulate the action. The action of vasopressin in regulating blood pressure is prominent only when other endocrine systems are deficient (e.g., in autonomic neuropathy).

VASOPRESSIN AND ADRENOCORTICOTROPIC HORMONE. Vasopressin in the parvicellular and paraventricular neurons that terminate on the pituitary portal system is released into the pituitary portal capillaries and carried to the anterior pituitary. Anterior pituitary corticotrophs are stimulated via V_{1a} receptors to release ACTH.

INTERACTION OF OSMOTIC AND VOLUME REGULATION. In physiologic regulation of water balance, osmotic regulation and volume regulation are usually synergistic. Dehydration causes an increase in osmolality and a decrease in volume, both of which stimulate the release of vasopressin. Similarly, excess administration of fluid causes both expansion of volume and a decrease in osmolality to inhibit vasopressin secretion. Pathologic situations may be characterized by hyponatremia with inadequate volume, as with diuretic use, or a sense of inadequate volume, as with cardiac failure or cirrhosis. In these situations, volume regulation is predominant and vasopressin levels are high. ANP, described in detail in Chapter 234, may affect the osmotic release and action of vasopressin. With volume expansion, ANP is released from atrial myocytes and acts at the kidney to induce natriuresis. ANP is also synthesized in the hypothalamus, where it may act to decrease vasopressin secretion.

PHYSIOLOGY OF OXYTOCIN. Oxytocin has similar concentrations in the posterior pituitary of men and women, but a physiologic function for oxytocin has been described only in women. Stimulation of the nipple during suckling causes release of oxytocin to induce myocontraction of ductile smooth muscle in the breast to eject milk. At parturition the uterus becomes increasingly sensitive to oxytocin, and pulses of oxytocin enhance uterine tone at term and delivery. The greatest release of oxytocin occurs with delivery of the infant, probably secondary to stretching of the vaginal wall. Oxytocin may be more important for its effect of inducing uterine

contraction to inhibit blood loss after delivery than for its role in initiating parturition. In animal studies, administration of oxytocin to males increases sperm transport, but this function has not been documented in humans. Similar to the receptors for vasopressin, the receptors for oxytocin in the breast and in the myometrium are different and independently regulated. At high levels, oxytocin will stimulate vasopressin receptors and vasopressin will stimulate oxytocin receptors.

No syndromes of increased or decreased secretion of oxytocin have been defined. Women with diabetes insipidus secondary to traumatic damage of the magnocellular neurons and presumed absence of oxytocin may have normal pregnancy and delivery and breast-feed their infants. Excessive administration of oxytocin to induce labor can stimulate V_2 receptors of the kidney and cause abnormal water retention and hyponatremia.

DIABETES INSIPIDUS

DEFINITION. Diabetes insipidus is the excretion of a large volume of hypotonic, insipid (tasteless) urine, usually accompanied by polyuria and polydipsia. The large volume, usually greater than 4 L/day, must be distinguished from increased frequency of small volumes and from large volumes of isotonic or hypertonic urine, both of which have other clinical significance. Three pathophysiologic mechanisms come into play in the differential diagnosis of diabetes insipidus: (1) *Hypothalamic diabetes insipidus* is the inability to secrete (and usually to synthesize) vasopressin in response to increased osmolality. No concentration of the dilute filtrate takes place in the renal collecting duct, and a large volume of urine is excreted. This situation produces an increase in serum osmolality with stimulation of thirst and secondary polydipsia. Levels of vasopressin in plasma are unmeasurable or low. (2) *Nephrogenic diabetes insipidus* is a disorder in which an otherwise normal kidney is unable to respond to vasopressin. As in hypothalamic diabetes insipidus, the dilute filtrate entering the collecting duct is excreted as a large volume of hypotonic urine. The rise in serum osmolality that occurs stimulates thirst and produces polydipsia. Unlike hypothalamic diabetes insipidus, however, measured levels of vasopressin in plasma are high. (3) *Primary polydipsia* is a primary disorder of thirst stimulation. Ingested water produces a mild decrease in serum osmolality that turns off the secretion of vasopressin. In the absence of vasopressin action on the kidney, urine does not become concentrated and a large volume of dilute urine is excreted. The amount of vasopressin measured in plasma is low. Although the pathophysiologic mechanisms for the three disorders are distinct, patients in each category usually have polyuria, polydipsia, and normal serum sodium because the normal thirst mechanism is sufficiently sensitive to maintain fluid balance in the first two disorders and the kidney is normally sufficiently responsive to excrete the water load in the third.

CLINICAL FEATURES. HYPOTHALAMIC DIABETES INSIPIDUS. The sudden appearance of hypotonic polyuria after transcranial surgery in the area of the hypothalamus or after head trauma with a basal skull fracture and hypothalamic damage obviously suggests the diagnosis of hypothalamic diabetes insipidus. In these situations, if the patient is unconscious and unable to recognize thirst, hypernatremia is a common accompaniment. However, even in patients with more insidious progression of a specific disease or in patients with idiopathic hypothalamic diabetes insipidus, the onset of polyuria is often relatively abrupt and occurs over a few days. The initial problem is the volume of urine and polydipsia, not the decrease in urine osmolality. Most patients do not complain of polyuria until urine volume exceeds 4 L/day, and as illustrated in Figure 238–2, urine volume is exponentially related to urine osmolality and to plasma vasopressin. Thus urine volume does not exceed 4 L/day until the ability to concentrate the urine is severely limited and plasma vasopressin is nearly absent. This same relationship has been observed in dogs with experimental lesions of the hypothalamus. Such dogs have little increase in urine volume until only 10% of the vasopressin cells remain, and then loss of the remaining 10% produces a rapid and marked increase in urine volume to 10 to 15 times normal. Urine volume seldom exceeds the amount of dilute fluid delivered to the collecting duct (about 18

L in humans), and in many cases urine volume is less because patients voluntarily restrict fluid intake, which causes some mild volume contraction and increased proximal tubular reabsorption of fluid. Patients often express a preference for cold liquids, which are probably more effective in assuaging thirst. Both thirst and urine output persist through the night. Patients with partial diabetes insipidus have some ability to secrete vasopressin, but this secretion is markedly attenuated at normal levels of plasma osmolality. Therefore, these patients have symptoms and urine volume only moderately different from patients with complete diabetes insipidus. Because most patients with hypothalamic diabetes insipidus have sufficient thirst to drink fluid to match urine output, few laboratory abnormalities are present at the time of initial evaluation. Serum sodium may be in the high-normal range, whereas blood urea nitrogen and uric acid may be low secondary to large urine volume.

A variant of hypothalamic diabetes insipidus is the syndrome of absent osmostat with intact volume receptors. This syndrome is referred to as essential hypernatremia because patients have increased sodium and absence of thirst. Physiologic maneuvers demonstrate that when these patients are euvolemic, an increase in plasma osmolality produces neither secretion of vasopressin nor sensation of thirst. However, vasopressin is synthesized by the hypothalamus and stored in the posterior pituitary because stimulation of baroreceptors results in prompt secretion of vasopressin, and the kidney is responsive because vasopressin release by volume receptor stimulation causes urinary concentration. Because patients lack thirst, they are chronically dehydrated with increased serum sodium. It is the dehydration and volume depletion, not the increased osmolality, that stimulate secretion of vasopressin. The amount of urine output depends on the degree of dehydration-induced secretion of vasopressin. If sufficient fluid replacement is given to return extracellular volume to normal, these patients are unable to regulate vasopressin by osmolality and they become markedly polyuric—manifesting the underlying diabetes insipidus.

Rarely, hypothalamic diabetes insipidus occurs as an autosomal dominant pattern of inherited disease. In reported families, the disorders are due to single nucleotide substitution or deletion in the vasopressin gene. Interestingly, in an animal model of hereditary diabetes insipidus (the Brattleboro rat), which is also due to a single nucleotide deletion, the diabetes insipidus is autosomal recessive. Diabetes insipidus is expressed only in the homozygote rat because both alleles of the gene are expressed, and 50% expression of vasopressin is adequate to allow normal water balance. In the human disorder, diabetes insipidus is not present at birth, which suggests normal synthesis of vasopressin presumably by the normal gene. However, by an as yet undetermined mechanism, the abnormal vasopressin translation product synthesized by the mutant allele causes the destruction of vasopressinergic neurons. Neuronal cell death produces diabetes insipidus later in childhood or early in adult years.

Diabetes insipidus with onset during pregnancy may be due to rapid catabolism of vasopressin. The placenta produces a cystine aminopeptidase (oxytocinase or vasopressinase) that enzymatically destroys vasopressin and thus increases the metabolic clearance rate of vasopressin. Polyuria becomes manifested in patients who have limited vasopressin reserve because of some underlying decreased ability to secrete vasopressin or to respond to vasopressin action, e.g., partial hypothalamic diabetes insipidus or compensated nephrogenic diabetes insipidus. Treatment may be required only during the pregnancy, and the patient may return to her previous baseline function without need for therapy when the pregnancy ends. In some patients, hypothalamic diabetes insipidus of any cause first becomes symptomatic during pregnancy and then persists with the usual course of diabetes insipidus.

Myxedema and adrenal insufficiency both impair the ability to excrete free water by renal mechanisms. The simultaneous occurrence of either of these diseases with diabetes insipidus (as may occur with a tumor of the hypothalamus or pituitary) may decrease the large urine output of diabetes insipidus. Replacement treatment for the anterior pituitary deficiency, especially glucocorticoids, may cause sudden and massive excretion of dilute urine. Similarly, the onset of either hypothyroidism or adrenal insufficiency during the course of diabetes insipidus may decrease the need for vasopressin replacement and even cause hyponatremia.

NEPHROGENIC DIABETES INSIPIDUS. The renal response to vasopressin may be impaired by abnormalities of the vasopressin V_2 receptor or the vasopressin-induced water channels aquaporin-2. The gene for the V_2 receptor has been localized to the Xq28 region of the X chromosome, and familial nephrogenic diabetes insipidus secondary to abnormalities in the V_2 receptor is a rare recessive X-linked disease. Symptoms are noted only in affected males who have excessive polyuria and dehydration from birth. Nephrogenic diabetes insipidus caused by abnormal aquaporin-2 is a rare autosomal recessive condition with few reported cases.

Nephrogenic diabetes insipidus may also be acquired during treatment with certain drugs such as demeclocycline (which is used to treat inappropriate secretion of vasopressin), lithium (used to treat bipolar disorders), and fluoride (previously used in fluorocarbon anesthetics) and from electrolyte abnormalities such as hypokalemia and hypercalcemia. Other diseases of the kidney produce polyuria and an inability to concentrate the urine secondary to altered renal medullary blood flow or to other disorders that inhibit maintenance of the hypertonic inner medulla. Renal manifestations of sickle cell disease, sarcoidosis, pyelonephritis, multiple melanoma, analgesic nephropathy, and the like are discussed in Chapter 107.

PRIMARY POLYDIPSIA. In some patients, primary polydipsia follows acute trauma to the hypothalamus and is severe and unremitting, but in most patients primary polydipsia has a slower onset and more erratic course. Virtually any of the pathologic processes described below as etiologies of hypothalamic diabetes insipidus can cause primary stimulation of thirst. Patients may drink even greater amounts of fluid (e.g., >20 L/day) than patients with hypothalamic diabetes insipidus, yet may sleep through the night with minimal disruption. The disorder may be exacerbated during times of stress and not bothersome during normal intervals. Sometimes a lifelong history of habitual excessive water drinking is noted in an entire family. Some patients have obvious psychiatric disorders that contribute to the polydipsia. The physician must always be alert to pharmacologic agents given to treat psychiatric disorders that may result in increased thirst by causing dry mouth, result in nephrogenic diabetes insipidus, or stimulate thirst. Laboratory studies in these patients are normal, although serum sodium may be at the low end of the normal range.

PHYSIOLOGIC DIAGNOSIS. Although osmotic diuresis secondary to hyperglycemia, an intravenous contrast agent, renal injury, and the like is a more common cause of polyuria, the medical history, isotonic urine osmolality, and routine clinical laboratory tests readily distinguish these disorders from diabetes insipidus. The diagnosis of diabetes insipidus is established when concentrations of plasma vasopressin are absent or low and urine osmolality is inappropriately low in the presence of elevated serum osmolality from increased serum sodium. These criteria may be met at the initial examination, especially in acute diabetes insipidus occurring after trauma or after surgery in which fluid replacement has not been adequate. In a patient with hypernatremia and hypotonic urine osmolality with normal renal function, diabetes insipidus is diagnosed. One need only administer a vasopressin agonist and document a renal response with decreased urine volume and increased urine osmolality to confirm the diagnosis of hypothalamic diabetes insipidus. Sometimes in the postoperative state a water diuresis occurs from water retention during the surgical procedure. Vasopressin is normally secreted in response to surgical stress, and fluid administered intravenously during the procedure may be retained. During recovery, when vasopressin levels fall, diuresis of the retained fluid occurs. If further fluid is administered to match the urine output, persistent polyuria might be mistaken for diabetes insipidus. In this situation the physician should decrease the rate of fluid administered and observe the urine output and serum sodium. If urine output decreases and serum sodium remains normal, no treatment is necessary. If serum sodium rises above the normal range and the urine is still hypotonic, the response to a vasopressin agonist will document the diagnosis of diabetes insipidus.

Most outpatients will have polyuria, polydipsia, and normal sodium. In these patients it is necessary to perform a test to increase serum osmolality and measure the urinary response. The best described and easiest to administer is the dehydration test with subsequent response to vasopressin (Fig. 238–3). The test should be

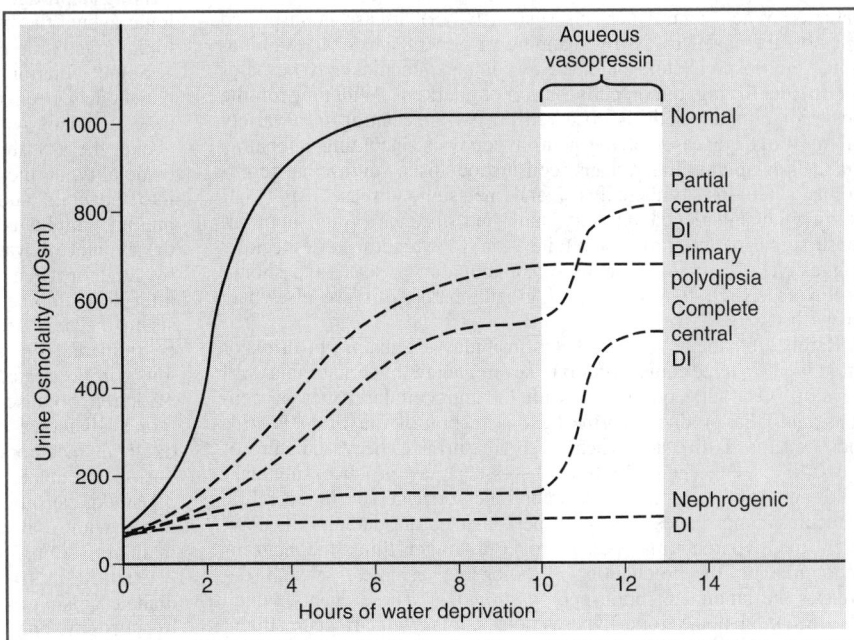

FIGURE 238–3 ■ Responses to the dehydration test described by Miller and associates (*Annals of Internal Medicine,* 1970) to differentiate various types of diabetes insipidus and primary polydipsia. The response to dehydration shows a plateau, and the subsequent change in urine osmolality in response to administered vasopressin is illustrated. See discussion in the text. *DI* = diabetes insipidus. (From Dennis VW: *In* Wyngaarden JB, Smith LH Jr, Bennett JC [eds]: Cecil's Textbook of Medicine, 19th ed. Philadelphia, WB Saunders, 1992, p 495.)

carried out under controlled observation in the hospital or an appropriately equipped outpatient area. The timing of the test depends on the symptoms of the patient. If the patient has marked polyuria during the night, it is best to begin the test during the day because the patient may readily become dehydrated. If the patient has only two or three episodes of nocturia per night, it may be best to begin the test in the evening so that the major part of the dehydration takes place when the patient is asleep. In either case the patient is weighed at the beginning of the test, and the volume and osmolality (usually determined by freezing point depression) of all excreted urine are measured. The patient is weighed after output of each liter of urine. When two consecutive urine samples have osmolality differing by no more than 10% and the patient has lost 2% of body weight, a blood sample is obtained for measurement of serum osmolality, sodium, and plasma vasopressin. The patient is then given 2 mg of desmopressin intravenously or intramuscularly. Patients with normal levels of vasopressin have less than a 5% increase in urine osmolality in response to the administered desmopressin. Patients with complete hypothalamic diabetes insipidus have minimal concentration of urine with dehydration and a marked increase in urine osmolality in response to administered desmopressin (usually greater than 50%).

Patients with nephrogenic diabetes insipidus usually have no urine concentration in response to administered vasopressin, although in some cases of acquired nephrogenic diabetes insipidus some urinary concentration may result. Nephrogenic diabetes insipidus is unequivocally distinguished from hypothalamic diabetes insipidus by measurement of vasopressin in plasma by radioimmunoassay. Vasopressin levels are usually elevated in nephrogenic diabetes insipidus, especially with dehydration.

In patients with partial hypothalamic diabetes insipidus and patients with primary polydipsia, the urine is somewhat concentrated in response to dehydration, but it cannot be expected to be concentrated to the maximum of a normal person because the chronically reduced levels of vasopressin decrease the number of aquaporin-2 water channels and the large urine volume, regardless of cause, washes out the medullary osmotic gradient that determines the maximum urine concentration. When vasopressin is administered, patients with partial hypothalamic diabetes insipidus have a further increase (usually greater than 10%) in urine osmolality, whereas patients with primary polydipsia have no further increase. The reliability of distinguishing these last two disorders with the controlled dehydration test described above is debated. Some patients with primary polydipsia may not become sufficiently dehydrated with the test to secrete maximum vasopressin and hence will have an increase in urine osmolality in response to administered desmo-

pressin. Alternatively, some patients with partial diabetes insipidus may become sufficiently dehydrated that their individual maximal concentration of urine is reached during the test and no further concentration is seen with administered desmopressin. When plasma vasopressin assays become sufficiently sensitive, reliable, and available, plasma vasopressin levels at the end of dehydration may better distinguish these two disorders. In the meantime, it is important to have adequate follow-up of patients with partial diabetes insipidus to ensure that during treatment with vasopressin a good therapeutic response is obtained, as would be expected, and that hyponatremia does not occur, as might be expected if the patient had primary polydipsia.

ETIOLOGIC DIAGNOSIS. The dehydration test will confirm that absence of vasopressin is responsible for the polyuria, but the cause of the lack of vasopressin must then be determined. As noted above, vasopressin is synthesized in paired paraventricular nuclei high on the walls of the third ventricle and in paired supraoptic nuclei lateral to and above the optic chiasm (see Fig. 238–1). Because diabetes insipidus is symptomatic only when 80 to 90% of the vasopressin cells are destroyed, a lesion must be quite large or strategically located where the paths from the four nuclear groups converge into the pituitary stalk just above the diaphragma sellae. Such lesions can be recognized by nuclear magnetic resonance (NMR) scans of the brain. An additional observation on NMR scans is that in about 80% of normal subjects the posterior pituitary on T1-weighted images is seen as a high intense signal (bright spot). Commonly in diabetes insipidus, the hyperintense signal of the posterior pituitary is lost, which is thought to be due to depletion of stored hormone. It is not known exactly what component of the hormone precursor store is responsible for the hyperintense signal.

Tumors that cause diabetes insipidus are most often benign primary intracranial tumors such as craniopharyngioma, ependymoma (suprasellar germinoma), or pinealoma that arises in the third ventricle. Primary tumors of the anterior pituitary cause diabetes insipidus only when suprasellar extension is present. Metastasis to the hypothalamus from lung, breast, melanoma, and such carcinomas may lodge in the portal capillaries of the median eminence, destroy the supraopticohypophysial tract, and thereby cause diabetes insipidus. Granulomatous diseases such as Langerhans' cell histiocytosis, sarcoidosis, or tuberculosis may destroy vasopressin cells in the hypothalamus. Leukemic infiltrates of the hypothalamus may cause diabetes insipidus. In diseases with peripheral manifestations, the diagnosis is usually suspected on the basis of general medical findings. Idiopathic diabetes insipidus is probably an autoimmune disease, and other autoimmune diseases are recognized in affected patients. When central nervous system (CNS) disease is suspected but not diagnosed by NMR scanning or general physical examination, cerebrospinal fluid obtained by lumbar puncture may be helpful in identifying tumor cells or tumor markers. Widening of the posterior pituitary stalk is observed on NMR scanning in a variety of infiltrative diseases of the neurohypophysis, including idiopathic diabetes insipidus, Langerhans' cell histiocytosis, suprasellar germinoma, sarcoidosis, tuberculosis, and metastatic disease. An NMR study with a widened pituitary stalk and absence of the hyperintense signal of the posterior pituitary on T1 weighting is especially suggestive of a granulomatous or inflammatory disease and should prompt a search for evidence of granulomatous disease elsewhere in the body.

Rarely, if patients with diabetes insipidus are unable to drink or are given a hypertonic solution, severe acute hypernatremia will develop. Osmotic equilibrium with the intracellular water of neurons and glia produces shrinking of the brain. The brain is in a closed vault (skull), and when the brain shrinks, the vasculature of the CNS is engorged. Rupture of vessels may produce subarachnoid hemorrhage, gross intracerebral hemorrhage, or intracerebral petechial hemorrhages producing permanent brain damage. If, however, the hypernatremia persists over a longer time, the neurons accommodate by production of "idiogenic osmoles," which decreases the amount of brain neuron shrinkage. These events, which also occur in non-ketotic hyperosmolar coma, will affect treatment recommendations.

TREATMENT. Water diuresis is the primary manifestation of diabetes insipidus, and water replacement in adequate quantities avoids metabolic complications. The aim of therapy is to reduce the amount of polyuria and polydipsia to a tolerable level while avoiding overtreatment, which might produce water retention and hyponatremia. The best therapeutic agent is the vasopressin agonist desmopressin. Desmopressin is different from vasopressin in that the terminal amino group of cystine has been removed to prolong the duration of action and D-arginine is substituted for L-arginine in position 8 to decrease the pressor effect. In therapeutic dosage, this agent acts on V_2, or antidiuretic, receptors with minimal action on V_1, or pressor, receptors. Desmopressin is available in tablets of 0.1 mg or 0.2 mg for oral administration and in either a spray bottle that delivers a fixed dose of 10 μg in 100 μL or in a bottle with a rhinal catheter that can deliver from 50 to 200 μL (5 to 20 μg for intranasal administration). When therapy is initiated, it is best to begin with a low dose, either ½ of an 0.1-mg tablet, a single spray of 10 μg (100 μL), or 5 μg (50 μL) by the rhinal tube, at night to allow the patient to sleep through the night and then determine the duration of action by quantifying the polyuria the next day. The duration of action of a single dose varies between patients from 6 to 24 hours, but in most patients a dosage can be determined that gives a good therapeutic response on an every-12-hour schedule for the nasal spray and an 8- or 12-hour schedule for the tablets. If patients are never polyuric on a fixed schedule, it may be advisable to delay administration of a dose once or twice a week to allow diuresis of any accumulated water. Desmopressin is also available for parenteral use in 2-mL vials of 4 μg/mL; 5 to 10% of an intranasal quantity administered intravenously, intramuscularly, or subcutaneously gives an equivalent response. Parenteral administration is especially useful postoperatively or when a patient is unable to take the nasal preparation.

Some orally administered pharmacologic agents are also useful in treating diabetes insipidus. Chlorpropamide in doses of 100 to 500 mg daily enhances the effect of vasopressin at the renal tubule and is especially useful in patients with partial hypothalamic diabetes insipidus. An antidiuretic effect is noted in 1 to 2 days, but maximum antidiuresis may not be achieved until after several days of administration. Carbamazepine (Tegretol) in doses of 200 to 600 mg/day causes release of vasopressin. Clofibrate also stimulates the release of endogenous vasopressin at doses of 500 mg every 6 hours. Thiazide diuretics cause sodium depletion and volume contraction and decrease urine volume by increasing the proximal tubular reabsorption of glomerular filtrate. Prostaglandin inhibitors (e.g., indomethacin) block the normal action of prostaglandin E to inhibit the action of vasopressin on the kidney. Although use of a prostaglandin inhibitor is not a primary treatment of diabetes insipidus, it may alter the antidiuretic response of other agents. Chloro-

thiazide, amiloride, or prostaglandin inhibitors may be useful in treating nephrogenic diabetes insipidus. For each of the pharmacologic agents the prescribing physician should be careful of potential toxicity and side effects.

Some situations require special attention during therapy. If the patient has been chronically hypernatremic and the brain has had time to adapt with production of idiogenic osmoles as described above, therapy should not be overly zealous. Too rapid lowering of osmolality in the extracellular fluid will produce a shift of water into the brain and cause cerebral edema. In this situation, desmopressin can be administered to produce constant antidiuresis, but the amount of water should be regulated to decrease the osmolality by no more than about 1 mEq every 2 hours. Postoperatively or after head trauma, diabetes insipidus may be transient (see prognosis in the next section), and long-term maintenance therapy cannot be immediately established. Pregnant patients with diabetes insipidus can be treated with desmopressin, which has a normal duration of action because it is not destroyed by vasopressinase. The additional advantage of desmopressin is that it has little action on the oxytocin receptors of the uterus. It should be noted, however, that during pregnancy normal plasma osmolality decreases by 10 mOsm/kg because of changes in serum sodium, and pregnant patients with diabetes insipidus require sufficient desmopressin to maintain serum sodium at this lower level.

COURSE AND PROGNOSIS. The prognosis of properly treated diabetes insipidus is excellent. Historical complications of bladder hypertrophy and hydroureter secondary to voluntarily decreasing urine frequency are largely unseen with modern therapy. When the diabetes insipidus is secondary to a recognized disease process, it is that disease that determines the ultimate prognosis. In some specific clinical situations the course is different and characteristic. Postoperative or post-traumatic diabetes insipidus is often due to rupture of the pituitary stalk and can follow a course referred to as "triphasic" (Fig. 238–4). The 1st phase is diabetes insipidus secondary to axon shock and lack of release of vasopressin. This phase lasts for 5 to 10 days and is followed by a second phase of antidiuresis, which is thought to be produced by uncontrolled release of vasopressin from the large storage pool in the axon terminals of the posterior pituitary. This store is sufficient to produce constant antidiuresis for an additional 5 to 10 days. The possibility of this course developing is one reason for closely monitoring desmopressin therapy in a postoperative or post-traumatic patient. Continued administration of desmopressin and especially continued forcing of fluids either orally or parenterally will produce profound hyponatremia during the second phase. Hyponatremia is often heralded by nausea or vomiting, and severe hyponatremia may cause cerebral edema and serious neurologic sequelae. Thus fluids may need to be restricted during this period, as they are in therapy for inappropri-

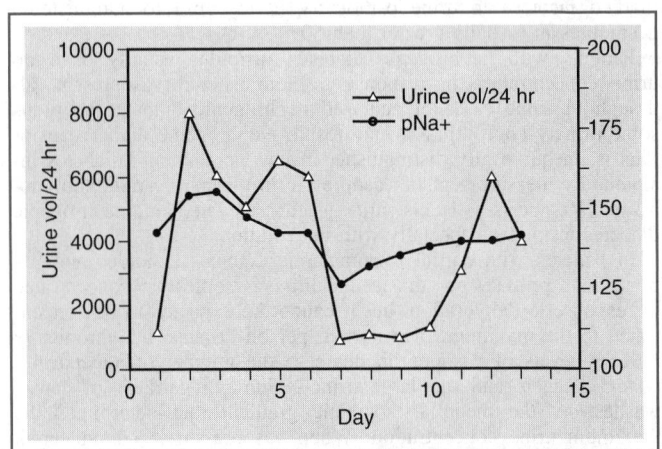

FIGURE 238-4 ■ Triphasic response of the pituitary stalk to trauma. Urine output (open triangles) and serum Na+ (solid dots) are illustrated. Note the onset of diabetes insipidus immediately after the head trauma and lasting for 6 days. On days 7 through 10 a marked decrease in diuresis (with elevated urine osmolality) occurred, typical of the second phase with inappropriate release of vasopressin. During this time the patient actually became hyponatremic and required fluid restriction to treat the hyponatremia. After day 10 a return of diabetes insipidus was noted.

ate secretion of antidiuretic hormone. The third or final phase is the return of diabetes insipidus after the pool of stored vasopressin has been exhausted. This phase may be permanent or transient. Eventually, sufficient vasopressin function may return to allow a lessening in intensity or discontinuation of treatment, which usually occurs within the first year of diabetes insipidus but has occurred as long as 10 years after the initiating event. Potential return of function is another reason for occasionally withholding therapy during long-term treatment. Interestingly, the second phase of excess vasopressin and hyponatremia has been reported without preceding or subsequent diabetes insipidus. This variation is reported as transient postoperative syndrome of inappropriate secretion of antidiuretic hormone. It is probably due to trauma to only some vasopressin axons. Sufficient functioning vasopressin neurons are present to prevent the diabetes insipidus of the first and third phases, but sufficient leakage of vasopressin occurs to cause the second phase. It is only the setting and timing that identify this phenomenon as an isolated second phase of the triphasic response.

Diabetes insipidus should not be considered idiopathic until after 4 years of follow-up. Over this interval, annual computed tomography or NMR scans are indicated to test for the appearance of a tumor or infiltrative process that may not have been detected at the initial examination.

SYNDROME OF INAPPROPRIATE SECRETION OF ANTIDIURETIC HORMONE

Excess secretion of vasopressin can be caused by abnormal secretion from the posterior pituitary or by ectopic synthesis and secretion of vasopressin by a tumor. The excess vasopressin causes water retention, volume expansion, and natriuresis, with consequent hyponatremia. This disorder is discussed in Chapters 101 and 102.

Fujiwara TJ, Morgan K: Molecular biology of diabetes insipidus. Annu Rev Med 46: 331, 1995. *A description of the various genetic causes of hypothalamic and nephrogenic diabetes insipidus.*

Martin PY, Schrier RW: Role of aquaporin-2 water channels in urinary concentration and dilution defects. Kidney Int 53(Suppl. 65):57, 1998. *A review of the clinical significance of water channels.*

Reeves WB, Bichet DG, Andreoli TE: The posterior pituitary and water metabolism. *In* Wilson JD, Foster DW, Kronenberg HM, Larsen PR (eds): Williams Textbook of Endocrinology, 9th ed. Philadelphia, WB Saunders, 1998, pp 341–387. *Extensively referenced chapter with a detailed description of the anatomy of the neurohypophysis, physiology of vasopressin and oxytocin, and abnormalities in water metabolism.*

Robertson GL: Diabetes insipidus. Endocrinol Metab Clin North Am 24:549, 1995. *A summary of many clinical research studies by this investigator. An especially good description of vasopressin levels in clinical conditions.*

Robinson AG, Verbalis JG: Diabetes insipidus. *In* Bardin CW (ed): Current Therapy in Endocrinology and Metabolism, 6th ed. St Louis, CV Mosby, 1997, pp 1–7. *Concise guide to acute and chronic therapy for diabetes insipidus.*

239 THE THYROID

Wolfgang H. Dillmann

Anatomy and Physiology

The thyroid, the largest endocrine gland in the body, weighs about 20 g, the right lobe usually being larger than the left. Adult size is reached at age 15. The two lateral lobes lie anterior to the thyroid cartilage and are connected by a small isthmus located just below the cricoid cartilage. The lobes have a pointed superior pole and a rounded inferior pole with a thickness of about 2 cm, a length of 4 to 5 cm, and a width of 2 to 3 cm. The lobes are divided by fibrous septa into pseudolobes composed of spherical structures called follicles. A dense capillary network surrounds the follicles, which are richly innervated by sympathetic and parasympathetic nerve endings. The follicles consist of a single layer of epithelial cells surrounding a lumen filled with a proteinaceous colloid material consisting of over 75% thyroglobulin. Thyroglobulin is formed by the epithelial thyroid cells, which both synthesize and store the hormone.

A feedback loop involving the hypothalamus, pituitary, and thy-

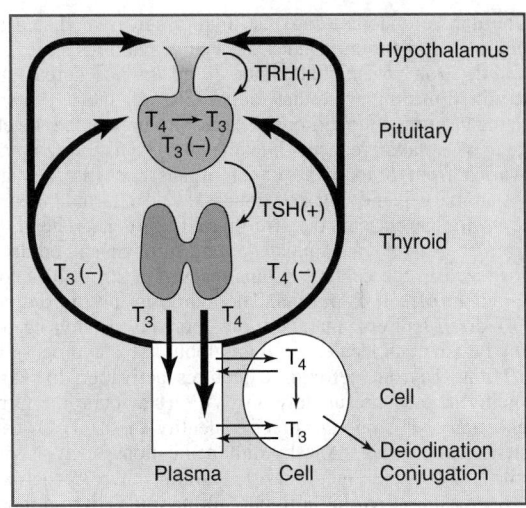

FIGURE 239–1 ■ Hypothalamic-pituitary-thyroid interrelationship. TRH exerts a positive stimulatory effect on TSH secretion, which stimulates thyroid hormone formation. T_4 is the primary thyroid secretory product, which is converted in the cells of specific organs, such as kidney and liver, to T_3. T_3 is the most biologically active thyroid hormone and is inactivated by further deiodination or conjugation and biliary excretion.

roid gland regulates the glandular secretion of thyroid hormone (Fig. 239–1). The hypothalamus generates thyroid-releasing hormone (TRH) to energize pituitary thyroid-stimulating hormone (TSH). TSH, in turn, stimulates thyroid hormonal output, which feeds back on both hypothalamus and pituitary to complete the regulatory circle.

Thyroid Hormone Formation

Thyroxine (T_4) is the major secretory product of the thyroid, with a daily production rate of 80 to 100 μg. T_4 is produced only by the thyroid gland. In contrast, only 20% of the daily production rate of triiodothyronine (T_3) is derived from thyroid secretion and 80% from peripheral T_4 conversion (Fig. 239–2). The daily production rate of T_3 is 30 to 40 μg. Normal thyroid hormone formation requires normal levels of TSH and an adequate but not excessive supply of iodine. Optimal iodine intake is 150 to 300 μg/day. In some mountainous areas of the world, daily iodine supplies can be as low as 20 to 30 μg. The United States population, however, has a high iodine intake, with a daily supply of 600 to 700 μg, much of which derives from food additives such as iodized salt and flour. The iodine intake in the United States has been declining recently. Iodine is reduced to iodide (I^-) in the gastrointestinal tract and readily absorbed. Iodide is removed from the bloodstream by uptake and concentration in the thyroid gland and excretion in the

FIGURE 239–2 ■ Structure of the thyroid hormones.

urine. The uptake of iodide into the thyroid cell is mediated by the sodium/iodide symporter. Under normal conditions, the kidney clears iodide from plasma at about 30 mL/min, whereas thyroid clearance is 8 mL/min, so that only 25% of intake enters the thyroid under normal conditions. Excess iodine intake levels the percentage of uptake; reduced intake raises it. Thyroid uptake of iodide varies from 5 to 30%. Other organs such as the salivary glands, mammary glands, gastric mucosa, and choroid plexus also can take up iodine but cannot form thyroid hormone. The ability of the thyroid to actively accumulate iodine through an iodide transporter localized in the cell membrane leads to a 20 to 40:1 concentration gradient of cell to plasma. The iodide in the thyroid cells is rapidly oxidized and enzymatically incorporated via thyroid peroxidase into tyrosine molecules of thyroglobulin by a process called organification. Thyroid peroxidase requires activation by H_2O_2. A flavoprotein enzyme, presumably an NAPDH cytochrome C reductase, generates H_2O_2, but the precise identity of the H_2O_2-generating system is uncertain. Antithyroid medications such as propylthiouracil (PTU) and methimazole inhibit thyroid peroxidase, thereby decreasing thyroid hormone formation. Thyroid hormone formation occurs on thyroglobulin, a 660-kd glycoprotein, with 25% of its tyrosine residues accessible to iodination. The monoiodinated tyrosine (MIT) and the deiodinated tyrosine (DIT) are coupled by the thyroid peroxidase enzyme to form T_4 by linking two DITs or, for T_3 formation, linking one MIT and one DIT molecule. Thyroglobulin contains only 3 or 4 T_4 and 0.2 to 0.3 T_3 residues. The organification and coupling reactions on thyroglobulin occur at the luminal border of the thyrocyte, which then exocytoses and stores it as colloid. Thyroid hormone secretion starts with endocytosis of a colloid droplet by the luminal cell membrane of the thyrocyte. The colloid droplet then combines with lysosomes to form phagolysosomes with thyroglobulin proteolysis and release of T_4 and T_3 at the basal border into the capillaries. Iodotyrosine and especially MIT and DIT, which are liberated from thyroglobulin, are deiodinated by a specific deiodinase. Iodide thus liberated mixes with iodide entering from the blood and is reused for organification. Decreased levels of this deiodinase rarely may cause goiter and hypothyroidism.

REGULATION OF THYROID HORMONE SYNTHESIS

Thyroid hormone synthesis is influenced by intrathyroidal factors, primarily the amount of iodide in the thyroid cell; by extrathyroidal factors, especially peptide hormones, which can occupy the TSH receptor especially under normal conditions; and by the thyroid-stimulating immunoglobulin (TSI) in Graves' disease. Under conditions of very low iodine intake, T_3 preferentially is formed instead of T_4. Iodide excess in the thyroid leads to a short-term inhibition of thyroid hormone formation. After about 48 hours, however, the iodide transporter system decreases and thyroid hormone formation returns to normal in spite of elevated circulating iodide levels. Excess iodide also inhibits thyroid hormone release. Increased iodination of thyroglobulin increases its resistance to proteolytic degradation, thereby freeing less T_4 and T_3. Paradoxically, excess iodide can also increase thyroid hormone formation, especially in abnormal thyroid glands. For these reasons, iodine should not be used to treat thyroid diseases except under special conditions. In addition to iodide, TSH influences thyroid function by stimulating all steps of thyroid hormone formation. TSH binding to TSH receptors stimulates cyclic adenosine monophosphate formation and subsequently protein kinase A activity. Such binding also stimulates the phospholipase C-based signaling system and the *ras* proto-oncogene kinase pathway. In addition to the marked influences that are exerted on thyroid hormone formation by iodide and TSH, IGF-1, EGF, prostaglandins, and cytokines such as interleukins and catecholamines modify thyroid function.

EXTRATHYROIDAL HORMONE PRODUCTION AND TURNOVER

Most T_3 is produced by extrathyroidal 5′ deiodination of T_4, which allows for alteration in T_3 production independent of changes in thyroid function. Because T_3 is three to four times as biologically active as T_4, extrathyroidal regulation of T_3 levels has

important consequences reflected by the non-thyroidal illness syndrome discussed below. The conversion of T_4 to T_3 is performed by two forms of 5′ deiodinases. Type I 5′ deiodinase contains the rarely used amino acid selenocysteine and is most active in liver and kidney. The activity of type I 5′ deiodinase declines with hypothyroidism and is inhibited by propylthiouracil and glucocorticoids. Type II 5′ deiodinase is active in the central nervous system (CNS), pituitary, brown adipose tissue, and placenta. It resists inhibition by PTU and increases with hypothyroidism, resulting in near-normal CNS T_3 levels. A third deiodinase, termed 5 deiodinase or type III 5 deiodinase, removes the inner ring iodide to form the biologically inactive reverse T_3 from T_4 and metabolizes T_3 to diiodothyronine (T_2). The thyroid hormone derivatives, including reverse T_3 and the di- and monothyronine compounds, have no currently recognized biologic importance.

In addition to deiodination, by which 80% of T_4 is metabolized, thyroid hormones are metabolized by transfer of glucoronyl and sulfate residues to the phenolic hydroxyl group of thyroid hormone and by biliary excretion. Deamination and decarboxylation of the alanine side chain and cleavage of the ether bridge also contribute to thyroid hormone metabolism. Certain specific differences in the metabolism of T_4 and T_3 have clinical importance. The half-life of T_4 is 1 week, and its total body store is 800 μg, in contrast to the half-life of 1 day for T_3, with total body stores amounting to 50 μg. These principles make T_4 more suitable than T_3 for chronic thyroid hormone replacement. Hyperthyroidism and vigorous exercise shorten the half-life of thyroid hormones, and hypothyroidism increases it. Drugs listed in Table 239–1 also influence thyroid hormone binding and metabolism.

Hormone Transport

T_4 and T_3 exist in plasma in free and protein-bound forms. T_4 is strongly protein bound, and only 0.03% is free. T_3, with its higher biologic activity, possesses 10 times less protein binding such that 0.3% is free. Only the free hormone enters cells, exerts its biologic action, and determines thyroid physiologic status. The most important binding proteins are thyroxine-binding globulin (TBG), transthyretin, and thyroxine-binding prealbumin albumin (TBPA); albumin and some lipoproteins play a minor role. TBG is a glyco-protein synthesized in the liver with a molecular weight of 55 kd. It has one binding site for either T_4 or T_3, with a 10-fold higher affinity for T_4. The serum concentration of TBG is about 20 mg/L to allow for binding of 20 μg of T_4 per deciliter. Transthyretin has two binding sites for T_4, but with an affinity 100-fold lower than that of TBG. T_3 binds weakly to transthyretin. The total binding capacity of transthyretin for T_4 is very large at 200 μg of T_4 per deciliter. Albumin has one binding site for T_4 or T_3, with a 50-fold lower affinity compared with TBG. In normal plasma, the T_4-binding distribution is 80% of T_4 binding to TBG, 15% to transthyretin, and 5% to albumin and lipoproteins. For T_3, the distribution is 90% bound to TBG and the rest to albumin and lipoproteins, with little binding to transthyretin. Table 239–1 lists conditions leading to alterations in TBG. Changes in total T_4 or T_3 resulting from such alterations may be confused with conditions leading to thyroid hormone excess or deficiency due to hyperthy-

Table 239–1 ■ FACTORS INFLUENCING THYROID HORMONE BINDING TO THYROXINE-BINDING GLOBULIN (TBG)

Increased TBG concentration
  Congenital abnormality
  Hyperestrogenic state
    Pregnancy, estrogen therapy
  Disease related
    Hepatitis, biliary cirrhosis, acute intermittent porphyria
  Drugs
    Tamoxifen, perphenazine, clofibrate
Decreased TBG concentration
  Congenital abnormality
  Drugs
    Glucocorticoids (large doses), androgenic steroids, asparaginase
  Severe systemic illness
    Nephrotic syndrome, chronic liver disease, protein malnutrition
Drugs interfering with binding to normal TBG
  Salicylates, diazepam, phenytoin, furosemide, high levels of free fatty acids

roidism or hypothyroidism. Elevated or decreased total T_4 or T_3 levels caused by abnormalities in binding proteins are always accompanied by normal free T_4 and free T_3 concentrations and a euthyroid state. Elevated levels of TBG as they occur, for example, in pregnant patients or patients with acute hepatitis lead to increased levels of total T_4 and T_3. Because more T_4 is bound, less T_4 is able to enter the tissue to be metabolized and inhibit TSH secretion. Slightly higher TSH levels result in increased thyroid hormone formation and a new steady state accompanied by normal free thyroid hormone concentrations. Specific drugs also can lower thyroid hormone concentrations without lowering thyroid hormone-binding proteins (see Table 239–1). For example, salicylic acid or phenytoin competes with thyroid hormone for binding to TBG. The effects of phenytoin are more complex in that they reduce both total serum T_4 levels and slightly lower free T_4 concentrations. TSH concentrations remain normal under such circumstances, and the patients are not hypothyroid. In contrast to alterations in binding proteins, increases or decreases in thyroid hormone production lead to abnormalities in both total and free hormone concentrations.

THYROID HORMONE ACTION

Most thyroid hormone effects are mediated by the binding of T_3 to nuclear thyroid hormone receptor proteins. T_3 has a 10-fold higher affinity for this nuclear receptor than T_4, accounting for the higher biologic activity of T_3. T_3 nuclear receptors belong to the c erbA proto-oncogene family and are encoded by the genes c erbA α and c erbA β. Each gene has several splice variants, only some of which bind T_3. The T_3 nuclear receptor is a T_3-activated transcription factor that binds to specific nucleotide sequences located upstream or downstream of the transcription start site of T_3-responsive genes. Many T_3-responsive genes show an increase in transcription upon T_3 binding to the nuclear T_3 receptor protein. This leads to increased formation of specific mRNAs and proteins such as those coding for growth hormone, malic enzyme, myosin heavy chain α and the calcium pump of the sarcoplasmic reticulum. T_3 suppresses transcription of other genes such as the gene coding for the TSH-α and TSH-β subunits. In this scenario, specific mutations of the c erbA β receptor lead to the generalized thyroid hormone resistant syndrome: The mutant $T_3\beta$ receptor interferes with the action of normal T_3 receptor proteins. In addition to its effects on transcription, T_3 influences the half-life of mRNA and proteins and affects the translation of mRNA, a step that may lead to rapid changes in ion transport.

Braverman LE, Utiger RD (eds): Werner and Ingbar's The Thyroid, 6th ed. Philadelphia, JB Lippincott, 1991. *A basic text.*

Lazar MA: Thyroid hormone receptors: Multiple forms, multiple possibilities. Endocrinol Rev 14:184, 1993.

Refetoff S, Weiss RE, Usala SJ: The syndromes of resistance to thyroid hormone. Endocrinol Rev 14:348, 1993.

Vassart G, Dumont JE: The thyrotropin receptor and the regulation of thyrocyte function and growth. Endocrinol Rev 13:596, 1992. *The titles of the above articles are self-explanatory.*

EVALUATION OF PATIENTS WITH THYROID DISEASE

The evaluation of patients with thyroid disease includes a physical examination of the thyroid, laboratory tests for thyroid function and, when indicated, specific other procedures including ultrasonography, radioactive iodine uptake and scan, and fine-needle aspiration.

Physical Examination

Palpation of the thyroid gland is an important part of the general physical examination, and abnormalities in size, consistency, and contour of the gland are a common finding. For example, 6% of women have thyroid nodules. An enlargement of the thyroid, however, may be a first clue for Graves' disease; or a firm thyroid nodule can represent thyroid cancer. Examination of the thyroid begins by having the patient swallow while observing the contour of the neck from the side. Thyroid enlargements and irregularities, like a nodule, moving up from the substernal area can be identified. Palpation of the thyroid can be performed by standing behind the patient and using the fingers of both hands to identify the isthmus lying just below the cricoid cartilage. Moving laterally, the second, third, and fourth fingers can palpate both thyroid lobes. By exerting

gentle pressure during swallowing, the surface of the thyroid moving past the fingers reveals enlargement or the presence of thyroid nodules. A thyroid examination should always include palpation of lateral and submandibular lymph nodes. The size of thyroid nodules can be recorded by measuring their two largest diameters.

Measurement of Thyroid Hormone Values

Techniques employed for measurement of T_4, free T_4, T_3, and TSH by radioimmunoassays or enzyme-coupled immunoassays are rapidly changing. The newer assays provide for increased assay sensitivity. Radioimmunoassays are progressively being replaced by enzyme-linked immunoabsorption assays, and new chemoluminescent compounds are available for supersensitive TSH assays. Serum thyroid hormone concentrations for T_4, free T_4, T_3, and TSH in normals and patients with thyroid disease are given in Table 239–2. These measurements accurately define thyroid function in most persons, making more specialized tests rarely needed.

TOTAL AND FREE T_4. Total T_4 values (4.5 to 12.5 μg/dL) are altered by changes in thyroid function or changes in the concentration affinities of thyroid hormone-binding proteins. Determination of free T_4 levels (non-protein-bound) corrects for these abnormalities. Current laboratory capacities involve quantitation of non-protein-bound T_4 by a two-step fluorometric enzyme immunoassay or by equilibrium dialysis. Normal values range from 0.9 to 2 ng/dL. Some of these assays occasionally falsely identify too high free T_4 values in patients with dysalbuminic hyperthyroxemia, but non-protein-bound T_4 measurement by the two-step immunoassay approach gives a good approximation of free T_4. This free T_4 index is constructed by multiplying the total T_4 by an estimated protein binding (usually the T_3 uptake test). The T_4 index does not adequately reflect the thyroid status in patients with the non-thyroidal illness syndrome, as discussed later.

Measurement of total T_3 levels by enzyme-coupled immunoassays has a normal range of 80 to 220 ng/dL and is also influenced by alterations in binding proteins, but to a lesser extent. The total T_3 assay should not be confused with the T_3 uptake or T_3 resin test, which is used to calculate the free thyroxine index.

SERUM REVERSE T_3. Reverse T_3 (rT_3) (normal range 20 to 40 ng/dL) should be determined only in special situations. Its level is elevated (40 to 120 ng/dL) in patients with various systemic illnesses, leading to the non-thyroidal illness syndrome (NTI). Because of decreased T_4, free T_4, and T_3 levels in some of these patients, its determination can help to distinguish NTI from hypothyroidism. In hypothyroid patients, reverse T_3 levels are decreased.

The levels of the thyroxine hormone-binding proteins, TBG, transthyretin, and albumin, can be directly measured by immunoassays. During pregnancy and with estrogen treatment, TBG levels are elevated 2- to 3-fold owing to a decreased metabolic clearance of TBG molecules, which have an increase in glycosylation. An albumin variant with increased affinity for T_4 exists in the familial dysalbuminic syndrome and leads to elevated T_4 levels with normal T_3 values and uptake. A transthyretin variant with similar effects on T_4 binding has also been described. Table 239–3 lists causes of increased T_4 levels.

SERUM THYROGLOBULIN. Thyroglobulin is produced only by thyroid tissue. Normal persons have low but detectable thyroglobulin levels. Total surgical removal of thyroid tissue for cancer should result in undetectable thyroglobulin levels. Determination of thyroglobulin levels by immunoassays has its most useful application after thyroid cancer surgery. The upper normal limit of thyroglobulin is 20 to 25 ng/dL, and levels above that range may indicate a return of thyroid cancer. Thyroglobulin levels also increase

Table 239–2 ■ SERUM THYROID HORMONE VALUES IN NORMAL PERSONS AND PATIENTS WITH THYROID DISEASE

	NORMAL	HYPERTHYROID	HYPOTHYROID
T_4 (μg/dL)	4.5–12.5	>12.5	<4.5
Free T_4 (ng/dL)	0.9–2	>2	<0.9
T_3 (ng/dL)	80–220	>220	<80
TSH (μU/mL)	0.3–6	<0.3	>6

Table 239–3 ■ CAUSES OF INCREASED SERUM TOTAL T₄ CONCENTRATION

THYROID STATE CONDITION	T$_4$	FREE T$_4$	T$_3$	TSH	COMMENTS
Hyperthyroid state	H	H	H or N	L	High T$_4$ combined with hypermetabolic state and hyperthyroidism
Euthyroid state					
Binding abnormalities					
Thyroxine-binding globulin levels increased	H	N	H	N	Autosomal dominant
T$_4$ binding to albumin increased (familial dysalbuminemic hyperthyroxinemia)	H	N,H*	N	N	*Same "free T$_4$" methods lead to erroneous results
T$_4$ binding by transthyretin increased (familial)	H	N	N	N	
T$_4$ antibodies present	H	N,H	N,L,*H*	N	*Method based, anti–T$_3$ antibody may also be present
Drug effects					
Inhibitors of 5′-deiodinase					
Oral cholecystographic contrast agents (ipodate, iopanoate)	H	H	L	H	Inhibition of T$_3$ formation
Amiodarone	H	H	L	L,N	
Propranolol	H	N	L,N	N,H	Only with large doses
Heparin	H	N,H	N	N	Temporary after IV doses
T$_4$ administration	H	H	N	L	Mild hyperthyroxinemia in patients on T$_4$ replacement
Various disorders					
Non-thyroidal illness syndrome	H,N	N,L	L	N,L,H	See text for detail
Hyperemesis gravidarum	H	H,N	N	L	During early part of pregnancy; remits
Acute psychiatric illness	H,N	H,N	N	L	During acute phase; remits without treatment
Extrathyroidal deiodinase defect	H	H	N	N	A few case reports but not completely documented
Thyroid hormone resistance syndrome (pituitary and generalized)	H	H	H	H	In generalized resistance syndrome, hypothyroid features can be present, especially related to central nervous system development. If only pituitary resistance, thyrotoxic symptoms

H = high; N = normal; L = low.
Sequence indicates frequency of occurrence; for example, free T$_4$ = HN—more frequently free T$_4$ is high, but normal levels can also be encountered.

when patients become hypothyroid, as occurs, for example, in preparation for radioactive iodine scanning and treatment. Determination of thyroglobulin levels at that time is strongly recommended. Normal thyroglobulin levels do not completely exclude the return of thyroid cancer because in about 10% of patients with thyroid cancer, thyroglobulin is normal in spite of the return of thyroid cancer. Intake of thyroid hormones leads to a decrease of thyroid tissue and thus lowers thyroglobulin levels. Patients with thyrotoxicosis factitia have, therefore, low thyroglobulin levels, in contrast to patients with thyroiditis. In both of these conditions, radioactive iodine uptake is low and thyroglobulin levels can help distinguish between these two conditions. In the presence of antithyroglobulin antibodies, accurate determination of thyroglobulin by immunoassays is not possible.

THYROID-STIMULATING HORMONE. Serum TSH levels correlate inversely with active thyroid hormone concentrations and represent the best single index to the presence of primary hyperthyroidism or primary hypothyroidism. In hypothyroidism with low thyroid hormone concentrations, TSH levels rise above the upper normal limit of 6 μU/mL. In hyperthyroidism with elevated thyroid hormone levels, TSH levels fall below the lower normal limit of 0.3 μU/mL. TSH levels as currently measured fall below the lower limit of normal in patients with hyperthyroidism, whatever the cause. Suppressed TSH levels also can accompany other conditions, including pituitary or hypothalamic disease; non-thyroidal illness; treatment with dopamine, glucocorticoids, and other drugs; and psychiatric illness or recent recovery from hyperthyroidism. In secondary hypothyroidism due to pituitary failure (< 5% of all hypothyroidism), the formation and secretion of thyroid hormone is low but TSH levels fail to rise. Similarly, in hypothalamic disease leading to decreased TRH formation, TSH levels are not elevated

in spite of decreased T$_4$ and T$_3$ concentrations. Elevated TSH levels rarely occur in the absence of hypothyroidism. TSH-producing pituitary tumors rarely cause hyperthyroidism. In the generalized thyroid hormone resistance syndrome, however, TSH levels are inappropriately elevated in proportion to the markedly elevated T$_4$ and T$_3$ levels. In hypothyroidism, markedly elevated TSH levels decline only slowly after thyroxine therapy achieves normal T$_4$ and T$_3$ concentrations. Hypothyroidism leads to an increase in the number of TSH-producing thyrotrophs, which decline only slowly after euthyroidism returns. Accordingly, 4 to 6 weeks should be allowed before increasing replacement doses of thyroxine above average on the basis of TSH levels. Severe long-standing hypothyroidism can lead to pituitary enlargement, mimicking pituitary tumors. The availability of sensitive TSH levels allows adequate assessment of pituitary reserves under such circumstances and makes TRH tests less useful.

ANTITHYROID ANTIBODIES. Antibody formation can occur against the thyroid peroxidase enzyme, thyroglobulin, and the TSH receptors T$_4$ and T$_3$. These antibodies can be present in serum. The most frequently occurring is the antimicrosomal antibody for which the thyroid peroxidase enzyme is the antigen. In Hashimoto's disease, elevated antibodies occur in more than 80% of patients with no specific therapeutic requirements resulting from high antiperoxidase antibody titers. Antithyroglobulin antibodies are positive in 60% of Hashimoto's disease. Occurrence of antithyroglobulin antibodies precludes using thyroglobulin levels to follow patients after thyroid cancer surgery or radioactive iodine treatment. Different types of TSH receptor antibodies occur, some of which stimulate thyroid hormone formation, whereas others only stimulate DNA synthesis or block TSH action. The TSI is a TSH receptor antibody that stimulates thyroid hormone formation and accompanies more than 90% of cases of Graves' disease. The TSI is related to, but not the same as, the long-acting thyroid-stimulating antibody (LATS), a previously used assay. In patients in whom the diagnosis of Graves' disease cannot be made clinically, determination of the TSI may be helpful, but routine TSI determination is not recommended. Persistent high levels of TSI in patients with Graves' disease on long-term antithyroid medication suggests but does not guarantee that stopping the antithyroid medication will not be followed by continuous euthyroidism. Anti-TSH antibodies can cross the placenta and produce neonatal Graves' disease or hypothyroidism. Circulating antibodies to T_4 and T_3 can interfere with the accurate determination of these hormones.

Evaluation of the Thyroid by Radioisotope Tests

RADIOACTIVE IODINE (RAI) UPTAKE. The epithelial cells of the thyroid actively transport iodide (I^-) and molecules of similar charge and configuration such as $^{99m}TcO_4^-$ pertechnetate and ^{201}Th. Only iodide is permanently retained in the thyroid cell by organification. Two separate tests use radioactive iodine: total radioactive uptake and thyroid scanning. Both are contraindicated during pregnancy. The radioactive iodine uptake only roughly indicates thyroid function. The 24-hour uptake ranges widely from 5 to 20%, and this, along with the marked decreased uptake in the presence of increased amounts of bodily cold iodine, makes it an unreliable indicator of thyroid function. Patients with subacute thyroiditis have a markedly reduced or absent uptake, whereas patients with active Graves' disease have a normal or increased uptake. Accordingly, the radioactive iodine uptake may be useful in diagnosing subacute thyroiditis. Its routine use for the diagnosis of Graves' disease is not recommended.

THYROID SCAN. Thyroid scans give graphic representations of the distribution of radioactive iodine in the gland. They are useful in identifying whether thyroid nodules show decreased ("cold") or increased ("hot") accumulation of radioactive iodine compared with normal paranodular tissue. Uptake also identifies thyroid tissue outside the gland. The isotopes ^{123}I, ^{131}I, and ^{99m}Tc can be used. ^{123}I is preferred because it provides a much smaller radiation dose to the thyroid than ^{131}I. With a ^{99m}Tc scan, good quality images can be obtained about 30 minutes after administration. Some thyroid nodules have a normal iodine transporter but lose the ability to organify iodine. Such nodules (about 10%) are not cold on ^{99m}Tc scans, a significant disadvantage of the technique. The ^{131}I isotope is sometimes preferred for identifying thyroid cancer metastases because it has a higher energy gamma ray and better penetrates the tissue. Scans in some patients fail to co-localize palpable nodules adjacent to areas of increased or decreased radioactive iodine retention. Such nodules may be autonomously either hot or cold. Because thyroid cancers exists in less than 1% of hot nodules compared with 20% of cold ones, the radioactive iodine uptake of thyroid nodules can be useful. In special cases, a suppression scan may be useful. After placing the patient on 150 to 200 μg of T_4 per day for 4 to 6 weeks, one repeats the thyroid scan. Thyroid hormone and TSH values should be normal before thyroxine is started. Autonomous nodules continue to show an increased iodine uptake (hot), whereas other nodules lose their radioactive iodine retention, becoming cold. Cold nodules need to be further evaluated with fine-needle aspiration, but this is not required for hot ones.

THYROID ULTRASONOGRAPHY. Ultrasonography gives a high-resolution image of the thyroid and can identify nodules 1 to 3 mm in diameter. Such small nodules are, however, not clinically relevant. Ultrasonography can distinguish solid from cystic lesions and determine changes in the size of the nodule in response to thyroid hormone suppression therapy. Ultrasound-guided fine-needle aspiration helps in obtaining cytologic material from nodules that are difficult to identify by palpation. Ultrasonography cannot distinguish between benign and malignant thyroid nodules, nor can the technique identify substernal extensions of the thyroid or spread of metastatic disease to this region. For the latter purpose, magnetic resonance imaging (MRI) or computed tomography (CT) can be useful.

Fine-Needle Aspiration of Thyroid Nodules

Aspiration of thyroid nodules with a fine needle (22 to 27 gauge) to obtain material for cytologic examination provides good diagnostic accuracy with minimal side effects. Bleeding into the aspirated nodule is the only unwanted effect and usually has no clinical

Table 239–4 ■ **RESULTS OBTAINED BY FINE-NEEDLE ASPIRATION OF THYROID NODULES**

	% OF PATIENTS
Adequate tissue obtained	90
Benign tumor	74
Malignant tumor	4
Suspicious or indeterminate	12
Correct diagnosis	<90
False-negative result	4
False-positive result	1

One fifth of these nodules are malignant after surgery by final pathology.

consequence. Results obtained with this procedure are listed in Table 239–4. Seeding of malignant cells along the needle track does not present a clinical problem with fine-needle aspiration. An experienced cytopathologist is crucial for the successful use of this procedure. Since the advent and wide use of fine-needle aspiration, surgical removal of benign nodules has substantially decreased.

Bayer MF: Effective laboratory evaluation of thyroid status. Med Clin North Am 75:1, 1991. *Provides a succinct guide to modern testing.*

Nicoloff JT, Spencer CA: The use and misuse of sensitive thyrotropin assays. J Clin Endocrinol Metab 71:493, 1990. *A valuable paper on the do's and don'ts of the subject.*

Stocklig JR: Serum thyrotropin and thyroid hormone measurements and assessment of thyroid hormone transport. *In* Braverman LF, Utiger RD (eds): The Thyroid, 7th ed. Philadelphia, JB Lippincott, 1996, p 377. *Comprehensively discusses the subject.*

NON-THYROIDAL ILLNESS SYNDROME

Severe systemic illness, physical trauma, and psychiatric disturbances can substantially alter thyroid hormone levels in patients without intrinsic thyroid disease. Various terms have been used for this condition, including the non-thyroidal illness syndrome, sick euthyroid syndrome, and low T_3 syndrome. The severity of the illness correlates roughly with the extent of thyroid hormone changes. A decreased serum T_3 concentration is the critical component of the syndrome. The frequent alterations of thyroid hormone levels in severe illness probably make NTI a more common cause of abnormal thyroid hormone values than intrinsic thyroid disease. NTI represents one end of a spectrum of endocrine responses to severe illness which include increases in adrenocorticotropic hormone (ACTH) and cortisol levels. Increases in cytokines, especially tumor necrosis factor and interleukin-1 and interleukin-6, also occur. The consequences, if any, of NTI for total body metabolism and the functional status of specific organs are unclear and therapy is not recommended. Diagnosing the simultaneous occurrence of hypothyroidism or hyperthyroidism in patients with NTI is a difficult diagnostic challenge. Different variants of NTI occur.

LOW T_3, NORMAL T_4 VARIANT. A marked decrease in serum total T_3 and free T_3 concentrations accompanied by normal serum T_4 and TSH levels is the most frequently encountered combination of thyroid hormone values in NTI. A rough correlation exists between the severity of the systemic illness and the decrease in T_3 levels. Decreased T_3 levels are most likely caused by an impairment of extrathyroidal T_4 to T_3 conversion. The decline is accompanied by an increase in rT_3 levels. Diminished 5' deiodinase activity accounts for this reciprocal change, with T_3 no longer being formed from T_4 and reverse T_3 not being metabolized to rT_2. The decrease in T_3 levels may decrease protein turnover and exert a sparing effect on body proteins, but the overall impact on metabolic and organ function is unclear. Because of normal T_4 and TSH levels, this variant of NTI can be clearly distinguished from hypothyroidism.

LOW T_3, LOW T_4 VARIANT. In addition to low T_3 levels, T_4 levels also decline in patients with more severe illness. Several changes contribute (1) decreases in thyroxine-binding proteins (TBG and transthyretin); (2) displacement of T_4 from proteins by fatty acids; and (3) decreased thyroid hormone production because of lowered TSH levels. The degree of lowered T_4 levels correlates with disease severity: Mortality increases in patients with T_4 levels below 4 μg/dL and approaches 80% in patients with T_4 levels below 2 μg/dL. T_4 administration does not influence outcome, and the low levels reflect the severity of the underlying illness but appear not to contribute directly to mortality. In addition to low T_3 and T_4 levels, T_4 indexes are low but dialysis-measured free T_4 levels remain normal or only minimally lowered. TSH levels are low but may be slightly elevated during recovery from severe illness. TSH levels above 20 μU/mL are not compatible with NTI and point to hypothyroidism.

Unusual Variants of Non-thyroidal Illness

Elevated T_4 levels with initially normal T_3 levels that subsequently decline occur with liver disease, especially acute hepatitis. Increased synthesis and release of TBG most likely accounts for the increased T_4 levels. A delayed fall in T_3 levels can affect patients with the acquired immunodeficiency syndrome (AIDS) indicating a poor prognosis; rT_3 levels are not elevated. In psychiatric illness, especially manic depressive disease, elevated T_4 levels occur during the initial disease phase, T_3 levels are normal, and TSH results vary. Elderly patients frequently show low T_3 levels; possible causes include chronic illness, medication intake, or an adjustment to increasing age. T_3 levels remain normal in selected healthy elderly individuals.

Diagnostic Considerations

The diagnosis of hypothyroidism or hyperthyroidism in severely ill patients with NTI can be difficult. Signs indicating the prior existence of thyroid disease such as a goiter, a thyroidectomy surgical scar, exophthalmos, or pretibial myxedema should be sought. Organ manifestations such as marked bradycardia for hypothyroidism or tachycardia and fine tremor for hyperthyroidism may provide important clues, especially if no other reason for these signs can be identified. As described earlier, NTI-induced alterations in thyroid function tests suppress the standard indices of hypothyroidism or hyperthyroidism, but certain guidelines can help. A TSH level above 20 μU/mL in an NTI patient makes a diagnosis of hypothyroidism highly likely, and thyroxine therapy is indicated. Similarly, TSH levels below 0.03 μU/mL and only moderately elevated T_3 and T_4 levels make hyperthyroidism likely. As systemic illness improves, T_3 and T_4 levels rise further and hyperthyroidism becomes evident. If Graves' disease causes the hyperthyroidism, a TSI determination can be helpful. The preferred treatment for such hyperthyroidism is by medical therapy using PTU or methimazole.

THYROTOXICOSIS

Thyrotoxicosis occurs when tissues are exposed to excess amounts of thyroid hormone, resulting in specific metabolic changes and pathophysiologic alterations in organ function. A distinction can be made between thyrotoxicosis and hyperthyroidism. Hyperthyroidism denotes increased formation and release of thyroid hormone from the thyroid gland, whereas thyrotoxicosis describes the clinical syndrome that results. Excess intake of exogenous thyroid hormone would lead to thyrotoxicosis but by the definition given above, such a patient would not be hyperthyroid. The terms, however, are frequently used interchangeably. Table 239–5 lists causes for thyrotoxicosis. The major ones are (1) increased occupancy of TSH receptors by TSI, TSH, or human chorionic gonadotropin (hCG); (2) autonomous overproduction of thyroid hormone by thyroid nodules; (3) increased release of thyroid hormone during specific phases of thyroiditis; (4) excessive thyroid hormone intake or ectopic thyroid hormone formation. The most frequent cause of thyrotoxicosis is Graves' disease, accounting for 60 to 90% of cases and occurring among women with a frequency of 1.9%. Men experience one tenth of the occurrence in women. Other causes in decreasing order of frequency include toxic thyroid nodules, thyroiditis, factitious thyrotoxicosis, iodine-induced thyrotoxicosis, and hCG- and TSH-induced hyperthyroidism.

Graves' Disease

Graves' disease, also termed Basedow's or Parry's disease, carries the hallmarks of excess formation and secretion of thyroid hormone and diffuse goiter. Additional characteristics include exophthalmos, dermopathy (especially pretibial myxedema), and

Table 239–5 ■ CAUSES OF THYROTOXICOSIS

Dependent on Increased Thyroid Hormone Production
Dependent on increased occupancy of the TSH receptor by:
  Thyroid-stimulating immunoglobulin (TSI)
    Graves' disease
    Hashitoxicosis
  Human chorionic gonadotropin (hCG)
    Hydatiform mole
    Choriocarcinoma
  Thyroid-stimulating hormone (TSH)
    TSH-producing pituitary tumor
Autonomous overproduction of thyroid hormone (independent of TSH)
  Toxic adenoma (TSH receptor mutant)
  Toxic multinodular goiter
  Follicular cancer (rare)
Jodbasedow effect (excess iodine-induced hyperthyroidism)
Independent of Increased Thyroid Hormone Production
Increased thyroid hormone release
  Subacute granulomatous thyroidits (painful)
  Subacute lymphocytic thyroidits (painless)
Non-thyroidal source of thyroid hormone
  Thyrotoxicosis factitia
  "Hamburger" thyrotoxicosis
  Ectopic production by:
    Ovarian teratoma (struma ovarii)
    Metastasis of follicular cancer

rarely thyroid acropathy. These supplementary manifestations seldom appear together and often run a divergent time course.

ETIOLOGY AND PATHOGENESIS. Graves' disease is most likely an autoimmune disorder with B lymphocytes producing immunoglobulins, some of which bind to and activate the TSH receptor, stimulating excess thyroid growth and hormone secretion. For these antibodies the TSH receptor appears to represent the antigenic site, and they act like TSH and are termed *thyroid-stimulating immunoglobulins* (TSI). Other antibodies occur in Graves' and other autoimmune diseases such as Hashimoto's disease. These antibodies bind to the TSH receptor but stimulate only thyroid growth without increasing thyroid hormone secretion. Some antibodies bind to the TSH receptor but block TSH action and lead to thyroid atrophy. A diversity of TSH antibodies occurs in autoimmune thyroid diseases, generating a spectrum of illnesses with Graves' disease and hyperthyroidism at one end and Hashimoto's disease and thyroid atrophy leading to hypothyroidism at the other. The role that specific antibodies play in causing the ophthalmopathy that occurs in 20 to 40% of patients with Graves' disease is less clear. Specific antibodies directed against non-TSH retro-orbital antigens localized on retro-orbital fibroblasts and muscle cells as well as antibodies directed at TSH-like antigens have been described. Retro-orbital fibroblasts appear to express a TSH receptor-like protein. Anti-TSH antibodies occur at a low frequency in Hashimoto's disease and in euthyroid relatives of patients with Graves' disease. The simultaneous occurrence of blocking TSH antibodies may prevent hyperthyroidism in such patients.

The precise sequence of events leading to TSH receptor antibody production and factors that initiate antibody formation have not been clearly identified. A genetically mediated antigen-specific defect in T lymphocyte suppressor function has been proposed. Such a defect in immune surveillance would allow T helper cell clones, which mistake part of the TSH receptor as a foreign antigen, to arise and persist. Such clones would then stimulate B cells to produce anti-TSH receptor antibodies. Alternatively, thyroid cells stimulated by specific cytokines produced in response to a viral infection may express on their cell surface Class II molecules of specific HLA-DR types that present fragments of the TSH receptor to T lymphocytes; these then would stimulate B lymphocytes to produce TSH receptor antibodies. The two mechanisms are not mutually exclusive and both could contribute to TSH receptor-directed antibody formation. The autoimmune response may be promoted by poorly defined factors including the following: (1) iodide excess; for example, the incidence of Graves' disease increases after iodine supplementation in deficient areas; (2) viral or bacterial infection; for example, outbreaks of Graves' disease can follow *Yersinia enterocolitica* infection; (3) glucocorticoid withdrawal or stress; the stress induction has been questioned and may relate to a worsening of symptoms by the combined occurrence of hyperthyroidism and physical or emotional stress, which brings the patients to medical attention; (4) parturition: a state of relative immune tolerance develops during pregnancy and reverses after delivery; (5) lithium therapy; this may modify immune responses.

PATHOLOGY. The thyroid gland in Graves' disease enlarges diffusely and contains increased vascularity. The parenchyma exhibits hypertrophy and hyperplasia, with follicular cells showing increased height, surrounding a lumen containing a decreased amount of colloid. Infiltration by lymphocytes indicates the autoimmune nature of the disease. These cells probably generate a considerable amount of TSH receptor antibody. Iodide administration increases the colloid accumulation and decreases vascularity, making the gland firmer. A gland that increases in size in patients receiving antithyroid medication indicates either excess medication, inducing hypothyroidism, or too low a dose, providing inadequate receptor blockade and continued thyroid hormone formation and growth. Severe thyrotoxicosis can lead to muscle atrophy with muscle fiber degeneration, cardiac hypertrophy, focal hepatic necrosis with lymphocyte infiltration, a decrease in bone density, and hair loss. In patients with Graves' disease ophthalmopathy, an increase in retro-orbital contents leads to protrusion of the globe. The retro-orbital tissues show marked infiltration by lymphocytes, mast cells, and plasma cells along with increased amounts of mucopolysaccharide, especially hyaluronic acid. Extraocular muscles show edema, round cell infiltration, and mucopolysaccharide deposition eventually resulting in muscle fibrosis. In patients with pretibial myxedema, the skin shows prominent lymphocyte infiltration and mucopolysaccharide deposition.

CLINICAL FEATURES. Excess thyroid hormone action due to any of the causes listed in Table 239–5 can lead to an increased metabolic rate and changes in the function of several organs. In addition, patients with Graves' disease have specific clinical manifestations resulting from the underlying autoimmune process. The thyrotoxicosis and autoimmune-related manifestations can show independent variations in intensity and time course, causing diagnostic difficulties.

FEATURES OF THYROTOXICOSIS. Table 239–6 lists common signs and symptoms of thyrotoxicosis. The typical patient with Graves' disease is a woman in her mid-20s to 30s experiencing recent onset of nervousness, difficulty in controlling emotions, and a state of agitated tiredness made worse by sleep disturbances. She speaks rapidly and cannot sit still. Problems of recent onset in interaction with others at home or at work are frequently reported. Questioning brings out feelings of intolerance with excess sweating, palpitations, muscle weakness, frequent bowel movements, and weight loss in spite of good appetite. Sometimes weight gain ensues because the increased appetite and caloric intake exceed the enhanced caloric consumption. Oligomenorrhea and amenorrhea occur in premenopausal women. On physical examination, the skin is warm and moist and has a fine velvety texture. The hair is fine and when combed, sheds substantial amounts, leading to thinning of the hair. Onycholysis with separation of the nail from the fingertip is frequent. Gynecomastia can occur in men because of increased estrogen production. Fine tremor is noted on the stretched-out hands, and tendon reflexes become hyperactive. The eye signs of thyrotoxicosis are most likely mediated by an increased sympathetic tone and include a widened distance between the upper and lower lid, lid lag on upward gaze, and frequent blinking. These signs do not indicate Graves' ophthalmopathy and are not accompanied by protrusion of the eyes. Cardiovascular manifestations can be marked, characterized by sinus tachycardia, a widened pulse pressure, and an often elevated systolic blood pressure. True hypertension is not frequent in hyperthyroidism but does occur in hypothyroidism. The heartbeat is vigorous with a hyperactive pericardium. On auscultation the first sound is increased and a third sound and frequently a systolic murmur are audible. A harsh to-and-fro sound can be audible and is most likely caused by the pleural and pericardial surfaces rubbing each other. Cardiac arrhythmia, especially atrial fibrillation, can contribute to the development of heart failure. Muscle atrophy and weakness develop, and hypokalemic periodic paralysis has a measurable incidence in males of Asian extraction. Bone turnover can be increased, leading to hypercalcemia of as much as 12 mg/dL. Unusual blood-detected abnormalities (<10% of patients) include elevated alkaline phosphatase levels, increased direct bilirubin, mild anemia, and moderate neutropenia. Renal tubular acidosis can occur, and immune complex nephritis has been reported.

In older patients, the manifestations of thyrotoxicosis can be considerably modified. Affected patients frequently appear apathetic rather than nervous. Cardiovascular signs, general muscle weakness, and marked weight loss are more prominent. Cardiac arrhythmias that are refractory to conventional treatment, unexplained heart failure, or the recent onset or marked worsening of pre-existing angina pectoris should lead to a determination of thyroid hormone values.

FEATURES SPECIFIC FOR GRAVES' DISEASE. Autoimmune processes mediate the enlargement of the thyroid gland, infiltrative ophthalmopathy, dermopathy, and acropachy, thereby distinguishing Graves' disease from other causes of thyrotoxicosis. Palpation most frequently reveals diffuse and symmetric thyroid enlargement (two to six times normal). Thyroid nodules can occur and should be sampled because, although unusual, thyroid cancer can coincide with Graves' disease. Auscultation of the thyroid frequently reveals a thyroid bruit, reflecting the increased blood supply. In a small number of patients, the thyroid remains of normal size. A hallmark finding of Graves' disease is infiltrative ophthalmopathy. Clinically detectable eye disease occurs in 20 to 40% of patients with Graves' disease, but severe ophthalmopathy requiring aggressive treatment affects only about 5%. Affected persons complain of easy tearing, photophobia, a feeling of sand in the eyes, diplopia, and decreased visual acuity. Ophthalmopathy affects the anterior soft tissue structures of the eye and with progressive severity involves more posterior structures as well. Periorbital edema and chemosis occur early and result from impaired drainage of the orbital veins. The swollen and fibrotic muscles cause lid retraction and restrict ocular movement, leading to diplopia. Upward gaze is most frequently impaired; with limitations of lateral gaze occurring less frequently. Tissue edema and accumulation of hydroscopic hyaluronic acid lead to engorgement of extraocular muscles and swelling of retro-orbital connective tissue, pushing the globe forward and resulting in proptosis and further restriction of eye movement. Proptosis and lid retraction prevent complete closure of the eyes, resulting in exposure keratitis and corneal ulceration. Adequate care to prevent drying and infection of the cornea is important. Compression of the optic nerve at the posterior apex by enlarged muscles may lead to blurring and impaired visual acuity, visual field defects, impairment of color vision, and papilledema. Optic nerve compression can occur in the absence of proptosis. Graves' ophthalmopathy that is clinically apparent in only one eye occurs in 5 to 14% of patients. Sensitive imaging techniques like CT, however, show that most of these patients have bilateral orbital disease. Most patients with Graves' ophthalmopathy are hyperthyroid, but dissociation can occur, with ophthalmopathy appearing in patients of euthyroid or hypothyroid status. More unusual manifestations include coexisting myasthenia gravis with Graves' disease. Other cases may include diffuse lymphadenopathy and splenomegaly. Rarely, other autoimmune disorders occur in patients with Graves' disease.

DIAGNOSIS AND DIFFERENTIAL DIAGNOSIS. In patients with severe Graves' disease showing typical signs of thyrotoxicosis and autoimmune-mediated manifestations such as ophthalmopathy, the

Table 239–6 ▪ **TISSUE-SPECIFIC SIGNS AND SYMPTOMS OF THYROTOXICOSIS**

TISSUE	SYMPTOMS AND SIGNS
Central nervous system	Nervousness and emotional lability Fine tremor of hands
Cardiovascular	Palpitations, tachycardia, atrial fibrillation, increased difference between systolic and diastolic blood pressure
Gastrointestinal	Hyperdefecation, gastrointestinal hypermotility, diarrhea
Muscle	Proximal muscle weakness, muscle atrophy, hyperreflexia
Skin	Warm moist smooth skin, onycholysis, fine hair, hair loss, excessive perspiration
Metabolic	Heat intolerance, weight loss usually with increased appetite
Thyroid	Enlargement of nodule(s)

diagnosis is not difficult (see Table 239–6). Gauging the degree of thyroid hormone overproduction guides subsequent therapy. Measurement of free T_4, T_3, and TSH levels constitutes a sufficient laboratory workup. In all patients with Graves' disease, T_3 levels are markedly elevated, and in most such patients free T_4 levels are elevated as well. In some patients, however, the marked stimulation of TSH receptors leads to higher hormone production rates of T_3 so that serum T_3 levels rise markedly whereas T_4 levels remain normal. This combination of laboratory values is termed T_3 toxicosis and is most frequently found during the initial phases or a relapse of Graves' disease. TSH levels are undetectable and serve to exclude TSH-producing tumors or thyroid hormone resistance as causes for the elevated thyroid hormone levels. In typical Graves' disease, radioactive iodine-based tests and a determination of the TSI are unnecessary. The clinical diagnosis becomes more difficult in patients with milder disease, in older patients manifesting apathetic thyrotoxicosis, and in patients with coexisting illnesses. Determination of free T_4, T_3, and TSH levels adequately establish the degree of thyrotoxicosis in patients with mild disease and older patients with an apathetic picture. Undetectable TSH levels using an ultrasensitive TSH assay are especially helpful in establishing that the body contains an excess amount of thyroid hormone. Intercurrent illness modifies thyroid hormone values by lowering T_3 levels and in some patients T_4 levels. Elevated reverse T_3 levels further implicate an intercurrent illness as a modifier of thyroid hormone values. Obtaining TSI values can be helpful in these patients because their elevation confirms the diagnosis of Graves' disease. Palpation of the thyroid revealing a nodule, a somewhat painful thyroid, or no palpable thyroid tissue is unusual and requires additional diagnostic procedures. A radioactive iodine scan is especially helpful in identifying a cold thyroid nodule surrounded by high uptake in surrounding tissue, a combination compatible with Graves' disease with a cold nodule requiring biopsy. Alternatively, the nodule may be hot, with surrounding areas showing decreased or absent uptake, which makes it more likely that the patient has a toxic adenoma. Very low uptake in patients who experience pain on palpation of the thyroid area indicates thyroiditis. In patients with no palpable thyroid tissue and absent thyroid uptake, ectopic production of thyroid hormone or factitious intake should be suspected. Thyroglobulin levels are very low in such patients.

Discrepancies between the degree of thyrotoxicosis and the extent of autoimmune abnormalities can complicate the diagnosis of Graves' disease. Some patients can exhibit marked bilateral or unilateral ophthalmopathy with minimal or no signs of thyrotoxicosis. In such instances, T_4 and T_3 levels are in the upper normal range and TSH levels are in the low normal or decreased range. The condition has been termed euthyroid ophthalmopathy or euthyroid Graves' disease. Thyrotoxicosis is mimicked by few clinical syndromes, and thyroid hormone values are normal in most of these. Pheochromocytomas can lead to heat intolerance, profuse sweating, palpitations, tachycardia, elevated glucose levels, and a state of anxiety. Anxiety states by themselves also lead to irritability, tremor, weakness, tachycardia, and weight loss. Thyroid hormone values are normal in these conditions.

TREATMENT OF GRAVES' DISEASE. The ophthalmopathy and dermopathy of Graves' disease require separate therapeutic approaches. The therapy for thyrotoxicosis is aimed at decreasing thyroid hormone formation and secretion. Three different therapeutic approaches are used: (1) antithyroid drugs that inhibit the thyroid peroxidase enzyme involved in thyroid hormone formation, (2) radioactive iodine, and (3) surgery. Both of the latter treatments decrease the amount of functional thyroid tissue. The most frequently used treatment modalities are antithyroid drugs or radioactive iodine, and the choice between them depends on the phase and severity of the disease, the specific situation of the patient, and the preference and experience of the physician. Spontaneously occurring increases and decreases of the underlying autoimmune abnormality lead to cycles of worsening and improvement of the thyrotoxic symptoms, making variable the natural history of Graves' disease. Consequently, life-long follow-up is recommended. Ten to 20 percent of patients with Graves' disease experience spontaneous remittance, and about half become hypothyroid after 20 to 30 years in the absence of therapy, most likely due to continued autoimmune destruction of the thyroid. Not treating patients and awaiting a spontaneous remission is not recommended. Therapy directed against the autoimmune process is currently not available.

TREATMENT OF THYROTOXICOSIS. ANTITHYROID DRUG THERAPY. Amelioration of thyrotoxic symptoms by decreasing thyroid hormone formation and release is the initial task in severe thyrotoxicosis. The thionamide derivatives, propylthiouracil (PTU) and methimazole (MMI), are the preferred initial treatment options in Graves' disease in the absence of contraindications. Radioactive iodine can lead to increased release of thyroid hormone and, infrequently, worsen the thyrotoxic symptoms to the point of inducing thyroid storm. Thyroid surgery is contraindicated in severely hyperthyroid patients. PTU and MMI, as well as carbimazole, which is used in Great Britain and is metabolized to methimazole, interfere with organification and iodotyrosine coupling by inhibiting the peroxidase enzyme. Both compounds may exert a mild immunosuppressive effect; a decrease in the level of TSI occurs after the drugs are started. This could be due to a mild immunosuppressive effect but also could result from decreased thyroid hormone secretion. Both drugs are rapidly absorbed from the gastrointestinal tract and concentrated in the thyroid. PTU inhibits peripheral conversion of T_4 to T_3, contributing 10 to 20% to the decrease in T_3 levels. This effect does not occur with MMI. MMI, however, is at least 10 times more potent than PTU and has a longer intrathyroidal residence time. MMI administered once a day is effective, whereas PTU must be given every 6 to 8 hours to exert its full effect. Both PTU and MMI cross the placenta; given in high doses they can interfere with fetal thyroid function. The choice between PTU and MMI and particular dosing schemes vary considerably between different centers. PTU is most useful for patients with severe thyrotoxicosis; those with moderate thyrotoxicosis are started on MMI, which comes in 5- and 10-mg tablets. Starting doses of 20 to 30 mg once daily are used. Improvement of thyrotoxic symptoms, in general, takes 2 to 3 weeks and can lag behind the normalization of thyroid hormone values. Euthyroidism can be achieved in 4 to 6 weeks. Thyroid hormone values are checked 4 weeks after the start of therapy and if no decrease in values occurs in spite of compliance, the dose may be increased to 30 to 40 mg a day. Once thyroid hormone levels normalize, the dose is decreased. A decrease in dose that is accompanied by an increase in free T_4 or T_3 levels and symptoms suggesting disease reactivation requires maintenance at higher dose levels for a longer time. Most patients can be maintained on low doses of 2.5 to 5 mg of MMI for 12 to 24 months.

A few patients with severe hyperthyroidism are started on PTU (100 to 150 mg every 8 hours). The choice is based on the faster decrease in T_3 levels with PTU than MMI. In some patients, higher doses of 200 to 300 mg every 6 hours are required. PU comes in 50-mg tablets and, when taken in doses of two or three tablets three times a day, can lead to compliance problems. With improvement, the physician can progressively lower PTU doses and switch to once-a-day MMI. Most patients are then maintained on the lower MMI dose (2.5 to 5 mg/day) for 12 to 24 months. It appears that longer duration of antithyroid therapy bodes well for patients staying euthyroid after the medication is stopped. Most relapses occur within the first 3 to 6 months after discontinuation of antithyroid therapy. In young adults, a second course of antithyroid drug therapy can be tried, but the chance of permanent remission declines.

Undesired occurrences during PTU and MMI therapy include an increase in thyroid size, which may result from overtreatment, shown by low T_4 levels and elevated TSH levels, or undertreatment and reactivation of disease. Unfavorable indicators of disease activity are a requirement for higher PTU and MMI doses and T_3 levels that increase excessively compared with T_4 levels. Favorable prognostic signs are continued normalization of thyroid hormone levels, especially a normal T_4 to T_3 ratio in spite of using lower PTU and MMI doses, and decreasing thyroid size and TSI levels. Routine monitoring of TSI is not recommended. One recent report suggests a different treatment protocol. Patients are treated initially with MMI until euthyroid. Subsequently a combination of MMI (10 to 20 mg) plus thyroxine (0.1 mg T_4 per day) is used for another 12 to 24 months, at which time all signs of active Graves' disease have disappeared. MMI is discontinued and the patient is continued on 0.1 mg T_4 for 1 more year. Long-term remissions have been reported to occur in more than 90% of patients treated with this regimen. Before such a protocol is adopted for routine use, however, confirmation of results in patients of a different ethnic background and iodine exposure should be obtained.

Table 239–7 lists side effects of thionamide compounds. These occur most frequently during the initial 3 to 6 months after the therapy is started. The most frequent complications are allergic in nature, and rashes occur in 2 to 3% of patients. The major toxic reaction is agranulocytosis, which develops suddenly and occurs in 0.2 to 0.5% of patients. Routine monitoring of leukocyte counts is not recommended, but a leukocyte count should be obtained before starting therapy. Patients need to be instructed to discontinue their medication and contact their physician when a fever occurs or infections develop, especially in the oropharynx. A white blood cell count below $0.5 \times 10^9/L$ indicates agranulocytosis and requires both discontinuation of antithyroid drugs and administration of broad-spectrum antibiotics as well as supportive therapy. Other treatment modalities such as radioactive iodine should be chosen for further treatment.

RADIOACTIVE IODINE. RAI therapy (^{131}I) is used most frequently to treat hyperthyroidism in adults in the United States, in contrast to Europe and Japan where antithyroid medication is the preferred approach. In either event, antithyroid drugs are the preferred initial therapy for thyrotoxicosis. RAI therapy is preferred for older patients with moderate hyperthyroidism and thyroid enlargement, for patients with a prior allergic or toxic reaction to the antithyroid medication, and when frequent medication intake cannot be guaranteed. ^{131}I is also used after a course of antithyroid medication has failed to induce a long-term euthyroid state. RAI treatment is contraindicated during pregnancy; the fetal thyroid becomes able to accumulate iodine at 10 to 12 weeks of gestation. RAI can induce a thyroiditis with glandular swelling leading to potential air-way obstruction in patients with large retrosternal goiters. A very low RAI uptake caused by excessive iodine exposure also precludes ^{131}I use.

Before ^{131}I administration, antithyroid drugs should be stopped for 3 or 4 days. Different dosing methods have been proposed for ^{131}I application. One approach is to aim at delivering 80 μCi ^{131}I per gram of thyroid tissue. The 80 μCi is then multiplied by the estimated weight of the gland and corrected for ^{131}I uptake. This delivers 6000 to 8000 rad to the thyroid and most frequently requires doses of 5 to 10 mCi. In patients with low uptake, large glands, and severe thyrotoxicosis leading to rapid intrathyroidal iodine turnover, larger doses often are chosen. Improvement in thyrotoxicosis occurs after 4 to 5 weeks, and 40 to 70% of patients regain normal thyroid functions within 6 to 8 weeks. Almost 80% of patients are cured with one dose. The remaining need a second dose, which should not be undertaken before 6 months have elapsed. After giving radioactive iodine, antithyroid drugs can be added at day 5 to reach a euthyroid state more quickly. In addition, β-sympathetic blockade is used to relieve associated symptoms. RAI can induce a painful thyroiditis and lead to acute thyroid hormone release and worsening of thyrotoxicosis. Severe thyroiditis

Table 239–7 ■ SIDE EFFECTS OF ANTITHYROID DRUGS

Severe
  Agranulocytosis (0.2–0.5%)
  Only rare cases reported
    Hepatitis (can result in hepatic failure)
    Cholestatic jaundice
    Thrombocytopenia
    Hypoprothrombinemia
    Aplastic anemia
    Lupus-like syndrome with vasculitis
    Hypoglycemia (insulin antibodies)
Less Severe
  Most frequent (1–5%)
    Rash
    Urticaria
    Arthralgia
    Decreased leukocyte level (drop in white blood cell counts by 2–3 × 10³)
    Fever
  Less frequent
    Arthritis
    Diarrhea
    Decreased sense of taste

can be treated with anti-inflammatory agents such as aspirin; rarely glucocorticoids are required. RAI treatment-induced worsening of Graves' ophthalmopathy has been reported in some studies but not in others. Administration of glucocorticoids concurrently with RAI treatment may be beneficial, but such treatment is not well enough established to be recommended for routine use. Conticosteroids, however, may be useful for patients with prominent eye disease in whom RAI therapy is the approach of choice. No increase of thyroid cancer, other malignancies, or malformations in subsequent pregnancies have been documented after RAI therapy. It is recommended, however, that pregnancy not occur for 6 to 12 months after RAI treatment. Hypothyroidism is a consequence of RAI treatment. More than 50% of patients become hypothyroid during the first year after therapy, with an additional 2 to 3% during each subsequent year. Unless otherwise treated, transient hypothyroidism occurs 2 to 3 months after radioactive iodine treatment, with subsequent spontaneous normalization of thyroid hormone values. Patients should be informed of this risk and be followed after the acute phase of treatment every 4 to 6 months and subsequently at least once a year.

SURGICAL THERAPY. Surgical removal of a large part of the thyroid (subtotal thyroidectomy) is indicated in patients with large obstructing glands or glands containing nodules that are identified as malignant or equivocal on fine-needle aspiration. Pregnant women with severe hyperthyroidism, which is difficult to control with antithyroid drugs, can be treated with thyroidectomy during the second trimester. In addition, young patients who are difficult to control on antithyroid drugs, patients with toxic reactions to antithyroid drugs, and patients who are not candidates for antithyroid drugs and refuse radioactive iodine are treated by surgery. Nevertheless, patients must be euthyroid before surgery is undertaken. This is achieved by using PTU or MMI for approximately 6 weeks. In patients on PTU or MMI, a saturated solution of potassium iodide (1 drop three times a day) can be administered daily for 10 days before surgery to reduce the vascularity of the gland. Subtotal thyroidectomy should be performed by an experienced thyroid surgeon. Complications including hypoparathyroidism, recurrent laryngeal nerve paralysis, and hemorrhage should occur in less than 1 to 2% of patients. In addition, transient hypocalcemia, wound infection, and keloid formation leading to unsightly scars may occur. Hypothyroidism occurs to a somewhat lower extent than after RAI, but its frequency may be underestimated. Recurrent hyperthyroidism occurs in about 10% of patients.

ALTERNATIVE AND SUPPORTIVE THERAPIES. In a small number of patients with Graves' disease, the conventional therapies listed earlier cannot be used. In some, toxic reactions preclude the use of antithyroid drugs and ^{131}I cannot be employed because a very low uptake occurs due to excess iodine exposure or because of pregnancy. Also, some patients may present a high surgical risk because of underlying medical problems. In such cases, the oral cholecystographic agent iopanoic acid or sodium iopodate (Oragrafin), administered at 1 g/day, inhibits T_4 to T_3 conversion and leads to rapid lowering of T_3 levels. In addition, because of release of iodine from the compound, T_4 levels fall. These compounds should be used for only 2 to 3 months because escape from their antithyroid effect occurs. The perchlorate ion (ClO_4^-) of $KClO_4$ is a competitive inhibitor of thyroidal iodide transport. In doses limited to 1 g/day, serious toxic effects such as anaplastic anemia and gastric ulcers can be avoided. The compound is especially effective in iodine-induced hyperthyroidism (jodbasedow) as occurs, for example, in patients treated with the antiarrhythmic compound amiodarone. Potassium perchlorate should be used for only a short duration and with careful supervision. The isolated use of iodine to treat thyrotoxicosis is ill advised because its inhibitory effects on thyroid hormone secretion often fail. Iodine should be used only in patients who are on antithyroid medication and are prepared for thyroid surgery or in the treatment of thyroid storm (see later).

β-Adrenergic blocking agents such as propranolol, 60 to 120 mg/day in three or four divided doses, help to provide relief of symptoms such as tachycardia, tremor, anxiety, and heat intolerance. The rationale for their use is based on an increased sensitivity of the β-sympathetic system in thyrotoxicosis and on a small inhibitory effect of T_4 to T_3 conversion. Patients with a history of asthma or congestive heart failure should not receive propranolol because it constricts bronchial smooth muscle and has a negative inotropic effect. Propranolol should not be used as a sole agent to treat hyperthyroidism because it neither directly inhibits thyroid hormone action nor induces a euthyroid state. Multivitamin supplementation is advisable in patients with severe thyrotoxicosis, especially if nutrition is not well balanced and adequate.

TREATMENT OF OPHTHALMOPATHY AND DERMOPATHY. Clinically apparent ophthalmopathy affects 20 to 40% of patients with Graves' disease, but severe symptoms occur in only a minority. For most patients with mild eye signs, only general supportive measures are needed. These include elevation of the head at night and wearing of tinted glasses to protect the eyes from sunlight and foreign bodies. Application of 1% methylcellulose drops to the eyes and taking a diuretic to decrease periorbital swelling provide further relief. Patients with more severe ophthalmopathy should be managed in close consultation between an endocrinologist and an ophthalmologist. Severe inflammatory reactions are treated with 60 to 100 mg of prednisone in divided doses for 2 to 4 weeks, with subsequent tapering of the dose over 8 to 12 weeks. Combinations of prednisone and cyclosporine have also been used. External x-ray therapy to the retro-orbital area may be helpful but is less well established as desirable therapy. The total dose is 20 Gy (2000 rad) given in 10 fractions over 2 to 3 weeks. Signs of optic nerve compression such as papillary edema, decreased color vision, and decreased visual acuity require surgical decompression, for which a transantral approach is frequently favored. After the active inflammatory process subsides, corrective surgical procedures may be beneficial. Retro-orbital muscle surgery may correct for eyeball misalignment and double vision. Eyelid surgery aimed at protecting the cornea, relieving discomfort, and cosmetic improvement should be the last surgical step.

Other Causes of Thyrotoxicosis

TOXIC ADENOMA AND TOXIC MULTINODULAR GOITER. Increased formation and secretion of T_3 and T_4 can occur in a single nodule or in multiple thyroid nodules. The latter condition is also termed *Plummer's disease.* In toxic adenomas several point mutations of the TSH receptor gene leading to constitutive activation have been described. A small number of toxic adenomas have mutations in G proteins also resulting in constitutive activation. Single nodules need to be larger than 2 to 3 cm in diameter to emgender hyperthyroidism. Histologically, these nodules are follicular adenomas. Frequently a large nodule is palpable on one side of the thyroid, with atrophy of the other side. In contrast, patients with toxic multinodular goiter may undergo general nodular enlargement. Such persons frequently are older and have had a goiter for a long time before autonomous overproduction of thyroid hormone ensues. The thyrotoxicosis can be precipitated by excess iodine intake (jodbasedow effect) and appears to occur particularly frequently in autonomous thyroid tissue, which functions independently of TSH stimulation. On physical examination, multinodular goiters range from small to large with possible substernal extension. Laboratory values show suppressed TSH levels and marked elevation of T_3 levels, with T_4 levels showing a lesser increase. Antibodies against the TSH receptor (TSI) and thyroid peroxidase (anti-TPO) are absent, in contrast to patients with Graves' disease. On RAI scan two patterns can be distinguished. Some patients show an irregular and patchy distribution of increased RAI uptake. In others, one or more distinct hot nodules occur with marked, localized increased RAI accumulation and no uptake between the hot nodules. Both patterns are compatible with toxic goiter. Clinically affected patients may be difficult to diagnose because the disease affects elderly patients, who tend to present with apathetic hyperthyroidism. As noted earlier, typical thyrotoxic signs can be minimal in such patients, who often show apathy, lethargy, a depressed mood, weight loss, and cardiac abnormalities.

RAI is the treatment of choice for most patients with one toxic adenoma or multinodular toxic goiter. Severely thyrotoxic patients may need a course of antithyroid medication several weeks before they receive RAI to forestall acute worsening and decompensation after ^{131}I administration. The ^{131}I dose is 150 μCi per gram of tissue, twice that used for Graves' disease. Permanent hypothyroidism infrequently develops because remaining thyroid tissue resumes

thyroid hormone secretion after ablation of toxic adenomas. Surgery can remove isolated adenomas, especially in younger patients.

RARE CAUSES. Thyrotoxicosis can be caused by TSH-producing pituitary tumors as well as by excess formation of hCG by hydatiform moles or choriocarcinoma. Surgical therapy is appropriate for both pituitary tumors and moles. Choriocarcinoma is treated by appropriate chemotherapy, and persistent thyrotoxicosis may require antithyroid drugs. Ectopic production of thyroid hormone by ovarian teratoma leads to mild thyrotoxicosis. Body scans detect RAI uptake in the location of the ovaries. Surgical removal is corrective. Follicular carcinoma of the thyroid with functioning metastases rarely leads to hyperthyroidism. Therapy is discussed in the section on thyroid cancer. Subacute or chronic thyroiditis can release high amounts of T_4 and T_3 and induce hyperthyroidism lasting for several weeks or months. RAI uptake is very low in such lesions. *Thyrotoxicosis factitia* results from inadvertent or planned ingestion of large amounts of thyroid hormone. It most frequently accompanies efforts at weight loss or occurs in patients with psychiatric problems. Many of these patients have easy access to thyroid hormone because they took it in the past, have relatives or acquaintances who are taking thyroid hormone, or are medical personnel. Ingestion of ground meat products prepared from neck trim containing thyroid tissue has also been reported (hamburger thyrotoxicosis). Patients with thyrotoxic symptoms, suppressed TSH levels, increased T_4 and T_3 levels, low RAI uptake, and suppressed thyroglobulin levels meet the diagnostic criteria for thyrotoxicosis factitia. Patients taking T_3 preparations have elevated T_3 levels but suppressed T_4 levels. Stopping thyroid hormone intake usually suffices. Additive β-sympathetic blockade or agents like ipodate to inhibit T_4 to T_3 conversion are rarely needed.

The term *jodbasedow effect,* as noted earlier, designates iodine-induced hyperthyroidism. It occurs most frequently in patients with toxic nodular goiter exposed to excess amounts of iodine but has also been reported in Graves' disease. Problems with the autoregulation of thyroid hormone formation usually exist before iodine exposure, however, some patients have been reported who exhibited completely normal thyroid function after iodine was withheld. The jodbasedow effect typically occurs in iodine-deficient areas after iodine supplementation is provided. Exposure to iodinated radiographic contrast media and iodinated drugs presents a frequent triggering event for the jodbasedow effect in the United States. The antiarrhythmic agent amiodarone, which contains 37% iodine, can induce the jodbasedow effect. The developing hyperthyroidism can worsen arrhythmias and lead to difficult management problems. In milder cases, antithyroid drugs such as MMI are used. Potassium perchlorate prevents further iodine uptake and inhibits thyroid hormone formation. The usual dose is 200 mg four times a day.

Special Therapeutic Problems

THYROID STORM. Thyroid storm or thyrotoxic crisis is a life-threatening form of decompensated hyperthyroidism. Thyroid storm occurs most frequently in patients with severe thyrotoxicosis who develop an intercurrent severe illness such as an infection or sepsis or undergo a major surgical procedure. The distinction between severe thyrotoxicosis with an additional intercurrent illness and thyroid storm cannot be clearly drawn. Patients with severe thyrotoxicosis developing an intercurrent illness should be aggressively treated by the approach outlined in Table 239–8 because the illness can quickly decompensate into thyrotoxic crisis. Thyrotoxic crisis requires no acute increase in thyroid hormone values, and it cannot be identified by laboratory tests. An acute increase in tissue availability of free thyroid hormones caused by a decrease in plasma-binding proteins may cause it, but equally likely are coincident increases in cytokines such as tumor necrosis factor-α and interleukin-6. Clinical signs compatible with thyrotoxic crisis are fever in excess of the temperature elevation expected from the intercurrent illness, with temperatures of 41° C (105° F) and even higher. In addition, marked tachycardia, extreme restlessness, agitation, and tremor occur. Patients may experience mental deterioration and become delirious, psychotic, obtunded, and even comatose. Hypotension with congestive heart failure and signs of an acute abdomen can develop. Table 239–8 outlines therapy, which includes high doses of antithyroid medication and iodine after starting antithyroid drugs. Cortisol turnover increases markedly, inducing enhanced formation of 11-keto compounds (cortisone), which are less metaboli-

Table 239-8 ■ MANAGEMENT OF THYROID STORM

Inhibition of Thyroid Hormone Formation and Secretion
PTU, 400 mg q8h PO or by nasogastric tube
Sodium iodide, 1 g IV in 24 hr, or saturated solution of KI, 5 drops q8h

Sympathetic Blockade
Propranolol, 20–40 mg q4–6h, or 1 mg IV slowly (repeat doses until heart rate slows); not indicated in patients with asthma or congestive heart failure that is not rate related

Glucocorticoid Therapy
Hydrocortisone, 50–100 mg IV q6h

Supportive Therapy
Intravenous fluids (depending on indication: glucose, electrolytes, multivitamins)
Temperature control (cooling blankets, acetaminophen; avoid salicylates)
O₂ if required
Digitalis for congestive failure and to slow ventricular response; pentobarbital for sedation
Treatment of precipitating event (e.g., infection)

cally active. Administration of 300 mg of hydrocortisone in divided doses is therefore indicated. Propranolol provides effective sympathetic blockade that has a favorable effect on rapid heart rate and induced cardiac failure. The compound, however, has a negative inotropic effect and should be used cautiously in patients with congestive heart failure. A history of asthma attacks precludes the use of β-sympathetic blockers. Treatment of precipitating events and supportive therapy must be started immediately.

THYROTOXICOSIS AND PREGNANCY. The most frequent cause of thyrotoxicosis during pregnancy is Graves' disease, but hyperthyroidism can result from toxic multinodular goiter and more rarely an excess of hCG production by hydatiform moles or choriocarcinoma. Hyperthyroidism may be difficult to recognize because pregnancy itself can lead to a hyperdynamic cardiovascular state and heat intolerance. Total T₄ and T₃ levels are increased owing to elevated thyroid hormone-binding protein levels, but T₄ values above 15 μg/dL strongly suggest hyperthyroidism. Hyperemesis gravidarum leads to elevated T₄ levels (hyperthyroxinemia), with normal T₃ values. In addition to medical problems of the mother resulting from severe thyrotoxicosis, slight increases in neonatal mortality rate and low birth weight in newborns have been reported. Antithyroid drugs are the initial therapy of choice. RAI is contraindicated, and the patient needs to be euthyroid before surgery can be considered. Because PTU inhibits T₄ to T₃ conversion, crosses the placenta less readily, and is concentrated to a lower extent in the mother's milk than MMI, use of PTU is preferred over that of MMI in pregnant patients. Isolated cases of aplastica cutis induced by MMI have been reported. At high doses, PTU can induce fetal hypothyroidism and goiter because it crosses the placenta. In contrast, thyroid hormone minimally crosses the placenta. PTU doses are therefore limited to 200 to 300 mg/day; the addition of thyroxine confers no advantage. PTU administered in this way during pregnancy is relatively safe and does not negatively affect either fetal development or the outcome of pregnancy. If adequate control of hyperthyroidism is not possible, subtotal thyroidectomy should be considered, which is best performed during the second trimester. Long-term treatment with propranolol is not recommended because low birth weight can result. In addition, postnatal bradycardia and poor responses to hypoxia have been noted in newborns of mothers treated with propranolol. During the postpartum period, the mother risks developing new Graves' disease, a recurrence of previously quiescent Graves' disease, or postpartum thyroiditis. A state of relative immunosuppression during pregnancy that disappears with delivery has been implicated. Newborns delivered of mothers with Graves' disease can have a state of transient hyperthyroidism due to placental passage of TSI or less frequently long-term Graves' disease because of a genetic propensity. Mild neonatal thyrotoxicosis requires no therapy because the disease is self-limiting. In severe and more long-term thyrotoxicosis, PTU at doses of 10 to 25 mg every 8 hours is given. Nursing mothers with thyrotoxicosis can safely receive PTU in doses of 200 to 300 mg/day; these doses do not lead to levels in the milk that impair a newborn's thyroid function. MMI is concentrated in the milk at higher levels and should not be used.

Cardiac Disease

Thyrotoxicosis in patients with pre-existing cardiac disease can worsen symptoms and induce cardiac decompensation. Rarely, however, does severe hyperthyroidism induce cardiac symptoms in patients without underlying cardiac disease. Nevertheless, angina pectoris or high output failure has been reported after resumption of a euthyroid state in patients with severe thyrotoxicosis without prior evidence of cardiac disease. An increased association exists between Graves' disease and mitral valve prolapse. Most patients with cardiac problems due to hyperthyroidism are elderly, and many have toxic multinodular goiter. It is important to restore a euthyroid state promptly in these patients. This is best achieved by adequate doses of PTU (300 to 600 mg/day). Atrial fibrillation occurs in 10 to 15%; signs of congestive heart failure may be due to the rapid ventricular response and the absence of atrial contraction. Prompt slowing of the ventricular heart rate with digitalis and inducing β-sympathetic blockade with propranolol or atenolol are important. Digitalis must be prescribed with care because thyrotoxic patients are somewhat digitalis resistant, and a narrow margin separates therapeutic and toxic doses. Similarly, β-sympathetic blockers with negative inotropic effects should be used with caution in patients with congestive heart failure. The presence of atrial fibrillation usually requires anticoagulant therapy with aspirin or warfarin sodium. Increased vitamin K metabolism, however, may require lower warfarin doses. Spontaneous reversion from atrial fibrillation to regular sinus rhythm occurs frequently as successfully treated patients achieve a euthyroid state. if sinus rhythm has not returned after a euthyroid period of 4 months, cardioversion should be considered. Angina pectoris can worsen sufficiently in hyperthyroid patients that preinfarction angina becomes a concern. In markedly hyperthyroid patients, interventional procedures such as coronary angioplasty or bypass surgery should not be undertaken without prior treatment with antithyroid drugs because of the danger of thyrotoxic crisis. Calcium channel blockers like diltiazem are useful in patients with contraindications to propranolol. Angiographic procedures using iodinated contrast agents can markedly worsen the thyrotoxicosis because of the induction of the jodbasedow effect, which especially endangers patients with toxic multinodular goiter. The antiarrhythmic compound amiodarone also can induce the jodbasedow effect, as described earlier.

Becks GP, Burrow GN: Thyroid disease and pregnancy. Med Clin North Am 75:121, 1991. *A useful article for physicians caring for pregnant women.*
Burch AB, Wartofsky L: Graves' opthalmopathy: Current concepts regarding pathogenesis and management. Endocr Rev 14:747; 1993. *A thorough exploration of this difficult clinical problem.*
Gavin LA: Thyroid crisis. Med Clin North Am 75:179; 1991. *Provides a clinically detailed consideration of the problem.*
Van Sande J, Parma J, Tonacchera M, et al: Somatic and germline mutations of the TSH receptor gene in thyroid diseases. J Clin Endocrinol Metab, 80:2577–2585, 1995.

HYPOTHYROIDISM

Hypothyroidism is the clinical syndrome that results from decreased secretion of thyroid hormone from the thyroid gland. It most frequently reflects a disease of the gland itself (primary hypothyroidism) but can also be caused by pituitary disease (secondary hypothyroidism) or hypothalamic disease (tertiary hypothyroidism). Hypothyroidism leads to a slowing of metabolic processes and in its most severe form to the accumulation of mucopolysaccharides in the skin, causing a non-pitting edema termed *myxedema*. The term *myxedema* is reserved by some for a severe form of hypothyroidism, whereas others use the terms interchangeably. The term *cretinism* is reserved for hypothyroidism dating from birth and leading to abnormalities of intellectual and physical development. The generalized thyroid hormone resistance syndrome (GTRS) results from an abnormality in the amino acid sequence of the β form of the nuclear thyroid hormone receptor, leading to decreased T₃ binding. Impairment of thyroid hormone effects in GTRS is partly overcome by increased thyroid hormone levels, thereby preventing significant hypothyroid symptoms in most patients. The condition is rare.

INCIDENCE, ETIOLOGY, AND PATHOGENESIS. The incidence of hypothyroidism varies somewhat with the geographic area. In areas of adequate iodine supply, like the United States, hypothyroidism occurs in 0.8 to 1.0% of the population. In iodine-deficient areas of the world, the incidence is 10- to 20-fold higher. Neonatal hypothyroidism occurs with a frequency of 0.02% in the white population, whereas among blacks it falls to 0.003%. Table 239–9 lists the causes of hypothyroidism.

Primary hypothyroidism accounts for 90 to 95% of all cases, the remainder being of pituitary or hypothalamic origin. Most patients with primary hypothyroidism develop thyroid hormone deficiency during adulthood. Only a minority of patients have congenital hypothyroidism resulting from defects in enzymes required for thyroid hormone synthesis, thyroid agenesis, dysgenesis, or ectopic thyroid tissue. Temporary congenital hypothyroidism can be induced by maternal iodine or antithyroid drug administration. Primary hypothyroidism can be of a thyroprivic form, with markedly reduced or absent thyroid tissue, or a goitrous form, with an enlarged thyroid. The most frequent cause of hypothyroidism in adults is autoimmune disease, with goitrous or thyroprivic Hashimoto's disease being the prime example. In autoimmune-based hypothyroidism, antibodies are directed against thyroperoxidase, thyroglobulin, and the TSH receptor. Antithyroglobulin and antiperoxidase antibodies probably serve only as markers of autoimmunity, but anti-TSH antibodies cause disease. TSH receptor antibodies can block TSH action and thus contribute to decreased thyroid hormone formation. In addition to antithyroid antibodies, antibodies can be directed against the proteins of other endocrine organs such as the pancreas, adrenals, parathyroids, and gonads. Affected patients suffer from polyglandular endocrine deficiency states (see Chapter 244). A strong family history can be identified in most of these conditions.

Thyroid autoimmune disease also has an increased association with non-endocrine abnormalities such as pernicious anemia, lupus erythematosus, rheumatoid arthritis, Sjögren's syndrome, chronic hepatitis, and myasthenia gravis. Thyroprivic hypothyroidism due to iatrogenic destruction of thyroid tissue by RAI, external beam radiation, or surgery is second only to autoimmune disease in causing hypothyroidism in the United States. Worldwide, hypothyroidism due to iodine deficiencies and goitrogens predominates. Goitrous hypothyroidism develops because TSH hypersecretion results in excessive thyroid growth. Iodine excess also can lead to goitrous hypothyroidism through iodine-induced inhibition of thyroid hormone formation (Wolff-Chaikoff effect). This occurs especially in patients with underlying thyroid disease. The thyroid is unable to reduce iodide uptake in spite of increased iodide stores,

Table 239–9 ■ CAUSES OF HYPOTHYROIDISM

Primary hypothyroidism
  Insufficient amount of thyroid tissue
    Destruction of tissue by autoimmune process
      Hashimoto's thyroiditis (atrophic and goitrous forms)
      Graves' disease—end-stage
    Destruction of tissue by iatrogenic procedures
      [131]I therapy
      Surgical thyroidectomy
      External radiation
    Destruction of tissue by infiltrative processes
      Amyloidosis, lymphoma, scleroderma
  Defects of thyroid hormone biosynthesis
    Congenital enzyme defects
    Congenital mutations in TSH receptor
    Iodine deficiency or excess
    Drug-induced: thionamides, lithium, sulfonamides, interleukins, tumor necrosis factor, and others
Secondary hypothyroidism
  Pituitary
    Panhypopituitarism (e.g., neoplasm, radiation, surgery, Sheehan's syndrome)
    Isolated TSH deficiency
  Hypothalamic
    Congenital
    Infection
    Infiltration (sarcoidosis, granulomas)
Transient hypothyroidism
  Silent and subacute thyroidits
  Thyroxine withdrawal
Generalized resistance to thyroid hormone

Table 239–10 ■ TISSUE-SPECIFIC SIGNS AND SYMPTOMS OF HYPOTHYROIDISM

TISSUE	SIGNS AND SYMPTOMS
Central nervous system	Forgetfulness, stoic appearance, myxedematous dementia, cerebellar ataxia
Cardiovascular	Bradycardia, pericardial effusion, hypertension
Respiratory	Depressed ventilatory drive, pleural effusion, sleep apnea
Gastrointestinal	Constipation, hypomotility
Muscle	Delayed tendon reflexes, muscle stiffness and cramps, increased muscle volume weakness
Skin	Dry, rough, hyperkeratosis; non-pitting puffiness due to mucopolysaccharide deposits
Metabolic	Basal metabolic rate decreased, cold intolerance, decreased T_4 and drug turnover, weight gain

and the inability to escape from the Wolff-Chaikoff effect leads to goitrous hypothyroidism.

Secondary hypothyroidism is due to destruction of pituitary thyrotrophs by pituitary or adjacent tumors or by necrosis, as in Sheehan's syndrome. Mutations in the TSH β-subunit can lead to biologically inactive TSH, resulting in secondary hypothyroidism. In addition, mutations in the TSH receptor leading to hypothyroidism are described. Hypothalamic hypothyroidism is due to decreased TRH secretion, resulting in diminished TSH synthesis. TSH produced in the absence of a TRH stimulus does not show normal glycosylation and has decreased biologic activity. In addition to permanent hypothyroidism, transient hypothyroidism affects patients with subacute or painless thyroiditis, including the postpartum variety. Withdrawal of long-time thyroid hormone replacement leads to several weeks of hypothyroidism until the pituitary thyrotroph population is replenished and normal thyroid-pituitary feedback resumes.

Pathologic changes in hypothyroidism depend on the cause. In patients with thyroprivic hypothyroidism, the thyroid atrophies and is replaced by fatty and fibrous tissue. By contrast, in iodine deficiency-induced goitrous hypothyroidism, the gland appears hyperplastic with tall columnar epithelium. Extrathyroidal pathology is more uniform and independent of the cause of hypothyroidism. It is characterized by increased accumulation of glycosaminoglycans in interstitial tissue, giving the skin a waxy appearance. Glycosaminoglycan accumulation occurs because of decreased removal of the substance. With severe long-standing hypothyroidism, increased capillary permeability leads to proteinaceous fluid accumulation, which may involve the pericardium.

CLINICAL MANIFESTATIONS. The different causes of hypothyroidism lead to similar symptoms, the most common of which are listed in Table 239–10. The slow and progressive onset in most patients can make clinical diagnosis difficult. This is especially true in elderly patients exhibiting changes such as dry skin, reduced body and scalp hair, and memory difficulties, all of which could be due to the aging process in the absence of hypothyroidism. Typical complaints in hypothyroid patients include increased tiredness and sleep requirement with a depressed mood, feeling cold, gaining weight on the same diet, constipation, increased forgetfulness and increased time needed to fulfill a task, and decreased exercise tolerance associated with muscle cramps on strenuous exercises. Affected patients relate these complaints in a low-pitched, hoarse voice with a slow speech pattern. Frequently the changes are only fully appreciated by the patient after thyroid hormone replacement and return to a euthyroid state. The facial appearance is frequently dull and apathetic with puffiness around the eyes and loss of lateral eyebrows. The skin takes on a yellow complexion due to carotene accumulation and becomes cold, dry, and rough with non-pitting edema (myxedema). The thyroid may be normal, enlarged, or absent, depending on the cause of hypothyroidism. Cardiovascular changes can include bradycardia and an enlarged cardiac silhouette primarily due to pericardial effusion. Hypertension occurs in 10% of hypothyroid patients and resolves after thyroid hormone replacement. Because of the increased occurrence of hypercholesterolemia and hypertension, hypothyroid patients have more coronary artery disease. Angina pectoris sometimes develops only after starting thyroid hormone replacement. Anemias of different causes accompany hypothyroidism and can contribute to angina symptoms. Iron deficiency anemia results from decreased iron absorption. Absorption of folic acid is decreased. Pernicious anemia results from gastric mucosa atrophy with antibodies directed against the gastric mucosa. The decreased oxygen consumption in the hypothyroid state leads to diminished erythropoietin production, resulting in a mild anemia that can be thought of as an adaptive state. Pulmonary function is characterized by shallow and slow breathing and a decreased respiratory response to hypercapnia and hypoxia. Patients are very sensitive to sedatives that can depress the respiratory drive and lead to CO_2 retention and coma. Gastrointestinal motility decreases markedly and can lead to paralytic ileus and the megacolon of myxedema. The kidneys not only have an impaired ability to excrete a free water load, but an inappropriate secretion of antidiuretic hormone syndrome (SIADH) can develop and intensify hyponatremia. Because of physical resistance in associated tissues, slow Achilles tendon reflexes are a hallmark of hypothyroidism. Similarly, severe hypothyroidism can lead to cerebellar ataxia and peripheral neuropathy. Endocrine and metabolic abnormalities include hyperprolactinemia leading to galactorrhea, heavy menstrual bleeding, menorrhagia, hypoglycemia, and SIADH. Long-standing and severe hypothyroidism can induce marked thyrotroph hyperplasia, resulting rarely in increased pituitary size and sella enlargement suggesting a pituitary tumor. Hypothyroidism in newborns needs to be treated immediately with thyroxine replacement; otherwise, severe retardation of mental development, short stature, and deaf mutism can develop.

DIAGNOSIS. Figure 239–3 gives an approach to the diagnosis of hypothyroidism. An elevated TSH combined with a below-normal free T_4 is diagnostic of primary hypothyroidism. T_3 levels are not useful in the diagnosis of hypothyroidism because they are frequently normal in mild hypothyroidism and are markedly lowered by the NTI syndrome. In pituitary or hypothalamic hypothyroidism, the TSH level is normal or decreased, and only below-normal T_4 or free T_4 levels are diagnostic. With third-generation sensitive TSH assays, the TRH stimulation test provides little additional information. Using the TRH stimulation test, an absent response of TSH indicates secondary hypothyroidism whereas a partial or delayed TSH response indicates partial pituitary deficiency or hypothalamic disease. Patients with pituitary hypothyroidism frequently show other signs of pituitary deficiency, including low follicle-stimulating hormone and luteinizing hormone levels in the face of low sex hormone levels. It is especially important to identify deficient ACTH secretion and resulting secondary adrenal insufficiency. When present, thyroid hormone replacement cannot be started before initiating cortisol replacement. Low TSH levels can also be found in patients who recently became hypothyroid after a prolonged period of hyperthyroidism that led to a decrease in the pituitary thyrotroph population. Other laboratory manifestations of hypothyroidism include elevated cholesterol, creatine kinase, lactate dehydrogenase, and aspartate transaminase levels.

The presence of antithyroid antibodies is compatible with Hashimoto's disease and presents a risk factor for developing hypothyroidism. During early phases of hypothyroidism, T_4 and free T_4 lie just below the lower normal range. T_3 is normal and TSH is barely elevated. This condition has been termed *subclinical hypothyroidism,* or *the failing gland syndrome.* Patients show minimal or no signs of hypothyroidism because a normal T_3 level maintains their metabolic status. Many such patients later develop clinical hypothyroidism with a further increase in TSH levels and a decrease in T_4 and free T_4 levels. In patients with Hashimoto's disease or after RAI treatment of Graves' disease, this pattern occurs frequently. Transient hypothyroidism frequently occurs in postpartum patients, with subacute thyroiditis, or after RAI treatment for Graves' disease. Changes in TSH levels lag behind alterations in T_4 and T_3 levels; careful follow-up is required to determine if permanent hypothyroidism ensues.

DIFFERENTIAL DIAGNOSIS. Fully developed hypothyroidism presents a distinct clinical picture with few imitations. Patients with renal disease resulting in a nephrotic syndrome and hypoalbuminemia can develop a puffy face, peripheral edema, a pale downy skin, anemia, and hypercholesterolemia. Goiter and thyroid nodules occur with increased frequency in patients with renal disease. Lowering of TBG levels leads to a decrease in total T_4 values. In contrast to hypothyroidism, however, free T_4 is not decreased and TSH is not increased. In children, Down syndrome can mimic hypothyroidism. Differential diagnosis is further complicated by an increased incidence of Hashimoto's thyroiditis and resultant hypothyroidism in patients with Down syndrome, but thyroid hormone values are normal in Down syndrome patients without thyroid disease.

TREATMENT. Hypothyroidism is preferentially treated with levothyroxine (T_4), with doses ranging from 0.05 to 0.2 mg/day and an average replacement dose of 1.6 µg/kg/day T_3 is formed from T_4 by intracellular conversion so that both T_4 and T_3 exist in the body. Synthetic T_4 has a long shelf life and uniform potency. Eighty percent is absorbed, and once-a-day intake leads to stable T_4, T_3, and TSH levels. Accordingly, thyroxine represents the preferred thyroid hormone preparation for chronic replacement. Patients should be informed that replacement probably is needed for the rest of their lives and that periodic evaluation is required. In young healthy adults without coronary artery disease, a starting dose of 75 to 100 µg/day can be used and then adjusted after 2- to 3-week intervals to reach the final replacement level. In elderly patients and those with coronary artery disease, the initial dose should be 12.5 to 25 µg/day and increased by 25 to 50 µg every 4 to 6 weeks to allow a slow increase in metabolic rates, avoiding a mismatch between coronary blood supply and metabolic demand. The aim is to achieve a euthyroid status with TSH, T_4, and T_3 levels in the normal range. Because in the complete absence of functioning thyroid tissue all T_3 is formed from the thyroxine medication and the 20% of thyroidal contribution to T_3 levels is missing, T_3 levels are frequently in the mid-normal range and T_4 levels are in the upper range of normal. A slight increase in T_4 levels occurs 2 to 6

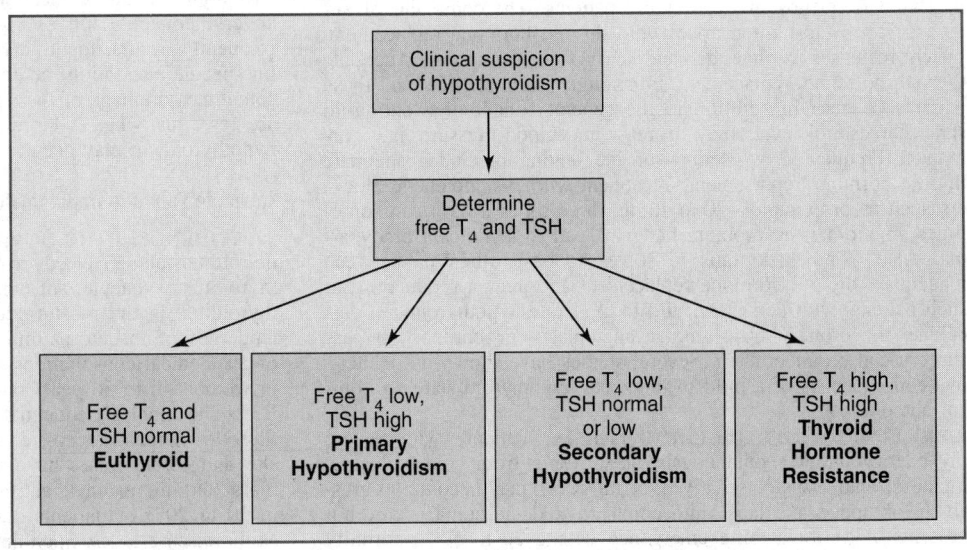

FIGURE 239–3 ■ Diagnostic approach to hypothyroidism.

hours after thyroxine intake so that blood for thyroid hormone determination should be drawn 20 to 24 hours later. The average replacement dose for thyroxine varies with age and to a lesser degree with the cause of hypothyroidism and the level of physical activity. Children (5 to 10 years), for example, require average replacement doses of 3 to 4 μg/kg. Required replacement doses in elderly persons, by contrast, are 20 to 30% lower (1.4μg/kg/day) than those needed in middle-aged adults. Patients with malabsorption or those taking aluminum preparations (antacids), cholestyramine, lovastatin, ferrous sulfate, and rifampin need higher replacement doses. During pregnancy, especially in the third trimester, thyroxine replacement needs increase by 30 to 50%. After delivery, thyroxine replacement is decreased to standard levels.

The ease of approach, virtual absence of side effects, and observance of a revitalized patient make thyroxine treatment of hypothyroid patients a satisfying therapeutic experience. Thyroxine and T_3 levels normalize within 2 to 3 weeks. TSH levels lag behind for 3 to 4 weeks or more because of the increased number of thyrotrophs in the pituitary after long-standing hypothyroidism. Clinical improvement begins 2 to 3 weeks after therapy, but complete resumption of a euthyroid state can take several months.

Patients receiving chronic T_4 replacement should be evaluated by physical examination and free T_4, T_3, and TSH determination once or twice a year. The TSH level is a good indicator of adequate replacement. In patients with primary hypothyroidism, TSH levels below the normal range indicate overreplacement and levels above the upper normal range indicate underreplacement. Chronic overreplacement with thyroxine can increase bone turnover, which is a special concern in women; however, no evidence currently exists for an increased bone fracture rate. Chronic T_4 overreplacement also can lead to cardiovascular abnormalities, especially arrhythmias and cardiac hypertrophy. The treatment of subclinical hypothyroidism is controversial. Enlargement of the thyroid gland, elevated cholesterol levels (especially with LDL:HDL ratios above 3) or signs of decreased exercise tolerance and mild congestive heart failure warrant treatment.

In addition to thyroxine, triiodothyronine T_3, combinations of T_4 and T_3, desiccated thyroid, and thyroxine plus iodine in one tablet are available. Only the use of T_3 is recommended in special situations. T_3 is useful for short-term treatment of patients with thyroid cancer after thyroid surgery and before RAI administration, because of its short half-life of 1 day versus the half-life of T_4 of 7 days (see section on thyroid cancer). Parenteral T_3 can be used to treat myxedema coma. In patients with the rare condition of 5′ deiodinase deficiency T_3 preparations are also useful. Other thyroid preparations have no advantage over thyroxine and are not recommended.

Special Clinical Conditions

ANGINA PECTORIS, CARDIAC SURGERY, AND THYROID HORMONE REPLACEMENT. Coronary artery disease occurs with increased frequency in hypothyroid patients. The complaint of angina pectoris most often arises with thyroid hormone replacement, which increases cardiac demand and O_2 consumption. Adequate thyroid hormone replacement is strongly recommended in these patients because in addition to the general benefit of a euthyroid state, cholesterol levels may decrease and blood pressure may normalize. Frequently, worsening of the angina precludes adequate thyroid hormone replacement. Treatment with β-sympathetic blockers such as propranolol (20 to 40 mg three times a day) can sometimes ameliorate the problem but may lead to significant bradycardia. Also, β-blockade fails to solve the basic dilemma between inadequate thyroid hormone replacement and angina production. In such patients with persistent mild to moderate hypothyroidism, percutaneous coronary transluminal angioplasty or coronary bypass surgery can be undertaken. Several studies have shown no deleterious consequences of a mild to moderate hypothyroid state on clinical outcome.

TREATMENT OF MYXEDEMA COMA. Patients with severe myxedema, either spontaneously or suffering from cold exposure, intake of analgesics or sedatives, or infection, may become progressively obtunded and lapse into coma. Myxedema coma is rare but presents a life-threatening emergency with a 20 to 50% mortality

Table 239–11 ■ TREATMENT OF MYXEDEMA COMA

Thyroid Hormone Administration
300 μg T_4 over 5–10 minutes initially, followed by 100 μg T_4 IV q24h until oral T_4 therapy can be started
Alternatively, 10 μg T_3 IV q4h until oral T_4 therapy can be started
Glucocorticoid Administration
Hydrocortisone, 100 mg IV bolus followed by 25 mg q6h by IV drip
Cover to conserve heat
Intravenous fluids, electrolytes, and glucose to correct electrolyte abnormalities and hypoglycemia
Tracheal intubation and mechanical ventilation as required
Treat precipitating conditions (infection)
Avoid sedatives, narcotics, and overhydration

that is best treated in an intensive-care unit. Treatment should be instituted immediately; and if T_4 and TSH levels cannot be readily obtained, therapy may be started on clinical suspicion. Increasing obtundation and elevated PCO$_2$ levels especially indicate the need for thyroid hormone administration. Assessment of adrenal function should also be undertaken because giving hydrocortisone can disturb pituitary-adrenal feedback and make subsequent diagnosis difficult. Vigorous thyroid hormone replacement is required. Thyroxine can be given as a single 300 μg T_4 bolus followed by daily 50- to 100-μg intravenous T_4 maintenance doses. A T_3 replacement schedule using 10 μg T_3 intravenously every 4 hours until the patient greatly improves and oral therapy can be resumed has been advocated. T_3 administration offers the potential advantage that no conversion of T_4 to T_3 is required, a step that may be impaired in severely ill patients. The treatment of myxedema coma is outlined in Table 239–11.

Arlot S, Debussche X, Lalau JD, et al: Myxedema coma: Response of thyroid hormone with oral and intravenous high-dose L-thyroxine treatment. Intensive Care Med 17:16, 1991.
Fisher DA: Management of congenital hypothyroidism. J Clin Endocrinol Metab 72:523, 1991.
Mandel SJ, Larsen PR, Seeley EW, Brent GA: Increased need for thyroxine during pregnancy in women with primary hypothyroidism. N Engl J Med 323:91, 1990.
Mitchell JM: Thyroid disease in the emergency department: Thyroid function tests and hypothyroidism and myxedema coma. Emerg Med Clin North Am 7:885, 1989.
Roti E. Minelli R. Gardini E, et al: The use and misuse of thyroid hormone. Endocr Rev 14:401, 1993.

THYROIDITIS

Thyroiditis includes infectious and autoimmune inflammatory diseases of the thyroid. Thyroiditis is divided into acute (suppurative), subacute painful (granulomatous), subacute painless (lymphocytic), chronic lymphocytic (Hashimoto's), and chronic fibrous (Riedel's) thyroiditis. Postpartum thyroiditis is classified as a variant of subacute painless lymphocytic thyroiditis.

Acute (Suppurative) Thyroiditis

Acute suppurative thyroiditis consists of a rare infection of the gland by bacteria, fungi, *Pneumocystis carinii*, or other organisms. Symptoms include tender swelling, sometimes with fluctuation and an erythematous skin overlying the area. Fever with leukocytosis frequently occurs. Identification of the microbial agent may require fine-needle aspiration of the lesion. Appropriate antibiotics and sometimes drainage of the abscess are required. Long-term sequelae are rare, but when a large part of the thyroid gland is involved, hypothyroidism may occur.

Subacute Painful (Granulomatous) Thyroiditis

INCIDENCE, ETIOLOGY, AND PATHOLOGY. Subacute painful thyroiditis, also referred to as de Quervain's thyroiditis, giant cell thyroiditis, subacute nonsuppurative thyroiditis, or granulomatous thyroiditis, is the most frequent cause of severe thyroid pain and tenderness. Subacute painful thyroiditis is not rare, resulting in 5% of all medical consultations for thyroid disease. It is most common in women 40 to 50 years old and shows an association with HLA-B35. The disease frequently follows a viral infection, and elevated titers to mumps, adeno-, entro-, echo-, influenza, coxsackie-, measles and other viruses have been found. Increased thyroid antibody titers (antimicrosomal, antithyroglobulin, anti-TSH receptor) occur in 10 to 20% of patients during the subacute phase and disappear as the disease fades. Such antibodies are polyclonal and most likely arise secondary to thyroid damage caused by viral infection. The thyroid is enlarged and edematous with destruction of follicular architecture and the presence of histocytes that coalesce into giant cells.

MANIFESTATIONS, DIAGNOSIS, AND TREATMENT. The disease frequently follows by 1 to 3 weeks the occurrence of viral pharyngitis, mumps, measles, or other viral syndromes. Severe pain develops over the thyroid area, radiates to the ear, and is enhanced by swallowing. A feeling of general malaise with muscle aches, pain, anorexia, and fever is present. On palpation, the thyroid is very tender and may be generally enlarged but can contain unilateral painful areas. Cervical lymphadenopathy rarely occurs. Characteristic laboratory findings are an elevated sedimentation rate, often above 100 mm/hr Westergren, and a markedly decreased RAI uptake ($< 2\%$ at 24 hours). The levels of free T_4 and TSH depend on the phase of the disease, with high T_4 levels occurring during the early stage owing to follicle disruption and hormone release. At later stages, transient hypothyroidism may follow, with elevated TSH levels. Rarely, permanent hypothyroidism ensues. Thyroglobulin levels are elevated during the acute phase.

Subacute thyroiditis is an inflammatory, self-limiting disorder that at most requires symptomatic therapy. In mild cases, no therapy or analgesics such as aspirin (2 to 3 g/day) are sufficient. Prednisone, 40 to 60 mg/day, can suppress more severe symptoms and bring relief. Within 8 to 10 days symptoms markedly decrease, and the dose can be tapered and completely stopped after 4 weeks. Sometimes symptoms flare up again and the prednisone taper needs to be reversed. In some patients, more than one attack may occur, leading to an increased risk of permanent hypothyroidism. During the initial phase, the patient may be thyrotoxic and need treatment with β-sympathetic blocking agents such as propranolol. Rarely hepatitis develops, requiring careful follow-up.

Subacute Painless (Lymphocytic) Thyroiditis with Transient Hyperthyroidism

INCIDENCE, ETIOLOGY, AND PATHOLOGY. Subacute painless thyroiditis with transient hyperthyroidism is also called subacute lymphocytic thyroiditis with spontaneously revolving hyperthyroidism and silent thyroiditis. The hallmark of the disorder is a self-limiting episode of thyrotoxicosis and a histologic picture of lymphocytic infiltration that differs from the changes found in Hashimoto's disease. Both postpartum thyroiditis and the sporadic disease occurring in the general population are forms of subacute lymphocytic thyroiditis. The incidence of sporadic subacute painless thyroiditis shows some geographic variability, with the sporadic form occurring more frequently in previously iodine-deficient areas that are now iodine replete, like the Great Lakes area of the United States, where the disease may account for 5 to 15% of all thyroiditis. Postpartum thyroiditis occurs in 2 to 6% of all pregnant women in the United States. The incidence is even higher in Sweden and Japan, reaching 7 to 12%. Eighty per cent of cases of the sporadic form affect women between the ages of 30 and 40 years. The disease is most likely autoimmune and independent of a preceding viral illness. Subacute lymphatic thyroiditis is distinguished from chronic lymphocytic thyroiditis (Hashimoto's disease) by a self-limiting course and a lower extent of lymphocyte infiltration with the absence of germinal centers.

MANIFESTATIONS, DIAGNOSIS, AND TREATMENT. Typical are an abrupt onset with signs of thyrotoxicosis such as nervousness, heat intolerance, tachycardia, and weight loss. A small, firm, but painless goiter is noted in about half the patients. Some may present in a hypothyroid state after the initial hyperthyroid phase was unnoticed. Postpartum thyroiditis usually occurs 3 to 6 months after delivery 5 and is probably due to a rebound of immune activity after it was suppressed during pregnancy, one finds an initial transient hyperthyroid phase followed by hypothyroidism. The latter lasts 1 to 3 months, and most patients make a spontaneous recovery. During the initial hyperthyroid phase, which can last 2 to 4 months. T_4 and T_3 are elevated, with relatively higher T_4 levels due to thyroid hormone release from damaged follicles. Thyroid antibodies, especially antiperoxidase, are frequently positive but at low titers. Sedimentation rate is normal or only slightly elevated, in contrast to the marked elevation occurring in subacute painful thyroiditis. The RAI uptake is suppressed. Signs of Graves' disease, such as ophthalmopathy and pretibial myxedema, are ab-

sent, and the level of TSI, which is the hallmark of Graves' disease, is normal. Thyroid biopsy shows a typical histologic picture with abundant lymphocyte infiltration, but the procedure is not required for routine diagnosis. Treatment aims at sympathetic blockade using, for example, propranolol to alleviate symptoms during the thyrotoxic phase. Glucocorticoids are not needed. Prolonged hypothyroid episodes may be treated with thyroxine replacement, but with subsequent tapering of the dose and final withdrawal because most patients regain euthyroid status. Increased incidences of goiter and persistent hypothyroidism have been noted in patients who continue to show antiperoxidase antibodies. Similarly, the recurrence of postpartum thyroiditis has been noted in some patients with continued presence of antiperoxidase antibodies after the initial phase of the disease.

Chronic Lymphocytic Thyroiditis (Hashimoto's Thyroiditis)

Chronic lymphocytic thyroiditis is the most prevalent form of thyroid autoimmune disease, affecting 3 to 4% of the population in the United States. It is three times more common in women and most frequently diagnosed between the third and fifth decade of life. A genetic propensity for the disease is demonstrated by an increased familial incidence and an association with major histocompatibility antigens such as HLA-B8. The goitrous variant of Hashimoto's thyroiditis occurs more frequently in patients positive for HLA-DR5, whereas the atrophic variant is associated with HLA-DR3. The presence of antiperoxidase and antithyroglobulin antibodies indicates the autoimmune nature of the disease. Very high levels of thyroid antibodies distinguish Hashimoto's thyroiditis from other forms. In addition, anti-TSH receptor antibodies can occur that are frequently of the blocking variety, impairing TSH action. Rarely, TSIs are present, leading to hyperthyroidism and the combined occurrence of Graves' disease and Hashimoto's disease called Hashitoxicosis. Thyroid pathology is dominated by heavy lymphocyte infiltration destroying the normal follicular architecture. Lymph follicles and germinal centers can be identified. The presence of copious lymphocytes is a hallmark of the disease that distinguishes it from other forms of autoimmune thyroiditis. Differential diagnosis between the abundant lymphocyte infiltrates of Hashimoto's disease and the occurrence of a primary thyroid lymphoma is sometimes difficult. Thyroid lymphomas occur with an increased frequency in Hashimoto's disease but overall are rare. Also, the pathology of the thyroid gland in Hashimoto's disease is characterized by extensive fibrosis throughout the gland. Different manifestations of Hashimoto's disease can be distinguished. The occurrence of a goitrous versus an atrophic variant may be explained by the prevailing autoimmune antibodies. For example, in patients with atrophic thyroiditis, high titers of TSH receptor-blocking antibodies are found. In other patients with Hashimoto's disease, a goiter and features of Graves' disease occur that results from the TSI presence.

CLINICAL MANIFESTATIONS AND DIAGNOSIS. In Hashimoto's thyroiditis, thyroid enlargement is the most frequent manifestation, with 75% of patients having a euthyroid goiter; the remainder have the atrophic variety and may not have a palpable gland. Hypothyroidism occurs as an initial manifestation in 20% of patients. Hyperthyroidism occurs in less than 5% of patients and can be either self-limiting or of long standing, representing Hashitoxicosis. The principal abnormalities in the immune system discussed for Graves' disease also apply to Hashimoto's disease. The prevalence of specific forms of TSH receptor antibodies with a predominance of the TSI in Graves' disease versus the occurrence of TSH receptor-blocking antibodies in Hashimoto's disease distinguishes the two autoimmune diseases. In addition, lymphocyte infiltration is much more destructive to the architecture of the normal gland than in Graves' disease. Other autoimmune diseases occur with increased frequency in Hashimoto's patients, including autoimmune diseases of the endocrine system with adrenal, parathyroid, pituitary, and gonad destruction and damage to β cells of the pancreas. Furthermore, an association occurs with pernicious anemia, Sjögren's syndrome, lupus erythematosus, and idiopathic thrombocytopenic purpura. Graves' disease can occur in conjunction with the same illnesses.

On physical examination, a painless symmetrically enlarged thyroid gland is noted that feels firm and rubbery with an irregular surface. The gland can reach a size and firmness that leads to pressure symptoms, impairing swallowing and resulting in inlet obstruction with tracheal compression. Sometimes only one firm lobe or a single firm thyroid nodule may be palpable, representing the only remnant, with other parts of the gland destroyed by the autoimmune process. On laboratory examination, 90% of patients have positive antiperoxidase antibodies and 50% have antithyroglobulin antibodies. T_4 and TSH levels can be normal. In patients with the hypothyroid form, TSH levels are elevated and T_4 and free T_4 levels are decreased. RAI scans are not required for routine workup and are not diagnostic. They can show normal, increased, or decreased overall uptake with local patchy areas of increased and decreased iodine accumulation. Fine-needle aspiration is not routinely used but can be helpful in differentiating a firm nodule as a thyroid remnant in Hashimoto's disease versus a benign thyroid adenoma or thyroid cancer. The incidence of thyroid cancer is not increased in Hashimoto's disease except for the increased occurrence of lymphomas, a rare event.

TREATMENT. The autoimmune abnormality underlying Hashimoto's disease is currently not amenable to therapy. Therapy is directed at achieving a euthyroid state and dealing with mechanical problems resulting from the goiter. Thyroxine replacement is initiated when T_4 levels are low and TSH levels are high. In some patients, only the TSH is slightly elevated and the T_4 is low-normal, with signs of hypothyroidism being absent. These patients can be treated with thyroxine replacement to forestall further thyroid gland enlargement and future clinical hypothyroidism. In some patients, thyroxine therapy cannot decrease the goiter size and obstructive symptoms may require surgery for relief. During the early phases of Hashimoto's disease, transient hyperthyroidism can occur and requires only symptomatic treatment with sympathetic β-blockers. Hyperthyroidism developing in well-established Hashimoto's disease is treated like Graves' disease, with antithyroid medication as the treatment of choice.

Fibrous Thyroiditis (Riedel's Thyroiditis)

In fibrous thyroiditis, thyroid tissue is replaced by dense, chronically inflamed fibrous tissue. The thyroid is rock hard on palpation, a finding that can be compatible with thyroid cancer. Thyroid aspiration can clarify the diagnosis. Tracheal obstruction can occur and may require surgery. Sclerosing mediastinitis, retroperitoneal fibrosis, sclerosis of the biliary tract, and pseudotumors of the orbit have been described in such patients. When hypothyroidism exists, thyroxine replacement is required.

Rapoport B: Pathophysiology of Hashimoto's thyroiditis and hypothyroidism. Ann Rev Med 42:91, 1991. *A thorough review of the subject.*
Singer PA: Thyroiditis. Acute, subacute, and chronic. Med Clin North Am 75:61, 1991. *Provides a thorough discussion of the condition.*

NON-TOXIC DIFFUSE AND NODULAR GOITER

The term *non-toxic* or *simple goiter* indicates an increase in the mass of the thyroid gland resulting from excessive replication of benign thyroid epithelial cells. In patients with non-toxic goiter, thyroid hormone values usually are normal. The increase in thyroid size is a slow process evolving over many years, starting with a diffuse initial enlargement, which frequently becomes multinodular with time. Non-toxic goiter is the most common thyroid disease in America, affecting about 5% of the population. Its incidence increases with age and affects women three to five times more frequently than men. Goiters have been classified according to the epidemiologic pattern in which they occur as endemic or sporadic goiters. Thyroid enlargement occurring in more than 10% of a population is termed *endemic goiter* and is presumed to result from environmental factors, such as iodine deficiency or the presence of goitrogens in the food chain that inhibit thyroid hormone formation. *Sporadic goiter* indicates thyroid enlargement in a small fraction of the population. The cause of sporadic goiter varies, with thyroid growth most frequently stimulated by extrathyroidal growth factors. TSH is the most frequent stimulator. The observation that goiters also occur in patients with adequate thyroid hormone levels and normal or low TSH levels indicates either that the sensitivity of thyroid cells to TSH can increase markedly or that other factors

drive thyroid cell growth. Stimulatory effects of IGF-I and EGF on thyroid cell growth have been reported. In addition, TSH receptor-directed antibodies that have only a growth-stimulating effect have been described. Different thyroid cells also have a varying propensity to grow and enter the mitotic cycle independent of stimulation by growth factors. Specific thyroid cells and their descendants that possess an increased noncancerous propensity to divide and grow can form new thyroid follicles. These different factors that contribute to goiter formation explain why not all goiters shrink or stop growing on thyroxine supplementation and resultant TSH suppression.

The pathology of the goitrous thyroid varies, depending on the stage and cause of the goiter. Initially, hypertrophic follicles with hypervascularity are prevalent throughout the gland. With increasing duration, follicle size varies. Some follicles become involuted, whereas others enlarge with colloid accumulation. Fibrotic areas sometimes separate hypertrophic from atrophic and involuted areas. This mixed pattern of follicle activity is reflected in RAI scans with patchy areas of increased and decreased uptake.

MANIFESTATIONS. Patients with non-toxic simple goiter can be asymptomatic or present with symptoms due to mechanical pressure exerted by the enlarged thyroid gland. Structures exposed to pressure are the trachea, esophagus, recurrent laryngeal nerve, and large cervical veins. Substernal goiters are most frequently responsible for tracheal pressure symptoms leading to deviation, narrowing, and chondromalacia. The trachea must be narrowed to 20 to 30% of its normal diameter to produce respiratory symptoms, especially inspiratory stridor. Pull and pressure on the laryngeal nerve leading to hoarseness can occur with benign goiters but should raise the suspicion of malignancy. The presence of a substernal goiter is made evident when patients raise both arms above the head, which pulls the goiter upward into the thoracic inlet. The resultant impediment of jugular venous return leads to a livid suffusion of the face and discomfort for the patient (Pemberton's sign). An acute painful enlargement of an area of the thyroid frequently reflects sudden bleeding into a thyroid nodule; symptoms improve as resorption of the hemorrhage occurs. In a slow and progressively developing dominant nodule, thyroid cancer must be excluded by cytologic examination of a fine-needle aspirate.

Congenital goiter in endemic areas results most frequently from insufficient thyroid hormone formation due to iodine deficiency or the presence of goitrogens and resultant TSH stimulation of the gland. Sporadic congenital goiter is often due to biosynthetic abnormalities in thyroid hormone formation resulting from defects in (1) iodide transport into the thyroid, (2) deficient peroxidase activity, (3) deficient iodotyrosine coupling, (4) formation of abnormal thyroglobulin, (5) impaired thyroglobulin proteolysis, or (6) deiodinases being deficient or absent and not allowing for intrathyroidal iodide conservation. These defects are rare and account for 10% of all congenital hypothyroidism. If these patients are left untreated, goiter and cretinism can result. In other patients, non-toxic goiter with mild hypothyroidism develops. The combination of congenital hypothyroidism and eighth nerve deafness has been termed *Pendred's syndrome.*

DIAGNOSTIC PROCEDURES. The most sensitive index to evaluate thyroid status in patients with goiter is the TSH level. TSH can be elevated in the face of normal or low-normal T_4 levels and mid-normal T_3 values. Most such patients benefit from thyroxine replacement, with TSH decreasing into the normal range and removing the thyroid growth stimulus. The thyroid status of patients with non-toxic goiter needs to be evaluated once or twice a year because some thyroid nodules develop autonomy over time, and toxic adenomas with resulting thyrotoxicosis can develop. In addition, ingestion of excess iodine can induce thyrotoxicosis due to the jodbasedow effect. With progressive involution of the goiter, TSH values increase progressively and hypothyroidism develops. The presence of pressure symptoms requires evaluation for substernal extension of the thyroid gland, which is best performed by CT or MRI. In the absence of such imaging, radiography reveals tracheal deviation, and pulmonary function tests can document inspiratory impairment. In patients with endemic goiter, especially due to iodine deficiency, laboratory values show low T_4, normal T_3, and elevated TSH levels stimulating the thyroid gland for further compensatory growth. The amount of iodine intake can be documented by determining iodide excretion in the urine, which is correspondingly low in iodine-deficiency regions.

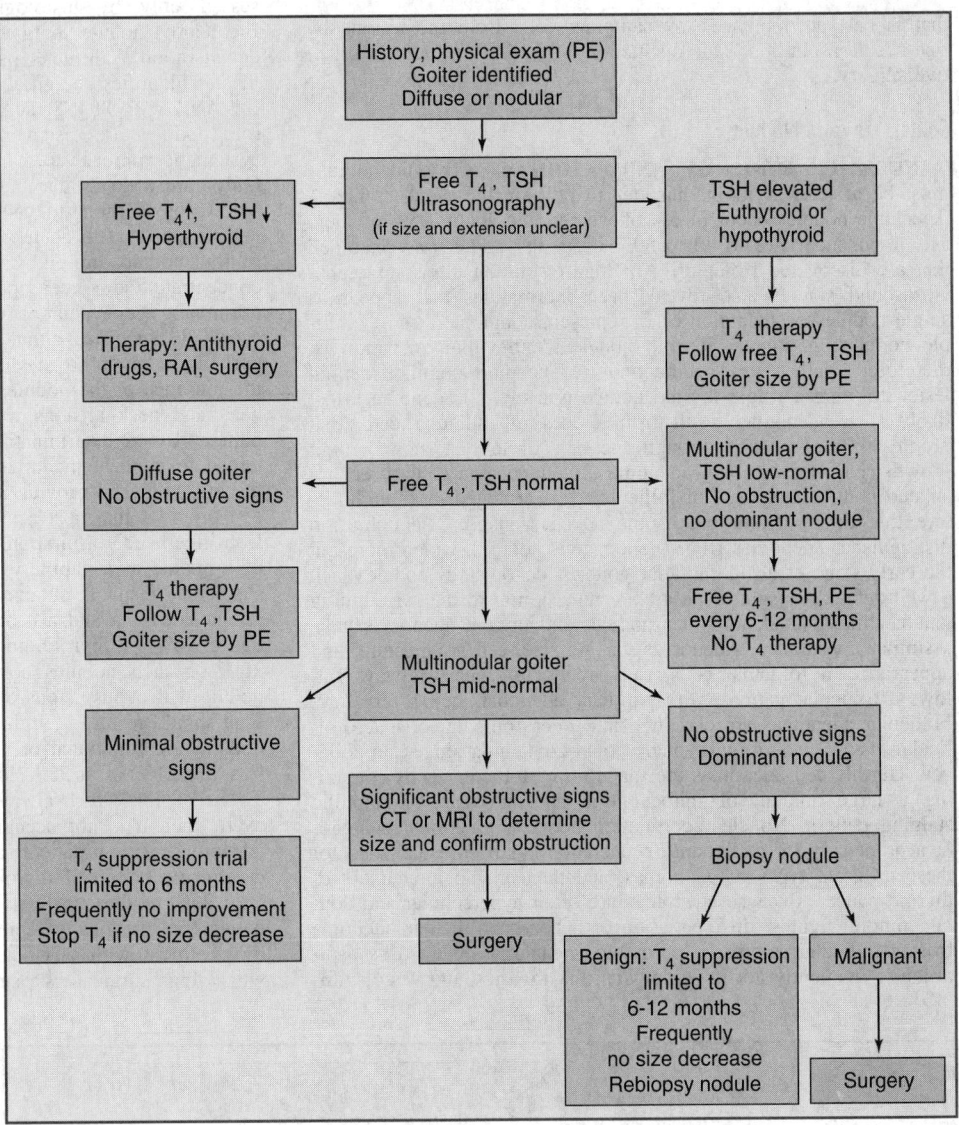

FIGURE 239–4 ▪ Evaluation and management of patients with non-toxic diffuse and nodular goiter and undetermined thyroid status.

TREATMENT. The aim of therapy is to decrease the size of the thyroid, relieve pressure-induced symptoms, and achieve a euthyroid state. The approach to the patient with a goiter is outlined in Figure 239–4. In patients with sporadic goiter and elevated TSH levels, a clear rationale for thyroxine therapy is given. Thyroxine is started at 100 μg/day with subsequent dose adjustments to bring TSH into the low-normal but not the undetectable range. In patients with large, nontoxic diffuse goiters and normal T_4 and TSH levels, the same approach is chosen. The efficiency of this approach is indicated by a 20% decrease in thyroid volume after 1 year of treatment. In patients showing a response to therapy, treatment may be indefinite.

Treatment of multinodular goiter, especially in older patients, provides a more difficult problem. The TSH level must be determined, and if it is suppressed or in the low-normal range, thyroxine therapy should not be started. Thyroxine therapy also can be guided by results of an RAI scan and the suppression test, as described earlier. Identification of autonomous areas excludes thyroxine therapy. In patients with multinodular goiter without autonomous areas and high-normal or elevated TSH levels, a trial of thyroxine therapy can be undertaken. In older patients, the initial dose of thyroxine should not be higher than 50 μg, and dose increases should be staggered at 25-μg steps at 4- to 6-week intervals. The results of thyroxine suppression therapy in patients with long-standing multinodular goiter are frequently disappointing, with little or no decrease in goiter size. Because thyroid tissue between nodules can decrease considerably, however, the nodules may appear more prominent. If no discernible decrease in size of

multinodular goiter occurs after 6 to 12 months, thyroxine therapy should be stopped. In such patients, symptoms of temporary hypothyroidism can occur 1 month after stopping the medication and last for an additional month.

Endemic goiter is best treated by iodine supplementation, providing approximately 200 μg of iodine per day, or by the removal of identifiable goitrogens. Iodine supplementation can induce thyrotoxicosis due to the jodbasedow effect. Surgical therapy of a goiter should be undertaken only if significant obstructive symptoms occur and goiter size cannot be reduced by thyroxine therapy. After partial thyroidectomy, thyroxine at 1.6 μg/kg/day should be supplied to prevent regenerative hyperplasia. RAI therapy for large goiters has been tried with modest success. ^{131}I can induce a thyroiditis and thyroid swelling, leading to an acute increase in obstructive symptoms, and should therefore be performed only in carefully observed patients.

Greenspan FS: The problem of the nodular goiter. Med Clin North Am 75:195, 1991. *Provides a detailed analysis of the problem.*

BENIGN AND MALIGNANT THYROID NODULES

A thyroid nodule is a single palpable abnormality in the thyroid gland that can be a benign adenoma or thyroid cancer. Thyroid nodules are frequent and occur in about 5% of the population. In contrast, thyroid cancer is much less frequent, and among 100 patients with thyroid nodules only 4 have thyroid cancer. Distinguishing between benign and malignant lesions is an important task that is best accomplished by sampling cells from the lesions by fine-needle aspiration. This distinction is required to perform selective surgery.

Solitary Thyroid Nodules

INCIDENCE, ETIOLOGY, AND PATHOLOGY. Thyroid nodules must be at least 1 cm in diameter to be palpable. Such clinically detectable nodules occur in 6% of women and about 1.5% of men. The prevalence rises to 40 to 50% if smaller nodules are included that are discovered by autopsy or high-resolution ultrasonography: Ultrasound studies also reveal that abnormalities that appear as single nodules on palpation often represent conglomerates of multiple nodules. A solitary thyroid nodule identified on palpation is, therefore, a rather non-specific finding. The most common benign lesion forming a single thyroid nodule is a thyroid adenoma. Most likely such adenomas result from clones of follicular cells that progress more quickly through the cell cycle but show benign growth characteristics. An adenoma is defined as a solitary encapsulated nodule composed of follicular cells arranged in an architecture that differs from that of the adjacent gland. The definition distinguishes adenomas from adenomatous nodules, which represent the early stage of a multinodular goiter. Adenomatous nodules lack a well-defined capsule or an architecture similar to the surrounding gland; clinically, adenomatous nodules and thyroid adenomas have a similar appearance. Adenomas vary in size, cell architecture, and appearance of follicular cells. Cell architecture nearly always follows a follicular pattern, with papillary adenomas being very rare. Follicular adenomas are classified into microfollicular or macrofollicular lesions and an embryonal variant containing almost no collagen. Hürthle cell adenomas are made up of follicular cells containing a large amount of mitochondria and have an eosinophilic staining pattern. No clear correlation between functional behavior or a propensity for malignant degeneration has been established for these different types of adenomas, and they are not precursors of thyroid cancer. Because adenomas are often hypercellular and contain mitotic figures, differentiation of a benign follicular adenoma from a follicular carcinoma on cytologic material obtained by aspiration is frequently not possible. Capsular invasion and vessel infiltration are hallmarks of a malignant lesion, and these can be assessed only by histologic examination of the entire nodule. Frequently, nodules outgrow their blood supply and undergo cystic degeneration. Ultimate pathologic evaluation of follicular neoplasms identifies benign adenomas in 85% and carcinomas in 15%.

MANIFESTATIONS, DIAGNOSIS, AND TREATMENT. Most thyroid nodules are discovered on routine physical examination. A systematic approach to thyroid nodules is outlined in Figure 239–5. Only rarely do solitary nodules become large enough or extend below the sternum to cause pressure symptoms. Bleeding into a nodule can lead to acute pain and enlargement. Most patients with thyroid nodules are euthyroid because 85 to 90% of the adenomas concentrate iodine very poorly and do not actively form thyroid hormone. The evaluation of a thyroid nodule includes a history, especially inquiries about the occurrence of specific risk factors such as radiation to the head and neck area. Examination reveals the presence of the nodule and should evaluate lymph nodes in the head and neck area as well as the clinical thyroid status of the patient. Blood determinations of free T_4 and TSH should be obtained to confirm the thyroid status. Fine-needle aspiration of the thyroid nodule to provide material for evaluation by a cytopathologist provides the most accurate assessment. Results to be expected from fine-needle aspiration are listed in Table 239–4. Identification of a nodule as a papillary carcinoma requires thyroid surgery. If a suspicious result is obtained and cannot distinguish between a follicular adenoma and a carcinoma, an RAI scan can be performed: 85 to 90% of thyroid nodules are non-functional or "cold" and 20% of such nodules contain a malignancy. Identification of a nodule with a suspicious cytologic result as non-functional on RAI scan should result in surgical removal. Ten to 15 percent of thyroid nodules are functional or "hot"; the incidence of thyroid cancer is less than 1% in such lesions. One report indicates that a mutant TSH receptor, which always stimulates thyroid hormone formation even when it is not occupied by TSH, is expressed in functional adenomas. If such patients are euthyroid, they can be followed with careful evaluation of thyroid size and functional status. Sooner or later 25% of these patients become hyperthyroid. Nodules in such patients are surgically removed after the patient is made euthyroid by treatment with PTU or MMI. In older patients or in patients with a high surgical risk, such nodules can be ablated with RAI.

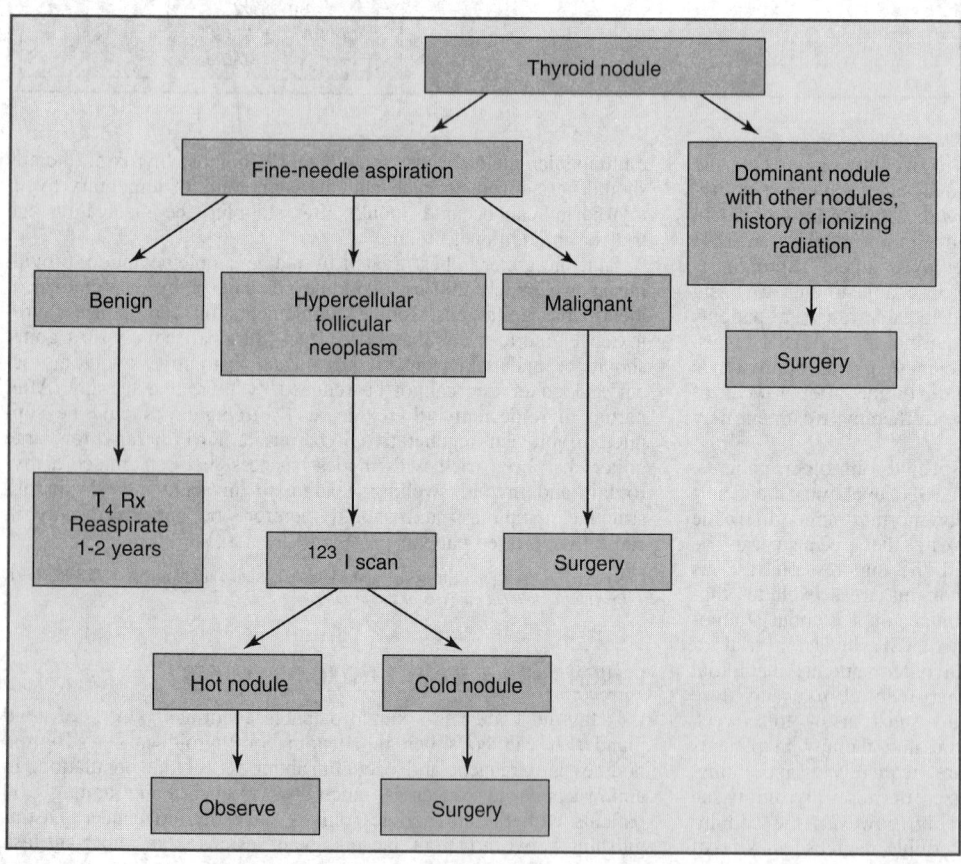

FIGURE 239–5 ■ Workup of thyroid nodules.

In about 75% of patients, a thyroid nodule aspirate indicates a benign thyroid nodule. Most such patients have few or no pressure symptoms. In patients with a normal TSH level, thyroxine should be given, starting at 100 μg/day but choosing lower doses in elderly patients and those having cardiovascular symptoms, as discussed earlier. Approximately a one-fifth reduction in the size of these nodules occurs in a majority of patients within 6 to 12 months. If no response to thyroxine occurs, the medication can be stopped. The size of the nodule should then be followed carefully, and a growing nodule should be reaspirated at 1- to 2-year intervals. Rapid growth of a nodule, especially in a patient on thyroxine, requires reaspiration. Increase in nodule size can be due to the accumulation of fluid in a cystic lesion. Although the cyst can be aspirated, fluid frequently reaccumulates and the nodule progressively enlarges. Benign enlarging nodules can be removed surgically.

Thyroid Cancer

INCIDENCE AND ETIOLOGY. Thyroid cancer almost always presents as a palpable thyroid abnormality. Although most thyroid nodules are benign, about 1 in 25 contains a thyroid cancer. In every 100,000 adults, about six women and two men each year develop thyroid cancer. Such cancers can progress aggressively, especially by local invasion, and lead to much suffering; about 9% are fatal. The incidence of clinically apparent thyroid cancer contrasts to reports that small (<10 mm in diameter), asymptomatic thyroid cancers are found in 5 to 10% of the population at autopsy. These small lesions are considered occult neoplasms of unclear clinical significance. Rarely, such small lesions metastasize to lymph nodes. The cause of thyroid cancer remains unknown, but activation of kinase genes *ret* and *trk* have been reported. In follicular cancer mutations of the *ras* kinase gene occur and in papillary cancer managements of the *ret* proto-oncogene have been described. Anaplastic cancer shows inactivating mutations of the *p53* repressor gene. Despite these beginnings, however, a conclusive relationship between specific gene alterations and particular forms of thyroid cancer has not been established. Certain risk factors for thyroid cancer can be identified. Radiation to the head and neck area, especially during early childhood, leads to a 30-fold increase in thyroid cancer with radiation doses up to 1500 rad. Higher radiation doses of 5000 rad or more, as they are delivered to the thyroid by ^{131}I therapy for Graves' disease, do not lead to an increased incidence of thyroid cancer. Other risk factors are primarily genetic and include familial forms of papillary cancer, Gardner's and Cowden's syndrome for papillary cancer, and the multiple endocrine neoplasia (MEN) type II syndrome for medullary cancer. Most thyroid cancers are of follicular epithelial cell origin; chronic TSH stimulation appears to play a permissive but not causative role in differentiated papillary and follicular thyroid cancers. Papillary cancer is the least aggressive malignancy and represents about 70% of all thyroid cancer, with follicular cancers representing 15%. The rest are made up of medullary cancer, anaplastic cancer, lymphomas, and other rare tumors. Metastases to the thyroid occur primarily from malignant melanomas and cancers of breast, lung, and kidney.

PATHOLOGY. Papillary cancer is the most common thyroid cancer in the United States, being two to three times more common in women and relatively more common in young patients. The absolute incidence is higher in the fourth to seventh decades. Papillary cancers occur most frequently in parts of the world where iodine supply is adequate. Papillary cancers generally are not encapsulated, and they grow slowly by infiltrative local spread, initially affecting other parts of the thyroid and extending to regional lymph nodes in the neck. Microscopically, papillary cancer is characterized by epithelial cells with large, irregular, frequently clear nuclei covering fibrovascular stalks. The papillae, which give the tumor its name, may not be present in parts of the tumor, and some parts may have a follicular structure. About half of papillary carcinomas contain laminated, calcified spherules called psammoma bodies. Variants of papillary cancer with good prognosis include the micropapillary encapsulated, solid, and follicular variants. A poor prognosis is associated with tall, columnar cells and diffuse sclerosis variants. Although one study has reported a higher mortality with lymph node metastases, local lymph node invasion is not necessarily a bad prognostic sign in papillary cancer because it occurs even

with occult tumors less than 1 cm in diameter, which have a favorable prognosis. In patients older than 50 years of age, papillary cancers undergo a more aggressive local spread, leading to death from local invasions in over half of the patients. Distant metastases are uncommon (2 to 3% of patients), with the lung more frequently involved than bone or the central nervous system.

Follicular carcinoma develops more frequently with increasing age, but its incidence remains only one fifth that of papillary cancer. Despite this lower incidence, however, follicular cancer accounts for more deaths than papillary cancer because of its early hematogenous spread to lung, bone, brain, and liver. Distant metastases occur in about one fifth of patients. Lymph node involvement occurs in less than 1% of patients. Follicular cancer presents as an encapsulated, expansible neoplasm with a microfollicular pattern. Its hallmark is invasion of the tumor capsule and extension into blood vessels at its periphery. These invasive features distinguish follicular carcinomas from follicular adenomas. Aspirates obtained from follicular carcinomas are hypercellular, containing cells with numerous mitotic figures with large nuclei. The diagnosis, however, can be difficult on frozen section. Cyst formation occurs in follicular cancer just as it does in benign thyroid nodules. Rarely, follicular cancer concentrates iodine actively and generates sufficient thyroid hormone to create hot nodules leading to thyrotoxicosis. In some forms of differentiated thyroid cancer, epithelial cells called Hürthle cells show oxyphilic staining and contain numerous mitochondria. Hürthle cell cancer is primarily a variant of follicular cancer but has also been rarely described with a papillary structure. Hürthle cell cancer appears to be more aggressive than papillary or follicular cancer.

Anaplastic cancer represents about 5% of thyroid cancer and occurs predominantly in persons older than 70 years. The spindle and giant cell variants are most frequent, and the rare small cell variant can be confused with lymphomas or medullary cancer. Almost one third of anaplastic cancers arise in pre-existing differentiated cancers. The prognosis is dismal, with a mean survival of 7 to 12 months. Death most commonly results from aggressive local invasion causing progressive tracheal obstruction or massive hemorrhage. Distant metastases occur, but the local spread is so rapid that metastatic foci have little clinical importance.

Medullary carcinoma is a malignant tumor of calcitonin-secreting C cells that accounts for 2 to 3% of all thyroid cancer. The tumor produces calcitonin, calcitonin-related peptide, chromogranin A, ACTH, prostaglandins, and carcinoembryonic antigen. Densely packed cells form solid masses separated by hyalinized tumor stroma. Amyloid deposits occur frequently. Several variants of the tumor have been described, with the sporadically occurring form accounting for 80% and genetic or familial variants making up the remainder. The familial variants can be subdivided into those occurring with MEN IIa, MEN IIb, and a familial non-MEN variant. In MEN IIa, the medullary cancer occurs together with pheochromocytomas and parathyroid adenomas; in MEN IIb, pheochromocytomas and ganglioneuromas occur. In the familial form, the tumor is multicentric in origin and C-cell hyperplasia precedes cancer development. The tumor metastasizes via the lymphatic route and the blood stream. The peak incidence of the sporadic form is in the sixth and seventh decades. At the time of diagnosis, lymphatic spread has frequently developed. Medullary carcinoma is quite aggressive and fewer than half its carriers survive for 10 years.

Thyroid lymphoma most frequently consists of the diffuse B-cell variant and occurs most frequently in patients with Hashimoto's disease. Such lymphomas present as rapidly growing masses replacing thyroid tissue and extending through the capsule into adjacent soft tissue. Secondary involvement of the thyroid by malignant lymphoma arising elsewhere occurs in about one fifth of patients with advanced generalized lymphoma.

MANIFESTATIONS, DIAGNOSIS, AND TREATMENT. Thyroid nodules are frequent, but only about 1 in 20 contains a thyroid cancer. Figure 239–5 outlines the approach to such lesions. The task is to identify the cancerous lesion in order to perform selective surgery. Specific features in the patient's history and symptoms and signs can point to the occurrence of cancer but are not conclusive. Thyroid cancer is more likely in a nodule developing in a child or a patient older than age 60, especially men. A single hard nodule showing rapid, painless growth is more likely to be a cancerous lesion. A history of radiation to the head and neck area during childhood, a family history of thyroid cancer, Gardner's syndrome, Cowden's syndrome, and MEN II syndrome all represent strong risk factors. A single hard nodule noted on palpation that is fixed to surrounding tissue and the identification of firm, poorly mobile lateral lymph nodes may indicate cancer spread.

Laboratory tests offer little in the diagnosis of thyroid cancer. In most patients with thyroid nodules, thyroid hormone values are normal. Elevated thyroid hormone levels indicate a follicular carcinoma markedly overproducing thyroid hormone. In the rare patients with medullary cancer, calcitonin-related peptides and calcitonin levels are elevated. The evaluation of patients with MEN type II is discussed in Chapter 244. Fine-needle aspiration of thyroid nodules and examination of the obtained material by a cytopathologist provide the highest diagnostic yield. The procedure is easy to perform and, aside from occasional bleeding in the thyroid nodule, is without serious risk. Results obtained by fine-needle aspiration are listed in Table 239–4. When a trained cytopathologist is not available, the evaluation needs to be modified. A ^{123}I scan is performed to determine if the thyroid nodule is cold. Because 20% of cold nodules coming to attention in a referral center contain thyroid cancer, such nodules are surgically removed. Thyroid ultrasonography can provide further detail, especially related to the presence of fluid and cystic lesions. Most fluid accumulation in thyroid nodules represents cystic degeneration of thyroid nodules, and the incidence of cancer in such lesions is not markedly different from that in solid nodules.

Thyroid surgery should be performed by an experienced thyroid surgeon. Some diversity of opinion exists related to the extent of the operation. For example, some thyroid surgeons treat a 1.5- to 2.0-cm papillary cancer only with a lobectomy, whereas others prefer a near-total thyroidectomy. I prefer the removal of such lesions by near-total thyroidectomy. In the hands of an experienced surgeon, complications from permanent hypoparathyroidism (2%) or vocal cord paralysis (2%) are no greater for a near-total thyroidectomy than for a lobectomy. A near-total thyroidectomy has the advantage that only small remnants of thyroid tissue remain, which can be ablated with RAI. Because normal thyroid tissue accumulates RAI much more avidly than any thyroid cancer, it is not possible to treat thyroid cancer successfully by ^{131}I therapy in the presence of a large amount of normal thyroid tissue. In addition, after near-total thyroidectomy the patient can be followed with thyroglobulin levels. Increases in the level of thyroglobulin indicate a return of thyroid cancer.

[131]I ablation is used in patients who undergo near-total thyroidectomy, especially if the primary lesion is a papillary cancer greater than 2 cm in diameter or a follicular cancer. The regimen goes as follows: One day after surgery, patients are started on triiodothyronine (Cytomel 25 μg every day or twice a day) and maintained on this dose of T_3 for 4 to 6 weeks. T_3 has a half-life of 1 day and the patient becomes hypothyroid much more quickly than with thyroxine treatment. When medication is stopped at the end of the 4- to 6-week healing period, the patient becomes markedly hypothyroid, documented by an elevated TSH level. After the TSH has attained levels of at least 40 μU/mL, a scanning dose of 3 mCi of ^{123}I is administered. If a small remnant of thyroid tissue is left in the bed of the thyroid, an ablative dose of 29 mCi of ^{131}I is administered. Identification of a larger amount of thyroid tissue or lymph node metastases leads to the administration of a higher dose of ^{131}I, ranging from 75 to 125 mCi according to the amount of remaining tissue. Seven to 10 days after treatment, a second RAI scan can be performed. This post-treatment scan identifies areas of ^{131}I uptake that were not detected by the initial lower-dose diagnostic scan. In the future, administration of human recombinant TSH will induce high TSH levels and stimulate ^{131}I uptake. This step will eliminate the need to achieve hypothyroidism before RAI is administered.

When patients become hypothyroid for RAI scanning, it is important to obtain a thyroglobulin level: elevated levels indicate that a sizable mass of thyroid tissue was left after surgery. Patients who had considerable thyroid tissue left or tumor spread to lymph nodes should be rescanned 6 months after the initial scan to ensure that the initial RAI treatment ablated all thyroid tissue. Patients who had only a small amount of tissue left can be rescanned within 1 year. Patients whose thyroglobulin levels remain normal should be

rescanned 3 years after surgery. If no evidence of RAI accumulation occurs, no subsequent rescanning is necessary and patients can be followed with thyroglobulin values. In about 10% of patients, thyroid cancer can differentiate, resulting in a discrepancy between a positive RAI scan and undetectable thyroglobulin levels. Similarly, patients with elevated thyroglobulin level and minimal or absent RAI uptake on scans have been identified. Such individuals need to be followed carefully and may require additional RAI treatment because the elevated thyroglobulin level can indicate the presence of thyroid cancer. The best initial treatment of patients with near-total thyroidectomy for papillary cancer consists of giving sufficient thyroxine to suppress TSH into the low-normal range combined with RAI therapy. This regimen markedly decreases the late recurrence of papillary cancer. Follicular carcinoma is more aggressive and should be treated more vigorously than papillary cancer. Medullary cancer does not respond to RAI therapy and must be treated with surgery plus external radiation and chemotherapy, especially if bone metastases occur. Anaplastic cancer has a poor prognosis; attempts to increase survival time by treatment with chemotherapy and external radiation therapy have been unsuccessful, although palliative external radiation can especially alleviate obstruction.

Clark OH, Duh Q-Y: Thyroid cancer. Med Clin North Am 75:211, 1991.
Mazzaferri EL: Papillary thyroid carcinoma: Factors influencing prognosis and current therapy. Semin Oncol 14:3l5, 1987.
Nikiforov YE, Fagin JA: Risk factors for thyroid carcinoma. Trends Endocrinol Metab 8:20–25, 1997.
Ridgeway EC: Clinician's evaluation of a solitary thyroid nodule. J Clin Endocrinol Metab 74:231, 1992.
Robbins J. Merino MJ, Boice JD Jr, et al: Thyroid cancer: A lethal endocrine neoplasm. Ann Intern Med 115:133, 1991.

240 THE ADRENAL CORTEX

D. Lynn Loriaux

The two adrenal glands lie either on top of or next to each kidney (Fig. 240–1). Each gland, between 6 and 8 g in weight, is composed of a cortex and medulla. The cortex makes steroid hormones and the medulla, in essence a sympathetic ganglion, makes catecholamines. The cortex is composed of three histologic zones in the adult: zona glomerulosa, zona fasciculata, and zona reticularis (Fig. 240–2). Each zone can be thought of as an independent organ. The outermost zona glomerulosa produces aldosterone, the primary mineralocorticoid in humans. The zona fasciculata primarily produces cortisol, the major glucocorticoid in humans, and the zona reticularis produces the "adrenal androgens." The adrenal androgens are in fact androgen and estrogen precursors, the parent compound being dehydroepiandrosterone and its sulfate conjugate. The biologic actions of these steroid hormones are effected via intracellular receptors, cytoplasmic or nuclear in location, that regulate gene transcription on binding with the appropriate ligand. Dehydroepiandrosterone has no known receptor. The distribution of these receptors defines the responsive tissues for each hormone. Aldosterone regulates sodium balance, primarily acting on the distal tubule of the nephron. Cortisol maintains physiologic integrity in ways that remain poorly understood, and its receptors are found in virtually every cell in the body. Dehydroepiandrosterone has no identifiable biologic action. The synthesis and secretion of each of these hormones are regulated, in the main, by a separate "feedback" system. The major trophic hormone for aldosterone secretion is renin, for cortisol, adrenocorticotropic hormone (ACTH); and for dehydroepiandrosterone, cortical androgen–stimulating hormone, which is not yet fully characterized. Thus in the case of the zona glomerulosa and the zona fasciculata, the functional status of each can be assessed by measuring two hormones: aldosterone and plasma renin for the former and cortisol and ACTH for the latter.

The adrenal medulla, in essence a sympathetic ganglion, produces catecholamines in response to neural input. Disorders of the adrenal medulla are discussed in Chapter 241.

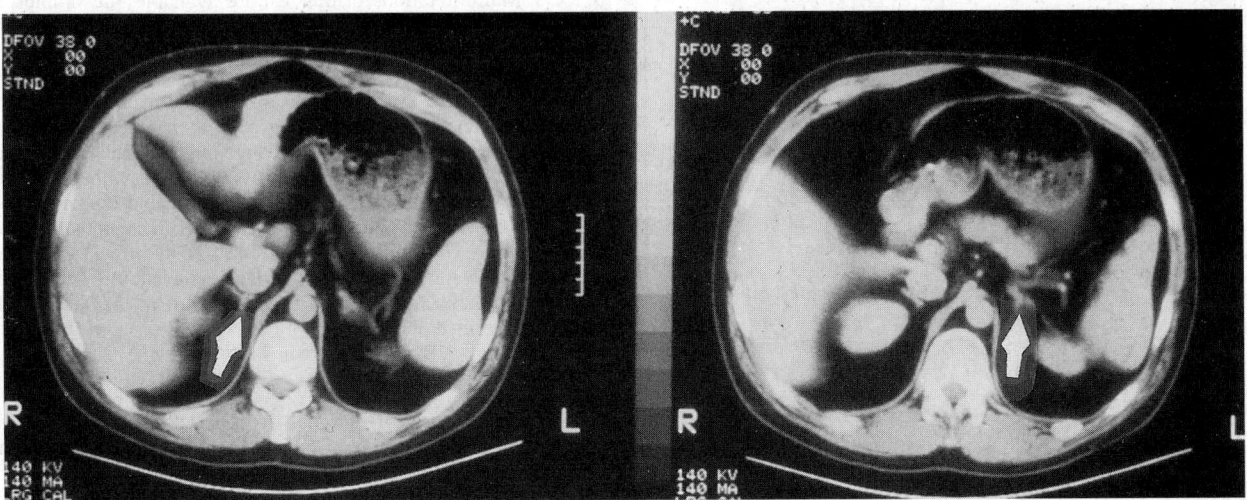

FIGURE 240–1 ▪ Magnetic resonance images of the abdomen showing the position and relative size of the normal adrenal glands.

DISORDERS OF ADRENOCORTICAL FUNCTION

Disorders of adrenocortical function can be thought of as disorders of overproduction or underproduction of the four classes of steroid hormones produced by the adrenal gland: cortisol, aldosterone, androgen, and estrogen. In addition, "mixed" disorders, the congenital adrenal hyperplasias, are characterized by a clinical picture of combined hormone excess and deficiency. These disorders are considered separately.

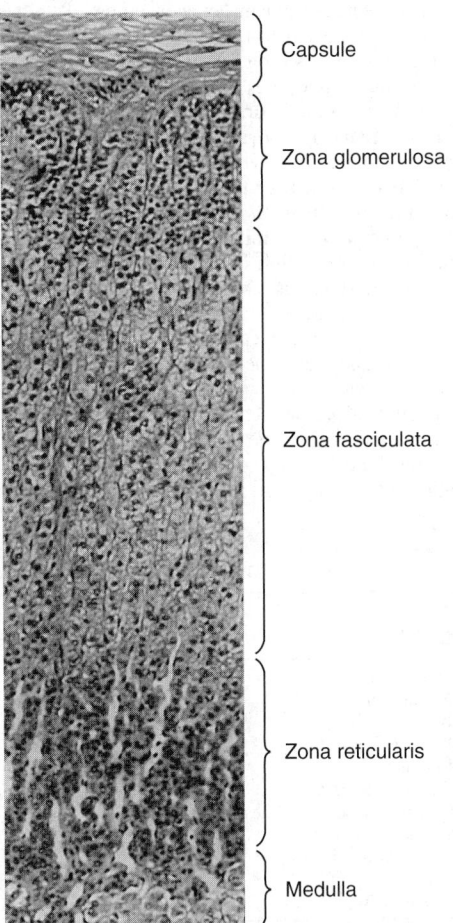

FIGURE 240–2 ▪ Histologic section through a normal adult adrenal gland showing the progression, outside in, of the zona glomerulosa, zona fasciculata, and zona reticularis.

The diagnosis of disorders of adrenocortical function, like that of other endocrine syndromes, requires a compatible clinical picture with biochemical confirmation of the associated underlying abnormality. In years past, the tests used in the diagnosis of adrenal disease were both confusing and many. Fortunately, the last several years have brought order and simplification to the process.

Tests of Adrenocortical Function

THE PORTER-SILBER CHROMOGENS. The three-carbon side chain of cortisol reacts with meta-dinitrobenzene to form a colored adduct with an absorption maximum at 410 μm. Other adrenal steroids having this configuration in the side chain include cortisone, 11-deoxycortisol, tetrahydrocortisone, tetrahydro-11-deoxycortisol, and tetrahydrocortisol (Fig. 240–3). This reaction, called the Porter-Silber chromogen reaction, was the basis of the first test to provide some measure of cortisol production. It is still in widespread use. Because urinary metabolites are, for the most part, conjugated to glucuronic acid and sulfuric acid, measurement of Porter-Silber chromogens initially involves acid hydrolysis to cleave these conjugates. This step is followed by lipid extraction with a solvent such as dichloromethane. The Porter-Silber reaction is performed on the steroids in the lipid extract. The absorption maximum is quantitated spectrophotometrically. The normal range for Porter-Silber excretion is 2 to 12 mg/day. Excretion of these steroids is markedly affected by body size, and the normal range is considerably narrowed by normalizing the measurement against urinary creatinine excretion. With this correction, the normal range is the same for all ages, 4.5 ± 1 (SD) mg/g of creatinine per day. The normal range includes the extinction point for the assay, which means that values below the normal range cannot be measured reliably with this assay.

URINE FREE CORTISOL. Urine free cortisol is that fraction of urinary cortisol that is neither conjugated to glucuronic or sulfuric acid nor bound to a protein. Accordingly, it is filtered by the renal glomerulus and can be extracted directly from urine with a lipid solvent. The detection limit of this assay also lies in the normal range of cortisol excretion and hence the assay is not a reliable test for adrenal insufficiency.

PLASMA CORTISOL. Intuitively, measurement of circulating plasma cortisol should provide the most direct assessment of adrenal cortisol secretion. The secretion of cortisol is pulsatile, with a steady frequency of about one pulse per hour in adults. The amplitude of these pulses, however, varies markedly, with 8 to 10 high-amplitude pulses clustering in the early morning hours. This pattern creates a diurnal secretory rhythm in plasma cortisol concentration. Cortisol circulates predominantly bound to a glycosylated 59-kd α_2-globulin, cortisol-binding globulin (transcortin). This binding protects circulating cortisol from hepatic clearance and gives cortisol a relatively long plasma half-life of 60 to 80 minutes. Normal plasma cortisol concentrations range between 5 and 20 μg/dL. At some

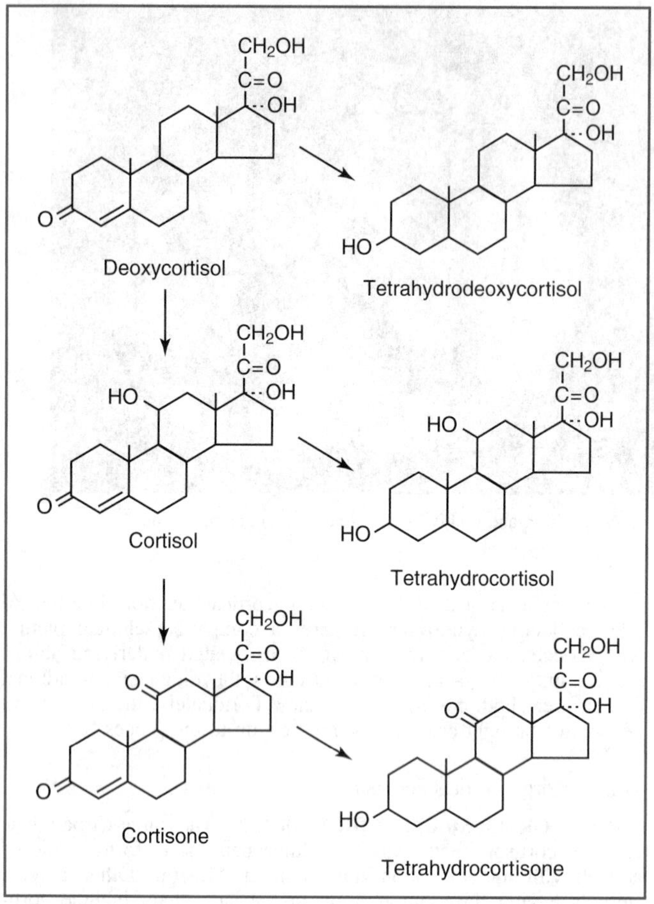

FIGURE 240–3 ■ Family of steroids known as the Porter-Silber chromogens, commonly referred to as the 17-hydroxysteroids.

time each day, normal subjects have plasma cortisol concentrations that cannot be differentiated from zero. These biologic complexities make interpretation of isolated plasma cortisol determinations hazardous. If cortisol is measured at frequent intervals (30 minutes) over a 24-hour period and the values are averaged, the mean plasma cortisol concentration amounts to 7.5 ± 1 μg/dL. To work within this narrow confidence interval, however, requires the measurement of a large number of plasma cortisol concentrations, which is prohibitive except in extraordinary circumstances.

PLASMA ACTH CONCENTRATION. Development of the two-site immunoradiometric assay for ACTH considerably simplified the differential diagnosis of adrenal disease. The normal range of plasma ACTH extends up to 100 pg/mL.

PROVOCATIVE TESTS OF ADRENAL FUNCTION. Three provocative tests of adrenal function are in common use. The *ACTH stimulation test* is the most reliable screening test for adrenal hypofunction. It is also the standard method by which suspected enzymatic deficiencies in adrenal steroidogenesis are examined. The test is performed by administering 250 μg of synthetic ACTH (Cortrosyn) intravenously and measuring the serum steroids of interest 45 and 60 minutes later. The normal adrenal gland produces plasma cortisol concentrations greater than 20 μg/dL in response to this challenge. *Corticotropin-releasing hormone,* the 41–amino acid hypothalamic secretagogue for ACTH, is a useful test for separating ACTH-dependent from ACTH-independent hypercortisolism and is an essential component of the inferior petrosal sinus sampling procedure for localizing the site of ACTH secretion (see Chapter 237). The test is performed by infusing corticotropin-releasing hormone, 1 μg/kg, intravenously over a period of 1 minute and measuring the ACTH response between 3 and 30 minutes thereafter.

The *dexamethasone suppression test* is widely used to screen for adrenal hyperfunction. The test has so many false-positive and false-negative results (sensitivity and specificity of about 0.8), however, that it is superseded by the tests mentioned above. The test

retains some value in the differential diagnosis of mineralocorticoid excess. Many iterations of this test are available, the simplest being 0.5 mg dexamethasone administered by mouth every 6 hours for 2 days.

Plasma and urine aldosterone and plasma renin activity are important tests to evaluate states of apparent mineralocorticoid excess and deficiency.

The differential diagnosis of congenital adrenal hyperplasia requires the measurement of specific steroid biosynthetic intermediates that accumulate proximal to the responsible enzymic deficiencies in the steroid biosynthetic cascade. The most commonly measured are 17-hydroxyprogesterone (21-hydroxylase deficiency) and 11-deoxycortisol (11-hydroxylase deficiency). These steroids are most reliably measured in the context of an ACTH stimulation test, as described above.

Adrenal Hyperfunction

Four syndromes of adrenal hyperfunction are differentiated: Cushing's syndrome, hypokalemic metabolic alkalosis, masculinization, and feminization. These syndromes result from the excessive secretion of cortisol, mineralocorticoid, androgen, and estrogen, respectively. These disorders can occur in isolation or, more commonly, in combination with one or more of the others.

GLUCOCORTICOID EXCESS—CUSHING'S SYNDROME. DIAGNOSIS. Cushing's syndrome is caused by glucocorticoid excess. The "classic" syndrome is defined clinically: weight gain, plethora, striae, hypertension, and proximal muscle weakness (Table 240–1). The weight gain is predominantly truncal, with increased fat deposited in a yoke-like pattern around the neck leading to the well-known dorsocervical fat pad (buffalo hump) and filling in of the supraclavicular fossae. Plethora is evident as a ruddy complexion. The striae of Cushing's syndrome are characteristically violaceous and occur in thin skin. Proximal muscle weakness is best assessed by testing the ability of the patient to rise unassisted from a squatting position. The biochemical diagnosis depends on the demonstration of an elevated plasma concentration of "bioactive" cortisol, which is best reflected in the excretion of urine free cortisol. If the clinical picture is "strong," urine free cortisol concentrations above the normal range are adequate for the diagnosis. If the clinical picture is "weak," urine free cortisol excretion must be above the levels found in "physiologic" causes of adrenal activation such as stress and depression. This level is generally taken to be 250 μg/day. This approach to the diagnosis of Cushing's syndrome occasionally identifies patients with an "atypical" picture. At one extreme are patients with minimal clinical manifestations of Cushing's syndrome but very high levels of free cortisol excretion. This constellation of findings is characteristic of Cushing's syndrome associated with systemic malignancy, typically a small cell carcinoma of the lung. The clinical picture is dominated by the "cachexia" of malignancy, and the typical "anabolic" features of Cushing's syndrome such as weight gain and dorsocervical fat distribution fail to develop. At the other extreme are patients with well-established clinical signs of Cushing's syndrome but without sufficient urine free cortisol excretion to confirm the diagnosis. This situation is usually the result of iatrogenic or surreptitious

Table 240–1 ■ CLINICAL FEATURES OF GLUCOCORTICOID EXCESS

FEATURE	FREQUENCY (%)
Weight gain	90
"Moon facies"	75
Hypertension	75
Violaceous striae	65
Hirsutism	65
Glucose intolerance	65
Proximal muscle weakness	60
Plethora	60
Menstrual dysfunction	60
Acne	40
Easy bruising	40
Osteopenia	40
Dependent edema	40
Hyperpigmentation	20
Hypokalemic metabolic alkalosis	15

ACTH-Dependent Causes
   ACTH-secreting pituitary tumor (Cushing's disease)
   Non-pituitary ACTH-secreting neoplasm (ectopic ACTH syndrome)
ACTH-Independent Causes
   Adrenal adenoma
   Adrenal carcinoma
   Micronodular adrenal disease
   Factitious or surreptitious glucocorticoid administration

ACTH = adrenocorticotropic hormone.

exogenous glucocorticoid administration. A careful history and review of systems usually reveal the source of the glucocorticoid. In the rare cases of surreptitious glucocorticoid abuse, measurement of the commonly prescribed synthetic glucocorticoids in randomly obtained serum samples is necessary for the diagnosis. Rarely, naturally occurring Cushing's syndrome can be cyclic or even intermittent. In this case, repeated measurement of urine free cortisol at frequent intervals of 3 to 5 days necessary to establish the diagnosis.

DIFFERENTIAL DIAGNOSIS AND TREATMENT. The causes of Cushing's syndrome are shown in Table 240–2. They can be conveniently divided into ACTH-dependent and ACTH-independent causes. This differentiation is made on the basis of the plasma ACTH concentration following the administration of corticotropin-releasing hormone. Values greater than 10 pg/dL indicate ACTH-dependent disease; values less than 10 pg/dL indicate ACTH-independent disease.

The causes of ACTH-dependent Cushing's syndrome include *Cushing's disease* caused by an ACTH-secreting pituitary tumor and the *ectopic secretion of ACTH* from a neoplasm not of pituitary origin. Cushing's disease, the most common cause of Cushing's syndrome, accounts for 70 to 80% of all non-iatrogenic cases (see Chapter 237). Ectopic secretion of ACTH by a non-pituitary neoplasm accounts for about 10% of cases. The common causes of ectopic ACTH secretion are listed in Table 240–3. More than 90% of these tumors are found in the chest. The most common cause is small cell cancer of the lung. Other neoplasms include bronchial carcinoid tumors, medullary cancer of the thyroid, islet cell tumors of the pancreas, and pheochromocytoma.

Two forms of the ectopic ACTH syndrome can be differentiated. In the first, Cushing's syndrome occurs as classically described by Harvey Cushing. It can be thought of as the *anabolic form* of ectopic ACTH secretion because it is associated with weight gain and the characteristic central obesity of the disorder. It is usually caused by slow-growing benign tumors such as bronchial carcinoid tumors. The second form, *the catabolic form,* has none of the anabolic features associated with "classic" Cushing's syndrome. Weight loss, hypertension, edema, and hypokalemia dominate the clinical picture. This form of the disease is commonly associated with advanced and widely metastatic tumors that impair caloric intake and prevent weight gain and the development of central obesity.

Differentiating the two ACTH-dependent forms of Cushing's syndrome from each other depends on localizing the source of the ACTH secretion. The most effective method of doing so is by sampling inferior petrosal sinus blood for the measurement of ACTH levels. Pituitary venous blood drains into the cavernous sinuses on either side of the sella turcica and thence into the internal jugular veins by way of the inferior petrosal sinuses. These sinuses can be readily cannulated via catheters inserted into the femoral vein. Blood sampled simultaneously from both sinuses and

Table 240–3 ■ COMMON CAUSES OF ECTOPIC ADRENOCORTICOTROPIC HORMONE SECRETION

Small cell carcinoma of the lung	50%
Endocrine tumors of foregut origin	35%
Thymic carcinoid	
Islet cell tumor	
Medullary carcinoma, thyroid	
Bronchial carcinoid	
Pheochromocytoma	5%
Ovarian tumors	2%

a peripheral vein allows the ratio of ACTH between the sites to be determined. The test is most precise when the blood is sampled after the administration of corticotropin-releasing hormone. The lowest central-peripheral ratio of ACTH compatible with Cushing's disease is 3. The highest ratio seen with ectopic ACTH-secreting tumors is 1.8.

When ACTH secretion is localized to the pituitary gland, therapeutic intervention is recommended without further delay (see Chapter 237). If the ACTH originates from an ectopic site, an attempt to define the specific lesion is undertaken. The most direct course is to examine the entire chest by computed tomography (CT) at 0.5-cm intervals. If this approach fails to identify a suspicious lesion, the test should be repeated with magnetic resonance imaging (MRI) because it is subject to less "vascular" artifact in the central lung fields. If this approach fails, CT or MRI of the abdominal cavity is indicated.

ACTH-secreting microadenomas of the pituitary gland should be surgically removed. In the hands of an experienced neurosurgeon, the cure rate for these tumors is between 90 and 95% with the first operation. In the case of a failed transsphenoidal procedure, a second procedure is successful in 50% of cases. The recurrence rate appears to be less than 5%. Ectopic tumors should be removed if found. If the tumor cannot be detected or is found to be widely metastatic, adrenal blockade with ketoconazole, up to 1200 mg by mouth in divided doses, is an effective treatment for the associated glucocorticoid excess. Ultimately, if the process appears to be headed to a protracted course, bilateral adrenalectomy via flank incision or laparoscopy is a useful adjunct to management.

The causes of ACTH-independent Cushing's syndrome, if iatrogenic and factitious disease is excluded, are adrenal in origin: adrenal adenoma, adrenal cancer, and micronodular adrenal dysplasia. They account for 10 to 20% of naturally occurring cases of Cushing's syndrome. Adrenal adenomas are the most common and account for about 15% of cases of Cushing's syndrome. The tumors are typically unilateral, are less than 4 cm in diameter, and produce only a single steroid hormone, in this case, cortisol. Adrenal cancers are rare, with an incidence of 1 in 600,000 per year. They are generally unilateral and large at the time of discovery, usually larger than 6 cm in diameter. Adrenal cancers typically produce more than one steroid hormone, the most common combinations being glucocorticoid and mineralocorticoid or glucocorticoid and androgen. Differentiation of an adenoma from a carcinoma is made clinically; histologic examination of the tissue is of little value. The most important indicators of malignancy are size at the time of diagnosis, the number of steroid hormones clinically apparent, and any evidence of spread at the time of surgical intervention. Micronodular adrenal dysplasia is characterized by normal or small adrenal glands that show scattered 1- to 3-mm hyperplastic nodules separated by atrophic adrenal cortex. This disease can be sporadic or part of a larger syndrome, Carney's complex, in which the adrenal disease is associated with pigmented lentigines, atrial myxoma, and germ cell tumors (see references).

The differential diagnosis of ACTH-independent Cushing's syndrome depends almost exclusively on the findings produced by CT or MRI. Small unilateral lesions with no evidence of metastasis should be removed by a unilateral flank excision or by a laparoscopic procedure. Large lesions should be removed via a transabdominal approach so that the abdominal organs can be carefully examined and the liver biopsied at the time of surgery. Treatment of micronodular adrenal dysplasia is bilateral adrenalectomy.

Metastases should be surgically excised until no longer feasible. The only known chemotherapy effective against this cancer is *ortho, para'*-dichlorodiphenyldichloroethane. It is given orally to tolerance, usually a dose between 6 and 10 g/day. Side effects are neuropsychiatric and gastrointestinal, with somnolence, ataxia, reduced attention span, nausea, and diarrhea predominating. One fourth of patients have an objective remission, and the remissions average 7 months in duration. No one has been cured of metastatic adrenocortical carcinoma.

MINERALOCORTICOID EXCESS. DIAGNOSIS. No reliable symptoms are known for mineralocorticoid excess. Signs include arterial hypertension and dependent edema. Laboratory findings are more specific. The mineralocorticoid effect on the distal nephron is sodium retention at the expense of potassium and hydrogen excretion.

Excess mineralocorticoid produces an expanded vascular volume in association with hypokalemia and metabolic alkalosis. Mineralocorticoid excess can be renin-angiotensin independent or dependent. The aldosterone-secreting tumor is an example of renin-angiotensin–independent disease. In renin-angiotensin–dependent disease, the mineralocorticoid is produced in response to the renin-angiotensin trophic signal. This trophic signal is commonly encountered in states of contracted arterial volume such as congestive heart failure or cirrhosis with ascites. The two forms of mineralocorticoid excess can be differentiated on the basis of plasma renin activity. If resting plasma renin activity is high, the mineralocorticoid excess is renin-angiotensin dependent. If plasma renin activity is low and cannot be stimulated by 4 hours of upright posture, the mineralocorticoid excess is renin-angiotensin independent.

RENIN-ANGIOTENSIN–INDEPENDENT MINERALOCORTICOID EXCESS. Differential Diagnosis and Treatment. Table 240–4 lists the causes of renin-angiotensin–independent mineralocorticoid excess. Aldosterone is the offending mineralocorticoid in most but not all of these disorders. The initial task is to differentiate cases caused by aldosterone excess from those caused by another mineralocorticoid. Urine and plasma aldosterone measurements provide the answers for this differentiation. If the aldosterone concentration is normal or above, aldosterone is the causative agent. If the aldosterone concentration is below the normal range or undetectable, the disorder is caused by a mineralocorticoid other than aldosterone.

Two common causes of aldosterone-mediated renin-angiotensin–independent mineralocorticoid excess are aldosterone-producing adenoma and bilateral hyperplasia of aldosterone-secreting cells. Dexamethasone-suppressible hyperaldosteronism is a rare cause of aldosterone-mediated renin-angiotensin–independent mineralocorticoid excess. It can be excluded by finding normal or high levels of circulating aldosterone after 2 days of giving dexamethasone, 2 mg/day by mouth in divided doses. The remaining causes of renin-angiotensin–independent aldosterone excess must be separated from one another to guide the appropriate therapeutic intervention. Aldosterone-secreting adenomas respond well to surgical removal, whereas bilateral hyperplasia does not. The most direct approach to this differentiation is to measure cortisol-aldosterone ratios in adrenal venous blood sampled simultaneously from both glands following the administration of ACTH. The diagnostic accuracy of this test approaches 100%. Aldosterone-secreting adenomas are characterized by high levels of aldosterone from one side and none from the other, the secretion from the non-affected side being suppressed by the volume-expanded state. Bilateral hyperplasia is characterized by comparable aldosterone levels from each gland, and therefore cortisol-aldosterone ratios in effluent adrenal blood are roughly equal on the two sides.

Unilateral adrenal adenomas should be surgically excised. In the hands of an experienced surgeon, the cure rate is very high. Bilateral hyperplasia does not respond well to surgery and is best treated with spironolactone to address the metabolic sequelae of mineralocorticoid excess and with antihypertensive medications if spironolactone inadequately controls blood pressure.

The causes of non–aldosterone-mediated renin-angiotensin–independent mineralocorticoid excess are rare (Table 240–5). The initial task is to exclude adrenocortical carcinoma, which is best done by imaging the adrenal glands with CT or MRI. Failure to find adrenal asymmetry and the presence of a dominant mass, usually larger than 4 cm in diameter, essentially exclude the diagnosis. Symmetrically enlarged adrenal glands of moderate degree suggest congenital adrenal hyperplasia. The two congenital adrenal

Table 240–4 ■ COMMON CAUSES OF RENIN-ANGIOTENSIN–INDEPENDENT MINERALOCORTICOID EXCESS

Aldosterone-secreting adenoma
Adrenal cancer
Congenital adrenal hyperplasia
  11-Hydroxylase deficiency
  17-Hydroxylase deficiency
11β-Hydroxysteroid dehydrogenase deficiency
Licorice intoxication
Glucocorticoid-suppressible hyperaldosteronism

Table 240–5 ■ COMMON CAUSES OF RENIN-ANGIOTENSIN–DEPENDENT MINERALOCORTICOID EXCESS

Vomiting
Diuretics
Edematous disorders
  Congestive heart failure
  Hepatic cirrhosis
  Nephrotic syndrome
Renal ischemia
Bartter's syndrome
Renin-secreting tumors

hyperplasias that lead to hypertension are 11-hydroxylase deficiency and 17-hydroxylase deficiency. The former can be diagnosed by measuring the circulating concentration of 11-deoxycortisol. Normally, this steroid does not circulate in plasma. 17-Hydroxylase deficiency is best diagnosed by a unique clinical picture (hypertension, pubertal delay, and genital ambiguity) coupled with an inappropriately elevated plasma progesterone concentration.

The enzyme 11β-hydroxysteroid dehydrogenase (11β-HSD) catalyzes the conversion of cortisol to cortisone. Cortisol interacts with the mineralocorticoid receptor as an agonist; cortisone does not. Because the circulating concentrations of cortisol are 1000 times those of aldosterone, cortisol can have considerable mineralocorticoid activity in humans. Excess activity is prevented by the action of 11β-HSD, which converts cortisol to its inactive metabolite cortisone. If the activity of this enzyme is impaired, cortisol assumes the role of aldosterone. Because cortisol secretion is not regulated by the renin-angiotensin system, a state of mineralocorticoid excess at normal plasma cortisol concentrations results. The appropriate treatment is to suppress cortisol secretion with an exogenous glucocorticoid having little or no mineralocorticoid activity, such as dexamethasone or prednisone.

The active ingredient in licorice, glycyrrhizic acid, is a competitive inhibitor of 11β-HSD. Thus licorice intoxication can cause hypertension by the same mechanism as spontaneously occurring 11β-HSD deficiency. Licorice intoxication can usually be excluded by history. The most common source of licorice in the United States is chewing tobacco.

All causes of non–aldosterone-mediated renin-angiotensin–independent mineralocorticoid excess except for malignancy should "respond" to adrenal suppression with dexamethasone, 2 mg/day. If this measure fails, especially in the presence of an adrenal mass, adrenal malignancy is suggested. When adrenal suppression is successful, hydrocortisone, 12 to 15 mg/m²/day, should be used for long-term treatment.

Adrenal Hypofunction

GLUCOCORTICOID DEFICIENCY. DIAGNOSIS. A broad spectrum of signs and symptoms can herald the presence of glucocorticoid deficiency (Table 240–6). At one extreme is the *"chronic syndrome,"* characterized by symptoms of malaise, anorexia, and orthostatic hypotension. Occasionally, vague abdominal pain can occur. Signs include weight loss, hypotension with an orthostatic component, and in certain cases, a melanin-based hyperpigmentation of the skin. The routine laboratory picture reveals a normochromic normocytic anemia, relative lymphocytosis often with an unexplained eosinophilia, mild pre-renal azotemia, and hyponatremia. If aldosterone secretion is impaired by the process, hyperkalemia can also be observed. At the other extreme is the *"acute syndrome,"* characterized by rapidly evolving agitation, confusion, fever, and abdominal pain, all associated with arterial hypotension. As the hypotension evolves into shock, it is relatively unresponsive to volume replacement and pressor agents and imitates the hemodynamic characteristics of "pump" failure in association with increased vascular volume. The laboratory findings are the same as those found in the chronic syndrome. Untreated, the acute syndrome quickly leads to coma and death. When initially seen, the symptoms and signs of most patients with adrenal insufficiency lie somewhere on the continuum between these two extremes.

The diagnosis of glucocorticoid deficiency is confirmed by the inability of the adrenal glands to respond normally to an ACTH challenge. Synthetic ACTH, 250 μg, is administered intravenously,

ACTH-Independent Causes
  Tuberculosis
  Autoimmune (idiopathic)
  Other rare causes
    Fungal infection
    Adrenal hemorrhage
    Metastases
    Sarcoidosis
    Amyloidosis
    Adrenoleukodystrophy
    Adrenomyeloneuropathy
    HIV infection
    Congenital adrenal hyperplasia
    Medications (ketoconazole, OP'DDD)
ACTH-Dependent Causes
  Hypothalamic-pituitary-adrenal suppression
    Exogenous
      Glucocorticoid
      ACTH
    Endogenous—cure of Cushing's syndrome
  Hypothalamic-pituitary lesions
    Neoplasm
      Primary pituitary tumor
      Metastatic tumor
    Craniopharyngioma
    Infection
      Tuberculosis
      Actinomycosis
      Nocardiosis
  Sarcoid
  Head trauma
  Isolated ACTH deficiency

ACTH = adrenocorticotropic hormone; HIV = human immunodeficiency virus; OP' = DDD-*ortho, para'*-dichlorodiphenyldichloroethane.

and plasma cortisol is determined 45 and 60 minutes later. The normal adrenal gland produces plasma cortisol concentrations of 20 μg/dL or more. Any value lower than 20 μg/dL implies a degree of adrenal compromise. Because the differential diagnosis of adrenal insufficiency relies on the plasma concentration of ACTH, it is prudent to draw a blood sample for ACTH before the administration of ACTH and "hold" the sample in the laboratory pending results of the plasma cortisol determination.

DIFFERENTIAL DIAGNOSIS AND TREATMENT. The initial task in the differential diagnosis of glucocorticoid deficiency is to define whether the process is ACTH dependent. ACTH-dependent glucocorticoid deficiency implies disordered function of the hypothalamus and/or pituitary gland leading to ACTH deficiency, whereas ACTH-independent glucocorticoid deficiency is caused by disordered adrenal function, such as destruction of the gland by an infectious process like tuberculosis. This distinction is best made on the basis of plasma ACTH concentrations measured at the time of glucocorticoid deficiency (i.e., before treatment with glucocorticoid has been initiated). ACTH concentrations in or below the normal range imply an ACTH-dependent process. ACTH concentrations above the normal range imply an ACTH-independent process.

Glucocorticoid Deficiency Related to Adrenal Suppression. The most common cause of ACTH-dependent glucocorticoid deficiency is hypothalamic-pituitary-adrenal "suppression" by exogenously administered glucocorticoids, either iatrogenic or factitious. Whether adrenal suppression develops as a result of exogenous glucocorticoid administration depends on three variables: the dose of the glucocorticoid administered, the duration of administration, and the schedule of administration. It is unusual for clinically manifested adrenal suppression to develop with doses of glucocorticoid equal to or less than the daily replacement dose of the preparation used—20 mg/day of hydrocortisone, 5 mg/day of prednisone or prednisolone, and 0.5 mg/day of dexamethasone. Given doses that exceed these limits, it is unusual for clinically manifested glucocorticoid deficiency to develop if the duration of administration is less than 3 weeks. Finally, the dosage schedule can affect the rapidity with which the final state of adrenal suppression is reached. Glucocorticoids given as a single dose upon awakening in the morning are the least suppressive; glucocorticoids given in divided doses throughout the day are the most suppressive. Thus at one extreme

are patients given decreasing doses of prednisone for 14 days to treat an acute inflammatory process such as poison ivy. Signs and symptoms of glucocorticoid deficiency following cessation of the medication are extremely unlikely. At the other extreme are patients treated with large doses of glucocorticoids given in divided doses for long periods for the treatment of disorders such as chronic obstructive pulmonary disease. Many of the stigmata of Cushing's syndrome develop in these patients, who manifest signs and symptoms of glucocorticoid deficiency within 48 hours if the glucocorticoid treatment is stopped for any reason. The clinical manifestations of this deficiency can range from the "chronic" syndrome at one extreme to the "acute" syndrome at the other.

Glucocorticoid Deficiency Caused by Hypothalamic-Pituitary Disease. Destructive lesions of the hypothalamus and pituitary gland are a rare cause of ACTH-dependent glucocorticoid deficiency. Although this condition is uncommon, diagnosis is imperative because early therapeutic intervention can prevent many of the serious sequelae of these tumors, including blindness. Examples include pituitary tumor, metastatic tumors to the region, sarcoid, amyloid, craniopharyngioma, and Rathke's pouch cyst. Pituitary infections such as actinomycosis and nocardiosis and vascular accidents such as Sheehan's syndrome can also lead to adrenal insufficiency. The most direct approach to the diagnosis of these lesions is imaging with CT scan using contrast enhancement or with MRI following gadolinium administration. A rare cause of ACTH-dependent glucocorticoid deficiency is *autoimmune lymphocytic hypophysitis*.

Treatment of chronic ACTH-dependent glucocorticoid insufficiency consists of replacing the missing hormone. Glucocorticoid should be replaced in the form of hydrocortisone, the naturally occurring glucocorticoid in humans, at a rate of 12 to 15 mg/m^2/day. Cortisol is secreted in bursts, between 7 and 10 per day, clustering in the morning hours. To reproduce this pattern with replacement steroid is impossible with the currently available methods. Empirically, however, it has been found that patients do as well with a single morning dose of cortisol as with divided doses, and compliance is simplified with this regimen. Clinical measures best monitor the adequacy of replacement: Anorexia, weight loss, and hyponatremia suggest underreplacement; weight gain, plethora, and supraclavicular fat deposition suggest overreplacement. The current standard of practice is to increase the cortisol dose in the context of "stress," actual or anticipated. The dose of cortisol is doubled for the duration of the stress and returned to replacement levels immediately upon cessation of the stress. Typical stresses include febrile illness; nausea and vomiting; trauma such as lacerations, contusions, and fractures; and surgical procedures, including dental extraction. Acute glucocorticoid deficiency is treated with large doses of cortisol given intravenously, 100 mg every 6 hours, coupled with emergency support of blood pressure plus volume expansion and pressors when indicated.

Primary Adrenal Insufficiency. The most common cause of primary adrenal insufficiency worldwide is tuberculosis. Tuberculosis causes adrenal insufficiency by destroying the adrenal cortex and replacing it with caseating granulomas. The most common cause of adrenal insufficiency in the industrialized West is an autoimmune process, usually as part of the polyglandular deficiency syndrome. In this disorder, an autoimmune "adrenalitis" leads to destruction of the adrenal cortex. This disease has two forms, types I and II. The relative features of the two forms are detailed in Table 240–7.

Table 240–7 ■ POLYENDOCRINE DEFICIENCY SYNDROMES

FEATURE	TYPE I	TYPE II
Age of onset	12 yr	24 yr
Adrenal insufficiency	+	+
Diabetes mellitus	–	+
Autoimmune thyroid disease	–	+
Hypoparathyroidism	+	–
Mucocutaneous candidiasis	+	–
Hypogonadism	+	+/–
Chronic active hepatitis	+	–
Pernicious anemia	+	–
Vitiligo	+	+

Type I is a disease of childhood with a mean age of onset of 12 years. Type II begins at an average age of 24 years. The dominant features of type I disease are adrenal insufficiency, hypoparathyroidism, and mucocutaneous candidiasis. The dominant features of type II disease are adrenal insufficiency, autoimmune thyroid disease, and insulin-dependent diabetes mellitus. Other important differences include the patterns of inheritance. Type I is transmitted as an autosomal recessive trait occurring across sibships, whereas type II has a "dominant" pattern of inheritance appearing in multiple generations of an affected family. Also, type I disease has no HLA association, whereas type II is associated with the DR3/DR4 haplotypes. Both disorders appear to be mediated by an autoimmune process. For example, circulating antibodies to one or more endocrine organs are found in most patients, and defects in T-lymphocyte function such as a decrease in "suppressor" activity are described.

All of the clinically important fungi except *Monilia* can cause adrenal destruction. The most common cause is histoplasmosis, which is due to an organism particularly prominent in the Ohio and Tennessee valleys and along the Piedmont Plateau of the Middle Atlantic states. South American blastomycosis is the next most common fungal cause of adrenal insufficiency, followed by North American blastomycosis, coccidioidomycosis, and cryptococcosis. The pathophysiology of fungal adrenalitis is much like that of tuberculosis—destruction leading to adrenal enlargement with caseating granuloma formation. If healing occurs, the adrenal glands can shrink in size, sometimes resuming a relatively normal volume. The healing process is often accompanied by calcification.

The advent of CT has revealed adrenal hemorrhage as a more frequent cause of adrenal insufficiency than had been recognized previously. The usual setting is a stressed individual receiving long-term anticoagulation for the prevention of pulmonary or cardiac emboli or other thrombotic phenomena. Typically, affected patients complain of back pain followed, in a few days, by onset of the initial signs and symptoms of adrenal insufficiency.

Metastases to the adrenal gland are common, with a frequency as high as 70% in patients with disseminated breast or lung cancer. Adrenal insufficiency as a result of metastases, however, is uncommon, although moderate abnormalities in adrenal function can often be detected in patients with bilateral adrenal metastases. Tumors commonly associated with adrenal insufficiency are cancers of the breast, lung, stomach, and colon; melanoma; and some, lymphomas.

The syndrome of acquired immune deficiency (AIDS) can be associated with adrenal insufficiency in its late stages. Cytomegalovirus infection of the adrenal glands commonly accompanies this condition, as does infection with *Mycobacterium avium-intracellulare* and the various fungi that can colonize and destroy the adrenal glands. The plasma cortisol response to ACTH administration is abnormal in 10 to 15% of patients with AIDS and its advanced complications.

Adrenoleukodystrophy is an inborn abnormality of long-chain fatty acids that causes adrenal insufficiency in association with several neurologically impaired phenotypes. Newborn adrenoleukodystrophy is transmitted as an autosomal recessive trait. Adrenoleukodystrophy, also known as brown Schilder's disease (brown being an adjective describing the hyperpigmentation of the skin) or sudanophilic leukodystrophy, is transmitted as an X-linked disease of children characterized by rapidly progressive central demyelination eventuating in seizures, dementia, cortical blindness, coma, and death. Death usually occurs before puberty is complete. X-linked adrenomyeloneuropathy is a disease of young adults characterized by a slowly progressive mixed upper and lower motor and sensory neuropathy leading to an ascending spastic paraparesis. Signs and symptoms of spinocerebellar degeneration appear in some cases. Both forms of the disease are associated with progressive failure of all steroid-secreting cells leading to adrenal and gonadal failure. The metabolic marker for these diseases is an elevated circulating level of very long chain fatty acids C-26 and greater in length. The cause of this abnormality seems to be an abnormal peroxisomal transporter protein that prevents appropriate metabolism of the very long chain fatty acids. Several treatments have been tried, but only autologous bone marrow transplantation appears to be successful.

Other rare causes of primary adrenal insufficiency include amy-loidosis, congenital unresponsiveness to ACTH, congenital adrenal hypoplasia, and familial glucocorticoid insufficiency.

Treatment of ACTH-independent glucocorticoid deficiency is the same as that outlined for ACTH-dependent glucocorticoid deficiency except that the addition of a mineralocorticoid is usually required because adrenal cortical destruction impairs both cortisol and aldosterone secretion. The available orally active mineralocorticoid is fludrocortisone acetate (Florinel). It is equipotent with aldosterone. The secretion rate of aldosterone in salt-replete humans is about 100 μg/day. Thus fludrocortisone, 100 μg/day, is the appropriate replacement dose. The drug has a wide therapeutic window, and no specific monitoring for treatment effect other than an occasional plasma potassium concentration is necessary.

MINERALOCORTICOID DEFICIENCY. DIAGNOSIS. The major clinical manifestations of mineralocorticoid deficiency are hyponatremia, hyperkalemia, and mild metabolic acidosis. These disorders can lead to profound muscle weakness and cardiac arrhythmias. Combined glucocorticoid and mineralocorticoid deficiency is a common cause of this picture and should initially be excluded with an ACTH stimulation test. If that test is normal, the diagnosis of isolated hypoaldosteronism depends on the demonstration of an inappropriately low circulating aldosterone level. The causes of isolated hypoaldosteronism are listed in Table 240-8.

DIFFERENTIAL DIAGNOSIS AND TREATMENT. Selective hypoaldosteronism was, until recently, believed to be rare. Recent studies, however, show that it accounts for as many as 10% of cases of unexplained hyperkalemia. The causes of hypoaldosteronism can be divided into renin-angiotensin–dependent (hyporeninemic) and renin-angiotensin–independent (hyperreninemic) causes. Differentiation is based on plasma renin activity. The usual test is a measurement of plasma renin activity following 4 hours of upright posture. Levels in the normal or low range identify cases that are renin-angiotensin dependent, whereas high levels identify cases that are renin-angiotensin independent.

Renin deficiency, overall, is the most common cause of selective aldosterone deficiency. It is usually found in elderly subjects with mild, non-oliguric renal disease. Many such patients have insulin-dependent diabetes, and diabetic nephropathy is thought to be an important contributing abnormality. Other causes of renin-angiotensin–dependent hypoaldosteronism include autonomic dysfunction associated with prolonged bed rest and, rarely, treatment with prostaglandin synthesis inhibitors such as indomethacin.

The causes of renin-angiotensin–independent hypoaldosteronism include all causes of ACTH-independent adrenal insufficiency listed in Table 240-6. In this setting, selective hypoaldosteronism can result if treatment is confined to glucocorticoid replacement. The other causes of this disorder center on alterations in the synthesis and secretion of aldosterone and include long-term heparin administration and the "salt-wasting" forms of congenital adrenal hyperplasia (21-hydroxylase deficiency, 3β-hydroxysteroid dehydrogenase deficiency, and 17-hydroxylase deficiency). Again, treating these disorders with glucocorticoid alone is a common cause of selective hypoaldosteronism. Finally, any defect in the conversion of corticosterone to aldosterone, such as 18-hydroxylase deficiency, leads to selective hypoaldosteronism.

Treating selective hypoaldosteronism of any cause is straightforward. Aldosterone deficiency does not produce clinical symptoms unless the subject is "salt deprived." This condition is unlikely to occur at levels of salt intake greater than 10 mEq/kg/day. For adults, this amount equals about 4 g of sodium chloride per day, which is routinely ingested in the average American diet. Thus a

Table 240-8 ■ **CAUSES OF ISOLATED HYPOALDOSTERONISM**

Renin-Angiotensin Dependent
   Hyporeninemic hypoaldosteronism
   Autonomic neuropathy
   Prostaglandin synthesis inhibitors
Renin-Angiotensin Independent
   Inhibition of aldosterone synthesis
     Heparin
     Cyclosporine
     Calcium channel blockers
   Following resection of an aldosterone-secreting adenoma
   18-Hydroxylase deficiency
   Aldosterone resistance (pseudohypoaldosteronism)

simple way to treat selective hypoaldosteronism is to ensure adequate dietary salt intake, which in the United States is not a problem in young and otherwise healthy subjects. This approach, however, fails in patients with "fetish" diets or those who cannot maintain an adequate oral intake of salt for any reason. Important in this regard are the dietary restrictions that frequently accompany old age and those often imposed on infants and toddlers. In these cases it is advisable to supply exogenous mineralocorticoid. Fludrocortisone is the only available preparation of orally active mineralocorticoid. It is equipotent with aldosterone and is given in doses that approximate the daily production rate of aldosterone in a salt-replete individual, 100 μg/day. The preparation can be given as a single daily dose with the morning meal. The drug's therapeutic window is wide, so overtreatment is unlikely. Thus an occasional serum potassium concentration measurement is adequate to monitor the efficacy of treatment.

Disorders of Combined Insufficiency and Excess

THE CONGENITAL ADRENAL HYPERPLASIAS. Defects in the synthesis of cortisol lead to compensatory stimulation of adrenal steroidogenesis to maintain normal plasma cortisol concentrations. Such stimulation inevitably leads to an accumulation of the steroid biosynthetic intermediate immediately before the enzymic defect in the biosynthetic cascade. Clinically, the result is expressed as glucocorticoid deficiency (which can be so mild as to be inapparent or so severe as to be life threatening) in association with mineralocorticoid excess or deficiency and androgen excess or deficiency. These disorders are usually classified as "salt wasting," "hypertensive," "virilizing," or "feminizing," depending on the combination of hormone excess and deficiency. They are presented in detail in Chapter 246. Only the attenuated or "non-classic" form of 21-hydroxylase deficiency is presented here.

21-Hydroxylase deficiency is one of the most prevalent autosomal recessive disorders, with a heterozygote frequency that may be as high as one in five. Although congenital in nature, the disorder usually makes its initial appearance with the onset of puberty. Hirsutism, oligomenorrhea, and cystic acne are the most common clinical manifestations. The disorder is identical in clinical features to idiopathic hirsutism–polycystic ovarian disease and cannot be differentiated from this disorder without specifically examining adrenal steroidogenesis to look for the 21-hydroxylase block. Such examination is best done in the context of an ACTH stimulation test performed in the usual way, with measurements of 17-hydroxyprogesterone made 45 and 60 minutes after administration of the ACTH. Normal subjects do not exceed 17-hydroxyprogesterone levels of 350 ng/dL, but patients with the disorder attain plasma levels greater than 1500 ng/dL. The incidence of this disorder in young hirsute patients varies between 1 and 30%, depending on ethnic background, and averages about 5% for the population as a whole.

As with the other congenital adrenal hyperplasias, treatment consists of exogenous glucocorticoid replacement to circumvent the deficiency in cortisol biosynthesis. The usual approach is to administer cortisol (Cortef), 12 to 15 mg/m²/day as a single morning dose. Care should be taken that the adrenal gland is not completely suppressed by the replacement regimen chosen, which can be assessed by an ACTH stimulation test 3 to 6 months following the initiation of treatment.

DISORDERS OF TISSUE RESPONSIVENESS: THE STEROID RESISTANCE SYNDROMES Two disorders of end-organ resistance are relevant to a discussion of disorders of adrenal function: glucocorticoid resistance and mineralocorticoid resistance.

Glucocorticoid resistance is rare, only 17 separate probands have been described to date. The disease is characterized by markedly elevated indices of cortisol production (increased urine free cortisol excretion) in the absence of any of the clinical stigmata of Cushing's syndrome. Occasionally, signs and symptoms of mineralocorticoid and androgen excess are responsible for bringing the patient to medical attention. Like the situation in congenital adrenal hyperplasia, androgen and mineralocorticoid concentrations are elevated in this syndrome as a by product of the increased adrenal steroidogenesis necessary to produce enough cortisol to maintain life. The cause of the disease, which has not been proved in all cases, is a defect in the ligand-binding domain of the glucocorticoid receptor. The disease is transmitted as an autosomal recessive trait, with

heterozygote subjects sometimes manifesting attenuated forms of the disorder.

The diagnosis is suggested by finding elevated rates of urine free cortisol excretion in a subject with none of the stigmata of Cushing's syndrome. The diagnosis is confirmed by demonstrating abnormal binding characteristics of the glucocorticoid receptor, usually in mononuclear leukocytes. Treatment should be reserved for persons manifesting signs and symptoms of androgen or mineralocorticoid excess and consists of the exogenous administration of a synthetic glucocorticoid, usually dexamethasone, in doses sufficient to bring the urine free cortisol excretion into the normal range. Such treatment is usually accompanied by remission of the associated steroid excess syndromes.

Mineralocorticoid resistance is characterized by elevated levels of aldosterone and increased plasma renin activity in association with signs and symptoms of mineralocorticoid deficiency. The disorder is generally referred to as pseudohypoaldosteronism. It is commonly divided into two subtypes, but only type I appears to fulfill the usual criteria for receptor-mediated end-organ resistance.

Type I pseudohypoaldosteronism is a rare inherited disorder characterized by salt loss and failure to thrive in infancy, most commonly between 5 and 7 days of age. The cause appears to be an abnormal mineralocorticoid receptor, with decreased binding affinity and decreased receptor number both described. Hyponatremia, hyperkalemia, and metabolic acidosis in association with elevated plasma and urine aldosterone and elevated plasma renin activity make the diagnosis. Treatment is to replace dietary salt at a rate of 10 to 40 mEq/kg/day.

Aubourg P, Blanche S, Jambaqué I: Reversal of early neurologic and neuroradiologic manifestations of X-linked adrenoleukodystrophy by bone marrow transplantation. N Engl J Med 322:1860, 1990. *Describes a successful outcome from a previously always progressive and often fatal disease.*

Carney JA, Young WF: Primary pigmented nodular adrenocortical disease and its associated conditions. Endocrinologist 2:6, 1992. *Describes an associated complex of abnormalities.*

Donovan DS, Dluhy RG: AIDS and its effect on the adrenal gland. Endocrinologist 1: 227, 1991. *The title says it all in this informative review.*

Friedman RB, Oldfield EH, Nieman LK: Repeat transsphenoidal surgery for Cushing's disease. J Neurosurg 71:520, 1989. *Describes the surgical approach when transnasal hypophysectomy fails to remove the tumor.*

Gill JR: Primary hyperaldosteronism: Strategies for diagnosis and treatment. Endocrinologist 1:365, 1991. *The title is self-explanatory.*

Javier E, Reardon GE, Malchoff CD: Glucocorticoid resistance and its clinical presentations. Endocrinologist 1:141, 1991. *A helpful discussion of a rare disorder.*

Miller J, Crapo I.: The biochemical analysis of hypercortisolism. Endocrinologist 4:7, 1994. *Brings order and simplification to the subject.*

Muir A, Maclaren NK: Autoimmune diseases of the adrenal glands, parathyroid glands, gonads, and hypothalamic-pituitary axis. Endocrinol Metab Clin North Am 20:619, 1991. *Detailed coverage of the mechanisms and treatment of the autoimmune syndrome.*

Schteingart DE: Treating adrenal cancer. Endocrinologist 2:149, 1992. *Describes treatment and outcome in greater detail.*

Veldhuis JD, Melby JC: Isolated aldosterone deficiency in man: Acquired and inborn errors in the biosynthesis of action of aldosterone. Endocrinol Rev 2:495, 1986. *A clearly stated description of the problem.*

241 THE ADRENAL MEDULLA, CATECHOLAMINES, AND PHEOCHROMOCYTOMA

Daniel T. O'Connor

The catecholamines (norepinephrine, epinephrine, and dopamine) serve as neurotransmitters and circulating hormones. Catecholamines acquire their name by the catechol (3,4-dihydroxyphenyl) modification of their aromatic (phenyl) rings. *Norepinephrine* is the amine neurotransmitter released from terminals of post-ganglionic axons of the sympathetic nervous system, as well as from central nervous system noradrenergic axons. Adrenal medullary chromaffin cells store both epinephrine and norepinephrine in catecholamine secretory vesicles.

Chromaffin cells derive embryologically from neuroectoderm. Precursor cells differentiate in the center of the adrenal gland in response to cortisol, after which the precursors again differentiate into sympathetic neurons in response to nerve growth factor. A few such cells also migrate to form paraganglia, collections of chromaffin cells on both sides of the aorta. The largest such periaortic cluster, often found near the level of the inferior mesenteric artery, is referred to as the organ of Zuckerkandl. Both chromaffin cells and post-ganglionic sympathetic axons are part of the effector limb of the sympathetic branch of the autonomic nervous system and are innervated by thoracolumbar pre-ganglionic axons emerging from the spinal cord.

Catecholamines are released from the adrenal medulla into the circulation through the adrenal vein. Norepinephrine from sympathetic neurons is released pre-synaptically and acts as a cell-to-cell neurotransmitter. Circulating plasma norepinephrine influences blood pressure and heart rate under only the most extreme circumstances of sympathetic activation. Relatively selective adrenal catecholamine release occurs during syncope and insulin-evoked hypoglycemia, whereas active, dynamic exercise selectively stimulates sympathetic neuronal norepinephrine release.

CATECHOLAMINE BIOSYNTHESIS AND METABOLISM

Catecholamine biosynthesis starts with the essential dietary amino acid phenylalanine, which is converted to tyrosine by phenylalanine hydroxylase. Tyrosine is hydroxylated to dihydroxyphenylalanine (DOPA) by the action of tyrosine hydroxylase, the rate-limiting enzymatic step in catecholamine biosynthesis. DOPA decarboxylase then converts DOPA to dopamine, which is carried by the vesicular monoamine transporter from the cytosol into the catecholamine storage vesicle, where dopamine β-hydroxylase converts it to norepinephrine. In sympathetic axons and in 15 to 20% of chromaffin cells, norepinephrine is the final catecholamine product. In 80 to 85% of chromaffin cells a further enzymatic step occurs: phenylethanolamine-N-methyltransferase, a cytosolic enzyme, catalyzes the N-methylation of norepinephrine to epinephrine.

Catecholamines in noradrenergic axons and chromaffin cells are sequestered from the cytosol in membrane-limited organelles called catecholamine storage vesicles (or chromaffin granules in chromaffin cells). Chromaffin granule cores contain not only catecholamines but also soluble proteins such as dopamine β-hydroxylase and chromogranin A.

The process of catecholamine discharge from chromaffin cells and sympathetic axons is *exocytosis,* wherein all soluble components of the granule are coreleased and ultimately make their way to the circulation.

Neuronal uptake ("reuptake") is the major route of norepinephrine removal from synaptic clefts (Fig. 241–1). Characteristics of this process are its location at the pre-synaptic axonal membrane, high affinity, stereoselectivity, saturability, dependence on extracellular sodium, and specific pharmacologic inhibition by agents such as tricyclic antidepressants (e.g., desipramine) and cocaine. After neuronal uptake, cytosolic catecholamines can be either retransported into storage vesicles or deaminated by the enzyme monoamine oxidase (MAO) to yield the catecholamine metabolite dihydroxymandelic acid. The enzyme catechol O-methyltransferase (COMT), which acts on both catecholamines and dihydroxymandelic acid, is present mainly in the cytosol of liver and kidney cells. COMT adds a methyl group to one of the hydroxyl oxygens on the catecholamines' dihydroxyphenyl rings to yield either metanephrine (or methoxyepinephrine from epinephrine), normetanephrine (or methoxynorepinephrine from norepinephrine), or methoxytyramine (from dopamine). The metanephrines can then be deaminated by MAO to yield vanillylmandelic acid, whereas deamination of methoxytyramine by MAO yields homovanillic acid. Dihydroxymandelic acid is also a substrate for COMT in the formation of vanillylmandelic acid. Thus, complete enzymatic degradation of catecholamines to vanillylmandelic acid (from epinephrine or norepinephrine) or homovanillic acid (from dopamine) involves the sequential action of two enzymes (MAO and COMT), either of which may initiate the process. In the blood stream, catecholamines have a very short half-life, 1 to 2 minutes. They are cleared from the circulation largely by neuronal uptake, but in addition are subject to direct renal excretion or sulfoconjugation of a ring hydroxyl group.

CATECHOLAMINE ACTION

Catecholamine receptors are specific for ligands and are classified as subtypes of the α ($\alpha_{1a,b,c}$, $\alpha_{2a,b,c}$) and β ($\beta_{1,2,3}$) classes. The hemodynamic effects of circulating norepinephrine require extreme concentrations. Whereas plasma norepinephrine may vary normally over a range of 200 to 1000 pg/mL during physiologic stimulation of sympathetic neuronal activity, far higher concentrations of infused norepinephrine (in excess of 1000 to 2000 pg/mL) are required to substantially affect the blood pressure or heart rate. At β-receptors, norepinephrine is a strong agonist at β_1 (cardiac, inotropic, and chronotropic) sites, although a relatively weak agonist at β_2 (vascular, vasodilatory) sites. At α-receptors, norepinephrine is an effective agonist at both α_1 (vascular, vasoconstrictive) and α_2 (neuronal and vascular) sites. Infused norepinephrine acutely raises both systolic and diastolic blood pressure by actions on both β_1- and α-adrenergic receptors, with vasoconstriction accompanied by reflex bradycardia. The hemodynamic effects of circulating epinephrine (50 to 500 pg/mL) differ from those of norepinephrine. At β-receptors, epinephrine is an agonist at both the β_1 and β_2-sites. It is also a more potent agonist than norepinephrine at both the α_1- and α_2-sites. During acute infusion, it increases systolic blood pressure, heart rate, and cardiac output, with a fall in diastolic blood pressure and systemic resistance, the latter effects resulting from actions at β_2-adrenergic receptors.

With chronic excess of circulating catecholamines, the hemodynamic profile may change substantially, in part as a consequence of desensitization of catecholamine target organs resulting from adaptive changes in both receptor and post-receptor responses.

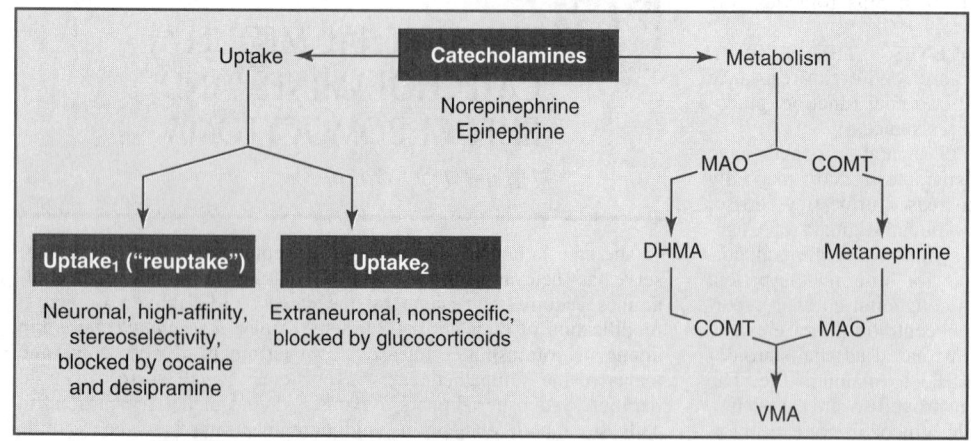

FIGURE 241–1 ■ Catecholamine disposition and metabolism. MAO = monoamine oxidase; COMT = catechol-O-methyltransferase; VMA = vanillylmandelic acid; DHMA = dihydroxymandelic acid.

Pheochromocytoma is a chromaffin cell neoplasm that typically causes symptoms and signs of episodic catecholamine release, including paroxysmal hypertension. The tumor is an unusual cause of hypertension and accounts for at most 0.1 to 0.2% of cases of high blood pressure. In population-based cancer studies, its frequency was about two cases per million population. The diagnosis of pheochromocytoma is typically made in young to middle-aged adults, most commonly in the 4th or 5th decade of life; about 10% of diagnoses are made in children (usually male). Autopsy series indicate that the incidence of pheochromocytoma increases progressively with age. In adults, no gender difference is seen in the incidence of pheochromocytoma.

About 90% of pheochromocytomas exist as solitary, unilateral, encapsulated adrenal medullary tumors. About 10% are bilateral, more commonly seen in several members of a family, 40 to 70% of whose members may have bilateral tumors. The tumors are vascular, and large ones often contain internal hemorrhagic or cystic areas. Reported sizes have ranged from less than 1 g to several kilograms; the average is about 40 g. About 10% of tumors are extra-adrenal (paragangliomas), and 90% of these are intra-abdominal, most commonly arising from chromaffin cells near the aortic bifurcation in the organ of Zuckerkandl or near the kidney. Other sites include the paravertebral sympathetic ganglia, the urinary bladder, other autonomic ganglia (celiac, superior, or inferior mesenteric), the thorax (including the posterior mediastinum, the heart, and paracardiac regions), and the neck (in sympathetic ganglia, the carotid body, cranial nerves, or the glomus jugulare). Bilateral and extra-adrenal tumors are more common in children. Histologically, oval groups of cells, in clusters or "nests," stain for chromogranin A; a less frequently used stain identifies neuron-specific enolase. Fewer than 10% of the tumors are malignant; malignancy occurs more frequently in extra-adrenal tumors and is diagnosed by local invasion or distant metastases but cannot be judged reliably from the histologic appearance. Local invasion commonly involves adjacent vascular structures such as the inferior vena cava. Distant metastatic sites include bone, lung, lymph nodes, and liver. Bilateral adrenal medullary hyperplasia has been reported in gene carriers from kindreds with multiple endocrine neoplasia (MEN) type II. This hyperplasia may be a precursor of pheochromocytoma.

The "rule of 10s" is useful to recall approximate frequencies of pheochromocytoma that vary from the usual: 10% bilateral, 10% extra-adrenal, 10% extra-abdominal, 10% malignant, 10% familial, 10% pediatric, and 10% without blood pressure elevation.

ETIOLOGY. *Familial* pheochromocytomas constitute 5 to 10% of the total and are more frequently bilateral and extra-adrenal, although less commonly malignant. A careful family history is essential, and relatives of patients with the familial syndromes should be screened for pheochromocytoma; biochemical screening is often not sufficient, and imaging studies are also recommended in this high-risk group.

Von Hippel-Lindau syndrome is an autosomal dominant disorder resulting from mutations at a tumor suppressor locus on chromosome 3p25-p26. Its manifestations include pheochromocytoma (in about 14% of gene carriers), retinal angioma, cerebellar hemangioblastoma, renal cysts and carcinoma, pancreatic cysts, and epididymal cystadenoma. Accordingly, all patients with pheochromocytoma deserve careful funduscopic examination.

MEN type IIA and type IIB (Sipple's syndrome) are autosomal dominant disorders arising from mutations on chromosome 10q11.2 in the region of the *RET* proto-oncogene, which encodes a receptor tyrosine kinase. The features of MEN type IIA include pheochromocytoma (in about 40% of gene carriers), medullary thyroid carcinoma, and primary hyperparathyroidism (adenoma or hyperplasia). Because of this syndrome, it is wise to screen all pheochromocytoma patients for medullary thyroid carcinoma with serum calcitonin. MEN type IIB features include pheochromocytoma, medullary thyroid carcinoma, multiple mucosal neuromas (of the lips, tongue, buccal mucosa, eyelids, conjunctivae, corneas, and gastrointestinal tract), and a marfanoid body habitus (but without lens or aortic abnormalities).

Hereditary neurofibromatosis (von Recklinghausen's disease), an autosomal dominant disorder resulting from mutations at the *NF1* (neurofibromin) locus on chromosome 17q11.2, is manifested as neurofibromas and café au lait spots; about 1% of patients with neurofibromatosis have pheochromocytoma. Familial pheochromocytoma may also occur in isolation; whether such families represent disease processes etiologically distinct from von Hippel-Lindau syndrome or MEN is not clear.

In the 90 to 95% of pheochromocytomas that are *sporadic,* the cause of the neoplastic process remains obscure, although loss of heterozygosity on chromosomes 1p, 3p, 17p, and 22q suggests somatic cell deletion mutation of one autosomal allele at as-yet-uncharacterized tumor suppressor loci.

DIAGNOSIS. Because pheochromocytoma is a potentially curable form of hypertension, the diagnosis is worth considering in each new case of hypertension. However, because hypertension is so commonly encountered in clinical practice (~20 to 25% of the adult population) and pheochromocytoma is so distinctly unusual (~0.1 to 0.2% of patients with hypertension), laboratory evaluation should be selective, guided by the degree of clinical suspicion, and based on criteria outlined below (Table 241–1).

SYMPTOMS AND SIGNS. Paroxysmal symptoms (such as the triad of episodic palpitations, diaphoresis, and headache) are the classic features of pheochromocytoma. These paroxysmal "attacks" characteristically begin abruptly, may last for minutes to hours, and subside gradually, with a frequency varying from many times daily to one or more per week (most commonly) or even every few months. Less common symptoms include apprehension or anxiety, tremulousness, pain in the chest or abdomen, weakness, or weight loss. In some series, more than 90% of patients have experienced paroxysmal symptoms of one or more of the classic triad. Autopsy series indicate that as many as 50 to 75% of pheochromocytomas may be undiagnosed during life, thus suggesting that many pheochromocytomas do not give rise to these classic symptomatic features. Patients older than 60 years with pheochromocytoma are especially likely to report minor or no symptoms.

Other features in the history may suggest pheochromocytoma. Affected patients may report an increase in blood pressure after receiving certain antihypertensive drugs, especially β-adrenergic antagonists and guanethidine, or they may experience a remarkable fall in blood pressure after receiving α_1-adrenergic antagonists such as prazosin. Hypertension in such patients is relatively refractory to medical management. A history of extreme blood pressure lability

---

Table 241–1 ■ DIAGNOSTIC APPROACH TO PHEOCHROMOCYTOMA

Clinical clues or "tipoffs"
  History
    Paroxysmal symptoms (classic triad is headache, diaphoresis, palpitations)
    History of extraordinarily labile or refractory hypertension
    Family history of pheochromocytoma, von Hippel-Lindau syndrome or multiple endocrine neoplasia
    Incidental adrenal abnormality on abdominal imaging test (rarely)
  Physical examination
    Labile, refractory hypertension
    Orthostatic hypotension
    von Hippel-Lindau syndrome–or multiple endocrine neoplasia–associated findings (retinal angiomas, thyroid enlargement, mucosal neuromas)
Biochemical confirmation (only after clue or tipoff; begin with urinary tests)
  Urinary catecholamines and metabolites (24-hr sample or 2-hr sample after a paroxysm; metanephrines, the initial screening test)
  Plasma catecholamines (if urinary values are equivocal; take care to obtain a basal, resting sample)
  Clonidine suppression test (if plasma catecholamines are in the equivocal 1000 to 2000-pg/mL range)
  Plasma chromogranin A (storage vesicle protein released with catecholamines; also elevated by renal failure)
Anatomic localization (only after biochemical confirmation)
  By morphology (most sensitive, less specific)
    Computed tomography (the imaging test most frequently obtained)
    Magnetic resonance imaging (may have advantages for extra-adrenal tumors)
  By function (most specific, less sensitive)
    Radiolabeled metaiodobenzylguanidine scanning (accumulates in functioning chromaffin tissue)

during intubation, surgery, or induction of general anesthesia also suggests possible pheochromocytoma. A family history of pheochromocytoma, von Hippel-Lindau syndrome, or MEN should prompt an evaluation for pheochromocytoma. Paroxysmal symptoms on micturition or bladder distention or painless, gross hematuria may suggest pheochromocytoma of the bladder; the diagnosis is confirmed by cystoscopy.

Hypertension (usually severe and refractory to antihypertensive medications) is the cardinal sign of pheochromocytoma, although it is non-specific and may be insensitive. In about half of patients, hypertension is sustained, with intermittent blood pressure surges in half or more of these; in about 40%, hypertension is paroxysmal, with relatively normal blood pressure between surges. Hypertensive surges may be precipitated by abdominal manipulation, but generally no antecedent is noted. The heart rate is usually elevated during blood pressure surges but may decline as a result of physiologic reflex bradycardia. Orthostatic hypotension is variably observed. As many as 15 to 20% of patients may have cholesterol gallstones.

LABORATORY DIAGNOSIS. Because hypertension is so common and pheochromocytoma so rare, further biochemical evaluation for pheochromocytoma in hypertensives should be selective and focused on subjects who display some relevant clue to pheochromocytoma on history, physical examination, or screening laboratory evaluation. If interpretation of urinary measurements is not clearcut, evaluation should proceed to plasma measurements, which require more careful sampling technique. The number and diversity of biochemical tests obtained should parallel the clinical index of suspicion. If suspicion is low, a single screening test may suffice, usually 24-hour urinary metanephrine excretion. If suspicion is high, multiple tests, both urine and plasma, are in order. Because anatomic or imaging studies may detect non-specific adrenal abnormalities in up to 2% of the population, such studies should not be undertaken unless biochemical tests are positive.

Routine Tests. Results of routine screening tests obtained for other purposes (such as general health maintenance) may provide tipoffs. Hyperglycemia is common, and about half of patients with pheochromocytoma manifest carbohydrate intolerance; frank diabetes requiring insulin is unusual. Lactic acidosis occurs rarely, even without shock. Serum lactate dehydrogenase activity may be elevated from adrenal isoenzyme 3. Rarely, pheochromocytoma may be an incidental finding on computed tomography (CT) or magnetic resonance imaging (MRI) of the abdomen undertaken for other indications.

Urine Tests. Widely available tests measure urinary free (unconjugated) catecholamines and catecholamine metabolites: the metanephrines and vanillylmandelic acid. A 24-hour urine sample is collected, and creatinine is measured in the same sample as an index of adequacy and completeness of collection. Of the available tests, increased urinary metanephrines have the highest diagnostic sensitivity and specificity for pheochromocytoma. Urinary excretion of metanephrines and vanillylmandelic acid remains normal until the very end stage of renal disease, so elevated levels validly diagnose pheochromocytoma.

Artifactual false-positive assay results have been greatly minimized in recent years with the introduction of more specific assay methods based on separation of catecholamines and metabolites in urine by high-pressure liquid chromatography. False-positive increases in free catecholamines may result from exogenous sources, such as catecholamines (which may be administered surreptitiously), α-methyldopa (but vanillylmandelic acid excretion is characteristically normal), L-DOPA, labetalol, sympathomimetic amines (which release endogenous catecholamines from their stores), and fluorescent drugs such as tetracycline. Misleading elevations of endogenous catecholamines may occur as a consequence of the sympathoadrenal responses to shock, hypoglycemia, physical exertion, increased intracranial pressure, or withdrawal of central α_2-agonists such as clonidine. False-positive metanephrine elevations may result from excessive catecholamines (exogenous or endogenous) or the use of MAO inhibitors or propranolol (which interferes with the spectrophotometric assay). False-positive elevations in vanillylmandelic acid may occur after ingesting carbidopa (a peripheral DOPA decarboxylase inhibitor) or MAO inhibitors.

Blood Tests. Biochemical tests on blood samples offer the advantage of patient convenience but the disadvantage that even minor physical or mental stress can result in false-positive elevations. Plasma catecholamines are best sampled from a supine, resting patient in whom an indwelling antecubital venous cannula has been in place for at least 15 minutes. Plasma assay methods generally provide reliable results with the usual normal resting norepinephrine value being 200 to 400 pg/mL and the normal resting epinephrine value being 20 to 60 pg/mL. Most patients with pheochromocytoma have markedly elevated (>2000 pg/mL) resting plasma catecholamine (norepinephrine plus epinephrine) values; plasma concentrations elevated beyond this point strongly suggest pheochromocytoma. The upper limit of normal (norepinephrine plus epinephrine) is less than 1000 pg/mL. Values between 1000 and 2000 pg/mL are equivocal and may represent either pheochromocytoma or sympathoadrenal activation by physical or mental stress. In these subjects the clonidine suppression test discussed below is of particular value.

False-positive plasma catecholamine elevations may result from the same factors that produce false-positive urinary elevations but are a more severe problem because measurements are made at only one point. These factors include physical stress, such as trauma, surgery, upright posture, acute venipuncture, hypoglycemia, hypovolemia, hypotension, cold, and sodium depletion, or mental stress, such as anxiety or pain. Drugs that increase plasma catecholamines include sympathomimetic amines, which release catecholamines from their stores; cocaine, which blocks catecholamine reuptake; and abrupt clonidine withdrawal. Illnesses known to elevate plasma catecholamines include both acute (e.g., myocardial infarction, diabetic ketoacidosis, or sepsis) and chronic conditions (e.g., congestive heart failure, anemia, respiratory failure, or hypothyroidism). Factors that diminish plasma catecholamines include drugs (clonidine, reserpine, and α-methylparatyrosine), autonomic neuropathy, and congenital deficiency of dopamine β-hydroxylase activity.

As with urine biochemical tests, plasma catecholamine sampling during a paroxysmal attack of hypertension is of value. A finding of normal plasma catecholamines when blood pressure is elevated is quite a useful negative result. Because only extreme elevations of plasma norepinephrine perturb blood pressure, the finding of normal plasma catecholamines while blood pressure is elevated argues strongly against pheochromocytoma as the cause.

Other components of the catecholamine storage vesicle core are released into the blood stream by pheochromocytomas. The plasma concentration of chromogranin A is elevated in patients with pheochromocytoma, with a diagnostic sensitivity of 83% and specificity of 96%. It is not substantially elevated by acute venipuncture, nor is it affected by drugs used in treatment or diagnosis of pheochromocytoma. Because chromogranin A is released by a variety of neuroendocrine secretory vesicles, its plasma concentration is also elevated in other neuroendocrine neoplasias. Chromogranin A values are also elevated in renal insufficiency because of retained immunoreactive fragments of the protein.

PHARMACOLOGIC DIAGNOSTIC TESTS: SUPPRESSIVE AND PROVOCATIVE. Pharmacologic tests for pheochromocytoma are generally not necessary because the diagnosis can usually be confirmed by urine and plasma biochemical measurements at rest or during spontaneous blood pressure surges.

The *clonidine suppression test* is of value if plasma catecholamine elevations in a patient with suspected pheochromocytoma are equivocal (that is, from 1000 to 2000 pg/mL). The rationale for the test is that pheochromocytoma chromaffin cells, unlike normal adrenal medullary chromaffin cells, are not innervated; hence catecholamine release from pheochromocytoma chromaffin cells is autonomous and not susceptible to manipulation by drugs that decrease efferent sympathetic outflow, such as the central α_2-agonist clonidine. Blood is obtained for plasma catecholamines before and 3 hours after a single oral dose of 0.3 mg clonidine. In a subject without pheochromocytoma, plasma norepinephrine should fall to less than 500 pg/mL after clonidine. A positive test (failure of catecholamines to decline after clonidine) is sensitive but may not be entirely specific for pheochromocytoma. Although catecholamine levels do not fall after clonidine administration in pheochromocytoma, the blood pressure fall is comparable to that seen in essential hypertensives. To prevent inordinate falls in blood pressure during the test, prior volume depletion should be avoided; the test is most safely done in subjects whose diastolic blood pressure before clonidine is 100 mm Hg or higher. Because β-blockers such as propranolol diminish circulating norepinephrine clearance (and hence plasma norepinephrine responses to clonidine), their use should be discontinued 48 hours before and during the test. The test remains valid during a blockade.

Catecholamine provocative tests (such as the glucagon test) are used in only a few centers because of the potential hazard posed by inordinate catecholamine release.

ANATOMIC LOCALIZATION. Tumor location must be known to plan the proper surgical route. Ninety-five per cent of pheochromocytomas are in the abdomen, and the great majority of these can be visualized by one of three modalities: CT MRI, or metaiodobenzylguanidine (MIBG) scintigraphy. CT and MRI are highly sensitive, although non-specific because they visualize any mass lesion, not just pheochromocytomas. MIBG scanning is highly specific for chromaffin tissue, although somewhat less sensitive than CT or MRI.

MIBG, a radiolabeled analogue of guanethidine, is transported into chromaffin cells by the reuptake cell membrane catecholamine carrier. Because it accumulates in chromaffin cells, an MIBG abnormality is extraordinarily specific (about 98%) for pheochromocytoma, although somewhat less sensitive (85 to 90%). MIBG imaging is especially useful for metastatic, recurrent, or extra-adrenal tumors. Abdominal ultrasonography is a safe imaging tool but is less sensitive than CT or MRI. Plain abdominal radiography, intravenous urography (pyelography), air insufflation retroperitoneal pneumography, arteriography, and venography are no longer done to localize pheochromocytoma. Indeed, arteriography or venography of the tumor may trigger hypertensive crises.

DIFFERENTIAL DIAGNOSIS. Because many conditions can mimic the diagnostic features of pheochromocytoma, as many as 90% of patients who have some feature of the tumor turn out not to have one after diagnostic testing. Examples include certain drugs, such as surreptitiously self-administered epinephrine or isoproterenol. Abrupt withdrawal from clonidine can provoke a sympathoadrenal discharge with "rebound" blood pressure elevation. Subjects treated with MAO inhibitors for depression may have hypertensive crises if they inadvertently ingest foods rich in tyramine.

Disease states causing or simulating catecholamine excess and hypertension include thyrotoxicosis; acute intracranial disturbances such as subarachnoid hemorrhage or posterior fossa masses; hypertensive crisis of paraplegia, which can be initiated by visceral manipulation or bladder distention; and hypoglycemia, especially in the presence of β-blockade. Damage to carotid sinus baroreceptors by surgery or tumor may result in baroreflex failure, with episodic blood pressure and plasma catecholamine surges; clonidine is the drug of choice. Episodic surges in plasma dopamine have been described in some patients with episodic blood pressure elevation but without pheochromocytoma; the mechanism has not been established.

PATHOPHYSIOLOGY AND COMPLICATIONS. Although circulating catecholamine excess is the ultimate cause of hypertension in pheochromocytoma, the correlation of blood pressure with plasma catecholamines is modest. Desensitization to catecholamine effects may contribute to underdiagnosis of the tumor in the elderly. In addition to catecholamines, pheochromocytomas also release a number of potentially vasoactive substances that may modify blood pressure. Hemodynamic studies suggest that elevations in systemic vascular resistance rather than cardiac output account for the blood pressure rise.

Acute norepinephrine infusion leads to plasma volume contraction, and a past mainstay of pheochromocytoma management has been an effort to re-expand plasma volume, either spontaneously after therapeutic α-blockade or with preoperative saline infusion. However, recent careful measurements of plasma volume indicate that on average it is not as contracted as once believed. Orthostatic hypotension is variably observed in pheochromocytoma. It cannot be clearly attributed to plasma volume contraction and probably reflects catecholamine desensitization, the effects of vasodilator peptides and catecholamines, and dysautonomia.

The major catecholamine secreted by most pheochromocytomas is norepinephrine. Small intra-adrenal tumors (especially early in the course of MEN type II) may secrete predominantly epinephrine. Pure epinephrine secretion by pheochromocytomas is rare.

Cardiomyopathy (myocarditis) occurs in a minority of patients

with pheochromocytoma, presumably as a consequence of catecholamine excess. This process is generally reversible after tumor removal, and congestive heart failure responds to preoperative α-adrenergic blockade. In most patients, however, the degree of myocardial left ventricular hypertrophy on cardiac ultrasonography is no different from that seen in essential hypertension.

MANAGEMENT. PREOPERATIVE PREPARATION AND DRUG TREATMENT. Once pheochromocytoma has been diagnosed, the patient is prepared for surgery with adrenergic blockade for a period of 1 to 4 weeks. During α-blockade, any catecholamine-induced plasma volume contraction is allowed to correct itself. α-Blockade is usually accomplished with oral phenoxybenzamine, an irreversible, non-competitive antagonist that acts predominantly at α_1-receptors. The drug is begun at 5 mg twice daily, and the dose is adjusted gradually upward by increments of 10 mg every 1 to 4 days to a maximum of 50 to 100 mg twice daily. The usual dose range required is 30 to 80 mg/day. Treatment goals are to normalize blood pressure ($\leq160/\leq90$ mm Hg), prevent paroxysmal hypertension, and abolish tachyarrhythmias (ventricular extrasystoles, <1 to 5 per minute) without inducing intolerable orthostatic hypotension (i.e., orthostatic falls of $>85/>45$ mm Hg). Side effects of an adequate phenoxybenzamine dosage include orthostatic hypotension, tachycardia, nasal congestion, dry mouth, diplopia, and ejaculatory dysfunction. In patients intolerant of phenoxybenzamine, one can use the α_1-selective antagonist prazosin in a dose range of 0.5 to 16 mg/day given orally two to four times daily.

If blood pressure of tachyarrhythmias, including sinus tachycardia, are not fully controlled by α-blockade, β-blockade is instituted with oral propranolol, 10 to 40 mg four times daily. β-blockade must not be undertaken before α-blockade has been instituted; after blockade of vasodilatory vascular β_2-adrenergic receptors, catecholamines' continued access to vasoconstrictive α_1-receptors may induce unopposed vasoconstriction and exacerbation of hypertension. β-Blockade may be especially useful for predominantly epinephrine-secreting tumors. Metoprolol and labetalol are alternatives to propranolol. In subjects with contraindications to β-blockade, lidocaine or amiodarone can be used for tachyarrhythmias.

If combined management with α- plus β-adrenergic antagonists is not fully effective, the tyrosine hydroxylase inhibitor α-methyl-paratyrosine is added at an oral dose of 0.25 to 1.0 g four times daily. Its use may be complicated by sedation, fatigue, anxiety, diarrhea, or extrapyramidal reactions.

For acute management of severe hypertensive crises, intravenous nitroprusside is effective. Intravenous non-selective α_1/α_2-blockade with phentolamine (1-mg bolus, then by continuous infusion) is also useful. Calcium channel blockade with sublingual nifedipine (10 mg broken under the tongue) has also been used.

Opiates (narcotic analgesics), narcotic antagonists (such as naloxone), histamine, adrenocorticotropic hormone, saralasin, glucagon, or indirect sympathomimetic amines (such as phenylpropanolamine or tyramine) should be avoided. All of these agents may provoke hypertensive surges by releasing catecholamines from the tumor. Drugs that block catecholamine reuptake, such as tricyclic antidepressants (e.g., desipramine), cocaine, or guanethidine, may worsen hypertension. β-Adrenergic antagonists, by blocking vasodilatory vascular β_2-receptors, may cause unopposed α-mediated vasoconstriction by circulating catecholamines and thereby result in severe hypertension, unless α-blockade is first instituted beforehand. Dopaminergic antagonists (such as metoclopramide or sulpiride) may result in hypertension. All should be avoided.

OPERATIVE AND PERIOPERATIVE MANAGEMENT. Autopsy series of pheochromocytoma indicate that even clinically unsuspected cases can be lethal. At least 90% of pheochromocytomas are benign, and surgical resection provides a cure, although up to 25% of patients may retain some lesser degree of hypertension. Residual tumor may be diagnosed by urinary catecholamine measurement 1 to 2 weeks postoperatively. The operative mortality of pheochromocytoma resection should not exceed 2 to 3%. In malignant pheochromocytoma, the individual course is highly variable, but long-term 50% survival is less than 5 years.

Several surgical approaches are feasible, depending on the particular characteristics of the pheochromocytoma; the experience of the surgeon is crucial. The entire adrenal gland harboring a pheochromocytoma is usually excised. Anesthetic management is guided by selection of agents that do not cause catecholamine release or potentiate catecholamines' dysrhythmic effects. Intravenous glucose replacement (5% dextrose in water or saline) should be given to prevent hypoglycemia, a frequent occurrence after tumor removal. Times at which hypertensive surges are likely to occur include anesthetic induction, intubation, tumor palpation, and ligation of tumor veins. If intraoperative hypotension occurs, the initial treatment should be saline infusion to expand intravascular volume. Only after plasma volume expansion to euvolemia is norepinephrine infusion appropriate.

For intraoperative blood pressure surges, intravenous nitroprusside is often used. Alternatively, α-blockade can be accomplished with intravenous phentolamine (an α_1- and α_2-antagonist), starting with a 1-mg dose and proceeding to infusion. The calcium channel antagonist nicardipine has also been used.

In the postoperative period, several problems occur with some frequency:

1. Hypotension. Most commonly, hypotension results from hypovolemia and responds to saline infusion; several liters may be required, often with the guidance of central pressure measurements. After volume repletion, norepinephrine can be infused if needed.
2. Hypertension. Plasma catecholamine levels remain elevated for several days after complete pheochromocytoma resection. Even 2 weeks postoperatively, up to one fourth of patients still have hypertension. At this time the differential diagnosis includes residual unresected tumor, essential hypertension, or hypertension secondary to renal damage caused by prior hypertension. A urine collection for catecholamines, obtained at least 1 to 2 weeks after tumor resection, will clarify matters.
3. Hypoglycemia. After correction of catecholamine excess, insulin release may be increased and end-organ responsiveness to insulin augmented, resulting in hypoglycemia. Hypoglycemia may masquerade as refractory hypotension. Infusion of glucose (5% dextrose in water or saline) during the intraoperative and immediate postoperative period is useful.

MALIGNANT PHEOCHROMOCYTOMA. Although most pheochromocytomas are well-encapsulated, localized growths, approximately 5 to 10% are malignant. Malignancy is diagnosed by the biologic behavior of the tumor in the form of adjacent tissue invasion or distant metastatic spread. Extra-adrenal tumors are more likely to metastasize than are primary adrenal ones. Catecholamine biosynthesis tends to be especially deranged in malignant tumors, with secretion of substantial amounts of DOPA and dopamine (metabolized to homovanillic acid, which can be detected in the urine). Increased plasma DOPA in pheochromocytoma suggests malignancy.

In patients with malignant pheochromocytoma, α- and β-adrenergic blockade with phenoxybenzamine and propranolol remains the mainstay of management of the symptoms and signs of catecholamine excess. If catecholamine effects are not controlled, the tyrosine hydroxylase inhibitor α-methylparatyrosine can be effective at 0.25 to 1.0 g four times daily.

Metastases tend to be slow growing, and the natural history of malignant pheochromocytoma is variable; the 5-year survival rate is less than 50%. Common sites of metastasis are the retroperitoneum, skeleton (bone), lymph nodes, and liver. Periodic surgical debulking may help control symptoms. The response to chemotherapy has generally been disappointing, but the combination of vincristine, cyclophosphamide, and dacarbazine shows promise in many patients. Skeletal metastases show some response to irradiation, although the neoplasm is not particularly susceptible to radiation therapy. High-dose (300 mCi) radiation therapy with intravenous ^{125}I-MIBG remains experimental but is of value in some patients.

CATECHOLAMINE DEFICIENCY DISEASE STATES

Loss of even both adrenal glands seldom produces a catecholamine deficiency state. In diabetics receiving insulin, the usual counterregulatory response to hypoglycemia involves the actions of epinephrine and glucagon to trigger hepatic glycogenolysis. In diabetics who also have autonomic neuropathy, deficient epinephrine

release during hypoglycemia coupled with deficient glucagon responses may result in impairment of the usual counterregulatory response to hypoglycemia and prolong its duration.

Several individuals have been described with an apparent congenital deficiency of dopamine β-hydroxylase; such individuals have greatly diminished or undetectable norepinephrine and epinephrine in blood, urine, and cerebrospinal fluid. The initial features of this lifelong syndrome include severe orthostatic hypotension, ptosis, nasal stuffiness, hyperextensible joints, and retrograde ejaculation. The diagnosis is made in patients with severe orthostatic hypotension, a plasma norepinephrine/dopamine ratio of less than 1, and undetectable plasma dopamine β-hydroxylase activity. During sympathoadrenal activation in these subjects, increments in efferent sympathetic nerve traffic occur, but sympathetic axons release the precursor dopamine instead of norepinephrine, perhaps compounding the hypotension.

THE INCIDENTAL ADRENAL MASS (OR "INCIDENTALOMA")

Up to 2% of all abdominal CT scans, as well as 9% of autopsies, incidentally discover minimal adrenal gland abnormalities. Rarely do these lesions require further attention.

Occasionally the appearance of an adrenal mass on CT or MRI is sufficiently characteristic for a firm diagnosis; an example is adrenal myelolipoma, a benign accumulation of bone marrow elements in an otherwise normally functioning adrenal gland with a characteristic fat-density image on CT or MRI. Myelolipoma requires no treatment.

If an adrenal mass is larger than 4 to 6 cm in span, its chance of malignancy (especially adrenocortical carcinoma) increases, and such masses should be resected unless they have a clearly benign appearance (such as myelolipoma) on CT or MRI. In smaller lesions, adrenal carcinoma is unlikely unless other signs or symptoms of adrenocortical hormone excess are apparent. Incidental masses smaller than 4 to 6 cm in span are monitored by periodic CT scanning. In subjects with known metastatic carcinoma, adrenal abnormalities are likely to be adrenal metastases. In subjects with recent major abdominal trauma, adrenal abnormalities probably represent hemorrhage and should resolve with time.

Because not all pheochromocytomas manifest hypertension at all times, all patients with incidental adrenal masses should be screened for pheochromocytoma with a 24-hour urine collection for catecholamine metabolites.

Virtually all patients with aldosterone-producing adrenal adenoma have hypertension and hypokalemia. If blood pressure and serum potassium are normal on a diet of greater than 200 mEq sodium per day and less than 100 mEq potassium per day (confirmed by 24-hour urine), no further evaluation is needed.

Cushing's disease is likely only if other signs or symptoms are suggestive. The diagnosis is made by giving 1 mg of oral dexamethasone at 11 P.M. and sampling serum cortisol the next morning at 8 A.M.

Cryer PE: Pheochromocytoma. West J Med 156:399, 1992. *A comprehensive review contrasting the diagnostic value of plasma versus urinary catecholamines.*

Grossman E, Goldstein DS, Hoffman A, et al: Glucagon and clonidine testing in the diagnosis of pheochromocytoma. Hypertension 17:733, 1991. *A large series evaluating the sensitivity and specificity of these provocation and suppression tests of catecholamine release.*

Hsiao RJ, Parmer RJ, Takiyyuddin MA, et al: Chromogranin A storage and secretion: Sensitivity and specificity for the diagnosis of pheochromocytoma. Medicine (Baltimore) 70:33, 1991. *The chromaffin storage vesicle protein chromogranin A, coreleased by exocytosis with catecholamines, is a sensitive and specific plasma marker of pheochromocytoma in hypertension patients.*

Jovenich JJ: Anesthesia in adrenal surgery. Urol Clin North Am 16:583, 1989. *Practical suggestions on anesthetics to use or avoid.*

Kailasam MT, O'Connor DT, Parmer RJ: The regulation and role of catecholamines in hypertension and pheochromocytoma. Curr Opin Endocrinol Diabetes 1:135, 1994. *A review emphasizing recent diagnostic developments.*

Malone MJ, Libertino JA, Tsapatsaris NP, et al: Preoperative and surgical management of pheochromocytoma. Urol Clin North Am 16:567, 1989. *Rationale for selection from several possible surgical approaches.*

Neumann HPH, Berger DP, Sigmund G, et al: Pheochromocytomas, multiple endocrine neoplasia type 2, and von Hippel-Lindau disease. N Engl J Med 329:1531, 1993. *This large series highlights the importance and yield of screening patients with pheochromocytoma for familial syndromes.*

Ross NS, Aron DC: Hormonal evaluation of the patient with an incidentally discovered adrenal mass. N Engl J Med 323:1401, 1991. *A sensible approach to this increasingly frequent and vexing clinical problem.*

242 DIABETES MELLITUS

Robert S. Sherwin

OVERVIEW

Diabetes mellitus is a chronic disorder characterized by impaired metabolism of glucose and other energy-yielding fuels, as well as the late development of vascular (involving small and large blood vessels) and neuropathic complications. Diabetes mellitus consists of a group of disorders involving distinct pathogenic mechanisms in which hyperglycemia is the common denominator. Regardless of the cause, the disease is associated with a common hormonal defect, namely, insulin deficiency, which may be total, partial, or relative when viewed in the context of coexisting insulin resistance. Lack of insulin plays a primary role in the metabolic derangements linked to diabetes, and hyperglycemia in turn plays a key role in the complications of the disease.

In the United States the number of diagnosed cases of diabetes mellitus has substantially increased in the last half of the 20th century. Diabetes mellitus is the fourth most common reason for patient contact with a physician, accounts for nearly 15% of health care costs in the United States, and is a major cause of premature disability and mortality. It is the leading cause of blindness among working-age people, of end-stage renal disease (ESRD), and of non-traumatic limb amputations. It increases the risk of cardiac, cerebral, and peripheral vascular disease two- to seven-fold and is a major factor contributing to neonatal morbidity and mortality. On the bright side, recent data indicate that most, if not all of the debilitating complications of the disease can be prevented or delayed by prospective treatment of hyperglycemia and other cardiovascular risk factors.

CLASSIFICATION

The newly revised classification of diabetes mellitus is summarized in Table 242–1. Clinical diabetes may be divided into four general subclasses, including (1) type 1 (caused by beta cell destruction and characterized by absolute insulin deficiency), (2) type 2 (characterized by insulin resistance and relative insulin defi-

Table 242–1 ■ CLASSIFICATION OF DIABETES

Clinical Diabetes

I. Type I diabetes, formerly called insulin-dependent diabetes mellitus (IDDM) or "juvenile-onset diabetes"
   A. Immune mediated
   B. Idiopathic
II. Type II diabetes, formerly called non–insulin-dependent diabetes (NIDDM) or "adult-onset diabetes"
III. Other specific types
   A. Genetic defects of β-cell function (e.g., maturity-onset diabetes of the young [MODY] types 1–3 and point mutations in mitochondrial DNA)
   B. Genetic defects in insulin action
   C. Disease of the exocrine pancreas (e.g., pancreatitis, trauma, pancreatectomy, neoplasia, cystic fibrosis, hemochromatosis, fibrocalculous pancreatopathy)
   D. Endocrinopathies (e.g., acromegaly, Cushing's syndrome, hyperthyroidism, pheochromocytoma, glucagonoma, somatostinoma, aldosteronoma)
   E. Drug or chemical induced (e.g., glucocorticosteroids, thiazides, diazoxide, pentamidine, vacor, thyroid hormone, phenytoin [Dilantin], β-agonists, oral contraceptives)
   F. Infections (e.g., congenital rubella, cytomegalovirus)
   G. Uncommon forms of immune-mediated diabetes (e.g., "stiff-man" syndrome, anti–insulin receptor antibodies)
   H. Other genetic syndromes (e.g., Down, Klinefelter's, Turner's syndrome, Huntington's disease, myotonic dystrophy, lipodystrophy, ataxia-telangiectasia)
IV. Gestational diabetes mellitus
   Risk categories
   I. Impaired fasting glucose
   II. Impaired glucose tolerance

ciency), (3) other specific types of diabetes (associated with various identifiable clinical conditions or syndromes), and (4) gestational diabetes mellitus. In addition to these clinical categories, two conditions—impaired glucose tolerance and impaired fasting glucose—refer to a metabolic state intermediate between normal glucose homeostasis and overt diabetes. These conditions significantly increase the later risk of diabetes mellitus and may in some instances be part of its natural history. It should be noted that patients with any form of diabetes may require insulin treatment at some point. For this reason the previously used terms insulin-dependent diabetes (for type 1 diabetes mellitus) and non–insulin-dependent diabetes (for type 2) have been eliminated.

TYPE 1 DIABETES MELLITUS. Patients with this disorder have little or no insulin secretory capacity and depend on exogenous insulin to prevent metabolic decompensation (e.g., ketoacidosis) and death. Commonly but not always, diabetes appears abruptly (i.e., over days or weeks) in previously healthy non-obese children or young adults; in older age groups it may have a more gradual onset. At the time of initial evaluation the typical patient often appears ill, has marked symptoms (e.g., polyuria, polydipsia, polyphagia, and weight loss), and may demonstrate ketoacidosis. Type 1 diabetes is believed to have a long asymptomatic pre-clinical stage often lasting years, during which pancreatic beta cells are gradually destroyed by an autoimmune attack that is influenced by HLA and other genetic factors, as well as the environment (Fig. 242–1). In some, an acute illness may speed the transition from the pre-clinical to the clinical stage. Initially, insulin therapy is essential to restore metabolism toward normal. However, a so-called honeymoon period may follow and last weeks or months, during which time smaller doses of insulin are required because of partial recovery of beta cell function and reversal of insulin resistance caused by acute illness. Thereafter, insulin secretory capacity is gradually lost (over several years). That type 1 diabetes is an autoimmune disease is supported by its association with specific immune response (HLA) genes and the presence of antibodies to islet cells and their constituents. This syndrome accounts for less than 10% of diabetes in the United States.

TYPE 2 DIABETES MELLITUS. Type 2, by far the most common form of the disease, is found in over 90% of the diabetic patient population. These patients retain a significant level of endogenous insulin secretory capacity. However, insulin levels are low relative to the magnitude of insulin resistance and ambient glucose levels. Type 2 patients are not dependent on insulin for immediate survival and ketosis rarely develops, except under conditions of great physical stress. Nevertheless, these patients may require insulin therapy to control hyperglycemia. Type 2 diabetes typically appears after the age of 40 years, has a high rate of genetic penetrance unrelated to HLA genes, and is associated with obesity. The clinical features of type 2 diabetes are much more insidious. The classic symptoms of diabetes may be mild (fatigue, weakness, dizziness, blurred vision, or other non-specific complaints may dominate the picture) or may be tolerated for many years before the patient seeks medical attention. Moreover, if the level of hyperglycemia is insufficient to produce symptoms, the disease may become evident only after complications develop.

OTHER SPECIFIC TYPES OF DIABETES. This category encompasses a variety of diabetic syndromes attributed to a specific disease, drug, or condition (see Table 242–1). Genetic research has provided new insights into the pathogenesis of maturity-onset diabetes of the young (MODY), which was formerly included as a form of type 2 diabetes. MODY encompasses several genetic defects of beta cell function, among which mutations at several genetic loci on different chromosomes have been identified. The most common forms—MODY type 3—is associated with a mutation for a transcription factor encoded on chromosome 12 named hepatocyte nuclear factor 1α (HNF-1α) and -MODY type 2 is associated with mutations of the glucokinase gene (on chromosome 7). Mutations of the HNF-4α gene (on chromosome 20) are responsible for type 1 of MODY. Each of these conditions is inherited in an autosomal dominant pattern. Two new rare forms of MODY are associated with mutations of the HNF-1β (on chromosome 17) and an insulin gene transcription factor termed PDX-1 or 1DX-1 (on chromosome 13).

It should be emphasized that severe illness (e.g., burns, trauma, sepsis) may also provoke stress hyperglycemia as a result of hypersecretion of insulin antagonistic hormones. Although some of

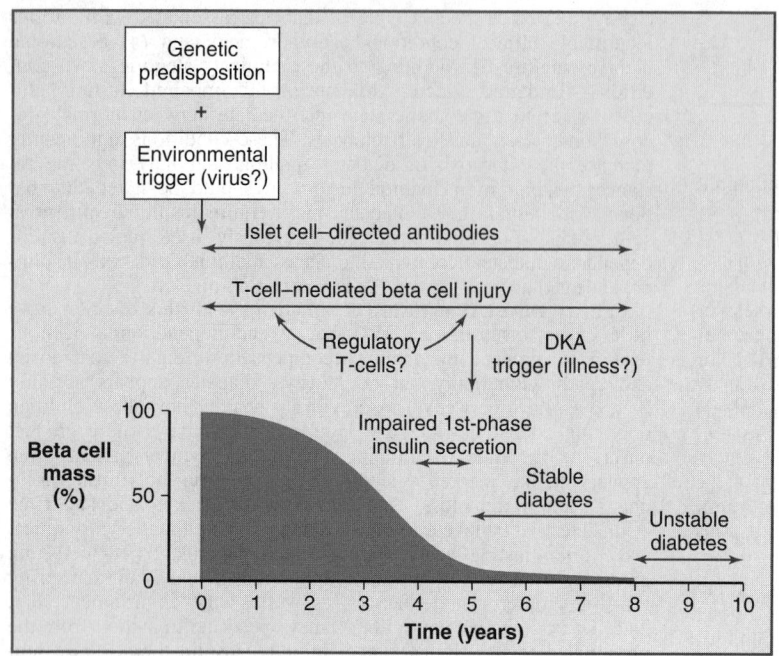

FIGURE 242-1 ■ A summary of the sequence of events that lead to beta cell loss and ultimately to the clinical appearance of type I diabetes.

these individuals may have underlying diabetes, the metabolic disturbance is often self-limited and should therefore not be classified as diabetes until the precipitating illness has fully resolved.

Distinction between the various subclasses of diabetes mellitus is usually made on clinical grounds. However, a small subgroup of patients are difficult to classify, that is, they display features common to both type 1 and 2 diabetes. Such patients are commonly non-obese and have reduced insulin secretory capacity that is not sufficient to make them ketosis prone. Many initially respond to oral agents but, with time, require insulin. Some appear to have a slowly evolving form of type 1 diabetes, whereas others defy easy categorization.

GESTATIONAL DIABETES. The term *gestational diabetes* describes women with impaired glucose tolerance that appears or is first detected during pregnancy. Women with known diabetes before conception are not considered to have gestational diabetes. Gestational diabetes usually appears in the 2nd or 3rd trimester, a time when pregnancy-associated insulin antagonistic hormones peak. After delivery, glucose tolerance generally (but not always) reverts to normal. However, within 5 to 10 years, type 2 diabetes develops in 30 to 40%. Occasionally, pregnancy may precipitate type 1 diabetes. Gestational diabetes occurs in about 2% of pregnant women. Although patients generally have only mild, asymptomatic hyperglycemia, rigorous treatment, often with insulin, is required to protect against hyperglycemia-associated fetal morbidity and mortality.

IMPAIRED GLUCOSE TOLERANCE AND IMPAIRED FASTING GLUCOSE. These terms are applied to individuals who have glucose levels that are higher than normal but lower than those accepted as diagnostic for diabetes mellitus. Both conditions are associated with an increased risk for cardiovascular disease but do not produce the classic symptoms or the microvascular and neuropathic complications associated with diabetes mellitus. In a subgroup of patients (about 25 to 30%), however, type 2 diabetes eventually develops.

DIAGNOSIS

The diagnosis is usually straightforward when the classic symptoms of polyuria, polydipsia, and weight loss are present. All that is required is a random plasma glucose measurement from venous blood that is 200 mg/dL or greater. Further diagnostic testing is unwarranted and delays treatment. Although glycosuria is strongly suggestive of diabetes, urine testing should never be used exclusively; a low renal threshold for glucose can produce a similar clinical picture. If diabetes is suspected but not confirmed by a random glucose determination, the screening test of choice is an overnight fasting plasma glucose level; it varies less from day to day and is more resistant to factors that non-specifically alter glucose metabolism. The diagnosis is established if fasting glucose is equal to or greater than 126 mg/dL on at least two separate occasions. This value is lower than the value previously used (i.e., 140 mg/dL) because it is now appreciated that it more closely reflects the level diagnostic of diabetes during oral glucose testing and the level at which diabetic complications appear. Fasting glucose levels less than 110 mg/dL generally do not warrant further testing. On the other hand, values between 110 and 126 mg/dL, although not diagnostic, should arouse suspicion. Results in this range are classified as impaired fasting glucose. Because individuals with impaired fasting glucose may exhibit severe postprandial hyperglycemia, further testing may be done with the oral glucose tolerance test (OGTT). The OGTT has the advantage of detecting diabetes at its earliest stage, when treatment is most effective. The disadvantage is that the test may lead to overdiagnosis unless the clinician recognizes its pitfalls. Common factors that non-specifically deteriorate the OGTT include (1) carbohydrate restriction (⟨150 g for 3 days), (2) bed rest (days) or severe inactivity (weeks), (3) medical or surgical stress, (4) drugs (e.g., thiazides, β-blockers, glucocorticoids, or phenytoin), (5) smoking during the test, or (6) anxiety from repeated needlesticks. As a result, its value in the clinical setting is limited. If the OGTT is used, some individuals neither meet the diagnostic criteria for diabetes nor show a normal glucose profile. They are classified as having impaired glucose tolerance if the fasting glucose is less than 126 mg/dL and the 2-hour OGTT level is between 140 and 200 mg/dL. Because no diagnostic markers can distinguish individuals with impaired fasting glucose or impaired glucose tolerance who will become diabetic, these individuals should be tested annually with a fasting glucose measurement. It is also prudent to prescribe the same lifestyle changes as offered to overtly diabetic patients because such patients (like those with diabetes mellitus) have a higher risk of premature cardiovascular disease.

Because many patients with type 2 diabetes have the disease years before symptoms are appreciated, it is important to screen (with a fasting glucose measurement) high-risk individuals every 3 years (Table 242-2). Mild glucose elevations may have adverse effects on the fetus, so a more aggressive approach aimed at detection of subtle diabetes is recommended for pregnant women who are older than 25 years, are obese, have a family history of diabetes, or are a member of an ethnic group with a high prevalence of diabetes. Such pregnant women should receive a screening 50-g OGTT between 24 and 28 weeks of gestation. If the fasting glu-

Table 242–2 ■ CANDIDATES FOR DIABETES SCREENING

1. Presence of suggestive symptoms
2. Obesity (especially if centrally distributed)
3. Positive family history
4. Women with a morbid obstetric history or with large babies (>9 lb)
5. Recurrent skin or genital infections
6. High-risk populations (blacks, Latinos, Native Americans, Asians)
7. Age older than 45 yr
8. Presence of other risk factors for atherosclerosis (hypertension, dyslipidemia)

cose is 105 mg/dL or the 1-hour OGTT value is greater than 140 mg/dL, an extended 100-g OGTT should be performed. Gestational diabetes is diagnosed if two values equal or exceed the upper limits of normal: fasting, 105 mg/dL; 1 hour, 190 mg/dL; 2 hour, 165 mg/dL; and 3 hour, 145 mg/dL.

PREVALENCE/EPIDEMIOLOGY

TYPE 1 DIABETES. Prevalence rates for type 1 diabetes are relatively accurate because patients invariably become symptomatic. Estimates for the United States are about 0.3 to 0.4%. Type 1 diabetes is more prevalent in Finland, Scandinavia, Scotland, and Sardinia, less prevalent in Southern Europe and the Middle East, and uncommon in Asian countries such as Japan. The annual incidence appears to have risen in the last half century, which implies the introduction of an unidentified environmental factor. Prevalence rates are strikingly different among different ethnic groups living in the same geographic environment, observations most likely explained by genetic differences in susceptibility.

The recognition that type 1 diabetes has a protracted pre-clinical phase has placed some epidemiologic characteristics of the disease in a new light. Its increased incidence in the winter months and its association with specific viral epidemics may in part be explained by the superimposition of illness-provoked insulin resistance in a patient with marginal beta cell function. Similarly, its common appearance during puberty may also be attributed to the appearance of insulin resistance; normal puberty is accompanied by impaired insulin-stimulated glucose metabolism. New methods for tracking islet-directed autoimmunity have led to a reappraisal of the age at which type 1 diabetes first appears. Although the age-specific incidence rises progressively from infancy to puberty and then declines, incidence rates appear to continue at a low level for many decades. The disease develops in approximately 30% of patients after the age of 20 years. In these patients the clinical syndrome evolves more slowly, islet-directed antibody titers may be lower, and HLA types may be different from those of their younger counterparts. As a result, type 2 diabetes mellitus is initially misdiagnosed in many of these patients.

TYPE 2 DIABETES. Systematic screening for asymptomatic diabetes is restricted to relatively small groups, which makes estimates of prevalence rates imprecise. The U.S. rate is at least 6%, with a prevalence increasing to 10 to 15% in persons older than 50 years. Often the disease is not diagnosed; it is estimated that there may be one undiagnosed case for every two diagnosed cases. Type 2 diabetes is more common and occurs at an earlier age in Native Americans, Mexican descendants, and blacks. In these minority populations the appearance of type 2 diabetes may occur as early as adolescence. Type 2 prevalence rates also vary worldwide, with a propensity for Asiatic Indians, Polynesians/Micronesians, and Australian Aborigines when they migrate to westernized surroundings. Similarly, type 2 diabetes has markedly increased in people of Asian descent who have emigrated to the United States. These changes have been attributed to an inability to metabolically adapt to the behavioral patterns of westernization, i.e., reduced activity and higher caloric intake.

Although little is known about the specific genetic abnormalities associated with most forms of type 2 diabetes, personal factors promoting disease expression are well established. Increasing age, reduced physical activity, and especially obesity promote disease expression in individuals with a genetic susceptibility to the disease. Type 2 diabetes is much more common in obese individuals with one or two diabetic parents. Also, the severity and duration of obesity enhance the risk of development of diabetes. Individuals

with higher waist-hip ratios (i.e., central or upper body obesity) are much more prone to diabetes in subsequent years.

IMPAIRED FASTING GLUCOSE AND IMPAIRED GLUCOSE TOLERANCE. Precise statistical data regarding the prevalence of these new diagnostic categories are lacking. However, it is estimated that these patients represent 6 to 8% of the U.S. population.

PATHOPHYSIOLOGY

INSULIN SECRETION AND ACTION. Insulin is initially synthesized in the pancreatic beta cells as a large single-chain polypeptide, proinsulin, and subsequent cleavage of proinsulin results in the removal of a connecting strand (C peptide) and appearance of the smaller, double-chain insulin molecule (51 amino acid residues). Insulin and the C-peptide remnant are packaged in membrane-bounded storage granules; stimulation of insulin secretion results in the discharge of equimolar amounts of insulin and C peptide and a small amount of unconverted proinsulin into the portal circulation. Because C peptide escapes hepatic metabolism, unlike insulin, its concentration provides a more precise marker of endogenous insulin secretion. The concentration of glucose is the key regulator of insulin secretion. For glucose to activate secretion, it must first be transported by a protein (GLUT 2) into the beta cell, phosphorylated by the enzyme glucokinase, and metabolized. The immediate triggering process is poorly understood but probably involves the activation of signal transduction pathways, closure of adenosine triphosphate (ATP)-sensitive potassium channels, and entry of calcium into the beta cell. Normally, when blood glucose rises even slightly above the fasting level of 75 to 100 mg/dL, beta cells secrete insulin, initially from pre-formed stored insulin and later from the synthesis of new insulin. The route of glucose entry as well as its concentration determines the magnitude of the response. Higher insulin levels are produced when glucose is given orally than when given intravenously because of the simultaneous release of gut peptides (e.g., glucagon-like peptide I, gastric inhibitory polypeptide). Other insulin secretagogues include amino acids and vagal stimulation. Once secreted into portal blood, insulin encounters the liver as its first target organ. The liver effectively removes approximately 50% of the insulin and degrades it. The consequence of this uptake is that portal vein insulin is always at least two- to four-fold higher than that in the peripheral circulation. Conversely, when blood glucose levels decline even slightly (e.g., to 70 mg/dL), insulin secretion promptly diminishes.

Insulin acts on responsive tissues by first passing through the vascular compartment and, on reaching its target, binding to its specific receptor. The insulin receptor is a heterodimer with two α- and β-chains formed by disulfide bridges. The α-subunit resides on the extracellular surface and is the site of insulin binding. The β-subunit spans the membrane and can be phosphorylated on serine, threonine, and tyrosine residues on the cytoplasmic face. The intrinsic protein tyrosine kinase activity of the β-subunit is essential for insulin receptor function. Rapid receptor autophosphorylation and tyrosine phosphorylation of cellular substrates (e.g., insulin receptor substrates 1 and 2) are important early steps in insulin action. Thereafter, a series of phosphorylation and dephosphorylation reactions are triggered that ultimately produce insulin's effects in insulin-sensitive tissues (liver, muscle, and fat). A variety of post-receptor signal transduction pathways are activated by insulin, including PI3 (phosphatidylinositol 3') kinase, an enzyme that appears to be critical for the translocation of glucose transporters (GLUT 4) to the cell surface and, in turn, glucose uptake.

A number of other hormones termed counterregulatory hormones (glucagon, growth hormone, catecholamines, and cortisol) oppose the metabolic actions of insulin. Among these, glucagon and to a lesser extent growth hormone have important roles in development of the diabetic syndrome. Glucagon is secreted by pancreatic alpha cells in response to hypoglycemia, amino acids, and activation of the autonomic nervous system. Its major effect is on the liver, where it stimulates glycogenolysis, gluconeogenesis, and ketogenesis via cyclic adenosine monophosphate–dependent mechanisms. It is normally inhibited by hyperglycemia but is absolutely or relatively increased in both type 1 and type 2 diabetes despite the presence of hyperglycemia. Growth hormone secretion by the anterior pituitary is also inappropriately increased in type 1 diabetes as a result, at least in part, of an attempt to overcome a defect in insulin-like growth factor type 1 generation caused by insulin deficiency. The major metabolic actions of growth hormone are on peripheral tissues, where it acts to promote lipolysis and inhibit glucose consumption. In type 1 diabetic patients with reduced portal vein insulin levels, growth hormone is also capable of stimulating hepatic glucose production.

METABOLIC EFFECTS OF INSULIN. Insulin's pivotal role in diabetes is best appreciated by first examining the extent to which it participates in fuel homeostasis in healthy subjects.

FASTED STATE. After an overnight fast, low basal levels of insulin diminish glucose uptake in peripheral insulin-sensitive tissues (muscle and fat). Most glucose uptake occurs in non–insulin-sensitive tissues, primarily the brain, which because of its inability to use free fatty acids is critically dependent on glucose for oxidative metabolism. Maintenance of stable blood glucose levels is achieved by release of glucose by the liver and to a small extent by the kidney at rates (7 to 10 g/hour) matching those of consuming tissues. The hepatic processes involved consist of glycogenolysis and gluconeogenesis, with gluconeogenesis contributing about half and glycogenolysis contributing the remainder. Both play a significant role, and both depend on the balance of insulin and glucagon in the portal circulation. Reduced insulin levels decrease glycogen synthesis, which allows glucagon's effect on glycogenolysis to prevail. Glucagon also stimulates gluconeogenesis, whereas the lowered insulin promotes peripheral mobilization of glucose precursors (amino acids, lactate, pyruvate, glycerol) and fuels (free fatty acids) for gluconeogenesis.

FED STATE. Ingestion of a large glucose load triggers multiple homeostatic mechanisms that minimize glucose excursions and restore normoglycemia. These mechanisms include (1) suppression of endogenous glucose production, (2) stimulation of hepatic glucose uptake, and (3) acceleration of glucose uptake by peripheral tissues, predominantly muscle. Each depends on insulin. In the liver, a meal-stimulated increase in insulin rapidly suppresses glucose production directly and indirectly via suppression of lipolysis and limits glucose entry into the circulation at a time when it is flooded by exogenous glucose. In addition, about 30% of the ingested glucose is deposited in the liver as a result of the combined effects of hyperglycemia and hyperinsulinemia in the portal circulation. Consequently, a substantial amount of glucose is retained in the liver as glycogen. The uptake of glucose by peripheral tissues is mediated predominantly by insulin. Insulin-stimulated glucose transport across the plasmalemma of both adipose and muscle tissue is attributable to the recruitment of glucose-transporting proteins (i.e., GLUT 4) from a cytosolic compartment to the plasma membrane. In muscle, glucose may be used for glycogen synthesis or undergo oxidative or non-oxidative metabolism. In adipose tissue, glucose is used for the formation of α-glycerophosphate, which is necessary for the esterification of free fatty acids to form triglycerides. Intracellular metabolic processes are also facilitated by the action of insulin. Insulin promotes glycogen formation by stimulating glycogen synthase and glucose oxidation by activating pyruvate dehydrogenase and decreasing lipolysis (free fatty acids compete with glucose for oxidative metabolism).

Ingestion of large quantities of glucose is not representative of conditions during the ingestion of ordinary meals. If the quantity of carbohydrate consumed and the resultant insulin response are small, glucose homeostasis is maintained largely by a reduction in hepatic glucose production rather than by an increase in glucose uptake because glucose production is much more sensitive than glucose uptake to the effects of small changes in insulin secretion. The rise in insulin that accompanies the consumption of mixed meals also facilitates protein and fat storage. Because muscle is in negative nitrogen balance in the fasting state, repletion of muscle nitrogen depends on a net uptake of amino acids in response to protein feeding. In muscle, insulin acts to promote positive nitrogen balance by inhibiting the breakdown of protein and to a lesser extent by stimulating the synthesis of new protein. Similarly, in adipose tissue the action of insulin accelerates triglyceride incorporation by stimulating lipoprotein lipase while simultaneously reducing the hormone-sensitive lipase that catalyzes the hydrolysis of stored triglycerides.

METABOLIC DEFECTS IN DIABETES. In type 2 diabetes, fasting hyperglycemia is accompanied by an inappropriate increase in hepatic glucose production that is generally proportionate to the blood glucose elevation. In type 1 diabetes, portal insulin deficiency is invariably present and thus hepatic glucose production is consistently elevated. In addition, insulin deficiency leads to hypersecretion of glucagon and growth hormone, which further accentuate glucose overproduction. Because basal glucose uptake occurs largely in non–insulin-sensitive tissues, total-body glucose uptake tends to be increased because of the mass action of hyperglycemia. This tendency underscores the crucial role that the liver plays in determining the fasting glucose level in diabetes. The increase in glucose production in both types of diabetes is due to an acceleration of gluconeogenesis. Loss of the restraining effect of insulin on the alpha cell leads to a relative increase in portal glucagon and, in turn, an increase in the uptake and conversion of glycogenic substrates to glucose within the liver. In the extreme situation of total insulin lack, excessive release of a variety of counterregulatory hormones causes gluconeogenesis to increase further and blocks compensatory increases in glucose disposal. The clinical correlate is profound hyperglycemia (Fig. 242–2). Fasting levels of free fatty acids are also frequently elevated because of accelerated mobilization of fat stores. In type 2 diabetes, elevations in free fatty acids occur in the presence of normal or increased insulin, which suggests resistance to insulin's inhibitory effect on lipolysis. Although free fatty acids are not directly converted to glucose, they promote hyperglycemia by providing the liver with energy to support gluconeogenesis and by interfering with glucose uptake by reducing glucose transport and utilization in muscle. Endogenous insulin secretion in type 2 diabetes provides sufficient levels of insulin in portal blood to suppress the conversion of free fatty acids to ketones in the liver. In type 1 diabetes, however, mobilized free fatty acids are more readily converted to ketone bodies. The combined effects of insulin deficiency and the presence of glucagon suppress fat synthesis in the liver. This suppression of fat synthesis reduces intrahepatic malonyl coenzyme A, which together with carnitine stimulates the activity of hepatic acylcarnitine transferase I and thereby facilitates the transfer of long-chain fatty acids into mitochondria, where they are broken down via β-oxidation and converted to ketone bodies. In addition, hypoinsulinemia, by decreasing ketone turnover, enhances the magnitude of the ketosis for any given level of ketone production. During diabetic ketoacidosis, ketone levels are further increased because of the concomitant release of counterregulatory hormones. The rise in glucagon accelerates

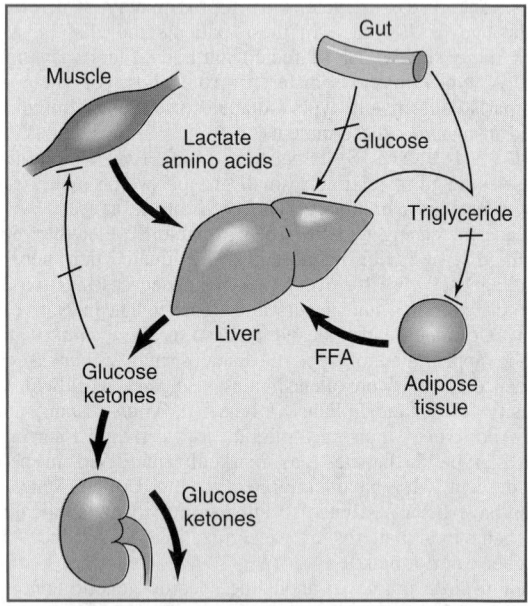

FIGURE 242–2 ■ The effects of severe insulin deficiency on body fuel metabolism. Lack of insulin leads to mobilization of substrates for gluconeogenesis and ketogenesis from muscle and adipose tissue, accelerated production of glucose and ketones by the liver, and impaired removal of endogenously produced and exogenous fuels by insulin-responsive tissues. The net result is severe hyperglycemia and hyperketonemia that overwhelm renal removal mechanisms.

hepatic ketogenesis, whereas elevations of catecholamines, growth hormone, and cortisol act in concert to increase lipolysis and, in turn, the delivery of free fatty acids to the liver (see Fig. 242–2). The increase in substrate delivery may become so pronounced that it saturates the oxidative pathway and leads to a fatty liver and severe hypertriglyceridemia.

Diabetes is characterized by marked postprandial hyperglycemia after carbohydrate ingestion. In type 2 diabetes, the combined effects of delayed insulin secretion and hepatic insulin resistance impair the suppression of hepatic glucose production and the ability of the liver to store glucose as glycogen. Hyperglycemia ensues, even though insulin levels may eventually rise to levels above those seen in non-diabetic individuals (insulin secretion remains deficient relative to the prevailing glucose level), because insulin resistance reduces the capacity of muscle to remove the excess glucose released from the liver and store it in the myocyte as glycogen. The normal increase in glucose-6-phosphate in muscle after insulin is markedly attenuated in diabetes, which implies that the block in glycogen synthesis precedes glucose-6-phosphate formation and is mediated at the level of either glucose transport or its conversion to glucose-6-phosphate (by hexokinase). These defects are more pronounced in patients with severe hyperglycemia, in whom insulin secretion is further reduced. Type 1 patients show the most marked and prolonged elevations in blood glucose after ingestion of carbohydrate. These individuals have low portal vein insulin levels, which are not reversed by conventional subcutaneous insulin therapy. Consequently, the liver fails to reduce its glucose production or to appropriately take up glucose and store it as glycogen. In addition, glucose uptake by peripheral tissues is impaired by the lack of insulin and the development of insulin resistance secondary to chronic insulin deprivation and the toxic effects of chronic hyperglycemia. The net result is a gross defect in glucose disposal that is only partially compensated by renal glycosuria. An insulin-deficient patient may exhibit defects in the disposal of ingested protein and fat as well. In the absence of a rise in insulin, meal ingestion may cause hyperaminoacidemia because of failure to stimulate the net uptake of amino acids in muscle and can cause hypertriglyceridemia because of reduced activity of lipoprotein lipase. Thus type 1 diabetes may be viewed as a disorder of protein and fat tolerance, as well as glucose tolerance.

PATHOGENESIS

Type 1 diabetes produces profound beta cell failure with secondary insulin resistance, whereas type 2 diabetes causes less severe insulin deficiency and a more severe impairment in insulin action. Given the similarity in the overall picture, it is not surprising that both forms of diabetes share many pathophysiologic features. However, despite the apparent phenotypic similarity, the underlying pathogenetic mechanisms leading to type 1 and type 2 diabetes are strikingly different.

TYPE 1 DIABETES. Type 1 diabetes results from an interplay of genetic, environmental, and autoimmune factors that selectively destroy insulin-producing beta cells (see Fig. 242–1).

GENETIC FACTORS. The role of genetic factors is underscored by data in identical twins showing concordance rates of 30 to 50%, rates much higher than those for non-identical twins or siblings. It has been assumed that because concordance rates are not 100%, environmental factors must be important for disease expression. Even identical twins, however, do not have identical T-cell receptor or immunoglobulin genes, and thus for autoimmune diseases such as type 1 diabetes, total concordance would not be expected. Although all the genes linked to the disease have not been identified, one is located within the insulin promoter region on chromosome 11 and another involves the HLA region on the short arm of chromosome 6. The HLA genes undoubtedly play the dominant role. In non-affected siblings, the risk of diabetes developing is 15 to 20% if they are HLA identical, about 5% if they share one HLA gene, and less than 1% if they are HLA non-identical. Specific HLA haplotypes are linked to type 1 diabetes: 90 to 95% express DR3 and/or DR4 class II HLA molecules, as compared with an incidence of 50 to 60% in the general population, and 60% of patients express both alleles, a rate more than 10-fold that of the general population. Another class II allele, HLA-DR2, has a negative association with disease. Specific class II DQ haplotypes (e.g.,

DQ8 and DQ2) even more strongly correlate with disease susceptibility in white individuals. Susceptibility is associated with polymorphisms of the allele encoding the β-chain of the DQ class II HLA molecule. The presence of aspartic acid at position 57 protects against disease, whereas substitution of a neutral amino acid at this position is associated with a much higher frequency of disease. Other polymorphisms, such as substitution of arginine at position 52 of the DQ α-chain, may confer additional risk. It is likely, however, that no single class II HLA gene accounts for HLA-associated susceptibility to disease and that significant genetic heterogeneity exists. Association of the disease with specific class II HLA genes implies the involvement of CD4+ T cells in the autoimmunity process because these molecules are critical for the presentation of antigenic peptides to CD4+ T cells and for selection of the CD4+ T-cell repertoire in the thymus. It has been suggested that the diabetes susceptibility gene in the insulin promoter region influences insulin gene expression in the thymus and therefore the thymic selection of insulin-reactive T cells.

ENVIRONMENTAL FACTORS. Although environmental factors such as diet and toxins have been proposed as initiating factors, most attention has focused on viruses. Epidemics of mumps, coxsackievirus, and congenital rubella have been associated with an increased frequency of type 1 diabetes. In one instance, coxsackievirus B4 was isolated from the pancreas of a child who died of diabetic ketoacidosis, and inoculation of the virus into mice caused disease, thereby fulfilling Koch's postulates. Viruses that produce acute, lytic infection, however, are probably responsible for only an occasional case. Instead, if viruses are involved, it is more likely that they trigger an autoimmune response. It has been postulated that if a virus contains an epitope that resembles a beta cell protein, infection with the virus could abrogate self-tolerance and trigger autoimmunity. Interestingly, sequence homology has been identified between a coxsackievirus B protein and the beta cell enzyme glutamic acid decarboxylase, which is an important autoantigen in type 1 diabetes.

AUTOIMMUNE FACTORS. About 80% of patients with new-onset type 1 diabetes have islet cell antibodies. A variety of antibodies with specificity against beta cell constituents have been identified, including insulin, isoforms of glutamic acid decarboxylase (GAD 65 and GAD 67), and the secretory granule protein ICA 512, which has a tyrosine phosphatase–like domain. The idea that type 1 diabetes is a chronic autoimmune disease with an acute manifestation has come from evidence that islet antigen-directed antibodies are present in approximately 3% of asymptomatic first-degree relatives of patients, and these individuals have a high risk of development of type 1 diabetes, often many years later. The likelihood of type 1 diabetes is greater than 50% if autoantibodies are present to more than one beta cell antigen (i.e., insulin, GAD 65, and ICA 512). Type 1 diabetes very rarely develops in islet antigen-directed antibody–negative relatives. These antibodies, however, appear to be markers for rather than the cause of beta cell injury. Beta cell destruction (by apoptotic and cytotoxic mechanisms) is probably mediated by a variety of cytokines released by T cells and macrophages or by the direct actions of T cells. In keeping with this view, type 1 diabetes has been transferred by bone marrow cells from a diabetic patient to a non-diabetic recipient, and patients dying soon after disease onset have monocytic cellular infiltrates restricted to islets (termed insulitis) that are composed of CD8+ and CD4+ T cells, macrophages, and B cells. However, as the disease progresses, the islets become completely devoid of beta cells and inflammatory infiltrates, with alpha, delta, and pancreatic polypeptide cells left intact, thus illustrating the exquisite specificity of the autoimmune attack. At the time of clinical diagnosis, about 5 to 10% of the beta cell mass remains (see Fig. 242–1).

A critical role for T cells is supported by studies involving pancreatic transplantation in identical twins. Monozygotic twins with diabetes who received kidney and pancreas grafts from their non-diabetic, genetically identical sibling required little or no immunosuppression for graft acceptance. Nevertheless, the islets were soon selectively invaded with mononuclear cells, predominantly CD8+ T cells, with the subsequent recurrence of diabetes. Thus decades after the original onset of disease, the immune system still had the ability to selectively destroy beta cells. Evidence implicating T cells also derives from clinical trials using immunosuppressive drugs. Drugs such as cyclosporine slow or prevent the progression of recent-onset diabetes, but immunosuppression must be administrated continuously to maintain the effect. Supporting data for a primary role for T cells derives from animal models in which diabetes spontaneously develops. Insulitis and islet autoantibodies develop at about 4 weeks of age in NOD mice, and diabetes ultimately develops after 12 to 24 weeks. A variety of treatments designed to deplete T cells prevent diabetes. Most importantly, adoptive transfer of T cells isolated from acutely diabetic mice donors into immune-incompetent NOD mice rapidly produces diabetes. Both CD4+ and CD8+ T cells are generally required for transfer of disease, which suggests that both are necessary for disease expression. The specific antigens recognized by these diabetogenic T cells remain uncertain. A potential role for glutamic acid decarboxylase and/or insulin is suggested by data showing that if NOD mice are made tolerant to glutamic acid decarboxylase or insulin (or peptides derived from these molecules) early in life, insulitis and diabetes fail to develop. The chronic smoldering nature of the disease suggests the presence of regulatory or protective influences. In keeping with this observation, T cells that protect the islet from immune attack have been isolated from the islets of NOD mice. Such findings suggest that the rate of appearance and clinical expression of disease may be modulated by the balance between diabetogenic and protective populations of T cells.

TYPE 2 DIABETES. Hyperglycemia in type 2 diabetes results from undefined genetic defect(s) (concordance rates in identical twins are nearly 100%), the expression of which is modified by environmental factors. Inasmuch as hyperglycemia itself impairs insulin secretion and action, a phenomenon termed "glucose toxicity" (Fig. 242–3), by the time that full-blown hyperglycemia has become manifested, nearly all patients exhibit both insulin resistance and defective insulin secretion. The sequence makes it difficult to determine which one started the vicious cycle leading to the disease.

INSULIN SECRETION. Fasting insulin levels in type 2 diabetes are generally normal or increased. Yet they are relatively low if one takes into account the coexisting presence of hyperglycemia. As hyperglycemia becomes more severe, basal insulin fails to increase or declines further. The insulin secretory defect usually correlates with the severity of fasting hyperglycemia and is more evident following carbohydrate ingestion. In its mildest form, the beta cell defect is subtle and involves loss of the acute (or 1st phase) insulin response to glucose and the normal regular oscillatory pattern of insulin secretion. Although the overall insulin response appears intact, when viewed in the context of simultaneous insulin resistance, a "normal" response is actually inadequate to maintain glucose tolerance. In these subjects the beta cell defect is specific for glucose, i.e., it is spared from affecting other secretagogues (e.g., amino acids). Insulin deficiency is thus less pronounced during the ingestion of mixed meals. Patients with more severe fasting hyperglycemia (>200 mg/dL) lose the capacity to respond to increases in circulating glucose. These observations suggest that a specific abnormality in recognition of glucose by the beta cell occurs in the earliest stages of type 2 diabetes and that this defect worsens as the disease progresses. Unfortunately the cause of beta cell failure is unknown.

Studies in rodents suggest that the loss of glucose-stimulated insulin secretion is followed by decreased expression of GLUT 2, the beta cell glucose transporter. Loss of GLUT 2 during transition to the diabetic state could accelerate further loss in glucose-stimulated insulin secretion. Pathology studies of patients with long-standing type 2 diabetes have demonstrated amyloid-like deposits within islets composed of islet amyloid polypeptide, or "amylin," a peptide synthesized in the beta cell and cosecreted with insulin. Chronic hypersecretion of islet amyloid polypeptide accompanying hyperinsulinemia may lead to precipitation of the peptide, which over time might contribute to impaired beta cell function. Recent experiments in gene knockout mice suggest a potential role for impaired insulin receptor signaling within the pancreatic beta cell in the development of impaired beta cell function. A link between insulin resistance and secretion is also suggested by data showing that accumulation of fat within the beta cell as a result of insulin resistance and increased fatty acid turnover over time reduces insulin secretion.

The mechanism for beta cell dysfunction has, however, been defined in a subgroup of patients with a related, but distinct disorder, MODY type 2. These patients share a mutation in the gene encoding glucokinase, the key enzyme responsible for the phosphorylation of glucose within the beta cell and liver. A variety of glucokinase mutations have been identified in different families, each capable of interfering with transduction of the glucose signal to the beta cell. Other MODY families have no detectable glucokinase gene mutations but instead carry mutations of two different genes encoding HNF-1α (MODY type 3), HNF-1β (MODY type 4), and HNF-4α (MODY type 1). Thus MODY appears to be a heterogeneous disorder much like the more common type 2 diabetes, which is not characterized by glucokinase or HNF gene mutations.

INSULIN RESISTANCE. With few exceptions (e.g., some black patients), type 2 diabetes is characterized by marked impairment in insulin action. The insulin dose-response curve for augmenting glucose uptake in peripheral tissues is shifted to the right (decreased sensitivity), and the maximal response is reduced, particularly with more severe hyperglycemia. Other insulin-stimulated processes such as inhibition of hepatic glucose production and lipolysis also show reduced sensitivity to insulin. The mechanisms responsible for insulin resistance remain poorly understood. Early studies focused on defects in insulin binding to its receptor. Mutations in insulin receptors result in the syndrome called leprechaunism, characterized by severe growth retardation and insulin resistance. Two other rare syndromes of extreme insulin resistance have been identified and are characterized by either a profound deficiency of insulin receptors (most often affecting young females with acanthosis nigricans, polycystic ovaries, and hirsutism) or the presence of anti–insulin receptor antibodies (associated with acanthosis nigricans and other autoimmune phenomena).

Although insulin receptors may be reduced in some type 2 diabetic patients, defects in more distal or "post-receptor" events play the predominant role in insulin resistance. An important component of this defect is reduced capacity for translocation of GLUT 4 to the cell surface in muscle cells. A separate defect in glycogen synthesis is also likely to be present. Whether the defects uncovered are primary or secondary to the disturbance in glucose metabolism is uncertain. Possibly, a variety of genetic abnormalities in cellular transduction of the insulin signal may individually or in concert produce an identical clinical phenotype. No evidence has shown that the mechanisms of insulin resistance in non-obese patients differ from those of their obese diabetic counterparts, but the coexistence of obesity accentuates the severity of the resistant state. In particular, upper body or abdominal as compared with lower body or peripheral obesity is associated with insulin resistance and diabetes. It is now believed that intra-abdominal visceral fat (detected by computed tomography or magnetic resonance imaging) may be a key culprit. Abdominal fat cells have a higher lipolytic rate and are more resistant to insulin than is fat derived from peripheral deposits. Cortisol hypersecretion and/or hereditary factors influence the distribution of body fat, the latter contributing an additional genetic influence on expression of the disease.

The adverse effects of increased free fatty acid levels include accelerated hepatic gluconeogenesis and impaired muscle glucose metabolism and beta cell function ("lipotoxicity"). The release of tumor necrosis factor α by adipocytes may also interfere with insulin-stimulated glucose uptake by altering the pattern of phosphorylation of insulin-signaling molecules.

GLUCOTOXICITY. Hyperglycemia per se impairs the beta cell response to glucose and promotes insulin resistance (see Fig. 242–3). The exact mechanism remains uncertain; however, glucosamine—a product of glucose metabolism via the hexosamine pathway—has

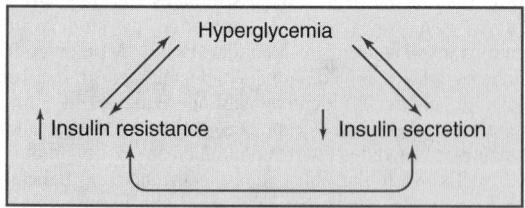

FIGURE 242–3 ■ Elevations of circulating glucose initiate a vicious cycle in which hyperglycemia begets more severe hyperglycemia.

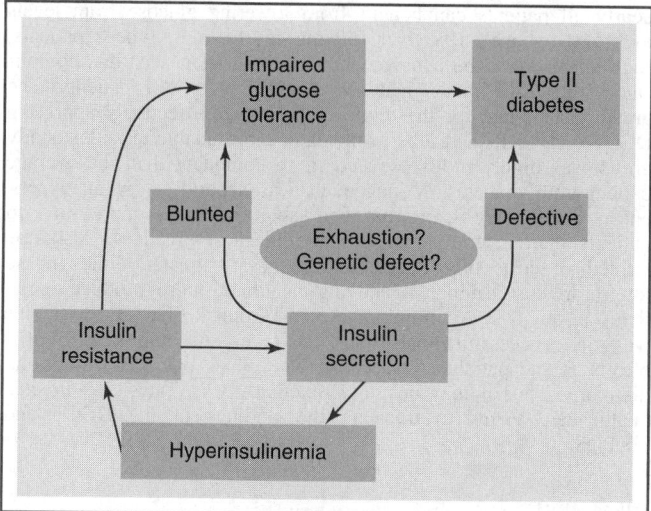

FIGURE 242–4 ■ A proposed sequence of events leading to the development of type 2 diabetes: insulin resistance resulting from genetic influences, central obesity, inactivity, or a combination of these factors leads over time to a progressive loss of the beta cell's capacity to compensate for this defect.

been implicated as a culprit. Glucosamine induces insulin resistance in animals by impairing insulin-induced GLUT 4 translocation to the cell membrane in isolated adipocytes and in skeletal muscles in vivo. Activation of protein kinase C may also be a contributing factor. Regardless of its molecular mechanism, reversal of glucotoxicity can disrupt the vicious cycle that perpetuates hyperglycemia, thereby facilitating therapeutic outcomes.

WHAT IS THE PRIMARY DEFECT? It remains uncertain whether insulin resistance or defective insulin secretion is the primary event leading to type 2 diabetes. Because it is difficult to resolve this issue once overt diabetes has developed, attention has focused on high-risk non-diabetic subjects. Studies in populations with high prevalence rates, such as Pima Indians and Mexican Americans, have found that insulin resistance is the initial predisposing defect. Similar results have been reported in non-diabetic 1st-degree relatives of type 2 diabetic patients and in healthy pre-diabetic offspring of two diabetic parents. Interestingly, hyperinsulinemia has been detected in pre-diabetic subjects one to two decades before the onset of diabetes, thus suggesting that development of the diabetic syndrome is exceedingly slow. Although these studies support the view that insulin resistance generally antedates insulin deficiency, its presence was insufficient to produce overt diabetes. The finding implies that for diabetes to become manifested, the additional factor of impaired insulin secretion is required (Fig. 242–4). It is unclear whether the appearance of a secretory defect is a secondary phenomenon (e.g., "beta cell exhaustion," increased fatty acid delivery, or islet amyloid polypeptide hypersecretion) or the result of a second independent defect that becomes evident only upon chronic beta cell stimulation (e.g., a subtle genetic defect in beta cell signal transduction). This sequence of events, although common, does not occur in all patients. The demonstration of functional glucokinase gene mutations in some patients with MODY clearly indicates that primary beta cell defects are capable of producing a similar phenotype. Furthermore, some blacks with type 2 diabetes exhibit little or no insulin resistance, and diminished glucose-stimulated insulin secretion has been reported to be a feature of the subgroup of women with gestational diabetes in whom type 2 diabetes later developed. Thus it is unlikely that a single pathogenetic mechanism is responsible for type 2 diabetes.

RELATIONSHIP BETWEEN DIABETES CONTROL AND ITS COMPLICATIONS

Whether the vascular and neuropathic complications of diabetes can be prevented or delayed by improved glycemic control was debated for more than a half century. To answer the question, the National Institutes of Health initiated the Diabetes Control and Complications Trial (DCCT), a 9-year multicenter study involving

1441 type 1 patients aged 13 to 39 years who were randomly assigned to either intensive insulin therapy or conventional care. Intensive care consisted of three or more insulin injections per day or an insulin pump, self-monitoring of blood glucose at least four times per day, and frequent contact with a diabetes health care team. Conventional care consisted of one or more, commonly two injections of insulin mixtures per day, less frequent monitoring, standard education, and less frequent visits. The target goals of therapy were markedly different. The intensive care group sought pre-meal blood levels of 70 to 120 mg/dL, postprandial blood levels of less than 180 mg/dL, and glycohemoglobin values as close to normal as possible. In the conventional care group the goal was clinical well-being. Patients were divided into two groups: (1) a primary prevention group with diabetes for 1 to 5 years and no detectable complications and (2) a secondary intervention group with diabetes for 1 to 15 years who had mild non-proliferative retinopathy. Remarkably, nearly 99% of the patients completed the trial.

The DCCT achieved a clear separation of glucose levels between the groups over the entire study period. Glycohemoglobin (Hb A_{1c}) and mean glucose levels in the intensive care group were 1.5 to 2.0% and 60 to 80 mg/dL lower than those receiving conventional care. Although considerable variability was noted among individual patients, most of the intensive care group failed to achieve normal glucose levels (glycohemoglobin averaged 1.1% above normal, or a glucose level of about 155 mg/dL). Nevertheless, intensive care reduced the development of retinopathy by 76% in the primary prevention group and the progression of retinopathy by 54% in the secondary intervention group (Fig. 242–5). The latter effect became apparent only after 4 years. In addition, intensive care reduced the

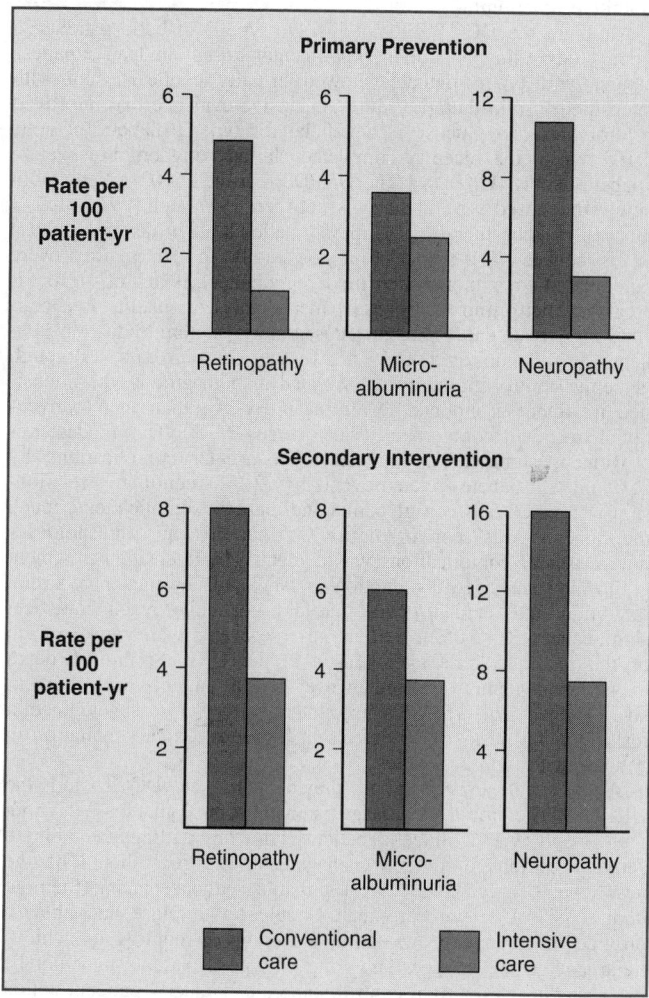

FIGURE 242–5 ■ A summary of the results of the Diabetes Control and Complications Trial (DCCT).

risk of microalbuminuria by 39%, frank proteinuria by 54%, and clinical neuropathy by 60% when compared with conventional care. The incidence of major cardiovascular events also tended to be lower, but the number of events was insufficient to provide statistical proof. At the least, intensive therapy did not pose a risk for macrovascular complications. The exponential relationship over time between the average blood glucose level as reflected by Hb A$_{1C}$ and the frequency with which retinopathy progressed in the intensive care group suggests that there may be no threshold level at which complications occur. The findings imply that any degree of improvement in glycemic control has benefit and that normalization is not required to slow the progression of complications.

The DCCT found that the benefits of intensive control were not without risk. The frequency of severe hypoglycemia requiring help from another person increased three-fold. Also, severe hypoglycemia often occurred without classic warning symptoms (often while the patient was asleep). These complications are in keeping with data showing suppression of adrenergic responses to hypoglycemia (1) in subjects treated with intensive insulin regimens that provoke iatrogenic hypoglycemia and (2) during stage 3 or 4 sleep. Weight gain was also more common. These changes indicate that in some patients the risks of intensive therapy may outweigh the benefits. Included are patients with recurrent severe hypoglycemia and hypoglycemic unawareness, patients in whom the dangers of hypoglycemia are greater because of other coexisting medical conditions or their occupation, patients with far-advanced complications, young children, the elderly, and patients who are unable or unwilling to participate in their management (e.g., self-monitoring of blood glucose). Such individuals are likely to benefit from less aggressive therapy designed to lower glucose levels without provoking hypoglycemia. It is noteworthy that despite a higher rate of hypoglycemia, intensive care did not have any detectable long-term effect on cognitive functioning.

Although the DCCT did not involve type 2 diabetic patients, a small study using a similar experimental design in lean Japanese patients with type 2 diabetes showed virtually identical results with intensified insulin therapy. More conclusive evidence that improved control of blood glucose is beneficial for type 2 diabetic patients derives from the recently completed United Kingdom Prospective Diabetes Study (UKPDS). The UKPDS recruited 5102 patients with newly diagnosed type 2 diabetes between 1977 and 1991. After 3 months of diet therapy, the 3,867 patients with fasting glucose levels between 6.1 and 15.0 mmol/L (110 to 270 mg/dL) were randomized to a more intensified regimen consisting of sulfonylurea and metformin (for obese patients only) or insulin or a conventional treatment regimen focused on symptom reduction. Patients were monitored for an average of 10 years. Although glycemic control gradually deteriorated in both groups, the intensified treatment group had lower mean Hb A$_{1c}$ than their conventional treatment counterparts (7.0% versus 7.9%). This modest improvement significantly reduced microvascular complications by 25% and all diabetes-related events by 12%. A continuous relationship was noted between glycemia and diabetic complications, much the same as was seen in the DCCT. No glycemic threshold for microvascular complications was evident. The intensified treatment group also had a 16% reduction in fatal and non-fatal myocardial infarction and sudden death that did not quite reach statistical significance ($P = .052$). Serious adverse events were rare for each of the pharmacologic agents used in the UKPDS; only 1 death from hypoglycemia occurred in over 27,000 patient-years of intensive therapy. This result is accounted for by more severe insulin resistance and less severe defects in hormonal counterregulation in patients with type 2 diabetes.

What conclusions can be drawn from the DCCT and the UKPDS? The primary message is that "control matters." In both type 1 and type 2 diabetic patients who are willing and able to actively participate in their management, the goal should be the best level of glycemic control possible without placing them at undue risk. A health care team should be in place and able to provide the resources, guidance, and support required to achieve treatment goals. A larger subgroup of type 2 patients may not be ideal candidates for tight control, particularly elderly patients with a shorter life expectancy, such those with coexisting severe cardiovascular disease. The DCCT and the UKPDS demonstrate that

nearly all patients can benefit from lowering glucose from levels over 200 to levels less than 150 mg/dL; for most type 2 patients, such changes can be achieved by diet, oral agents, or less complicated insulin regimens than are required in type 1 patients. The greatest challenge for the clinician is how to effectively apply the DCCT and UKPDS results in practice, a formidable task. The study group was highly motivated and more compliant than the average patient with diabetes. Management was supervised by an experienced health care team that was able to devote more time to patients than is commonly possible in most practices. Also, the immediate costs of intensive treatment are greater, although the long-term cost savings of having healthier, more productive patients is obvious. An important lesson from the DCCT experience was that successful treatment was largely accomplished by the efforts of the patients themselves, as well as nurse educators and dietitians. Thus it may be more practical to use physician-directed health care teams to translate the findings of the DCCT and UKPDS.

TREATMENT

Treatment of diabetes mellitus involves changes in lifestyle and pharmacologic intervention with insulin or oral glucose-lowering drugs. In type 1 diabetes, the primary focus is to replace insulin secretion; lifestyle changes are required to facilitate insulin therapy and optimize health. For most patients with type 2 diabetes, changes in lifestyle are the cornerstone of treatment, particularly in the early stages of the disease. Pharmacologic intervention is a secondary treatment strategy. Although therapeutic strategies for the two forms of diabetes differ, the short-term and long-term goals of treatment are identical (Table 242–3).

Type 1 Diabetes

INSULIN PREPARATIONS AND PHARMACOKINETICS. A variety of highly purified insulin preparations are commercially available that differ mainly in their time of onset and duration of action (Table 242–4). Pre-mixed preparations of insulin containing both intermediate- and rapid-acting insulin are available and may be a convenient form of therapy for some patients, particularly those with type 2 diabetes. Nearly all insulin preparations contain 100 U/mL (U-100), although a more concentrated regular insulin with a more prolonged action (500 U/mL or U-500) can be obtained for resistant patients. Pure insulin preparations result in fewer problems related to insulin antigenicity, such as insulin allergy, insulin resistance, and lipoatrophy. Human insulin is now the only form of insulin sold in North America and other industrialized countries. Human insulin is less antigenic than porcine and much less antigenic than bovine insulin. Because human insulin generates lower titers of insulin antibodies, it acts more rapidly after injection and the effects tend to persist for a shorter time. This combination allows for better synchrony between insulin peaks and meal absorption after injection of rapid-acting insulin with meals. The earlier peaks of intermediate-acting human insulin, however, fail to sustain its effects for a full 24-hour period, thereby necessitating twice-daily injections. It is noteworthy that the same insulin preparation may produce variable responses in a given patient because the peak and duration of action of most insulin preparations depend on (1) the route of administration, (2) the dose, and (3) the duration of the treatment with insulin.

RAPID-ACTING INSULIN PREPARATIONS. After subcutaneous injection, regular insulin begins to act in about 30 minutes and should therefore be given 20 to 30 minutes before a meal. Because it acts quickly, it is most effective in blunting elevations in glucose following meals and in allowing for rapid adjustments in insulin dosage based on measurements of blood glucose by the patient.

Table 242–3 ■ TREATMENT GOALS

Short term
Restore metabolic control to as close to normal as possible
Improve sense of well-being
Long term: Minimize risk of diabetic complications
Accelerated atherosclerosis
Microangiopathy (retinopathy, nephropathy)
Neuropathy

Table 242–4 ■ INSULIN PREPARATIONS: TIME COURSE OF ACTION AFTER SUBCUTANEOUS ADMINISTRATION

CLASS	PREPARATION	ONSET OF EFFECT	PEAK EFFECT (hr)	DURATION OF ACTION (hr)
Rapid acting	Regular	30 min	2–4	5–8
	Lispro	10–15 min	1–2	3–4
Intermediate acting	NPH or Lente	1–2 hr	6–10	16–24
Long acting	Ultralente	4–6 hr	8–20	24–28

This property is especially helpful in managing glucose elevations that occur during illness or with consumption of large meals.

Regular insulin preparations are predominantly in hexameric form and must dissociate into monomers, which accounts for the delay in its absorption from subcutaneous injection sites. Recently, lispro (an insulin analogue with reversed order of the amino acids in positions 28 [lysine] and 29 [proline] on the B chain) was developed by recombinant DNA technology, which can more easily dissociate into its monomeric form. Because it is absorbed more rapidly, lispro can be given just before eating, a feature that simplifies meal planning. Because its effects wane more rapidly, the risk of hypoglycemia if the next meal is delayed may be reduced. Rapid-acting insulins afford much greater flexibility and have therefore assumed a greater role in intensive treatment regimens.

INTERMEDIATE- AND LONG-ACTING INSULIN PREPARATIONS. Other insulin preparations are modified to delay their absorption from injection sites so that their action is prolonged. Either protamine is added, yielding intermediate-acting NPH insulin, or the size of the zinc-insulin crystal is enlarged by adjusting the preparation process. The latter yields Lente (intermediate-acting) and Ultralente (long-acting) insulin. The intermediate-acting insulins (NPH and Lente) have a similar time course of action. They offer the compromise of some degree of coverage for meals coinciding with their peak actions and provision of basal levels of insulin when given twice per day. Longer-acting insulins (Ultralente), because they have less evident "peaks," offer some advantages for basal insulin replacement but generally still require twice-daily dosing.

INSULIN REGIMENS. Insulin treatment of diabetes is complex; no universal and predictable algorithm can be uniformly applied to all patients. In general, treatment regimens may be divided into conventional insulin treatment and intensive insulin treatment (e.g., multiple subcutaneous injections and continuous subcutaneous insulin infusion).

CONVENTIONAL INSULIN THERAPY. During the first few years of type 1 diabetes some degree of beta cell function typically persists, which allows many patients to achieve glycemic control with less intensive effort. Because intermediate-acting insulins are not generally sustained over a 24-hour period and insulin requirements tend to increase early in the morning, most patients should start with two daily injections of a mixture of intermediate-acting and rapid-acting human insulin before breakfast and dinner. Although Lente insulin has a theoretic advantage over NPH insulin in that it does not contain a foreign protein (protamine), this difference appears to have negligible clinical significance. Some advantage is gained by using NPH if regular insulin is mixed with it because if NPH is mixed with Lente, the excess zinc may cause regular insulin to precipitate out of solution and delay its absorption. Initially, the doses of intermediate-acting insulin are adjusted to optimize pre-dinner and fasting glucose levels. Once this adjustment is accomplished, the doses of rapid-acting insulin are varied to optimize postprandial glucose peaks as well as pre-lunch and bedtime glucose values. Patients should inject in the same region but at different locations at the same time each day, i.e., in the abdomen in the morning to optimize insulin delivery and in the leg or buttock at night to slow absorption. Some patients may experience a brief "honeymoon" period during which beta cell function partially recovers and insulin doses need to be reduced. This improvement should not be used as a signal to reduce efforts aimed at glycemic control; optimized insulin therapy helps preserve residual beta cell function.

MULTIPLE SUBCUTANEOUS INJECTIONS. Several years after the onset of type 1 diabetes, residual insulin secretion typically ceases and twice-daily insulin injections no longer suffice despite control of diabetic symptoms. Optimal glycemic control requires that insu-

lin delivery be directed toward more closely simulating the normal pattern of insulin secretion, namely, continuous "basal" insulin secretion throughout the day and night and brief increases in insulin levels coinciding with the ingestion of meals. The major problem with regimens relying on twice-daily injections is that the glucose-lowering effect of pre-dinner intermediate-acting insulin is greatest at the time when requirements are lowest (i.e., 2:00 to 3:00 A.M.) whereas when requirements are increasing early in the morning (i.e., 5:00 to 8:00 A.M.), insulin levels decline. The result is a tendency to nocturnal hypoglycemia and/or fasting hyperglycemia.

Successful management begins with control of fasting glucose levels. Failure to do so commonly leads to perpetuation of hyperglycemia for the remainder of the day or attempts at corrective measures with supplemental insulin that miss the mark. The therapeutic obstacle imposed by fasting hyperglycemia is best appreciated in the context of its pathogenesis, namely, glucose overproduction. Once hepatic gluconeogenesis has been activated in the morning, it is not readily suppressed by subcutaneous injections of insulin, and hyperglycemia persists after breakfast. The key factors responsible for fasting hyperglycemia are inadequate overnight delivery of insulin and sleep-associated growth hormone release. The "dawn phenomenon" is most pronounced in patients with type 1 diabetes because of their inability to compensate by raising endogenous insulin secretion. The magnitude of the dawn phenomenon can be attenuated by designing insulin regimens to ensure that the effects of exogenous insulin do not peak in the middle of the night and become dissipated by morning. Several approaches can deal with the problem (Fig. 242–6). The simplest is to use three injections, i.e., mixtures of intermediate- and short-acting insulin before breakfast, short-acting insulin before dinner, and intermediate-acting insulin at bedtime. The primary disadvantage of this approach is that meal schedules must be fixed rather rigidly. Alternative multidose regimens include (1) Ultralente (twice daily) to replace basal insulin secretion and short-acting insulin before each meal or (2) short-acting insulin before each meal and intermediate-acting insulin at bedtime. Pen injectors containing cartridges filled with insulin make multidose insulin regimens more convenient.

CONTINUOUS SUBCUTANEOUS INSULIN INFUSION. An alternative that provides greater flexibility in insulin dosing while minimizing variation in absorption is continuous subcutaneous insulin infusion. In this method, rapid-acting insulin is administered around the clock via a battery-powered, externally worn, computer-controlled infusion pump (see Fig. 242–6). The pump delivers basal rates continuously and can be programmed to vary the flow rate automatically for set periods, such as reducing the flow rate at 1:00 to 4:00 A.M. and then increasing it to compensate for increased insulin requirements early in the morning (i.e., 5:00 to 8:00 A.M.). Boluses determined by self-monitoring of blood glucose are given before meals by manually activating the pump. Most pumps contain a syringe filled with insulin attached to an infusion set consisting of a catheter and a needle that is inserted subcutaneously, preferably in the abdomen, to optimize absorption. Unfortunately, the approach has problems that limit its use. The most obvious disadvantage is wearing the pump itself. Because continuous subcutaneous insulin infusion uses short-acting insulin, any interruption in flow (most commonly because of insulin precipitation within the catheter) leads to rapid deterioration in control. Local infections at the catheter site occasionally occur. Also, maintenance of the pump and appropriate infusion rates requires effort and sophistication.

The intensive treatment regimens described above are not for everyone. In patients appropriate for such care, however, intensive insulin therapy should be strongly encouraged to reduce the risk of late complications. An absolute indication for intensive therapy is pregnancy. To eliminate the excess neonatal morbidity and mortal-

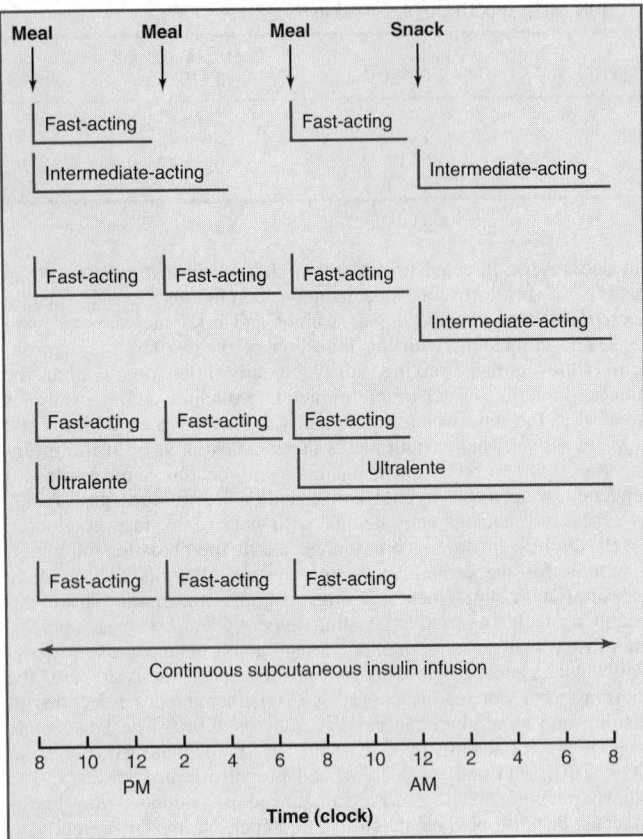

FIGURE 242–6 ■ Several intensive insulin regimens commonly used in the treatment of diabetes. Each is designed to provide a continuous supply of insulin around the clock and to make extra insulin available at the time of meals, thereby simulating more closely the normal physiologic pattern of insulin secretion.

ity that in the past were associated with diabetic pregnancy requires maintaining glycemic control. Ideally, intensive insulin therapy should be instituted before conception to minimize the higher risk of fetal anomalies. After conception, blood glucose targets are more stringently applied than at other times, with the aim of restoring glucose levels to those found in non-diabetic pregnant individuals.

LIFESTYLE CHANGES. Management of diet and exercise contribute importantly to the care of patients with type 1 diabetes (Table 242–5). The patient must be advised of the need for a careful balance between calorie intake and energy expenditure (exercise) while taking into account the availability of injected insulin.

DIET. The introduction of intensive insulin regimens has permit-

Table 242–5 ■ LIFESTYLE MODIFICATIONS FOR PATIENTS WITH DIABETES

I. Diet prescription
  1. Weight reduction, gain, or maintenance (as appropriate)
  2. Carbohydrates: 45–60% (depending on the severity of diabetes and triglyceride levels)
  3. Restriction of saturated fat (to <10% of calories)
  4. Increased monounsaturated fat (depending on the need to limit carbohydrate)
  5. Decreased cholesterol intake to <200 mg/d
  6. Sodium restriction in patients prone to hypertension
II. Exercise prescription*
  1. Aerobic strongly preferred. Avoid heavy lifting, straining, and Valsalva maneuvers that raise blood pressure
  2. Intensity: Increase pulse rate to at least 120–140, depending on the age and cardiovascular state of the patient
  3. Frequency: 3–4 d/week
  4. Duration: 20–30 min preceded and followed by stretching and flexibility exercises for 5–10 min

*Limitations are imposed by pre-existing coronary or peripheral vascular disease, proliferative retinopathy, peripheral or autonomic neuropathy, and poor glycemic control.

ted more flexibility in meal planning by allowing more latitude in varying the size, content, and timing of meals. This new approach offers the opportunity for a more normal lifestyle, thus minimizing compliance problems and optimizing patient acceptance. Meals should be nutritionally sound and provide sufficient calories to meet the energy needs of growing children, active young adults, or pregnancy. The 1800-kcal diet commonly used in type 2 patients is grossly insufficient in such active individuals. Furthermore, diets should be specifically aimed at minimizing long-term cardiovascular risk. Because type 1 patients depend on exogenous insulin, management is facilitated by using a meal plan designed to match the time course of the insulin dosage regimen selected. Patients should learn to compensate for departures from the meal plan by adjusting insulin doses or for periods of increased activity by consumption of extra food. Effort should be made to avoid long delays between meals; frequent small snacks may be needed at times of peak insulin action to avoid hypoglycemia. Most patients, regardless of their regimen, require a bedtime snack to reduce the risk of nocturnal hypoglycemia. The potential for weight gain requires special emphasis on portion control and appropriate (but not excessive) food intake for the treatment of hypoglycemia.

EXERCISE. Regular exercise is important to promote well-being and reduce vascular complications. Little evidence suggests, however, that exercise substantially improves glycemic control in type 1 diabetes, even though it reduces overall insulin requirements by enhancing insulin sensitivity. Exercise may rapidly reduce blood glucose levels, particularly when it coincides with the peak action of an insulin injection or if it accelerates insulin absorption from its injection site. Exercise also produces a marked increase in glucose uptake by muscle. Blood glucose levels nevertheless remain stable in normal subjects because there is a decrease in insulin levels that promotes increased hepatic glucose production to match the rate of glucose consumption. In a diabetic receiving insulin exogenously, this "finely tuned" homeostatic mechanism is disturbed. The continued presence of exogenous insulin further accelerates glucose uptake and, more importantly, blocks the compensatory increase in glucose production, so circulating glucose levels fall. Because the magnitude of the fall is not easily titrated, hypoglycemia may be a complication if the patient is unable to appropriately adjust diet and insulin.

Type 2 Diabetes

Non-pharmacologic Measures

In most type 2 diabetic patients, diet and exercise are the key or the only therapeutic intervention required to restore metabolic control (see Table 242–5), and therefore the temptation to use pharmacologic agents should be restrained at the outset unless hyperglycemia is severe. However, the clinician should also resist the temptation to stop at diet and exercise, if they are sufficient, only to eliminate symptoms.

DIET (see also Part XVI). For obese patients, modest weight reduction (e.g., 5 kg), irrespective of the starting weight, leads to a rapid decline in blood glucose levels. The dramatic impact of weight loss is mediated by changes in insulin-responsive tissues, as well as the beta cell: Insulin resistance diminishes, glucose production declines, and the resulting fall in glucose leads to improved glucose-stimulated insulin secretion. The effect of weight loss is not restricted to glucose; lipoprotein profiles and blood pressure also improve. In general, it matters little how weight loss is achieved provided that adequate nutrition is maintained. In sedentary diabetic patients, daily caloric requirements for weight maintenance are as low as 25 to 30 kcal/kg body weight per day. In such individuals, the classic 1800-kcal diet commonly prescribed is generally ineffective. It is sensible to begin with a nutritionally sound, individually tailored restrictive diet aimed at producing a caloric deficit of about 500 kcal/day. Because a caloric deficit of 3500 kcal is required to lose 1 lb of body fat, weight loss can be expected to be approximately 1 lb/week. For some very obese patients with a history of failed weight loss attempts, very low calorie diets (600 to 800 kcal/day) can be useful when done under medical supervision. Regardless of the method used, most patients are unable to maintain a diet for an extended period, and if they are successful, most regain the lost weight. Although reasons for the failure of most diet programs are unclear, confounding factors may make weight loss more difficult in type 2 diabetes. The normal decrease in basal metabolic rate during weight loss is accentuated in diabetic

Table 242-6 ■ CHARACTERISTICS OF ORAL GLUCOSE-LOWERING AGENTS

AGENT	TOTAL DAILY DOSE (mg/d)	DOSES PER DAY	METABOLISM AND EXCRETION*	DURATION OF ACTION (h)
Sulfonylureas				
First generation				
Chlorpropamide	100–750	1	K > L	60
Tolazamide	100–1000	1–2	L > K	12–14
Tolbutamide	500–3000	2–3	L > K	6–12
Sulfonylureas				
Second generation				
Glimepiride	1–8	1	L > K	24
Glyburide	1.25–20	1–2	L > K	Up to 24
Glyburide micronized	0.75–12	1–2	L > K	Up to 24
Glipizide	2.5–40	1–2	L > K	Up to 24
Glipizide GITS	5.0–20	1	L > K	24
Biguanide				
Metformin	500–2550	2–3	K	Up to 24
Thiazolidinedione				
Troglitazone	400–600	1	L	24
Pioglitazone	15–45‡	1	L	24
Rosiglitazone	4–8‡	1–2	L	Up to 24
α-Glucosidase inhibitors				
Acarbose	75–300	3†	gut/k**	N/A
Miglitol	75–300	3†	gut/k**	N/A
Benzoic acid derivatives				
Repaglinide	1–16	3†	L > K	short

*L = liver; K = kidney.
**The small fraction of the drug which is absorbed is eliminated via kidneys.
†To be taken with meals.
‡Pending FDA approval.

patients because the metabolic improvement produced by weight loss reverses the accelerated gluconeogenesis and futile cycling of substrates commonly seen in poorly controlled diabetes, both of which waste energy. Moreover, dieting reduces glycosuria and thus lessens urinary caloric loss. Success is best achieved by a combination of a supportive environment that emphasizes long-term goals (short-term weight changes mean little in the big picture), regular exercise to increase energy expenditure, and behavior modification.

Even when weight loss is not successful, the meal plan can remain a valuable tool to reduce the risk of cardiovascular disease in patients with diabetes. This benefit is best achieved by reducing saturated fat and in turn raising the content of carbohydrate or monounsaturated fat in the diet. Although it was originally thought that carbohydrate intake should be restricted, it is now appreciated that a diet higher in carbohydrate (50 to 60%) may improve insulin action and glycemic control, particularly in patients with mild hyperglycemia. In patients with more severe fasting hyperglycemia or with triglyceride elevations that may be aggravated by high-carbohydrate diets, reduced carbohydrate intake (45% of the total calories) and greater reliance on monounsaturated fats are preferable. It has been assumed that carbohydrate intake should be focused on complex carbohydrates (starches). Little evidence supports this assumption; simple sugars raise glucose levels to about the same extent as complex carbohydrates do when consumed by diabetic patients. Thus the total amount of carbohydrate in the diet rather than the source of carbohydrate should be the primary consideration. The optimal source of carbohydrate may be foods containing water-soluble fiber (e.g., oats, gums, legumes, fruit pectin). Such fiber blunts the meal-induced rise in blood glucose by delaying gastric emptying and, in turn, the rate of meal absorption. Mild lowering of triglyceride and low-density lipoprotein (LDL) cholesterol levels may occur as well. It is commonly believed that sucrose leads to excessive glycemic excursions and must therefore be omitted. Such is not the case when modest amounts of sucrose are eaten within the context of mixed meals. Glucose excursions are not significantly different when equivalent amounts of sucrose and complex carbohydrates are added to meals, possibly because other foods (e.g., protein and fat) act to delay absorption and promote insulin secretion. Thus it is unnecessary to forbid the use of foods containing sucrose, provided that sucrose is consumed in moderation. Such restrictions can lead to poor adherence to the meal plan.

A key component of the diabetic meal plan is to reduce or

change the composition of dietary fat. The typical diet of Western countries, high in saturated or animal fat, appears to contribute to the development of atherosclerosis in patients with diabetes. Although substituting monounsaturated fatty acids rather than carbohydrates for saturated fat in the diet has been advocated to reduce LDL cholesterol without raising triglyceride levels, the approach may be difficult to achieve inasmuch as the major sources of monounsaturated fatty acids are olive, canola, and peanut oils.

EXERCISE. Regular exercise is a useful adjunct in the treatment of diabetes (see Table 242-5). It can improve insulin action and facilitate weight loss, but its major advantage is to lower cardiovascular risk. In support of this view, regular exercise produces a fall in very-low-density lipoprotein triglyceride and a rise in high-density lipoprotein (HDL) cholesterol and fibrinolytic activity in type 2 diabetes. Limitations may be imposed by pre-existing coronary or peripheral vascular disease, proliferative retinopathy, peripheral or autonomic neuropathy, and poor control.

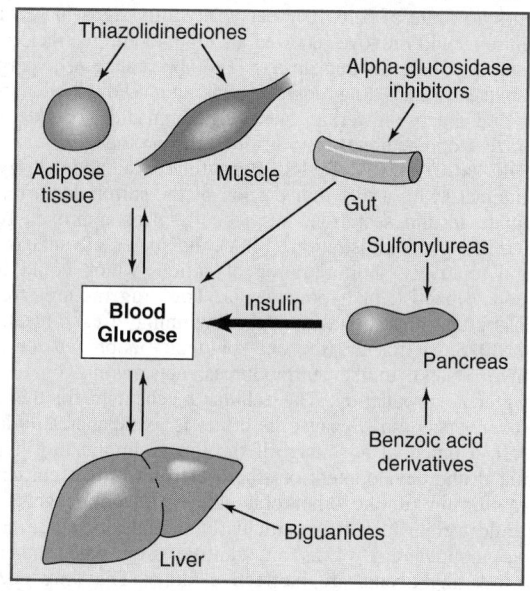

FIGURE 242-7 ■ Mechanism of action of oral glucose lowering agents.

Pharmacologic Intervention

ORAL GLUCOSE-LOWERING AGENTS. Several new classes of oral glucose-lowering agents have recently become available for the treatment of type 2 diabetes (Table 242–6, Fig. 242–7). These drugs are generally effective in patients in whom diet and exercise fail to achieve treatment goals. Oral agents tend to be favored as first-line therapy if hyperglycemia is mild, the patient is older, and obesity is more pronounced. The response cannot be predicted with certainty from clinical characteristics, and few circumstances contraindicate their use (e.g., severe insulin deficiency, allergy, pregnancy). Patients with severe hyperglycemia generally require insulin to lower glucose levels in the initial phases of treatment. Once glucose levels have stabilized and the "toxic" effects of severe hyperglycemia on beta cell function and insulin action have been minimized, many such patients become responsive to oral agents.

SULFONYLUREA. Sulfonylurea drugs were the only class of oral agents available in the United States before 1995. They act by enhancing insulin secretion by virtue of their ability to bind to their receptors associated with ATP-dependent potassium channels on the surface of the beta cell, thereby facilitating cellular depolarization. The reduction in glucose that follows is accompanied by a decline in insulin levels toward baseline. Insulin resistance commonly diminishes as a result of reversal of glucotoxicity. Because of their mechanism of action, sulfonylureas are totally ineffective in type 1 diabetes. Although the sulfonylureas differ in relative potency, effective dosage, duration of action, metabolism, and side effects, from a clinical standpoint these differences have marginal practical significance (see Table 242–6). Each drug has similar hypoglycemic effects when used in maximal doses. Drugs with a shorter duration of action that are metabolized by the liver have advantages in elderly patients with impaired renal function because such patients are more vulnerable to hypoglycemia, but they may be less effective because of problems with compliance with multiple dosing schedules. Longer-acting sulfonylureas require only once-per-day dosing but enhance the risk of hypoglycemia in patients who omit meals. Sulfonylureas with an intermediate duration of action may offer a reasonable compromise, although they still have a risk of producing severe hypoglycemia. These drugs may be given once per day, although twice-daily dosing may be required in patients with more severe hyperglycemia. After choosing an oral agent, treatment is initiated at low doses, with the dosage increased every 1 to 2 weeks until treatment goals or maximally effective doses are reached. Most patients initially respond with a lowering of glucose levels; however, about 15 to 20% of diabetic patients do not benefit (so-called primary failure). It is not uncommon to see loss of drug effect after years of therapy because of failure to sustain enthusiasm for diet and exercise, progression of beta cell failure, superimposition of other medical problems or drugs, or drug tolerance. The deteriorating glycemic control begets even poorer control as a result of glucotoxicity (see Fig. 242–4). Secondary drug failure occurs at a rate of 5 to 10% per year. Early signs of secondary drug failure should provoke renewed attempts to enforce diet, as well as a prompt increase in drug dosage. The appearance of hyperglycemia despite maximal drug doses signals the need to add another class of oral glucose-lowering agent (e.g., biguanide, or glucosidase inhibitor, thiazolidinedione) or to institute insulin therapy.

BENZOIC ACID DERIVATIVES. Repaglinide, a non-sulfonylurea which interacts with a different portion of the sulfonylurea receptor to stimulate insulin secretion, has recently been approved by the Food and Drug Administration (FDA). Its major advantage is its rapid and relatively short duration of action, which could potentially reduce the risk of hypoglycemia. The drug requires frequent daily dosing and must be taken at the beginning of each meal.

BIGUANIDES. Metformin (the only biguanide approved for use in the United States), unlike sulfonylureas, acts mainly by reducing hepatic glucose production. The cellular mechanism for this effect is, however, uncertain. Because its effect is extrapancreatic, insulin levels fall, a potential advantage if the theory implicating hyperinsulinemia in the development of atherosclerosis proves correct. Because metformin (unlike other oral glucose-lowering agents) may induce mild weight loss, it is particularly suitable for obese patients either as monotherapy or as an additive drug when other oral glucose-lowering agents are ineffective alone. The drug does not produce hypoglycemia when used as monotherapy; however, it can rarely produce lactic acidosis (approximately 0.03 cases per 1000 patient-years) and should therefore not be given to patients with renal insufficiency, liver disease, a history of congestive heart failure or chronic hypoxia, or alcohol abuse. The major side effects are gastrointestinal, particularly anorexia and nausea, which may contribute to its effect on weight loss. Metformin has a relatively short half-life (it is eliminated exclusively by the kidney), which generally necessitates administration as two or three divided doses given with meals.

THIAZOLIDINEDIONES. Thiazolidinediones reduce insulin resistance, most likely through activation of the peroxisome proliferator–activated receptor γ—a nuclear receptor that regulates the transcription of several insulin-responsive genes. Their biologic effect is mediated via stimulation of peripheral glucose metabolism. They have little effect on hepatic glucose production. Clinical studies demonstrate a reduction in both plasma glucose and insulin levels. Troglitazone was the first thiazolidinedione derivative approved for use in the United States. It is most effective when used in conjunction with insulin in type 2 diabetic patients who are not adequately controlled with insulin or in combination therapy with other oral hypoglycemic agents such as sulfonylureas. Troglitazone commonly requires 4 to 6 weeks for its glucose-lowering effect to be fully manifested. It has been reported to cause an increase in transaminases in about 2% of patients. Reports of cases of severe liver failure have led the FDA to recommend measuring liver enzymes at baseline every month for the first year of treatment and on a regular basis thereafter.

Recently, the FDA approved two new thiozolidinediones, rosiglitazone and pioglitazone, which are effective glucose-lowering agents either as monotherapy or in combination with other drugs. Preliminary data suggest that both drugs have a much lower risk of hepatotoxicity and therefore are more appropriate for use as monotherapy. Nevertheless, none of the thiozolidinediones should be used in patients with liver function abnormalities, and they should be discontinued if liver enzymes (e.g., ALT) become elevated. Hypoglycemia is rare when thiozolidinediones are used as monotherapy, but may occur when these drugs are used in conjunction with insulin or sulfonylureas. Weight gain and/or edema may also complicate thiozolidinedione therapy.

α-GLUCOSIDASE INHIBITORS. Acarbose and miglitolare, reversible inhibitors of α-glucosidases (the intestinal enzymes that break down complex carbohydrates into monosaccharides), delay the absorption of carbohydrates such as starch, sucrose, and maltose. It does not affect the absorption of monosaccharides such as glucose. To be effective, this class of drugs must be taken at the beginning of each carbohydrate-containing meal. In controlled trials performed in patients with type 2 diabetes, α-glucosidase inhibitors alone or as an adjunctive therapy to reduce postprandial hyperglycemia resulted in a small, but clinically meaningful reduction in glycosylated hemoglobin levels.

A major advantage is that α-glucosidase inhibitors do not have significant toxicity. The most common side effects are abdominal bloating, flatulence, and sometimes diarrhea. The adverse gastrointestinal effects are minimized by using a slowly escalating dose titration schedule in which treatment is initiated at the lowest dose.

INSULIN THERAPY. Insulin is most commonly used as 1st-line therapy for non-obese, younger, or severely hyperglycemic type 2 diabetic patients and is temporarily required during severe stress (e.g., injury, infection, surgery) or in pregnancy. Insulin should not be used as 1st-line therapy in poorly compliant patients who are unwilling to self-monitor glucose levels or for patients with a high risk of hypoglycemia. In patients with severe obesity, profound insulin resistance often necessitates the use of large doses of insulin, which sometimes interferes with efforts to restrict caloric intake to achieve weight loss. In patients with newly diagnosed diabetes or those with relatively mild fasting hyperglycemia who continue to maintain endogenous insulin secretory capacity, relatively small doses of insulin (e.g., 0.3 to 0.4 U/kg of body weight per day) given once or twice per day may be sufficient to achieve target goals. Such patients retain some degree of meal-stimulated endogenous insulin secretion and may therefore require less rapid-acting insulin. Although it is common practice to administer a single dose of intermediate-acting insulin in the morning, frequently its glucose-lowering effect does not extend over a full 24-hour period. Because a key element of successful insulin treatment is to dimin-

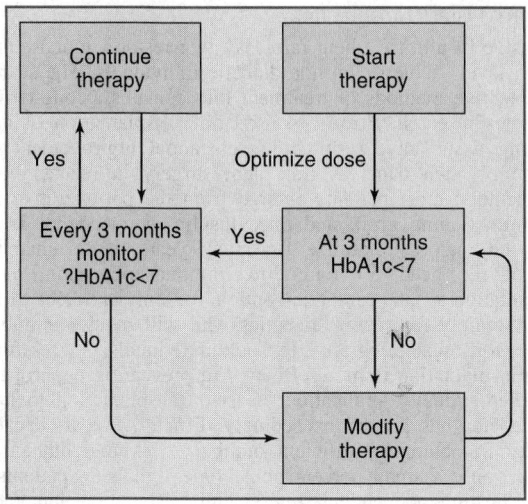

FIGURE 242–8 ■ Strategy for the treatment of type 2 diabetes.

ish accelerated rates of endogenous glucose production in the morning, it is generally more effective to split the dose and administer sufficient amounts of intermediate-acting insulin in the evening (before dinner or preferably at bedtime) to optimize control of the fasting glucose level. Alternatively, a single small dose of intermediate-acting insulin given at bedtime to control fasting hyperglycemia may be effective throughout the remainder of the day in patients who have retained the capacity to secrete insulin with meals. This approach has the advantage of greater simplicity and may be combined with oral glucose-lowering agents during the day to facilitate endogenous insulin release or action with meals.

In practice, most insulin-treated patients are obese, have more severe hyperglycemia, and have already failed oral therapy. These patients are more insulin deficient and insulin resistant. As a result, they often require multiple-dose regimens involving mixtures of rapid- and intermediate-acting insulin to control hyperglycemia. As in type 1 patients, it is best to distribute their insulin as evenly as possible throughout the day and to provide sufficient insulin overnight to control fasting hyperglycemia. The complexity of the regimen must be individualized according to the total clinical context of the patient's disease, the level of diabetes education and ability to perform self-care, and most importantly, the patient's motivation. In some cases, combinations of insulin and oral hypoglycemic drugs (particularly thiozolidinediones) may reduce insulin dose requirements and at the same time improve glycemic control. It should be noted that in such patients requiring insulin, combination therapy may be no more effective than giving larger doses of insulin alone in controlling blood glucose. The potential benefit of reducing circulating insulin levels with combination therapy on the development of atherogenesis remains to be established.

Experience with the use of intensified insulin treatment, including continuous subcutaneous insulin infusion pumps and multiple subcutaneous injection regimens, is limited in patients with type 2 diabetes. However, preliminary data suggest that they may be successfully applied in a select group of these patients.

TREATMENT STRATEGIES FOR TYPE 2 DIABETES. In contrast to type 1 diabetes, in which pharmacologic treatment is limited only to insulin, several pharmacologic options exist for the management of type 2 diabetes. In the UKPDS, the improved outcomes produced by intensified therapy were similar for patients given insulin or oral agents (sulfonylurea or metformin). However, the ability of the UKPDS to detect differences among the various pharmacologic agents used is limited because of drug crossovers and the common need for drug combinations as the study progressed. It should be noted that some discrepancies were noted in the results derived from the smaller subgroup of patients who received metformin. However, overall analysis of the results of the metformin-treated group suggests that intensified therapy with each pharmacologic agent was beneficial and that no specific therapy was superior. Thus regardless of whether type 2 patients are treated with insulin or oral hypoglycemics, the goals of therapy *should be the same*, namely, to lower blood glucose as close to normal as possible. Success at meeting target goals requires careful follow-up

and rapid therapeutic responses to the continuously progressing dysfunction of glucose homeostasis. For most patients, glycemic control deteriorates over time, thus necessitating more intensive pharmacologic interventions.

The decision regarding initial therapy for type 2 diabetes should be influenced by the severity of the fasting hyperglycemia, the presence of symptoms, and obesity. Other factors such as the patient's age, motivation, and coexistence of other diseases should be considered as well. To determine the effectiveness of the therapy selected, dosages should be adjusted over about a 3-month period based on glucose self-monitoring. Failure to meet established target glycemic goals within 3 months should prompt modification of treatment (e.g., combination therapy). In many cases, patients who were initially well controlled with only one drug will with time require combination therapy and may ultimately use insulin. Ultimately, if treatment glycemic targets are not met with oral agents, insulin remains an effective treatment option (Fig. 242–8).

Monitoring

SELF-MONITORING OF BLOOD GLUCOSE. Self-monitoring of blood glucose has revolutionized diabetes management. It actively involves patients in the treatment process, allows more rapid treatment adjustments, and reinforces diet therapy. Self-monitoring provides the patient with the tools necessary for crucial self-management and is especially useful in the care of patients receiving insulin or oral glucose-lowering agents during periods of stress and in patients susceptible to hypoglycemia. Urine glucose testing is unreliable and should be used only in patients who cannot or refuse to apply self-monitoring of blood glucose or in whom the treatment goal is only prevention of symptomatic hyperglycemia.

The newer glucose meters are small, portable, and accurate, give a digital readout, and have computerized memory to facilitate record keeping. These factors make them preferable to visual estimates from test strips. Blood sampling is facilitated and made less painful by automated spring-operated lancet devices. Self-monitoring of blood glucose is of value only if the patient performs tests on a regular basis, can accurately measure glucose levels, and can make use of the results. The patient must become familiar with what a normal glucose value is, what the glucose targets are, and how they may vary with changes in diet, activity, and insulin absorption. Day-to-day adjustments in short-acting insulin based on pre-meal values and a "sliding scale" can be readily accomplished by most patients. The patient also needs to examine the effects of longer-acting insulin and make small adjustments if glucose levels (e.g., pre-breakfast and pre-dinner values) are not within the target range. At a minimum, patients need to be able to adjust to repetitive patterns of hypoglycemia or hyperglycemia, as well as periods of illness ("sick days"). In the latter circumstance, urine testing for ketones should be done as well.

The success of insulin therapy depends on the frequency with which the patient performs self-monitoring. Patients with type 1 diabetes should be encouraged to monitor before each meal and at bedtime. Periodic checks 90 to 120 minutes after meals help control postprandial hyperglycemia, and patients may occasionally need to monitor blood levels in the middle of the night (e.g., 3 A.M.) to avoid nocturnal hypoglycemia. Currently, no clear guidelines have been established for the frequency of self-monitoring of blood glucose in type 2 diabetes. Type 2 patients who are treated with insulin should conduct self-monitoring daily, before breakfast and dinner and at bedtime. Here the aim is to meet target glycemic goals and reduce the risk of hypoglycemia. In patients taking oral agents, the frequency of blood glucose self-monitoring will depend on the duration of the therapy and the metabolic control achieved by it. Self-monitoring of blood glucose should be more frequent at the beginning of treatment and any time that deterioration in metabolic control is suspected. Type 2 patients maintained by diet therapy should, at the very least, learn self-monitoring of blood glucose to prevent metabolic decompensation. They often benefit from monitoring glucose levels periodically so that they can better appreciate how individual foods or deviations from the meal plan adversely affect their glycemic control.

GLYCOHEMOGLOBIN. Glycohemoglobin (or glycosylated hemoglobin) assays have emerged as the "gold standard" by which glycemic control is measured. The test does not rely on the patient's ability to monitor or accurately record blood glucose levels, and it is not influenced by acute changes in blood glucose or by the interval since the last meal. Glycohemoglobin is formed when glucose reacts non-enzymatically with the hemoglobin A molecule and is composed of several fractions, the major one being Hb A_{1c}. Total glycohemoglobin (Hb A_1) and Hb A_{1c} (expressed as the percentage of total hemoglobin) vary in proportion to the average level of glucose over the lifespan of the red blood cell (RBC), thereby providing an index of glycemic control during the preceding 6 to 12 weeks. Several assay methods have been developed that vary in their precision, yield different ranges for non-diabetic values, and lack common standardization procedures. Clinicians must therefore become familiar with the assays used in their own laboratory and use that specific assay when evaluating changes in glycemic control in individual patients. Although the ambient glucose level is the dominant factor influencing glycohemoglobin, other factors may confound interpretation of the test. For example, any condition that increases RBC turnover (e.g., pregnancy or hemolytic anemia) spuriously lowers glycohemoglobin, regardless of the assay used. Some assays yield spuriously low values in patients with hemoglobinopathies such as sickle cell disease or trait and hemoglobin C or D or spuriously high values when hemoglobin F is increased (e.g., thalassemia, myeloproliferative disorders) or large doses of aspirin are consumed. Thus for unexpectedly high or low values, factors that alter the specific test used should be excluded. In most cases, however, discrepancies between self-monitoring of blood glucose and glycohemoglobin results reflect problems with the former rather than the latter. Although glycohemoglobin provides the most accurate estimate of overall glycemic control, it is less valuable in determining what specific changes in therapy are indicated. Blood glucose measurements are essential to adjust the components of the regimen appropriately.

MANAGEMENT PLAN/TREATMENT GOALS. A management plan should take into consideration the life patterns, age, work and school schedules, psychosocial needs, educational level, and motivation of the individual patient. The plan should include medications, recommendations for lifestyle changes, a meal plan, monitoring instructions (including "sick day" management), and hypoglycemia prevention and treatment strategies. Each component of the plan must be understood and agreed upon by the patient. Active patient participation in problem solving plus ongoing, continued support from the health care team is critical for successful management. At each visit the management plan should be reviewed and an assessment made of the patient's progress in achieving target goals. If the goals are not met, the causes need to be identified and the plan modified accordingly. The history and physical examination should focus on early signs and symptoms of retinal, vascular, neurologic, and foot complications and reinforcement of the diet and exercise prescription. A complete ophthalmologic examination, an assessment of cardiovascular risk factors, and a timed urine collection for albumin should be obtained annually.

Formulation of individual target glycemic goals must take into account the results of the DCCT (type 1) and the UKPDS (type 2 diabetes) in the context of the patient's capacity to implement the treatment plan, the risk for hypoglycemia, and other factors that would alter the risk-benefit ratio. Table 242–7 presents target glycemic guidelines for non-pregnant diabetic patients and targets for other factors that increase the potential for diabetic complications.

Pancreas/Islet Transplantation

Intensive insulin treatment rarely, if ever restores glucose homeostasis to levels achieved in non-diabetic individuals. The search for more effective methods of treatment thus remains a long-term goal of diabetes research. Efforts focused on transplantation of insulin-producing tissue have resulted in substantial improvement in the outcome of such pancreas transplant surgery in recent years. In major centers, most patients emerge from the perioperative period with a functioning graft, and once insulin independence is established, the majority stabilize for many years. Unfortunately, because of the need for long-term immunosuppression, pancreas transplantation is at present an option for only a select group of patients, mainly for type 1 diabetics who will require immunosuppression for renal allografts. In such individuals, successful pancreas transplantation is more effective in preventing nephropathy in the grafted kidney. Application of islet transplantation to humans with diabetes has proved exceedingly difficult, in part because of difficulty in obtaining sufficient numbers of viable human islets. Thus far, only a small percentage of type 1 diabetic patients have become insulin independent. Interestingly, islet transplantation has been much more successful in patients with chronic pancreatitis who have undergone total pancreatectomy followed by intraportal injection of their own islets. The implication is that the use of immunosuppressive drugs, chronic low-grade rejection of the foreign islet grafts, and activation of an autoimmune response account for the high incidence of failure. If correct, the future of islet transplantation therapy may depend more on manipulation of the islet or the immune system than on technical surgical advances.

Prevention of Diabetes

As the pathogenesis of both types of diabetes becomes better understood, the potential for prevention of these diseases is more realistic. Multicenter disease prevention trials are already under way in the United States. In the Diabetes Prevention Trial Type 1, relatives of type 1 diabetic subjects who are at high risk (based on antibody screening and HLA typing for the disease) are given insulin, a therapy used in rodent models of spontaneous autoimmune diabetes to prevent disease expression. The Diabetes Prevention Program is designed to determine whether type 2 can be prevented or delayed with early introduction of lifestyle changes or oral glucose-lowering agents (metformin) in persons with impaired glucose tolerance.

ACUTE METABOLIC COMPLICATIONS

HYPERGLYCEMIC STATES. Metabolic decompensation in diabetes is manifested as severe hyperglycemia with or without ketoacidosis. Although diabetic ketoacidosis is generally seen in type 1 patients and non-ketotic hyperosmolar syndrome is generally seen in type 2 patients, exceptions occur. In both conditions mortality increases with age and is usually due to an associated catastrophic illness (e.g., myocardial infarction, cerebrovascular accident, sepsis) or acute complications (e.g., aspiration, arrhythmias, or cerebral edema). Thus treatment does not simply depend on insulin to reverse the metabolic abnormalities that dominate the picture; it also depends on detection and treatment of precipitating illnesses, as well as prompt attention to fluid and electrolyte disturbances.

DIABETIC KETOACIDOSIS. Diabetic ketoacidosis may herald the onset of type 1 diabetes, but it most often (>80%) occurs in established diabetic patients as a result of an intercurrent illness (e.g., infection), an inappropriate reduction in insulin dosage, or

---

Table 242–7 ■ THERAPEUTIC TARGETS FOR NON-PREGNANT DIABETIC PATIENTS

PARAMETERS	NORMAL	GOAL	SIGNALS POSSIBLE INTERVENTION*
Premeal glucose (mg/dL)	<110	80–120	<80 or >140
Bedtime glucose (mg/dL)	<120	100–140	<100 or >160
Hb A_{1c}† (%)	<6	<7	>8
LDL cholesterol (mg/dL)	<130	<100‡	>130‡
HDL cholesterol (mg/dL)	>35	>35	<35
Fasting triglycerides (mg/dL)	<150	<150	>250–300
Blood pressure (mm Hg)	<140/90	<130/85	>130/85

LDL = low-density lipoprotein; HDL = high-density lipoprotein.
*Targets may vary depending on assessment of risk-benefit ratio.
†Targets need to be adjusted for local laboratory differences in assay method and non-diabetic reference ranges.
‡Less than 100 for patients with coexisting cardiovascular disease.

missed injections (especially in adolescents). A common scenario is a patient who fails to increase insulin therapy and consume extra fluid during illness. Prevention requires education in "sick day" management and assessment of urine ketones whenever blood glucose monitoring shows severe hyperglycemia or physical illness is noted.

The two cardinal biochemical features of diabetic ketoacidosis—hyperglycemia and hyperketonemia—are caused by the combined effects of severe insulin deficiency and excessive secretion of counterregulatory hormones that interact synergistically to magnify the effects of insulin lack. These changes mobilize the delivery of substrates from muscle (amino acids, lactate, pyruvate) and adipose tissue (free fatty acids, glycerol) to the liver, where they are actively converted to glucose (via gluconeogenesis) or ketone bodies (β-hydroxybutyrate, acetoacetate) and ultimately released into the circulation at rates that greatly exceed the capacity of tissues to use them. The net result is hyperglycemia (>300 mg/dL), acidosis (pH <7.35), and an osmotic diuresis leading to marked dehydration. Typically, the history indicates deterioration over days with symptoms of increasing hyperglycemia. Other features may include abdominal pain, anorexia, and nausea. The pain is normally periumbilical and constant and can mimic the pain associated with surgical emergencies. Reduced motility of the gastrointestinal tract or, in severe cases, paralytic ileus may further contribute to the diagnostic confusion. Vomiting is a threatening symptom because it precludes oral replacement of the excessive fluid loss caused by the osmotic diuresis; severe volume depletion follows quickly. Physical findings are mainly secondary to dehydration and acidosis and include dry skin and mucous membranes, reduced jugular venous pressure, tachycardia, orthostatic hypotension, depressed mental function, and deep and rapid (termed Kussmaul) respirations. Ketosis is recognizable by a sweet, sickly smell on the patient's breath.

The diagnosis is usually straightforward and should be made promptly. The clinical picture and the presence of severe hyperglycemia should alert the clinician to test for serum ketones and, if possible, to measure arterial pH. The severity of hyperglycemia can vary from 250 to 300 to greater than 1000 mg/dL, serum bicarbonate is depressed, and there is an increase in the anion gap (the difference between the serum sodium and the sum of the chloride and bicarbonate concentrations) that is generally proportional to the decrease in serum bicarbonate. Hyperchloremia may be superimposed if the patient maintains an adequate glomerular filtration rate (GFR) and is able to exchange keto acid anions for chloride in the kidney. The depression in arterial pH depends on the degree of respiratory compensation; in mild cases pH ranges from 7.20 to 7.35, whereas in severe cases it may be as low as 6.8 to 6.9. Usually the severity of the clinical signs and symptoms depends more on the magnitude of the acidosis than the magnitude of the hyperglycemia. Occasionally, a degree of superimposed metabolic alkalosis (e.g., caused by vomiting or diuretic use) may obscure the true severity of ketoacidosis. An increase in the anion gap out of proportion to the level of bicarbonate should suggest this possibility. Because quantitative measurements of β-hydroxybutyrate and acetoacetate are not readily available, rapid diagnosis requires qualitative assessment of serum ketones by using dilutions of serum and reagent strips (Ketostix) or tablets (Acetest). These methods depend on a nitroprusside reaction with acetoacetate. Acetone, however, reacts weakly with nitroprusside and β-hydroxybutyrate reacts not at all, which makes the test sometimes misleadingly low. Because of the presence of intracellular acidosis, β-hydroxybutyrate levels are often much higher than acetoacetate, and the frequent presence of concomitant lactic acidosis farther reduces acetoacetate. Conversely, once insulin therapy begins, the nitroprusside reaction often remains "positive" and gives the false impression of sustained ketosis for many hours or days because some β-hydroxybutyrate is converted to acetoacetate and non-acidic acetone is cleared slowly from the body. Other laboratory abnormalities in diabetic ketoacidosis include reduced serum sodium (because of hyperosmolarity and shift of water from the extravascular to the intravascular space), prerenal azotemia, and hyperamylasemia, which is usually of non-pancreatic origin but can lead to the erroneous diagnosis of pancreatitis. Normal, elevated, or reduced concentrations of potassium, phosphate, and magnesium may exist when diabetic ketoacidosis is diagnosed. Nevertheless, large deficits of these electrolytes invariably accompany the osmotic diuresis and become apparent during the course of treatment. Mortality rates may be as high as 5 to 10%. For the most part, death occurs in elderly patients (>65 years) in whom diabetic ketoacidosis is initiated or complicated by a serious underlying illness. Diabetic ketoacidosis also remains a major cause of death in young children with type 1 diabetes, especially if complicated by the development of cerebral edema.

NON-KETOTIC HYPEROSMOLAR SYNDROME. Non-ketotic hyperosmolar syndrome is characterized by severe hyperosmolarity (greater than 320 mOsm/L), hyperglycemia (>600 mg/dL), and dehydration. The major reason that such severe hyperglycemia occurs is that patients cannot drink enough fluid to keep pace with the osmotic diuresis caused by hyperglycemia. The resulting impairment in renal function reduces glucose loss via the kidney, thereby leading to remarkable elevations in blood glucose. The history is usually one of an insidious onset with deterioration over weeks. Patients are often elderly with either mild or undiagnosed type 2 diabetes. They may be taking medications that contribute to the diuresis as well as the impairment in insulin secretion (e.g., thiazide diuretics), or they may be demented or institutionalized and unable to recognize thirst or have access to fluids. Unlike diabetic ketoacidosis, severe acidosis and ketosis are absent. However, some type 2 patients with depressed endogenous insulin secretion may be unable to suppress ketone production in the face of elevations in the counterregulatory hormones produced by physical illness. Because they have higher portal vein insulin concentrations than do type 1 diabetic patients, ketone production by the liver and in turn the severity of the acidosis are usually mild. The level of consciousness generally correlates with the severity and duration of hyperosmolarity. Only about 10% of patients are initially seen in coma, and an equal number show no signs of mental obtundation. A variety of often reversible neurologic abnormalities may exist, including grand mal or focal seizures (about 10% of cases), extensor plantar reflexes, aphasia, hemisensory or motor deficits, delirium, and exacerbation of a pre-existing organic mental syndrome. Clinical signs show profound dehydration; gastrointestinal symptoms are less frequent than in diabetic ketoacidosis. The laboratory picture is dominated by the effects of uncontrolled diabetes and dehydration; renal function is invariably impaired, hemoglobin is elevated, liver function tests may be abnormal because of fatty liver, and hypertriglyceridemia may lead to a falsely low serum sodium value ("pseudohyponatremia"). Although the severe hyperosmolarity would be expected to lower serum sodium as well, it is not uncommon to see "normal" or even elevated levels because of the severe dehydration. The severity of the hyperosmolar state can be measured directly or estimated according to a formula that excludes urea because it is freely diffusible throughout the body and therefore has little influence on the osmotic pressure gradient:

Effective osmolarity (mOsm/L):

$$= 2[Na^+ + K^+ \ (mEqL)] + \frac{plasma \ glucose \ (mg/dL)}{18}$$

A value greater than 320 mOsm/L reflects hyperosmolarity and greater than 350 mOsm/L indicates a severe hyperosmolar state. Recent data suggest that mortality is approximately 10 to 20%. Poor outcome is related to age as well as elevated blood urea nitrogen and sodium concentrations. The syndrome may be complicated by thromboembolic events, aspiration, and rhabdomyolysis.

MANAGEMENT. The goals of therapy for both diabetic ketoacidosis and non-ketotic hyperosmolar syndrome are to reverse the metabolic disturbance and replace fluid and electrolyte deficits (Table 242–8). This task requires the prompt delivery of water, electrolytes, and insulin, as well as attention to potential complications that might arise during therapy and treatment of underlying precipitating events.

In the initial stages of therapy, the primary consideration is to restore vascular volume and correct hypoperfusion. At this time a massive total-body deficit of water (5 to 12 L) and sodium (about 5 to 10 mEq/kg) requires prompt attention (deficits are usually more profound in non-ketotic hyperosmolar syndrome). Although water loss is greater than sodium loss, it is usually preferable to initially replace fluid deficits with isotonic normal saline (0.9% NaCl solution) to restore intravascular volume as quickly as possible. Fluid replacement regimens vary, but it is common to administer 1 L of normal saline within the 1st hour, followed by 1 L/hour over the next few hours to restore intravascular volume. Therefore, the regimen (normal or half-normal saline) and the rate of infusion (commonly 0.25 to 0.5 L/hour) should be adjusted over the next 6 hours

Table 242–8 ■ THERAPY FOR DIABETIC KETOACIDOSIS AND NON-KETONIC HYPEROSMOLAR SYNDROME

PARAMETER	INITIAL MANAGEMENT	CONTINUING MANAGEMENT
Volume	*IV fluids:* Initially use NS at 1 L/hr × 1–5 L to restore volume; thereafter, half NS or NS at 250–500 mL/hr	*Adjust rate of IV fluids:* Base on cardiovascular parameters (e.g., heart rate, blood pressure) and urine output
Acidosis	*Use bicarbonate if pH < 7.1, shock, coma, or severe hyperkalemia is present:* 1 ampule of NaHCO$_3$ (44 mEq) Check ABG after 1 hr: if pH > 7.1, stop	*Monitor* ABGs Bicarbonate Anion gap
Insulin	*Regular insulin:* Bolus: 0.1 U/kg IV drip: start at 0.1 U/kg	*Monitor blood glucose* Expected rate of fall, ~100 mg/dL/hr Initial goal: 200–300 mg/dL (to avoid hypoglycemia) *Blood glucose still elevated or falling slowly:* Increase insulin IV by 50–100% per hr
Glucose		*Blood glucose <250 mg/dL* Start IV dextrose infusion Start SC regular insulin Discontinue IV insulin 2 hr after giving SC insulin Begin clear liquid diet and progress as tolerated
Electrolytes	*Hyperkalemia* may be initially present *Hypokalemia* during insulin therapy should be anticipated	*Monitor* Serum K, Ca, Mg, phosphate; replace as needed ECG Urine output (should be at least >30 mL/hr)

IV = intravenous; NS = normal saline; ABG = arterial blood gases; SC = subcutaneous; ECG = electrocardiogram.

(and thereafter) according to the response to fluid replacement and the clinical status of the patient (e.g., underlying cardiovascular disease or oliguria). In general, normal saline and hypotonic solutions are alternated for diabetic ketoacidosis. For non-ketotic hyperosmolar syndrome or older patients with diabetic ketoacidosis, hypotonic solutions are more commonly used. In the latter circumstance, normal saline generally provides more sodium and chloride than the patient needs and may result in hypernatremia; in diabetic ketoacidosis, hypotonic solutions may accelerate the shift of water into the intracellular space and in turn contribute to the development of cerebral edema that may be seen in young patients. During the course of treatment, once blood glucose falls to 250 to 300 mg/dL, glucose should be added to the solution to avoid eventual hypoglycemia and to minimize the risk of cerebral edema.

Although insulin resistance is present in both diabetic ketoacidosis and non-ketotic hyperosmolar syndrome, large supraphysiologic doses of insulin are not necessary and are more likely to provoke hypokalemia, hypophosphatemia, and delayed hypoglycemia. A typical insulin replacement regimen is to give an intravenous bolus of 0.1 U of rapid-acting (regular) insulin per kilogram, followed by 0.1 U/kg/hour thereafter. Intravenous administration is the most predictable way of delivering insulin to target tissues, particularly in severely hypovolemic patients with reduced peripheral blood flow. If intravenous administration is not possible, the intramuscular site is preferred to the subcutaneous site because the latter predisposes to unpredictable absorption. It is ideal if blood glucose falls at a steady and predictable rate (about 100 mg/dL/hour), so it is important to monitor blood glucose closely after starting insulin to check that the rate of fall is appropriate. Blood glucose should not fall too rapidly, especially in young children, because a rapid fall may be associated with cerebral edema. A steady fall in blood glucose also means that the time at which glucose is added to the regimen may be predicted in advance. When reviewing the progress of treatment, it is important to consider a failure in insulin delivery if blood glucose fails to drop. In some, such failure is due to severe insulin resistance and necessitates an increase in the insulin dose. Because the primary mechanism for lowering plasma glucose in the early stages of treatment is disposal of glucose via the urine rather than by insulin-stimulated glucose consumption, the problem may reflect inadequate replacement of intravascular volume and restoration of GFR or the development of renal failure. After achieving a relatively stable blood glucose level at or below 250 mg/dL, subcutaneous administration of insulin can be started, and about 2 hours later the intravenous insulin infusion may be discontinued. To avoid return of hyperglycemia, a standing order for subcutaneous injections of regular insulin about every 4 to 6 hours should be given (the dosage and frequency will depend on the patient's condition). Adjustment of the intravenous glucose infusion should be based on frequent blood glucose monitoring to prevent the development of hypoglycemia.

Potassium replacement needs close attention because both hyperkalemia and hypokalemia are associated with cardiac arrhythmia. At the initial evaluation, patients have a severe total-body deficit of potassium (about 5 mEq/kg), yet serum potassium levels may be low, normal, or high (especially if acidosis or renal failure is present). Once intravenous fluid and insulin administration is started, serum potassium levels fall quickly because of an insulin-mediated shift of potassium into the intracellular space. In addition, fluid replacement causes extracellular dilution of potassium and increases potassium removal because of improved renal perfusion. This trend can be countered by potassium replacement based on serum levels. A low potassium level requires prompt treatment with 30 to 40 mEq/hour, whereas normal serum potassium signals the need to ensure adequate urine output before starting therapy at approximately 20 mEq/hour. In patients who may have lost potassium for other reasons such as diuretic use or gastrointestinal loss, one should anticipate the need for greater potassium supplementation. Patients with circulatory collapse or compromised renal function may not be able to tolerate a potassium load. Electrocardiograms may provide a more direct assessment of intracellular potassium and are recommended. Flat or inverted T waves suggest a low potassium level, and peaked T waves suggest high intracellular potassium. The intracellular potassium deficit in renal tubular cells further promotes potassium loss by the kidneys, and this abnormality does not correct immediately. As a result, excess potassium loss may continue for days or weeks.

In most patients with diabetic ketoacidosis, the acidosis disappears with standard therapeutic measures. Artificial correction with alkali (bicarbonate) is unnecessary. Suppression of lipolysis by insulin reduces free fatty acid flux to the liver and ketogenesis. The remaining keto acids are oxidized, with subsequent regeneration of bicarbonate. In severe acidosis, bicarbonate administration is indicated. The hyperventilatory drive of severe acidosis is uncomfortable, and severe acidosis has a negative inotropic effect and causes vasodilation. However, bicarbonate must be used with caution because it may provoke hypokalemia, which in the context of a falling serum potassium concentration may precipitate a cardiac arrhythmia. In addition, by causing a sudden left shift of the dissociation curve for oxyhemoglobin, bicarbonate may impair oxygen delivery to tissues. When the patient is first seen, the dissociation curve for oxyhemoglobin is approximately in the normal position because the expected right shift caused by acidosis is offset by a left shift as a result of reduced red cell 2,3-diphosphoglycerate. Sudden correction of acidosis moves the curve to the left because red cell 2,3-diphosphoglycerate levels recover only slowly during the course of therapy. If alkali is given, small amounts should be slowly administered (44 mEq every 1 to 2 hours) when there is evidence of severe acidosis (pH < 7.0 to 7.1). Therapy should be discontinued when the pH rises to about 7.1. Although substantial phosphate depletion occurs with both diabetic ketoacidosis and non-ketotic hyperosmolar syndrome, the prophylactic use of phosphate in diabetic ketoacidosis has failed to show any significant benefit. Hypocalcemic tetany may complicate phosphate therapy unless magnesium supplements are provided. Because the longer prodromal period associated with non-ketotic hyperosmolar syndrome may lead to more severe phosphate losses, they may need to be replaced as potassium phosphate together with magnesium.

The patient's fluid and cardiovascular status must be carefully monitored throughout treatment. When severe hypovolemia or renal dysfunction is present, central venous pressure monitoring is indicated. The presence of cardiac dysfunction or adult respiratory distress syndrome, both recognized complications in severe cases, calls for measuring pulmonary wedge pressure. Urinary catheterization is essential in unconscious or oliguric patients, and gastric decompression may be required to minimize the risk of aspiration. As in any intensive care situation, an accurate record of fluid input and output and key laboratory measurements (every 1 to 2 hours), such as plasma glucose, arterial pH, and electrolytes, allow an ongoing review of progress. Even more important is the need to search for a possible coexisting illness; serious medical illness may easily be overlooked for several hours during the early phases of therapy. In children, monitoring of mental status is crucial because of their risk of cerebral edema. Leukocytosis often accompanies diabetic ketoacidosis or non-ketotic hyperosmolar syndrome and should not be taken as a rationale for antibiotic prophylaxis. Table 242–8 outlines the principles of management of diabetic ketoacidosis and non-ketotic hyperosmolar syndrome.

ALCOHOLIC KETOACIDOSIS. Alcoholic ketoacidosis may be confused with diabetic ketoacidosis, particularly when hyperglycemia is present. It is typically seen in people who have consumed large amounts of alcohol and then abstain from food or drink for an extended period. Commonly, the patient is anorectic and has nausea and vomiting, thus prolonging the period of starvation. The syndrome is characterized by severe ketoacidosis and dehydration. Hyperglycemia is inconsistent; it may exist in association with underlying diabetes (or pancreatitis) or be mild in non-diabetic subjects. The stress of the illness, volume depletion, activation of the sympathetic nervous system following alcohol withdrawal, prolonged starvation, or probably a combination of these factors results in a fall in insulin and a rise in glucagon levels. The combination markedly accelerates ketogenesis. Hyperglycemia is probably limited because hepatic metabolism of alcohol leads to an increase in the ratio of reduced to non-reduced nicotinamide adenine dinucleotide, which inhibits gluconeogenesis despite insulin deficiency. Alcoholic ketoacidosis is rapidly reversed by the intravenous administration of fluids and glucose; insulin is rarely needed, except in diabetic persons.

HYPOGLYCEMIA. Severe hypoglycemia is the most frequent complication in type 1 diabetes. It symptomatically affects 10 to 25% of these patients at least once a year. The condition can vary widely, from requiring just the help of another person to being severe enough to require emergency medical assistance. The frequency of less disabling hypoglycemia is much higher. From a practical standpoint, data showing that near normoglycemia prevents the long-term vascular complications of diabetes have resulted in a much greater frequency of severe hypoglycemia in insulin-treated patients and have stimulated interest in its physiology and prevention. The less common event of hypoglycemia induced by oral glucose-lowering agents should not be overlooked. This problem tends to occur in elderly diabetics with impaired renal function and is more common with the longer-acting sulfonylureas. Its management is no different from the treatment of insulin-induced hypoglycemia, but because of the long-acting nature of oral agents, hypoglycemia may recur for 24 to 48 hours after drug withdrawal. Prolonged and very severe hypoglycemia can cause irreversible brain damage; it has been less clear, however, whether any neurologic damage is caused by milder episodes of hypoglycemia. Some studies have shown that electroencephalographic abnormalities are more prevalent in young children who have a history of recurrent hypoglycemia. The DCCT, on the other hand, reported no evidence of neuropsychological impairment after an average of 7 years of intensified treatment, even in patients with recurrent severe hypoglycemic episodes. Nevertheless, hypoglycemia may provoke seizures, accidental injury, and a catecholamine response that can induce arrhythmias or cardiac ischemia in patients with underlying cardiac disease. Hypoglycemia is thought to account for 3 to 4% of deaths in insulin-treated diabetic patients. It also has far-reaching social implications. At a personal level, it can become

the patient's greatest fear and lead the patient and clinician to aim deliberately for less than optimal glycemic control.

In normal persons, hypoglycemia provokes a response that returns blood glucose to normal. This process involves three defense mechanisms: (1) insulin dissipation, (2) counterregulatory hormone secretion and action, and (3) a subjective awareness of hypoglycemia resulting in carbohydrate ingestion. The brain cannot synthesize or store more than a few minutes' supply of glucose and, in the short term, is wholly dependent on a constant supply of glucose. If glucose efflux from the circulation exceeds exogenous and endogenous influx, hypoglycemia results. Spontaneous recovery of blood glucose involves a complex response that includes activation of endogenous glucose production and diminution of peripheral glucose uptake. These changes are triggered when plasma glucose begins to approach the hypoglycemic range (65 to 70 mg/dL). The rise in glucose production is initiated by the release of glucagon, as well as epinephrine, in conjunction with a fall in endogenous insulin release and, at the outset, probably reflects mainly the stimulation of hepatic glycogenolysis. When hypoglycemia is sustained, other hormones such as growth hormone and cortisol help ensure continued glucose production via gluconeogenesis. Multiple factors contribute to the diminution in glucose uptake, including epinephrine's inhibitory effect on insulin-stimulated glucose uptake, insulin disappearance, elevations of free fatty acids, and hypoglycemia per se.

Type 1 diabetic patients are much more prone to hypoglycemia for several reasons. Insulin enters the circulation from a non-physiologic source (e.g., a subcutaneous depot) that is unaffected by regulatory responses to a falling blood glucose level. In addition, these patients for unclear reasons have attenuated or absent glucagon secretion during hypoglycemia, although glucagon responses to other stimuli persist. Defective glucagon responses develop in most patients after 2 to 5 years, about the time that they become totally insulin dependent. Consequently, they must rely heavily on their ability to release epinephrine. Unfortunately, nearly half of type 1 patients with disease for over 10 years also undergo a stimulus-specific diminution in their epinephrine response to hypoglycemia that increases its risk. The ability of type 1 patients to recognize hypoglycemia and take corrective action may be impaired as well, further adding to the risk. Symptoms result from changes in autonomic activity and brain function. Autonomic symptoms, including sweating, tremor, and palpitations, are often the earliest subjective warning of hypoglycemia. Symptoms and signs of glucose deficiency in the central nervous system, termed neuroglycopenia, may be non-specific (e.g., fatigue or weakness) or more clearly neurologic (e.g., double vision, oral paresthesias, slurring of speech, apraxia, and behavioral disturbances). The irritability and confusion that occur during hypoglycemia may prevent a patient's awareness of their cause. Some diabetic patients lose their normal autonomic warning symptoms of hypoglycemia and may recognize the condition only when somatic neurologic function becomes impaired. Loss of awareness of symptoms is more likely to be found in patients with long disease duration and is associated with an absent or impaired sympathoadrenal response. The duration of diabetes, however, is not the only factor responsible for impaired adrenergic and symptomatic responses to hypoglycemia. Similar phenomena may also occur when patients are switched to intensive insulin regimens. The introduction of intensified treatment regimens can lower the specific glucose level that triggers epinephrine release and adrenergic symptoms (Fig. 242–9), which at least partly explains the increased frequency of severe hypoglycemia reported in the DCCT. The mechanism underlying the changes is the increased appearance of iatrogenic hypoglycemia during intensified insulin therapy; it has been shown that brief periods of antecedent hypoglycemia suppress counterregulatory hormone responses and symptoms during subsequent hypoglycemia for several days. The defective glucose counterregulation induced by intensive insulin regimens appears to be reversible by scrupulous avoidance of hypoglycemia and readjustment of treatment goals, which underscores the need to prevent iatrogenic hypoglycemia by improving self-management skills.

PATHOGENESIS OF CHRONIC DIABETIC COMPLICATIONS

The pathogenesis of the microvascular and neuropathic complications of diabetes remains poorly understood. Proteins are readily

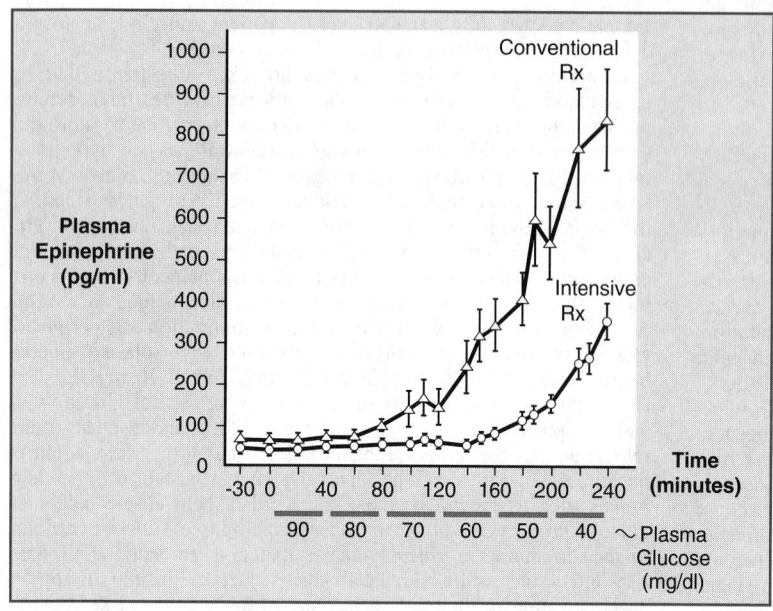

FIGURE 242–9 ■ Plasma epinephrine levels during a stepwise reduction in plasma glucose levels from 90 to 40 mg per deciliter over 4 hours in patients with type I diabetes before *(triangles)* and after several months of intensive insulin treatment *(circles).* (Adapted from Amiel SA, Sherwin RS, Simonson DC, Tamborlane WV: Diabetes 37:901, 1988.)

glycosylated in vivo in direct proportion to the prevailing levels of glucose. The relative non-specificity of the process is underscored by the fact that non-enzymatic glycosylation involves not only hemoglobin but also serum and membrane proteins, LDLs, peripheral nerve protein (tubulin), and structural proteins. Thus hyperglycemia induces widespread modifications in cellular and structural proteins that may contribute to long-term complications. Advanced glycosylation end products generated by the non-enzymatic glycosylation of long-lived proteins (e.g., collagen, laminin) have been found to accumulate in a variety of tissues, including the kidneys and blood vessels. In experimental diabetic animals, inhibition of advanced glycosylation end product formation not only reduces tissue deposition of these end products but also inhibits the expansion of glomerular volume and urinary protein excretion in the absence of changes in circulating glucose levels. These observations suggest that at least some complications may be amenable to agents that do not depend on reversing hyperglycemia. Other potential biochemical mechanisms through which hyperglycemia could impair cell function include (1) the polyol pathway through which non-phosphorylated glucose is reduced to sorbitol by aldose reductase, which in turn leads to changes in the intracellular oxidation-reduction state, and (2) increased diacylglycerol production with subsequent activation of specific isoforms of protein kinase C. Beneficial effects of aldose reductase inhibitors and specific protein kinase C inhibitors have been demonstrated in animal models of diabetes; however, such effects have not been convincingly shown in patients.

Hemodynamic changes in the microcirculation may also contribute to microangiopathy. In the kidney the GFR is increased out of proportion to plasma flow owing to an elevation in the transglomerular pressure gradient. It has been postulated that the raised glomerular pressures promote transglomerular passage of proteins and advanced glycosylation end products; with time their accumulation in the mesangium could trigger the proliferation of mesangial cells and matrix production, eventually leading to glomerulosclerosis. Compensatory hyperfiltration would develop in less affected glomeruli, but they would ultimately succumb because of progressive glomerular damage. Clinical studies support this view. Unilateral renal artery stenosis diminishes diabetic pathologic lesions in the affected kidney, and angiotensin-converting enzyme (ACE) inhibitors, which reduce intraglomerular pressure, slow the progression of diabetic nephropathy. The diabetes-associated increase in microcirculatory hydrostatic pressure may also contribute to the generalized capillary leakage of macromolecules in diabetic patients.

The above theories would predict the benefits of optimal glycemic control reported by the DCCT in patients with few or no complications. Whether similar benefits can be expected once severe damage has occurred is less clear. Extensive glycosylation of proteins with slow turnover rates would not be readily affected by correction of hyperglycemia. Moreover, the hemodynamic theory

for nephropathy predicts that once glomerular injury causes compensatory hyperfiltration, progressive injury may continue in the remaining glomeruli, regardless of the metabolic state.

Diabetic Retinopathy

Diabetes is the leading cause of blindness in persons aged 20 to 74 years. Blindness occurs 20 times more frequently in diabetic patients than others and is most often seen after the disease has been manifested for at least 15 years. Approximately 10 to 15% of type 1 diabetic patients become legally blind (visual acuity of 20/200 or worse in the better eye), whereas in type 2 diabetic patients the risk is less than half that value. The primary cause of visual loss is retinopathy.

The earliest retinopathy changes are classified as non-proliferative. The first sign is microaneurysms (small red dots 20 to 200 mm), which typically arise in areas of capillary occlusion. Microaneurysms develop after about 3 to 5 years of diabetes and are seen in most conventionally treated patients who have had diabetes for 10 years. Subsequently, retinal blot hemorrhages (round with blurred edges) and hard exudates (variable size, sharply defined and yellow) appear as a result, respectively, of extravasation of blood and lipoproteins. Infarctions of the nerve fiber layer, called "cotton-wool spots" or "soft exudates," may be observed as white or gray rounded swellings. These lesions generally do not affect visual acuity. Advanced non-proliferative lesions occur if retinal ischemia becomes more severe, including intraretinal microvascular abnormalities, dilated capillaries that are very permeable, and venous irregularities. They compose the "pre-proliferative phase" of retinopathy, which predicts a high risk for proliferative retinopathy within 1 to 2 years. Proliferative retinopathy is characterized by the growth of fine tufts of new blood vessels and fibrous tissue from the inner retinal surface or optic nerve head. The vessels and fibrous tissue begin on the retinal surface and later grow into the vitreous, eventually leading to retinal detachment and hemorrhage, the most important contributors to blindness. Occasionally, new vessels may invade the anterior chamber angle and cause intractable glaucoma, severe pain, and blindness. In some patients without proliferative changes, severe visual loss may also develop from vascular leakage (macular edema) and/or vascular occlusion in the area of the macula. Macular edema may be suggested by the presence of large deposits of hard exudates surrounding the macular area but is often undetectable by direct ophthalmoscopy. Maculopathy is more common in type 2 diabetes and is an important cause of decreased visual acuity in this group. Visual loss in diabetes is further complicated by the high prevalence rates of cataracts and open-angle glaucoma. Diabetic patients commonly report changes in vision resulting from osmotic swelling of the lens secondary to hyperglycemia. These changes are reversed by improved glycemic control and must be distinguished from more serious ocular pathology.

The eye provides a unique window through which to follow the appearance and progression of retinopathy. Regardless of the type of diabetes, the severity of retinopathy increases with increasing duration of the disease. The one exception is early childhood diabetes; before puberty, retinopathy (as well as other complications) is less common regardless of disease duration. Prevalence rates of both non-proliferative and proliferative retinopathy are higher in type 1 than in type 2 diabetes. In conventionally treated type 1 diabetes, patients rarely, if ever, exhibit retinopathy when diabetes is first diagnosed. Thereafter, the frequency of retinopathy rises to 20 to 25% at 5 years, 50 to 70% at 10 years, and greater than 95% after 15 years. Proliferative retinopathy is rare within the first 10 years of type 1 diabetes but increases to 50% after 20 years. Less common in type 2 diabetes, proliferative retinopathy appears in about 10 to 15% of patients after 20 years. Retinopathy affects about 15 to 20% of type 2 diabetic patients at the time of disease detection, which implies that the disease had previously been undetected.

Although retinopathy may be triggered by hyperglycemia, eventually retinal vascular perfusion diminishes, and this decline in perfusion is believed to accelerate the process. New vessels generally appear in areas of non-perfusion. Ischemia may provoke the local production of growth factors such as vascular endothelial growth factor, which stimulates retinal angioneogenesis in animals. Retinopathy and macular edema are accelerated by hypertension, nephropathy, and pregnancy. At present, medical therapy is restricted to optimization of glycemic control, which delays and slows the progression of non-proliferative retinopathy. Little evidence suggests that improving glycemic control benefits the more advanced stages of retinopathy. In addition, hypertension must be treated aggressively. Surgical therapy using retinal photocoagulation is the treatment of choice when progressive retinopathy threatens vision. Its value was established by the prospective Diabetic Retinopathy Study involving patients with proliferative retinopathy. The risk of severe visual loss in treated eyes was less than half of that in untreated eyes. The study also defined the advantage of panretinal photocoagulation for proliferative lesions (e.g., involving the disk, associated with hemorrhage), which posed the highest risk for visual loss. The more recent Early Treatment Diabetic Retinopathy Study involved patients at an earlier stage and showed an even more striking reduction in the risk of visual loss after laser therapy. It established the benefit of photocoagulation for nearly all patients with new vessels, regardless of severity, and for macular edema. The trial found that interventions at the non-proliferative stage had no detectable value. In more advanced proliferative retinopathy, vitrectomy may be required to remove vitreous hemorrhage or to cut extensive fibrous bands causing retinal detachment. In such cases, surgery may restore vision, although vitrectomy has risks, including retinal detachment, cataract formation, and glaucoma.

The above considerations make it imperative for physicians to prospectively identify patients at risk. Non-specialists, including house officers, internists, and diabetologists, have difficulty diagnosing proliferative retinopathy; in one study, proliferative retinopathy was correctly diagnosed in fewer than half the cases! Accordingly, diabetic patients should be advised to have annual ophthalmologic examinations. In type 1 diabetes, ophthalmologic visits should begin within 3 to 5 years, whereas type 2 diabetic patients should be seen from disease onset.

Diabetic Nephropathy

ESRD from diabetic nephropathy (see also Chapter 110) is a major cause of death, particularly in type 1 diabetes, in which it affects 30 to 35% of patients. Although it is less frequent (about 20%) in the type 2 diabetic population, in part because of their shorter life expectancy, type 2 diabetes still constitutes the majority of diabetic patients seeking therapy for ESRD. Overall, diabetes is the leading cause and accounts for one third of the ESRD cases in the United States.

The natural history of diabetic nephropathy has been well characterized in type 1 diabetes (Fig. 242–10); much fewer data are available for type 2. Soon after diagnosis, the GFR is commonly increased as a result of renal hypertrophy and an increase in glomerular volume and capillary surface area. Hyperfiltration depends, at least in part, on hyperglycemia because it is diminished by intensive treatment. After several years glomerulosclerosis appears and is characterized by thickening of the glomerular capillary basement membrane and expansion of collagen matrix material within

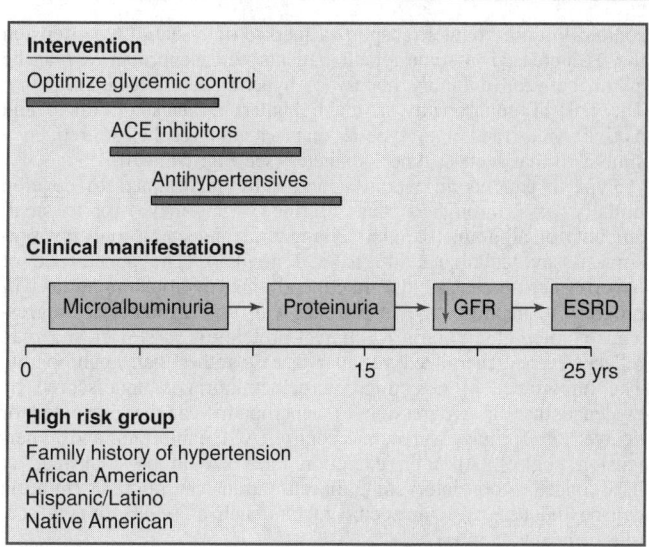

FIGURE 242–10 ■ The natural history of diabetic nephropathy and the time sequence of various medical interventions.

the mesangial region, as well as arteriolosclerosis. In the early years of this histologic evolution, renal function is not impaired and routine urinalysis test strips show no evidence of proteinuria. Although mesangial and capillary wall changes continue to develop in most patients as the duration of diabetes increases, sufficiently extensive glomerulosclerosis to cause ESRD develops in only a minority. Renal biopsy specimens from these individuals generally show more pronounced expansion of mesangial volume and diffuse deposits of mesangial matrix that presumably encroach on the glomerular filtering capacity. Accordingly, routine tests of renal function (e.g., serum creatinine and urinalysis) remain normal during a long "silent" period as glomerular compromise gradually progresses. Detection of renal disease requires sensitive assays of albumin excretion (microalbuminuria).

In patients in whom ESRD is destined to develop, gross proteinuria (>0.3 g of albumin per day) begins approximately 15 years after the diagnosis of type 1 diabetes. At this time, renal function remains normal, but hypertension is generally present. After a variable period, however (about 3 years), the GFR diminishes, as reflected by an increase in serum creatinine. The appearance of massive proteinuria and the nephrotic syndrome is common in this context and often heralds progression to renal insufficiency. Once serum creatinine rises (reflecting a 40 to 50% decline in GFR), ESRD develops in most patients within 10 years. The course is highly variable, however, particularly in type 2 diabetes, in which moderate proteinuria may persist for many years without substantive deterioration in renal function. A simple but useful method of monitoring progression of renal failure is to plot the reciprocal of the serum creatinine as a function of time. This technique allows better assessment of therapeutic interventions and the time when dialysis will be necessary.

Several potential complications accentuate renal dysfunction in diabetes. Azotemic patients are at higher risk for acute renal failure after the injection of contrast for diagnostic studies. When such tests are necessary, special attention should be given to ensure adequate hydration before and immediately after the procedure. Other types of renal disease are also more prevalent in diabetes. Asymptomatic bacteriuria and pyelonephritis are about twice as common, especially in women. Multiple factors, including autonomic bladder dysfunction, impaired perfusion, and glycosuria, enhance bacterial growth. Papillary necrosis is associated with diabetes in over half the cases, and renal artery stenosis is more common in patients with diabetes. Particularly in patients receiving ACE inhibitors, hyperkalemia may develop. A variety of other factors contribute to hyperkalemia, including insulin deficiency, metabolic acidosis, reduced GFR, tubulointerstitial disease, and the syndrome of hyporeninemic hypoaldosteronism commonly seen in older patients with impaired renal function.

A genetic predisposition to hypertension and persistent elevations in the GFR predict an increased risk of nephropathy. Erythrocyte sodium-lithium countertransport, a marker of essential hypertension that is increased in some type 1 patients with nephropathy, may be a link between a family history of hypertension and nephropathy. The risk of nephropathy is much higher in blacks, Latinos, and Native Americans with type 2 diabetes and reaches a frequency similar to that seen in type 1 diabetes (see Fig. 242–10).

Type 1 patients in whom nephropathy is destined to develop initially pass through a stage during which they excrete small amounts of albumin (or microalbuminuria) detectable only by sensitive assay techniques (40 to 300 mg/day). The appearance of hypertension increases the likelihood that microalbuminuria will progress to nephropathy. In patients with type 2 diabetes, progression of microalbuminuria to clinical proteinuria is slower and may reflect severe generalized vascular disease rather than nephropathy. The importance of detecting microalbuminuria is underscored by evidence that its progression to nephropathy can be prevented or delayed by optimized glycemic control, ACE inhibitors, and hypertension control. Albumin excretion rates should be confirmed at least once before intervening because transient microalbuminuria can be induced by non-specific factors such as severe hyperglycemia or heavy exercise.

Treatment of nephropathy varies depending on the stage of disease (see Fig. 242–10). Early in the course of diabetes (no microalbuminuria), primary efforts should focus on optimizing glycemic control, especially in higher-risk patients. Other measures should include aggressive treatment of coexisting hypertension, as well as routine screening for asymptomatic urinary tract infections and bladder dysfunction. We recommend strict glycemic control in conjunction with ACE inhibitors for patients with microalbuminuria. ACE inhibitors appear to have special value, with benefits, such as retarding proteinuria, that are independent of their blood pressure–lowering effects. Once clinical nephropathy becomes evident, aggressive efforts at glycemic control have marginal value; reducing hypertension and intraglomerular pressure with ACE inhibitors alone or in combination with other antihypertensive agents remains the only proven means of slowing progression. Dietary protein restriction (i.e., 0.8 g/kg of body weight) may add limited benefit once the GFR becomes subnormal. As ESRD approaches, long-term treatment plans should proceed much as they would in non-diabetic uremic patients, but therapy should be instituted earlier. Diabetic patients tolerate uremia poorly: Retinopathy and neuropathy deteriorate more rapidly, hypertension becomes more difficult to control, glycemic excursions increase, and protein wasting is aggravated. The acceleration in generalized atherosclerosis leads to significant morbidity during dialysis or following transplantation. The decision between transplantation and dialysis should be individualized. Renal transplantation represents the treatment of choice for most young patients, especially if one can find a matched living related donor. Survival rates for recipients of cadaver grafts remain high and are only about 10% less than those for non-diabetic graft recipients. Cardiovascular disease is the major cause of morbidity and mortality following transplantation. Accordingly, transplant candidates should be evaluated prospectively and treated for vascular insufficiency. Most older type 2 patients are offered dialysis. The preference between continuous ambulatory peritoneal dialysis and hemodialysis varies among centers. However, many diabetic patients have problems caused by the rapid shifts in blood volume that accompany hemodialysis. Although survival rates are considerably worse for dialysis than for transplantation, this difference may reflect the fact that the patients are older and have more severe underlying disease. Mortality is substantially higher in diabetic than non-diabetic patients receiving dialysis because of the more rapid development of vascular insufficiency.

Diabetic Neuropathy

Symptomatic, potentially disabling neuropathy affects nearly 50% of diabetic patients. It is usually symmetrical, but may be focal and often involves the autonomic nervous system as well. The prevalence of symmetrical neuropathy is similar in type 1 and 2 diabetes, whereas focal neuropathy is more common in older type 2 patients. Because it is a heterogeneous collection of clinical syndromes, multiple pathogenetic factors are probably involved. Hyperglycemia figures prominently; however, other factors may also be important, especially ischemia. The chronic, more insidious

neuropathic disorders may be mediated by a "metabolic" process, whereas the more acute, often self-limiting neuropathies may have a vascular cause. Nerve growth factor is diminished in the nerves of patients with neuropathy, perhaps limiting regenerative capacity. Autonomic nerve bundles and ganglia from type 1 diabetic patients with autonomic neuropathy show monocytic infiltration, and their sera may contain complement-fixing antibodies to sympathetic ganglia, thus suggesting that autoimmune mechanisms may also contribute to this complication. Because the mechanisms producing such a heterogeneous clinical picture are poorly understood, neuropathy is classified according to the areas affected (Table 242–9). Currently, therapy is mainly limited to improving glycemic control. This approach is, however, most effective mainly before clinical symptoms have developed.

DISTAL SENSORIMOTOR NEUROPATHY. This syndrome, characterized by axonal loss, is the most common manifestation of diabetic neuropathy. The process involves all somatic nerves but has a distinct predilection for distal sites, e.g., the distal sensorimotor nerves of the feet and hands. Patients complain of numbness and tingling in the extremities, especially the feet. Symptoms characteristically worsen at night, and function usually declines relentlessly with time. In early cases, the neuropathy can be asymptomatic and may be discovered only during clinical examination. Sometimes, distal neuropathy first expresses its presence via complications, such as foot ulceration or spreading cellulitis from a traumatic cut (see below). Bedside clinical testing typically demonstrates a symmetrical loss of sensation distally, with variable loss of distal reflexes (e.g., ankle) and muscle wasting of the intrinsic muscles of the hands and feet. Damage usually affects sensory more than motor fibers and usually encompasses both small (pain and temperature) and large (position and touch) sensory fibers. In less obvious cases, subtler deficits may be detected by testing with a 10-g Semmes-Weinstein monofilament, thermal discrimination, vibration sense thresholds, and nerve conduction. Because the clinical picture is not distinguishable from that of other forms of distal neuropathy (e.g., alcohol, heavy metal, uremia, amyloidosis), the diagnosis is one of exclusion.

ACUTE SENSORY NEUROPATHY. This less common form of neuropathy is symptomatically distressing but usually self-limiting. It may develop after a period of altered metabolic control, such as an episode of diabetic ketoacidosis. It is characterized by severe pain, hyperesthesias, and worsening of pain at night. The hyperesthesia can be so severe that even contact with bedclothes brings on distressing pain. Some cases are associated with weight loss and depression. Pathologic studies show a loss of small sensory fibers. Occasionally, small fiber injury is selective, with vibratory and position sense and motor function left intact.

PROXIMAL MOTOR NEUROPATHY. This syndrome, also known as diabetic amyotrophy or femoral neuropathy, affects males more than females and tends to occur in elderly type 2 patients. It is characterized by wasting and weakness of the major proximal muscle groups of the pelvis and may be accompanied by sensory defects, often with a femoral nerve distribution. The anterolateral muscles of the calf are less often involved. Occasionally an extension plantar response is present. Some overlap is seen with the clinical features of acute sensory neuropathy in that most such patients have suffered recent severe weight loss and many are depressed. Nerve biopsies show ischemic changes in keeping with a vascular cause. This form of neuropathy has a good prognosis; most cases resolve within 12 months.

MONONEUROPATHIES. The mononeuropathies are a collection of isolated lesions affecting the cranial or peripheral nerves. They usually have a sudden onset and occur most often asymmetrically. The oculomotor, trochlear, and abducens nerves mark the most common sites for a cranial nerve lesion, with lesions of the oculomotor nerve characteristically sparing the pupillary reflex. The me-

Table 242–9 ■ **CLASSIFICATION OF DIABETIC NEUROPATHY**

POLYNEUROPATHIES	MONONEUROPATHIES
Distal symmetrical	Isolated nerve lesions
Chronic sensorimotor	Peripheral
Acute sensory	Cranial
Proximal motor	Radiculopathy
Autonomic	

dian, radial, and lateral popliteal nerves are the most common sites of peripheral nerve lesions. The cause of such lesions is unknown, but their sudden onset suggests a vascular component. Nerve entrapment may contribute to peripheral nerve lesions. Painful radiculopathies may also occur in the distribution of one or a number of spinal roots and be manifested as an asymmetrical lesion in a well-defined dermatome(s) that may be confused with herpetic neuralgia or occasionally with abdominal or cardiac disease. The mononeuropathies and radiculopathies are symptomatically distressing, but all tend to resolve with time.

AUTONOMIC NEUROPATHY. Symptomatic, autonomic diabetic neuropathy produces a wide range of problems and carries a poor prognosis. It usually accompanies other chronic complications of diabetes and may play a role in their pathogenesis through disturbed regulation of local blood flow. Neuropathic lesions may result in abnormalities of the cardiovascular system, skin, gastrointestinal tract, bladder, and sexual function. In recent years a battery of tests of cardiac autonomic function based on reduced changes in the RR interval of the electrocardiogram following a Valsalva maneuver or standing have proved useful diagnostically. The most disabling cardiovascular effect is orthostatic hypotension, caused by an impaired sympathetic vasoconstrictor response and possibly impaired cardiac reflexes. Medications that cause volume depletion or vasodilation may worsen the hypotension. More commonly, cardiac denervation results in a rapid heart rate and an impaired heart rate response to stress. Patients with cardiovascular autonomic neuropathy are more likely to have silent myocardial ischemia or infarction, an abnormal prolongation of the QT interval, and defective heart rate and blood pressure responses to exercise, each of which is potentially capable of precipitating an acute cardiac event. Autonomic sudomotor dysfunction is characterized by distal anhidrosis, compensatory truncal and facial sweating, heat intolerance, and on occasion, gustatory sweating. Heat stroke and hyperthermia are the most serious risks, especially when vascular disease is present. It may also facilitate foot infections by creating breaks in the skin. Altered gastrointestinal function is frequent. The most common symptom is constipation, but diarrhea is often the most distressing. Diarrhea may have a variety of causes, including hypermotility secondary to impaired sympathetic inhibition, hypomotility leading to bacterial overgrowth, pancreatic insufficiency, or celiac sprue, which may occur in type 1 patients. The problem may be compounded by fecal incontinence from the loss of sphincter control and by intensification of diarrhea during sleep. Gastroparesis may lead to complaints such as bloating and early satiety after meals or nausea and vomiting. This problem affects patients receiving insulin, in whom unpredictable food absorption may adversely affect glycemic control and exacerbate hypoglycemia. Bladder dysfunction caused by neuropathy leads to infrequent urination, incomplete bladder emptying, dribbling, and overflow incontinence. Bladder residual volumes may exceed 150 mL and predispose to urinary tract infection. Psychologically, the most disturbing complication of autonomic neuropathy is impaired sexual function, which in males is characterized by impotence and retrograde ejaculation. The prevalence of sexual dysfunction may be as high as 50% in males and 25% in females at some point in the disease. One must exclude psychogenic or other organic causes of impotence resulting from medications, alcohol, or vascular insufficiency.

TREATMENT. In the absence of specific ways to reverse established neuropathy, pain control is the highest priority. Some patients respond to standard analgesic therapies. Anticonvulsants (e.g., gabapentin) and tricyclic antidepressants have shown some efficacy in prospective randomized trials. Intravenous lidocaine may be of benefit when pain is extremely severe. Occasionally, opiates are the only option. Autonomic neuropathy causes specific problems for which more therapeutic interventions are available. Stocking supports, 9α-fluorohydrocortisone, pindolol (a β-blocker with partial agonist properties), and clonidine have all been used with mixed success for orthostatic hypotension. Metoclopramide and cisapride can stimulate gastric emptying in cases of gastroparesis. Erythromycin also stimulates gastric emptying and may be helpful. These patients should avoid high-fiber diets, which interfere with treatment. Diarrhea may respond to broad-spectrum antibiotics, clonidine, or agents such as diphenoxylate or loperamide (Imodium), and bladder emptying may be enhanced by drugs such as bethanechol. Treatment of impotence in males includes vacuum erection aids, intracorporeal papaverine or phentolamine injections, and pe-

nile prosthetic implants. Sildenafil citrate, a new oral therapy, ameliorates erectile dysfunction in nearly half of diabetic patients. It acts by inhibiting a tissue-specific cyclic guanosine monophosphate (cGMP) phosphodiesterase, thereby increasing the concentration of cGMP in the corpus cavernosum, which in the presence of nitric oxide (released by sexual stimulation) leads to smooth muscle relaxation and erection.

Diabetic Foot

The "diabetic foot" results from a complex interplay of factors. The syndrome is characterized by plantar ulcers that heal slowly and follow apparently insignificant trauma. In severe cases, gangrene may be a complication and amputation the outcome. Diabetes accounts for about half of non-traumatic limb amputations. To varying degrees, the diabetic foot is characterized by chronic sensorimotor neuropathy, autonomic neuropathy, and poor peripheral circulation; visual loss may also contribute to difficulties with self-care. Sensorimotor neuropathy results in loss of normal sensation, which prevents the detection of traumatic events. Accordingly, sharp objects left in the sole of the shoe or ill-fitting shoes may erode the skin surface without signaling pain. Neuropathy also produces abnormal motor function of the intrinsic muscles of the foot and abnormal proprioception, thereby altering weight distribution on the sole. Unnatural weight bearing on the metatarsal heads and clawing of the metatarsophalangeal joints result. Also, callus formation occurs at these sites and may erode the softer underlying tissues. In severe cases the abnormal distribution of weight endured by the foot can result in repeated painless fractures and displacement of normal joint surfaces and produce the so-called Charcot joint. Impaired peripheral circulation often coexists. Atheromatous plaque in the descending aorta, major vessels of the leg, or distal sites compromises flow. Diminished cardiac output secondary to cardiovascular disease and/or disturbed autoregulatory mechanisms of the microcirculation may contribute to impaired peripheral blood flow. Characteristically, the diabetic foot, in the absence of severe atheromatous disease, appears to be well perfused with a skin surface that is normally warm and dry. This appearance of the foot is thought to be due to increased skin blood flow and reduced sweating, both features of impaired autonomic regulation. Treatment of the diabetic foot is aimed primarily at prevention, which involves education (Table 242–10) and regular checking of the state of the feet of patients at risk during routine visits and by foot care specialists. Proper preventive foot care can reduce the rate of amputations by 50%. In cases of deformed feet, orthotics to minimize abnormal weight bearing or orthopedically fitted shoes may be required. It is essential that ulcers be treated immediately with broad-spectrum antibiotics, dead tissue débridement, and appropriate dressings. Local application of growth factors may also be useful. Cast immobilization made for the foot may be a useful adjunct to the treatment of foot ulcers by redistributing weight away from an ulcerated area. Surgical removal or débridement is required for non-viable tissue such as gangrenous toes or deep soft tissue infections with evidence of gas gangrene. In extensive cases, foot or even leg amputation may be necessary; a compromised peripheral circulation makes this outcome more likely. If poor circulation is a dominant feature, one must attempt to improve distal flow by surgery or angioplasty.

Table 242–10 ■ **FOOT CARE PRESCRIPTION FOR HIGH-RISK PATIENTS***

Never walk barefooted
Do not apply hot water or heating pads to the feet
Inspect the feet daily (use a mirror for plantar surfaces)
Keep the feet clean, dry between toes
Lubricate dry skin with a non-greasy lotion or cream to avoid cracking
Wear properly fitting soft shoes
Break in new shoes slowly
Use a 2nd pair of shoes at night (larger size for edema)
Cut toenails straight across
Visit foot care specialist regularly
Stop smoking

*High-risk patients include those with neuropathy and/or vascular insufficiency.

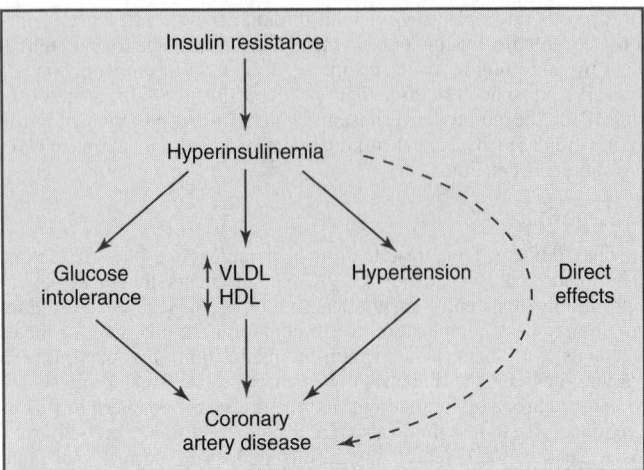

FIGURE 242–11 ■ Syndrome X, a hypothesis based on the premise that insulin resistance accounts for the clustering of cardiovascular risk factors within a given individual.

Atherosclerosis and Hypertension

Atherosclerosis involving the arteries of the heart, lower extremities, and brain is the major cause of death from diabetes. The atherosclerotic process is indistinguishable from that affecting the non-diabetic population but begins earlier and may be more severe. The predilection to atherosclerosis is observed over the entire spectrum of diabetes—from difficult-to-control insulin-dependent patients to patients with mild hyperglycemia not necessitating insulin. For unclear reasons, the disparity between diabetic and normal subjects is more pronounced in women.

Diabetes is an independent risk factor for accelerated atherosclerosis and not solely attributable to an increased frequency of the other recognized risk factors, e.g., hypertension or dyslipidemia. Abnormalities induced by the diabetic state could be responsible, such as small dense atherogenic LDL, oxidized or glycosylated LDL, increased platelet aggregation, hyperviscosity, endothelial cell dysfunction, decreased fibrinolysis, and increased clotting factors and fibrinogen. Clinical studies indirectly support the hypothesis that hyperinsulinemia per se may contribute to macrovascular disease in diabetes, perhaps by stimulatory effects on smooth muscle proliferation.

Diabetes may be accompanied by other risk factors for atherosclerosis that markedly increase the incidence of macrovascular complications. The prevalence of hypertension is increased at least 2-fold in patients with type 2 diabetes, partly because of the clustering of both disorders in patients with obesity and insulin resistance. Hypertension is not associated with type 1 diabetes in the absence of renal disease but develops in most patients with nephropathy. Although LDL cholesterol levels are commonly not higher in diabetes, dyslipidemia characterized by elevated triglycerides, decreased HDL cholesterol, and smaller, denser LDL cholesterol is often seen in type 2 diabetic patients and in poorly controlled type 1 diabetes. The presence of dyslipidemia is associated with the severity of macrovascular disease. Thus the major cardiovascular risk factors—hypertension, hypercholesterolemia, and smoking—interact with diabetes to further promote atherosclerosis. As a result, the risk of myocardial infarction is 2- to 3-fold greater in diabetes but increases to about 8-fold in the presence of hypertension and to nearly 20-fold if hypercholesterolemia coexists. Smoking enhances the risk even further. The diagnosis of diabetes should prompt a careful search for other risk factors for atherosclerotic vascular disease and initiation of aggressive preventive measures.

Because hypertension accelerates not only atherosclerosis but also nephropathy and retinopathy, even minimal elevations in blood pressure should be treated that in non-diabetics might be dismissed. It should be noted that the normal nocturnal fall in blood pressure may be lost in diabetic patients, thus leading to more sustained hypertension throughout the day. The importance of aggressive treatment of hypertension is clearly established by the results of the UKPDS (see above). In type 2 diabetic patients with coexisting hypertension in the study, blood pressure reduction (with ACE inhibitors or β-blockers) produced striking decreases in both cardiovascular and microvascular outcomes. Initially, non-pharmacologic treatment measures such as weight loss, exercise training, and sodium restriction may be tried. If blood pressure is not lowered below 130/85 mm Hg, drug therapy is indicated. The selection of drugs should be individualized, with other coexisting medical problems taken into consideration. Among the various therapeutic options, ACE inhibitors may offer special advantages, especially when concomitant renal disease and hyperkalemia are not present. Alternatively, β-blockers may be used. In the UKPDS, β-blocker therapy was just as effective as ACE inhibitors in reducing cardiovascular and microvascular outcomes. Moreover, β-blockers are known to be cardioprotective for patients who have had a myocardial infarction. β-Blockers should be avoided, however, in patients who are predisposed to hypoglycemia inasmuch as they may compromise counterregulatory defense mechanisms. Angiotensin II receptor blockers, α-adrenergic blockers, and vasodilators have no adverse metabolic effects and are therefore good therapeutic alternatives. Diuretics may be helpful as adjuncts if a volume component is associated with the hypertension. If thiazides are used, they should be given in small doses to minimize their adverse effects on glucose and lipid control. Recent data suggest that hypertensive treatment with calcium channel blockers, although effective in low-

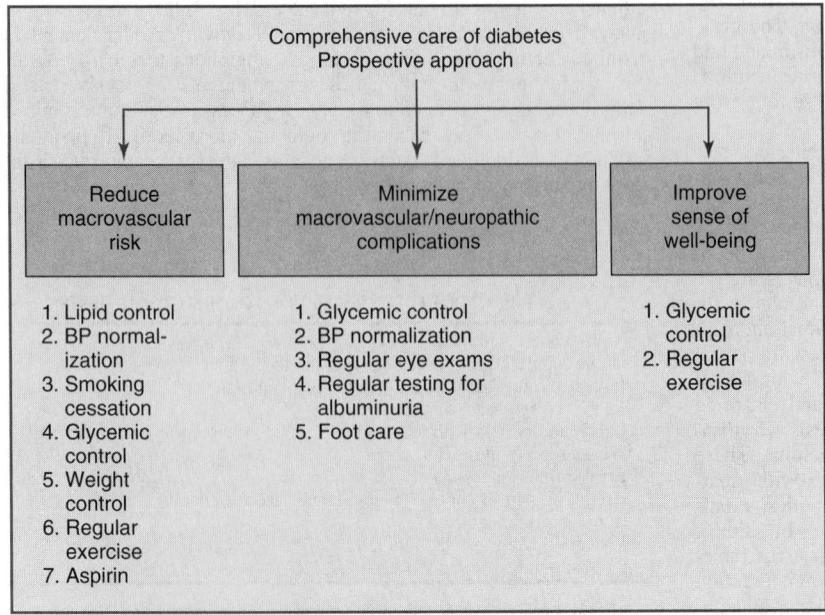

FIGURE 242–12 ■ The key elements of a comprehensive management plan for patients with diabetes.

ering blood pressure, may be less effective in reducing the risk of cardiovascular events in diabetic subjects.

Elevations in LDL cholesterol must also be treated. Because women with diabetes have a cardiovascular risk similar to that of men, all diabetic patients should be viewed as "high risk," regardless of gender. The minimum goals should be an LDL cholesterol level less than 130 mg/dL, but lower values should be the target if evidence of vascular disease is present (e.g., below 100 mg/dL). The 1st step lies in reinforcement of diet and optimization of glycemic control. If this measure fails, hepatic hydroxymethylglutaryl coenzyme A reductase inhibitors (or, alternatively, bile sequestrants) are recommended. Nicotinic acid is less useful because it increases insulin resistance and hyperglycemia. More commonly, diabetes is associated with elevations of very-low-density lipoprotein triglyceride and reductions in HDL cholesterol. These variables often respond to weight reduction, diet modification, regular exercise, and other measures aimed at improving glycemic control. If this option fails, drug therapy (e.g., fibric acid derivatives) should be considered. Unfortunately, drug treatment is more effective in lowering triglyceride than raising HDL cholesterol levels. Low-dose aspirin therapy should be routinely recommended because it reduces cardiovascular events in diabetic patients much like its effect in non-diabetic individuals. Large vessel disease in diabetics is as well treated surgically as it is in non-diabetic illness. Similarly, the frequency of multiple coronary vessel disease and the outcome of coronary vascular surgery differ only slightly between diabetic and non-diabetic persons. In contrast, the benefits of angioplasty for the treatment of multiple coronary artery occlusions are significantly reduced in diabetic patients.

The association of diabetes with premature atherosclerosis may only represent the "tip of the iceberg." Impaired insulin-stimulated glucose metabolism commonly affects seemingly healthy people living in industrialized Western countries, but it is generally counterbalanced by increased insulin secretion. Although this state of chronic hyperinsulinemia may successfully defend against the development of diabetes, it has been suggested that a price may be paid (Fig. 242–11). According to this hypothesis, compensatory hyperinsulinemia has adverse effects on other systems affected by insulin, such as sympathetic nervous system activity, renal sodium reabsorption, hepatic triglyceride synthesis, and arterial smooth muscle proliferation. Healthy, non-obese, non-diabetic individuals with hyperinsulinemia have higher blood pressure and glucose and triglyceride levels and lower HDL cholesterol concentrations than do subjects with normal insulin levels. The term syndrome X (or metabolic syndrome) has been coined to describe this phenomenon, namely, the clustering within the same person of hyperinsulinemia, mild glucose intolerance, dyslipidemia, and hypertension, each of which is a risk factor for atherosclerosis. Several prospective population studies have found that the presence of hyperinsulinemia is closely related to the subsequent appearance of cardiovascular disease. Although statistical associations of this sort do not prove causality, they suggest that insulin resistance could have a potential role in the pathogenesis of atherosclerosis. If true, it further underscores the importance of lifestyle changes that improve insulin action in the treatment of type 2 diabetes and suggests that the same approach could benefit insulin-resistant patients with more subtle metabolic abnormalities (syndrome X or impaired glucose tolerance and impaired fasting glucose). These data should not, however, be a signal to lower therapeutic insulin doses because the long-term adverse effects of hyperglycemia in diabetic patients are much greater than those caused by hyperinsulinemia. This point is clearly supported by the UKPDS. In that long-term trial, more intensive treatment with insulin or sulfonylurea agents that raise insulin levels tended to reduce and did not increase cardiovascular events.

SUMMARY

The long-term goals of diabetes care consist of minimizing vascular and neurologic complications and maintaining a sense of well-being. These goals are best attained by early detection and treatment. In view of the wide array of potential problems and their multifactorial nature, diabetes care must be comprehensive rather than limited to glycemic control. Attention should be devoted to risk factors that compound the adverse effect of diabetes on atherogenesis, the principal cause of mortality from the disease. Because the complications of diabetes develop slowly and are not readily reversible, it is crucial for clinicians to take a prospective approach, as summarized in Figure 242–12.

American Diabetes Association: Clinical Practice recommendations 1998. Diabetes Care 21(Suppl.):1, 1998. *An up-to-date summary of the current classification of diabetes and standards of care for the management of diabetic patients, including the goals of treatment.*

Diabetes Control and Complications Trial Research Group: The effect of intensive treatment of diabetes on the development and progression of long-term complications of insulin-dependent diabetes mellitus. N Engl J Med 329:927, 1993. *This report summarizes the results of the landmark multicenter prospective trial that evaluated the impact of intensive insulin therapy on its long-term complications.*

Kreisberg RA: Diabetic ketoacidosis. *In* Porte D Jr, Sherwin RS (eds): Ellenberg and Rifkin's Diabetes Mellitus, 5th ed. New York, Elsevier, 1997, p 827. *A thorough and current review of the pathogenesis and treatment of this disorder.*

Physician's Guide to Insulin Dependent (Type I) Diabetes: Diagnosis and Treatment, 2nd ed. Alexandria, VA, American Diabetes Association, 1998. *A monograph that provides a detailed review of the diagnosis and treatment of type 1 diabetes.*

Physician's Guide to Non–Insulin-Dependent (Type II) Diabetes: Diagnosis and Treatment, 3rd ed. Alexandria, VA, American Diabetes Association, 1998. *A monograph that reviews the diagnosis, pathogenesis, and treatment of type 2 diabetes.*

Turner RC, Holman RR, Cull CA, et al: Intensive blood-glucose control with sulphonylureas or insulin compared with conventional treatment and risk of complications in patients with type 2 diabetes (UKPDS 33). Lancet 352:837, 1998. *This report summarizes the results of the UKPDS, the longest and largest study of patients with type 2 diabetes. It showed that more intensive therapy aimed at lowering blood glucose reduces diabetes-related complications, particularly microvascular disease.*

243 HYPOGLYCEMIA/PANCREATIC ISLET CELL DISORDERS

Robert A. Rizza ■ *F. John Service*

HYPOGLYCEMIA

Hypoglycemia is a clinical syndrome of diverse causes in which low levels of plasma glucose eventually lead to neuroglycopenia.

Regulation of Carbohydrate Metabolism

Interactions Between Insulin and Counter-Insulin Hormones

Under normal circumstances, plasma glucose concentration averages 70 to 100 mg/dL before meals and rarely exceeds 140 to 150 mg/dL after meals. The brain is almost totally dependent on glucose for energy, although over the long term it can adapt to substrates other than glucose (e.g., ketone bodies). Because severe hypoglycemia can impair mental function and, if prolonged, can cause permanent brain damage, a series of well-developed, and at times redundant, homeostatic processes defend against hypoglycemia. Insulin suppresses glucose production by inhibiting both glycogenolysis and gluconeogenesis. Insulin also stimulates glucose uptake in muscle, liver, and fat. Glucagon, epinephrine, cortisol, and growth hormone, collectively referred to as the counter-regulatory or counter-insulin hormones, oppose the effects of insulin.

In healthy non-diabetic subjects, insulin concentration increases as glucose concentration increases and falls as glucose concentration falls. In contrast, counter-regulatory hormone concentrations change (in general) in the opposite direction of insulin, falling as glucose rises and rising as glucose falls. By so doing, insulin and the counter-insulin hormones act in concert to ensure that the amount of glucose entering and leaving the blood stream is closely matched in both the fed and fasted state. Excess amounts of insulin or insulin-like material (e.g., IGF-1 or IGF-2), inadequate secretion of counter-insulin hormones, insufficient substrate, or defects in the gluconeogenic or glycogenolytic pathways alone or in combination can disrupt this balance and cause hypoglycemia.

Regulation of Glucose Concentration in the Fed State

After an overnight fast (e.g., 8–10 hours), rates or glucose production and utilization average about 2 mg/kg/min. At this time, the majority of the glucose is released from the liver, with a small amount being produced by the kidney. Carbohydrate ingestion increases glucose concentration, which stimulates secretion of insulin from the pancreatic β cells and suppresses secretion of glucagon from the pancreatic α cells. The resultant rise in the insulin-to-glucagon ratio increases hepatic glycogen synthesis and inhibits both glycogenolysis and gluconeogenesis, thereby resulting in a decrease in hepatic glucose release and an increase in hepatic glycogen content. Glucose concentrations continue to rise until the rate of glucose uptake by peripheral tissues exceeds the net amount of glucose (meal-derived and endogenously produced) being released from the splanchnic bed. Glucose concentration then begins to fall toward preprandial levels. This results in a progressive fall in insulin and a progressive rise in glucagon concentrations, which in turn permits a gradual increase in endogenous glucose production and a gradual fall in glucose utilization to basal rates. Depending on the amount and type of food ingested, both glucose concentration and turnover are generally back to basal levels sometime between 4 and 6 hours after the start of a meal.

Thus, the rate of carbohydrate absorption, the timing as well as the amount of insulin and glucagon secreted, the ability of the liver to store and subsequently release glucose, as well as the response of the liver, muscle, and fat to insulin and counter-insulin hormones all interact to minimize the rise in glucose concentration after a meal as well as to ensure a smooth return of glucose concentrations to preprandial levels during the transition from the fed to the postabsorptive state.

Regulation of Glucose Concentrations in the Fasted State

The contribution of gluconeogenesis becomes progressively more important as the duration of fast is extended and hepatic glycogen stores are depleted. The rate of glycogen depletion depends on a variety of factors, including antecedent diet and exercise, but is nearly complete after 24 to 48 hours of fasting. Anything that lowers the demand for glucose lessens the need to break down protein stores. This is accomplished by changing from a primarily carbohydrate-based metabolism in the fed state to a primarily fat-based metabolism in the fasted state.

Insulin decreases and glucagon, growth hormone, and cortisol concentrations all increase as hepatic glycogen is depleted and the glucose concentration falls. This change in the hormonal milieu stimulates lipolysis and ketogenesis, which results in an increase in plasma glycerol, free fatty acid, and ketone body concentrations. Glycerol serves as a gluconeogenic substrate, thereby sparing amino acids. Free fatty acids are metabolized by muscle, liver, and other tissues in place of glucose. Free fatty acids also are converted by means of ketogenesis to acetoacetate and β-hydroxybutyrate, which can substitute for glucose as a fuel for the brain. These metabolic adaptations normally permit glucose to gradually decrease to 40 to 50 mg/dL during a fast without provoking symptoms of hypoglycemia.

Inadequate glycogen stores or breakdown, insufficient gluconeogenesis due to defects in enzyme activity, lack of substrate availa-

bility, or persistent elevations of insulin or insulin-like activity, alone or in combination, can cause or exacerbate hypoglycemia.

Recovery from Hypoglycemia

If counter-regulation is intact, hypoglycemia (regardless of the cause) will result in a decrease in insulin secretion and an increase in glucagon, epinephrine, cortisol, and growth hormone secretion. Glucagon provides the major defense against acute hypoglycemia. Epinephrine appears to become progressively more important when hypoglycemia is prolonged or severe. Permissive amounts of cortisol and growth hormone are required for a normal hepatic response to glucagon and epinephrine. Drugs or diseases that inhibit counter-regulatory hormone secretion or action predispose to hypoglycemia.

Symptoms of Hypoglycemia

Symptoms of hypoglycemia have been classified into two major groups: those arising from activation of the autonomic nervous system (autonomic) and those related to insufficient glucose supply to the brain (neuroglycopenic).

During acute insulin-induced hypoglycemia in healthy persons, autonomic symptoms are recognized at a threshold of approximately 60 mg/dL (3 mM) and impairment of brain function manifested by neuroglycopenic symptoms occurs at a threshold of approximately 50 mg/dL (2.8 mM) in arterialized venous blood (Fig. 243–1). Comparable venous levels would be about 3 mg/dL (0.16 mM) less. The rate of glucose descent does not influence the occurrence of symptoms and signs of hypoglycemia.

Variations among reports regarding allocation of symptoms to the autonomic and neuroglycopenic types may be ascribed to the types of patients examined, diabetic versus nondiabetic, type 1 versus type 2 diabetes, clinical versus experimental conditions, and, probably most importantly, differences among persons regarding their perceptions of symptoms. During experimentally induced hypoglycemia in 20 persons with and 25 persons without diabetes, a principal component analysis allocated sweating, trembling, warmness, anxiety, and nausea to the autonomic group and dizziness, confusion, tiredness, difficulty with speaking, headache, and inability to concentrate to the neuroglycopenic group. Hunger, blurred vision, drowsiness, and weakness could not be allocated to either group with any confidence. In another study of 10 non-diabetic persons, partitioning of symptoms during insulin-induced hypoglycemia allocated shaky/tremulous, heart pounding, nervous/anxious, sweaty, hungry, and tingling to the autonomic group and warm, weak, difficulty thinking/confused, and tired/drowsy to the neuroglycopenic group.

In a retrospective analysis of 60 patients with insulinoma, 85% had various combinations of diplopia, blurred vision, sweating, palpitations, and weakness; 80% had confusion or abnormal behav-

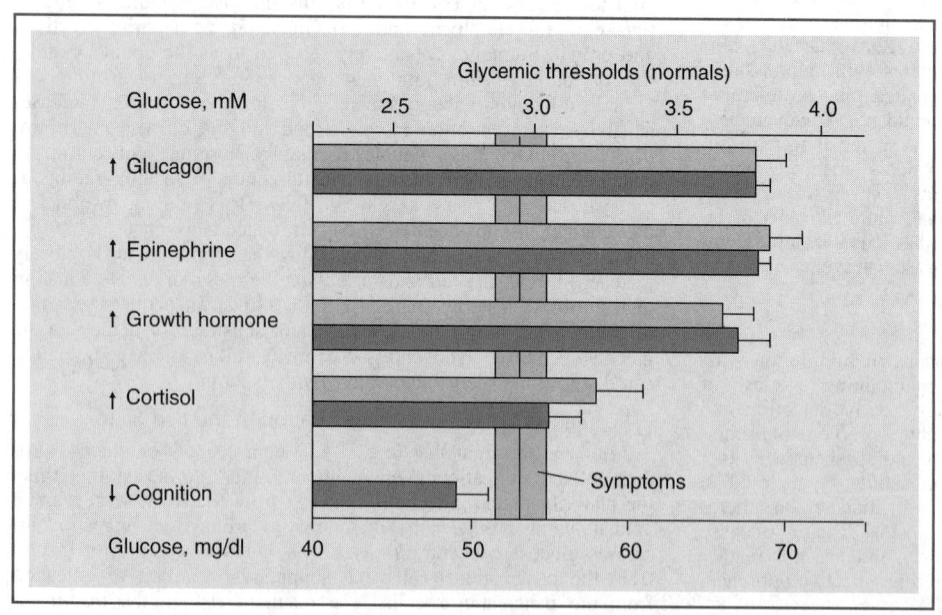

FIGURE 243–1 ■ Arterialized venous glycemic (M ± SE) thresholds for increments in plasma glucagon, epinephrine, growth hormone, and cortisol for symptoms of hypoglycemia and for impairment of cognitive function during decrements in plasma glucose in normal humans from two independent studies. (From Cryer PE: Glucose counterregulation: The physiological mechanisms that prevent or correct hypoglycemia. *In* Frier B, Fisher BM [eds]: Hypoglycaemia and Diabetes: Clinical and Physiological Aspects. London, Boston, Edward Arnold, 1993, pp 34–55 with permission.)

Table 243–1 ■ CLINICAL CLASSIFICATION OF HYPOGLYCEMIC DISORDERS

I. Patient Appears Healthy*
  A. No coexistent disease
    1. Drugs
      a. Ethanol
      b. Salicylates
      c. Quinine
      d. Haloperidol
    2. Insulinoma
    3. Islet hyperplasia/nesidioblastosis
    4. Factitial hypoglycemia from insulin or sulfonylurea
    5. Severe exercise
    6. Ketotic hypoglycemia
  B. Compensated coexistent disease
    1. Drugs
      a. Dispensing error
      b. Disopyramide
      c. β-Adrenergic blocking agents
      d. Sulfhydril- or thiol-containing drugs with autoimmune insulin syndrome
      e. Unripe ackee fruit and undernutrition
II. Patient Appears Ill
  A. Drugs
    1. Pentamidine and *Pneumocystis pneumonia*
    2. Sulfamethoxazole/trimethoprim and renal failure
    3. Propoxyphene and renal failure
    4. Quinine and cerebral malaria
    5. Quinine and malaria
    6. Topical salicylates and renal failure
  B. Predisposing illness
    1. Small-for-gestational-age infant
    2. Beckwith-Wiedemann syndrome
    3. Erythroblastosis fetalis
    4. Infant of diabetic mother
    5. Glycogen storage disease
    6. Defects in amino acid and fatty acid metabolism
    7. Reye's syndrome
    8. Cyanotic congenital heart disease
    9. Hypopituitarism
    10. Isolated growth hormone deficiency
    11. Isolated ACTH deficiency
    12. Addison's disease
    13. Galactosemia
    14. Hereditary fructose intolerance
    15. Carnitine deficiency
    16. Defective type 1 glucose transporter in the brain
    17. Acquired severe liver disease
    18. Large non–β cell tumor
    19. Sepsis
    20. Renal failure
    21. Congestive heart faliure
    22. Lactic acidosis
    23. Starvation
    24. Anorexia nervosa
    25. Postoperative removal of pheochromocytoma
    26. Insulin receptor antibody hypoglycemia
  C. Hospitalized patient
    1. Diseases predisposing to hypoglycemia
    2. Total parenteral nutrition and insulin therapy
    3. Questran interference with glucocorticoid absorption
    4. Shock

*Mutations in the β-cell sulfonylurea receptor gene, glutamate dehydrogenase gene, and glucokinase gene are rare causes of hyperinsulinemic hypoglycemia usually manifested in infancy or childhood.

ior; 50% were amnesic for the episode or had coma; and 12% had generalized seizures. None of the symptoms noted earlier, regardless of type, is specific for hypoglycemia.

Classification of Hypoglycemia

A useful approach for the practitioner is a classification based on clinical characteristics (Table 243–1). Persons who appear healthy are likely to have hypoglycemic disorders different from persons who are ill. Hospitalized patients are at additional risk for hypoglycemia often from iatrogenic factors.

Evaluation of Hypoglycemia

The direction and extent of evaluation is dependent on the clinical presentation. The healthy-appearing patient with no coexistent disease who has a history of episodic symptoms suggestive of hypoglycemia requires an approach quite different from the hospitalized patient with acute hypoglycemia.

Healthy-Appearing Patient

Plasma Glucose

Because symptoms from hypoglycemia are not specific, it is essential to document a low plasma glucose concentration at the time of the occurrence of spontaneous symptoms and relief of symptoms through correction of the low plasma glucose concentration (Whipple's triad) before concluding that a patient has a hypoglycemic disorder. Furthermore, reliance solely on a low blood glucose value to diagnose a hypoglycemic disorder fails to take into consideration the possibility of laboratory error, artifactual hypoglycemia, and, indeed, that normal persons may have plasma glucose levels well below 50 mg/dL (2.8 mM) during prolonged fasting. It is important to recognize that a normal plasma glucose concentration (when measured reliably) obtained during the occurrence of spontaneous symptoms absolutely eliminates the possibility of a hypoglycemic disorder; no further evaluation is required! Although hypoglycemic disorders are uncommon, symptoms suggestive of hypoglycemia are quite common.

Often measurement of plasma glucose is not feasible during the occurrence of spontaneous symptoms during ordinary life activities. Under such circumstances, a judgment whether to proceed with further evaluation depends on a detailed history. Elicitation of a history of neuroglycopenic symptoms or evidence for a confirmed low plasma glucose concentration warrants further testing.

72-Hour Fast

The prolonged supervised (72 hour) fast is the classic diagnostic test. It should be conducted in a standardized fashion. A suggested protocol is shown in Table 243–2. For patients who experience signs or symptoms of hypoglycemia and have simultaneously measured plasma glucose in the hypoglycemic range, the fast should be terminated at that point. Studies in patients who have neither should not be extended beyond 72 hours.

The decision to end the fast may not be easy. Some patients have slightly depressed glycemic levels without symptoms or signs of hypoglycemia. Other patients may reproduce during fasting the symptoms they experienced in ordinary life but may have plasma glucose levels that are sometimes within and sometimes above the hypoglycemic range. Young, lean, healthy women and, to a lesser degree, men, may have plasma glucose levels in the range of 40 mg/dL or even lower after 72 hours of fasting. Careful examination and testing for subtle signs or symptoms of hypoglycemia should be conducted repeatedly when the patient's plasma glucose level is near or in the hypoglycemic range. The prolonged supervised fast (72 hrs) may be ended when plasma glucose is ≤55 mg/dL if Whipple's triad had previously been demonstrated. Beta cell polypeptides are suppressed in healthy persons when plasma glucose is ≤55 mg/dL.

The interpretation of concentrations of β-cell polypeptides (insulin, C peptide, and proinsulin) during the prolonged supervised fast is predicated on the concomitant plasma glucose concentration. The

Table 243–2 ■ PROTOCOL FOR 72-HOUR FAST

1. Date onset of fast as of last ingestion of calories discontinue all nonessential medications.
2. May drink calorie-free and caffeine-free beverages.
3. Must be active during waking hours.
4. Measure plasma glucose, insulin, and C-peptide (on the same venipuncture specimen) every 6 hours until plasma glucose ≤60 mg/dL (3.3 mM) when frequency should be every 1 to 2 hours.
5. End the fast when the plasma glucose is ≤45 mg/dL (2.5 mM) and the patient has symptoms and/or signs of hypoglycemia, or plasma glucose ≤55 mg/dL if Whipple's triad had been demonstrated previously.
6. At the end of the fast, measure plasma glucose, insulin, C-peptide, β-hydroxybutyrate, and sulfonylurea (on the same venipuncture specimen); then inject glucagon 1 mg intravenously and measure plasma glucose q 10 min × 3. After this, feed the patient.
7. Under some circumstances measure plasma cortisol, growth hormone, or glucagon at the end of the fast.

normal overnight fasting ranges for these polypeptides do not apply when the plasma glucose is low (e.g., ≤ 55 mg/dL).

Insulin-mediated hypoglycemic disorders are characterized by plasma insulin concentrations greater than or equal to 6 μU/mL (limit of sensitivity 5 μU/mL using radioimmunoassay) and that persons with non–insulin-mediated hypoglycemic disorders and healthy persons with plasma glucose of less than or equal to 50 mg/dL have insulin concentrations of less than or equal to 5 μU/mL. (Fig. 243–2). Recently, an immunochemiluminometric assay for insulin has been developed that has sensitivity of less than or equal to 1 μU/mL. The criterion for hyperinsulinemia is 3 μU/mL or more using this assay.

Persons with insulinomas have insulin concentrations (radioimmunoassay), that rarely exceed 100-μU/mL range. Values of 1000 μU/mL or greater suggest recent insulin administration or the presence of insulin antibodies. Ratios of glucose to insulin, and vice versa, including the "amended ratio" have been used in an effort to identify relative hyperinsulinemia when the insulin concentration is in the normal overnight fasting range. Unfortunately, these ratios have very poor diagnostic utility.

Criteria for hyperinsulinemia using C-peptide and proinsulin (each measured by immunochemiluminometric assays) are 200 pmol/L or more and 5 pmol/L or more, respectively (see Fig. 243–2). The molar ratio of insulin to C-peptide is the same for patients with insulinomas and healthy individuals (approximately 0.2).

Because of the antiketogenic effect of insulin, plasma β-hydroxybutyrate measurement at the end of the fast (72 hours in normal individuals and at Whipple's triad in patients with a hypoglycemic disorder) is useful. This parameter is considered to be an insulin surrogate. Patients with insulin-mediated hypoglycemia have concentrations of less than 2.7 mmol/L, whereas others (normal individuals or those with non–insulin-mediated hypoglycemia) have higher levels (see Fig. 243–2). Another insulin surrogate is the response of plasma glucose to 1 mg of glucagon injected intravenously at the end of the fast. The rationale for this procedure is that insulin is glycogenic and antiglycogenolytic. Patients with in-

sulin-mediated hypoglycemia have a maximum increment of 25 mg/dL or more above the terminal fasting plasma glucose, whereas others (normal individuals or those with non–isulin-mediated hypoglycemia) have lower increments (see Fig. 243–2). When the plasma glucose concentration exceeds 60 mg/dL at the end of the fast, knowledge of the β-cell polypeptides and insulin surrogates is unnecessary.

Measurement of sulfonylureas in the plasma at the end of the fast is an essential component of the prolonged supervised fast. The pattern of plasma glucose and β-cell polypeptides in sulfonylurea-induced hypoglycemia is identical to that observed in persons with insulinoma. A liquid chromatographic mass spectrography method provides a sensitive measurement of second-generation sulfonylureas. See Table 243–3 for diagnostic interpretation.

Mixed Meal Test

For persons with a history of neuroglycopenic symptoms within 5 hours of food ingestion, a mixed meal test may be conducted. The patients should eat a meal that is similar to that which leads to symptoms during ordinary life activities. The test is positive when the patient experiences neuroglycopenic symptoms and a concomitant plasma glucose is low (e.g., ≤ 50 mg/dL). There are no standards for the interpretation of levels of β-cell polypeptides measured during this test. A positive mixed meal test in and of itself does not provide a diagnosis, only biochemical confirmation of the history. Because patients with insulinoma may have neuroglyopenic symptoms after meals, and in some instances only after meals, all patients with a positive mixed meal test should undergo a prolonged supervised fast. For those patients with a positive mixed meal test and a negative 72-hour fast, glucagon levels during the mixed meal test should be determined to ensure that there was an increase in response to the low plasma glucose concentration. Nuclear gastric emptying studies are done to look for accelerated transit as a cause of postprandial hypoglycemia; and if this is found, measurement of prokinetic gastrointestinal hormones may be indicated. This investigative area of positive mixed meal test and negative 72-hour fast is somewhat murky and very difficult clinically. If there is any guiding principle in the evaluation of such patients, it is that neuroglycopenia, regardless of when it happens,

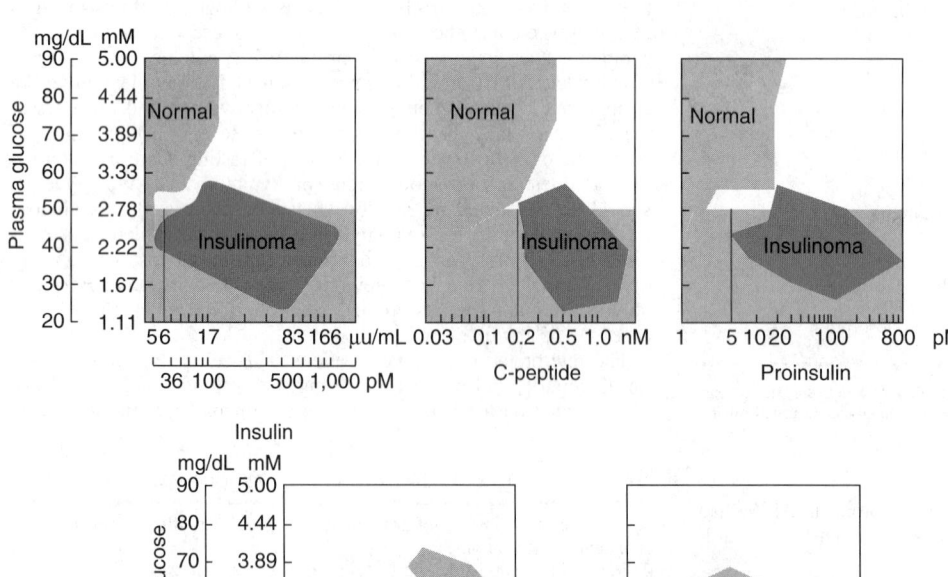

FIGURE 243–2 ■ Distributions of plasma insulin, C-peptide proinsulin, β-hydroxybutyrate, and plasma glucose (Δ glucose) response to intravenous glucagon versus plasma glucose at the end of the prolonged fast (72 hours in normal persons [N = 25] or at Whipple's triad for patients with histologically confirmed insulinoma [N = 40]) are shown. The shaded area represents plasma glucose level less than or equal to 50 mg/dL (2.8 mM). The vertical line represents the diagnostic level for insulinoma. Criteria for insulinoma are insulin greater than or equal to 6 μU/mL (36 pM), C-peptide greater than or equal to 200 pM, proinsulin greater than or equal to 5 pM, β-hydroxybutyrate less than or equal to 2.7 mM and Δ glucose greater than or equal to 25 mg/dL (1.4 mM).

Table 243–3 ■ DIAGNOSTIC INTERPRETATION OF THE RESULTS OF A 72-HOUR FAST*

	SIGNS AND SYMPTOMS	GLUCOSE† (mg/dL)	INSULIN§ (μU/mL)	C-PEPTIDE§¶ (nmol/L)	PROINSULIN§ ‖ (pmol/L)	β-HYDROXYBUTYRATE (mmol/L)	CHANGE IN GLUCOSE** (mg/dL)	SULFONYLUREA IN PLASMA
Normal	No	≥40	<6	<0.2	<5	>2.7	<25	No
Insulinoma	Yes	≤45	≥6††	≥0.2	≥5	≤2.7	≤25	No
Factitious hypoglycemia from insulin	Yes	≤45	≥6§§	<0.2	<5	≤2.7	≥25	No
Sulfonylurea-induced hypoglycemia	Yes	≤45	≥6	≥0.2	≥5	≤2.7	≥25	Yes‡‡
Hypoglycemia mediated by insulin-like growth factor	Yes	≤45	≤6	<0.2	<5	≤2.7	≥25	No
Non-insulin–mediated hypoglycemia	Yes	≤45	<6	<0.2	<5	>2.7	<25	No
Inadvertent feeding during the fast	No	≤45	<6	<0.2	<5	≤2.7	≥25	No
Non-hypoglycemic disorder	Yes	≥40	<6	<0.2	<5	>2.7	<25	No

*Measurements are made at the point the decision is made to end the fast.
†Sequential plasma glucose measurements in the hypoglycemic range fluctuate. Plasma glucose levels ≤ 45 mg/dL at the time a decision is made to end the fast may rise to as much as 56 mg/dL when the fast is actually ended approximately 1 hour later. Plasma glucose levels may be as low at 40 mg/dL during prolonged fasting in normal women.
‡Measured by double-antibody radioimmunoassay (lower limit of detection, 5 μU/mL) using ICMA criterion is ≥3 μU/mL.
§In normal subjects plasma insulin, C-peptide, and proinsulin levels may be higher if the plasma glucose level is > 60 mg/dL.
¶Measured by the immunochemiluminometric technique (lower limit of detection, 0.033 nmol/L).
‖ Measured by the immunochemiluminometric technique (lower limit of detection, 0.2 pmol/L).
**In response to intravenous glucagon (peak value minus value at end of fast).
††Ratios of insulin to glucose are of no diagnostic value in patients with insulinomas.
‡‡Unlike the first generation of sulfonylurea drugs, which were easily measured, second-generation drugs are difficult to measure.
§§Plasma insulin levels may be very high (>100 μU/mL or even ≥ 1000 μU/mL) in factitious hypoglycemia produced by insulin.
Reprinted with permission from Service FJ: Hypoglycemia Disorder. N Engl J Med 332:1144–1152, 1995. © 1995, Massachusetts Medical Society. All rights reserved.

requires intensive evaluation. The latter usually requires bringing to bear several dynamic diagnostic tests. The 5-hour oral glucose tolerance test should never be used as a diagnostic test for hypoglycemia because a substantial percentage of healthy persons may have a plasma glucose nadir less than or equal to 50 mg/dL.

The C-Peptide Suppression Tests

The C-peptide suppression test may be used to provide additional diagnostic information, especially if data from the 72-hour fast are not conclusive. These tests may also be used as screening tests: when the likelihood of a hypoglycemic disorder is not high, a normal result on these tests may obviate the need for a 72-hour fast. The C-peptide suppression test is based on the observation that β-cell secretion (as measured by levels of C-peptide) is suppressed during hypoglycemia to a lesser degree in persons with insulinomas than in normal persons. Interpretation of the C-peptide suppression test requires normative data appropriately adjusted for the patient's body mass index and age. This test should not be administered unless the immediate pre-test plasma glucose level exceeds 60 mg/dL.

Insulin Antibodies

The detection of insulin antibodies was once considered to be firm evidence of factitious hypoglycemia due to self-administered insulin, especially when animal insulin was the only commercially available type. Such patients currently have no detectable insulin antibodies, because of the use of human insulin, which is less antigenic than that derived from animals. Hypoglycemia that can be directly attributed to the spontaneous generation of antibodies to native insulin is a rare occurrence. The detection of low titers of insulin antibodies in a patient with hypoglycemia thus sometimes serves more to confuse than to clarify the diagnosis. However, it is important to test for the presence of insulin antibodies, because they may cause spurious results of the radioimmunoassay for insulin.

Glycated Hemoglobin

Although glycated hemoglobin concentrations are statistically significantly lower in patients with insulinomas than in control subjects, there is too much overlap to provide a diagnostic criterion.

Insulin Response to Selective Arterial Calcium Injection

The diagnosis of a hypoglycemic disorder is made entirely from biochemical evidence. Should the data point to insulinoma, then localization procedures are undertaken. Up to the present, standard radiologic tests have been done in an effort to localize a lesion rather than to provide a specific diagnosis. This position may change, somewhat, with the availability of the selective arterial calcium stimulation test. This test is conducted in a vascular radiology suite and requires access to various intra-abdominal vessels: hepatic vein, splenic artery, gastroduodenal artery, and superior mesenteric artery. This test may be viewed by purists as a dynamic biochemical test. A twofold to threefold increase in insulin concentration in response to calcium injection into one or more of the arteries noted earlier suggests that a region of the pancreas served by that artery harbors abnormally functioning β cells, either insulinoma or hyperplasia/nesidioblastosis.

Ill-Appearing Patient

Hypoglycemia in persons with coexistent disease sometimes occurs as a discrete episode, which may be asymptomatic if there is pre-existing blunting of consciousness. Recognition of the underlying disease and its propensity for hypoglycemia and action taken to minimize recurrence may be sufficient. Confirmation of the suspected mechanism for the hypoglycemia may be pursued, such as, low insulin and C-peptide levels in non–insulin-mediated hypoglycemia; ethanol hypoglycemia; elevated insulin-like growth factor II in non–β-cell tumor hypoglycemia; low level of cortisol in adrenal insufficiency; blunted plasma glucose responses to intravenous glucagon in hypoglycemia due to abnormal liver function; glycogen storage disease; sepsis; and congestive heart failure.

With the progressively restrictive limitations for admissions to hospital, those that are in hospitals constitute severely ill persons with multisystem disease. They are at risk for iatrogenic hypoglycemia in addition to the potential risk generated from the underlying disease. In one tertiary medical center, 1.2% of all patients admitted over a 6-month period experienced hypoglycemia (plasma glucose ≤ 49 mg/dL). The primary causes among persons without diabetes were renal insufficiency, malnutrition, liver disease, infection, and shock. Several patients had more than one risk factor. Not infrequently, non-diabetic patients become hyperglycemic because of treatment with enteral or parenteral nutrition or glucocorticoids.

Use of insulin to control hyperglycemia puts patients at risk of hypoglycemia, especially if feedings are interrupted, the dose of glucocorticoid is abruptly reduced or stopped or its availability is diminished through simultaneous administration of a bile acid sequestrant. In ferreting out the cause of hypoglycemia in the seriously ill hospitalized patient, diligent examination of the record is profitable.

Management

The treatment of hypoglycemic disorders encompasses two distinct components: (1) relief of neuroglycopenic symptoms by restoration of the low plasma glucose to the normal range and (2) correction of the underlying cause of the hypoglycemia. Unlike diabetes, in which restoration of euglycemia after hypoglycemia is the ideal goal, overtreatment of hypoglycemia in a non-diabetic person has no sequelae. For the as yet undiagnosed patient, blood by venipuncture should be obtained for measurement of glucose, β cell polypeptides, counter-regulatory hormones, and β-hydroxybutyrate before treatment. Both diagnosis and treatment may be achieved by intravenous injection of glucagon and the plasma glucose response monitored. Depending on the response, the patient may require intravenous glucose administration as a bolus of 50% or a continuous infusion of 5 or 10% or recover sufficiently to take oral nutrition.

Treatment of the underlying cause of the hypoglycemia depends on the specific cause. Once a biochemical diagnosis of insulinoma has been made, preoperative localization should be attempted. Because of the rarity of insulinoma, only a few referral centers have generated sufficient experience to assess the effectiveness of various localization procedures: computed tomography, magnetic resonance imaging, endoscopic and transabdominal ultrasonography, octreotide scan, celiac axis angiography, and selective arterial calcium stimulation and transhepatic portal venous sampling. Experts differ in their preferred approaches because of differences in experience and skill level. Ultrasonography has the advantage of precise localization especially in relation to the pancreatic duct. There is general agreement that intraoperative ultrasonography combined with careful palpation of the pancreas provides the highest success rate in localization.

Specific Causes

Insulinoma is a rare tumor, the incidence of which is estimated to be four cases per 1 million person-years, an incidence similar to that of pheochromocytoma. Insulinoma occurs at any age, is slightly more common in women (59%), and is associated with low rates of malignancy (6%), multiplicity (9%), multiple endocrine neoplasia syndrome (8%), and recurrence (8%). After successful removal of an insulinoma, the patient can look forward to normal life expectancy. Medical therapy for the patient whose insulinoma is missed at pancreatic exploration, for the patient unsuitable for surgery, or for the patient with metastatic insulinoma may include diazoxide, verapamil, phenytoin, propranolol, or octreotide. Insulinoma is occasionally suspected in patients with labile diabetes, especially when insulin therapy has apparently been suspended. There is one case of documented insulinoma in a person with type 1 diabetes and a few cases in type 2 diabetes.

Very rarely, adults with episodes of hyperinsulinemic hypoglycemia resulting in neuroglycopenia harbor islet hyperplasia/nesidioblastosis but no insulinoma. Their clinical features are predominant in males, postprandial neuroglycopenia, negative prolonged supervised foci; negative radiologic localization studies, positive selective arterial calcium stimulation test, and relief of symptoms with gradient guided partial pancreatectomy.

Insulin factitial hypoglycemia usually is manifested by neuroglycopenic symptoms that occur erratically. This disorder is observed more often in women, usually those in a health-related occupation. Once confronted with the diagnosis, about half of the patients admit to self-abuse and most cease this activity. Insulin autoimmune hypoglycemia may be very difficult to distinguish from insulin factitial hypoglycemia because of similar biochemical features. However, many patients of the former have evidence of other autoimmune disease.

Mutations in the β-cell sulfonylurea receptor gene, glutamate dehydrogenase gene, and glucokinase gene have been reported to cause hyperinsulinemic hypoglycemia, primarily at an early age and often in a familial pattern.

ISLET CELL TUMORS

Tumors of the endocrine pancreas generally are malignant. Insulin-producing tumors are the exception, because they are usually benign. Islet cell tumors are commonly referred to as either "functioning" or "non-functioning." "Functioning" tumors release one or more hormones in amounts sufficient to raise plasma concentrations. "Non-functioning" tumors may contain one or more hormones but, by definition, do not release substantial amounts into the systemic circulation. Functioning tumors generally present with symptoms relating to the hormone(s) being secreted whereas non-functioning tumors generally present as a pancreatic mass or as a metastasis. Non-functioning tumors tend to be larger and more advanced at the time of diagnosis.

Functioning islet cell tumors are commonly associated with one of five widely recognized syndromes (Table 243–4). The insulinoma, Zollinger-Ellison, glucagonoma, VIPoma, and somatostatinoma syndromes are believed to be due (at least in part) to excess secretion of insulin, gastrin, glucagon, vasoactive intestinal polypeptide (VIP), and somatostatin, respectively. However, a number of additional symptoms also can occur because these tumors frequently secrete more than one hormone (e.g., pancreatic polypeptide, adrenocorticotropin, calcitonin, neurotensin, human chorionic gonadotropin, growth hormone–releasing factor, prostaglandins, and parathyroid hormone) and the amount and type of the hormone being secreted can change over time. Islet cell tumors are either sporadic or can occur in association with other known genetic syndromes such as multiple endocrine neoplasia type 1. Sporadic tumors occur at any age but most commonly are detected between 40 and 60 years of age. The diagnosis can be confirmed by obtaining tissue during surgical resection or by means of a needle biopsy.

With the exception perhaps of insulinomas, the optimal treatment of islet cell tumors is currently not known because their rarity has made the conduct of randomized therapeutic trials extremely difficult. Furthermore, in the absence of metastases, there are no reliable histologic criteria that can distinguish benign from malignant lesions. Islet cell tumors most commonly metastasize to the liver and adjacent lymph nodes. Metastases to lung, bone, adrenal, kidney, and ovary also may occur. Fortunately, the rate of growth of malignant islet cell tumors is generally slow. Therefore, many clinicians would recommend surgery if the pancreatic tumor is resectable and if the extent of metastatic disease (if present) is limited. "Debulking" of metastases, whether by surgery or by hepatic embolization, may improve symptoms by lowering circulating hormone concentrations. Treatment with chemotherapeutic agents such as streptozotocin (alone or in combination with 5-fluorouracil), doxorubicin, dacarbazine or interferon-α also may improve symptoms and, in some instances, perhaps improve survival. Somatostatin is a potent inhibitor of hormone secretion. Treatment with long-acting analogues of somatostatin can result in a dramatic, albeit at times temporary, decrease in symptoms, particularly those associated with glucagonomas and VIPomas.

Insulin-Secreting Tumors

Insulinomas are the most common type of islet cell tumor. As discussed earlier in this chapter, these tumors cause hypoglycemia, are typically small, and are usually benign.

Gastrin-Secreting Tumors

Gastrin-secreting tumors are the second most common type of islet cell tumor. When untreated, these tumors are associated with high rates of gastric acid secretion and intractable peptic ulcer disease. Diarrhea also is common. This group of symptoms is usually referred to as the Zollinger-Ellison syndrome, which is discussed in detail in Chapter 130.

Glucagon-Producing Tumors

Glucagon is a 3500-kd polypeptide that is primarily secreted by the α cells of the pancreas. Glucagon stimulates glycogenolysis and gluconeogenesis, increases ketogenesis, and enhances hepatic amino acid uptake and oxidation. Glucagon-secreting tumors are rare (esti-

Table 243–4 ■ CHARACTERISTICS OF FUNCTIONING ISLET CELL CARCINOMAS

SYNDROME	CLINICAL PRESENTATION	BIOCHEMICAL DIAGNOSIS	RATE OF MALIGNANCY (%)	METASTASES AT DIAGNOSIS (%)	LOCALIZATION (RADIOGRAPHIC)	ECTOPIC SITES (NON-PANCREATIC)
Insulinoma	Neuroglyco-penia Andrenergic response	Blood glucose ≤45 mg/dL Insulin > 6μU/mL Absence of insulin antibodies Nl/elevated C-peptide	<10	<10	US, spiral CT, selective calcium stimulation test	Rare
Zollinger-Ellison syndrome	Dyspepsia/ulcer Diarrhea	Elevated basal gastrin Elevated basal acid output Positive secretin test	50–60	50–80	US, CT, angio, PVS	Duodenum Rarely other
WDHA (VIPoma)	Profuse, secre-tory diarrhea Hypokalemia Hypo/achlorhy-dria, hyper-calcemia, hy-perglycemia	Elevated VIP	50	50	CT, occas. angio, PVS	Retroperitoneum Lung
Glucagonoma	Dematitis Diabetes Weight loss Anemia	Elevated glucagon	75	60–70	CT	Rare
Somatostatinoma	Diabetes Cholelithiasis Diarrhea Steatorrhea	Elevated somatostatin	90–100	50–75	CT	Duodenum

WDHA = water diarrhea, hypokalemia, achlorhydria; VIP = vasoactive intestinal pepide; US = ultrasonography; angio-angiography; PVS = portal venous sampling; CT = computed tomography.

Modified from Grant CS: Surgical management of malignant islet cell tumors. World J Surg 17:498–503, 1993.

mated incidence about 1 in 20 million), are generally detected between 40 to 60 years of age, and are almost always malignant. They occur with equal frequency in men and women. Glucagon-secreting tumors are often accompanied by a characteristic rash called necrolytic migratory erythema (NME). This rash typically begins as small erythematous lesions involving the lower extremities and perineal and perioral regions. The lesions may take the form of pustules or blisters, which frequently crust and merge. Healing may occur in the center while spreading continues at the edges. NME is generally pruritic, tends to wax and wane, and leaves behind areas of scaring and increased pigmentation. It is frequently accompanied by weight loss, diabetes mellitus, stomatitis, and diarrhea. This constellation of symptoms has been referred to as the glucagonoma syndrome. Venous thrombosis, abdominal pain, peptic ulcer, and neurologic symptoms such as ataxia, fecal and urinary incontinence, and visual symptoms also may occur.

Glucagon-secreting tumors are diagnosed by the presence of elevated plasma glucagon concentrations. Glucagon concentrations at the time of diagnosis are usually greater than 500 pg/mL but, in some instances, may be only minimally elevated. The degree of elevation may depend on the specificity of the glucagon assay, in particular its cross reactivity with precursor hormones and other glucagon-like materials circulating in plasma. Although diabetes, sepsis, renal failure, and familial hyperglucagonemia all may increase plasma glucagon concentrations, these conditions rarely pose a diagnostic problem because the signs and symptoms of the glucagonoma syndrome are absent. Furthermore, clinically evident glucagon-secreting tumors are almost always large and are usually readily visualized with imaging techniques such as computed tomography.

Metastasis to the liver, lymph nodes, or bone are frequently present at the time of diagnosis. Fortunately, glucagon-secreting tumors tend to grow slowly and survival for many years is not uncommon. Although surgical resection of an malignant islet cell tumor may be curative, treatment is generally directed toward decreasing symptoms and improving quality of life. Reduction in the concentration of glucagon and other associated hormones by surgical debulking, hepatic embolization, chemotherapy, or use of a somatostatin analogue to inhibit hormone secretion can result in a marked improvement in symptoms. Although results are variable, all of these therapies have the potential to decrease the frequency and severity of NME, slow or prevent weight loss, improve glucose tolerance, and reverse the paraneoplastic neurologic manifestations of the syndrome. Regardless of therapy, the average 5-year survival is approximately 50%.

Vasoactive Intestinal Polypeptide (VIP)-Secreting Tumors

VIP is a 28-amino acid neuropeptide that is widely distributed throughout the body. It is a member of the glucagon family of hormones and has numerous effects on the gastrointestinal tract, including stimulation of chloride secretion in the small intestine and bicarbonate secretion in the colon. VIP also inhibits gastric acid release. VIP-secreting tumors can occur within the pancreas or along the autonomic nervous system, including the adrenal medulla. Pancreatic tumors are approximately 10 times more common then extrapancreatic tumors. Extrapancreatic tumors tend to be less aggressive and usually occur in children as neuroblastomas, ganglioneuromas, or ganglioblastomas.

Pancreatic VIPomas generally are malignant and are frequently associated with watery diarrhea, hypokalemia, hypochlorhydria, and acidosis, a group of symptoms referred to as the WDHA syndrome. The diarrhea is secretory and severe. Stool volume typically exceeds 3 L/day; a stool volume of less than 700 mL/day makes the diagnosis unlikely. The resultant hypokalemia, hypovolemia, and acidosis can be life threatening. VIPomas also can cause glucose intolerance and, occasionally, frank diabetes. Impaired insulin secretion due to hypokalemia and stimulation of hepatic glycogenolysis by VIP likely contribute to this association. Hypercalcemia and hypophosphatemia are common. This presumably results from the concomitant secretion of calcitropic hormones such as parathyroid-related peptide, because infusion of VIP in healthy volunteers does not alter calcium levels. Plasma VIP concentrations in excess of 200 pg/mL strongly suggest the presence of a VIP-secreting tumor. However, the WDHA syndrome can occur in the absence of elevated VIP levels, and VIPomas can secrete other potentially diarrheogenic hormones, including pancreatic polypeptide, neurotensin, calcitonin, prostaglandin, and peptide-histidine-methionine. These findings suggest that elevated VIP levels may be one of several factors responsible for the syndrome.

Pancreatic VIPomas usually are large at the time of diagnosis and readily visualized by standard imaging techniques. Catecholamines should be measured if an extrapancreatic VIPoma is suggested because a pheochromocytoma also may be present. Surgical resection of a VIPoma can be curative. "Debulking" by means of hepatic artery embolization also has been successful in relieving symptoms in individuals with liver metastasis. Streptozotocin alone or in combination with 5-fluorouracil may produce a prolonged remission. Remissions also have been observed after treatment with interferon-α. Somatostatin or its analogues can dramatically decrease diarrhea. Somatostatin analogues may be a particularly useful adjuvant in the treatment of severe electrolyte disturbances or during preparation of patients for surgery or chemotherapy.

Somatostatinoma

Somatostatin is a 1600-kd polypeptide that is secreted by the delta cells of the pancreas as well as by multiple other tissues, including the small intestine and central nervous system. Somatostatin tumors are extremely rare (incidence about 1 in 40 million). Both pancreatic and extrapancreatic somatostatin-secreting tumors have been reported. Pancreatic tumors most commonly involve the head of the pancreas. At the time of diagnosis, these tumors are generally large and usually metastatic to the liver, lymph nodes, and/or duodenum. Patients frequently present with non-specific complaints such as weight loss and abdominal pain. Some present with diabetes, hypochlorhydria, cholelithiasis, diarrhea, and steatorrhea, a constellation of symptoms referred to as the somatostatinoma syndrome. These symptoms are presumed to be due to inhibition of insulin, gastrin, cholecystokinin, and pancreatic enzyme secretion respectively by the high circulating levels of somatostatin. However, hyperglycemia is not invariable; glucose concentrations may be high, normal, or low depending on whether inhibition of insulin or counter-insulin hormone secretion (e.g., glucagon and growth hormone) predominate. Somatostatinomas may secrete a variety of other hormones, including insulin, parathyroid-related polypeptide, or adrenocorticotropin, resulting in an array of additional clinical presentations including hypoglycemia, hypercalcemia, or Cushing's syndrome.

Pancreatic somatostatinomas usually are large and readily visualized by ultrasound or computed tomography. Extrapancreatic somatostatin-secreting tumors tend to be smaller and to occur in the duodenum or the ampulla of Vater. These tumors, although commonly malignant, do not result in either elevated plasma somatostatin concentrations or symptoms typical of the somatostatinoma syndrome. Of note, duodenal carcinoids (see Chapter 245) may contain somatostatin and may be associated with neurofibromatosis and pheochromocytomas. Although resection of a localized pancreatic or extrapancreatic somatostatin-secreting tumor can result in long-term survival, the prognosis generally is poor.

Non-functioning Islet Cell Tumors

Non-functioning islet cell tumors, by definition, are not associated with any hormonal syndrome. They therefore are generally clinically silent until they reach a size sufficient to cause pain, weight loss, or obstruction of biliary or pancreatic drainage. By the time of detection, they are almost invariably malignant. As is typical of other endocrine tumors, there are no reliable histologic features that distinguish benign from malignant non-functioning tumors. These tumors tend to be slow growing and of low grade. Therefore, surgical resection may be of value. Although residual unresectable tumor may respond to chemotherapy, the effects on survival are unknown.

Cryer PE: Glucose counterregulation: The physiological mechanisms that prevent or correct hypoglycaemia. *In* Frier BM, Fisher BM (eds): Hypoglycaemia and Diabetes: Clinical and Physiological Aspects. London, Edward Arnold, 1993, pp 34–55.
Fischer KF, Lees JA, Newman JH: Hypoglycemia in hospitalized patients. N Engl J Med 315:1245–1250, 1986.
Palardy J, Havrankova J, Lepage R, et al: Blood glucose measurements during symptomatic episodes in patients with suspected post prandial hypoglycemia. N Engl J Med 321:1421–1425, 1989.
Service FJ, O'Brien PC, McMahon MM, Kao PC: C-peptide during the prolonged fast in insulinoma. J Clin Endocrinol Metab 76:655–659, 1993.
Service FJ, Natt N, Thompson GB, et al: Noninsulinoma pancreatogenous hypoglycemia: A novel syndrome of hyperinsulinemic hypoglycemia in adults independent of mutations in Kir6.2 and SUR1 genes. J Clin Endocrinol Metab 84:1999 (in press).
Wermers RA, Fatourechi V, Wynne AG, et al: The glucagonoma syndrome: Clinical and pathologic features in 21 patients. Medicine 75:53–63, 1996.

244 MULTIPLE-ORGAN SYNDROMES: POLYGLANDULAR DISORDERS

Henry M. Kronenberg

Internists need to recognize diseases that involve independent abnormalities of more than one endocrine gland for a number of reasons. First, the known patterns of multiglandular disease can alert the clinician to look for a second disorder when one is diagnosed. Second, the treatment of many of the individual diseases in polyglandular disorders may differ from the treatment appropriate for the same diseases when they present in isolation. Third, because many of these diseases appear in characteristic familial patterns, the recognition of the syndromes can lead to useful family screening. Fourth, an understanding of the pathogenesis of these unusual disorders is likely to clarify the pathogenesis of more common single-gland disorders as well. In this chapter the best-characterized polyglandular disorders are discussed with these four considerations as the primary focus. Other chapters should be consulted for more detailed discussions of the diseases of individual glands.

POLYGLANDULAR NEOPLASIA

Three mechanistically distinct neoplastic syndromes involve more than one endocrine gland. Although given a variety of different names in the past, they are now most frequently called multiple endocrine neoplasia type 1, multiple endocrine neoplasia types 2a and 2b, and McCune-Albright syndrome.

MULTIPLE ENDOCRINE NEOPLASIA TYPE 1. Multiple endocrine neoplasia type 1 (MEN 1) is an autosomal dominant disorder involving characteristically the parathyroid glands, the pancreatic islets, and the anterior pituitary. Less commonly, adrenal gland neoplasia, foregut carcinoids (primarily of thymus and lung), and lipomas occur. Because thyroid neoplasms are so common in the general population, their true association with MEN 1 is debated.

Parathyroid Disease (see also Chapter 264). Hyperparathyroidism is the most common abnormality in MEN 1, found in more than 90% of patients. Elevation of blood calcium concentration generally first appears between the ages of 20 and 40, considerably earlier than in sporadic primary hyperparathyroidism; this is not a disease of children, however. At first, the disease is asymptomatic, but then it can lead to all the expected consequences of primary hyperparathyroidism. Unlike sporadic hyperparathyroidism, the disease is relentlessly progressive and, as seen with prolonged follow-up, always involves all four parathyroid glands. The involvement is characteristically asymmetrical and asynchronous. This pattern can lead to inappropriately limited parathyroid surgery. If fewer than three parathyroid glands are removed, hypercalcemia always recurs, although not necessarily immediately. Surgical results in MEN 1 are generally less satisfactory than in sporadic four-gland parathyroid disease. At some centers, all four glands are removed and a portion of one gland is reimplanted in the easily accessible forearm in an attempt to avoid the hazards of too much or too little surgery. The difficulty in attaining long-term normocalcemia has led many clinicians to postpone surgery when the disease is asymptomatic. This strategy may need to be modified if the patient develops Zollinger-Ellison syndrome (see later), because hypercalcemia can dramatically increase the gastrin levels in such patients.

Pancreatic Islet Disease (see also Chapter 243). As many as 80% of patients have pancreatic abnormalities at autopsy; a large number correspondingly have increased blood levels of gastrin, insulin, pancreatic polypeptide, somatostatin, vasoactive intestinal polypeptide, or glucagon during stimulation or suppression tests. The pancreas is often diffusely involved with microadenomas and macroadenomas and apparently hyperplastic lesions. Characteristically, more than one islet hormone is secreted from these multiple tumors. Despite this underlying pattern of multiple cellular involvement, patients characteristically present with symptoms of only one hormonal disorder. The most common disease is Zollinger-Ellison syndrome, which is peptic ulcer disease associated with gastrin-producing tumors. Identification of disease-causing tumors has proven difficult. The gastrinomas in MEN 1 are often multiple, very small, and found in the duodenal wall. Macroadenomas observed in the pancreas by computed tomography or intraoperative ultrasonography may well synthesize hormones other than gastrin. Although some centers continue to experiment with aggressive attempts at surgical cure, the high recurrence rate after surgery has limited the role for surgery in this disease. Medical therapy with histamine-2 receptor antagonists and H^+,K^+-ATPase inhibitors can usually adequately control the secretion of stomach acid. The tumors are slow growing but frequently metastasize locally and to the liver. Chemotherapy is only partially effective and never cures the disease.

Insulinomas are the second most common clinically important islet tumor in MEN 1. These tumors are often small and multiple and are much less frequently malignant than the gastrinomas. Despite the frequently diffuse nature of the disease, dominant insulin-producing tumors can often be identified by selective portal venous sampling. Removal of the dominant tissue, or, if necessary, subtotal (80%) pancreatectomy is the primary therapeutic strategy.

Pituitary Disease (see also Chapter 237). As in sporadic disease, pituitary disease can present as a hypersecretion syndrome or as symptoms due to a sellar mass or hypopituitarism. Pituitary tumors occur in more than half of MEN 1 patients. Prolactinomas are the most common tumors. Adrenocortical hyperfunction can result from a pituitary adenoma or from production of adrenocorticotropic hormone (ACTH) or corticotropin-releasing hormone by a foregut carcinoid. Although non-functioning adrenal neoplasms are common in MEN 1, primary adrenal neoplasms causing glucocorticoid excess are rare. Acromegaly can result from a pituitary neoplasm or as a consequence of production of growth hormone–releasing hormone by pancreatic islet tumors. After consideration of ectopic hormone and releasing hormone production by non-pituitary tumors, the course and treatment of pituitary disease in MEN 1 resemble those of sporadic pituitary disease.

Pathogenesis. The gene for MEN 1 is located at chromosome 11, band 11q13, and encodes a 610-amino acid protein called menin. Menin is a nuclear protein expressed in most tissues. Although the normal function of menin is unknown, the pattern of menin gene abnormalities in MEN 1 suggests that the menin gene is a tumor suppressor gene. The inherited mutations in the menin gene, which vary widely and are found throughout the gene, often generate truncated, presumably non-functional, menin peptides. In addition to this genetic abnormality, inherited by all cells in the body, MEN 1 tumors usually harbor deletions of the normal allele of the menin gene. Presumably, loss of both copies of the tumor suppressor gene—one by inherited mutation and one by mutation of one particular cell—confers a selective advantage to the cell that proliferates to become a clonal tumor. Such clonal deletions have been found in 100% of parathyroid tumors removed at surgery from MEN 1 patients. Other acquired genetic abnormalities accumulate in these tumors; thus, the tumors in MEN 1 follow the pattern of multi-step tumorigenesis found in malignant tumors.

The two-hit, tumor suppressor model can explain many of the features of MEN 1. Clinical presentation of an inherited disorder in adulthood can be explained by the requirement for second mutations before clonal expansion. The asymmetrical but relentless nature of the parathyroid disease may be explained by asynchronous but inevitable somatic mutations in each of the parathyroid glands. Multiple islet tumors might result from the same process.

The menin gene is mutated in about 20% of sporadic parathyroid adenomas, a fraction of sporadic malignant endocrine tumors of the pancreas, and some sporadic carcinoid tumors of the lung as well. Because these mutations occur only in the tumor and not in the patient's normal cells, no familial clustering occurs.

Genetic screening for menin gene mutations is not routinely available and will be difficult to provide because of the wide variety of differing abnormalities in the menin gene in different families with MEN 1. Research laboratories can identify affected family members by characterizing closely linked genetic markers in blood cells if specimens from more than one affected family member are available. The most useful single test to complement a thorough history and physical examination is measurement of blood calcium concentration, particularly ionized calcium, at intervals after age 15. Prolactin, gastrin, and fasting blood sugar measurements can also be useful.

MULTIPLE ENDOCRINE NEOPLASIA TYPES 2A AND 2B. Multiple endocrine neoplasia type 2a is an autosomal dominant disease that presents as medullary carcinoma of the thyroid, pheochromocy-

toma, and, less commonly, hyperparathyroidism. MEN 2b is closely related to MEN 2a because it also presents with medullary carcinoma of the thyroid and pheochromocytoma and because both diseases involve mutations in the *RET* proto-oncogene (see later). MEN 2b presents as a number of abnormalities not found in MEN 2a, however. These include mucosal neuromas of the tongue, lips, eyelids, and gastrointestinal tract and a marfanoid habitus. Hyperparathyroidism rarely occurs in MEN 2b. MEN 2b is less common than MEN 2a; both diseases are rarer than MEN 1.

In MEN 2a and 2b, the medullary cancers and the pheochromocytomas often present bilaterally. Careful prospective analysis of MEN 2a families has demonstrated that diffuse C-cell hyperplasia precedes clinically obvious appearance of medullary cancer by decades. C-cell hyperplasia can be detected by measurement of calcitonin after administration of gastrin. With current sensitive assays, the median age at presentation with C-cell hyperplasia is 8 or 9 years. Virtually all MEN 2a patients eventually develop C-cell disease. Complete thyroidectomy of patients with C-cell hyperplasia has dramatically decreased the incidence of medullary cancer, which has been the major cause of death in MEN 2a.

Half the patients with MEN 2a develop pheochromocytomas. Family screening allows the detection of pheochromocytoma before the development of hypertension. The first laboratory abnormalities noted include an increase in urinary levels of epinephrine and in the ratio of epinephrine to norepinephrine in the urine. Increases in urinary metanephrine and norepinephrine come later. The tumors are usually found in the adrenal glands and can be documented preoperatively by computed tomography, magnetic resonance imaging, and ^{131}I-metaiodobenzylguanidine scanning.

Most patients with MEN 2a have been found to harbor point mutations in the *RET* proto-oncogene, found in the pericentromeric region of chromosome 10. *RET* encodes a member of the tyrosine protein kinase family of cell surface receptors. The gene is expressed in spinal cord, in certain cultured blood cell lines, and in all tested medullary cancer and pheochromocytoma lines (both from MEN 2 patients and from sporadic tumors). RET is the receptor for glial cell-derived neurotrophic factor, which controls the migration, proliferation, and survival of neural crest cells that populate the thyroid, adrenal, and the intrinsic nervous system of the gut. Mutations have been found in five different cysteines located in the portion of the receptor that forms the extracellular, ligand-binding domain. In contrast to the pattern in MEN 1, no evidence for somatic mutations in the RET region of chromosome 10 have been found in MEN 2a tumors. The mutant *RET* gene signals in a ligand-independent manner, thereby acting as an oncogene. The mutant *RET* genes can transform cultured cells and cause medullary cancer of the thyroid in transgenic mice.

The transition from diffuse hyperplasia of C cells or adrenal medullary cells to clonal neoplasms of the thyroid or adrenal probably requires subsequent somatic mutations. Such mutations include the loss of genetic markers on chromosomes 1p, 3p, 3q, and 22q that frequently occur in these tumors.

Patients with MEN 2b harbor a point mutation that changes Met918 to a threonine within the RET protein's intracellular kinase domain. Studies suggest that this mutation activates the kinase and may change its substrate specificity.

Familial medullary cancer of the thyroid, without tumors of the adrenal or parathyroid, is also caused by mutations of the *RET* gene. These mutations include the same mutations that cause MEN 2a, as well as unique mutations in the *RET* gene's kinase domain. Systematic analysis of the *RET* gene has demonstrated that inheritable *RET* gene abnormalities occur in patients with apparently sporadic medullary cancer of the thyroid, as well. Inherited *RET* gene abnormalities are not found in patients with isolated pheochromocytomas or parathyroid adenomas, however. Remarkably, some patients with familial Hirschsprung's disease, associated with absence of neurons in the enteric sympathetic nervous system, have inactive *RET* genes.

Direct genetic testing has now replaced calcitonin testing as a screening tool in MEN 2 families. These genetic studies have shown that calcitonin testing and even histologic analysis of thyroid tissue can lead to false-positive and false-negative assignment of disease within families. The limited number of sites in the *RET* gene that cause inherited disease make genetic testing now routinely feasible.

McCUNE-ALBRIGHT SYNDROME. The McCune-Albright syndrome is a non-inherited disorder consisting of the triad of polyostotic fibrous dysplasia, light brown pigmented skin lesions (café-au-lait spots), and endocrinopathy (usually precocious puberty). Multiple endocrine abnormalities can occur. The precocious puberty, more often seen in girls than boys, is gonadotropin independent. Hyperthyroidism is caused by autonomous thyroid nodules. Acromegaly is caused by pituitary adenomas that produce growth hormone and, usually, prolactin. Adrenocortical hyperfunction is caused by ACTH-independent adrenal adenomas. Hypophosphatemic rickets, with normal blood calcium concentrations, phosphate wasting, and low or inappropriately normal levels of 1,25-dihydroxyvitamin D_3, may result from release of a humoral factor from the dysplastic fibrous tissue.

This somewhat bewildering array of endocrine abnormalities has been rationalized by the observation that cells in the involved tissues harbor mutations in the α subunit of the G_S protein. The G_S protein links cell surface receptors to the activation of adenylate cyclase. The mutations in McCune-Albright syndrome are point mutations at Arg201 in the G_S subunit; these mutations lead to prolonged activity of G_S and inappropriate activation of adenylate cyclase. Increased levels of cyclic adenosine monophosphate lead to cellular proliferation and hormone secretion. Patients with McCune-Albright syndrome are genetic mosaics. Presumably, at an early stage in embryonic development, a point mutation occurs in the G_S gene of a cell that then proliferates, differentiates, and variably populates normal bone, skin, and endocrine tissues. In cell types in which elevations in cyclic adenosine monophosphate lead to proliferation, abnormal cells become predominant and lead to disease. Because the disease is never inherited, the mutation is presumably lethal when present in all cells of the embryo. In contrast, the very same mutations at Arg201 have been found in cases of isolated acromegaly and autonomous thyroid nodules. One can, therefore, speculate that McCune-Albright syndrome is the most dramatic example of a spectrum of disorders that vary in severity and presentation depending on the stage of development of the original mutant cell.

AUTOIMMUNE POLYGLANDULAR DYSFUNCTION

Organ-specific autoimmune disease, characterized by lymphocytic infiltration and organ-specific autoantibodies, commonly results in endocrine hypofunction or hyperfunction. Clinical manifestations of disease are usually limited to one gland. Not uncommonly, however, disorders of more than one endocrine gland appear in families or in individual patients. Characteristic patterns of disease presentation and genetic inheritance allow the definition of two syndromes with overlapping manifestations (Table 244–1).

AUTOIMMUNE POLYGLANDULAR SYNDROME TYPE 1. This rare disease presents typically in early childhood. Mucocutaneous candidiasis occurs in virtually all patients and is usually the first manifestation of disease. Hypoparathyroidism and Addison's disease are the most common endocrine manifestations; each of these diseases occurs in 70 to 80% of patients. Hypoparathyroidism usually precedes Addison's disease; both diseases typically present before age 15. Premature ovarian failure (in 60% of affected women) usually presents as secondary amenorrhea; testicular failure occurs less frequently. Insulin-dependent diabetes mellitus occurs in 12% of patients, usually in adulthood; hypothyroidism is uncommon.

Non-endocrine components of this syndrome, in addition to the mucocutaneous candidiasis, include alopecia, vitiligo, corneal opacities, autoimmune hepatitis, enamel hypoplasia of teeth, tympanic membrane calcification, nail dystrophy that correlates only loosely with obvious candidiasis, parietal cell atrophy and vitamin B_{12} malabsorption, and more general intestinal malabsorption with steatorrhea. Asplenism, with Howell-Jolly bodies on peripheral blood smears, has been noted in several patients.

Each of the disease components should be sought when any patient presents with hypoparathyroidism, primary adrenal insufficiency, or mucocutaneous candidiasis. The hypoparathyroidism is treated like the sporadic disease with oral calcium and 1,25-dihy-

Table 244–1 ▪ CLINICAL FEATURES OF AUTOIMMUNE POLYGLANDULAR SYNDROMES

	TYPE 1	TYPE 2
Mucocutaneous candidiasis	Very common	Not seen
Hypoparathyroidism	Common	Rare
Addison's disease	Common	Common
Primary hypogonadism	Common	Occurs
Autoimmune thyroid disease	Rare	Common
Autoimmune diabetes	Occurs	Common
Hypophysitis	Occurs	Occurs
Autoimmune hepatitis	Occurs	Not seen
Pernicious anemia	Occurs	Occurs
Vitiligo	Occurs	Occurs
Malabsorption syndrome	Occurs	Occurs in celiac disease
Alopecia	Common	Occurs
Myasthenia gravis	Not seen	Occurs
Keratopathy	Common	Not seen
Tympanic membrane calcification	Common	Not seen
Inheritance	Autosomal recessive	HLA association
Age at onset	Usually childhood	Usually adulthood

droxyvitamin D, although variable intestinal malabsorption can present a particular therapeutic challenge. The candidiasis can be satisfactorily controlled with ketoconazole.

Autoimmune polyglandular syndrome type 1 is an autosomal recessive disorder mapped to a small region within chromosomal region 21q22.3. The appearance of organ-specific autoantibodies precedes disease presentation and predicts the development of specific end organ damage. The role of these antibodies and the precise pathogenesis of the syndrome are unknown, however.

AUTOIMMUNE POLYGLANDULAR SYNDROME TYPE 2. This syndrome is considerably more common than the type 1 syndrome and typically presents in adulthood. Insulin-dependent diabetes mellitus and thyroid dysfunction—either autoimmune hypothyroidism or Graves' disease—are the most frequent manifestations. Addison's disease is the third major endocrine component of this disorder. Although most patients who present with autoimmune diabetes or thyroid disease have clinical involvement of only one gland, a large fraction of patients with autoimmune Addison's disease develop clinically evident disease in other endocrine glands. Less common components of the type 2 polyglandular syndrome include primary hypogonadism and hypophysitis. Pernicious anemia, vitiligo, celiac disease, alopecia, and myasthenia gravis are also associated with this syndrome.

The treatment of each component of this syndrome is identical to the treatment of each disorder in isolation, although possible clustering of diseases must be kept in mind during the evaluation and follow-up of all patients with each individual component disorder. Thyroid hormone therapy can precipitate symptoms of adrenal insufficiency in patients with both disorders, for example. Consequently, careful history, including family history, physical examination, and a low threshold for specific laboratory testing for adrenal insufficiency should be part of the evaluation of every patient with autoimmune hypothyroidism. Furthermore, combinations of hypothyroidism, adrenal insufficiency, and hypogonadism can mimic hypopituitarism, although specific hormonal testing can easily distinguish these disorders. Because multiple components of the syndrome can present asynchronously, periodic evaluation for early appearance of further disease components is indicated.

Autoimmune polyglandular syndrome type 2 is usually inherited in families with characteristic HLA associations. The HLA associations do not predict disease absolutely, even in identical twins, so environmental factors must contribute to disease presentation. Typically, several different autoimmune diseases occur in each family. Autoimmune vulnerability rather than specific organ disease is inherited. Diabetes, as part of the polyglandular syndrome, usually presents at an older age and develops more slowly than isolated autoimmune diabetes. The characteristic pattern of association with specific DQ loci does not differ between polyglandular and isolated diabetes, however. Presumably, genes not linked to the HLA complex modify the presentation of diabetes.

Organ-specific antibodies appear before clinical disease and predict subsequent disease. The role of these antibodies in organ hypofunction has not been established, however.

Agarwal SK, Kester MB, Debelenko LV, et al: Germline mutations of the *MEN1* gene in familial multiple endocrine neoplasia type 1 and related states. Hum Mol Genet 6: 1169–1175, 1997. *The first large series of menin gene abnormalities.*

Ahonen P, Myllärniemi S, Sipilä I, et al: Clinical variation of autoimmune polyendocrinopathy-candidiasis-ectodermal dystrophy (APECED) in a series of 68 patients. N Engl J Med 322:1829, 1990. *A large series with prolonged follow-up that presents a thorough summary of the clinical features of autoimmune polyglandular syndrome type 1.*

Eisenbarth GS, Verge CF: Immunoendocrinopathy syndromes. *In* Wilson JD, Foster DW, Kronenberg HM, Larsen PR (eds): William's Textbook of Endocrinology, 9th ed. Philadelphia, WB Saunders, 1998, p 1651. *An excellent general review stressing immune mechanisms.*

Eng C, Clayton D, Schuffenecker I, et al: The relationship between specific *RET* proto-oncogene mutations and disease phenotype in multiple endocrine neoplasia type 2. JAMA 276:1575–1579, 1996. *A thorough correlation of clinical presentation with specific RET gene mutations.*

Santoro M, Carlomagno F, Romano A, et al: Activation of *RET* as a dominant transforming gene by germline mutations of MEN 2A and MEN 2B. Science 267: 381, 1995. *Elegant demonstration that mutant RET genes are the first inherited disease-causing oncogenes.*

245 MULTIPLE-ORGAN SYNDROMES: CARCINOID SYNDROME

John A. Oates

Carcinoid syndrome incorporates the constellation of signs and symptoms associated with malignant neoplasms of enterochromaffin cells. Cutaneous flushing, diarrhea, and cardiac valvular lesions are the most common endocrine consequences of these tumors.

THE NEOPLASMS

Tumors that cause the carcinoid syndrome have the characteristics of neuroendocrine cells of the enterochromaffin type. These tumors typically contain 5-hydroxytryptamine (serotonin) and tachykinins such as substance P. The metastatic tumors associated with carcinoid syndrome usually arise from primary tumors in the ileum. The syndrome also can be produced by neoplasms arising from the remainder of the small intestine, from organs derived from the embryonic foregut (e.g., bronchus, stomach, pancreas, and thyroid), and from ovarian or testicular teratomas. The usual carcinoid tumor arising from the ileum has the histologic pattern of dense nests of cells with uniform size and nuclear appearance. Histochemically, they typically exhibit an argentaffin reaction in which the cells convert a silver salt to metallic silver. A positive argentaffin reaction is not required for the diagnosis, however, as carcinoid tumors arising from organs of the embryonic foregut may contain few if any argentaffin cells. Ultrastructural examination of carcinoid tumors reveals electron-dense secretion granules.

Carcinoid tumors have a proclivity to metastasize to the liver and may involve this organ extensively and predominantly. Extrahepatic metastases occur in bone, where they are often osteoblastic, and in the lung, pancreas, spleen, ovaries, adrenals, and other organs.

Primary carcinoid tumors of the appendix are common, but they rarely metastasize. Those from the large intestine may metastasize but almost never exhibit endocrine effects.

CLINICAL MANIFESTATIONS

Carcinoid tumors typically have a slow rate of growth, and many patients with carcinoid syndrome survive for a decade after the disease is recognized. For much of the duration of the illness, morbidity results largely from the endocrine functions of the tumor. Death usually is caused by cardiac or hepatic failure and by complications associated with tumor growth.

VASODILATOR PAROXYSMS. Cutaneous flushing is the most common clinical feature. The typical flush is erythematous and involves the head and neck (blush area). Some patients exhibit vivid color changes from red to violaceous to pallor. Prolonged flushing attacks may be associated with lacrimation and periorbital edema. The flush may be accompanied by tachycardia, and the blood pressure usually falls or does not change. A rise in blood pressure during flushing is rare, and carcinoid syndrome is not a cause of sustained hypertension. Flushing may be provoked by excitement, exertion, eating, and ethanol ingestion.

TELANGIECTASIA. In addition to paroxysms of cutaneous vasodilatation, some patients also develop telangiectasia, primarily on the face and neck, which is most marked in the malar area.

GASTROINTESTINAL SYMPTOMS. Intestinal hypermotility with borborygmi, cramping, and explosive diarrhea may accompany the episodic flushes. Chronic diarrhea is more common and may have a secretory component. When this is severe, malabsorption may occur.

CARDIAC MANIFESTATIONS. Plaquelike thickening of the endocardium of the valvular cusps and cardiac chambers occurs primarily on the right side of the heart but may involve the left side to a minimal degree. The endocardial thickening is composed of smooth muscle cells embedded in a stroma rich in mucopolysaccharides. The thickening and deformation of the valve cusps, chordae tendineae, and papillary muscles interfere with valvular function and may lead to regurgitation, stenosis, or combined functional lesions. The fibrosing process has a tendency to produce incompetence of the tricuspid valve and stenosis of the smaller pulmonary orifice, a deleterious hemodynamic combination. Cardiac dysfunction may be further compromised by impaired atrial and ventricular compliance and by the occasional occurrence of a high cardiac output that probably results from continuing release of a vasodilator.

PULMONARY. Bronchoconstriction, usually most pronounced during flushing attacks, is a less common feature of the syndrome, but it may be severe.

GENERAL. Intestinal obstruction may result from the primary tumor or from the desmoplastic reaction in the surrounding mesentery; infrequently, the primary tumors cause gastrointestinal bleeding. Necrosis of hepatic tumor masses may produce an acute syndrome of abdominal pain, tenderness, fever, and leukocytosis. Hepatomegaly from the metastatic disease is usually present, but extensive metastatic involvement of the liver by the slowly growing tumors may occur before liver function tests become abnormal. Generalized fatigue and debilitation are underappreciated features of carcinoid syndrome.

THE ENDOCRINE FUNCTION OF CARCINOID TUMORS

SEROTONIN. The most constant biochemical feature of carcinoid tumors is the presence of tryptophan hydroxylase, which catalyzes the formation of 5-hydroxytryptophan (5-HTP) from tryptophan (Fig. 245–1). The typical ileal carcinoid tumor also contains aromatic L-amino-acid decarboxylase, which catalyzes the conversion of 5-HTP to 5-hydroxytryptamine (serotonin). Gastric carcinoids, however, are frequently deficient in this decarboxylase and release 5-HTP from the tumor.

Following its release from the tumor, serotonin is inactivated primarily by monoamine oxidase; uptake in the platelets also contributes to removal of free serotonin from blood. Monoamine oxidase oxidizes serotonin to 5-hydroxyindoleacetaldehyde, which is rapidly converted to 5-hydroxyindoleacetic acid (5-HIAA) by aldehyde dehydrogenase (see Fig. 245–1). This acid is rapidly excreted into the urine, and almost all circulating serotonin can be accounted for as urinary 5-HIAA.

TACHYKININS. Peptides of the tachykinin family are stored in carcinoid tumors and are released during flushing. Several tachykinins are derived from a common precursor β-preprotachykinin; of these, neuropeptide K, neurokinin A, and substance P have been identified in tumors and blood from patients with the carcinoid syndrome.

OTHER BIOLOGICALLY ACTIVE SUBSTANCES. Some carcinoid tumors, particularly those of gastric origin, release excessive amounts of histamine. This can be detected by an increased urinary excretion of histamine or its metabolite, *N*-methylhistamine.

Carcinoid tumors have been associated with a number of ectopic endocrine syndromes, including hyperadrenocorticism that results

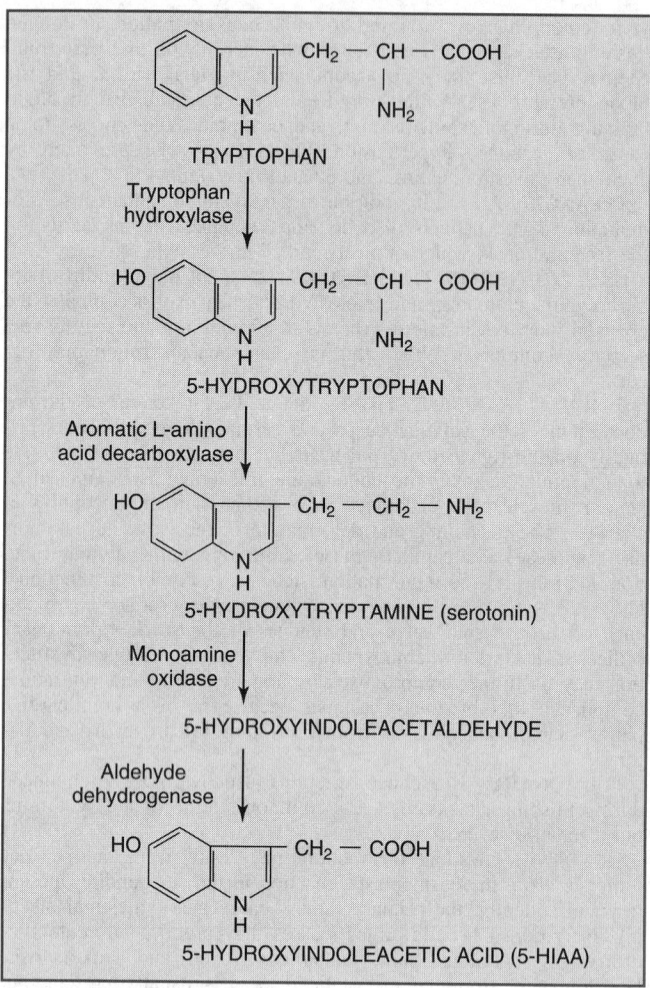

FIGURE 245–1 ■ Synthesis and degradation of serotonin.

from ectopic production of adrenocorticotropic hormone and acromegaly due to secretion of growth hormone-releasing hormone by the tumor.

MECHANISM OF THE FLUSH. Flushing can be triggered by catecholamines, and this probably accounts for the association of flushing with exercise and emotional stimuli. For experimental induction of flushing, injection of isoproterenol in amounts of as little as 0.5 μg may be effective. Pentagastrin, in doses as small as 0.25 μg, also can trigger flushing, an action that may explain the provocation of flushes by eating in some patients. As the hemodynamic changes associated with such pharmacologically induced attacks can be severe, epinephrine and other β-adrenergic amines as well as pentagastrin should be administered with great caution. Flushing episodes can be blocked by somatostatin.

Most of the evidence points to the tachykinins as mediators of the carcinoid flush. Tachykinins, particularly neuropeptide K, can be identified in plasma during flushing. Tachykinin levels have been shown to be increased during pentagastrin-induced flushing, and when pentagastrin-induced flushing is inhibited by somatostatin, the rise in tachykinin levels also is blocked. Tachykinins are known vasodilators.

Serotonin does not cause flushing. In patients with gastric carcinoids that secrete histamine, the flushing attacks can be attributed to histamine.

PATHOPHYSIOLOGY OF SEROTONIN OVERPRODUCTION. Serotonin contributes to the intestinal hypermotility and diarrhea. A secondary effect of serotonin overproduction occurs when a large fraction of dietary tryptophan is shunted into the hydroxylation pathway, leaving less tryptophan available for the formation of nicotinic acid and protein. When urinary excretion of 5-HIAA exceeds 100 mg daily, low levels of plasma tryptophan and evidence of nicotinic acid deficiency are seen.

DIAGNOSIS

When all of its clinical features are present, carcinoid syndrome is easily recognized. The diagnosis also must be considered when any one of its clinical manifestations is present.

The diagnostic hallmark consists of overproduction of 5-hydroxyindoles accompanied by increased excretion of urinary 5-HIAA. Normally, excretion of 5-HIAA does not exceed 9 mg daily. Ingestion of foods containing serotonin may complicate the biochemical diagnosis of carcinoid syndrome; both bananas and walnuts contain enough serotonin to produce abnormally elevated urinary excretion of 5-HIAA after their ingestion. When dietary 5-hydroxyindoles are excluded, urinary excretion of 25 mg of 5-HIAA daily is diagnostic of carcinoid. Elevation in the range of 9 to 25 mg may be seen with carcinoid syndrome, nontropical sprue, or acute intestinal obstruction. Measurement of serotonin in blood or platelets is of interest but has less diagnostic value than assay of the major metabolite of serotonin in the urine.

Assessment of the extent and localization of both primary and metastatic tumor is aided by computed tomographic scans of the abdomen and chest and by imaging with radionuclide-labeled somatostatin receptor ligands.

DIFFERENTIAL DIAGNOSIS. Attacks of flushing in a patient with normal urinary excretion of 5-HIAA raises other diagnostic possibilities. Systemic mastocyte activation disorders, including systemic mastocytosis and idiopathic anaphylaxis, produce flushing and diarrhea and should be considered when 5-HIAA excretion is not elevated. Flushing also occurs in genetically predisposed individuals following ethanol ingestion, in the postmenopausal state, and in conjunction with other neuroendocrine tumors such as VIPomas and medullary carcinoma of the thyroid.

VARIANTS OF THE CARCINOID SYNDROME. The origin of the tumor influences the biologically active substances produced and their storage and release. The typical carcinoid syndrome usually results from tumors of midgut origin, which almost invariably secrete serotonin. Tumor serotonin content is likely to be high, and the tumor usually contains dense nests of argentaffin-positive cells. In contrast, tumors arising from the embryonic foregut contain fewer argentaffin cells, have lower serotonin content, and may secrete 5-HTP. Ectopic hormone production (e.g., Cushing's syndrome and acromegaly) and multiple endocrine adenomas are more likely to be associated with tumors of embryonic foregut.

Patients with gastric carcinoids frequently exhibit unique flushing, which begins as a bright, patchy erythema with sharply delineated serpentine borders; these patches tend to coalesce as the blush heightens. Food ingestion is especially likely to produce flushes. The tumors are usually deficient in decarboxylase enzyme and secrete 5-HTP; histamine secretion is also common, as is a high incidence of peptic ulceration. In these patients, histamine is the principal factor causing flushing.

With carcinoid tumors arising from the bronchus, attacks of flushing tend to be prolonged and severe and may be associated with periorbital edema, excessive lacrimation and salivation, hypotension, tachycardia and tachyarrhythmias, anxiety, and tremulousness. Nausea, vomiting, explosive diarrhea, and bronchoconstriction may progress to a severe degree. This group is therapeutically unique in that severe flushes often can be prevented by corticosteroids.

TREATMENT

Treatment of the carcinoid syndrome is directed toward (1) pharmacologic therapy for humorally mediated symptoms and (2) the reduction of tumor mass.

The discovery that somatostatin can prevent the flushing and other endocrine manifestations of the carcinoid syndrome has provided the basis for a major advance in the treatment of these patients. The development of analogues of somatostatin, with longer biologic half-lives than the native hormone, has made subcutaneous administration a feasible route of therapy. One of the somatostatin analogues, octreotide, has been found to markedly improve the flushing and other endocrine manifestations of most patients with carcinoid syndrome. This is frequently associated with a reduction in urinary 5-HIAA excretion and in tachykinin levels in blood. With the improvement of these endocrine symptoms, including fatigue, a considerable improvement in quality of life may be achieved. Octreotide is administered subcutaneously at intervals of approximately 8 hours, usually beginning with 75 to 150 μg and titrating upward until maximum inhibition of flushing and other symptoms is achieved, which usually occurs at single doses of 750 μg or less. An uncommon but severe adverse effect of octreotide is hypoglycemia, probably as a result of the inhibition of glucagon and growth hormone secretion. The suppression of pancreatic exocrine function by octreotide can cause steatorrhea, and inhibition of the release of cholecystokinin can cause cholelithiasis. In patients receiving octreotide, about 5% achieve tumor regression, and in the group as a whole, less tumor progression and a longer median survival are seen in comparison with historical controls. Octreotide can prevent or treat carcinoid crises that accompany the massive release of mediators that sometimes occurs during operative procedures and tumor necrosis. In patients with histamine-secreting gastric carcinoids, blockade of both H_1- and H_2-histamine receptors markedly ameliorates flushing.

Early diagnosis of the carcinoid syndrome has led to complete surgical cure of a few patients with tumors arising in ovarian or testicular teratomas or in the bronchus. By releasing their humoral mediators directly into the systemic circulation, these tumors can produce the syndrome before metastatic disease occurs. In contrast, tumors that release humoral substances into the portal circulation to be largely metabolized by the liver usually produce the syndrome only after liver metastases occur. Given the slow progression of this neoplasm, however, effective reduction in tumor mass can ameliorate morbidity and improve the quality of life even after metastases have occurred. In selected patients, this can be achieved by surgical debulking of tumor, including hemihepatectomy for unilobar metastases, excision of large superficial hepatic metastases, and removal of the primary tumor together with regional lymph nodes containing metastases. Elective cholecystectomy during the surgical intervention will prevent the complications of cholelithiasis that may result from octreotide treatment. As the blood supply of hepatic metastases is largely arterial, percutaneous embolization of the hepatic arterial supply to the most involved hepatic lobe sometimes can reduce inoperable hepatic metastases; the procedure carries a high risk of complications. Chemotherapy with single or combination cytotoxic agents given acutely has produced little benefit except perhaps intra-arterially in conjunction with hepatic arterial embolization. For patients who exhibit tumor progression or whose clinical syndrome has failed to improve following cytoreduction and octreotide, interferon-alpha may be considered as adjunctive therapy.

A concerted strategy consisting of removal of the primary tumor, reduction in tumor bulk, and the administration of octreotide (with or without interferon-alpha) can lead to considerable amelioration of symptoms and improvement in the quality of life and also is intended to reduce the release of the humoral substances that engender the cardiac lesions.

Ahlman H, Wängberg B, Jansson S, et al: Management of disseminated midgut carcinoid tumors. Digestion 49:78, 1991. *Describes an approach to cytoreduction with surgical resection and hepatic arterial embolectomy in a well-studied series.*

Kvols LK, Reubi JC: Metastatic carcinoid tumors and the carcinoid syndrome. Acta Oncol 32:197, 1993. *A selective review that presents the results of octreotide therapy in 66 patients.*

Öberg K, Eriksson B, Janson ET: Interferons alone or in combination with chemotherapy or other biologicals in the treatment of neuroendocrine gut and pancreatic tumors. Digestion 55(suppl 3):64–69, 1994. *Describes treatment of carcinoid syndrome with interferons.*

246 DISORDERS OF SEXUAL DIFFERENTIATION*

Maria I. New ■ *Nathalie Josso*

Gonads, genital ducts, and external genitalia become sexually dimorphic during fetal life, depending on the presence or absence

*Significant sections of the work on which the data are reported herein were supported by USPHS Grant HD00072 and GCRC Grant 06020.

of genetic and endocrine factors, nearly all of which actively impose maleness. Female differentiation usually requires no specific stimulus and occurs constitutively in the absence of male-determining factors. This asymmetrical mechanism of sex differentiation has an important bearing on the pathogenesis of intersex disorders: Male pseudohermaphroditism, defined as incomplete virilization of a 46,XY male, results from defects in the synthesis, metabolism, or action of one or several masculinizing factors. In contrast, female pseudohermaphroditism results from inappropriate exposure of female anlagen to masculinizing agents.

ANATOMY OF NORMAL SEX DIFFERENTIATION

MALE SEX DIFFERENTIATION. TESTICULAR DIFFERENTIATION. The gonadal primordium is represented by the gonadal ridge, which is progressively colonized by extraembryonic primordial germ cells. The first recognizable event of testicular differentiation, at 7 weeks' gestation, is the development of primordial Sertoli cells, which aggregate to form seminiferous tubules and produce antimüllerian hormone (AMH). Leydig cells differentiate at 8 weeks of gestation and increase until 12 to 14 weeks, when they begin to degenerate. At birth, very few remain in the interstitial tissue; the Leydig cell population reappears at puberty.

SOMATIC SEX DIFFERENTIATION. After gonadal differentiation, the internal reproductive tract consists of two pairs of ducts: the wolffian ducts and the müllerian ducts. In males, müllerian duct regression begins at 8 weeks and is more or less complete at 10 to 12 weeks. The wolffian ducts develop into the vasa deferentia, epididymides, and seminal vesicles. Prostatic buds develop around the opening of the ducts at 10 to 11 weeks of gestation, and fusion of outgrowths of the urogenital sinus forms the prostatic utricle, the male equivalent of the vagina (Fig. 246–1). At 10 weeks, elongation of the genital tubercle and fusion of the urethral folds over the urethral groove lead to formation of the penile urethra, whereas the genital swellings move posteriorly and fuse to form the scrotum (Fig. 246–2). Male anatomic development is completed by 90 days of gestation, but penile growth occurs only between 20 weeks and term, at a time when, paradoxically, serum testosterone levels are declining.

FEMALE DIFFERENTIATION. OVARIAN DIFFERENTIATION. Slower than the testis to differentiate initially, the fetal ovary eventually reaches a more advanced stage of maturation. At 12 to 13 weeks, some oogonia located in the deepest layer of the cortex have entered the meiotic prophase. By 7 months' gestation, all germ cells have entered or completed the meiotic prophase. Fetal granulosa cells produce estrogen at the same developmental stage at which fetal testes produce testosterone, but ovarian production of AMH can be demonstrated only after birth.

SOMATIC SEX DIFFERENTIATION. Female fetal sex differentiation is characterized by degeneration of the wolffian ducts at 10 weeks, whereas the müllerian ducts develop into fallopian tubes, uterus, and the upper part of the vagina. The vagina differentiates at the level of the müllerian tubercle, between the openings of the wolffian ducts where the prostatic utricle forms in males. Whereas in males the prostatic utricle opens just beneath the neck of the bladder, in females, the lower end of the vagina slides down the posterior wall of the urethra to acquire a separate opening on the body surface (see Fig. 246–1). Feminization of the external genitalia begins with formation of the dorsal commissure between the genital swellings, which in the female do not migrate posteriorly or fuse and give rise to the labia majora. Because the genital folds do not fuse, they become the labia minora, and the genital tubercle becomes the clitoris. In the female, all these steps are constitutive and occur in the absence of hormonal stimulation.

MECHANISMS OF SEX DIFFERENTIATION

GENETICS OF SEX DETERMINATION: SRY AND ITS PARTNERS. Testicular differentiation is usually called sex determination because it determines whether testicular hormones, responsible for subsequent somatic sex differentiation, will be produced. Sex determination in mammals is governed primarily by SRY, a transcription factor expressed by Sertoli cells under the control of a gene

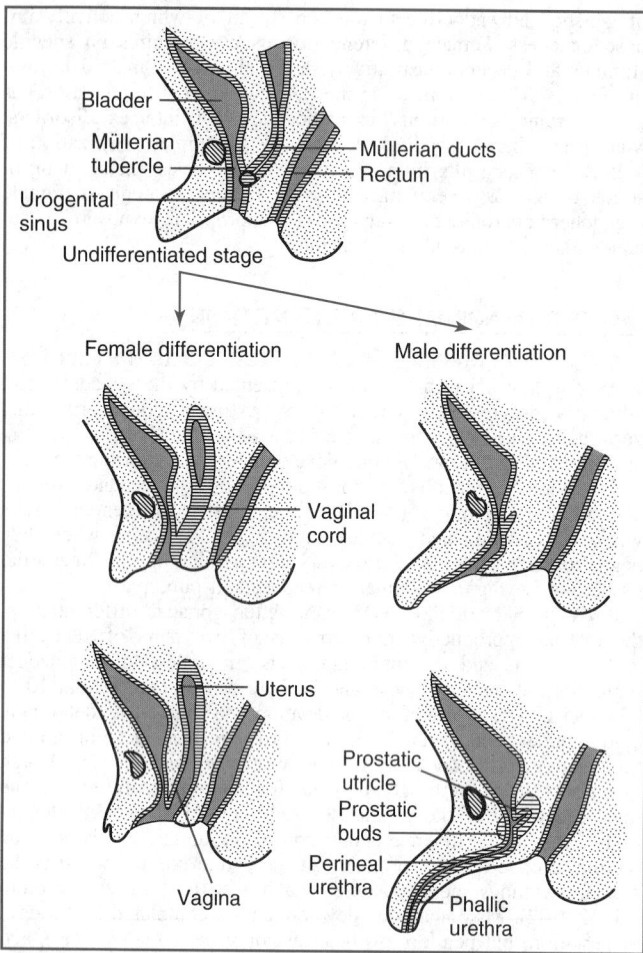

FIGURE 246–1 ■ Differentiation of the urogenital sinus. (From Josso N: Physiology of sex differentiation: A guide to the understanding and management of the intersex child. *In* Josso N [ed]: The Intersex Child. Basel, Karger, 1981, p 1.)

located on the Y chromosome proximal to the pseudoautosomal boundary. The pseudoautosomal regions of the sex chromosomes enter into homologous recombination at meiosis, and it is essential that the testis-determining gene be situated in the non-recombining Y-specific region. Mutations of *SRY* are encountered in approximately 15% of XY sex-reversed females, and conversely, translocation of *SRY* on an X chromosome leads to maleness in XX individuals.

However, normal SRY transcripts, although necessary, do not guarantee normal testicular differentiation. Wilms' tumor type 1 (WT-1), a tumor suppressor, and the orphan nuclear receptor SF-1 (steroidogenic factor type 1) are required for gonadal development irrespective of genotype, as shown by knockout experiments in mice. Dominant mutations of *WT-1* often lead to sexual ambiguity in XY patients. Another autosomal sex-determining locus, *SOX9* on chromosome 17q, is associated with campomelic dysplasia and sex reversal in XY individuals. Monosomy of 9p and 10q also lead to XY sex ambiguity. *DAX-1,* an Xp21 gene, is not required for testicular development but may be involved in ovarian differentiation because the duplication of a 160-kilobase region of Xp21 in males overrides the effect of *SRY* and results in XY sex reversal.

BIOSYNTHESIS AND ACTION OF TESTICULAR HORMONES. Virilization of the reproductive tract is mediated by AMH and testosterone; in their absence or inactivity, female differentiation proceeds unimpeded. AMH, a glycoprotein synthesized by immature Sertoli and postnatal granulosa cells, is responsible for müllerian regression. The gene, located on chromosome 19, is a member of the transforming growth factor β (TGF-β) family and acts via a type II AMH receptor whose gene is located on chromosome 12q13.

Androgens are responsible for maintenance of the wolffian ducts

and virilization of the urogenital sinus and external genitalia. Testosterone is produced from cholesterol by gonadotropin stimulation of fetal Leydig cells through the coordinated action of steroidogenic enzymes, most of which are also expressed in the adrenal gland. P-450 side-chain cleavage enzyme, which is responsible for the initial step in the steroidogenic pathway, is located at the inner mitochondrial membrane. Translocation of cholesterol into the mitochondrion is dependent on steroidogenic acute regulatory protein, a phosphoprotein coded by a gene located on chromosome 8p11.2. Steroidogenic acute regulatory protein, steroidogenic P-450 enzymes, and AMH are positively regulated by SF-1, whose action is opposed by DAX-1.

Testosterone production by the fetal testis is detectable at 9 weeks in the human fetus, increases to a peak at 15 to 18 weeks, and then falls sharply, so the serum concentrations of testosterone overlap in males and females in late pregnancy. When human chorionic gonadotropin (hCG) declines in the 3rd trimester, the hypothalamic-pituitary axis gains control over testicular functional activity.

Testosterone is the major steroid released by fetal testes in the blood stream and enters cells by passive diffusion or pinocytosis. A local source of androgen is important for wolffian duct development, which does not occur if testosterone is supplied only via the peripheral circulation, as in female pseudohermaphroditism caused by adrenal hyperplasia. Testosterone is converted intracellularly to dihydrotestosterone (DHT) by the enzyme 5α-reductase (Fig. 246–3). Two distinct isoforms of 5α-reductase have been cloned: Type 1 is present in very low levels in the prostate and the sebaceous glands; type 2 is present in high levels in the prostate and in the

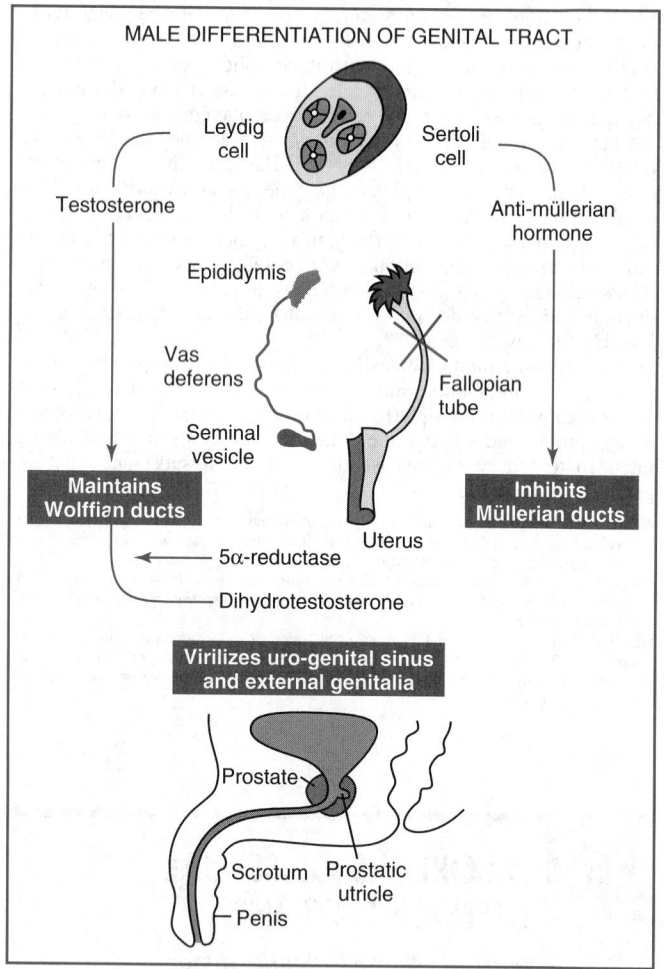

FIGURE 246–2 ■ Hormones involved in male differentiation of the reproductive tract. Testosterone, synthesized by Leydig cells, maintains the wolffian ducts and virilizes the urogenital sinus and external genitalia after reduction to dihydrotestosterone. Antimüllerian hormone, produced by fetal Sertoli cells, inhibits development of the müllerian ducts, which would otherwise develop into the uterus and fallopian tubes. (From Josso N: Physiology of sex differentiation: A guide to the understanding and management of the intersex child. *In* Josso N (ed): The Intersex Child. Basel, Karger, 1981, p 1.)

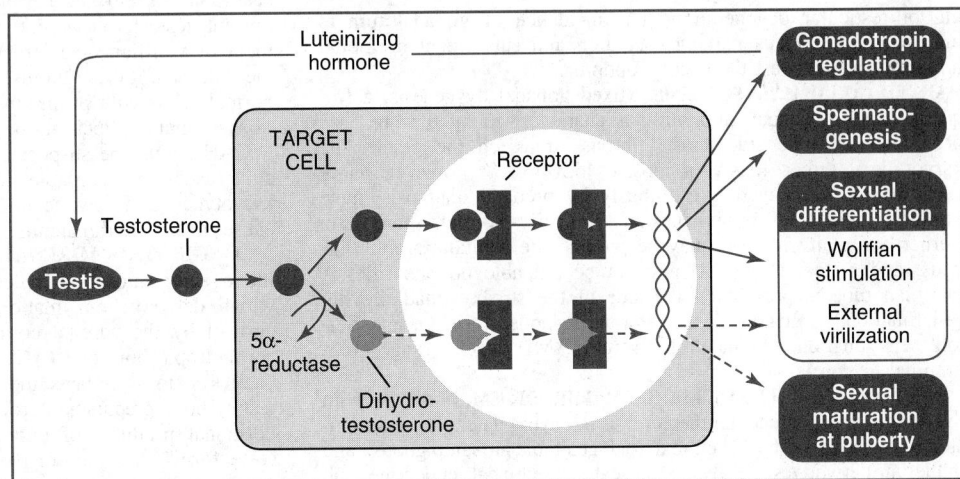

FIGURE 246-3 ■ General scheme of androgen action. (From Wilson JD: Syndromes of androgen resistance. Biol Reprod 46:168, 1992.)

area of the external genitalia. DHT binds to the androgen receptor with greater affinity and stability than does testosterone. Therefore, in tissues equipped with 5α-reductase at the time of sex differentiation, such as the prostate, urogenital sinus, and external genitalia, DHT is the active androgen. However, at high concentrations, testosterone interacts with the androgen receptor similarly to DHT. The gene coding for the androgen receptor is located on the long arm of the X chromosome.

CLASSIFICATION OF INTERSEX STATES

Normal sex differentiation occurs at various levels (Fig. 246-4). Genetic sex is established at fertilization by the nature of the sex chromosome donated by the spermatozoon. The presence or absence of sex-determining genes dictates gonadal sex, whereas the presence or absence of fetal testicular hormones determines somatic sex. Gender identity is established early in life by the sex of rearing but can be disrupted at puberty by hormonal factors.

Disorders of Gonadal Sex

Gonadal sex disorders may or may not be associated with sex chromosome abnormalities.

TURNER'S SYNDROME. Patients with Turner's syndrome have normal female genitalia, short stature, and typical dysmorphic features. The dysmorphism includes an increased carrying angle of the arms, sphinx-like neck, low hairline, shield chest, widely spaced

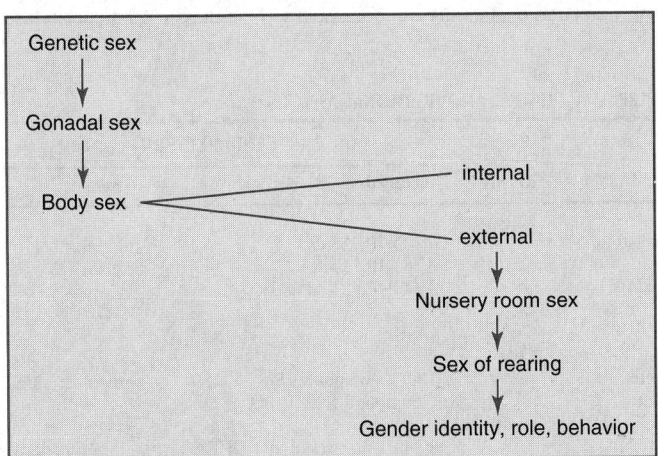

FIGURE 246-4 ■ Stages of sex differentiation. Genetic sex specified at fertilization determines gonadal sex, which in turn determines somatic and legal sex. Gender identity is usually determined by the sex of rearing. (From New MI, Levine LS: Congenital adrenal hyperplasia. In Harris H, Hirschhorn K [eds]: Advances in Human Genetics. New York, Plenum Press, 1973, p 251.)

nipples, and typical facies characterized by low-set ears and micrognathia. The chromosomal complement is 45,X, and the incidence is about 1 in 2500 births. Treatment with human growth hormone has improved the final height of patients with Turner's syndrome. The patients are infertile because the ovaries are dysgenetic and have become bilateral streaks without follicles. Thus these patients have primary amenorrhea and are infertile. Because the internal genitalia include a normal uterus and fallopian tubes, patients may benefit from *in vitro* fertilization.

KLINEFELTER'S SYNDROME. In this condition, males have normal development of the penis and scrotum, but the testes are small and firm. At adolescence, gynecomastia is frequent and infertility is common as a result of azoospermia. The usual karyotype is 47,XXY. Hormonal findings include elevated gonadotropin levels and a decreased serum testosterone concentration. Klinefelter's syndrome is a common disorder that occurs in 1 in 500 men.

XX MALE SYNDROME. Males with a 46,XX karyotype have normal external and internal male genitalia; however, they resemble patients with Klinefelter's syndrome in that they have small testes, azoospermia, and infertility. Translocation of the *SRY* gene on the X chromosome is detected in 90% of sporadic cases, but not when XX maleness and true hermaphroditism are transmitted as an autosomal recessive condition in the same family.

TRUE HERMAPHRODITISM. True hermaphroditism, a rare and usually sporadic disorder, is defined as the coexistence of seminiferous tubules and ovarian follicles in the same subject. Most patients have an ovotestis with either an ovary or a testis on the opposite side; a testis is usually in the scrotum, an ovotestis more seldom.

The genitalia are usually ambiguous; rare cases of completely masculine or feminine genitalia have been reported. The anatomy of the internal reproductive tract depends on the nature of the gonads. A uterus is present in approximately 90% of cases. Testosterone response to hCG is variable, and AMH levels are usually low. Most patients experience breast development, ovulation, and even menstruation at puberty; pregnancy and successful childbirth are possible if selective removal of testicular tissue is feasible. Unless gender has already been assigned, male orientation should be restricted to patients with no uterus and descended testicular tissue because testicular tissue is usually dysgenetic and prone to malignant degeneration. The majority of true hermaphrodites have a 46,XX karyotype. To resolve the discrepancy between the presence of testicular tissue and the lack of a Y chromosome, the DNA of 46,XX true hermaphrodites has been probed for SRY. True hermaphrodites usually lack SRY, which suggests that the condition, at least in familial cases, is due to constitutive activation of a gene normally triggered by SRY.

TESTICULAR DYSGENESIS. Testicular dysgenesis is characterized by seminiferous tubule degeneration and invasion by connective tissue arranged in whorls as in a streak gonad. Germ cells are rare or absent; the gonad is often maldescended and prone to malignant degeneration. The clinical picture, as in true hermaphroditism, combines defects of AMH- and testosterone-dependent steps of sex differentiation, depending on the extent and timing of testicular degeneration. The incidence of gonadal tumors may reach 30%, thus making castration and subsequent hormonal replacement the safest therapeutic option.

MIXED GONADAL DYSGENESIS. Mixed gonadal dysgenesis, a frequent cause of sexual ambiguity, is characterized by the presence of a testis on one side and a fibrous streak on the other. The karyotype is either 46,XY or mosaic 45,X/46,XY; however, many such mosaics, discovered fortuitously by prenatal diagnosis, have normally developed testes and are clinically normal. Otherwise, Turner-like malformations may be present, the genitalia are ambiguous, and a gonad may or may not be palpable on one side. A fallopian tube is present on the side of the streak gonad. Leydig cell function, evaluated by testosterone response to hCG, and Sertoli cell function, evaluated by serum AMH levels, range from minimal to normal.

DYSGENETIC MALE PSEUDOHERMAPHRODITISM. Patients with dysgenetic male pseudohermaphroditism have bilaterally differentiated dysgenetic testes. Their external genitalia are ambiguous, and müllerian derivatives are always present. The clinical, endocrine, and cytogenetic picture is similar to that of mixed gonadal dysgenesis.

PURE GONADAL DYSGENESIS, TESTICULAR REGRESSION SYNDROME. Patients with pure gonadal dysgenesis have a normal female phenotype, including uterus and fallopian tubes, but have fibrous streaks instead of gonads; they are free of Turner-like malformations and attain normal height. Familial cases have been described with either a 46,XX or, more frequently, a 46,XY karyotype; in the latter, mutations of the *SRY* gene have been identified in 15% of cases. Other 46,XY patients with absent gonads have various degrees of sexual ambiguity and no müllerian derivatives. The implication that some testicular tissue was functional at least up to 10 weeks and subsequently regressed has led to the name "fetal testicular regression syndrome." Testicular regression may occur in late pregnancy or even postnatally; these fully virilized males have only bilateral cryptorchidism. This condition is also known as *anorchia*.

Disorders of Phenotypic Sex

Female Pseudohermaphroditism

Female pseudohermaphroditism, defined as the sexual ambiguity of a 46,XX fetus with two normal ovaries, is the most frequent type of intersex. Rarely, the female fetus is masculinized because of transplacental transfer of androgens from an ovarian or adrenocortical tumor in the mother or from exogenous steroids. Most female pseudohermaphrodites have been exposed to endogenous androgens prenatally as a result of congenital adrenal hyperplasia (CAH).

Virilization caused by androgen excess is limited to the androgen-responsive external genitalia (the lower part of the vagina, genital folds and swellings, and phallus). Masculinization ranges from minimal clitoromegaly and a mild degree of posterior labial fusion to the formation of a urogenital sinus with the orifice lo-

cated distally along the urethral groove and ending, in extreme cases, at the tip of the phallus. Because no testicular tissue is present, testosterone is not produced locally to support the development of wolffian duct structures, nor is AMH produced; therefore the fallopian tubes, uterus, and upper portion of the vagina are normal. Thus with proper medical treatment and vaginal reconstruction, normal childbearing is possible.

CAH should be suspected in sexually ambiguous newborns with a uterus but no palpable gonadal tissue. Such patients should be karyotyped and have endocrine evaluation done immediately because of the life-threatening salt loss found in many cases of CAH.

CONGENITAL ADRENAL HYPERPLASIA. CAH is a family of monogenic autosomal recessive disorders of steroidogenesis in which defective enzymatic steps result in impaired synthesis of cortisol by the adrenal cortex (Table 246–1). Subsequent adrenocorticotropic hormone (ACTH) oversecretion via the negative-feedback system stimulates the adrenal to become hyperplastic. As a result, both precursor steroids proximal to the enzyme block and hormonal products of unimpeded pathways are overproduced. In some forms, diversion of precursor steroids into androgen pathways results in excessive levels of potent androgens and virilization of the female fetus. In other forms, underproduction of sex steroids in both the adrenal and the testes leads to ambiguous genitalia in genetic males. Abnormal secretion of mineralocorticoids in some cases results in disturbances in the regulation of electrolytes, plasma volume, and blood pressure, with the risk of decompensation and shock.

STEROID 21-HYDROXYLASE DEFICIENCY. CLASSIC 21-HYDROXYLASE DEFICIENCY. Steroid 21-hydroxylase deficiency is the most common enzymatic defect causing CAH. Classic 21-hydroxylase deficiency occurs in about 1 in 15,000 live births, but the incidence may vary by population and geographic area (Fig. 246–5). The classic disorder has two forms: salt wasting and simple virilizing (non–salt wasting); both result in sexual ambiguity in the newborn genetic female. In the salt-wasting form, which occurs in about three fourths of cases, adrenal production of aldosterone and cortisol is inadequate. Salt-wasting crises are associated with hyponatremia, hyperkalemia, and hypovolemia, with metabolic acidosis, loss of vascular tone, and in some cases, shock and death. Crises usually arise between 7 days and 2 weeks of life, after discharge from the hospital. Thus an affected first-born male who has normal genitalia is particularly at risk for a salt-wasting crisis at home. Ambiguous genitalia in a female usually prompt diagnostic procedures, thus placing females at lower risk. Salt wasting should be carefully ruled out even in newborns with mild genital ambiguity. Unlike salt wasters, simple virilizers can synthesize sufficient amounts of aldosterone for salt retention.

NON-CLASSIC 21-HYDROXYLASE DEFICIENCY. Non-classic 21-hydroxylase deficiency, a genetic variant of the classic form, is associated with a milder enzyme defect and does not cause prenatal virilization in a genetic female. However, signs of androgen excess may appear postnatally in both sexes. Non-classic 21-hydroxylase

---

Table 246–1 ■ FORMS OF CONGENITAL ADRENAL HYPERPLASIA: CLINICAL AND HORMONAL ASPECTS

DEFICIENCY	GENITAL AMBIGUITY	POSTNATAL VIRILIZATION	SALT METABOLISM	RENIN	STEROID PATTERN Increased	STEROID PATTERN Decreased
21-Hydroxylase				High		
A. Classic salt wasting	F	Yes	Salt wasting		17-OHP; Δ⁴-A	aldo; cortisol
Simple virilizing	F	Yes	Normal		17-OHP; Δ⁴-A	cortisol
B. Non-classic (symptomatic and asymptomatic)	No	Yes	Normal		17-OHP; Δ⁴-A	—
11β-Hydroxylase				Low		
A. Classic	F	Yes	Salt retention		DOC; compound S	cortisol ± aldo
B. Non-classic	No	Yes	Normal		Compound S ± DOC	
3β-Hydroxysteroid dehydrogenase				High		
A. Classic	M/F	Yes	Salt wasting		17-OH-pregnenolone; DHEA	aldo; cortisol; T
B. Non-classic	No	Yes	Normal		17-OH-pregnenolone; DHEA	—
17α-Hydroxylase	M	No	Salt retention	Low	DOC; compound B	cortisol; T
17,20-Lyase	M	No	Normal		None	DHEA; T; Δ⁴-A
Cholesterol desmolase	M	No	Salt wasting	High	None	All

17-OHP = 17-hydroxyprogesterone; Δ⁴-A = Δ⁴-androstenedione; aldo = aldosterone; DOC = deoxycorticosterone; compound S = 11-deoxycortisol; DHEA = dehydroepiandrosterone; T = testosterone; B = corticosterone.

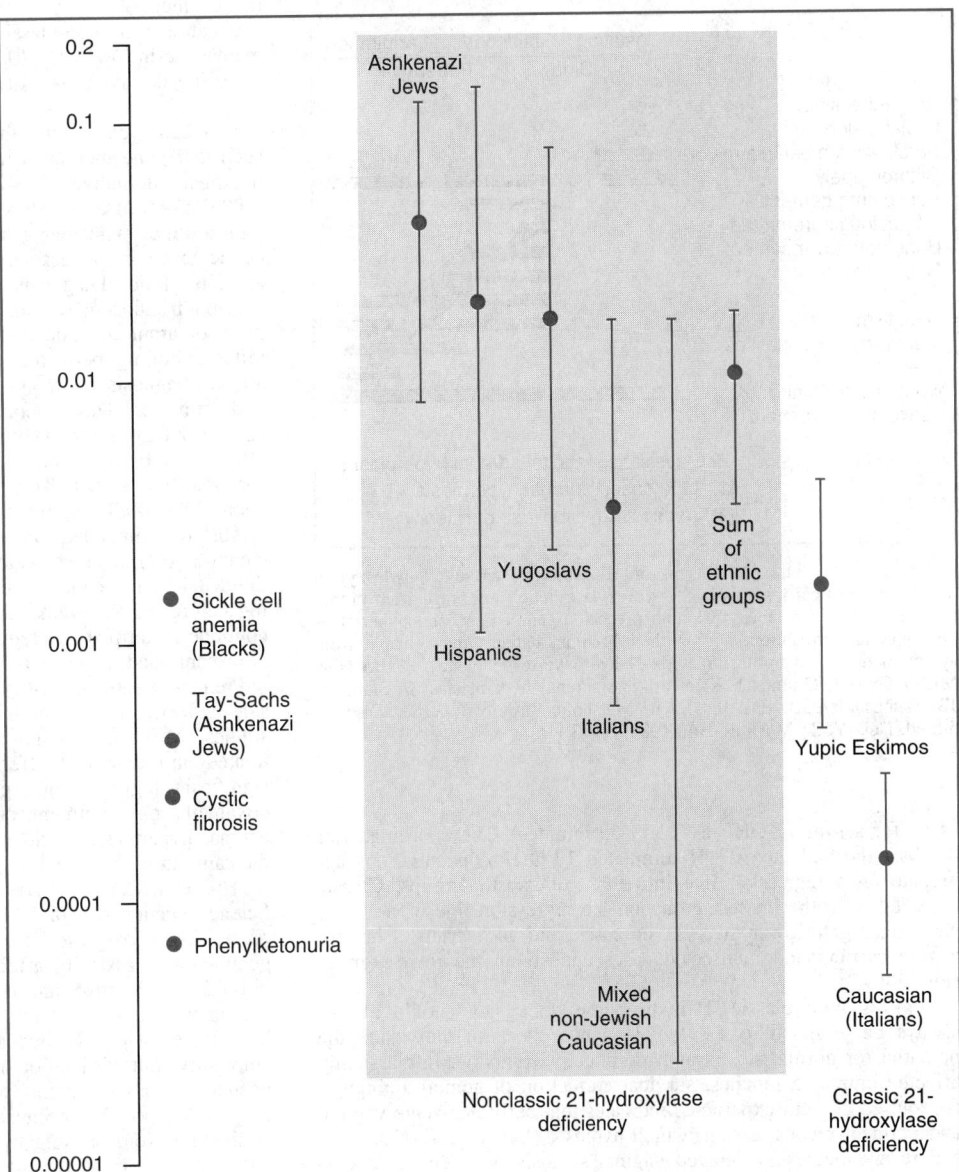

FIGURE 246–5 ■ Disease frequencies of classic 21-hydroxylase deficiency (in two populations), non-classic 21-hydroxylase deficiency (in five ethnic groups), and four other relatively common autosomal recessive disorders are compared. (From Speiser PW, DuPont B, Rubinstein P, et al: High frequency of nonclassical steroid 21-hydroxylase deficiency. Am J Hum Genet 37:650, 1985.)

deficiency occurs in 1 in 100 people in the general population, with a higher frequency in specific ethnic groups (e.g., 1 in 27 Ashkenazi Jews, 1 in 40 Hispanics, 1 in 50 Slavs, 1 in 300 Italians), which makes this deficiency the most frequent autosomal recessive disease in humans.

CLINICAL FEATURES. In 21-hydroxylase deficiency, 17α-hydroxy-progesterone (17-OHP) and progesterone are overproduced and are converted to the androgens dehydroepiandrosterone, Δ4-androstene-dione, and testosterone, which cause virilization. Postnatally, in children with untreated classic and non-classic 21-hydroxylase deficiency, growth accelerates in the early years but the epiphyses close prematurely, which results in a tall child but a short adult. Even when treated, most patients do not reach the height potential indicated by family height. Pubertal development under hypotha-lamic-pituitary control may be suppressed by excess adrenal andro-gens, and fertility potential may not be achieved until proper treat-ment is instituted to suppress ACTH and adrenal androgen secretion. Without treatment, males may have evidence of pseudo-puberty marked by phallic growth, small testes, and precocious growth of pubic, axillary, and body hair. Male internal and ex-ternal genital development is normal. Untreated females may suffer from excessive androgenic symptoms such as cystic acne, men-strual/ovulatory irregularities, or polycystic ovarian syndrome (Fig. 246–6).

MOLECULAR GENETICS. The gene encoding 21-hydroxylase is lo-

cated on the short arm of chromosome 6 within the human major histocompatibility complex. The gene locus for the 21-hydroxylase enzyme, termed *CYP21*, has a closely neighboring homologue, the pseudogene *CYP21P*, that is not expressed. Two forms of muta-tions observed are gene deletions, which result from chromosomal misalignment as well as unequal crossing over during meiosis, and gene conversions, which apparently involve the transfer of short sequences resident on the pseudogene to the active gene. Although in most patients the severity of the *CYP21* mutation correlates with the severity of disease and the disease type, among apparently mutation-identical groups, genotype does not always correlate with phenotype.

DIAGNOSIS AND TREATMENT. Screening of newborns for elevated serum 17-OHP identifies males and females with classic 21-hydrox-ylase deficiency irrespective of genital phenotype. In the United States, newborns are currently screened in 18 states. In suspected cases, the chromosomal or genetic sex should be determined by buccal smear for Barr bodies, karyotyping, fluorescent Y, or SRY analysis. Elevated 17-OHP, which may be several hundred times normal, confirms the enzyme defect. Routine screening at random does not detect the non-classic form of 21-hydroxylase deficiency. In the non-classic form, 17-OHP levels may be elevated in early morning readings but normal in midmorning and afternoon. Thus the deficiency is best diagnosed with an ACTH stimulation test (an intravenous bolus injection of 0.25 mg of synthetic ACTH and

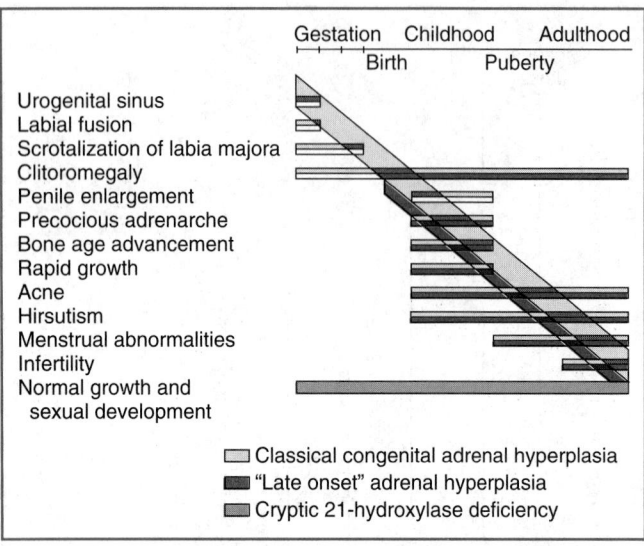

FIGURE 246–6 ■ Clinical spectrum of HLA-linked steroid 21-hydroxylase deficiency. Clinical features in 21-hydroxylase deficiency range from prenatal virilization with labial fusion to precocious adrenarche and pubertal or post-pubertal virilization. During their lifetime, patients may change from symptomatic to asymptomatic with 21-hydroxylase deficiency. (From New MI, DuPont B, Grumbach K, et al: The adrenal hyperplasias. *In* Stanbury JB, Wyngaarden JB, et al [eds]: The Metabolic Basis of Inherited Disease, 5th ed. New York, McGraw-Hill, 1983, p 973.)

assay for serum 17-OHP at 0 and 60 minutes). The coordinates of the baseline and the ACTH-stimulated 17-OHP concentrations aggregate on a regression line into three diagnostic groups. Classic cases fall into the highest group on the regression line, non-classic cases aggregate lower than classic cases, and an overlap of heterozygote carriers and unaffected cases appears in the lowest group (Fig. 246–7).

Females with classic 21-hydroxylase deficiency should almost always be assigned to the female gender because they have the potential for normal sexual and reproductive function. In classically affected untreated females, surgical correction of genital ambiguity is required. Recent experience indicates that early one-stage vaginal and perineal reconstruction, which avoids a 2nd-stage surgical procedure and decreases delayed vaginal stenosis, is effective in correcting the ambiguity in certain cases.

Postnatal management involves lifelong hormonal replacement. It is necessary to monitor the 17-OHP serum concentration (or daily urinary excretion of pregnanetriol) as well as plasma renin activity in the classic salt-wasting form. Hydrocortisone is generally given in infancy and childhood in a dose range of 10 to 25 mg/m²/day to maintain the serum 17-OHP concentration between 500 and 1000 ng/dL. Attempts to bring the 17-OHP concentration to normal will result in cushingoid features and retarded growth. In adolescence and adulthood, hydrocortisone may be replaced with dexamethasone or prednisone. Mineralocorticoid (9α-fluorohydrocortisone) administration and added salt to the diet are necessary in patients with salt-wasting disease and may improve hormonal control in simple virilizers. Unfortunately, in a sizable number of children with CAH, it has proved difficult to maintain satisfactory adrenal suppression without producing an unacceptable degree of hypercortisolism. Unfavorable outcomes include short stature, reduced fertility, polycystic ovaries, irregualar menses, acne, hirsutism, frontal balding, and progressive obesity. Although erratic compliance with prescribed substitution therapy is undeniably a major cause of escape from pituitary suppression, much of the problem is inherent in our limited ability to control ACTH secretion. For this reason, it has been suggested that the more severely affected children (severely virilized and salt wasting with double null mutations in the 21-hydroxylase gene) will have a better quality of life if they are adrenalectomized at an early age and reared as patients with Addison's disease would be, who require modest doses of daily steroids (with provision for increased dosages in the face of stress). To

date, this approach shows promise in the limited number of cases documented.

Treatment of non-classic 21-hydroxylase deficiency with dexamethasone in low doses (0.25 mg at bedtime) is usually effective in reversing the symptoms of androgen excess, including reduced fertility.

In recent years, gene therapy technology has greatly advanced such that gene therapy using CYP21 cDNA may become a viable treatment alternative.

PRENATAL MANAGEMENT. Prenatal diagnosis is best performed with a direct molecular genetic approach; in salt wasters it can also be achieved by assessment of 17-OHP or Δ⁴-androstenedione in amniotic fluid. Diagnosis by DNA testing requires sampling of chorion frondosum obtained by chorionic villus sampling or sampling of amniotic fluid cells obtained by amniocentesis. Chorionic villus sampling performed in the 8th to 10th week of gestation allows diagnosis earlier than does amniocentesis performed in the 2nd trimester. Direct examination of the *CYP21* gene locus is carried out by Southern blotting for identification of gene deletions (10 to 35% of cases) and with allele-specific oligonucleotide probes for point mutations. Together, these two tests routinely identify about 90% of all mutations.

The recommended prenatal treatment of 21-hydroxylase deficiency is oral dexamethasone, 20 μg/kg/day (pre-pregnancy weight) divided in three equal doses and administered to the mother starting before the 9th week of gestation (Fig. 246–8). Therapy should continue to term if the fetus is found to be an affected female but is discontinued if the fetus is male or an unaffected female.

Prenatal treatment with dexamethasone has been shown to be safe and effective for both mother and child in the largest human studies. Mean birthweight and fetal wastage were the same for treated and untreated affected females. Except for a statistically significant higher weight gain in mothers who received prenatal dexamethasone treatment, other maternal side effects such as striae, edema, hypertension, and gestational diabetes were reported to be the same in both groups.

11β-HYDROXYLASE DEFICIENCY. Steroid 11β-hydroxylase deficiency occurs in 1 in 100,000 to 1 in 200,000 births worldwide. As in 21-hydroxylase deficiency, masculinization of the external genitalia in classically affected females occurs in utero. The steroids 11-deoxycortisol and deoxycorticosterone are oversecreted, and precursors are shunted into uninhibited androgen pathways. Newborn males with 11β-hydroxylase deficiency do not have genital ambiguity, but virilization in untreated males and females ensues postnatally. Hypertension with or without hypokalemic alkalosis may occur, possibly because of excess deoxycorticosterone (a salt-retaining steroid causing hypokalemia), plasma volume expansion, and suppression of plasma renin activity. Non-classic manifestations of 11β-hydroxylase deficiency have also been recognized.

MOLECULAR GENETICS. Two genes located on the long arm of chromosome 8 encode the 11β-hydroxylase enzyme proteins CYP11B1 (expressed in the zona fasciculata) and CYP11B2 (expressed in the zona glomerulosa). Mutations in the *CYP11B1* gene, which has regulatory sequences responsive to ACTH, impair cortisol synthesis and cause CAH. Mutations in the *CYP11B2* gene, which normally expresses the enzyme aldosterone synthase, impair aldosterone synthesis but not cortisol synthesis. This rare condition, termed corticosterone methyloxidase type II deficiency (Persian salt-wasting disease), causes salt-wasting symptoms in early life that often resolve by adulthood. Because the *CYP11B* genes are homologues, splicing mutations create a chimeric gene having regulatory sequence features of *CYP11B1* and structural coding features of *CYP11B2*; the result is a rare form of low-renin hypertension called dexamethasone-suppressible hyperaldosteronism.

DIAGNOSIS AND TREATMENT. In 11β-hydroxylase deficiency, serum 11-deoxycortisol (compound S) and deoxycorticosterone are elevated. Plasma renin activity is suppressed and/or plasma aldosterone levels are very low. In genetic females with ambiguous genitalia, 11β-hydroxylase deficiency can be distinguished from 21-hydroxylase deficiency by elevated levels of compound S and deoxycorticosterone, as well as by suppressed plasma renin activity.

Treatment of 11β-hydroxylase deficiency with glucocorticoids leads to reduced levels of deoxycorticosterone with natriuresis, a rise in plasma renin activity, and normotension. Because the renin-angiotensin system is no longer suppressed, aldosterone levels rise to normal. Surgical correction may be necessary in untreated ge-

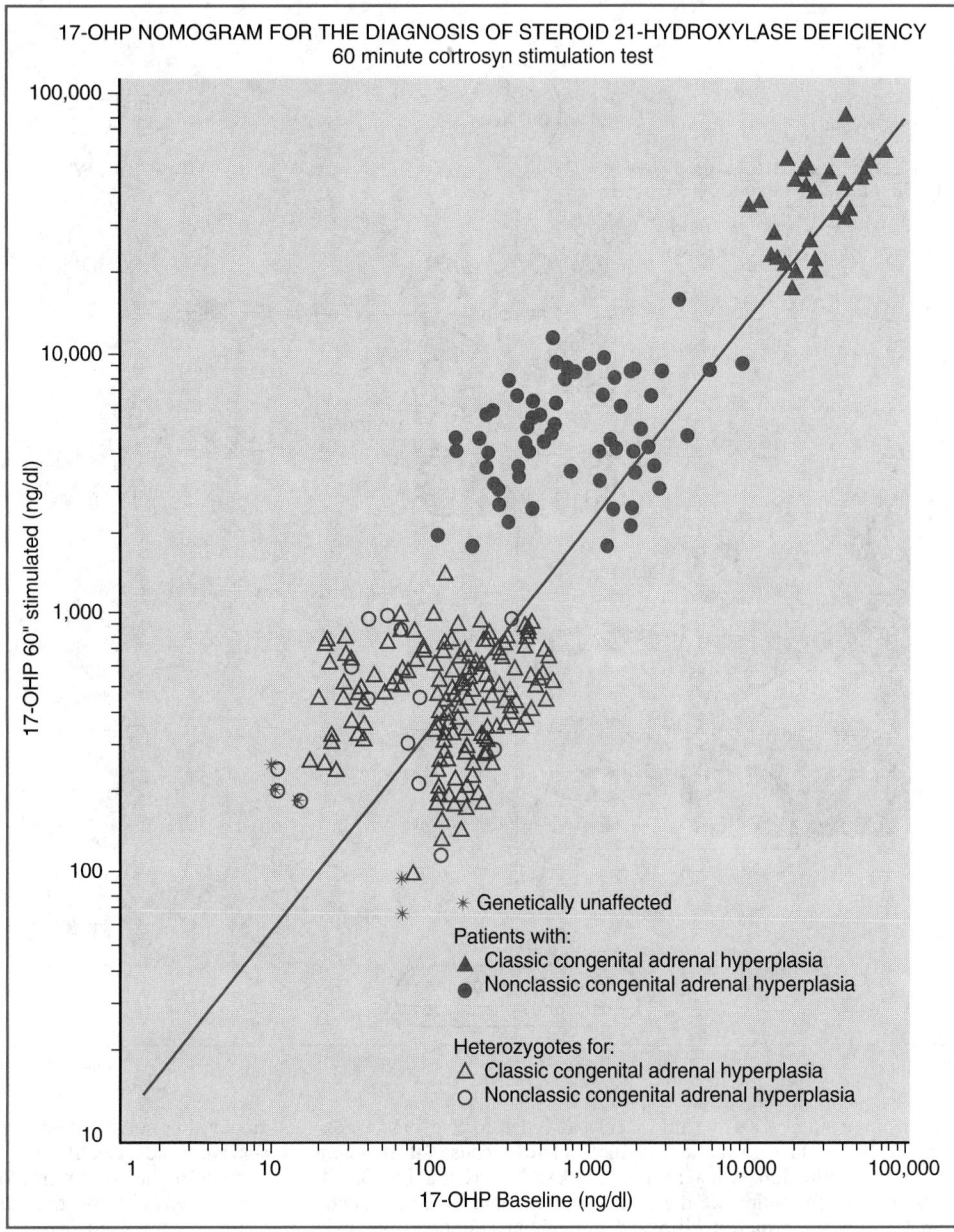

FIGURE 246–7 ▪ Nomogram relating baseline to adrenocorticotropic hormone–stimulated serum concentrations of 17-hydroxyprogesterone (17-OHP). The scales are logarithmic. A regression line for all data points is shown. The data for this nomogram were collected between 1982 and 1991 at the Department of Pediatrics, The New York Hospital–Cornell Medical Center, New York.

netic female genitalia. In recent years, prenatal diagnosis and treatment of 11β-hydroxylase deficiency have been carried out with the same protocol as in steroid 21-hydroxylase deficiency and have achieved the same success.

Male Pseudohermaphroditism

Male pseudohermaphroditism occurring in the absence of testicular dysgenesis is due to biochemical defects impairing the biosynthesis or action of either testosterone or AMH and is usually genetically transmitted in an autosomal recessive fashion, with the notable exception of androgen insensitivity, which is X-linked.

3β-HYDROXYSTEROID DEHYDROGENASE DEFICIENCY. A defect in 3β-hydroxysteroid dehydrogenase, an enzyme that acts early in the pathway of cortisol synthesis, impairs sex steroid synthesis in both the adrenal and the gonads. Because the synthesis of testosterone is impaired in 3β-hydroxysteroid dehydrogenase deficiency, males are incompletely masculinized and are born with ambiguous genitalia. In a genetic female fetus, Δ⁴-androgens formed peripherally from the excess secretion of dehydroepiandrosterone may produce mild clitoral enlargement. In the case of a severe enzyme deficiency in either sex, salt wasting secondary to aldosterone deficiency may develop.

A gene for the peripheral form of 3β-hydroxysteroid dehydro-

genase (type I) and a gene for the adrenal-gonadal form of 3β-hydroxysteroid dehydrogenase (type II) have been identified and mapped to chromosome 1. Mutations in the type II gene have been described only in the classic form of the disorder.

Steroid 3β-hydroxysteroid dehydrogenase deficiency is diagnosed by a high ratio of Δ⁵- to Δ⁴-steroids. Elevated levels of pregnenolone, 17-hydroxypregnenolone, and dehydroepiandrosterone are evident in serum; the urinary Δ⁵-metabolites pregnanetriol and 16-pregnanetriol are elevated. Steroid values in the newborn period may not be informative inasmuch as Δ⁵-steroid levels are normally high during this time in unaffected persons. Glucocorticoid administration, with the addition of a mineralocorticoid to correct salt wasting, is effective.

Some women exhibiting clinically significant signs of androgen excess show a pattern of elevated Δ⁵- to Δ⁴-steroids; this condition may represent an underlying mild (non-classic) 3β-hydroxysteroid dehydrogenase defect. No mutation has been identified to date in the non-classic form. The non-classic defect is diagnosed by 60-minute ACTH testing. Treatment consists of oral dexamethasone administration in small doses (0.25 mg at bedtime).

17α-HYDROXYLASE/17,20-LYASE DEFICIENCY. Combined 17α-hydroxylase/17,20-lyase deficiency, a rare form of CAH, impairs the synthesis of cortisol and sex steroids. Males at birth may have

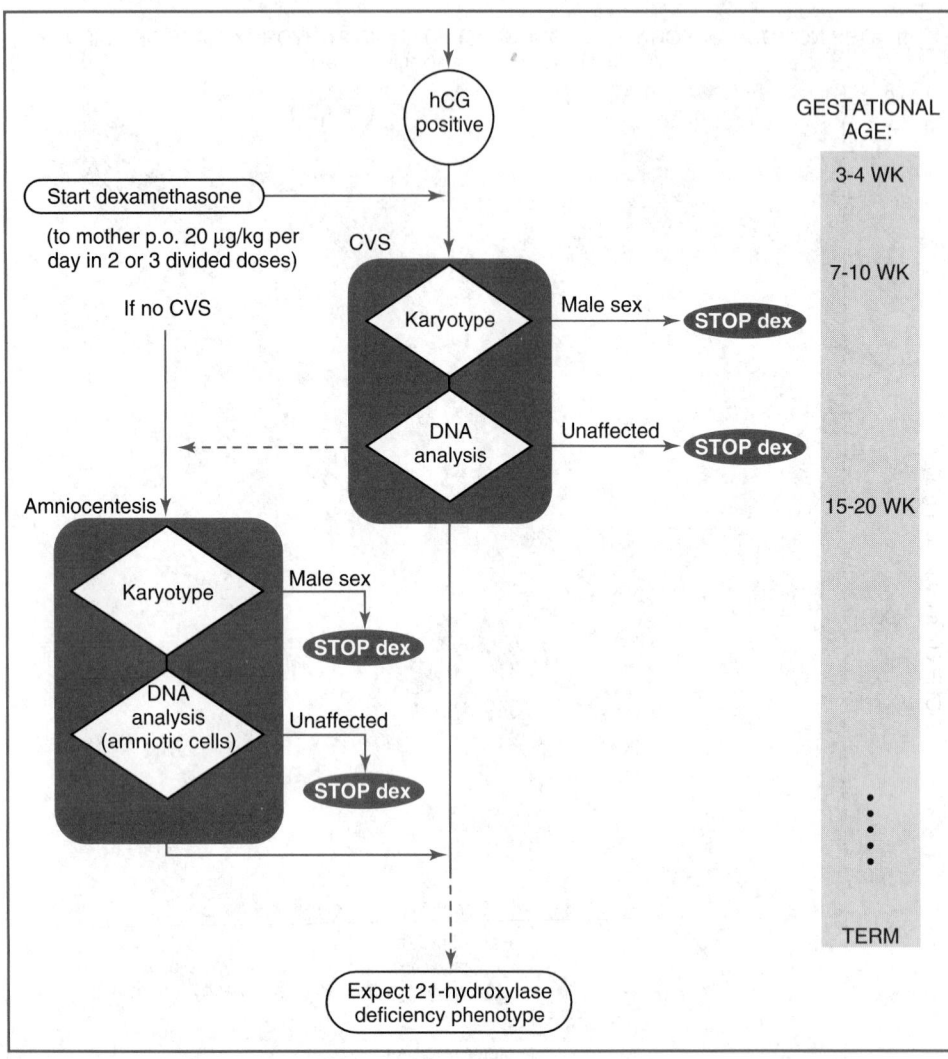

FIGURE 246–8 ■ Algorithm depicting prenatal management of pregnancy in families at risk for a fetus affected with 21-hydroxylase deficiency. hCG = human chorionic gonadotropin; CVS = chorionic villus sampling; 17-OHP = 17α-hydroxyprogesterone. (From Speiser PW, Laforgia N, Kato K, et al: First trimester prenatal treatment and molecular genetic diagnosis of congential adrenal hyperplasia [21-hydroxylase deficiency]. J Clin Endocrinol Metab 70:838–848, 1990. © The Endocrine Society.)

ambiguous genitalia and be mistakenly assigned to the female gender. Wolffian duct formation is incomplete because of deficient androgen production, whereas normal AMH secretion by Sertoli cells inhibits formation of the uterus and fallopian tubes. Genetic females appear normal at birth and throughout childhood but may have primary amenorrhea at puberty. Plasma gonadotropins are elevated in both sexes. Hypertension with hypokalemia secondary to excess deoxycorticosterone may develop and be seen clinically in childhood or may be found incidental to failure of puberty. The structural gene for P-450c17 is located on chromosome 10.

The deficiency is diagnosed by high serum deoxycorticosterone and extremely high corticosterone levels. Aldosterone levels are low because of suppressed renin and hypokalemia from excess deoxycorticosterone. Before puberty, 17α-hydroxylase/17,20-lyase deficiency is treated with glucocorticoids. Sex steroids appropriate to the gender of rearing are given at the age of puberty to induce the development of secondary sex characteristics. In genetic males raised as females, gonadectomy and vaginal reconstruction are required.

Isolated 17,20-lyase deficiency can also occur; the 17-hydroxylase function of the enzyme is intact and allows for the synthesis of cortisol, but C_{19}-steroid production is deficient.

CHOLESTEROL DESMOLASE DEFICIENCY. Cholesterol desmolase deficiency (lipoid adrenal hyperplasia or Prader's syndrome) is an extremely rare condition in which cholesterol is not converted to pregnenolone; this defect profoundly impairs the synthesis of all steroids and results in massive accumulations of cholesterol and cholesterol esters. Affected males and females have a female external genital phenotype. Biochemical findings include profound deficiencies of all steroids, low plasma volume, hyperkalemia, and hyponatremia. Neonatal mortality is high from total adrenal insuffi-

ciency, but some patients maintained by hormonal replacement can survive to adulthood.

Abnormalities in steroidogenic acute regulatory protein (STAR) are responsible for this disorder. Steroidogenic acute regulatory protein is involved in the transfer of cholesterol from the outer to the inner mitochondrial membrane, where it is then converted to pregnenolone. The gene encoding steroidogenic acute regulatory protein is on chromosome 8, region p11.2, where mutations were found that result in lipoid CAH.

17β-HYDROXYSTEROID DEHYDROGENASE TYPE 3. 17β-Hydroxysteroid dehydrogenase type 3 promotes the conversion of androstenedione to testosterone, the last step in the testosterone biosynthetic pathway. It is predominantly expressed in the testes and its gene is located on chromosome 9q22. Mutations in XY patients lead to isolated male pseudohermaphroditism without CAH. The external genitalia are usually unambiguously female. At puberty, marked virilization occurs because of the activity of the ubiquitously expressed type 1 isoform of 17β-hydroxysteroid dehydrogenase. Breast development occurs in half of the cases. At surgery, testes and epididymides are found in the inguinal canal, and the uterus and fallopian tubes are absent. The hallmark of the condition is elevated plasma androstenedione with testosterone levels in the lower male range; AMH levels are high. Male reconstruction of the genitalia is usually deemed impossible, and most patients are raised as girls and gonadectomized; however, a gender role change has been reported when the testes are left in place.

LEYDIG CELL APLASIA. Leydig cell aplasia or hypoplasia is a rare syndrome characterized by the absence of phenotypic virilization, high basal luteinizing hormone, normal follicle-stimulating hormone, high AMH, and low testosterone, even after hCG stimu-

Table 246–2 ▪ DISORDERS OF SEXUAL DIFFERENTIATION IN MALES

| DISORDER | DEFECTIVE PROTEIN | GENE LOCALIZATION | PHENOTYPE | | | | ENDOCRINOLOGY | |
			Müllerian Ducts	Wolffian Ducts	External Genitalia	Other	Testosterone	AMH
Defects in enzymes involved in testosterone synthesis or metabolism	Side chain cleavage	15q23–24	Absent	Present	Ambiguous		Low	Normal
	17α-Hydroxylase	10	Absent	Present	Female	Hypertension	Low	Normal
	3β-HSD type 2	1p13	Absent	Present	Ambiguous	Salt loss	Low	High*
	17β-HSD type 3	9q22	Absent	Present	Female		Low	Normal
	5α-Reductase type 2	2p23	Absent	Present	Ambiguous		High	Normal
Androgen insensitivity								
A. CAIS	Androgen receptor	Xq11–12	Absent	Absent	Female		Normal	High*
B. PAIS	Androgen receptor	Xq11–12	Absent	Present	Ambiguous		Normal	High*
Persistent müllerian duct syndrome	AMH	19p13	Present	Present	Male		Normal	Low
	AMH receptor	12q13	Present	Present	Male		Normal	Normal

AMH = antimüllerian hormone; HSD = hydroxysteroid dehydrogenase; CAIS = complete androgen insensitivity; PAIS = partial androgen insensitivity.
*In the neonatal and pubertal period; normal at other times.

lation. It is due to mutations of the luteinizing hormone receptor, whose gene is located on chromosome 2p21.

5α-REDUCTASE DEFICIENCY. Deficiency of 5α-reductase is a rare autosomal recessive disorder (Table 246–2). The membrane-bound enzyme 5α-reductase type 2 is responsible for the conversion of testosterone to DHT. A defect in 5α-reductase causes selective impairment of the DHT-dependent steps of male sex differentiation. Plasma testosterone levels are normal to elevated, whereas DHT levels are low. Luteinizing hormone levels are normal or slightly elevated. Most patients have severe perineoscrotal hypospadias, and a blind vaginal pouch may be present and open into the urogenital sinus or the urethra. Because the wolffian ducts are maintained by testosterone, patients have normal vasa deferentia, seminal vesicles, and epididymides. DHT-mediated virilization of the urogenital sinus and the external genitalia is impaired, and the prostate is small or absent. Patients have a female habitus without breast development but lack female internal genital structures. At puberty, testosterone-dependent masculinization occurs to a variable degree; rugation and hyperpigmentation of the scrotum, growth of the phallus, an increase in muscle mass, and deepening of the voice develop in affected males. Some may have testicular descent (Fig. 246–9A). Gender change from female to male in untreated affected subjects has been documented.

Patients in whom 5α-reductase deficiency is diagnosed in infancy and early childhood are best reared as males once the hypospadias and cryptorchidism are surgically corrected. Because DHT is not available for general use, adults are usually treated with high doses of testosterone esters. In the absence of 5α-reductase, 19-nortestosterone is active and can be given by injection in an esterified form.

5α-Reductase isoform 2 is the major isoenzyme expressed in genital tissues, and a deletion in the type 2 gene has been found in affected subjects. Eighteen different mutations have been identified in 25 families, and approximately 40% of affected individuals are compound heterozygotes.

ANDROGEN INSENSITIVITY. Masculinization of the reproductive tract depends on androgen binding to the androgen receptor protein. Mutations of the X-linked gene coding for the androgen receptor in subjects hemizygous for the mutated gene therefore lead to androgen insensitivity, formerly known as testicular feminization syndrome (see Table 246–2). Androgen insensitivity is one of the most frequent forms of male pseudohermaphroditism; estimates of incidence vary from 1 in 20,000 to 64,000 male births. It causes a spectrum of phenotypic abnormalities.

CLINICAL FEATURES. Subjects affected by the complete form of androgen insensitivity have a normal female phenotype. They are rarely discovered before puberty unless masses are palpated in the

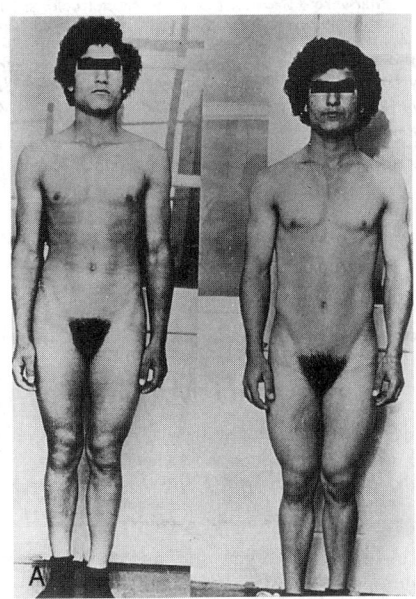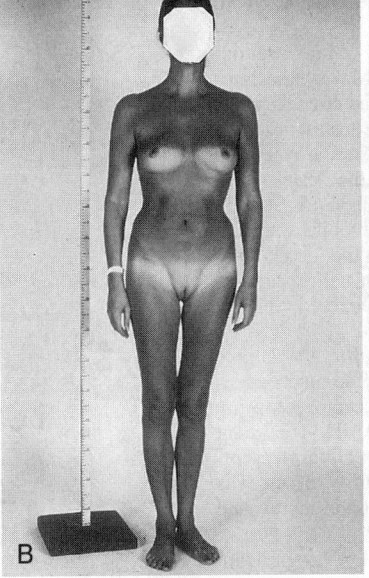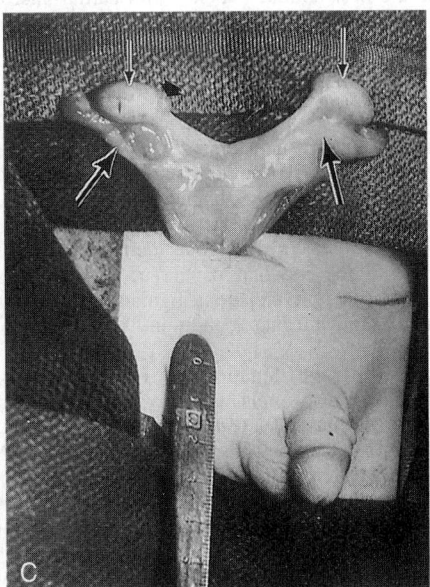

FIGURE 246–9 ▪ A, Pubertal virilization in brothers with 5α-reductase deficiency. (From Savage MO, Preece MA, Jeffcoate SL, et al: Familial male pseudohermaphroditism due to deficiency of 5α-reductase. Clin Endocrinol 12:397, 1980.) B, Patient with complete androgen insensitivity. C, A case of persistent müllerian duct syndrome—operative field. Above the normal, infantile male genitalia are the contents of the right hernia sac, which consists of the testes (small arrow) and fallopian tubes (large arrow) separated by the uterus. A portion of an epididymis (arrowhead) caps the right testis. The vas deferens was palpable posteriorly on both sides. (From Harbison MD, Magid MLS, Josso N, et al: Anti-müllerian hormone in three intersex conditions. Ann Genet 34:226, 1991.)

groin or labia and discovered to be testes at surgical exploration. The vagina is usually shallow and ends blindly. Internal genital structures are generally absent, although some cases with residual müllerian derivatives have been described. The testes may be located in the abdomen or in the labia majora and do not undergo spermatogenesis. Pubic and axillary hair is scant or absent (Fig. 246–9B). AMH levels are elevated during the 1st year and after puberty. Testosterone and luteinizing hormone levels are elevated as a result of defective-feedback regulation caused by androgen resistance at the level of the hypothalamus. Estrogen production is usually increased; when coupled with androgen insensitivity, the increased estrogen production results in an unopposed estrogen effect and is the most likely explanation for breast development at puberty.

Partial androgen insensitivity, also termed Reifenstein's syndrome, is characterized by a variable degree of genital ambiguity, and both virilization and breast development occur at puberty (see Table 246–2). Partial androgen insensitivity is also consistent with a male phenotype with gynecomastia and infertility as the sole manifestations.

MOLECULAR GENETICS AND PRENATAL DIAGNOSIS. The androgen receptor gene is located on the X chromosome between Xq12 and Xp11, consistent with the sex-linked recessive mode of inheritance observed in affected families. De novo cases are not uncommon and contribute to the negative family history exhibited by approximately one third of complete androgen insensitivity sufferers.

At the cellular level, androgen insensitivity can usually be recognized by studying the affinity of cultured genital skin fibroblasts for DHT, but mutations can affect DNA binding and other aspects of receptor function. Prenatal diagnosis of androgen receptor defects is possible with chorionic villus tissue biopsy and DNA analysis.

MANAGEMENT. Management depends on the severity of the androgen receptor defect. Patients with complete androgen insensitivity should be raised as girls, and the testes should be removed to avoid malignant degeneration, which occurs in 1 to 2% of cases. The optimal time for castration is controversial. Some physicians prefer to delay it until after adolescence to allow spontaneous feminization to occur. Estrogen treatment is then required to preserve breast development. Management of patients with partial androgen insensitivity is less straightforward because the diagnosis cannot always be confirmed by molecular studies in the neonatal period. When the phallus is very small and other causes of male pseudohermaphroditism have been excluded, female gender assignment is the best option. Patients with partial androgen insensitivity who are raised as girls should have their testes removed early to avoid unwanted virilization.

PERSISTENT MÜLLERIAN DUCT SYNDROME. Male pseudohermaphroditism caused by an isolated defect of AMH synthesis or action is a rare autosomal recessive disorder characterized by the presence of a uterus and tubes tightly linked to the testes in otherwise normally virilized males. When these structures are held in the pelvis by the round ligament, they prevent the testes from descending and lead to bilateral cryptorchidism (Fig. 246–9C). In most cases, however, müllerian derivatives are mobile and are dragged into the inguinal canal and scrotum by the descending testis; the result is an apparent inguinoscrotal hernia with contralateral cryptorchidism. The condition is usually discovered only at surgery.

A dozen different mutations of the gene coding for AMH have been described in patients with low or undetectable serum concentrations of the hormone. Mutations of the AMH receptor gene are involved in subjects with normal serum levels of AMH. Treatment should aim at preserving fertility through early correction of cryptorchidism while paying great attention to the integrity of the vas deferens, which is often incorporated in the wall of the uterus and cervix.

UNEXPLAINED MALE PSEUDOHERMAPHRODITISM. A significant number of cases of male pseudohermaphroditism are not explained by molecular analysis. They could be due to mutations of yet unknown genes specifically involved in sex differentiation. Alternatively, sex ambiguity could represent a malformation masquerading as a testosterone or AMH defect. Association of genital ambiguity with other developmental defects is frequently observed, sometimes as one of the several components of a recognized syndrome such

as Smith-Lemli-Opitz syndrome; the WAGR syndrome, which include Wilms' tumor, aniridia, gonadal abnormalities, and mental retardation; or the hand-foot-genital syndrome.

CONCLUSIONS AND GENERAL MANAGEMENT

Sexual ambiguity, at least in the newborn, should be treated as a pediatric emergency. It may threaten the life of the patient if, as in most cases, the intersex condition is due to CAH and is associated with salt loss. Even if such is not the case, it is important to assign gender as early as possible. Gender identity is established very early in life, certainly by the time that speech is established. Gender confusion because of indeterminant or wrong assignment of gender may lead to severe emotional disorders later in life.

Three diagnostic clues are helpful: gonadal location, presence of a uterus, and karyotype. If no gonads are palpable in a 46,XX chromatin-positive baby, CAH should be suspected before the possibility of true hermaphroditism or idiopathic female pseudohermaphroditism is entertained. In patients with at least one palpable gonad, if a uterus can be visualized by ultrasonography, the most likely diagnosis is testicular dysgenesis in 46,XY subjects and true hermaphroditism or XX maleness in 46,XX subjects. If no müllerian derivatives are present, male pseudohermaphroditism caused by testosterone defects or malformations should be considered. It is prudent to wait a few days to assign the gender until common causes of sexual ambiguity are investigated and the various issues have been thoroughly discussed with the parents. However, once gender has been assigned, there should be no ambiguity in the sex of rearing to avoid confusion of gender.

Carlson AD, Obeid JS, Kanellopoulou N, et al: Congenital adrenal hyperplasia: Update on prenatal diagnosis and treatment. Proceedings of the Xth International Congress on Hormonal Steroids, Quebec City, Canada. June 17–21, 1998. J Steroid Biochem Molec Biol, in press. *Update on prenatal dexamethasone treatment for CAH: demonstrated to be safe for both mother and child.*

Josso N, Picard JY, Imbeaud S, et al: Clinical aspects and molecular genetics of the persistent müllerian duct syndrome. Clin Endocrinol 47:137, 1997. *A review of the clinical and molecular aspects of AMH and AMH receptor defects.*

New MI, Crawford C, Wilson RC: Genetic disorders of the adrenal gland. *In* Rimoin DL, Connor JM, Pyeritz RE (eds): Emery and Rimoin's Principles and Practice of Medical Genetics, 3rd ed. New York, Churchill Livingstone, 1996, pp 1441–1476. *An overview of the molecular genetics of adrenal disorders.*

New MI, White PC: Genetic disorders of steroid hormone synthesis and metabolism. *In* Thakker R (guest editor): Genetic and Molecular Biological Aspects of Endocrine Disease. *In* Alberti KGMM, Burger HG, Cohen RD, Ranke MB (Series editors): Baillière's Clinical Endocrinology and Metabolism. London, Baillière Tindall, 1995, pp 525–554. *An overview of endocrine disorders: pathophysiology and clinical management.*

Quigley CA, De Bellis A, Marschke KB, et al: Androgen receptor defects: Historical, clinical, and molecular perspectives. Endocr Rev 16:271, 1995. *An excellent review of the clinical and molecular aspects of androgen insensitivity.*

VanWyk JJ, Gunther DF, Ritzen M, et al: The use of adrenalectomy as a treatment for congenital adrenal hyperplasia. J Clin Endocrinol Metab 81:3180, 1996. *Theoretic arguments for prophylactic adrenalectomy in CAH patients with CYP21 double-null alleles.*

Yu RN, Achermann JC, Ito M, Jameson JL: The role of DAX-1 in reproduction. Trends Endocrinol Metab 9:169, 1998. *A review of the roles of DAX-1 and SF-1 in reproduction.*

247 THE TESTIS AND MALE SEXUAL FUNCTION

Ronald S. Swerdloff ■ Christina Wang

The testis is a bi-functional organ serving as the site of sex steroid (i.e., testosterone synthesis) and sperm production in the male. Thus, the testis controls both sexuality and the perpetuity of the species (fertility). In addition, androgens and their metabolites (including estrogens) serve essential metabolic roles and may be important inducers and effectors of brain function in men. The discussion in this chapter focuses on the issues of male reproductive physiology and its disorders: androgen deficiency, sexual dysfunction, infertility, and androgen excess states.

The male reproductive axis consists of six main components: (1) extrahypothalamic central nervous system, (2) hypothalamus, (3) pituitary, (4) testes, (5) sex steroid–sensitive end organs, and (6) sites of androgen transport and metabolism (Fig. 247–1). The components of this system function in an integrative fashion to control the concentrations of circulating gonadal steroids required for normal male sexual development and function, for androgen- and estrogen-mediated metabolic effects on critical end organs such as brain, bone, muscle, liver, skin, bone marrow, and for immune systems. The reproductive axis is also responsible for normal germ cell maturation and sperm delivery necessary for male fertility.

Hypothalamic Pituitary Function (see Chapter 235)

The hypothalamus is the principal integrative unit responsible for the normal pulsatile secretion of gonadotropin-releasing hormone (GnRH), which is delivered through the hypothalamic-hypophyseal portal blood system to the pituitary gland. Although GnRH has been identified in many areas of the central nervous system (CNS), it is most concentrated in the medial basal, arcuate, and suprachiasmatic nuclei in the hypothalamus and travels by axonomic flow to the axon terminals of the median eminence. The pulsatile release of GnRH provides the signals for the timing of the release of luteinizing hormone (LH) and follicle-stimulating hormone (FSH), which in normal circumstances occurs approximately every 60 to 90 minutes. The secretion of GnRH is regulated in a complex fashion by neuronal input from higher cognitive and sensory centers and by circulating levels of sex steroids and peptide hormones such as prolactin, activin, inhibin, and leptin. The local effectors of GnRH synthesis and release include a number of neuropeptides, catecholamines, indolamines, nitric oxide and excitatory amino acids, γ-aminobutyric acid, dopamine, neuropeptide Y, vasoactive intestinal peptide (VIP) and corticotropion-releasing hormone (CRH). Testosterone either directly or through its metabolic products (i.e., estradiol and dihydrotestosterone) has predominantly inhibitory effects on the secretion and release of GnRH, LH, and FSH. Prolactin is a potent inhibitor of GnRH secretion, thus explaining its role in inhibiting LH and testosterone secretion in conditions of hyperprolactinemia.

LH and FSH are glycopeptides consisting of two subunits (α and β). They share the same α-subunit with specificity endowed by the β-subunit. The heterodimer is required for biologic activity; the subunits can be detected in serum and may be increased in certain pathologic conditions (e.g., α-subunit elevations in gonadotropin-secreting pituitary adenomas). LH and FSH are synthesized in the same pituitary cell (gonadotrophs) and secreted in a pulsatile pat-

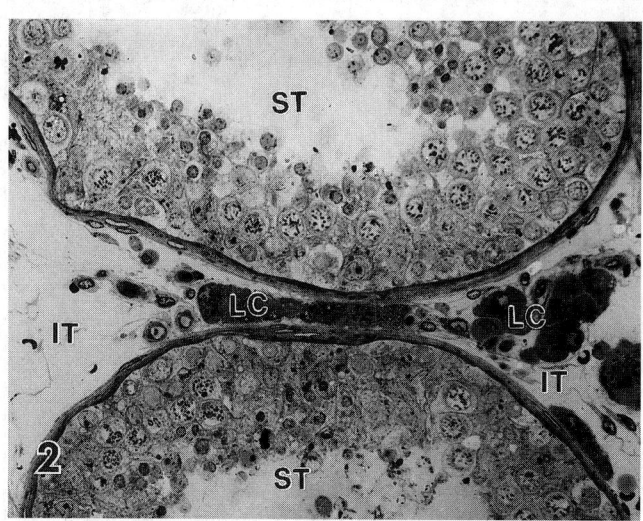

FIGURE 247–2 ■ Testis. Light micrograph of the glutaraldehyde-fixed, epoxy-embedded testicular section from a normal man showing seminiferous tubules (ST) and interstitium (IT). The seminiferous tubules contain Sertoli cells and germ cells at various phases of maturation. The interstitium consists of Leydig cells (LC), blood vessels, and lymphatic space.

tern. The clearance of the two gonadotrophic hormones (LH and FSH) differs, with LH having a shorter half-life than FSH. There is a diurnal rhythm of both gonadotropins (in young adult men) with higher circulating levels in the early morning and lowest levels in the evening. Puberty is heralded by night-time pulsatile serum patterns before obvious increases are noted in the daytime. A second level of feedback regulation of LH and FSH secretion occurs at the pituitary, with testosterone, dihydrotestosterone (DHT), and estrogens inhibiting the synthesis and/or release of both gonadotropins. Circulating testicular peptide products of the Sertoli cell (i.e., inhibin, activin) also produce selective inhibition or stimulation of FSH. LH and FSH circulate unbound to carrier proteins and act predominantly through specific cell surface receptors on the Leydig and Sertoli cells of the testes, respectively.

Testis Function

The testis is a complex organ consisting of (1) seminiferous tubules containing Sertoli cells and germ cells in various stages of maturation and (2) the interstitium where the steroid-secreting cells (Leydig), macrophages, and blood vessels reside (Fig. 247–2). The Leydig cells synthesize steroid hormones under the regulation of LH. The LH receptors on the cell surface of the Leydig cells lead to G protein/cyclic adenosine monophosphate–mediated events. This process involves a steroid acute regulatory protein essential for steroidogenesis in the gonads and adrenal glands (Fig. 247–3).

TESTOSTERONE SYNTHESIS. Testosterone is the principal male hormone secreted by the testes, with about 7 mg produced per day. Testosterone synthesis occurs in the human testes through either the delta 4 or delta 5 pathways (see Fig. 247–3), with the latter predominant. The enzymatic rate-limiting step in the process is the LH-inducible conversion of cholesterol to pregnenolone by the cholesterol side-chain cleavage enzyme.

TESTOSTERONE TRANSPORT IN BLOOD. Testosterone circulates mainly bound to two plasma proteins: sex hormone–binding globulin (SHBG, also known as testosterone-binding globulin) and albumin. In young adult men, about 54% of testosterone is bound to albumin, 44% is bound to SHBG, and 2 to 3% is unbound or free. The SHBG-testosterone fraction is tightly bound and serves a storage role. Bioavailable testosterone refers to the sum of albumin-bound and free testosterone and is measured by separating SHBG-bound testosterone from the total testosterone in the serum. Serum SHBG levels are increased in endogenous and exogenous hyperestrogenemic states, hyperthyroidism, aging, phenytoin treatment, anorexia nervosa, and prolonged stress. SHBG levels are lowered with androgen treatment, obesity, acromegaly, and hypothyroidism. In most instances, measurement of serum total testosterone will

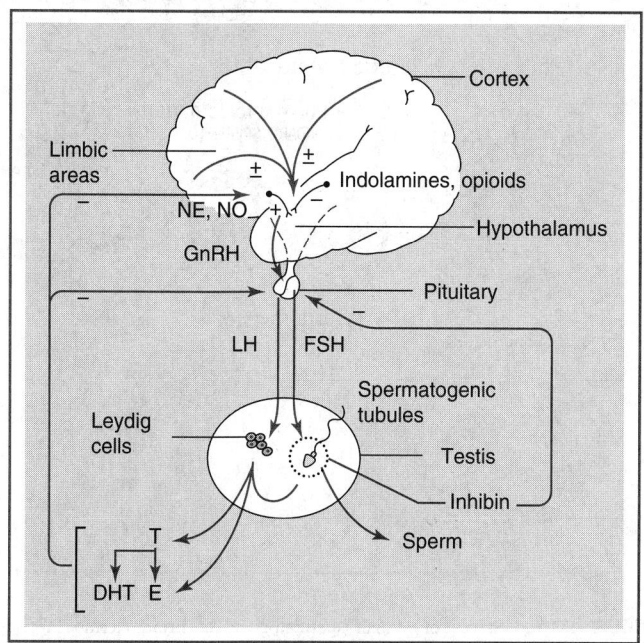

FIGURE 247–1 ■ The hypothalamic-pituitary-gonadal axis in the male.

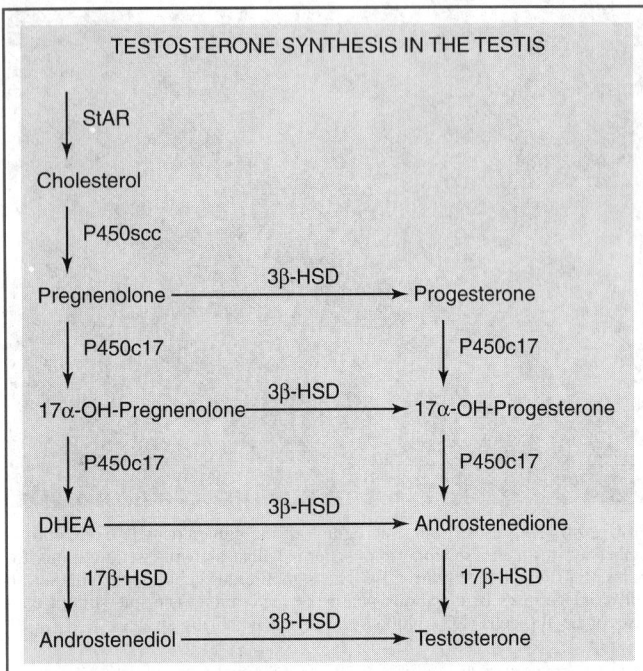

FIGURE 247-3 ■ STAR protein mobilizes cholesterol from cellular stores to the mitochondria. Intratesticular steroidogenic pathways for synthesis of testosterone. Whereas both the delta 5 (left) and delta 4 (right) pathways exist, the delta 5 pathway predominates in the testis.

detect individuals with androgen deficiency. In conditions with abnormal SHBG levels, the total testosterone measurement (usual laboratory test requested) may be misleading.

TESTOSTERONE ACTION. Testosterone exerts its effects at different end organs either through direct action or after conversion to an active metabolite such as DHT or estradiol (Fig. 247–4). Thus, testosterone can act as an androgenic hormone or as a precursor for DHT with effects mediated by the intracellular androgen receptor. It also can serve as a precursor for estradiol in some tissues where it binds the estrogen receptors (α and β) to induce estrogenic effects. Various end organs differ in their 5α-reductase and aromatase activity and in their requirements for conversion of testosterone to DHT for androgenic activity. Congenital and acquired de-

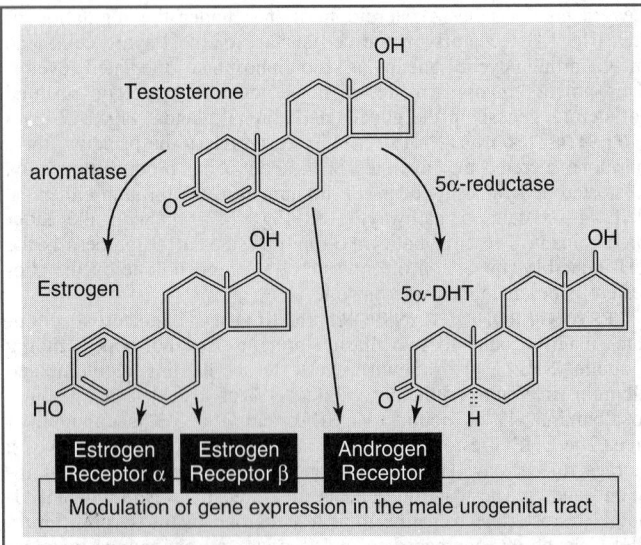

FIGURE 247-4 ■ Testosterone action is mediated either directly (androgen receptor), after conversion to estradiol (estrogen receptor α or β), or after conversion to DHT (androgen receptor). (From George GJ, Kuiper M, Carlquist M, Gustafson JA: Estrogen is a male and female hormone. Sci Med, July/August, 1998.)

fects in these two enzymes as well as in the estrogens and androgen receptors result in distinct syndromes with characteristic phenotypes (see Chapter 246).

SPERMATOGENESIS. The spermatogenic compartment consists of the Sertoli and germ cells and is intimately interactive with the interstitial compartment (Fig. 247–5). The Sertoli cells bridge the entire space between the basement membrane and the lumen of the tubules (see Fig. 247–2). They are the target of androgenic and FSH stimulation of spermatogenesis and also the source of a multitude of paracrine regulators of spermatogenesis, and gonadotropin secretion (e.g., inhibin, activin).

Germ cell maturation is dependent on the proper hormonal (FSH) and paracrine milieu (testosterone) for proliferation to occur. Not all germ cells reach maturity. Spontaneous death of certain germ cells is a constant feature of germ cell homeostasis. In fact, considerable data indicate that major effects of both testosterone and FSH are to limit the amount of germ cell death (apoptosis).

SPERM TRANSPORT. After spermatogenesis is completed, mature spermatozoa are released into the excretory system and travel through the rete testes and epididymis, where they functionally mature before traversing the vas deferens. The semen gains constituents from the seminal vesicles, prostate, and bulbourethral glands before ejaculation.

Normal Sexual Function and Erectile Physiology

Normal sexual function in men requires normal sexual desire (libido) and erectile, ejaculatory, and orgasmic capacity. The process is complex, involving cognitive, sensory, hormonal, autonomic neuronal, and penile vascular integrative actions for normal function. Defects occur at multiple levels. Although considerable progress has occurred in the past few years in therapeutic options, an understanding of the normal physiology is essential for proper assessment and treatment of men with sexual dysfunction.

The brain is the integrative center of the sexual response system. It processes sensory input, stored fantasy information, purposeful thoughts, spontaneous nocturnal reflex activity, and hormonal signals (e.g., testosterone) to create the hypothalamic neuronal message that traverses the spinal cord to the thoracic 9-12 sympathetic and sacral parasympathetic outflow tracts. The non-adrenergic, noncholinergic (NANC) autonomic plexus nerves initiate vasodilatation of the cavernosal arterial and corporal cavernosa sinusoids of the

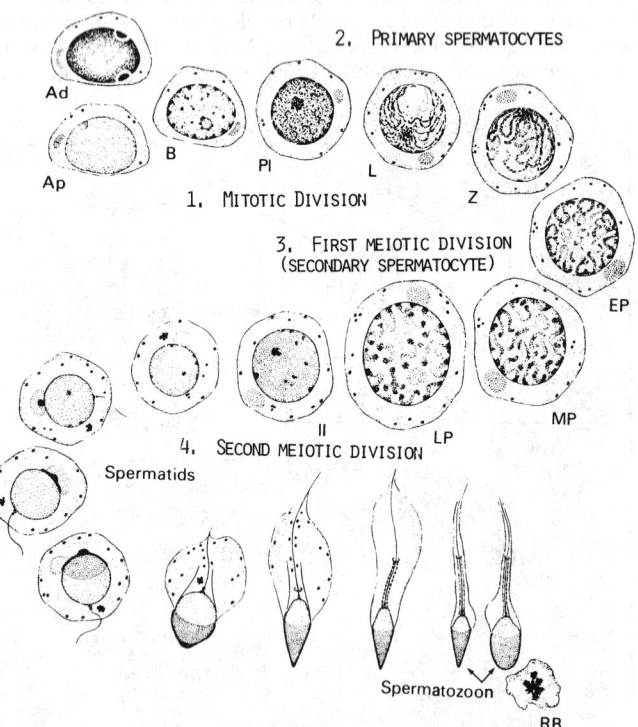

FIGURE 247-5 ■ Stages of human spermatogenesis. (From Hermo L, Clemont Y: How are germ cells produced and what factors control their production? *In* Robaine B, Pryor J, Trasler J [eds]: Handbook of Andrology. American Society of Andrology, 1995, pp 13–15.)

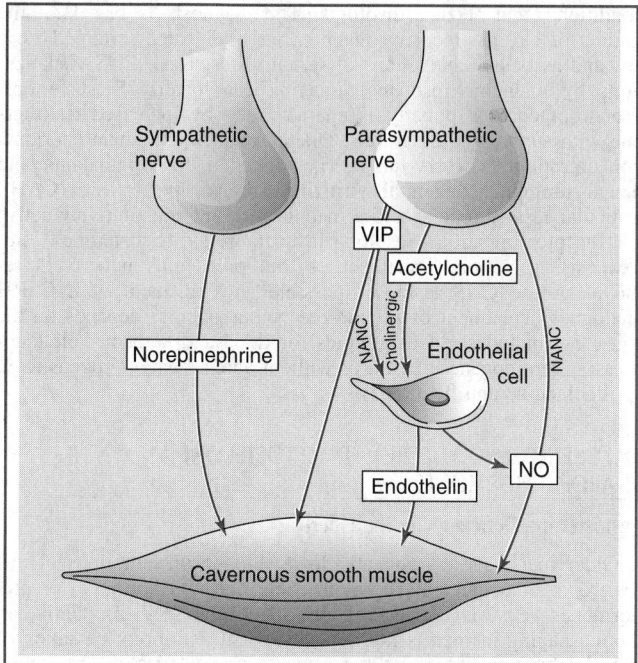

FIGURE 247–6 ■ The interaction among cholinergic, adrenergic and non-adrenergic, non-cholinergic (NANC) neuronal pathways and their contribution to penile smooth muscle contraction (patterned arrows) and dilation (open arrows). NO = nitric oxide; VIP = vasoactive intestinal polypeptide. (From Lue TF: Physiology of penile erection and pathophysiology of erectile dysfunction and priapism. *In* Walsh P, Retick A, Vaughn E, Wein A (eds): Campbell's Urology, 7th ed. Philadelphia, WB Saunders, 1998, p 1164.)

penis through release of local vasodilators such as nitric oxide (NO) and VIP from the vascular endothelium of and the smooth muscle cells of the sinusoids (Fig. 247–6). A family of enzymes (nitric oxide synthetases) regulates NO synthesis, which produces smooth muscle dilatation through activation of cyclic guanosine monophosphate (GMP) and modification of calcium flux. Cyclic GMP levels are rapidly reversible through inactivation by phosphodiesterase. The neurogenic mechanisms leading to vasodilatation of the cavernosal arterioles and sinusoids lead to a rapid increase in penile blood flow and expansion of the vascular channels; this, in turn, inhibits venous return through compression of the venous channels against the tunica albuginea and limits drainage of the obliquely penetrating veins. After orgasm, detumesence occurs, owing to less vasodilation (NO) and greater vasoconstrictive signals (α_2-adrenergic).

Testosterone seems to have its primary effect on erectile function by enhancing libido with secondary effects on penile NO synthase activity. Libido is highly sensitive to testosterone, thus explaining the preservation of erectile capacity in many men with partial androgen deficiency. In contrast, erectile dysfunction is common in older men despite normal serum testosterone levels; the latter effect appears to be the result of impaired penile vasodilatory capacity. This is often reversible through local (intracavernosal or transurethral) administration of potent vasodilators (prostaglandins, papaverine, and phentolamine) or by oral administration of penile-specific phosphodiesterase inhibitors (sildenafil). Combined androgen defi-

ciency with decreased libido and decreased penile responsiveness due to impaired NO synthesis activity may be common in elderly men. With the availability of effective penile vasodilatory medications to ensure erectile capacity, complaints of diminished libido may be effectively treated with androgen supplementation.

REPRODUCTIVE AXIS DURING FETAL DEVELOPMENT, CHILDHOOD, AND PUBERTY

Sexual Differentiation in the Fetus

Normal male sexual differentiation is complex and includes the establishment of genetic and phenotypic sex (see Chapter 246).

Adrenarche and Puberty

Adrenarche occurs at about 7 or 8 years of age when the zona reticularis of the adrenal undergoes maturation, leading to increased secretion of androgen precursors, such as androstenedione, dehydroepiandrosterone (DHEA), and DHEA sulfate (DHEA-S). Although the physiologic events initiating adrenarche are incompletely understood, the process is probably under the control of adrenocorticotropic hormone (ACTH) and independent of the control of LH and FSH. Adrenarche usually heralds subsequent activity in the hypothalamic-pituitary-gonadal axis. Androstenedione and DHEA are technically androgenic prehormones and do not bind to the androgen receptor. In part, the prepubertal growth spurt and the early development of pubic and axillary hair are mediated by conversion of these precursors to testosterone and DHT at the peripheral tissues sites.

Puberty occurs when a hypothalamic clock gets activated, resulting in increased GnRH and gonadotropin secretion. In the interval before the onset of puberty, LH and FSH are secreted in low amounts and are subject to feedback control by the small amounts of circulating testosterone from the testes. Initiation of puberty is determined by increase in the pulsatile pattern of hypothalamic GnRH secretion. As puberty progresses, feedback sensitivity of the hypothalamus and pituitary to circulating steroids lessens and increasing concentrations of both gonadal steroids and gonadotropin hormones ensue. The increasing concentrations of intratesticular testosterone and circulating FSH stimulate the Sertoli cell to produce factors leading to the maturation of spermatogenesis and inhibition of germ cell apoptosis. The phenotypic equivalents of the hormonal changes in puberty have been well documented. Pediatricians and endocrinologists routinely perform staging of the genital and pubic hair development (Table 247–1). The majority of the extratesticular end organ events of puberty are secondary to the increased circulating levels of testosterone and its metabolic products (DHT and estradiol). The penis and scrotum grow and become pigmented. As spermatogenesis advances the testes increase in size from 1 to 2 mL at the outset to 15 to 35 mL in adulthood. There is a progressive increase in facial, axillary, chest, abdominal, thigh, and pubic hair; frontal scalp hair regresses, and the voice deepens (Fig. 247–7). Genital and sexual hair development requires conversion of testosterone to DHT for its full effects.

Aberrations of Timing of Puberty

Delayed puberty in boys is usually defined as a temporary (physiologic) form of hypothalamic hypogonadotropic hypogonadism in which sexual development has not begun by age 13 ½ years. Once initiated, puberty should be completed within 4 ½ years. Although

Table 247–1 ■ PUBERTAL STAGES IN BOYS

	PUBIC HAIR STAGE	GENITAL STAGES
Stage 1	Absence of pubic hair	Childlike penis, testes, and scrotum (testes 2 mL).
Stage 2	Sparse lightly pigmented hair mainly at the base of the penis	Scrotum enlarged with early rugation and pigmentation. Testes begin to enlarge (3–5 mL).
Stage 3	Hair becomes coarse, darker, and more curled and more extensive	Penis has grown in length and diameter. Testes now 8–10 mL. Scrotum more rugated.
Stage 4	Hair adult in quality but distribution does not include medial aspect of thighs	Penis further enlarged with development of the glans. Scrotum and testes (10–13 mL) further enlarged.
Stage 5	Hair is adult and extends to thighs	Penis and scrotum fully adult. Testes 15 mL and greater.

Modified from Marshall WA, Tanner JM: Variation in pattern of pubertal changes in boys. Arch Dis Child 45:13–23, 1970.

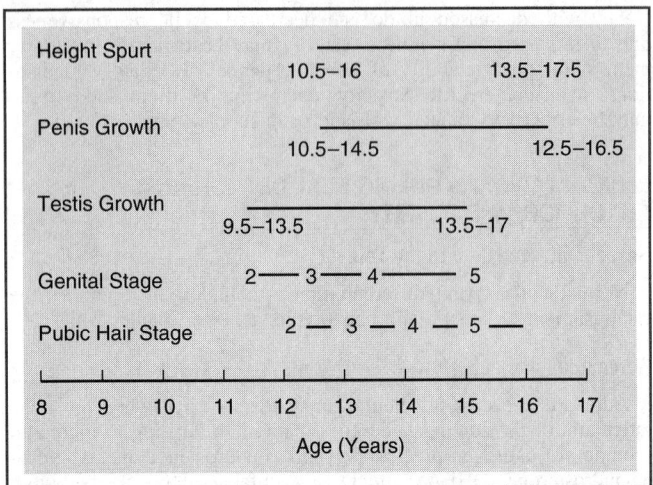

FIGURE 247–7 ▪ Diagram of the timing of the various components of puberty. The range of ages in which each parameter begins and is completed is shown for each bar. These data are from European children obtained 30 years ago. There may be a slight trend for earlier onset of puberty in the past 30 years. (From Marshall WA, Tanner JM: Variations in the pattern of pubertal changes in boys. Arch Dis Child 45:13–23, 1970.)

delayed sexual maturation is an inevitable component of prepubertal onset of hypogonadism or androgen resistance, the majority of boys with delayed development have a constitutional delayed physiologic clock and eventually attain full sexual adulthood. Careful documentation of changing physical findings and measurement of serum LH, FSH, and testosterone may prove valuable clues of the beginning of puberty. Inquiring and testing for hyposmia or anosmia may indicate a common variant of congenital hypogonadotrophic hypogonadism (Kallmann's syndrome). A family history of delay in puberty may encourage patience and observation. The decision of how early to treat depends on the perceived degree of psychological stress associated with the maturational delay. The major concern about treatment is early fusion of the epiphyses, which compromises optimal height. With proper dosing and monitoring of bone age this is unusual, because bone age is usually retarded in delayed puberty. In adolescent boys with delayed puberty and low levels of gonadotropins, periodic withdrawal of treatment is used to determine if testosterone therapy should be begun if spontaneous puberty has occurred. Many adult men diagnosed and treated for hypogonadotropic hypogonadism at ages 15 to 19 have proved to have normal reproductive function when taken off testosterone therapy many years later.

Precocious puberty in boys is defined as the onset of pubertal (genital and secondary sexual) development beginning before 9 (2.5 SD above the mean age of progression to stage 2) years of age. Sexual precocity can be subcategorized to true isosexual precocious puberty and incomplete isosexual precocity or pseudoprecocious puberty. The distinction is that true precocious puberty is associated with increases in GnRH-stimulated LH and FSH secretion (hypothalamic-pituitary origin) whereas pseudo-precocious puberty is independent of GnRH stimulation of LH and FSH secretion. True precocious puberty is often associated with CNS disease (two thirds of boys), including hypothalamic tumors, cysts, inflammatory

conditions, and seizure disorders. The diagnosis is based on the finding of sexual precosity, inappropriately elevated serum LH levels, and associated elevations of serum testosterone. CNS visualizations by magnetic resonance imaging can localize most lesions. Pseudo-precocious puberty is characterized by increased testosterone with suppressed LH levels. Diagnoses include human chorionic gonadotrophin secretory tumors (i.e., testes, liver, hypothalamic and pineal tumors), congenital virilizing adrenal hyperplasia (CAH), testicular testosterone-secreting neoplasms, and constitutively active LH receptor mutations, resulting in uncontrolled testosterone (testotoxicosis) secretion. Treatment of true precocious puberty is removal of the CNS lesion if possible and treatment with GnRH analogues. Treatment of pseudo-precocious puberty depends on the cause but includes glucocorticoids for CAH and ketoconazole (suppresses steroidogenesis) with or without adrenal antiandrogens (e.g., spironolactone and flutamide).

MALE SENESCENCE: DECREASED TESTOSTERONE AND OTHER ANABOLIC HORMONES

Testosterone Deficiency in the Elderly

Older men have significantly lower blood concentrations of testosterone, other anabolic hormones (e.g., growth hormone) or prehormones (e.g., DHEA and DHEA-S) (Table 247–2). Unlike in women, aging in men is not associated with an abrupt cessation of gonadal hormone secretion but rather a gradual decline, beginning as a young adult and progressing throughout life. Multiple cross-sectional and longitudinal studies have shown a progressive decrease in both total and free serum testosterone levels with aging (Fig. 247–8).

The effects of low testosterone levels in aging men are similar to those observed in younger hypogonadal men. These include decreases in muscle mass, muscle strength, bone mass, libido, and erectile function and impaired mood and sense of well-being. Older men have increased body fat, particularly visceral fat. The effect of reduced androgen levels on cognitive and memory are unknown, but it is possible that androgens may have similar positive effects on brain functions as estrogen does in older women. In recent years, a number of short-term studies have demonstrated the beneficial effects of testosterone replacement in elderly men with relatively low serum testosterone levels. Long-term, placebo-controlled studies are in progress. Testosterone replacement therapy, in most studies, decreases fat mass, increases lean body mass, and improves strength. Because erectile dysfunction in the older man is multifactorial, with impaired vasodilatory function in the penis predominating in many cases (see section on sexual dysfunction), testosterone replacement therapy in older men may enhance libido but erectile dysfunction is often not improved. Improved sense of well-being and increased energy levels are also generally observed after treatment with testosterone.

In older men, before androgen replacement therapy is considered, one must ascertain that the patient does not have an elevated hematocrit or a sleep-related breathing disorder.

Digital rectal examination should be performed and a prostate-specific antigen (PSA) level obtained to ensure there are no findings suggestive of severe benign prostatic hypertrophy or prostate cancer (nodules, irregularities).

Adrenal Deficiency of Androgen Precursors in Older Men

In recent years, marked decline in the circulating levels of adrenal androgens, especially DHEA and its sulfate DHEA-S, has been

Table 247–2 ▪ HORMONAL CHANGES ASSOCIATED WITH AGING

GNRH-LH/FSH/T	CRH-ACTH-DHEA(S)	GHRH-GH-IGH AXIS
↑ LH,* ↑ FSH	No change in ACTH	↓ GHRH message and receptor
↓ T (↓ Leydig cells)	↓ DHEA and DHEA-S	↓ GH secretory pulses
↓ Free T	↓ DHEA and DHEA-S	↓ Circulating GH
↑ SHBG	Response to ACTH	↓ Serum IGF-I

* ↓ LH pulse amplitude and ↓ responsiveness to GnRH.
GnRH = goandotropin-releasing hormone; LH = luteinizing hormone; FSH = follicle-stimulating hormone; T = testosterone; SHBG = sex hormone binding globulin; CRH = corticotropin-releasing hormone; DHEA = dehydroepiandrosterone; DHEA-S = DHEA sulfate; ACTH = adrenocorticotropic hormone; GHRH = growth hormone–releasing hormone; GH = growth hormone; IGF-I = insulin-like growth factor-I.

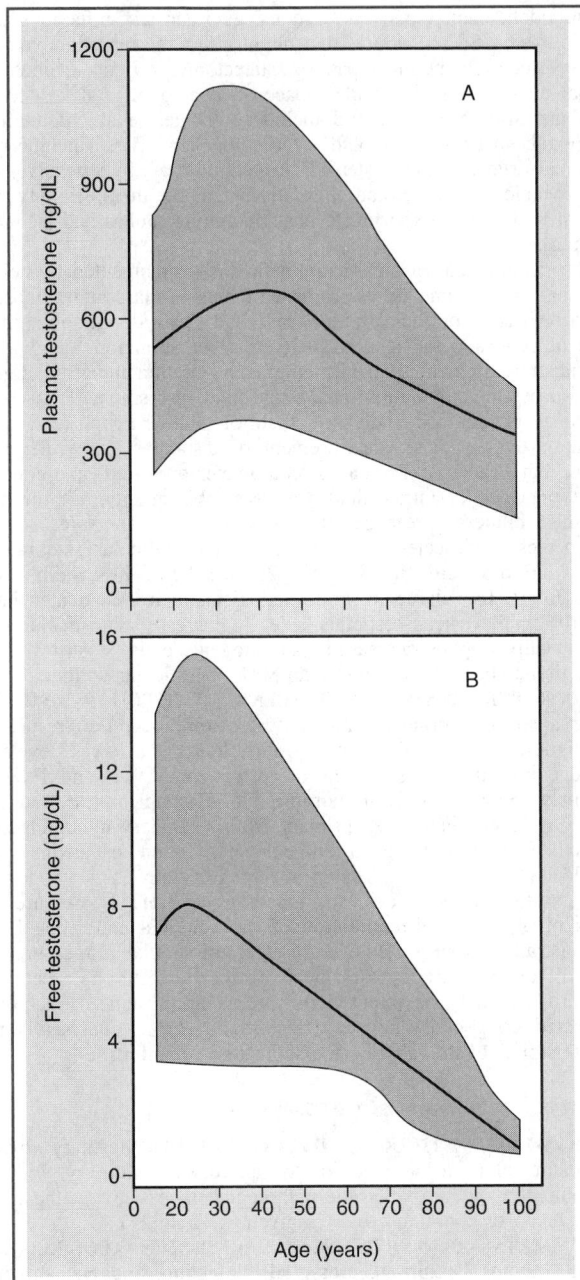

FIGURE 247-8 ■ Relationship between plasma testosterone (upper) and free testosterone (lower) levels and age in normal males. (From Baker HWG, Berger HG, DeKretser DM, et al: Changes in the pituitary-testicular system with age. Clin Endocrinol 5:349–372, 1996.)

small-scale, placebo-controlled, single-center study showed that oral administration of 50 mg of DHEA to older men improved the sense of well-being but did not change libido. In the United States, DHEA is available without prescription as a health supplement and is widely used, creating a situation in which large-scale multicenter, prospective, placebo-controlled trials are difficult to perform. Unless results from such studies are available, there is no substantial reason to administer DHEA to older men who may have low serum DHEA levels.

GH/IGF-1 Deficiency in Older Men

Hypothalamic growth hormone–releasing hormone (GHRH) messenger RNA, pituitary GHRH receptor concentrations, pituitary secretion of growth hormone (GH), and serum insulin-like growth factor-1 (IGF-1) levels decrease with aging (see Table 247–2). Part of the decline may be related to falling testosterone levels, because testosterone is known to enhance GH secretion. GH is an anabolic and lipolytic hormone, and many of its actions on peripheral tissues are mediated by IGF-1. GH deficiency in adults results in changes in body composition and mood (decreased muscle mass, increased body fat, decreased strength, and a decline in sense of well-being), which are very similar to those observed with aging. Studies show that although GH induced changes in body composition compared with placebo, the individual's muscle strength, exercise endurance, mood, and cognitive function remained unchanged. The side effects of GH treatment include edema of lower extremities, diffuse arthralgias, hand stiffness, and tiredness.

MALE HYPOGONADISM

DEFINITION. Hypogonadism refers to low circulating levels of testosterone. Most androgen-deficient men are infertile. Primary hypogonadism indicates that the abnormality originates in the testis; secondary hypogonadism indicates a defect at the hypothalamus or pituitary, resulting in decreased gonadotropins (LH and/or FSH) and secondary impairment of testicular function. Combined primary and secondary hypogonadism occurs in aging and in a number of systemic diseases, such as alcoholism, liver disease, and sickle cell disease. Decreased androgen action mimicking androgen deficiency may occur in patients with androgen receptor defects (androgen resistance), post-receptor signaling abnormalities, and inability to

recognized (Fig. 247–9) (see Chapter 246). Serum levels of DHEA and DHEA-S peak at about the third decade of life and then decline at about 2% per year, resulting in levels 10 to 20% of baseline by age 80. This decline in DHEA and DHEA-S is not accompanied by a decrease in ACTH. DHEA is a precursor to true androgens such as testosterone and DHT but does not bind to the androgen receptor itself. It is unclear whether DHEA binds to a unique nuclear receptor to initiate its action. Studies have been reported that DHEA administered to aging experimental animals and humans may improve sense of well-being, reduce anxiety and depression, enhance memory, prevent development of cancer, decrease body fat, decrease risk of cardiovascular disease, and provide other beneficial effects on immune function. Most studies in humans used oral doses of 1 to 5 mg/kg/day. An oral dose of 50 mg/day will increase testosterone and DHT to or above the normal physiologic range for women but not men. Much higher doses of DHEA can increase testosterone to male ranges but at the expense of very high serum DHEA concentrations. One short-term,

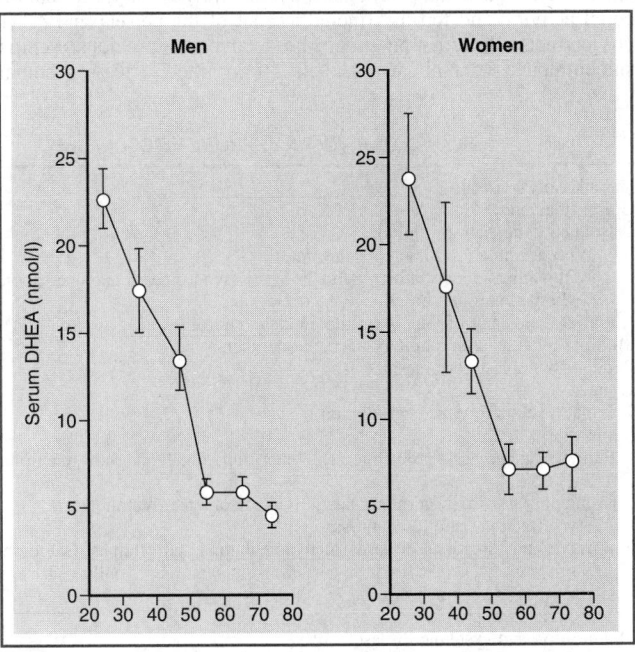

FIGURE 247-9 ■ Declining serum DHEA with aging. Serum DHEA-S levels (not shown) parallel the decrease in DHEA. (Adapted from Labrie F, et al: Marked decline in serum concentrations of adrenal C19 sex steroid precursors and conjugated androgen metabolites during aging. J Clin Endocrinol Metab 82:2396–2402, 1997. © The Endocrine Society.)

Table 247–3 ■ CAUSES OF PRIMARY TESTICULAR FAILURE AND END ORGAN RESISTANCE

Congenital disorders
  Chromosomal disorders
    Klinefelter's and related syndromes (e.g., XXY, XXY/XY, XYY, XX males)
  Testosterone biosynthetic enzyme defects
  Myotonia dystrophy
  Developmental disorders
    Prenatal diethylstilbestrol syndrome
    Cryptorchidism
Acquired defects
  Orchitis
    Mumps and other viruses
    Gramulomatous (e.g., tuberculosis leprosy)
    Human immunodeficiency virus
  Infiltrative diseases (i.e., hemochromatosis, amyloidosis)
  Surgical, traumatic injuries, and torsion of testis
  Irradiation
  Toxins (i.e., alcohol, fungicides, insecticides, heavy metals, cottonseed oil, DDT and other environmental estrogens)
  Drugs
    Cytotoxic agents
    Inhibitions of testosterone synthesis and antiandrogens (e.g., ketoconazole, cimetidine, flutamide, cyproterone, spironolactone)
    Ethanol and recreational drugs
  Autoimmune testicular failure
    Isolated
    Associated with other organ-specific disorders (i.e., Addison's disease, Hashimoto's thyroiditis, insulin-dependent diabetes)
  Systemic diseases (e.g., cirrhosis, chronic renal failure, sickle cell disease, acquired immunodeficiency syndrome, amyloidosis)
Androgen resistance syndromes
5α-Reductase deficiency

convert testosterone to the active metabolite DHT (5α-reductase abnormalities).

ETIOLOGY. Many of the causes of primary and secondary hypogonadism are listed in Tables 247–3 and 247–4 (see Chapter 246).

CLINICAL MANIFESTATIONS. CLINICAL HISTORY AND PHYSICAL EXAMINATION FOR HYPOGONADISM. The medical history should focus on testicular descent, pubertal development, shaving frequency, changes in body hair, and present and past systemic illnesses. A complete sexual history will include changes in libido, erectile and ejaculatory functions, and frequency of masturbation, coital activity, and fertility (including that of the present and previous partners). Information should be obtained on previous orchitis, sinopulmonary complaints, sexually transmitted diseases, human

Table 247–4 ■ CAUSES OF HYPOGONADOTROPIC HYPOGONADISM

Idiopathic or Congenital
GnRH deficiency
  Isolated deficiency of GnRH
    With anosmia (Kallmann's syndrome)
    With other abnormalities (Prader-Willi syndrome, Laurence-Moon-Biedl syndrome, basal encephalocele)
  Partial deficiency of GnRH (fertile eunuch syndrome)
Multiple hypothalamic/pituitary hormone deficiency
Pituitary hypoplasia or aplasia
Acquired
Trauma, post surgery, post irradiation
Neoplasic
  Pituitary adenomas (prolactinomas, other functional and non-functional tumors)
  Craniopharyngiomas, germinomas, gliomas, leukemia, lymphomas
Pituitary infarction, carotid aneurysm
Infiltrative and infectious diseases of hypothalamus and pituitary (sarcoidosis, tuberculosis, coccidioidomycosis, histoplasmosis, syphilis, abscess, histiocytosis X, hemochromatosis)
Autoimmune hypophysitis
Malnutrition and systemic disease
  Anorexia nervosa, starvation, renal failure, liver failure
Exogenous hormones and drugs
  Antiandrogens, estrogens, and antiestrogens, progestogens, glucocorticoids, cimetidine, spironolactone, digoxin, drug-induced hyperprolactinemia (metoclopramide, tranquilizers, antihypertensives)

immunodeficiency virus (HIV) status, genitourinary infections, and previous surgical procedures that might affect the reproductive tract (e.g., vasectomy, hernia repair, prostatectomy, varicocele ligation). Social history should include tobacco and alcohol intake. Medication and drug history should include any agent that could affect hormonal, spermatogenic, and erectile function. These include recreational drugs; anabolic steroids; psychiatric, antihypertensive, antiandrogenic, cytotoxic, and alternative medicine therapies; environmental toxins; and exposure to heat (including saunas and jacuzzis) and radiation.

The generalized physical examination is supplemented by height and span measurements; assessment of muscle mass and adiposity; characterization of facial, pubic, and body hair distribution; presence of acne and facial wrinkling; breast examination for gynecomastia; measurement of penile length and urethra integrity; digital rectal prostate examination; and visual field assessment. The scrotal examination should include assessment of midline fusion (e.g., bifid scrotum, hypospadias); measurement of testicular size (ruler will suffice but Prader or Takihara orchidometer preferred) and consistency; presence of intratesticular masses; abnormalities of the epididymis; bilateral presence of a vas deferens; and presence of varicoceles, hydroceles, or hernias. Normal testicular size ranges from 3.6 to 5.5 cm in length; 2.1 to 3.2 cm in width, and 15 to 35 mL in volume in white and black men. Asian men have slightly smaller mean testicular size. A decrease in testicular volume usually implies decreased spermatogenic cells because the tubular tissue accounts for more than 80% of testicular volume.

LABORATORY TESTS IN ASSESSMENTS OF HYPOGONADISM. Because a strong diurnal rhythm in testosterone secretion results in the highest serum levels in the morning hours and lowest levels in the evening, the measurement of testosterone, LH, and FSH is routinely determined from morning blood samples. Elevated LH and FSH levels distinguish primary from secondary hypogonadism (both have low serum testosterone levels). Serum prolactin levels should be measured in all cases of hypogonadotrophic hypogonadism, pituitary mass lesions, and galactorrhea. DHT is measured in cases of abnormal differentiation of the genitalia and when DHT administration is suspected. Serum estradiol should be measured in cases of gynecomastia. Assessment of other testosterone precursors and products may be required in special circumstances, including suspected congenital enzyme defects. The semen analysis is the "cornerstone" of the laboratory examination for infertility.

Hypogonadism and Androgen Resistance

PRIMARY TESTICULAR HYPOGONADISM. Primary hypogonadism refers to a condition of androgen deficiency with or without infertility in which the pathologic process lies at the testis level. A list of common causes is given in Table 247–3.

CONGENITAL DISORDERS (SEE CHAPTER 246). ACQUIRED DEFECTS. Mumps Orchitis, Leprosy, HIV Infection, and Hematochromatosis. After puberty, mumps is associated with clinical orchitis in 25% of cases and 60% of those affected will become infertile. During acute orchitis the testes are inflamed, painful, and swollen. After the acute inflammatory phase, the testes gradually decrease in size, although swelling can persist for months. The testes may return to normal size and function or undergo atrophy. Spermatogenic changes occur more often and earlier than Leydig cell dysfunction. Thus, patients with postorchitic infertility may have normal testosterone and LH levels with increased serum FSH levels. With time, elevations in LH and lowered serum testosterone levels may appear. Leprosy may also cause orchitis and gonadal insuffi-

Table 247–5 ■ INDICATIONS FOR ANDROGEN THERAPY

Androgen deficiency (hypogonadism)
Microphallus (neonatal)
Delayed puberty in boys
Elderly men with low testosterone levels
Angioneurotic edema
Other possible uses or under investigation:
  Hormonal male contraception
  Wasting disease associated with cancer/human immunodeficiency virus/chronic infection
  Postmenopausal female
  Aging men with borderline low testosterone levels

Table 247–6 ■ ANDROGEN PREPARATIONS

ROUTE	PREPARATION	DOSE AND FREQUENCY OF ADMINISTRATION
Oral*	Testosterone undecanoate (not available in United States; available in Canada, Mexico, Europe, Asia)	40 to 80 mg orally two to three times per day
Implants	Testosterone implants	200-mg pellets, three inserted once every 4 to 6 months
Transdermal	Scrotal patch	One patch delivers 4 or 6 mg testosterone per day
	Non-scrotal patch, Androderm	Two patches delivering 2.5 mg testosterone each per day or one patch delivering 5 mg testosterone per day.
	Testoderm TTS	One patch delivering 5 mg testosterone per day

*Oral modified 17α-alkylated androgens such as methyltestosterone, fluoxymesterone, oxymethalone, stanozolol, and oxandrolone are not recommended for use in treatment of androgen deficiency states because of potential hepatotoxicity and adverse effects on serum lipids.

ciency HIV infection is often associated with hypogonadism, which can be either hypogonadotropic or hypergonadotropic (see Chapter 417). Hemochromatosis and amyloidosis are examples of infiltrative diseases of the testis that can result in hypogonadism.

Trauma. The exposed position of the testes in the scrotum makes it particularly susceptible to injury. Surgical injury during scrotal surgery for hernias, varicocele, and vasectomy can result in permanent testicular damage.

Irradiation. Irradiation to the testes from accidental exposure in the treatment of an associated malignant disease will produce testicular damage.

Drugs. Chemotherapy, in particular with alkylating agents such as in busulfan, for malignant disorders frequently leads to irreversible germ cell damage. Toxins may also directly damage the testes. Many agents such as fungicides and insecticides (e.g., DBCP), heavy metals (lead, cadmium), and cottonseed oil (gossypol) produce damage to the germ cells. Leydig cells are relatively less susceptible to most chemotherapeutic drugs than Sertoli and germ cells. Serum testosterone levels are usually normal despite infertility in the exposed men.

Some medications may interfere with testosterone biosynthesis (e.g., ketoconazole, spironolactone, and cyproterone). Ethanol, independent of its effect in causing liver disease will inhibit testosterone biosynthesis. Marijuana, heroin, methadone, medroxyprogesterone acetate, and estrogens all lower testosterone, but mainly by decreasing the pituitary secretion of LH.

Autoimmune Testicular Failure. Antibodies against microsomal fraction of the Leydig cells may occur either as an isolated disorder or as part of a multiglandular disorder involving, to variable degrees, the thyroid, pituitary, adrenals, pancreas, and other organs.

Testicular Defects Associated with Systemic Diseases. Abnormalities of the hypothalamic-pituitary-testicular axis occur in a number of systemic diseases. These include liver failure, renal failure, severe malnutrition, sickle cell anemia, advanced malignancies, cystic fibrosis, and amyloidosis. About half of men undergoing chronic hemodialysis for renal failure experience decreased libido, infertility, and impotence. The effects of cirrhosis of the liver on testicular function are complex and may be both independent or associated with direct toxic effects of continued use of alcohol. Gynecomastia, testicular atrophy, and impotence are concomitant signs of cirrhosis. Decreased spermatogenesis with peritublar fibrosis occurs in at least 50% of the patients. In contrast to the decrease in serum testosterone levels, estradiol levels are usually elevated. This results in an increased ratio of serum estradiol to testosterone with an

increased proclivity for gynecomastia. Patients with sickle cell anemia often have impaired testicular function. Boys with sickle cell anemia may have impaired sexual maturation, and men are often infertile. The defect in sickle cell anemia seems to be ischemic in origin, probably with accelerated apoptosis; it may occur either at the testicular or the hypothalamic-pituitary level.

SECONDARY GONADAL INSUFFICIENCY (HYPOGONADOTROPIC HYPOGONADISM). Hypogonadotropic hypogonadism represents a deficiency in the secretion of gonadotropins (LH and FSH) due to an intrinsic or functional abnormality in the hypothalamus or pituitary glands (see earlier and Chapter 246). Such disorders result in the secondary Leydig cell dysfunction (see Table 247–4). The clinical manifestations depend on the age at onset of the disorder.

ACQUIRED HYPOGONADOTROPIC DISORDERS, FUNCTIONAL DISORDERS. Anorexia nervosa and weight loss are examples of functional defects resulting in low serum testosterone levels. Anorexia nervosa, predominantly a disorder of adolescent girls, is characterized by excessive weight loss as a result of dietary restriction and/or bulimia. Occasionally, this disorder is seen in men but in this instance usually implies a variant of a more severe psychiatric disorder. Men and women present with manifestations of hypogonadotropic hypogonadism. Starvation from other than a psychologic basis may also reduce gonadotropic secretion, although the female seems more susceptible to this disorder. Although strenuous exercise commonly produces reproductive dysfunction in female athletes (long-distance runners and dancers), it has minimal effects on testicular function in men. Severe stress and systemic illness also lowers gonadotropin and testosterone levels. Organic hypothalamic-pituitary disorders include neoplastic, granulomatous, infiltrative, and post-traumatic lesions in the region of the hypothalamus and pituitary.

Prolactinomas present differently in men and women (see Chapter 237). Unlike in women in whom small tumors are detected early because of symptoms of amenorrhea and galactorrhea, in men they are usually large (greater than 1 cm in diameter [macroadenomas]) by the time of their detection. It is unclear whether the large size of the adenoma at the time of presentation in men is due to the late diagnosis caused by failure of patients and physicians to appreciate early signs or to more rapid growth of these tumors in men. Male patients with prolactin-secreting macroadenomas usually present with hypogonadism, erectile dysfunction, and visual manifestations from suprasellar extension.

Large non–prolactin-secreting pituitary tumors (GH, ACTH, gly-

Table 247–7 ■ ANDROGEN THERAPY: RISKS VERSUS BENEFITS

BENEFITS	RISKS
Development or maintenance of secondary sex characteristics	Fluid retention
Improves libido and sexual function	Gynecomastia
Increases muscle mass and strength	Acne/oily skin
Increases bone mineral density	Increases hematocrit
Decreases body and visceral fat	Decreases HDL-cholesterol (cardiovascular risk ?)
Improves mood	Sleep apnea
Effect on cognition (?)	Prostate diseases
Effect on quality of life (?)	Benign prostate hyperplasia
	Carcinoma of prostate
	Aggressive behavior (?)

HDL = high-density lipoprotein.

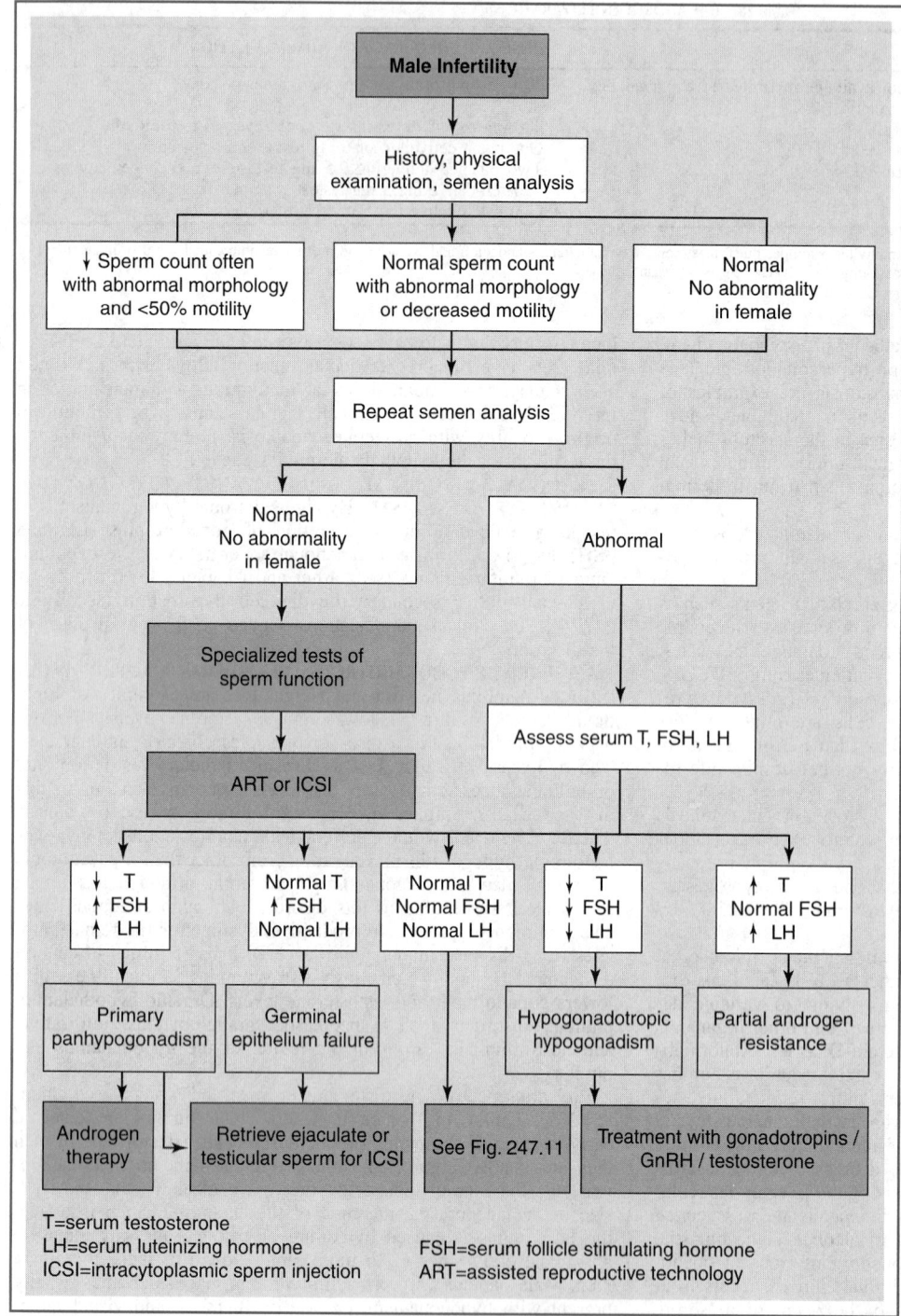

Male Infertility

History, physical examination, semen analysis

↓ Sperm count often with abnormal morphology and <50% motility

Normal sperm count with abnormal morphology or decreased motility

Normal No abnormality in female

Repeat semen analysis

Normal No abnormality in female

Abnormal

Specialized tests of sperm function

ART or ICSI

Assess serum T, FSH, LH

↓ T ↑ FSH ↑ LH

Normal T ↑ FSH Normal LH

Normal T Normal FSH Normal LH

↓ T ↓ FSH ↓ LH

↑ T Normal FSH ↑ LH

Primary panhypogonadism

Germinal epithelium failure

Hypogonadotropic hypogonadism

Partial androgen resistance

Androgen therapy

Retrieve ejaculate or testicular sperm for ICSI

See Fig. 247.11

Treatment with gonadotropins / GnRH / testosterone

T=serum testosterone
LH=serum luteinizing hormone
ICSI=intracytoplasmic sperm injection

FSH=serum follicle stimulating hormone
ART=assisted reproductive technology

FIGURE 247–10 ■ Algorithmic approach to the diagnosis and treatment of male infertility.

copeptide, and null cell) may also produce gonadotropin insufficiency from damage of the adjacent normal pituitary gland (see Chapter 237), resulting in decreased serum LH and testosterone levels.

ANDROGEN RESISTANCE (ANDROGEN-SENSITIVE END ORGAN DEFICIENCY). Certain conditions have clinical phenotypes mimicking testosterone deficiency in the absence of lowered testosterone levels. These are either drug induced (antiandrogens) or congenital defects in the androgen receptor, postreceptor defects, or 5α-reductase deficiency (see Chapter 246).

TREATMENT OF ANDROGEN DEFICIENCY

INDICATIONS. The main medical indication for androgen replacement therapy is male hypogonadism (Table 247–5). The diag-

nosis is based on clinical symptoms and signs and a reduced serum testosterone level. If a morning serum testosterone level is repeatedly less than 250 ng/dL (8.5 nmol/L), the patient is most probably hypogonadal and testosterone replacement is indicated. If the serum testosterone level is between 250 and 300 ng/dL with normal serum LH levels, the patient may not be hypogonadal and androgen replacement may not improve the symptoms (e.g., sexual dysfunction).

CONTRAINDICATIONS TO TESTOSTERONE THERAPY. Absolute contraindications for androgen replacement therapy include carcinoma of the prostate and the male breast. These cancers are androgen dependent for growth and proliferation. Androgens should be used with caution in older men with enlarged prostates and urinary symptoms.

ANDROGEN PREPARATIONS. Testosterone esters such as testosterone enanthate (or cypionate) are the most widely used prepara-

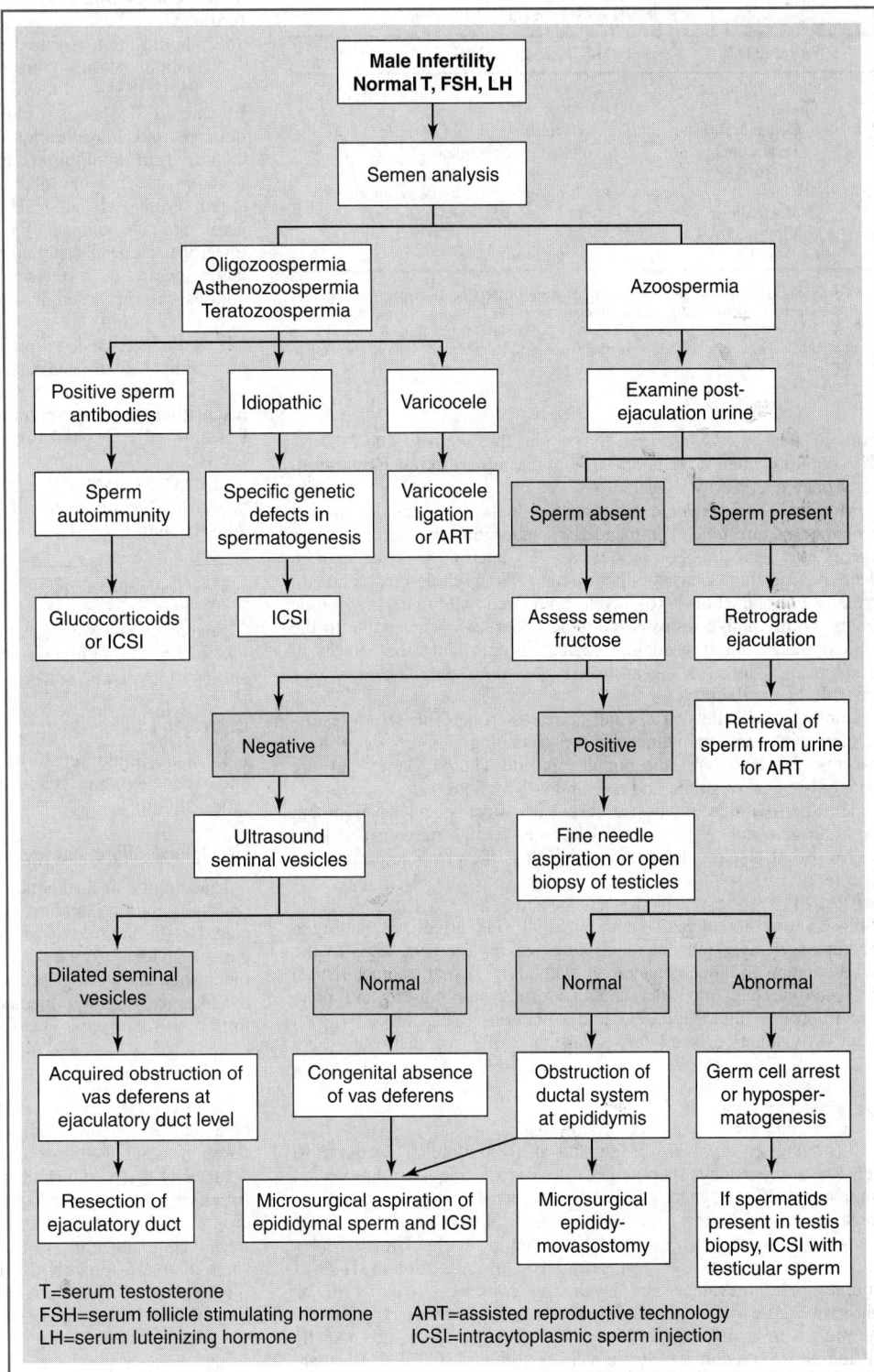

FIGURE 247–11 ■ Algorithmic approach to the diagnosis and treatment of male infertility in patients with normal serum hormone concentrations.

Table 247–8 ■ MALE INFERTILITY—BASIC LABORATORY TESTS

SEMEN ANALYSES	HORMONE ANALYSES (IN PATIENTS WITH ABNORMAL SEMEN ANALYSES)
Volume	Serum/luteinizing hormone/follicle-stimulating hormone
pH	Serum testosterone
Microscopy: agglutination, debris	If luteinizing hormone and testosterone low, serum
Sperm: concentration, motility, morphology, vitality	Prolactin
Leukocytes	
Immature germ cells	
Sperm autoantibodies	
(sperm/semen biochemistry sperm function tests)	

Table 247–9 ■ SEMEN ANALYSIS: REFERENCE RANGE

PARAMETER	REFERENCE RANGE
Semen volume	>2 mL
Sperm	
Concentration	>20 million/mL
Total count	>40 million/ejaculate
Motility	>50% motile
	>25% rapid progressively motile
Morphology	>15% normal*
Vitality (live)	>75%
Leukocytes	<1 million/mL

*This value is based on using the strict criteria for assessment of sperm morphology in studies using in vitro fertilization as an endpoint.

From World Health Organization Laboratory Manual for Examination of Human Semen and Sperm Cervical Mucus Interaction, 4th ed. Cambridge, Cambridge University Press, 1999.

tions in the United States and throughout the world (Table 247–6). The recommended dose is 150 to 200 mg administered intramuscularly once every 2 to 3 weeks.

Modified 17α-alkylated androgens, which are available in oral preparations, are not recommended as androgen replacement. These agents may lead to abnormalities in liver function tests and marked decreases in high-density lipoprotein (HDL) cholesterol and increases in total cholesterol levels compared with the testosterone esters. Orally active testosterone undecanoate is not available in the United States but is used in Canada, Europe, and other places in the world. This ester is absorbed into the lymphatics and has variable bioavailability.

Implants are pellets of crystalline testosterone. The serum testosterone levels are maintained in the physiologic range for 4 to 6 months. Implants are not popular in the United States but are widely used in Australia and the United Kingdom.

Transdermal skin patches represent the most recent development in androgen delivery system. The non-scrotal patch(es) deliver 5 or 6 mg of testosterone per day, which is the physiologic production rate.

BENEFITS VERSUS RISKS OF ANDROGEN THERAPY. Table 247–7 shows the benefits and potential side effects of androgen treatment. In hypogonadal men, androgen replacement leads to the development and maintenance of secondary sexual characteristics. Testosterone has important anabolic effects on muscle and bone and improves libido and sexual dysfunction. It has less effect on erectile dysfunction (see later section on sexual dysfunction).

MALE INFERTILITY

DEFINITION. *Infertility* is defined as the failure of a couple to achieve a pregnancy after at least 1 year of frequent unprotected intercourse. If a pregnancy has not occurred after 3 years, infertility most likely will be persistent without medical treatment.

PREVALENCE AND INCIDENCE. Studies in the United States and Europe showed a 1-year prevalence of infertility in 15% of couples. The prevalence in developing countries is likely to be higher because of the higher prevalence of genital tract infection. As shown in multicenter studies, 30 to 35% of subfertility can be attributed to predominantly female factors, 25 to 30% to male factors, and 25 to 30% to problems in both partners; and in the remaining no cause can be identified.

ETIOLOGY. Hypothalamic-pituitary disorders are infrequent causes of male infertility and are discussed in the section on hypogonadism and androgen deficiency. Primarily, testicular disorders are the most frequent identifiable cause of infertility (see Table 247–3).

APPROACH TO DIAGNOSIS OF MALE INFERTILITY. The approach to the diagnosis of an infertile couple includes the management of the male and female partner (Figs. 247–10 and 247–11).

Examination of the ejaculate is the cornerstone for the investigation of an infertile man (Table 247–8). Semen samples are collected when possible at the physician's office or at home, preferably, after 2 to 7 days' abstinence from sexual intercourse.

The generally accepted reference values for a semen analysis are

given in Table 247–9. A normal sperm concentration is greater than 20 million/mL; however, men with lower sperm counts can be fertile. Over 50% of the spermatozoa should be motile and over 25% should demonstrate a rapidly, progressive motility pattern.

In patients with abnormal semen analyses, measurements of serum FSH, LH, and testosterone are indicated (see Fig. 247–10). Elevated FSH levels usually indicate severe germinal epithelium damage and may be associated with guarded prognosis. A decreased serum inhibin B level also reflects poor Sertoli cell dysfunction and may be a marker of spermatogenic dysfunction. Elevated serum LH and FSH together with a low serum testosterone level indicate pantesticular failure. Low serum FSH, LH, and testosterone suggest hypothalamic pituitary dysfunction; a serum prolactin level should be measured and additional appropriate investigations (as discussed in the section on secondary hypogonadism) may be required. Presence of low sperm concentration, suppressed LH, with increased, normal, or low serum testosterone level (without clinical manifestations of androgen deficiency) may suggest exogenous androgen therapy. The hormonal pattern in androgen insensitivity (an uncommon cause of male infertility) is elevated LH, normal FSH, and high normal to increased serum testosterone levels.

MANAGEMENT OF MALE INFERTILITY. An algorithmic approach to the treatment of male infertility is illustrated in Figures 247–10 and 247–11.

SEXUAL DYSFUNCTION

Sexual dysfunction can be divided into four main categories: (1) loss of libido, (2) erectile dysfunction, (3) ejaculatory insufficiency, and (4) anorgasmic states.

Decreased Libido

Loss of libido refers to reduction in sexual interest, initiative, and frequency and intensity of responses to internal or external erotic stimuli.

Ejaculatory Failure and Impaired Orgasm

Ejaculatory insufficiency refers to absent or reduced seminal emission and/or impaired ejaculatory contraction. It is usually associated with neurologic conditions and medication therapy. Anorgasmic state is a distressing but relatively uncommon condition in men when the normal process of erection and ejaculation occurs in the absence of the subjective sensation of pleasure initiated at the time of emission and ejaculation.

Erectile Dysfunction

DEFINITION. Erectile dysfunction can be defined as the inability of a man to obtain rigidity sufficient to permit coitus of adequate duration to satisfy himself and his partner.

PREVALENCE. Current estimates suggest that 10 to 15% of all American males suffer from erectile dysfunction, with the incidence progressively increased as men get older. Data from the Massachusetts Aging Study report that 52% of men age 40 to 70 experience some degree of erectile dysfunction.

ETIOLOGY. The causes of erectile dysfunction are many but can be generally categorized in the following areas: psychological, endocrine, systemic illness, neurologic, iatrogenic, drug related, and aging.

CLINICAL MANAGEMENT OF ERECTILE DYSFUNCTION. ORAL MEDICATIONS FOR ERECTILE DYSFUNCTION. Yohimbine is an indolalquinolonic alkaloid with central-acting effects, including α₂-adrenergic blockade and cholinergic and dopaminergic stimulation. Despite its widespread use, placebo-controlled studies have failed to show a significant effect. Trazodone possesses both serotonin and α₂-adrenergic antagonistic properties. It appears to be moderately effective in approximately one third of patients, with the main side effect being sedation. Oral sildenafil has been approved by the U.S. Food and Drug Administration (FDA) and rapidly has become the most widely used and the most financially successful new drug for this disorder. Sildenafil is a competitive and selective inhibitor of cyclic GMP phosphodiesterase-5 (the primary phosphodiesterase in cavernosal tissue). Inhibition of phosphodiesterase-5 causes persistence of normally stimulated GMP in the corpora cavernosa, resulting in protracted cavernosal tumescence and rigidity. Early reports indicate that sildenafil is effective in 60 to 80% of treated men. The usual starting dose of sildenafil is 50 mg 1 hour before anticipated intercourse, increasing in 25-mg increments up to 100 mg when required. The most serious side effect is cardiovascular collapse, particularly in patients taking long-acting nitrate or nitroglycerin preparations. Because of its mechanism of action, sildenafil is used on demand, with administration of 20 to 60 minutes before intercourse. Apomorphine is a selective dopamine receptor agonist that stimulates the CNS, generating an arousal response that includes a penile erection. Apomorphine has not been approved by the FDA.

The intrauretheral prostaglandin E1 suppository (alprostadil) is believed to work locally on the corpora cavernosa as a vasodilatory agent. The suppository is apparently successful in improving erectile function in one third to two thirds of cases.

INTRACAVERNOSAL INJECTIONS OF VASODILATING DRUGS. Until the recent availability of oral sildenafil, intracavernosa injection with prostaglandin E_1 and other vasodilators (papaverin, phentolamin) was the mainstay of pharmacologic therapy for erectile dysfunction. The medications are injected using a 27- to 30-gauge needle.

Lue TF: Physiology of penile erection and pathophysiology of erectile dysfunction and priapism. *In* Walsh P, Retick A, Vaughn E, Wein A (eds): Campbell's Urology, 7th ed. Philadelphia, WB Saunders, 1998, p 1164. *Superb review of pathogenesis, evaluation and management of erectile dsyfunction.*

Swerdloff RS, Wang C: Clinical evaluation of Leydig cell function. *In* Payne, AH Hardy, MP Russell LD (eds): The Leydig Cell. Vienna, IL, Cache River Press, 1996, pp 663–694. *Detailed review of hypogonadism.*

Swerdloff RS, Wang C: Causes of male infertility; Treatment of male infertility; Diagnosis of infertility. *In* Rose BD (ed): UpToDate. Wellesley, MA, 1998. *On line UpToDate publication describing the pathogenesis approach to diagnosis and treatment of the male partner of infertile couples.*

Wang C, Swerdloff RS: Androgen replacement therapy. Ann Med 29:365–370, 1997. *Discussion on risks and benefits of androgen treatment with information on available androgen preparations.*

PART XVIII

WOMEN'S HEALTH

248 APPROACH TO WOMEN'S HEALTH

Janet B. Henrich ▪ *Wendy Levinson*

Over the past decade, women's health has emerged as a rapidly expanding field of scientific inquiry and knowledge with important implications for clinical practice and for the education and training of physicians. The increasing scientific information about the influence of gender differences on health and disease has expanded our concept of women's health beyond the traditional focus on reproductive organs and their function. Women's health can be viewed broadly as the study of the effect of sex and gender on health and disease that occurs across the spectrum of the biologic, behavioral, and social sciences. This broader interdisciplinary perspective of women's health has created an area of new knowledge and scholarship that is distinct from or more detailed than the knowledge base of existing disciplines. It has provided a new model by which to study the interactions between biologic mechanisms and psychosocial and environmental factors and their influence on human growth and development and response to health challenges. The clinical application of this information to women across all age groups highlights the interdisciplinary nature of this field.

BASIC PRINCIPLES UNDERLYING WOMEN'S HEALTH

The concept of women's health requires a reassessment of the importance of gender differences on health and disease. Complex interactions exist between sex hormones, normal and abnormal physiology, and the physical and emotional well-being of women. As early as the embryonic period, there are structural differences between female and male brains. Many of these differences are programmed during fetal life by hormones. During the reproductive years, the influence of sex hormones on sexual development and reproductive function differentiates a category of health issues that are unique to women. As women age and sex hormones decrease during the menopause, women's risk factors for disease change dramatically and become more similar to men's. Although women develop the diseases that affect men, biologic mechanisms and psychosocial factors influence the course of disease differently in women.

Until recently, most of the information used to make clinical decisions in women was based on studies conducted primarily in men. Women were excluded from research on diseases that are important to both sexes because of misconceptions about women's health, legal and ethical issues, and cultural biases. Because women, on average, live longer than men and are affected by major diseases at a later age, it was often perceived incorrectly that women were healthier than men. In fact, throughout life women experience poorer health than men, especially in the advanced years. The lack of information concerning women had important implications. Information based primarily on studies done in men was often applied inappropriately to women or resulted in different standards of care.

Efforts to increase our knowledge about women's health issues require an integrated approach that acknowledges the diversity among women and considers the social factors that influence their lives. One of the important social trends over the past 50 years is the increasing participation of women in the work force. Since World War II, the number of women who work has more than

doubled and is expected to exceed 80% by the end of the 20th century. The full effects of multiple roles, work stress, and new environmental exposures on women's health and reproductive status are largely unknown but are certain to have important health and social ramifications. Paralleling the growing numbers of women in the work force is the increasing number of single-parent families headed by women, especially minority women. Many of these families live in poverty. Increasing evidence indicates that socioeconomic factors are major indicators of health and that, for some health outcomes, poverty and lack of education are more important determinants of health than ethnicity. However, important ethnic and racial differences remain in women's susceptibility and response to certain diseases that cannot be explained wholly by socioeconomic status. For example, mortality rates for coronary heart disease, stroke, and breast cancer are higher in black than in white women, whereas death rates from lung cancer are higher in white women.

The increasing diversity of the population will affect health trends in the United States and the health status of women specifically. Regardless of their minority group, ethnic minority women have a lower life expectancy than white women and experience greater health problems. These differences are most pronounced in areas related to reproductive issues and childbearing, the occurrence and course of chronic disease, the incidence and outcome of cancer, and acts of interpersonal violence. Along with changes in our society, human immunodeficiency virus (HIV) infection and homelessness have become additional special health concerns of minority group women.

One of the most important factors underlying the current interest in women's health is the increasing number of women entering the health professions, especially the discipline of medicine. Since the early 1900s, the proportion of women represented in the physician population increased threefold, from 6 to 17%. According to projections, this proportion will increase to 30% early in the 21st century. Already, women comprise over 40% of entering medical students and over 50% of minority graduates from medical schools. Although significant barriers remain to their attaining equal professional and academic status, the potential for women to influence the structure of their profession, the delivery of health care, and the direction of medical research is considerable.

MORBIDITY AND MORTALITY IN WOMEN

At the turn of the century the average life span of women in the United States was 48 years, compared with 46 years in men. Since then the life expectancy in women has almost doubled and is now 79 years, compared with 73 years in men. Because of the gender gap in life expectancy, women currently comprise close to two thirds of the population older than age 65 and three fourths of the population older than age 85. The fastest-growing age group in the United States is the population aged 85 years and older. As a result, it is estimated that at the beginning of the 21st century, women will outnumber men by 2 to 1 in the age groups older than 65 and by 3 to 1 in the population older than 85. The reasons for the dramatic increase in overall life expectancy are thought to be related to the control of infectious diseases and progress in the treatment of chronic diseases such as diabetes and cardiovascular disease. The reasons for the disparity in life expectancy in women and in men are less well established but are thought to be primarily biologic.

Table 248–1 shows the leading causes of death in women of all ages and races. Despite a dramatic decline in mortality rates for heart disease that has occurred in both sexes over the past two

Table 248–1 ■ AGE-ADJUSTED DEATH RATES FOR LEADING CAUSES OF DEATH: U.S. FEMALES, 1995

CAUSE OF DEATH	RATE (PER 100,000 POPULATION)	PERCENT OF TOTAL DEATHS
All causes	847.3	100.0
Cardiovascular disease	278.8	32.9
Malignant neoplasms	191.0	22.5
Cerebrovascular disease	71.7	8.5
Chronic lung disease	36.4	4.3
Pneumonia/influenza	33.6	4.0
Diabetes	24.6	2.9
Accidents and adverse effects	23.7	2.8
Alzheimer's disease	10.1	1.2
All other causes	177.2	20.9

From Anderson RN, Kochanek KD, Murphy SL: Report of final mortality statistics, 1995. Monthly vital statistics report; vol 45, No. 11, Suppl. 2, table 7. Hyattsville, MD: National Center for Health Statistics, 1997.

decades, heart disease remains the leading cause of death in women and accounts for one third of all deaths in women. Heart disease occurs about 10 years later in women than in men. This delayed onset is thought to be due primarily to the protective effect of estrogens in premenopausal women and accounts for the fact that 90% of heart disease mortality in women occurs after the menopause. There are significant racial and ethnic differences in mortality among women. Black women are more likely to die of heart disease than white women up to age 75; thereafter, death rates are higher in white women. In contrast, Hispanic and Native American women have significantly lower rates of death from heart disease. Evidence suggests that heart disease, once it develops, is more serious in women than in men, resulting in higher mortality rates. In addition to biologic factors, the poorer survival of women may be due to the older age and increased prevalence of co-morbid conditions in women at the time of diagnosis, as well as to less well-defined social factors that influence the diagnosis and treatment of heart disease in women.

Cancer is the second leading cause of death in women and is the most common cause of premature death. The mortality rate for all cancers combined in women has changed little during the last part of the 20th century. Major advances in the diagnosis and treatment of cervical and uterine cancers in women have been offset by an increase in mortality rates for lung and breast cancer. Although breast cancer is still the most common cancer diagnosed in women, lung cancer is now the leading cause of cancer deaths. Unfortunately, most of these deaths can be attributed to cigarette smoking. Whereas deaths from lung cancer in men have begun to decline due to a decrease in male cigarette use, death rates for women increased between 1990 and 1995 and are expected to continue to rise.

Breast cancer is the second leading cause of cancer deaths in women. Although the incidence of breast cancer has risen over the past decade, mortality rates have remained relatively stable. This disparity is thought to be caused partly by the widespread use of screening mammography and the detection of earlier-stage cancers that have a more favorable prognosis. There are significant age and racial differences in breast cancer mortality. Declining mortality rates in younger women have been offset by an increase in mortality rates in older women. Although breast cancer incidence rates are 12% lower in black than in white women, mortality rates are 15% higher in black women. Reasons for racial differences in breast cancer incidence and mortality are unclear but may be related to socioeconomic and biologic factors as well as certain health behaviors, such as participation in screening mammography. Although it has been shown that breast cancer screening with mammography and clinical breast examination decreases mortality from breast cancer in women older than age 50 by approximately 30%, less than 50% of American women aged 50 years and older receive regular screening; and this figure is considerably lower in poor, minority, and elderly women.

Although stroke-related deaths have declined by almost 60% in the United States over the past 25 years, deaths from stroke still account for approximately 6% of all deaths in women and rank third as a cause of mortality. Striking racial differences exist in stroke mortality: death rates in black women are almost twice those for white women. Most of the stroke deaths in women result from thromboembolic disease and occur in older women. However, subarachnoid hemorrhage, the least common form of stroke, is more common in women than in men and contributes to stroke mortality, particularly in younger women.

Death rates from chronic pulmonary diseases have increased steadily for both women and men during the past 25 years; however, the increase has been greater in women. Because this increase has been linked to patterns in cigarette smoking, the increase in death rates in women for pulmonary disease, as well as for lung cancer, are expected to continue to rise. Death rates from pneumonia and influenza closely parallel pulmonary-related deaths and vary over time based on the epidemiology of these acute illnesses.

Diabetes has consistently ranked as a leading cause of death in women. Moreover, the reported death rate from diabetes most likely underestimates the impact of this disease on mortality because of its strong association with other life-threatening medical conditions, such as cardiovascular disease, stroke, and kidney failure. It is estimated that diabetes affects one in six women older than age 45; however, prevalence rates are higher in black, Hispanic, and Native American women. Separate from disease-related death rates, diabetes is a significant cause of morbidity and, in women of childbearing age, has important adverse effects on pregnancy outcome, resulting in an increased risk of fetal and perinatal mortality as well as congenital malformations.

Although HIV infection is not one of the 10 leading causes of death in women overall, it is responsible for the largest percent increase in death rates of all the major causes of mortality. HIV-related mortality rates are nine times higher for black than for white women. As a result, HIV infection ranks third as the leading cause of death in black women ages 15 to 24 and first in the age group 25 to 44 and in some geographic areas has become the number one cause of death. As the epidemiology of this epidemic changes, with heterosexual transmission accounting for an increasing proportion of HIV infection in women, these rates are expected to continue to rise.

Mortality rates alone do not provide a complete picture of women's health status. Although women live longer than men, overall measures of health status are worse in women (Table 248–2). Based on estimates from the National Health Interview Survey (NHIS), more women than men report symptoms or seek care for acute medical conditions, such as respiratory and digestive disorders, and are more disabled by these self-limited illnesses, as measured by number of days spent in bed or days lost from work. In addition, several chronic conditions occur more frequently in women and cause significant disability, such as arthritis, thyroid disease, migraine, bladder disorders, gastritis, colitis, and chronic constipation. Data from other sources show that affective disorders, especially major depressive episodes, and the anxiety disorders are significantly more prevalent in women. Most importantly, women's self-perceived health status is poorer than men's. According to estimates from the NHIS, only 36% of women describe their health as excellent, compared with 41% of men.

Table 248–2 ■ AGE-ADJUSTED SELECTED INDICATORS OF HEALTH STATUS AND MEDICAL CARE UTILIZATION, 1991

INDICATOR	FEMALE	MALE	FEMALE/MALE
Physician contacts (per person)	6.6	4.9	1.3
Acute conditions (per 100 persons)	204.7	178.1	1.2
Restricted activity days (per person)	8.2	6.4	1.3
Work loss days (per person ≥ age 18 years)	3.7	2.8	1.3
Hospitalization (excluding births)	5.4%	4.8%	1.1
Excellent health (self-report)	35.8%	41.4%	0.9

From Vital and Health Statistics: Current Estimates from the National Health Interview Survey, 1991, DHHS publication No. (PHS) 93–1512. Atlanta, Centers for Disease Control, National Center for Health Statistics, December 1992.

LIFE SPAN GROUPS

Many of the important health issues in women have their onset or greatest impact at certain ages and are intricately linked with women's psychosocial and sexual development. To develop a more integrated concept of women's health, it is instructive to look at the important health issues in women within the major life span groups. Several governmental and institutional sources were used to compile this information. Of these, the themes developed by the "Report of the National Institutes of Health: Opportunities for Research on Women's Health," known as the Hunt Valley Report, form the basis of this section.

BIRTH TO YOUNG ADULTHOOD. As young women reach puberty, the health issues that emerge are related primarily to developmental changes involving physical and sexual growth and changing relationships within and outside the family. Central to the psychosocial development of young women is the process of gender identification and orientation and the development of self-esteem. Intentional and unintentional injuries, including an increasing frequency of acts of physical and sexual violence, are the primary cause of death and disability in young women and account for half of all deaths in women in this age group. A small proportion of girls develop a chronic disease or disability. Most of these conditions are related to autoimmune disorders, such as lupus erythematosus, juvenile rheumatoid arthritis, and thyroid disease. Because of hormonal influences, many of these conditions first occur or are exacerbated during puberty.

AGES 15 TO 44 YEARS. During young adulthood, mortality rates in women are relatively low, and deaths due to injury predominate. As women progress through this age group, cancer of the breast and reproductive tract emerges as the leading cause of death, followed by unintentional injury and heart disease. Among the unintentional and intentional injuries in this age group, motor vehicle accidents, homicide, and suicide account for three fourths of all injury deaths. The death rate from motor vehicle accidents is highest in women aged 15 to 24; more than half of these deaths are alcohol-related. A major tragedy in the United States is the rapidly increasing death rate from homicide and suicide in young women. Black women, similar to black men, are most likely to be homicide victims, and firearms are used in more than half of these deaths. Because 30% of murders in women are perpetrated by a family member or acquaintance, the contribution of ongoing family violence to these fatal events is thought to be substantial.

The most dramatic trend in this age group has been the emergence and rapid rise of HIV infection as a major cause of death. Poor and minority women have experienced the greatest increase in death rates from this disease. The biologic and social aspects of HIV infection are difficult to separate; however, evidence suggests that HIV infection in women may have a different presentation and clinical course and worse prognosis than in men. The consequences of this disease for gynecologic care and reproductive counseling in women are unique. Because of the potential interrelationship between HIV disease, human papillomavirus infection, and cervical neoplasia, as well as recent questions about the accuracy of the Papanicolaou test in women with HIV disease, the Centers for Disease Control and Prevention recommend that HIV-infected women have a Papanicolaou smear performed annually. As a result of HIV transmission during pregnancy (see Chapter 254), HIV infection is the fourth leading cause of death among black children. The social consequences of this disease are enormous and result in loss of productive life, disruption of family structure, and premature death. The challenge to primary physicians to help control the transmission of HIV infection is an essential part of national prevention efforts.

An important role of physicians in the care of young women is to recognize and reduce risk-taking and other unhealthy behaviors. Health habits become established during early adulthood. Unhealthy behaviors not only place women at risk for life-threatening events but also have important implications for the development of illness later in life. For example, early or unprotected sexual activity increases women's risk for sexually transmitted diseases. Not only are these diseases transmitted more easily from men to women, but women are also disproportionately affected because of infectious complications that can lead to disorders of reproductive function,

such as pelvic inflammatory disease, ectopic pregnancy, and infertility. Unfortunately, efforts at risk reduction, particularly in the use of harmful substances, are hampered by industry and market forces and other social factors that influence women's lives. For example, the adverse effects of cigarette smoking on lung cancer and other respiratory diseases, heart disease, osteoporosis, and reproductive function are well documented, yet women become established smokers at an earlier age and have longer lifetime smoking histories than men. However, it is unclear what effect recent restrictions in advertising will have on women's tobacco use. Social values and cultural pressures have also contributed to the increasing prevalence of dieting and eating disorders. Using strict criteria, it is estimated that up to 5% of adolescent girls and young women suffer from bulimia and/or anorexia (see Chapter 227). These disorders are often refractory to treatment and can be life-threatening.

This life span group delineates women's reproductive years. In addition to traditional childbearing and family responsibilities, women are increasingly assuming new roles. The effect of multiple and often conflicting roles on women's mental and physical health remains to be determined but is closely linked to reproductive freedom and health. Thus, physicians need to understand the safety, effectiveness, and acceptability of current methods of contraception in culturally diverse women. Because of an increased understanding of many other common disorders of reproductive function, it is also clear that general physicians can no longer view these disorders as exclusively gynecologic problems. The association of polycystic ovary disease with insulin resistance and the hyperandrogenic state and the contribution of non-reproductive causes to chronic pelvic pain highlight the general medical nature of these disorders.

One of the themes that links together many of the medical disorders that have the highest prevalence in women in this age group is the role of autoimmunity. Most of the autoimmune diseases are more common in women than in men and cause greater morbidity. Many are influenced by changes in estrogen levels, particularly during pregnancy. Among the collagen vascular diseases, rheumatoid arthritis, systemic lupus erythematosus, and scleroderma have prevalence rates that are three to nine times higher in women. Many autoimmune-related endocrinopathies, such as Hashimoto's thyroiditis and Graves' disease, have a female-to-male ratio as high as 15:1. Other autoimmune diseases that are more prevalent in women are type 1 diabetes mellitus, idiopathic adrenal failure, multiple sclerosis, and myasthenia gravis. Less well recognized is the role of autoimmunity in recurrent pregnancy loss and infertility in women.

Among the mental disorders, depressive illnesses are twice as common in women as in men. An estimated 6% of women will experience a major depressive episode at some time during their lifetime, and twice that many will have chronic low-grade symptoms of depression. The excess risk of depression in women increases from childhood to adolescence and extends throughout life; however, the genetic, biologic, and environmental contributions to this gender effect are not fully understood. Women are also three times as likely as men to be diagnosed with an anxiety disorder, including agoraphobia, simple phobia, and panic disorder, as well as with somatization disorders. In addition, many women experience mood, cognitive, or behavioral changes associated with cyclic changes in hormone levels during the menstrual cycle or with marked changes in levels during the postpartum period or at the menopause.

A major cause of psychosocial morbidity in women is sexual and physical abuse. It is reported that 20% of adult women, 15% of college-age women, and 12% of adolescent girls have experienced sexual abuse and assault, and one in eight women in an ongoing relationship with a man has been assaulted by her partner. Pregnancy is a particularly high-risk factor for assault. Unfortunately, owing to lack of knowledge and training and misconceptions about domestic violence, physicians often fail to recognize or address symptoms of abuse. Adequate screening tools are especially crucial in the emergency department, where the proportion of women seeking care who have been abused can reach 30%. To ensure widespread detection of abuse, screening should become a regular part of the medical history in any setting.

AGES 45 TO 64 YEARS. Death rates for women in this age group have declined by 30% in the past 25 years. Previously, the leading cause of death was heart disease; however, cancer is now ranked number one, with lung cancer emerging as the leading cause of cancer deaths. These shifts in mortality rates reflect primarily a decline in death rates for heart disease that has been observed in both sexes and is attributed to changes in lifestyle, such as better control of hypertension and lower blood cholesterol levels.

Many of the important chronic conditions in women first appear in this age group, and the prevalence of some increases markedly during this time period. There are significant racial and ethnic differences in the prevalence of many of these conditions. The prevalence of obesity (see Chapter 228) especially is disproportionately high in minority women; 52% of black and 50% of Mexican American women are overweight compared with 33% of white women. Because obesity is a major risk factor for diabetes, heart disease, stroke, gallbladder disease, and some cancers, and may be a factor in osteoarthritis, weight control in women is an important public health issue.

The emergence of many of these conditions is inextricably linked to the menopause (see Chapter 256) and the marked decline in estrogen levels that occur during this age period. Decreased estrogen levels contribute to the development or progression of many of the disorders that are central to the aging process in women, such as heart disease, osteoporosis, and cancer. Because hormone replacement therapy (HRT) has been shown in observational studies to decrease the risk of developing some of these disorders, a woman's decision to use HRT reflects a consideration of the beneficial effects of HRT on menopausal symptoms, osteoporosis, and cardiovascular disease and of the reported risks associated with HRT, specifically an increased risk of uterine and breast cancer.

Whereas the menopause encompasses many of the physiologic changes that define this period, women also experience major transitions in social roles and life circumstances that profoundly affect their physical and mental health. Children leave home, many women become widowed or divorced, parenting roles change as women are called on to care for aging parents, and disabilities increase, making it difficult for some women to function within and outside the home. Not surprisingly, 3% of women will experience a major depressive episode during this period. An understanding of these life events is essential to the comprehensive care of mature women.

AGES 65 YEARS AND OLDER. Heart disease is the leading cause of death in older women, followed by cancer and stroke. Mortality rates for all three disorders rise steeply after age 65 and begin to approach the rates for men. Chronic pulmonary disease and pneumonia continue to cause high death rates because of the increase and severity of infections associated with an age-related decline in immune function. Injury is the sixth leading cause of death in older women; most of these deaths are related to falls.

After age 65, many other chronic illnesses, such as hypertension, diabetes, the arthritides, most digestive disorders, and thyroid disease, are more common in women than in men of the same age and cause significant morbidity. As women's longevity increases, they bear the burden of illnesses that are seen primarily in the very old. Of these, the neurologic degenerative diseases, such as dementia, sleep disorders, and neurosensory and movement disorders, are particularly common in women. Unfortunately, the added years of life in women are often spent in a frail or dependent state and often result in institutionalization. Currently, women residing in nursing homes outnumber men by 3 to 1. In particular, urinary incontinence (see Chapter 119) and osteoporosis (see Chapter 257) put women at high risk for institutionalization. Prevalence rates of urinary incontinence are twice as high in women as in men and affect up to one half of community-dwelling women. Osteoporosis is associated with deformity and pain secondary to vertebral fractures; however, hip fracture, usually the result of a fall, is the most serious consequence of osteoporosis in older women. According to the National Osteoporosis Foundation, one half of women with a hip fracture will never walk independently, one third will never live independently, and one fifth will die within a year of the fracture.

The social and psychological changes that women experience as they age add to the burden of illness. Social isolation increases as a result of death of loved ones, loss of financial stability, and increasing physical disabilities. In addition to an increasing incidence of dementia with age, mental health problems become more prevalent or serious. The role of the primary physician is to recognize

and help reduce the impact of these accumulated conditions on women's ability to function and on their quality of life.

WOMEN'S HEALTH EDUCATION AND TRAINING

Among academic medical institutions, there is increasing awareness of the importance of women's health. However, there is often uncertainty about what actually comprises women's health and the best way to train physicians to provide more comprehensive care to women. Broader clinical and educational issues exist, such as questions concerning the domain of women's health and how it differs from routine general medical or gynecologic care, the best way to train physicians to be more responsive to women's health concerns, and more practical considerations, such as which discipline(s) should be primarily responsible for curriculum development, clinical care, and training in this area.

Data from the National Ambulatory Medical Care Survey (NAMCS) provide insight into the complex nature of the way women receive care and the content and provision of that care. In an analysis by Bartman of differences in the delivery of medical care to women among physician specialties, family practitioners provided the majority of non-obstetric care to women aged 15 and older (57%); internists and gynecologists provided decreasing amounts of the remaining services (25% and 18%, respectively). Within internal medicine and gynecology, there was an age gradient in the provision of services; as women age, the proportion of care delivered by gynecologists decreased whereas that provided by internists increased. Gynecologists provided few services to women older than age 65. There were also specialty-specific differences in the type of service provided by each discipline. Family practitioners and internists provided services for both acute and chronic non-gynecologic disorders, whereas gynecologists provided little of this care. In contrast, over half of general medical examinations and two thirds of routine gynecologic services were provided by gynecologists.

When the realities of clinical practice are examined, the issues are more complex. There is considerable overlap between the practice parameters of family practice and general internal medicine and those of obstetrics and gynecology. In addition, many physicians in medical subspecialties provide some generalist care to women outside their subspecialty focus. Female patients seek care from one or a range of these providers over their lifetime, and the patterns of care vary depending on the age and the social, economic, and health status of each woman. Where women fall in this health care matrix determines to a large extent the type and comprehensiveness of care received.

These findings have important implications for the health care of women. The lack of uniform standards of care, especially regarding preventive services, and the splintering of routine care among disciplines, may result in poorly coordinated and incomplete care. The multiprovider approach that this system fosters does not necessarily mean improved services to women and is antithetical to the concept of primary care. Faced with overlapping but often inadequate services, women must increasingly take responsibility for directing and monitoring their health care.

In response to these findings, the Council on Graduate Medical Education recommends that all physicians, regardless of their educational level and specialty interest, be educated in the fundamentals of women's health and demonstrate competence in providing care to women. To implement these recommendations, women's health must have a form and a structure, a source of funding, and a recognized place in the medical community. Many of these objectives can be achieved by the establishment of collaborative interdisciplinary centers or programs in women's health within academic health centers. The Department of Health and Human Services through the Public Health Service Office on Women's Health funded six such vanguard centers in 1996 and an additional six in 1997. These centers are designed to facilitate the development of innovative clinical models, integrated curricula, and interdisciplinary research in women's health and to foster the development of female faculty.

There is also activity by some disciplines to expand residency training to address new national residency training requirements in women's comprehensive health care. In internal medicine, training programs must now include women's health topics as part of their core curricula; some offer additional clinical experience through multidisciplinary women's health centers. A few programs have developed separate residency tracks within sections of general internal medicine that focus on women's health. At the fellowship level, scattered programs in women's health exist as separate tracks in general medicine fellowship programs.

RECOMMENDATIONS FOR A CORE WOMEN'S HEALTH CURRICULUM

As a foundation for addressing women's health conditions, it is essential that physicians understand basic female physiology and reproductive biology. In addition, they need to appreciate the complex interaction between the environment and the biology and the psychosocial development of women. Among the conditions that are not specific to women, physicians need to be aware of those aspects of disease that are different in women or have important gender implications. The ability to apply this information requires that physicians adopt attitudes and behavior that are culturally and gender-sensitive. Women's relationship to the medical system is also changing and requires physicians to understand women's patterns of health seeking and forms of communication and interaction, as well as to appreciate gender differences in clinical decision making.

To assist academic medical institutions in implementing curricular changes, the Public Health Service Office on Women's Health, in collaboration with the National Institutes of Health Office of Research on Women's Health and the Health Resources and Services Administration, published a report in 1996 that provides the rationale for the development of a women's health curriculum and outlines the educational philosophy, scope, and content of a core curriculum. The report's recommendations are designed to augment and enhance rather than duplicate or replace existing curricula in the traditional disciplines. Although the report is directed to undergraduate medical education, its concepts and content can be applied broadly across the educational spectrum and may be helpful in modifying and updating residency training in the traditional medical disciplines.

Anderson RN, Kochanek KD, Murphy SL: Report of Final Mortality Statistics, 1995. Monthly Vital Statistics Report; vol 45, No. 11, Suppl. 2, table 7. Hyattsville, MD, National Center for Health Statistics, 1997. *The data in this report show the top ten causes of death for the white and black populations. The data are presented for several different subgroups, including all women–all ages, all women in specific age groups, and each race in separate age groups.*

Council on Graduate Medical Education: Fifth Report: Women and Medicine. DHHS publication No. HRSA-P-DM-91-1. July 1995. *A two-part report that presents the findings and recommendations of the Council regarding the status of women's health and women's health education and training and the status of women health professionals.*

Report of the National Institutes of Health: Opportunities for Research on Women's Health. NIH publication No. 92-3457. Bethesda, MD, U.S. Department of Health and Human Services, Public Health Service, National Institutes of Health, September 1992. *This historic document set forth the research agenda on women's health that is being implemented by the National Institutes of Health.*

Wingo PA, Ries LA, Rosenberg HM, et al: Cancer incidence and mortality, 1973–1995: A report card for the U.S. Cancer 82:1197–1207, 1998. *This report examines the annual percent changes in incidence and mortality during 1973–1990 and 1990–1995 for the most commonly occurring cancers. The authors also put forth potential explanations for the trends.*

Women's Health in the Medical Curriculum: Report of a Survey and Recommendations. U.S. Department of Health and Human Services, Health Resources and Services Administration, and the National Institutes of Health. HRSA-A-OEA-96-1. *A three-part document that reports on a national survey of women's health in the medical curriculum and outlines the educational philosophy, scope, and content of a core women's health curriculum.*

249 OVARIES AND DEVELOPMENT

Robert W. Rebar ■ *Gregory F. Erickson*

The ovaries episodically release female gametes (oocytes or eggs) and secrete sex steroid hormones, principally androstenedi-

one, estradiol, and progesterone. Oocytes are released only during the adult reproductive years, when sex steroid secretion is also greatest, but the ovaries are physiologically active throughout life.

Sex steroids affect the growth, differentiation, and function of a variety of tissues and organs throughout the body; therefore, abnormalities of the ovaries and of sex steroid secretion should be recognized by all physicians. A rational approach to the diagnosis and treatment of reproductive disorders in women requires an understanding of the functions of the ovaries and of their most important unit, the follicle, throughout life.

EMBRYOLOGY AND ANATOMY OF THE OVARIES

EMBRYOGENESIS AND DIFFERENTIATION. The primordial follicles represent a pool of non-growing follicles from which all dominant preovulatory follicles are selected. In this sense, primordial follicles are the fundamental reproductive units of the ovary. Morphologically, each primordial follicle is composed of an outer single layer of squamous epithelial cells that are termed *granulosa* or *follicle cells* and a small (approximately 15 μm in diameter), immature oocyte arrested in the dictyotene stage of meiosis; both the granulosa and the oocyte are enveloped by a thin, delicate membrane called the *basal lamina* (Fig. 249–1). By virtue of the basal lamina, the granulosa and the oocyte exist in a microenvironment in which direct contact with other cells does not occur. Although small capillaries are occasionally observed in proximity to primordial follicles, these follicles do not have an independent blood supply.

All the primordial follicles present in a woman's ovaries are formed before birth. Developmentally, the primordial follicles are formed in the cortical cords of the fetal ovaries between the sixth and ninth months of gestation (see Fig. 249–1). During this period, the oocytes are stimulated to initiate meiosis in an asynchronous manner. Because the oocytes in the primordial follicles have entered meiotic prophase, all oocytes that are capable of participating in reproduction during a woman's life are formed at birth. Soon after primordial follicle formation, some are recruited or activated to initiate growth. As successive recruitments proceed, the size of the pool of primordial follicles becomes smaller. Between the times of birth and menarche the number of primordial follicles (and thus oocytes) decreases from several million to several hundred thousand (Fig. 249–2). As a woman ages, the number of primordial follicles continues to decline, until at menopause they are difficult to find (Fig. 249–3).

THE ADULT OVARY: ANATOMY. During the reproductive years, the normal human ovaries are oval-shaped bodies that each measure 2.5 to 5.0 cm in length, 1.5 to 3 cm in width, and 0.6 to 1.5 cm in thickness. The medial edge of the ovary is attached by the mesovarium to the broad ligament, which extends from the uterus laterally to the wall of the pelvic cavity. The surface of the ovary is a layer of cuboidal cells resting on a basement membrane. This layer, termed the *germinal* or *serous* epithelium, is continuous with the peritoneum. Underlying the serous epithelium is a layer of dense connective tissue termed the *tunica albuginea.*

The ovary is organized into two principal parts: a central zone called the *medulla,* which is surrounded by a particularly prominent peripheral zone called the *cortex* (Fig. 249–4). A characteristic feature of the cortex is the presence of follicles containing the female gametes or *oocytes.* The number and size of the follicles vary depending on the age and reproductive state of the female. The existence of follicles of different sizes reflects specific changes associated with their growth and development. At the end of the follicular phase, the follicle that reaches maturity secretes its ovum into the peritoneal cavity (Fig. 249–4). After ovulation, the follicle wall develops into a *corpus luteum* (see Fig. 249–4). If implantation does not occur, the corpus luteum deteriorates and eventually becomes a nodule of dense connective tissue called the *corpus albicans.* Another class of cells in the cortex is the steroidogenic cells termed *interstitial cells.* These cells are found in nests or cords and are present throughout the life of the female. At the medial border of the cortex is a mass of loose connective tissue, the *medulla.* This tissue contains a network of convoluted blood vessels and associated nerves, which pass through the connective tissue toward the cortex.

The arterial supply to the ovary originates from two principal

3 mo 4 mo 7 mo 9 mo

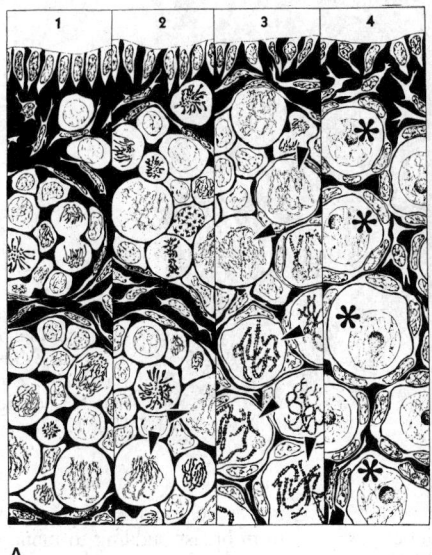

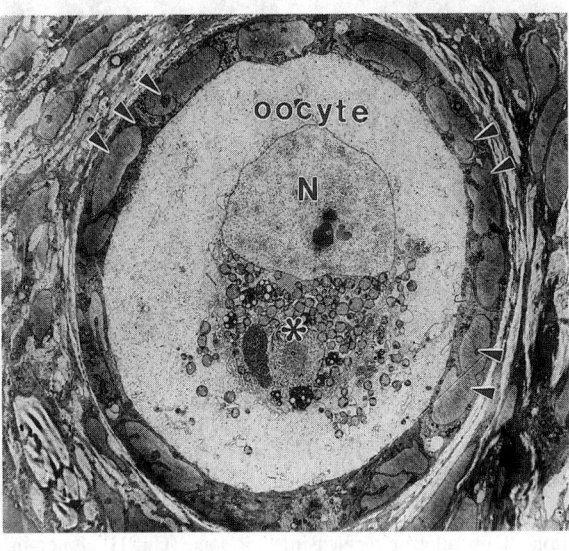

FIGURE 249-1 ■ *A*, Drawing of the initiation of meiosis in the cortex of the human fetal ovary, leading to the formation of the pool of primordial follicles. At 3 months (1), most of the oogonia are dividing mitotically. At 4 months (2), some oocytes deep within the cortical cords enter meiosis (arrowheads). At 7 months (3), the cords are no longer distinct, and all germ cells are in meiotic prophase I. At 9 months (4), the oocytes become associated with pregranulosa cells and appear as primordial follicles (asterisks). *B*, Electron micrograph of human primordial follicle. Granulosa cells (arrowheads), oocyte nucleus (N), and Balbiani body (asterisk) are shown. (From Erickson GF: The ovary: Basic principles and concepts. *In* Felig P, Baxter JD, Broadus AE, Froman LA [eds]: Endocrinology and Metabolism, 3rd ed. New York, McGraw Hill, 1995.)

A   B

sources: One, the ovarian artery, arises from the abdominal aorta; the other is derived from the uterine artery. These two vessels, which enter the mesovarium from opposite directions, form an anastomotic trunk and become a common vessel called the *ramus ovaricus* artery. At frequent intervals, this artery gives rise to a series of primary branches which enter the hilum like teeth on a rake. In the hilum, numerous secondary and tertiary branches are given off to supply the medulla (see Fig. 249–4).

Baker TG, Sum W: Development of the ovary and oogenesis. Clin Obstet Gynaecol 3: 3–26, 1976.

Fawcett DW: A Textbook of Histology. Philadelphia, WB Saunders, 1975.

OVARIAN FUNCTION IN CHILDHOOD AND PUBERTY

PHYSICAL CHANGES AT PUBERTY. Puberty extends from the earliest signs of sexual maturation until the attainment of physical,

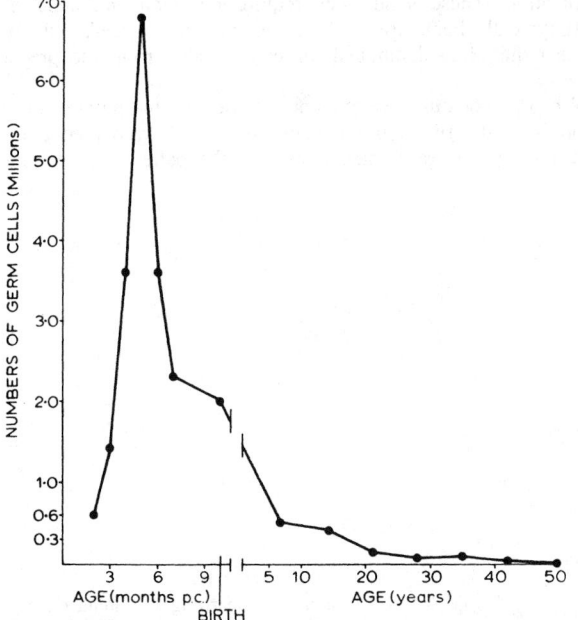

FIGURE 249-2 ■ Changes in the total number of germ cells in the human ovaries during aging. At early to midgestation, the number of germ cells increases to almost 7 million. Shortly thereafter, the number declines rapidly to about 2 million at birth. The number continues to decline until no oocytes are detected at 50 years of age. (Reproduced from Reban, RW: Semin Reprod Endocrinol 1:169–176, 1983.)

mental, and emotional maturity. Pubertal changes in girls result directly or indirectly from maturation of the hypothalamic-pituitary-ovarian unit. Hormonally, human puberty is characterized by a resetting of the negative gonadal steroid feedback loop, the establishment of new circadian and ultradian (frequent) gonadotropin rhythms, and the acquisition in the female of a positive estrogen feedback loop controlling the menstrual cycle as interdependent expressions of the gonadotropins and ovarian steroids. In girls, pubertal development generally occurs between 8 and 14 years of age. The age at onset and the rate of progress through puberty are variable and depend on genetic, socioeconomic, nutritional, physical, and psychological factors.

Physical changes occur in an orderly sequence over a definite time frame during puberty (Fig. 249–5). Breast budding in girls is usually the first pubertal change, followed shortly by the appearance of pubic hair, with menarche occurring late in pubertal development. The time from breast budding (median age at onset 9.8 years) to menarche approximates 2 years. Breast development results from increasing ovarian estrogen production and pubic and axillary hair from increasing ovarian androgen production. Estrogens are required for growth of pubic hair as well.

The ovarian sex steroids join with growth hormone and adrenal androgens to produce the adolescent growth spurt. Peak growth velocity is achieved relatively early with little growth observed following menarche. Lean body mass, skeletal mass, and body fat are equal in prepubertal boys and girls, but by maturity, women have twice as much body fat and less lean body mass and skeletal mass as men, as a result of differences in sex steroid secretion beginning at puberty. Estrogens are necessary for normal formation, mineralization, and maturation of bones. Well-established standards exist for determining radiographically, typically by examining radiographs of the bones of the wrist, whether bone age is appropriate for chronologic age. Estrogen deficiencies retard and excesses advance bone age in relation to chronologic age.

HORMONAL CHANGES. The ovaries function even in early childhood. The low levels of luteinizing hormone (LH) and follicle-stimulating hormone (FSH), which are normally present, increase if the ovaries are removed prior to puberty, just as they do later in life, indicating exquisite sensitivity of the hypothalamic-pituitary unit to extremely low circulating sex steroid levels. As puberty nears, there is a progressive decrease in sensitivity of the hypothalamic-pituitary unit to sex steroids, leading to increased secretion of pituitary gonadotropins, stimulation of sex steroid output, and the development of secondary sex characteristics. Increased secretion of both LH and FSH initially occurs at night with sleep and is associated with increased estradiol secretion the following morning (Fig. 249–6). As is true for most hormones, both LH and FSH are secreted in an episodic or pulsatile rather than a continuous fashion. It is possible that the sleep-entrained pulsatile secretion of

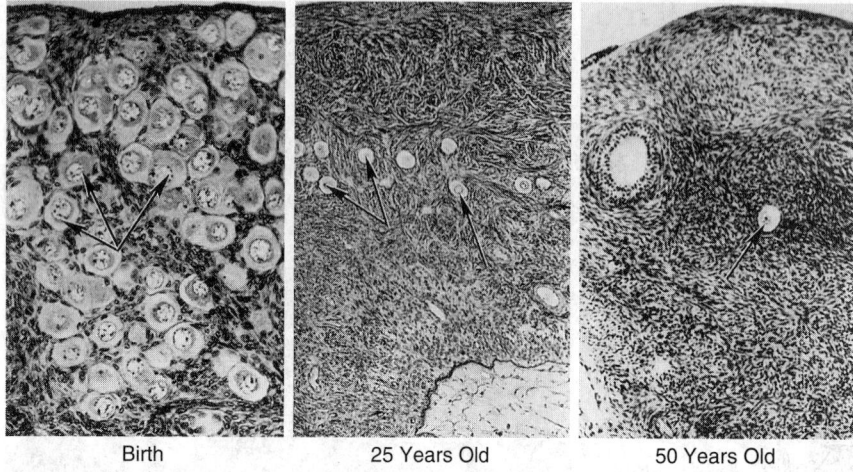

Birth   25 Years Old   50 Years Old

FIGURE 249-3 ■ Photomicrographs of sections through the cortex of human ovaries at different periods in life, showing the progressive decrease in the number of primordial follicles (arrows). (From Erickson GF: The ovary: Basic principles and concepts. *In* Felig P, Baxter JD, Broadus AE, Froman LA [eds]: Endocrinology and Metabolism, 3rd ed. New York, McGraw Hill, 1995.)

gonadotropins commences in response to increased pulsatile secretion of gonadotropin-releasing hormone (GnRH). Later in puberty, secretion of LH and FSH is increased, relative to childhood, throughout the 24-hour period, except during the early follicular phase when nighttime increases still occur. Basal levels of estradiol, the major estrogen secreted by the ovaries, increase throughout puberty. A "critical body mass" may be required for positive estrogen feedback and ovulation. During the first 2 years after menarche, up to 90% of menstrual cycles may be anovulatory because of a delay in the synchronization of the hypothalamic-pituitary-ovarian axis.

ABERRATIONS IN PUBERTAL DEVELOPMENT

DEFINITION. Abnormalities of pubertal development can be divided into four major categories (Table 249–1):

1. *Precocious puberty* represents any pubertal changes before the age of 8 years. The precocious development is *isosexual* when the development is common to the phenotypic sex of the individual and *heterosexual* when the development is characteristic of the opposite sex. *True* or *central precocious puberty* is due to premature maturation of the hypothalamic-pituitary axis. In the absence of increased hypothalamic-pituitary activity, *precocious pseudopuberty* (also known as precocious puberty of peripheral origin) exists.
2. *Delayed (or interrupted) puberty* is defined as the absence of any secondary sex characteristics by the age of 13 years or of

menarche by age 16 years or by passage of 5 or more years from breast budding to menarche.
3. *Asynchronous pubertal development* occurs when there is deviation from the normal pattern of pubertal development.
4. *Heterosexual pubertal development* is development that occurs at the appropriate time, but with some features characteristic of the opposite sex.

PRECOCIOUS PUBERTY. DIFFERENTIAL DIAGNOSIS. The temporal sequence in which the signs and symptoms of sex steroid hormone excess appear is most important. *Incomplete isosexual precocious puberty* indicates premature development of only a single pubertal feature. If breast budding occurs prior to the age of 8 years in the absence of any other development, the diagnosis may be *premature thelarche*. Premature thelarche is believed due to transient increases in estrogen secretion or increased breast sensitivity to the small quantities of circulating estrogens present prior to puberty. Simple ovarian cysts may be present in some girls with this disorder. If pubic and/or axillary hair develops alone and persists, *premature pubarche* and *adrenarche* must be considered. These abnormalities are associated with slight increases in adrenal androgen secretion, but not with clitorimegaly or other signs of virilization. These syndromes require no treatment, and affected girls typically begin true puberty at the usual age. Careful follow-up is required to distinguish these disorders from true precocious puberty.

When precocious development is isosexual, the purpose of evaluation is to determine if the cause is central (true precocious puberty) or not. Careful questioning of the patient and her parents

STRUCTURE OF THE HUMAN OVARY

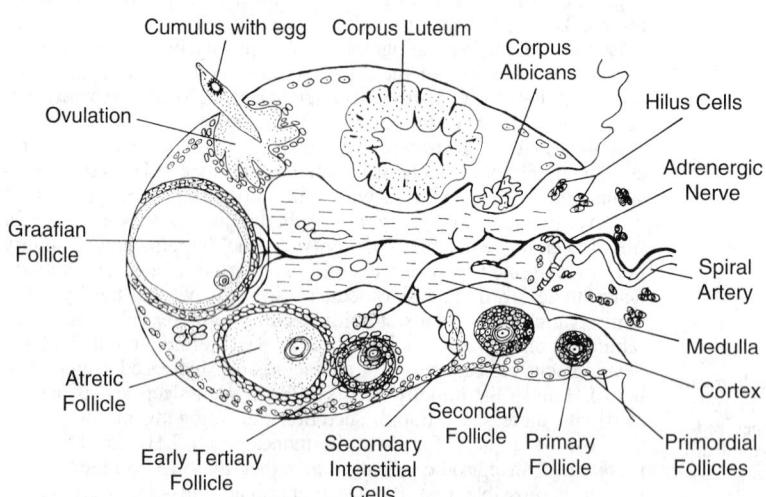

Cumulus with egg
Corpus Luteum
Corpus Albicans
Hilus Cells
Ovulation
Adrenergic Nerve
Graafian Follicle
Spiral Artery
Atretic Follicle
Medulla
Cortex
Early Tertiary Follicle
Secondary Interstitial Cells
Secondary Follicle
Primary Follicle
Primordial Follicles

FIGURE 249-4 ■ Diagram summarizing the architecture of the human ovary during the reproductive years. The follicles, corpora lutea, and interstitial cells are located in the outer cortex, whereas the hilus cells, autonomic nerves, and spiral arteries are found in the medulla. (From Erickson GF: The ovary: Basic principles and concepts. *In* Felig P, Baxter JD, Broadus AE, Froman LA [eds]: Endocrinology and Metabolism, 3rd ed. New York, McGraw Hill, 1995.)

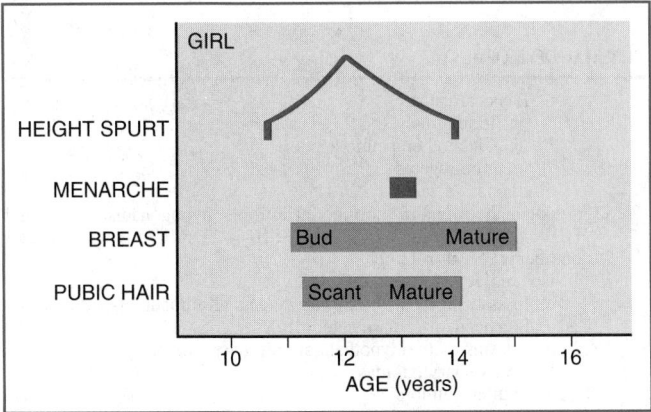

FIGURE 249-5 ■ Temporal sequence of events for the "average" girl during puberty. (From Rebar RW: *In* Yen SSC, Jaffe RB [eds]: Reproductive Endocrinology: Physiology, Pathophysiology, and Clinical Management, 4th ed. Philadelphia: WB Saunders, 1999, p 710.)

may indicate inadvertent ingestion or absorption of sex steroids (iatrogenic or factitious). About 10% of individuals with true precocious puberty have one of several organic brain diseases, including neoplasms, tuberous sclerosis, neurofibromatosis, encephalitis, meningitis, and hydrocephalus. The seriousness of intracranial lesions mandates that girls with precocious puberty have radiographic evaluation of the central nervous system, most effectively by magnetic resonance imaging (MRI). In almost 90% of girls with true precocious puberty, however, no cause is identified (idiopathic or constitutional).

The physical examination may also provide critical information about the cause of the precocious development. Cutaneous café-au-lait spots, facial asymmetry, polyostotic fibrous dysplasia and other skeletal abnormalities, cranial nerve deficits, and multiple ovarian follicular cysts suggest *McCune-Albright syndrome* in a girl with precocious puberty. It is now known that various clones of cells in the endocrine glands of girls with this disorder function autonomously with respect to cyclic AMP (cAMP) production as a consequence of a mutation within exon 8 of the G protein α subunit.

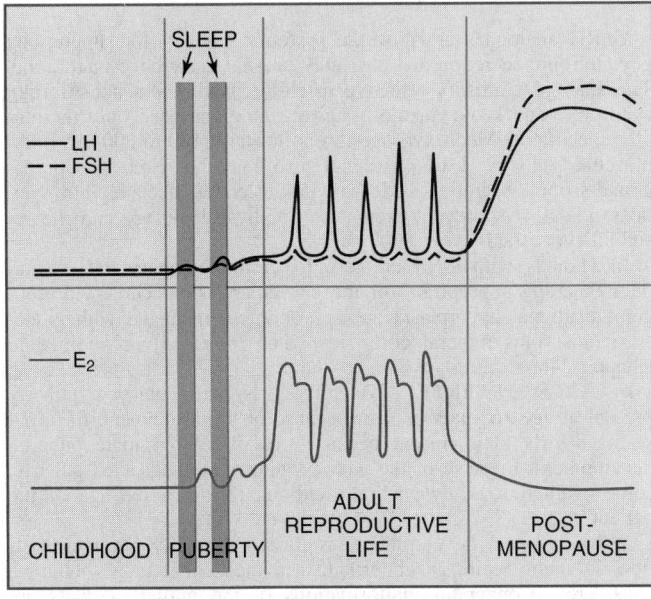

FIGURE 249-6 ■ The changing patterns of LH, FSH, and estradiol (E_2) concentrations in peripheral blood throughout the life of a woman. The elevated levels of LH and FSH present in the first several weeks of life are not shown, nor is the fact that both LH and FSH are secreted in a pulsatile fashion. The pubertal period has been expanded to illustrate the sleep-associated increases in LH and FSH followed by morning increases in E_2 that are observed during puberty. (Reprinted with permission from Endocrine and Metabolism Continuing Education Quality Control Program, 1982. Copyright American Association for Clinical Chemistry, Inc.)

This same mutation probably accounts for the bone lesions and café-au-lait hyperpigmentation. Precocious development associated with short stature, congenital bodily asymmetry, triangular facies, and clinodactyly suggests the *Silver-Russell syndrome*. Characteristic signs and symptoms may suggest the coexistence of primary hypothyroidism and precocious puberty, especially if galactorrhea is also present. In these patients, thyroid hormone replacement therapy halts progression of pubertal development until the expected age of puberty. (Enigmatically, primary hypothyroidism may also lead to delayed pubertal development. Thyroid hormone replacement permits the onset of puberty.)

Abdominal and rectal examination may reveal a mass, suggesting an adrenal or ovarian tumor. Because palpable ovarian cysts may develop rarely prior to ovulation in true precocious puberty, the presence of a mass need not confirm the diagnosis of precocious pseudopuberty.

When vaginal bleeding is the only sign of development, the diagnosis of sexual precocity should be suspect. Common causes of bleeding in this age group include irritation from a vaginal infection or foreign body, sexual assault, prolapse of the urethral meatus, and ingestion of estrogen-containing medications (most commonly oral contraceptive preparations). A vaginal or cervical neoplasm is also a rare possibility. Thus, vaginal bleeding dictates the need for vaginal examination, often best performed under anesthesia, before further evaluation is undertaken.

Heterosexual precocity in an apparent prepubertal female is almost always due to congenital adrenal hyperplasia or to an androgen-secreting adrenal or ovarian neoplasm. Only very rarely must another disorder of sexual differentiation be considered (see Chapter 246). It is important to examine the external genitalia carefully because congenital adrenal hyperplasia is usually associated with some degree of sexual ambiguity.

Excessive androgens produced endogenously by abnormal fetal adrenal glands in utero or diffusing across the placenta to the fetus from the mother can virilize the external genitalia and result in female pseudohermaphroditism. The extent of virilization varies from an enlarged clitoris only to sexual ambiguity sufficient to make gender assignment difficult.

Excessive maternal androgen secretion, typically from an ovarian or adrenal neoplasm, can lead to virilization of a female fetus. This occurs very rarely, because of the great capacity of the placenta to aromatize naturally occurring androgens to estrogens. Virilization of a female fetus is much more likely to occur if a pregnant woman has ingested a synthetic steroid preparation with androgenic properties because available synthetic compounds generally cannot be aromatized.

Excessive androgen secretion beginning in utero is usually associated with defective cortisol synthesis. As a consequence, pituitary corticotropin secretion is increased, resulting in congenital adrenal hyperplasia and excessive androgen secretion. The three different enzyme defects in the steroidogenic pathway that can lead to virilization of the female fetus are described in Chapter 246. 21-Hydroxylase deficiency is the most common form of congenital adrenal hyperplasia, accounting for the disorder in more than 90% of affected individuals. The defect may vary from partial to complete deficiency of the enzyme.

DIAGNOSTIC TESTS. MEASUREMENT OF PEPTIDE AND STEROID HORMONES. Increased levels of immunoreactive human chorionic gonadotropin (hCG) may suggest an hCG-secreting neoplasm, most commonly an ovarian teratoma or dysgerminoma. In such cases, the hCG, which is antigenically and biologically similar to LH, stimulates ovarian steroid secretion and pseudopubertal development. Because even specific LH immunoassays show some cross-reactivity with hCG, values for serum LH may be elevated in individuals with hCG-secreting tumors. Immunoreactive hCG is always elevated in the presence of such tumors. Levels and ratios of FSH and LH typical of pubertal as opposed to prepubertal girls help in diagnosing true precocious puberty. Timed urine collections rather than blood samples can be used to measure gonadotropin secretion if necessary. The use of exogenous GnRH to stimulate endogenous LH and FSH secretion can be useful in differentiating gonadotropin-dependent from gonadotropin-independent precocious puberty. Excessively high circulating levels of estrogen suggest an estrogen-producing neoplasm. High levels of serum testosterone

Table 249–1 ■ ABERRATIONS OF PUBERTAL DEVELOPMENT

I. **Precocious development (before age 8 yr)**
  A. Isosexual precocity
    1. Incomplete sexual precocity
      a. Premature thelarche
      b. Premature pubarche
      c. Premature adrenarche
    2. True (central) precocious puberty
      a. Idiopathic (constitutional)
      b. Due to CNS lesions
      c. Primary hypothyroidism
      d. Silver-Russell syndrome
    3. Precocious pseudopuberty (of peripheral origin)
      a. Ovarian neoplasms
      b. Adrenal neoplasms
      c. Iatrogenic (estrogen-containing preparations)
      d. hCG-secreting neoplasms distinct from CNS and ovarian tumors
      e. McCune-Albright syndrome
  B. Heterosexual precocity
    1. Ovarian neoplasms
    2. Adrenal neoplasms
    3. Congenital adrenal hyperplasia
    4. Other rare disorders of sexual differentiation
II. **Delayed pubertal development**
  (no development by age 13 yr; absence of menarche by age 16 yr; passage of 5 yr or more from breast budding without menarche)
  A. Anatomic abnormalities
    1. Müllerian agenesis or dysgenesis (Rokitansky-Küster-Hauser syndrome)
    2. Distal genital tract obstruction
      a. Transverse vaginal septum
      b. Imperforate hymen
      c. Vaginal agenesis
  B. Hypergonadotropic hypogonadism (FSH > 30–40 mIU/mL)
    1. Gonadal dysgenesis
      a. With stigmata of Turner's syndrome
      b. Pure (46,XX or 46XY)
      c. Mixed
    2. Ovarian failure with normal ovarian development
      a. Autoimmune disorders
      b. Gonadotropin receptor and/or postreceptor defects (?resistant ovary or Savage syndrome)
      c. Enzymatic defects (17α-hydroxylase deficiency, galactosemia)

    d. Physical causes
      i. Irradiation
      ii. Chemotherapeutic agents
      iii. Viral agents
    e. Idiopathic
  C. Hypogonadotropic or normogonadotropic hypogonadism (LH and FSH < 10 mIU/mL or LH and FSH 6–25 mIU/mL with at least one being > 10 mIU/mL)
    1. Isolated gonadotropin deficiency
      a. In association with midline defects (Kallmann's syndrome)
      b. Independent of associated disorders
    2. Neoplasms of the hypothalamic-pituitary axis
      a. Craniopharyngiomas
      b. Pituitary tumors
      c. Others
    3. Infiltrative processes (Langerhans-type histiocytosis)
    4. Idiopathic hypopituitarism
    5. "Hypothalamic" forms of amenorrhea
      a. Psychogenic
      b. Exercise associated
      c. Associated with malnutrition
      d. Anorexia nervosa
    6. Miscellaneous disorders
      a. Prader-Labhardt-Willi syndrome
      b. Lawrence-Moon-Bardet-Biedl syndrome
      c. Primary hypothyroidism
    7. Constitutional delayed puberty
III. **Asynchronous pubertal development**
  A. Incomplete forms of androgen insensitivity
  B. Complete forms of androgen insensitivity
IV. **Heterosexual pubertal development**
  A. Polycystic ovary syndrome
  B. Congenital adrenal hyperplasia (female pseudohermaphroditism)
    1. 21-Hydroxylase deficiency
    2. 11β-Hydroxylase deficiency
    3. 3β-ol-Hydroxysteroid dehydrogenase deficiency
  C. Male pseudohermaphroditism due to 5α-reductase deficiency
  D. Male pseudohermaphroditism due to partial androgen insensitivity
  E. Mixed gonadal dysgenesis
  F. Androgen-producing neoplasms
    1. Ovarian
    2. Adrenal
  G. Cushing's syndrome

suggest an ovarian source of excess androgen in girls with heterosexual development, whereas increased levels of dehydroepiandrosterone (DHEA) or its sulfate (DHEA-S) (the principal precursors of 17-ketosteroids) suggest an adrenal source. High levels of serum l7-hydroxyprogesterone imply congenital adrenal hyperplasia (CAH) secondary to 21-hydroxylase deficiency, whereas high levels of serum 11-deoxycortisol imply an 11β-hydroxylase deficiency. In CAH these hormone levels should decrease promptly following oral administration of suppressive doses of dexamethasone. Suppression in response to exogenous corticoids occurs much less consistently in individuals with adrenal cortical adenomas and carcinomas and rarely in those with ovarian androgen-secreting neoplasms (see Chapters 240 and 246).

Additional Studies. Ultrasonic scanning of the adrenals and ovaries and computed tomography (CT) of the adrenals may be indicated to confirm clinical suspicions. In girls with ovarian or adrenal neoplasms, the tumor can almost always be localized radiographically. Catheterization of the ovarian and adrenal veins and measurements of the effluent steroids from each gland should be pursued only when CT, ultrasonography, or MRI fails to identify what is suspected to be a neoplasm. Although plain skull films are of use in screening for pituitary and parapituitary tumors, CT or MRI of the skull is indicated in the presence of definite neurologic deficits or if true precocious puberty is suspected. Radiographic estimation of bone age is indicated in all cases and serves as a useful tool to follow the results of treatment.

TREATMENT. Treatment for precocious puberty should be initiated promptly so that (1) the patient's ultimate height is not compromised as a result of sex steroid-induced premature epiphyseal closure; and (2) emotional disturbances in the patient and her parents are prevented or attenuated.

GnRH analogues are now the preferred therapy for suppressing gonadotropin secretion and also may prevent early bone maturation. The analogues are not effective in children with McCune-Albright syndrome, and ketoconazole or testolactone has been only marginally successful. Medroxyprogesterone acetate (100 to 200 mg intramuscularly every 2 to 4 weeks) also may be used to suppress gonadotropin secretion. Medroxyprogesterone acetate, however, does not always prevent premature epiphyseal closure and the resultant short stature.

Individuals with CNS or steroid-secreting neoplasms must undergo therapy appropriate for the particular lesion. Girls with congenital adrenal hyperplasia are appropriately managed with glucocorticoids (plus mineralocorticoids when indicated) as outlined in Chapter 246.

DELAYED PUBERTY. Typically girls with delayed puberty present at age 16 years or later because of primary amenorrhea, but younger girls may present because of failure to initiate pubertal development. Because of the anxiety generated by delayed puberty, some evaluation is always indicated regardless of the age of the patient.

When pubertal development progresses normally but menstruation does not begin, an abnormality in the genital tract should be considered. Congenital malformations of the müllerian ducts are uncommon, occurring in 0.02% of all women. Most do not cause amenorrhea, and many do not impair reproduction. The anomalies associated with amenorrhea vary in severity from an imperforate hymen to complete aplasia of all müllerian duct derivatives with vaginal atresia. Although aplasia generally involves all of the müllerian duct derivatives, defects may involve only a single part of the distal genital tract.

A müllerian duct anomaly is suggested by (1) normal levels of serum gonadotropins and steroids, (2) an abnormal outflow tract, (3) a history of cyclic abdominal pain with or without a palpable mass, and (4) normal development of secondary sex characteristics. Normal ovarian function still induces endometrial growth and shedding after menarche if the uterus is normal. In the absence of a normal outflow tract, however, the menstrual effluent is retained and may or may not be able to escape into the abdominal cavity. Free in the abdominal cavity, the effluent may cause endometriosis. Constrained to the uterine cavity, the effluent causes hematometra and a large abdominal mass. In the absence of a mass or cyclic pain, a karyotype is indicated in girls with evidence of an abnormal genital tract to rule out any of several disorders of sexual differentiation (see Chapter 246). Such disorders, however, almost never occur together with completely normal pubertal development. In girls with a normal karyotype and a genital tract anomaly, examination under anesthesia and diagnostic laparoscopy should be undertaken to delineate the extent of the defect. When the abnormality consists of an imperforate hymen or transverse vaginal septum only, surgical restoration can be accomplished relatively simply. Attempts to provide an outflow tract for the uterus should not be undertaken if there is no cervix, because of the high risk of recurrent pelvic infection. Even with a functional cervix, the creation of an outflow tract that will permit successful pregnancy is unlikely. A functional vagina can be created surgically or by the daily use of ever-larger dilators. To prevent shrinkage and scarring, surgery should be deferred until the patient is willing to use dilators postoperatively on a daily basis or she is about to become sexually active.

Other causes of delayed puberty and primary amenorrhea are the same as those that may cause amenorrhea in older women (see below). When no apparent cause for delayed development is found, constitutional delayed puberty must be entertained as a diagnosis of exclusion. A strong family history of delayed maturation adds support to this presumption. Small doses of estrogen may be administered to induce some pubertal development but may obscure a pathologic cause for the delay and may compromise linear growth and ultimate height.

ASYNCHRONOUS PUBERTAL DEVELOPMENT. Asynchronous pubertal development is characteristic of male pseudohermaphroditism due to androgen insensitivity, especially complete testicular feminization. This syndrome of androgen insensitivity is inherited either as an X-linked recessive or as a sex-limited autosomal dominant trait. Despite the presence of intra-abdominal or inguinal testes, there is complete failure of virilization. Affected individuals develop breasts (but only to Tanner stage 3) and a typical female habitus with unambiguous female external genitalia but with absence of internal female structures, generally having only a foreshortened blind-ending vagina. Little or no pubic and axillary hair develops. The karyotype is obviously 46,XY in these individuals. Circulating testosterone levels are equivalent to or higher than those found in normal men, and LH levels are elevated while FSH levels are normal compared to those in menstruating women. This syndrome is further discussed in Chapter 246.

HETEROSEXUAL PUBERTAL DEVELOPMENT. *Polycystic ovary (PCO) syndrome,* by far the most common cause of heterosexual pubertal development, is associated with the development of some secondary sex features characteristic of males at the normal age of puberty. Feminization occurs in affected girls, and they develop normal breasts and a typical female habitus, but masculinization also occurs. (In contrast, girls with congenital adrenal hyperplasia generally show little if any female development at puberty.) A heterogeneous syndrome, PCO syndrome most typically begins at or near puberty with hirsutism and irregular menses from the time of menarche. Menarche may be delayed as well, so that young women may present with primary amenorrhea. Basal LH levels tend to be somewhat elevated in perhaps 80% of cases, and circulating levels of all androgens are elevated moderately.

Congenital adrenal hyperplasia is generally diagnosed prior to puberty, and heterosexual precocious pseudopuberty is typical. However, if the defect is mild and changes to the external genitalia are minimal, masculinization may occur at the expected age of puberty. This attenuated or nonclassic form of 21-hydroxylase deficiency seems to occur in families with a strong family history of hirsutism. Affected girls generally have some defeminization with flattening of the breasts, severe hirsutism, relatively short stature, and obesity.

Mixed gonadal dysgenesis designates asymmetrical gonadal development, with a germ cell tumor or a testis on one side and an undifferentiated streak, rudimentary gonad, or no gonad on the other. The extent of genital virilization prior to puberty is variable in this rare disorder. The vast majority are reared as girls, in whom virilization occurs at puberty; some may note breast development as well. Affected individuals generally have a mosaic karyotype, with 45,X/46,XY being most common. Short stature and other stigmata associated with a 45,X karyotype in Turner's syndrome are less common in patients with tumors than in patients with testes. Gonadectomy is indicated in all individuals with a Y chromosome to eliminate the increased neoplastic potential of such dysgenetic gonads and in all patients in whom virilization occurs at puberty to remove the source of androgen. Estrogen replacement therapy is warranted following gonadectomy. Other causes of male pseudohermaphroditism associated with heterosexual pubertal development are described in Chapter 246.

An androgen-producing neoplasm or Cushing's syndrome may occur rarely during the pubertal years and lead to heterosexual development.

Marshall WA, Tanner JM: Variations in the pattern of pubertal changes in girls. Arch Dis Child 44:291, 1969. *A classic article that is required reading for all serious students.*
Simpson JL, Rebar RW: Normal and abnormal sexual differentiation and development *In* Becker KL, et al (eds): Principles and Practice of Endocrinology and Metabolism, 2nd ed. Philadelphia, JB Lippincott, 1995, p 788. *A detailed discussion of the disorders of sexual differentiation organized similarly to the discussion in this chapter.*
Miller WL, Styne DM: Female puberty and its disorders. *In* Yen SSC, Jaffe RB, Barbieri RL (eds): Reproductive Endocrinology. Physiology, Pathophysiology, and Clinical Management, 4th ed. Philadelphia, WB Saunders, 1999, p 388. *A detailed and excellently referenced discussion of normal and abnormal pubertal development.*

---

250 MENSTRUAL CYCLE AND FERTILITY

Robert W. Rebar ▪ *Gregory F. Erickson*

THE NORMAL MENSTRUAL CYCLE

CHARACTERISTICS OF THE MENSTRUAL CYCLE. Between menarche at approximately age 12 years and the menopause at about age 51 years, the reproductive organs of normal women undergo a series of closely coordinated changes at approximately monthly intervals that together comprise the normal menstrual cycle. The menstrual cycle is the expression of the coordinated interactions of the hypothalamic-pituitary-ovarian axis, with associated changes in the target tissues (endometrium, cervix, vagina) of the reproductive tract.

A menstrual cycle begins with the first day of genital bleeding (day 1; menses) and ends just prior to the next menstrual period. The median menstrual cycle length is 28 days, but normal ovulatory menstrual cycles may range from about 21 to 40 days in length. Menstrual cycles vary most greatly in length in the years immediately following menarche and in the years immediately preceding menopause, largely because of an increased incidence of anovulatory cycles. Irregularities in menstrual cycle length also may be caused by abrupt changes in diet, exercise, or environment; serious emotional disturbances; and following parturition or abortion. The menstrual cycle can be divided into three distinct phases: *follicular, ovulatory,* and *luteal.*

THE FOLLICULAR OR PREOVULATORY PHASE. Variable in length, the follicular phase begins with the first day of menstrual bleeding and extends to the day prior to the preovulatory LH surge. A rise in serum FSH begins in the late luteal phase of the previous menstrual cycle, continues into the early follicular phase, and initiates growth and development of a group of follicles (Fig. 250–1). The preovulatory follicle destined for ovulation is selected from

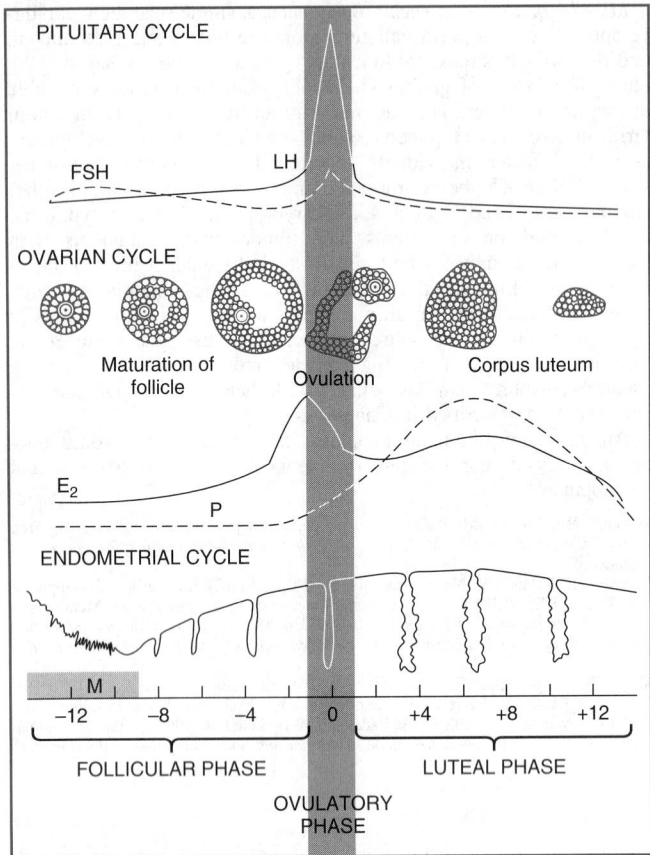

PITUITARY CYCLE

FSH   LH

OVARIAN CYCLE

Maturation of   Ovulation   Corpus luteum
follicle

E₂

P

ENDOMETRIAL CYCLE

M

−12   −8   −4   0   +4   +8   +12

FOLLICULAR PHASE   LUTEAL PHASE

OVULATORY
PHASE

FIGURE 250–1 ■ The idealized cyclic changes observed in gonadotropins, estradiol (E₂), progesterone (P), and uterine endometrium during the normal menstrual cycle. The data are centered on the day of the LH surge (day 0). Days of menstrual bleeding are indicated by M. (Reprinted with permission from Endocrine and Metabolism Continuing Education Quality Control Program, 1982. Copyright American Association for Clinical Chemistry, Inc.)

this cohort in a manner that is not yet understood. Circulating LH levels rise slowly throughout the follicular phase, but FSH levels fall after the early follicular phase increase. Approximately 7 to 8 days before the preovulatory LH surge, estradiol (E_2) and estrone (E_1) begin to increase, generally reaching a maximum on the day before or the day of the LH surge. The divergence in LH and FSH levels may be related to the follicular secretion of *inhibin* (folliculostatin), a hormone that specifically inhibits the release of FSH. Several days before the LH surge, plasma androgens (androstenedione and testosterone) and some progestins (17α-hydroxyprogesterone and 20α-dihydroprogesterone) begin to increase. They peak on the day prior to the LH surge. Progesterone itself does not increase until just prior to the onset of the LH surge.

THE OVULATORY PHASE. During this phase the ovum is released from the mature graafian follicle about 32 to 34 hours after the onset of the preovulatory surge of LH by the pituitary gland. The ovulatory phase extends from 1 day prior to the LH surge to 1 day following the LH surge. Some women experience brief (a few minutes to a few hours in length), dull, unilateral pelvic pain near the time of ovulation, termed *mittelschmerz.* The association of this pain to ovulation is unknown, but it may be due to leakage of follicular fluid into the abdominal cavity at ovulation. *Mittelschmerz* may occur before or after actual ovulation or not at all in ovulatory women. During the ovulatory phase a rapid rise in plasma LH results in response to positive estrogen feedback, leading to final maturation of the follicle and to ovulation. As peak LH levels are reached, E_2 levels drop, but progesterone levels continue to increase.

THE LUTEAL OR POSTOVULATORY PHASE. The more constant half of the menstrual cycle, the luteal phase, is approximately 14 days in length and ends with the onset of menses. This phase represents the functional lifespan of the corpus luteum ("yellow

body") of the ovary, which supports the released ovum by secreting progesterone. In the luteal phase, progesterone secretion increases to peak 6 to 8 days after the LH surge. Parallel but smaller increases in 17α-hydroxyprogesterone, E_2, and E_1 levels also occur. Progesterone levels decrease toward menses unless the ovum is fertilized and pregnancy results. The finding of serum progesterone levels greater than 10 ng/mL 1 week prior to menses is probably diagnostic of normal ovulation. Progestins increase basal morning body temperature so that a "thermogenic shift" of more than 0.3° C occurring after a nadir is a presumptive sign of ovulation and progesterone secretion. Unfortunately, taking basal temperatures on a daily basis is tedious, subject to error, and not very reliable.

CYCLIC CHANGES IN TARGET ORGANS. ENDOMETRIUM. During the menstrual cycle the endometrium undergoes remarkable histologic and cytologic changes, which culminate with menstrual bleeding when the corpus luteum ceases to secrete progesterone. The *basal layer of the endometrium,* which is not lost during menses, then regenerates the *superficial layer* of compact epithelial cells lining the uterine cavity and an *intermediate layer of spongiosa,* both of which are shed at each menstruation. Endometrial glands in these layers proliferate under the influence of estrogen in the follicular phase so that the mucosa thickens. In the luteal phase, under the influence of progesterone, the glands become coiled and secretory, with increased vascularity and edema of the stroma. As both E_2 and progesterone decline in the late luteal phase, the stroma becomes increasingly edematous, endometrial and blood vessel necrosis occurs, and endometrial bleeding ensues. Local release of prostaglandins may initiate vasospasm and ischemic necrosis in the endometrium as well as the uterine contractions accompanying menstrual flow. Thus prostaglandin synthetase inhibitors can relieve dysmenorrhea (menstrual cramping). Fibrinolytic activity in the endometrium also peaks at the time of menstruation, accounting for the noncoagulability of menstrual blood. Because the histologic changes during the menstrual cycle are so characteristic, endometrial biopsies are used to date the stage of the cycle and to assess the tissue response to gonadal steroids.

CERVIX AND CERVICAL MUCUS. During the follicular phase, cervical vascularity, congestion, and edema increase progressively under the influence of estrogen. The external cervical os opens to a diameter of 3 mm at ovulation and then decreases to 1 mm. Cervical mucus increases in quantity (10- to 30-fold) and in elasticity. "Palm leaf" arborization (ferning) becomes prominent just prior to ovulation (if cervical mucus is allowed to dry on a glass slide and is examined microscopically). Under the influence of progesterone during the luteal phase, cervical mucus thickens, becomes less watery, and loses its elasticity and ability to fern. The characteristics of cervical mucus are useful clinically to evaluate the stage of the cycle and the amount of estrogen present.

VAGINA. When ovarian estrogen secretion is low, as in the early follicular phase, vaginal epithelium is pale and thin. In the follicular phase under the influence of estrogens the epithelium thickens, and the number of mature cornified epithelial cells increases. During the luteal phase, progesterone causes a decrease in the percentage of cornified cells and an increase in the number of precornified intermediate cells and polymorphonuclear leukocytes. There is also increased cellular debris and clumping of shed desquamated cells. Histologic changes in the vaginal epithelium and in the cervical mucus are the most sensitive indicators of estrogen status in the body. However, the reliability of vaginal smears depends on the absence of infection or exogenously administered steroid hormones that have antiestrogenic effects. Steroid hormones also facilitate progression of spermatozoa toward the ovaries and of ova toward the uterine cavity through effects on the fallopian tubes.

OVARY. Physiologically, the human ovaries produce a single dominant follicle that secretes a mature egg into the oviduct to be fertilized at the end of the follicular phase of each menstrual cycle. Each dominant follicle begins with the recruitment of a primordial follicle into the pool of growing follicles. It is not known exactly how recruitment occurs, but it is independent of the pituitary and thus involves local autocrine/paracrine mechanisms. As a consequence of successive recruitments, the ovaries appear to always contain a pool of small graafian follicles from which a prospective dominant follicle can be selected. Once selected, a dominant follicle typically grows and develops to the preovulatory state. Those follicles that are not selected die by atresia by a programmed cell death mechanism called apoptosis.

Theca Interstitial Cell

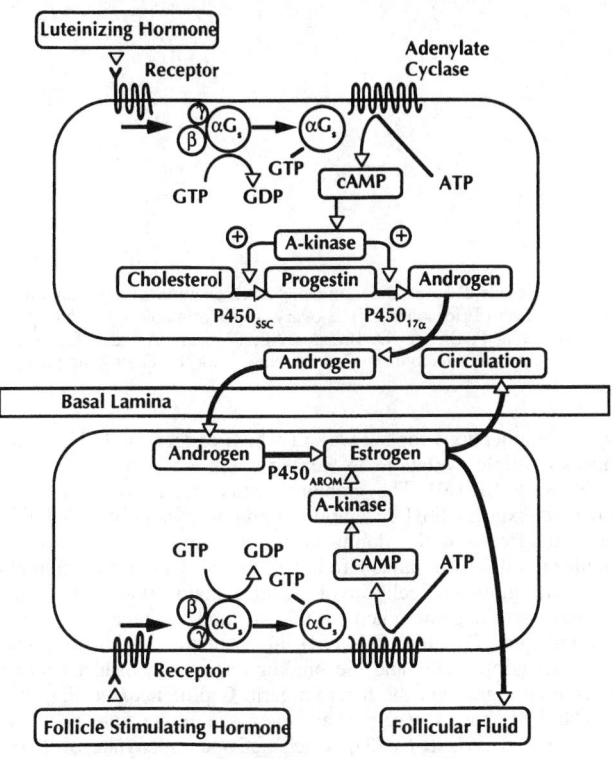

Granulosa Cell

FIGURE 250–2 ■ The two gonadotropin-two cell concept of follicle estrogen production. (From Kettel M, Erickson GF: Basic and clinical concepts in ovulation induction. *In* Rock J, Alvarez-Murphy A [eds]: Advances in Obstetrics and Gynecology, vol 1. St Louis, Mosby–Year Book, 1994.)

Endocrinology of Folliculogenesis. The signaling pathways activated by FSH and LH play a fundamental role in the expression of the differentiated state of a dominant follicle. The primary roles of these signal transduction pathways are to stimulate mitotic and differentiation responses in the granulosa and theca cells. Physiologically, these signaling pathways act in parallel to regulate the expression of a set of genes in a precise quantitative and temporal fashion. One endocrine response associated with the action of FSH and LH is the production of large amounts of estradiol by the dominant follicle. This gonadotropin-dependent mechanism is called the two gonadotropin-two cell concept (Fig. 250–2). Because the estradiol response appears to be specific to a dominant follicle, the levels of plasma estradiol can be used as an indicator for follicle differentiation during ovulation induction. What are the mechanisms that lead to dominant follicle development and estradiol production?

Chronology. In normal women, folliculogenesis is a very long process (Fig. 250–3). In each menstrual cycle, the dominant follicle that is selected to ovulate originates from a primordial follicle that was recruited to grow about 1 year earlier. The very early stages of folliculogenesis (class 1, primary and secondary; class 2, early tertiary) proceed very slowly. Consequently, it requires 300 days or more for a recruited primordial follicle to complete the preantral or hormone-independent period. The basis for the slow growth is the very long doubling time (~250 hours) of the granulosa cells. When follicular fluid begins to accumulate at the class 2 stage, the size of the graafian follicle begins to increase relatively rapidly (see Fig. 250–3). As the antral (hormone-dependent) period proceeds, the graafian follicle passes through the small (class 3, 4, and 5), medium (class 6 and 7), and large (class 8) stages. A dominant follicle that survives to the ovulatory stage requires about 40 to 50 days to complete the whole antral period. Selection of the dominant follicle is one of the last steps in the long process of folliculogenesis. The dominant follicle, which is selected from a cohort of class 5 follicles, requires approximately 20 days to develop to the stage at which it undergoes ovulation. Those follicles that are not selected become atretic. Atresia can occur at each stage

of graafian follicle development, but atresia appears most prominent in follicles at the class 5 stage (see Fig. 250–3).

Physiology of Selection. The results of morphometric studies indicate that the dominant follicle that will ovulate its egg the next cycle is selected from a cohort of healthy, small graafian follicles (4.7 ± 0.7 mm in diameter) at the end of the luteal phase of the menstrual cycle. Morphologically, each cohort follicle contains a fully grown egg, about 1 million granulosa cells, a theca interna containing several layers of theca interstitial cells, and a band of smooth muscle cells in the theca externa (Fig. 250–4).

Selection is characterized by a high sustained rate of granulosa mitosis. Shortly after the midluteal phase, the granulosa cells in all of the cohort class 4 and 5 follicles show a sharp increase (about twofold) in the rate of granulosa mitosis. This result suggests that luteolysis is associated with a sharp increase in division of the granulosa cells within the cohort follicles. The first indication that a cohort follicle has been selected is that the granulosa cells of the chosen follicle continue dividing at a fast rate while proliferation slows in the nondominant cohort follicles. Because this distinguishing feature is evident at the late luteal phase, it has been concluded that selection occurs at this point in the cycle. As mitosis and follicular fluid accumulation continue, the dominant follicle grows rapidly during the follicular phase, reaching 6.9 ± 0.5 mm at days 1 to 5, 13.7 ± 1.2 mm at days 6 to 10, and 18.8 ± 0.5 mm at days 11 to 14. In nondominant follicles, growth and expansion proceed more slowly, and with time, atresia becomes increasingly more evident. Rarely does an atretic follicle reach 9 mm or more in diameter, regardless of the stage in the cycle.

FSH is obligatory for follicle selection, and no other ligand by itself can serve in this regulatory capacity. Furthermore, once selected, the dominant follicle depends on FSH for its survival. Physiologically, the secondary rise in plasma FSH is crucial for follicle selection. The secondary rise in plasma FSH begins a few days before the progesterone levels reach basal levels at the end of luteal phase, and it continues through the first week of the follicular phase (Fig. 250–5). The importance of the secondary rise in FSH is demonstrated by the fact that the dominant follicle will undergo atresia if the FSH levels are decreased. One of the major consequences of the secondary FSH rise is that the FSH levels increase within the chosen follicle. In normal class 5 to 8 follicles, the mean concentration of follicular fluid FSH increases from about 1.3 mIU/mL (about 58 ng/mL) to about 3.2 mIU/mL (about 143 ng/mL)

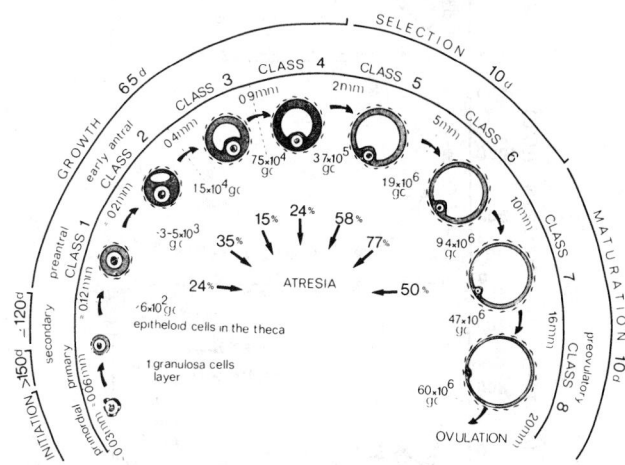

FIGURE 250–3 ■ The chronology of folliculogenesis in the human ovary. Folliculogenesis is divided into two major periods, preantral (gonadotropin-independent) and antral (FSH-dependent). In the preantral period, a recruited primordial follicle develops to the primary/secondary (class 1) and early tertiary (class 2) stage, at which time cavitation or antrum formation begins. The antral period includes the small graafian (0.9 to 5 mm, class 4 and 5), medium graafian (6 to 10 mm, class 6), large graafian (10 to 15 mm, class 7), and preovulatory (16 to 20 mm, class 8) follicles. Time required for completion of preantral and antral periods is approximately 300 and approximately 40 days, respectively. gc = number of granulosa cells; mm = follicle diameter; % = atresia indicated. (From Gougeon A: Dynamics of follicular growth in the human: A model from preliminary results. Hum Reprod. 2:81–87, 1986.)

HISTOLOGIC ARCHITECTURE OF GRAAFIAN FOLLICLE

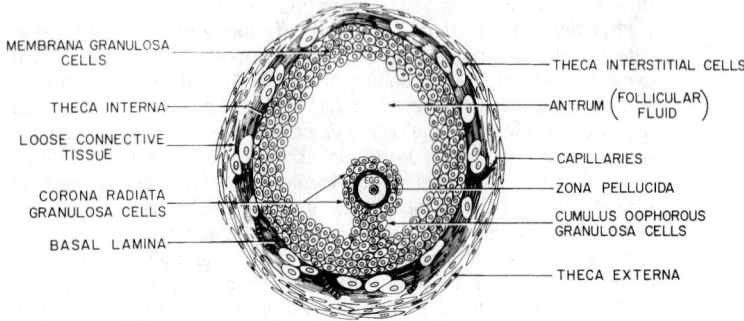

FIGURE 250–4 ■ Diagrammatic representation of graafian follicle. (From Erickson GF: The ovary: Basic principles and concepts. *In* Felig P, Baxter JD, Broadus AE, Froman LA [eds]: Endocrinology and Metabolism, 2nd ed. New York, McGraw-Hill 1987.)

through the follicular phase. In contrast, the levels of FSH are low or undetectable in the microenvironment of the nondominant cohort follicles. Thus, selection and growth of a dominant follicle involves a progressive increase in the concentration of FSH within its microenvironment.

The FSH triggers a marked activation of mitosis and differentiation of the granulosa cells, which in turn is reflected in a progressive increase in estradiol synthesis and follicular fluid accumulation. One of the effects of the increased estradiol production is that the secondary rise in FSH is suppressed (see Fig. 250–5). When this occurs, the concentration of FSH falls below threshold levels, and the development of the nondominant follicles stops. It is noteworthy that mitosis in these atretic follicles can be markedly stimulated by treatment with human menopausal gonadotropin (hMG) during the early follicular phase. Thus, if FSH levels within the microenvironment are increased, the nondominant follicles could perhaps be rescued from atresia. If this is the case, this phenome-

non has implications for the way in which exogenous FSH or hMG induces multiple ovulations in women.

THE ROLE OF FSH. The granulosa cells are the only cell types known to express FSH receptors. It follows, therefore, that FSH-mediated effects in the dominant follicle are at the level of the granulosa cells. In dominant follicles, the FSH-induced differentiation of the granulosa cells involves three major responses, namely increased steroidogenic potential, mitosis, and LH receptors.

Steroidogenic Potential. The FSH ligand interacts with its receptor on the granulosa cells, and the binding event is transduced into an intracellular signal via the heterodimeric G proteins (see Fig. 250–2). The FSH-bound receptor activates the alpha subunit of the stimulatory G protein (αGS), which activates adenylate cyclase to generate increases in cyclic adenosine monophosphate (cAMP), which in turn triggers protein kinase A (PKA) to phosphorylate cAMP–responsive element-binding protein (CREB) or other related DNA binding proteins. After phosphorylation, these proteins bind to upstream DNA regulatory elements called cAMP response elements (CRE), where they regulate gene transcription. In this regard, the FSH signal mechanisms stimulate the expression of specific genes that control the level of estradiol production by the granulosa cells. The major steroidogenic genes induced by FSH include the P450 aromatase ($P450_{arom}$) and 17β-hydroxysteroid dehydrogenase (17β-HSD) (see Fig. 250–2). The temporal pattern of expression of these genes has an important role in generating the normal pattern of estradiol production by the dominant follicle during the follicular phase of the cycle.

Mitosis. The granulosa cells in the dominant follicle have the ability to divide at a relatively rapid rate throughout the follicular phase of the cycle, increasing from about 1×10^6 cells at selection to more than 50×10^6 cells at ovulation. Despite its overall importance to ovarian physiology, it remains unclear how granulosa proliferation is controlled. Evidence in humans indicates that FSH stimulates the rate of granulosa cell division in vivo and in vitro, but the mechanism by which FSH stimulates mitosis is not understood.

Induction of LH Receptor. The ability of LH–human chorionic gonadotropin (hCG) to generate the ovulatory sequence in the dominant follicle is dependent on the expression of a large number of LH receptors on the granulosa cells. Studies have clearly demonstrated an obligatory role of FSH in the induction of LH receptor. A key feature of LH receptor expression in the granulosa layer is that it is suppressed throughout most of folliculogenesis. That is, the number of LH receptors remains low in granulosa cells during the early and intermediate stages of dominant follicle growth, but then the number increases sharply to very high levels at the preovulatory stage. The acquisition of LH receptors implies that when the LH ligand enters the microenvironment of the dominant follicle in the late follicular phase, it can act on the granulosa cells to regulate their function, perhaps even replacing FSH as the principal regulator of granulosa cytodifferentiation.

THE ROLE OF LH. Throughout the life of a woman, an interplay between LH and the interstitial tissue results in changes in ovarian androgen biosynthesis. The LH-receptor interacting in the interstitial cells are critically important in estradiol production by virtue of their ability to promote the production of $P450_{arom}$ substrate, androstenedione. The activation of the LH-receptor signaling pathway is

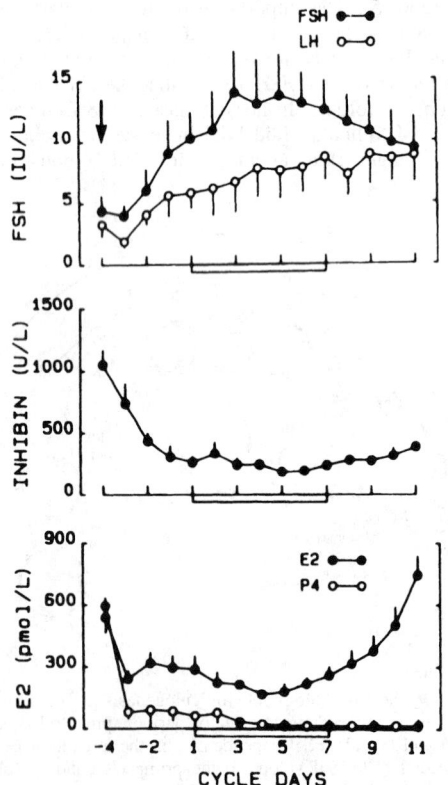

FIGURE 250–5 ■ The endocrinology of the luteal-follicular transition in women. Data are mean ± SE of daily serum concentrations of FSH, LH, estradiol (E$_2$), progesterone (P$_4$), and immunoreactive inhibin in women with normal cycles. Note the secondary rise in plasma FSH in the late luteal phase (−2 days before menses). (From Bangah ML, Kettel LM, Vale W, et al: Dynamic changes in circulating inhibin levels during the luteal follicular transition of the human menstrual cycle. J Clin Encocrinol Metab 69:1033–1039, 1989. © The Endocrine Society.)

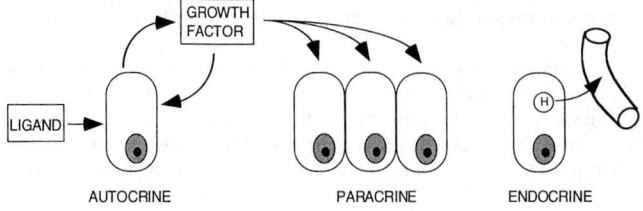

FIGURE 250-6 ■ Comparison of the autocrine-paracrine and endocrine concepts. *H* = hormone. (From Erickson GF, Danforth DR: Ovulation control of follicle development. Am J Obstet Gynecol 172:736–747, 1995.).

associated with the expression of a battery of genes leading to increased androgen synthesis. The role of LH in stimulating androgen production has been intensively studied in women because of its involvement in infertility and hyperandrogenism, such as in polycystic ovary syndrome.

There are four families of interstitial cells in the human ovaries, the theca interstitial cells (TIC), secondary interstitial cells (SIC), theca lutein cells (TLC), and hilus cells (HC). The TIC, SIC, and TLC are related to each other during a developmental sequence occurring during folliculogenesis and luteogenesis, a process called thecogenesis. The formation of the TIC, SIC, and TLC involves a developmental process which encompasses both proliferation and differentiation. Since thecogenesis is accompanied by mitosis, it contributes to total interstitial mass and therefore total androgen potential. HC are found in the hilus and adjacent mesovarium. They appear as nests of differentiated steroidogenic cells juxtaposed to nerves and blood vessels. HC appear to be specialized Leydig cells, that is, they express relatively high levels of P450c17 and 17β-hydroxysteroid dehydrogenase and respond to LH by producing testosterone. The physiologic significance of the HC is totally obscure; however, it is clear that overexpression of HC activity results in hyperandrogenism.

The Endocrine Regulators. Two hormones, LH and insulin, regulate steroidogenesis in the interstitial tissue, and both function as stimulators of androgen production. Each hormone interacts with a transmembrane receptor and the binding event is transduced into an intracellular signal that stimulates transcription and translation of specific steroidal genes.

LH Signal Transduction. LH promotes androgen synthesis through activation of the LH/hCG receptor/cAMP-dependent PKA signal transduction pathway (see Fig. 250–2). The heterotrimeric guanine-nucleotide proteins (G proteins) act as transducers that couple LH/hCG-bound receptors to adenylate cyclase, which forms the second messenger, cAMP. The cAMP activates PKA, which in turn phosphorylates specific serine and threonine residues on substrate proteins. The phosphorylated proteins generate cytoplasmic and nuclear responses that can lead to increased steroidogenesis.

Biological Response. Androstenedione is the principal steroid produced by TIC, and treatment with LH increases its production in a time- and dose-dependent manner. This concept explains in part the regulated production of androstenedione in normal women and its overexpression in women with chronically elevated levels of plasma LH. At the molecular level, activation of the LH signaling cascade leads to the stimulation of gene transcription, most notably P450c22 and P450c17. The fact that the level of transcription and translation of these genes increases during folliculogenesis argues that LH-induced differential gene expression plays a physiologic role in androstenedione production by human TIC over the menstrual cycle.

It has been known for many years that the rate-limiting step in steroidogenesis involves the translocation of cholesterol from the

Table 250–1 ■ THE AUTOCRINE AND PARACRINE CONTROL SYSTEMS IN THE OVARY

GROWTH FACTOR FAMILIES
Insulin-like growth factor (IGF)
Transforming growth factor-α/epidermal growth factor (TGF-αEGF)
Transforming growth factor-β (TGF-β); activin/inhibin
Fibroblast growth factor (FGF)
Cytokine family

outer mitochondrial membrane to the inner mitochondrial membrane, where it is metabolized by pregnenolone by P450c22. Recently this protein, called *s*teroidogenic *a*cute *r*egulatory protein (StAR) has been isolated and cloned. An important concept is that StAR is obligatory for LH-induced steroidogenesis. Further work is necessary to determine the details of StAR expression in human TIC. In this regard it will be interesting to determine whether alterations in StAR activity in any way relate to hyperandrogenism.

Insulin Receptor Signal Transduction. Convincing evidence has been offered that insulin signaling plays a role in regulating interstitial cell function in women. Insulin receptors with protein tyrosine kinase (PTK) activity have been demonstrated in human ovaries. In situ hybridization and immunohistochemical studies have revealed that insulin receptors are expressed in TIC of graafian follicles (both dominant and cohort) and in SIC. Insulin stimulates androgen production by isolated TIC and SIC, and the stimulation is believed to be mediated by the insulin receptor. Activation of the insulin receptor signaling pathway can function alone to increase TIC/SIC androgen production and, importantly, the pathway can synergize with the LH receptor pathway to further enhance the signals evoked by each receptor. The cross-talk between the insulin and LH receptor pathways may be the cause of the development of hyperandrogenism in women with hyperinsulinemia.

INTRAOVARIAN CONTROL OF FOLLICULAR DEVELOPMENT. As discussed, the development of a dominant follicle is under the control of the endocrine hormones FSH and LH. These ligands bind to receptors that are coupled to the cAMP/PKA signal transduction pathways, which in turn are coupled to differential gene activity required for selection and growth of preovulatory follicles. An important concept to emerge in the past decade is that growth factors (GF), which are themselves products of the ovary, modulate (either amplify or attenuate) FSH and LH action. All growth factors are ligands that act in an autocrine/paracrine manner to modify the timing and degree of hormone-dependent folliculogenesis. This is the autocrine/paracrine or growth factor concept (Fig. 250–6). There are five different classes of growth factors, and all five classes have been described within follicles of human ovaries (Table 250–1). The principle that arises from all of the evidence is that growth factors act by autocrine and paracrine mechanisms to cause positive and negative changes that determine whether a follicle lives or dies. The current challenges are to understand how specific GF families exert control of ovary functions and how these modulations are integrated into the overall pattern of physiology and pathophysiology during the life of a woman.

Adashi E, Leung PCK: The Ovary: Comprehensive Endocrinology. New York, Raven Press, 1993.

Erickson GF: The Ovary: Basic Principles and Concepts. *In* Felig P, Baxter JD, Broadus AE, Frohman LA (eds): Endocrinology and Metabolism, 3rd ed. New York, McGraw-Hill, 1995, pp 973–1015.

Erickson GF, Danforth DR: Ovarian control of follicle development. Am J Obstet Gynecol 172:736–747, 1995.

Gougeon A: Regulation of ovarian follicular development in primates: Facts and hypotheses. Endocrinol Rev 17:121–155, 1996.

NEUROENDOCRINE REGULATION OF THE OVARIES. Neurons containing various peptide hormones that can release or inhibit secretion of the gonadotropins are found in the hypothalamus (see Chapter 235). Specifically, cells containing GnRH occur in the area including the arcuate nucleus and median eminence and the preoptic area. Axons from these neurons run in the tuberoinfundibular tract and terminate on capillaries within the median eminence; this allows for delivery of their products through the portal vascular system to the anterior pituitary gland. It appears that classic neurotransmitters, including norepinephrine, dopamine, and serotonin, as well as neuromodulators, such as endogenous opiates and prostaglandins, influence secretion of GnRH by the hypothalamus. In addition, estrogens and androgens bind to cells in the hypothalamus and the anterior pituitary, and progestins bind to cells in the hypothalamus to influence hypothalamic-pituitary regulation of ovarian function.

GnRH is secreted in a pulsatile fashion (perhaps because of an inherent oscillator within the arcuate nucleus) and is responsible for pulsatile release of gonadotropins. Pulsatile gonadotropin release in turn appears to account for the pulsatile secretion of sex steroids from the ovaries. The ovarian sex steroids then feed back on the hypothalamic-pituitary unit to modulate both the frequency and

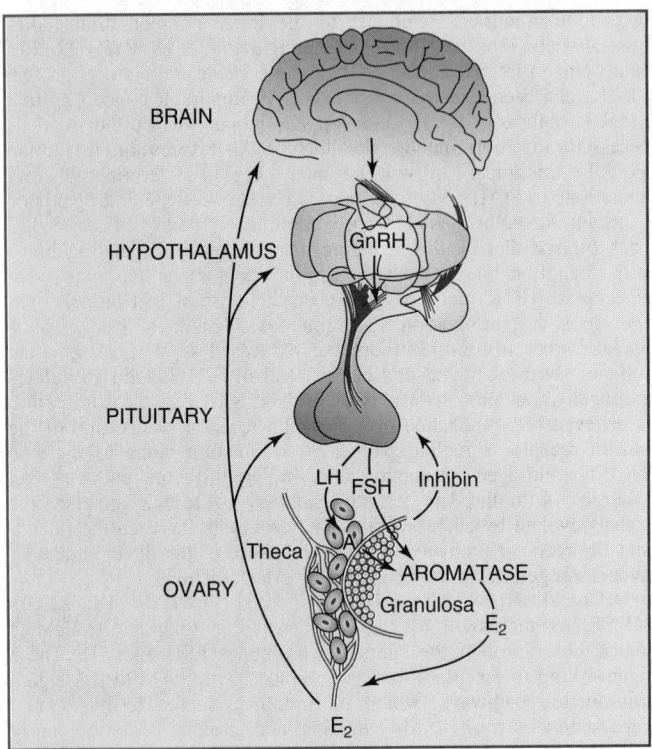

FIGURE 250-7 ■ The hypothalamic-pituitary-ovarian axis in the regulation of follicular maturation and steroidogenesis. A = androgens; E_2 = estradiol. (Modified from Endocrine and Metabolism Continuing Education Quality Control Program, 1982. Copyright American Association for Clinical Chemistry, Inc.)

amplitude of the gonadotropin pulse (Fig. 250–7). Thus, gonadotropin pulses vary throughout the menstrual cycle. Pulses occur at approximately 60- to 90-minute intervals in the follicular phase and at intervals of more than 180 minutes in the luteal phase.

Gonadal steroids can exert both negative and positive feedback effects on gonadotropin secretion. Among ovarian steroids, 17β-estradiol is the most potent inhibitor of gonadotropin secretion, acting on both the hypothalamus and the pituitary. For women to ovulate, E_2 must also elicit a positive feedback effect on gonadotropin release. The feedback effects are both time and dose dependent. In the normal menstrual cycle the positive feedback action of E_2 leading to the LH surge is preceded by a period when lower E_2 levels are present with their negative feedback effects.

It appears that the ovary is the "clock" for the timing of ovulation, with the hypothalamus stimulating pulsatile release of the gonadotropins. The follicle complex and corpus luteum develop in response to gonadotropin stimulation. For appropriate ovarian regulation of reproductive function in women, three biologic characteristics are necessary: (1) an appropriate balance and sequence of negative and positive feedback actions; (2) differential feedback effects on the release of LH and FSH; (3) local intraovarian controls on follicular growth and maturation, separate from but interrelated to the effects of gonadotropins on the ovaries.

ABNORMALITIES OF THE REPRODUCTIVE YEARS

DYSMENORRHEA AND ENDOMETRIOSIS. Dysmenorrhea, perhaps the most common of all gynecologic disorders, affects about 50% of postpubertal women. Dysmenorrhea can be classified as primary or secondary.

Primary dysmenorrhea occurs only in ovulatory cycles. Prostaglandins that are released from the endometrium just prior to and during menstruation cause contraction of uterine smooth muscle and produce dysmenorrhea by initiating painful, exaggerated uterine contractions and myometrial ischemia. Associated systemic symptoms include nausea, diarrhea, headache, and emotional changes.

Primary dysmenorrhea is much more common than is secondary dysmenorrhea.

In *secondary dysmenorrhea* there is a pathologic cause for the dysmenorrhea. Endometriosis, the ectopic occurrence of endometrial tissue generally within the abdominal cavity, is the most common cause in severe cases. Other possible causes include pelvic inflammatory disease, congenital abnormalities such as atresia of a portion of the distal genital tract and cystic duplication of the paramesonephric ducts, and cervical stenosis.

Prostaglandin synthetase inhibitors such as naproxen, ibuprofen, mefenamic acid, and indomethacin are the mainstays of treatment. If the dysmenorrhea is still severe, addition of an oral contraceptive preparation to inhibit ovulation and limit prostaglandin release is generally effective. In cases in which the pelvic pain still remains intractable, additional evaluation is warranted. If thorough evaluation of the gastrointestinal and urinary tracts fails to reveal a definitive cause, examination under anesthesia and diagnostic laparoscopy may be indicated.

If endometriosis is diagnosed at laparoscopy, treatment varies, depending on the severity of the disease and the goals of the patient regarding fertility. It may be possible to fulgurate implants or lyse adhesions through the laparoscope. In general, endometriosis should be treated medically, with additional surgery deferred until infertility (if present) becomes manifest. Medical therapy can consist of continuous suppression with GnRH analogues, progestins, oral contraceptive agents, or danazol for 3 to 6 months. GnRH analogues are rapidly becoming the most frequent form of medical suppressive therapy. After a course of therapy, use of oral contraceptive agents probably should be continued until fertility is desired. Conservative surgical resection of endometriotic tissue should almost always be deferred until it is established as the cause of infertility. Surgery may be required, however, for continuing severe pain, severe endometriosis, or large ovarian cysts containing endometriosis (endometriomas). If symptoms continue despite adequate treatment or if psychological overlay is suspected, psychiatric evaluation may be indicated. Medical causes of dysmenorrhea, however, should be eliminated first.

PREMENSTRUAL SYNDROME. Premenstrual syndrome (PMS), also known as premenstrual tension (PMT), is a complex of physical and/or emotional symptoms that occur repetitively in a cyclic fashion before menstruation and that diminish or disappear with menstruation. Typically these cyclic symptoms are sufficiently severe to interfere with some aspects of life. Women with established psychiatric disturbances probably should not be included among those with PMS. More than 150 different symptoms are now thought to vary with the menstrual cycle (Table 250–2). Estimates of the prevalence of PMS range from 25 to 100%. For most women the syndrome is merely annoying; it is likely that PMS causes serious difficulties for no more than 5 to 10%. The diagnosis is best established by requiring patients to keep prospective daily records of symptoms over a 2- to 3-month period. Fewer than 50% of women complaining of PMS are found to have the syndrome when such records are examined.

Most women seek help for PMS in their 30s after 10 or more

Table 250–2 ■ COMMON SYMPTOMS OF CYCLIC PREMENSTRUAL SYNDROME

Somatic Symptoms	
Abdominal bloating	Constipation or diarrhea
Acne	Headache
Alcohol intolerance	Peripheral edema
Breast engorgement and tenderness	Weight gain
Clumsiness	

Emotional and Mental Symptoms	
Anxiety	Insomnia
Change in libido	Irritability
Depression	Lethargy
Fatigue	Mood swings
Food cravings (especially salt and sugar)	Panic attacks
Hostility	Paranoia
Inability to concentrate	Violence toward self and others
Increased appetitie	Withdrawal from others

years of symptoms. Many report that their symptoms began at menarche; approximately half state that symptoms followed childbirth. Severity and duration of symptoms are often reported to increase following each successive pregnancy, and to become more severe with advancing age. Women with severe longstanding PMS almost always describe associated psychological reactions, including social difficulties, such as marital discord, difficulty relating to their children, difficulty maintaining friendships, and withdrawal from social activities.

The cause of PMS is unknown and patients should be informed that no one therapy has been effective in all women. Women with mild premenstrual symptoms often benefit from simple changes in lifestyle, including addition of mild aerobic exercise each day; reduction in intake of xanthine-containing beverages, salt, and refined sugar in the day, particularly in the luteal phase; stress reduction; and adequate rest. Women with more severe PMS may benefit from treating predominant complaints symptomatically. Thus bromocriptine* (generally 2.5 mg twice a day) or danazol (100 to 400 mg/day in two divided doses) may be given continuously for relief of mastalgia, with the understanding that both may have unpleasant side effects. Prostaglandin synthetase inhibitors may help reduce dysmenorrhea and may benefit headaches. Mild sedatives and tranquilizers may help reduce insomnia and anxiety. Low doses of fluoxetine (20 mg) and other selective serotonin reuptake inhibitors, either administered daily or for the last 2 weeks of each menstrual cycle, have been reported to reduce the emotional symptoms associated with PMS. Mild diuretics (especially spironolactone at doses up to 100 mg each morning) may benefit cyclic edema if such can be confirmed.

Because PMS requires the occurrence of cyclic ovulation, oophorectomy is occasionally considered for patients with particularly intractable symptomatology. However, oophorectomy may create new problems related to estrogen deficiency for women with PMS treated in this permanent fashion. Several recent trials employing a GnRH agonist together with exogenous steroids (so-called add-back therapy) have been described as reducing PMS. Whether such therapy can be utilized long-term remains to be determined.

Natural progesterone, particularly in the form of vaginal suppositories given at doses of up to 800 mg/day, has been used, but results of double-blind placebo-controlled trials have provided no evidence of efficacy. Likewise, the use of large quantities of multiple vitamins or of oil of evening primrose, containing the essential fatty acid γ-linolenic acid, a precursor of prostaglandins, is unsubstantiated.

Keye WR Jr (ed): The Premenstrual Syndrome. Philadelphia, WB Saunders, 1988. *A simple multiauthored text detailing what is known about this disorder.*

Littman BA, Smotrich DB, Stillman RJ: Endometriosis. *In* Becker KL (ed.): Principles and Practice of Endocrinology and Metabolism, 2nd ed. Philadelphia, JB Lippincott, 1995, p 906. *A succinct summary of this enigmatic disorder.*

ABNORMAL UTERINE BLEEDING. DIFFERENTIAL DIAGNOSIS.

The causes of abnormal uterine bleeding in the reproductive years include complications from the use of oral contraceptive preparations; complications of pregnancy (especially threatened, incomplete, or missed abortion and ectopic pregnancy); coagulation disorders (most commonly idiopathic thrombocytopenic purpura and von Willebrand's disease); and pelvic disease such as intrauterine polyps, leiomyomas, and tumors of the vagina and cervix. Clear-cell adenocarcinoma of the vagina or cervix may occur in women exposed to diethylstilbestrol (DES) during fetal life as a result of maternal ingestion. Affected women also may have congenital abnormalities of the upper vagina, cervix, and uterus. Because a history of DES exposure is not always obtained and because this malignant tumor may be fatal, clinical suspicion should remain high. Women with a history of DES exposure should be reassured, however, that the incidence of malignancy is extremely low. Trauma (coital or otherwise), foreign bodies, systemic illnesses including various endocrinopathies (such as diabetes mellitus, hypothyroidism and hyperthyroidism, Cushing's syndrome, and Addison's disease), leukemia, and renal disease may also be associated with abnormal bleeding as the presenting manifestation.

Dysfunctional uterine bleeding (DUB), abnormal uterine bleeding with no demonstrable organic genital or extragenital cause (75% of cases), is most frequently associated with anovulation. Postmenar-

chal bleeding in adolescents secondary to immaturity of the hypothalamic-pituitary-ovarian axis accounts for about 20% of all cases, and premenopausal bleeding consequent to incipient ovarian failure constitutes more than half of the cases. Most anovulatory bleeding is due to either estrogen withdrawal or estrogen breakthrough bleeding. In anovulatory women, estrogen stimulates the endometrium unopposed by progesterone. As a consequence, the endometrium proliferates, becomes thicker, and may shed irregularly, especially if estrogen levels drop. Anovulatory bleeding tends to occur at less frequent intervals, while organic lesions tend to cause bleeding more frequently than cyclic menses.

EVALUATION AND TREATMENT. All cases of abnormal bleeding should be evaluated, including obtaining a thorough history with special emphasis on the amount and duration of blood loss. Prospective charting of the days on which bleeding occurs may be required to evaluate the bleeding pattern. Complications of pregnancy or a bleeding diathesis must always be ruled out.

The physical examination (including the Papanicolaou smear) is normal in dysfunctional bleeding except for signs of anemia in the more severe cases. Laboratory tests should include a complete blood count, platelet count, coagulation studies, thyroid function tests, and fasting blood glucose. DUB must be a diagnosis of exclusion. Management of DUB depends on the age of the patient and the extent of the bleeding. A sample of the endometrium should be obtained by biopsy or by dilatation and curettage from all women over age 35 years and from those at increased risk of developing endometrial carcinoma because of prolonged anovulatory bleeding.

Even profuse bleeding in anovulatory women can almost always be successfully treated by administering one combination oral contraceptive pill every 6 hours for 5 to 7 days. Bleeding should cease within 24 hours, but patients should be warned to expect heavy bleeding 2 to 4 days after stopping therapy. If anemia and signs of acute blood loss are profound, blood transfusion may be necessary. If the bleeding continues despite therapy, curettage can be carried out. Recurrence can be prevented by giving the patient combination oral contraceptive agents cyclically for 3 or more months. If spontaneous cyclic menses do not resume and pregnancy is not desired, the patient can be treated with cyclic progestin (medroxyprogesterone acetate, 5 to 10 mg for 10 to 14 days each month) or oral contraceptive agents. If pregnancy is desired, ovulation can be induced, as discussed subsequently.

Acute episodes of anovulatory bleeding also can be treated with conjugated estrogens administered intravenously (25 mg every 4 hours for up to three doses) until bleeding ceases. Progestin therapy (medroxyprogesterone acetate, 5 to 10 mg orally for 10 days) should be started simultaneously. Withdrawal bleeding will occur after cessation of therapy, and the patient can then be treated with oral contraceptive agents for at least three cycles.

For individuals with anovulatory bleeding without an episode of profuse bleeding, treatment with cyclic oral contraceptive agents or progestin can be provided unless pregnancy is desired, in which case ovulation must be induced.

Speroff L, Glass RH, Kase NG: Dysfunctional uterine bleeding. *In* Clinical Gynecologic Endocrinology and Infertility, 5th ed. Baltimore, Williams & Wilkins, 1994, p 531. *A detailed and logical approach to the treatment of abnormal uterine bleeding.*

AMENORRHEA. DEFINITION AND ETIOLOGY.

Amenorrhea is the absence of menstruation for 3 or more months in women with past menses (*secondary amenorrhea*) or the absence of menarche by the age of 16 years regardless of the absence or presence of secondary sex characteristics (*primary amenorrhea*). If an intact genital outflow tract exists and there is no primary disease of the uterus, amenorrhea is a sign of failure of the hypothalamic-pituitary-ovarian axis to produce cyclically the hormones necessary for menses. Amenorrhea is a sign of any of several disorders involving different organ systems. Amenorrhea is physiologic in the prepubertal girl, during pregnancy and early in lactation, and after the menopause. At any other time it is pathologic and demands evaluation. Use of the term *post-pill amenorrhea* to refer to failure to resume menses within 3 months of discontinuing oral contraceptives is inappropriate. Women so affected should be evaluated in the same manner as for any woman with amenorrhea. Similarly, individuals

---

*This use is not listed in the manufacturer's directive.

Table 250-3 ■ CRITERIA FOR DISTINGUISHING TANNER STAGES 1 TO 5 DURING PUBERTAL MATURATION

TANNER STAGE	BREAST	PUBIC HAIR
1 (Prepubertal)	No palpable glandular tissue or pigmentation of areola; elevation of areola only	No pubic hair; short, fine vellous hair only
2	Glandular tissue palpable with elevation of breast and areola together as a small mound; areolar diameter increased	Sparse, long, pigmented terminal hair chiefly along the labia majora
3	Further enlargement without separation of breast and areola; although more darkly pigmented, areola still pale and immature; nipple generally at or above midplane of breast tissue when individual is seated upright	Dark, coarse, curly hair, extending sparsely over mons
4	Secondary mound of areola and papilla above breast	Adult-type hair, abundant but limited to mons and labia
5 (Adult)	Recession of areola to contour of breast; development of Montgomery's glands and ducts on areola; further pigmentation of areola; nipple generally below midplane of breast tissue when individual is seated upright; maturation independent of breast size	Adult-type hair in quantity and distribution; spread to inner aspects of the thighs in most racial groups

Data from Ross GT: Disorders of the ovary and female reproductive tract. *In* Wilson JD, Foster DW (eds): Textbook of Endocrinology, 7th ed. Philadelphia, WB Saunders, 1985, p 206; Speroff L, Glass RH, Kase N: Clinical Gynecologic Endocrinology and Infertility, 3rd ed. Baltimore, Williams & Wilkins, 1983, p 377; and Kustin J, Rebar RW: Menstrual disorders in the adolescent age group. Primary Care 14:139, 1987.

with menses occurring at infrequent intervals of greater than 40 days or having fewer than nine menses per year, termed *oligomenorrhea*, should be evaluated identically to women with amenorrhea.

CLINICAL EVALUATION. In patients with amenorrhea, even subtle hormonal abnormalities may be manifested by obvious signs and symptoms. Breast development indicates exposure to estrogens, and the presence of pubic and axillary hair indicates androgenic stimulation.

Patients should be questioned especially closely for evidence of psychological disturbances, dietary and exercise habits, lifestyle, environmental stresses, a family history of genetic anomalies, and abnormal growth and development. Patients should also be asked about and examined for the presence of any signs of hyperandrogenism, including hirsutism, temporal balding, deepening of the voice, increased muscle mass, clitoromegaly, and increased libido, as well as for any signs of defeminization, including decreasing breast size and vaginal atrophy. Any history of galactorrhea, the nonpuerperal secretion of milk from the breasts, should be determined (see Chapter 237). A history of symptoms related to thyroid and adrenal dysfunction should also be sought.

The physical examination should focus on evaluating (1) body dimensions and habitus, (2) the extent and distribution of body hair, (3) breast development and secretions, and (4) the genitalia.

In normal adult women the arm span is similar to the height, whereas in hypogonadal women the span is generally more than 5 cm greater than the height. The general appearance of the patient should be evaluated to determine if the habitus is that of an adult female. The distribution and quantity of body hair should be considered in view of the family history. The extent of any hirsutism should be recorded, preferably by photographs. Other signs of virilization should be sought carefully. Breast development should be graded according to the method of Tanner (Table 250–3). Breast secretion should be sought by applying pressure to the breasts while the patient is seated. Any secretion should be examined microscopically for the presence of perfectly round fat globules of varying size, which are always present in milk and indicate galactorrhea. Finally, the female genitalia should be examined carefully because they are such sensitive indicators of hormonal milieu. The Tanner stage of pubic hair development should be noted (see Table 250–3). Because the sensitivity of the genitalia to androgens decreases onward from early in fetal development, the extent of any virilization is important. Fusion of the labia and enlargement of the clitoris with or without formation of a penile urethra are observed in women exposed to androgens during the first 3 months of fetal development (see Chapter 246). Significant clitoromegaly in the absence of other signs of sexual ambiguity and in the presence of other signs of virilization requires marked androgenic stimulation and strongly implicates an androgen-secreting neoplasm in the absence of a history of ingestion of exogenous steroids. The development of the labia minora in postpubertal women indicates the influence of estrogens. Overt anomalies of the distal genital tract and especially any evidence of obstruction to the escape of menstrual blood should be sought in the remainder of the pelvic examination. The vaginal mucosa and the cervical mucus are exquisitely sensitive to estrogen. Under the influence of estrogen the vaginal mucosa changes during sexual maturation from a tissue with a shiny, bright red appearance with sparse, thin secretions to a dull, gray-pink rugated surface with copious, thick secretions.

The history and physical examination quickly differentiate among several causes of amenorrhea, regardless of the age of the patient (Table 250–4). The various disorders of sexual differentiation and the other peripheral causes are often apparent on inspection. Distal genital tract obstruction should be identified at the time of pelvic examination even if the specific abnormality is not obvious. The physical stigmata of Turner's syndrome, discussed subsequently, generally make the diagnosis simple. Any sexual ambiguity indicates the need for chromosomal analysis and the measurement of 17α-hydroxyprogesterone to rule out congenital adrenal hyperplasia. Pregnancy and gestational trophoblastic disease may be suspected and confirmed by measuring circulating concentrations of hCG. The possibility of intrauterine synechiae or adhesions (Asherman's syndrome) must be considered in individuals developing amenorrhea following curettage or endometritis. Tuberculous endometritis, especially in younger women, may also lead to this disorder. Without hormonal measurements it may be impossible to distinguish among individuals with chronic anovulation, in whom hypothalamic-pituitary-ovarian function is insufficiently coordinated to produce cyclic ovulation, and those with ovarian failure, in whom in most cases the ovaries are devoid of oocytes. Still, it is generally possible to form some strong clinical impressions about the cause of the amenorrhea. It can be noted if the patient has absence of, incomplete, or complete development of secondary sex characteristics. The presence of excess body hair or galactorrhea may provide clinical evidence of the pathogenesis of the amenorrhea. Signs and symptoms of adrenal or thyroid dysfunction may be important as well.

The administration of a progestin (typically medroxyprogesterone acetate, 5 to 10 mg given orally for 5 to 10 days, or progesterone

Table 250-4 ■ CAUSES OF AMENORRHEA

Disorders of sexual differentiation
    Distal genital tract obstruction (müllerian agenesis and dysgenesis)
    Gonadal dysgenesis
    Ambiguity of external genitalia (male and female pseudohermaphroditism)
Other peripheral causes
    Pregnancy
    Gestational trophoblastic disease
    Amenorrhea traumatica (Asherman's syndrome)
Chronic anovulation or ovarian failure
    Due to CNS-hypothalamic-pituitary dysfunction
    Due to inappropriate feedback (e.g., polycystic ovary syndrome)
    Due to thyroid and adrenal disorders
    Presumptive ovarian failure (i.e., primary hypogonadism)

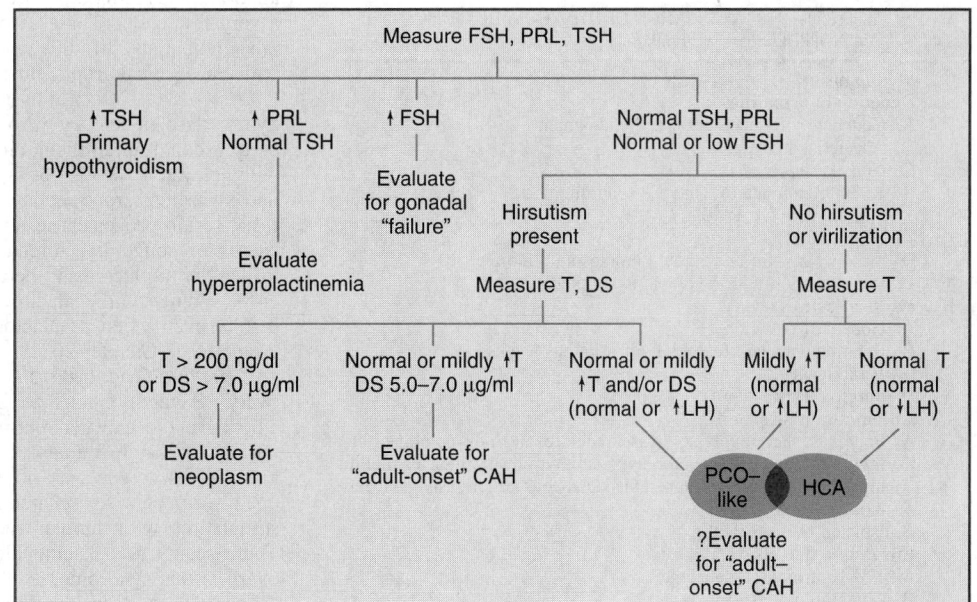

FIGURE 250–8 ■ Biochemical evaluation of amenorrhea. This schema must be considered as an adjunct to the clinical evaluation of the patient. See text for details. Abbreviations: FSH = follicle-stimulating hormone; PRL = prolactin; TSH = thyroid-stimulating hormone; T = testosterone; DS = dehydroepiandrosterone sulfate; LH = luteinizing hormone; PCO-like = polycystic ovarian-like; HCA = hypothalamic chronic anovulation; CAH = congenital adrenal hyperplasia.

in oil, 100 mg given intramuscularly) has been advocated to assess the level of endogenous estrogen. This test is of limited value, however, because almost half the young women with premature ovarian failure experience withdrawal bleeding in response to progestin.

To ascertain if the outflow tract is intact, an orally active estrogen, such as 2.5 mg of conjugated estrogen daily for 21 days, with 5 to 10 mg of oral medroxyprogesterone acetate for the last 5 to 10 days, may be administered. Withdrawal bleeding should occur if the endometrium is normal. Still, hysterosalpingography and hysteroscopy may be required to diagnose Asherman's syndrome because some patients do continue to have some withdrawal bleeding.

LABORATORY EVALUATION. Basal levels of FSH, prolactin, and TSH should be measured in all amenorrheic and oligomenorrheic women to confirm the clinical impression (Fig. 250–8).

Increased TSH levels with or without increased levels of prolactin imply primary hypothyroidism, and further evaluation for this disorder is indicated (see Chapter 237). Although hypothyroidism commonly results in anovulation, amenorrhea occurs in only some hypothyroid women. Menorrhagia and oligomenorrhea may occur as well. The very sensitive immunoassays for TSH permit identification of women with hyperthyroidism as well because TSH levels are suppressed in those individuals.

If the prolactin concentration is increased (typically >20 to 30 ng/mL) and the TSH level is normal (generally <5 μU/mL), measurement of the prolactin concentration in the basal state should be repeated before more extensive evaluation is undertaken. This is the case because prolactin levels are increased by nonspecific stressful stimuli, sleep, and food ingestion. Prolactin levels may be elevated in as many as one third of women with amenorrhea.

Increased FSH levels (generally >30 to 40 mIU/mL) imply ovarian failure and require further evaluation. Chromosomal evaluation is indicated in all individuals with elevated FSH levels who are under the age of 30 years at the time the amenorrhea begins.

If prolactin and TSH concentrations are within normal ranges and FSH levels are low or normal, the measurement of total testosterone levels may be helpful whether or not there is any evidence of hirsutism or virilization. Hyperandrogenic women need not be hirsute because some have relative insensitivity of the hair follicles to androgens. Mildly increased levels of testosterone (and perhaps DHEA-S as well) suggest PCO syndrome. However, total circulating androgen levels are rarely not elevated because of the alterations in metabolic clearance rate and SHBG that are present in PCO syndrome. Consequently, some clinicians prefer to measure circulating free testosterone levels. Circulating levels of LH and FSH may aid in differentiating PCO syndrome from hypothalamic-pituitary dysfunction. LH levels are frequently elevated in PCO

syndrome such that the ratio of LH to FSH is increased; however, LH levels may be identical to those observed in normal women in the follicular phase. In contrast, levels of LH and FSH are normal or slightly reduced in hypothalamic-pituitary dysfunction. There is some overlap between women with "PCO-like" disorders and those with hypothalamic-pituitary dysfunction. Radiographic assessment of the sella turcica is indicated in all amenorrheic women in whom both LH and FSH levels are very low (both <10 mIU/mL) to exclude a pituitary or parapituitary neoplasm. Other pituitary functions should be evaluated in any individual with significantly impaired LH and FSH secretion, as detailed subsequently. Both total testosterone and DHEA-S levels should be measured in hirsute or virilized women. Testosterone levels of >200 ng/dL should lead to investigation for an androgen-producing neoplasm, most likely of ovarian origin. DHEA-S levels >7.0 μg/mL should lead to evaluation for an adrenal neoplasm, and DHEA-S levels between 5.0 and 7.0 μg/mL should lead to evaluation for "adult-onset" congenital adrenal hyperplasia (see Chapter 246).

HYPERGONADOTROPIC AMENORRHEA (PRESUMPTIVE OVARIAN FAILURE, PRIMARY HYPOGONADISM). Differential Diagnosis. Gonadal failure may begin at any time during embryonic or postnatal development and may result from many causes (Table 250–5). Normally the ovaries fail at menopause when virtually no functioning follicles remain. However premature loss of oocytes prior to age 40 years may occur and lead to premature ovarian failure, possibly from abnormalities in the recruitment and selection of oocytes. Because FSH is the principal regulator of folliculogenesis, most causes of premature ovarian failure may somehow involve FSH secretion or action. Circulating gonadotropin levels increase whenever ovarian failure occurs because of decreased negative estrogen feedback to the hypothalamic-pituitary unit.

Genetic Abnormalities. Several pathologic conditions with dysgenetic gonads have elevated gonadotropin levels and amenorrhea. The term *gonadal dysgenesis* refers to individuals with undifferentiated streak gonads without any association with either extragonadal stigmata or sex chromosomal aberrations. Because individuals with gonadal dysgenesis have the normal complement of oocytes at 20 weeks of fetal age but virtually none by birth, this disorder is a form of premature ovarian failure.

Turner's syndrome describes patients with streak gonads composed of fibrous stroma and four cardinal features: (1) a female phenotype, (2) sexual infantilism, (3) short stature, and (4) several physical abnormalities, sometimes including a webbed neck, low-set ears, multiple pigmented nevi, double eyelashes, micrognathia, epicanthal folds, shieldlike chest with microthelia, short fourth metacarpals, an increased carrying angle of the arms, and certain renal and cardiovascular defects (most commonly coarctation of the

Table 250–5 ■ CLASSIFICATION OF HYPERGONADOTROPIC AMENORRHEA (FSH > 30 mIU/mL)

I. Menopause
II. Genetic abnormalities
   A. Genetically reduced germ cell endowment
   B. Accelerated atresia
   C. Gonadal dysgenesis
      1. With stigmata of Turner's syndrome (45,X)
      2. Pure (46,XX or 46,XY)
      3. Mixed
   D. Trisomy X with or without chromosomal mosaicism
   E. In association with myotonia dystrophica
III. Physical causes
   A. Gonadal irradiation
   B. Chemotherapeutic (especially alkylating) agents
   C. Viral agents
   D. Surgical extirpation
IV. Autoimmune disorders
   A. Polyglandular, involving ovarian failure and any combination of thyroiditis, hypoadrenalism, hypoparathyroidism, diabetes mellitus, myasthenia gravis, vitiligo, mucocutaneous candidiasis, and pernicious anemia
   B. Isolated ovarian failure
V. Enzymatic defects
   A. 17α-Hydroxylase deficiency
   B. Galactosemia
VI. Defective gonadotropin secretion and/or action
   A. Resistant ovary or Savage syndrome
   B. Secretion of biologically inactive forms
   C. α or β subunit defects
VII. Congenital thymic aplasia
VIII. Circulating gonadotropin antibodies
IX. Idiopathic premature ovarian failure

aorta and aortic stenosis). The diagnosis can sometimes be made at birth because of unexplained lymphedema of the hands and feet. The syndrome is associated with an abnormality of sex chromosome number, morphology, or both. Most commonly the second sex chromosome is absent (45,X). This is the single most common chromosomal disorder in humans, but more than 95% of such fetuses are aborted, so that the incidence in newborns is approximately 1 in 3000 to 5000. Chromosomal breakage and mosaicism occur frequently as well. In mosaic individuals with a normal 46,XX cell line, sufficient follicles may persist postnatally to initiate pubertal changes and to cause ovulation so that pregnancy is possible.

Pure gonadal dysgenesis is the term given to phenotypically female individuals with streak gonads who are of normal stature and have none of the physical stigmata associated with Turner's syndrome. Such individuals have either a 46,XX or 46,XY karyotype. The 46,XX defect may be inherited as an autosomal recessive, with 10% having associated nerve deafness. The 46,XY defect may be inherited as an X-linked recessive, with clitoromegaly occurring in 10 to 15% and gonadal tumors developing in 25% if the gonads are not removed.

Trisomy X (46,XXX karyotype) is also associated with premature menopause, while many such individuals actually have normal reproductive lives. Premature menopause can also occur in mosaic individuals with cell lines with excess X chromosomes. When gonadal abnormalities occur in women with excess X chromosomes, they seem to occur after ovarian differentiation so that some ovarian function is possible. Only later in life do such women develop secondary amenorrhea and premature ovarian failure.

Other Causes. *Physical, Chemical, and Infectious Causes.* Irradiation and chemotherapeutic agents, especially alkylating agents, utilized to treat various malignant diseases also may cause premature ovarian failure. Ovulation and cyclic menses return in some of these patients even after prolonged intervals of hypergonadotropic amenorrhea associated with signs and symptoms of profound hypoestrogenism. Rarely, mumps affects the ovaries and causes ovarian failure.

Autoimmune Disorders. Premature ovarian failure may occur in conjunction with a variety of autoimmune disorders. The most well-known syndrome involves hypoadrenalism, hypoparathyroidism, and mucocutaneous candidiasis together with ovarian failure

(see Chapter 244). Thyroiditis is the most commonly associated abnormality. Antibodies to the FSH receptor have been identified in a very few cases. These associations make it mandatory to rule out other potentially life-threatening endocrinopathies in young women with hypergonadotropic amenorrhea.

Enzymatic Defects. In girls with the rare syndrome of 17α-hydroxylase deficiency who survive until the expected age of puberty, sexual infantilism and primary amenorrhea occur together with elevated levels of gonadotropins. Increased synthesis of desoxycorticosterone leads to hypertension with hypokalemic alkalosis; serum progesterone levels are elevated as well. As with other causes of congenital adrenal hyperplasia, the hypertension is controlled by replacement therapy with glucocorticoids (see Chapter 246). Women with galactosemia also develop ovarian failure early in life, even when a galactose-restricted diet is introduced early in infancy (see Chapter 202).

Defective Gonadotropin Secretion and/or Action. The resistant ovary (Savage) syndrome occurs in young amenorrheic women who have (1) elevated peripheral gonadotropin concentrations, (2) normal (although immature) follicles present on ovarian biopsy, (3) a 46,XX karyotype with no evidence of mosaicism, (4) fully developed secondary sex characteristics, and (5) ovarian resistance to stimulation with human menopausal or pituitary gonadotropins. There seems to be some block to gonadotropin action within the ovary in this syndrome.

Therapeutic Considerations. Women with hypergonadotropic amenorrhea and ovarian failure should be treated identically whether or not they have signs of hypoestrogenism or desire pregnancy. Ovarian biopsy is not indicated to document the existence of follicles because only a small portion of each ovary can be sampled and because pregnancies have resulted in patients who had biopsies devoid of follicles. Estrogen replacement is warranted to prevent the accelerated bone loss known to occur in affected women (see Chapter 257). The estrogen should be given sequentially with a progestin to prevent endometrial hyperplasia. Young women with ovarian failure may require twice as much estrogen as postmenopausal women for relief of signs and symptoms of hypoestrogenism.

Women with hypergonadotropic amenorrhea are rarely able to become pregnant. It is not clear why pregnancy may rarely occur in such women, but the pregnancy rate is less than 10%. The most successful treatment of young women with hypergonadotropic amenorrhea involves hormone replacement to mimic the normal menstrual cycle and embryo transfer utilizing donor oocytes. Pregnancy rates are higher than in other women undergoing in vitro fertilization and typically exceed 30% per cycle.

DIFFERENTIAL DIAGNOSIS AND TREATMENT OF CHRONIC ANOVULATION. Chronic anovulation, the most frequent form of amenorrhea encountered in women of reproductive age, implies that functional ovarian follicles remain and that cyclic ovulation can be induced or reinitiated with appropriate therapy (Table 250–6). Appropriate management requires that the cause of the anovulation be determined. The pathophysiologic bases for several forms of anovulation are unknown, but the anovulation can be interrupted transiently by nonspecific induction of ovulation in the majority of affected women. It is important to recognize that anovulation can result in either amenorrhea or irregular (generally less frequent) menses.

Hypothalamic Chronic Anovulation (HCA). HCA represents a heterogeneous group of disorders with similar manifestations. Emotional and physical stress, exercise, diet, weight loss, body composition, malnutrition, environment, and other unrecognized factors may contribute in varying proportions to the anovulation. Abrupt cessation of menses in women under 30 years of age who have no anatomic abnormalities of the hypothalamic-pituitary-ovarian axis and no other endocrine disturbances suggests a diagnosis of HCA. Affected individuals tend to be bright, educated, and engaged in intellectual occupations and may well give a history of psychosexual problems and socioenvironmental trauma. HCA is characterized by low to normal levels of gonadotropins and relative hypoestrogenism. Rarely, however, do affected women present with signs and symptoms of estrogen deficiency. Psychological counseling and/or a change in lifestyle, especially for those women engaged in strenuous exercise programs, may be effective in inducing cyclic ovulation and menses. For women desiring pregnancy, ovulation can also be induced with clomiphene citrate (50 to 100 mg/day for

I. Chronic anovulation of hypothalamic-pituitary origin
  A. Hypothalamic chronic anovulation
    1. Psychogenic
    2. Exercise associated
    3. Associated with diet, weight loss, and/or malnutrition
    4. Anorexia nervosa and bulimia
    5. Pseudocyesis
  B. Forms of isolated gonadotropin deficiency (including Kallmann's syndrome)
  C. Due to hypothalamic-pituitary damage
    1. Pituitary and parapituitary tumors
    2. Empty-sella syndrome
    3. Following surgery
    4. Following irradiation
    5. Following trauma
    6. Following infection
    7. Following infarction
  D. Idiopathic hypopituitarism
  E. Hypothalamic-pituitary dysfunction or failure with hyperprolactinemia (multiple causes)
  F. Due to systemic diseases
II. Chronic anovulation due to inappropriate feedback (i.e., polycystic ovary syndrome)
  A. Excessive extraglandular estrogen production (i.e., obesity)
  B. Abnormal buffering involving sex hormone–binding globulin (including liver disease)
  C. Functional androgen excess (adrenal or ovarian)
  D. Neoplasms producing androgens or estrogens
  E. Neoplasms producing chorionic gonadotropin
III. Chronic anovulation due to other endocrine and metabolic disorders
  A. Adrenal hyperfunction
    1. Cushing's syndrome
    2. Congenital adrenal hyperplasia (female pseudohermaphroditism)
  B. Thyroid dysfunction
    1. Hyperthyroidism
    2. Hypothyroidism
  C. Prolactin and/or growth hormone excess
    1. Hypothalamic dysfunction
    2. Pituitary dysfunction (microadenomas and macroadenomas)
    3. Drug induced
  D. Malnutrition

Modified from Rebar RW: Chronic anovulation. *In* Serra GB (ed.): The Ovary. New York, Raven Press, 1983, p 217.

5 days beginning on the fifth day of withdrawal bleeding). Treatment with exogenous purified or synthetic gonadotropins to induce follicular maturation followed by human chorionic gonadotropin (hCG) to induce follicular rupture or GnRH administered in a pulsatile fashion may be effective in women who do not ovulate in response to clomiphene. Most physicians advocate the use of exogenous steroids to prevent osteoporosis. A regimen can be used consisting of oral conjugated or esterified estrogens (0.625 to 1.25 mg), ethinyl estradiol (20 μg), or micronized estradiol-17β (1 to 2 mg) or transdermal estradiol-17β (0.05 to 0.10 mg) daily, with oral medroxyprogesterone acetate (5 to 10 mg) added for the first 12 to 14 days of each month. Sexually active women can be given oral contraceptive agents as an alternative. If steroid therapy is administered, patients must be informed that the amenorrhea probably will be present when therapy is discontinued. Other physicians believe only periodic observation is indicated, with barrier methods of contraception recommended for fertility control. Adequate ingestion of calcium should be ensured regardless of therapy. Contraception is needed for sexually active women with HCA, because the functional defect is mild in these disorders and may resolve spontaneously at any time, with ovulation occurring prior to any episode of menstruation.

Individuals with amenorrhea and significant weight loss should be examined for the possibility of *anorexia nervosa* (see Chapter 227). This disorder may be the most severe form of functional HCA, or it may be a distinct entity.

Kallmann's syndrome (isolated gonadotropin deficiency or familial hypogonadotropic hypogonadism) is a familial disorder consisting of gonadotropin deficiency, anosmia or hyposmia, and color blindness in men or, more rarely, in women. Other midline defects such as cleft lip and palate can occur in the affected individual or in family members. The trait is transmitted as an X-linked reces-

sive or a male-limited autosomal dominant trait, but genetic heterogeneity may occur. Partial or complete agenesis of the olfactory bulb is present on autopsy, accounting for use of the term *olfactogenital dysplasia*. The disorder affects only gonadotropin secretion, and all other pituitary hormones are secreted normally. Isolated gonadotropin deficiency in the absence of anosmia occurs as well. Sexual infantilism with a eunuchoid habitus is the clinical hallmark of this disorder, but moderate breast development may occur. Circulating LH and FSH levels are quite low, but almost always detectable. Ovulation induction requires use of exogenous gonadotropins and hCG or pulsatile GnRH. Estrogen replacement therapy is indicated in these women until such time as pregnancy is desired. It may not be possible to distinguish between partial isolated gonadotropin deficiency and functional HCA in all cases.

Hypopituitarism may be obvious on cursory inspection or sufficiently subtle to require endocrine testing (see Chapter 237). The clinical presentation depends on the age of onset, the cause, and the nutritional status of the individual. Failure of development of secondary sex characteristics or for development to progress once puberty is initiated must always raise the question of hypopituitarism. Ovulation can be induced successfully with exogenous gonadotropins when pregnancy is desired and after the hypopituitarism is treated appropriately. Replacement therapy with estrogen is indicated to prevent signs and symptoms of estrogen deficiency.

Galactorrhea associated with hyperprolactinemia, whatever the cause, almost always occurs together with amenorrhea caused by hypothalamic-pituitary dysfunction or failure. Many conditions can cause excess prolactin secretion (see Chapter 237). Hirsutism may be observed occasionally in association with amenorrhea-galactorrhea and hyperprolactinemia. Elevated levels of the adrenal androgens DHEA and DHEA-S may be observed and may account for the PCO-type ovaries present in some hyperprolactinemic women.

The hypothalamic-pituitary unit also may fail to function normally in a number of stressful, debilitating, systemic illnesses that interfere with somatic growth and development. Chronic renal failure, liver disease, and diabetes mellitus are the most prominent examples.

Chronic Anovulation Due to Inappropriate Feedback. PCO syndrome, which causes anovulation because of inappropriate feedback signals to the hypothalamic-pituitary unit, is a heterogeneous disorder in which there is considerable clinical and biochemical variability among affected individuals. Although patients usually present with amenorrhea, hirsutism, and obesity, affected women may instead complain of irregular and profuse uterine bleeding, may not have hirsutism, and may be of normal weight. Excess androgen from any source or increased extraglandular conversion of androgens to estrogens can lead to the typical findings of PCO syndrome. Included are such diverse disorders as Cushing's syndrome, mild congenital adrenal hyperplasia, virilizing tumors of adrenal or ovarian origin, hyperthyroidism and hypothyroidism, obesity, and primary PCO syndrome with no other recognizable cause. In the primary syndrome the irregular menses, mild obesity, and hirsutism begin during puberty and typically become more severe with time. Obesity alone can lead to a PCO-like syndrome, with the degree of obesity required to cause anovulation varying widely from individual to individual. All such patients are well estrogenized regardless of whether they present with primary or secondary amenorrhea or dysfunctional bleeding. As noted, LH concentrations tend to be elevated, with relatively low and constant FSH levels, but both may be in the normal range compared with levels in women in the follicular phase of the menstrual cycle. Levels of most circulating androgens, especially testosterone, tend to be mildly elevated. The cause of PCO syndrome is unknown, but current evidence suggests that the hypothalamic-pituitary unit is intact and that a functional derangement, perhaps involving insulin-like growth factors such as insulin-like (IGF-I) within the ovary, results in abnormal gonadotropin secretion. There is increasing evidence of specific genetic abnormalities in some women with PCO.

The aim of the diagnostic evaluation is to rule out any causes (such as neoplasms) that require definitive therapy. Hirsutism should be evaluated as detailed in Chapter 255. PCO syndrome itself is a benign disorder. Patients generally require therapy for hirsutism, for induction of ovulation if pregnancy is desired, and for prevention of estrogen-induced endometrial hyperplasia and cancer. No ideal therapy exists, but rather the therapeutic approach must be individualized to the needs of each patient. In addition, the risks of cardiovascular disease and of diabetes mellitus are increased in women with PCO, presumably at least in part because of the increased androgens invariably present.

In the anovulatory woman not desiring pregnancy who is not hirsute, therapy with intermittent progestin administration (such as medroxyprogesterone acetate, 5 to 10 mg orally for 10 to 14 days each month) or oral contraceptives can be provided to reduce the increased risk of endometrial carcinoma that is present in such a woman with unopposed estrogen. All women utilizing intermittent progestin administration should be cautioned about the need for effective contraception if they are sexually active, because these agents do not inhibit ovulation when administered intermittently.

The approach to the hirsute anovulatory woman not desiring pregnancy is detailed in Chapter 255. Oral contraceptive agents are the first line of therapy for such women with mild hirsutism and offer protection from endometrial hyperplasia.

In women with PCO syndrome desiring pregnancy, clomiphene citrate is the first approach to inducing ovulation because of its simplicity and high success rate. Approximately 75 to 80% conceive with such therapy. Other possible methods of inducing ovulation include use of exogenous gonadotropins and hCG, pulsatile GnRH, wedge resection of the ovaries at laparotomy, and laser or cautery destruction of follicles at laparoscopy. Surgical treatment is warranted only rarely and only in women in whom all other methods fail, in whom there is a question of an ovarian tumor because of ovarian size or circulating androgen levels, and in whom fertility is not an issue (because of the risk of pelvic adhesions from the surgery leading to infertility).

A particularly severely affected subset of women present with marked obesity, anovulation, mild glucose intolerance and high levels of circulating insulin with insulin resistance, acanthosis nigricans, hyperuricemia, and severe hirsutism with markedly elevated circulating androgen levels. These women have *hyperthecosis of the ovaries* in which the androgen-producing cells in the stromal, hilar, and thecal components of the ovaries are increased greatly in number. Although considered a separate entity by some clinicians, hyperthecosis probably should be viewed as a part of the spectrum of disorders constituting PCO syndrome.

CHRONIC ANOVULATION DUE TO OTHER ENDOCRINE AND METABOLIC DISORDERS. Adrenal hyperfunction appears to cause chronic anovulation by inducing a PCO-like syndrome secondary to increased adrenal androgen secretion, but other possible mechanisms also exist.

Both hyperthyroidism and hypothyroidism are associated with a variety of menstrual disturbances, including dysfunctional uterine bleeding and amenorrhea as a result of alterations in the metabolism of androgens and estrogens. These metabolic changes in turn result in inappropriate steroid feedback and chronic anovulation.

Rebar RW: Premature ovarian failure. *In* Lobo RA (ed): Treatment of the Postmenopausal Woman: Basic and Clinical Aspects. New York, Raven Press, 1994, p 25. *A detailed discussion of the diagnosis and treatment of premature ovarian failure.*

Yen SSC, Jaffe RB, Barbieri RL (eds): Reproductive Endocrinology, 4th ed. Philadelphia, WB Saunders, 1999. *Detailed chapters describe practical evaluation of hormonal status and chronic anovulation caused by peripheral endocrine disorders as well as by CNS-hypothalamic-pituitary dysfunction.*

DISORDERS OF FOLLICULOGENESIS. Recognized disorders of folliculogenesis cannot be identified before ovulation begins. They are believed to reflect abnormalities in follicular development.

LUTEINIZED UNRUPTURED FOLLICLE (LUF) SYNDROME. The LUF syndrome describes development of a dominant follicle without its subsequent disruption and release of the ovum. The abnormality can be diagnosed by ultrasonography or by the absence of evidence of ovulation when the ovary is viewed at laparoscopy. The disorder is believed to occur infrequently and sporadically and is probably not a significant cause of infertility. Menstrual cycles in which no ovum is released are characterized by presumptive evidence of ovulation, including biphasic basal body temperatures, secretory endometrium, a normal LH surge, and normal progesterone production in the luteal phase. In fact, although the syndrome is believed to occur, data to substantiate its existence are only circumstantial (although strongly suggestive) at present.

LUTEAL PHASE DYSFUNCTION. Progesterone secretion in the lu-

teal phase may be reduced in duration (termed luteal phase insufficiency) or in amount (termed luteal phase inadequacy). More rarely the endometrium may be unable to respond to secreted progesterone because of the absence of progesterone receptors. These disorders are believed to represent causes for infertility (because of inability of fertilized ova to implant) in approximately 5% of infertile couples. Abnormalities of the follicular phase, especially in the frequency of gonadotropin pulses, may account for most luteal phase defects. Luteal phase defects also may occur sporadically in normally ovulating women approximately once each year.

Luteal phase dysfunction may be associated with several clinical entities, including mild or intermittent hyperprolactinemia (of any cause), strenuous physical exercise, inadequately treated 21-hydroxylase deficiency, and habitual abortion. Luteal dysfunction occurs more commonly at the extremes of reproductive life and in the first menstrual cycles following full-term delivery, abortion, or discontinuation of oral contraceptives. It also may occur during ovulatory cycles induced with clomiphene citrate or exogenous gonadotropins and hCG.

The diagnosis of luteal phase dysfunction can be made either by endometrial biopsy or by serial progesterone determinations. Endometrial biopsies obtained from the uterine fundus in the late luteal phases of two different cycles must be at least 2 days out of phase from the expected date of bleeding, as judged from the subsequent menstrual cycle, for the diagnosis to be made. The absolute concentration that progesterone must achieve and the length of time progesterone must be increased in the luteal phase to exclude luteal dysfunction are unclear. Luteal dysfunction is extremely rare in women with menstrual cycles greater than 25 days in length in whom a single random progesterone determination is greater than 15 ng/mL.

Treatment of luteal dysfunction is controversial. Any underlying defect should be treated. If subsequent luteal function depends on prior follicular development, modification of follicular development with either clomiphene citrate (25 to 100 mg daily by mouth for 5 days beginning on cycle day 3 to 5) or FSH (75 to 300 IU intramuscularly for 3 to 5 days beginning on cycle day 3 to 5) is reasonable. hCG (2500 to 5000 IU intramuscularly at 2- to 3-day intervals beginning with the shift in basal body temperature) or progesterone (12.5 mg intramuscularly in oil daily or 25 mg twice a day as rectal or vaginal suppositories) can be utilized as well. Bromocriptine may correct the abnormality in individuals with hyperprolactinemia. Synthetic progestational agents should not be used to treat luteal phase defects because of their possible (although unproven) association with congenital anomalies. Furthermore, the synthetic progestins produce an abnormal endometrium. None of these agents has been shown to increase the pregnancy rate.

Soules MR: Luteal phase deficiency: A subtle abnormality of ovulation. *In* Keye WR Jr, Chang RJ, Rebar RW, Soules MR (eds): Infertility: Evaluation and Treatment. Philadelphia, WB Saunders, 1995. *A complete consideration of the etiology, diagnosis, and treatment of luteal phase abnormalities.*

INFERTILITY. *Infertility* may be defined as involuntary inability to conceive. *Sterility* is total inability to reproduce. In either case the situation may or may not be correctable, especially for each particular couple. Failure to reproduce thwarts a basic human instinct and causes anger, guilt, and depression. More than 10% of couples in the United States seek medical assistance for infertility.

The requirements for pregnancy to occur are several:

1. The male must produce adequate numbers of normal, motile spermatozoa.
2. The male must be capable of ejaculating the sperm through a patent ductal system.
3. The sperm must be able to traverse an unobstructed female reproductive tract.
4. The female must ovulate and release an ovum.
5. The sperm must be able to fertilize the ovum.
6. The fertilized ovum must be capable of developing and implanting in appropriately prepared endometrium.

Infertility is too frequently viewed primarily as a problem of the female. In fact, in approximately 40% of cases, infertility is caused by the male (Table 250–7). In perhaps one third of couples, more than one cause contributes to the infertility.

Peak age for fertility in the female is 25 years. For nulliparous

I. Male factors (40%)

A. Decreased production of spermatozoa
1. Varicocele
2. Testicular failure
3. Endocrine disorders
4. Cryptorchidism
5. Stress, smoking, caffeine, nicotine, recreational drugs

B. Ductal obstruction
1. Epididymal (postinfection)
2. Congenital absence of vas deferens
3. Ejaculatory duct (postinfection)
4. Postvasectomy

C. Inability to deliver sperm into vagina
1. Ejaculatory disturbances
2. Hypospadias
3. Sexual problems (i.e., impotence), medical or psychological

D. Abnormal semen
1. Infection
2. Abnormal volume
3. Abnormal viscosity

E. Immunologic factors
1. Sperm-immobolizing antibodies
2. Sperm-agglutinating antibodies

II. Female factors

A. Fallopian tube pathology (20–30%)
1. Pelvic inflammatory disease or puerperal infection
2. Congenital anomalies
3. Endometriosis
4. Secondary to past peritonitis of nongenital origin

B. Amenorrhea and anovulation (15%)

C. Minor ovulatory disturbances (<5%?)

D. Cervical and uterine factors (10%)
1. Leiomyomas and polyps
2. Uterine anomalies
3. Intrauterine synechiae (Asherman's syndrome)
4. Destroyed endocervical glands (postsurgery or postinfection)

E. Vaginal factors (<5%)
1. Congenital absence of vagina
2. Imperforate hymen
3. Vaginismus
4. Vaginitis

F. Immunologic factors (<5%)
1. Sperm-immobilizing antibodies
2. Sperm-agglutinating antibodies

G. Nutritional and metabolic factors (5%)
1. Thyroid disorders
2. Diabetes mellitus
3. Severe nutritional disturbances

III. Idiopathic or unexplained (<10%)

women of this age, the average time during which unprotected intercourse occurs until conception is 5.3 months. For parous women, the average duration of intercourse until conception is 2.7 months. The reproductive performance of couples is influenced by the ages of the female and male partners, the frequency of intercourse, and the length of time the couple has been attempting to conceive. There is a decline in both female and male reproductive performance after age 25 years.

Couples who complain of infertility merit evaluation regardless of the length of infertility. If the couple believes there is a problem, it is the physician's responsibility to reassure them by appropriate evaluation and subsequent explanation of all findings and the prognosis.

The evaluation begins with a detailed history obtained from both partners and physical examinations of both individuals. The couple should be seen together for the first visit. Each couple should be questioned together and separately because separate interviews may uncover information that would not be imparted in the presence of the partner.

Initial evaluation for infertility generally includes (1) assessment of semen, (2) documentation of ovulation by basal body temperature, serum progesterone determination approximately 6 to 8 days before menses, or endometrial biopsy less than 3 days before onset of menses, and (3) evaluation of the female genital tract by hysterosalpingography. Basal serum levels of prolactin and thyroid hormones should be measured. Diagnostic laparoscopy with tubal dye instillation should be performed if results of all previous tests are normal because 30 to 50% of women are found to have endo-

metriosis or tubal disease on surgical evaluation. Treatment must be predicated on the findings of the infertility evaluation.

Barbieri RL: Infertility. *In* Yen SSC, Jaffe RB, Barbieri RL (eds): Reproductive Endocrinology, 4th ed. Philadelphia, WB Saunders, 1999, p 562. *A summary of the approach to the infertile couple.*

INDUCTION OF OVULATION. Induction of ovulation should never be attempted until serious disorders precluding pregnancy are ruled out or treated. Furthermore, ovulation induction should be utilized only in women with chronic anovulation, because women with ovarian failure are unresponsive to any form of ovulation induction. In general, the use of pharmaceutical agents does not improve the quality of an ovum, and thus the chance of pregnancy is not improved in women who ovulate regularly.

Clomiphene citrate is the agent that usually induces ovulation most easily. Clomiphene should be utilized in individuals without hyperprolactinemia who have the ability to release LH and FSH. A typical course of clomiphene therapy is begun on the fifth day following either spontaneous or induced uterine bleeding. The initial dosage is 50 mg daily for 5 days. Clomiphene appears to act as an anti-estrogen and stimulates gonadotropin secretion by the pituitary gland to initiate follicular development. If ovulation is not achieved in the very first cycle of treatment, the daily dosage is increased to 100 mg. If ovulation is still not achieved, dosage is increased in a stepwise fashion by 50-mg increments to a maximum of 200 to 250 mg daily for 5 days. The highest dose should be continued for 3 to 6 months before the patient is regarded as a clomiphene failure. The quantity of drug and the length of time that it can be used, as suggested here, are greater than those recommended by the manufacturers, but conform with published series.

The ovulatory surge of LH may occur 5 to 12 days (average, 7 days) after the completion of the last day of clomiphene treatment in each course. Couples are advised to have intercourse every other day during this interval. Ovulation can be documented by monitoring changes in basal body temperature or preferably by measuring serum progesterone approximately 14 days after the last clomiphene tablet is taken. In addition, menses should occur about 3 weeks after the last day of therapy. Withdrawal bleeding with progestin can be induced if the patient fails to bleed within 4 weeks of therapy and if a serum hCG level documents that the patient is not pregnant. Testing the urine for an LH surge with any of several commercially available tests may also be useful in timing ovulation.

Some clinicians give 5,000 to 10,000 IU of hCG intramuscularly 7 days after the last day of clomiphene therapy to trigger ovulation, but this approach has not been established to increase effectiveness. The administration of hCG, however, does serve to time ovulation and may be helpful in selected couples. Ovulation can be expected to occur approximately 36 hours after hCG administration.

Of appropriately selected patients, 75 to 80% will ovulate and 40 to 50% can be expected to become pregnant. About 15% of pregnancies can be expected with each ovulatory cycle. The multiple pregnancy rate is about 8%, with almost all being twins. The incidence of congenital anomalies is not increased.

Side effects of clomiphene are uncommon and rarely serious. The most serious ones include vasomotor flushes (10%), abdominal discomfort (5%), breast tenderness (2%), nausea and vomiting (2%), visual symptoms (1.5%), and headache (1%). Ovarian enlargement may occur but is rare (5%). Concern has recently been raised about the potential for clomiphene to increase the risk of epithelial ovarian cancer. The evidence is insufficient to change current practices but suggests that clomiphene be administered prudently and for only a limited number of cycles.

The addition of dexamethasone, 0.5 mg orally at bedtime to blunt the nighttime secretion of ACTH, may be useful in hyperandrogenic women with an adrenal component who fail to ovulate in response to clomiphene. Other individuals failing to respond to clomiphene typically require exogenous gonadotropins and hCG or perhaps pulsatile GnRH to induce ovulation.

Both bromocriptine and cabergoline, two dopamine agonists, are effective in inducing ovulation in hyperprolactinemic women. The drug should be stopped once pregnancy is confirmed. Ovulatory menses and pregnancy are achieved in about 80% of patients with galactorrhea and hyperprolactinemia. The majority of women with prolactin-secreting pituitary tumors remain asymptomatic during pregnancy. It is rare for a patient with either a microadenoma or a macroadenoma to develop a problem related to the tumor that affects either the mother or the fetus during pregnancy. Monitoring during pregnancy need consist only of questioning the patient about the development of visual symptoms and headaches. Formal assessment of visual fields and CT or MRI should be carried out in any patient developing suspicious symptoms. Symptoms generally abate with institution of therapy with a dopamine agonist. No adverse effects of dopamine agonists on fetuses or pregnancies have been reported.

Several preparations of purified and synthetic biochemically engineered gonadotropins for use for induction of ovulation now exist. Synthetic preparations consist entirely of FSH, whereas most purified preparations contain some LH as well. Each vial typically contains 75 U of the appropriate gonadotropin. Individuals with gonadotropin deficiency will require a preparation containing some LH. Exogenous gonadotropins are typically administered at doses of two to four vials for 5 to 12 days to achieve follicular development as monitored by ultrasonography and serum or urinary E_2, concentrations, hCG, 5,000 to 10,000 IU, is administered as a single intramuscular dose when follicular maturation is apparent. The hCG should be withheld if more than three follicles mature together. GnRH analogues are now being utilized to suppress endogenous follicular activity before initiating therapy with exogenous gonadotropins and continued until hCG is given in older women and those with poor responses to exogenous gonadotropins. Use of the analogues necessitates administration of larger quantities of exogenous gonadotropins. Success rates, however, seem to be somewhat improved with this combined therapy.

Because of the expense and the complication rate, thorough evaluation should be carried out to exclude other causes of infertility before exogenous gonadotropins and hCG are used. Ovulation can be induced in almost 100% of patients, but pregnancy occurs in only 50 to 70%. There is no increased risk of congenital anomalies with exogenous gonadotropins and hCG. Concerns have been raised that exogenous gonadotropins may increase the risk of ovarian epithelial cancer, but the data are too tenuous to require any change in current practice.

The rate of multiple pregnancies with exogenous gonadotropins hCG may approach 30%, with 5% being triplets or more. Ovarian hyperstimulation is the major side effect and may be life threatening. The ovaries enlarge remarkably in this treatment-induced syndrome, and multiple follicle cysts, stromal edema, and multiple corpora lutea are present. There is a shift of fluid from the intravascular space into the abdominal cavity with resultant hypovolemia and hemoconcentration. The cause of the ascites is unknown. Treatment is conservative, with monitoring of fluid and electrolyte status. Pelvic examinations should not be performed for fear of rupturing the ovaries. The hyperstimulation generally resolves slowly over about 7 days.

GnRH, administered intravenously or less effectively subcutaneously at doses of 5 to 20 μg every 60 to 120 minutes, also can be used to induce ovulation in women with an intact pituitary gland. It is most effective in individuals with hypothalamic chronic anovulation. hCG can be administered to support the corpus luteum after ovulation at a dose of 1500 IU intramuscularly every 3 days for three to four doses. The advantage of GnRH rests in the fact that hyperstimulation is extremely unlikely. However, reported pregnancy rates have been no greater than those achieved with exogenous gonadotropins and hCG. Furthermore, some patients do not tolerate wearing the infusion pump that must be utilized.

Speroff L., Glass RH, Kase NG: Induction of ovulation. *In* Clinical Gynecologic Endocrinology and Infertility, 5th ed. Baltimore, Williams & Wilkins, 1994, p 897. *A detailed and practical survey of how to induce ovulation.*

SEXUAL FUNCTION AND DYSFUNCTION. Although sexual responses begin following puberty, they can continue for the duration of a woman's life. Sexual responses generally are divided into four phases: excitement, plateau, orgasm, and resolution.

With sexual arousal and excitement, vasocongestion and muscular tension increase progressively, primarily in the genitals, manifested by vaginal lubrication in the female. The lubrication is due to formation of a transudate in the vagina. Sexual excitement is initiated by any of a variety of psychogenic or somatogenic sexual stimuli and must be reinforced to result in orgasm. With continued stimulation, the excitement phase increases in intensity into a plateau phase during which a high state of sexual interest is maintained. The plateau phase may be short or long, and it is from this phase that an individual can shift to orgasm. The orgasmic phase tends to be brief and is characterized by rapid release from the developed vasocongestion and muscular tension. The orgasmic release is also known as the climax because peak psychological and physical intensity is achieved and there is an attendant feeling of satisfaction. Copious secretions and transudate may flow during orgasm in women. Although women may resolve toward sleep following orgasm, many remain responsive to sexual stimulation and may return to plateau and subsequent orgasm.

Characteristic genital and extragenital responses occur during these phases. Estrogens magnify the sexual responses, but responses may occur in estrogen-deficient women. For women these changes occur in the breasts and in the pudendal region and are variable from one response cycle to another. For some women, excitement proceeds quickly through plateau to orgasm, and orgasm is explosive and accompanied by vocalization and involuntary contractions of the pelvic skeletal muscles. For other women, the responses are slow in building, controlled in amplitude, and long-lasting. For a few women orgasm never occurs; for many it is intermittently absent.

The somatic sensate focus enabling orgasmic release is variable and may include stimulation of the breasts, vagina, or clitoris. The psychological aspect of coitus may involve concentration on the current partner or act or fantasies about other times and persons. Although orgasms may vary in physiologic intensity, what is important is psychological satisfaction. Satisfaction for both men and women may be had without orgasm.

Women may seek consultation because of disturbances in normal sexual arousal or orgasm. Such sexual dysfunction may be due to either organic or functional disturbances.

A variety of diseases affecting neurologic function, including diabetes mellitus and multiple sclerosis, may prevent sexual arousal. So, too, may local pelvic disorders, such as endometriosis and vaginitis, which cause dyspareunia and lead to sexual avoidance. Estrogen deficiency causing vaginal atrophy and dyspareunia is a relatively common cause of sexual dysfunction. Debilitating systemic diseases such as malignant disease may also affect sexual function indirectly.

In most cases the cause of sexual dysfunction is psychological. For instance, vaginismus involves involuntary contractions of the muscles surrounding the introitus and leads to dyspareunia. It is a conditioned response engendered by a previous imagined or real traumatic sexual experience. Feelings of guilt, caused by incest or rape as examples; of inadequacy, caused by hysterectomy or mastectomy; or of depression or anxiety may lead to failure to be aroused. Failure to achieve orgasm may be viewed as a dysfunction if the woman is frustrated or dissatisfied.

Treatment of sexual dysfunction is best accomplished by eliminating functional causes and providing the patient, often together with her partner, with appropriate psychological counseling. Behavioral modification is effective in treating many women with psychological sexual dysfunction.

Kaplan HS: The Evaluation of Sexual Disorders: Psychological and Medical Aspects. New York, Brunner-Mazel, 1983. *A good general text detailing sexual disorders.*
Kaplan HS: The Illustrated Manual of Sex Therapy, 2nd ed. New York. Brunner-Mazel, 1987. *A simple text graphically detailing the therapeutic techniques first introduced by Masters and Johnson.*
Levine SB: Sexual Life: A Clinician's Guide. New York, Plenum Press, 1992. *A widely used text detailing sexual problems and their therapy.*
Masters W, Johnson V: Human Sexual Response. Boston, Little, Brown and Company, 1966. *The classic work detailing human sexual response. Required reading for all individuals seriously interested in this field.*

251 CONTRACEPTION

Daniel R. Mishell, Jr.

CONTRACEPTIVE USE AND EFFECTIVENESS

Reversible contraception, the temporary prevention of fertility, includes all contraceptive methods except sterilization. Sterilization should be considered to be permanent, despite the possibility of surgical reversal. There are advantages and disadvantages for each contraceptive method. During contraceptive counseling these advantages and disadvantages should be thoroughly explained so the individual will choose the most acceptable method and not discontinue use prematurely and have an unwanted pregnancy.

In the United States in 1995 there were about 60 million women in the reproductive age group (15 to 44) and 39 million (65%) were using a method of contraception. Of the remainder, about 5% were sterile (prior hysterectomy), 9% were pregnant or trying to conceive, 11% were never sexually active, and 6% had no recent sexual activity. Only 5% who were sexually active were not using a method of contraception.

In the United States in 1995 the most common methods of fertility prevention were female sterilization and oral contraceptives (OCs), each used by about 10 million women. Next in frequency of use was the male condom followed by male sterilization (Table 251–1). The injectable progestin was used by about 1 million women, but the intrauterine device (IUD) and progestin implants, the two most effective methods of reversible contraception were used by less than 1 million women. Since 1982 there has been a marked decrease in diaphragm and IUD use and a continuous increase in condom use. Nearly 80% of reproductive age women have used OCs at some time.

Despite an increased use of contraceptive methods by U.S. women since 1982, more than half the pregnancies that occur are unwanted. Of the 6.3 million pregnancies that occurred in the United States in 1994, 3.1 million were unwanted and 1.4 million

Table 251–1 ■ PERCENTAGE OF WOMEN EXPERIENCING A CONTRACEPTIVE FAILURE DURING THE FIRST YEAR OF TYPICAL USE AND THE FIRST YEAR OF PERFECT USE

METHOD	% OF WOMEN EXPERIENCING AN ACCIDENTAL PREGNANCY WITHIN THE FIRST YEAR OF USE	
	Typical Use	Perfect Use
Chance	85	85
Spermicides	21	6
Periodic abstinence	20	
Calendar		9
Ovulation method		3
Symptothermal		2
Postovulation		1
Withdrawal	19	4
Cap		
Parous women	36	26
Nulliparous women	18	9
Diaphragm	18	6
Condom		
Female	21	5
Male	12	3
Pill	3	
Progestin only		0.5
Combined		0.1
IUD		
Progesterone T	2.0	1.5
Copper T380A	0.8	0.6
Depo-Provera	0.3	0.3
Norplant (6 capsules)	0.09	0.09
Female sterilization	0.4	0.4
Male sterilization	0.15	0.10

From Trussell J, Hatcher RA, Cates W, et al:, Contraceptive failure in the United States: An update. American Health Consultants, Contraceptive Technology Update 17(2):13, 1995.

Table 251–2 ■ PERCENTAGE DISTRIBUTION AND NUMBER (IN 000s) OF CONTRACEPTIVE USERS AGED 15–44, BY CURRENT METHOD, 1982–1995

METHOD	1982 %	1982 No.	1988 %	1988 No.	1995 %	1995 No.
Sterilization	34.1	10,295	39.2	13,686	38.6	14,942
Female	23.2	6,998	27.5	9,614	27.7	10,727
Male	10.9	3,298	11.7	4,069	10.9	4,215
Pill	28.0	8,431	30.7	10,734	26.9	10,410
Implant	NA	NA	NA	NA	1.3	515
Injectable	NA	NA	NA	NA	3.0	1,146
IUD	7.1	2,153	2.0	703	0.8	310
Diaphragm	8.1	2,436	5.7	2,000	1.9	720
Male condom	12.0	3,608	14.6	5,093	20.4	7,889
Foam	2.4	711	1.1	371	0.4	161
Periodic abstinence	3.9	1,166	2.3	806	2.3	883
Withdrawal	2.0	588	2.2	778	3.0	1,178
Other*	2.5	754	2.1	733	1.3	508
Total	100.0	30,142	100.0	34,912	100.0	38,663
Sample n	NA	4,242	NA	5,176	NA	7,145

*Other consists of douche, sponge, jelly or cream alone, and other methods.
From Piccinini LJ, Mosher WD: Trends in contraception use in the United States 1982–1995. Fam Plann Perspect 30:4–10 and 46, 1998. With permission of The Alan Guttmacher Institute.

of them were terminated by elective abortion. Of the women with an unwanted pregnancy, 50% stated they were using a method of contraception in the month they conceived.

The terms *method effectiveness* and *use effectiveness* (or *method failure* and *patient failure*) were previously used to describe the frequency of conceptions that occurred while the method was being used correctly or incorrectly. These terms have been replaced by the terms *typical* and *perfect use*. Methods used at the time of coitus have failure rates in the first year of use of about 5%, or more, whereas OCs, implants, injections, the IUD, and sterilization have first-year typical use failure rates of 3% or less (Table 251–2). Cumulative failure rates for use of long-acting methods are low. The pregnancy rate for 5 years of use of the progestin implants is 1.1%, and for 10 years use of the Copper T380 IUD it is 2.2%. The cumulative failure rate of all types of tubal sterilization is 1.31% during the first 5 years after the procedure and 1.85% after 10 years, being highest for tubal fulguration and lowest for segmental resection. When women conceive while using these long-acting methods, the ectopic pregnancy rates are high: about 30% with tubal sterilization failure, 25% with implant failure, and 5% with copper IUD failure.

SPERMICIDES AND BARRIERS

All spermicidal agents contain a surfactant, usually nonoxynol 9, that immobilizes or kills sperm on contact. They also provide a mechanical barrier and need to be placed into the vagina before each coital act. There is no increased risk of birth defects in the offspring of women who conceive while using spermicides.

A diaphragm must be carefully fitted by the health care provider. The largest size that does not cause discomfort or undue pressure on the vagina should be used. The diaphragm should not be left in place for more than 24 hours, because it may cause ulceration of the vaginal epithelium. Diaphragm users have an increased risk of urinary infection.

The cervical cap, a cup-shaped plastic or rubber device that fits around the cervix can be left in place longer than the diaphragm and is more comfortable. The various types of caps are manufactured in different sizes and should be fitted to the cervix by a clinician. The cap should be left on the cervix for no more than 48 hours, and a spermicide should always be placed inside the cap before use.

Use of the male condom by individuals with multiple sex partners should be encouraged because it is the most effective way to prevent sexually transmitted diseases.

The female condom consists of a soft, loose-fitting prelubricated sheath and two flexible polyurethane rings. The female condom can be inserted before beginning sexual activity and be left in place for a longer time period after ejaculation occurs than the male condom. Because the female condom covers the external genitalia it may prevent transmission of genital herpes. Because polyurethane is stronger than the latex used in male condoms the female condom is less likely to rupture. Polyurethane does not allow virus transmission and should reduce the risk of acquiring human immunodeficiency virus infection.

ORAL STEROID CONTRACEPTIVES

There are three major types of OC formulations: fixed-dose combination, combination phasic, and daily progestin. The combination formulations are the most widely used and most effective. They consist of tablets containing both an estrogen and a progestin given continuously for 3 weeks. No steroids are given for the next 7 days (except for one formulation in which estrogen alone is given for an additional 5 days) after which time the active combination is given for an additional 3 weeks. The endometrium usually begins to slough 1 to 3 days after stopping steroid ingestion causing withdrawal bleeding, which usually lasts 3 to 4 days. The uterine blood loss with OC use averages about 25 mL per cycle, less than the 35-mL average for ovulatory cycles.

All formulations are made from synthetic steroids. There are two major types of synthetic progestins: derivatives of 19-nortestosterone (which are used in OCs) and derivatives of 17α-acetoxyprogesterone (pregnanes). Pregnanes are structurally related to progesterone but are not used in OCs.

The 19-nortestosterone progestins used in OCs are of two major types, estranes and gonanes, and both have androgenic activity. The estranes currently used in several OCs are norethindrone and its acetates or norethindrone acetate and ethynodiol diacetate. Gonanes have greater progestational activity per unit weight than estranes, and thus a smaller amount of these progestins are used in OC formulations. The parent compound of the gonanes is dl-norgestrel, but only the levo isomer is biologically active. Gonanes used in OCs include both norgestrel and levonorgestrel and three less androgenic derivatives of levonorgestrel: desogestrel, norgestimate, and gestodene.

With the exception of two daily progestin-only formulations, the progestins are combined with varying dosages of two estrogens, ethinyl estradiol and its 3-methyl ether, called mestranol. All the older higher-dosage OC formulations contained mestranol, and this steroid is still present in some 50-μg formulations. All formulations with less than 50 μg of estrogen (20–35 μg) contain ethinyl estradiol.

The estrogen-progestin combination is the most effective type of OC formulation because these preparations consistently inhibit the mid-cycle gonadotropin surge and thus prevent ovulation. The progestin-only formulations have a lower dose of progestin than the combined agents and do not consistently inhibit ovulation even though they are ingested every day. Both types of formulations also act on the cervical mucus and tubal motility to interfere with sperm transport. Progestins also alter the endometrium to interfere with implantation if fertilization occurs. To maintain contraceptive effectiveness with the combination formulations it is very important that the pill-free interval be limited to no more than 7 days. This is best accomplished by ingesting either a placebo or iron tablet daily during the steroid-free interval.

METABOLIC EFFECTS. The synthetic steroids in OC formulations have many metabolic effects in addition to their contraceptive actions. These effects can cause the more common, less serious side effects as well as the rare, serious complications. The magnitude of these effects is directly related to the dosage and potency of the steroids in the formulations. The most frequent symptoms produced by the estrogen component include nausea, breast tenderness, and fluid retention. The progestins can produce certain androgenic effects, such as weight gain, acne, and nervousness. Because estrogens decrease sebum production, women who have acne should be given a formulation with a low progestin-estrogen ratio. Unscheduled (breakthrough) bleeding is usually produced by insufficient estrogen, too much progestin, or a combination of both. This problem is more common with formulations containing 20 μg of estrogen than 30 to 35 μg and is increased in women who also smoke cigarettes.

The synthetic estrogens used in OCs cause an increase in the hepatic production of several proteins. The progestins do not affect protein synthesis except to reduce levels of sex hormone–binding globulin. Some of the proteins that are increased by ethinyl estradiol, such as factors V, VIII, and X and fibrinogen, may enhance thrombosis, whereas an increase in angiotensinogen levels may elevate blood pressure in some users. Blood pressure should be monitored in all users of OCs and the agent discontinued if there is a clinically significant increase. The incidence of both venous and arterial thrombosis in OC users is directly related to the dose of estrogen. Changes in the coagulation parameters with most low-dose OCs are very small or non-existent.

The effect of OCs on glucose metabolism is directly related to the dose, potency, and type of progestin. Although high-progestin dose formulations caused peripheral insulin resistance, the low-progestin formulations in current use do not significantly alter levels of glucose, insulin, or glucagon after a glucose load. The risk of developing diabetes mellitus is not increased in women with a history of gestational diabetes who take OCs compared with controls. The risk of development of type 2 diabetes is not increased among current or post OC users compared with age-matched controls.

The estrogen component of OCs causes an increase in high-density lipoprotein cholesterol (HDL-C), a decrease in low-density lipoprotein levels (LDL-C), and an increase in total cholesterol and triglyceride levels. The progestin component causes a decrease in HDL levels, an increase in LDL levels, and a decrease in total cholesterol and triglyceride levels. High-progestin dose formulations have an adverse effect on the lipid profile; but because of the direct beneficial effect of estrogen on the arterial wall, users of these agents do not have an increased risk of cardiovascular disease. The newer combination formulations with less androgenic progestins have a more favorable effect upon the lipid profile.

COMPLICATIONS AND RISK FACTORS. The cause of the increased incidence of both venous and arterial cardiovascular disease in users of OCs is thrombosis, not atherosclerosis. The background rate of venous thrombosis and embolism in women of reproductive age is about 0.8 per 10,000 woman-years. Among users of OCs with 30 or 35 μg ethinyl estradiol, it is 3 per 10,000 woman-years, about four times the background rate, but one half of the rate of 6 per 10,000 woman-years that occurs in association with pregnancy. Although the risk of venous thrombosis and embolism is higher among women ingesting OCs with 50 μg of ethinyl estradiol than 30 to 35 μg, studies to date indicate the risk of venous thrombosis and embolism with OCs containing 20 μg ethinyl estradiol is similar to that of OCs with 30 to 35 μg ethinyl estradiol. In the presence of an inherited coagulopathy disorder the risk is increased severalfold. Because only 1 in 300 women with activated protein C resistance will develop venous thrombosis with OC use, it is not recommended that screening for coagulation deficiencies be undertaken before starting OC use unless the woman has a personal or strong family history of thrombotic events.

The use of high-dose OCs by cigarette smokers significantly increases the risk of myocardial infarction. Therefore, combination OCs should not be prescribed to women older than 35 years who smoke cigarettes or use alternative forms of nicotine. Recent epidemiologic studies indicate that use of low-dose OCs by non-smoking women without hypertension is not associated with a significantly increased incidence of either myocardial infarction or hemorrhagic or thrombotic stroke.

For about 2 years after the discontinuation of contraceptives, the rate of return of fertility is slightly lower for users of OCs than for users of barrier methods. OCs do not cause permanent infertility or adversely affect pregnancies that occur after their discontinuation. OCs are not teratogenic if accidentally ingested during pregnancy.

The risk of breast cancer diagnosis is increased by about 25% in young women who are currently using OCs. Because there is no relation between dose or duration of use of estrogen it is *unlikely that OCs initiate breast cancer.* Furthermore, there is no significant increase in risk of breast cancer with initiation of OC use at a very young age, use before a first birth, or use by women with a family history of breast cancer (see Chapter 258).

The epidemiologic data regarding the risk of invasive cervical cancer as well as cervical intraepithelial neoplasia and OC use is conflicting. Nonetheless, the majority of well-controlled studies indicate that there is no change in risk of cervical intraepithelial neoplasia and OC use. However, it is likely that a causal relation exists between OC use and a reported increased risk of cervical adenocarcinoma. OC users need annual cervical cytology screening (see Chapter 259).

Several studies have shown that the use of OCs has a protective effect against endometrial cancer. This decrease in risk persists for many years after stopping OCs. Women who use OCs for at least 1 year have a 50% reduced risk of endometrial cancer development between ages 40 and 55 compared with non-users. This protective effect is related to duration of use, increasing from a 20% reduction with 1 year of use to a 60% reduction with 4 years of use.

OCs reduce the risk of developing epithelial ovarian cancer as well as those with low malignant potential. The magnitude of the decrease in risk is directly related to the duration of OC use, increasing from about a 40% reduction with 4 years of use to a 60% reduction with 12 years of use. The protective effect continues for at least 20 years after the use of OCs ends. As with endometrial cancer, the protective effect occurs only in women of low parity (≤ 4), who are at greatest risk for this type of cancer.

The development of a benign hepatocellular adenoma was a rare occurrence in long-term users of high-dose OCs containing mestranol but is not increased by use of ethinyl estradiol OCs. There is no increased risk of liver cancer associated with OC use. OC use also does not increase the risk of development of malignant melanoma or prolactin-secreting pituitary adenomas.

OCs can be prescribed for the majority of women of reproductive age. Absolute contraindications include a history of vascular disease, including systemic diseases that affect the vascular system, such as lupus erythematosus or diabetes with retinopathy or nephropathy. Cigarette smoking by OC users older than age 35 and uncontrolled hypertension are also contraindications, as are a personal history of cancer of the breast or endometrium and cholestatic jaundice of pregnancy. Pregnancy and any undiagnosed cause of uterine bleeding are also contraindications. Women with functional heart diseases should not use OCs because the fluid retention could result in congestive heart failure. There is no evidence, however, that individuals with asymptomatic mitral valve prolapse should not use OCs. Women with active liver disease should not take OCs. However, women who have recovered from liver disease, such as viral hepatitis, and whose liver function test results have returned to normal, can safely take OCs. Relative contraindications to OC use include classic but not common migraine headaches, undiagnosed causes of amenorrhea, and depression. Use of OCs does not cause enlargement of prolactin-secreting pituitary microadenomas or worsen functional prolactinoma (see Chapter 237) as was previously believed.

INITIATION OF THERAPY AND SURVEILLANCE

If a healthy woman has no contraindications to OC use, it is unnecessary to perform any laboratory tests, including cervical cytology, before use unless these are necessary for routine health maintenance. Routine use of laboratory tests is not indicated unless the woman has a family history of diabetes or arterial vascular disease at a young age, in which case a fasting glucose or lipid panel should be obtained. After the first three cycles of OC use a non-directed history should be obtained and blood pressure measured. After this visit the woman should be seen annually, at which time a non-directed history should again be taken, blood pressure and body weight measured, and a physical examination (including breast, abdominal, and pelvic examination with cervical cytology) performed. It is not necessary to measure lipids, other than the routine cholesterol screening every 5 years, in women with no cardiovascular risk factors, even if they are older than age 35. If the woman has history of liver disease, a liver panel should be obtained to make certain that liver function is normal before OCs are started. There is no reason to discontinue OC use unless pregnancy is desired. Intermittent discontinuation is unnecessary and may result in an unwanted pregnancy.

Although synthetic sex steroids can retard the biotransformation of certain drugs (e.g., phenazone and meperidine) as a result of substrate competition, such interference is not important clinically. OC use has not been shown to inhibit the action of other drugs. However, some drugs can interfere clinically with the action of OCs by inducing liver enzymes that convert the steroids to more polar and less biologically active metabolites. These drugs include barbiturates, sulfonamides, cyclophosphamide, and rifampin. There

is a high incidence of OC failure in women ingesting rifampin, and these two agents should not be given concurrently. There is no reliable evidence that other antibiotics, analgesics, or barbiturates inhibit OC effectiveness. Women taking medication for epilepsy should be treated with 50-μg estrogen formulations, because many antiepileptic medications lower ethinyl estradiol levels and cause breakthrough bleeding, which may cause premature discontinuation of use. Because of their many health benefits, including reduction in risk of endometrial and ovarian cancer and induction of regular cyclic uterine bleeding, the continued use of OCs until menopause should be encouraged in women without contraindications.

LONG-ACTING CONTRACEPTIVE STEROIDS

Several types of long-acting steroid injectable suspensions and subdermal implant formulations are being used for contraception. Because most of the long-acting steroid formulations contain only a progestin, without an estrogen, endometrial integrity is not maintained and uterine bleeding occurs at irregular and unpredictable intervals. Therefore, women wishing to use these methods need to be counseled about the development of irregular bleeding before their use to enhance continuity of use.

Several types of injectable steroid formulations are in use for contraception throughout the world. These include depo-medroxyprogesterone acetate (DMPA), given in a dose of 150 mg every 3 months; norethindrone enanthate, given in a dose of 200 mg every 2 months, and several once-a-month injections of combinations of different progestins and estrogens. DMPA has a low failure rate, 0.1% at 1 year and 0.4% at 2 years. Then major contraceptive action consists of inhibition of ovulation, sperm transport by keeping the cervical mucus thick, and inhibition of endometrial growth and glycogen production. Serum DMPA levels rise steadily to contraceptively effective blood levels (> 0.5 ng/mL) within 24 hours after the injection. Levels plateau for about 3 months, after which there is a gradual decline until levels become undetectable 7 to 9 months after the injection. Endogenous estradiol levels remain above the postmenopausal range, and symptoms of estrogen deficiency do not occur.

Because of the lag time it takes to clear DMPA from the circulation, resumption of ovulation is delayed for a variable period of time after the last injection. It may take as long as 1 year for ovulatory cycles to return. After this initial delay, fecundity resumes at a rate similar to that found after discontinuing a barrier contraceptive.

The major side effect of DMPA is complete disruption of the menstrual cycle. The bleeding is usually light in amount and does not cause anemia. As duration of therapy increases, the incidence of frequent bleeding steadily declines and the incidence of amenorrhea steadily increases, so that at the end of 2 years about 70% of users are amenorrheic. Women who use this method of contraception should be counseled that with time the irregular bleeding episodes will cease and amenorrhea will most likely occur. Most DMPA users gain between 1.5 to 4 kg in their first year of use and continue to gain weight thereafter. If weight gain occurs, caloric intake should be decreased. Because there is no estrogen in DMPA, its use does not cause hypertension or thromboembolism.

In cycling women, the initial injection should be given no later than day 5 of the cycle to be certain to inhibit ovulation in the initial treatment cycle. The first injection should be given within 5 days after delivery in non-lactating women but not until after 6 weeks in lactating women.

Because the major reason for discontinuance of all progestin-injectable contraceptives is menstrual irregularity, several combined progestin-estrogen injectables that are given once monthly and produce regular withdrawal bleeding have been developed. A combination of medroxyprogesterone acetate, 25 mg, and estradiol cypionate 5 mg will soon be marketed in the United States. In addition to a more regular bleeding pattern, this agent has the advantage of being as effective as DMPA with a much more rapid rate of clearance and resumption of ovulatory cycles after stopping use.

SUBDERMAL IMPLANTS. Subdermal implants of six 3.4-cm polydimethylsiloxane (Silastic) capsules each containing 36 mg of levonorgestrel are very effective long-term contraceptives. Subcutaneous insertion in the upper arm is performed in an outpatient setting utilizing a small skin incision with local anesthesia. The capsules need to be removed when desired by the user, or at the end of 5 years, which is the duration of maximal contraceptive effectiveness. Return to ovulation is prompt after implant removal.

After insertion, blood levels of levonorgestrel rise rapidly to 1 to 2 ng/mL/24 hr. These levels then fall during the first month, after which they plateau during the first year. Levels then gradually fall so at the end of 5 years, levels range between 170 and 350 pg/mL. Annual pregnancy rates for the first 5 years of use are about 0.2 per 100 women, whereas the cumulative 5-year pregnancy rate is 1.1%.

The major side effect is the totally irregular pattern of uterine bleeding. Bleeding episodes are more prolonged and irregular during the first year of use, after which they become more regular as ovulatory cycles occur.

EMERGENCY CONTRACEPTION. For a woman not using contraception, if emergency contraception is given within 72 hours after a single coitus in mid cycle, about 75% of pregnancies will be prevented. If more than one episode of coitus has occurred, or if treatment is initiated later than 72 hours after coitus, the method is less effective. The most common currently used regimen is ingestion of four tables of the OC containing 50 μg of ethinyl estradiol, and 0.5 mg dl-norgestrel, in doses of two tablets 12 hours apart. The pregnancy rate with this regimen is 1.5% about one-fourth that of the 8% expected rate.

INTRAUTERINE DEVICES. The main benefits of IUDs are (1) a high level of effectiveness, (2) a lack of systemic metabolic effects, and (3) the need for only a single act of motivation for long-term use. Despite these advantages, less than 1% of married women of reproductive age use the IUD for contraception in the United States, compared with 15% to 30% in most European countries and Canada. The Copper T380A IUD is the only copper-bearing IUD currently marketed in the United States, but the Multiload CU 375 is widely used in Europe. The Copper T380A is approved for use in the United States for 10 years and maintains its effectiveness for at least 12 years. A progesterone-releasing IUD that is also marketed in the United States allows 65 mg of progesterone to diffuse into the endometrial cavity each day. Because of the progestational effect on the endometrium, the amount of uterine bleeding is reduced with use of this device, and it has been used therapeutically to treat menorrhagia. The progesterone-releasing IUD needs to be replaced annually, but a levonorgestrel-releasing IUD that is currently marketed only in Europe is effective for 7 years.

The main mechanism of contraceptive action of copper-bearing IUDs is spermicidal. This effect is caused by a local sterile leukocytic response produced by the copper as well as the plastic IUD itself. Because of the spermicidal action of IUDs, very few, if any, spermatozoa reach the oviducts, and the ovum usually does not become fertilized. The progesterone-releasing IUD acts mainly by preventing transport of spermatozoa through the cervical mucus and slowing tubal transport of the embryo. After removal of the IUD, the inflammatory reaction rapidly disappears and resumption of fertility is prompt. In general, in the first year of use, copper IUDs have less than a 1% pregnancy rate, a 10% expulsion rate, and a 15% rate of removal for medical reasons, mainly bleeding and pain. The incidence of each of these events, especially expulsion, diminishes steadily in subsequent years. Mefenamic acid ingested in a dosage of 500 mg three times a day during the days of menstruation has been shown to significantly reduce the amount of uterine bleeding in IUD users.

Development of acute salpingitis more than a month after insertion of the IUD is due to infection with a sexually transmitted pathogen and is unrelated to the presence of the device. All IUD-related upper genital tract infections occur only during the insertion process. If there is clinical suspicion that cervicitis is present, the endocervix should be cultured and the insertion delayed until the results reveal no pathogenic organisms are present. It is not cost-effective to routinely administer antibiotics with IUD insertion.

The IUD is not associated with an increased incidence of either endometrial or cervical carcinoma. The IUD is a particularly useful method of contraception for women who have completed their families and do not wish permanent sterilization and have contraindications to, or do not wish to use, other effective methods of reversible contraception. A recent analysis reported that after 5 years of use the IUD was the most cost effective of all methods of contraception, including sterilization.

Piccinini LJ, Mosher WD: Trends in contraception use in the United States 1982–1995. Fam Plan Perspect 30(1):4–10 and 46, 1998.

Trussell J, Hatcher RA, Cates W, et al: Contraceptive failure in the United States: An update. American Health Consultants, Contraceptive Technology Update, February 1995, vol 17(2), pp 13–24.

252 PREGNANCY: NEOPLASTIC DISEASES

Edward C. Grendys, Jr.

Although uncommon in a relative sense, cancer remains a leading cause of death in women of reproductive age (Table 252–1). Overall cancer-related deaths account for 13% of mortality in women between the ages of 15 and 34 years and 38% in women aged 35 to 54. In this reproductive age-group, cancer is expected to complicate approximately 3500 pregnancies in the United States, with an incidence of 1 in 1000. However, it has been suggested that as women continue to delay childbearing this incidence may begin to rise in concordance with the direct relationship of age on cancer incidence (Fig. 252–1).

Given these statistics it is imperative that primary care physicians (i.e., family practitioners, internists, and obstetricians/gynecologists) be knowledgeable in current screening recommendations, especially regarding the cervix, colon, and breast malignancies. Subtle signs of malignancy can occasionally be mistaken for side effects of pregnancy, thus possibly leading to diagnostic and treatment delay.

When a cancer occurs in a gravid woman it obviously carries with it enormous pressures on both the patient, her family, as well as the treating team of physicians. The diagnosis alone is certainly anxiety provoking enough without the burden of the treatment decision that is about to affect two lives.

The approach to a pregnant patient diagnosed with a concomitant malignant process requires a concerted multidisciplinary approach. This team should include, at a minimum, obstetricians with experience in high-risk pregnancies as well as oncologists with a keen understanding of fetal development and maturation. Also, significant input from psychosocial, religious, and even legal personnel can be invaluable to maximize the outcome of mother, fetus, and family. An integrated care plan should be formulated, and communication between all team members must be encouraged. The medical and psychologic sequelae of this process are complex and not to be taken lightly. Decisions ranging from pregnancy preservation, type and timing of diagnostic and therapeutic interventions, use of antepartum lung-maturing corticosteroids, as well as timing and mode of delivery must all be carefully planned and executed.

The most common malignancies encountered during pregnancy are uterine/cervical cancer, breast cancer, melanoma, ovarian cancer, thyroid cancer, leukemia, lymphoma, and colorectal cancer (Table 252–2). Specific reviews of these common malignancies encountered in this population are presented, along with various strategies employed in their management.

Two fundamental issues must be contemplated when one approaches the care of a gravid patient diagnosed with a malignant process. The impact of the disease state on the patient is of obvious paramount importance, and an understanding of the natural history of the disease is therefore critical. Treatment options, success rates, and risk of treatment modifications or delays must be

Table 252–1 ■ **REPORTED DEATHS IN U.S. WOMEN AGED 15–54**

CAUSE	NO. CASES/YEAR
Cancer	34,361
Cardiac disease	13,900
Trauma	12,154

Data from American Cancer Society, Cancer Statistics, 1998.

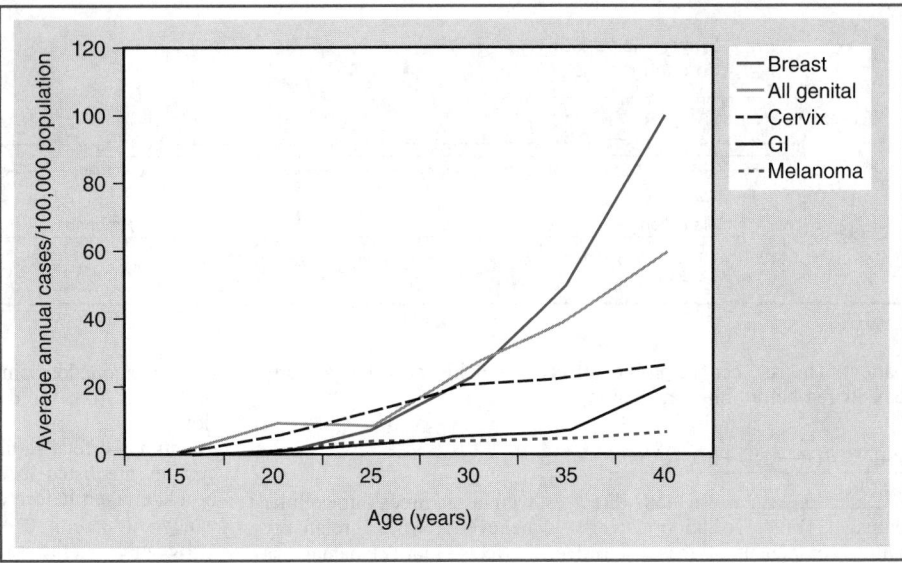

FIGURE 252–1 ■ Incidence of common malignancies seen in pregnancy. (Data from American Cancer Society, Cancer Statistics, 1998.)

considered. Equally important is the maternal and paternal desires of pregnancy preservation and the risk of the chosen treatment regimens on fetal health, including sequelae resulting from elective, early delivery or potential for in utero fetal harm from toxic side effects of therapy. Patients need to be presented with unbiased information regarding risks to both mother and fetus and with all potential options of intervention, including pregnancy termination if it is required and desired. Most likely, these management issues are best left to a tertiary care center with a high-risk neonatal nursery (level III) that can adequately manage a preterm yet viable infant if necessary.

FETAL DEVELOPMENT

Physicians involved with the treatment of cancer in the pregnant patient must possess an in-depth understanding of embryonic development as well as of the disease process and the available therapeutic options. The terminology adopted by embryologists and clinical obstetricians must also be understood.

Fetal age is the most critical in terms of prediction of fetal survival and subsequent morbidity. In clinical obstetrics, estimated gestational age (EGA) is defined as the time from the last day of the last menstrual period (LMP) (Fig. 252–2). Embryonic age from a developmental biologist's viewpoint begins at fertilization and is thus 2 weeks shorter in duration. This 2-week differential is critical and potentially legally important when considering fetal viability and age at which termination (abortion) can be legally performed. It must be remembered that ovulation and subsequent fertilization does not occur until approximately 2 weeks after the LMP. Thus, the normal gestation is 40 weeks and clinical viability generally has been defined as greater than 25 weeks' EGA. For accurate clinical communication, fetal age should be documented in terms of EGA (in weeks). Gestation is further subdivided into 14-week trimesters, as shown in Figure 252–2. In most states abortion can

legally be performed in the first trimester whereas some states allow termination until 24 weeks (late abortion).

The most vulnerable portion of development is believed to be during the embryonic period (see Fig. 252–2). During this time, major organ systems are forming (organogenesis) and it appears that the conceptus is susceptible to outside teratogenic influences. For this reason, most clinicians believe that therapeutic intervention is best delayed until after this period to lessen fetal risk in a patient desirous of preserving her pregnancy.

After the embryonic period, fetal development is focused on organ growth and maturation. Certain basic physical and metabolic capabilities appear to be required to maintain extrauterine life. Most commonly, viability is defined as 25 weeks of EGA although reports of fetal survival before this age have been noted. Subsequent fetal morbidity and mortality are linearly correlated with gestational age (Table 252–3). Obviously, preterm infants require care in a specific neonatal unit prepared for such complicated management (level III nurseries). A review of 600 preterm infants without associated congenital anomalies demonstrated a mortality rate of approximately 32% for a fetus delivered at 26 weeks' EGA compared with 2.7% when the fetus was allowed to develop to 34 weeks of age (Table 252–4). Significant literature support the concept of maximizing in utero fetal life to decrease fetal morbidity, mortality, and long-term developmental delay.

Although the short-term major risk to the fetus appears to be secondary to poor lung development, subsequent development of hyaline membrane disease (HMD), and bronchopulmonary dysplasia (BPD) (see Table 252–3), recent reports are confirming increased risk of intraventricular hemorrhage and significant long-term motor and neurologic sequelae associated with surviving a preterm delivery. Infants weighing less than 1500 g at birth appear to suffer from significant long-term deficiencies in intelligence quotient, visual motor integration, and reading performance. Similar data reveal significant neurologic impairment in infants documented with intraventricular hemorrhage (IVH). In one study, only 26% of low-birth-weight children with subsequent IVH had normal developmental abilities at the time of preschool testing. It appears that predelivery use of corticosteroids decreases the risk of pulmonary complications as well as IVH. It is important for parents to understand the potential ramifications of early delivery on their child and realize that survival can be associated with significant long-term morbidity.

DIAGNOSTIC AND THERAPEUTIC PROCEDURES IN THE PREGNANT PATIENT WITH CANCER

Commonly accepted practices of diagnostic imaging, surgery, therapeutic radiation therapy, as well as chemotherapy, have profoundly different implications in the pregnant versus non-pregnant

Table 252–2 ■ INCIDENCE OF CANCER IN PREGNANCY

SITE/TYPE	ESTIMATED INCIDENCE/ 1000 PREGNANCIES
Cervix uteri	
Non-invasive	1.3
Invasive	1.0
Breast	0.33
Melanoma	0.14
Ovary	0.10
Colorectal	0.02
Leukemia	0.01
Lymphoma	0.01

From Allen HH, Nisker JA (eds): Cancer in Pregnancy: Therapeutic Guidelines. Mt. Kisco, NY, Futura, 1986.

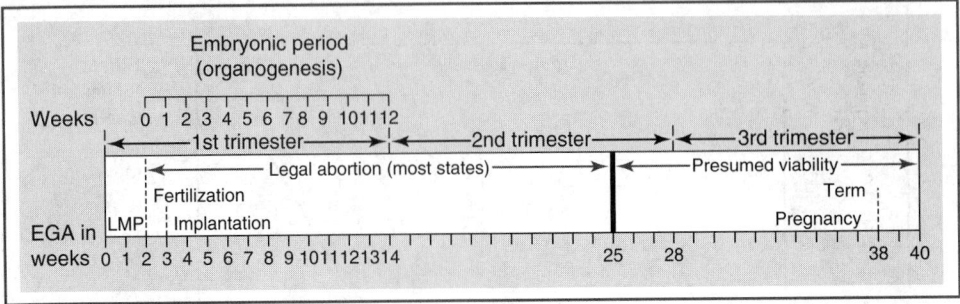

FIGURE 252–2 ■ Fetal development.

patient. The risk-benefit profiles of each modality must be carefully considered before implementation.

RADIATION AND PREGNANCY

Radiation can cause both direct as well as indirect intracellular damage. Direct radiation damage is believed to be a relatively minor component of these detrimental effects. Indirect damage is initiated by free water radiation-induced ionization. This leads to free radical formation with subsequent chemical intracellular reaction and damage. Because the major component of cells is water this is believed to be the major mechanism of action. In vitro studies indicate that dividing cells specifically near the mitotic phase appear to be most vulnerable.

At therapeutic doses, radiation does not significantly directly damage cellular microstructures, membranes, or metabolic processes. The primary toxic effects appear to result primarily from free radical induced damage at the DNA level. The damage is most likely secondary to double-stranded breaks in DNA leading to replication errors, which are presumably lethal or perhaps teratogenic.

At doses of radiation below 100 cGy cellular death results from direct inhibition of cell division and is most prevalent in cells undergoing active division. The induction of radiation-induced mutations increases as a linear function of single doses up to 400 to 600 cGy. Because of the acute toxicity to cells, radiation is considered a weak teratogen as opposed to long-term birth defects. Clinical retrospective studies suggest some association of spontaneous abortion with early fetal irradiation.

The fetal effects of radiation appear to be related to the gestational age at the time of exposure, as well as total dose received. An analysis of children exposed in utero to atomic bomb–produced radiation revealed most long-term neurologic sequelae occurred in children exposed between 8 to 15 weeks' EGA with no cases reported before 8 weeks' EGA. Exposure at an earlier age most likely resulted in miscarriage.

Fetal exposure to radiation between ages 11 to 16 weeks appears to result in an increased risk of microcephaly and mental retardation. Exposure in the third trimester may be associated with longer-term developmental abnormalities (Tables 252–5 and 252–6). In general, third-trimester fetal doses should not exceed 100 cCy.

The maternal effects of radiation are well documented. Direct ovarian exposures of 1000 cGy are associated with permanent sterilization in more than 90% of women. Lower doses also result in sterility but appear to be dependent on patient age and menstrual and reproductive history. Ovarian suppression with oral contracep-

tives or gonadotropin hormone antagonists do not appear to be protective from the damaging effects of radiation on ovarian function.

Estimated fetal radiation exposures for standard radiographic procedures are listed in Table 252–7. A risk-benefit assessment must be undertaken before obtaining any radiographic evaluation in pregnancy.

Because of the relatively high fetal exposure associated with pelvic abdominal computed tomography (CT), it is not recommended especially in early pregnancy. The limited use of CT pelvic imaging to evaluate pelvic outlets for term vaginal delivery has been used, but fetal risk should be minimal at this gestational age.

Mammography, as noted in Table 252–7, presents essentially no risk to the developing fetus. Therefore, its use as a diagnostic modality in the patient with a clinically suspicious breast lesion is recommended.

Perhaps the most commonly employed imaging procedure in the pregnant patient is real-time ultrasonography. Its use in fetal anatomic observation and age determination has been well studied and is considered safe throughout the gestational period.

It can also be an important instrument for evaluation of suspected renal, abdominal, pelvic hepatic, cardiac, vascular, and breast tissues. Hepatic ultrasound evaluation can detect occult liver metastasis with a sensitivity of 76% without fetal risk. Breast ultrasonography is a useful adjunct in characterizing breast lesion architecture noted on physical examination or mammography (see section on Breast Carcinoma in Pregnancy).

Magnetic resonance imaging (MRI), due to its lack of ionizing radiation, is believed to be acceptable in pregnancy.

Therapeutic megavoltage radiation therapy has a pivotal role in the management of many malignancies, such as breast and cervical cancer and lymphoma etc. Depending on the specific anatomic area to be treated, the fetal exposure can range from minimal to substantial (Table 252–8).

SURGERY IN PREGNANCY

Of the common solid tumors cancers affecting the pregnant patient most are treatable and many curable by a surgical approach. Fetal risk appears to be most dependent on the anatomic location

Table 252-3. ■ INCIDENCE OF FETAL MORTALITY, HYALINE MEMBRANE DISEASE (HMD), BRONCHOPULMONARY DYSPLASIA (BPD), AND INTRAVENTRICULAR HEMORRHAGE (IVH) AS ASSOCIATED WITH FETAL AGE

EGA(WEEKS)	MORTALITY (%)	HMD (%)	BPD (%)	IVH (%)
24–25	66	93	59	36
26–27	32	86	59	32
28–29	20	71	34	34
30–31	9	46	13	7
32–33	1.2	33	2.4	1.8

EGA = Estimated gestational age.

Table 252-4. ■ SURVIVAL STATISTICS IN RELATION TO ESTIMATED GESTATIONAL AGE (EGA)

EGA(WEEKS)	% SURVIVAL
25	24.0
26	57.1
27	66.7
28	84.9
29	82.9
30	80.7
31	94.2
32	92.1
33	92.2
34	94.8
35	98.1
36	98.1
37	93.3
38	97.7

Table 252-5 ■ CRITICAL PERIODS FOR FETAL IRRADIATION

DISORDER/PROBLEM	RADIATION DOSE	
	100 to 500 cGy	500 to 1000 cGy
Embryonic death		0–1 week
Malformation	1–8 weeks	1–8 weeks
Microcephaly	1–15 weeks	1–15 weeks
Mental retardation	8–15 weeks	8–25 weeks
Growth retardation	1–15 weeks	1–25 weeks
Late-onset cancer		1–39 weeks
Genetic aberrations		

Table 252-7 ■ ESTIMATED FETAL DOSE FROM COMMON DIAGNOSTIC RADIOGRAPHIC PROCEDURES

EXAMINATION	FETAL DOSE IN cGY (RAD)
Chest (posteroanterior/lateral)	0.00006
Abdomen	0.15–0.26
Lumbar spine	0.65
Pelvis	0.2–0.35
Hip	0.13–0.2
Intravenous pyelography	0.47–0.82
Upper gastrointestinal tract	0.17–0.48
Barium enema	0.82–1.14
Mammography	Undetectable
CT of head	0.007
CT of abdomen (early pregnancy)	0.04
CT of pelvis	2.5
^{99m}Tc-MDP bone scan	0.15

of the neoplasm and the risk of subsequent stimulation of preterm labor, which is most affected by timing of the procedure. Pelvic and abdominal radical procedures can be safely undertaken if appropriate planning is used.

Surgical approaches to breast, ovarian, gastrointestinal, thyroid, melanoma, neurologic, and vulvar cancer have been well described, along with a multitude of benign surgical conditions. The current anesthetic agents in common use are believed to be without risk of fetal teratogenicity, and certainly minor procedures with local or regional analgesia (epidural, spinal, nerve block) are essentially without risk. Exclusive of cesarean section, it has been estimated that approximately 35,000 pregnant women will undergo some surgical procedure per year.

An issue that should be considered is the critical nature of the uteroplacental unit that is susceptible to blood pressure changes and intavascular volume depletion. Major changes in blood flow to the placenta can lead to subsequent fetal hypoxia and potential precipitate neurologic sequelae. Therefore, the supine position is best avoided in the gravid patient (especially after 20 weeks' EGA) owing to decreased cardiac return associated with uterine compression on the inferior vena cava. Patients are best maintained in the left lateral decubitus position (30°) to decrease this compressive effect. Diagnostic procedures including fine-needle aspiration, core biopsy, and/or surgical removal of suspicious lesions should rarely, if ever, be deferred due to pregnancy. As described earlier, a surgeon and anesthesiologist with appropriate understanding of uteroplacental dynamics should be sought to provide optimal care.

Equally critical is the increased thrombogenic state associated with pregnancy as brought about by decreases in plasma fibrinolytic activity, increases in coagulation factors, as well as increased pelvic and lower extremity stasis. These factors combine for a five to six times increased risk of thromboembolic phenomena in the pregnant patient, and thus appropriate thromboprophylaxis should be undertaken. Current acceptable techniques include subcutaneous heparin 5000 units three times a day, low-molecular-weight heparin (enoxaparin, 40 mg/day), or inflatable compression stockings. Non-custom fit elastic stockings (TedHose) have no role in thromboprophylaxis.

CHEMOTHERAPY IN PREGNANCY

Chemotherapy has an integral role in the management of many of the cancers encountered during pregnancy. Some agents are used as adjuvant therapy after primary surgery (e.g., breast), whereas others are the primary treatment modality (e.g., Hodgkin's disease). The potential toxicity to the developing fetus must be considered when discussing potential treatment regimens in the pregnant patient.

Table 252-6 ■ TOTAL RADIATION EXPOSURE RESULTING IN MAJOR ABNORMALITIES

GESTATION (MONTHS)	RADIATION DOSE (cGy)
1	40
2	90
3	140
4	200
5	250
6	350
8	500
9	600

All chemotherapeutic agents, by virtue of their mechanism of action, have the ability to be both mutagenic as well as teratogenic to the actively dividing cells of the embryo and fetus. Unfortunately, controlled data on their effects on the developing fetus are limited. Most information has come from retrospective reviews as well as laboratory experiments on gravid animals.

It appears that the first trimester is the most susceptible to deleterious chemotherapy influences. Overall, it appears that approximately 20% of fetuses exposed to cytotoxic agents in the first trimester will manifest major anomalies, as compared with 3% in an unexposed population.

Chemotherapeutic agents primarily act by interrupting various portions of vital cell processes. This reproductive cell cycle is divided into five phases, each with specific actions leading to cell duplication (Table 252-9). Cancer cells are thought to replicate at a higher rate and therefore should be more susceptible to the cytotoxic or cytostatic effects of chemotherapy. Specific chemotherapeutic agents are often categorized by their interaction within the cell cycle and are traditionally classified into alkylating agents, antitumor antibiotics, antimetabolites, *Vinca* alkaloids, biologic response modifiers, hormones, and taxanes. Specific agents and their actions are listed in Table 252-10 (see Chapter 198)

The timing of chemotherapy administration in relationship to anticipated delivery must be carefully planned to avoid delivery around the time of the maternal hematopoietic nadir. Hematopoietic suppression (anemia, leukopenia, and thrombocytopenia) may occur in the fetus as a result of transplacental passage of cytotoxic agents from the mother to the fetus, and the neonatology team should be advised accordingly.

One of the most active new agents in the treatment of solid tumors is paclitaxel. To date no reasonable experience of its use in pregnancy has been reported; therefore, its use cannot be advocated. Given its activity of microtubular assembly, concern for its effect on fetal development is significant.

Breast-feeding is contraindicated during chemotherapeutic administration because these systemically administered antineoplastic agents may reach significant levels in breast milk.

SPECIFIC MALIGNANCIES IN PREGNANCY

Cervical Cancer

Cervical cancer remains the most common malignancy encountered during pregnancy. It occurs with an incidence of approximately 1.2 cases/10,000 pregnancies. With the expanded knowledge of the natural history of this disease, the majority of patients with early cervical carcinoma can be managed with fetal preservation (if desired) without undo maternal morbidity or mortality.

A routine part of initial prenatal evaluation should include a Papanicolaou (Pap) smear. This simple, inexpensive, and extremely effective screening procedure has significantly decreased the incidence of invasive squamous cell carcinoma of the cervix in the United States. In countries where this procedure is not widely practiced, cervical cancer remains one of the leading causes of death. After intense investigation and numerous clinical observa-

Table 252–8 ■ ESTIMATED FETAL DOSES FROM EXTRAPELVIC AND EXTRA-ABDOMINAL MATERNAL IRRADIATION

RADIATION SITE/PRESCRIBED DOSE	ESTIMATED GESTATIONAL AGE	FETAL DOSE
Tibia sarcoma/50 Gy	25 weeks	1.5 cGy
Brain glioblastoma/60 Gy	13 weeks	3.9 cGy
Hodgkin's disease (mantle fields)/38 Gy	34 weeks	42 cGy
Hodgkin's disease with mediastinum/neck/40 Gy	18–31 weeks	20 cGy
Breast cancer/50 Gy	Ovarian dose	9 cGy

Data from Greer BE, Goff BA, Kuh W, et al: Cancer in the pregnant patient. *In* Hoskins WJ, Perez CA, Young RC (eds): Principles and Practice of Gynecologic Oncology, 2nd ed. Philadelphia, Lippincott-Raven, 1997, pp 463–485.

tions, the natural progression from a preinvasive dysplastic lesion to overt invasive cervical carcinoma is well understood. The purported rationale of the Pap smear is as a screening, and not a diagnostic, procedure. The success of Pap smear screening has been in its ability to diagnose dysplastic lesions, thus allowing for simple ablative and curative measures.

All clinicians who practice Pap smear screening should have an understanding of the Bethesda system of Pap smear interpretation as well as diagnostic and treatment algorithms. The Bethesda classification system is listed in Table 252–11. In general, a diagnosis of atypical squamous cells of undetermined significance (ASCUS) on an initial Pap smear can usually be managed with a simple repeat smear in 3 months. A Pap smear diagnosis of atypical glandular cells (AGUS) is, however, significantly different. (Persistent ASCUS smears, squamous intraepithelial lesions, or evidence of carcinoma mandates colposcopic evaluation of the cervix and vagina.) AGUS Pap smears are associated with a high incidence (11%) of invasive cancer and must be evaluated aggressively.

Cytologic finding of squamous intraepithelial lesions is most commonly evaluated with cervical colposcopy. Colposcopy during pregnancy is safe and effective and in the far majority (>90%) provides adequate diagnostic information. Similar in the non-pregnant patient, any area of gross abnormality, even in the presence of a normal Pap smear, requires biopsy.

Given the knowledge of the natural history of cervical dysplasia, observational strategies have been developed to allow the pregnancy to continue without need for intervention. Even in the patient with biopsy-proven carcinoma in situ, excision or cervical ablation can most commonly be deferred until after delivery. Importantly, a diagnosis of cervical dysplasia is not an indication for cesarean delivery because there has been no demonstrable increased risk to mother or fetus with vaginal delivery.

Locally advanced cervical carcinoma, not amenable to surgical resection, requires treatment with radical radiation therapy. The standard external high-energy teletherapy radiation often exceeds 4500 cGy and is not compatible with fetal life. Again, decision regarding fetal age, risk of early delivery versus waiting, as well as parental desires must be weighed, given the curability of this disease. With most lesions confined to the cervix, careful observation and expedited delivery after fetal maturation followed by radical treatment appears reasonable.

Ovarian Carcinoma

The lifetime risk of ovarian carcinoma for an American woman is approximately 1 in 70, with an age-adjusted annual incidence of approximately 13.7 cases per 100,000 women. This results in approximately 21,000 new cases of ovarian cancer and 12,500 deaths per annum.

These malignancies can occur at any age, including infancy and childhood; however, the overall age-specific incidence increases

dramatically with age. In women 40 years of age there are approximately 10 cases per 100,000, increasing to a peak incidence of approximately 45 cases per 100,000 women between the ages of 60 and 65 years.

The incidence of adnexal masses associated with pregnancy has been reported to range from 1 in 81 to 1 in 2500. With the use of ultrasound for routine fetal surveillance, the detection of previously unrecognized adnexal masses in both early and late gestation is likely to increase.

Of the adnexal masses noticed in pregnancy, approximately 50% will be less than 5 cm in diameter, whereas 25% are between 5 and 10 cm and 25% will be greater than 10 cm at the time of discovery. Ninety-five per cent of these also will be unilateral.

Unilateral, mobile, non-complex masses less than 5 cm, noticed in the first trimester, will resolve in greater than 90% of cases. It therefore is reasonable to observe non-suspicious neoplasms conservatively with repeat ultrasound into the second trimester (when elective surgical intervention is safest) to document spontaneous resolution.

A subgroup of patients undergoing assisted reproductive therapy with various ovulation-inducing medications present a unique situation. Because of the induced ovarian hyperstimulation and increased ultrasound surveillance, these patients will commonly have ovarian cysts noted in the first trimester. Spontaneous resolution of benign-appearing ovarian cysts can be expected in greater than 90% of patients who have undergone ovulation induction. Recent reports of possible associations between ovulation induction and an increased incidence of ovarian neoplasms should, however, be kept in mind, although this is considered to most likely be a long-term effect.

Adnexal masses can originate from multiple sources, and the differential diagnosis is complex, including multiple gynecologic and non-gynecologic entities. Fortunately, modern pelvic imaging, especially ultrasonography, aids greatly in differentiating the primary origins of these masses. The common types of neoplastic and non-neoplastic ovarian masses noticed during pregnancy are described in Tables 252–12 and 252–13. Most ovarian tumors occurring during early pregnancy are benign, with the most common neoplastic ovarian mass being a benign cystic teratoma.

EVALUATION OF PELVIC MASSES IN PREGNANCY

Pelvic Imaging

The key to evaluation of the pelvic/adnexal mass in pregnancy is to attempt to differentiate benign versus malignant process, to avoid unnecessary intervention.

Two to 5 per cent of adnexal masses persisting after the first trimester will be pathologically confirmed as being malignant, resulting in an overall malignancy rate of 1 in 5,000 to 18,000 live births.

Other than the acute presentation of abdominal pain associated with ovarian torsion, most common between the 6th and 14th weeks of gestation, these masses often are clinically inapparent and may be accompanied only with the vague non-specific abdominal discomfort common to pregnancy.

Real-time ultrasonography has revolutionized obstetrics and has become the most commonly used diagnostic tool in pregnancy.

Tumor Markers (see Chapter 192)

The use of CA-125 to differentiate malignant versus benign adnexal masses has been well described. Unfortunately, in the pre-

Table 252–9 ■ CELL CYCLE

CELL PHASE	APPROXIMATE TIME (HOURS)	ACTIVITY
G1 (gap 1)	Variable	RNA manufacture, preparation for DNA synthesis
S (synthesis)	8	DNA duplication
G2 (gap 2)	3	Spindle apparatus formation
M (mitosis)	1	Mitosis
G0 (gap 0)		Resting (quiescent)

Table 252-10 ■ SPECIFIC CHEMOTHERAPEUTIC AGENTS AND THEIR ACTIONS

AGENT	CELL-CYCLE ACTION	POTENTIAL FETAL TOXICITY
Alkylating agent: cyclophosphamide, ifosfamide, chlorambucil, nitrogen mustard, cisplatin	Non-specific	14% fetal malformations in first trimester; chlorambucil syndrome of renal aplasia, cleft palate, skeletal anomalies
Antitumor antibiotics: dactinomycin, mitomycin C, bleomycin, doxorubicin	Variable	None reported
Antimetabolites: 5-fluorouracil methotrexate, cytarabine	Cell Cycle specific	Multiple defects: cranial dysostocia, hypertelorism, micrognathia, cleft palate; contraindicated in pregnancy
Taxanes: paclitaxel	Cell cycle specific	No data in pregnancy
Biologic response modifiers: interleukins, interferons	Non-specific	Contraindicated in pregnancy
Hormones: tamoxifen, megestrol	Non-specific	Contraindicated in pregnancy

menopausal woman, the high rate of false-positive serum elevations in CA-125 makes this a relatively poor screening test.

MANAGEMENT OF THE PELVIC MASS IN PREGNANCY

The discovery of an asymptomatic adnexal mass in the first trimester should be viewed with cautious optimism. As described earlier, many of these are functional in nature (corpus luteum) and most will resolve spontaneously. Observation of non-suspicious (simple, non-complex, without excrescences, without ascites) lesions into the second trimester with repeat ultrasonographic assessment is appropriate.

Pelvic Surgery in Pregnancy

The timing of the surgical intervention cannot always be controlled and emergent situations occasionally arise.

If laparotomy is required during the first trimester, spontaneous abortion is more likely, possibly because of disruption of the delicate corpus luteum. After 7 to 10 weeks of gestation the trophoblast is capable of supplying sufficient quantities of specific steroid hormones for the maintenance of the gestation.

Should surgical extirpation of the corpus luteum be required in the first trimester, progestin support is recommended. A daily intramuscular injection of 100 mg of progesterone in oil or a 100-mg transvaginal suppository every 12 hours provides adequate progestin replacement. A mass that is first noted in the third trimester is best managed by awaiting fetal maturity if the clinical suspicion of malignancy is low.

The optimal timing of elective surgical intervention is during the second trimester. Apparent risk of preterm labor with subsequent fetal morbidity seems to be lessened. Uterine size at this gestational age does not preclude appropriate aortic and upper abdominal surgical exposure. Severe third-trimester complications are associated with failure to remove significant ovarian masses during mid pregnancy.

BREAST CANCER IN PREGNANCY (See Chapter 258)

Cancer of the breast occurring during pregnancy or within the first year after delivery is considered pregnancy-associated breast carcinoma (PABC). Breast carcinoma remains the second most common malignancy occurring in the pregnant patient and impacts approximately 1 in 3000 pregnancies in the United States.

Traditionally, PABC has been thought to carry a poorer prognosis; however, recent matched controlled data do not support this claim. Unfortunately, women with PABC are more commonly diagnosed with locally advanced node positive disease at time of diagnosis (61% vs. 38%). The obvious adverse effect of advanced disease is reflected by a decrease in 5-year survival from 82% (node negative) to 47% in the node-positive group. Pregnant patients are also two and one-half times more likely to present with distant metastatic disease at the time of diagnosis as compared with their non-pregnant counterparts.

Both the patient as well as the clinician must be continually vigilant to subtle breast changes. Most PABCs initially present as a painless mass and more than 90% are detected during patient self-breast examination. Similar diagnostic algorithms should be applied in both the pregnant and non-pregnant patient with a suspicious breast lesion. Fine-needle aspiration, diagnostic mammography, ultrasonography and open-breast biopsy pose no documented fetal risk. The historical reluctance to aggressively pursue histologic diagnosis of breast masses in pregnancy is unwarranted and perhaps detrimental.

A recent series of 134 breast biopsies performed during pregnancy revealed a 21% incidence of malignancy, thereby confirming the need for aggressive measures. As in non-pregnant women, infiltrating ductal carcinoma continues to be the most common histologic subtype encountered.

Breast ultrasonography is an important adjunct in the evaluation of the palpable or mammographically demonstrated breast lesion. Its ability to differentiate cystic versus solid lesions can provide useful information and can guide subsequent diagnostic decisions. On characterization of a breast mass the most common initial diagnostic modality of choice is the fine-needle aspiration.

Management of Breast Carcinoma in Pregnancy

The initial approach to breast carcinoma is most commonly surgical. Depending on the clinical stage, either breast-conserving

Table 252-11 ■ COMPARISON OF PAPANICOLAOU SMEAR CYTOLOGIC NOMENCLATURE

BETHESDA SYSTEM	CIN SYSTEM	HISTOLOGY
Normal	Normal	Normal
Benign cellular changes; requires specific annotation	Inflammatory atypia	Atypical cells
Squamous cell abnormalities		
Atypical squamous cells of undetermined significance (ASCUS)	CIN I	Mild dysplasia
Low-grade squamous intraepithelial lesion	CIN I	Mild dysplasia
High-grade squamous intraepithelial lesion	CIN II or III	Moderate or severe dysplasia

Table 252-12 ■ DIFFERENTIAL DIAGNOSIS OF THE PELVIC MASS

Gynecologic
  Ovary
    Benign (Functional)
    Neoplastic (Benign, malignant)
  Fallopian tube
    Hydrosalpinx
    Tubo-ovarian abscess
    Ectopic pregnancy
  Uterine
    Benign (Leiomyomata)
    Malignant (Sarcoma)
Non-gynecologic
  Gastrointestinal
    Colon (including stool, diverticular disease)
    Small bowel
    Appendix
  Mesothelial tumors
  Lymphoma
  Retroperitoneal neoplasm
  Pelvic kidney
  Urachal cyst
  Mesenteric cyst
  Metastatic disease
  Sacral meningocele
  Distended bladder

Table 252–13 ■ HISTOLOGIC TYPE OF NON-NEOPLASTIC OVARIAN TUMORS IN PREGNANCY

HISTOLOGIC TYPE	FREQUENCY (%)
Endometriotic	14.0
Paraovarian	11.0
Simple cyst	12.0
Corpus luteal	50.0
Unknown	6.0
Miscellaneous	
Luteoma	1.0
Ovarian edema	1.0
Thecal lutein	5.0

Data from Stedman C, Kline R: Intraoperative complications and unexpected pathology at the time of cesarean section. Obstet Gynecol Clin North Am 15:756, 1988.

lumpectomy or mastectomy both with axillary lymph node dissection is undertaken.

After surgical resection and lymph node evaluation a decision on adjuvant therapy must be made. In surgically documented, early-stage disease, a complete metastatic work-up is not warranted given the low yield. Therefore, decisions regarding the need for adjuvant therapy are usually based on the initial choice of surgical procedure. Again given the potential harm of radiation therapy to the developing fetus, a radical mastectomy with lymph node dissection is usually the procedure of choice, thereby eliminating the need for postoperative radiation therapy.

Chemotherapeutic intervention has been advocated in cases of locally advanced and advanced carcinoma of the breast. As described previously it is prudent to avoid chemotherapeutic intervention during the critical period of organogenesis in a desired pregnancy (see section on chemotherapy in pregnancy).

MELANOMA IN PREGNANCY (See Chapter 520)

The overall incidence of cutaneous melanoma appears to be increasing, and it has been estimated that 1 in 90 persons will be diagnosed with this neoplasm in 2000. Some literature suggests that the incidence of melanoma complicating pregnancy will exceed that of cervical carcinoma.

Risk factors documented to increase the risk of melanoma development are outlined in Table 252–14. Increased awareness among both physicians and patients as well as improved screening appears to have led to a tendency toward earlier diagnosis. These lesions tend to occur in sun-exposed areas; however, it must be recalled that 17% of melanomas diagnosed in the female population are found on the vulva and perineum. This high incidence provides the basis for aggressive biopsy of suspicious pigmented vulvar lesions.

Initial treatment of a melanotic lesion is the same in a pregnant or non-pregnant patient. Wide local excision with adequate surgical margins remains the procedure of choice.

The fetal risk of maternal melanoma is not well defined. It remains the most common malignancy to metastasize to the placenta and fetus. Although overall the incidence appears to be extremely low (approximately 60 cases reported), careful pathologic examination of the placenta is warranted. In documented cases of placental spread the fetal risk appears to be as high as 40 to 50%. Data suggesting an altered clinical course in the pregnant patient with melanoma has also been suggested. This observational data implies a potential hormonal influence on the melanotic process. Given the well-documented cutaneous manifestations of pregnancy, including increased pigmentation of the vulva, areola, as well as

Table 252–14 ■ RISK FACTORS ASSOCIATED WITH DEVELOPMENT OF CUTANEOUS MELANOMA

Fair complexion
Tendency toward easy sunburning
Early age of first sunburn
Inability to tan
Familial history of malignant melanoma
Personal history of melanoma
Environmental exposure to ultraviolet B irradiation

linea nigra, some have postulated that the increased levels of estrogen, progesterone, adrenocorticotropic hormone, as well as melanin-stimulating hormone may somehow influence melanoma growth.

THYROID CANCER IN PREGNANCY (See Chapter 239)

Thyroid cancer is the most commonly diagnosed endocrinologic malignancy, with approximately 16,100 cases noted in 1997 of which about 11,000 were in women. Of these cases almost half were documented in reproductive-aged women (ages 15–44 years); thus, thyroid carcinoma complicating pregnancy is not uncommon. Thyroid nodules are common and are often encountered during initial prenatal evaluation (they represent benign entities in approximately 90% of cases).

The diagnostic evaluation of the thyroid nodule in the pregnant patients is usually limited to physical examination, laboratory studies, and thyroid ultrasonography followed by fine needle or excisional biopsy. Specifically, nuclear medicine scintigraphy scans are omitted due to concerns of radioactive ^{123}I or ^{131}I effects on the fetal thyroid. Transplacental passage of iodine is well documented.

After an appropriate diagnosis, surgical resection remains the primary mode of treatment. The timing of this intervention remains an important decision. A recent retrospective review suggests equivalent outcomes in the patients who undergo thyroidectomy during pregnancy when compared with waiting until the postpartum state. Radionuclide thyroid ablation is contraindicated during pregnancy.

COLORECTAL CANCER IN PREGNANCY (See Chapter 139)

The lifetime risk of colorectal carcinoma in women is 1 in 17 (6%), with the vast majority of these being diagnosed after age 50. Only 8% of cases are noted in the reproductive age group (< age 40). A similar increase in incidence may be noted as childbearing is delayed.

More than 80% of colorectal carcinomas associated with pregnancy occur in the rectum (commonly below the peritoneal reflection and thus palpable on digital rectal examination). Diagnostic delays are usually attributed to the increased frequency of rectal bleeding episodes common to pregnancy (usually hemorrhoid related) and thus decreased clinical suspicion. Symptoms associated with advanced disease such as abdominal pain, distention, and constipation are rarely encountered.

The diagnosis of colorectal carcinoma includes a detailed history of risk factors such as history of polyps or family history of carcinoma (including gastrointestinal, breast, etc.), a complete lymph node survey, a digital rectal examination with Hemoccult testing, as well as a sigmoidoscopy or colonoscopy. A serum marker such as carcinoembryonic antigen determination is of no value in pregnancy because it is elevated in the normal gestation.

Management of colorectal carcinoma is most commonly surgical, and similar surgical practices as outlined previously should be followed.

The prognosis for a woman diagnosed with colorectal carcinoma in pregnancy is similar to that of matched non-pregnant controls. Postoperative local adjuvant pelvic radiation therapy is obviously contraindicated in a desired pregnancy.

HEMATOLOGIC MALIGNANCY IN PREGNANCY
(See Chapters 179 and 180)

Hematologic malignancies complicating pregnancy are rare. Hodgkin's disease, considered a primary lymph node malignancy, commonly affects young adults and is the most common hematologic malignancy associated with pregnancy. An incidence of 1 in 5000 live births has been reported. Specific histologic subtypes, epidemiology, as well as proposed etiologic agents are discussed elsewhere in this text (see Chapter 180).

More than 70% of patients diagnosed with Hodgkin's disease initially present with painless lymphadenopathy, commonly noted in the cervical, submaxillary, or axillary chains. Systemic signs often associated with advanced disease include night sweats, fever, weight loss, and fatigue. Diagnosis depends on appropriate lymph node biopsy and documentation of the pathognomonic Reed-Sternberg cell.

Staging modalities include physical examination; CT of chest, abdomen, and pelvis; lymphangiography; as well as occasional staging laparotomy with splenectomy. The use of abdominopelvic CT is not recommended in pregnancy, although magnetic resonance imaging can be done safely. Both the surgeon as well as oncologist must carefully consider decisions on risk versus benefit of staging laparotomy on both fetus and mother.

Chemotherapy can be toxic to ovarian function, and its risk seems to be related to patient age. Commonly used protocols consisting of mechlorethamine, vincristine, procarbazine, and prednisone (MOPP) result in amenorrhea in one third of patients, with permanent ovarian failure occurring in 75% of patients older than age 30 at the time of treatment. It appears that the doxorubicin, bleomycin, vinblastine, dacarbazine (ABVD) regimen is potentially less toxic, with an approximate risk of amenorrhea being 5%.

PHEOCHROMOCYTOMA IN PREGNANCY (See Chapter 241)

While only rarely encountered in pregnancy, a pheochromocytoma represents a unique neoplastic event with significant morbidity and mortality to both mother and fetus. It most commonly represents a non-malignant entity, although malignant differentiation can occur. They are most commonly found within the adrenal medulla, although they can also arise from the chromaffin cell within sympathetic ganglia.

In pregnancy the syndrome is usually manifested by severe episodes of hypertension usually not associated with significant proteinuria. It can be easily confused with an atypical presentation of preeclampsia. Associated signs and symptoms include tachycardia, palpitations, headache, diaphoresis, and anxiety. Given its rarity, the diagnosis is often unsuspected. If the pheochromocytoma is undiagnosed and therefore not treated, maternal and fetal mortality rates exceed 16 and 26%, respectively.

CONCLUSION

The diagnosis of cancer in pregnancy presents a unique management dilemma that ultimately affects two patients. The decision process is complicated by the significant risks to the fetus in terms of developmental abnormalities and preterm delivery and to the mother in terms of the malignant process itself. Multiple social, ethical, moral, and religious issues also play an important part in the decision tree.

The treatment of these patients should remain unbiased, well researched, and, above all, multidisciplinary. Basic aspects of cancer screening must be maintained even during pregnancy, and signs and symptoms of serious neoplastic processes must not be overlooked.

Chez RA (ed): Cancer in pregnancy. Clin Consult Obstet Gynecol 7(4), 1995. *Good review of radiation effects in pregnancy and fetal development.*

Hoskins WJ, Perez AC, Young RC: Principles and Practice of Gynecologic Oncology, 2nd ed. Philadelphia, Lippincott–Raven 1997. *General reference on management of carcinoma in pregnancy.*

Sorosky JI (ed): Cancer complicating pregnancy. Obstet Gynecol Clin North Am 25;2, 1998. *Excellent review of specific gynecologic and nongynecologic malignancy in pregnancy, including ethical issues.*

253 PREGNANCY: HYPERTENSION AND OTHER COMMON MEDICAL PROBLEMS

Diane L. Elliot

Caring for women of reproductive age requires understanding how to diagnose pregnancy and manage medical problems during gestation. For the latter, considerations are the pregnancy's influence on the illness, the condition's effects on the pregnancy, and appropriate management to optimize the well-being of both mother and fetus.

DIAGNOSIS AND MANAGEMENT OF PREGNANCY

Laboratory testing for pregnancy is suggested for women with suspected pregnancy, amenorrhea, pelvic pain, and scheduled radiographic studies. Historical information (e.g., last menses, sexual activity, contraceptive practices) has limited use in excluding pregnancy, which is especially true among teenage girls. When seen in an acute setting, approximately 10% of pregnant adolescents reported no sexual activity.

Serum and urine pregnancy tests use monoclonal antibodies for the intact human chorionic gonadotropin (hCG) molecule or its β-subunit. hCG is synthesized by the placenta. Two weeks after conception, the hCG level is approximately 80 mIU/mL, with comparable serum and urine values. During a normal intrauterine pregnancy, the level doubles every 2 days. Monoclonal assays can detect hCG at a level of 20 mIU/mL, resulting in a sensitivity for pregnancy of more than 90% at the time of the first missed menses. Several home urine tests, also using monoclonal antibodies, are available. Although these claim to be 99% accurate, when assessed, the user accuracy was only 77%, with a sensitivity of 80% and a specificity of 68% for diagnosing pregnancy.

Transabdominal ultrasonography can detect a gestational sac 5 to 6 weeks after conception. Before that time, sequential hCG levels may be needed to distinguish an ectopic from an intrauterine pregnancy. A fetal heartbeat is detectable by ultrasound by 7 to 8 weeks and is audible with Doppler at 10 to 12 weeks. Quickening and fetal heart tones by fetoscope both occur between 16 and 20 weeks of gestation.

When pregnancy is diagnosed, important issues to address include the woman's feelings about the pregnancy and the importance of early and continuous prenatal care. The clinician should assess the patient's nutrition, review her medications for contraindicated drugs, and emphasize discontinuing smoking and alcohol. Supplemental folic acid before and early in gestation halves the risk of neural tube defects, such as spina bifida and anencephaly. All women of childbearing age should receive additional folate, either as a daily multivitamin or fortified breakfast cereal. Laboratory tests such as a complete blood cell count, Rh determination, Papanicolaou smear and vaginal cultures, and screening for rubella, hepatitis, cytomegalovirus, and toxoplasmosis antibodies usually are deferred until the first visit with the health care provider who will care for the woman during pregnancy and delivery.

HYPERTENSION

DEFINITION AND EPIDEMIOLOGY. Hypertension (see also Chapter 55) is the most common medical problem during pregnancy, with a prevalence of 7 to 12%. It is diagnosed when the blood pressure is greater than 140/90 mm Hg (in the sitting position) on two occasions. Previously, an increase of more than 30/15 mm Hg during pregnancy also was considered criteria, but this finding alone has poor predictive value.

DIAGNOSTIC CLASSIFICATION. Hypertension during pregnancy can be classified as (1) preeclampsia, (2) transient gestational or pregnancy-induced hypertension, (3) chronic hypertension, and (4) chronic hypertension plus preeclampsia. *Pregnancy-associated hypertension* is a more generic term and includes preeclampsia and transient gestational hypertension. During a normal pregnancy, blood pressure declines during the first and second trimesters, rising to pre-pregnancy levels near term. Because of the initial blood pressure decrement, when readings before pregnancy are not known, an elevation during the third trimester could represent either pre-existing or pregnancy-associated hypertension.

Preeclampsia and Transient Gestational Hypertension

DEFINITION AND EPIDEMIOLOGY. Preeclampsia usually develops during the third trimester, often after 32 weeks. Its incidence varies in different groups of women, with a prevalence of 6 to 10% in Western countries. Risks include prior preeclampsia, chronic hypertension, multifetal gestation, and diabetes. Typically, diastolic pressure increases more than systolic, and systolic levels often are less than 160 mm Hg (which should not be considered reassuring). Severe organ system dysfunction can occur with what would be only moderate hypertension among non-pregnant women. In addition to hypertension, criteria for preeclampsia are rapid weight gain (>2 kg/week), generalized edema, and proteinuria (>0.3 g/24 hours or >1+ on a random specimen). However, the spectrum of manifestations varies, and none of these indicators is required for the diagnosis. Among women with eclampsia (preeclampsia plus seizures), 20% did not have proteinuria and 40% did not have edema.

Hypertension without other manifestations of preeclampsia is termed *transient gestational* or *pregnancy-induced hypertension*. By definition, transient gestational hypertension resolves by 3 months post partum. It is not clear whether this is an early manifestation of preeclampsia or exposure of a predisposition for essential hypertension. This group is at increased risk for preeclampsia, and approximately one fourth with transient gestational hypertension will go on to preeclampsia during the pregnancy.

PATHOGENESIS. During a normal pregnancy, the implanted placenta replaces the endothelium and internal elastic lamina of the maternal uterine spiral arteries with fetal trophoblastic tissue. These altered arteries dilate to five times their pre-pregnant state and are no longer responsive to circulating vasoconstrictors. This trophoblastic invasion does not occur with preeclampsia, and the arteries do not dilate. Accordingly, the placenta is chronically underperfused. This is thought to result in the secondary widespread endothelial dysfunction, with activation of platelets and the coagulation cascade. In addition, women with preeclampsia fail to develop the normal increased blood volume and reduced systemic vascular resistance of pregnancy. Women develop an imbalance of vasoactive prostaglandins, with an increase in the ratio of thromboxane A_2 (vasoconstriction) to prostacyclin (vasodilation), leading to vasospasm. The rationale for low-dose acetylsalicylic acid is its inhibition of cyclooxygenase and selective reduction in thromboxane synthesis.

CLINICAL MANIFESTATIONS. Clinical criteria subdivide preeclampsia into severe and non-severe, based on the degree of blood pressure elevation and the presence of seizures (eclampsia) or other end-organ damage (renal dysfunction, pulmonary edema, thrombocytopenia, hepatic abnormalities, or central nervous system effects). Intravascular coagulation and hepatic ischemia can cause a constellation of findings, called the HELLP (*h*emolysis, *e*levated *l*iver functions and *l*ow *p*latelets) syndrome. Although delivery is the treatment of preeclampsia, a small percentage of manifestations are seen immediately post partum.

Laboratory tests do not reliably predict development of preeclampsia, nor do they differentiate among the different hypertensive disorders. Serum uric acid levels were considered useful in identifying preeclampsia. However, when evaluated in a nested-case control study, an individual's level could not be used to classify her hypertension.

MANAGEMENT. Transient gestational hypertension is treated with bed rest, close monitoring, and medications, when necessary. When to initiate antihypertensive drug treatment is controversial. Many authorities recommend drug therapy when the blood pressure persistently exceeds 140/90 mm Hg. Drug therapy reduces perinatal deaths and severe maternal hypertension. However, for women with pre-existing hypertension, it has not been shown to affect development of preeclampsia. The experience with antihypertensive medication in pregnancy appears in Table 253–1. The definitive treatment of preeclampsia and transient gestational hypertension is delivery. Before 34 weeks of gestation, that benefit is weighed against the fetal advantages of prolonging intrauterine development.

PREVENTION. Supplemental calcium (2 g/day) reduces the incidence of preeclampsia, without any recognized maternal or fetal adverse effects. Epidemiologic studies had suggested an inverse relationship between calcium intake and preeclampsia, which led to prospective trials of its use. Current studies suggest that low-dose acetylsalicylic acid (60 to 81 mg/day) may be preventive when at higher risk of preeclampsia, but its use is not justified for all pregnant women.

Chronic Hypertension and Chronic Hypertension with Preeclampsia

ETIOLOGY AND EPIDEMIOLOGY. Most of the 1 to 5% of women of reproductive age with hypertension have essential hypertension. For the unusual individual with secondary hypertension, causes include intrinsic renal disease, renal artery stenosis, aortic coarctation, connective disease diseases, and Cushing's disease.

Although there are fewer than 250 reported cases, pheochromocytoma during pregnancy produces significant morbidity and mor-

Table 253–1 ■ ANTIHYPERTENSIVE DRUG USE DURING PREGNANCY*

MEDICATION	SAFETY OF USE DURING PREGNANCY	COMMENTS
Methyldopa (central sympatholytic)	++++	Extensive use; best studied antihypertensive used during pregnancy. It reduces vascular resistance while preserving maternal cardiac output and uteroplacental perfusion.
α- and β-blockers (labetalol)	++++	Agents block both α- and β-receptors. α-Blocking results in vasodilation (including uteroplacental blood vessels), and β-blockade prevents reflex tachycardia. Cardiac output is unchanged.
β-blockers (atenolol, pindolol, metoprolol, oxprenolol)	+++	Probably safe for third trimester use, but neonatal bradycardia, respiratory distress, and hypoglycemia have been reported. Use earlier in gestation may result in intrauterine growth retardation.
Hydralazine (direct arterial vasodilator)	++++	Extensively used during pregnancy. It causes vascular dilatation and a reflex tachycardia. Primarily used parenterally for acute management of hypertension or with methyldopa or a β-blocker for treatment of pregnancy-associated hypertension.
Calcium-channel blockers (nifedipine most commonly used, owing to its having primarily peripheral effects)	+++	Probably safely used in the third trimester. Their use maintains uteroplacental perfusion; may also have tocolytic effects. Avoid use with magnesium sulfate, because combination risks profound hypotension.
Diuretics	+	Use during pregnancy is controversial. Often discontinued as blood pressure decreases, early in pregnancy. If used before pregnancy, it can be continued, but its use should not be initiated during pregnancy.
Clonidine	++	Although it has been used safely, it is not a first-line antihypertensive agent during pregnancy. It has the potential for rebound when discontinued abruptly.
Angiotensin-converting enzyme inhibitors and angiotensin II receptor antagonists	0	Use is contraindicated during pregnancy, because miscarriage, fetal death, malformations, and neonatal renal failure can result. No reports of adverse effects from brief use, limited to the first trimester.

*Drugs listed have established effects during pregnancy. Antihypertensive agents not listed may be safe during pregnancy; however, until that is known, those drugs should be switched to one of the safely used listed agents.

tality. Its features (headache, excessive perspiration, and palpitations) overlap with those of pregnancy, and evaluation with urinary catecholamines is indicated for all women with newly diagnosed hypertension before 34 weeks of pregnancy.

MANAGEMENT. Among women with pre-existing hypertension, the usual blood pressure decrease during the first trimester may allow gradual discontinuation of antihypertensive medications. Pharmacologic treatment can be reinstituted during the third trimester, at a threshold of 140/90 to 100 mm Hg. Chronic hypertension, newly diagnosed during pregnancy, can be differentiated from transient gestational hypertension, because the former persists for more than 3 months post partum.

PROGNOSIS AND PREVENTION. Eighty-five per cent of hypertensive women have uncomplicated pregnancies. Chronic hypertension is associated with an increased risk of preeclampsia. Its fetal risks directly relate to the maternal blood pressure and include abruptio placentae, intrauterine growth restriction, and fetal death. Women with pre-existing hypertension are followed more closely during gestation, often with additional home blood pressure monitoring. The use of calcium and low-dose acetylsalicylic acid for preeclampsia prevention has not been established for women with pre-existing hypertension.

CARDIAC DISEASE (See also Part VII)

ETIOLOGY AND EPIDEMIOLOGY. The prevalence of heart disease during pregnancy is approximately 1%. In Western countries, congenital lesions have surpassed rheumatic heart disease as its most common etiology.

PATHOGENESIS. Understanding the hemodynamic changes during normal pregnancy permits interpretation of history and physical examination findings and anticipation of pregnancy's effect on pre-existing cardiac abnormalities. During gestation, cardiac output increases 30 to 50%, peaking near week 27. This increase is due to greater heart rate and stroke volume, plus a decrease in systemic vascular resistance. Blood volume also expands, with a greater plasma than red blood cell mass increase, resulting in the physiologic anemia of pregnancy.

A woman's previous cardiac functional status is a guide to pregnancy's effects. Women with New York Heart Association Functional Class I or II heart disease (no symptoms with normal daily activities) usually can withstand pregnancy. Because of the decreased systemic vascular resistance, regurgitant lesions are tolerated better than stenotic left-sided abnormalities. At greatest risk are women with pulmonary hypertension (either primary or Eisenmenger's syndrome), with limitations in right-sided output. The mortality during pregnancy among this last group approaches 50%.

CLINICAL MANIFESTATIONS AND MANAGEMENT. Normal pregnancy results in findings that can simulate heart disease. More than 50% of normal pregnant women complain of dyspnea. Physical findings of congestive heart failure also are common during pregnancy. The increased stroke volume results in approximately 90% having a systolic flow murmur, and an S_3 is audible in a significant percentage of normal pregnant women. The electrocardiogram can show anterior T-wave changes, owing to leftward myocardial rotation late in gestation. Echocardiography retains its utility during pregnancy and may be needed to characterize abnormal findings during pregnancy.

Pregnancy is proarrhythmic, and both atrial and ventricular ectopy increase. Among women with structurally normal hearts, these are benign and managed expectantly. The therapy for most arrhythmias is not altered during pregnancy. Drug therapy is needed only for intolerable symptoms or threats to maternal or fetal well-being. Cardioversion does not present increased risk for the mother or fetus, and most antiarrhythmic drugs are not contraindicated during pregnancy. Adenosine can be used safely for terminating atrioventricular node–dependent tachyarrhythmias. Most class I agents also are safe. Digoxin dosage usually requires an increase, owing to the reduced protein binding and increased renal excretion during pregnancy. Amiodarone should be avoided during gestation. As with most antiarrhythmic drugs, it crosses the placenta and can cause fetal goiter, growth retardation, and neonatal hypothyroidism. β-Blocker and calcium channel blocker use is discussed in the preceding section on hypertension.

Certain cardiac abnormalities pose unique considerations. For women with Marfan syndrome, pregnancy's connective tissue changes and hyperdynamic state can increase the risk for aortic dissection. However, the risk is acceptably low when the pre-pregnancy aortic diameter is less than 40 mm. Women with repaired aortic coarctation have successful pregnancies, with a pre-eclampsia incidence similar to the general population when the arm:leg blood pressure difference is less than 20 mm Hg. Ischemic cardiac disease is rare during gestation, with a prevalence of 1 in 10,000 pregnancies. When present, it usually is associated with cocaine use or accelerated atherosclerotic vascular disease (e.g., long-standing type I diabetes or hyperlipidemia).

Peripartum cardiomyopathy is defined as onset of a global dilated cardiomyopathy during the third trimester to 6 months post partum. Its prevalence is 1 in 4000 pregnancies. Because the changes of pregnancy may unmask a pre-existing cardiomyopathy, it is difficult to secure a uniform patient cohort. Risk factors for peripartum cardiomyopathy include obesity, African American heritage, and multiple prior pregnancies. Its cause is not understood, and prognosis is variable. Overall, approximately one third stabilize, one third progress, and one third improve. Both recurrence and normal outcomes have been described with subsequent pregnancies.

PROGNOSIS. A retrospective study of 276 pregnancies among 221 women with heart disease (excluding isolated mitral valve prolapse) showed that 96% of individuals were functional Class I or II. Approximately 25% of pregnancies resulted in a maternal and/or neonatal cardiac adverse event. Based on clinical and echocardiographic assessment, independent predictors of cardiac events were prior cardiac events, previous arrhythmias, functional Class more than II, left-sided heart obstruction, and myocardial dysfunction. With no, one, or more than one factor, maternal events were 3, 30, and 66%, respectively. These predictors have not been prospectively validated, and few women with certain cardiac problems were included in the cohort. However, the results are consistent with pregnancy's hemodynamic changes and can be combined with lesion-specific considerations when advising women with heart disease about the risk of pregnancy.

An additional prognostic consideration for women with congenital heart disease is their offsprings' recurrence rate. The rate of congenital heart disease is increased tenfold above normal. However, because this rate varies with different abnormalities, referral for genetic counseling is appropriate.

THROMBOEMBOLIC DISEASE

EPIDEMIOLOGY. Thromboembolism (deep venous thrombosis and pulmonary emboli) is uncommon during pregnancy, with a prevalence of 1 per 2000 pregnancies. However, when they occur, maternal morbidity is high and thromboemboli are the leading non-obstetric cause of maternal mortality.

PATHOGENESIS. Pregnancy results in physical and biochemical changes that increase clot formation approximately fivefold. During gestation, the venous system dilates and stasis is increased further by obstruction from the gravid uterus. The plasma concentration of coagulation factors, fibrinolysis inhibitors, and procoagulants shift to promote coagulation. Those women with a hereditary thrombophilic disorder (activated protein C resistance, protein C and S deficiency, and antithrombin deficiency) have high rates of thrombosis during pregnancy.

Antiphospholipid antibodies result in platelet activation and, despite these patients' prolonged partial thromboplastin times, lead to thrombosis. During pregnancy, these patients are prone to placental thrombosis and infarction, causing recurrent pregnancy loss, intrauterine growth retardation, fetal death, severe preeclampsia, and maternal arterial and venous thromboemboli.

CLINICAL MANIFESTATIONS. The symptoms and signs of deep venous thrombosis (DVT) and pulmonary emboli retain their low sensitivity and specificity during pregnancy, and findings are limited further by the lower extremity edema that is a feature of many normal pregnancies. During gestation, the distribution of DVTs is altered, and they are much more common in the left leg.

In addition, for unexplained reasons, the pulmonary alveolar-arterial oxygen gradient may be normal in more than 50% of pregnant women with documented pulmonary emboli. That percentage is much greater than that rate among non-pregnant patients (2 to 20%). (During the third trimester, arterial Po_2 is altered by position, with sitting values approximately 15 mm Hg higher than when supine.)

DIAGNOSIS. Diagnostic options include non-invasive studies (e.g., compression ultrasonography, Doppler studies, and impedance plethysmography), lung ventilation-perfusion scan, and pulmonary angiography. The operating characteristics of non-invasive studies of the lower extremities appear similar to non-pregnant results, provided women are evaluated in the lateral decubitus position. Magnetic resonance imaging can be used to detect iliac and ovarian vein thrombosis.

Fetal radiation exposure is a consideration when selecting diagnostic tests for pulmonary emboli. However, most procedures can be performed with minimal risk. Ventilation and perfusion scanning result in fetal radiation of 0.01 and 0.015 rad, respectively. Pulmonary angiography (by the brachial route) exposes the fetus to 0.05 rad. These are low amounts of radiation, because fetal risk is thought to increase after approximately 5 rad of radiation exposure.

MANAGEMENT. Initial anticoagulation usually is with intravenous heparin, followed by adjusted dose subcutaneous low-molecular-weight (LMW) heparin. The intravenous heparin requirements are variable, and higher than the usual doses may be required for anticoagulation during pregnancy. Heparins, including LMW forms, are large, charged molecules that do not cross the placenta or cause fetal problems. Warfarin (Coumadin) causes an embryopathy, and its use is avoided during pregnancy.

LMW heparin has a longer half-life and more uniform dose response than unfractionated heparin. Although studies during pregnancy are few, as with non-pregnant patients, subcutaneous LMW heparin is as effective as intravenous or adjusted-dose subcutaneous unfractionated heparin therapy. Treatment must be adjusted during labor and delivery, either by holding the subcutaneous dosing, switching to lower-dose subcutaneous prophylaxis, or initiating intravenous heparin. Eight hours after delivery, subcutaneous heparin therapy can be resumed and continued for 6 to 12 weeks post partum.

Risks of heparin therapy include thrombocytopenia and osteopenia. Heparin-induced thrombocytopenia develops in 2% of those treated with unfractionated heparin. Despite the thrombocytopenia, the disorder is characterized by arterial and venous thromboses. It can be suspected when platelets decrease and confirmed by assaying for the causative heparin-induced antibody. The disorder's risk is less with LMW heparin, but LMW heparin cannot be substituted, when heparin-induced thrombocytopenia develops while on unfractionated heparin. Heparin-associated osteoporosis can occur when individuals receive more than 20,000 U/day for more than 3 months; this risk also may be less with LMW heparin.

PREVENTION. When a woman has experienced a DVT during pregnancy, has a hereditary thrombophilic disorder, or has antiphospholipid antibodies, her DVT risk during a subsequent pregnancy is increased significantly. The indications for and preferred method of prophylaxis are not established. Subcutaneous unfractionated heparin, at a dose of 5000 units twice a day, has been used. For prophylaxis, the heparin level should be 0.08 to 0.20 U/mL, 3 hours after an injection. Often, the dose must be increased by 2500 units each trimester to achieve that level. More recently, LMW heparin has been replacing that therapy, using a fixed dose slightly less than used for DVT treatment and compara-

ble to the prophylactic dose used in surgical patients. The management of pregnant women with antiphospholipid antibodies is dependent of the presence of prior problems and associated conditions. At a minimum, low-dose acetylsalicylic acid is administered. Aspirin and prophylactic heparin are given if the woman has experienced thromboembolic problems during a prior pregnancy. When heparin is contraindicated (e.g., with thrombocytopenia), low-dose acetylsalicylic acid plus prednisone and intravenous IgG may be used.

ASTHMA (See also Chapter 74)

EPIDEMIOLOGY. Asthma is the most common chronic respiratory illness during pregnancy, with a prevalence of 1 to 7%.

PATHOGENESIS AND CLINICAL MANIFESTATIONS. Pregnancy is accompanied by changes that alleviate reactive airway disease and others that exacerbate bronchoconstriction, with little net alteration of pulmonary function during gestation. The course of asthma during pregnancy is variable and cannot be predicted from patient characteristics. In general, half of the women remain stable, one fourth improve, and one fourth worsen. Those with more severe disease and a history of prior exacerbations during pregnancy are at greatest risk for deterioration during gestation.

MANAGEMENT. Management is similar to that of asthma in non-pregnant individuals. Table 253–2 lists therapies commonly prescribed for asthma, with comments about their use during pregnancy. Up to 50% of women with asthma do not require drug treatment during pregnancy. When indicated, medication use is similar to use by the non-pregnant individual. Inhaled and oral β_2-agonists can be used during pregnancy. These are tocolytic agents and rarely have been reported to inhibit labor. Inhaled cromolyn sodium can be continued. Aminophylline crosses the placenta, but, other than rare reports of newborn jitteriness, it is safe during pregnancy; however, its clearance is reduced in the third trimester, and levels should be monitored. There are little data on use of inhaled ipratropium during pregnancy, although it probably is safe.

Maternal hypoxia, hypocapnia, and alkalemia are detrimental to the fetus. Exacerbations should be treated early and aggressively; oxygen is needed if PaO_2 is less than 75 mm Hg. The typical exacerbation triggers are respiratory infections and gastroesophageal reflux. During pregnancy, bronchopulmonary infections can be treated with erythromycin (avoiding the estolate esters), penicillins, and first- and second-generation cephalosporins. Tetracycline and trimethoprim/sulfamethoxazole are contraindicated.

Corticosteroids, both inhaled and systemically administered, can be used during pregnancy. The use of inhaled corticosteroids decreases the number of asthma exacerbations during pregnancy. Among inhaled corticosteroids, beclomethasone has been used most extensively and is the preferred agent. The risk of an asthma exacerbation compromising pregnancy far outweighs any potential corticosteroid risk. In addition, prednisone is metabolized by the placenta, which limits fetal exposure to the active drug. Women using oral corticosteroids near term require "stress doses" at the time of delivery.

PROGNOSIS. With current therapy and avoidance of hypoxia, the additional maternal and fetal morbidity associated with asthma usually is low. Risk of antepartum and postpartum hemorrhage is increased slightly, and women requiring corticosteroids are more likely to develop pregnancy-associated hypertension. Offspring of asthmatic women are more subject to hyperbilirubinemia.

Table 253–2 ■ **DRUG TREATMENT OF ASTHMA DURING PREGNANCY**

THERAPY	COMMENTS
Desensitization or immunotherapy ("allergy shots")	Do not begin desensitization during pregnancy, but ongoing therapy can be continued.
Disodium cromoglycolate	Less than 10% of drug is absorbed. No reported adverse effects from use during pregnancy.
Aminophylline	Distribution and clearance altered during pregnancy, and levels should be checked monthly. It crosses the placenta; and, rarely, neonatal toxicity has been reported, despite therapeutic maternal levels.
β-Agonists	Use is safe during pregnancy. Rare report of tocolytic effects.
Inhaled corticosteroids	Regular use reduces asthma exacerbations during pregnancy.
Oral corticosteroids	May be used safely, when indicated. Ninety per cent of prednisone is inactivated by the placenta, reducing fetal exposure. Betamethasone does not undergo placental 11-oxidation and is the preferred corticosteroid when promoting fetal lung maturation.
Anticholinergics	Experience is limited, but use is believed to be safe.

Fetal thyroid gland development is independent of maternal hormone levels, because the placenta is impermeable to thyroid hormones and thyroid-stimulating hormone (TSH). The critical period for thyroid hormone's effects on fetal brain maturation is 1 month before birth through the first year of life. Although thyroid hormones do not cross the placenta, antithyroid therapeutic agents do. Both situations must be considered when managing maternal thyroid illness.

Pregnancy alters certain indices of maternal thyroid function. Thyroid binding globulin increases during pregnancy, leading to an elevation of total thyroxine and a decreased T_3 resin uptake. However, free thyroxine and the calculated thyroid index accurately reflect thyroid function during pregnancy. TSH levels are altered only slightly and remain a useful means of screening for hypothyroidism and for assessing the adequacy of thyroid hormone replacement.

Hypothyroidism

EPIDEMIOLOGY. Hypothyroidism frequently is associated with anovulation, resulting in reduced fertility. Hence, the coexistence of untreated hypothyroidism and pregnancy is rare.

MANAGEMENT. Women on thyroid replacement should have their TSH levels monitored each trimester. Approximately 20% will require a dose increase during pregnancy. The absorption of levothyroxine is inhibited by iron, and women should be reminded not to take thyroid replacement with prenatal vitamins.

Hyperthyroidism

EPIDEMIOLOGY. Hyperthyroidism develops during 0.02 to 0.3% of pregnancies, and it follows diabetes as the most common endocrine disorder during pregnancy.

ETIOLOGY. Hyperthyroid pregnant women are presumed to have Graves' disease, and thyroid scanning is contraindicated during pregnancy. hCG and TSH share the same α-subunit, and hCG weakly cross-reacts with TSH. A molar pregnancy, with high hCG levels, is a rare cause of hyperthyroidism.

CLINICAL MANIFESTATIONS. Certain findings of hyperthyroidism (e.g., tachycardia, sensation of warmth, fatigue) are features of a normal pregnancy. Rather than the traditional symptoms of weight loss, hyperthyroidism during pregnancy can cause an inappropriately low weight gain. Although the usual clinical findings are limited during pregnancy, treating gestational hyperthyroidism significantly improves maternal and fetal outcomes. Accordingly, a low threshold for obtaining thyroid function tests during pregnancy is appropriate.

MANAGEMENT. The hyperthyroid pregnant woman is treated medically with propylthiouracil (PTU). Radioactive iodine is absolutely contraindicated during pregnancy, because it will also affect the fetus. Surgical treatment of hyperthyroidism is reserved for the unusual individual with complications from medical therapy.

Medical therapy usually is initiated with a PTU dose of 100 mg three times a day, with tapering based on measured thyroid hormone levels. PTU is preferred because of the rare report of aplasia cutis with methimazole and PTU's lower placental permeability. β-Blockers may be necessary transiently to control initial symptoms.

PTU treatment usually reduces the thyroid hormone level within 3 to 4 weeks, at which time the dose is tapered to 50 mg three times a day. Thyroid function is monitored monthly, and the therapeutic goal is the lowest PTU dose needed to maintain maternal thyroid hormone levels in the high-normal range. PTU crosses the placenta, whereas thyroid hormones and TSH do not. Infants are at risk for a neonatal goiter when prenatal PTU dosage is more than 100 mg/day. Because of the "immunosuppression" of pregnancy, tapering the PTU dose usually is possible, and approximately one third of women can discontinue PTU therapy in the last trimester.

PROGNOSIS. Graves' disease may worsen postpartum; and because fetal exposure is no longer a consideration, many clinicians empirically increase the PTU dose after delivery. Neonatal Graves' disease is uncommon and occurs in approximately 2% of offspring. Because of residual effects of PTU, the disorder may not become apparent until 2 weeks post partum.

Postpartum Thyroid Dysfunction

EPIDEMIOLOGY. Postpartum thyroid dysfunction occurs in 5 to 10% of women in the year after delivery. Most affected women have goiters (which are not normally present during pregnancy). Additional risk factors include a family or personal history of postpartum thyroid dysfunction and the presence of antimicrosomal antibodies. The recurrence rate in subsequent pregnancies is approximately 50%.

PATHOGENESIS, MANAGEMENT, AND PROGNOSIS. Postpartum thyroid dysfunction is associated with a "flare" of the woman's pre-existing autoimmune thyroid disease. Affected individuals typically develop transient hyperthyroidism, associated with a low iodine uptake, 6 to 12 weeks post partum. Treatment is symptomatic with β-blockers. Hyperthyroidism is followed by reduced thyroid hormone levels. Hypothyroidism also usually is temporary and managed with several months of thyroid replacement, with an attempt to stop therapy after 6 months. For some individuals, the hypothyroidism will be permanent.

DIABETES MELLITUS (See also Chapter 242)

DEFINITION, DIAGNOSIS, AND EPIDEMIOLOGY. Diabetes is present during 3% of all pregnancies. More than 90% of pregnant diabetics have gestational diabetes mellitus (GDM). GDM is defined as glucose intolerance detected during pregnancy. Risk factors for GDM include obesity, age older than 35 years, family history of type II diabetes, and prior delivery of a large (>9 lb) infant.

Gestational diabetes is asymptomatic when diagnosed. The decision to screen for GDM remains controversial. The Centers for Disease Control and Prevention recommends screening all pregnant women at 24 to 28 weeks' gestation with a glucose measurement obtained 1 hour after 50 g of oral glucose. A serum glucose level greater than 140 mg/dL or whole blood glucose level greater than 170 mg/dL is considered positive. This cutoff value is 90% sensitive and 80% specific. A 100-g 3-hour glucose tolerance test confirms the presence of GDM.

White's classification stratifies diabetes during pregnancy based on duration of diabetes, therapy, and the presence of retinopathy, nephropathy, or heart disease. Class A refers to women with GDM. Classes B and C include women requiring insulin but without other complications from diabetes. Those women in classes D (benign retinopathy), F (nephropathy), R (proliferative retinopathy), and H (heart disease) have the greatest potential for complications during pregnancy.

PATHOGENESIS. Organogenesis occurs early in the first trimester. Because "tight" blood glucose control during this interval decreases congenital malformations and miscarriages, optimal blood glucose especially is appropriate when diabetic women are considering pregnancy and early in gestation. Hemoglobin A_{1c} should be normal for 2 months before conception. Women taking oral hypoglycemic agents should be switched to insulin before conception, because these agents cross the placenta, may be teratogenic, and can cause prolonged fetal hyperinsulinemia.

MANAGEMENT. The therapeutic goal is "tight" glucose control, with fasting and preprandial levels of 60 to 90 mg/dL, and 1-hour postprandial values less than 140 mg/dL. Women must be able to monitor their blood glucose and obtain several values per day (fasting, following breakfast, late afternoon, and evenings). Ketonemia adversely affects the fetus, and care must be taken to prevent starvation ketosis and weight loss. Hospitalization for intense patient education and glucose control may be appropriate early in gestation. Additional indications for hospitalization include nausea and vomiting, poor glucose control that is unresponsive to insulin adjustments, and persistent ketonuria.

The recommended diet is 30 to 35 kcal/kg/day based on ideal body weight, with a composition of 60% carbohydrate, 15 to 20% protein, and 20 to 25% fat. Calories are divided as three meals and two snacks a day: 20% breakfast, 30% lunch, 35% dinner, 10% evening snack, and 5% midmorning snack. Low-intensity aerobic exercise is being studied for its benefits for GDM, and obese women with GDM may be advised to use a mild caloric restriction (e.g., 25 kcal/kg/day).

Approximately 15% of women with GDM will require insulin

Table 253–3 ■ ETIOLOGY OF NEW-ONSET JAUNDICE DURING PREGNANCY

DIAGNOSIS	PREVALENCE	WHEN	SYMPTOMS	SIGNS	ASPARTATE AMINOTRANSFERASE	ALKALINE PHOSPHATASE	BILIRUBIN	OTHER LABORATORY STUDIES	MATERNAL OUTCOME	FETAL OUTCOME	THERAPY	RECURRENCE RATE
Viral hepatitis (leading cause of jaundice during pregnancy [50% of total])	Acute hepatitis A or C in 1 per 1000 pregnancies; Acute hepatitis B in 2 per 1000 pregnancies	Any trimester	Usual symptoms of viral hepatitis	Usual signs of viral hepatitis	Typical of non-pregnant individuals with viral hepatitis	Typical of non-pregnant individuals with viral hepatitis	Typical of non-pregnant individuals with viral hepatitis	Serologic diagnosis is typical of non-pregnant individuals with viral hepatitis	Comparable to nonpregnant individuals	Potential for transmission at delivery is an indication for passive (hepatitis B immunoglobulin) and active (hepatitis B vaccine) immunization; utility passive immunization for hepatitis C not established	Supportive and similar to general guidelines for viral hepatitis	Natural history of viral hepatitides is unchanged by pregnancy
Intrahepatic cholestasis of pregnancy (IHCP) (second leading cause of jaundice during pregnancy)	Varies with ethnicity (0.1% in United States–20% in Chile)	Third trimester	Pruritus of entire body, usually beginning with palms and soles	30% become jaundiced ≈2 weeks after onset of pruritus	2–10 × ⇑	4 × ⇑	⇑ but <6 mg/dL	⇑ bile acids 30–100×	No increase in morbidity	⇑ Prematurity, fetal distress, and peripartum fetal death	Vitamin K + cholestyramine; limited study of ursodeoxycholic acid, dexamethasone, and S-adenosyl-L-methione	Resolves 2 d–2 wk after delivery; recurs in most subsequent pregnancies
Preeclampsia's HELLP (hemolysis, elevated liver functions, and low platelets) syndrome	4–12% of women with preeclampsia	Late second-third trimester (usually earlier in gestation than AFLP)	Nausea, vomiting, right upper quadrant pain; other findings of preeclampsia	Right upper quadrant tenderness, hypertension, diffuse edema, hyperreflexia	2–10 × ⇑	1–2 × ⇑	⇑ but <5 mg/dL	Platelets <100,000, microangiopathic hemolytic anemia, disseminated intravascular coagulation	Maternal mortality 2%, ⇑ risk of hemorrhage and need for blood products	⇑ Prematurity and perinatal mortality 5–30%	Delivery and other therapeutic measures for preeclampsia	May transiently worsen, then improve over several days; recurrence rate 5%
Hepatic rupture (80% is associated with preeclampsia)	Five per 10,000 pregnancies	Third trimester and postpartum	Acute abdominal pain, nausea, vomiting	Right upper quadrant tenderness, shock; preexisting findings of preeclampsia	2–100 × ⇑	1–2 × ⇑	⇑ but <5 mg/dL	May see subcapsular hematoma on ultrasonography	Mortality 60%	Mortality 60%	Delivery, surgery when indicated	Data inadequate to predict outcome, one report of recurrence
Acute fatty liver of pregnancy (AFLP)	One per 13,000 pregnancies	Third trimester	Malaise, nausea, vomiting, epigastric pain	Right upper quadrant tenderness; may be findings of hepatic encephalopathy	1–5 × ⇑, usually <500 U/L	2–8 × ⇑	⇑ but <10 mg/dL	White blood cell count >15,000; platelets often <100,000; hypoglycemia; disseminated intravascular coagulation	Mortality 10–18%	Mortality 18–25%	Delivery and supportive care	Normal liver function restored post partum; usually does not recur during next pregnancy

Additional considerations are drug-induced hepatitis, cholelithiasis with common duct obstruction, Budd-Chiari syndrome, and chronic liver disease.

therapy during pregnancy. Insulin therapy usually is initiated when the fasting blood glucose level is greater than 105 mg/dL or 2 hours postprandial glucose exceeds 120 mg/dL on two occasions within 2 weeks. The initial human insulin dose is 0.3 to 0.7 units/ kg (based on prepregnancy weight). Human insulin is administered in two or three injections per day. In general, insulin requirements decrease slightly during the first trimester, then increase until term, when requirements are approximately 50% greater than preconception. However, these are general guidelines, and individual requirements are variable. Insulin requirements decrease after delivery and are reduced by approximately 50% at 1 week post partum.

PROGNOSIS. Most women with uncomplicated type I diabetes (White's classes B and C) do well during pregnancy, although maternal risks (preeclampsia, pyelonephritis) and perinatal mortality are increased slightly. Despite careful management, congenital malformations complicate 6 to 10% of diabetic women's pregnancies.

Risk factors for maternal morbidity and relative contraindications to pregnancy include established renal disease (creatinine >2.0 mg/ dL or proteinuria >2 g/day), uncontrolled hypertension, severe gastroparesis, and atherosclerotic vascular disease. If the creatinine clearance is less than 80 mL/min or urine protein more than 2 g/ day, up to 50% of women will experience permanent further renal impairment during pregnancy. Because diabetic retinopathy progresses in 10 to 50%, patients should be examined by an ophthalmologist each trimester.

Women with GDM usually normalize their blood glucose immediately post partum. Follow-up fasting glucose values should be obtained approximately 2 months post partum. Two thirds of these women will have GDM in subsequent pregnancies, and up to 50% will develop diabetes over the next 15 years.

HEPATIC DISEASE (See also Part XII)

Most liver function tests are unchanged by pregnancy. The mean levels of alanine aminotransferase, aspartate aminotransferase, γ-glutamyl transpeptidase, and bilirubin are slightly lower during pregnancy. Alkaline phosphatase, coming primarily from the placenta, increases slowly during the first and second trimester and rises to four times the prepregnant values at term. Because of the expanded plasma volume, the serum albumin value decreases 10 to 50%.

New-Onset Jaundice During Pregnancy

ETIOLOGY AND EPIDEMIOLOGY. Jaundice occurs in approximately 1 in 2000 pregnancies. Evaluation of the jaundiced pregnant patient is altered, owing to conditions unique to pregnancy and urgency to confirm and treat the pregnancy-associated life-threatening hepatic disorders. The features of the usual causes for new-onset jaundice during pregnancy are listed in Table 253–3.

CLINICAL MANIFESTATIONS, DIAGNOSIS, AND MANAGEMENT. Viral hepatitis is the most common cause of gestational jaundice, accounting for 50% of jaundice among pregnant women. Its occurrence is distributed evenly among trimesters. All the viral hepatitides have natural histories that are not altered by pregnancy nor are their serologic diagnoses changed. Neonates may need therapy to reduce their acquiring the infection at delivery.

The pregnancy-associated causes of jaundice are intrahepatic cholestasis of pregnancy, preeclampsia, and the HELLP syndrome, acute fatty liver of pregnancy, and hepatic rupture. Each typically presents in the third trimester. During the first trimester, hyperemesis gravidarum also may cause jaundice. However, its clinical manifestations usually suggest this diagnosis and abnormalities resolve within days of improved nutrition.

Ultrasonography is an important non-invasive assessment tool during pregnancy. It can detect biliary tract disease, duct dilatation, and hepatic subcapsular hematomas. In addition, the liver's appearance can suggest fatty infiltration, mass lesion, and cirrhosis. However, although findings of acute fatty liver are helpful when present, ultrasonography and computed tomography have low sensitivity in detecting acute fatty liver of pregnancy, and liver biopsy may be needed to confirm that diagnosis.

Burrow GN, Duffy TP (eds): Medical Complications During Pregnancy, 4th ed. Philadelphia, WB Saunders, 1995. *Excellent text on medical disorders during pregnancy; the fifth edition is due out in the spring of 1999.)*

Elkayam U, Gleicher N (eds): Cardiac Problems in Pregnancy: Diagnosis and Management of Maternal and Fetal Disease, 3rd ed. New York, Wiley-Liss, 1998. *More than 750 pages, this text is a comprehensive resource for maternal cardiac disease.*

Saphier CJ, Repke JT: Hemolysis, elevated liver enzymes, and low platelets (HELLP) syndrome: A review of diagnosis and management. Semin Perinatol 22(2):118–133, 1998. *Article from an issue devoted to liver disease and pregnancy. The authors discuss the condition's manifestations, differentiation from other causes of jaundice, and management.*

254 HIV IN PREGNANCY

Stephen A. Spector

The World Health Organization estimated that by the end of 1998 more than 33 million people were living with human immunodeficiency virus (HIV) infection, including 1 in every 100 adults in the sexually active ages of 15 to 49 years. Overall, approximately 16,000 new HIV infections occur daily, of whom 40% affect women and more than 90% are in developing countries. In the United States, approximately 15% of the more than 600,000 cases of the acquired immunodeficiency syndrome (AIDS) reported to the Centers for Disease Control and Prevention (CDC) were in females, and AIDS is the third most common cause of death in women between 24 and 44 years of age (see also Chapter 409).

Pregnant women are at risk of transmitting HIV to their newborns, with approximately 25% of exposed infants becoming infected unless intervention occurs. The exact timing of HIV transmission from mother to infant is unknown. Best estimates are that approximately one third of infections occur in utero whereas two thirds occur intrapartum. Risk factors for increased mother-to-infant transmission include women with low CD4+ lymphocyte counts, high HIV RNA loads, the presence of active sexually transmitted diseases, rupture of amniotic membranes beyond 4 hours, and prematurity. Women may also transmit HIV through their breast milk. Therefore, HIV-infected women should be strongly discouraged from breast-feeding their newborns.

USE OF ANTIRETROVIRAL AGENTS DURING PREGNANCY

Treatment recommendations for HIV-infected pregnant women are based on the premise that therapies known to be of benefit should not be withheld during pregnancy unless they are known to be harmful to the mother or fetus (see also Chapter 418). Thus, unless there are specific reasons for withholding antiretroviral therapy, pregnant women should be given optimal combination therapy usually including two reverse transcriptase inhibitors and a protease inhibitor. When possible, one of the reverse transcriptase inhibitors should include zidovudine because, at present, it is the only drug demonstrated to decrease vertical transmission and to be safe for mother and infant. In a controlled trial conducted by the Pediatric AIDS Clinical Trials Group (PACTG 076), HIV infection occurred in 25% of infants when the mother and infant received placebo compared with 8% of infants when mother and infant received zidovudine. The treatment regimen used for the PACTG 076 study is summarized in Figure 254–1. The intervention involves three parts: (1) treatment of the mother with oral zidovudine during pregnancy, (2) administration of intravenous zidovudine during labor, and (3) 6 weeks of oral zidovudine administered to the infant after birth. The contribution of each of these three parts to decreasing transmission is unknown; thus, all parts of the intervention should be administered whenever possible.

In another study (PACTG 185), mother-to-infant transmission with zidovudine intervention was shown to be even more effective, decreasing mother-to-infant transmission to approximately 5%. The use of HIV specific immune globulin provides no additional benefit to the use of zidovudine alone. A study in Thailand found that mother-to-infant transmission can be decreased when women receive zidovudine only in their last month of pregnancy. These data indicate that HIV-infected women identified at any stage of preg-

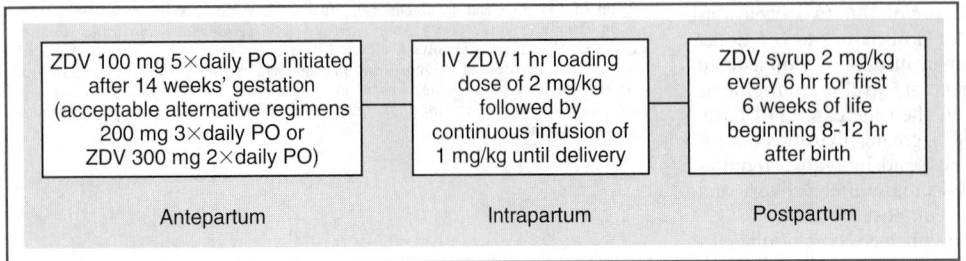

ZDV 100 mg 5×daily PO initiated after 14 weeks' gestation (acceptable alternative regimens 200 mg 3×daily PO or ZDV 300 mg 2×daily PO)	IV ZDV 1 hr loading dose of 2 mg/kg followed by continuous infusion of 1 mg/kg until delivery	ZDV syrup 2 mg/kg every 6 hr for first 6 weeks of life beginning 8-12 hr after birth
Antepartum	Intrapartum	Postpartum

FIGURE 254–1 ■ PACTG 076 zidovudine (ZDV) regimen for prevention of mother-to-infant transmission of HIV.

nancy should still receive zidovudine to decrease the risk of perinatal transmission. However, this approach is suboptimal, and women and infants should receive the full PACTG 076 regimen whenever possible.

The treatment regimen of zidovudine, 100 mg, administered five times daily in the PACTG 076 study was based on the standard dose of zidovudine for adults in 1989. The current recommended dosing for zidovudine of 200 mg three times daily, or 300 mg twice daily, has been associated with a comparable clinical response and is the recommended dosing schedule for use by pregnant women.

The impact of combination therapy on mother-to-infant transmission is unknown, but combination therapy has the potential to decrease transmission even further. However, the possible long-term risk to children after in utero exposure to combination antiretrovirals is unknown. Thus, a decision to use any antiretroviral therapy during pregnancy should be made by the woman after a thorough discussion of risks and benefits with her health care provider. Infants born to HIV-infected women should be followed by or in consultation with health care providers experienced in the care of HIV-infected children. Infants identified as infected should be treated as outlined in the CDC's "Guidelines for the Use of Antiretroviral Agents in Pediatric HIV Infection."

SCENARIOS THAT MAY REQUIRE ADJUSTMENTS TO THE STANDARD CARE OF HIV-INFECTED WOMEN

HIV-INFECTED PREGNANT WOMEN WITHOUT PRIOR ANTIRETROVIRAL THERAPY. The recommendation for antiretroviral therapy should be made after standard clinical, immunologic, and virologic evaluation. The three-part zidovudine chemoprophylaxis regimen should be recommended for all pregnant women. If the woman's HIV status indicates that more aggressive antiretroviral therapy is warranted, decisions regarding combination antiretroviral treatment should be made after a full review of risks and benefits of treatment. At present, most HIV experts recommend combination antiretroviral therapy including zidovudine. In a woman with more than 500 CD4+ lymphocytes/μL and an HIV plasma RNA load less than 10,000 copies/mL, some HIV experts recommend beginning antiretroviral therapy after the first trimester (the period of organogenesis) in an attempt to minimize risk to the fetus.

HIV-INFECTED WOMEN RECEIVING ANTIRETROVIRAL THERAPY DURING THE CURRENT PREGNANCY. Women receiving antiretroviral therapy identified as being pregnant should continue their antiretroviral therapy. Women who are identified as pregnant during the first trimester should be counseled regarding the potential risks of antiretroviral agent administration during this period. If therapy is discontinued, all drugs should be stopped and reintroduced at the same time to avoid the development of resistance. If the current antiretroviral regimen does not include zidovudine, substituting zidovudine or adding it to the regimen should be considered after 14 weeks' gestation.

HIV-INFECTED PREGNANT WOMEN IN LABOR WHO HAVE HAD NO PRIOR THERAPY. Administration of intrapartum intravenous zidovudine is recommended, followed by the 6-week zidovudine regimen for the newborn. Cesarean section prior to rupture of amniotic membranes is recommended by some experts for this situation to prevent transmission. The benefit to the infant must be weighed relative to the potential risk to the mother of performing a casarean section. After delivery, the woman should have a full

evaluation of her HIV status and have antiretroviral therapy recommended for her own health.

INFANTS BORN TO MOTHERS WHO HAVE RECEIVED NO ANTIRETROVIRAL THERAPY DURING PREGNANCY OR INTRAPARTUM. The 6-week neonatal course of zidovudine is recommended as soon after birth as possible for infants born to HIV-infected women. Many HIV experts recommend three-drug combination regimens, including two reverse transcriptase inhibitors and an antiprotease compound for 6 weeks.

TESTING AND SUPPORTIVE CARE

After delivery, HIV-infected women should receive comprehensive care and support services required for management of their HIV infection and for care of their family. This care should begin before pregnancy, with continuity of care ensured throughout pregnancy and post partum.

HIV testing and counseling are essential to any successful plan for identification of treatment of pregnant women. All pregnant women regardless of their sexual or social history should be offered HIV antibody testing (see Chapter 407). Patients who test negative should be informed that false (positive/negative) results may occur owing to the latent phase between HIV exposure and development of antibody. The false-negative rate depends on the prevalence of risk-related behavior in the tested population. Patients who test negative should be encouraged to practice low-risk behavior to minimize their risk of infection. A pregnant woman who tests positive should have a confirmatory test performed. After confirmation, the patient should have counseling regarding whether to continue the pregnancy, potential risks to the fetus, and benefits of antiretroviral intervention and treatment for herself and her newborn. After identification of HIV infection, care for the infected woman should be the same as for any other person newly identified as HIV positive. Prophylaxis for opportunistic pathogens and treatment of infections should be as recommended for others infected with HIV.

Centers for Disease Control and Prevention. U.S. Public Health Service recommendations for the use of antiretroviral drugs during pregnancy for maternal health and reduction of perinatal transmission of human immunodeficiency virus type 1. MMWR 47(RR-2), 1998. *Reviews current guidelines for the use of antiretroviral agents during pregnancy for the health of the mother and for reduction of mother-to-infant transmission of HIV.*

Centers for Disease Control and Prevention. U.S. Public Health Service guidelines for the use of antiretroviral agents in pediatric HIV infection. MMWR 47(RR-4), 1998. *Reviews guidelines for treatment of HIV-infected infants and children.*

Centers for Disease Control and Prevention. U.S. Public Health Service report of the NIH panel to define principles of therapy of HIV infection and guidelines for the use of antiretroviral agents in HIV-infected adults and adolescents. MMWR 47(RR-5), 1998. *Reviews principles and guidelines for treatment of HIV-infected adults and adolescents.*

Connor EM, et al: Reduction of maternal-infant transmission of human immunodeficiency virus type 1 with zidovudine treatment. N Engl J Med 331:1173–1180, 1994. *Demonstrated that when HIV-infected pregnant women were given a regimen of zidovudine ante partum and intrapartum and when the newborn was treated for 6 weeks the risk of mother-to-infant transmission was reduced by approximately two thirds.*

Landesman SH, et al: Obstetrical factors and the transmission of human immunodeficiency virus type 1 from mother to child. N Engl J Med 334:1617–1623, 1996. *Demonstrated that the risk of transmission of HIV from mother-to-infant increases when the fetal membranes rupture for more than 4 hours before delivery.*

Sperling RS, et al: Maternal viral load, zidovudine treatment, and the risk of transmission of human immunodeficiency virus type 1 from mother to infant. N Engl J Med 335:1621–1629, 1996. *Demonstrated that a high maternal plasma concentration of HIV RNA is a risk factor for mother-to-infant transmission. However, women transmit the virus at every level of plasma HIV RNA. To prevent HIV transmission, initiating maternal treatment with zidovudine is recommended regardless of the plasma HIV RNA level or CD4+ lymphocyte count.*

255 HIRSUTISM

Roger S. Rittmaster

DEFINITION. NORMAL HAIR GROWTH. Most body hair can be classified as vellus or terminal. Vellus hairs are fine and unpigmented, such as those that cover the face of children. Terminal hairs, pigmented and coarser, may be sex hormone-dependent (such as those over the chin and abdomen of men) or sex hormone-independent (such as eyebrows and eyelashes) (Fig. 255–1). Androgens convert vellus hair to terminal hair in sex hormone-dependent areas.

HIRSUTISM. Hirsutism is the presence of excess hair in women. This is usually an androgen-dependent process. Twenty-five to 35% of young women have terminal hair over the lower abdomen, around the nipples, or over the upper lip. Most women gradually develop more androgen-dependent body hair with age. Nevertheless, "normal" patterns of female hair growth are unacceptable to many women. At the other extreme, severe hirsutism may rarely be the earliest sign of masculinizing diseases. More often, however, severe hirsutism reflects only increased androgen production in women with no serious underlying disorder.

ETIOLOGY. Hirsutism may be divided into androgen-dependent and androgen-independent causes. Androgen-dependent hirsutism is restricted to areas where men typically become hirsute and often begins with adolescence. In women, androgens arise from the ovaries, the adrenal glands, or exogenous sources such as anabolic steroids (Table 255–1). Often, no definite abnormality exists; the hirsutism simply results from modestly increased androgen production and/or increased skin sensitivity to androgens.

Androgen-independent hirsutism (also termed "hypertrichosis") is caused by drugs (cyclosporine, glucocorticoids, minoxidil, diazoxide, and possibly phenytoin) or starvation (anorexia nervosa); it may be associated with the skin lesions of porphyria; or it may be an inherited condition. Androgen-independent hirsutism is characterized by long, fine hairs occurring over much of the body, including such areas as the forehead and flanks. Androgens may exacerbate androgen-independent hirsutism, giving rise to a clinically confusing presentation. The pathophysiology of androgen-independent hirsutism is unknown.

PATHOPHYSIOLOGY OF ANDROGEN-DEPENDENT HIRSUTISM. To be active in skin, testosterone, the major circulating androgen, must first be converted to dihydrotestosterone by the enzyme 5α-reductase. Hirsute women have elevated skin 5α-reductase compared with nonhirsute women. They may also have polymorphisms of the androgen receptor leading to increased androgen effect.

Hirsute women as a group also have increased androgen production from the adrenal glands, the ovaries, or both. Either testosterone itself is secreted, or androgen precursors such as androstenedione are secreted, which are then converted in the liver or skin to active androgens. Many hirsute women simply fall at one end of the normal spectrum of androgen production and skin sensitivity to androgens.

The ovarian and adrenal causes of hirsutism listed in Table 255-1 lead to increased androgen production. Virilizing tumors secrete androgens directly. The pituitary adenomas in Cushing's disease release ACTH, which stimulates the adrenals to secrete both cortisol and androgens (see Chapter 240). The virilizing forms of congenital adrenal hyperplasia involve enzyme defects that impair cortisol synthesis, leading to increased ACTH secretion (see Chapter 240). The enzyme block causes shunting of cortisol precursors to androgens. The most common form, 21-hydroxylase deficiency, leads to an overproduction of 17-hydroxyprogesterone. Whereas severe forms of 21-hydroxylase deficiency cause ambiguous genitalia in female infants, milder forms may lead only to hirsutism and/or irregular menses. This "non-classical" form of 21-hydroxylase deficiency is present in about 1% of hirsute women.

In the polycystic ovarian syndrome, both the ovaries and adrenals secrete excess androgens, although the majority of the androgens are usually of ovarian origin (see Chapter 250).

CLINICAL MANIFESTATIONS. Androgen-induced hirsutism of benign origin usually begins in adolescence and becomes gradually worse with time. Family history is often positive. The hirsutism may vary from mild to severe. Usually hair growth begins over the lower abdomen, on the breasts, and over the upper lip. Widespread hirsutism over the upper back, upper abdomen, and upper chest implies severe hyperandrogenism. Some women have only facial hair or other unusual patterns of hirsutism, probably due to local variation in skin 5α-reductase activity.

Severe, rapidly progressive hirsutism, beginning in childhood or beyond adolescence, suggests an androgen-secreting tumor. Such tumors can cause signs of virilization: deepening of the voice, excess muscle development, and marked clitoral enlargement. Signs of virilization, however, simply imply severe hyperandrogenism and can occasionally be seen with all causes of hirsutism. Androgen-secreting tumors are rare, and most severely hirsute women have either polycystic ovarian syndrome or hirsutism alone.

Non-classical congenital adrenal hyperplasia is clinically indistinguishable from simple hirsutism or polycystic ovarian syndrome, and the diagnosis must be made biochemically. Cushing's disease may be suspected when the patient presents with central obesity, hypertension, diabetes, and/or thinning of the skin (see Chapter 237).

DIAGNOSIS. The diagnostic evaluation of hirsutism is directed at ruling out a significant underlying cause. Important historical points include a drug history, age of onset and rate of progression of hirsutism, presence of thinning of scalp hair or deepening of the voice, menstrual history, history of obesity, and family history of hirsutism. The physical examination should include an assessment of the quality and distribution of hair growth, signs of virilization or Cushing's syndrome, and presence of abdominal or pelvic masses in women suspected of having an androgen-secreting tumor.

Table 255–1 ■ CAUSES OF ANDROGEN-DEPENDENT HIRSUTISM

Ovarian causes
Severe insulin resistance
Virilizing ovarian tumors
Adrenal causes
Congenital adrenal hyperplasia
   21-Hydroxylase deficiency
   3β-Hydroxysteroid dehydrogenase deficiency
   11-Hydroxylase deficiency
Cushing's disease
Ectopic ACTH-producing tumors
Virilizing adrenal tumors
Combined ovarian and adrenal causes
Polycystic ovary syndrome
"Idiopathic" hirsutism
Exogenous androgens
"Anabolic" steroids
Danazol
Postmenopausal hormone replacement formulations containing androgens

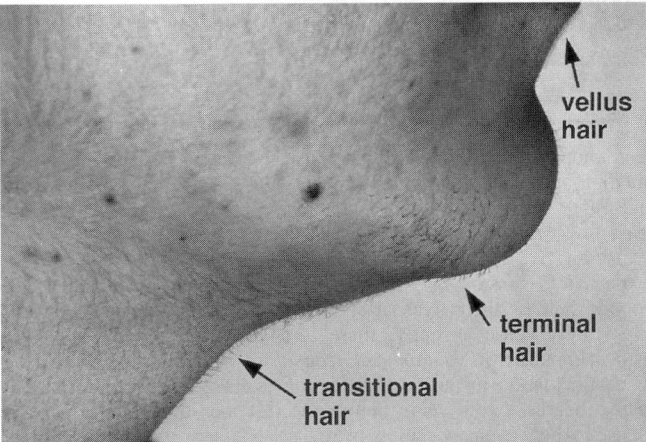

FIGURE 255–1. ■ Facial hair growth in a hirsute woman. Vellus hair is fine, unpigmented hair. Terminal hair is coarse and pigmented. Transitional hair is intermediate between vellus and terminal. This woman also has mild acne, another androgen-dependent process. (Reprinted with permission from Rittmaster RS: Hirsutism. Med Clin North Am 14:2686, 1987.)

vellus hair

terminal hair

transitional hair

LABORATORY EVALUATION. In women with androgen-dependent hirsutism, regular ovulatory menses, and no physical signs of Cushing's syndrome, hormonal evaluation is usually unnecessary. Virilizing tumors have not been reported in such patients, and hirsutism associated with non-classical congenital adrenal hyperplasia need not be treated differently from other benign forms of hirsutism (see Treatment section).

In hirsute women with irregular menses, a reasonable laboratory evaluation includes measurement of serum testosterone, 17-hydroxyprogesterone, prolactin, LH, and FSH. A testosterone level <170 ng per deciliter (6 nmol per liter) makes an androgen-secreting tumor highly unlikely, although re-evaluation may be necessary if the hirsutism continues to progress or signs of virilization appear. Testosterone levels above 170 ng per deciliter may also be seen with polycystic ovarian syndrome. To rule out attenuated 21-hydroxylase deficiency, serum 17-hydroxyprogesterone should be measured between 7 and 9 A.M. during the first week of the menstrual cycle (values may be elevated during the luteal phase). Values <200 ng per deciliter (6 nmol per liter) rule out this diagnosis. Mildly elevated values (<1000 ng per deciliter) (30 nmol per liter) may be seen in both heterozygous and homozygous 21-hydroxylase deficiency (the heterozygous disorder is not associated with hirsutism) and in polycystic ovarian syndrome. To distinguish between these conditions, 17-hydroxyprogesterone should be measured 30 to 60 minutes after the intravenous administration of 250 μg synthetic ACTH. Levels are usually >1500 ng per deciliter (45 nmol per liter) in homozygous 21-hydroxylase deficiency. Other forms of attenuated congenital adrenal hyperplasia are too rare to justify routine hormonal screening. Serum prolactin, LH, and FSH are used to evaluate the possibility that a prolactinoma, ovarian failure, or polycystic ovarian syndrome is contributing to the irregular menses. These tests are not directly relevant to the evaluation of hirsutism itself. Measurement of dehydroepiandrosterone sulfate (DHEAS) as an index of adrenal androgen production is generally unhelpful.

TREATMENT. Hirsutism is a cosmetic problem that may have severe psychosocial consequences. Because it is not a disease in itself, the benefits and risks of any therapy should be carefully weighed and the treatment individualized.

MECHANICAL HAIR REMOVAL. For mild hirsutism, bleaching and mechanical hair removal are adequate and safe. Shaving is the easiest method of temporarily removing visible hair. Although shaving does not increase hair growth rates, it may leave a stubble and is unacceptable to many women. Plucking and waxing may control mild hirsutism, but they also do not resolve the problem and may lead to scarring. Electrolysis can provide a safe, effective alternative for localized mild to moderate hirsutism and is a useful adjunct to medical therapy in more severe cases. Electrolysis is expensive, however, and long-term treatment may be necessary.

DRUG TREATMENT. Successful medical therapy results in a gradual return of terminal hair to finer, less pigmented vellus hair. Younger women with mild hirsutism of brief duration respond best to medical therapy. More severe hair growth can be prevented, and resolution of the hirsutism is possible. Nevertheless, drug treatment is not a cure, and lifelong therapy may be necessary to prevent recurrence. Generally, 6 months is needed to judge the efficacy of a given therapy, although improvement may continue indefinitely. No drug is approved by the Food and Drug Administration for treatment of hirsutism.

Antiandrogens. Antiandrogens (spironolactone, cyproterone acetate, flutamide) block the androgen receptor and are the drug treatment of choice for hirsutism. They are effective in reducing hair growth in at least 70% of women, and hirsutism stabilizes in the remaining ones. Spironolactone is usually given in a starting dose of 50 mg twice daily. The most common side effect is increased frequency of menses, which can be controlled by combining spironolactone with an oral contraceptive. Spironolactone should not be given to women with renal insufficiency. Cyproterone acetate, a potent antiandrogen and progestin, is often given as 25 to 50 mg daily for the first 10 days of a birth control pill cycle. Although widely used in Europe and Canada, it is not available in the United States. Flutamide is given as 125 to 250 mg twice daily. Both flutamide and cyproterone acetate can cause a drug-induced hepatitis,

and all antiandrogens should be avoided in pregnant women. Flutamide is more expensive than other antiandrogens.

5α-Reductase Inhibitors. Finasteride, the only such inhibitor available at the time of publication, blocks the formation of dihydrotestosterone and is approved for treatment of benign prostatic hyperplasia and male pattern baldness. Several studies suggest that it also effectively treats hirsutism. All studies to date have used 5 mg daily, although 1 mg daily should be as effective. It would be expected to cause ambiguous genitalia in the male offspring of women taking the drug during pregnancy.

Ovarian Suppression. Although oral contraceptives are often used to control menstrual cycles in women given antiandrogens, they are usually ineffective for treating hirsutism when used alone (although they may prevent the hirsutism from becoming worse). Birth control pills differ in the androgenicity of the progestational component, but this difference has never been shown to have clinical significance in the treatment of hirsutism. For treatment of women with polycystic ovary syndrome, a progestin-dominant pill is likely to be of more benefit by causing a greater reduction in ovarian testosterone production. Gonadotropin-releasing hormone analogues suppress the ovary by suppressing LH and FSH secretion. They are effective in treating hirsutism associated with polycystic ovarian syndrome but are expensive and lead to menopausal symptoms unless estrogens are given concurrently.

Glucocorticoids. Glucocorticoids suppress adrenal cortisol and androgen secretion. They are frequently ineffective in low doses, and higher doses can cause Cushing's syndrome. They also can cause a drug-induced hirsutism in some women and cannot be recommended as a routine treatment. Although glucocorticoids have traditionally been used to treat congenital adrenal hyperplasia, antiandrogens are more effective in treating the hirsutism associated with this disorder.

PROGNOSIS. Untreated, hirsutism usually becomes gradually worse with time, and most therapies need to be continued indefinitely. However, worsening hirsutism is easily prevented with antiandrogen therapy, and most women experience a satisfactory improvement with the judicious use of mechanical and medical therapies.

Dunaif A, Givens J, Merriam G, Haseltine F (eds): Polycystic Ovary Syndrome (Current Issues in Endocrinology and Metabolism). Cambridge, MA. Blackwell Scientific Publications, 1992. *A collection of excellent reviews on polycystic ovary syndrome.*

Jeffcoate W: The treatment of women with hirsutism. Clin Endocrinol 39:143, 1993. *A somewhat different approach (from mine) to the evaluation and treatment of hirsutism.*

Rittmaster RS: Hyperandrogenism. *In* Copeland LJ (ed): Textbook of Gynecology. Philadelphia, WB Saunders, 1993, p 414. *A detailed review of the pathophysiology, evaluation, and treatment of hyperandrogenism.*

Rittmaster RS: Treating hirsutism. Endocrinologist 3:211, 1993. *An overview of recent advances in the evaluation and treatment of hirsutism.*

256 MENOPAUSE

Rogerio A. Lobo

Menopause is defined as the last menstrual period and has a median age of 51.4 years and a Gaussian distribution ranging from age 40 to 58 years. Age at menopause has not changed over the past few centuries while there has been a gradual increase in life expectancy. Thus, whereas in previous centuries women were not expected to live beyond menopause, women now spend one third to one half of their lives after menopause. Because menstrual cycles rarely cease abruptly, there is a period of time, termed the *perimenopause* or *menopausal transition*, during which there is a wide fluctuation in the hormonal profiles. In general, the perimenopause begins a few years before the last menstrual period (menopause) when cycles become irregular and there are often, but not always, symptoms suggesting a declining estrogen status. Although estrogen levels can be higher than normal early in the perimenopause, an abrupt decline in estrogen occurs 6 months before menopause. The perimenopause also extends for a few years beyond the menopause, a time during which transient and episodic bursts of ovarian activity may occur that may result in some vaginal bleeding.

The total group of postmenopausal women in the United States is increasing. In 2000, it is estimated that there will be 31.2 million women older than age 55, compared with 28.7 million in 1990. By 2020, the size of this group is estimated to be 45.9 million.

REPRODUCTIVE DECLINE AND MENOPAUSE

The time from the decline in reproductive capacity onward is often referred to as the *climacteric*. Reproductive aging occurs rapidly after the third decade, and fecundity is extremely low before menopause. Thus, reproductive aging precedes menopause by 5 to 10 years, at a "young" chronologic age. This is signified by an increase in serum follicle-stimulating hormone (FSH) level in the early follicular phase of regular cycles. These values may be elevated only intermittently before they continue to rise at the time of menopause. Decreasing ovarian estrogen, but particularly inhibin B, is responsible for the rise in FSH (see Chapter 237).

HORMONAL CHANGES WITH ESTABLISHED MENOPAUSE

Depicted in Figure 256–1 are the typical hormonal changes of postmenopausal women compared with those of ovulatory women in the early follicular phase. The most significant findings are the marked reductions in estradiol (E_2) and estrone (E_1). Serum E_2 is reduced to a greater extent than E_1. Serum E_1, on the other hand, is produced primarily by peripheral aromatization from androgens, which are not affected as dramatically. Levels of E_2 average 15 pg/mL and range from 10 to 25 pg/mL. In oophorectomized women, values are usually 10 pg/mL or less. Serum E_1 values average 30 pg/mL but may be higher in obese women because aromatization increases as a function of the mass of adipose tissue. Estrone sulfate (E_1S) is an estrogen conjugate that serves as a stable-circulating reservoir of estrogen, and its levels are the highest of any estrogen. In premenopausal women, values are usually above 1000 pg/mL; and in PM women, levels average 350 pg/mL. Apart from elevations in FSH and luteinizing hormone (LH), pituitary hormones are not affected. Specifically, growth hormone, thyroid-stimulating hormone, and adrenocorticotropic hormone (ACTH) levels are normal. Serum prolactin levels may be very slightly decreased because prolactin is somewhat influenced by estrogen status. Both the postmenopausal ovary and the adrenal gland continue to produce androgen. The ovary continues to produce androstenedione and testosterone but not E_2, and this production has been shown to be at least partially dependent on LH. Androstenedione and testosterone levels are lower in women who have experienced bilateral oophorectomy, with values averaging 0.8 ng/mL and 10 ng/dL, respectively. The adrenal gland also continues to produce androstenedione, dehydroepiandrosterone, and dehydroepiandrosterone sulfate; and, primarily as a function of aging, these values decrease somewhat (adrenopause), although cortisol secretion remains unaffected.

Whether an androgen "deficiency" occurs after menopause is still debated. Cross-sectional data obtained across the perimenopause have suggested very little early change in secreted androstenedione and testosterone. However, 24-hour mean values have been shown to decline with age and were shown to decrease between the second and fourth decades. The decline in androstenedione after menopause also is greater than that of testosterone; and it is clear that several years after the menopause, levels of androstenedione and testosterone are significantly lower than values in premenopausal women.

EFFECTS OF DECLINING ESTROGEN

Estrogen receptors are abundant throughout the body; and, therefore, the absence of estrogen potentially influences virtually all systems in some way.

BRAIN AND CENTRAL NERVOUS SYSTEM. In the brain, because estrogen receptors are abundant and estrogen is known to influence many brain processes, the absence of estrogen can result in symptomatic as well as physiologic changes. Estrogen is important for blood flow, synaptic activity, neuronal growth, the survival of cholinergic neurons, and many other functions, including cognition. Hot flushes are an early and acute symptom of estrogen deficiency. This can occur in the perimenopause when levels characteristically fluctuate widely. It is the rapid fall in estrogen levels that precipitates the symptoms. Although the proximate cause of the flush remains elusive, the episodes result from a hypothalamic response (probably mediated by catecholamines) as a result of a change in estrogen status. The flush has been well characterized physiologically. It results in heat dissipation by an increase in peripheral temperature (finger, toe); a decrease in skin resistance, associated with diaphoresis; and a reduction in core body temperature (Fig. 256–2). There are hormonal correlates of flush activity such as an increase in serum LH and plasma pro-opiomelanocortin peptides (ACTH, β-endorphin) at the time of the flush, but these occurrences are thought to be epiphenomena that result as a consequence of the flush and are not related to its etiology.

In general, estrogen has a positive effect on mood and contributes to a sense of well-being. In an estrogen-deficient state such as occurs after the menopause, a higher incidence of depression (clini-

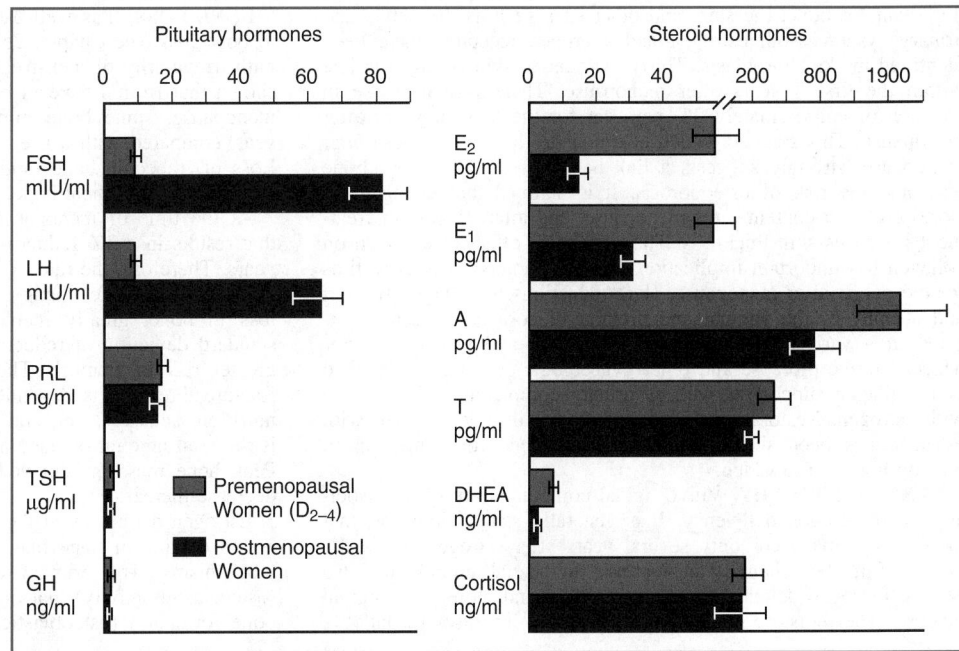

FIGURE 256–1 ■ Circulating levels of pituitary and steroid hormones in postmenopausal women compared with levels in premenopausal women studied during the first week (days 2 to 4 [*D2-4*]) of the menstrual cycle. FSH = follicle-stimulating hormone; LH = lutenizing hormone; PRL = prolactin; TSH = thyroid-stimulating hormone; GH = growth hormone; E_2 = estradiol; E_1 = estrogen; A = androstenedione; T = testosterone; DHEA = dehydroepiandrosterone. (From Yen SSC: The biology of menopause. J Reprod Med 18:287, 1977.)

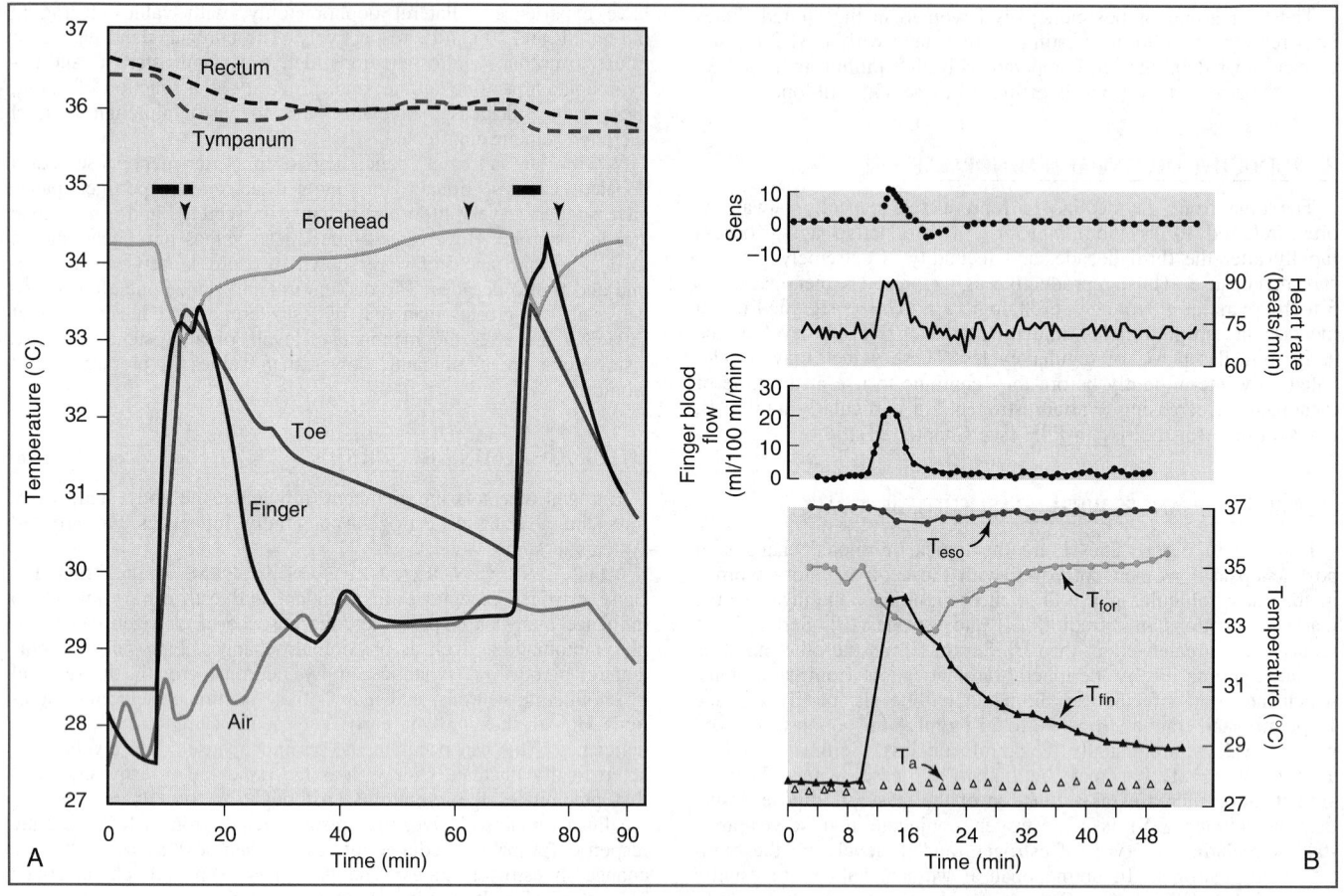

FIGURE 256–2 ■ Temperature responses to two spontaneous flushes (−) and evoked flush (=). Down arrow indicates finger stab for blood sample. (Data adapted from Molnar GW: Body temperatures during menopausal hot flashes. J Appl Physiol 38:499–503, 1975.)

cal or subclinical) is manifest. Dementia increases as a function of age and has a higher prevalence in women compared with men. Some of this trend may be related to estrogen deficiency. Thus, the risk of Alzheimer's disease may be reduced with estrogen in postmenopausal women. Estrogen is also thought to have an overall positive effect on memory.

COLLAGEN. Estrogen has a positive effect on collagen that is important for bone, the skin, and other sites such as the pelvis and urinary system. Both estrogen and androgen receptors have been identified in skin fibroblasts. Thirty per cent of skin collagen is lost within the first 5 years after menopause. There is a decrease in collagen of approximately 2% per year for the first 10 years after menopause. This statistic, which is similar to that of bone loss after menopause, strongly suggests a link between skin thickness, bone loss, and the risk of osteoporosis. It is claimed that estrogen restores collagen content after menopause, and after 2 years of treatment improves skin thickness. The supportive effect of estrogen on collagen has important implications for bone homeostasis as well as for the pelvis after menopause. Here reductions in collagen support and atrophy of the vaginal and urethral mucosa have been implicated in a variety of symptoms of prolapse and urinary incontinence. Uterine prolapse and other gynecologic symptoms related to poor collagen support as well as urinary complaints may improve with estrogen. Restoration of bladder control in older women with estrogen has been shown to decrease the need for admission to nursing homes in Sweden.

GENITAL ATROPHY. Vulvovaginal complaints are often associated with estrogen deficiency. It is generally stated, however, that these symptoms occur only several years after estrogen levels decline. With this change, an increase in sexual complaints also occurs. Estrogen deficiency results in a thin and more pale vaginal mucosa. The moisture content is low, the pH increases (usually >

5), and the mucosa may exhibit inflammation and small petechiae. With estrogen treatment, it has been documented that vaginal cytology changes from a profile of predominantly parabasal cells to one with an increased number of superficial cells. Along with this, the vaginal pH decreases, vaginal blood flow increases, and the electropotential difference across the vaginal mucosa increases to premenopausal levels.

BONE LOSS. It is well established that estrogen deficiency leads to bone loss (see Chapter 257). This can be noted for the first time with irregularity of menstrual cycles before menopause. It has been shown that from 1.5 years before the menopause to 1.5 years after menopause, spine bone mineral density decreases by 2.56% per year, compared with a premenopausal loss rate of 0.13% per year. Loss of trabecula bone (spine) is greater with estrogen deficiency than is loss of cortical bone.

At the time of menopause there is an accelerated loss of bone that results in a 3% reduction in bone mass per year for the first 5 years. Therefore, the rate of loss of bone is in the range of 1 to 2% per year. Dramatic changes in bone architecture accompany this loss in bone, greatly increasing the risk of fracture. For every standard deviation of reduction in bone mass there is a twofold or greater risk of fracture. The rate at which a woman reaches the fracture threshold is dependent on many factors, such as genetics, nutrition, activity level, and lifestyle; but also extremely important is the total amount of bone a woman has at the time of menopause. Peak bone mass is achieved by the second decade and begins to decrease thereafter.

Estrogen deficiency at the time of menopause results in an accelerated decline in bone mass, and this is mediated by a variety of mechanisms. The primary deficit is one of increased resorption (osteoclastic activity) that outsteps and is therefore uncoupled from bone formation (osteoblastic activity). In old age, bone formation also lags further. Estrogen action on bone is both directly on bone, through receptor and cellular membrane effects, and on collagen. There is also an indirect effect by opposing the resorptive effects of parathyroid hormone and cytokines. Positive influences also involve growth factors, calcitonin, vitamin D metabolism, and calcium absorption. In an estrogen-deficient state these positive effects are diminished.

Osteoporosis is a devastating and debilitating disease. The only way to accurately access bone mass is by direct measurements. Historical information about risk factors and biochemical urinary analyses are only partially helpful. Dual x-ray absorptiometry remains the best approach at present and has high precision, reproducibility, and low radiation exposure (see Chapter 241).

CARDIOVASCULAR EFFECTS. It appears clear that estrogen deprivation increases the risk of cardiovascular disease in women. Data from the Framingham study have been used to compare the incidence of cardiovascular disease in men and women as they age. Although the incidence is three times lower in women than in men before the menopause (3.1/1000 per year in women aged 45 to 49), it is approximately equal in men and women aged 75 to 79, being 53 and 50.4/1000 per year, respectively. This trend also pertains to gender differences in mortality due to cardiovascular disease. Coronary artery disease is the leading cause of death in women, and the lifetime risk of death is 31% in postmenopausal women versus a 3% risk of dying of breast cancer.

Although cardiovascular disease becomes more prevalent only in later years following a natural menopause, premature cessation of ovarian function (before menopause) constitutes a significant risk. Premature menopause, occurring before age 35, has been shown to increase the risk of myocardial infarction twofold to threefold, and premature oophorectomy (before age 35) increases the risk sevenfold.

When the possible reasons for the increase in cardiovascular disease are examined, the most prevalent finding is that of the rise in total cholesterol at an accelerated rate in postmenopausal women. Although changes with age, weight, blood pressure, and blood glucose levels are not thought to be substantially different in men and women, the rate of rise in total cholesterol after menopause is significantly different. This increase in total cholesterol is explained by increases in levels of low-density lipoprotein cholesterol (LDL-C). The oxidation of LDL-C is also enhanced, as are levels of very low density lipoproteins and Lp(a) lipoprotein. HDL-C levels trend downward with time, but these changes are small relative to the increases in LDL-C.

Coagulation balance is not altered significantly as a counterbalance of changes occurs; some procoagulation factors increase (Factor VII, fibrinogen) but so do factors such as antithrombin III and plasminogen. Blood flow in all vascular beds decreases after menopause; prostacyclin production decreases, endothelin levels increase, and vasomotor responses to acetylcholine challenges are constrictive. With estrogen, all these parameters improve and coronary arterial responses to acetylcholine are dilatory with a commensurate increase in blood flow. Circulating plasma nitric oxide has also been shown to increase and levels of angiotensin-converting enzymes to decrease. Estrogen and progesterone receptors have been found in vascular tissues, including coronary arteries. Overall, the direct vascular effects of estrogen are viewed to be as important, or more important, than the changes in lipid and lipoproteins after menopause.

In normal, non-obese postmenopausal women, carbohydrate tolerance also decreases as a result of an increase in insulin resistance. This, too, is partially reversed by estrogen. Biophysical and neurohormonal responses to stress (stress reactivity) are exaggerated in postmenopausal women compared with premenopausal women, and this heightened reactivity is blunted by estrogen replacement as well. Whether these changes influence cardiovascular risk with estrogen deficiency is not known, but clearly estrogen replacement returns many parameters into the range of premenopausal women.

There are probably subtle effects of estrogen on the musculoskeletal system, the eyes, the ears, and the sensory organs, but these systems have been incompletely studied. It is known, however, that the rate of macular degeneration increases after menopause, and this rate may be attenuated in users of estrogen. Similarly, there is an important effect of estrogen on immune function, but this, too, warrants further investigation.

THE DECISION TO USE ESTROGEN

Whether or not hormonal "replacement" should be considered is a very individual decision. This takes into account symptoms, risk factors, and individual preferences and needs. Alternatives should also be considered. If hormonal therapy is chosen, there should be flexibility in prescribing because there is no ideal regimen for every women.

RISK-BENEFIT ASSESSMENT. Estrogen "replacement" therapy, is often referred to as ERT. ERT is indicated for the relief of hot flushes and urogenital atrophy and for the prevention of osteoporosis. For these indications, a titration of dose is important, with the most common dose being 0.625 mg of conjugated equine estrogen (CEE) or its equivalent. ERT may be divided into short-term relief of symptoms such as hot flushes, for which a larger dose may be required, and long-term prophylaxis against the morbidity and mortality from osteoporosis and cardiovascular disease. Cognitive effects, risk of Alzheimer's disease, and quality of life are also reasons to consider long-term therapy. These long-term benefits are sustained as long as ERT is prescribed, and the benefits decrease after cessation. For osteoporosis and fractures, ERT reduces the risk by 30 to 60% (RR 0.4-0.7) with a dose equivalent of 0.625 mg CEE. The relative risk for the effect of estrogen in a large number of epidemiologic trials in women using estrogen (average RR 0.5) is shown in Figure 256-3. The dose again is the equivalent of 0.625 mg of CEE. Although estrogen use appears to be protective, the magnitude of its effect must ultimately be determined in prospective, randomized clinical trials. The protective effect is likely to range from 0.3 to 0.8. This range is wide, and any small change in relative risk results in a great reduction in mortality. Therefore, an ERT-associated reduction in mortality from cardiovascular disease may be relatively minor to very large.

The cardiovascular effect of estrogen is partially due to an improvement in lipids and lipoproteins (30-40%), with the remaining effect due to vascular changes, insulin sensitivity, and so on, as described above previously. For cardiovascular disease mortality, a protective effect 10-fold greater than that for osteoporosis is estimated. The annual economic benefit on cardiovascular disease is estimated at $60 billion, and that for osteoporosis is $10 billion. Not estimated here is the potential protective effect of estrogen of developing Alzheimer's disease. Observational studies have been consistent in finding a 50 to 60% protective effect (RR 0.5-0.6). The protective effect is also greater with a longer duration of ERT.

CHANGES IN MORTALITY WITH ESTROGEN USE. Ischemic heart disease, osteoporotic fractures, breast cancer, and endometrial cancer are four events that are potentially affected by estrogen use. The case-fatality rate for ischemic heart disease is greater than that for osteoporotic fractures and both types of cancer combined. It has been calculated that the ERT-related change in relative risk has a greater impact on mortality from ischemic heart disease than on other events for estrogen use in women aged 50 to 75 years. A

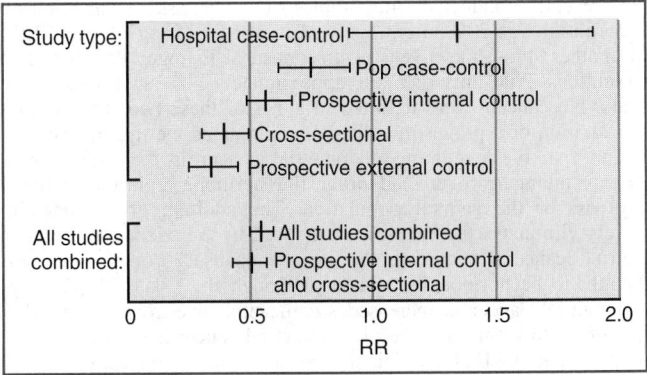

FIGURE 256-3 ■ Summary of relative risk (RR) and 95% confidence interval estimates for epidemiologic studies of ERT and risk of coronary heart disease, by study design (P < 0.001). (From Stampfer MJ, Colditz GA: Estrogen replacement therapy and coronary heart disease: A quantitative assessment of the epidemiologic evidence. Prev Med 20:47-63, 1991.)

relative risk of 0.4 for osteoporotic fracture represents a cumulative change in mortality of 563 lives saved per 100,000 estrogen users. For gallbladder disease, a relative risk of 1.5 results in a net loss of only two lives per 100,000 estrogen users. Although the magnitude of the association between estrogen and endometrial cancer is controversial, these figures reflect a relative risk of only 2.0 and a case-fatality rate of 0.05, resulting in an excess mortality of 63 lives per 100,000 estrogen users. Another controversial issue is the risk of breast cancer with estrogen use, if we assume, a risk of 1.1, or a 10% increase in incidence, this would result in a net increase of 187 lives lost per 100,000 estrogen user (see Chapter 258).

Clearly, the change in mortality with estrogen use is greatest for ischemic heart disease. For a relative risk of 0.5, there are 5250 lives saved per 100,000 estrogen users. In calculating the cumulative change in mortality, approximately 41% of women benefited by taking estrogen. Overall, the net change of 5,561 lives saved per 100,000 estrogen users is largely explained by estrogen's protective effect on ischemic heart disease. Thus, a change in relative risk anywhere in the range of 0.3 to 0.8 dramatically changes the estimate.

Although these were calculated data, these findings have been corroborated in several cohort studies. Each has demonstrated an overall 40% reduction in all-cause mortality with estrogen. Two studies have shown that the benefit in mortality is related to the duration of use; but one has suggested that the effect is decreased beyond 10 years of use because of an increase in breast cancer mortality that was present in this cohort (nurses). These data are not consistent with these reports, which have shown either no change in breast cancer mortality with estrogen use or actually a decrease in mortality.

Mortality from stroke has also been shown to decrease by approximately 40% with estrogen use. However, the literature is less consistent about stroke than the effect on ischemic heart disease. Data have also shown a protective effect of ERT on colon cancer mortality. This protection of approximately 50% (RR 0.5) is also greater with a longer duration of use.

There have been several models to help guide decision making regarding estrogen. In general, the data are consistent in showing decreased mortality and an increased longevity (1 to 2.5 years); it is suggested that these years of life are of improved quality. The benefit is greatest for those with cardiovascular risk factors and is least for those with significant risk factors for breast cancer.

RISKS ASSOCIATED WITH ERT. Among the risks that have been associated with ERT are endometrial disease, breast cancer, side effects such as vaginal bleeding, somatic complaints, and idiosyncratic reactions, including hypertension and thrombosis. Endometrial disease occurs with unopposed estrogen therapy in women who have a uterus. Although a woman's risk of developing endometrial cancer with unopposed estrogen use is twofold to eightfold higher than that for the general population, in most patients, precursor lesions, primarily endometrial hyperplasia, signal the presence of an abnormality (see Chapter 259). Thus, the risk is far less for endometrial cancer than it is for varying degrees of hyperplasia. One recently conducted study showed that the risk of endometrial hyperplasia was 20% after 1 year of use of 0.625 mg of oral CEE. In another study, the 3-year postmenopausal Estrogen/Progestin Interventions Trial, this risk was approximately 40% at the end of 3 years. No cancers were reported in either of these two studies, and the addition of a progestin essentially eliminated the hyperplasia.

The risk of developing endometrial cancer is the same for a woman taking estrogen and progestin (hormone replacement therapy) as for the general population. The addition of a progestin merely eliminates the excess risk induced by estrogen. Other endometrial cancers occurring in postmenopausal women are not thought to be hormonally related. Although the risk of developing endometrial cancer is increased significantly in estrogen users, the risk of death from this type of endometrial cancer does not increase proportionately. Endometrial cancers associated with estrogen use are thought not to be as aggressive as spontaneously occurring cancers or that tumors in women taking estrogen are likely to be discovered and treated at an earlier stage, thus improving survival rates.

More controversial is the risk of breast cancer with ERT. In the previous models, a relative risk of 1.1 was ascribed to all estrogen use, suggesting a 10% increase in risk over the baseline rate. Several meta-analyses have suggested either no significantly increased risk, a relative risk hovering around 1.0, or a risk as high as 1.6. It has also been suggested that there is no additional risk for women with a family history of breast cancer. Admittedly, a slightly increased surveillance bias exists for women who see their doctors regularly. It is also possible that estrogen use causes breast cancer to occur earlier in some women, but it is not clear which women are at greatest risk. However, breast cancer–related mortality has not been shown consistently to be increased, and indeed there are data to suggest that it may be lower among estrogen users.

Although we can expect to see more analyses on the association between ERT and breast cancer risk, new data are not likely to be any more illuminating. Thus, we are left with the question of whether estrogen use carries any increased relative risk for breast cancer or a real risk that may be relatively small. Both the estrogen dose and the duration of use are implicated in risk estimates. For moderate doses of estrogen, the risk of breast cancer is probably in the range of 20 to 30% in those women who are susceptible. Unfortunately, such women cannot be identified before therapy is initiated. Recent trends in prescribing have suggested lowering the dose of estrogen for long-term use, as both dose and duration are associated with risk.

One of the greatest concerns of women receiving estrogen is the return of menstrual bleeding. Somatic complaints such as breast tenderness and bloating may also occur with ERT but can be alleviated by alterations in dose and type of preparation. Such concerns should be discussed with the patient, and the choice of regimen should remain flexible.

Idiosyncratic reactions including hypertension, thrombosis, and allergic manifestations have also been observed in users of estrogen, particularly oral estrogen. Hypertension with estrogen use, the cause of which is not entirely clear, occurs in about 5% of oral contraceptive users. Estrogen usually causes no change in blood pressure; it may actually reduce blood pressure, a finding that has relevance for normotensive as well as hypertensive individuals. However, an increase in both diastolic and systolic blood pressure has been noted in susceptible individuals and is rapidly reversible with discontinuation of ERT. A different form of estrogen may eliminate the problem. Alterations in the route of estrogen administration and dose have resulted in improved blood pressure in such individuals.

In non-susceptible individuals, ERT does not increase procoagulant factors, and for many years, ERT was considered not to increase the risk of venous thrombosis unlike oral contraceptive use. However, several recent observational studies have suggested a twofold increase in venous thromboembolic phenomena with oral estrogen. This did not increase mortality, and the rate is low (background prevalence of 11 per 100,000 women). Although it is unclear if this level of risk is real, it would be prudent to inform patients of these findings. In women with the history of thrombosis, however, there is an increased risk with estrogen administered orally, a risk that is not easily identifiable except by reviewing the patient's history and by measuring coagulation factors. Women who have a family history of thrombosis or have had thrombotic events with oral contraceptives or any prior estrogen use should be counseled very carefully and monitored closely. Non-oral estrogen is a consideration for these patients and can be used judiciously.

HORMONAL REGIMENS. The aim of ERT is to provide "replacement" in a fashion that is as physiologic as possible. Follicular phase levels of E_2 during the normal menstrual cycle range between 40 and 100 pg/mL. Threshold levels of E_2 for achieving benefit for osteoporosis and cardiovascular disease are in the range of 50 to 60 pg/mL for most women. Nevertheless, any increment of estrogen levels from baseline is expected to exert some significant effect, thus leading to the concept of a minimal effective dose.

Oral ERT results in higher levels of E_1 than E_2. This is true for oral estradiol as well as estrone products. CEE is a mixture of at least 10 conjugated estrogens derived from equine pregnant urine. Estrone sulfate is the major component, but the biologic activities of equilin, 17α-dihydroequilin, and several other B-ring estrogens, including Δ dihydroestrone, have been documented. Table 256–1 compares the standard doses of the most frequently prescribed oral estrogens and the levels of E_1 and E_2 achieved.

Synthetic estrogens, given orally, are vastly more potent. Ethinyl

Table 256–1 ■ MEAN SERUM ESTRADIOL (E_2) AND ESTRONE (E_1)

| ESTROGEN DOSE (mg) | LEVEL (pg/mL) | |
	E_2	E_1
CEE (0.3)*	18	76
CEE (0.625)	39	153
CEE (1.25)	60	220
Micronized E_2 (1)	35	190
Micronized E_2 (2)	63	300
E_1 sulfate (0.625)	34	125
E_1 sulfate (1.25)	42	220

*Conjugated equine estrogen (CEE) contains biologically active estrogens other than E_2 and E_1.

estradiol is used in oral contraceptives. A dose of 5 µg is equivalent to the standard ERT doses used (0.625 mg CEE or 1 mg micronized estradiol). Standard ERT doses are five or six times less than the amount of estrogen used in oral contraceptives.

Oral estrogens have a potent hepatic ("first pass") effect that results in the loss of approximately 30% of its activity with a single passage after oral administration. However, this results in stimulation of hepatic proteins and enzymes. Some of these changes are not particularly beneficial (an increase in procoagulation factors), whereas other changes are beneficial (an increase in high density lipoprotein cholesterol (HDL-C) and a decrease in fibrinogen and plasminogen activator inhibitor-1.

Non-oral estrogen delivers estrogen in the form in which it is formulated. E_2 is administered in patches, gels, and subcutaneously. This synthetic administration is not subject to major hepatic effects as with oral therapy. Standard doses in the United States of alcohol-based or matrix patches are 0.05 or 0.1 mg. Lower-dose patches of 0.025 mg are also available for administration once a week or twice a week. Matrix patches are preferable because there is less skin reaction and estrogen delivery is more reliable. Whereas levels of E_2 vary widely among women, levels with transdermal therapy are more constant in individual women than with oral ERT. With the 0.05-mg patch, E_2 levels are in the 40 to 50-pg/mL range; and with the 0.1-mg patch, levels are typically 70 to 100 pg/mL. It is not unusual, however, for some women to have levels in excess of 200 pg/mL.

In women with vulvovaginal or urinary complaints, vaginal therapy is most appropriate. Creams of estradiol or CEE are available. Systemic absorption occurs but with levels that are one fourth of that achieved after similar milligram doses administered orally. Absorption is less the more estrogenized the mucosa is. For CEE, only 0.5 g (0.3 mg) is necessary; and for micronized E_2, doses as low as 0.25 mg are sufficient. Other products (tablets and rings) are available that have been designed to limit systemic absorption. A silastic ring of E_2 is now available that delivers E_2 to the vagina for 3 months with only minimal systemic absorption.

With oral and transdermal methods, estrogen is administered every day, although it is still acceptable to consider cyclic regimens of every 25 to 26 days of therapy.

USE OF A PROGESTIN. In women with a uterus, a progestin is necessary to "oppose" the proliferative effects of estrogen on the endometrium. A regimen that includes progestins is usually referred to as hormonal replacement therapy (HRT) rather than ERT. Progestins are usually administered orally but may be used vaginally or as an intrauterine device. The dose of progestins should be kept low to prevent attenuating the beneficial effects of ERT on the cardiovascular system and brain.

There are many ways to administer progestins. The most commonly used oral progestins are medroxyprogesterone acetate (MPA) in doses of 5 to 10 mg, norethindrone in doses of 0.3 to 1 mg, and micronized progesterone in doses of 100 to 300 mg. Equivalent doses to prevent hyperplasia when administered for at least 10 days in a woman receiving ERT (equivalent to 0.625 mg CEE) are as follows: MPA, 5 mg; norethindrone, 0.7 mg; and micronized progesterone, 200 mg. Larger doses of estrogen may require larger doses and more prolonged regimens of progestins. In sequential administration of progestins, the number of days (length of exposure) is more important than the dose. Thus, if a woman is receiving oral ERT continuously, a regimen of at least 10 to 12 days of exposure is preferable to a 7-day regimen.

When progestins are administered sequentially (10–14 days each month), withdrawal bleeding occurs in about 80% of women. Continuous administration of both estrogen and progestin (continuous combined therapy) was developed to achieve amenorrhea. In the first 3 to 6 months, breakthrough bleeding and spotting is common. In some women on this regimen, amenorrhea is never completely achieved. The most common combination, in the United States, is a single tablet containing 0.625 mg CEE and 2.5 mg MPA. A similar tablet with 5 mg MPA is also available. Currently, the only marketed sequential regimen is one that contains 0.625 mg CEE and 5 mg MPA, whch is added for 14 days each cycle. Other regimens are under review by the Food and Drug Administration.

Progesterone administered vaginally (in low doses) avoids systemic effects and results in high concentrations of progesterone in the uterus. Intrauterine delivery of progestins is ideal for targeting the uterus but is not approved in the United States.

Progestins, particularly when taken orally, may lead to problems of continuance or compliance because of side effects, including mood alterations and bleeding. These have to be dealt with effectively and usually require more flexibility in prescribing habits. Most short-term clinical trials have demonstrated an attenuating effect of progestins on cardiovascular end points that are improved with estrogen. These include lipoprotein changes (an attenuation of the rise in HDL-C) as well as arterial and metabolic effects. A reduction in blood flow and some brain effects may also be found. Nevertheless, observational cohort studies have not demonstrated any difference in benefit between ERT and HRT. It would be prudent, however, to use the lowest dose of progestin necessary to prevent hyperplasia until more data are available. Except in rare circumstances (e.g., previous endometrial cancer, recent diagnosis of endometriosis) progestins should not be prescribed in women who have undergone hysterectomy.

ANDROGEN THERAPY. In a very subtle way, women are relatively androgen deficient. Clinicians have proposed adding androgen to ERT or HRT for complaints on problems relating to libido and energy. Although well-controlled trials using parenteral testosterone have shown benefit in younger oophorectomized women, there are few data showing any benefit using more physiologic therapy, particularly in older women. As newer forms and doses of androgen become available, perhaps more women may benefit from this approach. At present, androgen therapy should be individualized and considered for those women who have symptoms that are not adequately relieved with traditional ERT or HRT. At lower doses, androgenizing side effects are very infrequent but should be discussed before prescribing testosterone. At present, small doses of methyltestosterone (1.25 and 2.5 mg) added to esterified estrogens are available in tablets, as are testosterone patches that are available for men (and therefore require dose reductions) and testosterone subcutaneous pellets. Administration of dehydroepiandrosterone at 25 to 50 mg/day may also be an option.

SELECTIVE ESTROGEN RECEPTOR MODULATORS (SERMs) AND OTHER ALTERNATIVES. If women chose not to receive estrogen or should not because of an estrogen-responsive disease such as breast cancer, there are several alternatives. For osteoporosis, bisphosphonates are an effective therapy. Alendronate, in doses of 5 and 10 mg, may be highly beneficial as a primary agent but may also be used as an adjunctive to estrogen for women with low bone mass. Obviously, calcium, vitamin D, and exercise are important adjuncts as well but when used alone are not as effective as other measures discussed here. Nevertheless, all postmenopausal women should receive adequate vitamin D and ingest at least 1000 mg of calcium and up to 1500 mg if not receiving other measures.

SERMs such as tamoxifen and raloxifene have mixed agonist and antagonistic properties. Both of these first- and second-generation SERMs antagonize estrogen action in the breast and induce hot flushes. Raloxifene, but not tamoxifen, is also antagonistic to the uterus (endometrium). Both have agonistic properties on bone and liver. This leads to a protective effect against osteoporosis and beneficial lipid and lipoprotein effects. Table 256–2 provides an appreciation of the current agonistic and antagonistic effects that are important for postmenopausal health.

Raloxifene has been shown to be beneficial for the prevention of bone loss, although the effects are less than those of ERT at

Table 256–2 ■ EFFECTS OF ESTRADIOL AND SERMS ON VARIOUS ORGAN SYSTEMS AS PERTINENT TO POSTMENOPAUSAL USE

	BRAIN	UTERUS	VAGINA	BREAST	BONE	CARDIOVASCULAR SYSTEM
E₂	++	++	++	++	++	++
Pure antiestrogen	−	−	−	−	−	−
"Ideal"	++	−	++	−	++	++
Tamoxifen	−	+	−	−	+	+
Raloxifene	−	−	−	−	+	+
Isoflavones	+	−	+−	−	+	+

standard doses. Both tamoxifen and raloxifene, while having beneficial effects on bone resorption, also reduce cholesterol and LDL-C but do not increase HDL-C. Raloxifene, as a more potent estrogen antagonist, may not have beneficial vascular effects. The agonistic hepatic effects, in addition to the beneficial effects on lipoproteins, increase the risk of venous thrombosis. Raloxifene may be viewed to be an alternative that is keenly suited for the women with a uterus who is asymptomatic but needs protection against osteoporosis. More long-term data on these alternatives will be available shortly.

For prevention of cardiovascular disease, diet and exercise as well as use of statins and possibly the use of aspirin are all important measures. Data also point to the beneficial effects of isoflavanoids in dietary phytoestrogens such as soy. Data, primarily in the monkey, have provided evidence for beneficial cardiovascular, brain, and bone effects while having minimal, if any, effects on reproductive tissue such as the breast and uterus.

Col NF, Eckman, MH, Karas RH, et al: Patient-specific decisions about hormone replacement therapy in postmenopausal women. JAMA 277:1140–1147, 1997. *Up-to-date review of epidemiologic evidence to help decision making about the use of hormones.*

Lindsay R, Bush TL, Grady D, et al: Therapeutic controversy: Estrogen replacement in menopause. J Clin Endocrinol Metab 81:3829–3838, 1996. *Concise evaluation of the risks of osteoporosis and the benefits of various treatments.*

Lobo RA: Benefits and risks of estrogen replacement therapy. Am J Obstet Gynecol 173(Suppl.):982–989, 1995. *Assessment of risks and benefits of hormone replacement with a focus on changes in mortality and quality of life.*

Stampfer MJ, Colditz GA: Estrogen replacement therapy and coronary heart disease: A quantitative assessment of the epidemiologic evidence. Prev Med 20:47–63, 1991. *Most definitive meta-analysis of observational data showing a protective effect of estrogen on heart disease.*

257 OSTEOPOROSIS

Joel S. Finkelstein

Osteoporosis, the most common type of metabolic bone disease, is characterized by a parallel reduction in bone mineral and bone matrix so that bone is decreased in amount but is of normal composition. Osteoporosis affects 20 million Americans and leads to approximately 1.3 million fractures in the United States each year. During the course of their lifetime, women lose about 50% of their trabecular bone and 30% of their cortical bone, and 30% of all postmenopausal white women eventually sustain osteoporotic fractures. By extreme old age, one third of all women and one sixth of all men will have a hip fracture. The annual cost of health care and lost productivity due to osteoporosis is nearly $14 billion in the United States.

ETIOLOGY AND PATHOGENESIS

At any point in time, bone density in adults depends on both the peak bone density achieved during development and the subsequent bone loss (Fig. 257–1). Thus, osteopenia can result either from deficient pubertal bone accretion, accelerated adult bone loss, or both.

DETERMINANTS OF PEAK BONE DENSITY. Bone density increases dramatically during puberty in response to gonadal steroids

and eventually reaches values in young adults that are nearly double those of children. Other factors that influence peak bone density are listed in Table 257–1. Of these, genetic factors account for up to 80% of the variance in peak bone mass. The impact of genetic factors on bone density has been demonstrated in several ways. For example, bone density is lower in the daughters of women with osteoporosis than in those without osteoporosis. Moreover, the concordance of bone density is much higher among monozygotic than dizygotic twins. Several genes, including the vitamin D receptor gene, the estrogen receptor gene, and the type I procollagen genes, have been implicated as determinants of bone density.

Men have higher bone density than women and blacks have higher bone density than whites. These differences may account for a lower incidence of osteoporotic fractures in men and in blacks. Men with histories of constitutionally delayed puberty have decreased peak bone density, a finding that may be important in the pathogenesis of osteoporosis in some men. Similar findings have been reported in women with delayed menarche. Studies in identical twins suggest that moderate calcium supplementation can enhance prepubertal bone accretion. Associations between peak bone density and physical activity during development have also been reported.

PHYSIOLOGIC CAUSES OF ADULT BONE LOSS. After peak bone density is reached, bone density remains stable for years and then declines. Bone loss begins before menses cease in women, although the precise time of onset is unknown. Once menses cease, the rate of bone loss is accelerated severalfold in women. During the first 5 to 10 years of the menopause, trabecular bone is lost faster than cortical bone, with rates of 2 to 4% and 1 to 2% per year, respectively. A woman can lose 10 to 15% of her cortical bone and 25 to 30% of her trabecular bone during this time, a loss that can be prevented by estrogen replacement therapy. Furthermore, rates of bone loss vary considerably between women. It is not clear why some postmenopausal women are "fast losers" of bone. A subset of women in whom osteopenia is more severe than expected for their age are said to have type I or "postmenopausal" osteoporosis (Fig. 257–2). Clinically, type I osteoporosis often presents as vertebral "crush" fractures or Colles' fractures. The mechanism whereby estrogen deficiency leads to bone loss is still

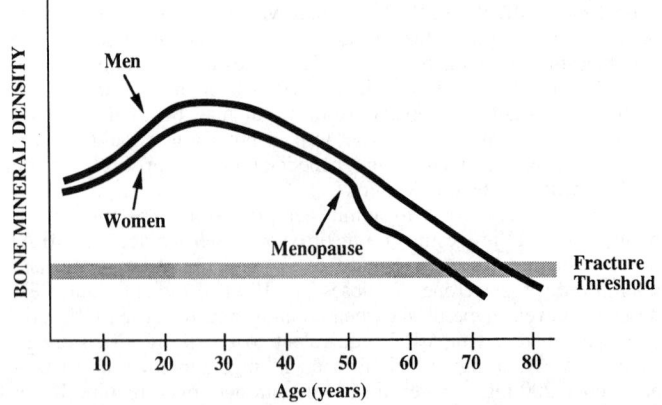

FIGURE 257–1 ■ Cortical bone mineral density versus age in men and women. Women have lower peak cortical bone density than men and experience a period of rapid bone loss at the time of the menopause, thus reaching the fracture threshold (the level of bone density at which the risk of developing osteoporotic fractures begins to increase) earlier than men.

Table 257–1 ■ FACTORS THAT MAY AFFECT PEAK BONE MASS

Gender
Race
Genetic factors
Gonadal steroids
Growth hormone
Timing of puberty
Calcium intake
Exercise

not established. Evidence suggests that estrogen deficiency may increase skeletal production of bone-resorbing cytokines such as interleukin-1 (IL-1), interleukin-6 (IL-6), and tumor necrosis factor. Estrogen deficiency may also decrease production of osteoprotegerin, a soluble member of the tumor necrosis receptor family that normally reduces osteoclastogenesis and bone resorption. Estrogen deficiency may also reduce skeletal production of growth factors that stimulate bone formation, such as insulin-like growth factor-1 and transforming growth factor-β. Estrogen deficiency increases the skeleton's sensitivity to the resorptive effects of parathyroid hormone. Estrogen deficiency therefore leads to a small increase in serum calcium levels. According to one hypothesis, increased calcium levels suppress parathyroid hormone secretion, thereby decreasing renal 1,25-dihydroxyvitamin D formation, which then limits intestinal calcium absorption (see Fig. 257–2). Finally, the discovery of estrogen receptors on osteoblasts suggests that estrogen deficiency may also alter bone formation directly.

Once the period of rapid postmenopausal bone loss ends, bone loss continues at a more gradual rate throughout life. The osteopenia that results from normal aging, which occurs in both women and men, has been termed *type II* or *"senile" osteoporosis* (Fig. 257–3). Because type II osteoporosis is associated with a more balanced decrease in cortical and trabecular bone mass, fractures of the hip, pelvis, wrist, proximal humerus, proximal tibia, and vertebral bodies all occur commonly. Factors that may be important in the pathogenesis of type II osteoporosis include (1) a primary defect in the ability of the kidney to make 1,25-dihydroxyvitamin D and/or decreased intestinal sensitivity to 1,25-dihydroxyvitamin D, leading to diminished calcium absorption and mild secondary

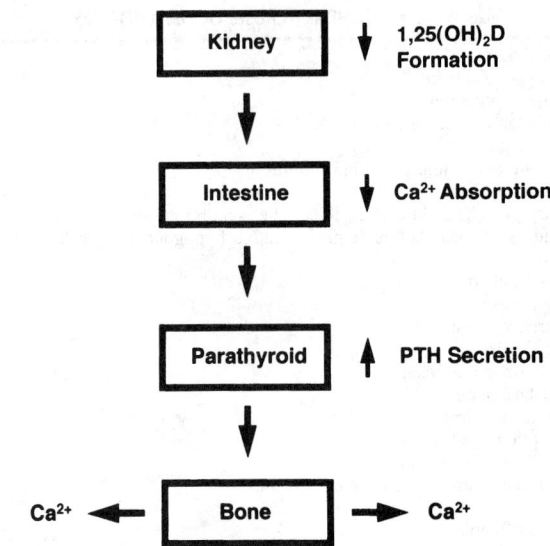

FIGURE 257–3 ■ Physiologic alterations in women with type II ("senile") osteoporosis.

hyperparathyroidism, and (2) a decrease in osteoblastic bone formation with aging. Finally, the distinctions between type I and type II osteoporosis are often quite arbitrary and there may be considerable overlap between these syndromes.

SECONDARY CAUSES OF ADULT BONE LOSS. A large number of disorders can lead to osteoporosis independent from the normal effects of the menopause in women and aging in both women and men (Table 257–2). For example, young women who develop estrogen deficiency due to hyperprolactinemia, anorexia nervosa, or hypothalamic amenorrhea frequently lose bone in a manner similar to that which occurs at the onset of the natural menopause. Hypogonadism is also an important secondary cause of osteoporosis in men. Other endocrine disorders such as hyperthyroidism, hyperparathyroidism, hypercortisolism, and growth hormone deficiency are important secondary causes of osteoporosis primarily due to increased bone resorption in the former two disorders and decreased bone formation and intestinal calcium absorption in the last disorder. Patients with hepatobiliary disorders most often have low-turnover osteoporosis, although some have osteomalacia or secondary hyperparathyroidism due to calcium and/or vitamin D malabsorption. Bone density is decreased in women with histories of major depression, possibly because of increased cortisol production. The osteoporosis in patients with marrow-related disorders may be due to local effects of cytokines on bone remodeling or to the release of systemic factors that activate bone resorption. Peak adult bone mass is compromised in individuals with certain connective tissue disorders, such as osteogenesis imperfecta. Many drugs such as ethanol, heparin, glucocorticoids, cyclosporine, suppressive doses of thyroxine, and anticonvulsants can cause osteoporosis. Ethanol is toxic to osteoblasts, whereas heparin and cyclosporine increase osteoclastic bone resorption. In patients receiving anticonvulsant therapy, the combined effects of reduced 25-hydroxyvitamin D levels, secondary hyperparathyroidism, direct inhibition of intestinal calcium transport, and suppression of osteoblast function can lead to osteoporosis and/or osteomalacia. Bone resorption is accelerated in patients who are immobilized and in patients with rheumatoid arthritis. Finally, bone formation may be diminished in individuals with insulin-dependent diabetes mellitus.

CLINICAL MANIFESTATIONS

Osteoporosis is asymptomatic unless it results in a fracture—usually a vertebral compression fracture or a fracture of the wrist, hip, ribs, pelvis, or humerus. Vertebral compression fractures often occur with minimal stress, such as with sneezing, bending, or lifting a light object. The middle and lower thoracic and upper lumbar regions are most frequently involved. Back pain usually begins acutely and produces pain that often radiates laterally to the

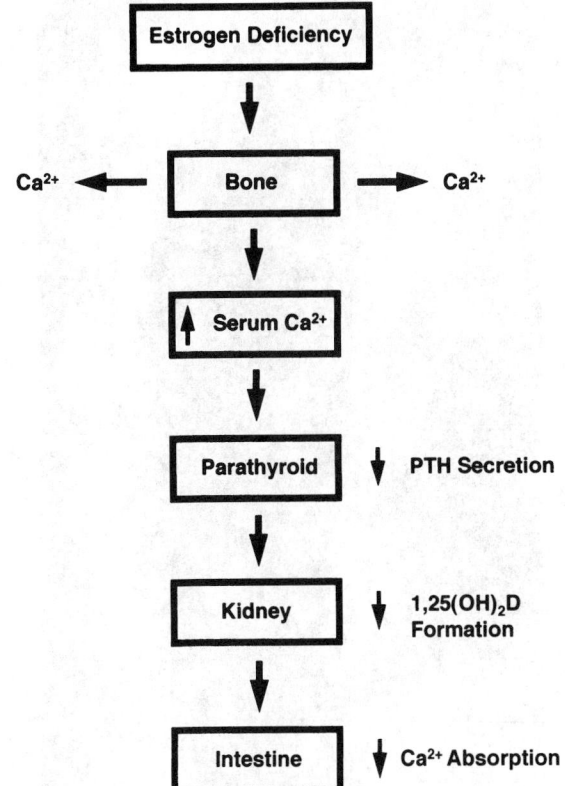

FIGURE 257–2 ■ Physiologic alterations in women with type I ("postmenopausal") osteoporosis.

Table 257–2 ■ SECONDARY CAUSES OF OSTEOPOROSIS

Endocrine Diseases
Female hypogonadism
  Hyperprolactinemia
  Hypothalamic amenorrhea
  Anorexia nervosa
  Premature and primary ovarian failure
Male hypogonadism
  Primary gonadal failure (e.g., Klinefelter syndrome)
  Secondary gonadal failure (e.g., idiopathic hypogonadotropic hypogonadism)
  Delayed puberty
Hyperthyroidism
Hyperparathyroidism
Hypercortisolism
Growth hormone deficiency
Gastrointestinal Diseases
Subtotal gastrectomy
Malabsorption syndromes
Chronic obstructive jaundice
Primary biliary cirrhosis and other cirrhoses
Alactasia
Bone Marrow Disorders
Multiple myeloma
Lymphoma
Leukemia
Hemolytic anemias
Systemic mastocytosis
Disseminated carcinoma
Connective Tissue Diseases
Osteogenesis imperfecta
Ehlers-Danlos syndrome
Marfan syndrome
Homocystinuria
Drugs
Alcohol
Heparin
Glucocorticoids
Thyroxine
Anticonvulsants
Gonadotropin-releasing hormone agonists
Cyclosporine
Chemotherapy
Miscellaneous Causes
Immobilization
Rheumatoid arthritis

flanks and anteriorly. The pain subsides gradually over a period of weeks to months and recurs with the occurrence of new fractures. Patients with fractures that result in spinal deformity may have a chronic backache that is made worse by standing. Such patients lose height and may develop the characteristic dorsal kyphosis and cervical lordosis known as the "dowager's hump." In some patients, vertebral collapse can occur slowly and without symptoms. Fractures of the femoral neck and intertrochanteric region are the most devastating complication of osteoporosis. The type of hip fracture is best predicted by the bone density of the trochanter. Hip fractures are associated with falls, occurring either as a result of modest trauma, or, in some instances, before the fall. The likelihood of suffering a hip fracture during a fall is also related to the direction of the fall so that fractures are more likely to occur when falling to the side, probably because there is less soft tissue available to dissipate the impact. Secondary complications of hip fractures, such as pulmonary thromboembolism or nosocomial infections, carry a mortality rate of 15 to 20% in elderly patients, and an additional 30% of hip fracture victims require long-term nursing home care.

A characteristic radiograph of osteoporosis of the spine is shown in Figure 257–4. With the loss of trabecular bone in the vertebral bodies, the vertebral end plates appear to be accentuated. Loss of horizontal trabeculae causes the vertical trabeculae to appear more prominent. The normal contrast between the radiodensity of the spinal column and the adjacent soft tissues also may be lost. Vertebral deformity may take the form of collapse (reduction in both anterior and posterior height), anterior wedging (reduction in anterior height), or the so-called codfish deformity (due to weakening of the subchondral plates and expansion of the intervertebral disks).

Protrusion of the intervertebral disks in the vertebral bodies produces Schmorl's nodules. In the absence of fractures, radiographs are insensitive indicators of bone loss because a substantial reduction in bone mass is required before it is visible on radiographs.

DIAGNOSIS

The diagnosis of osteopenia can be made by either documenting a typical fragility fracture or measuring bone mineral density, in which case a bone density value below the lower limit of normal for sex-matched young adults establishes the diagnosis. The World Health Organization nomenclature uses the term *osteopenia* to refer to individuals whose bone mineral density is between 1 and 2.5 standard deviations below peak bone mass and the term *osteoporosis* to refer to individuals whose bone mineral density is more than 2.5 standard deviations below peak bone mass. Although this terminology may have clinical utility, the term *osteopenia* is actually a generic term that refers to decreased bone mass, regardless of the severity or the histopathology. A true diagnosis of osteoporosis requires a histomorphometric analysis of bone because some individuals with low bone mineral density have osteomalacia.

BONE DENSITOMETRY. Several techniques are available for measuring bone mineral density in the axial and appendicular skeleton (Table 257–3). Large prospective studies have demonstrated that bone density measurements of the distal and proximal radius, os calcis, proximal femur, or spine can predict the development of the major types of osteoporotic fractures, including hip fractures. In general, for every one standard deviation that bone mineral density decreases, the risk of all future osteoporotic fractures increases by about 50%, regardless of the technique or the site used to assess bone density. However, a bone density measurement at a specific skeletal site predicts fractures at that site better than bone density measurements made at a different skeletal site. Moreover, techniques for assessing bone density differ greatly in their reproducibility, radiation exposure, examination time, cost, and sensitivity for detecting osteopenia. Because it measures trabecular bone in the vertebral bodies, quantitative computed tomography (QCT) of the spine is the most sensitive method for diagnosing osteopenia. However, because the expense and radiation dose of QCT are high and

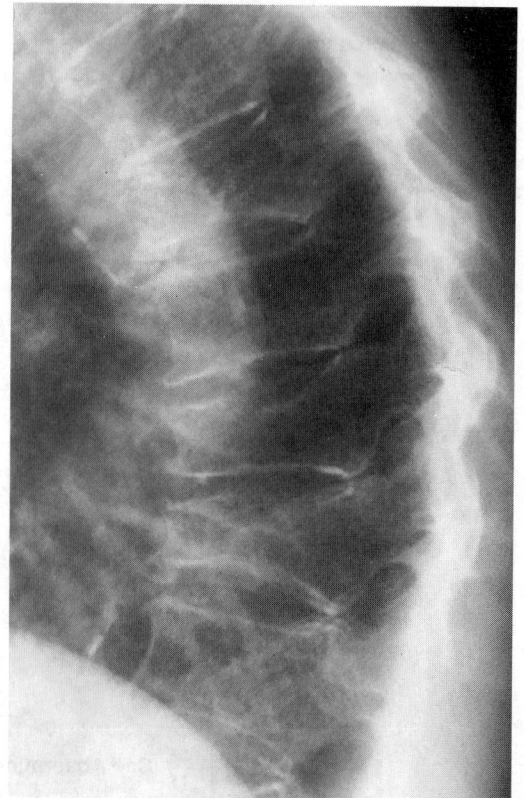

FIGURE 257–4 ■ Radiograph showing radiolucency, compression fractures, and kyphosis in the spine of a patient with osteoporosis.

Table 257-3 ■ TECHNIQUES FOR MEASURING BONE MINERAL DENSITY

SITES MEASURED*	PRECISION (%)	ACCURACY (%)	SCAN TIME (minutes)	RADIATION DOSE (mrem)
Quantitative computed tomography (QCT) Lumbar spine Proximal radius Distal radius	2–10	5–20	10–15	100–1000
Single-photon absorptiometry (SPA) Proximal radius Distal radius Calcaneus	1–3	4–6	3–5	10–20
Dual-photon absorptiometry (DPA) Lumbar spine (anteroposterior) Lumbar spine (lateral) Proximal femur Total body	2–6	4–10	20–40	10–15
Dual-energy x-ray absorptiometry (DXA) Lumbar spine (anteroposterior) Lumbar spine (lateral) Proximal radius Distal radius Proximal femur Total body	1–2	3–5	2–8	1–3

*For SPA, numbers refer to measurements of the proximal radius. For QCT, numbers refer to measurements of the lumbar spine. For DPA and DXA, numbers refer to anteroposterior measurements of the lumbar spine.

its reproducibility is relatively poor, it is not an ideal technique when repeat measurements aimed at detecting small changes in bone density are needed. Single-photon absorptiometry of the proximal forearm has good precision and low radiation exposure but is relatively insensitive for detecting osteopenia because it measures cortical bone, which is lost more slowly than trabecular bone in the early menopause. Dual-photon absorptiometry (DPA), which measures bone density in the axial skeleton and proximal femur, is limited by poor reproducibility, long examination times, and artifacts caused by vascular calcifications and changes in the radioactive source. For most patients, dual-energy x-ray absorptiometry (DXA) of either the lumbar spine or the proximal femur is the method of choice for measuring bone mineral density. Because DXA scans of the spine in the anteroposterior projection include both the trabecular-rich vertebral bodies and the cortical-rich posterior spinal elements, DXA measurement of the spine is not as sensitive as QCT for detecting early trabecular bone loss. However, its far greater precision, low radiation dose, rapid examination time, and lower cost make DXA preferable to QCT in most situations, particularly when serial scans are planned to assess changes in bone mineral density. Some DXA scanners can measure spinal bone mineral density in both the anteroposterior and lateral projections. Lateral spine DXA is more sensitive than anteroposterior spine DXA for detecting osteoporosis, although its reproducibility is somewhat lower. DXA measurements of the proximal femur predict hip fractures better than measurements made at other sites and may also be preferred in elderly patients in whom focal osteosclerosis associated with degenerative changes of the posterior spine can mask decreases in bone mineral density of the vertebral bodies.

BIOCHEMICAL MARKERS OF BONE TURNOVER. In recent years, there has been considerable interest in tests for biochemical markers of bone formation (serum osteocalcin, bone-specific alkaline phosphatase, or type-1 procollagen carboxy-terminal peptide) and bone resorption (urine hydroxyproline, urine pyridinium cross links, or urine cross-linked N-telopeptides of type 1 collagen). In theory, a simple blood or urine test that could predict rates of bone loss or the response to therapy would be of great value. However, the clinical utility of routine measurements of these biochemical markers of bone turnover has not been established. Some data suggest that measurements of bone formation or resorption markers, either alone or in combination, can predict rates of bone loss in postmenopausal women receiving calcium or other antiresorptive agents whereas other data do not. Moreover, correlations between bone turnover markers and changes in bone mineral density may not be strong enough to be useful in individual patients. Bone turnover markers may also be independent predictors for osteoporotic fracture after adjusting for bone mineral density. At

the present time, routine use of bone turnover measurements should be discouraged. Specialized current or potential future uses for bone turnover marker measurements are shown in Table 257–4.

SECONDARY CAUSES OF OSTEOPOROSIS. Secondary causes of osteoporosis should be sought in patients with an established diagnosis of osteoporosis, particularly when the bone density is significantly lower than that of age- and sex-matched individuals. A history and a physical examination that focus on the factors that may affect peak bone mass (see Table 257–1) and secondary causes of osteoporosis (see Table 257–2), and selected laboratory tests, are sufficient in most patients. Levels of serum calcium, inorganic phosphate, and alkaline phosphatase are usually normal in patients with osteoporosis, although the latter may be elevated transiently after a fracture. A sustained elevation of the alkaline phosphatase level, in the absence of liver disease, may suggest osteomalacia, Paget's disease, or skeletal metastases. Other routine chemistry tests can help exclude renal or hepatic diseases, and a complete blood cell count may help uncover a hematologic or myeloproliferative disorder. Because multiple myeloma can mimic involutional osteoporosis, it should be considered when evaluating patients with osteoporosis, particularly those with unexpectedly severe disease. Measuring serum parathyroid hormone and 25-hydroxyvitamin D levels is recommended to exclude hyperparathyroidism and vitamin D deficiency. A serum thyroid-stimulating hormone level should be checked when thyroid disease is suspected. In men with unexplained osteoporosis, a serum testosterone level should be measured. The clinical utility of measuring biochemical markers of bone turnover has not been established. Measurements of bone turnover markers may, however, be useful to evaluate patients with osteoporosis of unknown cause or of unexplained severity. Moreover, it is possible that these markers may

Table 257-4 ■ POTENTIAL USES OF BIOCHEMICAL MARKERS OF BONE TURNOVER

1. Evaluation of osteoporosis of unknown cause
2. Evaluation of osteoporosis of unexplained severity
3. Monitoring therapy in patients who cannot tolerate standard doses of antiresorptive agents
4. Monitoring therapy in patients with questionable absorption of antiresorptive agents
5. To assess mechanisms of bone loss in clinical trials
6. Predicting rates of bone loss in patients not receiving antiresponsive therapy
7. Predicting changes in bone density in patients receiving antiresorptive therapy
8. To provide adjunctive information to predict risk of fractures
9. Selection of patients for anabolic vs. antiresponsive therapies

help classify patients into high and low bone turnover states in the future and thereby provide a more rational basis for selecting therapies. Finally, in selected patients, iliac crest bone biopsy after double tetracycline labeling may be useful, particularly for distinguishing osteoporosis from osteomalacia.

TREATMENT

At present, it is not possible to reverse established osteoporosis. Early intervention, however, can prevent osteoporosis in most people and later intervention can halt the progression of osteoporosis once it has developed. The choice of treatment for osteoporosis depends on its cause and the stage of the illness. If a secondary cause of osteoporosis is present, specific treatment should be aimed at correcting the underlying disorder. During the acute phase of vertebral compression, attention is directed toward relieving pain with analgesics, muscle relaxants, heat, massage, and/or rest. Many patients with discomfort related to osteoporotic fractures or deformity benefit from a well-designed program of physical therapy. Some patients appear to benefit from a corset or an orthopedic back brace. Both weight-bearing and non–weight bearing exercises appear to have beneficial effects on bone mass. For most patients, exercises to strengthen the abdominal and back muscles are appropriate and referral to a physical therapist with expertise in treating osteoporotic patients is often helpful. Precautions to prevent falls should be taken. Pharmacologic therapy is aimed at preventing further bone loss and decreasing the likelihood of future fracture.

CALCIUM. Both dietary calcium intake and fractional intestinal calcium absorption decrease with age. Most postmenopausal women consume less than 500 mg of calcium each day, far below the U.S. Recommended Dietary Allowance (RDA) of 1000 to 1500 mg. The effects of calcium supplementation on bone mass in early postmenopausal women have been examined in several prospective, randomized trials. The results are inconsistent. In general, it appears that calcium can retard, but not arrest, cortical bone loss from the forearm in women who are within the first several years of the menopause. Calcium supplementation, however, is clearly less effective than estrogen. Most studies have failed to demonstrate a protective effect of calcium on spinal bone loss in early postmenopausal women. Calcium therapy appears to be more effective in arresting bone loss in late postmenopausal women, although some studies indicate that administering calcium does not halt their bone loss completely. Overall, it appears that calcium therapy is somewhat beneficial in both early and late postmenopausal women. Additional therapy, however, is needed if the goal of therapy is to prevent bone loss completely. In the United States, the recommended daily calcium intake for adolescents and young adults between the ages of 11 and 24 years is 1200 to 1500 mg. The recommended daily calcium intake for men between 25 and 65 years and women between 25 and 50 years is 1000 mg. Postmenopausal women up to the age of 65 years should consume 1000 mg of calcium per day if they are also on hormone replacement therapy and 1500 mg of calcium per day in the absence of estrogen replacement. Adults older than age 65 should consume 1500 mg of calcium daily.

ESTROGEN. Estrogen replacement therapy inhibits osteoclastic bone resorption. It prevents both cortical and trabecular bone loss in estrogen-deficient women and is effective if administered orally or topically. Estrogen replacement therapy prevents bone loss in both early and late postmenopausal women, although its efficacy has not been tested adequately in women older than age 75. On average, spinal bone mineral density increases 3 to 5% during the first 3 years of estrogen therapy and significant bone loss is rare among women who are compliant with their treatment regimen. Because bone loss is most rapid in the first years of the menopause, the benefits of estrogen therapy probably are greater if started during this time before a substantial amount of bone loss has occurred. Case-control studies suggest that estrogen therapy significantly reduces the risk of forearm, vertebral, pelvic, and hip fractures in postmenopausal women. The minimally effective doses of estrogen to prevent bone loss are 0.625 mg/day of conjugated estrogens, 2 mg/day of estradiol, 20 μg/day of ethinyl estradiol, or 50 μg/day of transdermal estrogen, although some studies have shown that lower doses of conjugated estrogens (0.3 mg/day) prevent bone loss when combined with sufficient calcium intake. How long a women should remain on estrogen replacement therapy has not been established.

Although the beneficial effects of estrogen replacement therapy on bone mass are well established, less than 15% of postmenopausal women in the United States take estrogen replacement. The decision to treat with estrogen is influenced by other factors and should be individualized. In some women, estrogen is prescribed to alleviate menopausal symptoms. In others, the prospect of adhering to a treatment program that may produce menstruation is unacceptable. The relationships between estrogen replacement therapy and endometrial cancer, breast cancer, and ischemic heart disease have been the subjects of numerous investigations. When given without concomitant progestin, estrogen replacement therapy increases the risk of endometrial carcinoma. Thus, in a woman whose uterus in intact, estrogen replacement therapy should be combined with a progestin, administered either cyclically (e.g., 5 to 10 mg medroxyprogesterone acetate for 10 to 14 days each month) or continuously (e.g., 2.5 mg medroxyprogesterone acetate per day). The latter regimen often eliminates menstrual bleeding after an initial period of 3 to 6 months during which irregular bleeding may occur. Progestins may also enhance the osteoprotective effect of estrogens. In a woman who has had a hysterectomy, unopposed estrogen should be given daily. Estrogen therapy is generally contraindicated in women with histories of endometrial cancer.

The relationships between estrogen replacement therapy and breast cancer or cardiovascular disease have been the subject of many case-control and cohort studies yet remain unclear. Although many studies, including at least one meta-analysis, have concluded that long-term (greater than 15 years) estrogen replacement is associated with an increase in the risk of breast cancer in postmenopausal women, other studies have failed to detect such a relationship. It has also been suggested that the risk of developing breast cancer is increased in women who take higher doses of estrogen (at least 1.25 mg of conjugated estrogen) and among women with a family history of breast cancer. A recent large prospective cohort study, however, did not detect an increase in the risk of estrogen-induced breast cancer in postmenopausal women with a family history of breast cancer. The risk of breast cancer appears to be restricted to current estrogen users and there appears to be little, if any, increase in the risk of breast cancer if estrogen therapy is used for less than 5 years. Because the relationship between estrogen replacement therapy and breast cancer remains uncertain, estrogen replacement therapy is generally contraindicated in women with a history of breast cancer and all postmenopausal women receiving estrogen therapy should have regular breast examinations and annual mammograms. Numerous case-control and cohort studies have reported that estrogen replacement therapy decreases the risk of major coronary disease by approximately 50%. The potential for bias due to patient selection or uneven diagnostic surveillance in these nonrandomized studies of breast cancer and cardiovascular disease cannot, however, be excluded completely. In fact, the first large randomized controlled trial to assess the effects of estrogen/progestin replacement therapy on the occurrence of non-fatal myocardial infarction or cardiovascular death in postmenopausal women with established coronary disease failed to detect any overall difference between treated and untreated women. The potential beneficial effect of estrogen on coronary heart disease is often attributed to its ability to lower low-density lipoprotein (LDL) cholesterol and raise high-density lipoprotein (HDL) cholesterol. Still, because the reduction in cardiac events appears to be limited to current estrogen users and exceeds that attributable to changes in blood lipids, other mechanisms, including direct effects of estrogens on vascular wall function and coagulation factors, may be important. Finally, estrogen replacement therapy may increase the risk of venous thromboembolic disease.

SELECTIVE ESTROGEN RECEPTOR MODULATORS. Tamoxifen, a mixed estrogen receptor antagonist and agonist, prevents bone loss from the spine and proximal femur in women with breast cancer and lowers serum LDL cholesterol levels. Tamoxifen blocks the actions of estrogen on the breast but acts like an estrogen agonist on the endometrium. Data suggest that tamoxifen reduces the risk of breast cancer in women at high risk for developing breast cancer, although it increases the risk of endometrial cancer and venous thromboembolic disease.

Raloxifene, a selective estrogen receptor modulator (SERM) that is closely related to tamoxifen, prevents bone loss from the spine, proximal femur, and total body in early postmenopausal women and reduces serum total and LDL cholesterol levels. Like tamoxifen, raloxifene blocks the effect of estrogen on the breast. In contrast to tamoxifen, however, raloxifene does not cause endometrial hyperplasia. In woman with established postmenopausal osteoporosis, raloxifene reduces the risk of spine fractures and the incidence of estrogen receptor positive cases of breast cancer. The molecular basis for the differential effects of raloxifene on estrogen-responsive tissues is reasonably well understood. Both estrogen and raloxifene bind to the same site of the estrogen receptor. When estrogen binds to its receptor, the complex assumes a conformation that allows binding of specific co-activator proteins. When raloxifene binds to the estrogen receptor, however, the receptor folds in such a way that prevents binding of these proteins and may recruit binding of additional co-repressor proteins. Differential expression of these co-activator and co-repressor proteins in tissues may be involved in the tissue-specific effects of raloxifene and estrogen. Raloxifene is approved by the U.S. Food and Drug Administration (FDA) for prevention of bone loss in early postmenopausal women and is under review for women with established osteoporosis. The recommended dosage is 60 mg/day. It is well tolerated by most women. Controlled studies have not demonstrated an increase in vasomotor flushes in raloxifene-treated women, although anecdotal reports suggest that this may occur. Like estrogen and tamoxifen, raloxifene does increase the risk of venous thromboembolic disease. Studies are being done to determine if raloxifene reduces the risk of fractures in postmenopausal women with established osteoporosis and to determine whether raloxifene reduces the risk of breast cancer in women. Several other SERMs are under development.

BISPHOSPHONATES. Bisphosphonates are carbon-substituted analogues of pyrophosphate that bind tightly to hydroxyapatite crystals and inhibit osteoclastic bone resorption. Several bisphosphonates have been reported to increase bone mineral density in postmenopausal women, although alendronate is the only bisphosphonate that has been approved by the FDA for prevention of bone loss or treatment of established osteoporosis in postmenopausal women. Alendronate is a second-generation animobisphosphonate that is much more potent than etidronate, a first-generation bisphosphonate. Oral alendronate, in a dose of 5 mg/day, increased bone mineral density of the lumbar spine, proximal femur, and total body in early postmenopausal women, although the increases were slightly smaller than in women who received hormone replacement therapy. In contrast to hormone replacement therapy, alendronate did not prevent cortical bone loss from the radius. In late postmenopausal women with pre-existing spine fractures, alendronate, in a dose of 10 mg/day, increased bone mineral density of the lumbar spine and proximal femur and reduced the incidence of osteoporotic fractures, including hip fractures and symptomatic vertebral fractures, by approximately 50%. Although bone loss resumes after alendronate therapy is discontinued, there is no evidence that the rate of bone loss is accelerated. Because alendronate is poorly absorbed in the presence of food, it must be given by itself after an overnight fast and patients should remain fasting for at least 30 minutes. Occasional patients may develop esophagitis or other gastrointestinal problems during alendronate therapy. The symptoms of esophagitis usually begin within 1 to 2 months after alendronate therapy is started. To decrease the incidence of these side effects, alendronate should be taken with at least 8 oz of water and patients should remain upright for at least 30 minutes after taking the medication.

Like alendronate, cyclic etidronate administration increases spinal bone mineral density and decreases the incidence of vertebral fractures in late menopausal women. Etidronate is less potent, however, than alendronate and inhibits normal bone mineralization when given continuously for many months. Although initial reports suggested that cyclic etidronate administration reduced the incidence of spine fractures by 50%, further follow-up of these patients indicates that the reduction in vertebral fracture risk may be considerably less and that the benefits of etidronate therapy may be restricted to a subgroup of women at particularly high risk for fracture. Etidronate is well tolerated. The best documented effects of etidronate are with a dose of 400 mg/day for the first 2 weeks of every 3-month period. To ensure adequate absorption, patients should not eat for 2 hours before or after etidronate administration.

Other bisphosphonates, including risedronate and ibandronate, are being investigated for treatment of osteoporosis.

CALCITONIN. Calcitonin is a 32-amino-acid peptide that is normally produced by the thyroid C cells. Osteoclasts have calcitonin receptors and calcitonin rapidly inhibits osteoclastic bone resorption. Calcitonin from salmon is more potent than human calcitonin and is therefore preferred in most circumstances. The effects of salmon calcitonin therapy on bone loss in women who are within the first 5 years of the menopause have been inconsistent. Some groups have demonstrated that intranasal salmon calcitonin therapy prevents spinal bone loss for up to 3 years whereas others have been unable to demonstrate such an effect. Salmon calcitonin appears to prevent spinal bone loss in late postmenopausal women, although appendicular (i.e., cortical) bone loss continues. Overall, calcitonin appears to have a smaller beneficial effect on bone mass than most other therapies for osteoporosis. Moreover, the effect of calcitonin therapy on the rate of osteoporotic fractures has not been well studied. Calcitonin is approved by the FDA for treatment of late postmenopausal women with low bone mineral density and is available for both parenteral and intranasal use. The recommended dose is 100 IU subcutaneously or 200 IU intranasally each day, given with adequate calcium and vitamin D. Side effects of injected calcitonin administration, including nausea, flushing, and local inflammatory reactions, occur in 10 to 15% of patients and can often be minimized by administering the medication at bedtime, starting at low doses (i.e., 25 IU), and increasing the dosage gradually over a period of several weeks. Side effects are uncommon with intranasal calcitonin. In occasional patients, calcitonin may have significant analgesic effects. Thus, it may be particularly useful in patients with osteoporosis who have chronic musculoskeletal pain related to fractures or skeletal deformity.

VITAMIN D AND ITS METABOLITES. Vitamin D is important for absorption of calcium from the gastrointestinal tract. Vitamin D deficiency is common yet rarely diagnosed in the United States. Data indicate that over half of general medical inpatients have hypovitaminosis D. Most Americans consume diets whose vitamin D content is well below the recommended daily intake. Elderly people are at particular risk for vitamin D deficiency because calcium absorption decreases with age and the ability of the skin to synthesize vitamin D is reduced. Furthermore, the ability to convert 25-hydroxyvitamin D to 1,25-dihydroxyvitamin D is impaired in many elderly people. Decreased vitamin D formation and calcium absorption may lead to secondary hyperparathyroidism and accelerated bone loss.

Small doses of vitamin D (800 IU/day) plus calcium dramatically reduce the incidence of hip fractures and other non-spine fractures in elderly women with hypovitaminosis D. Similar results have been found in a group of men and women older than the age of 63 years in the United States. Because toxicity from such doses of vitamin D has not been reported, this therapy can be recommended to virtually all postmenopausal women. Smaller doses of vitamin D (400 IU/day) may not produce the same benefit. The current recommended daily intake of vitamin D is 200 IU for adults 19 to 50 years old, 400 IU for adults 51 to 70 years old, and 600 IU for adults over age 70. Some experts, however, recommend that all adults should consume 800 IU of vitamin D each day.

The role of 1,25-dihydroxyvitamin D therapy in postmenopausal osteoporosis is more controversial. At high doses (0.8 μg/day), 1,25-dihydroxyvitamin D plus calcium administration increases bone mass but most patients develop hypercalciuria and/or hypercalcemia. At doses of 0.5 to 0.6 μg/day, 1,25-dihydroxyvitamin D plus calcium administration preserves bone mass and decreases the rate of both vertebral and non-vertebral fractures with little toxicity. It is unclear, however, whether 1,25-dihydroxyvitamin D therapy is superior to treatment with small doses of vitamin D. Because the therapeutic index of 1,25-dihydroxyvitamin D therapy is small, its use should probably be reserved for patients who are not candidates for other forms of pharmacological therapy. Other analogues of vitamin D are being investigated as potential therapies for postmenopausal osteoporosis.

FUTURE THERAPIES. Several new types of therapeutic agents are in clinical trials. It is well known that sodium fluoride increases spinal bone density. Bone formed in response to fluoride, however, is qualitatively abnormal and cortical bone density sometimes decreases. A randomized controlled trial demonstrated that a standard formulation of sodium fluoride therapy failed to reduce the risk of vertebral fractures and actually increased the incidence of fractures of the appendicular skeleton despite large increases in spinal bone mineral density. One recent study suggested that sodium fluoride reduces the risk of vertebral fractures without accelerating cortical bone loss when administered in a lower dose as a slow-release preparation. The risk of vertebral fractures was not reduced, however, in a second study that used a similar dose of sodium fluoride. Parathyroid hormone, when given intermittently in low doses, is a potent stimulator of osteoblastic bone formation. In contrast to sodium fluoride, the bone formed in response to parathyroid hormone administration is histologically normal and its strength is increased. Many animal studies have demonstrated that parathyroid hormone can prevent or reverse estrogen-deficiency osteoporosis. Parathyroid hormone increases bone mineral density of the spine and prevents bone loss from the proximal femur and total body in young women with estrogen deficiency induced by gonadotropin-releasing hormone analogue therapy. In women with postmenopausal osteoporosis, parathyroid hormone increases trabecular bone density of the spine but does not increase cortical bone mass and may even accelerate cortical bone loss. In osteoporotic women who are also receiving estrogen replacement, parathyroid hormone increases bone mineral density of the lumbar spine, proximal femur, and total body progressively over 3 years. Further investigation of the therapeutic potential of parathyroid hormone is needed. Other future potential therapies to prevent or reverse osteoporosis include growth factors (insulin-like growth factors, transforming growth factor-β, fibroblast growth factor, platelet-derived growth factor, and bone morphogenetic proteins), agents that suppress or antagonize the effects of bone-resorbing cytokines, vitamin D analogues, prostaglandin E_2, strontium salts, agents that interfere with osteoclast attachment to bone such as integrin antagonists, and phytoestrogens, particularly the isoflavones like ipriflavone.

OSTEOPOROSIS IN MEN

Although osteoporosis is less common in men, men lose about 30% of their trabecular bone and 20% of their cortical bone during the course of their lifetimes. Thirty percent of all hip and vertebral fractures occur in men. By extreme old age, one in every six men will have a hip fracture.

Secondary causes of osteoporosis in men are similar to those in women. Epidemiologic studies suggest that hypogonadism, prior glucocorticoid use, gastric resection, or ethanol abuse are among the most common identifiable causes of osteoporosis in men. Between 15% and 25% of men with hip or vertebral fractures are androgen deficient. Androgens have important effects on skeletal development. Peak bone mass is reduced in men who were androgen deficient during adolescence due to idiopathic hypogonadotropic hypogonadism or Klinefelter's syndrome and in men with histories of constitutionally delayed puberty. In adult men, castration or induction of androgen deficiency with long-acting gonadotropin-releasing hormone analogues increases bone resorption and leads to rapid bone loss. Osteoporosis is frequently observed in men with primary gonadal failure, hemochromatosis, hyperprolactinemic hypogonadism, or other disorders of the pituitary-hypothalamic axis.

Androgens may stimulate bone formation directly since osteoblastic cells possess androgen receptors. Androgens stimulate osteoblastic cell proliferation and differentiation, an effect that may be mediated by transforming growth factor-β or fibroblast growth factor. Androgens also inhibit bone resorption, probably through mechanisms that involve alterations in the local production of bone-resorbing cytokines such as interleukin-1 and interleukin-6. In the majority of eugonadal osteoporotic men, bone formation and osteoblastic cell proliferation are decreased.

Aromatization of testosterone into estrogens may be essential for many of the effects of testosterone on bone. Estrogen therapy can maintain bone mass in castrated male-to-female transsexuals. More importantly, severe osteopenia has been reported both in a man with estrogen resistance due to a genetic defect in his estrogen receptor and in a man with estrogen deficiency due to a mutation

in aromatase P-450 despite normal or high serum testosterone levels in both men. No clear effects of androgens on calcium regulatory hormones have been demonstrated. Further studies are needed to clarify the physiologic roles of androgens and estrogens on bone metabolism in men.

In men with androgen-deficiency osteoporosis, androgen replacement is usually indicated. Beneficial effects of androgen therapy on bone mass have been demonstrated in men with hyperprolactinemic hypogonadism, idiopathic hypogonadotropic hypogonadism, and acquired hypogonadism. A notable exception, however, is men with prostatic carcinoma in whom androgen replacement is contraindicated. The degree of androgen deficiency that leads to bone loss is unknown. In men with primary gonadal failure, testosterone can be administered parenterally or transdermally. In men with secondary hypogonadism, treatment with human chorionic gonadotropin or pulsatile gonadotropin-releasing hormone may also be considered. The efficacy of antiresorptive agents, such as calcitonin, raloxifene, or bisphosphonates, on osteoporosis in men has not been investigated.

GLUCOCORTICOID-INDUCED OSTEOPOROSIS

Bone loss is a common complication of glucocorticoid excess, whether due to endogenous Cushing's syndrome or administering exogenous glucocorticoids. The most important adverse effects of glucocorticoids on bone metabolism appear to be suppressed osteoblast activity and a vitamin D–independent inhibition of intestinal calcium absorption. The ability of glucocorticoids to suppress bone formation appears to be mediated, at least in part, by suppression of local secretion of insulin-like growth factor-1 in bone and by accelerated osteoblastapoptosis.

The predominant effect of administering glucocorticoids on the skeleton is a loss of trabecular bone, although cortical bone mass also decreases. Bone loss is most rapid in the first 6 to 12 months of therapy, but accelerated bone loss appears to continue as long as therapy is continued.

Because the bone loss associated with glucocorticoids is largely irreversible, the decision to administer them should be made carefully. When used, the dosage should be maintained as low as possible. If it is anticipated that glucocorticoid therapy will be maintained for several months or longer, treatment to prevent bone loss should be considered, particularly in estrogen-deficient women and when a high dosage of glucocorticoids is needed. Large randomized controlled trials have now demonstrated that bisphosphonate therapy (i.e., etidronate, alendronate, or risedronate) prevents bone loss from the spine and hip in patients receiving glucocorticoid therapy and may reduce the risk of spine fractures. Alendronate, at a dose of 5 mg daily, was recently approved for treatment of glucocorticoid-induced osteoporosis although a higher dosage (10 mg daily) may be required in estrogen-deficient women. Smaller studies suggest that calcitonin therapy also prevents bone loss in patients receiving glucocorticoid therapy. Studies of the effects of vitamin D and its metabolites on glucocorticoid-induced bone loss have produced inconsistent results. One controlled study demonstrated that 0.5 to 1.0 μg of calcitriol plus 1000 mg of calcium per day prevents spinal bone loss for at least 1 year in patients who are starting treatment with glucocorticoids. Because of the potential for hypercalciuria and/or hypercalcemia, patients receiving calcitriol therapy require careful monitoring. Calcitriol therapy seems most logical in patients with low urinary calcium excretion, suggesting poor intestinal absorption of calcium, and should be avoided in patients with hypercalciuria. Physiologic vitamin D replacement (400 to 800 IU/day) can be safely recommended in all patients receiving glucocorticoids and calcium supplementation (1000 mg/day) should be added unless the urinary calcium excretion is excessive.

American College of Rheumatology Task Force on Osteoporosis Guidelines: Recommendations for the prevention and treatment of glucocorticoid-induced osteoporosis. Arthritis Rheum 39:1791–1801, 1996. *A consensus statement developed by the American College of Rheumatology for management of glucocorticoid-induced osteoporosis.*

Calvo MS, Eyre DR, Gundberg CM: Molecular basis and clinical application of biological markers of bone turnover. Endocrinol Rev 17:333–368, 1996. *The most thorough review of this complex, rapidly-emerging field.*

Eastell R: Drug therapy: Treatment of postmenopausal osteoporosis. N Engl J Med 338:736–746, 1998. *A recent review of current and future therapies with a focus on trials that have used fractures as the therapeutic end point.*

Klein RF, Orwoll ES: Bone loss in men: Pathogenesis and therapeutic considerations. Endocrinologist 4:252–269, 1994. *A thorough, clinically oriented review of the epidemiology, etiology, diagnosis, and therapy of osteoporosis in men.*

Neer RM: Osteoporosis. *In* DeGroot LJ (ed): Endocrinology, vol 2. Philadelphia, WB Saunders, 1994, pp 1228–1258. *A thorough, scholarly review of osteoporosis that carefully discusses the limitations of many prior studies. Virtually every significant reference is cited.*

Riggs BL, Melton III LJ: The prevention and treatment of osteoporosis. N Engl J Med 327:620–627, 1992. *A concise review of practical therapeutic options for women with postmenopausal osteoporosis.*

258 BREAST CANCER AND DIFFERENTIAL DIAGNOSIS OF BENIGN NODULES

Hyman B. Muss

EPIDEMIOLOGY/STATISTICS

Breast cancer is the most common cancer affecting American women. In the United States in 1998, 180,000 new cases of breast cancer will be diagnosed and 44,000 will die of breast cancer. Breast cancer will occur in 12.5% (1 of every 8 women) during their lifetime and accounts for 32% of cases of female cancer; it is the second leading cause of female cancer death after lung cancer. Male breast cancer accounts for about 1% of all new cases and, stage for stage, has a natural history similar to that in females. The incidence of breast cancer may now be slowly decreasing, but the mortality rate has remained constant for the last several decades.

It is estimated that worldwide almost 1 million new cases of breast cancer will be diagnosed yearly by the year 2000. The incidence and mortality rates for breast cancer differ dramatically among nations. In general, more affluent Western nations have the highest incidence rates whereas developing nations have the lowest. Although racial factors may play a role in its incidence, the differing rates of breast cancer among nations are more likely related to sociodemographic and dietary factors, including per capita income, nutritional status, and dietary composition.

PATHOGENESIS AND RISK FACTORS

The causes of breast cancer remain elusive, but numerous risk factors have been defined (Table 258–1). The incidence of breast cancer increases dramatically with increasing age; more than 50% of women with breast cancer in the United States are older than 60 years, and the number of older women with breast cancer is increasing dramatically as the population ages. Several risk factors such as younger age at menarche and older age at menopause are indirect measures of the number of menstrual cycles that a women has in her lifetime. Increasing the number of cycles might predispose women to greater DNA damage in the proliferating breast ductal tissue and thus increase the risk of mutations that directly lead to breast cancer. The Western and especially the American lifestyle may predispose women to breast cancer by increasing the frequency of known risk factors. Western cultures are characterized by younger age at menarche, older age at menopause, later age of childbearing or being nulliparous, increased obesity, more sedentary lifestyles, and increased use of hormone replacement therapy. Although it is a major concern that exposure to environmental pollutants (dichlorodiphenyltrichloroethane [DDT], polychlorinated biphenyls [PCBs] and others) increases the risk of breast cancer, studies to date have failed to confirm such a relationship.

The available data suggest that the risk of breast cancer is not affected by dietary saturated fat intake during adulthood or by vitamin A, C, and E consumption. Dietary composition, however, may be important; populations with high intake of soy proteins, rich sources of plant estrogen-like compounds (phytoestrogens), have lower rates of hormonally related cancers such as breast, endometrial, and prostate cancer. Alcohol intake is also related to breast cancer, with women who have several drinks daily having a moderately higher risk than those who abstain. Oral contraceptive use increases breast cancer risk minimally if at all. The use of hormone replacement therapy for 5 or more years in postmenopausal women increases the risk of breast cancer about 1.5 times when compared with non-use. The greatest increase in risk associated with the use of hormone replacement therapy is in leaner postmenopausal women. Women with Hodgkin's disease who have been treated with chest irradiation have a risk of breast cancer at least 2 to 3 times normal.

The judicious use of risk factor data can provide women with reliable information concerning their risk of development of breast cancer. Not all risk factors are independent predictors. The Gail model is an excellent tool for assessing risk in women without an extensive family history of breast cancer but who undergo yearly mammography; graphs that calculate the risk of breast cancer over specific time spans can be quickly used to accurately inform women of their risk. For patients with a strong family history of breast cancer, the model developed by Claus and colleagues is more accurate and is also available in tabular form.

Twenty per cent of women with breast cancer have a positive family history, and a clear pattern of autosomal dominant inheritance is noted in about 5% of all breast cancer patients. The majority of these patients have mutations of either the *BRCA1* or *BRCA2* gene (Table 258–2). More than 100 mutations have already been described for these putative tumor suppressor genes. The *BRCA1* and *BRCA2* genes can be carried and passed to offspring by males as well as females. Specific genetic abnormalities appear to be characteristic of specific ethnic groups. For example, only 3 specific mutations account for 95% of *BRCA1* and *BRCA2* carriers among Ashkenazi Jewish women. The Li-Fraumeni syndrome is a

Table 258–1 ▪ RISK FACTORS FOR BREAST CANCER

RISK FACTOR	RELATIVE RISK
Any benign breast disease	1.5
Postmenopausal hormone replacement (estrogen±progestin)	1.5
Proliferative breast disease without atypia	2.0
Menarche <12 yr	1.1–1.9
Moderate alcohol intake (2–3 drinks per day)	1.1–1.9
Menopause >55 yr	1.1–1.9
Sedentary lifestyle and lack of exercise	1.1–1.9
Age at first birth >30 yr or nulliparous	2.0–4.0
First-degree relative with breast cancer	2.0–4.0
Postmenopausal obesity	2.0–4.0
Upper socioeconomic class	2.0–4.0
Personal history of endometrial or ovarian cancer	2.0–4.0
Significant radiation to chest	2.0–4.0
Older age	>4.0
Personal history of breast cancer (in situ or invasive)	>4.0
Proliferative breast disease with atypia	>4.0
Two 1st-degree relatives	5.0
Atypical hyperplasia and 1st-degree relative	10.0

Table 258–2 ▪ CHARACTERISTICS OF THE BRCA1 and BRCA2 GENES

CHARACTERISTIC	BRCA1	BRCA2
Accounts for what percentage of breast cancer in the population	2–3%	2–3%
Frequency in population	1/345	Unknown
Jewish individuals	1%	1.2%
Chromosome location	17	13
Breast cancer risk if woman carries gene and has		
Strong family history	50% by age 50 70–90% by age 70	Same as *BRCA1*
Limited pedigree or no family history	Uncertain; probably about 50%	Same as *BRCA1*
Ovarian cancer risk if woman carries gene and has		
Strong family history	30% by age 50 20–45% by age 70	About 15%
Limited pedigree or no family history	Unknown	Unknown
Risk of male breast cancer	Low	6–7%

rare disorder of the *p53* gene; affected patients have a high incidence of breast cancer, brain tumors, sarcomas, and leukemias.

Genetic tests for *BRCA1* and *BRCA2* are now commercially available (see Chapter 192). Consideration of genetic testing is appropriate for women in whom breast cancer develops at a young age, women with a family history of breast or ovarian cancer in 1st-degree relatives, or women who are blood relatives of those with known *BRCA1* or *BRCA2* mutations. All women who have testing for genetic abnormalities should have genetic counseling. In addition to psychosocial issues related to testing, issues concerning insurance coverage and potential job discrimination are unresolved. Management of women who carry the *BRCA1* and *BRCA2* genes is controversial. Prophylactic mastectomy will eliminate the likelihood of breast cancer in 90% or more of these patients, but it is not possible to remove all breast tissue with mastectomy. Prophylactic oophorectomy after completion of childbearing is also recommended and will also substantially lower the likelihood of ovarian cancer; areas of embryonic epithelial tissue in the peritoneal cavity remain a potential source of ovarian cancer even after oophorectomy.

SCREENING AND PREVENTION

The routine use of annual screening mammography in women older than 50 years has been shown to lower the likelihood of dying of breast cancer by 20 to 30%. In women 40 to 49 years of age, the use of screening mammography remains controversial. It is this author's opinion that screening mammography saves lives in this younger age group but that the probable magnitude of this improvement is only about 10%. About 15 to 25% of palpable breast cancers are not imaged by mammography; this phenomenon is most common in premenopausal women. The sensitivity and specificity of mammography are also diminished in postmenopausal women taking hormone replacement therapy. Newer imaging methods, including digital mammography, magnetic resonance imaging of the breast, radionuclide imaging with sestamibi, and high-resolution ultrasonography are currently in clinical trials, but as yet none has been shown to be convincingly superior to mammography for routine screening.

Physical examination by a health professional should be part of all screening programs. Breast self-examination may be helpful, but available clinical trials have not shown any convincing effect of this practice on reducing breast cancer mortality; nevertheless, a substantial number of women are still the first to detect a cancerous breast mass and most screening recommendations advise breast self-examination. The role of screening mammography in women older than 70 years has not been rigorously tested in clinical trials, but most experts recommend screening mammography for all older women who are in reasonably good health. Current screening recommendations of the American Cancer Society are listed in Table 258–3.

Most experts have recommended that women with a strong family history of breast cancer have screening performed at an age 5 to 10 years younger than that of the youngest relative in whom breast cancer has developed. This approach appears to be a prudent recommendation, although no evidence has shown that this strategy saves lives.

Prevention trials have just begun. The most exciting lead concerning a preventive agent is tamoxifen. In clinical trials of women with early-stage breast cancer, 2 years or more or tamoxifen treatment lowered the risk of subsequent contralateral breast cancer by about 40%. The results of the Breast Cancer Prevention Trial (National Surgical Adjuvant Breast and Bowel Project P-1) that randomized 13,388 high-risk women to either tamoxifen, 20 mg daily

or a placebo have recently been published. Tamoxifen reduced the risk of both invasive and noninvasive breast cancer by about 50%, and benefits were seen for all age groups. Women at high risk should be informed of the potential benefits and risks of tamoxifen and should be offered such treatment when appropriate. Two smaller randomized trials similar in design have not shown any benefit for tamoxifen but both were smaller than the P-1 trial and both had different eligibility criteria. In addition, several new selective estrogen receptor modulators that have similar antiestrogen effects as tamoxifen on breast ductal epithelium but that lack tamoxifen's estrogen agonist effects on the endometrium are currently in development. One such agent (raloxifene) has recently been approved by the Food and Drug Administration for use in the prevention of postmenopausal osteoporosis. A new prevention trial comparing tamoxifen with raloxifene (study of tamoxifen and raloxifene—"STAR") will open shortly in the United States (see Chapter 257). These new selective estrogen receptor modulators have excellent potential as preventive agents. In addition, new retinoic acid derivatives, aromatase inhibitors, and phytochemicals have promise as preventive agents, and several are being evaluated in clinical trials.

DIAGNOSIS

SIGNS AND SYMPTOMS. Breast cancer is usually first detected as a palpable mass or as a mammographic abnormality, but it can also be manifested by nipple discharge, breast skin change, or breast pain. Palpable masses, including discrete masses and areas of asymmetric thickening of breast glandular tissue, remain the most common manifestation of breast cancer and are often first detected by the patient. Paget's disease of the nipple is a form of adenocarcinoma involving the skin and lactiferous sinuses of the nipple; it is usually seen as an eczematous lesion of the skin of the nipple and is frequently associated with excoriation of the skin and discharge.

Spontaneous bloody or watery nipple discharge is commonly associated with underlying breast malignancy. Milky discharge almost always has a benign etiology. Patients with a clear or bloody discharge require breast examination and mammography. If the results of mammography and breast examination are normal and the discharge is located within a single or a few well-defined ducts, excisional biopsy of the involved ducts is indicated. A bloody discharge is frequently caused by an intraductal papilloma; a ductogram may help locate such lesions.

Breast pain is a common symptom in many women and is reported in about 10% of patients with breast cancer. When associated with breast cancer, breast pain will typically be associated with a palpable lump or mammographic abnormality. In premenopausal women, breast pain is commonly noted as a premenstrual symptom. In these patients, pain that is well localized to a specific region of the breast and that occurs throughout the menstrual cycle is the type most likely to be associated with an underlying malignancy. All patients with non-cyclic breast pain should have a breast examination and bilateral mammography. If no abnormalities are found, ultrasound evaluation of the painful area may help rule out the small possibility of a malignancy.

In a small percentage of patients, breast cancer is manifested as an axillary mass without any breast lesion detected on physical examination, mammography, or other breast imaging. These patients characteristically have axillary node involvement by adenocarcinoma; the history, physical examination, and appropriate studies to detect other potential primary lesions are negative. Such patients are best managed by axillary node dissection, ipsilateral breast irradiation (mastectomy is not necessary and, even when performed, fails to detect a primary lesion in 30% of patients), and appropriate systemic adjuvant therapy. The natural history of such patients may be somewhat better than that of node-positive patients with palpable breast lesions.

EVALUATING A BREAST MASS. Most breast masses, especially those found in young premenopausal women, are benign. All breast masses require evaluation. In a premenopausal woman, if the mass is small and likely to be a cyst, it can be observed for 2 to 4 weeks until after the next menstrual period. If the mass persists, biopsy is indicated; all masses in postmenopausal women require prompt investigation.

Mammograms and/or ultrasound evaluation may help character-

Table 258–3 ■ SCREENING RECOMMENDATIONS (AMERICAN CANCER SOCIETY)

AGE GROUP	EXAMINATION	FREQUENCY
20–39 yr	Breast self-examination	Every month
	Clinical breast examination	Every 3 yr
40 yr and over	Breast self-examination	Every month
	Mammography	Every year
	Clinical breast examination	Every year

ize a mass as well as detect abnormalities in non-involved breast tissues, but all persistent masses require biopsy—even when all imaging studies are normal. As many as 15 to 25% of all palpable breast cancers are not detected with mammography. Fine-needle aspiration should be considered for lesions likely to be cysts; aspiration of the fluid with resolution of the mass is adequate treatment. If the cystic fluid is clear, cytologic evaluation is not usually necessary. Currently, core biopsy is replacing fine-needle aspiration as a diagnostic tool for solid masses. Core biopsies provide larger tissue samples and most importantly are frequently able to distinguish in situ from invasive lesions. Because management may be quite different for these lesions—axillary dissection is not indicated for in situ lesions—treatment planning can be greatly facilitated by core biopsy. A negative fine-needle or core biopsy of a persistent breast mass should be followed by a repeat biopsy, preferably an excisional biopsy.

PATHOLOGY, PATHOGENESIS, AND PROGNOSTIC FACTORS

Invasive breast cancer accounts for approximately 75 to 85% of lesions, with the remaining 15 to 25% being carcinoma in situ. Infiltrating ductal carcinoma accounts for 85% of invasive lesions, infiltrating lobular carcinoma for 5 to 10%, medullary carcinoma for 5 to 7%, mucinous or colloid carcinoma for 3%, and tubular carcinoma for 2%. When matched for stage, infiltrating ductal and infiltrating lobular carcinoma have a similar prognosis and are more likely to metastasize than medullary carcinoma. Tubular and colloid carcinomas are usually associated with an excellent prognosis. The histologic grade is important in determining the prognosis for women with infiltrating ductal carcinoma; when matched by stage, patients with high-grade lesions are more likely to be affected by metastatic disease. A small percentage of patients, mainly premenopausal, initially have inflammatory carcinoma. This lesion is associated with an almost 95% risk of distant metastases and is characterized clinically by redness and erythema involving more than half the breast or pathologically by tumor involvement of the dermal lymphatics of the breast.

Carcinoma in situ is characterized by the proliferation of malignant cells within the ducts or lobules of the breast without invasion of stromal tissue. The two major subtypes are ductal carcinoma in situ (DCIS) and lobular carcinoma in situ (LCIS). Differences in the clinical features of these lesions are noted in Table 258–4.

Metastases from invasive breast cancer probably develop early during growth of the primary lesion, proliferate in distant metastatic sites as occult "micrometastases," and after about 30 tumor cell doublings become clinically detectable (about 1 cm³). The axillary lymph nodes are not barriers to metastases; the number of axillary nodes involved by tumor is directly correlated with the risk of both locoregional and distant metastases. The most common metastatic sites are locoregional, i.e., the chest wall and/or regional lymph nodes (20 to 40%); bone (60%); lung, i.e., malignant effusion and/or parenchymal lesions (15 to 25%); and the liver (10 to 20%).

PROGNOSTIC FACTORS. Numerous prognostic factors have been identified but few have proved to be independent predictors of outcome when subjected to multivariate analysis. The essential prognostic factors remain (1) invasion—DCIS and other non-invasive tumors have excellent prognoses; (2) the number of involved ipsilateral axillary nodes; and (3) tumor size. Estrogen and progesterone receptor expression is only marginally related to prognosis, although in most series patients whose primary lesions express either estrogen and/or progesterone receptors have a 5 to 10% improvement in survival. Estrogen and progesterone receptors are

now also regarded as predictive factors; they help predict the response to endocrine therapy. Axillary dissection, with removal of at least six lymph nodes, should be performed in almost all patients for both therapeutic and prognostic purposes. Clinical examination of the axilla correlates poorly with pathologic findings. Patients without palpable ipsilateral axillary nodes on physical examination display pathologic tumor involvement in up to 40% of cases, whereas palpable axillary nodes exhibit no tumor involvement in up to 40% of patients. The risk of recurrence in the axilla is extremely low (⟨5%) when adequate dissection is performed.

The major use of prognostic factors has been to predict the risk of distant metastases in women with node-negative breast cancer. For node-negative patients, tumor size, estrogen and progesterone receptor status, and histologic grade remain the key prognostic indices. Primary tumors with an invasive component 1 cm in largest diameter or smaller generally have an excellent prognosis with an overall survival rate of 90% or more. Poorly differentiated tumors tend to have more aggressive growth patterns and are associated with a poorer prognosis. Calculation of the number of breast cancer cells synthesizing DNA (S phase) is commonly performed on node-negative lesions; tumors with a low percentage of cells in S phase have a more favorable prognosis. Currently, a variety of potential predictive factors are under investigation. The HER-2/neu (c-erb-b2) oncogene is expressed in about 25% of all breast cancers; patients with HER-2 expression tend to have a poorer prognosis but more importantly may be more likely to respond to anthracycline-containing chemotherapy. Most prognostic and predictive factors can be assayed on paraffin-embedded tissue with immunohistochemical methods, which allows the clinician to request specific assays after primary treatment.

PRIMARY TREATMENT OF MALIGNANT LESIONS

CARCINOMA IN SITU. Historically, patients with both LCIS and DCIS but without any invasive component have been treated with mastectomy. More recently, patients with DCIS have been managed with lumpectomy (excision of the tumor mass with a clear margin around the tumor) and irradiation and, in selected patients, with lumpectomy alone. Lumpectomy with or without irradiation allows for breast preservation and is preferred by most patients. At present the best predictor of recurrence following lumpectomy alone is the extent of normal tissue around the tumor. Patients with DCIS in which the closest margin is 1 cm or more have a local recurrence rate following lumpectomy alone that is about 10%. Breast irradiation following lumpectomy lowers the risk of breast recurrence irrespective of the size of the primary lesion, but the major benefits of breast irradiation are in patients with larger lesions. Patients with lesions greater than 2.5 cm in largest diameter and those with multifocal DCIS may be best treated with mastectomy. Metastatic disease occurs in only 1 to 3% of patients with DCIS. Axillary nodes are rarely involved, so axillary dissection is not indicated. In spite of the better prognosis of DCIS than invasive breast cancer, primary treatment of DCIS remains controversial and such patients should be managed by surgeons and radiation oncologists with expertise in breast cancer management. LCIS is not considered a malignant lesion but a marker of increased risk for subsequent breast cancer; patients with LCIS alone are currently managed by physical examination and yearly mammography without additional surgery or irradiation and have a 25% risk of invasive ductal cancer developing in either breast.

INVASIVE BREAST CANCER. Patients with smaller tumors (less

Table 258–4 ■ CARCINOMA IN SITU—DUCTAL VERSUS LOBULAR

FEATURE	LOBULAR CARCINOMA IN SITU	DUCTAL CARCINOMA IN SITU
Age	Younger	Older
Palpable mass	No	Sometimes
Mammographic appearance	Not detected on mammography	Microcalcifications, mass
Usual manifestation	Incidental finding on breast biopsy	Microcalcifications on mammography or breast mass
Bilateral involvement	Common	Probably low
Risk and site of subsequent breast cancer	About 15–25% risk for invasive breast cancer in either breast	At site of initial lesion
Treatment	Yearly mammography and breast examination	Lumpectomy alone or with breast radiation; mastectomy for large or multifocal lesions

than 4 to 5 cm) are best managed with lumpectomy followed by radiation therapy to the involved breast. This treatment is as effective as mastectomy, is associated with similar survival, and results in breast preservation. Breast irradiation following lumpectomy reduces the risk of ipsilateral breast tumor recurrence (which usually occurs at the lumpectomy site) from 40% to less than 10% without affecting cosmetic results. For patients with larger lesions or those with skin involvement, mastectomy is still preferred but preoperative chemotherapy may cause tumor shrinkage and make the majority of these patients suitable candidates for lumpectomy and irradiation. Patients with stage IIIB breast cancer (see Staging below) or inflammatory breast cancer are best treated with preoperative ("neoadjuvant") chemotherapy, mastectomy, and post-mastectomy chest wall irradiation. Patients with DCIS in addition to invasive breast cancer are managed like patients with invasive breast cancer. Tumor size in patients with lesions that contain both in situ and invasive components is defined as the largest diameter of the invasive lesion.

Axillary node dissection should be performed on almost all women who are suitable candidates for preventive (adjuvant) therapy (see below). Exceptions include patients with small, well-differentiated primary lesions (5 mm or less) or patients with small tubular carcinomas. Newer techniques such as the "sentinel node" biopsy may minimize the need for extensive axillary staging in most patients. The sentinel node is identified by injecting a blue dye, a radioactive isotope, or both around the primary lesion. The sentinel node is identified visually (blue dye) or by a gamma detector (radioisotope) and is defined as the first node (or nodes) draining the primary lesion. In 95% of breast cancer patients the sentinel node is in the ipsilateral axilla. Patients whose sentinel node is histologically negative have less than a 5% chance of having histologically positive nodes higher in the axilla. In 60% of patients with a positive sentinel node, only the sentinel node is involved by tumor.

Preoperative chemotherapy—the use of three to four courses of an active chemotherapy regimen or a single agent before definitive treatment of the primary tumor—is effective in causing tumor regression in as many as 90% of patients. Five to 10% of these patients demonstrate complete regression of the tumor pathologically as well as clinically. Recent data suggest that patients who achieve a complete or nearly complete response to preoperative chemotherapy have better survival rates than do patients who have significant residual disease in the primary site or lymph nodes after primary therapy. This observation suggests that the response to preoperative chemotherapy may be a "predictive factor" for breast cancer recurrence. Another advantage of preoperative chemotherapy is its ability to convert a large primary lesion unsuitable for lumpectomy to a smaller lesion that is amenable to lumpectomy and breast conservation. Preliminary data suggest that preoperative endocrine therapy may be as effective as chemotherapy in causing tumor shrinkage in patients with estrogen or progesterone receptor–positive lesions.

Adaptation to a diagnosis of breast cancer is frequently difficult. A wealth of information concerning psychosocial support suggests that psychological counseling and support groups can help patients better cope with breast cancer, especially during the first several years after diagnosis. Moreover, several controlled trials have suggested that such support is associated with improved survival. Patients should be offered psychosocial support shortly after diagnosis. Many women may wish to become more involved in breast cancer issues through advocacy. The National Alliance of Breast Cancer Organizations (1-800-719-9154, see Table 258–9) is an outstanding resource for information on organizations interested in breast cancer.

RECONSTRUCTION. In many women, mastectomy is associated with a loss of self-esteem and body image, sexual dysfunction, and difficulty dressing. Breast reconstruction provides an opportunity for women to overcome the psychological damage that frequently follows mastectomy and helps relieve the patient's sense of deformity. Several procedures are available, including implants and the use of flaps from autogenous tissue. Implants are less costly and generally easier to perform, whereas flaps eliminate the need for the foreign materials contained in the implants; flaps are more suitable for the repair of large mastectomy defects. No evidence

has demonstrated that silicone implants increase the risk of breast cancer. Reconstruction is usually performed after mastectomy; more recently, however, immediate reconstruction, done concurrently with mastectomy, has become more popular. The remaining breast frequently requires surgery to match its size and configuration to the reconstructed site. Although reconstruction is frequently associated with excellent cosmetic results, the results of lumpectomy and breast irradiation are far superior.

STAGING

A complete history and physical examination, complete blood count and chemistry profile, and chest radiograph constitute an appropriate preoperative work-up for asymptomatic women with breast cancer. Women with bone pain, abdominal pain, or other symptoms should have appropriate studies of symptomatic sites. Bilateral mammograms should be performed in all women with biopsy-proven breast cancer to look for other lesions in the involved breast as well as the opposite breast.

Staging of breast cancer is based on tumor size, the extent of breast involvement, axillary lymph node involvement, and distant metastases (the TNM system). Determination of tumor size is made by the pathologist on review of biopsy, lumpectomy, or mastectomy specimens. The staging system currently in use has been developed by the American Joint Committee on Cancer and is presented in Table 258–5. Survival rates based on the TNM stage are listed in Table 258–6. Currently, about 50 to 60% of women with newly diagnosed breast cancer are node negative and 25 to 40% are node positive; of those who are node positive, about 60% have involvement of only one to three nodes. Fewer than 10% of patients are initially seen with distant metastases.

ADJUVANT THERAPY

Adjuvant therapy is defined as the use of chemotherapy, hormonal therapy, and/or immunotherapy either before, during, or after definitive treatment of the primary breast cancer. The objective of adjuvant therapy is to destroy small, clinically occult, distant micrometastases. Breast cancer metastases composed of microscopic distant foci can be eliminated by adjuvant therapy, with a subsequent reduction in the odds of dying of breast cancer of about 20 to 25% within each stage group. In addition, adjuvant therapy probably delays recurrence for a median of 2 to 3 years in the majority of women treated.

The rationale of adjuvant chemotherapy is based on the observations that (1) smaller tumors have a larger component of dividing cells, (2) most chemotherapeutic agents are most effective in destroying proliferating cells, (3) smaller tumors are less likely to be

Table 258–5 ■ STAGING OF BREAST CANCER—THE TNM SYSTEM

Tumor Size—T (Largest Diameter)
TX   Primary tumor cannot be assessed
T0   No evidence of primary tumor
Tis Carcinoma in situ: intraductal carcinoma, lobular carcinoma in situ, or Paget's disease of the nipple with no tumor
T1   Tumor <2 cm in greatest dimension
T2   Tumor >2 cm but not >5 cm in greatest dimension
T3   Tumor >5 cm in greatest dimension
T4   Tumor of any size with direct extension to chest wall* or skin (includes inflammatory carcinoma)

Nodal Involvement—N (Nodal Status)
NX   Regional lymph nodes cannot be assessed (e.g., previously removed, not removed)
N0   No regional lymph node metastases
N1   Metastasis to movable ipsilateral axillary nodes
N2   Metastasis to ipsilateral axillary nodes fixed to one another or to other structures
N3   Metastases to ipsilateral internal mammary lymph nodes

Metastases
M0   No evidence of distant metastasis
M1   Distant metastases (including metastases to ipsilateral supraclavicular lymph nodes)

*The chest wall includes the ribs, intercostal muscles, and serratus anterior but not the pectoral muscle.
From American Joint Committee on Cancer: AJCC Cancer Staging Handbook. Philadelphia, Lippincott-Raven, 1998.

Table 258-6 ■ TNM STAGE AND SURVIVAL

STATE	TNM CATEGORY*	PER CENT RECURRENCE FREE AT 10 YEARS
0	Tis, N0, M0	98
I	T1, N0, M0	80 (all stage I patients)
	T ≤ 1 cm	90
	T > 1–2 cm	80–90
IIA	T0, N1, M0; T2, N0, M0	60–80
IIA	T1, N1, M0	10–60
	1–3 positive nodes	50–60
	4–9 positive nodes	20–30
	≥10 positive nodes	5–20
IIB	T2, N1, M0	5–10% worse than IIA above and based on node
IIB	T3, N0, M0	30–50
IIIA	T0 or T1 or T2, N2, M0; or T3, N1 or N2, M0	10–40
IIIB	T4, any N, M0; any T, N3, M0	5–30
IV	Any T, any N, M1	<5%

*See Table 258–5 for TNM definitions.

drug resistant, (4) the immunologic status of patients is most favorable early in the course of their disease when they are asymptomatic, and (5) asymptomatic patients are better able to tolerate therapy than those who are ill. Response to adjuvant therapy is based on recurrence-free (relapse-free) survival and overall survival. Recurrence in these patients indicates treatment failure. Because micrometastases cannot be detected clinically, both patients who are cured (by their primary treatment) and those with micrometastases will be treated. Careful estimation of the risks versus benefits of therapy, by both the patient and the physician, is mandatory before placing patients on such treatment regimens.

Recommendations for adjuvant therapy are based on menopausal status, tumor size, the presence of lymph node involvement, and the estrogen and progesterone receptor status of the tumor. It is an area with much controversy, and all patients with primary breast cancer should be seen by a surgical or medical oncologist to discuss the risks and benefits of adjuvant therapy. Current recommendations for adjuvant therapy are presented in Table 258–7. The proportional decrease in risk of recurrence is similar for all patients irrespective of the presence of lymph node involvement. For instance, if risk of dying of breast cancer is 30% and adjuvant therapy decreases this risk by 25%, the overall survival rate for patients given adjuvant therapy is 77.5% (70% survival without adjuvant therapy + 7.5% [0.25 × 30%] with adjuvant therapy). Similarly, if the risk of dying of breast cancer is 80% without adjuvant therapy, the use of adjuvant therapy increases survival to 40% (20% survival without adjuvant therapy + 20% (0.25 × 80%) with adjuvant therapy).

In general, combinations of several chemotherapeutic agents given concurrently are superior to single-drug treatment, and short courses of chemotherapy (3 to 6 months) are as effective as longer treatments. The most effective chemotherapy regimens include either cyclophosphamide, methotrexate, and fluorouracil or cyclophosphamide and doxorubicin. Oophorectomy and chemotherapy are equally effective in improving survival in premenopausal women with estrogen or progesterone–positive tumors.

Tamoxifen is the most widely used endocrine agent and, when added to chemotherapy, improves survival in both premenopausal and postmenopausal patients who are estrogen or progesterone positive. For patients given tamoxifen, 5 years is superior to shorter or longer times of administration. The estrogen agonist effects of tamoxifen on bone and liver result in maintenance of bone density and lowering of cholesterol in postmenopausal women; this latter effect may lower the risk of cardiovascular disease. In premenopausal women, tamoxifen has been associated with bone loss. The agonist effects of tamoxifen on the uterus result in a 1% risk of endometrial cancer for every 5 years of use. A 1% incidence of deep venous thrombosis is also noted. Tamoxifen can cause or exacerbate hot flashes in 10 to 30% of postmenopausal women because of its estrogen antagonist effects in the hypothalamus.

The results of current adjuvant regimens must be improved. Current research approaches for patients at high risk for recurrence (for example, those with four or more involved lymph nodes) include high-dose chemotherapy and autologous bone marrow or stem cell transplantation (see below). Other research strategies include administering larger doses of single agents sequentially as opposed to concurrently, decreasing the interval between chemotherapy treatments with the use of growth factors, and using new highly active agents such as the taxanes in addition to standard regimens. When eligible, patients with early-stage breast cancer should be offered participation in clinical trials.

The use of radiation therapy to the chest wall following mastec-

Table 258-7 ■ ADJUVANT TREATMENT FOR PATIENTS WITH EARLY STAGE BREAST CANCER

NODE NEGATIVE PATIENTS			
Patient group	Minimal or low risk*	Intermediate risk**	High risk***
Premenopausal, ER or PR+	None or tamoxifen	Tamoxifen ± chemotherapy	Chemotherapy + tamoxifen
Premenopausal, ER and PR−	Not applicable	Not applicable	Chemotherapy
Postmenopausal, ER or PR+	None or tamoxifen	Tamoxifen ± chemotherapy	Tamoxifen + chemotherapy
Postmenopausal, ER and PR−	Not applicable	Not applicable	Chemotherapy
Elderly	None or tamoxifen	Tamoxifen ± chemotherapy	Tamoxifen, if ER− and PR− then chemotherapy

NODE POSITIVE PATIENTS	
Patient group	Treatment
Premenopausal, ER or PR+	Chemotherapy + tamoxifen or ovarian ablation
Premenopausal, ER and PR−	Chemotherapy
Postmenopausal, ER or PR+	Tamoxifen + chemotherapy
Postmenopausal, ER and PR−	Chemotherapy
Elderly	Tamoxifen, if ER− and PR− then chemotherapy

*All the following factors: invasive tumor less than or equal 1 cm in largest diameter, ER or PR+, low grade, age 35 years and greater.
**All of the following; invasive tumor ≥1–2 cm in largest diameter, ER or PR+, low to intermediate grade.
***At least one of the following: invasive tumor ≥2 cm in largest diameter, ER and PR−, grade 2–3, less than age 35 years.
Modified from Goldhirsch et al: Natl Cancer Inst 90:1601, 1998.
ER or PR+, estrogen or progesterone receptor positive.

tomy has been shown to decrease the rate of local recurrence at the mastectomy site and in the regional nodes. Recently, two prospective randomized trials in node-positive women with early-stage breast cancer, all of whom received mastectomy and adjuvant chemotherapy, have shown a 10% survival advantage with the use of post-mastectomy chest wall irradiation versus no further treatment. Post-mastectomy chest wall irradiation should be offered to all women with large primary lesions (5 cm or larger irrespective of nodal involvement) and those with extensive nodal involvement (four or more positive lymph nodes). The use of routine post-mastectomy chest wall irradiation in patients with one to three positive nodes is controversial and should be readdressed in new clinical trials. Although routine post-mastectomy chest wall irradiation is generally well tolerated, it increases the risk of lymphedema in the upper extremity on the side of the mastectomy and is associated with a very small risk of radiation-induced malignancy.

FOLLOW-UP OF EARLY-STAGE PATIENTS

The underlying assumption for intensive follow-up of asymptomatic patients after the diagnosis and treatment of early-stage breast cancer is that early detection of metastases improves survival. Detection by routine laboratory tests, tumor marker assessment (carcinoembryonic antigen, CA-15.3, and CA-27.29), and imaging studies (for example, chest radiographs, bone scans, and computed tomography or ultrasound of the liver) may occasionally precede the development of signs and symptoms of metastases by 3 to 6 months, but at present early detection by these means has not been translated into improved survival. Two large randomized trials have directly compared routine visits alone with routine visits plus intensive follow-up testing with frequent imaging and laboratory tests. In both trials, asymptomatic recurrence was noted in about 30% of the intensively monitored patients and 21% of controls. Of note, 30 to 40% of the recurrences were noted between routinely scheduled visits. Survival was identical in both groups, and quality of life was not affected by the follow-up method.

About 75% of recurrences, even when frequent imaging and laboratory testing are performed, are detected by the physician or the patient from signs and symptoms. Locoregional recurrence on the chest wall or in regional lymph nodes accounts for 19 to 39% of initial recurrences, bone for 16 to 63%, lung for 16 to 25%, and liver for 5 to 22%. Of note, almost a third of initial recurrences occur in soft tissue and nodal areas; physical examination remains the mainstay of such detection.

Routine follow-up visits provide a forum for patients to discuss their fears and concerns and for physicians to provide reassurance and obtain annual mammography. The American Society of Clinical Oncology has recently published evidence-based guidelines for follow-up (Table 258–8). These guidelines should be used for patients outside the clinical trial setting. Patient education concerning the limitations of follow-up is mandatory; patients should be informed that the use of extensive imaging and laboratory studies does not improve survival.

TREATMENT OF METASTATIC DISEASE

SYSTEMIC THERAPY: ENDOCRINE THERAPY AND CHEMOTHERAPY. Almost all patients with metastatic breast cancer are incurable. One to 3% of patients treated with standard endocrine therapy or chemotherapy regimens may attain long-term remission and may never have further recurrence, but the median survival for all patients after recurrence is about 2 to 3 years. Breast cancer may recur in any site; clinically detectable metastatic disease indicates a substantial amount of body tumor burden. Responses are defined as complete (complete disappearance of all metastatic lesions irrespective of location or means of measurement), partial (50% reduction in tumor mass based on comparing products of perpendicular diameters of measurable lesions before and after treatment), stable (less than 50% reduction or a 25% increase in measurable lesions for 3 to 4 months), and progressing (continued growth during therapy). New lesions at any time during therapy indicate treatment failure. Tumor reduction must last for at least 1 month to be considered a complete or partial response.

Patients whose tumors are positive for estrogen or progesterone receptors are good candidates for endocrine therapy. Women who are older, who have a long disease-free interval (time from diagnosis to recurrence), or who have bone or soft tissue lesions are most likely to respond. Response to endocrine therapy is seen in 30 to 70% of women who are hormone receptor positive and in up to 10 to 20% who are receptor negative. The antiestrogen tamoxifen is appropriate therapy for both premenopausal and postmenopausal women. In premenopausal women, tamoxifen and oophorectomy are the treatments of choice. Oophorectomy can be done surgically, with external beam irradiation, or medically with luteinizing hormone–releasing hormone agonists such as goserelin or leuprolide. In postmenopausal women, newer aromatase inhibitors (letrozole and anastrozole) and progestins (megestrol and medroxyprogesterone acetate) and, in selected patients, androgens and estrogens can be used. Responses to initial hormonal therapy last an average of 12 months, and patients responding to one agent have a fair chance of responding to a second hormonal agent after failure of initial therapy.

Chemotherapy is best reserved for women who have tumor progression on hormonal therapy or those who have cancers lacking hormone receptors. In general, 40 to 80% of patients have a complete or partial response to their initial chemotherapy regimen. Initial responses generally last for 6 to 12 months. Responses to second-line chemotherapy are frequently seen but usually last only several months. Chemotherapy using combinations of drugs has previously been shown to be superior to single-agent therapy, but new agents, especially the taxanes (paclitaxel [Taxol] and docetaxel [Taxotere]) have displayed response rates similar to those of combination regimens. High-dose chemotherapy with autologous bone marrow or stem cell transplantation is currently being studied in the research setting in patients with metastatic disease (see below).

SPECIFIC ISSUES RELATED TO METASTATIC DISEASE. CNS, SPINAL CORD, AND LEPTOMENINGEAL METASTASES. Radiation therapy can be an extremely effective therapy for palliation of central nervous system (CNS) metastases and spinal cord compression. Dexamethasone in doses of 4 to 10 mg every 6 hours should be used in conjunction with irradiation. Spinal cord compression is most commonly seen in patients with bone metastases, and almost all patients have back pain. Magnetic resonance imaging is currently the imaging method of choice to establish the diagnosis. For patients with rapid loss of function or progression of symptoms while receiving radiation therapy, surgical decompression is necessary to lower the probability of paraplegia. Patients with leptomeningeal metastases frequently have headache and cranial nerve and peripheral nerve lesions. The diagnosis is best made with lumbar puncture and examination of cerebrospinal fluid for malignant cells. Gadolinium-enhanced magnetic resonance scans of the brain or spinal cord may show enhancement of the meninges in about 70% of patients with leptomeningeal spread. Intrathecal methotrexate can lead to brief remission, but the general outlook for such patients is exceedingly poor.

SKELETAL METASTASES. The use of bisphosphonates can signifi-

Table 258–8 ■ FOLLOW-UP GUIDELINES FOR PATIENTS WITH EARLY-STAGE BREAST CANCER: AMERICAN SOCIETY OF CLINICAL ONCOLOGY GUIDELINES*

PROCEDURE OR TEST	FREQUENCY
History and physical examination* (eliciting of symptoms of breast cancer)	Every 3–6 mo for 1st 3 yr, every 6–12 mo for next 2 yr, then yearly
Mammography	
Mastectomy patients	Yearly
Lumpectomy patients	Yearly
Pelvic examination	Yearly
Breast self-examination	Monthly
Other	†, ‡

*Limited evaluation: Assess for pain, dyspnea, weight loss, and other major changes in function. The limited examination should include an assessment of nodes, axillae, lumpectomy or mastectomy site, chest, and abdomen. Patients should be instructed regarding symptoms of recurrence.

†The literature does not support the use of complete blood counts and chemistry studies.

‡Chest radiography, bone scans, liver imaging, and tumor marker studies are not recommended for routine follow-up in asymptomatic patients. Patient education regarding signs and symptoms of recurrence is recommended.

cantly reduce the complications of skeletal metastases in both pre-menopausal and postmenopausal patients. Such treatment does not improve survival. Pamidronate (Aredia) given intravenously every 3 or 4 weeks has been shown to be effective in this setting and can be given at the same time as endocrine therapy or chemotherapy. In addition, radioisotopes that localize in bone such as strontium-89 may be effective. External beam irradiation will result in significant palliation in patients with moderate to severe bone pain at specific metastatic sites. Hypercalcemia is a common complication of meta-static breast cancer and more likely to occur in patients with skele-tal metastases. Initial treatment of symptomatic patients includes hydration and diuresis. Calcitonin can also be effective in patients who need rapid reduction of their serum calcium. Bisphosphonates and glucocorticoids are also effective. Ultimate control depends on the response to systemic therapy.

SURGERY. Patients with isolated or minimal metastatic disease (one to three lesions) to the CNS or lung and who have limited or no other metastatic disease may benefit from surgical resection of metastatic lesions. Also, patients with locoregional recurrence are best managed by surgical resection of chest wall lesions when feasible, followed by external beam irradiation of the involved area. Chest tube drainage and sclerotherapy are successful in about 70% of patients with persistent or recurrent malignant effusions that have not been controlled by systemic therapy. Patients with ipsilat-eral breast tumor recurrence after lumpectomy alone or with breast irradiation for early-stage breast cancer are usually best managed by mastectomy, although further lumpectomy may be appropriate in patients with smaller recurrences.

OTHER ISSUES

GETTING INFORMATION. Never has high-quality medical in-formation been more accessible to the practicing clinician. In addi-tion to journals and textbooks, the Internet has now become a major resource for a wealth of up-to-date information derived from multiple sources. Several major information resources are listed in Table 258–9. The National Cancer Institute Physician Data Query (PDQ) system is a major resource for both patients and physicians seeking general or specific information about cancer and available clinical trials. PDQ is updated monthly by an editorial board of physician scientists. Physicians may also contact the National Can-cer Institute's Cancer Information Service for access to PDQ by calling 1-800-4-CANCER.

BREAST CANCER AND PREGNANCY. The diagnosis of breast cancer during pregnancy is extremely traumatic. Such patients are usually first seen at higher stages, probably because of difficulties in diagnosis. After the 1st trimester, definitive surgical procedures can usually be performed with minimal risk to the mother and fetus. Chemotherapy administered after the 1st trimester has not been associated with increased fetal loss or birth defects. Limited data suggest that childhood development is normal in children of mothers who have received chemotherapy during pregnancy. Alky-lating agents given during pregnancy will frequently cause subse-quent infertility. Hormonal agents should be avoided during preg-nancy. Pregnancy following breast cancer, especially 2 to 3 years

after diagnosis, does not appear to increase the risk of metastatic disease. Major considerations relating to childbearing after breast cancer should be based on the risks of recurrence.

HIGH-DOSE CHEMOTHERAPY AND STEM CELL SUPPORT. The use of autologous blood progenitor cells (stem cells) obtained from bone marrow or peripheral blood is capable of rescuing pa-tients from potentially lethal myelosuppression caused by the use of chemotherapeutic agents given in dosages several times higher than normal. The use of peripheral blood stem cells as opposed to bone marrow and the introduction of granulocyte-stimulating growth factors (filgrastim and others) have greatly reduced the costs as well as the morbidity and mortality of this technique. Current mortality rates associated with high-dose therapy are about 2 to 3%. Although widely used in breast cancer, the benefits of high-dose chemotherapy and stem cell support remain controversial. A large randomized trial in the adjuvant setting comparing standard with high-dose therapy and stem cell support in women with early-stage breast cancer and 10 or more positive axillary lymph nodes is close to completion. One randomized trial in the metastatic setting showed a survival benefit for a high-dose regimen versus a lower-dose regimen, but both groups did poorly. From 10 to 25% of patients with metastatic breast cancer have shown relapse-free sur-vival in excess of 5 years after high-dose programs; critics believe that patient selection accounts for a major proportion of these long-term survivors. Ongoing clinical trials in both the adjuvant and metastatic settings should help define the magnitude of benefit, if any, of commonly used high-dose regimens.

HORMONE REPLACEMENT THERAPY AFTER BREAST CAN-CER. The use of hormone replacement therapy in women with a diagnosis of breast cancer is an area of heated controversy. Current data suggest that the use of estrogens alone in patients with hyster-ectomy or the use of estrogens and progestins in patients with an intact uterus for 5 years or longer is associated with a relative risk of breast cancer 1.5 times greater than that of non-users. The major concerns related to the use of hormone replacement therapy after breast cancer are (1) whether such therapy will substantially in-crease the risk of a new primary breast cancer in a patient group already at higher risk for breast cancer and (2) whether such ther-apy might stimulate the growth of occult breast cancer metastases. The benefits of hormone replacement therapy in postmenopausal women are substantial and include slowing the rate of bone loss, lowering the risk of cardiovascular disease, limiting or eliminating vasomotor symptoms, and possibly lowering risks of dementia and colon cancer. In young premenopausal women, the frequent toxicity of chemotherapy-induced amenorrhea increases the long-term risk of osteoporosis and heart disease. Newer bisphosphonates (alen-dronate) or selective estrogen receptor modulators (raloxifene) are effective in lowering the risks of osteoporosis, and several non-hormonal agents can favorably affect lipid profiles. No highly ef-fective methods of controlling vasomotor symptoms other than en-docrine therapy have been described. Clonidine, vitamin E, and other agents are of little to no benefit but should be considered in patients with major symptoms. About 25% of patients with moder-ate to severe vasomotor symptoms have had major relief with a placebo in randomized, blinded clinical trials. Newer antidepres-sants such as venlafaxine may be helpful in reducing hot flashes and other menopausal symptoms, and trials are in progress. Meges-trol acetate, an oral progestin, is as effective as estrogen in reduc-ing vasomotor symptoms, but its long-term risks in patients with early-stage breast cancer, especially those receiving tamoxifen, are unknown. Selective estrogen receptor modulators that have no ago-nist effects on the CNS (tamoxifen and raloxifene are both associ-ated with hot flushes) and no agonist effects on the endometrium would be ideal agents for such patients. At present, this investiga-tor would only consider hormone replacement therapy after early-stage breast cancer for patients with disabling vasomotor symp-toms. The bone and cardiovascular benefits of hormone replacement therapy can be accomplished with non-endocrine agents. Hormone replacement therapy, however, does not appear to increase the risk of breast cancer in women with other major risk factors such as a strong family history.

LYMPHEDEMA. Lymphedema of the ipsilateral arm develops in about 15% of women with breast cancer following primary therapy. The incidence of this complication may be slightly higher in

Table 258–9 ■ INFORMATION RESOURCES

WEB ADDRESS OR NUMBER	DESCRIPTION
1-800-4-CANCER	Access number for the NCI Cancer In-formation Service
http://cancernet.nci.nih.gov	Information service of the NCI. Includes PDQ and summaries on treatment, screening, prevention, supportive care, and ongoing clinical trials. Also access to CANCERLIT, NCI's biblio-graphic database
http://www.nabco.org	The National Alliance of Breast Cancer Organizations is the leading non-profit resource for information about breast cancer events and activities and has links to other key sites
http://www.breastcancernet.net	Excellent general site with many helpful links

NCI = National Cancer Institute; PDQ = Physician Data Query.

women treated with lumpectomy and radiation and may be less in women who are staged via sentinel lymph node procedures. In some affected women symptom are mild, but in many they are persistent, and slowly progressive edema can lead to functional loss. Early recognition is key, and patients should be asked about this complication at each clinic visit. Affected patients should be referred to physical therapists and other health professionals skilled in lymphedema management. Treatment consists of avoidance of trauma, special exercises, elevation of the extremity, and the use of compression pumps and specially fitted compression stockings. Recently, manual lymphatic drainage procedures have gained wide use and may be more effective than compression pumping. No effective medications have as yet been identified; diuretics are rarely effective and should be avoided.

American Society of Clinical Oncology: Recommended breast cancer surveillance guidelines. J Clin Oncol 15:2149, 1997. *Evidence-based review of follow-up procedures by an expert panel.*

Benichou J, Gail MH, Mulvihill JJ: Graphs to estimate an individualized risk of breast cancer. J Clin Oncol 14:103, 1996. *A collection of excellent graphs that allows accurate estimation of risk in women without a strong history of breast cancer and who receive yearly mammography.*

Claus EB, Risch N, Thompson WD: Autosomal dominant inheritance of early-onset breast cancer. Cancer 73:643, 1994. *An excellent series of tables to estimate breast cancer risk in women with strong family histories.*

Genetic Testing Guidelines: Statement of the American Society of Clinical Oncology: Genetic testing for cancer susceptibility. J Clin Oncol 14:1730, 1996. *Practical guidelines for the practicing clinician.*

Harris JR, Lippman ME, Morrow M, Hellman S (eds): Diseases of the Breast. Philadelphia, JB Lippincott, 1996. *Best all-around text with excellent reviews on all aspects of breast cancer biology and management.*

259 CERVICAL AND UTERINE CANCER SCREENING

Ralph M. Richart ■ *Edyta C. Pirog*

SCREENING FOR CERVICAL CANCER AND ITS PRECURSORS

Virtually all, if not all cervical squamous and glandular neoplasms are caused by a sexually transmitted, tightly coiled, circular virus called "human papillomavirus" (see also Chapter 361).

Productive human papillomavirus infections of the cervix are accompanied by cytologic atypia, binucleation, hyperchromatism, alterations in chromatin distribution, and perinuclear clearing, which when accompanied by nuclear atypia is known as "koilocytosis." A trained cytopathologist can recognize and distinguish papillomavirus-altered cells from normal epithelial cells. This difference forms the basis for screening with the Papanicolaou (Pap) smear.

Screening for cervical cancer and its precursors is one of the most successful and cost-effective methods of cancer detection yet devised. The Pap smear is the standard screening test and relies on microscopic examination of a glass slide onto which exfoliated cells from the lower female genital tract have been placed. The usual technique in preparing a Pap smear is to scrape the squamocolumnar junction and immature transformation zone of the cervix with a wooden spatula and sample the endocervical canal with a small brush. Cells from both of these sampling instruments are then transferred onto a glass slide and stained and examined by a cytopathologist. Pap smears have a high degree of specificity (95% or greater), but the sensitivity is in the range of 70 to 80%.

Because the Pap smear is a screening test—not a diagnostic test—and is designed to be relatively inexpensive and cost-effective, its efficacy in detecting cervical neoplasms is dependent on repeating the test at regular intervals. Considerable debate surrounds the appropriate Pap smear screening interval. The debate centers principally on the balance between cost and undetected neoplasms. In the United States the screening standard for the Pap smear endorsed by the American College of Obstetricians and Gy-

necologists and other organizations dealing with women's health issues is that "All women who are or have been sexually active or who have reached age 18 should have an annual Papanicolaou test and pelvic examination. After a woman has had three or more consecutive, satisfactory, normal, annual examinations, the Papanicolaou test may be performed less frequently at the discretion of her physician." For all practical purposes, this statement is interpreted in the United States as mandating annual screening. The screening strategy in much of the rest of the world varies. In many countries in Europe, Pap smear screening is not begun until age 25, and the re-examination interval generally varies from 3 to 5 years.

In the United States only 15,000 new invasive cancers of the cervix are seen yearly and only 5000 patients die of this disease despite the fact that the population has a high incidence rate of cervical pre-cancerous lesions. These figures attest to the effectiveness of conventional screening by Pap smear. However, cervical cancer is potentially completely preventable if the precursors are detected and treated before their transit to invasive cancer. A high proportion of invasive cervical cancer develops in women because they are not screened. Many such women have little contact with the health care system, and others are not screened because the clinician failed to include a pelvic examination and Pap smear as part of the patient's regular health care. It is important that physicians caring for elderly patients in nursing homes, treating disabled patients in whom a pelvic examination may be difficult, and acting as the primary care physician for women not seeing a gynecologist perform Pap smears on a regular basis or ensure that another physician has done so. Simple attention to this mandate could substantially reduce the already low incidence of invasive cancer in U.S. women.

SCREENING FOR ENDOMETRIAL CANCER AND ITS PRECURSORS

No mass screening method is available for the detection of endometrial cancer or its precursors.

Screening for endometrial cancer precursors has been attempted via a cytologic approach, but endometrial cancer precursors lack the easy-to-identify cytologic alterations that permit cervical cancer screening to be carried out with relative ease. Most attempts at screening (which, by definition, is carried out in an asymptomatic population), either by cytology or by endometrial biopsy, have foundered because of the low detection rate in asymptomatic women and because of the high false-positive rate when endometrial cytology is used as a screening technique. For these reasons, organized programs for endometrial cancer screening have not been promulgated on a population-wide basis. Even in high-risk groups such as obese, hypertensive, or estrogen-treated patients, endometrial cancer screening is not generally recommended.

Detection of endometrial cancers and their precursors has instead concentrated on educating physicians and patients about the need for biopsy in any patient who has signs and symptoms that may point to an abnormality in the endometrial cavity. Because endometrial hyperplasia and cancer are commonly associated with abnormal patterns of uterine bleeding, it is universally recommended that any patient with menorrhagia, metrorrhagia, or postmenopausal or other unexplained vaginal bleeding be evaluated and that the evaluation include at least an endometrial biopsy. Ultrasonography, with its ability to identify the thickness of the endometrium, has also been used to examine patients with abnormal uterine bleeding and, in some instances, has been suggested as a potential screening procedure for endometrial cancer and its precursors. Ultrasonography has a high false-positive rate, however.

A diagnosis of endometrial cancer or its precursors is most commonly established after patient self-referral for postmenopausal, intermenstrual, or excessive uterine bleeding. Despite the fact that bleeding is a non-specific symptom of endometrial pathology, about 10% of postmenopausal women who bleed have endometrial cancer. To detect as many cancers and their precursors as possible, even a transient episode of vaginal bleeding or spotting in postmenopausal women or any abnormal vaginal bleeding pattern in perimenopausal women must be evaluated in timely fashion. In such patients, endometrial biopsy is usually used as the initial diagnostic procedure, and the patient is generally only monitored if it is negative. If the patient continues to be symptomatic, however, hysteroscopy and endometrial curettage are advocated as the next diagnostic procedure, and other causes of bleeding should be evaluated.

Kurman R, Soloman D: The Bethesda System for Reporting Cervical/Vaginal Cytologic Diagnoses. Definitions, Criteria, and Explanatory Notes for Terminology and Specimen Adequacy. New York, Springer-Verlag, 1994.
Richart RM: Screening: The next century. Cancer 76:1919, 1995.
Richart RM, Masood S, Syrjanen KJ, et al: Human papillomavirus: IAC Task Force Summary. Acta Cytol 42:50, 1998.

260   OVARIAN CARCINOMA
Howard W. Jones, III

Ovarian carcinoma is the most deadly of the gynecologic malignancies. The age-specific incidence gradually rises and reaches a peak at about age 70, at which time the incidence is 55 per 100,000 among white women. The rate is somewhat lower in black women. The lifetime risk of ovarian cancer for women in the United States is about 1.4%, but women with one 1st-degree relative appear to have an increased risk of 3 to 5%. The cause of ovarian cancer is unknown; except for some relatively rare familial groups, it has not been possible to identify any clinically useful high-risk groups for increased surveillance. *BRCA1* gene mutations are found in about 10% of women with epithelial ovarian cancer. However, the risk of ovarian cancer in women with *BRCA1* mutations is not yet known. Rare familial groups with a high incidence of ovarian, breast, and colon cancer have been described. Multiple pregnancies and the use of oral contraceptives may be protective because of decreased ovulation and hormonal influences.

PATHOLOGY

Four types of ovarian tumors require separate consideration because of their clinical characteristics and prognoses: (1) Common *epithelial tumors* of the ovary include serous, mucinous, endometrioid, clear cell, and otherwise unspecified adenocarcinomas. These tumors account for almost 90% of ovarian cancers and are most commonly found in postmenopausal women. (2) *Germ cell tumors,* which arise from the totipotent oocytes, are usually benign ("dermoid cysts"). They often occur in young women and are almost always unilateral. When malignant (e.g., dysgerminoma, teratoma), they are highly aggressive but respond very well to combination chemotherapy. (3) *Stromal tumors* are generally low grade, and because they arise from the granulosa, theca, and Sertoli-Leydig cells of the ovary, they may be hormonally functional. These tumors are usually unilateral and may occur in any age group, but most typically in the 4th and 5th decades. Surgical excision alone may be all the therapy required, but combination chemotherapy is effective for metastatic or recurrent disease. (4) Malignancies of other sites that are metastatic to the ovary must always be considered in the evaluation of patients with a pelvic mass. In some cases, a pelvic mass is the 1st indication of a primary gastrointestinal or endometrial carcinoma. Breast cancer also commonly metastasizes to the ovary.

DIAGNOSIS

CLINICAL CHARACTERISTICS. Early ovarian cancer is usually asymptomatic. Occasionally, ovarian enlargement is found on routine examination, and cancer may be discovered incidentally at the time of abdominal or pelvic surgery for other indications. In two thirds of patients, however, widespread intra-abdominal metastases are present by the time the diagnosis is made. Symptoms of abdominal swelling, bloating, and pelvic fullness or pressure are common. It is not unusual for the patient to have had vague abdominal complaints or non-specific gastrointestinal symptoms. Ascites or a palpable abdominopelvic mass may be found on examination. The presence of an irregular mass in the pelvis or cul-de-sac nodularity accompanied by ascites is often diagnostic. Malignant pleural effu-

sions develop in some patients, and they initially seek medical attention for shortness of breath.

SCREENING TESTS. Screening tests for ovarian cancer remain controversial. Transvaginal ultrasonography, although quite effective for diagnosing ovarian cysts and tumors, is non-specific and its use for screening results in surgical exploration of a large number of women with benign ovarian cysts. Serum levels of the tumor-associated antigen CA-125 above 35 U/mL are highly correlated with ovarian cancer in postmenopausal women. Unfortunately, many ovarian tumors do not cause elevated levels of CA-125, whereas endometriosis, pelvic inflammatory disease, and some benign ovarian tumors may do so. The relative rarity of ovarian cancer, combined with the non-specific nature and relative sensitivity of currently available tests, makes ovarian cancer screening unsatisfactory. The risk of ovarian cancer developing in women with various genetic mutations has not been determined.

DIFFERENTIAL DIAGNOSIS. A pelvic mass can be caused by either a benign or a malignant tumor of the ovary, as well as by inflammatory conditions, physiologic cysts, and malignancies of other pelvic organs and structures. Initially, a careful history and physical examination are most helpful in suggesting possible primary sites. Pelvic ultrasonography may allow the dimensions and character of the mass to be determined. Smooth-walled, unilocular ovarian cysts are almost always benign, whereas malignancies are most commonly described as echogenically "complex," with both cystic and solid components. The possibility of ectopic pregnancy must always be considered, and a pregnancy test is therefore normally the first laboratory study done in women in the reproductive age group. A careful contraceptive history is important because functional ovarian cysts, including both follicle cysts and corpus luteum cysts, are common in ovulating women. Inflammatory masses and endometriosis can be confused with ovarian cancer and can cause elevated CA-125 levels in addition to a complex adnexal mass. In the older age group, diverticular abscesses and carcinoma of the colon must be considered in the differential diagnosis.

Once a complete history and physical examination have been done and the size and character of the mass have been confirmed by ultrasonography, several additional studies may be helpful. A chest radiograph is useful to rule out pulmonary metastases and pleural effusions. An abdominal and pelvic computed tomography scan can identify evidence of upper abdominal metastases or ureteral obstruction, and a barium enema or colonoscopy is almost always indicated before surgery to rule out a primary lesion or secondary involvement of the colon.

Additional studies (e.g., brain scans, bone scans) should generally be reserved for patients whose symptoms or physical findings suggest involvement of the areas to be studied.

TREATMENT

SURGERY. In almost all cases of suspected ovarian carcinoma, an exploratory laparotomy is the ultimate diagnostic procedure. If the diagnosis is confirmed, tumor debulking, including total abdominal hysterectomy and bilateral salpingo-oophorectomy, if possible, should be done. At this point a definitive diagnosis can be made and the extent of the disease accurately staged (Table 260–1). Aggressive tumor debulking, even when all cancer cannot be removed, improves the length and quality of survival. Ideally, this initial surgery should be done by a gynecologic oncologist whose special training and experience should provide the optimal surgical and postoperative management.

The goal of the initial operation for ovarian cancer is two-fold. First, all tumor should be removed, if possible, to provide the greatest possibility of cure. In approximately two thirds of patients, however, widespread intra-abdominal metastases prevent complete surgical debulking. The second goal of surgery is accurate staging (see Table 260–1). In addition to patients with early-stage disease, a more favorable prognosis is seen in women who have minimal residual disease, well-differentiated cancers, and mucinous or endometrioid histology and in patients younger than 50 years.

Careful staging evaluation with peritoneal cytology and multiple biopsies of the upper region of the abdomen (the omentum, diaphragm, and retroperitoneal nodes) is especially important in early-

Table 260–1 ■ **DEFINITIONS OF THE STAGES IN PRIMARY CARCINOMA OF THE OVARY***

Stage I	Growth limited to the ovaries
Stage Ia	Growth limited to one ovary; no ascites No tumor on the external surface; capsule intact
Stage Ib	Growth limited to both ovaries; no ascites No tumor on the external surfaces; capsules intact
Stage Ic	Tumor either stage Ia or Ib, but with tumor on the surface of one or both ovaries, with the capsule ruptured, with ascites present containing malignant cells, or with positive peritoneal washings
Stage II	Growth involving one or both ovaries with pelvic extension
Stage IIa	Extension and/or metastases to the uterus and/or tubes
Stage IIb	Extension to other pelvic tissues
Stage IIc	Tumor either stage IIa or IIb, but with tumor on the surface of one or both ovaries, with capsule(s) ruptured, with ascites present containing malignant cells, or with positive peritoneal washings
Stage III	Tumor involving one or both ovaries with peritoneal implants outside the pelvis and/or positive retroperitoneal or inguinal nodes. Superficial liver metastases equal stage III Tumor limited to the true pelvis but with histologically proven malignant extension to small bowel or omentum
Stage IIIa	Tumor grossly limited to the true pelvis with negative nodes but with histologically confirmed microscopic seeding of abdominal peritoneal surfaces
Stage IIIb	Tumor involving one or both ovaries with histologically confirmed implants of abdominal peritoneal surfaces, none exceeding 2 cm in diameter. Nodes are negative
Stage IIIc	Abdominal implants greater than 2 cm in diameter and/or positive retroperitoneal or inguinal nodes
Stage IV	Growth involving one or both ovaries with distant metastases. If pleural effusion is present, cytology must be positive to assign stage IV Parenchymal liver metastases equal stage IV

*Nomenclature of the International Federation of Gynecology and Obstetrics. Staging is based on findings at clinical examination and surgical exploration

stage disease because microscopic metastases often escape clinical detection. Accurate staging guides the most appropriate postoperative management.

In patients with advanced disease, aggressive surgical debulking includes bowel resection or colostomy in as many as 25% of patients. Whether such extensive surgical resection actually improves 5- and 10-year survival rates is still controversial. It is agreed, however, that optimal tumor debulking (《1-cm residual) results in prolongation of good-quality survival. This setting is where the skills and experienced judgment of the gynecologic oncologist are most important.

CHEMOTHERAPY. Except for some patients with stage IA disease, chemotherapy is usually recommended postoperatively for most women with ovarian cancer. Cisplatin or carboplatin, usually combined with paclitaxel, is the most effective and widely used initial chemotherapy regimen for ovarian cancer. Following primary surgery, patients are usually treated with six cycles of 3-week intervals of chemotherapy. The mean disease-free interval for women with stage III and IV disease is about 18 months, but only 20 to 30% of these patients will be long-term survivors. Other active drugs include cisplatin, cyclophosphamide, and altretamine (Hexalen). Intraperitoneal chemotherapy has been used in some clinics for patients with minimal residual disease. This chemotherapy is well tolerated and quality of life is quite satisfactory in most patients until late in the course of the disease.

RADIATION THERAPY. Postoperative external radiation therapy to the whole abdomen may be as effective as chemotherapy for patients with minimal residual tumor. The toxicity of such therapy, especially gastrointestinal obstruction, is greater than that associated with chemotherapy, so chemotherapy has been favored in most cases.

Intraperitoneal radioactive colloidal chromic phosphate is also used to treat some women with stage I or II disease and no gross residual tumor. Only patients with very early disease are good candidates for this therapy, which requires a complete and uniform intraperitoneal distribution of the radioactive suspension.

Table 260–2 ■ **CARCINOMA OF THE OVARY: DISTRIBUTION BY STAGE AND 3- AND 5-YEAR SURVIVAL RATES IN THE DIFFERENT STAGES***

	PATIENTS TREATED		SURVIVAL	
STAGE	**No.**	**%**	**3-yr**	**5-yr**
I	5,559	46.5%	87.5%	82.1%
II	3,364	28.1%	72.1%	64.5%
III	2,530	21.2%	47.0%	38.1%
IV	492	4.2%	20.7%	14.0%
Total	11,945	100%	71.6%	65.4%

*Data from Percorelli S, Odicino F, Maisonneuve P, et al: Carcinoma of the ovary. *In* Percorelli S (ed): Annual report on the results of treatment in gynaecological cancer. J Epidemiol Biostat 3:75, 1998. The "annual report" is published at regular intervals by the International Federation for Gynecology and Obstetrics and contains vast quantities of statistics generated from institutions that submit their treatment results from throughout the world.

"SECOND-LOOK" SURGERY. A planned re-exploration to evaluate the extent of disease following a course of therapy and to resect any residual malignancy has been called "second-look" surgery. This approach allows an excellent research evaluation of the effect of the primary therapy, but it has not proved to be of significant clinical benefit to patients with ovarian cancer. Measurements of tumor-associated antigens such as CA-125, used in conjunction with periodic physical examinations and selected radiographic studies, have been helpful in monitoring the disease status of treated patients. Until more effective salvage therapy is available, second-look surgery in asymptomatic patients with a normal physical examination is probably not indicated.

TREATMENT OF RECURRENT, METASTATIC DISEASE. The overall survival rate of patients treated for ovarian cancer is only about 40%; progressive disease develops in many women despite appropriate primary therapy. Salvage chemotherapy protocols for recurrent disease produce a 10% response rate. Although almost all women with recurrent disease will succumb to cancer, many women will live 3 to 5 years with a good quality of life. Eventually, widespread intra-abdominal metastases with bowel obstruction often occur, but reoperation with resection, bypass, or enterostomy may provide significant palliation. Pleural effusion may require thoracentesis and pleural sclerotherapy. With the relative effectiveness of current primary chemotherapy, patients may survive to the development of late metastases to the liver, brain, and meninges. Localized irradiation has been helpful in some of these patients.

PROGNOSIS

The long-term survival rate of patients treated for epithelial ovarian cancer is still disappointing (Table 260–2). Almost 60% of patients have stage III or IV disease at the time of diagnosis. Although the majority of women with advanced disease live 2 years with a reasonable quality of life, recurrent cancer eventually becomes symptomatic in most, and by 5 years only about 15% still survive. The results are much better for patients in whom ovarian cancer is diagnosed at an earlier stage. Almost three fourths of women with stage I ovarian cancer survive 5 years.

Collins WP, Bourne TH, Campbell S: Screening strategies for ovarian cancer. Curr Opin Obstet Gynecol 10:33, 1998. *A good review of the current status of ovarian cancer screening with an emphasis on ultrasound.*

Gotlieb WH, Flikker S, Davidson B, et al: Borderline tumors of the ovary; fertility treatment, conservative management, and pregnancy outcome. Cancer 82:141, 1998. *This article emphasized the possibility of conservative management of borderline ovarian tumors with subsequent pregnancy.*

Grann VR, Panageas KS, Whang W, et al: Decision analysis of prophylactic mastectomy and oophorectomy in BRCA1-positive or BRCA2-positive patients. J Clin Oncol 16:979, 1998. *An excellent review indicating the rather minimal benefits of prophylactic surgery in most women with BRCA gene mutations.*

Le T, Krepart GV, Lotocki RJ, Heywood MS: Does debulking surgery improve survival in biologically aggressive ovarian carcinoma? Gynecol Oncol 67:208, 1997. *The importance of aggressive primary surgical therapy in advanced ovarian cancer is supported in this paper from Canada.*

Munoz KA, Harlan LC, Trimble EL: Patterns of care for women with ovarian cancer in the United States. J Clin Oncol 15:3408, 1997. *Current management of ovarian cancer is examined in this review of the Surveillance, Epidemiology and End Results (SEER) database.*

Rubin SC, Blackwood MA, Bandera C, et al: BRCA1, BRCA2, and hereditary nonpolyposis colorectal cancer gene mutations in an unselected ovarian cancer population; relationship to family history and implications for genetic testing. Am J Obstet Gynecol 178:670, 1998. *A good discussion of the role of genetic mutation in ovarian cancer.*

PART XIX

DISEASES OF BONE AND BONE MINERAL METABOLISM

261 MINERAL AND BONE HOMEOSTASIS

Stephen J. Marx

DIVERSE ROLES FOR CALCIUM, PHOSPHATE, AND MAGNESIUM

Calcium, phosphorus, and magnesium, three of the principal body elements, have diverse roles. The calcium ion is particularly versatile. In the crystalline phase, it contributes to the varied structural roles of bone. In a supersaturated solution in blood, it contributes to plasma membrane excitability, plasma enzyme activities, and accretion of all minerals in extracellular matrix of bone. In the cytoplasmic fluid, its extraordinarily low concentrations allow rapid rises of its local concentrations to transmit information among cell compartments via its interactions with high-affinity calcium-binding proteins, such as calmodulin or protein kinase C. Phosphorus in the form of phosphate is the principal intracellular anion, with central roles in cytoplasm as a buffer, energy carrier (mainly via the high-energy phosphate bonds of adenosine triphosphate [ATP]), and molecular switch (through phosphorylation and dephosphorylation). Magnesium is the principal divalent cation in cytoplasm, functioning as a cofactor in many chemical reactions (for example, as a magnesium-ATP complex or as a cofactor in many steps of DNA or RNA metabolism).

MINERALS IN BLOOD

The States of Calcium, Phosphate, and Magnesium in Blood

Total calcium concentration in blood is tightly regulated so that typical diurnal fluctuations are not more than 5% from the mean value. Calcium in blood is divided among protein-bound, complexed, and ionized fractions (Table 261–1). Protein binding of calcium in blood is principally to albumin, and this binding is decreased by acid pH. The ionized calcium fraction is the focus for metabolic control by the parathyroid gland, and measurements of ionized calcium in blood give the most valid index of pathologic disruptions of calcium homeostasis.

Phosphate and magnesium in blood are principally unbound (see Table 261–1), and the concentration of each is regulated over a broader relative variation from its mean than that for calcium. Neither phosphate nor magnesium has a unique endocrine system dedicated to its control. Rather, their blood concentrations are sus-

tained indirectly by the hormones directed at calcium control and directly by poorly understood local processes in bone, kidney, and other organs.

Steady-State Flow of Minerals to and from Blood

Only 0.1% of the total body calcium is in blood and extracellular fluid (Table 261–2). This calcium pool is in a rapidly exchanging equilibrium with large calcium pools controlled by three organs (bone, intestine, and kidney), each of which is an important site for the regulation of mineral metabolism. The rate of these daily fluxes (Fig. 261–1) is sufficiently large that disturbance of mineral flux to or from any of these three organs can result in abnormally high or low concentrations of one of these minerals in blood.

ORGANS EXCHANGING MUCH MINERAL WITH BLOOD

Bone

Bone Function and Architecture

Major functions of bone include support, locomotion, encasement of hematopoietic or central nervous system tissue, and reservoir for calcium, phosphate, and magnesium. The architecture of bone responds dynamically to changes in mechanical load. Mature bone adopts one of two macroscopic organizations (Fig. 261–2). The cortices of all bones and the interior of certain bones have a continuous structure termed cortical or lamellar bone. Lamellar bone, which is predominant in the long bones, is characterized by little metabolic activity and few cells. It has a highly organized extracellular matrix of mineral and parallel bundles of type I collagen. During embryonic development or in states with pathologic increase of bone turnover, bone assumes a less organized "woven" architecture. Within the vertebral bodies and in portions of the interior of other bones, bone is organized as a series of thin, interdigitating plates; this is termed trabecular, cancellous, or spongy bone. Its ratio of surface to volume is higher than that found in cortical bone and is thus better suited to rapid turnover.

Extracellular Matrix

Newly deposited osteoid, the organic component of the extracellular matrix, must undergo a poorly understood maturation process for 1 to 3 weeks until it is able to accumulate minerals. The mineral phase of bone extracellular matrix is a mixture of multiple amorphous and crystalline states, the latter principally as hydroxyapatite crystals: $Ca_5(OH)(PO_4)_3$. Ninety to 95% of osteoid is composed of bundles of type I collagen, a long triple helix of two alpha$_1$ (type I) chains and one alpha$_2$ (type I) chain. The principal

Table 261–1 ■ CONCENTRATIONS AND STATES OF CALCIUM, MAGNESIUM, AND PHOSPHATE IN NORMAL HUMAN PLASMA OR SERUM*

STATE	CALCIUM (mM)	MAGNESIUM (mM)	PHOSPHATE (mM)
Protein-bound	1.15 (47)	0.26 (31)	0.15 (13)
Filterable or free†			
Complexed	0.25 (10)	0.06 (7)	0.40 (35)
Ionized	1.06 (43)	0.52 (62)	0.60 (52)

*Number in parentheses indicates percentage of total for that mineral.
†Filterable or free = complexed + ionized.

Table 261–2 ■ DISTRIBUTION OF CALCIUM, MAGNESIUM, AND PHOSPHATE IN THE BODY OF A 70-KG ADULT*

COMPARTMENT	CALCIUM (g)	MAGNESIUM (g)	PHOSPHATE (g)
Bone and teeth	1300 (99)	14.0 (54)	600.0 (86)
Extracellular fluid	1 (0.1)	0.3 (1)	0.2 (0.03)
Cells	7 (1.0)	12.0 (46)	100.0 (14)

*Most of calcium is in bone; almost half of magnesium is in cells. Phosphate, as the principal counterion to calcium and magnesium in their dominant pools, has an intermediate proportional distribution. Number in parentheses is the percentage of total for that mineral.

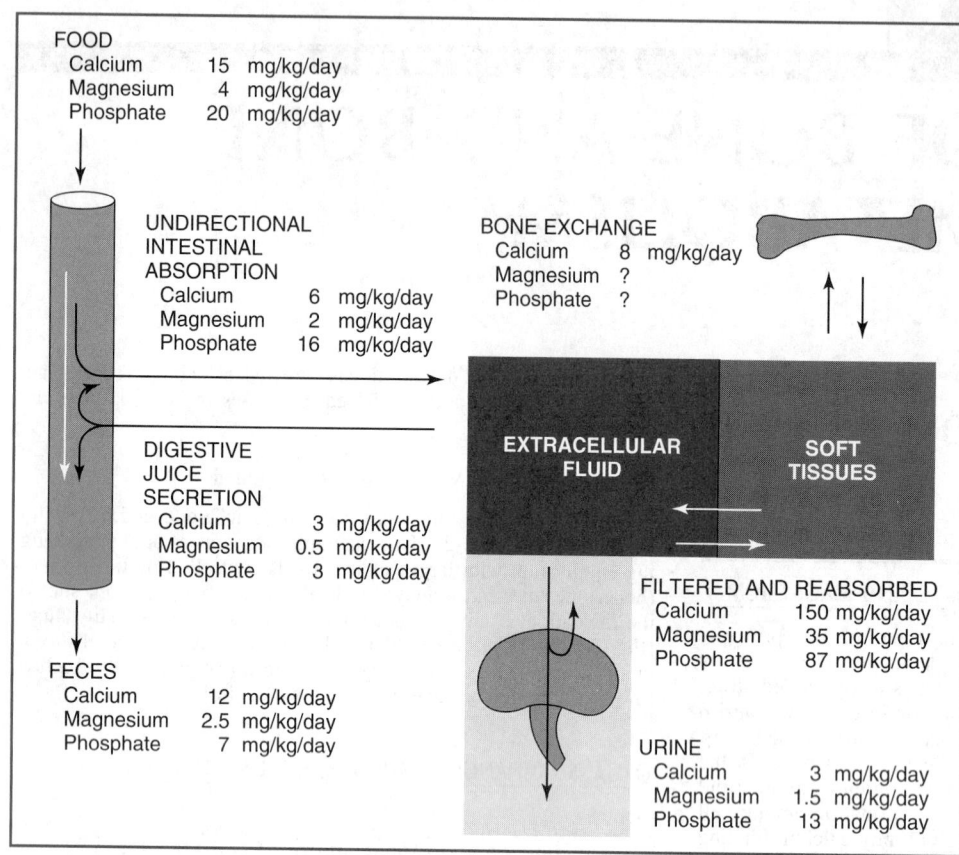

FOOD
Calcium	15	mg/kg/day
Magnesium	4	mg/kg/day
Phosphate	20	mg/kg/day

UNDIRECTIONAL
INTESTINAL
ABSORPTION
Calcium	6	mg/kg/day
Magnesium	2	mg/kg/day
Phosphate	16	mg/kg/day

BONE EXCHANGE
Calcium	8	mg/kg/day
Magnesium	?	
Phosphate	?	

DIGESTIVE
JUICE
SECRETION
Calcium	3	mg/kg/day
Magnesium	0.5	mg/kg/day
Phosphate	3	mg/kg/day

EXTRACELLULAR FLUID

SOFT TISSUES

FILTERED AND REABSORBED
Calcium	150	mg/kg/day
Magnesium	35	mg/kg/day
Phosphate	87	mg/kg/day

FECES
Calcium	12	mg/kg/day
Magnesium	2.5	mg/kg/day
Phosphate	7	mg/kg/day

URINE
Calcium	3	mg/kg/day
Magnesium	1.5	mg/kg/day
Phosphate	13	mg/kg/day

FIGURE 261–1 ■ Typical mineral fluxes in adults. (Modified from Aurbach GD, Marx SJ, Spiegel AM: Parathyroid hormone, calcitonin, and the calciferols. *In* Wilson JD, Foster DW [eds]: Williams Textbook of Endocrinology, 7th ed. Philadelphia, WB Saunders, 1985, p 1144.)

collagen of cartilage matrix is type II as a homotrimer of three alpha$_1$ (type II) chains. Fibrils of collagen play a major role in the strength of bone (type I collagen), cartilage (type II collagen), and elastic tissues (type III collagen). Their disruption results in characteristic disturbances (osteogenesis imperfecta [type I collagen], chondrodysplasia [type II collagen], Ehlers-Danlos syndrome or arterial aneurysms [type III collagen], and even certain variants of familial osteoarthritis [type II collagen]). The second most prominent protein in bone matrix is osteocalcin (or bone Gla-protein); it has a molar content of three residues of gamma-carboxyglutamic acid, an unusual amino acid that confers to the molecule high affinity for calcium on bone crystals. The roles of osteocalcin are unknown, but its concentration in blood is a potential index of osteoblast activity. Many other proteins, phosphoproteins, glycoproteins, and so on, in bone matrix have been identified in the search for molecules regulating bone mineral accumulation and bone growth.

Bone Cells

Several cells are highly characteristic of bone. A flat bone-lining cell (perhaps derived from marrow stroma) with few organelles covers many bone surfaces thought not to be undergoing modification. This cell is perhaps one precursor of the osteoblast. The osteoblast is a cuboidal bone matrix-synthesizing cell. It lines any periosteal, endosteal, or trabecular surface at which bone formation takes place. Its plasma membrane is highly enriched with a bone-specific isoform of the alkaline phosphatase enzyme. This enzyme promotes bone mineralization by catalyzing, in supersaturated extracellular fluid of bone, the hydrolysis of pyrophosphate and other inhibitors of calcium-phosphate crystallization. The osteocyte is the principal stable cell inside mature bone. It is probably derived from an osteoblast that has encased itself in bone. Osteocytes are interconnected with one another via long processes that traverse bone canaliculi. The role of the osteocyte is unknown, but the osteocyte is appropriately located to modulate local mineral fluxes.

The chondrocyte is the dominant cell of cartilage; it releases to the extracellular matrix type II collagen and vesicles that are rich in alkaline phosphatase and that may be a central organelle for accumulating calcium in preparation for mineralizing cartilage.

The osteoclast is the main bone-resorbing cell. It is derived from precursors of the premonocyte lineage. It is a highly motile, multinucleated giant cell with several specialized features for bone. These include organelles that mediate cell attachment to bone surface (podosomes), a strikingly redundant ruffled border at the bone face for ion transport, many enzymes that can function in bone resorption, and a high concentration of carbonic anhydrase II, which helps acidify the extracellular pocket between the osteoclast ruffled border and the skeletal resorption surface.

Local Regulators of Bone Cells

Bone cells are under systemic and local regulation. Known systemic regulators include parathyroid hormone (PTH), calcitonin, and calcitriol, which are considered later in this chapter. There is also a highly complex network of local controls. The term osteoclast-activating factors was applied in the 1980s to components in incompletely characterized fluids that could activate bone resorption in vitro. some of their active components have been identified. For example, interleukin-1 and lymphotoxin/tumor necrosis factor–beta are potential stimulators of bone resorption that seem to be released locally by some tumors in bone. They cannot act directly on mature osteoclasts but can act through nearby cells, such as osteoblasts or marrow stromal cells, that communicate with osteoclasts. Parathyroid hormone–related protein (PTH-RP) is a local mediator of diverse functions in many tissues. For example, it regulates chondrocyte differentiation. When oversecreted from a tumor into blood, PTH-RP can be the principal cause of humoral hypercalcemia of malignancy. Like the activators of bone resorption, the activators of bone formation are poorly understood, particularly because this process involves a complex interplay of osteoblast proliferation and differentiation. Some other contributors to this process include type 1 insulin-like growth factor and transforming growth factor-beta; the latter is present selectively and at high concentrations in osteoblasts and osteocytes. In addition, bone morphogenetic proteins are a family of major embryo pattern determinants (homologues of transforming growth factor–beta) that can induce bone formation in soft-tissue sites. Prostaglandins can stimulate bone formation or bone resorption, and they may be important mediators in inflammatory processes of the skeletal system.

Bone Remodeling

Bone growth or modeling occurs initially within a membrane or along the edge of cartilage (e.g., periosteum or epiphyseal growth plate). Although it contains few cells, cortical bone is constantly going through slow and orderly cycles of localized resorption and then rebuilding. This process is mediated by the local remodeling unit (alternately termed osteon or basic multicellular unit). Remodeling begins with osteoclasts excavating a cavity; as this resorption tunnel advances, osteoclasts are replaced by other cells. Over an interval of several months, new bone is deposited in cylindrical lamellae around the rim of the cavity until it is refilled to complete this cycle. This cycle is an important example of the normal, coordinated relation between the bone resorption and bone formation processes. Most perturbations that modify one component of these two processes also modify the other in the same direction. The determinants of this coupling between bone resorption and formation are not known, but they probably include a host of growth factors present at high local concentrations in bone extracellular matrix and exposed or released by the skeletal resorption process.

Intestines

Mineral Absorption

The intestinal absorption of magnesium and phosphate is not subject to fine regulation and has not been studied intensively. By contrast, intestinal absorption of calcium is tightly regulated, and its quantitation has been analyzed in detail. Most calcium absorption is accomplished in the small bowel. Over a wide range of intakes, approximately 10% of dietary calcium is absorbed passively; the remainder of net intestinal absorption of calcium is regulated by active vitamin D metabolites, especially $1\alpha,25(OH)_2D$, in blood. With a normal diet, approximately 30% of calcium is absorbed. With low dietary calcium, the secondarily high blood $1\alpha,25(OH)_2D$ level can drive fractional calcium absorption to approach 90%.

Kidney

Ion Filtration and Reabsorption

The non-protein-bound fractions of calcium, magnesium, and phosphate from plasma cross the glomerulus. The distal portions of the nephron have efficient and selective systems that can complete the reabsorption from tubular fluid of more than 99% of any one of these minerals. Tubular calcium reabsorption is stimulated principally by PTH; thiazides or lithium can also increase tubular calcium reabsorption. Saline loading with or without loop diuretics can inhibit this. Tubular phosphate reabsorption is mainly under negative influence by PTH. The determinants of tubular reabsorption of magnesium are incompletely understood.

Integrated Fluxes: Mineral Balance and Nutrition

Skeletal growth is maximal throughout childhood, nearing completion during adolescence. Until this time, the rate of skeletal calcium accretion is typically 200 to 400 mg (5 to 10 mmol)/d. Fetal mineralization during the last trimester or milk secretion during lactation imposes similar total daily increments on calcium efflux from maternal blood. The skeleton remains in a state of approximately 0 mineral balance between ages 20 and 35 years, after which it slowly loses mass. This loss is greatest in the trabecular bone of the vertebrae, attaining peak rates about the menopause (3 to 10% per year during the first 1 to 4 years after surgically induced menopause).

Normal adults can sustain 0 calcium balance with daily calcium

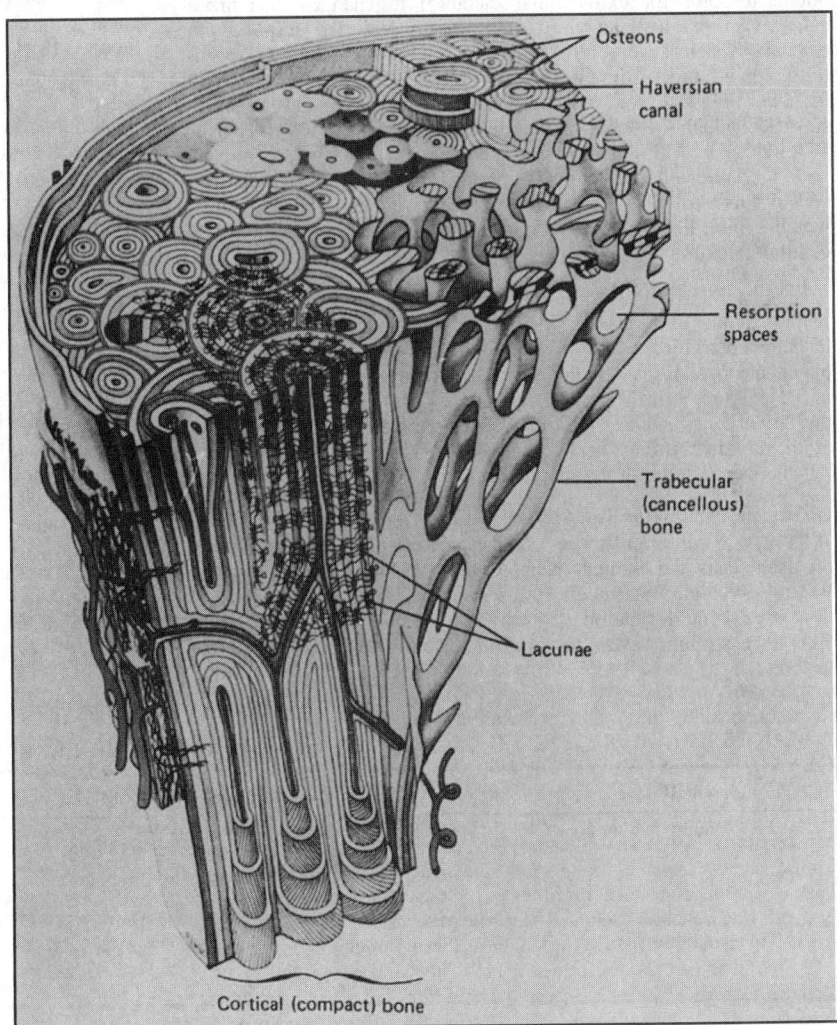

FIGURE 261–2 ■ Bone organization. Microstructure of mature bone; areas of cortical (lamellar) and trabecular (cancellous) bone are shown. The central area in the transverse section shows differences in mineral density as degrees of shading. Note the organization of osteons, the distribution of osteocyte lacunae, and the organization of bone lamellae. (Adapted from Warwick R, Williams PL [eds]: Gray's Anatomy, 35th ed. Edinburgh, Churchill Livingstone, 1973, p 217.)

intakes between 400 and 1500 mg (10 to 37.5 mmol), mainly as dairy products. Typical daily calcium intakes in the United States are 500 to 800 mg (12.5 to 20 mmol), and there is uncertainty over the minimal level for optimal skeletal health. With a typical daily calcium intake of 700 mg (17.5 mmol), about one-fourth, or 175 mg (4.37 mmol), is absorbed; during skeletal balance, this amount must equal the amount lost in urinary excretion (disregarding the small amount of calcium lost from skin).

Because of the large mineral fluxes between blood and three principal pools (bone, renal tubular lumen, and intestinal lumen), it is often difficult to assign mild disruptions to one pool. For example, there is uncertainty whether the slow bone losses with idiopathic age-associated osteoporosis reflect primary disturbances of calcium flux in bone, in the intestine, or in combinations of these.

HORMONAL REGULATORS OF MINERAL HOMEOSTASIS

Parathyroid Hormone

Synthesis, Secretion, and Metabolism

PTH is a rapidly regulated hormone that sustains calcium and $1,25(OH)_2D$ in blood and depresses phosphate in blood (Table 261–3). PTH is stored in the parathyroid cell mainly as a native peptide of 84 amino acids. The parathyroid cell secretes PTH as the native molecule or as fragments, only some of which are biologically active. Fragments of PTH are also generated from its metabolism after secretion into blood. The amino terminus of PTH (residues 1 to 34) contains the requirements for receptor binding and biologic activity.

Blood Calcium Effect on the Parathyroid Gland

The parathyroid gland, as the coordinator of blood levels of PTH and $1\alpha,25(OH)_2D$, is exquisitely sensitive (through its membrane-bound receptor for extracellular calcium) to changes of ionized calcium in extracellular fluid. The parathyroid cell responds to calcium in at least three different ways. First, low calcium concentration is a direct stimulus for the gradual increase in size and numbers of parathyroid cells (secondary hypertrophy and hyperplasia). Second, low calcium stimulates the biosynthesis of PTH over 1 to 2 days. Third, depression of the calcium level stimulates within seconds the secretion of preformed PTH. The parathyroid cell differs strikingly from most other hormone secretory cells, which exhibit decreased secretion in response to decreases of extracellular calcium.

Parathyroid Hormone Mechanisms of Action

PTH binds to a plasma membrane receptor; activation of the PTH receptor then causes a rise of cyclic 3',5'-adenosine monophosphate (cAMP) and other second messengers in the cytoplasm of PTH target cells. The consequence is rapid effects of PTH on the target cells in bone and kidney. PTH-RP has homology to PTH at the amino terminus and is secreted by many cancers, causing hypercalcemia through its interactions with PTH receptors.

Parathyroid Hormone Action in Bone

PTH in bone stimulates osteoblasts and osteoclasts. The effects on osteoclasts are indirect because these cells lack receptors for PTH. Very high PTH levels result in clear excess of bone resorption over bone formation. Controversy exists over whether mild PTH excess might have a net anabolic effect selectively in trabecular bone.

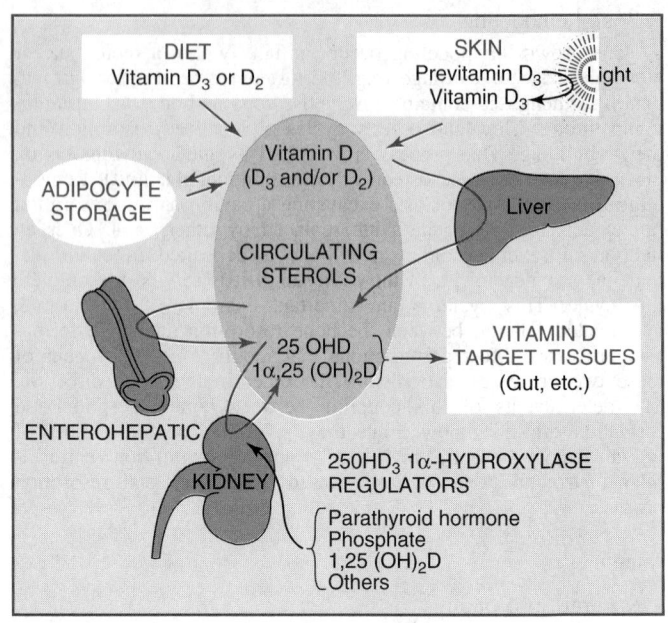

FIGURE 261–3 ■ The vitamin D activation pathway. This involves steps in many different organs. Dysfunction at any step can have clinically important consequences.

Parathyroid Hormone Action in Kidney

PTH acts in the kidney to stimulate the synthesis of $1,25(OH)_2D$ by increasing the activity of $25OHD_31\alpha$-hydroxylase in the proximal tubules. PTH acts in the distal portions of the nephron to increase tubular reabsorption of calcium. In addition, PTH inhibits phosphate reabsorption in the distal, and perhaps also the proximal, tubules. PTH also inhibits bicarbonate reabsorption.

Parathyroid Hormone Action on Intestine

PTH has no important direct action on the intestine. However, the direct renal effect of PTH to increase serum $1\alpha,25(OH)_2D$ causes highly important secondary effects in the intestine (see the later section on Intestinal Actions of Calcitriol).

Calcitonin

Calcitonin Synthesis and Secretion

Calcitonin is a peptide of 32 amino acids that is normally synthesized and secreted by the parafollicular or C cells, which are neuroectodermal cells within the thyroid gland. Calcitonin secretion is stimulated by calcium and also by certain intestinal peptides (gastrin and glucagon) (see Chapter 265).

Calcitonin Actions

Calcitonin, at high concentrations, can directly inhibit osteoclast function. Calcitonin can also act in the kidney to cause mild natriuresis. These calcitonin actions have not been shown to be important in normal physiology. The principal interests in calcitonin are as a tumor marker, particularly for familial parafollicular or C-cell neoplasia, or as a pharmacologic agent to treat osteolytic bone disorders, such as Paget's disease.

Table 261–3 ■ EFFECTS OF PRINCIPAL CALCIOTROPIC HORMONES

HORMONE	PRINCIPAL TARGET TISSUES	ACTION
Parathyroid hormone	Renal proximal convoluted tubule	Increase serum $1\alpha,25 (OH)_2D$
	Renal distal convoluted tubule	Increase calcium reabsorption
	Renal proximal and distal convoluted tubules	Decrease phosphate reabsorption
	Bone	Increase calcium and phosphate resorption
Calcitonin	Bone	Decrease calcium and phosphate resorption
$1\alpha,25(OH)_2D$	Small bowel	Increase calcium absorption
	Bone	Increase calcium and phosphate resorption
	Parathyroid gland	Decrease synthesis of PTH

Vitamin D and Its Metabolites

Synthesis of Vitamin D

Vitamin D_3 is a secosteroid (i.e., a steroid with one ring opened) synthesized from 7-dehydro-cholesterol in the skin (Fig. 261–3) in a reaction catalyzed by ultraviolet light derived from the sun. Vitamin D_2, produced synthetically from the plant sterol ergosterol, is a vitamin D_3 analogue used as a dietary supplement or drug. The metabolism and actions of vitamin D_3 and vitamin D_2 are similar in humans (see Chapter 262).

Hydroxylations of Vitamin D Metabolites

Vitamin D ("D" refers to combinations of the D_3 and D_2 isoforms) is converted to 25OHD in hepatocytes. This reaction is not under metabolic control and is determined principally by the serum levels of its substrate, vitamin D. 25OHD is normally converted to $1\alpha,25(OH)_2D$ (calcitriol) only in the renal proximal tubule by an enzyme system stimulated by PTH. A similar PTH-independent 1a-hydroxylation occurs in the normal placenta and abnormally in granuloma tissues, as in sarcoidosis. 25OHD and $1\alpha,25(OH)_2D$ are bioactive; they can also be hydroxylated at other residues (C-23, C-24, C-26), but these and other conversions probably serve mainly to inactivate vitamin D metabolites.

Absorption and Transport of Vitamin D Metabolites

Vitamin D metabolites enter the bloodstream like other sterols, and a small fraction of all vitamin D metabolites undergoes an enterohepatic recirculation. When cutaneous synthesis of vitamin D is marginal, any cause of intestinal malabsorption can result in vitamin D deficiency. Vitamin D metabolites are lipid-soluble; they circulate in plasma bound to a specific 25OHD binding protein and, to a lesser degree, to other carriers.

Mechanism of Actions of Vitamin D Metabolites

Vitamin D is an inactive precursor; 25OHD and $1\alpha,25(OH)_2D$ are both active. Although the concentration of 25OHD is about 1000-fold higher than that of $1\alpha,25 (OH)_2D$ in blood, the latter has far higher affinity for the vitamin D receptor and normally determines the degree of vitamin D receptor activation. Calcitriol binds to intracellular receptors in target cells and causes gradual changes in the nuclei of those cells. The vitamin D receptor is highly homologous to the receptors for other steroids and to those for thyroid hormone and retinoic acid. All are DNA-binding regulators of transcription from selected genes.

Intestinal Actions of Calcitriol

Calcitriol—$1,25(OH)_2D$—increases the flux of calcium from the intestinal lumen to blood. Calcitriol, to a much lesser extent, increases the flux of phosphate and magnesium from intestinal lumen to blood.

Skeletal Effects of Calcitriol

The principal effects of calcitriol on bone (antirachitic effects) are indirect results of its action to promote calcium influx from intestinal lumen to blood. The deficient bone mineralization in vitamin D deficiency states is the consequence of the combination of low calcium in blood and low phosphate in blood, the latter resulting from the renal phosphate-wasting effects from secondary hyperparathyroidism.

Although physiologic calcitriol levels help move calcium to bone, the supraphysiologic concentrations of vitamin D metabolites sometimes reached during pharmacotherapy can raise blood calcium in part by increasing osteoclast numbers and activity and thereby increasing bone resorption and calcium flux from bone to blood.

Other Effects of Calcitriol

Calcitriol can inhibit PTH biosynthesis and secretion; the direct negative effects of calcitriol might contribute a form of short-loop negative feedback to parathyroid function, independent of blood calcium. Calcitriol exerts direct effects on the renal enzymes that hydroxylate 25OHD; calcitriol inhibits the $25OHD_3 1\alpha$-hydroxylase and stimulates the other hydroxylases that catabolize 25OHD in the renal tubule and in other tissues. Possibly important effects of calcitriol in skin and hair are suggested by its protective effect on psoriatic skin at pharmacologic doses and by the striking association of total alopecia with the rare syndrome of severely defective

vitamin D receptors. Vitamin D receptors are present in many additional organs, but no role for them has been identified in normal physiology.

Other Hormones

Sex Steroids

Sex steroids, particularly estrogens, have slow but extremely important anabolic effects on bone. The effects are exerted directly on the bone organ, perhaps through receptors in the osteoblast. Estrogen deficiency results in accelerated bone remodeling with disproportionate bone resorption, particularly in trabecular bone.

Glucocorticoids

Glucocorticoids affect many of the cells that contribute to mineral metabolism. The most striking effect is bone thinning that results from high glucocorticoid concentrations. This thinning is probably a consequence mainly of inhibited osteoblasts. In addition, glucocorticoids antagonize the actions of vitamin D metabolites by unknown mechanisms.

Thyroid Hormone

Thyroid hormones also have direct effects on bone cells. Excess of thyroid hormones causes increased release of calcium from bone. The skeletal consequences of deficient thyroid hormone are most evident in the disordered growth of cartilaginous epiphyses associated with congenital hypothyroidism.

Growth Hormone

Growth hormone stimulates the growth of bone and cartilage, in part by stimulating local production of IGF-1 by osteoblasts and chondrocytes.

ADAPTATIONS TO DISRUPTIONS OF MINERAL METABOLISM

Two principal calciotropic hormones, PTH and $1\alpha,25(OH)_2D$, interact with each other and with multiple target tissues to control the metabolism of calcium, phosphate and, to a lesser degree, magnesium (Fig. 261–4; see Table 261–3). These hormones allow for adaptations over intervals that are short (minutes) or long (months).

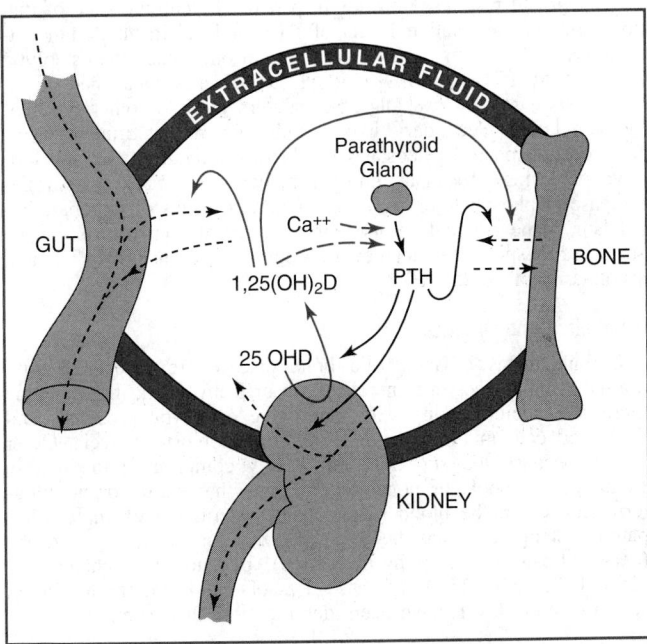

FIGURE 261–4 ■ Integrated control of secretion and actions of parathyroid hormone (PTH) and calcitriol ($1\alpha,25(OH)_2$ vitamin D = $1\alpha,25(OH)_2D$) with emphasis on calcium fluxes. Solid lines show secretion and targets of PTH and calcitriol. Interrupted black lines are calcium fluxes. Solid red or black lines show stimulatory effects; interrupted red lines show inhibitory effects.

Blood levels of ionized calcium are sustained at nearly invariant levels, with minimal diurnal changes reflecting mainly the sudden rises of calcium influx with meals. Serum levels of PTH and $1\alpha,25(OH)_2D$ also show only modest diurnal changes under normal conditions. Serum phosphate typically has broad diurnal fluctuations, with a nadir around 9:00 A.M. and peaks at around 6:00 P.M. and 4:00 A.M.

Calcium Excess States

States with long-term excess or deficiency of calcium are associated with deviations at multiple steps of the integrated mineral homeostasis system. The most common calcium excess state in adults is primary overfunction of the parathyroid gland. Of course, this has the potential to distort most of the normal calcium regulatory processes. Primary hyperparathyroidism results in high blood levels of PTH and often of $1\alpha,25(OH)_2D$ as well. The results are combinations of increased calcium influx to blood dependent on the evoked dysfunctions in intestinal, skeletal, and renal lumenal pools of calcium. A different integrated metabolic pattern results when calcium excess is caused by dysfunction outside the parathyroid; for example, with osteolytic metastases, skeletal immobilization, or dietary calcium overload (milk-alkali syndrome). In the latter disturbances, the parathyroid gland reacts appropriately and becomes suppressed by the increase of ionized calcium in blood; blood concentrations of PTH and $1\alpha,25(OH)_2D$ become low. The abnormally high filtered load of calcium without the anticalciuric effects of PTH results in severe hypercalciuria; with such hypercalciuria, irreversible renal damage can occur over a period of only a few weeks.

Calcium Deficiency States

Calcium deficiency states generally result in the parathyroid gland's recognizing the signal of a low ionized calcium level in blood. Increased PTH secretion (within seconds), increased PTH biosynthesis (within days), and parathyroid cell hyperplasia (within weeks) activate the homeostatic pathways. The consequences of this secondary hyperparathyroidism are increased renal tubular secretion of $1\alpha,25(OH)_2D$ (if there is not underlying deficiency of 25OHD or of the 25OHD 1α-hydroxylase)) and increased net calcium flux into blood from the intestinal lumen, from bone, and from the renal tubular lumen. The relative contribution of each calcium pool to this integrated response depends in part on the chronic state of that pool and on the relative levels of PTH and calcitriol. Serum calcium typically begins to fall below normal only when the osteolytic response to PTH or to $1\alpha,25(OH)_2D$ becomes weakened (from depletion of readily exchangeable calcium pools or other types of tachyphylaxis). Secondary hyperparathyroidism has important effects on phosphate homeostasis by directly affecting bone and kidney, increasing phosphate influx from bone, and causing a similar increase in phosphate efflux into urine. With forms of hypoparathyroidism, some residual components of mineral homeostasis can be sustained despite a deficiency or complete absence of PTH and secondarily of $1\alpha,25(OH)_2D$.

Metabolic Bone Diseases

Certain forms of metabolic bone disease are associated with dramatic imbalances in mineral flux to or from blood; these include increased calcium influx with aggressive osteolytic processes and decreased calcium influx with many forms of osteomalacia. Other forms, because they do not dramatically compromise the readily exchangeable pools of bone mineral, may have little or no long-term impact on the blood homeostatic system. For example, idiopathic osteoporosis has been categorized into two major forms (perimenopausal and aging-associated), but no clear changes in blood PTH or $1\alpha,25(OH)_2D$ as causes of or adaptations to altered serum calcium levels have been identified in either form.

USES OF LABORATORY TESTING

Electrolytes in Blood

Calcium in Blood

To stabilize blood albumin concentration, total calcium should be measured in the fasting patient who is seated or recumbent. Most laboratories measure it inexpensively and with high precision. A high or low calcium value from multichannel screening is often the first indication of a treatable disorder. Serum calcium has traditionally been expressed in the United States in units of milligrams per deciliter, with a typical normal range being 8.8 to 10.2 mg/dL. Because calcium has a molecular weight of 40 and is divalent, this can be easily converted into milliequivalents per liter (divide milligrams per deciliter by 2.0) or into millimolar units (SI units) (divide milligrams per deciliter by 4.0). Simple equations allow measurements of total calcium in serum to be "corrected" (to better reflect ionized calcium) for distortions by deviation of albumin concentration (for example, total calcium can be adjusted upward by 1 mg/dL [0.25 mM] for each gram per deciliter that serum albumin is below the normal mean and vice versa). When uncertainty exists about the direction or severity of an abnormality of blood calcium, the ionized calcium fraction should be evaluated as it is a more valid and direct reflection of pathophysiology. This is a more demanding laboratory procedure than is total calcium, and the reproducibility is generally worse. An abnormality of blood calcium can arise from an abnormal flux to or from the major sites of calcium turnover—bone, gut, and renal luminal fluid.

Phosphate in Blood

Phosphate measurements in serum represent only the 30% that is in inorganic compounds. By convention, phosphate is reported in units of elemental phosphorus. These conventions avoid some of the confusion that would result from efforts to consider molar anion content (phosphate in serum is in a variable equilibrium between its monobasic and dibasic states). Its principal determinants are PTH, age, gender, food ingestion, and diurnal rhythm. Serum phosphate is only a weak index of intracellular phosphate stores. Its fractional swings about its average are far wider than those for calcium. Thus the morning fasting state is preferred.

Magnesium in Blood

Serum magnesium, like phosphate, is determined by its threshold for renal excretion and by total body pools. Primary disturbance of magnesium in blood is unusual, but important abnormalities can occur during major illnesses; for example, in association with chemotherapy or with extensive burns, tissue necrosis may increase blood magnesium levels, or large fluid losses could depress it.

Hormones in Blood

Parathyroid Hormone

PTH is often the first regulator that should be examined when evaluating a possible disturbance of mineral homeostasis. A two-site assay can give a result that is a valid indicator of intact, biologically active PTH. Clinical correlations are excellent with this assay, and only small adjustment is generally needed for renal compromise.

Calcitonin

Calcitonin is measured by radioimmunoassay (RIA). Clinical uses are limited. When the RIA is used in family screening for early stages of C-cell neoplasia, it is particularly important to use normal ranges, adjusted for the selected C-cell challenge protocol and the patient's age.

25-Hydroxyvitamin D

Vitamin D itself is rarely measured in clinical settings. Two different vitamin D metabolites can be measured in clinical settings. It is essential to understand that these two metabolites, 25OHD and $1\alpha,25(OH)_2D$, are usually indicators of two entirely different types of process. Serum 25OHD is a useful index of vitamin D nutritional status. It is also a good index of sterol absorption. Low levels can arise from deficiency of sunlight, from deficiency of vitamin D nutritional supplementation, from fat malabsorption, and from accelerated hepatic catabolism of vitamin D metabolites. Because the body easily compensates for concentrations above normal, dangerously high levels occur only with intake of pharmacologic doses of vitamin D or of 25OHD.

$1\alpha,25$-Dihydroxyvitamin D

$1\alpha,25(OH)_2D$ measurement in serum gives an index of the steroid hormone whose renal production is usually finely regulated by blood PTH. Even with vitamin D intoxication and high blood

25OHD, the serum levels of $1\alpha,25(OH)_2D$ may be appropriately low because of this regulatory system. Serum $1\alpha,25(OH)_2D$ has only limited diagnostic use. However, certain states can be associated with otherwise unexplainable mineral disturbances that reflect high levels of $1\alpha,25(OH)_2D$ (sarcoidosis and other granulomas) or low levels (certain renal tubular disorders, such as X-linked hypophosphatemia).

Blood Indices of Bone Disturbance

Alkaline phosphatase enzyme in serum is an index of its sources in bone, liver, and placenta and of its excretion by the biliary tree. With increased osteoblastic activity, the amount of skeletal alkaline phosphatase enzyme in serum can rise dramatically. Skeletal alkaline phosphatase can be measured selectively through its physicochemical properties (it is the heat-labile component of total alkaline phosphatase) or otherwise (e.g., by RIA, a topic for research in several centers). High skeletal alkaline phosphatase levels can point to high bone turnover (hyperparathyroidism, Paget's disease). Specific portions of procollagen type I and other bone-specific proteins are also under investigation as possible specific indicators of skeletal processes. Osteocalcin (sometimes called bone Gla-protein) is another osteoblast-specific protein that has been useful in some long-term studies of bone turnover, but its insensitivity to diffuse bone pathology has compromised its broad clinical use.

Measurements on the Skeleton

Bone Radiograms and Scans

Standard radiography is often the starting point in evaluating bone disorders. Images can be specific for numerous conditions or can direct further diagnostic procedures (i.e., bone biopsy) to sites of focal disturbance. A bone scan with technetium-99m diphosphonate may identify a local disturbance that is not accompanied by radiographic change; the label adsorbs to bone mineral, and increased local blood flow without fracture is sufficient to give a positive signal.

Bone Mass Indices

Bone mass can be measured noninvasively with a variety of techniques. These include dual-channel radiographs, single- and dual-channel photon absorptiometry, radiographs with computed tomography, and other methods under development. The choice of one over another should depend largely on local expertise. For sequential studies in a patient, these methods are compromised, to varying degrees, by high cost, lack of precision, and poor correlation between institutions.

Bone Biopsy

Bone biopsy can be the final diagnostic tool in identifying local or generalized bone disturbances. It can be particularly useful in distinguishing osteomalacia from osteoporosis. Maximal information about the bone formation process can be obtained by prior administration of two pulses of tetracyclines 14 days apart (tetracyclines selectively adsorb to the mineralization front of osteoid and provide a fluorescent signal in the biopsy sample). When considering this test, the clinician should consult persons knowledgeable about its indications and the details of its processing.

Analyses of the Intestines in Mineral Metabolism

Specific tests of intestinal function are rarely used in current clinical practice. Metabolic balance studies are time-consuming and expensive. Calcium absorption studies with radioactive or stable isotopes are not applied outside research settings. General indices of intestinal function are considered in other chapters.

Analyses of the Kidney and Urine

Renal biopsy should be done only for the standard indications related to intrinsic or systemic diseases in the kidney. Urinary excretion of hydroxyproline and other collagen metabolites is a useful index of bone resorption rates because 60% of urinary hydroxyproline is normally derived from collagen in bone. Pyridinium cross-links, another collagen by-product in urine, may prove to be a more useful index of bone resorption.

Urinary excretion of calcium, magnesium, or phosphate is useful in screening for total body excess or deficiency of any of these minerals. Urinary excretion of calcium is central in the evaluation of urolithiasis. More detailed discussion of the work-up of urolithiasis is presented elsewhere (see Chapter 114).

Bilezekian JP, Raisz LG, Rodan GA (eds): Principles of Bone Biology. New York, Academic Press, 1996. *A multi-authored book, particularly strong on basic principles of bone pathophysiology.*

DeGroot LJ (ed): Endocrinology, 3rd ed. Philadelphia, WB Saunders, 1995. *Section IV on the parathyroids has 20 very detailed chapters covering the parathyroids and metabolic bone disease. Other textbooks on endocrinology and bone disorders cover the same topics in more or less detail.*

Favus MJ (ed): Primer on Metabolic Bone Diseases and Disorders of Mineral Metabolism, 4th ed. New York, Lippincott-Raven Publishers, 1999. *Concise chapters that quickly advance the reader to current research on a topic.*

262 VITAMIN D

Bess Dawson-Hughes

Vitamin D, originally described as a fat-soluble vitamin that would prevent rickets, is a steroid hormone. Natural forms of the vitamin include cholecalciferol, or vitamin D_3, produced in the skin of humans and other vertebrates, and ergocalciferol, or vitamin D_2, derived from plants and fungi. These forms are metabolized similarly in humans, and the term *vitamin D* in this chapter applies to both forms. To become biologically active, vitamin D is hydroxylated first in the liver to 25-hydroxyvitamin D (25 [OH] D) and then in the kidney to form 1,25-dihydroxyvitamin D (1,25 [OH]$_2$D).

SOURCES

Rich dietary sources of vitamin D include fish oil, cod liver oil, egg yolks, and fortified milk and cereals. Vitamin D from food and supplements is absorbed in the distal ileum by a process that requires bile salts. Gastrointestinal disorders of mixing and fat emulsification, decreased transit time, and fat malabsorption reduce vitamin D absorption. Adults in the United States, Europe, and Japan typically consume 100 to 150 IU of vitamin D daily. The Institute of Medicine recommends an intake of 200 IU/day for adults up to age 51 years, 400 for adults age 51 through 70 years, and 600 for those older than 70 years.

Vitamin D_3 is produced in the epidermal layer of the skin on exposure to ultraviolet sunlight of wavelength 294 to 310 nm by photoconversion of the prohormone 7-dehydrocholesterol to previtamin D. The latter spontaneously isomerizes to vitamin D_3 during the 3 or 4 days following sun exposure and enters the circulation bound to vitamin D binding protein. Sunscreens and the skin pigment melanin reduce cutaneous production of vitamin D_3 because they absorb solar ultraviolet light, leaving fewer photons available to initiate photosynthesis. Photoproduction declines with aging because of a twofold age-related reduction in epidermal 7-dehydrocholesterol concentration. Thinning of the skin and reduced sun exposure may also contribute to decreased vitamin D_3 production in the elderly.

In the heavily populated temperate zone, season and latitude regulate cutaneous vitamin D_3 production because they determine the intensity of ultraviolet rays reaching earth's surface. At 42 degrees North, the latitude of Boston, very little photosynthesis occurs between October and March, and in the winter, 25(OH)D levels typically decline by about 30% in ambulatory adults. This decline is accompanied by an increase in circulating levels of the bone-resorbing agent, parathyroid hormone (PTH) and, in older adults, increased wintertime bone loss.

METABOLISM

LIVER. Vitamin D is hydroxylated by a hepatic microsomal cytochrome P-450 mixed-function oxidase to form 25(OH)D. This process is not tightly regulated and depends on the combined skin

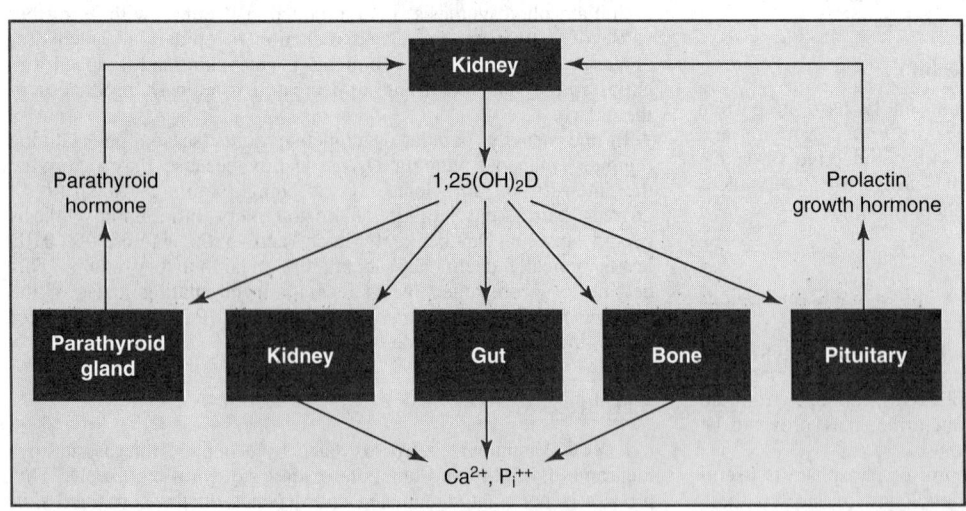

FIGURE 262–1 ■ Activation of vitamin D. Estrogen, growth hormone, prolactin, placental lactogen, calcitonin, and insulin stimulate 1α-hydroxylase, but their role in the day-to-day regulation of 1,25(OH)₂D production is uncertain.

and dietary supplies of vitamin D. Several medications and diseases alter 25(OH)D metabolism. Anticonvulsants, rifampin, primidone, and other drugs that induce microsomal enzymes accelerate metabolism of 25(OH)D to inactive metabolites, thereby increasing the requirement for vitamin D. Cholestyramine increases the vitamin D requirement by binding 25(OH)D in the gut. Production of 25(OH)D is compromised by liver disease only when the disease is advanced.

RENAL. In the final step of activation, 25(OH)D is hydroxylated at the 1α-position in the proximal renal convoluted tubule to form 1,25(OH)₂D. Extrarenal production occurs in the normal placenta and sometimes in sarcoid and other granulomas. PTH and low blood levels of calcium and phosphorus promote renal 1,25(OH)₂D production. High blood levels of calcium and phosphorus, and also 1,25(OH)₂D itself, limit 1,25(OH)₂D production (Fig. 262–1). When 1α-hydroxylase is inhibited, 25(OH)D is metabolized by an alternate renal pathway to 24,25-dihydroxyvitamin D, a compound with no established function in humans. Advanced renal disease compromises 1α-hydroxylase, but the stage in renal failure at which 1,25(OH)₂D production starts to decline varies with calcium and phosphorus intake levels.

ACTIONS OF 1,25(OH)₂D

This hormone is part of the vitamin D endocrine system that regulates blood calcium and bone mineralization by its actions on the intestine, bone, kidney, and other tissues (Fig. 262–2). 1,25(OH)₂D promotes absorption of intestinal calcium and phosphorus by acting on mucosal cell nuclear receptors to initiate the production of separate calcium- and phosphorus-binding proteins. These proteins ferry calcium and phosphorus across the intestinal mucosa. 1,25(OH)₂D is essential for both the formation and resorption components of bone remodeling. In concert with PTH, 1,25(OH)₂D stimulates bone resorption, perhaps by increasing the number of osteoclasts that are formed from macrophage stem cells. In addition to providing calcium for bone mineralization through increased intestinal absorption, 1,25(OH)₂D may also play a role in regulating osteoblast function. In vitro, 1,25(OH)₂D acts on osteo-

blast receptors to enhance production of alkaline phosphatase, osteocalcin, and several bone growth factors. In other actions, an elevated 1,25(OH)₂D level decreases PTH synthesis and release, and in concert with PTH, 1,25(OH)₂D reduces renal excretion of calcium.

PHARMACOLOGY

Selected properties of the major vitamin D metabolites are given in Table 262–1. Up to 99% of these three compounds circulates bound to vitamin D-binding protein, an α-globulin that protects them from rapid renal clearance. In nephrotic syndrome, the bound portion of each metabolite is reduced. Serum 25(OH)D reflects the solar and dietary contributions of vitamin D and is the best clinical measure of vitamin D status. Serum levels vary with sun exposure and intake, but typical values are vitamin D, 1.5 ng/mL; 25(OH)D, 35 ng/mL; and 1,25(OH)₂D, 30 pg/mL.

HYPOVITAMINOSIS D

Vitamin D insufficiency contributes to osteoporosis (see Chapter 257), and more severe deficiency results in osteomalacia (see Chapter 263).

HYPERVITAMINOSIS D

Vitamin D toxicity causes hypercalcemia and/or hypercalciuria because of increased calcium absorption. In animals, vitamin D also enhances bone resorption, but this has not yet been confirmed in people. The clinical manifestations of vitamin D intoxication are associated with hypercalcemia (see Chapter 264). Hypervitaminosis D can result from excess intake or from altered metabolism of the vitamin.

EXCESS INTAKE. The Institute of Medicine has identified a safe upper limit of 2,000 IU/day. Toxicity may result from dietary excess but more often occurs when vitamin D is given therapeutically, as for hypoparathyroidism. A study of six patients with vitamin D intoxication from drinking overfortified milk revealed

FIGURE 262–2 ■ The vitamin D endocrine system. The hormone 1,25(OH)₂D acts principally on the gut, bone, and kidney but also on other tissues to help regulate calcium (Ca²⁺) and inorganic phosphorus (P_i) homeostasis. Parathyroid hormone regulates Ca²⁺ and P_i homeostasis by direct actions on bone and kidney.

Table 262-1 ■ PHARMACOLOGIC PROPERTIES OF VITAMIN D METABOLITES

METABOLITE	TIME TO PEAK SERUM CONCENTRATION (hr)	ONSET OF HYPERCALCEMIC ACTION (hr)	DURATION OF ACTION
Ergocalciferol or cholecalciferol	—	12–14*	≥6 mo
Calcifediol [25(OH)D]	4	12–24	15–20 days†
Calcitriol [1,25(OH)$_2$D]	2	2–6	1–2 days

*Therapeutic effect may take 10 to 14 days.
†Increased two to three times in renal failure.
From Dawson-Hughes B: Metabolic bone disease. *In* Bayliss TM (ed): Current Therapy in Gastroenterology and Liver Disease, 4th ed. St. Louis, CV Mosby, 1994.

that the homeostatic regulation of 1α-hydroxylase is sometimes overridden by very high levels of the substrate 25(OH)D. Two of the six patients had elevated levels and four maintained normal serum levels of 1,25(OH)$_2$D. The basis for hypercalcemia/hypercalciuria in the latter four is uncertain, although these findings demonstrate that at least one other vitamin D metabolite, perhaps 25(OH)D in very large amounts, influences calcium metabolism.

ALTERED VITAMIN D METABOLISM. Disordered calcium homeostasis sometimes occurs in granulomatous diseases, especially sarcoidosis, as a result of 1,25(OH)$_2$D production by macrophages in the granulomas. This hormone production is not regulated by factors that modulate renal synthesis of 1,25(OH)$_2$D. Hypercalcemia occurs in about 10% of patients with sarcoidosis and can be the presenting feature. Sun exposure produces more substrate for 1,25(OH)$_2$D synthesis and can exacerbate the hypercalcemia.

TREATMENT. Hypervitaminosis D of any origin is treated by restricting calcium intake, rehydration, and administration of glucocorticoids. Up to 60 mg/day of prednisone may be needed to normalize serum calcium levels in vitamin D intoxication. If fat stores of vitamin D are large, toxicity can persist for well beyond 1 year. Intoxication from treatment with excess 25(OH)D or 1,25(OH)$_2$D resolves more rapidly. Glucocorticoids in low to moderate doses inhibit 1,25(OH)$_2$D production in granulomas and promptly reverse hypercalcemia in sarcoidosis and related diseases.

Dietary Reference Intakes: Calcium, Phosphorus, Magnesium, Vitamin D, and Fluoride. Washington, DC, Institute of Medicine, National Academy Press, 1997. *Describes the scientific basis for setting the vitamin D intake requirements.*
Jacobus CH, Holick MF, Shao Q, et al: Hypervitaminosis D associated with drinking milk. N Engl J Med 326:1173, 1992. *A careful documentation of clinical and biochemical aspects of vitamin D intoxication.*

263 OSTEOMALACIA AND RICKETS

Marc K. Drezner

DEFINITION. Rickets and osteomalacia are diseases characterized by defective bone and cartilage mineralization in children and bone mineralization in adults. The abnormal calcification of cartilage occurs at epiphyseal growth plates, which also exhibit delayed maturation of the cartilage cellular sequence and disorganization of cell arrangement. The resultant profusion of disorganized, nonmineralized, degenerating cartilage causes widening of the epiphyseal plates with flaring or cupping and irregularity of the epiphyseal-metaphyseal junctions. The abnormal calcification of bone is restricted to the organic matrix at the bone-osteoid interfaces of remodeling tissue. The insufficient mineralization of newly formed matrix paradoxically results in enhanced bone volume and increased susceptibility to fractures or bone deformities. The various disorders associated with rickets and osteomalacia that have been identified and characterized to date are numerous (Table 263–1). Although the phenotypic expression of the defective bone and cartilage mineralization is similar in each of these, the associated biochemical abnormalities and the therapeutic approaches differ according to the pathogenetic defect. Therefore, when diagnosing

rickets and/or osteomalacia, further systematic analysis is needed to determine cause and appropriate therapy for the disorder.

ETIOLOGY AND PATHOGENESIS. Mineralization of cartilage and bone is a complex process in which the calcium-phosphorus inorganic mineral phase is deposited in an organic matrix in a highly ordered fashion. Such mineralization depends on (1) the availability of sufficient calcium and phosphorus from the extracellular fluid; (2) adequate metabolic and transport function of chondrocytes and osteoblasts to regulate the concentration of calcium, phosphorus, and other ions at the mineralization sites; (3) the presence of collagen with unique type, number, and distribution of cross-links, remarkable patterns of hydroxylation and glycosylation; and abundant phosphate content, which collectively permits and facilitates deposition of mineral at gaps, hole zones, and between the distal ends of two collagen molecules; (4) maintenance of an optimal pH (approximately 7.6) for deposition of calcium-phosphorus complexes; and (5) low concentration of calcification inhibitors (e.g., pyrophosphates, proteoglycans) in bone matrix.

Many of the disorders of mineralization occur secondary to known defects in these control steps. In this regard, most diseases resulting in rickets and/or osteomalacia result from abnormalities in the vitamin D endocrine system (see Chapter 262). Traditionally, a direct role has been assumed for vitamin D or, more properly, its active metabolite, 1,25-dihydroxyvitamin D, on production of normal collagen matrix and regulation of bone mineralization. However, it is more likely that the abnormal mineralization in these disorders results from an associated calcium and phosphorus deficiency that diminishes the driving force for calcification. Primary disorders of phosphate homeostasis also underlie a large number of the rachitic/osteomalacic disorders. Diminished gastrointestinal absorption or renal wasting of phosphorus limits this essential mineral in such disorders. The isolated deficiency of phosphorus alone or in conjunction with a frequently occurring aberration in vitamin D metabolism underlies defective mineralization. In accord with the complex regulation of bone mineralization, however, decreases in calcium or phosphorus do not account for the rickets and osteomalacia in all forms of the disease. Indeed, certain forms of rickets and osteomalacia occur in spite of a normal or even elevated calcium-phosphate product. In such diseases, altered pH, abnormal collagen matrix, or excessive concentration of calcification inhibitors underlies the abnormal mineralization. In other forms of the disease, the precise mechanism causing the defective mineralization remains unknown.

Inadequate mineralization in rickets occurs in the matrix of cartilage in the growing epiphyseal plate. These characteristic changes are confined to the maturation zone of the cartilage, whereas the resting and proliferative zones of the epiphyses exhibit normal histologic features. In the maturation zone, the height of the cell columns is increased and the cells are closely packed and irregularly aligned. Moreover, calcification in the interstitial regions of this hypertrophic zone is defective.

In bone, the abnormal mineralization results in accumulation of excess osteoid, a sine qua non for the diagnosis of osteomalacia in most instances (Fig. 263–1). A supranormal amount of osteoid, however, may also occur in disease states associated with accelerated bone turnover, such as hyperparathyroidism. In addition, reduced mineralization activity may be observed without hyperosteoidosis in osteoporosis. Establishing the diagnosis of osteomalacia histopathologically, therefore, requires documenting abnormal mineralization with excess osteoid. These defects are manifest in bone

Table 263–1 ■ THE RICKETS AND OSTEOMALACIA SYNDROMES

I. Disorders of the vitamin D endocrine system
  A. Decreased bioavailability of vitamin D
    1. Deficient endogenous production
      a. Inadequate sunlight exposure
      b. Aging
    2. Nutritional deficiency
    3. Loss of vitamin D metabolites
      a. Nephrotic syndrome
      b. Peritoneal dialysis
  B. Vitamin D malabsorption
    1. Gastrointestinal disorders
      a. Partial/total gastrectomy
      b. Small bowel disease (e.g., celiac disease)
      c. Intestinal bypass
    2. Pancreatic insufficiency
    3. Hepatobiliary disease
      a. Biliary atresia
      b. Biliary obstruction
      c. Biliary fistula
      d. Cirrhosis
  C. Abnormal vitamin D metabolism
    1. Impaired hepatic 25-hydroxylation of vitamin D
      a. Liver disease
      b. Anticonvulsant therapy
    2. Impaired renal 1α-hydroxylation of 25-hydroxyvitamin D
      a. Hereditary vitamin D-dependent rickets type 1 (pseudo-vitamin D deficiency)
      b. Chronic renal failure
      c. Pseudohypoparathyroidism
  D. Target organ resistance to vitamin D and metabolites
    1. Hereditary vitamin D-dependent rickets type 2
      a. Hormone binding negative
      b. Defect in hromone-binding capacity
      c. Defect in hormone-binding affinity
      d. Deficient hormone-receptor nuclear localization
      e. Decreased affinity of the hormone-receptor complex
II. Disorders of phosphate homeostasis
  A. Dietary
    1. Low phosphate intake
    2. Ingestion of phosphate-binding antacids
  B. Impaired renal tubular phosphate reabsorption
    1. Hereditary
      a. X-linked hypophosphatemic rickets/osteomalacia
      b. Hereditary hypophosphatemic rickets/osteomalacia with hypercalciuria
      c. Autosomal dominant hypophosphatemic rickets
      d. Hypophosphatemic bone disease (nonrachitic hypophosphatemic osteomalacia)
      e. Adult-onset hypophosphatemic rickets
      f. Autosomal recessive hypophosphatemic rickets (X-linked hypercalciuric nephrolithiasis)
      g. X-linked recessive hypophosphatemic rickets (X-linked hypercalciuric nephrolithiasis)
    2. Acquired
      a. Tumor-induced osteomalacia (oncogenous osteomalacia)
        (1) Mesenchymal, epidermal, and endodermal tumors
        (2) Fibrous dysplasia of bone
        (3) Neurofibromatosis
        (4) Linear nevus sebaceous syndrome
        (5) Light chain nephropathy
      b. Sporadic hypophosphatemic osteomalacia
  C. General renal tubular disorders
    1. Fanconi's syndrome type 1
      a. Hereditary
        (1) Familial idiopathic
        (2) Cystinosis (Lignac-Fanconi disease)
        (3) Hereditary fructose intolerance
        (4) Tyrosinemia
        (5) Galactosemia
        (6) Glycogen storage disease
        (7) Wilson's disease
        (8) Oculocerebral renal syndrome (Lowe's syndrome)
      b. Acquired
        (1) Renal transplantation
        (2) Multiple myeloma
      c. Intoxication
        (1) Cadmium
        (2) Lead
        (3) Tetracycline (outdated)
    2. Fanconi's syndrome type 2
III. Metabolic acidosis
  A. Distal renal tubular acidosis
    1. Primary
      a. Sporadic
      b. Familial
    2. Secondary
      a. Galactosemia (after galactose ingestion)
      b. Hereditary fructose intolerance with nephrocalcinosis (after chronic fructose ingestion)
      c. Hypergammaglobulinemic states
      d. Medullary sponge kidney
    3. Acquired
      a. Ureterosigmoidostomy
      b. Drug-induced
        (1) Acetazolamide
        (2) Ammonium chloride
IV. Disorders of calcium homeostasis
  A. Dietary calcium deficiency
V. Abnormal bone matrix
  A. Fibrogenesis imperfecta ossium
  B. Axial osteomalacia
VI. Primary mineralization defects
  A. Hereditary
    1. Hypophosphatasia
      a. Perinatal disease
      b. Infantile disease
      c. Childhood disease
      d. Adult-onset disease
      e. Pseudohypophosphatasia
VII. Mineralization inhibitors
  A. Etidronate
  B. Fluoride
  C. Aluminum

by an increase in the forming surface covered by incompletely mineralized osteoid, an increase in osteoid volume and thickness, and a decrease in the mineralization front (the percentage of osteoid-covered bone-forming surface undergoing calcification) or the mineral apposition rate. The amount of osteoid in bone and the mineralization dynamics are determined in 3- to 5-μm thick sections of un-decalcified bone by special stains and the fluorescence of previously ingested tetracycline that is deposited at calcification fronts (see Fig. 263–1).

CLINICAL MANIFESTATIONS. The clinical features of rickets, although variable to some degree according to the underlying disorder, are primarily related to skeletal pain and deformity, bone fractures, slipped epiphyses, and abnormalities of growth. In addition, hypocalcemia, when present, may be severe enough to produce tetany, laryngeal spasm, and seizures.

In infants and young children, symptoms include listlessness, irritability, and, in some forms of metabolic rickets, profound hypotonia and proximal muscle weakness. Indeed, as the disease progresses and muscle weakness is present, children often are unable to walk without support. Throughout early life, classic skeletal deformities appear. By age 6 months, frontal bossing with flattening at the back is evident. Later, a lateral collapse of both chest walls (Harrison's sulcus) and rachitic rosary may appear. If untreated, progressive bony deformities result in bowing—particularly in the tibia, femur, radius, and ulna—and fractures. In addition, dental eruption may be delayed and, in those forms of the disease with hypocalcemia or hereditary hypophosphatemia, enamel defects and inadequate dentin calcification occur, respectively.

In contrast, clinical signs of osteomalacia are nondescript. Indeed, the disease-specific abnormalities may be overlooked and features of an underlying disorder (e.g., malabsorption) may predominate. Symptoms, when present, may include diffuse skeletal pain and muscular weakness. The pain, often described as dull and aching, is generally worsened by activity and prominent around the hips, resulting in an antalgic gait. The muscle weakness is primarily proximal and frequently associated with wasting, hypotonia, and a waddling gait. This myopathy is seen in almost all forms of rickets and osteomalacia, X-linked hypophosphatemic rickets and

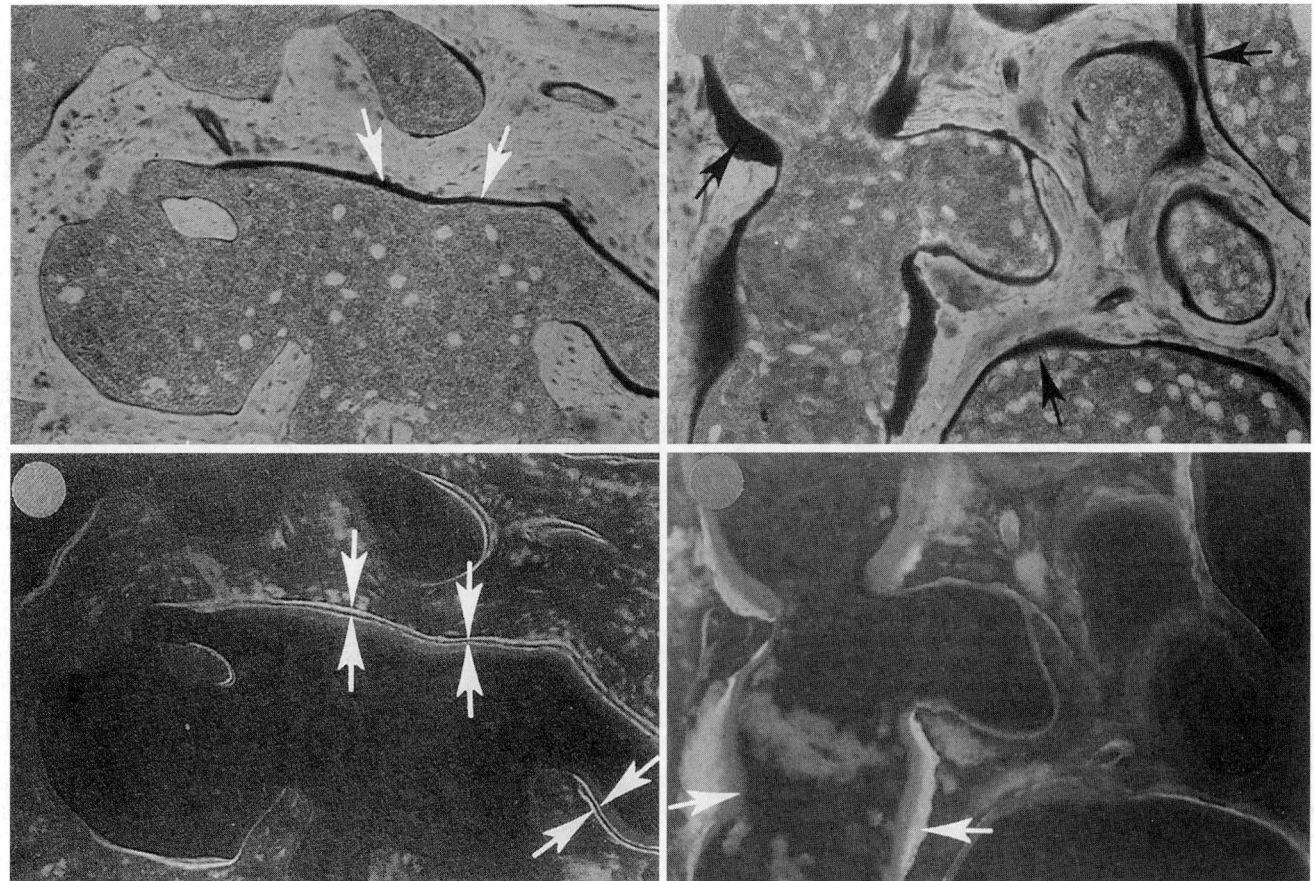

FIGURE 263-1 ■ Microscopic appearance of bone biopsy sections from a normal patient and one with osteomalacia. In the upper panels the Villanueva-stained sections exhibit mineralized bone *(white tones)* covered by unmineralized osteoid seams *(black tones).* Thin osteoid seams are distributed over a limited portion of the bone surface in normal bone *(white arrows).* In contrast, osteomalacic bone is covered almost completely with thick osteoid seams *(black arrows).* In the lower panels, the same bone sections are viewed under ultraviolet light to estimate mineralization activity by visualizing tetracycline labels. The normal bone reveals that the majority of the osteoid has crisp double tetracycline labels *(white arrows),* indicative of normal mineralization activity. The osteomalacic bone, however, has evidence only of smeared tetracycline labels without the double label *(white arrows).* Moreover, the tetracycline labels do not occupy the majority of the osteoid-bone interface. Such observations are representative of the abnormal mineralization that characterizes the osteomalacic bone disorder.

osteomalacia notably excepted. Clinical improvement in the myopathy usually results from specific therapy, such as vitamin D repletion in nutritional osteomalacia, phosphate supplementation in disorders marked by renal phosphate wasting, or correction of acidosis. Fractures of the ribs, vertebral bodies, and long bones may occur and lead to progressive deformities as well as point tenderness on palpation.

The radiographic abnormalities in both rickets and osteomalacia reflect the histopathologic changes. In rickets, alterations are most evident at the growth plate, which is wide and flared and displays an irregular hazy appearance at the diaphyseal line secondary to uneven invasion of the recently calcified cartilage by adjacent bone tissue. The trabecular pattern of the metaphyses is also abnormal, the cortices of the diaphyses are thinned, and the shafts frequently are bowed.

In osteomalacia, a moderate decrease in bone density is usually associated with coarsening of trabeculae and blurring of their margins. When secondary hyperparathyroidism is present, subperiosteal resorption in the phalanges and metacarpals, erosion of the distal ends of the clavicles, and bone cysts may be observed. A more specific radiographic abnormality is the presence of Looser's zones, also called pseudofractures or Milkman's fractures, in the shafts of long bones. These are ribbon-like zones of rarefaction, ranging from a few millimeters to several centimeters in length and usually oriented perpendicular to the bone surface. Often, they occur symmetrically and most commonly are present at the medial aspect of the femurs near the femoral heads, in the metatarsals, or in the pelvis. Long-standing osteomalacia may also result in additional

characteristic radiographic abnormalities, including biconcave collapsed vertebrae and a trefoil (or triangular) pelvis.

In patients with renal tubular disorders (see Chapter 109), increased rather than decreased bone density may be present. Despite the increased bone mass, histopathologic evaluation of biopsies reveals an abundance of unmineralized osteoid, and bones remain subject to fracture. Thus, the increased density likely reflects replacement of marrow air space with osteoid.

Biochemical abnormalities in patients with rickets and osteomalacia vary with the cause of the disorder. However, the rachitic and osteomalacic syndromes may be divided into calciopenic and phosphopenic forms, as well as those in which mineral availability is apparently normal. In general, patients with the calciopenic diseases exhibit a low or marginally normal serum calcium level, a decreased serum phosphorus concentration, and (secondary) hyperparathyroidism. If vitamin D deficiency prevails, the serum 25(OH)D levels are characteristically low, generally less than 3 ng/mL. In contrast, the serum $1,25(OH)_2D$ concentration may not be overtly decreased secondary to the prevailing hyperparathyroidism. Alternatively, a defect in vitamin D metabolism often results in an isolated deficiency of $1,25(OH)_2D$, whereas end-organ resistance to this active vitamin D metabolite increases the circulating level of calcitriol.

A primary abnormality of transepithelial phosphate transport in the nephron, resulting in renal phosphate wasting, underlies the majority of the phosphopenic disorders. As a rule, patients with these disorders maintain a normal serum calcium concentration, whereas the serum phosphorus level is characteristically low. In contrast to the calciopenic forms of disease, the serum 25(OH)D and parathyroid hormone levels are normal in patients with hypophosphatemic disease. Moreover, affected subjects commonly maintain a normal (or mildly decreased) serum 1,25(OH)$_2$D level despite the prevailing hypophosphatemia, which should increase production of this active vitamin D metabolite. However, an elevated serum 1,25(OH)$_2$D concentration was recently reported in several rare genetic phosphopenic disorders, hereditary hypophosphatemic rickets with hypercalciuria, Fanconi's syndrome, type 2 and X-linked recessive hypophosphatemic rickets. Whereas the elevated calcitriol level underlies increased gastrointestinal absorption of calcium and hypercalciuria in these diseases, the impact of abnormal vitamin D metabolism on the phenotypic expression of the phosphopenic disorders is less certain. In those diseases with normal serum calcium and phosphorus concentrations, laboratory abnormalities are unique to each form of the disease. Nevertheless, alkaline phosphatase activity in plasma is generally elevated in all forms of rickets and osteomalacia. Even severe forms of disease, however, particularly those due to renal tubular disorders, may be associated with normal or only marginally elevated enzyme activity.

DISORDERS OF THE VITAMIN D ENDOCRINE SYSTEM

Rickets and osteomalacia due to disorders of the vitamin D endocrine system comprise a wide variety of calciopenic diseases. The variable biochemical abnormalities associated with these disparate disorders are summarized in Table 263–2. Although many of these diseases are no longer common causes of rickets and osteomalacia, others are often hidden causes of bone disease in a varying population of patients.

DECREASED BIOAVAILABILITY OF VITAMIN D. INADEQUATE SUNLIGHT AND NUTRITIONAL VITAMIN D DEFICIENCY. Adequate exposure to sunlight and fortification of dairy products with vitamin D have eliminated vitamin D deficiency secondary to inadequate endogenous production or nutrition in the majority of countries. However, in several populations, such as Asian immigrants in Britain, rickets and osteomalacia secondary to vitamin D deficiency occurs in neonates and infants, adolescents during pubertal growth, and less frequently among adults. Insufficient vitamin D intake secondary to using unfortified foods, racial pigmentation (which interferes with ultraviolet transmission through the skin), genetic factors, and social customs (such as avoiding sun exposure) contribute to the development of disease in these subjects. Moreover, in the United States and other developed countries, a surprisingly frequent occurrence of vitamin D deficiency osteomalacia has been recognized recently in alcoholics, institutionalized patients, and the elderly. Poor diet, in some cases including avoiding milk and milk products due to lactose intolerance, lack of sunlight exposure, and an age-related decline in the dermal synthesis of 7-dehydrocholesterol are among the factors predisposing to the vitamin D deficiency and consequent bone disease.

The clinical sequelae of decreased vitamin D bioavailability are generally preceded by a fall in circulating 25(OH)D levels. Mea-

surement of this metabolite therefore serves to identify populations at risk for and facilitates early detection of vitamin D deficiency rickets and osteomalacia. Introducing vitamin D supplements (400 U/day) may, under these circumstances, prevent development of clinically significant disease.

Regardless, treating clinically evident vitamin D–deficient rickets and osteomalacia invariably results in healing of the bone disease. The disorder is best treated with vitamin D and restoration of normal dietary calcium and phosphorus intake. Ergocalciferol (vitamin D$_2$) is preferred because it provides the missing substrate that submits to physiologic regulation of vitamin D metabolite production.

VITAMIN D MALABSORPTION. Gastrointestinal malabsorption associated with diseases of the small intestine, hepatobiliary tree, and pancreas may result in decreased absorption of vitamin D and/or depletion of endogenous 25(OH)D stores due to abnormal enterohepatic circulation. In general, malabsorption of vitamin D occurs as a consequence of steatorrhea, which disturbs fat emulsification and chylomicron-facilitated absorption (see Chapter 134). Such abnormalities often are associated with rickets and/or osteomalacia. However, most affected patients are asymptomatic, and many exhibit only reduced bone volume rather than evidence of defective bone mineralization. Intestinal bypass surgery and adult celiac disease are common examples of disorders in which vitamin D malabsorption occurs and in which the suspicion for osteomalacia should remain high. In contrast, patients with cholestatic liver disease, extrahepatic biliary obstruction, and diseases of the distal portions of the small intestine, such as regional enteritis, may develop bone disease secondary not only to poor vitamin D absorption but to disruption of enterohepatic circulation as well.

Osteomalacia may also develop in patients who have had partial or total gastrectomy for peptic ulcer disease or other indications. Loss of gastrointestinal acidity or malfunction of the proximal small bowel underlies the vitamin D malabsorption in such circumstances. Absence of sufficient absorbing surface or failure of intestinal mucosal cells to respond to vitamin D or its metabolites may also cause vitamin D malabsorption and consequent bone disease.

The prevalence of osteomalacia in patients with gastrointestinal malabsorption varies widely from country to country. However, as many as 25 to 50% of British and European patients with partial gastrectomy, inflammatory bowel disease, and cholestatic liver disease have bone biopsy–proven osteomalacia.

Treatment of established disease generally requires pharmacologic amounts of vitamin D or its metabolites to overcome the defective absorption and the aberrant enterohepatic circulation or to offset end-organ resistance at the intestinal mucosa. Most patients respond well to calcium supplements, 1 to 1.5 g/day, and ergocalciferol, 1250 to 5000 μg/day. If the severity of malabsorption makes oral vitamin D ineffective, parenteral ergocalciferol, 12,500 to 25,000 μg, given intramuscularly once a month, is a practical alternative. Because magnesium deficiency often co-exists in malabsorptive diseases and may slow healing of the osteomalacia, adjunctive therapy with magnesium oxide may facilitate bone mineralization.

ABNORMAL VITAMIN D METABOLISM. LIVER DISEASE. Be-

Table 263–2 ■ BIOCHEMICAL ABNORMALITIES OF THE CALCIOPENIC RACHITIC/OSTEOMALACIC DISORDERS

	VDDR	CRF	HVDDR 1	HVDDR 2	HP	PSH
Biochemical findings						
Calcium	⇓	⇓	⇓	⇓	⇓	⇓
Phosphorus	N/⇓	⇑	N/⇓	N/⇓	⇑	⇑
Alkaline phosphatase	⇑	⇑	⇑	⇑	N/⇑	N/⇑
Parathyroid hormone	⇑	⇑	⇑	⇑	⇓	⇑
25(OH)D	⇓	N/⇓	N	N	N	N
1,25(OH)$_2$D	⇑	⇓	⇓	⇑	⇓	⇓
Renal function						
Urinary phosphorus	⇑	⇓	⇑	⇑	⇓	⇓
Urinary calcium	⇓	⇓	⇓	⇓	⇓	⇓
Gastrointestinal function						
Calcium absorption	⇓	⇓	⇓	⇓	⇓	⇓
Phosphorus absorption	⇓	⇓	⇓	⇓	⇓	⇓

VDDR = Vitamin D-deficiency rickets (including sunlight or nutritional deficiency, vitamin D malabsorption, inhibition of 25-hydroxylation); CRF = chronic renal familure; HVDDR 1 = hereditary vitamin D-dependent rickets type 1; HVDDR-2 = hereditary vitamin D-dependent rickets type 2; HP = hypoparathyroidism; PSH = pseudohypoparathyroidm; N = normal; ⇓ = decreased; ⇑ = increased; N/⇓ = normal or decreased; and N/⇑ = normal or increased.

cause vitamin D is hydroxylated in the liver to form 25(OH)D, patients with severe parenchymal or obstructive hepatic disease (see Chapter 145) may have reduced production of this metabolite. These patients, however, rarely manifest biochemical or histologic evidence of osteomalacia. Indeed, an overt decrease of 25(OH)D generally requires concomitant nutritional deficiency or interruption of the enterohepatic circulation. Consequently, therapy for biopsy-proven osteomalacia, when present, is similar to that secondary to malabsorption of vitamin D.

DRUG-INDUCED DISEASE. Decreased circulating levels of 25(OH)D may also occur in patients treated with drugs such as phenytoin or phenobarbital. This defect in vitamin D metabolism is due to induction of hepatic microsomal enzymes that metabolize 25(OH)D to inactive metabolites. Secondary to this abnormality and/or to the direct inhibitory effects of these drugs on intestinal calcium absorption and parathyroid hormone (PTH)–mediated calcium mobilization from bone, treated subjects often exhibit a decreased level of ionized calcium. These multiple influences commonly result in a bone disorder that may be mild osteomalacia or hyperparathyroid bone disease. Treatment of the bone disease and hypocalcemia generally requires modest vitamin D supplementation (150 to 400 μg/week).

VITAMIN D–DEPENDENT RICKETS TYPE 1 (PSEUDOVITAMIN D DEFICIENCY). Limited production of 1,25(OH)$_2$D due to hereditary or acquired diseases represents another abnormality of vitamin D metabolism that invariably results in rickets or osteomalacia. Vitamin D-dependent rickets type 1 is such a genetic disorder, transmitted as an autosomal recessive trait and characterized by hypocalcemia, hypophosphatemia, and elevated alkaline phosphatase activity. As a result of the hypocalcemia, PTH levels are elevated and, consequently, urinary excretion of amino acids and phosphate enhanced. In addition to these biochemical abnormalities, within the first year of life patients exhibit muscle weakness and hypotonia, motor retardation, and stunted growth. With progression, patients develop the classic radiographic signs of vitamin D-deficiency rickets and bone biopsy evidence of osteomalacia. Further, affected subjects have a decreased serum 1,25(OH)$_2$D concentration, due to missense and null mutations in the 1α-hydroxylase gene, localized to chromosome 12q13.3, which abolish enzyme activity and limit production of this active vitamin D metabolite. This abnormality has been substantiated by (1) experiments in humans that demonstrate serum calcitriol levels do not increase in response to classic stimuli of enzyme activity, and (2) the absence of enzyme activity in renal cortical homogenates from the porcine homologue of this disease. Consistent with these observations, a physiologic dose of calcitriol (1 μg/day) generally promotes complete healing of the bone disease and resolution of the biochemical abnormalities, whereas a pharmacologic dose of vitamin D (20,000 to 100,000 U/day) or 25(OH)D (0.1 to 1.0 mg/day) is required to achieve similar effects. Regardless of the therapy used, in the majority of affected patients, therapy with vitamin D or its metabolites must be continued for life to prevent relapse. However, in a minority of subjects with a syndrome clinically identical to vitamin D-dependent rickets type 1, stopping treatment does not result in reappearance of biochemical or radiographic signs of the disease.

CHRONIC RENAL FAILURE. Osteomalacia is common in patients with chronic renal failure and often tends to be the predominant type of renal osteodystrophy in younger patients (see Chapter 266). The defect in mineralization almost certainly results in part from a decreased conversion of 25(OH)D to 1,25(OH)$_2$D. Such abnormal vitamin D metabolism occurs secondary to either insufficient viable renal cortical tissue or the inhibitory effects of hyperphosphatemia on renal 25(OH)D-1α-hydroxylase activity. In addition, in some patients aluminum accumulated in bone underlies the abnormal mineralization. Indeed, the presence of aluminum may render the bone abnormality vitamin D-resistant. Under such circumstances, treatment with deferoxamine may be necessary to mobilize the aluminum from bone and other tissues and improve mineralization.

HYPOPARATHYROIDISM. Osteomalacia only rarely occurs in patients with hypoparathyroidism (see Chapter 264). Hypocalcemia and low or low-normal serum 1,25(OH)$_2$D are usually present and appear important in the pathogenesis of the bone disease. However, the underlying reason for the variable occurrence of bone pathology remains uncertain. The low serum 1,25(OH)$_2$D concentration results from the PTH deficiency. Bone pain suggests the diagnosis, and

generally the diagnosis depends on histomorphometric analysis of a bone biopsy. The majority of patients respond well to treatment with vitamin D and calcium supplements, but for reasons that are not clear, some require therapy with 1,25(OH)$_2$D.

PSEUDOHYPOPARATHYROIDISM. In pseudohypoparathyroidism apparent bone and kidney resistance to PTH results in hypocalcemia, retention of phosphate, and low serum 1,25(OH)$_2$D levels (see Chapter 264). Surprisingly, however, affected patients often manifest bone disease marked by increased resorptive activity and osteomalacia. Indeed, severe demineralization, including frank osteitis fibrosa cystica and occasionally rickets or osteomalacia, has been observed in 24 patients with pseudohypoparathyroidism. More commonly, the bone disease is silent and diagnosis often depends on histomorphometric analysis of a bone biopsy. Undoubtedly, hypocalcemia, secondary hyperparathyroidism, and low serum 1,25(OH)$_2$D levels are important cofactors in the pathogenesis of the disease. Patients respond well to pharmacologic amounts of vitamin D or replacement doses of 1,25(OH)$_2$D.

TARGET-ORGAN RESISTANCE TO CALCITRIOL. VITAMIN D-DEPENDENT RICKETS, TYPE 2. Patients with clinical and biochemical abnormalities similar to those of subjects with vitamin D-dependent rickets type 1, but elevated 1,25(OH)$_2$D levels, have recently been described. They have not only calciopenic rickets and/or osteomalacia but variably associated abnormalities, including alopecia (in 60% of patients) and, in a minority of subjects, additional ectodermal anomalies, such as multiple milia, epidermal cysts, and oligodontia. The disease is a rare autosomal recessive disorder due to mutations in the DNA and ligand-binding domains of the vitamin D receptor, which results in a decreased target-organ responsiveness to 1,25(OH)$_2$D through heterogeneous mechanisms. The genetic defects identified to date consist largely of point mutations in the conserved zinc finger region that reduce or abolish the affinity of the receptor for the DNA response element and, less often, point mutations that introduce a premature stop codon in the hormone-binding domain of the receptor, which limits binding of 1,25(OH)$_2$D to the receptor. As a consequence, affected patients manifest (1) failure of 1,25(OH)$_2$D binding to available receptors; (2) a reduction in 1,25(OH)$_2$D receptor-binding sites; (3) abnormal binding affinity of 1,25(OH)$_2$D to receptor; (4) inadequate translocation of 1,25(OH)$_2$D-receptor complex to the nucleus; and (5) diminished affinity of the 1,25(OH)$_2$D-receptor complex for the DNA-binding domain secondary to changes in the structure of receptor zinc-binding fingers. The role of the vitamin D receptor in the pathogenesis of this disorder has been confirmed in mice by targeted ablation of the DNA binding domain of the receptor, which results in hypocalcemia, hyperparathyroidism, and alopecia within the first month of life. Effective treatment of this disease likely depends on the nature of the underlying abnormality. Thus, patients with deficient affinity of 1,25(OH)$_2$D to receptor and inadequate nuclear translocation respond to high-dose vitamin D or 1,25(OH)$_2$D with complete clinical and biochemical remission. In contrast, patients with other forms of the disease generally remain refractory to treatment with vitamin D or its analogues. However, every patient should receive a 6-month trial of therapy with supplemental calcium (1 to 3 g/day) and vitamin D (400,000 to 1,200,000 U/day), 25(OH)D (0.05 to 1.5 mg/day), or, in more severe cases, 1,25(OH)$_2$D (5 to 60 μg/day). If the abnormalities of the syndrome do not normalize in response to this treatment, clinical remission may be achieved by administering high-dose oral calcium or long-term intracaval infusion of calcium.

DISORDERS OF PHOSPHATE HOMEOSTASIS (See Chapter 222)

Rickets and osteomalacia occur in association with a variety of disorders in which phosphate depletion predominates. Most typically, these diseases have in common abnormal proximal renal tubular function, which results in an increased renal clearance of inorganic phosphorus and hypophosphatemia. However, the biochemical abnormalities characteristic of these disorders are quite variable (Table 263–3).

IMPAIRED RENAL TUBULAR PHOSPHATE REABSORPTION. X-LINKED HYPOPHOSPHATEMIC RICKETS/OSTEOMALACIA. X-linked hypophosphatemic (XLH) rickets/ostemalacia represents the proto-

Table 263–3 ■ BIOCHEMICAL ABNORMALITIES OF THE PHOSPHOPENIC RACHITIC/OSTEOMALACIC DISORDERS

	XLH	HHRH	ADHR	XRHR	FS 1	FS 2	TIO
Biochemical findings							
Calcium	N	N	N	N	N	N	N
Phosphorus	⇓	⇓	⇓	⇓	⇓	⇓	⇓
Alkaline phosphatase	N/⇑	N/⇑	N/⇑	N/⇑	N/⇑	N/⇑	N/⇑
Parathyroid hormone	N	⇓	N		N	⇓	N
25(OH)D	N	N	N	N	N	N	N
1,25(OH)₂D	(⇓)	⇑	(⇓)	⇑	(⇓)	⇑	⇓
Renal function							
Urinary phosphorus	⇑	⇑	⇑	⇑	⇑	⇑	⇑
Urinary calcium	⇓	⇑	⇓	⇑	⇓	⇑	⇓
Gastrointestinal function							
Calcium absorption	⇓	⇑	⇓	⇑	⇓	⇑	⇓
Phosphorus absorption	⇓	⇑	⇓	⇑	⇓	⇑	⇓

XLH = X-linked hypophosphatemic rickets; HHRH = hereditary hypophosphatemic rickets with hypercalciuria; XRHR = autosomal recessive hypophosphatemic rickets; FS I = Fanconi's syndrome type I; FS 2 = Fanconi's syndrome type II; TIO = tumor-induced osteomalacia; N = normal; ⇓ = decreased; ⇑ = increased; (⇓) = decreased relative to the serum phosphorus concentration; N/⇑ = normal or increased.

Modified from Econs MJ, Drezner MK: Bone disease resulting from inherited disorders of renal tubule transport and vitamin D metabolism. *In* Coe FL, Favus MJ: Disorders of Bone and Mineral Metabolism. New York, Raven Press, 1992, p 937.

typic phosphate-wasting disorder, characterized in general by progressively severe skeletal abnormalities, growth retardation, and X-linked dominant inheritance. However, the clinical expression of the disease varies widely. The mildest abnormality is hypophosphatemia without clinically evident bone disease, and the most common clinically evident manifestation is short stature. Nevertheless, the majority of children with the disease exhibit enlargement of the wrists and/or knees secondary to rickets, as well as bowing of the lower extremities. Additional early signs of the disease may include late dentition, tooth abscesses secondary to poor mineralization of the interglobular dentine, and premature cranial synostosis. Despite marked variability in the clinical presentation, bone biopsies in affected children and adults invariably reveal osteomalacia, the severity of which has no relationship to gender, the extent of the biochemical abnormalities, or the severity of the clinical disability. In untreated youths and adults, the serum 25(OH)D levels are normal and the concentration of 1,25(OH)₂D is in the low-normal range. The paradoxical occurrence of hypophosphatemia and normal serum calcitriol levels is due to aberrant regulation of renal 25(OH)D-1α-hydroxylase activity, most likely caused by the abnormal phosphate transport. Indeed, studies in *Hyp* mice, the murine homologue of the human disease, have established that defective regulation is confined to enzyme localized in the proximal convoluted tubule, the site of the abnormal phosphate transport.

A primary inborn error that results in an expressed abnormality in the renal proximal tubule (and perhaps the intestine), which impairs phosphate reabsorption (and absorption), underlies the pathogenesis of XLH. Although controversy exists regarding the character of the inborn error, studies in *Hyp* mice suggest that elaboration of a humoral factor underlies the observed inhibition of phosphate transport in affected patients. In this regard, recent investigations resulted in the cloning and identification of the disease gene as PHEX, a phosphate regulating gene with homologies to endopeptidases located on the X chromosome. Deactivating mutations of this membrane-localized gene clearly underlie the phenotypic expression of XLH by a mechanism that is as yet poorly understood. However, recognition of a humoral factor as essential to the pathogenesis of the disease suggests that the PHEX gene product may function normally to inactivate phosphatonin, a presumed phosphaturic hormone. An excess of this hormone would occur secondary to PHEX protein dysfunction and result in renal phosphate wasting.

Choice of therapy for this disease has been remarkably influenced by an increased understanding of the pathophysiologic factors that affect its phenotypic expression. Thus, current treatment strategies for children directly address the combined calcitriol and phosphorus deficiency characteristic of the disease. Generally, the regimen includes a period of titration to achieve a maximum dose of calcitriol, 40 to 60 ng/kg/day in two divided doses and phosphorus, 1 to 2 g/day in four or five divided doses. Although youths occasionally prove refractory to such therapeutic intervention, com-

bined therapy often improves growth velocity, normalizes lower extremity deformities, and induces healing of the attendant bone disease. Of course treatment involves a significant risk of toxicity that is generally expressed as abnormalities of calcium homeostasis and/or detrimental effects on renal function. Therapy in adults is reserved for episodes of intractable bone pain and refractory nonunion of bone fractures. Recent observations that long-term growth hormone administration in affected youths may benefit growth, phosphate retention, and bone density suggest that a subgroup of patients may benefit from adjunctive treatment with this hormone.

HEREDITARY HYPOPHOSPHATEMIC RICKETS WITH HYPERCALCIURIA (HHRH). This rare genetic disease is marked by hypophosphatemic rickets with hypercalciuria. In contrast to other diseases in which renal phosphate transport is limited, patients with HHRH exhibit increased 1,25(OH)₂D production. The resultant elevated serum calcitriol levels enhance the gastrointestinal calcium absorption, which in turn increases the filtered renal calcium load and inhibits PTH secretion. The clinical expression of the disease is heterogeneous, although initial symptoms generally consist of bone pain and/or deformities of the lower extremities. Additional features of the disease include short stature, muscle weakness, and radiographic signs of rickets or osteopenia. The various symptoms and signs may exist separately or in combination and may be present in a mild or severe form. Relatives of patients with evident HHRH may exhibit an additional mode of disease expression. These subjects manifest hypercalciuria and hypophosphatemia, but the abnormalities are less marked and occur in the absence of discernible bone disease. The preponderance of evidence indicates that HHRH is inherited by autosomal recessive transmission.

Patients with HHRH have been treated successfully with high-dose phosphorus (1 to 2.5 g/day in five divided doses) alone. In response to therapy, bone pain disappears and muscular strength improves substantially. Moreover, the majority of treated subjects exhibit accelerated linear growth, and radiologic signs of rickets are completely absent within 4 to 9 months. Despite this favorable response, limited studies indicate that such treatment does not heal the associated osteomalacia. Therefore, further studies are necessary to determine if phosphorus alone is truly sufficient for this disorder.

AUTOSOMAL DOMINANT HYPOPHOSPHATEMIC RICKETS (ADHR). Although many investigators assume that all familial renal phosphate wasting disorders are X-linked, several studies have documented an autosomal dominant inheritance of a hypophosphatemic disorder similar to XLH. The phenotypic manifestations of this disorder include the expected hypophosphatemia due to renal phosphate wasting, lower extremity deformities, and rickets/osteomalacia. Affected patients also demonstrate normal serum levels of parathyroid hormone and 25(OH)D, while maintaining an inappropriate normal concentration of 1,25(OH)₂D, in the presence of hypophosphatemia. Long-term studies indicate that a few of the affected female patients demonstrate delayed penetrance of clinically apparent disease and an increased tendency for bone fracture, uncommon occurrences in XLH. In addition, among patients who manifest disease in childhood, rare individuals lose the renal phosphate-wasting defect after puberty. Limited information is available regarding other aspects of the disease. However, recent studies have identified the gene locus for this disease on chromosome 12p13 in an 18-cM interval between the flanking markers D12S100 and D12S397.

An apparent *forme fruste* of ADHR (autosomal dominant) hypophosphatemic bone disease has many of the characteristics of XLH and ADHR, but recent reports indicate that affected children display no evidence of rachitic disease. Because this syndrome is described in only a few small kindreds, and radiographically evident rickets is not universal in children with familial hypophosphatemia, these families may have ADHR. Further observations are necessary to discriminate this possibility.

X-LINKED RECESSIVE HYPOPHOSPHATEMIC RICKETS (X-LINKED HYPERCALCIURIC NEPHROLITHIASIS). The initial description of X-linked recessive hypophosphatemic rickets involved a family in which males presented with rickets or osteomalacia, hypophosphatemia, and a reduced renal threshhold for phosphate reabsorption. In contrast to patients with XLH, affected subjects exhibited hypercalciuria, elevated serum 1,25(OH)₂D levels, and proteinuria of up to 3 g/day. Patients also developed nephrolithiasis and nephrocalcinosis with progressive renal failure in early adulthood. Female carriers in the family were not hypophosphatemic and lacked any biochemical abnormalities other than hypercalciuria. Three related syndromes have been reported independently: X-linked recessive nephrolithiasis with renal failure, Dent's disease, and low-molecular-weight proteinuria with hypercalciuria and nephrocalcinosis. These syndromes differ in degree from each other, but common themes include proximal tubular reabsorptive failure, nephrolithiasis, nephrocalcinosis, progressive renal insufficiency, and, in some cases, rickets or osteomalacia. Identification of mutations in the voltage-gated chloride-channel gene *CLCN5* in all four syndromes has established that they are phenotypic variants of a single disease and are not separate entities. However, the varied manifestations that may be associated with mutations in this gene, particularly the presence of hypophosphatemia and rickets/osteomalacia, underscore that environmental differences, diet, and/or modifying genetic backgrounds may influence phenotypic expression of the disease.

TUMOR-INDUCED OSTEOMALACIA (ONCOGENOUS OSTEOMALACIA). Since initial recognition of this disease, reports have been published of approximately 90 patients in whom rickets and/or osteomalacia have been associated with a coexisting tumor. The coexistent tumors have been of mesenchymal origin in the majority of patients. The cardinal feature of this disease is remission of the unexplained bone disease after tumor resection. In general, affected patients present with bone and muscle pain, muscle weakness, and, occasionally, recurrent fractures of long bones. Biochemical abnormalities include renal phosphate wasting marked by an abnormally low renal tubular maximum for the reabsorption of phosphate per liter of glomerular filtrate, decreased gastrointestinal absorption of phosphate, and consequent hypophosphatemia. In general, serum 25(OH)D levels are normal and serum calcitriol is profoundly decreased or inappropriately normal relative to the hypophosphatemia. Generalized osteopenia, pseudofractures, and coarsened trabeculae, as well as widened epiphyseal plates in children, comprise the common radiographic abnormalities of the syndrome.

Most investigators agree that tumor production of a humoral factor or factors that may affect multiple functions of the proximal renal tubule, particularly phosphate reabsorption (resulting in hypophosphatemia), underlies the pathogenesis of this syndrome. This possibility is supported by (1) the presence of phosphaturic activity in tumor extracts in patients with tumor-induced osteomalacia; (2) the absence of parathyroid hormone, parathyroid hormone-related peptide, and calcitonin from these extracts, and an apparent cyclic adenosine monophosphate (cAMP)–independent mode of action of the extracts from a majority of affected patients; (3) the occurrence of hypophosphatemia and increased urinary phosphate excretion in heterotransplanted tumor-bearing athymic nude mice; (4) the demonstration that extracts of the heterotransplanted tumor inhibit renal 25-hydroxyvitamin D-1α-hydroxylase activity in cultured kidney cells; and (5) the coincidence of aminoaciduria and glycosuria with renal phosphate wasting in some affected subjects, indicative of complex alterations in proximal renal tubular function. Indeed, par-

tial purification of "phosphatonin" from a cell culture derived from a sclerosing hemangioma causing tumor-induced osteomalacia has reaffirmed this possibility. These studies reveal that the putative phosphatonin is a peptide with molecular weight of 8 to 25 kd that does not alter glucose or alanine transport but inhibits sodium-dependent phosphate transport in a cAMP-independent fashion. Moreover, the activity of the phosphatonin is not blocked by a parathyroid hormone receptor antagonist. However, recent studies that document the presence in various disease states of additional phosphate transport inhibitors indicate that the tumor-induced osteomalacia syndrome is heterogeneous and that "phosphatonin" may be a family of hormones. In fact, additional recent observations indicate that some mesenchymal tumors from affected subjects do not secrete phosphaturic factors into culture medium. Thus, the pathogenesis of the disorder may be more complicated than is currently appreciated.

Adding to the complexity of the syndrome, patients with tumor-associated osteomalacia secondary to hematogenous malignancy exhibit abnormalities of the syndrome secondary to a distinctly different mechanism. In these subjects, the nephropathy associated with light-chain proteinuria results in decreased renal phosphate reabsorption and consequent hypophosphatemia. At least 15 patients with this form of the disorder have been reported.

The primary treatment of this disorder is complete resection of the associated tumor. However, recurrence or metastases of tumors often preclude such definitive therapy. In such cases, calcitriol (1.5 to 3.0 μg/day) alone or combined with phosphorus supplementation (2 to 4 g/day) completely heals the attendant bone disease or significantly improves the biochemical and histologic abnormalities. Careful serial assessment of parathyroid function, serum and urinary calcium, and renal function are essential to ensure safe therapy in affected subjects.

FANCONI'S SYNDROME (SEE CHAPTER 109). Rickets and osteomalacia are frequently associated with Fanconi's syndrome, a disorder characterized by phosphaturia and consequent hypophosphatemia, aminoaciduria, renal glycosuria, albuminuria, and proximal renal tubular acidosis. Although a wide diversity of congenital and acquired diseases are associated with this syndrome (see Table 263–1), damage to the proximal renal tubule represents the common underlying mechanism of disease. Resultant dysfunction results in renal wasting of those substances primarily reabsorbed at the proximal tubule. The associated bone disease in this disorder is likely secondary to hypophosphatemia and/or acidosis, abnormalities that occur in association with aberrantly (Fanconi's syndrome, type 1) or normally regulated (Fanconi's syndrome, type 2) vitamin D metabolism. In any case, regardless of the underlying cause, osteomalacia associated with adult acquired Fanconi's syndrome appears to respond well to treatment with phosphate and vitamin D replacement. In fact, these patients do not appear to necessarily require 1,25(OH)₂D.

METABOLIC ACIDOSIS

Osteomalacia occurs secondary to renal tubular acidosis and the acidosis that follows ureterosigmoidoscopy. The bone disease results from the multifactorial influence of acidosis, which decreases the conversion of amorphous calcium phosphate to hydroxyapatite at the mineralization front, induces renal phosphate wasting, and possibly interferes with calcitriol production. Systemic acidosis also enhances dissolution of bone and results in hypercalciuria. Affected patients have a normal serum calcium level, a low normal or decreased serum phosphorus level, and an elevated alkaline phosphatase level. Secondary to hypercalciuria, nephrocalcinosis and renal lithiasis often occur. Bicarbonate therapy alone effectively treats the osteomalacia associated with metabolic acidosis, although administering vitamin D and calcium when starting therapy facilitates healing of the bone disease.

PRIMARY DISORDERS OF BONE MATRIX

Intrinsic disorders of bone in which apparently abnormal matrix is produced but is not normally mineralized are extremely rare and are poorly understood. These diseases may result from presumed abnormalities of collagen or other proteins in the matrix or aberrant enzyme activity essential for normal mineralization.

ABNORMAL BONE MATRIX. FIBROGENESIS IMPERFECTA OSSIUM. Fibrogenesis imperfecta ossium is a rare, sporadically occurring disorder characterized by the gradual onset of intractable skeletal pain in middle-aged men and women. Pathologic fractures are a prominent clinical feature, and patients typically become bedridden. Although the serum calcium and phosphorus levels are normal, alkaline phosphatase level is invariably elevated. The bones have a dense, amorphous, mottled appearance radiologically and a disorganized arrangement of collagen with decreased birefringence histologically. Most likely, the disorganized collagen matrix limits normal bone mineralization.

AXIAL OSTEOMALACIA. Axial osteomalacia is another unusual sporadically occurring disorder that generally affects only middle-aged men. The majority of patients present with only vague, dull, chronic axial discomfort that typically affects the cervical region most severely. Abnormal radiographic findings are limited to the pelvis and spine, where the coarsened trabecular pattern is characteristic of osteomalacia. Although the alkaline phosphatase may be increased, histopathologic studies reveal a normal lamellar pattern of collagen. However, the osteoblasts appear flat and inactive, suggesting that an osteoblastic defect, and perhaps an attendant abnormal matrix, inhibits normal mineralization.

ABNORMAL ENZYME ACTIVITY. HYPOPHOSPHATASIA. Hypophosphatasia is a heritable disorder characterized by a deficiency of the tissue nonspecific (liver, bone, kidney) isoenzyme of alkaline phosphatase, increased urinary excretion of phosphorylethanolamine, and skeletal disease that includes osteomalacia and rickets. The severity of clinical expression is remarkably variable and spans intrauterine death from profound skeletal hypomineralization at one extreme to lifelong absence of symptoms at the other. As a consequence, six clinical disease types are distinguished (see Table 263–1). The age at which skeletal disease is initially noted delineates, in large part, the perinatal (lethal), infantile, childhood, and adult variants of the disorder. However, affected children and adults may manifest only the unique dental abnormalities of the syndrome and, accordingly, are classified as having odontohypophosphatasia. Finally, patients with the rare variant, pseudohypophosphatasia, have the clinical-radiologic-biochemical features of the classic disease without a decrease in the circulating levels of alkaline phosphatase. These individuals have defects in cellular localization and substrate specificity of the enzyme.

Affected infants exhibit hypercalcemia, hypercalciuria, enlarged sutures of the skull, craniosynostosis, delayed dentition, enlarged epiphyses, and prominent costochondral junctions. Genu valgum or varum may develop subsequently. In older children, disease may be limited to rickets. Surprisingly, the disorder in adults is mild despite the presence of osteopenia. Indeed, the disease may be limited to slowly healing metatarsal fractures or loss or fracture of teeth. Nevertheless, 50% of patients have an history of early exfoliation of deciduous teeth and/or rickets, and disease may reflect re-expression of the childhood disorder.

The perinatal and infantile forms of disease are inherited as autosomal recessive traits. The mode(s) of inheritance for odontophosphatasia, adult, and childhood hypophosphatasia remains unclear, although an autosomal dominant disease transmission has been described in some kindreds with mild disease. The physiologic basis for the bone disease likely relates to the role of alkaline phosphatase in cleaving pyrophosphate, an inhibitor of bone mineralization. Failure to hydrolyze this physiologic substrate results in inorganic pyrophosphate elevated to levels sufficiently high to inhibit the mineralization process. The consequence of this pathophysiologic process is a block of the vectorial spread of mineral from initial nuclei within matrix vesicles outward into the matrix of growth cartilage and bone.

Therapy of this disease has been generally unrewarding. Thus, supportive treatment is important and may include craniotomy in children (to manage craniosynostosis) and, in adults, insertion of load-sharing intramedullary rods to treat fractures. Expert dental care is also crucial to minimize tooth loss and prevent consequent malnutrition in youths.

MINERALIZATION INHIBITORS

DRUGS. ETIDRONATE. Disturbances in mineralization may be seen in patients consuming etidronate daily at doses greater than 5 mg/k of body weight. The etidronate is deposited at the bone surface and inhibits osteoblast function; it also directly inhibits calcium-phosphate crystallization.

FLUORIDE. Although multiple studies document that fluoride stimulates new bone formation, administering the drug in high doses without adequate calcium supplementation results in poorly mineralized bone, consistent with osteomalacia. The mechanisms by which fluoride alters osteoblast function and/or directly inhibits mineralization remains unknown.

ALUMINUM. Excess aluminum accumulation in bone inhibits mineralization and is a potential mechanism for the osteomalacia observed in patients with chronic renal failure, as discussed above. In addition, accumulation of aluminum in bone likely underlies the osteomalacia observed in patients treated with total parenteral nutrition. In such cases aluminum contamination of casein hydrolysate, as well as albumin, phosphate, and calcium solutions, provides the major source of the mineral. Changing total parenteral nutrition solutions from those with casein hydrolysate to those with purified amino acids has markedly reduced the incidence of clinically evident bone disease.

Cai Q, Hodgson SF, Kao PC, et al: Inhibition of renal phosphate transport by a tumor product in a patient with oncogenic osteomalacia. N Engl J Med 330:1645, 1994. *Presentation of evidence that tumor-induced osteomalacia is caused by ectopic secretion of a heat-labile factor with a mass between 8000 and 25,000, which inhibits renal tubular reabsorption of phosphate.*

Econs MJ, Drezner MK: Bone disease resulting from inherited disorders of renal tubule transport and vitamin D metabolism. *In* Coe FL, Favus MJ: Disorders of Bone and Mineral Metabolism. New York, Raven Press, 1992, p 935. *Extensive review of the classic vitamin D-resistant rachitic and osteomalacic disorders. Discussion includes clinical features, differential diagnosis, genetics, and therapy.*

Friedman NJ, Drezner MK: Osteomalacia, genetic. *In* Bardin CW: Current Therapy in Endocrinology and Metabolism, 4th ed. Philadelphia, BC Decker, 1991, p 421. *Review of the underlying concepts and the specific details of treatment for hypophosphatemic rickets in all its varieties of clinical presentation.*

Scheinman SJ: X-linked hypercalciuric nephrolithiasis: Clinical syndromes and chloride channel mutations. Kidney Int 53:3, 1998. *Review of the interrelationships and common themes (including rickets/osteomalacia) between the various X-linked recessive syndromes that are caused by mutations in the chloride channel gene.*

---

264 THE PARATHYROID GLANDS, HYPERCALCEMIA, AND HYPOCALCEMIA

Allen M. Spiegel

THE PARATHYROID GLANDS

EMBRYOLOGY AND ANATOMY. Normally, there are four parathyroids, averaging 120 mg in total weight, but as many as 5% of normal individuals may have more than four glands. The superior parathyroids are derived from the fourth (more caudal) branchial pouches and remain almost stationary during embryologic development. Their typical final location is near the upper poles of the thyroid. Aberrant locations include the tracheoesophageal groove and the retroesophageal space. The inferior parathyroids develop (in association with the thymus) from the third branchial pouches. During normal development, they migrate caudally, assuming a final position near the lower poles of the thyroid. The inferior parathyroids may fail to descend, remaining near the angle of the jaw or, at the other extreme, may descend into the anterior mediastinum in association with the thymus.

SYNTHESIS AND SECRETION OF PARATHYROID HORMONE. Parathyroid hormone (PTH), together with vitamin D (see Chapter 262), is the principal regulator of ionized calcium in extracellular fluid. PTH is synthesized in the parathyroid glands as "preproparathyroid hormone," a precursor composed of 115 amino acids. A hydrophobic "leader" peptide of 25 amino acids is first cleaved from the amino-terminus to yield the prohormone, followed by cleavage of a basic, amino-terminal hexapeptide to yield the mature 84-amino-acid hormone. The latter is the principal secreted form of the hormone. There is no evidence for secretion of either the preprohormone or the prohormone. The prohormone possesses <0.2% of the biologic activity of the native 84-amino-acid hormone. The full biologic activity of the intact hormone resides within the amino-terminal 1–34 fragment, whereas fragments from the midregion and carboxy-terminal regions lack biologic activity (Fig. 264–1).

Secretion of PTH is regulated primarily by the concentration of ionized calcium in the extracellular fluid. Normally, PTH secretion is regulated at a "set point" that maintains serum ionized calcium within a relatively narrow range. Deviations below the set point stimulate, and deviations above the set point inhibit, hormone secretion. Effects of calcium on hormone secretion occur acutely (within minutes); low calcium levels have a slower stimulatory action on hormone synthesis. At high calcium concentrations, there is evidence for intracellular degradation of synthesized hormone and possible release of biologically inactive fragments. High magnesium ion concentrations in extracellular fluid, like high calcium concentrations, inhibit PTH secretion, but hypomagnesemia, unlike hypocalcemia, may inhibit hormone secretion and action. The active metabolite of vitamin D, 1,25(OH)$_2$D (dihydroxycholecalciferol), suppresses both secretion and synthesis of PTH. Reduction in 1,25(OH)$_2$D is a major factor contributing to increased PTH secretion in renal failure.

FORMS OF PARATHYROID HORMONE IN PLASMA. PTH circulates in plasma as the intact hormone secreted from the gland and as fragments derived either from glandular secretion (particularly in hypercalcemic states) or from peripheral metabolism of the intact hormone. Most, if not all, of these fragments lack biologic activity but may, depending on antibody specificity, contribute to immunoreactivity in plasma (see Fig. 264–1).

PARATHYROID HORMONE ACTION. PTH acts directly on kidney and bone, and indirectly on the gut, to maintain the normal concentration of serum ionized calcium (see Chapter 261 for a complete discussion of mineral homeostasis). In the kidney, PTH (1) enhances reabsorption of calcium, and also magnesium, from the glomerular filtrate; (2) increases excretion of phosphate and of bicarbonate; (3) activates the enzyme (1α-hydroxylase) that forms the active metabolite, 1,25(OH)$_2$D, of vitamin D. In bone, PTH causes the release of calcium and phosphate into the extracellular

fluid. The hormone acts directly on osteoblasts, which secondarily affect osteoclast activity. The hypercalcemic action on bone and the anticalciuric action on kidney combine to raise the serum calcium level. The phosphatemic action on bone tends to blunt the hypercalcemic effect of the hormone owing to formation of calcium phosphate complexes, but the phosphaturic action counteracts the tendency to hyperphosphatemia. Stimulation of 1,25(OH)$_2$D formation promotes enhanced intestinal absorption of calcium, which also serves to maintain a normal serum calcium level (see Chapter 262). The clinical consequences of PTH excess (or in the opposite direction, hormone deficiency) follow directly from the actions of the hormone: (1) hypercalcemia, (2) a tendency to hypophosphatemia, (3) a tendency to reduced serum bicarbonate levels and hyperchloremia, (4) increased serum levels of 1,25(OH)$_2$D, and (5) relative reduction in urinary calcium excretion and increase in urinary phosphate excretion for a given filtered load.

MECHANISM OF PARATHYROID HORMONE ACTION. The first step in PTH action is binding to specific plasma membrane–bound receptors on target cells in bone and kidney. Such receptors are coupled to guanosine triphosphate (GTP)—binding proteins—in particular, the Gs protein that links receptors to stimulation of adenylyl cyclase (for a more general description of the mechanism of polypeptide hormone action, see Chapter 232). Adenylyl cyclase catalyzes the formation of the "second messenger," cyclic adenosine monophosphate (cAMP), which mediates hormone action by stimulating the phosphorylation of critical intracellular proteins. A diagnostically useful peculiarity of PTH action on proximal renal tubular cells is that not only are cAMP levels increased intracellularly but, because of overflow into the extracellular fluid, urinary cAMP excretion is also increased. "Second messengers" other than cAMP may also mediate certain actions of PTH.

ASSAY OF PARATHYROID HORMONE IN PLASMA. Normally, the concentration of biologically active PTH circulating in plasma is quite low (<50 pg/mL). Bioassays sensitive enough to detect such low levels include a renal cytochemical assay and several assays based on stimulating cAMP formation in bone or kidney cells. Unfortunately, such assays are too cumbersome for routine clinical use. Total urinary cAMP excretion (normalized to creatinine clearance by simultaneously measuring serum and urinary creatinine) is an easily measured and sensitive index of circulating PTH bioactivity. It is elevated in primary hyperparathyroidism, is

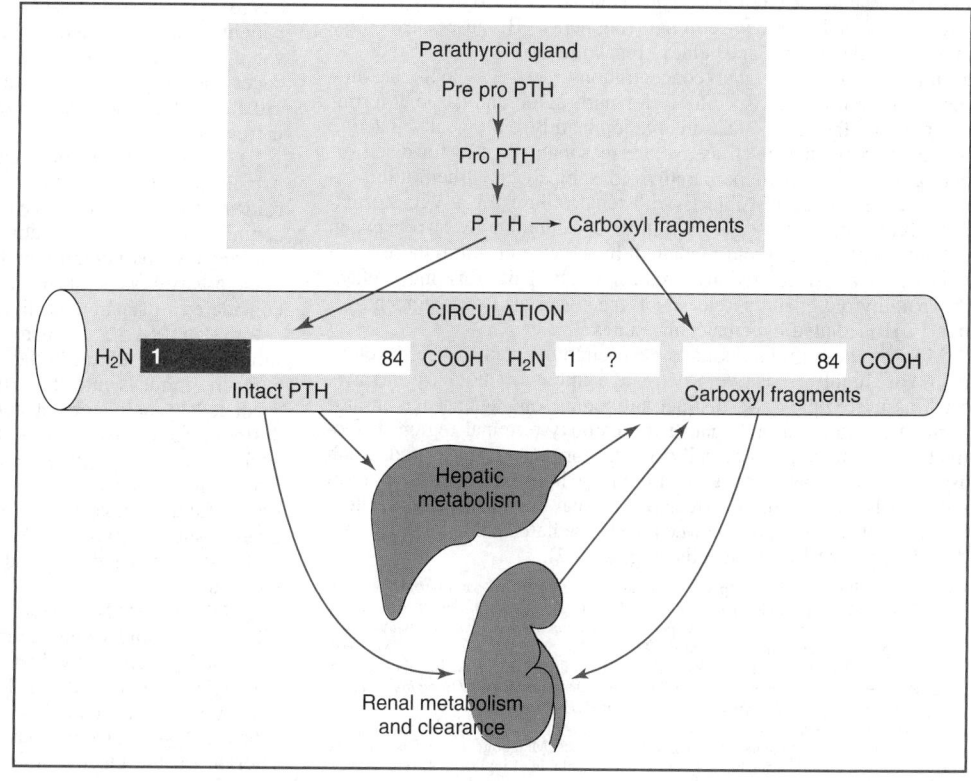

FIGURE 264–1 ■ Secretion, metabolism, and clearance of parathyroid hormone (PTH). *Top.* PTH is synthesized as a preprohormone and undergoes successive cleavages within the parathyroid to the mature (1–84), major secreted form of the hormone. Under certain conditions (e.g., hypercalcemia), some of the hormone is cleaved intracellularly into biologically inactive, carboxy-terminal fragments, which are also secreted. *Middle.* The major circulating forms of the hormone are the intact 1–84 species (the shaded region corresponds to the amino-terminal 1–34 portion possessing full biologic activity) and biologically inactive carboxy-terminal fragments. The presence of amino-terminal fragments in the circulation is unclear (indicated by "?"). *Bottom.* Peripheral metabolism of the hormone occurs in liver and kidney. The kidney also clears intact hormone and carboxy-terminal fragments from the circulation. (From Endres DE, Villanueva R, Sharp CF Jr, et al: Measurement of parathyroid hormone. Endocrinol Metab Clin North Am 18:611, 1989.)

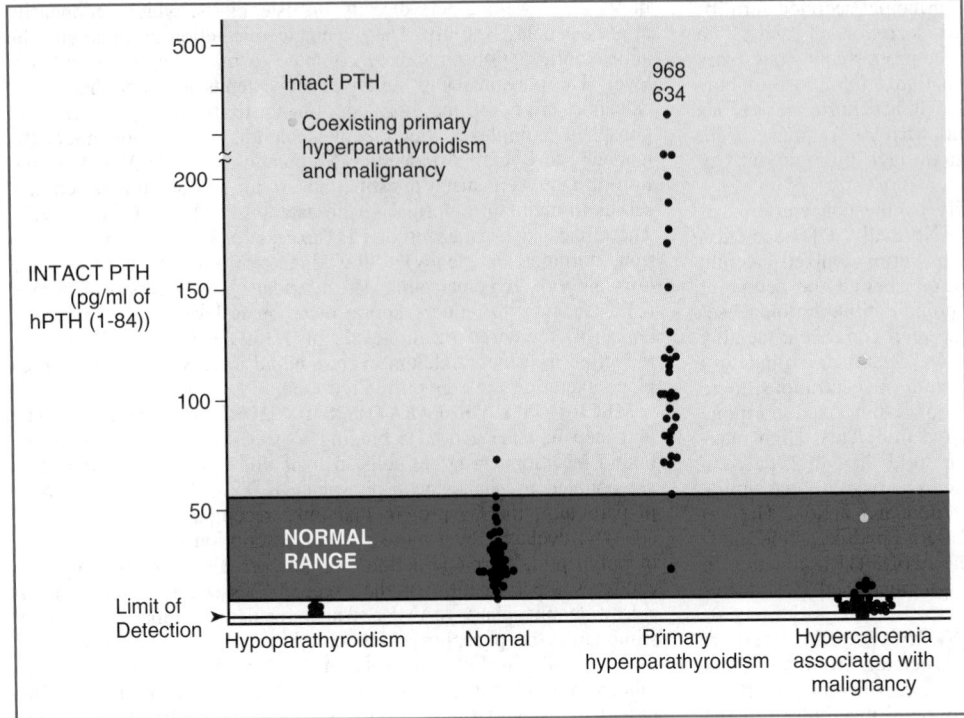

FIGURE 264–2 ■ Two-site immunoassay for parathyroid hormone (PTH) in serum. The two-site method measures exclusively intact PTH. The hormone is detectable in the majority of normal subjects and undetectable in patients with various forms of hypoparathyroidism. Almost all patients with primary hyperparathyroidism show values outside the normal range. In contrast, values are low to undetectable in patients with malignancy-associated hypercalcemia, except for four individuals with coexistent primary hyperparathyroidism. (From Endres DB, Villanueva R, Sharp CF Jr, et al: Measurement of parathyroid hormone. Endocrinol Metab Clin North Am 18:611, 1989.)

low in hypoparathyroidism, and falls within 1 hour of successful parathyroidectomy in patients with hyperparathyroidism. Increased urinary cAMP excretion, however, is not absolutely specific for PTH hypersecretion; parathyroid hormone–related peptide, secreted by many malignancies, similarly increases urinary cAMP excretion, and this must be taken into account when interpreting urinary cAMP measurements in subjects with hypercalcemia (see Hypercalcemia Associated with Malignancy, below).

Radioimmunoassays are sufficiently sensitive and practical for routinely measuring circulating PTH. Interpretation of assay results requires an understanding of what a particular antiserum is measuring. Immunoreactivity need not correlate with biologic activity. Indeed, the bulk of circulating PTH consists of biologically inactive mid-region and carboxy-terminal fragments. Because such fragments are cleared by the kidney, renal impairment causes them to accumulate at even higher concentrations (see Fig. 264–1). Antisera with predominant specificity for mid-region and carboxy-terminal regions, therefore, measure predominantly biologically inactive hormone fragments. Such assays are reasonably useful for discriminating normal from hyperparathyroid subjects, but their utility is much more limited in subjects with renal failure. Even with normal renal function, such assays may show considerable overlap between patients with parathyroid-mediated hypercalcemia and those with non-parathyroid-mediated hypercalcemia. In part, this may reflect the parathyroid gland's release of inactive hormone fragments in non-PTH-mediated hypercalcemic states.

Most of these problems have been circumvented by the development of highly sensitive "two-site" immunoradiometric assays. Such assays employ two distinct antibodies, one against the amino-terminal region and one against the carboxy-terminal region. Effectively, only intact, biologically active hormone is measured. Such assays allow measurement of circulating hormone in most normal individuals, are scarcely affected by renal impairment, and allow excellent discrimination between PTH-mediated and non-PTH-mediated causes of hypercalcemia (Fig. 264–2).

Endres DB, Villanueva R, Sharp CF Jr, et al: Measurement of parathyroid hormone. Endocrinol Metab Clin North Am 18:611, 1989. *Complete discussion of methods for PTH assay, including comparison of two-site versus mid-region immunoassays.*
Kronenberg HM: Parathyroid hormone: Mechanism of action. *In* Favus MJ (ed): Primer on the Metabolic Bone Diseases and Disorders of Mineral Metabolism, 3rd ed. Philadelphia, Lippincott-Raven, 1996, p 68. *Description of PTH action at cellular and molecular level including discussion of PTH receptor.*
Segre GV, Brown EM: Secretion, circulating heterogeneity, and metabolism of parathyroid hormone. *In* Favus MJ (ed): Primer on the Metabolic Bone Diseases and Disorders of Mineral Metabolism, 3rd ed. Philadelphia, Lippincott-Raven, 1996, p

63. *Detailed description of basic aspects of PTH secretion and metabolism including discussion of role of calcium-sensing receptor.*

HYPERCALCEMIA

DEFINITION. Hypercalcemia is defined as an abnormal elevation in serum ionized calcium concentration. Because total, rather than ionized, calcium is generally measured, one must be aware of factors that influence the fraction of total serum calcium that is ionized. Of these, serum albumin concentration is of greatest clinical relevance because albumin is the chief circulating calcium-binding protein. "Normal" total serum calcium concentration associated with a significant reduction in serum albumin (e.g., in patients with malignancy) may actually represent abnormally elevated levels of serum ionized calcium. Acid-base status also influences the proportion of total serum calcium that is protein bound (alkalosis decreases the ionized calcium concentration, and acidosis increases it).

ETIOLOGY. Many different diseases are potential causes of hypercalcemia. Of these, the most common are primary hyperparathyroidism (particularly in asymptomatic individuals whose hypercalcemia is detected by routine serum chemistry measurement) and malignancy (particularly in hospitalized individuals). These disorders, as well as some of the rarer causes of hypercalcemia, are considered in separate sections below.

PATHOGENESIS. Hypercalcemia results from excessive calcium influx into the extracellular fluid from bone and decreased efflux from the kidneys into the urine. Calcium mobilization from bone is mediated by activators of bone resorption. These activators include systemic factors (e.g., PTH, $1,25(OH)_2D$) and locally acting factors, such as various lymphokines. Reduced renal calcium excretion may lead to hypercalcemia, particularly in states of increased bone turnover. Renal impairment, volume depletion, and anticalciuretic agents, such as thiazide diuretics and PTH, are clinically relevant factors that can reduce renal calcium excretion and provoke hypercalcemia.

CLINICAL MANIFESTATIONS. Many manifestations are not specific to the underlying cause (specific disease manifestations are discussed under individual disease headings). Extreme hypercalcemia leads to coma and death. Neurologic manifestations in less severe cases may include confusion, lethargy, weakness, and hyporeflexia. Hypercalcemia may be detected by shortening of the QT interval on the electrocardiogram. Arrhythmias are rare, but bradycardia and first-degree heart block have been reported. Acute hypercalcemia may be associated with significant hypertension. Gastrointestinal manifestations include constipation and anorexia; in severe cases, there may be nausea and vomiting. Acute pancreatitis has been reported in association with hypercalcemia of various causes. Hypercalcemia interferes with antidiuretic hormone action, thereby leading to polyuria and polydipsia. Reversible reduction in renal function associated with significant hypercalcemia is followed by more permanent damage if hypercalcemia persists. Particularly if serum phosphorus is also increased, hypercalcemia can lead to nephrocalcinosis and interstitial nephritis. Hypercalciuria and nephrolithiasis may also occur. Deposition of calcium in other soft tissues, including skin and cornea, is most likely to occur in patients with associated hyperphosphatemia.

DIFFERENTIAL DIAGNOSIS. Potential causes of hypercalcemia are listed in Table 264–1. These may be divided into PTH-mediated (primary hyperparathyroidism) and non–PTH-mediated diseases (all others). Although ectopic secretion of PTH by tumors was long considered a potential cause of PTH-mediated hypercalcemia, there is now general agreement that ectopic secretion of authentic PTH (as opposed to PTH-related peptides; see below) by tumors is extremely rare. The first step in the differential diagnosis of hypercalcemia is to establish whether or not PTH hypersecretion is present because subsequent diagnostic maneuvers and definitive therapy critically depend on this distinction.

Readily measured blood and urine chemistries may offer some clues to diagnosis. In theory, PTH hypersecretion should be reflected by hypophosphatemia, hyperchloremia, hypobicarbonatemia, increased urinary phosphate excretion, and urinary calcium excretion that is relatively low for the filtered load. PTH secretion suppressed by hypercalcemia of non-parathyroid etiology should, in theory, reverse these parameters. In practice, there is considerable overlap in each of these parameters between patients with parathyroid-mediated forms of hypercalcemia and those with non-parathyroid-mediated forms. This situation may reflect confounding variables, such as vomiting, diuretic treatment, and renal failure, as well as the ability of certain hypercalcemic agents to mimic many actions of PTH. Most important in this respect is parathyroid hormone–related peptide, first isolated from tumors associated with the syndrome of humoral hypercalcemia. This peptide mimics all of the known actions of PTH on kidney and bone, including increasing urinary cAMP excretion and stimulating renal formation of $1,25(OH)_2D$. Decreased urinary cAMP excretion (with normal renal function) strongly suggests non–PTH-mediated hypercalcemia, but increased urinary cAMP excretion is compatible with both primary hyperparathyroidism and tumor secretion of parathyroid hormone-related peptide. Serum $1,25(OH)_2D$ concentration also does not allow definitive diagnosis. It may be elevated in primary hyperparathyroidism and vitamin D–related causes of hypercalcemia and may be reduced in other non–parathyroid-mediated causes of hypercalcemia. For reasons that are not entirely clear, the serum $1,25(OH)_2D$ level is often low in patients with malignancies secret-

Table 264–1 ■ CAUSES OF HYPERCALCEMIA

Parathyroid hormone–mediated causes
  Primary hyperparathyroidism
    Sporadic, familial (multiple endocrine neoplasia types I and II)
  Familial hypocalciuric hypercalcemia*
  Ectopic secretion of parathyroid hormone by tumors (very rare)
Non-parathyroid hormone–mediated causes
  Malignancy associated
    Local osteolytic hypercalcemia
    Humoral hypercalcemia of malignancy
  Vitamin D–mediated
    Vitamin D intoxication
    Excessive production of $1,25(OH)_2D$ in granulomatous disorders
  Other endocrinopathies
    Thyrotoxicosis
    Hypoadrenalism
Immobilization with increased bone turnover, e.g., Paget's disease
Acute renal failure with rhabdomyolysis
Calcium carbonate ingestion (milk-alkali syndrome)
Jansen-type metaphyseal chondrodysplasia (activating mutation of parathyroid hormone receptor)

*Parathyroid hormone secretion is necessary for hypercalcemia but is not the primary defect.

Table 264–2 ■ DIAGNOSTIC APPROACH TO HYPERCALCEMIA

1. Distinguish parathyroid hormone (PTH)–mediated forms of hypercalcemia from non–PTH-mediated forms: *PTH immunoassay (preferably two-site type) is the definitive test.*
2. If the PTH level is elevated, primary hyperparathyroidism is the most likely diagnosis: *Family history for hypercalcemia should be checked to distinguish sporadic from familial (multiple endocrine neoplasia syndromes and hypocalciuric hypercalcemia) disease. Marginal elevation in PTH levels, particularly in young, asymptomatic individuals, should prompt urine calcium measurement to exclude familial hypocalciuric hypercalcemia. In patients with coexisting malignancy, selective venous sampling can be done to exclude ectopic PTH secretion, but the latter is extremely rare.*
3. If PTH is low or undetectable, further laboratory tests (in addition to complete history, physical, and radiologic studies) are needed to distinguish among the various forms of non–PTH-mediated forms of hypercalcemia: *Increased urinary cAMP excretion suggests tumor secretion of PTH-related peptide (direct radioimmunoassays for this peptide are now available). Increased $1,25(OH)_2D$ suggests granulomatous disease (including some types of lymphoma).*

cAMP = cyclic adenosine monophosphate.

ing PTH-related peptide, despite the ability of the peptide to stimulate $1,25(OH)_2D$ formation.

Definitive distinction between parathyroid- and non–parathyroid-mediated causes of hypercalcemia relies primarily on PTH immunoassay. As discussed earlier, this distinction is best made with the two-site type of assays that measure intact PTH and are unaffected by renal function (see Fig. 264–2). An elevated PTH level secures the diagnosis of primary hyperparathyroidism. In selected cases with coexistent malignancy, the unlikely possibility of ectopic PTH secretion may be excluded by selective venous sampling and assay of PTH, but generally this testing is unnecessary. Hormone levels in the normal range suggest the possibility of familial hypocalciuric hypercalcemia. This entity is discussed further in the section on hyperparathyroidism. Low to undetectable values for PTH place the patient in the non–parathyroid-mediated category. Additional testing is necessary to establish a specific diagnosis within this group. Immunoassays for parathyroid hormone–related peptide have been developed, and these may allow the diagnosis of hypercalcemia caused by a tumor secreting this agent. Complete clinical evaluation, including history (e.g., vitamin ingestion, chronicity of symptoms), physical examination (masses, lymphadenopathy), radiologic studies, and other blood tests (e.g., thyroid and adrenal function), may point to a diagnosis. An unusual cause of non–PTH-mediated hypercalcemia is Jansen-type metaphyseal chondrodysplasia, in which an activating mutation of the PTH receptor mimics the effects of excess PTH. The diagnostic approach to hypercalcemia is summarized in Table 264–2.

TREATMENT. The definitive treatment of hypercalcemia depends on the specific diagnosis and treatment of the underlying disease, e.g., parathyroidectomy for primary hyperparathyroidism, chemotherapy for a malignancy. The initial treatment of hypercalcemia can be instituted (and in acute hypercalcemic crisis, often *must* be instituted) without a specific diagnosis, but cumulative toxicity and loss of efficacy preclude long-term nonspecific treatment. Measures aimed at reducing the serum calcium level act by increasing urinary calcium excretion and by decreasing bone resorption. General measures applicable to every patient include mobilization as soon as feasible (because immobility increases bone resorption) and hydration (because significant hypercalcemia causes dehydration). Volume depletion, by limiting renal calcium excretion, perpetuates a vicious circle that can lead to acute hypercalcemic crisis. Volume expansion with isotonic saline often significantly reduces the serum calcium level by enhancing renal calcium excretion. Only after volume repletion should diuretics be used to enhance sodium and thereby calcium excretion. With a vigorous saline diuresis, calcium excretion in the range of 1 to 2 g/day can be achieved as a temporary measure to reduce the serum calcium level. In patients with renal failure, dialysis can be employed almost as effectively to remove calcium from extracellular fluid. Careful monitoring of cardiac function and serum electrolytes is necessary with both saline diuresis and dialysis treatment.

Measures aimed at reducing bone resorption by inhibiting osteoclast function are most effective in treating hypercalcemia, irrespective of the specific factor causing increased bone resorption. Available agents include calcitonin, bisphosphonates (diphosphonates), plicamycin (mithramycin), and gallium nitrate. Calcitonin has low toxicity and acts most rapidly, but even in doses up to 32 MRC U/kg/day by intravenous infusion, lowering of serum calcium is generally limited and transient. Bisphosphonates must be given parenterally, and their effect is both significant and often prolonged (days). Initially, only etidronate (7.5 mg/kg/day intravenously) was available, but this is being replaced by pamidronate (dose 30 to 90 mg intravenously over 24 hours), which is more potent and effective. Plicamycin (25 μg/kg intravenously) quite effectively lowers serum calcium, but it has cumulative toxicity in liver, kidney, and platelets and can no longer be justified as initial therapy. Gallium nitrate is an effective calcium-lowering agent and has recently been approved by the FDA, but it has potential nephrotoxicity and its place in treating hypercalcemia is not yet clear. Intravenous phosphate poses a serious danger of metastatic calcification in the hypercalcemic patient and should probably no longer be used, given availability of other safer and effective agents. Oral phosphate is safer and useful in patients with significant hypercalcemia who are awaiting definitive treatment and in whom hypercalcemic crisis should be prevented. Dosages in the range of 2 g/day of elemental phosphorus (10 g of phosphate salts) in divided doses can be given. Serum phosphate and renal function should be carefully monitored.

Glucocorticoids are highly effective in treating hypercalcemia caused by vitamin D-related mechanisms (vitamin D intoxication, overproduction of $1,25(OH)_2D$ in granulomatous disorders) and by certain malignancies (cytokine release associated with myeloma) but are ineffective in most other forms of hypercalcemia, including hyperparathyroidism and most malignancies. Forty to 100 mg/day of prednisone or the equivalent is the usual dose range.

PRIMARY HYPERPARATHYROIDISM

DEFINITION. Primary hyperparathyroidism is a disorder in which hypercalcemia is due to hypersecretion of PTH.

ETIOLOGY. In most cases (about 85%), hyperparathyroidism is caused by sporadic, solitary adenomas. Hyperplasia of all four glands occurs in about 10% of cases, and these are most often familial, in the context of three distinct autosomal dominant inherited diseases: multiple endocrine neoplasia (MEN) types I and II and familial hypocalciuric hypercalcemia. Carcinoma occurs rarely (<5% of cases). The gene for MEN type I on chromosome 11q13 has recently been identified. Enlarged glands in this disease contain monoclonal tumors with germline loss-of-function mutations in one allele of the MEN I gene and somatic loss of the second, normal allele. This suggests that the MEN I gene is a "tumor suppressor" whose loss leads to tumorigenesis. About 30% of sporadic parathyroid tumors also show allele loss at 11q13, and in a subset, somatic loss-of-function mutations of the MEN I gene have been identified, suggesting a similar pathogenesis. The gene for MEN type II has been identified as the *RET* proto-oncogene on chromosome 10q11. Identification of the MEN type I and type II genes facilitates genetic diagnosis and studies of pathogenesis. Very rarely, a rearrangement involving the PTH gene on the short arm of chromosome 11 and a cell cycle control gene termed cyclin D or PRAD 1 on the long arm of chromosome 11 appears to cause parathyroid adenoma formation. Epidemiologic evidence suggests that a history of neck irradiation predisposes to parathyroid tumor formation. Specific molecular defects have not been identified. Finally, longstanding secondary hyperparathyroidism (e.g., in response to renal failure) may evolve into autonomous hypersecretion, so-called tertiary hyperparathyroidism.

INCIDENCE. The incidence of hyperparathyroidism has increased substantially, largely as a result of routine blood calcium measurement. Age-adjusted incidence rates are between 25 and 50 per 100,000, based on recent surveys. A prevalence between 0.1 and 0.5% has been estimated, with females affected about twice as commonly as males. The incidence rises sharply after age 40 years.

PATHOLOGY. Microscopic distinction between adenoma and hyperplasia is difficult, if not impossible. The distinction between single-gland and multigland disease relies on gross surgical identification of more than one enlarged gland. In MEN types I and II, there is always multigland involvement, although asymmetrical gland enlargement is often present. The chief cell generally predominates in parathyroid tumors; oxyphil cell tumors are much rarer.

PATHOPHYSIOLOGY. The primary disturbance is inappropriate secretion of PTH for the level of serum calcium. Studies (in vitro) with isolated parathyroid cells show that most adenomas either fail to suppress secretion at high calcium levels or show an altered setpoint, i.e., a higher calcium level is required to suppress secretion than for normal cells. Cells from hyperplastic glands may show a normal calcium setpoint for secretion. Hypersecretion of PTH in such cases may be due to a primary defect causing cellular proliferation and to an inability to suppress hormone secretion completely because of increased cell mass.

Slight increases in PTH secretion act on bone to increase turnover and may reduce cortical rather than trabecular bone density. At very high levels, PTH causes radiographically detectable subperiosteal bone resorption and, eventually, marrow fibrosis and cystic, reparative bone lesions termed "brown tumors." This is the classic form of the disease called "osteitis fibrosa cystica." PTH increases renal calcium reabsorption, but nonetheless, at high filtered loads of calcium, hypercalciuria develops. Enhanced $1,25(OH)_2D$ formation by the kidneys is prominent in some patients and is associated with increased intestinal calcium absorption. Such patients may be at particular risk for renal stones.

CLINICAL MANIFESTATIONS. Most patients either are asymptomatic at presentation (discovered through incidental blood calcium measurement) or have vague, nonspecific symptoms, such as fatigue, weakness, and mental disturbance. Patients with significant hypercalcemia show many of the signs and symptoms of hypercalcemia discussed above. Nephrolithiasis, with or without renal colic, is not specifically associated with hyperparathyroidism but is most commonly seen in this setting. Subperiosteal bone resorption is rarely seen, and osteitis fibrosa cystica even less commonly. Neuromuscular abnormalities, particularly proximal muscle weakness affecting the lower limbs, may be prominent. Joint manifestations include chondrocalcinosis that may lead to pseudogout. It has been claimed that hypertension and peptic ulcer disease are manifestations of hyperparathyroidism, but these are common, and there is no firm evidence for a causal relationship. No specific physical findings are present in hyperparathyroidism. A neck mass, if present, most commonly represents a coincidental thyroid nodule, less commonly a benign or malignant parathyroid tumor. "Band keratopathy," calcification at "3 and 9 o'clock" of the cornea, is best seen by slit-lamp examination and occurs most often when hypercalcemia is accompanied by hyperphosphatemia—thus less commonly in hyperparathyroidism than in other hypercalcemic disorders. Radiologic findings include subperiosteal resorption, which, when present, is best seen at the radial sides of the phalanges, distal phalangeal tufts, and distal clavicles. Lucent bone lesions, representing brown tumors, are seen in rare, severely affected patients. Soft tissue calcification may be evident in the joints, kidneys, and lungs. The calcification is best appreciated on bone scans.

DIAGNOSIS. The differential diagnosis of hypercalcemia is discussed above. PTH immunoassay, preferably one of the newer two-site assays, is the key to diagnosis. In distinguishing between hyperparathyroid and normal states (e.g., in patients presenting with nephrolithiasis), repeated careful serum calcium and PTH (including the mid-region type of assay) measurements are most useful. Hypercalcemic subjects taking lithium or thiazides should be retested for hyperparathyroidism after discontinuing the drug (this may not be feasible in some patients on lithium), because both drugs may alter serum calcium and PTH secretion. In relatively young, asymptomatic individuals, or if the serum PTH level is marginally elevated, hypercalcemia may be due to familial hypocalciuric hypercalcemia rather than hyperparathyroidism (see discussion below under Familial Hypocalciuric Hypercalcemia).

PROGNOSIS AND TREATMENT. Surgical parathyroidectomy is the only definitive treatment for hyperparathyroidism. Oral phosphate treatment can lower the serum calcium level, but the long-term safety and efficacy of this approach are unclear. In mildly affected, older women, estrogen treatment has been advocated, particularly to blunt bone resorption, but, again, long-term efficacy is unknown. Thus, the only alternative to surgery at present is conservative medical follow-up. Most experts recommend surgery for all patients with symptomatic disease and even for asymptomatic patients meeting other, somewhat arbitrary, criteria, such as age younger than 40 years or a serum calcium level > 11.5 mg/d. The appropriate management of patients not fitting any of these criteria is controversial; some advocate surgery for all, and others conservative follow-up. The long-term course of untreated hyperparathyroidism is unknown. Controlled studies comparing surgery versus medical follow-up have not been performed. Small series of patients followed conservatively for several years suggest that mild biochemical disease rarely progresses to severe symptomatic disease. Bone densitometry is an important component of the evaluation of patients with hyperparathyroidism, because it is much more sensitive than plain radiographs. Reduction in cortical bone density (measured in the forearm) greater than 2 SD below the mean of age-matched controls is an indication for surgery. Evidence exists for a substantial increase in bone density following parathyroidectomy in a subset of patients with low vertebral bone density at presentation, so surgery may be indicated in such patients as well. Because definitive treatment recommendations are not possible, therapy must be individualized. The author personally follows a policy of recommending surgery for all but older patients with only mild biochemical disease.

If the decision is to perform surgery, a highly experienced parathyroid surgeon must be found. A success rate as high as 95% can be expected for initial neck exploration by a skilled surgeon. The success rate is substantially lower with inexperienced surgeons. Preoperative localization is not needed by the skilled surgeon performing initial exploration. Neither localization studies nor neck exploration itself should serve as *diagnostic* maneuvers. Only after the diagnosis has been established biochemically (by PTH assay) should one recommend surgery. In patients undergoing repeat neck exploration for recurrent or persistent disease, localization studies are extremely helpful. Noninvasive studies include ultrasonography, technetium 99m sestamibi scanning, computed tomography (CT), and magnetic resonance imaging. Invasive techniques include fine-needle aspiration of imaged lesions for PTH assay, selective arteriography, and selective venous catheterization for hormone assay. The latter techniques are best performed by radiologists with specialized experience.

After successful surgery, hypocalcemia is generally mild and transient and rarely requires treatment. In the rare case of subjects with extensive bone disease, severe, prolonged hypocalcemia secondary to "bone hunger" occurs. Persistent relative hypophosphatemia suggests that bone hunger, rather than hypoparathyroidism, is the cause of hypocalcemia in this setting. Acute treatment with calcium infusions and long-term treatment with vitamin D and oral calcium may be needed. Eventually, treatment can be discontinued if normal parathyroid tissue remains. In patients without residual normal parathyroid tissue, life-long vitamin D therapy is necessary. Autotransplantation of parathyroid tissue in the forearm is an experimental alternative in such cases. Successful surgery generally halts formation of renal stones in patients with nephrolithiasis and allows skeletal remineralization in patients with bone disease. There is no definitive evidence that surgery corrects hypertension or other nonspecific manifestations of hyperparathyroidism.

FAMILIAL HYPOCALCIURIC HYPERCALCEMIA

DEFINITION. This is an autosomal dominant genetic disease with essentially complete penetrance that causes hypercalcemia and relatively low urinary calcium excretion for the filtered load.

ETIOLOGY. The disease is caused by mutations in a gene on the long arm of chromosome 3 encoding a calcium-sensing receptor. In some families, the disease may be caused by a gene localized to a different chromosome.

INCIDENCE. The disorder is relatively rare, but it is over-represented among patients presenting with unsuccessful neck exploration because of the difficulty in achieving normocalcemia by surgery.

PATHOPHYSIOLOGY. The primary disturbance appears to be in divalent cation transport and/or "sensing" in at least the kidneys and parathyroids. The kidneys show an exaggerated reabsorption of

filtered calcium (and magnesium) that leads to hypercalcemia. The parathyroids, however, fail to suppress fully hormone secretion despite hypercalcemia. The process is PTH-dependent because totally parathyroidectomized subjects become hypocalcemic, but even small amounts of parathyroid tissue are sufficient to maintain hypercalcemia. Parathyroid gland mass is generally only mildly increased.

CLINICAL MANIFESTATIONS. The disease leads to few, if any, clinical manifestations—hence its other name, "familial benign hypercalcemia." Nephrolithiasis and bone disease are, in general, not seen. Pancreatitis has been reported, but the specificity of this association is unclear. Hypercalcemia is present at birth. In some neonates, a clinically severe form of the disease is present. This severe form may be due to inheritance of a double dose of the abnormal gene. Otherwise, the main morbidity is that resulting from unsuccessful neck exploration that has failed to distinguish this disorder from conventional hyperparathyroidism. There is no evidence of associated endocrinopathies, as in the MEN syndromes.

DIAGNOSIS. A high index of suspicion is needed to recognize this disease. Hypercalcemia associated with relatively young age, with only slight elevation in the serum PTH level, or with a family history of unsuccessful neck exploration should trigger further evaluation. Hypermagnesemia is suggestive; urinary calcium-creatinine ratios <0.01:1 strongly support the diagnosis. Screening first-degree relatives for hypercalcemia may also be helpful. For those families in which the disease gene is localized to chromosome 3q, specific genetic diagnosis is possible by screening for mutations in the calcium-sensing receptor gene. Distinct mutations in this gene have already been identified in several kindreds.

PROGNOSIS AND TREATMENT. Because the disease is compatible with normal life expectancy and is associated with little, if any, morbidity, neck exploration appears to be contraindicated. Successful surgical treatment, moreover, is quite difficult, with permanent hypoparathyroidism or, more commonly, recurrent hypercalcemia, the usual result.

HYPERCALCEMIA ASSOCIATED WITH MALIGNANCY

ETIOLOGY AND PATHOGENESIS. Malignancies can cause hypercalcemia through two non-mutually exclusive mechanisms. First, local osteolytic hypercalcemia is caused by tumor metastatic to bone. Tumor cells may release bone-resorbing factors or so-called osteoclast-activating factors which indirectly lead to bone resorption. Cytokines such as lymphotoxin and interleukin-1 are potent osteoclast-activating factors. Second, humoral hypercalcemia of malignancy is caused by tumor-secreting factors into the circulation that act systemically to increase bone resorption. Such factors may show other PTH-like actions, including increasing urinary cAMP and phosphate excretion and decreasing renal calcium excretion. This condition leads to a syndrome with biochemical features closely resembling those of primary hyperparathyroidism. One such factor commonly associated with many tumors has recently been identified as a polypeptide roughly twice as large as PTH and homologous in amino acid sequence to the biologically active amino-terminus of PTH. This so-called PTH-related peptide may also be secreted by tumors metastatic to bone, so that humoral and local osteolytic mechanisms may combine to cause hypercalcemia. Some tumors cause hypercalcemia through excessive synthesis of $1,25(OH)_2D$, in a manner analogous to that seen in sarcoidosis (see below). A role for additional, as yet unidentified, bone-resorbing agents secreted by tumors has not been excluded.

INCIDENCE. Malignancy-associated hypercalcemia occurs most commonly in patients with bone metastases. Breast carcinoma is one of the most frequent causes. Most subjects with bone metastases are not hypercalcemic because of adequate renal compensatory mechanisms. Slight renal impairment may then provoke hypercalcemia. Treatment of women with breast cancer metastatic to bone with tamoxifen has been associated with acute sharp increases in the serum calcium level. Certain hematogenous neoplasms, such as myeloma and human lymphotropic virus type I-associated leukemia/lymphoma, are frequently associated with hypercalcemia. Humoral hypercalcemia of malignancy is much rarer. It is seen most frequently with squamous carcinomas, but biochemical evidence indicates that almost any tumor type, including breast carcinoma, can produce PTH-related peptide.

CLINICAL MANIFESTATIONS. Malignancy-associated hypercalcemia often develops acutely, may be quite severe (hypercalcemic crisis), and is frequently a grave prognostic sign. In most cases, particularly of the local osteolytic hypercalcemia variety, the underlying neoplasm is clinically evident. An otherwise occult neoplasm may occasionally manifest with humoral hypercalcemia of malignancy. Accurate and rapid diagnosis is critical in such cases because successful tumor removal may be feasible.

DIAGNOSIS. As discussed earlier, PTH radioimmunoassay is the crucial test for excluding coexistent primary hyperparathyroidism. PTH-related peptide fails to cross-react in such assays. Specific immunoassays for this peptide have been developed, and these facilitate diagnosis of tumor secretion of the peptide. Increased urinary cAMP excretion (coupled with low or undetectable PTH measurement) also favors tumor secretion of PTH-related peptide. If both PTH and urinary cAMP levels are low, one is dealing with a vitamin D–mediated or local osteolytic hypercalcemia.

TREATMENT AND PROGNOSIS. Acute, nonspecific treatment of hypercalcemia is instituted if the diagnosis is unclear (see Chapter 194). Definitive treatment must be directed at the underlying neoplasm, if feasible. When tumor treatment is not possible, vigorous treatment of hypercalcemia may be irrelevant. In those cases mediated by vitamin D or lymphokine release, glucocorticoids are often uniquely effective in lowering the serum calcium level.

HYPERCALCEMIA DUE TO GRANULOMATOUS DISEASES

ETIOLOGY AND PATHOGENESIS. Hypercalcemia is caused by unregulated formation of $1,25(OH)_2D$ in granuloma-associated macrophages. Normally, 1-hydroxylation takes place in the kidney and is sensitive to feedback suppression by high serum calcium levels. Unregulated synthesis of $1,25(OH)_2D$ in patients with granulomatous diseases renders them hypersensitive to vitamin D (from the diet or through sun exposure).

INCIDENCE AND PREVALENCE. This form of hypercalcemia has been observed in almost any disease capable of causing granulomas. These diseases include sarcoidosis, tuberculosis, fungal infections, berylliosis, and some lymphomas, such as Hodgkin's disease. Overt hypercalcemia may be seen in only about 10% of patients with sarcoidosis, but hypercalciuria and intestinal hyperabsorption of calcium may occur in almost half of such individuals.

CLINICAL FEATURES. Manifestations are those of the underlying disease, as well as the superimposed effects of hypercalcemia. Because this form of hypercalcemia often coexists with relatively higher serum phosphorus levels than those seen in hyperparathyroidism, soft tissue calcification, nephrocalcinosis, and renal impairment are more common. Patients may present with hypercalcemia and relatively few other findings (e.g., subtle hilar adenopathy in sarcoidosis).

DIAGNOSIS. PTH and urinary cAMP are suppressed. The serum level of $1,25(OH)_2D$ is elevated (in cases of vitamin D intoxication, the serum $1,25(OH)_2D$ level may be normal and only serum $25(OH)D$ is increased).

TREATMENT AND PROGNOSIS. The prognosis depends on that of the underlying disease. Glucocorticoids are extremely effective in lowering the serum calcium level in such cases. Chloroquine has been used effectively in subjects who cannot tolerate glucocorticoid treatment.

Aurbach GD, Marx SJ, Spiegel AM: Parathyroid hormone, calcitonin, and the calciferols. *In* Wilson JD, Foster DW (eds): Williams Textbook of Endocrinology, 8th ed. Philadelphia, WB Saunders, 1992, p 1429. *Detailed description of primary hyperparathyroidism and malignancy-associated and other forms of hypercalcemia, including differential diagnosis and treatment.*

Deftos LJ, Parthemore JG, Stabile BE: Management of primary hyperparathyroidism. Annu Rev Med 44:19, 1993. *Brief review focusing on managing "asymptomatic" patients. Encompasses recommendations from 1991 Consensus Conference on Hyperparathyroidism.*

Edelson GW, Kleerekoper M: Hypercalcemic crisis. Med Clin North Am 79:79, 1995. *Discusses pathogenesis, diagnosis, and treatment of this endocrine emergency.*

Mundy GR, Guise TA: Hypercalcemia of malignancy. Am J Med 103:134, 1997. *Description of pathogenesis, differential diagnosis, and management of various forms of malignancy-associated hypercalcemia.*

Pearce SHS, Brown EM: Disorders of calcium ion sensing. J Clin Endocrinol Metab 81:2030, 1996. *Evidence that distinct mutations in the calcium-sensing receptor gene cause familial hypocalciuric hypercalcemia in heterozygotes and that neonatal*

severe hyperparathyroidism can be caused by mutations in both alleles of the same gene.

Silverberg SJ, Bilezikian JP: Evaluation and management of primary hyperparathyroidism. J Clin Endocrinol Metab 81:2036, 1996. *Recommendations for evaluation, treatment, and follow-up based on extensive personal experience with this disease.*

Singer FR, Adams JS: Abnormal calcium homeostasis in sarcoidosis. N Engl J Med 315:755, 1986. *Reviewed derangements in vitamin D metabolism causing hypercalcemia and hypercalciuria in granulomatous disorders.*

HYPOCALCEMIA

DEFINITION. Hypocalcemia is an abnormal reduction in serum ionized calcium concentration.* Reduction in total serum calcium, as may occur in patients with hypoalbuminemia, does not necessarily reflect a reduction in ionized calcium. Ionized, not total, serum calcium affects neuromuscular function and is therefore the clinically relevant parameter.

ETIOLOGY AND PATHOGENESIS. Normal serum ionized calcium concentration is maintained by the direct actions of PTH on kidney and bone and by the indirect actions (through $1,25(OH)_2D$) on the intestine (see Chapter 261). Hypocalcemic disorders can be divided according to pathogenesis into two broad categories: (1) primary hypoparathyroidism, in which hypocalcemia is due to deficient secretion and/or action of PTH (specific subtypes are discussed under individual headings below); and (2) hypocalcemia due to target organ malfunction (e.g., renal failure, intestinal malabsorption, vitamin D deficiency). Hypocalcemia occurs in this category despite normal or even increased PTH secretion (secondary hyperparathyroidism). In hypoparathyroidism, there is reduced mobilization of calcium from bone, reduced renal reabsorption of calcium, lowered phosphaturia, and reduced $1,25(OH)_2D$ formation with a resultant decrease in intestinal calcium absorption. The end results are hypocalcemia and hyperphosphatemia. Renal failure (see Chapter 103) and acute phosphate loads (as may occur with chemotherapy of certain tumors, such as Burkitt's lymphoma) are other causes of hypocalcemia with hyperphosphatemia. With vitamin D deficiency or malabsorption, hypocalcemia occurs with normal or low serum phosphorus levels (the latter reflecting secondary hyperparathyroidism). Hypocalcemia with low or normal serum phosphorus levels is also seen in acute pancreatitis (attributed to calcium soap formation, but this is unproved) and in some patients with osteoblastic tumor metastases. Table 264–3 summarizes the causes of hypocalcemia.

CLINICAL MANIFESTATIONS. Hypocalcemia of any cause is associated with certain typical signs and symptoms. Most prominent among these is increased neuromuscular excitability. Paresthesias of the fingers, toes, and circumoral region are mild manifestations; in more extreme cases there may be muscle cramping, carpopedal spasm, laryngeal stridor, and convulsions. Symptoms reflect not only the degree of hypocalcemia but also the acuteness of the fall in serum calcium concentration. Patients with long-standing severe hypocalcemia may show surprisingly few symptoms. Factors that acutely alter the balance between ionized and protein-bound calcium may precipitate symptoms. For example, alkalosis lowers ionized calcium; thus hyperventilation may provoke symptoms of tetany. Signs of latent tetany include Chvostek's sign (twitching of the upper lip after tapping on the facial nerve below the zygomatic arch) and Trousseau's sign (carpal spasm after inflating a cuff on the upper arm above systolic blood pressure for 2 to 3 minutes).

Various mental disturbances, such as irritability, depression, and even psychosis, have been attributed to hypocalcemia. Papilledema and other signs of increased intracranial pressure have been reported. Intracranial calcifications, particularly of the basal ganglia, may be seen on plain radiographs and even more frequently on CT. Increased sensitivity to the dystonic effects of phenothiazines has been attributed to basal ganglia calcification. Long-standing hypocalcemia may lead to cataract formation. Cardiac effects of hypocalcemia include a prolonged QT interval and, rarely, congestive heart failure. Dental anomalies depend on age of onset; in children hypocalcemia can cause enamel hypoplasia and failure of the adult teeth to erupt.

DIFFERENTIAL DIAGNOSIS. Measuring serum calcium, phosphorus, and creatinine levels allows one to categorize the form of

---

*See Chapter 261 and Part XXVIII for calcium and phosphorus reference range values.

Hypoparathyroidism
Deficient parathyroid hormone secretion
  Idiopathic (autoimmune)
  Parathyroid hormone gene mutation
  Activating calcium-sensing receptor mutation (autosomal dominant hypo-
    parathyroidism)
  Surgical
  Infiltrative (iron overload, Wilson's disease)
  Functional
    Hypomagnesemia
    Transient postoperative
Deficient parathyroid hormone action (hormone resistance)
  Pseudohypoparathyroidism types Ia and Ib
Normal or Increased Parathyroid Hormone Function
Renal failure
Intestinal malabsorption
Acute pancreatitis
Osteoblastic metastases
Vitamin D deficiency or resistance

hypocalcemia. Hypocalcemia and hyperphosphatemia with normal renal function are pathognomonic of hypoparathyroidism. Low or undetectable PTH by immunoassay despite hypocalcemia confirms the diagnosis. (Rare forms of PTH-resistant hypoparathyroidism show elevated levels of PTH and are discussed further below.) Hypocalcemia and hyperphosphatemia caused by renal failure pose no diagnostic problem. Hypocalcemia with normal or low serum phosphorus levels should prompt measurement of vitamin D metabolites and assessment of gastrointestinal function to check for vitamin D deficiency and malabsorption, respectively. Measurements of PTH should show increased values in such patients, as the normal parathyroids attempt to compensate for hypocalcemia.

TREATMENT. Acute, symptomatic hypocalcemia requires emergency treatment in the form of intravenous calcium infusion. Ten to 20 mL of 10% calcium gluconate solution (contains 10 mg of elemental calcium per milliliter) may be given over 10 to 20 minutes (this may be hazardous in patients taking cardiac glycosides). In less urgent settings, a slow intravenous infusion (over 4 to 8 hours) of 20 mg of elemental calcium per kilogram of body weight may be given. As with hypercalcemic disorders, definitive resolution of hypocalcemia requires treating the underlying disease. In patients with hypoparathyroidism, life-long therapy with vitamin D (with or without oral calcium) is required. This is discussed further under treatment of hypoparathyroidism, below.

HYPOPARATHYROIDISM

DEFINITION. Hypoparathyroidism is defined as deficient PTH secretion and/or action. This condition may lead to overt hypocalcemia and hyperphosphatemia, as discussed above, or may only predispose to hypocalcemia (decreased parathyroid reserve) in times of increased calcium demand, such as pregnancy.

ETIOLOGY AND PATHOGENESIS. **PERMANENT DEFICIENCY IN PARATHYROID HORMONE SECRETION.** This deficiency may result from surgical removal of the parathyroids, from glandular destruction by iron overload (e.g., transfusions in thalassemia) or copper overload (Wilson's disease), and from glandular destruction through a presumed autoimmune mechanism. The latter often has a genetic basis. The parathyroids may fail to develop as part of the DiGeorge syndrome. Some cases termed "idiopathic hypoparathyroidism" may be due to inherited mutations in the PTH gene that prevent synthesis and secretion of PTH. Activating mutations of the calcium-sensing receptor lead to inhibition of PTH secretion at inappropriately low serum ionized calcium levels and are a cause of autosomal dominant hypoparathyroidism.

TRANSIENT DEFICIENCY IN PARATHYROID HORMONE SECRETION. Reversible hypoparathyroidism can be caused by hypomagnesemia. The latter may compromise both PTH secretion and action. Magnesium replacement corrects the defect. Transient hypoparathyroidism may also result from suppression of normal parathyroids by parathyroid adenomas or other causes of hypercalcemia. This condition rarely lasts more than 1 week. Surgical injury to the parathyroids is another postulated cause of transiently reduced hormone secretion.

DEFICIENCY IN PARATHYROID HORMONE ACTION. Secretion of a biologically inactive form of PTH is a theoretical, but unproven, cause of deficient PTH action. Target-organ resistance to PTH appears to be the major cause of this form of hypoparathyroidism, which was termed "pseudohypoparathyroidism" by Albright, who described it as the first example of a hormone-resistance disorder. Subsequent studies indicated that the defect in this disease occurs before formation of cAMP (a second messenger of PTH action) because affected subjects lack the normal brisk increase in urinary cAMP excretion observed after infusing PTH in normal individuals. There are at least two forms of pseudohypoparathyroidism. In type Ia disease, a 50% deficiency has been found in the Gs protein that couples PTH (and many other) receptors to the enzyme that forms cAMP, adenylyl cyclase. This deficiency may limit normal cAMP production in response to PTH as well as to other hormones, such as thyroid-stimulating hormone. As a result, patients with this form of the disease show many abnormalities (e.g., hypothyroidism, hypogonadism) in addition to hypoparathyroidism. In affected subjects from several families with type Ia disease, distinct mutations that prevent synthesis of normal Gs protein have been found in the gene encoding the Gs protein. Inheritance of the mutation is autosomal dominant. In subjects with type Ib disease, the Gs protein is normal, and resistance is limited to PTH. A defective PTH receptor is a theoretical but unproven basis for this disease. In some subjects, hypocalcemia and hyperphosphatemia are associated with radiographically evident osteitis fibrosa cystica. This finding suggests selective renal, as opposed to skeletal, resistance to PTH action. The pathogenesis is unclear.

INCIDENCE. All forms of hypoparathyroidism are relatively rare. The incidence of surgical hypoparathyroidism varies widely as a function of the skill of the surgeon.

CLINICAL MANIFESTATIONS. The manifestations generally associated with hypocalcemia have been discussed above. The clinical features unique to each form of hypoparathyroidism reflect the underlying disease. In autoimmune forms, there may be associated endocrine deficiency, most frequently Addison's disease, as well as a T-cell defect predisposing to mucocutaneous candidiasis. Alopecia and vitiligo may also be seen. In pseudohypoparathyroidism type Ib, the appearance is normal, but in type Ia disease, affected individuals show a constellation of abnormal physical findings termed Albright's hereditary osteodystrophy (Fig. 264-3). These findings include obesity, short stature, round face and short neck, metacarpal and metatarsal shortening (most often fourth and fifth), shortening and broadening of the distal phalanges, and subcutaneous calcifications. Such individuals often show slight mental retardation and associated endocrine abnormalities, most commonly hypothyroidism (without goiter) and hypogonadism. First-degree relatives of patients with pseudohypoparathyroidism type Ia may show the physical features of Albright's osteodystrophy without evidence of hormone resistance. This condition has been termed pseudopseudohypoparathyroidism. Rarely, individuals with pseudohypoparathyroidism (more often of the Ib type) have radiographic evidence of osteitis fibrosa cystica and elevated serum levels of bone-derived alkaline phosphatase.

DIFFERENTIAL DIAGNOSIS. Low or undetectable serum PTH in the face of hypocalcemia, hyperphosphalemia, and normal renal function establishes the diagnosis of hormone-deficient hypoparathyroidism. Diagnosis of the underlying disease depends on history (e.g., neck surgery), physical findings (e.g., candidiasis, alopecia), and additional laboratory tests (e.g., evidence for hypoadrenalism). Inappropriately elevated urine calcium in subjects with hypoparathyroidism (with or without a family history) suggest the diagnosis of autosomal dominant hypoparathyroidism caused by activating mutation of the calcium-sensing receptor. Such mutations not only cause inappropriate suppression of PTH secretion but also inappropriate increase in renal calcium excretion. DNA diagnosis is possible but is not routinely available for clinical use. Antibodies to parathyroid antigens have been detected in the autoimmune form of the disease, but this test is not available for routine clinical use. An elevated level of serum PTH measured by immunoassay in a subject with hypocalcemia, hyperphosphatemia, and normal renal function suggests hormone-resistant hypoparathyroidism. PTH infusion (at present with commercially available synthetic 1–34 peptide) and measurement of urinary cAMP excretion can be performed to

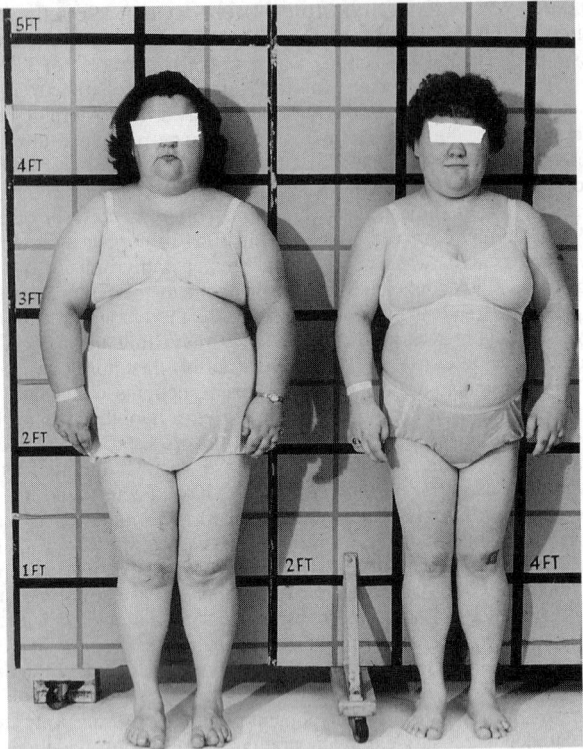

FIGURE 264–3 ■ Phenotypic features of Albright's hereditary osteodystrophy. A mother (left) and daughter display many of the features of Albright's osteodystrophy, including obesity, short stature, round face, and short neck. Metacarpal and metatarsal shortening manifest as shortened fourth and fifth fingers (right hands of both subjects) and shortened fourth toes (left feet of both subjects), respectively. Both subjects show resistance to parathyroid hormone (PTH) and thyroid-stimulating hormone, as well as deficient Gs protein activity, characteristic of pseudohypoparathyroidism type Ia. (From Spiegel AM: Pseudohypoparathyroidism. *In* Scriver CR, Beaudet AL, Sly WS, Valle D (eds). The Metabolic Basis of Inherited Disease, 6th ed. New York, McGraw-Hill, 1989, p 2013.)

confirm PTH resistance. Physical appearance can help distinguish type Ia from type Ib pseudohypoparathyroidism, as can testing for other endocrinopathies, such as hypothyroidism. Measurement of Gs protein and detection of mutations in the corresponding gene are not routinely available tests.

TREATMENT. Transient forms of hypoparathyroidism may not require treatment. Reversible forms should be treated appropriately, i.e., magnesium replacement for hypomagnesemia. In permanent hormone-deficient hypoparathyroidism, hormone replacement therapy is not practical. Parathyroid autografting is effective in some patients with surgical hypoparathyroidism. When this is not feasible, and also in subjects with pseudohypoparathyroidism, life-long treatment with oral vitamin D is required. Vitamin D$_2$ ergocalciferol (generally 50,000 U/day), is inexpensive by comparison with the active metabolite, 1,25(OH)$_2$D (generally 0.25 μg/day). The latter has the theoretical advantage of more rapid onset (and in case of toxicity, offset) of action, but with appropriate monitoring, vitamin D$_2$ can be used very effectively. Oral calcium salts (1 to 2 g of elemental calcium per day in divided doses) may be added for individuals whose dietary calcium intake is highly variable or inadequate. The goal of treatment is the lowest serum calcium concentration compatible with avoidance of symptoms, because without PTH, urinary calcium excretion (and the possibility of nephrolithiasis) is increased at any filtered load of calcium. Both serum and urine calcium levels, as well as renal function, must be monitored. In patients with autosomal dominant hypoparathyroidism due to calcium-sensing receptor mutation, particular care must be taken to avoid overcorrecting hypocalcemia, because such patients are particularly susceptible to renal calcification and nephrolithiasis given the tendency to hypercalciuria in this disease. In forms of hypoparathyroidism that have associated endocrinopathies, appropriate hormone replacement therapy should be instituted.

Aurbach GD, Marx SJ, Spiegel AM: Parathyroid hormone, calcitonin, and the calciferols. *In* Wilson JD, Foster DW (eds): Williams Textbook of Endocrinology, 8th ed. Philadelphia, WB Saunders, 1992, p 1456. *Detailed description of clinical and pathophysiologic features of hypocalcemic disorders and the multiple forms of hypoparathyroidism.*

Pearce SHS, Williamson C, Kifor O, et al: A familial syndrome of hypocalcemia with hypercalciuria due to mutations in the calcium-sensing receptor. N Engl J Med 335: 1115, 1996. *Description of gain-of-function mutations in this receptor that cause a unique form of hypoparathyroidism.*

Spiegel AM: Pseudohypoparathyroidism. *In* Scriver CR, Beaudet AL, Sly WS, et al (eds): The Metabolic Basis of Inherited Disease, 6th ed. New York, McGraw-Hill, 1989, p 2013. *Extensive discussion of clinical features and pathogenesis of hormone-resistant forms of hypoparathyroidism.*

265 CALCITONIN AND MEDULLARY THYROID CARCINOMA

Leonard J. Deftos ■ *Robert F. Gagel*

Calcitonin (CT) is a 32-residue peptide secreted primarily by the thyroidal C-cells in mammals and by the embryologically related ultimobranchial gland in submammals. The main biologic effect of CT is to decrease bone resorption by inhibiting the osteoclast. This effect decreases the concentration of blood calcium, with a nadir directly related to bone turnover; thus, the hypocalcemia may be slight in normal adults but considerable when bone resorption is increased pathologically in disease states or physiologically during bone growth. This property of CT makes it an effective drug for hyperresorptive diseases, such as Paget's disease, osteoporosis, and hypercalcemia. The physiologic significance of other reported effects of CT is not well established. The calciuric effect of CT is seen primarily with pharmacologic doses of the hormone. A stimulatory effect on bone formation may be attributed to a CT-related molecule rather than to CT itself. However, an analgesic effect of CT continues to receive considerable attention and may be related to neuroendocrine features of the hormone. In addition to its role in skeletal physiology and treatment, CT is a serum and tumor marker for medullary thyroid carcinoma (MTC), which is the signal tumor of multiple endocrine neoplasia (MEN) type 2 (Table 265–1) and its variants (Table 265–2).

CALCITONIN

BIOCHEMISTRY. The 32-residue structure of CT, determined for nine species, reveals a common 1,7 amino-terminal disulfide bridge and carboxy-terminal proline. Seven of the nine amino-terminal residues are identical in all CT molecules. The interspecies structural differences in the rest of the molecule cause the submammalian (ultimobranchial) CT molecules to be more potent in mammals than the mammalian CT molecules. Thus, the potent salmon form of the hormone is widely used for treatment in humans. The greater chemical basicity of these submammalian CT species probably accounts for their increased potency. In contrast to the other major skeletal peptide hormone, parathyroid hormone (PTH), a biologically active fragment of CT has not been identified, and the entire molecule seems to be necessary for biologic activity.

SECRETION AND PRODUCTION. The most important secretory regulation of CT is mediated by ambient calcium. An acute increase in blood calcium concentration increases the secretion of

Table 265–1 ■ COMPONENTS OF MULTIPLE ENDOCRINE NEOPLASIA TYPE 2 AND THEIR FREQUENCY BASED ON AVERAGE FIGURES FROM THE LITERATURE

COMPONENT	MEN TYPE 2A (%)	MEN TYPE 2B (%)
Medullary thyroid carcinoma	97	90
Pheochromocytoma	30	45
Hyperparathyroidism	50	Rare
Mucosal neuroma syndrome	—	100

MEN 2A (Sipple syndrome): MTC, pheochromocytoma, parathyroid hyperplasia, or adenomas
MEN 2A with Hirschsprung's disease
MEN 2A with cutaneous lichen amyloidosis (CLA) over the upper back
Familial medullary thyroid carcinoma (FMTC): Hereditary MTC alone
MEN 2B: MTC, pheochromocytoma, mucosal neuromas, marfanoid features

CT, and an acute decrease in blood calcium level decreases the secretion of CT. The effects of chronic changes in blood calcium concentration on secretion have not been as well defined. Chronic hypercalcemia may stimulate CT production, but this compensatory response may be limited. Chronic hypocalcemia seems to increase CT storage in C-cells. Although a variety of other factors have been reported to stimulate CT secretion, only pentagastrin and its related peptides are consistent additional secretagogues. The high concentration of pentagastrin necessary to stimulate secretion does not support the presence of a normal entero–C-cell secretory pathway. Nevertheless, pentagastrin and calcium are clinically important agents for evaluating CT secretion by both normal and malignant C-cells.

The effect of gonadal steroids and age on CT production remains controversial. It is well established that blood concentrations of CT are higher in males than females and in children than adults. Some studies report a decline in CT secretion during adulthood and a stimulation of CT secretion by estrogens and testosterone. These observations have led to the hypothesis that age- and menopause-related declines in CT production contribute to the corresponding declines in bone mass seen in the elderly, especially postmenopausal women. These observations support the use of CT in treating osteoporosis, but more complex hormonal abnormalities underlie this skeletal disorder.

MEDULLARY THYROID CARCINOMA

Medullary thyroid carcinoma is a tumor of the CT-producing C-cells of the thyroid gland. These cells migrate from the neural crest to the thyroid gland and to other sites of the diffuse neuroendocrine system during embryogenesis in mammals. In submammals, these cells form their own distinct organ, the ultimobranchial gland. The neural crest origin of C-cells accounts for their production of a variety of biologically active substances. This embryologic origin may also explain the common association of MTC with other neuroendocrine tumors. Thus, MTC can occur as part of MEN type 2 or sporadically.

PATHOLOGY. A palpable tumor is the most common physical finding in the patient with MTC. The tumor is usually firm and located in the middle or upper lobes of the gland. Bilateral tumors are common in MEN. Calcification can be present in the tumor, and this may result in a radiographic pattern that is characteristic enough to help diagnose it clinically. Similarly, amyloid present in the tumor can assist in histologic diagnosis. However, cytologic diagnosis is made difficult by the fact that the cells of MTC can be arranged in a variety of patterns. Therefore, the diagnosis of MTC is conclusively made by demonstrating CT in the tumor by immunohistology. Hyperplasia of the C-cells antedates the frank malignancy of MTC, especially in the familial forms of the tumor. C-cell hyperplasia is often too subtle to be appreciated by light microscopy, and immunohistology for CT is necessary to make this diagnosis. The advent of genetic testing for MEN provides additional impetus for distinguishing MTC from other thyroid tumors.

TUMOR BEHAVIOR. The clinical behavior of MTC is usually intermediate between that of aggressive anaplastic thyroid cancer and that of indolent papillary and follicular thyroid cancer. Local lymph node spread is common, and metastases to lung and bone can occur. MTC in which all or most of the cells produce CT may have a better prognosis than a more heterogeneous tumor in which CT production is not uniform. Even in the most aggressive tumors, CT production is usually sufficient to serve as a specific marker for this thyroid cancer. However, there may be rare instances in which CT production has ceased. The 5-year survival of those with metastatic MTC approximates 50%. Survival can vary from several months to three decades after diagnosis. Patients under age 2 years with metastatic disease and over age 50 years with only localized

disease have been reported. C-cell hyperplasia can occur in those as young as age 2 years and as old as 45 years. Therefore, the tumor can be rapidly aggressive, leading to death within months after diagnosis, or it can be indolent and compatible with survival for decades.

MULTIPLE ENDOCRINE NEOPLASIA (MEN) (See Chapter 244)

MTC can occur in association with other endocrine tumors as part of a multiple endocrine neoplasia, designated MEN type 2, to distinguish it from MEN type 1, which consists of parathyroid, pancreatic, and pituitary tumors. MEN type 2 is an autosomal dominant syndrome that can be clinically classified into two subtypes, type 2A and 2B (see Table 265–1).

PHEOCHROMOCYTOMA. Pheochromocytoma is a component of MEN type 2A and 2B. Bilateral and multifocal pheochromocytomas are very common in this clinical setting, with an incidence of more than 70%. This figure contrasts with a bilateral incidence of usually less than 10% for sporadic pheochromocytomas and only 20 to 50% for familial pheochromocytomas. Other hereditary forms of bilateral pheochromocytoma include von Hippel-Lindau disease and isolated hereditary pheochromocytoma. Pheochromocytomas are rarely seen in MEN 1. Adrenal medullary hyperplasia is a predecessor of the pheochromocytomas seen with MTC. The increase in adrenal medullary mass results from diffuse or multifocal proliferation of adrenal medullary cells, primarily those found within the head and body of the glands. The biochemical as well as clinical manifestations of this tumor may be subtle, so diagnostic tests for pheochromocytoma should be pursued vigorously in MEN type 2.

HYPERPARATHYROIDISM. Hyperparathyroidism is much more common in MEN type 2A than in MEN type 2B (and it also occurs in MEN type 1). The presence of hyperparathyroidism thus should always make one consider the possibility of MEN. The differential diagnosis of hereditary hypercalcemia includes familial hypercalcemic hypocalciuria, familial parathyroid adenoma-jaw tumor syndromes, familial parathyroid hyperplasia, MEN 1, and MEN 2A. Parathyroid hyperplasia is more common than adenoma, an important consideration for surgical treatment. Although a calcium-mediated functional relationship between hyperparathyroidism and MTC has been suggested, the two neoplasias are probably linked to the same gene.

MULTIPLE MUCOSAL NEUROMAS. The presence of neuromas with a centrofacial distribution is the most consistent component of MEN type 2B. The most common location of neuromas is the oral cavity. The oral lesions are almost invariably present by the first decade and in some cases even at birth. Mucosal neuromas can also be present in the eyelid, conjunctiva, and cornea. The most prominent microscopic feature of neuromas is an increase in the size and number of nerves. These hypertrophied nerve fibers are readily seen with a slit lamp and occasionally by direct ophthalmologic examination.

Gastrointestinal tract abnormalities are part of the multiple mucosal neuroma syndrome. The most common of these is gastrointestinal ganglioneuromatosis, which usually occurs in the small and large intestines but has also been noted in the esophagus and stomach. The lesions are sometimes associated with swallowing abnormalities, megacolon, diarrhea, and constipation. The diarrhea may also be due to excess production of bioactive substances by the MTC. In any case, diarrhea is the most common symptom of MTC.

MARFANOID HABITUS. Patients with this component have a tall, slender body with long arms and legs, an abnormal ratio of upper to lower body segments, and poor muscle development. Other features associated with the marfanoid habitus may include dorsal kyphosis, pectus excavatum or pectus carinatum, pes cavus, and high-arched palate. In contrast to patients with true Marfan's syndrome, these patients do not have aortic arch abnormalities, ectopia lentis, homocystinuria, or mucopolysaccharide abnormalities.

PATHOGENESIS. HEREDITARY MTC (FAMILIAL MTC AND MEN 2). Genetic linkage studies mapped the gene for MEN 2 to a centromeric chromosome 10 locus, and c-ret proto-oncogene mutations were subsequently identified for the associated clinical syndromes (see Tables 265–1 and 265–2). Two broad classes of mutations have been identified (Fig. 265–1). Six specific codons (609, 611, 618, 620, 630, and 634) in the extracellular domain of the tyrosine kinase receptor encoded by c-ret change a conserved cysteine to another amino acid. Codon 634 mutations, and by inference other extracellular domain mutations, cause receptor dimerization and activation and initiate the transformation of C-cells. The second class of mutations are intracellular domain mutations, with the most common located at codon 918 (see Fig. 265–1). This coding change results in receptor activation in the absence of dimerization. Other intracellular domain mutations occur at codons 768, 790, 791, 804, 891, and 883. The clinical syndromes associated with each of these mutations is described in Figure 265–1. Mutations of other components of the Ret signaling system (glial cell–derived neurotrophic factor [GDNF] and the GDNF-alpha receptor) have not been identified in MTC (see Fig. 265–1).

In familial MTC, the earliest identified histologic abnormality associated with the c-ret proto-oncogene mutations is C-cell hyperplasia. It is unclear whether additional mutations are required for the development of MTC, but mutations at other chromosomal locations (1p, 3q, 13q, 22q) could be involved in the progression of this malignant tumor, analogous to the progression observed in hereditary forms of colon carcinoma.

GERMLINE MUTATIONS IN APPARENTLY SPORADIC MTC. The discovery of c-ret proto-oncogene mutations in MTC has uncovered unidentified kindreds with hereditary MTC in which the proband masqueraded as sporadic MTC. Approximately 6% of patients with apparently sporadic MTC have germline c-ret mutations indicative of familial MTC. Although most are members of previously unidentified kindreds, some are examples of de novo mutations, most commonly of codon 634. This has led to the identification of additional family members at risk for development of MTC. These studies recommend c-ret proto-oncogene testing all patients with apparently sporadic MTC.

SOMATIC MUTATIONS IN SPORADIC MTC. Somatic mutations (non-germline mutations acquired during cell growth and differentiation) of codon 918 are found in approximately 25% of sporadic tumors (see Fig. 265–1) and evidence suggests that sporadic MTCs with this mutation are more aggressive and associated with shorter survival. In tumors with a codon 918 mutation, it is not clear whether the mutations is the initiating abnormality or one that is acquired in the progression from a less to a more malignant phenotype.

DIAGNOSIS. GENETIC TESTING. Genetic testing is used to identify individuals, especially children, at risk for development of familial MTC and MEN 2. These tests are available from a variety of commercial sources (http://endocrine.mdacc.tmc.edu). The test can be performed on a single peripheral blood sample. The presence of a specific mutation and the propensity to develop the clinical syndrome of MEN 2 or FMTC essentially indicates full concordance. Genetic testing can be complicated by a variety of laboratory or sampling errors. It is thus prudent to repeat the genetic test on a separate peripheral blood sample, preferably in more than one laboratory. It is reasonable to exclude an individual with two or more negative genetic test results from further screening efforts. Although genetic testing will have a great impact on the diagnosis and treatment of MTC, it will have little impact on management of adrenal medullary and parathyroid disease, which manifestations generally develop later. Appropriate screening recommendations for these neoplasia should be followed.

CALCITONIN. Overexpression of the CT gene is the molecular hallmark of MTC. This overexpression results in the increased production of CT by the tumor and increased secretion of the hormone into blood. As a result, most patients with MTC have an increased circulating concentration of CT that can be detected by radioimmunoassay and increased tumor concentrations that can be demonstrated directly by immunohistology or through increased messenger RNA (mRNA) expression by in situ hybridization. Usually, the basal blood concentration of CT is sufficiently elevated to be diagnostic of the presence of the tumor. In the early stages of the diseases, however, the basal concentrations of CT cannot be readily distinguished from normal. In these circumstances, provocative testing of CT secretion can reveal the presence of the abnormal C-cells. Such testing is also clinically indicated for the relative of a patient with familial MTC when early diagnosis is sought. Screening is also recommended for apparently sporadic tumors because family history can be unreliable. The two most commonly used provocative agents for CT secretion are calcium and the synthetic gastrin analogue pentagastrin, alone or in combination. Most tumors respond to either agent with a diagnostic increase in CT secretion. CT blood measurements can also be used to evaluate therapy and monitor tumor recurrence. Interpretation must be made according to the specific parameters of the procedure used.

The primary genetic abnormality in MEN type 2A and 2B have been localized to chromosome 10. For MEN 2A, the genetic defect has been localized to the *RET* oncogene, which encodes a tyrosine kinase. Molecular genetic techniques allow gene carrier status to be assigned in a patient at risk and with a well-documented pedigree. However, confounding factors such as mistaken diagnoses and nonpaternity can complicate genetic analysis. The ethical considerations that surround all genetic screening should be considered in the light of the effective and curative treatment that is available for

Clinical Syndrome	Codon of Ret Mutated
MEN 2A FMTC	609
	611
	618
	620
	630
	634
	790
FMTC	768
	791
	804
	891
MEN2A/CLA	634
MEN 2/ Hirschsprung	609
	618
	620
MEN2B	883
	918
Sporadic MTC (Somatic)	630 (rare)
	768 (rare)
	883 (rare)
	918 (25%)

FIGURE 265–1 ■ The Ret proto-oncogene (RET)/glial cell-derived neurotrophic factor receptor (GDNFR)-alpha complex. Mutations of the c-ret proto-oncogene receptor are causative for multiple endocrine neoplasia type 2A (MEN 2A), familial medullary thyroid carcinoma (FMTC), MEN 2A/cutaneous lichen amyloidosis (MEN 2A/CLA), MEN 2 associated with Hirschsprung's disease, or MEN 2B. Mutations of the extracellular cysteine-rich region of the receptor (Cys) and intracellular tyrosine kinase domain (TK) have been identified as germline mutations in the indicated syndromes. Somatic mutations of the c-ret proto-oncogene have also been identified in sporadic MTC. GDNF = glial cell-derived neurotrophic factor, which is a small peptide ligand for the RET/GDNF receptor complex.

the components of MEN type 2A and 2B. Nevertheless, genetic diagnosis represents a substantial advance in management of the inherited forms of MTC.

TREATMENT. SURGERY. Surgery is the treatment of choice for the three neoplasia in MEN 2. Because all are potentially lethal, especially MTC and pheochromocytoma, but can be cured in their early stages, aggressive therapy is warranted. Management of the individual components of MEN 2 generally follows the accepted procedures for each neoplasm. The sequence of treatment, however, is guided by several important principles. In adults with the fully formed MEN 2A syndrome, pheochromocytomas, commonly bilateral, should be treated first because they can be life threatening. Management of thyroid and parathyroid disorders follows. Accepted surgical procedures include unilateral or bilateral adrenalectomy for diseased glands by anterior, posterior, or laparoscopic approaches or unilateral cortical sparing adrenalectomy in an attempt to preserve adrenal cortical function. Bilateral adrenalectomy at an early age is mandatory in the rare kindred with malignant pheochromocytoma. In adults with palpable MTC (> 1 cm) metastasis to local lymph nodes is common, and a total thyroidectomy and compartment oriented lymph node dissection should be performed to enhance the likelihood of complete removal of all tumor. Hyperparathyroidism may be managed by either subtotal parathyroidectomy or total parathyroidectomy with transplantation of parathyroid tissue to the non-dominant forearm.

GENETIC TESTING AND MANAGEMENT. The identification of a mutation of the c-ret proto-oncogene indicates that the affected individual has a greater than 90% probability of development of MTC at some point during life. Thyroidectomy should be based on genetic testing and performed early in childhood. The identification of metastatic disease in children as young as 6 years suggests it is appropriate to perform thyroidectomy before this age in children with MEN 2A or FMTC. An alternative approach is to initiate calcium or pentagastrin testing on gene carriers at age 5 years with removal of the thyroid gland at the time of a positive test, an approach which has been the mainstay of diagnosis and management for the past 25 years. However, this approach fails to identify C-cell disease before development of microscopic MTC in more than 50% of children. In children with MEN 2B (codon 883 or 918 c-ret mutations), thyroidectomy should be performed in the first months of life because of reports of early metastasis in these children. A small percentage of kindreds with proven germline transmission of MTC have no identifiable mutation of the c-ret proto-oncogene. CT testing should be continued in these kindreds.

MANAGEMENT OF PERSISTENT POSTOPERATIVE CALCITONIN MEASUREMENTS IN PATIENTS WITH MTC. A vexing problem for clinicians is the persistence of calcitonin elevations following primary surgical management. The major question is whether reoperation to remove all identifiable lymph nodes in the neck (compartment-oriented dissection) has value. A recent body of experience has accumulated regarding reoperative strategy in patients with persistent disease. In the selection of these patients it is important to perform a careful search for distant metastatic disease and to exclude hepatic, bone, and pulmonary metastasis by appropriate imaging studies. Some perform laparoscopy with direct hepatic visualization or selective catheterization of the arterial and venous supply of the liver with measurement of pentagastrin-stimulated CT in hepatic venous effluent to exclude hepatic metastasis. In patients with no evidence of distant metastatic disease, reoperative compartment-oriented lymphadenectomy may be appropriate. Approximately one of five carefully selected patients will have the serum CT normalized following microsurgical dissection (CT values nondetectable following pentagastrin). No long-term follow-up studies in this group of patients has been performed to determine whether this type of surgical intervention affects morbidity or mortality related to MTC, yet the lack of other effective therapy for this disease makes it a reasonable consideration.

Burns DM, Birnbaum RS, Roos BA: A neuroendocrine peptide derived from the amino terminal half of rat procalcitonin. Mol Endocrinol 3:140, 1989. *An exposition of the complexities of CT gene expression.*

Deftos LI: Radioimmunoassay for calcitonin in medullary thyroid carcinoma. JAMA 227:403, 1974. *Early study of the application of CT radioimmunoassay to the diagnosis of MTC.*

Deftos LI, Roos BA: Medullary thyroid carcinoma and calcitonin gene expression. Bone Miner Res 6:267, 1989. *A detailed exposition of multiple endocrine neoplasia and the regulation of calcitonin-gene products.*

Eng C, Clayton D, Schuffenecker I, et al: The relationship between specific RET proto-oncogene mutations and disease phenotype in multiple endocrine neoplasia type 2. International RET mutation consortium analysis. J Am Med Assoc 276:1575, 1996. *Genotype/phenotype correlation of clinical syndromes with specific mutations of the c-ret proto-oncogene.*

Gagel RF, Cote GJ, Martins Bugalho MJG, et al: Clinical use of molecular information in the management of multiple endocrine neoplasia type 2A. J Intern Med 238:333, 1995. *Discussion of problems and pitfalls of genetic testing in MEN 2.*

Mulligan LM, Kwok JBJ, Healey CS, et al: Germ-line mutations of the *RET* protooncogene in multiple endocrine neoplasia type 2A. Nature 363:458, 1993. *Identification of the genetic abnormality in MEN IIA.*

Wohllk N, Cote GJ, Bugalho MMJ, et al: Relevance of RET proto-oncogene mutations in sporadic medullary thyroid carcinoma. J Clin Endocrinol Metab 81:3740, 1996. *Identification of germline c-ret proto-oncogene mutations in patients with sporadic MTC.*

266 RENAL OSTEODYSTROPHY

Marie-Claude Monier-Faugere
■ *Hartmut H. Malluche*

Renal osteodystrophy is a metabolic bone disease that develops secondary to chronic failure of the kidneys' excretory and endocrine functions. Renal osteodystrophy encompasses a wide variety of derangements in mineral and bone metabolism.

INCIDENCE AND PREVALENCE

The earliest histologic abnormalities of bone are seen after a relatively mild reduction in the glomerular filtration rate (creatinine clearances between 70 and 40 mL/min). Histologic changes are found in virtually all patients with end-stage renal disease (ESRD). The incidence of ESRD in the United States is 56,600 patients per year (215 per million per year) and the prevalence is 218,000 patients (825 per million).

PATHOGENESIS AND HISTOPATHOLOGY

Pathogenetic Factors

The kidneys have a well-established pivotal role in maintaining mineral homeostasis and hormonal balance. With progressive loss of excretory kidney function, abnormalities in divalent ions and secondary hyperparathyroidism typically develop early.

FACTORS IMPLICATED IN THE DEVELOPMENT OF SECONDARY HYPERPARATHYROIDISM. In advanced renal failure a variety of factors have been identified as direct stimulators of parathyroid hormone (PTH) secretion, including hypocalcemia, low levels of circulating calcitriol (the active vitamin D metabolite), and more recently, hyperphosphatemia. However, most patients with mild chronic renal failure exhibit increased serum PTH levels without alterations in serum levels of calcium, phosphorus, and calcitriol.

EARLY RENAL FAILURE. The early sequence of events is still not fully elucidated. However, the early stages of renal failure are marked by some signs of end-organ resistance to vitamin D, such as a mild decrease in intestinal calcium absorption and an altered calciuric response to oral supplementation of calcitriol. Calcitriol exerts its action by binding to vitamin D receptors, which interact with specific sequences of nuclear DNA, the vitamin D response elements that control genomic synthesis of many proteins, including PTH. In early renal failure, binding of the hormone–vitamin D receptor complex to the vitamin D response element has been found to be reduced, which could lead to less suppressive effects of physiologic blood levels of calcitriol on PTH synthesis and therefore PTH overproduction. The exact mechanisms implicated in impaired binding of the hormone-vitamin D receptor complex to the vitamin D response element are not fully elucidated. In experimental studies on rats, alterations in the vitamin D receptor heterodimer partner (retinoid X receptor) have been observed; however, this mechanism has not been proved in humans. Other alterations in accessory nuclear factors, abnormal phosphorylation, and changes in conformation of the vitamin D receptor or chemical alteration of the DNA binding domain may be involved in the impaired vitamin D receptor response to calcitriol.

ADVANCED RENAL FAILURE. With more advanced nephron loss, the phosphate load of the remaining functioning nephrons progressively increases. This increased load results in inhibition of C1-α-hydroxylase, the enzyme responsible for the conversion of 25-hydroxyvitamin D to its active metabolite 1,25-dihydroxyvitamin D (calcitriol). Calcitriol deficiency in turn further decreases intestinal calcium absorption and thus results in hypocalcemia. Calcitriol deficiency in advanced renal failure is associated with a decreased number of vitamin D receptors, in particular, receptors in parathyroid glands. Because calcitriol has been shown to suppress the expression of pre-pro-PTH mRNA, lower circulating calcitriol levels together with a low number of vitamin D receptors in patients with ESRD result in stimulation of both synthesis and secretion of PTH. Low blood ionized calcium levels rapidly stimulate PTH secretion, whereas high calcium concentrations suppress it. The relationship between ionized calcium and PTH follows a sigmoidal pattern. The action of calcium on parathyroid gland cells is associated with modulation of intracellular cyclic adenosine monophosphate (cAMP). The short-term stimulation induced by low calcium is due to release of stored pre-formed hormone and an increase in the number of cells that secrete PTH. More prolonged hypocalcemia induces changes in intracellular PTH degradation with reutilization of degraded hormone and mobilization of the secondary storage pool. Within days or weeks of the onset of hypocalcemia, pre-pro-PTH mRNA expression is stimulated. This effect is exerted through a recently described negative calcium response element located in the upstream flanking region of the gene for PTH. Calcium exerts its effects on parathyroid gland cells through a recently isolated G protein–coupled calcium-sensing receptor located on the cell membrane. Expression of the calcium receptor has been shown to be suppressed by calcitriol deficiency and stimulated by calcitriol administration, thus suggesting an additional regulatory mechanism of the active vitamin D metabolite on PTH production. The decreased number of calcium-sensing receptors with low circulating calcitriol may, at least in part, explain the relative insensitivity of parathyroid gland cells to calcium in patients undergoing dialysis (higher set point).

When the glomerular filtration rate reaches levels of less than 25% of normal, the serum phosphorus content rises. At this level of reduced renal function, the ability of the remaining nephrons to increase phosphate excretion is exhausted. Increased serum phosphorus levels further decrease serum calcium through physicochemical binding and suppress C1-α-hydroxylase activity, which results in further lowering of the circulating levels of calcitriol. Moreover, a direct stimulatory effect of phosphorus on parathyroid gland cells, independent of calcium and calcitriol, has recently been observed in patients with ESRD. The mechanism of the direct action of phosphorus on PTH secretion has not been fully elucidated.

All the mechanisms described above result in increased production of PTH and increased parathyroid gland mass. The size of the parathyroid glands progressively increases with time in dialyzed patients and parallels serum PTH levels. This increase in size is mainly due to diffuse cellular hyperplasia. Monoclonal cell growth may also develop and result in the formation of tumor-like nodules that have less or no vitamin D and calcium-sensing receptors and that promote parathyroid gland resistance to calcitriol and calcium.

FACTORS AFFECTING PARATHYROID HORMONE PRODUCTION AND ITS EFFECTS ON BONE. Other systemic factors such as α-adrenergic agonists, dopamine, prostaglandin E, secretin, and phosphodiesterase inhibitors that alter the cAMP content of parathyroid cells may increase PTH secretion. Recently, the inflammatory cytokine interleukin-8 has been found to stimulate PTH secretion. The effect of magnesium in regulating PTH secretion is similar to that of calcium, but not as potent. Moreover, peripheral degradation of PTH is reduced in uremia, and numerous PTH fragments circulate, thus prolonging the effects of PTH on target organs.

Accumulation of aluminum in bone and other organs such as the parathyroid glands may occur in patients undergoing dialysis or before the initiation of dialysis. Aluminum accumulation in the parathyroid glands results in decreased secretion of PTH and sup-

pression of bone turnover. In addition, aluminum inhibits renal and intestinal C1-α-hydroxylase activity and may thus further contribute to reduced levels of calcitriol. Possible sources of aluminum include high concentrations in the water used for dialysis, prescription of aluminum-containing phosphate binders, and aluminum in drinking water, infant formula, and other liquids or solid food.

Bone is an important buffer for excess acid production in patients with ESRD. Metabolic acidosis has been shown to stimulate bone resorption and suppress bone formation, thereby resulting in negative bone balance.

Patients with ESRD are in a hypogonadal state, and some of them are treated with glucocorticoids, which have an impact on bone metabolism. Patients maintained on chronic dialysis have retention of β_2-microglobulin and alterations in cytokines, growth factors, PTH, and vitamin D receptors that may be involved in the regulation of bone remodeling, thus affecting the histologic pattern of renal osteodystrophy.

Histologic Pattern

Renal osteodystrophy is not a uniform bone disease. Depending on the relative contribution of the different pathogenic factors, patients with ESRD will have different histologic patterns.

PREDOMINANT HYPERPARATHYROID BONE DISEASE. Excess parathyroid hormone results in a marked increase in bone turnover. Osteoclasts, osteoblasts, and osteocytes are found in abundance (Fig. 266–1). Disturbed osteoblastic activity results in a disorderly production of collagen, which is deposited not only toward the trabecular surface but also in the marrow cavity, thereby causing peritrabecular and marrow fibrosis. The non-mineralized component of bone, i.e., osteoid, is increased, and the normal three-dimensional architecture of osteoid is frequently lost. Osteoid seams no longer exhibit their usual birefringence under polarized light; instead, a disorderly arrangement of woven osteoid and woven bone with a typical crisscross pattern under polarized light is seen. The mineral apposition rate and number of actively mineralizing sites are increased, as documented under fluorescent light after the administration of time-spaced tetracycline markers.

LOW-TURNOVER BONE DISEASE. Low-turnover uremic osteodystrophy is the other end of the spectrum of renal osteodystrophy. The histologic hallmark of this group is a profound decrease in bone turnover, i.e., low number of active remodeling sites resulting in bone resorption and suppressed bone formation. The majority of trabecular bone is covered by lining cells, with few osteoclasts and osteoblasts. Bone structure is predominantly lamellar. The extent of mineralizing surfaces is markedly reduced. Usually only a few thin single labels of tetracycline are observed. Two histologic subgroups can be identified in this type of renal osteodystrophy, depending on the sequence of events leading to a decline in the number and/or

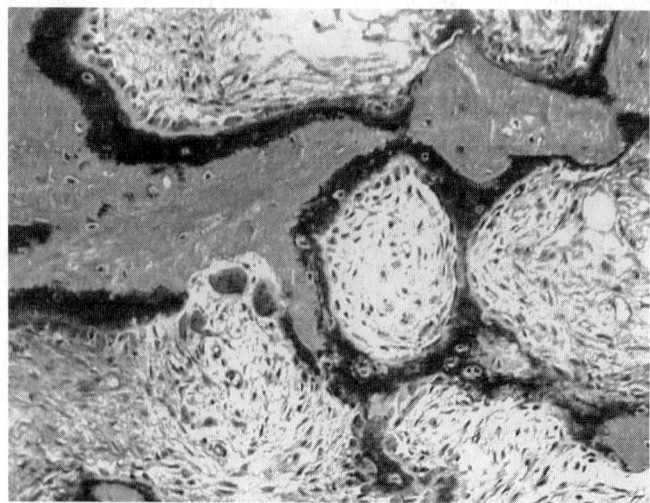

FIGURE 266–1 ■ Predominant hyperparathyroid bone disease with a high fraction of the trabecular surface covered by osteoid seams, many osteoblasts and osteoclasts, and marrow fibrosis; undecalcified 3-μm-thick section of iliac bone (brightfield light microscopy; modified Masson-Goldner stain; original magnification, ×125).

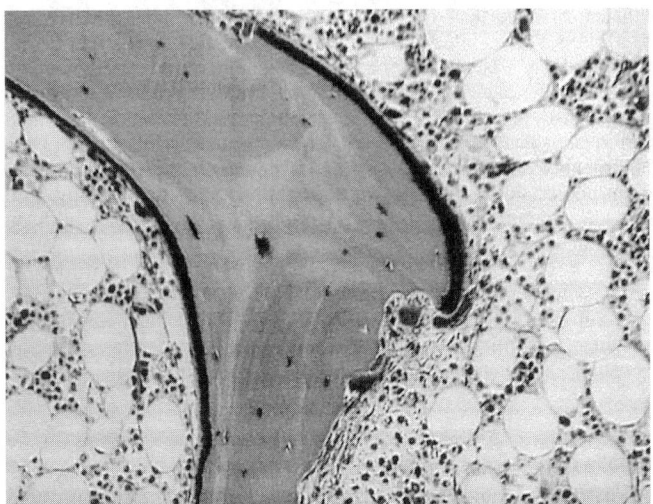

FIGURE 266–2 ■ Low-turnover osteomalacia demonstrating an accumulation of osteoid, a high osteoid surface–bone surface ratio, thick osteoid seams, and absence of active osteoblasts or osteoclasts; undecalcified 3-μm-thick section of iliac bone (brightfield light microscopy; modified Masson-Goldner stain; original magnification, ×160).

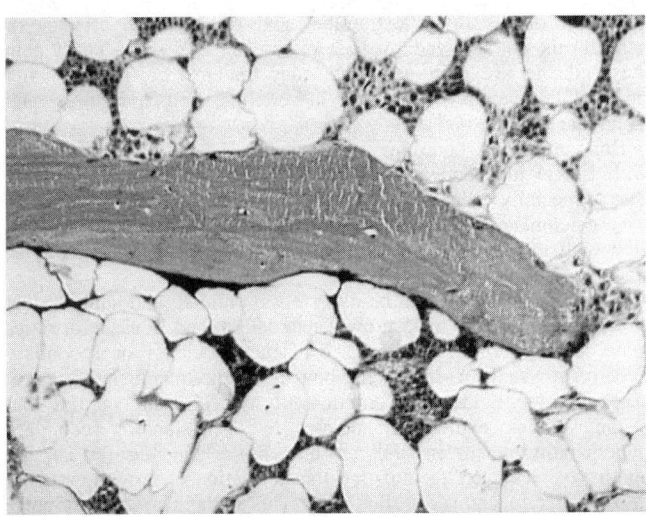

FIGURE 266–4 ■ Mixed uremic osteodystrophy. Few osteoblasts, several osteoclasts, and mild peritrabecular fibrosis; and an undecalcified, 3-μm-thick section of human iliac bone (brightfield light microscopy; modified Masson-Goldner stain; original magnification, ×125).

activity of the osteoblasts: low-turnover osteomalacia and adynamic bone disease.

Low-turnover osteomalacia is characterized by an accumulation of unmineralized matrix in which a diminution in mineralization precedes or is more pronounced than the inhibition of collagen deposition. Unmineralized bone represents a sizable fraction of trabecular bone volume. The increased lamellar osteoid volume is due to the presence of wide osteoid seams that cover a large portion of the trabecular surface (Fig. 266–2). The occasional presence of woven bone buried within the trabeculae indicates past high bone turnover. When osteoclasts are present, they are usually seen within trabecular bone or at the small fraction of trabecular surface left without osteoid coating.

With adynamic uremic bone disease, the reduction in mineralization is coupled with a concomitant and parallel decrease in bone formation. Adynamic uremic bone disease is characterized by few osteoid seams and few bone cells (Fig. 266–3).

MIXED UREMIC OSTEODYSTROPHY. Mixed uremic osteodystrophy is caused primarily by hyperparathyroidism and defective mineralization with or without increased bone formation. These features may coexist in varying degrees in different patients. Increased numbers of heterogeneous remodeling sites can be seen (Fig. 266–4). The number of osteoclasts is usually increased. Be-

cause active foci with numerous cells, woven osteoid seams, and peritrabecular fibrosis coexist next to lamellar sites with a more reduced activity, greater production of lamellar or woven osteoid causes an accumulation of osteoid with normal or increased thickness of osteoid seams. Whereas active mineralizing surfaces increase in woven bone with a higher mineralization rate and diffuse labeling, mineralization surfaces may be reduced in lamellar bone with a decreased mineral apposition rate.

ASSOCIATED FEATURES. BONE ALUMINUM ACCUMULATION. Aluminum accumulates in bone at the mineralization front, at the cement lines, or diffusely. The extent of stainable aluminum at the mineralization front correlates best with histologic abnormalities in mineralization. Aluminum deposition is most severe in cases of low-turnover osteomalacia. However, it can be observed in all histologic forms of renal osteodystrophy. In patients in whom an increased aluminum burden develops, bone mineralization and bone turnover progressively decrease. These abnormalities are reversed with removal of the aluminum.

OSTEOPOROSIS AND OSTEOSCLEROSIS. With progressive loss of renal function, cancellous bone volume is increased along with a loss of cortical bone. Patients undergoing chronic dialysis might have a loss or gain in bone volume depending on bone balance. In the case of negative bone balance, bone loss occurs in cortical and cancellous bone and is more rapid when bone turnover is high. When the bone balance is positive, osteosclerosis may be observed when osteoblasts are active in depositing new bone, thus superseding bone resorption. When bone turnover is low, however, positive bone balance results in hypercalcemia and possibly extraosseous calcification.

CLINICAL MANIFESTATIONS

Patients with mild to moderate renal insufficiency are rarely symptomatic. Symptoms appear in patients with advanced renal failure. Clinical manifestations are preceded, however, by an abnormal biochemical profile that should alert the physician and prompt steps to prevent more severe complications. When symptoms occur, they are usually insidious, subtle, non-specific, and slowly progressive. Patients with ESRD are prone to a variety of symptoms related to alterations in bone and mineral metabolism.

BONE PAIN, FRACTURES, AND SKELETAL DEFORMITIES. Bone pain is usually vague, ill defined, and deep seated. It may be diffuse or localized in the lower part of the back, hips, knees, or legs. Weight bearing and changes in position commonly aggravate it. Bone pain may progress slowly to the degree that patients are completely incapacitated. Bone pain in patients with ESRD usually does not cause physical signs; however, local tenderness may be apparent with pressure. Occasionally, pain can occur suddenly at

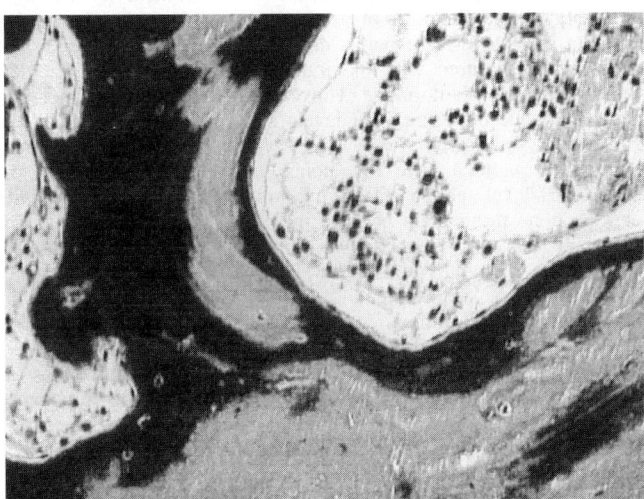

FIGURE 266–3 ■ Adynamic bone disease with no accumulation of osteoid, and absence of osteoblasts and osteoclasts; undecalcified 3-μm-thick section of iliac bone (brightfield light microscopy; modified Masson-Goldner stain; original magnification, ×125).

one joint of the lower extremities and mimic acute arthritis or periarthritis not relieved by heat or massage. A sharp chest pain may indicate rib fracture. Spontaneous fractures or fractures after minimal trauma may also occur in vertebrae (crush fractures) and in tubular bones.

Bone pain and bone fractures can be observed in all patients with ESRD independently of the underlying histologic bone disease, especially when osteoporosis is present. However, low-turnover osteomalacia and aluminum-related bone disease are associated with the most severe bone pain and the highest incidence of fractures and incapacity.

Skeletal deformities can be observed in children and adults. Most children with ESRD have growth retardation, and bone deformities may develop from vitamin D deficiency (rickets) or secondary hyperparathyroidism. In rickets, bowing of the long bones is seen, especially the tibiae and femora, with typical genu valgum that becomes more severe with adolescence. Long-standing secondary hyperparathyroidism in children may be responsible for slipped epiphyses secondary to impaired transformation of growth cartilage into regular metaphyseal spongiosa. This complication most commonly affects the hips, becomes obvious in pre-adolescence, and causes limping but is usually painless. When the radius and ulna are involved, ulnar deviation of the hands and local swelling may occur. In adults, skeletal deformities can be observed in cases of severe osteomalacia or osteoporosis and include lumbar scoliosis, thoracic kyphosis, and recurrent rib fractures.

MYOPATHY. Proximal muscle weakness is fairly common in dialysis patients, particularly those with aluminum toxicity, severe hyperparathyroidism, or osteomalacia. Its onset is usually gradual and mainly affects the lower extremities. Proximal myopathy is manifested by difficulty rising out of a chair or climbing stairs. Patients may have a characteristic waddling gait.

PRURITUS. Itching affects 40 to 90% of patients with ESRD. Pruritus can occur before the institution of dialysis and can disappear after regular dialytic therapy. However, symptoms more often begin about 6 months after the start of dialysis and persist thereafter. Pruritus may be localized and mild or generalized and severe and prevent sleep and interfere with the patient's normal activities.

The mechanisms underlying pruritus in patients with ESRD are poorly understood. Several possible factors have been implicated (alone or in combination), such as secondary hyperparathyroidism, hypercalcemia, and increased calcium phosphate production, in addition to dry skin (xeroderma), intradermic microprecipitation of divalent ions, peripheral neuropathy, allergic reactions, hypersensitivity, histamine, proliferation of skin mast cells, hypervitaminosis A, iron deficiency, and abnormal fatty acid metabolism.

SOFT TISSUE CALCIFICATIONS, TUMORAL CALCINOSIS, AND CALCIPHYLAXIS. Asymptomatic vascular calcification is common in patients with ESRD. Soft tissue calcification may occur in the eyes and be manifested as band keratopathy in the sclerae or induce an inflammatory response known as the red eye syndrome in the conjunctiva. These types of calcifications are usually associated with hyperparathyroidism or increased calcium phosphate product. Calcium deposits are also found in the lungs and lead to restrictive lung disease. Deposits in the myocardium might cause arrhythmias, annular calcifications, or myocardial dysfunction. Most soft tissue calcifications are attributed to secondary hyperparathyroidism or to the increased calcium phosphate product associated with it. However, they have also been described in patients with adynamic bone disease. This diversity could be explained by increased calcium and/or phosphate release from bone in patients with severe hyperparathyroidism and an inability to maintain normal mineral accretion in patients with adynamic bone disease.

Tumoral calcinosis is a form of soft tissue calcification that usually involves the periarticular tissues. Calcium deposits may grow to enormous size and interfere with the function of adjacent joints and organs. Although this type of calcification is usually associated with high calcium phosphate product, its exact pathogenesis is poorly understood. It may also be associated with certain ill-defined intrinsic factors. Similar to soft tissue calcification, it is observed with severe hyperparathyroidism and low-turnover bone disease.

The syndrome of calciphylaxis is characterized by vascular calcification in the tunica media. These calcifications induce painful violaceous skin lesions that progress to ischemic necrosis. This syndrome is associated with serious complications and often death. Calciphylaxis has been associated with high serum calcium phosphate product and severe secondary hyperparathyroidism. However, it can also be seen in patients with normal or mildly elevated serum phosphate or PTH levels. The pathogenesis of calciphylaxis is probably multifactorial because hyperparathyroidism, high calcium phosphate production, steroid therapy, vitamin D therapy, iron overload, aluminum toxicity, and protein C deficiency have all been implicated.

DIALYSIS DEMENTIA. Clinically, dialysis dementia is a form of progressive neurologic abnormality and includes dysarthria, dysphagia, amnesia, apraxia, mutism, myoclonic jerks, facial grimacing, seizures, and ultimately, severe dementia and death. This condition is usually associated with severe aluminum accumulation.

DIAGNOSIS

The only unequivocal tool for the exact diagnosis of renal osteodystrophy is bone biopsy for mineralized bone histology after tetracycline double labeling and aluminum staining. It determines, on the same bone sample, the precise level of bone formation, mineralization, bone resorption, bone turnover, and extent of bone aluminum deposition, if present. The results serve as a basis for appropriate use of tailored therapeutic regimens.

In the absence of bone biopsy, the physician needs to estimate the level of bone turnover, the presence of osteomalacia, and the possibility of bone aluminum toxicity. Abnormalities in serum calcium, phosphorus, and alkaline phosphatase levels indicate severe renal osteodystrophy but are useless when used alone to indicate bone turnover or osteomalacia. Hypercalcemia may be observed in severe hyperparathyroidism or adynamic bone disease, especially with vitamin D therapy. Hyperphosphatemia is an indication of non-compliance with phosphate binders and/or severe hyperparathyroidism secondary to increased release of phosphorus from bone. High serum levels of alkaline phosphatase are usually seen in both osteomalacia and predominant hyperparathyroidism.

Skeletal radiographic abnormalities are seen when the disease is advanced and include erosive cortical defects in the skull (pepper pot skull), acro-osteolysis of the clavicula, and erosion of the terminal finger phalanges. A rugger-jersey appearance of the spine and a ground-glass appearance of the skull, ribs, pelvis, and metaphysis of tubular bones reflect advanced cancellous changes. In severe hyperparathyroid bone disease, pseudocysts or brown tumors may be observed. However, signs of increased bone resorption may be seen on radiographs reflecting past resorption activity, which may have been succeeded by the accumulation of osteoid. Because osteoid is radiolucent, the superimposed osteomalacia will be missed by x-ray examination. Looser zones that are straight bands of radiolucency abutting onto the cortex and running perpendicular to the long axis of bone are of relatively low sensitivity and low specificity for the diagnosis of osteomalacia.

Serum PTH levels are better indicators of bone turnover, especially when measured with the immunoradiometric assay that detects only the intact hormone. However, careful assessment of the predictive value of serum PTH levels for bone turnover shows that all patients with serum PTH levels within or below the normal range (<65 pg/mL) have low bone turnover and that values of serum PTH levels above 450 pg/mL are 100% and 95.5% specific for high bone turnover in patients maintained on hemodialysis and peritoneal dialysis, respectively. For the majority of dialyzed patients, i.e., those with serum PTH levels between 65 and 450 pg/mL, bone turnover cannot be predicted accurately. In addition to serum PTH values, certain risk factors for low bone turnover have been isolated and include peritoneal dialysis, diabetes, advanced age, high calcium content in the dialysate, high doses of phosphate binders, aggressive vitamin D therapy, or previous parathyroidectomy. However, in individual patients, discrepancies between risk factors, PTH levels, and bone turnover are frequent, and this situation calls for bone biopsy.

Aluminum accumulation may be seen at any level of bone turnover or any serum PTH level. Although correlations exist between random serum aluminum levels and the extent of stainable aluminum in bone, no threshold value allows a clear-cut distinction between patients with and patients without aluminum-related bone disease. The deferoxamine infusion test is advocated to improve the sensitivity of random serum aluminum levels. An increase in serum aluminum levels of greater than 200 μg/L 48 hours after a standardized infusion constitutes a positive result. This test does improve the sensitivity of predicting aluminum-related bone disease, but the specificity is greatly reduced. Both a positive deferoxamine test and a PTH level less than 200 pg/mL will make the diagnosis of aluminum-related bone disease with almost absolute certainty. However, the sensitivity is greatly reduced and many patients will have false-negative results.

PREVENTION AND THERAPY

Therapeutic intervention should begin before far-advanced bone disease develops, that is, not later than at the time of institution of dialysis. Secondary hyperparathyroidism can be prevented by avoiding deviations of serum phosphorus and calcium levels from normal.

CONTROL OF SERUM PHOSPHORUS AND CALCIUM. None of the available dialytic methods is efficient in removing phosphorus because of compartmentalization and slow efflux of phosphorus from the intracellular space. Dialysis removes approximately 3 g of phosphorus per week. Therefore, in patients with ESRD, dietary phosphate restriction has to be implemented. However, because phosphate is present in most protein-containing food products, phosphate restriction is limited by the need for appropriate dietary protein intake. With the current recommendations, the protein intake of dialyzed patients should be at least 1 g/kg/day, which provides a minimum of 1 g of phosphorus per day. Therefore, the addition of phosphate binders is needed in most patients. Currently used phosphate binders are calcium carbonate and calcium acetate. They are most effective when given with meals and in proportion to the size of the meal. Calcium citrate should be avoided because it promotes intestinal aluminum absorption. Aluminum-containing phosphate binders, even though more potent than calcium salts, should not be used because of the risk of aluminum-related bone disease. However, in severe cases of hyperphosphatemia, when calcium-containing phosphate binders have proved to be insufficient, low doses of aluminum-containing phosphate binders can be used in addition to calcium salts for a limited period.

Hypocalcemia in chronic renal failure may be corrected by control of serum phosphorus and also by administration of calcium salts between meals.

USE OF VITAMIN D AND ITS METABOLITES. Replacement of the missing hormone calcitriol in patients with chronic renal failure is an established practice. Calcitriol therapy is effective in suppressing secondary hyperparathyroidism. In moderate hyperparathyroidism with or without mineralization defects, daily oral administration of calcitriol (0.25 to 2.0 μg/day of Rocaltrol) usually decreases serum PTH levels, suppresses bone turnover, and improves mineralization. It is advisable to start with low doses and increase the daily dose in steps of 0.25 μg if serum calcium levels do not increase (at least 0.5 mg/dL) after 2 weeks of therapy. However, episodes of hypercalcemia may occur but can be circumvented by decreasing oral calcium salts and/or by lowering the dialysate calcium content. Despite these measures, however, hypercalcemia may persist. Alternative approaches have been developed and include pulse oral (Rocaltrol) or intravenous (Calcijex) calcitriol administration two or three times per week at doses as high as 3 μg. Both measures are effective even though the positive response is clearly reduced if deposits of stainable aluminum are present in bone or when the parathyroid glands undergo monoclonal growth transformation and become refractory to the action of calcitriol. Newly developed vitamin D analogues with similar potency to calcitriol but with less hypercalcemic effects are currently under investigation. 19-Nor-1-α-25-dihydroxyvitamin D_2 (Zemplar) has recently been introduced as a less hypercalcemic vitamin D analogue for control of secondary hyperparathyroidism. However, its effects on bone are not known at this time.

To prevent severe osteomalacia, deficiency in the parent vitamin D, 25(OH)-vitamin D should be ruled out and corrected if found abnormally low.

PARATHYROIDECTOMY. Despite treatment, overt secondary hyperparathyroidism develops in some patients and may necessitate parathyroidectomy. Indications for parathyroidectomy include

(1) persistent hypercalcemia despite no vitamin D treatment and modulation of the dialysate calcium concentration, (2) persistent hyperphosphatemia and high calcium phosphate production despite aggressive dietary counseling and compliance with prescriptions, (3) progressive and symptomatic soft tissue calcification with high bone turnover (including calciphylaxis), (4) severe progressive and symptomatic hyperparathyroidism when rapid reduction in PTH is required and vitamin D pulse therapy has failed, and (5) refractory pruritus. Before parathyroidectomy, histologic evidence of severe hyperparathyroidism and absence of aluminum accumulation need to be documented.

The most frequently used surgical approaches to parathyroidectomy are subtotal parathyroidectomy and total parathyroidectomy with parathyroid autotransplantation. Subtotal parathyroidectomy risks the possibility of inadequate reduction in parathyroid gland mass or the recurrence of hyperparathyroidism in the remaining tissue. These complications might require re-exploration of the neck, which can be difficult because of the formation of scar tissue. Re-exploration may be facilitated by marking the remaining gland with a metallic clip or a suture. Total parathyroidectomy with parathyroid autotransplantation in the forearm allows easy access to the residual parathyroid tissue if necessary. However, migration of the transplanted cells into the venous circulation and the muscles of the forearm has been reported. The success of both techniques relies on the expertise and experience of the surgeon.

Patients undergoing parathyroidectomy require careful follow-up and meticulous management. Postoperative hypocalcemia should be anticipated and treated with oral and intravenous calcium. The use of calcitriol may minimize the need for large doses of calcium salts; however, it may interfere with successful uptake of the transplanted gland. A reasonable approach would be the use of intravenous calcitriol administered at the end of each dialysis treatment for two to three treatments before parathyroidectomy, followed by the lowest dose of oral calcitriol needed.

REMOVAL OF ALUMINUM. Any therapeutic maneuver that lowers plasma aluminum levels and creates a concentration gradient across the bone–extracellular fluid membrane will be able to move aluminum from bone to blood. Aluminum is 80% protein bound; therefore, only 20% of total aluminum is ultrafilterable. Elimination of aluminum from bone through normal turnover and by completely withdrawing aluminum sources is very slow and may take years. However, aluminum removal is greatly enhanced by use of the chelator agent deferoxamine (Desferal*). Deferoxamine increases the complex bound fraction of aluminum and facilitates its removal through dialysis. An appropriate dose range appears to be 5 to 15 mg/kg one to three times per week infused slowly over a 2-hour period. Deferoxamine is relatively safe, but rare ocular complications such as cataracts, altered color vision, night blindness, or scotoma have been reported. Episodes of hypotension caused by a vasodilatory effect of the drug can occur during deferoxamine therapy. Hypotension can be precipitated by rapid infusion ($>$15 mg/kg/hour) and the use of low-calcium dialysate. This condition is usually easily reversible; however, in some cases angina has been reported. Nausea, vomiting, and neuromuscular excitability are usually transient. The association between deferoxamine therapy and infection has been a subject of controversy. Although numerous case reports of bacteremia and mucormycosis occurring with deferoxamine therapy have been published, a large survey did not confirm that deferoxamine increases the risk of bacteremia in dialysis patients. The possible relationship between deferoxamine therapy and mucormycosis—although rare—represents a very serious complication. Therefore, unequivocal documentation of aluminum overload is required before long-term deferoxamine therapy is begun.

TREATMENT OF ADYNAMIC BONE DISEASE. When adynamic bone disease is not the result of bone aluminum toxicity, measures to avoid oversuppression of PTH and bone turnover are indicated. These measures include discontinuation of vitamin D therapy and reduction in calcium-containing phosphate binders and/or the dialysate calcium content. However, no specific treatment is available for adynamic bone disease at present. Thus preventive measures

---

*Note: Deferoxamine is approved by the Food and Drug Administration for the chelation and thus removal of iron but not for aluminum removal.

should be carefully considered because of the morbidity and risk of hypercalcemia associated with this condition.

Bushinsky DA (ed): Renal Osteodystrophy. Philadelphia, Lippincott-Raven, 1998. *A compilation of chapters on all aspects of renal osteodystrophy. Virtually every significant reference is cited.*

Malluche HH, Faugere MC: Atlas of Mineralized Bone Histology. New York, Karger, 1986. *A well-illustrated presentation of information obtained from bone biopsies for mineralized bone histology and histomorphometry, in particular, in patients with renal osteodystrophy.*

Malluche HH, Faugere MC: Renal bone disease 1990: An unmet challenge for the nephrologist. Kidney Int 38:193, 1990. *A concise description of current knowledge, contemporary challenges, and future directions of management of patients with renal osteodystrophy.*

Qi Q, Monier-Faugere MC, Geng Z, Malluche HH: Predictive value of serum parathyroid hormone levels for bone turnover in patients on chronic maintenance dialysis. Am J Kidney Dis 26:622, 1995. *Presents information on the limitations of serum parathyroid hormone levels in predicting bone turnover in dialyzed patients. Useful for practicing nephrologists.*

267 PAGET'S DISEASE OF BONE (OSTEITIS DEFORMANS)

John A. Kanis

DEFINITION. Paget's disease of bone is a focal disorder of skeletal metabolism in which all the elements of skeletal remodeling (resorption, formation, and mineralization) are increased. Increased bone formation results in the disorganized assembly of collagen, which give rise to bony enlargement and deformity.

ETIOLOGY. The cause is unknown. A viral infection of osteoclasts is postulated on the basis of finding viral nucleocapsids of the Paramyxoviridae in affected osteoclasts. Such findings are, however, not specific and are seen in some other rare disorders of bone turnover (pycnodysostosis and some cases of osteopetrosis [see Chapter 268]). Canine distemper is caused by a member of the Paramyxoviridae, and an association between owning dogs and Paget's disease has been reported. A positive family history in approximately 10% of patients suggests a dominant pattern of susceptibility, with weak associations with the HLA Dqwl antigens in the United States and with A9 and B15 in the United Kingdom (see Chapter 278).

PREVALENCE AND EPIDEMIOLOGY. Paget's disease is the 2nd most common disorder of bone, outstripped only by osteoporosis. It is most commonly found in the United Kingdom, where the prevalence is 5% of the population older than 55 years and is roughly equal between genders. The frequency of symptomatic disease rises with age. The paucity of evidence for the occurrence of new lesions in symptomatic disease, however, suggests a high modal incidence in early middle age that declines rapidly thereafter, but with a variable latency between onset of the disorder and its radiographic or clinical expression.

Although most common in the United Kingdom, it is also common in places such as Australia, New Zealand, South Africa, and the United States, where significant British immigration occurred in the past, but the disease occurs with a lower frequency in native-born individuals than in immigrants. The disorder is extremely rare in the Nordic countries, the Arab Middle East, China and Japan and among Australian aboriginals. Intermediate rates are found in France, Germany, Italy, and Spain. Some evidence suggests that the incidence of Paget's disease is falling.

PATHOPHYSIOLOGY AND HISTOPATHOLOGY. The disease is characterized by increased metabolic activity of bone surfaces. Bone remodeling normally occupies 10 to 15% of bone surfaces, and at affected sites this activity may be increased 5- to 10-fold. Osteoclast numbers are increased, as is their size, and they may contain up to 100 nuclei. Osteoclast competence is decreased, but their plethora results in an increase in bone resorption with crenated erosion cavities subsequently filled in by the activity of osteoblasts. The irregular cement lines give rise to a mosaic patchwork appearance at bone histologic examination. New bone that is formed is often woven rather than lamellar and is thus structurally less competent and occupies more space. Mineralization rates are normal, but because abnormally large volumes of bone are undergoing mineralization, the surface covered with unmineralized osteoid is increased. Marrow fibrosis and hypervascularity are also features.

Remodeling throughout the cortex increases its porosity and blurs the distinction between cortical and cancellous bone. An imbalance between formation and resorption characteristically results in increased bone size and deformity.

CLINICAL AND LABORATORY MANIFESTATIONS. The extent of disease involvement is markedly heterogeneous. Paget's disease may involve only one bone. More frequently, multiple sites are involved, typically in an asymmetrical distribution. The most common sites are the pelvis, lumbar spine, and femur; one or more of these sites are affected in more than 75% of cases.

More than 95% of patients with Paget's disease are asymptomatic. The most common problems encountered are bone pain, skeletal deformity, and fracture (Table 267–1). Apart from fracture, the onset is insidious and 30% of patients have had symptoms for more than 10 years before diagnosis. It may be difficult to distinguish bone pain arising from Paget's disease from that caused by arthritis, particularly of the hip and the spine. Deformity is an initial complaint in one fifth of patients. Obvious bone enlargement is seen, particularly in the limbs and also in the skull and facial bones. Bone enlargement contributes significantly to the neurologic complications and more uncertainly to joint disease. The most frequent deformity of long bones is bowing, which is characteristically lateral in the case of the femur and anterior in the case of the tibia.

The incidence of fissure fractures is significantly greater in patients with bowing. Fissure fractures may be symptomatic and may herald complete fractures, but many patients have indolent pain, particularly on weight bearing associated with local tenderness. Complete fractures of the long bones occur most commonly in the femur, followed by the tibia and the forearm, which together account for up to 90% of pathologic fractures of long bones. They commonly follow trivial injury, and unlike the case in osteoporosis, femoral fractures are less frequently cervical and more usually subtrochanteric or involve the shaft.

Neurologic complications are common and are among the more serious clinical problems. A variety of neurologic problems arise from platybasia. Cranial disease also results in deafness, vertigo, and tinnitus. Spinal syndromes most frequently occur when Paget's disease affects the thoracic spine. They are usually associated with enlarged vertebrae and decreased diameter of the spinal canal with

Table 267–1 ■ **CLINICAL FEATURES AND COMPLICATIONS OF PAGET'S DISEASE**

Common
  Bone pain—pagetic, articular
  Fracture—long bones, vertebral bodies
  Neurologic—deafness
  Deformity and enlargement of bones
Uncommon
  Pain—fissure fracture
  Spinal neurologic syndromes
  Hypercalciuria of immobilization or fracture
  Vascular bleeding from bone during surgery
  Extraskeletal (aortic) calcification
  Osteosarcoma and other bone tumors
Rare
  Cardiovascular disease
  Cranial nerve lesions (except VIII)
  Brain stem and cerebellar lesions
  Hypercalcemia of immobilization
  Extramedullary hematopoiesis
  Epidural hematoma
Significance uncertain
  Gout
  Pseudogout
  Angioid streaks
  Hyperparathyroidism
  Urolithiasis

From Kanis JA: Pathophysiology and Treatment of Paget's Disease of Bone, 2nd ed. London, Martin Dunitz, 1998.

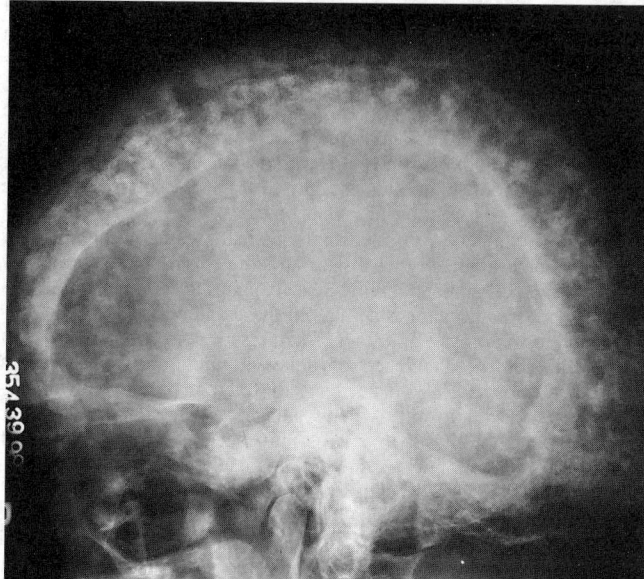

FIGURE 267-1 ■ Advanced involvement of the skull with marked thickening of the entire vault, areas of osteolysis, and patchy new bone formation resulting in a "cotton-wool" appearance.

cord or root compression. Also, the highly vascular pagetic bone may divert the blood supply from neural tissue.

Cardiac output may be increased and give rise to high-output failure in patients with extensive disease when 30% or more of the skeleton is involved. Sarcoma arising in pagetic bone, a rare but serious complication of the disorder, accounts for most cases of sarcoma in the population 50 years or older. The pelvis and femora are common sites, followed by the humerus, face, and skull. Benign and malignant giant cell tumors may also occur. New pain developing in a patient with long-standing Paget's disease not attributable to microfractures should arouse a high degree of suspicion. Other manifestations include the development of a large mass or pathologic fracture.

RADIOGRAPHIC FEATURES. The early phase of osteolytic activity is sometimes seen clearly in the skull as osteoporosis circumscripta or as a V-shaped advancing front in a long bone. A 2nd mixed

phase shows evidence of patchy osteolysis and sclerosis, which is the most common radiographic finding. The 3rd phase is that of predominant bone sclerosis (Fig. 267–1). Thickening of the cortices is characteristic, along with enlargement of the long bones (Fig. 267–2). Intracortical resorption results in a loss of the corticomedullary junction and accentuation of trabecular markings. The combination of all these features is virtually diagnostic, so bone biopsy is rarely required. The average patient has six lesions affecting 14% of the skeleton. In approximately 10 to 20% of symptomatic patients, the disorder is mono-ostotic. As a general rule, scintigraphy is more sensitive than radiography, but 2 to 3% of radiographically overt lesions may not be associated with increased scintigraphic uptake (so-called burnt-out Paget's disease).

The pelvis is the most common site affected; evidence is found in approximately two thirds of patients. Narrowing of the joint space of the hip is common. Most patients show medial or concentric narrowing of the joint space; degenerative osteoarthrosis more frequently causes narrowing of the superior aspect. Computed tomography is also useful to assess the cause of pain at the spine and in the investigation for osteosarcoma.

BIOCHEMICAL MANIFESTATIONS. Extracellular calcium homeostasis is almost invariably normal despite the massive increase in bone turnover. Hypercalciuria and more rarely hypercalcemia may occur with prolonged immobilization or fracture. Serum activity of alkaline phosphatase, in part derived from osteoblasts, is most often used to measure the extent of skeletal involvement. Increased bone resorption can be assessed by the urinary excretion of hydroxyproline, which in Paget's disease is derived largely from the collagen destruction of bone. Urinary excretion of pyridinoline cross-links is a more specific and sensitive marker. In untreated patients, serum activity of alkaline phosphatase and urinary excretion of hydroxyproline are closely correlated, and both correlate with the extent of disease. Up to 10% of patients with symptomatic Paget's disease have values of alkaline phosphatase within the laboratory reference range, and this figure is even higher in the case of hydroxyproline.

TREATMENT. Data are insufficient to recommend medical treatment to asymptomatic patients, except in the presence of rapidly advancing osteolytic disease in the long bones of the lower limb, where the risk of pathologic fracture is high. Medical treatment has centered on specific inhibitors of osteoclast-mediated bone resorption, including the bisphosphonates, calcitonins, mithramycin, and gallium nitrate.

CALCITONINS. A variety of calcitonins have been used. The most

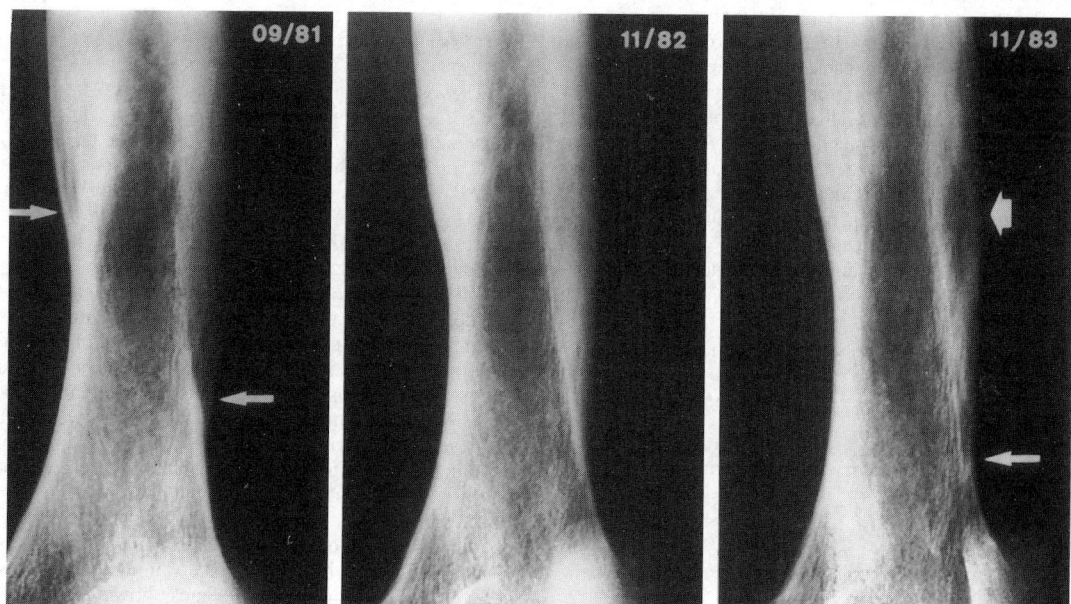

FIGURE 267-2 ■ Sequential radiographs of the distal end of the femur at the dates shown. *Left,* Distinction between Paget's and normal bone *(arrows),* the osteolytic front, and expansion of bone diameter at the affected site. Treatment with a bisphosphonate *(center)* induced infilling of the resorption font. Relapse after treatment *(right)* was associated with a new area of osteolysis *(thick arrow)* and progression of the resorption front. (From Kanis JA: Pathophysiology and Treatment of Paget's Disease of Bone, 2nd ed. London, Martin Duntiz, 1998.)

common is synthetic salmon calcitonin (salcatonin), which may be given by subcutaneous injection, 50 to 100 U daily or on alternate days. In several European countries salcatonin is available as a nasal spray. Treatment results in an early decrease in bone resorption, which can be monitored by the fall in urinary excretion of hydroxyproline and, after several weeks, a decrease in the serum activity of alkaline phosphatase. On average, these indices fall to 40 to 50% of pre-treatment values. Treatment is associated with relief of bone pain, healing of osteolytic lesions, decreased cardiac output, and improvement of neurologic disease. Deafness is rarely reversed, but progression may be prevented.

Disease, activity recurs once treatment is stopped, so if long-term control is required, calcitonin must be given indefinitely. In the case of bone pain, relief may occur for many months or years after treatment is stopped, and therefore intermittent treatment is worthwhile. The escape phenomenon describes failure to maintain a biochemical response despite continued treatment or even increasing the dose. In some cases this acquired resistance appears to be associated with the development of salcatonin antibodies, in which case a biochemical response is elicited with an alternative calcitonin. No serious side effects of calcitonin are reported, but transient nausea or flushing develops in up to one third of patients, and in 5 to 10% of patients long-term treatment cannot be tolerated.

BISPHOSPHONATES. These pyrophosphate analogues are adsorbed onto hydroxyapatite, particularly at sites of resorption. As with calcitonin, an early effect of treatment is to decrease bone resorption, followed by a later decrease in bone formation, as marked by alkaline phosphatase. Unlike the calcitonins, their effects persist for many months or years when treatment is stopped, so the bisphosphonates (Table 267–2) have largely replaced the use of calcitonin. Etidronate has activity comparable to that of calcitonin, and higher doses may impair the mineralization of bone. Other bisphosphonates induce more complete effects on disease activity, symptoms, and radiographic abnormalities (see Fig. 267–2) than in the case of the calcitonins or elidronate. Other non-approved treatments include mithramycin, gallium nitrate, and the combination of calcium with thiazide diuretics.

SURGICAL MANAGEMENT. Elective surgery is often undertaken despite effective medical treatment to decrease bone vascularity and provide a more normal environment for prosthetic implants. Apart from fractures, the most common indication for surgery is joint disease at the hip. In the case of hip pain and some of the spinal neurologic syndromes, surgery can be avoided by medical treatment. Osteotomy has a role in managing deformities or the pain associated with fissure fractures in the presence of deformity.

PROGNOSIS. Pagetic bone pain almost invariably responds to medical treatment. In practice it may be difficult to distinguish the pain in Paget's disease from pain caused by coexisting osteoarthropathy or joint pain arising from deformity. In patients in whom pain at the hip is not controlled by analgesics or specific treatment, replacement arthroplasty is the treatment of choice.

Long-term treatment results in the resumption of lamellar bone formation, and in the case of the calcitonins and newer bisphosphonates, more normal radiographic appearances. Overall, there appears to be good correlation between the degree of biochemical control and attaining clinical improvement, so biochemical monitor-

ing of disease activity is of value. Decreased bone enlargement and deformity have been reported following long-term treatment with the bisphosphonates. Effective medical management improves spinal neurologic syndromes when they are slowly progressive. The long-term results are as good as those from surgery without the mortality of the latter. The rate of neurologic improvement seen with drug treatment is often more rapid than can be accounted for by remodeling of bone but is due to a decrease in soft tissue swelling and redistribution of blood flow.

No good evidence indicates that medical treatment significantly alters the natural history of fissure fractures. These fractures may be indolent, occasionally giving rise to pain and complete fracture. Limited experience suggests that in these patients pain decreases following osteotomy. Pathologic fractures of long bones generally heal well, but the incidence of delayed union and non-union is higher than normal. The occurrence of fracture provides an opportunity to correct deformity when managed either conservatively or with surgery. Long-term treatment may decrease the frequency of pathologic fracture, but this potential advantage has not been assessed by long-term prospective studies.

The prognosis of patients with osteosarcoma is extremely poor, and no evidence indicates that medical treatment alters its natural history. Indeed, the role of radiation therapy, chemotherapy, or surgical intervention has not been established except for symptomatic treatment.

Anderson DC: Paget's disease. *In* Mundy GR, Martin TJ (ed): Physiology and Pharmacology of Bone. New York, Springer-Verlag, 1993. p 419. *A general account of Paget's disease.*

Kanis JA: Pathophysiology and Treatment of Paget's Disease of Bone, 2nd ed. London, Martin Duntiz, 1998. *A comprehensive monograph of Paget's disease of bone.*

Singer FR, Wallach S (ed): Paget's Disease of Bone: Clinical Assessment, Present and Future Therapy. New York, Elsevier, 1991. *A collection of review articles and recent abstracts of scientific contributions.*

---

268 OSTEONECROSIS, OSTEOSCLEROSIS/HYPEROSTOSIS, AND OTHER DISORDERS OF BONE

Michael P. Whyte

OSTEONECROSIS

Osteonecrosis (aseptic, avascular, or ischemic necrosis of bone) refers to skeletal infarction. Bone infarcts may be asymptomatic, cause self-limited discomfort, or engender painful collapse of subarticular bone leading to joint destruction.

ETIOLOGY. Many conditions are associated with osteonecrosis (Table 268–1). In adults, the most common causes are ethanol abuse and long-term glucocorticoid therapy, both of which demonstrate dose-dependent effects.

PATHOGENESIS. Skeletal infarction may result from blood vessel destruction (e.g., joint dislocation, fracture), obstruction (e.g., thromboemboli, sickle cell disease, fat emboli, caisson disease), or hypothetically, compression from local expansion of fatty tissue (e.g., ethanol abuse, glucocorticoid treatment, diabetes mellitus). However, symptoms may not occur unless, weeks later, resorption of dead bone during skeletal repair leads to pathologic fracture. Certain skeletal sites (often subarticular) are predisposed to osteonecrosis but differ for traumatic and non-traumatic processes and for children and adults. *Osteochondrosis* refers to necrosis of ossification centers; more than 50 eponymic types are recorded. The susceptibility of children to osteochondrosis and its pathogenesis are poorly understood. At all ages, however, the femoral head is especially prone to infarction. Non-traumatic osteonecrosis also commonly affects the femoral condyles, distal end of the tibia, humeral head, and talus.

CLINICAL FEATURES. Pain occurs acutely upon skeletal col-

Table 267–2 ■ BISPHOSPHONATES USED IN THE TREATMENT OF PAGET'S DISEASE

AGENT	ROUTE	DOSE (mg/day)	DURATION
Alendronate	Oral	40	6 mo
Clodronate*	Oral	1600	3–6 mo
	IV	300	5 d
Etidronate	Oral	400	6 mo
Pamidronate	IV	30–60†	3 d
Risedronate	Oral	30	2 m
Tiludronate*	Oral	400	3 m

*Has not been approved by the Food and Drug Administration at the time of publication.
†Lower dose approved, higher dose used by investigators.

Endocrine/metabolic
  Ethanol abuse
  Glucocorticoid therapy
  Cushing's disease
  Diabetes mellitus
  Hyperuricemia
  Osteomalacia
  Hyperlipidemia
Storage diseases (e.g., Gaucher's disease)
Hemoglobinopathies (e.g., sickle cell disease)
Trauma (e.g., dislocation, fracture)
Dysbaric conditions (e.g., caisson disease)
Collagen-vascular disorders
Irradiation
Pancreatitis
Organ transplantation
Hemodialysis
Idiopathic, familial
Burns
Intravascular coagulation

lapse. Chronic arthralgia results from desquamated necrotic tissue and articular destruction.

DIAGNOSIS. Magnetic resonance imaging (MRI) demonstrating marrow edema is especially sensitive for detecting early osteonecrosis. Bone scintigraphy discloses skeletal reconstitution with or without fracture. Relatively late in the pathologic process, radiographs first show patchy areas of osteopenia and osteosclerosis that reflect skeletal repair. A linear subchondral radiolucency (crescent sign) indicates bony collapse.

TREATMENT. Non–weight bearing is advisable for an affected limb. Decompression by trephine insertion is used for some sites. Arthrotomy to remove debris, transpositional osteotomy, arthroplasty, or joint replacement may be necessary.

OSTEOSCLEROSIS/HYPEROSTOSIS

Many conditions are associated with radiographic evidence of increased bone density. Skeletal dysplasias, metabolic disturbances, and a variety of other disorders can cause generalized or focal increases in bone mass (Table 268–2). Aberrations in skeletal growth, modeling (shaping), and/or remodeling (turnover) may be at fault. *Osteosclerosis* refers to thickening of trabecular (spongy, cancellous) bone. *Hyperostosis* describes widening of cortical (compact) bone. Increases in trabecular or cortical bone or both may augment skeletal density.

Osteosclerosis

Neoplastic, hematologic, and metabolic disorders may preferentially cause sclerosis in trabecular bone because it houses marrow and remodels more rapidly than cortical bone.

FIBROGENESIS IMPERFECTA OSSIUM. This rare, sporadic condition features generalized osteopenia, but coarsening of remaining trabeculae places it among disorders of increased bone mass.

ETIOLOGY AND PATHOGENESIS. The cause is unknown. Subperiosteal bone formation and collagen synthesis in non-osseous tissues seem to be normal.

CLINICAL FEATURES. Typically, intractable skeletal pain begins gradually during middle age or later and then rapidly increases with a debilitating course and immobility. Spontaneous fractures are a prominent complication. Physical examination reveals marked bony tenderness.

DIAGNOSIS. On radiographic study, only the skull is spared. Initially, osteopenia and a slightly abnormal appearance of trabecular bone are noted. Subsequently, the changes suggest osteomalacia. Corticomedullary junctions become indistinct as compact bone is replaced by an abnormal cancellous pattern. Generalized osteopenia causes the remaining spongy bone to appear coarse and dense in a fish-net pattern of mixed lytic and sclerotic areas.

Alkaline phosphatase activity in serum is increased.

HISTOPATHOLOGIC FINDINGS. The skeletal lesion is a localized form of osteomalacia that varies considerably in severity from area to area. In diseased regions, polarized light microscopy shows col-

lagen fibrils that lack birefringence, and electron microscopy reveals that they are thin and randomly organized.

Hyperostosis

PROGRESSIVE DIAPHYSEAL DYSPLASIA (CAMURATI-ENGELMANN DISEASE). This skeletal dysplasia affects all races and is inherited as an autosomal dominant trait with variable penetrance. New bone formation gradually envelops both the periosteal and endosteal surfaces of long bone diaphyses. With severe disease, osteosclerosis also occurs in the axial skeleton.

ETIOLOGY AND PATHOGENESIS. The gene defect has not been mapped. Osteoblast differentiation may be deranged.

CLINICAL FEATURES. During childhood, limping or a broad-based and waddling gait is noted. Muscular dystrophy can be diagnosed erroneously. Severely affected individuals may have a characteristic body habitus featuring an enlarged head with prominent forehead, proptosis, and thin limbs with little subcutaneous fat or muscle mass and tender thickened bones. Cranial nerve palsies and raised intracranial pressure can occur. Some patients have hepatosplenomegaly, Raynaud's phenomenon, and additional findings suggestive of vasculitis. Symptoms may remit during puberty.

DIAGNOSIS. Irregular hyperostosis of the diaphyses of the major long bones slowly develops as a result of periosteal and endosteal new bone formation. Femora and tibiae are most commonly af-

Table 268–2 ■ DISORDERS THAT CAUSE DENSE BONES

Dysplasias
Central osteosclerosis with ectodermal dysplasia
Craniodiaphyseal dysplasia
Craniometaphyseal dysplasia
Dysosteosclerosis
Endosteal hyperostosis
  van Buchem's disease
  Sclerosteosis
Frontometaphyseal dysplasia
Infantile cortical hyperostosis (Caffey's disease)
Lenz-Majewski syndrome
Melorheostosis
Metaphyseal dysplasia (Pyle's disease)
Mixed sclerosing-bone dystrophy
Oculodento-osseous dysplasia
Osteodysplasia of Melnick and Needles
Osteoectasia with hyperphosphatasia (hyperostosis corticalis)
Osteopathia striata
Osteopetrosis
Osteopoikilosis
Progressive diaphyseal dysplasia (Engelmann's disease)
Pycnodysostosis
Metabolic
Carbonic anhydrase II deficiency
Fluorosis
Heavy metal poisoning
Hepatitis C–associated osteosclerosis
Hypervitaminosis A, D
Hyperparathyroidism, hypoparathyroidism, and pseudohypoparathyroidism
Hypophosphatemic rickets or osteomalacia
Milk-alkali syndrome
Renal osteodystrophy
Other
Axial osteomalacia
Fibrogenesis imperfecta ossium
Ionizing radiation
Lymphoma
Mastocytosis
Multiple myeloma
Myelofibrosis
Osteomyelitis
Osteonecrosis
Paget's disease
Sarcoidosis
Skeletal metastases
Tuberous sclerosis

From Whyte MP: Skeletal disorders characterized by osteosclerosis or hyperostosis. *In* Avioli LV, Krane SM (eds): Metabolic Bone Disease, 3rd ed. San Diego, Academic Press, 1998.

fected. Metaphyses may eventually become involved. The age of onset, rate of progression, and severity are variable. Clinical, radiographic, and bone scan findings are generally concordant. Routine biochemical parameters of bone and mineral metabolism are typically normal, although serum alkaline phosphatase activity, urinary hydroxyproline levels, and the erythrocyte sedimentation rate can be elevated. Histopathologic study reveals newly formed woven bone that matures and becomes incorporated into cortical bone. Electron microscopy of muscle may show myopathic changes and vascular abnormalities.

TREATMENT. Glucocorticoid therapy (typically a low dose of prednisone on alternate days) can relieve bone pain and may normalize skeletal histology.

ENDOSTEAL HYPEROSTOSIS. Sclerosteosis and van Buchem's disease, autosomal recessive disorders, are the principal types of endosteal hyperostosis.

ETIOLOGY AND PATHOGENESIS. Sclerosteosis and van Buchem's disease probably involve defects in the same gene, but the molecular pathology is unknown. Van Buchem's disease has recently been mapped to chromosome 17q12-q21. Clinical differences could be due to the effects of modifying genes. Enhanced osteoblast activity with failure of osteoclasts to compensate for the increased bone formation seems to explain the skeletal changes.

CLINICAL FEATURES. Sclerosteosis (cortical hyperostosis with syndactyly) occurs primarily in Afrikaners of South Africa. Elsewhere, Dutch ancestry is also common. Gender distribution appears equal. Patients are tall and heavy beginning in childhood, have a prominent mandible of square configuration, and suffer deafness and facial nerve palsy from cranial nerve entrapment. Raised intracranial pressure and headache may reflect a small cranial cavity that can shorten life expectancy. Van Buchem's disease causes progressive asymmetric enlargement of the jaw during puberty, but prognathism is not a feature. Patients may be symptom free or, beginning as early as infancy, have recurrent facial nerve palsy, deafness, and optic atrophy from narrowing of cranial foramina. Long bones may hurt with applied pressure but are not fragile.

DIAGNOSIS. In sclerosteosis, the skeleton is radiographically normal in early childhood except when bony syndactyly is present. Syndactyly, most often involving the index and 3rd fingers, is common. Progressive bony thickening widens the skull and causes prognathism. Long bones have thickened cortices. The pelvis, vertebral pedicles, ribs, and other tubular bones may become dense. Computed tomography has shown fusion of ossicles and narrowing of the internal auditory canals and cochlear aqueducts. In van Buchem's disease, endosteal thickening homogeneously widens diaphyseal cortices and narrows medullary canals. Bones are properly modeled. Osteosclerosis involves the skull base, facial bones, vertebrae, pelvis, and ribs.

Serum alkaline phosphatase activity can be increased from enhanced skeletal formation.

TREATMENT. Surgical decompression of narrowed foramina may alleviate cranial nerve palsies.

PACHYDERMOPERIOSTOSIS. Pachydermoperiostosis (hypertrophic osteoarthropathy, primary or idiopathic) is an autosomal dominant disorder that features clubbing of the digits, hyperhidrosis with thickening of the skin (especially of the face), and periosteal new bone formation prominently in the distal ends of the limbs. Autosomal recessive inheritance also seems to occur. Not all patients manifest all three principal features.

ETIOLOGY AND PATHOGENESIS. The genetic defect is unknown. A controversial hypothesis suggests that initially some circulating factor acts on the vasculature to cause hyperemia and thereby alters soft tissues, but later blood flow is reduced.

CLINICAL FEATURES. Men appear to be more severely affected than women and blacks more commonly than whites. Symptoms typically begin during adolescence, intensify during the next decade, but then become quiescent. Arthralgia and fatigue are common. Stiffness and limited mobility occur in both the appendicular and the axial skeleton. Clubbing with slowly progressive enlargement of the hands and feet results in a paw-like appearance. Cutaneous changes include thickening, furrowing, pitting, and oiliness, especially of the scalp and face.

RADIOLOGIC FEATURES. Periostitis thickens the distal portions of the tibia, fibula, radius, and ulna. Clubbing is obvious, and acro-

osteolysis can occur. Ankylosis of joints, especially in the hands and feet, may trouble older patients. Periosteal proliferation is exuberant, with irregular texture, and often involves the epiphyses, whereas secondary hypertrophic osteoarthropathy (pulmonary or otherwise) typically causes a smooth and undulating periosteal reaction. Bone scanning in either condition reveals symmetric, diffuse, regular uptake along the cortical margins of long bones, especially in the legs, called a "double stripe" sign.

TREATMENT. Painful synovial effusions may respond to non-steroidal anti-inflammatory drugs. Contractures or neurovascular compression by osteosclerotic lesions may require surgical intervention.

Osteosclerosis with Hyperostosis

OSTEOPETROSIS. Osteopetrosis (marble bone disease) occurs in two major clinical forms—the autosomal recessive or "malignant" type, which kills during infancy or early childhood if untreated, and the autosomal dominant or "benign" type, which causes few or no symptoms. Other autosomal recessive types feature intermediate severity, neuronal storage disease, stillbirth, or renal tubular acidosis with cerebral calcification secondary to carbonic anhydrase II isoenzyme deficiency.

ETIOLOGY AND PATHOGENESIS. The defective gene for autosomal dominant osteopetrosis has recently been mapped to chromosome 1p21. In carbonic anhydrase II deficiency, mutations in the candidate gene encoding the carbonic anhydrase II isoenzyme have been identified.

Histopathologic studies show that all true forms of osteopetrosis feature profound deficiency of osteoclast action. Primary spongiosa (calcified cartilage deposited during endochondral bone formation) persists away from growth plates and constitutes the pathognomonic finding. Defective endosteal bone resorption impairs the formation of marrow space. Quiescent skeletal remodeling leads to bone fragility from diminished interconnection of osteons, and the conversion of immature (woven) bone to mature (compact) bone is delayed. Studies of animal models of osteopetrosis suggest that patients may have abnormalities as distal as the marrow microenvironment, with effects on osteoclast precursor cell growth and differentiation, or abnormalities as proximal as bone tissue itself, with resistance to degradation. Neuronal storage disease (ceroid lipofuscin) could reflect a lysosomal defect. Deficient superoxide production (necessary for bone resorption) may also be a pathogenetic factor. Viral-like inclusions in osteoclasts are of uncertain significance.

CLINICAL FEATURES. Malignant osteopetrosis can be manifested during infancy as nasal "stuffiness" from underdeveloped mastoid and paranasal sinuses. Small cranial foramina may cause optic, oculomotor, or facial nerve palsy. Failure to thrive, delayed dentition, and fracture are common. Hypersplenism and recurrent infection, bruising, and bleeding reflect myelophthisis. Short stature, large head, frontal bossing, nystagmus, hepatosplenomegaly, and genu valgum are characteristic physical features. Untreated children usually die during the 1st decade of life from hemorrhage, pneumonia, severe anemia, or sepsis. Benign osteopetrosis occasionally causes fracture, facial palsy, deafness, mandibular osteomyelitis, impaired vision, psychomotor delay, carpal tunnel syndrome, or osteoarthritis. Carbonic anhydrase II deficiency can result in failure to thrive, fracture, developmental delay, mental subnormality, and short stature. Cerebral calcification develops during childhood, but defective skeletal modeling and osteosclerosis may correct spontaneously. Both proximal and distal renal tubular acidosis has been described.

DIAGNOSIS. A generalized increase in bone density is the radiographic hallmark. In severe disease, modeling defects in long bones produce an "Erlenmeyer flask" deformity (Fig. 268–1). Alternating dense and lucent bands commonly occur in the metaphyses and pelvis. The cranium is usually thickened and dense, especially at the base, and the paranasal and mastoid sinuses are underpneumatized. Vertebrae may show, on lateral view, a "bone-in-bone" (endobone) configuration or end-plate sclerosis causing a "rugger-jersey" appearance. Skeletal scintigraphy can disclose fractures and osteomyelitis. MRI helps monitor the response to bone marrow transplantation because successful engraftment normalizes marrow signals.

Serum levels of acid phosphatase and creatine kinase (brain isoenzyme), apparently from osteoclasts, are abnormal. In malignant

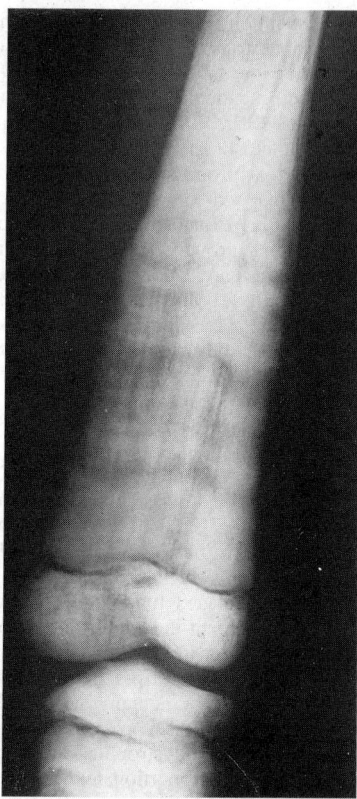

FIGURE 268-1 ■ *Osteopetrosis.* An anteroposterior radiograph of the distal end of the femur shows a widened metadiaphyseal region with characteristic alternating dense and lucent bands. (From Whyte MP, Murphy WA: Osteopetrosis and other sclerosing bone disorders. *In* Avioli LV, Krane SM [eds]: Metabolic Bone Disease, 2nd ed. Philadelphia, WB Saunders, 1990.)

osteopetrosis, hypocalcemia with secondary hyperparathyroidism and elevated serum concentrations of calcitriol can accompany radiologic changes that resemble rickets. In benign osteopetrosis, biochemical indices of mineral homeostasis are typically unremarkable, although serum parathyroid hormone levels may be increased.

TREATMENT. Because the etiology, pathogenesis, and prognosis of the osteopetroses differ, correct classification is crucial. It may be necessary to evaluate disease progression and study the family. For the malignant form, HLA-identical bone marrow transplantation to supply functional osteoclasts has remarkably benefited some children. Calcium-deficient diets have been used but may be limited by hypocalcemia and rickets. Massive oral doses of calcitriol (1,25-dihydroxyvitamin D) together with dietary calcium restriction (to prevent hypercalciuria/hypercalcemia) or human interferon-γ, which enhances superoxide production, have been given to stimulate osteoclast activity. Prednisone with a low-calcium, high-phosphate diet may also be effective. Glucocorticoid therapy stabilizes pancytopenia and hepatosplenomegaly. Hyperbaric oxygenation helps treat osteomyelitis. Surgical decompression of optic and facial nerves can be beneficial. Early prenatal diagnosis, radiographically or by ultrasound, has not been successful.

PYCNODYSOSTOSIS. Pycnodysostosis is believed to have troubled the French impressionist painter Henri de Toulouse-Lautrec (1864–1901). Most descriptions have come from Europe and the United States, but the disorder seems to be especially common in Japan.

ETIOLOGY AND PATHOGENESIS. This autosomal recessive condition is caused by defects in the gene that encodes cathepsin K. Diminished rates of collagen degradation and skeletal turnover are reported. In chondrocytes and osteoblasts, abnormal inclusions have been described.

CLINICAL FEATURES. Characteristic features seen during infancy or early childhood are a disproportionate short stature, relatively large cranium, fronto-occipital prominence, proptosis, bluish sclerae, a beaked and pointed nose, small facies and chin, obtuse mandibular angle, a high-arched palate, and dental malocclusion with retention of primary teeth. Cranial sutures remain open. Fingers are short and clubbed from acro-osteolysis or aplasia of the terminal phalanges, and the hands are small and square. Repeated fractures cause knock-knee deformity. Mental retardation is noted in approximately 10% of patients. Adult height ranges from 4 ft 3 inches to 4 ft 11 inches. Life expectancy can be shortened by recurrent respiratory infections and right-sided heart failure from chronic upper airway obstruction secondary to micrognathia.

LABORATORY FINDINGS. Osteosclerosis is uniform, first becoming apparent in childhood and increasing with age. Skeletal modeling defects do not occur, although long bones appear to have thick cortices because of narrow medullary canals. Clavicles are gracile and hypoplastic at their lateral segments. The calvarium and base of the skull are sclerotic, orbital ridges are dense, and wormian bones are present. Serum calcium and inorganic phosphate levels and alkaline phosphatase activity are typically normal. Anemia is not a problem.

TREATMENT. No effective medical therapy is available. Fractures of the long bones usually mend satisfactorily. Internal fixation of long bones is formidable because of their hardness. Tooth extraction is difficult. Osteomyelitis of the mandible may require antibiotic, surgical, and/or hyperbaric therapy.

HEPATITIS C–ASSOCIATED OSTEOSCLEROSIS. Rarely, achy and tender limbs develop in individuals who are infected with hepatitis C virus. Radiographic studies reveal a marked generalized increase in bone mass from osteosclerosis and hyperostosis. Disturbances in the insulin-like growth factor system may explain the enhanced bone formation. Calcitonin or biphosphonate therapy has benefited some patients.

Focal Osteosclerosis/Hyperostosis

OSTEOPOIKILOSIS. Osteopoikilosis ("spotted bones") is a radiologic curiosity inherited as a highly penetrant autosomal dominant trait. The bony lesions are asymptomatic. Incorrect diagnosis may lead to confusion with serious conditions, including metastatic disease. Some patients have connective tissue nevi called *dermatofibrosis lenticularis disseminata*, i.e., Buschke-Ollendorff syndrome.

RADIOLOGIC FEATURES. Numerous small round or oval foci of bony sclerosis appear in cancellous bone in the tarsal, carpal, pelvic, and metaepiphyseal regions of tubular bones.

OSTEOPATHIA STRIATA. This autosomal dominant curiosity features linear striations in the metaphyseal regions of long bones and in the ilium. Clinically important syndromes include osteopathia striata with cranial sclerosis or with focal dermal hypoplasia (Goltz's syndrome). Goltz's syndrome is an X-linked recessive condition featuring widespread linear areas of dermal hypoplasia and various bony defects in the limbs of affected males.

MELORHEOSTOSIS. Melorheostosis causes changes likened to melted wax dripping down a candle. No mendelian basis for this disorder has been found. The anatomic distribution suggests a segmentary embryogenic defect.

CLINICAL FEATURES. Usually, monomelic involvement is noted; bilateral disease is generally asymmetric. Cutaneous changes over affected bones are not uncommon (e.g., linear scleroderma-like areas and hypertrichosis). Soft tissue abnormalities are often noted before the hyperostosis. Symptoms typically begin during childhood, with pain and stiffness being the major complaints. Joints may become contracted and deformed. Leg length inequality results from soft tissue contractures and premature fusion of epiphyses. Skeletal changes appear to progress most rapidly throughout childhood. During adult life, melorheostosis may or may not gradually spread, although pain is especially common.

RADIOLOGIC FEATURES. Irregular, very dense, eccentric periosteal and endosteal hyperostosis affects a single bone or several adjacent bones. The lower limbs are most commonly involved. Endosteal thickening predominates during infancy and childhood and periosteal new bone formation during adulthood. Ectopic bone formation may occur, particularly near joints.

TREATMENT. Surgical correction of contractures is difficult; recurrent deformity is common.

MIXED SCLEROSING-BONE DYSTROPHY. This typically sporadic disorder features combinations of osteopoikilosis, osteopathia striata, melorheostosis, cranial sclerosis, or other skeletal defects in one individual. Patients may experience problems associated with the individual patterns of osteosclerosis or hyperostosis, e.g., nerve palsy with cranial sclerosis, bone pain with melorheostosis.

OTHER DISORDERS OF BONE

FIBROUS DYSPLASIA. This sporadic, developmental disorder features an expansile fibrous lesion(s) within bone. Polyostotic disease is typically seen before the age of 10 years; monostotic disease begins in adolescence or early adult life. McCune-Albright syndrome refers to polyostotic fibrous dysplasia, café au lait spots (Color Plate 8*F*), and endocrine hyperfunction.

ETIOLOGY AND PATHOGENESIS. Somatic mosaicism for activating mutations in the gene that encodes the α subunit of the receptor/adenylate cyclase–coupling G protein causes fibrous dysplasia and the McCune-Albright syndrome. Imperfect bone forms because mesenchymal cells do not fully differentiate to osteoblasts. Endocrinopathy generally results from end-organ hyperactivity.

CLINICAL FEATURES. Monostotic fibrous dysplasia is more common than polyostotic disease. The skull and long bones are affected most often. The skeletal lesions can deform bone, cause fractures, and occasionally entrap nerves. Sarcomatous degeneration is rare (incidence, <1%), but typically occurs within the facial bones or femur and is more frequent when polyostotic disease is present. Pregnancy may "reactivate" previously quiescent lesions. McCune-Albright syndrome usually causes pseudoprecocious puberty in girls. Less commonly there is pseudoprecocious puberty in boys or thyrotoxicosis, Cushing's disease, acromegaly, hyperprolactinemia, or hyperparathyroidism. In some patients, acquired renal phosphate wasting causes hypophosphatemic rickets or osteomalacia.

RADIOLOGIC FEATURES. In the long bones, lesions are found in either the metaphysis or the diaphysis. They are typically well defined with thin cortices and have a ground-glass appearance (Fig. 268–2). Occasionally, the defects are lobulated with trabeculated areas of radiolucency.

TREATMENT. With mild disease, bone lesions may not expand. In severe cases, individual defects can progress and new ones appear. Spontaneous healing does not occur, but pathologic fractures generally mend well. Stress fractures, however, can be difficult to detect and treat. When the skull is involved, nerve compression may

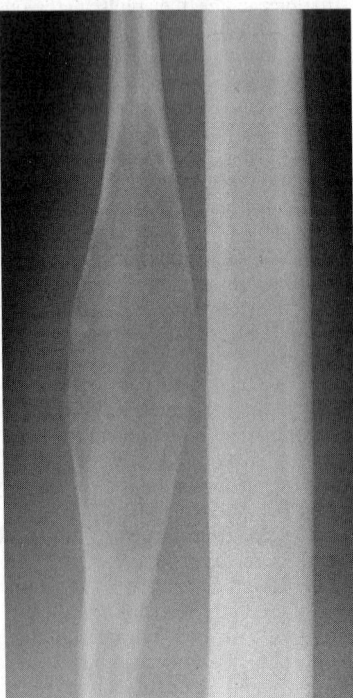

FIGURE 268–2 ■ *Fibrous dysplasia.* A characteristic expansile lesion with a ground-glass appearance has caused thinning of the cortex in the mid-diaphysis of the fibula. (From Whyte MP: Fibrous dysplasia. *In* Favus MJ [ed]: Primer on the Metabolic Bone Diseases and Disorders of Mineral Metabolism, 3rd ed. Philadelphia, Lippincott–Raven Press, 1996.)

require surgical intervention. In the McCune-Albright syndrome, the aromatase inhibitor testolactone helps control pseudoprecocious puberty in girls. Intravenous infusions of the biphosphonate pamidronate have helped some patients.

HEREDITARY MULTIPLE EXOSTOSES. This relatively common, highly penetrant, autosomal dominant disorder features irregular bony excrescences that protrude from expanded metaphyses. A gene defect has been mapped to chromosome 8 in some affected families. Osteocartilaginous exostoses arise from growth plates and increase in size until linear growth ceases. Lesions may or may not become detached from the parent bone. Their structure is relatively unremarkable, with an outer cortex and an inner spongiosa. Disability results primarily from limb length discrepancies when linear bone growth suffers at the expense of transverse expansion. Compression of nerves, the spinal cord, or the vascular system occurs occasionally. Sarcomatous degeneration (0.5 to 2% of patients) should be suspected when an exostosis enlarges rapidly, especially during adult life.

ENCHONDROMATOSIS (DYSCHONDROPLASIA, OLLIER'S DISEASE). This sporadic disorder features cartilaginous masses within the trabecular bone that arise from growth plates. The condition begins in childhood with localized swelling and interferes with linear bone growth. At puberty, expansion of cartilage masses ceases, and they can be replaced by mature bone. Enchondromas appear radiographically as lucent defects in flat bones or in metaphyses of tubular bones, often with central calcific stippling. When enchondromatosis occurs with multiple hemangiomas (Maffucci's syndrome), the enchondromas or hemangiomas undergo malignant transformation in about 15% of cases.

ACHONDROPLASIA. Chondrodystrophies are disorders of cartilage growth that result in disproportionately short stature. Achondroplasia is the most common. Defects in the gene that encodes fibroblast growth factor receptor type 3 cause this dysplasia. About 80% of cases are new mutations for this autosomal dominant defect, which increases in frequency with increasing paternal age. Short, tubular bones form because of abnormal endochondral ossification in the limbs. In the chondrocranium, membranous ossification is undisturbed—thus the skull vault is normal. However, the cranial base and foramen magnum are small. Lumbar lordosis is greatly exaggerated, and the spinal canal narrows from the upper to lower segments of the vertebral column. This disturbance is revealed radiographically by decreasing interpeduncular distance. The head is large with frontal bossing and midface hypoplasia. The trunk is of relatively normal length, but the limbs show rhizomelic shortening and the hands have a trident configuration. The long bones appear massive owing to their disproportionately normal width. Surprisingly, growth plates are not grossly disorganized in achondroplasia, and chondrocytes appear normal. Complications can include hydrocephalus or compression of the brain stem, spinal cord, or nerve roots. Minimal impingement by a disk or osteophyte on the small spinal canal can cause neurologic disturbances. Despite its problems, achondroplasia is compatible with good health and a normal lifespan.

Chang CC, Greenspan A, Gershwin ME: Osteonecrosis: Current perspectives on pathogenesis and treatment. Semin Arthritis Rheum 23:47, 1993. *Overview of osteonecrosis.*

McKusick VA: Mendelian Inheritance in Man: A Catalog of Human Genes and Genetic Disorders, 12th ed. Baltimore, Johns Hopkins University Press, 1998. *Clinical features, patterns of inheritance, and molecular bases of heritable diseases.*

Taybi H, Lachman RS: Radiology of Syndromes, Metabolic Disorders, and Skeletal Dysplasias, 4th ed. St. Louis, Mosby, 1996. *Concise summaries with clinical and radiologic illustration.*

Whyte MP: Skeletal disorders characterized by osteosclerosis or hyperostosis. *In* Avioli LV, Krane SM (eds): Metabolic Bone Disease, 3rd ed. San Diego, Academic Press, 1998. *Overview of disorders that increase bone mass.*

269 BONE TUMORS

Daniel I. Rosenthal

Tumors may involve bone as the result of (1) neoplastic transformation of bone or bone marrow cells, (2) metastatic dissemination of neoplasms arising in other organs, or (3) local invasion from contiguous tissues.

Of these three mechanisms, metastatic involvement is by far the most frequent.

METASTATIC TUMOR

Several common cancers frequently involve the skeleton. In women, breast cancer is the most common primary tumor to result in skeletal metastases. Lung cancer is a distant second, although increasing in frequency. In men, prostate cancer is the most common primary tumor, followed by tumors arising in lung, kidney, gastrointestinal tract, and thyroid.

Whenever a destructive lesion of the skeleton is encountered, an effort should be made to determine whether it is primary or secondary. Metastatic bone lesions usually produce an infiltrative pattern of bone destruction on radiographic or other imaging studies. Compared with primary tumors, metastatic disease is usually accompanied by little or no soft tissue mass. Cancers arising in breast or prostate usually produce mixed lytic and blastic change within bone, whereas lung and renal cancers are purely lytic. A radioisotope bone scan is recommended to determine whether the lesion is solitary, because metastatic lesions will often be multiple at presentation. Isotope bone scans are generally more sensitive than plain films for detecting metastasis. The addition of single-photon emission computed tomography further increases the sensitivity of the isotope scan. Magnetic resonance imaging (MRI) is probably even more sensitive, especially for lesions involving the spine. Unfortunately, imaging of the entire skeleton by MRI is a time-consuming and cumbersome process, despite the recent progress in rapid-imaging pulse sequences. When more than one focus is present, the primary tumor is probably extraskeletal. Although bone sarcomas may metastasize to other parts of the skeleton, this is generally a phenomenon that occurs late in the course of the disease, after lung metastases are present.

If multiple lesions are present, and the primary tumor is not apparent, it may be desirable to consider biopsy for diagnosis rather than engage in an extended search for the primary lesion. Needle biopsy can be accomplished safely for most skeletal sites and is the most direct approach to diagnosis. Unfortunately, in a certain percentage of cases presenting as metastatic carcinoma, the primary tumor remains unknown despite all efforts.

Whether chemotherapy or hormonal therapy will be useful in treating metastatic disease depends on the primary tumor. Most metastatic lesions can be palliated with radiation. The new class of bisphosphonate drugs has also been shown to be effective in ameliorating the symptoms and perhaps slowing the progression of disease. If there is important structural compromise of the skeleton and the patient's life expectancy justifies it, surgical stabilization should be considered to preserve function.

DIRECT INVASION

Direct invasion of bone by contiguous visceral or soft tissue tumors is uncommon. The most frequent cause of this complication is lung cancer invading ribs or vertebrae. Paravertebral lymphadenopathy may sometimes involve the vertebrae. Deeply situated soft tissue sarcomas may also invade bone, but this event is relatively rare considering the frequent proximity of these lesions to the skeleton. The radioisotope bone scan is useful to exclude bone involvement. However, a positive bone scan must be viewed with caution, because reactive changes at the margins of the tumor may cause the bone scan to be "hot." Confirmation of involvement by computed tomography (CT) or MRI is desirable.

PRIMARY BONE TUMORS

Primary bone tumors may arise from any of the cellular elements that are present. Tumors may be either malignant or benign. However, tumors of the mesenchymal tissues usually fall into a more or less continuous spectrum that extends from benign to malignant. Not all lesions are clearly characterizable as either one or the other. For this reason, adequate diagnosis of most lesions requires not only the name of the tumor but also its histologic grade. Furthermore, individual tumors commonly exhibit a variety of cell types

and grades. Features on imaging studies reflect the most abundant histologic elements, whereas clinical behavior is shaped by the most aggressive or malignant components. In general, the better differentiated the lesion (lower grade), the more it resembles the tissue from which it arose. Highly malignant lesions exhibit considerable similarity to each other on imaging studies.

Tumors may arise sporadically, as part of a generalized (and sometimes inherited) tendency to neoplasia, or by degeneration of precursor lesions. Almost any condition that causes a prolonged period of accelerated bone remodeling may lead to tumor formation. Some examples include Paget's disease, infections, irradiation, bone infarctions, and benign bone lesions.

Adequate staging requires four pieces of information: tumor type, histologic grade, local extent, and presence of metastases. Tissue type and grade are learned from biopsy. Biopsy of these lesions requires considerable sophistication to avoid complicating future therapy. Biopsy should be performed in such a way as to obtain representative tissue, preserve structural integrity, and permit curative resection should that prove to be desirable. Such resection usually requires that the biopsy track be excised along with the tumor.

Local extent can be determined by imaging studies. Plain radiographs are important in all cases. Either CT or MRI may be used to evaluate soft tissue and marrow extent. If the lesion is suspected of being malignant, a radioisotope bone scan is used to determine whether the lesion is solitary, and either chest radiography or CT of the chest is desirable to exclude pulmonary metastases.

Benign bone tumors are usually relatively small and often painless. Of these, the most common (and least significant) is the bone island. These asymptomatic lesions arise during adult life, may slowly enlarge, and eventually regress. They are usually incidental findings on radiographs. Bone islands are not usually detected on isotope scans, although large lesions may show some uptake. Benign cartilage tumors, including osteochondroma and enchondroma, are next in order of frequency. These lesions are not generally painful unless complicated by pathologic fracture, adjacent soft tissue inflammation (bursitis), or malignant degeneration. Some painful benign tumors include osteoid osteoma, chondroblastoma, giant cell tumor, and chondromyxoid fibroma. Treatment by limited resection is adequate for these tumors. If the diagnosis is certain from imaging studies and resection is not required to relieve symptoms, observation may be adequate.

The most common malignant bone tumor is multiple myeloma, which is considered separately elsewhere (Chapter 181). Osteosarcoma (or osteogenic sarcoma) is next in order of frequency and much more common than any of the others. Osteosarcoma exhibits two age incidence peaks, one in the second decade of life and another in the fifth and sixth decades, when it frequently represents a complication of a precursor lesion such as Paget's disease. It is most common in the distal femur and proximal tibia. Although low-grade osteosarcoma exists, most lesions are highly malignant. Ten per cent of patients have metastases at the time of presentation, and if the disease is not treated, death ensues in less than 1 year. The alkaline phosphatase level is usually elevated, and levels correlate with prognosis. Contemporary treatment uses combination chemotherapy and amputation or, if possible, limb-sparing surgery. With this approach, survival rates of 85 to 90% are possible. Even for those patients presenting with pulmonary metastases, a combination of resection of the pulmonary lesion and chemotherapy may produce a 20% salvage rate.

Ewing's sarcoma is classified in a group of round cell lesions because of similar histologic and radiographic features. Lymphoma is another member of this group. Ewing's sarcoma tends to occur in children and young adults, whereas primary lymphoma of bone (usually non-Hodgkin's type) is seen in older individuals. The two entities may be difficult to differentiate. Ewing's sarcoma is of unknown pathogenesis and is highly malignant. It is remarkable for a tendency to produce both local and systemic symptoms that may simulate infection including fever, malaise, and chills. Chemotherapy and surgery produce 60% cure rates.

Chondrosarcoma is usually a disease of people in the fourth, fifth, and sixth decades of life. Unlike osteosarcoma and Ewing's sarcoma, chondrosarcoma is of more variable grade, with most lesions of low or intermediate malignancy. Irradiation and chemotherapy are relatively ineffective, but surgery may produce cure rates of 85%.

Goorin AM, Anderson JW: Experience with multi-agent chemotherapy for osteosarcoma. Clin Orthop Rel Res 270:22–28, 1991. *Current status of chemotherapy.*

O'Connor MI, Pritchard DJ: Ewing's sarcoma: Prognostic factors, disease control and the re-emerging role of surgical treatment. Clin Orthop Rel Res 262:78–87, 1991. *Improvements in survival related to local and systemic treatment.*

Schajowicz F: Tumors and Tumorlike Lesions of Bone and Joints. New York, Springer-Verlag, 1981. *A good general textbook that provides incidence and age distribution for most lesions.*

Springfield DS (ed): Limb salvage in the treatment of musculoskeletal tumors. Orthop Clin North Am 22:1–180, 1991. *A comprehensive multiauthor review of the status of limb-sparing surgery.*

PART XX

DISEASES OF THE IMMUNE SYSTEM

270 APPROACH TO THE PATIENT WITH IMMUNE DISEASE

J. Claude Bennett

The immune system consists of an integrated constellation of various cell types, each with a specifically designated functional role (Fig. 270–1). In addition, secreted-molecules (cytokines) are responsible for interactions, modulations, and regulation of the system. These molecules and cells participate in specific interactions with immunogenic epitopes present on foreign materials (i.e., antigens introduced from the exterior world and foreign to the host). Recognition events are the beginning of the physiologic steps that make up the immune response; they initiate a series of processes causing a wide range of effects within the host. These include the pathways through which inflammation takes place, the killing of invading microbial agents, and the disposal of foreign toxic compounds.

Events leading to specific molecular interactions depend on the differentiation and expansion of the cell clones that are involved. These include production of specific cell-bound receptor molecules (TCR, T-cell receptors) and secreted or cell-bound immunoglobulins (antibodies). The cellular network (see Fig. 270–1) results in an enormous array of specific molecular events. Abnormal regulation of the immune system may prevent the host from handling antigenic stimuli, resulting in a state of immune deficiency (see Chapter 272). At the other extreme it may allow the host to react to its own tissues, resulting in an autoimmune process (see Chapter 289).

In an immunocompetent individual, the immune response is initiated when introduced to an external agent that possesses an immunogenic structural epitope. The appropriate response depends on the recognition by surface receptors of B and T lymphocytes of the foreignness of the introduced agent. These interactions lead to events that allow proliferation and differentiation of the antigen-stimulated cells. To appreciate the exquisite degree of specificity expressed by this remarkable system, one must understand the molecular interactions that result in antigen processing, presentation, and cellular proliferation, B lymphocytes differentiate to produce specifically directed immunoglobulins (antibodies). All such immunoglobulins share an overall structure, but each contains its own antigen-binding area (Fab region) and within any class (e.g., IgG, IgM) a similar constant region (Fc) (Fig. 270–2). Therefore, the product of any given clone of B cells has a unique specificity distinct from that of all other clonal lines of B cells. This provides the enormous diversity in the recognition properties of the immune system. Furthermore, each of the classes of immunoglobulins is imbued with structural elements that set it apart and define its distinct function in biologic effector mechanisms (Table 270–1).

As the immune process is triggered, T lymphocytes respond to antigen on the surface of macrophages or other specialized antigen-presenting cells (APC) (see Figs. 270–1 and 270–3). T cells then differentiate as they express various functions, such as cytotoxic potential, enhanced expression of immunity (helper T cells), or down-modulation of the immune response. Therefore, the T lymphocyte becomes pivotal in the development of both *humoral immunity* by way of its stimulation of B lymphocytes and the development of *cellular immunity* and regulation by virtue of its own intrinsic properties and its role in elaborating cytokines for cellular communication processes.

Reactions of the immune system may activate the complement cascade (see Chapter 271) and the production of arachidonic acid derivatives such as prostaglandins and leukotrienes (see Chapter 29), which play key roles in expressing inflammation. Both lymphocytes and macrophages secrete a variety of cytokines, which modulate the immune response and the induction of inflammation (Table 270–2).

Immunologic events can be regulated through networks of antibody-forming cells, helper/suppressor mechanisms, and cytokine mediation, or through specific mechanisms of immunologic tolerance. Immunodeficiency states and autoimmune diseases represent the end points of either a genetically incompetent or a poorly regulated immune system.

B LYMPHOCYTE LINEAGE AND ANTIBODY PRODUCTION

Secreted antibodies are produced by plasma cells, which represent the terminal phase of differentiation of B lymphocytes. The latter are found in all peripheral lymphoid tissues and also in the circulating pool of lymphocytes. Within their surface membranes, B cells have receptors that allow them to recognize foreign antigenic determinants. These receptors are immunoglobulin molecules, and in the initial stages of differentiation are generally of the IgM and IgD classes. When stimulated by a specific antigen, in conjunction with appropriate cytokines, these B cells proliferate and secrete antibody (see Fig. 270–1).

In the earliest stages of differentiation (Fig. 270–4), B lymphocytes lack membrane immunoglobulin (mIg). However, these cells begin to express in their cytoplasm the μ chain, which is the heavy (H) chain of IgM. Later they produce the light (L) chain (either kappa [κ] or lambda [λ]) which allows IgM molecules to be expressed on the surface. The binding region on the mIg of each cell line is unique in its specificity and is identical to that of the antibody molecule that is to be secreted. This means that at a very early developmental stage, a given cell is locked into its own specificity). This process involves several gene rearrangements (see below).

B-cell activation, proliferation, and differentiation require a variety of cytokines. Perhaps the most important in humans is interleukin-2 (IL-2), which seems to play a central role in these events and thus facilitates the production of immunoglobulins of all isotypes. Although other cytokines (e.g., IL-4 and TGF-β) are identified as being able to amplify and modify antibody production, generally they cannot do this unless IL-2 is present (see Table 270–2).

IMMUNOGLOBULIN FUNCTION AND STRUCTURE

The basic structure of all immunoglobulin molecules (see Fig. 270–2) is similar among the various classes. Essentially they consist of two types of polypeptide chains—the larger, called the *heavy* (H) *chain,* and the smaller, known as the *light* (L) *chain.* Each immunoglobulin subunit consists of two identical H and two identical L chains and would therefore have the molecular formula H_2L_2. The H and L chains are connected to each other by disulfide bonds, and similarly there are disulfide bridges between the two H chains (which vary in number for the different classes and subclasses). They are generally located in the center of the H chain

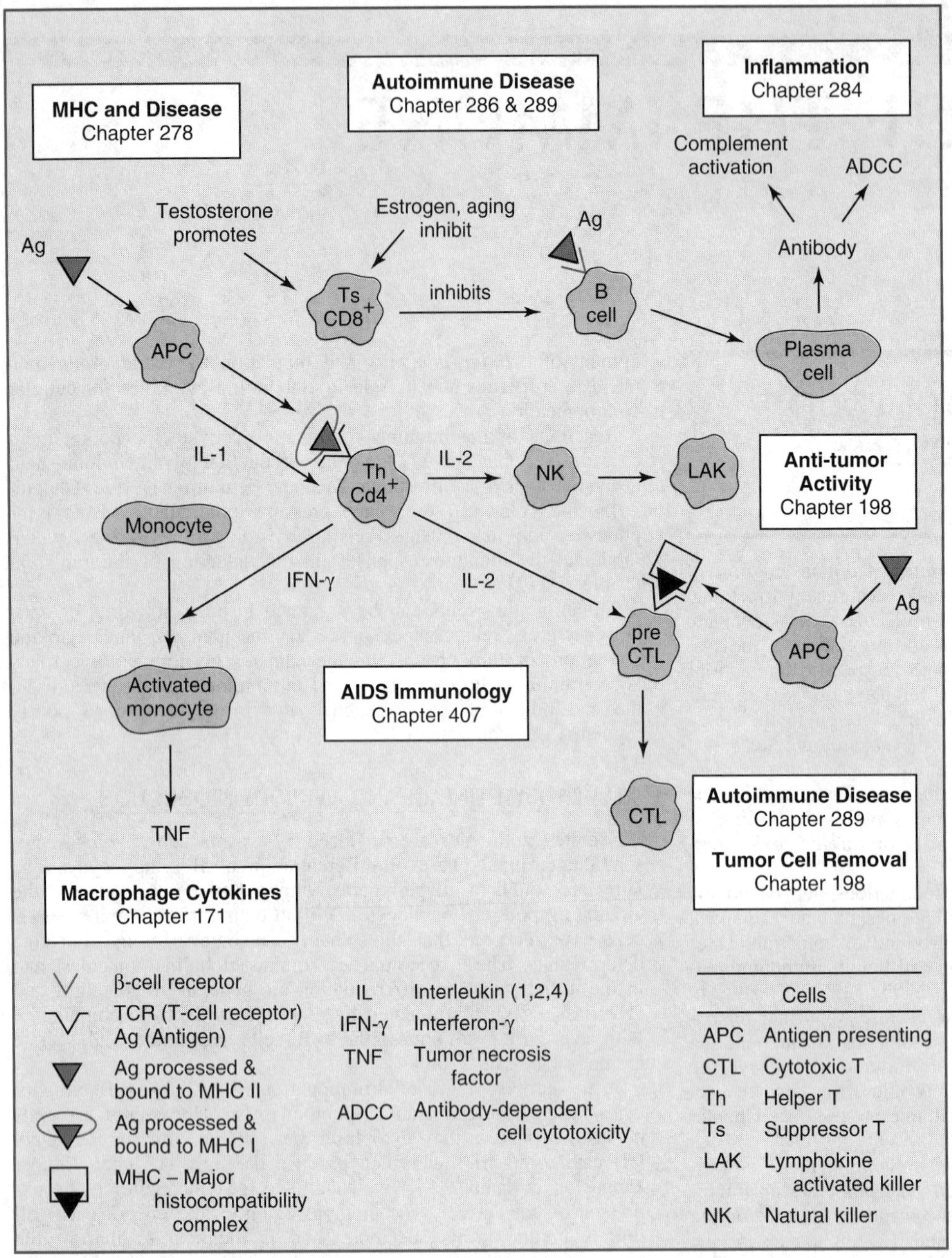

MHC and Disease
Chapter 278
Autoimmune Disease
Chapter 286 & 289
Inflammation
Chapter 284
Complement activation
ADCC
Antibody
Testosterone promotes
Estrogen, aging inhibit
Ag
Ts CD8+
inhibits
B cell
Plasma cell
APC
IL-1
Th Cd4+
IL-2
NK
LAK
Anti-tumor Activity
Chapter 198
Monocyte
IFN-γ
IL-2
pre CTL
APC
Activated monocyte
AIDS Immunology
Chapter 407
TNF
CTL
Autoimmune Disease
Chapter 289
Tumor Cell Removal
Chapter 198
Macrophage Cytokines
Chapter 171
β-cell receptor
TCR (T-cell receptor)
Ag (Antigen)
Ag processed & bound to MHC II
Ag processed & bound to MHC I
MHC – Major histocompatibility complex
IL Interleukin (1,2,4)
IFN-γ Interferon-γ
TNF Tumor necrosis factor
ADCC Antibody-dependent cell cytotoxicity
Cells
APC Antigen presenting
CTL Cytotoxic T
Th Helper T
Ts Suppressor T
LAK Lymphokine activated killer
NK Natural killer

FIGURE 270–1 ■ The molecular events involved in antigen presentation to the T cell. Shown are the interactions among the various cell surface molecules, including the major histocompatibility complex (MHC-II), the T-cell Receptor/CD3 complex, and the CD4. In the case of cytotoxic T cells (not shown) MHC-I and CD8 are involved. Co-stimulatory events take place via B7 on the antigen-presenting cell and CD28 on the T cell.

region, known as the "hinge" region, which is unusually rich in cysteine and proline. The L chain has a molecular weight of about 25,000 daltons; the H chain varies between 50,000 and 65,000 daltons. H chain size is related to differences in the structure of the hinge region or to the presence of an extra globular domain, as in the case of the μ and ϵ H chains (in IgM and IgE, respectively). Globular domains, formed by intrachain disulfide bonds, each consist of about 110 amino acid residues; and there are four or five such domains in each H chain and two in each L chain. The domains are separated by extended regions, known as *interdomain stretches.* These domain structures may have evolved to execute specialized biologic functions.

The amino-terminal 110 to 120 residues of each immunoglobulin chain are known as the *variable* (V) region because the amino acid sequences of those molecules produced from a single clonal line differ from those of other lines. The remaining part of the immunoglobulin chain is identical for any given class and is referred to as the *constant* (C) region. Many direct lines of evidence indicate that the variable region contains the antibody-binding site into which antigen fits and that "hypervariable regions" are in the most intimate contact with the structural elements of the antigen. X-ray crystallography has confirmed these three-dimensional structures. The hypervariable regions are also largely responsible for the *idiotypic* determinants on an antibody molecule and tend to be similar on all antibodies that share specificities. The structures throughout the remainder of the V segments, which show less sequence variability, are referred to as the "framework" areas.

Although the amino acid sequences of the constant regions of the H chains show homologies among the Ig classes and subclasses, there are also very significant differences. The structural features appear to be important in giving the molecule its particular biologic function that distinguishes one class from another. Complement fixation, for example, seems to depend on a structural determinant in the IgG CH2 domain, whereas features of the CH3 domain seem to be important for interacting with a variety of cells by way of the Fc receptors. More than one domain in the Fc region of the IgG H chain is required to react with the binding sites on rheumatoid factors (see Chapter 286).

Since Porter's original work on the structure of antibodies, much has been learned about their molecular structure by using proteolytic enzymes. For example, papain cleaves IgG into an Fc fragment and two Fab fragments, whereas pepsin degrades the Fc fragment and yields the two Fab fragments still joined by a disulfide bridge $(Fab)_2$ (see Fig. 270–2). Different enzymes cleave the various classes in different ways, and this approach has been important in defining structural corollaries to biologic properties.

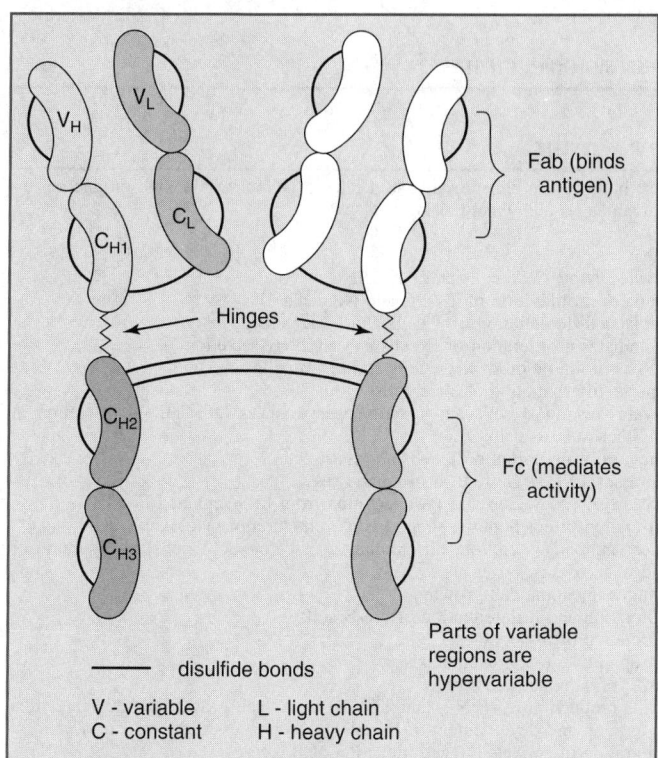

FIGURE 270-2 ■ Diagram of the overall structure of immunoglobulin G, the basic structural pattern for all immunoglobulins (see text), which highlights the various reactive areas and emphasizes the globular domain features of the immunoglobulin molecule.

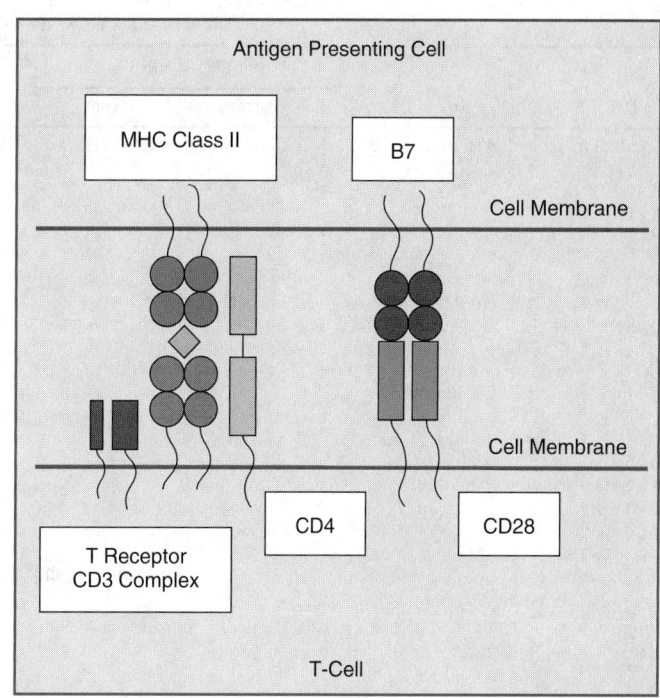

FIGURE 270-3 ■ The molecular events involved in antigen presentation to the T cell. Shown are the interactions among the various cell surface molecules, including the major histocompatibility complex (MHC-II), the T-cell Receptor/CD3 complex, and the CD4. In the case of cytotoxic T cells (not shown) MHC-I and CD8 are involved. Co-stimulatory events take place via B7 on the antigen-presenting cell and CD28 on the T cell.

Comparisons among the various classes of immunoglobulin are shown in Table 270-1. Certain immunoglobulins appear very different from IgG. for example, IgM is a large molecule but consists of five subunits of the same basic immunoglobulin pattern. It has 10 H and 10 L chains and, therefore, 10 antibody-binding sites per molecule. However, because of steric factors, when IgM reacts with large protein antigens, it tends to bind with a valence of five. This can best be seen in the case of IgM rheumatoid factor binding to IgG, which yields a 22 s complex with a formula $(\mu_2L_2)5$-(IgG)5.

IMMUNOGLOBULIN GENETICS AND GENE ORGANIZATION

Human immunoglobulin genes are contained on chromosomes 2, 14, and 22 (Table 270-3). Several sequences of events must take place for immunoglobulin genes to be expressed. This requires a random process of gene reorganization. As shown in Figure 270-5, each C region is coded by a single gene, but many gene segments are necessary to form the repertoire of V genes. The latter are formed by rearrangement of DNA to bring one V gene into proximity with a J (junction) gene in the case of the L chains; and in the case of the H chains, the V must be brought into proximity with a D (diversity) region and a J region. For any given H-chain gene, the total V region is formed from a single V region, a single D, and a single J (Fig. 270-5). Combination with a given constant region would determine the Ig class. Recombination activating genes (RAG) facilitate the V-D-J recombination, and this suggests that they may encode enzymes that have the properties of being V-D-J recombinases. The C region genes are located in tandem, so a switching process must occur in order to allow a given assembled V-D-J region to attach to any constant region. This process deletes all intervening genes from that particular clone (Fig. 270-6). In some B lymphocytes both IgD and IgM are present on the cell membrane at the same time, and this occurs through alternative RNA splicing.

Table 270-1 ■ PROPERTIES OF IMMUNOGLOBULINS BY CLASS AND SUBCLASS

CLASS	IgG		IgA		IgM	IgD	IgE
Molecular weight	160,000		17,000 or polymer		900,000	80,000	90,000
Sedimentation constant	7S		7S (9, 11, 13)		19S	7S	8S
Serum concentration	1000–5000		250–300		100–150	0.3–30	0.0015–0.2
Valence	2		2 (monomer)		10	2	2
Molecular formula	γ_2L_2		$(\alpha_2L_2)_n$		$(\gamma_2L_2)_5$	δ_2L_2	ϵ_2L_2

SUBCLASS	IgG1	IgG2	IgG3	IgG4	IgA1	IgA2	IgM	IgD	IgE
Subclass percent of class, in serum	65	20	10	5	90	10			
Complement fixation	++	+	++	−	−	−	++	−	−
Alternative complement fixation					+	+	+	±	±
Placental passage	+	+	+	+	−	−	−	−	−
Fixing to mast cells or basophils	−	−	−	−	−	−	−	−	+
Binding to									
Macrophages	+	±	+	±	−	−	−	−	−
Neutrophils	+	+	+	+	+	+	−	−	−
Platelets	+	+	+	+					
Lymphocytes	+	+	+	+			+		
Half-life (days)	23	23	8–9	23	6	6	5	3	2.5
Synthesis rate (mg/kg/day)	25	?	3.5	?	44	22	7	0.4	0.02

Table 270–2 ■ CYTOKINES AND THEIR BIOLOGIC ACTIVITIES

| CYTOKINE | CELL SOURCE | | | MAJOR ACTIVITIES |
	T	Macrophages	Other	
Interleukin-1α and β (IL-1α and β)		+	+	Fever; bone resorption; prostaglandin release; stimulate cytokine production by macrophages and T cell
IL-1α		+		
IL-1β			+	Same
IL-2	+			Activates cytotoxic T cells and NK cells
				Stimulates proliferation of T cells and NK cells
				Stimulates differentiation of T cells and LAK cells
				Costimulates proliferation of B cells and antibody secretion
IL-3	+	+	+	Supports proliferation of mast cells and pre-B cells
				Supports differentiation of stem cells
IL-4	+		+	Activates resting B cells and macrophages; induces IgG and IgE secretion in LPS-activated B cells
				Stimulates proliferation of T cells and mast cells
				Suppresses TNF-α, IL-1, IL-6 in monocytes
IL-5	+			Induces IgA production and IgM secretion from LPS-activated B cells
				Proliferation of eosinophils; supports differentiation of cytotoxic T cells
IL-6	+	+	+	Induces antibody secretion; differentiation of cytotoxic T cells; proliferation of megakaryocytes
				Promotes myeloma cell growth
IL-7			Thymic strand cells	Proliferation and differentiation of pre-B cells
				Proliferation of thymocytes
IL-8		+		Neutrophil and T-cell chemotaxis
IL-9	+			Growth of T-helper cell clones
IL-10	+	+	+	Inhibits production of (IFN-γ and TNF-α) and B-cell growth and differentiation
IL-11			+	Proliferation and development of B cells, macrophages, and megakaryocytes
IL-12		+		Proliferation of activated T cell induction of IFN-γ
IL-13			Mast cells	Induces IgE production in B cells
IL-15	+			Shares many activates with IL-2
IL-16	+			Chemotactic for and activation of CD4+ cells
IL-17	+			Contributes to IL-6 production by synoviocytes (in rheumatoid arthritis)
IL-18		+		Induces IFN-γ production in spleen cells
Tumor necrosis factor-α (TNF-α) (cachectin)	+	+		Fever; shock; activates macrophages; stimulates PMN chemotoxin; angiogenesis, bone resorption; cytotoxic to many cells
Tumor necrosis factor-β (TNF-β) (lymphotoxin)	+			Activates endothelial cells, granulocytes, and B cells
				Inhibits angiogenesis; cytotoxic to many cells
Inteferon-γ (IFN-γ)	+		NK cells	Activated NK cells, cytotoxic T cells, endothelial cells, and macrophages; has antitumor activity
				Stimulates LAK activity; co-stimulates B-cell proliferation; inhibits T-cell proliferation

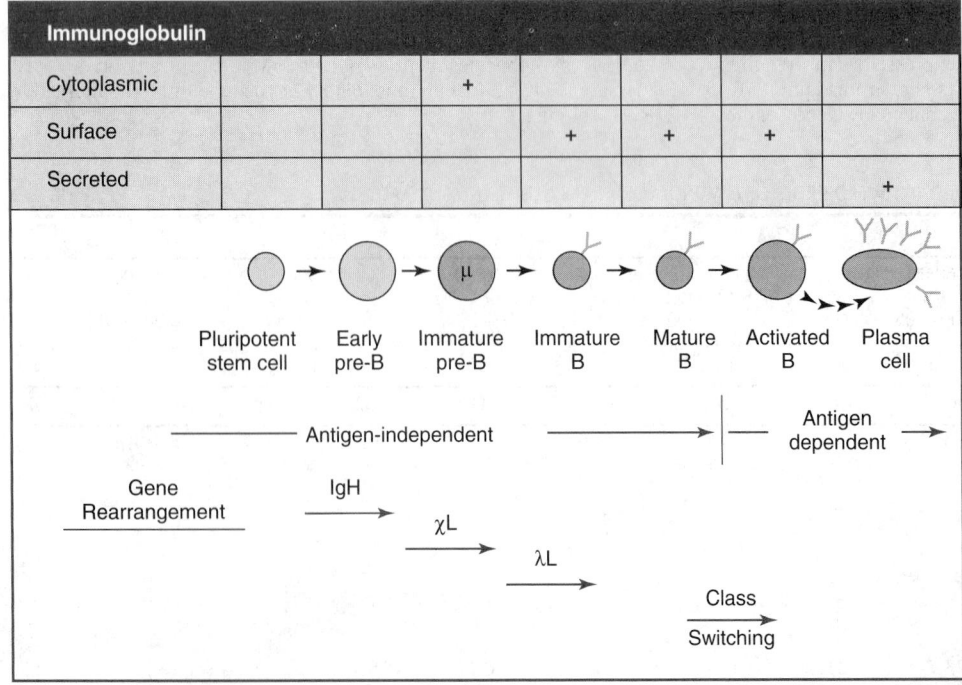

FIGURE 270–4 ■ Presentation of B-cell pathway development in a sequential form, which indicates when immunoglobulin appears in the cytoplasm or on the surface or is secreted. The gene rearrangements that take place at various stages of the differentiation pathway are indicated.

Table 270–3 ■ CHROMOSOMAL LOCATIONS OF THE HUMAN IMMUNOGLOBULIN AND T-CELL RECEPTOR GENES

CHAIN	SYMBOL	LOCUS
Immunoglobulin		
Heavy chain	H	14q32
Kappa light chain	κ	2p12
Lambda light chain	λ	22q11
T-cell receptor		
Alpha and delta chains	α, δ	14q11–12
Beta chain	β	7q32–35
Gamma chain	γ	7p15

There are several mechanisms that generate antibody diversity which are inherent in the somatic process of forming Ig genes.

1. *Combinatorial diversity,* which results from the combination of various gene segments as described above
2. *Junctional diversity,* which results at the joining site because of some imprecision in codon formation
3. *Junctional insertion,* by which diversity may arise because of insertion of extra nucleotides
4. *Somatic mutational events*
5. *Exchange rearrangement* of the H segments
6. The *combination of associated H and L chains*

This process allows an essentially random extrapolation of combinations into the millions of possibilities, (i.e., it *generates* antibody diversity).

T LYMPHOCYTES

T-Cell Receptors

The most common form of T-cell receptor consists of a disulfi-delinked heterodimer of α and β chains. Both of these chains contain amino-terminal *variable* regions and carboxy-terminal *constant* regions, just as occur in immunoglobulins. These chains contain carbohydrate and are bound within the surface of the T cell with membrane-spanning regions. A subset of T cells possesses similar receptors made up of γ and δ chains that seem to be highly specialized and located in certain regions of the body, such as the gastrointestinal tract. A molecule called the T3 complex bears the CD3 determinant and is non-covalently linked to the T-cell receptor heterodimer (see Fig. 270–3). It is of special note that variable regions of the T-cell receptor genes are assembled from V-D-J segment joining just as the immunoglobulin V region genes are assembled. Much less if any somatic hypermutation occurs in the T-cell receptor V region genes. Thus, rearrangement occurs during the process of differentiation, and once it has occurred it produces a stable clone with a fixed specificity.

ANTIGEN PRESENTATION AND THE MAJOR HISTOCOMPATIBILITY COMPLEX

Certain cell types such as macrophages, dendritic cells, and epidermal Langerhans cells are able to take up antigens nonspecifically and, when they express major histocompatibility class I or II (MHC I or II) molecules, present antigen to T cells (see Fig. 270–3). In some cases other cells, including activated B cells that may express class II MHC molecules, may also act as antigen-presenting cells. The antigen presented has often been processed so that only a relatively small peptide determinant is bound to the MHC for presentation (see Chapter 278). This event appears to involve the MHC molecule in conjunction with the processed antigen peptide on the surface of the antigen-presenting cell so that it can react with the T-cell receptor, and the CD4 molecule in the case of MHC-II, or with CD8 in the case of MHC-I, on the membrane of the T cell (see Chapter 278).

Similar membrane recognition events take place when cytotoxic

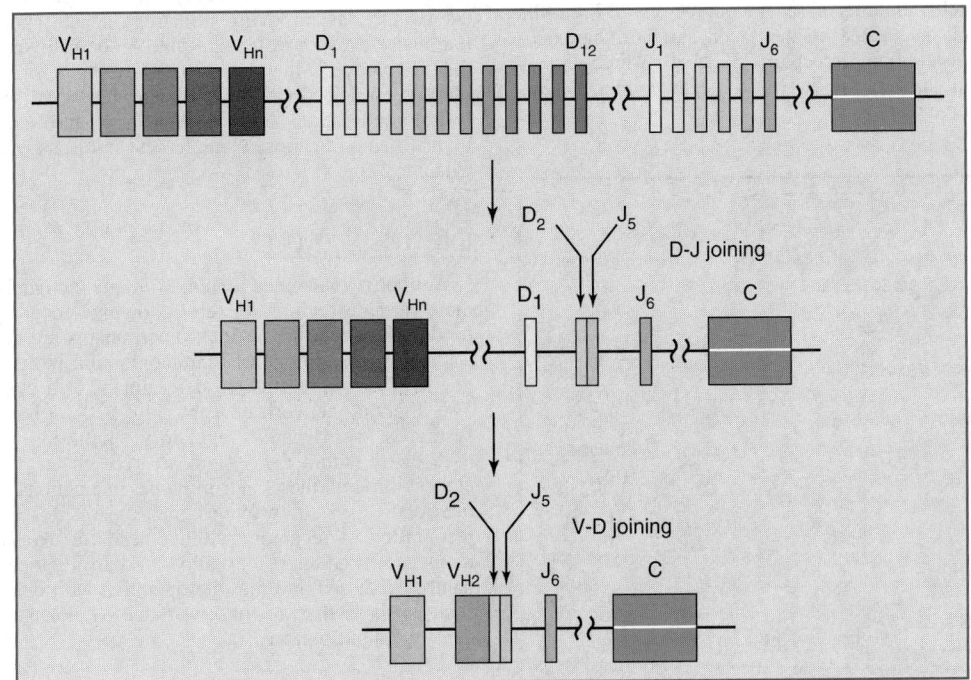

FIGURE 270–5 ■ The mechanisms for the joining of DJ and VD to form the entire variable region of the heavy chain. Note that intervening gene sequences at each step of joining are deleted, giving rise to the final finished product of an entire V region with the constant region at some distance. This event would be followed by a messenger RNA developing and splicing to form the entire translatable message sequence (see text for details).

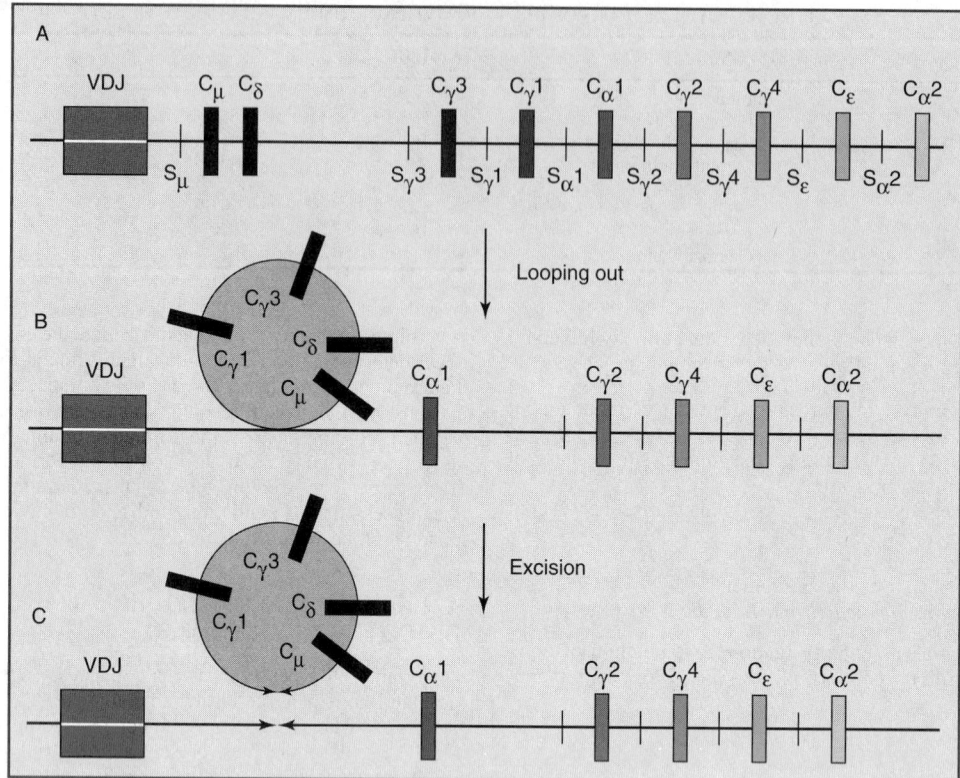

FIGURE 270–6 ■ A diagrammatic representation of class switching to produce IgA₁. The switch sequence regions (S) identify places where looping can occur. This results ultimately in excision of the loop containing $C\mu$, $C\delta$, $C\gamma_3$, and $C\gamma_1$, and brings $C\alpha_1$, into close juxtaposition to the rearranged VDJ regions. (Adapted from von Schwedler V, Jack HM, Wabl M: Circular DNA is a product of the immunoglobulin class switch rearrangement. Nature 345:452–454, 1990. Copyright 1990, Macmillan Magazines Ltd.)

T cells recognize and interact with cells bearing specific foreign antigens. In this case, the cytotoxic T cell may recognize the foreign antigen in conjunction with a class I MHC molecule, and it does so by virtue of its T-cell receptor in the presence of the CD8 molecule.

Activation of T cells requires a second signal via B7 on the antigen-presenting cell and CD28 on the T-cell surface. Once activated they express an additional receptor (CTLA-4), which closely resembles CD28 and appears to deliver a negative signal, thus limiting the proliferative response.

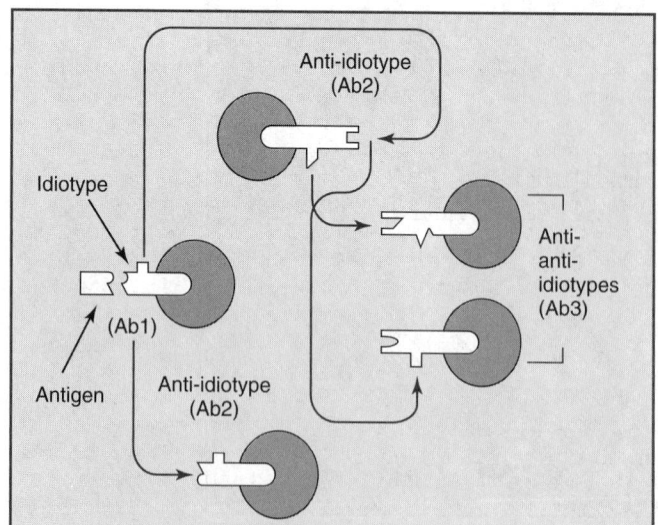

FIGURE 270–7 ■ Diagrammatic representation of the idiotypic network showing the development of anti-idiotypes and anti-anti-idiotypes in sequential processes. This complementary fit mechanism provides the structural basis for the feedback network.

REGULATION AND MODULATION OF THE IMMUNE PROCESS

Complement

The complement cascade is important to modify the effector arm of the immune system. Activating complement allows important events such as removing infectious agents and expressing the inflammatory response to take place. These involve active fragments of the pathway that enhance chemotaxis of macrophages, alter blood vessel permeability, change blood vessel diameters, cause lysis to cells, alter blood clotting, and cause numerous other subtle points of modification. Complement is discussed in greater detail in Chapter 271.

IDIOTYPIC NETWORKS

Antibody molecules express unique antigenic determinants on their variable regions, thereby allowing secondary antibodies to be produced against them. Such determinants are designated *idiotopes*. Therefore, an idiotope of immunoglobulin is functionally equivalent to the *clonotypic* antigenic determinant of a clonal line of T cells. The idiotypic network concept (Fig. 270–7) holds that the immune system is in a dynamic regulatory equilibrium so that members of each clone within the system are recognized by members of other clones through these anti-idiotope interactions. Conceptually, this interrelated system provides mechanisms for regulation based on recognition of receptors without need for exogenous antigen. This method of regulation may allow certain idiotopes to become dominantly expressed and may be operative with unique *clonal markers*, such as those that are observed due to clonal expansion in malignant lymphoid diseases.

HELPER T-CELL SYSTEM

Helper T-cells may be divided into Th1 and Th2 populations. A feedback control mechanism regulates these subsets. Generally, Th1 cytokines promote Th1 activity and inhibit Th2 activity. The reverse is also true. Th1 cytokines are IL-1, IL-12, and IFN-γ and enhance the cellular immune response. Th2 cytokines are IL-4, IL-5, and IL-6 and enhance the humoral immune response.

CYTOKINES

A growing array of molecules have been identified as products of cells that serve to regulate the immune system and to evoke responses in other cells, such as blood vessel endothelial cells and precursor cells in the bone marrow. Cytokines can regulate levels of response or induce differentiation and proliferation of cells. Table 270–2 summarizes the properties of some of these molecules that may be encountered in immune regulation (see also Chapters 158 and 312).

SUMMARY

The immune system is a highly orchestrated and coordinated system that allows a rapid response to foreign substances in a highly specific manner. The organization occurs at the level of the gene, the cell, and the mediator. Therefore, any qualitative or quantitative change in this system can produce profound effects. This is evident in diseases of the immune system, such as those that occur as the result of altered immune regulation (see Chapters 286 and 289).

Inflammation, often immunologically mediated and often resulting in tissue damage, is a key feature of diseases of virtually any organ system. Therefore, a knowledge of basic immunology is critical to a clear understanding of the nature of these abnormalities. A student of medicine must be prepared to apply immunology to every branch of internal medicine and to recognize its importance in understanding disease and, hence, the care of the patient.

Javeway C.H. Jr., Travers P.:, *Immunobiology*, 3rd ed. London, Current Biology Ltd/Garland. 1997. *An excellent introductory textbook, easy to read, with good visual aide.*

271 COMPLEMENT

John E. Volanakis

Complement is a major effector system of host defense against invading pathogens. It comprises more than 30 proteins that on activation elaborate protein fragments and protein-protein complexes that interact with specific cellular receptors or directly with cell membranes to mediate acute inflammatory reactions, clearance of foreign cells and molecules, killing of pathogenic microorganisms, and regulation of immune responses. In their native state, complement proteins are either serum soluble or associated with cell membranes (Table 271–1). Most of the serum-soluble proteins are synthesized in the liver. Complement proteins exhibit extensive structural homologies among themselves, remarkably conserving a

small number of repeated structural motifs, indicating that multiple gene duplication events marked the evolution of the system. Functionally, complement proteins are categorized as those participating in the activation sequences, those regulating the activation and activities of the system, and those serving as receptors for biologically active fragments. Some complement proteins overlap these functional categories.

NOMENCLATURE

Eleven proteins originally described as components of the classic pathway are designated by the capital letter C and a number from 1 to 9. C1 is a complex of three distinct proteins named C1q, C1r, and C1s. Two proteins participating in the activation of the alternative pathway are termed *factors* and are designated by the capital letters B and D. Proteins of the recently described lectin pathway are designated by their abbreviated descriptive names: MBL (mannose-binding lectin) and MASP (MBL-associated serine protease). An overbar indicates the enzymatically active form of a complement protein or protein complex, as in C1. Proteolytic cleavage fragments of complement proteins are symbolized by lower case letters, as in C2a and C2b, and inactive fragments by the letter i, as in C2ai. Regulatory proteins are designated by capital letters, as in H and I, or by their abbreviated descriptive names, as in DAF for decay-accelerating factor. Four of the complement receptors are symbolized by the letters CR, for complement receptor, and a number from 1 to 4. The remaining receptors are denoted by the symbol of the protein or protein fragment they bind followed by the letter R, as in C5aR.

COMPLEMENT ACTIVATION

The complement system must be activated to express biologic activity and is characterized by operational simplicity and economy of design. The most important host defense activities are derived from two proteins, C3 and C5, which are structurally similar and probably represent gene duplication products. Expression of activity requires that C3 and C5 be cleaved by highly specific proteases termed *convertases* (Fig. 271–1). There are two C3 and two C5 convertases. They are assembled during activation of the three pathways of complement, which are termed *classic, lectin,* and *alternative.* The activation pathways use different proteins to form these enzymes. In addition, the assembly of the convertases is initiated by different activators in the three pathways. However, the resulting enzymes have identical substrate and peptide bond specificity, giving rise to identical biologically active fragments. Characteristic of the simplicity and economy of design of complement activation is the fact that C5 convertases are derivatives of C3 convertases (see Fig. 271–1). Furthermore, C3 and C5 are activated by their respective convertases in similar fashion: a single peptide bond near the NH₂ terminus of the α polypeptide chain of either C3 or C5 is cleaved to generate a small peptide, C3a or C5a, and a large two-polypeptide fragment, C3b or C5b. Each of these four fragments, as well as further cleavage fragments of C3b, expresses at least one activity important to host defense.

Table 271–1 ■ PROTEINS OF THE COMPLEMENT SYSTEM*

| PREVALENT FORM IN NATIVE STATE | FUNCTIONAL GROUP | | |
	Participating in Activation Sequences	Regulatory	Receptors
Serum soluble	C1q, MBL C1r, C1s, MASP-1, MASP-2, D C2, B C4, C3, C5 C6, C7, C8, C9	C1INH, C4bp, H, I, P C3a/C5a INA S protein, SP 40/40	
Membrane associated		CR1, DAF, MCP CD59	C1qR C3aR, C5aR CR1, CR2 CR3, CR4

*Established symbols have been used for most complement proteins. In addition, the following generally accepted abbreviations have been used: MBL, mannose-binding lectin; MASP, MBL-associated serine protease; INH, inhibitor; C4bp, C4b-binding protein; INA, inactivator; R, receptor, e.g., CR1, complement receptor type 1; DAF, decay accelerating factor; MCP, membrane cofactor protein.

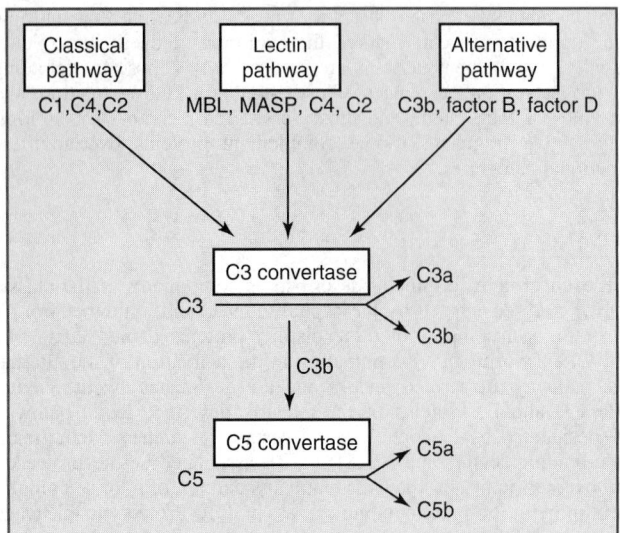

FIGURE 271–1 ■ Activation of the complement system.

ASSEMBLY OF COMPLEMENT CONVERTASES

CLASSIC PATHWAY. In the classic pathway, assembly of the convertases is usually initiated by antibodies of the IgG or IgM class complexed with antigen. Several other substances, including C-reactive protein complexes, certain viruses, and gram-negative bacteria, can also activate this pathway. Activators are recognized by C1q, one of the three proteins in the C1 complex. Binding to an activator induces a change in the conformation of C1q that causes the autoactivation of C1r, which in turn activates proenzyme C1s to enzymatically active C1s (Fig. 271–2). In the next step, C1s cleaves C4, resulting in the covalent attachment of its major fragment, C4b, to the surface of the activator. C4b is attached through a transacylation reaction similar to that leading to covalent binding of C3b to activating surfaces (see later). C2 binds to C4b and is also cleaved by C1 into two fragments, the larger of which, C2a, remains bound to C4b, completing the assembly of the C4b2a complex, which is the C3 convertase of the classic pathway. Cleavage of C3 by the C3 convertase results in the covalent binding of many C3b fragments to the surface of the activator and the eventual binding of one C3b to the C4b subunit of the C3 convertase. This leads to the formation of the $\overline{C3b4b2a}$ complex, which is the C5 convertase of the classic pathway.

LECTIN PATHWAY. This is a newly described antibody- and C1-independent pathway of complement activation that like the classic pathway leads to the formation of the $\overline{C4b2a}$, C3 convertase. In the lectin pathway a protein complex between MBL and two distinct serine proteases, MASP-1 and MASP-2, is the structural and functional equivalent of C1 in the classic pathway. MBL has binding specificity for bacterial pathogens expressing terminal mannose or N-acetylglucosamine on their surface. Binding of MBL to carbohydrates on pathogens results in activation of MASP-1 and MASP-2, which in turn sequentially activates C4 and C2, resulting in the assembly of pathogen-bound $\overline{C4b2a}$, C3 convertase and the subsequent formation of the $\overline{C3b4b2a}$, C5 convertase (Fig. 271–3).

ALTERNATIVE PATHWAY. Alternative pathway activation is initiated by a variety of cellular surfaces, including those of certain bacteria, parasites, viruses, and fungi. Antibodies can also activate this pathway, but they are not usually required. Assembly of the convertases depends on certain structural features of the multifunctional protein C3. C3 is the most abundant complement protein in blood and is characterized by the presence on its α-chain of an unusual, for blood proteins, thioester bond. Under physiologic conditions, this bond is relatively stable, being hydrolyzed at very slow rates to give rise to $C3_{H_2O}$, which can initiate the formation of the short-lived *initiation* C3 convertase. This is accomplished by the formation of a complex between $C3_{H_2O}$ and factor B and the subsequent cleavage of B by factor D to generate the $\overline{C3_{H_2O}Bb}$ complex, the initiation C3 convertase (Fig. 271–4). This series of reactions, starting with the hydrolysis of the thioester bond in native C3 and concluding with the cleavage of C3 into C3a and C3b by the initiation C3 convertase, is considered to occur in the blood continuously at slow rates. Thus, a constant supply of small amounts of freshly generated C3b is available at all times. The initiation C3 convertase is quickly inactivated by the control proteins H and I.

Cleavage of C3 by a C3 convertase induces a change in the conformation of C3b associated with an extremely labile (mestastable) thioester bond that reacts either with water or with hydroxyl or amino groups on the surface of cells or proteins. Thus, C3b can become covalently attached by means of an ester or amide bond to surfaces in the immediate vicinity of its generation. The fate of surface-bound C3b depends entirely on the chemical nature of the surface. C3b bound to a non-activator of the alternative pathway (e.g., the host's red cells) is quickly inactivated by the action of control proteins. In contrast, C3b bound to an activator (e.g., *Escherichia coli*) preferentially binds factor B, which is then cleaved by factor D, generating the $\overline{C3bBb}$ complex, which is the C3 convertase of the alternative pathway. This enzyme is labile, but it is stabilized by the binding of P and is termed the *amplification* C3 convertase because it generates many C3b fragments and thus additional molecules of C3 convertase. Binding of a single C3b molecule to the C3 convertase gives rise to the $(C3b)_2Bb$ complex,

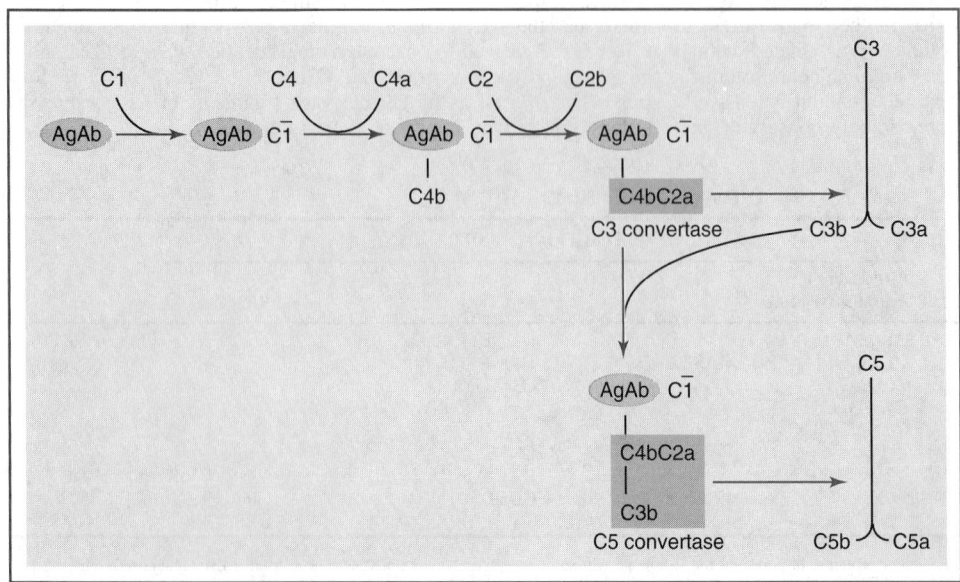

FIGURE 271–2 ■ Formation of complement convertases in the classic pathway of activation.

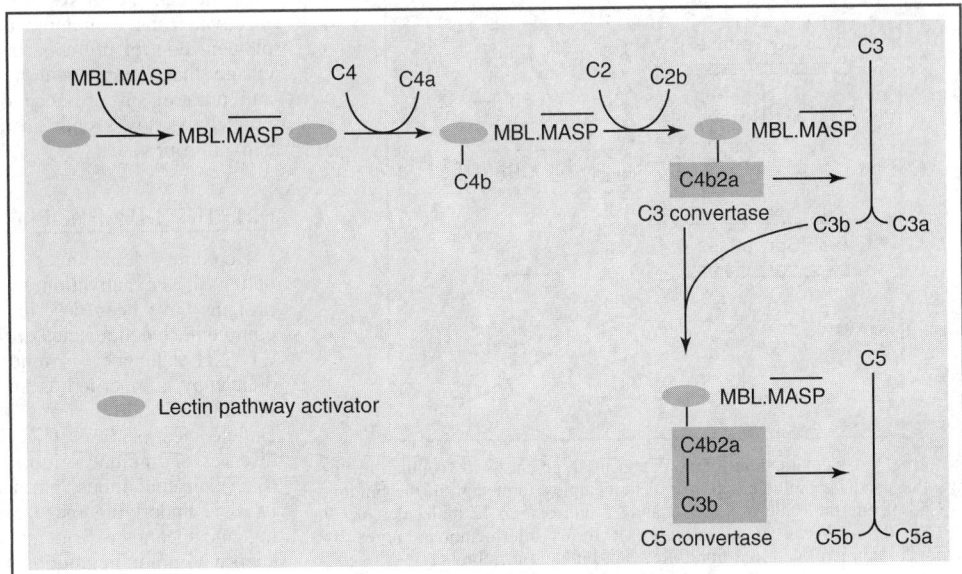

FIGURE 271-3 ■ Formation of complement convertases in the lectin pathway of activation.

which is the C5 convertase of the alternative pathway (see Fig. 271–4).

BIOLOGIC ACTIVITIES OF COMPLEMENT

With the exception of C5b, the fragments produced by the action of the convertases carry out their biologic functions by interacting with specific cellular receptors (Fig. 271–5). The complement *anaphylatoxins,* C3a and C5a, react with specific receptors to stimulate the release of histamine from mast cells and basophils mediating smooth muscle contraction and increased vascular permeability. In the presence of interleukin-3 or interleukin-5, C5a also causes release of leukotrienes from basophils. In addition, C5a evokes neutrophil and monocyte responses, including up-regulation of cellular

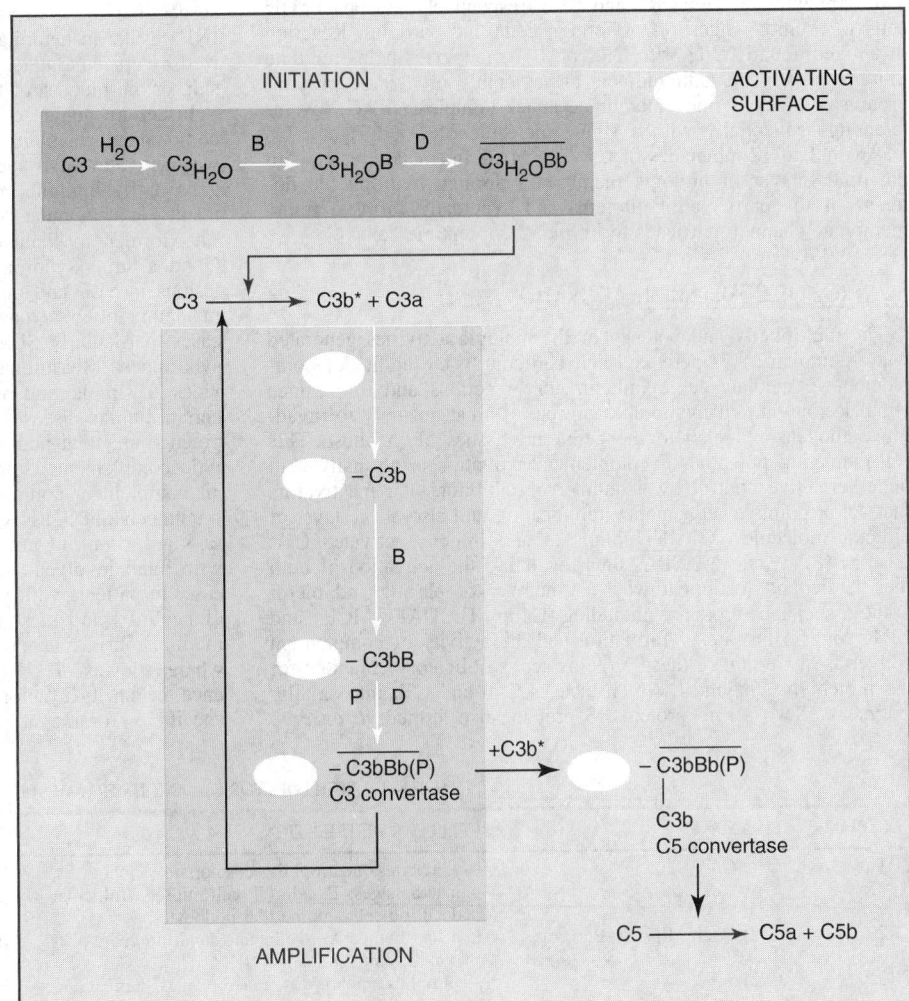

FIGURE 271-4 ■ Formation of complement convertases in the alternative pathway of activation. Assembly of the *initiation* C3 convertase occurs at low levels continuously. When an activator is present, metastable C3b (C3b*) binds covalently to the activating surface and, because it is protected from the action of the regulatory proteins, initiates the assembly of the stable, *amplification* C3 convertase, which forms additional C3 convertase complexes and also the C5 convertase.

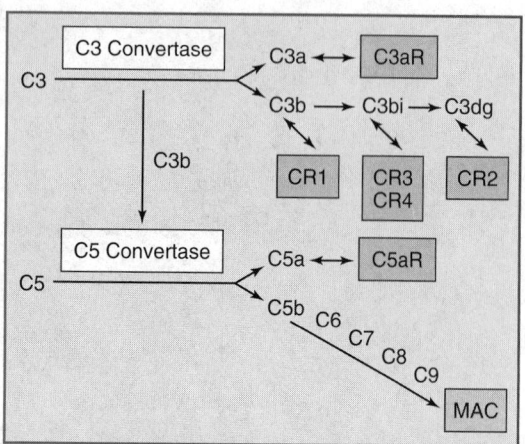

FIGURE 271–5 ■ Interactions of complement fragments with cellular receptors that mediate biologic activities. The complex formed from the binding to C5b of one molecule of C6, C7, and C8 and of 1 to 12 molecules of C9 is termed *membrane attack complex*. It forms transmembrane pores by interacting directly with the lipid bilayer of biologic membranes.

receptors, adherence to vascular endothelia, chemotaxis, release of lysosomal enzymes, and generation of oxygen free radicals. Collectively, the anaphylatoxins allow for the recruitment of host defense molecules and cells to tissue sites invaded by pathogens. C3b and its further cleavage fragments, C3bi and C3dg, react with multiple receptors distributed in a variety of cells (Table 271–2). C3b convalently attached to immune complexes binds to CR1 receptors on erythrocytes, which transport the complexes to the liver, where they are taken up by Kuppfer cells and cleared from the circulation. C3b and C3bi interact with CR1 and CR3, respectively, on phagocytic cells to promote ingestion of foreign cells and particles. Reaction of antigen-bound C3dg with CR2 on B lymphocytes helps regulate immune responses. C5b initiates the assembly of a large protein-protein complex, termed membrane attack complex (MAC), by interacting sequentially with a single molecule of C6, C7, and C8 and with 1 to 12 molecules of C9. The MAC interacts directly with the lipid bilayer of biologic membranes through hydrophobic domains of the participating proteins and eventually forms a transmembrane channel that leads to killing of susceptible cells.

CONTROL OF COMPLEMENT ACTIVATION

The multiplicity and potency of the biologic activities generated when complement is activated and particularly the ability of complement to mediate acute inflammatory reactions and to produce lethal lesions in cell membranes present a threat not only to invading pathogens but also to the cells and tissues of the host. This self-damaging potential of complement activation is normally kept under effective control by a number of inhibitors and inactivators that act at points of enzymatic amplification and also at the level of effector molecules. C1 INH binds to and inhibits activated C1r, C1s, MASP-1, and MASP-2, thus regulating the activation of both the classic and lectin pathways. A number of plasma and membrane-associated proteins, including C4bp, H, DAF, MCP, and CR1, control the rate of formation and the activity of complement convertases. Certain of these proteins act as obligatory cofactors for the proteolytic enzyme I, which cleaves C4b and C3b into smaller fragments. Two serum proteins, S protein, also termed *vitronectin*,

and SP 40/40, and a cell-associated protein, CD59, inhibit the formation of the MAC. Finally, C3a/C5a INA, a carboxypeptidase, inactivates the complement anaphylatoxins. Collectively, the complement control proteins perform two important functions: (1) they ensure that complement activation is proportional to the amount and duration of presence of complement activators and (2) they protect the host's cells from the harmful potential of complement activation products.

INHERITED DEFICIENCIES OF COMPLEMENT PROTEINS

Hereditary deficiencies of almost all complement proteins participating in the activation sequences and of several of the control proteins have been described (Table 271–3). With two exceptions, complement deficiencies are inherited as autosomal recessive traits. C1 INH deficiency is inherited as an autosomal dominant and P deficiency is inherited as an X-linked trait. A rather limited number of clinical syndromes are associated with complement deficiencies. Deficiencies of C1q, C1r, C1s, C4, and C2 are associated with diseases of immune origin, including systemic lupus erythematosus (SLE), discoid lupus, glomerulonephritis, and non-specific vasculitis. The underlying mechanisms are unclear, but impaired processing and clearance from the circulation of immune complexes and aberrant immunoregulation have been implicated in the pathogenesis of these syndromes. Clinically, systemic lupus erythematosus in complement-deficient individuals is characterized by early-onset, extensive skin lesions and low levels of antinuclear and anti-DNA antibodies. Deficiencies of C3, H, I, or P predispose to severe recurrent infections with encapsulated pyogenic bacteria. Lack of or inefficient opsonization of the bacteria by C3b/C3bi apparently causes the susceptibility to infection. Individuals deficient in C5, C6, C7, or C8 are susceptible to disseminated neisserial infection, most commonly meningococcal meningitis. Direct lysis by complement is probably required for effective defense against gonococci and meningococci. Individuals with C9 deficiency are usually less susceptible to neisserial infections. Heterozygous deficiency of C1 INH results in hereditary angioedema (see Chapter 273), characterized by episodic attacks of circumscribed, non-pruritic edema of the skin or the mucosa of the respiratory or gastrointestinal tract.

In certain human diseases, uncontrolled or aberrant activation of complement plays an important pathogenetic role. The classic pathway activated at tissue sites by autoantibodies against tissue antigens or by immune complexes deposited at basement membranes results in accumulation of inflammatory cells and tissue damage. The former mechanism is exemplified by the renal lesions of Goodpasture's syndrome and the second by the vascular and renal lesions in SLE and other immune complex diseases. Hypocomplementemia often is present in patients with immune complex diseases, particularly SLE, but is also found in various other clinical syndromes. Measurement of serum complement levels thus provides a simple and widely used tool to diagnose and manage certain human diseases. The most commonly used assays in clinical practice are total hemolytic complement, C4, and C3. Total hemolytic complement, expressed in CH_{50} units, reflects the activity of all complement components. C4 and C3 are usually measured by immunochemical assays. Low complement levels by all three assays are often but not always seen in SLE, particularly in patients with renal involvement and during acute exacerbations of the disease. In patients with partial lipodystrophy with or without glomerulonephritis and in some patients with membranoproliferative glomerulonephritis, levels of total complement and C3 are very low, whereas levels of C4 are usually normal. This is due to the presence of an IgG autoantibody, termed *C3 nephritic factor*, with specificity for the amplification C3 convertase. This autoantibody

Table 271–2 ■ **RECEPTORS FOR C3b AND ITS FRAGMENTS**

RECEPTOR	LIGANDS	CELLULAR DISTRIBUTION	FUNCTIONS
CR1	C3b, C4b, C3bi	Erythrocytes, neutrophils, eosinophils, monocytes, macrophages, B cells, T cell subsets, follicular dendritic cells, glomerular podocytes	Immune complex clearance, endocytosis, phagocytosis
CR2	C3dg, C3bi, Epstein-Barr virus	B cells, thymocytes, follicular dendritic cells, pharyngeal epithelial cells	Immunoregulation
CR3	C3bi	Neutrophils, monocytes, macrophages, large granular lymphocytes	Phagocytosis, leukocyte adhesion, enhanced cytotoxicity
CR4	C3bi	Neutrophils, monocytes, macrophages	Unknown

DEFICIENT PROTEIN	DISEASES
Clq, Clr, Cls, C4, C2	SLE, SLE-like syndrome, discoid lupus, glomerulonephritis, vasculitis
C3, H, I, P	Recurrent pyogenic infections
C5, C6, C7, C8, C9	Recurrent disseminated neisserial infections
C1 INH	Hereditary angioedema

binds to C3bBb and creates a stable complex that is not regulated by control proteins and thus continuously cleaves C3. The alternative pathway is also activated during circulation of the blood through pump oxygenators or hemodialysis machines. The C5a generated during these procedures causes aggregation of neutrophils, leading to their sequestration in the pulmonary vasculature. In some patients this is manifested by symptoms of pulmonary dysfunction and hypoxemia. Complement activation may also play a role in the pathogenesis of myocardial reperfusion injury.

Colten HR, Rosen FS: Complement deficiencies. Annu Rev Immunol 10:809, 1992. *An excellent review of genetic abnormalities of the complement system.*
Davies KA, Walport MJ: Processing and clearance of immune complexes by complement and the role of complement in immune complex diseases. *In* Volanakis JE, Frank MM (eds): The Human Complement System in Health and Disease. New York, Marcel Dekker, 1998, p 423. *An enlightening review of a complex subject of medical significance.*
Fearon DT, Carter RH: The CD19/CR2/TAPA-1 complex of B lymphocytes: Linking natural to acquired immunity. Annu Rev Immunol 13:127, 1995. *An analysis of molecules and functions involved in the regulation of B lymphocyte responses by complement activation.*
Volanakis JE: Overview of the complement system. *In* Volanakis JE, Frank MM (eds): The Human Complement System in Health and Disease. New York, Marcel Dekker, 1998, p 9. *A comprehensive description of complement protein structure and complement activation.*

272 PRIMARY IMMUNODEFICIENCY DISEASES

Rebecca H. Buckley

Since the first genetic defect in immunity was described in 1952, more than 70 primary immunodeficiency syndromes have been reported. Such diseases may involve any component of the immune system, including lymphocytes, phagocytic cells, and the complement proteins. This chapter focuses on abnormalities of lymphocytes. Deficiencies of the complement system (see Chapter 271) are mentioned briefly. A review of neutrophil dysfunction syndromes is presented in Chapter 171 and an overall review of the compromised host is given in Chapter 314. The acquired immunodeficiency syndrome (AIDS) is described in Part XXIII.

Until recently, there was little insight into the fundamental problems underlying most of these conditions. However, the molecular defects have now been identified in a growing number of primary immunodeficiency diseases (Table 272-1). Most are recessive traits, some caused by mutations in genes on the X chromosome, others in genes on autosomal chromosomes. Table 272-1 also lists the most prominent functional abnormalities in a number of these primary immunodeficiency syndromes.

Primary immunodeficiencies are rare. The incidence of agammaglobulinemia is estimated at 1 in 50,000; severe combined immunodeficiency at 1 in 100,000. Selective absence of serum and secretory immunoglobulin A (IgA), the most common, has a reported prevalence of 1 in 333 to 1 in 700.

APPROACHES TO THE PATIENT WITH SUSPECTED IMMUNODEFICIENCY

The number of patients suspected of having primary immunodeficiency will far exceed the incidences of these diseases. It is thus important that the tests selected for immunologic assessment be broadly informative, reliable, and cost-effective. Familiarity with certain clinical guidelines aids in the initial selection. Patients with antibody, phagocytic cell, or complement deficiencies have recurrent infections with high-grade encapsulated bacteria. Therefore, those with only repeated viral respiratory infections are not likely to have any of these disorders. By contrast, patients with deficiencies in T-cell function usually manifest opportunistic infections. Most defects can be ruled out at little cost if the proper choice of screening tests is made. Among the most informative are the complete and differential blood counts and the sedimentation rate. Examining red cells for Howell-Jolly bodies helps exclude asplenia. A normal platelet count rules out the Wiskott-Aldrich syndrome. If the sedimentation rate is normal, chronic bacterial or fungal infection is unlikely. If the absolute neutrophil count is normal, congenital and acquired neutropenia and severe chemotactic defects are eliminated. If the absolute lymphocyte count is normal, a severe T-cell defect is unlikely. Beyond this, one should keep in mind that tests of immune function are far more informative and cost effective than those measuring immunoglobulin concentrations or counting lymphocyte subpopulations.

In assessing B-cell function, determinations of antibody titers to proteins (such as tetanus and diphtheria toxoids) and polysaccharides (such as pneumococcal antigens) after immunization are the most useful tests. As a rule, patients with B-cell defects for which there is an effective or indicated treatment do not produce antibodies normally. However, the presence of such antibodies does not exclude IgA deficiency, which would also be missed on a serum electrophoretic analysis. The quantification of serum IgA is particularly cost effective. If the IgA concentration is normal, this finding rules out not only IgA deficiency but all of the permanent types of agammaglobulinemia, because the IgA level is usually very low or absent in those conditions as well. A particularly uneconomical study is IgG-subclass measurement. It is far more helpful to know whether a patient can produce protein and polysaccharide antibodies normally, because there are well-documented cases of antibody deficiency despite normal concentrations of all immunoglobulin classes and subclasses.

The most cost-effective test for assessing T-cell function is an intradermal skin test with 0.1 mL of a 1:1000 dilution of a known potent *Candida albicans* extract. If the test result is positive, as defined by erythema and induration ≥10 mm at 48 hours, virtually all primary T-cell defects are excluded and the need for more expensive in vitro tests, such as lymphocyte phenotyping or assessments of responses to mitogens, is obviated. Killing defects of phagocytic cells, which should be suspected if the patient has problems with staphylococcal or gram-negative infections, can be screened for by tests measuring the neutrophil respiratory burst after phagocytosis or phorbol ester stimulation. Complement defects can be most effectively screened for in a CH_{50} assay, which measures the intactness of the entire complement pathway. If results of these tests are abnormal, or even if they are normal and clinical features of the patient still strongly suggest a host defect, the patient should be evaluated at a center where more definitive immunologic studies can be done before any type of immunologic treatment is begun.

ANTIBODY DEFICIENCY DISORDERS

Patients with antibody deficiency are usually recognized because they have recurrent infections, but some individuals with selective IgA deficiency or infants with transient hypogammaglobulinemia may have few or no infections.

X-LINKED AGAMMAGLOBULINEMIA (XLA). Patients with X-linked agammaglobulinemia remain well during the first 6 to 9 months of life as a result of maternally transmitted immunoglobulin. Thereafter, they acquire infections with high-grade extracellular pyogenic organisms such as pneumococci, streptococci, and *Haemophilus* spp. unless given prophylactic antibiotics or intravenous immunoglobulin (IVIG) therapy. The most common infections are sinusitis, pneumonia, otitis, septic arthritis, meningitis, and septicemia. Chronic fungal infections are usually not present, and *Pneumocystis carinii* pneumonia rarely occurs unless there is an associated neutropenia. Viral infections and live virus vaccines are also usually handled normally, with the notable exceptions of hepatitis and enterovirus infections. Several cases of paralysis after receiving polio vaccine have occurred, and chronic, eventually fatal central nervous system disease echovirus infections have occurred in more than 40 patients.

The diagnosis of XLA is suspected if serum concentrations of IgG, IgA, and IgM are below the 95% confidence limits for appropriate age- and race-matched controls (usually there is <100 mg/dL total immunoglobulin). Results of tests for natural antibodies to blood group substances, for antibodies to antigens given during standard courses of immunization, and for antibodies to and ability to clear bacteriophage φX174 are markedly abnormal. Polymorphonuclear functions are usually normal, but some patients with this condition have had transient, persistent, or cyclic neutropenia.

Lymphopenia is uncommon, and blood T cells are increased in number. In contrast, blood B lymphocytes are absent or are present in very low numbers. Hypoplasia of adenoids, tonsils, and peripheral lymph nodes is the rule; germinal centers are not present, and plasma cells are rarely found. Conversely, some pre-B cells are found in the bone marrow. The abnormal gene in XLA was discovered in 1993 by two groups, one through positional cloning and the

other through discovery of a B-cell-specific tyrosine kinase encoded by a gene on the X chromosome (see Table 272–1 and Figure 272–1). The tyrosine kinase has been named Bruton tyrosine kinase (or BTK) in honor of Dr. Bruton. BTK is a member of the Src-related non-receptor cytoplasmic tyrosine kinase family, which includes Lck, Fyn, and Lyn, thought to be involved in signal transduction in many hematopoietic cells. BTK is expressed at high levels in all B-lineage cells, including pre-B cells; it has not been detected in any cells of T lineage, but it has in cells of the myeloid series. To date more than 250 different mutations in the human BTK gene have been recognized. Mixed lymphocyte responsiveness and lymphocyte responses to antigens and mitogens are normal. Cell-mediated immune responses can be detected in vivo, and the thymus has appeared normal in autopsied cases.

Except in those unfortunate patients in whom polio, persistent echovirus infection, or lymphoreticular malignancy develops, the overall prognosis is reasonably good if IVIG therapy is instituted early. Systemic infection can be prevented by 400 mg/kg IVIG every 3 to 4 weeks. Such preparations are known to be free of human immunodeficiency virus (HIV) and hepatitis viruses. Many patients go on to experience crippling sinopulmonary disease de-

Table 272–1 ■ ABNORMAL GENES KNOWN TO CAUSE HUMAN PRIMARY IMMUNODEFICIENCY

CHROMO-SOME	GENE PRODUCT	DISORDER	FUNCTIONAL IMMUNODEFICIENCIES
1q	RFX5*	MHC class II antigen deficiency	Low immunoglobulin level, lack of T-cell responses to antigens, CD4 deficiency
1q25	p67phox*	Autosomal recessive CGD	Lack of bacterial and fungal killing by phagocytic cells
1q42-43	Vesicle membrane component	Chediak-Higashi syndrome	Lack of intracellular killing, T-cell or NK cell cytotoxicity; giant lysosomes
2p11	κ Chain*	κ Chain deficiency	Absence of immunoglobulins bearing κ chains
2q12	ZAP70*	CD8 lymphocytopenia	Failure of CD4+ T cells to respond to usual signals
5p13	IL-7Rα*	T-B+NK+ SCID	Absence of T- and B-cell functions
6p21.3	TAP*	MHC class I antigen deficiency	Marked deficiency of CD8+ T cells; combined B- and T-cell defects
6p21.3	Unknown	IgA deficiency; CVID	Low or absent serum IgA level; low concentrations of all immunoglobulins in CVID
q22-q23	IFN-γR1*	Disseminated mycobacterial infections	Failure of macrophages and other cells to produce TNF-α in response to IFN-γ
7q11.23	p47phox*	Autosomal recessive CGD	Lack of bacterial and fungal killing by phagocytic cells
8q21	Unknown	Nijmegen breakage syndrome	Combined B- and T-cell defects; resemble patients with A-T
9p21-p13	Unknown	Cartilage–hair hypoplasia	Combined T- and B-cell defects of varying severity
10p13	Unknown	DiGeorge/velocardiofacial syndrome	Low numbers of T cells and impaired T-cell function
10p14-15	IL-2Rα*	Lymphoproliferative syndrome	Poor T-cell responses; impaired apoptosis; increased bcl-2; autoimmunity
11	CD3 γ* or ε*	CD3 deficiency	Poor T-cell responses to mitogens; lack of cytotoxic T cells; IgG subclass deficiency
11p13	RAG-1 or RAG-2*	T-B-NK+SCID	Absence of T- and B-cell functions
11q22.3	DNA-dependent kinase*	Ataxia-telangiectasia	Selective IgA deficiency; T-cell deficiency
13q	RFXAP*	MHC class II antigen deficiency	Low immunoglobulin level; lack of T-cell responses to antigens; CD4 deficiency
14q13.1	Purine nucleosidase*	PNP deficiency	Severe T-cell deficiency; may have immunoglobulins
14q32.3	Immunoglobulin heavy chains*	B-cell-negative agammaglobulinemia (μ) or selective deficiencies of other isotypes	Absence of antibody production and lack of B cells in μ chain mutations; subclasses missing but B cells present in others
15q21	myosin-Vα*	Griscelli's disease (partial albinism)	Partial combined T- and B-cell immunodeficiencies
16p13	CIITA*	MHC class II antigen deficiency	Low immunoglobulin level; lack of T-cell responses to antigens; CD4 deficiency
16q24	p22phox*	Autosomal recessive CGD	Lack of bacterial and fungal killing by phagocytic cells
19p13.1	JAKIII*	T-B+NK-SCID	Absence of T-, B-, and NK cell functions
20q13.11	ADA*	T-B-NK-SCID	Absence of T- and B-cell functions
21q22.3	CD18*	Leukocyte adhesion deficiency, type 1 (LAD 1)	Absence of cytotoxic T and NK lymphocyte function; lack of phagocytic cell adhesion
22q11.2	Unknown	DiGeorge/velocardiofacial syndrome	Low numbers of T cells and impaired T-cell function
Xp21.1	p21phox*	X-linked CGD	Lack of bacterial and fungal killing by phagocytic cells
Xp11.23	WASP*	Wiskott-Aldrich syndrome	Thrombocytopenia; poor antipolysaccharide antibody production; T-cell deficiency
Xp11.3-p21.1	Properdin*	Properdin deficiency	Lack of complement alternate pathway function
Xq13.1	Common γ chain (γc)*	T-B+NK-SCID	Absence of T-, B-, and NK cell functions
Xq22	Bruton tyrosine kinase (BTK)*	X-linked (Bruton's) agammaglobulinemia	Absence of antibody production; lack of B cells
Xq24-26	SAP(SLAM-associated protein)	X-linked lymphoproliferative syndrome	Lack of anti-EBNA and long-lived T-cell immunity to EBV; low immunoglobulin level
Xq26	CD154 (CD40 ligand)*	X-linked hyper-IgM syndrome	Failure to produce IgG, IgA, and IgE antibodies

*Gene cloned and sequenced, gene product known. ZAP 70 = zeta-associated protein 70 IL-7Rα = α chain of interleukin 7 receptor; TAP = MHC = major histocompatibility complex; CGD = chronic granulomatous disease; T-B+NK+SCID = severe combined immunodeficiency; IFN-γR1 = interferon γ receptor 1; RAG-1 = recombinase activating gene 1; IgA = immunoglobulin A; CVID = common variable immunodeficiency; TNF-α = tumor necrosis factor α; A-T = ataxia-telangiectasia; CIITA = class II transactivator; JAK3 = Janus Kinase 3; ADA = adenosine deaminase deficiency; PNP = purine nucleoside phosphorylase; WASP = Wiskott-Aldrich syndrome protein; EBNA = Epstein-Barr nuclear antigen.

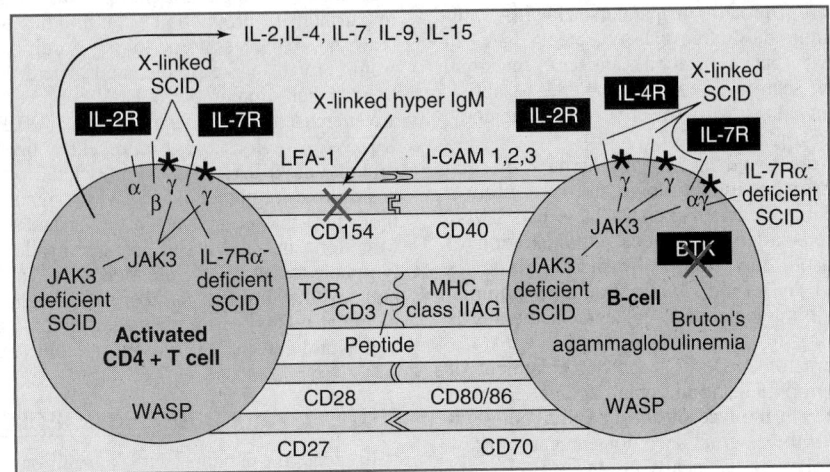

FIGURE 272–1 ■ Schematic of molecules involved in T- and B-cell interaction and signal transduction, showing the location of newly defined molecular defects in four X-linked primary immunodeficiency diseases. Mutations in the gene encoding the cytoplasmic non-receptor tyrosine kinase lead to Bruton's or X-linked agammaglobulinemia by preventing B-cell maturation beyond the pre-B cell stage. Mutations in the gene for the CD40 ligand, CD154, prevent expression of this crucial molecule necessary for T cells to activate B cells by interacting with CD40 on their surface. These mutations are responsible for the defect in X-linked immunodeficiency with hyper-IgM that prevents the B cells from isotype switching. Mutations in the common γ chain (γc) for several cytokine receptors (interleukin 2 [IL-2], IL-4, IL-7, IL-9, and IL-15) in infants with X-linked severe combined immunodeficiency (X-SCID) prevent the binding of those cytokines to their receptors, resulting in profound deficiencies in T, B, and natural killer (NK) cell development and function. Mutations in a novel gene encoding a 501-amino-acid cytoplasmic proline-rich protein (WASP) important in actin polymerization result in the Wiskott-Aldrich syndrome. Mutations in Janus kinase 3 (JAK3), the primary signal transducer for γc, result in autosomal recessive SCID that resembles X-SCID phenotypically. Finally, mutations in the α chain of the IL-7 receptor (IL-7Rα) also result in autosomal recessive SCID.

spite this therapy, because no effective means exists for replacing secretory IgA at the mucosal surface. Chronic antibiotic therapy is then also necessary for managing such patients.

COMMON VARIABLE IMMUNODEFICIENCY (CVID). Patients who have common variable immunodeficiency (formerly known as acquired hypogammaglobulinemia) may appear similar in many respects to those with XLA. Although this disorder may occur in children, most patients present with a history of recurrent infections beginning several years after birth. CVID is distinguished from XLA by later age of onset, somewhat less severe susceptibility to infections, and almost equal gender distribution. In contrast to patients with XLA, patients with CVID may have normal sized or enlarged tonsils and lymph nodes, and the latter may have cortical follicles. Additionally, such patients often have normal or nearly normal numbers of circulating B lymphocytes. Nevertheless, the serum immunoglobulin and antibody deficiencies are usually just as profound, and the bacterial etiologic agents are the same as in XLA. Echovirus meningoencephalitis is rare in patients with CVID.

This condition has been variably associated with a sprue-like syndrome, with or without nodular follicular lymphoid hyperplasia of the intestine; thymoma; alopecia areata; and autoantibody formation leading to hemolytic anemia, gastric atrophy, achlorhydria, and pernicious anemia. Frequent complications include giardiasis (seen far more often here than in XLA), bronchiectasis, gastric carcinoma, lymphoreticular malignancy, and cholelithiasis. Lymphoid interstitial pneumonia, pseudolymphoma, amyloidosis, and non-caseating sarcoid-like granulomas of the lungs, spleen, skin, and liver have also been seen.

Despite normal numbers of circulating B lymphocytes, the B cells do not differentiate into immunoglobulin-producing plasma cells. Because CVID occurs in first-degree relatives of patients with selective IgA deficiency (A Def), and some patients with A Def later become panhypogammaglobulinemic, it is possible that these diseases have a common genetic basis. This concept is supported by the finding of a high incidence of C4-A gene deletions and rare C2 gene alleles in the Class III major histocompatibility complex (MHC) region in individuals with either A Def or CVID, suggesting that there is a susceptibility gene in this region on chromosome 6 (see Table 272–1). However, the abnormal gene has not yet been identified. These studies have also shown that a small number of human leukocyte antigen (HLA) haplotypes are shared by individuals affected with CVID and A Def, with at least one of two

particular haplotypes being present in 77% of those affected. In one large family with 13 members, 2 had A Def and 3 had CVID. All of the immunodeficient patients in the family had at least one copy of a major histocompatibility complex (MHC) haplotype shown to be abnormally frequent in A Def and CVID: HLA-DQB1 *0201, HLA-DR3, C4B-Sf, C4A-deleted, G11-15, Bf-0.4, C2a, HSP70-7.5, tumor necrosis factor α (TNF-α-5), HLA-B8, and HLA-A1. However, four immunologically normal members of the pedigree also possessed this haplotype, indicating that its presence alone is not sufficient for expression of the defects. Environmental factors, particularly drugs such as phenytoin, have been suspected to provide the triggers for disease expression in individuals with the permissive genetic background. The treatment of CVID is the same as that for the X-linked disorder.

SELECTIVE IGA DEFICIENCY (A DEF). An isolated near-absence (i.e., <10 mg/dL) of serum and secretory IgA is the most common primary immunodeficiency disorder, with a frequency of 1:333 reported among some blood donors. Although A Def has been observed in apparently healthy individuals, it is commonly associated with ill health. The kinds of health problems experienced often reflect the type of clinic from which the patients are drawn. Among 75 from an allergy-immunology clinic, there were high frequencies of chronic or recurrent respiratory tract infection and atopic diseases. In contrast, 30 A Def patients drawn from a rheumatology clinic had a high frequency of autoimmune and/or collagen vascular disease.

IgA is the major immunoglobulin of external secretions. As would be expected, its deficiency is associated with infections occurring predominantly in the respiratory, gastrointestinal, and urogenital tracts. Bacterial agents responsible are essentially the same as in other types of antibody deficiency syndromes. Patients with this disorder do not appear to have an undue susceptibility to viral infections. Serum concentrations of other immunoglobulins are usually normal in patients with A Def, although an IgG₂ subclass deficiency has been reported in some, and IgM (level usually increased) may be of the low-molecular-weight variety. The defect may not always be permanent. Results of studies of T-cell function have been normal in most patients.

In addition to limiting the attachment of infectious agents to mucosal surfaces, secretory IgA antibodies probably act to prevent absorption of other foreign antigens, such as those in the diet. There is a high incidence of allergy and of IgG antibodies against cow's milk and ruminant serum proteins in patients with IgA deficiency. The antiruminant antibodies often falsely detect "IgA" in immunoassays that use goat (but not rabbit) antisera. Intestinal nodular hyperplasia has been seen in a few such patients. A sprue-like syndrome may occur in adults with selective IgA deficiency, and it sometimes responds to a gluten-free diet.

Serum antibodies to IgA are found in as many as 44% of such patients. This observation is of possible etiologic and great clinical significance. At least seven IgA-deficient patients have had severe or fatal anaphylactic reactions after intravenous administration of blood products. For this reason, only multiply washed erythrocytes or blood products from other A Def individuals should be administered to these patients, and immunoglobulin replacement therapy is contraindicated.

Currently the only therapy for A Def is vigorous treatment of specific infections with appropriate antimicrobial agents. Even if serum IgA could be replaced (in the face of anti-IgA antibodies), it would not be transported into the external secretions, because transport is an active process involving only locally produced IgA.

IMMUNODEFICIENCY WITH ELEVATED IgM LEVEL (HYPER-IgM). Immunodeficiency with elevated IgM level is characterized by very low serum levels of IgG and IgA but elevated level of polyclonal IgM. Some patients have low-molecular-weight IgM molecules. Like patients with XLA, those with this defect commonly become symptomatic during infancy with recurrent pyogenic infections, including otitis, sinusitis, pneumonia, and tonsillitis. In contrast to patients with XLA, in those with hyper-IgM the frequent presence of lymphoid hyperplasia often leads away from a diagnosis of immunodeficiency. There is an increased frequency of autoimmune disorders, such as hemolytic anemia and thrombocytopenia; and transient, persistent, or cyclic neutropenia is common. Normal or only slightly reduced numbers of B lymphocytes have been found in the blood of these patients. In the mid-1980s, cultured B cells from patients with X-linked hyper-IgM were shown to be capable of synthesizing IgA and IgG when co-cultured with a "switch" T-cell line, suggesting that the defect lay in T-lineage cells. The abnormal gene in X-linked hyper-IgM was localized to Xq26 and isolated in 1993. The gene product (now designated CD154) is the ligand for CD40 and is present on the surface of B cells (see Table 272–1 and Figure 272–1). It is found only on activated T cells, primarily of the CD4 phenotype. Cross-linking of CD40 on either normal or hyper-IgM B cells by reacting them with a monoclonal antibody to CD40 or by allowing CD40 to interact with CD154 on normal activated T cells in the presence of certain cytokines (interleukin 2 [IL-2], IL-4, or IL-10) causes the B cells to undergo proliferation and isotype switching and to secrete various types of immunoglobulins. CD154 is a Type II integral membrane glycoprotein with significant sequence homology to TNF. Mutations in CD154 on activated T cells from hyper-IgM patients result in failure of signaling of B cells to undergo isotype switching; thus, hyper-IgM B cells produce only IgM. However, mutations in CD154 are not the only cause of the hyper-IgM syndrome. A number of male and female hyper-IgM patients who have been identified have normal T cell CD154 but appear to have intrinsic B-cell defects that prevent isotype switching. *The molecular defect(s) in these patients remain unknown.*

Because hyper-IgM patients are unable to make IgG antibodies, treatment with IVIG is given as in agammaglobulinemia.

X-LINKED LYMPHOPROLIFERATIVE DISEASE. X-linked lymphoproliferative disease (XLP) is a recessive trait characterized by an inadequate immune response to infection with Epstein-Barr virus (EBV). The affected are healthy until they experience infectious mononucleosis. Through use of restriction fragment length polymorphism (RFLP) probes in linkage with XLP, it has recently become possible to identify affected males before primary EBV infection develops. Immunologic studies demonstrated elevated IgA or IgM level and/or variable deficiency of IgG, IgG1 and IgG3 in 13/13 RFLP-positive but in none of 14 RFLP-negative, EBV-negative males. The mean age of presentation is less than 5 years. The most common form of presentation (75%) is severe mononucleosis, of which 80% of cases are fatal, primarily because of extensive liver necrosis caused by polyclonally activated alloreactive cytotoxic T cells that recognize EBV-infected autologous B cells. In most patients surviving the primary infection global cellular im-

mune defects involving T, B, and natural killer (NK) cells, lymphomas, and/or hypogammaglobulinemia developed. There is a marked impairment in production of antibodies to the EBV nuclear antigen (EBNA), whereas titers to the viral capsid antigen have ranged from zero to markedly elevated. There is also a deficiency in long-lived T-cell immunity to EBV; numbers of blood CD8+ T cells are increased. The defective gene in XLP has been localized to the Xq26-q27 region and has recently been identified. It encodes a protein called SAP (SLAM-associated protein) that normally acts as a negative regulator of SLAM (signaling lymphocyte activation molecule) that is present on the surfaces of activated T and B cells. Mutations in SAP result in uncontrolled lymphocyte activation of lymphocytes in EBV infection (see Table 272–1). Approximately half of the limited number of patients with XLP given HLA-identical related or unrelated unfractionated bone marrow transplantations are currently surviving without any sign of the disease.

CELLULAR IMMUNODEFICIENCY DISORDERS

In general, patients with partial or absolute defects in T-cell function have infections or other clinical problems for which there is no effective treatment. It is rare that such individuals survive beyond infancy or childhood.

THYMIC HYPOPLASIA (DIGEORGE SYNDROME). Thymic hypoplasia results from dysmorphogenesis of the third and fourth pharyngeal pouches, leading to hypoplasia or aplasia of the thymus and parathyroid glands. Other structures forming at the same age are also frequently affected, resulting in anomalies of the great vessels (right-sided aortic arch), esophageal atresia, bifid uvula, congenital heart disease (atrial and ventricular septal defects), a short philtrum of the upper lip, hypertelorism, an antimongoloid slant to the eyes, mandibular hypoplasia, and low-set (often notched) ears. The diagnosis is usually first suggested by the presence of hypocalcemic seizures during the neonatal period.

A variable degree of hypoplasia of the thymus and parathyroid glands is more frequent than total aplasia. Some children with the features of this syndrome have little trouble with infections and show evidence of some cell-mediated immunity. They are often referred to as having partial DiGeorge syndrome. Those with marked thymic hypoplasia may resemble infants with severe combined immunodeficiency in their susceptibility to infection with low-grade or opportunistic pathogens (i.e., fungi, viruses, and *Pneumocystis carinii*) and to graft-versus-host disease (GVHD) from non-irradiated blood transfusions.

Serum immunoglobulin levels are usually normal for age, but those of some fractions, particularly IgA, may be diminished and the IgE level may be elevated. T-cell numbers are decreased, and there is an increased number of B cells. Responses of peripheral blood lymphocytes following mitogen stimulation have been absent, reduced, or normal. Careful postmortem studies have sometimes revealed tiny nests of thymic tissue containing Hassall's corpuscles and a normal density of thymocytes. Lymphoid follicles usually appear normal, but lymph node paracortical areas and thymus-dependent regions of the spleen show variable degrees of depletion, depending upon the degree of thymic hypoplasia. DiGeorge syndrome has occurred in both males and females. Familial occurrence is rare, but three cases of apparent autosomal dominant inheritance have been reported. Microdeletions of specific DNA sequences from chromosome 22q11.2 (the DiGeorge chromosomal region [DGCR]) have been shown in a majority of patients and there appears to be an excess of 22q11.2 deletions of maternal origin (see Table 272–1). Polymerase chain reaction– (PCR)-based genotyping using microsatellite DNA markers permits rapid detection of such microdeletions. Other deletions associated with DiGeorge and velocardiofacial syndromes have been identified on chromosome 10p13 (Table 272–1). The immune deficiency in the complete DiGeorge syndrome has been corrected by thymic tissue transplantation and by unfractionated HLA-identical bone marrow transplantation.

SEVERE COMBINED IMMUNODEFICIENCY (SCID) DISORDERS

The syndromes of severe combined immunodeficiency (SCID) are caused by diverse genetic mutations that lead to absence of all adaptive immune function and, in many cases, of natural killer cell function as well. Within the first few months of life, infants affected with all forms of SCID have frequent episodes of otitis, pneumonia, sepsis, diarrhea, and cutaneous infections. Growth may appear normal initially, but extreme wasting soon develops. Persistent infections with opportunistic organisms such as *Candida albicans, Pneumocystis carinii,* varicella, measles, parainfluenza virus 3, cytomegalovirus, and bacille Calmette-Guérin (BCG) frequently lead to death. SCID infants also lack the ability to reject foreign tissue and are, therefore, at risk for GVHD. GVHD can result from maternal T cells' crossing the placenta while the infant is in utero or from the post-natal administration of blood products or bone marrow containing viable T lymphocytes. Immunologic evaluation reveals lymphopenia in all forms of SCID. In addition, serum immunoglobulin concentrations are diminished, and no antibody formation occurs after immunization. Lymphocytes fail to respond to mitogens or allogeneic cells in vitro, and there is delayed cutaneous anergy in vivo. Despite the uniformly profound lack of T cells (except transplacentally transferred maternal T cells), there are variable numbers of B and NK cells, depending on the different SCID-causing mutations (see Table 272–1 and late discussion). Typically, patients with all forms of SCID have a very small thymus (<1 g), which usually fails to descend from the neck. They lack thymic lymphocytes and Hassall's corpuscles but have normal thymic epithelium. Tonsils, adenoids, lymph nodes, and Peyer's patches are small or absent.

IVIG fails to halt the progressively downhill course of SCID. Transplantation of bone marrow cells from HLA genotypically identical donors has resulted in apparent complete correction of the immunologic defect in more than 125 of these patients. More importantly, since 1982 techniques to deplete all post-thymic T cells from donor marrow have also allowed the use of haploidentical (half-matched) bone marrow cells for correction of SCID. To date, more than 270 infants with SCID who would have died because of lack of an HLA identical donor have been treated successfully with T-cell-depleted haploidentical parental bone marrow with transient or no GVHD. It is important to point out that neither pre-transplantation chemoablation nor GVHD prophylaxis is required for successful engraftment of either T-cell-depleted or unfractionated allogeneic bone marrow in SCID infants. Use of these agents only heightens the likelihood of death from opportunistic infection. SCID is a medical emergency, and, therefore, early diagnosis and transplantation are essential. It can be diagnosed on cord blood by the finding of lymphopenia. Unless immunologic reconstitution can be achieved through immunocompetent tissue transplantation, death from infection usually occurs before the patient's first birthday. The major genetic forms of this disorder are discussed below.

X-LINKED RECESSIVE SEVERE COMBINED IMMUNODEFICIENCY DISEASE (XSCID). X-linked recessive severe combined immunodeficiency syndrome is the most common form of SCID in the United States, accounting for approximately 47% of cases. Clinically, immunologically, and histopathologically, these patients appear similar to those with other forms of SCID except for uniformly low percentages of T and NK cells and an elevated percentage of B cells, a feature they share with Janus kinase III (Jak 3)-deficient SCID patients. The abnormal gene in XSCID was mapped to Xq13 and cloned in 1993. It encodes the common gamma chain (γ_c) for several cytokine receptors, including interleukin-2 (IL-2), IL-4, IL-7, IL-9, and IL-15 (see Table 272–1 and Figure 272–1). The shared γ chain functions both to increase the affinity of the receptor for the respective cytokine and to enable the receptors to mediate intracellular signaling. Incapacitation of the receptors for all of these developmentally crucial cytokines by genetic mutations in γ_c provides an explanation for the severity of the immunodeficiency in XSCID. Of the first 136 patients studied, 95 distinct mutations spanning all 8 IL-2RG exons were identified, most of them consisting of small changes at the level of one to a few nucleotides. These mutations resulted in abnormal γ_c chains in two thirds of the cases and absent γ_c protein in the remainder. Carriers can be detected by demonstrating non-random X-chromosome inactivation or the deleterious mutation in their T, B, and/or NK lymphocytes.

AUTOSOMAL RECESSIVE SEVERE COMBINED IMMUNODEFICIENCY DISEASES. An autosomal recessive severe combined immunodeficiency disease pattern of inheritance of SCID was reported initially by Swiss workers in 1958. It is less common in the United States than in Europe. Mutated genes on autosomal chromosomes have been identified in four forms of SCID—adenosine deaminase (ADA) deficiency, JAK3-deficiency, IL-7 receptor α chain (IL-7Rα) deficiency, and recombinase activating gene (*RAG-1* or *RAG-2*) deficiencies—and there are likely other causes yet to be discovered (see Table 272–1 and Figure 272–1).

WITH ADENOSINE DEAMINASE (ADA) DEFICIENCY. (SEE ALSO CHAPTER 207). An absence of the enzyme ADA occurs in approximately 15% of patients with SCID (see Table 272–1). Patients with ADA deficiency have the same clinical problems of susceptibility to opportunistic bacterial, viral, and parasitic diseases as those with the other forms. However, there are certain distinguishing features of ADA deficiency, including the presence of rib cage abnormalities similar to a rachitic rosary and multiple skeletal abnormalities of chondro-osseous dysplasia seen on radiographic examination; these occur predominantly at the costochondral junctions, at the apophyses of the iliac bones, and in the vertebral bodies.

ADA-deficient patients usually have a much more profound lymphopenia than infants with other types of SCID, with mean absolute lymphocyte counts of less than 500/mm³; they rarely have elevated percentages of B or NK cells. They have normal NK function and, after T-cell function is conferred by bone marrow transplantation without pre-transplantation chemotherapy, generally have excellent B-cell function. This is due to the fact that ADA deficiency affects primarily T-cell function. Milder forms of this condition have been reported, leading to delayed diagnosis of immunodeficiency even to adulthood.

The gene encoding ADA was mapped to chromosome 20q13ter and was cloned and sequenced nearly two decades ago (see Table 272–1). ADA deficiency results in marked accumulations of adenosine, 2'-deoxyadenosine, and 2'-O-methyladenosine. The latter directly or indirectly leads to T-cell apoptosis, which causes the immunodeficiency.

As with other types of SCID, ADA deficiency can be cured by HLA-identical or haploidentical T-cell-depleted bone marrow transplantation without the need for pre- or post-transplantation chemotherapy; this remains the treatment of choice. Enzyme replacement therapy is much less effective than bone marrow transplantation and should not be initiated if bone marrow transplantation is at all possible, because it will confer graft-rejection capability upon the infant. Gene therapy has been attempted but has thus far been unsuccessful. A spontaneous in vivo reversion to normal of a mutation in the ADA gene has been reported.

WITH JANUS KINASE 3 (JAK3) DEFICIENCY. SCID patients who have the recently discovered defect JAK3 deficiency resemble all other types clinically. However, they have a lymphocyte phenotype similar only to that of patients with X-linked SCID, i.e., an elevated percentage of B cells and very low or no T and NK cells. Because JAK3 is the only signaling molecule known to be associated with γ_c, it was a candidate gene for mutations leading to autosomal recessive SCID not due to ADA deficiency (see Table 272–1 and Figure 272–1). Thus far it appears to account for approximately 7% of SCID cases. Even after successful T-cell reconstitution by transplantation of haploidentical stem cells, some JAK3-deficient SCID patients fail to develop NK cells or normal B-cell function despite their high numbers of B cells. The reason for this is unknown but is thought to be related to the defective function of the multiple types of cytokine receptors that share γ_c.

WITH RAG-1 OR RAG-2 DEFICIENCIES. Infants with *RAG-1* or *RAG-2* deficiency, a recently discovered cause of SCID, have a different lymphocyte phenotype from that of patients with SCID, which is due to γ_c, JAK3, or ADA deficiencies in that they lack both B and T lymphocytes (so-called T-B-SCID) and have primarily NK cells. This suggested a problem with their antigen receptor genes that led to the discovery of mutations in the recombinase activating genes (*RAG-1* and *RAG-2*) (see Table 272–1). Such mutations result in a functional inability to form antigen receptors through genetic recombination. Recently, mutations in these same genes have also been found in a variant form of SCID, Omenn's syndrome.

WITH IL-7Rα DEFICIENCY. SCID patients with IL-7Rα deficiency, another newly discovered defect, also have a distinctive lymphocyte phenotype in that they have normal or elevated numbers of both B and NK cells. The prevalence of this form of SCID is as yet unknown. In contrast to γ_c- and JAK3 deficient SCID patients, in these patients the immunologic defect is completely correctable by T-cell-depleted haploidentical bone marrow stem cell transplantation.

SEVERE COMBINED IMMUNODEFICIENCY WITH LEUKO-PENIA (RETICULAR DYSGENESIS). In 1959, identical twin male infants who exhibited a total lack of both lymphocytes and granulocytes in their peripheral blood and bone marrow were described. Seven of eight infants reported died between ages 3 and 119 days from overwhelming infections; the eighth underwent complete immunologic reconstitution from bone marrow transplantation. The thymus glands have all weighed less than 1 g, no Hassall's corpuscles have been present, and few or no thymocytes have been seen. The molecular basis of this autosomal recessive disorder is unknown.

COMBINED IMMUNODEFICIENCY DISORDERS (CIDs)

Combined immunodeficiency, or CID, is distinguished from SCID by low but not absent T-cell function. Like SCID, however, it is a syndrome of diverse genetic causes. Patients with CID present during infancy with recurrent or chronic pulmonary infections, failure to thrive, oral or cutaneous candidiasis, chronic diarrhea, recurrent skin infections, gram-negative sepsis, urinary tract infections, and/or severe varicella infection. Although they usually survive longer than infants with SCID, they fail to thrive and die early in life.

Serum immunoglobulin numbers may be normal or elevated for all classes, but selective IgA deficiency, marked elevation of IgE, and elevated IgD level have been found in some cases. Antibody-forming capacity has been impaired in a majority. Other findings may include neutropenia and eosinophilia.

Studies of cellular immune function have shown delayed cutaneous anergy to ubiquitous antigens, lymphopenia, and extremely low but not absent lymphocyte proliferative responses to mitogens and allogeneic cells in vitro. CID patients may have profound deficiencies of CD3-positive T cells or they may have defective signaling of phenotypically normal T cells. Peripheral lymphoid tissues usually demonstrate paracortical lymphocyte depletion. The thymus is very small and has a paucity of thymocytes and usually no Hassall's corpuscles. Some patients with CID have attained successful reconstitution through unfractionated matched sibling or unrelated adult donor bone marrow or cord blood transplantation; however, they often require chemoablation prior to transplantation to achieve graft acceptance. T-cell-depleted haploidentical marrow stem cell transplantation has not been very successful in these patients because of opportunistic infections made worse by the need to chemoablate and to give GVHD prophylaxis and the time needed for T cells to mature from the transplanted stem cells.

CID WITH PURINE NUCLEOSIDE PHOSPHORYLASE DEFICIENCY. More than 40 patients with CID have been found to have purine nucleoside phosphorylase (PNP) deficiency (see Table 272–1). Although ADA and PNP are both purine salvage pathway enzymes, PNP deficiency leads to a less severe immunodeficiency than ADA deficiency does. In further contrast to ADA deficiency, in PNP deficiency no characteristic physical or skeletal abnormalities have been noted. Deaths have resulted from generalized vaccinia and varicella infections, lymphosarcoma, and GVHD mediated by T cells from non-irradiated allogeneic blood or bone marrow.

Most patients have normal or elevated concentrations of all serum immunoglobulins. PNP-deficient patients are as profoundly lymphopenic as those with ADA deficiency, with absolute lymphocyte counts usually less than 500/mm³. Analyses of lymphocyte subpopulations with monoclonal antibodies have demonstrated a marked deficiency of T cells and of T-cell subsets but increased numbers of cells with NK phenotype and function. T-cell function is low but not absent.

The gene encoding PNP is on chromosome 14q13.1, and it has been cloned and sequenced. Prenatal diagnosis is possible. Unlike in ADA deficiency, serum and urinary uric acid levels are markedly deficient, because PNP is needed to form the urate precursors, hypoxanthine and xanthine.

This condition is invariably fatal in childhood unless immunologic reconstitution can be achieved. Bone marrow transplantation is the treatment of choice but has thus far been successful in only three such patients.

CID DUE TO INTERLEUKIN-2 RECEPTOR α CHAIN (IL-2Rα, CD25) MUTATION. In a male infant born of a consanguineous union cytomegalovirus pneumonia, persistent candidiasis, adenoviral gastroenteritis, failure to thrive, lymphadenopathy, hepatosplenomegaly, and chronic inflammation of the lungs and mandible developed. Biopsies revealed extensive lymphocytic infiltration of his lung, liver, gut, and bone. Serum IgA level was low. He had T-cell lymphocytopenia and the T cells responded poorly to anti-CD3, PHA, and other mitogens, and to IL-2. He was found to have a mutation of the IL-2Rα chain (CD25) leading to truncation (Table 272–1). He had no CD1 in his thymus and an elevation of the level of the anti-apoptotic protein bcl-2. This defect reveals that some components of cytokine receptors normally have a negative regulatory role. Mutations in those components can result in unchecked lymphoproliferation and autoimmunity.

CID DUE TO T DEFECTIVE CELL ACTIVATION. T-cell activation defects are characterized by the presence of normal or elevated numbers of blood T cells that appear phenotypically normal but fail to proliferate or produce cytokines in response to stimulation with mitogens, antigens, or other signals delivered to the T-cell antigen receptor (TCR), as a result of defective signaling from the TCR to intracellular metabolic pathways.

One example of a T-cell activation defect is *CD8 lymphocytopenia due to ZAP 70 deficiency*. Patients with this condition have severe, recurrent, often fatal infections during infancy similar to SCID patients. A majority of reported cases have been Mennonites. They have normal or elevated numbers of circulating CD3+CD4+ T lymphocytes, but essentially no CD8+ T cells. These CD3+CD4+ T cells fail to respond to mitogens or to allogeneic cells in vitro or to generate cytotoxic T lymphocytes. By contrast, NK activity is normal, and they have normal or elevated numbers of B cells and low to elevated serum immunoglobulin concentrations. The thymus of one patient exhibited normal architecture; there were normal numbers of double-positive (CD4+CD8+) thymocytes, but an absence of CD8 single-positive thymocytes. This condition has been shown to be due to mutations in the gene encoding ZAP-70, a non-src family protein tyrosine kinase important in T-cell signaling. The gene is on chromosome 2 at position q12 (Table 227–1). ZAP-70 has been shown to have an essential role in both positive and negative selection in the thymus.

DEFECTIVE EXPRESSION OF MAJOR HISTOCOMPATIBILITY COMPLEX (MHC) ANTIGENS. There are two main forms of defective expression of MHC antigens: (1) class I MHC antigen deficiency (bare lymphocyte syndrome) and (2) class II MHC antigen deficiency.

MHC CLASS I ANTIGEN DEFICIENCY. An isolated deficiency of MHC class I antigens is rare, and the resulting immunodeficiency is much milder than in SCID, explaining a later age of presentation. Class I MHC antigens are not detected on any cells in the patient, but they are in the serum, along with β_2-microglobulin. There is a deficiency of CD8+ but not of CD4+ T cells. Recently, a non-sense mutation in *TAP2*, one of two genes (*TAP1* and *TAP2*) within the MHC locus on chromosome 6 that encode the protein TAP (see Table 272–1), has been discovered. TAP functions to transport antigenic peptides from the cytoplasm across the Golgi apparatus membrane to join the α chain of MHC class 1 antigens and β_2-microglobulin. These are then all assembled into an MHC class I complex that can then move to the cell surface. If the assembly of the complex cannot be completed because there is no antigenic peptide, the MHC class I complex is destroyed in the cytoplasm.

MHC CLASS II ANTIGEN DEFICIENCY. Many affected with MHC class II antigen deficiency, an autosomal recessive syndrome, are of North African descent. Patients present with persistent diarrhea in early infancy. The latter is often associated with cryptosporidiosis; infections with enteroviruses (poliovirus, echoviruses and coxsackievirus) and herpes or other viral agents; and oral candidiasis. They also experience bacterial pneumonia, pneumocystis infection, and septicemia. Nevertheless, their immunodeficiency is not as severe as in SCID, as evidenced by failure to develop BCG infection or GVHD from non-irradiated blood transfusions.

MHC class II–deficient patients have a very low number of

CD4⁺ T cells but normal or elevated numbers of CD8⁺ T cells. Lymphopenia is only moderate. The MHC class II antigens, HLA-DP, -DQ, and -DR, are undetectable on blood B cells and monocytes, even though B cells are present in normal number. The patients are hypogammaglobulinemic as a result of impaired antigen-specific responses caused by the absence of these antigen-presenting molecules. In addition, MHC antigen-deficient B cells fail to stimulate allogeneic cells in mixed leukocyte culture. Lymphocyte proliferation studies show normal responses to mitogens but no response to antigens. The thymus and other lymphoid organs are severely hypoplastic, and the lack of class II molecules results in abnormal thymic selection. The latter results in circulating CD4⁺ T cells that have altered CDR3 profiles. The associated defects of both B- and T-cell immunity and of HLA expression emphasize the important biologic role for HLA determinants in effective immune cell cooperation.

MHC class II antigen deficiency is genetically heterogeneous; at least four different complementation groups have been reported. The molecular defects thus far described affect the regulation of expression of class II genes rather than causing abnormalities of the coding regions for HLA-DP, -DQ, or -DR, and they do not segregate with the MHC genes on chromosome 6. Three different molecular defects that impair the coordinate expression of MHC class II molecules on the surface of B cells and macrophages have been identified. In one, there is a mutation in the gene on chromosome 1q that encodes a protein called RFX5, a promoter protein that binds to the MHC class II gene promoter region X-box (Table 272–1). A second such factor, RFXAP, is encoded by a gene on chromosome 13q. In the third, there is a mutation in the gene on chromosome 16p13 that encodes a novel MHC class II transactivator (CIITA), which coordinates the binding of proteins to the MHC class II gene promoter region.

IMMUNODEFICIENCY WITH THROMBOCYTOPENIA AND ECZEMA (WISKOTT-ALDRICH SYNDROME). Wiskott-Aldrich syndrome is an X-linked recessive syndrome characterized clinically by eczema, thrombocytopenic purpura, and undue susceptibility to infection. Often there is prolonged oozing from the circumcision site or bloody diarrhea during infancy. Megakaryocytes are present in the bone marrow, but the few platelets produced from them are small and abnormal in their function. Atopic dermatitis and infections caused by pneumococci and other bacteria with polysaccharide capsules develop during the first year of life, resulting in episodes of otitis media, pneumonia, meningitis, and sepsis. Later, infections with *Pneumocystis carinii* and the herpesviruses become more frequent. Survival beyond the teens is rare; major causes of death are infections, bleeding, vasculitis, and EBV-induced malignancy.

Serum immunoglobulin measurement usually reveals a low IgM, elevated IgA and IgE, and a normal or slightly low IgG concentration. Studies of immunoglobulin metabolism have shown an accelerated rate of synthesis—as well as hypercatabolism—of albumin, IgG, IgA, and IgM, resulting in highly variable immunoglobulin concentrations. Absent or markedly diminished isohemagglutinin titers are found uniformly, and poor or no responses are seen after immunization with polysaccharide antigens. Anamnestic antibody responses to protein antigens are also often poor or absent. Lymphocyte responses to mitogens are depressed, and there are moderately reduced percentages of T cells. The mutated gene responsible for this defect was mapped to Xp11.22-11.23 (Figure 272–1; Table 272–1). It was found to be limited in expression to lymphocytic and megakaryocytic lineages. The gene product, a 501-amino-acid proline-rich protein that lacks a hydrophobic transmembrane domain, was designated WAS protein (WASP). It has been shown to bind CDC42H2 and rac, members of the Rho family of guanosine triphosphates important in actin polymerization. A large and varied number of mutations in the WASP gene have been identified in WAS patients. Isolated X-linked thrombocytopenia is also caused by mutations in the WASP gene. Carriers can be detected by the finding of non-random X chromosome inactivation in several hematopoietic cell lineages or by detection of the mutated gene (if known in the family). Prenatal diagnosis of WAS can also be made by chorionic villus sampling or amniocentesis if the mutation is known in that family. Recently two families with apparent autosomal inheritance of a clinical phenotype similar to WAS have been reported.

A number of patients with WAS have had complete corrections of both their platelet and immunologic abnormalities by HLA-identical sibling bone marrow transplantation after being conditioned with irradiation or busulfan and cyclophosphamide. Success has been minimal with T-cell-depleted haploidentical stem cell transplantations in WAS. Recently, some success has been achieved in the treatment of WAS with matched unrelated donor (MUD) transplantations of patients below the age of 5 years. Several patients who required splenectomy for uncontrollable bleeding had impressive rises in their platelet counts and have done well clinically while on prophylactic antibiotics and IVIG. The higher platelet counts also permitted the use of high-dose aspirin or other non-steroidal anti-inflammatory agents in the control of vasculitis.

ATAXIA-TELANGIECTASIA. Ataxia-telangiectasia is a complex syndrome with neurologic, immunologic, endocrinologic, hepatic, and cutaneous abnormalities. The most prominent clinical features are progressive cerebellar ataxia, oculocutaneous telangiectasias, chronic sinopulmonary disease, a high incidence of malignancy, and variable humoral and cellular immunodeficiency. Ataxia typically becomes evident soon after the child begins to walk. Telangiectasias usually develop by age 3 to 6. Recurrent, usually bacterial, sinopulmonary infections occur in roughly 80% of these patients; varicella infection was fatal in one of the author's patients.

The most frequent humoral immunologic abnormality is selective absence of IgA, found in 50 to 80% of these patients. IgG2 or the total IgG concentration may also be decreased. IgE concentrations are usually low, and IgM may be of the low-molecular-weight variety. Specific antibody levels may be decreased or normal. In vivo, there is impaired but not absent cell-mediated immunity, as evidenced by delayed cutaneous anergy and prolonged allograft survival. Death from GVHD has not been reported. Enumeration of blood T cells and subsets reveals reduced percentages of total T cells. In vitro studies of lymphocyte function have shown moderately depressed proliferative responses to mitogens. The thymus is very hypoplastic and lacks Hassall's corpuscles. No satisfactory treatment has been found. The malignant tumors reported have usually been of the lymphoreticular type, but others have been seen. Cells from patients and heterozygous carriers have increased sensitivity to ionizing radiation, defective DNA repair, and frequent chromosomal abnormalities.

The mutated gene (*ATM*) responsible for this defect was mapped to the long arm of chromosome 11 (11q22-23) and has now been cloned (Table 272–1). The gene product is a DNA-dependent protein kinase localized predominantly to the nucleus. It is involved in mitogenic signal transduction, meiotic recombination, and cell cycle control.

CARTILAGE HAIR HYPOPLASIA. In 1965, an unusual form of short-limbed dwarfism with frequent and severe infections was reported among the Pennsylvania Amish; non-Amish cases have since been described. These patients have short and pudgy hands with redundant skin; metaphyseal chondrodysplasia; hyperextensible joints of hands and feet but an inability to extend the elbows completely; and fine, sparse light hair and eyebrows. These features led to the name *cartilage-hair hypoplasia* (CHH). Radiographically, the bones show scalloping and sclerotic or cystic changes in the metaphyses. In contrast to ADA deficiency, in which the predominant changes are in the apophyses of the iliac bones, the ribs, and the vertebral bodies, in CHH the chondrodysplasia principally affects the limbs. Severe and often fatal varicella infections, progressive vaccinia, and vaccine-associated poliomyelitis have been observed. Associated conditions include deficient erythrogenesis, Hirschsprung's disease, and an increased risk of malignancies.

Three patterns of immune dysfunction have emerged: defective antibody-mediated immunity, defective cellular immunity (most common form), and severe combined immunodeficiency. NK cells, however, are increased in number and function. CHH is an autosomal recessive condition, and the defective gene has recently been mapped to chromosome 9p21-p13 in Amish and Finnish families (Table 272–1). The gene has not been identified as yet, however, so the fundamental molecular abnormality is unknown. In vitro studies have shown decreased numbers of T cells and defective T-cell proliferation, due to an intrinsic defect related to the G1 phase, resulting in a longer cell cycle for individual cells. This abnormality also occurs in fibroblasts from these patients and in in vitro colony formation in erythroid, myeloid, and megakaryocytic lineages, suggesting a common cell proliferation defect in CHH. Bone marrow transplantation has resulted in immunologic reconstitution in some CHH patients with the SCID phenotype. Those with milder types of immune deficiency have lived to adulthood, some even to old age.

IFN-γR1 AND IL-12Rβ1 MUTATIONS. Disseminated BCG infections occur in patients with severe T-cell defects. However, in approximately half of cases no specific host defect is found. Recently, other possible explanations for this predilection were found. The first was found in a 2.5-month-old Tunisian female infant, who had fatal idiopathic disseminated BCG infection, and in four children from Malta who had disseminated atypical mycobacterial infection in the absence of a recognized immunodeficiency. There was consanguinity in all, who were each found to have a functional defect in the up-regulation of tumor necrosis factor α (TNF-α) production by their blood macrophages in response to stimulation with interferon-γ (IFN-γ). Each was found to have a mutation in the gene on chromosome 6q22-q23 that encodes the IFN-γ receptor (IFN-γR1) (Table 272–1). A second type of defect was discovered in other patients with disseminated mycobacterial infections, who were found to have mutations in the β 1 chain of the IL-12 receptor (IL-12Rβ1). IL-12 is a powerful inducer of IFN-γ production by T and NK cells. The mutated receptor chain resulted in unresponsiveness of these patients' cells to IL-12 and inadequate IFN-γ production. Interestingly, both the IFN-γR1 and IL-12Rβ1-deficient patients appeared not to be susceptible to infection with agents other than mycobacteria. TH1 responses appeared to be normal in these patients. The susceptibility of these patients to mycobacterial infections thus apparently results from an intrinsic impairment of the IFN-γ pathway response to these particular intracellular pathogens, showing that IFN-γ is obligatory for efficient macrophage antimycobacterial activity.

HYPERIMMUNOGLOBULINEMIA E SYNDROME. The hyperimmunoglobulinemia E (hyper-IgE) syndrome is a primary immunodeficiency characterized by recurrent staphylococcal abscesses and markedly elevated serum IgE concentrations. These patients all have lifelong histories of severe recurrent staphylococcal abscesses involving the skin, lungs, joints, and other sites. Persistent pneumatoceles develop as a result of their recurrent pneumonias. The pruritic dermatitis that occurs is not typical atopic eczema and does not always persist; respiratory allergic symptoms are usually absent. An autosomal-dominant form of inheritance with incomplete penetrance seems possible. Laboratory features include exceptionally high serum IgE concentrations but usually normal IgG, IgA, and IgM concentrations; pronounced blood and sputum eosinophilia; abnormally low anamnestic antibody responses; and poor antibody- and cell-mediated responses to neoantigens. Percentages of blood T, B, and NK lymphocytes are normal, as are lymphocyte responses to mitogens, but responses to antigens or to related allogeneic cells have been absent or very low. Histologic sections of lymph nodes, spleen, and lung cysts show striking eosinophilia.

Phagocytic cell ingestion, metabolism, and killing mechanisms and total hemolytic complement have been normal in all patients. Results of chemotaxis studies have been mostly normal; thus, defective chemotaxis is not the basic problem in this syndrome. Indeed, the fundamental biologic error remains to be identified.

The most effective therapy is chronic administration of therapeutic doses of a penicillinase-resistant antibiotic, adding other agents as required for specific infections.

LEUKOCYTE ADHESION DEFICIENCY 1 (LAD 1 OR CD11/CD18 DEFICIENCY). Leukocyte adhesion deficiency 1 is due to an autosomal-recessively inherited mutation in the gene encoding the 95-kd molecular weight (MW) subunit (CD18) shared by three adhesive heterodimers: leukocyte function antigen (LFA-1) on B, T, and NK lymphocytes; complement receptor type 3 (CR3) on neutrophils, monocytes, macrophages, eosinophils, and NK cells; and p150, 95 (another complement receptor). Because these cells cannot adhere to vascular endothelium, there is a significant leukocytosis, even in the absence of infection. Patients have histories of delayed separation of the umbilical cord, omphalitis, gingivitis, recurrent skin infections, repeated otitis media, pneumonia, peritonitis, perianal abscesses, and impaired wound healing. Severe widespread and life-threatening bacterial and fungal infections account for the high mortality rate. All cytotoxic lymphocyte functions are

markedly impaired as a result of a lack of the adhesion protein LFA-1; deficiency of LFA-1 also interferes with immune cell interaction and immune recognition. CR3 binds fixed iC3b fragments of C3 and glucans; its absence causes abnormal phagocytic cell adherence and chemotaxis and a reduced respiratory burst with phagocytosis. Deficiencies of these glycoproteins can be screened for by cytofluorography of blood leukocytes with appropriate monoclonal antibodies to CR3 (OKM1, MO1, MAC-1). The disease can be corrected by bone marrow transplantation.

LEUKOCYTE ADHESION DEFICIENCY 2 (LAD 2). LAD type 2 is due to the absence of the neutrophil Sialyl-Lewis X ligand for E-selectin on vascular endothelium. This disorder was discovered in two unrelated Israeli boys, aged 3 and 5 years, each the offspring of consanguineous parents. Both have severe mental retardation, short stature, a distinctive facial appearance, and the Bombay (hh) blood phenotype, and both are secretor- and Lewis-negative. They both have had recurrent severe bacterial infections similar to those seen in patients with LAD 1, including pneumonia, peridontitis, otitis media, and localized cellulitis. Similarly to patients with LAD 1, they have had infections accompanied by marked leukocytosis (30,000 to 150,000/mm³) but an absence of pus formation at sites of recurrent cellulitis. In vitro studies revealed a marked defect in neutrophil motility. Because the genes for the red cell H antigen and for the secretor status encode for distinct α1,2-fucosyl transferases and the synthesis of Sialyl-Lewis X requires an α1,3-fucosyl transferase, the authors have postulated a general defect in fucose metabolism as the basis for this disorder.

PRIMARY DEFICIENCIES OF THE COMPLEMENT SYSTEM

In addition to congenital or hereditary disorders of lymphoid cells, there are several well-defined primary immune defects involving the complement system. Genetically determined deficiencies have been described for all of the components of complement, and undue susceptibility to infection is a characteristic of deficiencies of C2, C3, C5, C6, and C7. The types of infections experienced in C2 and C3 deficiencies and in some with C5 deficiency are with gram-positive encapsulated organisms, whereas those in patients with deficiencies of the terminal components are usually meningococcal or gonococcal. A normal CH$_{50}$ finding would exclude all heritable complement deficiencies. The complement system is discussed in detail in Chapter 271.

Buckley RH, Schiff RI, Schiff SE, et al.: Human severe combined immunodeficiency (SCID): Genetic, phenotypic and functional diversity in 108 infants. J Pediatr 130: 378–387, 1997. *Unique characteristics of a large group of U.S. patients with SCID, according to the underlying genetic cause.*

Buckley RH, Schiff SE, Schiff RI, et al: Hematopoietic stem-cell transplantation for the treatment of severe combined immunodeficiency. N Engl J Med 340:508–516, 1999. *A 17-year experience in which outcomes of transplants in 89 patients are reported.*

Puck JM, Pepper AE, Henthorn PS, et al.: Mutation analysis of IL2RG in human X-linked severe combined immunodeficiency. Blood 89:1968–1977, 1997. *Mutations detected to date in the common γ chain gene, IL-2 RG.*

WHO Scientific Group Primary immunodeficiency diseases: Report of a WHO scientific group. Clin Exp Immunol 99:1–24, 1997. *The most recent published report of the World Health Organization's classification and discussion of the diagnosis and treatment of primary immunodeficiency diseases.*

273 URTICARIA AND ANGIOEDEMA

Michael M. Frank

Urticaria (Table 273–1) is defined as the transient appearance of elevated, erythematous pruritic wheals (hives) or serpiginous exanthem, usually surrounded by an area of erythema. It commonly involves the trunk and extremities, sparing palms and soles, but it may involve any epidermal or mucosal surface. The wheals are thought to result from local subcutaneous and intradermal leakage of plasma filtrate from postcapillary venules. In most cases there is associated increased blood flow to the localized area of swelling, resulting in a surrounding erythema or flare. The lesions blanch on pressure, reflecting this pathogenetic process. The appearance of

Table 273–1 ■ CLASSIFICATION OF URTICARIA/ANGIOEDEMA

I. Manifestation of Hypersensitivity to a Defined Agent
  A. Drug reactions
  B. Foods and food additives
  C. Inhaled and contact allergens
II. Presumed Immune Complex–Induced
  A. Collagen disease
  B. Endocrine disease (thyroid disorders)
  C. Serum sickness
  D. Transfusion-induced
  E. Malignancy (tumor antigen–induced)
  F. Infectious agents
  G. Urticarial vasculitis
III. Physical Urticarias
  A. Dermatographism
  B. Familial and acquired cold urticaria
  C. Localized heat urticaria
  D. Cholinergic urticaria
  E. Exercise-induced anaphylaxis/urticaria
  F. Delayed pressure urticaria/angioedema
  G. Familial and acquired vibratory angioedema
  H. Solar urticaria
  I. Aquagenic urticaria
IV. Urticaria Pigmentosa and Systemic Mastocytosis
V. Chronic Urticaria and Angioedema
VI. Defined Complement-Related Disorders
  A. Hereditary angioedema
  B. Acquired C1 inhibitor deficiency
  C. Complement Factor I deficiency
VII. Angioedema Induced by Angiotensin-Converting Enzyme Inhibitors and Interleukin-2

urticaria is believed to reflect in most cases an ongoing immediate hypersensitivity reaction.

Angioedema is formed by a similar extravasation of fluid, but in this case the leakage of fluid involves deeper dermal and subdermal sites. Because of its location in deeper cutaneous structures, it appears as brawny non-pitting edema, usually without well-defined margins. Although urticaria is almost always pruritic, indicating stimulation of nociceptive nerves in the region, angioedema may be unassociated with itching. Unlike other forms of edema, angioedema is not commonly distributed in dependent areas of the body. It often involves the lips, tongue, eyelids, genitalia, or hands or feet but also may involve any epidermal or mucosal surface. The transient nature of involvement is important in defining both urticaria and angioedema; these manifestations appear and peak in minutes to hours and disappear over hours to days.

INCIDENCE AND PREVALENCE

Acute episodes of urticaria/angioedema are arbitrarily defined as those lasting less than 6 weeks. More prolonged episodes are defined as chronic. Acute urticaria and angioedema are very common clinical problems, occurring in as much as 10 to 20% of the population at one time or another. The acute episodes may occur at any age and are the most common form seen in childhood. They occur in persons of either gender and of all races and occupations and at all seasons of the year. Chronic urticaria/angioedema also can occur in individuals of any age, but the peak incidence is noted in young adults.

In general, symptoms of urticaria are more striking and are more easily recognized than those of angioedema, and these symptoms are often the presenting complaint. At presentation, about 50% of patients are found to have both urticaria and angioedema, approximately 40% have urticaria alone, and about 10% have only angioedema. Although in the majority of patients the lesions clear spontaneously or respond rapidly to treatment with H_1 antihistamines, a minority of patients continue to have lesions over a period that may last years. It has been reported that of patients with chronic urticaria and angioedema, 75% have symptoms for longer than 1 year, 50% have symptoms for longer than 5 years, and 20% have symptoms for decades. At times, these symptoms can be quite debilitating. This clinical syndrome represents a final common pathway of multiple initiating stimuli, and the natural course of disease reflects multiple initiating factors.

PATHOGENESIS AND PATHOLOGY

Urticaria/angioedema results from dilatation of small vessels with associated leakage of plasma from local postcapillary venules. Experimentally, such leakage can be induced by multiple stimuli. Degranulation of cutaneous mast cells is thought to be the most frequent cause of disease. Mast cells are found in high frequency within the subcutaneous tissues and dermis. Their distribution is particularly rich around blood vessels. These cells stain poorly with the commonly used histopathologic stains and often must be visualized by specific staining techniques. On being activated by any of a number of stimuli, these cells degranulate, releasing over a period of seconds pre-formed mediators present in the granules, like histamine, that induce capillary permeability. They also synthesize various mediators in response to the activation signal that increase capillary permeability, including prostaglandins, hydroxyeicosatetraenoic acids (HETEs), leukotrienes C, D, and E, and platelet-activating factor (PAF). With appropriate stimuli, cellular regulatory factors such as cytokines are synthesized and released without degranulation and release of pre-formed mediators by the cells; these cytokines may control the function of other cells within the lesion. The various activation factors lead to up-regulation of various cellular adhesion molecules that promote the immigration of immune and inflammatory cells, resulting in the formation of longer-lasting lesions.

Many stimuli induce mast cells to degranulate. Probably most important is the interaction of mast cell membrane-bound IgE antibody with specific antigen. Mast cells have on their surface a high-affinity receptor for IgE (Fc_eRI) and in tissues are often found coated with IgE antibody derived from plasma. Interaction of IgE antibody with its specific multivalent antigen cross-links IgE receptors, a required step in initiating the degranulation process by antigen-mediated cell activation. In fact, anything that cross-links IgE receptors can cause the cells to degranulate. This includes IgG autoantibody to the IgE receptor (discussed later). In addition, a series of peptides derived from various plasma mediator molecules can interact with specific receptors for them on mast cells, triggering degranulation. For example, peptides derived from activated complement proteins including C3a, C4a, and C5a and small fragments of C2 can induce mast cell degranulation. Similarly, peptides such as bradykinin, derived from activation and cleavage of proteins of the kinin-generating system, neuropeptides such as substance P, and formation of PAF can induce mast cell degranulation. Leukotrienes were originally identified by their ability to induce delayed smooth muscle contraction in test systems and were encompassed by the term "slow releasing substance of anaphylaxis." Incompletely defined cellular products derived from circulating mononuclear cells and neutrophils can cause mast cell degranulation as well. Moreover, toxic products from neutrophils and monocytes, whose release is induced by many factors including mast cell products, can on injection induce a typical hive.

Inducing an immediate hypersensitivity response in an allergic individual by intradermally injecting a sensitizing antigen leads to rapid mast cell degranulation and the immediate appearance of a wheal and flare response that gradually fades. In many individuals 4 to 6 hours later a "late-phase" response is noted with an increase in local inflammation and swelling. Biopsy of such a late-phase reaction reveals that neutrophils, some lymphocytes, and eosinophils are accumulated in the inflamed area and later are gradually replaced by mononuclear cells. The factors that induce the late-phase reaction are not completely defined, but the recent demonstration that chemotactic cytokines are produced some hours after mast cell triggering suggests that these factors may contribute to late-phase inflammation.

An understanding of these experimental findings helps explain biopsy findings in patients with acute and chronic urticaria/angioedema. Although the disease may be chronic, individual lesions usually are evanescent, lasting hours to days. On biopsy, subcutaneous edema is prominent, with flattened rete pegs, widened dermal papillae, and swollen collagen fibers also seen. There is increased histamine content of skin, and some studies demonstrate an increased number of cutaneous mast cells noted when compared with normal individuals. Even uninvolved skin from a patient with urticaria may show higher histamine content than does the skin of normal persons. Mast cell degranulation is seen on biopsy of lesions, and in chronic urticaria a modest mononuclear cell infiltrate around vessels containing lymphocytes (predominantly CD4+ helper T cells) and a few monocyte/macrophages is noted. An increase in eosinophils may be seen. Patients with physical urticarias tend to have more neutrophils and eosinophils on biopsy than are observed in chronic urticaria/angioedema. In a minority of cases with typical urticarial lesions, a typical leukocytoclastic vasculitis is observed. This latter finding, reported to be associated with the formation of IgG anti-C1q autoantibody, indicates that the underlying diagnosis is vasculitis and places the patient in a different diagnostic and therapeutic group.

Causes of urticaria/angioedema are listed in Table 273–1. However, in most reported series the cause of urticaria/angioedema is never found. In several large series, approximately 70% of all cases remained in the idiopathic group after all other urticarial syndrome complexes were eliminated. It is believed that most acute urticaria/angioedema cases represent hypersensitivity reactions to drugs, foods, or, less commonly, inhalants, because when a cause is defined it commonly involves one of these sensitizing agents. Penicillin is the drug still most commonly associated with acute urticaria; aspirin and other non-steroidal anti-inflammatory agents (NSAIDs) may rarely exacerbate urticaria, possibly by inhibiting prostaglandin synthesis, and diuretics, radiocontrast dyes, food additives, sulfonamides, and muscle relaxants all are associated with acute urticaria. Opioids can trigger direct mast cell release of histamine and cause urticarial lesions. Among foods, nuts, milk, eggs, chocolate, citrus fruits, tomatoes, fish, shellfish, and food dyes have all been associated with onset of acute urticaria in some individuals. Nevertheless, so many different antigens, including food additives, drugs, foods, and food contaminants, have been defined as causative in individual cases and so little antigen may be required to precipitate attacks that it may be difficult or impossible to define the causative agent. In many cases in which the disease becomes chronic, the patient is asked to keep a diary to determine whether a particular food or commercial product is involved in an attack. If it proves impossible to define the precipitating agent by this means, a severely restricted elimination diet, limiting foods to boiled rice and lamb, may be tried for several weeks to see if eliminating an offending ingested agent will terminate attacks. Too often these attempts are unsuccessful.

There are defined clinical situations in which urticaria and/or angioedema is a common presenting problem: patients undergoing immune complex–mediated reactions, as occur in active systemic lupus erythematosus and serum sickness, may experience waves of urticarial lesions, in this case believed to be due to activation of mediator pathways by circulating immune complexes with generation of kinins and complement-derived anaphylatoxins.

Autoantibodies of various sorts interacting with antigen may induce urticarial reactions. Reports suggest that as many as 50% of patients with chronic urticaria have IgG autoantibody to the IgE Fc receptor Iα chain. This receptor is a four-chain molecule present on mast cells and eosinophils to which IgE binds with high affinity, setting the stage for an allergic attack. Multivalent antigen interacting with cell-bound IgE triggers the release of mediators. IgG autoantibody to the high-affinity IgE receptor, perhaps augmented by the action of complement, is thought to trigger receptor aggregation, releasing mediators in the absence of an allergic reaction. IgG anti-IgE is also present in a small number of patients; this autoantibody also cross-links receptors that have IgE bound to them, causing release of mediators from IgE-coated mast cells. Thyroid autoantibodies have been singled out as a cause of urticaria; in one study, 90 of 624 patients with chronic urticaria had antithyroglobulin or antimicrosomal antibodies, the patients being either hyperthyroid or hypothyroid. Similarly, blood transfusions and infusions of fresh frozen plasma (FFP) are often associated with hives caused by antibodies in the plasma encountering host antigen or circulating host antibodies binding antigens in the blood products. Some cancers—for example, lymphomas—may be associated with urticarial lesions, thought to be due to an antibody response to tumor antigens. A similar mechanism is clearly responsible for the hives associated with some infectious agents, particularly viral agents. Here, antigens on or released from infectious

agents are bound to antibodies induced in the patient and hives result. Hives are a frequent response to the antibodies formed in the early response to hepatitis A and B and Epstein-Barr virus infection. There are several recent anecdotal reports of *Helicobacter* infection leading to the release of antigens that cause chronic hives. These reports require confirmation in a controlled study. Rarely, fungal antigens such as those derived from *Candida albicans* may precipitate hives or angioedema. Given the rarity of this latter observation, nystatin treatment is inappropriate in patients with chronic urticaria/angioedema unless a clear association with a hypersensitivity response to candidal antigens can be demonstrated. Although rare in the United States, many parasitic diseases can, at times, be associated with urticaria/angioedema with or without hypereosinophilia. Presumably, the presence of the urticaria/angioedema reflects an ongoing immediate hypersensitivity reaction to parasite antigens.

The complex of urticaria, bone pain, and lymphadenopathy is termed *Schnitzler's syndrome.* Affected patients often have greatly increased IgM levels, suggesting an ongoing immunologic reaction, but the cause of the syndrome is unknown.

PHYSICAL URTICARIAS AND ANGIOEDEMAS. It is important to consider the physical urticaria/angioedema complex when evaluating patients with chronic recurrent urticaria or angioedema because in one large series, these represented 16% of all chronic urticaria/angioedema patients seen. In some cases a highly specific diagnosis can be made, a clear precipitating factor can be defined, and the patient can learn to avoid attacks. Moreover, specific therapy may be available. When one lists these causes of urticaria/angioedema, they appear to be so easily defined that it appears unlikely that they could be missed. However, in practice this is not the case; a detailed history is required to identify these factors. Indeed, it is common for these patients to go years before a correct diagnosis is made. The physical urticarias have in common urticaria/angioedema precipitated by a known physical cause. The response may follow exposure to cold, heat, elevated body temperature, pressure, vibration, specific-wavelength ultraviolet rays, or, rarely, even water on the skin. In some cases, these reactions are believed to be IgE-mediated, because they can be passively transferred with serum of an affected donor to the skin of an unaffected recipient. In other cases the cause is unknown.

SYMPTOMATIC DERMATOGRAPHISM. As many as 2 to 5% of the general population may be dermatographic, with the appearance of blanching followed by a linear streak of edema and erythema within 2 to 5 minutes of stroking the skin. A small proportion of such individuals have sufficiently severe dermatographism that they become symptomatic. In some cases the symptoms can be transferred to a normal recipient by passive transfer of plasma, suggesting that in some way IgE antibody plays a role. In general, these individuals can be treated successfully with H_1 and H_2 antihistamines.

COLD URTICARIA. Patients with cold urticaria experience urticaria/angioedema on exposure to cold and may become hypotensive on diving into a cold swimming pool. Careful studies have shown that mast cell degranulation with histamine release occurs in these patients on cold exposure. Degranulation may be even more extensive when the patient's tissues are warmed after cold exposure. Placing an ice cube on the skin for 5 minutes and then removing it reveals an area of blanching in the shape of the cube followed by edema formation in the same area surrounded by an erythematous flare caused by local hyperemia. During attacks, blood histamine and tumor necrosis factor-α levels are elevated. In some of these patients, passive transfer of the sensitivity to the skin of normal persons has been demonstrated. It has been suggested that on cold exposure, certain dermal antigens undergo a conformational change that allows specific IgE autoantibody to bind and initiate mast cell degranulation. These patients are typically treated with cyproheptadine, sometimes with the addition of hydroxyzine. Cold urticaria has been described in a number of diseases associated with pathologic globulins, such as cryoglobulins, or cryofibrinogens. The symptom complex, however, is not associated with the presence of cold agglutinins. When cold urticaria is associated with underlying disease, treatment of those diseases is an essential part of therapy.

In some patients, disease manifestations are atypical in that the patient gives a history of typical urticarial symptoms but the ice cube test is negative. In occasional patients, dermatographism is brought out by cold exposure; in others, exercise-induced urticaria is noted only in the cold. There is a rare familial type of cold urticaria inherited as an autosomal dominant trait in which patients develop urticarial lesions 9 to 18 hours after cold exposure. This cannot be passively transferred with plasma, and the cause is unknown.

CHOLINERGIC OR GENERALIZED HEAT URTICARIA. Typically, these patients, representing about 4% of all patients with chronic urticaria, develop small (several millimeters), intensely pruritic wheals on an erythematous base on their upper trunk and arms after exercise with sweating or after hot showers. A rise in core body temperature is essential for the development of lesions. It is generally believed that the parasympathetic nervous system supply to cutaneous vessels releases acetylcholine as well as a neuropeptide such as vasoactive intestinal peptide, causing mediator release. There is no evidence of an IgE-mediated reaction. In support of this hypothesis is the fact that some of these patients (30 to 50%) develop typical lesions as well as a series of local satellite lesions when intracutaneously injected with methacholine. Atropine may inhibit the skin test but does not successfully treat the disease. These patients are typically highly responsive to hydroxyzine therapy. There is a subset of patients who respond to heat exposure, developing large urticarial lesions rather than the typical lesions of cholinergic urticaria. These patients tend not to develop their hives with exercise and are less responsive to hydroxyzine therapy.

Localized heat urticaria has been described with a wheal-and-flare response noted 2 to 5 minutes after applying localized heat to the skin.

EXERCISE-INDUCED URTICARIA ANAPHYLAXIS. These patients note urticarial lesions appearing 5 to 30 minutes after the onset of exercise that last for 1 to 3 hours. In severe cases, anaphylactic reactions may be noted. This is an illness generally of young adults. At times, symptoms are difficult to distinguish from those of cholinergic urticaria; however, these patients do not develop urticaria on raising core body temperature as in a hot bath and tend to respond poorly to antihistamines. A β agonist or mast cell–stabilizing agent, such as cromolyn, taken before exercise may prevent attacks.

PRESSURE-INDUCED URTICARIA. For unknown reasons, urticarial lesions are common at pressure points on the body, such as where clothing is tight. Some patients note that marked urticarial lesions develop 4 to 6 hours after pressure is applied to the body. For example, these individuals may note urticarial lesions on buttocks after sitting for a long time on a hard chair or angioedema or urticaria on their feet after prolonged standing in one place. The lesions may be provoked by placing over the shoulders for 20 minutes a 1-inch strap weighted at the ends with 15-pound weights. A systemic response with malaise and even fever may be noted. The response to antihistamines is often poor. The urticaria but not the systemic toxicity may respond to antihistamine therapy. The most severely affected of these patients may require every-other-day glucocorticoid administration for partial relief. In general, these patients are unresponsive to NSAIDs.

Similarly, some patients respond to local vibration by developing urticarial lesions. Typically, symptoms are induced by placing a vibrator or vortex mixer on the arm for 5 minutes. Urticaria appears in 1 to 5 minutes.

SOLAR URTICARIA. In general in these patients urticarial responses develop shortly after exposure to sunlight; the patients are divided into subgroups by the wavelength of light that provokes attacks. Patients whose attacks are provoked by light at 280 to 320 nm (type 1) and 400 to 500 nm (type 4) typically have disease that can be passively transferred with serum to non-affected recipients, suggesting the presence of an IgE-dependent mechanism. Type 6, provoked by light at 400 nm, is present in some patients with erythropoietic protoporphyria. Glass absorbs light with a wavelength below 320 nm, and patients with urticaria in response to light wavelengths below 320 nm are protected by a pane of glass. Preparations containing zinc oxide or titanium dioxide block all light transmission but are white and present cosmetic difficulties. The erythema-causing band of the solar spectrum, UVB, is at wavelength 290 to 320 nm, and these patients can sometimes be helped considerably by para-aminobenzoic acid (PABA)-containing sunscreens, which absorb light in this range. However, many of these persons are not protected by the PABA sunscreens. Sunscreen preparations containing butyl methoxydibenzoyl methane or terephthalylidene dicamphor sulfonic acid absorb light in the ultraviolet

A range and may be more useful for this patient group. There are many types of light sensitivity, and sorting these out may be confusing. They range from metabolic abnormalities (erythrogenic porphyria), in which products of metabolism absorb light energy and undergo chemical alteration that renders them toxic, to photoallergic reaction, in which skin-sensitizing drugs induce allergic reactions when acted on by sunlight, to phototoxic reactions, in which drugs localized in cutaneous tissues directly cause tissue-damaging reactions when exposed to light of the proper wavelength. In many of these cases the light energy is absorbed by a complex ring structure in the drug, which subsequently releases photons and electrons that lead to local generation of toxic products such as singlet oxygen, hydrogen peroxide, and chloramines. Obviously, in each case, the clinician attempts to identify the cause of the urticaria and eliminate the offending agent.

AQUAGENIC URTICARIA. These patients respond within 2 to 30 minutes with urticaria when water is applied to the skin. Typically, this is noted in the course of baths or showers, even with water at tepid temperature. In most cases these individuals are probably exquisitely sensitive to additives in the water (e.g., chlorine), but it is reported that rare individuals develop urticaria in response to distilled water.

CHRONIC URTICARIA/ANGIOEDEMA. It should be clear from the material presented that chronic urticaria/angioedema has many causes, and identifying the causative agent may be difficult or impossible. Often, after attempts at identifying the cause of the urticaria have failed, we are left with a patient who requires treatment. H_1 antihistamines are usually the agents of first choice. Some examples of therapeutic agents are listed earlier in the chapter; in patients with chronic disease, high-dose hydroxyzine and cyproheptadine are often effective. These agents make patients drowsy and may not be well tolerated initially, but drowsiness may pass if the drug is continued. Optimally, the dose is increased until drowsiness persists and then the dosage is reduced slightly. It is common to find patients who, because the drugs have not been used properly, claim to have been unresponsive to these agents. Many more conveniently used and less sedating antihistamines have become available in the past few years and have been shown in controlled studies to be effective in chronic angioedema/urticaria. These include terfenadine, astemizole, loratadine, and cetirizine. H_2 inhibitory drugs are often added to H_1 inhibitors if the clinical response is not adequate. Other agents have also reported to be beneficial in individual cases, including doxepin, a tricyclic antidepressant with anti-H_1 and anti-H_2 properties; nifedipine, a calcium-channel blocker; and ketotifen, a drug shown to be efficacious in the physical urticarias. If these agents fail, a course of glucocorticoids may be required. In general, therapy begins with 40 to 60 mg of prednisone per day in divided doses for 1 week. The dosage is then consolidated to a single dose a day, and then the drug is rapidly tapered on an every-other-day schedule until the patient is receiving glucocorticoids once every other day. The dose of glucocorticoids should be tapered to the lowest dose that will maintain the patient with minimal symptoms. After a course of glucocorticoid therapy, patients often remain in remission for a prolonged time. The illness may recur at a later time or when glucocorticoids are tapered.

DIFFERENTIAL DIAGNOSIS

This set of diseases is multifactorial. Usually the diagnosis of urticaria/angioedema does not present a problem in the patient with clear episodes of pruritic wheals or localized brawny edema. Because many agents can cause these lesions, considerable detective work is required to define these diseases and to develop a suitable specific therapy. During the initial evaluation a number of points must be explored. A history of a fixed rather than evanescent eruption or the presence of burning, bruising, or vesiculating lesions should prompt early biopsy. Similarly, fever or systemic signs and symptoms, including arthralgias, pulmonary symptoms, and abdominal pain, suggest that further exploration is needed. Patients with idiopathic chronic urticaria typically have a normal sedimentation rate, white blood cell count, and differential count; and these should be determined. In appropriate cases, antinuclear antibodies (ANA), heterophile, STS, rheumatoid factor level, cryoglobulins and cryofibrinogen, cold hemolysin, C4, and C1 inhibitor levels should be studied for further clues to the underlying diagnosis. In the patient who responds poorly to therapy or who has atypical disease, a biopsy is clearly indicated. Patients with urticarial vasculitis are treated for the underlying vasculitis.

THERAPY

The use of antihistamines and glucocorticoids is discussed under the various entities and in the section on chronic urticaria/angioedema. Anecdotal reports of patients responding to leukotriene antagonists exist. Epinephrine is clinically useful in acute management of urticaria/angioedema. In this case the drug is administered as a series of injections (0.2 to 0.3 mL) of 1:1000 dilution subcutaneously, repeated at half-hour intervals two or three times until symptoms are controlled. Obviously, the use of epinephrine is contraindicated in certain patient groups, such as patients with severe cardiovascular disease. Longer-acting epinephrine preparations such as epinephrine in oil (Sus-Phrine) may be useful.

URTICARIA PIGMENTOSA AND SYSTEMIC MASTOCYTOSIS

Urticaria pigmentosa is characterized by the local accumulation of intradermal masses of infiltrating mast cells (see Chapter 280). The lesions may resemble freckles superficially but are raised, as might be expected of infiltrative lesions, and may be somewhat erythematous. They may urticate when stroked (Darier's sign). Systemic mastocytosis is associated with massive accumulation of mast cells in other organs, particularly the bone marrow and gastrointestinal tract. Although some affected patients may present with acute or chronic urticaria, that presentation is quite rare; systemic signs of histamine toxicity, gastrointestinal disorders, or disorders consequent to destruction of bone marrow or bone are more common.

HEREDITARY ANGIOEDEMA

Hereditary angioedema (HAE) presents clinically as episodic attacks of brawny non-pitting edema that usually involve the extremities but may affect any external body surface including the genitalia. Mucosal surfaces are affected as well, and patients frequently have attacks of severe abdominal pain due to swelling of the submucosa of the gastrointestinal tract. On rare occasions, attacks may affect the airway, where they can cause respiratory obstruction and asphyxiation. Although attacks are sporadic, about half the patients note that trauma, particularly associated with local pressure, precipitates an attack, and half the patients note a marked increase in attack frequency at times of emotional stress. About one third of patients note an erythema marginatum–like rash at the onset of attacks that they often describe as non-raised, nonpruritic circles on the skin. In general, attacks become progressively more severe over about 1.5 days and then regress over a similar time period, but the duration of an attack may be longer, with swelling moving from region to region of the body.

Although relatively rare (incidence about 1:10,000), this disease has received a great deal of attention because of the high incidence of lethal complications, because its pathophysiologic basis is best understood of all of the angioedemas, and because adequate therapy is available for most patients. Presence of this disease is associated with either low levels or abnormal function of a plasma regulatory protein, the C1 inhibitor (see Chapter 271). This protein controls activation of the complement, kinin-generating, fibrinolytic, and intrinsic clotting pathways. Although the precise cause of the capillary leakage is unknown, it is believed that a peptide formed during activation of either the complement or the kinin-generating mediator pathway is the responsible factor. HAE has an autosomal dominant inheritance pattern, affecting 50% of the offspring of a patient and occurring with equal frequency in males and females. This autosomal dominant inheritance reflects the presence of one normal and one abnormal gene for C1 inhibitor on chromosome 11. This abnormal gene may yield no gene product (85% of patients; type 1) or may code for a non-functional protein (15% of patients; type 2).

HAE tends to be mild in childhood, becoming more severe at puberty. The factors that initiate attacks are unknown. There is no direct relationship between the level or activity of C1 inhibitor and the severity of disease. Patients are described who presumably had the defect from birth but whose attacks began at age 70. Diagnosis is established by finding low levels of C1 inhibitor antigen (type I) or function (all patients) and low levels of the complement protein C4 and/or C2. C1 inhibitor inhibits the function of activated C1 of the classic complement pathway. C1 inhibitor acts by binding to the substrate to be inhibited, and the product of one normal gene is insufficient to control mediator activation. When activated, C1 cleaves the next two proteins in the cascade, C4 and C2. Because the function of activated C1 is unregulated in the presence of a relative C1 inhibitor deficiency, C1 continues to cleave C4 and C2. Patients always have low levels of circulating C4 and C2 during attacks and usually have low levels between attacks. Interestingly, because of the presence of other control proteins, the levels of C3, the most commonly measured complement protein, are always normal. Presumably because of the constant complement activation present in these patients, they have an immune dysregulation shown by the higher-than-normal incidence of autoimmune diseases. These include endocrinopathies, granulomatous bowel disorders, arthritides, and systemic lupus erythematosus.

Patients' angioedema attacks respond poorly to epinephrine, antihistamines, and glucocorticoids, the mainstays of treatment of urticaria and angioedema caused by immediate hypersensitivity reactions. Nevertheless, acute attacks are treated with epinephrine, both nebulized racemic epinephrine in the airway (1:1000 given by nebulization), and subcutaneous injections (0.2 to 0.3 mL 1:1000 repeated q20–30 min × 3). Epinephrine administered very early in an attack often produces some improvement. Patients also receive antihistamines for sedation. Patients often relate that intravenously administered FFP to supply the missing inhibitor protein terminates attacks. Nevertheless, a rare patient becomes more edematous after FFP, presumably reflecting increased availability of mediator substrates, and FFP, therefore, is not recommended for treating life-threatening laryngeal edema. In this circumstance, nasotracheal intubation in the operating room under conditions in which tracheostomy can be performed is indicated. FFP can be given in non-emergency situations, such as for preoperative patients to prevent attacks. The usual dose of FFP is 2 units, an arbitrary amount that has been used extensively and has proved to be effective. Evidence suggests that infusions of purified C1 inhibitor reliably terminate attacks; it is likely that this protein will be available for treatment of acute attacks within the next several years. Although short-term therapy and therapy for acute attacks of HAE have not been generally satisfactory, long-term therapy has been quite successful. Patients respond to all of the acetylated artificial androgens with increased C1 inhibitor levels that, in some cases, approach normal values, a correction of serum C4 and C2, and a marked amelioration of symptoms. In the rare patient in whom the drug is ineffective or in whom drug toxicity is a problem, plasmin inhibitors, such as ϵ-aminocaproic acid, have also been found to be effective. Their mechanism of action is unknown, and there is no change in the extent of complement activation reflected in the persistent reduction in the serum level of C4 and C2. With all of these agents there is a high degree of patient-to-patient variation in drug dosage, and the lowest dose that controls symptoms is chosen. Women are often treated with danazol (200 to 600 mg/day) or stanozolol (2–6 mg/day); danazol and stanozolol are impeded androgens that have few masculinizing side effects. Men are often treated with the less expensive but more androgenic agent methyltestosterone (10 to 30 mg/day orally). A number of agents, given to patients for other conditions, greatly increase the severity and number of HAE attacks. These include estrogens (often given in birth control agents) and angiotensin-converting enzyme inhibitors given for control of hypertension.

ACQUIRED C1 INHIBITOR DEFICIENCY

A number of syndromes have been recognized that are associated with a typical HAE symptom complex but are a reflection of acquired disease. Certain patients with malignancies, including lymphosarcoma, leukemia, lymphoma, and paraproteinemia, develop circulating or cellular factors that activate C1 and deplete the C1 inhibitor activity in serum. Also, rare patients with circulating immune complexes induce massive activation of the complement cascade, with C1 inhibitor utilization and an HAE-like clinical picture. Patients have been described with multiple myeloma and anti-idiotypic antibody causing the same symptom complex. Perhaps the most common of these rare individuals are recently described patients who form monoclonal or polyclonal autoantibodies to the C1 inhibitor, which destroy its activity. Clinically, these patients cannot be distinguished from patients with HAE. However, their laboratory test results are unique. All of these patient groups have profound depressions in functional C1, C4, and C2. Patients with HAE commonly have normal C1 levels. Although their plasma C1 inhibitor antigen level may be normal, these patient groups have marked depression of C1 inhibitor function. Their treatment focuses on the underlying disease when possible. Some of these patients respond to danazol or other anabolic steroids. Several of the patients with the anti–C1 inhibitor autoantibody have responded to glucocorticoid therapy, and several of these patients have responded to cytotoxic therapy. There is one report that plasmin inhibitors are more effective than the androgens in patients with anti–C1 inhibitor antibody.

FACTOR I DEFICIENCY

Factor I is one of the control proteins of the complement activation pathway. The rare individuals with an inherited deficiency of this protein continuously activate and cleave C3, generating the anaphylatoxins C3a and perhaps C5a. In vitro, these cleavage peptides induce mast cell degranulation and cause chronic urticaria that disappears when the patient is infused with Factor I. In general, this form of urticaria is relatively mild and is treated symptomatically with antihistamines.

ANGIOEDEMA INDUCED BY ANGIOTENSIN-CONVERTING ENZYME INHIBITORS AND INTERLEUKIN-2

Within hours to 1 week of therapy with angiotensin-converting enzyme inhibitors, or more rarely later, patients may note angioedema that becomes life-threatening. Angiotensin-converting enzyme plays an important role in the degradation of bradykinin and the neuropeptide substance P, and these mediators may be important in angioedema formation. Patients are treated with antihistamines and/or epinephrine as appropriate, and the angiotensin-converting enzyme inhibitor is discontinued. Recently, a patient has been described with congenital angiotensin-converting enzyme deficiency. This patient presented as an adult with recurrent angioedema of the upper airway, emphasizing the importance of this enzyme in the proper metabolism of mediators of edema. It will be of importance to determine whether other such patients exist. Just as patients exist with acquired autoantibodies to C1 inhibitor who present with recurrent angioedema, patients with antibody to angiotensin-converting enzyme may exist who have recurrent angioedema. It has also been noted that systemic capillary leak or angioedema may follow the systemic infusion of interleukin-2 used to treat malignancy. It is reported that this cytokine activates both the complement- and kinin-generating pathways. It also activates T cells, and it has been suggested that these activated cells directly damage the endothelium.

Beltrani VS: Urticaria and angioedema. Dermatol Clin 14:171–198, 1996. *Excellent general review of pathophysiology, diagnosis, and management.*

David AE III: C1 inhibitor gene and hereditary angioedema. *In* Volanakis JE, Frank MM (eds): The Human Complement System in Health and Disease. New York, Marcel Decker, 1998, pp 455–480. *Review of molecular biology, genetic defects, and pathophysiology of hereditary angioedema.*

Gonzalez E, Gonzalez S: Drug photosensitivity, idiopathic photodermatoses and sunscreens. J Am Acad Dermatol 35:871–885, 1996. *Discussion of all aspects of light sensitivity.*

Kontou-Fili K, Borici-Mazi R, Kapp A, et al: Physical urticaria: Classification and diagnostic guidelines. Allergy 52:504–513, 1997. *Excellent practice guide to the physical urticarias.*

Pillans PI, Coulter DM, Black P: Angioedema and urticaria with angiotensin converting enzyme inhibitors. Eur J Clin Pharmacol 51:123–126, 1996. *Discussion of this important cause of urticaria.*

Waytes AT, Rosen FS, Frank MM: Treatment of hereditary angioedema with a vapor-heated C1 inhibitor concentrate. N Engl J Med 334:1630–1634, 1996. *Use of purified inhibitor protein to treat disease, with reference to other therapies.*

274 ALLERGIC RHINITIS

Richard D. deShazo

DEFINITION. Allergic rhinitis is a symptom complex characterized by paroxysms of sneezing, itching of the eyes, nose, and palate, rhinorrhea, and nasal obstruction. It is often associated with post-nasal drip, cough, irritability, and fatigue. Symptoms develop when persons inhale airborne antigens (allergens) to which they have previously been exposed and have made IgE antibodies. These IgE antibodies bind to IgE receptors on mast cells in the respiratory mucosa and to basophils in the peripheral blood. When IgE molecules on their surface are bridged by allergen, mast cells release pre-formed and granule-associated chemical mediators. They also generate other mediators and cytokines that lead to nasal inflammation and, with continued allergen exposure, chronic symptoms.

EPIDEMIOLOGY. Allergic rhinitis is common and accounts for at least 2.5% of all physician visits, 2 million lost school days per year, 6 million lost work days, and 28 million restricted work days per year. Allergic rhinitis results in the expenditure of $2.4 billion on prescription and over-the-counter medications for allergy and $1.1 billion in physician billings per year. Between 10 and 20% of the U.S. population is affected, and the prevalence in urban areas is increasing. The prevalence is lowest in children younger than 5 years, rises to a peak in early adulthood (as high as 24% in the United States), and declines thereafter. The 4-year remission rate is reported to be 10% in males and 5% in females.

PHYSICAL FINDINGS AND ASSOCIATIONS. The swollen nasal mucosa of patients with acute allergic rhinitis is pale and blue but becomes erythematous and indurated with chronic allergen exposure. Clear rhinorrhea may be visible anteriorly or, with nasal obstruction, dripping down a cobblestone-appearing posterior pharynx. Giemsa or Hansel's stains of these nasal secretions show cell populations to be predominately eosinophils. A transverse nasal crease, a highly arched palate, mouth breathing, and dental malocclusion are common, especially in children. Venous dilation of the subcutaneous skin beneath the eyes may produce "allergic shiners."

Chronic allergic rhinitis may be associated with sleep disorders, sinusitis, secretory otitis media, and anosmia. Allergic rhinitis is also associated with other common allergic conditions, including allergic conjunctivitis, allergic asthma, and atopic dermatitis (eczema). Twenty-eight to 50% of patients with asthma and up to 30% with eczema have allergic rhinitis. These conditions have been termed "atopic diseases," and patients who have them are often called "atopic."

DIFFERENTIAL DIAGNOSIS. Syndromes of rhinitis may be divided into allergic, infectious, perennial non-allergic, and miscellaneous categories (Table 274–1). Allergic rhinitis should be differentiated from other forms of rhinitis because the approach to management is different. Episodic exposure to inhaled allergens such as cat salivary proteins, horse dander, murine urinary proteins, pollen, or house dust mite feces may provoke acute allergic symptoms that are easily diagnosed as *acute allergic rhinitis*. If allergen exposure is seasonal—for instance, tree and grass pollen in the spring (rose fever) or ragweed pollen exposure in the fall (hay fever)—symptoms are predictable and reproducible and thus *seasonal allergic rhinitis* may be diagnosed by the history (Fig. 274–1). When allergen exposure is chronic, *perennial allergic rhinitis* may result. This form is common in subtropical regions with long pollinating seasons and ever-present mold and dust mite allergens and with occupational allergen exposure. Perennial allergic rhinitis may be difficult to distinguish from non-allergic forms and could require certain testing (discussed later) for accurate diagnosis. Of all patients with rhinitis, 11% have seasonal symptoms, with 78% of these patients having an apparent allergic cause. Thirty-three per cent of patients with rhinitis have perennial symptoms with a seasonal exacerbation, and 68% of these patients have a probable allergic cause. Fifty-six per cent of patients with rhinitis have perennial symptoms alone, but only about 50% of them have

Table 274–1 ■ **CLASSIFICATION OF RHINITIS**

Allergic
Seasonal
Perennial
Occupational
Infectious
Acute: Viral, bacterial
Chronic:
   Specific: Bacterial, fungal
   Non-specific: Associated with immune deficiency (antibody deficiency, ciliary abnormalities)
Perennial Non-allergic
Idiopathic (vasomotor rhinitis)
Non-allergic rhinitis with eosinophilia (NARES)
Miscellaneous Forms
Hormonal: Pregnancy, hypothyroidism, etc.
Drug induced: Associated with aspirin and antihypertensives (rhinitis medicamentosa)
Food: Gustatory, IgE mediated, preservative induced
Atrophic rhinitis (*Klebsiella ozaenae*)
Mechanical: Hypertrophied turbinates, deviated nasal septum, foreign body, nasal polyps

symptoms that can be attributed to allergens. Most patients with allergic rhinitis have allergic symptom triggers, eosinophil-rich nasal secretions, allergen-specific IgE to inhalant allergens, and a family history of allergic disease.

Nasal eosinophilia is not diagnostic for allergic rhinitis because nasal eosinophilia occurs in the non-allergic rhinitis with nasal eosinophilia syndrome (NARES). NARES occurs in as many as 15% of patients with rhinitis and is characterized by perennial symptoms, an older average age than in patients with allergic rhinitis (39 versus 25 years), and milder symptoms of nasal itching and sneezing. The clear nasal secretions contain greater than 25% eosinophils, but the role of eosinophils in the disorder is unclear. Fifty per cent of patients with NARES have sinusitis, 33% have nasal polyps, and 14% have asthma. IgE to inhalant allergens is usually absent. Another frequent form of perennial non-allergic rhinitis is commonly called vasomotor rhinitis. Patients with this disorder complain predominantly of chronic nasal congestion intensified by rapid changes in temperature and relative humidity, odors, or alcohol. Several lines of evidence suggest that they have nasal autonomic nervous system dysfunction. For instance, they have abnormal nasal responses to temperature stimuli applied to the skin and excess nasal sensitivity to topically applied acetylcholine congeners. They have little nasal itching or sneezing, but headaches, anosmia, and sinusitis are common. A family history of allergy or

allergic symptom triggers is uncommon. Positive immediate hypersensitivity skin tests to inhalant allergens and nasal eosinophilia are unusual. Atrophic rhinitis is a syndrome of progressive atrophy of the nasal mucosa in elderly patients, who report chronic nasal congestion and constantly perceive a bad odor. Rhinitis medimentosa is a complication of chronic use of vasoconstrictor nasal sprays or intranasal cocaine abuse. Chronic nasal obstruction and nasal inflammation develop and are manifested as beefy red nasal membranes on physical examination. Rhinitis of pregnancy and rhinitis associated with birth control pills or hypothyroidism reflect nasal obstruction that occurs on a hormonal basis. Nasal obstruction may also be a side effect of antihypertensive drugs. Unilateral rhinitis or nasal polyps are uncommon in uncomplicated allergic rhinitis. Unilateral rhinitis suggests the possibility of nasal obstruction by a foreign body, tumor, or polyp, and the presence of nasal polyps suggest chronic sinusitis, aspirin hypersensitivity, or cystic fibrosis.

MECHANISMS OF ALLERGIC REACTIONS. The expression of allergic diseases reflects an autosomal dominant pattern of inheritance with incomplete penetrance. This inheritance pattern is manifested as a propensity to respond to inhalant allergen exposure by producing high levels of allergen-specific IgE. The IgE response appears to be controlled by immune response genes located within the major histocompatibility complex (MHC) on chromosome 6 (see Chapter 278). The immunologic mechanisms for atopy have been studied in murine models and in humans and appear to center on the expression of a repertoire of responses associated with the T_H2 type of T-helper lymphocyte, which is summarized below.

PRODUCTION OF IgE. Sensitization to allergen is necessary to elicit an IgE response (Fig. 274–2). After inhalation, the allergen must first be internalized by antigen-presenting cells, which include macrophages, dendritic cells, activated T lymphocytes, and B lymphocytes. After allergen processing, peptide fragments of the allergen are presented with class II (MHC) molecules of host antigen-presenting cells to CD4+ T lymphocytes. These lymphocytes have receptors specific for the particular MHC-peptide complex. This interaction results in the release of cytokines by the CD4+ cell.

T-helper lymphocytes (CD4+) appear to be of two classes: T_H1 and T_H2. If the CD4+ cells that recognize the allergen are of the T_H2 class, a specific repertoire of mediators are released, including interleukin-4 (IL-4), IL-5, and IL-9. Other cytokines, including IL-2, IL-3, IL-10, IL-13, and granulocyte-macrophage stimulating factor (GM-CSF), are also released in the process of antigen recognition but are not specific to activation of the T_H2 class. IL-4, IL-5, and IL-6 are cytokines involved in B-cell proliferation and differentiation. Activated B lymphocytes, having bound allergen via their allergen-specific IgM variable-region binding sites, are stimulated by these cytokines to proliferate and secrete IgM. IL-4, IL-6, IL-10,

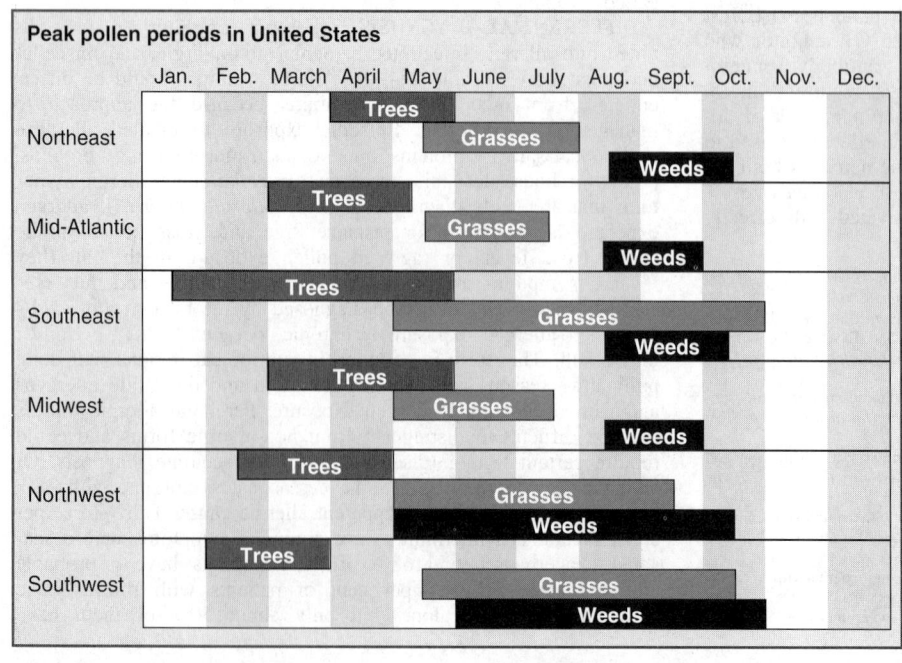

FIGURE 274–1 ■ Peak pollen periods in the United States. (Reproduced with permission from Fisons Pharmaceuticals. © 1989, Fisons Corporation.)

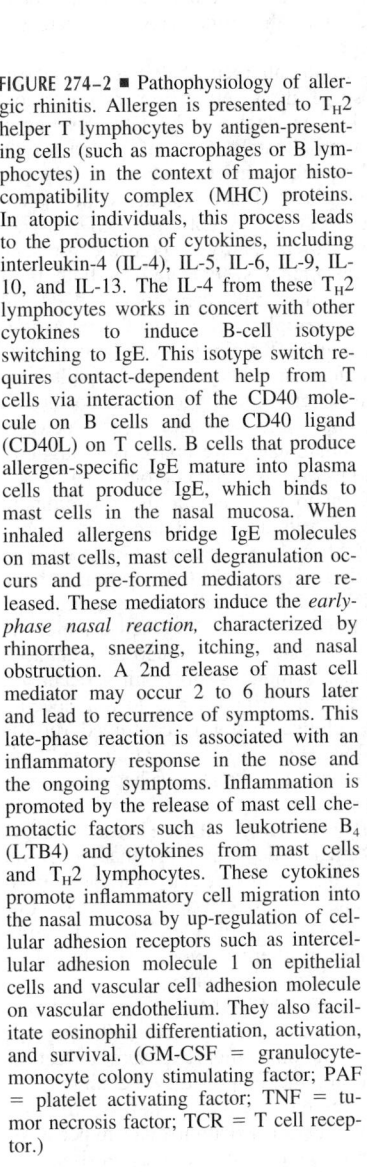

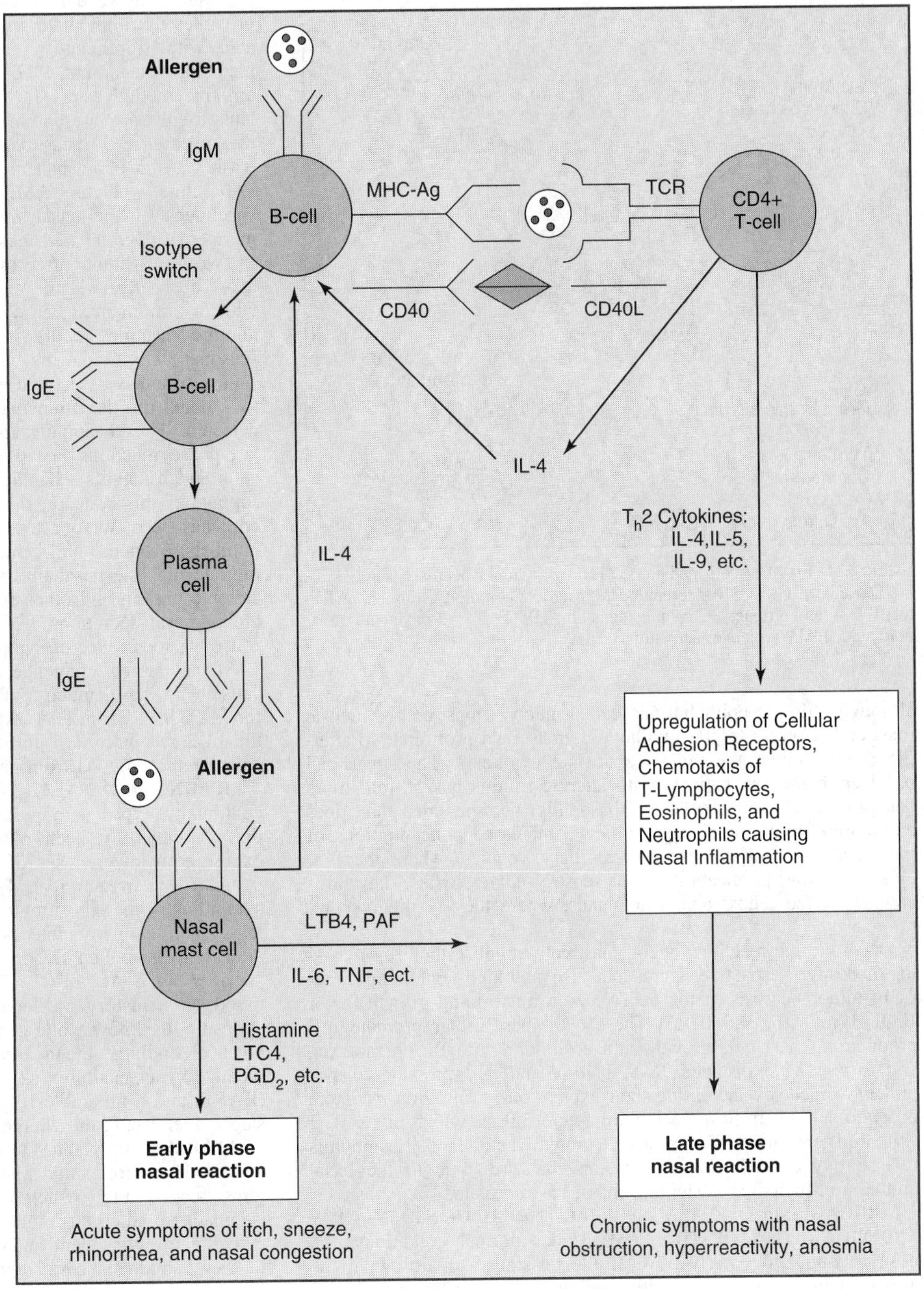

FIGURE 274–2 ▪ Pathophysiology of allergic rhinitis. Allergen is presented to T_H2 helper T lymphocytes by antigen-presenting cells (such as macrophages or B lymphocytes) in the context of major histocompatibility complex (MHC) proteins. In atopic individuals, this process leads to the production of cytokines, including interleukin-4 (IL-4), IL-5, IL-6, IL-9, IL-10, and IL-13. The IL-4 from these T_H2 lymphocytes works in concert with other cytokines to induce B-cell isotype switching to IgE. This isotype switch requires contact-dependent help from T cells via interaction of the CD40 molecule on B cells and the CD40 ligand (CD40L) on T cells. B cells that produce allergen-specific IgE mature into plasma cells that produce IgE, which binds to mast cells in the nasal mucosa. When inhaled allergens bridge IgE molecules on mast cells, mast cell degranulation occurs and pre-formed mediators are released. These mediators induce the *early-phase nasal reaction*, characterized by rhinorrhea, sneezing, itching, and nasal obstruction. A 2nd release of mast cell mediator may occur 2 to 6 hours later and lead to recurrence of symptoms. This late-phase reaction is associated with an inflammatory response in the nose and the ongoing symptoms. Inflammation is promoted by the release of mast cell chemotactic factors such as leukotriene B_4 (LTB4) and cytokines from mast cells and T_H2 lymphocytes. These cytokines promote inflammatory cell migration into the nasal mucosa by up-regulation of cellular adhesion receptors such as intercellular adhesion molecule 1 on epithelial cells and vascular cell adhesion molecule on vascular endothelium. They also facilitate eosinophil differentiation, activation, and survival. (GM-CSF = granulocyte-monocyte colony stimulating factor; PAF = platelet activating factor; TNF = tumor necrosis factor; TCR = T cell receptor.)

and IL-13 from T_H2 cells promote B-cell isotype switching to IgE antibody synthesis. Thus atopy appears to be the result of a predisposition toward T_H2-type responses, which result in the formation of large quantities of allergen-specific IgE.

BINDING TO MAST CELLS AND EOSINOPHILS. After IgE antibodies specific for a certain allergen are synthesized and secreted, they bind to mast cells and basophils. When allergen is inhaled into the nose, the allergen or a hapten-allergen complex cross-links these allergen-specific cell-bound IgE antibodies on the mast cell surface, whereupon rapid degranulation and mediator release occur.

Mast cell mediators are either pre-formed, associated with granules, formed during degranulation, or generated after transcription (Fig. 274–3). The most important pre-formed mediator is histamine, which reproduces all of the symptoms of acute allergic rhinitis when sprayed nasally into normal volunteers. Histamine causes vasodilation, which leads to nasal congestion, mucus secretion, and increased vascular permeability, which in turn leads to tissue edema and sneezing through stimulation of sensory nerve fibers. The cross-linking of IgE antibody on mast cells activates phospholipase A_2 and releases arachidonic acid from the A_2 position of cell membrane phospholipids. Mast cells then metabolize arachidonic acid—either via the cyclooxygenase pathway to form prostaglandin and thromboxane mediators or via the lipoxygenase pathway to form leukotrienes. Prostaglandin D_2 (PGD_2), the sulfidopeptide leukotrienes LTC_4, LTD_4, and LTE_4 (slow reacting substance of anaphylaxis) platelet-activating factor (PAF), and bradykinin are formed during degranulation. PGD_2 is synthesized by mast cells but not basophils and appears to be more potent than histamine in causing nasal congestion. PAF is a potent chemotactic factor, and the sulfidopeptide leukotrienes and bradykinins are vasoactive. One leukotriene, LTB_4, is the most potent chemotactic factor in humans.

Mast cells are present in concentrations of $7000/mm^3$ in the normal nasal submucosa but only $50/mm^3$ in the nasal epithelium. The total number of nasal epithelial mast cells remains constant during the allergy season. Nasal mast cells are predominately located in the nasal lamina propria as connective tissue mast cells,

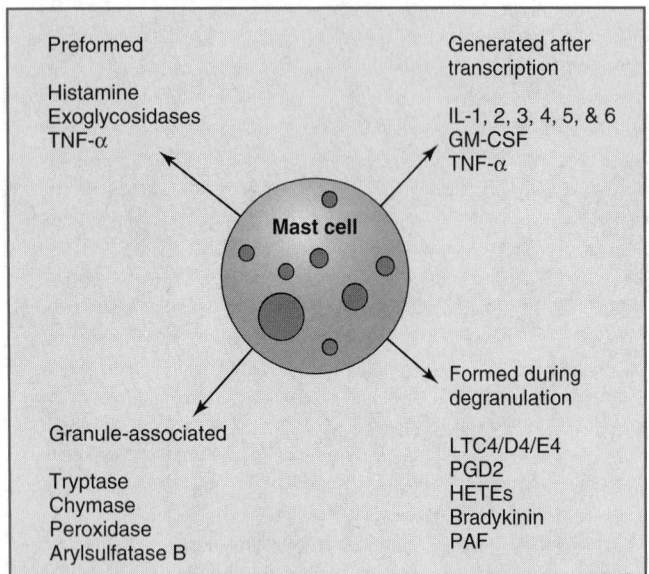

Preformed

Histamine
Exoglycosidases
TNF-α

Mast cell

Generated after transcription

IL-1, 2, 3, 4, 5, & 6
GM-CSF
TNF-α

Granule-associated

Tryptase
Chymase
Peroxidase
Arylsulfatase B

Formed during degranulation

LTC4/D4/E4
PGD2
HETEs
Bradykinin
PAF

FIGURE 274–3 ■ Mast cell mediators. (TNF-α = tumor necrosis factor α; IL = interleukin; GM-CSF = granulocyte-macrophage colony-stimulating factor; LT = leukotriene; PG = prostaglandin; HETE = hydroxyeicosatetraenoic acid; PAF = platelet-activating factor.)

although 15% are epithelial and called mucosal mast cells. Mucosal mast cells express tryptase without chymase and proliferate in allergic rhinitis under the influence of T_H2 cytokines. The superficial nasal epithelium in patients with allergic rhinitis has 50-fold more basophilic cells (mast cells and basophils) per specimen than does epithelium from non-allergic subjects. Increased concentrations of mast cells are found near post-capillary venules, where they increase vascular permeability; near sensory nerves, where they initiate the sneeze reflex; and near glands, where they facilitate secretion.

Once allergic reactions begin, mast cells amplify them by releasing not only vasoactive agents but also cytokines, including GM-CSF, tumor necrosis factor α (TNF-α), transforming growth factor β, IL-1 to IL-6, and IL-13. These cytokines further promote IgE production, mast cell growth, and eosinophil growth, chemotaxis, and survival. For instance, IL-5, TNF-α, and IL-1 promote eosinophil movement by increasing their expression of adhesion receptors on endothelium. In turn, eosinophils secrete IL-1, which favors T_H2 cell proliferation and the mast cell growth factor IL-3. Eosinophils release oxygen radicals and proteins that are toxic to the nasal epithelium, including eosinophil major basic protein.

MECHANISMS OF NASAL ALLERGIC REACTIONS. ANATOMY AND PHYSIOLOGY OF THE NOSE. Under normal conditions, the nose accounts for nearly 50% of the resistance to airflow in the airway. It is lined by pseudostratified epithelium resting on a basement membrane that separates it from deeper submucosal layers. The submucosa contains mucous, seromucous, and serous glands. The small arteries, arterioles, and arteriovenous anastomoses determine regional blood flow. Capacitance vessels consisting of veins and cavernous sinusoids determine nasal patency. The cavernous sinusoids lie beneath the capillaries and venules, are most dense in the inferior and middle turbinates, and contain smooth muscle cells controlled by the sympathetic nervous system. Withdrawal of sympathetic tone or, to a lesser degree, cholinergic stimulation causes this sinusoidal erectile tissue to become engorged. Cholinergic stimulation causes arterial dilation and promotes the passive diffusion of plasma protein into glands and active secretion by mucous glands in cells.

Novel neurotransmitters, including substance P, calcitonin gene–related peptide, and vasointestinal peptide, have been detected in nasal secretions after nasal allergen challenge of patients with allergic rhinitis. Antidromic stimulation of sensory nerve fibers in the nose can release a variety of neurotransmitters, including substance P, a chemical that increases vascular permeability. Because neurotransmitters also produce changes in regional blood flow and glandular secretion, their role in rhinitis may be important.

IMMEDIATE AND LATE NASAL REACTIONS. Exposing the nasal mucosa to ragweed in ragweed-sensitive subjects (nasal challenge) provokes the immediate onset of sneezing and nasal itching associated with significantly increased concentrations of inflammatory mediators. Histamine, PGD_2, the kininogen product toluenesulfonyl-arginine methyl ester (TAME), tryptase, kinins, and sulfidopeptide leukotrienes are present in nasal washes. Sneezing correlates with the appearance of measurable histamine, TAME, and PGD_2 in nasal washes. After about half an hour, PGD_2 and histamine levels return to baseline, whereas TAME concentrations remain elevated. Biopsy specimens of the nasal mucosa at this time show an increased number of degranulated mast cells.

Two to 6 hours after the initial allergen challenge, symptoms may recur after a 2nd release of mast cell mediators coincident with maximum mast cell cytokine production. This late-phase nasal allergic reaction occurs in approximately 50% of patients with seasonal rhinitis who are undergoing nasal challenge with allergen. This reaction is associated with elevated levels of the same mediators noted in the immediate reaction, except that PGD_2 is not detected. Thus basophils appear to be partly responsible for such late-phase reactions because histamine is generated by both mast cells and basophils whereas only mast cells can produce PGD_2. In support of this concept, marked basophil influx into the nasal mucosa has been noted 3 to 11 hours after allergen challenge. Large numbers of neutrophils, mononuclear cells, and eosinophils also migrate into the nasal mucosa at this time. Increases in eosinophil cationic protein and other eosinophil products also become detectable in nasal secretions. This inflammatory response is thought to cause the recurrence of symptoms and to induce chronic ones.

After allergen challenge, lymphocytes remain the predominant cells in the nasal mucosa. These cells actively transcribe messages for IL-3, IL-4, IL-5, and GM-CSF and have increased expression of the IL-2 receptor. IL-1 through IL-5 and GM-CSF, among others, have been recovered from nasal washes after allergen challenge.

PRIMING AND NASAL HYPERREACTIVITY. When a patient is continually exposed to pollen, persistent nasal mucosal inflammation develops. In such patients, symptoms of rhinitis occur on exposure to lower doses of allergen (priming) and to non-specific irritants (hyperreactivity). The clinical result is continued rhinitis symptoms with exposure to low allergen concentrations and irritants such as particulate pollution and volatile substances, even after the peak pollen season has passed.

MANAGING ALLERGIC RHINITIS. DIAGNOSIS. The diagnosis is based on a history of the characteristic symptoms that occur on exposure to known allergens. It is supported by the associated physical findings, by the presence of allergen-specific IgE on immediate hypersensitivity skin tests, or by radioallergosorbent testing (RAST) and a favorable response to allergen avoidance. The initial step is identifying the allergens that produce symptoms.

ALLERGEN IDENTIFICATION AND AVOIDANCE. A careful home and work environmental history is often informative. When symptoms occur acutely, such as symptoms after exposure to cat or occupational allergens, identifying the culprit may be simple. In perennial rhinitis, identifying allergens by history may be difficult. In these circumstances, carefully performed immediate hypersensitivity skin testing (prick skin tests) is a quick, inexpensive, and safe way to identify the presence of allergen-specific IgE. In sensitive patients, testing with selected extracts of tree, grass, or weed pollen, mold, house dust mite, and/or animal allergens results in a weal-and-flare reaction at the skin test site within 20 minutes. Although less sensitive and more expensive, the RAST is a surrogate test that gives similar information from a serum sample. Neither total serum IgE levels, elevated in only 30 to 40% of patients, nor peripheral blood eosinophil counts are sensitive enough to routinely diagnose allergic rhinitis. Stained nasal smears detect eosinophilia, which is helpful in narrowing the diagnosis to allergic rhinitis or NARES; and neutrophilia (>50%) associated with sinusitis.

Simple measures to avoid allergens include maintaining the relative humidity at 50% or less to limit house dust mite and mold growth and avoiding exposure to irritants such as cigarette smoke. Air conditioners decrease concentrations of pollen, mold, and dust mite allergens in indoor air. Avoiding exposure to the feces of the house dust mite—the most common cause of perennial allergic rhinitis—is facilitated by covering mattresses, box springs, and pillows with plastic and washing bedding in water hotter than 70° F once weekly. Synthetic pillows should also be used. Furry pets

Table 274–2 ▪ REPRESENTATIVE ANTIHISTAMINES*

DRUG	SEDATIVE EFFECTS	ANTIHISTAMINE EFFECTS	DOSING INTERVALS (hr)
Ethanolamines			
Clemastine (Tavist)	2+	1–2+	12
Diphenhydramine (Benadryl)	3+	1–2+	6–8
Ethylenediamines			
Pyrilamine (Histadyl)	1+	1–2+	6–8
Alkylamines			
Chlorpheniramine (Chlor-Trimeton)	1+	2+	4–6
Phenothiazines			
Promethazine (Phenergan)	3+	3+	6–24
Piperidines			
Astemizole (Hismanal)	±	2–3+	24
Loratadine (Claritin)	±	2–3+	24
Fexofenadine (Allegra)	±	2–3+	12–24
Azatadine (Optimine)	2+	2+	12
Cyproheptadine (Periactin)	3+	2+	8
Piperazines			
Hydroxyzine (Atarax)	3+	3+	12
Cetirizine (Zyrtec)	1+	2–3+	24
Miscellaneous			
Azelastine†	±	2–3+	12
Levocabastine†	±	2–3±	12

*Antihistamines in this listing have specific contraindications that require review before prescribing.
†Nasal spray.
©1993 by Facts and Comparisons. Used with permission and modified from Drug Facts and Comparisons. 1993 ed. St Louis, Facts and Comparisons, a division of the JB Lippincott Company. Effects were graded 1 to 4.

should be removed from the home unless testing shows they are not the source of symptoms.

PHARMACOLOGIC TREATMENT. If avoiding allergens does not result in improvement, antihistamine therapy is a reasonable next step. Antihistamines help control sneezing, rhinorrhea, and itching but may provide inadequate relief from nasal obstruction (Table 274–2). In this case, an oral antihistamine that contains a decongestant such as pseudoephedrine, phenylpropanolamine, or phenylephrine has been shown to be of added benefit. Because the latter agents may cause palpitations, insomnia or irritability, exacerbation of glaucoma, and urinary retention and are contraindicated in patients receiving monoamine oxidase therapy, they should be used cautiously. With use for more than 5 to 7 days, tachyphylaxis develops to nasal (decongestant) sprays of these drugs and rebound nasal congestion results. Continued use leads to rhinitis medimentosa.

The 1st-generation H_1-receptor antagonists produce sedation and other central nervous system symptoms in 20% of patients and may cause drying of the mouth and urinary hesitancy. Newer 2nd-generation antihistamines have sedative effects comparable to those of placebo. Some of these antihistamines, such as astemizole, have been associated with the induction of complex ventricular tachyarrhythmias when used concomitantly with ketoconazole, itraconazole, macrolide antibiotics, or metronidazole, which share hepatic

metabolic pathways. Some of the 2nd-generation H_1 antihistamines inhibit mast cell mediator release and inflammatory cell movement and function. This feature makes them effective in inhibiting not only the immediate but also the late nasal reaction to allergen challenge. However, these 2nd-generation agents have not yet been demonstrated to be clinically superior to other 2nd-generation antihistamines. There is no evidence that pharmacologic tolerance develops to antihistamines. Thus rotating from one antihistamine to another is not beneficial. Furthermore, clinical studies do not support the use of combinations of H_1 and H_2 antagonists to treat allergic rhinitis.

Cromolyn and nedocromil inhibit mast cell degranulation and mediator release from mast cells and have other anti-inflammatory actions. They thus inhibit both immediate and late-phase nasal reactions. Both appear to be as effective as antihistamines in treating allergic rhinitis, with nedocromil the more effective. Both agents must be used frequently (three or more times a day), take 2 to 6 weeks to reach full efficacy, and have few side effects.

Corticosteroids given orally or parentally usually abolish all symptoms of allergic rhinitis. The potential complications of such therapy make them unacceptable for treating allergic rhinitis except in very unusual circumstances. By contrast, topical intranasal steroid therapy causes few side effects when used at recommended doses (Table 274–3). In experimental nasal allergen challenge, they

Table 274–3 ▪ INTRANASAL STEROIDS AVAILABLE IN THE UNITED STATES

NAME/TRADE NAME	DOSE	APPROVED FOR CHILDREN (yr)
Dexamethasone sodium phosphate (Decadron, Turbinaire*)	2 sprays (168 μg) in each nostril b.i.d.–t.i.d.; max, 1008 μg/d	>6
Flunisolide (Nasalide)	2 sprays (50 μg) in each nostril b.i.d.–t.i.d.; max, 400 μg/d	>6
Beclomethasone dipropionate (Beconase, Vancenase, Beconase AQ, Vancenase AQ)	1 spray (42 μg) in each nostril b.i.d.–q.i.d.; max, 336 μg/d	>6
Triamcinolone acetonide (Nasacort)	2 sprays (110 μg) in each nostril once a day; max, 440 μg/d	>6
Budesonide (Rhinocort)	2 sprays (64 μg) in each nostril once a day; max, 256 μg/d	>6
Fluticasone (Flonase)	2 sprays (100 μg) in each nostril once a day; max, 200 μg/d	>12
Mometasone furoate monohydrate (Nasonex)	2 sprays (50 μg) in each nostril once a day; max, unclear	>12

*For short-term use only.
©1993 by Facts and Comparisons. Used with permission and modified from Drug Facts and Comparisons. 1993 ed. St Louis, Facts and Comparisons, a division of the JB Lippincott Company.

decrease the amount of histamine released in the early nasal response to allergen by 75% and increase the threshold dose for a positive response to allergen. With regular use, they inhibit both immediate and late-phase nasal reactions. Their maximal therapeutic effects are seen as quickly as 3 to 5 days. Corticosteroids have both vasoconstrictor and anti-inflammatory effects, including inhibition of mediator release and inflammatory cell chemotaxis. Topical nasal steroids are more effective than cromolyn and some second-generation antihistamines and improve the symptoms of seasonal asthma in patients with both seasonal allergic rhinitis and seasonal allergic asthma. These preparations are available in both aqueous and Freon-propelled preparations. The aqueous preparations may be particularly useful in patients in whom Freon preparations cause mucosal drying, crusting, or epistaxis. Rarely, nasal steroids are associated with nasal septal perforation, probably secondary to nasal septal wall damage from inappropriately using the pressurized aerosol. Mucosal atrophy has not been noted even after years of usage. Treatment failures occur if mucus or other debris is not cleaned from the nose before application. This cleaning can be facilitated by saline nasal sprays or washes.

Ipratropium bromide, a congener of atropine, has been found to reduce rhinorrhea when used intranasally. It does not block sneezing or nasal obstruction and is thus of greater use in non-allergic rhinitis with predominantly rhinorrhea.

ALLERGEN IMMUNOTHERAPY. Allergen immunotherapy is the subcutaneous administration of increasing concentrations of allergen to which the patient has demonstrated sensitization and symptoms by skin test (or RAST) and history, respectively. Immunotherapy should be considered when pharmacotherapy and avoidance of allergens fail to resolve the symptoms or when pharmacotherapy produces unacceptable side effects or is not cost-effective. High-dose immunotherapy for allergic rhinitis has been shown to effectively relieve symptoms of allergic rhinitis in controlled studies. It should be strongly considered in patients with perennial symptoms, perennial rhinitis with seasonal exacerbations, or constitutional symptoms (such as severe fatigue) or in patients with associated sinusitis, allergic conjunctivitis, or asthma. It is time consuming and associated with a risk of anaphylaxis, especially when administered by health care professionals not properly trained in its use.

Allergen immunotherapy blocks both the immediate and the late-phase nasal reaction. The specific mechanism by which it relieves symptoms is unclear, although it increases allergen-specific IgG, reduces allergen-specific IgE, decreases allergen-induced mediator release, decreases eosinophil chemotaxis, and appears to favor a shift to cytokine profiles associated with T_H1 responses to allergen.

Badhwar AK, Druce HM: Allergic rhinitis. Med Clin North Am 76:789, 1992. *A practical and well-written review of the diagnostic approach and treatment of rhinitis.*

Baraniut JN: Pathogenesis of allergic rhinitis. J Allergy Clin Immunol 99(Suppl.):763, 1997. *An excellent review article with an extensive discussion of the pathophysiology of allergic disease.*

Meltzer ED: The pharmacological basis for treatment of perennial allergic rhinitis and nonallergic rhinitis with topical corticosteroids. Allergy 52(Suppl. 136):33, 1997.

Naclerio R, Solomon W: Rhinitis with inhaled allergens. JAMA 278:1842, 1997. *An excellent review article covering all aspects of the topic.*

Webber RW: Immunotherapy with allergens. JAMA 278:1881, 1997. *A well-written review of the rationale and mechanism of action of allergen immunotherapy in allergic respiratory disease.*

275 ANAPHYLAXIS

Allen P. Kaplan

The term *anaphylaxis* arose from the experiments of Richer and Portier in the early 1900s and meant the opposite of prophylaxis, i.e., a lack of protection rather than the expected immunity. Nevertheless, the reaction is indeed immune in nature and depends on the formation of IgE antibody, the immunoglobulin responsible for typical allergic reactions. The initial sensitization step induces the formation of IgE specifically directed to the initiating substance. In anaphylaxis, the reaction is systemic in nature, occurs rapidly after the administration of minute concentrations of the offending material, and is potentially fatal. How the allergen is given can dictate the manifestations and magnitude of the ensuing allergic reaction; although all routes can lead to anaphylaxis, parenteral administration is more likely than inhaled or ingested allergens to cause elevated circulating levels of unaltered allergen and a systemic reaction. Thus parenteral administration of medication and insect sting reactions (injected into cutaneous vessels) are among the most common causes of anaphylaxis. Anaphylactoid reactions are defined as systemic reactions that have the same symptoms as anaphylaxis but are not due to an IgE-dependent mechanism and are not usually immune. Examples include reactions to radiographic contrast agents and non-steroidal anti-inflammatory drugs (e.g., acetylsalicylic acid, indomethacin, ibuprofen).

EPIDEMIOLOGY AND ETIOLOGY. The occurrence of anaphylaxis in the early 1900s was largely due to the use of serum from animals immunized with various toxins or bacteria to treat human illness. Most were due to diphtheria antitoxin injection. In the antibiotic era, penicillin and sulfa drugs have become the leading causes of fatal anaphylaxis. In recent years, between 100 and 500 deaths per year in the United States have been attributed to penicillin. The insect order Hymenoptera is responsible for about 40 deaths each year and is estimated to cause 1 significant reaction per 10,000 individuals per year, with a mortality of 0.2 per million in the United States. Estimates of penicillin-induced anaphylaxis are 10 to 40 per 100,000 injections. Most recently, allergy to the latex in surgical gloves has been seen in health care workers or patients undergoing frequent procedures, e.g., children with meningomyelocele, spina bifida, or congenital urogenital anomalies.

Although a history of atopy (allergic rhinitis, extrinsic asthma, atopic dermatitis) might be expected to be associated with an increased likelihood of anaphylactic reactions, atopic individuals appear to have, at worst, only a slightly greater risk than non-atopics do. Thus anyone can have an IgE response and clinical symptoms to the agents responsible for anaphylaxis. In addition, no evidence has shown that race, gender, age, occupation, or season intrinsically predisposes an individual to anaphylaxis.

Proteins, polysaccharides, and haptens are capable of eliciting systemic reactions in humans (Table 275–1). Proteins are the largest and most diverse group and include antiserum, hormones, seminal plasma, enzymes, latex, Hymenoptera venom (e.g., phospholipase A_2), pollen allergens administered for immunotherapy ("allergy shots"), and foods. Polysaccharides such as dextrans are rarer causes. The most common etiologic agents are low-molecular-weight drugs, which are not antigenic themselves but act as haptens and become antigenic on reaction with host proteins. Such drugs include antibiotics, local anesthetics, vitamins, and diagnostic reagents. Food-induced anaphylaxis and anaphylactic reactions to an orally administered drug can occur in very sensitive individuals.

Table 275–1 ■ AGENTS CAUSING ANAPHYLAXIS

TYPE	COMMON	RARE
Proteins	Venom (Hymenoptera)	Hormones, (insulin, ACTH, vasopressin, parathormone)
	Pollen (ragweed, grass, etc.)	Enzymes (trypsin, penicillinase)
	Food (eggs, seafood, nuts, grains, beans, cottonseed oil, chocolate)	Human proteins (serum proteins, seminal fluid)
	Horse and rabbit serum (antilymphocyte globulin)	
	Latex	
Haptens and other low-molecular-weight substances	Antibiotics (penicillins, sulfonamides, cephalosporins, tetracyclines, amphotericin B, nitrofurantoin, aminoglycosides)	Vitamins (thiamine, folic acid)
	Local anesthetics (lidocaine, procaine, etc.)	
Polysaccharides		Dextrans, iron-dextran

ACTH = adrenocorticotropic hormone.

CLINICAL MANIFESTATIONS. IgE-mediated reactions can cause symptoms involving the cutaneous, respiratory, cardiovascular, gastrointestinal, and hematologic systems (Fig. 275–1). The onset and manifestations vary according to the route of administration, dose, release of and sensitivity to vasoactive substances, and differing sensitivities of the organs to these substances. These parameters can vary from person to person, and individuals tend to react in a characteristic pattern. The initial manifestations can begin in seconds or take as long as an hour to develop; in severe reactions the onset usually occurs within 5 to 10 minutes of exposure. Initial manifestations often include skin erythema, pruritus, a generalized feeling of warmth and/or impending doom, light-headedness, shortness of breath, nausea, vomiting, or a lump in the throat. Urticaria is the most common manifestation of anaphylaxis. The rash is generalized and intensely pruritic and consists of well-circumscribed, erythematous, raised wheals with serpiginous borders and blanched centers. Angioedema may accompany urticaria and is typically manifested as swelling of the face, eyes, lips, tongue, pharynx, or extremities. The respiratory tract is commonly involved in fatal anaphylaxis. The early stages of upper airway edema consist of hoarseness, stridor, and/or dysphoria. Angioedema of the epiglottis and larynx can cause mechanical obstruction and death by suffocation. The swelling can extend to the hypopharynx and trachea. Between 25 and 50% of patients dying of anaphylaxis have pathologic changes consistent with severe asthma. Pulmonary hyperinflation, peribronchial congestion, submucosal edema, edema-filled alveoli, and eosinophilic infiltration are noted. The patient experiences shortness of breath, chest tightness, and wheezing. Severe hypoxemia and hypercapnia can occur rapidly.

Cardiovascular collapse is among the most severe clinical manifestations of anaphylaxis. The exact extent of fatal anaphylaxis is unknown inasmuch as anaphylaxis can be associated with myocardial ischemia and ventricular arrhythmias, each of which can cause or be caused by hypotension. Decreased blood pressure may be caused by diffuse peripheral vasodilatation from the release of vasodilatory mediators, decreased effective blood volume secondary to leakage of fluid into tissues, hypoxemia, or primary cardiac dysfunction.

Gastrointestinal manifestations can include nausea, vomiting, cramps, and diarrhea. Central nervous system abnormalities can include delirium and seizures, each of which may be due to hypoxemia and/or hypotension.

DIFFERENTIAL DIAGNOSIS. The diagnosis of systemic anaphylaxis may be obvious when a typical history of antecedent exposure to foreign antigenic material and a sequence of events consistent with the syndrome are present. Confirmation usually requires demonstration of IgE antibody to the substance by skin or radioallergosorbent testing. When a history of exposure is absent or when only a portion of the full syndrome is present, it may be difficult to exclude a vascular, cardiac, or neurologic disorder. Possibilities to be considered include acute myocardial infarction, pulmonary embolism, acute asthma, hereditary angioedema, the exercise-induced anaphylactic syndrome, cold urticaria, seizure disorder, anaphylactoid or idiosyncratic reaction, transfusion reaction, or vasovagal reaction. Vasovagal reactions may occur after an injection (e.g., penicillin, lidocaine [Xylocaine]) and include symptoms such as pallor, sweating, bradycardia, nausea, and hypotension, which can be confused with anaphylaxis. No cutaneous manifestations or evidence of respiratory difficulty is present, and the diagnosis hinges on the cause of the hypotension. In such instances, skin testing is negative. Hereditary angioedema is due to the absence or dysfunction of C1 inhibitor and is associated with laryngeal edema, peripheral angioedema, and acute abdominal pain. It is typically an autosomal dominant disorder with a family or prior history of typical episodes. Trauma and infections may precipitate attacks of swelling. Patients with cold urticaria may have systemic symptoms caused by water immersion, such as while swimming; diffuse urticaria, angioedema, and hypotension may ensue. Anaphylactoid reactions can occur to substances causing direct non-immune release of mast cell products (opiates, tubocurare, dextrans, sulfobromophthalein), which can induce urticaria, angioedema, chest tightness, wheezing, and hypotension. Aspirin and other non-steroidal agents can cause upper and lower airway obstruction, urticaria, and/or angioedema with no IgE involvement. These agents all inhibit prostaglandin synthetase (cyclooxygenase) and shunt arachidonate toward leukotriene synthesis. IgG–anti-IgA immune complexes may cause anaphylaxis-like symptoms when IgA-deficient patients receive blood. Complement activation appears to have a major role in such instances. Finally, radiocontrast media reactions occur in about 1% of patients when such agents are used. The mechanism is unknown but may relate to their osmolarity. Newer agents seem to markedly diminish the incidence. A syndrome of recurrent, apparently spontaneous episodes of anaphylaxis without an identifiable exogenous agent is known as "idiopathic anaphylaxis."

PATHOGENESIS. Antigenic induction of IgE formation requires antigenic processing (see Chapter 270) by dendritic cells or macrophages, T-cell help, and switching of B lymphocytes from IgG synthesis to IgE synthesis. Interleukin-4 and interleukin-13 are critical for the latter switch and function as T-cell helper factors for IgE formation. Subsequent combination of antigen with IgE bound

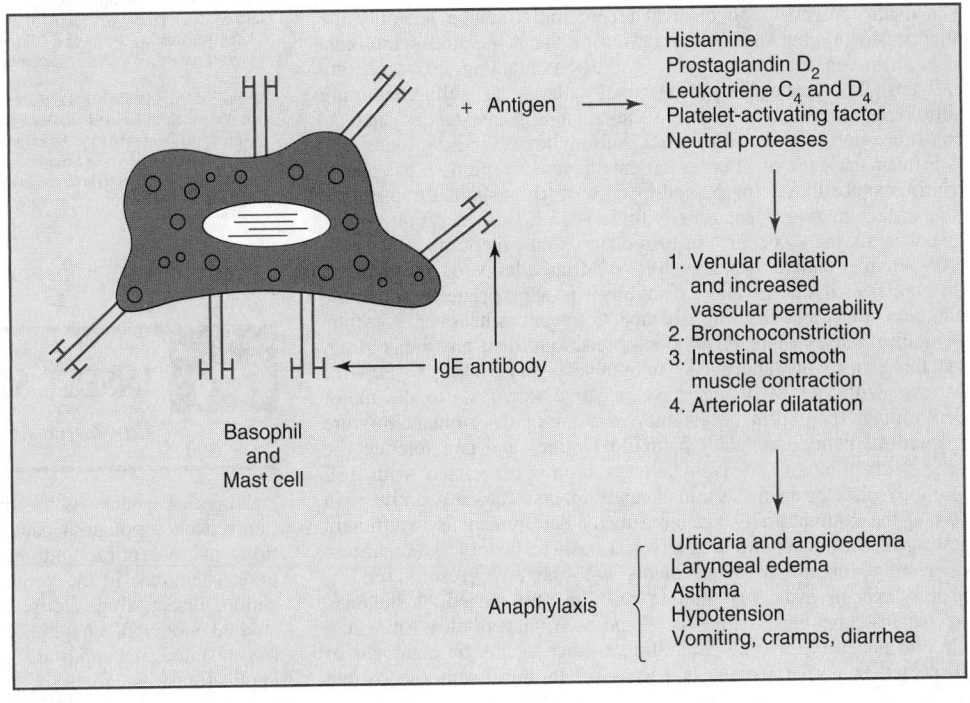

FIGURE 275–1 ■ Acute anaphylaxis.

to high-affinity receptors on mast cells and basophils (see Fig. 280–2) causes the secretion of a variety of vasoactive substances that may be responsible for the symptoms of anaphylaxis (see Fig. 275–1). These substances include histamine, prostaglandin D_2, leukotrienes C_4 and D_4, and platelet activating factor (1-O-alkyl-2-acetyl-sn-glyceryl-3-phosphorylcholine). Histamine is the major secretory product of basophils and mast cells. It causes venular and arterial vasodilation, increases vascular permeability, and causes a decrease in diastolic blood pressure when systemic levels of approximately 2.5 ng/mL are reached. Histamine has direct inotropic and chronotropic action when injected directly into cardiac muscle, effects that are prevented by H_1- plus H_2-receptor antagonists. Prostaglandin D_2 is synthesized by mast cells but not by basophils. It is a peripheral vasodilator. Leukotrienes C_4 and D_4 are produced by basophils and mast cells and profoundly constrict the peripheral arterial and coronary circulation and cause bronchoconstriction and decreased dynamic compliance. They also cause venular dilation and increase vascular permeability. Platelet activating factor is synthesized by mast cells but not basophils and causes venular dilatation and an increase in cutaneous vascular permeability. When infused into rabbits, it causes profound hypotension. Tryptase, a mast cell granule constituent released with histamine, can be assayed in blood as an indicator of anaphylaxis.

Bradykinin is a nine–amino acid peptide that may also contribute to the symptoms of anaphylaxis and is generated by kininogen cleaved by enzymes known as *kallikreins*. Kinins are peripheral vasodilators, cause systemic hypotension, and constrict coronary vessels. Basophils and mast cells have a kallikrein-like enzyme; organs containing glands (lung, nasal mucosa) secrete a tissue kallikrein that digests low-molecular-weight kininogen to release bradykinin. Plasma kinin formation is associated with contact activation of Hageman factor, conversion of plasma prekallikrein to kallikrein, and digestion of high-molecular-weight kininogen.

Anaphylaxis is associated with depletion of clotting Factors V, VII, and fibrinogen, activation of complement, and depletion of high-molecular-weight kininogen, consistent with acute intravascular coagulation. Clotting defects such as a prolonged partial thromboplastin time are commonly seen. Activation or depletion of these proteins is probably caused by enzymes released from cells, including not only mast cells and basophils but also monocyte-macrophages, eosinophils, and platelets. The latter group of cells possesses high- and low-affinity receptors for IgE, which may mediate cell secretion on contact with antigen.

PREVENTION AND TREATMENT. Patients who have previously experienced anaphylactic episodes should wear a Medic-Alert bracelet and be instructed regarding the importance of relating details of their specific drug reactions before taking medications. The medical history and medical record must include not only the allergic history but also a description of the associated symptoms. The physician must be aware of drugs containing cross-reacting antigens. For example, patients with allergy to sulfa-containing antibiotics should avoid other sulfa-containing substances such as chlorthiazide diuretics, furosemide, sulfonylureas, and dapsone.

Fifteen per cent of allergic patients have a reaction if a cephalosporin is substituted for penicillin because they share the presence of a β-lactam ring. Reactions with 2nd- and 3rd-generation cephalosporins may also occur, but aztreonam is an exception.

When the patient has a history of drug allergy or of taking a drug suspected of causing a reaction, it is appropriate to substitute another non–cross-reacting therapeutic agent whenever possible. Penicillin causes more anaphylactic reactions than any other drug, yet the history of "allergy" is unreliable because close to 80% of patients with such a history have negative skin tests to the major determinant (penicillin polylysine) or a minor determinant mixture (penicillin, penicilloic acid, penicilloylamine) and can tolerate the drug with impunity. Anaphylaxis is highly associated with IgE antibody directed to these minor determinants. Thus a negative skin test to the commercially available major determinant is insufficient testing to administer the drug given a positive history. The addition of testing for minor determinants with negative results renders anaphylaxis or even any allergic reaction rare indeed. Avoidance, in sensitive patients, is the best approach; nevertheless, in some circumstances the use of penicillin or other agents by a known or suspected sensitive patient is necessary. In this event the patient

can be desensitized by gradually administering increasing concentrations of the drug via specific oral/parenteral protocols. Such a procedure should be carried out by experienced personnel in an intensive care unit setting in which anaphylactic reactions can be effectively treated.

If an anaphylactic reaction is encountered, epinephrine given early quickly reverses most manifestations. When administered at a 1:1000 dilution (0.01 mL/kg with a maximum dose of 0.5 mL subcutaneously repeated every 20 minutes as necessary), it is initial treatment once an adequate airway is in place. Further exposure to the inducing substance should be limited. When an anaphylactic reaction is initiated by an injection into the arm or leg, a tourniquet may be applied to limit antigen absorption. In the case of a honeybee sting, care should be taken to remove the stinger without compressing the venom sac. Upper airway obstruction must be differentiated from asthma because laryngeal and epiglottic edema may require endotracheal intubation or emergency tracheostomy to provide an airway. Asthma can be treated with epinephrine or the administration of an inhaled β_2-sympathomimetic and/or intravenous aminophylline at a 6-mg/kg loading dose over a period of 20 to 30 minutes, followed by 0.5 to 1 mg/kg/hour.

If any respiratory, vascular, or cardiac complications occur, an intravenous line should be placed promptly and a sample of arterial blood obtained for pH, Po_2, and Pco_2. Supplemental oxygen should be given to reduce hypoxemia. The pulse, blood pressure, and respiratory rate are monitored, and an electrocardiogram is obtained. Hypovolemic shock requires rapid intravenous fluid administration. Additionally, 5 mL of a 1:10,000 solution of epinephrine repeated every 5 to 10 minutes can be given intravenously to patients in severe shock. A vasopressor such as dopamine (2 to 20 μg/kg/minute) is indicated to manage hypotension unresponsive to volume expansion. This approach may increase cardiac output and improve blood flow to the coronary, cerebral, renal, and mesenteric vascular beds. Higher doses of dopamine or norepinephrine yield significant α-receptor stimulation, which may increase blood pressure but constrict distal vascular beds. In case of significant cardiac dysfunction, an arterial line and a Swan-Ganz catheter should be placed.

Giving antihistamines at the onset of the acute episode may relieve pruritus, urticaria, and angioedema. Once an intravenous line is placed, 50 to 100 mg of diphenhydramine can be given slowly as a bolus. An H_2-receptor blocker may aid in the treatment of hypotension. Corticosteroids have no value during the acute episode, yet steroids are often also administered intravenously. It takes many hours before their first effect is seen. Thus administration of steroids helps treat protracted asthma and late reactions that can ensue 1 to 2 days beyond the initial insult.

Bochner BS, Lichtenstein LM: Anaphylaxis—Current concepts. N Engl J Med 324: 1785, 1991. *An additional review including approaches to therapy.*
Gold M, Swartz JS, Braude BM, et al: Intraoperative anaphylaxis: An association with latex sensitivity. J Allergy Clin Immunol 87:662, 1991. *Description of an increasingly recognized cause of anaphylactic reactions—namely, exposure to latex products.*
Sampson HA, Mendelson L, Rosen JP: Fatal and near fatal anaphylactic reactions to foods in children and adolescents. N Engl J Med 327:380, 1992. *Description of dangerous anaphylactic reactions to foods in children, including the course and confirmation by tryptase assay.*
Wasserman SI: Anaphylaxis. *In* Kaplan AP (ed): Allergy, 2nd ed. Philadelphia, WB Saunders, 1997, p 565. *Textbook review of etiology, pathogenesis, and treatment.*

276 INSECT STING ALLERGY

Lawrence M. Lichtenstein

Stings of insects of the order Hymenoptera have long been recognized as a potential cause of severe, often life-threatening reactions in susceptible individuals. These reactions are unrelated to toxic chemicals in the venom, instead being due to allergic sensitization. Insect sting allergy has recently become the most intensely studied model of anaphylaxis in humans, and study of this model has resulted in important advances that have had rapid clinical applications.

EPIDEMIOLOGY. The incidence of immediate hypersensitivity to insect stings based on history is 3%; more than 20% of the population, however, has positive skin test reactions to insect venom. Other allergies do not seem to predispose to insect sting sensitivity. The frequency varies with exposure and is therefore greater in children and males, as well as those inclined to outdoor activities. Systemic reactions to insect stings cause few fatalities, but the morbidity, fear, and change in lifestyle caused by these reactions are significant. A large number of people suffer prolonged and unusually severe local inflammatory reactions to insect stings that are allergic in nature. As with other allergies, there appears to be an inherited predisposition inasmuch as multiple family members are often affected.

ETIOLOGY. The only insects possessing true stingers are those of the order Hymenoptera. The two families of importance are the bees (honeybees, bumblebees) and the vespids (yellow jackets, hornets, wasps). Bees have barbed stingers that remain in the skin after a sting. Yellow jackets are the most common culprits, but honeybees are more commonly implicated in the western United States. Wasps are more common in the south central United States (especially Texas). Sensitivity develops to antigens in the insect venom, most of which have enzymatic activity. A major allergen in both insect families is phospholipase A, but these allergens do not cross-react with one another.

PATHOGENESIS. Injection of foreign proteins commonly causes the production of specific antibodies of the IgE and IgG classes. Venom-specific IgE antibodies may develop after any sting, this response sometimes persisting for less than 3 months and in other instances persisting for more than 25 years. Tissue mast cells and circulating basophils bind IgE antibody, thereby becoming sensitized so that a repeat encounter with the offending allergen triggers release of the mediators of anaphylaxis (see Chapter 275). Initiation and persistence of this sensitization are related to inheritable and other unknown determinants. Sensitization may occur at any time in life, even after many uneventful stings. The sensitizing sting itself causes no unusual reaction and is often so remote as to evade recollection.

Generalized mediator release from sensitized basophils and mast cells (see Table 280–2) causes the many manifestations of anaphylaxis. Localization of symptoms to specific target tissues is not well understood. The pathology observed in fatal cases includes upper airway edema and obstruction, the visceral consequences of hypotension, or, occasionally, no discernible abnormality (see Chapter 275 for a discussion of anaphylaxis).

Large local reactions are IgE dependent; their prolonged time course is characteristic of the so-called late-phase response to antigen. These reactions involve a cascade of events beginning with mediator release from mast cells and culminating in local inflammation involving many cell types and numerous mechanisms. The potential roles of eosinophils, basophils, lymphocytes, and cytokines and chemokines are being elucidated.

The venom-specific IgG antibody response to a sting is usually short lived, lasting only a few months. Repeated stings (as in beekeepers) are associated with high titers of IgG antibodies, which protect against allergic reactions. Beekeepers who do not have anaphylactic reactions have high IgG titers, as do affected individuals immunized with venom. Passive transfer of these IgG antibodies protects sensitive patients from a sting. These protective antibodies are thought to block the allergic reaction by competing with IgE for the allergenic venom proteins and have therefore been termed "blocking" antibodies.

CLINICAL MANIFESTATIONS. Allergic reactions to insect stings are either generalized (systemic) or large local reactions. *Systemic sting reactions* present the classic manifestations of anaphylaxis described in Chapter 275. The observed frequency of the most common symptoms in adult patients is presented in Table 276–1. The risk of a fatal outcome increases, as might be expected, with age and the use of certain drugs, especially antagonists of β-adrenergic receptors. Fatal anaphylaxis may occur without a history of sting allergy.

The onset of systemic symptoms is rapid, within 2 to 3 minutes, and rarely occurs more than 30 minutes after a sting. Symptoms occurring hours later (except large local reactions) are not usually associated with immediate hypersensitivity or IgE antibodies. Unusual reactions such as vasculitis, nephropathies, encephalitis, and other neurologic manifestations have been reported, but no causal

Table 276–1 ■ SYMPTOMS REPORTED BY 245 PATIENTS

SYMPTOM	PERCENTAGE
Cutaneous only	14
Urticaria-angioedema	78
Dizziness-hypotension	61
Dyspnea-wheezing	53
Throat tightness–hoarseness	40
Loss of consciousness	33

relationship has been established. Allergic respiratory symptoms may occur in beekeepers and their families through sensitization to the dust in the hives, which contains bee body protein. This sensitivity is unrelated to sting reactions.

Large local reactions are slow in onset and occur with or without concomitant early systemic reaction. The area of induration increases in size progressively for the first 24 to 48 hours and then resolves gradually over several days. These reactions may be so large as to immobilize an entire limb and are a significant cause of morbidity in sensitive individuals. Red streaks resembling lymphangitis may be observed and are often treated with antibiotics despite a lack of evidence for true cellulitis.

NATURAL HISTORY. The natural history of insect sting allergy has been incompletely documented. The prevalence of venom sensitization in the general population was noted above. It is estimated that about 20% of those at risk by virtue of positive skin tests (but with no history of a systemic reaction) will react on sting. There is considerable variability in the reaction to a sting among those who are clearly allergic as demonstrated by positive skin tests and a history of a previous reaction. Recent studies indicate that 25 to 60% of adults had a systemic reaction when stung by the appropriate insect. In children, on the other hand, a repeat sting causes a reaction in only 8%. The incidence in adolescents and young adults must lie between these extremes. This variability confounds the prediction of risk associated with sensitization.

Although many patients and physicians believe that allergic sting reactions become progressively more severe with every sting, such is not true. Most of those affected maintain a similar pattern of symptoms with every sting. Factors favoring a systemic reaction include multiple stings, as well as stings in close temporal proximity (only weeks apart).

Sensitization generally decreases or disappears in time, much more so in children than in adults. However, resensitization has been observed upon re-sting.

DIAGNOSIS. Acute anaphylaxis is easily diagnosed by the presence of classic symptoms and signs. The insect sting may be inapparent. The differential diagnosis is more difficult in localized reactions such as acute chest pain and dyspnea or syncope without urticaria.

The diagnosis of insect sting allergy currently rests on a convincing history and positive skin tests. Demonstration in vitro of venom-specific IgE by the radioallergosorbent test (RAST) is less sensitive than skin tests but is equally accurate when positive.

Skin tests are performed intradermally with venom diluted to concentrations in the range of 1 to 1000 ng/mL. Five types of venom are used: honeybee, yellow jacket, yellow hornet, white-faced hornet, and *Polistes* wasp. A positive intradermal skin test—a wheal larger than 5 mm in diameter with at least 20 mm of erythema—develops within 20 minutes. The degree of skin test sensitivity does not correlate with clinical sensitivity. Within a few months after a systemic sting reaction, skin tests are almost uniformly positive. Stings more remote in time are more commonly associated with an apparent loss of sensitivity (similar to the situation in penicillin-related anaphylaxis).

Honeybee venom sensitivity occurs independent of other venom allergies, but about 10% of patients are sensitive to both bee and vespid venom. Vespid venom is highly cross-reactive, so almost all vespid-sensitive patients have positive yellow jacket, yellow hornet, and white-faced hornet skin tests, even though most have been stung only by yellow jackets. Half of these patients are also sensitive to *Polistes* venom. Very few individuals are allergic to only one or two of the vespid venoms. In vitro RAST inhibition techniques are useful to distinguish cross-reactivity from specific sensitivity. This issue is clinically relevant in patients with a positive skin test to *Polistes,* which is often due to cross-reactivity, and the patient may be spared considerable expense and unnecessary immunization by RAST inhibition analysis.

TREATMENT. The treatment of choice for anaphylactic reactions is subcutaneous epinephrine, 1:1000, 0.5 mL initially and repeated twice at 10-minute intervals, if necessary, to reverse the progression of symptoms. Antihistamines and glucocorticoids do not contribute to the management of life-threatening symptoms but may reduce the duration and severity of cutaneous manifestations. Their use should not be considered until the acute episode has ended. Intravenous volume expansion or airway maintenance may be necessary. In a few individuals, the process is resistant to epinephrine; in such instances an α-adrenergic agent (i.e., norepinephrine) may be tried. Affected persons not yet protected by immunotherapy are advised to carry and are instructed in the use of a kit containing a syringe device pre-loaded with one or two recommended doses of epinephrine.

Venom immunotherapy is successful in virtually all patients. Fewer than 2% of those immunized have any systemic symptoms after a challenge sting, and these are uniformly less severe than their previous reactions. The indications for venom immunotherapy are now based on an improved understanding of the natural history of the disease. Those with a history of life-threatening reactions should be treated. The risk of progression from strictly cutaneous to life-threatening respiratory or vascular reactions is rare (<1%) in adults and children. Cutaneous reactors who are more likely to be stung in their daily activities or who for a variety of reasons (location, age, cardiovascular disease) can ill afford a reaction should be treated. The cost and inconvenience of treatment may deter other cutaneous reactors from undergoing immunotherapy. Children, much more commonly than adults, have cutaneous symptoms only. These children may be left untreated. Venom immunotherapy is usually contraindicated in the absence of positive venom skin tests or RAST. Although some rare individuals are sensitive without positive tests, current treatment recommendations are to use all venoms that cause a positive skin test (for *Polistes,* see above). Although other mechanisms may contribute, induction of increased serum levels of venom-specific IgG antibodies is the most apparent mechanism of protection for venom immunotherapy; less than 3 mg/mL is associated with an increased risk of sting anaphylaxis. In many European centers the patient is re-stung in the hospital before therapy is begun.

Rapid immunization in six to eight weekly visits is recommended to take advantage of a significantly greater and more rapid immune response with fewer adverse reactions than a slower (>20 weeks) regimen. The maintenance dose of 100 μg of each venom is repeated monthly for at least 6 months and then continued at 6- to 8-week intervals for 5 years. If treatment is interrupted for more than 3 months, it is likely that protection will diminish to inadequate levels. Loss of venom sensitivity during maintenance immunotherapy occurs in some patients during the initial 3 to 5 years of treatment. Skin tests should therefore be repeated every 2 years. After 5 years it appears that patients can stop therapy and suffer a sting without serious sequelae. Possible exceptions include patients with extremely severe reactions or those with complicating medical conditions. After stopping venom immunotherapy, venom sensitivity continues to decline and is not increased even after stings.

Adverse reactions to venom immunotherapy may be early or late. Immediate reactions include all the manifestations of anaphylaxis. During the initial course of treatment, 10 to 15% of patients report systemic complaints, only half of which require epinephrine. At maintenance doses, systemic reactions occur rarely. After a systemic reaction the dose should be reduced by up to 50% on the subsequent visit and then increased gradually toward 100 μg again.

Large local reactions occur frequently—50% of treated patients experience at least one such reaction. These reactions occur after 10 of every 100 injections in the induction phase, most commonly in the midrange of doses (10 to 50 μg) and much less often at maintenance doses. Large local reactions do not presage systemic reactions and require a reduction in dose only for the most severe reactions. Long-term side effects have not been observed with venom immunotherapy or in beekeepers stung frequently for over 30 years.

Golden DBK, Addison BI, Gadde J, et al: Prospective observations on patients who discontinue Hymenoptera venom immunotherapy. J Allergy Clin Immunol 88:162, 1989. *Studies of when and how to discontinue venom immunotherapy.*

Golden DBK, Lawrence ID, Hamilton RH, et al: Clinical correlation of the venom-specific IgG antibody level during maintenance venom immunotherapy. J Allergy Clin Immunol 90:386, 1992. *The relevance of IgG "blocking" antibodies in venom immunotherapy.*

Golden DBK, Marsh DG, Kagey-Sobotka A, et al: Epidemiology of insect sting allergy. JAMA 262:240, 1989. *A review of diagnostic and therapeutic problems in insect allergy.*

Hunt KJ, Valentine MD, Sobotka AK, et al: A controlled trial of immunotherapy in insect hypersensitivity. N Engl J Med 299:157, 1978. *A comparison of venom immunotherapy with whole-body extract and placebo. Demonstrates efficacy of venom therapy and the clinical consequences of challenge stings.*

Valentine MD, Schuberth KC, Kagey-Sobotka A, et al: The value of immunotherapy with venom in children with allergy to insect stings. N Engl J Med 323:1601, 1990. *A prospective study of the epidemiology and immunotherapy of insect sting allergy in children indicating that repeat reactions are rare and virtually never of increased severity.*

277 IMMUNE COMPLEX DISEASES

Richard D. deShazo

DEFINITION. Immune complex diseases are a group of conditions resulting from inflammation induced in tissues where immune complexes are formed or deposited. The clinical consequences may be local when immune complexes form in the tissues of a specific organ or systemic when complexes circulate and are widely deposited. A variety of antigens have been associated with the induction of immune complex disease in humans (Table 277–1) (see Chapter 270).

PATHOPHYSIOLOGY. In their studies, von Pirquet and Schick observed that a "serumkranheit" (serum sickness) developed in some children 1 to 2 weeks after being injected subcutaneously with horse-derived diphtheria antiserum. The syndrome was characterized by fever, lymphadenopathy, arthralgias or arthritis, leukopenia, proteinuria, and cutaneous findings including urticaria. They postulated that the illness was caused by newly formed host antibody reacting to horse serum and resulting in the deposition of antigen-antibody complexes in tissue. Much later, Germuth and Dixon developed rabbit models of serum sickness that confirmed this hypothesis.

In the model of acute serum sickness, rabbits receive a single injection of radiolabeled foreign serum, e.g., bovine serum albumin. Initially, levels of antigen measured in serum decrease rapidly as the antigen equilibrates in the animal's intravascular and extravascular fluid compartments over several days. Thereafter, the serum antigen concentration falls at a steady rate in association with degradation. About 10 to 12 days after injection, a second rapid decrease in the concentration of free antigen in serum is noted. This decrease coincides with the development of host antibody to the antigen and the formation and clearance of antigen-containing immune complexes by the reticuloendothelial system. At this time, serum complement levels drop, proteinuria develops, and histopathologic studies show inflammation in the rabbit's glomeruli, synovium, and arteries. Host immunoglobulin, complement, and antigen are deposited in a granular pattern along the glomerular basement membrane and near the internal elastic lamina of the coronary arteries. These findings occur when immune complexes of intermediate weight (>19S) are present in serum and resolve rapidly after these complexes are no longer detectable. If additional doses of antigen are given, chronic symptoms develop.

The relative amounts of antigen and antibody detectable in this model of serum sickness form a "precipitin curve" (Fig. 277–1). The curve may be divided into zones of "free antigen" on the left, "equivalence" in the center, and "antibody excess" on the right. In antigen excess, the very small antigen complexes produced (Ag_1: Ab_{1-3}) do not activate complement or induce inflammation. In antibody excess, the very large complexes present have difficulty diffusing across the endothelial barrier and are rapidly cleared by the reticuloendothelial system. Near the point of equivalence and in the area of slight antigen excess, little if any non-complexed anti-

Table 277–1 ■ REPRESENTATIVE ANTIGENS KNOWN TO CAUSE IMMUNE COMPLEX DISEASE IN HUMANS

ANTIGENS	SYNDROME
Therapeutic Agents	
Horse serum products:	Serum sickness
Antilymphocyte globulin	
Snake venom antiserum	
Monoclonal antibody products	
Streptokinase	
Drugs:	
Cephalosporins, penicillin,	
amoxicillin,	
trimethoprim-sulfamethoxazole,	
fluoxetine, iron-dextran,	
carbamazepine, and others	
Quinidine, chlorpromazine,	Hemolytic anemia (innocent bystander
sulfonamides	reaction)
Autologous (Self) Antigens	
DNA	Vasculitis and glomerulonephritis of
	systemic lupus erythematosus
IgG, IgM	Vasculitis of rheumatoid arthritis and
	mixed cryoglobulinemia
Tumor antigens: Colon carcinoma	Glomerulonephritis
(carcinoembryonic antigen)	
Microbial Antigens	
Hepatitis B	Systemic vasculitis
Plasmodium malariae	
Schistosoma mansoni	Glomerulonephritis
β-Hemolytic streptococci	
Staphylococcus epidermidis	

gen or antibody is detectable and intermediate-size (Ag_{2-3}:Ab_{2-6}) (>19S) soluble immune complexes circulate. At this point, a lattice of antigen and antibody molecules forms. This lattice results from non-covalent bonding between antigen and antibody and between the Fc portions of adjacent antibody molecules. The structure of this lattice depends on the valence of the antibody and the number of antigenic determinants on the antigen. In general, low-affinity antibodies form smaller immune complexes than do higher affinity antibodies.

BIOLOGIC PROPERTIES OF IMMUNE COMPLEXES. The biologic properties of antigen-antibody complexes depend on the nature of the antibodies and the degree of lattice formed and include (1) their ability to activate the complement system, (2) their ability to interact with cell receptors, and (3) their propensity to be deposited in tissues.

Immune complexes may fix complement by either the classic or alternative complement pathway (see Chapter 271). Immune complexes that contain antibodies of the IgG (usually IgG1 or IgG3) or IgM class in an appropriate lattice structure activate the classic complement pathway by binding C1q, the first subunit of the first component of complement. Antibodies of the IgG4 subclass are less efficient at activating complement than those of the other three subclasses. Immune complexes containing IgA may activate the alternative complement pathway but not the classic one.

Phagocytic cells and certain lymphocytes possess receptors for antibody molecules. Of these, the Fcγ receptors on these cells react with IgG molecules. The Kupffer cells of the liver possess a specific type of Fcγ receptor (Fcγ RIII) that helps remove IgG-containing immune complexes from serum. Very large latticed immune complexes containing IgG may bind to this Fcγ receptor without activating complement. Once bound, they condense or rearrange to form even larger lattices that undergo phagocytosis.

Human erythrocytes have receptors for C3b, called complement receptor type 1 (CR1). CR1 binds to immune complexes that contain molecules of C3b, iC3b, or C4b. When these erythrocytes circulate through the liver, Kupffer cells effectively remove the large, complement-containing immune complexes without damaging the erythrocytes. This action is accomplished by using their Fc receptors, which have a greater affinity for the complexes than does CR1 (Fig. 277–2). A similar phenomenon occurs in the spleen. Although platelets have receptors for complement, they are less important than erythrocytes in the clearance of immune complexes.

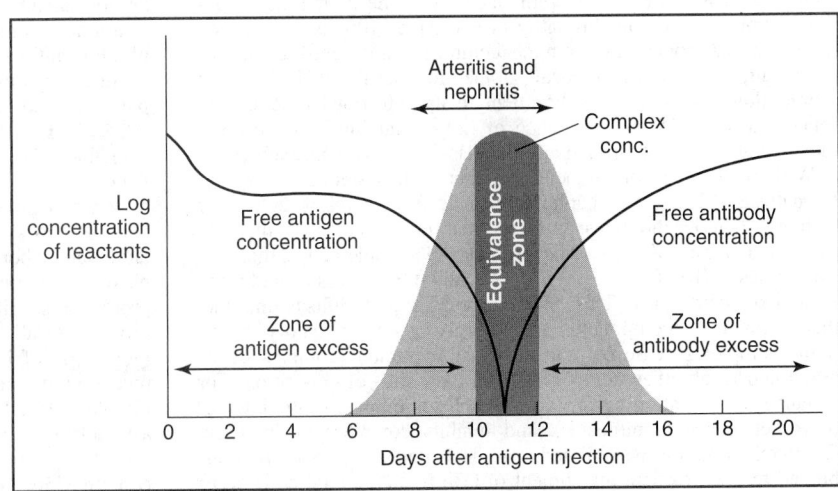

FIGURE 277–1 ■ Natural history of acute serum sickness in rabbits following a single injection of radiolabeled bovine serum albumin as antigen. The disease occurs when large quantities of soluble immune complexes are present in the circulation. (From Rich RR: Immune complex diseases. *In* Wyngaarden JB, Smith LH Jr, Bennett JC (eds): Cecil Textbook of Medicine, 19th ed. Philadelphia, WB Saunders, 1992, p 1468.)

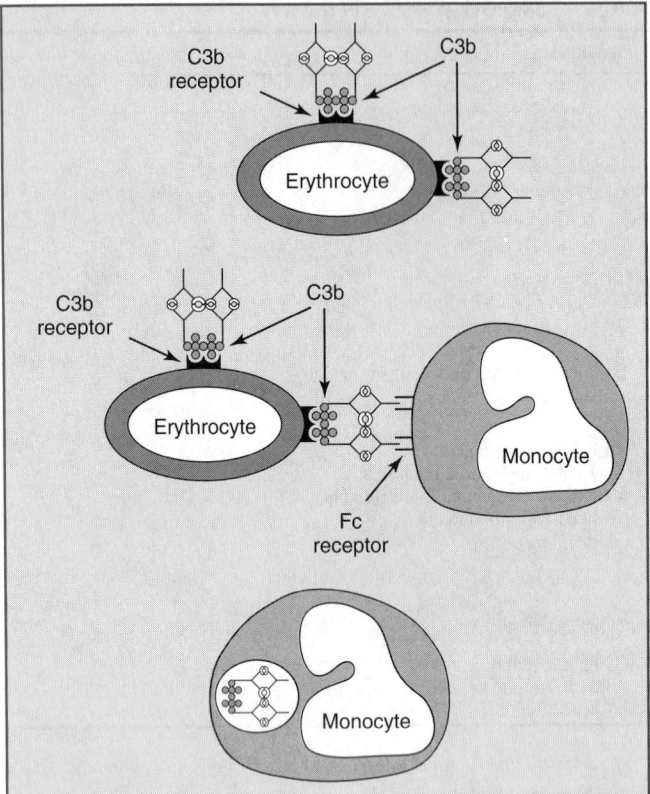

FIGURE 277–2 ■ Role of hepatic mononuclear phagocytes (Kupffer cells) in removal of immune complexes from the circulation. Circulating complexes are bound to erythrocytes by the CR1 receptors for C3b. The complexes are removed from the erythrocytes by the Fc receptors of Kupffer cells, which have a greater affinity for the complexes. (From Virella G: Immune complex disease. Immunol Ser 58:379, 1993.)

The fate of immunocomplexes that contain IgA is less clear in humans. In experimental animals, immune complexes containing eight or more IgA antibodies are rapidly taken up by the liver.

FACTORS AFFECTING HOW IMMUNE COMPLEXES ARE DEPOSITED. Experimental studies suggest that a number of factors determine the fate of immune complexes. These factors include the lattice structure, the presence of complement in the complex, the characteristics of antibodies and antigen in the complex, the numbers and functions of receptors on reticuloendothelial and other cells, and the charge of the immune complex. As far as *antibodies* are concerned, positive charges seem to facilitate the deposition of immune complexes in the glomeruli. Moreover, certain non-glomerular cationic antigens such as DNA appear to bind to glomeruli. They then serve as a nidus for immune complexes to form locally and be deposited in the subepithelial area of the glomerular capillary membrane. IgA nephropathy (see Chapter 106) is a condition in which IgA-containing immune complexes are deposited in the glomeruli, with resultant focal glomerulonephritis. This form of glomerulonephritis, often subsequent to an infectious illness, may reflect the less efficient clearance of IgA-containing immune complexes that are unable to activate the classic complement pathway.

With respect to complement, patients with systemic lupus erythematosus (SLE) (see Chapter 289) have fewer CR1 receptors for C3b on their erythrocytes, a factor that may predispose them to immune complex disease. The presence of complement deficiency syndromes (C1q, C1r, C1s, C4, C2, and C3) is associated with lupus-like syndromes. This phenomenon in part reflects the fact that complement components are not only pro-inflammatory in immune complex disease but can also inhibit immune complex deposition and resolubilize complexes from their sites of deposition. For instance, C1q fixation by immune complexes inhibits Fc-Fc interactions between IgG molecules and inhibits complex precipitation. Complex formation is inhibited, and deposited complexes are solubilized by the covalent attachment of C3b to antigen-antibody complexes. That Fc receptors can bind immune complexes to reticulo-

endothelial cells appears to influence their rate of clearance. In immune complex disease, Fc receptor function is often diminished. Finally, certain cells have receptors that facilitate interaction with immune complexes. Glomerular epithelium has receptors for C3, endothelial cells have receptors for C1q, and renal interstitial cells, damaged endothelial cells, and platelets have Fc receptors.

INDUCTION OF INFLAMMATION BY IMMUNE COMPLEXES. Inflammation associated with immune complexes results when circulating phagocytic cells move into tissue sites where the complexes are deposited. This movement is influenced by several processes. Tissue mast cells release vasoactive amines after antigen reacts with IgE or on contact with the anaphylatoxins C3a and C3b. These amines increase vascular permeability, which facilitates the movement of phagocytes responding to the chemotactic and adhesion-promoting factors, including C5a, that are released when immune complexes activate complement. This fact may explain why antihistamines may attenuate some of the cutaneous findings in experimental and human serum sickness. Subsequently, binding of immune complexes to neutrophils and/or monocytes by their C3b and Fcγ receptors results in cell activation and phagocytosis of the immune complexes. The activated phagocytes degranulate and release proteolytic enzymes and oxygen-derived free radicals. Cellular damage and loss of blood to local tissues result, and ischemic injury follows.

IMMUNE COMPLEX DISEASES IN HUMANS. Serum sickness occurs in humans, and the clinical and laboratory findings are much like those seen in the rabbit model. Serum sickness most commonly occurs after using horse serum products, including antivenin, which is used to treat rattlesnake bites, and antithymocyte globulin, which is used to treat aplastic anemia. The initial sign of the syndrome in patients with serum sickness from antithymocyte globulin is a curious band of erythema located laterally on the hands, feet, fingers, and toes. Circulating immune complexes and decreases in serum C3, C4, and CH50 concentrations occur at the time of symptoms of serum sickness. Serum sickness also occurs with certain drugs, including β-lactam antibiotics, sulfonamides, thiouracil, hydantoin, thiazide diuretics, and para-aminosalicylic acid. Fever, malaise, arthralgia and arthritis, abdominal pain sometimes associated with melena, and urticaria and/or urticarial vasculitis may develop. Similar symptoms may be noted in patients with mixed cryoglobulinemia, such as that associated with hepatitis C infection, rheumatoid arthritis with high titers of rheumatoid factor, and SLE with high titers of antibody to double-stranded DNA.

Another immune complex disease in humans is the syndrome of leukocytoclastic (hypersensitivity) vasculitis. It is associated with the characteristic physical finding of recurrent episodes of palpable purpura. Findings are usually, but not always limited to the skin and may occur as a reaction to drugs or in association with specific infections such as hepatitis B, in certain connective tissue diseases such as SLE, in cryoglobulinemia, or for no distinguishable cause. The histopathologic feature of a predominant polymorphonuclear cell infiltrate in post-capillary venules is associated with "nuclear dust" from leukocytoclasis, endothelial cell damage and proliferation, and distal infarction of tissues. Subendothelial electron-dense deposits in post-capillary venules appear in association with circulating immune complexes, which are detectable in a high percentage of patients.

Immune complexes may form locally within solid tissue at sites of high antigen concentration. Autoimmune thyroiditis and Goodpasture's syndrome are examples of such localized immune complex formation called the Arthus reaction.

TESTS TO DETECT CIRCULATING IMMUNE COMPLEXES. No available laboratory test detects all circulating immune complexes. *Complement assays,* including CH50, C3, and C4, are depressed only when large quantities of immune complexes that activate the complement system are present. *Physical methods* such as precipitation are laborious because they require separating immune complexes from other serum components. Each physical method has problems specific to it; for example, cryoprecipitation is not a property of all immune complexes. *Biologic methods* depend on the interaction of immune complexes with complement components or receptors on cells. The binding plus subsequent precipitation of radiolabeled C1q with immune complexes by polyethylene glycol is a widely used method that detects as little as 10 mg of aggregated IgG. Conglutinin assays detect only those immune complexes that contain C3bi. The most commonly used assay for immune complexes uses lymphoblastoid B cells, called *Raji cells.* These cells were derived from a patient with Burkitt's lymphoma. They lack surface immunoglobulins and have low-affinity receptors for IgG and high-affinity receptors for complement components.

Because immune complex assays are not antigen specific, they provide little insight into the cause of various immune complex diseases and do not provide a specific diagnosis. Some reports suggest that the presence of concentrations of immune complexes may correlate with the activity or prognosis of some diseases. Others suggest that they may be useful in the diagnosis of clinical diseases when immune complex deposition is a prominent component.

TREATMENT OF IMMUNE COMPLEX DISEASE. As with all diseases, the seriousness of the clinical syndrome determines the therapy. If the particular antigen that causes immune complex disease can be identified and avoided, for instance, a drug, immune complex disease can be expected to resolve. When immune complex disease is a feature of an autoimmune disease such as SLE, controlling the disease with anti-inflammatory and/or immunosuppressive therapy usually resolves the related symptoms.

Serum sickness following drug therapy or therapeutic use of autologous serum proteins, such as rattlesnake horse antiserum, usually resolves spontaneously over 7 to 14 days. Symptoms usually respond to antihistamine therapy with or without corticosteroid treatment. Although controlled treatment studies are not available, moderate doses of prednisone (20 to 40 mg) given twice a day for 3 to 5 days followed by a tapering dose of corticosteroids over 10 to 14 days usually resolve the symptoms in severe cases. The utility of plasmapheresis in immune complex disease is unproven.

Gauthier VJ, Abrass CK: Circulating immune complexes in renal injury. Semin Nephrol 12:379, 1992. *An extensive review of the mechanisms of immune complex–mediated renal disease.*

Hebert LA: The clearance of immune complexes from the circulation of man and other primates. Am J Kidney Dis 17:352, 1991. *A review of studies pertaining to the fate of immune complexes.*

Moxley G, Ruddy S: Immune complexes and complement. *In* Kelley W (ed): Textbook of Rheumatology. Philadelphia, WB Saunders, 1997, p 228.

278 THE MAJOR HISTOCOMPATIBILITY COMPLEX AND DISEASE SUSCEPTIBILITY

Robert R. Rich

It has been more than 30 years since the first report that susceptibility to a disease was associated with inheritance of a specific HLA gene. Since the discovery of a statistically significant increase in the incidence of Hodgkin's disease in patients inheriting certain HLA-B genes, such associations have been recorded for more than 500 different diseases. In many of these cases, the increase in susceptibility is quite weak and, in some, may represent faulty statistical analysis or a chance occurrence. In others, however, the association is very strong and impels a conclusion that genes within the HLA complex have a role in disease pathogenesis.

The importance of HLA genes in predisposition to disease is commonly expressed as "relative risk," or the ratio of the frequency with which a disease occurs in individuals carrying a particular HLA gene divided by its frequency in those not carrying it. As illustrated in Table 278–1, the relative risk between particular diseases and HLA molecules is reported to vary from marginally significant (e.g., ~2.0 for Hodgkin's disease in individuals who express the HLA molecule DP3) to a preponderant role in determining disease susceptibility (e.g., a relative risk of greater than 80 of ankylosing spondylitis developing in individuals who are HLA-B27). Inspection of a table of HLA inheritance and disease susceptibility reveals some general conclusions and a few surprises. Among the conclusions are that HLA-associated disease has been identified in virtually every major organ system and, additionally, the substantial majority of these diseases are regarded as autoimmune. A 2nd conclusion is that the majority of disease associations are with the HLA-DR and HLA-DQ molecules of the HLA complex, but with some notable exceptions, particularly the class I gene HLA-B27. Among the surprises is the observation that a role of the immune system is not apparent in certain of the highly associated diseases, most dramatically, the association of narcolepsy with inheritance of HLA-DR2, DQ6, which has a relative risk of nearly 130. Furthermore, in some cases inheritance of a specific HLA allele is associated with protection from rather than susceptibility to a disease. The best known of these cases is the negative association of HLA-DR2 and DQ6 with susceptibility to insulin-dependent diabetes mellitus (IDDM). Overall, however, the weight of these observations leads to a conclusion that the genes of the HLA complex are critically involved in the pathogenesis of autoimmune diseases. A logical corollary is that the role of HLA molecules in pathogenesis probably relates to their role in normal functioning of the immune system.

STRUCTURE AND FUNCTION OF HLA MOLECULES

HLA (for *Human Leukocyte Antigen*) is the designation in humans for the major histocompatibility complex (MHC). The MHC is a series of linked genes, present in all vertebrates studied, that are critically important in the presentation of antigens to T lymphocytes and the discrimination by T cells of molecules that are self constituents from those of non-self (see Chapter 270). It is in this manner that the immune system differentiates molecules and tissues that must be protected from immunologic attack from those that are possibly derived from pathogenic organisms and are thus appropriate targets. Based on this concept, it is a reasonable conclusion that ambiguity or mistakes in self/non-self discrimination could lead to autoimmunity, namely, immunologic attack directed against one or more of the body's own molecular constituents. To understand how this process might occur it is important to appreciate the basic molecular principles underlying T-cell recognition of antigen, which differ dramatically from those that determine antigen recognition by antibodies.

HLA GENES. The HLA complex resides on the short arm of the 6th chromosome, where it is distributed over more than 3.5 megabases of DNA (approximately the size of the *Escherichia coli* genome). At defined loci within this large amount of DNA are two classes of genes critically involved in T-cell recognition (Fig. 278–1). This activity is based on the capacity of the gene products (HLA molecules) to bind antigen fragments (which are, with few exceptions, oligopeptides) and then to present them on the surface of antigen-presenting cells (APCs) to T cells. Three genetic loci encode distinct class I-a MHC genes (HLA-A, HLA-B, HLA-C, hereafter designated class I for simplicity), and three loci encode the class II genes involved in antigen presentation (HLA-DR, HLA-DQ, and HLA-DP). In addition to the six class I-a and class II loci, the HLA complex includes many other genes, some of which are involved in effector functions of the immune system (e.g., tumor necrosis factor α; the C4, C2, and properdin factor B components of the complement system; and heat shock protein HSP-70). Others have no specific known role in the immune system, such as the 21-hydroxylase genes involved in steroid biosynthesis.

The HLA complex also contains a series of class I-b genes that are thought to serve a more specialized role (e.g., HLA-G, which is distinguished by its limited placental expression and has been hypothesized to be involved in protection of the maternal-fetal interface against immune attack), as well as a series of pseudogenes. At least one group of class I–like molecules, designated CD1, are not encoded on the 6th chromosome, but they nevertheless probably play an important role in defenses through binding and presentation of non-peptide (particularly glycolipid) antigens. At least two sets of class II–like genes, HLA-DM and HLA-DO, encode for products involved in the intracellular loading of exogenous peptide antigens into the classic class II molecules. Also within the class II region are several genes, designated LMP and TAP, that encode molecules that lack structural features of MHC molecules but play an important role in the hydrolysis and transport, respectively, of intracellular (endogenous) antigens to class I molecules.

CLASS I MOLECULES. A major conceptual advance in understanding the biologic function of MHC molecules was accomplished in 1987 with the solution by x-ray crystallography of the structure of a class I HLA molecule (Fig. 278–2). A 45-kd heavy

Table 278–1 ■ SELECTED HLA AND DISEASE ASSOCIATIONS

DISEASE	HLA MOLECULE	APPROXIMATE RELATIVE RISK*
Ankylosing spondylitis	B27	70–150†
Reiter's syndrome	B27	37–40
Acute anterior uveitis	B27	8–20
Hereditary hemochromatosis	A3, B14‡	90
Behçet's disease	B5	3–6
Sporadic narcolepsy	DR2, DQ6	130
Multiple sclerosis	DR2	3–6
	DR2, DQ6	12
Celiac disease	DR3	10–13
	DQ2	>250
Graves' disease	DR3	4
Idiopathic membranous glomerulonephritis	DR3	6–12
Chronic active hepatitis	DR3	7–9
Systemic lupus erythematosus	DR3	3–6
Insulin-dependent diabetes mellitus	DR3	3–5
	DR4	3–6
	DR3/DR4§	14–20
	DR3, DQ8	35–100
	DR2	0.2
	DQ6	0.02
Seropositive rheumatoid arthritis	DR4	4–10
Pauciarticular juvenile rheumatoid arthritis	DR5	3–5
Pemphigus vulgaris	DR4	14–21
	DR8	5–8
Dermatitis herpetiformis	DR3	15–18
Goodpasture's syndrome	DR2	16–20
Hodgkin's disease	DP3	2

*Relative risk = $\dfrac{(\% \text{ of patients with disease-associated HLA molecule}) (\% \text{ of controls lacking disease-associated HLA molecule})}{(\% \text{ of patients lacking disease-associated HLA molecules})(\% \text{ of controls with disease-associated HLA molecules})}$

†Ranges of relative risk are from different studies in the published literature, with significant differences commonly reflecting studies in different ethnic populations, perhaps with differing frequency of disease-associated molecular subtypes.

‡Denotes relative risk of extended haplotype.

§Denotes relative risk in heterozygotes.

(A) chain of these molecules consists of three extracellular domains of approximately 90 amino acids each connected to a transmembrane segment and a short intracytoplasmic tail (Fig. 278–3A). The class I heavy chains are non-covalently associated with a light chain (~12 kd), designated β_2-microglobulin, that is not genetically encoded within the MHC. Both β_2-microglobulin and the membrane-proximal α_3-domain of the heavy chain have structural features that define them as members of the immunoglobulin superfamily, including an intrachain disulfide bond and a secondary structure of antiparallel β-pleated sheets with loop connections. The crystallographic surprise, and new insight, derived from the structure of the α_1- and α_2-domains. Together these domains form a β-pleated sheet platform surmounted by two α-helical loops. Moreover, the initial crystal revealed the presence of an amorphous material bound within the cleft formed by the opposing helical loops.

It has since been shown that this cleft at the exterior-most surface of the class I molecule does indeed serve as a binding site for peptide fragments of partially digested proteins eight to nine amino acids in length. These peptides are loaded into newly synthesized class I molecules and then, together with β_2-microglobulin, are presented to T cells at the surface of APCs. More specifically, MHC class I molecules are now known to present oligopeptide antigens to T cells that express the accessory molecule CD8. The peptide thus presented may be derived either from self proteins, in which case it is either not recognized or is tolerated, or from a non-self protein, in which case it may lead to activation of CD8+ T cells of appropriate binding specificity. Antigens presented by

Human Major Histocompatibility Complex (Chromosome 6)

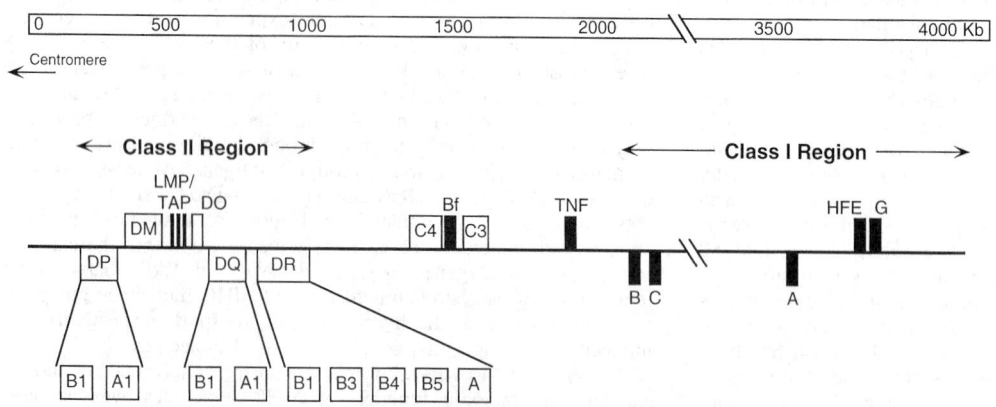

FIGURE 278–1 ■ Simplified schematic of the HLA complex. Illustrated below the line are MHC class I and class II genes, the products of which are involved in presentation of antigen to T lymphocytes. Above the line, within the class II region are genes involved in antigen processing, between the class II and class I regions are several genes involved in effector functions of the immune system, and in the class I region are two class I-b genes HLA-G and HFE (also known as HLA-H—a candidate gene for hereditary hemochromatosis). Not shown are several additional expressed class I-b genes, as well as a large number of class I and class II pseudogenes. Approximate genetic distances are given in thousands of base pairs (Kb).

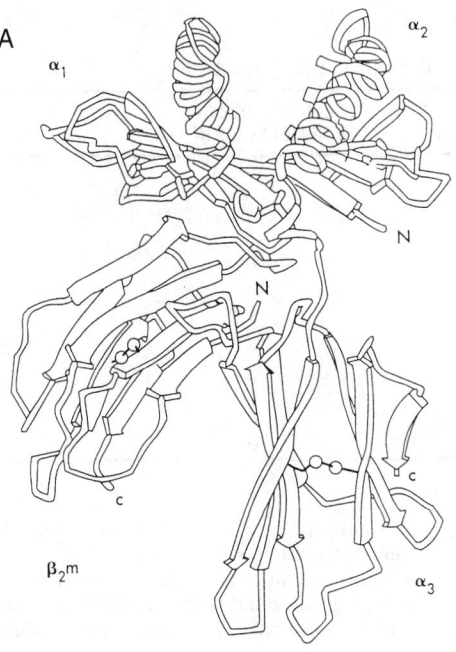

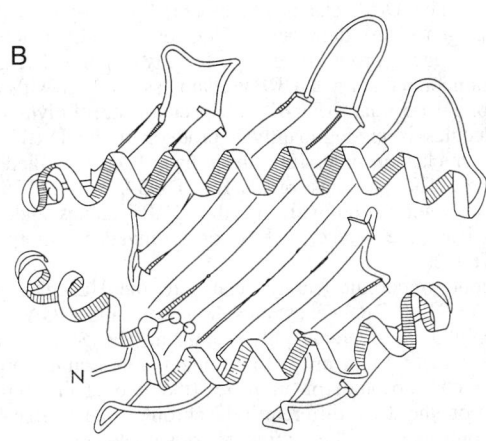

FIGURE 278-2 ■ Crystallographic structure of an HLA class I molecule. β-Strands are depicted as thick arrows in the amino-to-carboxy direction, and α-helices are presented as helical ribbons with connecting loops shown as thin lines. The disulfide bonds are illustrated as connected spheres. *A,* Side view of the molecule showing the three domains of the heavy chain non-covalently associated with β₂-microglobulin. *B,* Top view of the antigen binding cleft with the α-helices on top of a β-pleated sheet platform. (Reprinted by permission from *Nature,* Volume 329, p. 506. Copyright 1987 McMillian Magazines, Limited.)

class I molecules are usually derived from endogenous proteins (i.e., proteins synthesized within the APC). Foreign endogenous antigens include viral proteins and proteins from intracytosolic bacteria. T-cell receptors for antigen have been selected within the thymus gland to recognize, within a single binding site, specific elements of both the self-MHC molecule and the peptide within the antigen binding groove. Consequently, antigens presented (in an experimental system) by non-self MHC molecules are not recognized, a phenomenon known as "MHC restriction" of antigen recognition by T cells.

CLASS II MOLECULES. The overall structure of MHC class II molecules is very similar to that of class I molecules (Fig. 278–3*B*). Class II molecules also are composed of two non-covalently associated chains, A and B. In contrast to class I molecules, however, both chains of class II molecules are encoded within the MHC and both are integral membrane proteins that penetrate the cell membrane. The A and B class II polypeptide chains are of approximately equal size (about 34 and 29 kd, respectively) and consist of two rather than three extracellular domains. The membrane-proximal α₂- and β₂-domains, like the α₃-domain of the class

I heavy chain, are composed of antiparallel β-pleated sheets and contain a single intrachain disulfide bond. The α₁ and β₁ (amino terminal) domains come together to form an intermolecular β-pleated sheet platform that is also surmounted by two α-helical coils, one of which is contributed by each chain. These coils together with the β-pleated sheet floor again form an antigen binding cleft into which peptide fragments are bound for presentation to T lymphocytes. In the case of class II molecules, however, antigen presentation is exclusively to T cells for which the antigen receptor is characterized by coexpression of the accessory molecule CD4. Moreover, the proteins from which class II binding peptides are derived are generally synthesized extracellularly (e.g., most bacterial pathogens). They are then processed into oligopeptides and bound into a ternary complex with the class II A and B chains within endosomal granules, whereupon the complex is transported to the cell surface. The newly synthesized class II molecules are transported from the endoplasmic reticulum to the granules by a process that protects their antigen binding grooves from premature (endogenous) antigen-peptide encounter before arrival within the granules, where exogenous peptides are available.

The peptides that bind to MHC class II molecules are longer than those binding to class I molecules, usually 13 to 20 amino acids in length, because the ends of the helices are open to allow the peptide to extend outside the groove in either direction and also to slip back and forth to accomplish binding of the highest possible affinity. In contrast, the helices of class I molecules come together to close the antigen binding groove at both ends. Recognition of oligopeptide antigens bound to class II molecules is also MHC restricted and requires the T-cell receptors of CD4+ T cells to simultaneously recognize the self class II MHC molecule and the peptide antigen. Furthermore, again like class I molecules, although peptides derived from both self and non-self exogenous proteins may bind to class II molecules, processes of receptor selection normally ensure that only T cells with receptors that recognize a foreign peptide are available for activation.

HLA POLYMORPHISM

The HLA genes are the most polymorphic of the human genome, particularly in the case of molecules that have a major role in antigen presentation, namely, the class I molecules HLA-A and HLA-B and the class II molecules HLA-DR and HLA-DQ. Moreover, polymorphism defined serologically by antibodies has proved on subsequent typing by DNA sequencing to substantially underestimate true molecular polymorphism (Table 278–2). The definition of molecular subtypes is quite relevant to understanding of HLA and disease associations inasmuch as most such associations were initially based on serologic associations with a specific HLA type. Thus determination of associations with specific molecular variants

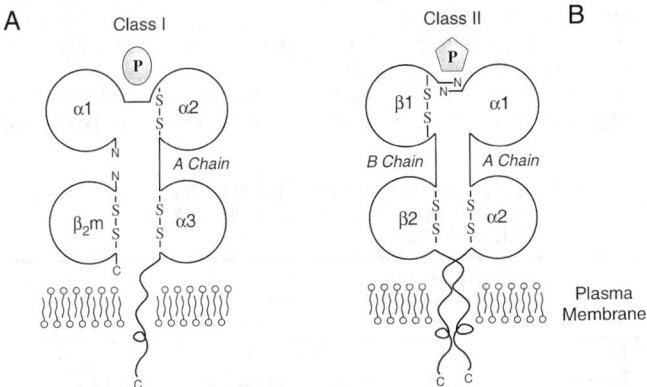

FIGURE 278-3 ■ Schematic representation of HLA molecules. *A,* A class I molecule illustrating the three-domain heavy chain, which penetrates the cell membrane and is non-covalently associated with β₂-microglobulin. An antigenic peptide (P) is illustrated in the antigen binding groove formed by the α₁ and α₂ domains. *B,* A class II molecule illustrating the non-covalently associated A and B chains of the molecule. Both chains are integral membrane proteins. The amino terminal domains of both chains together form an intermolecular antigen binding groove.

Table 278–2 ■ COMPARISON OF HLA ALLELES DETECTED BY SEROLOGIC AND MOLECULAR TECHNOLOGIES

	HLA ISOTYPE	ALLELES DEFINED BY DNA SEQUENCING	ALLELIC PRODUCTS DEFINED SEROLOGICALLY
Class I	HLA-A	50	39
	HLA-B	97	46
	HLA-C	34	15
Class II	HLA-DRA	2	0
	HLA-DRB1	106	14
	DRB3	4	1
	DRB4	5	1
	DRB5	5	1
	HLA-DQA1	15	0
	HLA-DQB1	26	7
	HLA-DPA1	8	0
	HLA-DPB1	59	6

has often resulted in a significant increase in relative risk (Table 278–3). A new nomenclature has been developed to distinguish related molecular subtypes of major alleles. The specific gene designated is separated by an asterisk from a four-digit number, the first two digits of which denote the major allelic specificity and the last two, the molecular subtype. For example, DRB1 *0301 defines the B chain of a molecular variant (split) of HLA-DR3 (which is also described by serologic typing as HLA-DR17).

For both class I and class II molecules, polymorphism is largely restricted to amino acid residues on the floor or the surrounding α-helices of the antigen binding groove. Polymorphism thus serves two distinct purposes. First, polymorphisms within the binding groove determine the peptide binding specificity (motif). This motif defines which few peptides any given MHC molecule will bind from among the many available in the cellular microenvironment. Second, polymorphisms within the α-helices also serve as the markers of "self" upon which T-cell receptors are selected. Polymorphisms of MHC molecules outside the antigen binding groove are far more limited.

The high degree of polymorphism at the HLA gene loci has several consequences. First, it is only rarely that two unrelated individuals are HLA identical with one another. Second, the vast majority of individuals are heterozygous at each HLA locus, having inherited one set of alleles from their mother and a 2nd (different) set from their father. Third, because all of the genes of the HLA complex are inherited as a single unit on the 6th chromosome, termed a haplotype, the likelihood of any two siblings being HLA identical with one another is 25%, in accord with Mendel's laws of inheritance. This situation would occur when both siblings inherited the same 6th chromosome from both parents. Similarly, the likelihood of two siblings sharing one such chromosome, termed haplo-identical, is 50%, and the lifelihood of sharing neither 6th chromosome, or HLA non-identical, is again 25%. The exception to this simple haplotype inheritance is the occasional interchromosomal crossing-over. Within the HLA complex, crossing-over is observed in approximately 3% of meioses.

Because HLA molecules are the most important elements in recognition of the foreignness of grafted tissues, tissue typing for

Table 278–3 ■ EFFECT OF MOLECULAR SUBTYPING OF HLA HAPLOTYPES ON RELATIVE RISK OF INSULIN-DEPENDENT DIABETES MELLITUS

HAPLOTYPE			RELATIVE RISK
DRB1	DQA1	DQB1	
0403	0301	0302	0.7
0406	0301	0302	0.2
0405	0301	0302	34.0
0405	0301	0301	2.1
0405	0301	0401	2.5
0401	0301	0302	3.0
0301	0501	0201	7.7
0901	0301	0303	1.2
1201	0501	0301	0.2

Data predominantly from Chinese subjects, abstracted from She J-X; Susceptibility to type I diabetes: HLA-DQ and DR revisited. Immunol Today 17:323, 1996.

HLA identity is generally performed to identify the most favorable donor-recipient pairs for grafting of bone marrow and solid organ transplantation, which for living related donors, often means identification of an HLA-identical sibling; for unrelated (usually cadaveric) donors, the intent is to maximize the number of shared HLA specificities.

For class II molecules, understanding of polymorphism requires appreciation of two additional phenomena. The first applies to DR molecules. The DRA chains are essentially non-polymorphic and the DRB genes are duplicated. Thus every individual expresses products on each chromosome of at least two sets of DR genes, the DRA chain paired with a DRB1 chain, as well as with a DRB3, DRB4, or DRB5 chain (DRB2 is a pseudogene). Polymorphism of DR molecules is predominantly a product of the DRB1 polypeptide, for which more than 100 alleles have been identified by DNA sequencing. The products of DRB3, DRB4, and DRB5 are expressed in combination with specific DRB1 alleles and, although differing from one another, exhibit only limited polymorphism (see Table 278–2).

A second important feature relates to the HLA-DQ genes. In contrast to HLA-DR, genes encoding both the DQA and DQB chains exhibit considerable polymorphism. The gene products can associate equally either in cis (both chains representing products of the same chromosome) or in trans (the two chains representing products of the two different 6th chromosomes). Because both chains contribute to the antigenic specificity of the assembled HLA-DQ molecule, novel assemblages expressed by neither parent can arise in offspring (e.g., an A chain from the mother and a B chain from the father yields a DQ molecule of antigenic specificity that is expressed by neither parent).

THE ANTIGEN BINDING GROOVE AND PEPTIDE MOTIFS

MHC molecules are one of three basic types involved in antigen binding and recognition, the others being immunoglobulins and T-cell receptors. The capacity of immunoglobulin and T-cell receptor molecules to bind a virtually limitless array of antigens is based on the construction of their antigen binding site through a process of DNA rearrangements between two or three gene segments that encode the site, together with nucleotide insertions at junctions between rearranged segments. MHC molecules, in contrast, do not rearrange. The capacity of MHC molecules to present a large number of different antigens thus depends on different strategies. First, the high degree of polymorphism at the various loci along with the multiplicity of loci within the HLA complex provides an organism with a considerable number of distinct antigen-presenting MHC molecules. The heart of the strategy, however, is that each MHC molecule has a distinct peptide binding "motif" that consists of pockets into which antigen-peptide amino acid side chains of a particular type (e.g., aromatic, hydrophobic, or charged) can be anchored (Fig. 278–4). Most peptides will be bound by two to three high-affinity major anchors and a similar number of minor anchors (of lower affinity). Thus a large number of different peptides derived from different proteins can be presented by any particular MHC molecule. The peptides interact with different T-cell receptors via side chains of amino acids other than the anchors that

A

HLA-A2 Peptides

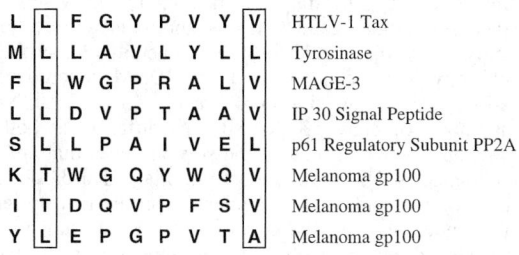

L	L	F	G	Y	P	V	Y	V		HTLV-1 Tax
M	L	L	A	V	L	Y	L	L		Tyrosinase
F	L	W	G	P	R	A	L	V		MAGE-3
L	L	D	V	P	T	A	A	V		IP 30 Signal Peptide
S	L	L	P	A	I	V	E	L		p61 Regulatory Subunit PP2A
K	T	W	G	Q	Y	W	Q	V		Melanoma gp100
I	T	D	Q	V	P	F	S	V		Melanoma gp100
Y	L	E	P	G	P	V	T	A		Melanoma gp100

B

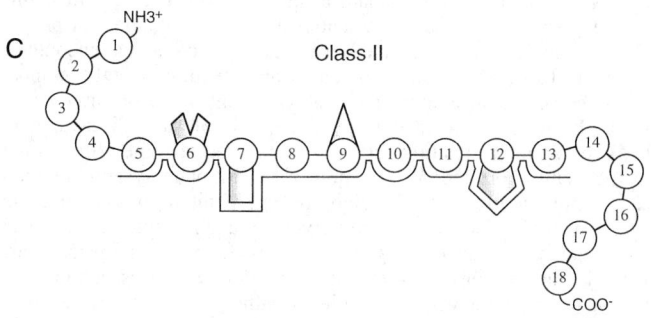

FIGURE 278–4 ■ Peptide binding motifs of HLA molecules. *A,* Nonamer peptides, which have been shown to bind into the antigen binding groove of HLA-A2, illustrate the strong anchors at positions 2 (leucine) and 9 (valine or leucine). The high degree of variability of peptides available for interacting with the T-cell receptor is apparent. Proteins from which these peptides are derived are listed to the right of the sequence. Sequences are denoted with the single letter amino acid code. Also shown are three peptides from the melanoma gp 100 antigen that appear to violate the canonic motif with a threonine at position 2 or an alanine at position 9. In these exceptional cases, weak anchors, illustrated in *B* as interactions with amino acids 1 and 3, are thought to contribute importantly to peptide binding. *B,* Peptide binding of HLA-A2 showing strong anchors at positions 2 and 9, minor anchors at positions 1 and 3, and closure of the binding groove ends with electrostatic interactions at both the NH_3^+ and COO^- termini. Side chains of residues at positions 5 and 8 are shown pointing up for interaction with the T-cell receptor. *C,* Peptide binding motif of a typical class II MHC molecule with strong anchors at positions 7 and 12 and weak anchors at positions 6, 10, and 11 and with positions 6 and 9 directing the side chain outward for interaction with the T-cell receptor. In contrast to class I, the ends of the class II binding groove are open, which allows for binding of a longer peptide and for movement back and forth to optimize interaction with MHC pocket anchors.

point out of the groove. As a consequence, any particular protein is highly likely to generate one or more peptides that can bind to one or more MHC molecules expressed by an individual. Nevertheless, the T-cell response to a complex protein antigen may be dominated by the response to one or a few specific peptides derived from that antigen.

The fact that peptides derived from single proteins have limited immunogenicity for T cells has obvious consequences when considering the design of T-cell vaccines. Thus the antigenic epitopes for one individual may differ from those of another, depending on the peptide binding specificity of their particular MHC molecules. When dealing with highly complex antigenic structure (e.g., from attenuated viral vaccines), such specificity is not of particular importance because there are almost always some antigen peptides that can bind to one or more MHC molecules from every individual. As antigens are simplified, however, specificity does become a matter of practical concern. For example, with recombinant hepati-

tis B surface antigen vaccines, 4 to 10% of vaccine recipients fail to mount a substantial immune response. This failure is associated with the inheritance of specific HLA haplotypes.

EXPRESSION AND DISTRIBUTION OF HLA MOLECULES

HLA genes are codominantly expressed. Thus cells display the products of both 6th chromosomes on their surface. This codominance is another important distinction from the products of immunoglobulin and T-cell receptor genes, which are subject to allelic exclusion and thus express the products of only one or the other chromosome. Moreover, cells express complete haplotypes of MHC molecules. That is, the products of both complete haplotypes (HLA-A, B, C and HLA-DR, DQ, and DP) are displayed. A fully competent APC thus expresses at least 6 different class I molecules and 10 different class II molecules (the larger number of class II molecules reflecting multiple DRB chains and *trans*-complementation of DQ).

The distribution of class I and class II molecules differs considerably. Class I molecules are expressed on almost all nucleated cells of the body (exceptions being very low or absent expression on neurons and spermatozoa). Expression of class II molecules is much more limited. Under normal circumstances (in the absence of an acute inflammatory process), class II molecules are expressed only on cells that are specialized for antigen presentation (i.e., APCs), including such cells as monocytes, macrophages, dendritic cells (including Langerhans' cells in skin), B lymphocytes, and (in humans) activated T lymphocytes. APCs are distinguished not only by their capacity to present peptide antigens to CD4+ T cells but also by their surface expression of costimulatory molecules essential to T-cell activation (see Chapter 270). In the presence of acute inflammation, however, other cell types can be induced by the T-cell cytokine interferon-γ to express class II molecules. Induced expression on endothelial cells and on the parenchymal cells of endocrine organs may be important in the pathogenesis of immunologic diseases involving such tissues.

LINKAGE DISEQUILIBRIUM

Analysis of HLA susceptibility to diseases is complicated by the phenomenon of linkage disequilibrium, which is the observation of an increased frequency with which a specific allele at one HLA locus is inherited in combination with a specific allele or alleles at some other HLA locus. Linkage disequilibrium results in considerable difficulty in determining which specific HLA locus is causally associated with a given disease because more than one locus may show a statistically significant association. The phenomenon is most consistently observed with closely linked genes, such as the association of DRB1 alleles determining DR3, DR5, DR6, and DR8 with the DRB3 alleles that determine DRw52 and the association of DRB1 alleles encoding DR4, DR7, and DR9 with the DRB4 allele that encodes DRw53. A very high level of association is also noted between certain DR and DQ specificities, such as DR2 with DQ1 and DQ6, DR3 with DQ2, DR7 with DQ2, and DR4 with DQ3. Linkage disequilibrium can operate over the substantial genetic distance of the entire HLA complex. For example, the frequent haplotypes of HLA-A1, B8, DR3 and A3, B7, DR2 are several times more frequent in white populations than their individual allelic gene frequencies would predict.

The mechanism of linkage disequilibrium is not well understood but may include such (non-mutually exclusive) explanations as (1) insufficient evolutionary time since emergence of the alleles that are in linkage disequilibrium to have come into equilibrium by the process of crossing-over, (2) selective advantage of certain combinations of allelic products in defenses against specific pathogens, and (3) possible physical impediments to DNA crossing-over between chromosomes bearing specific alleles.

MOLECULAR DEFINITION OF HLA-ASSOCIATED DISEASE SUSCEPTIBILITY

The availability of molecular subtyping of serologically related HLA specificities during the past decade has enabled definition of HLA-associated disease susceptibility in considerably greater detail.

Disease association defined at a molecular level can generally be associated with polymorphisms at specific sites within the HLA antigen binding groove. For example, in IDDM (see Chapter 242), the protective effect associated with DQ6 (as well as several other DQ alleles) is highly associated with the presence of an aspartic acid at residue 57 of the DQB chain. In contrast, IDDM susceptibility is highly associated with an alanine at this position, and valine and serine are associated with a modest increase in susceptibility. In fact, DQ8, which has an alanine in this position, is associated with IDDM in 65 to 70% of cases. Moreover, individuals inheriting the DQ7 molecule do not have an increase in IDDM susceptibility despite the fact that DQ7 and DQ8 share an identical DQA chain and differ in only four amino acids in the peptide binding portion of their B chain, including position 57, which is an aspartic acid in DQ7 and a non-charged amino acid (alanine) in DQ8. DQB57 lies on the α-helix of the B chain in pocket 9 of the peptide binding cleft, which implies a specific role of this pocket in the binding and presentation of a peptide involved in the pathogenesis of IDDM.

Disease association for IDDM, however, is more complex than simply the definition of a critical amino acid at DQB position 57. Of particular interest is the observation that heterozygosity for HLA-DR3/4 is more highly associated with disease than is homozygosity at either allele. This observation may reflect DR/DQ linkage disequilibrium and the formation of DQ trans-dimers in heterozygotes that are responsible for the increased susceptibility. Certain molecular polymorphisms of the DRB1 chain are also independently associated with disease susceptibility. This role of DRB1 alleles is illustrated in Table 278–3, which demonstrates significant differences in the susceptibility of individuals with identical DQ genes who differ for DRB1.

Molecular studies of disease association in seropositive rheumatoid arthritis have focused attention on a specific segment of the DRB1 chain. DRB1 *0401, *0404, *0405, and *0408 are all strongly associated with the development of rheumatoid arthritis. Indeed, approximately 70% of patients with rheumatoid arthritis are HLA-DR4+. On the other hand, DR4+ individuals with the molecular subtype DRB1*0402 are not at increased risk for rheumatoid arthritis. Each of the rheumatoid arthritis–associated HLA-DR molecules has an identical or very similar sequence of amino acids in positions 67 to 74 of the 3rd hypervariable region of the B chain of the molecule. Most notably, at position 71 the disease-associated genes encode the positively charged amino acids lysine or arginine. In contrast, DRB1*0402 encodes a negatively charged glutamic acid at this site. Because DRB1 position 71 is an important constituent of pocket 4 of the peptide binding cleft, this observation provides strong evidence of the role of a negatively charged peptide that may be accommodated into pocket 4 in the pathogenesis of rheumatoid arthritis.

Similar molecular studies have been carried out or are in progress for other HLA-associated diseases, particularly those for which molecular subtyping has revealed significant differences in susceptibility associated with minor molecular variants. Because such studies will also clarify the true disease-associated allele or alleles for isotypes in linkage disequilibrium, it is likely that future analyses of HLA and disease susceptibility will reveal increases in relative risk associated with specific HLA subtypes that are substantially greater than those based on analysis of serologically defined specificities.

INTERPRETATION OF HLA AND DISEASE ASSOCIATIONS

Observations of HLA and disease association lead to several conclusions and to theoretic speculation regarding pathogenetic mechanisms. First, it must be appreciated that none of the HLA-associated diseases occur as mendelian monogenic diseases (see Chapter 31). Indeed, the vast majority of individuals inheriting a specific disease-associated allele never exhibit manifestations of the disease. Such is the case even with the associations of greatest statistical significance. For example, ankylosing spondylitis or one of the other HLA-B27–associated diseases do not develop in most patients inheriting HLA-B27. Second, inheritance patterns within families with certain of the HLA-associated diseases demonstrate not only the important role of the HLA genes but also the impor-

tance of non-genetic (presumably environmental) etiologic factors. This point is clearly illustrated with IDDM, for which disease concordance for monozygotic twins is approximately 35 to 50%, thus strongly supporting a role for a non-genetic factor or factors in disease etiology. On the other hand, the IDDM concordance rate for HLA-identical siblings is approximately 15 to 25%, as compared with approximately 1% for siblings differing at both HLA haplotypes, thus indicating that of the several genes that are important in pathogenesis, HLA is the most important. Third, understanding of the biologic role of HLA molecules in antigen presentation to T lymphocytes leads to the conclusion that the pathogenesis of HLA-associated diseases involves T-cell activation in the vast majority of such diseases with a clear inflammatory component.

An interesting exception to the latter conclusion is narcolepsy, one of the most highly HLA-associated diseases, inasmuch as evidence for an inflammatory component in the pathogenesis of this disease is lacking. An interesting alternative suggestion is the possibility that the associated DQ6 molecule may act as a receptor for a neuropeptide of importance in maintaining wakefulness and promoting sleep. A 2nd exception is hereditary hemochromatosis, the candidate gene for which is a defective class I–like gene HFE (or HLA-H). The mutant allele of this gene, which is encoded approximately 300 kilobases telomeric of HLA-A, is in linkage disequilibrium with the haplotype HLA-A3, B14.

The molecular mechanisms involved in the pathogenesis of HLA-associated diseases remain a matter of speculation. Most immunologists believe that an essential non-genetic element is probably a specific peptide derived from an environmental encounter, either as food, as an allergen, or as an infectious agent. In most cases, however, no convincing etiologic agent has been discovered. It has been suggested that the pathogenesis of such diseases may involve common infectious agents encountered at some critical time in the maturation and/or activation of the immune system. In such cases, immunologic attack might not be limited to the etiologic agent; it might also be directed perversely against autologous tissue constituents. Recent data suggesting a possible role for Epstein-Barr virus in the etiology of systemic lupus erythematosus support the notion of infection with a ubiquitous pathogen leading to development of an autoimmune disease in a small minority of susceptible individuals.

A specific etiologic antigen has been implicated in at least one disease, celiac disease. In this case the antigen is the gliadin component of gluten, present as a dietary component derived from wheat and several other cereal grains. Patients with celiac disease have been shown to have gliadin-reactive T cells that are specifically activated when the antigen is presented by the disease-associated HLA-DQ molecule (DQ2 or DQ8, depending on the allele expressed by the specific patient).

An important mystery is the pathogenetic basis of an inflammatory lesion following encounter with an etiologic environmental peptide. To re-emphasize, the vast majority of DQ2 and DQ8 individuals ingest gluten-containing foods throughout their lives and celiac disease never develops. Moreover, it remains unclear in the case of tissue-specific autoimmune diseases why a particular etiologic event is associated with destruction of the specific target tissue. A frequently advanced hypothesis is that of "molecular mimicry," in which the structure of a particular autologous peptide is antigenically cross-reactive with an etiologic peptide when bound by chance by a disease-associated HLA molecule. In such cases, it is argued, T-cell tolerance for self tissues may be broken by an ambiguity in self/non-self discrimination, with an immune response initiated against the etiologic peptide, and then being directed (and perhaps amplified and perpetuated) as an immunologic response against the autologous self-peptide/MHC complex. Such a hypothesis gains credence with the recognition that tolerance for self proteins is not only determined by T-cell receptor selection in the thymus but also involves mechanisms of anergy or active suppression of potentially self-reactive T cells in peripheral lymphoid organs. It is further supported by the recent concept that with minor structural changes a T-cell–activating peptide bound to a particular MHC molecule can be converted from a T-cell agonist to antagonist and vice versa.

DIAGNOSTIC CONSIDERATIONS

With the very strong association between HLA inheritance and disease susceptibility for a considerable number of diseases, it is reasonable to ask whether HLA tissue typing has a role in the diagnostic tool kit or in assessing the future likelihood of development of an HLA-associated disease. Because HLA-associated disease does not develop in most individuals with the appropriate HLA inheritance, the general answer to this question is emphatically no. Moreover, in no instance can the presence of an appropriate HLA allele positively establish a diagnosis. For example, one cannot make the diagnosis of ankylosing spondylitis in an HLA-B27+ patient with low back pain in the absence of compatible radiologic findings (see Chapter 287). On the other hand, in selected cases, the *absence* of a highly associated marker may be of diagnostic usefulness. Thus a B27-negative patient with low back pain and equivocal or absent radiologic findings is unlikely to have incipient ankylosing spondylitis as an explanation for the symptoms. Similarly, a patient complaining of excessive daytime sleepiness in the absence of HLA-DQ6 is unlikely to have sporadic narcolepsy as an explanation.

One intriguing possibility for future diagnostic use is the identification of individuals at risk within families with an HLA-associated disease in which evidence of immunologic attack predictably antedates the development of clinical disease. For example, in IDDM, several studies are now in progress in families in whom HLA-identical siblings of a patient with disease are being monitored for immunologic signs of pancreatic β-cell destruction, which may occur years before the development of clinical diabetes. It is hoped that with the development of increasingly safe and effective immunosuppressive agents, the possibility of therapeutic intervention in the pre-clinical phase of such diseases may make prevention a possibility.

Lopez de Castro JA: The pathogenetic role of HLA-B27 in chronic arthritis. Curr Opin Immunol 10:59, 1998. *A brief review of a classic HLA-disease association with an excellent annotated bibliography.*

Nepom GT: Major histocompatibility complex–directed susceptibility to rheumatoid arthritis. Adv Immunol 68:315, 1998. *A comprehensive review, with a molecular emphasis, of an important HLA-disease association, by an important investigator in the field.*

Thosby E: Invited anniversary review: HLA associated diseases. Hum Immunol 53:1, 1997. *An excellent introduction to HLA and disease susceptibility, written by a pioneer in the field on the 30th anniversary of the first discovery of an HLA-disease association.*

279 DRUG ALLERGY

James R. Bonner

The designation "drug allergy" should be reserved for adverse drug reactions caused by immunologic mechanisms. Although drug allergies are responsible for only a minority of adverse drug effects, the possibility of such reactions is a daily concern of most physicians. Drug allergy has a great variety of clinical manifestations and has been attributed to most categories of therapeutic agents. Because specific diagnostic tests are not usually available, physicians most often base decisions on probabilities and the patient's need for treatment. This chapter provides an overview of drug allergy with an emphasis on pathogenic mechanisms, diagnostic considerations, and preventive measures. Non-allergic reactions are discussed in Chapter 26.

EPIDEMIOLOGY/ETIOLOGY

Complications of drug therapy are the most common adverse events among hospitalized patients, and 10 to 14% of such drug reactions have an allergic basis. An estimated 5% of adult patients have at least one drug allergy, and many more patients incorrectly believe that they are allergic to medications. Drug allergy may be more common in women and may be expected to occur more frequently in patients given multiple courses of treatment. Atopic patients are not predisposed to drug allergy but may have more severe reactions. Drug allergy appears to be less common at the extremes of age—a reflection of fewer sensitizing exposures in the very young and a decline in immune responsiveness in the very old. Risk factors for drug allergy are complex and include individ-

Table 279–1 ■ DRUGS FREQUENTLY CAUSING ALLERGIC AND PSEUDOALLERGIC REACTIONS

Antimicrobials
  β-Lactams
  Sulfonamides
  Vancomycin
  Nitrofurantoin
  Antituberculous drugs
  Quinolones
Anticonvulsants
  Phenytoin
  Carbamazepine
  Barbiturates
Cardiovascular agents
  Procainamide
  Hydralazine
  Quinidine
  Methyldopa
  ACE inhibitors
Macromolecules
  Heterologous antisera
  Enzymes
  Hormones
Anti-inflammatory agents
  Aspirin
  Other non-steroidal anti-inflammatory drugs
  Gold salts
  Penicillamine
Antineoplastic agents
  Azathioprine
  Procarbazine
  Asparaginase
  Cis-platinum
Other
  Allopurinol
  Radiographic contrast media
  Opiates
  Sulfasalazine
  Neuromuscular blocking drugs
  Antithyroid drugs

ACE = angiotensin-converting enzyme.

ual genetic differences in drug metabolism, as well as immunologic reactivity.

Most drugs are capable of causing allergic reactions; the agents listed in Table 279–1 are among the most frequent offenders. Table 26–1 provides a more comprehensive listing of individual drugs by type of reaction.

Topical application of drugs is associated with a higher risk of sensitization than is oral or parenteral administration, although reactions occur most frequently when medications are given parenterally.

PATHOGENIC MECHANISMS

The process by which patients become immunologically sensitized to therapeutic agents is complex and for most drugs poorly understood. It is generally accepted that to be an effective immunogen, a drug must have a molecular weight greater than 4000 or, for polypeptides, have at least seven amino acids. Some large-molecular-weight therapeutic agents such as antisera, vaccines, enzymes, and hormones are potentially immunogenic, but most drugs are much smaller and to elicit an immune response must form large hapten-carrier complexes by binding to tissue proteins. These carrier proteins may be free in plasma, intracellular, or incorporated into cell-surface membranes. A high hapten density on the carrier proteins strengthens the immune response, which can be directed against the haptenated drug itself, a complex of hapten and protein, or a tissue protein conformationally changed by the binding of hapten. The binding of hapten to carrier proteins must be covalent rather than the reversible binding by which drugs are usually associated with plasma proteins. Indeed, allergy to β-lactam antibiotics may occur frequently because these drugs and the products of their spontaneous *in vivo* degradation can readily form covalent bonds with proteins. Most drugs do not bind well to proteins and must initially be enzymatically metabolized to reactive forms by pro-

Table 279–2 ■ CLINICAL MANIFESTATIONS OF DRUG ALLERGY

Generalized
Anaphylaxis
Serum sickness
Drug fever
Vasculitis
Drug-induced systemic lupus erythematosus
Organ Specific
Cutaneous
    Urticaria, angioedema, exanthems, hypersensitivity, vasculitis, fixed eruptions, contact dermatitis, exfoliative dermatitis, erythema multiforme, toxic epidermal necrolysis, Stevens-Johnson syndrome
Renal
    Acute interstitial nephritis, glomerulonephritis
Pulmonary
    Asthma, acute infiltrates
Hematologic
    Hemolytic anemia, granulocytopenia, thrombocytopenia, eosinophilia
Hepatic
    Cholestatic hepatitis, hepatocellular damage

cesses such as oxidation. Reactive forms can lose their ability to bind proteins by undergoing further metabolism through processes such as acetylation and conjugation with glutathione. Therefore, risk factors for drug allergy in individual patients may include not only the ability to respond immunologically to hapten-carrier complexes but also the balance of genetically variable, drug-metabolizing enzymes.

All categories of immunologic hypersensitivity, as classified by Gell and Coombs, have been implicated in drug allergy (see Chapter 270); however, for many presumed allergic reactions the mechanism is unknown. Most hypersensitivity reactions require multivalent antigens to cross-link antibody such as IgE molecules bound to the high-affinity receptors on the surface of mast cells. Large-molecular-weight drugs may be inherently multivalent, and smaller drugs become effectively multivalent by binding to tissue proteins. To cause a generalized anaphylactic reaction, small drugs must bind *rapidly* to protein. Rapid protein binding is not as important in eliciting a primary immune response, which might explain why some drugs that frequently evoke an antibody response are less commonly associated with clinical reactions. The specific organ location of some reactions may be due to hapten binding to particular tissue proteins or the production of reactive drug metabolites in specific locations such as the liver.

Some drug reactions that clinically resemble an allergic response have been shown not to involve specific immune recognition. Such *pseudoallergic* reactions can result from direct histamine release from mast cells and basophils, complement activation, generation of inflammatory mediators from arachidonic acid metabolism, or activation of the contact coagulation system. Examples of pseudoallergic reactions include aspirin-induced asthma, anaphylactoid reactions to radiographic contrast media, and angioedema attributed to angiotensin-converting enzyme (ACE) inhibitors (see below).

CLASSIFICATION

Allergic drug reactions can be classified as generalized or organ specific (Table 279–2). Descriptions of these reactions can be found elsewhere in this text. Urticaria, eosinophilia, cutaneous exanthems, contact dermatitis, and drug fever are the most common clinical manifestations of drug allergy.

DIAGNOSIS

The following criteria should be considered when diagnosing drug allergy:

1. Enough time has elapsed for an immune response. For the initial use of most drugs, sufficient time is at least 7 to 10 days. Reactions with a more rapid onset are considered pseudoallergic or depend on prior sensitization during previous administration of the drug or a cross-reacting agent.
2. The character of the reaction does not suggest a pharmacologic or toxic effect of the drug.

3. The reaction does not appear to be dose dependent and is not caused by drug interaction or abnormalities of absorption or elimination.
4. The reaction has characteristics that suggest a hypersensitivity response such as skin rash, fever, and eosinophilia.
5. Clinical improvement occurs promptly after use of the suspect drug is discontinued. For most reactions, improvement is evident within 48 to 72 hours after stopping use of the drug.

Although it is not necessary that all these criteria be met, all should be considered when a patient is evaluated for possible drug allergy.

Patients suspected of having drug allergy are often receiving multiple drugs, and identifying the agent responsible can be difficult. It is sometimes helpful to make a flow chart listing the starting dates and times of all medications, including drug therapy that has recently been discontinued. The likely allergen may then be recognized by considering the above criteria and the drug categories most commonly implicated in allergic reactions (see Table 279–1). An allergic reaction to drugs that have been given continuously for long periods is much less likely than a reaction to recently introduced therapy. If the offending drug cannot be confidently identified, it may be necessary to discontinue all non-essential therapy and substitute treatment with chemically unrelated drugs.

Specific tests to evaluate drug allergy include skin tests, measurement of serum antibody levels, and challenge administration of suspect drugs. Skin testing to detect specific IgE involves pricking the skin or intradermal injection with dilute solutions of the drug in question. If the test solution contains antigen able to cross-link IgE molecules on cutaneous mast cells, histamine and other mediators of inflammation will be released and produce a wheal-and-flare response. The significance of a skin response must be evaluated by comparison with control testing using both histamine and diluent solutions. This testing method can be used only to predict or confirm drug reactions of the immediate hypersensitivity type, such as urticaria or systemic anaphylaxis. To get valid results, testing must be done with relevant antigens, which for most low-molecular-weight drugs are unknown metabolites. The lack of knowledge of the immunochemistry of most drugs severely limits the usefulness of skin testing. Negative tests are often uninterpretable, and false-positive reactions can result from non-specific skin irritation. Skin testing has proved useful for evaluating penicillin allergy in cases in which the relevant antigens are well known (see below) and for allergic reactions associated with anesthetic agents. Large-molecular-weight therapeutic agents such as heterologous antisera, peptide hormones (e.g., insulin), and vaccines are complete antigens that can appropriately be used for skin testing. Treatment with antihistamines must be discontinued before skin testing, and for safety, testing should always begin with the prick method. *In vitro* tests for drug-specific IgE, such as the radioallergosorbent test, are also limited by our incomplete knowledge of drug immunochemistry. Skin tests are generally more sensitive than measurement of specific IgE and have the advantage of immediately available results.

Challenge administration of a suspect drug offers the possibility of specific diagnosis or exclusion of drug allergy. However, challenges are inherently dangerous and should usually be avoided, especially if possible anaphylaxis or other potentially life-threatening complications such as exfoliative dermatitis are of concern. When the drug in question is considered essential and the history is vague or suggests a mild reaction, challenge testing might be justified. Challenges should begin with a very low dose considered unlikely to cause a reaction.

MANAGEMENT

Discontinuing use of the responsible drug is often the only treatment necessary. Some reactions may require supportive measures directed at relieving symptoms and reducing inflammation. Antihistamines such as diphenhydramine, 25 to 50 mg every 4 to 6 hours, or hydroxyzine, 25 mg four times daily for adults, can relieve pruritus and may lessen the duration of some reactions. Corticosteroids should be reserved for the most severe or prolonged reactions. Treatment of anaphylaxis is discussed in Chapter 275.

In exceptional circumstances it may be acceptable to continue drug treatment despite mild reactions such as delayed-onset urticaria, exanthems, and fever. Patients who continue to take the drug should receive supportive measures and should be monitored closely; if the reaction increases in severity, use of the drug should be stopped.

Patients with a history of allergic reactions to multiple drugs, particularly antibiotics, present a difficult management problem. These reactions can sometimes be attributed to immunologic cross-reactivity, but often patients claim sensitivity to chemically dissimilar agents. In some cases a careful history reveals that allergy has been confused with other types of adverse drug reactions, such as side effects or drug toxicity. Some patients who have experienced severe allergic reactions become fearful of all drug use and experience reactions attributable to anxiety. However, the possibility of true allergy to multiple, chemically dissimilar drugs must also be considered. A prospective study demonstrated that patients with a history of allergic reactions to any antimicrobial agent were 10 times more likely to react to unrelated antimicrobial drugs than were history-negative controls. This finding suggests the existence of a group of patients predisposed to respond immunologically to drug haptens. Special care should be taken for patients with a history of multiple drug allergy, including administering the initial dose of any new drug in a physician's office or other supervised environment.

Another group of patients at risk for multiple drug sensitivities are individuals with human immunodeficiency virus (HIV) infection (see Part XXIII). Patients with acquired immune deficiency syndrome (AIDS) are reported to be at increased risk for reaction to multiple antimicrobial agents, including sulfonamides, amoxicillin, pentamidine, clindamycin, dapsone, quinolones, acyclovir, probenecid, thalidomide, and antituberculosis drugs. Most drug reactions in HIV-infected patients are manifested by delayed onset of maculopapular rash and fever rather than the early onset of urticaria or cardiorespiratory symptoms that characterize type I hypersensitivity. The predisposition to drug reactions in HIV-infected patients may be due to immune dysregulation or changes in drug metabolism caused by the retroviral infection. The risk of drug reactions in HIV-infected patients can create difficult management problems. Successful rechallenge or desensitization of AIDS patients has been reported with trimethoprim-sulfamethoxazole, acyclovir, and dapsone. Although such procedures are inherently dangerous and have caused severe systemic reactions, the risk is sometimes justified for patients with opportunistic infections. Sensitivity to multiple antimicrobial agents has also been reported in patients with humoral immunodeficiency and patients with systemic lupus erythematosus.

PREVENTION

The most effective preventive measures are taking a careful history of previous drug reactions and avoiding unnecessary drug use. The history should be adequate to allow classification of the type of reaction experienced, and physicians should educate patients to distinguish allergy from other types of adverse reactions (see Chapter 26). Reactions attributable to drug toxicity or side effects do not necessarily preclude future use of the same or chemically similar agents.

Before prescribing any new drug, physicians should again inquire about past drug reactions. Skin tests can predict a type I hypersensitivity response to some drugs and should be done routinely before heterologous antisera is given. Patients should be kept under observation for 20 to 30 minutes after receiving parenteral medication.

When newly marketed drugs are used, physicians should be alert for unexpected complications, including allergic reactions. New drugs are not routinely evaluated for immunogenicity, and animal studies may not predict human hypersensitivity. Pre-marketing clinical trials seldom include adequate numbers of patients to detect problems of low incidence such as drug allergy.

When treatment is considered essential despite well-documented allergic hypersensitivity, the drug can sometimes be administered by following a desensitization protocol. Successful desensitization regimens have been published for β-lactam antibiotics (see below), trimethoprim-sulfamethoxazole, vancomycin, allopurinol, tetanus toxoid, acyclovir, sulfasalazine, insulin, aspirin, and heterologous antisera. These regimens start with a very low drug dose, which is

slowly increased as the patient is closely monitored. Reactions often occur during desensitization, and it is frequently necessary to drop back and repeat tolerated doses before proceeding. The mechanism of desensitization is uncertain but for some drugs may involve the gradual neutralization of IgE antibody with low drug doses. Desensitization is always a high-risk procedure that is undertaken only after obtaining informed consent from the patient or family and only by physicians who are prepared to treat severe reactions.

SPECIFIC DRUG ALLERGIES

β-LACTAM ANTIBIOTICS. β-Lactam antibiotics—including penicillins, carbapenems, cephalosporins, and monobactams—are the most common cause of drug-induced immediate hypersensitivity reactions. The immunochemistry of penicillin is the best studied of any drug. Most protein-bound penicillin is in the form of penicilloyl, which is designated the major determinant. Other products of penicillin degradation, including penicilloate and penilloate, and penicillin itself are designated the minor determinants, which indicates that these haptens are present in relatively small amounts. This terminology is somewhat confusing because the majority of patients who have had immediate reactions to penicillin are found to have IgE antibody to minor determinants rather than penicilloyl alone.

Most patients with a history of penicillin allergy have no reaction if given the drug. This observation can be attributed to both inaccurate histories and the loss of sensitivity with time. The significance of a history of penicillin allergy can be clarified by skin testing. If skin testing is performed with both penicilloyl (available as Pre-Pen) and minor determinants, the results are highly accurate in identifying patients at risk for immediate-type reactions, the sensitivity being approximately 99%. Although minor determinants other than penicillin itself are not commercially available, skin testing with just penicilloyl and penicillin will identify about 93% of patients at risk. Details of penicillin skin testing are given in Table 279-3.

Whenever possible, alternative antimicrobial agents should be chosen for patients with a history of penicillin allergy of any type. If, however, use of a penicillin or another β-lactam agent is considered essential for patient care, the decision to use a β-lactam can usually be based on the patient's history and skin test results. If the prior reaction is recalled as a delayed appearance of a morbilliform rash, the most common manifestation of penicillin sensitivity, a β-lactam may be cautiously administered starting with a low dose. If the history is one of rapid-onset urticaria or anaphylaxis, skin testing can help determine the risk. Patients with a history of immediate-type hypersensitivity in the distant past and negative skin testing with penicillin and penicilloyl can be given a β-lactam agent starting with a low dose under physician observation. For patients with positive skin tests or a recent history of anaphylaxis with penicillin, a formal desensitization protocol should be used. Examples of parenteral and oral desensitization regimens are given

---

Table 279-3 ▪ PENICILLIN SKIN TESTING

Testing materials
Penicilloyl polylysine (Pre-Pen)
Penicillin G, 10,000 U/mL
Histamine, 1 mg/mL (positive control)
Diluent (negative control)
Procedure
Testing is usually done on the volar surface of the forearm or lateral surface of the upper part of the arm. Begin the prick test by using a 26-gauge needle to prick through a drop of test material. If the prick test is negative, proceed with intradermal testing and raise a bleb by intradermal injection of 0.02 mL of test material. Read the test results at 15 min. For a patient with a history of a recent severe reaction to penicillin, begin testing with a 100-fold dilution of test antigens
Interpretation
Skin tests can be interpreted only if the histamine control produces a wheal-and-flare response. A positive reaction includes a wheal of at least 4 mm accompanied by erythema. If the patient has dermatographism, manifested by a significant response to the diluent control, skin test results may not be interpretable. Questionable results should be repeated.

in Table 279–4. Oral desensitization may be safer and is preferred in most situations.

The reliability of skin testing with β-lactam antibiotics other than penicillin has not been established, and the degree of cross-reactivity among different classes of β-lactams varies. Published reports of patients with a history of penicillin allergy and positive penicillin skin tests who were given a cephalosporin antibiotic indicate a reaction risk of less than 10%, but most reported reactions have been anaphylaxis. The carbapenem antibiotic imipenem has considerable cross-reactivity with penicillin, but the monobactam antibiotic aztreonam has no significant cross-reactivity and can be safely used in patients with penicillin allergy. Aztreonam and the 3rd-generation cephalosporin ceftazidime have the same side chain on the β-lactam ring and may have significant clinical cross-reactivity.

INSULIN. The incidence of significant allergic reactions to insulin has declined with the availability of recombinant human insulin. Most patients suspected of insulin allergy are found to have idiopathic urticaria or sensitivity to other medications. However, true immediate-type hypersensitivity reactions to human insulin do occur; such reactions are particularly likely in patients whose insulin therapy has been interrupted by attempts at management with diet and oral hypoglycemic agents. Sensitive patients usually have rapid-onset local reactions at insulin injection sites, and the presence of specific IgE antibody can be confirmed by skin testing. Effective desensitization regimens are available and after desensitization patients should receive insulin treatment continuously.

LOCAL ANESTHETICS. Immediate-type hypersensitivity to local anesthetics is rare. Most adverse reactions to these agents can be attributed to toxicity, anxiety, contact dermatitis, or coadministration of other drugs such as epinephrine. True allergy to local anesthetics is perhaps more common with benzoic acid esters such as procaine and benzocaine. When the history of past reactions is

unclear or suggests immediate-type hypersensitivity, skin testing with dilute solutions of local anesthetics can be diagnostically useful. Skin testing is usually done with one of the amide local anesthetics such as lidocaine and mepivacaine. If skin tests are negative, incremental challenge doses of the anesthetic are usually well tolerated.

ANGIOTENSIN-CONVERTING ENZYME INHIBITORS. Angioedema of the face and oropharyngeal structures is an important complication of ACE inhibitor therapy. Patients with such reactions appear to be sensitive to alternative ACE inhibitors that have the same pharmacologic action but different chemical structures. Such response suggests a pseudoallergic reaction not mediated by a specific immune response but possibly resulting from the drug's effect on kinin metabolism. The angioedema is characterized by nonpruritic swelling that is usually not accompanied by urticaria. Most reactions occur within the initial week of therapy, but reactions have been reported as long as 7 years after the start of drug use. These reactions may be more common in women, blacks, and patients who have experienced idiopathic angioedema. Fatal episodes have been reported, and therapy with alternative ACE inhibitor drugs should not be attempted. The angioedema associated with these drugs is unrelated to ACE inhibitor induced cough.

ASPIRIN AND OTHER NON-STEROIDAL ANTI-INFLAMMATORY DRUGS. Two to 6% of asthma patients have a history of aspirin-induced symptoms, and challenge studies have demonstrated airflow obstruction in up to 20% of unselected asthmatics. Asthma patients with chronic rhinosinusitis and nasal polyps are at particularly high risk for aspirin sensitivity. Aspirin can also cause symptom exacerbation in patients with chronic urticaria. Aspirin-sensitive patients with asthma or chronic urticaria also react to most other non-steroidal anti-inflammatory drugs (NSAIDs). This cross-reactivity between drugs with chemically different structures but similar pharmacologic action suggests that these reactions are not immunologically mediated. Reactions in asthmatics may be related to inhibition of cyclooxygenase with concomitant enhancement of leukotriene synthesis or to hyperresponsiveness to leukotrienes, which are potent bronchoconstrictors. Desensitization regimens have been effective for patients with aspirin-induced bronchospasm and produce cross-desensitization to other NSAIDs. Pre-medication with the 5-lipoxygenase inhibitor zileuton, which reduces production of leukotrienes, has been demonstrated to prevent bronchoconstriction in aspirin-sensitive asthmatics. For most sensitive asthma patients, aspirin and NSAIDs are easily avoided. Patients with both asthma and chronic rhinosinusitis/polyposis should probably avoid these drugs regardless of the past history of aspirin sensitivity. NSAIDs have been associated with other idiosyncratic inflammatory reactions, including acute aseptic meningitis and hypersensitivity pneumonitis.

Beall G, Sanwo M, Hussain H: Drug reaction and desensitization in AIDS. Immunol Allergy Clin North Am 17:319, 1997. *Features specific desensitization protocols.*

de Shazo, RD, Kemp SF: Allergic reactions to drugs and biologic agents. JAMA 278:1895, 1997. *A recent review with useful algorithms.*

DeSwarte RD, Paterson R: Drug Allergy. *In* Patterson R, Grammer LC, Greenberger PA (eds): Allergic Diseases Diagnosis and Management, 5th ed. Philadelphia, JB Lippincott, 1997, p 317. *A comprehensive review with 395 references.*

Table 279–4 ■ β-LACTAM DESENSITIZATION

PENICILLIN ORAL DESENSITIZATION PROTOCOL*

Dose*	Penicillin V Elixir (U/mL)	Amount mL	Amount U	Cumulative Dose (U)
1	1,000	0.1	100	100
2	1,000	0.2	200	300
3	1,000	0.4	400	700
4	1,000	0.8	800	1,500
5	1,000	1.6	1,600	3,100
6	1,000	3.2	3,200	6,300
7	1,000	6.4	6,400	12,700
8	10,000	1.2	12,000	24,700
9	10,000	2.4	24,000	48,700
10	10,000	4.8	48,000	96,700
11	80,000	1.0	80,000	176,700
12	80,000	2.0	160,000	336,700
13	80,000	4.0	320,000	656,700
14	80,000	8.0	640,000	1,296,700

Patients should be observed for 15 minutes between doses and for 30 minutes after the last dose before parenteral drug administration.

β-LACTAM INTRAVENOUS DESENSITIZATION PROTOCOL†

Dose No.	Concentration of Stock Solution (mg/mL)	Concentration of Infused Solution (mg/mL)	Amount of Antibiotic Administered (mg)
1	0.0005	0.00001	0.0005
2	0.005	0.0001	0.005
3	0.05	0.001	0.05
4	0.5	0.01	0.5
5	5	0.1	5
6	50	1	50
7	500	10	500

Stock solution is prepared by solubilizing the antibiotic with non-bacteriostatic saline to a final concentration IgE 500 mg/mL. Dilutions are prepared by adding 1 mL of each preceding dilution to 9 mL of diluent. One milliliter of stock solution is further diluted into 50 mL of saline and infused over 20 minutes.

*From Wendel GD Jr, Stark BJ, Jamison RB, et al: Penicillin allergy and desensitization in serious infections during pregnancy. N Engl J Med 312:1229, 1985.

†From Borish L, Tamir R, Rosenwasser LJ: Intravenous desensitization to beta-lactam antibiotics. J Allergy Clin Immunol 80:314, 1987.

280 ■ MASTOCYTOSIS

Dean D. Metcalfe

Mastocytosis is a rare disease characterized by an abnormal increase in mast cells in the bone marrow, liver, spleen, lymph nodes, gastrointestinal tract, and skin. Mastocytosis may occur in any age group and demonstrates a slight male preponderance (1.5:1.0). The prevalence of the disease is unknown, and familial occurrence is unusual.

The disease is divided into four categories on the basis of clinical features, pathologic findings, and prognosis (Table 280–1). Patients in the 1st category have a good prognosis, whereas patients in the other three groups do poorly. *Indolent mastocytosis* is di-

Table 280–1 ■ CLASSIFICATION OF MASTOCYTOSIS

280 Mastocytosis ■ 1467

Table 280–1 ■ CLASSIFICATION OF MASTOCYTOSIS

Indolent mastocytosis
  Skin only
    Urticaria pigmentosa
    Diffuse cutaneous mastocytosis
  Systemic
    Marrow
    Gastrointestinal
    ±Urticaria pigmentosa
Mastocytosis with an associated hematologic disorder (±urticaria pigmentosa)
  Dysmyelopoietic syndrome
  Myeloproliferative disorders
  Acute non-lymphocytic leukemia
  Malignant lymphoma
  Chronic neutropenia
Mast cell leukemia
Aggressive mastocytosis

vided into two subgroups: those with isolated skin involvement and those with systemic disease. In most cases such patients gradually accrue more mast cells with progression of symptoms but can be managed successfully for decades with medications that provide symptomatic relief. The 2nd most common form of mastocytosis is that associated with a *hematologic disorder,* in which examination of the bone marrow and peripheral blood reveals the hematologic abnormality. The prognosis in these patients is determined by the associated hematologic disorder. The 3rd category of mast cell disease is *mast cell leukemia;* it is the rarest form and has the most fulminant behavior. Mast cell leukemia is distinguished by its unique pathologic and clinical picture. The peripheral blood smear shows immature mast cells. The 4th category of patients has an *aggressive form* of mastocytosis; these individuals experience a rapid increase in mast cell numbers and have poor prognostic features but do not have a distinctive hematologic disorder or mast cell leukemia.

ETIOLOGY AND PATHOGENESIS. Mast cells originate from pluripotent bone marrow stem cells and migrate through the blood stream and lymphatics to specific sites, where they mature into fully granulated cells. Targeting of mast cells to defined locations is determined by the sequential expression of cell-surface adhesion molecules. Mast cells are often found along endothelial and epithelial basement membrane, along nerves, and around glandular structures. Tissues at interfaces between the external and internal environment, i.e., the skin and gastrointestinal tract, are particularly rich in mast cells.

Mast cell number and differentiation are regulated by factors produced both in the hematopoietic marrow and by cells in the tissues in which mast cells finally reside. Mast cell growth and differentiation depend on c-kit ligand, or stem cell factor, and are inhibited by granulocyte-macrophage colony-stimulating factor.

Table 280–2 ■ REPRESENTATIVE MAST CELL PRODUCTS AND THEIR BIOLOGIC EFFECTS

Granule Associated	
Histamine	Pruritus, increased vasopermeability, gastric hypersecretion, bronchoconstriction
Heparin	Local anticoagulation
Tryptase, chymotryptic proteases	Degradation of local connective tissues
Lipid Derived	
Sulfidopeptide leukotrienes	Increased vasopermeability, bronchoconstriction, vasoconstriction (LTC_4); increased vasopermeability, bronchoconstriction, vasodilation (LTD_4 and LTE_4)
Prostaglandin D_2	Vasodilation, bronchoconstriction
Platelet-activating factor	Increased vasopermeability, vasodilation, bronchoconstriction
Cytokines	
Pro-inflammatory factors	Fibrosis (TGF-β); activation of vascular endothelial cells, cachexia (TNF-α); IgE synthesis (IL-4)
Growth enhancing	Colony-stimulating factor (IL-3), eosinophilia (IL-5)

LTC_4 = leukotriene C_4; TGF-β = transforming growth factor β; TNF-α = tumor necrosis factor α; IL-4 = interleukin-4.

Mutations in *c-kit* that lead to ligand-independent phosphorylation of this receptor have been described in patients with mastocytosis. The most common of these mutations is a point mutation (Asp816Val) in the catalytic domain of *c-kit.*

Regardless of the cause of the increased burden of mast cells, the pathogenesis of the disease is largely the result of the increased production of mast cell mediators, which have effects both at the site of their production and at remote sites. Mast cell mediators are of three categories, all of which produce biologic effects typical of those observed in patients with mastocytosis (Table 280–2).

CLINICAL FEATURES. The categories of mastocytosis in general share similar clinical features, although some patterns of disease may predominate in a specific category. The skin, gastrointestinal tract, liver, spleen, lymph nodes, bone marrow, and skeletal system yield the most significant management problems. The respiratory tract and endocrine system are generally spared. Patients with mastocytosis do not suffer from recurrent infections.

The most common skin manifestation of mastocytosis is urticaria pigmentosa (Fig. 280–1). It is seen in more than 90% of patients with indolent mastocytosis and in fewer than 50% of patients with mastocytosis and an associated hematologic disorder or those with aggressive mastocytosis. The lesions of urticaria pigmentosa appear as scattered small reddish brown macules or slightly raised papules. Scratching or rubbing the lesions usually causes urtication and erythema around the macules, a phenomenon known as Darier's sign. Urticaria pigmentosa is associated with pruritus, which may be exacerbated by changes in climatic temperature, skin friction, ingestion of hot beverages or spicy foods, ethanol, and certain drugs. The diagnosis is confirmed by characteristic skin histopathologic findings. Diffuse cutaneous mastocytosis consists of a diffuse mast cell infiltration of the skin. Solitary lesions called *mastocytomas* do occur but are quite rare. Young children with urticaria pigmentosa or diffuse cutaneous mastocytosis may have bullous eruptions.

Gastrointestinal disease often develops in patients with mastocy-

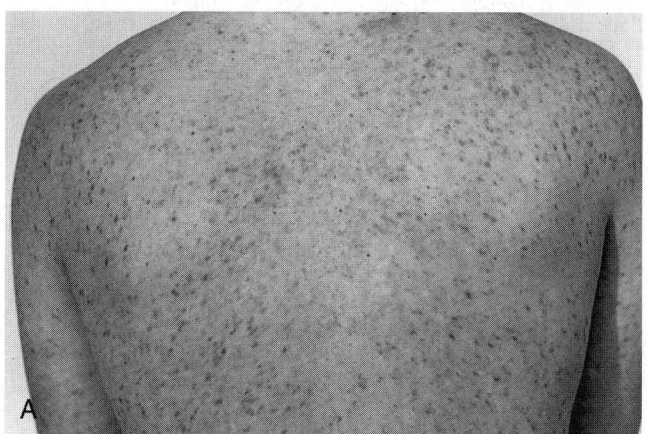

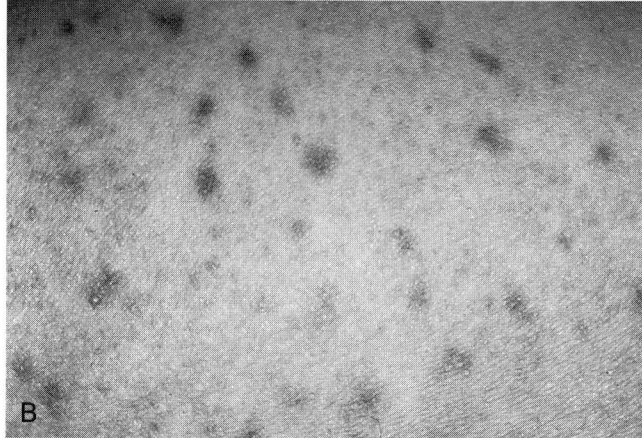

FIGURE 280–1 ■ *A,* Urticaria pigmentosa in a patient with indolent systemic mastocytosis. *B,* Close-up view of urticaria pigmentosa.

tosis. The most common problem is gastric hypersecretion caused by elevated plasma histamine with resultant gastritis and peptic ulcer disease. Diarrhea and abdominal pain are common and are followed by the onset of malabsorption in approximately one in three patients. Radiographic abnormalities fall into three major categories: peptic ulcers; abnormal mucosal patterns such as mucosal edema, multiple nodular lesions, coarsened mucosal folds, or multiple polyps; and motility disturbances. Histopathologic examination of jejunal biopsy specimens has shown moderate blunting of the villi; however, significant mast cell hyperplasia is uncommon.

Hepatic and splenic involvement in indolent systemic mastocytosis is relatively common, although liver function tests are usually normal. The most common chemical abnormality is an elevated alkaline phosphatase concentration, which must be distinguished from bone-derived alkaline phosphatase, levels of which may also be elevated. The most serious manifestation of hepatic and splenic involvement is portal hypertension and ascites associated with fibrosis of the liver and spleen. These conditions appear most commonly in patients who have mastocytosis with an associated hematologic disorder or in those with aggressive mastocytosis.

Bone marrow lesions consist of focal aggregates of spindle-shaped mast cells, often mixed with eosinophils, lymphocytes, and occasional plasma cells, histiocytes, and fibroblasts (Fig. 280–2). Anemia, leukopenia, thrombocytopenia, and eosinophilia may occur in association with systemic disease. Bone marrow infiltration with mast cells may induce bone changes that cause radiographically detectable lesions in up to 70% of patients. The proximal long bones are most often affected, followed by the pelvis, ribs, and skull. Bone pain is the most common symptom and is present in 19 to 28% of patients. Skeletal scintigraphy (bone scan) is more sensitive than radiographic surveys in detecting and locating active lesions. In severe or advanced disease, pathologic fractures do occur.

Patients with every category of mastocytosis sometimes experience flushing or frank anaphylaxis. In occasional patients, anaphylaxis may be provoked by alcohol, aspirin, exercise, or infections.

Neuropsychiatric abnormalities have been reported. Problems include a decreased attention span, memory impairment, and irritability. Depression as a consequence of chronic disease or possibly mediated by mast cell products is a possibility.

DIAGNOSIS. The diagnosis of mastocytosis rests on histology, supported by clinical, biochemical, and radiographic data. Mast cells may be overlooked on histologic sections depending on the fixation and/or stain used. The most useful stains for mast cells include metachromatic stains, such as toluidine blue and Giemsa, and enzymatic stains, such as chloroacetate esterase and aminocaproate esterase. These procedures highlight the granules in the cyto-

plasm of the mast cell. In trephine core bone marrow biopsies, decalcification interferes with subsequent attempts to visualize mast cell granules.

The majority of patients with mastocytosis have urticaria pigmentosa. This diagnosis should be confirmed by skin biopsy. Blind skin biopsies are not recommended inasmuch as other skin conditions, including eczema, are associated with an increase in dermal mast cells.

In the absence of skin lesions, mastocytosis may be suspected in patients with one or several of the following: unexplained ulcer disease or malabsorption, radiographic or ^{99m}Tc bone scan abnormalities, hepatomegaly, splenomegaly, lymphadenopathy, peripheral blood abnormalities, and unexplained flushing or anaphylaxis. Elevated levels of plasma or urinary histamine or histamine metabolites, prostaglandin D_2 metabolites in the urine, or plasma mast cell tryptase are not diagnostic but do raise the index of suspicion of mastocytosis. Reliable tests for these substances, however, are not generally available except in research laboratories.

Patients suspected of having mastocytosis in the absence of skin lesions should have a bone marrow biopsy and aspirate for diagnosis. Patients with urticaria pigmentosa or diffuse cutaneous mastocytosis should also have this procedure if they have peripheral blood abnormalities, hepatomegaly, splenomegaly, or lymphadenopathy to determine whether they have an associated hematologic disorder. Other tissue specimens such as lymph nodes, liver, and gastrointestinal mucosa define the extent of mast cell involvement but are obtained only as necessary.

Patients suspected of having mastocytosis should have 24-hour urine 5-hydroxyindoleacetic acid (5-HIAA) measured to help eliminate the possibility of a carcinoid tumor. Patients with mastocytosis do not excrete increased amounts of 5-HIAA. Idiopathic anaphylaxis and flushing must also be considered. Patients with these disorders do not have histologic evidence of significant mast cell proliferation.

TREATMENT. In all categories of mastocytosis, a primary objective of treatment is to control mast cell mediator–induced signs and symptoms such as anaphylaxis, gastrointestinal cramping, and pruritus. H_1 receptor antagonists such as hydroxyzine and doxepin are helpful in reducing pruritus, flushing, and tachycardia. If insufficient relief occurs, adding an H_2 antagonist such as ranitidine or cimetidine may be beneficial. However, many patients continue to complain of bone pain, headaches, and flushing, which result in part from the inability to block other mast cell mediators. Disodium cromoglycate (cromolyn sodium) inhibits the degranulation of mast cells and may have some efficacy in the treatment of mastocytosis. Epinephrine is used to treat episodes of anaphylaxis. Patients should be prepared to self-administer this drug. If subcutaneous epinephrine is insufficient, intensive therapy for anaphylaxis should be instituted. Patients with recurrent episodes of anaphylaxis may have H_1 and H_2 antihistamines prescribed to lessen the severity of attacks. Episodes of profound anaphylaxis may be spontaneous but have also been observed following stings from insects or the administration of radiocontrast media.

Treatment of gastrointestinal disease is directed at controlling peptic symptoms, diarrhea, and malabsorption. Gastric acid hypersecretion leading to peptic symptoms and ulcerations is controlled with H_2 antagonists and proton pump inhibitors. Diarrhea is difficult to manage, and H_2 antagonists are generally not effective. Anticholinergics may give partial relief. In patients with severe malabsorption, systemic steroids have been shown to be effective. Ascites is also difficult to manage. One patient with portal hypertension was successfully managed with a portacaval shunt. Another patient with exudative ascites was treated successfully with systemic steroid therapy.

Patients with mastocytosis and an associated hematologic disorder are treated as dictated by the specific hematologic abnormality. In mast cell leukemia, chemotherapy has not yet been shown to produce remissions. Chemotherapy has no place in the treatment of indolent mastocytosis. A recent study suggested that splenectomy may improve survival in patients with poor prognostic forms of mastocytosis.

PROGNOSIS. Prognosis must be addressed separately for each category of mastocytosis. One study found seven variables that were strongly associated with poor survival, including constitutional symptoms, anemia, thrombocytopenia, abnormal liver function tests, lobated mast cell nucleus, a low percentage of fat cells in the

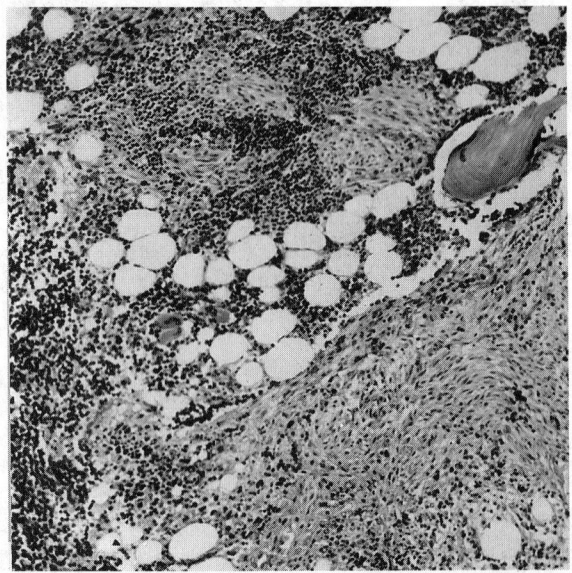

FIGURE 280–2 ■ Bone marrow biopsy shows a characteristic lesion of systemic mastocytosis with a nodular, paratrabecular infiltrate of mast cells.

bone marrow biopsy, and an associated hematologic disorder. Other poor prognostic variables include the absence of urticaria pimentosa, male gender, absence of skin and bone symptoms, hepatomegaly, splenomegaly, and normal bone radiographic findings.

As a group, patients with indolent mastocytosis and skin involvement alone have the best prognosis. Among children with isolated urticaria pigmentosa, at least 50% improve by adulthood. Adults with urticaria pigmentosa usually progress gradually to systemic disease and may rarely convert to type II disease. Diffuse cutaneous mastocytosis is usually associated with indolent systemic disease. Patients with mastocytosis and an associated hematologic disorder have a variable course, depending on the prognosis of their hematologic disorder. With mast cell leukemia, mean survival is less than 6 months. Survival with lymphadenopathic mastocytosis and eosinophilia is 2 to 3 years without therapy. The prognosis appears to improve with aggressive symptomatic management.

Cherner JA, Jensen RT, Dubois A, et al: Gastrointestinal dysfunction in systemic mastocytosis: A prospective study. Gastroenterology 95:657, 1988. *Describes patterns of gastrointestinal disease in mastocytosis and the implications for clinical management.*

Garriga MM, Friedman MM, Metcalfe DD: A survey of the number and distribution of mast cells in the skin of patients with mast cell disorders. J Allergy Clin Immunol 82:425, 1988. *A study of the value of determining mast cell numbers in skin biopsies.*

Lawrence JB, Friedman BS, Travis WD, et al: Hematologic manifestations of systemic mast cell disease. A prospective study of laboratory and morphologic features and their relation to prognosis. Am J Med 91:612, 1991. *An excellent review of the histopathologic and clinical features of mastocytosis.*

Mican JM, Di Bisceglie AM, Fong T-L, et al: Hepatic involvement in mastocytosis: Clinicopathologic correlations in 41 cases. *Hepatology* 22:1163, 1995. *A survey of liver histopathology in mastocytosis.*

Nagata H, Worobec AS, Oh CK, et al: Identification of a point mutation in the catalytic domain of the proto-oncogene c-kit in the peripheral blood mononuclear cells of patients with mastocytosis. Proc Natl Acad Sci U S A 92:10560, 1995. *Initial report of a mutation in c-kit in patients with mastocytosis and aggressive disease.*

Schwartz LB, Sakai K, Bradford TR, et al: The α form of human tryptase is the predominant type present in blood at baseline in normal subjects, and is elevated in those with systemic mastocytosis. *J Clin Invest* 96:2702, 1995. *Demonstration of mast cell tryptase in the serum of mastocytosis patients.*

281 DISEASES OF THE THYMUS

Max D. Cooper ■ *Barton F. Haynes*

NORMAL DEVELOPMENT AND FUNCTION. The essential role of the thymus is to generate clonally diverse T lymphocytes that can recognize a vast array of foreign proteins presented as peptides on host cells. An essential parallel thymic function is eliminating self-reactive T-cell clones that could damage normal tissue.

The embryonic thymus is formed initially from epithelial cells lining the 3rd and 4th pharyngeal pouches. These specialized epithelial cells migrate through the neck region to form bilateral thymic lobes in the upper anterior mediastinum. The epithelial thymus begins to attract hematopoietic stem cells from the circulation around the 8th week of fetal life. Within the epithelial thymus these precursor cells are influenced to proliferate and differentiate along T-lymphocyte lines. This lifelong process begins in the outer cortex of the thymus and the immature thymocytes migrate toward the medullary region as they proliferate and mature. Cortical regions of the lobules that collectively form the bilateral thymic lobes thus become filled with immature T lymphocytes, the extraordinary clonal diversity of which is manifested by differences in their T-cell receptor (TCR) specificities. Each developing T cell is selected for survival or death depending on the affinity of its receptor for self-peptides, which are presented initially on the surface of cortical epithelial cells. As maturing thymocytes approach the corticomedullary junction, they encounter macrophages or dendritic cell immigrants that can also present peptide fragments of antigenic proteins. Thymocytes that fail to receive any TCR-mediated signal are programmed to die. Immature thymocytes also receive a death signal if their TCR has relatively high affinity for a self-peptide, whereas moderate affinity for a self-peptide selects for survival. Only 1% or so of the thymic T cells survive this selection

process to seed the peripheral lymphoid tissues. After binding to dendritic cells and macrophages via TCR/major histocompatibility complex (MHC) interactions, thymocytes that are negatively selected become sensitive to death signals delivered by *fas* molecules (CD95) and undergo *apoptosis* (a term for programmed cell death). Mouse strains defective in fas expression (MRL/lpr) or fas ligand (gld/gld) have large thymuses and lymph nodes and defective negative selection of thymocytes and are prone to autoimmune syndromes. A molecule important for positive thymocyte selection is the oncogene product *bcl-2*. High levels of expression of bcl-2 in thymocytes promote cell survival by conferring resistance to programmed cell death.

Thymocytes also possess an array of non-TCR cell-surface glycoproteins that they use to interact with their environment. Progression of thymocyte maturation can be conveniently monitored by the expression of CD4 and CD8 molecules. The most immature thymocytes lack detectable CD4 and CD8. Intermediate-stage thymocytes express both CD4 and CD8; these double-positives predominate in the thymic cortex. Clonal selection occurs during this stage of differentiation, and the CD4 and CD8 molecules play key roles in the selection process. The peptide fragments of antigenic proteins are presented within the α-helical grooves of MHC class II and class I molecules. CD4 has an affinity for MHC class II molecules on specialized antigen-presenting cells, whereas the CD8 molecules can bind class I molecules present on all nucleated cells. The CD4 or CD8 molecules thus serve as coreceptors in the positive clonal selection, which leads to the development of either mature CD4+ cells with helper potential or CD8+ T cells with cytotoxic potential. Most of the positively selected helper or cytotoxic T cells exit the thymus via the small blood vessels in the corticomedullary region and via thymic lymphatics. The cellular debris of dying thymocytes undergoes phagocytosis by cortical and medullary macrophages, many of which migrate to epithelial cell swirls of terminally differentiated epithelium called *Hassall's bodies* located in the thymic medulla. Thymic function can be monitored throughout life by a surrogate marker for recent thymic emigrants in the circulation, namely the levels of DNA excision circles that are created in the thymus during TCR V(D)J gene rearrangements.

The lymphoid thymus reaches its maximal size of approximately 30 g by around age 1, and it gradually decreases in size thereafter to 3 g or less in most older individuals. Because the thymus-derived T-cell clones may have lifespans of several decades, normally there is little need for constant thymic replenishment. Nevertheless, thymocyte differentiation persists throughout life, albeit usually at low levels, which may vary according to an individual's hormonal balance and need for T-cell replenishment.

CENTRAL AND PERIPHERAL THYMIC COMPARTMENTS. The thymus can be thought of as a chimeric organ composed of a central lymphoid compartment that lies within the true epithelial thymus and a peripheral lymphoid compartment located in the extrathymic perivascular space (Fig. 281–1). At birth the thymic epithelial component is filled with developing thymocytes, whereas the thymic perivascular space contains only vessels and scattered peripheral lymphoid and myeloid cells (Fig. 281–1A). From early childhood onward the thymic perivascular space begins to accumulate peripheral lymphoid and myeloid cells, as well as gradually increasing numbers of mature adipose cells (Fig. 281–1B). The aging process within the thymus leads to progressive atrophy of the true epithelial thymus, loss of peripheral cells within the thymic perivascular space, and eventual filling of the perivascular space with adipocytes (Fig. 281–1C). An appreciation of the central and peripheral compartmentalization of the thymus and the age-related changes in these compartment is essential for the interpretation of disease-related alterations in thymic histology and function.

DEVELOPMENTAL DEFECTS OF THE THYMUS. *DiGeorge syndrome,* also called the 3rd and 4th pharyngeal pouch syndrome, features hypoplastic thymus and parathyroid development in addition to facial and cardiac abnormalities, which may include a ventricular septal defect and aortic abnormalities. DiGeorge syndrome occurs in both males and females, a majority of whom may have submicroscopic deletions of chromosome 22q11. The initial clinical manifestations are neonatal seizures secondary to hypocalcemia or cyanosis and other signs of cardiac insufficiency. Immunodeficiency is a later manifestation, the severity of which depends on the

The Newborn Thymus

The Adolescent Thymus

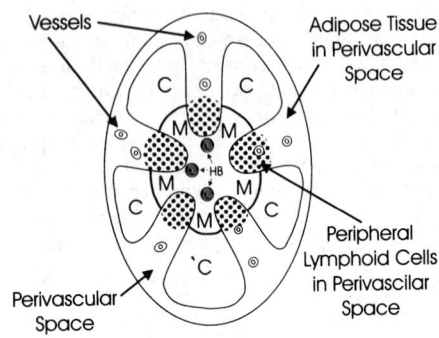

The Geriatric Thymus

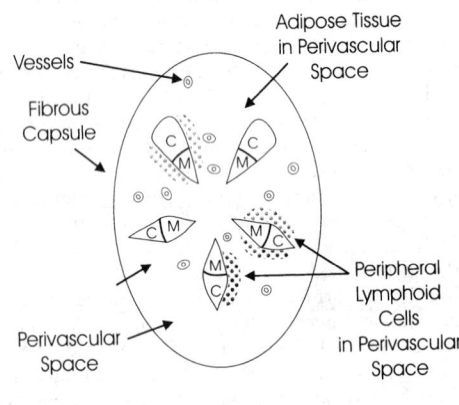

The Thymus in Myasthenia Gravis

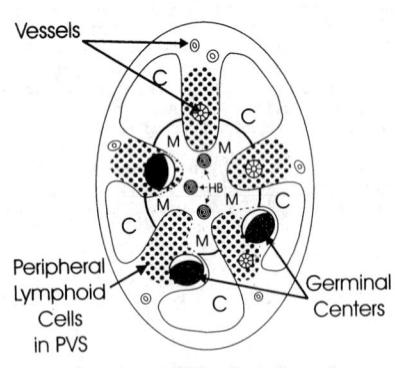

The Thymus in Early AIDS

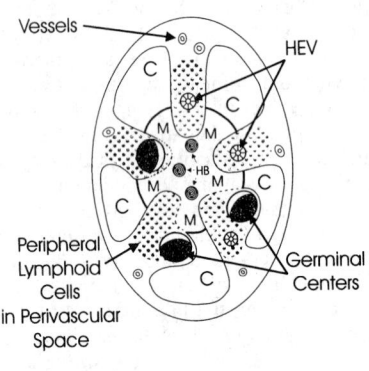

The Thymus in Late AIDS

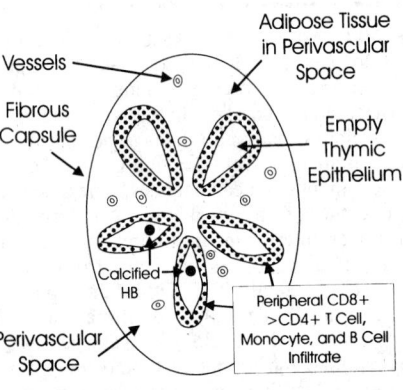

FIGURE 281–1 ■ Morphology of the human thymus during normal aging and in myasthenia gravis and HIV infection. Panels *A, B,* and *C* show schematic representations of a thymic lobule at birth (*A*), during adolescence and young adulthood (*B*) and in old age (*C*). At birth, the epithelial thymus contains most of the thymus tissue, and the perivascular space has only vessels and scattered peripheral lymphoid and myeloid cells (*A*). From age 5 to approximately age 25 the thymic perivascular space normally contains infiltrations of peripheral T and B cells and macrophages, as well as foci of adipocytes (*B*). As thymic atrophy progresses, the perivascular space fills up with adipocytes, peripheral immune cells decrease, and the true epithelial thymus lobes shrink in volume (*C*). Panels *D, E,* and *F* show schematic representations of the human thymus in myasthenia gravis (*D*), early HIV infection (*E*), and late HIV infection (*F*). The changes seen in myasthenia gravis are similar to those seen in early HIV infection and include germinal center formation in the thymic perivascular space, as well as perivascular space expansion of peripheral lymphoid and myeloid infiltrations (*D* and *E*). In late HIV infection, the true epithelial thymus can be depleted of developing thymocytes and is surrounded by large cellular infiltrates containing peripheral B cells, macrophages, and CD8+ cytotoxic effector T cells (*F*). (From Haynes BF, Hale LP: The human thymus: A chimeric organ comprised of central and peripheral lymphoid components. Immunol Res 18:175, 1998.)

degree of thymic hypoplasia. Most affected individuals have a small ectopic but functionally normal thymus that can seed T cells to the periphery in numbers that may or may not be sufficient for immune defense. In rare instances, affected infants have no detectable thymus or peripheral T cells, and thymic transplantation must be considered in these cases. Thymic grafts and all blood products given to these patients need to be rigorously depleted of donor T cells by high-dose irradiation or other means because of the threat of lethal graft-versus-host disease.

Ataxia-telangiectasia is a hereditary disorder in which thymic hypoplasia and variable T-cell deficiency are seen in association with oculocutaneous telangiectasia and truncal ataxia (see Chapter 272).

ACQUIRED ABNORMALITIES OF THYMIC FUNCTION. THYMIC HYPERPLASIA. Striking variability in thymic size can occur in apparently normal adults. The physiologic basis for thymic enlargement may include hormonal influences on thymopoietic activity. Pituitary hormones that can enhance thymic growth include growth hormone, luteinizing hormone, and follicle-stimulating hormone, whereas thyrotropin may inhibit thymic growth. Interleukin-7 (IL-7), a product of thymic stromal cells, is an important thymocyte growth factor. Other locally produced factors, including epithelial growth factor and transforming growth factor α, may regulate thymic epithelial cell production of cytokines that can affect T-cell proliferation, such as IL-1 and IL-6. Thymic enlargement can occur in adults without demonstrable pathology and rarely in patients with thyrotoxicosis or Addison's disease or following orchidectomy.

THYMIC INVOLUTION. Thymic involution is a well-known consequence of stressful illnesses, including severe infections, burns, and other conditions that result in elevated levels of adrenal corticosteroids. The involution is due to the relative susceptibility of immature thymocytes to lysis by corticosteroids of endogenous or exogenous origin. Temporary thymic involution also occurs as a consequence of irradiation or treatment with cytotoxic drugs. Thymic involution is a physiologic consequence of pregnancy and elevated levels of estrogen.

MYASTHENIA GRAVIS AND THE THYMUS. Myasthenia gravis is characterized by muscle weakness attributable to an autoimmune response against acetylcholine receptors (see Chapter 511). Improvement in this disease is frequently observed after thymectomy, thus implying a causal link between the thymus and the autoreactive T- and B-cell clones. Germinal center formation is seen in the thymic perivascular space of most patients with myasthenia gravis, and the morphology of the thymus in myasthenia is very similar to that seen in early human immunodeficiency virus (HIV) infection (Fig. 281–1*E* and *F*). Thymic B cells make anti–acetylcholine receptor antibodies. However, the precise reason why thymectomy works in the treatment of myasthenia gravis is not known because after thymectomy, serum anti–acetylcholine receptor antibody levels frequently do not decrease. Thymic epithelial tumors (thymomas) are diagnosed in approximately 10% of individuals with myasthenia gravis.

INFECTION. HIV infection can affect thymic function by several mechanisms. First, thymocyte maturation can be diminished because of infection of activated CD4+, chemokine receptor 5–bearing (CCR5+) developing thymocytes. Second, thymic myeloid cells, such as macrophages and dendritic cells, also express CD4 and CCR5 and are infectable by HIV. Third, macrophages, B cells, and CD8+ cytotoxic effector T cells migrate into the thymic perivascular space, with the formation of perivascular space germinal centers (Fig. 281–1*F*) and eventual migration of CD8+ cytotoxic T cells into the true epithelial thymus. Peripheral perivascular space CD4+ cells (mature T cells as well as macrophages) and developing thymocytes within the true epithelial thymus become infected with HIV. Active thymocyte development decreases over time in HIV-induced acquired immune deficiency syndrome (AIDS), which can result in empty thymic epithelium encased in CD8+ cytotoxic T-cell infiltrates (Fig. 281–1*F*).

Thus the capacity for production of CD4+ T cells is severely compromised in both pediatric and adult HIV-infected patients and may eventually be lost entirely. Consequently, severe immunodeficiency may occur relatively early in congenital HIV infection. In contrast, in adults, the peripheral pool of memory T cells becomes well established by adolescence. The extraordinary regenerative capacity of peripheral T cells in adults is temporarily able to compensate for the accelerated rate of T-cell death induced by HIV. After an average of 8 to 10 years, however, HIV infection can destroy the generative peripheral (lymph node and spleen) and central (thymus) microenvironments, and CD4+ T-cell lymphopenia with severe immunodeficiency and full-blown AIDS results (see Chapter 408).

THYMECTOMY. Removal of the thymus after the peripheral lymphoid compartments have been seeded with T-cell clones may have no discernible effects for many years, presumably because T-cell clones normally have very long lifespans. Thymectomy is rarely complete, moreover, in part because approximately 30% of individuals have extramediastinal thymic rests. Nevertheless, the potential need for thymic function later in life dictates careful consideration before undertaking thymectomy.

THYMOMA. The term *thymoma* is usually reserved for thymic epithelial cell tumors which, although rare, are the most commonly diagnosed tumors of the anterior superior mediastinum. Thymomas are frequently associated with myasthenia gravis. They also occur in rare individuals with acquired hypogammaglobulinemia who stop producing B-lineage cells; bone marrow insufficiency in these individuals may also extend to the erythroid and myeloid lineages.

The diagnosis of thymoma is suggested when these associated conditions occur or when an anterior mediastinal mass is detected, which may be an incidental finding because approximately one third of affected individuals are asymptomatic. Others with thymoma may have chest pain, dysphagia, signs of tracheal impingement, or superior vena cava obstruction. The extent of the tumor mass can be estimated by imaging procedures, but accurate diagnosis depends on obtaining thymic tissue for histologic assessment. Even when an adequate sample is available, the diagnosis may be difficult, however. No reliable markers for neoplastic epithelial clones are known, and thymomas are rarely composed of obviously neoplastic epithelial cells. Instead, they are usually formed by a mixture of apparently normal lymphoid thymocytes and epithelial cells that are either spindle shaped or ovoid. Consequently, the most reliable prognostic indication is evidence for or against invasiveness by the epithelial tumor. For this reason, direct tumor visualization by thoracotomy is favored for both diagnosis and treatment. In the case of well-encapsulated thymomas, tumors rarely occur after surgical removal. When the thymoma has invaded the capsule or surrounding tissue, surgical removal and irradiation or intensive chemotherapy may prevent 5-year recurrences in more than half of affected patients.

OTHER TUMORS OF THE THYMUS. Lymphomas. Thymic involvement may be a prominent feature in lymphoblastic neoplasms of T-cell origin. Hodgkin's disease, usually of the nodular sclerosing type, may primarily affect the thymus. Histiocytic lymphomas may also be manifested as an anterior mediastinal mass in adults.

Carcinoid Tumors. (See Chapter 245) Carcinoid tumors rarely arise in the thymus: those associated with elevated levels of adrenocorticotropic hormone–like hormones and Cushing's syndrome (approximately one third) are particularly invasive. Complete excision may be curative.

Germ Cell Tumors. Germ cell tumors occur rarely in the thymus but include seminoma, teratoma, embryonal cell carcinoma, and choriocarcinoma.

Douek DC, McFarland RD, Keiser PH, et al: Changes in thymic function with age and during the treatment of HIV infection. Nature 396:690, 1998.

Haynes BF, Hale LP, Weinhold KJ, et al: Analysis of the role of the adult thymus in reconstitution of peripheral T lymphocytes in human immunodeficiency virus type I infection. J. Clin Invest 103:453, 1999. *Describes the relationship of the true thymic epithelial component of the thymus to the perivascular space peripheral infiltrates of CD8+ cytotoxic T cells in HIV-infected thymus. This paper also describes HIV infection in previously thymectomized adults.*

Haynes BF, Hale LP: The human thymus: A chimeric organ comprised of central and peripheral lymphoid components. Immunol Res. 18:175, 1998. *A review of the status of the thymus in normal development, myasthenia gravis, and HIV-1 infection.*

Mackall CL, Hakim FT, Gress RE: T cell regeneration: All repertoires are not created equal. Immunol Today 18:245, 1997. *An excellent review of the respective roles of the thymus and peripheral immune microenvironments in maintaining T-cell immunity.*

Steinmann GG: Changes in the human thymus during aging. Curr Top Pathol 75:43, 1986. *Classic paper describing the normal morphogenesis and function of the thymus during aging.*

PART XXI

MUSCULOSKELETAL AND CONNECTIVE TISSUE DISEASES

282 APPROACH TO THE PATIENT WITH MUSCULOSKELETAL DISEASE

Duncan A. Gordon

Diseases of the musculoskeletal system are common, disabling, and costly to the economy. This chapter provides a guide for approaching patients with musculoskeletal symptoms by outlining the components necessary for identifying the patient's problems, formulating the diagnosis, and initiating treatment.

The pain, stiffness, and joint swelling of musculoskeletal disorders may be inflammatory, metabolic, degenerative, or combinations thereof. For the patient, however, it is the functional interference with daily activities that determines the impact of the condition. The value of a general medical approach to patients with musculoskeletal complaints is paramount, and specialized assessment should be kept in perspective. At times, a limited work-up may suffice, whereas in other instances, assessment by a number of laboratory, imaging, and other disciplines may be necessary. Before clinical approaches are considered, it is helpful to review the anatomy and pathophysiology of the structures affected.

ANATOMY. Knowledge of the anatomic structures will answer the question "Where is the lesion?" In the case of musculoskeletal diseases, the joints are primarily affected. The structures that may be involved are shown in Figure 282–1 *(top),* the articular structures of the musculoskeletal system. Foremost is the joint cavity and lining membrane known as the synovium. Hyaline cartilage overlying the bony end-plates provides the lubricating surface for the joint. An intact bony end-plate is required to support the cartilage. The joint capsule and ligaments provide further support and blend with the periosteum.

The non-articular anatomy of the musculoskeletal system is equally important (see Fig. 282–1, *top*) and includes local structures such as tendons, bursae, or muscles associated with various joint regions or, more generally, the collagen, elastin, and ground substance known as the connective tissue system. These latter tissues are so widespread that any organ system of the body may be involved.

PATHOPHYSIOLOGY. After determining which anatomic structures of the musculoskeletal system are involved, one must answer the question "What is the lesion?" The usual pathology is either inflammatory, metabolic, degenerative, or some combination thereof (see Fig. 282–1, *bottom*). Joint neoplasms are exceptional. With inflammatory disorders such as rheumatoid arthritis (RA) or septic arthritis, the joint cavity and synovial membrane are primarily affected, whereas with degenerative conditions such as osteoarthritis, the cartilage is primarily affected. Cartilage loss may also be secondary to synovial inflammation or trauma. Metabolic crystal deposition disorders such as gout or pseudogout also cause articular inflammation, whereas avascular necrosis of bone is associated with cartilage damage after bony end-plate collapse. Moreover, the same pathologic processes may affect extra-articular systems such as skin, muscle, and vasculature.

ROLE OF THE CLINICIAN. HISTORY. The interview should provide a detailed chronology of the illness; anatomic location of the pain, whether local or referred; its occurrence with activity, rest, or sleep; type of onset, whether sudden or insidious; the pattern of joint involvement, symmetrical or not and whether predominantly the upper or lower limbs; influence of previous and current treatments; systemic symptoms such as fatigue, weight loss, fever, and duration of morning stiffness; an up-to-date account and systematic review of all the joints of the body; and a psychosocial history. A non-restorative sleep pattern may be associated with morning stiffness and other diffuse aching. Symptoms should be interpreted in terms of the patient's functional ability to perform self-care and other daily activities. General weakness and fatigue reflect the presence of many musculoskeletal conditions affecting the patient's body as a whole and not just the joints.

FUNCTIONAL DISABILITY INDICES. A number of self-report questionnaires such as the Stanford Health Assessment Questionnaire, Functional Disability Index, Arthritis Impact Measurement Scales, or modifications of these instruments have been developed for ongoing evaluation of patients with arthritis (Table 282–1). These instruments document the patient's functional status with results comparable to traditional measures of joint disease activity such as tender joint count, radiographic joint erosion score, and erythrocyte sedimentation rate.

DEMOGRAPHY. An appreciation of the age, gender, marital status, and occupation of the patient is helpful. The age of the patient is relevant to developmental and heritable disorders of connective tissue. For example, arthritis is a major manifestation of hemophilia with onset during childhood. Juvenile RA refers to polyarthritis coming on before 16 years of age. In young adults, seropositive, seronegative, and septic arthritic conditions may arise, whereas osteoarthritis is exceptional. The onset of RA is the middle years, whereas the elderly are more prone to osteoarthritis. RA and the collagen diseases are more common in women, whereas ankylosing spondylitis and the other HLA-B27 spondyloarthropathies are more common in men. Gouty arthritis is more common in men and rarely attacks women before menopause. Arthritis in the elderly is often assumed to be degenerative, when in fact the patient may suffer from an inflammatory process such as polymyalgia rheumatica, RA, or systemic lupus erythematosus. Occupation is also important because of associated physical and psychological stresses. The clinician should find out exactly what the patient does to determine how demanding the job is. Occupational factors are important with repetitive joint trauma in individuals susceptible to osteoarthritis. Symptoms may be associated with jogging or trauma from sports activities.

PHYSICAL EDUCATION. Because many musculoskeletal/rheumatic disorders are systemic, physical examination may document the presence of extra-articular features. In RA these features include subcutaneous nodules, digital vasculitis, and other systemic findings described in Chapter 286. Any of these findings may be mistaken for a non-rheumatic condition, and their presence may indicate more ominous disease. Any number of systemic features may be the result of an adverse drug reaction. The joints shown in Figure 282–2 should be examined systematically to determine whether any are inflamed or damaged. The pattern of joint involvement, whether symmetrical, axial, or peripheral, should be recorded on the diagram.

JOINT INFLAMMATION. Key signs are tenderness and swelling. These signs may be associated with local heat, but erythema is not a feature of rheumatoid inflammation, whereas tenderness, heat, and erythema may be seen with septic or gouty arthritis. A joint is considered *active* if it is tender on pressure or passive movement with stress. Joint swelling may be periarticular or intra-articular. The latter is associated with a joint effusion detected by showing fluctuation (Fig. 282–3). It is important to note the difference between *tender joints* and deep referred *tender points* characteristic of a non-articular syndrome known as "fibromyalgia" (see Chapter 306).

JOINT DAMAGE AND DESTRUCTION. Damage and destruction of joints may be assessed clinically or radiologically. Common observations include loss of range of movement, collateral instability, malalignment, subluxation, or cartilage loss causing bone-on-bone crepitus. A separate count of damaged joints should be recorded, as with actively inflamed joints.

DIAGNOSIS. Clinical evaluation enables us to establish which musculoskeletal structures are inflamed, which are damaged, and

how function is impaired. Nine specific types of musculoskeletal involvement can be identified as a framework for considering various diagnostic possibilities or hypotheses (see Fig. 282–1, *bottom*). The nine categories presented in the following paragraphs are listed in Table 282–2, along with typical diseases, examples of laboratory tests, and treatment. Table 282–2 and the descriptions below provide the basis for more detailed information contained in the following chapters of this section.

SYNOVITIS. Inflammation of the synovial membrane lining of the joint is typical of inflammatory polyarthritis such as RA. If the synovitis is persistent, irreversible joint damage results. The polyarthritis of RA is like that found in the diffuse connective tissue diseases associated with autoantibodies. These autoimmune colla-

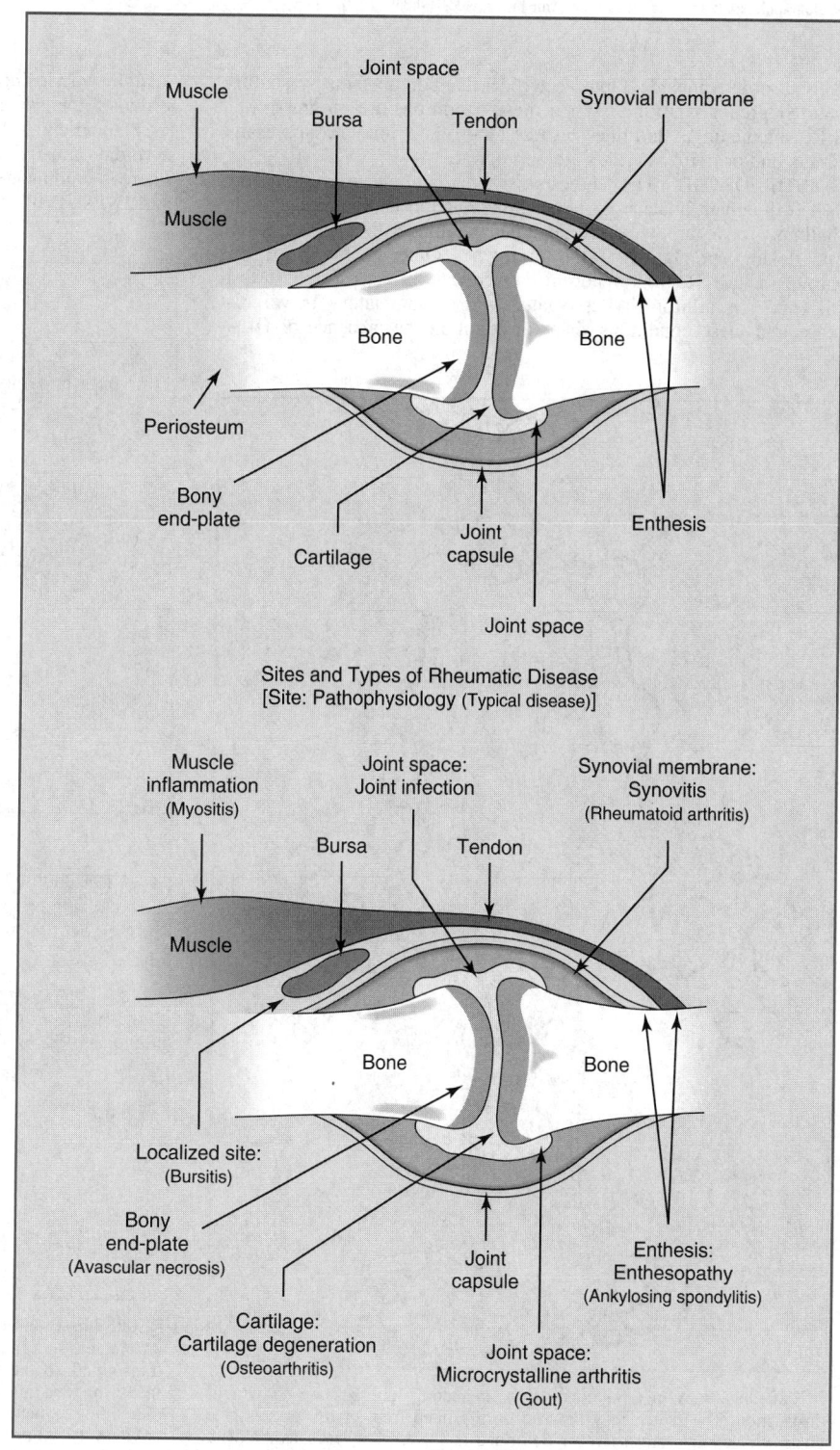

FIGURE 282–1 ▪ *Top,* Anatomic structures of the musculoskeletal system. *Bottom,* Location of musculoskeletal disease processes.

Table 282–1 ■ **SELF-REPORT QUESTIONNAIRE FOR ARTHRITIS**

Please check (√) the ONE best answer for your abilities.

At this moment, you are able to:	WITHOUT ANY DIFFICULTY	WITH SOME DIFFICULTY	WITH MUCH DIFFICULTY	UNABLE TO DO
a. Dress yourself, including tying shoelaces and doing buttons?				
b. Get in and out of bed?				
c. Lift a full cup or glass to your mouth?				
d. Walk outdoors on flat ground?				
e. Wash and dry your entire body?				
f. Bend down to pick up clothing from the floor?				
g. Turn regular faucets (taps) on and off?				
h. Get in and out of a car?				

Reproduced with permission from Pincus T, Callahan LF, Brooks RH, et al: Self-report questionnaire scores in rheumatoid arthritis compared with traditional physical, radiographic, and laboratory measures. Ann Intern Med 100:259, 1989.

gen disorders include lupus, scleroderma, polymyositis, vasculitis, and Sjögren's syndrome. When these conditions are progressive or life threatening, 2nd-line disease-modifying immunosuppressive drugs and/or corticosteroids are appropriate.

ENTHESOPATHY. The enthesis is the anatomic transition zone where ligament attaches to bone. Inflammation in this region is the hallmark of a family of seronegative rheumatic diseases, of which ankylosing spondylitis is the prototype. Other members of this group include Reiter's syndrome, reactive arthritis, psoriatic arthritis, and the arthropathy associated with inflammatory bowel disease. All these conditions share in common the presence of HLA-

B27. In ankylosing spondylitis, the sacroiliac joints and apophyseal joints of the spine show characteristic inflammation with a tendency to bony ankylosis. An exercise program along with non-steroidal anti-inflammatory drugs (NSAIDs) is usually effective, whereas prednisone is rarely needed.

CRYSTAL-INDUCED SYNOVITIS. Crystals of monosodium urate,

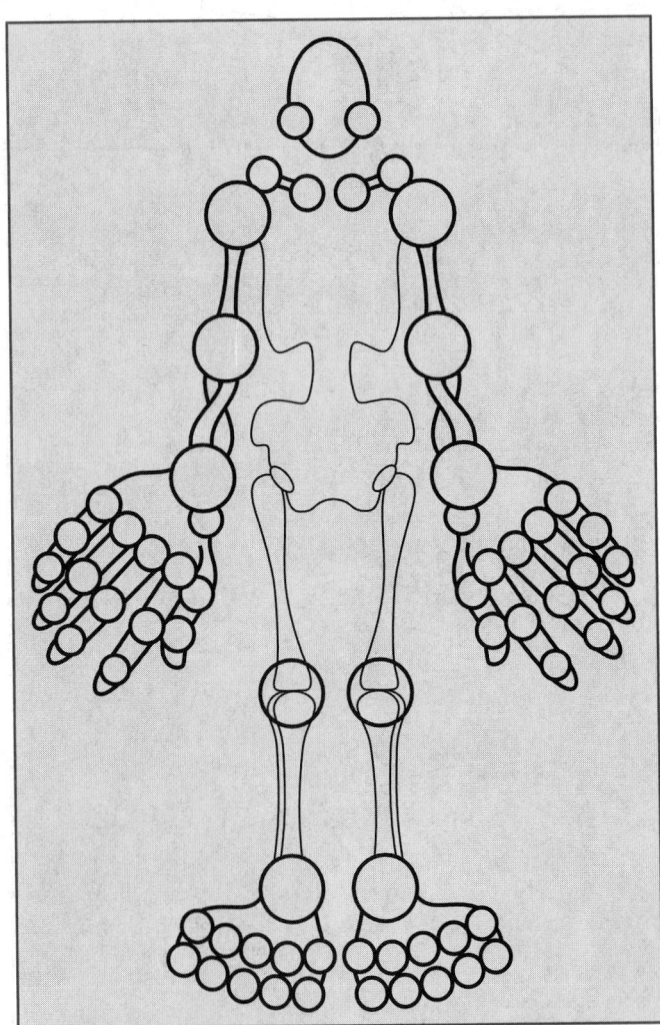

FIGURE 282–2 ■ A pictorial method for indicating joint disease activity or destruction. The sketch may be used on a printed form or rubber stamp to chart which joints are active or deformed at the time of each assessment. (Courtesy of Dr. Hugh A. Smythe, Toronto.)

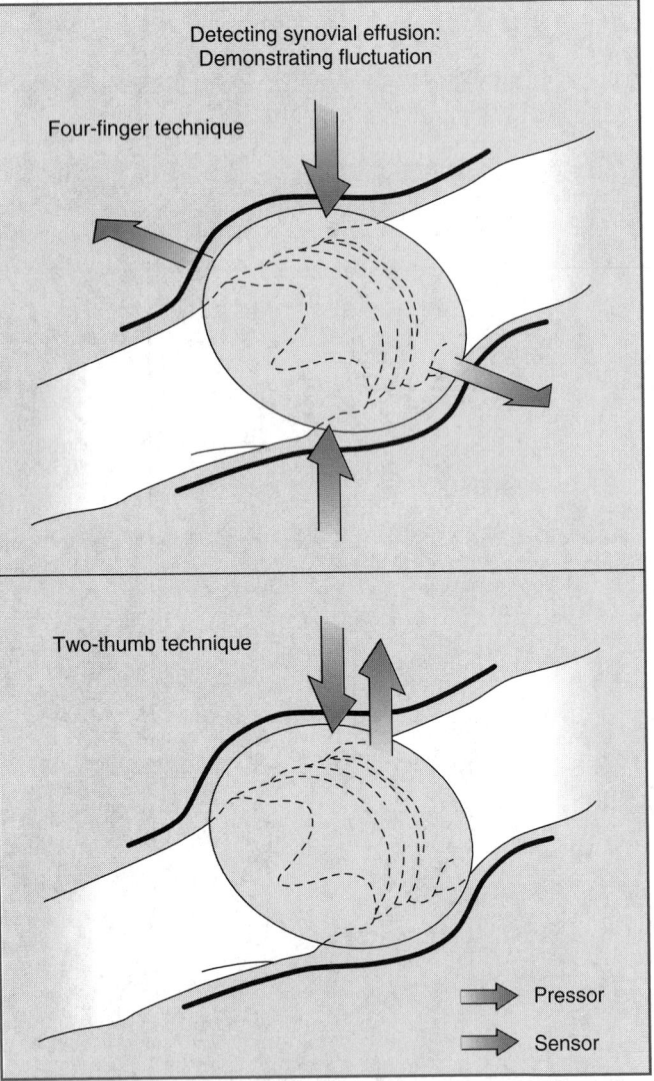

FIGURE 282–3 ■ Demonstration of fluctuation for detecting synovial effusion. An increase in fluid tension induced by finger pressure in one area is transmitted so that the sensor fingers can detect it elsewhere. In the two-thumb or four-finger technique, the pressure should be in a slightly different direction to the sensor finger to avoid false-positive results. (Reprinted courtesy of Klippel JH, Dieppe PA: Rheumatology, 2nd ed. Mosby, London, 1998, section 5, p 3.7.)

Table 282-2 ■ CLASSIFICATION OF RHEUMATIC DISEASE

CATEGORY	PROTOTYPES	USEFUL TESTS	TREATMENTS
Synovitis	Rheumatoid arthritis	Latex, erythrocyte sedimentation rate	Methotrexate
	Autoimmune collagen diseases	ANA test	Prednisone
Enthesopathy	Ankylosing spondylitis	Sacroiliac radiographs	Indomethacin
	HLA-B27 spondyloarthropathies		
Crystal-induced synovitis	Gout	Joint fluid crystal examination	Indomethacin
	Pseudogout	Radiographic chondrocalcinosis	Indomethacin
		Joint fluid crystal examination	
Joint space disease	Septic arthritis	Joint fluid culture	Antibiotics
Cartilage degeneration	Osteoarthritis	Radiographs of affected area	Physical therapy
			Analgesics
Osteoarticular disease	Avascular necrosis bone	Radiographs, magnetic resonance imaging	Prosthetic joint replacement
Polymyositis	Dermatomyositis	Muscle enzymes, EMG, muscle biopsy	Corticosteroids
	Inclusion body myositis		
Local conditions	Tendinitis	None, radiographs of affected area	Local
General conditions	Fibromyalgia	Erythrocyte sedimentation rate	Fitness exercises

ANA = antinuclear antigen; EMG = electromyogram.

calcium pyrophosphate, or hydroxyapatite are capable of inducing an acute inflammatory reaction in synovial fluid and joint lining. Although inflammation from these crystals may clear spontaneously, treatment with NSAIDs is effective. Crystal arthritis usually affects only one or at most a few joints at a time. Joint fluid aspiration and synovianalysis for crystals with polarized light microscopy will establish the diagnosis. Calcium pyrophosphate deposition disease is often associated with the radiologic appearance of chondrocalcinosis of hyaline cartilage.

JOINT SPACE. Septic arthritis may develop from hematogenous spread of microorganisms into the joint space. This condition is associated with intense pain even at rest, and the diagnosis is confirmed by joint aspiration and Gram stain and culture of synovial fluid. A joint prothesis increases susceptibility to infection in that joint. Although systemic antibiotics are usually sufficient, arthroscopic débridement and surgical drainage may be required.

Blood in the joint space, known as "hemarthrosis," may result from microfractures, coagulopathy, or tumor.

CARTILAGE DEGENERATION. Loss of articular cartilage with bony repair leading to the formation of osteophytosis is known as osteoarthritis. It should be considered a final pathway for persistent inflammatory conditions such as RA, ankylosing spondylitis, septic arthritis, and metabolic disorders with chondrocalcinosis. Joint hypermobility and previous trauma are other mechanical factors that may predispose to osteoarthritis. Although hereditary osteoarthritis may affect the distal interphalangeal joints of the fingers, it usually involves only one or two larger joints such as a hip or knee. For this reason, osteoarthritis disability can be more readily controlled by physical or orthopedic measures than can the disability associated with RA. Although NSAIDs and analgesics may provide pain relief, they are largely palliative.

OSTEOARTICULAR CONDITIONS. Avascular necrosis results after collapse of the bony end-plate from vascular insufficiency. The consequence is collapse and fragmentation of cartilage. Avascular necrosis may be idiopathic or associated with systemic conditions such as sickle cell disease or fatty liver after high-dose corticosteroids. Osteopenia/osteoporosis may complicate many rheumatic conditions and is dealt with in Chapter 257.

Inflammation of the periosteum, known as "periostitis," may be associated with hypertrophic pulmonary osteoarthropathy and clubbing. This syndrome may be a clue to underlying lung cancer.

POLYMYOSITIS. Inflammation and weakness of the proximal skeletal muscles are characteristic of polymyositis; with rash, it is called dermatomyositis. Elevated creatine kinase, electromyographic abnormalities, and histologic abnormalities of muscle biopsy specimens are characteristic. Corticosteroids and immunosuppressives may control polymyositis, but older patients with dermatomyositis may have hidden malignancy and steroid resistance.

LOCAL CONDITIONS. Non-articular disorders such as tendinitis, bursitis, and neck and low back strains are common problems. Local signs of inflammation are characteristic of these conditions and usually respond to physical therapy, protective splints, or injection of corticosteroids.

GENERAL CONDITIONS. Non-articular or extra-articular disorders are not usually associated with arthritis. This group includes polymyalgia rheumatica, sympathetic reflex dystrophy, and fibromyalgia. Polymyalgia rheumatica affects the elderly and causes persistent neck, shoulder, and hip pain, chronic fatigue, and a high erythrocyte sedimentation rate. Sometimes it is associated with underlying giant cell and temporal arteritis. In the latter case, corticosteroids are mandatory because of the risk of blindness from ophthalmic arteritis.

"Fibromyalgia" refers to a common syndrome of widespread polyarthralgias associated with chronic fatigue and a non-restorative sleep pattern. It is characterized by the presence of deep referred tender points, described in Chapter 306.

TREATMENT. Therapy should be based on a correct diagnosis, which may not be initially obvious (see Table 282–2). Also important is whether the patient's problem is urgent or whether treatment can be postponed until the diagnosis is established. For example, acute monarthritis secondary to sepsis or gout requires immediate attention, whereas widespread smouldering polyarthritis does not. However, a patient with polyarthritis who is systemically ill requires prompt investigation to exclude a diffuse connective tissue disease, underlying infection, or hidden malignancy.

Regardless of the diagnosis, educating the patient and family is crucial to successful management of any chronic musculoskeletal illness. An informed patient is more likely to comply with treatment and hold realistic expectations of outcome. For patients with musculoskeletal disease, the goal of management is to control pain and maintain independence. For this reason, treatment should be individualized and based on early identification of problems, a firm diagnosis, and continued monitoring of response to treatment.

Gordon DA, Inman RD: Musculoskeletal disability and rheumatology. J Rheumatol 21: 387, 1994. *This editorial draws attention to the frequency, types, risk factors, and economic impact of musculoskeletal disorders in the general population.*

Klippel JH (ed): Primer on the Rheumatic Diseases, 11th ed. Atlanta, Arthritis Foundation, 1997. *Classic, authoritative, current descriptions of all rheumatic diseases and of all rheumatology, available as a public service at nominal cost.*

Pincus T, Callahan LF, Brooks RH, et al: Self-report questionnaire scores in rheumatoid arthritis compared with traditional physical, radiographic, and laboratory measures. Ann Intern Med 100:259, 1989. *Illustrates the value of self-report questionnaires in providing quantitative data that reflect traditional disease activity measures in arthritis patients.*

283 CONNECTIVE TISSUE STRUCTURE AND FUNCTION

Steffen Gay ■ Renate E. Gay

One of the fundamental characteristics of all connective tissues is the relatively large proportion of extracellular matrix in relation to cells. Until recently, the extracellular matrix was viewed as a passive framework serving mainly as an inert scaffolding for stabilization of the physical structure of tissues. In addition to maintaining this three-dimensional form during morphogenesis and tissue repair, it is now recognized as a dynamic milieu in which cells become organized, exchange signals, and differentiate. In this regard, the composition of the extracellular matrix determines the gradients of diffusible cytokines and thereby modulates pivotal biologic processes such as proliferation, differentiation, and apoptosis. Study of these processes has led to the discovery of a plethora of new matrix components, matrix receptors, and cell-matrix interactions. The extracellular matrix is composed of multidomain macromolecules that are linked together by covalent and non-covalent bonds to form a highly intricate composite. Two major types of matrices exist: the *interstitium,* which is synthesized by mesenchymal cells and forms the stroma of organs, and the *basement membranes,* which are produced by epithelial and endothelial cells. These matrices comprise four major classes of extracellular macromolecules: (1) collagens, (2) elastin, (3) non-collagenous glycoproteins, and (4) glycosaminoglycans, which are usually covalently linked to proteins to form proteoglycans.

COLLAGENS. The collagens are the most abundant class of proteins in the human organism and constitute almost 30% of the body's total protein. The central feature of all collagen molecules is the stiff structure resulting from lengthy domains of triple-helical conformation. Three polypeptide chains called α-chains are wound around one another to generate a rope-like fold. An absolute requirement for the formation of this triple helix, as well as the most distinctive feature of the α-chains, is the presence of lengthy sequences of repeating Gly-X-Y triplets in which the X and Y positions are frequently occupied by prolyl and hydroxyprolyl residues.

Studies based on protein chemistry and complementary DNA (cDNA) sequencing have revealed a genetically determined heterogeneity with as many as 19 homopolymeric or heteropolymeric collagen types. They all share a triple-helical segment of variable length (100 to 450 mm) but differ considerably in the size and nature of their globular domains. It is of interest that 33 genes coding for the different chains are distributed mostly on different chromosomes in the human genome (Table 283–1). Even simultaneously expressed genes, such as those coding for the two $\alpha_1(I)$

and one $\alpha_2(I)$ chains of the heteropolymeric type I molecule, are located on different chromosomes.

Functional diversity of the various collagen types is accomplished by the formation of distinct extracellular aggregates. The most obvious are the interstitial linear polymers of fibrils derived from collagen types I, II, and III. These fibrils have characteristic banding patterns and can be readily visualized by electron microscopy. Type I collagen fibers are found in supporting elements of high tensile strength (e.g., tendon and cornea), whereas fibers formed from type II collagen molecules are restricted to cartilaginous structures. The fibrils derived from type III collagen are prevalent in more distensible tissues such as blood vessels and parenchymal organs. In addition, collagen types V, VI, IX, and XII are also involved in fiber formation, but largely as adducts. This finding is illustrated by the association of collagen types IX, X, and XI with type II collagen in hyaline cartilage. Knockout experiments of the $\alpha_1(IX)$ gene in transgenic mice indicate that a lack of functional type IX collagen results in the development of a mild chondrodysplasia and osteoarthritis in these animals. Adaptation for a special function is shown by type VII collagen molecules, which aggregate as antiparallel overlapping dimers to form the anchoring fibrils required to stabilize the dermoepithelial junction of the skin. In contrast to the interstitial types of collagen, type IV molecules form large polygonal aggregates fulfilling the structural and support requirements of basement membranes.

ELASTIN. Elastic fibers are composed of two morphologically and structurally distinct components: elastin and the microfibrils. Elastin, whose gene has now been characterized, is an insoluble protein polymer. The biosynthetic precursor of elastin, tropoelastin, is a linear polypeptide composed of about 700 amino acids and is rich in non-polar amino acids: glycine (>30%), valine, leucine, isoleucine, and alanine. Tropoelastin is synthesized by vascular smooth muscle cells and skin fibroblasts and subsequently incorporated into elastic fibers. Elastic fiber formation involves lysyl oxidase–mediated formation of intermolecular cross-links, called *desmosine* and *isodesmosine.* Because these cross-links do not exist in other proteins and are therefore elastin specific, determination of these two amino acid derivatives in a tissue sample reflects the amount of elastin present. The microfibrillar components of interstitial elastic fibers are not fully characterized. However, disulfide-rich glycoproteins such as *fibrillin* and *microfibril-associated glycopro-*

Table 283–1 ■ POLYMORPHISM OF THE COLLAGEN TYPES

TYPE	CHAIN(s)	MAJOR MOLECULAR SPECIES	MAJOR DISTRIBUTION
I	$\alpha_1(I)$ $\alpha_2(I)$	$[\alpha_1(I)]_2\alpha_2(I)$	Skin, tendon, bone, organ capsules
II	$\alpha_2(II)$	$[\alpha_1(II)]_3$	Hyaline cartilage
III	$\alpha_1(III)$	$[\alpha_1(III)]_3$	Blood vessels, parenchymal organs
IV	$\alpha_1(IV)$ $\alpha_2(IV)$ $\alpha_3(IV)$ $\alpha_4(IV)$ $\alpha_5(IV)$	$[\alpha_1(IV)]_2\alpha_2(IV)$	Basement membranes
V	$\alpha_1(V)$ $\alpha_2(V)$ $\alpha_3(V)$	$[\alpha_1(V)]_2\alpha_2(V)$	Smooth muscle associated with type I
VI	$\alpha_1(VI)$ $\alpha_2(VI)$ $\alpha_3(VI)$	$[\alpha_1(VI),\alpha_2(VI),\alpha_3(VI)]$	Minor collagen of stroma matrices
VII	$\alpha_1(VII)$	$[\alpha_1(VII)]_3$	Anchoring fibrils of the dermoepidermal junction
VIII	$\alpha_1(VIII)$	$[\alpha_1(VIII)]_3$	Descemet's membrane, sclera, dura mater
IX	$\alpha_1(IX)$ $\alpha_2(IX)$ $\alpha_2(IX)$	$[\alpha_1(IX),\alpha_2(IX),\alpha_3(IX)]$	Hyaline cartilage
X	$\alpha_1(X)$	$[\alpha_1(X)]_3$	Hypertrophic cartilage
XI	$\alpha_1(XI)$ $\alpha_2(XI)$ $\alpha_1(II)$	$[\alpha_1(XI),\alpha_2(XI),\alpha_3(XI)]$	Hyaline cartilage
XII	$\alpha_1(XII)$		Tendons, ligaments, periosteum, skin, cartilage
XIII	$\alpha_1(XIII)$		Skin, gut
XIV	$\alpha_1(XIV)$/undulin		Bone marrow, placenta
XV	$\alpha_1(XV)$		Fibroblasts, myoblasts
XVI	$\alpha_1(XVI)$		Placenta, fibroblasts, smooth muscle cells
XVII	$\alpha_1(XVII)$		BP180 autoantigen in bullous pemphigoid
XVIII	$\alpha_1(XVIII)$/endostatin		Collagen/heparan sulfate, proteoglycan of basement membranes
XIX	$\alpha_1(XIX)$		Vascular, neuronal basement membrane zone

tein have been identified and may serve as a scaffold onto which tropoelastin is deposited.

STRUCTURAL GLYCOPROTEINS. The major non-collagenous glycoprotein present in the extracellular matrix is *fibronectin*. Fibronectins are dimeric cell adhesion glycoproteins composed of two disulfide-bonded subunits and found in rather large quantities in blood plasma (~0.3 mg/mL). The functions of fibronectin in cell adhesion are illustrated in Figure 283–1. Some of these functions can be mimicked by synthetic peptides that contain the sequence Arg-Gly-Asp (RGD sequence). Similar sequences are found in other cell adhesion proteins such as vitronectin, laminin, and collagen type VI. Because fibronectin plays a major role in morphogenesis and tissue remodeling, regulation of fibronectin biosynthesis by growth factors and cytokines has been studied. For example, it is established that interferon-γ and transforming growth factor β (TGF-β) stimulate fibronectin synthesis, whereas tumor necrosis factor and interleukin-1 inhibit synthesis.

Vitronectin is a 75-kd protein that is considerably smaller than the 250-kd fibronectin polypeptide present in plasma and tissue. Vitronectin, also termed "serum spreading factor" and "complement S-protein," promotes cell attachment and spreading, inhibits cytolysis by the complement C5b–9 complex, and modulates antithrombin III–thrombin action in blood coagulation.

The *thrombospondins* consist of three or five disulfide-bonded subunits that, comparable to fibronectin, contain a number of distinct domains with specific binding sites for macromolecules occurring at cell surfaces or in extracellular matrices. The gene family comprises at least five members. Thrombospondin-1 has been shown to modulate cell attachment, migration, and proliferation.

Tenascin is another large glycoprotein of the extracellular matrix. The previous other name *hexabrachion* refers to its disulfide-linked six-armed structure. Tenascin mediates cell attachment through an RGD-dependent receptor and is expressed in association with mesenchymal-epithelial interactions during morphogenesis and development of undifferentiated tumors. The same protein has also been referred to as myotendinous antigen, GP 250 protein, glial mesenchymal extracellular matrix protein, cytotactin, J1-protein, and brachionectin. Gene knockout experiments suggest that tenascin might be a superfluous non-functional protein and that other tenascin-like proteins, such as major histocompatibility complex (MHC)-tenascin encoded in the human MHC class III regions, may compensate for the absence of tenascin.

The leucine-rich repeat proteins constitute an important group of matrix proteins. They have a major central domain with consecutively repeated, leucine-rich sequence motifs folded into a regular pattern in which several short "β-sheet" structures are aligned to expose a surface well suited for protein-protein interactions. *Decorin, biglycan, fibromodulin,* and *lumican* are four widely distributed leucin-rich repeat proteins. All four of them are recognized as small interstitial proteoglycans (see below). Their special leucin-rich repeat protein structure is involved in binding to collagens, as well as to the different variants of TGF-β.

CARTILAGE GLYCOPROTEINS. A number of structural glycoproteins have been isolated from various types of cartilage. The 550-kd cartilage oligomeric matrix protein *COMP*, which is made up of five identical subunits, is particularly abundant in articular cartilage. It shows sequence homology to members of the thrombospondin family and is also called thrombospondin-5. Mutations in the calcium-binding domain of COMP have been found in cases of pseudoachondroplasia or multiple epiphyseal dysplasia. The symptoms of these skeletal dysplasias arise either because of the lack of a structurally important protein within the extracellular matrix or because of abnormal retention of protein inside the chondrocyte with effects on cellular metabolism. Other cartilage matrix components are the 58-kd protein PRELP and the 36-kd protein chondroadherin, both of which are leucin-rich repeat proteins with a potential to interact with cell-surface macromolecules. A 148-kd cartilage matrix protein leucin-rich repeat is prominent in tracheal cartilage and growth cartilage but not present in normal articular cartilage.

PROTEOGLYCANS. Proteoglycans are proteins that carry one or more glycosaminoglycan side chains. Glycosaminoglycans are long, unbranched polysaccharide chains composed of repeating disaccharide units. One of the two sugar residues in the repeating disaccharide is always an amino sugar (*N*-acetylglucosamine or *N*-acetylgalactosamine). Glycosaminoglycans are highly negatively charged owing to the presence of sulfate and carboxyl groups on multiple sugar residues. Hyaluronic acid, also called *hyaluronan* is an exception among the glycosaminoglycans because this polymer of glucuronic acid and glucosamine is not sulfated and not attached covalently to a protein core connected via a link protein. Proteoglycans of almost all sizes and shapes have been biochemically identified. However, because cloning and sequence analysis have often identified the same core proteins, the number of distinct proteoglycans is limited (Table 283–2). With respect to their function, they have been referred to as a "multipurpose glue." Proteoglycans not only tie extracellular matrix components together and mediate cell binding to the matrix but also serve fundamental roles in binding water and restrain soluble molecules such as growth factors in the matrix and at cell surfaces. Heparan sulfate proteoglycan, for example, binds basic fibroblast growth factor released from injured endothelial cells. The role of proteoglycans in cell adhesion is best exhibited by a membrane-intercalated proteoglycan termed *syndecan*. This molecule binds to collagen and fibronectin through its heparan sulfate chains and mediates cell adhesion. Certain proteoglycans contain functional domains that are common for all members of the aggrecan/versican family. These domains share further functional domains with other important proteins and include an immunoglobulin-like, epidermal growth factor (EGF)-like, and complement regulatory protein–like sequence.

BASEMENT MEMBRANES. Basement membranes are thin, sheet-like structures deposited by endothelial and epithelial cells but also found surrounding nerve and muscle cells. They provide mechanical support for resident cells, function as a semipermeable filtration barrier for macromolecules in organs such as the kidney and the placenta, and act as regulators of cell attachment, migration, and

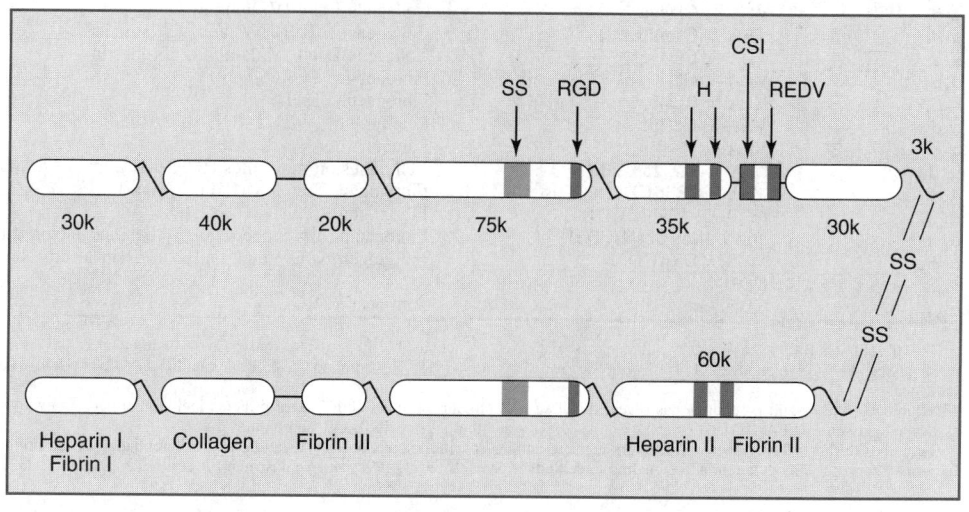

FIGURE 283–1 ■ Multiple cell recognition sites in fibronectin. The fibronectin molecule contains a series of functional domains that bind the indicated ligands. The thick vertical bars indicate cell adhesive recognition sequences. SS = putative synergistic second site; RGD = Arg-Gly-Asp site; H = putative sites in the heparin-binding domain; CS1 = the CS1 site in the alternatively spliced IIICS region; REDV = the Arg-Glu-Asp-Val site. (Reprinted with permission from Yamada KM: Fibronectins: Structure, functions and receptors. Curr Opin Cell Biol 1:956, 1989. Copyright 1989 by Current Science.)

Table 283–2 ■ STRUCTURAL FEATURES OF PROTEOGLYCANS

LOCATION	PROTEOGLYCAN	GAG (NUMBER)
Extracellular matrix	Aggrecan	CS/KS (>100)
	Versican	CS/DS (20)
	Decorin	CS or DS (1)
	Biglycan	CS or DS (2)
	Fibromodulin	KS (4)
	Lumican	KS (4)
	Epiphycan	CS or DS (1)
Cell surface	Syndecan	HS/CS (4)
	Betaglycan	HS/CS (2)
	CD44	HS or CS
	Glypican	HS
	Fibroglycan	HS
Intracellular	Serglycin	CS or Hep (8)
Basement membrane	Perlecan	HS (3)
	Bamaecan	CS
	Agrin	HS
Brain	Brevican	CS/DS (3)
	Neurocan	CS (7)
	Cerebroglycan	HS (5)
	Phosphaecan	CS (4)

GAG = Glycosaminoglycan; CS = chondroitin sulfate; KS = keratan sulfate; DS = dermatan sulfate; HS = heparan sulfate; Hep = heparin.

differentiation. The major constituents are collagen type IV, laminin, nidogen (entactin) and heparan sulfate proteoglycans. Collagen type IV molecules are $[\alpha_1(IV)]_2 \; \alpha_2(IV)$ heterotrimers consisting of an N-terminal rod 30 μm long (7S), a linear triple helix containing over 20 non-collagenous sequences, and a C-terminal globular domain (NCl). These molecules can spontaneously aggregate into a network consisting of N-terminal tetramers (7S), lateral associations between the triple-helical rods, and C-terminal dimers (NCl). The network is eventually stabilized by disulfide- and lysyl oxidase–derived intramolecular and intermolecular cross-links, which may provide the scaffold for basement membrane formation. Self-assembly has also been observed with *laminin,* a major basement membrane–associated glycoprotein. The typical features of the laminin molecule are a thread-like long arm terminating in a globular domain and three short arms, each consisting of two globular domains separated by short linear segments. The different laminins (1 to 11) serve in very specialized basement membranes such as the dermo-epidermal and myotendinous junctions. Collagen type IV and laminin appear to be highly integrated in the basement membrane matrix and are closely associated with nidogenes-1 and -2 in a stable non-covalent complex. Amino acid sequence data of nidogen have revealed EGF-like cysteine-rich motifs, segments showing homology to the EGF precursor, the low-density lipoprotein receptor, and

thyroglobulin. *Heparan sulfate proteoglycans* occur as an integral component in all basement membranes but play different roles in specific tissues. They control permeability of the glomerular basement membranes and have also been implicated in the anchorage of acetylcholinesterase to the neuromuscular junction.

CONNECTIVE TISSUE MATRIX IN CELL REGULATION

It is well established that matrix components influence the maintenance of cellular phenotypes mediated through matrix receptors.

RECEPTORS FOR EXTRACELLULAR MATRIX COMPONENTS. Adhesive interactions between cells and their surrounding extracellular matrix are not only important in most developmental events but also essential for maintaining fundamental life processes. Cell proliferation, polarization, migration, differentiation, and protein synthesis depend on interactions between cells and supporting matrix. Diverse families of structurally similar receptors for matrix components have been identified and include the transmembrane integrin superfamily, peripheral membrane glycoproteins, glycosyltransferases, and proteoglycans. *Integrins* are a group of α/β-heterodimers involved in cell binding, some of which involve recognition of an RGD sequence present in their ligands. Integrins consist of an α-subunit with a molecular mass of 130 to 210 kd and non-covalently associated β-subunits (95 to 130 kd). The cytoplasmic domain of the β-subunit reveals homologies to EGF, the insulin receptor, and the *neu* oncogene protein. Both subunits define the integrin subfamilies described in Table 283–3.

Because integrins localize in known junctional regions where actin bundles and myofibrils terminate at the cell surface, the major function of integrin receptors appears to be the linkage of extracellular matrix molecules with the intracellular cytoskeletal network. The connection is thereby mediated through the cytoplasmic domain of the subunits. That extracellular matrix components may influence gene expression by signal transduction is shown by the finding that fibronectin degradation products induce, via the fibronectin receptor, collagenase and stromelysin gene expression. The latter pathway may play a major role in inflammatory tissue destruction. The pivotal role of these receptors related to infectious diseases is further illustrated by the observation that bacteria use specific receptors to adhere to host connective tissue. For example, it has been shown that certain strains of *Escherichia coli* express a fibronectin receptor that is involved in colonization.

The most provocative question remains: How do matrix receptors transmit information from the extracellular structure to affect gene expression? Figure 283–2 illustrates a model of "dynamic reciprocity," in which the extracellular matrix is postulated to influence gene expression at all levels, including transcription, messenger RNA processing, and translation, via transmembrane and cytoskeletal components. Elucidating the molecular mechanisms of this message system remains one of the key challenges in cell biology.

Table 283–3 ■ THE INTEGRIN FAMILY OF CELL RECEPTORS*

SUBUNITS	DESIGNATION	LIGANDS	DISTRIBUTION
$\alpha_1\beta_1$	VLA-1; CD49a	Collagens I and IV, laminin	F, BM, aT
$\alpha_2\beta_1$	VLA-2; CD49b	Collagens I, III, IV, V, and VI, laminin	F, En, Ep, aT, Pl
$\alpha_3\beta_1$	VLA-3; CD49c	Collagens I and IV, laminin, fibronectin	F, Ep
$\alpha_4\beta_1$	VLA-4; CD49d	Fibronectin, VCAM-1	F, Nc, T, B, M
$\alpha_5\beta_1$	VLA-5; CD49e	Fibronectin (RGD)	F, En, Ep, aT, Th
$\alpha_6\beta_1$	VLA-6; CD49f	Laminin	En
$\alpha_7\beta_1$	VLA-7	Laminin	En
$\alpha_L\beta_2$	LFA-1; CD11a/CD18	Cell adhesion molecules (ICAM-1, 2, 3)	T, B, M, G
$\alpha_M\beta_2$	Mac-1; CR3; CD11b/CD18	Fibrinogen, Factor X, C3bi, ICAM-1	M, G
$\alpha_X\beta_2$	p150,95; CD11c/CD18	Fibrinogen, C3bi	M, G
$\alpha_{IIb}\beta_3$	gpIIb, IIIa; CD41/CD61	Fibronectin, fibronogen, von Willebrand factor, thrombospondin	Pl
$\alpha_V\beta_3$	VNR; CD51/CD61	Fibrinogen, von Willebrand factor, vitronectin, thrombospondin	En
$\alpha_6\beta_4$	CD104	—	Ec
$\alpha_V\beta_5$	CD51	Vitronectin (RGD)	Ca

F = fibroblasts; BM = basement membrane–associated; aT = activated T lymphocytes only; En = endothelial cells; Ep = epithelial cells; Pl = platelets; Nc = neural crest melanocytes; T = T lymphocytes; B = B lymphocytes; M = monocytes; Th = thymocytes; G = granulocytes; Ca = UCLA-P3 lung adenocarcinoma cells; RGD = Arg-Gly-Asp sequence.

*Cloning of the α- and β-subunits has revealed cell surface proteins on other cells. These proteins include the very late activation (VLA) antigens and the lymphocyte function–associated antigen 1 (LFA-1)/Mac-1/p 150,95 on leukocytes and the platelet IIb/IIIa glycoprotein.

Data from Springer TA: Adhesion receptors regulate antigen-specific interactions, localization, and differentiation in the immune system. Prog Immunol 7:121, 1989; Hynes RO: Integrins: Versatility, modulation, and signaling in cell adhesion. Cell 69:11, 1992; and Schlossman SF et al: CD antigens 1993. J Immunol 52:1, 1994.

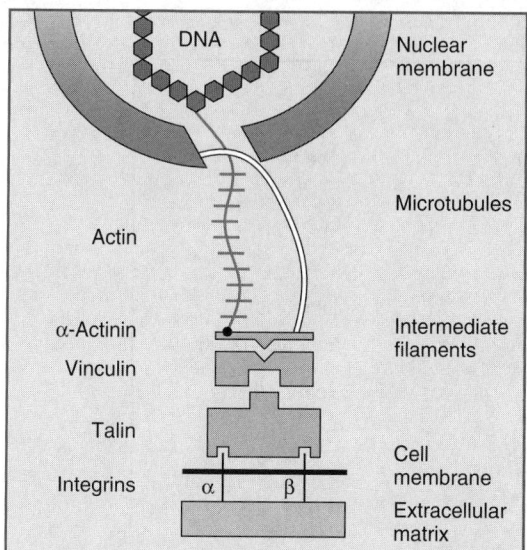

FIGURE 283-2 ■ This refined model of the ultrastructural interaction of cells with extracellular matrix is based on a model of "dynamic reciprocity" whereby the extracellular matrix is postulated to exert an influence on gene expression via transmembrane proteins and cytoskeletal components: the model was originally proposed by Bissell and Carcellos-Horf (J Cell Sci Suppl 8:327, 1987).

PATHOPHYSIOLOGY OF CONNECTIVE TISSUE

Some confusion remains about the role of collagen in a variety of diseases involving connective tissue. Historically, the term "collagen disease"—describing a heterogeneous group of acute and chronic diseases, including rheumatoid arthritis, systemic lupus erythematosus, progressive systemic sclerosis, polymyositis, dermatomyositis, Sjögren's syndrome, arteritis, rheumatic fever, ankylosing spondylitis, and amyloidosis—was based on the erroneous notion that "collagen" was equivalent to "connective tissue." However, as outlined above, the different types of collagen and the macromolecular aggregates derived from them are now recognized as distinct structural and histologic entities that exist within a meticulously intercalated connective tissue matrix along with structural glycoproteins and proteoglycans. Consequently, no justification exists for using the anachronistic term "collagen disease" to encompass a group of such diseases initiated by vastly different pathomechanisms and affecting distinct connective tissue entities. The term "collagen diseases" now exclusively pertains to inherited conditions in which the primary defect has been demonstrated to be at the gene level and to affect collagen biosynthesis, post-translational modification, or extracellular processing directly. Recent technologies of gene cloning and gene analysis have led to the delineation of mutations in the fibrillar collagen genes. Collagen type I is the target of certain genetic mutations associated with classic clinical variants of dwarfing syndromes, osteogenesis imperfecta, and Ehlers-Danlos syndrome (types IV and VII) (see Chapters 201, 216, and 217). Moreover, polymerase chain reaction amplification of a series of overlapping segments encoding for the entire helical and telepeptide regions of human $\alpha_1(I)$ collagen cDNA is expected to potentially identify all mutations and polymorphisms.

The acquired disorders of connective tissue involving collagen include conditions that result in repair from overt trauma; in diseases characterized by excessive deposition of collagenous matrix, e.g., fibroproliferative disorders; or in pathologic loss of tissue matrix, including the breakdown of basement membranes in tumor invasion and rheumatoid joint destruction.

Although connective tissue repair after trauma largely depends on the type of injury and is therefore quite variable, the repair of various connective tissue lesions in wound healing follows a characteristic sequence of events. The initial events involve the synthesis of pericellular and basement membrane collagens in the proliferating epithelial and/or endothelial cells. Subsequently, a loose fibrillar network largely consisting of fibronectin, collagen types III and V, and single interspersed fibers derived from type I collagen

is deposited. Finally, with the formation of scar tissue, the lesions become more fibrous and dense owing to the deposition of collagen fiber bundles derived largely from type I molecules. It is striking that the patterns of collagen deposition in fibroproliferative diseases show certain similarities. For example, liver damage is characterized by an initial accumulation of basement membrane collagens in the sinusoidal space of Disse, followed by a fine fibrillar material composed largely of type III collagen and, subsequently, in the case of the development of hepatic fibrosis (cirrhosis, see Chapter 153), by an augmented deposition of type I collagen. A similar pattern appears in the development of fibrotic plaque in atherosclerosis (see Chapter 158) or in cyclosporine-induced myocardial fibrosis in the transplanted human heart.

The major disease almost exclusively affecting the matrix of basement membranes is diabetes mellitus (see Chapter 242). The histopathologic hallmark of diabetic microvascular disease is generalized basement membrane thickening. In the kidney, these changes include an increase in glomerular basement membrane permeability, followed by decreased glomerular filtration. Evidence exists that accelerated non-enzymatic glycosylation plays an important role in the development of diabetic microangiopathy.

The loss of specialized connective tissue matrix plays a pivotal role in tumor progression and metastasis. With proliferation, malignant tumor cells acquire the capability to invade basement membranes actively and to migrate through the interstitial stroma. Despite the fact that tumor invasion requires a complex sequence of steps, such as the expression of receptors for basement membrane components by the malignant cells, invasion ultimately results in a loss of basement membrane integrity (Fig. 283-3). Severe recessive dystrophic epidermolysis bullosa features a loss of collagen type VII anchoring filaments, which normally connect the epidermal basement membrane to the interstitial matrix of the dermis. In Goodpasture's syndrome, basement membranes are damaged by circulating autoantibodies against basement membrane collagen (see Chapter 78). The Goodpasture antigen has been mapped to the C-terminal globular domain of type IV collagen, which explains the high cross-reactivity of the anti–glomerular basement membrane antibodies with alveolar basement membranes.

CONNECTIVE TISSUE MARKERS

The enormous progress in our knowledge of the structure and biology of the connective tissue matrix has caused considerable interest in the development of assays for diagnosis and monitoring of therapy in diseases involving connective tissue. Historically,

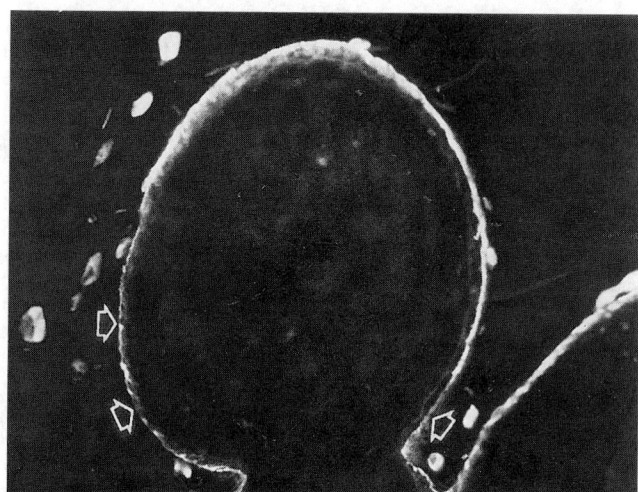

FIGURE 283-3 ■ Frozen section of carcinoma in situ of the breast stained with monoclonal antibodies against human collagen type IV and fluorescence-labeled immunoglobulin antimouse G (IgG). In contrast to other atypical hyperplastic lesions, thinning and focal loss of basement membrane integrity (arrows) are frequently observed in carcinoma in situ and suggest foci of preceding microinvasion.

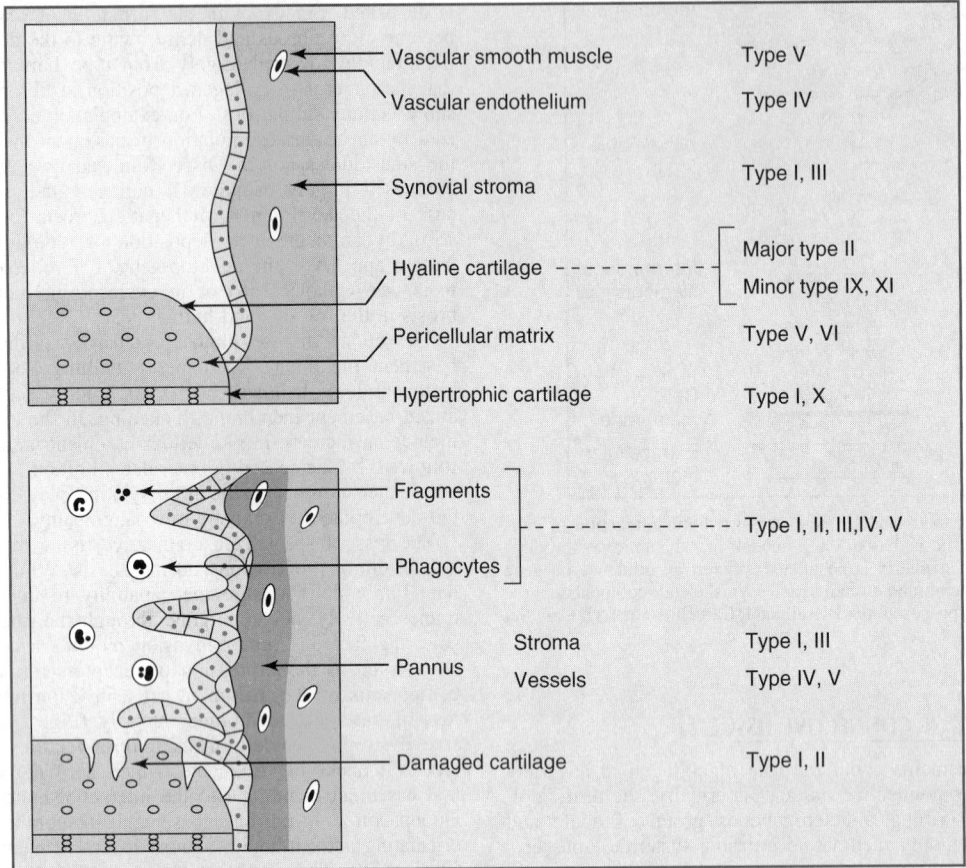

FIGURE 283–4 ■ Distribution of collagen types in a normal and rheumatoid joint. The normal synovial lining cell layer is supported by a loose fibrillar network composed of interstitial collagen types I and III but lacking a continuous basement membrane. Basement membrane collagen type IV is restricted to the vascular endothelium. Vascular smooth muscle cells and pericytes are surrounded with fine, filamentous collagen type V, which is further associated with the interstitial fibers. The vast majority of the interstitial cartilaginous matrix is derived from type II collagen. Collagen types V, IX, and XI are distinctly associated with the hyaline articular interstitium. Synovial fluid normally does not contain collagen. Therefore, detection of collagen in synovial fluid and phagocytes indicates erosive and/or inflammatory joint disease. Detection of type IV collagen suggests endothelial damage and if found concomitantly with type V collagen, implicates actual necrosis of the vessel walls, i.e. vasculitis. Detection of type I collagen indicates a high level of proteolytic breakdown of synovial stroma and/or bone matrix. Because type II collagen is restricted to cartilage, the appearance of type II collagen epitopes in synovial fluid and serum represents a sensitive indicator of cartilage destruction and may serve as a tool for monitoring the effects and side effects of antirheumatic drug therapy. (Reprinted with permission from Gay S, Gay RE: Cellular basis and oncogene expression of rheumatoid joint destruction. Rheumatol Int 9: 105, 1989.)

determination of hydroxyproline as a measure of total collagen content or turnover has been a useful technique in connective tissue research. However, with the discovery of collagen polymorphism and a variety of molecules containing collagenous sequences, measurement of hydroxyproline now appears to be of only limited value. This observation is based on the fact that different collagens have varying levels of hydroxylation. For example, the type III collagen molecule contains about 30% more hydroxyproline than does type I, and other proteins such as Clq. acetylcholinesterase, and elastin also contain hydroxyproline. Specific immunohistologic and immunoserologic assays have been used to evaluate the complexity of collagenous proteins in normal and pathologic samples. As illustrated in Figure 283–3, using a monoclonal antibody specific for collagen type IV has been advantageous in studies assessing the integrity of basement membranes in neoplastic lesions. Several markers of collagen assembly and turnover have been used to detect injury to a specific parenchymal organ or to diagnose organ fibrosis by non-invasive immunoserologic assays. The most widely applied test so far has been a radioimmunoassay to detect the N-terminal propeptide of type III procollagen in body fluids. The utility of this test was based on the notion that the propeptide is removed from type III procollagen molecules after synthesis to form new collagen fibrils. However, procollagen molecules may retain their propeptide as part of the normal extracellular matrix. Thus the presence of the propeptide in serum may be related not only to neosynthesis but also to degradation from a pre-existing matrix. Because both processes affect the results of this assay, increased levels of type III procollagen peptide have been reported in fibrotic diseases such as liver cirrhosis, myelofibrosis, and lung fibrosis and have also been correlated with destructive inflammation, such as that in acute viral hepatitis.

The development of molecular markers for joint diseases has focused on the immunochemical quantification of cartilage components by using specific antibodies. In this regard, cartilage oligomeric protein (COMP) has been studied in serum and synovial fluid from patients with various arthritides. Keratan sulfate has been assayed as a marker of cartilage metabolism, and collagen type II, as a marker of cartilage destruction (Fig. 283–4).

Aszodi A, Pfeiffer A, Wendel M, et al.: Mouse models for extracellular matrix diseases. J Mol Med 76:238, 1998. *This review article provides new insight regarding the role of extracellular matrix during development and disease.*

Brown JC, Timpl R: The collagen superfamily. Int Arch Allergy Immunol 107:484, 1995. *A concise review of new collagen types, including collagen type XIX.*

Howe A, Aplin AE, Alahari SK, Juliano RL: Integrin signaling and cell growth control. Curr Opin Cell Biol 10:220, 1998. *Concise review of the extracellular matrix–mediated regulation of integrin-cytoskeletal complexes and integrin-modulated growth factor signaling.*

Iozzo RV: Matrix proteoglycans: From molecular design to cellular function. Annu Rev Biochem 67:609, 1998. *Provides the most updated information on the structure and biologic functions of proteoglycans.*

Miller EJ, Gay S: Collagen structure and function. *In* Wound Healing—Biochemical and Clinical Aspects. Philadelphia, WB Saunders, 1992, pp 130–151. *An in-depth review of the biochemistry of the major collagens.*

284 TISSUE INJURY IN RHEUMATIC DISEASES

Gerald Weissmann

Acute inflammation and tissue injury in the rheumatic diseases are caused by host defense mechanisms that are designed to attack bacteria or viruses but instead become diverted into attacking the tissues of the host. The two major inflammatory diseases of rheumatology are rheumatoid arthritis (RA) and systemic lupus erythematosus (SLE), and we understand their pathophysiology thanks to three well-studied models of experimental pathology. Whereas some of their *acute* lesions resemble the Arthus and the Shwartzman reactions, in which neutrophils play the key role, the *chronic* features of RA mimic another model of experimental pathology, the tuberculin reaction and its late granuloma formation, in which cytokines, growth factors, and activated macrophages predominate. Joint injury and cartilage degradation result when synovial cells with activated proto-oncogenes form an invasive lesion called pannus.

THE ARTHUS LESION AS A MODEL FOR RHEUMATOID ARTHRITIS. Following the prescient observation of Magendie in 1839 that the 2nd and 3rd intravenous injections of foreign protein into rabbits were followed by increasing distress, Richet coined the word "anaphylaxis" in 1902 to describe acute catastrophes mediated by repeated intravenous injections of antigens. Arthus, in 1903, then provoked "local anaphylaxis" in rabbits by repeated injections of antigen intradermally; inflammation and necrosis resulted. Opie, in 1924, confirmed that the lesions of Arthus were local antigen-antibody reactions in which inflammation was mediated by white cells and that proteolysis was crucial. Indeed, it was found that the Arthus lesions could also be provoked by planting antigen in the skin, followed by specific antibody intravenously (the "passive Arthus reaction"), or by injecting antibody in the skin, followed by antigen intravenously (the "reversed passive Arthus reaction") (Fig. 284–1). In each case, one was dealing with the interactions at a surface of neutrophils that had been attracted by immune complexes localized beneath the endothelium of blood vessels. Complement, activated by immune complexes, releases anaphylatoxins (C5a and C3a) that liberate histamine. Histamine, in turn, causes reversible gaps to appear between endothelial cells, and once breached, the junctions permit egress of neutrophils. Stimulated by discrete receptors for C5a, C3a, and IgGs (FcγRII, FcγRIII), neutrophils release mediators of inflammation: reactive oxygen-derived products (O_2^-, H_2O_2), eicosanoids (see Chapter 29), and lysosomal enzymes. These products—especially superoxide (O_2^-), peroxide (H_2O_2), and proteases—cause irreversible tissue injury. Predictably, Arthus reactions can be abolished by rendering animals deficient in complement or in neutrophils. Antiproteases or antihistamines are somewhat less effective inhibitors of the Arthus lesion; antiplatelet agents or anticoagulants are useless. It is generally agreed that the local Arthus lesion is one model of immune complex vasculitis in humans that is also due to the interactions of neutrophils with immune complexes and complement. In generalized vasculitis of the Arthus type, the homotypic clumping of neutrophils to each other and their heterotypic sticking to endothelial cells are mediated by receptors for iC3b (CD11b/CD18), whereas the secretory responses of neutrophils are triggered by receptors for C5a and FcγRII. The central role of neutrophils in this lesion is mirrored by their abundance in the synovial fluid of patients with RA. Their role in periarteritis nodosa, leukocytoclastic vasculitis, some of the vasculitides of SLE, and allergic angiitis is equally important. Although the raison d'être for the preponderance of neutrophils in rheumatoid synovial fluid is not yet clear, their sheer number is impressive. Neutrophils represent over 90% of the cells found in the synovial fluid of patients with RA, and it has been estimated that the daily turnover of neutrophils in 30 mL of a rheumatoid joint effusion is greater than a billion cells per joint. The cells take up self-associating complexes of IgG-IgG rheumatoid factor, as well as the more common IgM/IgG complexes; complement is predictably activated. Rheumatoid vasculitis is another extra-articular problem mediated by neutrophils in seropositive RA patients.

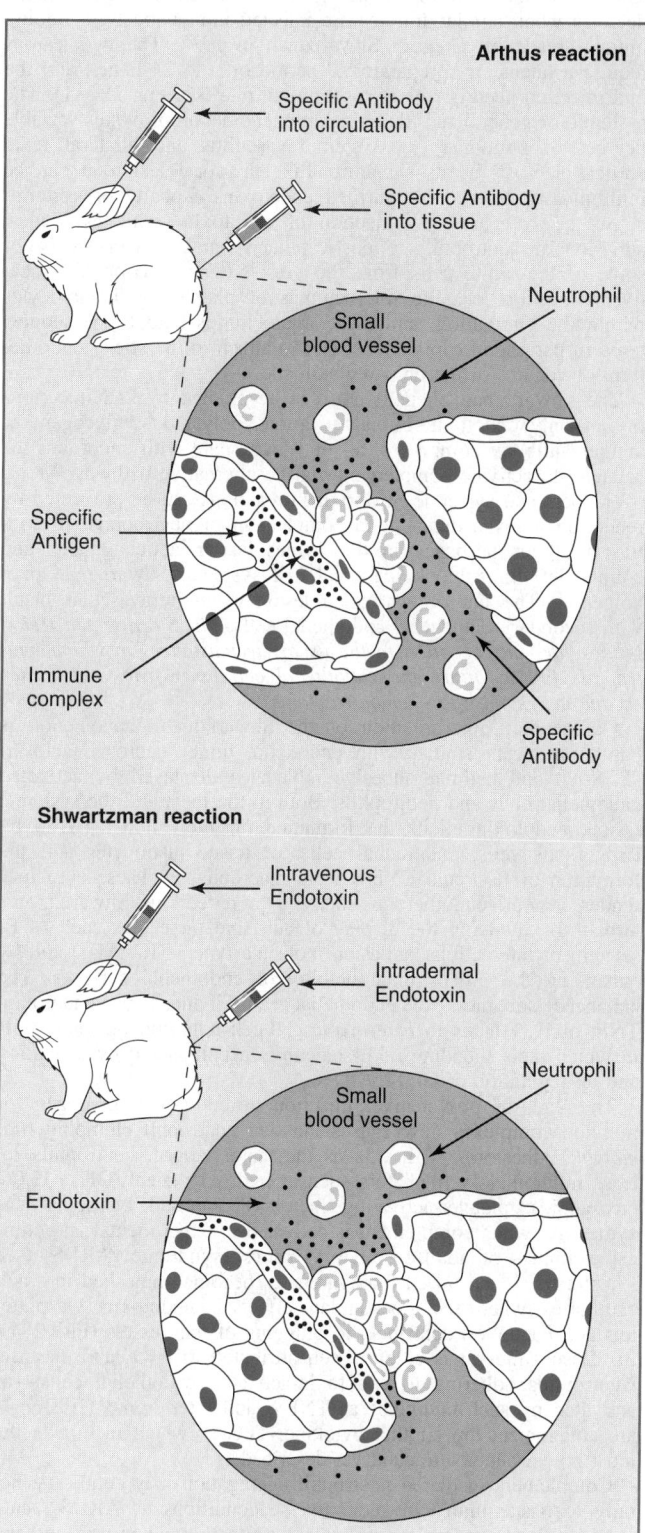

FIGURE 284–1 ■ In the Arthus model of vascular injury in systemic lupus erythematosus (*top*), intradermal injection of an antigen following intravenous injection of specific antibody leads to immune complex deposition in vessel walls at the intradermal injection site, which triggers local complement activation, inflammation, neutrophil infiltration, and tissue destruction. In the Shwartzman model (*bottom*), intradermal injection of the antigen leads to intravascular alternative pathway complement activation. Antibody is not required, and no immune complexes are formed. Instead, neutrophils, primed by endotoxin and activated by complement, aggregate within small blood vessels at the intradermal injection, plug them, and cause distal ischemia.

THE SHWARTZMAN PHENOMENON AS ANOTHER MODEL OF VASCULITIS. Culture filtrates of gram-negative bacteria injected into the skin of rabbits prepare the site for hemorrhagic necrosis when similar filtrates are injected intravenously, a finding initially made by Gregory Shwartzman in 1937. The two lesions require a latent, or "preparatory," period of 6 to 24 hours, and the 2nd injection need not be of the same filtrate (see Fig. 284–1). The systemic or generalized Shwartzman phenomenon provokes variable degrees of pulmonary or systemic vasculitis and bilateral renal cortical necrosis as its signature. Like the local lesion, it can be faithfully reproduced by purified endotoxins. Locally or systemically, the "preparatory" injection of endotoxin promotes modest adhesion of neutrophils to post-capillary venules, with escape of some of the white cells from the vessels. The 2nd, or "provocative," injection leads to microclumps of platelets and leukocytes within the circulation, and these microclumps tend to be sequestered in peripheral capillary beds or to attach to the sticky endothelium of venules of the prepared skin site.

The Shwartzman phenomenon can be elicited by 2nd injections of not only endotoxin but also various polyanions, glycogen, or antigen/antibody complexes, all of which share with endotoxin the capacity to activate complement via the alternative pathway. Moreover, local and systemic Shwartzman reactions can be prevented by rendering animals deficient in complement or neutrophils. In contrast to their inefficacy in the Arthus lesion, anticoagulants and antiplatelet drugs block the local and systemic Shwartzman phenomenon. The final Shwartzman lesion is an intravascular insult with secondary damage to endothelial cells. *The Shwartzman lesion is therefore an exception to the usual circumstances in which neutrophils fail to injure the endothelial cell layer from which they escape in response to chemoattractants.*

Our modern interpretation of the Shwartzman phenomenon is based on recent studies with endotoxin, tumor necrosis factor α (TFN-α), and cellular adhesive molecules displayed by activated endothelial cells and neutrophils. Both in the local and the systemic lesion, endotoxin elicits the formation of interleukin-1 (IL-1) by Langerhans cells, endothelial cells, or tissue histiocytes and the formation of IL-1 and TNF-α from macrophages. These cytokines render venous endothelium sticky—"prepared" in Shwartzman's terms—by inducing the display of adhesive molecules such as E-selectin or intercellular adhesion molecule type 1 (ICAM-1) and by enhancing the procoagulant activity of endothelial surfaces. The enhanced stickiness of endothelial cells induced by endotoxin, TNF, or IL-1 leads to *heterotypic* cell-cell adhesion of neutrophils in which their shedding of E-selectin is accompanied by activation and up-regulation of CD11b/CD18.

The 2nd, or provocative, injection of endotoxin, glycogen, or immune complexes now causes massive neutrophil clumping (*homotypic* adhesion). With C5a as the major culprit, neutrophils release inflammatory mediators such as hydroxl radical (OH⁻) H$_2$O$_2$, eicosanoids, platelet-activating factor (PAF), and lysosomal enzymes. As when complement is activated in experimental and clinical examples of adult respiratory distress syndrome (ARDS) (see Chapters 271 and 94), leukoaggregates become enmeshed in small capillaries, where the procoagulant effects of endotoxin (via platelets and Factor X) contribute to plugging of the vessels (Fig. 284–2). Tissue injury has chiefly been attributed to H$_2$O$_2$ and elastase. Neutrophils adhering to endotoxin-activated endothelial cells—or activated by such cytokines as TNF-α and interferon-γ (IFN-γ)—are antagonized by another cytokine, TFG-β, which in turn is the most potent chemoattractant yet described.

Complement-mediated neutrophil aggregation may contribute not only to tissue injury in such diverse conditions as ARDS, acute pancreatitis, Purtscher's retinopathy, acute thermal injury, and the extension of myocardial infarction but also—especially in SLE—to florid vascular crises. Sera from patients with active SLE contain several factors (among them C5a) that cause normal neutrophils to aggregate. Neutrophil aggregating activity correlates with the activity of the disease and is most pronounced in patients with central nervous system involvement. Levels of circulating C3a, C5a, and the C5b-9 membrane attack complex are sharply elevated in patients with active SLE. Indeed, elevated C3a levels may predict flares of SLE arising 2 months before the disease becomes clinically apparent. Moreover, the complement split products Ba and Bb

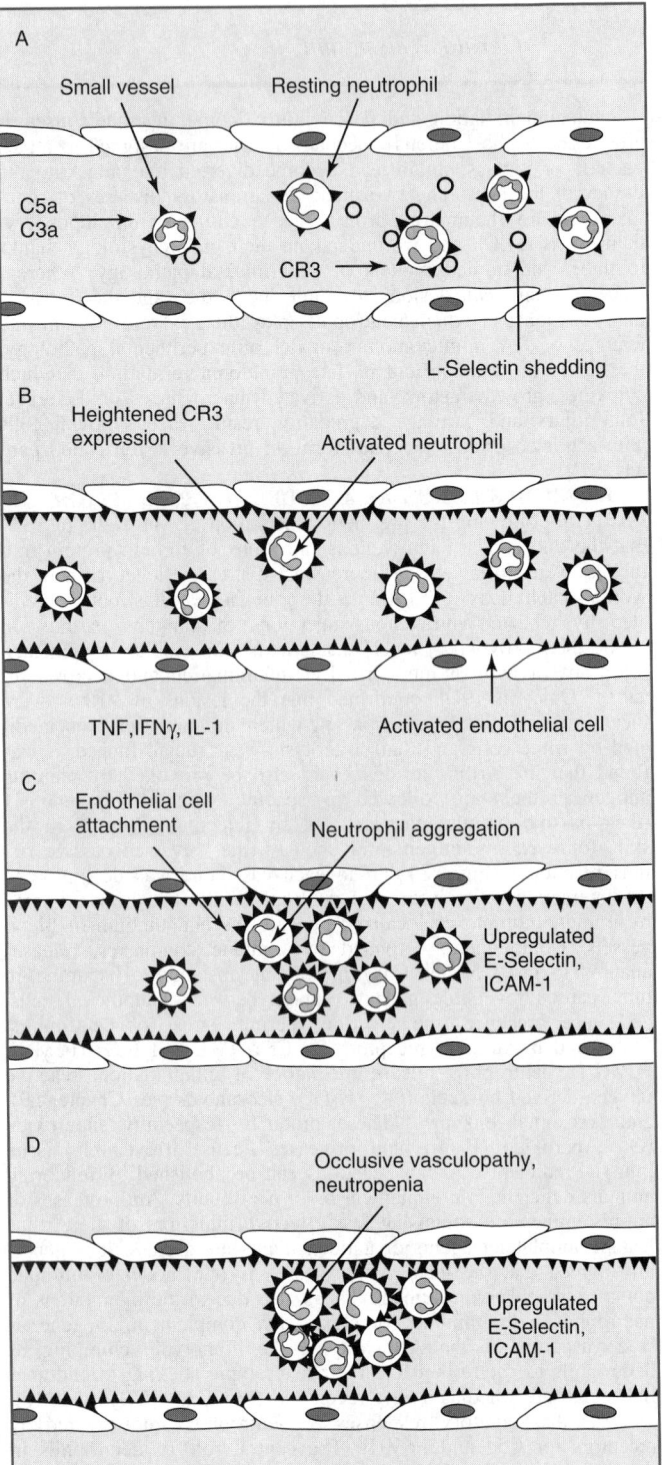

FIGURE 284–2 ■ In active systemic lupus erythematosus (SLE), the process of intravascular complement activation, complement split product release, and neutrophil activation involves C5a/C3a stimulation of neutrophil CR3 (CD11b/CD18 integrin) expression (*A* and *B*), as well as shedding of L-selectin. A hallmark of the activated neutrophil is heightened expression and activation of surface CR3, which makes the cell stickier; this change can be induced in vitro by a variety of chemoattractants, e.g., leukotriene B$_4$ and interleukin-8 (IL-8). Neutrophils with increased numbers of activated surface CR3 then aggregate and adhere to an equally activated vascular endothelium (*C*), which leads to neutropenia and occlusive vasculopathy (*D*). In SLE, endothelial cells have their own adhesive molecules (E-selectin, intercellular adhesion molecule type 1) up-regulated, thereby rendering them more sticky, a process in which interferon-γ, IL-1, and tumor necrosis factor have been implicated.

(generated exclusively by the alternative pathway) are also elevated in active SLE; elevated levels of Ba and Bb are better predictors of clinical disease than are conventional assays of total C3 and C4 or CH50.

With C5a and C3a active in plasma, it is not surprising that cell receptors for complement become activated and up-regulated; the integrin CD11b/CD18 has been best studied. As expected, increased expression of CD11b/CD18 on neutrophils was found in patients with active, but not inactive, SLE. The highest levels of neutrophil CD11b/CD18 were found in patients with the most severe disease, especially cerebritis. CD11b/CD18 expression returns to control levels with improvement in clinical disease after these episodes of "acute cerebral distress syndrome." *In sum, whereas the normal emigration of neutrophils from endothelium does little injury to the vessel wall, the unique circumstances of the Shwartzman lesion—in which C3a and C5a are activated in the circulation—permit cytokine-activated endothelial cells to become susceptible to damage by complement-activated neutrophils.*

RELEASE OF MEDIATORS OF INFLAMMATION FROM THE NEUTROPHIL. ADHESION AND ACTIVATION. After engagement of its surface receptors by immune complexes (via the FcγRII and FcγRIII receptors CD32 and CD16, respectively) or chemoattractants (receptors for C5a, IL-8), neutrophils are armed to seek and destroy microbes by chemotaxis and phagocytosis. Neutrophils are activated not only by particles (opsonized microbes, crystals) but also by diffusible chemoattractants such as bacterial signal peptides (formyl-methionylleucylphenyl alanine [fMLP]), complement split products (C5a), chemokines (IL-8), and eicosanoids such as leukotriene B$_4$ (LTB$_4$). Each chemoattractant engages a G-protein–linked receptor, and each stimulates intracellular proton and calcium fluxes; subplasmalemmal actin assembly; activation of phospholipases A$_2$, C, and D and phosphatidylinositol 3-kinase; formation of inositol 1,4,5-triphosphate, phosphatidylinositol 4,5-biphosphate, and phosphatidylinositol 4,5-triphosphate; release of arachidonate; and de novo synthesis of phosphatidate and diacylglycerol, followed by activation of protein kinase C. These intracellular events mediate the several functional responses of neutrophils in inflammation: (1) integrin (CD11b/CD18)-mediated neutrophil aggregation (homotypic cell adhesion), (2) integrin- and selectin-dependent sticking of neutrophils to vascular endothelium (heterotypic cell adhesion), (3) directed migration to the source of the signal (chemoattraction), (4) phagocytosis with or without release of granule contents (degranulation), and (5) the generation of O$_2^-$ and other toxic oxygen metabolites (the respiratory burst). Specific neutrophil functions appear to be regulated, at least in part, via distinct mechanisms because pharmacologic manipulators can inhibit some neutrophil responses without affecting others.

The mitogen-activated protein kinases p44^{Erk1} and p42^{Erk2} are serine/threonine protein kinases that in mitotic cells play roles in cell growth and differentiation. Exposure of synoviocytes, macrophages, or fibroblasts to protein tyrosine kinase receptor agonists (e.g., epidermal or nerve growth factor) results in Erk activation via a pathway dependent on the low-molecular-weight guanosine triphosphate (GTP) binding protein Ras and sequential activation of the kinases Raf-1, Mek, and the two Erks. Whereas circulating human neutrophils are post-mitotic and terminally differentiated, fMLP, LTB$_4$, and other chemoattractants nevertheless activate neutrophil Erk by pathways similar to those initiated by protein tyrosine kinase receptors, i.e., via activation of Ras, Raf-1, and Mek. A tight correlation exists between chemoattractant stimulation of Erk and neutrophil adhesion, but not between Erk activation and O$_2^-$ generation. *Homotypic cell-cell adhesion is a specific, non-mitotic response signaled by Ras $\rightarrow$ Raf $\rightarrow$ Mek $\rightarrow$ Erk in neutrophils.*

DEGRANULATIONS. During their maturation in the bone marrow, neutrophils acquire their characteristic populations of intracellular granules. These reservoirs, essentially lysosomes, serve as the main sources of the enzymes responsible for destroying foreign substances and—by error, as it were—the tissue injury of inflammation. As they mature, neutrophils also acquire the enzymatic equipment with which to produce superoxide anion (O$_2^-$) and other mediators of tissue injury such as PAF or LTB$_4$. Primary (azurophil) granules, so named because of their early appearance in neutrophil maturation (or staining properties), contain myeloperoxidase, lysozyme, acid hydrolases, and several serine proteases, including elastase. Elastase is particularly important in connective tissue degradation because it is capable of breaking down not only elastin but

also proteoglycans and collagen types III and IV. Secondary or specific granules are acquired later in maturation. These granules, like primary granules, also contain lysozyme, vitamin B$_{12}$ binding protein, lactoferrin, and the neutral proteinase collagenase. They also contain a reservoir of surface integrins (CD11b/CD18) and low-molecular-weight GTP binding proteins. Collagenase has been detected in rheumatoid synovial fluid and degrades collagen types I, II, and III. Gelatinase, a 3rd collagenolytic enzyme released by the neutrophil, has been localized to the C-particle compartment, an additional granule subclass. Gelatinase can degrade types IV, V, 1α2α3α, and denatured collagen. Thus neutrophil granules contain three enzymes—elastase, collagenase, and gelatinase—each with different substrate specificity and intracellular origin, that are capable of destroying collagen.

Neutrophils discharge the contents of their intracellular granules either overtly or covertly. During uptake of particles, the neutrophil plasma membrane initially invaginates to engulf particles such as immune complexes into a phagocytic vacuole. The vacuole then fuses with lysosomal granules to form a chamber called the "phagolysosome," and the granule contents are released into this chamber in a process called "covert degranulation." Sometimes, however, if the particle is too large or the opening of the chamber has not yet closed, lysosomal enzymes are freely discharged into the extracellular milieu, where they may attack host tissue (Fig. 284–3). This "overt degranulation," a mechanism for extracellular secretion, has been termed "regurgitation during feeding," or when the material is too large to be ingested (e.g., immune complexes trapped in the matrix of cartilage), it has also been given the picturesque name of "frustrated phagocytosis."

Antiproteases such as α_2-macroglobulin and α_1-antitrypsin may prevent the tissue damage caused by degradative proteases released inappropriately during overt degranulation. However, the effects of these antiproteases are readily overcome when they are exposed to hypochlorous acid, which inactivates them. Because hypochlorous acid is formed in the neutrophil after the interaction of myeloperoxidase, chloride anion, and H$_2$O$_2$ derived from O$_2^-$ via the reduced

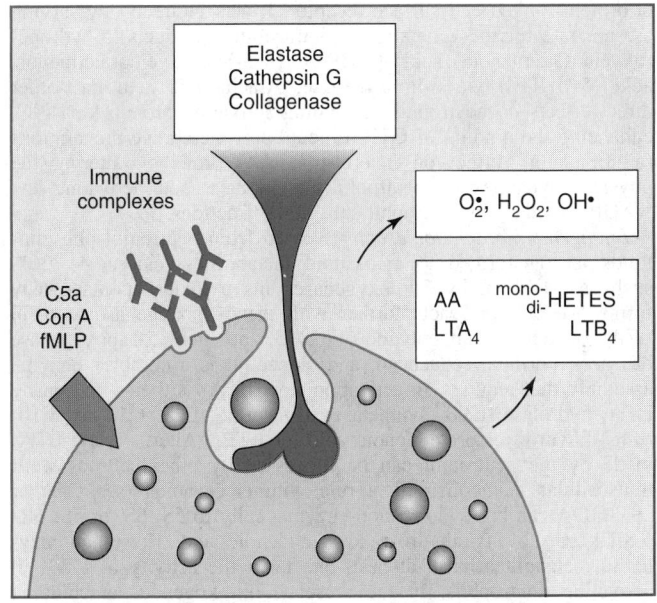

FIGURE 284–3 ■ Release of mediators of inflammation by the human neutrophil. When neutrophils are engaged by chemoattractants of bacterial origin (formyl-methionylleucyl-phenylalanine, a bacterial peptide analogue), by chemoattractants from the complement sequence (C5a), or by immune complexes, they release lysosomal enzymes from intracellular granules to the outside (overt degranulation), assemble and activate the reduced nicotinamide-adenine dinucleotide phosphate oxidase that forms toxic oxygen species (O$_2^-$, H$_2$O$_2$ etc.), and turn over membrane phospholipids. These are the precursors for arachidonic acid (AA), which is transformed by an activated 5-lipoxygenase to agonists such as 5-hydroxyeicosatetraenoic acids (HETEs) and the intermediate leukotriene A$_4$ (LTA$_4$), which can be used by neutrophils or shuttled to other cells to form other potent mediators such as leukotrienes (e.g., LTB$_4$). Con A = concanavalin A.

nicotinamide-adenine dinucleotide phosphate (NADPH) oxidase of the cell, hypochlorous acid is an important mediator of not only bacterial killing (see Chapter 29) but also tissue injury. The unfortunate interaction of granule enzymes and oxygen metabolites released by neutrophils permits proteases to act unopposed and elicit the inadvertent tissue injury that accompanies brisk phagocytosis.

RELEASE OF TOXIC OXYGEN PRODUCTS AND LIPID MEDIATORS. The H_2O_2 used in the reaction just described is one of several oxygen metabolites, including $O_2^{\cdot -}$ and $OH^{\cdot -}$, released during neutrophil activation. Generation of these toxic compounds is governed by a membrane-associated NADPH oxidase system. In addition to contributing to the formation of hypochlorous acid, oxygen metabolites can also damage connective tissue directly. For example, $O_2^{\cdot -}$ is capable of degrading bovine synovial fluid and depolymerizing purified hyaluronic acid. Neutrophils respond to the engagement of receptors for chemoattractants or immune complexes by mobilizing arachidonate from the sn-2 position of phospholipids. Arachidonate, a fatty acid with 20 carbons and 4 unsaturated double bonds, is mobilized from membrane stores directly via a phospholipase A_2 or indirectly via a phospholipase C, followed by the action of a diacylglycerol lipase on diacylglycerol. The phospholipase A_2 esterases, which are associated with both neutrophil granules and the plasma membrane, have two pH optima (5.5 and 7.5). Purified preparations of phospholipase A_2 esterases require high concentrations of calcium for activity. Neutrophils appear to contain at least two types of phospholipase C, one that acts specifically on phosphatidylinositol and a 2nd that acts on phosphatidylcholine to yield diacylglycerol. Data on the remodeling of lipids show that not only phospholipase A_2 activity but also the activity of phospholipase C and D can explain these changes (see below). After treatment with calcium ionophore or zymosan particles opsonized by C3b, neutrophils release arachidonate from phosphatidylinositol and phosphatidylcholine to an almost equivalent extent.

Exogenous arachidonic acid added to neutrophils mimics the engagement of G-protein–dependent chemoattractants: The cells aggregate, degranulate, and generate $O_2^{\cdot -}$. Moreover, some effects of exogenous arachidonic acid are inhibited by pertussis toxin. However, arachidonic acid does not engage its own specific G-protein–linked cell surface receptor. It acts indirectly by serving as substrate for the generation of intracellular products (5-hydroperoxyeicosatetraenoic acid [5-HPETE], 5-hydroxyeicosatetraenoic acid [5-HETE]) via 5-lipoxygenase. Arachidonic acid has other direct effects on neutrophils, including activating protein kinase C, enhancing the binding of GTP to neutrophil membrane preparations (a stimulatory effect on heterotrimeric G proteins), altering the physical dynamics of neutrophil membranes, and activating the NADPH oxidase in neutrophil subcellular fractions.

Endogenous arachidonic acid released from neutrophil phospholipids is transformed to eicosanoid metabolites (eicosa = "20") such as 5-HPETE by 5-lipoxygenase; this peroxide spontaneously forms 5-HETE or reacts further with the 5-lipoxygenase to form LTA_4, which has an epoxide at the 5,6-position. 5-Lipoxygenase has been purified, sequenced, and cloned. It is a complex enzyme assembly that requires an activation step. LTA_4 is then acted on by LTA_4 hydrolase (LTB_4 synthetase) to form 5S, L2R, 6,14-*cis*, 8,10-*trans*-dihydroxyeicosatetraenoic acid, or LTB_4. Alternatively, LTA_4 made by the neutrophil can be processed by other cells as well; transcellular metabolism is a rule with eicosanoids (see Chapter 29). LTA_4 can break down non-enzymatically to 5S, 6S, or 5S, 6R-6,8,10-*trans*-14-*cis*-dihydroxyeicosatetraenoic acid. These non-enzymatic metabolites have, at best, one tenth the activity of LTB_4 in activating neutrophils. In the presence of exogenous arachidonic acid, neutrophils also show 15-lipoxygenase activity, which in a parallel manner produces 15-HPETE and 15-HETE. These products, in turn, are acted on by an LTA_4 synthetase–like enzyme to make a 14,15-dihydroxy product and finally, in concert with 5-lipoxygenase, to yield the trihydroxy compounds lipoxins A and B. Mononuclear cells, in contrast, produce stable prostaglandins (prostaglandin E_2) and the sulfidopeptide leukotrienes LTC_4, LTD_4, and LTE_4.

The major inflammatory mediators made via lipoxygenase from neutrophils are LTB_4, 5-H (P)ETE, and lipoxin A (see Fig. 284–3). LTB_4 is a potent chemoattractant that promotes the adhesion of neutrophils to endothelial cells from a variety of arterial and ve-

nous sites of several species—an effect not shared with other eicosanoids. Like LTB_4, 5-HETE (acting via G-protein–linked receptors) provokes robust neutrophil aggregation and superoxide generation. Acting in an autacoid fashion, it is a major agonist in arachidonate-mediated inflammation. Indeed, 5-HPETE is metabolized, independently of 5-lipoxygenase, to 5-HETE, which diffuses to the extracellular face of the plasma membrane to engage a G-protein–linked receptor. G-protein activity then initiates Erk activation via Ras → Raf → Mek, as above. *Generation of 5-HPETE and 5-HETE via lipoxygenase is coupled to the mitogen-activated protein kinase cascade via extracellular, autacoid engagement of a G-protein–coupled receptor.*

SIGNAL TRANSDUCTION AND CELL ACTIVATION IN INFLAMMATION. LIPID REMODELING. When chemoattractants such as fMLP, C5a, C3a, IL-8, or LTB_4 engage their receptors, neutrophils respond by generating inositol trisphosphate and DAG. Signaling via Fcγ receptors and receptors for chemoattractants differs with respect to some details, but the general process of stimulus-response coupling is similar, and neutrophils do not differ in these general pathways from other cells of inflammation. Cellular inositol triphosphate and diacylglycerol concentrations substantially increase within seconds after the fMLP receptor is engaged. By 5 seconds, inositol triphosphate levels begin to decline. In contrast, both diacylglycerol and phosphatidic acid continue to increase over the course of the next 120 to 300 seconds. For neutrophils or macrophages to respond over time and in space, two signals must be generated: a short "triggering" signal with an immediate increase in intracellular messengers (e.g., inositol triphosphate) and sustained "activation" signals (e.g., diacylglycerol or phosphatidic acid) required for the longer processes of chemotaxis and phagocytosis. However, lipid remodeling provides only some of the messengers needed for signal transduction. Calcium plays another key role. When treated with chemoattractants such as C5a or fMLP, neutrophils increase their levels of cytosolic calcium and a peak is reached by 2 to 5 seconds. Over the next 2 minutes, cytosolic calcium slowly decreases and then returns toward—but not to—baseline. The peak levels (from 300 to 500 nm) are achieved primarily by inositol triphosphate–induced mobilization from intracellular stores inasmuch as similar levels are achieved in the absence of extracellular Ca. Influx of extracellular Ca begins approximately 5 seconds after Ca has been released from intracellular sites and while inositol triphosphate levels are still dropping. Although IP_4 (phosphatidy inositol triphosphate) may in part regulate Ca channels, it is also possible that phosphatidic acid helps maintain Ca-dependent Ca influx.

GTP BINDING PROTEINS AND SIGNAL TRANSDUCTION. Both the classic chemoattractants (fMLP, C5a, LTB_4, and PAF) and the more recently recognized α-chemokines (IL-8, GRO, NAP-2, ENA-78, and GCP-2) bind to receptors on neutrophils that are members of a large family of receptors that interact with G proteins. The cDNAs reveal that each receptor contains seven hydrophobic α-helices predicted to form seven transmembrane-spanning domains and a series of extracellular and cytoplasmic loops, analogous to the deduced structure of the best studied receptor of this class, the β-adrenergic receptor. In addition to the chemoattractant receptors, other receptors of this class expressed on neutrophils include receptors for β-adrenergic agents, prostaglandin E, and adenosine. Guanine nucleotide regulatory binding proteins, or G proteins, are α/β/γ-heterotrimeric proteins associated with the inner leaflet of the plasma membrane that transduce signals from transmembrane receptors to effector molecules by cycling between a guanosine diphosphate (GDP)-bound; inactive and a GTP-bound, active conformation. Receptor occupancy leads to a conformational change that allows the receptor to interact with a G protein and thereby stimulate the dissociation of GDP from G_α, the GTP binding subunit. Binding of GTP then leads to a dissociation of G_α from $G_{B/\gamma}$, each of which plays a role in activating effector molecules. The signal is terminated by the intrinsic GTPase activity of G_α. At least 16 α- as well as multiple β- and γ-subunits have been identified. Some of the α-subunits serve as substrates for the adenosine diphosphate ribosyltransferases contained in pertussis and cholera toxins. Human neutrophil plasma membranes contain substrates for both pertussis and cholera toxins. Because pertussis toxin inhibits much, but not all, of fMLP-stimulated neutrophil function, it has been deduced that neutrophils contain both pertussis-sensitive and pertussis-insensitive G proteins. Immunoblot analysis with subunit-specific antisera have identified $G_{\alpha i2,3}$, $G_{\alpha 8}$, $G_{\beta 1,2}$, and $G_{\gamma 2}$ in human neutrophil membranes. $G_{\alpha i2}$ is most intimately involved in neutrophil activation by chemoattractants.

MONOMERIC GTPases. Regulatory GTPases related to the proto-oncogene product $p21^{ras}$ control a wide variety of cellular processes. *Ras*-related GTPases are monomeric GTP binding proteins that undergo conformational changes when they cycle between their GTP-bound inactive and GTP-bound active states. The *ras* superfamily of GTPases can be divided into the *ras* family involved in signal transduction for growth and differentiation, the *rho* family involved in signaling for actin cytoskeleton remodeling, and the *rab* and *ARF* families involved in regulating vesicular trafficking. Members of each of these families have been identified in human neutrophils. Notable examples are $p21^{rac}$, which activates NADPH oxidase; $p21^{rap1}$, which is associated with cytochrome b_{558} but is not required for in vitro NADPH oxidase activity; $p21^{rho}$, which is involved in actin stress fiber formation in fibroblasts; $p21^{CDC42}$, which activates a specific kinase; and ARF, which activates phospholipase D, whose product, phosphatidic acid, may be involved in vesicular fusion. Chemoattractants activate $p21^{ras}$, Raf-1, and mitogen-activated protein kinase in neutrophils, although the pathway(s) coupling G-protein–linked receptors to the $p21^{ras}$ signaling pathway are undefined. Both *ras*-related GTPases and heterotrimeric G proteins are intrinsically hydrophilic proteins that exert their biologic effects at membranes. Both *ras*-related proteins and the γ-subunit of G proteins are targeted to membranes by a series of post-translational modifications of their carboxyl termini that involves prenylation (addition of a 15- or 20-carbon polyisoprene lipid), proteolysis, and carboxyl methylation. Carboxyl methylation, the only reversible step in this processing, is associated with neutrophil activation and plays a key regulatory role in signal transduction.

SIGNALING VIA Fcγ RECEPTORS: THE RESPONSE TO IMMUNE COMPLEXES. Three major classes of receptors have been described for the constant Fcγ region of human IgGs. FcγRI is a high-affinity receptor for monomeric IgG (K_a = ~10^{-8} mol/L, 72 kd) found mainly on mononuclear cells; recognized by monoclonal antibody 32, it is up-regulated in response to interferon. Neutrophils also have two low-affinity receptors (K_a = ~10^{-6} mol/L) that bind aggregated IgGs or immune complexes much more avidly than monomeric IgG. FcγRII (or CD32) of approximately 40 kd is present at 15,000 sites per cell (as recognized by monoclonal antibody IV-3) and is also present on B cells, macrophages, and platelets. FcγRII (1) is resistant to elastase, (2) is not linked to the plasmalemma via phosphotidylinositol, (3) is present on neutrophils from patients with paroxysmal nocturnal hemoglobinuria, (4) appears to mediate O_2^- generation and degranulation, and (5) transduces all the signal for O_2^- generation and some of the signal for degranulation by means of a pertussis-sensitive G protein. FcγRIII (or CD16) also prefers multimeric IgG and is expressed in heterogeneous fashion on neutrophils, macrophages, and natural killer (NK) cells. FcγRIII has a broad molecular weight range of 50,000 to 70,000, is present at approximately 120,000 sites per neutrophil, and is recognized by monoclonal antibody 3G8. The FcγRIII receptors on neutrophils and NK cells differ with respect to mass and

are products of different, but very homologous, genes. FcγRIII receptors of the neutrophil are (1) elastase sensitive, (2) linked to the external plasmalemma via phosphatidylinositol, (3) reduced to 90% of control levels at the plasmalemma—but not the Golgi region—of cells from patients with paroxysmal nocturnal hemoglobinuria, (4) an ineffective trigger of cells for O_2^- or enzyme release, and (5) polymorphic with respect to structure and antigenicity because they have two alleles (CNA1 and NA2). FcγRIII receptors are shed into the supernatant of neutrophils exposed to FMLP, whereas macrophages and NK cells—in which FcγRIII is a transmembrane structure—do not shed this receptor.

Like T-cell receptors, Fcγ receptors signal through tyrosine activation domains on the cytoplasmic portions of aggregated receptor complexes, which in turn activate Src-family tyrosine kinases such as $p72^{syk}$. FcγRIIIB, abundantly expressed on neutrophils, has a glycosylphosphatidylinositol anchor that lacks a cytoplasmic domain and must therefore signal through an accessory molecule, i.e., the ζ-homodimer associated with the T-cell receptor and FcγRIIIA, a transmembrane isoform. FcγRII is linked to GTP binding proteins, whereas FcγRIII is not; indeed, it appears that FcγRIII accumulates at the interface between neutrophils and immune complexes trapped in the subendothelium. Moreover, signaling via Fcγ receptors differs from signaling via chemoattractant receptors in that the former is dependent on the integrity of cytoplasmic microtubules whereas chemoattractant-induced signaling is independent of microtubules. *Colchicine* therefore inhibits FcγR signaling.

ADHESION MOLECULES AND INFLAMMATION. Three major families of proteins expressed on the surface of leukocytes and endothelium play a role in leukocyte-endothelial interactions. *Integrins* are a large family of heterodimeric adhesive proteins expressed on leukocytes and other cell types. All leukocytes express one or more of the β_2-integrins, which share a common β-chain (CD18) but differ with respect to their α-chains (CD11a, b, c). Integrins bind to a specific amino acid motif in their counterligands, and peptides containing this specific sequence of amino acids (RGD or arginine-glycine-aspartate) block many integrin-dependent functions. Their counterligands on endothelium (and other cells) belong to the *immunoglobulin superfamily* (ICAM-1, ICAM-2), which constitutes a 2nd major group of adhesion molecules. *Selectins,* the 3rd family of adhesive proteins, bind to carbohydrate residues on glycoproteins and glycolipids and consist of P-, E-, and L-selectin. P-selectin is expressed on stimulated platelets and endothelium, L-selectin on leukocytes (neutrophils, monocytes, and a subset of lymphocytes), and E-selectin on stimulated endothelium. The genes encoding these molecules are all located on chromosome 1. The selectins share an extracellular C-type (Ca^{2+}-dependent) selectin domain (responsible for binding to their cognate ligands), an epidermal growth factor–related domain of unknown function with variable numbers of short consensus repeats (complement regulatory protein domains) in their extracellular portions, a hydrophobic transmembrane domain, and a short cytoplasmic tail. E-selectin and P-selectin both bind to glycoproteins and glycolipids that con-

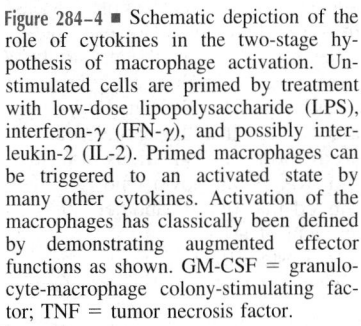

Figure 284–4 ■ Schematic depiction of the role of cytokines in the two-stage hypothesis of macrophage activation. Unstimulated cells are primed by treatment with low-dose lipopolysaccharide (LPS), interferon-γ (IFN-γ), and possibly interleukin-2 (IL-2). Primed macrophages can be triggered to an activated state by many other cytokines. Activation of the macrophages has classically been defined by demonstrating augmented effector functions as shown. GM-CSF = granulocyte-macrophage colony-stimulating factor; TNF = tumor necrosis factor.

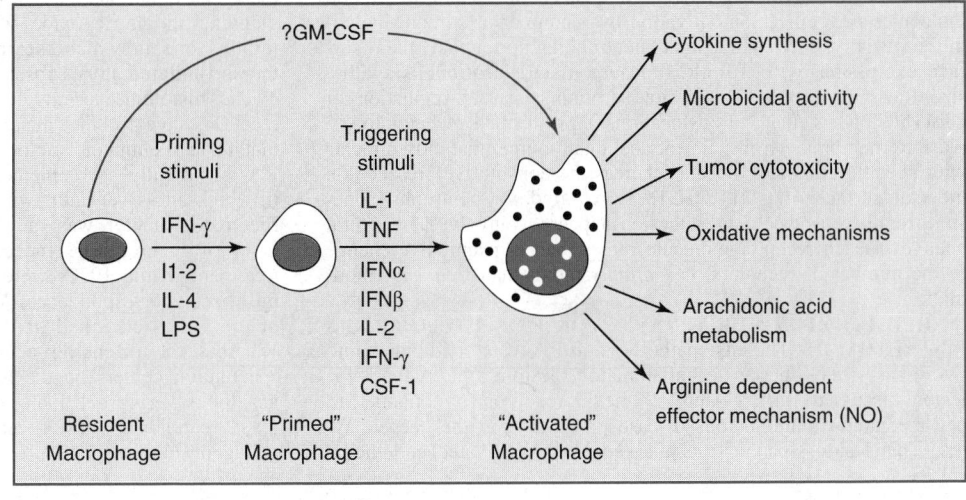

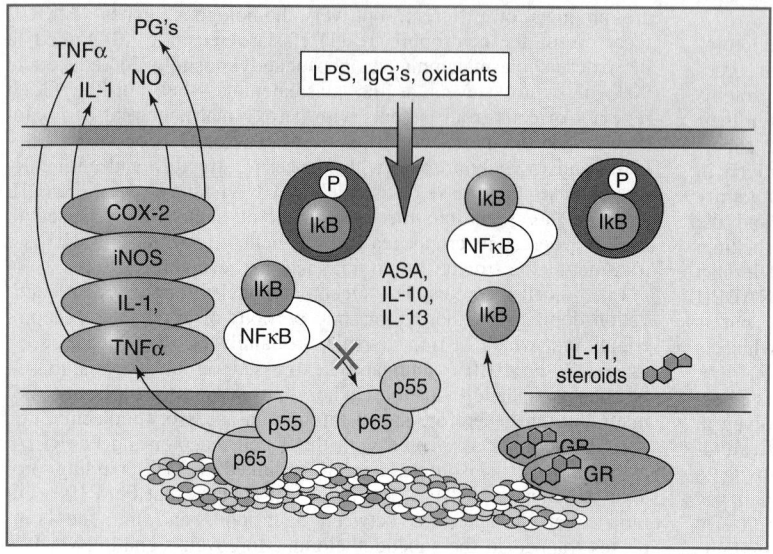

FIGURE 284–5 ■ In many cells of the inflamed synovium, increased levels of proteins and mRNAs for cyclooxygenase 2 (COX 2), inducible nitric oxide synthetase (iNOS), tumor necrosis factor (TNF), and interleukin-1 (IL-1) can be demonstrated. The gene expression of these mediators of inflammation is governed in good part by translocation of NFκB (65- and 55-kd subunits) from the cytoplasm to the nucleus. Increased synthesis of the NFκB inhibitor IκB, as induced by glucocorticoids and IL-11, or decreased breakdown of phosphorylated IκB (IκB.P) via the ubiquitin/proteosome pathway—an effect of salicylates, IL-10, and IL13—regulates the activation state of phagocytes, synoviocytes, and endothelial cells.

tain sialyl Lewis X antigen—a complex carbohydrate. Sialyl Lewis X antigen is expressed predominantly on the surface of neutrophils. Similarly, signaling from the extracellular matrix through integrins involves protein tyrosine phosphorylation, although the other integrin-mediated functions, including cell-cell adhesion and actin cytoskeleton organization, may be regulated independently. Like bacterial lipopolysaccharide, the cytokines TNF-α, granulocyte-macrophage colony-stimulating factor, and INF-γ do not stimulate neutrophil responses directly, but prime neutrophils to respond to lower concentrations of chemoattractants. Signaling from cytokine receptors in mitotic cells such as monocytes or synoviocytes involves hetero-oligomerization of the receptors with signaling molecules such as members of the JAK and STAT families, which leads to the transcription of specific sets of genes, but cytokine signaling in neutrophils has not been extensively studied.

The endothelial cell plays an active role in adhesion and displays inducible E-selectin to inflammatory cells, thereby facilitating their adhesion and transmigration. IL-1, TNF, lymphotoxin, and endotoxin induce the expression of E-selectin on endothelial cells. Endothelial ICAM-1 (ELAM-1) is the ligand for LFA-1 and is therefore one of several molecules that direct lymphocyte binding to high endothelial cells, especially those of a chronically inflamed rheumatoid joint. Endothelial cell activation is antagonized by TGF-β, and IL-10, IL-11, and IL-13, as well as by such anti-inflammatory agents as salicylates and corticosteroids (see below). TGF-β inhibits the adherence of human neutrophils not only to normal endothelium but also to endothelial cells rendered sticky by ELAM-1, as induced by TNF-α.

The CD11b/CD18 integrin is involved in homotypic *and* heterotypic adhesion. CD11b/CD18 is constitutively expressed on the surface of resting neutrophils at a density of 10,000 to 20,000 molecules per cell. Upon activation by a number of stimuli, including especially chemoattractants, neutrophils up-regulate their surface expression 5- to 10-fold. Because mature neutrophils synthesize few new proteins, it is not surprising that up-regulation of CD11b/CD18 is due to translocation of pre-formed receptor to the plasma membrane from an intracellular source that cosediments with specific granules. Indeed, whereas the constitutive presence on the cell surface of CD11b/CD18 is required for neutrophil adhesion, regulation of cell-cell adhesion appears to involve a structural change in each receptor molecule rather than a quantitative change in the number of receptors, i.e., *affinity* rather than *frequency* modulation.

RHEUMATOID ARTHRITIS AS A FORM OF THE TUBERCULIN REACTION. The histopathology of RA can be divided into two phases: (1) the acute inflammatory lesion—the Arthus-type lesion discussed earlier—and (2) the more chronic, mononuclear, cell-mediated granulomatous disease proceeding in the deeper layers. This lesion—pannus—is marked by (1) activated endothelial

cells, (2) focal collections of B lymphocytes and plasma cells that synthesize rheumatoid factors locally, (3) various subsets of T lymphocytes, (4) activated macrophages, and (5) proliferation of other mesenchymal cells of the synovium where genes for proto-oncogenes have been activated (Fig. 284–4). B-cell–derived plama cell clusters are nourished by local increments of IL-2; *indeed IL-2 is critical to B-cell activation, proliferation, and differentiation, thus playing a central role in keeping patients with RA "seropositive."*

In many cells of the inflamed synovium, mRNAs for cyclooxygenase 2, inducible nitric oxide synthetase, TNF, and IL-1 can be demonstrated; both transcription and translation of adhesion molecules such as ICAM-1 and E-selectin are also markedly elevated. The levels of inflammatory cytokines, their gene expression, and mRNAs and proteins are regulated, in good part, by the response of inflammatory cells to several interacting transcription factors: the cytoplasmic NFκB and glucocorticoid receptors (Fig. 284–5), as well as the nuclear transcription factors fos/jun (homodimers and heterodimers) acting at AP-1 sites. Translocation of NFκB from the cytoplasm to the nucleus is critical to the activation of synoviocytes, phagocytes, and endothelial cells, as well as B cells. Increased synthesis of the NFκB inhibitor IκB, which is induced by glucocorticoids, or decreased breakdown of phosphorylated IκB via the ubiquitin/proteosome pathway, an effect of salicylates, is important not only for the release of inflammatory stimuli such as cytokines or eicosanoids but also for the maintenance of B-cell function. *Thus NFκB controls both immunoglobulin synthesis and phagocyte activation.*

Two of these activated cell types, macrophages and synoviocytes, generate cytokines that cause chondrocytes to participate in their own destruction not only by releasing proteases and specific collagenase but also by up-regulating their production of prostaglandins and nitric oxide. The cytokine profile of the rheumatoid joint is one in which the inflammatory subset predominates over the anti-inflammatory subset (Fig. 284–6).

The histologic lesions resemble those found in the tuberculin reaction, save for the clusters of B lymphocytes and plasma cells that form rheumatoid factor locally. These cells yield the clue that RA is basically a complement-dependent immune complex disease in which an as yet unknown antigen is the culprit. However, before rheumatoid factor was on the horizon, RA was thought to be a form of tuberculosis. Indeed, the gold salts that were used for treatment in the 1920s were initially used for RA on the basis of this fuzzy correspondence. We may note that the earliest editions of this text classified RA as a form of "infectious arthritis." Whereas the offending agent of RA is unknown, most modern speculation centers on the likelihood that one or another self-antigen looks very much like the product of a bacterium or virus. The major candidates have been (1) Epstein-Barr virus, (2) type II collagen, (3) cartilage proteoglycan, and (4) heat shock (stress)

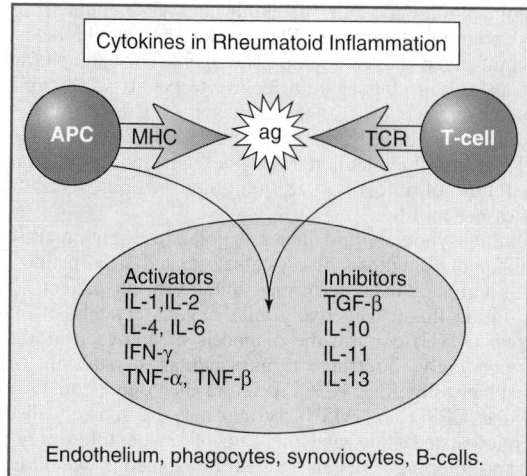

Cytokines in Rheumatoid Inflammation

Activators
IL-1, IL-2
IL-4, IL-6
IFN-γ
TNF-α, TNF-β

Inhibitors
TGF-β
IL-10
IL-11
IL-13

Endothelium, phagocytes, synoviocytes, B-cells.

FIGURE 284–6 ■ Schematic depiction of the role of pro- and anti-inflammatory cytokines in rheumatoid synovitis. Both classes of cytokines are provoked when T cells respond via their T-cell receptor (TCR) to antigen (ag) processed by antigen-presenting cells (APC) in the context of their major histocompatibly complex (MHC). Unstimulated APCs and T cells can also be primed by treatment with low-dose endotoxin. The synovium of patients with active rheumatoid arthritis usually contains an excess of activating over inhibitory cytokines, but so does an active tuberculin lesion. Consequently, the pathogenetic importance of IL2-driven synthesis of immune complexes (IgG-IgM rheumatoid factors) by plasma cells and subsequent complement activation should not escape our notice.

proteins—especially a 65-kd species against which many patients with RA mount a humoral and cellular immune response. Indeed, there is good evidence that stress proteins are present at the surface of antigen-presenting cells, and recently it was found that a helper T-cell clone derived from a patient with tuberculous leprosy reacted with a synthetic peptide found in the 3rd-type variable region of the major histocompatibility complex—DR2 β-chain. The observation that cartilage proteoglycans share epitopes with acetone-extracted fractions of the tubercle bacillus suggests that when humans get RA, they respond to their own tissues as though these tissues were products of the tubercle bacillus or Epstein-Barr virus.

Abramson SB, Weissmann G: Complement split products and the pathogenesis of SLE. Hosp Pract 23:45, 1988. *How the Arthus phenomenon and the Shwartzman reaction apply to vasculitis in SLE.*

Baeuerli PA, Henkel T: Function and activation of NFκB in the immune system. Annu Rev Immunol 12:141, 1994. *How this important transcription factor of inflammation regulates the expression of both cytokines and imunoglobulins.*

Capodici C, Pillinger MH, Han G, et al: Integrin-dependent homotypic adhesion of neutrophils; arachidonic acid activates Raf-1/Mek/Erk via a 5-lipoxygenase–dependent pathway. J Clin Invest 102:165–175, 1998. *Shedding light on how the 5-lipoxygenase pathway generates HETE in the course of cell-cell adhesion.*

Crofford LJ, Wilder RL, Ristimake AP, et al: Cyclooxygenase-1 and -2 expression in rheumatoid synovial tissues: Effects of interleukin-1, phorbol ester, and corticosteroids. J Clin Invest 93:1095, 1994. *How the two cyclooxygenases are influenced by interleukins and anti-inflammatory drugs in inflammation.*

Cronstein BN, Kimmel SC, Levin RI, et al: A mechanism for the anti-inflammatory effects of corticosteroids: The glucocorticoid receptor regulates leukocyte adhesion to endothelial cells and expression of ELAM-1 and ICAM-1. Proc Natl Acad Sci U S A 89:9991, 1992. *A description of how corticosteroids influence the display of adhesive molecules.*

Cronstein BN, Weissmann G: Targets for antiinflammatory drugs. Annu Rev Pharmacol Toxicol 35:449, 1995. *The role of adhesion molecules and receptors for prostaglandins and adenosine in leukocyte/endothelial interactions. Sites of action of salicylates, glucocorticoids, and methotrexate.*

Feldmann M, Brennan FM, Maini RN: Role of cytokines in rheumatoid arthritis. Annu Rev Immunol 14:397, 1995. *The outline of how specific inhibitors of proinflammatory cytokines might be used in treating rheumatoid arthritis, based on an analysis of the cytokine network pertinent to rheumatology.*

Harris ED Jr: The rationale for combination therapy of rheumatoid arthritis based on pathophysiology. J Rheumatol Suppl 44:2, 1996. *A brief summary of the complex, tuberculin-like lesion of rheumatoid arthritis and how combination therapy can interrupt the self-sustaining cytokine-driven cycle of tissue injury.*

Krane SM: Clinical importance of metalloproteinases and their inhibitors. Ann N Y Acad Sci 732:1, 1994. *A summary of how the proteinases of connective tissue are regulated in the course of tissue injury and remodeling.*

Mantovani A, Bussolino F, Dejana E: Cytokine regulation of endothelial cell function. FASEB J 6:2591, 1992. *How cytokines of the sort found in rheumatoid synovium or fluid affect the adhesive properties of endothelium.*

Pillinger MH, Philips MR, Feoktistov A, Weissmann G: Crosstalk in signal transduction via EP receptors: Prostaglandin E₁ inhibits chemoattractant-induced mitogen activated protein kinase activity in human neutrophils. Adv Prostaglandin Thrombox-

ane Leukot Res 23:311, 1995. *How G-protein–linked receptors communicate with ras-related signal transduction pathways in inflammatory cells and how these pathways are regulated by eicosanoids.*

Serhan CN, Haeggstrom JZ, Leslie CC: Lipid mediator networks in cell signaling: Update and impact of cytokines. FASEB J 10:1147, 1996. *How eicosanoids and other novel lipid mediators are influenced by the balance of pro- and anti-inflammatory cytokines. The discovery of new eicosanoids after aspirin blockade of the cyclooxygenases.*

Weissmànn G: The role of neutrophils in vascular injury: Signal transduction mechanisms in cell-cell interactions. Springer Semin Immunopathol 11:235, 1989. *A review of the Arthus and Shwartzman models and how they relate to the vascular lesions of rheumatic diseases.*

Winfield JB: Stress proteins and autoimmunity. Arthritis Rheum 32:1497, 1989. *How heat shock proteins may be the link between autoantigens and microbial products in perpetuating RA.*

285 SPECIALIZED PROCEDURES IN THE MANAGEMENT OF PATIENTS WITH RHEUMATIC DISEASES

Robert W. Ike ■ *William J. Arnold*

Rheumatic diseases can account for an array of clinical presentations that range from signs and symptoms reflecting multiorgan involvement to pain and compromised function in a single anatomic area. Correct diagnosis of a suspected rheumatic process and optimal management of the patient with an established rheumatic disease rest on the physician's ability to identify the site(s) from which the patient's symptoms arise, ascertain the pathologic process affecting the identified site(s), determine why the process is occurring, and find measures to gauge the activity of the disease so that response to treatment can be followed. A directed history and physical examination provide the bedrock for this exercise, with suspicions regarding anatomy, process, and diagnosis supported or refuted by appropriate laboratory tests, imaging modalities, and invasive procedures. The number of specialized procedures applicable to rheumatic diseases continues to grow. Testing for relevant immunologic phenomena becomes ever more complex as the molecular bases for the measured phenomena become appreciated. Certain anatomic abnormalities that had previously escaped detection can now be identified by imaging procedures—both direct (arthroscopy) and indirect (ultrasonography and magnetic resonance imaging)—although these procedures present hurdles of cost, availability, and operator expertise. These tests and the other procedures discussed below must always be interpreted in the context of a thorough, comprehensive, multifaceted evaluation.

ASPIRATION OF SYNOVIAL JOINTS AND BURSAE

In any patient with undiagnosed arthritis and an associated joint effusion, examination of the synovial fluid is mandatory. Gross appearance of the synovial fluid can provide an initial clue to the underlying process, and certain disorders such as crystalline arthropathies and bacterial infection are quickly confirmed by specialized microscopic examination. Successful joint or bursal aspiration depends on a thorough familiarity with certain principles.

Both the physician and the patient must be comfortable. The physician should have some experience and confidence concerning the particular joint to be tapped. Although most general internists can aspirate the knee or the olecranon bursa, other commonly inflamed structures, such as the shoulder, ankle, elbow, first metatarsophalangeal joint, and subdeltoid bursa, require special expertise for successful aspiration. The patient should be positioned to allow relaxation of muscles on both sides of the joint to be aspirated. For the knee, the patient should be supine with the knee in slight flexion, accomplished by resting it on a pillow. Palpation identifies landmarks for entry, discerns the region of the largest "bulge" in the joint capsule (critical for small joints), and confirms relaxation of periarticular muscles. If the patella cannot be moved side-to-side, entry to the knee will be painful and difficult, if not impossible.

After preparing the skin with iodine solution, the gloved aspirating hand determines point of entry. Most physicians find the knee easiest to enter from the medial aspect, just posterior to midpoint of the patella edge. Except for very large effusions that can be entered quickly with the aspirating needle, the skin and subcutaneous path to the joint capsule should be anesthetized with lidocaine, delivered while advancing slowly with the smallest gauge needle available. This promotes patient comfort and marks the path to be taken into the joint. The joint space is entered with an 18-gauge needle to which a syringe of up to 20 mL is attached, depending on the size of the effusion. Failure to obtain fluid from a clinically swollen joint space can result from several processes, including presence of synovial fluid too thick to be withdrawn through the needle used, presence of intra-articular debris clogging the needle, a swollen space composed mainly of tissue, or sequestration of fluid away from the needle point. When aspiration of fluid is critical, such as in suspected septic arthritis, ultrasonography or arthrography can help guide the needle to the fluid-containing section of the joint. A 5-mL sample of synovial fluid is more than adequate for all routine studies, including cultures.

Synovial fluid analysis begins with a look at the fluid in the heparinized tube. Fluid that transmits light and can be read through (determined by holding the tube in front of a sample of printed text) will generally prove to have fewer than 2,000 white blood cells (WBC)/mL and is associated with "non-inflammatory" disorders, most commonly osteoarthritis (Table 285–1). Translucent fluid that blurs print will have more than 2,000 WBC/mL but less than 100,000/mL and is associated with a wide array of "inflammatory" conditions, such as rheumatoid arthritis. Opaque fluid, usually quite thick, carries the usual concerns of pus obtained from any other body cavity and should place acute infection as the leading diagnosis until proven otherwise. Usually, such fluid will show 50,000 to 100,000 WBC/mL, but other compounds in high concentrations (cholesterol, monosodium urate) can produce opaque synovial fluid that is relatively acellular. Bloody-appearing fluid carries a specific differential diagnosis but does not always connote true hemarthrosis, because it takes but a small amount of blood within the joint space to make synovial fluid appear bloody. Viscosity of the joint fluid is determined largely by molecular weight and concentration of hyaluronate, a proteoglycan polymer. Elaboration of enzymes that depolymerize hyaluronate can accompany synovial tissue inflammation in the absence of fluid-phase inflammation. Hence, "non-inflammatory fluid" that appears "thin" and leaves a very short "string" when dripped from syringe into test tube can be due to synovitis that has not produced fluid phase inflammation and cloudy fluid. Bursal fluid cannot be classified by the same parame-

ters as joint fluid. As a rule of thumb, the WBC count from bursal fluid is about one-tenth the WBC count that would be expected from a joint given the same phlogistic agent. For example, in gouty bursitis, an average bursal fluid leukocyte count is 2,800/mL compared to an average of 21,000/mL in synovial fluid from an acute gouty joint. Thus, bursal fluid with a leukocyte count of only a few hundred per milliliter should raise the same concerns—including the possibility of infection—as joint fluid with several thousand leukocytes per milliliter.

Examining synovial fluid under a polarized light microscope is essential for the diagnosis of crystal-associated arthropathies (Color plate 3C) and should be performed initially in all patients. Needle-shaped, intracellular, negatively birefringent crystals of monosodium urate (MSU) confirm the diagnosis of gouty arthritis. Rhomboidal, positively birefringent intracellular crystals of calcium pyrophosphate dihydrate (CPPD) define the pseudogout syndrome. Intracellular CPPD and MSU crystals may be sparsely distributed on the microscope slide, and they are often identified only after a careful and thorough search guided by someone well versed in using the polarized microscope. Because other processes such as infection can "liberate" crystals into the joint fluid, identifying crystals in an acutely inflamed joint should not be taken as a complete explanation, particularly when CPPD is present. Other crystals and compounds identified by the polarized microscope include calcium oxalate (a positively birefringent tetrahedron found in some dialysis patients), corticosteroids from previous intra-articular injections (small and bright with variable birefringence characteristics), talc (positively birefringent clumps, transferred from gloved hand to slide), lipid (round "Maltese crosses" derived from bone marrow fat and indicative of fracture), and cholesterol (plate-like and brilliantly birefringent without a definite axis, associated with long-standing inflammatory effusions, especially when accompanied by bleeding, as in hemophilia).

Bacterial infection should be considered in all patients with acute arthritis and in patients with established rheumatic disorders with exacerbation in one or several joints. Purulent, opaque synovial fluid is not present in all cases, and early-stage bacterial arthritis may not even produce "inflammatory" fluid. The most common pathogen is *Staphylococcus aureus*. Findings on Gram stain of synovial fluid can help guide initial therapy, but a negative study does not rule out infection. In situations in which clinical suspicion of septic arthritis is strong but not confirmed by initial studies of synovial fluid, antibiotics should be given empirically until culture results are available.

Arthritis due to other infectious agents may be more difficult to confirm. *Neisseria gonorrhoeae* is the most common gram-negative organism associated with infectious arthritis but is identified by Gram stain of synovial fluid in only a minority of cases. Chances for isolation of the gonococcus are improved if synovial fluid is plated directly onto chocolate agar and similar cultures are made from swabs of any skin lesions and of all potential portals of entry

Table 285–1 ▪ SYNOVIAL FLUID ANALYSIS

	NON-INFLAMMATORY (GROUP I)	INFLAMMATORY (GROUP II)	PURULENT (GROUP III)	HEMORRHAGIC (GROUP IV)
Color	Yellow	Yellow	Yellow-green	Red
Clarity	Transparent	Translucent	Opaque	Opaque
Leukocyte count (WBC/mL)	<2000	2000–50,000*	>50,000	*
% Polymorphonuclear leukocytes	<25%	>50%	>75%	*
Disease examples	Osteoarthritis	Rheumatoid arthritis	Bacterial infections	Trauma
	Trauma	Reiter's syndrome	Tuberculosis	Neuropathic joint
	Osteochondritis dissecans	Crystal synovitis, acute	RA (rare)	Coagulation disorders
	Osteonecrosis	(gout, pseudogout)	Reiter's (rare)	Hemophilia
	Amyloidosis	Psoriatic arthritis	Pseudogout (rare)	von Willebrand's disease
	Scleroderma	Viral arthritis		Heparin or warfarin
	Systemic lupus†	Rheumatic fever		Sickle cell disease
	Polymyalgia rheumatica†	Behçet's syndrome		Chondrocalcinosis
	Hypertrophic pulmonary osteoarthropathy	Lyme disease		Scurvy
		Some bacterial infections		Tumor, especially pigmented villonodular synovitis, hemangioma

RA = rheumatoid arthritis.
*Wide range; WBC count should be interpreted in light of peripheral blood WBC and RBC counts.
†Sometimes inflammatory.

for the organism (urethra, cervix, anus, throat). *Mycobacteria* (*M. tuberculosis* and others) can cause an indolent monarthritis from which an inflammatory, mainly monocytic, synovial fluid is obtained. Synovial fluid cultures are usually sterile, and signs of active extra-articular disease are minimal. A prompt, accurate diagnosis of tuberculous arthritis requires a high degree of suspicion and culture of synovial biopsy specimens. Extensive joint destruction is often present before a diagnosis of tuberculous arthritis is made.

Reduction in synovial fluid glucose to less than 50% of simultaneous serum measurement should raise suspicion for the diagnosis of infectious arthritis. In a patient with infectious arthritis, serial measurement of synovial fluid glucose can be one of the several parameters used to gauge the effectiveness of therapy.

ERYTHROCYTE SEDIMENTATION RATE AND ACUTE PHASE RESPONSE PROTEINS

The systemic response to tissue injury, regardless of cause, is characterized by a cytokine-mediated alteration in the hepatic synthesis of a number of different plasma proteins, known collectively as "acute phase reactants" (see Chapter 313). These proteins, which include fibrinogen, haptoglobin, ceruloplasmin, α_1-antitrypsin, complement components C3 and C4, serum amyloid A protein, and C-reactive protein (CRP), rise in proportion to the severity of tissue injury, although the magnitude of rise in each component varies. Because some systemic rheumatic disorders cause chronic tissue inflammation and injury, assessment of the acute phase response is an important facet of rheumatic disease diagnosis and management (because the effectiveness of treatment is gauged by the extent to which the acute phase response is suppressed).

Measuring the *erythrocyte sedimentation rate* (ESR) has been a time-honored and simple method to approximate the acute phase response. "Extreme" elevation of the ESR (>100 mm/hour) has come to have diagnostic significance, associating with polymyalgia rheumatica, giant cell arteritis, multiple myeloma, lymphoma, metastatic cancer, severe chronic infections such as subacute bacterial endocarditis and tuberculosis, and chronic renal failure. Reduction or normalization of the ESR is a goal of treatment for those treatable disorders associated with a rapid ESR. Sedimentation of erythrocytes is facilitated by certain plasma proteins that neutralize the negative charge on the erythrocyte surface, thus permitting the erythrocytes to aggregate and "fall" as a clump rather than as individual cells. Fibrinogen is among the plasma proteins capable of this action; thus the level of fibrinogen—which varies according to the intensity of the acute phase response—substantially affects the ESR. However, other proteins not associated with the acute phase response—notably immunoglobulin (particularly when present as a single paraprotein) and certain "middle molecules" in patients with chronic renal failure—also accelerate the ESR. Normal values for ESR span a wide range, slightly higher in women than men and increasing with age in both sexes. Many individuals aged 70 and older may have ESRs in the range of 40 to 50 mm/hour without apparent inflammation or tissue injury. This confounds the usefulness of the ESR in supporting a suspected rheumatic disease diagnosis such a polymyalgia rheumatica in an elderly person. Finally, not all patients with clinically active rheumatic diseases will have raised ESRs because of individual differences in hepatic function, alterations in erythrocytes, or abnormalities of other plasma proteins that counteract effects of acute phase reactants that speed the ESR.

Of the several acute phase reactants that can be measured directly, CRP, named for its binding of pneumococcal C-polysaccharide, is the most extensively studied and clinically useful. Most rheumatic diseases, including rheumatoid arthritis, juvenile chronic arthritis, ankylosing spondylitis, polymyalgia rheumatica, systemic vasculitis, Behçet's syndrome, Reiter's disease, and psoriatic arthritis are associated with high levels of CRP (1 to 10 mg/dL) when they are active, with falling or undetectable levels when improving or inactive. For diseases in the spondyloarthropathy family (ankylosing spondylitis, Reiter's, psoriatic arthritis), the CRP is far more sensitive to fluctuations in disease activity than is the ESR. Systemic lupus (SLE) disease activity, in the majority of patients, raises the CRP only slightly if at all (1 to 3 mg/dL); concurrent infection in SLE will raise the CRP, and extreme CRP elevation

(>10 mg/dL) in a lupus patient should provoke a hunt for infection.

AUTOANTIBODIES

Rheumatoid factors are immunoglobulins directed against the Fc portion of immunoglobulin G (IgG) (see Chapter 286). Measuring rheumatoid factor by tests that determine the highest dilution of serum capable of agglutinating IgG-coated latex particles has been replaced in most laboratories by automated methods such as nephelometry and enzyme-linked immunosorbent assays. Thus, the reporting of rheumatoid factor "titer" is often replaced by reporting an absolute concentration. Rheumatoid factor positivity with titers up to 1:320 may be found in otherwise normal people older than age 70. Whereas rheumatoid factor can be found in 70 to 80% of patients with rheumatoid arthritis, it is also present in other rheumatic diseases (Sjögren's syndrome, cryoglobulinemia, SLE) and non-rheumatic diseases, such as chronic infections (hepatitis, subacute bacterial endocarditis). In patients with rheumatoid arthritis, the presence of rheumatoid factor is associated with more severe disease, manifested by rheumatoid nodules, rheumatoid vasculitis, and bone erosions.

Testing serum for presence of *antinuclear antibodies* (ANAs) is useful primarily in the evaluation of suspected SLE (see Chapter 289). Many different antigen-antibody reactions underlie the various patterns detected by the ANA test, and identification of antibody to a specific antigen is diagnostically useful in several instances (Table 285–2). Antibodies to double-stranded DNA (particularly if raised one or more standard deviations above normal test range) and to the Smith (Sm) antigen are highly specific for lupus but not present in all cases. Antibodies to U1-nRNP, particularly if high titer, identify mixed connective tissue disease, an overlap syndrome in which features of lupus, scleroderma, and myositis are likely to persist. An ANA pattern displaying fluorescence over centromeres in dividing cells associates with a range of scleroderma syndromes, usually with the milder CREST variant (but also with diffuse scleroderma) and sometimes identifies patients with isolated Raynaud's disease who will progress to a scleroderma syndrome (see Chapter 290). Tests for specific antibodies that associate with subsets of polymyositis (such as Jo-1) or scleroderma (ScL-70) are associated with good diagnostic specificity.

Most positive ANAs occur for reasons other than a rheumatic disease, because 1 to 2% of the normal population shows a positive, if low-titer, test. The frequency increases with age, with 20 to 25% of persons age 60 or older showing a positive test, and is higher in family members of patients with a rheumatic disease. Many drugs can produce a positive ANA without inducing a lupus-like syndrome, although the list of responsible agents is similar for both. Chronic liver diseases, pulmonary disorders (pulmonary fibrosis, primary pulmonary hypertension), and endocrine syndromes (type I diabetes mellitus, autoimmune thyroid disease) show positive ANAs in a high proportion in patients, which in some instances can be taken as an overlap with a forme fruste rheumatic disorder (such as the patient with primary biliary cirrhosis and a positive ANA). Certain leukemias, lymphomas, and solid tumors can be associated with ANAs; because paraneoplastic phenomena can mimic rheumatic disease, the diagnosis of malignancy should be kept in mind when encountering serologic tests suggesting a rheumatic disorder in a perplexing multisystem illness that does not fit well with any rheumatic disease diagnosis. Finally, a number of infections raise ANAs. These include chronic parasitic infestations such as malaria, schistosomiasis, trypanosomiasis, and liver flukes, along with tuberculosis, leprosy, and certain bacterial infections due to *Salmonella* and *Klebsiella*. In many affected patients, classic Epstein-Barr virus infection (infectious mononucleosis) shows ANAs that disappear with resolution of the illness. Some patients infected with the human immunodeficiency virus have ANA, but the prevalence and significance of this phenomenon remains to be determined.

Use of human granulocytes as substrates for immunofluorescence testing has identified a group of antibodies directed against particles in the neutrophil cytoplasm (anti-neutrophil cytoplasmic antibodies [ANCAs]) that are of growing diagnostic significance. Antibodies against a serine protease contained in cytoplasmic granules

Table 285–2 ■ ASSOCIATIONS BETWEEN SELECTED NUCLEAR AND CYTOPLASMIC AUTOANTIBODIES AND CERTAIN RHEUMATIC DISEASES

SUBSTRATE AND IM-MUNOFLUORESCENCE PATTERN	ANTIBODY	ANTIGEN	DISEASE ASSOCIATION(S)	COMMENTS
Human epithelial cells (Hep-2)				
Homogeneous ANA	Anti-histone	Histones H1, H2A, H2B, H3, H4	Drug-induced lupus (>95%), infectious mononucleosis (5–10%), normals (1–2%)	Low titer (<1:320) in "normals"
Rim ANA	Anti-native DNA	Double-stranded DNA	SLE (50%)	Antibodies to double-stranded DNA highly specific for SLE; "RiM ANA" is rare pattern on Hep-2 cells
Speckled ANA	Anti-Sm	Non-histone proteins DEFG complexed with small nuclear RNAs	SLE (30%)	Highly specific for SLE
	Anti-U1-nRNP	U1 small nuclear ribonucleo-protein	SLE (35%); MCTD (>95%)	High titer in MCTD
	Anti-Ro (SS-A)	Two proteins complexed with small RNAs Y1–Y5	SLE (35%); Sjögren's (70–80%)	Often missed on Hep-2 ANA; common in "ANA-negative" lupus
	Anti-La (SS-B)	Single protein + RNA polymerase III transcript	SLE (15%); Sjögren's (50–70%)	
	Anti-Ku	DNA binding protein	SLE (10%)	May identify SLE/PSS/myositis overlap
	Anti-Scl-70	DNA topoisomerase I	PSS (40–70%); CREST (10–20%)	
Nucleolar ANA	Anti-PM-Scl	Nucleolar protein complex	PSS (3%); PM (8%)	May identify "sclerodermato-myositis" overlap
	Anti-Mi-2	Nuclear protein complex	DM (15–20%)	Rare in PM
	Anti-RNA polymerase I	Subunits of RNA polymerase I	PSS (4%)	
Dividing cell–specific patterns	Anticentromere	Centromere/kinetochore protein	CREST (80%), PSS (30%)	In patients with isolated Raynaud's, may predict progression to CREST
	Anti–proliferating cell nuclear antigen	Auxiliary protein of DNA polymerase δ	SLE (3%)	
Cytoplasmic staining	Antisynthetases:			
	Anti–Jo-1	Histidyl tRNA synthetase	PM/DM (18–25%)	Often with ISLD
	Anti–PL-7	Threonyl tRNA synthetase	PM/DM (3%)	Often with ISLD
	Anti–PL-12	Alanyl tRNA synthetase	PM/DM (3%)	Often with ISLD
	Anti-SRP	Signal recognition particle	PM (4%)	No Raynaud's, rare ISLD, poor prognosis
	Antiribosomal P	Large ribosomal subunit	SLE (10%)	May associate with CNS manifestations
	Antimitochondrial	E2 component of pyruvate dehydrogenase complex at inner mitochondrial membrane	Primary biliary cirrhosis (PBC, 90–95%; normals, <1%)	PCB may show CREST, Sjögren's features
Alcohol-fixed human neutrophils				
Cytosol staining	c-ANCA	Serine protease 3 (PR-3)	Wegener's granulomatosis (90%)	
Perinuclear staining	p-ANCA	Myeloperoxidase	Microscopic polyarteritis (necrotizing glomerulonephritis with or without extrarenal small vessel vasculitis); Churg-Strauss syndrome, miscellaneous vasculitides	
	p-ANCA (atypical)	Lysozyme, lactoferrin, cathepsin G, bactericidal/permeability increasing protein (BPI)	Ulcerative colitis (40–80%), Crohn's disease (10–40%), primary sclerosing cholangitis (65-84%)	

ANA = antinuclear antibody; SLE = systemic lupus erythematosus; MCTD = mixed connective tissue disease; PSS = progressive systemic sclerosis (diffuse scleroderma); CREST = calcinosis, Raynaud's phenomenon, esophageal dysmotility, sclerodactyly, and telangiectasia; PM = polymyositis; DM = dermatomyositis; ISLD = interstitial lung disease; ANCA = antineutrophil cytoplasmic antibody.

(c-ANCA) can be found in 90% of patients with Wegener's granulomatosis (see Chapter 294) and in patients with chronic inflammation isolated to one or a few sites (e.g., sinuses, lung, or kidney) who do not have full-blown Wegener's granulomatosis. Although ANCA disappears in some patients with Wegener's granulomatosis with successful treatment, and may reappear before a clinically evident flare, these fluctuations have not proven sufficiently reliable to guide treatment. Other ANCA patterns, mostly due to reaction with myeloperoxidase, associate with a range of nephritic and vasculitic syndromes. However, these associations are not strong enough for ANCA to be considered a "vasculitis test," and a positive ANCA should not be substituted for biopsy confirmation of Wegener's granulomatosis or vasculitis when cytotoxic therapy is being considered.

Antiphospholipid antibodies are encountered in many patients with SLE and can be detected in patients without SLE who present with sequelae of thrombosis in vessels of different sizes (e.g., livedo reticularis, gangrene, venous thrombosis, pulmonary emboli, strokes, transverse myelitis, recurrent spontaneous abortions). Results of several other tests in which phospholipids play an important role can be altered by antiphospholipid antibodies. The partial thromboplastin time (PTT) is prolonged by interference with the prothrombin activator complex (coagulation Factors V and Xa, platelet factor 3, and calcium), and this in vitro anticoagulation is not completely corrected by normal plasma (defining the "lupus anticoagulant"). Recognizing the phospholipid-rich cardiolipin-cholesterol-phosphatidylcholine target antigen in the Venereal Disease Research Laboratories (VDRL) test turns this (and other tests for syphilis) falsely positive. Thrombocytopenia and a positive Coombs test may occur. A solid-phase immunoassay for IgG and IgM antibodies to cardiolipin is the most widely used test to confirm presence of antiphospholipid antibodies. Risk for future thrombosis in patients with cardiolipin antibodies is strongly predicted by a prolonged dilute Russell viper venom time.

Plain radiographs of the joints are relatively inexpensive and widely available. For many rheumatic diseases, information provided by plain radiographs (e.g., the presence, character, and distribution of bone erosions; soft tissue calcification or swelling; alignment of bones; reaction of bone adjacent to joint surfaces; and space between joint surfaces indicating cartilage space) is sufficient to define the problem and can serve as a baseline assessment for judging response to treatment of a chronic process. Plain radiographs may be normal or non-specific at baseline yet become diagnostic as characteristic features evolve. However, the pathologic processes of many rheumatic disorders often occur in structures not defined by x-rays, and other means of imaging must be employed. Arthrography has mostly been replaced by less invasive techniques for assessing such features as suspected loose bodies, meniscal derangements, or abnormalities of the rotator cuff; however, the technique still provides the standard for determining intra-articular volume and can be useful to guide entry into a difficult-to-aspirate joint.

Computed tomography (CT) provides excellent spatial resolution of bone and soft tissue structures in an axial plane and is most useful in defining abnormalities of the spine, including herniated disks, sacroiliac joint abnormalities, narrowing of spinal canal or neural foramina by bony outgrowths (spinal stenosis), and trauma. Magnetic resonance imaging (MRI) also provides superb spatial resolution of anatomic structures and characterizes tissue according to its morphologic appearance and physical properties. MRI has become the procedure of choice to delineate abnormalities of intra-articular and periarticular soft tissue structures in large joints, especially the shoulder (rotator cuff tears, glenoid labrum abnormalities) and knee (derangements of menisci and ligaments). For disorders of the spine, MRI can show structural abnormalities and discern their effect on the adjacent spinal cord. Although most bony abnormalities are better shown by plain radiographs or CT, MRI can show features of osteonecrosis (dead marrow secondary to ischemia) and osteomyelitis (increased focal marrow signal indicating edema) before they can be seen on any other imaging study. Because of the high cost and limited availability of MRI, its use should be limited to situations in which patient management will be significantly altered by possible findings.

Scintigraphy differs from other imaging techniques by providing information that pertains more to function than to structure of the abnormalities shown. The distribution of tracer is a function of local blood flow, vascular permeability, and tissue uptake. Technetium-99m-pyrophosphate is taken up by metabolically active bone and thus localizes where this is increased (fractures, blastic skeletal metastases, Paget's disease, periostitis, and "actively" degenerating joints); because initial distribution of this radionuclide is dependent on blood flow, scintigraphy, which measures activity at several time points (triple-phase scan), will show uptake initially at sites of increased vascularity (e.g., synovitis, infection, or neoplasia) and then localize to bone later. While ^{99m}Tc-labeled scanning is nonspecific, it can image the entire skeleton at modest cost and be used to screen for bone and joint abnormalities and metastatic disease. Gallium-67 binds to serum and cellular transferrin and lactoferrin and is preferentially taken up by neutrophils and some neoplastic tissues (e.g., lymphoma). Indium-111–labeled leukocyte scans permit more specific assessment of focal bone or joint infection. Site of tracer localization can be determined with some precision by subjecting the scanned image to single photon emission computed tomography (SPECT), which generates a virtual three-dimensional reconstruction of the image.

Ultrasonography (US) can discern boundaries between the various soft tissue structures comprising the musculoskeletal system and can evaluate pathology within these structures. That US can localize a fluid-containing structure can be useful in identifying a joint or bursa for aspiration that may have been difficult to enter using standard landmarks. Lesions of tendons, ligaments, and muscle can be identified and characterized. US is more operator dependent than other imaging modalities but in experienced hands is the procedure of choice for defining the pathologic anatomy of a painful periarticular region when physical examination and plain radiographs are not explanatory.

ARTHROSCOPY

Identifying and repairing traumatic injuries to specific intra-articular structures remain the major focus of arthroscopy. However, the use of arthroscopy as a tool for investigating and treating rheumatic disorders could grow considerably as more rheumatologists take up the procedure by using smaller "needle" arthroscopes that can be employed in an office setting.

Arthroscopy has three generic capabilities: direct inspection of intra-articular anatomy, visually guided sampling (biopsy) of tissues, and modification/resection of pathologic tissue under direct visualization using specially designed instruments. During the procedure, the joint is distended and irrigated with a physiologic salt solution to clear away blood and debris that might otherwise cloud the view. Conventional arthroscopy is usually done in a sterile operating room, using a rigid glass lens magnifying scope coupled to a small camera that projects the intra-articular view to a video screen. Other instruments placed into the joint through additional punctures can be used to manipulate, cut, shave, and remove various tissues. Virtually all major joints can be arthroscoped, with the knee by far the most commonly entered, followed by the shoulder, ankle, elbow, wrist, and hip.

Some differential diagnostic possibilities that can be confirmed or refuted by arthroscopy include processes that are treatable but lead to joint destruction if undetected, such as tuberculosis; and arthroscopy should be considered when these processes are even remotely possible. Closed synovial biopsy can be used if arthroscopy is not available, but it may miss areas of pathology sparsely distributed in the joint.

Arthroscopy can be used in the management of patients with a diagnosed inflammatory arthropathy (such as rheumatoid arthritis) who have persistent knee symptoms not responding to conventional medical management. Patients with persistent synovitis can be treated by removing visibly inflamed or proliferative synovial tissue from all compartments of the knee under arthroscopic guidance (arthroscopic synovectomy). In other patients whose features do not suggest ongoing synovitis (pain with minimal swelling, "locking" or "giving way"), arthroscopy can show pathology—focal collections of proliferative synovium, areas of synovial scarring, or other consequences of prior inflammation such as softened and torn menisci or attenuated and eroded cruciate ligaments—for which arthroscopically guided resection can often be therapeutic.

In contrast to the "inflamed" knee, the painful knee with non-inflammatory synovial fluid usually is diagnosed by defining a particular derangement of the intra-articular anatomy. The most common "derangement" is that of the articular cartilage surface, which is often suggested by grating or *crepitus* of the joint surfaces moving past one another and confirmed with some certainty by finding other features of osteoarthritis on plain radiographs (osteophytes, joint space narrowing, subchondral sclerosis). Other intra-articular abnormalities—torn or degenerated meniscal cartilage, loose bodies, focal synovial collections—can be identified and treated by arthroscopy. Some processes that disrupt joint surfaces through changes in underlying bone cannot be seen or modified at arthroscopy; these processes—osteonecrosis, stress fracture, malignancy—are often not apparent on plain radiographs and thus require more extensive imaging, such as MRI.

Casiano CA, Tan EM: Recent developments in the understanding of antinuclear autoantibodies. Int Arch Allergy Immunol 111:308–313, 1996. *Review of evolving concepts in the ANA response associated with various diseases, including the characteristic ANA spectrum with each systemic autoimmune disease, functionally important subcellular particles against which ANAs are directed, and role of apoptosis in releasing potentially immunostimulatory self-antigens from cells.*

Ike RW: Diagnostic arthroscopy. Baillières Clin Rheumatol 10:495–517, 1996. *A review of the various situations in rheumatology where diagnostic arthroscopy can be useful and why.*

Scott WW Jr: Evaluation of the patient: Imaging techniques. *In* Klippel JH (ed): Primer on the Rheumatic Diseases, 11th ed. Atlanta, Arthritis Foundation, 1997, pp 106–115. *Concise, well-illustrated synopsis of capabilities and limitations of available imaging procedures applicable to situations encountered in rheumatology.*

Ward MM: Laboratory testing for systemic rheumatic diseases. Postgrad Med 103:93–100, 1998. *The accuracy and utility of tests available for diagnosis and follow-up evaluation of systemic rheumatic diseases are discussed, with attention to the specificity, sensitivity, and predictive values of various tests, along with explanation of which tests are most helpful for specific situations.*

286 RHEUMATOID ARTHRITIS

Frank C. Arnett

Rheumatoid arthritis (RA) is a chronic systemic inflammatory disease predominantly affecting diarthrodial joints and frequently a variety of other organs. The American College of Rheumatology revised the classification criteria for RA to guarantee uniformity in investigative and epidemiologic studies (Table 286–1). Although these seven items include the most characteristic clinical features of RA, a variety of other disorders may mimic the disease (see Differential Diagnosis and Table 286–3).

RA occurs worldwide in all ethnic groups. Prevalence rates range from 0.3 to 1.5% in most populations, but frequencies of 3.5 to 5.3% have been found in several Native American tribes (Yakima, Chippewa, Inuit). The peak incidence of onset is between the 4th and 6th decades, but RA may begin at any time from childhood (see Juvenile Chronic Arthritis) to later life. Females are two to three times more likely to be affected than males.

ETIOLOGY. Despite intensive research over many decades, the cause of RA remains unknown. Three areas of interrelated research are currently most promising: (1) host genetic factors, (2) immunoregulatory abnormalities and autoimmunity, and (3) a triggering or persisting microbial infection.

Genetic susceptibility to RA has been clearly demonstrated. The disease clusters in families and is more concordant in monozygotic (30%) than dizygotic (5%) twins. Certain major histocompatibility complex (MHC) class II alleles (and their encoded HLA, or human leukocyte antigens) occur with increased frequency in affected individuals. Among white people of western European origin, HLA-DR4 occurs in 60 to 70% of seropositive patients with RA as compared with 25 to 30% of normal individuals. HLA-DR1 is found in the majority of HLA-DR4–negative patients and is most strongly associated with the disease in several other ethnic groups (Israelis, Asian Indians). Several subtypes of HLA-DR4 were initially defined by mixed lymphocyte culture and more recently by DNA sequencing (Table 286–2). Only certain HLA-DR4 subtypes predispose to RA (Dw4 or DRB1*0401, Dw14 or DRB1*0404, and Dw15 or DRB1*0405), whereas others do not (Dw10 or DRB1*0402 and Dw13 or DRB1*0403). HLA-DR4 subtypes result from only a few amino acid differences in the 3rd hypervariable region of the HLA-DR β-chain. HLA-DR1 shares this same amino acid sequence, as do several other HLA alleles that have more recently been associated with RA in some populations (see Table 286–2). Thus a "shared epitope" among several MHC class II molecules appears to predispose to RA. Moreover, homozygosity for the amino acid sequence, especially if carried on HLA-DR4 molecules, has been shown to correlate with disease severity, including more destructive joint disease, subcutaneous nodules, and extra-articular manifestations, especially rheumatoid lung disease and Felty's syndrome. The crucial region for the shared epitope on HLA-DR molecules appears to be a combining site for the T-cell antigen receptor (TCR). Because MHC class II molecules present processed antigen to the TCR on helper (CD4+) T lymphocytes (see Chapter 270) it appears likely that an abnormal antigen-specific cellular and/or humoral immune response is inherent to the

etiology of RA. The nature of the antigen, whether self or foreign, remains unknown, although candidates include type II collagen, microbial antigens or heat shock proteins, and immunoglobulins. Other genes are also necessary for RA, and genome mapping studies are in progress.

RA appears to be an "autoimmune" disease, similar to other MHC class II–associated disorders (see Chapter 278). Autoantibodies to the Fc portion of IgG molecules, or rheumatoid factors are present in the blood and synovial tissues of 80% of RA patients. Such cases are termed "seropositive." High titers of serum rheumatoid factor typically of the IgM isotype, are associated with more severe joint disease and with extra-articular manifestations, especially subcutaneous nodules.

Despite the extremely strong association of rheumatoid factors with RA, they clearly do not cause the disease. Production of rheumatoid factor commonly occurs in other disorders characterized by chronic antigenic stimulation, such as bacterial endocarditis, tuberculosis, syphilis, kala-azar, viral infections, intravenous drug abuse, and cirrhosis. Normal individuals occasionally produce rheumatoid factor, especially with increasing age.

An infectious origin for RA has been a continuing hypothesis. A variety of bacterial and viral candidates have been proposed and later discarded because of lack of definitive evidence. Viral infections such as rubella, Ross River virus, and parvovirus B19 have been shown to produce an acute polyarthritis, but no evidence exists that they initiate chronic RA. Epstein-Barr virus (EBV) remains a viable but unproven candidate for a pathogenetic role because several unusual immune responses to it are found in patients with RA. An EBV protein has also been shown to share the same five amino acids as the HLA-DR4 (Dw14) and HLA-DR1 molecules, which are implicated in susceptibility to RA, thus raising the possibility of "molecular mimicry" as a mechanism. A similar homology with an *Escherichia coli* heat shock protein has also been found.

PATHOLOGY AND PATHOGENESIS. The pathologic hallmark of RA is synovial membrane proliferation and outgrowth associated with erosion of articular cartilage and subchondral bone. Often likened to a malignant tumor, proliferating inflammatory tissue (pannus) may subsequently lead to destruction of intra-articular and periarticular structures and result in the joint deformities and dysfunction seen clinically.

The events initiating the process are unknown (Fig. 286–1). The earliest findings include microvascular injury and proliferation of synovial cells, accompanied by interstitial edema and perivascular infiltration by mononuclear cells, predominantly T lymphocytes. Continuation of the process leads to further hyperplasia of lining cells, both DR-positive type A (macrophage-like) and DR-negative type B (fibroblast-like), and the normally acellular subsynovial stroma becomes engorged with mononuclear inflammatory cells, which may collect into aggregates or follicles, especially around post-capillary venules. The composition of cellular infiltrates varies, with some being predominantly T cells, usually CD4+ (helper/inducer), and others having a mixed population of lymphocytes (often CD8+ cytotoxic T cells), plasma cells, macrophages, and interdigitating (dendritic) cells. Occasionally, germinal centers rich in B lymphocytes can be seen. The proliferating synovium (pannus) becomes villous and is vascularized by arterioles, capillaries, and venules.

Roles for both *cellular* and *humoral* immune mechanisms in the rheumatoid synovium are supported by molecular and immunopathologic findings. T lymphocytes, chiefly of the T_H1 type, appear to be activated, presumably by some unknown antigen(s) presented by DR-positive cells (type A synoviocytes, macrophages, dendritic cells, B lymphocytes). Studies of TCR gene expression suggest restricted $V\beta$ usage and oligoclonality, but this area is controversial. Collectively, these interacting immune cells produce a variety of cytokines that promote further synovial proliferation and inflammation, as well as bone and cartilage destruction. Important *proinflammatory cytokines* appear to be linked in a cascade, with tumor necrosis factor α (TNF-α) at the apex promoting the subsequent elaboration of interleukin-1 (IL-1), IL-6, IL-8, and granulocyte-macrophage colony-stimulating factor (GM-CSF). IL-1 induces the production of metalloproteinases (collagenase and stromelysin) and prostaglandin E_2 by synoviocytes. This cytokine also promotes the degradation and inhibits the synthesis of proteoglycan by chondrocytes, as well as enhances resorption of calcium from bone. At

---

Table 286–1 ■ CLASSIFICATION CRITERIA FOR RHEUMATOID ARTHRITIS*

1. Morning stiffness (≥ 1 hr)
2. Swelling (soft tissue) of 3 or more joints
3. Swelling (soft tissue) of hand joints (PIP, MCP, or wrist)
4. Symmetrical swelling (soft tissue)
5. Subcutaneous nodules
6. Serum rheumatoid factor
7. Erosions and/or periarticular osteopenia in hand or wrist joints seen on radiograph

PIP = proximal interphalangeal; MCP = metacarpophalangeal.
*Criteria 1 to 4 must have been continuous for 6 weeks or longer and criteria 2 to 5 must be observed by a physician. A diagnosis of rheumatoid arthritis requires that four of the seven criteria be fulfilled.

PLATE 7   MUSCULOSKELETAL AND CONNECTIVE TISSUE DISEASES

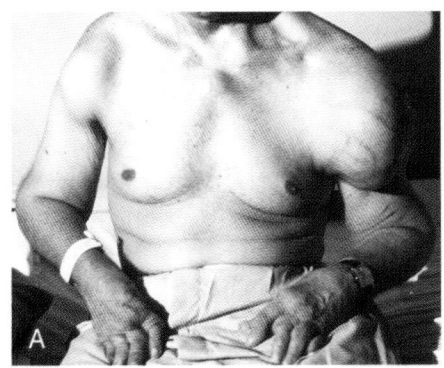

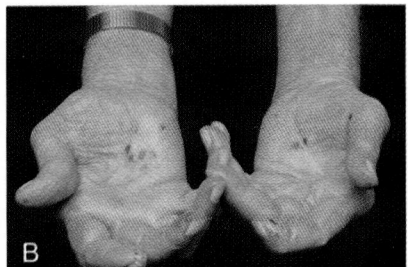

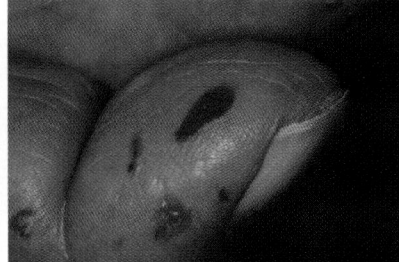

B, Left and *right.* Rheumatoid vasculitis with small brown infarcts of palms and fingers in chronic rheumatoid arthritis. (Courtesy of Dr. Martin Lidsky.)

A, Large synovial cysts of the shoulders, especially on the left, in a patient with chronic deforming rheumatoid arthritis.

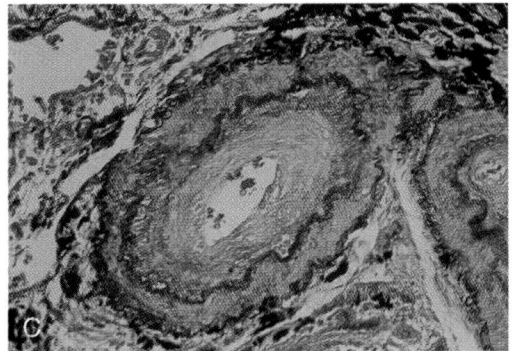

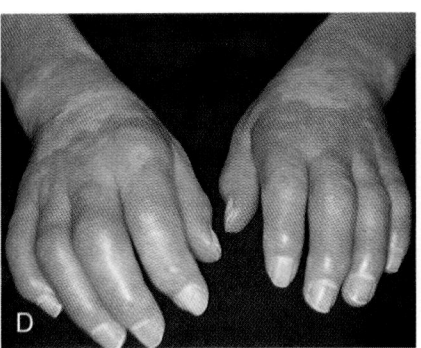

C, Scleroderma. Pathological slide of small artery in the lung. Marked proliferation of the intimal layer of the vessel narrows the lumen and alters local blood flow. Endothelial cell dysfunction is also known to occur.

D, Scleroderma involving the hands. *Left,* Edematous phase with diffuse swelling of fingers. *Right,* Atrophic phase with contracture and thickening sclerodactyly (thick skin over the fingers).

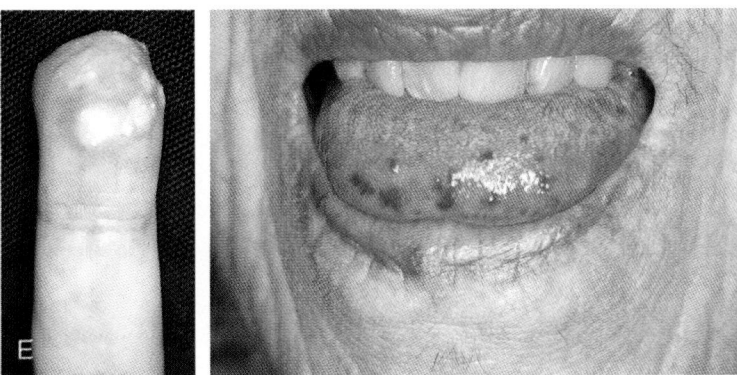

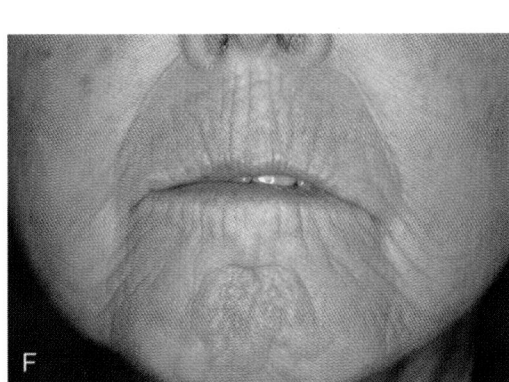

E, Features of CREST syndrome. *Left,* Subcutaneous calcinosis on tip of finger. *Right,* Telangiectasia on mucous membrane/tongue.

F, Facial features in scleroderma. Note the vertical lines or furrowing around the mouth in this patient with diffuse scleroderma.

PLATE 7   MUSCULOSKELETAL AND CONNECTIVE TISSUE DISEASES *Continued*

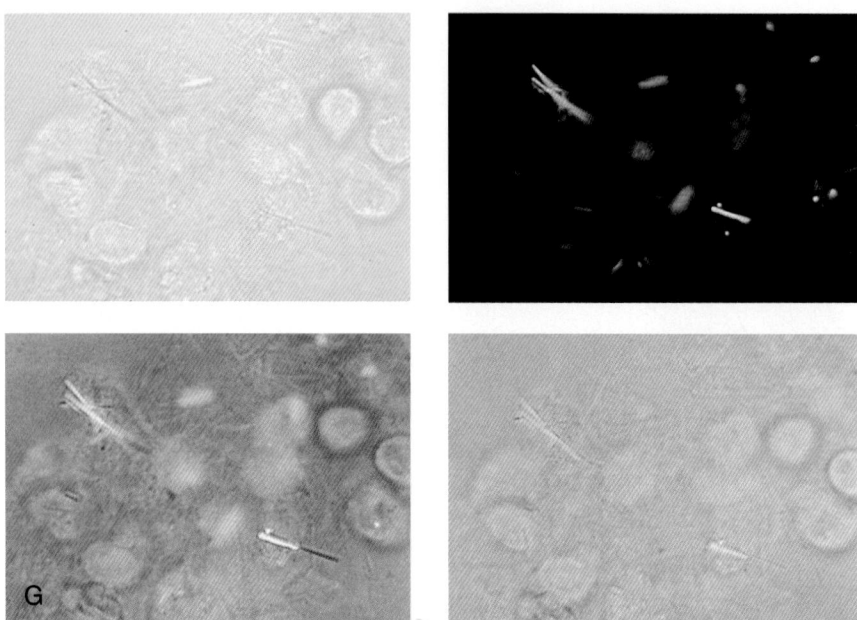

G, Monosodium urate crystals in synovial fluid aspirate. *Top left,* Plain light microscopy. *Top right,* Polarized light. *Bottom left,* First-order red compensator with axis of vibration perpendicular to crystals (2 o'clock to 7 o'clock). *Bottom right,* First-order red compensator with axis of vibration parallel to crystals (11 o'clock to 4 o'clock).

PLATE 8   INFECTIOUS, MUSCULOSKELETAL, AND PROTOZOAN DISEASES

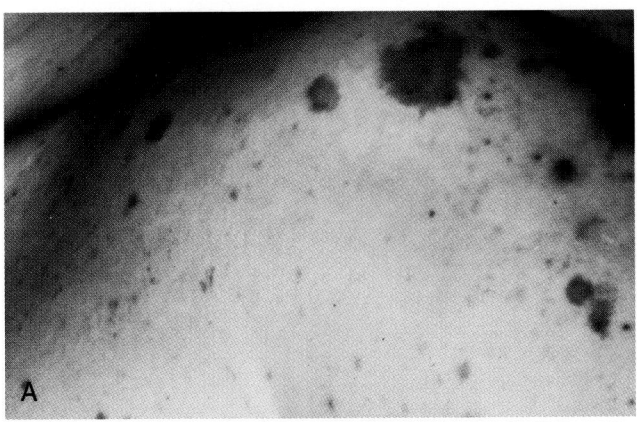

A, A patient with advanced meningococcemia who has multiple petechiae and ecchymoses on the shoulders, chest, and arm.

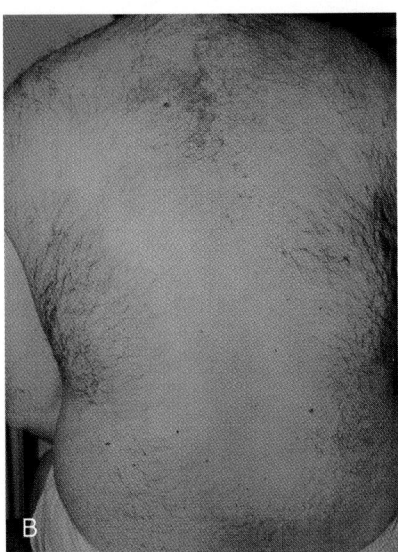

B, Erythema migrans (EM) is the major dermatologic manifestation of Lyme disease. Four days after onset of EM, this patient has developed secondary annular lesions; some of their borders have merged. (From Steere AC, Bartenhagen NH, Craft JE, et al.: The early clinical manifestations of Lyme disease. Ann Intern Med 99:76–82, 1983; with permission.)

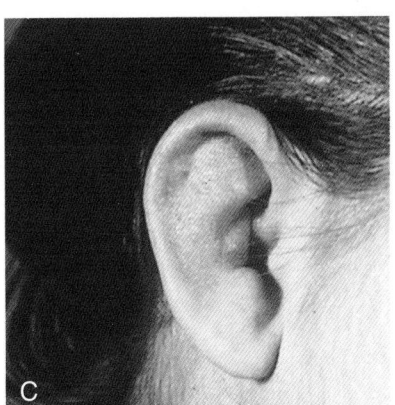

C, Polychondritis. Note nodularity of ear.

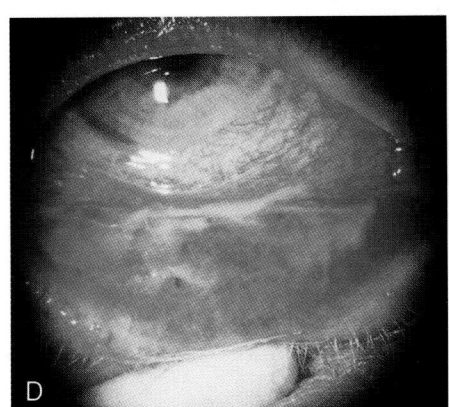
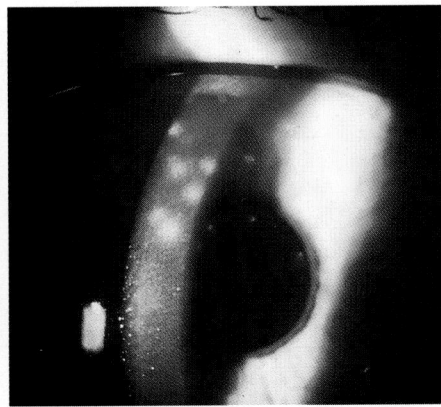

D, Left, Severe, hemorrhagic pseudomembranous conjunctivitis due to adenovirus. When lymphoid follicles are present, they are suggestive of a viral etiology. *Right,* Slit lamp examination 1 month after presentation shows subepithelial opacities composed of lymphocytic infiltrates. The opacities can persist for as long as 1 year. (Courtesy of Dr. Steven Ching.)

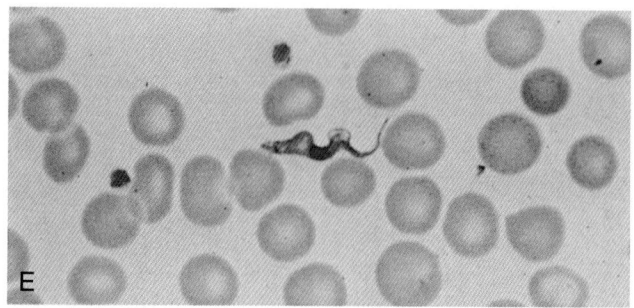

E, Trypanosoma rhodesiense in the peripheral blood. It has a nucleus, posterior kinetoplast, undulating membrane, and flagellum (×1500).

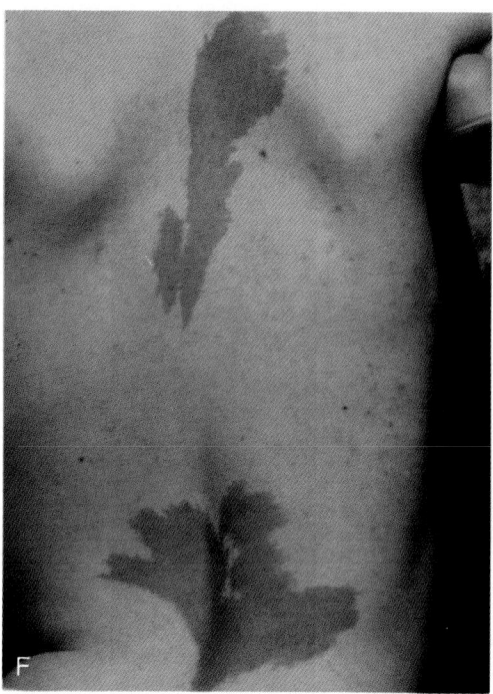

F, McCune-Albright syndrome. Typical rough-border ("coast-of-Maine") pigmented cafe au lait spot. (From Whyte MP: Metabolic and dysplastic disorders. *In* Coe FL, Favus MJ [eds]: Disorders of Bone and Mineral Metabolism. New York, Raven Press, 1992.)

Table 286–2 ■ HLA ASSOCIATIONS WITH RHEUMATOID ARTHRITIS

	HLA TYPES (ALLELES) AND METHODS OF DETECTION			THIRD HYPERVARIABLE REGION AMINO ACID SEQUENCES					MOST COMMON ETHNIC GROUPS
	Alloantisera (DR)	MLC (Dw)	DNA (DRB1)	70	71	72	73	74	
Associated with RA	DR4	Dw4	*0401	Q	K	R	A	A	Whites (west Europe)
	DR4	Dw14	*0404	·	R	·	·	·	Whites (west Europe)
	DR4	Dw15	*0405	·	R	·	·	·	Japanese, Chinese
	DR1	Dw1	*0101	·	R	·	·	·	Asian Indians, Israelis
	DR6 (14)	Dw16	*1402	·	R	·	·	·	Yakima Native Americans
	DR10	—	*1001	R	R	·	·	·	Spanish, Greeks, Israelis
Not associated with RA	DR4	Dw10	*0402	D	E	·	·	·	Whites (East Europe)
	DR4	Dw13	*0403	·	R	·	·	E	Polynesians
	DR2	Dw2	*1501	D	A	·	·	·	Whites
	DR3	Dw3	*0301	·	·	·	G	R	Whites

Q = glutamine, K = lysine, R = arginine, A = alanine, D = aspartic acid, E = glutamic acid; · = the same amino acid in that position as DRB1*0401.

the same time, there appears to be an attempt by unregulated *anti-inflammatory cytokines,* such as soluble TNF receptor, transforming-growth factor β (TGF-β), IL-10, and IL-1 receptor antagonist, to counterbalance these destructive effects.

Humoral mechanisms are supported by the demonstration of local rheumatoid factor production within the synovium, the formation of IgM-activated B cells and IgG immune complexes, and activation and consumption of complement via the classic pathway. The sequelae of complement activation include increased vascular permeability and phagocytosis of the immune complexes by phagocytic cells. Aggregates of immune complexes within polymorphonuclear leukocytes are often seen in rheumatoid synovial fluid and have been termed "RA cells" or "ragocytes." Antigen-antibody complexes formed within the joint cavity can become trapped in hyaline cartilage and fibrocartilage, where they cause changes in matrix macromolecules. Within the synovial fluid, immune complexes activate the complement system, kinins, phagocytic cells, and the release of lysosomal enzymes and oxygen free radicals. Mediators produced in this process stimulate synovial cells to proliferate and produce proteinases and prostaglandins. These products cause dissolution of connective tissue macromolecules, as well as articular cartilage. They may also activate fibroblasts to produce a denser connective tissue matrix (fibrosis).

The ultimate destruction of cartilage, bone, tendons, and liga-

ments probably results from a combination of proteolytic enzymes, metalloproteinases, and soluble mediators. Collagenase, produced at the interface of pannus and cartilage, is probably largely responsible for the typical bony erosions.

CLINICAL FEATURES. The mode of onset of RA is highly variable. In the majority of cases, joint pain and/or stiffness develops insidiously over several weeks to months. One or more small joints of the hands, wrists, shoulders, or knees and/or the metatarsophalangeal (MTP) joints are frequently the 1st symptomatic areas. Malaise and fatigue, occasionally with low-grade fever, may accompany musculoskeletal discomfort. As the disease progresses, joint swelling, tenderness, and a red or bluish discoloration become apparent (Fig. 286–2). The pattern of joint involvement is typically polyarticular and symmetrical and involves the proximal interphalangeal (PIP), metacarpophalangeal (MCP), wrist, elbow, shoulder, knee, ankle, and MTP joints. The distal interphalangeal (DIP) joints of the fingers are usually spared. Joint stiffness, especially if lasting more than 1 hour in the morning and after inactivity, is prominent. So characteristic is this symptom that the duration of morning stiffness is often used as a quantitative guide to the activity of the inflammatory process in both clinical practice and research studies. Over time the patient may experience increasing difficulty with pain and stiffness, as well as impaired joint function. The simple activities of daily living may be severely compromised, and the

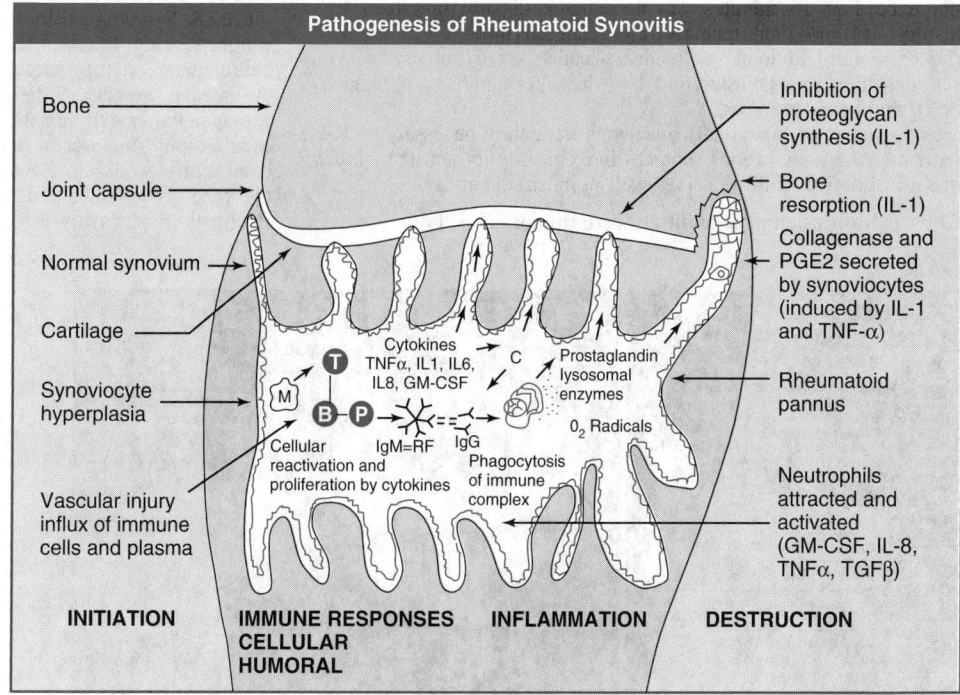

FIGURE 286–1 ■ Events involved in the pathogenesis of rheumatoid synovitis progress from left to right. M = macrophage; T = T lymphocyte; B = B lymphocyte; P = plasma cell; IL = interleukin; TNF-α = tumor necrosis factor α; TGF-β = transforming growth factor β; GM-CSF = granulocyte-macrophage colony-stimulating factor; RF = rheumatoid factor; PGE$_2$ = prostaglandin E$_2$; C = complement.

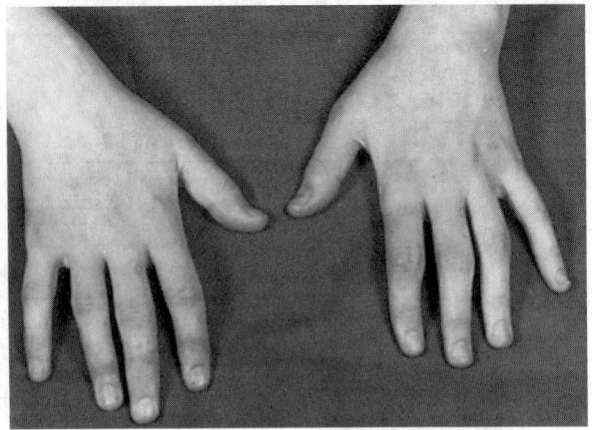

FIGURE 286–2 ■ Early rheumatoid arthritis manifested as symmetrical swelling and slight flexion deformities of the proximal interphalangeal joints of the hands. Radiographs were normal except for evidence of soft tissue swelling.

ability to continue a productive occupation is threatened. Sleep habits become disturbed, and the patient may experience depression and weight loss.

An "acute" onset occurring over 1 or several days is seen in about 20% of patients. Occasionally, an individual retires in the evening with no symptoms and awakens with acute, generalized RA. Such a rapid onset of pain involving the joints, surrounding soft tissue, and muscle can mimic and must be differentiated from acute myositis, viral syndromes, or if focal, even septic or crystal-induced arthritides. Rare patients experience recurrent (palindromic) episodes of acute monarthritis, often so severe as to mimic gout, yet lasting only 24 to 48 hours. Such patients, especially if seropositive, eventually contract the typical chronic, symmetrical polyarthritis of RA.

The course of RA, like its onset, varies widely. Fluctuating disease activity early in the disease process is usual. Ultimately, joint deformities and variable degrees of disability occur in most patients (Fig. 286–3). Some patients have a relentlessly progressive course leading to early disability or even death, but repeated periods of some degree of remission are the rule. The American College of Rheumatology has proposed criteria for clinical remission in RA. At least five of the following requirements must be fulfilled for at least 2 consecutive months: (1) duration of morning stiffness not exceeding 15 minutes, (2) no fatigue, (3) no joint pain (by history), (4) no joint tenderness or pain on motion, (5) no soft tissue swelling in joints or tendon sheaths, or (6) an erythrocyte sedimentation rate (Westergren) less than 30 mm/hour for females or 20 mm/hour for males.

Assessment of functional capacity is frequently necessary in RA patients. Although various schemes have been proposed, the simple classification that follows serves well in most situations:

Class I: No restriction of ability to perform normal activities.

Class II: Moderate restriction, but with an ability to perform most activities of daily living.

Class III: Marked restriction, with an inability to perform most activities of daily living and occupation.

Class IV: Incapacitation with confinement to bed or a wheelchair.

DIFFERENTIAL DIAGNOSIS. Considerations in the differential diagnosis of RA are numerous (Table 286–3). Early RA, especially that of acute onset, is more difficult to diagnose than is the typical established case. The finding of subcutaneous nodules and the presence of rheumatoid factor are useful but not absolutely specific differential features. Therefore, a complete medical evaluation, often including synovial fluid analysis, is indicated in all patients with significant joint manifestations.

ARTICULAR MANIFESTATIONS. RA can affect any diarthrodial joint. Those most commonly involved are the small joints of the hands, wrists, knees, and feet. With time, the disease may also affect the elbows, shoulders, sternoclavicular joints, hips, and ankles. The temporomandibular and cricoarytenoid joints are less frequently involved. Spinal involvement in RA is generally limited to the upper cervical articulations. In contrast to the spondyloarthropathies, RA does not cause sacroiliitis or clinically significant disease in the lumbar or thoracic spinal areas.

HANDS. Swelling of the PIP joints with a fusiform or spindle-shaped appearance of the fingers is one of the most common early signs. Bilateral and symmetrical swelling of the MCP joints is also frequent (see Fig. 286–2). The DIP joints are usually spared, which is a useful sign in discriminating RA from osteoarthritis and psoriatic arthritis. Soft tissue laxity gives rise to ulnar deviation of the fingers at the MCP joints (Fig. 286–3A). Swan neck deformities develop from hyperextension of the PIP joints in conjunction with flexion of the DIP joints (Fig. 286–3B). Boutonnière (buttonhole) deformities result from flexion contractures of the PIP joints in association with hyperextension of the DIP joints. These changes result in a loss of strength and dexterity in the hands, as well as the ability to maintain a good pinch. Synovial erosions of extensor tendons, usually at the dorsum of the wrist, may lead to sudden rupture and loss of the ability to extend one or more fingers.

WRISTS. The wrists are almost invariably involved in RA and frequently demonstrate easily palpable, boggy synovium, especially over the ulnar styloid. Loss of wrist motion, both flexion and extension, usually occurs to some degree. The median nerve on the volar side often becomes compressed by proliferating synovium, the result being carpal tunnel syndrome (Fig. 286–4). The patient notes paresthesias or pain in the thumb, 2nd and 3rd digits, and radial side of the 4th digit. Symptoms are typically worse at night or with other activities associated with sustained flexion of the wrist. *Tinel's* (Fig. 286–4) and *Phalen's* (Fig. 286–5) signs can usually be elicited, and thenar muscle wasting may be evident.

KNEES. Synovial proliferation and effusion are common in these weight-bearing joints. Effusions may be detected by performing ballottement on the patella or by observing a "bulge sign" along the medial aspect of the patella when fluid is pushed into the suprapatellar pouch and then expressed back into the joint. Quadriceps atrophy may occur, and a flexion contracture of the knee may compromise walking. Eventually, destruction of soft tissue around the knee can produce marked joint instability and valgus deformity. Popliteal (Baker's) cysts may form as a result of effusion or syn-

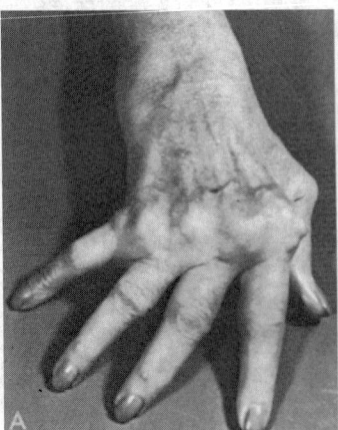
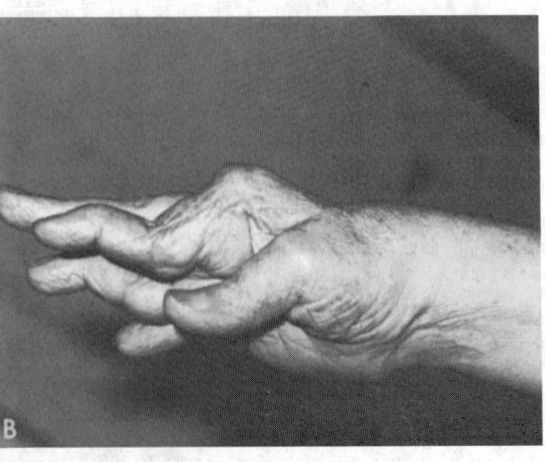

FIGURE 286–3 ■ Hand deformities characteristic of chronic rheumatoid arthritis. *A,* Subluxation of the metacarpophalangeal joints with ulnar deviation of the digits. *B,* Hyperextension ("swan neck") deformities of the proximal interphalangeal joints.

Table 286–3 ■ DIFFERENTIAL DIAGNOSIS OF RHEUMATOID ARTHRITIS

DISORDER	SUBCUTANEOUS NODULES	RHEUMATOID FACTOR
Acute viral arthritis (rubella, hepatitis B, parvovirus)	−	−
Bacterial endocarditis	+/−	+
Acute rheumatic fever	+	−
Serum sickness	−	−
Sarcoidosis	+	+
Reactive arthritis (Reiter's disease)	−	−
Psoriatic arthritis	−	−
Inflammatory bowel disease	−	−
Whipple's disease	−	−
Systemic lupus erythematosus	+	+
Sjögren's syndrome	−	+
Systemic sclerosis (scleroderma)	−	+/−
Polymyositis	−	+/−
Vasculitis syndromes	−	+
Polymyalgia rheumatica	−	−
Polyarticular gout	+ (tophi)	−
Calcium pyrophosphate disease	−	−
Amyloidosis	+/−	−
Paraneoplastic syndromes	−	−
Multicentric reticulohistiocytosis	+	−
Osteoarthritis (erosive)	−	−

− = not present; + = frequently present; +/− = occasionally present.

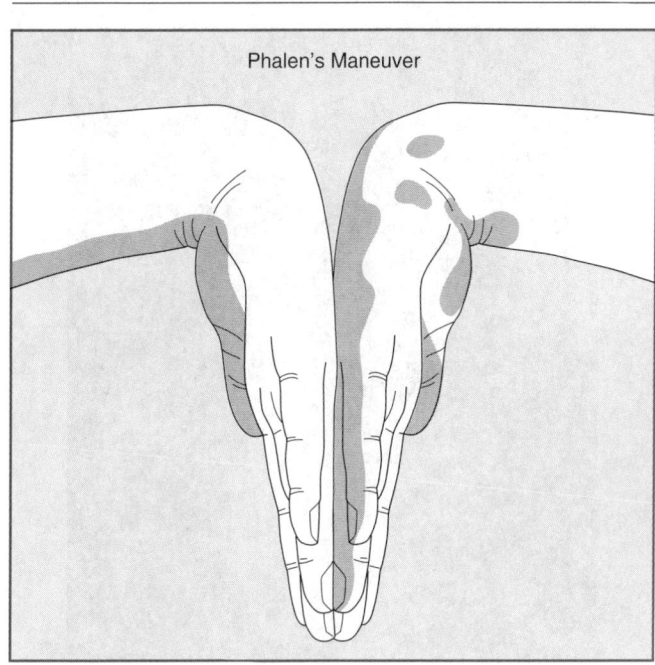

FIGURE 286–5 ■ Pain and/or paresthesias are produced in the distribution of the median nerve (see Fig. 286–4) when the hands are held in forced flexion for 30 to 60 seconds (Phalen's maneuver).

ovial proliferation into the semimembranous bursa (Fig. 286–6). Such synovial cysts may dissect or rupture into the calf and produce symptoms and signs mimicking those of thrombophlebitis. Ultrasonography and Doppler studies of the popliteal fossa and calf are useful in confirming the diagnosis, as well as in excluding venous thrombosis, which may occur from venous compression by a large cyst.

FEET AND ANKLES. The MTP joints are the most commonly involved sites. Subluxation of the metatarsal heads into the soles, often with cock-up and valgus deformities of the toes, results in painful walking and difficulty with footwear. Ankle and/or tarsal collapse may result in painful valgus deformity and/or pes planus.

NECK. Neck pain and stiffness are common. As in other joints, the rheumatoid process can lead to erosion of bone and ligaments in the cervical spine. Atlantoaxial subluxation (C1 on C2) can be seen radiographically in up to 30% of cases (Fig. 286–7). Spinal cord compression with neurologic manifestations occurs infre-

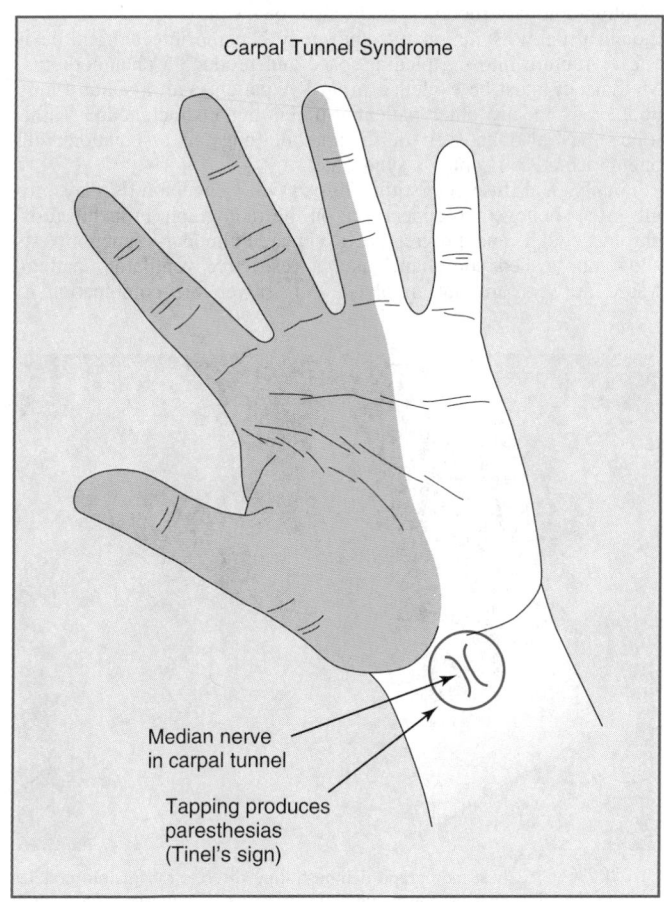

FIGURE 286–4 ■ Distribution of pain and/or paresthesias (shaded area) when the median nerve is compressed by swelling in the wrist (carpal tunnel).

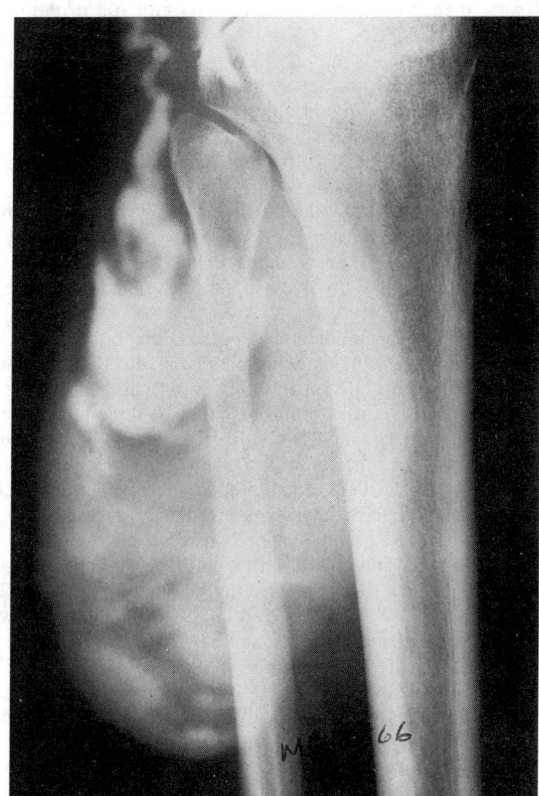

FIGURE 286–6 ■ Arthrogram with a radiocontrast agent injected into the knee. The dye flows into the popliteal space and through a narrow channel into a large synovial cyst (Baker's cyst) that has dissected into the soft tissues of the calf.

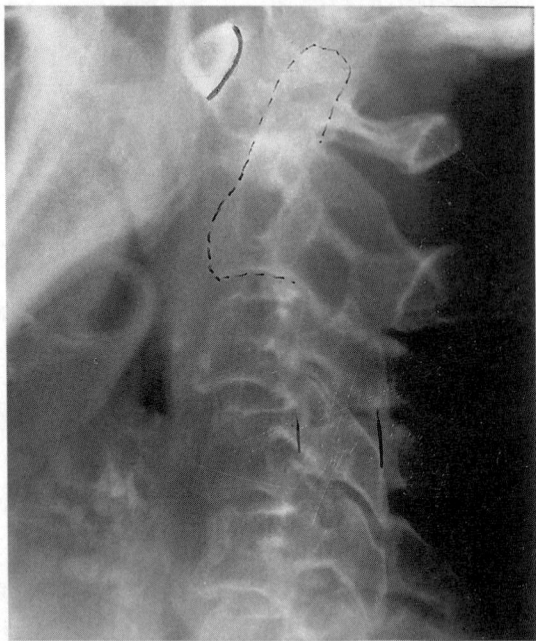

FIGURE 286-7 ■ Lateral radiograph of the cervical spine in flexion. The body of C2 and its odontoid process are outlined by broken lines, and the posterior aspect of the anterior segment of C1 is indicated by a solid line. Normally, a space of only 2 to 3 mm separates C1 from C2. The space between C1 and the odontoid of C2 is markedly increased, indicative of subluxation of C1 on C2. At a lower level, C3 is also displaced anteriorly because of rheumatoid erosion of articular and ligamentous structures.

quently but is a neurosurgical emergency. Occipital and/or frontal headache is a common premonitory sign of weakness in the extremities, bladder or bowel incontinence, or frank quadriplegia. Vertebral arteries may also be compressed and lead to vertebrobasilar insufficiency with vertigo or syncope, especially on downward gaze. Head tilt may occur from lateral mass collapse of the C1 and C2 vertebrae.

ELBOWS. Proliferative synovitis in the elbow often causes flexion contractures, even early in the disease. Supination of the hand may be impaired, especially if shoulder motion is concomitantly decreased. Rarely, ulnar or radial nerves may become entrapped.

SHOULDERS. Involvement of the glenohumeral, acromioclavicular, and thoracoscapular joints is common in advanced but not early RA. Limited motion and tenderness just below and lateral to the coracoid process are typical symptoms. Noticeable swelling is rare; however, large synovial cysts may occur (see Color Plate 3D). Joint destruction usually involves rupture of the joint capsule and subluxation of the humerus.

HIPS. Pain in the groin, lateral aspect of the buttock, or lower part of the back may indicate hip involvement. Because the hip joint capsule has poor distensibility, severe pain can result if a large effusion occurs. Arthrocentesis should be done to relieve pain and exclude infection in such cases. Rarely, extreme hip destruction results in protrusion of the femur into the pelvis.

CRICOARYTENOID JOINTS. Synovitis of the cricoarytenoid joints may result in dysphagia, hoarseness, or anterior neck pain. The sudden onset of stridor and dyspnea in a patient with RA is an emergency. Prompt administration of intra-articular or parenteral corticosteroids and/or tracheostomy may be necessary.

EXTRA-ARTICULAR MANIFESTATIONS. Constitutional symptoms, including malaise, fatigue, weakness, low-grade fever, and mild lymphadenopathy, are common in RA. All the extra-articular complications occur almost exclusively in seropositive patients.

SKIN. Subcutaneous nodules occur in 20 to 25% of RA patients and are almost always associated with serum rheumatoid factor and more severe articular disease. They occur most commonly in periarticular structures and areas subject to pressure, such as the elbows, extensor and flexor tendons of the hands and feet, Achilles tendons, and less commonly, the occipital and sacral areas. They may occasionally become infected but are usually asymptomatic.

Palmar erythema and fragility of the skin resulting in easy bruising are common manifestations. Rheumatoid vasculitis occurs in two major forms. The 1st is manifested by small, splinter-shaped brown infarcts in the nail folds and digital pulp, often also present over subcutaneous nodules (see Color Plate 3E). Histologic examination may reveal leukocytoclastic vasculitis or a mild venulitis. This process is benign in most patients and does not indicate serious systemic disease. The 2nd form is a severe necrotizing vasculitis of small and medium arteries indistinguishable from periarteritis nodosa. Digital infarcts, mononeuritis multiplex, fever, and other manifestations of systemic disease should prompt aggressive therapy.

CARDIAC MANIFESTATIONS. Pericardial disease is the most common cardiac feature of RA. Evidence of pericardial involvement with old fibrinous lesions is found in approximately 40% of patients at autopsy. A similar frequency of pericardial abnormalities can be detected by echocardiography in asymptomatic RA patients. Clinically evident pericarditis in RA, however, is infrequent. Large pericardial effusions with cardiac tamponade and death are rare. Constrictive pericarditis is somewhat more common and is typically manifested as dyspnea, right-sided heart failure, and peripheral edema. Pericardial fluid characteristics include a low glucose concentration, increased level of lactate dehydrogenase, elevated immunoglobulin levels, and low complement activity.

Rheumatoid nodules may occasionally develop in the myocardium or heart valves, and vasculitis may involve the coronary arteries. Conduction abnormalities, valvular incompetence or stenosis, and myocardial infarction are all rare clinical sequelae of rheumatoid heart disease.

PULMONARY MANIFESTATIONS. Rheumatoid pleural disease, although frequently found at autopsy, is most commonly asymptomatic. Occasionally a pleural effusion may cause respiratory limitation. Neoplasm and infection should be ruled out by a pleural tap. Typically the pleural fluid is exudative, and white cell counts vary greatly but are generally less than 5000 per microliter. Glucose levels tend to be low, and the lactate dehydrogenase level is high. Total hemolytic complement, C3, and C4 levels are low. Immune complexes and rheumatoid factor are frequently found in the pleural fluid.

Intrapulmonary nodules may also be seen (Fig. 286–8). Although usually asymptomatic, they may become infected and cavitate or rupture into the pleural space and produce a pneumothorax. Malignancy must be excluded in an RA patient with a solitary lung nodule, as in any other patient. Similar but distinct nodular infiltrates may also be seen in rheumatoid lungs in association with pneumoconiosis (Caplan's syndrome).

Finally, a diffuse interstitial fibrosis with pneumonitis may progress to a honeycomb appearance on the radiograph, bronchiectasis, chronic cough, and progressive dyspnea. Pulmonary function tests show diminished compliance and a restrictive ventilatory pattern. Large airways are not involved. An irreversible combination of

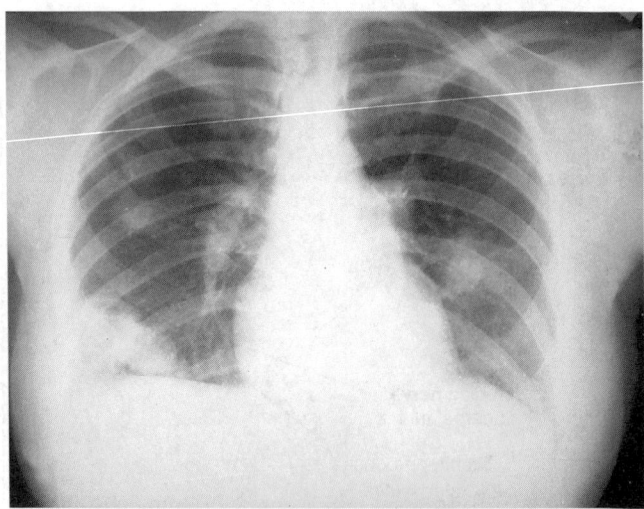

FIGURE 286-8 ■ Chest radiograph demonstrating discrete rheumatoid nodules in both the right and left lower lobes of the lungs. (Courtesy of Dr. Martin Lidsky, Houston.)

respiratory insufficiency and resultant right-sided cardiac failure is possible. Rarely, small airway obstruction may develop into a necrotizing bronchiolitis. This complication also may result from treatment with gold and D-penicillamine.

NEUROLOGIC MANIFESTATIONS. Peripheral neuropathies can be produced by proliferating synovium causing compression of nerves. Carpal tunnel syndrome (median neuropathy) (see under Articular Manifestations) is common, and a similar entrapment of the anterior tibial nerve (tarsal tunnel syndrome) can result in paresthesias with footdrop. Rheumatoid vasculitis may cause a mononeuritis multiplex condition with patchy sensory loss in one or more extremities, often in association with wristdrop or footdrop. Cervical myelopathy can result from atlantoaxial subluxation (see under Articular Manifestations). The central nervous system is usually spared, although cerebral vasculitis and rheumatoid nodules in the meninges have been described.

OPHTHALMOLOGIC MANIFESTATIONS. Sjögren's syndrome is the most frequent ocular complication and may cause corneal damage associated with dryness of the eyes. Xerostomia and/or parotid gland enlargement may accompany ocular dryness. Episcleritis is a self-limited condition associated with redness of the eye and only mild pain. Scleritis is more painful and may result in visual impairment. If this condition progresses to thinning of the tissue allowing the dark blue color of the choroid below to show through, it is termed "scleromalacia perforans." The histologic picture is similar to that of a rheumatoid nodule.

FELTY'S SYNDROME. This triad of chronic RA, splenomegaly, and neutropenia is often accompanied by lymphadenopathy, hepatomegaly, fever, weight loss, anemia, and thrombocytopenia. Hyperpigmentation and leg ulcers may also occur. The syndrome typically appears late in the course of a seropositive, destructive arthritis, often after joint disease is believed to be "burnt out." Recurrent infections with gram-positive organisms constitute the most serious clinical problems and do not correlate with the severity of neutropenia. The bone marrow is typically hyperplastic. Hypersplenism and immune-mediated destruction of white blood cells are believed to cause the neutropenia. Splenectomy may correct the neutropenia and prevent further infections in some patients, but many do not improve. The "large granular lymphocyte syndrome," which is probably a pre-malignant disorder of T lymphocytes, may mimic Felty's syndrome in RA patients. Splenectomy should not be performed for this disorder because it may hasten the onset of malignancy.

LABORATORY FEATURES. A chronic normocytic, normochromic anemia with hematocrit values from 30 to 35% is usual. Typically, both serum iron levels and iron-binding capacity are low. The anemia does not respond to administration of iron, but erythropoietin may be effective when the anemia is severe. The white blood cell count and differential are typically normal, but eosinophilia may occur in severe systemic disease. The platelet count may be moderately elevated because of chronic inflammation. The erythrocyte sedimentation rate is elevated in most patients but only roughly parallels disease activity. The presence of rheumatoid factor is detected in more than 80% of cases and is useful in clinical diagnosis. Antinuclear antibodies detected by immunofluorescence, usually in low titer, can be found in 30 to 40% of cases. DNA typing of RA-associated HLA-DRB1 alleles (DR4, DR1, others; see Table 286–2) has no diagnostic utility because these genes occur in high frequencies in the normal population. However, detection of patients homozygous for these DRB1 "susceptibility/severity" alleles early in disease may predict the worst prognosis, in which case early, aggressive therapy is indicated.

Synovial fluid analysis usually shows a poor mucin clot test and white cell counts in the range of 5000 to 20,000 per cubic millimeter, with 50 to 70% as polymorphonuclear leukocytes (Table 286–4). The synovial fluid glucose concentration is usually normal, but very low values occur occasionally, even in the absence of a superimposed infectious arthritis. Complement levels are typically low.

DISEASE COURSE AND PROGNOSIS. Although once considered a relatively benign disease, RA is now known to result in considerable disability and a higher than expected mortality rate. Approximately 20% of patients will improve spontaneously or even achieve remission, especially in the 1st year of disease; however, chronic disease progression and functional deterioration occur in the majority. Long-term studies have shown RA patients to have 6 times the probability of severe limitations in activity, 4 times as many restricted activity days, and 10 times the work disability rate as the general population, and approximately 50% are forced to stop working within 10 years of diagnosis. A higher mortality rate also correlates with the degree of disability and results from infections, systemic manifestations, and gastrointestinal bleeding or perforation. The economic impact on the health care system is also substantial.

THERAPEUTIC MANAGEMENT. Objectives of management include (1) relief of pain and stiffness, (2) reduction of inflammation, (3) minimization of undesirable drug side effects, (4) preservation of muscle strength and joint function, and (5) maintenance of as normal a lifestyle as possible. The basic initial program that achieves these objectives for the great majority of patients consists of (1) adequate rest, (2) adequate anti-inflammatory therapy, and (3) physical measures to maintain joint function. An additional objective, (6) to attempt to modify the disease course with early, aggressive drug therapies, has recently been advocated because of prognosis studies and the findings that rheumatoid pannus invades and irreversibly damages articular cartilage within 1 to 2 years of disease onset. Identification of patients at highest risk for a poor outcome may be possible by detecting high serum levels of rheu-

Table 286–4 ∎ SYNOVIAL FLUID FINDINGS IN RHEUMATOID ARTHRITIS AND OTHER FORMS OF ARTHRITIS

SYNOVIAL CHARACTERISTICS	RHEUMATOID ARTHRITIS	GOUT/PSEUDOGOUT	REITER'S/PSORIATIC ARTHRITIS	SEPTIC ARTHRITIS	OSTEOARTHRITIS, TRAUMATIC ARTHRITIS
Color	Yellow	Yellow-white	Yellow	White	Clear, pale yellow, or bloody
Clarity	Cloudy	Cloudy-opaque	Cloudy	Opaque	Transparent
Viscosity	Poor	Poor	Poor	Poor	Good
Mucin clot	Poor	Poor	Poor	Poor	Good
White blood cell count/mm^3	3000–50,000	3000–50,000 or higher	3000–50,000 or higher	50,000–300,000	<3000
% Polymorphonuclear leukocytes	>70	>70	>70	>90	<25
Glucose levels	10–25% less than serum*	10–25% less than serum	10–25% less than serum	70–90% less than serum	5–10% less than serum
Total protein	>3.0 g/dL	>3.0 g/dL	>3.0 g/dL	>3.0 g/dL	1.8–3.0 g/dL
Complement	Low	Normal	High	High	Normal
Microscopic features	"RA cells"†	MSU and CPPD crystals	"Reiter's cells"†	Microbes (Gram stain)	Cartilage fibrils†
Culture	Negative	Negative	Negative	Positive	Negative
IF, EM, and/or PCR for bacteria	Negative	Negative	Positive	Positive	Negative

MSU = monosodium urate; CPPD = calcium pyrophosphate dihydrate; IF = immunofluorescence; EM = electron microscopy; PCR = polymerase chain reaction.
*Rarely, glucose levels are very low, as in rheumatoid pleural effusions.
†These are not disease specific or diagnostic.

matoid factor and by DNA typing of HLA-DRB1 alleles; however, this approach is currently unproven. Moreover, it is unclear that the current armamentarium of disease-modifying drugs can achieve this goal.

Any confusion arising from the complementary requirements of rest and exercise should be promptly dispelled. Bed rest tends to decrease the general systemic inflammatory response, and most patients soon learn that their midafternoon fatigue is significantly reduced by a period of rest. During acute attacks, longer rest periods and perhaps even remaining in bed for the duration of the attack may be required to treat the inflammation.

At the same time, full range of joint motion should be maintained, which can usually be accomplished by the patient through graded exercise programs. However, during acute attacks, passive range-of-motion exercises by a physical therapist or instructed layperson may be indicated. Physical overexertion increases synovitis and inflammation in joints affected by RA, but this limitation does not contradict the usefulness of appropriate exercise. Exercise, as well as heat treatments such as showers, baths, warm pools, paraffin baths, or hot packs, should be used to loosen the joints and relieve stiffness. Exercise following the heat treatment maintains the motion of affected joints and prevents muscle atrophy.

NON-STEROIDAL ANTI-INFLAMMATORY DRUGS. Anti-inflammatory therapy is crucial to the basic program. Salicylates are inexpensive, generally well tolerated, and demonstrably effective in controlling RA inflammation. The patient needs to understand that a larger dose is required than would be used for analgesia alone. A constant blood level of 20 to 30 mg/dL is needed, which for most patients requires between 3 and 6 g of aspirin per day. All patients should be monitored for toxic levels by blood tests and should be alerted to report deafness, ringing in the ears, or gastrointestinal intolerance. With the availability of buffered and coated aspirin, a suitable salicylate preparation can be found for almost any patient.

Many other non-steroidal anti-inflammatory drugs (NSAIDs) that are effective against pain, fever, and inflammation in RA are available. These cyclooxygenase (COX)-1 and -2 inhibitors include ibuprofen, ketoprofen, flurbiprofen, oraprozin, naproxen, nabumetone, tolmetin, indomethacin, sulindac, piroxicam, diclofenac, diflunisal, and etodolac. Most of these drugs may be beneficial in RA but do not modify disease progression. Clinical experience suggests an occasional need to change from one to another of these drugs to minimize side effects and to give maximal symptomatic benefit to individual patients. Non-acetylated salicylates (sodium or choline) may be useful at times in patients intolerant of other NSAIDs or those with aspirin (and NSAID) hypersensitivity.

NSAIDs often cause silent gastrointestinal bleeding that is usually minimal and tolerable. Overt gastrointestinal tract hemorrhage or ulceration is infrequent, but when it occurs it dictates discontinuation of the drug. Concomitant administration of proton pump inhibitors (omeprazole, lansoprozole) or misoprostal has been shown to significantly reduce NSAID-induced gastrointestinal tract toxicity. Moreover, the recent introduction of NSAIDs that selectively inhibit COX-2 (celecoxib) will likely minimize the gastrointestinal and platelet dysfunction effects of other NSAIDs but not potential renal toxicity. In fact, all NSAIDs should be avoided or used with extreme caution in patients with poor renal function.

CORTICOSTEROIDS. Because of its side effects, long-term corticosteroid therapy should be reserved for patients with unresponsive and aggressive joint disease whose ability to function is threatened. When necessary, the smallest possible dose should be used, i.e., prednisone, 5 to 10 mg every other day or daily. Higher doses are necessary for patients with neuropathy, vasculitis, pleuritis, pericarditis, scleritis, and related conditions. Local steroid injections can sometimes be helpful in relieving persistent effusions and are the treatment of choice for Baker's cyst of the knee.

DISEASE-MODIFYING THERAPIES. The more slowly acting drugs include antimalarials, methotrexate, gold, penicillamine, sulfasalazine, and minocycline. Antimalarials are usually given as hydroxychloroquine (Plaquenil), 200 mg once or twice daily. This drug, or chloroquine, may cause retinal lesions and loss of vision; therefore, the patient should be examined by an ophthalmologist at least twice a year.

Currently, the most widely used and effective form of long-term therapy for RA appears to be methotrexate. An oral dosage of

7.5 to 15 mg one time per week is usually efficacious, and a therapeutic response can be anticipated in several weeks. Side effects include hepatotoxicity and possibly cirrhosis, bone marrow suppression, oral ulcers, and a potential life-threatening pneumonitis. Methotrexate may also cause a leukocytoclastic vasculitis and may promote the formation of rheumatoid nodules, including systemic nodulosis. Concomitant treatment with folic acid, 1 mg/day, reduces toxicity from methotrexate without impairing efficacy. Sulfonamides must be avoided because of potentiation of hematologic side effects.

Leflunomide (Arava), a pyrimidine antagonist that selectively inhibits activated T lymphocytes, has been recently introduced for long-term treatment of RA. The drug given with an oral loading dose of 100 mg for each of 3 days, followed by 20 mg daily thereafter, has shown considerable efficacy and little toxicity, although liver function tests require regular monitoring.

Sulfasalazine given in a dose of 2 to 3 g daily may be effective in some patients. Headache and gastrointestinal upset are the most common side effects. Another antibiotic, minocycline in a dosage of 100 mg twice daily, has also recently been found to be effective in RA. The most common side effect is gastrointestinal upset.

Gold salts, especially weekly intramuscular injections, produce remission in many cases. An oral gold salt, auranofin, appears to be therapeutically effective and to have less toxicity than do intramuscular injections. A dose of 3 mg two to three times per day is recommended. A therapeutic effect should not be expected before 4 to 6 months. Common side effects include pruritic skin rashes and painful mouth ulcers. Severe manifestations include bone marrow suppression, usually leukopenia or thrombocytopenia, renal damage with proteinuria, and rarely a nephrotic syndrome. Therefore, frequent urinalysis and blood counts must be performed, especially during the early phases of treatment.

Penicillamine is also effective in inducing improvements and sometimes even remissions. Like gold, however, its effects are slow in coming, and it may affect both the bone marrow and the kidneys, so careful monitoring for toxicity is required. In addition, it may induce other autoimmune diseases such as myasthenia gravis, Goodpasture's syndrome, or lupus erythematosus.

Immunosuppressive agents such as azathroprine, cyclophosphamide, chlorambucil, and cyclosporine have been used to treat especially severe, unremitting RA. A soluble recombinant TNF-α receptor, etanercept (Embrel), has recently been introduced for patients with severe RA who have failed other disease-modifying agents. Short-term clinical trials have shown it to be quickly, highly effective in a majority of patients. Toxicity appears to be low shortterm, but concerns about potential oncogenesis or infectious complications from TNF-α blockade with time remain to be determined. Other disadvantages include high cost and need for biweekly subcutaneous injections.

Combinations of certain long-lasting agents are increasingly being advocated for severe RA and may prove beneficial in some patients. The likelihood of serious side effects is significantly increased, however, and close consultation with a rheumatologist is strongly recommended.

Finally, reconstructive orthopedic surgery is of very great importance. Prosthetic devices for hip and knee joints have given excellent results, and devices for ankle, elbow, and shoulder replacement are improving.

JUVENILE CHRONIC ARTHRITIS. A chronic arthritis beginning in childhood and for which no underlying cause is apparent has been termed *juvenile rheumatoid arthritis*. Because the majority of these cases do not resemble adult RA, the term *juvenile chronic arthritis* is a more appropriate designation. Several subgroups of juvenile chronic arthritis are recognized on the basis of modes of onset, other clinical features, and immunogenetic differences.

Arthritis of systemic onset, or Still's disease, accounts for about 20% of patients. It can begin at any age. Rheumatoid factor and antinuclear antibodies are generally not found. Clinical characteristics include high, spiking daily fevers; an evanescent, salmon-colored rash usually appearing with fever; lymphadenopathy; hepatosplenomegaly; polyserositis; leukocytosis; thrombocytosis; and anemia. Serum ferritin levels may be extremely high. Although the disease is rarely life threatening, it can be confused with leukemia or infection. It tends to run a self-limited course in the majority of patients but may recur. Chronic polyarthritis and joint deformities occur in only about 10% of patients.

Disease characterized by polyarticular onset occurs in approximately 40% of patients, with a female preponderance. The majority of patients are seronegative. Seropositive patients have the worst prognosis, and the disease usually follows a chronic course similar to that in adult RA. HLA-DR4 is strongly associated with seropositive disease, but HLA-DR8 and DP3 are significantly increased in the seronegative group.

Disease with a pauciarticular onset accounts for the remaining 40% of patients with juvenile chronic arthritis. At least two subgroups are recognized within this group. One is characterized by early age of onset and female preponderance. The serum is usually positive for antinuclear antibodies but not rheumatoid factor. Patients in this subgroup are at risk for chronic iridocyclitis, which may progress to blindness. Therefore, frequent ophthalmologic evaluations should be performed. The arthritis usually resolves without deformity. HLA-DR5, HLA-DR8, and HLA-DP2 are significantly increased in this subgroup. A second subgroup with pauciarticular onset has a strong male preponderance and later age of onset. HLA-B27 occurs in the majority of these patients. The disease in these children follows a course consistent with spondyloarthropathy.

Treatment must be determined on the basis of disease severity. Aspirin is a basic standby, but tolmetin and naproxen can be used safely in children. Physical therapy and psychosocial support are also indicated.

ADULT-ONSET STILL'S DISEASE. Still's disease is one form of juvenile-onset chronic arthritis that may begin in adulthood. Cases have been recognized that span the entire adult age spectrum, including the elderly. The clinical features are the same as those described above. Acute symptoms often respond to salicylates or other NSAIDs, but prednisone may be necessary for short periods. The prognosis for complete recovery is good in the majority of patients.

Arnett FC, Edworthy SM, Block DA, et al: The American Rheumatism Association 1987 revised criteria for the classification of rheumatoid arthritis. Arthritis Rheum 31:315, 1988. *An in-depth discussion of the development, recommended uses, and potential pitfalls of criteria for RA.*

Conaghan PG, Lehman T, Brooks P: Disease-modifying antirheumatic drugs. Curr Opin Rheumatol 9:183, 1997. *A good update on currently used disease-modifying agents in RA.*

Feldman M, Brennon FM, Maini RN: Rheumatoid arthritis. Cell 85:307, 1996. *An excellent review of cytokines in rheumatoid synovitis and their implications for future therapies.*

Pincus T: The paradox of effective therapies but poor long-term outcomes in rheumatoid arthritis. Semin Arthritis Rheum 21(Suppl. 3):2, 1992. *An analysis of morbidity and mortality in RA patients.*

Weyand CM, Hicok KC, Conn DL, Goronzy JJ: The influence of HLA-DRB1 genes on disease severity in rheumatoid arthritis. Ann Intern Med 117:801, 1992. *A clinical-molecular study showing homozygosity for disease-associated HLA alleles correlates with RA severity.*

287 THE SPONDYLOARTHROPATHIES

John J. Cush ■ *Peter E. Lipsky*

The spondyloarthropathies are a heterogeneous group of disorders that share a number of clinical, radiographic, and genetic features. These disorders include ankylosing spondylitis, Reiter's syndrome, reactive arthritis, psoriatic arthritis, and the enteropathic arthropathies.

The spondyloarthropathies share a constellation of characteristic clinical, radiographic, and immunogenetic manifestations that suggest a common or related etiopathogenesis (Table 287-1). Distinctive features include a propensity for axial arthritis (sacroiliitis and spondylitis); peripheral arthritis (often asymmetrical and oligoarticular); inflammation at tendinous, ligamentous, or fascial insertions (enthesitis); and a familial pattern of inheritance based on the presence of the class I major histocompatibility complex (MHC) antigen HLA-B27. These disorders can manifest extra-articular features that suggest a particular spondyloarthropathy. Extra-articular manifestations may involve periarticular structures (enthesitis), eyes (conjunctivitis, uveitis), the gastrointestinal tract (oral ulcerations, asymptomatic gut inflammation), the genitourinary tract (urethritis,

prostatitis, cervitis), the heart (aortitis, heart block), skin (keratoderma blennorrhagicum), or nails (onycholysis, nail pitting). Often, patients will demonstrate overlapping features of more than one condition or will be HLA-B27+ and possess a constellation of symptoms that do not meet the strigent diagnostic criteria of a particular spondyloarthropathy. In such patients the more generic term "spondyloarthropathy" may be more accurate. This distinction allows the clinician to approach these conditions as a group of related disorders and permits the early diagnosis and treatment of affected individuals (Fig. 287-1).

New diagnostic criteria for the spondyloarthropathies have been proposed (Table 287-2) because previous diagnostic criteria have been shown to exclude many patients with spondyloarthropathy. The broader definitions used these criteria allow for earlier diagnosis and more liberal inclusion of many patients with spondyloarthropathy.

HLA-B27. The human leukocyte class I MHC antigen HLA-B27 was first linked with ankylosing spondylitis in 1973. This genetic marker is found in nearly 8% of North American white individuals. The actual risk of ankylosing spondylitis developing in an HLA-B27+ person is estimated to be 1 to 2%. A reactive arthropathy will develop in only 20% of HLA-B27+ individuals infected with arthritogenic bacteria (Table 287-3). Moreover, in only 20% of HLA-B27+ first-degree relatives of HLA-B27+ spondylitis patients will ankylosing spondylitis develop, which suggests that factors other than HLA-B27 must play a crucial role in determining disease susceptibility. The prevalence of HLA-B27 varies greatly among different ethnic groups. A higher prevalence is seen in the Haida and Pima Indians, and the lowest prevalence is seen among Africans and Asians. When North American whites are compared with blacks, HLA-B27 is found in 90 versus 60% of those with ankylosing spondylitis and 75 versus 50% of those with Reiter's syndrome, respectively.

Seven serologically defined subtypes of HLA-B27 have been defined, and six of these (B*2701, B*2702, B*2703, B*2704, B*2705, and B*2707) are associated with ankylosing spondylitis. Other class I MHC antigens are termed the HLA-B27 cross-reactive antigens and include HLA-B7, Bw22, -B39, -B40, -B42, and -B60, which are often present in HLA-B27−patients with spondyloarthropathy.

HLA-B27 has shown to influence disease expression for most of the spondyloarthropathies, especially those with Reiter's syndrome. HLA-B27+ individuals are more likely to have an earlier disease onset, sacroiliitis, spondylitis, a severe clinical course, or acute anterior uveitis. By contrast, in HLA-B27− patients, peripheral arthropathy, skin and nail disease, and inflammatory bowel disease or undifferentiated spondyloarthropathy are more likely to develop.

Strong evidence for the role of HLA-B27 in disease pathogenesis has been derived from experiments in which human HLA-B27 has been transfected into rats. Typical features of spondyloarthropathy, including gut inflammation, spondylitis, peripheral arthritis, psoriasiform skin and nail changes, uveitis, and orchitis, spontaneously develop in these transgenic rats. The role of environmental factors in disease pathogenesis is emphasized by the observation that many of these features do not develop when these animals are bred in a germ-free environment.

ANKYLOSING SPONDYLITIS. Ankylosing spondylitis is the most common inflammatory disorder of the axial skeleton. Epidemiologic studies have suggested that the prevalence of ankylosing spondylitis in a white population is 0.02 to 0.23%. Ankylosing spondylitis commonly affects young men more frequently than women, with an estimated male-female ratio ranging from 2.5 to 5:1. Ankylosing spondylitis in women is often underdiagnosed, primarily because of milder axial disease and occult extra-articular manifestations. Women with ankylosing spondylitis tend to have a delayed disease onset, less hip involvement, less aggressive axial disease, more peripheral arthritis, severe osteitis pubis, and a higher incidence of isolated cervical spine disease.

Ankylosing spondylitis often begins in young adulthood. Up to 15% of children with juvenile chronic arthritis are classified with juvenile spondylitis. These children between ages 9 and 16 are often HLA-B27+ and manifest low back pain or an asymmetrical oligoarthritis years before fully expressed spondyloarthropathy develops. In contrast, late-onset spondyloarthropathy has been de-

Table 287–1 ■ COMPARISON OF THE SPONDYLOARTHROPATHIES

FEATURE	ANKYLOSING SPONDYLITIS	POST-URETHRAL REACTIVE ARTHRITIS	POST-DYSENTERIC REACTIVE ARTHRITIS	ENTEROPATHIC ARTHRITIS	PSORIATIC ARTHRITIS
Sacroiliitis	+++++	+++	++	+	++
Spondylitis	++++	+++	++	++	++
Peripheral arthritis	+	++++	++++	+++	++++
Articular course	Chronic	Acute or chronic	Acute > chronic	Acute or chronic	Chronic
HLA-B27	95%	60%	30%	20%	20%
Enthesopathy	++	++++	+++	++	++
Common extra-articular manifestations	Eye Heart	Eye GU Oral/GI Heart	GU Eye	GI Eye	Skin Nails Eye
Other names	von Bechterev's Marie-Strümpell	Reiter's syndrome, SARA, NGU, chlamydial arthritis	Reiter's syndrome	Crohn's disease, ulcerative colitis	

GU = genitourinary; GI = gastrointestinal; SARA = sexually acquired reactive arthritis; NGU = non-gonococcal urethritis.

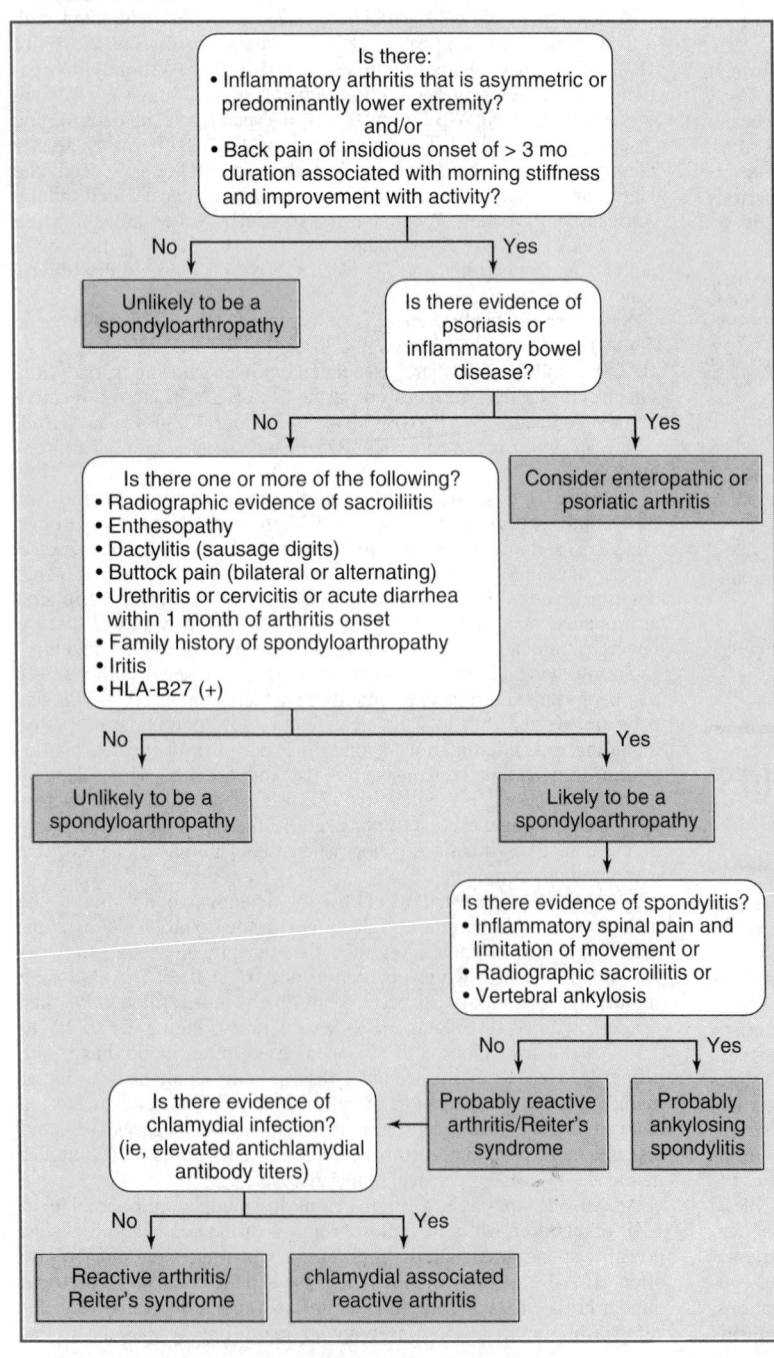

FIGURE 287–1 ■ Algorithm for diagnosis of the spondyloarthropathies.

Table 287–2 ■ DIAGNOSTIC CRITERIA FOR THE SPONDYLOARTHROPATHIES

Rome Criteria for Ankylosing Spondylitis (1961)	1981 ARA Criteria for Reiter's Syndrome
1. Low back pain and stiffness >3 mo, not relieved by rest 2. Pain and stiffness in the thoracic region 3. Limited motion of the lumbar spine 4. Limited chest expansion 5. History of iritis 6. Radiograhic evidence of bilateral sacroiliitis	Peripheral arthritis >1 mo in association with urethritis and/or cervicitis *Criteria for Psoriatic Arthritis* Cutaneous evidence of psoriasis plus inflammatory peripheral arthritis or spondylitis ≥6 wk
Diagnosis requires 4 of the 1st 5 criteria or sacroiliitis plus 1 of the clinical criteria	

ESSG Criteria for Spondyloarthropathy (1992)	Criteria for Diagnosing Spondyloarthropathies by Amor et al. (1993)	SCORE
Inflammatory spinal pain *or* peripheral synovitis (asymmetrical or lower limbs) Plus one or more of the following: Alternate buttock pain Sacroiliitis Enthesopathy Positive family history Psoriasis Inflammatory bowel disease Urethritis, cervicitis, or acute diarrhea occurring within 1 mo of the onset of arthritis	Lumbar pain at night or morning stiffness	1
	Asymmetrical oligoarthritis	2
	Buttock pain	1
	Alternating buttock pain	2
	Sausage-like toe or digit(s)	2
	Heel pain or enthesitis	2
	Iritis	2
	Non-gonococcal urethritis/cervicitis within 1 mo of onset	1
	Acute diarrhea within 1 mo of arthritis onset	1
	Psoriasis, balanitis, or inflammatory bowel disease	2
	Sacroiliitis (bilateral grade 2 or unilateral grade 3)	2
	HLA-B27+ or positive family history of a spondyloarthropathy	2
	Rapid (<48 hr) response to NSAIDs	2
	Diagnosis requires score ≥6	

Note: Older criteria *(top)* are being replaced by newer, more liberal criteria *(bottom)* for the spondyloarthropathies.

ARA = American Rheumatism Association; ESSG = European Spondyloarthropathy Study Group; NSAIDs = non-steroidal anti-inflammatory drugs.

scribed in several HLA-B27+ individuals older than 50 years, in whom sacroiliitis (without spondylitis), oligoarticular arthritis, an elevated erythrocyte sedimentation rate, and evidence of skeletal hyperostosis developed.

The insidious onset of low back pain and/or stiffness is often the initial symptom of ankylosing spondylitis. The hallmark of ankylosing spondylitis is symmetrical sacroiliitis that is often bilateral (Fig. 287–2). Sacroiliitis develops early but may take 7 to 10 years to become evident by conventional radiography. Pain is anatomically localized over the sacroiliac joints and less commonly radiates down the posterior of the thigh. Patients usually complain of inflammatory back-pain—prolonged spinal stiffness each morning that is relieved only by increased activity or anti-inflammatory

Table 287–3 ■ INFECTIOUS ORGANISMS ASSOCIATED WITH THE ONSET OF REITER'S SYNDROME

ENTERIC PATHOGENS	UROGENITAL PATHOGENS
Shigella flexneri (serotypes 2a, 1b) *Salmonella typhimurium* *Salmonella enteritidis* *Salmonella paratyphi* *Salmonella heidelberg* *Yersinia enterocolitica* (serotypes 0:3, 0:8, 0:9) *Yersinia pseudotuberculosis* *Campylobacter jejuni* *Campylobacter fetus*	*Chlamydia trachomatis* *Chlamydia psittaci* *Ureaplasma urealyticum*

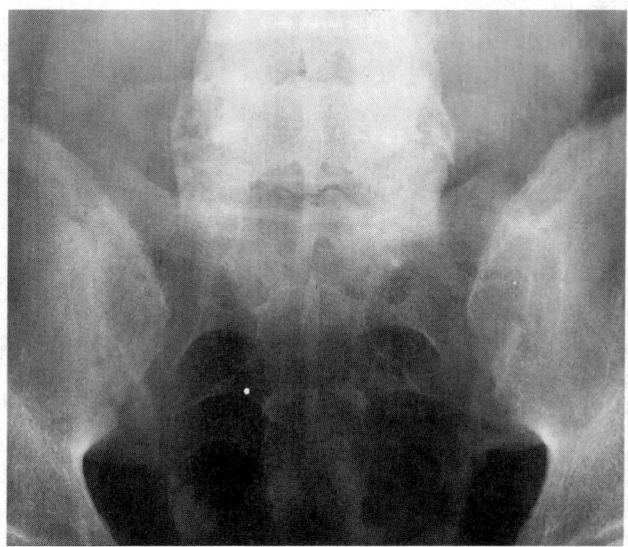

FIGURE 287–2 ■ Bilaterally symmetrical sacroiliitis in ankylosing spondylitis.

therapy. Other constitutional features (e.g., fever, anorexia, weight loss) are not uncommon at the onset. With progressive axial involvement, pain and stiffness result in difficulty with ambulation and activities of daily living. The cervical spine is involved late in the disease.

A peripheral asymmetrical oligoarthropathy is seen in up to 30% of patients with ankylosing spondylitis. Synovitis of the hip can be destructive and may lead to concentric loss of joint space, especially in men. Other involved joints include the ankles, wrists, shoulders, elbows, and small joints of the hands or feet.

Extra-articular disease in ankylosing spondylitis primarily affects the eye. Ocular involvement is seen in up to 40% of patients and is more frequently observed in HLA-B27+ individuals. Uveitis is manifested as acute, unilateral orbital pain accompanied by photophobia and progressive loss of vision if untreated. Aortitis, aortic insufficiency, and conduction defects are uncommon. Other uncommon manifestations include mitral valve disease, myocardial dysfunction, pericarditis, pulmonary fibrosis, and amyloidosis.

Restricted spinal movement results from the axial stiffness and paraspinal muscular spasm that accompany inflammatory spondylitis, with or without intervertebral or zygapophyseal ankylosis. A loss of normal lumbar lordosis is a frequent observation in early disease. Fixed forward flexion, especially at the hip and neck, is seen after years of progressive disease. Chest expansion, as measured by the inspiratory minus expiratory chest circumference, is normally greater than 5 cm. Patients with ankylosing spondylitis demonstrate diminished expansion (< 4 cm). Schober's test is performed to examine lumbar spine mobility. While the patient stands upright with heels together, a 10-cm span is marked from the 5th lumbar vertebra cephalad. Upon maximal forward flexion, the distance between marks is remeasured. Normal spinal flexion expands the skin surface area over the flexed spine to greater than 15 cm. Flexion in patients with spondylitis and limitation of spinal motion measures 14 cm or less.

Laboratory tests support the inflammatory nature of the disease: an elevated erythrocyte sedimentation rate or C-reactive protein, anemia of chronic disease, or mild elevations in alkaline phosphatase. Elevated IgA may be present, but other autoantibodies are noticeably absent. HLA-B27 determination is seldom necessary to establish the diagnosis. However, in questionable cases without distinctive radiographic changes, the presence of HLA-B27 may be of diagnostic value.

Radiographs demonstrate normal mineralization before the onset of ankylosis. Once present, ankylosis results in marked immobility and subsequent generalized osteoporosis. Sacroiliitis is indicated by erosions (leading to "pseudowidening"), ileal sclerosis, or fusion of the inferior synovial-lined portion of the sacroiliac joint (see Fig. 237–1). These findings are easily observed on plain radiographs of the pelvis and seldom require computed tomography or magnetic

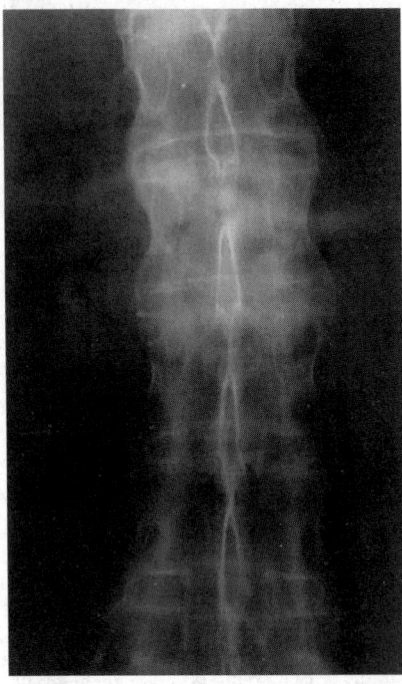
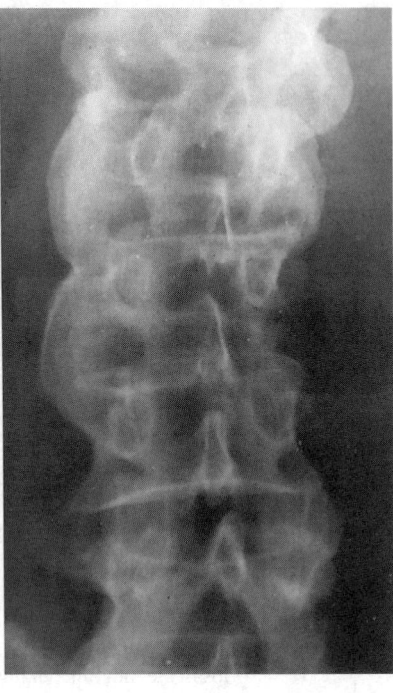

FIGURE 287–3 ▪ *Left*, Lumbar spondylitis in ankylosing spondylitis with symmetrical, marginal bridging syndesmophytes and calcification of the spinal ligament. *Right*, The bulky, non-marginal, asymmetrical syndesmophytes of Reiter's syndrome with lumbar spondylitis.

resonance imaging (MRI) for diagnosis. In selected instances, MRI may accurately diagnose periarticular disease such as plantar fasciitis. Axial radiographic findings also include marginal bridging syndesmophytes, interapophyseal joint fusion, and "squaring" of lumbar and thoracic vertebrae. Collectively, these findings may produce the classic appearance of a "bamboo spine" (Figs. 287–3 and 287–4).

The clinical course and disease severity are highly variable. Inflammatory back pain and stiffness are prominent early in the disease, whereas chronic, aggressive disease may produce pain and marked axial immobility or deformity. In patients with new, refractory spinal pain, intervertebral fracture should be considered. An earlier age of onset and diagnosis portends a more severe outcome. Moreover, patients with ankylosing spondylitis are at risk for complications, some of which may be life threatening. These complications include restrictive lung disease, cauda equina syndrome, posttraumatic intervertebral fractures, osteoporotic compression fractures, or spondylodiscitis.

The diagnosis of ankylosing spondylitis is suggested by (1) young age at onset, (2) strong family history of low back pain, (3) low back pain lasting more than 3 months, (4) prolonged morning stiffness, and (5) symptomatic improvement with activity or exercise. Ankylosing spondylitis must be distinguished from other causes of mechanical or degenerative low back pain. The differential diagnosis also includes other spondyloarthropathies, osteitis condensans ilii, diffuse idiopathic skeletal hyperostosis, and other causes of hyperostosis (Table 287–4).

REITER'S SYNDROME. Reiter's syndrome is defined by the classic triad of arthritis, urethritis, and conjunctivitis. It most often affects young people, with a peak onset during the 3rd decade of life. Like ankylosing spondylitis, however, it has also been reported in children and the elderly. Although men are most commonly affected, this preponderance is often overestimated because Reiter's syndrome in women may be associated with asymptomatic genitourinary disease and milder disease expression. Whereas post-venereal Reiter's syndrome is more common in males, post-dysenteric Reiter's syndrome affects the sexes equally. Reiter's syndrome is one of the most common causes of acute inflammatory arthritis in young men. Case studies of epidemic dysentery suggest an estimated incidence of Reiter's syndrome of approximately 4 cases per 1000 dysenteric subjects per year. Analysis of epidemic dysentery secondary to arthritogenic bacteria suggests that Reiter's syndrome develops in 2 to 3% of infected individuals whereas arthritis may develop in as many as 20% of HLA-B27+ infected individuals. Similarly, arthritis will develop in 1 to 3% of patients with non-gonococcal urethritis secondary to *Chlamydia trachomatis* infection. In Houston, the point prevalence of Reiter's syndrome was reported to be 33 per 100,000 men, and in Rochester, Minnesota, the age-adjusted incidence rate for males younger than 50 years was noted to be 3.5 cases per 100,000 per year. More recent studies suggest that the incidence of Reiter's syndrome has markedly decreased in the human immunodeficiency virus (HIV) era, presumeably because of increased condom use.

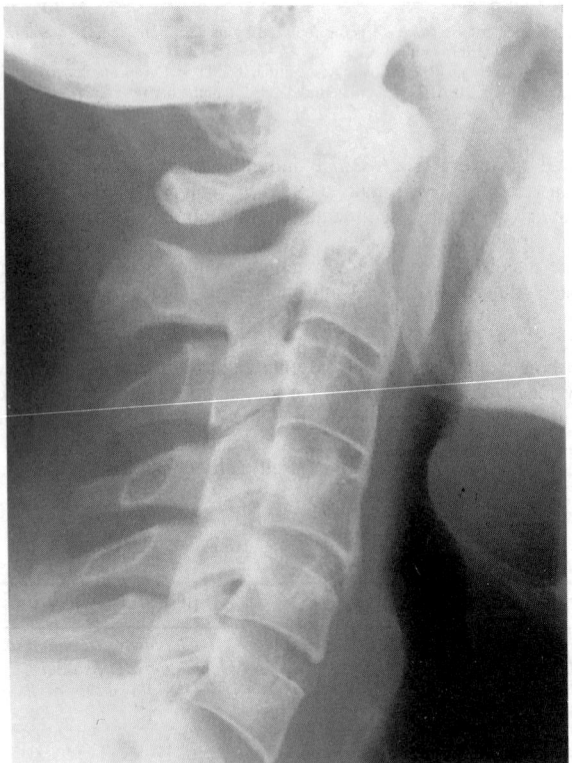

FIGURE 287–4 ▪ A 34-year-old male who had ankylosing spondylitis for 9 years and neck pain. Radiographs demonstrate narrowing of the C2–C3 apophyseal joints posteriorly and anterior bridging marginal syndesmophytes extending from C2 to C5.

Spondyloarthropathies (ankylosing spondylitis, Reiter's syndrome, psoriatic arthritis, reactive arthritis)
Diffuse idiopathic skeletal hyperostosis (Forestier disease)
Vitamin A intoxication, retinoid therapy (e.g., etretinate)
Hypoparathyroidism
Familial hyperphosphatemia
SAPHO syndrome
Pachydermoperiostitis
Hypertrophic osteoarthropathy
Plasma cell dyscrasia (POEMS syndrome)
Neurofibromatosis
Melorheostosis
Infantile cortical hyperostosis (Caffey's disease)
Fluorosis

SAPHO = synovitis, acne, pustulosis, hyperostosis, osteitis; POEMS = polyneuropathy, organomegaly, endocrinopathy, M protein, skin changes.

The clinical triad of urethritis, conjunctivitis, and arthritis is observed in only 33% of patients with Reiter's syndrome. Thus many will not have evidence of prodromal enteric or urethral inflammation. Such patients are often designated as having "incomplete Reiter's" or "sexually acquired reactive arthritis." In the remaining individuals the diagnosis can be made by the presence of an acute, additive lower extremity oligoarthritis accompanied by extra-articular features. The earliest features of Reiter's syndrome most frequently appear within 1 to 4 weeks of a putative microbial exposure. Disease onset is usually heralded by the development of one or more of the extra-articular features. Early genitourinary tract involvement may be manifested as dysuria, urethral discharge, prostatitis in men, or cervicitis or vaginitis in women. Fever, malaise, fatigue, anorexia, weight loss, and ocular symptoms (e.g., conjunctivitis) are also common at the onset.

The arthritis is often the last feature to appear and is manifested as an acute asymmetrical or ascending inflammatory oligoarthritis. Involvement of the lower extremity (first metatarsophalangeal joints, ankles, knees, and toes) is most common. Upper extremity involvement is rarely present at the onset. However, with chronicity, upper extremity involvement may occur. Involvement of the toes and fingers may result in dactylitis, or the so-called sausage digit. Dactylitis is the net result of inflammatory changes affecting the joint capsule, entheses, periarticular structures, and/or periosteal bone.

Low back pain and other axial findings are present in up to 50% of individuals with Reiter's syndrome. However, radiographic evidence of sacroiliac or axial involvement is observed only with chronic and severe disease. About 20% of the most severely affected individuals demonstrate radiographic sacroiliitis.

EXTRA-ARTICULAR MANIFESTATIONS. Extra-articular manifestations are frequently seen in Reiter's syndrome. *Enthesitis* most commonly affects the insertion of the Achilles tendon and/or plantar fascia on the calcaneus with resultant heel pain. *Mucocutaneous features* may affect the genitourinary or gastrointestinal tract. Genitourinary involvement includes transient mucopurulent urethral discharge, urethritis, circinate balanitis, cervicitis, or vaginitis. Circinate balanitis appears as painless vesicles or large, shallow, serpiginous ulcerations or plaques on the glans or shaft of the penis. Painless lingual or palatal oral ulcerations may be seen in up to 50% of patients. Keratoderma blennorrhagicum is the most common of the cutaneous manifestations and is seen as a painless papulosquamous eruption frequently found on the soles or palms and uncommonly on the penis, trunk, extremities, or scalp (Fig. 287–5). Patients with chronic disease may demonstrate nail changes of onycholysis or subungual hyperkeratosis. *Ocular manifestations* occur early in the disease and include conjunctivitis, uveitis, and rarely, keratitis. Conjunctivitis tends to be bilateral, painful, and recurrent and lasts days rather than weeks. Acute uveitis is most often characterized by unilateral ocular pain. *Other uncommon features* may include an asymptomatic conduction disturbance, prolonged PR interval, complete heart block, aortitis, aortic regurgitation, amyloidosis, central nervous system involvement, serositis, or pulmonary infiltrates.

Radiographic abnormalities in Reiter's syndrome are commonly seen in the peripheral joints, primarily in an asymmetrical distribution affecting the feet, ankles, and knees. The sacroiliac and hip

joints are less frequently involved. Soft tissue swelling, juxta-articular osteopenia, joint space narrowing, and/or ill-defined erosions are seen. Areas of periostitis or reactive new bone formation are common. Although bilaterally asymmetrical sacroiliitis is common (Fig. 287–6), unilaterally symmetrical inflammatory changes or ankylosis has also been observed. Involvement of the lumbar spine differs from ankylosing spondylitis by the presence of non-marginal syndesmophytes or "bulky" osteophytes that are often unilateral or asymmetrical and tend to spare the anterior surface of the spine (see Fig. 287–3). Involvement of the cervical spine is uncommon in Reiter's syndrome.

Reiter's syndrome can usually be distinguished from rheumatoid arthritis (see Chapter 286) by evolution, pattern of involvement, associated extra-articular features, clinical course, and absence of serum rheumatoid factor. Reiter's syndrome should also be distinguished from septic arthritis (especially gonococcal arthritis), crystal-induced arthritis, sarcoidosis, and erythema nodosum on clinical grounds and after appropriate laboratory and synovial fluid analyses. It is more difficult to distinguish Reiter's syndrome from the other spondyloarthropathies and other reactive arthritides such as that seen with *Yersinia, Chlamydia,* or acquired immune deficiency syndrome (AIDS)-associated reactive arthritis. In such instances, a diagnosis of Reiter's syndrome is made after a careful history, identification of extra-articular features, appropriate use of serologic testing, and most important, observation over time.

The prognosis and course of Reiter's syndrome are varied and unpredictable. The majority of patients have an initial episode usually lasting 2 to 3 months, but it may last up to a year. Recurrent attacks and prolonged disease-free intervals are common. A chronic peripheral arthropathy is observed in 20 to 50% of patients. These individuals have the greatest potential for axial progression and spondylitic changes. Death is rare and may be ascribed to cardiac complications or amyloidosis.

REACTIVE ARTHROPATHIES. "Reactive arthritis" refers to the occurrence of an acute, non-suppurative, sterile inflammatory arthropathy arising after an infectious process but at a site remote from the primary infection. Reiter's syndrome is one of the most common examples of reactive arthritis. The microbial pathogens commonly associated with reactive arthritis are *Shigella, Salmonella, Yersinia, Campylobacter,* and *Chlamydia.* The reactive nature of these arthritides has been debated, inasmuch as *Chlamydia, Yersinia,* and *Salmonella* microbial antigens have been identified at sites of tissue inflammation, thus suggesting that an ongoing immune response to disseminated material, rather than a reactive condition, may be the pathogenic mechanism. Many reactive arthritides occur after a known infection and have therefore been termed "post-infectious." Although the pathologic processes appear to be similar, this distinction may be important with regard to potential responsiveness to antibiotic therapy.

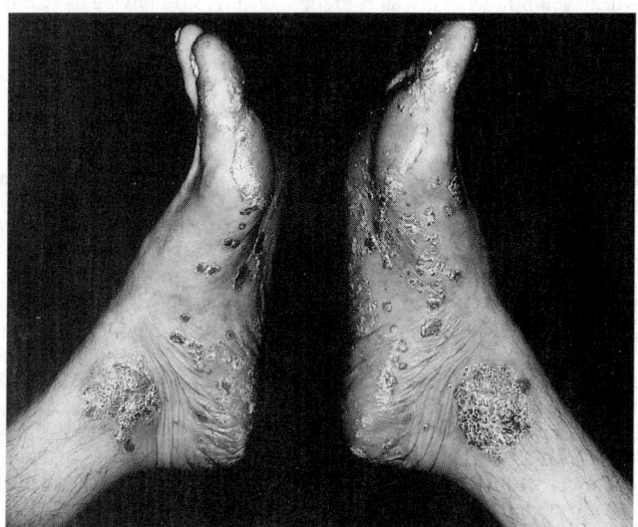

FIGURE 287–5 ■ Keratoderma blennorrhagicum of the feet in Reiter's syndrome.

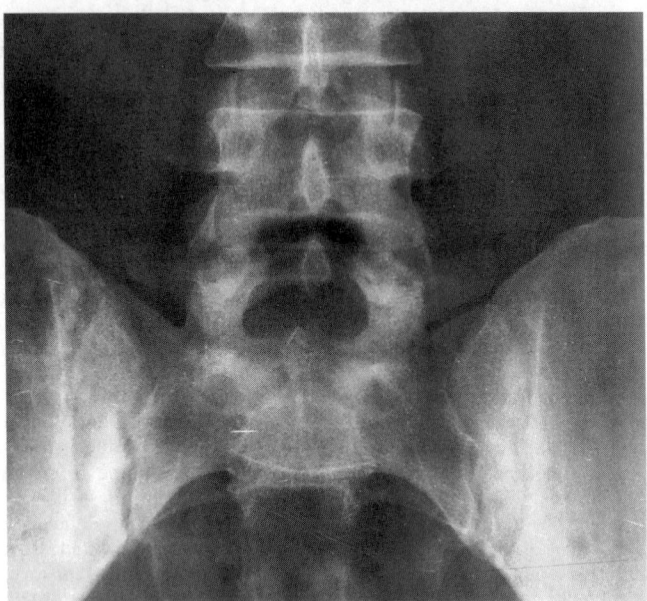

FIGURE 287-6 ■ Bilaterally asymmetrical sacroiliitis in Reiter's syndrome. Erosions, pseudowidening, and ileal sclerosis are present.

Reactive arthritis begins as an asymmetrical oligoarthritis, often preceded by an identifiable infectious event by 1 to 4 weeks. The temporal sequence suggests that these reactive disorders are triggered by an antecedent infectious process. Many patients without an identifiable infectious trigger have a similar constellation of signs and symptoms. The findings of sterile inflammatory synovial effusions, lymphocytes at sites of tissue inflammation, responsiveness to anti-inflammatory and immunosuppressive regimens, and the association with HLA-B27 suggest a common immunopathogenesis. Extra-articular manifestations may be a prominent feature of the reactive arthropathies. Although frequently self-limiting, these disorders have the potential for chronicity and serious articular damage to the peripheral or axial joints.

SHIGELLA. The occurrence of reactive arthritis after epidemics of Shigella dysentery has documented the arthritogenicity of this organism. Several reports suggest that Reiter's syndrome develops in 0.2 to 2% of infected individuals following epidemic shigellosis. Infections with Shigella flexneri trigger Reiter's syndrome, whereas the more frequent Shigella sonnei does not. In most cases, the diarrheal illness resolves before the articular symptoms appear.

SALMONELLA. Salmonella typhimurium is the most common Salmonella species inducing reactive arthritis. A sterile arthropathy will develop in as many as 6 to 10% of infected individuals within 3 weeks of a Salmonella outbreak. Nearly 60% of patients will possess HLA-B27 or one of the cross-reactive antigens. (HLA-B7 or HLA-B60). No clinical differences between Shigella- and Salmonella-induced reactive arthritis have been observed.

YERSINIA. Yersinia enterocolitica is a common cause of reactive arthritis in epidemic areas such as Scandinavia but is rarely encountered in England or the United States. Yersinia arthritis most commonly affects young adults as an acute, self-limiting gastrointestinal illness that may have associated joint complaints in 50% of cases. Chronicity, severity, sacroiliitis, and ocular inflammation are more likely in HLA-B27+ individuals. The arthritis is predominantly oligoarticular, usually affects the lower extremities and hands, and may run a chronic or relapsing course. Chronic low back pain and sacroiliitis are seen in one third of patients, but severe spinal ankylosis is rare. Extra-articular features occur in 20 to 30% of individuals. Erythema nodosum and glomerulonephritis have been described in HLA-B27− individuals. Sustained elevations of IgA antibody titers correlate with persistent infection, chronic arthritis, and occult enteritis. Treatment is similar to that for other reactive arthropathies. However, appropriate antibiotic therapy should be used in patients with persistently positive stool cultures for Yersinia.

CHLAMYDIA. C. trachomatis is thought to be responsible for up to 10% of all cases of early inflammatory arthritis (see Chapter 370). Arthritis will develop in as many as 1 to 3% of patients with chlamydial urethritis. The incidence of Chlamydia-induced arthritis has been estimated to be 5 cases per 100,000 per year. The diagnosis is suggested by the presence of persistent arthritis in at least one joint, symptoms of genitourinary infection, detection of IgG or IgA anti-Chlamydia antibodies, or Chlamydia found in genitourinary swabs or urine culture. Alternatively, chlamydial infection can be documented by enzyme immunoassay, direct fluorescent antibody testing or by using a DNA probe for chlamydial RNA. More than half of patients with Reiter's syndrome, non-gonococcal arthritis, or sexually acquired reactive arthritis will have antibodies to C. trachomatis, although positive cultures are seldom observed in patients with active disease.

The manifestations of Chlamydia-related reactive arthritis are similar to those described for classic Reiter's syndrome. However, only 20% of patients meet criteria for the diagnosis of Reiter's syndrome. Up to 15% of patients, especially women, have no urogenital manifestations at all. A chronic arthropathy develops in more than half, with nearly one third having inflammatory low back pain, enthesitis, or radiographic sacroiliitis. Fewer than 50% of patients are HLA-B27+. Chlamydia-induced arthritis apparently responds to antibiotic therapy, which is indicated in culture, serologic (IgM or IgA), or polymerase chain reaction–positive patients. A prolonged course (i.e., 12 weeks) of doxycycline, minocycline, or lymecycline may improve the symptoms.

AIDS AND REACTIVE ARTHRITIS. An aggressive form of Reiter's syndrome may develop in patients with AIDS (see Chapter 417). Early reports suggested that Reiter's syndrome developed in many HIV-infected individuals after profound immunosuppression. Although it has been suggested that AIDS patients are at increased risk of reactive arthritis, a number of prospective analyses of HIV-infected populations failed to reveal an increased incidence or prevalence of Reiter's syndrome when compared with that observed in an HIV-negative population matched for other risk factors. It seems clear that HIV infection alters the clinical expression of Reiter's syndrome. The vast majority of AIDS patients with Reiter's syndrome are HLA-B27+ and have incomplete symptoms and signs of Reiter's syndrome. The arthritis evolves in two main patterns: (1) an additive, asymmetrical polyarthritis or (2) an intermittent oligoarthritis that most commonly affects the lower extremities. Enthesitis, fasciitis, conjunctivitis, and urethritis are early and prominent symptoms. Although sacroiliitis does occur, HIV-associated reactive arthritis is rarely associated with axial disease or uveitis. HIV-associated disease also differs from classic Reiter's syndrome in the severity and chronicity of disease, prominent enthesitis, and a poor response to non-steroidal anti-inflammatory drugs (NSAIDs).

PSORIATIC ARTHRITIS. Psoriatic arthritis develops in 5 to 7% of patients with cutaneous psoriasis. Although most cases arise in patients with established, active cutaneous disease, other patients (especially children) have articular disease that antedates the development of psoriasis. Although the extent of psoriatic skin disease correlates poorly with the onset of arthritis, the risk of psoriatic arthritis increases with a family history of spondyloarthropathy or extensive nail pitting. The age of onset is usually between 30 and 55 years, and psoriatic arthritis has been shown to affect men and women equally. Psoriatic spondylitis, however, has a male-female ratio of 2.3:1.

The genetic associations with psoriatic arthritis are heterogeneous. Cutaneous psoriasis is associated with HLA-B13, HLA-Bw17, and HLA-Cw6. By contrast, HLA-B39 and HLA-B27 have been associated with sacroiliitis and axial involvement, and HLA-Cw6, HLA-Bw38, HLA-DR4, and HLA-DR7 have been associated with peripheral arthropathy. No etiologic agent or reactive process has been proved, although stress, trauma, the expression of heat shock proteins, and antecedent infection with Streptococcus or Staphylococcus have been suggested to play a role. The histopathology of psoriatic synovitis is similar to that seen in other inflammatory arthritides, with a notable lack of intrasynovial immunoglobulin and rheumatoid factor production and a greater propensity for fibrous ankylosis, osseous resorption, and heterotopic bone formation. Like HIV-associated Reiter's syndrome, disease severity in psoriatic arthritis is enhanced by coexistent HIV infection.

Psoriatic arthritis has an insidious onset and a progressive course. Five major variants of psoriatic arthritis have been described. These variants are not mutually exclusive, and patients

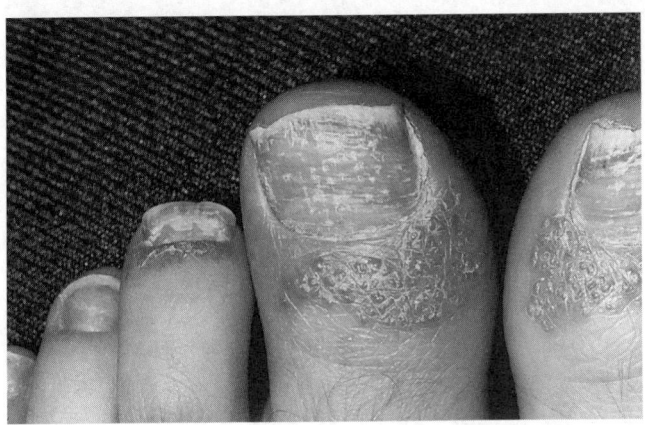

FIGURE 287–7 ■ Nail pitting, onycholysis, and transverse ridging in psoriatic arthritis. Dactylitis of the second toe is present.

may progress from one form to another. The 1st form is an asymmetrical oligoarthritis that is observed in 30 to 50% of patients and may involve both large and small joints. Dactylitis, or "sausage digits," may be seen in the fingers or toes. In this group, cutaneous features may be minimal and are often missed. The 2nd variant involves the distal interphalangeal joint and is seen in 10 to 15% of patients. It is strongly associated with nail changes of pitting, onycholysis, subungual hyperkeratosis, transverse ridging, and/or leukonychia (Fig. 287–7). Periungual erythema may reflect the extent of nail and joint disease. The 3rd variant is a rheumatoid arthritis–like symmetrical polyarthritis that is seen in 15 to 30% of patients who lack serum rheumatoid factor and rheumatoid nodules. The 4th variant is psoriatic spondylitis, which is seen in approximately 20% of psoriatic arthritis patients, 50% of whom are HLA-B27+. Finally, arthritis mutilans is seen in 5% of patients and is manifested as a destructive, erosive, polyarticular arthritis affecting the hands, feet, and spine. It often leads to progressive deformity and substantial disability.

Extra-articular features and laboratory findings are similar to those seen in Reiter's syndrome, although keratoconjunctivitis sicca, and mitral valve prolapse are less common. Hyperuricemia may be found and often correlates with the severity of cutaneous psoriasis.

Radiographic changes in psoriatic arthritis are similar to those seen in Reiter's syndrome and include soft tissue swelling ("sausage digits"), erosions, periostitis, asymmetrical sacroiliitis, and Reiter's-like spondylitis with asymmetrical non-marginal bulky syndesmophytes (see Fig. 287–3). The typical "pencil and cup" deformity may develop in patients with distal interphalangeal joint disease or arthritis mutilans. Acro-osteolysis, paravertebral ossification, and pericapsular calcification have also been described.

The diagnosis of psoriatic arthritis depends on finding typical cutaneous or nail changes in association with one of the recognized articular variants. Cutaneous psoriasis should be distinguished from seborrheic dermatitis, fungal infection, exfoliative dermatitis, eczema, keratoderma blennorrhagicum, and palmoplantar pustulosis. The arthritis of psoriasis is often misinterpreted as erosive osteoarthritis, gout, rheumatoid arthritis, pauciarticular juvenile arthritis, ankylosing spondylitis, or Reiter's syndrome. A minority of cases of psoriatic arthritis may exhibit clinical and radiographic features of Reiter's syndrome.

ENTEROPATHIC ARTHROPATHIES. "Enteropathic arthritis" refers to the arthropathies associated with Crohn's disease or ulcerative colitis (see Chapter 135). These disorders are unified by clinical and histologic gut inflammation, altered intestinal permeability, and the development of an inflammatory peripheral or axial arthritis. Peripheral arthritis is observed in nearly 20% and axial arthritis in 10 to 15% of patients. Peripheral arthropathy more frequently occurs in those with extraintestinal manifestations (e.g., erythema nodosum). Peripheral arthritis affects men and women equally. All age groups are affected, and although the onset of arthritis usually follows established intestinal inflammation in adults, the converse is true in children. Disease onset is sometimes heralded by low-grade fever, painful oral ulceration, ocular manifestations, cutaneous manifestations (e.g., erythema nodosum, pyoderma gangreno-

sum), or enthesitis. Rarely, a patient may have occult high fever, anemia, or weight loss. Peripheral arthritis is manifested as an inflammatory, non-erosive, asymmetrical oligoarthritis or monarthritis affecting the large joints (i.e., knees, ankles, elbows). Initially, the arthropathy may be migratory and resolve in weeks or months. Peripheral articular activity often parallels gut inflammation. Thus measures to control colitis may prove beneficial for managing peripheral arthritis. With chronicity, peripheral arthritis may be misdiagnosed as seronegative rheumatoid arthritis, particularly when symmetrical joint disease or quiescent gut inflammation is present.

In contrast, with peripheral arthritis, axial disease may precede or coincide with the onset of colitis and is more common in men. Axial arthropathy is clinically and radiographically indistinguishable from ankylosing spondylitis. The course of sacroiliitis and spondylitis is independent of active bowel inflammation. Whereas no association between HLA-B27 and colitic peripheral arthritis has been noted, HLA-B27 is found in 50% of patients with spondylitic colitis. Therefore, inflammatory bowel disease should be considered in the setting of HLA-B27− ankylosing spondylitis.

The association between enteritis and arthritis is supported by the findings of ileocolonoscopic evidence of subclinical gut inflammation in a variety of spondyloarthropathies. Histologic evidence of "acute" colitis (similar to bacterial enteritis) or "chronic" colitis (resembling chronic idiopathic inflammatory bowel disease) is commonly observed. Acute intestinal changes are commonly found in patients with post-dysenteric reactive arthritis, whereas chronic lesions are more typical of ankylosing spondylitis and patients in whom enteropathic arthritis will ultimately be diagnosed.

TREATMENT OF THE SPONDYLOARTHROPATHIES. Current therapies cannot cure the spondyloarthropathies; therefore, treatment should be aimed at reducing pain and stiffness. An aggressive approach to patient education and joint protection will contribute to the maintenance of optimal function and the patient's sense of well-being and may slow progression to immobility, joint deformity, or axial malalignment. All patients should be counseled regarding a rational program of exercise, rest, physical therapy, and diet and receive vocational counseling. Patients with axial disease should engage in lifelong physical therapy to maintain posture and prevent slow deformity. Once the diagnosis has been established, specific treatment can be initiated. Therapeutic options are largely the same for most of the spondyloarthropathies and as such are considered together (Fig. 287–8).

NSAIDs. NSAIDs have replaced the use of salicylates because they have more convenient dosaging and are more efficacious. NSAIDs effectively control the pain, stiffness, and/or joint swelling. Although these agents modify symptoms, they are not thought to retard the underlying inflammatory disease or suppress disease progression. NSAIDs are the mainstay of therapy in ankylosing spondylitis, Reiter's syndrome, reactive arthritis, and psoriatic arthritis. Their use in the enteropathic arthropathies is infrequently hampered by their potential to alter bowel permeability and/or induce exacerbations of colitis.

Although all NSAIDs are potentially useful in the spondyloarthropathies, only a few are of proven benefit and approved by the Fodd and Drug Administration for use in ankylosing spondylitis and/or Reiter's syndrome. These agents include indomethacin, diclofenac, naproxen, sulindac, and phenylbutazone. Of these, indomethacin, especially the sustained-release formula (1 to 2 mg/kg/day) is recommended because of its prolonged duration of effect and anti-inflammatory potency. Other NSAIDs are used according to individual tolerability and efficacy. Phenylbutazone is seldom used and no longer marketed in the United States but may be found in special compound in pharmacies. It is a very effective agent but should be reserved for intractable cases, primarily because of the risk of aplastic anemia.

CORTICOSTEROIDS. Systemic corticosteroids are seldom used in the spondyloarthropathies. They are most effective for controlling localized disease. They are used primarily as local therapy by intra-articular injection (e.g., monarthritis or oligoarthritis), topical management of ocular complications (conjunctivitis or uveitis), and on occasion, intralesionally to control enthesitis. Systemic low-dose or high-dose "pulse" corticosteroids should be reserved for severe disease flares.

ANTIBIOTICS. Antibiotic therapy may be indicated in certain indi-

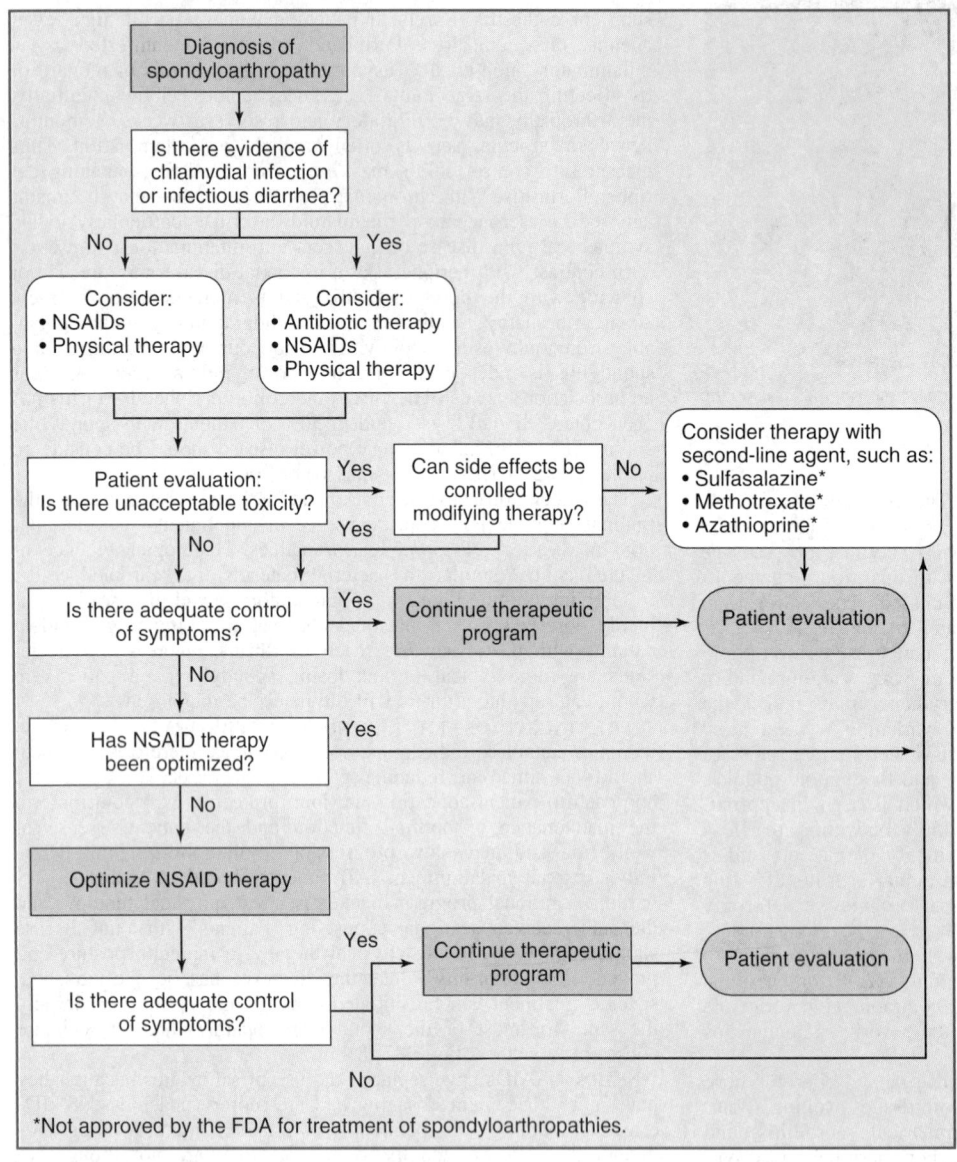

FIGURE 287–8 ■ Treatment algorithm for patients with a spondyloarthropathy.

*Not approved by the FDA for treatment of spondyloarthropathies.

viduals with reactive arthritis or Reiter's syndrome. Patients with culture-proven infectious diarrhea (e.g., *Shigella, Salmonella, Yersinia*) may benefit from appropriate antibiotic therapy. If chlamydial-induced arthritis is documented by serology, culture, or DNA probe, prolonged (e.g., 3 months) antibiotic therapy with doxycycline or lymecycline should be initiated. Studies have shown disappointing results with short-term tetracycline therapy.

SLOW-ACTING ANTIRHEUMATIC DRUGS. Slow-acting antirheumatic drugs (e.g., sulfasalazine, methotrexate) should be considered, when chronic NSAID-unresponsive peripheral arthritis, enthesitis, or spondylitis exists. These agents have a delayed onset of action (2 to 6 months), and their efficacy in the spondyloarthropathies is based on limited numbers of controlled trials and numerous anecdotal reports.

Placebo-controlled trials of sulfasalazine indicate that efficacy is greatest in patients with peripheral arthropathy and enthesopathy. Equivocal results have been observed in patients with long-standing disease and evidence of severe radiographic destruction or spinal ankylosis. At a dose of 2 to 4 g/day, it is most effective in patients with Reiter's syndrome, reactive arthritis, and enteropathic arthritis. The value of sulfasalazine in treating inflammatory axial disease has not been established but warrants consideration in poorly controlled spondylitis patients.

Methotrexate (7.5 to 20 mg/week) may also be effective in many patients with spondyloarthopathy. It is particularly effective for treating both cutaneous and articular disease in psoriasis, but higher

doses and prolonged use may be associated with unacceptable hepatotoxicity. Azathioprine (1 to 2 mg/kg/day) should be reserved for those unresponsive to or intolerant of other slow-acting antirheumatic drugs.

Additional therapeutic options exist for patients with psoriatic arthritis. Both methotrexate and sulfasalazine may be effective for managing articular and skin disease associated with psoriasis. Other patients may benefit from therapy with gold salts, antimalarials, etretinate, or cyclosporine. Newer agents (e.g., leflunomide) and proinflammatory cytokine inhibitors (e.g., etanercept, infliximab) have not been studied in spondyloarthropathy patients. Although immunosuppressive regimens should be avoided in HIV-associated arthritis, agents such as sulfasalazine or etretinate may be considered.

SURGERY. Surgery should be considered when pain and immobility markedly interfere with patient lifestyle. Total joint replacement is commonly performed in the hip or knee. The success of arthroplasty may be limited by postoperative heterotopic bone formation. Surgical correction of spinal deformities and/or fractures should be undertaken with extreme caution.

Amor B, Dougados M, Khan MA: Management of refractory ankylosing spondylitis and related spondyloarthropathies. Rheum Dis Clin North Am 21:117, 1995. *Review of the diagnosis and treatment of patients with refractory or severe spondyloarthropathy.*

Bardin T, Enel C, Cornelis F, et al: Antibiotic treatment of venereal disease and Reiter's syndrome in a Greenland population. *Arthritis Rheum* 35:190, 1992. *Suggested guidelines and treatment outcomes of patients with Reiter's syndrome treated with antibiotics.*

Cush JJ, Lipsky PE: Reiter's syndrome and reactive arthritis. In Koopman WJ (ed): Arthritis and Allied Conditions—A Textbook of Rheumatology, 13th ed. Baltimore, Williams & Wilkins, 1996, pp 1209–1227. *A comprehensive overview of Reiter's syndrome and reactive arthropathies.*

Hammer RE, Malka SD, Richardson JA, et al: Spontaneous inflammatory disease in transgenic rats expressing HLA-B27 and human b2m: An animal model of HLA-B27–associated human disorders. Cell 63:1099, 1990. *Describes the spectrum of clinicopathologic manifestations induced by introducing HLA-B27 into transgenic rats.*

Kettering JM, Towers JD, Rubin DA: The seronegative spondyloarthropathies. Semin Arthritis Rheum 31:220, 1996. *Review of the seronegative spondyloarthropathies with an emphasis on the clinical and radiographic features that distinguish these disorders from other arthritides.*

Lipsky PE, Alarcon GS, Bombardier C, et al: Algorithms for the diagnosis and management of musculoskeletal complaints. Am J Med 103 (Suppl. 6A): 49, 1997. *Overview of the diagnosis and management of several musculoskeletal disorders, including the spondyloarthropathies.*

Tay-Kearney ML, Schwam BL, Lowder C, et al: Clinical features and associated systemic diseases of HLA-B27 uveitis. Am J Ophthalmol 121:47, 1996. *Retrospective review of HLA-B27–associated uveitis in clinical practice, its manifestations, and clinical associations.*

Table 288–1 ▪ MOST COMMON MICROORGANISMS IN ACUTE NONGONOCOCCAL BACTERIAL ARTHRITIS (ALL AGES)

MICROORGANISM	FREQUENCY (%)
Gram positive	**60–90**
Staphylococcus aureus	50–70
Group B streptococci	15–30
Streptococcus pneumoniae	1–3
Gram negative	**5–25**
Salmonella spp.	
Pseudomonas aeruginosa	
Escherichia coli	
Kingella kingae	
Haemophilus influenzae	
Brucella	
Anaerobes	**1–2**
Fusobacterium necrophorum	
Anaerobic cocci	
Bacteriodes fragilis	

288 INFECTIOUS ARTHRITIS

Luis R. Espinoza

Infectious arthritis is a topic of great relevance in clinical medicine, and despite major advances in diagnostic approaches and the development of newer and more powerful antibiotics, its impact in terms of human morbidity and mortality has remained unchanged in the past 25 years.

The term infectious or septic arthritis refers to microbial invasion of the joint space (see also Parts XXII and XXIII) not associated with bone involvement. Regardless of age, bacterial septic arthritis is the most common form of infectious arthritis. Prompt diagnosis followed by appropriate therapeutic intervention is imperative to avoid destruction of the articular cartilage and permanent disability.

NON-GONOCOCCAL BACTERIAL ARTHRITIS. EPIDEMIOLOGY, PATHOGENESIS, AND RISK FACTORS. The incidence of septic arthritis is not well characterized, although it has been estimated to be 10 per 100,000 in northern Europe, and approximately 6.5% of all childhood arthritides may have a bacterial etiology. Septic arthritis occurs in all age groups but is more common in children than adults. Men are affected twice as often as women.

The microbial etiologic agent of septic arthritis varies with age. *Staphylococcus aureus* is the most common bacterial agent in both adults and children, followed by group B streptococci and *Streptococcus pneumoniae* (Table 288–1). Gram-negative microorganisms, including *Pseudomonas aeruginosa* and *Salmonella* species, frequently cause septic arthritis in immunosuppressed, sickle cell, and intravenous drug abusing patients. In neonates and infants younger than 2 months, *S. aureus*, group B streptococci, and gram-negative enteric bacilli are the usual pathogens. The frequency of *Haemophilus influenzae* infection has experienced a significant decrease since introduction of the Hib vaccine, and presently it is a less common pathogen than *S. aureus*.

Hematogenous spread is the most common cause of septic arthritis. Other less common routes include direct inoculation during diagnostic or therapeutic arthrocenteses or arthroscopies, trauma, and by contiguous osteomyelitis, cellulitis, abscesses, tenosynovitis, and/or septic bursitis. Once the microbial agent penetrates the joint space, it initiates a series of inflammatory reactions that may lead to joint destruction and permanent joint damage. Synovial membrane proliferation, granulation tissue, neovascularization, and infiltration by polymorphonuclear (PMN) cells may progress, if untreated, to cartilage and bone destruction. Expression of the collagen-binding protein adhesin by *S. aureus* and probably other microorganisms may play an important role in the initial steps of invasion into the joint space and adherence to collagen. Once microbial invasion into the joint is well established, bacterial endotoxin stimulates the release of inflammatory cytokines, including tumor necrosis factor and interleukin-1. Enzymes such as elastase and collagenase liberated from PMN cells and synovial cells also degrade the cartilage. Pressure necrosis from the accumulation of purulent synovial fluid further contributes to the destruction of cartilage.

Important risk factors for the development of septic arthritis include diabetes mellitus, immunodeficiency states, pre-existent joint damage (particularly rheumatoid arthritis), skin infection, debilitated conditions, hemoglobinopathy, intravenous drug use, and joint prostheses.

CLINICAL MANIFESTATIONS. Most patients have constitutional complaints that include chills, fever, malaise, and anorexia. In the majority of cases (80 to 90%), the symptoms are acute and monoarticular, with the knee joint being affected most commonly. On physical examination, the affected joint(s) can be extremely painful, warm, swollen, and filled with fluid. These inflammatory signs, however, may be masked in debilitated, severely ill patients or in those receiving corticosteroids or immunosuppressive agents. Polyarthritis may occur in patients with underlying connective tissue disease, particularly rheumatoid arthritis, or an immunosuppressive state and carries a worse prognosis, with a mortality rate of approximately 30%.

DIAGNOSIS. Early recognition of infection is the most important step in the management of septic arthritis. Arthrocentesis is mandatory in the presence of joint effusion, particularly when an infectious process is considered. All fluid aspirated should be sent for a Gram stain, aerobic and anaerobic bacterial cultures, and cell count with a leukocyte differential. The synovial fluid leukocyte count is usually between 40,000 and 50,000 cells per cubic millimeter, with a predominance (>80%) of PMN cells. Glucose, protein, and lactate levels are not very helpful and for the most part non-specific. The yield of organisms from joint fluid culture is approximately 50 to 60%. The erythrocyte sedimentation rate and C-reactive protein levels are elevated in most patients, and the latter may be helpful in the follow-up of patients. Plain radiographs are seldom useful early in the disease, although they may reveal joint abnormalities, e.g., loss of articular cartilage and bone erosions in untreated patients or in patients with aggressive disease. In patients suspected of deep-seated joint infections such as sacroiliac or facet joint involvement, scintigraphy, computed tomography, or magnetic resonance imaging studies may be helpful.

MANAGEMENT. Prompt institution of appropriate antibiotic therapy and joint drainage is essential in the management of septic arthritis. Antibiotics should be given to all patients suspected of having septic arthritis, even before results of bacteriologic studies become available. Initial antibiotic therapy should be based on Gram stain results of joint fluid or other body fluids or secretions. If no microorganisms are identified, empirical treatment should be given with the age, risk factors, and clinical picture of the patient taken into consideration. Normal individuals should be treated initially for infections with gram-positive organisms, whereas broad-spectrum antibiotics are indicated in debilitated, severely ill, and immunocompromised individuals. Once culture results become available, antibiotics can be changed if indicated. Parenteral, not intra-articular, therapy with either a β-lactamase–resistant penicillin or 1st-generation cephalosporin should be given for 2 to 4 weeks or more. Vancomycin should be used to treat methicillin-resistant *S. aureus* infection. Gram-negative organisms should be treated with a 3rd-generation cephalosporin such as cefotaxime or ceftriaxone or an aminoglycoside. Long-term administration of oral antibiotics is recommended in patients with chronic bone and joint infections (i.e., prosthetic joints). Closed needle aspiration on a daily basis or as often as necessary is an important part of medical management. Most patients can be treated in this manner, although in deep-seated joints, including the hips and shoulders, joints with pre-existent damage, joints not responding to appropriate medical management, or joints with loculated effusion or contiguous osteomyelitis, surgical drainage is indicated. Arthroscopic surgery rather than open surgery is recommended. Joint immobilization is not indicated except in patients with incapacitating pain or after surgical drainage. Joint mobilization and functional splinting of the affected joint(s) are recommended to prevent muscle atrophy and contracture and preserve joint function.

GONOCOCCAL ARTHRITIS. Gonorrhea is the most commonly reported communicable disease in the United States, and disseminated gonococcal infection remains the most common cause of acute septic arthritis in young sexually active individuals. Women are affected two to three times as often as men. The incidence of gonorrhea has decreased in the United States in the past few years, and this decrease has been observed for all racial and ethnic groups. The reduction appears to be related to the changes in sexual behavior that have occurred since the beginning of the human immunodeficiency virus (HIV) epidemic. Disseminated gonococcal infection occurs in between 0.5% and 3% of cases of mucosal infection and is the most common reason for hospital admission caused by infectious arthritis in the Unites States, with an estimated incidence of 2.8 cases per 100,000 population per year.

Disseminated gonococcal infection is always preceded by mucosal infection with *Neisseria gonorrhoeae*. The infection commonly involves the endocervix or urethra but may involve the pharynx and rectum and may or may not be symptomatic.

The risk for gonococcal dissemination following a mucosal infection depends on the status of the patient's immune system and on the virulence of the microorganism (Table 288–2).

CLINICAL MANIFESTATIONS. Monoarthralgia, oligoarthralgia, or polyarthralgia, the most common symptom of disseminated gonococcal infection, occurs in a diffuse, migratory, or additive pattern within a few days of onset. Tenosynovitis, with or without arthritis, commonly develops in the wrists, fingers, ankles, or toes in two thirds of patients. Any joint may be involved, but the knees, wrists, hands, and ankles are usually affected. Fever and chills are common. Skin involvement occurs in approximately two thirds of patients with disseminated gonococcal infection. Rash is manifested as macules, papules, necrosis, or pustules and may develop up to 48 hours after initiation of antibiotic therapy. Unusual clinical manifestations include pericarditis, meningitis, aortitis, endocarditis, myocarditis, and osteomyelitis.

Most patients with disseminated gonococcal infection have asymptomatic primary gonococcal infection of the genitourinary tract. The major differential diagnoses include Reiter's syndrome, bacterial arthritis, juvenile rheumatoid arthritis, meningococcemia, bacterial endocarditis, and acute rheumatic fever.

DIAGNOSIS. In most patients, the diagnosis is made indirectly by finding a positive culture from the genitourinary tract or, much less frequently, from the rectum or pharynx. *N. gonorrhoeae* is rarely found in synovial fluid, blood, or skin lesions. If Gram stains and cultures are negative, a presumptive diagnosis is made by the typical clinical findings associated with a rapid response to antibiotics. Polymerase chain reaction may be helpful in this situation and allows identification of the organism in synovial fluid. Other laboratory findings are non-specific.

MANAGEMENT. Hospitalization is recommended for initial therapy for disseminated gonococcal infection, particularly if complications such as endocarditis and meningitis are present. A 3rd-generation β-lactamase–resistant cephalosporin such as ceftriaxone, 1 g intramuscularly or intravenously every 24 hours, is initially recommended. Alternative initial regimens include cefotaxime or ceftizoxime, 1 g intravenously every 8 hours. For individuals allergic to β-lactam drugs, spectinomycin, 2 g intramuscularly every 12 hours, is the treatment of choice. If organisms are sensitive to penicillin, treatment may be switched to ampicillin, 1 g intravenously every 6 hours, or penicillin G, 10 million U intravenously daily in divided doses. Ceftriaxone and spectinomycin are safe and effective for the treatment of gonorrhea in pregnancy. Parenteral therapy should be given until evidence of clinical improvement is seen, usually 2 to 4 days, and then oral antibiotics can be substituted; a penicillin derivative and cephalosporin should be given for another 7 to 10 days. Concomitant use of oral doxycycline or another tetracycline should also be given because of the high prevalence of coexistent *Chlamydia* infection. Following completion of therapy, the patient should be evaluated, repeat cultures obtained, and tests for syphilis, *Chlamydia*, and HIV infection considered.

MYCOPLASMA ARTHRITIS. *Mycoplasma*-induced monoarthritis or oligoarthritis is relatively common in children, although its exact prevalence is unknown. It also occurs frequently in immunocompromised patients, particularly those with agammaglobulinemia.

VIRAL ARTHRITIS. This group of arthritides constitutes the second most common cause of infectious arthritis after bacterial arthritis. The most important viral infections associated with rheumatic complaints are hepatitis viruses, parvovirus, rubella virus, and HIV. Hepatitis B and C and to a lesser degree hepatitis A virus may cause immune complex–mediated rheumatic syndromes. Acute and, much less commonly, chronic arthritis and vasculitis, including forms with essential mixed cryoglobulinemia, have all been described during the course of hepatitis infection. Hepatitis C infection is responsible for over half of cases of essential mixed cryoglobulinemia. In general, arthritis associated with hepatitis is self-limiting and lasts less than 4 weeks, affects small joints, follows a migratory pattern, and can be either additive or non-additive. Arthritis subsides as jaundice appears in hepatitis B virus infection. Patients with hepatitis C virus infection may exhibit a more chronic, symmetric arthritis of the small and large joints, with positive rheumatoid factor indistinguishable from rheumatoid arthritis. Most patients respond to conventional analgesic and/or anti-inflammatory therapy. Prednisone, cytotoxic therapy, interferon-α, specific antiviral agents, and plasmapheresis alone or in combination have been shown to be beneficial for the most serious rheumatic syndromes.

Rheumatic manifestations are relatively frequent during the course of HIV infection. They may occur at any time during the natural course of the disease, although they tend to be more common in late stages. Arthralgia, usually of moderate intensity, intermittent, and oligoarticular, is the most frequent rheumatic manifestation of HIV disease. It occurs in approximately 35% of cases and predominantly affects the knees, shoulders, and elbows. Other distinct syndromes seen include Reiter's syndrome, psoriatic arthritis, undifferentiated spondyloarthropathy, vasculitis, myositis, Sjögren's syndrome, and fibrositis. Septic arthritis and myositis are also seen. Treatment of these conditions includes conventional anti-inflammatory therapy. Methotrexate, prednisone, and other immunosuppressive drugs may be indicated in patients with refractory arthritis, myositis, and/or vasculitis. These agents should be used in combination with antiretroviral therapy and antimicrobial prophylaxis to minimize the likelihood of serious complications, including the precipitation of acquired immune deficiency syndrome and Kaposi's sarcoma. Zidovudine therapy may induce a toxic mitochondrial myopathy, with the appearance of "ragged reed fibers." Clinical and biochemical abnormalities are similar to those of myositis, and a rapid response follows withdrawal of zidovudine therapy.

Rubella-associated arthritis occurs within days of the appearance

Table 288–2 ■ **MICROBIAL AND HOST FACTORS ASSOCIATED WITH DISSEMINATED GONOCOCCAL INFECTION**

HOST	MICROBIAL
Delayed diagnosis and treatment in women	Pili variation
Menses and pregnancy	Outer membrane proteins I, II, III
Cytokines	Lipo-oligosaccharide
Inherited complement deficiency	Proteoglycan
	IgA proteases

of skin rash in natural infection or 2 to 4 weeks after vaccination. The pattern of joint involvement is frequently that of a migratory polyarthralgia and less often polyarthritis. It may mimic rheumatoid arthritis, and the wrist, small joints of the hands, and knees are affected more commonly. The acute episode usually lasts 3 to 21 days, but it may persist for months. Rubella virus has been isolated from peripheral blood and synovial fluid from affected patients, but its role as an etiologic agent in rheumatoid arthritis is questionable.

Human parvovirus B19 is a DNA virus that is also associated with an inflammatory articular syndrome that can mimic rheumatoid arthritis at times. In most patients, joint symptoms subside in a few weeks without sequelae. B19 infection is seldom accompanied by a positive rheumatoid factor, subcutaneous nodules, or joint erosions. Elevated titer of specific IgM antibodies confirms the diagnosis, and treatment is symptomatic.

Other viruses less commonly causing arthralgia and polyarthritis include herpes zoster, cytomegalovirus, Epstein-Barr virus, echovirus, adenovirus, and coxsackievirus. Chikungunya, o'nyong-nyong, and Ross River viruses are all alphaviruses responsible for major epidemics of febrile polyarthritis in Africa, Australia, Europe, and Latin America.

MISCELLANEOUS FORMS OF INFECTIOUS ARTHRITIS. LYME DISEASE. Lyme disease (see also Chapter 368) is associated with monoarthritis or oligoarthritis and involves the large joints in a remitting fashion lasting months or years. Arthritis is the most common manifestation of late (persistent) or stage 3 infection. The knee joint is involved in almost all cases. Symmetric or rheumatoid arthritis–like joint involvement in association with HLA-DR4 usually does not respond to antibiotic therapy. Laboratory diagnosis is based on serologic techniques. Treatment with appropriate antibiotics is effective in most patients with the correct diagnosis. Some patients are refractory to conventional therapy, and in these patients newer modalities such as vaccination may be required.

SYPHILIS. Joint involvement may occur at any stage of congenital, secondary, and tertiary syphilis (see also Chapter 365). It is important to recognize the rheumatic manifestations of syphilis, principally because of its resurgence in recent years in association with HIV infection. A variety of musculoskeletal manifestations may occur, including osteochondritis, osteitis, periostitis, bilateral hydrarthrosis usually involving the knees and painless joints (Clutton's joints) in children with congenital syphilis, polyarthralgias, polyarthritis, tenosynovitis (not as common or as painful as in disseminated gonococcal infection), unilateral sacroiliitis, spondylitis in patients with secondary syphilis, and Charcot's joints, gummatous arthritis and osteitis, and chronic arthritis in patients with tertiary syphilis. Diagnosis can be difficult, especially in the setting of HIV infection, in which case repeated serologic analysis is often necessary. Penicillin remains the agent of choice and usually provides good results.

TUBERCULOUS ARTHRITIS. Tuberculosis is a rare cause of arthritis in the Western world. The increase in the incidence of pulmonary tuberculosis and its association (including the atypical forms) with HIV infection compel one to consider this etiology, especially in patients with chronic monoarthritis or oligoarthritis of the large joints. Active pulmonary involvement is often not detected, but the skin test is usually positive. Direct histologic evidence and culture of synovial tissue are required for diagnosis. Joint involvement with atypical *Mycobacterium* infection should be considered in immunocompromised patients, after repeated intra-articular steroid injections, and in certain occupations, e.g., fisherman. Long-term therapy with isoniazid, ethambutol, and/or rifampin is indicated.

FUNGAL ARTHRITIS. Musculoskeletal involvement secondary to fungal infection is rarely seen, although an increased incidence of pathogenic and opportunistic fungal infections and the emergence of new species, particularly in immunosuppressed patients, have been noted. Chronic evolution and delayed diagnosis are common.

The most common organisms affecting the musculoskeletal system are *Coccidioides immitis, Histoplasma capsulatum, Blastomyces dermatitidis, Sporothrix schenckii,* and in immunocompromised patients, *Candida, Aspergillus, Cryptococcus,* and *Histoplasma*. Diagnosis requires identification of the organism in synovial tissue or isolation from synovial fluid or tissue. Long-term therapy with amphotericin B and the newer antimycotic agents, with or without surgical débridement, is often effective.

Cucurull E, Espinoza LR: Gonococcal arthritis. Rheum Dis Clin North Am, 24:305, 1998. *An in-depth review of diagnostic and therapeutic modalities of disseminated gonococcal infection.*

Espinoza LR: Infectious arthritis. Rheum Dis Clin North Am 24:287, 1998. *An up-to-date review of the most common infectious disorders affecting the musculoskeletal system.*

Shetty AK, Gedalia A: Septic arthritis in children. Rheum Dis Clin North Am 24:305, 1998. *A comprehensive review of septic arthritis.*

289 SYSTEMIC LUPUS ERYTHEMATOSUS

Peter H. Schur

Systemic lupus erythematosus (SLE) is a disease of unknown cause that may produce variable combinations of fever, rash, hair loss, arthritis, pleuritis, pericarditis, nephritis, anemia, leukopenia, thrombocytopenia, and central nervous system (CNS) disease. The clinical course is characterized by periods of remissions and acute or chronic relapses. Characteristic immune abnormalities, especially antibodies to a number of nuclear and other cellular antigens, develop in patients with SLE. The diagnosis is facilitated by determining whether the patient has 4 of the 11 clinical and/or laboratory criteria developed for the classification of SLE (Table 289–1).

EPIDEMIOLOGY. SLE can occur at any age but has its onset primarily between ages 16 and 55. It occurs more frequently in women. In children, the female-male ratio is 1.4 to 5.8:1; in adults, it ranges from 8:1 to 13:1; and in older individuals, the ratio is 2:1. The prevalence of SLE is estimated to be between 4 and 250 cases per 100,000 population. In the United States, the highest incidence is among Asians in Hawaii, blacks, and certain Native Americans (Sioux, Crow, Arapahoe). The risk of SLE developing in a black American female has been estimated to be 1:250. The prevalence is about the same worldwide; the disease appears to be common in China, in Southeast Asia, and among blacks in the Caribbean, but is seen infrequently in blacks in Africa. Limited observations suggest that the incidence of discoid lupus erythematosus is the same as that for SLE.

ETIOLOGY. The cause of SLE remains unknown, although many observations suggest a role for genetic, hormonal, immune, and environmental factors. The evidence for a genetic role is summarized in Table 289–2. Some of these genetic marker associations are found more frequently in SLE patients of different races and ethnicities. It has been calculated that at least four genes are involved in predisposing individuals to SLE. Each gene presumably affects some aspect of immune regulation, protein degradation, peptide transport across cell membranes, immune response, complement, the reticuloendothelial system (including phagocytosis), immunoglobulins, apoptosis, and sex hormones. Thus combinations of dissimilar gene defects may result in distinct abnormal responses and produce separate pathologic processes and different clinical expression.

The evidence for hormonal abnormalities is based primarily on the observation that SLE is much more common among women in their childbearing years. In addition, SLE has been observed in some males with Klinefelter's syndrome, and some abnormalities of estrogen metabolism have been noted in both men and women with SLE. However, the clinical expression of SLE is the same in men and women. Furthermore, a lupus-like disease of New Zealand mice is more common and more severe and has an earlier onset in females—and is ameliorated by oophorectomy or treatment with male hormones. However, in other strains of mice with a lupus-like disease, this gender difference is not noted.

Numerous immune abnormalities occur in patients with SLE, the etiology of which remains unclear; nor do we know which are primary and which are secondary. Some of these immune defects are episodic, and some correlate with disease activity. SLE is pri-

Table 289–1 ■ **CRITERIA FOR CLASSIFICATION OF SYSTEMIC LUPUS ERYTHEMATOSUS***

CRITERION		DEFINITION
1. Malar rash		Fixed erythema, flat or raised, over the malar eminences, tending to spare the nasolabial folds
2. Discoid rash		Erythematous raised patches with adherent keratotic scaling and follicular plugging; atrophic scarring may occur in older lesions
3. Photosensitivity		Skin rash as a result of unusual reaction to sunlight, by patient history or physician observation
4. Oral ulcers		Oral or nasopharyngeal ulceration, usually painless, observed by a physician
5. Arthritis		Non-erosive arthritis involving two or more peripheral joints and characterized by tenderness, swelling, or effusion
6. Serositis	a.	Pleuritis—convincing history of pleuritic pain or rub heard by a physician or evidence of pleural effusion
		OR
	b.	Pericarditis—documented by electrocardiogram or rub or by evidence of pericardial effusion
7. Renal disorder	a.	Persistent proteinuria >0.5 g/day or >3+ if quantitation not performed
		OR
	b.	Cellular casts—may be red cell, hemoglobin, granular, tubular, or mixed
8. Neurologic disorder	a.	Seizures—in the absence of offending drugs or known metabolic derangements, e.g., uremia, ketoacidosis, or electrolyte imbalance
		OR
	b.	Psychosis in the absence of offending drugs or known metabolic derangements, e.g., uremia, ketoacidosis, or electrolyte imbalance
9. Hematologic disorder	a.	Hemolytic anemia with reticulocytosis
		OR
	b.	Leukopenia <4000/mm³ total on two or more occasions
	c.	Lymphopenia <1500/mm³ on two or more occasions
		OR
	d.	Thrombocytopenia <100,000/mm³ in the absence of offending drugs
10. Immunologic disorder	a.	Positive tests for antiphospholipid antibodies
		OR
	b.	Anti-DNA: antibody to native DNA in abnormal titer
		OR
	c.	Anti-Sm: presence of antibody to Sm nuclear antigen
		OR
	d.	False-positive serologic test for syphilis known to be positive for at least 6 mo and confirmed by *Treponema pallidum* immobilization or fluorescent treponemal antibody absorption test
11. Antinuclear antibody		An abnormal titer of antinuclear antibody by immunofluorescence or an equivalent assay at any point and in the absence of drugs known to be associated with "drug-induced lupus" syndrome

*The classification is based on 11 criteria. For the purpose of identifying patients in clinical studies, a person shall be said to have systemic lupus erythematosus if any 4 or more of the 11 criteria are present, serially or simultaneously, during any interval of observation.

marily a disease with abnormalities of immune regulation. These abnormalities are thought to be secondary to a loss of "self" tolerance; that is, SLE patients (either before or during disease evolution) are no longer totally tolerant of all their "self" antigens and consequently an immune response develops to these antigens. The number of suppressor T cells also decreases; these would normally be down-regulating (maintaining homeostasis) immune responses.

Furthermore, mice with lupus and possibly humans with SLE have a (genetic) defect in apoptosis that results in abnormal programmed cell death. As a result of these defects, cells break down abnormally; certain (especially nuclear) antigens are processed by antigen-presenting cells (i.e., macrophages, B lymphocytes, dendritic cells) into peptides. The peptide–major histocompatibility complex stimulates the expansion of helper (i.e., CD4) autoreactive T cells that through release of cytokines (i.e., interleukin-6 [IL-6], IL-4, and IL-10), cause autoreactive B cells to become activated, proliferate, and differentiate into antibody-producing cells and make an excess of antibodies to many nuclear antigens (Fig. 289–1). Thus a characteristic immune profile develops in patients with SLE—the development of elevated levels of antinuclear antibodies (ANAs) especially to DNA, Sm, RNP, Ro, La, and others (see Chapter 285) (Table 289–3). ANAs are made to molecules involved in essential cellular functions (e.g., RNA splicing); antigens are active sites on these molecules. With continued pressure over time from "self" antigens, the immune response switches from low-affinity, highly cross-reactive IgM antibodies—via somatic (hyper)mutation—to high-affinity IgG antibodies and to more limited epitopes on "self" antigens. Unique idiotypes of antibodies may stimulate autoreactive T cells to expand, thereby helping unique clones of B cells to expand and thus making more specific ANAs with unique idiotypes. Female hormones promote B-cell hyperactivity, whereas androgens may have the opposite effect. Environmental factors such as microorganisms (i.e., viruses) may stimulate specific cells in this immune network. Furthermore, ultraviolet (UV) light—known to exacerbate lupus skin lesions—may stimulate keratinocytes to secrete more IL-1, which in turn stimulates B cells to make more antibody. Not all autoantibodies cause disease. In fact, all normal individuals make autoantibodies, albeit in low levels. The variability in clinical disease (different organs in specific patients) may thus reflect variability in the quality and quantity of the immune response. Although these observations suggest possible triggering factors for disease, it remains unclear what causes exacerbations—although clinically they often follow infections and other stressful events—and what causes perpetuation of the immune abnormalities and waxing and waning of the disease.

PATHOGENESIS. Many manifestations are mediated by antibodies. The classic example is that of diffuse proliferative glomerulonephritis. Immune complexes, which consist of nuclear antigens (especially DNA) and high-affinity complement-fixing IgG (especially IgG1 and IgG3) and ANAs (especially antibodies to DNA), form in the circulation and are deposited in the glomerular basement membrane (GBM) or form in situ; histone may facilitate immune complex deposition. The complement system is then activated and chemotactic factors are generated. These factors induce the attraction and infiltration of leukocytes, which then phagocytose immune complexes and cause the release of mediators (such as activators of the clotting system), which further perpetuate the glomerular inflammation. With continuing immune complex deposition, chronic inflammation may ensue, ultimately leading to fibrinoid necrosis and scarring (crescents) and loss of renal function. In lupus membranous glomerulonephritis, similar mechanisms occur, although immune complex–containing, poorly complement-fixing IgG2 and IgG4 form primarily in situ on the GBM; there is no cellular infiltrate. The mechanism for the GBM protein leakage, which results in the nephrotic syndrome, is not clear. In lupus mesangial glomerulonephritis, mesangial cells (macrophage-like

Table 289–2 ■ **GENETIC RISK FACTORS FOR SYSTEMIC LUPUS ERYTHEMATOSUS**

High concordance rate (14–57%) in monozygotic twins
Increased frequency (5–12%) of LE, autoantibodies, suppressor cell defects in 1st-degree relatives
Increased frequency: HLA-B8, DR2, DR3, DQA1, DQB1
             C2, C4 (especially C4A), CR1 deficiency
             Certain genetic markers on IgG (Immunoglobulin G)
             T-cell receptor genes
             Chromosome markers in the 1q41–q42 region
Anti-DNA associated with DR2, DR3, DR7, DQB1
Anti-Sm associated with DR4, DR7, DQw6
Anti-RNP associated with DQw5, DQw8
Anti-Ro (SS-A) associated with DR2, DR3, DQA1/DQB1, C2D
Anti-La (SS-B) associated with DR3, DQw2.3
Antiphospholipid associated with DR4, DR7, DR53, DQw7

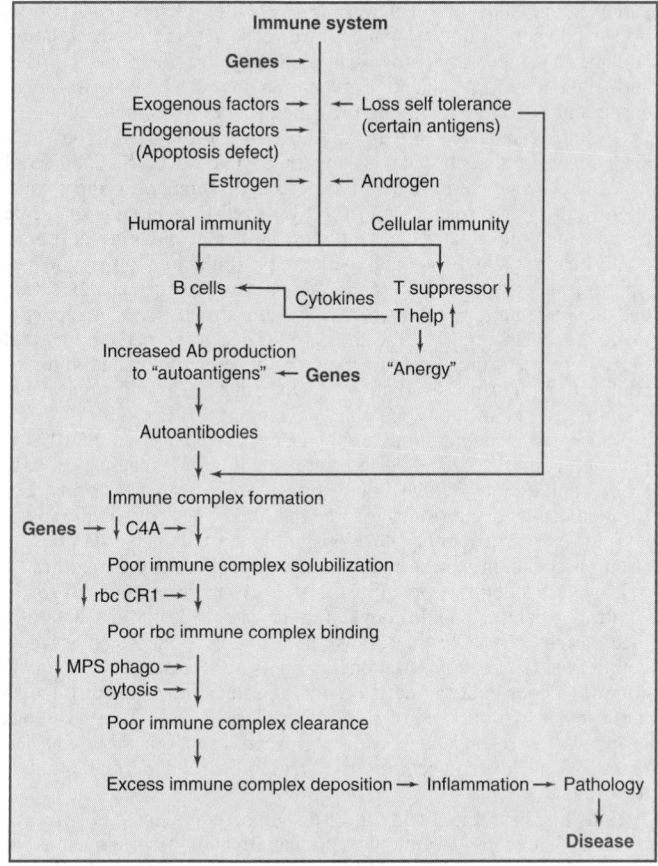

Immune system

FIGURE 289-1 ■ Pathogenetic events in systemic lupus erythematosus.

cells) have phagocytosed immune complexes, thus preventing them from being deposited on the GBM. Immune complexes have been detected (by immunofluorescence and/or electron microscopy) at the dermal-epidermal junction in both skin lesions and normal skin, in the choroid plexus, in the pericardium, and in the pleural cavity. The pathogenic potential of immune complexes depends on the antibody (its specificity, affinity, charge, ability to activate complement or other mediators of inflammation), the nature of the antigen (size, charge), the ability of the immune complex to be solubilized by complement or bound to and cleared by red blood cells (RBCs) (both systems may be defective in SLE), the clearance ability of the mononuclear phagocytosis system, and other factors.

Patients with SLE also make antibodies to cell-surface antigens. RBCs, white blood cells (WBCs), and platelets coated with such

Table 289-3 ■ AUTOANTIBODIES IN PATIENTS WITH SYSTEMIC LUPUS ERYTHEMATOSUS

TEST	SENSITIVITY (%)	SPECIFICITY (%)	PREDICTIVE VALUE (%)
ANA	99	80	15–35
dsDNA	70	95	95
ssDNA	80	50	50
Histone	30–80	Moderate	Moderate
Nucleoprotein	58	Moderate	Moderate
SM	25	99	97
RNP (U1-RNP)	50	87–94	46–85
Ro (SS-A)	25–35		
La (SS-B)	15		
PCNA	5	95	95

Cytoplasm: mitochondria, lysosomes, microsomes, ribosomes. RNA: dsRNA, ssRNA, rRNA. Cell membranes: red cells, white blood (T and B) cells, platelets, brain. Other: clotting factors (antiphospholipid antibodies), thyroid, rheumatoid factors, biologic false-positive serologic test for syphilis. In SLE, anti-DNA and anti-Sm are associated with renal disease, anti-RNP with Raynaud's, and anti-Ro with photosensitivity. Anti-RNP is seen in SLE, rheumatoid arthritis, scleroderma, Sjögren's syndrome, and mixed connective tissue disease. Anti-Ro (SS-A) is seen in SLE, Sjögren's syndrome, primary photosensitivity, and primary biliary cirrhosis. Anti-La (SS-B) is seen in SLE and Sjögren's syndrome.

antibodies are cleared from the circulation either through (Fc) receptors on macrophages of the reticuloendothelial system, by complement-mediated cytotoxicity, or by antibody-dependent cellular cytotoxicity—resulting in (hemolytic) anemia, leukopenia, and thrombocytopenia. Antibodies to endothelial cells have been implicated in vasculitis, antibodies to neuronal cells have been associated with neuropsychiatric lupus, and antibodies to renal glomerular and tubular antigens have been implicated in lupus nephritis. Of recent particular interest are antibodies to the phospholipid–β_2-glycoprotein I complex. These antibodies appear to interfere with the normal anticoagulant effect of β_2-glycoprotein I and are thus implicated in the arterial and venous thromboses (causing strokes and thrombophlebitis) and placental infarcts (causing miscarriages) complicating SLE.

Skin lesions are thought to be multifactorial in origin. UV light (1) damages DNA (the patient makes antibodies to DNA, immune complexes form, complement is activated, and a local inflammatory response ensues); (2) increases binding of anti-Ro, anti-La, and anti-RNP to UV-activated keratinocytes; (3) alters cellular membrane phospholipid metabolism; (4) increases IL-1 release from cutaneous keratinocytes and Langerhans' cells; and (5) affects suppressor T cells.

PATHOLOGY. Few unique pathologic features are associated with SLE. In patients with arthritis, the synovial histopathology tends to be non-specific, with superficial fibrin-like material and local or diffuse cell lining proliferation. Vascular changes include perivascular mononuclear cells, lumen obliteration, enlarged endothelial cells, and thrombi, but fibrinoid necrosis is uncommon. Biopsies of the malar erythema may reveal some minor basal layer abnormalities, as well as immune complex deposits at the dermal-epidermal junction. Discoid skin lesions are characterized by hyperkeratosis, follicular plugging, and more basal cell layer changes, including immune complexes at the dermal-epidermal junction. Pleura and pericardium are infiltrated by mononuclear cells. Lupus pneumonitis is characterized by alveolar wall injury, hemorrhage, and edema; hyaline membrane formation; and immune complex deposits. Coronary arteries often demonstrate premature-onset atherosclerosis. Libman-Sacks endocarditis is characterized by the accumulation of immune complexes, mononuclear cells, hematoxylin bodies, and fibrin and platelet thrombi. Pathologic examination of the spleen often reveals an "onion skin" appearance of the splenic arteries, which is thought to represent healed arteritis.

RENAL DISEASE. Minimal disease (type IIA mesangial disease) of glomeruli has immune complex deposits only in mesangial cells. Type IIb mesangial nephritis also has mesangial hypercellularity. Focal proliferative nephritis (type III) has segmental proliferation in glomerular tufts and in the mesangium and immune complex deposits in the mesangium and scattered granular deposits in the subendothelial, subepithelial, and intrabasement GBM. Active diffuse proliferative glomerulonephritis (type IV) affects more than 50% of glomeruli with cellular proliferation, necrosis, "wire loops," subendothelial deposits, and hematoxylin bodies. When chronic, the process involves sclerosis, adhesions, crescents, and (tubular) atrophy. Extensive "lumpy and bumpy" deposits of immune complexes are present. In membranous nephritis (type V) diffuse, uniform thickening of the GBM is seen, with a fine granular deposition of immune complexes in the subendothelial region beneath fused foot processes. Tubular degenerative changes with interstitial mononuclear cells are not uncommon. Extensive crescent formation, representing scarring, indicates a poor prognosis.

The brain is notable for the paucity of pathologic changes. Some minor blood vessel abnormalities, an occasional microinfarct, and some perivascular infiltration have been noted.

CLINICAL MANIFESTATIONS. SLE is highly variable in onset as well as course. The initial symptoms may be non-specific (Table 289–4) and include myalgia, nausea, vomiting, headaches, depression, easy bruising, or more specific symptoms or any combination thereof. These symptoms may be mild or severe, fleeting or persistent.

GENERAL SYMPTOMS. Fatigue occurs in virtually all patients with SLE. Fatigue may parallel the onset of SLE or its relapse but should be distinguished from the fatigue associated with other factors such as increased workload, sleep disturbance, depression, unhealthful habits, stress, deconditioning, anemia, the use of certain

Table 289–4 ■ CLINICAL FEATURES IN SYSTEMIC LUPUS ERYTHEMATOSUS

MANIFESTATION	APPROXIMATE FREQUENCY (%)	
	At Onset	At Any Time
Non-specific		
Fatigue	—	90
Fever	36	80
Weight loss	—	60
Arthralgia/myalgia	69	95
Specific		
Arthritis	—	90
Skin		
Butterfly rash	40	50
Discoid LE	6	20
Photosensitivity	29	58
Mucous ulcers	11	30
Alopecia	—	71
Raynaud's phenomenon	18	30
Purpura	—	15
Urticaria	—	9
Renal	16	50
Nephrosis	—	18
Gastrointestinal	—	38
Pulmonary	3	50
Pleurisy	—	45
Effusions	—	24
Pnemonia	—	29
Cardiac	—	46
Pericarditis	—	48
Murmurs	—	23
ECG changes	—	34
Lymphadenopathy	7	50
Splenomegaly	—	20
Hepatomegaly	—	25
Central nervous system	12	75
Functional	—	Most
Psychosis	—	20
Seizures	—	20
Hematologic	—	90

medications (including prednisone), and any intercurrent disease. Fever is seen in 80% of patients; it is usually episodic. Infections, which occur commonly in SLE patients, must always be considered.

MUSCULOSKELETAL MANIFESTATIONS. Arthralgia and arthritis have been noted in 95% of patients with SLE. Symptoms tend to be asymmetrical and migratory, with complaints in a particular joint often gone in 1 to 3 days. Fingers, hands, wrists, knees, and less frequently, ankles, elbows, shoulders, and hips are affected. Morning stiffness is generally measured in minutes, in contrast to hours in rheumatoid arthritis. Although joint deformities are considered to be more a feature of rheumatoid arthritis, damage to periarticular tissue can cause flexion deformities, ulnar deviation, soft tissue laxity, and swan neck deformities, particularly in those with long-standing disease who are receiving corticosteroids. Joint erosions are rare. Tenosynovitis is noted in 10 to 13% of patients. Synovial effusions are infrequent and usually small.

Avascular necrosis may occur, especially in the femoral head and less frequently in the humeral head, tibial plateau, and scaphoid naviculare. Involvement is often bilateral. High prednisone dosage, prolonged use, and pulse steroids are risk factors. The first symptom of hip involvement may be groin pain. Radiography may be negative or equivocal, but magnetic resonance imaging (MRI) is usually diagnostic. Osteoporosis is common, especially in trabecular bones, and may not be worsened by corticosteroids. Muscle weakness may represent myositis (uncommon) or be due to medications (corticosteroids, antimalarials). Myalgia is very common.

MUCOCUTANEOUS LESIONS. Photosensitivity, implying a rash after exposure to UVB light (e.g., sunlight, fluorescent light), occurs in more than 50% of patients. Some patients are also sensitive to UVA light—the clue, rash after exposure to sun filtered through glass. Fair-skinned individuals tend to be more susceptible. Photosensitivity may develop at any time or vary in intensity during the course of SLE. The classic butterfly rash, i.e., erythema over the cheeks and nose, develops after UV exposure in more than 50% of

patients. The skin may feel warm and slightly edematous. Application of alcohol, found in many sunscreens, may cause vasodilation and thereby more erythema. The rash may last for hours or days and often recurs. A maculopapular eruption with fine scaling may ensue and last longer, although it generally heals without residue.

Discoid lesions develop in 25% of patients with SLE but may also occur in the absence of any other feature of SLE. Discoid lesions are characterized by discrete round, annular, erythematous, slightly infiltrated plaques covered by a well-formed adherent scale that extends into dilated hair follicles. Follicular plugging is prominent. Lesions slowly expand with active inflammation at the periphery, and in their wake are left depressed scars, telangiectasia, and depigmentation; central scarring with atrophy is characteristic. Lesions tend to occur on the face, scalp, neck, and ears and around the shoulders. Some lesions may be hyperkeratotic and thus be confused with psoriasis. Patients with isolated discoid lupus have about a 10% chance of eventually developing SLE.

Subacute cutaneous lupus erythematosus occurs in about 10% of patients with SLE. The lesions are small, erythematous, slightly scaly papules that evolve into psoriasiform or annular forms. Lesions appear typically on the forearms and upper part of the torso; atrophy or scarring rarely develops, although telangiectasia does. A strong association is seen with HLA-DR3 and anti-Ro antibodies.

Lupus profundus/panniculitis is a rare manifestation of SLE. Typically, painful nodules develop under a skin lesion on the scalp, face, arms, chest, back, thighs, and buttocks and resolve as a depression. Ulcerations are uncommon. The presence of immune complex deposits at the dermal-epidermal junction helps distinguish these lesions from those of the Weber-Christian syndrome. Bullous lesions are rare and can be distinguished from other bullous diseases by the difference in serum antibodies and dermal immune deposits.

Hair loss, on the scalp or elsewhere, occurs in 71% of SLE patients. The most common is premature hair loss (telogen effluvium) characterized by a diffuse thinning of the scalp. Such hair loss may follow a flare of SLE, stress, pregnancy, or the use of steroids; the hair generally grows back. Some patients have "lupus hair," hair that easily fractures and is thin and unruly. Discoid lesions of the scalp usually result in permanent hair loss.

Mucous membranes are frequently affected. Discoid lesions may appear on the lip. The soft or hard palate may be involved by discoid plaques, by areas of erythema, and especially by painful ulcers. These lesions should be distinguished from lichen planus, candidiasis, aphthous stomatitis, bites, leukoplakia, and malignancy—by biopsy. Nasal ulcers have been noted in 20% of patients.

VASCULAR LESIONS. Livedo reticularis, secondary to spasm of the dermal ascending arterioles, is often seen on the forearms, legs, and even the torso. Occlusion may result in ulcers. A strong association is seen with Raynaud's phenomenon and with antiphospholipid antibodies. Telangiectases are found commonly on the face and elsewhere. They represent dilated blood vessels and *not* an active inflammatory lesion. Telangiectases appear more prominent when the patient blushes, is in a hot environment (shower), or takes a vasodilator (e.g., alcohol, calcium channel blocker). Telangiectases may also be associated with solar damage, aging, hypertension, diabetes, and other rheumatic diseases.

Raynaud's phenomenon occurs in 17 to 30% of patients. It is characterized by blanching of the nail beds, fingers, toes, and occasionally the ears, nose, and tongue. The vasospasm of small to medium-sized arteries may be induced by cold, cigarette smoke, caffeine, decongestants, stress, and other factors. After ischemia, there may be bluing and graying followed by vasodilation with warming and reddening. Gangrene is rare.

Vasculitis of post-capillary venules with neutrophil or lymphocyte accumulation develops in 20% of patients and is manifested as urticaria or purpura. When small arteries are affected, microinfarcts of the fingertips, toes, nail cuticles, forearms, or ankles may develop; the lesions about the ankle may ulcerate. The blood vessels typically have fibrinoid necrosis, thrombosis, and a variable cellular infiltrate. Patients with vasculitis have low serum complement and high serum immune complex levels and may have antiphospholipid antibodies.

Other less common vascular lesions include Janeway's spots on the palms, Osler's nodes on the fingertips, atrophie blanche lesions, and chilblain lupus (pernio) on the fingers and toes.

PULMONARY MANIFESTATIONS. Pulmonary involvement occurs in most patients and is manifested as pleurisy, coughing, dyspnea, abnormal pulmonary function tests, or chest radiographic abnormalities. Pleurisy occurs in over 50% of patients; the most common cause is chest wall pain on local pressure and/or movement. Pleuritis (inflammation of the pleura) also causes pleurisy. It is diagnosed by the presence of a pleural friction rub and/or the radiographic presence of a pleural effusion. Effusions typically have low complement and protein levels, few WBCs (the pleura has mononuclear cells), glucose levels approximating plasma levels (by contrast, they are low in rheumatoid arthritis), and LE cells. Cough usually represents an infection, but pulmonary edema secondary to cardiac or renal failure or fluid overload in a patient receiving corticosteroids should be considered.

Acute lupus pneumonitis occurs in 5 to 12% and is characterized by fever, cough (even hemoptysis), pleurisy, and dyspnea. Radiography shows diffuse acinar infiltrates, especially in the lower lobes. Subsequently, interstitial infiltrates and fibrosis may develop, with pulmonary function abnormalities. The prognosis is poor.

Pulmonary hypertension may complicate SLE but is more frequent with scleroderma or mixed connective tissue disease. Raynaud's phenomenon is common. Late findings include dyspnea, hypoxemia, restricting lung disease, and reduced CO_2 diffusing capacity.

The shrinking or vanishing lung syndrome has been described in some patients. It is believed to result from weakening and elevation of the diaphragm (lung fields are radiographically clear).

CARDIOVASCULAR MANIFESTATIONS. Pericardial effusion is observed by echocardiography in most patients, and clinical pericarditis, manifested as substernal chest pain, a pericardial rub, and electrocardiographic (ECG) changes, has been noted in up to 48% of patients. Tamponade and restrictive pericarditis are rare. The fluid has characteristics similar to SLE pleural fluids.

Myocarditis, characterized by resting tachycardia, arrhythmias, ECG non-specific ST-T wave abnormalities, and unexplained cardiomegaly with congestive heart failure, has been noted in 8 to 78% of large series.

Coronary artery disease is being recognized increasingly, particularly in patients with long-standing disease, especially those receiving chronic corticosteroids. As a result, a greater number of younger patients with angina, myocardial infarctions, and congestive heart failure are being seen. The cause of the premature atherosclerosis remains unclear, but steroid-induced lipid abnormalities, immune complex deposition along blood vessels, and hypertension may all play a role. Hypertension is common, especially with flares of nephritis, chronic renal disease, and steroid use.

Valvular disease has been noted in up to 25% of patients; most common is mitral valve prolapse. Murmurs are even more common and may represent valvular disease or be due to anemia, fever, and/or cardiomegaly. Echocardiography is very useful to detect Libman-Sacks verrucous endocarditis. Verrucae are typically near the edge of the valve. Bacterial endocarditis may develop on damaged valves.

Thrombophlebitis occurs in more than 10% of patients with SLE. It most commonly affects the lower part of the leg and is often associated with antiphospholipid antibodies and oral contraceptives. The renal veins and inferior vena cava are rarely involved, but their involvement may cause nephrotic syndrome; pulmonary embolisms are uncommon.

HEMATOLOGIC CONSIDERATIONS. Abnormalities of the formed elements of blood and the clotting and fibrinolytic systems are common. Anemia occurs in at least 50% of patients. The most common cause is chronic disease; RBCs are normochromic and normocytic, the reticulocyte count is low, and iron stores are adequate. Anemia may reflect chronic gastrointestinal blood loss secondary to the use of non-steroidal anti-inflammatory drugs (NSAIDs) and/or steroids—or secondary to excessive menstrual bleeding. Hemolytic anemia frequently occurs, and the reticulocyte count is elevated, haptoglobin levels are low, and the Coombs' test is positive. A positive Coombs' test with both immunoglobulin and complement on RBCs is associated with hemolysis, whereas a positive complement Coombs' test and no other findings rarely features hemolysis. Antibodies are usually anti-Rh and are "warm." Medications, especially immunosuppressives, may induce anemia—here, reticulocyte counts will be low and haptoglobin levels normal.

Leukopenia with a WBC count under 4500 has been noted in over 50% of patients, whereas counts under 4000 occur in only 17%. Granulocytes are affected more than lymphocytes. Leukopenia usually results from immune mechanisms (i.e., antineutrophil antibodies, immune complexes) or medications. Lymphocytopenia (which may be due to complement-fixing IgM or cold-reactive antibodies) may occur during active disease. Leukocytosis, or an excess of neutrophils, generally reflects infection or steroid use. An increase in activated T cells and a decrease in natural killer cells are noted, especially during active disease.

Thrombocytopenia with platelet counts under 150,000 per cubic millimeter has been noted in over 50% of patients, whereas counts under 50,000 have been noted in only 10%. Thrombocytopenia may reflect myeloproliferative diseases, ineffective thrombopoiesis (e.g., megaloblastic anemia), abnormal platelet distribution (e.g., splenomegaly), and abnormal immune mechanisms (antiplatelet antibodies, disseminated intravascular coagulation, and idiopathic thrombocytopenic purpura [ITP]). ITP may be the first manifestation of SLE. Most patients with both hemolytic anemia and ITP (Evans' syndrome) have SLE. In SLE-associated ITP, platelets are sensitized by IgG antibodies, which then bind to (splenic) macrophage Fc receptors with resulting phagocytosis—thrombocytopenia ensues when production fails to keep up with accelerated destruction. Platelet counts under 50,000 may rarely cause symptomatic bleeding, whereas counts under 20,000 per cubic millimeter may cause petechiae, purpura, nosebleeds, and gum bleeding.

Lymphadenopathy occurs in 50% of patients, especially during active disease. Nodes are typically small, soft, non-tender, and discrete in the neck, axillary, and inguinal areas. Biopsies may reveal follicular hyperplasia. Infection and malignancy should always be considered. When in doubt, a biopsy should be done.

Splenomegaly occurs in 10 to 20% of patients, especially during active disease and in association with lymphadenopathy. Splenomegaly does not necessarily cause hemolytic anemia but is usually associated with leukopenia. A slight increase in lymphoproliferative malignancies is observed in patients with SLE.

Antibodies to many clotting factors have been described in patients with SLE, including Factors VIII, IX, XI, XII, and XIII. These antibodies may induce bleeding. Antiphospholipid antibodies are found in about 25% of patients with SLE (see Chapter 187). They should be suspected when the patient has a prolonged partial thromboplastin time, arterial and venous thromboses, thrombocytopenia, false-positive tests for syphilis, or recurrent midtrimester miscarriages. Weaker associations have been noted with livedo reticularis, renal disease, pulmonary hypertension, and cardiac valvular disease. Some individuals with antiphospholipid antibodies do not have SLE. Antiphospholipid antibodies can be detected as a lupus anticoagulant and as anticardiolipin antibodies. Clinical risks increase with higher titers.

False-positive tests for syphilis have been noted in 25% of SLE patients and in fact may precede SLE by years. The "false" nature is confirmed when a *Treponema pallidum* immobilization test or fluorescent treponemal antibody absorption test is negative. There is no rationale for performing tests for syphilis in patients with SLE unless syphilis is suspected.

The erythrocyte sedimentation rate is elevated in most patients with SLE and is thought by some observers to correlate with clinical activity (see Chapter 282).

RENAL MANIFESTATIONS. Clinical lupus nephritis is observed in about 50% of SLE patients and is characterized by either urinary or functional (e.g., clearance) abnormalities. Also, many more patients have electron microscopic and/or immunofluorescence evidence of immune complex deposits in the glomeruli, even in the absence of light microscopic abnormalities. The presence of clinical lupus nephritis is of concern because of its potential for morbidity and mortality.

Minimal or mesangial nephritis (type II) develops in about 24% of patients. Patients may have some urinary abnormalities, the glomerular filtration rate is usually normal, complement levels may be somewhat depressed, and anti-DNA antibodies may be somewhat elevated. The prognosis is very good. Focal proliferative nephritis (type III) develops in 15% of patients; the clinical picture is similar to that of mesangial (type IIB) disease but is somewhat more severe. The prognosis is good.

Diffuse proliferative glomerulonephritis (type IV) occurs in about

Table 289–5 ■ NEUROPSYCHIATRIC MANIFESTATIONS—DIAGNOSTIC MANEUVERS

FUNCTIONAL ETIOLOGY	FUNCTIONAL OR ORGANIC	ORGANIC ETIOLOGY
Depression	Psychosis	Seizures
Hypomania/mania	Cognitive defects	Neuropathy
Anxiety	Dysesthesia	Stroke
Conversion reaction	Headache	Movement disorder
Affective disorder		Organic brain syndrome
Mood swings		Coma
Adjustment disorder		Transverse myelitis
		Meningitis
Psychiatric testing	EEG—evoked potentials	MRI
	CT	Angiography
	Brain scan	Antineuronal Ab
		Antiphospholipid Ab
		Lumbar puncture

EEG = electroencephalogram; MRI = magnetic resonance imaging; CT = computed tomography; Ab = antibody.

43% of patients. Active urinary sediment is noted, proteinuria may be marked, glomerular clearance is diminished, complement levels are significantly diminished, anti-DNA antibody and immune complex levels are elevated (especially during active nephritis), and patients are usually hypertensive. Initial creatinine levels greater than 1.2 mg/dL have a poor prognosis with regard to long-term renal function.

Membranous glomerulonephritis (type V) occurs in about 15% of patients. Proteinuria is marked with little urinary sediment; complement, anti-DNA antibody, and immune complex levels are normal; glomerular filtration is normal; lipid levels are elevated; and hypertension is a late event. Mild proteinuria has a good prognosis, but nephrotic syndrome with persistent edema and high lipid levels has a poor prognosis.

Biopsies are useful in patients with clinical nephritis to determine the pathologic type of nephritis, to detect whether active inflammation (which has the potential for reversal) is present versus fibrosis and sclerosis, and to distinguish lupus nephritis from other forms of renal disease.

Urinary tract infections are common. Azotemia (slight) may result from NSAIDs.

GASTROINTESTINAL MANIFESTATIONS. The gastrointestinal tract may be involved in 50% of patients. Up to 25% of patients have esophageal complaints, including difficulty swallowing. The lack of

Table 289–6 ■ LUPUS-INDUCING DRUGS

DEFINITE	POSSIBLE	UNLIKELY
Hydralazine	Phenytoin	Griseofulvin
Procainamide	Penicillamine	Phenylbutazone
Minocycline	Isoniazid	Oral contraceptives
	Chlorpromazine	Gold salts
	α-Methyldopa	Penicillins
	Quinidine	Hydrazine
	Sulfonamides	L-Canavanine
	Propylthiouracil	Aminosalicylic acid
	Practolol	Streptomycin
	Acebutolol	Other tetracyclines
	Lithium carbonate	Methylthiouracil
	p-Aminosalicylate	Oxyphenisatin
	Nitrofurantoin	Tolazamide
	Tartrazine	Methysergide
	Atenolol	Reserpine
	Metoprolol	Isoquinazepan
	Oxprenolol	
	Mephenytoin	
	Primidone	
	Trimethadione	
	Ethosuximide	
	Methimazole	
	Captopril	
	Chlorthalidone	
	Carbamazepine	
	Phenylethylacetylurea	

Table 289–7 ■ CLINICAL AND LABORATORY FEATURES OF DRUG-INDUCED LUPUS

CLINICAL FEATURES	SPONTANEOUS SLE (%)	DRUG-INDUCED LUPUS (%)
Age	20–40	50
Sex (F:M)	9	1
Race	All	"No blacks"
Acetylation type	Slow–fast	Slow
Onset of symptoms	Gradual	Abrupt
Constitutional symptoms (fever, malaise, myalgia)	90	50
Arthritis/arthralgia	95	95
Pleuropericarditis	50	50
Skin rash	74	10–20
Renal disease	50	5
CNS disease	75	0
Hematologic disease	Common	Unusual
Immune abnormalities		
ANA	95	95
LE cells	90	90
Anti-dsDNA	80	Rare
Anti-ssDNA	80	Common
Anti-histone	25	90
Anti-Sm	20–30	Rare
Anti-RNP	40–50	Rare
Complement	Reduced	Normal
Immune complexes	Elevated	Normal

SLE = systemic lupus erythematosus; ANA = antinuclear antibody.

radiographic abnormalities suggests stress, whereas if positive, scleroderma-overlap syndrome should be considered. In addition, dysphagia may result from hiatal hernia and gastric reflux. Dyspepsia is common, especially with stress and with NSAID and steroid use. Abdominal pain, nausea, and vomiting are also common. In the absence of peptic ulcers and adverse medication effect, a cause is rarely determined. On the other hand, one should always consider mesenteric vasculitis, which is characterized by intermittent lower abdominal pain eventually progressing to an acute abdomen. The diagnosis is usually confirmed by angiography. Pancreatitis (8% of patients) should also be considered in the presence of upper abdominal pain, nausea, and vomiting. Pancreatitis may reflect vasculitis and/or the use of steroids. Hepatomegaly is uncommon, but liver chemistry abnormalities (lactic dehydrogenase, serum glutamate pyruvate transferase) are common, especially in patients with active disease or those taking NSAIDs. Persistent liver chemistry abnormalities may suggest cirrhosis; chronic, active, or persistent hepatitis; granulomatous hepatitis; cholestasis; infection (e.g., hepatitis); or drug toxicity—and may warrant a liver biopsy.

NEUROPSYCHIATRIC MANIFESTATIONS. These symptoms occur in virtually all patients (Table 289–5). Many patients manifest anxiety and/or depression, often in response to their illness and the threat of loss of health, family, and job, disfigurement, disability, dependency, and death. Symptoms may include psychosomatic complaints such as insomnia, anorexia, constipation, myalgia, arthralgia, fatigue, palpitations, diarrhea, dizzy spells, hyperventilation, memory loss, emotional lability, confusion, decreased concentration, headaches, and cognitive defects. Frank psychosis may develop and be manifested as compulsive-obsessive behavior, phobias, and even suicide. These symptoms may also precede a diagnosis of SLE by

Table 289–8 ■ DISORDERS RESEMBLING SYSTEMIC LUPUS ERYTHEMATOSUS

COMMON	LESS COMMON
Drug-induced lupus	Polymyositis/dermatomyositis
Scleroderma	Rheumatic fever
Wegener's granulomatosis	Sarcoidosis
Cutaneous (discoid) lupus	Relapsing polychondritis
Rheumatoid arthritis	Weber-Christian disease
Chronic active hepatitis (lupoid hepatitis)	Mixed cryoglobulinemia
Vasculitis	Whipple's disease
Felty's syndrome	Familial Mediterranean fever
Juvenile (rheumatoid) arthritis	
Sjögren's syndrome	
Mixed connective tissue disease	
Fibromyalgia chronic fatigue syndrome	

Table 289–9 ■ CONDITIONS ASSOCIATED WITH ANTINUCLEAR ANTIBODIES

Lupus erythematosus
Sjögren's syndrome
Rheumatoid arthritis
Juvenile arthritis
Leprosy
Infectious mononucleosis
Scleroderma
Liver disease
Primary pulmonary fibrosis
Vasculitis
Dermatomyositis/polymyositis
Mixed connective tissue disease
Mixed cryoglobulinemia
Aging
Medications

years and leading to frustration by the patient and physician regarding the correct diagnosis. These psychological responses to illness should be differentiated from organic brain disease, which may cause the same symptoms. Most useful in discriminating functional from organic disease are tests of cognitive function and psychological tests (e.g., the Minnesota Multiphasic Personality Inventory); other tests such as MRI, electroencephalography (EEG) with evoked potentials, and antiribosomal P-protein antibody determinations may also be useful. Cerebrospinal fluid (CSF) analysis is most useful to exclude infection, although some physicians note a correlation of IL-6, elevated protein levels, and antineuronal antibodies with CNS activity.

Psychosis is said to occur in about 24% of patients. Psychosis can also be caused by renal failure (uremic encephalopathy), hypertension (with multiple cerebral infarcts), metabolic abnormalities, infection, or drugs (tranquilizers, antidepressants, narcotics, β-blockers, NSAIDs, cimetidine, antimalarials, alcohol, caffeine, benzodiazepine, and others). Steroids may cause or help clear a psychosis; clearing of a psychosis after steroid therapy suggests that the psychosis had an organic etiology. Medications may cause other problems: aseptic meningitis from azathioprine, ibuprofen, and other NSAIDs and, rarely, headaches, hallucinations, mental confusion, psychosis, seizures, and neuromyopathy from antimalarials.

Headaches are a frequent complaint and are usually due to stress and tension; migraine has been noted in 10 to 37% of patients. Other causes of headache include cold food, hangover, nitrites, monosodium glutamate, hunger, sinusitis, dental or eye disease, and malignancies.

Seizures are said to occur in 15 to 20% of patients and include grand mal, petit mal, temporal lobe, focal, and jacksonian seizures. Seizures may reflect an old scar or an acute inflammatory episode or may be due to metabolic imbalances, uremia, hypertension, infections, tumors, head trauma, or vasculopathy. When associated with other aspects of a lupus exacerbation, a CNS etiology should be suspected. CNS vasculitis is rare.

Cranial or peripheral neuropathies develop in 10 to 15% of patients. They usually occur coincident with lupus exacerbation. Cranial neuropathies include those affecting eye muscles, trigeminal neuralgia, facial weakness, and vertigo. Peripheral neuropathy is usually asymmetrical and mild and affects more than one nerve (mononeuritis multiplex).

Stroke has been noted in up to 15% of patients secondary to hemorrhage or thrombosis, antiphospholipid antibodies, hypertension, ITP, and thrombocytopenia. Less common are movement disorders (e.g., ataxia, choreoathetosis, hemiballismus) and transverse myelitis. Meningitis is not uncommon and may be due to either microorganisms or medication.

The eye is frequently involved by rash involving the eyelid, conjunctivitis, or keratoconjunctivitis. A characteristic finding is retinal "cotton wool" exudates (cytoid bodies), usually near the disk. They reflect a microangiopathy of retinal capillaries and localized microinfarction of the superficial nerve fiber layers of the retina. Whereas old textbooks cited a frequency of 10 to 25%, they are now seen only rarely.

MENSES AND PREGNANCY. Some patients think that their SLE flares with menses. Some patients have heavy menses, which may reflect antiphospholipid antibodies, the use of NSAIDs or steroids, or hormonal abnormalities. Lupus often becomes less active after menopause.

Approximately 25 to 30% of SLE pregnancies result in miscarriage; overall fetal loss approaches 35%, and patients are more likely to have a premature delivery. Increased fetal mortality is more likely (three times) to occur in the presence of major organ involvement, especially renal disease. Antiphospholipid antibodies predispose to recurrent midtrimester fetal loss. Preeclampsia is a frequent complication and is difficult to distinguish from a lupus flare.

Neonatal lupus is a rare condition characterized by typical skin lesions shortly after exposure to UV light in a nursery. The rash generally clears within months; SLE rarely develops later in life. Sera from the infants (and their mothers) have antibodies to Ro and La. The risk of neonatal lupus developing is about 1 to 5% in mothers with anti-Ro antibodies. If the mothers have other specific antibodies, hemolytic anemia or thrombocytopenia may ensue. Congenital heart block is very rare but is associated with anti-Ro, anti-La, and HLA-DR3 in the mother.

DRUG-INDUCED LUPUS. Some medications such as sulfonamides, penicillin, and oral contraceptives may exacerbate lupus. Hydralazine and procainamide can induce a lupus-like disease, especially in those who are slow acetylators and/or HLA-DR4+. Other medications may possibly induce lupus or just ANAs, but the evidence is less convincing (Table 289–6). The symptoms and serology of drug-induced lupus are quite similar to those of SLE, with notable differences (Table 289–7). Furthermore, the disease tends to be mild, is not life threatening, and is reversible. ANAs develop in between 50 and 100% of patients taking procainamide, whereas lupus develops in only 25% of those with ANAs. Therefore, the presence of a positive ANA test does not preclude continued use of these medications. The mechanism for drug-induced lupus is unknown.

DIFFERENTIAL DIAGNOSIS. SLE usually begins with the nonspecific or specific symptoms and signs listed in Table 289–4, but can also first present with easy bruising, splenomegaly, peripheral neuritis, myoendocarditis and endocarditis, interstitial pneumonitis, aseptic meningitis, or a positive Coombs' test. The presence of anemia (71%), leukopenia (56%), thrombocytopenia (11%), proteinuria, hematuria, pyuria, azotemia, hypergammaglobulinemia, immune complexes, cryoglobulins, antiphospholipid antibodies, and the Biologic False-Positive Serologic Test for Syphilis should also make one suspect SLE. On first examination, patients are often thought to have other connective tissue, rheumatic, or immune disorders (Table 289–8). Children tend to have more renal disease; older-onset patients have less rash, arthritis, and renal disease but more sicca; and males tend to have more serositis and less arthritis.

Most physicians use the American Rheumatism Association criteria for the classification of SLE (see Table 289–1) to help make a diagnosis—it should be noted that these criteria were developed for the *classification* of SLE, not for individual diagnoses. The sensitivity and specificity of these criteria are approximately 96% when compared with other rheumatic syndromes when patients

Table 289–10 ■ SYMPTOMS AND SIGNS SUGGESTING ACTIVE SYSTEMIC LUPUS ERYTHEMATOSUS

SYMPTOMS	SIGNS
Malaise	Anemia
Poor appetite	Leukopenia
Weight loss	Thrombocytopenia
Fatigue	Hematuria
Pallor	Pyuria
Abnormal menses	Proteinuria
Fever	Azotemia
Arthritis	ESR elevation
Seizures	Decreased complement (C3, C4, CH50)
Chest pain	Immune complexes
Edema	Anti-dsDNA
Hair loss	
Oliguria	
Rashes	
Mouth sores	

ESR = erythrocyte sedimentation rate.

Table 289–11 ■ **TREATMENT OF SPECIFIC PROBLEMS IN LUPUS**

Fever: NSAIDs → antimalarials → steroids
Arthralgia/myalgia: NSAIDs → acetaminophen → amitriptyline
Arthritis: NSAIDs → antimalarials → steroids (alternate day) or methotrexate
Rashes: Sunscreens → topical steroids → antimalarials → injection
Oral ulcers: Antimalarials
Raynaud's: No smoking, caffeine, decongestants → warm clothing → biofeedback → (long-acting) nifedipine → prazosin
Serositis: Indomethacin → steroids
Pulmonary: Steroids
Hypertension: Diuretics → ACE inhibitors → calcium channel blockers → β-blockers → vasodilators
Thrombocytopenia/hemolytic anemia: Steroids → IV γ-globulin → immunosuppressives → splenectomy
Renal disease: Steroids → pulse steroids → immunosuppressives
CNS disease
  Organic: Steroids → antiseizures drugs → immunosuppressives
  Functional: Antianxiety/antidepression drugs

NSAIDs = non-steroidal anti-inflammatory drugs; ACE = angiotensin-converting enzyme; CNS = central nervous system.

have four of these criteria; however, their predictive value is less. The diagnosis in patients with three criteria should be "probable" SLE, and in those with two criteria, "possible" SLE.

The ANA test is a useful screening test. If the test is negative, the patient has a 0.14% probability of having SLE. A positive test has a 15 to 35% predictive value for SLE (see Table 289–3)—see Table 289–9 for a list of other diseases associated with a positive ANA test. Low titers (i.e., 1/40 to 1/80) have less predictive value. If the ANA test is positive, it is useful to test for antibodies to double-stranded DNA and the Sm, RNP, Ro (SS-A), and La (SS-B) nuclear RNA proteins. Their sensitivity, specificity, and predictive value for SLE (as well as for some other specific ANAs) are detailed in Table 289–3.

Determining serum complement levels is also often helpful, both diagnostically and to assess lupus activity. Complement levels are rarely depressed in other rheumatic diseases. Levels of CH50 (total hemolytic complement), C4, and C3 tend to parallel or even precede activity, especially renal disease.

THERAPY. Treatment must be individualized for each patient. Not all patients require steroids; steroids have the potential of doing more harm than good. The goals for each therapy and the potential of each for benefit and risk should be considered carefully. The goal is to maintain organ function and prevent permanent organ injury. The threat of a chronic disease can be very stressful, as can visiting a physician frequently and having many laboratory tests—and waiting for the results. Thus emotional support is essential, as well as counseling and the provision of written

(and other) material. Patients should be assured that SLE is mild in most patients, that it is rarely life threatening, and that serious organ involvement can usually be prevented. Support by family, friends, and organizations such as the Lupus Foundation of America and the Arthritis Foundation is often helpful.

It is important to determine whether the symptoms and signs are due to SLE or something else (Table 289–10). For instance, fever is more likely to be due to an infection and fatigue due to lack of sleep. Low complement levels, high anti-DNA levels, and/or high immune complex levels suggest active SLE.

Preventive measures are useful. Patients should avoid using sulfonamides, penicillin, and high-estrogen birth control pills, which may exacerbate the lupus. Exercise has been demonstrated to ameliorate the fatigue associated with SLE. Patients should be questioned regarding their degree of photosensitivity; not all patients have photosensitivity, and the degree may vary, including variation over time. Photosensitive patients should use sunscreens daily with an SPF of at least 15; for those who are very photosensitive, sunscreen should be used twice daily. Photosensitizing medications (e.g., tetracyclines, psoralens) should be avoided. In postmenopausal women, estrogen is recommended for its benefit regarding osteoporosis and coronary artery disease (women with SLE are at excess risk for these conditions), unless the patient has contraindications or the SLE relapses. Immunization with flu and pneumococcal vaccines is advisable.

In treating SLE one should consider which organ is involved and to what degree ("severity"). Table 289–11 provides an outline of therapy based on organ involvement; treatment starts conservatively and, if the response is inadequate, becomes more aggressive.

Treatment of lupus nephritis (Table 289–12) should be based on whether the disease is considered active, the type of nephritis (see earlier), and the severity. The goal of treatment should be to improve, maintain, and prevent deterioration in renal function. For mesangial or focal glomerulonephritis, bed rest or a short course of prednisone (30 mg/day) will usually suffice to clear the urinary and serologic abnormalities. For diffuse proliferative glomerulonephritis, more vigorous treatment is usually given. Patients are generally treated with 1 mg/kg of prednisone. If azotemia is present (especially if the creatinine level is greater than 1.2 mg/dL), an immunosuppressive should be added, either azathioprine in doses of 50 to 200 mg/day (a dose to achieve slight leukopenia) or cyclophosphamide. Pulse steroids (1 g of IV methylprednisolone per day for 1 to 3 doses) may be useful acutely until the immunosuppressives start working (which may be 7 to 10 days). Cyclophosphamide given intravenously (in the morning) once monthly (for 6 months) and then every 3 months (for eight doses) appears to be as effective, and less toxic than the same drug given by mouth. The risks of this therapy (malignancy, infections, hair loss, infertility) should be discussed with patients. The initial dose is 0.85 g/1.7 m² body surface area. The WBC count is determined 7 to 10 days later, and the next dose is adjusted (to a maximum of 2 g/1.7 m²) to achieve

Table 289–12 ■ **TREATMENT OF RENAL LUPUS**

PATHOLOGY		SYMPTOMS	URINE	GFR	COMPLEMENT	TREATMENT	GOAL
Mesangial		0	RBC, WBC, protein	nl	± ↓	Monitor	Watch for progression
Membranous		Edema	Protein	nl	nl	Trial of prednisone immunosuppression, diuretic	Decrease proteinuria and edema
Focal	Active	0	RBC, WBC, protein	↓	↓	Prednisone	Improve renal function
	Chronic	BP ↑	Protein	↓	nl	Antihypertensive	
Proliferative							
Diffuse	Active	Edema BP	RBC, WBC, protein	↓ ↓	↓ ↓	Prednisone (pulse) Azathioprine, 50–200 mg Cyclophosphamide, 0.85–2 g/1.7 m²	Improve renal function
	Chronic	Uremia	Protein	↓ ↓	nl	Antihypertensive	Prevent deterioration of renal function
Failure		Uremia	None	0	nl	Dialysis transplant	Decrease uremia

GFR = glomerular filtration rate; RBC = red blood cell; WBC = white blood cell; nl = normal; BP = blood pressure.

a WBC count of about 4000. Acute membranous glomerulonephritis usually responds to high doses of prednisone (1 mg/kg of prednisone per day) or pulse steroids. If not, a trial of immunosuppressives should be instituted. Hypertension should be treated vigorously; angiotensin-converting enzyme inhibitors appear to help proteinuria. Diuretics are useful to control edema and hypertension. There is no evidence that plasmapheresis benefits the management of lupus nephritis. For active renal disease, patients should be monitored once a week with urinalysis, serum creatinine determination, and immune function tests (complement, anti-DNA). When the disease becomes inactive, monitoring will be less frequent, depending on the degree of residual damage—patients with nephrotic-range proteinuria or those with azotemia need to be monitored more closely.

Acute neuropsychiatric lupus should be treated aggressively and quickly in the hope of reversing the process, which usually means high doses of prednisone (1 to 2 mg/kg), as well as antipsychotics. Once the psychosis has cleared, the dosage of steroids should be tapered rapidly because patients are at high risk for infection; adding immunosuppressives, particularly cyclophosphamide, may be beneficial. Steroids themselves may induce psychosis; therefore it is important to serially monitor the patient with objective measures, including EEG, MRI, and some antibrain antibodies, as well as CSF protein. However, often one must rely on clinical judgment. Seizure disorders are treated with anticonvulsants (e.g., phenytoin, phenobarbital, carbamazepine); no evidence exists that these medications exacerbate SLE. Multiple small strokes may be due to antiphospholipid antibodies.

Treatment of the antiphospholipid antibody syndrome remains controversial. Low levels of this antibody rarely cause symptoms. Patients with high levels and no symptoms should be treated with low-dose aspirin (81 mg/day); with symptoms, chronic warfarin (Coumadin) therapy is used at a dosage to maintain an International Normalized Ratio between 3 and 4.

Patients started on prednisone therapy should receive high doses only until the inflammation has subsided—thus the patient should be assessed frequently regarding specific organ function, as well as immune status (complement, anti-DNA antibodies). For acute, severe lupus, split doses are recommended, then a switch to a daily morning dose. For long-term management, the benefit-risk issue needs to be discussed. The prednisone dosage should then be tapered, the rate depending on the severity of organ inflammation and damage, the maximum dose, and side effects from prednisone (i.e., psychological changes, insomnia, weight gain, hypertension, diabetes, peptic ulcer, infections such as acne, cushingoid features, adrenal suppression, osteonecrosis, myopathy, impaired wound and fracture healing, skin atrophy, cataracts, atherosclerosis, growth retardation). Once a dose of about 10 to 20 mg/day is achieved and the disease is "quiet," the patient can start every-other-day prednisone therapy by decreasing the dosage progressively on alternate days. Patients receiving long-term steroids should be monitored for osteoporosis and treated aggressively for it with either estrogen, calcium, vitamin D, bisphosphonates, or combinations thereof. Patients taking antimalarials should have an ophthalmologic examination every 6 months; those taking NSAIDs should be watched for gastrointestinal and renal toxicity.

PROGNOSIS. The prognosis for SLE patients in the United States has improved dramatically since the 1950s, when the survival rate was approximately 50% at 5 years; in 1994, it was approximately 90% at 10 years. The prognosis is worse for those with CNS involvement, hypertension, azotemia, and early age of onset. The major cause of death is infection. Although there is an impression of greater awareness of the disease, its clinical expression has not changed in 20 years; nor is there evidence that it is being diagnosed earlier.

Cervera R, Khamashta MA, Font J, et al: Systemic lupus erythematosus: Clinical and immunologic patterns of disease expression in a cohort of 1000 patients. Medicine (Baltimore) 72:113, 1993. *The largest cohort described in a cooperative European anthology—percentage of clinical and immunologic features.*

Hahn B, Wallace D (eds): Dubois' Lupus Erythematosus. Malvern, PA, Lea & Febiger, 1993. *An excellent source.*

Lahita RG (ed): Systemic Lupus Erythematosus. New York, Churchill Livingstone, 1992. *A comprehensive series of chapters on both mechanism and treatment arranged by organ systems.*

Schur PH (ed): The Clinical Management of Systemic Lupus Erythematosus, 2nd ed. Philadelphia, JB Lippincott, 1996. *A book for internists and generalists on practical management of SLE patients.*

290 SCLERODERMA (SYSTEMIC SCLEROSIS)

Fredrick M. Wigley

DEFINITIONS

Scleroderma (systemic sclerosis) is a chronic, systemic disease that targets the skin, lungs, heart, gastrointestinal tract, kidneys, and musculoskeletal system. The disorder is characterized by three features: (1) tissue fibrosis; (2) small blood vessel vasculopathy; (3) a specific autoimmune response associated with autoantibodies. Because thickening of the skin is the most prominent clinical feature, *scleroderma* ("hard skin") has become the most popular name for this disease. Scleroderma is classified into two major subsets, which are distinguished by the extent of skin thickening: (1) limited and (2) diffuse cutaneous scleroderma (Table 290–1). Patients with diffuse disease have widespread skin involvement, including areas proximal to the elbows or knees and/or the trunk. In limited scleroderma, the skin changes are restricted to the face, neck, and areas distal to the elbows and/or knees, sparing the trunk. The CREST syndrome (an acronym for subcutaneous calcinosis, Raynaud's phenomenon, esophageal dysfunction, sclerodactyly [scleroderma limited to the fingers] and telangiectasia) is a form of limited scleroderma that is associated with anticentromere antibodies. CREST syndrome generally follows a more benign disease course than does diffuse cutaneous disease.

Overlap syndromes, defined as features of two or more rheumatic diseases occurring in the same patient, frequently include findings suggestive of scleroderma. The most common overlap syndromes involve scleroderma with inflammatory polymyositis; Sjögren's syndrome; symmetrical polyarthritis; and lupus-like reactions. Mixed connective tissue disease (MCTD) is an overlap syndrome with features of scleroderma, polymyositis, lupus-like rashes, and rheumatoid-like polyarthritis. Patients with MCTD have a specific antibody response to ribonuclear protein (anti-U1snRNP). Either severe interstitial lung disease or isolated pulmonary hypertension may develop in these patients, which is similar to what occurs in patients with diffuse and limited scleroderma, respectively.

Table 290–1 ■ CRITERIA AND CLASSIFICATION FOR SCLERODERMA (SYSTEMIC SCLEROSIS)

Definite scleroderma. Scleroderma skin changes proximal to the metacarpophalangeal joints or metatarsophalangeal joints *OR* (2 of 3): (1) sclerodactyly (scleroderma limited to the fingers); (2) digital pitting scars or loss of finger pad; (3) bi-basilar pulmonary fibrosis

Diffuse cutaneous scleroderma. Scleroderma skin changes above the elbows or knees and/or on the trunk (abdomen or chest)

Limited cutaneous scleroderma. Scleroderma skin changes distal to the elbow, knees, and above the clavicles
  CREST syndrome. Subcutaneous calcinosis, Raynaud's phenomenon, esophageal dysfunction, sclerodactyly, and telangiectasia (3 of 5 must be present)

Overlap syndromes: Diffuse or limited scleroderma plus typical features of one or more of another connective tissue or autoimmune disease
  Mixed connective tissue disease: Features of scleroderma, systemic lupus erythematosus, polymyositis, rheumatoid arthritis, and the presence of anti-U1snRNP

Systemic sclerosis sine scleroderma. Systemic features without skin involvement

Undifferentiated connective tissue disease. Features of scleroderma but no definite clinical or laboratory findings to make a definite diagnosis

Localized scleroderma. Asymmetrical plaques of fibrotic skin without systemic disease
  Morphea. limited (single plaque); generalized (multiple plaques)
  Linear scleroderma. Longitudinal fibrotic bands
  Nodular scleroderma. Keloid-like nodules

Table 290–2 ■ CHARACTERISTICS OF SUBSETS OF SCLERODERMA

Diffuse Scleroderma
Widespread skin thickening involving distal and proximal body
Rapid onset (within 1 yr) of skin and other features following appearance of Raynaud's phenomenon
Significant visceral involvement including the heart, lungs, gastrointestinal tract, or kidneys
High scores on disability and organ damage indices secondary to extensive fibrosis of tissues
Poor prognostic signs include later age at onset, female sex, black or Native American race, absence of Raynaud's phenomenon, presence of large pericardial effusion, or tendon friction rubs
Associated with antinuclear antibodies and the absence of anticentromere antibody
Highly variable disease course but overall poorer prognosis with 10-yr survival of 40–60%

Limited Scleroderma
Limited to no skin thickening
Several year interval or slow progression of disease from the onset of Raynaud's phenomenon
Late visceral disease with unique features of isolated pulmonary hypertension and digital amputations secondary to severe ischemic vascular disease
CREST is a variant of limited scleroderma
Associated with primary biliary cirrhosis
Associated with anticentromere antibody
Relatively good prognosis with 10-yr survival of >70%

Localized scleroderma is a non-systemic skin disease that is primarily seen in children. The most common form of localized scleroderma is an isolated circular patch of thickened skin called *morphea*. Multiple morphea lesions can occur, and they occasionally coalesce, mimicking the skin changes of systemic sclerosis. Active morphea lesions present as enlarging geographic lesions with raised violaceous borders and ivory-white sclerotic centers. Infiltration of the dermis with lymphocytes and collagen deposition is seen in the morphea lesion. Some patients with morphea have antinuclear antibodies directed against histones, suggesting underlying autoimmunity. Localized scleroderma can also present as a linear streak (*linear scleroderma*) that crosses dermatomes and is associated with tracking of fibrosis from the skin into deeper tissues, including muscle and fascia. In severe cases, linear scleroderma leads to dramatic growth deformities of affected regions. Hemifacial atrophy caused by linear scleroderma has been called a *coup de sabre* ("sword stroke") lesion. Although localized scleroderma may be disfiguring and disabling, it is generally a self-limited process not associated with a systemic illness.

ETIOLOGY

Autoimmunity, genetics, hormones, and environmental factors may all play a role in the development of scleroderma. The presence of specific autoantibodies (anti-topoisomerase in the diffuse form; anticentromere in the limited form) places scleroderma separately in the family of autoimmune disorders. Furthermore, autoimmune diseases are frequently evident in the family members of scleroderma patients (e.g., systemic lupus erythematosus, rheumatoid arthritis, and Hashimoto's thyroiditis). Scleoderma-like skin changes are seen in patients with chronic graft-versus-host disease, suggesting a role for a cellular immune process in scleroderma. A genetic basis for scleroderma has been suggested, but familial clustering is rare (<2% of cases). A recent survey of 20 pairs of monozygotic twins (among whom one twin was a scleroderma proband) found 18 of 20 pairs discordant for the disease. Although no clear HLA association with scleroderma is defined, genealogy data suggest Oklahoma Choctaw Native Americans with scleroderma inherited a common haplotype, making them susceptible to the disease. Women are more likely than men to get scleroderma, as they are other autoimmune diseases, which suggests some hormonal influence. Finally, environmental factors may trigger the disease in the susceptible host. For example, silica exposure among miners has been associated with typical scleroderma. Certain chemical exposures (e.g., vinyl chloride, organic solvents) can cause scleroderma-like reactions.

INCIDENCE AND PREVALENCE

Scleroderma is a rare disease, with an incidence of approximately 20 per million population per year and a prevalence of 100 to 300 per million population. The average age at onset is between 35 and 50 years, and it is more common among women (3 to 7:1 female-to-male ratio). Although well described in the elderly, it is uncommon for the disease to become manifest before age 25 years, particularly the CREST variant. Scleroderma is found in all races and in various geographic areas. No urban to rural differences in occurrence are apparent. The prevalence of scleroderma is higher in Native Americans and it appears to be more severe in expression among both blacks and Native Americans. Females have a higher mortality rate than males; this finding has not changed over decades of follow-up.

NATURAL HISTORY

The natural history of this disease is variable, but scleroderma is typically a *chronic disease* that evolves over many months or years (Fig. 290–1). Scleroderma tends to be a monophasic disease that rarely relapses after remitting. The initial phase is active imflammation and is associated with progressive fibrosis of the skin and other organs; it lasts from several months to several years. As the disease activity remits, patients encounter a variety of complications resulting from skin and internal organ fibrosis. The degree of skin involvement predicts the subsequent course of events (Table 290–2). Patients with diffuse scleroderma (arms, legs, and trunk) have a worse prognosis than those with limited scleroderma (distal arms and legs only). Patients with limited disease have normal life expectancies, with the exception of those who develop severe isolated pulmonary hypertension (approximately 10%). In contrast to the CREST syndrome, patients with diffuse scleroderma have a rapid progression of skin disease over several months to involve the fingers, hands, arms, trunk, and legs with thickened, immobile skin. In concert with skin disease, patients with diffuse scleroderma frequently develop signs of pulmonary, musculoskeletal, gastrointestinal, cardiac, and renal dysfunction, some of which may lead to organ failure and/or death.

PATHOGENESIS

Raynaud's phenomenon (episodic color changes of the skin triggered by cold exposure or emotional stress) is a nearly universal

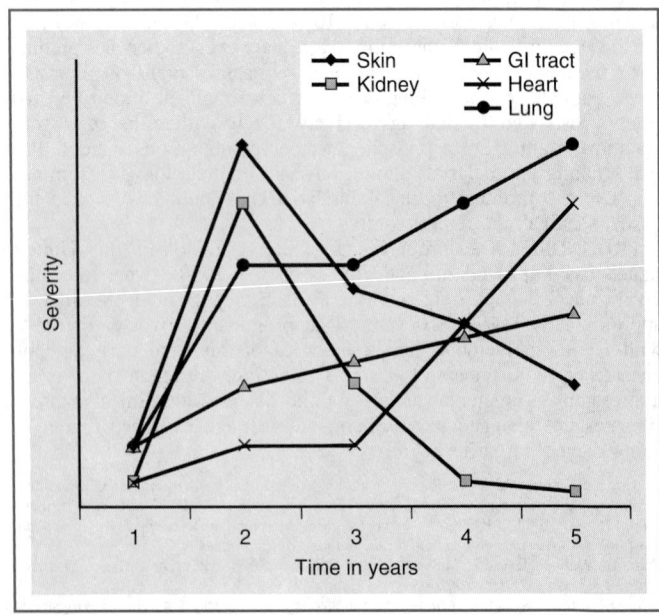

FIGURE 290–1 ■ Graphic depiction of the course of organ involvement in scleroderma. Skin, gastrointestinal tract, and lung disease are early manifestations. Serious lung and heart disease occur late as the skin improves. Kidney disease can present as a hypertensive crisis early in diffuse scleroderma.

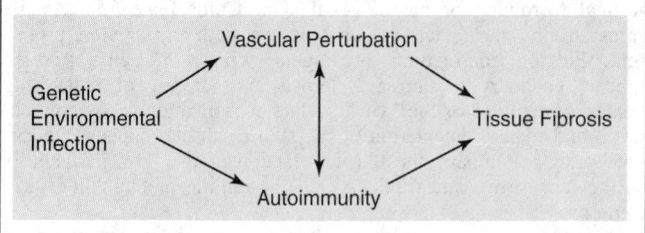

Figure 290–2 ■ Schematic diagram of the major pathophysiologic processes thought to occur in scleroderma: vascular disease with abnormal regional blood flow, autoimmunity, and tissue fibrosis.

symptom of scleroderma. Raynaud's phenomenon occurs early in the disease process, sometimes years before the diagnosis is suspected. The universality of Raynaud's phenomenon in scleroderma suggests that vascular perturbation is an early event in the pathogenesis of scleroderma (Fig. 290–2). Although the cause of this abnormality remains unknown, blood vessels in scleroderma patients are overly sensitive to cold temperatures and other sympathetic stimuli. In vitro studies of cutaneous vessels from patients with scleroderma show a 300-fold increase in α_2-adrenergic smooth muscle activity compared to normal vessels. Blood vessels in scleroderma also show evidence of endothelial cell dysfunction, including defects in the control of intravascular coagulation and platelet activation; enhanced trafficking of inflammatory cells into tissues; and increased production of inflammatory mediators (e.g., oxygen radicals and cytokines). Dysfunctional endothelium also causes an imbalance in the secretion of important vasoconstrictors (e.g., endothelin-1) or vasodilators (e.g., nitric oxide and prostacyclin). Events of ischemia-reperfusion, evidenced by the clinical occurrence of Raynaud's phenomenon, are associated with cutaneous ulcers or, on occasion, digital amputation. Digital ischemia is the most overt manifestation of widespread microvascular dysfunction affecting not only the skin, but *all* of the organs targeted in scleroderma. For example, disease of the pulmonary vessels may cause severe pulmonary hypertension and progressive right-sided heart failure. Episodic vasospasm and disease of the endomyocardial vessels of the heart causes *contraction-band necrosis,* or focal areas of fibrosis that can result in arrhythmia or cardiomyopathy. Vasospasm of the small arteries of the kidneys may be associated with severe hypertension, renal infarction, and, occasionally, renal failure. Gastrointestinal dysfunction is also thought to be secondary to small artery disease in the vessels to the esophagus and lower gastrointestinal tract coupled with neuromuscular abnormalities. Histologic examination of these organs demonstrates endothelial disruption, intimal proliferation, excessive collagen deposition, and overabundant extracellular matrix, all of which narrow the vessel lumen. This vasculopathy of small and medium arteries is fundamental in most pathologic findings in scleroderma (see Color Plate 7C).

Almost every patient with scleroderma develops a fibrotic reaction in tissue ranging from the skin to the heart. This fibrosis results from excessive production of collagen and other extracellular molecules by activated tissue fibroblasts. Excess tissue collagen causes decreased flexibility and malfunction of the affected organ. Most evidence suggests that the fibroblast is an innocent bystander, activated by profibrotic cytokines made during other biologic events. For example, cytokines made by activated T cells or other immune or inflammatory cells (e.g., macrophages, mast cells, or platelets) activate fibroblasts (see Fig. 290–2). Platelet-derived growth factor (released by activated platelets), transforming growth factor-β, and interleukin-1 are examples of profibrotic cytokines implicated in scleroderma. Endothelin-1, produced by the activated endothelium of injured blood vessels, also activates fibroblasts. Finally, fibroblasts may be activated by tissue hypoxia or oxygen radicals produced during the ischemic-reperfusion events associated with the vascular disease of scleroderma.

Scleroderma patients also have evidence of ongoing autoimmunity: namely, disease-specific autoantibodies (Table 290–3). In diffuse scleroderma, autoantibodies are directed against topoisomerase (formerly called Scl-70) as well as fibrillarin and RNA polymerases I, II, and III. In the CREST syndrome, the antibodies are directed against centromere structures (CENP A–C). The immune response

Table 290–3 ■ AUTOANTIGENS IN SCLERODERMA

Topoisomerase I (SCL-70/TOPO1). 25–40% of patients with diffuse scleroderma; Associated with severe lung disease and is seen more frequently in blacks than in whites

Centromere (ACA). 55–96% of patients with the CREST syndrome; targets CENP-B (100%) and CENP-C (50%); associated with Raynaud's phenomenon and is seen in 10% of patients with biliary cirrhosis; presence of ACA and anti-TOPO1 is mutually exclusive

Nucleolar Antigens
 RNA polymerase I, II, and III. 4–20% of patients; associated with diffuse skin disease, renal involvement, and less lung or muscle disease
 Fibrillarin (U3snRNP). 8–10% of patients; high frequency in blacks and Native Americans and associated with muscle and cardiopulmonary disease
 Th RNP (Endoribonuclease). 10% of patients with limited scleroderma
 Nor-90 (Nucleolus Organizer Protein). Rare
 PM–Scl (A Nucleolar Complex). Associated with inflammatory muscle disease in scleroderma
 Nucleolin. Rare

U1snRNP (U1 RNA and Polypeptides). Associated with the overlap syndrome mixed connective tissue disease

in scleroderma is driven by self-antigens and is T cell–dependent. T cells (both CD4 and CD8) are found in abnormal numbers in the tissue (e.g., skin, heart, lungs) of patients with scleroderma. However, it is conceivable that the autoimmune process in scleroderma is a biologic process that amplifies rather than causes the principal disease process.

Accumulating data indicate that naive autoreactive T cells are present and available to react with newly exposed self-antigens. Fragmentation of scleroderma autoantigens by reactive oxygen species (ROS) has been shown. The scleroderma autoantigens are unified by their ability to bind metals and by their unique susceptibility to fragmentation by ROS. Granzymes released by T cells also alter or cleave scleroderma autoantigens, revealing cryptic antigens and inducing an autoantibody response.

CLINICAL MANIFESTATIONS

Raynaud's Phenomenon

The diagnosis of Raynaud's phenomenon is based on clinical criteria. The patient must give a history of excessive cold sensitivity and have recurrent events of sharply demarcated pallor and/or cyanosis of the skin of the digits. Although a number of methods exist to quantitate attacks of Raynaud's phenomenon objectively, no test is considered practical or reproducible enough to replace the clinical criteria in diagnosis. Raynaud's phenomenon occurs in 5 to 15% of the general population. It is more common among females (3 to 4 : 1) and is likely to begin before age 20 years. During cold exposure (particularly during shifting temperatures and winter months) Raynaud's attacks increase in frequency and intensity. Primary Raynaud's phenomenon occurs when no disease process is associated with the events. Distinguishing primary Raynaud's from that associated with an underlying disorder is frequently challenging. Young age at onset (<30 years); symmetrical manifestation of symptoms; mild to moderate severity and no association with tissue gangrene; normal nailfold capillary examination; and a negative antinuclear antibody (ANA) titer are all indicative of primary Raynaud's phenomenon. Secondary Raynaud's phenomenon occurs in a variety of settings, including connective tissues diseases (e.g., systemic lupus erythematosus, mixed connective tissue disease, vasculitis), occupational trauma (e.g., hypothenar hammer syndrome), the use of certain drugs, disorders that alter normal flow properties of blood, and other conditions that damage vessels. The presence of intense Raynaud's attacks, especially when accompanied by skin gangrene or ulceration, warrants a thorough diagnostic evaluation for secondary causes.

In scleroderma, Raynaud's phenomenon and digital ischemia are the clinical manifestations of both fixed structural vascular disease and abnormal regulation of local blood flow. The intima of small and medium vessels proliferates with an increase collagen content, causing a loss of vessel flexibility and obliteration of its lumen

(Color Plate 7C). Despite significant structural disease, there remains sufficient vascular reserve to provide adequate blood flow and nutrition during periods of rest and in a warm ambient temperature. Digital pitting with loss of fingertip tissue and small, painful, superficial ulcerations are very common and are usually secondary to disease in the small arteries and arterioles of the skin. Large, deep ulceration of the distal finger is a consequence of larger-vessel (e.g., digital artery) occlusion associated with severe vasospasm. The latter events usually present as sharp demarcation of the distal digit with intense, localized pain secondary to ischemia. Failure to reverse these events may lead to loss of the whole digit or limb with deep tissue infarction.

The most important therapeutic intervention for Raynaud's phenomenon is the maintenance of *warmth*. A warm ambient temperature reduces the frequency and severity of Raynaud's phenomenon. All patients with Raynaud's phenomenon should understand that clothing should be layered and loose-fitting, with the goal of maintaining a warm core body temperature, not just warmth of the affected extremities. Avoidance of aggravating factors, including smoking, sympathomimetic drugs (e.g., preparations for the common cold), nonselective β-blockers (e.g., propranolol), and narcotics, is also crucial. Biofeedback alone is not helpful for Raynaud's phenomenon. Drug therapy for Raynaud's phenomenon includes oral or systemic vasodilators, antiplatelet agents, and antioxidants. The calcium-channel blockers are first-line therapy for severe Raynaud's phenomenon. Short-acting nifedipine administered three times per day reduces the severity of Raynaud's attacks and the number of ischemic digital ulcers. Sustained-release calcium-channel blockers have become popular (e.g., nifedipine, amlodipine, diltiazem) because of ease of administration and general safety. Although the calcium-channel blockers are the agents most likely to be effective, a host of other vasodilators have been used, including nitrates (topical and oral) and sympatholytic agents (e.g., prazosin, phenoxybenzamine, and others). Combinations of agents are tried in refractory cases, but this strategy is generally disappointing.

Intravenous vasodilating prostaglandins (prostaglandin E$_1$, epoprostenol, iloprost) reduce the severity and frequency of Raynaud's attacks and are most helpful during periods of sustained critical ischemia. Oral prostaglandins, nitric oxide, and inhibitors of endothelin are other experimental approaches to the problem. Patients with critical digital ischemia should be hospitalized to reduce activity, maintain warmth, and permit the rapid initiation of vasodilator therapy. Antiplatelet therapy with low-dose aspirin may be useful, but its benefit is unproven. Heparinization may be considered during acute ischemic crises of the digits, but chronic anticoagulation in scleroderma is not recommended. For refractory cases, temporary cervical or lumbar sympathectomy can reverse vasospasm. Chemical sympathectomy of the affected digit, performed by local infiltration with either lidocaine or bupivacaine, may be very effective. If temporary chemical sympathectomies prove efficacious, a surgical approach to sympathectomy may have merit. Local digital surgical sympathectomies may be more useful than proximal procedures; long-term responses to local sympathectomies have been reported. Ischemic digital lesions should be treated with topical antibiotics and daily cleansing with soap and water. Digits that progress to dry gangrene should be permitted to undergo autoamputation. Surgical amputation usually results in the loss of comparatively more viable tissue.

Skin Involvement

The most overt clinical manifestation of scleroderma, particularly in patients with diffuse disease, is cutaneous fibrosis. Cutaneous involvement with scleroderma begins with an edematous phase that is associated with an active inflammatory process. This phase persists for several weeks and is characterized by non-pitting edema of the affected limbs, erythema of the skin, and intense pruritus (Color Plate 7D). The edematous phase eventually gives way to a fibrotic stage, which may last months or years. Excessive collagen in the dermis thickens the skin, making it inflexible and causing dysfunction of skin appendages. Sweating is decreased, and hair growth on limbs ceases. In the late stages of disease, atrophy and permanent contractures develop (Color Plate 7E). Patients with diffuse cutaneous scleroderma develop masked facies, small oral apertures, and

vertical furrowing of the peri-oral skin (Color Plate 7F). As the gums atrophy and facial skin tightens, the teeth appear more prominent. Flexion contractures of fingers, wrists, and elbows often appear secondary to dermal sclerosis and atrophy of underlying tissues. Ulceration of the skin is a late complication. Hypopigmentation and hyperpigmentation of the skin ("salt-and-pepper" appearance) may accompany the fibrotic reaction of the skin, particularly on the face, arms, and trunk. A general tanning of the skin is also common.

Despite evidence of active inflammation in the edematous phase, corticosteroids are not effective. In the early active stage of diffuse scleroderma, pruritus can be the most distressing symptom. Antihistamines, analgesics, or cyclic antidepressants are often used but are not particularly effective. Topical corticosteroids can be helpful. After some weeks to months the skin becomes thickened, losing its natural lubrication secondary to damaged skin appendages. Pruritus secondary to surface drying can be improved by the use of the frequent application of topical emollients that contain lanolin or petroleum. Scratching and trauma to the skin can cause cutaneous ulcerations and secondary skin infections. Topical antibiotics and periodic cleansing with soap and water best treat traumatic ulcers. Ischemic leg ulceration occurs in a subset of patients. Conservative management with local dressing and periodic cleansing is appropriate.

Telangectasias of the skin appear as erythematous spots that blanch on pressure and are a manifestation of abnormal capillary function. Telangiectasias on the face, fingers, palms, and mucous membranes are prominent in the CREST syndrome (Color Plate 7E) and may resemble Osler-Weber-Rendu disease (hereditary hemorrhagic telangiectasia). Nailfold capillary abnormalities can be viewed using microscopy done after applying immersion oil to the skin surface. In early scleroderma, the nailfold capillaries appear enlarged. In later stages of scleroderma, the nailfold capillaries are attenuated and irregular.

Gastrointestinal Involvement

Almost every scleroderma patient will have symptoms or signs of gastrointestinal disease. Patients may complain that chewing is difficult because of decreased facial flexibility, a decreased oral aperture, or dry mucous membranes. Poor dental health may result from difficulty with routine dental care. Upper pharyngeal function is usually normal, but dysphagia resulting from esophageal disease sometimes mimics neuromuscular disease. Approximately 90% of patients will have symptoms of esophageal disease. Heartburn, regurgitation, or dysphagia for pills and solids (more than liquids) is caused by the loss of normal smooth muscle function and dysmotility of the lower two thirds of the esophagus. If untreated, gastrointestinal reflux may lead to esophagitis, bleeding, esophageal strictures, and Barrett's esophagus. The severity of symptoms may not accurately reflect the seriousness of the esophageal disease.

Barium swallows and cine-esophagograms are both sensitive tests for esophageal strictures. However, direct measurement of esophageal motility via esophageal manometry may be needed if the cause of symptoms is not clear. Direct endoscopy may be appropriate to rule out Barrett's esophagus. Most patients benefit from an aggressive antireflux program. Education about standard non-drug antireflux measures is critical. Patients often do well by eating frequent, smaller meals. Treatment of esophagitis by suppression of gastric acid with H$_2$-blockers has been disappointing in scleroderma. However, protein-pump inhibitors (e.g., omeprazole or lansoprazole) can be very effective and may need to be used long term. Acid suppression should be coupled with a prokinetic drug when symptoms of dysphagia or endoscopic findings of esophagitis are present. Metaclopramide or cisapride are more effective in early disease, but less likely to help in later, advanced esophageal dysfunction.

Delayed gastric emptying often causes early satiety, anorexia, or the sensation of bloating. Occasionally, dilatation of the gastric microvasculature gives the mucosa a "watermelon stomach" appearance on endoscopy. Laser therapy may be necessary to control bleeding from these abnormal vessels.

Bloating, abdominal distention, diarrhea, and/or constipation are common complaints caused by dysmotility of the small and large bowel. Sluggish or atonic bowel function allows bacterial overgrowth to result in serious diarrhea with malabsorption, weakness, and progressive loss of weight. Management includes the use of cyclic antibiotics and pro-kinetic drugs. Recurrent bouts of pseudo-obstruction are one of the most serious bowel problems in scleroderma. These episodes are sometimes mistaken for surgical emergencies. Pseudo-obstruction is the manifestation of profound loss of bowel muscle and bowel wall fibrosis causing regions of dysmotility. Pneumatosis cystoides intestinalis sometimes complicates scleroderma of the bowel when gas leaks into the diseased intestinal wall and tracks into the mesentery of the gut or the peritoneal cavity, mimicking a bowel perforation. Asymptomatic large-mouthed diverticula, pathognomonic of scleroderma, also result from fibrosis and atrophy of the bowel wall. Volvulus, stricture, or perforation are uncommon complications of severe bowel involvement. Incontinence of stool can result from fibrosis of both upper and lower rectal sphincters. Total parenteral nutrition may be necessary for patients who have severe scleroderma-related bowel disease without response to other medical therapy.

Pulmonary Involvement

Pulmonary disease has become one of the most difficult-to-treat end-organ manifestations of scleroderma. It is associated with significant morbidity and is now the leading cause of mortality in this disease. Lung injury in scleroderma results from one of two processes in scleroderma: (1) fibrosing alveolitis (leading to restrictive lung disease) or (2) obliterative vasculopathy of medium and small pulmonary vessels (associated in some cases with pulmonary hypertension). Both interstitial fibrosis and pulmonary vascular disease are present to some degree in most patients. However, interstitial lung disease is more characteristic of diffuse scleroderma, and isolated pulmonary hypertension is more closely associated with limited disease. Obstructive airway disease and pleural reactions are uncommon in scleroderma. Spontaneous pneumothorax, adult respiratory distress syndrome, and pulmonary hemorrhage have been reported rarely.

The most common symptom of scleroderma lung disease is dyspnea in the absence of chest pain. Nonproductive cough is a late manifestation. Active fibrosing alveolitis may be asymptomatic and undetectable by chest x-ray. Pulmonary function testing is the most sensitive method for detecting early lung dysfunction but may be normal during the early phase of active disease. Eventually, lung function testing is abnormal in more than 60% of patients. Isolated low diffusing capacity and reduced lung volume are the most common findings in early disease. A major challenge is to accurately gauge the activity of alveolitis. Activity can be defined by serial pulmonary function testing, by high-resolution computed tomography, or by analysis of cell counts from bronchoalveolar lavage (BAL) fluid. Patients with an excess percentage of neutrophils or eosinophils (>3%) on BAL tend to have worsening lung function over several months, whereas those with normal BAL findings generally do not show progressive worsening. If alveolitis is present, treatment with immunosuppressive drugs (cyclophosphamide and corticosteroids) is indicated. Uncontrolled studies suggest that daily oral cyclophosphamide (2 mg/kg) reduces the alveolitis and prevents progressive lung disease in scleroderma. The outcome of untreated alveolitis is pulmonary fibrosis, severe restrictive ventilatory defects, and ineffective gas exchange. Progressive restrictive disease occurs in 20 to 30% of patients and is more likely to occur in patients with diffuse scleroderma, those of black race, and those with antibodies to topoisomerase I (Scl-70 antibodies).

Severe isolated pulmonary hypertension (PHTN) (i.e., pulmonary hypertension in the absence of interstitial lung disease) occurs in 10% of patients with the CREST syndrome but is uncommon in diffuse scleroderma. The natural history of mild to moderate PHTN is not well defined in scleroderma. Detection of PHTN is most difficult until it has progressed to an advanced stage. Echocardiography is a sensitive and useful noninvasive method of detecting mild to moderate PHTN early. Mild PHTN can be treated with oral vasodilators. Moderate to severe PHTN (mean pulmonary artery pressure >35 mm Hg) should be managed more aggressively. Right-sided heart catheterization provides confirmation of the diagnosis and permits the measurement of pulmonary hemodynamics with and without a vasodilator challenge (e.g., adenosine, nitric oxide, or epoprostenol). Patients who respond to the challenge with a fall in pulmonary vascular resistance or pulmonary artery pressure are candidates for treatment with oral calcium-channel blockers. The dose of calcium-channel blockers in such patients should

be increased to the maximum dose tolerated. Patients who do not respond to a vasodilator challenge are candidates for continuous infusion of epoprostenol via a centrally placed intravenous line. Prognosis for patients with severe PHTN with or without fibrosis remains poor. Patients with PHTN in the setting of severe lung fibrosis are unlikely to respond to any vasodilator therapy. Lung transplantation may be necessary for patients with progressive, severe, isolated pulmonary hypertension.

Cardiac Involvement

Symptoms of cardiovascular disease in scleroderma are nonspecific and usually present as dyspnea on exertion or as congestive heart failure. Although symptoms of the cardiac involvement are often appreciated in later stages of the disease, objective noninvasive testing can demonstrate heart involvement early in the disease course. Asymptomatic pericardial effusions or clinically silent arrhythmias may be demonstrated, particularly in diffuse scleroderma. Pericardial disease is symptomatic in approximately 10% of patients, whereas pericardial disease can be demonstrated by echocardiography or at postmortem in 40 to 60% of cases. Acute pericarditis usually presents with chest pain, fever, and dyspnea. Tamponade is rare. Although pericardial disease may be present without symptoms, the presence of a large pericardial effusion is associated with poor overall prognosis.

Myocardial fibrosis can lead to a cardiomyopathy and heart failure. The fibrosis is distributed in patches of contraction band necrosis on both sides of the heart. Coronary circulation vasospasm has been demonstrated during attacks of cold-induced Raynaud's phenomenon. This suggests that myocardial fibrosis is associated with reversible vasospasm of the coronary circulation and repeated bouts of ischemia-reperfusion injury. Echocardiography demonstrates myocardial disease in approximately 50 to 70% of cases, but in most patients, cardiac dysfunction is clinically silent until late in the disease. Myocarditis associated with diffuse inflammatory polymyositis may affect the heart function in scleroderma patients.

Defects in conduction and cardiac rhythm occur as a consequence of myocardial fibrosis. Estimates of the prevalence of electrocardiographic abnormalities suggest that 50% of scleroderma patients will have some conduction defect or arrhythmia, most of which are asymptomatic. Scleroderma-related syncope is an ominous symptom of either late-stage pulmonary hypertension or an important arrhythmia. Valvular heart disease and coronary artery disease is not part of scleroderma; therefore, typical angina should make one consider atherosclerosis of the coronary vessels or another process. Atypical chest pain is usually caused by musculoskeletal problems, esophageal reflux disease, or pulmonary hypertension mimicking cardiac disease.

Renal Involvement

Before the discovery of angiotensin-converting enzyme (ACE) inhibitors, hypertensive renal crisis was the leading cause of death in scleroderma. In contrast, death or end-stage renal disease resulting from scleroderma renal crisis is now rare. Mild proteinuria or microscopic hematuria without loss of renal function or evidence of glomerular disease is the most common sign of renal disease. Approximately 10% of patients with diffuse scleroderma have a renal crisis that mimics malignant hypertension. Microangiopathic hemolytic anemia, thrombocytopenia, and rapidly progressive loss of renal function also accompany scleroderma renal crisis. Studies demonstrate high levels of renin associated with vasospasm and intrinsic renal vessel disease. Neither microscopic urinary findings nor baseline serum renin levels are predictors of a renal crisis. However, new anemia or thrombocytopenia, with or without hypertension, should alert the physician to scleroderma kidney disease. A renal crisis may be precipitated by the use of corticosteroids or situations that compromise renal blood flow (e.g., dehydration). Any hypertension in a scleroderma patient should be carefully evaluated because a renal crisis can be life-threatening. Indeed, the patients presenting with serum creatinine level of 3.0 mg/dL or greater have a poor prognosis. The key to successful therapy is early detection and rapid intervention. Most patients respond to aggressive use of ACE inhibitors, but other agents can be used to normalize the blood pressure. Some patients continue to have progressive renal failure despite control of blood pressure. Patients who progress to renal failure and dialysis can recover renal function after months of therapy. Successful renal transplantation has been done in patients with scleroderma.

Musculoskeletal Involvement

Musculoskeletal symptoms are almost always present in scleroderma and are often the initial symptom of the disease. The most common symptoms are pain, stiffness, and diffuse muscular discomfort that mimics a "flu-like" syndrome. The pain is more intense around joints, including the fingers, wrists, elbows, shoulders, knees, and ankles, yet inflammatory signs of synovitis are infrequent. A sense of weakness in the muscles of the hands, arms, and legs can be subtle or profound. On physical examination, a coarse rub can be palpated or auscultated over the wrists, knees, or ankles. These "tendon friction rubs" are secondary to fibrin deposition and fibrosis in the tissues. They occur exclusively in diffuse scleroderma and are predictive of a poor overall prognosis. Musculoskeletal symptoms in scleroderma often fail to respond to anti-inflammatory medications.

The muscle disease of scleroderma may be multifactorial. Weakness is often caused by muscle atrophy secondary to the inflexibility of fibrotic skin and lack of normal exercise. It can also occur because of malnutrition resulting from scleroderma bowel disease. Finally, muscle weakness in scleroderma may be secondary to direct muscle disease. In diffuse scleroderma, skin fibrosis can extend into the striated muscle, causing muscle atrophy and clinical weakness. More inflammatory muscle disease can follow the same course as polymyositis and other forms of idiopathic inflammatory myopathy.

Other

Dry eyes (keratoconjunctivitis sicca) and/or mucous membranes (xerostomia) occur in 25% of patients. Minor lip biopsy can demonstrate fibrosis or the lymphocytic infiltration typical of Sjögren's syndrome. The central nervous system is generally spared in scleroderma. Unilateral or bilateral trigeminal neuralgia is known to occur.

Psychosocial aspects are most important and are often overlooked. Scleroderma is a disfiguring disease that alters virtually every aspect of the patient's life. The chronic nature of the disease and the threat of death have significant psychological impact on the patient. Evidence suggests that depression in scleroderma patients is related more to the patient's personality and social support than to disease severity. Sexual performance is often affected significantly, particularly in patients with diffuse disease. Impotence in scleroderma may result from neurovascular disease.

DIAGNOSIS (WITH DIFFERENTIAL DIAGNOSIS)

The early symptoms of scleroderma, unexplained fatigue, arthralgia, myalgia, and the new onset of Raynaud's phenomenon are nonspecific and mimic other rheumatic diseases such as systemic lupus erythematosus, polymyositis, rheumatoid arthritis, and Sjögren's syndrome. Some patients ultimately diagnosed with scleroderma defy classification at the time of presentation. These patients' conditions are best classified as "undifferentiated connective tissue disease" with features of scleroderma. The presence of severe Raynaud's phenomenon with digital ulcers, nailfold capillary changes, gastrointestinal symptoms (e.g., esophageal reflux), and cutaneous changes begin to distinguish scleroderma from other rheumatic diseases.

A number of disorders mimic scleroderma. *Scleredema* is characterized by thick, indurated skin that begins on the trunk, especially over the upper back and shoulders, and can spread to arms, legs, and face. Scleredema can be a transient condition following infection or a more persistent disorder associated with insulin-dependent diabetes. Eosinophilic fasciitis (EF), also called Shulman's syndrome, can also mimic scleroderma. Eosinophilic fasciitis is more common in males and presents as a progressive stiffening of the arms, legs, and trunk. Inflammation and fibrosis within fascia create puckering of the skin and deep venous tracks (the "groove sign"). Because the inflammatory process is deep to cutaneous tissues, skin

may be pinched readily in EF, in contrast to skin involved in scleroderma. *Scleromyxedema* (papular mucinosis) closely mimics the cutaneous manifestations of scleroderma. Patients are usually between 30 and 70 years old and have an associated paraproteinemia that consists of IgG type with λ light chains. Scleroderma-like skin changes have been reported in a number of other disorders, including the carcinoid syndrome, chronic graft-versus-host disease, porphyria cutanea tarda, POEMS syndrome (*p*olyneuropathy, *o*rganomegaly, *e*ndocrinopathy, *m*onoclonal gammopathy, and *s*cleroderma-like skin changes), bleomycin exposure, Werner's syndrome, and phenylketonuria. Eosinophilia-myalgia syndrome and toxic oil syndrome are toxin-induced disorders that have scleroderma-like features.

TREATMENT

No drug or treatment has proved safe and effective in altering the underlying disease process in scleroderma. Treatment should be done during the early, inflammatory stage of the disease, before irreversible sclerosis has been established. The natural course of the disease is highly variable, and most effective therapy targets disease in specific organs. Strategy for treatment has included antifibrotic agents, anti-inflammatory drugs, immunosuppressive therapy, vascular drugs, and a variety of agents without clear mechanisms of action.

The most popular drug has been D-penicillamine, thought to work as an antifibrotic and immunosuppressive agent. A recent controlled trial of D-penicillamine found no difference between high and low doses, suggesting that D-penicillamine is not effective treatment. Low-dose weekly methotrexate has become popular for many inflammatory diseases including scleroderma. Although methotrexate may control myositis or inflammatory arthritis, evidence that it prevents or reverses sclerosis is lacking. Colchicine, potassium para-aminobenzoate, interferon, antithymocyte globulin, cyclosporin, Tacrolimus (FK-506), dimethyl sulfoxide, and corticosteroids have all been reported to be beneficial for scleroderma, but evidence of clear benefit is either lacking or a control trial negates initial enthusiasm. New agents under study include immunosuppressive therapy (e.g., cyclophosphamide), oral tolerance therapy, thalidomide, relaxin, autologous bone marrow transplantation, and long-term prostaglandin infusion. The long list of agents under study points out that no single strategy has proved satisfactory.

PROGNOSIS

The prognosis for patients with diffuse scleroderma may be improving. Estimates have suggested that the 5-year survival has improved from 60 to 70% to greater than 80%, and the 10-year survival from 40 to 50% to 60%. Patients with limited scleroderma generally have a normal survival, unless severe pulmonary hypertension is present. Patients with later age at onset, diffuse skin disease, presence of tendon friction rubs, and anti-topoisomerase antibody have a worse prognosis.

Arnett F: HLA and autoimmunity in scleroderma (systemic sclerosis). Intern Rev Immunol 12:107–128, 1995.
Casicola-Rosen L, Wigley F, Rosen A: Scleroderma autoantigens are uniquely fragmented by metal-catalyzed oxidation reactions: Implications for pathogenesis. J Exp Med 185:1–9, 1997.
Clements PJ, Furst DE (eds): Systemic Sclerosis. Baltimore, Williams & Wilkins, 1996.
Harley J, Neas B: Oklahoma Choctaw and systemic sclerosis: The founder effect and genetic susceptibility editorial. Arthritis Rheum 41:1725–1728, 1998.
Roca RP, Wigley FM, White B: Depressive symptoms associated with scleroderma. Arthritis Rheum 39:1035–1040, 1996.
Wigley FM, Flavahan NA: Raynaud's phenomenon. Rheum Dis Clin North Am 22: 765–781, 1996.

291 SJÖGREN'S SYNDROME

Marc C. Hochberg

DEFINITION. Sjögren's syndrome is a chronic immune-mediated inflammatory disorder characterized by lymphocytic infiltration of the exocrine glands, especially the lacrimal and salivary glands, associated with the clinical features of keratoconjunctivitis sicca and xerostomia. Sjögren's syndrome exists in both a primary and secondary form; the former comprises keratoconjunctivitis sicca and xerostomia with tissue confirmation of lymphocytic infiltration of the minor salivary glands, whereas the latter is either keratoconjunctivitis sicca or xerostomia occurring with a well-defined connective tissue disease, usually rheumatoid arthritis, systemic lupus erythematosus (SLE), systemic sclerosis, or polymyositis.

HISTORY. In 1933 Henrik Sjögren, a Swedish ophthalmologist, reported keratoconjunctivitis sicca with detailed histopathologic studies of the involved glands, the common occurrence of the disorder in postmenopausal women, its relationship with rheumatoid arthritis, and the ability to measure tear secretion with Schirmer's test.

EPIDEMIOLOGY. CLASSIFICATION. Numerous criteria were proposed for the classification of Sjögren's syndrome at the 1st International Conference on Sjögren's syndrome in 1986; however, none of these criteria were universally accepted. In 1993 the European Community Study Group proposed preliminary criteria to classify Sjögren's syndrome (Table 291–1); the presence of four or more of six clinical and laboratory features classifies primary Sjögren's syndrome with a sensitivity of 93.5% and a specificity of 94%. These preliminary criteria are currently undergoing validation.

PREVALENCE. The results of four small surveys suggest that between 2 and 5% of people aged 60 and older have primary Sjögren's syndrome. A large population-based study found that the prevalence of keratoconjunctivitis sicca and xerostomia, defined as symptoms and objective evidence of reduced glandular function, was 3.5 and 3.8%, respectively, whereas the prevalence of Sjögren's syndrome was less than 1%.

PATHOGENESIS AND PATHOLOGY. Sjögren's syndrome is an autoimmune disorder with a multifactorial etiology. Immunogenetic studies of patients with primary Sjögren's syndrome suggest a role for the HLA class II alleles DR3 and DQ2 and a disease-associated haplotype, DRB1*0301, DRB3*0101, DQA1*0501, DQB1*0201, in white persons, especially those with antibodies to Ro (SS-A) and La (SS-B). Although different genes may be involved in patients of other racial/ethnic groups, they share a sequence homology in the 1st hypervariable region of the DQB1 gene from positions 58 to 69.

The role of viral infection as a trigger for the development of primary Sjögren's syndrome remains controversial; candidate viruses include Epstein-Barr virus and retroviruses, including a human intracisternal A–type particle and human T-cell lymphotropic virus type 1. Increased attention has been directed to this area because a Sjögren's syndrome–like illness, diffuse infiltrative lymphocytosis syndrome, was recognized in patients infected with human immunodeficiency virus. Patients with diffuse infiltrative lymphocytosis syndrome differ from those with primary Sjögren's syndrome in that they are more likely to be male, have an absence of characteristic autoantibodies, have CD8+ rather than CD4+ T cells in biopsy specimens of lacrimal and minor salivary glands, and have an increased frequency of the HLA class II alleles DR5 and DR6 and DRB1*1102 and DRB1*1301.

Studies of biopsies of the lacrimal and minor salivary glands of patients with Sjögren's syndrome demonstrate infiltration by lymphocytes, predominantly the CD4+ subset of T cells bearing the CD45RO phenotype and expressing the $\alpha\beta$ T-cell antigen receptor, which is associated with destruction of acinar tissue and the resulting decrease in tear and saliva production, respectively. Destruction of acinar tissue may also be related to *fas*-mediated apoptosis. Based on the frequent discordance between the amount of acinar damage on biopsy and the physiologic decrease in fluid production, there appears to be a role for antisecretory cytokines produced by these T cells, particularly interferon-γ and interleukin-2 and interleukin-10. In addition, a neurogenic component is suggested by the presence of nerve fibers containing vasoactive intestinal peptide that innervate the acini and by the therapeutic efficacy of pilocarpine, which augments neural stimulation.

CLINICAL MANIFESTATIONS. The typical patient with primary Sjögren's syndrome is a perimenopausal or postmenopausal white woman; however, the disease affects both sexes and all ages and races.

OPHTHALMOLOGIC. Patients usually complain of dry eye symptoms, including burning, itching, or a foreign body (gritty, sandy) sensation; these symptoms are worse at the end of the day than on awakening. Patients may also notice blurred vision, redness of the eye, ocular discomfort, photophobia, and a mucinous discharge.

SALIVARY. Oral dryness may range in severity; many patients describe difficulty chewing and swallowing, oral soreness, changes in tasting or smelling, fissures of the tongue and lips (angular cheilitis), and an increase in dental caries. Often patients carry a bottle of water with them during the day and keep a glass of water or other liquid at their bedside at night. A helpful finding on the history is a positive "cracker test," i.e., the patient reports difficulty chewing and swallowing a packet of crackers without fluids. Bilateral parotid and submandibular gland enlargement may be present.

OTHER. Dryness may also affect other mucous membranes, including the nose, pharynx, tracheobronchial tree, and larynx; the skin; and the vulva and vagina. Involvement of pancreatic exocrine glands may lead to a decrease in pancreatic secretions and intestinal malabsorption; acute pancreatitis is rare. Dysphagia and noncardiac chest pain from gastroesophageal reflux are presumably due to decreased salivary production and, possibly, altered esophageal motility.

Joint involvement, particularly arthralgias and non-deforming arthritis, is common. Symmetrical inflammatory polyarthritis with deformity and radiographic erosions implies the existence of rheumatoid arthritis with concomitant secondary Sjögren's syndrome rather than primary disease.

Extraglandular manifestations of Sjögren's syndrome are more common in patients with primary than secondary Sjögren's syndrome, especially those with antibodies to Ro (SS-A) and La (SS-B); the spectrum of extraglandular manifestations is summarized in Table 291–2. Skin features include non-thrombocytopenic palpable purpura of the lower extremities, sometimes with leukocytoclastic vasculitis on biopsy, and photosensitive lesions indistinguishable from those of subacute cutaneous lupus erythematosus. Raynaud's phenomenon affects about one fifth of patients. Pulmonary features include lymphocytic pneumonitis, interstitial pulmonary fibrosis, and pseudolymphoma; pleurisy and pulmonary vasculitis are rare.

Table 291–1 ■ PRELIMINARY CRITERIA FOR THE CLASSIFICATION OF SJÖGREN'S SYNDROME, EUROPEAN COMMUNITY STUDY GROUP

1. Ocular symptoms: A positive response to at least one of these questions:
   a. Have you had daily, persistent, troublesome dry eyes for more than 3 months?
   b. Do you have a recurrent sensation of sand or gravel in the eyes?
   c. Do you use tear substitutes more than three times a day?
2. Oral symptoms: A positive response to at least one of these questions:
   a. Have you had a daily feeling of dry mouth for more than three months?
   b. Have you had recurrent or persistently swollen salivary glands as an adult?
   c. Do you frequently drink liquids to aid in swallowing dry foods?
3. Ocular signs: Objective evidence of ocular involvement determined on the basis of a positive result on at least one of the following tests:
   a. Schirmer's test (≤5 mm in 5 min).
   b. Rose Bengal score (≥4, according to the van Bijsterveld scoring system).
4. Histopathologic features: Focus score of 1 or more on minor salivary gland biopsy (focus defined as an agglomeration of at least 50 mononuclear cells; focus score defined as the number of foci per 4 mm² of glandular tissue).
5. Salivary gland involvement: Objective evidence of salivary gland involvement determined on the basis of a positive result on at least one of the following tests:
   a. Salivary scintigraphy
   b. Parotid sialography
   c. Unstimulated salivary flow (≤1.5 mL in 15 min)
6. Autoantibodies: Presence of at least one of the following serum autoantibodies:
   a. Antibodies to Ro (SS-A) or La (SS-B) antigens
   b. Antinuclear antibodies
   c. Rheumatoid factor

Exclusion criteria: Pre-existing lymphoma, acquired immune deficiency syndrome, sarcoidosis, or graft-versus-host disease.

Modified from Vitali C, Bombardieri S, Moutsopoulos HM, et al: Preliminary criteria for the classification of Sjögren's syndrome: Results of a prospective concerted action supported by the European Community. Arthritis Rheum 36:340, 1992.

Table 291–2 ▪ EXTRAGLANDULAR CLINICAL FEATURES IN PATIENTS WITH PRIMARY SJÖGREN'S SYNDROME

Skin and Mucous Membranes
Xerosis
Lower extremity purpura associated with hyperglobulinemia and/or leukocytoclastic vasculitis on biopsy
Photosensitive lesions indistinguishable from those of subacute cutaneous lupus erythematosus
Pulmonary
Chronic bronchitis secondary to dryness of the tracheobronchial tree
Lymphocytic interstitial pneumonitis, interstitial pulmonary fibrosis, chronic obstructive lung disease, bronchiolitis obliterans organizing pneumonia, pseudolymphoma with intrapulmonary nodules
Musculoskeletal
Polymyositis
Polyarthralgias, polyarthritis
Renal
Tubulointerstitial nephritis, type 1 renal tubular acidosis
Central Nervous System
Focal defects including multiple sclerosis, stroke
Diffuse deficits including dementia, cognitive dysfunction
Spinal cord involvement including transverse myelitis
Peripheral Nervous System
Peripheral sensorimotor neuropathy
Reticuloendothelial System
Splenomegaly
Lymphadenopathy and development of pseudolymphoma
Liver
Hepatomegaly
Primary biliary cirrhosis
Vascular
Raynaud's phenomenon
Small vessel vasculitis with either a mononuclear perivascular infiltrate or leukocytoclastic changes on biopsy
Endocrine
Hypothyroidism secondary to Hashimoto's thyroiditis
Other autoimmune endocrinopathies

Renal involvement secondary to lymphocytes infiltrating the cortex is manifested as type 1 distal renal tubular acidosis; the finding of glomerulonephritis should raise the question of coexistent SLE or cryoglobulinemia. Central nervous system involvement has been recognized over only the past decade, and its true frequency varies according to definition and referral patterns. Reported features include focal and diffuse defects, including multiple sclerosis, progressive dementia, and cognitive dysfunction, and spinal cord involvement similar to transverse myelitis. Sjögren's syndrome has also been associated with liver disease secondary to primary biliary cirrhosis and, recently, hepatitis C infection.

DIAGNOSIS. OPHTHALMOLOGIC. Keratoconjunctivitis sicca is demonstrated by decreased tear production with 5 mm or less wetting on Schirmer's test and the finding of devitalized cells and conjunctival and corneal defects with Rose Bengal staining observed during slit-lamp examination by an ophthalmologist. Other ocular tests, including measurement of tear lysozyme and lactoferrin and impression cytology, have only a limited role in routine clinical diagnosis. The main differential diagnosis for the ocular findings is blepharitis; other conditions include reduced tear production after using antihistamines, diuretics, and antidepressant medications.

ORAL. Salivary production can be evaluated by measuring unstimulated or stimulated flow rates; however, these tests lack specificity for Sjögren's syndrome because many conditions cause decreased production. Salivary gland scintigraphy, secretory sialography, ultrasound, and magnetic resonance imaging of the parotid glands, although useful for demonstrating glandular function and anatomy, have only a limited role in routine clinical practice. The major diagnostic tool is labial salivary gland biopsy; the characteristic finding is focal lymphocytic infiltration. Lymphocyte infiltration is measured semiquantitatively by the number of foci, defined as 50 or more round cells, and a score of greater than 1 focus per 4 mm² of tissue is diagnostic of Sjögren's syndrome. Biopsy is also useful in excluding other conditions that can cause xerostomia and bilateral glandular enlargement, including sarcoidosis, amyloidosis, hemochromatosis, and diffuse infiltrative lymphocytosis syndrome.

LABORATORY. Abnormalities in the complete blood count are common and include normochromic, normocytic anemia, leukopenia, and an elevated erythrocyte sedimentation rate; these abnormalities are all non-specific. Rheumatoid factor is present in half to three quarters of patients, especially with secondary Sjögren's syndrome. Antinuclear antibodies are present in over three quarters of patients, and antibodies to Ro (SS-A) and La (SS-B) are found in about one half to two thirds and one quarter to one third of patients with primary Sjögren's syndrome respectively. Other immunologic abnormalities include a polyclonal hyperglobulinemia and positive tests for cryoglobulins; these cryoglobulins may contain monoclonal IgMκ proteins. Patients with myalgias and fatigue should have thyroid function tests performed because of an increased frequency of hypothyroidism secondary to Hashimoto's thyroiditis.

TREATMENT. Treatment of dry eyes is largely symptomatic and includes artificial tears and lubricant ointments. Preservative-free artificial tears, packaged in unit-dose vials, are preferred, although they are more expensive than conventional eyedrops. Lubricant ointments should be instilled at bedtime. Occasionally, patients may require surgical punctal occlusion by an ophthalmologist to block tear drainage.

Managing the oral component of Sjögren's syndrome requires using saliva substitutes, stimulating salivary flow from functioning acinar tissue with pilocarpine hydrochloride at doses of 5 mg three times daily, treating oral candidiasis (a frequent complication of dry mouth) with nystatin or clotrimazole vaginal troches three times daily, and aggressively managing dental caries through both prevention and treatment.

Patients with arthralgias or myalgias may be treated with non-steroidal anti-inflammatory drugs and hydroxychloroquine; those with more severe extraglandular manifestations are usually treated with systemic corticosteroids. Patients with secondary Sjögren's syndrome should receive appropriate therapy for their associated connective tissue disease. Patients with lymphoma should be treated in consultation with an oncologist.

PROGNOSIS. The ophthalmologic and oral manifestations of Sjögren's syndrome are generally non-progressive. Patients with primary Sjögren's syndrome are at increased risk for lymphoproliferative disorders, including non-Hodgkin's lymphoma; the relative risk was estimated to be greater than 40, and the cumulative incidence was 2.5% in a large prospective study. Patients with splenomegaly, bilateral parotid enlargement, and a history of radiation treatment to shrink these enlarged glands were at especially high risk. The lymphomas are B cell derived, and the majority are IgMκ; recent studies have demonstrated a translocation of the *bcl*-2 t(14;18) proto-oncogene.

Young women with primary Sjögren's syndrome, especially those with antibodies to Ro (SS-A), should be counseled about the increased risk of delivering a child with neonatal SLE and congenital complete heart block; such women, when pregnant, should be monitored closely by an obstetrician expert in high-risk pregnancies.

Creamer P, Hochberg MC: Sjögren's syndrome. *In* UpToDate in Medicine. Wellesley, MA, UpToDate, 1998. *This CD-ROM includes four cards dealing with the classification and diagnosis, pathogenesis, clinical manifestations, and treatment of Sjögren's syndrome.*
Fox RI, Maruyama T: Pathogenesis and treatment of Sjögren's syndrome. Curr Opin Rheumatol 9:393, 1997. *This review article cites over 100 papers dealing with various aspects of Sjögren's syndrome.*
Manthorpe R, Jacobsson LH: Sjögren's syndrome. Baillieres Clin Rheumatol 9:483, 1995. *This chapter reviews classification criteria for Sjögren's syndrome.*
Parke AL: VIth International Symposium on Sjögren's Syndrome. J Rheumatol 24(Suppl. 50):1, 1997. *This supplement includes six keynote papers and abstracts presented at the VIth International Symposium on Sjögren's Syndrome held in October 1997.*

292 THE VASCULITIC SYNDROMES

Lanny J. Rosenwasser

Vasculitis is a clinicopathologic process characterized by inflammation and necrosis of the blood vessel wall. Associated with this inflammation may be compromise of the vessel lumen that results in ischemic changes in the tissues supplied by the vessel. Any size, location, and type of blood vessel may be involved, including large muscular arteries, medium-sized and small arteries, arterioles, capillaries, post-capillary venules, and veins. This heterogeneous category of diseases comprises unique syndromes as well as diseases with overlapping clinical and pathologic features. The vasculitis may be the primary process, or it may be a component of another underlying disease. Rarely, certain vasculitic disorders are life threatening (e.g., the hypersensitivity vasculitic syndromes in which cutaneous involvement usually predominates). Other vasculitic syndromes may be fulminant and, if untreated, rapidly fatal (e.g., Wegener's granulomatosis and polyarteritis nodosa).

The vasculitic syndromes are generally thought to result from immunopathogenic mechanisms; however, the evidence for such mechanisms varies among the different syndromes. Among these mechanisms, deposition of circulating immune complexes with subsequent vessel damage has emerged as a major immunopathologic event associated with most of the vasculitic syndromes (see Chapters 270 and 277). The presence of circulating immune complexes does not prove that the associated vasculitis is caused by them, and complexes per se need not result in vasculitis, even in diseases in which vasculitis is present.

The mechanism of tissue damage from immune complexes is thought to be similar to serum sickness. In this model, soluble immune complexes are formed in the presence of antigen excess and deposited in blood vessel walls in areas of increased vascular permeability. The increased permeability is attributed to release of vasoactive amines from platelets or mast cells under the influence of specific IgE. Following deposition of complexes, various components of complement are activated, particularly C5a, which is strongly chemotactic for neutrophils. The neutrophils infiltrate the vessel wall at the site of immune complex deposition and release intracytoplasmic enzymes such as collagenase and elastase that directly damage the vessel wall. Compromise of the lumen occurs with resulting ischemic changes.

Certain of the vasculitides are characterized by granulomatous inflammation in and around the blood vessels. Although granulomatous responses are generally of the delayed hypersensitivity type, immune complexes themselves can trigger granuloma formation and thereby produce granulomatous vasculitis. Recently it has been found that the vessel wall itself, in addition to being a target for immune complex deposition, may actively participate in inflammation in the blood vessel by locally producing cytokines that are pro-inflammatory and that will attract other inflammatory cells, including cells that are involved in cell-mediated immunity. Hence the mechanisms by which granulomatous inflammation may occur on the basis of immune complex initiation will clearly still involve the potential role of T cells, macrophages, and cytokines usually associated with delayed-type hypersensitivity.

CLASSIFICATION OF THE VASCULITIC SYNDROMES

The heterogeneity and the obvious overlap among the vasculitic syndromes have led to difficulties in classification of this group of diseases. The first report of a vasculitic syndrome was in 1866 by Kussmaul and Maier, who described the clinicopathologic features in a patient with what is now recognized as classic polyarteritis nodosa. It became evident that there were numerous vasculitic syndromes with diverse clinical and pathologic manifestations, but diagnostic criteria were controversial. More precise and accurate classification schemes now have emerged and are based on re-examination of clinical, pathologic, and immunologic features, as well as responses to certain therapeutic regimens. Table 292–1 is one such classification scheme.

The first group of vasculitides is the polyarteritis nodosa group. This syndrome is described in detail in Chapter 293. It is the prototype of the serious systemic necrotizing vasculitides and manifests features such as small and medium-sized muscular artery involvement, hypertension, visceral vessel involvement, and a noticeable lack of lung involvement. Eventually, physicians recognized a systemic vasculitis that resembled classic polyarteritis nodosa except that lung involvement was a prominent feature and the patients generally manifested eosinophilia, granulomatous reactions, and a strong allergic diathesis, usually severe asthma. Most of

Table 292–1 ■ CLINICAL SPECTRUM OF VASCULITIS

Polyarteritis Nodosa Group

Classic polyarteritis nodosa
Allergic angiitis and granulomatosis (Churg-Strauss disease)
Overlap syndrome
Hypersensitivity Vasculitis

Henoch-Schönlein purpura
Serum sickness and serum sickness–like reactions
Vasculitis associated with infectious diseases
Vasculitis associated with neoplasms
Vasculitis associated with connective tissue diseases
Vasculitis associated with other underlying diseases
Congenital deficiencies of the complement system
Granulomatous Vasculitides

Wegener's granulomatosis
Angiocentric immunoproliferative lesions (lymphomatoid granulomatosis)
Giant cell arteritides
    Cranial or temporal arteritis
    Takayasu's arteritis
Other Vasculitic Syndromes

Mucocutaneous lymph node syndrome (Kawasaki syndrome)
Behçet's disease
Vasculitis isolated to the central nervous system
Thromboangiitis obliterans (Buerger's disease)
Erythema nodosa
Erythema multiforme
Erythema elevatum diutinum
Miscellaneous vasculitides

these patients had what is now referred to as allergic angiitis and granulomatosis of the Churg-Strauss type. This disease is quite similar to classic polyarteritis nodosa except for the divergent features just mentioned. Many systemic necrotizing vasculitides manifest clinicopathologic characteristics that overlap with these two syndromes, as well as the hypersensitivity group of vasculitides (discussed below). This subgroup has been referred to as the overlap syndrome of systemic necrotizing vasculitis.

In addition to the polyarteritis nodosa group of systemic necrotizing vasculitides, certain other vasculitides are systemic and involve multiple organ systems. However, they are referred to by different names because they possess characteristic clinical and/or pathologic features. Such is true of diseases such as Wegener's granulomatosis (see Chapter 294), lymphomatoid granulomatosis, and the giant cell arteritides. In the last group, the two major subcategories—cranial or temporal arteritis (see Chapter 295) and Takayasu's arteritis—are systemic diseases involving large muscular arteries with mononuclear cell and often giant cell infiltration within the walls of the involved arteries. Despite the predisposition for certain vessels in these diseases (temporal artery in cranial arteritis and subclavian artery in Takayasu's arteritis), these diseases are systemic and involve multiple arteries. Lymphomatoid granulomatosis is generally considered in the differential diagnosis of systemic necrotizing vasculitis with lung involvement such as Wegener's granulomatosis. However, it is not, strictly speaking, an inflammatory response in vessels, but an infiltration of blood vessel walls with atypical and often neoplastic-looking lymphoid cells. Lymphomatoid granulomatosis will often evolve into a lymphoma, and it has been suggested that these cases be classified as angiocentric proliferative lesions.

Other vasculitic syndromes can be considered under the category of miscellaneous for want of a better term and include Kawasaki's disease and Behçet's disease, the major pathologic feature of which is a true vasculitis (see Chapter 298), and thromboangiitis obliterans, which is an inflammatory and occlusive disease of arteries and veins, although its true vasculitic character has been questioned. In addition to the granulomatous vasculitis of the central nervous system (CNS), which is seen in association with certain lymphoproliferative malignant neoplasms, a rare syndrome of isolated vasculitis of the CNS also occurs in the apparent absence of systemic vasculitis or other systemic disease. Finally, erythema nodosum, erythema multiforme, and erythema elevatum diutinum are dermal vasculitides in this category.

HYPERSENSITIVITY VASCULITIS

Hypersensitivity vasculitis is a term applied to a heterogeneous group of disorders that are thought to represent a hypersensitivity reaction to an antigenic stimulus such as a drug or an infectious agent—hence the word hypersensitivity. Although the antigenic stimuli associated with this group are heterogeneous, these disorders generally involve the small vessels. They can be subdivided into two basic groups. The vast majority of patients manifest involvement of the post-capillary venules and hence have a venulitis. A smaller group of patients fall into the 2nd category, in which arterioles are predominantly involved (arteriolitis). Most important, predominant and often exclusive involvement of the vessels of the skin is noted. Confusion in the literature generally resulted from grouping this category of vasculitis with the more serious systemic varieties, such as classic polyarteritis nodosa and related diseases. It is true that the hypersensitivity vasculitides may have variable degrees of organ system involvement other than the skin. However, such involvement is usually less severe than that of the typical systemic vasculitis of polyarteritis nodosa and Wegener's granulomatosis. Most frequently the skin is exclusively involved, or if other organ systems are involved, the cutaneous disease still dominates the clinical picture.

ETIOLOGY. As indicated by the terminology, the cause is usually a recognizable antigenic stimulus such as a drug, microbe, toxin, or foreign or endogenous protein. Etiologically the hypersensitivity vasculitides segregate into two distinct groups, depending on the source of the sensitizing antigen. In the classic original group, the antigen is foreign to the host. In the 2nd group the antigen is endogenous.

INCIDENCE AND PREVALENCE. It is difficult to determine an accurate incidence for the hypersensitivity group of vasculitides because of the marked heterogeneity among these diverse syndromes. However, the hypersensitivity group of vasculitides is much more common than the polyarteritis group and other syndromes such as Wegener's granulomatosis and Takayasu's arteritis. The disease can be seen at any age and in both genders; however, this characteristic varies considerably with the particular subgroup in question.

PATHOLOGY AND PATHOGENESIS. The histopathologic hallmark of the hypersensitivity vasculitides is leukocytoclastic venulitis. The term *leukocytoclasis* refers to nuclear debris derived from the neutrophils that have infiltrated in and around the involved vessels. In skin biopsies, this type of involvement is most common in the post-capillary venules just beneath the epidermis. When biopsies are obtained in the acute phase of active disease, the typical pattern of neutrophil infiltration is readily observed. In the subacute or chronic stages, biopsies often reveal mononuclear cell infiltration. In the 2nd and smaller category of hypersensitivity vasculitis, arterioles and capillaries are predominantly involved. In the typical case of hypersensitivity vasculitis with a predominance of cutaneous involvement, the lesions are usually found in the lower extremities or in dependent areas such as the sacrum in supine patients, most probably because of the increase in hydrostatic pressure within the post-capillary venules in these areas.

Although immune complex deposition is widely considered to be the pathogenic mechanism of this group of vasculitides, not every case of hypersensitivity vasculitis has had immune complexes demonstrated, even when carefully sought, as mentioned above.

CLINICAL MANIFESTATIONS. Just as the broad group is etiologically heterogeneous, so too are the clinical manifestations. However, the hallmark of the group is the predominance of cutaneous involvement. The skin lesions may appear as classic palpable purpura resulting from extravasation of erythrocytes into the tissue surrounding the involved venules. In addition, one may see macules, papules, vesicles, bullae, subcutaneous nodules, ulcers, and even recurrent or chronic urticaria.

Even though skin lesions generally dominate, various organ system involvement can be seen. Certain constellations of clinicopathologic findings define relatively distinct syndromes. For example, in Henoch-Schönlein purpura the typical syndrome consists of palpable purpura (usually over the buttocks), arthralgias, gastrointestinal symptoms, and glomerulonephritis. Henoch-Schönlein purpura is usually seen in children; however, adults of any age may be af-

fected. The disease usually remits spontaneously after 1 week. However, the disease is remarkable for its tendency to recur a number of times over weeks to months before remission is complete. The characteristic skin lesions are present in virtually all patients, with most having arthralgias involving multiple joints, but frank arthritis is rare. The gastrointestinal involvement is usually manifested as colicky abdominal pain that may mimic an "acute surgical abdomen." Patients may experience nausea, vomiting, diarrhea, constipation, and occasionally the passage of blood and mucus per rectum. In more severe and rare cases bowel intussusception may occur. Renal disease is a glomerulitis (see Chapter 106) that is usually expressed as microscopic hematuria without significant renal functional impairment. However, in rare cases, renal failure can occur. Most frequently, patients recover spontaneously and completely.

Other groups within the hypersensitivity category include serum sickness and serum sickness–like reactions. The classic manifestations are fever, urticaria, arthralgias, and lymphadenopathy occurring 7 to 10 days after primary exposure to the antigen in question, which for serum sickness is usually a heterologous serum protein and for serum sickness–like reactions is usually a drug such as penicillin. Very careful studies of serum complement levels demonstrate consumption of serum complement components C3 and C4 during the height of heterologous protein-related serum sickness. This depression of serum C3 and C4 is associated with increases in the plasma level of C3a and other products that are indicative of complement activation. These alterations in serum complement correlate with the presence of immune complexes in the serum in these models of serum sickness. In addition, cases may occasionally progress to a typical systemic necrotizing vasculitis involving multiple organ systems.

A number of disorders have vasculitis as a manifestation of an underlying primary disease. Included in these diseases are systemic lupus erythematosus (SLE), rheumatoid arthritis, mixed cryoglobulinemia, and other connective tissue diseases. In these disorders the manifestations of the underlying disease usually predominate. When vasculitis is observed, it is generally of the small vessel cutaneous type, which is virtually indistinguishable from the vasculitis seen in the hypersensitivity group with recognized exogenous antigens. However, in patients with these disorders, particularly SLE and rheumatoid arthritis, a systemic necrotizing vasculitis may also develop that closely resembles the polyarteritis nodosa group in manifestations and severity. Nevertheless, in the typical case, the cutaneous vasculitis usually dominates the clinical picture with respect to the vasculitic process.

Other diseases that may fall into this category are the vasculitis associated with congenital deficiencies of various complement components, such as Clr, Cls, and C2; erythema elevatum diutinum; hypocomplementemic vasculitis; the vasculitis associated with certain neoplasms, particularly of the lymphoid type; and the vasculitis associated with other primary disorders such as ulcerative colitis, Crohn's disease, biliary cirrhosis, and retroperitoneal fibrosis.

DIAGNOSIS. The diagnosis of hypersensitivity vasculitis rests on demonstration of vasculitis by biopsy. Since the predominant organ involved is the skin, histopathologic material is usually readily available. Because cutaneous involvement is often present in severe systemic vasculitides, one should undertake a systematic work-up of other organ systems in patients with apparently isolated cutaneous vasculitis. Recently it has been suggested that the presence of antibodies against the cytoplasm of neutrophils is supportive evidence for a diagnosis of Wegener's granulomatosis (see Chapters 294 and 285).

TREATMENT AND PROGNOSIS. Therapy for the hypersensitivity group of vasculitides has in general been unsatisfactory. Because most cases resolve spontaneously, the lack of response to therapeutic regimens is of less importance. However, in patients in whom persistent cutaneous disease or serious organ system involvement develops, several regimens have been tried with variable results. In cases in which a recognized antigenic stimulus is present, the sensitizing drugs or responsible organisms should be removed by appropriate antibiotic therapy when possible. In situations in which the disease appears to be self-limited, no specific therapy is indicated. However, when disease persists or results in organ system dysfunction, a glucocorticoid is the drug of choice. Prednisone is usually administered in doses of 1 mg/kg/day with rapid tapering when possible, in some instances directly to discontinuation or initially to an alternate-day regimen followed by ultimate discontinuation. In cases that prove refractory to corticosteroid therapy, cytotoxic agents such as cyclophosphamide have been used. The efficacy of these regimens has not yet been fully evaluated in hypersensitivity vasculitis.

The prognosis of most of these diseases is generally excellent, with spontaneous and complete remissions in most patients. However, persistent and debilitating cutaneous disease may develop in some patients, and some cases may evolve into typical systemic vasculitis with a serious prognosis.

Calabrese LH, Michel BA, Bloch DA, et al: The American College of Rheumatology 1990 criteria for the classification of hypersensitivity vasculitis. Arthritis Rheum 33: 1108, 1990. *This paper is from an issue of* Arthritis and Rheumatism *that identified the American College of Rheumatology criteria for diagnosis of vasculitis using algorithms for patient symptoms and pathologic findings.*

Cupps TR, Fauci AS: The Vasculitides. Philadelphia, WB Saunders, 1981, pp 1–21. *Comprehensive treatise on the entire spectrum of the vasculitis syndromes that discusses pathogenesis, clinicopathologic manifestations, and updated therapeutic approaches.*

Fries JF, Hunder GG, Bloch DA, et al: The American College of Rheumatology 1990 criteria for the classification of vasculitis: Summary. Arthritis Rheum 33:1135, 1990.

Hiltz RE, Cupps TR: Cutaneous vasculitis. Curr Opin Rheumatol 6:20, 1994. *Reviews in detail the various mechanisms and forms of cutaneous vasculitis and provides an interesting summary of cutaneous manifestations of hypersensitivity vasculitis.*

Lawley TJ, Bielory L, Gascon P, et al: A prospective clinical and immunologic analysis of patients with serum sickness. N Engl J Med 311:1407, 1984. *Elegant description of changes in immune complexes and serum complement levels associated with horse antithymocyte globulin–induced serum sickness.*

Lipford EH Jr, Margolick JB, Longo DL, et al: Angiocentric immunoproliferative lesions: A clinicopathologic spectrum of post-thymic T-cell proliferations. Blood 72: 1674, 1988. *Detailed description of various stages of lymphomatoid granulomatosis.*

Michel BA: Classification of vasculitis. Curr Opin Rheumatol 4:3, 1992. *Provides algorithms and overviews necessary for differential diagnosis of a number of vasculitic syndromes and gives a very concise overview of all the vasculitic syndromes.*

293 POLYARTERITIS NODOSA GROUP

Lanny J. Rosenwasser

DEFINITION. In 1866 Kussmaul and Maier described a patient with polyarteritis nodosa and introduced the term *periarteritis nodosa* to describe segmental nodules of medium-sized muscular arteries. Because swelling of the arterial walls often leads to occlusion, many of the clinical manifestations are secondary to necrosis. Hence polyarteritis nodosa is often classified as one of the systemic necrotizing vasculitides. Classic polyarteritis does not involve the lung, as do the allergic angiitis and granulomatosis of Churg-Strauss (see Chapter 292). Polyarteritis associated with hepatitis B antigenemia was described in 1970 by Gocke and colleagues. The association of hepatitis B antigen-antibody complexes and polyarteritis provides strong support for the hypothesis that the vasculitides in general are secondary to the deposition of soluble immune complexes.

Some patients have manifestations of both classic polyarteritis nodosa and the allergic angiitis and granulomatosis of Churg-Strauss. Such patients are classified in the group with the so-called overlap syndrome. Diagnosis, work-up, and management are no different from those in other patients in the polyarteritis nodosa group. Polyarteritis nodosa occurs from infancy to old age, with a peak incidence in the 5th and 6th decades of life; the male-female ratio has been estimated to be 2 to 3:1.

PATHOLOGY. The lesions of polyarteritis affect arteries of medium and small caliber, especially at bifurcations and branchings. The segmental process involves the media, with edema, fibrinous exudation, fibrinoid necrosis, and infiltration of polymorphonuclear neutrophils, and extends to the adventitia and intima. Thrombosis and infarction or hemorrhage occur at this stage. Subsequently the regions of fibrinoid necrosis are replaced by granulation tissue, and the intima proliferates. Finally, the involved segment is replaced by scar tissue with associated intimal thickening and periarterial fibrosis. These changes produce partial occlusion, thrombosis and infarction, and palpable or visible aneurysms with occasional rupture.

In allergic angiitis and granulomatosis the acute fibrinoid necrosis with cellular infiltration involves arterioles and venules as well as medium-sized muscular arteries. It is characteristic of the polyarteritis nodosa group for the vascular lesions to be in different stages of evolution, i.e., acute, subacute, and healed. In allergic angiitis and granulomatosis, the pulmonary granulomatous lesions in vascular and extravascular sites are accompanied by intense eosinophilic infiltration.

CLINICAL MANIFESTATIONS AND DIAGNOSIS. The widespread distribution of the arterial lesions produces diverse clinical manifestations that reflect the particular organ systems in which the arterial supply has been impaired. Among the early symptoms and signs of polyarteritis nodosa are fever, weight loss, and pain in viscera and/or the musculoskeletal system. Striking and specific initial signs may relate to abdominal pain, acute glomerulitis, polyneuritis on occasion, or myocardial infarction. Pulmonary manifestations, especially intractable bronchial asthma, would indicate allergic angiitis and granulomatosis rather than classic polyarteritis nodosa.

RENAL. Renal involvement in two forms, renal polyarteritis and glomerulitis, may occur separately or together. Approximately 70% of patients with polyarteritis nodosa and renal disease have renal vasculitis, whereas the other 30% have glomerulitis. Renal polyarteritis is the most common lesion seen at post-mortem examination. Manifestations of the renal involvement include intermittent proteinuria and microscopic hematuria with occasional hyaline and granular casts. The glomerulitis is manifested by microscopic and even macroscopic hematuria, proteinuria, cellular casts, and progressive renal failure. Hypertension is common. Renal involvement is the cause of death in about two thirds of patients with classic polyarteritis nodosa and about one third with allergic angiitis and granulomatosis.

GASTROINTESTINAL. Arterial lesions are commonly found in one or more abdominal viscera. The principal manifestation is pain; anorexia, nausea, and vomiting are less prominent. Impaired arterial blood supply to the bowel can produce mucosal ulceration, perforation, or infarction with melena or bloody diarrhea. Involvement of the appendix, gallbladder, or pancreas can simulate appendicitis, cholecystitis, or hemorrhagic pancreatitis. Liver involvement can range from hepatomegaly with or without jaundice to signs of extensive hepatic necrosis. Splenomegaly is uncommon. No consistent relationship has been seen between the development of necrotizing vasculitis and the appearance of liver disease in patients with hepatitis B antigenemia. Some of the combinations observed include necrotizing vasculitis as the initial clinical finding superimposed on chronic active hepatitis or appearing simultaneously with acute hepatitis.

CENTRAL AND PERIPHERAL NERVOUS SYSTEM. Central nervous system (CNS) manifestations are generally late occurrences in the course of polyarteritis nodosa, and their particular manifestation reflects the specific area of the brain that is compromised. Headache, seizures, and retinal hemorrhage and exudate occur with or without localizing signs referable to the cerebrum, cerebellum, or brain stem; meningeal irritation may occur as a result of subarachnoid hemorrhage. Multiple mononeuropathy, i.e., involvement of several or even many individual nerves at the same or different times, is common and attributed to arteritis of the vasa nervorum. The peripheral neuropathy is usually asymmetrical, with both sensory and motor distribution. The former can be extremely painful, but the latter has attendant muscular degeneration that can be so severe that it dominates the clinical picture.

ARTICULAR AND MUSCULAR. Arthralgias and myalgias are frequent in polyarteritis nodosa. Arthralgias are migratory, generally without swelling, and thought to be due to small, localized arterial lesions. Muscle pain or weakness reflects either direct involvement of the arterial supply or a peripheral neuropathy.

CARDIAC. Polyarteritis of the coronary arteries and their branches has a frequency approaching that of renal polyarteritis, and heart failure is responsible for or contributes to death in one sixth to one half of the cases. Clinical manifestations are partial or complete arterial occlusion, as modified by the superimposition of renal hypertension and an appreciable incidence of acute pericarditis without effusion. Whereas the combination of infarction and hypertension commonly leads to left-sided failure, an occasional patient with allergic angiitis and granulomatosis has predominantly right-sided decompensation.

GENITOURINARY. Involvement of the ovaries, testes, and epididymis is frequent, although usually asymptomatic. Mucosal ulceration in the bladder can occasionally precipitate gross hematuria with dysuria.

CUTANEOUS. Cutaneous involvement of some form is believed to occur in more than 25% of those affected. The acute cutaneous manifestations include polymorphic exanthemas—purpuric, urticarial, and multiform in character—and severe subcutaneous hemorrhage resulting from necrotizing arteritis, with secondary gangrene. Ulcerations and a persistent livedo reticularis are associated with the more chronic stage. A most characteristic but uncommon finding is cutaneous and subcutaneous nodules; these nodules occur at any time in the disease course. The nodules tend to group, appear in crops, are usually movable, may regress in days or persist for months, range in size from a pea to a walnut, and may cause the overlying skin to become reddened or ulcerate.

PULMONARY. Although the bronchial arteries can be involved in classic polyarteritis, only allergic angiitis and granulomatosis involving the pulmonary arteries and parenchyma with granulomatous lesions give rise to clinical manifestations. Asthma, when present, is intractable and associated with marked peripheral eosinophilia. Pneumonic episodes are transient or progressive and may be accompanied by hemoptysis and/or pleuritic pain. Respiratory involvement accounts for about 50% of deaths, with the remainder being attributable to arteritis in other organs.

COURSE WHEN UNTREATED. The course of polyarteritis nodosa is progressive, with destruction of vital organs. Intermittent acute episodes resulting from thrombosis of vital or non-vital structures are prominent. Death is most frequently attributed to renal involvement in cases of classic polyarteritis nodosa and to pulmonary lesions in cases classified as allergic angiitis with granulomatosis. Cardiac failure caused by a combination of infarction and renal hypertension is an additional frequent cause of death in both groups, and acute vascular accidents of the gastrointestinal tract or CNS account for much of the remaining mortality. In the retrospective post-mortem study of Rose and Spencer, the 5-year survival rate was about 10% in classic polyarteritis nodosa and about 25% in allergic angiitis and granulomatosis if onset was dated from the start of respiratory symptoms. The report of the British Medical Research Council in 1960 placed the 54-month survival rate in polyarteritis nodosa at nearly 50%. Rare patients with polyarteritis limited to non-vital sites have been reported to experience an unusually long course or even a lasting remission.

LABORATORY FINDINGS. Leukocytosis, predominantly polymorphonuclear, is apparent in more than 75% of cases of polyarteritis nodosa or allergic angiitis and granulomatosis, eosinophilia often being marked in the latter group. Hypocomplementemia, which has not been observed in classic polyarteritis nodosa, has been present in patients with hepatitis B antigenemia. The erythrocyte sedimentation rate is customarily elevated. Abnormalities in the urine sediment, especially hematuria and proteinuria, reflect renal involvement. Abnormalities of the electrocardiogram and electroencephalogram are those common to arterial occlusive disease or secondary to the metabolic disturbances of uremia. Lesions apparent on chest radiographs are the rule in patients with allergic angiitis and granulomatosis. The findings range from transient or progressive infiltration to consolidation, cavitation, or scarring; upper and lower lobes are involved with equal frequency. Inasmuch as none of these findings are specific, antemortem diagnosis of polyarteritis depends on biopsy. Because the arterial involvement is segmental and spotty in distribution, it is advisable to obtain tissue from a symptomatic site, and it is essential to section the entire specimen completely. A deep, open surgical biopsy sample, including subcutaneous tissue and underlying muscle, should be obtained whenever possible from a skeletal muscle exhibiting pain and tenderness. Involvement of the epididymis and testes is sufficiently common to make this a useful biopsy site if palpation reveals the typical nodularity of segmental vascular lesions. Needle and surgical biopsies of internal organs with clinical involvement, such as the liver or kidney, are gaining in favor. As an alternative or

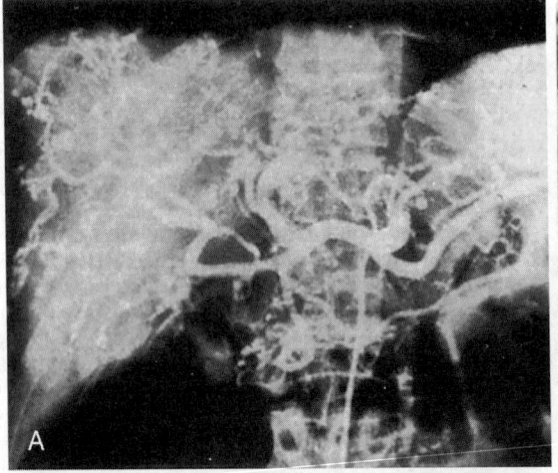
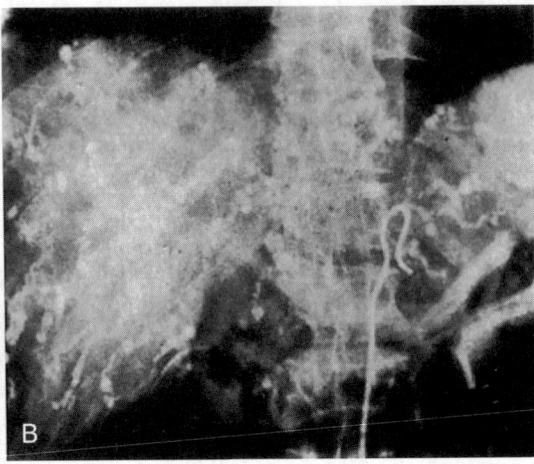
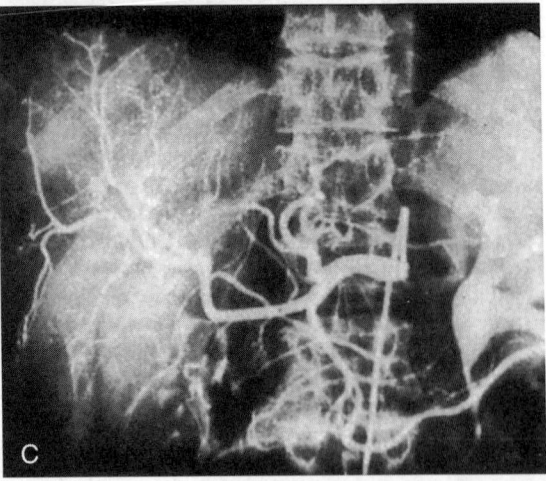

FIGURE 293–1 ■ A selective celiac arteriogram demonstrates large hepatic arteries *(A)* and multiple aneurysms *(A and B)* throughout the liver. Resolution of the aneurysms is seen after therapy *(C)*. (From Fauci AS, Doppman JL, Wolff SM: Cyclophosphamide-induced remissions in advanced polyarteritis nodosa. Am J Med 64:891, 1978.)

additional procedure, angiography to detect aneurysms of medium-sized muscular arteries in renal, hepatic, or intestinal sites may be helpful.

DIFFERENTIAL DIAGNOSIS. The differential diagnosis includes not only the constituent syndromes but also all conditions associated with systemic necrotizing vasculitis. The key differences between classic polyarteritis nodosa and other causes of necrotizing vasculitis include the absence of extravascular granulomas, sparing of the pulmonary arteries, failure of venous involvement except by contiguous spread, and predilection for medium-sized arteries. For allergic angiitis and granulomatosis, the striking granulomatous response excludes all but Wegener's granulomatosis. The prominence of bronchial asthma and peripheral eosinophilia and the usual absence of necrotizing lesions in the upper respiratory tract permit tentative clinical distinction between allergic angiitis with granulomatosis and Wegener's granulomatosis. Recently, an association with allergic angiitis and granulomatosis was described in patients receiving the leukotriene receptor antagonist zafirlukast. Whether this association is due to unmasking of vasculitis as steroid therapy is withdrawn in moderately severe asthma or due to intrinsic pathogenetic effects of the drug is not yet clear. Underlying connective tissue diseases are still recognized by their clinical characteristics even when necrotizing arteritis becomes prominent. For example, patients with rheumatoid arthritis with ulcerating cutaneous lesions and peripheral neuropathy often exhibit prominent rheumatoid nodules and a high titer of rheumatoid factor. The specificities of the immunoglobulins that accompany active systemic lupus erythematosus or mixed cryoglobulinemia are distinctive; in addition, in the presence of active renal disease both entities manifest a reduced serum complement level not generally observed in classic polyarteritis nodosa. The giant cell arteritides (i.e., temporal arteritis, Takayasu's arteritis) lack the glomerulitis, peripheral neuropathy, and cutaneous manifestations notable in polyarteritis nodosa. The combination of progressive nephritis and pulmonary hemorrhage seen in Goodpasture's syndrome is unlike polyarteritis nodosa. The drug-induced hypersensitivity vasculitis group may be difficult to separate on purely clinical grounds, although a history of antecedent drug administration, infrequency of gastrointestinal manifestations, and absence of nodules along arteries are useful points. The clinical findings in Henoch-Schönlein purpura are distinctive.

TREATMENT. The commonly used non-steroidal anti-inflammatory agents have no specific therapeutic role in polyarteritis nodosa; thus corticosteroids have been used most widely. Large doses, in the range of 40 to 60 mg of prednisone per day, afford symptomatic relief but probably have little effect on 1-year survival statistics. In a series of 17 patients within the polyarteritis group, including 2 with allergic angiitis and granulomatosis and 6 with hepatitis B–associated polyarteritis, 14 experienced dramatic remission with 2 mg/kg/day of cyclophosphamide. It was subsequently possible to reduce the cyclophosphamide and taper the steroid dose to every other day and yet maintain remission, and in some instances resolution of microaneurysms was noted on repeat celiac axis angiography (Fig. 293–1).

In patients who have polyarteritis nodosa associated with hepatitis B virus infection, recent reports from a European collaborative group have identified significant responses to treatment regimens that include the cytokine interferon-α2b and plasma exchange. When these approaches are taken in conjunction with short-term steroid therapy and potential antiviral treatment with vidarabine (Vira-A), a significant number of patients had long-term remission and seroconversion in terms of hepatitis. Obviously, initial interest in treating this subgroup of polyarteritis nodosa patients, those who have documented hepatitis B virus infection, with alternative treatments to cytotoxic drugs and steroids is promising.

Fauci AS, Katz P, Haynes BF, et al: Cyclophosphamide therapy of severe systemic necrotizing vasculitis. N Engl J Med 301:235, 1979. *Most important contribution dealing with cyclophosphamide therapy effectiveness in management of a series of patients within the polyarteritis group and including such subgroups as allergic angiitis and granulomatosis and hepatitis B–associated polyangiitis.*

Guillevin L, Lhote F, Leon A. et al: Treatment of polyarteritis nodosa related to hepatitis B virus with short term steroid therapy associated with antiviral agents and plasma exchanges. A prospective trial in 33 patients. J Rheumatol 20:289, 1993.

Guillevin L, Lhote F, Sauvaget F, et al: Treatment of polyarteritis nodosa related to hepatitis B virus with interferon-alpha and plasma exchanges. Ann Rheum Dis 53:334, 1994. *This and the preceding report prospectively identify the response of patients with interferon-α2b and plasma exchange. The data in these two trial suggest that cytokine and antiviral therapy as well as plasmapheresis may have a*

role as a potential 1st line treatment in proven virus-induced vasculitis and polyarteritis nodosa.

Wechsler ME, Garpestad E, Flier SR, et al: Pulmonary infiltrates, eosinophilia, and cardiomyopathy following corticosteroid withdrawal in patients with asthma receiving zafirlukast. JAMA 279:455, 1998. *This report highlights the association of allergic angiitis and granulomatosis with institution of the leukotriene receptor antagonist zafirlukast in moderately severe asthma requiring steroid therapy. Whether the pathogenesis is due to a reduction in steroid dose unmasking vasculitis or due to pathogenetic effects of the drug are as yet unknown.*

294 WEGENER'S GRANULOMATOSIS

Nancy B. Allen

Wegener's granulomatosis falls within the spectrum of systemic vasculitides as a clinicopathologic syndrome involving the upper and lower respiratory tract and kidneys and less commonly the eyes, joints, skin, and neurologic and cardiac tissue. Described in 1931 and 1936 by H. Klinger and F. Wegener, respectively, necrotizing granulomatous vasculitis is the hallmark disorder in the lower respiratory tract, and focal segmental glomerulonephritis and small vessel or granulomatous vasculitis are found elsewhere. The disease is now known to be associated with the cytoplasmic pattern of antineutrophil cytoplasmic antibody (c-ANCA) and more specifically with antibodies against proteinase 3 (PR-3), a serine protease found in neutrophils.

ETIOLOGY. The cause of Wegener's granulomatosis is not yet known, but much research is being done. Because of the almost universal upper and/or lower airway involvement, inhaled antigen(s) stimulating granuloma formation and altered immune reactivity with features of immune complex deposition and altered cellular immune responses are believed to play significant roles, along with host factors and/or genetic predisposition. As of this writing, no single genetic marker, environmental agent, microorganism, or other factor can be identified as initiating this syndrome. Rare familial reports of Wegener's granulomatosis in 1st degree relatives exist.

INCIDENCE AND PREVALENCE. The demographics of Wegener's granulomatosis may be changing with the presence of new laboratory markers (c-ANCA), enhanced education of physicians regarding this diagnosis, and expansion of the spectrum of clinical features and manifestations. In the United States the disease frequency is approximately 1 in 30,000. In recent studies the mean age of onset is approximately 40, equal in men and women, predominant in white individuals, and occurring from childhood into older adulthood.

PATHOLOGY AND PATHOGENESIS. The classic histopathology in Wegener's granulomatosis is necrotizing granulomatous vasculitis involving small arteries and veins, most reliably found on biopsies of the lung (Table 294–1). This typical pathology has been seen in many other tissues, including unusual clinical locations such as muscle, prostate, and breast. Upper respiratory tract biopsies, including the nasal septum, sinus, and trachea, most often show non-specific acute and chronic inflammation with or without giant cells and generally without true vasculitis.

Renal biopsies typically show focal segmental glomerulonephritis, with crescent formation and necrosis in more severe forms. Generally, immunofluorescent staining yields pauci-immune deposits, but these findings are not specific to Wegener's granulomatosis because they can be seen in polyarteritis nodosa, other vasculitides, and some non-vasculitic conditions. Biopsy does help exclude other conditions such as systemic lupus erythematosus (SLE), post-streptococcal disease, Goodpasture's syndrome, and cryoglobulinemia.

In the initial phase of Wegener's granulomatosis, bronchoalveolar lavage shows neutrophilic alveolitis, phagocytosis of neutrophils by monocytes, and higher levels of c-ANCA in lavage fluid than in serum. A current theory about the pathogenesis of Wegener's granulomatosis involves a stimulus (inhalant) of some type, activation of neutrophils, transfer of PR-3 to the cell membrane, and in-

Table 294–1 ■ PATHOLOGIC FINDINGS IN WEGENER'S GRANULOMATOSIS

LOCATION	PATHOLOGY
Upper airways (sinus, nasal septum)	Acute and chronic inflammation, giant cells, necrotizing granulomas, rarely vasculitis
Lung	
Transbronchial	Acute and chronic inflammation, giant cells, granuloma, rarely vasculitis
Thorascopic or open	Necrotizing granulomatous vasculitis* (negative special stains and cultures), eosinophils, hemosiderin-laden macrophages, capillaritis
Kidney	Focal segmental glomerulonephritis with or without crescent formation, pauci-immune deposits, rarely vasculitis (<1%)
Orbital/ocular	Acute and chronic inflammation with or without granuloma and/or vasculitis
Skin	Leukocytoclastic vasculitis, occasionally granulomatous vasculitis with or without necrosis
Sural nerve/muscle	Acute axonopathy, denervation and/or renervation, occasionally vasculitis of vasa nervorum, myopathy with or without inflammation
Liver/spleen	Granulomatous hepatitis, triaditis, granulomatous vasculitis in the spleen
Cardiac	Pericardial inflammation; rarely true coronary arteritis or granulomatous inflammation in the myocardium or conduction system

*"Diagnostic" pathologic triad in Wegener's granulomatosis.

creased levels of c-ANCA, rheumatoid factor, γ-globulins, and circulating immune complexes. Both cellular and humoral immune factors then lead to vasculitis, tissue destruction, and granuloma formation, which contribute to the clinical features of the disease.

CLINICAL MANIFESTATIONS. The spectrum of clinical features and organ system involvement in Wegener's granulomatosis is broad (Table 294–2). As a multisystem disorder predominantly involving the upper and lower respiratory tracts and the kidneys, clinical manifestations vary from "classic," with sinusitis, serous otitis media, rhinitis with nasal ulcerations, cough, hemoptysis, and constitutional symptoms, to "fulminant," with rapidly progressive renal failure and respiratory failure requiring intensive care unit management, to "mild," with arthralgias, polymyalgia rheumatica–type symptoms, or inflammatory eye disease as examples. Astute clinicians must carry Wegener's granulomatosis as a potential diagnosis in their differential diagnosis list for multisystem disease or unexplained illness, much as one keeps SLE or subacute bacterial endocarditis in mind. With greater understanding of the systemic vasculitic syndromes and education of primary care providers, this diagnosis may be considered in more individuals than previously and thereby lead to earlier diagnosis and selection of appropriate management.

Nearly three fourths of patients in whom Wegener's granulomatosis is eventually diagnosed initially seek help because of upper and/or lower respiratory complaints. These complaints include seasonal allergic rhinitis symptoms, recurrent epistaxis, oral or nasal ulcerations, ear pain, cough, fever, or hearing abnormalities. Some patients experience months or years of these symptoms before diagnosis. Constitutional symptoms with fever, weight loss, anorexia, fatigue, arthralgias, and myalgias, although non-specific, are common in this condition.

Lung involvement may be symptomatic, with cough, dyspnea, pleuritic chest pain, and hemoptysis, or may be totally asymptomatic, with abnormalities found only on chest radiographs. Fleeting or persistent pulmonary infiltrates are more commonly found in the upper lobes and may be due to pulmonary hemorrhage or granulomatous inflammation along with vasculitis. Solitary or multiple pulmonary nodules and, less commonly, bibasilar interstitial changes may be seen. Some patients with lower respiratory symptoms but normal chest radiographs may have endobronchial lesions found only at bronchoscopy.

Renal involvement is certainly one of the most serious clinical aspects of Wegener's granulomatosis. The involvement may be asymptomatic such that urinalysis and serum creatinine measurements are important and must be monitored closely in patients suspected to have Wegener's granulomatosis. Rapidly progressive renal insufficiency with or without hypertension, edema, and nephrotic syndrome requires prompt evaluation and management. Irreversible renal failure requiring dialysis may be part of the initial clinical findings or may slowly develop during therapy or with recurrent disease.

Musculoskeletal manifestations occur in the majority of patients. Observations have included diffuse polyarthralgias, an arthritis ranging from monarticular to oligoarticular, and a rheumatoid arthritis–like picture with polyarthritis involving the wrists, metacarpophalangeal and proximal interphalangeal joints, knees, ankles, and other large or small joints. When rheumatoid factor occurs along with symmetrical polyarthritis, the initial diagnosis may be rheumatoid arthritis; however, attention to extra-articular symptoms and/or signs and laboratory data may lead to a diagnosis of Wegener's granulomatosis instead. Diffuse myalgias are often present, and in patients older than 50 years, a polymyalgia rheumatica–type onset of Wegener's granulomatosis and/or overlap of Wegener's granulomatosis and temporal arteritis has been described. True myositis, with creatine phosphokinase, aldolase, or aminotransferase elevations, proximal muscle weakness, and findings of granulomatous vasculitis or less specific myositis, has been observed in Wegener's granulomatosis.

Ocular involvement occurs in one half to two thirds of patients with Wegener's granulomatosis on the basis of either vasculitis or tracking granulomatous tissue through the lamina papyracea into the medial aspect of the orbit. Vasculitis is responsible for conjunctivitis, scleritis-episcleritis, uveitis, retinal vasculitis, and corneoscleral ulceration. Granulomatous mass lesions contribute to proptosis, orbital masses, optic nerve compression, diplopia, and nasal lacrimal duct obstruction.

Cutaneous involvement is most typically seen as palpable purpura, predominantly in the lower extremities, but it may occur in the upper extremities and over bony prominences. Vesicles, verru-

Table 294–2 ■ CLINICAL MANIFESTATIONS OF WEGENER'S GRANULOMATOSIS

REGION/ORGAN	SIGN OR SYMPTOM
Upper airway (90–95%)	Sinusitis, serous otitis media, rhinitis, nasal ulcerations/septal perforation, epistaxis, oral ulcerations, saddle nose deformity (later), headaches
Lower airway (90–95%)	Cough, dyspnea, hemoptysis, pulmonary infiltrates (may be fleeting or persistent), nodules, cavities, pleural effusions/pleuritis, subglottic stenosis, endobronchial lesions, interstitial lung disease
Kidneys (75%)	Urinary sediment abnormalities (microscopic hematuria, casts, proteinuria), with or without renal insufficiency, nephrotic syndrome, hypertension
Musculoskeletal (70–90%)	Polyarthralgias, myalgias, mono-, oligo-, or polyarthritis (may be in a rheumatoid pattern), myositis, muscle weakness
Eye (50–65%)	Conjunctivitis, scleritis/episcleritis, uveitis, proptosis, nasolacrimal duct obstruction, orbital mass lesions, retinal vasculitis, corneoscleral ulceration
Skin (50%)	Palpable purpura, subcutaneous nodules, petechiae, vesicles, ulcers, Raynaud's phenomenon, digital ischemia, livedo reticularis, necrotic papules, pyoderma gangrenosum–type lesions (rare)
Neurologic (20–25%)	Mononeuritis multiplex, peripheral neuropathy, cranial neuropathy, central nervous system vasculitis (cerebral hemorrhage, cerebritis, syncope, diabetes insipidis)
Cardiac (20%)	Pericarditis, pancarditis, cardiomyopathy, arrhythmias, coronary arteritis
Gastrointestinal (15–30%)	Alkaline phosphatase and/or aminotransferase elevations, granulomatous hepatitis/triaditis, small bowel vasculitis, ascites, splenic granulomatous vasculitis
Miscellaneous (<1–5%)	Involvement of the breast, prostate, testicle, pinnae, urethra, ureter, lymph nodes, parotid, pulmonary or temporal artery, vagina, other
Constitutional	Fatigue, weight loss, fever, malaise, anorexia

cous/necrotic papular lesions, subcutaneous nodules, petechiae, and more severe pyoderma gangrenosum–type lesions have been described. Raynaud's phenomenon, digital ischemia/necrosis, and livedo reticularis are present in some patients with acute and fulminant disease, with small vessel vasculitis with or without vasospasm being the predominant cause. Biopsy of the skin most commonly shows leukocytoclastic vasculitis.

Neurologic involvement is most typical with mononeuritis multiplex and footdrop and/or wristdrop, with patchy sensory and/or motor abnormalities. A diffuse peripheral neuropathy and cranial neuropathy, particularly of cranial nerves I, VII, and VIII, have been described. Headaches, hypothalamic or pituitary disease with clinical diabetes insipidus, and cerebral or subarachnoid hemorrhage have been reported infrequently.

Cardiovascular manifestations include pericarditis, pericardial effusions, and rarely, coronary vasculitis, myocarditis, congestive heart failure (other than observed secondary to acute renal failure), valvular abnormalities, and arrhythmias. Miscellaneous clinical features are listed in Table 294–3.

DIAGNOSIS. The diagnosis is based on supportive clinical, pathologic, and laboratory confirmation. The diagnosis should be strongly suspected when a patient has multisystem illness involving upper and/or lower respiratory tract disease, glomerulonephritis, and vasculitis in any organ system. (See Table 294–3 for a listing of typical, occasional, and rare laboratory abnormalities in Wegener's granulomatosis.) The gold standard for a diagnosis of Wegener's granulomatosis has been the pathologic finding of necrotizing granulomatous vasculitis, particularly at open lung biopsy. However, active lung involvement is not always present initially. Localized disease may lead the clinician to entertain biopsy of other tissues, and thus knowledge of the array of pathologic findings in other organ systems is necessary.

Until fairly recently, laboratory features of Wegener's granulomatosis were relatively non-specific. A typical laboratory profile included normocytic normochromic anemia, unelevated erythrocyte sedimentation rate, leukocytosis, and positive rheumatoid factor in 30 to 40% of patients, with or without urine sediment abnormalities or elevated serum creatinine. In the past 15 years, c-ANCA and its relationship to Wegener's granulomatosis have been studied. Clearly, this test is helpful in Wegener's granulomatosis, particularly during active generalized disease, and may be confirmatory. Because reports of false positives are increasing and because sensitivity varies from 30 to 90% in a clinician's diagnosis of Wegener's granulomatosis, depending on the extent of disease and disease activity level, the test cannot be used as a sole diagnostic criterion for Wegener's granulomatosis. c-ANCA and more specific antibodies against PR-3 are somewhat analogous to a combination of antinuclear antibodies in SLE as a disease marker and anti-DNA in lupus as a disease activity marker. This topic continues to attract much attention.

Radiologic imaging studies are helpful in diagnosing Wegener's granulomatosis, including chest and sinus radiographs and computed tomography. The differential diagnosis is quite broad and depends on the patient's signs and symptoms. When the classic triad of involvement occurs, with confirmatory tissue biopsy and a positive c-ANCA, the diagnosis is easy. When the process is early and/or limited to the upper airway or kidney, the diagnosis is clinically challenging. Destructive upper airway disease needs to be differentiated from infection such as fungal, mycobacterial, staphylococcal, or syphilitic; substance abuse (particularly cocaine); malignancy (particularly T-cell lymphoma and squamous cell carcinoma); or rarely, self-mutilating trauma. In the past, *idiopathic midline granuloma* or idiopathic midline destructive disease was included in the differential diagnosis. Current investigators place this condition in the spectrum of *angiocentric immunoproliferative lesions,* believed to be a prelude to lymphoma (see Part XIII).

The differential diagnosis of pulmonary involvement is broad but, particularly in combination with renal disease, should include Goodpasture's syndrome, SLE, lymphomatoid granulomatosis (also in the spectrum of angiocentric immunoproliferative lesions), infection (fungal, mycobacterial, bacterial), and malignancy.

TREATMENT AND PROGNOSIS. Optimal treatment of active Wegener's granulomatosis, particularly with multisystem involvement, including renal disease, entails cyclophosphamide and corticosteroids. Cyclophosphamide therapy is started at a dose of 1 to 2 mg/kg/day, with initially weekly monitoring of complete blood counts to keep the total white count above 3.0 and the neutrophil count above 1.0 to limit complications of infection secondary to neutropenia. The dose is adjusted according to blood counts, particularly as corticosteroid use is tapered. The drug is generally continued for approximately 1 year beyond clinical remission, followed by discontinuation and close observation of the patient's clinical status and laboratory features, including blood counts, erythrocyte sedimentation rate, renal parameters, chest radiographs, and c-ANCA. This drug or alternative therapy is reinstituted in the case of recurrence or relapse. Complications include hemorrhagic cystitis (and thus patients should be instructed to drink at least 1.5 L of liquids per day), bone marrow toxicity, infections, hair loss, nausea, infertility, and increased risk of malignancy (bladder carcinoma, leukemia, lymphoma).

Corticosteroids are used at the time of diagnosis for severe disease, initially at 1 mg/kg/day (may be used in divided dose, intravenous methylprednisolone for fulminant disease, followed by consolidation to daily or alternate-day therapy). Prednisone equivalent doses of 60 mg/day are then tapered to alternate-day therapy over 1 month and then to the lowest possible level to control upper airway and/or musculoskeletal symptoms, preferably discontinuing use of this drug by 3 to 6 months.

Whereas Wegener's granulomatosis was once an invariably fatal disease, the combination of cyclophosphamide and prednisone has provided remission in 75% of all patients and improvement in 90%, as evidenced in the National Institutes of Health (NIH) series of long-term follow-up studies. However, relapses occur in at least 50% of those achieving remission at any time from several months to 15 to 20 years after stopping cytotoxic therapy. Thus Wegener's granulomatosis is a chronic disease and patients deserve close follow-up, patient and provider education, and sometimes creative therapeutic strategies.

Table 294–3 ■ LABORATORY ABNORMALITIES IN WEGENER'S GRANULOMATOSIS

	TYPICAL	OCCASIONAL	RARE
Hematologic	Normochromic, normocytic anemia Leukocytosis Eosinophilia Elevated erythrocyte sedimentation rate	Thrombocytosis	Microangiopathic hemolytic anemia
Urine sediment	Microhematuria Proteinuria Cellular casts	Sterile pyuria	
Chemistries	Hypoalbuminemia Renal insufficiency (mild to severe)	Elevated alkaline phosphatase +/or aminotransferases, elevated creatine phosphokinase and aldolase	
Serologic	Positive c-ANCA Positive rheumatoid factor Hypergammaglobulinemia Elevated C-reactive protein	Positive ANA (any pattern) Positive p-ANCA Elevated circulating immune complexes	

ANCA = antineutrophil cytoplasmic antibody; ANA = antinuclear antibody.

Table 294–4 ▪ TREATMENT OF WEGENER'S GRANULOMATOSIS

DRUG	INDICATIONS	INITIAL DOSE	MONITORING	DURATION
Cyclophosphamide	Moderate to severe	1–2 mg/kg/day PO	CBC weekly; keep WBC >3000, PMN >1000, and monitor liver tests; urine cytology and/or cystoscopy if prolonged therapy	Approximately 1 yr beyond clinical remission
	Fulminant	3–4 mg/kg/day IV for 2–3 day, then reduce to 2 mg/kg/day po or IV		
Corticosteroids	Moderate to severe	1 mg/kg/day prednisone equivalent (IV initially or PO)	Glucose, lipids, bone density	Taper to low dose (5–10 mg/day) or alternate-day therapy over 2 mo
Methotrexate	Mild to moderate upper airway or diffuse disease without significant renal involvement	Up to 15– 25 mg once weekly	Monitor CBC and liver tests every 4–8 wk	Taper to lowest dose controlling features; possibly a trial of no methotrexate 1 yr past clinical remission; close follow-up
Antibiotics	Adjunctive, not primary, to treat secondary bacterial infections; consider chronic suppression in chronic upper airway disease (sulfa may be contraindicated with methotrexate)			Intermittent or chronic low-dose "prophylaxis"
Cyclosporine	Refractory disease, dialysis dependent, patients awaiting renal transplant	3–5 mg/kg/day	BP, chemistries (Cr, Mg)	1 yr beyond clinical remission or until transplant

CBC = complete blood count; WBC = white blood cell count; PMN = polymorphonuclear leukocytes; BP = blood pressure.

Even though mortality from Wegener's granulomatosis and/or its therapy has improved significantly, disease-related morbidity occurs in the majority of patients, with chronic renal insufficiency, hearing loss, nasal deformity, tracheal stenosis, and ocular abnormalities leading the list. These complications are also reviewed thoroughly in the NIH series. More recently, alternative treatment strategies have been reported. Weekly low-dose (15 to 25 mg) oral or intramuscular methotrexate has provided hope and, because of experience in the management of rheumatoid arthritis, may provide a less toxic alternative to cyclophosphamide in patients who relapse, particularly with significant upper airway disease. Azathioprine, pulse monthly cyclophosphamide, intravenous immunoglobulin, cyclosporine, and immune modulators have all been used in individual cases. Because of the relative infrequency of the disease, controlled, double-blind studies have not yet been performed.

An overview of treatment strategies is listed in Table 294–4. Antibiotic therapy has a role, but at present it is considered adjunctive, not primary therapy. Because of necrotic upper airway tissue, staphylococcal and other infections are quite common and could be part of the "chicken and egg" perpetuation of this condition. In patients with Wegener's granulomatosis who are taking immunosuppressives, fever, new pulmonary infiltrate, new headache, hematuria, and pyuria deserve careful evaluation for infection before the symptoms are ascribed to disease flare.

Thus Wegener's granulomatosis is a multisystem, inflammatory, autoimmune disorder with a spectrum of clinical, laboratory, radiographic, and pathologic features; c-ANCA has been helpful diagnostically. Careful diagnosis, thoughtful management, and close follow-up are necessary for optimal outcome.

Gross WL (ed): ANCA-Associated Vasculitides: Immunologic and Clinical Aspects. New York, Plenum Press, 1993. *Compilation of papers presented at the 2nd International Colloquium on Wegener's Granulomatosis and Vasculitic Disorders in Lubeck, Germany, in May 1992.*
Hoffman GS: Treatment of Wegener's granulomatosis: Time to change the standard of care? Arthritis Rheum 40:2099, 1997. *Excellent update of controversis of care.*
Hoffman GS, Kerr GS, Leavitt RY, et al: Wegener's granulomatosis: An analysis of 158 patients. Ann Intern Med 116:488, 1992. *Updated review of NIH series on focusing on Wegener's granulomatosis clinical manifestations, disease spectrum, chronicity, and morbidity/mortality issues.*
Hoffman GS, Leavitt RY, Kerr GS, et al: The treatment of Wegener's granulomatosis with glucocorticoids and methotrexate. Arthritis Rheum 35:1322, 1992. *First article reviewing and significant number of patients with Wegener's granulomatosis treated with methotrexates.*
Lieberman K, Churg A: Wegener's granulomatosis. *In* Churg A, Churg J (eds): Systemic Vasculitides. New York, Igaku-Shoin, 1991, p 77. *A concise review of the topic with an emphasis on pathologic findings. Beautiful color photomicrographs.*

295 POLYMYALGIA RHEUMATICA AND GIANT CELL ARTERITIS
Gene G. Hunder

Polymyalgia rheumatica and giant cell arteritis are common rheumatic diseases of middle-aged and older persons. Although the etiology of these conditions is unknown, it is clear that they are closely related. Recent studies suggest that a single agent causes both conditions and that host and other unknown factors determine whether one or both processes will develop. A strong association with HLA-DR4 has been observed, thus indicating a hereditary link.

POLYMYALGIA RHEUMATICA

Polymyalgia rheumatica is characterized by aching and morning stiffness in the shoulder and hip girdles, the proximal ends of the extremities, the neck, and the torso. Usually it is accompanied by evidence of an inflammatory reaction. The mean age at onset is about 70 years, and it nearly always occurs after age 50, with women affected twice as commonly as men.

CLINICAL FINDINGS. Polymyalgia rheumatica may begin abruptly but usually develops gradually over a number of weeks. In mild or early cases, the symptoms may subside 1 to 2 hours after the patient arises in the morning, only to return later after a period of inactivity. Generally, the discomfort becomes severe enough to interfere with usual activities and may confine the patient to bed. Fatigue, loss of weight, and a low-grade fever may be present. Joint inflammation has been demonstrated in some cases, which supports the contention that polymyalgia rheumatica is a form of synovitis of the proximal joints and periarticular structures. Marked tenosynovitis may cause diffuse distal extremity swelling with pitting edema. Upon careful testing, muscle strength is found to be normal or nearly normal.

LABORATORY TESTS. Normochromic anemia is typical. Usually the erythrocyte sedimentation rate is markedly elevated, averaging 70 to 80 mm in 1 hour (Westergren). Other acute-phase protein

Age older than 50 yr
Aching and morning stiffness in at least two of the following areas:
 Neck
 Shoulder girdle
 Pelvic girdle
Erythrocyte sedimentation rate greater than 40 mm in 1 hr
Duration of symptoms for 1 mo
No other disease present

levels are also elevated. Some patients have mild hepatic dysfunction that reverts to normal with treatment. Other tests are normal.

INCIDENCE. White individuals appear to be affected more frequently than other groups. The highest recorded incidence rates are from northern Europe and the northern United States. In one population study, the prevalence found was approximately 1 in 200 persons in the population aged 50 or older. Recent reports on incidence rates in Europe show similar findings.

DIAGNOSIS. Several criteria sets for diagnosing polymyalgia rheumatica have been suggested. Most are similar to those in Table 295–1. Morning stiffness should last at least one-half hour. The erythrocyte sedimentation rate is an indicator of systemic inflammation. An additional criterion of rapid response to 10 to 20 mg of prednisone per day is suggested by some. These criteria are only guidelines because patients occasionally have normal sedimentation rates at onset and symptoms may develop slightly before age 50.

DIFFERENTIAL DIAGNOSIS. Some patients with early rheumatoid arthritis lack the more characteristic distal joint involvement and serum rheumatoid factor and have prominent proximal symptoms. In polymyositis, limitation is due to a lack of muscle strength; in polymyalgia rheumatica, limitation is due to pain. In polymyositis, muscle biopsy shows an inflammatory myopathy; in polymyalgia rheumatica, biopsy is normal or shows only atrophy (Table 295–2).

Fibromyalgia usually affects younger individuals and tends to be associated with tender spots; laboratory tests are normal. When encouraged to do so, patients with fibromyalgia can move the joints through a full range of motion without great difficulty. Wakefulness in polymyalgia rheumatica is due to discomfort caused by movement in bed. In fibromyalgia, however, a more generalized, persistent discomfort that is less tangible is characteristic.

Other conditions that occasionally need to be distinguished from polymyalgia rheumatica include chronic infections such as subacute bacterial endocarditis or viral infections, malignancies, hypothyroidism, and other connective tissue diseases.

GIANT CELL ARTERITIS

Giant cell (temporal) arteritis affects large and medium-sized arteries, especially those branching from the proximal aorta that supply the neck, the extracranial structures of the head, and the arms. The lesions tend to be scattered irregularly along the involved vessels. A focal or diffuse granulomatous inflammatory infiltration is present along with multinucleated histiocytic and foreign body giant cells, histiocytes, lymphocytes, and fibroblasts. Lymphocytes tend to be predominantly helper T cells.

CLINICAL FINDINGS. Giant cell arteritis affects the same population subject to polymyalgia rheumatica. The manifestations of giant cell arteritis are diverse, and many clinical features have been described.

In most patients, symptoms or signs related to the vascular system develop at some time during the course of the disease (Table 295–3). Headache may be mild or severe. The scalp may be tender over the arteries of the head or at other sites.

Visual symptoms are present in about one third of patients; half are transient and half are permanent. The former includes amaurosis fugax and diplopia. Permanent visual loss may be partial or complete and may occur without warning; about half are unilateral and half are bilateral. The vision loss is due to narrowing or occlusion of the ophthalmic or posterior ciliary arteries.

Intermittent claudication occurs in about one half of patients, with the jaw muscles most frequently involved. During chewing of firm foods such as meat, fatigue or discomfort is noted. In a small percentage of patients, claudication of the tongue or throat develops with eating and repeated swallowing. Nervous system alterations are found in up to 30%; 14% have either mononeuritis or polyneuropathy, and 7% have transient ischemic attacks or strokes.

Polymyalgia rheumatica occurs in about 40% of patients with giant cell arteritis. It may precede other symptoms or become manifested only during the withdrawal of corticosteroid therapy given for the arteritis. Diffuse or asymmetrical myalgias, arthralgias, or joint swelling may be present in other patients with giant cell arteritis.

PHYSICAL EXAMINATION. The temporal, occipital, or other scalp or cervical arteries may be enlarged, tender, and erythematous. Bruits or pulse deficits may be present over the carotid, subclavian, or brachial arteries. Large artery involvement may be present initially or later as part of an exacerbation. Findings in the eyes of patients with recent visual loss include papilledema, hemorrhage, and exudates; later, optic atrophy develops.

LABORATORY TESTS. Blood test results are similar to those seen in polymyalgia rheumatica. The platelet count is generally increased. The erythrocyte sedimentation rate averages 80 to 100 mm in 1 hour (Westergren) but is occasionally normal.

INCIDENCE. Reported annual incidence rates have varied considerably and are highest (20 per 100,000) in persons aged 50 and older in northern Europe and the United States. Although the reasons for the variable rates are unknown, ethnic and geographic factors have been suggested. Familial cases of giant cell arteritis and polymyalgia rheumatica have been reported. Giant cell arteritis appears to be one third as common as polymyalgia rheumatica.

DIAGNOSIS. Giant cell arteritis should be considered in any older person with transient or sudden visual changes, unexplained fever, polymyalgia rheumatica or new headaches, and an elevated erythrocyte sedimentation rate. The arteries of the head, neck, and extremities should be examined carefully. Distinct tenderness, redness, and a palpable but non-pulsatile temporal artery are important

Table 295-2 ■ DIFFERENTIAL FEATURES IN POLYMYALGIA RHEUMATICA AND SIMILAR DISORDERS

SIGNS/SYMPTOMS	POLYMYALGIA RHEUMATICA	GIANT CELL ARTERITIS	RHEUMATOID ARTHRITIS	DERMATOMYOSITIS	FIBROMYALGIA
Morning stiffness >30 min	+	±	+*	±	Variable
Headache and/or scalp tenderness	0	+	0	0	Variable
Pain with active joint movement	+	0	+*	0	Inconstant
Tender joints	±	0	+*	0	Tender spots
Swollen joints	±	±	+	0	0
Muscle weakness	±†	0	+*	+	0
Normochromic anemia	+	+	+	0	0
Elevated erythrocyte sedimentation rate	+	+	+	±	0
Elevated serum creatine kinase	0	0	0	+	0
Serum rheumatoid factor	0	0	70%	0	0
Distinct electromyographic abnormality	0	0	0	+	0
Response to non-steroidal anti-inflammatory drug	±	0	+	0	0

0 = absent; + = present; ± = present in minority of cases.
*Associated with affected joints.
†Pain inhibits movement. Disuse atrophy may occur.

Table 295-3 ■ GIANT CELL ARTERITIS: CLINICAL FINDINGS IN 94 PATIENTS

CLINICAL MANIFESTATION	FREQUENCY (%)
Headache	77
Abnormal temporal artery	53
Jaw claudication	51
Scalp tenderness	47
Constitutional symptoms	48
Polymyalgia rheumatica	34
Fever	27
Respiratory symptoms	23
Facial pain	14
Diplopia/blurred vision	12
Transient vision loss	5
Blindness (partial or complete)	13
Hemoglobin <11.0 g/dL	24
Erythrocyte sedimentation rate >40 mm/hr	97

After Machado EBV, Michet CJ, Ballard DJ, et al: Trends in incidence and clinical presentation of temporal arteritis in Olmstead County, Minnesota, 1950–1985. Arthritis Rheum 31:745, 1988.

clues to the presence of arteritis. In the absence of similar changes in the lower extremities, pulse changes or bruits over the axillary and brachial arteries are more likely to be caused by vasculitis than by arteriosclerosis.

Temporal artery biopsy is recommended for all patients suspected of having giant cell arteritis. A biopsy should be performed on the most clinically abnormal artery segment. When the arteries appear normal on examination, a segment several centimeters long should be removed from one temporal artery, and histologic sections should be examined at multiple levels in an effort to find an involved area. In the author's experience, if the first temporal artery biopsy is normal, the second side will yield approximately 10 to 15% additional positive cases.

Some patients with polymyalgia rheumatica may be monitored carefully without a temporal artery biopsy. If no signs or symptoms of vasculitis are present and the symptoms and laboratory test parameters respond completely to low-dose corticosteroids, biopsy may be deferred and the patient monitored closely.

DIFFERENTIAL DIAGNOSIS. Conditions that have been confused with giant cell arteritis include systemic infections, amyloidosis with prominent vascular involvement, neoplasms, arteriosclerotic vascular disease in patients with an elevated erythrocyte sedimentation rate that is due to some other cause, arteriovenous fistulas, and other forms of vasculitis.

Follow-up studies of patients who have had a negative temporal artery biopsy have shown that in only approximately 10% do findings of giant cell arteritis develop; these patients require long-term corticosteroid therapy.

MANAGEMENT

Therapy for polymyalgia rheumatica is aimed at alleviating systemic symptoms and musculoskeletal discomfort. Corticosteroids are recommended for most patients, with an initial daily dose of 10 to 20 mg of prednisone (or the equivalent dose of another corticosteroid). Prednisone acts rapidly, and the patient should notice significant improvement within 24 hours. The corticosteroid dose can be reduced as tolerated after 1 month or earlier. Non-steroidal anti-inflammatory drugs may be added to control the mild discomfort that may occur while corticosteroids therapy is being withdrawn and discontinued.

In giant cell arteritis, the recommended dosage of prednisone is 40 to 60 mg/day. Vascular complications seldom occur after corticosteroids have been started. If the response to the initial dose of prednisone is incomplete, the dosage should be increased by 20 to 30 mg/day. Usually, if symptoms subside and laboratory values return to normal with a given dose, the disease process is adequately suppressed. Prednisone for both conditions may be administered as a single morning dose or in two to three divided doses per day.

The overall goal of therapy is to administer the lowest dose of corticosteroid that adequately controls the arteritis and prescribe it for the shortest necessary time. The dose needed to achieve control

varies among patients and must be determined empirically. There is no evidence that corticosteroid therapy alters the natural course of the disease.

In a small proportion of cases, the corticosteroid dose cannot be reduced without an exacerbation of the disease. Cyclophosphamide, azathioprine, dapsone, and methotrexate have been reported as steroid-sparing drugs in some instances. The average duration of both polymyalgia rheumatica and giant cell arteritis is about 2 years, during which time the intensity of the process may flare up at times but appears to resolve slowly. The course in individual patients, however, varies considerably, and some may continue with active symptoms for several years. Thoracic aortic aneurysm is a late complication of giant cell arteritis.

Aiello PD, Trautmann JC, McPhee TJ, et al: Visual prognosis in giant cell arteritis. Ophthalmology 100:550, 1993. *A study of the ocular effects and outcome of vision in giant cell arteritis.*

Salvarani C, Gabriel SE, O'Fallon WM, et al: The incidence of giant cell arteritis in Olmsted County, Minnesota: Apparent fluctuations in a cyclic pattern. Ann Intern Med 123:192, 1995. *A cyclic occurrence of giant cell arteritis suggests a possible infectious link.*

Weyand CM, Tetzloff N, Björnsson J, et al: Disease patterns and tissue cytokine profiles in giant cell arteritis. Arthritis Rheum 40: 19, 1997. *Manifestations in giant cell arteritis correlated with cytokines found in temporal arteries.*

296 IDIOPATHIC INFLAMMATORY MYOPATHIES

Robert L. Wortmann

DEFINITION. The term "idiopathic inflammatory myopathy" designates a group of rare diseases of unknown cause that are characterized by symmetrical proximal muscle weakness and non-suppurative inflammation of skeletal muscle. Specific diagnoses characterized by this term include polymyositis, dermatomyositis, cancer-associated myositis, myositis associated with another connective tissue disease (overlap syndromes), and inclusion body myositis. Patients with any idiopathic inflammatory myopathy generally fulfill the criteria used to define polymyositis originally proposed in 1975 by Bohan and Peter (Table 296–1).

INCIDENCE. The idiopathic inflammatory myopathies are rare conditions, with an annual incidence ranging between 0.5 and 8.4 cases per 1 million population. The incidence is highest in blacks and lowest in Japanese. Women are generally more often affected than men, with female preponderance most pronounced between the ages of 15 and 44 and in persons having myositis associated with other connective tissue diseases. The gender ratio is equal in older age groups and in myositis associated with malignancy, but it is reversed in inclusion body myositis. Overall, the age of onset has a bimodal distribution, with peaks in children between 10 and 14 and in adults between 45 and 54. The mean age of onset for the subset of myositides with other connective tissue diseases is similar to that for the associated condition. Individuals with myositis associ-

Table 296-1 ■ CRITERIA USED TO DEFINE IDIOPATHIC INFLAMMATORY MYOPATHY*

1. Symmetrical weakness of limb girdle muscles and anterior neck flexors with or without dysphagia
2. Elevation in serum of skeletal muscle enzymes, especially creatine phosphokinase
3. Electromyographic changes consistent with inflammatory myopathy: short, small polyphasic motor units; fibrillations; positive waves; and bizarre, high-frequency repetitive discharges
4. Muscle biopsy evidence of fiber necrosis, phagocytosis, and regeneration; variation in fiber size; and inflammatory exudate

Note: Patients are classified as having definite disease with four, probable disease with three, and possible disease with two criteria.

*These criteria were orginally proposed in 1975 by Bohan and Peter to define polymyositis. At that time the term "polymyositis" was used to represent a specific disease, as well as being a general term representing all the recognized forms of inflammatory myopathy.

ated with malignancy or inclusion body myositis have a mean age older than 60 years.

PATHOLOGY AND PATHOGENESIS. Abnormalities in skeletal muscle indicative of an idiopathic inflammatory myopathy include muscle fiber degeneration, regeneration, necrosis, phagocytosis, and mononuclear cell infiltration. In polymyositis, necrosis of single muscle fibers is common, and some non-necrotic fibers are invaded by T cells and macrophages. Collections of lymphocytes, plasma cells, and histiocytes are found primarily in the endomysium. Inflammatory aggregates contain high percentages of T cells but few B cells. Over time, fiber diameter variation increases, and interstitial fibrosis develops. Dermatomyositis can be distinguished histologically by the presence of perifascicular atrophy. This characteristic feature results from degeneration of fibers at the periphery of the fascicles secondary to microvascular damage. Analysis of these areas reveals focal capillary depletion and deposition of IgG, IgM, C3, and the complement membrane complex in and around microvascular endothelium. The inflammatory cells are grouped in the perimysium with a perivascular distribution and contain a higher percentage of B cells. In inclusion body myositis, light microscopy reveals inflammatory changes similar to those in polymyositis but with the additional feature of characteristic intracellular vacuoles. The vacuoles are lined with basophilic granules on cryostat sections and eosinophilic material on paraffin sections. Intracytoplasmic or intranuclear tubulofilamentous inclusions are also seen with electron microscopy. These inclusions are straight and rigid and have periodic striations resembling paramyxovirus. Ubiquitin and β-amyloid protein (two proteins that have been identified in the plaques in brains from patients with Alzheimer's disease) have been identified in the vacuoles and tubulofilamentous inclusions.

The idiopathic inflammatory myopathies are believed to be immune-mediated processes triggered by environmental factors in genetically susceptible individuals. This concept is in part based on the prevalence of autoantibodies, inflammatory pathology, association with other autoimmune diseases, and response to corticosteroid therapy.

Many patients with idiopathic inflammatory myopathies have circulating autoantibodies (Table 296–2). Some are termed "myositis-specific autoantibodies" and are seen only in patients with polymyositis or dermatomyositis; others are those associated with other connective tissue diseases. Most myositis-specific autoantibodies are directed against cytoplasmic antigens and bind to evolutionarily conserved epitopes. The percentage of patients with polymyositis and dermatomyositis who have circulating myositis-specific autoantibodies is uncertain, but estimates range between 10 and 50%. Eight different myositis-specific autoantibodies have been described, but no more than one has been found in an individual

Table 296–2 ■ AUTOANTIBODIES FOUND IN PATIENTS WITH IDIOPATHIC INFLAMMATORY MYOPATHY

AUTOANTIBODY	CLINICAL ASSOCIATION
Myositis-Specific Autoantibodies	
Anti-tRNA synthetases	PM with interstitial lung disease,
Anti–Jo-1	arthritis, and fever; less common
Anti–PL-7	in DM
Anti–PL-12	
Anti-OJ	
Anti-EJ	
Anti-SRP	PM with poor prognosis
Anti-MAS	PM after alcoholic rhabdomyolysis
Anti–Mi-2	DM
Antinuclear Antibodies Associated with Other Connective Tissue Diseases	
Anti-SM	SLE
Anti-RNP	SLE, MCTD
Anti-SSA (anti-Ro)	SLE, Sjögren's syndrome
Anti-SSB (anti-La)	SLE, Sjögren's syndrome
Anti-centromere	CREST syndrome
Anti-SCL70	Scleroderma
Anti–PM-1	Scleroderma
Anti-Ku	Scleroderma
Anti–PM-Scl	Scleroderma

Anti-SRP = anti–signal recognition particle; PM = polymyositis; DM = dermatomyositis: SLE = systemic lupus erythematosus; MCTD = mixed (undifferentiated) connective tissue disease; CREST = *c*alcinosis, *R*aynaud's phenomenon, *e*sophageal dysmotility, *s*clerodactyly, *t*elangiectasia.

patient. The more common myositis-specific autoantibodies are directed against aminoacyl-tRNA (transfer RNA) synthetases and inhibit the activity of the respective antigenic enzyme protein in vitro. The most prevalent antisynthetase antibody is directed against histidyl-tRNA synthetase and is called "anti–Jo-1." Certain picornaviruses can substitute for tRNA and interact with aminoacyl-tRNA synthetase enzymes. Interestingly, amino acid sequences near the active site of histidyl-tRNA synthetase (Jo-1) have some homology with certain capsid proteins in encephalomyocarditis virus, a picornavirus that induces a mouse model of polymyositis. Thus antibodies initially directed against virus or a virus-enzyme complex could cross-react with homologous areas of host proteins or the enzyme itself. This process is termed "molecular mimicry" and could explain the autoantibody production.

Several observations emphasize the importance of genetic factors in general and class II antigens in particular in the pathogenesis of inflammatory myopathy (see Chapter 278). Almost 50% of patients with polymyositis, dermatomyositis, and inclusion body myositis have the HLA-DR3 phenotype. This phenotype is almost always linked with HLA-B8 and is most common in patients with anti–Jo-1 antibodies. HLA-DR52 is found in over 90% of patients who have myositis and anti–Jo-1 antibodies.

Viruses, particularly picornaviruses, have been implicated as causes of myositis. Several viruses, especially Coxsackie A9, have been associated with myositis in individual cases; elevated titers to coxsackievirus have been found in childhood dermatomyositis; mumps virus antigen has been demonstrated in inclusions in inclusion body myositis; and certain viral infections can induce inflammatory myopathy in mice, with inflammation persisting long after virus can be detected.

The pathologic changes in polymyositis and inclusion body myositis appear to result from cell-mediated, antigen-specific cytotoxicity. Cell adhesion molecules participate in target-effector cell interactions in cell-mediated cytotoxicity and leukodiapedesis. One of these molecules, intercellular adhesion molecule type 1 (I CAM-1), is strongly induced on the surface of non-necrotic muscle fibers. In these disorders, non-necrotic muscle fibers are surrounded by and invaded by CD8+ mononuclear cells, with cytotoxic cells outnumbering suppressor cells by a ratio of 4:1. About 50% of the CD8+ antoinvasive T-cells are HLA-DR positive and express the RD form of the leukocyte common antigen CD45, which suggests that they are activated memory cells. Different immune mechanisms are evident in dermatomyositis. Mononuclear cell invasion of non-necrotic fibers is rare, ICAM-1 is strongly expressed on endothelial cells of perimysial arterioles and venules and on some perifascicular capillaries, cellular infiltration is predominantly perivascular, B cells outnumber T cells, and the CD4/CD8 ratio is higher. These findings indicate that humoral mechanisms play a significant role in the pathogenesis of dermatomyositis.

Loss of muscle fibers as a result of the immune response may contribute to muscle weakness in some patients with an idiopathic inflammatory myopathy. However, other factors must also be involved because weakness can occur in the absence of an inflammatory infiltrate or fiber necrosis. These observations suggest that abnormalities of the contractile process may underlie the muscle weakness. Energy (adenosine triphosphate [ATP]) is required for normal muscle contraction and relaxation, as well as the maintenance of membrane integrity. Altered muscle energy metabolism has been demonstrated *in vitro* in a coxsackievirus B1–induced mouse model of inflammatory myopathy. Muscles from these mice have increased glycolytic activity when compared with controls, as well as decreased activity of myophosphorylase and myoadenylate deaminase. A secondary deficiency of myoadenylate deaminase activity has been observed in muscle from some patients with polymyositis. *In vivo* ^{31}P magnetic resonance spectrographic studies of patients with polymyositis and dermatomyositis have shown lower levels of high-energy phosphate–containing compounds at rest, faster depletion of ATP with exercise, and slower recovery rates than seen in normal individuals. These abnormalities reverse as patients improve with therapy, particularly in dermatomyositis. Such studies support the hypothesis that metabolic changes contribute to the muscle weakness in the inflammatory myopathies.

CLINICAL MANIFESTATIONS. The onset of an idiopathic inflammatory myopathy is usually insidious, with no identified precipitating event. The cardinal feature of any inflammatory myopathy is symmetrical muscle weakness of the shoulder and pelvic girdles, at times accompanied by mild pain and tenderness. Weakness of proximal leg and arm muscles, neck flexors, and pharyngeal muscles may follow. Early symptoms include difficulty getting up from a chair, climbing stairs, and using one's hands above shoulder level. Dysphagia, dysphonia, and dysarthria may develop when the disease affects the pharynx. Morning stiffness, fatigue, and other systemic symptoms are common. Arthralgias are noted with active disease, but frank synovitis is quite rare. With progression, weakness can become so severe that patients cannot lift their extremities against gravity, involved muscles become atrophic, and contractures develop. An explosive onset with rhabdomyolysis, myoglobinuria, and renal failure is rare. Typically, the neurologic examination is normal except for the motor component. Deep tendon reflexes are normal or appear slightly decreased because of muscle weakness. Cranial nerve function is normal. Dysphagia is primarily due to weakness of striated musculature in the posterior of the pharynx and is often associated with a poor prognosis. Patients may have difficulty swallowing liquids, are prone to aspiration, and may have nasal speech. These symptoms may be accentuated by spasm or fibrosis of the cricopharyngeal muscles and may require surgical treatment. Esophageal dysfunction may occur but is often clinically insignificant.

Pulmonary manifestations develop in some patients as a result of hypoventilation secondary to muscle weakness, swallowing abnormalities with aspiration, and infection. Interstitial lung disease develops in approximately 5 to 10%. Some patients with interstitial pneumonitis have no respiratory symptoms, but others experience non-productive cough and dyspnea, which may precede the onset of muscle weakness. The restrictive lung disease is associated with bibasilar fine crackles on chest auscultation and reduced diffusion capacity. Symptomatic cardiac problems are unusual, although conduction abnormalities and tachyarrhythmias may be seen on electrocardiograms. Congestive heart failure can result from hypoxemia, pulmonary hypertension, or cardiomyopathy. Raynaud's phenomenon is reported in a small percentage of patients.

Periorbital edema may develop in patients with polymyositis. When other cutaneous manifestations are seen, the disease is termed "dermatomyositis." Typically, the rash is erythematous and appears on the face, neck, chest, and extensor surfaces of the extremities. The name "Gottron's patches" is given to raised, red to violet, scaly patches seen over the knuckles, elbows, and knees. A heliotrope rash on the upper eyelids is very characteristic. The term "mechanic's hands" is applied to the darkened or dirty-appearing horizontal lines that develop across the lateral and palmar aspects of the fingers (because of the similarity to changes seen in the hands of people who do manual labor). Capillary nail fold changes are present in some individuals, especially those with Raynaud's phenomenon. These changes include dilated or distorted capillary loops sometimes alternating with avascular areas. Dermatomyositis in children is sometimes referred to by the specific term "childhood dermatomyositis." Childhood dermatomyositis is similar to dermatomyositis in adults, except that vascular involvement is more prominent. Fever, weight loss, and subcutaneous calcifications are more common, and gastrointestinal tract hemorrhage or perforation may occur.

When myositis occurs in association with another connective tissue or autoimmune disease, the associated conditions may dominate the clinical picture. The most frequently associated disease is systemic lupus erythematosus (SLE), but others include scleroderma, rheumatoid arthritis, polyarteritis nodosa, giant cell arteritis, autoimmune thyroid disease, insulin-dependent diabetes mellitus, dermatitis herpetiformis, myasthenia gravis, and primary biliary cirrhosis.

Approximately 20% of adults with polymyositis or dermatomyositis also have cancer. Although this figure may seem higher than expected for the general population, there appears to be no significant difference in the frequency of malignancy when compared with appropriate age-matched control populations. Most often the myositis and malignancy are diagnosed within a year of each other. In general, the type of neoplasm is that expected for the patient's age. Overall, the most commonly associated tumors are of the breast and lung. Ovarian and stomach cancers occur more

frequently than in the general population; rectal and colon cancers are less frequent. Neoplastic disease is less common in patients with interstitial lung disease or in those with an associated connective tissue disease.

Inclusion body myositis occurs most commonly in older men and can differ from polymyositis by the additional features of distal muscle weakness, asymmetrical muscle involvement, and neuropathic findings on physical examination and electromyography (EMG).

CLINICAL COURSE AND PROGNOSIS. The overall 5-year survival rate is approximately 80%, with children having the best prognosis. About half of surviving patients with polymyositis or dermatomyositis essentially recover completely. Older patients, those with associated neoplasms, or those with significant pulmonary, cardiac, or gastrointestinal involvement have a poorer prognosis. Patients with antibodies to aminoacyl-tRNA synthetases (i.e., anti–Jo-1) have a very high prevalence of interstitial lung disease, arthritis, and fever and do not respond well to therapy. Those with circulating anti-SRP (signal recognition particle) antibodies have a high prevalence of Raynaud's phenomenon and the worst prognosis of any subset. Although most patients with inclusion body myositis do not improve with therapy, their survival rate appears to be good. Typically the weakness progresses very slowly and may become fixed in some cases.

LABORATORY DATA. Serum levels of muscle-derived enzymes are elevated at some time during the course of the disease in 99% of patients. Creatine phosphokinase (CPK) levels are the most sensitive, but levels of aldolase, aspartate and alanine aminotransferase, and lactate dehydrogenase are also useful. CPK levels can be used as an index of disease activity or therapeutic response in some but not all patients. When normal CPK values are encountered in the presence of active disease, possible explanations include circulating enzyme inhibitors, a possible associated malignancy, or longstanding disease with severe muscle atrophy. The MB isoenzyme of CPK may be increased in the absence of cardiac involvement because of expression of that isoform in regenerating skeletal muscle fibers.

The erythrocyte sedimentation rate remains normal in over half the patients and, when elevated, does not correlate with the degree of weakness. Complete blood count, urinalysis, and other laboratory studies are usually normal unless an associated connective tissue disease or neoplasm is present.

Circulating autoantibodies are common in patients with idiopathic inflammatory myopathies (see Table 296–2). The most common myositis-specific autoantibody, anti–Jo-1, is found in polymyositis and less commonly in dermatomyositis. Certain antinuclear antibodies may herald an associated connective tissue disease: anti-SM and anti–double-stranded DNA for SLE; anti–SS-A and anti–SS-B for Sjögren's syndrome; anti-centromere for CREST syndrome (calcinosis, Raynaud's phenomenon, esophageal dysmotility, sclerodactyly, telangiectasia); and anti–PM-1, anti-Ku, anti–PM-Sc1, and anti-SCL70 for scleroderma.

The EMG is abnormal in 90% of patients. Classic changes include the triad of (1) small-amplitude, short-duration, polyphasic motor unit potentials; (2) fibrillation, positive waves, and increased insertional irritability; and (3) spontaneous, bizarre high-frequency discharges. The complete triad may be found in only 40% of patients, and in some patients changes are restricted to the paraspinal muscles.

DIAGNOSIS AND DIFFERENTIAL DIAGNOSIS. Criteria are useful in establishing the diagnosis of an idiopathic inflammatory myopathy (see Table 296–1). These criteria can be used only after other causes are excluded because no change or test is specific for the diagnosis. CPK elevation can occur in a wide number of conditions, as well as with blunt or sharp trauma, aerobic exercise, EMG studies, muscle biopsies, or drugs that retard the elimination of CPK from the serum such as barbiturates or narcotics. Normal blacks have higher levels of CPK than whites do, frequently with values above the normals established for large populations. The EMG changes seen in polymyositis are not specific. Even in the classic case, the change can only be considered myopathic and consistent with inflammation. The EMG is useful in identifying areas of abnormality to be biopsied, but biopsy should not include the actual site of EMG needle insertion. Because of the symmetrical nature of this disease, it is best to limit the EMG to one side of the body and perform biopsy on the other side. Magnetic resonance imaging may provide an effective, non-invasive means for identifying the site for biopsy and for monitoring the course of the disease, especially in dermatomyositis. Although the possibility of malignancy should be considered in each patient with myositis, extensive undirected testing is not advised. Clues to the coexistence of neoplastic disease are almost always apparent on the history, physical examination, or routine laboratory tests. Routine screening should be appropriate for the patient's age and sex.

A variety of other diseases may cause muscle weakness (Table 296–3), and patients with these conditions may fulfill some or all four criteria for polymyositis (see Table 296–1); thus these diagnoses must be excluded before the diagnosis of an idiopathic inflammatory myopathy can be made. A careful history and physical examination coupled with the judicious use of laboratory tests allow one to sort through the extensive differential list efficiently. For example, a careful review of medication use may reveal an agent that induces muscle injury such as alcohol, corticosteroids, cimetidine, colchicine, lovastatin, or zidovudine (AZT). On physical examination, asymmetrical weakness and distal extremity involvement, as well as abnormal reflexes, altered sensation, or cranial nerve abnormalities, should suggest a neurologic disease. Patients with inclusion body myositis may prove the exception because some have distal or asymmetrical muscle involvement.

Table 296–3 ■ DIFFERENTIAL DIAGNOSIS OF MUSCLE WEAKNESS

Immunologic	*Neurologic*
Polymyositis	Denervating disorders
Dermatomyositis	Amyotrophic lateral sclerosis
Inclusion body myositis	Neuromuscular junction disorders
Polymyalgia rheumatica	Myasthenia gravis
Temporal arteritis	Eaton-Lambert syndrome
Rheumatoid arthritis	Muscular dystrophies
Systemic lupus erythematosus	Limb-girdle
Polyarteritis nodosa	Becker's syndrome
Scleroderma	Duchenne's syndrome
Adult Still's disease	Neuropathies
Eosinophilic fasciitis	Guillain-Barré syndrome
Graft-versus-host disease	Diabetes mellitus
Endocrine	Porphyria
Hypothyroidism	*Metabolic-Nutritional*
Hyperthyroidism	Uremia
Hyperparathyroidism	Hepatic failure
Hypocalcemia	Hypercalcemia
Cushing's disease	Hypocalcemia
Addison's disease	Hyperkalemia
Aldosteronism	Hypokalemia
Malabsorption	Hypernatremia
Diabetic amyotrophy	Hyponatremia
Infectious	Hypomagnesemia
Influenza, Coxsackie, HIV, and	Hypophosphatemia
other viruses	Periodic paralysis
Infectious mononucleosis	Vitamin D deficiency
Rickettsia	Vitamin E deficiency
Toxoplasmosis	*Carcinomatous*
Trichinella	Neuropathy
Schistosomiasis	Neuromyopathy
Bacterial toxins	Myositis
Staphylococcal	Microembolization
Streptococcal	Eaton-Lambert syndrome
Clostridial	*Inherited Deficiency States*
Toxic (Drug Related)	Glycogen storage diseases
Alcohol	McArdle's syndrome (myophos-
Chloroquine/hydroxychloroquine	phorylase)
Clofibrate	Phosphofructokinase
Cocaine	Debrancher enzyme
Colchicine	Brancher enzyme
Cromolyn	Phosphoglycerate kinase
Cyclosporine	Phosphoglycerate mutase
Emetine	Lactate dehydrogenase
Gemfibrozil	Acid maltase
L-Tryptophan	Lipid disorders
Lovastatin	Carnitine (primary and second-
Penicillamine	ary)
Zidovudine (AZT)	Carnitine palmitoyltransferase
Miscellaneous	Purine disorders
Hypereosinophilic syndromes	Myoadenylate deaminase
Rhabdomyolysis	Mitochondrial myopathies
Sarcoidosis	*Psychosomatic*
Fibromyalgia	Hysterical (?)

Table 296–4 ■ PROTOCOL FOR FOREARM ISCHEMIC EXERCISE TESTING

Procedure
Venous blood samples are drawn for ammonia and lactate levels from the non-dominant arm, preferably without a tourniquet.
A sphygmomanometer is inflated around the upper part of the dominant arm to at least 20 mm Hg above systolic pressure.
The subject then squeezes the dominant hand as vigorously as possible at a rate of one squeeze every 2 seconds for 2 minutes.
After 2 minutes of exercise, the cuff is deflated.
Two minutes after the cuff is deflated, venous samples are taken from the dominant arm for lactate and ammonia levels.

Interpretation
Normal individuals exercising with maximal effort increase lactate and ammonia levels at least three-fold over baseline values. Individuals with a glycogen storage disease elevate ammonia levels normally but cannot raise lactate levels. Myoadenylate deaminase–deficient individuals raise lactate levels, but ammonia levels remain at baseline values. Falsely abnormal results may be obtained if the subject does not exercise with sufficient intensity. Abnormal results must be supported by a muscle biopsy to confirm the putative diagnosis.

Inclusion body myositis may be difficult to separate from some cases of muscular dystrophy.

Serum electrolytes (sodium, potassium, calcium, phosphorus, and magnesium) should be measured. An abnormality in any electrolyte may interfere with normal functioning of muscle fibers and result in weakness or myalgias. Uncovering an electrolyte abnormality usually reveals a reversible myopathy, especially if the cause of the electrolyte disturbance is identified. Some inherited metabolic myopathies can mimic inflammatory myopathy. Individuals with glycogen storage diseases such as myophosphorylase deficiency (McArdle's disease) or phosphofructokinase deficiency, as well as some with carnitine deficiency or myoadenylate deaminase deficiency, have proximal muscle weakness, elevated CPK levels, and myopathic EMG abnormalities. A forearm ischemic exercise test can be used to screen for the glycogen storage diseases and myoadenylate deaminase deficiency (Table 296–4).

TREATMENT. During the active stage of the disease, bed rest is essential, and physical therapy with passive range-of-motion exercises should be performed to maintain function and avoid contractures. Smoking is prohibited, and the head of the bed should be elevated in patients at risk for aspiration. Antacids or H$_2$ antagonists may also be useful to raise the pH of gastric fluids.

Treatment with corticosteroids is empirical but the standard. Initially, prednisone is used in single daily doses of 1 to 2 mg/kg. In responsive patients, muscle strength usually improves in 1 to 2 months, and the CPK normalizes in 3 months. Daily high-dose prednisone should be continued until strength has remained normal for 3 to 6 weeks. Once remission is attained, steroid use is tapered very gradually, a process that may require up to 2 years. Alternate-day use is recommended only when the disease is under excellent control.

Steroid failures may be attributed to an inadequate initial dosage, tapering too quickly, inaccurate diagnosis, or an associated malignancy, refractory disease, or coincident steroid myopathy. Improvement in muscle strength when the steroid dose is raised indicates active disease; improved strength with a lower dose of steroid implicates steroid myopathy. Immunosuppressive agents are used in patients who do not respond adequately to corticosteroids. Daily oral azathioprine and weekly oral or parenteral methotrexate are the usual next choices. Cyclophosphamide, chlorambucil, cyclosporine, and intravenous immunoglobulin have been used in refractory cases. Only a small percentage of patients with inclusion body myositis achieve remission with steroid or other immunosuppressive therapy. Despite this poor prognosis, a therapeutic trial is indicated because remission occurs in some cases and progression may be delayed in others. However, if some benefit is not observed, drug therapy should be discontinued to avoid side effects and toxicity.

Drake LA, Dinehart SM, Farmer ER, et al: Guidelines of care for dermatomyositis: American Academy of Dermatology. J Am Acad Dermatol 34:824, 1996. *Recent recommendations for the management of dermatomyositis by a large consensus group.*

Oddis C: Idiopathic inflammatory myopathy. *In* Wortmann RL (ed): Diseases of Skeletal Muscle. Philadelphia, Lippincott–Williams & Wilkins, 1999. *Recent comprehensive discussion that includes historical perspective.*

Targoff IN: Immune manifestations of inflammatory muscle disease. Rheum Dis Clin North Am 20:857, 1994. *Detailed review of the myositis-specific antibodies as well as autoantibodies associated with other connective tissue diseases.*

Wortmann RL: Inflammatory diseases of muscle. *In* Kelley WN, Harris ED Jr, Ruddy S, et al (eds): Textbook of Rheumatology, 5th ed. Philadelphia, WB Saunders, 1997, p 1177. *In-depth review of the inflammatory myopathies.*

Wortmann RL: Inflammatory muscle disease. *In* Weisman M, Weinblatt M (eds): Drug Therapy for the Rheumatic Diseases. Philadelphia, WB Saunders, 1994. *Current status of treatments used.*

297 THE AMYLOID DISEASES

Louis W. Heck

DEFINITION. Amyloidosis is not one clinical entity but a group of diverse, structurally driven protein deposition diseases. They are similar in that protein deposition occurs extracellularly and these deposits stain eosinophilic with standard tissue histologic stains, bind Congo red dye, and emit an apple-green birefringence when examined under polarized light microscopy; they also exhibit metachromasia with crystal violet and have an array of 75- to 100-Å non-branching fibrils by electron microscopy and a twisted, β-pleated sheet, antiparallel configuration by x-ray crystallography. They differ, however, in the biochemical nature of the proteinaceous deposits, the "etiology" of the associated diseases (neoplastic, inflammatory, degenerative, hereditary), the tropism of protein deposition, and the spectrum of disease manifestations. Thus amyloidosis is not a single disease but a variety of diseases ranging from asymptomatic conditions with focal deposits discovered as an incidental finding to generalized involvement with severe multiorgan failure.

Before the early 1970s, all amyloid deposits were thought to be chemically identical despite the clinical observations that systemic amyloidosis occurred in certain patients with either plasma cell myeloma or diverse chronic inflammatory states such as tuberculosis, osteomyelitis, rheumatoid arthritis, ankylosing spondylitis, and Crohn's disease. The major breakthrough in the physicochemical characterization of amyloid proteins resulted from the discovery that many of the non-amyloid proteins in amyloid-laden tissue could be extracted with physiologic saline and the insoluble amyloid fibrils solubilized by using dilute aqueous solutions and/or chaotropic agents such as urea and guanidine, isolated by column chromatography, and biochemically defined by amino acid sequence analyis. By studying amyloid-laden tissues and using the aforementioned techniques, many different amyloid proteins and precursor proteins associated with clinical syndromes or specific diseases have been identified (Table 297–1).

All the monomeric amyloidogenic proteins have a β-pleated sheet conformation in solution, and many have been demonstrated to form insoluble β-pleated sheet fibrils in vitro. The known properties of tissue amyloid deposits such as binding to Congo red, resistance to proteolysis, and insolubility in physiologic solutions are directly attributed to the periodic β-pleated sheet motif. The formation of β-pleated sheets in vivo is an extremely complex process involving crucial ion concentrations and hydrogen bonding between many similar monomeric polypeptide chains at high focal concentrations, as well as molecular interactions with the myriad extracellular matrix components. Furthermore, most amyloid deposits contain P component, an acute-phase circulating serum protein.

No clinical classification of the amyloidoses is satisfactory. One method is to consider three major systemic forms—AA, AL, and ATTR; two major localized forms—Aβ_2 and Aβ; and several miscellaneous forms (see Table 297–1). Each form has many clinical features.

PATHOGENESIS AND CLINICAL MANIFESTATIONS. PRIMARY (AL) AMYLOIDOSIS. AL amyloid was the first amyloid protein defined biochemically and shown to be identical to the variable region of immunoglobulin light chain (Bence Jones protein). AL amyloidosis is the most common of the systemic amyloidoses in the United States and is associated with plasma cell myeloma (20%) or plasma cell dyscrasias (80%), with involvement of skin and subcutaneous tissue, nerve, liver, spleen, heart, kidney, and lung. In a large retrospective series of patients with AL protein, approximately 50% had initial symptoms of fatigue and weight loss; less frequent symptoms included peripheral edema, dyspnea, paresthesias, lightheadedness, hoarseness, purpura, and bone pain (usually related to bone lesions in plasma cell myeloma). The initial physical findings revealed a palpable liver and peripheral edema in one third of the patients. Orthostatic hypotension, purpura, macroglossia, a palpable spleen, skin papules, ecchymoses, and lymphadenopathy were found less commonly. The signs and symptoms result from amyloid infiltration of organs and tissues with subsequent dysfunction. Examples of syndromes include those related to nerve tissue such as carpal tunnel syndrome, peripheral neuropathy with paresthesias of the fingers and toes, and sympathetic dysfunction manifested by orthostatic hypotension, impotence, sweating abnormalities, and gastrointestinal disturbances secondary to autonomic nerve involvement; other syndromes include those related to congestive heart failure and characterized by either

Table 297–1 ■ NOMENCLATURE AND CLASSIFICATION OF THE AMYLOIDOSES, 1990

	AMYLOID PROTEIN	CLINICAL STATE(S)	MAJOR ORGAN/TISSUE INVOLVEMENT*
Major systemic amyloidoses	1. AA	1. Chronic inflammatory conditions	K, L, S, GI, Sc
		a. Infectious: tuberculosis, osteomyelitis, etc.	H, unusual
		b. Non-infectious: juvenile rheumatoid arthritis, ankylosing spondylitis, Crohn's disease, etc.	N, rare
		2. Familial Mediterranean fever	
	2. AL	Plasma cell dyscrasia	H, L, S, T
		10% multiple myeloma/macroglobulemia	N, GI, Sc
		90% idiopathic; "primary"	
	3. ATTR	Various familial polyneuropathies and cardiomyopathies	N, H, K, E, GI, Sc
Major localized amyloidoses	4. Aβ_2M	Chronic dialysis usually longer than 8 yr	B, Sy, Ts
	5. Aβ	1. Alzheimer's disease	
		2. Down syndrome	
		3. Hereditary cerebral hemorrhage, Dutch	C, CV
		4. Non-traumatic cerebral hemorrhage of the elderly	
Miscellaneous amyloidoses	6. A Apo AI	Familial polyneuropathy, Iowa	N, K
	7. A Gel	Familial amyloidosis, Finnish	CN, E, skin
	8. A Cys	Hereditary cerebral hemorrhage, Icelandic	C, CV
	9. A Scr	Creutzfeldt-Jakob disease	C
	10. A Cal	Medullary carcinoma of the thyroid	Th
	11. AANF	Atrial amyloid	H
	12. AIAPP	Diabetes mellitus, insulinomas	P

*B = bone; C = cerebrum; CN = cranial nerves; CV = cerebral vessels; E = eye; GI = gastrointestinal; H = heart; K = kidney; L = liver; N = nerve; P = pancreas; S = spleen; Sc = subcutaneous tissue; T = tongue; Th = thyroid; Ts = tenosynovium; Sy = synovium.

predominantly right-sided failure with restrictive cardiomyopathy (see Chapter 64) secondary to stiff noncompliant ventricles and a thick intraventricular septum (multiple discrete 3- to 5-mm highly refractile echoes with a "speckled" pattern on two-dimensional echocardiography) or, rarely, a dilated cardiomyopathy with biventricular failure. Both forms may be associated with conduction disturbances. Renal involvement consisting of albuminuria, full expression of the nephrotic syndrome (see Chapter 106), and slow progressive renal failure may be seen. Finally, ecchymoses and "pinch purpura" may result from minor skin trauma caused by increased fragility from amyloid infiltration of the small blood vessels.

SECONDARY (AA) AMYLOIDOSIS. AA amyloidosis was the 2nd systemic type of amyloidosis shown to be due to protein deposition—in this case the precursor protein is a serum component (serum amyloid A) synthesized in the liver that may increase 100- to 200-fold following an inflammatory stimulus. Certain monocyte/macrophage cytokines such as interleukin-1 (IL-1), tumor necrosis factor, and IL-6 may up-regulate hepatic gene expression of this protein. Secondary amyloidosis usually involves the liver, spleen, and kidneys; heart involvement is less frequent than seen in primary amyloidosis, and nerve involvement is very infrequent. Some of the associated infectious diseases include osteomyelitis, tuberculosis, and bronchiectasis, and some of the non-infectious inflammatory states include rheumatoid arthritis, juvenile rheumatoid arthritis, ankylosing spondylitis, Crohn's disease, and familial Mediterranean fever. Curiously, the renal disease may be slow and indolent, with progressive proteinuria evolving into nephrotic syndrome and persisting for 5 to 10 years before end-stage renal disease. In Europe, renal amyloidosis has been reported as the major cause of death in patients with juvenile rheumatoid arthritis, but this associated complication has not been seen in the United States. Another interesting observation is that AA may be resorbed in vivo, as manifested by reduction of an enlarged liver or spleen or reduction in proteinuria without defined treatment of the underlying disorder. Finally, the successful use of colchicine to reduce the attacks and development of amyloidosis in patients with familial Mediterranean fever, decrease proteinuria, and improve renal function in some cases mandates that AA be considered carefully and ruled out in all amyloid patients.

FAMILIAL (ATTR) AMYLOIDOSIS. ATTR amyloidosis was the 3rd systemic amyloidosis to be defined and shown to be associated with the presence of an abnormal plasma pre-albumin protein that normally functions to transport thyroxine and retinol-binding protein and was subsequently termed *transthyretin*. It was originally defined as an autosomal dominantly inherited peripheral neuropathy (see Chapter 500) occurring in middle to late life that was progressive over the next several decades with additional autonomic neuropathy and variable organ involvement, primarily in Portuguese patients. Subsequently, many clinical manifestations defining different kindreds in Europe and the United States have resulted from mutations (greater than 50) in the gene for transthyretin; amino acid substitutions in this transport molecule have been associated with variable amyloid infiltration in the heart, bowel, and kidney. A recent report has defined an increased prevalence of late-onset cardiac amyloidosis in elderly blacks with variant-sequence transthyretin (isoleucine 122).

DIALYSIS-RELATED (β_2-MICROGLOBULIN) AMYLOIDOSIS ($A\beta_2M$). This localized amyloidosis occurs in most patients undergoing maintenance hemodialysis or peritoneal dialysis for longer than 8 years and is due to the deposition of β_2-microglobulin amyloid in periarticular, joint, bone, and carpal tunnel tissue. Some of the rheumatic complaints/findings include chronic shoulder pain with tenderness over the subacromial bursae, pain and swelling of the wrist and finger joints, proliferative tenosynovium over the wrist extensor tendons, and radiographic evidence of subchondral erosions of the carpal bones, femur, and humerus. Pathologic fractures of the humerus and femur have been described.

β_2-Microglobulin is the non-covalently associated chain of class I major histocompatibility complex molecules and is present on virtually all human nucleated cells. Catabolism of this small protein depends on normal kidney filtration and excretion. In dialysis patients and those with end-stage renal disease, plasma levels of β_2-microglobulin are elevated. Efforts to effectively remove this protein with conventional dialysis membranes of cellulose acetate or cuprophane have not been successful because of poor protein clearance. Furthermore, these membranes induce complement activation and generation of IL-1, which may result in β_2-microglobulin accumulation.

β-PROTEIN (ALZHEIMER'S DISEASE) AMYLOIDOSIS. Alzheimer's disease, the most common cause of dementia in elderly patients, afflicts 5 to 10% of the population older than 65 years (see Chapter 449). In neuropathologic studies of the brains of patients with Alzheimer's disease, neurofibrillary tangles and neuritic plaques are frequently found in the amygdala, hippocampus, and frontal, temporal, and parietal lobes. In addition, acellular thickening of the small and medium-sized arteries of the leptomeninges and cerebral cortex have been seen in aged patients and those with Alzheimer's disease. By standard histologic techniques, the amorphous material in the walls of meningeal vessels and the central region of neuritic plaques has the characteristic staining property for amyloid. The chemical nature of both amyloid deposits has been identified as a novel 40–amino acid protein (β-protein) that is generated by proteolysis of a much larger transmembrane glycoprotein termed "β-amyloid precursor protein." In some forms of familial Alzheimer's disease, point mutations have resulted in single–amino acid substitutions in this precursor protein. Recent studies have reported that most patients with late-onset sporadic Alzheimer's disease have a strong association of ApoE$_4$ alleles and Aβ deposits within the cerebrum and cerebral vessels, which suggests the possibility that bimolecular complexes between ApoE$_4$ and Aβ may be important in the extracellular deposition and formation of cerebral amyloid.

There is evidence that cerebrovascular deposition of β-protein amyloid is an important etiology of non-traumatic/non-hypertensive brain hemorrhage in the elderly, usually manifested as cerebral lobe hemorrhage involving the cortex and subcortical white matter. In addition, a familial syndrome defined in a Dutch kindred in which certain family members died in their 40s or 50s of cerebral hemorrhage (hereditary cerebral hemorrhage with amyloidosis, Dutch type) has been shown to be due to an amino acid substitution in the protein.

CLINICAL MANIFESTATIONS. The signs and symptoms suggestive of the amyloidoses result directly from tissue/organ infiltration with subsequent dysfunction. As can be seen in Table 297–1, multiple organ involvement is common but variable in degree, which necessitates formulating a list of differential diagnoses to exclude other localized or systemic diseases. For example, carpal tunnel syndrome is a common clinical entity that is seen very frequently in patients undergoing hemodialysis for longer than 8 to 10 years; it is due to $A\beta_2M$ deposition in the tenosynovium of the carpal tunnel. Such deposition is also commonly found in the AL and ATTR forms and in non-amyloid diseases such as hypothyroidism, rheumatoid arthritis, and diabetes mellitus. Thus many disorders must be considered and subsequently excluded. The AA, AL, and ATTR forms may be associated with significant proteinuria or nephrotic syndrome, and many primary glomerular diseases must be excluded. The AL and ATTR forms may also be the cause of vexing unexplained congestive heart failure with cardiomyopathy in patients who have had repeated heart catheterization and coronary angiography without a clear answer. Clues to cardiac amyloidosis may be present on the standard 12-lead electrocardiogram and include decreased QRS voltage, first-degree atrioventricular block with intraventricular conduction defects, and Q waves in precordial leads V$_1$ to V$_3$ (pseudoinfarction); findings of a "speckled" pattern of intraventricular septum/myocardium on two-dimensional echocardiography also provide clues to cardiac amyloidosis. Peripheral neuropathies may be the initial and dominant expression primarily in the ATTR and other familial forms (see Table 297–1). Generally, the onset of symptoms occurs in early middle age (30 to 40 years old) in the lower extremity, with progressive sensorimotor involvement including the proximal and truncal sensory nerves. Foot ulcers with secondary infections may occur. An autonomic neuropathy with orthostatic hypotension, impotence, and diminished peristalsis with pseudo-obstruction, diarrhea, or malabsorption may be present. Gastrointestinal bleeding and/or perforation may be associated with amyloid infiltration of the lamina propria and submucosal blood vessels. Often, many interacting variables come into play; for example, orthostatic hypotension in an amyloid patient may result from the combination of restrictive cardiomyopathy with diastolic dysfunction, diminished intravascular volume, and sympathetic dysfunction.

Two uncommon syndromes may be easily confused with amyloidosis. The POEMS syndrome (polyneuropathy, organomegaly, endocrinopathy, monoclonal gammopathy, skin findings) (see Chapter 244) is a plasma cell dyscrasia with a constellation of diverse features similar to the systemic/localized amyloid syndrome, but no amyloid deposits have been described in these patients. Immunotactoid glomerulopathy (fibrillary renal deposits) is characterized by progressive proteinuria, microscopic hematuria, and hypertension. Renal biopsy tissue has variable glomerular deposits containing IgG, IgM, C3, C4, and λ and κ light chains (immunotactoid). On electron microscopy, fibrillary material is deposited within the mesangium and capillary walls and can be differentiated from typical amyloid fibrils in that the fibrils are thicker and do not stain with Congo red.

DIAGNOSIS. The diagnosis is made by detecting amyloid deposits in tissue preparations stained with Congo red; polarized light microscopy discloses an apple-green birefringence. If a patient is suspected of having one of the systemic amyloidoses (AL, AA, ATTR), aspiration and staining of abdominal subcutaneous fat tissue should be performed and can be done rapidly and safely at the bedside. Fat tissue is obtained with a 16-gauge needle fixed to a 20- to 30-mL syringe—repeated movement of the needle with gentle pulling of the syringe barrel to produce negative pressure is done to obtain fragments of the fatty tissue. The fatty fluid and fragments are placed on alcohol-cleaned glass slides, air-dried, and submitted for Congo red staining. Because variable false-negative results have been reported, repeat biopsy of the subcutaneous tissue or an alternative site such as the rectal mucosa is warranted. The redundant mucosal folds (valves of Houston) may be visualized directly and tissue (including the vascular submucosa) obtained by pincer forceps with bleeding controlled by cautery. Other biopsy sites include carpal tunnel tissue, kidney, sural nerve, heart (endomyocardial biopsy of the right ventricle), bone, and synovium. Staining of amyloid deposits in the synovial fluid of patients with the AL and $A\beta_2M$ forms has been described. In general, biopsy of the liver should be avoided because of the risk of bleeding. Attempts to define the chemical amyloid type should be made. For example, specific antisera to λ and κ light chains, serum amyloid A, β_2-microglobulin, and transthyretin are commercially available to stain the tissue via immunofluorescent or immunoperoxidase methods.

In patients with suspected AL amyloidosis with or without myeloma, agarose gel electrophoresis of serum and concentrated urine may be done easily. The monoclonal paraprotein is separated from other serum components by electrophoresis; interacted with separate antisera to λ and κ light chains, IgM, IgA, and IgG (immunofixation); and identified by protein staining. Bone marrow aspiration and biopsy are usually done to quantify the number of plasma cells, which can be stained for amyloid. Scintigraphy using radiolabeled P component, which binds to all amyloid types, remains experimental and cannot be justified as a screening or routine test.

TREATMENT. AL amyloidosis is treated with chemotherapy as a plasma cell neoplasm, even though only 10 to 20% of patients have plasma cell myeloma. Some have used a treatment protocol of melphalan, 0.15 mg/kg/day in two divided doses, and prednisone, 0.8 mg/kg/day in four divided doses. The duration of each treatment is 7 days, with repeated cycles every 6 weeks. Diuretics may be necessary to treat fluid retention. Every patient with AL amyloidosis should be given a trial with this regimen, even though the response rate is disappointingly low at approximately 20%. However, dramatic resolution of multiorgan dysfunction/amyloid infiltration with cyclic prednisone and melphalan treatment has been reported.

Newer treatments involving dose-intensive melphalan therapy with either allogeneic bone marrow transplantation or autologous growth factor–mobilized blood stem cells have been performed in a few patients with AL amyloid; complete remission of the plasma cell dyscrasia and organ-specific disease was noted after a 1-year follow-up. Clearly, further long-term studies need to be done to assess efficacy.

Successful prevention and treatment of the amyloidosis of familial Mediterranean fever with low-dose colchicine, 0.6 mg once or twice daily, have been dramatic developments in the treatment of AA amyloidosis. If the amyloidosis is related to an infectious process such as tuberculosis, it must be defined and treated aggressively. Likewise, any non-infectious inflammatory condition should be treated and patients given colchicine concomitantly.

Since 1993, several hundred patients have received liver transplants for the treatment of ATTR amyloidosis; the abnormal transthyretin protein in the blood disappeared, and the severity of neuropathy improved in some patients. However, guidelines for hepatic transplatation have not been defined and results of long-term outcome have not been published.

$A\beta_2M$ is a very common localized amyloidosis that is thought to result from poor clearance of β_2-microglobulin by conventional dialysis membranes, with subsequently high levels of this protein in serum and tissues enhancing fibril formation. A new group of synthetic high-flux, highly permeable dialysis membranes (polycarbonate, polymethylmethacrylate, polyacrylonitrile) are currently available but very expensive. Long-term studies are necessary to determine whether these new synthetic membranes will prevent dialysis-related $A\beta_2M$ amyloidosis.

No preventive therapy for Alzheimer's disease is currently available. Research is currently being performed to understand the the role of ApoE-Aβ complexes in the formation of neuritic plaques.

Benson MD: Amyloidosis: *In* Beaudet AL, Scriver CR, Sly WS (eds): The Metabolic Basis of Inherited Disease. New York, McGraw-Hill, 1994. *A superb review of amyloidosis focusing primarily on the ATTR forms.*

Falk RH, Comenzo RL, Skinner M: The systemic amyloidoses. N Engl J Med 337: 898, 1997. *A review of the clinical features of AL, AA, and ATTR amyloid and recent progress in pathogenesis and new treatments of these disorders.*

Jacobson DR, Pastore RD, et al: Variant-sequence transthyretin (isoleucine 122) in late-onset cardiac amyloidosis in black Americans. N Engl J Med 336:466, 1997. *A newly described senile cardiac amyloidosis primarily in older blacks that is underrecognized.*

298 BEHÇET'S DISEASE

Eugene V. Ball

Behçet's disease is idiopathic and multisystemic and can closely resemble sarcoidosis. Its symptoms appear insidiously, one by one, or dramatically and involve several organs. They commonly wax and wane. Although no invariable symptom of Behçet's disease can be found, certain symptoms occur often enough to define the syndrome and serve as the basis for diagnostic criteria. One set of criteria in common use requires the presence of recurrent oral ulcers and any two of the following: genital ulcers, uveitis, cutaneous or large vessel inflammation, arthritis, and meningoencephalitis. An "incomplete" form has been defined as recurrent aphthous ulcers and any one of the other features. Although oral ulcers are the linchpin of diagnostic criteria, a diagnosis of probable Behçet's disease is tenable when several of these symptoms occur together in the absence of aphthous ulcers and when other known causes can be excluded. Diagnosis has been possible in some patients only after as many as 20 years of minor symptoms. No laboratory tests are diagnostic.

CLINICAL MANIFESTATIONS. Table 298–1 lists manifestations of the disease in one group of 60 patients. Constitutional signs such as fever and weight loss were noted in 63%. At least 24 patients from Mediterranean areas have had both Behçet's disease and secondary (AA) amyloidosis.

Painful oral ulcers are round or oval and usually multiple. Recur-

Table 298–1 ■ **MAJOR MANIFESTATIONS OF BEHÇET'S DISEASE**

MANIFESTATION	PREVALENCE (%)
Mouth ulcers	97
Genital ulcers	83
Uveitis	48
Joint pain	48
Phlebitis	17

rent oral ulcers may be the only sign of Behçet's disease; for example, of 67 patients with recurrent ulcers only who were monitored in a Behçet's disease clinic in Korea, other signs of the disease eventually developed in 52%. On the other hand, isolated genital ulcers are seldom indicative of Behçet's disease. Ulcers occur elsewhere on the skin, and an assortment of non-ulcerative skin lesions can be found such as erythema, erythema nodosum, photosensitivity, and spontaneous pustules. The pustular reaction of the skin to intradermal needle prick (sometimes referred to as "pathergy") was once thought to be pathognomonic of Behçet's disease, but this reaction occurs in no more than 70% of patients, usually in those with extensive disease. In a group of 85 Saudi patients, the pathergy test was positive in only 15 (17.6%). Furthermore, it is non-specific in that it was positive in 7% of one group of healthy control subjects.

Eye involvement is common: 10 to 15% of cases of acquired blindness among Japanese are thought to be due to the uveoretinitis of Behçet's disease, which is characterized by waves of repeated attacks and spontaneous improvement. Decreased visual acuity results from retinal veno-occlusive disease, inflammation with secondary glaucoma, cataracts, or vitreous hemorrhage; retinal vein thrombosis leading to sudden blindness is not rare.

As many as a quarter of all patients will have phlebitis or arteritis predisposing to thrombosis and aneurysms; for example, 10% of a group of 450 Tunisians had arterial aneurysms, large artery occlusions, or both. Thromboses occur in almost any vessel, including the superior vena cava, and Behçet's disease was found in 7 of 44 patients with cavernous transformation of the portal vein. Aneurysms are particularly common in pulmonary arteries and are most often single, but as many as 14 have occurred in 1 patient in less than 1 year. Pulmonary arteritis produces dyspnea, chest pain, cough or hemoptysis and is a significant cause of death. Its radiographic signs include scattered infiltrates and pleural effusions.

The arthritis of Behçet's disease is usually intermittent, self-limited, and localized to the knees and ankles; however, bone erosions have been observed in hip, heel, wrist, knee, ankle, and foot radiographs.

Aseptic meningitis and transverse myelitis are common in neurologic Behçet's disease; other manifestations include encephalopathy, seizures, bulbar palsy, ataxia, transient ischemic attacks, strokes, and pseudotumor cerebri. These complications may be acute or gradual in onset and cause persistent neuropathies or death, or they may resolve completely. Focal intracranial abnormalities are detected by imaging studies.

Small and large ulcers in the gut produce symptoms of inflammatory bowel disease and perforation and are more common in Japanese than in Turkish patients.

PREVALENCE. Behçet's disease is rare in the Americas and Europe. It is more prevalent—and more virulent—in Turkey and the Middle and Far East. Evidence of Behçet's disease was found in 19 of 1531 persons aged 10 or older in a field survey conducted in rural Turkey. On Hokkaido, Japan, its estimated prevalence was 1 in 1000 persons, but Behçet's disease is less common in ethnic Japanese living in Hawaii. Its prevalence was estimated at 1 in 25,000 in Olmsted County, Minnesota.

GENETICS AND PATHOLOGY. Although not considered hereditary, Behçet's disease was present in members of four HLA-B51–positive families. HLA-B51, a split antigen of HLA-B5, has been detected in 51% of patients with Behçet's disease versus 16% of control subjects in Japan and in 62% with the disease versus 29% of control subjects in Iraq. The HLA-B5101 allele of B51 was found in all 46 HLA–B51-positive Japanese patients with Behçet's disease; 80% of 31 Greek patients were also B5101 positive.

The histopathologic characteristics of Behçet's disease are non-specific. Despite its classification as a vasculitis, fibrinoid necrosis of vessels is not usually apparent. Mononuclear cells, found in the epidermis and around small vessels in early lesions, are later replaced by neutrophils and plasma cells. Arteritis, which may be catastrophic, is due to inflammation of the vasa vasorum. Many of the attributes of autoimmune disease are missing, and abnormalities of the immune system have been found inconsistently, thus providing few clues to the cause and pathogenesis of Behçet's disease. Experiments showing the induction of uveitis in Lewis rats by heat shock protein T-cell peptide epitopes specific for T lymphocytes from subjects with Behçet's disease offer some support for the view that peptide T-cell determinants may be involved in neutrophil hyperfunction and the pathogenesis of Behçet's disease.

TREATMENT. Treatment is based on symptoms, and the spontaneous ebb and flow of these make treatment evaluation difficult. For example, pentoxifylline has been advocated as treatment of uveitis, but improvement in the few reported patients may have been spontaneous. More conventional treatment of eye disease has included colchicine, corticosteroids, azathioprine, cyclosporine, and laser photocoagulation. Corticosteroids are given for life-threatening complications, although in general the response to these drugs is disappointing. Allowing for proscriptions against its use in women of childbearing age, thalidomide appears to be particularly useful in the treatment of mucocutaneous ulcers. Interferon-α and -γ have been advocated for arthritis and mucocutaneous lesions, and, on the assumption that streptococcal antigens may play a role in pathogenesis, benzathine penicillin has been used for the latter. Thromboses are treated with anticoagulants, and arterial aneurysms may require surgical treatment or embolization. Specialty sources should be consulted for details of treatment.

Akman-Demir G, Baykan-Kurt B, Serdaroglu P, et al: Seven year follow-up of neurologic involvement in Behçet syndrome. Arch Neurol 53:691, 1996. *Fifteen patients with neuro-Behçets were re-evaluated 7 years after the appearance of neurologic signs; the course was stationary in 7 and progressive in 8. The 3 deaths emphasize the investigators' conclusions that neuro-Behçets is less favorable than had been thought.*

Hamurydan V, Mat C, Saip S, et al: Thalidomide in the treatment of the mucocutaneous lesions of the Behçet syndrome. Ann Intern Med 128:443, 1998. *Thalidomide was moderately effective in suppressing ulcers, follicular lesions, and erythema nodosum; however, polyneuropathy was detected in 6.3% of treated patients.*

Mizuki N, Inoko H, Ando H, et al: Behçet's disease associated with one of the HLA-B51 subantigens, HLA-B*5101. Am J Ophthalmol 116:406, 1993. *Of three HLA-B51 alleles, only B05101 was found in 46 HLA-B51–positive Behçet's patients.*

Nussenblatt RB: Uveitis in Behçet's disease. Int J Immunol 14:67, 1997. *An authoritative review of the manifestations of uveitis and its treatment.*

299 GOUT AND URIC ACID METABOLISM

Michael S. Hershfield

Gout refers to the *inflammatory arthritis* induced by microscopic *crystals* of monosodium urate monohydrate and to the pathognomonic deposition of aggregated monosodium urate crystals (*tophi*) in various tissues and some organs. Chronic *hyperuricemia* is necessary for the development of gout, although not sufficient. *Urolithiasis* (renal stones composed of uric acid) may accompany gout or occur independently when renal urate excretion is excessive. Gout is chiefly a disease of adult men. It is mostly *idiopathic* and multifactorial in etiology. A few rare, inherited metabolic disorders markedly enhance urate production, with urolithiasis and gout as primary manifestations. Other genetic and acquired disorders and some drugs cause secondary hyperuricemia and gout by impairing renal urate excretion or by indirectly increasing urate production (Table 299–1).

If untreated, gout can lead to painful, destructive arthropathy, and urolithiasis can lead to renal failure. Correcting hyperuricemia and hyperuricosuria prevents these consequences and is achievable in most cases. However, because neither gout nor renal insufficiency will develop in most hyperuricemic individuals and because therapy is not without risk and expense, *asymptomatic hyperuricemia* per se generally does not require therapy; observation and in some cases a search for a contributing, treatable disease are warranted.

PREVALENCE AND INCIDENCE. Surveys made in the 1960s estimated the prevalence of gout at about 0.5 to 0.7% for men and about 0.1% for women. The prevalence has been increasing over the past two decades. Gout is the most common inflammatory arthritis in men older than 40 years in the United States. A 1986 U.S. Health Interview Survey estimated 2.2 million cases of self-reported gout, about twice the physician-reported prevalence.

Table 299–1 ■ CLASSIFICATION OF HYPERURICEMIA AND GOUT

TYPE	DISTURBANCE IN URIC ACID, PURINE METABOLISM	INHERITANCE
Primary		
I. Idiopathic (>99% of primary gout)		
A. Normal urinary excretion (80–90% of primary gout)	Decreased renal clearance ± overproduction of urate	Polygenic
B. Increased urinary excretion (10–20% of primary gout)	Overproduction ± decreased renal clearance of urate	Polygenic
II. Due to specific inherited metabolic defects (>1% of primary gout)		
A. PP-ribose-P synthase overactivity	Increased de novo purine synthesis	X-linked
B. Hypoxanthine-guanine phosphoribosyltransferase deficiency	Impaired purine salvage + increased de novo purine synthesis	X-linked
Secondary		
I. Glucose-6-phosphatase deficiency	Increased catabolism of adenine nucleotides + secondary increase in purine synthesis de novo	Autosomal recessive
II. Chronic hemolysis; erythroid, myeloid, and lymphoid proliferative disorders	Increased cell and nucleic acid turnover	—
III. Renal mechanisms		
A. Familial progressive renal insufficiency	Reduced renal functional mass and various defects in renal tubular function	Variable
B. Acquired chronic renal insufficiency	Reduced renal functional mass	—
C. Drugs (diuretics, cyclosporine, toxins, including lead)	Inhibited urate secretion or enhanced reabsorption	—
D. Endogenous metabolic products (lactate, ketoacids, β-hydroxybutyrate)	Inhibited urate secretion	—

PP-ribose-P = phosphoribosylpyrosphosphate.

As Hippocrates observed, gout rarely occurs before puberty in males and seldom before menopause in females. Serum urate values are consistent with this pattern. In normal children of both sexes, serum urate averages 3.6 mg/dL. Levels rise at puberty, more so in males than in females. In the United States, the central 95% segment of the serum urate distribution ranges from 2.2 to 7.5 mg/dL in adult men and from 2.1 to 6.6 mg/dL in adult premenopausal women. Serum urate values increase with age; after menopause, mean values in women approach levels in men. Epidemiologic surveys have noted a trend toward increasing serum urate values in the United States in recent decades and significant variations among population groups, which is a reflection of genetic and environmental factors. Obesity, alcohol consumption, and diuretic use are associated with hyperuricemia.

The incidence of gout increases with the degree and duration of hyperuricemia; age, obesity, hypertension, and alcohol intake show much weaker relationships when serum urate is factored out. Although lower levels are occasionally found during an attack, serum urate exceeds 7 mg/dL at some time in virtually all patients with gout. Nevertheless, the risk of gout is modest, even at higher serum urate levels. Among about 2000 initially healthy white males monitored over a 15-year period, annual incidence rates for gout were 0.1% at less than 7 mg/dL, 0.5% at 7.0 to 8.9 mg/dL, and 4.9% at ≥9 mg/dL. At levels over 9 mg/dL (the highest 1.8% of values observed), the cumulative incidence of gout after 5 years was 22%. Incidence rates were about three-fold higher for hypertensive men than for normotensive men in all age groups because of the hyperuricemic effect of diuretics. The incidence of gout was about two-fold greater among black than white male physicians monitored for 26 to 34 years after graduation from medical school; this difference was partly explained by a greater incidence of hypertension among the blacks.

PATHOGENESIS AND PATHOLOGY. Serum urate levels are low and gout is nonexistent in species that possess urate oxidase (*uricase*), which converts urate to allantoin, a more soluble and efficiently excreted compound. Mutational inactivation of the uricase gene occurred during evolution of *Homo sapiens* and several hominoid species. From this perspective, *hyperuricemia* in humans is due to an inborn error of urate catabolism. Urate (in solution) may be of benefit as a scavenger of reactive oxygen species, including peroxynitrite derived from nitric oxide and superoxide. Because gout is caused by urate crystals rather than urate in solution, "hyperuricemia" is defined by the solubility of urate in body fluids, not by statistical distributions of urate levels. Producing more urate than can be disposed of or maintained in solution over time leads to extracellular deposition of monosodium urate crystals. Urate solubility is much lower at the temperature of peripheral joints (about 32° C in the knee and 29° C in the ankle). Gout ensues when an inflammatory response is triggered.

URATE PRODUCTION AND ELIMINATION. The total-body urate pool, with which sodium urate in plasma is miscible, is determined by rates of uric acid production and disposal and is expanded in patients with gout (Table 299–2A). Urate arises from the action of *xanthine oxidase* on its substrates, the purine bases hypoxanthine

Table 299–2 ■ URIC ACID PRODUCTION AND ELIMINATION

A. URATE KINETICS	MILLIGRAMS (mmol)
Total miscible pool	1200 (7.2)
Daily turnover	600–900 (3.6–5.4)
Daily production	750 (4.5)
Daily intestinal uricolysis	100–365 (0.6–2.2)
Daily urinary excretion	500–1000 (3–6) on normal diet
	420 ± 75 (2.5 ± 0.5) on a purine-restricted diet

B. RENAL CLEARANCE (FOUR-COMPONENT, BIDIRECTIONAL TRANSPORT MODEL)	RELATIVE AMOUNT
1. *Glomerular filtration* • Complete • ↓ By diuretics, renal failure	100
2. *Tubular reabsorption* • Active, linked to Na⁺ reabsorption • Inhibited by *uricosuric drugs:* probenecid, sulfinpyrazone, benzbromarone, high-dose aspirin (>2 g/d)	98–100
3. *Tubular secretion* • Active process • Inhibited by agents that cause *hyperuricemia:* pyrazinamide, low-dose aspirin, lactate, β-hydroxybutyrate, branched-chain keto acids	50
4. *Post-secretory reabsorption*	40–44
Net clearance	6–10

Note. Gouty individuals have shown enlarged urate pools and in some cases increased urate turnover. Daily urinary excretion of uric acid is an index of urate production, provided that renal function is normal. About 10% of patients with idiopathic gout are "urate overexcretors," defined as a daily urinary excretion exceeding the normal mean + 2 SD (i.e., >600 mg on a purine-restricted diet or >800 mg on an ordinary diet).

and xanthine (Fig. 299–1). Dietary purines are largely degraded to urate by catabolic enzymes located in the intestinal epithelium, including xanthine oxidase. Purine restriction can modestly reduce serum urate by 0.6 to 1.8 mg/dL, but variation in absorption has not been implicated as a cause of hyperuricemia. Most urate is produced by hepatic xanthine oxidase acting on hypoxanthine and xanthine derived from nucleic acids of senescent cells and from the metabolic turnover of cellular purine nucleotides. The latter arise from two biosynthetic pathways termed "de novo" and "salvage" (or "reutilization") (see Fig. 299–1).

Most urate is eliminated by renal excretion (see Table 299–2B). About one third is degraded by bacteria in the gut, but bacterial degradation of urate increases substantially in renal insufficiency. Uricosuric agents act by blocking urate reabsorption, whereas other drugs and weak organic acids raise serum urate levels by blocking renal urate secretion (see Table 299–2B). The latter mechanism contributes to the hyperuricemia associated with fasting, alcohol metabolism, and ketoacidosis.

MECHANISMS OF HYPERURICEMIA. About 10% of patients with gout show evidence of urate overproduction, as indicated by uri-

nary excretion of uric acid exceeding the normal mean plus 2 SD (>600 mg per 24 hours on a purine-restricted diet, >800 mg on an ordinary diet). The highest overproduction occurs in patients with either of two rare inherited defects in the regulation of purine nucleotide synthesis, deficiency of the salvage enzyme hypoxanthine-guanine phosphoribosyltransferase and overactivity of phosphoribosylpyrophosphate synthetase (see Fig. 299–1).

In the majority of patients with idiopathic gout, renal function is normal, but reduced clearance of filtered urate results in hyperuricemia. No specific renal abnormality has been identified to account for this action. Urate excretion diminishes with the onset of renal insufficiency, but in general, gout is uncommon in patients with chronic renal failure. Several kindreds have been reported in which early-onset hyperuricemia, gout, and progressive renal failure (with or without hypertension) are linked (see Table 299–1). Chronic lead nephropathy, alcohol abuse, diuretics, and certain other drugs have been implicated in causing hyperuricemia and gout through renal mechanisms (see Tables 299–1 and 299–2B). In renal and

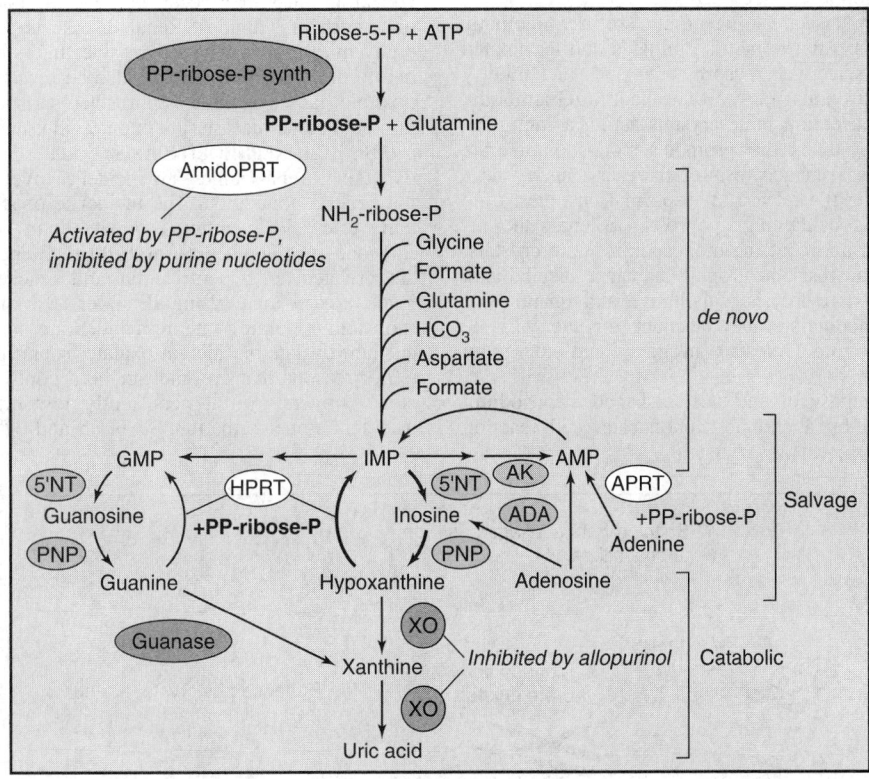

FIGURE 299–1 ■ Intracellular purine metabolism and the basis for "metabolic" hyperuricemia. In the "de novo" pathway, the purine ring (hypoxanthine) of inosinic acid (IMP) is constructed from precursors on a ribose-5'-phosphate backbone derived from phosphoribosylpyrophosphate (PP-ribose-P). At IMP the pathway branches and gives rise to adenosine monophosphate (AMP) and guanosine monophosphate (GMP) and their derivatives. In the *"salvage"* pathway, the pre-formed purine bases hypoxanthine, guanine, and adenine, derived from turnover of IMP, GMP, and AMP, are directly condensed with PP-ribose-P by hypoxine-guanine phosphoribosyltransferase (HPRT) and adenine phosphoribosyltransferase (APRT) to regenerate these ribonucleotides. Some of the hypoxanthine formed by nucleotide turnover is divereted to the liver and catabolized by xanthine oxidase (XO) to uric acid; the remainder is salvaged by HPRT.

Operation of the salvage pathway (the more economical in terms of energy required) reduces de novo activity because (1) HPRT and APRT have greater affinity for PP-ribose-P than amidophosphoribosyltransferase does AmidoPRT, the first committed enzyme of the de novo pathway, (2) base salvage lowers the concentration of PP-ribose-P and AmidoPRT is converted to an inactive form, and (3) the nucleotide end products of the HPRT and APRT reactions directly inhibit AmidoPRT. Allopurinol, by blocking XO, enhances salvage of hypoxanthine, further inhibiting de novo activity; this action reduces purine excretion more than expected from inhibition of uric acid formation alone.

Deficiency of HPRT causes an obligatory loss of all hypoxanthine and guanine as urate and also allows a compensatory increase in de novo pathway activity because of reduced formation of inhibitory nucleotides and increased concentration and availability of PP-ribose-P for the AmidoPRT reaction. In individuals with inherited "overactive" variants of PP-ribose-P synthase, increased formation of PP-ribose-P stimulates AmidoPRT and thereby markedly enhances de novo purine synthesis. The excess IMP formed is degraded to urate.

Increased nucleotide breakdown can cause hyperuricemia by increasing the production of XO substrates and by releasing inhibition of AmidoPRT. This mechanism has been implicated in the hyperuricemia and gout associated with glucose-6-phosphatase deficiency (glycogen storage disease type I): Glucose-6-phosphate accumulates at the expense of hepatic adenosine triphosphate (ATP), with degradation of AMP to urate. Hyperuricemia may occur acutely in various conditions that result in nucleotide catabolism: hypoxia, metabolism of some sugars, vigorous exercise in normal individuals, and moderate exercise in patients with metabolic myopathies. (5'NT = 5'-nucleotidase; PNP = purine nucleoside phosphorylase; ADA = adenosine deaminase; AK = adenosine kinase.)

cardiac transplant patients, the use of cyclosporine has been associated with severe hyperuricemia and accelerated development of gout.

Hyperuricemia and idiopathic gout are associated with both obesity and hypertriglyceridemia. In some gouty patients, weight reduction and abstinence from alcohol reverse the hypertriglyceridemia, hyperuricemia, and evidence of both overproduction and impaired renal clearance of urate.

MECHANISM OF THE ACUTE GOUTY ATTACK. The neutrophil is an essential mediator of acute inflammation in gout (Fig. 299–2). Ingestion of monosodium urate crystals causes neutrophils to release leukotrienes, interleukin-1, and the glycoprotein "crystal chemotactic factor"; these substances further amplify neutrophil infiltration into the involved joint. Activated neutrophils also produce superoxide and release lysosomal enzymes as a result of crystal-induced rupture of lysosomal membranes and cell lysis. The resulting cleavage of complement peptides and kinins from precursors induces pain, vasodilation, and vascular permeability. Released lysosomal and cytoplasmic enzymes, as well as collagenase and prostaglandins produced by joint mesenchymal cells, contribute to chronic articular destruction and tissue necrosis.

Extracellular urate crystals are often found in asymptomatic joints of gouty individuals. Attacks may be initiated and terminated by plasma proteins that selectively adsorb to crystals and modify their interaction with neutrophils. Early in an attack, IgG antibody, possibly induced by monosodium urate crystals acting as antigens, may serve as a nucleating agent that promotes monosodium urate crystallization and increases phagocytosis of these crystals by neutrophils, thereby enhancing the release of lysosomal enzymes. Late in an attack, lipoproteins containing apoprotein B enter the inflamed joint from plasma and coat the monosodium urate crystals; this action inhibits phagocytosis, neutrophil oxidative metabolism, superoxide production, and cytolysis. Qualitative and quantitative differences in protein modulators may account for the variable inflammatory response to urate crystals in gouty and non-gouty individuals.

TOPHI. A tophus is a deposit of fine, needle-shaped monosodium urate crystals surrounded by a chronic mononuclear cell reaction and a foreign body granuloma of epithelial and giant cells, which may be multinucleate (see Fig. 299–2). Tophi are commonly found in articular and other cartilage, synovia, tendon sheaths, bursae and other periarticular structures, epiphyseal bone, subcutaneous tissues, and the kidney interstitium.

When compared with an acute gouty attack, tophi evoke little inflammatory response and generally develop silently. In some gouty individuals, tophi may be detected radiographically in bone and articular cartilage but may be absent in subcutaneous tissues. In the joint, tophi gradually enlarge and cause degeneration of cartilage and subchondral bone, proliferation of synovium and marginal bone, and sometimes fibrous or bony ankylosis. The punched-out lesions of bone commonly seen on radiographs represent marrow tophi, which may communicate with the urate crust on the articular surface through defects in cartilage. In vertebral bodies, urate deposits involve the marrow spaces adjacent to the intervertebral disks.

THE GOUTY KIDNEY. Interstitial deposits of monosodium urate crystals in the medulla or pyramids, with surrounding mononuclear and giant cell reaction, are found commonly in gouty patients at autopsy and have been referred to as "urate nephropathy." Crystalline deposits of uric acid (not urate) within distal tubules and collecting ducts may occur and lead to dilatation and atrophy of the more proximal tubules. Renal disease is common in gout but generally mild and slowly progressive. Interstitial nephropathy may be due to urate deposits but can also be present in their absence. Other possible causes include nephrosclerosis secondary to hypertension, uric acid stone disease, infection, aging, and lead toxicity.

URIC ACID NEPHROLITHIASIS. About 10 to 25% of gouty patients experience renal stones, an incidence over 200-fold higher than in the general population. The incidence of stones exceeds 20% when daily uric acid excretion is greater than 700 mg (see Table 299–2A), and it is about 50% at 1100 mg. The prevalence of stones is also related to hyperuricemia and reaches 50% at serum urate levels greater than 12 mg/dL. Over 80% of the stones are uric acid (not sodium urate); the remainder are mixtures of uric acid and calcium oxalate or calcium oxalate or phosphate alone.

For reasons that are unclear, both gouty and non-gouty uric acid stone formers exhibit persistently low urinary pH, which favors uric acid stone formation. At pH 5 and 37° C, free uric acid has a

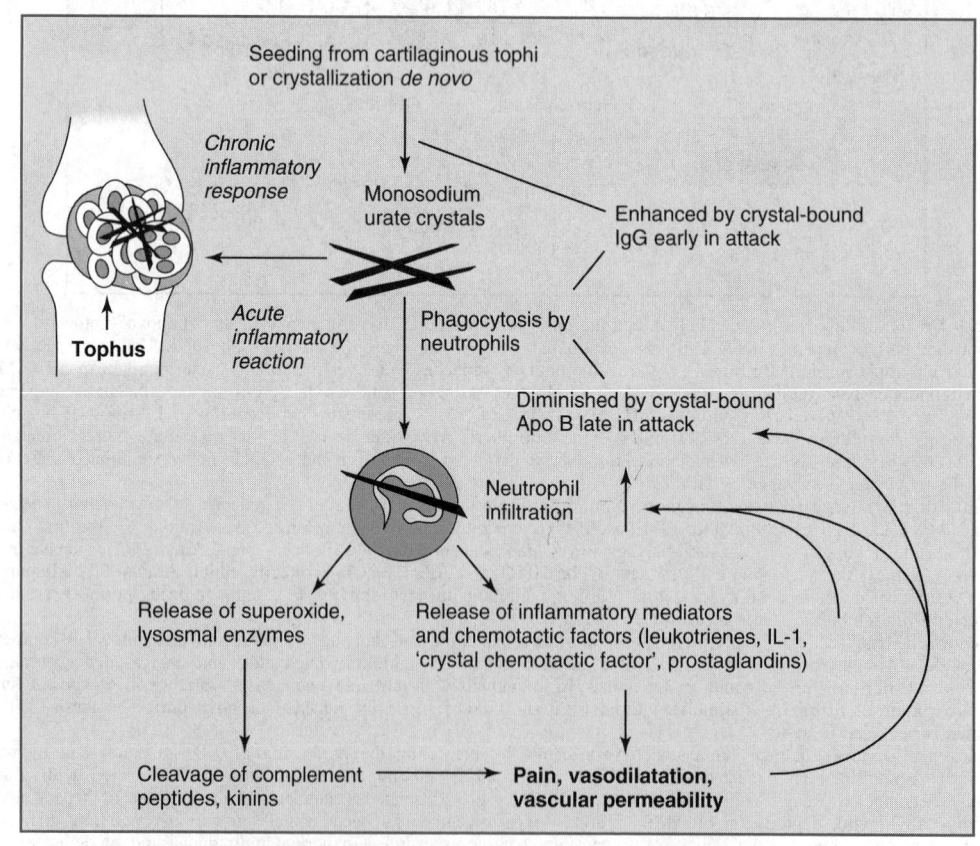

FIGURE 299–2 ■ Inflammatory responses to monosodium urate crystals.

solubility of only 15 mg/dL. Thus supersaturation is required to excrete an average uric acid load in a normal urine volume. The solubility increases more than 10-fold at pH 7 and more than 100-fold at pH 8.

CLINICAL MANIFESTATIONS. The peak age of onset of gout is about 45 years in men, by which time the average gouty male has been exposed to 20 or 30 years of asymptomatic hyperuricemia and to varying degrees of tissue urate deposition. In predisposed women, gout usually occurs some years after menopause, when they become hyperuricemic.

ACUTE GOUTY ARTHRITIS. Gout is usually initially manifested as a fulminating arthritic attack affecting the lower extremity. Over 75% of initial attacks are monarticular; at least half involve the metatarsophalangeal joint of the great toe (podagra). Next in order are the instep, ankle, heel, knee, wrist, finger, and elbow. Tenosynovitis, bursitis, or cellulitis may also occur. Minor episodes of "ankle sprain" or twinges of pain in the great toe may precede the first attack, sometimes by several years. More often the attack occurs explosively during apparent good health, often at night. Within minutes to hours the affected joint becomes hot, dusky red, and exquisitely tender and painful. Very severe attacks may be manifested as fever, leukocytosis, and an increased erythrocyte sedimentation rate, suggestive of infection. The course of an untreated attack is variable, with resolution in hours or a few days when mild and lasting many days to several weeks when severe. As the attack subsides, desquamation of inflamed skin over the affected joint may occur. Once the attack has broken, recovery is generally rapid and complete. The patient then re-enters an asymptomatic phase, often termed "intercritical" or "interval" gout.

The subsequent course is variable, but commonly a pattern of recurrences develops. Attacks often follow a precipitating event such as a long walk, trauma, surgery, alcohol or dietary overindulgence, starvation, infection, or the start of hypouricemic drug therapy. In an untreated patient, attacks often increase in frequency, and they may become more severe, last longer, and are more often polyarticular. Later attacks may involve the shoulder or hip or rarely the sacroiliac, sternoclavicular, or mandibular joints or even the spine. The more distal the site, the more typical the attack. Eventually, attacks may be refractory to usually effective measures; they resolve incompletely, and disability may become permanent.

CHRONIC TOPHACEOUS GOUT. Progressive inability to dispose of urate results insidiously in tophaceous crystal deposition in and around joints. Tophi may first appear as superficial yellowish white infiltrates on the fingertips, palms, and soles and later as irregular, asymmetrical enlargement of joints, fusiform or nodular enlargements of the Achilles tendon, or saccular distentions of the olecranon bursa (Fig. 299–3). A classic, although relatively infrequent, site of tophi is the helix or anthelix of the external ear. Visible tophi develop in 10 to 25% of gouty patients and in over 50% of those who are non-compliant; the time of appearance after the initial attack is correlated with the degree and duration of hyperuricemia and with renal insufficiency. In rare patients, often those with gout secondary to a myeloproliferative disease or in organ transplant recipients receiving cyclosporine, tophi are present at the time of the initial attack.

Although tophi themselves are relatively painless, they often result in stiffness and persistent aching that limit the use of affected joints. Destruction of cartilage and bone by tophi leads to radiolucent "punched-out" lesions and to cortical erosions with characteristic "overhanging margins" (see Fig. 299–3). Eventually, extensive destruction of joints may be disabling, and large subcutaneous tophi may cause grotesque deformities. The stretched, thin skin over tophi may ulcerate and extrude white chalky or pasty "milk of urate" composed of a myriad of fine, needle-like crystals. The olecranon bursa may be massively distended with this material, which may be mistaken for pus if not examined by polarized light microscopy. Rarely, tophi may involve the tongue, larynx, corpus cavernosum and prepuce of the penis, aortic or mitral valves, and cardiac conducting system and cause rhythm disturbances. They do not involve the liver, spleen, lungs, or central nervous system.

GOUTY NEPHROPATHY. Progressive renal failure secondary to urate nephropathy may occur in patients with inherited metabolic disorders that cause extreme urate overproduction and possibly in rare forms of inherited renal disease and chronic lead poisoning. Isosthenuria and mild intermittent proteinuria occur in about one third of patients with idiopathic gout. The decline in renal function correlates with aging, hypertension, renal calculi, pyelonephritis, or independently occurring nephropathy. Hyperuricemia per se is not a risk factor for renal insufficiency.

Acute oliguric renal failure can result from bilateral tubular obstruction by uric acid crystals. This disorder occurs in several clinical settings, including untreated leukemia and lymphoma or during chemotherapy for these disorders (tumor lysis syndrome), and in the presence of severe dehydration and acidosis. This condition is preventable by maintaining a high urine volume, with alkalinization, and by pre-treating with allopurinol. Daily infusions of fungal urate oxidase have also been effective (this drug has not been approved by the Food and Drug Administration at the time of publication).

DIAGNOSIS. The sudden onset of severe inflammatory arthritis in a peripheral joint, especially a joint of the lower extremity, suggests gout. A history of discrete attacks separated by completely asymptomatic periods is helpful for diagnosis. The diagnosis is established by demonstrating brilliant, negatively birefringent, needle-shaped monosodium urate crystals by polarized light microscopy in the leukocytes of synovial fluid (see Chapter 285) (Fig. 299–4; Color Plate 7G). The synovial fluid leukocyte count ranges from 5000 to over 50,000 per cubic millimeter, depending on the acuteness of inflammation. A Gram stain and culture of synovial fluid should always be obtained to evaluate infection, which may coexist.

Determining the 24-hour urinary excretion of uric acid can be informative, particularly in a young, markedly hyperuricemic patient in whom a metabolic etiology may be suspected. The sample should be collected after 3 days of moderate purine restriction, during an intercritical period. Values greater than 600 mg/1.72 m²/day under these conditions suggest overproduction, and those over 800 mg/day warrant additional studies for a specific subtype of primary gout, such as hypoxanthine-guanine phosphoribosyltransferase deficiency or phosphoribosylpyrophosphate synthetase overactivity, or for a subtype of secondary gout, such as a myeloproliferative disorder. Elevated urinary uric acid excretion also predicts a higher risk for renal stones and is an indication for allopurinol rather than uricosuric drug therapy for gout.

DIFFERENTIAL DIAGNOSIS. Acute gout must be differentiated from pseudogout, acute rheumatic fever, rheumatoid arthritis, traumatic arthritis, osteoarthritis, pyogenic arthritis, sarcoid arthritis, cellulitis, bursitis, tendinitis, and thrombophlebitis. Gout can coexist with most of these conditions. Podagra, the most common initial manifestation of gout, can be mimicked by trauma, degenerative arthritis, acute sarcoidosis, psoriatic arthritis, pseudogout, Reiter's syndrome, and infection, and in the immediate postoperative period following parathyroidectomy, podagra can be caused by hydroxyapatite crystals. Pseudogout (see Chapter 300), which is manifested by acute attacks of arthritis of the knees and other joints, is often accompanied by calcification of joint cartilage; the synovial fluid contains non-urate crystals of calcium pyrophosphate. When gout and pseudogout coexist, both types of crystals will be found in synovial leukocytes.

TREATMENT. Understanding of the rationale for treatment by both the physician and patient is essential for long-term success. One aspect is aimed at terminating the acute inflammatory gouty attack, and the other is aimed at correcting the underlying metabolic problem (Table 299–3).

ACUTE ATTACK. The affected joint(s) should be kept at rest and therapy begun promptly with full doses of an oral non-steroidal anti-inflammatory drug (NSAID). Salicylates should not be used because of their effects on urate excretion (see Table 299–2). The typical monarticular acute attack responds within 24 hours and resolves in 48 to 72 hours; established or polyarticular attacks may require longer treatment. Once the attack subsides, the NSAID dose is tapered over several days and treatment discontinued. Hypouricemic therapy should not be initiated during an acute attack because it is ineffective in relieving inflammatory symptoms and in some patients (estimated at 10 to 24%) may induce a recurrent attack by mobilizing urate from tissues.

Oral colchicine is effective therapy for acute gout but has a low therapeutic index; relief of pain often coincides with gastrointestinal toxicity. If an attack does not respond in 48 hours, alternative therapy should be used. If oral medication is precluded, intravenous colchicine may be used *with caution*. Colchicine is a microtubule

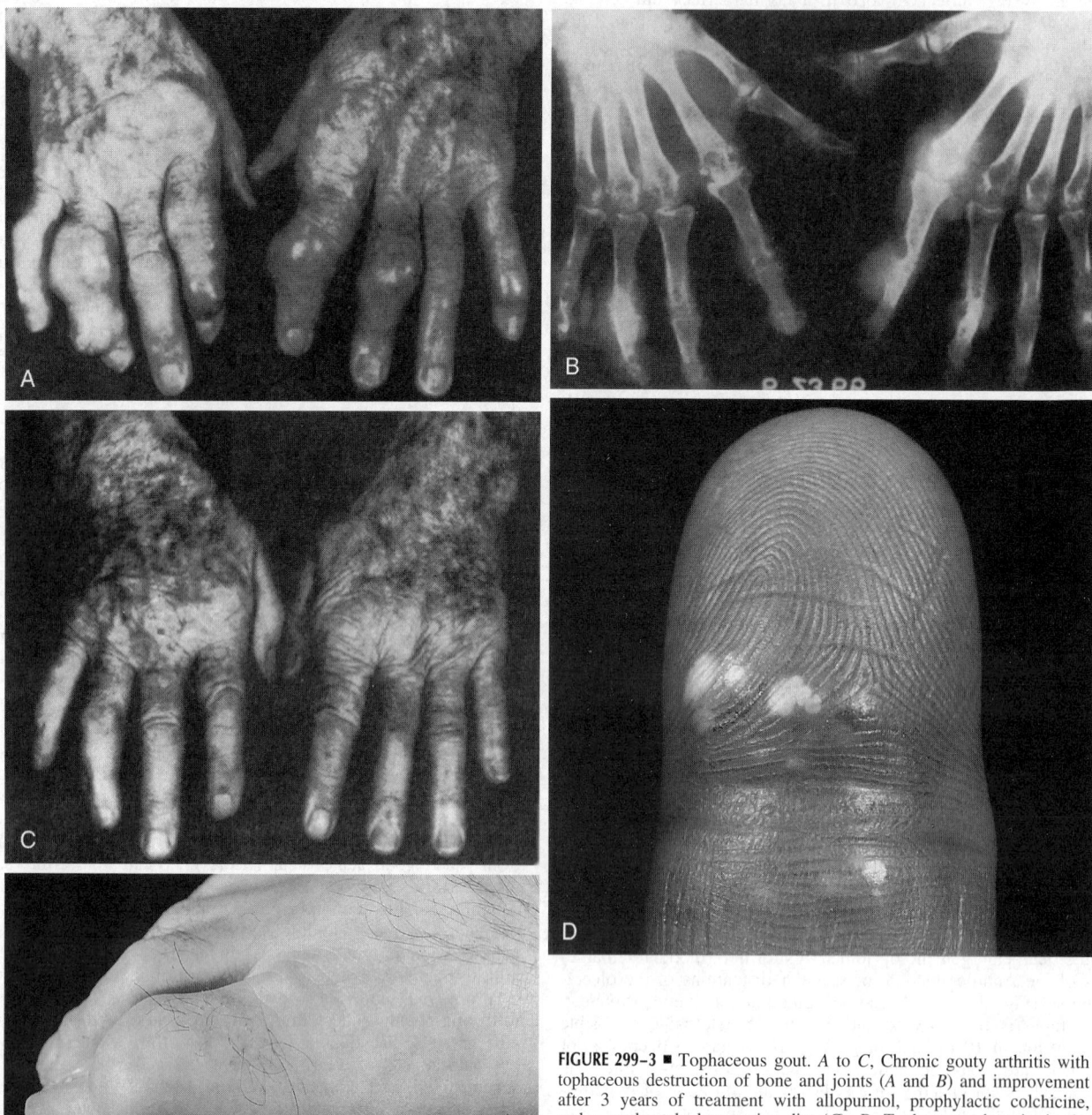

FIGURE 299–3 ■ Tophaceous gout. *A* to *C*, Chronic gouty arthritis with tophaceous destruction of bone and joints (*A* and *B*) and improvement after 3 years of treatment with allopurinol, prophylactic colchicine, and a moderately low purine diet (*C*). *D*, Tophaceous deposits in the digital pad of a 28-year-old man with systemic lupus erythematosus under treatment with diuretics. A single attack of gout had occurred 2 years earlier. *E*, Tophaceous enlargement of the great toe in a 44-year-old man with a 4-year history of recurrent gouty arthritis.

poison; it is retained in cells (half-life, about 30 hours) and is not dialyzable. Dose-related toxicity includes alopecia, bone marrow suppression, and hepatocellular damage. Deaths from overdosage have been reported. Blood counts should be monitored during intravenous use of colchicine and periodically during long-term oral therapy. The dosage should be reduced in the presence of renal or hepatic disease, and it should not be used in patients with advanced disease. Reversible myopathy has occurred in elderly patients undergoing daily colchicine prophylaxis who have been treated with larger doses for an acute attack.

In patients with peptic ulcer disease or renal insufficiency, in whom NSAIDs and colchicine may be contraindicated, various steroid preparations such as intramuscular injection of triamcinolone acetonide can be effective in treating the acute attack.

INTERVAL PHASE. Patients should be warned that acute attacks may still occur, particularly in the first 6 months or so after beginning hypouricemic therapy. Oral colchicine is effective prophylaxis to prevent recurrent attacks, but an NSAID should be taken at the initial sign of prodromal symptoms, if recognizable. Although hy-

pouricemic therapy is not usually initiated during an acute attack, once begun, it should not be interrupted during subsequent attacks. Hypertension should be treated vigorously; if hyperuricemia worsens, antihyperuricemic drug therapy can be initiated or appropriately increased.

LONG-TERM MANAGEMENT. Use of a drug to lower the serum uric acid level to less than 6 mg/dL is indicated in all patients with visible tophi or radiographic evidence of urate deposits or in patients with a history of two or more major attacks of gouty arthritis per year. Allopurinol is preferred unless the patient is already well managed with a uricosuric agent. With either type of agent, the number of acute attacks may increase during the initial few months (this situation may be prevented with prophylactic colchicine); after 12 to 18 months, the frequency of attacks should decline.

Allopurinol reduces urate production by inhibiting xanthine oxidase, with secondary reduction of de novo purine synthesis (see Fig. 299–1). Its major active metabolite, oxypurinol, has a long half-life (about 28 hours) and is primarily responsible for these effects during maintenance. In contrast to uricosuric agents, allopu-

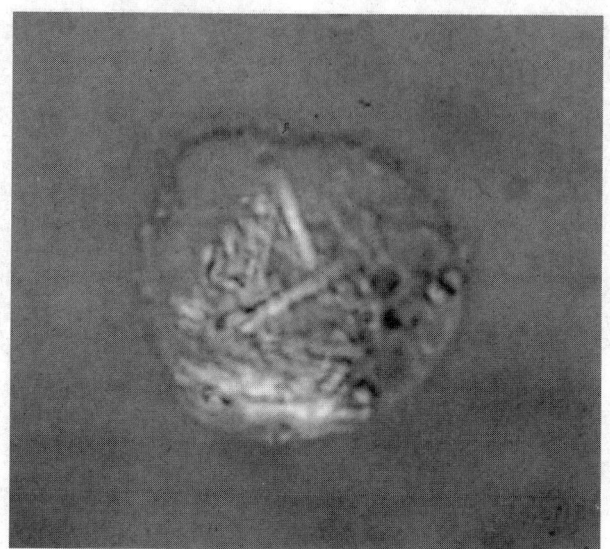

FIGURE 299–4 ■ Sodium urate monohydrate crystals phagocytosed by a leukocyte in synovial fluid from acute gouty arthritis, examined by polarized light.

rinol reduces urinary uric acid excretion and is effective in renal failure and in controlling urolithiasis, and its action is not blocked by salicylate. In the presence of renal insufficiency, the maintenance dose of allopurinol should be reduced because the half-life of oxypurinol is prolonged. Allopurinol-induced xanthinuria has resulted in xanthine renal stones on rare occasion in patients with hypoxanthine-guanine phosphoribosyltransferase deficiency and during chemotherapy for leukemias.

Allopurinol is well tolerated but may cause gastric irritation,

diarrhea, or skin rash in about 3% of patients. In about 0.4%, allopurinol causes a serious hypersensitivity syndrome, with worsening renal function, hepatitis, and severe dermatologic injury (epidermal necrolysis, exfoliative dermatitis, erythema multiforme, Stevens-Johnson syndrome), often with fever, leukocytosis, and eosinophilia. Patients with renal insufficiency are at higher risk, particularly if the dosage has not been appropriately reduced. Allopurinol interferes with the metabolism and increases the half-life of azathioprine and 6-mercaptopurine used to treat leukemia and to prevent allograft rejection, conditions in which significant hyperuricemia and gout may be associated with renal insufficiency.

If the serum urate level can be maintained at less than 6 mg/dL, some tophi resolve and bone erosions may be reduced. In selected patients, surgical treatment of chronically draining tophi or removal of large extra-articular urate deposits may be advisable. Effective treatment of severe gout is difficult in certain situations, particularly in patients with renal failure and allopurinol hypersensitivity and if allopurinol may interfere with drug therapy necessary for allograft rejection or malignancy. Desensitization to allopurinol has been used in some patients with mild allergic reactions but is considered dangerous in those who have had severe hypersensitivity reactions.

ASYMPTOMATIC HYPERURICEMIA. Asymptomatic hyperuricemia is frequent in family members of patients with gout and in the general population. In fewer than a fifth of hyperuricemic individuals does gout ever develop, and effective therapy can be begun when attacks do occur. In patients with a strong family history of tophaceous diseases or gout and renal problems, treatment with allopurinol should be begun before articular or renal complications develop.

Arellano F, Sacristan JA: Allopurinol hypersensitivity syndrome: A review. Ann Pharmacother 27:337, 1993. *Reviews over 100 reports of a serious potential complication of allopurinol therapy.*
Hochberg MC, Thomas J, Thomas DJ, et al: Racial differences in the incidence of

Table 299–3 ■ **TREATMENT OF GOUT**

ACUTE GOUT	INTERVAL GOUT	LONG-TERM TREATMENT
Therapeutic goal: Terminate acute inflammatory attack.	**Therapeutic goal:** Prevent recurrent attacks.	**Therapeutic goals:** Prevent attacks, resolve tophi, maintain serum urate at ≤6 mg/dL.
NSAIDs (*preferred*): Indomethacin, 50 mg qid, or ibuprofen, 800 mg tid (or other NSAIDs in full doses) (*lower dose in renal insufficiency; contraindicated with peptic ulcer disease*).	**Colchicine, oral:** 0.6–1.2 mg daily as prophylaxis against recurrent attacks.	**Colchicine, oral:** 0.6–1.2 mg daily for 1–2 weeks before initiating hypouricemic therapy and for several months afterward to prevent recurrent attacks during initial period of hypouricemic therapy (see text for discussion of colchicine toxicity).
OR		
Colchicine, oral (*used infrequently*): 0.6–1.2 mg (1–2 tablets), then 0.6 mg (1 tablet) q1–2h until attack subsides or until nausea, diarrhea, or GI cramping develops. Maximum total dose, 4–6 mg. If ineffective in 48 hr, do not repeat (see text for discussion of colchicine toxicity).	**Hypouricemic agent:** Start only if indicated by frequent attacks, severe hyperuricemia, presence of tophi, urolithiasis, or urate overexcretion.	**Allopurinol:** Dose variable; usually 300 mg once daily, but up to 900 mg may be needed in occasional patient; dose should be reduced to 100 mg daily or every other day in patients with renal insufficiency (see text for discussion of allopurinol hypersensitivity).
Colchicine, IV (*only if oral medication is precluded*): 1–2 mg in 20 mL 0.9% saline infused slowly (*extravasation causes tissue necrosis*); dose may be repeated once in 6 hr. Few GI symptoms with IV use. Maximum total dose, 4 mg per attack. Monitor blood counts.	**Other:** Diet—moderate protein, low fat; avoid excessive alcohol. Treat hypertension if present. High fluid intake to promote uric acid excretion in a dilute urine (for uric acid overexcretors).	**OR**
		Uricosuric agent (*reduced efficacy if creatinine clearance <80 mL; ineffective if <30 mL*): Probenecid, 0.5–1 g bid, or sulfinpyrazone, 100 mg tid or qid; usually well tolerated, but may cause headache, GI upset, rash.
Steroids (*if NSAIDs or colchicine is contraindicated or if oral medication is precluded, e.g., postoperatively*): Triamcinolone acetonide, 60 mg IM, *or* ACTH, 40 U IM *or* 25 U by slow IV infusion, *or* prednisone, 20–40 mg daily. Intra-articular steroids may be used to treat a single inflamed joint: triamcinolone hexacetonide, 5–20 mg, or dexamethasone phosphate, 1–6 mg.		**Other:** Diet—moderate protein, low fat; avoid excessive alcohol. Treat hypertension if present. For uric acid overexcretors or when initiating uricosuric agent: high fluid intake, particularly at night, to promote uric acid excretion in a dilute urine. Acetazolamide, 250 mg at bedtime, may be used to keep urine pH >6.
Hypouricemic agents: Of no benefit for inflammatory attack and may initiate recurrent attack. Should not be started until attack has resolved, but *ongoing use should not be interrupted during an attack.*		

NSAIDs = non-steroidal anti-inflammatory drugs; qid = four times daily; tid = three times daily; q1–2h = every 1 to 2 hours; IV = intravenously; GI = gastrointestinal; bid = twice daily; ACTH = adrenocorticotropic hormone; IM = intramuscularly.

gout. The role of hypertension. Arthritis Rheum 38:628, 1995. *Analyzes the incidence of gout in cohorts of black and white male physicians.*

Hooper DC, Spitsin S, Kean RB, et al: Uric acid, a natural scavenger of peroxynitrite, in experimental allergic encephalomyelitis and multiple sclerosis. Proc Natl Acad Sci U S A 95:675, 1998. *Intriguing study suggesting that multiple sclerosis and gout are mutually exclusive diseases because hyperuricemia protects against free radical injury.*

Pui C-H, Relling MV, Lascombes F, et al: Urate oxidase in prevention and treatment of hyperuricemia associated with lymphoid malignancies. Leukemia 11:1813, 1997. *A fungal urate oxidase infused daily for 6 days was effective in preventing hyperuricemia caused by tumor lysis syndrome.*

Rosenthal AK, Ryan LM: Treatment of refractory crystal-associated arthritis. Rheum Dis Clin North Am 21:151, 1995. *A helpful discussion of the management of gout in difficult situations.*

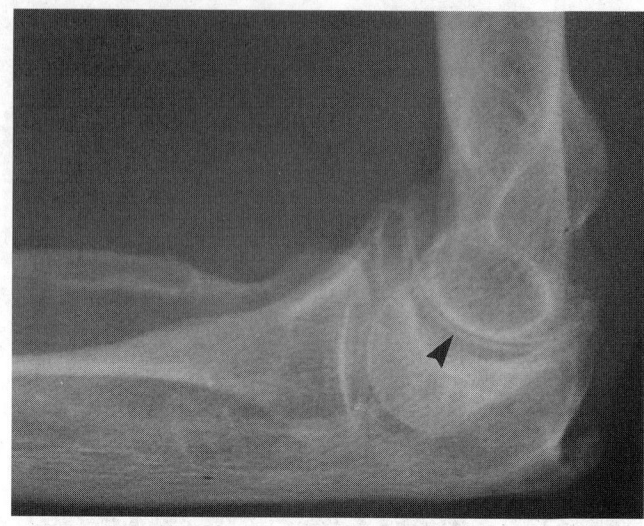

FIGURE 300–1 ■ Chondrocalcinosis (arrow) at the elbow joint of a patient with calcium pyrophosphate dihydrate deposition disease.

300 CRYSTAL DEPOSITION ARTHROPATHIES

H. Ralph Schumacher, Jr.

At least three different calcium-containing crystals are now known to be deposited in joints and are associated with a variety of patterns of arthritis, in much the same way as urate crystals cause the various features of gouty arthritis. Calcium pyrophosphate and occasionally calcium oxalate produce linear or punctate calcifications in menisci and articular cartilage that can be readily seen on radiographs (Fig. 300–1). These calcifications are termed "chondrocalcinosis." Both these crystals and calcium apatite can also be deposited diffusely in synovium and periarticular tissues and produce a soft tissue pattern on radiographs. Moreover, radiographs may not show obvious calcifications when crystals are relatively few. Definitive diagnosis is made only by aspiration of synovial fluid for identification of crystal type. In addition to the crystals discussed below, others of various implications may be seen in joint fluid (Table 300–1).

Schumacher HR, Reginato AJ: Atlas of Synovial Fluid Analysis and Crystal Identification. Philadelphia, Lea & Febiger, 1991. *An extensively illustrated compendium of all joint fluid findings, including less common crystals and artifacts.*

CALCIUM PYROPHOSPHATE DIHYDRATE CRYSTAL DEPOSITION DISEASE (PSEUDOGOUT SYNDROME)

Calcium pyrophosphate dihydrate (CPPD) crystals are rod- or rhomboid-shaped, 2- to 20-μm-long weakly birefringent crystals with positive elongation. CPPD crystals can be present without symptoms or can cause several patterns of arthritis. They are most frequent in the elderly. Up to 27% of nursing home patients in their 80s have radiographic evidence of chondrocalcinosis. Familial cases have been described in populations of various ethnic origins. Both genders are affected.

The cause of CPPD crystal deposition is not established, but local overproduction of pyrophosphate related to excessive activity of nucleoside triphosphate pyrophosphohydrolase, deficiency of phosphatases, and local changes in matrix proteoglycans and collagen are probably important. CPPD crystals are deposited only in joints and adjacent tendons or bursae, where they produce hematoxyphilic clumps replacing the normal tissue. Virtually any joint can be involved, but the knees, wrists, and second and third metacarpophalangeal joints are most common, so chronic cases can be confused with rheumatoid arthritis. Acute bouts of crystal-induced arthritis at one or more joints can mimic gout and lead to "pseudogout." Fever with bouts of arthritis can mimic infection. Recent reports have emphasized occurrence of symptomatic CPPD disease at rare sites such as the spine, temporomandubular joint, and sacroiliac joints. CPPD crystal deposition often complicates osteoarthritis; this association is more prominent at the knees than the hips. Whether crystals contribute to cartilage degeneration in osteoarthritis or are purely an epiphenomenon is not yet clear. Occasional severe arthritis mimics the destruction seen in neuropathic joints. Radiographic evidence of calcification can be present in some cases

Table 300–1 ■ DIFFERENTIAL DIAGNOSTIC FEATURES FOR SOME OF THE CRYSTAL-ASSOCIATED ARTHROPATHIES

	CRYSTAL SIZE (μm)	CRYSTAL SHAPE	CRYSTAL BIREFRINGENCE AND ELONGATION	OTHER POINTS	X-RAY FINDINGS
Calcium pyrophosphate	2–20	Rods, rhomboids	Weak positive	Elderly and consider associated metabolic diseases	Chondrocalcinosis, bony sclerosis
Apatite	2–25	Chunks or globules*	Non-birefringement	Clumps stained with alizarin red S	Soft tissue calcification
Oxalate	2–15	Rods, bipyramids	Positive	Renal failure	Chondrocalcinosis or soft tissue calcification
Monosodium urate	2–20	Rods, needles	Bright negative	Middle-aged men and elderly women	Cysts and erosions; tophi may calcify
Liquid lipid crystals	2–12	Maltese crosses	Positive	Unexplained acute arthritis	
Cholesterol	10–80	Notched rectangles	Positive or negative	May complicate RA and OA	
Depot corticosteroids	4–15	Irregular or rods	Bright positive or negative	Can cause iatrogenic inflammation	
Immunoglobins, other proteins	3–60	Rods or irregular	Positive or negative	Cryoglobulinemia	
Charcot-Leyden	10–25	Spindles	Positive or negative	Eosinophilic synovitis	

RA = rheumatoid arthritis; OA = osteoarthritis.

*Aggregates are seen by light microscopy. Individual needle-shaped crystals are seen only by electron microscopy.

Hyperparathyroidism
Hemochromatosis
Hypophosphatasia
Hypomagnesemia
Myxedematous hypothyroidism
Ochronosis

for years without inducing any symptoms. Others may have crystals in joint fluid with osteoarthritis-like radiographic changes but no visible chondrocalcinosis.

Synovial effusions may have leukocyte counts up to 100,000 per cubic millimeter and with 80 to 90% neutrophils during acute attacks. Between attacks or in osteoarthritis, crystals can be seen in clear, non-inflammatory joint effusions.

CPPD crystal deposition can be an important clue to a number of associated diseases, many of which have specific treatments that can control systemic features if not the arthropathy. Some clearly associated diseases are shown in Table 300–2. CPPD crystal deposition is increased in knees after meniscectomy and may complicate advanced arthritides.

Treatment of inflammatory episodes with thorough aspiration and use of non-steroidal anti-inflammatory drugs (NSAIDs) is generally successful. Intra-articular steroid injections may provide relief in refractory involvement of individual joints. Intravenous colchicine may also be helpful. Chronic therapy with 0.6 to 1.2 mg of colchicine per day can decrease the frequency of acute attacks but may be accompanied by neuropathy or myopathy if patients have liver or kidney disease. Hydroxychloroquine or methotrexate can be tried in the presence of chronic synovitis. Otherwise the prognosis is for slow progression. Joint replacement has been successful when needed.

Rahman MU, Shenberger KN, Schumacher HR: Initially unrecognized calcium pyrophosphate dihydrate deposition disease as a cause of fever. Am J Med 89:115, 1990. *Even mild crystal-induced joint findings can cause potentially confusing fever.*
Roane DW, Harris MD, Carpenter MT: Prospective use of intramuscular triamcinolone acetonide in pseudogout. J Rheumatol 24:1168, 1997. *In polyarticular disease, systemic steroids may occasionally be needed as in gout to control attacks.*

APATITE CRYSTAL DEPOSITION DISEASE

Individual apatite crystals can be seen only by electron microscopy, but clumps of these crystals appear as 2- to 25-μm shiny (but not generally birefringent) globules that can suggest the diagnosis. Apatite crystal deposition and crystal-induced inflammation are common factors in bursitis and periarthritis. Apatite crystals also occur in some cases of otherwise unexplained acute arthritis and in osteoarthritic joint effusions. Most joints or bursae can be involved, with more common sites including the shoulders, hips, knees, and digits (including the first metatarsophalangeal joint). Joint or periarticular inflammation can be acute or chronic. An extremely destructive arthritis has been noted especially at the shoulders ("Milwaukee shoulder"), hips, and knees in elderly patients. Radiographs can show soft tissue calcifications with or without bone erosions. Definitive diagnosis of the crystal type is only possible by electron microscopy with electron probe elemental analysis, x-ray diffraction, or infrared spectroscopy. Other calcium phosphates, such as octacalcium phosphate, can be seen along with the apatite; the significance of amounts of other associated calcium phosphates is not known. Synovial or bursal effusions can have many or few leukocytes. Serum studies are generally normal except that phosphate levels are often elevated in renal dialysis patients, who are at high risk of apatite deposition, and in tumoral calcinosis caused by renal retention of phosphate.

Apatite deposition can also be associated with scleroderma and other connective tissue diseases, repeated depot corticosteroid injections, central nervous system injury, and high-dose vitamin D therapy. In most instances, the cause of soft tissue apatite deposition is not known. Treatment of acute arthritis or periarthritis is with NSAIDs or colchicine. Aspiration of crystals and local injection with depot corticosteroids can also be effective. Diltiazam has recently been suggested to be able to slowly resorb the chronic calcinosis seen with collagen disease.

Paul H, Reginato AJ, Schumacher HR: Alizarin red S staining as a screening test to detect calcium compounds in synovial fluid. Arthritis Rheum 26:191, 1983. *This article describes a simple office screening test for apatite and other calcium-containing crystals.*
Pinals RS, Short CL: Calcific periarthritis involving multiple sites. Arthritis Rheum 9:566, 1966. *This recurrent calcific periarthritis is related to apatite crystals.*
Zakraouil, Schumacher HR, Rothfuss S: Idiopathic destructive arthropathies: Clinical, light and electron microscopic studies. J Clin Rheumatol 219, 1996. *The very destructive osteoarthritis at large joints of the elderly is invariably associated with apatite or CPPD crystals and must be distinguished from joint infections.*

OXALATE CRYSTAL DEPOSITION DISEASE

Calcium oxalate deposition can occur in joints along with other tissues of patients with renal failure who are maintained on chronic hemodialysis or peritoneal dialysis and can produce radiographic evidence of soft tissue calcification or chondrocalcinosis. Acute or chronic joint effusions with intracellular crystals can be seen. Oxalate deposits in vessels can mimic vasculitis. Masses of vertebral oxalates can cause spinal cord compression. The diagnosis is made by identification of typical bipyramidal crystals in joint fluid or biopsy specimens. When less characteristic crystals are seen, other techniques as described under apatite deposition can be used. Vitamin C may potentiate oxalate deposition, so it might be avoided.

Hoffman EC, Schumacher HR, Paul H, et al. Calcium oxalate microcrystalline–associated arthritis in end stage renal disease. Ann Intern Med 97:36, 1982. *Three cases with oxalosis and arthritis are described. Methods to identify oxalate crystals are included.*
Reginato AJ, Kurnik BRC: Calcium oxalate and other crystals associated with kidney disease and arthritis. Semin Arthritis Rheum 18:198, 1989. *Extensive oxalosis can involve the skin, bursae, tendon sheaths, vessel walls, and joints, as well as the kidneys and various viscera.*

GOUT

Monosodium urate crystal deposition (see Color Plate 7*G*) in joints and other connective tissue accounts for the most frequent clinical manifestations of gout. The complex genetic, metabolic, and renal factors that interact to produce hyperuricemia and eventually gout are described in detail in Chapter 299. Gouty arthropathy and the gross tophaceous deposits in chronic gout are also described in Chapter 299 but are summarized here because gout is the most common and prototypic of the crystal deposition diseases.

Monosodium urate crystals are rods or needles up to 15 to 20 μm in length and are brightly birefringent with negative elongation when viewed with compensated polarized light. Those from visible tophi or synovial microtophi tend to be more often needle-like, whereas some in acute arthritis can be very short. At least some crystals are intracellular during gouty arthritis. Leukocyte counts during attacks usually range from 10,000 to 50,000 per cubic millimeter, with 80 to 90% neutrophils. Gout is most common in middle-aged men but is increasingly seen in women after menopause. It is very rare in premenopausal women but may occur with chronic renal failure. A variety of lower extremity joints are commonly involved, in addition to the classic first metatarsophalangeal joint, but any joint or bursa, including those in the upper extremities, can be affected by either acute or chronic arthritis. Chronic or recurrent acute gout can be polyarticular, can mimic rheumatoid arthritis, and may be misdiagnosed, especially if the typical dramatic early short-lived attacks are not appreciated and synovial fluid is not examined. Tophaceous gout can slowly destroy joints. Crystals are often present in joint fluid even between attacks and may contribute to low-grade inflammation and joint damage.

Radiographs show only soft tissue swelling early in gout but can later reveal cystic erosions with thin, overhanging edges of bone suggestive of gout. Soft tissue tophi are common around joints, in bursae, in Achilles tendons, and at the extensor surface of the forearm. Gout should be recognized as a syndrome resulting from the many possible causes noted in Chapter 299. Cyclosporine causes an especially rapidly progressive form of gout in transplant patients.

Treatment of acute gouty arthritis can be with NSAIDs (although relatively high doses are needed), oral or intravenous colchicine, adrenocorticotropic hormone, or prednisone. The latter two agents may be needed in complicated patients with renal failure, liver disease, or gastrointestinal disease. Colchicine is most effective early in attacks (see also Chapter 299). Joint aspiration with instillation of depot corticosteroids may also be used if a single joint is involved and infection is excluded. If recurrent attacks develop, chronic low doses of NSAIDs or colchicine can suppress inflammation, but crystal accumulation will probably continue. Thus with more frequent attacks or visible tophi, patients should be considered for long-term lowering of urate levels with a uricosuric agent such as probenecid (if renal function is good and the patient is not overexcreting uric acid) or, in other cases, allopurinol, a xanthine oxidase inhibitor. Either urate-lowering agent must be given in sufficient dosage to lower serum uric acid levels below 6.0 mg/dL, a level at which tophi can dissolve and attacks eventually cease.

Moreland LM, Ball GV: Colchicine and gout. Arthritis Rheum 34:782, 1991. *Some of the complex situations involved in colchicine use for acute and chronic gout are reviewed. There are risks both from disease progression and from drug toxicities. Colchicine, NSAIDs, and allopurinol all require care in appropriate use.*

301 RELAPSING POLYCHONDRITIS

H. Ralph Schumacher, Jr.

The uncommon disease relapsing polychondritis is characterized by recurrent inflammation and destruction of cartilaginous and other connective tissue structures. Frequently involved cartilagenous structures are the pinnae of the ears, nasal cartilage, and tracheal rings. Polychondritis occurs nearly equally in both genders and at any age, but with a peak in onset between the ages of 40 and 60.

The pathologic lesion seen by light microscopy consists of loss of matrix staining, predominantly superficial infiltration with polymorphonuclear neutrophils or lymphocytes, and eventual destruction of normal structures followed by fibrosis. Electron microscopy in addition shows alterations of superficial chondrocytes, matrix, and elastic fibers. The cause of polychondritis is unknown, but the location of lesions and frequency of associated systemic diseases suggest the importance of systemic factors. Antibodies to types II, IX, and X collagen and the presence of cell-mediated immunity to proteoglycan and type II collagen are evidence of immunologic aberrations. An association with HLA-DR4 has been noted.

Inflammation of the cartilaginous structures of the ears is the most common initial finding (see Color Plate 8C). An acute onset of pain and tenderness may be seen along with erythema and swelling of one or both helices. The lobe is spared. Inner and middle ear involvement can occur and cause hearing loss or vertigo. Hearing loss can also result from edema of the external canal. Nasal cartilage involvement can produce a saddle nose. Laryngeal and tracheal disease can cause hoarseness or life-threatening upper respiratory obstruction. Ocular manifestations are common and include conjunctivitis, episcleritis, iridocyclitis, proptosis, and, rarely, other problems such as optic neuritis.

Cardiac involvement, especially involvement of the aortic root with aortic insufficiency, is seen in up to one fourth of cases. Aortic aneurysms, arrhythmias, and mitral regurgitation may also be present. Arthritis is reported in about three fourths of cases but is generally non-destructive. Fever, rashes, oral or genital ulcers, and renal disease can occur. Renal involvement can include glomerulonephritis and IgA nephropathy. Aseptic meningitis has been reported.

No laboratory tests are diagnostic, although the erythrocyte sedimentation rate is often elevated. Antineutrophil cytoplasmic antibodies have been reported. Anemia and leukocytosis may be present. Radiographs can detect advanced tracheal narrowing. Computed tomographic scans or magnetic resonance imaging and pulmonary function tests can detect more subtle airway obstruction.

Relapsing polychondritis is associated with other diseases in one third or more of cases, including rheumatoid arthritis, systemic lupus erythematosus, Sjögren's syndrome, thyroid disease, inflammatory bowel disease, psoriasis, spondyloarthropathies, Behçet's disease, vasculitis of various types, cryoglobulinemia, diabetes mellitus, biliary cirrhosis, panniculitis, malignancies, myelodysplastic syndromes, sinusitis, and mastoiditis. Wegener's granulomatosis and infections can cause potentially confusing chondritis.

In mild cases, non-steroidal anti-inflammatory agents can be used for symptomatic treatment, although adrenocorticosteroids in the range of 30 to 60 mg of prednisone per day are generally needed for acute inflammatory episodes and severe respiratory involvement. Methotrexate can be steroid sparing. Other immunosuppressives and cyclosporine have also been used with apparent benefit. Dapsone has been used with variable results. Tracheostomy or stents may be life saving if tracheal collapse occurs.

The course is unpredictable, with about 55% of subjects surviving for 10 years. Infection and systemic vasculitis caused more deaths than did airway obstruction in a recent series. Remissions do occur. Aortic valve disease has required surgery.

Chang-Miller A, Okamura M, Torres VE, et al: Renal involvement in relapsing polychondritis. Medicine (Baltimore) 66:202, 1987. *Glomerulonephritis often responds to corticosteroids or cytotoxic agents.*
Michet CJ, McKenna Ch, Luthra HS, et al: Relapsing polychondritis. Survival and predictive role of early disease manifestations. Ann Intern Med 104:74, 1986. *Anemia, saddle nose deformity, and vasculitis appear to be poor prognostic signs.*
Park J, Gowin KM, Schumacher HR: Steroid-sparing effect of methotrexate in relapsing polychondritis. J Rheumatol 23:937, 1996. *Methotrexate may be the easiest to use and safest steroid-sparing agent.*
Yang CL, Brinkmann J, Rui HF, et al: Autoantibodies to cartilage collagens in relapsing polychondritis. Arch Dermatol Res 285:245, 1993. *Immune mechanisms appear to be important.*
Zeuner M, Straub RH, Rauh G, et al: Relapsing polychondritis: Clinical and immunogenetic analysis of 62 patients J Rheumatol 24:96, 1987. *HLA-DR4 and other autoimmune diseases are frequently associated with polychondritis.*

302 OSTEOARTHRITIS (DEGENERATIVE JOINT DISEASE)

Thomas J. Schnitzer

Osteoarthritis is a disorder of diarthrodial joints characterized clinically by pain and functional limitations, radiographically by osteophytes and joint space narrowing, and histopathologically by alterations in cartilage integrity. The most common of all joint diseases, its importance derives from its economic impact, in terms of both productivity (single greatest cause of days lost from work) and cost of treatment (chronic use of analgesics and anti-inflammatory drugs). Although the etiology of the disorder is still not clearly understood, osteoarthritis has been shown to be a family of disorders with cartilage as a target organ in which biomechanical factors play a central role and with risk factors such as age, weight, and occupation also of major importance. Because no treatment can currently prevent or ameliorate the basic disease process, medical treatment is aimed primarily at relieving pain, with orthopedic intervention largely reserved for situations that cannot be controlled with more conservative therapy.

EPIDEMIOLOGY. Osteoarthritis is by far the most common joint disorder, one of the most common chronic diseases in the elderly, and a leading cause of disability. Because osteoarthritis can be defined both radiographically and clinically and because there is little correlation between the two, the prevalence of this condition has been variously estimated in epidemiologic studies. If radiographic criteria are used, the prevalence of joint findings steadily increases from less than 2% in women younger than 45 years to 30% in those aged 45 to 64 and to 68% in those older than 65. Its prevalence in men is slightly higher in the younger age groups (younger than 45), whereas women are affected more commonly at ages older than 55, except for disease of the hip.

The pattern of joint involvement in osteoarthritis is strikingly affected by age, gender, and previous occupational history. Before age 55, little difference in joint pattern is noted between men and women. In older men, hip osteoarthritis is more common, whereas older women tend to have more involvement of the proximal interphalangeal (PIP) joints and the base of the thumb. Joints subjected to repeated trauma or overuse demonstrate a higher prevalence of osteoarthritis. Cotton and mill workers have increased osteoarthritis of the hand and involved fingers, miners demonstrate increased knee and spine involvement, and pneumatic drill workers experience increased elbow and wrist disease.

Racial and genetic factors are also important in the prevalence and pattern of osteoarthritis. Chinese, Jamaican blacks, South African blacks, and Asian Indians have been shown to have a lower incidence of osteoarthritis of the hip than do whites, whereas Japanese have an increased incidence, apparently related to the more frequent occurrence of congenital hip dysplasia. Black American women have a higher prevalence of knee osteoarthritis than do white women, but a lower prevalence of involvement of the distal interphalangeal (DIP) joints of the hand (Heberden's nodes). Involvement of the DIP joints of the hands is particularly common in women and is often found to have a familial pattern of inheritance, with the female relatives of the proband having similar joint findings with a two- to five-fold increased prevalence.

Modifiable risk factors for osteoarthritis have also been identified in recent studies. Weight demonstrates by far the strongest association with osteoarthritis, and importantly, weight reduction has been shown to correlate with a reduction in the risk of later osteoarthritis. Certain types of repetitive activities have been correlated with increased osteoarthritis in the stressed joint (see above), whereas, interestingly, others have not. In particular, marathon runners appear to have no increased prevalence of knee osteoarthritis, but this observation may be due to a self-selection process, with those experiencing knee pain unable to continue the activity. Smoking and osteoporosis have both been shown to be negatively associated with osteoarthritis, but the explanation for this association is unknown.

PATHOLOGY. The hallmarks of osteoarthritis on gross or arthroscopic examination are focal ulcerated areas of cartilage exposing underlying eburnated (ivory-appearing) bone that occur at the load-bearing areas of the joint surface, as well as juxta-articular osteophytes growing at the joint margins. It is important to understand that these states represent the end stage of a continuum and that osteoarthritis is a pathologic *process*. At its earliest stage, it appears as a softening of the cartilage surface that progresses to fibrillation of the surface layers, loss of cartilage thickness, development of clefts into the depth of the cartilage, and eventual loss of cartilage integrity with release of shards of cartilage. Bone participates in this process as well, with reactive changes (bony sclerosis) underlying the areas of cartilage loss, development of subchondral bone cysts that may communicate with the joint space and expand into geodes, and marginal osteophytes (new cartilage and bone growth) at non–weight-bearing areas.

The earliest histologic changes reveal loss of extracellular cartilage matrix, loss of chondrocytes in the surface layers of articular cartilage, and reactive changes in the deeper chondrocytes manifested by cellular division and "cloning" in an apparent attempt at repair. Later, progressive loss of chondrocytes is seen at all levels, with marked thinning of the cartilage matrix and, in some instances, development of fibrocartilage in place of lost hyaline cartilage. The surrounding synovium is largely unaffected, although in later disease cartilage fragments may incite focal inflammatory lesions without the progressive and destructive pannus seen in typical inflammatory arthropathies.

PATHOGENESIS. Articular cartilage serves two major functions: (1) to permit nearly frictionless joint motion and (2) to act as a "shock absorber" and transmit loads across joint surfaces to the surrounding tissue. The requisite properties of elasticity and high tensile strength are imparted by proteoglycans and collagen in the extracellular matrix, which account for over 90% of the cartilage macromolecules. The proteoglycan elements of the matrix are actively being metabolized and turned over with a half-life of weeks. The highly negatively charged sulfated glycosaminoglycan components of the proteoglycans impart the elastic properties to cartilage. The collagen component is characterized by a unique structure (type II collagen), provides the tensile strength, and tightly constrains the proteoglycan molecules in a three-dimensional framework. The collagen fibers are covalently linked by other matrix molecules believed to provide the "glue" to hold the matrix intact. Collagen itself is extremely slowly metabolized (half-life of many years) in the normal state.

Osteoarthritis begins with an initial phase in which chondrocytic metabolic activity is up-regulated (enhanced proteoglycan synthesis), followed by eventual chondrocytic loss (apoptosis). The reason for failure of repair is unclear but may relate to the inability to re-form, once disrupted, the three-dimensional architecture of cartilage in mature individuals.

The processes responsible for degrading collagen and proteoglycans in osteoarthritis are driven by proteolytic enzymes being synthesized and released from the chondrocytes themselves. Subsequent activation of these potent enzymes overwhelms the natural matrix defenses and ultimately results in collagen breakdown and proteoglycan cleavage. Fragments from these molecules are then released into the synovial fluid and enter the circulation, where they provide "markers" that can be used as a means to detect and measure the degradative process.

The factors responsible for activating chondrocytes to degrade matrix in osteoarthritis are not known. However, certain conditions causing biomechanical alteration of cartilage are known to lead to osteoarthritis: joint injury, abnormal joint loading because of neuropathic changes (Charcot joint) or ligamentous damage (anterior cruciate ligament or meniscus injuries), altered joint surface congruity as in dysplasias, and muscle atrophy in the elderly. A number of metabolic conditions are known to predispose to the early onset of osteoarthritis; e.g., ochronosis with the deposition of homogentisic acid and hemochromatosis with the deposition of iron. Gene defects affecting matrix structures would be expected to possibly lead to osteoarthritis, but thus far genetic factors have played a role only in the development of dysplasias with secondary osteoarthritic changes. The pathogenetic mechanisms and feedback loops associated with altered cartilage structure and biomechanics are demonstrated in Figure 302–1.

CLINICAL FEATURES. The initial stages of the osteoarthritic process are clinically silent, which explains the high prevalence of radiographic and pathologic signs of osteoarthritis in clinically asymptomatic patients. Even in the later stages of osteoarthritis, clinical symptoms and alterations in cartilage and bone integrity, defined arthroscopically or by indirect imaging techniques (radiography, magnetic resonance imaging [MRI]), are poorly correlated. The factors or events that make the osteoarthritic process clinically apparent are unknown but are likely to be heterogeneous in nature and invoke processes within the synovium, bone, and surrounding supporting structures (muscle, ligaments) that produce pain rather than involve cartilage itself, a completely aneural tissue.

Pain is the predominant symptom that prompts the diagnosis of osteoarthritis and initially often involves only one joint, with others becoming painful subsequently. The pain is most often described as a deep ache frequently accompanied by joint stiffness that follows periods of inactivity (upon arising in the morning, after sitting). Pain is aggravated by using the involved joints, may radiate or be referred to surrounding structures, and in the early stages of the disease is commonly relieved by rest. With more severe disease, pain may be persistent and interfere with normal function. and prevent sleep, even with medical management. Even in severe disease, systemic manifestations such as fever, weight loss, anemia,

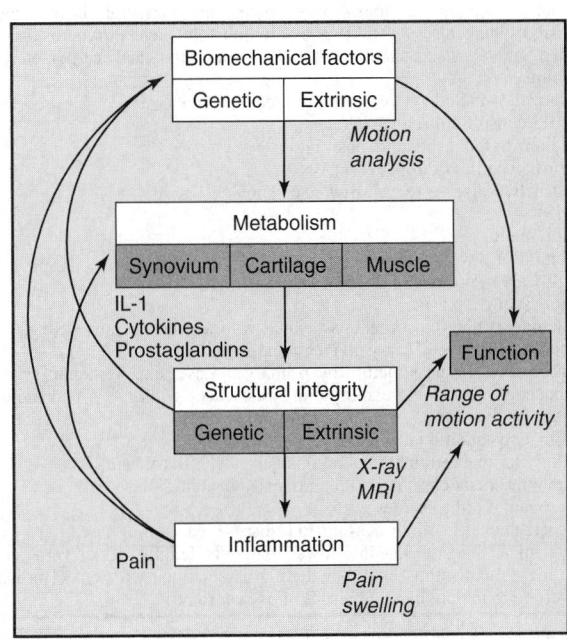

FIGURE 302–1 ■ Pathogenetic pathways in osteoarthritis. IL-1 = interleukin-1; MRI = magnetic resonance imaging.

and an elevated erythrocyte sedimentation rate (ESR) are not present.

The joints most commonly involved in osteoarthritis are the metatarsophalangeal joint of the great toe (hallux valgus or "bunion"), the PIP and DIP joints of the fingers, the carpometacarpal joint of the thumb, and the hips, knees, and both the lumbar and cervical spine. Interestingly, other joints, even major weight-bearing joints such as the ankle, are regularly spared unless involved in secondary forms of osteoarthritis (Table 302–1). On physical examination the joints may demonstrate tenderness, crepitus, and limited range of motion. Joint swelling may be due to an accompanying synovial effusion or bony enlargement and osteophytes. Joint instability is seen only in severe disease or after internal derangement of the knee with disruption of one or more of the major supporting structures (e.g., anterior cruciate ligament, medial collateral ligament). Patients with far-advanced disease exhibit gross deformity with subluxation of the involved joints. Although osteoarthritis is thought to be a uniformly progressive disease that invariably leads to joint replacement, such is not the case. The disease appears to stabilize in many patients with no worsening of signs or symptoms and actual improvement in some.

SPECIFIC JOINT INVOLVEMENT. HAND. Firm, slowly progressive bony enlargements of the DIP joints are called Heberden's nodes and represent marginal osteophytic spurs. Occasionally, the onset of symptoms is acute with sudden redness and tenderness in the involved joint. These changes can lead to deformity at these joints with lateral and flexor deviation. A related disorder, erosive osteoarthritis, is associated with repetitive episodes of acute symptoms and is differentiated by the additional finding of erosive changes on radiographs of the involved joints and a tendency to bony ankylosis. A genetic basis for Heberden's nodes appears to exist, the condition demonstrating a distinct female-dominant familial tendency (women are affected 10 times more commonly than men) (Fig. 302–2). Changes similar to those in the DIP joints occur in the PIP joints and are termed Bouchard's nodes. The only other joint to be commonly involved is the carpometacarpal joint of the thumb, often eliciting complaints of pain on use (wringing out

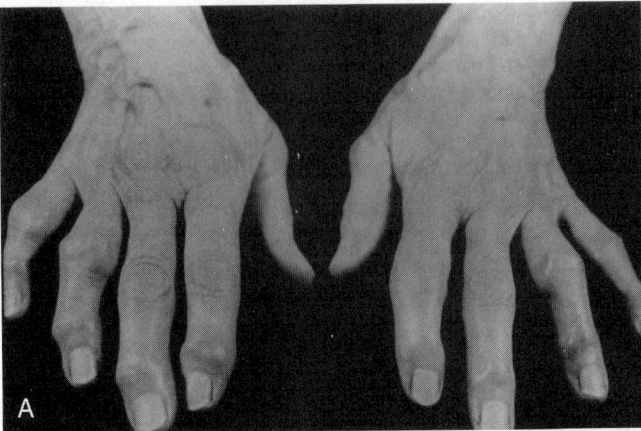
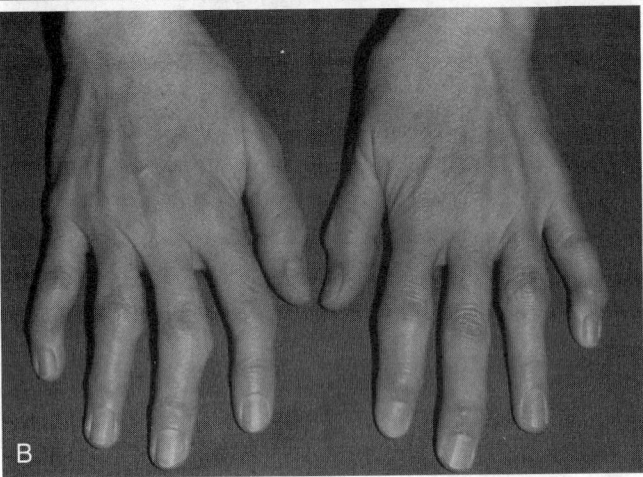

FIGURE 302–2 ■ Typical hand deformities in osteoarthritis. *A,* Typical Heberden's and Bouchard's nodes represent hypertrophic bony enlargement of the distal and proximal interphalangeal joints, respectively. *B,* Prominent Bouchard's nodes and minor subluxations may cause a misdiagnosis of rheumatoid arthritis.

Table 302–1 ■ ETIOLOGIC CLASSIFICATION OF OSTEOARTHRITIS

Idiopathic (Primary)
Localized
  Hands: Heberden's nodes, erosive interphalangeal arthropathy
  Feet: hallux valgus, hammer toes; talonavicular osteoarthritis
  Knees: medial, lateral, patellofemoral compartments
  Hips: sites of cartilage loss—eccentric (superior), concentric (axial, medial), diffuse
  Spine: zygapophyseal joints, osteophytes, intervertebral disks (spondylosis); ligaments, e.g., disseminated idiopathic skeletal hyperostosis
  Other single sites: shoulder, temporomandibular and carpometacarpal joints
Generalized—includes three or more areas listed above
Mineral deposition diseases
  Calcium pyrophosphate deposition disease
  Hydroxyapatite arthropathy
  Destructive disease (e.g., Milwaukee shoulder)
Secondary
Post-traumatic
Congenital or developmental
  Legg-Calvé-Perthes hip dislocation
  Epiphyseal dysplasias
  Articular cartilage disorders associated with a gene deficiency (e.g., association with type II procollagen gene mutation)
Disturbed local tissue structure by primary disease, e.g., ischemic necrosis, tophaceous gout, hyperparathyroid cysts, Paget's disease, rheumatoid arthritis, osteopetrosis, osteochondritis
Miscellaneous additional diseases
  Endocrine: diabetes mellitus, acromegaly, hypothyroidism
  Metabolic: hemochromatosis, ochronosis, Gaucher's disease
  Neuropathic arthropathies
  Miscellaneous: frostbite, Kashin-Bek disease, caisson disease
  Mechanical: obesity, unequal lower extremity length; valgus/varus deformities, ligamentous laxity (including associations with type I procollagen gene mutations of Ehlers-Danlos syndrome)

Compiled in part by the Osteoarthritis Diagnostic Criteria Committee, American Rheumatism Association, 1983.

clothes [washerwoman's hands] and grasping objects such as screwdrivers and doorknobs) and leading to a squared appearance of the base of the hand.

KNEE. Idiopathic knee osteoarthritis is a leading cause of painful ambulation and its prevalence has a direct relationship to weight; it is more common in women than in men. The medial compartment of the femorotibial joint space is more frequently affected and results in varus deformity (bowlegs). Lateral compartment disease may lead to valgus (knock-knee) deformity. Patellofemoral disease has recently been shown to be common and may represent a substantial portion of knee pathology in patients with knee pain. It is important to exclude other causes of knee pain such as internal derangements of the knee (which may lead to secondary knee osteoarthritis), soft tissue sprains, bursal inflammation, and Baker's cysts (which may coexist with knee osteoarthritis). In young women, the possibility of chondromalacia patellae should always be considered. Its cause is not known, but it is almost always self-limited and is not thought to lead to osteoarthritis. In idiopathic knee osteoarthritis, physical examination of the involved joint often elicits crepitus, pain, and decreased range of motion. Effusions are not infrequently present but are often small and may be difficult to appreciate.

HIP. Although congenital (Legg-Calvé-Perthes disease) and developmental (slipped femoral capital epiphysis) abnormalities have long been implicated in secondary hip osteoarthritis, the majority of primary hip osteoarthritis is now believed to be the consequence of mild dysplasia of the femoral head and/or acetabulum resulting in incongruity of the articulating surfaces. Use of the joint leads to progressive cartilage degeneration and secondary bony productive changes typical of osteoarthritis. Pain is typically referred to the groin, with anterior thigh and knee symptoms occasionally predominant. The majority of patients with pain in their "hip" are suffering from osteoarthritis of the lumbar spine. The earliest physical finding in hip osteoarthritis is loss of internal rotation; with progressive disease, range of motion is limited further in all directions, and significant functional limitation occurs, often necessitating surgery.

FOOT. The 1st metatarsophalangeal joint is the primary joint involved with associated bony swelling and deformity (bunion). Significantly more common in women than in men, these changes have been attributed to abnormal stresses imposed on the joint by footwear. In extreme cases, the joint space may be destroyed and result in a condition known as "hallux rigidus," which may interfere with normal ambulation and necessitate surgical correction.

SPINE. Technically, osteoarthritis of the spine relates strictly to changes in synovial-lined joints (apophyseal and uncovertebral joints) that can lead to localized pain as well as irritation of adjacent nerve roots with referred pain in the form of radiculopathy. Nerve root compression resulting from apophyseal joint subluxation, prolapse of an intervertebral disk, or osteophytic spurring may occur and be manifest as muscle weakness, hyporeflexia, and paresthesia or hypoesthesia. In the cervical region, spinal involvement can lead to cord impingement with long tract signs or may affect the vertebral artery and produce posterior circulation insufficiency with associated symptoms. Osteoarthritis of the spine should be differentiated from diffuse skeletal hyperostosis, which is characterized by marked calcification of the paraspinous ligaments and sparing of the arthrodial spinal joints.

PRIMARY GENERALIZED OSTEOARTHRITIS. The pattern of involvement of three or more joints or joint groups with osteoarthritis has been given the name primary generalized osteoarthritis and is seen most commonly in older women. Typically, the DIP and PIP joints of the hand, the knees, and the spine are involved. Whether this pattern represents a distinct subset of osteoarthritis is not known but has been suggested.

LABORATORY FINDINGS. Osteoarthritis involves a pathologic process that appears to be largely limited to cartilage and surrounding tissues with no evidence of systemic involvement. Typically, the ESR is normal, and levels of acute-phase reactants are not elevated. The hemoglobin and leukocyte counts remain within normal limits. The synovial fluid itself demonstrates no evidence of an inflammatory reaction, with few leukocytes (typically less than 3000 per cubic millimeter) and good viscosity. Occasionally, fragments of cartilage and crystals of calcium hydroxyapatite or calcium pyrophosphate dihydrate are seen. Rheumatoid factor is absent in the majority affected, but a significant number of older individuals will exhibit low-titer elevations that are not diagnostic of rheumatoid arthritis but are a common accompaniment of aging.

Cartilage matrix components unique to the joints have been identified, and sensitive assays have been developed to detect these "markers" in synovial fluid, serum, and urine. Further clinical correlations will need to be performed to determine the relationship of these markers to the disease process, activity, and state and their utility for earlier diagnosis and management of osteoarthritis.

RADIOLOGY AND IMAGING TECHNIQUES. Pathognomonic findings on plain radiography of involved joints include the presence of osteophytes at the margins of involved joints, associated joint space narrowing representing areas of cartilage thinning or loss, and evidence of bony reaction marked by subchondral sclerosis and bone cysts in more progressive disease. Some patients may lack one or more of these findings.

Radiography has been shown to be very insensitive to the pathologic processes occurring in the cartilage, with many patients having normal radiographs but destructive cartilage changes documented by arthroscopy. Other techniques have therefore been developed with greater potential sensitivity to detect cartilage change. In particular, MRI has the advantage of demonstrating cartilage as a positive image and has been widely used to document major cartilage injury such as meniscal tears. Further refinement of this technology will enhance the resolution possible, as well as increase the sensitivity to detect changes in hydration, which mark the earliest changes in osteoarthritis. It is anticipated that such technology will be important in assessing disease progression in the future.

Other technologies being developed to evaluate osteoarthritic joints include scintigraphy and ultrasound.

TREATMENT. People with osteoarthritis seek pain relief and improvement in physical functioning. Because no therapy in humans is known to affect the basic disease process (inhibit cartilage degradation or enhance synthesis), medical therapy has focused on pro-

viding symptomatic relief. Largely because of ease of administration and acceptance by patients, unwarranted reliance has been placed on pharmacologic intervention, particularly non-steroidal anti-inflammatory drugs (NSAIDs), as initial therapy at the expense of physical measures that have less morbidity and may provide longer-term benefit. The American College of Rheumatology has recently formulated evidence-based guidelines for progressive, stepwise treatment of patients with knee and hip osteoarthritis that incorporates this approach.

PHYSICAL MEASURES. Although often overlooked, physical therapy and exercise programs provide important benefit and should be prescribed as baseline therapy for all patients with osteoarthritis. Muscle atrophy commonly accompanies osteoarthritis. Because muscles serve to reduce load on cartilage, maintaining muscle function is crucial for cartilage integrity and can reduce pain. Both muscle strength and range of motion can be improved with appropriate physical therapy. Isometric exercises are preferred to isotonic ones because they place less stress on the involved joint.

Heat and cold are both used with varying effectiveness to provide symptomatic relief to patients and as an important adjunct to physical therapy regimens. The use of transcutaneous nerve stimulation, particularly to relieve back pain, is effective in some patients and provides an attractive alternative to pharmacologic intervention.

Periods of rest throughout the day may be an important adjunct in the routine of patients with osteoarthritis. Reduction in joint loading, either by resting or appropriately using a cane, will often permit increased periods of activity with reduced pain. Using cushioned shoes (commercial running or walking shoes) may also help lower extremity joint symptoms. Back pain may be reduced by muscle-strengthening exercises, as well as a well-fitted brace.

PHARMACOLOGIC THERAPY. Symptomatic relief of pain in patients with osteoarthritis is best achieved with simple analgesic agents such as acetaminophen. The effectiveness of NSAIDs is due primarily to their analgesic rather than their anti-inflammatory properties. Recent controlled studies have demonstrated that acetaminophen is as effective as NSAIDs and has considerably fewer serious side effects. Particularly in the elderly, with decreased renal reserve and an increased risk of upper gastrointestinal bleeding, acetaminophen and other simple analgesics should be the drugs of initial choice. If inflammation is present (erosive osteoarthritis) or symptoms are not well controlled with simple analgesics, low (analgesic) doses of NSAIDs may prove effective. A new class of NSAIDs (COX-2 inhibitors) that inhibit inflammatory-mediated production of prostaglandins (cyclooxygenase 2 mediated) but permit constitutive prostaglandin production (cyclooxygenase 1 mediated) are now available. If the gastrointestinal and overall safety of these agents is adequately demonstrated, their use will be preferred to nonselective NSAIDs, particularly in patients at high risk of GI side effects.

Intra-articular injection of both various steroid and hyaluronan preparations can also control joint symptoms. Controlled studies of intra-articular steroid injections have demonstrated only short-term relief of symptoms. Intra-articular injections of steroids should not be repeated more than three to four times per year in any given joint because of the possibility of the steroids potentiating cartilage breakdown. Systemic use of steroids has no place in the treatment of osteoarthritis. In knee osteoarthritis, intra-articular hyaluronan has been shown to produce modest clinical benefit that may persist for months.

Other approaches to therapy are under investigation. Topical treatment with capsaicin, a substance P inhibitor, has been shown to relieve localized pain in some patients with osteoarthritis. The development of agents that can stimulate cartilage synthesis or prevent degradation is actively being pursued and should provide the next generation of agents to treat this condition.

ORTHOPEDIC SURGERY. Joint replacement surgery has been the single biggest advance in the treatment of osteoarthritis in the past half century. Patients in whom optimal medical management has failed and who continue to have pain that interferes with sleep or activity or have significant limitations of joint function are candidates for an operation. Some individuals, those with altered limb alignment and early osteoarthritis of a hip or knee, may benefit from osteotomy. Most patients have more advanced disease and require total joint replacement. Ideal candidates for total joint arthroplasty have well-maintained muscle strength and should be older than 60 years. Younger patients are discouraged from undergoing joint replacement because of the small but real incidence of long-term failure of joint implants, mainly from loosening. Revision arthroplasty is possible but has a higher failure rate and can be avoided by delaying the initial arthroplasty as long as possible and putting less load on the replaced joint.

Arthroscopic surgery is useful for removing loose bodies and repairing intrinsic defects of the knee, as well as for shoulder (rotator cuff) and ankle pathology. Arthroscopic lavage (flushing of saline to remove cartilage debris) in patients with knee osteoarthritis may provide pain relief. Abrasion arthroplasty (chondroplasty) has been widely used in patients with knee osteoarthritis, but no data have demonstrated its efficacy, and it cannot currently be recommended.

Koopman WJ: Arthritis and Allied Conditions: A Textbook of Rheumatology. Baltimore, Williams & Wilkins, 1996. *Comprehensive overview of all aspects with illustrations.*
Kuettner K, Goldberg V (eds): Osteoarthritis Disorders. Rosemont, IL, American Academy of Orthopedic Surgeons, 1995. *Current understanding of cartilage biology and the pathogenesis of osteoarthritis.*
Moskowitz W, Howell DS, Goldberg VM, et al: Osteoarthritis: Diagnosis and Medical/Surgical Management. Philadelphia, WB Saunders, 1992. *In-depth coverage of all aspects of osteoarthritis.*
Silman AJ, Hockberg MC (eds): Epidemiology of the Rheumatic Diseases. New York, Oxford Press, 1993. *A comprehensive review of the definition, incidence, and prevalence of rheumatic disease.*

303 THE PAINFUL SHOULDER

Dennis W. Boulware

Shoulder pain can originate from many anatomic sites, including the structures comprising the glenohumeral joint and the periarticular soft tissue structures, or be referred from the cervical spine, the thorax, the diaphragm, and the upper abdominal cavity. Although non-musculoskeletal causes of shoulder pain are important, the focus in this chapter is on the musculoskeletal causes of isolated shoulder pain.

The more common causes of shoulder pain are due to disorders of the surrounding periarticular soft tissue structures: the biceps and rotator cuff tendons, the subacromial and subdeltoid bursae, and the

articular capsule (Fig. 303–1). Infrequently, diseases of the bone and the glenohumeral joint can be responsible for isolated shoulder pain.

With a fundamental knowledge of the anatomy of the shoulder joint and the physical examination of these specific structures, a proper diagnosis can be made. Once a proper diagnosis is made, appropriate treatment can be prescribed, ensuring greater success for improvement.

TENDONS. In general, tendon lesions are painful only during active use. A bicipital tendinitis will elicit anterior shoulder pain during active flexion of the elbow or forward flexion of the shoulder, and a rotator cuff lesion will cause more diffuse pain on active abduction of the shoulder. On examination, active testing of the myotendinous unit results in more tenderness than passive range of motion. Isometric loading of the tendon by active resistance without joint motion will often pinpoint a tendinous cause of pain rather than an articular cause. Passive range of motion is preserved in isolated tendinitis.

THE ROTATOR CUFF. *All lesions of the rotator cuff* will precipitate pain on active abduction of the shoulder, particularly the initial 90 degrees of motion. This pain is usually focused over the lateral aspect of the shoulder and frequently a problem during sleep. On examination of the shoulder, active abduction will elicit more tenderness than passive abduction done by the examiner. A "drop

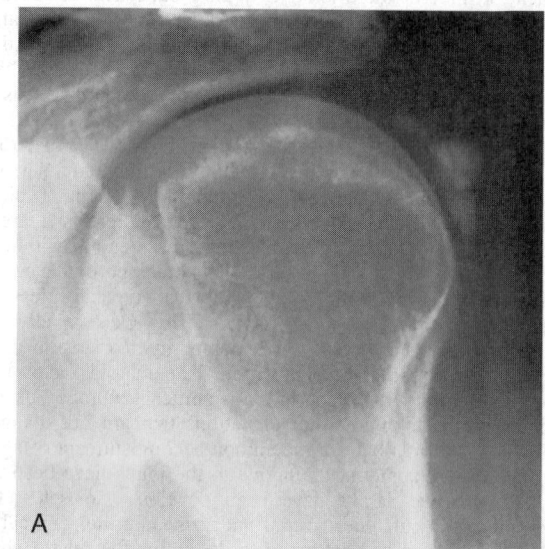

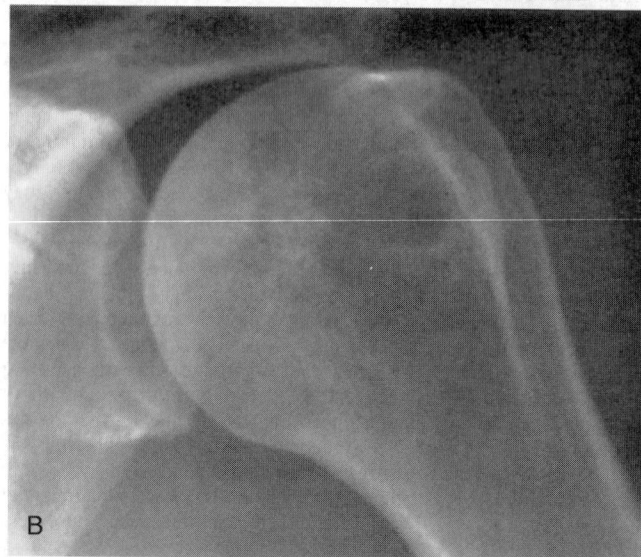

FIGURE 303–2 ■ Calcific tendinitis. *A,* Two distinct deposits of calcium are present on the internal rotation view. *B,* External rotation projects the supraspinatus calcification above the greater tuberosity and superimposes the larger collection (within the infraspinatus tendon) over the humeral head. (From Forrester DM, Brown JC: The Radiology of Joint Disease, vol 2. Philadelphia, WB Saunders, 1987, p 364.)

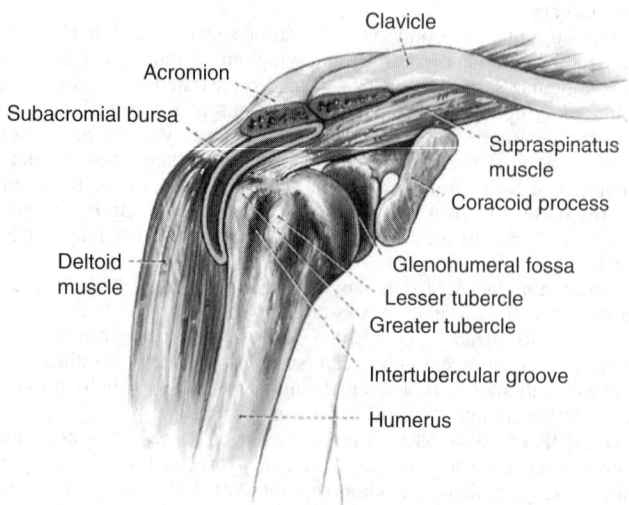

FIGURE 303–1 ■ Anterior aspect of the shoulder joint showing palpable landmarks and their relationship to the subacromial bursa. (From Polley HF, Hunder GG [eds]: Rheumatologic Interviewing and Physical Examination of the Joints, 2nd ed. Philadelphia, WB Saunders, 1978, p 63.)

sign" is helpful in identifying the rotator cuff as the source of pain and can be accomplished by passively placing the patient's arm at full abduction. The patient will experience severe pain when the arm is slowly adducted from 120 to 60 degrees and the arm will reflexively "drop."

Rotator cuff tendinitis is the most common cause of shoulder pain and is usually due to unaccustomed overuse of the arm in overhead activities. This abducted position impinges the cuff between the acromion and the humeral head, resulting in injury. An acute impingement can also occur during a fall on the arm or shoulder, trapping the cuff between the humeral head and the acromion. Occasionally, this injury can lead to a partial or complete tear. Chronic impingements also can occur from inferior osteophytes of the acromioclavicular joint encroaching into the acromiohumeral space. With time, chronic impingements can result in attenuation of the rotator cuff and an eventual tear.

Injury, overuse, or degenerative processes can lead to *rotator cuff tears* in the shoulder. The tear can exist as a complete rupture of the rotator cuff or as incomplete tears. Similar to tendinitis, the pain is worse with active abduction of the shoulder, particularly the initial 90 degrees. A complete tear of the cuff will make abduction of the initial 90 degrees impossible when the patient is upright. Differentiating tendinitis from a tear requires diagnostic imaging, but this should be reserved for suspected complete tears because the initial treatment of incomplete tears and tendinitis is similar.

The diagnosis of *calcific tendinitis* is made in the clinical setting of a rotator cuff tendinitis coupled with the radiographic appearance of calcification of the rotator cuff, usually the supraspinatus tendon near its insertion on the humerus (Fig. 303–2).

Diagnostic plain radiography is helpful in chronic rotator cuff lesions. Chronic impingements with tendinitis will reveal degenerative sclerotic and cystic changes of the humeral greater tuberosity. Significant attrition or complete tears of the cuff will be demonstrated as narrowing or obliteration of the acromiohumeral space. Magnetic resonance imaging and ultrasonography are useful but expensive and difficult to interpret except by experienced musculoskeletal radiologists. Arthrography is the best study to document complete ruptures and often can detect incomplete tears (Fig. 303–3).

The diagnosis of a rotator cuff lesion often can be made by instilling an intralesional local anesthetic agent. When 2 to 4 mL of a local anesthetic is properly placed inferolaterally to the acromial process in the subacromial bursa, the patient should experience significant relief of pain and be capable of active, painless abduction. The exception will be the complete rupture of the rotator cuff,

which will have pain relief but still be incapable of unassisted abduction.

The treatment of lesions of the rotator cuff is similar for all types of problems except a complete tear, which will require a surgical referral. Initial management with heat, physical therapy, and non-steroidal anti-inflammatory drugs (NSAIDs) is more effective when prescribed early. If this therapy is ineffective, intralesional corticosteroid agents placed in the subacromial bursa may be required. Recalcitrant cases of impingement may eventually require surgery in the form of acromioplasty. Job modification is essential for individuals with chronic impingement from occupational overuse.

BICIPITAL TENDON. In *bicipital tendinitis*, the tendon of the long head of the biceps becomes inflamed as it traverses the bicipital groove of the humerus. Clinically, the patient experiences pain in the anterior aspect of the shoulder, especially on actively using the biceps. Clinical examination can confirm the presence of bicipital tendinitis by one of several techniques. Tenderness elicited by directly palpating the tendon within the bicipital groove is a very helpful sign. Further confirmation of bicipital tendinitis can be demonstrated by Yergason's sign. The examiner should place the shoulder in the initial position of full adduction, the elbow in full flexion, and the wrist in supination. Then the patient is asked to resist an attempt to suddenly extend the elbow and pronate the wrist. Tenderness in the anterior shoulder would be indicative of bicipital tendinitis.

Chronic problems can cause attrition of the tendon and eventual rupture. Complete rupture will cause mild weakness of the biceps and a prominent bulge of the muscle belly. Integrity of the rotator cuff should be assessed in chronic bicipital tendinitis, because the two entities frequently occur concomitantly.

Treatment of bicipital tendinitis is initially conservative with rest and NSAIDs. Physical therapy and intralesional corticosteroids are reserved for refractory cases. Successful treatment is more likely when initiated early. Surgery is essential for complete rupture and may be required for intractable cases of tendinitis.

BURSAE. The subacromial or subdeltoid bursa is the largest and most frequently inflamed bursa of the shoulder. Located between the acromion process and the rotator cuff, and extending beneath the deltoid muscle, *subacromial* or *subdeltoid bursitis* will cause pain in the lateral aspect of the shoulder similar to that caused by rotator cuff tendinitis. It differs from a rotator cuff tendinitis by the presence of tenderness on direct palpation beneath the acromion

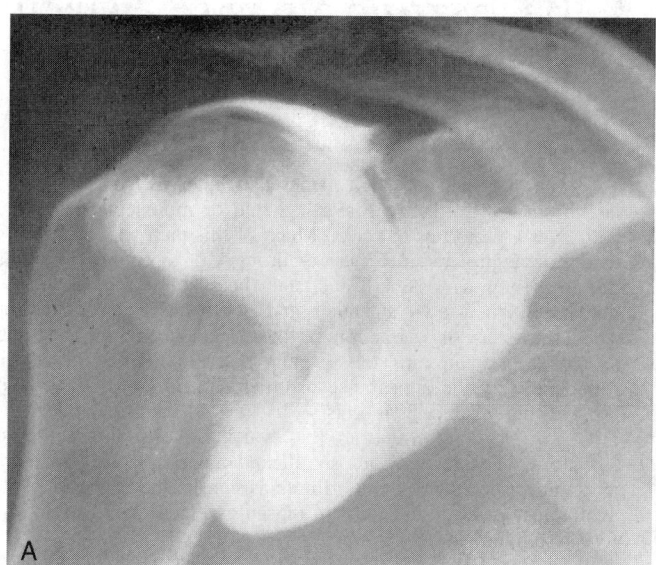
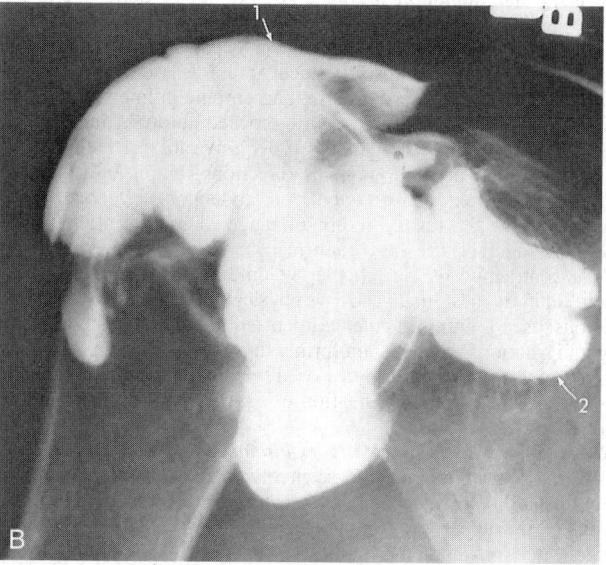

FIGURE 303–3 ▪ *A*, Arthrogram of normal shoulder. The extent of the joint capsule is delineated by contrast material. A prominent subscapular extension of the capsule is seen projecting toward the axilla. Filling of the subacromial bursa may occasionally occur normally. Extension of the capsule as a pouch around the long head of the biceps demarcates the intertubercular groove. *B*, Rotator cuff tear. Filling of (1) the subacromial bursa superiorly and (2) the subcoracoid bursa inferiorly indicates tear of the rotator cuff. The normal hyaline articular cartilage is seen as a radiolucent crescent over the head of the humerus. (From Forrester DM, Brown JC: The Radiology of Joint Disease, vol 2. Philadelphia, WB Saunders, 1987, pp 362, 363.)

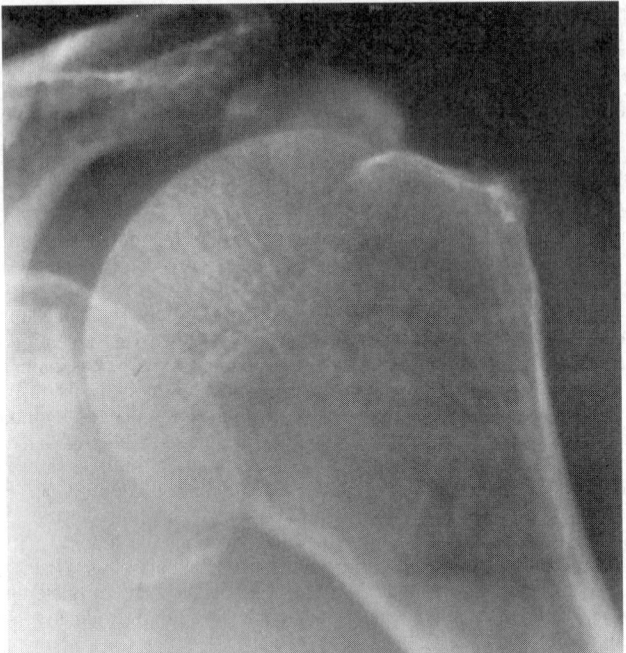

FIGURE 303–4 ■ Calcific bursitis. A large amorphous collection of calcium lies within the subacromial bursa. In addition, a small fleck of calcium just above the greater tuberosity represents supraspinatus tendinitis. (From Forrester DM, Brown JC: The Radiology of Joint Disease, vol 2. Philadelphia, WB Saunders, 1987, p 369.)

process. Similar to tendinitis, isolated bursitis will have full passive range of motion. Plain radiography is typically not helpful but sometimes can demonstrate calcification in chronic subacromial bursitis (Fig. 303–4).

Treatment of subacromial or subdeltoid bursitis is conservative, with rest, physical therapy, and NSAIDs. Patients whose cases are refractory to initial conservative management can receive intralesional corticosteroids given directly into the subacromial bursa, which are quite effective.

ARTICULAR CAPSULE. Disorders of the articular capsule often cause diffuse shoulder pain radiating into the brachium. It will be evident by the limitation of range of motion by both active and passive abduction. *Adhesive capsulitis,* also known as "frozen shoulder," is a common entity that can occur in association with diabetes mellitus, tuberculosis, cervical spine disease, upper extremity injuries, coronary artery disease, and chronic pulmonary disease. Initially a painful condition, it will proceed through an adhesive phase characterized by the painless progressive loss of both passive and active range of motion in all directions, but usually starting with a loss of external rotation and abduction. Eventually, the shoulder "thaws," with the return of range of motion after several years. The diagnosis is best confirmed by arthrography, which reveals a contracture of the articular volume and loss of the axillary pouch. Pain is best managed by physical therapy, NSAIDs, and judicious use of intra-articular corticosteroids. Early restoration of range of motion has been uniformly unsuccessful even when attempted by physical therapy, closed manipulation under general anesthesia, and hydraulic distention using large-volume intra-articular injections.

Reflex sympathetic dystrophy syndrome is similar to adhesive capsulitis except for more diffuse involvement with pain and vasomotor instability of the hand, wrist, and arm. More common after trauma of the upper extremity, it occurs in association with some clinical situations similar to adhesive capsulitis. This condition can occur bilaterally and responds more favorably to early therapy. Treatment should include aggressive physical therapy to maintain range of motion, non-narcotic analgesia for pain management, and a short, rapidly tapering course of corticosteroids. Best results have occurred when corticosteroids are started at 40 to 60 mg of prednisone per day and tapered over a 3-week period. Stellate ganglion

blocks and intra-articular corticosteroids are sometimes helpful, but with less uniform improvement.

BONE. Primary diseases of the bone can manifest themselves as shoulder pain. *Avascular necrosis of bone* can affect the humeral head, although it is not as common as avascular necrosis of the femoral head. If avascular necrosis of bone is suspected, early diagnosis is best made by magnetic resonance imaging. Plain radiographic changes occur late in the disease process and should not be required to confirm the diagnosis.

GLENOHUMERAL JOINT. Arthritis of the glenohumeral joint is common and like adhesive capsulitis has diffuse shoulder pain often radiating into the upper arm. Glenohumeral arthritis is easily detected on physical examination by the presence of tenderness on passive rotation of the fully adducted shoulder. Soft tissue swelling is not easily perceived on routine examination, and tenderness on active rotation will not discriminate glenohumeral arthritis from lesions of the rotator cuff. Although painful for the patient, passive range of motion should be determined because it will be near normal in acute arthritis but not in adhesive capsulitis.

Because the glenohumeral joint is a common site of involvement for many forms of the polyarthritides, most episodes of glenohumeral arthritis are part of a polyarthritis. Alternatively, an isolated severe destructive degenerative glenohumeral arthritis seen in the elderly should make the clinician suspect *Milwaukee shoulder.* Predisposing factors for this condition include chronic renal failure, local calcium pyrophosphate dihydrate deposition, chronic joint overuse, and large tears of the rotator cuff. The long-term disruption of the rotator cuff and chronic shoulder instability seem to be the key factors in allowing this problem to occur.

Biundo JJ, Torres-Ramos FM: Common shoulder problems. Primary Care Rheumatol 4:1, 1991. *A practical approach to examination of the shoulder and diagnosing common problems.*

Boublik M, Hawkins RJ: Clinical examination of the shoulder complex. J Orthop Sports Phys Ther 18:379, 1993. *A comprehensive approach to the examination of the shoulder.*

Kozin F: Painful shoulder and the reflex sympathetic dystrophy syndrome. *In* Koopman WJ (ed): Arthritis and Allied Conditions, 13th ed. Baltimore, Williams & Wilkins, 1997, pp 1887–1922. *A detailed and comprehensive resource of etiology, diagnosis, and treatment with 315 references.*

Thornhill TS: Shoulder pain. *In* Kelley WN, Harris ED, Ruddy S, et al (eds): Textbook of Rheumatology, 5th ed. Philadelphia, WB Saunders, 1997, pp 413–438. *A detailed and comprehensive resource of etiology, diagnosis, and treatment with 157 references.*

304 SYSTEMIC DISEASES IN WHICH ARTHRITIS IS A FEATURE

Eugene V. Ball

Eleven per cent of adult Americans interviewed in a national health survey claimed to have had one or more episodes of joint pain over a period of 6 weeks. Much of this pain was probably due to fibromyalgia and soft tissue syndromes, or to common rheumatic diseases such as osteoarthritis and rheumatoid arthritis, that are defined by their own attributes and not by associated symptoms. The arthralgias of a fraction of these persons might have represented early symptoms of systemic diseases that could be diagnosed only by the appearance of other clinical signs or by laboratory testing. Table 304–1 is a list of selected general medical laboratory tests of value in the evaluation of non-specific joint symptoms. The tests afford significant diagnostic clues for certain systemic diseases in which arthralgias can be the earliest and only symptoms. Brief descriptions of musculoskeletal manifestations of a few systemic disorders follow.

PRIMARY BILIARY CIRRHOSIS (see Chapter 153). More than half of women with primary biliary cirrhosis may have rheumatoid factors and antinuclear antibodies, in addition to antimitochondrial antibodies. A large percentage of these have joint pains or outright rheumatic disease, mainly rheumatoid arthritis, Sjögren's syndrome, or limited scleroderma. An asymmetrical, non-deforming arthritis has been described in as many as 30% of patients. Other defined

TEST	DISEASE
Liver function tests	Primary biliary cirrhosis; hepatitis B and C; chronic active hepatitis
Calcium and phosphorus	Hyperparathyroidism
Serum protein electrophoresis	Hypogammaglobulinemic arthritis; primary amyloidosis; hyperimmunoglobulin D
Serum iron and total iron-binding capacity; ferritin	Hemochromatosis
Lipase or amylase	Pancreatic-arthritis syndrome
Thyroid-stimulating hormone; thyroxine	Thyroid myopathy or arthritis
Complete blood cell count	Leukemia; sickle cell disease
Lipid analysis	Hyperlipidemia-associated arthritis
Partial thromboplastin time; rapid plasma reagin (RPR) or VDRL	Hemophilia Syphilis
Anti–human immunodeficiency virus (HIV)	HIV arthritis
Antiparvovirus antibody	Parvovirus arthritis

causes for bone or joint pains in primary biliary cirrhosis include osteomalacia and hypertrophic osteoarthropathy.

HEMOCHROMATOSIS (see Chapter 221). Arthritis is frequently the first sign of hemochromatosis and eventually develops in as many as half of all persons with the disease. Typically occurring between the ages of 40 and 50, the arthritis of hemochromatosis has been reported in persons younger than age 30 and is easily overlooked or confused with primary osteoarthritis, even though their distributions often differ. It also may be dismissed as idiopathic tendinitis or bursitis. Pain and stiffness frequently appear first in the metacarpophalangeal joints; other joints that are involved frequently include wrists, hips, and knees. Signs of inflammation are negligible except during episodes of pseudogout. Chondrocalcinosis is common on radiographs, as are subchondral cysts, sclerosis, and joint space narrowing. The arthritis is not altered by phlebotomy; treatment is symptomatic and may necessitate arthroplasties, particularly in the hips.

SICKLE CELL DISEASE AND OTHER HEMOGLOBINOPATHIES (see Chapter 169). Almost all persons with sickle cell disease experience musculoskeletal symptoms. Large joint arthritis lasting a few days to a few weeks results from small vessel occlusion caused by local sickling. Osteonecrosis occurs in both SS and SC disease, often in the head of the femur; however, multiple areas may be infarcted. Osteomyelitis is much more common in persons with sickle cell disease than in normal persons and is often caused by *Salmonella*. Hyperuricemia attributable to SS disease has culminated in gout in older patients. Pain due to microfractures in the lower leg, ankle, or foot, lasting up to 1 to 2 years, has been described in almost one half of a group of 50 patients with β-thalassemia.

HYPOGAMMAGLOBULINEMIA (see Chapters 272 and 305). Arthritis as a complication of hypogammaglobulinemia is most typical of the X-linked variety (Bruton's disease) in children; however, it also occurs in other types of primary hypogammaglobulinemia. Septic arthritis is caused by common pathogens or by mycoplasmal organisms such as *Ureaplasma urealyticum*. Non-erosive oligoarthritis, without evidence of infection or other demonstrable cause, often resolves after institution of immunoglobulin therapy. Its resolution with treatment does not necessarily constitute a priori evidence of an infectious etiology. Intravenous gamma globulin treatment might suppress arthritis through its complex modulating effect on the immune system.

WHIPPLE'S DISEASE (see Chapters 134 and 136). The arthritis of Whipple's disease mimics that of rheumatic fever in some respects. It is painful, and there is often warmth, redness, and swelling; it favors large joints, and subcutaneous nodules have been noted in a few patients. Recurrences are common, and the disease can be migratory. Less often, small joints of the hands and feet are inflamed, and the arthritis becomes chronic and resembles rheumatoid arthritis. The synovial fluid white blood cell count is some-

times elevated to 50,000/mm³, and rod-shaped bacilli (*Tropheryma whippelii*) have been identified, usually by electron microscopy, in synovial biopsy specimens. These organisms are also seen attached to circulating erythrocytes. Diagnosis is facilitated by polymerase chain reaction analysis of tissue or blood. The arthritis may antedate gastrointestinal and other symptoms by years. Rheumatoid factors and antinuclear antibody are not features of Whipple's disease.

HYPERLIPOPROTEINEMIA (see Chapter 206). An association exists between type II familial hypercholesterolemia (both homozygous and heterozygous forms) and musculoskeletal symptoms such as Achilles tendinitis, oligoarthritis, and polyarthritis. Transient pain in the Achilles tendon appears to be more common than frank inflammatory tendinitis, which can last a few days and recur two or three times a year. A few patients have acute painful monoarthritis or pauciarthritis of the knees, ankles, or small joints that lasts a week or more and recurs frequently. Less common is an incapacitating polyarthritis resembling rheumatic fever, persisting a month or more. In one study, 40% of 73 heterozygous patients were symptomatic; articular manifestations appeared at times before the xanthomas that are the major diagnostic sign of familial hypercholesterolemia.

ENDOCRINE DISORDERS (see Chapters 237, 239, and 264). Aches and stiffness simulating fibromyalgia may appear early in hypothyroidism; if untreated, this may progress to proximal myopathy with elevated creatine kinase levels, simulating polymyositis, or to a syndrome of synovial thickening and joint effusions, simulating rheumatoid arthritis. Carpal tunnel syndrome is a recognized manifestation of hypothyroidism, and there appears to be an association with calcium pyrophosphate deposition disease. Hyperthyroidism can cause myopathy without elevations of the creatine kinase level but with muscle wasting, which can be severe. Thyroid acropachy, seen rarely in association with pretibial myxedema and Graves' disease, is characterized by diffuse swelling of the fingers and clubbing.

Hyperparathyroidism is a rare cause of diffuse, vague musculoskeletal pains resembling those of fibrositis. The other musculoskeletal complications of hyperparathyroidism include back pain due to vertebral body fractures, an erosive arthritis predominantly in the hands and wrists, and chondrocalcinosis (with pseudogout occurring most often after parathyroidectomy).

Carpal tunnel syndrome has been reported in almost one half of persons with acromegaly. Raynaud's phenomenon is rare. The arthritis of acromegaly is clinically indistinguishable from osteoarthritis.

SARCOIDOSIS (see Chapter 81). Joint or juxta-articular pains are experienced by as many as one third of patients with acute sarcoidosis and may be the only symptom of the disease; however, erythema nodosum often accompanies the arthritis and, together with hilar adenopathy, suggests the diagnosis (one should be aware that arthritis may accompany erythema nodosum of any cause). Arthritis often begins in the ankles and spreads symmetrically. The distal interphalangeal joints are typically spared, but any of the other peripheral joints, as well as the heels, may be painful out of proportion to signs of inflammation, which are meager. Episodes last a few days to a few months, and the arthritis usually resolves completely. The erythrocyte sedimentation rate is often elevated; antinuclear antibodies and rheumatoid factors may be present in high titer. Treatment with salicylates, non-steroidal anti-inflammatory drugs (NSAIDs), or prednisone is based on the severity of the arthritis. Progressive, deforming arthritis is a feature of chronic sarcoidosis, as are bone lesions, both lytic and sclerotic. Clinically significant sarcoid myopathy is rare.

FAMILIAL MEDITERRANEAN FEVER (see Chapters 171 and 297). Serositis, fever, and arthritis are the major signs of familial Mediterranean fever. Arthritis occurs in as many as one half of patients; it is usually monoarticular and confined to large joints in the lower extremities. Although the arthritis usually lasts less than 1 week, it has been reported to persist for several months. Synovial fluid contains large numbers of granulocytes, and there is intense infiltration of granulocytes and hyperemia in synovial tissue. Diagnosis is suggested by demographic and other clinical features of the disease; criteria for diagnosis have been proposed and are based on the clinical features. In the absence of these, familial Mediterranean fever is easily confused with juvenile rheumatoid arthritis. Colchicine often prevents arthritis as well as amyloidosis.

Livneh A, Langevitz P, Zemer D, et al: Criteria for the diagnosis of familial Mediterranean fever. Arthritis Rheum 40:1879, 1997. *The authors propose diagnostic criteria based on the major clinical manifestations of pleuritis, pericarditis, peritonitis, fever, and arthritis.*

Totemchokchyakarn K, Ball G: Sarcoid arthropathy. Bull Rheum Dis 46:3, 1997. *A review of the various rheumatologic manifestations of sarcoidosis.*

305 MISCELLANEOUS FORMS OF ARTHRITIS

Eugene V. Ball

NEUROPATHIC JOINT DISEASE (CHARCOT'S JOINTS). Recognition of neuropathic joint disease and its association with syphilis preceded reports of its association with diabetes mellitus by 64 years, but syphilis has been surpassed by the latter as the leading cause of this disorder. In syphilis, subacute combined degeneration of the spinal cord, paraplegia, and Charcot-Marie-Tooth disease, weakness, decreased pain sensation, and impaired position sense contribute to the massive destruction of the knee (or less often the hip, ankle, or spine) that typifies the disorder. In syringomyelia, the shoulder or upper limb is most often involved. Neuropathic disease of the knee or ankle is suggested by effusions, crepitus, enlargement, and relatively little pain, although pain may become worrisome late in the disease. Neuropathic joint disease in diabetes mellitus (Fig. 305–1) causes painless swelling of one or both feet in patients with long-standing disease and sensory neuropathy. For mechanical reasons, the tarsometatarsal and the metatarsophalangeal joints are most frequently involved. Destruction also occurs in the talus, the calcaneus, the ankle joints, and the distal tibia. Radiographs characteristically show loss of joint space, sclerosis, multiple irregular bodies representing chip fractures, and new bone formation; comparable changes are seen in osteomyelitis. Differen-

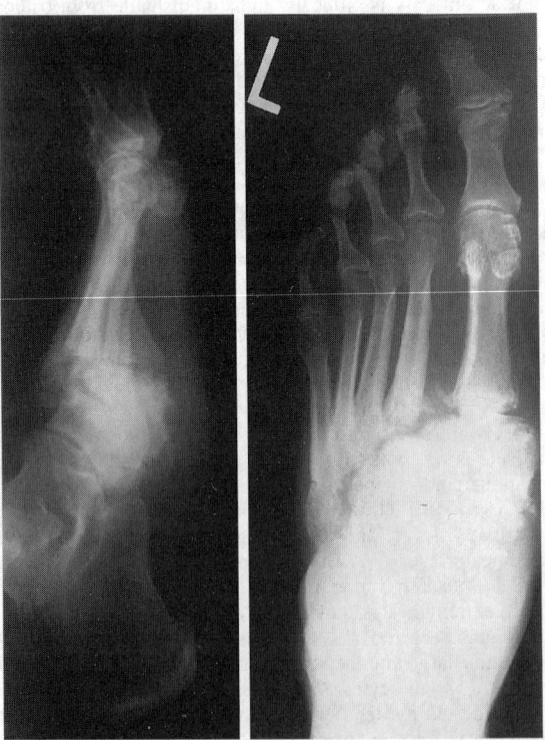

FIGURE 305–1 ■ Diabetes mellitus and neuropathic arthritis. Note lateral displacement of metatarsals *(left)* and fragmentation and osseous debris *(right)*.

tiation of these two disorders can be difficult; magnetic resonance imaging may help identify them. (Less severe, but similar, changes have been reported in calcium pyrophosphate deposition disease.) It is thought that excess osteoclast activity is responsible for early bone changes in diabetes. Treatment of acute arthropathy requires prompt reduction in weight bearing. Attempts at stabilizing the involved joint with various orthotic devices are often unsatisfactory, and surgical fusion is difficult. Total knee or hip arthroplasty may be useful.

HEMARTHROSIS. Although trauma accounts for most hemarthrosis, hemophilia A and B (see Chapter 185) are its major medical cause. The severity of hemarthrosis in hemophilia is related to the levels of clotting factors. For example, infants with factor VIII or IX levels less than 1% often experience hemarthrosis before the age of 1. By age 15, virtually all persons with severe, inadequately treated factor deficiencies have some form of chronic joint impairment.

Acute bleeding into a joint (most often the knees, elbows, or ankles) or muscle is frequently signified by stiffness or discomfort, followed by pain, swelling, and redness. The joint should be immobilized, and adequate factor replacement should be started as early as possible, preferably during the prodromal phase. The joint changes stimulated by repeated intra-articular bleeding resemble those of rheumatoid arthritis. Hyperplastic synovium appears to be the source of proteases and other enzymes that destroy cartilage and bone, culminating in the absence of articular cartilage, joint disorganization, and fibrous contractures. Education of the patient and family, as well as home treatment, prevents or attenuates chronic, destructive arthritis. Joint replacements have been done successfully to relieve pain and restore function.

Bleeding into a muscle, which also should be treated with replacement factor, can lead to necrosis and fibrotic scarring. Pseudotumors are cystic bone swellings resulting from intraosseous bleeding and necrosis.

Von Willebrand's disease can produce hemarthrosis and joint destruction comparable to that of hemophilia.

Painful but non-destructive intra-articular bleeding is a common feature of scurvy, and intra-articular tumors such as pigmented villonodular synovitis frequently cause monoarticular bleeding.

MULTICENTRIC RETICULOHISTIOCYTOSIS. The chief manifestations of multicentric reticulohistiocytosis are arthritis and red to purple skin nodules varying in size from 1 to 10 mm. The nodules are found in any part of the skin but tend to concentrate on the face and hands and uncommonly coalesce. The arthritis is most often symmetrical and polyarticular. Unlike adult rheumatoid arthritis, it does not spare the distal interphalangeal joints. It can be severely destructive, and in one third of cases it progresses to arthritis multilans. Systemic signs include fever and weight loss; less often, pericarditis and myositis are present, and it is frequently associated with malignancy.

The disorder also has been termed *lipoid dermatoarthritis* because of the glycolipids contained within the histiocytes and granulomas that constitute the basic lesion. In the absence of a serum or lesional lipid abnormality, lipid deposition is now thought to be non-specific. Improvement, which may be spontaneous, has been reported more consistently with alkylating agents and methotrexate than with prednisone.

HYPERTROPHIC OSTEOARTHROPATHY AND CARCINOMA POLYARTHRITIS. Hypertrophic osteoarthropathy is a systemic disorder distinguished by clubbing of the digits as a result of edema and collagen deposition and by periostitis of the distal ends of tubular bones. The lesions presumably begin with increased blood flow and periosteal edema and with fibroblast proliferation, followed by new bone formation. Radionuclide bone scans are positive at an early stage, often preceding radiographic evidence of periosteal new bone. Hypertrophic osteoarthropathy frequently involves the tibiae, ulnae, radii, femora, metatarsals, and metacarpals. Painful articular swelling appears in approximately 30% of patients and may be debilitating; other variable features of the syndrome include gynecomastia and thickening and furrowing of the facial skin. Intrathoracic malignancies, especially squamous cell carcinoma, have supplanted pulmonary infections as the most common cause. Pleural and diaphragmatic neoplasms and nasopharyngeal carcinomas are strongly associated with hypertrophic osteoarthropathy. Less common causes include chronic liver disease, inflammatory bowel disease, and cyanotic heart disease. There is also a hereditary form termed *pachydermoperiostosis*, with strong male predominance and a curious bimodal distribution of disease onset during the first year of life or the midteens. No satisfactory unifying theory of pathogenesis exists, although there is some evidence that platelet activation of endothelial cells, and excess platelet-derived growth factor and fibroblast growth factors, may cause the changes seen clinically. Successful treatment of the underlying disorder results in regression of the disorder. In fact, thoracotomy for cancer-causing pulmonary hypertrophic osteoarthropathy may result in a marked decrease in pain and swelling within 24 hours. Pamidronate and subcutaneous octreotide have been reported to reduce pain, which can be severe.

The "sudden" onset of polyarthritis resembling rheumatoid arthritis in an older adult should prompt suspicion of an associated malignancy. Carcinoma polyarthritis may appear months before, or after, detection of malignancy of many types, particularly lung and breast. Its incidence is unknown; in one small series it was almost as common as carcinomatous hypertrophic osteoarthropathy and more common than cancer-related dermatomyositis. Palmar fasciitis has been noted in association with ovarian cancer.

Holmes GB, Hill N: Fractures and dislocations of the foot and ankle in diabetics associated with Charcot joint changes. Foot Ankle Int 15:182–185, 1994. *A report of foot and ankle fractures and their management in 18 patients with diabetes mellitus.*

Hoyer LW: Hemophilia A. N Engl J Med 330:38, 1994. *A review of the structure and function of factor VIII, the molecular genetics of hemophilia A, its clinical manifestations, and treatment.*

Speden D, Nicklason F, Ward FHJ: The use of pamidronate in hypertrophic pulmonary osteoarthropathy (HPOA) Aust NZ J Med 27:307–310, 1997. *Pain was relieved in three patients given pamidronate.*

306 NON-ARTICULAR RHEUMATISM
Eugene V. Ball

FIBROMYALGIA (FIBROSITIS). Primary fibromyalgia (FM) has been defined as chronic, widespread musculoskeletal pain and tenderness at multiple sites (e.g., at 11 of 18 specific sites in the criteria of the American College of Rheumatology). (The tender point count has been referred to as a "sedimentation rate" for distress.) Implicit in this definition is the absence of signs of connective tissue or other musculoskeletal disease. Because of its subjective nature and its frequent association with disturbed sleep, chronic fatigue, headaches, and irritable bowel syndrome, the validity of classifying FM as a disease rather than a "syndrome of being out of sorts" has been challenged. Patients often appear anxious and depressed, and studies have shown that they may feel dissatisfied with all aspects of their lives and it is claimed there is strong evidence for an association between FM and major depressive disorder. Nevertheless, the specific characteristics of anxiety and depression have not been identified consistently on psychological testing, and it has been suggested that chronic pain and fatigue of any cause can engender anxiety and depression. Despite their subjectivity, symptoms of FM tend to be constant over many years; exceptionally, FM has been found to be premonitory of psychosis or hypothyroidism. Decreased threshold to pain on pressure over certain sites and increased skin fold tenderness have led to numerous attempts to demonstrate localized peripheral abnormalities and to speculation that FM is a disorder of pain modulation. There have been no irrefutable biochemical, immunologic, or anatomic abnormalities detected in FM; however, studies of biopsied muscle samples have found decreased levels of adenosine triphosphate and phosphocreatine. These findings have been confirmed by magnetic resonance spectroscopy in a small number of patients. Other findings such as decreased regional cerebral blood flow have been cited as evidence for functional dysregulation of central pain pathways.

Functional disability in FM may exceed that of rheumatoid arthritis; and in 1989, FM was the most frequent single reason for disability pensions among women in Norway, accounting for 7.2% of new pensions. (The prevalence in Norway has been estimated to be as high as 10% in women.) Patients whose FM begins acutely after a specific traumatic event are more likely to be disabled than those in whom the disorder evolves insidiously. FM is significantly less common in men than in women and is either underreported or uncommon in developing countries. Treatment is often frustrating for both patient and physician. It should emphasize the non-destructive nature of FM, and the physician should be wary of overusing drugs to allay anxiety or induce sleep. Low-dose amitriptyline and fluoxetine are valuable for decreasing pain and improving sleep in some patients. It has been the author's experience that patients are often either intolerant of medications or they have a short-lived response to any intervention.

BURSITIS. Bursae are small, synovial-lined, fluid-filled sacs located between tendons and bones which serve to reduce friction between opposing muscles or tendons. Most bursae are present from birth; however, others form in response to repeated pressure.

Of the approximately 80 bursae located on each side of the body, only a few are common sources of pain. The subdeltoid is the largest of the bursae around the shoulder (see Chapter 303); it is located between the deltoid muscle and the shoulder capsule and extends under the acromion. Acute inflammation of this or nearby bursae and tendons may be exceedingly painful, resulting in restricted shoulder movement and tenderness over the rotator cuff. Intrabursal injection of lidocaine is diagnostic and often curative; however, recurrences are common. Bursal calcification predisposes to more frequent attacks. Infection is most common in the olecranon bursa.

Trochanteric bursitis is believed to occur as a result of chronic strain on weak quadricep muscles or overuse of hip and thigh muscles. Pain is often perceived to be in the lateral aspect of the thigh and the low back and is aggravated by abducting the affected leg and by lying on the affected side. Tenderness is present at the edge of the greater trochanter. Injections of lidocaine and depot corticosteroids often abolish the pain.

TENDINOUS LESIONS. Tendinous lesions include tenosynovitis, a lesion of the gliding surfaces of a tendon and its sheath; tendinitis, painful scarring within a tendon; and trigger lesions, which are localized enlargements of the tendon that engage a constricted part of the sheath (as in "trigger finger"). Flexor digital tenosynovitis may cause pain in the metacarpophalangeal or proximal interphalangeal joints. Tendinous lesions are common, occurring in many areas of the musculoskeletal system. An example is de Quervain's disease, which is stenosing tenosynovitis of the abductor pollicis longus and extensor pollicis brevis at the medial styloid. Pain can localize or radiate into the hand or back to the shoulder. This and carpal tunnel syndrome occur frequently during pregnancy.

CARPAL TUNNEL SYNDROME. The symptoms of carpal tunnel syndrome are paresthesias and pain in the palmar side of the first three fingers and at times the radial half of the fourth finger; the pain may radiate proximally to the shoulder, creating confusion with a cervical disk syndrome. Physical findings include sensory loss, weakness on abduction and opposition of the thumb, and atrophy of the thenar eminence. Carpal tunnel syndrome is caused by an array of conditions that result in pressure on the median nerve as it passes through the bony flexor compartment of the wrist. Some of these are listed in Table 306–1. Patients with fibromyalgia often have symptoms of carpal tunnel syndrome.

Diagnosis is confirmed by electrophysiologic nerve tests. (The clinical tests commonly used are of questionable value.) Magnetic resonance imaging may be useful in defining the cause and thus directing treatment, which might include splinting of the wrist, corticosteroid injections, and surgical release of the transverse carpal ligament.

TENNIS ELBOW. "Tennis elbow" refers to a lesion of the wrist extensor muscles causing pain at the outer elbow, along the back of the forearm, or, less commonly, into the shoulder. The burning or

Table 306–1 ■ CONDITIONS CAUSING CARPAL TUNNEL SYNDROME

Trauma
Occupation
Infections (e.g., Lyme disease and rubella)
Rheumatoid arthritis and gout
Pregnancy
Hypothyroidism and acromegaly
Amyloidosis
Median artery aneurysm
Ganglion cyst, increased fat, hypertrophy of abductor pollicis muscle

aching pain is produced by resisted extension of the wrist, as in grasping and lifting, and rarely is felt as sudden, searing twinges of intensity sufficient to cause momentary grip paralysis. Tennis elbow usually results from repeated forceful extension of the wrist. A tear or area of degeneration most often occurs at the origin of the common extensor tendon from the lateral humoral epicondyle; much less frequently, the tear is in the muscle belly. Treatment includes exercise of wrist extensor muscles, injection of triamcinolone into the painful scar, manipulation, or partial tenotomy.

Like tennis elbow, "golfer's elbow" is a misnomer in that both conditions occur frequently in people who do not play either sport. Golfer's elbow is less painful than tennis elbow; it represents a lesion of the common flexor tendon at the medial epicondyle. Pain is usually localized to the inner side of the elbow and is produced by resisted flexion of the wrist. Treatment includes triamcinolone injection and massage.

TIETZE'S SYNDROME. Tietze's syndrome is an uncommon cause of chest pain that can be mistaken for visceral pain. There is tender, most often unilateral, swelling at one or more costosternal junctions. Biopsy samples of involved areas have revealed chronic inflammatory fibrosis. The syndrome may result from prolonged coughing or hyperventilation, but it is often idiopathic. Injections into the painful area with triamcinolone are sometimes curative. Tietze's syndrome may be differentiated from the more common costochondritis, in which there are no signs of inflammation. Chest wall pain and tenderness are common in patients with fibromyalgia.

Aaron LA, Bradley LA, Alarcon GS, et al: Perceived physical and emotional trauma as precipitating events in fibromyalgia: Associations with health care seeking and disability status but not pain severity. Arthritis Rheum 40:453–460, 1997.
Kennedy M, Felson DT: A prospective long-term study of fibromyalgia syndrome. Arthritis Rheum 39:682–685, 1996.
Park JH, Phothimat P, Oates CT, et al: Use of P-31 magnetic resonance spectroscopy to detect metabolic abnormalities in muscles of patients with fibromyalgia. Arthritis Rheum 41:406–413, 1998.

307 ARTICULAR TUMORS

Eugene V. Ball

Articular tumors can be classified as those that arise within the synovium; those that arise from cartilage, bone, or contiguous structures; and neoplasms that are non-articular in origin but that metastasize to joints or develop in multiple areas, including joints. Benign tumors include lipomas, neuromas, fibromas, and hemangiomas. The most common of these are probably synovial chondromas, which develop as cartilaginous synovial plaques that sometimes calcify. These plaques cause episodic pain or swelling in a single knee, hip, elbow, or shoulder and osteoarthritis. The joint may lock if the plaques become detached, forming loose bodies. Radiographs reveal multiple opacities if ossification has occurred; arthroscopy may be useful for both diagnosis and treatment, which is surgical.

Pigmented villonodular synovitis (PVNS) is a non-malignant proliferative disorder of unknown cause that usually affects the entire synovium of a single joint. This condition occurs most often in early middle age and in the knee in 80% of cases. Uncommonly, two or more joints are involved; similar lesions occur in tendons and bursae. Pain and swelling are characteristic, as is serosanguineous synovial fluid. Radiographic signs include soft tissue swelling, osteolysis, subchondral cysts (particularly in the hip), and pressure erosions. One of two major cell types exhibit features associated with osteoclasts. Treatment is synovectomy. Hemangiomas, lipomas, and xanthomas may simulate PVNS.

Synovial sarcomas (synoviomas) are rare, aggressive tumors of young adults. They usually originate in the extremities adjacent to, but not within, a joint. Primary tumors histologically identical to synoviomas have been found in the head and neck, abdominal wall, retroperitoneum, heart, and mediastinum, supporting the view that the tumor originates from mesenchyme rather than synovium. An SYT-SSX fusion gene is detectable in almost all synovial sarco-

mas. These tumors are usually discovered as deep swellings within a tendon sheath, a bursa, or a joint capsule. A few have been described with extensive osteoid and bone formation, simulating the radiographic appearance of benign lesions. Pain and tenderness are variable, as are effusions. These tumors metastasize early to lungs, bone, and lymph nodes. Tumor size more than 4 cm, a high mitotic rate, and local recurrence after excision convey a poor prognosis. Metastatic synovial sarcomas appear to be sensitive to multiagent chemotherapy.

Chondrosarcomas and fibrosarcomas are other malignancies arising within or near joints, and intrasynovial myeloma and lymphoma are rare causes of a swollen or painful joint.

Thorough investigation is required for unexplained pain or swelling within or adjacent to a single joint.

Kawai A, Woodruff J, Healey JH, et al: SYT-SSX gene fusion as a determinant of morphology and prognosis in synovial sarcoma. N Engl J Med 338:153–160, 1998. *The authors found that SYT-SSX fusion transcripts are a diagnostic marker, and have prognostic implications, for synovial sarcomas.*
Neale SD, Kristelly R, Gundle R, et al: Giant cells in pigmented villonodular synovitis express an osteoclast phenotype. J Clin Pathol 50:605–608, 1997. *The authors found evidence in one patient that the multinucleated giant cells of PVNS were phenotypically similar to osteoclasts, including their ability to cause bone resorption.*

308 ERYTHROMELALGIA

Eugene V. Ball

Erythromelalgia (erythermalgia) is a syndrome of episodic burning pain and redness in the extremities. Attacks may be confined to feet or, if severe and prolonged, may spread to hands, or they may begin simultaneously in hands and feet. They are often provoked by increasing ambient temperatures, although a few persons experience attacks only with febrile illnesses. The combination of increasing warmth and exercise often induces symptoms. To avoid attacks, some persons maintain environmental temperatures at levels that are uncomfortably low for themselves, as well as others. Relief may require immersing the feet in ice water. The feet appear normal between attacks, except in those persons who habitually walk barefoot because their attacks are provoked by wearing shoes.

Some clinicians use the terms *erythromelalgia* and *erythermalgia* for the symptom-complex, which they classify into primary erythromelalgia, erythromelalgia associated with thrombocythemia, and secondary erythromelalgia associated with a potpourri of unrelated medications and disorders. The primary form is sometimes familial. In one paradigmatic kindred, the disorder is autosomal dominant, and it has afflicted 29 members. Most often beginning between ages 2 and 8, it has been responsible for severe adjustment problems in youth, engendered in part by an inability to sit comfortably in a heated classroom or to participate in physical activities. In this kindred, the disorder has been frequently misdiagnosed as arthritis, reflex sympathetic dystrophy, or Raynaud's phenomenon. Its pathogenesis is unknown, but it is not related to thrombocythemia.

The most common recognized cause of non-familial erythromelalgia is thrombocythemia, which is usually a feature of a myeloproliferative disorder. In essential thrombocythemia, erythromelalgia has been noted with platelet counts as low as $400–500 \times 10^9/L$. It can be prevented by aspirin but not by oral anticoagulant or heparin therapy. Arteriolar inflammation and thrombotic occlusions are found on skin punch biopsy samples. Erythromelalgia disappears for 3 or 4 days after a single dose of aspirin, which is the duration of its inhibition of platelet aggregation; and studies by van Genderen and associates confirm that the erythromelalgia is caused by intravascular activation and aggregation of platelets, leading to endothelial cell damage.

Other reported associations with erythromelalgia include diabetes mellitus, pregnancy, neurologic disorders, and gout and connective tissue diseases. Nifedipine and bromocriptine can cause an erythromelalgia-like disorder. In the absence of thrombocythemia, aspirin is ineffective for treating or preventing erythromelalgia. Although there is no proven treatment, examples of those agents for which effectiveness has been claimed for non-thrombocythemic erythromelalgia include intravenous nitroprusside, cyproheptadine, and, counterintuitively, capsaicin ointment.

Finley WH, Lindsey Jr, Fine J-D, et al: Autosomal dominant erythromelalgia. Am J Med Genet 42:310, 1992. *Clinical description of erythromelalgia in a large kindred.*

Millard FE, Hunter CS, Anderson M, et al: Clinical manifestations of essential thrombocythemia in young adults. Am J Hematol 33:27, 1990. *Essential thrombocythemia was identified in 13 patients whose median age was 26. Erythromelalgia was the most common complication, occurring in 7 of the 13, of whom 7 were males.*

Van Genderen PJJ, Lucas IS, van Strik V, et al: Erythromelalgia in essential thrombocythemia is characterized by platelet activation and endothelial cell damage but not by thrombin generation. Thromb Haemost 76:333, 1996. *Studies show that the generation of thrombin is not essential for formation of platelet thrombi in this condition and that aspirin-induced remission was accompanied by a significant decrease in β-thromboglobulin and thrombomodulin.*

309 MULTIFOCAL FIBROSCLEROSIS

H. Ralph Schumacher, Jr.

In rare instances, the delicate fibrous areolar tissue in a certain anatomic region becomes the site of a chronic low-grade inflammatory process leading to deposition of dense sclerotic plaques that may obstruct or limit the movement of adjacent viscera. When the process is in the active phase, characteristic findings of chronic or granulomatous inflammation are present and featured by mononuclear cell infiltration, plasma cells, some eosinophils, and occasional giant cells. In the end stages the pathologic lesion is simply that of scar tissue, so by the time that this process causes clinical manifestations, little evidence of the initial inflammatory reaction may remain. At least some cases have an accompanying vasculitis. As a general rule, the process tends to originate in the midline, around the great vessels, and to then spread laterally. In most cases a clue to the inciting mechanism is lacking.

Syndromes that have been considered as manifestations of multifocal fibrosclerosis include retroperitoneal fibrosis, mediastinal fibrosis, sclerosing cholangitis (see Chapter 157), Riedel's thyroiditis (see Chapter 239), pseudotumor of the orbit, Peyronie's disease (sclerotic induration of the corpora cavernosa of the penis), pachymeningitis, and sclerosing peritonitis. Other sites of a similar fibrosis, such as the testes and vagina, have also been reported. Pulmonary and myocardial fibrosis syndromes have not generally been seen as being related to multifocal fibrosclerosis, although pleural fibrosis along with retroperitoneal fibrosis can be seen with ergotamine use.

Although most of these syndromes have been described as separate entities, several anatomic areas may become affected in one person. For example, retroperitoneal fibrosis and sclerosing mediastinitis may be present at the same time along with varying combinations of sclerosing cholangitis, Riedel's thyroiditis, and pseudotumor of the orbit. A possible genetic predisposition is suggested by familial cases and by an association between fibrosing syndromes and α_1-antitrypsin deficiency. Familial mediastinal or retroperitoneal fibrosis may also be associated with HLA-B27 and seronegative spondyloarthrophaties.

Comings DE, Skubi KB, Van Eyes J, et al: Familial multifocal sclerosis. Ann Intern Med 66:884, 1967. *Description of multiple sites of fibrosis in two brothers.*

Goldbach P, Mohsenifar Z, Salick Al: Familial mediastinal fibrosis associated with seronegative spondyloarthropathy. Arthritis Rheum 26:221, 1983. *Two siblings with both diseases.*

RETROPERITONEAL FIBROSIS. In retroperitoneal fibrosis, the process usually begins over the promontory of the sacrum and extends laterally across the ureters and as high as the 2nd or 3rd lumbar vertebra. Less commonly, the lesion develops in other extraperitoneal areas, e.g., contiguous with the kidneys, duodenum, descending colon, or urinary bladder. Some cases have an associated vasculitis in the skin and subcutaneous tissue manifested by the formation of nodules, erythematous discoloration, and ulceration. Similarly, inflammatory changes in small vessels at the sites of the sclerosis have been noted. Glomerulonephritis has been seen in a few patients.

The occurrence of retroperitoneal fibrosis in patients taking methysergide for migraine has been reported with greater frequency than could be due to chance. Occasional cases have been reported after the use of other drugs such as ergotamine, pergolide, various β-adrenergic blocking agents, hydralazine, and methyldopa. Associated diseases in patients with retroperitoneal fibrosis have included systemic lupus erythematosus; vasculitis with one patient positive for cytoplasmic antineutrophil cytoplasmic antibody; scleroderma; eosinophilic fasciitis; biliary cirrhosis; juvenile and rubella-associated arthritis; renal, uterine, and other cancers; and carcinoid. Trauma, surgery, and, occasionally, ruptured echinococcal cysts have been reported as apparent causes. One patient with associated periarticular fibrosis had elevated plasma levels of a platelet-derived growth factor.

The disorder is about twice as common in males as in females, and the peak incidence is in the 5th and 6th decades. Cases have been reported in children. The manifestations are variable, depending on the anatomic location of the process. Pain is the most common symptom; it tends to be located in the low back region and may be accompanied by symptoms referable to the gastrointestinal tract. The patient is likely to lose weight and have low-grade fever. Some anemia and an elevated erythrocyte sedimentation rate may be present. Although the ureter is the structure most often affected, symptoms referable to the urinary tract are uncommon until obstructive uropathy has led to azotemia and other clinical manifestations of renal insufficiency. The fibrosing process may surround the inferior vena cava, but obstruction of that vessel is uncommon. Thromboembolism and hypertension can be complications. Arterial invasion has been described, and portal hypertension or bile duct obstruction with pseudotumor of the pancreas may occur. Retroperitoneal fibrosis occasionally develops in association with definable abdominal aortic aneurysm or aortitis and is considered in some cases to begin as a periaortitis. A possible element of reaction to atheromatous components has been described.

The diagnosis of retroperitoneal fibrosis has been most often suggested by findings at intravenous pyelography: displacement of the ureters toward the midline and evidence of obstruction, usually at the level of the pelvic brim. One or both ureters may be affected. In rare instances a mass can be palpated in the pelvis or on the posterior abdominal wall. Ultrasonography, computed tomographic scanning, and magnetic resonance imaging can also identify the fibrosing masses. Gallium scintigraphy may help assess activity of inflammation. Once a mass has been disclosed, the main problem in the differential diagnosis lies in distinguishing retroperitoneal fibrosis from retroperitoneal tumor. Multiple deep biopsies should be made at the time of laparotomy. Fine-needle aspiration biopsy may be suggestive if laparoscopy or laparotomy are not possible.

Surgical treatment, if performed before severe renal damage, is often highly successful. Inasmuch as the fibrosing process is seldom invasive, the constricted organ can usually be freed by blunt dissection so that normal movement or flow is restored. Relief of ureteral obstruction is usually achieved by bringing the ureter out on the anterior surface of the sclerotic mass. Occasionally, however, the obstruction recurs months or years after such treatment. Some surgeons wrap the ureters in omentum to decrease recurrent obstruction. Steroid therapy may be helpful in the rare case detected early or may be used as an adjunct to surgical measures. Azathioprine or cyclophosphamide has been used successfully in a few cases. Progesterone and tamoxifen have been reported to produce regression of fibrosis. When the inferior vena cava is obstructed, surgical relief is technically difficult and risky; here it may be preferable to temporize in the hope that development of collateral pathways may alleviate the circulatory block.

The long-term outlook is fairly good if the disease is recognized and its obstructive consequences can be treated by surgical means. The disease often tends to run its course and subside. Most deaths have been caused by renal failure.

Bonnet C, Arnavel M, Bertin P, et al: Idiopathic retroperitoneal fibrosis with systemic manifestations. J Rheumatol 21:360, 1994 *Panniculitis occurred along with mesenteric, pulmonary, and perhaps periarticular fibrosis.*

Cohle SD, Leil JT: Inflammatory aneurysm of the aorta, aortic note and coronary arteritis. Arch Pathol Lab Med 112:1121, 1988. *Inflammatory aneurysms of the aorta and other vasculitis may be associated with retroperitoneal fibrosis.*

Owens LV, Cance WG, Huth JF: Retroperitoneal fibrosis treated with tamoxifen. Am Surg 61:842, 1985. *Tamoxifen is an increasingly reported therapeutic choice.*

MEDIASTINAL FIBROSIS. Taut bundles of collagenous tissue form in the superior and anterior mediastinum, with impingement on the aorta, trachea, bronchi, esophagus, and pericardium. Patients may have thoracic pain, but the predominant manifestations are those caused by obstruction of the superior vena cava: puffy, suffused appearance of the face and conjunctivae; non-pitting edema of the face, neck, and upper extremities: and distended veins in the neck and upper extremities. Rarely, the principal vessels affected are the pulmonary arteries, with subsequent pulmonary hypertension. More frequently, the pulmonary veins are involved, and here severe hemoptysis may be the most prominent manifestation. Pericardial fibrosis can lead to constrictive pericarditis. The main task in the differential diagnosis is to distinguish this relatively benign condition from obstruction caused by tumor. Radiographic examination of the chest may reveal little or no abnormality or some pleural thickening. Angiographic studies show obstruction of the affected vessels. Thoracotomy may be required for histologic diagnosis.

Histoplasmosis and possibly tuberculosis may cause some mediastinal fibrosis. Mediastinal hemorrhage can lead to fibrosis, and cases have been associated with methysergide use. An interesting recent association has been with the SAPHO syndrome (*s*ynovitis, *a*cne, *p*ustulosis, *h*yperostosis, and *o*steomyelitis). Some patients with this syndrome have shown gradual improvement over months or years, presumably because of the development of collateral circulation. Successful superior vena cava bypass surgery has been described. Corticosteroid therapy was ineffective in some reported cases.

Cunningham T, Farrell J, Veale D, et al: Anterior mediastinal fibrosis with superior vena caval obstruction complicating the synovitis-acne-pustulosis-hyperostosis-osteo-myelitis syndrome. Br J Rheumatol 32:408, 1993. *This idiopathic sterile inflammatory reaction most often involves the anterior chest wall.*

Mathiesen DJ, Grillo HC: Clinical manifestation of mediastinal fibrosis and histoplasmosis. Ann Thorac Surg 54:1053, 1992. *Histoplasma was still stainable in some resected specimens.*

Papandreou L, Panagou P, Bouros D: Mediastinal fibrosis and radiofrequency radiation exposure: Is there an association? Respiration 59:181, 1992. *Hemoptysis can be an initial symptom. This and other reports raise the question of radiation as a cause.*

SCLEROSING PERITONITIS. A fibrotic syndrome has been observed in patients treated for prolonged periods with the now withdrawn β-adrenergic blocking drug practolol and very rarely with other β-blockers. Some cases developed years after cessation of therapy. The peritonitis consists of thick fibrous encasement of the small intestine, and symptoms include abdominal fullness, back pain, ascites, weight loss, and signs of subacute intestinal obstruction. Surgery may be needed to peel away the fibrous tissue. Sclerosing peritonitis with many similarities has also been seen in idiopathic forms in association with systemic conditions, including drug abuse, sarcoidosis, and sicca syndrome, and now most importantly in patients treated with continuous ambulatory peritoneal dialysis and in women with ovarian tumors, most often luteinized thecomas. A variety of factors used in dialysis have been suggested to contribute. Hemoperitoneum and peritoneal calcification have been reported along with intestinal obstruction and ultrafiltration failure. Ultrasound findings can suggest the diagnosis. Some recent cases have responded to immunosuppresive or corticosteroid therapy.

Lo WK, Chan KT, Leung AC, et al: Sclerosing peritonitis complicating prolonged use of chlorhexidine in alcohol in the connection procedure for continuous ambulatory peritoneal dialysis. Peritoneal Dialysis Int 11:166, 1991. *A mechanism is suggested and improvement noted with continued chronic ambulatory peritoneal dialysis without the chlorhexidine.*

Mori Y, Matsco S, Sutch IT et al: A case of a dialysis patient with sclerosing peritonitis successfully treated with corticosteroid therapy alone. Am J Kidney Dis 30:275, 1997. *Surgery may be avoided in some cases.*

PART XXII

INFECTIOUS DISEASES

310 INTRODUCTION TO MICROBIAL DISEASE

Gerald L. Mandell

Infectious diseases have profoundly influenced the course of human history. The black plague (caused by *Yersinia pestis*) changed the social structure of medieval Europe. The outcomes of military campaigns have been altered by outbreaks of diseases such as dysentery and typhus. Malaria influenced the geographic and racial pattern of distribution of hemoglobins and erythrocyte antigens. The development of *Plasmodium falciparum* is inhibited by the presence of hemoglobin S, and Duffy blood group–negative erythrocytes are resistant to infection with *Plasmodium vivax*. Thus, populations with these erythrocyte factors are found in areas where malaria is common. Infections are the major cause of morbidity and mortality in the developing world. The acquired immunodeficiency syndrome (AIDS) threatens to disrupt the social fabric in some countries of Africa and is severely stressing the health care system in the United States and other parts of the world.

Infection may be defined as multiplication of microbes (viruses, bacteria, fungi, protozoa, or multicellular parasites) in the tissues of the host. The host may or may not be symptomatic. For example, infection with the human immunodeficiency virus (HIV) may cause no overt signs or symptoms of illness for years. The definition of infection also should include instances of multiplication of microbes on the surface or in a lumen of the host, causing signs and symptoms of illness or disease.

Toxin-producing strains of *Escherichia coli* may multiply in the gut and cause a diarrheal illness without invading tissues. Microbes can cause diseases without actually coming in contact with the host by virtue of toxin production. *Clostridium botulinum* may grow in certain improperly processed foods and produce a toxin that can be lethal on ingestion. A relatively trivial infection such as that caused by *Clostridium tetani* in a small puncture wound can cause devastating illness because of a toxin released from the organism growing in the tissues.

We live in a virtual sea of microorganisms, and all our body surfaces have an indigenous bacterial flora. This normal flora actually protects us from infection. Reduction of gut colonization increases susceptibility to infection by pathogens such as *Salmonella typhimurium*. The normal florae are thought to exert their protective effect by several mechanisms: (1) utilizing nutrients and occupying an ecologic niche, thus competing with pathogens; (2) producing antibacterial substances that inhibit the growth of pathogens; and (3) inducing host immunity that is cross-reactive and effective against pathogens. In addition to the normal flora, transient colonization may be seen with known or potential pathogens. This may be a special problem in hospitalized patients (see Chapter 315).

Only a very small proportion of microbial species may be considered to be primary or professional pathogens, and even among these species only a relatively small number of clones have been shown to cause disease. This supports the concept that pathogenic organisms are highly adapted to the pathogenic state and have developed characteristics that enable them to be transmitted, to attach to surfaces, to invade tissue, to avoid host defenses, and thus to cause disease. In contrast, opportunistic pathogens cause disease principally in impaired hosts. Organisms that may be harmless members of the normal flora in healthy persons may act as virulent invaders in patients with severe defects in host defense mechanisms.

Pathogenic organisms may be acquired by several routes. Direct contact has been implicated in the acquisition of staphylococcal disease. Airborne spread, usually by droplet nuclei, occurs in respiratory diseases such as influenza. Contaminated water is the usual vehicle in *Giardia* infection and typhoid fever. Food-borne toxin illnesses may be caused by extracellular toxins produced by *Clostridium perfringens* and *Staphylococcus aureus*. Blood and blood products may be vectors for transmitting hepatitis B virus and HIV. Sexual transmission is also important for these latter two agents and for a variety of pathogens, including *Treponema pallidum* (syphilis), *Neisseria gonorrhoeae* (gonorrhea), and *Chlamydia trachomatis* (non-specific urethritis). The fetus may be infected in utero, and this may be devastating if the infective agent is rubella virus or cytomegalovirus. Arthropod vectors may be important, as illustrated by mosquitoes for malaria, ticks for Lyme disease, and lice for typhus.

Pathogens are able to cause disease because of a finely tuned array of adaptations. These include the ability to attach to appropriate cells, often mediated by specialized structures such as the pili on gram-negative rods. Microbes such as *Shigella* species have the ability to invade cells and cause damage in that way. Toxins may act at a distance or may intoxicate only infected cells. Pathogens have the ability to thwart host defenses by a variety of ingenious maneuvers. The antiphagocytic capsular coat of the pneumococcus is an example. Organisms may change their surface antigen display so as to outmaneuver the host immune system. This can be seen with influenza virus and trypanosomes. Certain pathogens have the ability to inhibit the respiratory burst of phagocytes (*Toxoplasma gondii*), and others can destroy phagocytic cells that have engulfed them (*Streptococcus pyogenes*). The environment plays an important role in infection, both in transmission and in the ability of the host to combat the invader. The humidity and temperature of air may affect the infectivity of airborne pathogens. The sanitary state of food and water is an important factor for the acquisition of enteric pathogens. The "bad air" of swamps associated with malaria turned out to be due to the mosquitoes, but the environmental association was appropriate. The nutritional status of the host clearly is a significant factor in certain infectious diseases. The establishment of infection is a complicated interplay of factors involving the microbe, the host, and the environment.

Host reaction to infection may result in illness. For example, recent data suggest that prior infection with *Campylobacter jejuni* is responsible for about 40% of cases of Guillain-Barré syndrome. The mechanism is thought to be production of antibodies against *C. jejuni* lipopolysaccharides that cross react with gangliosides in peripheral nerves.

With rare exceptions, infections are treatable and often curable diseases. Thus, it is important to make an accurate etiologic diagnosis and promptly institute appropriate therapy. In acute infections such as pneumonia, meningitis, or gram-negative sepsis, rapid institution of therapy may be lifesaving, and thus a *presumptive* etiologic diagnosis should be established before a *definitive* diagnosis. This presumptive diagnosis can be based on the history, physical examination, epidemiology of illness in the community, and rapid techniques such as microscopic examination of appropriate gram-stained specimens. Antimicrobial therapy can then be instituted for the presumptive etiologic agents but must be re-evaluated as more definitive diagnostic information becomes available (see Chapters 318 and 374).

311 THE FEBRILE PATIENT

David C. Dale

Fever, or "pyrexia," is an elevation of body temperature to a level above normal, i.e., to greater than 37.5° C (99.5° F), caused by resetting of the thermoregulatory center in the medulla. To detect fever, oral, rectal, tympanic membrane, and pulmonary artery measurements are more reliable than axillary temperatures. Fever is a useful marker of inflammation; usually the height of the fever reflects the severity of the inflammatory process. Anorexia, malaise, myalgias, headache, and other constitutional symptoms often occur concomitantly. When the body temperature changes rapidly, chills and sweats are also observed. Fever with night sweats is a feature of many chronic inflammatory conditions. *Hyperthermia* is a term for fever caused by a disturbance in thermal regulatory control: excessive heat production (e.g., with vigorous exercise or as a reaction to some anesthetics), decreased dissipation (e.g., with dehydration), or loss of regulation (e.g., from injury to the hypothalamic regulatory center).

Most febrile patients have pain, tenderness, redness, and swelling at the site of inflammation, and the cause of the fever is readily identified. In a general medical practice, the most common causes of fever are upper respiratory illnesses, urinary tract infections, cellulitis, superficial abscesses, and pneumonia. In otherwise healthy individuals, fever alone is not a cause for hospitalization unless it is quite high (>39° C or 102° F) or accompanied by shaking, chills, hypotension, a change in sensorium, or other symptoms suggesting bacteremia. However, in immunosuppressed individuals, the elderly, and patients with recent surgery, greater caution is indicated.

FEVER OF UNEXPLAINED ORIGIN. A unexplained fever is usually defined in adults as an illness lasting more than 3 weeks with temperatures greater than 101° F (38.3° C) in which a diagnosis has not been made despite a good hospital or office evaluation. Ordinarily, by this time the work-up has included a history, physical examination, routine blood and urine tests and cultures, radiographs, and some specialized serologic tests. With careful further evaluation a diagnosis can be made in 70 to 90% of these cases.

Diagnoses for unexplained fevers fall into six general categories: infections, non-infectious inflammatory conditions, neoplastic diseases, drug fevers, factitious illnesses, and a group of less common causes (Table 311–1). The pattern of fever is only occasionally helpful in pointing to a specific diagnosis, e.g., the alternate-day fever in established *Plasmodium vivax* infections, the sustained fever in untreated *Salmonella typhi* infections and other continuous bacteremias, and the relapsing (Pel-Ebstein) fever in Hodgkin's disease and other lymphomas.

EVALUATION OF THE PATIENTS WITH UNEXPLAINED FEVER. In patients with persisting fever, it is important initially to review carefully the medical history and repeat the physical examination. New clues may be found in the social, occupational, travel, and medication history. On physical examination, special attention should be given to the skin, lymph nodes (including epitrochlear, post-auricular, axillary), mucous membranes (including the conjunctivae), and abdominal region (masses, tenderness, and size of the liver and spleen). Usually the basic laboratory tests—complete blood count, differential, sedimentation rate, urinalysis, liver function tests, skin tests for delayed hypersensitivity (e.g., purified protein derivative, mumps), and stool for occult blood—should be repeated. Most patients with active inflammation are anemic, and the leukocyte differential can provide valuable clues. Neutrophilia suggests an occult bacterial infection. Monocytosis suggests tuberculosis, brucellosis, inflammatory bowel disease, or other chronic inflammatory conditions. Severe lymphopenia suggests immunodeficiency or a malignancy. A very elevated sedimentation rate suggests giant cell/temporal arteritis, polymyalgia rheumatica, Still's disease, bacterial endocarditis, or other occult infections, and a normal test rarely occurs with any of these illnesses. If the alkaline phosphatase level is elevated, obstructive or infiltrative disease of the liver is the most likely cause, although non-specific elevation is

Table 311–1 ■ CAUSES OF FEVER OF UNKNOWN ORIGIN

Infections
Abscesses—hepatic, subhepatic, gallbladder, subphrenic, splenic, periappendiceal, perinephric, pelvic, and other sites
Granulomatous—extrapulmonary and miliary tuberculosis, atypical *mycobacterial* infection, fungal infection
Intravascular—catheter-related endocarditis, meningococcemia, gonococcemia, *Listeria, Brucella*, rat-bite fever, relapsing fever
Viral, rickettsial, and chlamydial—infectious mononucleosis, cytomegalovirus, human immunodeficiency virus, hepatitis, Q fever, psittacosis
Parasitic—extraintestinal amebiasis, malaria, toxoplasmosis

Non-infectious Inflammatory Disorders
Collagen vascular diseases—rheumatic fever, systemic lupus erythematosus, rheumatoid arthritis (particularly Still's disease), vasculitis (all types)
Granulomatous—sarcoidosis, granulomatous hepatitis, Crohn's disease
Tissue injury—pulmonary emboli, sickle cell disease, hemolytic anemia

Neoplastic Diseases
Lymphoma/leukemia—Hodgkin's and non-Hodgkin's lymphoma, acute leukemia, myelodysplastic syndrome
Carcinoma—kidney, pancreas, liver, gastrointestinal tract, lung, especially when metastatic
Atrial myxomas
Central nervous system tumors

Drug Fevers
Sulfonamides, penicillins, thiouracils, barbiturates, quinidine, laxatives (especially with phenolphthalein)

Factitious Illnesses
Injections of toxic material, manipulation or exchange of thermometers

Other Causes
Familial Mediterranean fever, Fabry's disease, cyclic neutropenia

not uncommon. Other tests, e.g., antinuclear antibodies, febrile agglutinins, complement assays, may be positive but are rarely helpful in evaluation of unexplained fever.

A definitive diagnosis is usually made through a combination of imaging studies, microbiologic tests, and/or biopsies. Previous radiographs should be carefully reviewed for evidence of sinusitis, apical inflammation or small nodules in the lungs, hilar adenopathy, or an intra-abdominal mass. Abdominal ultrasonography, gallium and radioisotopically labeled leukocyte scans, computed tomography, and magnetic resonance imaging are very helpful to examine the liver, gallbladder, spleen, and pelvic areas for tumors and abscesses. These tests have reduced, but not completely eliminated, the need for exploratory laparotomies.

Cultures of blood (including for *Myobacterium avium* in human immunodeficiency virus–infected patients), urine (including mycobacterial cultures if tuberculosis is suspected), and other body fluids (e.g., cerebrospinal, peritoneal, pleural) should be obtained if at all suggested by the clinical examination. It is useful to perform anaerobic cultures of material from suspected abscess cavities and to examine blood cultures for fastidious bacteria, yeast, and fungi in difficult cases. A tissue diagnosis can often be made from a biopsy of abnormal skin or lymph nodes or the bone marrow. Biopsy or needle aspiration of liver, lung, bone, or other deep tissue sites is also valuable when abscesses or tumors are suspected.

THERAPY. Therapeutic trials with antibiotics, corticosteroids, or antipyretics before the diagnosis is clear can confuse the evaluation. In some instances, a trial may be justified but should be time limited, i.e., about 2 weeks. In patients with deep tissue abscesses, fever usually persists despite antibiotics. In patients with non-infectious inflammatory diseases, e.g., sarcoidosis, Still's disease, or vasculitis, a good clinical diagnosis can usually be made before such therapies are begun. In patients with malignancies, rational therapy depends on a tissue diagnosis. Patients with factitious illness often have serious underlying psychiatric disorders. Care in confrontation is essential to prevent desperate acts, including suicide.

Extensive work-ups of unexplained fevers can be very expensive. In every patient the need for hospital care and testing should be continually reassessed. When the patient is not severely ill, it is frequently worthwhile to use observation alone as a diagnostic tool. Sometimes even a short period of observation allows an obscure diagnosis to become obvious. In other cases, the fever disappears without the necessity for further diagnostic tests.

Arnow PM, Flaherty JP: Fever of unknown origin. Lancet 350:575, 1997. *A succinct summary of the causes of unexplained fever category by category.*

de Kleijn EM, van Lier HJ, van der Meer JW: Fever of unknown origin (FUO). II. Diagnostic procedures in a prospective multicenter study of 167 patients. The Netherlands FUO Study Group. Medicine (Baltimore) 76:401, 1997. *A report on the value of diagnostic tests and procedures in a series of 167 patients recently evaluated for unexplained fever.*

Sullivan, M, Fineberg, J, Bartlett, JG: Fever in patients with HIV infection. Infect Dis Clinic North Am 10:149, 1996. *A good summary of the causes of fever in patients with HIV infection. This issue also contains a series of other excellent articles on evaluating patients with fever.*

312 THE PATHOGENESIS OF FEVER

Bruce Beutler ■ *Steven M. Beutler*

DEFINITION. *Fever* (pyrexia) is defined as an elevation of core body temperature above the level normally maintained by the individual. Under normal circumstances, core body temperature (the temperature of blood in the right atrium) is tightly regulated, with circadian variations over a range that usually does not exceed 1° F (0.6° C) and a mean value of 98.6° F (37° C) (the normal "setpoint"). An array of thermoregulatory mechanisms, described in detail below, ensure that this temperature is maintained. During episodes of fever, the thermoregulatory set-point is shifted such that the same thermoregulatory mechanisms are used to maintain an abnormally elevated temperature.

It is important to realize that fever is not equivalent to an elevated core temperature but to an elevated set-point. Under many circumstances ranging from intense physical exertion to immersion in hot liquids, core temperature may be elevated yet fever does not exist because the body is attempting to cope with the departure from homeostasis. Failure of thermoregulation may also be associated with elevated core temperature; this problem too (which occurs in malignant hyperthermia) is distinct from fever.

THERMOREGULATORY MECHANISMS. Core body temperature is determined by two opposing processes, each of which is regulated by the central nervous system. On the one hand, energy in the form of heat is generated by living tissues ("thermogenesis"). Energy may be passively absorbed from the environment as well. On the other hand, energy is inevitably lost to the environment, chiefly through the emission of infrared radiation and through transfer of energy to the surrounding medium. The temperature at which tissues are maintained is related to heat capacity (e.g., to the amount of energy required to elevate temperature by a defined increment) and to the quantity of energy lost or gained by the system.

Metabolic reactions proceed more rapidly at an elevated temperature. Therefore, the passive warming effect of a febrile state leads to accelerated energy production in the form of heat: for each temperature increment of 1° F (0.6° C), the basal metabolic rate increases by approximately 10%. This increase may at times be quite significant from a nutritional point of view.

Muscle is a particularly flexible transducer of chemical energy. "Shivering thermogenesis" refers to the unconscious process whereby muscles are recruited to produce energy through the exercise of activity. Such induction of energy leads to enhanced metabolic demand, which is one mechanism responsible for the rise in body temperature in fever. Hence a sharp "chill" often heralds the onset of fever.

Conservation of energy is effected through piloerection in mammals other than humans. In humans, "gooseflesh" is the equivalent response. "Flushing" represents a redistribution of circulation to dermal vessels and facilitates heat loss; a blanched appearance of the skin indicates an attempt to conserve heat.

INITIATION OF FEVER. The neural pathways responsible for thermoregulation originate in the hypothalamus. A local sensing mechanism exists wherein the temperature of blood is coupled to the development of autonomic discharge. Elevation of body temperature depends primarily on sympathetic outflow and leads to shivering thermogenesis and dermal vasoconstriction, whereas cooling mechanisms (sweating and dermal vasodilation) involve a mixture of sympathetic and parasympathetic pathways.

Certain neurotropic drugs can disrupt the hypothalamic thermo-sensory mechanism—or blunt the hypothalamic response—and thus may interfere with the development of fever. Among these drugs phenothiazines are the best known for their "poikilothermic" effect. These agents are not specifically active in febrile states; rather, they act to disable thermoregulatory mechanisms.

CLINICAL MANIFESTATIONS. Although fever patterns tend to be non-specific, they may sometimes provide diagnostic clues (Table 312–1). Intermittent fevers are seen in many conditions and are therefore of little help in discriminating between various disorders. Intermittent fever may also occur when a continuous fever is interrupted with antipyretics or cooling measures; such interventions must be taken into account in analysis of a temperature curve.

In addition to considering patterns of pyrexia, it is worthwhile to note the relationship between core temperature and other vital signs. For example, dissociation between the temperature and pulse is sometimes seen in cases of typhoid fever, Legionnaires' disease, psittacosis, and brucellosis. Factitious fever is also accompanied by an inappropriately low pulse. In addition, the respiratory rate may remain unchanged and normal, superimposed diurnal variations in temperature may be absent in factitious fever.

Drug fever may occur in association with nearly any medication. No fever pattern is characteristic. Fevers caused by drug allergy tend to be well tolerated and may be accompanied by other allergic phenomena such as rash, nephritis, or neutropenia in 20 to 60% of patients.

Extreme pyrexia (characterized by a core temperature higher than 106° F) often indicates failure of a distal mechanism of thermoregulation occurring alone or in combination with infection. Examples of non-infectious causes of such extreme pyrexia include heat stroke (see Chapter 97), neuroleptic malignant syndrome (see Chapter 451), and malignant hyperthermia associated with succinylcholine.

CYTOKINES AND FEVER. Hypothalamic dysregulation and fever are triggered by proteins released from cells of the immune system (Fig. 312–1). This communication between the immune system and the nervous system is perhaps the most thoroughly studied "neuroimmunoendocrine" link. In response to invasive stimuli, including components of various microorganisms (e.g., lipoteichoic acid, lipopolysaccharides, and other constituents collectively termed "exogenous pyrogen") or certain chemical agents (e.g., amphotericin and perhaps other drugs), cells of the immune system (principally macrophages and, to a lesser extent, lymphocytes) produce proteins that behave as "endogenous pyrogens." These proteins are designated "monokines" and "lymphokines," respectively, and are often denoted under the more general heading of "cytokines." During the past decade, several of the cytokines active in the pathogenesis of fever have been isolated, and their structures have been determined by molecular cloning. As of this writing, 11 proteins with pyrogenic activity have been identified (Table 312–2); it is likely that many others exist. Although mononuclear phagocytes are the principal source of pyrogenic cytokines, the same proteins may sometimes originate from non-immune cells of neoplastic tissue through autonomous production and secretion.

The pyrogenic cytokines are structurally diverse proteins with well-established effects in hematopoiesis, inflammation, and regulation of cell metabolism. Individual agents are often markedly pleiotropic in their actions. In addition to their involvement in mediating fever, cytokines mediate the "acutephase-response" (see Chapter 313), which is characterized by increased production of "acutephase reactants" in the liver (fibrinogen, C-reactive protein, comple-

Table 312–1 ■ **FEVER PATTERNS AS DIAGNOSTIC CLUES**

FEVER PATTERN	CAUSE
Alternate-day fever	*Plasmodium vivax, P. ovale*
Fever every 3rd day	*P. malariae*
Relapsing fever: daily for 3–6 d; fever-free interval for about 1 wk supervenes	*Borrelia* spp., rat-bite fever (*Streptobacillus moniliformis; Spirillum minus*)
Continuous "undulating fever"	Brucellosis; typhoid
Periodic pyrexia (Pel-Ebstein phenomenon) with variable cycles	Hodgkin's disease

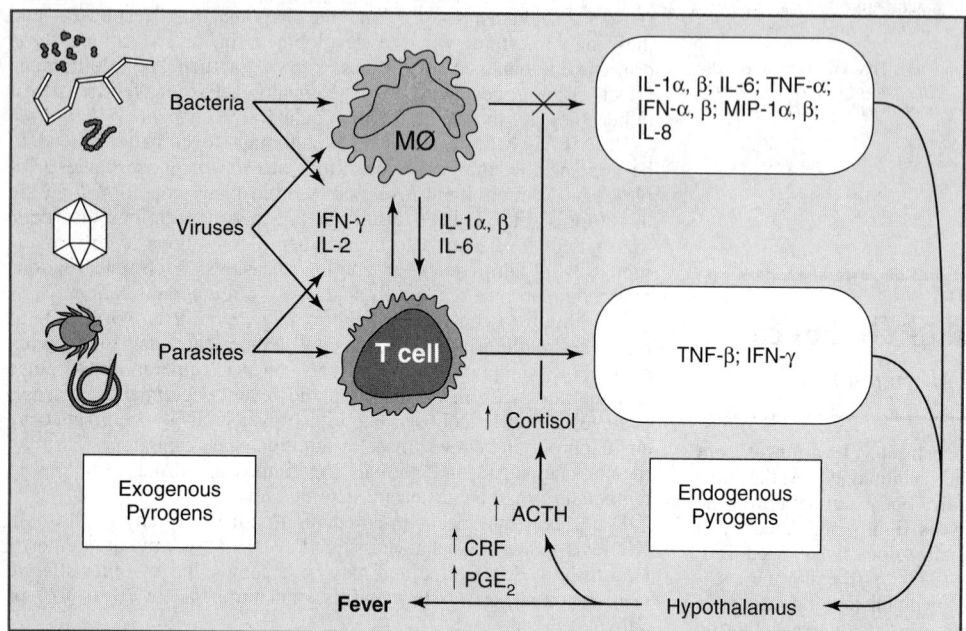

FIGURE 312–1 ■ Production of endogenous pyrogens by macrophages and T lymphocytes. A variety of microbial pathogens produce molecules that function as exogenous pyrogens and trigger the release of endogenous pyrogens from mononuclear cells. ACTH = adrenocorticotropic hormone: CRF = corticotropin-releasing factor; PGE_2 = prostaglandin E_2; other abbreviations are defined in the text and Table 312–2.

ment proteins B, C3, C4, α_2-acid glycoprotein, serum amyloid A, and a variety of proteinase inhibitors among them), decreased production of albumin and transferrin, hypoferremia, hypertriglyceridemia, and other metabolic changes.

Pyrogenic cytokines are presumed to bind to receptors present on vascular endothelial cells that lie within the hypothalamus. They act to reset the hypothalamic thermoregulatory center by prompting an elevation in core body temperature. The resetting is believed to depend largely on endothelial cells producing prostaglandins (PGE_2 and perhaps $PGF_{2\alpha}$). Thromboxanes and lipooxygenase products may also affect the set-point. Cytokines can also interact directly with neural tissues; some evidence suggests that the release of corticotropin-releasing factor may trigger thermogenesis in response to at least one cytokine (interleukin-1 β [IL-1β]).

Although no single cytokine is capable of provoking fever of a magnitude equivalent to that elicited by endotoxin, it is probable

Table 312–2 ■ PROTEINS WITH PYROGENIC ACTIVITY

ENDOGENOUS PYROGEN	OTHER NAMES/ ABBREVIATIONS	PRINCIPAL SOURCE	INDUCED BY	PRINCIPAL EFFECTS IN ADDITION TO PYROGENESIS	PHYSICAL CHARACTERISTICS
Cachectin/tumor necrosis factor α	TNF-α	Macrophages	Lipopolysaccharide (LPS), other microbial products	Fever, shock, anorexia, wasting, tumor necrosis, bone resorption, ↓ adipocyte lipoprotein lipase, neutrophil activation, ↑ endothelial cell adhesiveness/procoagulant effect	Homotrimer; 17 kd subunit size (nonglycosylated) ↕ 26% identity
Lymphotoxin/tumor necrosis factor β	TNF-β; LT	Lymphocytes (T & B)	Antigenic/mitogenic stimulation		Homotrimer; 20–25 kd subunit size (glycosylated)
Interleukin-1α (IL-1α)	Leukocyte activity factor (LAF), leukocyte endogenous mediator (LEM), mononuclear cell factor (MCF), endogenous pyrogen (EP)	Macrophages and many other cell types	LPS, other microbial products, TNF	Fever, IL-2 production, bone resorption, pannus formation, neutrophil activation, ↑ endothelial cell adhesiveness/procoagulant effect	Monomer; 17 kd (glycosylated) ↕ 26% identity
Interleukin-1β (IL-1β)					Monomer; 17 kd (glycosylated)
Interferon-α	IFN-α; leukocyte interferon	Leukocytes (esp. monocyte-macrophages)		Induction of antiviral state	22 kd (glycosylated) ↕ 23% identity
Interferon-β	IFN-β; fibroblast interferon	Fibroblasts	LPS, viral infection, double-stranded RNA		22 kd (glycosylated)
Interferon-γ	IFN-γ; immune interferon; type 2 interferon	T lymphocytes		Macrophage activation Up-regulation of class I and class II MHC molecules	20–25 kd (glycosylated)

Table 312–2 ■ PROTEINS WITH PYROGENIC ACTIVITY *Continued*

ENDOGENOUS PYROGEN	OTHER NAMES/ ABBREVIATIONS	PRINCIPAL SOURCE	INDUCED BY	PRINCIPAL EFFECTS IN ADDITION TO PYROGENESIS	PHYSICAL CHARACTERISTICS
Interleukin-6 (IL-6)	Interferon-β_2, hepatocyte-stimulating factor (HSF), B-cell stimulating factor-2 (BSF-2), B-cell differentiation factor (BCDF)	Many cell types	LPS, TNF	↑ Synthesis of acute-phase reactants Weak antiviral effect Terminal differentiation of B cells; T-cell activation	21–26 kd (glycosylated)
Macrophage inflammatory protein 1α	MIP-1α				7.9 kd (non-glycosylated)
		Macrophages	LPS	Neutrophil chemotaxis	↕ 57% identity
Macrophage inflammatory protein 1β	MIP-1β				7.8 kd (non-glycosylated)
Interleukin-8 (IL-8)	Monocyte-derived neutrophil chemotactic factor (MDNCF)		LPS, TNF, IL-1		8.0 kd (non-glycosylated)

that the combined production of several cytokines is sufficient to explain most fevers.

One monokine known as tumor necrosis factor α (TNF-α) seems capable of reproducing many of the physiologic derangements observed in septic shock and thus appears to mediate most of the deleterious effects of bacterial endotoxin, including fever. A lymphokine known as lymphotoxin (also referred to as tumor necrosis factor β) is homologous to TNF-α, binds to the same receptor as TNF-α, and elicits many of the same effects. Two other cytokines (IL-1α and IL-1β), although incapable of causing shock by themselves, produce many effects similar to those of TNF-α, and in some instances, synergistic responses have been noted.

Many of the cytokines are mutually inducing, and the concept of a "cytokine cascade" has been offered to describe the production of several factors occurring in response to the elaboration of one member of the group. The temporal sequence of induction may be reflected in the course of fever *in vivo*. For example, injecting a bolus of TNF-α into a rabbit will immediately raise body temperature and cause a delayed rise, apparently related to secondary production of IL-1.

MECHANISMS OF ANTIPYRESIS. Non-steroidal antipyretic agents inhibit fever by blocking the synthesis of prostaglandins (see Chapter 29) within the endothelium of the hypothalamic vasculature, which is accomplished through inhibition of cyclooxygenase. However, they do not diminish the elaboration of endogenous pyrogens and may actually increase the production of some of these proteins (notably TNF-α). Non-steroidal antipyretics do not produce poikilothermic effects; they can reduce fever but cannot lower body temperature beneath its normal set-point. It may reasonably be inferred from this observation that prostaglandins do not normally act to maintain core body temperature.

Glucocorticoid hormones directly impede the production of endogenous pyrogens by mononuclear phagocytic cells. Cytokine synthesis is inhibited at more than one level and has been studied most thoroughly in the case of TNF-α biosynthesis. Both transcription of the TNF-α gene and translation of TNF-α mRNA are down-regulated by glucocorticoid agonists.

The cyclic (often circadian) course followed in many febrile illnesses has not been fully explained. In some instances (e.g., in malaria), a clear relationship to the life cycle of the pathogen has been demonstrated. Cyclicity may, in other cases, follow from the fact that cells constituting the chief source of endogenous pyrogens are rendered refractory by continued exposure to the stimulatory agent and must recover or be replaced.

TREATMENT. In the absence of specific knowledge concerning the benefits of fever, a conservative approach to the treatment of fever is advisable. Core temperatures beneath 105° F are well tolerated by most individuals. Moreover, when its source has been defined, fever often serves as an important indicator of therapeutic effect.

Under certain circumstances, aggressive treatment of fever is warranted. Patients with myocardial ischemia, patients predisposed to seizures, and pregnant women may require treatment with antipyretics because elevation of core temperature increases cardiac output and myocardial oxygen demand, increases the likelihood of seizures, and may exert a teratogenic effect. Acetaminophen or non-steroidal anti-inflammatory agents prove adequate for this purpose in the majority of cases. Physical methods for increasing heat dissipation may also be used.

Temperatures that exceed 106° F are life threatening and must be lowered immediately. Antipyretics are often ineffective in such instances because pyrexia of this degree does not result from an aberrant hypothalamic set-point. It is advisable, in such cases, to lower the temperature by any means possible; the most effective action to be taken is to immerse the patient in ice water while monitoring core temperature to be certain that a state of hypothermia is not induced.

Moltz H: Fever: Causes and consequences. Neurosci Biobehav Rev 17:237, 1993. *An excellent review analyzing the neurochemistry and neuroanatomy of fever.*
Rothwell NJ: CNS regulation of thermogenesis. Crit Rev Neurobiol 8:1, 1994. *A current appraisal of the pyrogenicity of various cytokines.*

313 THE ACUTE-PHASE RESPONSE

Charles A. Dinarello

ACUTE-PHASE CHANGES. Infections, trauma, inflammatory processes, and some malignant diseases induce a constellation of host responses collectively referred to as the "acute-phase response." The response is associated with characteristic metabolic changes in liver protein synthesis, but on closer examination, changes also occur in several other systems and are responsible for various hematologic, endocrinologic, and immunologic dysfunctions. These changes are called "acute" because most are observed within hours or days following the onset of infection or injury, although some acute-phase changes also indicate chronic disease. The full spectrum of the response includes dramatic increases in the synthesis of several unique hepatic proteins that are not produced in health. One of these, C-reactive protein, is a marker of the acute-phase response and can be used to indicate disease. The increased plasma concentrations of acute-phase hepatic proteins, glycoproteins, and globulins are responsible for elevated erythrocyte sedimentation rates. Although the liver is producing increasing amounts of a variety of proteins, hepatic albumin synthesis is decreased. Increases in gluconeogenesis, energy expenditure, and muscle proteolysis occur and contribute to weight loss. However, anorexia is often present and may account for most of the weight loss. Fever may be present, and increased sleep and lethargy are frequent clinical complaints. Leukocytosis with increased numbers of circulating immature neutrophils is common, and serum iron and zinc levels are depressed, whereas increased ceruloplasmin levels result in elevated serum copper. Thyroid dysfunction can be present, and glucose tolerance and lipid metabolism are often abnormal. In addition, anemia develops despite adequate stores of iron, and hypergammaglobulinemia often occurs.

Although the most florid manifestation of the acute-phase response is observed in patients with bacterial infections, burns, or multiple injuries, clinicians also encounter acute-phase changes in patients with occult infections or chronic illnesses such as rheumatoid arthritis, Crohn's disease, and several autoimmune diseases. The presence of acute-phase changes can also serve as an indicator of silent disease and some cancers, particularly renal cell carcinoma and Hodgkin's disease. The acute-phase response has the outstanding characteristic of being a generalized host reaction irrespective of the localized or systemic nature of the inciting disease. The various components of the response are remarkably consistent despite the considerable variety of pathologic processes that induce it. For example, plasma levels of several acute-phase proteins are elevated following myocardial infarction, fracture of a bone, or bacterial pneumonia.

INDUCTION OF ACUTE-PHASE CHANGES. How are infections, injuries, and immunologic and inflammatory reactions able to elicit acute-phase changes in the host? Initiation of the acute-phase response is linked to the production of hormone-like polypeptide mediators, now called cytokines. Several cytokines induce acute-phase changes: interleukin 1 (IL-1), tumor necrosis factor, interferon-γ, IL-6, leukemia inhibitory factor, ciliary neurotropic factor, oncostatin M, and 1L-11. These last five cytokines induce hepatic acute-phase protein synthesis via glycoprotein cell receptor 130. The ability of microbial and inflammatory substances to stimulate the production of these mediators in strategically located, specialized cells appears to be part of local pathologic changes in many diseases, as well as the systemic characteristics of the acute-phase response.

Interferon-α is produced primarily during viral infections. Although it shares with IL-1 and tumor necrosis factor the ability to produce fever, sleep, and lethargy, interferon-α does not induce certain other acute-phase changes, and hence elevated erythrocyte sedimentation rates and neutrophilia are not commonly observed during viral infections.

A patient with a localized bacterial infection represents an excellent example of development of the acute-phase response. At the onset of the infection, blood monocytes and tissue macrophages become activated either by phagocytosis of the invading microbe or by exposure to its products or toxins; the process results in the synthesis and release of various cytokines within 1 to 2 hours. These mediators enter the circulation and reach the brain, where they initiate fever. Whereas fever is clearly one of the most obvious signs of the acute-phase response, other components of the response can be present without apparent clinical manifestations. One of the most sensitive measures of the acute-phase response is an increase in the number and immaturity of circulating neutrophils. In human subjects injected with small doses of IL-1 or related cytokines, neutrophilia can be measured in the absence of fever. Although not routinely measured, serum zinc and iron levels are depressed. Low serum iron associated with anemia in the face of adequate iron stores is characteristic of the acute-phase response.

Within 8 to 12 hours after the onset of infection or trauma, the liver increases the synthetic rate of the so-called acute-phase proteins. The response includes increases in proteins normally found in health, as well as the appearance of new proteins that serve as markers of a pathologic event. Several normal plasma proteins increase several-fold during the acute-phase response, including haptoglobin, certain protease inhibitors, complement components, ceruloplasmin, and fibrinogen. However, true acute-phase reactants increase several hundred-fold. These reactants include serum amyloid A protein, a precursor of the amyloid fibril in secondary amyloidosis, and C-reactive protein. C-reactive protein was named for its ability to interact with the C polysaccharide of pneumococci and was the first acute-phase protein described. Table 313–1 lists

Table 313–1 ■ PLASMA PROTEINS THAT INCREASE DURING THE ACUTE-PHASE RESPONSE

C-reactive protein
Serum amyloid A protein
α_1-Glycoprotein
Ceruloplasmin
α-Macroglobulins
Complement components (C1–C4, factor B, C9, C11)
α_1-Antitrypsin
α_1-Antichymotrypsin
Fibrinogen
Prothrombin
Factor VIII
Plasminogen
Haptoglobin
Ferritin
Immunoglobulins
Lipoproteins

the characteristic pattern of increased plasma proteins observed during the acute-phase response. Note one exception: The plasma concentration of albumin is decreased.

Of all the acute-phase proteins, C-reactive protein is clinically the most important because its presence serves as an indicator of disease. C-reactive protein is particularly useful as a marker of the hepatic acute-phase protein response and can be measured easily in most hospital clinical laboratories.

Despite the anabolic processes of the liver, the acute-phase response is accompanied by pronounced catabolism of muscle protein associated with loss of body weight and overall negative nitrogen balance. Fever increases oxygen and caloric demands (usually 7% per degree F), and most of the negative nitrogen balance results from the oxidation of amino acids from skeletal muscle, which contributes to wasting. These amino acids are largely used for gluconeogenesis. Although the metabolic demands of elevated temperature contribute to the increased need for energy substrates, the host also requires a large supply of amino acids to synthesize new protein at a time when food intake may be impaired or appetite reduced. Amino acids are required for immunologic and reparative processes such as the clonal expansion of lymphocytes and the proliferation of fibroblasts. Also, they are needed for synthesis of hepatic acute-phase proteins, immunoglobulins, and collagen. The mechanism of providing ample amino acids for these cellular functions seems to be well orchestrated during the acute-phase response. The catabolism during infection and inflammation differs from that of starvation. Unlike starvation, in which large amounts of ketones are spilled into the urine, an individual with an infectious or inflammatory disease excretes protein with small amounts of ketones. IL-1, tumor necrosis factor, and IL-6, the primary mediators of acute-phase changes, inhibit lipoprotein lipase and suppress appetite. In addition, these cytokines and interferons directly stimulate hepatic lipogenesis, thereby contributing to the hypertriglyceridemia observed in patients with either acute or chronic disease.

MEASUREMENT OF ACUTE-PHASE CHANGES IN CLINICAL MEDICINE. The acute-phase response is non-specific. However, the presence of certain acute-phase changes in an otherwise healthy individual can alert the physician to hidden disease. Increased peripheral neutrophils and erythrocyte sedimentation rate are often used to detect an acute-phase response. Measurement of C-reactive protein can help the physician determine the presence of disease in patients with vague constitutional complaints. C-reactive protein levels are usually less than 100 μg/L but increase within hours 10- to 1000-fold. In severe bacterial infections, the serum level can rise from undetectable to over 100 mg/L in 48 hours. The presence of elevated levels of C-reactive protein or serum amyloid A protein, even in the absence of fever or neutrophilia, may indicate occult infection or malignant change. Increases in C-reactive protein and serum amyloid A protein occur in patients of any age and also in immunocompromised patients with opportunistic infections.

Not all inflammatory diseases are associated with elevated C-reactive protein. A refractory state can develop in certain diseases such as scleroderma, ulcerative colitis, and lupus erythematosus. Failure of hepatic protein changes and the neutrophilia of the acute-phase response to develop seems to be related to the presence of circulating inhibitors of cytokines, e.g., the IL-1 receptor antagonist.

TREATMENT OF ACUTE-PHASE RESPONSES. Measurements of fever, acute-phase plasma proteins, and peripheral leukocyte numbers are well-established procedures for monitoring many disease states. Although non-steroidal anti-inflammatory agents are used to treat the fever and associated myalgias of acute-phase responses, these drugs do not affect other acute-phase changes in the liver, various endocrinologic parameters, or the bone marrow response. Antipyretic blood levels of aspirin and therapeutic concentrations of drugs such as indomethacin or ibuprofen do not reduce the production of cytokines. On the other hand, corticosteroids are highly effective in reducing cytokine synthesis, as well as the effect of these mediators on various tissue targets. Patients receiving therapeutic doses of corticosteroids have blunted acute-phase responses with ongoing infections, inflammatory processes, or immunologic reactions.

The role of acute-phase proteins in host defense and repair is not entirely clear. Studies suggest that the major role of C-reactive protein is to bind serum lipids or opsonize pneumococci, whereas serum amyloid A is thought to be immunosuppressive. Ceruloplasmin scavenges toxic free oxygen radicals that are injurious to many tissues. What is clear, however, is that the production and physical structure of these acute-phase proteins have been conserved through 400 million years of evolution, and therefore they have presumably been useful to the host. The *Limulus* crab and fish make C-reactive protein that is nearly identical to human C-reactive protein, which argues that the acute-phase response plays a role in survival.

Beisel WR: Magnitude of the host nutritional responses to infection. Am J Clin Nutr 30:1236, 1977. *Discussion of the metabolic imbalances seen in patients with infection and injury.*

Dinarello CA, Wolff SM: The role of interleukin-1 in disease. N Engl J Med 328:106, 1993. *Clinical role for IL-1 and IL-1 receptor antagonist in disease.*

Feingold KR, Soued M, Serio MK: Multiple cytokines stimulate hepatic lipid synthesis *in vivo.* Endocrinology 125:267, 1989. *Evidence that IL-1, tumor necrosis factor, and interferon may account for the hyperlipidemias observed in patients with acute or chronic inflammatory disease.*

Kushner I, Gewurz H, Benson MD: C-reactive protein and the acute-phase response. J Lab Clin Med 97:739, 1981. *A brief discussion of the usefulness of measuring C-reactive protein levels in clinical practice.*

Pepys MB, Baltz ML: Acute phase proteins with special reference to C-reactive protein and related proteins (pentaxins) and serum amyloid A protein. *In* Dixon FJ, Kunkel HG (eds): Advances in Immunology, vol 34. New York, Academic Press, 1983, pp 141–211. *A comprehensive discussion of the hepatic acute-phase protein pattern observed during the acute-phase response, with special attention to various autoimmune diseases.*

314 THE COMPROMISED HOST

Philip A. Pizzo

"Compromised host" is used to describe patients who have an increased risk for infectious complications as a consequence of a congenital or acquired qualitative or quantitative abnormality in one or more components of the host defense matrix (Table 314–1). Until the early 1980s, this term was largely restricted to patients with congenital immunodeficiencies (see Chapter 272) those who became immunocompromised as a consequence of cancer or its treatment, bone marrow failure, or treatment with immunosuppressive therapy. The advent of acquired immune deficiency syndrome (AIDS) has given the term "compromised host" a new meaning and relevance. The compromised host with AIDS is discussed in detail in Part XXIII. In this chapter the focus is on non-AIDS patients with altered immune defenses. However, many of the complications and approaches to diagnosis and management are generic.

PHYSICAL DEFENSE BARRIERS

The skin and mucosal surfaces represent the primary defense against both endogenous and exogenous sources of infection. Disruption of skin and mucosa may result from trauma, tumor invasion, the cytotoxic effects of chemotherapy or radiotherapy, the use of invasive diagnostic or therapeutic procedures (e.g., intravenous catheters), and effects of locally destructive infections such as oral herpes simplex. Such mucosal alterations provide a nidus for microbial colonization, a focus for localized infection, and a portal of entry for systemic invasion.

The skin and various mucosal surfaces are normally colonized by aerobic and anaerobic bacteria. However, in patients who have been hospitalized, who are neutropenic, or who have received prior broad-spectrum antibiotics, the normal gram-positive flora of the skin can be replaced by other gram-positive organisms such as Centers For Disease Control and Prevention (CDC) group JK *Corynebacterium* or *Bacillus* species or by gram-negative organisms (e.g., pseudomonads, enteric gram-negative rods), fungi (e.g., *Candida albicans* or *Aspergillus* species), and atypical *Mycobacterium* species such as *M. chelonei* or *M. fortuitum.*

Similarly, the gastrointestinal tract is normally colonized by an array of aerobic and anaerobic bacteria, as well as some fungi, and disruption of its mucosa may lead to infection by a variety of pathogens, including polymicrobial infections. A common cause of disruption of gastrointestinal mucosal integrity is cytotoxic chemotherapy to patients with malignancy, particularly cytarabine, the anthracyclines (daunorubicin and doxorubicin), methotrexate, 6-mercaptopurine, and 5-fluorouracil. Although stomatitis is usually the most clinically recognizable manifestation of gastrointestinal toxicity, diffuse gastrointestinal involvement is also likely. Frequently the differentiation between chemotherapy-induced stomatotoxicity and localized infection (e.g., necrotizing gingivitis from anaerobic bacteria or mucosal lesions from herpes simplex virus [HSV]) can be difficult, particularly in neutropenic patients.

In addition to mucosal breakdown, mechanical obstruction of body passages can also increase the risk of serious localized infection as a result of stasis of local body fluids and resultant overgrowth of potentially pathogenic colonizing organisms. Common sites of secondary infection resulting from obstruction include the lung, urinary tract, biliary tract, and eustachian tube. One should consider an obstructive process when infection at any of these sites fails to respond to appropriate antibiotics.

Anatomic changes can also contribute to the risk of infection. For example, in patients with sickle cell disease, macrophage and splenic dysfunction predispose to the development of certain bacteremias, especially by *Streptococcus pneumoniae* and *Salmonella* species. Anatomic abnormalities of bones and joints as a result of vaso-occlusive crises caused by infarction of bone marrow, bony cortex, or synovium in patients with sickle cell disease can also predispose to the development of infections caused by these organisms such as osteomyelitis or arthritis.

PHAGOCYTE DEFECTS

The polymorphonuclear leukocyte (PMN) and the monocyte are the two most important components of cellular host defense that protect against invasive bacteria and fungi. Both quantitative and qualitative defects affecting PMNs and monocytes may occur in compromised patients.

Quantitative Abnormalities of Phagocytes

Granulocytopenia is among the most important risk factors for serious infection in a compromised host. However, it is important to keep in mind that except for congenital neutropenias, other alterations of the host defense matrix often occur in concert with granulocytopenia and can further alter the risk for infection, as well as the types of infectious complications that occur.

Granulocytopenia is most commonly associated with malignant disease and its treatment with cytotoxic therapy. This category includes patients with hematologic malignancies and lymphomas, as well as the increasing number of patients with solid tumors who receive cytotoxic chemotherapy. Patients with primary or secondary bone marrow failure also have neutropenia as their predominant risk for infection. In addition to the neutropenia *per se*, the patterns of infection are also influenced by the other disease- or treatment-related immune abnormalities. For example, despite equivalent degrees of granulocytopenia, a patient with acute myelogenous leukemia may have a different pattern of infection than a patient with aplastic anemia. Disruption of a mucosal defense barrier in a pa-

Table 314–1 ■ PREDOMINANT PATHOGENS IN COMPROMISED PATIENTS; ASSOCIATION WITH SELECTED DEFECTS IN HOST DEFENSE

HOST DEFENSE IMPAIRMENT/PHAGOCYTIC DYSFUNCTION	BACTERIA	FUNGI	VIRUSES	OTHER

Neutropenia	Gram-negative
	  Enteric organisms
	    Escherichia coli, Klebsiella pneumoniae, Enterobacter spp., *Citrobacter* spp.
	    Pseudomonas aeruginosa
	Gram-positive
	  Staphylococci
	    Coagulase-negative, coagulase-positive
	  Streptococci, including viridans enterococci
	  Anaerobes
	    Anaerobic streptococci, *Clostridium* spp., *Bacteroides* spp.
		Candida species
		  C. albicans > C. tropicalis > other species
		Aspergillus species
		  A. fumigatus, A. flavus
		Other opportunistic fungi
		  Mucor, Trichosporon		

Abnormal cell-mediated immunity	*Legionella* *Nocardia asteroides* *Salmonella* spp. Mycobacteria *M. tuberculosis* and atypical mycobacteria Disseminated infection from live bacteria vaccine (BCG)	*Cryptococcus neoformans* *Histoplasma capsulatum* *Coccidioides immitis* *Candida*	Varicella-zoster virus Herpes simplex virus Cytomegalovirus Epstein-Barr virus Herpesvirus 6 Disseminated infection from live virus vaccines (vaccinia, measles, rubella, mumps, yellow fever, live polio)	*Pneumocystis carinii* *Toxoplasma gondii* *Cryptosporidium* *Strongyloides stercoralis*

Immunoglobulin abnormalities	Gram-positive
	  Streptococcus pneumoniae, Staphylococcus aureus
	Gram-negative
	  Haemophilus influenzae
	  Neisseria spp., enteric organisms
			Enteroviruses
			Disseminated infection from live virus vaccines (vaccinia, measles, rubella, mumps, yellow fever, polio)
				Giardia lamblia

Complement abnormalities
  C3, C5
	Gram-positive
	  S. pneumoniae, staphylococci
	Gram-negative
	  H. influenzae, Neisseria spp., Enteric organisms			

C5–C9	*Neisseria* species *N. gonorrhoeae, N. meningitidis*			

Anatomic disruption
  Oral cavity
	α-Hemolytic streptococci, oral anaerobes
	  Peptococcus, Peptostreptococcus
		Candida	Herpes simplex virus	

Esophagus	Staphylococci, other colonizing organisms	*Candida*	Herpes simplex virus Cytomegalovirus	

Lower gastrointestinal tract	Gram-positive
	  Enterococci
	Gram-negative
	  Enteric organisms
	Anaerobes (*Bacteroides fragilis, Clostridium perfringens*)
		Candida		*S. stercoralis*

Skin (IV catheter)	Gram-positive
	  Staphylococci, streptococci
	  Corynebacterium, Bacillus spp.
	Gram-negative
	  P. aeruginosa, enteric organisms
	Mycobacteria
	  M. fortuitum, M. chelonei
		Candida
		Aspergillus		

Urinary tract	Gram-positive
	  Enterococci
	Gram-negative
	  Enteric organisms
	  P. aeruginosa
		Candida		

Splenectomy	Gram-positive
	  S. pneumoniae
	Gram-negative
	  Capnocytophaga
	  H. influenzae
	  Salmonella (sickle cell disease)
				Babesia

BCG = bacille Calmette-Guérin.

From Rubin M, Walsh TJ, Pizzo PA: Clinical approach to the compromised host. *In* Hoffman R, Benz EJ Jr, Shattil SJ, et al (eds): Hematology: Basic Principles and Practices, 2nd ed. New York, Churchill Livingstone, 1994.

tient with acute myelogenous leukemia who is receiving cytotoxic therapy appears to increase the risk for infection with enteric gram-negative bacteria, α-hemolytic streptococci, or anaerobes. In contrast, a patient with aplastic anemia who does not have impaired mucosal integrity may be able to sustain longer periods of granulocytopenia without a systemic bacterial infection developing. On the other hand, if a patient with aplastic anemia is treated with steroids or cyclosporine, the risk for viral or fungal infection may be increased.

Regardless of these modifying factors, the relationship between granulocytopenia and serious infection has been unequivocally established by the classic study of Bodey and colleagues (Table 314–2). This study demonstrated that the risk of infection begins to increase significantly when granulocyte counts fall below 1000 per microliter and is most marked when the counts are 100 per microliter or lower. In addition to the absolute granulocyte count, the duration of granulocytopenia is also directly related to the direction of granulocytopenia as well as whether the counts are rising or falling.

For practical purposes, granulocytopenia is usually defined as a count of 500 or fewer PMNs and band forms per microliter. However, a patient with an absolute granulocyte count of 500 to 1000 per microliter that is rapidly falling is probably at greater risk for infection than a patient with a count of 200 per microliter that is rising. Thus the absolute granulocyte count, the duration of granulocytopenia, and whether the neutrophil count is falling or rising must all be considered when assessing the risk to any individual patient. Some clinicians also include the monocyte count in this equation to generate an absolute phagocyte index.

Granulocytopenia primarily predisposes patients to bacterial and fungal infection and does not of itself appear to increase the incidence or severity of viral and parasitic infections. In the 1950s and 1960s, when cytotoxic therapy was initially being developed, gram-positive bacteria (especially *Staphylococcus aureus*) predominated. In the early 1970s, with the availability of antibiotics to control gram-positive bacteria (e.g., methicillin), gram-negative organisms (e.g., *Escherichia coli*, *Klebsiella*, *Pseudomonas aeruginosa*) emerged as the predominant pathogens in neutropenic patients, perhaps because of the increasing use of more aggressive chemotherapy regimens and the use of broader-spectrum antibiotics. During the 1980s, gram-positive organisms re-emerged as common bacterial isolates, and at many centers they now represent the most frequently encountered organisms.

In addition to these changes in the pattern of infection, institutional and geographic variations in the causes of infection and the antibiotic sensitivity patterns of isolates cannot be overemphasized, and it is imperative that physicians have a working knowledge of the specific isolates encountered at their own clinical setting.

The gram-negative organisms encountered most commonly in granulocytopenic patients are *E. coli*, *Klebsiella pneumoniae*, and *P. aeruginosa*. Together, these organisms have generally accounted for approximately 90% of the gram-negative isolates at most centers. A precise source for gram-negative bacteremia is identified in only a minority of cases, but the gastrointestinal tract, respiratory tract, soft tissue, and urinary tract are the most probable sources for infection. Of these three organisms, *P. aeruginosa* is often the most virulent in neutropenic hosts, although in most developed countries the incidence of infection by *Pseudomonas* declined in neutropenic patients during the 1980s. As a general rule, however, virtually any organism can be pathogenic if host defenses are severely impaired. *Enterobacter* species, *Citrobacter* species, and *Serratia marcescens*

are less frequently encountered but are notable because they rapidly become resistant to β-lactam antibiotics through the induction of chromosomally mediated β-lactamases. Of concern, an increase in *Enterobacter* sepsis has been observed at a number of treatment centers. Other less common gram-negative isolates include *Acinetobacter* species, *Haemophilus* species (usually non-typable *H. influenzae*), and non-*aeruginosa* pseudomonads (often catheter related and antibiotic resistant).

The gram-positive organisms most frequently encountered are the coagulase-negative staphylococci (most commonly *S. epidermidis*), coagulase-positive staphylococci (*S. aureus*), enterococci, and α-hemolytic streptococci (e.g., *S. mutans* or viridans group streptococci). Both coagulase-positive and coagulase-negative staphylococci are most commonly isolated from the blood, often from patients with indwelling intravenous catheters or from those with foreign bodies such as prosthetic heart valves or orthopedic implants. *S. aureus* tends to be significantly more virulent, and its sensitivity to β-lactam antibiotics (e.g., methicillin, oxacillin, or nafcillin) can vary from center to center, thus making it imperative for physicians to be aware of the frequency of methicillin-resistant *S. aureus* at their institutions. In contrast, coagulase-negative staphylococci tend to be relatively indolent. During the last decade, coagulase-negative staphylococci have become increasingly resistant to β-lactam antibiotics, and the majority (50 to 80%) are methicillin resistant and generally require treatment with vancomycin. Notable are the recent reports of α-hemolytic viridans streptococci that have been associated with septic shock and adult respiratory distress syndrome in patients who are receiving high-dose cytosine arabinoside and in whom oral mucosal disruption occurs. Other gram-positive bacteria that may be encountered in neutropenic patients include *Bacillus* species (often catheter related), and group CDC-JK *Corynebacterium* (often catheter related and relatively antibiotic resistant). *Enterococcus* has emerged as a cause of serious infection in some centers and is particularly important because of the increased resistance to vancomycin (e.g., *E. faecium*).

Infections caused solely by anaerobic bacteria are less common and usually associated with a concomitant abnormality in gastrointestinal mucosal integrity. Although *Bacteroides fragilis* and *Clostridium perfringens* are the most common organisms, other *Bacteroides* species, as well as other *Clostridium* species (e.g., *C. tertium*, *C. septicum*), which are often clindamycin resistant, can be clinically important. Anaerobes are frequent components of intra-abdominal infections, including peritonitis, intra-abdominal abscesses, and perirectal cellulitis or abscesses. *Clostridium difficile* is a common cause of colitis in neutropenic patients treated with antibiotics or cytotoxic agents.

Although infections by *Mycobacterium tuberculosis* have not been significantly increased in non-AIDS immunocompromised hosts, the increases in the incidence of tuberculosis (especially with multidrug-resistant strains) in homeless persons and people with AIDS raises serious concern that these infections will occur in other immunocompromised hosts. Patients with hairy cell leukemia, who have profound monocytopenia in addition to neutropenia, appear to have an increased risk for atypical mycobacterial infection (e.g., *M. kansasii*, *M. fortuitum*, *M. chelonei*, and *M. avium-intracellulare* complex). Rapidly growing mycobacteria (*M. fortuitum* and *M. chelonei*) may also cause exit site infections in patients with indwelling intravenous catheters or wound infections following surgery.

In contrast to bacterial infections, which are often associated

Table 314–2 ■ ASSOCIATION OF GRANULOCYTE LEVEL AND CHANCE OF SIGNIFICANT INFECTION DEVELOPING

GRANULOCYTE LEVEL (per mm³)		PERCENTAGE OF SERIOUS INFECTIONS (DURATION OF GRANULOCYTOPENIA IN WEEKS)							
Initial	Change	1	2	3	4	6	10	12	14
Any level	Any fall	12							
Any level	Fall to 2000	2							
Any level	Fall to 1500	5							
Any level	Fall to 1000	10	30	45	50	65	70	85	100
Any level	Fall to 500	19							
Any level	Fall to <100	28	50	72	85	100			

Adapted from Bodey GP, Buckley M, Sathe YS, Freireich EJ: Quantitative relationships between circulatory leukocytes and infection in patients with acute leukemia. Ann Intern Med 61: 328, 1966.

with the onset of fever in neutropenic patients, fungal infections only rarely cause primary infection (i.e., initial infection in patients not yet receiving antibiotics). More commonly, fungal infections occur as a secondary process in patients receiving antibacterial agents. Although a variety of fungal infections may be encountered in a neutropenic host, *Candida* and *Aspergillus* species predominate.

The vast majority of infections with *Candida* are caused by *C. albicans,* with other potential pathogens including *C. tropicalis, C. parapsilosis, C. krusei,* and *C. glabrata* (previously known as *Torulopsis glabrata*). In neutropenic patients, *Candida* infections may include candidemia, catheter-related infections, invasive mucosal infections (e.g., oral, esophageal, or lower gastrointestinal), and disseminated disease, in which the most commonly affected organs are the liver and spleen (so-called hepatosplenic candidiasis), the eye (endophthalmitis), and the skin.

Aspergillosis is usually due to *A. fumigatus* and *A. flavus,* although *A. niger* and *A. terreus* can also result in infection. The upper airways (e.g., oral cavity, nasal cavity, or sinuses) and lung are the primary sites involved with *Aspergillus,* and spread is usually by direct invasion into contiguous areas, although widespread dissemination has been described in various sites, including the brain, liver and spleen, gastrointestinal tract, heart, and kidneys. However, positive blood cultures virtually never occur.

Other fungal pathogens that may occur in neutropenic patients include Mucoraceae organisms (*Mucor, Rhizopus, Absidia,* and *Cunninghamella*—often clinically resembling *Aspergillus* infections), *Trichosporon beigelii* (which may cause disseminated visceral and cutaneous disease), *Fusarium, Drechslera, Pseudallescheria boydii,* and *Malassezia furfur.*

Qualitative Abnormalities of Phagocytes

The microbicidal activity of granulocytes and monocytes involves complex interactions between the cell and the organism or inflammatory site. Some of the major functions important for microbicidal activity include migration of the cell to the inflammatory site (or chemotaxis), cell activation, phagocytosis, and intracellular and extracellular killing via both oxygen-dependent and oxygen-independent pathways. Qualitative abnormalities in microbicidal function can be operationally divided into the following categories: (1) those associated with the malignant or myeloproliferative disease itself (2) those associated with diseases that do not primarily affect leukocytes, (3) iatrogenic causes (such as administration of pharmacologic agents or radiation), and (4) primary disorders of phagocytes.

PATIENTS WITH MALIGNANT DISORDERS AND MYELODYSPLASIA. Significant functional defects in mature PMNs can occur in patients with acute myelogenous leukemia and acute lymphoblastic leukemia before therapy. Although it has largely been assumed that granulocytes from patients with chronic myelogenous leukemia have normal microbicidal activity, some studies have documented significant impairment in the neutrophil function of morphologically mature PMNs from patients with chronic myelogenous leukemia, including abnormalities in phagocytosis, random migration, chemotaxis, and bactericidal activity. Nevertheless, during the stable chronic phase of the disease, infectious complications are rarely seen in these patients.

In addition to immunoglobulin deficiencies that impair opsonization, patients with chronic lymphocytic leukemia and multiple myeloma may also have such abnormalities as defective granulocyte adherence, decreased granulocyte migration, a decrease in the number of granulocyte receptors for C3b and IgG, and decreased chemotaxis of monocytes.

Significant defects in granulocyte function have also been found in PMNs from patients with myelodysplastic syndromes and pre-leukemic states. The clinician should probably assume that neutrophils from patients with myelodysplastic syndromes or pre-leukemia are functionally defective, and thus patients with "borderline" granulocyte counts should be approached as though they had an absolute neutropenia.

NON-MALIGNANT HEMATOLOGIC DISEASE. Although the predominant defect in host defense in most patients with aplastic anemia is neutropenia, followed by immune suppression as a result

of therapy (e.g., steroids, antithymocyte globulin, or cyclosporine), deficient production of superoxide and a deficiency of myeloperoxidase can sometimes be observed. Patients with paroxysmal nocturnal hemoglobinuria appear to have an increased susceptibility to bacterial infection. Impaired chemotaxis despite normal phagocytosis and bacterial killing has been described in patients with paroxysmal nocturnal hemoglobinuria, and Fc receptor type III (the major Fc receptor in blood and on neutrophils) has also been shown to be deficient in such patients.

In addition to splenic dysfunction, abnormal complement activation, and defective serum opsonizing capacity, defective phagocytic function has been described in patients with sickle cell anemia, although the significance of this relationship is unclear. Neutrophils from infection-prone children with sickle cell disease have been shown to have defective bactericidal activity, perhaps second to zinc deficiency.

Some patients with severe glucose-6-phosphate dehydrogenase deficiency appear to have an increased susceptibility to infections caused by catalase-positive bacteria. The clinical picture resembles that of chronic granulomatous disease of childhood, although only rarely are infections reported in the 1st decade of life. The granulocytes show normal phagocytosis and chemotaxis but defective bactericidal activity.

Although most studies address disseminated intravascular coagulation secondary to overwhelming bacterial infection, the potential role of fibrinogen degradation products (FDPs) in modifying PMN function has been suggested by the finding that two FDPs (FDP D and FDP E) can cause substantial *in vitro* inhibition of PMN chemotaxis, oxidative metabolism, and killing of *E. coli.* Disseminated intravascular coagulation associated with infection, then, may represent a vicious circle in which the organism triggers the coagulation abnormalities, which in turn may result in neutropenia and defective PMN function, thus worsening the infection.

PHARMACOLOGIC AGENTS AND RADIOTHERAPY. Most cytotoxic drugs used for the treatment of malignant and autoimmune diseases or transplantation have antiproliferative effects resulting in neutropenia and monocytopenia. Among the antineoplastics, the most commonly implicated agents include methotrexate, 6-mercaptopurine, vincristine, vinblastine, anthracyclines, cyclophosphamide, carmustine, and platinum compounds.

Glucocorticoids are associated with increased susceptibility to infection. As a general rule, the signs and symptoms of even severe infections may be masked or greatly reduced in patients receiving steroids. Steroids impair neutrophil chemotaxis, and at high dosages, PMN phagocytosis, microbicidal activity, and antibody-dependent cytotoxicity may also be altered. In addition, steroids may cause monocytopenia as well as defects in monocyte chemotaxis, phagocytosis, and killing of bacteria and fungi. In addition to their action on granulocytes and monocytes, steroids may enhance susceptibility to infection by impairing wound healing, increasing skin fragility, and depressing lymphocyte function, the production of cytokines, and humoral immune responses.

Biologic agents (e.g., colony-stimulating factors, interleukins, interferons) have become an increasingly routine component of therapy for immunocompromised patients. Granulocyte-macrophage colony-stimulating factor (GM-CSF) or granulocyte colony-stimulating factor (G-CSF) not only increases cell number but may also enhance a number of neutrophil functions, including oxidative metabolism, phagocytosis, microbicidal activity, and antibody-dependent cytotoxicity. The appropriate use of these hematopoietic cytokines in neutropenic cancer patients has been the topic of debate and is best guided by the recommendation from the American Society of Clinical Oncologists that restricts use to high-risk patients with a greater than 40% likelihood of fever associated with a neutropenic episode. It must be underscored that the use of new biologic agents in clinical practice should be guided by carefully conducted clinical trials.

PRIMARY DISORDERS OF PHAGOCYTE FUNCTION. Chronic granulomatous disease has served as a prototype for diseases characterized by defective oxidative metabolism of phagocytes. Although chronic granulomatous disease represents a heterogeneous group of disorders from a molecular and genetic perspective, the common denominator is that phagocytes lack essential components of oxidative metabolism and fail to generate the respiratory burst in response to various stimuli, including certain pathogenic organisms. The organisms that cause serious infections in patients with chronic granulomatous disease are most often those that contain the enzyme catalase. In the absence of cellular production of H_2O_2, the peroxide generated by non–catalase-containing organisms is enough to ameliorate the neutrophil deficiency and allow microbicidal activity. However, if the organism also contains catalase, the H_2O_2 it produces is rapidly degraded and is not available for participation in oxidative-based killing. The majority of infections in patients with chronic granulomatous disease are caused by *S. aureus,* although serious infections can also result from enteric gram-negative bacilli (e.g., *E. coli, K. pneumoniae,* or *Serratia* species), *Pseudomonas cepacia, Nocardia asteroides,* and *Aspergillus* species.

Serious recurrent infections usually begin in the 1st year of life in children with chronic granulomatous disease. The lung is the most common site of infection (pneumonias and abscesses), with other common infections including skin and soft tissue abscesses, visceral abscesses (particularly hepatic), osteomyelitis (especially of the small bones in the hands and feet), and suppurative lymphadenopathy. Uncommonly, chronic granulomatous disease can occur in adolescence or adulthood, although with a careful history, infectious complications often date back to childhood.

Antibiotic prophylaxis with trimethoprim-sulfamethoxazole has been advocated by many investigators. Interferon-γ has also been shown to reduce the incidence of serious infection and the number of hospital days for patients with chronic granulomatous disease.

Myeloperoxidase deficiency is perhaps the most common of all granulocyte disorders, with an estimated frequency ranging from 1 in 2000 to 1 in 4000. Myeloperoxidase is a lysosomal enzyme that catalyzes the formation of hypochlorous acid from H_2O_2 produced in the respiratory burst. Interestingly, most individuals identified with myeloperoxidase deficiency are healthy, and infectious complications are exceedingly rare. Systemic *Candida* infections have occurred in a small number of myeloperoxidase-deficient patients who also had diabetes mellitus.

Chédiak-Higashi syndrome is a rare disorder characterized by autosomal recessive inheritance, recurrent infections, partial oculocutaneous albinism, central and peripheral neuropathy, and increased bleeding time. Neutropenia can also be present. Infections result from the combined effects of neutropenia and functional defects in phagocytes, which include impaired degranulation and defective chemotaxis. Infections frequently involve the skin, respiratory tract, and mucous membranes and are most commonly caused by *S. aureus* or gram-negative bacilli. Deficiency of the iC3b receptor (also known as CR3, Mol, and MC-1), which is important for adherence and phagocytosis, is a rare disorder. Accordingly, neutrophils demonstrate defects in aggregation, margination, chemotaxis, and phagocytosis. The most common infections are skin and subcutaneous tissue infections, otitis, mucositis, gingivitis, and periodontitis.

A number of disorders have been described that are characterized by defects in the chemotaxis of granulocytes and/or monocytes. Infections in these patients tend to be cutaneous, and the most common pathogens are *S. aureus,* streptococci, *C. albicans, E. coli,* and *Trichophyton rubrum.* Depending on the specific syndrome, deep-seated infections may also occur. The "lazy leukocyte" syndrome may also be associated with neutropenia and is characterized by gingivitis, recurrent otitis media, rhinitis, and stomatitis. Hyperimmunoglobulin E syndrome (Job's syndrome) is usually associated with multiple cutaneous abscesses caused by staphylococci, but deep-seated infections and infections by other organisms such as pseudomonads and *Candida* have also been reported. Wound healing does not appear to be a problem, as it is in chronic granulomatous disease. Chemotaxis defects have been reported in patients with congenital ichthyosis and recurrent *T. rubrum* infections.

DEFECTS IN CELL-MEDIATED IMMUNITY

Cellular immune dysfunction may either be primary, as in a number of congenital immunodeficiency states; or may occur secondary to other disorders or therapeutic interventions. Defective cell-mediated immunity may lead to infections caused by bacteria, fungi, viruses, and protozoa. The predominant pathogens are intracellular organisms (those microbes that survive inside macrophages) and include mycobacteria (both *M. tuberculosis* and atypical mycobacteria), *Legionella, N. asteroides, Salmonella* species, *Cryptococcus neoformans, Histoplasma capsulatum, Coccidioides immitis,*

varicella-zoster virus (VZV), HSV, cytomegalovirus, Epstein-Barr virus, *Pneumocystis carinii, T. gondii, Cryptosporidium,* and *Strongyloides stercoralis.*

Patients with Malignant Disorders

Hodgkin's disease and the non-Hodgkin's lymphomas are associated with altered cell-mediated immunity not only when the malignancy is active but also in some instances even when the malignancy is in remission.

Cell-mediated immunity defects have been postulated to help explain the incidence of atypical mycobacterial infections in patients with hairy cell leukemia and also occur in relatively rare T-cell malignancies such as mycosis fungoides and T-cell chronic lymphocytic leukemia. Cell-mediated immunity defects exist in children with acute lymphocytic leukemia, as evidenced by their increased susceptibility to infections by *P. carinii* or disseminated VZV, but it is likely that concurrent therapy plays a major role. Clinically significant impairment in cell-mediated immunity has not been well established for other malignancies.

Patients with Non-malignant Hematologic Disorders

Impaired cell-mediated immunity is not a prominent feature for non-malignant hematologic disorders unless associated with therapy or acquisition of human immunodeficiency virus type 1 (HIV-1) infection. Abnormalities in cell-mediated immunity have been best described in patients with hemophilia who have received Factor VIII concentrates even in the absence of apparent HIV-1 infection. Patients with sickle cell anemia have been found to be anergic in association with zinc deficiency and decreased nucleoside phosphorylase activity.

A number of infections may produce impaired cell-mediated immunity either directly (e.g., by infecting key cellular components such as T lymphocytes or macrophages) or by affecting other immunoregulatory mechanisms. The most notable viral infection associated with impaired cell-mediated immunity is HIV-1. Other viral infections that are also associated with cell-mediated immunity defects include cytomegalovirus, Epstein-Barr virus, respiratory syncytial virus, hepatitis B, and influenza. Other non-viral infections that have been variably associated with impaired cell-mediated immunity by *in vitro* testing have included tuberculosis, leprosy, bacterial pneumonia, brucellosis, typhoid fever, coccidioidomycosis, syphilis, and a variety of parasitic diseases.

Non-infectious conditions that have been linked to abnormal cell-mediated immunity include chronic protein-calorie malnutrition, uremia, diabetes mellitus, surgery, anesthesia, sarcoidosis, and cystic fibrosis.

Pharmacologic Agents

Corticosteroids are the pharmacologic agents most often associated with abnormalities in cell-mediated immunity although they may also cause immune suppression as a result of effects on other host defense mechanisms. The degree of immunosuppression and the relative risk of infection depend on the dose and duration of corticosteroids, as well as the underlying disease. Patients receiving pharmacologic doses of steroids (e.g., brain tumor patients, those with inflammatory bowel disease, and patients with autoimmune disorders) may have impaired cell-mediated immunity and should be considered at risk for mycobacterial, viral, and parasitic infections. Patients to be treated with corticosteroids who have a known history of tuberculosis or a positive purified protein derivative skin test should be given prophylactic isoniazid to prevent reactivation and potential dissemination of disease.

A number of cytotoxic agents are also associated with impaired cell-mediated immunity including methotrexate, cyclophosphamide, 6-mercaptopurine, and azathioprine. Cyclosporine is an immunosuppressant used to suppress transplant rejection and is associated with alterations in helper T cells, effector T cells, and natural killer cells. It has not been established, however, that cyclosporine *per se* is associated with an increased risk of infection.

Radiotherapy also may result in impaired cell-mediated immunity, especially when used in combination with other immunosuppressive agents or to treat patients with underlying diseases associated with intrinsic defects in cell-mediated immunity (e.g., as a component of the preparatory regimen for bone marrow transplantation or for treatment of Hodgkin's disease).

Primary Disorders of Cell-Mediated Immunity

Defects in cell-mediated immunity are found as components of mixed primary B- and T-cell abnormalities, including severe combined immunodeficiency disease, Wiskott-Aldrich syndrome, ataxia-telangiectasia, and certain purine pathway enzyme deficiencies (see Chapter 207). Infections in patients with these disorders tend to begin early in life and may be caused not only by pathogens associated with abnormalities in cell-mediated immunity but also by pathogens seen with humoral defects such as the encapsulated bacteria.

Severe combined immunodeficiency disease is associated with a marked decrease in both B- and T-cell numbers and extremely low levels of immunoglobulins. Patients fail to react to skin tests and have a negligible antibody response following immunizations. Failure to thrive and recurrent infections are seen within the initial few months of life. Infections are due to *S. aureus, S. pneumoniae, H. influenzae, P. carinii, Candida,* and herpes group viruses. Affected infants usually die by 2 years of age. A variant of severe combined immunodeficiency disease has been described that is associated with chronic skin eruption, hepatosplenomegaly, eosinophilia, and histiocytic infiltration of the lymph nodes (Omenn's disease). *P. carinii* pneumonia may be a common initial symptom in this disorder.

In patients with Wiskott-Aldrich syndrome, the major abnormality is an inability to respond to polysaccharide antigens. Infections are caused by polysaccharide-encapsulated bacterial pathogens such as *S. pneumoniae* and *H. influenzae.* However, patients may also lose T-cell functions and have increased susceptibility to pathogens such as HSV and certain fungi and protozoa.

Ataxia-telangiectasia is associated with absent serum and secretory IgA. The thymus is hypoplastic, and thymus-dependent zones in lymph nodes are empty or unoccupied. Infection with encapsulated bacteria predominates, especially recurrent sinopulmonary infections. Many patients progressively lose T-cell function over time and may become susceptible to associated pathogens.

Purine pathway enzyme deficiencies (adenosine deaminase deficiency or nucleoside phosphorylase deficiency) may be associated with either combined B- and T-cell defects or isolated B- or T-cell abnormalities. The type of infection depends on the predominant immune defect. Infections may not appear until 6 to 12 months of age.

The primary cellular immunodeficiencies associated with T-cell abnormalities include thymic hypoplasia (DiGeorge syndrome), combined immunodeficiency with predominant T-cell defects (Nezelof syndrome), purine nucleoside phosphorylase deficiency, and chronic mucocutaneous candidiasis.

DiGeorge syndrome develops when the 3rd and part of the 4th pharyngeal pouches fail to develop during embryogenesis, thereby resulting in absence of the thymus and parathyroid glands. Children with DiGeorge syndrome can lack T lymphocytes and may have severe depression of cell-mediated immunity, which makes them susceptible to overwhelming infections by variety of organisms, including HSV, VZV, *C. albicans,* and *P. carinii.* Nezelof syndrome can be differentiated from DiGeorge syndrome by the absence of parathyroid and cardiac involvement.

Cartilage-hair hypoplasia is a form of short-limbed dwarfism associated with a virtual absence of T-cell function. Interestingly, susceptibility to infection is not as pronounced as in other T-cell deficiencies. Overwhelming viral infections from vaccinia or varicella viruses may occur.

Chronic mucocutaneous candidiasis involves impairment in cell-mediated immunity, and infection is almost always limited to the skin and mucous membranes.

ABNORMALITIES OF HUMORAL DEFENSE MECHANISMS—IMMUNOGLOBULINS AND COMPLEMENT

Immunoglobulins and complement are among the most important components of the humoral immune system, and defects or deficiencies in either may be associated with serious infections. Other proteins that have been classified as part of the humoral defense system include lysozyme, lactoferrin, tuftsin, and fibronectin. Immunoglobulins may be opsonic (enhance phagocytosis), or neutralizing (inhibit replication of viruses) or, with complement, may lyse microbes or cells. The humoral system functions predominantly against bacterial infections. Patients with either primary or secondary defects or deficiencies in these proteins are at highest risk for serious infections from encapsulated bacteria and to a lesser extent the enteroviruses and *Giardia lamblia.*

Patients with Malignant Disorders

The degree of humoral impairment in multiple myeloma appears to be related to the stage of the disease and is primarily caused by malignant plasma cell induction of a protein that is synthesized by macrophages and that selectively suppresses B-cell function. Myeloma patients are most susceptible to recurrent infections from encapsulated bacteria such as *S. pneumoniae* or *H. influenzae* early in the course of the disease. Infections caused by enteric gram-negative rods and staphylococci are also encountered, especially in patients with refractory or advanced disease. Recurrent infection most often occurs in the upper respiratory tract, urinary tract, or skin.

Patients with B-cell chronic lymphocytic leukemia appear to have unbalanced immunoglobulin chain synthesis and resultant hypogammaglobulinemia. The incidence of infection correlates with the duration and stage of the disease, as well as serum levels of immunoglobulins (particularly IgG). Encapsulated bacteria predominate, although infections by staphylococci and enteric gram-negative bacilli also occur. Upper and lower respiratory tract infections are encountered most commonly, although other sites such as the urinary tract and skin are frequently involved.

Non-malignant states (e.g., nephrotic syndrome, burns, protein-losing enteropathy) can be associated with increased immunoglobulin catabolism or loss and may lead to decreased antibody levels and enhanced susceptibility to infection. Clinically significant acquired complement defects are unusual.

Primary Deficiencies

Isolated B-cell immunodeficiency states and their associated risks for infection in children include transient hypogammaglobulinemia of infancy, which is not usually associated with serious infections; sex-linked hypogammaglobulinemia, which is associated with recurrent pyogenic infections and septicemia from *S. pneumoniae, H. influenzae, S. aureus, Neisseria meningitidis,* and *P. aeruginosa;* hypogammaglobulinemia associated with hyperimmunoglobulin M, in which patients have recurrent respiratory, soft tissue, and gastrointestinal infections; selective IgM deficiency, in which patients have severe recurrent infections secondary to pyogenic bacteria; and selective IgA deficiency, in which certain patients may have increased numbers of upper respiratory tract infections whereas others appear not to be at increased risk. Chronic diarrhea caused by *G. lamblia* is also associated with IgA deficiency. Common variable hypogammaglobulinemia is associated with respiratory tract infections with *S. pneumoniae, H. influenzae,* and *S. aureus.* Diarrhea caused by *G. lamblia* also occurs.

Many patients with B-cell deficiencies, particularly those with congenital hypogammaglobulinemia, appear to be at risk for chronic central nervous system infections by enteroviruses.

A number of primary defects in complement components have also been described. Although deficiencies of the early classic pathway components (C1, C2, C4) have been reported, associated infection is rare, probably because the alternative pathway remains functional and is able to compensate. Deficiencies of C3 or C5, on the other hand, often lead to severe infections with encapsulated organisms, enteric gram-negative bacteria, and staphylococci. Absence of the later components (C5b, C6, C7, C8, C9) leads to an increase in infections, primarily with *Neisseria* species, both *N. gonorrhoeae* and *N. meningitidis.* Although the defects in these later components may be present from birth, infectious episodes do not typically begin until the teenage years. Indeed, any patient with recurrent infections by *Neisseria* species should be investigated for complement deficiency.

SPLENECTOMY AND SPLENIC DYSFUNCTION

Splenectomy may be performed either as a part of staging or as a therapeutic intervention in a number of disorders, including

Hodgkin's disease, agnogenic myeloid metaplasia, paroxysmal nocturnal hemoglobinuria, hereditary spherocytosis, thalassemia, and a variety of autoimmune disorders.

The spleen probably plays an adjunctive role in host defense by removing organisms from the blood that have been ineffectively opsonized by complement. In addition, it participates in the primary immunoglobulin response and is involved in regulation of the alternative complement pathway, with low levels of immunoglobulins and properdin reported in patients following splenectomy. A decrease in the opsonic peptide tuftsin has also been reported following splenectomy, and alternative pathway defects may be important in patients with sickle cell disease and splenic dysfunction.

The risk of development of serious infection, as well as the types of infections, may vary depending on the reason for abnormal splenic function and the presence or absence of other immune abnormalities. Patients who undergo post-traumatic splenectomy appear to be at a lower risk for infection. An increased risk of *Salmonella* infection appears to be unique for the sickle cell population. Most asplenic patients or patients who have undergone splenectomy are at increased risk for serious bacterial infections, primarily with *S. pneumoniae* and *H. influenzae*, as well as *Neisseria* species and *Capnocytophaga*. The initial manifestation of even overwhelming infection may be deceptively subtle, with fever often being the only sign of infection. Asplenic patients with an underlying hematologic disease who have fever should be managed initially as potentially septic.

EVALUATING AND MANAGING THE FEBRILE GRANULOCYTOPENIC PATIENT: A PARADIGM FOR THE COMPROMISED HOST

A classic tenet of infectious disease is that antibiotic therapy is based on isolating and identifying a specific organism or on reliably predicting a specific organism from a clinically involved site of infection. The overall management of neutropenic patients is based on the use of empirical antibiotics directed against a wider array of potential pathogens. Indeed, it is well accepted that when a new fever develops in a neutropenic patient (usually defined as one oral temperature of ≥38.5° C or more than two successive readings of ≥38° C in a 12-hour period), an empirical broad-spectrum antibacterial regimen should be started expeditiously. The rationale for this approach evolved from the observation that bacteremias in neutropenic patients were rapidly lethal, especially those caused by gram-negative organisms, if antibiotic therapy was delayed until an organism was isolated or a site of infection identified. Although the goal of pre-antibiotic evaluation of a newly febrile neutropenic patient is to identify potential sources, the majority of patients will not have a source of infection identified to explain the fever. It is also important to underscore that the absence of fever does not preclude the presence of a serious or life-threatening infection if a neutropenic patient manifests localizing signs or symptoms otherwise compatible with an infectious etiology.

The standard initial evaluation should include a careful physical examination with particular attention to areas that may "hide" an infection, notably the oral cavity and the perianal area. Examination of the perirectal area, including deep palpation, should be performed, and only if findings suggestive of a localized inflammatory site (e.g., pain or fluctuance) are noted should a judicious digital examination be performed. At a minimum, two sets of blood samples for culture should be obtained. If the patient has an indwelling intravenous catheter, at least one set should be drawn through the catheter and another from a peripheral vein. For patients with multilumen intravenous catheters, a culture should be obtained through *each* lumen and the specific lumen clearly identified on the culture bottle. Such practice is important because catheter infection may be limited to a single lumen. Because of the absence of granulocytes, microscopic examination of the urine may be normal even in the presence of a urinary tract infection. A chest radiograph can serve as a valuable baseline, although some investigators have questioned the use of this procedure in patients without pulmonary symptoms. In addition, accessible sites of potential infection should be aspirated or biopsied, with appropriate material sent for Gram stain, culture, and histologic examination.

Even with a comprehensive evaluation, an infectious cause for the initial pre-antibiotic fever is found in only 30 to 50% of

patients. Nonetheless, even subtle indications of inflammation must be considered as sites of potential infection in the presence of granulocytopenia. For example, minimal perirectal erythema and tenderness may be harbingers of perirectal cellulitis. Minimal erythema or serous discharge at the exit site of an indwelling intravenous catheter may herald a tunnel or exit site infection.

Colonization with microorganisms often precedes the development of significant infection. However, routine "surveillance" cultures are not of practical benefit in a neutropenic patient because colonization of a single body site is not consistently predictive and multiple potential pathogens are usually isolated from any single site, thus making it difficult to predict the organism responsible for infection. Moreover, because empirical broad-spectrum antibiotics are administered under any circumstance, the expense of routine surveillance cannot be justified.

Tests such as nuclear scanning have also been used to define occult sites of infection. Although gallium citrate accumulates in inflammatory lesions because of its avid binding to lactoferrin, this test has not been shown to be useful in granulocytopenic patients. Autologous or allogeneic leukocytes labeled *in vitro* with indium-111 or indium-111 linked to IgG have been used by some investigators in the evaluation of febrile granulocytopenic patients.

Because of these diagnostic difficulties, even fevers that are temporally associated with the administration of blood products or with fever-producing antineoplastic agents should be considered potentially infectious and treated as such. In sum, virtually all new fevers in the neutropenic population warrant careful clinical and microbiologic evaluation, followed by prompt initiation of empirical antibiotic therapy. Conversely, any clinically evident site of potential infection mandates expeditious broad-spectrum therapy, even in the absence of fever.

Because the goal of empirical antibiotic therapy is to protect against the early morbidity and mortality that result from untreated bacterial infections, regimens have been formulated to maximize activity against commonly encountered organisms that are particularly virulent. However, empirical regimens cannot realistically be designed to cover every potential bacterial pathogen. Moreover, no regimen is capable of completely eliminating the risk of subsequent infections in persistently neutropenic patients.

Management of Indwelling Intravenous Catheters

Although gram-positive bacteria (especially staphylococci) are the most frequent causes of catheter-related infections, other bacterial and non-bacterial species can be encountered, particularly in a neutropenic patient. These species include resistant *Corynebacterium*, *Bacillus* species, gram-negative organisms, and fungi. In evaluating a patient with catheter-related infection, it is important to consider the specific type of infection, its location (i.e., bacteremia versus exit site versus tunnel), the type of access device (e.g., Hickman versus implantable subcutaneous reservoir), and the duration of symptoms.

In general, the vast majority of simple catheter-related bacteremias and exit site infections can be cleared by using appropriate antibiotics and do not require catheter removal. This observation applies to both neutropenic and non-neutropenic patients. If multilumen devices are used, the antibiotic infusion should be rotated among the ports because infection may be limited to one lumen (failure to do so can be a cause of persistent infection despite antibiotics). If bacteremia persists after 48 hours of appropriate therapy, the catheter should be removed. Failure of therapy is more common when the infections are due to certain organisms such as *Bacillus* species or *C. albicans,* and when these organisms are isolated, the catheter should usually be removed.

Infections extending to involve the tunnel of a Hickman catheter also mandate prompt removal of the device because antibiotics alone rarely cure this "closed-space" infection, particularly in a granulocytopenic host. Likewise, infections around the reservoir of an implantable subcutaneous device may be difficult to eradicate without catheter removal. Patients with recurrent catheter infections (despite a history of appropriate therapy) are also candidates for prompt catheter removal.

It is unresolved whether a non-neutropenic patient with an indwelling catheter who becomes newly febrile should receive antibiotics empirically. The safest policy is to begin antibiotics (using a

3rd-generation cephalosporin such as ceftriaxone or an aminoglycoside plus vancomycin) and continue them pending culture results and clinical response. This approach protects against rapid progression of undetected yet virulent infections (such as *S. aureus*) and may minimize the need for ultimate catheter removal. If by 72 hours the cultures are negative and the patient is stable, antibiotic therapy can be discontinued.

Initial Management of the Neutropenic Patient Who Becomes Febrile

Although gram-negative bacteria still predominate at some institutions, in recent years the trend has been toward more gram-positive infections, which now represent the majority of isolates at many centers. In general, gram-negative infections tend to be more virulent, and early empirical regimens have been formulated to provide protection primarily against these organisms while maintaining a broad spectrum of activity against other potential pathogens. Indeed, adequate coverage of these gram-negative organisms is still an essential property of any empirical regimen.

Although no single best regimen or recipe is known, a number of options are appropriate. Selection of a specific antibiotic regimen depends on many factors, including institutional sensitivity patterns, individual and institutional experience, and clinical parameters.

The standard approach to the empirical management of a febrile neutropenic patient has been to use combination antibiotic regimens. Until recently, combination regimens have been the only way to provide coverage broad enough to encompass the predominant gram-positive and gram-negative organisms. Moreover, some combinations have been thought to provide synergy and to have the potential for decreasing the emergence of resistant isolates. Aminoglycoside–β-lactam combinations were the first empirical regimens with acceptable efficacy in the setting of fever and neutropenia. Such combination regimens are still widely used and represent a standard against which newer regimens are tested. Many variations have been studied and include aminoglycosides combined with either an extended-spectrum penicillin or a cephalosporin or as a component of a triple-drug regimen. If an aminoglycoside-containing combination regimen is to be used, the choice of specific antibiotics should be based primarily on the institutional antibiotic sensitivity patterns and secondarily on toxicity and cost differences.

Non–aminoglycoside-containing combination regimens have also been studied. These regimens have consisted of combinations of two β-lactam antibiotics, or so-called double β-lactam regimens, usually consisting of an expanded-spectrum carboxypenicillin or ureidopenicillin plus a 3rd-generation cephalosporin (e.g., piperacillin and ceftazidime).

New or Novel Antibiotics for Neutropenic Patients

The advent of β-lactam antibiotics with broad-spectrum activity that achieve high serum bactericidal levels has made monotherapy another option for the initial empirical treatment of a febrile neutropenic patient (Table 314–3). The 3rd-generation and "4th-generation" cephalosporins and the carbapenems are the two classes that include potential candidates for empirical single-agent therapy. Ceftazidime has been the most extensively studied of the 3rd-generation cephalosporins as monotherapy because of its superior activity against *P. aeruginosa*.

A large, randomized study evaluating 550 consecutive episodes of fever and neutropenia was conducted at the National Cancer Institute (NCI). In this study, patients with fever and granulocytopenia underwent a standard initial evaluation and were then randomized to receive either a combination of antibiotics (cephalothin, gentamicin, and carbenicillin) or ceftazidime as a single agent. The overall results show that monotherapy compared favorably with a standard combination regimen. Approximately two thirds of the episodes in both groups were treated successfully for the entire duration of their granulocytopenia without requiring *any* changes in their initial regimen. The other third of the episodes required some change or modification (such as the addition of an antibacterial, antifungal, or antiviral drug) to ensure a successful outcome (see indications for modifications below), and an equally low number in both groups (about 5%) died of infection. None of the deaths were attributable to a specific deficiency in one regimen that was not present in the other.

Two subgroups of patients were identified who required more

Table 314–3 ■ MEDICATIONS IN PATIENTS WITH NEUTROPENIA AND FEVER

AGENT	COMMENTS
Antibiotic	
Third-generation cephalosporins	Only ceftazidime and cefepine are appropriate for coverage of *Pseudomonas aeruginosa*
Carbapenems	If *P. aeruginosa* is suspected or cultured, an aminoglycoside should be added
Extended-spectrum penicillins	Because of the potential for resistance, piperacillin, azlocillin, or mezlocillin should be administered with either an aminoglycoside or a 3rd-generation cephalosporin
Monobactams	Aztreonam is an important alternative for patients allergic to β-lactam antibiotics, but it should be combined with vancomycin for empirical therapy
Quinolones	Important for gram-negative infection and possibly for use in low-risk patients with neutropenia; to avoid resistance, do not use for prophylaxis
Vancomycin	Pathogen-directed therapy generally suffices. Empirical use can be restricted to centers with a high incidence of methicillin-resistant *Staphylococcus aureus*. Of concern, strains of vancomycin-resistant enterococci have been described
Antifungal	
Amphotericin B	Still the best treatment. A dose of 0.6 mg/kg of body weight per day suffices for *Candida albicans* and *Cryptococcus,* 1 mg/kg/day is preferred for *Candida tropicalis,* and 1.5 mg/kg/day is preferred for *Aspergillus*
Lipid preparations of amphotericin	Similar to and slightly greater benefit than amphotericin B with less toxicity albeit more expense
Ketoconazole	Not an alternative to amphotericin B for empirical therapy. Useful for thrush or esophagitis.
Fluconazole	Very effective for thrush or esophagitis. Value for systemic mycoses, including hepatosplenic candidiasis; requires additional study
Itraconazole	Activity against *Aspergillus,* although absorption can be unpredictable
Antiviral	
Acyclovir	Oral therapy is not advised for severely immunocompromised patients with varicella-zoster infections. For such patients, parenteral therapy (1500 mg/m² of body surface area per day in 3 divided doses) is indicated. For patients with herpes simplex, oral or parenteral therapy (750 mg/m² day in 3 divided doses) is satisfactory
Ganciclovir	Of value for cytomegalovirus retinitis, prevention of pneumonitis, and combined with an intravenous immunoglobulin for pneumonitis
Foscarnet	Of value for cytomegalovirus retinitis in patients in whom ganciclovir is ineffective
Antiparasitic	
Trimethoprim-sulfamethoxazole	Best drug for *Pneumocystis carinii* prophylaxis. Not required in all cancer patients. Thrice-weekly schedule is satisfactory (150 mg of trimethoprim/m²/day in 2 divided doses)
Aerosolized pentamidine	Expensive and not as effective as trimethoprim-sulfamethoxazole in adults with HIV infection

Modified from Pizzo PA: Management of fever in patients with cancer and treatment-induced neutropenia. N Engl J Med 328:1323, 1993. Copyright by the Massachusetts Medical Society.

frequent modifications of the initial regimen to achieve a successful outcome: (1) those with a documented source of infection to account for the initial fever and (2) those having relatively protracted periods of granulocytopenia (≥ 1 week). The need for modification in these subgroups was identical for episodes treated with monotherapy and those treated with combination therapy. In this study, these modifications did not represent a failure of either regimen *per se* but instead were reflective of the limitations of any regimen in treating patients who are at high risk for subsequent infections.

An international cooperative study that enrolled 676 patients (83% with acute leukemia) with 876 episodes of fever and neutropenia in a recently reported randomized trial comparing ceftazidime monotherapy with the combination of piperacillin and tobramycin demonstrated comparable efficacy with both regimens but less toxicity with ceftazidime monotherapy.

Concerns regarding the use of ceftazidime as a single agent for fever and neutropenia include the lack of synergy against documented gram-negative infections, lack of activity against certain gram-negative isolates, poor antianaerobic activity, and the potential for development of resistance. Cefepime, a "third-generation" cephalosporin, overcomes some of these limitations.

In addition to the 3rd-generation cephalosporins, other antibiotics have been evaluated in neutropenic patients. Imipenem, for example, is a member of the carbapenem class of antibiotics. It is formulated in fixed combination with cilastatin, which inhibits a renal enzyme that can degrade imipenem. Overall, it has the broadest spectrum of activity of any available antibiotic. Of note is its excellent *in vitro* activity against enterococci and many anaerobes.

The results of two randomized studies appear to corroborate its efficacy in this setting—one comparing it with an aminoglycoside-containing combination and another performed at the NCI comparing it with monotherapy with ceftazidime. Interestingly, neither of these studies demonstrate superior efficacy for imipenem. Two potential drawbacks to its use include a relatively high incidence of the development of resistant *P. aeruginosa,* as well as its potential to decrease the seizure threshold in patients with central nervous system pathology. In addition, in the NCI trial, a higher than expected frequency of nausea and vomiting as well as a significantly higher incidence of diarrhea, especially with *C. difficile,* have been found with imipenem.

Because of the increasing incidence of gram-positive infections in cancer patients during the 1980s and their increased resistance to β-lactam antibiotics, some authorities initially recommended that vancomycin be added to empirical regimens. Conversely, because of the increasing incidence of vancomycin-resistant enterococci, the Infectious Disease Society of America's expert panel on the care of neutropenic patients recommended that vancomycin not be used empirically. Rather, its use should be guided by institutional microflora and sensitivity patterns. For example, in a center with a high incidence of methicillin-resistant *S. aureus,* routine use of vancomycin is clearly warranted because *S. aureus* may be a particularly virulent organism if not treated. In addition, fluctuations in patterns of infecting microorganisms may occur over time. Furthermore, penicillin-resistant α-hemolytic streptococci have recently been identified as particularly virulent pathogens in some centers (perhaps related to the use of high-dose cytosine arabinoside). However, for most centers, these conditions will not apply. Clearly, the emergence of new pathogens or pathogens with altered sensitivity profiles may force dramatic changes in how we use antibiotics in the future.

The appropriate role for quinolones in a neutropenic patient has yet to be fully defined. Because of their relatively poor activity against certain gram-positive organisms, they should not be used for empirical therapy alone. They may, however, be beneficial in "low-risk" neutropenic patients (i.e., duration of neutropenia, < 10 days) and may include the combination with agents that expand the gram-positive and anaerobic spectrum of selected quinolones (e.g., ciprofloxacin plus amoxicillin/clavulanate or clindamycin) and expanded spectrum quinolones such as levofloxacin and trovofloxacin. They may be useful to complete therapy in patients who initially respond to intravenous antibiotics and who have had either an unexplained fever or a susceptible bacterial isolate.

A particularly useful feature of the monobactam aztreonam is its apparent lack of cross-reactivity with the other β-lactams in patients who have penicillin or β-lactam allergies. In this group of patients, empirical therapy might begin with a combination of vancomycin, aztreonam, and an aminoglycoside.

Also beneficial are combinations of β-lactams with β-lactamase inhibitors (i.e., clavulanic acid and sulbactam). Three preparations are available, including amoxicillin plus clavulanic acid (oral formulation only), ticarcillin plus clavulanic acid, and ampicillin plus sulbactam. A number of studies have documented the efficacy of ticarcillin plus clavulanic acid combined within aminoglycoside for initial empirical treatment of fever in neutropenic patients. The expanded gram-positive coverage may obviate additional anti–gram-positive agents.

APPROACH TO THE PATIENT WITH PROLONGED GRANULOCYTOPENIA

How Long Should Antibiotics Be Continued?

A question of practical importance is how long empirical antibiotic therapy should be continued in persistently neutropenic pa-

tients. Should they always be continued until the granulocyte count recovers, or can they be safely discontinued before that?

The question of duration of therapy can be approached by placing patients in two categories: those whose initial work-up (at the time of evaluation for fever and neutropenia) did not reveal a source of infection (i.e., unexplained fever; see Chapter 311) and those whose initial work-up revealed an infection to account for the fever (i.e., a positive culture, a clinically infected site, or both). Approximately 60% fall into the unexplained fever category, although this figure varies with the institution, the therapy, and the patient population (Fig. 314–1).

PATIENTS WITH UNEXPLAINED FEVER Only limited data specifically address the issue of duration of empirical therapy in neutropenic patients with unexplained fever. For patients with an expected short duration of granulocytopenia (e.g., < 1 week) and those with evidence of hematologic recovery, abbreviated courses of empirical therapy are safe and appropriate. However, the real dilemma arises in the population with more prolonged granulocytopenia.

In a study from the NCI, patients with unexplained fever and persistent granulocytopenia were randomized either to discontinue antibiotics on day 7 of therapy or to continue them until resolution of the neutropenia. Recurrent fever and hypotensive episodes developed in nearly 40% of afebrile patients in whom antibiotic when use was stopped. It was concluded that day 7 was too early to discontinue antibiotics in this group of afebrile patients with persistent and profound neutropenia. However, other studies have demonstrated that empirical antibiotics can be safely discontinued in patients with unexplained fever who have some evidence of hematologic recovery.

In contrast, patients with persistent and profound neutropenia who remain febrile despite empirical antibiotics should keep taking antibiotics until resolution of the granulocytopenia. These "high-risk" patients may also require the addition of one or more antimicrobial agents during their course of neutropenia (see below)

PATIENTS WITH DOCUMENTED INFECTIONS. Even fewer data address the issue of duration of antibiotics in patients with defined sites of infection. For persistently neutropenic patients who have had clinical and microbiologic resolution of their infection and who are afebrile at day 14 (for a minimum of 7 days), antibiotic use should be discontinued. The ultimate decision of whether to continue or discontinue therapy rests on a number of clinical parameters, such as the degree of or potential for antibiotic toxicity, the predicted duration of neutropenia, the seriousness of the initial infection, and the presence or absence of a continued site of infection or other factors predisposing to subsequent infection. It should be emphasized that any neutropenic patient whose antibiotic therapy is discontinued requires careful, meticulous follow-up to quickly detect new fevers or infection.

Modifications of Antibiotic Therapy During the Course of Granulocytopenia

Empirical antibiotics have their greatest impact early in the course of neutropenia. However, it is during prolonged granulocytopenic episodes that patent are at highest risk for multiple types of secondary infections or superinfections. Many of these conditions dictate specific modifications of the initial regimen (Table 314–4).

Bacterial isolates that are resistant to the initial empirical regimen are invariably encountered when managing neutropenic patients. For example, at most centers the majority of coagulase-negative staphylococci are resistant to β-lactams, and breakthrough infections might be anticipated. Fortunately, coagulase-negative staphylococci are relatively indolent, and the risk for secondary infection can be balanced accordingly. Thus for patients with evidence of gram-positive infection while receiving β-lactam therapy or with evidence of a catheter site infection, vancomycin is an appropriate addition to the initial antibiotic regimen. Similarly, if the coverage of the initial regimen has limited antianaerobic activity, secondary infection with anaerobics might be anticipated.

The appearance of "secondary" resistance is seen more frequently with certain organisms. For example, *Enterobacter* species, *Citrobacter* species, and *Serratia* have inducible β-lactamases, and the appearance of a clinically significant clustering of resistant *Enterobacter* in a neutropenic population has been observed re-

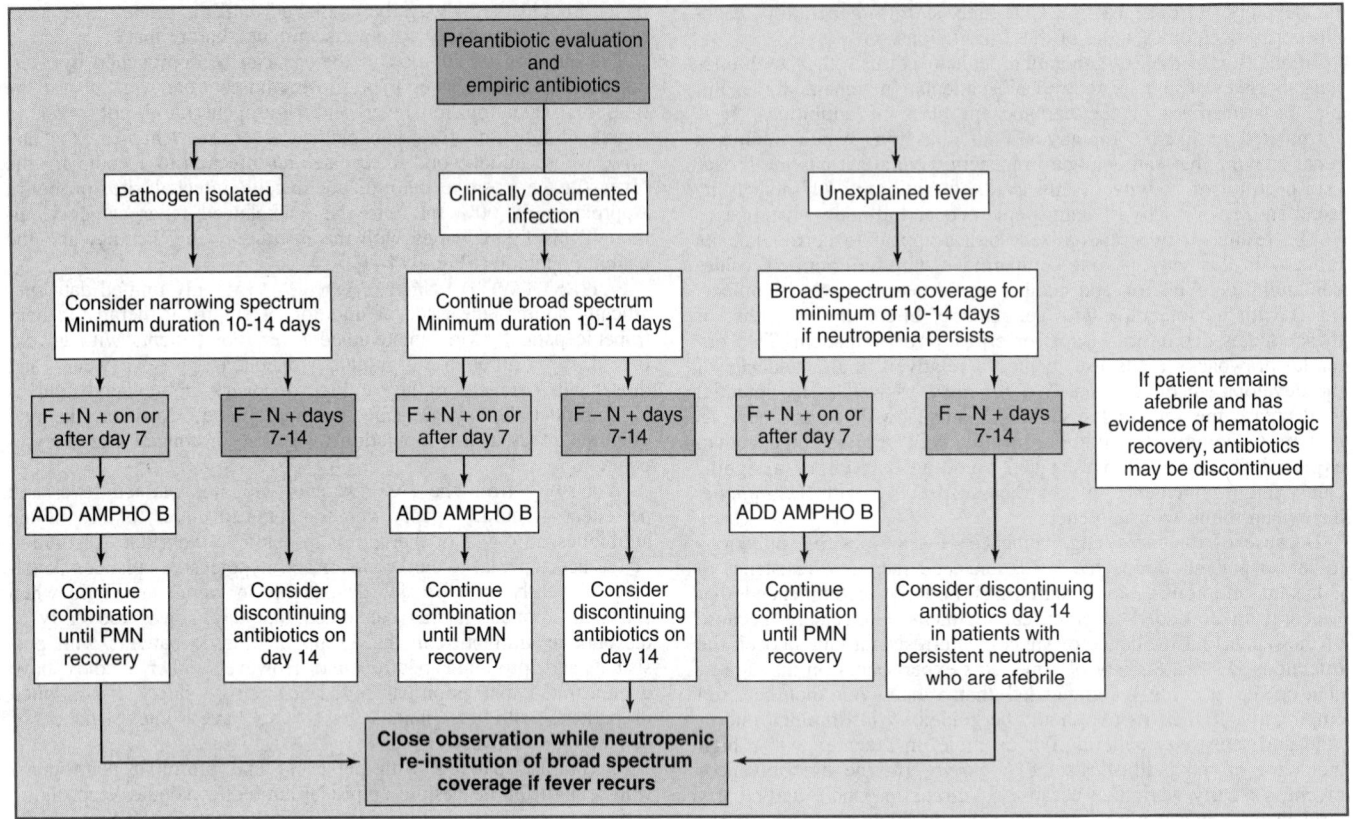

FIGURE 314–1 ■ Management of fever and neutropenia. F + N + = febrile, neutropenic; F − N + = afebrile, neutropenic; AMPHO B = amphotericin B. (From Rubin M, Walsh TJ, Pizzo PA: Clinical approach to the compromised host. *In* Hoffman R, Benz EJ Jr, Shattil SS, et al (eds): Hematology: Basic Principles and Practices, 2nd ed. New York, Churchill Livingstone, 1994.)

cently. Accordingly, when these organisms are isolated from a patient, careful observation for emergence of resistance is warranted, and for patients receiving monotherapy with a broad-spectrum β-lactam, an aminoglycoside should be added. *P. aeruginosa* may become resistant to imipenem through a relatively novel mechanism involving a change in the porins. Hence patients receiving single-agent therapy for *P. aeruginosa* infection should also have an aminoglycoside added to their regimens. Secondary development of resistance by gram-positive organisms is somewhat rarer, although it has been increasingly described. Of considerable concern, a number of recent studies have documented the emergence of vancomycin-resistant coagulase-negative staphylococci and enterococci in patients receiving vancomycin.

The appearance of a new site of infection (e.g., cellulitis or pneumonia) or the progression of a previously documented site of infection is an additional reason for modification of the antimicrobial regimen. For example, the development of marginal or necrotizing gingivitis is relatively common in patients who have received intensive cytotoxic therapy. Anaerobic organisms contribute to this process, and an antianaerobic agent such as clindamycin or metronidazole should be added to the empirical regimen if gingivitis is diagnosed.

The most common pathogens contributing to perianal cellulitis are the aerobic gram-negative bacilli, enterococci, and bowel anaerobes. Therefore, when perianal cellulitis occurs in a patient already receiving broad-spectrum antibiotics, the addition of an antianaerobic agent as well as a change in broad-spectrum coverage may be necessary. Similarly, any suspected intra-abdominal site of infection should prompt the addition of antibiotics active against aerobic gram-negative bacilli, enterococci, and bowel anaerobes.

The development of a new site of infection may also warrant the addition of antimicrobial agents directed at fungi, viruses, or parasites. The appearance of burning retrosternal pain is frequently an indicator of esophagitis, most often caused by cytotoxic therapy, *Candida,* or herpes simplex. The development of pulmonary infiltrates might raise suspicion of not only resistant bacteria but also

P. carinii, fungi, or a viral pneumonia. A new localized infiltrate in a neutropenic patient whose white blood count is rising while receiving broad-spectrum antibiotics with the "new" infiltrate may simply represent an inflammatory reaction at a previously unrecognized site of infection. Close observation without any modification may be appropriate. If, however, the granulocyte count is not rising and the patient has been neutropenic for only a short time (≤ 1 week), a bacterial process is most likely. If the patient has been persistently neutropenic for longer, fungal pneumonia should also be strongly considered and amphotericin B added while a diagnostic work-up is initiated.

Patients who become hypotensive while receiving broad-spectrum antibiotics should be presumed septic with a resistant organism or breakthrough infection. In such patients, changes in the empirical regimen should be made expeditiously and continued for the duration of treatment if an organism is not recovered. So-called culture-negative sepsis may occur when the growth of resistant organisms is suppressed by marginally effective antibiotics or when samples for culture are not drawn during the bacteremic episode.

Empirical Antifungal Therapy

The diagnosis of a disseminated fungal infection is difficult in an immunocompromised patient. Neutropenic patients who remain persistently febrile despite a 4- to 7-day trial of broad-spectrum antibacterial therapy are particularly likely to have a fungal infection. Empirical antifungal therapy might be expected to have a dual effect: preventing fungal overgrowth in patients with prolonged neutropenia and treating "subclinical" fungal disease early.

To date, the only proven agent for empirical therapy has been amphotericin B. Amphotericin B should be begun at 0.6 mg/kg/day and administered along with antibiotics until the resolution of neutropenia. If *Aspergillus* or *Mucor* is suspected, the dosage of amphotericin should be increased to 1 to 1.5 mg/kg/day. Liposome-encapsulated amphotericin B appears to be at least as effective as amphotericin B and has the advantage of significantly fewer sys-

Table 314-4 ■ COMMON MODIFICATIONS TO INITIAL EMPIRICAL ANTIBIOTIC THERAPY IN PATIENTS WITH NEUTROPENIA AND FEVER

STATUS OR SYMPTOMS	MODIFICATIONS OF PRIMARY REGIMEN
Fever	
Persistent for >1 wk	Add empirical antifungal therapy with amphotericin B
Recurrence after 1 wk or later in patient with persistent neutropenia	Add empirical antifungal therapy
Persistent or recurrent fever at time of recovery from neutropenia	Evaluate liver and spleen by CT, ultrasonography, or MRI for hepatosplenic candidiasis and evaluate need for antifungal therapy
Blood Stream	
Cultures before antibiotic therapy	
Gram-positive organism	Add vancomycin pending further identification
Gram-negative organism	Maintain regimen if patient is stable and isolate is sensitive. If *Pseudomonas aeruginosa, Enterobacter,* or *Citrobacter* is isolated, add an aminoglycoside or an additional β-lactam antibiotic
Organism isolated during antibiotic therapy	
Gram-positive organism	Add vancomycin
Gram-negative organism	Change to new combination regimen (e.g., imipenem plus gentamicin or vancomycin, or gentamicin plus piperacillin)
Head, Eyes, Ears, Nose, Throat	
Necrotizing or marginal gingivitis	Add specific antianaerobic agent (clindamycin or metronidazole) to empirical therapy
Vesicular or ulcerative lesions	Suspect herpes simplex infection. Culture and begin acyclovir therapy
Sinus tenderness or nasal ulcerative lesions	Suspect fungal infection with *Aspergillus* or *Mucor*
Gastrointestinal Tract	
Retrosternal burning pain	Suspect *Candida,* herpes simplex, or both. Add antifungal therapy and, if no response, acyclovir. Bacterial esophagitis also a possibility. For patients who do not respond within 48 hr, endoscopy should be considered
Acute abdominal pain	Suspect typhlitis, as well as appendicitis, if pain in right lower quadrant. Add specific antianaerobic coverage to empirical regimen and monitor closely for need for surgical intervention
Perianal tenderness	Add specific antianaerobic drug to empirical regimen and monitor need for surgical intervention, especially when patient is recovering from neutropenia
Respiratory Tract	
New focal lesion in patient recovering from neutropenia	Observe carefully; may be a consequence of inflammatory response in concert with neutrophil recovery
New focal lesion in patient with continuing neutropenia	Aspergillosis is the chief concern. Perform appropriate cultures and consider biopsy. If patient is not a candidate for procedure, administer high-dose amphotericin B (1.5 mg/kg/day)
New interstitial pneumonitis	Attempt diagnosis by examination of induced sputum or bronchoalveolar lavage. If not feasible, begin empirical treatment with trimethoprim-sulfamethoxazole or pentamidine. Consider non-infectious causes and the need for open-lung biopsy if condition has not improved after 4 d of therapy
Central Venous Catheters	
Positive culture for organisms other than *Bacillus* species or *Candida*	Attempt to treat. Rotate antibiotic administration in patients with multilumen catheters
Positive culture for *Bacillus* species or *Candida*	Remove catheter and treat appropriately
Exit site infection with *Mycobacterium* or *Aspergillus*	Remove catheter and treat appropriately
Tunnel infection	Remove catheter and treat appropriately

From Pizzo PA: Management of fever in patients with cancer and treatment-induced neutropenia. N Engl J Med 328:1323, 1993. Copyright by the Massachusetts Medical Society.

temic and renal side effects. A number of new azole and triazole antifungal agents (fluconazole, itraconazole, variconazole) also offer less toxic alternatives to amphotericin B for certain patients.

Patients who remain febrile after the resolution of neutropenia should be evaluated for hepatosplenic candidiasis. The diagnosis is suggested by "bull's-eye" lesions on computed tomography or ultrasonography of the liver and spleen. Magnetic resonance imaging of the liver may be even more sensitive. Biopsy and histologic examination are essential. Patients with hepatosplenic candidiasis may require extended courses of antifungal therapy. The average amount of amphotericin B required to resolve these lesions is approximately 5 g, often in conjunction with 5-flucytosine (100mg/kg/day). These patients can be treated successfully with liposomal formulations of amphotericin and some may respond to oral therapy with fluconazole after an initial response to parenteral treatment has been observed.

PREVENTION OF INFECTIONS

Because bacteria account for the majority of infections in compromised patients, prophylactic strategies have focused on these pathogens. Strategies that have been explored include mechanical techniques to prevent the acquisition of new pathogens, absorbable or non-absorbable oral antibiotic regimens to either prevent the acquisition of decrease the number of potentially pathogenic colonizing organisms, and methods to improve the host defense matrix,

including immunization and, more recently, biologic agents (e.g., the colony-stimulating factors) (Table 314–5).

Perhaps the most important infection prevention strategy of all, however, is handwashing. Although taken for granted, this simple procedure is frequently overlooked to the detriment of the patient.

Neutropenic Patients

MECHANICAL TECHNIQUES. Reverse isolation (i.e., single room with gowns, masks, and gloves) following the onset of neutropenia does not prevent infection because most of the infections arise from the patient's endogenous microbial flora. In addition, having patients wear a surgical mask outside their room does little to protect against subsequent infection. Although some authorities have recommended that all foods he thoroughly cooked and that fresh fruits and vegetables be avoided to decrease the acquisition of gram-negative bacteria, the value of these measures in preventing infection remains unproven.

The total protective environment is a comprehensive regimen designed to reduce the patient's endogenous microbial burden as well as the acquisition of new organisms. A total protective environment includes a high-efficiency particulate air (HEPA)-filtered laminar airflow room together with an aggressive program of surface decontamination, including the sterilization of all objects that enter the room, and an intensive regimen to disinfect the microbial diet. A number of studies have documented that such program can

Table 314-5 ■ METHODS STUDIED FOR PREVENTING
INFECTION IN HIGH-RISK PATIENTS

PREVENT ACQUISITION AND/OR SUPPRESS OR ELIMINATE MICROBIAL FLORA	IMPROVE OR MODIFY HOST DEFENSES
Isolation	Immunization
Simple or reverse isolation	Active
Isolation with HEPA air filtration	*Pneumococcus*
Prophylactic antibiotics	VZV
Non-absorbable antibiotics	Passive
Trimethoprim-sulfamethoxazole,	J-5 core glycolipid
erythromycin	Pooled immunoglobulins
Selective decontamination	Hyperimmune globulins
Quinolones	Monoclonal antibodies
Prophylactic antivirals	Cell component replacement
Acyclovir	Leukocyte transfusions
Amantadine	Accelerate granulocyte recovery
Prophylactic antifungals	G-CSF
Nystatin	GM-CSF
Imidazoles	Immunomodulations
Triazoles	Interferons
Amphotericin B	Interleukins
Prophylactic antiparasitics	
Thiabendazole	
Trimethoprim-sulfamethoxazole	
Combination-comprehensive	
Total protective isolation	

VZV = varicella-zoster virus; G-CSF = granulocyte colony-stimulating factor; GM-CSF = granulocyte-macrophage colony-stimulating factor.

Modified from Pizzo PA; Considerations for the prevention of infectious complications in patients with cancer. Rev Infect Dis 11(Suppl): 1551, 1989.

reduce infections in profoundly granulocytopenic individuals. However, a total protective environment is expensive, and because of the improvement in treating established infections, it does not offer a current survival advantage to most patients. Thus a total protective environment is not necessary for routine care of the majority of granulocytopenic patients.

ORAL ANTIBIOTIC REGIMENS. Numerous studies have evaluated both non-absorbable antibiotics (such as gentamicin, vancomycin, polymyxin, or colistin) and antibiotics that are absorbed from the gastrointestinal tract (e.g., trimethoprim-sulfamethoxazole. erythromycin, or quinolones). The goal of antibiotics has ranged from "total decontamination" of the alimentary tract with oral non-absorbable antibiotics to "selective decontamination," in which the goal is to eliminate the potentially pathogenic aerobic flora (mostly the enteric gram-negative bacteria) while preserving the majority of anaerobic organisms and thus preserving "colonization resistance." Although the introduction of each new prophylactic regimen has been met with enthusiasm, over time these strategies have failed because of the emergence of resistant organisms.

The fluoroquinolones (mostly norfloxacin and ciprofloxacin) have been used in recent years for prophylaxis in neutropenic patients. These agents are well absorbed, and their use may really represent "early treatment" rather than prophylaxis. Although studies evaluating quinolones have demonstrated a reduction in gram-negative infections in the patients who receive them, organisms resistant to the quinolones have been increasingly described, and indiscriminate use of these agents only accelerates this process. Thus the Infectious Disease Society of America recommends against the use of quinolone for routine antibiotic prophylaxis in neutropenic patients.

PATIENTS WITH SICKLE CELL ANEMIA. Because patients with sickle cell anemia are prone to infections with encapsulated organisms (e.g., *S. pneumoniae, H. influenzae*), especially young children, pneumococcal vaccine and prophylactic penicillin have been used to prevent these infections. Unfortunately, the vaccination has not resulted in an effective antibody response. Prophylactic penicillin can, however, significantly reduce the incidence of infection, and it is recommended that penicillin prophylaxis be begun by 4 months of age in children with sickle cell anemia and that it be continued beyond the 3rd birthday.

Prevention of Fungal Infections

Although the increasing incidence of fungal infection makes a preventive strategy desirable, to date no clear evidence of benefit has been demonstrated with the possible exception of fluconazole prophylaxis for patients undergoing allogeneic bone marrow transplantation. It is hoped that newer azole and triazole antifungal agents may improve the ability to control these opportunistic pathogens.

Prevention of Viral Infections

HERPES SIMPLEX. Herpes simplex is a frequent cause of morbidity in compromised patients, particularly in association with bone marrow or renal transplantation or intensive chemotherapy regimens. Several studies have demonstrated that acyclovir administered either orally or intravenously at dosages of 250 mg/m^2 every 8 hours can reduce the incidence of herpetic gingivostomatitis. Accordingly, it seems reasonable to administer prophylactic oral or intravenous acyclovir in patients who are HSV seropositive (titers ≥1:16) or who have a prior history of infection and are undergoing bone marrow transplantation or intensive therapy for acute leukemia.

VARICELLA-ZOSTER VIRUS. One of the most important ways to prevent VZV transmission is to prevent contact of immunosuppressed individuals with infected individuals, including patients with either primary VZV (chickenpox) or secondary VZV (zoster). If a seronegative individual has had contact with an infected individual, passive immunization with zoster immune globulin has been shown to reduce the incidence of pneumonitis and encephalitis. Administration of zoster immune globulin (1 vial per 15 kg) must occur within 72 hours after exposure.

A varicella vaccine has been shown to reduce infection in children with leukemia. The live vaccine has recently been licensed for administration to normal healthy children and, if appropriately used, should reduce the overall population of infected individuals.

CYTOMEGALOVIRUS. Successful strategies aimed at preventing cytomegalovirus infection have included the use of seronegative blood products in seronegative patients, passive immunization, and chemoprophylaxis with acyclovir or ganciclovir.

Prevention of Parasitic Infections

P. carinii pneumonia can largely be prevented with trimethoprim-sulfamethoxazole. The decision to administer prophylaxis for *P. carinii* should be influenced by the patient's underlying disease, the intensity or immunosuppression of the therapy being delivered, and the center where the treatment is being administered. Recent studies have demonstrated that trimethoprim-sulfamethoxazole can be effective and safe at a dosage of 75 mg/m^2 twice a day given on 3 consecutive days each week. Alternatives include aerosolized pentamidine or atovaquone.

Improving Host Defense

Immunization against bacterial and viral pathogens has played an extremely important role in decreasing the incidence and/or severity of many infectious diseases. Unfortunately, active immunization is generally unsuccessful in immunocompromised hosts because of their inability to mount or sustain an antibody response to most vaccines.

Passive immunization, on the other hand, involves the administration of pre-formed antibodies to high-risk patients. Zoster immune globulin, for example, is effective in preventing infection and decreasing the incidence of morbidity and mortality associated with primary chickenpox in susceptible hosts. Pooled immunoglobulin preparations do not appear to offer benefit for neutropenic hosts but are of benefit to patients who have either congenital or acquired (e.g., chronic lymphocytic leukemia, multiple myeloma) hypogammaglobulinemia. Monoclonal antibodies have recently been evaluated but were accompanied by unanticipated toxicity, thus impeding the use of current formulations.

An exciting area of investigation has been the prophylactic and therapeutic use of cytokines and lymphokines to enforce the host defense repertoire. A number of studies have demonstrated that both GM- and G-CSF can shorten the duration of chemotherapy-induced neutropenia, abbreviate the duration of hospitalization and decrease the need for antimicrobial therapy although a clear benefit on survival or outcome from defined infection has not been definitively demonstrated. The American Society of Clinical Oncology has recommended, on the basis of published data, that hematopoietic cytokines be used when the likelihood of a chemotherapy regimen resulting in fever and neutropenia, is greater than 40%, when the interest is not in reducing the dose intensity of chemotherapy after a prior episode of fever and neutropenia, and when they are needed following autologous bone marrow transplantation. Conversely, these colony-stimulating factors are not indicated for patients with low-risk (i.e., short-duration) neutropenia. Clearly, as new factors become defined, the prospect for restoring function in the compromised host stands as the opportunity for the next decade.

American Academy of Pediatrics: Immunization in special circumstances. *In* Peter G (ed): 1997 Redbook: Report of the Committee on Infectious Diseases, 24th ed. Elk Grove Village, IL, American Academy of Pediatrics, 1997, pp 50–58.

Armitage JO: Bone marrow transplantation. N Engl J Med 330:327, 1994.

Chanoch SJ, Pizzo PA: Infectious complications of patients undergoing therapy for acute leukemia: Current states and future prospect. Semin Oncol 24:132, 1997.

Denning D: Invasive aspergillosis. Clin Infect Dis 26:781, 1998.

Freifeld AG, Walsh TJ, Pizzo PA: Infectious complications in the pediatric cancer patient. *In* Pizzo PA, Poplack DG (eds): Principles and Practice of Pediatric Oncology, 3d ed. Philadelphia, JB Lippincott, 1997, pp 1069–1114.

Hathorn JW: Critical appraisal of antimicrobials for prevention of infections in immunocompromised hosts. Hematol Oncol Clin North Am 7:1051, 1993.

Hughes WT, Armstrong D, Bodey GP, et al: Guidelines for the use of antimicrobial agents in neutropenic patients who have unexplained fever. Clin Infect Dis 25:551, 1997.

Pizzo PA: Management of fever in patients with cancer and treatment induced neutropenia. N Engl J Med 328:1323, 1993.

315 NOSOCOMIAL INFECTIONS

John A. Jernigan

The word *nosocomial* is derived from the Greek *nosos* (disease) and *komeion* (to take care of) and is defined as "belonging or pertaining to a hospital." Infections acquired within a hospital or other health care facility have therefore been termed nosocomial infections.

Nosocomial infections have plagued hospitalized patients since the very inception of institutionalized medical care. Records from medieval hospitals in Western Europe contain frequent descriptions of pestilence and "visitations" of disease, attributed by some at the time to infectious "miasmas." By the early 19th century, the concept that infection could be transmitted between patients led to the formation of special fever hospitals in England intended to segregate patients with communicable illnesses. In the mid-19th century, Florence Nightingale's studies of mortality in military hospitals dramatically demonstrated that far more soldiers died of hospital-acquired infection than from the primary effects of battle. At about the same time a Hungarian obstetrician named Ignaz Semmelweis gave birth to the discipline of infection control and hospital epidemiology when he recognized that puerperal fever could be spread from patient to patient via the hands of health care workers in an obstetrics ward and demonstrated that washing hands between patient contacts prevented infections. Later in the 19th century, Joseph Lister's insight into the role of bacteria in surgical wound infections led to the concept of surgical antisepsis and asepsis.

Although many advances have been made in hospital infection control since these seminal observations were made more than a century ago, nosocomial infections continue to be a significant source of morbidity and mortality. About 5% of patients hospitalized in the United States acquire an infection during their hospitalization, or between 2 and 4 million nosocomial infections annually. These infections result in average excess durations of hospital stay of up to 24 days, directly account for up to 100,000 deaths per year, and result in many billions of dollars in excess health care costs annually.

NOSOCOMIAL PATHOGENS

Sources of Nosocomial Pathogens

Nosocomial pathogens can originate from either endogenous or exogenous sources. Endogenous pathogens originate from the commensal flora of the patient's skin or gastrointestinal or respiratory tract. Exogenous pathogens are transmitted to the patient from external sources after admission to the hospital.

Numerous factors contribute to increased susceptibility to infection in hospitalized patients, including immunocompromising underlying diseases, immunosuppressive medications, extremes of age (young or old), and perhaps most importantly, compromise of the most basic and first lines of host defense, i.e., the skin and mucosal surfaces, by drugs, irradiation, trauma, invasive diagnostic and therapeutic procedures, and invasive indwelling devices (intravenous catheters, endotracheal tubes, etc.)

The makeup of a patient's endogenous flora may change as a result of being hospitalized. Several studies suggest that after admission to a hospital the oropharyngeal flora changes from normal respiratory bacteria to predominantly gram-negative bacilli. The stool and skin may also become colonized with bacteria not normally found in non-hospitalized individuals. Thus many nosocomial infections arising from "endogenous" flora may be caused by microorganisms acquired following admission to the hospital.

Exogenous sources of nosocomial pathogens commonly include health care workers, other patients, visitors, and contaminated environmental sources such as equipment, water, air, and occasionally medications.

Modes of Transmission of Nosocomial Pathogens

The five major routes by which nosocomial pathogens can be transmitted are contact transmission, droplet transmission, airborne transmission, common vehicle transmission, and vector-borne transmission. Some pathogens may be transmitted by more than one route.

Contact transmission occurs through direct contact and physical transfer of microorganisms between an infected or colonized person and a susceptible host or, indirectly, when a susceptible host touches contaminated objects such as equipment, clothing, or the unwashed hands of health care workers. Contact transmission is probably the most common and important mode of nosocomial transmission. Pathogens transmitted in this way include multidrug-resistant bacteria; enteric pathogens such as *Clostridium difficile*, *Shigella*, or rotavirus; skin and soft tissue pathogens such as *Staphylococcus aureus* and *Streptococcus pyogenes*; and viral pathogens such as adenovirus and varicella-zoster virus.

Droplet transmission occurs via droplets of respiratory secretions generated during coughing, sneezing, and talking and during instrumentation of the respiratory tract such as suctioning or bronchoscopy. Transmission occurs when droplets containing microorganisms are propelled a short distance through the air and are deposited on a susceptible host's conjunctivae, nasal mucosa, or mouth. Examples of pathogens transmitted in this way include the bacterial pathogens *Haemophilus influenzae* type B and *Neisseria meningitidis* and the viral pathogens influenza, adenovirus, mumps, rubella, and parvovirus B19.

Airborne transmission occurs by dissemination of either airborne droplet nuclei (small particle residue [≤5 μm in size] of evaporated droplets containing microorganisms that remain suspended in the air for prolonged periods) or dust particles containing the infecting agent. Transmission occurs when a susceptible host inhales air containing contaminated droplet nuclei or dust particles. Examples of pathogens transmitted in this way include *Mycobacterium tuberculosis*, measles virus, and varicella virus.

Common vehicle transmission has been described in a number of point source outbreaks involving contaminated medications or infusions. Vector-borne transmission of nosocomial infectious disease is rare in developed countries.

Strategies for Preventing Transmission of Nosocomial Pathogens

In 1994 the Hospital Infection Control Practices Advisory Committee of the Centers for Disease Control and Prevention issued general guidelines designed to prevent the transmission of infectious agents within hospitals. These guidelines recommend a two-tiered approach for controlling transmission of nosocomial pathogens.

The first tier, termed "standard precautions," is designed to prevent the transmission of microorganisms from moist body substances, including blood. Standard precautions are designed to be used by health care workers during all patient contacts, even when the patient is not known to be infected or colonized with an important nosocomial pathogen. The basic components of standard precautions include thorough hand washing after patient contact; using gloves when touching blood, body fluids, secretions, or contaminated items; and wearing a mask, eye protection, or gown during patient care activities and procedures that are likely to generate splashes or sprays of blood, body fluids, secretions, or excretions. To prevent percutaneous injury, standard precautions also call for preventive measures in handling needles, scalpels, or other sharp devices.

An additional tier of control measures termed "transmission-based precautions" may be used (in addition to standard precautions) during care of patients known to be infected or colonized with an infectious agent that can be transmitted via contact, airborne, or droplet transmission. For example, when a patient is infected or colonized with epidemiologically important microorganisms transmitted primarily by contact (e.g., multidrug-resistant bacteria, C. difficile, or S. aureus), "contact precautions" (placing the patient in a private room, wearing gloves with each patient room entry, and wearing a gown if contact with the patient or other environmental surfaces is expected) may be used to supplement standard precautions. "Airborne precautions" may be used when patients are known to be infected with pathogens transmitted by the airborne route (e.g., tuberculosis, measles, or varicella). Airborne precautions involve the use of protective respiratory masks by health care workers and private patient rooms equipped with negative-pressure ventilation systems that discharge air either to the outdoors or through high-efficiency air filtration systems. "Droplet precautions," used in the care of patients infected with microorganisms transmitted primarily by larger respiratory droplets (influenza virus, H. influenza, N. meningitidis), require a private room and use of a mask when in close proximity (3 ft) to the patient.

Nosocomial Pathogens by Category

BACTERIA. The Enterobacteriaceae as a group are the most common bacterial pathogens isolated in U.S. hospitals. This group includes Escherichia coli, Klebsiella spp., Enterobacter spp., Proteus spp., and Citrobacter spp. (Table 315–1). The non-fermentative gram-negatives Pseudomonas aeruginosa (and other Pseudomonas spp.), Acinetobacter spp., Stenotrophomonas spp., Flavobacterium spp., and Alcaligenes spp. are also major nosoco-mial pathogens. Gram-positive bacteria have become increasingly prominent nosocomial pathogens in recent years. S. aureus is now the single most common nosocomial pathogen isolated in U.S. hospitals, but coagulase-negative staphylococci and enterococci are nearly as common. Other bacterial nosocomial pathogens of note include Legionella pneumophila, an important cause of nosocomial pneumonia, and C. difficile, an important cause of nosocomial diarrhea.

The rapid emergence of antibiotic-resistant bacteria in recent years is having an important impact on the morbidity and mortality associated with nosocomial infections. The high prevalence of methicillin resistance among the two most common gram-positive nosocomial pathogens, S. aureus (up to 40% of U.S. isolates) and coagulase-negative staphylococci (>80% of U.S. isolates), has led to widespread increases in vancomycin use. The resultant increase in selective pressure has contributed to the emergence of vancomycin resistance in the 1990s, particularly among enterococci. Even more disturbing is the recent appearance of clinical isolates of S. aureus that have decreased susceptibility to vancomycin. The emergence of vancomycin resistance in S. aureus could result in lack of effective antibiotic therapy for this common and virulent nosocomial pathogen and is a matter of serious public health concern. The Enterobacteriaceae, Pseudomonas species, and other gram-negative bacilli are now frequently resistant to many frontline antibiotics, and some isolates are resistant to all available therapy. Strategies that successfully optimize antibiotic usage and prevent transmission of antibiotic-resistant bacteria within health care settings are badly needed.

FUNGI. In the last two decades, fungi have played an increasingly important role in nosocomial infections. Their emergence is related to several factors, including advances in cancer therapy and organ transplantation, which have led to highly immunocompromised inpatient populations, and the widespread use of broad-spectrum antibiotics, which provide a selective advantage for opportunistic fungi. Candida species are now the fourth most common cause of nosocomial bloodstream and urinary tract infections in the United States, and they account for almost 75% of all nosocomial fungal infections. Risk factors for candidemia include the use of broad-spectrum antibiotics, parenteral hyperalimentation, presence of a central venous catheter, neutropenia, and colonization with Candida species at other body sites.

Aspergillus species are a major cause of nosocomial fungal infection in patients with hematologic malignancy, prolonged neutro-

Table 315–1 ■ PER CENT DISTRIBUTION OF NOSOCOMIAL PATHOGENS BY INFECTION SITE IN HOSPITALS CONDUCTING HOSPITAL-WIDE SURVEILLANCE, NATIONAL NOSOCOMIAL INFECTION SURVEILLANCE SYSTEM, JANUARY 1990 TO MARCH 1996

PATHOGEN*	ALL INFECTION SITES	URINARY TRACT	SURGICAL SITE	BLOODSTREAM	PNEUMONIA	OTHER
Staphylococcus aureus	13	2	20	16	19	18
Escherichia coli	12	24	8	5	4	4
Coagulase-negative staphylococci	11	4	14	31	2	14
Enterococcus spp.	10	16	12	9	2	5
Pseudomonas aeruginosa	9	11	8	3	17	7
Enterobacter spp.	6	5	7	4	11	4
Candida albicans	5	8	3	5	5	4
Klebsiella pneumoniae	5	8	3	5	8	3
Gram-positive anaerobes	4	0	1	1	0	19
Proteus mirabilis	3	5	3	1	2	2
Other Streptococcus spp.	2	1	3	3	1	2
Other Candida spp.	2	3	1	3	1	1
Other fungi	2	3	0	1	1	1
Acinetobacter spp.	1	1	1	2	4	1
Serratia marcesclens	1	1	1	1	3	1
Citrobacter spp.	1	2	1	1	1	1
Other non-Enterobacteriaceae—aerobes	1	0	1	1	4	1
Group D streptococci	1	2	2	1	0	1
Group B streptococci	1	1	1	2	1	1
Haemophilus influenzae	1	0	0	0	5	1
Other Klebsiella spp.	1	1	1	1	1	1
Other Enterobacteriaceae—aerobes	1	1	1	0	1	1
Other gram-positive aerobes	1	0	2	1	1	1
Viruses	1	0	0	0	1	2
Bacteroides fragilis	1	0	2	1	0	0

*Pathogens with fewer than 1% of the isolates at all sites are not shown.

penia, or other highly immunocompromising conditions (e.g., prolonged corticosteroid therapy). These fungi are transmitted by inhalation of airborne fungal conidia and usually cause necrotizing bronchopneumonia, sinusitis, or rhinocerebral disease. Hospital reservoirs of *Aspergillus* include unfiltered air, ventilation systems, and contaminated dust generated during hospital construction.

Other emerging fungal pathogens include the yeast *Malassezia furfur* (a cause of fungemia often associated with infusion of intravenous lipids because it requires exogenous lipid for growth), *Trichosporon* spp., *Fusarium* spp., *Acremonium* spp., and *Pseudallescheria boydii.*

VIRUSES. Influenza is an important cause of morbidity and mortality in health care institutions, not only acute care hospitals but also long-term care facilities such as nursing homes. Control measures include new case surveillance, droplet (some prefer airborne) precautions for known or suspected cases, vaccination of health care workers, and in outbreak situations, prophylactic antiviral therapy with rimantadine or amantadine.

The varicella-zoster virus is highly contagious. It represents a potentially lethal threat to susceptible immunocompromised patients, in whom it can cause pneumonia, encephalitis, and disseminated infections. In cases of varicella infection, the virus can be transmitted either by direct contact or by the airborne route, so a combination of airborne and contact precautions is used to interrupt transmission. In cases of localized zoster, the active skin lesions are the only source of virus, and standard precautions are usually adequate to contain transmission. Susceptible health care workers are an important potential reservoir of infection and should therefore be immunized against varicella.

Other significant nosocomial respiratory viral pathogens, particularly in children and immunosuppressed adults, include respiratory syncytial virus (spread primarily by contact), measles virus (spread by the airborne route), and adenovirus (spread by either respiratory droplets or direct contact). Adenovirus is also a common cause of acute keratoconjunctivitis that is transmitted by direct contact and can spread rapidly in health care settings. Personnel with adenoviral keratoconjunctivitis should be restricted from patient care for the duration of the illness.

Enteric viral pathogens can be transmitted within health care settings. Rotavirus is a common cause of both endemic and epidemic nosocomial diarrhea in pediatric populations. Nosocomial hepatitis A infection does occur, although rarely. Both are transmitted primarily by contact.

Nosocomial transmission of herpes simplex virus is infrequent but does occur. Infants and burn patients are at greatest risk. Transmission occurs through contact with other patients, parents, or health care workers with mucosal or digital herpes simplex lesions. Nosocomial transmission of cytomegalovirus most commonly occurs via blood transfusion, although patient-to-patient transmission occurs rarely, usually through direct contact with the urine or saliva of acutely infected patients. Transmission of cytomegalovirus from patients to health care workers is probably rare.

The blood-borne pathogens hepatitis B, hepatitis C, and human immunodeficiency virus (HIV) are transmitted in the nosocomial setting primarily by direct percutaneous inoculation (e.g., needlestick) or by exposure of mucosal surfaces or non-intact skin to contaminated blood or body fluids. Nosocomial transmission is more common with hepatitis B than with other blood-borne pathogens, probably because of its ability to remain viable on environmental surfaces at room temperature for days. Thus in clinical settings with significant blood exposure (e.g., dialysis units), the risk of hepatitis B virus transmission is considerable.

Nosocomial transmission of blood-borne pathogens from patients to health care workers is an area of serious concern. The risk is highest with hepatitis B, especially when the source patient is seropositive for hepatitis B e antigen. The risk of infection in non-immune individuals is at least 30% after percutaneous exposure to blood from a hepatitis B e antigen–positive source if no post-exposure prophylactic measures are taken. All health care workers involved in direct patient care should be vaccinated against hepatitis B infection. The risk of transmission of hepatitis C is lower than for hepatitis B and ranges from 1 to 10% after percutaneous exposure to blood from a hepatitis C–infected patient. Transmission of HIV from patient to health care worker by percutaneous exposure is rare, as low as 0.3% per exposure. Recent studies

suggest that post-exposure prophylactic treatment with antiretroviral agents may lower the risk even further.

The risk posed to patients from health care personnel infected with blood-borne pathogens such as hepatitis B virus and HIV has been the subject of much concern and debate. No data indicate whether infected workers who do not perform invasive procedures pose a risk to patients. Some reports of apparent transmission of blood-borne pathogens from health care worker to patient during invasive procedures have appeared, but this event is most likely extremely rare.

MYCOBACTERIA. Respiratory disease caused by *M. tuberculosis* represents a major threat to patients, visitors, and health care workers because it is readily transmitted by the airborne route unless proper precautions are taken. Nosocomial transmission can be effectively controlled through programs promoting early recognition of tuberculosis, prompt initiation of airborne precautions, use of protective respirators when caring for tuberculosis patients, and surveillance for *M. tuberculosis* infection in health care workers through regular skin testing.

Nosocomial infections caused by non-tuberculous mycobacteria are being reported with increasing frequency. They most commonly involve the rapidly growing mycobacteria *M. chelonei, M. abscessus,* and *M. fortuitum* and have been described in surgical site infections (often following cardiovascular or plastic surgery), infections from implantable prosthetic devices, and contamination of bronchoscopes and endoscopes.

OTHER PATHOGENS. The ectoparasites *Sarcoptes scabiei* (scabies) and *Pediculus* spp. (lice) are common nosocomial pathogens and can spread quite rapidly, primarily by contact. In immunosuppressed populations, scabies in particular can cause significant morbidity.

Creutzfeldt-Jakob disease, a transmissible neurodegenerative disease caused by a prion, has rarely been acquired in hospitals. Nosocomial transmission has been associated with contaminated neurosurgical instruments, transplantation of infected central nervous system tissue (corneal transplants, dura mater transplants), and injection of hormonal products derived from central nervous tissue (growth hormone, gonadotropin).

NOSOCOMIAL INFECTIONS BY SITE

Bloodstream Infections

EPIDEMIOLOGY. An estimated 250,000 nosocomial bloodstream infections occur each year in U.S. hospitals. They are an important cause of morbidity and mortality, prolong hospital stays by an average of 7 days, and cause an estimated 62,500 deaths annually.

About 30 to 40% of all nosocomial bloodstream infections originate from infections at other body sites (e.g., urinary tract, surgical site, pulmonary, etc.) and are thus termed "secondary" bloodstream infections. Nosocomial bloodstream infections that cannot be attributed to a specific anatomic site are termed "primary" bloodstream infections. Intravascular device–related nosocomial bloodstream infections are included in this category and in fact account for most nosocomial primary bloodstream infections. About 90% of intravascular device–related nosocomial bloodstream infections are associated with central venous catheters.

PATHOGENS. Over the last two decades an increasing proportion of nosocomial bloodstream infections have been caused by gram-positive cocci and *Candida* species. The most common causes of primary bloodstream infection in U.S. hospitals, in decreasing order of frequency, are coagulase-negative staphylococci, *S. aureus, Enterococcus* spp., *Candida* spp., *E. coli,* and *Klebsiella pneumoniae* (see Table 315–1).

The pathogens found in secondary bloodstream infections reflect the distribution of organisms causing the underlying primary infections and commonly include *E. coli, S. aureus, K. pneumoniae,* and *P. aeruginosa.*

PATHOPHYSIOLOGY. Catheter-related bloodstream infections originate from migration of microorganisms from the skin insertion site into the cutaneous catheter tract and along the external surface of the catheter until the intravascular catheter tip becomes colonized or from migration of organisms from a contaminated hub through the lumen of the catheter. Many factors play a role, includ-

Table 315–2 ■ FACTORS THAT INFLUENCE SURGICAL SITE INFECTION RISK

INTRINSIC—Patient-Related Risk Factors
Age
Nutritional status
Diabetes
Smoking
Obesity
Remote infections
Endogenous mucosal microorganisms
Altered immune response
Preoperative stay/severity of illness
EXTRINSIC—Operation-Related Risk Factors
Duration of surgical scrub
Skin antisepsis
Preoperative shaving
Preoperative skin preparation
Surgical attire
Sterile draping
Duration of surgery
Exogenous microorganisms
Antimicrobial prophylaxis
Ventilation
Sterilization of instruments
Wound class
Foreign material
Surgical drains
Surgical technique
  Poor hemostasis
  Failure to obliterate dead space
  Tissue trauma

ing the type of catheter material (Teflon or polyurethane is more resistant to colonization than polyvinyl chloride or polyethylene) and the adherence properties of a given microorganism. For example, *S. aureus* can bind to host fibronectin, which is commonly deposited on catheters; coagulase-negative staphylococci and possibly *Candida* spp. can produce an extracellular polysaccharide "slime" matrix that enhances catheter colonization.

The pathophysiology of secondary bloodstream infection depends on the primary infection from which it originates, discussed below under site-specific nosocomial infections.

PREVENTIVE STRATEGIES. The most effective way to prevent primary nosocomial bloodstream infections is to prevent intravascular catheter–related infections because these account for most primary bloodstream infections.

The risk of catheter-related bloodstream infection varies with the site of catheter insertion. Peripheral venous catheters have a much lower risk of bloodstream infection and should be used in lieu of a central venous catheter whenever possible. Among central venous catheters, subclavian catheters have a lower risk of infection than do those inserted in either the internal jugular or femoral veins, and therefore a subclavian insertion should be used whenever possible.

Certain types of central venous catheters are associated with a lower risk of infection. Among central venous catheters intended for short-term use, those equipped with a silver-chelated collagen cuff attached to the subcutaneous portion of the catheter have been shown to decrease the risk of catheter-related bloodstream infection. In addition, catheters impregnated with chlorhexidine or silver sulfadiazine have been shown in randomized trials to decrease the risk of catheter-related bloodstream infection. The risk of bloodstream infection associated with tunneled central venous catheters (e.g., Hickman, Broviac, Groshong) has been compared with that of non-tunneled catheters. Although the data are conflicting, tunneled catheters may have no advantage over non-tunneled catheters with regard to infection risk. Totally implantable intravascular devices appear to have the lowest reported rates of catheter-related bloodstream infection among devices used for long-term central venous access.

Prospective studies have demonstrated that using barrier precautions during catheter insertion significantly lowers the risk of catheter-related bloodstream infection. Mask, sterile gloves, gown, and a large drape should be used during catheter placement, even if the catheter is being inserted while in an operating room.

Skin cleansing with antisepsis of the insertion site is one of the most important measures for preventing catheter-related bloodstream infection. Agents such as 2% aqueous chlorhexidine, 10% povidone-iodine, and 70% alcohol are acceptable alternatives. Routine application of antimicrobial ointments to central venous catheter insertion sites is not generally recommended.

Insertion and maintenance of intravascular catheters by inexperienced staff may increase the risk of catheter-related bloodstream infection. A number of studies suggest that using teams of personnel specially trained and designated with the responsibility for inserting and maintaining intravascular catheters reduces catheter-related bloodstream infection and costs.

Surgical Site Infections

EPIDEMIOLOGY. Surgical site infections account for nearly 20% of all nosocomial infections in the United States. An estimated 27 million surgical procedures are performed in the United States each year, and surgical site infections develop in an estimated 2 to 5%. They prolong hospitalizations by an average of 7 days and are an important cause of mortality in hospitalized patients.

PATHOGENS. The distribution of pathogens isolated from surgical site infections has not changed significantly in the last decade. The most frequently isolated pathogens are *S. aureus*, coagulase-negative staphylococci, *Enterococcus* spp., and *E. coli* (see Table 315–1).

PATHOPHYSIOLOGY. Surgical site infections result from microbial contamination of the incision, usually at the time of surgery. The reservoir for contamination is most often endogenous patient flora, but pathogens can also originate from exogenous sources such as the environment, hospital personnel, or distant foci of infection. Factors that influence whether microbial wound contamination leads to surgical site infection include the size of the bacterial inoculum (larger numbers of bacteria increase the risk), the presence of foreign material within the wound (foreign material decreases the inoculum required to cause surgical site infection), and virulence properties of individual pathogens (e.g., endotoxins, cytolytic exotoxins, bacterial surface components that can inhibit phagocytosis, etc.)

RISK FACTORS AND PREVENTIVE STRATEGIES. Factors that influence the risk for surgical site infection can be divided into intrinsic (related to the underlying patient condition) and extrinsic (related to the operative procedure) and are listed in Table 315–2. Some intrinsic risk factors are amenable to preoperative interventions that may decrease the risk of surgical site infection. Such interventions include enhancement of nutritional status, cessation of smoking, and delay in surgery until other existing infections can be adequately treated.

A number of preoperative interventions are designed to decrease extrinsic risk factors for surgical site infection. Preoperative antiseptic showers or baths with agents such as chlorhexidine or povidone-iodine have been shown to reduce microbial colony counts on the skin but have not been definitively shown to reduce surgical site infection rates.

Hair removal at the operative site has traditionally been used to decrease the risk of surgical site infection. Recent studies suggest that some methods of hair removal such as preoperative shaving with a razor actually increase the risk of surgical site infection when compared with alternatives such as hair clipping or the use of depilatory agents. Some studies even suggest that preoperative hair removal by any method may increase the risk, although further study is required.

The skin at the operative site is usually prepared before the incision by application of an antiseptic agent such as povidone-iodine, alcohol-containing products, or chlorhexidine gluconate.

Members of the surgical team are advised to wash their hands and forearms with an antiseptic agent before surgery (the "surgical scrub"). Povidone-iodine or chlorhexidine gluconate are most commonly used. Although traditionally the recommended duration of the surgical scrub has been 10 minutes, recent studies suggest that a 3- to 5-minute scrub is equally effective in reducing bacterial colony counts.

The use of preoperative antibiotic prophylaxis has been shown to decrease the risk of surgical site infection in certain settings, particularly operations resulting in wounds classified as clean-contaminated (an operative wound in which the respiratory, alimentary, genital, or urinary tract is entered). The choice of antibiotic agent is based on its activity against pathogens that might be expected as common contaminants for a particular operation. Antibiotic prophylaxis is most effective if administered within 30 minutes before the incision, with additional doses administered intraoperatively as needed to maintain therapeutic serum levels for the duration of the procedure. There is no evidence that antibiotics given after closure of the incision have any beneficial prophylactic effect on clean or clean-contaminated surgical wounds.

Intraoperative risk factors amenable to intervention include airflow in the operating room, sterilization of surgical instruments, attire of the surgical team, and surgical technique. Operating room air may contain vectors for microorganisms such as dust, lint, skin cells, and respiratory droplets shed from operating room personnel. The microbial density in operating room air is directly proportional to the number of people in the room. Therefore, personnel traffic should be kept to a minimum during the procedure. Although few studies have evaluated the efficacy of surgical attire in preventing surgical site infection, the use of scrub suits, masks, caps, gloves, and gowns minimizes exposure of the patient to the skin, mucous membranes, or hair of the surgical team and may prevent shedding of contaminated particles into the air. Optimal surgical technique such as maintaining effective hemostasis, gently handling tissues, removing devitalized tissue, eradicating dead space, using drains and sutures appropriately, and minimizing the duration of the procedure are all believed to be important in reducing the risk of surgical site infection. Adequate sterilization of surgical instruments by an approved method such as pressurized steam, dry heat, or ethylene oxide is essential.

Pneumonia

EPIDEMIOLOGY. Pneumonia accounts for about 15% of all nosocomial infections. It has an attributable mortality of up to 30%, prolongs the mean duration of hospitalization by up to 9 days, and results in estimated excess costs of $1.2 billion annually in the United States. Patients at highest risk for nosocomial pneumonia include postoperative patients (particularly after thoracoabdominal procedures) and patients with endotracheal tubes, depressed levels of consciousness, chronic underlying lung disease, and age older than 70 years.

PATHOGENS. Nosocomial pneumonia is often polymicrobial. The most frequently isolated pathogens in nosocomial pneumonia are gram negative and include *P. aeruginosa*, *Enterobacter* spp., *K. pneumoniae*, *E. coli*, *Serratia marcescens*, and *Acinetobacter* spp. Gram-positive pathogens, especially *S. aureus*, have also emerged as important causes of nosocomial pneumonia (see Table 315–1).

PATHOPHYSIOLOGY. Microorganisms most often invade the lower respiratory tract through aspiration of oropharyngeal secretions or inhalation of aerosols containing bacteria. Small-volume aspiration is very common even among healthy individuals, but aspiration is even more likely in patients with depressed mental status, patients with endotracheal or upper gastrointestinal intubation or instrumentation, and postoperative patients. The predominance of gram-negative pathogens in nosocomial pneumonia probably reflects colonization of the upper respiratory and gastrointestinal tracts with gram-negative bacilli, which commonly occurs following admission to the hospital.

The stomach may be an important reservoir for nosocomial pneumonia pathogens. Hospitalized patients often have an increased gastric pH because of either medication or underlying illness (achlorhydria, ileus, tube feedings, antacids, histamine antagonists). In the absence of normal acidic gastric conditions, bacteria are able to multiply freely within the stomach. Aspiration of gastric fluid in this setting may deliver high concentrations of microorganisms to the lower respiratory tract.

Other potential sources of pathogens in nosocomial pneumonia include inhalation of contaminated aerosols generated by respiratory therapy or anesthesia equipment. Rarely, pathogens may reach the lung by hematogenous spread from a distant focus of infection.

PREVENTIVE STRATEGIES. Strategies designed to prevent aspiration of oropharyngeal or gastric secretions are central in preventing nosocomial pneumonia. Patients at high risk for aspiration (e.g., depressed level of consciousness) should be positioned with the head of the bed elevated 30 to 45 degrees if possible. Enteral tubes, endotracheal tubes, and tracheostomy tubes should be re-

moved promptly when no longer clinically indicated. It has been suggested that pooled secretions above the cuff of endotracheal tubes may leak into the lower respiratory tract and serve as an important source of lower respiratory tract contamination. The use of specially designed endotracheal tubes with a separate suction lumen allowing for removal of these secretions has shown benefit in one study, but this finding requires further investigation.

Preventive strategies designed to decrease bacterial concentrations of gastric and oropharyngeal secretions have been attempted. In several studies, avoidance of medications that raise gastric pH seemed to prevent bacterial proliferation in gastric fluid and protect against nosocomial pneumonia in mechanically ventilated patients. Using agents that do not raise gastric pH should therefore be considered in patients requiring stress ulcer prophylaxis. Several investigators have demonstrated benefit from the use of combinations of prophylactic antimicrobial agents designed to decontaminate and prevent bacterial colonization of the gastrointestinal tract, thereby preventing pneumonia in mechanically ventilated patients. However, lack of consistent results in other studies and concern about antibiotic resistance preclude the routine use of this approach at present.

Preventing contamination of instruments that come into contact with the respiratory tract is an important preventive strategy. Attention to hand washing and glove use is critical in preventing cross-transmission of potential pathogens among patients. Reusable respiratory equipment that comes into contact with mucous membranes of the lower respiratory tract must be adequately disinfected or sterilized. Frequent changing of ventilator breathing circuits results in more frequent contamination of circuit tubing and increases the risk of pneumonia. These circuits should therefore not be changed more frequently than every 48 hours. Some studies suggest that even less frequent breathing circuit changes may be safe, but the optimal duration for leaving a breathing circuit unchanged has yet to be determined. Periodically draining and discarding the condensate that collects in breathing circuit tubing is likely to decrease the risk of pneumonia.

Postoperative patients, particularly those who have had thoracoabdominal procedures, usually have impairment in normal diaphragmatic excursion that results in decreased functional residual capacity, closure of airways, atelectasis, and increased risk of pneumonia. Deep-breathing exercises, incentive spirometry, intermittent positive-pressure breathing, and control of pain that interferes with coughing and deep breathing are likely to decrease the risk of pneumonia in postoperative patients.

Interventions directed at environmental sources may be indicated for certain nosocomial pneumonia pathogens, particularly *Legionella* and *Aspergillus* species. The appearance of nosocomial cases of legionellosis should prompt an investigation of the hospital water system for possible contamination with *Legionella*. *Aspergillus* spp. are transmitted by inhalation of airborne fungal conidia. Reservoirs of these fungi in hospitals may include unfiltered air, ventilation systems, and contaminated dust generated during hospital construction. Patient care areas in which highly immunocompromised patients are housed should optimally have high-efficiency air filtration, positive air pressure in the patient's room in relation to the corridor, and a high rate of change in room air. Additional preventive measures may be required during construction or renovation activities within the health care facility.

Urinary Tract Infections

EPIDEMIOLOGY. The urinary tract, the single most common site of nosocomial infection in the United States, accounts for nearly 35% of all nosocomial infections. Despite its frequency, the attributable mortality for urinary tract infections is low, about 0.1%. Nosocomial urinary tract infections are nevertheless an important cause of morbidity, including secondary bacteremia, perinephric abscess, epididymo-orchitis, and prostatitis. About 80% of all nosocomial urinary tract infections are associated with indwelling urinary catheters. The cumulative risk of bacteriuria with indwelling catheters increases 3 to 6% per day of catheterization, and bacteriuria develops in up to 30% of all catheterized patients.

PATHOGENS. The most common nosocomial urinary tract pathogens include gram-negative bacilli (*E. coli*, *P. aeruginosa*, *K. pneu-*

moniae, Proteus mirabilis), enterococci, and *Candida* species (see Table 315–1).

PATHOPHYSIOLOGY. Under normal conditions, the urinary tract above the distal portion of the urethra is sterile. Even if bacteria are introduced into the bladder, defense mechanisms such as urine acidity and osmolality, urinary immunoglobulins, local mucosal defenses, bladder emptying, and urinary flow usually prevent sustained colonization or infection. In the presence of a urinary catheter, microorganisms are able to gain access to the bladder by either direct inoculation during catheter insertion, migration along the inner lumen of indwelling catheters, or migration along the outer surface of indwelling catheters in the periurethral mucous sheath. The presence of the catheter provides a focus for continued bacterial growth and seeding of bladder urine and destroys some of the natural defense mechanisms by damaging epithelium and preventing complete bladder drainage (the retention balloon obstructs the bladder outlet and creates a small pool of residual urine). In not all patients with catheter-associated bacteriuria, however, do symptomatic urinary tract infections develop. About 70% of bacteriuric episodes will resolve spontaneously while the catheter is in place or shortly after removal.

PREVENTIVE STRATEGIES. The primary means of preventing nosocomial urinary tract infection is avoiding urinary catheterization except when absolutely necessary and removing the catheter as soon as possible. Alternatives to indwelling urinary catheters such as intermittent catheterization, suprapubic catheterization, and condom drainage are often used. No definitive controlled trials have compared indwelling urethral catheters with either intermittent urethral catheterization or suprapubic catheterization, but these approaches may have advantages over indwelling urethral catheters in some clinical settings. Condom drainage is associated with bacteriuria and urinary tract infections, and data showing advantages over indwelling urethral catheters are sparse.

The single most important advance in the prevention of nosocomial urinary tract infections has been the introduction of closed sterile catheter drainage systems. Early catheters with open drainage systems (i.e., the distal end of the drainage tube was open to the environment) resulted in bacteriuria in almost all patients within 4 days of insertion. When closed sterile drainage systems were introduced (i.e., the distal end of the drainage tube has a closed connection to a sterile collection receptacle), the rate of catheter-associated urinary tract infections was reduced substantially, thus suggesting that migration of microorganisms along the lumen of the catheter is a major route of infection with open drainage systems.

With widespread use of closed sterile drainage systems, migration of periurethral microorganisms along the external surface of the catheter is now the most common route of infection. Interventions designed to prevent periurethral colonization with pathogenic bacteria are therefore important in controlling nosocomial urinary tract infections. These interventions include attention to aseptic technique during catheter insertion, attention to hand washing during catheter care, proper securing of the catheter, and the use of aseptic technique when obtaining urine specimens. Routine meatal care such as daily cleansing or application of antibiotic ointments may actually increase the risk of catheter-associated urinary tract infection and is therefore not recommended. Some studies suggest that prophylactic antibiotic administration at the time of catheterization may be beneficial, but this practice cannot be routinely recommended without further study. Silver-coated urinary catheters, which take advantage of the bactericidal effect of silver ions, have been shown to reduce the risk of catheter-associated urinary tract infection in some studies, but other trials have produced conflicting results.

INFECTION CONTROL PROGRAMS

Although infections in hospitalized patients are inevitable given underlying host factors and the invasive nature of current medical care, many nosocomial infections are preventable. The combination of surveillance and preventive interventions based on the epidemiology and pathophysiology of particular infections can substantially reduce the rate of nosocomial infections in health care institutions.

The Study on the Efficacy of Nosocomial Infection Control Project, a national controlled study initiated by the Centers for Disease Control and Prevention in the early 1970s, examined the effectiveness of nosocomial infection control programs in the United States. This study found that hospitals with infection surveillance and control programs reduced their nosocomial infection rates by approximately 32% in comparison to those that did not have such programs, with significant savings in morbidity, mortality, and cost. The Joint Commission on Accreditation of Healthcare Organizations now requires the presence of an infection surveillance and control program for accreditation of U.S. hospitals. The key components of an effective nosocomial infection control program include systematic surveillance for the occurrence of nosocomial infections, development and implementation of policies and procedures designed to reduce the risk of nosocomial infections, education of hospital personnel about institutional policies regarding communicable diseases, and an employee health program that manages occupational exposure to infectious diseases and ensures that employees are free of communicable disease.

The evolution of medical practice in recent decades has produced important changes in the epidemiology of nosocomial infections that directly affect infection control programs. Economic pressures have resulted in an increase in the delivery of medical care outside traditional hospital settings, and now only the most severely ill persons are hospitalized; thus inpatient populations are more susceptible to infection than in previous decades. In addition, procedures and treatments that predispose to infection are now commonly performed in outpatient centers, subacute/chronic care facilities, and even the home. Surveillance and control measures originally designed for the hospital must now be adapted to various inpatient and outpatient health care settings.

The current economic environment demands that health care delivery systems fulfill two often competing objectives: provide the highest-quality health care at the lowest possible cost. Perhaps in no other discipline of medical care are these goals more compatible than in infection control and health care epidemiology. Investment in the judicious application of preventive strategies based on an understanding of the epidemiology and pathophysiology of nosocomial infections undoubtedly leads to more efficient, less expensive, and higher-quality patient care.

Centers for Disease Control and Prevention: Draft guideline for the prevention of surgical site infections. Fed Reg 63:33168, 1998. *Reviews current understanding of the epidemiology and pathogenesis of surgical site infections. Provides comprehensive recommendation regarding preventive and surveillance strategies.*

Garner JS, The Hospital Infection Control Practices Advisory Committee: Guideline for isolation precautions in hospitals. Infect Control Hosp Epidemiol 17:54, 1996. *Reviews the history of isolation precautions in U.S. hospitals and recommends a unified approach to controlling nosocomial transmission of pathogens. Contains specific recommendations for a comprehensive list of nosocomial pathogens.*

Pearson ML, The Hospital Infection Control Practices Advisory Committee: Guideline for prevention of intravascular device–related infections. Infect Control Hosp Epidemiol 17:438, 1996. *Excellent review of the epidemiology and pathogenesis of catheter-related bloodstream infections. Provides specific recommendations regarding preventive strategies.*

Tablan OC, Anderson LJ, Arden NH, et al: Guideline for prevention of nosocomial pneumonia. Infect Control Hosp Epidemiol 15:587, 1994. *A very thorough review of the problem of nosocomial pneumonia and strategies for prevention. Includes separate sections for legionellosis, aspergillosis, and viral pneumonia.*

316 ADVICE TO TRAVELERS

Richard D. Pearson

Millions of North Americans and Europeans travel to developing areas of the world each year. Modern air transportation has brought even the most exotic sites within easy reach. Most travelers go for vacation or business and are away for a few weeks or less, but some spend extended periods abroad. In addition, thousands of American troops are deployed at various times in tropical or developing areas.

The risks associated with international travel depend on the locations visited, the duration of the trip, and the traveler's health status and activities. Persons visiting Australia, Canada, western

Europe, Japan, New Zealand, and the United States require no special prophylactic measures. In contrast, visitors to developing areas, particularly in the tropics, may be exposed to serious infectious and non-infectious risks.

Specific prophylactic health measures should be tailored to the traveler's itinerary and individual needs. They can be separated into the following areas: pre-travel health assessment, diseases prevented by immunization, prevention and treatment of traveler's diarrhea, malaria prophylaxis, and behavioral modifications that reduce the risk of infectious or non-infectious hazards. Information about risks and recommendations for travel to specific geographic locations is provided by the Centers for Disease Control and Prevention (CDC) through its publications (see References), International Traveler's Hotline ([404] 332-4559), and World Wide Web site (www.cdc.gov/travel/travel.html); other publications (see References); and several commercially available travel information systems.

PRE-TRAVEL HEALTH ASSESSMENT

It is important to review the past medical history, active medical problems, allergies to antibiotics or vaccine components, and pregnancy status before embarking on prophylactic measures. Special arrangements may be necessary for those with insulin-dependent diabetes, chronic renal failure, or other medical problems. Women who are pregnant and persons infected with the human immunodeficiency virus (HIV) or otherwise immunocompromised also require special attention as discussed below.

For long-term travelers, it is important to address routine health maintenance issues. Their purified protein derivative (PPD) status should be determined because tuberculosis is prevalent in many developing areas. Some countries now require HIV testing before issuing long-term visas. Travelers should check with the appropriate embassies to determine whether such testing is required.

IMMUNIZATIONS

GENERAL CONSIDERATIONS. A number of infectious diseases can be prevented by immunization. It is important to review the traveler's immunization status. Vaccines can be grouped into those that everyone should receive, whether they travel or not, those recommended for travelers to tropical or developing areas (see information from the CDC for specific recommendations by location), and those legally required for entrance into a country (see Table 316–1). No immunizations are required for American citizens entering the United States. Some countries require that all

Table 316–1 ■ IMMUNIZATION OF INTERNATIONAL TRAVELERS

Routine Vaccines that Should Be Up-to-Date in All Travelers
Diphtheria/tetanus
Pertussis (children <7 yr)
Poliomyelitis
Measles
Mumps
Rubella
Haemophilus influenzae (children)
Hepatitis B
Varicella

Routine Vaccines Indicated in Special Populations
Influenza
Pneumococcal

Vaccines Potentially Indicated for Travelers to Developing Areas*
Cholera (seldom used)
Hepatitis A (or immune serum globulin)
Japanese B encephalitis
Meningococcal
Poliomyelitis
Rabies
Typhoid
Yellow fever†

*The choice of specific vaccines depends on the itinerary, activities, and duration of travel, as well as cost, efficacy, and potential side effects of the vaccines.
†Required for entry by some countries. See Centers for Disease Control and Prevention: Health Information for International Travel and "Summary of Health Information for International Travel" for a listing of countries requiring vaccination for entry.

visitors be immunized against yellow fever, whereas others require it only for those who have traveled in yellow fever–endemic areas. Countries that require the yellow fever vaccine are listed in the CDC information. Cholera immunization is no longer necessary to enter any country, but local officials may still require it in a few areas. Administration of the yellow fever vaccine and other immunizations should be documented in the small booklet "International Certificate of Vaccination," which should be carried during the trip.

Before vaccination, persons should be questioned about allergies. A history of hypersensitivity to egg protein is important because many viral vaccines (e.g., yellow fever, mumps, measles, and influenza) are prepared in embryonated eggs or chicken embryo cell cultures. In general, anyone who can eat eggs will tolerate these vaccines. On rare occasion, persons may be hypersensitive to thimerosal, neomycin, or other trace vaccine components.

The precise indications, contraindications and potential side effects of each vaccine are outlined in the package insert and summarized elsewhere (see References). In general, multiple vaccines can be given simultaneously at different sites without adversely affecting their efficacy. Exceptions include the yellow fever and cholera vaccines, which reciprocally inhibit antibody responses to one another, and immune serum globulin, which inactivates some live vaccines. If used, immune serum globulin should be given at least 3 weeks after or 5 months before most live vaccines are administered. Immune serum globulin has no apparent adverse effect on the efficacy of oral poliomyelitis vaccine or yellow fever vaccine, but when possible, it should be given at a separate time. If live viral vaccines are not administered simultaneously, it is recommended that they be spaced 4 weeks apart to avoid immune interference. Vaccination should also be delayed in persons with acute febrile diseases.

Live viral and bacterial vaccines are generally contraindicated in travelers with HIV or immunocompromised by chemotherapy, but there are exceptions. The measles vaccine can be administered to persons with asymptomatic HIV infection. The yellow fever vaccine has been used in situations where the benefits are deemed to outweigh the risk of vaccine-related encephalitis. It is safe to administer inactivated vaccines to immunocompromised persons, but the immune responses that they elicit may be impaired and leave the traveler at risk. Live vaccines are generally contraindicated during pregnancy, and the safety of many inactivated vaccines has not been assessed in pregnant women.

IMMUNIZATIONS TO PROTECT INTERNATIONAL TRAVELERS. CHOLERA. (See Chapter 344) The currently available, nonviable, parenteral cholera vaccine provides approximately 50% protection for 3 to 6 months. Few experts recommend the vaccine, but travelers are strongly urged to follow food and water precautions (see below) and to institute rehydration and antibiotic treatment immediately if diarrhea develops. Cholera immunization is no longer necessary for entrance into any country, but documentation of immunization may be required by some local officials. A live, oral cholera vaccine has been licensed in Canada and Europe, but not in the United States. It is not protective against the non-01 strain of Bengal cholera.

HEPATITIS A. (See Chapter 149) Hepatitis A constitutes a major risk for travelers to areas where sanitation and hygiene are poor. The likelihood of acquiring hepatitis A has been estimated to be as high as 1 in 1000 travelers per 2- to 3-week trip in some areas. Symptomatic hepatitis A infection can be prevented by immunization with one of the inactivated hepatitis A vaccines or immune serum globulin, 0.02 mL/kg given intramuscularly for travel less than 3 months and 0.06 mL/kg for travelers going for 3 to 5 months. Transmission of HIV is not a concern with immune globulin preparations manufactured in North America. In some instances it is cost-effective to determine the immune status of travelers who may have been previously infected. The presence of anti–hepatitis A IgG antibodies indicates that the traveler is immune.

HEPATITIS B. (See Chapter 149) The hepatitis B vaccine is recommended for long-term travelers (>6 months), health care workers, and others likely to be exposed to blood or body fluids while abroad. It can be argued that everyone should receive the vaccine whether or not they travel abroad.

JAPANESE B ENCEPHALITIS. (See Chapter 392) The Japanese B encephalitis vaccine is indicated for travelers who have intense and/

or prolonged (>4 weeks) exposure in rural endemic areas in China, Korea, Southeast Asia, India, the lowlands of Nepal, Sri Lanka, and to a limited degree, Japan and other areas of Asia and Oceania. This mosquito-borne disease is most common in rural rice and pig farming areas. It occurs from June through September in temperate regions and throughout the year in tropical areas. Travelers to urban sites are usually at low risk of infection. Unfortunately, the vaccine is not without side effects. Allergic reactions, including rash, urticaria, anaphylaxis, and on rare occasion sudden death, occur in 0.1 to 10 per 100,000 vaccinations. Persons with a history of hypersensitivity responses to other allergens seem to be at greatest risk. Vaccine recipients should be observed in the office for 30 minutes after immunization; however, reactions can occur days to weeks later, most within 10 days of immunization.

MENINGOCOCCAL DISEASE. (See Chapter 329) Meningococcal vaccine (A/C/Y/W-135) should be considered for travelers going to Mecca, Saudi Arabia during the Moslem Hajj, Kenya, Tanzania, Burundi, Nigeria and other countries in sub-Saharan Africa during the dry season, or other sites where travel advisories have been issued. Type A is the principle cause of meningococcal disease in those areas.

POLIOMYELITIS. (See Chapter 476) Everyone should be immunized against poliomyelitis whether or not they travel. A single booster once in adulthood is recommended for travelers to developing areas, with the exception of those staying in the western hemisphere, where no cases of wild-type poliomyelitis have been identified since 1991. The inactivated polio vaccine is preferred by many physicians because it is not associated with a risk of vaccine-related paralytic disease in recipients or their contacts.

RABIES. (See Chapter 478.) Rabies is endemic in many areas. Travelers should be warned about the disease and advised to avoid dogs and other animals. In general, long-term travelers (30 days or more) who live in areas where rabies is a threat should receive pre-exposure immunization with a rabies vaccine propagated in human diploid cells. Any short-term traveler who plans to have close contact with dogs, wild animals, or bat-infested caves should also be immunized. Simultaneous administration of chloroquine—and possibly mefloquine—can decrease the immunogenicity of intradermally administered rabies vaccine. If such drug therapy cannot be stopped, the vaccine should be given intramuscularly. The high cost of the rabies vaccine has limited its use for pre-exposure prophylaxis.

All persons, regardless of whether they have received pre-exposure immunization, who are bitten by a potentially rabid animal, should be advised to wash the site thoroughly with water and detergent and to seek medical evaluation. Those who have received pre-exposure prophylaxis need additional doses of the human diploid cell vaccine; those who have not been previously immunized require full immunization plus human rabies immune globulin.

TYPHOID. (See Chapter 340.) Typhoid is common in developing areas where sanitation is poor. The risk is relatively low among short-term travelers to urban areas who adhere to food and water precautions. The oral, live Ty21a typhoid vaccine and injectable Vi capsular polysaccharide vaccine are well tolerated and have largely replaced the crude killed vaccine, which was frequently associated with local pain, erythema, and constitutional symptoms. The oral typhoid vaccine should not be given to HIV-infected persons or those taking antibiotics or mefloquine, which can inactivate it. It is recommended that the oral series be repeated at 5-year intervals and the Vi capsular polysaccharide vaccine boosted at 2-year intervals.

YELLOW FEVER. (See Chapter 391.) Yellow fever is endemic in tropical areas of Africa and Latin America in a band ranging from approximately 15 degrees north to 15 degrees south of the equator. The yellow fever vaccine is a live, attenuated strain (17D). It is available only at licensed centers, which can be identified by calling local or state health offices. The vaccine is boosted at 10-year intervals. The yellow fever vaccine should not be given to HIV-infected or other immunocompromised travelers unless the risk of yellow fever exceeds the risk of vaccine-related encephalitis. If possible, they should avoid travel in endemic areas. If they must travel, they should do all that they can do to minimize mosquito bites and carry with them written evidence of medical exemption.

OTHER VACCINES. (See Chapter 15.) The plague vaccine can be used for persons with intense field exposure in endemic areas, but it is seldom recommended for travelers. Typhus and tick-borne encephalitis vaccines are not available in the United States. Currently, no vaccines protect against a number of important viral diseases, including dengue, and against parasitic diseases such as malaria.

TRAVELER'S DIARRHEA

Traveler's diarrhea (see Chapter 346) is the most common problem encountered by North Americans who visit developing areas. The incidence is as high as 40 to 60% among short-term travelers to many developing areas if appropriate food and water precautions are not followed.

The risk of traveler's diarrhea can be reduced approximately four-fold by following the commandment "Cook it, boil it, peel it, or forget it" and by eating only foods served piping hot. Even when these recommendations are followed, diarrhea may occur. The duration and severity can be reduced by early self-treatment. Travelers should be instructed in oral rehydration with solutions containing glucose and electrolytes. They should also have available and take an appropriate antibiotic; ciprofloxacin (500 mg twice a day for 3 days) is widely used in healthy, non-pregnant adults. Use of an antimotility agent such as loperamide can further reduce the duration of secretory diarrhea, but it should not be used in those with bloody diarrhea, high fever, or other evidence of inflammatory colitis.

PREVENTING MALARIA

Malaria (see Chapter 421) poses a major health hazard for travelers to endemic tropical areas, and the risk of exposure varies greatly throughout the tropics. The frequency of transmission is high in sub-Saharan Africa; more than 80% of cases of falciparum malaria diagnosed in the United States are acquired in East Africa. The mortality of falciparum malaria in the United States is approximately 4%. Fortunately, malaria transmission is infrequent in most urban areas of Latin America and Asia.

Every effort should be made by travelers to minimize contact with *Anopheles* mosquitoes—the vector of malaria—which prefer to feed in the evening, at night, and in the early morning. Travelers' outdoors at those times should wear long-sleeved clothing and apply insect repellents that contain *N,N*-diethylmethyltoluamide (DEET) at a concentration of 30 to 35% to exposed skin. DEET should be used cautiously in young children because of the potential for seizures and other neurologic side effects from percutaneous absorption. Clothing and mosquito netting can be treated with permethrin, which confers further protection against mosquitoes for weeks.

Even with these measures, chemoprophylaxis is necessary (Table 316–2). For a full discussion of the efficacy and toxicity of these drugs and alternatives, see Chapter 318.

Table 316–2 ■ CHEMOPROPHYLAXIS FOR MALARIA*

Travelers to Areas with Chloroquine-Sensitive Plasmodium *Species*
Chloroquine phosphate, 300 mg base (500 mg salt) orally once a week†

Travelers to Areas with Chloroquine Resistance
Mefloquine, 250 mg orally once a week†
  or
Doxycycline, 100 mg orally daily†

Prevention of Late Relapses with P. vivax *and* P. ovale‡
Primaquine phosphate, 15 mg base (26.3 mg salt) orally each day for 14 d

*Insect repellents, insecticide-impregnated bed nets, and proper clothing are important adjuncts for preventing malaria. The potential toxicities and contraindications of antimalarial medications are discussed in Chapter 421 and should be reviewed before use. Chloroquine has been used extensively and safely in pregnancy, but other prophylactic medications are either contraindicated during pregnancy (doxycycline and primaquine) or their safety is uncertain (mefloquine). No prophylactic regimen guarantees protection, and travelers should be warned about the possibility of malaria during travel or after return.

†Adult dose: start 1 week before departure with chloroquine and mefloquine, 1 to 2 days before with doxycycline, continue during travel and for 4 weeks after return.

‡Occasional relapses have been reported with this regimen. Some experts prescribe primaquine during the last 2 weeks of malaria prophylaxis for travelers with prolonged exposure to P. vivax or P. ovale. Others avoid primaquine and rely on early detection and treatment of P. vivax or P. ovale malaria if it occurs.

INFECTIOUS DISEASES TO BE AVOIDED. SEXUALLY TRANSMITTED DISEASES. (See Chapters 361, 149 and Part XXIII). A surprising number of U.S and European travelers have sexual relations with local residents or casual contacts among other travelers while abroad and therefore are at risk for HIV infection and other sexually transmitted diseases. These risks must be explicitly discussed with all travelers. Abstinence is the only fully effective way to avoid sexually transmitted diseases. Those who choose to have sex abroad should use latex condoms purchased before departure because condoms manufactured abroad may not be protective. Some countries now require HIV testing before granting long-term visas.

ARTHROPOD-BORNE DISEASES. (See Chapters 391, 392, and 420.) A number of infectious diseases can be avoided by taking appropriate precautions. Every effort should be made to minimize exposure to arthropod vectors with clothing, insect repellents, and mosquito nets. Travelers to Latin America should not sleep in mud or adobe dwellings in areas where reduviid bugs transmit *Trypanosoma cruzi,* the cause of Chagas' disease.

WATER AND SOIL CONTACT. (See Chapter 420.) Travelers should not walk barefoot where hookworms and *Strongyloides stercoralis* are endemic. Persons visiting areas where *Schistosoma* species are found should avoid swimming or bathing in fresh or brackish water. People should not lie directly on beaches where dogs may have defecated and left *Ancylostoma brazilienes,* the cause of cutaneous larva migrans. Travelers should avoid streams and mud in areas with leptospirosis.

OTHER IMPORTANT ISSUES

CHRONIC MEDICAL PROBLEMS. Special attention should be directed to patients with pre-existing medical problems. They should wear medical alert identification. Travelers requiring medications should always keep these with them because luggage may be unavailable, lost, or stolen. It is wise to keep a list of all medications. An extra set of glasses often comes in handy.

LONG-TERM TRAVEL. Those who plan to reside abroad for prolonged periods frequently face special challenges. They should be counseled about the difficulties of adapting to a different language, culture, and climate. Routine health maintenance measures should be addressed before they leave. It is advisable to determine their PPD status and, in selected cases, HIV status before and after the trip.

JET LAG. When travelers cross multiple time zones, the following few days are frequently disrupted by jet lag. Dietary measures have not been rigorously evaluated, but it is thought that the symptoms may be minimized by avoiding excessive amounts of alcohol and food during flight. Short-acting benzodiazepines have been recommended by some to help with the adaptation to new time zones, but they can result in confusion.

MOTION SICKNESS. Travelers with motion sickness may gain relief with short-term, over-the-counter preparations of diphenhydramine. For longer trips or cruises, sustained-release transdermal scopolamine may be preferred.

ALTITUDE SICKNESS. Travelers to high elevations are at risk of acute mountain sickness, particularly if they ascend rapidly to heights greater than 9000 ft. Gradual ascent over a period of days is the best way to acclimatize. Acetazolamide, 250 mg two or three times a day, beginning 1 to 2 days before and continued during ascent, has been recommended for those who do not have time to acclimatize, but it is a diuretic, causes tingling and paresthesias that may interfere with climbing, and is contraindicated in persons with sulfonamide allergies. If mountain sickness develops, the safest course of action is to descend. Steroids and pressurizing bags are helpful. Anyone going to extreme elevations should seek advice from a mountaineering expert before the trip.

VENOMOUS SNAKES, SPIDERS, AND SCORPIONS. In tropical areas it is advisable to hike on clear paths, to avoid thick grass or brush, and to check the inside of shoes, closets, and drawers before extending feet or hands into them. Hikers should always wear shoes or boots.

ACCIDENTS AND CRIME. Automobile and other accidents are important causes of morbidity and mortality among travelers. They should wear seat belts and avoid motorcycles. Travelers frequently have a false sense of security. They should inquire about potential risks to their safety before exploring new areas or swimming, particularly in the ocean, where tides may be dangerous. Information about civil unrest and political instability can be obtained from the Department of State ([202] 647-5225; http://travel.state.gov/travel_warnings.html).

ILLNESS ABROAD. Before departure, travelers should review the status of their health insurance and what to do if they become ill. Self-limited traveler's diarrhea and upper respiratory tract infections are common and seldom require medical intervention. Travelers should seek expert medical evaluation if a high fever develops because it may herald malaria or another life-threatening tropical infection, bloody diarrhea, or other severe symptoms. Lists of reputable physicians can be obtained from American embassies or consulates or from travel insurance companies. Travelers should beware of previously used needles that might transmit HIV or other viruses. In the United States, physicians with special expertise in tropical diseases are available in traveler's clinics and many academic medical centers.

Centers for Disease Control and Prevention: CDC Health Information for International Travel 1999. HHS Publication No. (CDC) 99-8280. Atlanta, U.S. Department of Health and Human Services, Public Health Service, 1999. *For sale by the US Government Printing Office, Superintendent of Documents, P.O. Box 371954, Pittsburgh, Pa 15250-7954. Excellent source of information on health risks in overseas locations, as well as key information on vaccines and drugs. It is updated yearly. (Information available at http://www.cdc.gov/travel/travel.html.)*

Centers for Disease Control and Prevention: Summary of Health Information for International Travel. HHS Publication No. 396. Atlanta, U.S. Department of Health and Human Services. *Published biweekly, listing countries or areas reporting yellow fever, cholera, and plague.*

Hill DR, Pearson RD: Health advice for international travel. *In* Reece RE, Betts RF (eds): A Practical Approach to Infectious Diseases, 4th ed. Boston, Little, Brown, 1996, pp 812–845. *A comprehensive review of health issues related to international travel.*

International Travel and Health. Vaccination Requirements and Health Advice. Geneva, World Health Organization, 1998. *Summarizes the WHO recommendations for vaccinations and malaria prophylaxis, as well as other health advice for travelers. (Information available at http://www.who.int/ith/english/welcome.html.)*

Thompson RF: Travel and Routine Immunizations: A Practical Guide for the Medical Office. Milwaukee, WI, Shoreland, 1997. *A summary of guidelines for travel and routine immunization with detailed information about vaccines.*

■ BACTERIAL DISEASES

317 INTRODUCTION TO BACTERIAL DISEASE

Gerald L. Mandell

Bacteria are classified in the kingdom Procaryotae and contain DNA in a double-stranded loop not bounded by a membrane. The success of bacteria as life forms can be illustrated by the fact that fossils of bacteria 3.5 billion years old have been found. Bacteria are ubiquitous and can grow at temperatures as low as 0° C and as high as 110° C. All bacteria have a bilayered cytoplasmic membrane, and most bacteria (*Mycoplasma* are exceptions) have an outer cell wall containing muramic acid. Morphologic features are often used to categorize bacteria. Bacilli are rods or cylinders, with about half the species being motile, whereas cocci are spherical and non-motile. It is useful to distinguish bacteria by their ability to retain a basic dye (crystal violet) after iodine fixation and alcohol decolorization (the Gram reaction). Gram-positive organisms retain the dye and contain teichoic acids in their cell walls, whereas gram-negative bacteria have an additional outer membrane containing lipopolysaccharide (endotoxin) (Fig. 317–1). Capsules may serve as major virulence factors by interfering with the ability of phagocytes to ingest the encapsulated organisms. The capsules of the pneumococcus and *Haemophilus influenzae* are important factors for the virulence of the organisms. Other virulence factors include exotoxins released from the microbe, such as tetanus toxin and cholera toxin. Some bacteria, such as *Shigella flexneri,* can invade and damage host cells. Many gram-negative bacteria contain potent endotoxins that are important mediators of the sepsis syndrome. Pili or fimbriae are small hairlike structures that mediate bacterial attachment to various tissues and body surfaces. Only a very small proportion of species are pathogenic for humans, and new data suggest that even among those pathogenic species only certain clones are true pathogens.

Bacteria may be separated by their ability to reside and replicate intracellularly. Examples of intracellular bacteria include *Salmonella typhi, Legionella* species, mycobacteria, and chlamydiae. Extracellular pathogens include streptococci (including pneumococci), staphylococci, and most gram-negative enteric rods, such as *Escherichia coli, Klebsiella* species, and *Pseudomonas* species. The main technique used for identification of bacteria in patient specimens is culture on artificial media. The ability to grow on the surface of such media in air defines aerobic organisms. Anaerobes cannot grow under such conditions, and facultative organisms can grow either aerobically or anaerobically. Microscopy can be a very useful technique, especially when combined with appropriate staining procedures, such as acid-fast stains for mycobacteria or Gram stain to differentiate gram-positive from gram-negative organisms. Newer techniques use direct immunofluorescence (e.g., for *Chlamydia trachomatis*), DNA probes (e.g., for *Legionella* species), and tests to detect antigen (e.g., for pneumococcal capsular antigen in spinal fluid or legionella antigen in urine). Assays using the polymerase chain reaction are now employed. Tests for antibodies are less useful but may be helpful in some diseases (e.g., Lyme disease).

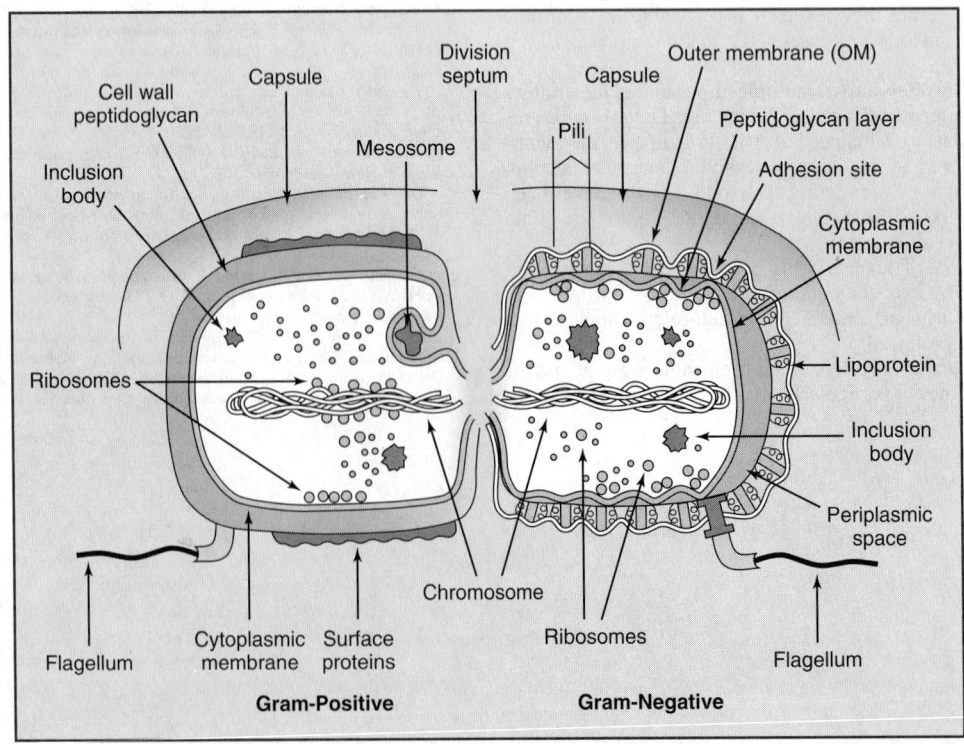

FIGURE 317–1 ■ Cross-section through a generalized bacterial cell. The left half of this figure depicts the structure of a gram-positive bacterium; the right half shows the structure of a gram-negative bacterium. (From Basic bacteriology, concepts of virulence and technologic advances in clinical microbiology: An overview. *In,* Koneman E, Allen SD, Janda WM, et al [eds]: Color Atlas and Textbook of Diagnostic Microbiology, 5th ed. Philadelphia, Lippincott–Raven, 1997.)

Table 317–1 ■ CLASSIFICATION OF SELECTED BACTERIA THAT CAUSE DISEASE IN HUMANS

AEROBES
Gram-Positive Cocci
Catalase-positive
   Staphylococcus aureus
   Staphylococcus epidermidis
   Other coagulase-negative staphylococci
Catalase-negative
   Enterococcus faecalis
   Enterococcus faecium
   Leuconostoc species
   Streptococcus agalactiae (group B *Streptococcus*)
   Streptococcus bovis
   Streptococcus pneumoniae
   Streptococcus pyogenes (group A *Streptococcus*)
   Viridans group streptococci
      S. anginosus
      S. mutans
Gram-Negative Cocci
Moraxella catarrhalis
Neisseria gonorrhoeae
Neisseria meningitidis
Gram-Positive Bacilli
Bacillus anthracis
Corynebacterium diphtheriae
Corynebacterium jeikeium
Erysipelothrix rhusiopathiae
Gardnerella vaginalis
Acid-Fast Organisms
Mycobacterium avium-complex
Mycobacterium kansasii
Mycobacterium leprae
Mycobacterium tuberculosis
Nocardia species
Gram-Negative Rods
Enterobacteriaceae
   Citrobacter species
   Enterobacter aerogenes

Escherichia coli
Klebsiella species
Morganella morganii
Proteus species
Providencia rettgeri
Salmonella typhi
Other *Salmonella* species
Serratia marcescens
Shigella species
Yersinia enterocolitica
Yersinia pestis
Fermentive Non-Enterobacteriaceae
   Aeromonas hydrophila
   Chromobacterium violaceum
   Plesiomonas shigelloides
   Pasteurella multocida
   Vibrio cholerae
   Vibrio vulnificus
Non-fermentive Non-Enterobacteriaceae
   Acinetobacter calcoaceticus
   Alcaligenes xylosoxidans
   Eikenella corrodens
   Flavobacterium meningosepticum
   Pseudomonas aeruginosa
   Stenotrophomonas maltophilia
   Other *Pseudomonas* species
Gram-Negative Coccobacilli
Actinobacillus actinomycetemcomitans
Bartonella bacilliformis
Bartonella henselae
Bartonella quintana
Brucella species
Bordetella species
Other *Campylobacter* species
Haemophilus influenzae
Haemophilus species
Helicobacter pylori

Legionella species
Chlamydiae
   Chlamydia trachomatis
   Chlamydia pneumoniae
   Chlamydia psittaci
Rickettsiae
   Rickettsia prowazekii
   Rickettsia rickettsii
Mycoplasmas
   Mycoplasma pneumoniae
Treponemataceae (spiral organisms)
   Borrelia burgdorferi
   Leptospira species
   Treponema pallidum
ANAEROBES
Gram-Negative Bacilli
Bacteroides fragilis
Other *Bacteroides* species
Fusobacterium species
Prevotella species
Gram-Negative Cocci
Veillonella species
Non-Spore-Forming Gram-Positive Bacilli
Actinomyces species
Bifidobacterium species
Eubacterium species
Proprionibacterium species
Endospore-Forming Gram-Positive Bacilli
Clostridium botulinum
Clostridium perfringens
Clostridium tetani
Other *Clostridium* species
Gram-Positive Cocci
Peptostreptococcus species
Gemella morbillorum
Peptococcus niger

Adapted from Bruckner DA, Colonna P: Nomenclature for aerobic and facultative bacteria. Clin Infect Dis 25:1–10, 1997; Jousimies-Somer H, Summanen P: Microbiology terminology update: Clinically significant anaerobic gram-positive and gram-negative bacteria [excluding spirochetes]. Clin Infect Dis 25:11–14, 1997. University of Chicago.)

Classification of bacteria has an historic basis and is based in large part on morphology and Gram-stain reaction; however, new genetic information results in frequent changes in nomenclature. Table 317–1 is a much-abbreviated summary of potentially pathogenic microbes.

318 ANTIBACTERIAL THERAPY

Adolf W. Karchmer

Modern antibacterial therapy has markedly reduced the morbidity and mortality of infections, has prevented disease, and has contributed significantly to the development of modern surgery, trauma therapy, and organ transplantation. The broad application of antimicrobial agents in modern medicine has not, however, been problem-free. These agents occasionally cause major adverse reactions, interact with other classes of pharmacologic agents, and exert a major selective pressure for widespread antimicrobial resistance among bacteria.

MECHANISMS AND TYPES OF ANTIBACTERIAL ACTIVITY

By selectively acting on targets in bacteria that are either absent from mammalian cells or are more vulnerable to the antimicrobial agent than are the analogous mammalian targets, an ideal antimicrobial agent kills or inhibits the growth of a bacterium without injuring the human host. For example, the peptidoglycan rigid cell

wall is unique to bacteria and thus a target for selective activity by β-lactam antibiotics. In contrast to humans who can use exogenous folic acid, bacteria cannot use exogenous tetrahydrofolic acid (folinic acid) in the synthesis of nucleic acids and must synthesize folinic acid from *p*-aminobenzoic acid. Inhibition of this pathway by sulfonamides or trimethoprim, independently or together, thus results in selective antibacterial activity. Antimicrobial agents that inhibit the growth of microorganisms are *bacteriostatic,* whereas those that kill bacteria at physiologically achievable concentrations are *bactericidal.* Growth inhibition and killing in general are the product of the drug's mechanism of action but, on occasion, are concentration dependent or unique to the interaction of a drug and a particular bacterial species. For example, chloramphenicol, which is generally bacteriostatic even at high concentrations, is bactericidal for *Haemophilus influenzae* at concentrations achieved in patients with standard doses. Conversely, penicillin G is generally bactericidal for susceptible organisms but is only bacteriostatic against *Enterococcus faecalis* and *E. faecium.* The site of action and antibacterial effect of major classes of antimicrobial agents are shown in Table 318–1. Combinations of antibiotics may produce an antibacterial effect greater than the sum of the agents' independent activities; this is called *synergism.* The sequential inhibition of tetrahydrofolic acid by a sulfonamide and trimethoprim may cause synergism. Also, facilitated penetration of aminoglycosides to their intracellular target in enterococci by penicillin, ampicillin, or vancomycin can result in bactericidal synergism.

MECHANISMS OF BACTERIAL RESISTANCE TO ANTIMICROBIALS

In considering bacterial resistance to antimicrobial agents, it is useful to consider both the mechanisms of action of individual antibacterial compounds and the general properties of antibiotics that are necessary for efficacy. Antimicrobial agents must be able

Table 318–1 ■ **MECHANISMS OF ACTION OF ANTIMICROBIAL AGENTS**

AGENT	SITE OF ACTION	EFFECT	CIDAL	STATIC
Penicillins, cephalosporins, other β-lactams	Penicillin-binding proteins (peptidoglycan synthetic enzymes)	Inhibits cross-linking of peptidoglycan (transpeptidation); impairs cell wall synthesis	+	Occasionally
Vancomycin, teicoplanin	Terminal D-alanyl-D-alanine of pentapeptide peptidoglycan precursor	Inhibits polymerization of disaccharide precursors to peptidoglycan (transglycosylation); impairs cell wall synthesis	+	Occasionally
Aminoglycosides	Ribosome, 30S subunit	Complex; inhibits peptide elongation; causes misreading of genetic code	+	
Tetracycline	Ribosome, 30S subunit	Inhibits binding of transfer RNA; inhibits protein synthesis		+
Chloramphenicol	Ribosome, 50S subunit	Blocks transfer of amino acids to peptide chains; inhibits protein synthesis	Occasionally	+
Erythromycin, new macrolides, azalides	Ribosome, 50S subunit	Inhibits translocation of ribosome on messenger RNA; inhibits protein synthesis	Occasionally	+
Clindamycin	Ribosome, 50S subunit	Blocks transfer of amino acids to peptide chain; inhibits protein synthesis	Occasionally	+
Quinupristin/dalfopristin	Ribosome, 50S subunit	Blocks extrusion of peptide chains; inhibits protein synthesis	+	+
Rifampin	DNA-dependent RNA polymerase	Impairs RNA synthesis	+	
Metronidazole	Nucleic acids	Damages nucleic acid structure	+	
Quinolones	DNA gyrase, topoisomerase IV	Impairs supercoiling of DNA, prevents decatenation of linked DNA molecules after replication	+	
Sulfonamides	Dihydropteroate synthetase	Competitive inhibition of synthesis of dihydrofolate from p-aminobenzoic acid		+
Trimethoprim	Dihydrofolate reductase	Inhibits reduction of dihydrofolate to tetrahydrofolic acid		+

to (1) reach the molecular targets, which are primarily intracellular, in sufficient amounts; (2) interact with a target molecule in a manner that initiates an antibacterial effect; and (3) avoid inactivation by drug-modifying enzymes in the extracellular environment or within the bacterial cell. The mechanism used by individual bacteria to resist specific antimicrobials can be viewed as a strategy to subvert these requirements for antimicrobial efficacy (Table 318–2). Frequently, bacteria use more than one strategy; multiple mech-

Table 318–2 ■ **MECHANISMS OF ANTIBIOTIC RESISTANCE**

ANTIMICROBIAL	MECHANISM	REPRESENTATIVE ORGANISM
β-Lactam (penicillins, cephalosporins, carbapenems, carbacephems, monobactams)	Altered target (penicillin-binding protein)	*Enterococcus faecium, Streptococcus pneumoniae*, methicillin-resistant *Staphylococcus aureus*
	Reduced permeability	*Enterobacter* species, *Pseudomonas aeruginosa*
	β-Lactamase	*S. aureus*, gram-negative bacilli, *Haemophilus influenzae, Neisseria gonorrhoeae, E. faecalis, Moraxella catarrhalis*
Aminoglycosides	Modifying enzymes (acetylation, adenylation, phosphorylation)	*S. aureus*, enterococci, *P. aeruginosa*, Enterobacteriaceae
	Reduced permeability or energy-dependent uptake	Enterobacteriaceae, *P. aeruginosa, S. aureus* (small cell variant), enterococci
	Decreased ribosomal binding	*S. aureus, Enterococcus faecalis* (streptomycin)
Chloramphenicol	Active efflux	*H. influenzae*
	Reduced permeability	Enterobacteriaceae
	Inactivating enzyme (acetylation)	*S. aureus*, enterococci, Enterobacteriaceae
Erythromycin, clindamycin, new macrolides, azalide, quinupristin	Decreased ribosomal binding (methylation of ribosomal RNA)	*S. aureus, S. pneumoniae*, streptococci, *Bacteroides fragilis*
	Reduced permeability	Enterobacteriaceae, *Staphylococcus epidermidis*
	Modifying enzymes	*E. coli, Klebsiella pneumoniae, S. aureus*
Quinolones	Target alteration (DNA gyrase, topoisomerase IV)	Enterobacteriaceae, *S. aureus*
	Reduced permeability	Enterobacteriaceae, *P. aeruginosa*
	Active efflux	*Escherichia coli*
Tetracyclines	Altered target (ribosome)	*N. gonorrhoeae*, streptococci
	Active efflux	*E. coli*
	Permeability barriers	Enterobacteriaceae
	Drug detoxification	*B. fragilis*
Rifampin	Reduced RNA polymerase binding	*E. coli, S. aureus*
Sulfonamides, trimethoprim	Altered dihydropteroate synthetase or dihydrofolate reductase	Enterobacteriaceae, *Moraxella catarrhalis*
	Increased p-aminobenzoic acid	*S. aureus, N. gonorrhoeae*
	Reduced permeability	*P. aeruginosa*, Enterobacteriaeceae
Vancomycin	Altered peptidoglycan precursor binding site	*E. faecium*

anisms acting in concert may produce markedly enhanced antimicrobial resistance. Resistance to an antimicrobial agent may be an intrinsic property of a bacterial species or an acquired capability. To acquire resistance, a bacterium must alter its DNA by mutating native DNA or by introducing foreign DNA. Resistance genes are often part of extrachromosomal plasmid DNA, which can transfer among organisms by conjugation, transduction, or transformation. Some resistance genes are part of DNA units called *transposons* that move between chromosomes and transmissible plasmids. Foreign DNA may be acquired through transformation, resulting in exchanges of chromosomal DNA among species and subsequent interspecies recombination. Genetic mechanisms of resistance function constitutively (at a constant rate) or may be induced on exposure to antimicrobial agents, which may confound detection of resistance by laboratory tests.

Exclusion of effective amounts of an antibiotic from intracellular compartments is a common mechanism of intrinsic resistance. Limited permeability is a property of the lipopolysaccharide outer cell membrane of gram-negative bacteria. The permeability of this membrane resides in special proteins, *porins,* which provide specific channels through which substances can pass to the periplasmic space and thereafter into the cell. Limited permeability accounts for the intrinsic resistance of gram-negative bacilli to penicillin, erythromycin, clindamycin, and vancomycin; *Pseudomonas aeruginosa* to trimethoprim; and streptococci as well as enterococci to aminoglycosides. Additionally, bacteria use this strategy in acquiring resistance. Thus, a mutational change in the specific porin of the outer cell membrane of *P. aeruginosa* through which imipenem usually diffuses can exclude the antibiotic from its target and render the *P. aeruginosa* resistant to imipenem. In general, however, mutations to decrease porin channels and reduce permeability are inefficient mechanisms for bacterial resistance and require a second mechanism (e.g., a coexisting β-lactamase) to generate higher-level resistance. The active pumping of antimicrobial agents from the intracellular milieu (i.e., active efflux) in effect excludes antibiotics from their targets and causes bacterial resistance. Plasmid-encoded resistance to tetracyclines among *Escherichia coli* results from active efflux.

Alteration of the target site at which an antimicrobial agent acts, such that an inhibitory or killing effect no longer occurs, constitutes a second major mechanism of resistance. Bacteria may acquire a gene, or a complex of genes, that encodes a new antibiotic-resistant product that now substitutes for the original target. Thus, new forms of dihydropteroate synthetase and dihydrofolate reductase with lower affinity to sulfonamides and trimethoprim, respectively, mediate resistance to these drugs. Methicillin-resistant *Staphylococcus aureus* and coagulase-negative staphylococci have acquired the chromosomal gene *mecA* and produce a β-lactam–resistant penicillin-binding protein (PBP), called 2a or 2′, which is sufficient to maintain cell wall integrity during growth when other essential PBPs are inactivated by β-lactam antibiotics. Alternatively, a newly acquired gene may act to modify a target, rendering it less vulnerable to an antimicrobial. Thus, a plasmid- or transposon-borne gene encodes an enzyme that methylates the 23S rRNA of the 50s ribosome and impairs the binding of macrolides, azalide, streptogramin B, and clindamycin to their target. The resistance to these antimicrobials that results may be constitutive or inducible. Mutations in existing genes or homologous DNA acquired by transformation may result in antibiotic-resistant targets. Mutations leading to amino acid changes in RNA polymerase decrease the binding of rifampin to this enzyme and result in rifampin resistance. Similarly, mutations in the *gyrA* gene that alters amino acids in the A subunit of DNA gyrase or in the par C gene that alters the A subunit of topoisomerase IV have resulted in resistance to the fluoroquinolones among various bacteria. Alterations of essential high molecular mass PBPs of gonococci, meningococci, *E. faecium,* and pneumococci result in the decreased binding of penicillin to these targets and penicillin-resistance. Among pneumococci, the acquisition by transformation of homologous DNA has resulted in mosaic genes, which in turn give rise to the penicillin-resistant hybrid PBPs. The resultant pneumococci have relative or high-level resistance to penicillin and also may be relatively resistant to third-generation cephalosporins. Vancomycin resistance is acquired by *E. faecalis* and *E. faecium* through a series of seven linked genes that interact to ultimately alter the pentapeptide cell wall peptidoglycan precursors. D-Alanyl-D-alanine, the site at which vancomycin binds

and inhibits cell wall synthesis, is replaced by D-alanyl-D-lactate, which serves as a functional peptidoglycan precursor but to which vancomycin can no longer effectively bind. Of great concern is the location of the vancomycin resistance genes on a self-transferable plasmid that could ultimately spread to *S. aureus.*

Perhaps the most commonly used mechanism by which bacteria are resistant to antibiotics entails the enzymatic alteration and inactivation of an antimicrobial agent. β-Lactamases hydrolyze the amide bond of the β-lactam ring, thus destroying the site whereby β-lactam antibiotics bind to bacterial PBPs to exert their antibacterial effect. The many different β-lactamases are encoded chromosomally or extrachromosomally through plasmids or transposons and may be either produced constitutively or induced. The almost universal resistance of *S. aureus* to penicillin, ampicillin, the carboxypenicillins, and the ureidopenicillins is mediated by a plasmid-encoded, inducible β-lactamase. Staphylococcal β-lactamase, which is secreted into the surrounding environment, does not inactivate the penicillinase-resistant penicillins (oxacillin, nafcillin), the cephalosporins, or the carbapenems (imipenem, meropenem). Although occasionally hyperproduction of β-lactamase by *S. aureus* has engendered borderline resistance to oxacillin and nafcillin, these antibiotics retain antistaphylococcal activity in the presence of this β-lactamase. β-Lactams with minimal antibacterial activity that can bind and irreversibly inhibit β-lactamases have been developed. These so-called β-lactamase inhibitors (clavulanic acid, sulbactam, tazobactam) have been combined with the penicillins to restore antistaphylococcal activity despite the presence of β-lactamase.

In gram-negative bacteria the role of β-lactamases in bacterial resistance is both complex and extensive. There are numerous structurally unique enzymes that inactivate a broad range of β-lactam antibiotics. The genes encoding some of these β-lactamases are subject to mutations that expand enzymatic activity and are both relatively easily transferred and widely distributed. In addition, in gram-negative bacteria β-lactamases are secreted into the limited confines of the periplasmic space, where they act in concert with the permeability barrier of the outer cell wall to produce clinically significant antibiotic resistance. Among the more common of the plasmid-mediated β-lactamases are the TEM-1 and TEM-2 enzymes, the SHV-1 of *Klebsiella pneumoniae,* and the PSE-1 of *P. aeruginosa.* These confer resistance to penicillin, ampicillin, carbenicillin, ticarcillin, cephalothin, and cefamandole but not to the cephamycins (cefoxitin, cefotetan), third-generation cephalosporins, monobactams, or carbapenems. Plasmid-mediated, extended-spectrum β-lactamases (ESBLs) that inactivate third-generation cephalosporins and monobactams result from mutations in the *TEM* and *SHV* genes. β-Lactam/β-lactamase inhibitor combinations and carbapenems remain active against organisms producing ESBLs. Overproduction of TEM-1 β-lactamase by genes on multicopy plasmids has been encountered in *E. coli* that are resistant to β-lactam/β-lactamase inhibitor combinations. Chromosomally mediated β-lactamases are produced at low levels by *P. aeruginosa, Enterobacter cloacae, Citrobacter freundii, Serratia marcescens,* and other gram-negative bacilli; when these organisms are exposed to β-lactam antibiotics, high levels of these β-lactamases are either induced, or due to an *ampD* mutation, produced constitutively, causing resistance to the broad-spectrum cephalosporins, cephamycins, and the β-lactam/β-lactamase inhibitor combinations. Although third-generation cephalosporins are relatively resistant to hydrolysis by these enzymes, the limited entry of most of these cephalosporins into the periplasmic space allows even these β-lactamases to effectively mediate resistance. Cefepime, a cephalosporin with zwitterionic properties that allows it to reach greater concentrations in the periplasmic space, and the carbapenems, which are not hydrolyzed by the chromosomal β-lactamases, remain active against these organisms. The metallo-β-lactamases produced by *Stenotrophomonas maltophilia,* some *Bacteroides fragilis,* and other gram-negative rods hydrolyze a broad array of β-lactam antibiotics, including the carbapenems.

Resistance to aminoglycosides can result from constitutively produced modifying enzymes that acetylate amino groups and phosphorylate or adenylate hydroxyl groups on these compounds. Permeability barriers to aminoglycosides may enhance this type of resistance. Several genes that encode different aminoglycoside-modifying enzymes may exist simultaneously in a bacterium. They are commonly on a plasmid, the chromosome, or a transposon. Modifying enzymes commonly cause aminoglycoside resistance in gram-negative bacilli. A bifunctional acetylating and phosphorylating enzyme that results in resistance to all clinically available aminoglycosides except streptomycin has been found increasingly in *Staphylococcus aureus,* coagulase-negative staphylococci, and enterococci. In enterococci, this enzyme prevents the combination of penicillin, ampicillin, or vancomycin plus any aminoglycoside, except streptomycin, from exerting a bactericidal effect. The frequent coexistence in enterococci of this enzyme and a streptomycin-adenylating enzyme renders strains resistant to all bactericidal combinations.

To effectively treat infection, physicians must be aware of resistance profiles for pathogens generally as well as in their immediate practice environment. For example, as a result of the frequency of pneumococci that are relatively or highly resistant to penicillin, empirical therapy for pneumococcal meningitis is now ceftriaxone plus vancomycin rather than penicillin. Similarly, in any given hospital a physician must know the frequency with which the *S. aureus* causing wound infections are resistant to methicillin in order to choose between vancomycin and oxacillin as empirical therapy. Additionally, physicians must attempt to reduce the emergence of antimicrobial resistance among bacteria. Treatment with multiple antimicrobial agents, an effective strategy to decrease mutational resistance among *Mycobacterium tuberculosis,* is less applicable to controlling antibiotic resistance among bacteria because bacteria become resistant to the multiple antimicrobial agents through acquiring a single plasmid or transposon rather than by multiple mutations. Antibiotics do not cause mutations and create resistant bacteria; nevertheless, their indiscriminate use provides enormous selective pressure to sustain and enrich resistant bacteria. Expanded antibiotic use is followed by increased frequency of resistant bacteria, which are then disseminated by poor sanitation and hygiene. Improved sanitation and hygiene and enhanced infection control in hospitals can reduce the dissemination of resistant organisms. Although antimicrobial use cannot be eliminated, optimal antibiotic use not only requires judicious selection of an agent and duration of therapy but also avoidance of inappropriate use.

SELECTING ANTIMICROBIAL THERAPY

IDENTIFYING THE INFECTING AGENT. Effective therapy requires that the causative agent either be recovered and its antimicrobial susceptibility identified or be reliably anticipated on the basis of the clinical presentation. Recovering the pathogen(s) by culture and subsequently determining antimicrobial susceptibility is highly desirable. Culture results, however, are usually not available when initial therapy is being selected, particularly for patients with more acute or severe infections. There are a few non–culture-based tests used to identify bacterial pathogens (e.g., group A streptococci in the pharynx, gonococci from genital secretions, pneumococci and *H. influenzae* in cerebrospinal fluid [CSF], and *Legionella pneumophila* antigen in urine). Examination of a Gram stain, or acid-fast stain, of material obtained from an infected site allows rapid assessment of the types of bacteria present and the inflammatory response.

Physicians commonly initiate antimicrobial therapy empirically; and even when knowing the pathogen, they must select antibacterial therapy without having specific antimicrobial susceptibility information. Various scenarios prompt empirical therapy: (1) the infection is immediately life-threatening; (2) a less threatening infection is likely to worsen if therapy is delayed until culture results become available; (3) considering the predictability of the pathogens causing a syndrome, the inconvenience or hazards of acquiring a culture are unjustified; (4) the causative agent is predictable, therapy is relatively simple, and the hazards of failed therapy are low. Meningitis with a polymorphonuclear CSF response (presumably bacterial) or clinical findings suggestive of septic shock mandates empirical therapy immediately after cultures are obtained. In contrast, pneumonia, even when not life-threatening, is likely to progress if therapy is delayed. Hence, it is prudent to obtain blood and sputum cultures, examine a sputum Gram stain, and initiate empirical therapy. In contrast, the treatment of otitis media or acute bacterial sinusitis is initiated empirically based on the high probability that the bacterial infection is likely to be caused by pneumococci, *H. influenzae, Moraxella catarrhalis,* or, less commonly, group A streptococci. Tympanocentesis or aspiration of the sinus for material to culture is reserved for patients in whom empirical therapy fails. Empirical treatment of recurrent uncomplicated cystitis in a young, otherwise healthy woman is an example of the fourth scenario. Although urine is easily cultured, the infection is probably due to *E. coli* or *Staphylococcus saprophyticus,* and successful empirical therapy with trimethoprim/sulfamethoxazole or a fluoroquinolone for 3 days will have been completed before culture results are available.

Culture results must be interpreted in the clinical context. Does the *E. coli* recovered from an abscess due to a ruptured appendix reflect the true microbiology or were the anticipated anaerobic bacteria not isolated because the specimen was mishandled? Furthermore, all isolates are not necessarily causing the infection; some may be contaminants or reflect colonizing flora. Thus, interpretation of the culture results is important, particularly if the specimen has been obtained across non-sterile surfaces. Some isolates from normally sterile material must be questioned. The coagulase-negative *Staphylococcus* or *Corynebacterium* species recovered from a blood culture is possibly a contaminant, but in the patient with indwelling vascular catheters or leukopenia and fever after cancer chemotherapy, these isolates may be pathogens. Repetitively isolating small numbers of organisms, even those commonly considered contaminants from sequential specimens (e.g., *S. epidermidis* from a dysfunctional prosthetic joint), strongly suggests infection.

Whether one is treating an infection empirically or on the basis of microbiologic data, the antimicrobial regimen should be as targeted as possible. Empirical therapy often necessitates broader-spectrum antimicrobial therapy; nevertheless, judgment must be exercised to focus initial and subsequent (after culture data are available) antimicrobial therapy. Using multiple antimicrobial agents or broad-spectrum therapy where more narrow-spectrum therapy will suffice inevitably exposes the patient to increased risks of adverse effects and selects for increasingly resistant organisms.

EVALUATING ANTIMICROBIAL SUSCEPTIBILITY. Appropriate antimicrobial therapy is founded on laboratory-documented inhibition of growth or actual killing of the organism by concentrations of antibiotics that can be achieved in a patient's serum using acceptable doses. Excretion by the kidney results in striking urine concentrations for some antibiotics; for an agent used only to treat urinary tract infection (e.g., nitrofurantoin), susceptibility is based on concentrations achieved in urine.

For most bacteria, antibiotic susceptibility cannot be adequately predicted and should be determined with in vitro tests. The predictable susceptibility of a few organisms obviates the need for their testing. Group A streptococci are universally susceptible to penicillin and cephalosporins, and *Neisseria meningitidis* is susceptible to penicillin, ampicillin, and chloramphenicol. The susceptibility of these organisms to other antimicrobial agents is less predictable, and if other agents were used for therapy, testing would be required (e.g., erythromycin or tetracycline against group A streptococci or sulfonamides against meningococci).

PHARMACOLOGIC AND PHARMACODYNAMIC CONSIDERATIONS. Successful therapy requires that an antibiotic with in vitro activity be delivered to the site of infection in adequate concentration without inducing adverse reactions. Knowledge of the major pharmacologic and pharmacokinetic properties of the antimicrobial agent is necessary. The major pharmacologic properties of commonly used antibiotics are shown in Table 318–3. Penetration of antibiotics into some tissues and fluids is limited and drug specific. Lipid-soluble agents such as chloramphenicol, rifampin, sulfonamides, trimethoprim, metronidazole, and isoniazid penetrate into the CSF well, whereas penicillins, third-generation cephalosporins, and vancomycin penetrate adequately only when there is meningeal inflammation. Treatment of infection occurring in the CNS or other sites where antibiotic penetration is limited (e.g., the prostate or vitreous humor of the eye) requires special consideration and, on occasion, direct instillation. Most antibiotics are excreted primarily through the kidneys. Biliary excretion can be an advantage in treatment of biliary tract infection; however, excretion is markedly reduced if the biliary tract is obstructed. To achieve meaningful serum concentrations, aminoglycosides, carbapenems, and glyco-

Table 318–3 ▪ DOSAGE, PHARMACOLOGIC FACTORS, AND ADJUSTMENT IN RENAL AND HEPATIC FAILURE

CLASS/AGENT	DOSE* Systemic Infection	ORAL FORMU-LATION	PEAK SERUM CONCENTRA-TION (µg/mL)	PROTEIN BINDING (%)	NORMAL SERUM HALF-LIFE (hr)	DOSE ADJUSTMENT Hepatic Failure	DOSE ADJUSTMENT Renal Failure	SERUM LEVELS AFFECTED BY DIALYSIS‡
Aminoglycosides								
Amikacin	5–7 mg/kg/q8h	—	35	0	2–3	No	Major	Yes (H, P)
Gentamicin	1.7 mg/kg/q8h	—	7	0	2–3	No	Major	Yes (H, P)
Netilmicin	1.7 mg/kg/q8h	—	7	0	2–3	No	Major	Yes (H, P)
Tobramycin	1.7 mg/kg/q8h	—	7	0	2–3	No	Major	Yes (H, P)
Antituberculous Agents								
Ethambutol	15 mg/kg/d (PO)	Yes	2	10	1.5	No	Major	Yes (H, P)
Isoniazid	5 mg/kg/d (PO)	Yes	4.5	10	3	Yes	Minor	Yes (H, P)
Pyrazinamide	10 mg/kg/q8h (PO)	Yes	39	—	10	Yes	Yes	Yes (H)
Rifampin	10 mg/kg/d (PO)	Yes	7	70	3	Yes	Minor	No (H)
First-Generation Cephalosporins								
Cefadroxil	15 mg/kg/q12h (PO)	Yes	16	20	1.2	No	Yes	Yes (H)
Cefazolin	15 mg/kg/q8h	—	80	80	2	No	Major	Yes (H) No (P)
Cephalexin	7 mg/kg/q6h (PO)	Yes	18	15	1	No	Yes	Yes (H, P)
Cephapirin	30 mg/kg/q6h	—	150	50	0.6	No	Yes	Yes (H, P)
Cephradine	30 mg/kg/q6h	Yes†	140	10	0.7	No	Yes	Yes (H, P)
Second-Generation Cephalosporins								
Cefaclor	7 mg/kg/q6h (PO)	Yes†	13	20	1	No	Yes	Yes (H)
Cefmetazole	30 mg/kg/q12h	—	140	65	1.1	No	Yes	Yes (H)
Cefotetan	30 mg/kg/q12h	—	230	85	3	No	Major	Yes (H)
Cefoxitin	30 mg/kg/q6h	—	150	70	0.7	No	Yes	Yes (H) No (P)
Cefprozil	15 mg/kg/q12h (PO)	Yes	10	42	1.2	No	Yes	Yes (H)
Cefuroxime	15–20 mg/kg/q12h	—	100	50	1.5	No	Yes	Yes (H, P)
Cefuroxime axetil	7.5 mg/kg/q12h (PO)	Yes	9	50	1.2	No	Yes	Yes (H, P)
Third-Generation Cephalosporins								
Cefepime	30 mg/kg/q12h	—	193	20	2.1	No	Yes	Yes (H, P)
Cefixime	8 mg/kg/d (PO)	Yes	3.9	67	3.7	No	Yes	No (H, P)
Ceftibuten	3–5 mg/kg/q12h (PO)	Yes	9.9	60	2.5	No	Yes	Yes (H)
Cefdinir	5–7 mg/kg/q12h (PO)	Yes	2.9	60	1.7	No	Yes	Yes (H)
Cefotaxime	30 mg/kg/q6h	—	130	50	1.2	Some	Minor	Yes (H) No (P)
Cefpodoxime proxetil	3–6 mg/kg/q12h (PO)	Yes	3.9	25	2.5	No	Minor	Yes (H) No (P)
Ceftazidime	30 mg/kg/q8h	—	160	60	2	No	Major	Yes (H, P)
Ceftizoxime	30 mg/kg/q6–8h	—	130	50	1.3	No	Minor	Yes (H) No (P)
Ceftriaxone	30 mg/kg/q12–24h	—	250	90	8	No	No	No (H)
Penicillins								
Amoxicillin	7 mg/kg/q6h (PO)	Yes	6	20	1	No	Yes	Yes (H) No (P)
Ampicillin	30 mg/kg/q6h	Yes†	100	20	1	No	Yes	Yes (H) No (P)
Cloxacillin	7 mg/kg/q6h (PO)	Yes†	9	95	0.5	No	No	No (H, P)
Dicloxacillin	7 mg/kg/q6h (PO)	Yes†	18	97	0.5	No	No	No (H, P)
Mezlocillin	50 mg/kg/q6h	—	260	50	1	Yes	Major	Yes (H) No (P)
Nafcillin	30 mg/kg/q4–6h	—	160	90	0.5	Yes	No	No (H, P)
Oxacillin	30 mg/kg/q4–6h	—	200	90	0.5	Yes	No	Yes (H, P)
Penicillin G	3–4 million U q4–6h	Yes†	60	60	0.5	No	Yes	Yes (H) No (P)
Penicillin V	7 mg/kg/q6h (PO)	Yes	4	80	1	No	No	Yes (H) No (P)
Piperacillin	40 mg/kg/q6h	—	240	50	1	Minor	Major	Yes (H)
Ticarcillin	40 mg/kg/q4–6h	—	220	50	1	Minor	Major	Yes (H, P)
Quinolones								
Ciprofloxacin	7 mg/kg/q12h (PO)	Yes†	2–2.8	30	3	No	Yes	No (H, P)
Lomefloxacin	6 mg/kg/q24h	Yes	4	10	8		Yes	No (H, P)
Ofloxacin	6 mg/kg/q12h	Yes†	3–5	30	7		Yes	No (H, P)
Levofloxacin	7 mg/kg/q24h	Yes	5.7	35	6–8	No	Yes	No (H, P)
Sparfloxacin	400 mg load, 200 mg q24h (PO)	Yes	1.3	45	16–20	No	Yes	No (H)
Grepafloxacin	8.5 mg/kg q24h (PO)	Yes	2.4	50	12	Yes	No	No (H, P)
Trovafloxacin	3–4 mg/kg q24h	Yes	3.1	70	12	Yes	No	No (H, P)
Tetracyclines								
Doxycycline	1.5 mg/kg/q12–24h	Yes	1.8–2.9	90	15–20	Avoid	No	No (H, P)
Minocycline	1.5 mg/kg/q12–24h	Yes	2.2	90	15	No	Avoid	No (H, P)
Tetracycline	7 mg/kg/q6h	Yes†	4	50	7	Avoid	Avoid	No (H, P)
Sulfonamides								
Sulfadiazine	15 mg/kg/q6h	Yes	30	50	3	Avoid	Avoid	Unknown
Sulfamethoxazole	12 mg/kg/q8h (IV)	Yes	100	50	6	Avoid	Major	Yes (H) No (P)
Trimethoprim (used with sulfa-methoxazole)	2.3 mg/kg/q8–12h (IV)	Yes	3–9	60	10	No	Avoid	Yes (H) No (P)
Macrolides-Lincosamides								
Azithromycin	4 mg/kg/q24h (PO)	Yes†	0.4	50	57 (tissue)	Unknown	Unknown	Unknown
Clarithromycin	7.5 mg/kg/q12h (PO)	Yes	2–3	70	7	No	Yes	Yes (H) No (P)
Clindamycin	7 mg/kg/q6h	Yes	15	90	2.5	Some	No	No (H, P)
Erythromycin	7 mg/kg/q6h (PO)	Yes†	1.8	20	1.5	Some	No	No (H, P)
Other Agents								
Aztreonam	30 mg/kg/q8h	—	250	60	2.0	No	Major	Yes (H, P)
Chloramphenicol	7–15 mg/kg/q6h (PO)	Yes	8–14	30	1.5	Some	No	Yes (H) No (P)
Imipenem	7.5 mg/kg/q6h	—	40	15	1	No	Avoid	Yes (H)
Loracarbef	15 mg/kg/q12h (PO)	Yes†	18	25	1.2	No	Yes	Yes (H)
Meropenem	15 mg/kg/q8h	—	40		1.0	Unknown	Yes	Yes (H)
Metronidazole	7 mg/kg/q6h	Yes	25	20	8	Yes	No	Yes (H) No (P)
Nitrofurantoin	1 mg/kg/q6h (PO)	Yes	nil	60	0.3	No	Avoid	Yes (H)
Spectinomycin	30 mg/kg/d	—	100	0	2	No	Avoid	Unknown
Vancomycin	15 mg/kg/q12h	Yes§	35	10	6	No	Major	No (H, P)
Quinupristin/dalfopristin (30:70)	7.5 mg/kg/q8h	—	2.5/6.8 ‖	90/30	0.8/0.6 ‖	Some	No	No (P)

*mg/kg body weight at hour interval in patients with normal renal function; all doses are parenteral unless specified PO.
†Do not administer with food—absorption is decreased or delayed.
‡H = hemodialysis; P = peritoneal dialysis.
§Orally administered vancomycin is not absorbed; gastrointestinal tract lumen therapy only.
‖Extensive non-enzymatic degradation to active metabolites that are not included.

peptides (vancomycin and teicoplanin) must be administered parenterally. Although parenterally administered antimicrobials are preferred for treatment of severe infections, the availability of well-absorbed potent penicillins, cephalosporins, quinolones, macrolides, and metronidazole allows early transition from parenteral to less costly oral therapy in many patients.

Antibiotic penetration into cells, particularly polymorphonuclear leukocytes and macrophages, and intracellular antibacterial activity are necessary to effectively treat some infections (e.g., *M. tuberculosis, L. pneumophila, Listeria monocytogenes, Brucella* species, and *Salmonella typhi*).

The serum and tissue concentrations over time of an antimicrobial administered by a given route and the microbiologic activity of that antimicrobial when viewed together describe the pharmacodynamic properties of the agent. Bacterial killing by β-lactam antibiotics and vancomycin does not increase after antibiotic concentrations exceed an organism's minimal inhibitory concentration (MIC) by several multiples. Also, the post-antibiotic effect (inhibition of an organism's growth resulting from immediately prior exposure to an antibiotic) of these antimicrobial agents is negligible. These considerations suggest that administration of β-lactam antibiotics and vancomycin to achieve sustained concentrations (four to five times the MIC) over a greater proportion of the interval between doses is likely to result in more profound antibacterial action than is dosing to achieve a transient higher concentration but a less sustained concentration above the MIC. Sustained concentrations may be achieved by more frequent dosing, by using higher doses, by using antibiotics with a long half-life, or by continuous infusion. Aminoglycosides and fluoroquinolones, as well as metronidazole against anaerobic gram-negative bacteria, exhibit concentration-dependent killing, wherein higher concentrations exert an increasingly bactericidal effect and cause a prolonged post-antibiotic effect. Accordingly, for these agents higher ratios of the maximum antibiotic plasma concentration to organism MIC or the area under the concentration (AUC) versus time curve to organism MIC correlates with increased antibiotic efficacy. These interactions suggest that for antibiotics exhibiting concentration dependent killing larger doses administered less frequently each day provide greater antibacterial activity. Aminoglycoside therapy given as a single daily dose is as effective and less ototoxic and nephrotoxic than the same quantity of aminoglycoside divided in the standard multiple daily-dose regimen. In both animal models of infection and clinical trials, the clinical and microbiologic efficacy of fluoroquinolone therapy has been correlated with peak plasma concentration:MIC and the 24-hour AUC:MIC ratios.

PATIENT-RELATED CONSIDERATIONS. Unique aspects of the patient and site of the specific infection are important in selecting an optimal antimicrobial agent, as well as the appropriate dose, route of administration, and duration of therapy. Recent treatment with an antibiotic, for example, increases the risk that the subsequent infection is caused by residual antibiotic-resistant bacteria. Residing in an environment that has an extensive antibiotic-resistant flora (e.g., an intensive-care unit, a skilled nursing care facility, or a day care center) increases the risk for colonization and subsequent infection by antibiotic-resistant bacteria.

The patient's physiologic and metabolic status must be considered when therapy is selected. Premature infants and neonates have incompletely developed renal function and hepatic metabolism pathways requiring adjustment of antibiotic doses. Because tetracyclines deposit in growing bones and teeth and quinolones may damage cartilage, they are not used in children. Genetically determined drug metabolism also affects antibiotic selection. Antimicrobial agents, including sulfonamides, sulfones (dapsone), nitrofurantoin, chloramphenicol, and pyrimethamine, may cause hemolysis in patients with deficient glucose-6-phosphate dehydrogenase. Pyridoxine is routinely given with isoniazid treatment or prophylaxis of tuberculosis to prevent the peripheral neuropathy that occurs among those who are "slow" acetylators of isoniazid.

Hypersensitivity to one member of an antibiotic class usually extends to all other compounds in that class and, if the reaction was severe, contraindicates their use. However, if the hypersensitivity reaction to penicillin, for example, was not an immediate or accelerated anaphylactic or urticarial reaction, cautious treatment with a cephalosporin is acceptable. From 3 to 7% of patients with a history of penicillin allergy experience an allergic reaction when treated with a cephalosporin, a rate one and one half to two times that noted among patients who do not report a penicillin allergy.

Most antimicrobial agents cross the placenta and reach therapeutic concentrations in fetal tissues; thus, antibiotics, in general, should be administered during pregnancy only if absolutely required. The fetus should not be exposed to trimethoprim or rifampin, both of which are teratogens in animals; to metronidazole, which is mutagenic; or to clarithromycin, which has been associated with fetal toxicity in primates. Tetracyclines cause fetal bone changes and in pregnant women are associated with increased risk for hepatotoxicity. If antimicrobial therapy is required during pregnancy, penicillins, β-lactam/β-lactamase inhibitor combinations, cephalosporins, and erythromycin are preferred. Data indicating safety during pregnancy are insufficient for clindamycin, vancomycin, azithromycin, and the aminoglycosides; hence, these agents should be avoided, if possible. Many antibiotics appear in breast milk; antibiotics that pose a risk to the neonate or infant (chloramphenicol, sulfonamides, tetracyclines, and quinolones) must not be administered to nursing mothers. Generally, mothers are advised to temporarily discontinue nursing during periods of antimicrobial therapy.

The pharmacokinetics of antibiotics that are primarily excreted by the kidneys are significantly altered in patients with moderate to severe renal dysfunction. If antibiotic accumulation and potential toxicity are to be avoided, dosage adjustments, after an initial standard dose, are necessary when the antibiotics are administered to patients with renal dysfunction (see Table 318–3).

Antibiotics that are metabolized in the liver or excreted in the bile should be used with caution when treating patients with severe liver failure (see Table 318–3). The potential for antibiotics to interact with other drugs that the patient is receiving is yet another important consideration that affects the selection of antimicrobial therapy (Table 318–4).

SPECIFIC ANTIMICROBIAL AGENTS

Although oversimplifying the process of selecting appropriate therapy, Table 318–5 lists the agents of choice and some of the alternative agents recommended for the treatment of infections caused by specific bacteria. Table 318–6 details the relative antibacterial activity of specific antimicrobial agents against organisms that commonly cause infections. Because gram-negative bacilli and enterococci commonly acquire resistance genes, antimicrobial susceptibility testing is required when treating serious infection caused by these organisms.

BROAD-SPECTRUM PENICILLINS AND RELATED COMPOUNDS. Selected side chains added to the β-lactam ring of the penicillin nucleus result in broad-spectrum penicillins that, although still inactivated by staphylococcal β-lactamase, possess enhanced activity against gram-negative bacilli. The aminopenicillins—ampicillin and amoxicillin—have expanded the penicillin spectrum to include many of the gram-negative bacilli. However, subsequent acquisition of β-lactamase genes by many of these species, except *Proteus mirabilis*, has limited the use of aminopenicillins. Notably, 25% of *E. coli* and at least 15% of *H. influenzae* are resistant to these agents. Bacteria that are susceptible to penicillin G remain susceptible to ampicillin and amoxicillin. Amoxicillin is more fully absorbed from the gastrointestinal tract than ampicillin. Amoxicillin is the recommended antimicrobial agent for prophylaxis against endocarditis at the time of dental procedures. Aminopenicillins are effective therapy for early Lyme disease (*Borrelia burgdorferi* infection) as are doxycycline, cefuroxime axetil, clarithromycin, and azithromycin.

The carboxypenicillins—carbenicillin and ticarcillin—and the ureidopenicillins—azlocillin, mezlocillin, and piperacillin—comprise the remaining broad-spectrum penicillins available in the United States. Carbenicillin and ticarcillin extended the antibacterial spectrum of penicillins to include indole-positive *Proteus* species, some *Enterobacter* species, *Acinetobacter*, and, importantly, *Pseudomonas aeruginosa*. The spectra of antibacterial activity of carbenicillin and ticarcillin are similar; however, the potency of ticarcillin against *P. aeruginosa* is twice that of carbenicillin. Mezlocillin and piperacillin are more active against the Enterobacteriaceae than are carbenicillin, ticarcillin, and azlocillin. Piperacillin and azlocillin are the most potent antipseudomonal penicillins. In treating serious gram-negative infection, the carboxypenicillins and ureidopenicillins are combined with an aminoglycoside because of their inactivation by various β-lactamases and the potential emergence of resistance.

318 Antibacterial Therapy ■ 1597

Agents from each group of broad-spectrum penicillins have been combined with a β-lactamase inhibitor. The β-lactamase inhibitors inhibit staphylococcal β-lactamase, many plasmid-mediated β-lacta-

Table 318–4 ■ IMPORTANT ANTIBIOTIC-DRUG INTERACTIONS*

ANTIMICROBIAL AGENT	INTERACTING DRUG	EFFECT
Aminoglycosides	Amphotericin B, cyclosporine, vancomycin	Increased nephrotoxicity
	Loop diuretics (bumetanide, furosemide, ethacrynic acid)	Increased ototoxicity (avoid)
	Carboxy/ureidopenicillins	Decreased aminoglycoside activity (renal failure only)
Cephalosporins		
MTT side chain†	Warfarin, dicumarol, heparin, thrombolytics, platelet inhibitors	Increased anticoagulation, bleeding
MTT side chain†	Alcohol	Disulfiram-like reaction
All	Loop diuretics	Nephrotoxicity
Chloramphenicol	Warfarin	Increased warfarin activity, increased anticoagulation
	Phenytoin	Increased serum phenytoin, phenytoin toxicity
	Sulfonylureas	Increased sulfonylurea, hypoglycemia
Clarithromycin,‡ Erythromycin	Carbamazepine	Increased serum carbamazepine (avoid)
	Cyclosporine, tacrolimus	Increased serum tacrolimus, cyclosporine, nephrotoxicity
	Digoxin	Increased serum digoxin, toxicity
	Terfenadine, astemizole, loratadine, cisapride	Increased cisapride or antihistamine level, arrhythmia (avoid)
	Theophylline	Increased theophylline level, toxicity
	Ergot alkaloids	Increased ergot alkaloid
Isoniazid	Warfarin	Increased warfarin activity, increased anticoagulation
	Alfentanil	Prolonged alfentanil activity
	Phenytoin	Increased serum phenytoin, phenytoin toxicity
	Disulfiram	Psychosis, behavioral change (avoid)
	Carbamazepine	Increased carbamazepine, toxicity (avoid)
	Rifampin	Additive hepatotoxicity
Metronidazole	Alcohol	Disulfiram-like reaction
	Disulfiram	Psychosis (avoid)
	Warfarin, dicumarol	Increased anticoagulation
	Phenobarbital	Decreased metronidazole
Penicillins		
Ampicillin/amoxicillin	Allopurinol	Increased rash
Ampicillin/carboxypenicillins, ureidopenicillins	Oral contraceptives	Decreased contraceptive effect
	Probenecid	Increased serum penicillins
Fluoroquinolones		
All	Cimetidine	Increased antibiotic concentration
	Cyclosporine	Increased serum cyclosporine, nephrotoxicity
	Multivalent cations (Ca²⁺, Mg²⁺, Fe²⁺, Zn²⁺, Al³⁺ orally)	Decreased absorption quinolones
	Sucralfate, didanosine	Decreased absorption quinolones
	Warfarin	Increased anticoagulation
	Probenecid	Increased fluoroquinolone
All except trovafloxacin	Non-steroidal anti-inflammatory drugs, carbapenems	Increased central nervous system stimulation, seizure risk
Grepafloxacin, ciprofloxacin, enoxacin	Theophylline	Increased serum theophylline, toxicity
Grepafloxacin, norfloxacin, pefloxacin, ciprofloxacin, trovafloxacin	Caffeine	Increased serum caffeine, insomnia, restlessness
Grepafloxacin, sparfloxacin	Cardiac antiarrhythmics	Increased QT interval, risk of torsades de pointes
Rifampin, rifabutin§	Corticosteroids	Decreased corticosteroid, supplement dose
	Cyclosporine, tacrolimus	Decreased cyclosporine, tacrolimus
	Methadone	Decreased serum methadone, withdrawal
	Phenytoin	Decreased serum phenytoin
	Warfarin, dicumarol	Decreased anticoagulation, need large doses
	Oral contraceptives	Decreased contraceptive effect
	Sulfonylureas	Decreased sulfonylurea, hyperglycemia
	Theophylline	Decreased serum theophylline
	Quinidine, β-blocker	Decreased quinidine, β-blocker
	Clarithromycin	Uveitis
Sulfonamides	Cyclosporine	Decreased serum cyclosporine
	Phenytoin	Increased serum phenytoin, toxicity
	Warfarin	Increased warfarin effect
	Sulfonylureas	Increased sulfonylurea, hypoglycemia
Trimethoprim	Azathioprine, methotrexate	Increased leukopenia
	Dapsone	Increased serum dapsone and trimethoprim, increased methemoglobinemia
	Potassium-sparing diuretics	Increased potassium
Tetracycline	Multivalent cations (Ca²⁺, Al³⁺, Mg²⁺, Bi²⁺, Zn²⁺, Fe²⁺)	Decreased tetracycline absorption
	Barbiturates, carbamazepine	Decreased doxycycline
	Digoxin	Increased digoxin, toxicity
	Phenytoin	Decreased doxycycline
	Methoxyflurane (Penthrane)	Severe nephrotoxicity (avoid)

*Not all interactions have been listed.
†MTT = methylthiotetrazole ring (cefamandole, cefotetan, cefmetazole, cefoperazone, moxalactam, cefmenoxime); decreases vitamin K–dependent clotting factors.
‡Interactions with azithromycin not adequately studied.
§Multiple other rifampin and rifabutin interactions mediated through cytochrome system.

Table 318–5 ■ ANTIBACTERIAL DRUGS OF CHOICE FOR INFECTIONS CAUSED BY SELECTED BACTERIA

INFECTING ORGANISM	AGENT OF CHOICE*	ALTERNATIVE AGENT†
Gram-Positive Cocci		
S. aureus/coagulase-negative staphylococci		
Non-penicillinase producing	Penicillin G or V	Cephalosporin,‡ vancomycin, clindamycin, erythromycin
Penicillinase producing	Nafcillin, oxacillin	Cephalosporin,‡ vancomycin, clindamycin, erythromycin, imipenem, β-lactam/β-lactamase inhibitor combinations
Methicillin-resistant§	Vancomycin	Trimethoprim-sulfamethoxazole, minocycline, teicoplanin (investigational)
β-Hemolytic streptococci (groups A, B, C, G)	Penicillin G or V	Cephalosporin,‡ erythromycin, vancomycin, clindamycin
Viridans streptococci, *Streptococcus bovis*	Penicillin G	Cephalosporin,‡ vancomycin, erythromycin
Enterococci ‖		
Uncomplicated urinary tract infection	Ampicillin, amoxicillin	Nitrofurantoin, quinolone,¶ fosfomycin
Moderately severe wound infection	Ampicillin	Penicillin G, vancomycin
Serious infection: Endocarditis or meningitis	Ampicillin plus gentamicin or streptomycin	Vancomycin plus gentamicin or streptomycin (test for high-level aminoglycoside resistance)
Vancomycin-resistant *Enterococcus faecium*	Quinupristin/dalfopristin**	
Streptococcus pneumoniae ‖		
Pneumonia, upper respiratory tract infection	Penicillin G, amoxicillin	Cephalosporin,‡ macrolide, azithromycin, clindamycin, vancomycin, new fluoroquinolones††
Meningitis	Ceftriazone, cefotaxime	Ceftriaxone plus vancomycin ± rifampin, vancomycin + rifampin (penicillin G only if MIC <0.1 µg/mL)
Gram-Negative Cocci		
Neisseria gonorrhoeae	Ceftriaxone, cefixime	Second- or other third-generation cephalosporins,‡‡ quinolones,¶ spectinomycin, trimethoprim/sulfamethoxazole, azithromycin (choices vary by sites of infections)
N. meningitidis	Penicillin G	Third-generation cephalosporin,‡‡ chloramphenicol, sulfonamide (if susceptible)
Moraxella catarrhalis	Trimethoprim/sulfamethoxazole	Amoxicillin/clavulanate, third-generation cephalosporin,‡‡ cefuroxime, clarithromycin, azithromycin, new fluoroquinolones††
Gram-Positive Bacilli		
Bacillus anthracis (anthrax)	Penicillin G	Erythromycin, tetracycline
Corynebacterium diphtheriae	Erythromycin	Penicillin G
Corynebacterium species	Penicillin + gentamicin	Vancomycin
Listeria monocytogenes	Ampicillin or penicillin G ± gentamicin	Trimethoprim/sulfamethoxazole, vancomycin, tetracycline
Clostridium perfringens	Penicillin G	Metronidazole, chloramphenicol, imipenem, tetracycline
Clostridium difficile	Metronidazole	Vancomycin (oral only), bacitracin
Gram-Negative Bacilli ‖		
Acinetobacter species	Imipenem ± gentamicin	Ureidopenicillin; aminoglycoside
Bordetella pertussis (pertussis)	Erythromycin	Trimethoprim/sulfamethoxazole
Brucella species (brucellosis)	Tetracycline + gentamicin or streptomycin	Tetracycline + rifampin, chloramphenicol ± streptomycin, trimethoprim/sulfamethoxazole ± gentamicin
Campylobacter fetus spp. *jejuni*	Erythromycin, quinolone¶	Tetracycline
Enterobacter species	Imipenem, aminoglycoside	Quinolone,¶ third-generation cephalosporin,‡‡ cefepime, trimethoprim/sulfamethoxazole
Eikenella corrodens	Penicillin G, ampicillin	Tetracycline, cefoxitin, third-generation cephalosporin,‡‡ ampicillin-sulbactam
Escherichia coli		
Uncomplicated urinary tract infection	Fluoroquinolone¶	Ampicillin, trimethoprim/sulfamethoxazole, trimethoprim, quinolone,¶ tetracycline
Systemic infection	Third-generation cephalosporin	Aminoglycoside,§§ β-lactam/β-lactamase inhibitor, aztreonam, trimethoprim/sulfamethoxazole, fluoroquinolone
Helicobacter pylori	Tetracycline + metronidazole + bismuth subsalicylate	Amoxicillin + metronidazole + bismuth subsalicylate Teracycline + clarithromycin + bismuth subsalicylate
Francisella tularensis (tularemia)	Streptomycin, gentamicin	Tetracycline, chloramphenicol
Haemophilus influenzae		
Meningitis, bacteremia	Ceftriaxone, cefotaxime	Meropenem (ampicillin only if β-lactamase negative and susceptible)
Other infection	Ampicillin/clavulanate, amoxicillin/clavulanate	Trimethoprim/sulfamethoxazole, cefuroxime, quinolone,¶ third-generation cephalosporin‡‡
Haemophilus ducreyi (chancroid)	Ceftriaxone	Azithromycin, erythromycin, amoxicillin/clavulanate, quinolone¶
Klebsiella pneumoniae/oxytoca	Aminoglycoside,§§ third-generation cephalosporin‡‡	First- or second-generation cephalosporin, quinolone,¶ ureidopenicillin, imipenem, aztreonam, β-lactam/β-lactamase inhibitor
Legionella pneumophila	Levofloxacin, azithromycin	Erythromycin ± rifampin, clarithromycin
Nocardia asteroides	Trimethoprim/sulfamethazole	Sulfisoxazole, imipenem, meropenem, minocycline
Pasteurella multocida	Penicillin G	Tetracycline, amoxicillin/clavulanate, third-generation cephalosporin‡‡
Proteus mirabilis	Ampicillin	Cephalosporin,‡ trimethoprim/sulfamethoxazole, aminoglycoside,§§ fluoroquinolone¶
Proteus (indole positive)	Third-generation cephalosporin	Imipenem, aminoglycoside,§§ trimethoprim/sulfamethoxazole, quinolone¶
Bartonella henselae/quintana	Erythromycin	Tetracycline, clarithromycin, azithromycin
Salmonella sp.	Ceftriazone, quinolone¶	Chloramphenicol, trimethoprim/sulfamethoxazole
Serratia marcescens	Aminoglycoside,§§ third-generation cephalosporin‡‡	Imipenem, quinolone,‡‡ aztreonam
Shigella sp.	Quinolone¶	Trimethoprim/sulfamethoxazole, ceftriaxone, chloramphenicol
Pseudomonas aeruginosa		
Urinary tract infection	Ciprofloxacin, ureidopenicillin	Aminoglycoside,§§ ceftazidime, imipenem, aztreonam
Pneumonia, bacteremia	Aminoglycoside§§ + ureidopenicillin or ceftazidime	Imipenem + aminoglycoside,§§ aztreonam + aminoglycoside,§§ ciprofloxacin + ceftazidime
Vibrio vulnificus	Tetracycline + ceftazidime	Chloramphenicol
Stenotrophomonas maltophilia	Trimethoprim/sulfamethoxazole	Ticarcillin/clavulanate, quinolone,¶ ceftazidime
Yersinia pestis (plague)	Streptomycin, gentamicin	Tetracycline, chloramphenicol
Anaerobic Gram-Negative		
Bacteroides sp.	Metronidazole	Clindamycin, cefoxitin, cefotetan, cefmetazole, chloramphenicol, β-lactam/β-lactamase inhibitor Cefoxitin, cefotetan, clindamycin, imipenem, β-lactam/β-lactamase inhibitor, chloramphenicol

MIC = minimum inhibitory concentration.
*Dose and route of administration must be adjusted for severity of illness and host characteristics (organ dysfunction, allergy).
†List of alternative agents is not fully inclusive; confirm susceptibility in vitro.
‡First-generation cephalosporin preferred (cephalothin, cephapirin, cephradine, cephalexin, cefazolin).
§Must test for susceptibility for alternative agents; methicillin resistance implies resistance to penicillins, cephalosporins, and carbapenems.
‖Must test susceptibility; resistant strains are increasingly frequent.
¶Ciprofloxacin, lomefloxacin, ofloxacin (or for urinary tract infection, norfloxacin).
**Investigational in United States, available from Rhone-Poulenc Rorer.
††Levofloxacin, trovafloxacin, grepafloxacin, sparfloxacin; penicillin-resistant *S. pneumoniae* susceptible to these.
‡‡Third-generation cephalosporins for this indication include ceftriaxone, cefotaxime, and ceftizoxime.
§§Aminoglycosides for this indication include gentamicin, tobramycin, netilmicin, and amikacin.

mases of gram-negative bacilli, the ESBLs, and the chromosomal β-lactamases of *Klebsiella* and *Bacteroides* species. They do not inhibit the chromosomal β-lactamases (cephalosporinases) of *Enterobacter* species, *Serratia,* and *P. aeruginosa.* Ampicillin/sulbactam, ticarcillin/clavulanate, and piperacillin/tazobactam are available for parenteral use, and amoxicillin/clavulanate is available for oral administration.

CEPHALOSPORINS. The cephalosporins contain a nucleus in which the β-lactam ring is fused to a six-membered dihydrothiazine ring (in contrast to the five-membered thiazolidine ring in the analogous position in penicillins). Substituent side chains are added to the β-lactam ring to alter antimicrobial activity and to the dihydrothiazine ring to alter metabolic and pharmacokinetic properties. A widely accepted system classifies the cephalosporins into "three generations" on the basis of their spectrum of microbiologic activity. With each successive generation, cephalosporins have increasing antibacterial activity against gram-negative bacilli and, to a degree, decreasing activity against gram-positive bacteria. For treatment of serious *S. aureus* infections in patients intolerant of antistaphylococcal penicillins, first-generation cephalosporins are preferred. The cephamycins (cefoxitin, cefotetan, and cefmetazole) are grouped with the second-generation cephalosporins and are active against many gram-negative anaerobic bacteria, including *B. fragilis.* All cephalosporins are inactive against enterococci, methicillin-resistant staphylococci, and *L. monocytogenes.* Ceftazidime and cefepime possess clinically significant antipseudomonal activity; and cefepime and cefpirome, which have been called fourth-generation compounds, are active against *Enterobacter* species and related organisms that produce chromosomal β-lactamases. Organisms producing an ESBL are resistant to third-generation cephalosporins. Ceftriaxone, cefotaxime, and cefepime retain clinically relevant activity against *S. pneumoniae* that are resistant to penicillin; however, some of these strains have become relatively resistant to even these cephalosporins. Cefazolin is widely used for perioperative prophylaxis in surgical procedures involving foreign body implantation and for many clean and clean-contaminated operations, except those involving the colon. Cefotaxime or ceftriaxone with vancomycin is recommended for empirical therapy for presumed pneumococcal meningitis, and these cephalosporins with an aminoglycoside are used to treat meningitis due to enteric gram-negative bacilli (except *Enterobacter* species and organisms producing chromosomal cephalosporinases, whereupon cefepime or meropenem would be preferred). Ceftazidime is the agent of choice for meningitis caused by *P. aeruginosa.* Ceftriaxone is the drug of choice for treatment of late stages of Lyme disease.

Adverse reactions caused by the cephalosporins are independent of their antibacterial spectra (Table 318–7). Hypersensitivity cross-reactions between cephalosporins are not universal; nevertheless, they occur more frequently than penicillin-cephalosporin cross-reactions. There are no skin test reagents that predict cephalosporin hypersensitivity, and testing with the drug in question is not recommended. Whereas aztreonam can be administered to most patients with hypersensitivity to penicillins and cephalosporins, use of imipenem or meropenem may result in cross-reactions.

QUINOLONES. The quinolones have a bicyclic aromatic core in which the right-hand side is a pyridone ring. Current quinolones contain a fluorine atom at the 6 position, which yields increased gram-negative potency and gram-positive activity; as a result they are referred to as fluoroquinolones. Among the multiple fluoroquinolones developed for clinical use, ciprofloxacin remains the most potent against gram-negative bacilli, particularly *P. aeruginosa.* Levofloxacin, the L-isomer of ofloxacin, retains excellent activity against Enterobacteriaceae and has enhanced activity against gram-positive cocci. Trovafloxacin is uniquely active against anaerobic gram-negative bacteria. The newer quinolones, levofloxacin, sparfloxacin, grepafloxacin, gatifloxacin, trovafloxacin, and moxifloxacin (listed in order of increasing potency) have significantly increased activity against *S. pneumoniae* (as well as *S. aureus* and streptococci) and are also active against *Chlamydia pneumoniae, Mycoplasma pneumoniae,* and *Legionella* species. Methicillin-resistant *S. aureus* is commonly resistant to the fluoroquinolones.

Given a broad spectrum of activity, a high degree of bioavailability after oral administration, and demonstrated efficacy against many clinical infections, fluoroquinolones are used extensively. Fluoroquinolones have proven highly effective treatment for urinary tract infections (except trovafloxacin and grepafloxacin, which have non-urinary clearance mechanisms); prostatitis; complicated skin and soft tissue infection; and enteric infections, including typhoid fever; and as single-dose therapy for uncomplicated gonococcal infection (susceptible strains). Fluoroquinolones are the agents of choice for osteomyelitis caused by gram-negative bacilli. The newer fluoroquinolones (noted earlier), which are highly active against both penicillin-susceptible and penicillin-resistant pneumococci as well as *Haemophilus influenzae, Moraxella catarrhalis,* and the agents causing atypical pneumonia, are agents of choice for mild to moderate community-acquired pneumonia. High-dose ciprofloxacin and trovafloxacin have been effective therapy for nosocomial pneumonia but should not be used alone if the infection is caused by *P. aeruginosa.*

COMBINATION ANTIMICROBIAL THERAPY

There are several rationales for administering antibiotics in combination: (1) a broader, more comprehensive antibacterial effect when treating a severe infection of unknown cause may be achieved; (2) the bacteria causing mixed infection may exceed the antibacterial range of a single agent; (3) combination therapy may decrease the opportunity for the emergence of resistant bacteria; and (4) antibiotics administered concurrently may interact to exert an enhanced (synergistic) or additive antibacterial effect. An improvement in outcome of infection achieved by the enhanced antibacterial effect of combination therapy is seen in ampicillin/gentamicin therapy for enterococcal endocarditis and antipseudomonal penicillin/tobramycin therapy for *P. aeruginosa* endocarditis.

In spite of laudable goals, the end result of the combination therapy is not always favorable. Antibiotics administered in combinations may interact in antagonistic fashion (the net effect of the combination is less than that of the most effective of the agents acting individually). Although difficult to demonstrate clinically, antagonism must remain a concern. Additionally, administering multiple antibiotics may increase the risk for adverse events and increase selective pressure, leading to colonization or secondary infection by resistant bacteria or fungi. Thus, effective targeted single-antibiotic therapy is preferred whenever possible.

DURATION OF THERAPY

There is no easy formula to determine optimal duration of therapy. One must weigh the site of infection, the patient as a host, the pathogen involved, the pharmacodynamics of the selected antimicrobial therapy, the response to treatment, the toxicity of the regimen, and the hazards of failure occasioned by terminating therapy prematurely. When the infecting organisms are not proliferating, as in the vegetation of endocarditis, more prolonged therapy is required to eradicate the bacteria. Patients with impaired host defenses are treated with longer courses of therapy, assuming that host defenses will play less of a role in terminating infection. Superficial mucosal infection can be cured by single-dose therapy, as noted with ceftriaxone, cefixime, or fluoroquinolone treatment of uncomplicated genitourinary gonorrhea. Single-dose therapy is also effective for bacterial cystitis, although 3-day short-course therapy is now preferred. Decisions regarding duration of therapy often are based on studies in which the goal was not to examine the impact of duration of therapy on outcome but rather to assess a predefined regimen. It is likely that antibiotic therapy is often excessive in length. This exacerbates costs of treatment, increases the risks of adverse events, and exerts unnecessary selective pressure on bacteria to become resistant.

ANTIBIOTIC TOXICITY AND UNTOWARD REACTIONS

Antibiotics commonly cause adverse drug reactions (see Table 318–7). The majority of adverse events are mild and resolve when the offending drug is withdrawn. Untoward reactions also result from interactions between an antimicrobial agent and another medication that the patient is receiving (see Table 318–4).

FAILURE OF THERAPY

The persistence of fever and other signs of infection during antibiotic therapy calls for careful reassessment of the patient. Anti-

Table 318-6 ■ ACTIVITY OF MAJOR ANTIBIOTICS AGAINST SELECTED ORGANISMS*

	STREPTOCOCCI	STREPTOCOCCUS PNEUMONIAE†	ENTEROCOCCI‡	STAPHYLOCOCCUS AUREUS (MS)	STAPHYLOCOCCUS AUREUS (MR)	STAPHYLOCOCCI COAGULASE-NEGATIVE‡	LISTERIA MONOCYTOGENES	NEISSERIA GONORRHOEAE	NEISSERIA MENINGITIDIS	MORAXELLA CATARRHALIS	HAEMOPHILUS INFLUENZAE	ESCHERICHIA COLI	ENTEROBACTER sp.	KLEBSIELLA sp.	PROTEUS MIRABILIS	PROTEUS VULGARIS	SALMONELLA sp.	SERRATIA sp.	SHIGELLA sp.	ACINETOBACTER sp.	PSEUDOMONAS AERUGINOSA	STENOTROPHOMONAS MALTOPHILIA	PASTEURELLA MULTOCIDA	VIBRIO VULNIFICUS	LEGIONELLA sp.	CHLAMYDIA sp.	MYCOPLASMA PNEUMONIAE	RICKETTSIA sp.	BACTEROIDES FRAGILIS group#	CLOSTRIDIUM sp. (not C. difficile)	PREVOTELLA MELANINOGENICUS	ACTINOMYCES sp.
Penicillin G	+	+	+	0	0	0	+	±	+	0	0	0	0	0	±	0	0	0	0	0	0	0	+	±	0	0	0	0	0	+	+	+
Oxacillin[1]	+	±	0	+	0	±	0	0	0	0	0	0	0	0	0	0	0	0	0	0	0	0	0	0	0	0	0	0	0	0	0	0
Ampicillin[2]	+	+	+	0	0	0	+	±	+	0	±	±	0	0	+	0	+	0	±	0	0	0	+	+	0	0	0	0	0	+	+	+
Ampicillin/sulbactam[2]	+	+	+	+	0	±	+	+	+	+	+	+	±	+	+	0	+	0	±	+	0	0	+	+	0	0	0	0	+	+	+	+
Ticarcillin	+	+	+	0	0	0	+	+	+	0	±	±	±	0	+	+	+	+	+	+	+	0	+	+	0	0	0	0	0	+	+	+
Ticarcillin/clavulanate	+	+	+	+	0	±	+	+	+	+	+	+	±	+	+	+	+	+	+	+	+	±	+	+	0	0	0	0	+	+	+	+
Piperacillin	+	+	+	0	0	±	+	+	+	0	+	+	±	+	+	+	+	±	+	+	+	±	+	+	0	0	0	0	+	+	+	+
Piperacillin/tazobactam	+	+	+	+	0	±	+	+	+	+	+	+	±	+	+	+	+	±	+	+	+	±	+	+	0	0	0	0	+	+	+	+
Aztreonam	0	0	0	0	0	0	0	+	0	+	+	+	±	+	+	+	+	+	+	0	+	0	+	ND	0	0	0	0	0	0	0	0
Imipenem	+	+	±	+	0	±	+	+	+	+	+	+	+	+	+	+	+	+	+	+	+	0	+	ND	ND	0	0	0	+	+	+	+
Cefazolin[3]	+	+	0	+	0	±	0	±	0	0	0	+	±	+	+	0	+	0	0	0	0	0	+	0	0	0	0	0	0	0	±	+
Cefotetan[4]	+	+	0	+	0	±	0	+	+	+	+	+	0	+	+	+	+	+	+	0	0	0	+	ND	0	0	0	0	±	+	+	+
Cefoxitin	+	+	0	+	0	±	0	+	0	+	+	+	±	+	+	0	+	0	+	0	0	0	+	0	0	0	0	0	+	+	+	+
Cefuroxime	+	+	0	+	0	±	0	+	+	+	+	+	±	+	+	0	+	0	+	0	0	0	+	0	0	0	0	0	0	+	+	+
Cefotaxime	+	+	0	+	0	±	0	+	+	+	+	+	±	+	+	+	+	+	+	±	0	0	+	+	0	0	0	0	0	+	+	+
Ceftriaxone	+	+	0	+	0	±	0	+	+	+	+	+	±	+	+	+	+	+	+	±	0	0	+	+	0	0	0	0	0	+	+	+
Ceftazidime	±	±	0	±	0	±	0	+	+	+	+	+	±	+	+	+	+	+	+	±	+	±	+	+	0	0	0	0	0	+	+	+
Cefepime	+	+	0	+	0	±	0	+	+	+	+	+	+	+	+	+	+	+	+	±	+	0	ND	ND	0	0	0	0	0	ND	ND	ND
Cephalexin[3]	+	+	0	+	0	±	0	0	0	±	0	±	0	+	+	0	+	0	0	0	0	0	0	0	0	0	0	0	0	ND	ND	ND
Cefuroxime axetil	+	+	0	+	0	±	0	+	+	+	+	+	0	+	+	0	+	0	+	0	0	0	0	ND	0	0	0	0	0	ND	+	+
Cefixime	+	+	0	0	0	0	0	+	+	+	+	+	0	+	+	+	+	+	+	0	0	0	+	0	0	0	0	0	0	0	+	+
Cefpodoxime proxetil	+	+	0	+	0	±	0	+	+	+	ND	+	±	+	+	±	+	+	+	0	0	0	ND	ND	0	0	0	0	0	ND	ND	ND
Gentamicin[5]	C/S	ND	C/S	C/S	C/S	C/S	C/S	0	0	ND	ND	+	+	+	+	+	0	+	ND	±	+	0	0	+	0	0	0	0	0	0	ND	0
Clindamycin	+	+	0	+	0	±	0	0	0	±	0	0	0	0	0	0	0	0	0	0	0	0	0	0	0	ND	0	0	+	+	0	+
Clarithromycin[6]	+	+	0	+	0	±	ND	+	+	+	+	0	0	0	0	0	0	0	0	0	0	0	ND	ND	+	+	+	ND	0	+	+	+
Erythromycin	+	+	0	±	0	±	±	±	±	+	±	0	0	0	0	0	0	0	0	0	0	0	0	±	+	+	+	±	0	±	+	+
Doxycycline[7]	±	±	±	±	±	±	+	+	+	+	+	±	0	0	0	0	0	0	0	0	0	±	+	+	+	+	+	+	0	+	+	±
Vancomycin	+	+	+	+	+	+	+	0	0	0	0	0	0	0	0	0	0	0	0	0	0	0	0	0	0	0	0	0	0	0	0	±
Ciprofloxacin	±	±	±	+	±	±	0	+	+	+	+	+	+	+	+	+	+	+	+	±	+	0	+	+	+	0	0	0	0	0	0	ND
Ofloxacin	±	±	±	+	±	±	ND	+	+	+	+	+	+	+	+	+	+	+	+	±	±	0	+	+	+	+	+	ND	0	+	0	ND
Trovafloxacin	+	+	±	+	+	+	ND	+	+	+	+	+	+	+	+	+	+	+	+	+	0	0	ND	+	+	+	+	+	+	+	0	ND
Levofloxacin	+	+	0	+	±	±	ND	+	0	+	+	+	+	+	+	0	+	+	+	+	±	0	ND	0	+	+	+	+	0	+	0	ND
Metronidazole	0	0	0	0	0	0	0	0	0	0	0	0	0	0	0	0	0	0	0	0	0	0	0	0	0	0	0	0	+	+	+	0
Trimethoprim/sulfamethoxazole	+	+	0	+	±	±	+	±	±	ND	+	+	±	+	+	0	+	+	+	ND	0	+	±	+	+	0	0	0	ND	ND	ND	ND
Rifampin[8]	ND	C/S	ND	C/S	+	+	+	ND	+	+	+	ND	0	ND	ND	ND	ND	ND	ND	ND	ND	ND	ND	ND	C/S	ND	ND	±	ND	ND	ND	ND

*Activity estimate is based on in vitro susceptibility and, where available, the results of treatment; activity against individual gram-negative facultative bacilli within a given species is difficult to predict. Discrepancies may exist between in vitro antimicrobial activity and clinical efficacy (especially for intracellular pathogens); review of disease-specific therapeutic recommendations is advised.

0 = uniformly or frequently resistant.

± = variable susceptibility.

+ = usually susceptible.

C/S = used in combination or for synergy.

ND = insufficient or no data.

[1]Similar activity for methicillin, nafcillin, cloxacillin, dicloxicillin.

[2]Similar activity for amoxicillin and amoxicillin/clavulanate, respectively.

[3]Similar activity for other first-generation cephalosporins.

[4]Similar activity for cefmetazole.

[5]Similar activity against gram-negative bacilli for tobramycin, netilmicin; resistance of gram-negative rods to amikacin less frequent.

[6]Similar activity for azithromycin.

[7]Similar activity for other tetracyclines.

[8]Broad spectrum of activity but resistance emerges rapidly; limit use to combination therapy or eradication of meningococcal and *H. influenzae* pharyngeal carriage.

†Relative and full resistance to penicillin increasingly prevalent; resistant to first- and second-generation cephalosporins parallels that to penicillin.

‡*E. faecium* intrinsically more resistant than *E. faecalis*; resistance to penicillin, ampicillin, vancomycin, and aminoglycosides (high level) increasingly frequent.

§Many nosocomially acquired strains are methicillin resistant.

#Some of the *B. fragilis* group (*B. thetaiotaomicron, B. distasonis, B. ovatus, B. vulgatus*) are more resistant than *B. fragilis.*

Table 318–7 ■ UNTOWARD EFFECTS OF ANTIMICROBIAL AGENTS*

AGENT	TARGET—MANIFESTATION						
	General	Skin	Gastrointestinal Tract	Blood Cells	Kidney	Nervous System	Other
Sulfonamides	Hypersensitivity, anaphylaxis, serum sickness, fever	Rash, Stevens-Johnson syndrome, photosensitivity	Hepatitis	Hemolysis (G6PD deficiency), agranulocytosis, marrow suppression	Crystalluria	Neuropathy	Vasculitis
Trimethoprim with/without sulfamethoxazole†	Fever	Rash, erythema multiforme, Stevens-Johnson syndrome, TEN	Hepatitis, pancreatitis	Marrow suppression	Hyperkalemia, acute renal failure		
Penicillin	Hypersensitivity, anaphylaxis, Jarisch-Herxheimer reaction (syphilis), serum sickness	Rash, urticaria, erythema multiforme	Diarrhea (ampicillin, amoxicillin/clavulanate), hepatitis (oxacillin)	Coombs' test positive, impaired platelet function (carbenicillin, ticarcillin), leukopenia, thrombocytopenia	Nephritis (methicillin), hypokalemia, alkalosis (carboxy/ureidopenicillins)	Seizures, twitching (high doses, renal failure)	Inactivate aminoglycosides when admixed, possible with concurrent therapy in renal failure
Cephalosporins	Serum sickness (cefaclor), hypersensitivity, anaphylaxis (rare)	Rash, urticaria	Diarrhea (cefoperazone), hepatitic dysfunction, precipitates in bile (ceftriaxone), mild increase in LFT	Neutropenia, increased prothrombin time, bleeding (relates to MTT side chain), impaired platelet function (moxalactam), Coombs' test positive	Enhance aminoglycoside toxicity, acute renal failure (rare), nephritis		Disulfiram-like reaction with concurrent alcohol use (MTT side chain)
Carbapenems	Hypersensitivity	Rash, urticaria, erythema multiforme	Nausea, vomiting, abnormal LFT	Bone marrow suppression, Coombs' test positive	Renal dysfunction	Seizures, myoclonus (reduced with meropenem)	
Chloramphenicol	Fever			Marrow suppression (dose related), aplastic anemia		Optic neuritis, neuropathy	Circulatory collapse (gray baby syndrome—neonate)
Tetracyclines	Allergy	Photosensitization (doxycycline, demeclocycline)	Hepatotoxicity in azotemia or pregnancy, gastrointestinal discomfort		Catabolic aggravation of azotemia (except doxycycline)	Vertigo (minocycline)	Deposition in bone (dysplasia) and teeth (staining)
Erythromycin	Fever	Rash	Gastrointestinal discomfort, nausea, cholestatic jaundice (erythromycin estolate)			Decreased hearing	Phlebitis if given through peripheral veins
Metronidazole	Headache, allergy		Nausea, metallic taste, pancreatitis	Leukopenia		Peripheral neuropathy, ataxia	Mutagenic, carcinogenic in rodents; disulfiram-like reaction with alcohol
Vancomycin	Allergy, fever	Rash		Leukopenia, thrombocytopenia	Nephrotoxic with aminoglycoside	Decreased hearing (serum > 50 μg/mL), neuropathy	Histamine release with flushing and hypotension (infusion < 1 hr—antihistamines prevent)
Aminoglycosides	Fever	Rash			Renal failure	Irreversible vestibular toxicity (streptomycin, gentamicin, tobramycin), irreversible auditory damage (kanamycin, netilmicin, amikacin)	Neuromuscular blockade (with anesthetics and myasthenia—calcium reverses)
Quinolones	Headache, allergy, anaphylaxis (rare)	Rash, photosensitization (pefloxacin, sparfloxacin, fleroxacin), urticaria	Gastrointestinal distress, LFT abnormalities			Dizziness, insomnia, nervousness, tremors, visual changes, seizures, pseudotumor cerebri	Cartilage deposition and arthropathy (animal studies), tendinitis and rupture (Achilles), electrocardiogram QT prolongation (sparfloxacin, grepafloxacin)

TEN = toxic epidermal necrolysis; MTT = methylthiotetrazole ring (see Table 318–4); LFT = liver function tests.
*Not all reactions are listed; check other sources for unusual reactions.
†Reactions to sulfonamides are not repeated.

microbial therapy must be evaluated in the light of available microbiologic data and new culture data sought to explain the failure of therapy. Explanations for fever other than failure of antimicrobial therapy must be considered; these range from a new superimposed infection to a non-infectious complication or a drug reaction. Additionally, reasons for the failure of appropriate therapy must be considered. These include (1) the presence of anatomic abnormalities or an obstructed drainage system; (2) an undrained abscess; (3) the presence of a foreign body or the equivalent (renal calculus, osteomyelitic sequestrum) at the site of infection; (4) impaired host defenses; (5) infection in infarcted tissue; (6) emergence of resistance in the original pathogen or a resistant superinfecting organism; and (7) suboptimal antibiotic therapy because of poor penetration to the site or physical inactivation (local pH) of the antibiotic. The physician must search diligently to explain and correct the antibiotic failure.

Acar JF, Kaplan EL, O'Brien TF (eds): Monitoring and management of bacterial resistance to antimicrobial agents: A World Health Organization symposium. Clin Infect Dis 24(Suppl 1), 1997. *A careful examination by international experts of the mechanisms of antimicrobial resistance, the extent of resistance among major pathogens, and global challenge of antimicrobial resistance.*

Andriole VT (ed): The Quinolones, 2nd ed. San Diego, Academic Press, 1998. *An authoritative monograph detailing the chemistry, pharmacology, and clinical use of this important class of antimicrobial agents.*

Craig WA: Pharmacokinetic/pharmacodynamic parameters: Rationale for antibacterial dosing of mice and men. Clin Infect Dis 26:1, 1998. *A detailed explanation of the concepts of pharmacodynamics as applied to antimicrobial therapy and an illustration of the scientific principles that give rise to effective antibiotic dosing.*

Davies J: Inactivation of antibiotics and the dissemination of resistance genes. Science 264:375, 1994. *Detailed discussion of the major mechanisms whereby bacteria inactivate antibiotics. The original sources of the genes conveying these abilities are considered.*

Gilbert DN, Moellering RC Jr, Sande MA: The Sanford Guide to Antimicrobial Therapy 1998. Vienna, VA, Antimicrobial Therapy, Inc, 1998. *Pocket guide to antibiotic use that is remarkably detailed. It is updated and published annually.*

Kucers A, Crowe SM, Grayson ML, Hoy JF (eds): The Use of Antibiotics: A Clinical Review of Antibacterial, Antifungal and Antiviral Drugs, 5th ed. Oxford, UK: Butterworth-Heinemann, 1997. *An extensively referenced definitive text on antimicrobial agents including antibacterial, antiviral, and antifungal drugs.*

Nikaido H: Prevention of drug access to bacterial targets: Permeability barriers and active efflux. Science 264:382, 1994. *Detailed consideration of permeability and active efflux mechanisms as used by bacteria in resisting antibiotics. Special attention is directed toward active efflux systems increasingly recognized as important in antibiotic resistance.*

Spratt BG: Resistance to antibiotics mediated by target alterations. Science 264:388, 1994. *Readable discussion of antibiotic resistance that results from changes in targets and resulting reductions in the affinity of antibiotics for their sites of action. Major focus is alterations in penicillin-binding proteins.*

Gold HS, Moellering RC Jr: Antimicrobial-drug resistance. N Engl J Med 335:1445, 1996. *A readable lucid examination of selected aspects of antimicrobial resistance, including that due to β-lactamases, penicillin resistance in S. pneumoniae, and vancomycin resistance in enterococci.*

319 PNEUMOCOCCAL PNEUMONIA

Richard J. Duma

DEFINITION. Pneumococcal pneumonia is an acute, suppurative infection of the lungs produced by an encapsulated bacterium, *Streptococcus pneumoniae* (pneumococcus). It is the most commonly occurring bacterial pneumonia in the world; in the United States, an estimated 150,000 to 570,000 cases occur annually.

MICROBIOLOGY. Virulent *S. pneumoniae* organisms are encapsulated, gram-positive cocci about 0.8 μm in diameter that occur in chains (streptococci) or pairs (diplococci) (see Color Plate 9E). When in pairs, cocci are characteristically lancet shaped; i.e., each coccus is pointed at the end like the tip of a lance, and the bases are in juxtaposition. The capsule, which is a complex polysaccharide that varies in chemical composition and thickness, is not seen with Gram staining but may be recognized by negative staining (e.g., with India ink or methylene blue). In purulent clinical specimens, some pneumococci stain negatively rather than positively with Gram stain because aging, exposure of the cell wall to a variety of destructive host enzymes (e.g., lysozyme), and/or inhibition of cell wall synthesis by antibiotics (e.g., penicillin) result in incomplete or abnormal bacterial cell walls that no longer retain the iodine-fixed crystal violet stain.

Pneumococci are fastidious, facultative bacteria that grow best in the presence of blood or serum and in air supplemented with 10% carbon dioxide. Because they are fermentative and lactic acid is the usual end product, concentrations of glucose in the culture media must be controlled and should not exceed 1%. In addition, because they produce hydrogen peroxide (H_2O_2) but not catalase, the addition of a catalase source (e.g., red blood cells) enhances growth. Viability is reduced by drying, a low pH (<6.5), and prolonged incubation.

On blood agar after overnight incubation at 37° C, colonies generally appear mucoid, glistening, and dome shaped and are surrounded by an area of greening (α-hemolysis) within the blood agar. With continued incubation, as aged bacteria undergo autolysis, the colony domes of highly encapsulated strains collapse centrally and appear umbilicated. An important biologic feature that distinguishes *S. pneumoniae* from other streptococci is its bile solubility or susceptibility to surface-active agents such as sodium deoxycholate and ethyl hydrocuprein chloride (optochin). The latter agent (optochin) is incorporated into a standardized 5-μg disk and used worldwide to identify pneumococci rapidly. However, because optochin-resistant pneumococci occasionally occur and some nonpneumococcal α-hemolytic streptococci are optochin sensitive, for purposes of species determination, the usefulness of this biologic property may be questioned.

Pneumococcal virulence is often studied in the mouse because this animal is highly sensitive to encapsulated pneumococci (with the exception of type 14). Indeed, the sensitivity of mice to encapsulated pneumococci may be used for rapidly and selectively isolating virulent pneumococci from sputum specimens or from clinical materials containing other bacteria. If injected into the peritoneal cavity of the mouse, an exudate containing pneumococci may be harvested in 24 hours.

Unlike many other streptococci, particularly those belonging to Lancefield group A, and unlike other pyogenic bacteria that produce pneumonia, *S. pneumoniae* does not produce any major toxins, particularly none that are tissue destructive. Some strains may elaborate hyaluronidase, and all contain pneumolysin, a hemolytic cytotoxic protein, released when the organism undergoes autolysis, that disrupts the respiratory epithelium and slows ciliary movement.

The most important factor defining virulent *S. pneumoniae* is the presence of a high-molecular-weight complex polysaccharide capsule, which is a potent inhibitor of neutrophil phagocytosis. At least 84 different immunogenic types of capsules exist, and two different nomenclatures (Danish and American) are used to number them (which is often a source of confusion). Antigenically distinct capsules are easily identified with polyvalent antisera in an agglutination or precipitin test or by the Neufeld quellung reaction, a rapid test based on visualization of refractile swelling of the capsule after application of a polyvalent or monovalent type-specific antiserum to the bacterium in question. Non-encapsulated pneumococci, which are generally avirulent, do not react with antipolysaccharide antisera. Although identification of pneumococcal capsular antigen in certain body fluids or secretions may suggest active pneumococcal infection (see below), immunologic tests to detect such antigens must be interpreted with caution because antibodies against some pneumococcal capsular serotypes cross-react with polysaccharides of other streptococci (particularly group B), *Haemophilus influenzae* type B, *Escherichia coli, Klebsiella pneumoniae, Salmonella* species, and even human ABO blood group isoantigens.

Capsular polysaccharides consist of repeating di- or penta-oligosaccharides, some of which contain large proportions of acid constituents such as cellobiuronic, hexuronic, and pyruvic acid. Most are linear, although some are branched, and their antigenicities result principally from oligosaccharide epitopes of no more than six or seven sugar residues. The frequency of capsular types observed varies with time, geography, and the age of the patient; for example, types 6, 14, 18, 19, and 23 are common in infants and children, whereas types 1, 2, 3, 5, and 8 are common in adults.

The susceptibility of pneumococci to most chemotherapeutic antibacterials, especially to the β-lactams (except the monobactams), is generally good; however, this pattern appears to be rapidly changing. For penicillin G, the antibiotic against which all other antibacterials are compared, *susceptibility* is defined as inhibition of growth of pneumococci at a concentration of less than 0.1 μg/mL

Table 319–1 ■ MIC$_{90}$ OF SOME COMMONLY USED β-LACTAM ANTIBIOTICS AGAINST PENICILLIN-RESISTANT PNEUMOCOCCI

| ANTIBIOTIC | MIC$_{90}$ (μg/mL) | |
	Intermediate Penicillin Resistance	High-Level Penicillin Resistance
Ampicillin	0.5	8
Oxacillin	4.0	31
Methicillin	—	64
Carbenicillin	32.0	64
Ticarcillin	64.0	128
Piperacillin	1.0	8–16
Mezlocillin	1.0–2.0	8–15
Azlocillin	1.0	16
Cephalothin	1.0	8–31
Cefaclor	4.0–16.0	16
Cefonicid	16.0	16
Cefoxitin	4.0–8.0	32–125
Cefamandole	0.5–2.0	8–31
Cefuroxime	0.25–0.44	—
Cefotaxime	0.125–1.0	1–4
Ceftriaxone	0.12–0.5	1
Ceftazidime	3.2–32.0	64
Cefoperazone	1.0–2.0	2–16
Moxalactam	2.0–4.0	128
Imipenem	0.06–1.0	1–2

MIC$_{90}$ = minimal inhibitory concentration at which 90% of strains are susceptible.
Adapted with permission from Klugman KP: Pneumococcal resistance to antibiotics. Clin Microbiol Rev 3:171, 1990.

(referred to as the *minimum inhibitory concentration* [MIC]). However, since 1968, when penicillin-resistant strains were first identified in clinical isolates from Australia, a significant but variable percentage of isolates are defined as *intermediately* (i.e., MIC, ≥ 0.1 to < 2.0 μg/mL) or *highly resistant* (i.e., MIC, ≥ 2.0 μg/mL). Strains that are highly resistant to penicillin G are resistant to a wide array of other β-lactams (Table 319–1) but may be susceptible to the 3rd-generation cephalosporins ceftriaxone and cefotaxime and to the carbapenems. Presently, all pneumococci are susceptible to vancomycin and teicoplanin, agents generally reserved for serious, life-threatening infections (e.g., meningitis).

Other effective antibacterials often used clinically include the macrolides (e.g., erythromycin), lincosines (e.g., clindamycin), some of the newer fluoroquinolones (e.g., levofloxacin), chloramphenicol, and the rifamycins (e.g., rifampin). However, strains that are highly resistant to penicillin G (see Table 319–1) are often resistant to many of these antibacterials, especially the macrolides. Resistance of pneumococci to β-lactams is *not* due to bacterial production of a β-lactamase or a cephalosporinase and is *not* plasmid mediated; rather, it results from transformation of previously susceptible strains by DNA from penicillin-resistant, related streptococci and from point mutations of host chromosomal elements and/or newly acquired transposons. These newly formed genetic elements dictate the production of aberrant target membrane, penicillin-binding proteins that have little or no affinity for penicillin G or other β-lactams, thus rendering the penicillins ineffective.

Pneumococci are relatively resistant to aminoglycosides; in fact, gentamicin may be incorporated into primary culture media for selective isolation of pneumococci from sputum because it suppresses the growth of concurrent bacteria. Furthermore, in some studies more than 50% of pneumococcal isolates are resistant to tetracyclines.

EPIDEMIOLOGY. Pneumococcal pneumonia is generally a community-acquired, sporadic disease that occurs most often during the coldest months of the year. More recently, it has been recognized as an occasional cause of nosocomial pneumonia. The vast majority of cases occur after aspiration of "normal" oropharyngeal secretions that may contain encapsulated pneumococci, followed by an inability to clear such secretions; thus oropharyngeal carrier rates of pneumococci are important in the dynamics of acquiring pneumococcal pneumonia, its spread, and its frequency of occurrence within a population.

Because most data referable to oropharyngeal carrier rates were obtained before the use of pneumococcal vaccine, colonization rates with (or carriage of) certain serotypes and the relative importance

of factors that have an impact on carriage must be interpreted with caution. Nevertheless, in longitudinal, pre-vaccine studies of pneumococcal oropharyngeal carriage by people living in temperate zones, serotypes with USA numbers of 23 or less are most frequently encountered, further suggesting that humans are infected by their own endogenous flora inasmuch as more than half the cases of pneumococcal pneumonia and bacteremia are caused by these strains. Clustering of one serotype within a family commonly occurs, and carriage rates do not appear to be affected by gender. Rates of carriage are higher in children, particularly those of pre-school age, than in adults; and among adults, rates are highest in those intimately exposed to pre-school children. Oropharyngeal carriage appears to be highest during the coolest months of the year (fall, winter, and early spring), when respiratory infections are common, and spread may be enhanced during respiratory tract infections by pneumococcus or certain respiratory viruses such as rhinovirus. Although the prevalence of oropharyngeal carriage in the surrounding community or within households affects the risk of individual acquisition, crowding does not appear to be important. The duration of oropharyngeal carriage of a particular serotype ranges from 2 weeks to years, the mean being 6 to 8 weeks. Reacquisition of the same serotype commonly occurs. In children but not usually adults, initial acquisition within a family setting is frequently associated with rises in homotypic serum antibody and occasionally with illness.

Although epidemics of pneumococcal pneumonia may occur, they are *rare* and generally appear in special populations at high risk for pneumococcal disease, such as domiciliary populations of alcoholics, institutionalized elderly, Navajo Indians, New Guinea highlanders, Alaskan natives, and South African gold miners. In studies of ambulatory adult populations, a variety of risk factors appear to predispose to the development of pneumococcal infections (Table 319–2).

IMMUNOLOGY. In non-immunized, untreated patients, specific anticapsular humoral antibody (IgM and IgG) can be detected in the blood 5 to 10 days after infection and correlates with the clearance of pneumococci and eventual recovery. Both classic and alternative-pathway complement (C'3) and type-specific opsonizing antibody, principally IgG (IgG1 in children and IgG2 and IgG4 in adults), enhance the phagocytosis and intracellular killing of pneumococci by polymorphonuclear leukocytes and alveolar macrophages, the major host defense mechanism for eradicating pneumococci. Patients with deficiencies of biologically active IgM, IgG, and to a lesser degree, IgA (particularly secretory) are more susceptible to pneumococcal pneumonia and other pneumococcal infections than are normal persons without such deficiencies. In normal persons, once specific anticapsular antibodies form, they generally persist for life.

If pneumococci escape this host defense mechanism, they may

Table 319–2 ■ **RISK FACTORS OR UNDERLYING CONDITIONS PREDISPOSING TO THE DEVELOPMENT OF PNEUMOCOCCAL PNEUMONIA OR SERIOUS PNEUMOCOCCAL INFECTIONS**

Age (extremes)
Alcoholism
Bone marrow transplantation
Bronchiectasis
Cerebrovascular occlusions or severe neurologic impairment
Chronic bronchitis
Chronic lymphocytic leukemia
Chronic obstructive pulmonary disease
Cirrhosis or chronic liver disease
Complement deficiency (particularly C'3 and C'4)
Conditions associated with aspiration (e.g., seizures)
Congestive heart failure
Dementia
Diabetes mellitus
Immunologic deficiencies (acquired, hereditary, or iatrogenic)—humoral (IgG or IgA) or cellular (e.g., AIDS)
Institutionalization, homelessness, day care centers
Malignancy (particularly solid tumors of the lung)
Multiple myeloma
Nephrotic syndrome
Neutropenia
Smoking
Splenic dysfunction (e.g., in sickle cell disease) or asplenia
Viral diseases, especially influenza

enter the blood stream via lymph channels and the thoracic duct and produce bacteremia. Clearance from the blood also depends on opsonization via type-specific antibodies and activated complement; however, liver and spleen macrophages rather than polymorphonuclear leukocytes are principally responsible for removing pneumococci from the blood. Thus splenectomy or cirrhosis of the liver rather than neutropenia increases the risk for pneumococcal bacteremia, dissemination, and death.

PATHOGENESIS AND PATHOLOGY. Most cases of pneumococcal pneumonia result from the aspiration of oropharyngeal material containing indigenous, virulent pneumococci into terminal bronchioles and alveoli, followed by atelectasis and an inability to clear bacteria from these sites. Although microaspiration is a natural event that occurs commonly, pneumonia in normal individuals seldom results because pulmonary bacterial clearance and/or local host defense mechanisms are generally adequate and intact and are not defective or suppressed. These important defense mechanisms, which serve as either a barrier against or a clearance for bacteria, are the epiglottic reflex, ciliary escalator and mucous blanket, secretory and humoral immunoglobulins, surfactant, alveolar macrophage and polymorphonuclear leukocyte activity, and lymphatic drainage. When these mechanisms are blunted or overwhelmed by aspirated noxious material, by large inocula of pneumococci, by a highly virulent strain, and/or by material containing additional pathogens, pneumonia may result. In addition, once infection occurs, further atelectasis from inspissated material may result.

After pneumococci establish themselves in the lung, the first visible evidence of an inflammatory response is localized capillary dilatation and hyperemia, the appearance of serous edema within alveoli, followed by margination, diapedesis, and chemotaxis of polymorphonuclear cells induced by immunoglobulins and/or activated complement. In addition, pneumococci produce a soluble, oxygen-labile 53-kd toxin, pneumolysin, that is cytotoxic to pulmonary endothelial cells and may be important in the early phases of pneumonia and entry of *S. pneumoniae* into the blood. Fluid-filled alveoli enhance the passage of bacteria through the pores of Kohn and into terminal bronchioles, with spread to contiguous, uninfected alveoli forming the advancing margins of the disease. If clearance and host immune mechanisms are adequate at this stage, the infection may resolve. However, if not, the disease may spread until the pleura and interlobar fissures are reached and consolidation with dense infiltrates of polymorphonuclear leukocytes and extravasated red blood cells occurs (see Color Plates 9A to 9C).

Pneumococcal pneumonia may involve an entire lobe (lobar pneumonia), multiple lobes (multilobar pneumonia), or just segments of a lobe and produce a patchy area (or areas) of pneumonia (pneumonitis). At times, infection spreads concentrically from bronchi (bronchopneumonia), a pattern occasionally seen in infants and the elderly. In the central and oldest portions of infection, consolidation with massive numbers of polymorphonuclear leukocytes predominates, whereas peripheral to this are new areas of hemorrhage, infiltrating polymorphonuclear cells, and edema. Early pathologists referred to these areas in the lung as "gray hepatization" and "red hepatization," respectively, because of the gross resemblance of involved lung to liver tissue (see Color *Plate 9A*). In fully developed, untreated pneumococcal pneumonia, all stages of the cellular inflammatory process may be present.

In 5 to 10% of patients, infection may extend into the pleural space and result in an *empyema,* or in 15 to 25% of patients, bacteria may enter the blood stream (*bacteremia*) via the lymphatics and thoracic duct. Invasion of the blood stream by pneumococci may lead to serious metastatic disease at a number of extrapulmonary sites (Table 319–3), the most important and most frequent of which is the subarachnoid space (*meningitis.*) Other infections that may occur from bacteremic spread are *septic arthritis, pericarditis, endocarditis* (infection of the heart valves), and in patients with ascites, *peritonitis (spontaneous bacterial peritonitis.)* In addition, pneumococci may concurrently infect other tissues or organs such as the sinopulmonary system, air sinuses (*sinusitis*), mastoids (*mastoiditis,*) ears (*otitis media,*) conjunctivae (pyogenic *conjunctivitis*), epiglottis (*epiglottiditis,* particularly in infants), or rarely the soft tissues of the neck or retropharyngeal area (*Ludwig's angina.*)

CLINICAL FINDINGS. The features of acute bacterial pneumonia caused by *S. pneumoniae* may be highly variable, depending on when the patient is seen by the physician in the course of the disease, whether or not bacteremia and/or dissemination has occurred, the patient's age, whether or not effective antibiotics were

Table 319–3 ■ CONCURRENT OR COMPLICATING PNEUMOCOCCAL INFECTIONS OCCURRING IN PNEUMOCOCCAL PNEUMONIA
Otitis media
Sinusitis/mastoiditis
Conjunctivitis (suppurative)
Epiglottiditis
Tracheobronchitis
Pleuritis (empyema)
Soft tissue cellulitis (Ludwig's angina)
Pericarditis*
Endocarditis*
Meningitis*
Arthritis (septic)*
Peritonitis (in presence of ascites)*

*Usually blood-borne.

previously administered, the presence or absence of satisfactory host defenses, and the existence of risk factors for dissemination of pneumococci (e.g., asplenia, neutropenia, and agammaglobulinemia). The manifestations may be mild or explosive and rapidly lethal. Classically, the onset of acute pneumococcal pneumonia is sudden and characterized by an abrupt occurrence of cough, chills, high fever (up to 40 °C), myalgias, tachypnea, shallow respirations, tachycardia, weakness, and often frank rigors. Initially the cough may be productive of scant mucopurulent or blood-streaked sputum; later (after 24 to 48 hours) it may be thick, purulent, frankly bloody or rust-colored, and consistent with an alveolar, hemorrhagic, exudative process. If the infecting pneumococcus is highly encapsulated, a gelatinous, blood-tinged sputum may be seen. The presence of pleuritic pain is specific clinical evidence that the pneumonia is probably bacterial and, in the presence of most of the above findings, probably pneumococcal.

Patients with pneumococcal pneumonia are generally diaphoretic and, in addition, may be dehydrated and hypotensive. Anorexia, nausea, and vomiting are common. If allowed to continue untreated, single-lobe disease may progress to multilobe involvement, and the patient may become dusky, cyanotic, and confused. If bacteremia occurs, chills and rigors may persist, and rarely shock, disseminated intravascular coagulopathy (DIC), and/or adult respiratory distress syndrome may supervene and ultimately lead to the patient's death.

A history is frequently elicited of a recent upper respiratory or viral-like illness that has occurred before the appearance of clinical pneumonia, especially during the winter months, when influenza is common. Risk factors for aspiration, such as alcoholism, seizures, or vomiting, or for acquiring pneumococcal pneumonia may be present (see above).

On physical examination, the acutely ill patient is tachypneic and may be observed to use accessory muscles for respiration (intercostal, abdominal, and sternocleidomastoid) and even to exhibit nasal flaring. If pleuritic pain is severe, reflex splinting of the ipsilateral thorax is observed. Fever and tachycardia are present, and although hypotension may occur, frank shock is unusual, except in the later stages of infection or DIC.

Auscultation of the chest reveals bronchovesicular or tubular breath sounds and wet rales over the involved lung. As consolidation occurs, vocal and tactile fremitus is increased; however, if a concurrent pleural effusion is present, breath sounds and fremitus may be diminished or absent. A localized, grating pleural friction rub may occasionally be heard.

Examination of the upper respiratory passages may be helpful in suggesting a diagnosis of pneumococcal pneumonia. For example, in children the absence of exudative pharyngitis and the presence of otitis media might suggest pneumococcal involvement. In older children and adults, the air sinuses and/or mastoids may be acutely infected. (However, these infections can also occur with streptococcal, staphylococcal, and *H. influenzae* pneumonia.)

Evidence of extrapulmonary infections may be present, particularly in untreated disease lasting more than 48 hours; for example, signs of meningeal irritation (stiff neck, Kernig's or Brudzinski's sign) with abnormalities in mentation may suggest meningitis; the appearance of pathologic heart murmurs, splenomegaly, and heart failure may be evidence of endocarditis; or the presence of pain, swelling, tenderness, heat, and possibly redness in one or more joints may point toward a septic arthritis of hematogenous origin.

Additional findings unrelated to pneumonia per se but related to sepsis and/or toxicity may be noted: a paralytic ileus with abdominal pain, distention, and loss of bowel sounds; mild jaundice from reactive hepatitis or intrapulmonary hemorrhage; frank shock; purpuric lesions resulting from DIC; or symmetrical gangrene and purpura of the fingers and/or toes (*purpura fulminans*) associated with bacteremia.

LABORATORY FINDINGS. The peripheral white blood cell (WBC) count is often two to three times the normal value; however, in alcoholics or immunosuppressed patients, it may be normal or low. Of more value is the WBC differential, which consists predominantly of bands and polymorphonuclear leukocytes (left shift). If DIC is suspected, thrombocytopenia, pleomorphism of red blood cells (schistocytes and helmet cells), prolonged prothrombin and partial thromboplastin times, and hypofibrinogenemia and circulating fibrin split products may be present.

In some patients, total bilirubin and hepatic cellular enzyme levels may be slightly elevated. Because dehydration and hypovolemia commonly occur (secondary to fever, diaphoresis, nausea, and vomiting), the hemoglobin, hematocrit, and serum sodium level may be elevated. When pneumonia is the dominant clinical event, arterial blood gas studies, which reflect pulmonary function and compensatory events, usually reveal hypoxemia (low PO_2), hypocapnia (low PCO_2), and alkalosis (blood pH >7.4) resulting from hyperventilation and shunting. However, if frank shock intervenes, a metabolic acidosis may result (blood pH <7.4); if it is not corrected, death may follow.

Good posteroanterior and lateral chest radiographs are important to obtain, initially to confirm the presence and to ascertain the extent and radiographic character of the pneumonia and secondly, to determine whether underlying predisposing pulmonary diseases are present such as bronchiectasis, bronchial obstruction, emphysema, tumor, or tuberculosis. In severely dehydrated or profoundly neutropenic or immunodeficient patients, early inflammatory infiltrates may not be seen radiographically or may be patchy and irregular in appearance, but after hydration or restoration of circulating levels of inflammatory cells, patterns of lobar consolidation may become apparent.

Characteristically, in immunocompetent patients with untreated, frank pneumococcal pneumonia, chest radiographs reveal a lobar distribution and an air space (or alveolar exudative) pattern of disease with an air bronchogram effect. However, if prior, partially effective antibiotic usage has occurred, the pattern may be atypical, and a lobar distribution may be the exception rather than the rule. Interlobar fissures may bulge because of the considerable fluid content within the involved lung associated with large amounts of capsular material. In severe cases, more than one lobe may be involved (multilobar pneumonia). In 30% of cases, a pleural effusion may be present and may be readily detected by a lateral decubitus film. Such effusions may be sterile and represent parapneumonic collections of fluid, or occasionally they may be infected with pneumococci, in which case they are called *empyemas*.

If blunting of the costophrenic angle is noted radiographically and the finding is believed to represent an effusion, at least 300 to 500 mL of fluid is probably present and thoracentesis is indicated. Unless contraindicated, *every pleural effusion associated with an acute bacterial pneumonia in which the etiology of the pneumonia is unclear should be tapped and the fluid studied for microorganisms* (see Color Plate 9D). Ordinarily, fluid removed from the pleural space is sterile, so any bacteria seen on a Gram stain or cultured from the fluid represent pathogens until proved otherwise.

Other important laboratory studies *that must be obtained early in the patient's work-up* are routine cultures of the blood, microscopic examination of a Gram stain and culture *of purulent material from the site of infection* (alveoli, bronchi, or lung), and examination of any infected material that can be removed from a secondarily infected extrapulmonary focus. Results of blood cultures may not be available for 18 to 24 hours and thus cannot assist the physician in making a presumptive diagnosis or in selecting appropriate initial chemotherapy. Often, in asplenic patients a high-grade bacteremia occurs, so examination of the peripheral WBC smear or the buffy coat for pneumococci may be useful.

Microscopic examination and cultures of expectorated purulent sputum from a patient with acute bacterial pneumonia are essential if a correct presumptive etiologic diagnosis is to be made and an appropriate antibiotic is to be given. Ideally, these tests should be done before therapy is initiated; however, significant delay in instituting therapy should not be permitted. Attention must be given to obtaining a diagnostically useful sputum sample; that is, material must be purulent to be presumed to be from the site of infection. Salivary or oropharyngeal gross contamination of the sample should be avoided.

In a patient with the clinical picture of acute bacterial pneumonia, the finding of gram-positive diplococci in expectorated sputum that contains ≥ 50 polymorphonuclear cells per $100\times$ field (purulent sputum) and few (<10 squamous cells per $100\times$ field) or no squamous epithelial cells (which indicates little or no oropharyngeal contamination of the specimen) is strong presumptive evidence of pneumococcal pneumonia.

Cultures of expectorated sputum are also important but are not without problems; for example, because *S. pneumoniae* is fastidious, it may fail to grow in culture, but negative culture results do not exclude its presence. In addition, pneumococci may be overlooked because they may be overgrown by other organisms or mixed with similar-appearing, non-pneumococcal, α-hemolytic streptococci, which are normally present in oropharyngeal secretions. On the other hand, because *S. pneumoniae* is often present normally in the oropharynx, its growth from sputum, especially from expectorated sputum, may not be indicative of pneumococcal disease. Perhaps the main value of securing a sputum culture is to confirm or question observations made from the Gram stain and, if pneumococci (and/or other bacteria) are ultimately isolated, to perform antibiotic susceptibility testing.

If the patient is unable to expectorate purulent sputum for microscopic examination and culture and if other infected materials (e.g., pleural or joint fluid) are not available or are negative for pneumococci, various procedures for obtaining pus from the infected lung must be considered. Cough can be induced by having the patient inhale an aerosol of warm 3% NaCl; a plastic catheter can be inserted into the trachea via the nose or throat and suction applied; a direct transtracheal needle and catheter aspiration may be performed (a procedure not without complications); the patient may undergo endoscopy (provided that arterial PO_2 is ≥ 50 mm Hg), and alveolar washings or bronchial brushings may be obtained; or rarely, direct aspiration of the pneumonic infiltrate through the chest wall with a long, "skinny" needle (22 gauge) may be used (a procedure also not without risks). Open-lung biopsies for pneumococcal pneumonia are not indicated, although they may be for certain complications, ill-defined superinfections, or underlying diseases. In any acute bacterial pneumonia, the guiding principles for deciding what procedure, if any, to use for obtaining purulent sputum from the involved lung for diagnostic study are as follows: (1) if expectorated sputum is satisfactory (i.e., purulent and relatively free of contaminating oropharyngeal material), further efforts to obtain pus from the deeper recesses of the lung are probably not necessary; (2) if additional procedures are necessary, one should initially select the procedure that is least traumatic and invasive and is risk-free and then proceed, if necessary, in stepwise fashion to the next least invasive, risk-free procedure until satisfactory material is obtained; (3) one should not delay more than several hours before beginning chemotherapy, and if the patient is extremely ill, one must rely on clinical judgment and probabilities and not delay treatment, and (4) one must make every effort to identify the etiologic agent (or agents) responsible for the pneumonia early in the course of the illness because once this goal is realized, the chances of managing the patient successfully are markedly enhanced.

A variety of other tests may be applied to sputum specimens to identify pneumococci in acute bacterial pneumonia, but in skilled hands, few, if any, are better, less costly, easier to do, and more informative than the Gram stain. All tests done on sputum possess a similar problem in interpretation, namely, determining whether the bacteria present in the sample are responsible for the pneumonia observed. If blood or pleural fluid cultures are subsequently positive for *S. pneumoniae,* the etiologic agent is confirmed, although the presence of additional pathogenic bacteria within the lung may not be entirely excluded because blood or pleural fluid cultures may rarely yield other bacteria (polymicrobial infection) in addition to pneumococci.

Detection of pneumococcal capsular antigen generally requires the presence of approximately 10^5 bacteria per milliliter, about the same concentration required to observe an average of one bacterium per $1000\times$ field (or an oil-immersion field on a standard light microscope) on a Gram stain. Cross-reactions with other antigens of other bacteria are frequent, and with certain serotypes, false-positive results are common. Perhaps the greatest value of capsular antigen detection is to confirm the presence of pneumococci in patients who have been partially treated and in whom sputum cultures may be negative and a Gram stain may reveal few, if any, intact bacteria.

Colony counts of bacteria from bronchoalveolar lavage washings obtained during endoscopy are seldom available early in the course of illness. Specimens must be obtained with a special cuffed endoscope so that oropharyngeal contamination does not occur with insertion of the scope. Generally, counts of colony-forming units of bacteria higher than 10^3 to 10^5 per milliliter of fluid removed are considered significant, but such counts are not invariably found.

DNA hybridization studies may be performed directly on the sputum, but as with capsular antigen detection, adequate numbers of bacteria must be present for the test to be positive. Use of the polymerase chain reaction may amplify pneumococcal DNA and improve the potential for detection; however, such enhanced sensitivity may lead to false-positive results caused by very small numbers of contaminating pneumococci.

Elastase or elastin fibers in sputum may suggest the presence of a gram-negative bacillary necrotizing pneumonia, particularly that caused by *Pseudomonas,* but this test is of little value in the diagnosis of pneumococcal pneumonia (other than that the test should be negative) because necrosis of tissue is not produced by pneumococci.

DIFFERENTIAL DIAGNOSIS. (See also Chapter 82 and chapters dealing with the specific organisms.) The clinical picture and many of the routine laboratory and radiographic features associated with pneumococcal pneumonia are often indistinguishable from those of other acute bacterial pneumonias. Thus collecting appropriate microbiologic data is essential if the correct etiologic diagnosis is to be made.

In adults, the second most common community-acquired, acute bacterial pneumonia is that caused by *H. influenzae.* Gram stain of purulent sputum from such patients often reveals myriads of tiny gram-negative coccobacilli, with the observation of an occasional filamentous form. Such an infection often occurs in a patient with chronic bronchitis or chronic obstructive pulmonary disease and is usually due to non-encapsulated *H. influenzae* (as opposed to highly encapsulated, serotype B strains commonly associated with young children).

Staphylococcus aureus is another bacterium occasionally producing acute pneumonia, but when this kind of pneumonia is community-acquired, it usually occurs during or just after an epidemic of viral influenza. In the hospital setting, *S. aureus* may be seen year-round because it is a commonly occurring nosocomial infection. If a highly virulent, toxin-producing strain is responsible, the "toxic shock syndrome" may be observed. On a Gram stain of purulent sputum, clusters and characteristic tetrads of gram-positive cocci are seen. Late in the clinical course, abscess formation or destruction of the lung occurs.

Group A streptococci (*S. pyogenes*) also produce acute pneumonia, and in such instances the patient may be more toxic appearing than the extent of involvement of the lung might suggest. Classically, a small, peripherally located, wedge-shaped infiltrate is seen, and a thin, watery, serosanguineous, pleural effusion is present. A radiograph of the chest may suggest pulmonary infarction. An upper respiratory tract infection, particularly an exudative or erythematous pharyngitis or tonsillitis (especially in children), may be present, and an erythematous rash produced by streptococcal erythrogenic toxin (scarlet fever) may be seen. Gram staining of purulent sputum usually reveals numerous short chains of gram-positive cocci or diplococci. Thus the Gram stain may not differentiate group A streptococcal from pneumococcal pneumonia.

Branhamella catarrhalis may produce acute pneumonia, but this pneumonia usually occurs in the elderly, particularly in those with chronic bronchitis or obstructive lung disease. It is a relatively benign infection when compared with those produced by other pyogenic bacteria and is rarely, if ever associated with bacteremia. A Gram stain of purulent sputum is again important, and the diagnosis should probably be made only when numerous gram-negative coccobacilli are seen in the absence of other potentially pathogenic bacteria. *Neisseria meningitidis* (meningococci) is morphologically similar to *B. catarrhalis* and must also be included in the differential diagnosis. However, in meningococcal disease, patients are generally young adults, and the infection is associated with significant toxicity.

Gram-negative bacilli, particularly those belonging to the family Enterobacteriaceae (e.g., *E. coli, Klebsiella, Enterobacter, Serratia,* and *Proteus*), must also be considered as causative agents in the differential diagnosis of pneumococcal pneumonia, particularly if the patient is debilitated and residing in a nursing home or similar institution and certainly if the patient is hospitalized. Aerobic gram-negative bacilli are often responsible for nosocomial pneumonias but infrequently for community-acquired pneumonias, because gram-negative bacilli rarely colonize the oropharynx of otherwise healthy people in the community but they are common oropharyngeal residents in debilitated, hospitalized, or institutionalized patients. In addition, the patient in question may exhibit certain risk factors associated with invasion by gram-negative bacilli, such as the receipt of prior antibiotics, corticosteroids, inhalation therapy, or tracheostomy, and the existence of profound neutropenia or severe debilitation. The pneumonic process is usually necrotizing, and gas formation may be detected on radiographs. A Gram stain of purulent sputum usually reveals many large, bipolar-staining gram-negative rods. Elastin fibrils may also be seen on a KOH preparation of sputum from the site of infection.

Anaerobic bacteria may also produce acute suppurative pneumonia. Those most frequently involved are *Bacteroides* species (usually *B. melaninogenicus*), *Peptostreptococcus,* and *Fusobacterium.* Frequently, anaerobic infections are polymicrobial and may include bacteria other than strict anaerobes (e.g., *S. aureus*). The occurrence of anaerobic infection is usually preceded by gross aspiration and is enhanced if the individual has anaerobic oral infections or solid tumors of the oropharyngeal structures or tracheobronchial tree. The clinical features of anaerobic pleuropneumonic disease may be indolent rather than abrupt, and it may be accompanied by pus that has a fetid and nauseating odor. Necrosis of the lung with gas formation is often noted.

Mycoplasma pneumoniae, Chlamydia, and *Legionella* may also produce acute pneumonias, which are usually best described as atypical. With mycoplasmal pneumonia, patients are ordinarily young, and prolonged communicability, especially within households, may often be documented. The clinical, radiographic, and pathologic features are usually those of an interstitial pneumonia rather than lobar consolidation and an alveolar exudative process. Serum cold agglutinin levels may be elevated, and the disease is rarely, if ever fatal. Chlamydial pneumonia, especially that caused by *C. psittaci,* is contracted from infected psittacine birds, whereas *C. pneumoniae* or the TWAR agent is acquired from other infected humans. *C. pneumoniae* is the most common species producing chlamydial pneumonia in humans, and the clinical picture is usually that of pharyngitis, often with laryngitis, and segmental pneumonia of a single lobe without pleural effusion. Seroepidemiologic studies reveal a higher prevalence of antibodies in males than females and in older adults than children. Legionnaires' disease, which may be produced by a variety of *Legionella* species but principally by *L. pneumophila,* is associated with considerable systemic toxicity (nausea, vomiting, and diarrhea) and may be very difficult to differentiate from pneumococcal pneumonia. However, in the temperate zones, community-acquired Legionnaires' disease usually occurs in the warmer months or summer; patients are typically male construction workers and smokers in their 50s whose clinical manifestations include fever, chills, myalgias, headache, dry non-productive cough, and non-specific pulmonary infiltrates. Anti-*Legionella* fluorescein-labeled antibodies, which may be used to examine sputum for *Legionella,* as well as antigen detection techniques applied to the urine, may be helpful in the early diagnosis of this disease.

Patients with the acquired immune deficiency syndrome (AIDS) and acute pneumonia present considerable diagnostic problems. Although pneumococcal pneumonia and infections from other encapsulated bacteria occur with greater frequency in patients with AIDS than in normal individuals, pneumocystosis and cytomegalovirus pneumonia, as well as tuberculosis, occur frequently and must thus be excluded.

Finally, not only does pneumonia caused by microbes other than the pneumococcus have to be considered in the differential diagnosis, but also a variety of non-infectious conditions may mimic the clinical picture of pneumococcal pneumonia. Pulmonary infarction, with emboli (e.g., in right-sided endocarditis) or without emboli (e.g., in sickle cell anemia), may present a considerable diagnostic challenge, even after differential lung scanning and pulmonary angiography. Chemical pneumonitis, localized or diffuse (Mendelson's syndrome) and often caused by aspiration of gastric juice of low pH, may also be difficult to differentiate from pneumococcal or other bacterial pneumonias; however, in the absence of antibiotic therapy, a Gram stain of purulent sputum consistently reveals few or no bacteria.

TREATMENT. All patients with suspected pneumococcal pneumonia should be treated as promptly as possible with an effective antimicrobial agent. One should not wait for cultural confirmation of the diagnosis to initiate therapy. Although some patients may recover without antibacterial therapy, effective antimicrobial agents reduce morbidity, mortality, and complications.

If penicillin resistance, especially high-level resistance, is not considered a problem, penicillin G is considered the therapy of choice. Blood and tissue levels of penicillin G in excess of the MIC for susceptible strains (< 0.1 μg/mL) are easily achieved with doses of 1.2 to 2.4 million U/day. If the infecting strain is of intermediate resistance (MIC ≥0.1 to <2.0 μg/mL), penicillin G can still be successfully used; however, doses approximating 6 to 12 million U/day need to be used. For patients who are believed to be allergic to penicillin, one may select a first- or second-generation cephalosporin or erythromycin, clindamycin, or a fluoroquinolone.

With the advent of high-level penicillin resistance, different strategies of therapy may have to be devised on the basis of susceptibility to non–penicillin G, β-lactams (see Table 319–1) and to non–β-lactam antibacterials (Table 319–4). In many parts of the United States and the world, cefotaxime and ceftriaxone resistance is approaching 25% in respiratory tract pneumococcal isolates. Nevertheless, if the presence of high-level penicillin resistance is considered a good possibility, ceftriaxone, 1 to 2 g every 24 hours, or cefotaxime, 1 to 2 g every 6 hours, perhaps combined with a macrolide, fluoroquinolone, rifamycin, or lincomycin, may need to be used until susceptibility data become available. However, if a serious, life-threatening infection such as meningitis caused by high-level penicillin-resistant pneumococci is present, vancomycin plus ceftriaxone or cefotaxime need to be used.

Initial therapy should be parenteral to ensure delivery and adequate serum and tissue levels. If the patient is in shock or has heart failure, the route of delivery should be intravenous. Later in the course of therapy, if the patient's progress is good, the route of administration may be changed to oral. Treatment with any effective agent should be given for at least 5 to 7 days.

Table 319–4 ■ CRITERIA FOR RESISTANCE OF
STREPTOCOCCUS PNEUMONIAE TO SOME COMMONLY USED
ANTIBIOTICS*

ANTIBACTERIAL AGENT	MIC (μg/mL)
Penicillin G	
Intermediate	≥0.1 to <2.0
High level	≥2.0
Erythromycin	≥1.0
Clindamycin	≥1.0
Levofloxacin	≥8.0
Rifampin	≥4.0
Chloramphenicol	≥8.0

MIC = minimum inhibitory concentration.
*Based on criteria established by the National Committee for Clinical Laboratory Standards (NCCLS), Document M100-58, vol 18; No 1, Jan 1998, pp 68–69, Wayne, PA.

If effective antibacterial therapy is used, the patient's temperature usually falls to or below normal by crisis within 24 hours. However, in some instances, perhaps because of the nature of the pathology or complications that occur (e.g., pleural effusion), the patient's temperature may fall by lysis over 2 to 3 days. Resolution and recovery from pneumococcal pneumonia generally result in restoration of normal pulmonary architecture. Occasionally, healing may be via fibrosis, in which instance persistence of pulmonary infiltrates on radiographs may be evident for months after clinical recovery.

In addition to effective antibacterial therapy, a variety of supportive measures are generally used in the initial management of acute pneumococcal pneumonia; such measures include bed rest, monitoring vital signs and urine output, inserting a Swan-Ganz catheter to monitor cardiac output, administering an occasional analgesic to relieve pleuritic pain to permit effective breathing and coughing, replacing fluids if the patient is dehydrated, correcting electrolytes, oxygen therapy, and relieving an ileus with nasal gastric suctioning. When relieving pleuritic pain or providing sedation in situations requiring it (e.g., in delirium tremens), care should be taken to not use excessively high doses of analgesics or sedatives that might depress the respiratory center. Intercostal nerve blocks, which do not interfere with the respiratory drive, may be used. If possible, antipyretics should also be avoided because these agents interfere with the evaluation of fever as a measurement of the patient's progress (or lack of).

COMPLICATIONS. Empyema develops in approximately 5% of patients with pneumococcal pneumonia, although sterile pleural effusions commonly develop in a larger percentage (up to 30%). Most effusions resolve with successful antibacterial therapy, although empyemas often require drainage. Empyemas usually consist of thick pus composed of fibrin, serous proteins, large numbers of leukocytes and/or their products, and pneumococci. Initially, such collections may be drained by needle aspiration; however, later, as loculations occur, drainage via chest tubes is usually necessary. Chest radiographs with lateral decubitus films are often useful in the early recognition of pleural effusions; however, at a later time and in the course of removal and follow-up, ultrasonography and/or computed tomography may be necessary. In any acute bacterial pneumonia, pleural fluid that is removed should be subjected to Gram stain, aerobic and anaerobic cultures, pH determination, cell count and differential, protein and sugar analysis, and a lactate dehydrogenase test to determine whether an empyema is present.

If pneumococcal bacteremia occurs, extrapulmonary complications such as *meningitis, septic arthritis,* and *endocarditis* must be excluded because their therapy generally requires higher dosages of antibiotics and, in the case of septic arthritis, may require drainage. A spinal tap with examination of cerebrospinal fluid should be done if meningitis is suspected, and multiple pre-treatment blood cultures and echocardiography of the heart valves should be obtained if endocarditis is suspected. Other complications that might occur are *pyogenic pericarditis,* which may produce tamponade and require drainage, and *peritonitis* in those with ascites (e.g., cirrhosis or nephrotic syndrome).

PROGNOSIS. The case fatality rate for untreated pneumococcal pneumonia is about 25%, whereas in those treated promptly with an appropriate antibiotic, it may be less than 5%. Fatality rates differ considerably among patient groups, depending on such factors as the presence or absence of bacteremia, multilobe or single-lobe involvement, the presence or absence of neutropenia or asplenism, underlying diseases (particularly of the heart or lung), age of the patient (the prognosis being poor at the extremes), complicating extrapulmonary pneumococcal infections (e.g., meningitis), the occurrence of shock, the serotype of pneumococcus responsible (type 3 being highly virulent), delayed therapy, penicillin susceptibility or resistance, and prior immunization with polyvalent pneumococcal vaccine. However, since the advent of penicillin G in the 1940s, despite the advent of a variety of antibiotics, the case fatality rate of pneumococcal pneumonia and bacteremia remains essentially unchanged.

PREVENTION. The most important preventive tool available is polyvalent pneumococcal vaccine. This type-specific vaccine contains 23 antigenic capsular polysaccharides, which in the United States account for up to 90% of bacteremic infections. In immunocompetent populations, it is estimated to be 79% protective and induces antibodies of the IgG2 and IgG4 subclasses in adults, which enhance opsonization, phagocytosis, and killing of pneumococci by polymorphonuclear leukocytes and fixed macrophages. It is virtually free of life-threatening side effects and obviously cannot produce a pneumococcal infection because it contains no viable, intact pneumococci. Fever, localized swelling, and/or pain at the injection site may develop in about 15 to 30% of patients who receive the vaccine. As with all polysaccharide vaccines, it is not immunogenic below ages 18 to 24 months and is poorly immunogenic in the very elderly and in those with a variety of conditions generally associated with decreased vaccine responsiveness. In normal individuals, if antibodies result from vaccination, colonization, or natural infection, they usually persist for several years and then progressively decline. The vaccine is not associated with a booster effect, probably because it functions as a thymus-independent type 2 antigen. At present, highly immunogenic vaccines in which the capsular antigens are conjugated to proteins are under development. Revaccination of the elderly and other high-risk groups needs to be considered at 3- to 5-year intervals.

The U.S. Public Health Service specifically recommends the currently available pneumococcal vaccine for patients with underlying conditions associated with increased susceptibility to pneumococcal infections or increased risk of mortality from such infections, namely, healthy adults 65 years or older and those with chronic cardiac or pulmonary diseases, anatomic or functional asplenia, chronic liver disease, alcoholism, diabetes mellitus, and cerebrospinal fluid leaks. Perhaps the greatest value of vaccination against pneumococci is to reduce bacteremia, dissemination, and mortality, especially in those with hepatic or splenic dysfunction. Type-specific antibody can be elicited with pneumococcal polysaccharides by subcutaneous vaccination even in splenectomized patients. In addition, recommendations for receiving the vaccine are also made for those with chronic renal failure or those undergoing hemodialysis; for those with Hodgkin's disease, chronic lymphocytic leukemia, multiple myeloma, or AIDS; or for those receiving or about to receive chemotherapy for cancer, organ transplantation, or splenectomy.

Antibiotic prophylaxis with penicillin G or similar agents in otherwise healthy patients with viral upper respiratory infections is not routinely indicated, is not cost-effective, and may only lead to superinfections with antibiotic-resistant bacteria or to adverse side effects from the antibiotic itself. However, in individuals with seriously compromised pulmonary, cardiac, or immune function, an appropriate, narrow-spectrum antibacterial agent (the selection of which depends on anticipated antibiotic susceptibility patterns) may be given in moderate dosages during a viral syndrome for a limited time to reduce the risk of morbidity and mortality from potentially invasive pneumococci. Such prophylaxis may especially apply to those in households where pneumococcal infections recently occurred.

Finally, it should be appreciated that pneumococcal infections, including pneumonia, are not generally acquired by otherwise normal people from exposure to other patients with pneumococcal pneumonia; thus patients with pneumococcal pneumonia do not require isolation, and prophylaxis for medical staff exposed to such infections is not indicated.

Austrian R: Life with the Pneumococcus. Notes from the Bedside, Laboratory, and Library. Philadelphia. University of Pennsylvania Press, 1985. *An array of interesting observations, both clinical and laboratory, on pneumococcal infections by an outstanding authority and the father of the modern capsular polysaccharide pneumococcal vaccine.*

Doern GV, Pfaller, MA, Kugler K, et al: Prevalence of antimicrobial resistance among respiratory tract isolates of *Streptococcus pneumoniae* in North America: 1997 results from the SENTRY Antimicrobial Surveillance Program. Clin Infect Dis 27:764, 1998. *Update on the prevalence of pneumococcal resistance among 1047 isolates from 27 U.S. and 7 Canadian institutions.*

Friedland IR, McCracken GH Jr: Management of infections caused by antibiotic-resistant *Streptococcus pneumoniae*. N Engl J Med 331:337, 1994. *An excellent review of clinical responsiveness of infections caused by penicillin-resistant pneumococci to various antibiotics with suggested therapeutic strategies.*

Musher DM, Groover JE, Rowland JM, et al: Antibody to capsular polysaccharides of *Streptococcus pneumoniae*: Prevalence, persistence and response to revaccination. Clin Infect Dis 17:66, 1993. *Presents new and reviews previously published data on the appearance, persistence, and fall of anticapsular antibodies against pneumococci after colonization, natural infections, and immunization.*

Rubins JB, Duane PG, Charbonneau D, et al: Toxicity of pneumolysin to pulmonary endothelial cells in vitro. Infect Immun 60:1740, 1992. *Thorough study of pneumoly-*

sin and projection of its importance in the pathogenesis of pneumonia and perhaps complicating bacteremia.

320 MYCOPLASMAL INFECTION

David Schlossberg

BACKGROUND. The mycoplasmas associated with humans include species from the genera *Mycoplasma, Ureaplasma,* and *Acholeplasma.* Because these genera all belong to the order Mycoplasmatales in the class Mollicutes, they are collectively called "mollicutes" or, more commonly, "mycoplasmas." Over 150 species are recognized, and they are found in humans, animals, plants, and insects. Most of these organisms are commensals, but some of the human strains are pathogenic; rarely, some of the animal strains infect humans as well.

Mycoplasmas are the smallest free-living organisms. At 200 nm, they approximate the size of the larger viruses. Bound by a triple-layered cell membrane, they have no cell wall (thus the name "mollicute," Greek for "soft skin") and are therefore not seen on Gram stain and cannot be treated with cell wall–active antibiotics such as the β-lactams or vancomycin.

Most mycoplasmas are facultative anaerobes. They grow down into agar and produce a dark center with a light periphery on the surface, the so-called fried-egg colonies. Mycoplasmas are distinguished from bacteria in that they lack a cell wall and cannot produce cell wall precursors and are distinguished from viruses, chlamydiae, and rickettsiae in that the mycoplasmas can grow on cell-free media.

The mycoplasmas of humans are listed in Table 320–1. Some are established pathogens, some are commensals, and some infect immunocompromised patients.

IMMUNOLOGY. Mycoplasmas have a wide range of immunomodulatory effects, including stimulation of T- and B-lymphocyte proliferation, induction of cytolytic activity of macrophages and cytotoxic T cells, stimulation of cytokine production, induction of major histocompatibility complex expression in macrophages and B cells, and production of chemotactic factors, Fc factors, Fc receptors, superantigens, and immunoglobulin proteases. This explosive and varied immunologic activity may contribute to disease expression. It is well known that rheumatoid factor, biologic false-positive tests for syphilis, antinuclear antibodies, and other antibodies sometimes appear in the course of mycoplasmal infection.

MYCOPLASMA PNEUMONIAE. *M. pneumoniae* accounts for 10 to 20% of all pneumonias and for at least half of all pneumonias in children and young adults. Although most cases occur in the first two decades of life, mycoplasmal infection is seen at all ages. *M. pneumoniae* typically causes community-acquired pneumonia, but rare cases of nosocomial acquisition are reported.

Infection with *M. pneumoniae* can occur in any season, with a 4-year periodicity for outbreaks. Because epidemics of pneumonia secondary to other agents usually peak in the winter, it is diagnostically helpful when *Mycoplasma* pneumonia occurs in other sea-

Table 320–1 ■ HUMAN MYCOPLASMAS

ESTABLISHED PATHOGENS	OPPORTUNISTS	COMMENSALS
M. pneumoniae	M. salivarium	M. buccale
M. hominis	M. orale	M. faucium
M. fermentans	M. genitalium	M. lipophilum
M. urealyticum	M. pirum	M. primatum
	M. penetrans	M. spermatophilum
	M. arginini	A. laidlawii
	M. felis	A. oculi
	M. edwardii	

sons. College epidemics of *Mycoplasma,* for example, tend to peak in the fall.

The incubation period for *M. pneumoniae* averages 2½ weeks but ranges from 4 days to over 3 weeks. This longer incubation period furnishes an important diagnostic clue inasmuch as incubation periods for most of the respiratory viruses are measured in days, not weeks. Spread is person to person via droplet nuclei after close and prolonged contact.

The attack rate of *M. pneumoniae* diminishes with age. Second infections can occur (especially if a patient is immunocompromised), but the second case is usually milder than the first. Extremely severe disease is seen in patients who have SS or SC hemoglobinopathy, Down syndrome, or hypogammaglobulinemia. Furthermore, patients with humoral deficiency are more likely to become chronic carriers; most normal patients shed the organism by 6 weeks, although in some it may persist for 3 to 4 months.

CLINICAL FINDINGS. (See Fig. 320–1). Most patients with *M. pneumoniae* infection are older children, adolescents, and young adults with a minor respiratory illness. In general, 75% of patients have tracheobronchitis, 5% have an atypical pneumonia, and 20% are asymptomatic. Children younger than 5 years tend to have coryza and wheezing, whereas the age of maximum risk for the development of pneumonia is 5 to 15 years. Bronchospasm may develop in asthmatics. In many patients, a sequence of symptoms occurs: The illness begins insidiously over days or a week with constitutional symptomatology (e.g., fever, myalgia, headache, and malaise); then upper respiratory signs and symptoms appear, with combinations of sore throat, cervical adenopathy, hoarseness, earache, coryza, and non-productive cough; less commonly, croup or bronchiolitis may supervene, and in a small percentage, pneumonia ensues. At this point, the cough becomes productive.

Many patients report chilliness but not rigors. Protracted coughing results in tracheal tenderness and a sore chest, but actual pleuritic pain is rare. A prolonged illness with paroxysmal cough followed by vomiting may occur in children and mimic pertussis. Signs include fever, an erythematous pharynx without exudate, and

rarely, bullae on the tympanic membrane. The illness is usually self-limited and mild.

The insidious onset is followed by gradual recovery. The upper respiratory symptoms may last for 2 to 3 weeks, and signs of pneumonia may persist for 4 to 6 weeks. Laboratory abnormalities are not specific; a slight leukocytosis (<15,000 per cubic millimeter) is seen in 25% of patients, with a normal differential count. Sputum Gram stain is very helpful in demonstrating inflammatory cells (polymorphonuclear leukocytes or lymphocytes) but a paucity of bacteria.

Radiographic findings are manifold. Most patients have unilateral lower lobe segmental abnormalities on the right. The earliest signs are an interstitial accentuation of markings with subsequent patchy air space consolidation and thickened bronchial shadows. Additional findings are plate-like atelectasis, Kerley B lines, perihilar accentuations of markings, and nodular infiltrates. Hilar adenopathy is seen only occasionally in adults but in 30% of children and may be unilateral or bilateral. A small effusion is seen in one fourth of patients, but even in these patients pleuritic pain is rare. Complications seen on chest radiographs include pneumothorax, pneumatoceles, abscess, and in the rare case of fulminant disease, changes compatible with respiratory distress syndrome (see Chapter 88). In convalescence, an area of hyperlucent lung may persist on chest radiographs, but most of the changes resolve. Rarely, bronchiectasis, bronchiolitis obliterans, and progressive fibrosis are permanent sequelae.

Extrapulmonary complications are common and are usually superimposed on pulmonary disease, so a mycoplasmal etiology can be suspected. The most frequent extrapulmonary complication is neurologic.

Neurologic symptoms are seen as early as several days after the onset of respiratory symptoms or 2 weeks or more after the respiratory symptoms subside. Respiratory disease may be absent in as many as 50% of patients at the initial evaluation. Thus both infectious and immunologic mechanisms seem to be involved. *Mycoplasma* has been isolated rarely from cerebrospinal fluid (CSF), although not from brain biopsy. Polymerase chain reaction (PCR) may be positive in CSF, especially in early central nervous system

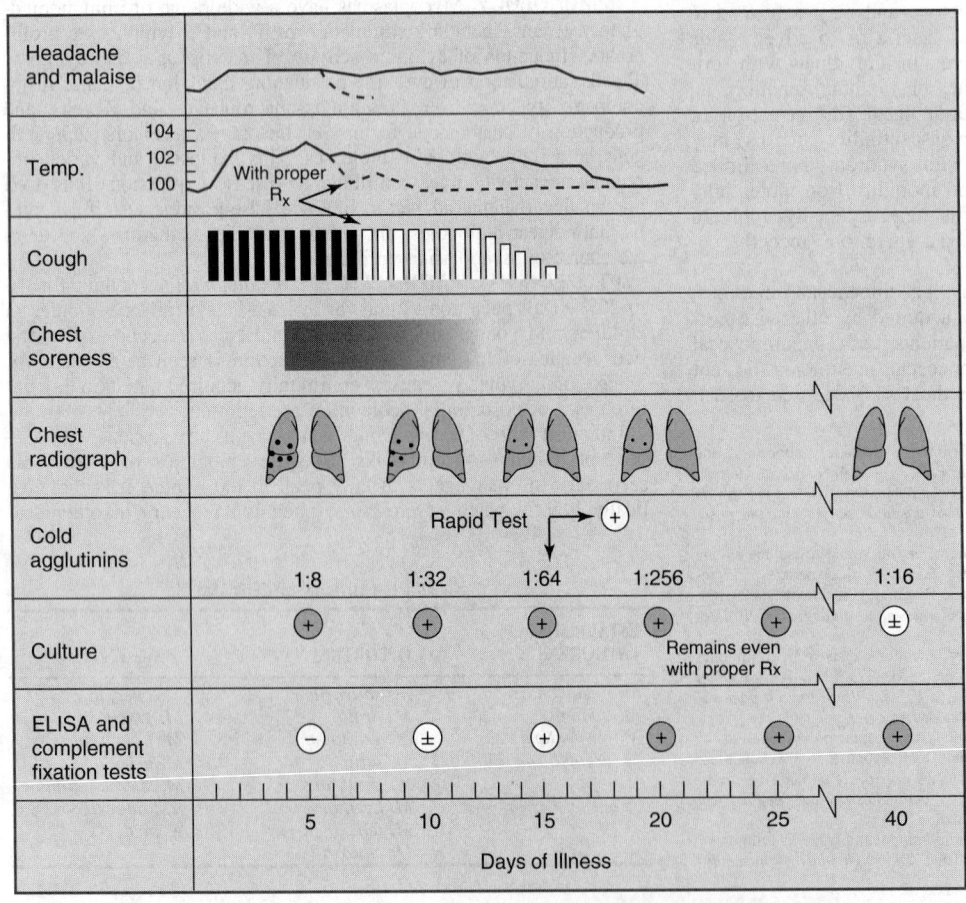

FIGURE 320–1 ■ Major clinical and laboratory manifestations of mycoplasmal pneumonia. ELISA = enzyme-linked immunosorbent assay.

disease. Most neurologic complications occur in children, and mycoplasmal infection accounts for 10 to 15% of childhood encephalitis. CSF typically displays a small number of lymphocytes (50 to 100) with normal or slightly elevated protein and occasionally lowered glucose levels.

Encephalitis may result in coma or psychosis or more focal phenomena such as stroke, ataxia, choreoathetosis, and non-convulsive status epilepticus. An acute brain stem syndrome and bilateral striatal necrosis have been described, as has post-infectious leukoencephalitis. Patients may also have clinically characteristic meningitis. A number of types of myelitis are seen including transverse myelitis and a polio-like syndrome. Peripheral neuropathy may involve the peripheral or cranial nerves; it is believed that *M. pneumoniae* accounts for 5% of cases of Guillain-Barré syndrome, and the Miller Fisher variant has been documented. More limited peripheral neuropathies have been manifested as mononeuritis multiplex with brachial plexopathy and as acute sensorineural hearing loss. Sequelae of neurologic involvement range from mental retardation to movement disorders and epilepsy.

Rashes are seen in 10 to 20% of patients. Most are maculopapular, but they may also be vesicular, petechial, or urticarial, most commonly on the trunk and extremities. Less frequently, the face, buttocks, genitalia, hands, and feet are included. Rash usually begins during the acute illness but may precede or follow it. Most patients have obvious respiratory disease, and some have an associated conjunctivitis or an enanthem in the oropharynx. Other exanthemata associated with *M. pneumoniae* infection include pityriasis rosea, leukocytoclastic vasculitis, toxic epidermal necrolysis, erythema nodosum, and erythema multiforme or Stevens-Johnson syndrome. In fact, 15 to 20% of patients with erythema multiforme have been shown to have *M. pneumoniae* infection.

M. pneumoniae is the most common cause of rash and pneumonia, a combination also produced by viruses (herpes simplex, varicella-zoster, Epstein-Barr virus, enterovirus, adenovirus, and measles), *Chlamydia psittaci*, *Mycobacterium tuberculosis*, fungi (*Histoplasma, Cryptococcus, Coccidioides*), and meningococci.

Hematologic complications are well-known features of mycoplasmal infection. Anemia, hemolytic anemia, thrombocytopenia, disseminated intravascular coagulation, thromboembolism, thrombotic thrombocytopenic purpura, Pelger-Huët abnormality (polymorphonuclear leukocytes with a monolobed or bilobed appearance), and hemophagocytic histiocytic syndrome are all described, but the most common hematologic complication is the formation of cold agglutinins. These antibodies agglutinate red blood cells and are seen in a variety of infections (influenza, mononucleosis, psittacosis, rubella, adenovirus, measles, and others) but usually occur at higher titer in mycoplasmal infection. If the titer is high enough, they may bind complement and cause hemolysis. These cold agglutinins are IgM antibodies directed against the I antigen of the red blood cell. They are seen in up to 70% of patients, especially those with severe disease. Appearing in the second week of illness, they peak at 4 weeks and disappear by 2 months. Thus at the time that the cold agglutinin titer is highest and hemolysis most likely to occur, the clinical disease is abating. A simple bedside test may be performed by adding 1 to 2 mL of the patient's blood to an anticoagulated tube. This tube is placed in a cup of ice water and tilted after 2 to 3 minutes to detect clumping, which represents agglutination of red blood cells. The tube is then warmed by holding it in the hands, and if the clumps redissolve, the test is positive and correlates with a titer of cold agglutinins of 1:64 or greater. Hemolysis is treated with corticosteroids as well as antibiotics.

Cardiac complications include pericarditis with occasional hemopericardium, myocarditis with congestive heart failure, complete heart block, or atrioventricular block with atrial tachycardia. A migratory arthritis involving medium-sized joints and occasionally resembling rheumatoid arthritis may be seen. Ophthalmologic complications include iritis and conjunctivitis, as well as optic neuritis with optic nerve atrophy. On occasion, retinal hemorrhage and exudates are seen. A number of other organ systems may be involved, with resultant bullous myringitis, glomerulonephritis, tubulointerstitial nephritis, hepatitis, pancreatitis, splenomegaly, polymyositis, tubo-ovarian abscess, pediatric priapism, and Raynaud's phenomenon.

The differential diagnosis of *M. pneumoniae* infection includes most causes of the atypical pneumonia syndrome (Table 320–2). This syndrome refers to a generally benign febrile illness with prominent systemic complaints, non-productive cough, and interstitial abnormalities on chest radiography. The differential diagnosis includes many diseases with clinical or epidemiologic clues. For example, psittacosis should be suspected if a patient has had contact with birds, Q fever follows exposure to farm animals or cats, and *Legionella* tends to infect older men who smoke. *Chlamydia pneumoniae* (see Chapter 370) infection often causes a biphasic illness, with sore throat and hoarseness followed by cough. True viruses cause a more fulminant pneumonia. Early in the course of bacterial pneumonia, a cough may be non-productive, but eventually sputum is produced with neutrophils and bacteria on Gram stain, in association with rigors and pleuritic pain. Tularemia follows exposure to an infected animal carcass or arthropod. Other illnesses that rarely mimic *M. pneumoniae* infection include acute fungal infection, such as histoplasmosis, and tuberculosis, particularly primary disease, or reactivation in a compromised host.

Factors suggesting a mycoplasmal etiology are sore throat, headache, fever, rash, an indolent course, a paucity of physical findings on examination, and a chest radiograph more abnormal than the physical examination predicted. Although rare, bullous myringitis is a helpful clue. *Against* a mycoplasmal etiology is a fulminant course, extreme leukocytosis, pre-existing disease, and recurrent infection. Although both coryza and hoarseness may be seen with mycoplasmal infection, they are more common in viral disease.

DIAGNOSIS. *Mycoplasma* can be cultured, but this capability is not widely available, and recovery of the organism from sputum does not prove the diagnosis because it can persist for a long time after infection. Thus most diagnoses are made by serology. The most widely available serologic test has been the complement fixation test, although a growing number of diagnostic laboratories are using enzyme-linked immunosorbent assay. With either test, 90% of patients have either a four-fold rise in antibody titer (2 to 3 weeks apart) or a single titer of 1:32 or greater. There are problems with these serologic tests: First, the complement fixation titer can remain elevated for a year after the infection. Second, the glycolipid antigen used in the complement fixation test is not specific for *Mycoplasma* and is found in a variety of tissues, including human heart muscle, brain, and pancreas, as well as in some streptococci and leafy vegetables. Thus false-positive results may be seen, for example, in certain neurologic syndromes and pancreatitis. Third, false-negative reactions are seen with both tests. Fourth, some adults form only IgG antibody. Thus the complement fixation test, which detects primarily IgM, is more likely to be falsely negative. Fifth, antibody appears only after 7 to 10 days of illness, thus providing no diagnostic help early in the cause of infection. Finally, detection of IgM does not prove current infection because IgM may persist for months and could thus indicate a recent rather than current infection.

Methods of direct detection include antigen detection techniques, DNA probes, and PCR. Of these, the most promising in terms of speed, sensitivity, and specificity is PCR, although cost and lack of general availability limit its routine use. Also, the relevance of detecting *Mycoplasma* in respiratory secretions is limited in view of the prolonged carrier state. Thus the diagnosis is generally *proved* by a four-fold rise in antibody titer and is strongly *supported* by a single antibody titer of 1:32 or greater, a titer of cold agglutinins of 1:64 or greater, or a single IgM determination.

THERAPY. From a practical standpoint, therapy for *M. pneumoniae* infection is empirical because culture takes time and may be misleading and serologic investigation is not diagnostic early in the course. Thus a compatible illness in a susceptible patient should be treated on the basis of clinical suspicion. A definite clinical response is seen to tetracyclines and erythromycin, although treat-

Table 320–2 ▪ DIFFERENTIAL DIAGNOSIS OF
MYCOPLASMA PNEUMONIAE INFECTION

COMMON	RARE
Chlamydia pneumoniae pneumonia	Q fever
Legionnaires' disease	Psittacosis
Viral pneumonia	Acute fungal infection
Early bacterial pneumonia	Tularemia
	Tuberculosis

ment does not influence the carrier state, and the organism may persist in respiratory secretions despite appropriate antibiotic therapy.

Currently, erythromycin or tetracycline (either as 2 g daily in divided doses) is standard therapy (Table 320–3). Doxycycline and the newer macrolides (azithromycin and clarithromycin) can substitute for tetracycline and erythromycin, respectively, and offer the advantage of greater patient convenience, but at increased cost. Although most recommendations are for 10 to 14 days of therapy, longer courses of treatment (e.g., 2 to 3 weeks) may avoid the relapse that occurs in 5 to 10% of patients. Prophylaxis of contacts does not prevent infection but can prevent clinical disease. Tetracyclines should be avoided in children younger than 8 years and pregnant patients but are preferable if the differential diagnosis includes psittacosis, Q fever, or *Mycobacterium fermentans* (see below). Correspondingly, erythromycin is preferred if the differential diagnosis includes legionellosis. Quinolones show good in vitro activity (see Table 320–3), but clinical experience is limited and they can not be recommended at this point as primary therapy. These drugs should be avoided in children and adolescents under 18 and in woman who are nursing or pregnant.

OTHER MYCOPLASMAS AND UREAPLASMAS. *Mycoplasma hominis* is a commensal of the genitourinary tract, especially in women. It is seen in up to 50% of sexually active women and 30% of sexually active men. Occasionally it is found in the pharynx. *M. hominis* may produce several different syndromes. A known pathogen of the female urogenital tract, it causes Bartholin's gland abscess, pelvic inflammatory disease, and pyelonephritis. It also causes post-abortal and postpartum fever, wound infection following cesarean section, and postpartum retroperitoneal obscess. *M. hominis* can infect the fetus in utero or during birth and result in neonatal infection and stillbirth. Scalp wound infection may complicate fetal monitoring devices.

M. hominis also causes extragenital infection in adults, often following genitourinary manipulation in an immunosuppressed patient. Some infections caused by *M. hominis* follow trauma, e.g., orbital abscess complicating sinus trauma. *M. hominis* pneumonia in organ transplant patients has resulted both from indigenous and donor *M. hominis*. Infection of surgical wounds should be suspected if a purulent exudate is negative on Gram stain and culture. Other sites of extragenital infection include the brain, lung, prosthetic devices, skin, peritoneum, and joints (especially in patients with hypogammaglobulinemia). Although these organisms are not visible on Gram stain, some investigators have identified them in infected joint fluid with acridine orange stain and immunofluorescent staining. The organism may grow on routine media but is easily overlooked, and if it is suspected, the laboratory should be alerted. Because *M. hominis* is resistant to erythromycin, tetracycline is the drug of choice, with clindamycin and the quinolones as alternatives (see Table 320–3).

Another definite pathogen has been recognized in *M. fermentans*. This organism has been recovered from the lower genital tract of men and women, the oropharynx, and the lower respiratory tract. Although associated with immunosuppression (leukemia, acquired immune deficiency syndrome [AIDS], and chemotherapy), it has also been described in normal patients in whom a febrile illness

with fever, vomiting, and diarrhea developed, with progression to fulminant disease with respiratory distress syndrome, multiple organ failure, and death. *M. fermentans* may also play a role in inflammatory arthritides. This organism is resistant to erythromycin and should be treated with doxycycline or a quinolone (see Table 320–3).

A growing number of other mycoplasmas are thought to possibly cause disease, especially in immunosuppressed patients; *M. orale* has been isolated from the blood and marrow of children with leukemia; *M. pirum* has been recovered from lymphocytic cells from patients with AIDS; *M. genitalium* causes urethritis and arthritis in hypogammaglobulinemic patients and may be an important cause of non-gonococcal urethritis; *M. penetrans* is strongly associated with homosexual activity and has been isolated from the urine of patients with AIDS; *M. felis* has caused septic arthritis in a patient with hypogammaglobulinemia; *M. salivarium* causes periodontitis and septic arthritis in hypogammaglobulinemic patients; *M. edwardii* has caused septicemia in a patient with AIDS; and *M. arginini*, an animal strain of *Mycoplasma*, has caused septicemia and pneumonia in an immunocompromised patient with lymphoma. Like *M. fermentans*, this strain of *Mycoplasma* is resistant to erythromycin and should be treated with tetracycline if suspected (see Table 320–3). Other human mycoplasmas, as noted in Table 320–1, are presently considered commensals.

Recent interest has focused on the relationship between mycoplasmas and human immunodeficiency virus (HIV) infection. A role of cofactor with HIV has been suggested for several strains of mycoplasmas, including *M. fermentans*, *M. genitalium*, *M. pirum*, and *M. penetrans*, all of which have been isolated from HIV-infected patients and are potent immunomodulators.

Ureaplasma urealyticum colonizes the genital tract of 75% of women and 45% of men who are sexually active (see Chapter 361). In an adult, it may cause non-gonococcal urethritis, as well as salpingitis and pelvic inflammatory disease; outside the genitourinary tract, it can infect joints (especially in patients with hypogammaglobulinemia), transplant sites, and surgical wounds. In the neonate, it is associated with chorioamnionitis and with chronic lung disease of prematurity, but it is not strongly associated with prematurity, and treatment to eradicate it during pregnancy does not reduce the incidence of premature birth or low birth weight. It may account for some acute respiratory illnesses in children. Tetracyclines are agents of choice, with erythromycin or possibly quinolones as alternatives (see Table 320–3).

Koskiniemi M: CNS manifestations associated with *Mycoplasma pneumoniae* infections: Summary of cases at the University of Helsinki and review. Clin Infect Dis 17(Suppl. 1):52, 1993. *An excellent and thorough review of neurologic complications.*

McMahon DK, Dummer JS, Pasculle AW, et al: Extragenital *Mycoplasma hominis* infections in adults. Am J Med 89:275, 1990. *Good concise review with helpful references.*

Taylor-Robinson D: Infections due to species of *Mycoplasma* and *Ureaplasma*: An Update. Clin Infect Dis 23:671, 1996. *A detailed review of clinical aspects of infection by* Mycoplasma *and* Ureaplasma.

Table 320–3 ■ ANTIBIOTIC SUSCEPTIBILITY

MYCOPLASMA	ERY	TCN	CLN	QUN
M. pneumoniae	sens	sens	res	sens*
M. fermentans	res†	sens	sens	sens
M. hominis	res	sens‡	sens	sens*
U. urealyticum	sens‡	sens‡	res	sens
M. arginini	res	sens		
M. penetrans	sens	sens‡	sens	sens
M. pirum	res†	sens‡	sens	sens

ERY = erythromycin; TCN = tetracycline; CLN = clindamycin; QUN = quinolones; sens = sensitive; res = resistant.

*Sensitivity to quinolones is adequate for the earlier quinolones, e.g., ciprofloxacin and ofloxacin, but it is greatest for newer agents of this class, e.g., sparfloxacin and trovafloxacin.

†Sensitive to azithromycin and clarithromycin.

‡Some resistance seen.

321 PNEUMONIA CAUSED BY AEROBIC GRAM-NEGATIVE BACILLI

Waldemar G. Johanson, Jr.

Gram-negative enteric bacilli (GNB) rarely cause pneumonia in previously healthy hosts. These organisms are not highly virulent respiratory pathogens but strike instead individuals whose defense mechanisms have been diminished by acute or chronic disease. The typical patient would be in an intensive-care unit (ICU), intubated, and receiving mechanical ventilation after surgery, trauma, or life-threatening illness. Antimicrobial therapy, usually with multiple agents, would have been used for several days before GNB appeared to colonize the oropharynx or tracheal secretions. Over the next 1 or 2 days secretions become more purulent, gas exchange worsens, and new infiltrates appear on the chest radiograph.

PATHOGENESIS. Pneumonias due to GNB are generally caused by aspiration of contaminated oropharyngeal secretions and are preceded by colonization, either of the respiratory or upper gastrointestinal tract. Colonization of the upper respiratory tract with GNB is present in 10% or fewer of normal persons, but its prevalence is markedly increased among patients with acute or chronic diseases. Colonization increases swiftly among healthy persons undergoing elective surgical procedures from essentially zero to 35 to 50% within 24 hours after surgery. Similarly, approximately 50% of ICU patients become colonized within a few days of admission. The organisms responsible for colonization vary from one study to another but are only rarely attributable to demonstrable environmental sources. Instead, colonization appears to be caused by a translocation of the patient's fecal flora or the transfer of organisms from one patient to another on the hands of personnel. Colonization rates among populations with chronic disease, such as alcoholics and residents of skilled nursing facilities, may approach 50%. The root cause of this colonization is the great susceptibility of ill patients to acquire GNB from the immediate environment.

Once established in the oropharynx, GNB multiply, achieve high concentrations in secretions, and are aspirated in small liquid boluses into the lungs (see Chapter 82). Because lung defenses are often impaired by the same underlying conditions that promote changes in cell resistance to adherence and colonization, the ability of the lungs to handle this bacterial inoculum is insufficient, and pneumonia results. The specific lung defense mechanism that might be impaired in a given patient varies with the nature of underlying illness. For example, patients with chronic airway obstruction have impaired mucociliary transport and alveolar hypoxia that hinders the effectiveness of phagocytic cells. Patients who are neutropenic are remarkably predisposed to develop pneumonias with GNB, a clinical observation that correlates nicely with the experimental finding that swift recruitment of circulating neutrophils into the lungs is a crucial aspect of host defense against *Pseudomonas aeruginosa* infection. Alcoholism seems to predispose to GNB pneumonias in several ways. Malnutrition promotes colonization of the upper tract by GNB, aspiration is facilitated by episodes of impaired consciousness, and acute alcohol intoxication hinders the ability of phagocytes to migrate to the site of inflammation.

GNB may appear first in the gastric contents and only subsequently be found in the oropharynx or tracheal secretions. This phenomenon has been associated with the presence of nasogastric tubes, which allow reflux of gastric material into the esophagus. The role of gastric acid neutralization for prophylaxis of stress ulceration is controversial; bacterial concentrations in the stomach increase dramatically as the pH rises, and some studies have associated such prophylaxis with higher rates of pneumonia, although this has been an inconstant finding.

Of the many species of aerobic GNB that colonize human hosts, only *Haemophilus influenzae* can be classified as a true respiratory pathogen, if the ability of the organism to produce infections in previously normal individuals is accepted as a reasonable criterion of pathogenicity. All the others together, including Enterobacteriaceae (*Escherichia coli, Klebsiella, Enterobacter, Serratia,* and *Proteus*), *Pseudomonas,* and *Acinetobacter,* account for 10 to 20% of community-acquired pneumonias, and these occur almost exclusively in patients with serious underlying disease. The genus *Klebsiella* contains seven species, of which only *K. pneumoniae* and *K. oxytoca* cause pneumonia; infections due to *K. pneumoniae* are by far the most common.

Pneumonia caused by *Klebsiella* has been held separate from that caused by other GNB, largely for historical reasons. It was the first such organism to be recognized as a pulmonary pathogen, and the pneumonia it caused was distinct from that caused by the pneumococcus, especially in its lack of response to early forms of treatment and its predilection to cause upper lobe pneumonias in alcoholic men. However, the classic features of *Klebsiella* pneumonia as described in the earlier literature, such as "currant jelly" sputum (a mixture of blood and mucus), the bulging fissure associated with upper lobe consolidation, and the syndrome of "chronic cavitary pneumonia," are rarely observed today. Although *Klebsiella* remains an important pulmonary pathogen, the illness it causes cannot be clinically differentiated from that caused by other aerobic

GNB; thus, the treatment of *Klebsiella* infection is similar to that of infections with other aerobic GNB.

Contamination of respiratory therapy equipment by GNB, usually *P. aeruginosa,* was recognized as a major cause of nosocomial pneumonias in the 1960s. With the advent of disposable nebulizers and other control strategies, this problem has been largely eliminated.

CLINICAL MANIFESTATIONS. Pneumonias caused by GNB may be community acquired or hospital acquired (nosocomial). Virtually all patients with community-acquired pneumonias caused by GNB have serious underlying chronic illnesses, especially chronic obstructive pulmonary disease, alcoholism, or malignancy. Nosocomial pneumonias resulting from GNB occur principally in patients with severe, acute illnesses whether or not they have underlying chronic disease as well. Thus, these infections are most likely to be found in postoperative patients or patients who require intensive care for other reasons. The clinical manifestations of infection are influenced by the nature of the associated processes.

Community-acquired GNB pneumonias share the common features of all bacterial pneumonias—fever, cough productive of purulent sputum, chest pain, and shortness of breath. The illness tends to be abrupt and associated with prominent systemic signs and symptoms, such as mental confusion, vomiting, and hypotension. Physical examination reveals rales in most patients, but the classic findings of dense consolidation are uncommon. Pleural effusion is present in 15 to 20% of patients. Radiographic infiltrates may involve any lobe and are bilateral in about one third of patients. Although cavitation is most likely to occur in pneumonia caused by *Klebsiella,* it also occurs commonly with *Pseudomonas* infections and occasionally with other organisms. Laboratory features include leukocytosis or leukopenia, either of which is characteristically associated with a marked left shift. Leukopenia is a poor prognostic sign.

Nosocomial pneumonia produced by GNB can be an explosive illness similar to the community-acquired form but frequently proceeds with a more indolent but seemingly inexorable course. Often the patient is in respiratory failure, intubated, and receiving mechanical ventilation. GNB are initially found colonizing the oropharynx, and over the subsequent few days appear in tracheal secretions, followed by increasing numbers of neutrophils. Finally, the patient becomes febrile and develops new radiographic infiltrates and worsening hypoxemia. Another common presentation is fever on the second or third postoperative day. Postoperative pneumonias are most common after lateral thoracotomies (especially combined thoracoabdominal procedures) and upper abdominal incisions. When nosocomial GNB pneumonia complicates the course of an already seriously ill patient, it is frequently associated with evidence of multiple organ failures. For a variety of reasons, these patients are usually receiving antibiotics when new GNB appear in the respiratory tract. As a result, the organisms are often resistant to antimicrobial agents used frequently in that particular hospital, reflecting acquisition of nosocomial strains such as *Acinetobacter, Pseudomonas,* and *Stenotrophomonas.* These and other organisms have shown the capacity to develop high-level resistance to virtually all antimicrobial agents in frequent use, an observation that supports the concept of restricting the use of certain antibiotics for periods of time.

A deteriorating clinical course associated with GNB bacteremia is usually not due to GNB pneumonia. Pulmonary infiltrates in that instance usually represent non-cardiogenic pulmonary edema or the adult respiratory distress syndrome (see Chapters 88 and 92) and not actual pneumonia, with bacteremia arising from a non-pulmonary source such as the gastrointestinal or urinary tract.

DIAGNOSIS. Confirmation that GNB are responsible for pneumonia is a difficult clinical problem created largely by colonization of proximal airways by these organisms. Thus, GNB are often present in the secretions of ill patients whether they have pneumonia or not and whether or not the GNB are the cause of pneumonia. Blood cultures are positive in 20 to 30% of patients with community-acquired infections but in as few as 8% of those with nosocomial pneumonias. Nevertheless, because the information gained from a positive blood culture regarding the causative organism and its antimicrobial susceptibility is so important in patient management, blood cultures should always be obtained when GNB pneumonia is suspected. Similarly, although pleural effusion is usually not present, the yield of positive cultures from such fluid when it is present is about 30%, and a diagnostic thoracentesis should be performed if a sufficient volume of fluid is identified radiographically.

The usefulness of invasive sampling remains somewhat controversial. Transthoracic needle aspiration is rarely used in critically ill patients because of concern about complications, especially pneumothorax. Sampling by means of the fiberoptic bronchoscope using either bronchoalveolar lavage (BAL) or the protected specimen brush (PSB) technique offers a safe alternative. Both techniques have been studied extensively and accurately portray the lung's bacterial flora in the absence of antibiotic therapy. BAL has the added advantage of providing specimens for special staining and cytology and is especially useful in the diagnosis of infections in immunocompromised hosts. The finding of bacteria phagocytosed by more than 7% of lavaged cells seems to have predictive importance and has been used to guide empirical therapy until culture results are known. A reasonable strategy has emerged in recent years as experience has been gained with these techniques. If the patient has had no changes of antibiotic therapy in the past 72 hours, any new infection will presumably be due to resistant organisms and either PSB or BAL or both specimens should be obtained and quantitatively cultured. In other circumstances, the yield is too low to be recommended. Despite the ready availability of bronchoscopy, the etiology of nosocomial pneumonias is often frustratingly difficult to establish with certainty.

TREATMENT. Patients who are susceptible to infection by GNB are at even greater risk of pulmonary infection by more virulent organisms, such as the pneumococcus, *Haemophilus,* and *Staphylococcus aureus.* Thus, despite the presence of GNB in sputum, initial treatment of these pneumonias—particularly those acquired outside the hospital or in the absence of concomitant antibiotic therapy—should include coverage of the usual respiratory pathogens. Evaluation of the efficacy of treatment is confounded by the severity of underlying disease present in most of these patients; mortality rates of 20 to 30% are not uncommon among patients treated with agents that have demonstrated in vitro activity against the infecting organism.

Table 321–1 provides therapeutic options for the patient with a suspected GNB pneumonia. Agents other than fluoroquinolones must be given parenterally and in adequate dosage. The results of monotherapy rival those of multidrug regimens when broad-spectrum agents such as third-generation cephalosporins (ceftazidime or cefotaxime), carbepenems (imipenem or meropenem), β-lactam/β-lactamase inhibitor combinations (piperacillin/tazobactam or ticarcillin/clavulanate), or fluoroquinolones (ciprofloxacin or alatrofloxacin) are used. *P. aeruginosa* infections are best treated with a combination of drugs.

Table 321–1 ■ EMPIRICAL ANTIBIOTIC THERAPY FOR AEROBIC GRAM-NEGATIVE BACILLARY PNEUMONIA*

Monotherapy
Consider in mild to moderately ill patients in whom *Pseudomonas aeruginosa* is unlikely.
Cefuroxime, 1.5 g every 8 hours
Cefotaxime, 2 g every 8 hours
Ticarcillin/clavulanate, 3.1 g every 4 hours
Piperacillin/tazobactam, 4.5 g every 6 hours
Ciprofloxacin, 400 mg every 12 hours
Alatrofloxacin, 300 mg every 24 hours
Combination Therapy
Consider in patients with severe illness, immunosuppression, neutropenia, and those with a high likelihood of *P. aeruginosa*
Aminoglycoside† or ciprofloxacin, 400 mg every 12 hours, plus one of the following:
  Ceftazidime, 2 g every 8 hours
  Cefepime, 2 g every 12 hours
  Piperacillin/tazobactam, 4.5 g every 6 hours
  Imipenem/cilastatin, 500 mg every 6 hours
  Aztreonam, 2 g every 8 hours
Ciprofloxacin, 400 mg every 12 hours plus aminoglycoside

*Recommendations for adults with normal renal function.
†Dosages of 5 mg/kg every 24 hours for gentamicin and tobramycin; 15 mg/kg every 24 hours for amikacin.

Treatment of nosocomial infection is made more difficult by previous antimicrobial therapy, and drug susceptibility studies are critically important. However, empirical therapy usually must be initiated before the results of such studies are available. Factors to consider when selecting appropriate therapy include knowledge of local resistance patterns, previous culture results, and prior treatment. For example, resistance of *P. aeruginosa* to gentamicin may approach 50% in some hospitals. If *P. aeruginosa* is strongly suspected on the basis of previous cultures or the clinical setting (respiratory failure, neutropenia), a β-lactam agent or fluoroquinolone with antipseudomonal activity should be combined with an aminoglycoside (see Table 321–1). Amikacin is often used in this setting because of less frequent resistance to this agent. A single daily dose of an aminoglycoside has been shown to be equally as effective as more frequent dosing and may be less nephrotoxic. Doses must be adjusted in the presence of impaired renal function.

Prospective studies have shown that carefully chosen empirical regimens are inadequate in up to 73% of cases when invasive sampling techniques are used to determine the etiologic organisms. Causes of inadequacy are the presence of resistant organisms singly or in polymicrobial infections; up to 40% of nosocomial pneumonias are polymicrobial. When the pathogenic organisms have been identified and the susceptibility patterns are known, modifications can be made to optimize antibiotic therapy. Ideally, antibiotics with the narrowest spectrum of activity, the least toxicity, and the best lung penetration should be chosen. In neutropenic patients and in seriously ill patients with pneumonia caused by resistant organisms such as *P. aeruginosa, Serratia marcescens,* and *Acinetobacter,* continued combination therapy with an appropriate β-lactam agent and an aminoglycoside is recommended. Duration of therapy should be based on clinical response, but a minimum of 2 to 3 weeks is usually required.

PROGNOSIS. A number of studies have compared outcomes of GNB pneumonias when antimicrobial therapy was judged to be either adequate or inadequate; in most, adequate therapy reduced the overall mortality rate. The observed level of mortality depends on the population studied and has been reported as high as 91%, but it is more commonly in the range of 20 to 50%. That adequate therapy did not reduce mortality in some studies is explained by the fact that underlying disease is the main predictor of survival for many patients. Early, broad-spectrum therapy that covers all of the organisms present in the lung is important for patients with survivable illnesses.

COMPLICATIONS. Pneumonias caused by GNB are more likely than other pneumonias to be complicated by one or more adverse events. Important complications include empyema, lung necrosis, superinfections, and multiple organ failure; metastatic seeding of infection to other sites is an uncommon complication.

Empyema occurs in perhaps as many as 30% of patients with GNB pneumonias. Criteria for the diagnosis of empyema, besides the presence of gross pus, include the presence of bacteria on Gram stain, pleural fluid pH less than 7.2, or a pleural fluid white blood cell count greater than 30,000/dL. Each of these criteria indicates a condition that is unlikely to respond to antimicrobials alone and that usually requires drainage of the pleural space as well. Thus the term *complicated effusion* has gained favor over *empyema* to identify pleural fluid collections for which drainage needs to be considered. The occurrence of a complicated effusion generally prevents the recovery of the patient until it is recognized and effectively treated. Signs and symptoms of continuing illness, such as fever, persistent leukocytosis, and the onset of multiple organ failure, in a patient undergoing treatment for a GNB pneumonia should raise suspicion of a complicated effusion. If pleural fluid is identified on upright posteroanterior and lateral chest radiographs, thoracentesis should be performed; useful studies of the fluid obtained include measurements of pH and glucose, white blood cell count, Gram stain, and cultures for aerobic and anaerobic organisms.

If the fluid qualifies as a complicated effusion, prompt placement of a thoracostomy tube should be considered. Alternative approaches (principally, repeated thoracentesis) are less successful, owing to loculation of the pleural space. Surgical drainage of the pleural space, using localized resection of an overlying rib with creation of a larger drainage tract, is reserved for patients who do not respond to tube drainage and are not candidates for a larger operation. Decortication of the pleura may be necessary if the clinical signs of uncontrolled infection are not ameliorated by simple drainage plus antimicrobial therapy. In such patients, radiographic evidence of effusion persists, along with continued fever and leukocytosis. At surgery, the pleural space is found to contain numerous loculated pockets of pus. The timing of intervention with these techniques requires excellent clinical judgment, because the patients are usually seriously ill and poor candidates for surgical treatment of any kind; on the other hand, they will not recover unless the pleural space is adequately drained.

Extensive lung necrosis has been termed *lung gangrene* because of the rapid occurrence of pulmonary cavitation associated with marked systemic toxicity and the appearance of extensive devitalization of lung tissue at necropsy. Occasionally, an entire lung appears to dissolve within a few days, leaving multiple cavities with air-fluid levels. This complication occurs with all of the common GNB, although perhaps more commonly in infections produced by *K. pneumoniae* and *P. aeruginosa*. Lung necrosis may be caused by the extracellular products of these organisms. *P. aeruginosa* makes a number of "virulence factors," including exotoxin A, exoenzyme S, elastase, and a neutral protease. However, *K. pneumoniae* makes none of these, and the propensity of this organism to cause lung necrosis remains unexplained. Extensive lung necrosis may be followed by massive hemoptysis, continued suppuration because of inadequate drainage of the massively disrupted lung parenchyma, or bronchopleural fistula caused by extension of the necrotizing process through the pleura. The last must be promptly treated by placing a chest tube because of the attendant pneumothorax. However, the definitive treatment of extensive lung necrosis is surgical resection of the involved lobe or lobes.

Assessment of the patient with multiple organ failure in the context of a serious illness complicated by a GNB pneumonia is always difficult. The major question is usually whether a new complication such as oliguria is due to the underlying disease, to the current treatment, or to the infection. Each of the common manifestations of multiple organ dysfunction—altered liver function, acute renal failure, hematopoietic abnormalities, upper gastrointestinal bleeding, and altered mental state—may be multifactorial, and the antimicrobial agents used to treat GNB pneumonia may cause most of them. The guiding principles are to treat the infection aggressively and to correct life-threatening complications as they occur.

Superinfections may develop during the treatment of GNB pneumonia, just as GNB pneumonia may occur as a superinfection of a previous pneumonia. Unfortunately, treatment of the patient's pneumonia does not prevent colonization of the oropharynx and tracheobronchial tree by additional GNB or fungi. Thus, the clinician is often faced with evaluating a new set of microorganisms recovered from the patient's secretions. The guiding principle here is to treat patients, not culture results. If the patient is responding well and appears to be improving, the new culture results can be disregarded for the time being. On the other hand, if the new cultural data correspond to a worsening clinical course, the process of evaluation and revision of treatment must be begun again.

Kollef MH, Ward S: The influence of mini-BAL cultures on patient outcomes: Implications for the antibiotic management of ventilator-associated pneumonia. Chest 113: 412–420, 1998. *Results of BAL cultures were used to assess the adequacy of empirical antimicrobial therapy for suspected nosocomial pneumonia in 130 ICU patients. Empirical therapy was judged to be inadequate in 73% of 60 cases with positive cultures, leading to a later change in treatment.*

Kollef MH, Vlasnik J, Sharpless L, et al: Scheduled change of antibiotic classes: A strategy to decrease the incidence of ventilator-associated pneumonia. Am J Respir Crit Care Med 156:1040–1048, 1997. *This study shows that a control strategy consisting of intentional rotation of drugs used as empirical therapy for nosocomial pneumonia in an ICU was followed by reductions in both prevalence of resistance and the frequency of pneumonia.*

Yinnon AM, Butnaru A, Raveh D, et al: *Klebsiella* bacteremia: Community versus nosocomial infection. Q J Med 89:933–941, 1996. *This study reports an analysis of 241 cases of Klebsiella bacteremia, emphasizing the frequent presence of severe underlying disease and overall poor response to therapy.*

322 ASPIRATION PNEUMONIA

Waldemar G. Johanson, Jr.

Aspiration of oropharyngeal liquids into the lungs is a key step in the pathophysiology of many pulmonary disorders. Most of the important syndromes are dealt with elsewhere in this volume: gastric acid aspiration (see Chapter 80), anaerobic pneumonias and lung abscess (see Chapter 83), lipoid pneumonia (see Chapter 80), and hydrocarbon aspiration (see Chapter 80). Most bacterial pneumonias are initiated by the aspiration of minute quantities of secretions, a process termed *microaspiration,* which occurs in normal individuals during sleep. In this chapter the focus is placed on an infrequent but difficult problem—that of recurrent bacterial pneumonias in the context of diseases that lead to frequent and usually documentable aspiration of oropharyngeal secretions. Such pneumonias are defined as recurring clinical illnesses characterized by fever, purulent sputum, and new radiographic infiltrates in the lungs in a patient with known or suspected chronic aspiration of oropharyngeal contents.

ETIOLOGY. Most patients afflicted with this problem have serious problems with swallowing, an altered level of consciousness, or both. Common predisposing conditions are carcinoma of the esophagus with obstruction, tracheobronchial fistula (usually after treatment for cancer), and neurologic diseases affecting deglutition. Strokes are certainly the most common cause of the last condition, but amyotrophic lateral sclerosis (including bulbar palsy), multiple sclerosis, and the myopathies may be responsible. Recurrent nocturnal aspiration of gastric contents by patients with esophageal reflux represents the one situation in which the swallowing mechanism may be intact in this syndrome.

Impaired swallowing due to neural or myopathic causes is most pronounced when the patient attempts to swallow liquids. By contrast, dysphagia caused by obstruction is always worst with solid foods. Thus, it is not surprising that the patient with myoneural deficits of the pharyngeal musculature repeatedly aspirates oropharyngeal secretions. In patients with esophageal obstruction, secretions accumulate proximal to the obstruction, especially at night, and are aspirated. Gastric contents are normally sterile. However, as the patient with reflux aspirates gastric contents, a certain volume of oropharyngeal secretions is necessarily carried along.

Oropharyngeal secretions are massively contaminated, containing 10^6 to 10^8 aerobic bacteria per milliliter and about 10 times as many anaerobic organisms. Although the majority of organisms composing the normal flora of this region have little invasiveness for the normal host, highly pathogenic organisms, including *Streptococcus pneumoniae, Staphylococcus aureus,* and *Haemophilus influenzae,* may be present in the secretions of normal people. Because most of the patients susceptible to recurrent aspiration have serious underlying diseases, their upper respiratory tracts are likely to be colonized by enteric gram-negative bacilli and *Pseudomonas* as well.

Normal individuals aspirate small volumes of oropharyngeal secretions during sleep but do not develop recurrent pneumonias. The difference between normal people and those who do develop recurrent pneumonias is probably the volume of material aspirated and the underlying chronic illnesses of the latter patients; differences in the bacterial flora of secretions may play a role as well.

CLINICAL MANIFESTATIONS. Episodes of recurrent pneumonia associated with aspiration tend not to be acute, fulminant illnesses but rather are characterized by progressive fever, purulent sputum production, shortness of breath, and systemic symptoms (such as loss of appetite and malaise) over a period of days.

Physical findings include those related to the underlying illness and the presence of coarse rhonchi over dependent lung zones. Rales and signs of consolidation may or may not be present. Fever and leukocytosis are regularly present. Radiographs of the chest reveal infiltrates of varying intensity, with a preponderance of change in the dependent zones, that is, posterior aspects of the lower lobes and posterior segments of the upper lobes. Pleural effusion is uncommon unless anaerobic infection is present.

DIAGNOSIS. A high index of suspicion, based on the patient's underlying disease, is the first step. The presence of food particles in tracheal secretions is clear evidence of aspiration. In patients receiving enteral feedings, the presence of glucose in secretions may be demonstrable by bedside tests. Because glucose cannot be detected in normal secretions, a positive result is highly specific for aspiration. Dietary lipids form large intracellular deposits when ingested by phagocytic cells, and examination of sputum with a lipid stain may confirm the clinical impression of chronic aspiration. The microscopic appearance of the large lipid deposits is important in differentiating this type of lipid inclusion from the foamy deposit that occurs in macrophages due to the accumulation of endogenous lipid distal to an obstructing lesion in the airways. The sputum of such patients is intensely purulent, with a wide spectrum of bacterial forms present on Gram stain. Culture yields upper respiratory flora, and the clinical problem is to discern which of several pathogenic organisms should be treated. Culture may be useful because knowledge of the sensitivity of the organisms present may be needed to guide therapy. Blood cultures are rarely positive.

Several techniques may be used when the diagnosis of recurrent aspiration is in doubt (Table 322–1). Cineradiographic studies of the patient swallowing a thin, water-soluble contrast material can demonstrate abnormalities of deglutition and may actually show aspiration. Thick barium should be avoided because aspiration of this material compounds the patient's problems, and a thick solution is less likely to identify the swallowing difficulty. A prolonged pharyngeal transit time may be the best predictor of subsequent pneumonia. Radionuclide salivagrams utilize isotopes for the same purpose and may be particularly useful in children because of lesser radiation exposure. Documentation of impaired sensory function in the posterior pharynx and larynx are highly predictive of later aspiration, especially when combined with the aforementioned techniques.

The relationship between esophageal reflux and pneumonia may be difficult to determine. If aspiration is suspected on clinical grounds, monitoring of the pH in the upper esophagus during sleep can confirm it. Reflux into the upper esophagus is marked by a sudden fall in pH, an event that is easily captured on a long-term strip chart recorder for review the next morning. However, prospective studies have shown that it is difficult to predict which patients will experience aspiration pneumonias except in the most obvious situations, indicating that the fact of aspiration does not necessarily lead to clinical pneumonia.

TREATMENT. Initial antibiotic therapy should provide coverage for gram-positive and gram-negative organisms as well as oral anaerobes. Pending the results of culture and susceptibility studies, empirical therapy with intravenous penicillin or clindamycin and an aminoglycoside or aztreonam is reasonable. Alternatively, monotherapy with a second- or third-generation cephalosporin, imipenem, trovafloxacin, or a drug combining a β-lactam antibiotic with a β-lactamase inhibitor such as ampicillin-sulbactam, ticarcillin-clavulanate, or piperacillin-tazobactam can be used. Supportive care, including aggressive tracheobronchial toilet, is required. Nutrition must not be overlooked despite the difficulties encountered in many of these patients. If swallowing is impossible and a small feeding tube cannot be placed in the intestinal tract through the nose or mouth, parenteral nutrition should be provided while a long-term solution to the patient's problem is sought. Failure to address the nutritional deficits of these patients is a common cause of protracted and often lethal complications.

Bypassing the mouth to facilitate feeding can be accomplished with a gastrostomy placed surgically or, more commonly, a percutaneous endoscopic gastrostomy. In some patients, cessation of swallowing food diminishes the frequency and severity of aspiration and successfully ameliorates the clinical problem. However, in many it does not because patients must still handle their own secretions. Drug therapy aimed at reducing the volume of secre-

tions in this situation is usually not successful. Tracheostomy does not eliminate the possibility of aspiration because secretions pool above the cuff. Continuous suction of these supra-cuff secretions has been shown to reduce the incidence of nosocomial pneumonia in intubated, mechanically ventilated patients, but that approach is not practical in other situations. Separation of the airway from the esophagus is the only certain way to prevent aspiration in some patients. Studies have shown that this can be accomplished by closing the supraglottic space at the level of the false cords. Wound healing is promoted by inactivity of the laryngeal musculature, which can be accomplished by injections of botulinum toxin. This closure can be reversed at a later date if the condition leading to aspiration improves. These procedures should not be contemplated in all patients with the syndrome of recurrent aspiration, because many patients have underlying conditions that will be lethal in a short time. However, if the patient has a reasonable chance of long-term survival in the absence of recurrent episodes of pneumonia, these steps should be considered.

Feinberg MJ, Knebl J, Tully J: Prandial aspiration and pneumonia in an elderly population followed over 3 years. Dysphagia 11:104–109, 1996. *This prospective study found that episodes of aspiration pneumonia were more common in patients with documented swallowing difficulty. However, tube feedings did not decrease the incidence of pneumonia but were actually associated with an increase.*
Jacobson K, Griffiths K, Diamond S, et al: A randomized controlled trial of penicillin vs. clindamycin for the treatment of aspiration pneumonia in children. Arch Pediatr Adolesc Med 151:701–704, 1997. *This is one of the few studies in which penicillin is compared directly with alternative agents in an adequate experimental design; no differences were found.*
Johnson ER, McKenzie SW, Sievers A: Aspiration pneumonia in stroke. Arch Phys Med Rehabil 74:973, 1993. *This study found that nearly 50% of stroke victims with dysphagia developed aspiration pneumonia within the first year. Pharyngeal transit time, as assessed by videofluoroscopy, was the best predictor of the subsequent development of pneumonia.*
Pototschnig CA, Schneider I, Eckel HE, Thumfart WF: Repeatedly successful closure of the larynx for the treatment of chronic aspiration with the use of botulinum toxin A. Ann Otol Rhinol Laryngol 105:521–524, 1996. *These investigators used botulinum toxin A to paralyze the intrinsic musculature of the larynx to achieve immobility while an approximation of the false cords healed.*

323 LEGIONELLOSIS

Paul H. Edelstein

DEFINITION. "Legionellosis" is the term used to describe infections caused by bacteria of the genus *Legionella*. The most important of these diseases is pneumonia, called "legionnaires' disease." Either as part of legionnaires' disease or distinct from it, legionellae may cause infections elsewhere in the body, usually in the form of abscesses. Pontiac fever, which is a self-limited mild febrile illness, is assumed to be caused by legionellae, although this assumption is unproven.

HISTORY. Legionnaires' disease was initially recognized when it caused epidemic pneumonia among members of the American Legion attending a convention in Philadelphia in 1976; this outbreak resulted in 29 deaths and 182 cases of pneumonia. Charles McDade and William Shepard of the U.S. Centers for Disease Control and Prevention determined that this disease was caused by an ostensibly newly discovered bacterium, which was named *Legionella pneumophila*. Neither the disease nor the bacterium is new. The first documented epidemic of legionnaires' disease occurred in a meat packing plant in Minnesota in 1957, and the first recorded isolation of the bacterium was in 1943. In fact, three different *Legionella* species had been isolated from humans before 1976, although they were thought to be rickettsia-like agents. Several unsolved epidemics of pneumonia, including one in Philadelphia in 1974, were recognized to have been due to legionnaires' disease.

BACTERIOLOGY. Thirty-nine *Legionella* species have been recognized to date. About half of them have been isolated from patients with legionnaires' disease, and about half have been isolated only from the environment. The species that most commonly cause disease are *L. pneumophila*, *L. micdadei*, *L. bozemanii*, *L. dumoffii*, and *L. longbeachae*. Fifteen serogroups are recognized for *L. pneumophila*, whereas several other species contain up to two sero-

Table 322–1 ■ DIAGNOSTIC TESTS FOR CHRONIC ASPIRATION

TEST	FINDING
Cineradiography	Vallecular and/or pyriform pooling; delayed pharyngeal transit*; laryngeal transit of contrast medium†
Radionuclide imaging	Activity over the trachea*; activity over the lungs†
Esophageal pH monitoring	Nocturnal decrease of pH in upper esophagus
Bronchoscopy	Bronchial inflammation; lipid-laden macrophages†

*Correlated with increased risk of pneumonia.
†Confirms a diagnosis of aspiration.

groups. *L. pneumophila* serogroup 1 causes 70 to 90% of cases of legionnaires' disease in non-immunocompromised individuals. *L. micdadei* is probably the second most common cause of legionnaires' disease and frequently causes legionnaires' disease in immunocompromised patients.

Legionellae are small, gram-negative, obligately aerobic bacilli. *Legionella* requires complex growth media because of an absolute nutritional requirement for L-cysteine. Optimal growth occurs on a buffered charcoal yeast extract medium supplemented with iron, L-cysteine, and α-ketoglutarate. These bacteria do not grow on conventional bacteriologic media such as trypticase soy broth agar, MacConkey agar, or unsupplemented chocolate agar. Their usual habitat is natural and treated waters such as lakes, ponds, and tap water. Legionellae are found in the highest concentration in warm water, especially in water heaters, hot water plumbing fixtures, and cooling towers. They appear to be obligate or facultative parasites of freshwater amoebae such as *Hartmannella* and *Acanthamoeba*. Humans are very likely accidental hosts of these bacteria.

Virulence factors have been examined for relatively few strains of *L. pneumophila* and *L. micdadei* and are not well understood. The bacteria produce endotoxins and exotoxins, which may cause tissue damage independently or in concert with the host immune system.

PATHOGENESIS. Legionnaires' disease is acquired by inhaling aerosolized water containing *Legionella* organisms or possibly by pulmonary aspiration of contaminated water. The contaminated aerosols are derived from humidifiers, shower heads, respiratory therapy equipment, industrial cooling water, and cooling towers. Aerosols formed by contaminated water in plumbing systems and in cooling towers are the most common sources of infection. Inhaled organisms undergo phagocytosis by pulmonary alveolar macrophages, which are unable to kill the bacteria. The bacteria multiply within the phagosome. Eventually, the multiplying bacteria, which produce cytotoxins, kill the macrophage and are released extracellularly. The intracellular infection cycle is reinitiated in another macrophage. Continuing bacterial multiplication and consequent lung damage produce symptoms 2 to 10 days after the initiation of infection. Bacterial uptake and multiplication are curtailed by the action of cytokines (e.g., interferon-γ) produced by macrophages and lymphocytes. Natural killer and lymphokine-activated killer cells probably lyse infected macrophages and thereby abort the intracellular infection cycle. The role of polymorphonuclear phagocytes is unclear, although they probably have some part in eliminating bacteria, especially after activation by interleukin-2 and tumor necrosis factor. Antibody appears to have little function in host immunity or defense, whereas T lymphocytes play a major role in the immune process. The actual mechanism of pulmonary damage is not well understood and could be due to bacterial toxins, immune reactions to infection, or both. The bacteria may spread to extrapulmonary sites via the lymphatic system and blood stream; they are probably transported in the blood by infected blood mononuclear cells. The mechanism whereby the pneumonia exerts systemic effects is unknown but could be the result of disseminated bacterial infection, the effect of toxin, or production of host factors such as tumor necrosis factor.

The pathogenesis of Pontiac fever is a mystery. Inhalation of water contaminated with many different types of bacteria, including *Legionella* species, produces the disease. The incubation period of the disease, 12 to 36 hours, is too short to allow for bacterial infection and multiplication. It is possible that bacterial or fungal toxins present in the water produce this illness, as has been hypothesized for a closely related disease, "humidifier fever." Another possibility is an immune response to one or more of the multiple microorganisms found in the water. Antibody to *Legionella* species found in contaminated water is present in most disease victims, but it is unclear what this immune response means.

EPIDEMIOLOGY. Legionnaires' disease occurs worldwide but is primarily a disease found in technically advanced countries. Case reports from underdeveloped countries are rare, perhaps because of limited diagnostic facilities and also perhaps because of the infrequent use of air conditioning and complex plumbing systems. Normal children rarely acquire this disease. Major risk factors for acquisition of legionnaires' disease are given in Table 323-1. Legionnaires' disease is an uncommon disease in patients with the acquired immune deficiency syndrome (AIDS), although they are at increased risk of acquiring the disease. Males get legionnaires'

Table 323-1 ■ RISK FACTORS FOR LEGIONNAIRES' DISEASE

Altered Local and Systemic Host Defenses
Glucocorticosteroid administration or Cushing's disease (5–10)*
Cytotoxic chemotherapy (5)
Cigarette smoking (2–5)
Diabetes (2)
Male gender or age older than 50 yr (>2)
AIDS (40)
Immune suppressive therapy for solid organ transplantation (>2)
Chronic heart or lung disease (>1)
Renal failure requiring dialysis (20)
Lung or hematologic cancer (especially hairy cell leukemia) (7–20)
Increased Chance of Exposure to Environmental Legionella *Bacteria*
Recent travel away from home (2)
Use of domestic well water (2)
Recent plumbing work in home or at work (2)
Exposure to poorly maintained hot tub spas
Recent surgical procedure

*Numbers in parentheses represent the approximate relative risk of acquiring legionnaires' disease over that for someone without the risk, where known.

disease about twice as often as females, although this difference does not hold true for several epidemics of legionnaires' disease. No good evidence exists for person-to-person spread of legionnaires' disease.

Legionnaires' disease may occur in epidemics originating in a single building or area. Outbreaks of the disease have occurred among hotel guests, hospital inpatients and outpatients, office building workers, and factory workers. People with occupational water exposure appear to have little, if any increased risk of disease acquisition. About 80% of cases of legionnaires' disease are non-epidemic. Of these, perhaps 10% may be acquired in the home and the remainder through other exposure.

It is estimated that from 1 to 5% of all pneumonias requiring hospitalization in adults are due to legionnaires' disease, which represents about 10,000 cases of legionnaires' disease per year in the United States. In some geographic regions, community-acquired legionnaires' disease is more common, such as in western Pennsylvania and Ohio. When the disease occurs in endemic or epidemic nosocomial form, 1% to as many as 20% of hospitalized patients with pneumonia have this disease.

Pontiac fever has been recognized primarily as an epidemic illness, with attack rates in excess of 90%. It has been noted to occur in office and factory workers and in recreational bathers using spa or whirlpool-type baths. The disease very likely has a sporadic form, but the lack of specific diagnostic tests makes diagnosis of this form very difficult.

PATHOLOGY. Specific pathologic changes are found only in the lung in the vast majority of fatal cases of legionnaires' disease. Intense inflammation is present in alveoli, alveolar ducts, respiratory bronchioles, and alveolar septa. The inflammatory process consists of bacteria, polymorphonuclear leukocytes, and macrophages. On occasion, pleuritis, pleural empyema, pericarditis, and cavitary lung disease are found. Very rarely, abscess formation occurs outside the chest cavity.

CLINICAL FEATURES. Legionnaires' disease is manifested as a febrile systemic illness with pneumonia. Several prospective and retrospective studies of patients with different types of pneumonia have shown that legionnaires' disease has few, if any characteristic clinical features and that it cannot be clinically distinguished from pneumococcal pneumonia. However, clinical observations during epidemics of legionnaires' disease have often documented characteristic clinical findings. It is probable that the spectrum of clinical findings is wide, ranging from a "typical" form of legionnaires' disease to one indistinguishable from other causes of pneumonia. This chapter describes the "typical" form of legionnaires' disease, which in reality may be present in the minority of patients. A prodromal illness consisting of malaise, low-grade fever, and anorexia may develop several days before the onset of more severe symptoms. Myalgia, extreme fatigue, and high fever then develop. Gastrointestinal complaints are common, such as generalized or localized abdominal pain, nausea, vomiting, and diarrhea; the diarrhea is generally watery and not dehydrating. Recurrent rigors and prostration may occur. Symptoms referable to the respiratory tract may not develop until later. It is this paucity of respiratory tract symptoms, despite evidence of a systemic febrile illness, that can either be a clue to diagnosis or mislead clinicians. When the patient is pressed for details regarding symptoms, a history of a non-productive cough or one productive of non-purulent, sometimes bloody secretions is usually obtained. Production of large amounts of grossly purulent sputum is unusual. Pleuritic chest pain, sometimes in concert with hemoptysis, may occur and can mislead the clinician into considering pulmonary infarction. Mental confusion is commonly reported in some series; obtundation, seizures, and focal neurologic findings may also occur less frequently.

Fever is almost uniformly present in cases of legionnaires' disease, although short (days) afebrile periods have been reported in some immunosuppressed patients with *L. micdadei* pneumonia. Chest examination early in the disease may reveal only scattered rales or evidence of pleural effusion. However, later in the course, most patients have classic findings of consolidating pneumonia. Abdominal examination may reveal generalized or local tenderness and, in rare cases, evidence of peritonitis. Splenomegaly is uncommon. Findings of pericarditis, myocarditis, and focal abscesses are rare. No rash is associated with this disease, except that caused by other factors such as drug therapy.

The fatality rate of untreated legionnaires' disease is about 3 to 30% in non-immunosuppressed patients and up to 80% in immuno-compromised ones. The majority of previously healthy people recover from untreated legionnaires' disease after 7 to 10 days of severe illness; those who do not recover die of progressive respiratory and multisystem failure.

Clinically significant extrapulmonary infection in patients with legionnaires' disease is quite rare (Table 323–2).

Pontiac fever is a non-fatal influenza-like disease, with symptoms of myalgia, fever, headache, and malaise occurring in 60 to 90% of patients. Arthralgia occurs with variable frequency, as do cough, anorexia, and abdominal pain. The illness is generally not severe enough or long enough in duration to cause most patients to seek medical attention. Not much is known about its physical findings early in the disease; findings after 3 to 5 days of illness are generally normal except for fever and possibly tachypnea. Pneumonia does not occur. The illness lasts about 3 to 5 days, although some patients may have persistent fatigue or non-focal neurologic complaints for weeks to months afterward.

CHEST RADIOGRAPHIC FINDINGS. Legionnaires' disease causes alveolar-filling infiltrates that usually eventuate in consolidation. Interstitial infiltrates are rare, although they may occur early in the course of disease and then progress to consolidating infiltrates. The infiltrates may be unilateral or bilateral and can spread very quickly to involve the entire lung. Pleural effusion, usually small in volume, occurs commonly and may be the sole abnormal radiographic finding in early disease.

DIAGNOSIS. The results of multiple non-specific laboratory tests may be abnormal in patients with legionnaires' disease. These abnormal findings include proteinuria, pyuria, hematuria, leukocytosis, leukopenia, and thrombocytopenia. Disseminated intravascular coagulation may be seen in patients with respiratory failure caused by

Table 323–2 ■ **EXTRAPULMONARY INFECTIONS CAUSED BY** *LEGIONELLA*

Dialysis shunt infection
Sinusitis
Pericarditis
Prosthetic valve endocarditis
Peritonitis
Abscesses
Skin
Brain
Bowel
Rectum
Kidney
Myocardium

legionnaires' disease. Hyponatremia, hypophosphatemia, hyperbilirubinemia, and elevated serum alanine transminase, serum aspartate transaminase, and alkaline phosphatase concentrations may also be found. Elevation of creatine kinase (MM isoenzyme) is common, and myoglobinuria and renal failure develop in some patients. Cerebrospinal fluid is usually normal, although rare patients may have 25 to 100 white blood cells per microliter of cerebrospinal fluid.

Legionnaires' disease can be diagnosed by using specific laboratory tests (Table 323–3). The most sensitive and specific test is culture of respiratory tract secretions, such as sputum. Sputum culture for *Legionella* should be performed on every patient suspected of having this disease. Serologic testing is more useful to epidemiologists than to clinicians because of cross-reactions with antibodies to unrelated organisms. No laboratory test currently available is 100% accurate for the diagnosis of legionnaires' disease. Thus empirical therapy must be considered in appropriate clinical settings.

The diagnosis of Pontiac fever is based on demonstration of legionellae in water to which the patient was exposed, significant increases in antibody to the isolated *Legionella* species, and a clinical course compatible with this diagnosis. To be certain about the diagnosis of Pontiac fever, it is almost always necessary to perform extensive studies of unaffected people and their environments because recovery of legionnellae from water and the elevation of antibodies to *Legionella* are relatively common events. Thus it is nearly impossible to diagnose non-epidemic cases of Pontiac fever specifically.

The differential diagnosis of legionnaires' disease is broad because the disease is usually manifested as a non-specific pneumonia. Mycoplasmal pneumonia is generally much less severe and causes significant respiratory system complaints. Pneumococcal pneumonia, in contrast to legionnaires' disease, is usually penicillin responsive. Psittacosis and Q fever can have clinical features quite similar to those of legionnaires' disease.

THERAPY. Erythromycin (Table 323–4) is considered the drug of choice for this disease on the basis of retrospective studies, which show that the case fatality rate is lowered about two-fold by prompt administration of erythromycin. Intravenous drug therapy should be given until clinical improvement is seen, which usually occurs in 2 to 4 days. Afterward, oral drug therapy is continued.

Table 323–3 ■ **SPECIFIC DIAGNOSTIC TESTS FOR** *LEGIONELLA*

TYPE	SUITABLE SPECIMENS	SENSITIVITY* (%)	SPECIFICITY (%)	NOTES
Culture	Sputum, lung, pleural fluid, blood, abscess contents	—	100	Use of special and selective media required; 3 to 5 d required for growth
Immunofluorescent microscopy	Sputum, lung, pleural fluid, abscess contents	25–75	95–99.9	Species-specific monoclonal antibody available; not helpful for diagnosis of all species; highest specificity for *L. pneumophila;* relatively low specificity for other species; 2 to 3 hr required for testing
Urine antigen detection	Urine	90–95	99.9	Useful only for detection of *L. pneumophila* serogroup 1, the most common cause of legionnaires' disease; 2 to 3 hr required for testing; may be positive despite antimicrobial therapy
Antibody	Serum	60–70	90–99	Requires testing of paired specimens; seroconversion may not occur until 2 to 3 mo after infection; most specific for *L. pneumophila* serogroup 1; cross-reactions with antibodies to many other bacteria

*Sensitivity versus culture. Culture is the most sensitive diagnostic technique, but its absolute sensitivity is unknown; reasonable estimates are 80 to 90%.

Table 323-4 ■ ANTIMICROBIAL DRUG THERAPY FOR LEGIONNAIRES' DISEASE

PATIENT TYPE	DISEASE SEVERITY*	FIRST CHOICES	DOSAGE	ALTERNATIVES	DOSAGE
Normal host	Mild to moderate	Erythromycin†	500 mg to 1 g IV, 500 mg orally each four times daily; 14–21 d	Levofloxacin†‡	500 mg IV or orally once daily; 7–10 d
		or Doxycycline	200 mg IV or orally once daily; 14–21 d	*or* Azithromycin†	500 mg IV or orally once daily; 3 d
	Severe	Levofloxacin†‡	500 mg IV or orally once daily; 7–10 d	Azithromycin†	Same dosage as above; 5 d
Immunosuppressed	Any type	Levofloxacin†‡	Same as above	Azithromycin†	Same dosage as above; 5 d

*Severe disease is that causing respiratory failure, bilateral pneumonia, or rapidly worsening pulmonary infiltrates, or the presence of at least two of the following three: blood urea nitrogen ≥30 mg/dL (11 mmol/L); diastolic blood pressure <60 mm Hg; respiratory rate >30/min.
†Approved by the Food and Drug Administration for the treatment of legionnaires' disease.
‡Acceptable alternatives include trovafloxacin,† 200 mg once daily IV or orally and ofloxacin, 500 mg twice daily IV or orally, both for 7 to 10 days.

Mild cases of legionnaires' disease can be treated with oral therapy exclusively. Quinolone antimicrobials (especially levofloxacin, trovafloxacin, and sparfloxacin) and the newer macrolide antimicrobials (clarithromycin and especially azithromycin) are more effective than erythromycin or doxycycline in experimental laboratory studies. The more active quinolone drugs (levofloxacin, trovafloxacin, and sparfloxacin) are preferred for organ transplant patients because of their very high activity in experimental legionnaires' disease and lack of interference with cyclosporine levels. In addition, most immunocompromised patients and most patients with severe legionnaires' disease should receive one of the more active quinolone antimicrobials or perhaps azithromycin rather than erythromycin. Because of its potent activity in experimental legionnaires' disease, many clinicians add rifampin to an erythromycin or doxycycline regimen for treatment of severe cases of legionnaires' disease. No clinical data have indicated the superiority of such combination therapy. The availability of newer and more active drugs makes such combination therapy less desirable. Penicillins, cephalosporins (first, second, and third generation), and aminoglycosides are ineffective for the treatment of legionnaires' disease. In fact, failure of pneumonia to respond to these agents should prompt consideration of legionnaires' disease and perhaps initiation of specific anti-*Legionella* therapy. No effective therapy for Pontiac fever is known.

Most patients with legionnaires' disease respond within 1 to 4 days to specific antimicrobial therapy. The symptoms clearing most rapidly are rigors, mental confusion, myalgia, anorexia, fatigue, and abdominal complaints. Fever may persist for a week after the initiation of therapy but starts a downward trend within a few days. Despite this clinical evidence of improvement, other findings may falsely imply disease progression, such as evidence of increased pulmonary consolidation on physical examination and on radiography. Weeks to months are required for the resolution of pulmonary infiltrates. Patients with respiratory failure have a relatively poor prognosis and tend to have a much slower response to therapy.

Edelstein PH: Antimicrobial chemotherapy for legionnaires' disease: A review. Clin Infect Dis 21 (Suppl.):265, 1995. *Detailed review of antimicrobial therapy.*

Fang GD, Fine M, Orloff J, et al: New and emerging etiologies for community-acquired pneumonia with implications for therapy: A prospective multicenter study of 359 cases. Medicine (Baltimore) 69:307, 1990. *Excellent survey of community-acquired pneumonia, including legionnaires' disease.*

Stout JE, Yu VL: Legionellosis. N Engl J Med 337:682, 1997. *Good recent clinical review.*

324 STREPTOCOCCAL INFECTIONS

Dennis L. Stevens

CLASSIFICATION AND IDENTIFICATION OF STREPTOCOCCI

Streptococci are gram-positive globular or coccoid bacteria that grow in chains. Streptococci colonize the skin and mucous membranes of animals, produce catalase, and may be aerobic, anaerobic, or facultative. Streptococci require complex media containing blood products for optimal growth. On blood agar plates, streptococci may cause complete (β), incomplete (α) or no hemolysis (γ). The exhaustive work of Rebecca Lancefield has allowed hemolytic streptococci to be classified into types A through O based on acid-extractable carbohydrate antigens of cell wall material. The availability of rapid latex agglutination kits provides even small clinical laboratories with the means to identify streptococci according to Lancefield group. Bacitracin susceptibility, bile esculin hydrolysis, and the CAMP (Christie-Atkins-Munch-Peterson) test (flame-type synergistic hemolysis on a *Staphylococcus aureus* blood agar streak) are useful presumptive tests for classifying groups A, D, or B streptococci, respectively. Modern schemes of classification of hemolytic and non-hemolytic streptococci use complex biochemical and genetic techniques.

GROUP A STREPTOCOCCAL INFECTIONS EPIDEMIOLOGY. HOST RANGE. The concept of group A streptococcus as a pure human pathogen is supported by the observations that (1) natural group A streptococcus infection in animals is rare; (2) laboratory animals are not useful models of streptococcal pharyngitis, scarlet fever, erysipelas, rheumatic fever, or post-streptococcal glomerulonephritis; (3) the inoculum needed to cause infection in laboratory animals is orders of magnitude greater than that estimated to cause infection in humans; and (4) streptococci have developed highly sophisticated defensive molecules that bind, inactivate, or destroy human immune response molecules (e.g., IgG antibody and complement [C5a]).

AGE-RELATED ATTACK RATES. All group A streptococcal infections have the highest incidence in children younger than 10 years. The asymptomatic prevalence is also higher (15 to 20%) in children than in adults (<5%). Age is not the only factor; crowded conditions in temperate climates during the winter months are also associated with epidemics of pharyngitis in school children, as well as in military recruits. Impetigo is most common in children aged 2 to 5 and may occur year-round in tropical areas but largely in the summer in temperate climates. Similarly, 90% of cases of scarlet fever occur in children 2 to 8 years old and, like pharyngitis, it is most common in temperate regions during winter. An experiment of nature in the Faeroe Islands (Denmark) suggested that susceptibility to scarlet fever is not dependent on young age *per se*. Briefly, scarlet fever had disappeared from that isolated island group for several decades until it was reintroduced by a visitor with unsuspected scarlet fever. An epidemic of scarlet fever ensued, with significant attack rates in all age groups, thus suggesting that other factors, such as the lack of protective antibody against scarlatina toxin or the introduction of a new strain, rather than age predisposed those individuals to clinical illness.

In contrast to pharyngitis, impetigo, and scarlet fever, bacteremia has had the highest age-specific attack rate in the elderly and in neonates. However, between 1986 and 1988, the prevalence of bacteremia increased 800 to 1000% in adolescents and adults in western countries. Although some of this increase is attributable to intravenous drug abuse and puerperal sepsis, most of the increase is due to cases of streptococcal toxic shock syndrome, in which a defined portal of entry is not apparent in 50% of cases.

TRANSMISSION OF GROUP A STREPTOCOCCUS. Human mucous

membranes and skin serve as the natural reservoirs of *S. pyogenes*. Pharyngeal and cutaneous acquisition is by person-to-person spread via aerosolized microdroplets or by direct contact, respectively. Epidemics of pharyngitis and scarlet fever have also occurred after the consumption of contaminated, non-pasteurized milk or food. Epidemics of impetigo have been reported, particularly in tropical areas, in day care centers, and among underprivileged children. Group A streptococcal infections in hospitalized patients occur during childbirth (puerperal sepsis), times of war (epidemic gangrene), and surgical convalescence (surgical wound infection, surgical scarlet fever) or as a result of burns (burn wound sepsis). Thus in most clinical streptococcal infections, the mode of transmission and portal of entry are easily ascertained. In contrast, among patients with streptococcal toxic shock syndrome, the portal of entry is obvious in only 50% of cases.

PATHOGENESIS. Adherence of cocci to the mucosal epithelium is necessary but not sufficient to cause disease in all cases inasmuch as prolonged asymptomatic carriage is well documented. Complex interactions between host epithelium and streptococcal factors such as M protein, lipoteichoic acid, and fimbriae are necessary for adherence. Fibronectin binding protein (protein F) also contributes to adherence because protein F–deficient mutants are incapable of binding to epithelial cells. Protein F is up-regulated by oxygen and decreased in anaerobic conditions.

Within the tissues, streptococci may evade opsonophagocytosis by virtue of a hyaluronic acid capsule, a C5a peptidase that destroys or inactivates complement-derived chemoattractants and opsonins, or by immunoglobulin binding protein. Expression of M protein, in the absence of type-specific antibody, also protects the organism from phagocytosis by polymorphonuclear leukocytes (PMNs) and monocytes. In tissues, streptolysin O secreted in high concentration destroys approaching phagocytes. Distal to the focus of infection, lower concentrations of streptolysin O stimulate PMN adhesion to endothelial cells, effectively preventing continued granulocyte migration and promoting vascular damage. In a non-immune host, streptolysin O, streptococcal pyrogenic exotoxins (SPE A, B, C, MF, and SSA), and other streptococcal components stimulate host cells to produce tumor necrosis factor (TNF) and interleukin-1 (IL-1), cytokines that mediate hypotension, stimulate leukostasis, and eventually result in shock, microvascular injury, multiorgan failure, and if excessive, death. A unique feature of the pyrogenic exotoxins and some M protein fragments is their ability to interact with certain V_β regions of the T-cell receptor in the absence of classic antigen processing by antigen-presenting cells (Fig. 324–1). This interaction results in massive clonal proliferation of T lymphocytes. SPE type B, a cysteine protease, may play a role in the pathogenesis of necrotizing fasciitis and shock through its ability to cleave pre–IL-1β into active IL-1β, activation of endogenous metalloproteases, and cleavage of high-molecular-weight kininogen into bradykinin. Thus in streptococcal toxic shock syndrome, lymphokines (TNF-β, interferon-γ, and IL-2), monokines (TNF-α, IL-1, and IL-6), and bradykinin may be crucial in the mediation of shock and organ failure.

BACTERIAL CELL STRUCTURE AND EXTRACELLULAR PRODUCTS. CAPSULE. Some strains of *S. pyogenes* possess capsules of hyaluronic acid and form large mucoid colonies on blood agar. Luxuriant production of M protein may also impart a mucoid colony morphology, and this trait has been associated with M-18 strains. An operon promoter sequence is the key element in both the constitutive and dynamic regulation of hyaluronic acid synthesis in group A streptococci, and its activity is increased during ideal growth conditions and log-phase growth. It plays an important role in pharyngitis, soft tissue infection, and invasive disease by binding to CD44 on epithelial cells and by serving as an antiphagocytic factor.

CELL WALL. The cell wall is composed of a peptidoglycan backbone with integral lipoteichoic acid components. The function of lipoteichoic acid is not well known, but both peptidoglycan and lipoteichoic acid have important interactions with the host.

M PROTEINS. Over 80 different M protein types of group A streptococci are currently described. The protein is a coil structure consisting of four regions of repeating amino acids (A to D), a proline/glycine-rich region that serves to intercalate the protein into the bacterial cell wall, and a hydrophobic region that acts as a

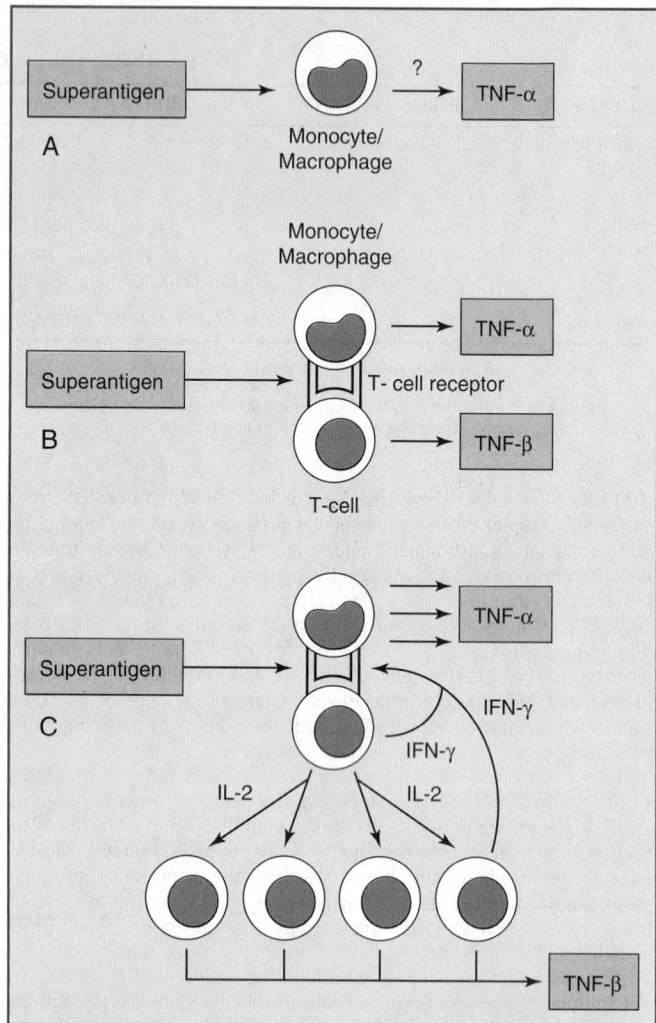

FIGURE 324–1 ■ Superantigen-induced production of tumor necrosis factor α (TNF-α) and lymphotoxin (TNF-β) by periperal blood mononuclear cells. *A*, Superantigens induce human monocytes to produce TNF-α; however, it is unclear whether such production results solely from direct stimulation of the monocyte by the superantigen. *B*, In mixed mononuclear cell populations, superantigens stimulate TNF-α synthesis in monocytes and, by binding to specific V_β regions of the T-cell receptor, induce the synthesis of lymphotoxin (TNF-β) from T cells. *C*, The T-cell response to superantigen stimulation includes the production of interleukin-2 (IL-2), which results in clonal proliferation with concordant production of interferon-γ (IFN-γ) and TNF-β. IFN-γ can then amplify monocyte synthesis of TNF-α, IL-1, and IL-6. (From Stevens DL, Bryant AE, Hackett SP: Sepsis syndromes and toxic shock syndromes: Concepts in pathogenesis and a perspective of future strategy. Current Opin Infect Dis 6:374, 1993.)

membrane anchor. Region A near the *N* terminus is highly variable, and antibodies to this region confer type-specific protection. Within the more conserved B to D regions lies an area that binds one of the complement regulatory proteins (factor H), stearically inhibiting antibody binding and complement-derived opsonin deposition and effectively camouflaging the organism against humoral immune surveillance. M protein inhibits the phagocytosis of *S. pyogenes* by PMNs, although this property can be overcome by type-specific antisera. Observations by Lancefield suggest that the quantity of M protein produced decreases with passage on artificial media and conversely increases rapidly with passage through mice. The quantity of M protein produced by an infecting strain progressively decreases during convalescence and during prolonged carriage.

STREPTOLYSIN O. Streptolysin O belongs to a family of oxygen-labile, thiol-activated cytolysins (TAC) and causes the broad zone of β-hemolysis surrounding colonies of *S. pyogenes* on blood agar plates. TAC toxins bind to cholesterol on eukaryotic cell membranes and create toxin-cholesterol aggregates that contribute to cell lysis via a colloid-osmotic mechanism. Cholesterol inhibits toxicity in isolated myocytes and hemolysis of red blood cells *in vitro.* In situations in which serum cholesterol is high, i.e., nephrotic syndrome, falsely elevated antistreptolysin O titers may occur because both cholesterol and antistreptolysin O antibody will "neutralize streptolysin O." Striking amino acid homology exists between streptolysin O and other TAC toxins.

STREPTOLYSIN S. Streptolysin S is a cell-associated hemolysin that does not diffuse into the agar media. Purification and characterization of this protein have been difficult, and its only role in pathogenesis may be in direct or contact cytotoxicity.

DEOXYRIBONUCLEASES A, B, C, AND D. Expression of deoxyribonucleases (DNases) *in vivo* elicits the production of anti-DNase antibody following both pharyngeal and skin infection; this response is most true for DNase B with group A streptococci. Dnases may also contribute to cytokine production, although their importance in pathogenesis has not been established.

HYALURONIDASE. This extracellular enzyme hydrolyzes hyaluronic acid in deeper tissues, thereby facilitating the spread of infection along fascial planes. Antihyaluronidase titers rise following *S. pyogenes* infections, especially those involving the skin.

PYROGENIC EXOTOXINS. SPE types A, B, and C, also called scarlatina toxin and erythrogenic toxins, induce lymphocyte blastogenesis, potentiate endotoxin-induced shock, induce fever, suppress antibody synthesis, and act as superantigens. Identification of these three different types of SPEs may in part explain why some individuals may have multiple attacks of scarlet fever. The gene for pyrogenic exotoxin A *(speA)* is transmitted by bacteriophages, and stable production depends on lysogenic conversion in a manner analogous to diphtheria toxin production by *Corynebacterium diphtheriae.* Control of SPE A production is not yet understood, although the quantity of SPE A produced varies dramatically from decade to decade. Historically, SPE A–producing strains have been associated with severe cases of scarlet fever and, more recently, with streptoccal toxic shock syndrome.

Although all strains of group A streptococci are endowed with genes for SPE B *(speB)*, like SPE A, the quantity of toxin produced varies greatly.

Pyrogenic exotoxin type C (SPE C), like SPE A, is bacteriophage mediated, and expression is likewise highly variable. Mild cases of scarlet fever in England and the United States have been associated with SPE C–positive strains. Recently, two other pyrogenic exotoxins, streptoccal superantigen (SPE SSA) and mitogenic factor (SPE MF), have been described and their role in pathogenesis is being studied.

CLINICAL INFECTIONS. PHARYNGITIS AND THE ASYMPTOMATIC CARRIER. Patients with streptococcal pharyngitis have an abrupt onset of sore throat, submandibular adenopathy, fever, and chilliness but not usually frank rigors. Cough and hoarseness are rare, but pain on swallowing is characteristic. The uvula is edematous, tonsils are hypertrophied, and the pharynx is erythematous with exudate that may be punctate or confluent. Acute pharyngitis is sufficient to induce antibody against M protein, streptolysin O, DNase, hyaluronidase, and if present, pyrogenic exotoxins. Depending on the infecting strain, pharyngitis may progress to scarlet fever, bacteremia, suppurative head and neck infections, rheumatic fever, post-streptococcal glomerulonephritis, or streptococcal toxic shock syndrome. Pharyngitis is usually self-limited, and pain, swelling, and fever resolve spontaneously in 3 to 4 days even without treatment.

Definitive diagnosis is difficult when based only on clinical parameters, especially in infants, in whom rhinorrhea may be the dominant manifestation. Even in older children with all the preceding physical findings, the correct clinical diagnosis is made in only 75% of patients. Absence of any one of the classic signs greatly reduces the specificity. Rapid antigen detection tests in the office setting have a sensitivity and specificity of 40 to 90%. A popular approach in clinical practice is to obtain two throat swab samples from the posterior of the pharynx or tonsillar surface. A rapid strep test is performed on the 1st, and if it is positive, the patient is treated with antibiotics and the 2nd swab discarded. If the rapid strep test is negative, the 2nd sample is sent for culture, and treatment is withheld pending a positive culture.

SCARLET FEVER. During the last 30 to 40 years, outbreaks of scarlet fever in the western world have been notably mild, and the illness has been referred to as "pharyngitis with a rash" or "benign scarlet fever." In contrast, in the latter half of the 19th century,

mortalities of 25 to 35% were common in the United States, western Europe, and Scandinavia. The fatal or malignant forms of scarlet fever have been described as either septic or toxic. "Septic scarlet fever" refers to the development of local invasion of the soft tissues of the neck and complications such as upper airway obstruction, otitis media with perforation, meningitis, mastoiditis, invasion of the jugular vein or carotid artery, and bronchopneumonia. "Toxic scarlet fever" is rare today, but historically, severe sore throat, marked fever, delirium, skin rash, and painful cervical lymph nodes initially developed. In severe toxic cases, temperatures of 107° F, pulses of 130 to 160 beats per minute, severe headache, delirium, convulsions, little if any skin rash, and death within 24 hours were common. These cases occurred before the advent of antibiotics, antipyretics, and anticonvulsants, and sudden deaths were the result of uncontrolled seizures and hyperpyrexia. In contrast, children with septic scarlet fever had prolonged courses and succumbed 2 to 3 weeks after the onset of pharyngitis. Complications of streptococcal pharyngitis and malignant forms of scarlet fever have been less common in the antibiotic era. Even before antibiotics became available, necrotizing fasciitis and myositis were not described in association with scarlet fever.

ERYSIPELAS. Erysipelas is caused exclusively by *S. pyogenes* and is characterized by an abrupt onset of fiery red swelling of the face or extremities. Distinctive features are well-defined margins, particularly along the nasolabial fold, scarlet or salmon-red rash, rapid progression, and intense pain. Flaccid bullae may develop during the 2nd to 3rd day, yet extension to deeper soft tissues is rare. Surgical débridement is not necessary, and treatment with penicillin is effective. Swelling may progress despite treatment, although fever, pain, and the intense redness diminish. Desquamation of the involved skin occurs 5 to 10 days into the illness. Infants and elderly adults are most commonly afflicted, and historically erysipelas, like scarlet fever, was more severe before 1900.

STREPTOCOCCAL PYODERMA (IMPETIGO CONTAGIOSA). Impetigo is most common in patients with poor hygiene or malnutrition. Colonization of the unbroken skin occurs first, and then intradermal inoculation is usually initiated by minor abrasions or insect bites. Single or multiple thick-crusted, golden-yellow lesions develop within 10 to 14 days. Penicillin orally or parenterally and bacitracin or mupirocin topically are effective treatments for impetigo and also reduce the transmission of streptococci to susceptible individuals. None of these treatments, including penicillin, prevents post-streptococcal glomerulonephritis.

CELLULITIS. Group A streptococcus is the most common cause of cellulitis; however, alternative diagnoses may be obvious when associated with a primary focus such as an abscess or boil *(S. aureus),* dog bite *(DF-2),* cat bite *(Pasteurella multocida),* freshwater injury *(Aeromonas hydrophila),* seawater injury *(Vibrio vulnificus),* and so on (see Chapters 372 and 437). Clinical clues to diagnosis are important because aspiration of the leading edge or punch biopsy yields a causative organism in only 15 and 40% of cases, respectively. Patients with lymphedema of any cause such as lymphoma, filariasis, or sequelae of regional lymph node dissection (as in mastectomy or carcinoma of the prostate) are predisposed to streptococcal cellulitis, as are patients with chronic venous stasis. Recently, recurrent saphenous vein donor site cellulitis has been attributed to group A, C, or G streptococci. Group A streptococci may invade the epidermis and subcutaneous tissue and cause local swelling, erythema, and pain. The skin becomes indurated and, unlike the brilliant redness of erysipelas, is pinkish. Streptococcal cellulitis responds quickly to penicillin, although when staphylococcus is of concern, nafcillin or oxacillin may be a better choice. If fever, pain, or swelling increases, if bluish or violet bullae or discoloration appears, or if signs of systemic toxicity develop, a deeper infection such as necrotizing fasciitis or myositis should be considered (see Necrotizing Fasciitis). When an elevated serum creatine phosphokinase level suggests deeper infection, prompt surgical inspection and débridement should be performed.

LYMPHANGITIS. Cutaneous infection with bright red streaks ascending proximally is invariably due to group A streptococcus. Prompt parenteral antibiotic treatment is mandatory because bacteremia and systemic toxicity develop rapidly once streptococci reach the blood stream via the thoracic duct.

NECROTIZING FASCIITIS. Necrotizing fasciitis, originally called "streptococcal gangrene," is a deep-seated infection of the subcutaneous tissue that results in progressive destruction of fascia and fat but may spare the skin itself. Subsequently, "necrotizing fasciitis" has become the preferred term because *Clostridium perfringens,* *Clostridium septicum,* and *S. aureus* can produce a similar pathologic process. Infection may begin at the site of trivial or inapparent trauma. Within the initial 24 hours, swelling, heat, erythema, and tenderness develop and rapidly spread proximally and distally from the original focus. During the next 24 to 48 hours, the erythema darkens, changing from red to purple and then to blue, and blisters and bullae form that contain clear yellow fluid. On the 4th or 5th day, the purple areas become frankly gangrenous. From the 7th to the 10th days, the line of demarcation becomes sharply defined, and the dead skin begins to reveal extensive necrosis of the subcutaneous tissue. Patients become increasingly prostrated and emaciated and may become unresponsive, mentally cloudy, or even delirious. Aggressive fasciotomy and débridement ("bearclaw fasciotomy") and irrigations with Dakan's solution achieved mortality rates as low as 20%, even before antibiotics were available. Since 1989, the mortality rate of necrotizing fasciitis despite antibiotics, surgical débridement, and intensive care unit treatment is higher than that reported by Meleney in 1924, probably because of the increased virulence of streptococci (see Streptococcal Toxic Shock Syndrome below).

MYOSITIS. Historically, streptococcal myositis has been an extremely uncommon infection, only 21 cases being documented from 1900 to 1985. Recently, the prevalence of streptococcal myositis has increased in the United States, Norway, and Sweden. Translocation of streptococci from the pharynx to the deep site of trauma (muscle) must occur hematogenously. Symptomatic pharyngitis or penetrating trauma are uncommon. Severe pain may be the only symptom, and swelling and erythema may be the only signs of infection. In some cases a single muscle group is involved; however, because patients are frequently bacteremic, multiple sites of myositis or abscess can occur. Distinguishing streptococcal myositis from spontaneous gas gangrene caused by *C. perfringens* or *C. septicum* may be difficult, although the presence of crepitus or gas in the tissue would favor clostridial infection. Myositis is easily distinguished from necrotizing fasciitis anatomically by surgical exploration or incisional biopsy, although the clinical features of both conditions overlap. Many cases of necrotizing fasciitis have associated myositis and myonecrosis. In published reports, the case fatality rate of necrotizing fasciitis is between 20 and 50%, whereas that of streptococcal myositis is between 80 and 100%. Aggressive surgical débridement is extremely important because of the poor efficacy of penicillin described in human cases, as well as in experimental models of streptococcal myositis (see the section on antibiotic efficacy).

PNEUMONIA. Pneumonia caused by group A streptococcus is most common in women in the 2nd and 3rd decades of life and causes large pleural effusions and empyema that develop rapidly. Chest tube drainage is mandatory even though management is complicated by multiple loculations and fibrinous effusions resulting in restrictive lung disease. Prolonged penicillin therapy, thoracoscopy, and decortication of the pleura may be necessary to prevent adhesive pleuritis, fibrosis, and subsequent restrictive lung disease.

STREPTOCOCCAL TOXIC SHOCK SYNDROME. Epidemiology. In the late 1980s, invasive group A streptococcal infections occurred in North America and Europe in previously healthy individuals aged 20 to 50. This illness is associated with bacteremia, deep soft tissue infection, shock, multiorgan failure, and death in 30% of cases. Although streptococcal toxic shock syndrome occurs sporadically, minor epidemics have been reported. Most patients have either a viral-like prodrome, a history of minor trauma, recent surgery, or varicella infection. The prodrome may be due to a viral illness predisposing to toxic shock syndrome, or these vague early symptoms may be related to the evolving infection. In about 50% of cases associated with necrotizing fasciitis, the infection begins deep in the soft tissue at a site of minor trauma that frequently did not result in a break in the skin. Surgical procedures, viral infections such as varicella and influenza, penetrating trauma, insect bites, slivers, and burns may provide portals of entry in the remaining cases.

Symptoms and Physical Findings. The abrupt onset of severe pain

Table 324–1 ■ CLINICAL AND LABORATORY FEATURES OF STREPTOCOCCAL TOXIC SHOCK SYNDROME

Symptoms
  Viral-like prodrome
  Severe pain
  Confusion
  Nausea
  Chills
Signs
  Fever
  Soft tissue swelling and tenderness
  Tachycardia
  Tachypnea
  Hypotension
Laboratory Findings
  Hematologic tests
    Marked left shift
    Red cell hemolysis
    Thrombocytopenia
  Chemistry tests
    Azotemia
    Hypocalcemia
    Hypoalbuminemia
    Creatine phosphokinase elevation
  Urinalysis
    Hematuria
  Blood gases
    Hypoxia
    Acidosis
  Radiographic
    ARDS
    Soft tissue swelling
Complications
  Profound hypotension
  ARDS
  Renal failure
  Liver failure
  Necrotizing soft tissue infections
  Bacteremia
  Death (30%)

ARDS = adult respiratory distress syndrome.

is a common initial symptom of streptoccal toxic shock syndrome (Table 324–1). The pain most commonly involves an extremity but may also mimic peritonitis, pelvic inflammatory disease, acute myocardial infarction, or pericarditis. Treatment with non-steroidal anti-inflammatory agents may mask the initial symptoms or predispose to more severe complications such as shock.

Fever is the most common initial sign, although some patients have profound hypothermia secondary to shock (see Table 324–1). Confusion is present in over half the patients and may progress to coma or combativeness. On admission 80% of patients have tachycardia, and over half have systolic blood pressure lower than 110 mm Hg. Of those with normal blood pressure on admission, most become hypotensive within 4 hours. Soft tissue infection evolves to necrotizing fasciitis or myositis in 50 to 70% of patients, and these conditions require emergency surgical débridement, fasciotomy, or amputation. An ominous sign is progression of soft tissue swelling to violaceous or bluish vesicles or bullae. Many other clinical pictures may be associated with streptococcal toxic shock syndrome including endophthalmitis, myositis, perihepatitis, peritonitis, myocarditis, meningitis, septic arthritis, and overwhelming sepsis. Patients with shock and multiorgan failure without signs or symptoms of local infections have a worse prognosis because definitive diagnosis and surgical débridement may be delayed.

Laboratory Abnormalities. Hemoglobinuria is present and serum creatinine is elevated in most patients at the time of admission. Serum albumin concentrations are moderately low (3.3 g/dL) on admission and drop progressively over 48 to 72 hours. Hypocalcemia, including ionized hypocalcemia, is detectable early in the hospital course. The serum creatinine kinase level is a useful test to detect deeper soft tissue infections such as necrotizing fasciitis or myositis.

The initial hematologic studies demonstrate only mild leukocytosis, but a dramatic left shift (43% of white blood cells may be band forms, metamyelocytes, and myelocytes). The mean platelet count is normal on admission but may drop rapidly by 48 hours,

Table 324–2 ■ ANTIBIOTIC THERAPY FOR GROUP A STREPTOCOCCAL INFECTIONS

CONDITION	ROUTE	DOSAGES
Pharyngitis and impetigo		
Benzathine penicillin	IM	1.2 million U (>27 kg)
Penicillin G (or V)	PO	200,000 U qid for 10 d
Erythromycin	PO	40 mg/kg/d (up to 1 g/d)
Recurrent streptococcal pharyngitis/tonsillitis		
Same as above, *or*		
Ampicillin plus clavulanic acid	PO	20–40 mg/kg/d
Oral cephalosporin		Check *PDR*
Clindamycin	PO	10 mg/kg/d
Cellulitis and erysipelas		
Penicillin G or V	PO	200,000 U qid for 10 d
Dicloxacillin*	PO	500 mg qid for 10 d (adults)
Necrotizing fasciitis/myositis/ streptococcal toxic shock syndrome		
Clindamycin	IV	1800–2100 mg daily (adults)
Penicillin	IV	2 million U q4h (adults)
Prophylaxis for rheumatic fever (see Chapter 325)		

PDR = *Physicians' Desk Reference.*
*Alternative to penicillin if *Staphylococcus aureus* is of concern. Cephalosporins could be used; however, most (except ceftriaxone) have less activity than penicillin G against streptococci.

even in the absence of criteria for disseminated intravascular coagulopathy.

Clinical Course. Shock is apparent early in the course, and fluid management is complicated by profound capillary leak. Adult respiratory distress syndrome occurs frequently (55%), and renal dysfunction that precedes hypotension in many patients may progress in spite of treatment. In patients who survive, serum creatinine levels return to normal within 4 to 6 weeks; many require dialysis. Overall, 30% of patients die despite aggressive treatment including intravenous fluids, colloid, pressors, mechanical ventilation, and surgical interventions such as fasciotomy, débridement, exploratory laparotomy, intraocular aspiration, amputation, and hysterectomy.

Characteristics of Clinical Isolates. Group A streptococcus is isolated from blood in 60% of cases and from deep tissue specimens in 95% of cases. M types 1, 3, 12, and 28 are the most common strains isolated but account for only 60 to 70% of the isolates, the remaining being a wide variety of M typable and non-typable strains. Pyrogenic exotoxins A and/or B have been found in isolates from the majority of patients with severe infection, although the quantities of these toxins that are produced in vitro varies widely. Infections in Norway, Sweden, and Great Britain have been primarily due to M type 1 strains that produce pyrogenic exotoxin B. Other novel pyrogenic exotoxins are also being described and may explain the recent enhanced virulence of group A streptococcus.

NON-SUPPURATIVE COMPLICATIONS. The non-suppurative complications of streptococcal disease are acute rheumatic fever and acute glomerulonephritis. These conditions are discussed in Chapters 106 and 325, respectively.

TREATMENT OF GROUP A INFECTIONS. PROPHYLAXIS. During epidemics, particularly when rheumatic fever or post-streptococcal glomerulonephritis is prevalent, treatment of asymptomatic carriers may be necessary. Studies by the U.S. military have shown that monthly injections of benzathine penicillin greatly reduce the incidence of streptococcal pharyngitis and rheumatic fever in young soldiers living in crowded conditions.

EMERGENCE OF RESISTANCE. Erythromycin resistance of *S. pyogenes* is currently 4% in western countries; however, in Japan in 1974 the rate reached 72%, and reports of 100% resistance have emanated from Scandanavia. Sulfonamide resistance is currently reported in fewer than 1% of group A streptococcal isolates.

THERAPEUTIC FAILURE OF PENICILLIN. The recommended antibiotic therapies for group A streptococcal diseases are shown in Table 324–2. Resistance to penicillin has not been described, yet in some settings a lack of in vivo efficacy is seen despite in vitro susceptibility to penicillin. Three mechanisms may explain this lack of efficacy.

1. *β-Lactamase production by coinfecting organisms.* Penicillin failure in pharyngitis, tonsillitis, or mixed infections may be due to inactivation of penicillin in situ by β-lactamases produced by cocolonizing organisms such as *Bacteroides fragilis, Haemophilus influenzae,* or *S. aureus.* For example, the failure rate of penicillin treatment of group A streptococcal pharyngitis may approach 25%, and if such patients are treated with a 2nd course of penicillin, the failure rate may approach 80%, perhaps because of selection of β-lactamase–producing bacteria. In contrast, cure rates of 90% have been achieved when treatment consisted of amoxicillin plus clavulanate or clindamycin.

2. *Genotypic tolerance.* Genotypic tolerance to penicillin may also contribute to penicillin's lack of efficacy in tonsillitis or pharyngitis. In fact, penicillin-tolerant strains have also caused epidemics of pharyngitis. Tolerant strains demonstrate a slower rate of growth, a slower rate of bacterial killing by penicillin, and an absence of β-lactam–induced cell lysis. The role of tolerance in antibiotic treatment failure is not fully understood.

3. *Inoculum effect.* Studies in animals infected with group A streptococcus demonstrate that penicillin is effective only if given early or if small numbers of streptococci are used to initiate infection. It is likely that streptococci are not in a logarithmic phase of growth when the clinical diagnosis of necrotizing fasciitis or myositis is made. Penicillin is most effective against streptococci in log-phase growth, a stage in their life cycle when five penicillin binding proteins are expressed. Conversely, during the stationary phase, the two penicillin binding proteins with the greatest affinity for penicillin are absent. In contrast, clindamycin has much greater efficacy than penicillin even if treatment is delayed up to 16 hours. Clindamycin's greater efficacy could be due to its ability to suppress M-protein and toxin synthesis, its longer post-antibiotic effect, an indifference to the in vivo inoculum effect, or its effects on the host's immune system such as suppression of TNF synthesis.

NON-GROUP A STREPTOCOCCAL INFECTIONS (Table 324-3)

ENTEROCOCCUS FAECALIS AND ENTEROCOCCUS FAECIUM. These gram-positive, facultatively anaerobic bacteria are usually non-hemolytic but may demonstrate α- or β-hemolysis. Enterococci were previously classified as group D streptococci because they hydrolyze bile esculin and possess the group D antigen. Based on nucleic acid hybridization studies, they are now designated *Entero-*

Table 324-3 ■ NON-GROUP A STREPTOCOCCAL INFECTIONS

ORGANISM	LANCEFIELD GROUP	TYPE OF INFECTION	THERAPY
S. agalactiae	B	Neonatal sepsis Postpartum sepsis Septic arthritis Soft tissue infection Osteomyelitis	Ampicillin or penicillin
Enterococcus faecalis	D	Endocarditis Bacteremia UTI Abscesses, GI	Ampicillin + gentamicin
S. milleri	A, C, F, G, and non-typable	Abscesses Bacteremia	Penicillin
S. bovis	D	Bacteremia Abscesses	Penicillin
S. equi	C	Bacteremia Cellulitis Pharyngitis	Penicillin
S. canis	G	Bacteremia Cellulitis Pharyngitis	Penicillin
"Viridans" *S. salivarius*	Non-typable	Non-pathogen	
S. mutans		Endocarditis Caries	Penicillin
S. sanguis		Endocarditis	Penicillin
S. mitior		Endocarditis	Penicillin

UTI = urinary tract infection; GI = gastrointestinal.

coccus. Enterococci are commonly isolated from the stool, urine, and sites of intra-abdominal and lower extremity infection. Enterococci cause subacute bacterial endocarditis and have become an important cause of nosocomial infection, not because of increased virulence but because of antibiotic resistance. First, person-to-person transfer of multidrug-resistant enterococci is a major concern to hospital epidemiologists. Second, superinfections and spontaneous bacteremia from endogenous sites of enterococcal colonization are described in patients receiving quinolone or moxalactam antibiotics. Last, conjugational transfer of plasmids and transposons between enterococci in the face of intense antibiotic pressure within the hospital mileu have created multidrug-resistant strains, including those with vancomycin and teicoplanin resistance. Acquired resistance to glycopeptide in enterococci is due to the production of peptidoglycan precursors ending in the dipeptide D-alanine-D-lactate (D-ala-D-lac) instead of the dipeptide D-ala-D-ala, which is found in susceptible bacteria. This substitution prevents the formation of complexes between glycopeptides and peptidoglycan precursors at the cell surface that are responsible for inhibition of cell wall synthesis. Acquired glycopeptide resistance by this mechanism is conferred by two classes of genetic elements (Van A or Van B), often carried by mobile elements (transposons), that encode a dehydrogenase (Van H or Van HB) for reduction of pyruvate into D-lactate and a ligase (Van A or Van B) for synthesis of D-ala-D-lac. The majority of enterococci harboring Van B–type gene clusters are inducibly resistant to vancomycin but remain susceptible to teicoplanin because induction occurs only in the presence of vancomycin. Serious enterococcal infections such as endocarditis or bacteremia require a synergistic combination of antimicrobials such as ampicillin or vancomycin, together with an aminoglycoside. Teicoplanin may be substituted for vancomycin if Van B–type resistance is present. Unfortunately, some strains of enterococci are resistant to all known antibiotics. β-Lactamase–positive (Nitrocefin disk positive) strains can be treated with ampicillin and sulbactam.

STREPTOCOCCUS BOVIS. *S. bovis* is also a cause of subacute bacterial endocarditis and bacteremia in patients with underlying gastrointestinal pathology or malignancy. Unlike the enterococcus, it remains highly sensitive to penicillin.

GROUP C AND G STREPTOCOCCI. These organisms may be isolated from the throats of both humans and dogs, produce streptolysin O, and resemble group A in colony morphology and spectrum of clinical disease. Before rapid identification tests were developed, many infections caused by groups C and G were mistakenly attributed to group A, such as pharyngitis, cellulitis, skin and wound infections, endocarditis, meningitis, osteomyelitis, and arthritis. Rheumatic fever following group C or G infection has not been described. These strains also cause recurrent cellulitis at the saphenous vein donor site in patients who have undergone coronary artery bypass surgery. Both organisms are susceptible to penicillin, erythromycin, vancomycin, and clindamycin.

STREPTOCOCCUS MILLERI. *S. milleri* bacteria are usually β-hemolytic but may also be non-hemolytic or α-hemolytic and produce minute colonies on blood agar plates. They normally colonize the oropharynx, upper gastrointestinal tract, and appendix. Infections are most commonly related to contiguous abscess formation such as a tooth abscess or periapendiceal abscess. Primary bacteremia with or without endocarditis and metastatic abscesses of the brain, lung, bone, joints, liver, and spleen are characteristic of *S. milleri.*

STREPTOCOCCUS AGALACTIAE. *S. agalactiae* (group B streptococci) colonizes the vagina, gastrointestinal tract, and occasionally the upper respiratory tract of normal humans. These organisms are recognized as gray-white colonies, slightly larger than group A streptococci, but with a narrower zone of hemolysis. They are resistant to bacitracin, do not hydrolyze bile esculin, demonstrate a positive CAMP test, and hydrolyze sodium hippurate. Definitive identification is made with group-specific antiserum or commercial kits that use agglutination end points. The polysaccharide capsule is the prime virulence factor in group B streptococci and is instrumental in the evasion of phagocytosis. Currently, six different capsular polysaccharide types of group B are recognized and designated Ia, Ib, II, III, IV, and V. Immunity results from the development of opsonic type-specific antibody.

Group B streptococci are the most common cause of neonatal pneumonia, sepsis, and meningitis in the United States and western Europe, with an incidence of 1.8 to 3.2 cases per 1000 live births. Preterm infants born to mothers with premature rupture of membranes who are colonized with group B streptococci are at highest risk for early-onset pneumonia and sepsis. The mean time of onset is 20 hours, and symptoms are respiratory distress, apnea, fever, and hypothermia. Ascent of the streptococcus from the vagina to the amniotic cavity causes amnionitis. Infants may aspirate streptococci either from the birth canal during parturition or from amniotic fluid in utero. Radiographic evidence of pneumonia and or hyaline membrane disease is present in 40% of neonates with infection, and meningitis occurs in 30 to 40% of cases. Type III group B streptococcus causes most cases of meningitis.

Late-onset neonatal sepsis occurs 7 to 90 days postpartum, with symptoms of fever, poor feeding, lethargy, and irritability. Bacteremia is common, and meningitis occurs in 80% of cases.

Adults with group B infections include postpartum women and patients with peripheral vascular disease, diabetes, or malignancy. Soft tissue infection, septic arthritis, and osteomyelitis are the most common findings. Although penicillin is the treatment of choice, in practice many neonates are empirically treated with ampicillin (300 to 400 mg/kg/day) plus gentamicin. Once the diagnosis is established, penicillin at 200 to 500,000 U/kg/day should be given. Adults should receive 10 to 12 million U of penicillin per day for bacteremia, soft tissue infection, or osteomyelitis, but the dose should be increased to 18 to 24 million U/day for meningitis. Vancomycin and a 1st-generation cephalosporin are alternatives for penicillin-allergic patients. Intrapartum administration of ampicillin to women colonized with group B streptococcus who also had premature labor or prolonged rupture of membranes prevents group B neonatal sepsis. Infants should continue to receive ampicillin for 36 hours postpartum. It is imperative that women during the 3rd trimester be screened for risk factors for premature labor, and those at high risk should undergo culturing for streptococci. Women in labor who have not had such studies could be screened with a rapid antigen detection kit, even though the false-negative rate may be 10 to 30%. Passive immunization with intravenous immune globulin or active immunization with multivalent polysaccharide vaccine shows promise and will probably be the best approach to prevent neonatal sepsis, as well as postpartum infection of the mother.

Arthur M, Depardieu F, Gerbaud G, et al: The VanS sensor negatively controls VanR-mediated transcriptional activation of glycopeptide resistance genes of Tn1546 and related elements in the absence of induction. J Bacteriol 179:97, 1997.

Bisno AL, Stevens DL: Streptococcal infections in skin and soft tissues. N Engl J Med 334:240, 1996. *A general clinical review of soft tissue infections caused by group A streptococci.*

Herwald H, Collin M, Muller-Esterl W, Bjorck L: Streptococcal cysteine proteinase releases kinins: A novel virulence mechanism. J Exp Med 184:1, 1996. *This paper describes a novel mechanism for generation of potent endogenous mediators by group A streptococci.*

Kiska DL, Thiede B, Caracciolo J, et al: Invasive group A streptococcal infections in North Carolina: Epidemiology, clinical features, and genetic and serotype analysis of causative organisms. J Infect Dis 176:992, 1997. *A description of a recent epidemic of invasive group A streptococcal infections in North Carolina.*

Stevens DL: Invasive group A streptococcus infections. Clin Infect Dis 14:2, 1992. *A review article describing the changing epidemiology of scarlet fever, necrotizing fasciitis, myositis, bacteremia, and the streptococcal toxic shock syndrome.*

Stevens DL, Bryant AE, Hackett SP: Sepsis syndromes and toxic shock syndromes: Concepts in pathogenesis and a perspective of future treatment strategies. Curr Opin Infect Dis 6:374, 1993. *Compares the cellular basis of cytokine- and lymphokine-mediated shock caused by gram-negative and gram-positive bacteria.*

Stevens DL, Tanner MH, Winship J, et al: Severe group A streptococcal infections associated with a toxic shock–like syndrome and scarlet fever toxin A. N Engl J Med 321:1, 1989. *Reports clinical and laboratory features and complications of 20 patients with streptococcal toxic shock syndrome. An analysis of strains reveals that most were M types 1 and 3 and most strains produced pyrogenic exotoxin type A.*

325 RHEUMATIC FEVER

Alan L. Bisno

DEFINITION. Rheumatic fever is an inflammatory disease that occurs as a delayed, non-suppurative sequela of upper respiratory infection with group A streptococci. Its clinical manifestations include polyarthritis, carditis, subcutaneous nodules, erythema marginatum, and chorea in varying combinations. In its classic form the disorder is acute, febrile, and largely self-limited. However, damage to heart valves may be chronic and progressive and cause cardiac disability or death many years after the initial episode.

ETIOLOGY. The development of acute rheumatic fever requires antecedent infection with a specific organism, the group A *streptococcus,* at a specific body site, the upper respiratory tract. Cutaneous streptococcal infection, a precursor of post-streptococcal acute glomerulonephritis, has never been shown to cause rheumatic fever.

A substantial body of evidence indicates that individual strains of group A streptococci vary in their rheumatogenic potential. In discrete epidemics of acute rheumatic fever, a limited number of group A streptococcal serotypes tend to predominate (e.g., 3, 5, 18, 24, and others), and the infecting organisms are often heavily encapsulated, as evidenced by their growth as mucoid colonies on blood agar plates. Strains of the most common rheumatogenic serotypes share a specific surface-exposed epitope of the M-protein molecule, and elevated levels of IgM antibodies to this epitope are present in the majority of patients with acute rheumatic fever.

PATHOGENESIS. The mechanism by which group A streptococci elicit the connective tissue inflammatory response that constitutes acute rheumatic fever remains unknown. Various theories have been advanced, including (1) toxic effects of streptococcal products, particularly streptolysins S and O, both of which can initiate tissue injury; (2) inflammation mediated by antigen-antibody complexes, perhaps localized to sites of tissue injury; and (3) "autoimmune" phenomena induced by the similarity of certain streptococcal and human tissue antigens ("molecular mimicry").

Efforts to discriminate among these potential pathogenetic mechanisms have been hampered by the lack of an animal model of rheumatic fever. Most authorities currently favor the theory that the tissue damage in acute rheumatic fever is mediated by the host's own immunologic responses to the antecedent streptococcal infection. This theory is rendered more credible by the relatively long latent period between the onset of pharyngitis and acute rheumatic fever and by the demonstration of numerous examples of antigenic similarity between somatic constituents of group A *streptococci* and human tissues. The most intensively studied of these cross-reactions is that between streptococci and human heart tissue. Many patients with acute rheumatic fever (as well as patients with uncomplicated streptococcal infections) have in their sera antistreptococcal antibodies that cross-react with heart tissue in a variety of test systems. Components of the streptococcal cell wall (including group A carbohydrate and M protein) and the cell membrane contain epitopes that share antigenic determinants with certain constituents of the human heart.

Antibodies to the cytoplasm of neurons located in the caudate and subthalamic nuclei of the brain have been identified in the sera of patients with Sydenham's chorea, and such antibodies cross-react with group A streptococcal membranes. Streptococcal extracellular products appear to be present in immune complexes circulating in the blood of patients with acute rheumatic fever. Taken together, these and other reported immunologic cross-reactions and toxic phenomena could theoretically account for most of the manifestations of acute rheumatic fever. As yet, however, there is no direct evidence that any of these manifestations are pathogenetically significant.

Patients with acute rheumatic fever have, on average, higher titers of antibodies to streptococcal extracellular and somatic antigens than do patients with uncomplicated streptococcal infections. Data relating to cellular immunity are more limited. Patients with acute rheumatic fever exhibit an exaggerated cellular reactivity to streptococcal cell membrane antigens, as demonstrated by *in vitro* inhibition of migration of peripheral blood lymphocytes. During active rheumatic carditis, both the number of helper (CD4) lymphocytes and the ratio of CD4 to CD8 cells are increased in heart valves and peripheral blood.

Several observations suggest that development of rheumatic fever may be modulated, at least in part, by the specific genetic constitution of the host. These observations include (1) the tendency of rheumatic fever to affect more than one member of a given family, (2) the fact that acute rheumatic fever develops in only a small percentage of all individuals experiencing an immunologically significant streptococcal infection, (3) the tendency of rheumatic individuals to experience recurrent attacks, (4) the propensity of rheu-

matic subjects to exhibit exaggerated immunologic responses to streptococcal antigens, and (5) the fact that certain class II histocompatibility antigens are encountered significantly more frequently in patients with acute rheumatic fever than in controls. Recently, a unique non-HLA alloantigen has been found to be strongly expressed on the B cells of virtually all patients with acute rheumatic fever but in fewer than 20% of controls.

EPIDEMIOLOGY. The epidemiology of acute rheumatic fever mirrors that of streptococcal pharyngitis. The peak age of incidence is 5 to 15 years, but both primary and recurrent cases occur in adults. Acute rheumatic fever is rare in children younger than 4 years, a fact that has led some observers to speculate that repetitive streptococcal infections are necessary to "prime" the host for the disease. No clear-cut gender predilection has been observed although certain manifestations such as Sydenham's chorea and mitral stenosis are more likely to develop in females.

The frequency with which acute rheumatic fever develops following untreated group A streptococcal upper respiratory infection differs with the prevalence of highly rheumatogenic strains in the population and the epidemiologic circumstances. In the years following World War II, careful prospective studies were conducted among personnel in military camps suffering from exudative tonsillitis or pharyngitis caused by M-typable group A streptococci. Under such circumstances, in which cases of streptococcal pharyngitis tend to be clinically severe and to appear in epidemics, acute rheumatic fever developed in approximately 3% of untreated patients. Studies of endemically occurring streptococcal infection among open populations of children are complicated by the difficulties of differentiating cases of streptococcal pharyngitis from viral pharyngitis occurring in streptococcal carriers; nevertheless, the acute rheumatic fever attack rate in such circumstances is clearly lower than in the military experience, with an overall attack rate of less than 1%.

Certain features of the antecedent streptococcal infection are associated with an increased risk of acute rheumatic fever. Among these features are the magnitude of the antistreptolysin O titer rise and the persistence of the infecting organism in the pharynx. Although acute rheumatic fever is more likely to occur following clinically severe exudative pharyngitis than following mild nonexudative illness, one third or more of cases occur after streptococcal infections that are asymptomatic or so mild as to have been forgotten by the patient.

Patients with a history of acute rheumatic fever have a greatly increased risk of recurrent disease following an immunologically significant streptococcal infection. In one long-term prospective study of rheumatic subjects at a rheumatic fever sanitarium, one of every five documented streptococcal infections gave rise to a recurrence of acute rheumatic fever. The risk of recurrence is greater in patients with pre-existing rheumatic heart disease and in those experiencing symptomatic throat infections; the risk declines with advancing age and with increasing interval since the most recent rheumatic attack. Nevertheless, rheumatic patients remain at increased risk well into adult life, perhaps indefinitely.

Rheumatic fever occurs in all parts of the world, without any racial predisposition. In temperate climates, acute rheumatic fever peaks in the cooler months of the year, in the winter and early spring or shortly after schools open in the fall. The major environmental factor favoring occurrence appears to be crowding, as in military barracks or similar closed institutions and large households. Crowding favors interpersonal spread of group A streptococci and perhaps enhances streptococcal virulence by frequent human passage.

Acute rheumatic fever remains rampant in developing areas such as the Middle East, the Indian subcontinent, and many nations of Africa and South America. It has been estimated that more than 1 million people have rheumatic heart disease in India. Extremely high acute rheumatic fever attack rates occur among indigenous populations such as the Maoris of New Zealand and the Australian aborigines. In striking contrast, the incidence of acute rheumatic fever and the prevalence of rheumatic heart disease have declined both in North America and in western Europe during the course of the 20th century. Rates of fewer than 2 per 100,000 school children have been reported from several areas of the United States. The disease has become extremely uncommon in the affluent suburbs of many U.S. cities while persisting among lower socioeconomic groups, particularly in the densely populated core areas of major urban centers. The higher incidence rates reported for blacks than whites appears to be due to socioeconomic rather than genetic factors.

The mid-1980s, however, witnessed some startling developments in the epidemiology of acute rheumatic fever in the United States. Outbreaks of the disease were reported in Salt Lake City, Utah, Columbus and Akron, Ohio, Pittsburgh, Pennsylvania, Nashville and Memphis, Tennessee, and a number of other communities. The largest outbreak was in Salt Lake City and its environs, where approximately 500 cases occurred between 1985 and 1988 (Veasy LG; personal communication). Equally surprising was the fact that in many of these outbreaks, the victims were predominantly white, middle-class children dwelling in the suburbs. Moreover, epidemics of acute rheumatic fever occurred in military training bases in Missouri and California, a phenomenon that had not been observed for two decades. Group A streptococci recovered from patients with acute rheumatic fever, their families, and community and training camp surveys were generally highly mucoid and belonged to well-established rheumatogenic serotypes (e.g., serotypes 3 and 18). These outbreaks appear to have subsided during the 1990s.

PATHOLOGY. Acute rheumatic fever is characterized by exudative and proliferative inflammatory lesions in connective tissue, especially connective tissue of the heart, joints, and subcutaneous tissue. The early lesions consist of edema of the ground substance, fragmentation of collagen fibers, cellular infiltration, and fibrinoid degeneration. In the heart, diffuse degeneration and even necrosis of muscle cells may be observed. At a slightly later stage, focal perivascular inflammatory lesions develop. These so-called Aschoff nodules, considered virtually pathognomonic of rheumatic fever, consist of a central area of fibrinoid surrounded by lymphocytes, plasma cells, and large basophilic cells, some of them multinucleate. Many of these cells have elongated nuclei with a distinctive chromatin pattern, sometimes called "caterpillar" or "owl-eye" nuclei, depending on their orientation in microscopic cross-section. Cells containing these nuclei are called "Anitschkow myocytes" despite the fact that most authorities believe them to be of mesenchymal origin.

Cardiac findings may include pericarditis, myocarditis, and endocarditis. Foci of coronary arteritis may also be observed. A thickened and roughened area ("MacCallum's patch") is frequently present in the left atrium above the posterior leaflet of the mitral valve. Valvular lesions appear early as small verrucae along the line of closure. Later, as healing occurs, the valves may become thickened and deformed, the chordae shortened, and the commissures fused. These changes result in valvular stenosis or insufficiency. The mitral valve is involved most commonly, followed by the aortic, the tricuspid, and rarely, the pulmonic valves.

Pathologically, the arthritis of acute rheumatic fever is characterized by a fibrinous exudate and sterile effusion without erosion of the joint surfaces or pannus formation. The subcutaneous nodules have many histologic features in common with Aschoff nodules and consist of central zones of fibrinoid necrosis surrounded by histiocytes, fibroblasts, occasional lymphocytes, and rare polymorphonuclear cells. Inflammation of the smaller arteries and arterioles may occur throughout the body. Despite pathologic evidence of diffuse vasculitis, aneurysms and thrombosis are not typical features of acute rheumatic fever.

CLINICAL MANIFESTATIONS. Rheumatic fever may involve a number of different organ systems, most notably the heart, joints, skin, subcutaneous tissue, and central nervous system. The clinical picture of the disease may thus be quite variable (Table 325–1),

Table 325–1 ■ THE MANY FACES OF ACUTE RHEUMATIC FEVER: POSSIBLE FEATURES

High fever, prostration, crippling polyarthritis
Lassitude, tachycardia, new cardiac murmurs
Acute pericarditis
Fulminant heart failure
Sydenham's chorea without fever or toxicity
Acute abdominal pain mimicking appendicitis
Varying combinations of the above

depending on which systems are attacked, whether they are involved singly or in combination, and the severity of the involvement. Five clinical features of the disease are so characteristic that they are recognized as "major manifestations" according to the revised Jones' criteria (see below) for the diagnosis of acute rheumatic fever: carditis, polyarthritis, chorea, subcutaneous nodules, and erythema marginatum. Certain other findings, frequently present but non-specific, have been designated "minor manifestations." These manifestations include arthralgia, fever, and certain laboratory findings (see below).

In cases in which it can be determined, the latent period between the antecedent streptococcal infection and the onset of symptoms of acute rheumatic fever ranges between 1 and 5 weeks. The average latent period is 19 days for both primary and recurrent attacks. When acute polyarthritis is the initial complaint, the onset is often rather abrupt and may be marked by high fever and toxicity. If isolated carditis is the initial manifestation, the onset may be insidious or even subclinical. Between these two extremes, diverse gradations exist in the initial features of acute rheumatic fever (see Table 325–1). In most attacks, fever and joint involvement are the earliest clinical manifestations, although occasionally they may be preceded by abdominal pain localized to the periumbilical or infraumbilical areas. At times, the location and severity of the pain, as well as fleeting signs of peritoneal inflammation, may lead to a misdiagnosis of acute appendicitis. Carditis, if it is to appear, usually does so within the initial 3 weeks of the illness. In contrast, chorea tends to occur later in the course of the disease, sometimes after all other manifestations have subsided. Fortunately, chorea and polyarthritis almost never occur simultaneously. Epistaxis may be a feature of acute rheumatic fever occurring both at the onset and throughout the acute phase of the illness; it may be quite severe.

The incidence of major manifestations varies in reported series. Overall, however, arthritis occurs in approximately 75% of initial attacks of acute rheumatic fever, carditis in 40 to 50%, chorea in 15%, and subcutaneous nodules and erythema marginatum in fewer than 10%. The frequency of individual manifestations varies with age. Carditis is more frequent in the youngest age groups and is relatively uncommon in initial attacks occurring in adults. Chorea occurs primarily in persons between age 5 and puberty. It is seen more frequently in females and virtually never occurs in adult males. Thus the majority of acute rheumatic fever attacks occurring in adults are manifested primarily by arthritis.

ARTHRITIS. Joint involvement ranges from arthralgia alone to acute, disabling arthritis characterized by swelling, warmth, erythema, severe limitation of motion, and exquisite tenderness to pressure. The larger joints of the extremities are usually involved—most frequently the knees and ankles but also the wrists and elbows. The hips and small joints of the hands and feet are affected occasionally. Involvement of shoulders and lumbosacral, cervical, sternoclavicular, and temporomandibular joints occurs in a relatively small percentage of cases. The synovial fluid contains thousands of white blood cells, with a marked preponderance of polymorphonuclear leukocytes; bacterial cultures are sterile. Characteristically, the articular involvement in acute rheumatic fever assumes a pattern of migratory polyarthritis. Migratory does not mean that inflammation in one joint disappears before the next is attacked. Rather, a number of joints are affected in succession, and the periods of involvement overlap. Inflammation in one joint may subside while another is becoming symptomatic, so the process seems to migrate from joint to joint. In untreated cases, as many as 16 joints may be affected, and arthritis develops in more than 6 joints in about half the patients. When effective anti-inflammatory therapy is administered early in the course of the disease, the involvement not infrequently remains monarticular or pauciarticular.

In most instances, inflammation in any one joint begins to subside spontaneously within a week, and the total duration of involvement is no more than 2 or 3 weeks. The entire bout of polyarthritis rarely lasts more than 4 weeks and resolves completely, with no residual joint damage left. Some authors have described the rare occurrence of Jaccoud's arthritis, so-called chronic post–rheumatic fever arthropathy of the metacarpophalangeal joints, following repetitive bouts of rheumatic polyarthritis. This entity is not a true arthritis but a form of periarticular fibrosis; its relationship to rheumatic fever remains unresolved.

Murmurs*
    Apical systolic
    Apical mid-diastolic (Carey Coombs murmur)
Basal diastolic
Pericarditis
Cardiomegaly
Congestive heart failure

*At least one of the characteristic murmurs is almost always present in acute rheumatic carditis (see text for details).

CARDITIS. Rheumatic fever may involve the endocardium, myocardium, and pericardium (Table 325–2), and thus the disease is capable of inducing a true pancarditis. Carditis is the most important manifestation of acute rheumatic fever because it is the only one that can cause significant permanent organ damage or death. Although the clinical picture may at times be fulminant, it is more frequently mild or even asymptomatic and may escape notice in the absence of more obvious associated findings such as arthritis or chorea. The diagnosis of carditis requires the presence of one of the following four manifestations: (1) organic cardiac murmurs not previously present, (2) cardiomegaly, (3) pericarditis, or (4) congestive heart failure. In practice, the characteristic murmurs of acute rheumatic fever are almost always present in cases of rheumatic carditis, unless the ability to hear them is obscured (e.g., loud pericardial friction rub, large pericardial effusion, low cardiac output, severe tachycardia). The diagnosis of carditis should be made with caution in the absence of one of the following three murmurs: apical systolic, apical mid-diastolic, and basal diastolic. Such murmurs, if they are destined to develop, do so usually within the 1st week and almost always within the 1st 3 weeks of illness. (An exception to this rule may occur in patients with "pure" chorea; see later discussion.) The apical systolic murmur of mitral regurgitation encompasses most of systole. It is blowing, relatively high pitched, and heard best at the apex; it radiates to the axilla and at times to the base of the heart or the back. It must be carefully distinguished by quality, location, and radiation from a variety of functional precordial systolic murmurs heard in normal individuals, especially in children. The apical mid-diastolic (Carey Coombs) murmur is a low-pitched sound replacing or immediately following the 3rd heart sound and ending distinctly before the 1st heart sound. It may be heard in a variety of conditions associated with increased flow across the mitral valve and is thus not pathognomonic of acute rheumatic fever. It may be differentiated from the diastolic rumble of mitral stenosis by the absence of an opening snap, pre-systolic accentuation, or accentuated 1st sound at the mitral area. The high-pitched, decrescendo basal diastolic murmur of aortic regurgitation is best heard along the upper left sternal border or over the aortic area. It may be brief and faint but is best heard after expiration with the patient leaning forward. Some patients with ARF have echocardiographic evidence of mitral regurgitation in the absence of an audible murmur. This finding is not considered diagnostic of rheumatic carditis for the purpose of fulfilling the Jones criteria, and its prognostic significance remains uncertain.

Other prominent auscultatory findings in patients with active rheumatic carditis include tachycardia, which persists during sleep; protodiastolic, pre-systolic, or summation gallops; an indistinct or "mushy" quality to the 1st heart sound (resulting in some cases from 1st-degree heart block); pericardial friction rub; or muffling of heart tones caused by pericardial effusion. In the early stages of congestive heart failure, rapid distention of the hepatic capsule may lead to right upper quadrant aching and tenderness over the liver. All the usual clinical findings of pericarditis or congestive failure may be observed.

A number of different rhythm disturbances may occur during the course of acute rheumatic fever. By far the most common is 1st-degree atrioventricular block. Second- and 3rd-degree heart block, nodal rhythm, and premature contractions may also be observed; atrial fibrillation, on the other hand, is usually a feature of chronic rather than acute rheumatic involvement. Conduction disturbances do not in themselves indicate acute carditis, and their presence or absence is unrelated to the subsequent development of rheumatic heart disease.

In cases of acute rheumatic fever with severe carditis, areas of patchy pneumonitis are sometimes seen. Many observers believe that these pulmonary infiltrates represent a specific rheumatic pneumonia. The case is difficult to prove, however, because of the confusion induced by such confounding clinical entities as pulmonary edema, pulmonary embolization, superimposed bacterial pneumonia, and acute respiratory distress syndrome in these severely ill and toxic patients.

SYDENHAM'S CHOREA (CHOREA MINOR, "ST. VITUS' DANCE"). This neurologic syndrome occurs after a latent period that is variable but on average longer than that associated with the other manifestations of acute rheumatic fever. It frequently occurs in "pure" form, either unaccompanied by other major manifestations or, after a latent period of several months, at a time when all other evidence of acute rheumatic activity has subsided. Chorea is characterized by rapid, purposeless, involuntary movements, most noticeable in the extremities and face. The arms and legs flail about in erratic, jerky, uncoordinated movements that may sometimes be unilateral (hemichorea). Facial tics, grimaces, grins, and contortions are evident. The speech is usually slurred or jerky. The tongue, when protruded, retracts involuntarily, and asynchronous contractions of lingual muscles produce a "bag of worms" appearance. The involuntary motions disappear during sleep and may be partially suppressed by rest, sedation, or volition.

Patients with chorea display generalized muscle weakness and an inability to maintain a tetanic muscle contraction. Thus when the patient is asked to squeeze the examiner's fingers, a squeezing and relaxing motion occurs that has been described as "milkmaid's grip." The knee jerk may have a pendular quality. No cranial nerve or pyramidal involvement occurs, and sensory modalities are unaffected. The electroencephalogram may display abnormal slow wave activity.

Emotional lability is characteristic of Sydenham's chorea and may often precede other neurologic manifestations, with teachers and parents left puzzled over apparently inexplicable personality changes.

SUBCUTANEOUS NODULES. These nodules are firm, painless subcutaneous lesions that vary in size from a few millimeters to approximately 2 cm. The skin overlying them is freely movable and not inflamed. The lesions tend to occur in crops over bony surfaces or prominences and over tendons. Sites of predilection include the extensor surfaces of the elbows, knees, and wrists, the occiput, and the spinous processes of the thoracic and lumbar vertebrae (Fig. 325–1). Nodules are virtually never the sole major manifestation of acute rheumatic fever; they almost always appear in association with carditis, and the cardiac involvement in such cases tends to be clinically severe. Nodules ordinarily do not appear until at least 3 weeks after the onset of an attack, which usually lasts 1 to 2 weeks. They may appear in repeated crops in patients with protracted carditis. Similar nodules may be seen in systemic lupus erythematosus (SLE) and in rheumatoid arthritis. Subcutaneous nodules in the latter disease are larger and more persistent than those in rheumatic fever.

ERYTHEMA MARGINATUM. The rash begins as an erythematous macule or papule and then extends outward while the skin in the center returns to normal. Adjacent lesions coalesce and form circinate or serpiginous patterns. The lesions may be raised or flat, are neither pruritic nor indurated, and blanch on pressure. They vary greatly in size and appear mostly on the trunk and proximal parts of the extremities, with the face being spared. The lesions are evanescent, migrating from place to place, at times changing before the observer's eyes, and leaving no residual scarring. The erythema may be brought out by applying heat. Individual lesions may come and go in minutes to hours, but the process may go on intermittently for weeks to months uninfluenced by anti-inflammatory therapy; its persistence is not necessarily an adverse prognostic sign. In the great majority of cases, erythema marginatum is accompanied by carditis; it also tends to be associated with subcutaneous nodules.

LABORATORY FINDINGS. No specific laboratory test is diagnostic of acute rheumatic fever. Usually, leukocytosis with an increase in the proportion of polymorphonuclear leukocytes is observed. A mild to moderate normocytic, normochromic anemia is the rule. In some patients, the serum aspartate aminotransferase level is elevated. Evidence of acute inflammation is prominent, including elevated serum levels of C-reactive protein and elevation

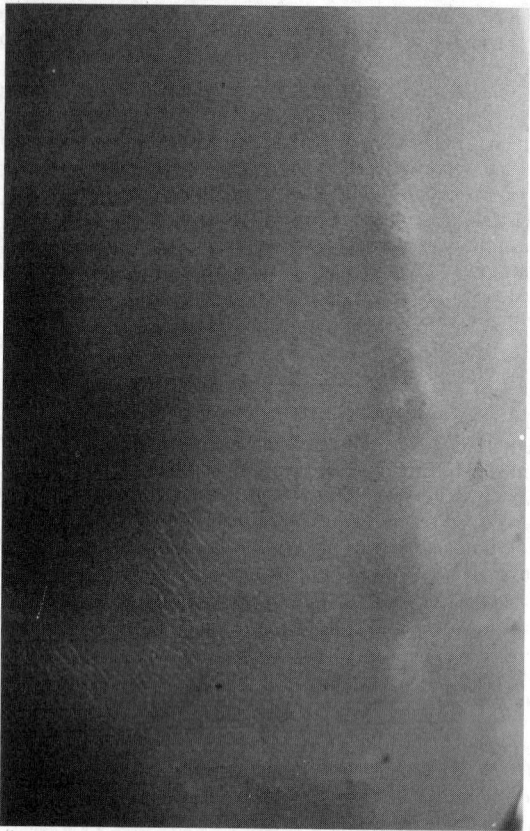

FIGURE 325-1 ■ Subcutaneous nodules over spinous processes on the back of a patient with acute rheumatic carditis. (Courtesy of S. Levine, M.D.)

of the erythrocyte sedimentation rate. An exception is "pure" chorea, which may appear long after indices of inflammation have returned to normal.

The urine may contain protein, white cells, and red cells. Biopsy studies have revealed a variety of renal abnormalities, but the classic proliferative glomerular abnormalities that characterize post-streptococcal acute glomerulonephritis occur quite rarely in acute rheumatic fever. Electrocardiographic and radiographic studies may reveal evidence of rhythm disturbances, pericarditis, or congestive heart failure. Echocardiography may document myocardial and valvular dysfunction and pericardial effusion.

The major laboratory contribution to the diagnosis of acute rheumatic fever is the documentation of recent group A streptococcal infection. Throat culture should always be performed but is positive in only a minority of cases. The low rate of culture positivity remains unexplained, although it may be due in part to the time lapse of several weeks between the onset of the pharyngeal infection and the throat culture. The serum titer of antistreptolysin O is elevated in 80% or more of patients with acute rheumatic fever. If two streptococcal antibody tests, e.g., antistreptolysis O plus either anti-DNase B or antihyaluronidase, are performed, an elevated titer of at least one will be found in 90% of patients with acute rheumatic fever. A battery of three tests establishes the presence of recent, immunologically significant streptococcal infection in more than 95% of individuals experiencing an acute rheumatic attack. The definition of an "elevated" titer varies, depending on the test used, the patient's age, and the geographic locale. Antistreptolysin O titers of greater than 200 Todd units per milliliter in adults and 320 Todd units in children are generally considered elevated. At times, serial sampling may detect a rising titer of streptococcal antibodies in patients seen early in the course of a rheumatic attack.

COURSE AND PROGNOSIS. The average duration of an untreated attack of acute rheumatic fever is approximately 3 months. The duration tends to be longer, up to 6 months, in patients with severe carditis. Fewer than 5% of patients have continuing rheumatic activity for longer than 6 months. In a few of these patients

the disease is limited to chorea and is otherwise benign. Other patients exhibit evidence of persistent inflammatory activity, including arthritis, carditis, and subcutaneous nodules. "Chronic rheumatic fever" occurs more frequently in patients who have had one or more previous attacks; cardiac involvement in chronic rheumatic fever tends to be frequent and severe.

Death from intractable myocarditis during the acute phase of acute rheumatic fever is now very rare. Once the acute attack has subsided, the only long-term sequela is that of rheumatic heart disease, manifested primarily by scarring and/or calcification (Fig. 325–2) of the mitral and aortic valves (see Chapter 63) and leading to insufficiency and/or stenosis. The prognosis from a cardiac standpoint very much depends on the clinical findings when the patient is initially seen. In one large study, for example, 347 patients were examined during an acute rheumatic attack and again 10 years later. Among patients who had been free of carditis during their acute attack, only 6% had residual heart disease on follow-up. Patients with no pre-existing heart disease and with mild carditis during their acute attack (i.e., apical systolic murmur without pericarditis or heart failure) had a relatively good prognosis in that only approximately 30% had heart murmurs 10 years later. About 40% of subjects with apical or basal diastolic murmurs and 70% of subjects with failure and/or pericarditis during their acute attacks had residual rheumatic heart disease. The prognosis was worse in patients with pre-existing heart disease and in those who had experienced recurrent attacks of acute rheumatic fever in the 10-year interval.

These data indicate that patients in whom carditis does not develop during an acute attack and who are protected from recurrences of acute rheumatic fever are most unlikely to suffer from rheumatic heart disease. Patients with "pure" chorea represent an exception to this rule. Some patients who have no evidence of carditis when initially examined may have rheumatic valvular disease on prolonged follow-up. Although the explanation for this phenomenon is unknown, it is conceivable that in view of the long latent period associated with chorea, signs of carditis might have been present earlier but subsided by the time that the neurologic abnormality became evident.

DIAGNOSIS. Although acute rheumatic fever is readily recognized in individuals with multiple major manifestations or in epidemic circumstances, at other times the disease may be extraordinarily difficult to diagnose with confidence because of the variability of its clinical features, the frequency with which only a single major manifestation is detected, and the fact that no definitive diagnostic laboratory test is available. Nevertheless, precise diagnosis is especially important in this disease because of the need

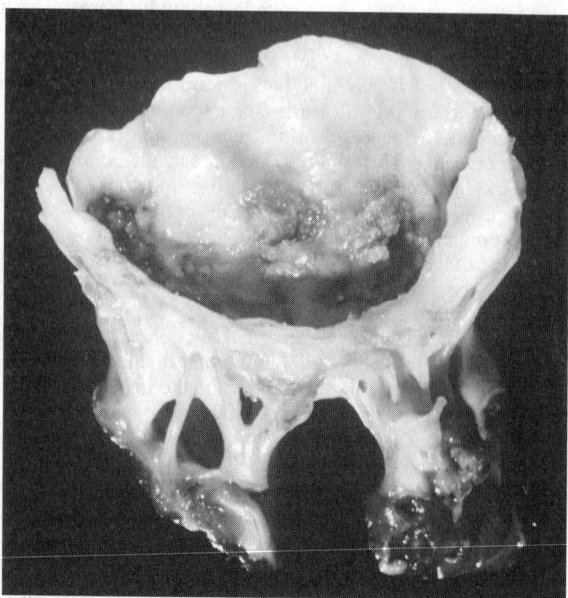

FIGURE 325-2 ■ Calcified mitral valve from a patient with rheumatic heart disease. (Courtesy of A. Morales, M.D., from Bisno AL: Rheumatic fever. *In* Kelley WN, et al [eds]: Textbook of Rheumatology, 4th ed. Philadelphia, WB Saunders, 1993, p 1214.)

to advise the patient regarding prolonged antimicrobial prophylaxis (see below).

The diagnostic criteria of T. Duckett Jones, initially proposed in 1944 and subsequently modified by committees of the American Heart Association, attempt to minimize overdiagnosis and underdiagnosis (Table 325–3). The most recent (1992) revision specifies that the guidelines be designed to assist in the diagnosis of the initial attack of acute rheumatic fever. Although most patients with recurrent acute rheumatic fever fulfill the criteria, in some cases the diagnosis of a recurrence may be less apparent.

Two major manifestations or one major and two minor manifestations indicate a high probability of acute rheumatic fever provided that supporting evidence of recent streptococcal infection is present. Although a positive throat culture or rapid antigen test for group A streptococci technically satisfies this requirement, streptococcal carriage rates of 15% are not uncommon among school-aged children during the fall and winter. Elevated titers of antibodies to streptococcal extracellular products, although not diagnostic of acute rheumatic fever, do indicate a recent, immunologically significant streptococcal infection. Conversely, if a battery of streptococcal antibody tests fail to reveal any evidence of recent infection, the diagnosis of acute rheumatic fever must be considered unlikely.

The modified Jones' criteria are, of course, only guidelines. They are most difficult to apply confidently when polyarthritis is the single major manifestation. Under such circumstances, the diagnosis of acute rheumatic fever should be made only after excluding other causes of polyarthritis such as rheumatoid arthritis, Still's disease, Lyme disease, viral arthritides (e.g., rubella, hepatitis B), the early pre-purpuric phase of Henoch-Schönlein purpura, and septic arthritis, including gonococcal arthritis. The latter diagnosis cannot be excluded unequivocally by negative cultures of blood and synovial fluid. Therefore, if the clinical and epidemiologic picture is compatible with disseminated gonococcal infection, a trial of antigonococcal therapy should precede initiation of treatment with anti-inflammatory drugs.

Some patients have been described as manifesting polyarthritis that is atypical in time of onset and duration, does not respond dramatically to salicylate therapy, and is unassociated with other clinical features of acute rheumatic fever. Such individuals have on occasion been categorized as having "post-streptococcal reactive arthritis." The existence of this entity as a distinct syndrome, however, and its relationship to rheumatic fever remain uncertain. Pending further clarification, such individuals should be considered to have acute rheumatic fever if they fulfill the Jones' criteria and alternative diagnoses have been excluded.

Serum sickness is frequently a serious consideration, particularly if the patient has received penicillin or other antibiotics for a preceding respiratory infection. SLE, sickle cell hemoglobinopathies, and infective endocarditis may involve the joints and the heart. Other differential diagnostic considerations include congenital heart lesions, viral and idiopathic forms of myocarditis and pericarditis, and functional heart murmurs. Non-familial forms of chorea have been described in SLE, rarely in association with the use of birth control pills, and in patients with neoplasms involving the basal ganglia. The involuntary jerks of Gilles de la Tourette syndrome may be confused with chorea. It remains uncertain how often episodes of chorea occurring during pregnancy ("chorea gravidarum") represent attacks of rheumatic fever. Other disorders that

may at times be confused with acute rheumatic fever are gout, sarcoidosis, Hodgkin's disease, and acute leukemia.

In certain circumstances, acute rheumatic fever can be diagnosed even when the guidelines set forth in Table 325–3 have not been met. Patients whose only rheumatic manifestation is Sydenham's chorea may not fulfill the Jones' criteria. Because of the long latent period between the antecedent streptococcal infection and appearance of the neurologic abnormalities, evidence of inflammation encompassed in the minor manifestations may no longer be present, and previously elevated antibody titers may have declined to normal. A similar situation occasionally occurs in patients with indolent carditis, who may not come to medical attention until months after the onset of rheumatic fever. In patients with established rheumatic heart disease, it may be difficult to distinguish new from pre-existing cardiac involvement unless the patient has been under careful prospective follow-up, a previously undamaged valve is involved, or pericarditis is evident. Thus the diagnosis of recurrent acute rheumatic fever must be strongly entertained in the presence of suggestive clinical findings, provided that evidence of recent group A streptococcal infection is present.

TREATMENT. Antibiotics neither modify the course of a rheumatic attack nor influence the subsequent development of carditis. Nevertheless, it is conventional to give a course of antibiotics designed to eradicate any rheumatogenic group A streptococci remaining in the tonsils and pharynx to prevent spread of the organism to close contacts. The recommended regimens are those conventionally used for the treatment of acute streptococcal pharyngitis (see Chapter 324). Benzathine penicillin G is preferred in non–penicillin-allergic patients. Following completion of this therapy, continuous antistreptococcal prophylaxis should commence (see below).

Treatment with anti-inflammatory agents is effective in suppressing many of the signs and symptoms of acute rheumatic fever. These agents do not "cure" the disease, nor do they prevent the subsequent evolution of rheumatic heart disease. They should be avoided in very mild or equivocal cases because by suppressing the clinical manifestations, they may obscure the diagnosis. The two drugs most widely used are aspirin and corticosteroids. The former is used in patients with acute polyarthritis, provided that carditis is either absent or mild and no evidence of congestive heart failure is found. Aspirin is very effective in decreasing fever, toxicity, and joint inflammation. It should be given in a dosage of 90 to 100 mg/kg/day in children and 6 to 8 g/day in adults administered in equally divided doses every 4 hours for the initial 24 to 36 hours; thereafter it may be given in four doses during waking hours. A salicylate level of 25 mg/dL is usually satisfactory. The incidence of nausea and vomiting may be minimized by starting somewhat below the optimal dosage level and gradually increasing over a few days. The patient should be observed for evidence of significant gastrointestinal bleeding and for signs and symptoms of salicylism (see Chapter 29). After 2 weeks, the dosage is reduced to 60 to 70 mg/kg/day for an additional 6 weeks. These dosage schedules represent general guidelines only. The precise aspirin dose must be determined by the patient's clinical response, blood salicylate levels, and tolerance of the drug.

Corticosteroids are generally reserved for patients who have se-

Table 325–3 ■ GUIDELINES FOR DIAGNOSIS OF THE INITIAL ATTACK OF RHEUMATIC FEVER (JONES CRITERIA, UPDATED 1992)*

MAJOR MANIFESTATIONS	MINOR MANIFESTATIONS	SUPPORTING EVIDENCE OF ANTECEDENT GROUP A STREPTOCOCCAL INFECTIONS
Carditis	Clinical findings	Positive throat culture or rapid streptococcal antigen test
Polyarthritis	Arthralgia	Elevated or rising streptococcal antibody titer
Chorea	Fever	
Erythema marginatum	Laboratory findings	
Subcutaneous nodules	↑ Acute-phase reactants	
	↑ Erythrocyte sedimentation rate	
	↑ C-reactive protein	
	Prolonged PR interval	

*If supported by evidence of preceding group A streptococcal infection, the presence of two major manifestations or one major and two minor manifestations indicates a high probability of acute rheumatic fever.

Reprinted from Special Writing Group of the Committee on Rheumatic Fever, Endocarditis and Kawasaki Disease, American Heart Association. Guidelines for the diagnosis of rheumatic fever: Jones criteria, 1992 update. JAMA 268 15:2069, 1992 with permission. Copyright, 1992, American Medical Association.

vere carditis manifested by congestive heart failure, who are unable to tolerate large doses of salicylates, or whose signs and symptoms are inadequately suppressed by aspirin. As with aspirin, the dosage must be individualized. Prednisone, 40 to 60 mg/day in divided doses, may be used initially. After 2 to 3 weeks it should be withdrawn slowly over an additional 3-week period. In cases of fulminating carditis with profound heart failure, intravenous corticosteroids may be used. As is the case for other patients receiving corticosteroids, the physician should be alert to problems such as gastrointestinal bleeding, sodium and water retention, and impaired glucose tolerance. Suppression of the pituitary-adrenal axis or the host immune system is a potential problem but not ordinarily a major one during this relatively short course of treatment. Although non-steroidal anti-inflammatory agents have proved highly effective in various types of acute arthritides, published experience regarding the use of these agents in patients with acute rheumatic fever is extremely limited.

After cessation of anti-inflammatory therapy, clinical or laboratory evidence of acute rheumatic fever may reappear. Such therapeutic "rebounds" occur more frequently after corticosteroid therapy than after treatment with aspirin. They may be minimized by prolonging salicylate therapy for 9 to 12 weeks and, when corticosteroids have been required, by continuing aspirin for a month after corticosteroid use has been discontinued. Congestive heart failure is managed by conventional measures. If digitalis is used, the potential risk of drug-induced arrhythmias in patients with active myocarditis must be kept in mind. Patients with Sydenham's chorea require a quiet environment, and sedatives such as phenobarbital or diazepam may be helpful. Trials of plasmapheresis and intravenous immunoglobulin in the management of severe and intractable chorea are currently in progress.

Once the acute attack has subsided completely, the patient's subsequent level of physical activity depends on cardiac status. Patients without residual heart disease may resume full and unrestricted activity. It is important that patients not be subjected to unwarranted invalidism because of either their own inaccurate perceptions of the nature of the rheumatic process or those of parents, teachers, or employers.

PREVENTION. "Primary prevention" of acute rheumatic fever consists of accurate diagnosis and appropriate treatment of streptococcal sore throat (see Chapter 324). Although straightforward in theory, primary prevention is often frustratingly difficult to achieve. In many of the densely populated indigent communities in which the risk of acute rheumatic fever is greatest, children with self-limited illnesses such as sore throats may never come to medical attention, and throat culture services are usually unavailable to aid in diagnosis. Moreover, in one third or more of cases, acute rheumatic fever may arise after a clinically inapparent streptococcal infection.

Perhaps the most effective strategy for avoiding the mortality and chronic cardiac disability associated with acute rheumatic fever is that of "secondary prevention." This strategy focuses on the group of persons who have already suffered a rheumatic attack and who are inordinately susceptible to a recurrence following an immunologically significant streptococcal upper respiratory infection. Recurrent attacks tend to be mimetic in nature, so patients who

Table 325–4 ■ SECONDARY PREVENTION OF RHEUMATIC FEVER (PREVENTION OF RECURRENT ATTACKS)

AGENT	DOSE	MODE
Benzathine penicillin G	1,200,000 U every 4 wk* *or*	Intramuscular
Penicillin V	250 mg twice daily *or*	Oral
Sulfadiazine	0.5 g once daily for patients ≤27 kg (60 lb) 1.0 g once daily for patients >27 kg (60 lb)	Oral
For Individuals Allergic to Penicillin and Sulfadiazine		
Erythromycin	250 mg twice daily	Oral

*In high-risk situations, administration every 3 weeks is justified and recommended.
Reproduced by permission of Pediatrics 96:758, copyright American Academy of Pediatrics 1995.

Table 325–5 ■ DURATION OF SECONDARY RHEUMATIC FEVER PROPHYLAXIS

CATEGORY	DURATION
Rheumatic fever with carditis and residual heart disease (persistent valvar disease*)	At least 10 yr since last episode and at least until age 40 yr, sometimes lifelong prophylaxis
Rheumatic fever with carditis but no residual heart disease (no valvar disease*)	10 yr or well into adulthood, whichever is longer
Rheumatic fever without carditis	5 yr or until age 21 yr, whichever is longer

*Clinical or echocardiographic evidence.
Reproduced by permission of Pediatrics 96:758, Copyright American Academy of Pediatrics 1995.

have suffered carditis with their previous attack are likely to have repetitive cardiac involvement and progressive cardiac damage. Because carditis with recurrent attacks of acute rheumatic fever may develop even in patients who experienced only arthritis or chorea, all patients who have experienced a documented attack of acute rheumatic fever should receive continuous antimicrobial prophylaxis to prevent either symptomatic or asymptomatic streptococcal infections. The specific regimens to be used are indicated in Table 325–4. By far the most effective of these regimens is intramuscular benzathine penicillin G every 4 weeks. Rheumatic recurrences are very unusual in compliant patients receiving an injection every 4 weeks. In areas of the world where incidence of acute rheumatic fever and the risk of recurrence are extremely high, however, injections every 3 weeks provide more complete protection.

The total duration of intramuscular or oral rheumatic fever prophylaxis remains unresolved. The risk of rheumatic recurrence is known to diminish with increasing age and increasing interval since the most recent rheumatic attack. Patients who escape carditis during their initial attack are less likely to experience rheumatic recurrences and less prone to the development of carditis if a recurrence does ensue. These facts suggest that prophylaxis need not be perpetual for all rheumatic subjects. Recommendations of the American Heart Association for the duration of secondary prophylaxis are given in Table 325–5. The decision to remove a rheumatic subject from continuous prophylaxis should be an individualized one based on the physician's assessment of the risk and probable consequences of recurrence and taken with the patient's informed consent. Particular care should be taken with those at high risk of streptococcal acquisition (e.g., parents of school children, school teachers, military recruits, nurses, pediatricians, or residents of areas with a high incidence of acute rheumatic fever). Patients taken off prophylaxis must be instructed to return immediately for medical follow-up whenever symptoms of pharyngitis occur.

Patients with rheumatic valvular heart disease must receive prophylaxis designed to avoid bacterial endocarditis whenever they undergo dental or surgical procedures likely to evoke bacteremia. Such prophylaxis is not necessary in a rheumatic subject who is free of residual heart disease. Regimens to prevent endocarditis (see Chapter 326) are different from those prescribed for preventing acute rheumatic fever, and the fact that a patient is receiving rheumatic fever prophylaxis does not exempt that patient from endocarditis prophylaxis. This concept is a frequent point of confusion not only among patients but among physicians and dentists as well.

Berrios X, Del Campo E, Guzman B, Bisno AL: Discontinuance of rheumatic fever prophylaxis in selected adolescents and young adults. Ann Intern Med 118:401, 1993. *Presents new data, along with a review of previous studies, on the circumstances under which rheumatic fever prophylaxis might be discontinued.*

Bisno AL: Group A streptococcal infections and acute rheumatic fever. N Engl J Med 325:783, 1991. *Review of the biology of the group A streptococcus as it relates to civilian and military outbreaks of acute rheumatic fever in the 1980s and the more recent resurgence of life-threatening streptococcal infections.*

Marcus RH, Sareli P, Pocock WA, Barlow JB: The spectrum of severe rheumatic mitral valve disease in a developing country. Ann Intern Med 120:177, 1994. *A detailed analysis of the demographic, pathologic, and hemodynamic profiles of more than 700 South African patients with severe rheumatic valvular disease.*

Stollerman GH: Rheumatic Fever and Streptococcal Infection. New York, Grune & Stratton, 1975. *A comprehensive, extremely readable summary of rheumatic fever. Detailed descriptions of clinical manifestations will be particularly valuable to physicians unfamiliar with the disease.*

Veasy LG, Tani LY, Hill HR: Persistence of acute rheumatic fever in the intermountain area of the United States. J Pediatr 124:9, 1994. *A summary of the demographic and clinical data on 274 patients with acute rheumatic fever hospitalized in Salt Lake City between 1985 and 1992.*

326 INFECTIVE ENDOCARDITIS

Matthew E. Levison

Endocarditis is characterized pathologically by the "vegetation," a lesion that results from deposition of platelets and fibrin on the endothelial surface of the heart. Infection is the most common cause, the usual pathogen being one of a variety of bacterial species, including rickettsia and chlamydia, microscopic colonies of which are buried beneath the surface of fibrin. However, other types of microorganisms, e.g., fungi, may be involved, so the more general term *infective* rather than *bacterial* endocarditis is preferred. Usually the heart valve is the site of the vegetation, but in certain instances vegetations may occur on other parts of the endocardium. Involvement of extracardiac intravascular sites, which can produce an illness clinically similar to endocarditis, is properly termed *endarteritis.*

PATHOGENESIS

Endocarditis is the result of interaction among (1) host factors that predispose the endothelium to infection, (2) circumstances that lead to transient bacteremia, and (3) the tissue tropism and virulence of the circulating bacteria.

HOST. In population-based studies, the age- and gender-adjusted incidence of endocarditis is about 5 per 100,000 person-years. The incidence rates that have been reported range from 1.7 to 9.3 per 100,000 person-years. This variation is likely the consequence of the prevalence of certain risk factors in the population, e.g., the highest rate reported, 9.3, probably reflects the high prevalence of intravenous drug use in that particular population studied. Advancing age and male gender are significant risk factors; the incidence rate for those 65 years or older is almost 9 times that of those younger than 65 years and for males 2.5 times that of females. The greater frequency in the aged is due in part to the increased prevalence of predisposing cardiac lesions (e.g., degenerative cardiac lesions and prosthetic cardiac valves) and circumstances that may lead to bacteremia (e.g., invasive urologic procedures, anorectal and colonic disease, and intravascular catheterization) in this age group and, in males, the increased prevalence of certain cardiac lesions such as bicuspid aortic valves.

LOCAL HOST FACTORS. Non-bacterial Thrombotic Endocarditis. The normal endothelium is non-thrombogenic, but when damaged or denuded the endothelium is a potent inducer of blood coagulation. Certain types of congenital or acquired heart disease can result in a high-velocity jet stream from a high- to a low-pressure chamber (aortic or mitral insufficiency, ventricular septal defect, or patent ductus arteriosus) or create a pressure gradient across a narrowed orifice between two chambers (aortic stenosis or coarctation of the aorta). The high-velocity jet stream can lead to turbulent blood flow distal to the pressure gradient, which is thought to damage the valvular and endocardial endothelium in a predictable pattern distal to the pressure gradient (Fig. 326–1). Damage to the endothelium can be induced in an experimental animal by passing a catheter into the heart across the aortic or tricuspid valves, and intracardiac catheters can induce similar lesions in humans. Platelets are deposited on the surface of the damaged endothelium. The adherent platelets then degranulate and stimulate local deposition of fibrin. In the process, a sterile thrombus is formed on the endothelial surface, so-called non-bacterial thrombotic endocarditis (NBTE). For unknown reasons, NBTE is also found in some patients with chronic wasting illnesses (marantic endocarditis) and systemic lupus erythematosus (SLE) (Libman-Sacks endocarditis). NBTE can dislodge fibrin, embolize to block peripheral arteries, and produce sterile infarction of distal organs. The resultant clinical manifestations of NBTE in cachetic illnesses or SLE may simulate those of infective endocarditis (see below).

NBTE is the point of attachment and subsequent proliferation for certain microorganisms once they have gained access to the circulation. Following induced bacteremia in experimental animals without pre-existing NBTE, the endothelial surface is resistant to bacterial attachment and the subsequent development of infective endocarditis. The left side of the heart is apparently more susceptible to infection than the right side is. For example, the left side

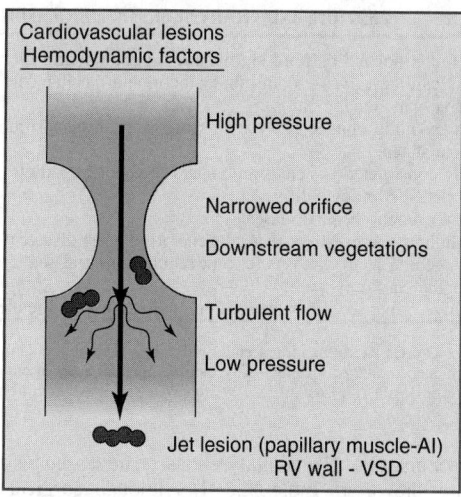

FIGURE 326–1 ■ Schematic diagram of hemodynamic factors favoring the development of non-bacterial thrombotic endocarditis. AI = aortic insufficiency; RV = right ventricular; VSD = ventricular septal defect.

is infected more readily with relatively avirulent microorganisms such as α-hemolytic streptococci, whereas the right is infected only by virulent pathogens such as *Staphylococcus aureus*: bacteria reach higher densities on the left side (e.g., 10^{10} to 10^{11} colony-forming units [CFU] per gram) than on the right (e.g., 10^8 CFU per gram). Right-sided lesions tend to respond more readily to antimicrobial therapy than do left-sided lesions; right-sided lesions may even heal spontaneously, in contrast to persistence of infection on the left. Responsible factors may include differences between the left and right side of the heart in blood PO_2, and intracardiac pressure. Spontaneous resolution of right-sided endocarditis is probably also a consequence of bacterial clearance on the right side by polymorphonuclear leukocytes, a factor not operative to the same extent on the left for unknown reasons. Pre-existing cardiac lesions that are believed to promote the formation of NBTE are identified in about three fourths of patients with infective endocarditis. The cardiac defects most frequently found in patients with endocarditis are mitral valve prolapse, degenerative heart disease, congenital heart disease, rheumatic heart disease, and prosthetic cardiac valves. However, the degree of risk that each type of cardiac lesion poses for subsequent endocarditis cannot be inferred from their relative frequency because the prevalence of these cardiac defects in the general population varies widely. The absolute risk is indicated by the incidence rate of endocarditis for each cardiac lesion (when the frequency of the cardiac defect in the general population is known), and the relative risk is indicated by the incidence rate with reference to the incidence rate of endocarditis in the general population (Table 326–1).

Prosthetic cardiac valves are a major risk factor for endocarditis. Endocarditis occurs in 1 to 5% of patients with prosthetic valves over the lifetime of the valve, with an incidence rate of about 300 to 600 per 100,000 patient-years. The risk is greatest during the first few months after implantation. Mechanical prosthetic cardiac valves probably have about the same risk as bioprostheses (e.g., porcine heterografts), and risk probably does not vary by site of prosthetic valve replacement but is greater when valves are placed in the presence of active endocarditis. Prior native valve endocarditis poses a significant risk factor for subsequent episodes as a consequence of both the continued presence of the risk factors that contributed to the initial episode (e.g., intravenous drug use or periodontitis) and the additional risk posed by the damage to the valve sustained in the initial episode. The decreasing relative frequency of valvular rheumatic heart disease among patients with endocarditis in the United States reflects the decreasing prevalence of rheumatic heart disease in this country. Nevertheless, valvular rheumatic heart disease is a major risk factor for endocarditis, with an incidence rate only slightly lower than that for prosthetic valves. Valvular rheumatic heart disease remains a frequent predisposing lesion for endocarditis in the developing world because of persistence of rheumatic heart disease

Table 326–1 ■ ABSOLUTE AND RELATIVE RISK FOR ENDOCARDITIS AMONG VARIOUS CARDIAC LESIONS (INCIDENCE RATE, CASES PER 100,000 PATIENT-YEARS)

High risk for endocarditis (and significant morbidity and mortality if endocarditis complicates the underlying cardiac condition)		
Prosthetic cardiac valves—both bioprosthetic and mechanical	300–630	(61–129)*
Prior native valve endocarditis	300–740	(61–151)
Complex cyanotic congenital heart disease (e.g., transposition of the great arteries, tetralogy of Fallot, single ventricle states)	120†	(25)
Surgically constructed systemic pulmonary shunts or conduits		
Moderate risk for endocarditis		
Valvular rheumatic heart diseases	380–440	(78–90)
Other acquired heart disease (e.g., degenerative heart disease)		
Other congenital heart diseases (except secundum atrial septal defect)		
Hypertrophic cardiomyopathy		
Mitral valve prolapse with regurgitation and/or thickened leaflets	52	(11)

*Incidence rate relative to the rate of endocarditis in a normal population, 4.9/100,000 patient-years (the list is not meant to be all-inclusive).
†Overall incidence rate for a variety of types of congenital heart disease.
Adapted from Dajani AS, Taubert KA, Wilson W, et al: Prevention of bacterial endocarditis. Recommendations of the American Heart Association. JAMA 277:1794, 1997.

in those populations. Congenital defects at increased risk for endocarditis are shown in Table 326–1. Although surgical correction of congenital defects such as ventricular septal defect lowers risk, it does not eliminate it. Nevertheless, the American Heart Association does not recommend preventive antibiotic therapy for patients 6 or more months after corrective surgery without residua. As a general rule, cardiac lesions not associated with turbulent blood flow, such as cardiac lesions in a relatively low-pressure system (e.g., on the right side of the heart) or abnormal flow through a wide orifice (e.g., secundum type of atrial septal defect), are less likely to be complicated by endocarditis. Because of its high prevalence in the population (2 to 22%), mitral valve prolapse is the most frequent lesion predisposing to endocarditis. However, the absolute risk for endocarditis among patients with mitral valve prolapse and an audible murmur of mitral insufficiency is considerably lower than that of other cardiac abnormalities listed in Table 236–1, i.e., about 10 times that of the general population. Cardiac lesions that rarely predispose to endocarditis are shown in Table 326–2. Endocarditis can occur on structurally normal native valves in 25% or more of patients. In these patients, endocarditis is more likely to be nosocomial or caused by more virulent organisms such as *S. aureus,* or the patient is more likely to be an intravenous drug user.

SYSTEMIC HOST FACTORS. Systemic host defenses (e.g., granulocytes, T lymphocytes, antibody, complement) most likely play a minor role in the development or maintenance of endocarditis, except perhaps for granulocytes in right-sided endocarditis. Various immunodeficiency states, including human immunodeficiency virus (HIV) infection, do not seem to place the patient at increased risk for endocarditis, although endocarditis-related morbidity and mortality rates for HIV-infected patients with acquired immune deficiency syndrome (AIDS) defining illness exceed those of HIV-infected patients without AIDS.

CIRCUMSTANCES THAT LEAD TO TRANSIENT BACTEREMIA. Transient bacteremia is a common event and occurs as a consequence of trauma to the skin or mucosal surfaces, which are normally laden with endogenous flora. The bacteremia is characterized by a low number of organisms per milliliter of blood (usually <10 CFU per milliliter) and very short duration (15 to 30 minutes). The intensity of the bacteremia is directly related to the magnitude of the trauma, the density of the microbial flora, and the presence of inflammation or infection at the site of skin or mucosal injury.

Mucosal sites that have a dense endogenous flora include the gingival crevice, oropharynx, terminal ileum and colon, distal part of the urethra, and vagina. Bacteremia may follow certain medical or surgical procedures that traumatize the skin or mucosal surfaces (Table 326–3). Indeed, cases of endocarditis occurring soon after tooth extraction, tonsillectomy, and other types of surgery were initially reported in the 1930s. A history of such procedures is found in 25% of patients with viridans streptococcal endocarditis within the preceding 2 months and 40% of patients with enterococcal endocarditis. However, these procedures (particularly dental procedures) are common in the general population, which makes assessment of the risk of the procedure per se difficult. A history of a recent dental procedure in a patient with endocarditis does not necessarily mean that the procedure was the proximate cause of the infection. One study of patients with endocarditis that used age- and sex-matched population-based controls sought to quantify the risk attributable to various procedures but, with few exceptions, failed to demonstrate a relationship between these procedures and endocarditis. Nevertheless, interest in preventive strategies has focused on specific procedures because these procedures are predictably followed by episodes of transient bacteremia with organisms of the type likely to cause endocarditis.

Minor mucosal trauma as routine as bowel movements, brushing

Table 326–2 ■ CARDIAC LESIONS THAT RARELY PREDISPOSE TO ENDOCARDITIS*

Isolated secundum type of atrial septal defect
Previous coronary artery bypass graft
Physiologic, functional, or innocent heart murmurs
Mitral valve prolapse without murmur
Previous Kawasaki's or rheumatic heart disease without valvular dysfunction
Permanent cardiac pacemakers and implanted defibrillators
Surgical repair, without residua, of atrial septal defect, ventricular septal defect, patent ductus arteriosus after 6 mo

*Low-risk for endocarditis; no chemoprophylaxis is recommended (the list is not meant to be all inclusive).
Adapted from Dajani AS, Taubert KA, Wilson W, et al: Prevention of bacterial endocarditis. Recommendations of the American Heart Association. JAMA 277:1794, 1997.

Table 326–3 ■ CIRCUMSTANCES LIKELY TO LEAD TO TRANSIENT BACTEREMIA THAT CAN PRECEDE ENDOCARDITIS

Chemoprophylaxis Recommended for High- and Medium-Risk Patients
Dental procedures
  Dental and periodontal procedures known to induce mucosal bleeding
    Dental extractions
    Periodontal procedures, including surgery, scaling and root planing, probing, and recall maintenance
  Dental implant placement and reimplantation of avulsed teeth
  Endodontic instrumentation or surgery only beyond the apex
  Subgingival placement of antibiotic fibers or strips
  Initial placement of orthodontic bands but not brackets
  Intraligamentary local anesthetic injections
Respiratory tract
  Tonsillectomy and adenoidectomy
  Bronchoscopy with a rigid bronchoscope
  Surgery on respiratory mucosa
Genitourinary tract
  Prostate surgery
  Cystoscopy or urethral dilatation
Chemoprophylaxis Recommended for High-Risk, Optional for Medium-Risk Patients
Gastrointestinal tract
  Esophageal dilatation or sclerotherapy for esophageal varices
  Biliary tract surgery
  Endoscopic retrograde cholangiography with biliary obstruction
  Surgery on intestinal mucosa
Chemoprophylaxis Optional for High-Risk Patients
Bronchoscopy with a flexible bronchoscope with or without biopsy
Transesophageal echocardiography
Endoscopy with or without gastrointestinal biopsy
Vaginal hysterectomy
Vaginal delivery

Adapted from Dajani AS, Taubert KA, Wilson W, et al: Prevention of bacterial endocarditis. Recommendations of the American Heart Association. JAMA 277:1794, 1997.

Table 326–4 ■ FREQUENCY OF INFECTING MICROORGANISMS IN ENDOCARDITIS (%)

NATIVE VALVE		PVE			ENDOCARDITIS IN IVDU	
			Early	Late		
Streptococci	50	Coagulase-negative staphylococci	33	29	*S. aureus*	57
Enterococci	10	*S. aureus*	15	11	Streptococci	13
Staphylococcus aureus	20	Gram-negative bacilli	17	11	Gram-negative bacilli	8
HACEK	5	Fungi	13	5	Enterococci	7
Other	10	Streptococci	9	36	Fungi	5
Culture negative	5	Diphtheroids	9	3	Polymicrobial	5
		Other	4	5	Culture negative	5

PVE = prosthetic valve endocarditis; IVDU = intravenous drug user; HACEK = *Haemophilus,* Actinobacillus, Cardiobacterium, Eikenella, and *Kingella.*

teeth, chewing hard candy, or other everyday experiences also causes transient bacteremia. Although transient bacteremia is a common, everyday event and each event is associated with only a very small risk for endocarditis, the cumulative risk of these transient episodes of low-grade bacteremia is sufficient to account in large part for the 75% of patients with viridans streptococcal endocarditis or 60% of patients with enterococcal endocarditis who fail to recall a medical or dental procedure that preceded the onset of their endocarditis. Spontaneous bacteremia is also likely to be responsible even for some of those cases in patients who give a history of a preceding procedure because the mere temporal association of a rare disease like endocarditis with a particularly common procedure such as a dental procedure does not necessarily infer causation. It seems increasingly apparent that spontaneous bacteremia, especially as a consequence of poor dental hygiene, accounts for the great majority of cases of viridans streptococcal endocarditis.

Transient bacteremia likely to lead to endocarditis can also result from illicit intravenous drug use and nosocomial procedures. The source of bacteremia can be identified in more than 90% of cases of nosocomial endocarditis. However, some of these procedures may be associated with subsequent endocarditis only in the presence of high-risk underlying cardiac lesions such as prosthetic valve or previous native valve endocarditis. The prosthetic valve is usually infected at the time of surgical insertion of the valve or following transient bacteremia in the postoperative period. Rarely the source is a prosthetic valve that was contaminated before insertion.

INFECTING MICROORGANISMS. Trauma to the skin or mucosal surfaces that harbor a prolific endogenous flora releases into the blood stream many different microbial species. The array of microorganisms entering the circulation varies with the unique endogenous microflora at the particular traumatized site. Staphylococci and diphtheroids are characteristic for skin; oral anaerobes and streptococci for the oropharyngeal mucosa; and colonic anaerobes, enteric aerobic gram-negative bacilli, and enterococci for the genitourinary and lower intestinal mucosa. However, only a few of these species, e.g., most commonly oral streptococci, staphylococci, and enterococci, are likely to cause endocarditis. The frequency with which a particular organism causes endocarditis depends on how frequently it can gain access to the circulation and its ability to survive in the blood stream and adhere to components of NBTE, exposed subendothelial structures, or the endothelial surface itself.

A predictable array of microorganisms cause endocarditis for each of the specific conditions that predispose patients to infective endocarditis (Table 326–4). For example, in community-acquired endocarditis in non–intravenous drug users, a variety of α-hemolytic streptococci (*S. mitis, S. sanguis, S. mutans,* and *S. intermedius*) and enterococci are the usual pathogens. *Streptococcus bovis,* a streptococcal species that contains group D polysaccharide capsular material, as do enterococci, causes endocarditis in patients who are likely to have an underlying gastrointestinal lesion. Isolation of *S. bovis* from blood cultures should prompt a complete evaluation of the gastrointestinal tract, especially the colon, in that patient. Less frequent are fastidious gram-negative bacilli, the so-called HACEK microorganisms (*Haemophilus* species, *Actinobacillus, Cardiobacterium, Eikenella,* and *Kingella*). The *Haemophilus* species are usually *H. aphrophilus, H. paraphrophilus,* or *H. parainfluenzae* and rarely *H. influenzae. S. aureus* causes more than 50% of cases of endocarditis occurring in intravenous drug users and in

many geographic locations the strains of *S. aureus* are resistant to all β-lactam antibiotics (i.e., usually designated as methicillin-resistant strains). Streptococci and enterococci are less frequent pathogens in intravenous drug users. Gram-negative bacilli (usually *Pseudomonas aeruginosa, Pseudomonas cepacia,* and *Serratia marcescens*) and fungi (usually non-*albicans Candida* species), unusual in non–intravenous drug use–associated native valve endocarditis, occur in about 8 and 5% of case of endocarditis caused by intravenous drug use, respectively. Although uncommon in patients without prosthetic valves, coagulase-negative staphylococci, usually of the methicillin-resistant variety, are the predominant pathogen of prosthetic valve endocarditis within 2 months after surgery, designated as early prosthetic valve endocarditis. Indeed, the frequency of methicillin-resistant coagulase-negative staphylococci remains constant over the entire first 12 months, which suggests that a similar pathogenesis may extend over the initial year after surgery, not just the first 2 months. After the first year the array of organisms in prosthetic valve endocarditis tends to resemble that of native valve endocarditis, i.e., streptococci. However, fungi, usually *C. albicans,* and aerobic enteric gram-negative bacilli occur more frequently in both early and late prosthetic valve endocarditis than in native valve endocarditis.

DEVELOPMENT OF VEGETATION. Microorganisms adherent to the vegetation stimulate further deposition of platelets and fibrin on their surface. Within this secluded focus, the buried microorganisms then begin multiplying as rapidly as they would in broth cultures, apparently uninhibited by host defenses, e.g., phagocytes, antibody, and complement, to reach maximally dense populations of 10^8 to 10^{11} CFU per gram of vegetation. Over 90% of the microorganisms in these established vegetations are metabolically inactive and non-growing, i.e., in a phase least susceptible to the bactericidal effects of β-lactam and aminoglycoside antibiotics.

Sustained bacteremia that is characteristic of endocarditis results from an equilibrium between the rate of release of microorganisms as the vegetation fragments and the rate of clearance of the circulating microorganisms by the reticuloendothelial system in the liver, spleen, and bone marrow. The vegetation enlarges as circulating bacteria are redeposited on the surface of the vegetation, which in turn stimulates further deposition of fibrin on the surface (Fig. 326–2). The resultant vegetation is composed of successive layers of fibrin and clusters of bacteria, with rare red cells and leukocytes, almost always covered by a layer of fibrin on the luminal surface.

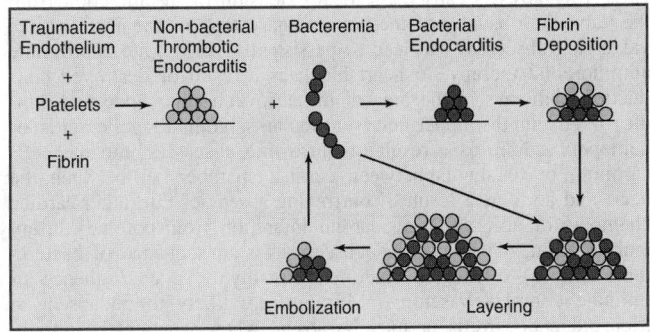

FIGURE 326–2 ■ Schematic diagram of the pathogenetic events leading to the development of infective endocarditis.

Enlargement of the vegetation tends to be counterbalanced by continued fragmentation. The ultimate size of the vegetation can vary from small sessile granular protuberances to a large pedunculated mass. The size of the vegetation itself and the fragments that break off depend to some extent on the type of infecting microorganism: for example, *H. parainfluenzae* and *C. albicans* tend to produce large friable vegetations and large emboli.

With effective antimicrobial therapy the vegetation becomes progressively organized as the edematous, vascular, and fibrogenic granulation tissue grows in from the base and is replaced by mature fibrous tissue with varying degrees of calcification. Healed vegetations are re-endothelialized, but the associated valve leaflet may become progressively more distorted as the healing proceeds. Thus despite bacteriologic response, distortion of the healing valve may lead to hemodynamic decompensation and a highly susceptible site for development of repeated episodes of infective endocarditis in the future.

CLINICAL FEATURES (See Color Plates 11*A* Through 11*D*

Clinical manifestations include fever and cardiac and extracardiac findings that are the result of either (1) the valvular infection itself, (2) embolization of fragments of the vegetation, (3) suppurative complications caused by hematogenous spread of infection, or (4) immunologic response to the infection in the form of immune complex vasculitis.

NATIVE VALVE ENDOCARDITIS. Symptoms usually begin within 2 weeks of the inciting bacteremia. In the pre-antibiotic era, when endocarditis was uniformly fatal, a short duration of illness of less than 6 weeks before death was used to characterize acute endocarditis: in contrast, subacute and chronic endocarditis had a more indolent course until death at 6 weeks to 2 years. Chronicity is now used in reference to the duration of illness before medical attention is sought. Acute endocarditis is usually (50 to 70%) caused by *S. aureus,* especially when accompanied by marked signs of general infection and suppurative embolic phenomena, and has a rapidly fatal course if treatment is delayed. *S. aureus* infection may develop on a previously normal valve. In a non–intravenous drug user, the aortic valve is usually involved. Therefore a diagnosis of acute endocarditis can serve as an effective guide to empirical antibiotic therapy, even before results of blood cultures are available. Subacute endocarditis, commonly caused by streptococci and enterococci, in contrast often develops on previously damaged endocardium, has less dramatic clinical manifestations of general infection, and is characterized by non-suppurative peripheral vascular phenomena.

Systemic manifestations of endocarditis include fever most commonly and other symptoms that may accompany fever, such as drenching night sweats, arthralgias, myalgias (especially in the lower part of the back and thighs), and weight loss. Fever, especially in subacute endocarditis, is usually low grade, the temperature peaks rarely exceeding 39.4° C. Fever may be absent in a few patients, e.g., those who are very elderly or severely debilitated, have significant renal or heart failure, or are taking antipyretics or antibiotics.

Cardiac manifestations include (1) murmurs of valvular insufficiency caused by a destroyed or distorted valve and its supporting structures or valvular stenosis caused by large vegetations; (2) valve ring abscess caused by local extension of the infection from the valve ring usually of the non-coronary cusp of the aortic valve; valve ring abscesses can lead to persistent fever despite appropriate antimicrobial therapy, to heart block as a result of destroyed conduction pathways in the area of the atrioventricular node and bundle of His in the upper interventricular septum, to pericarditis or hemopericardium as a result of burrowing abscesses into the pericardium, or to shunts between cardiac chambers or between the heart and aorta as a result of burrowing abscesses into other cardiac chambers or aorta; (3) myocardial infarction from coronary artery embolization; (4) myocardial abscess as a consequence of bacteremia; and (5) diffuse myocarditis, possibly as a consequence of immune complex vasculitis. Murmurs are likely to be absent in tricuspid endocarditis or may be absent when a patient is initially seen with acute endocarditis. Congestive heart failure (CHF), the most common complication of endocarditis, develops in about 60%

of patients as a consequence of valvular or myocardial involvement or may precede the onset of endocarditis as a consequence of the underlying cardiac lesion. CHF may be present on admission in patients with subacute or streptococcal endocarditis but may also develop dramatically in patients with acute *S. aureus* endocarditis with an aortic diastolic murmur or sudden rupture of mitral valve chordae, valvular obstruction from a bulky vegetation, sudden intracardiac shunt from a fistulous tract, or dehiscence of a prosthetic cardiac valve. CHF occurs more frequently with left-sided than right-sided endocarditis and with aortic more than mitral involvement.

Extracardiac manifestations include (1) embolic events that result in infarction of numerous organs, such as the lung in right-sided endocarditis or the brain, spleen, or kidneys in left-sided endocarditis; (2) suppurative complications that include abscesses, septic infarcts, and infected mycotic aneurysms; and (3) immunologic reactions to the valvular infection, including glomerulonephritis, sterile meningitis, and polyarthritis, and a variety of vascular phenomena such as mucocutaneous petechiae (see Color Plates 10*A* and 10*C*), splinter hemorrhages, Roth's spots (see Color Plate 10*B*), and Osler's nodes. Systemic embolization, often a devastating complication when it involves the cerebral circulation, occurs in about 20 to 40% of patients with left-sided endocarditis. Frank cerebral abscess is rare, except in *S. aureus* endocarditis, where it occurs in 1 to 5% of patients. Septic pulmonary emboli commonly occur in patients with right-sided endocarditis. On chest radiograms, these emboli appear as multiple round infiltrates that may undergo cavitation or be complicated by empyema. Emboli can occur at any time during the course of illness, although the frequency of embolization decreases as the vegetation heals. Most emboli occur before or within the first few days after initiation of appropriate antibiotic therapy. Emboli are less frequent in viridans streptococcal endocarditis than endocarditis due to more virulent organisms, e.g., *S. aureus.* Mycotic aneurysms are an unusual but important complication of endocarditis. Mycotic aneurysms (see Color Plate 10*D*) are commonly asymptomatic but can become clinically evident in 3 to 5% of patients, even months or years after completion of successful therapy. These aneurysms characteristically develop at arterial bifurcations, e.g., in the middle cerebral, splenic, superior mesenteric, pulmonary, coronary, and extremity arteries, the abdominal aorta, and the sinus of Valsalva. In a patient with endocarditis, unremitting headache, visual disturbance, or cranial nerve palsy suggests an impending rupture of a cerebral mycotic aneurysm. Signs of blood loss at any site in a patient with endocarditis should suggest rupture of a mycotic aneurysm once the aneurysm has enlarged beyond a critical size.

The development of clinically apparent splenomegaly and many of the various non-suppurative peripheral vascular phenomena is related to the duration of illness before diagnosis. The frequency of these clinical manifestations (<50%) is currently less than in the past as a result of shorter durations of illness before antimicrobial therapy is given.

ENDOCARDITIS IN INTRAVENOUS DRUG USERS. Intravenous drug users with endocarditis tend to be younger than non–intravenous drug users with endocarditis, the disease is usually acute, and a previously normal tricuspid valve is generally involved. In tricuspid endocarditis, murmurs and heart failure are usually absent, but septic pulmonary complications occur in about 75% of these patients and *S. aureus* is the usual pathogen. Left-sided endocarditis in intravenous drug users resembles that in non–intravenous drug users and is manifested by aortic or mitral murmurs, heart failure, neurologic damage, systemic embolization, peripheral mucocutaneous stigmata of endocarditis, or systemic metastatic infection such as osteomyelitis and septic arthritis. The pathogens isolated to intravenous drug users with left-sided endocarditis are similar those isolated from non-users although *S. aureus* is probably disproportionately involved in users. Fever, the usual initial manifestation of endocarditis in an intravenous drug user, also accompanies other major and minor illnesses in this population. Indeed, only about 10% of febrile intravenous drug users coming to the emergency room actually have endocarditis. In most febrile intravenous drug users with a major infectious disease such as cellulitis, endocarditis, pneumonia, or osteomyelitis, the cause of the patient's fever is obvious at initial evaluation. However, in about one third of febrile intravenous drug users with endocarditis the cause of the patient's fever will be not immediately apparent.

NOSOCOMIAL ENDOCARDITIS. Nosocomial endocarditis,

which is defined as endocarditis resulting from a hospital-based procedure performed within 4 weeks preceding the onset of symptoms, accounts for 10 to 30% of cases of endocarditis, the frequency varying with the types of patients. Patients with nosocomial native valve endocarditis tend to be elderly and have predisposing cardiac lesions, usually on the left side of the heart. The major predisposing cardiac lesion for nosocomial endocarditis is a prosthetic cardiac valve (present in up to 50% of cases). The most important bacteremia-inducing event during hospitalization that results in endocarditis is use of an intravascular device, present in up to 50% of cases. Nosocomial *S. aureus* bacteremia is much more frequently complicated by endocarditis (up to 25% of the time) than is enterococcal bacteremia (<1%). The clinical features of nosocomial endocarditis are similar to those of community-acquired endocarditis. In patients with prosthetic valve endocarditis, fever is usually present, although the classic clinical features of endocarditis, such as peripheral vascular phenomena, are frequently absent, especially in early infection. Although blood cultures are usually positive, the diagnosis is frequently delayed because of failure to recognize the significance of the positive blood cultures.

ELECTROCARDIOGRAPHIC MANIFESTATIONS. A baseline electrocardiogram (ECG) should be obtained to assess the presence of conduction abnormalities, which develop in about 10 to 20% of patients with endocarditis as a consequence of burrowing valve ring abscesses. A prolonged PR interval may be the initial indication of the sudden development of more severe conduction abnormalities such as complete heart block. Other abnormalities that can be detected by ECG include myocardial infarction and pericarditis.

HEMATOLOGIC MANIFESTATIONS. In patients with subacute endocarditis, progressive anemia of chronic disease with normochromic, normocytic indices routinely develops, and platelet, white cell, and differential counts are relatively normal. In acute endocarditis of short duration caused by *S. aureus,* anemia may initially be absent, although the white blood cell count is usually elevated with a shift to the left and the platelet count is often low. Prosthetic valve endocarditis with an unstable prosthesis may cause acute hemolysis. The erythrocyte sedimentation rate is routinely elevated in endocarditis except when hypofibrinogenemia secondary to disseminated intravascular coagulation or CHF is present.

RENAL MANIFESTATIONS. Proteinuria and microscopic hematuria are common findings that occur in up to 50% of patients. Renal emboli or focal glomerulonephritis can cause microscopic hematuria, but gross hematuria usually indicates renal infarction. Renal failure that develops in a patient with endocarditis is usually due to diffuse immune complex glomerulonephritis (see Color Plate 11*E*).

OTHER LABORATORY MANIFESTATIONS. Serologic evidence of circulating immune complexes may by found in endocarditis, the frequency of which is related to the duration of illness. Occasional false-positive non-treponemal serologic tests for syphilis occur. The cerebrospinal fluid may show polymorphonuclear leukocytes and a moderately elevated protein concentration in up to 15% of patients. Frank bacterial meningitis, although unusual, occurs in *S. aureus* endocarditis.

DIAGNOSIS

Definitive diagnosis depends on microbiologic or pathologic proof of infection by histology or culture of vegetations obtained at surgery or autopsy or when an arterial embolus is surgically removed. In lieu of surgery or autopsy, a definitive diagnosis can be established by demonstrating (1) a characteristic vegetation, valve ring abscess, or new prosthetic valve dehiscence with echocardiography and (2) intravascular infection with multiple blood cultures obtained over an extended period that are positive for a microorganism consistent with endocarditis. However, a blood culture or echocardiography is usually obtained only after the diagnosis is suspected from the history and physical findings. The diagnosis can be ranked in order of the probability that endocarditis is present by distinction between major and minor criteria; such criteria allow for weighting of clinical findings, echocardiographic findings, the type of microbial species isolated from blood, the frequency of positive blood cultures, and the absence of another source of infection (Table 326–5).

MICROBIOLOGIC INVESTIGATION. Isolating a pathogen from several blood cultures that are obtained over an extended period is

Table 326–5 ▪ CRITERIA FOR THE DIAGNOSIS OF INFECTIVE ENDOCARDITIS (DUKE UNIVERSITY ENDOCARDITIS SERVICE)

1. Definitive diagnosis
   a. Pathology/microbiology of vegetations or embolized vegetations obtained at surgery or autopsy
   b. 2 major criteria
   c. 1 major/3 minor
   d. 5 minor
2. Possible diagnosis: Findings consistent with infective endocarditis that fall short of a definitive diagnosis of endocarditis, but not rejected
3. No endocarditis: No pathology at surgery or autopsy, clinical resolution with ≤4 d of antimicrobial therapy, or firm alternative diagnosis

Major Criteria
1. Blood culture
   a. 2 separate blood cultures positive for
      i. Viridans streptococci, *Streptococcus bovis,* HACEK
      ii. Community-acquired *Staphylococcus aureus* or enterococci in the absence of a primary focus
   b. Positive blood cultures >12 hr apart
   c. Positive blood cultures: 3 of 3, majority of ≥4 with 1st and last ≥1 hr apart
2. Endocardial involvement
   a. Echocardiography: Oscillating intracardiac mass on a valve or supporting structure, in the path of a regurgitant jet stream, or on implanted material in the absence of an alternative anatomic explanation, valve ring abscess, or new dehiscence of a prosthetic valve
   b. New valvular regurgitant murmur

Minor Criteria
1. Predisposing heart condition or IVDU
2. Fever (≥38° C)
3. Systemic or pulmonary emboli, mycotic aneurysm, intracranial hemorrhage, conjunctival hemorrhages, Janeway lesions
4. Immunologic phenomena: glomerulonephritis, Roth's spot, Osler's node, rheumatoid factor
5. Echocardiography findings consistent with but not definitive of endocarditis
6. Microbiologic/serologic findings consistent with but not definitive of endocarditis

HACEK = *Haemophilus, Actinobacillus, Cardiobacterium, Eikenella,* and *Kingella;* IVDU = intravenous drug user.

Adapted from Durack DT, Lukes AS, Bright DK, et al: New criteria for diagnosis of infective endocarditis: Utilization of specific echocardiographic findings. Am J Med 96:200, 1994. With permission from Excerpta Medica Inc.

important both to confirm the diagnosis of endocarditis and to enable determination of the antibiotic regimen that is optimal for therapy. Bacteremia in endocarditis is characterized by a constant number of organisms per milliliter of blood (usually 20 to 200 CFU per milliliter), unrelated to the height of the patient's temperature or the site of blood sampling (e.g., arterial versus venous blood), except for a slight fall in numbers across the hepatic or splenic circulation. Fewer than 5% of patients with endocarditis have sterile blood cultures if adequate blood culture methods are used. Three blood cultures should be obtained at least 1 hour apart to demonstrate that the bacteremia is continuous. If the cultures remain negative for 48 hours, two additional cultures should be obtained. However, in the absence of prior antibiotic therapy, the first three blood cultures are expected to be positive in more than 95% of patients with positive cultures. Prior antibiotic therapy, fastidious bacteria (such as the nutritionally deficient streptococci, now called *Abiotrophia* species, the HACEK group of organisms, *Neisseria, Brucella,* and *Legionella*), fungi, chlamydial, *Bartonella (Rochalimaea)* spp., *Coxiella burnetii,* and rickettsial can result in negative cultures. Additional use of a lysis-centrifugation system for blood cultures can enhance the recovery of fungi, mycobacteria, and *Bartonella.* In acute endocarditis, when empirical antibiotic therapy should be initiated as soon as possible, two or three blood cultures should be drawn 1 hour apart before starting empirical therapy. In the face of a preceding course of antibiotics, further antibiotic therapy should be withheld and blood cultures repeated until positive, if clinical conditions permit. The longer the time since the last dose of antibiotic or the shorter the preceding course of antibiotic, the more likely that the blood cultures will be positive. When fastidious bacteria and fungi are suspected, the clinical microbiology laboratory should be consulted for advice on the optimal methods to isolate these microorganisms, which may require more prolonged incubation (e.g., up to 3 weeks) or special media for isolation. Gram stain of the cultures may identify some pathogens not otherwise apparent in the blood cultures. Fungal endocarditis, which is likely to have negative blood cultures, tends to be complicated by large vegetations and embolization, in which case the organisms can be identified by Gram stain and culture of the surgically removed emboli. Serology techniques are needed to diagnose endocarditis caused by *Chlamydia psittaci, Chlamydia trachomatis,* or *C. burnetii* and may be helpful for *Brucella* endocarditis. Bacteriuria with either enterococci or *S. aureus* occurs in endocarditis caused by the respective organism. Several in vitro tests must be done on the pathogen isolated from blood to assess susceptibility to potential bactericidal drugs (Table 326–6).

CARDIAC IMAGING PROCEDURES. Echocardiography has become second only to culture of blood for investigating patients who are clinically suspected to have endocarditis. Echocardiography can visualize valvular vegetations, satellite vegetations, flail valves, ruptured chordae, perivalvular abscesses, fistulas, valvular perforations, and mycotic aneurysms. Echocardiography can be used to define the causes and severity of CHF by assessment of ventricular size, wall motion, and dynamic function. Echocardiography can also identify predisposing cardiac lesions. Two-dimensional transthoracic echocardiography (TTE) and transesophageal echocardiography (TEE), the two currently performed types of echocardiography, are safe and portable to the bedside. TTE is rapid, non-invasive, and relatively inexpensive (see Chapter 43).

TEE uses high ultrasonic frequencies, which improves spatial resolution, eliminates interference from interposed tissues, and therefore results in much higher sensitivity and specificity. Small vegetations and intracardiac complications such as ring abscesses may be detected only by TEE. Visualization of the extent and mobility of vegetations can be improved by imaging with TEE in two or more planes. Placement of the TEE transducer in the esophagus gives better views of the left side of the heart because of its close proximity to the aortic root, basal septum, and the left side of the heart, whereas TTE and TEE give equivalent views of the more anteriorly placed right side of the heart.

OTHER INVESTIGATIVE PROCEDURES. Although other studies may be suggestive, angiography is required for the definitive antemortem diagnosis of a mycotic aneurysm. Cardiac catheterization can provide important information and should not be avoided when indicated in selected patients with endocarditis for fear of dislodging emboli. Coronary angiography is used to assess the presence of significant coronary artery disease before elective placement of prosthetic cardiac valves in patients who are older than 40 years and have additional atherogenic risk factors. Computed tomography or magnetic resonance imaging is used to define the cause of focal neurologic findings and identify metastatic suppurative infection or embolic events that can impede clinical or bacteriologic therapeutic responses.

DIAGNOSTIC STRATEGIES IN SPECIAL SITUATIONS. INTRAVENOUS DRUG USERS. (See Chapter 17) Because outpatient follow-up in this population is rarely possible, admitting febrile intravenous drug users without a clinically apparent source for their fever

is indicated for at least 1 week until the results of blood culture are available. Blood cultures become positive within 1 week in most patients if *S. aureus,* fungi, fastidious gram-negative bacilli or streptococci, or anaerobes are involved or the patient has recently taken antibiotics. After obtaining blood cultures, empirical antimicrobial therapy should be initiated. Once the blood cultures are found to be positive, evidence of endocarditis should be sought initially by TTE and, if TTE is negative, by TEE. If echocardiography reveals vegetations, valvular destruction or its hemodynamic effects, valve ring abscess or a fistula, or a predisposing valvular lesion and/or clinical evidence of left-sided or right-sided endocarditis (e.g., septic pleuropulmonary complications) exists, the diagnosis of endocarditis is made. Vegetations detected by TTE indicate a group of patients at greater risk of morbidity, i.e., prolonged fever or development of CHF. Evidence of CHF on echocardiography defines a group of patients who may subsequently require valve replacement. Even if another potential source for the bacteremia is present and no echocardiographic or clinical evidence of endocarditis but the organism isolated is likely to cause endocarditis, such as *S. aureus* or a streptococcus, the diagnosis of endocarditis should nevertheless be suspected. If no apparent source is found for the bacteremia, even if echocardiographic and clinical evidence is lacking, the patient should still be considered to possibly have endocarditis. With negative echocardiography, if the clinical course dictates and another diagnosis is still not apparent, TEE should be repeated in about 1 week. If blood cultures remain negative after 1 week of incubation, the patient may be discharged from the hospital without echocardiography, unless clinical evidence of left-sided or right-sided endocarditis is present, in which case the diagnosis of endocarditis should nevertheless be suspected.

NOSOCOMIAL NATIVE VALVE ENDOCARDITIS. In patients with bacteremia related to intravascular devices, such as an arteriovenous fistula or graft for hemodialysis, indwelling central intravenous line, cardiac assist balloon pump, or pacemaker wire, the device should be removed, especially with *S. aureus* bacteremia or fungemia or if an indwelling catheter is associated with a tunnel or exit site infection. In nosocomial, as in community-acquired *S. aureus* bacteremia, especially early in the course of the disease when clinical evidence of endocarditis or metastatic foci of infection are likely to be absent, or even if there is an obvious primary focus of *S. aureus* infection (e.g., intravenous catheter) or a normal TTE, TEE has been reported to detect otherwise unsuspected endocarditis or its intracardiac complications in a high percentage of patients (up to 25%). Catheter-associated coagulase-negative staphylococcal nosocomial bacteremia, which rarely eventuates in native valve endocarditis, should not be investigated with echocardiography after antibiotics are begun unless a prosthetic cardiac valve is present. Indeed, catheter removal may not be necessary to cure coagulase-negative staphylococcal catheter-associated bacteremia. Catheter-associated nosocomial fungemia should probably be investigated with echocardiography after the catheter is removed and antifungal chemotherapy begun, regardless of whether clinical evidence of endocarditis is present.

PROSTHETIC VALVE ENDOCARDITIS. The diagnosis of pros-

Table 326–6 ■ IN VITRO ASSAYS

Viridans streptococci	Broth dilution test	Penicillin MIC
Enterococci	Broth dilution test	Penicillin MIC
		Vancomycin MIC
	Growth in	High-level resistance to
	500 μg/mL	Gentamicin
	1000 μg/mL	Streptomycin
	Nitrocefin	β-Lactamase production
Staphylococcus aureus, coagulase-negative staphylococci	Nitrocefin	β-Lactamase production
	Oxacillin/methicillin sensitivity	MRSA/MRCNS
	Broth dilution test	Vancomycin MIC
		Rifampin MIC
		TMP-SMX MIC
Other pathogens	Broth dilution tests	Antibiotic MIC/MBC
All pathogens	Serum bactericidal activity*	Bactericidal activity at peak
	Serum antibiotic level	Peak and trough gentamicin and vancomycin levels

MIC = minimal inhibitory concentration; MBC = minimal bactericidal concentration; MRSA = methicillin-resistant *S. aureus;* MRCNS = methicillin-resistant coagulase-negative staphylococci; TMP-SMX = trimethoprim-sulfamethoxazole.
*May be useful for non-standard antimicrobial regimens or unusual pathogens.
From Levison ME: *In vitro* assays. *In* Kaye D (ed): Infective Endocarditis, 2nd ed. New York, Raven Press, 1992, p 151.

thetic valve endocarditis is usually suspected because of fever and confirmed by the presence of multiple blood cultures positive for the same microorganism. Echocardiography, in particular TEE, is helpful in the diagnosis of prosthetic valve endocarditis and its complications, such as prosthetic valvular insufficiency, perivalvular extension of infection, and fistulas. In a recent study, 43% of patients with a prosthetic valve in whom fever and bacteremia developed had or subsequently acquired prosthetic valve endocarditis. Any organism in blood cultures in these patients must be taken seriously as a potential cause of endocarditis. In those with clinical evidence suggestive of prosthetic valve endocarditis, empirical antibiotic therapy can be initiated after three or four sets of blood cultures are obtained. After antimicrobial therapy is started, blood cultures should be repeated to assess for clearance of bacteremia. In bacteremic patients with no evidence of endocarditis despite these studies, antimicrobial therapy has traditionally been recommended for 2 weeks, but new data suggest that even therapy continued beyond 2 weeks may not prevent prosthetic valve endocarditis from occurring as a result of the initially transient bacteremia.

ANTIBIOTIC THERAPY

PRINCIPLES. Effective antimicrobial therapy for endocarditis optimally requires identification of the specific pathogen and assessment of its susceptibility to various antimicrobial agents. Therefore, every effort must be made to isolate the pathogen before initiating antimicrobial therapy, if clinically feasible. In patients who are in immediate danger of death, empirical antibiotic therapy should be started as soon as possible after obtaining blood cultures. Empirical therapy should be targeted at the most likely pathogens in that particular clinical setting (see Table 326-4). The minimal requirements for an effective antimicrobial regimen include the following:

1. BACTERICIDAL ACTIVITY. Bacteriostatic agents are not able to clear the pathogen from infected tissues unaided by host defenses such as polymorphonuclear leukocytes, antibody, and complement. Because host defenses are thought to not operate within vegetations (except in tricuspid valve vegetations, in which polymorphonuclear leukocytes may aid the effect of an antimicrobial agent), clearing bacteria from these vegetations requires bactericidal action from antibiotics. In fact, complete eradication of pathogens from the vegetation by the antimicrobial drug is thought to be essential to cure endocarditis. If any bacteria remain after completion of antibiotic therapy, the residual organisms regrow and result in relapse. If the pathogen cannot be eliminated completely by antimicrobial therapy, e.g., if relapse occurs or the patient has persistent bacteremia, the infected vegetation may need to be excised surgically for cure. Table 326-7 shows the various antimicrobial agents that have bactericidal activity. For microorganisms without predictable susceptibility, the bactericidal activity of an antimicrobial agent for the particular patient's pathogen must be assessed by determination of the minimal inhibitory (MIC) and minimal bactericidal concentrations of the antimicrobial agents in vitro (see Table 326-6).

The enterococcus illustrates the problems in selecting appropriate bactericidal therapy for endocarditis. Enterococci are relatively resistant to penicillin. In contrast to many viridans streptococci, which are inhibited by 0.1 μg/mL or less of penicillin G, most *Enterococcus faecalis* strains require up to 6.3 μg/mL to be inhib-

ited. Unlike viridans streptococci, which are killed by relatively low concentrations of penicillin, penicillin G alone, even at concentrations of up to 1000 μg/mL, is only inhibitory or at best slightly bactericidal against enterococci. The aminoglycosides are also poorly effective at low concentrations (<500 to 1000 μg/mL) because of inadequate permeability of the bacterial cell. Antibiotic synergism does occur, however, as the result of enhanced intracellular uptake of the aminoglycoside in the presence of a β-lactam (such as penicillin, ampicillin, or piperacillin) or a glycopeptide (such as vancomycin or teicoplanin), the so-called cell wall–active antibiotics. The definition of synergism requires that the reduction in bacterial count at 24 hours with the drug combination be at least 100-fold greater than that with the cell wall–active antibiotic alone. Synergism is predicted on routine screening of strains by inhibition of growth with 500 μg/mL of gentamicin or 1000 μg/mL of streptomycin (see Table 326-6). In addition to determination of susceptibilities to high levels of streptomycin and gentamicin, all enterococci causing endocarditis should be tested for β-lactamase production and susceptibility to penicillin and vancomycin to select optimal therapy. If the strain is β-lactamase positive (detected by a nitrocefin strip because MIC testing of β-lactamase–positive strains may fail to disclose this type of penicillin resistance), ampicillin/sulbactam or vancomycin must be used alone for 8 to 12 weeks because most strains are also high-level aminoglycoside resistant. If the MIC of penicillin is greater than 16 μg/mL vancomycin can be used in combination with an aminoglycoside if the strain is high-level aminoglycoside susceptible. If vancomycin resistant (MIC, >4 μg/mL), infectious disease consultation should be sought because these strains are usually multidrug resistant. No bactericidal therapy exists for strains that exhibit high-level resistance to both gentamicin and streptomycin or strains that exhibit high-level resistance to both β-lactam (penicillin MIC, >16 μg/mL) and glycopeptide (vancomycin MIC, >4 μg/mL) antibiotics.

2. HIGH CONCENTRATIONS OF THE ANTIMICROBIAL AGENT IN THE VEGETATION. Doses of the antimicrobial agent must achieve blood concentrations of the antimicrobial agent high enough to facilitate passive diffusion of the antimicrobial agent into the depths of the vegetation where microcolonies of the pathogen are located. Dosing sufficiently large to attain bactericidal activity in a 1:8 or greater dilution of the patient's serum against the patient's pathogen at the peak time after administrating the antimicrobial agent has traditionally guided therapy (although more recent data suggest that dilutions of 1:64 or greater have more predictive accuracy for bacteriologic cure).

3. PROLONGED DURATION OF ANTIMICROBIAL THERAPY. Over 90% of the microbial population in the vegetation is non-growing and metabolically inactive once the infection has become well established. Non-growing organisms are more likely to be found in the central portions of the microcolonies in the deeper regions of the vegetation. As a result, microorganisms in vegetations for the most part are not susceptible to commonly used antibiotics such as the β-lactams and aminoglycosides, which are effective only against actively growing bacteria. Optimally, the antimicrobial agent should be active against non-growing microorganisms. However, when the drug is active only against growing microorganisms, each dose of the bactericidal drug is able to effect a reduction in the microbial count only in that minor portion (<10%) of the population that happens to be growing at the time of drug administration. The duration of drug therapy must therefore be prolonged to completely clear the pathogen from the vegetation.

The duration of therapy varies with the specific pathogen, the site of the infection, and the type of antibiotic. For example, bacterial clearance is more rapid for viridans streptococci than for staphylococci, in tricuspid than in aortic vegetations, with antistaphylococcal β-lactams than with vancomycin, or with combinations of cell wall–active agent plus aminoglycoside than with single drugs. More rapid clearance in these special circumstances may permit a shorter course of therapy to achieve cure.

4. DOSING SHOULD BE FREQUENT ENOUGH TO PREVENT REGROWTH OF MICROORGANISMS BETWEEN DOSES. The organisms that remain after brief in vitro exposure to an aminoglycoside or a β-lactam antibiotic frequently exhibit a post-exposure delay in further in vitro growth, the so-called post-antibiotic effect. Unfortunately, no such effect occurs with some organisms such as entero-

Table 326-7 ■ BACTERICIDAL AGENTS

β-Lactams	Penams (e.g., penicillin, ampicillin, amoxicillin, nafcillin, ticarcillin, piperacillin)
	Penems (none as yet marketed)
	Carbapenems (imipenem, meropenem)
	Cephems (cephalosporins, cefoxitin)
	Carbacephems (loracarbef)
	Monobactams (aztreonam)
Aminoglycosides	Gentamicin, tobramycin, amikacin, etc.
Quinolones	Ciprofloxacin, ofloxacin, trovafloxacin, levofloxacin, etc.
Glycopeptides	Vancomycin, teicoplanin
Other	Trimethoprim-sulfamethoxazole
	Metronidazole
	Rifampin

Adapted from Levison ME: *In vitro* assays. *In* Kaye D (ed): Infective Endocarditis, 2nd ed. New York, Raven Press, 1992, p 151.

cocci or *P. aeruginosa* in vegetations. Thus even though a bactericidal effect can be achieved in the vegetation in the early portions of a dosing interval when levels of the drug are high, if antibiotic levels are not maintained in the vegetation at least above the MIC during the rest of the dosing interval, the residual organisms may regrow and efficacy may be compromised.

Standardized regimens have been recommended for the most common pathogens—viridans streptococci, enterococci, and staphylococci on native and prosthetic valves (Table 326–8). Standardized regimens are not available for more unusual pathogens, includ-

Table 326–8 ■ ANTIBIOTIC THERAPY (ADULT DOSES)[a] FOR INFECTIVE ENDOCARDITIS

REGIMEN	DOSE AND DURATION[a]

Highly penicillin-susceptible streptococci (MIC, ≤0.1 μg/mL)

1. Aqueous penicillin, 12–18 million U daily IV, cefazolin,[b] 1 g IV q8h, ceftriaxone,[b] 2 g IV q24h, or vancomycin,[c] 15 mg/kg (max 2 g/day unless serum levels are monitored[d]) IV q12h for 4 wk (this regimen is preferred in patients ≥65 yr and those with 8th nerve or renal impairment)

2. Aqueous penicillin, 12–18 million U daily IV, or ceftriaxone,[b] 2 g IV q24h, plus streptomycin[e,f] 7.5 mg/kg (max, 500 mg/dose) q12h, or gentamicin,[e,f] 1 mg/kg IV or IM q8h for 2 wk (this regimen is appropriate for uncomplicated cases of endocarditis in patients at low risk for adverse events from aminoglycosides. If streptomycin is preferred, susceptibility to high levels of this aminoglycoside must be determined in vitro. Isolates from patients with endocarditis rarely have been reported that are resistant to high levels of streptomycin (MIC, >1000 μg/mL) and lack penicillin-streptomycin synergy in vitro. Endocarditis from these high-level streptomycin-resistant strains that are susceptible to high levels of gentamicin in vitro (MIC, ≤500 μg/mL) can be treated with a penicillin-gentamicin combination)

Relatively penicillin-resistant streptococci (MIC, >0.1 and <0.5 μg/mL)

Aqueous penicillin, 18 million U daily IV, cefazolin,[b] 1 g IV q8h, ceftriaxone,[b] 2 g IV q24h, or vancomycin,[c,g] 15 mg/kg (max 2 g/day unless serum levels are monitored[d]) IV q12h for 4–6 wk, plus streptomycin,[e,f] 7.5 mg/kg (max 500 mg/dose) q12h, or gentamicin,[e,f] 1 mg/kg IV or IM q8h for the 1st, 2 wk (This regimen gives high cure rates for endocarditis secondary to highly penicillin-susceptible streptococci but is now reserved for endocarditis secondary to relatively resistant strains. For patients with streptococcal prosthetic valve endocarditis, a 6-wk course of penicillin plus gentamicin for at least the first 2 wks is recommended)

Penicillin-resistant streptococci (MIC, ≥0.5 μg/mL), enterococci, or nutritionally variant streptococci or for streptococcal prosthetic valve endocarditis

Aqueous penicillin 18–30 million U daily IV, or vancomycin,[c,h] 15 mg/kg (max, 2 g/day unless serum levels are monitored[d]) IV q12h, plus streptomycin,[e,f] 7.5 mg/kg (max, 500 mg/dose) q12h, or gentamicin,[e,f] 1 mg/kg IV or IM q8h for 4–6 wk (Because of technical difficulties in susceptibility testing of nutritionally variant streptococci, many experts recommended treating endocarditis caused by these strains with the standard regimen recommended for enterococci. Six wks of therapy is recommended for patients with streptococcal prosthetic valve endocarditis or for patients with enterococcal endocarditis and more than 3 mo of symptoms before therapy)

Methicillin/gentamicin-susceptible staphylococci—Uncomplicated,[i] Right sided, native valve only

Nafcillin or oxacillin,[j] 2 g q4h IV for 2 wk
　　with
Gentamicin,[e] 1 mg/kg q8h IV/IM for 2 wk

Methicillin-susceptible staphylococci—Native valve

Nafcillin or oxacillin,[j] 2 g q4h IV for 4–6 wk
　　with or without
Gentamicin,[k] 1 mg/kg q8h IV/IM for the 1st 3–5 d only

Methicillin-susceptible staphylococci—Native valve, penicillin-allergic patient

Cefazolin,[b] 2 g IV q8h for 4–6 wk
　　with or without
Gentamicin,[k] 1 mg/kg q8h IV/IM for the 1st 3–5 d only
　　or
Vancomycin,[c,j] 30 mg/kg daily (max, 2 g/day unless serum levels are monitored[d]) divided q12h for 4–6 wk

Methicillin-resistant staphylococci—Native valve

Vancomycin, 30 mg/kg daily (max, 2 g/day unless serum levels are monitored[d]) divided q12h for 4–6 wk

Methicillin-resistant staphylococci—Prosthetic device

Vancomycin, 30 mg/kg daily (max, 2 g/day unless serum levels are monitored[d]) divided q12h 6 wk or longer
　　plus
Rifampin,[l] 300 mg q8h for 6 wk or longer
　　plus
Gentamicin,[e,m] 1 mg/kg q8h IV/IM for the 1st 2 wk

Methicillin-susceptible staphlococci—Prosthetic device

Nafcillin or oxacillin,[j,n] 2 g q4h IV for 6 wk or longer
　　plus
Rifampin,[l] 300 mg q8h for 6 wk or longer
　　plus
Gentamicin,[e,m] 1 mg/kg q8h IV/IM for the 1st 2 wk

[a]Antibiotic doses are for adults with normal renal function.

[b]Cephalosporins or vancomycin could be used in patients with penicillin allergy. However, cephalosporins should not be used in individuals with an immediate-type hypersensitivity reaction (urticaria, angioedema, or anaphylaxis) to penicillin.

[c]Vancomycin is preferred if immediate-type hypersensitivity to penicillin is suspected. Vancomycin use may enhance the nephrotoxicity of gentamicin.

[d]Vancomycin peak serum levels should be obtained 1 hr after completion of a 1- to 2-hour infusion and should be in the range of 30 to 45 μg/mL.

[e]Gentamicin peak serum levels obtained 1 hour after start of a 20 to 30-min IV infusion or IM injection should be about 3 μg/mL and trough level should be less than 1 μg/mL. The streptomycin peak serum level 1 hour after IM administration is about 20 μg/mL.

[f]The choice of an aminoglycoside should be based on in vitro high-level aminoglycoside susceptibility testing. If the strain is susceptible to high levels of gentamicin, gentamicin is preferred because determination of gentamicin serum levels is more generally available.

[g]When vancomycin is chosen, the addition of gentamicin is not recommended by the American Heart Association.

[h]For treatment of enterococcal endocarditis, penicillin desensitization should be considered if penicillin allergy is not suspected to be of the immediate type; cephalosporins are not acceptable alternatives.

[i]No evidence of metastatic pleuropulmonary or systemic infection or left-sided endocarditis and the isolate is gentamicin susceptible.

[j]Vancomycin is less rapidly bactericidal than antistaphylococcal β-lactam antibiotics, as reflected by slower clearance of staphylococci from the vegetations and blood. Consequently, vancomycin is not effective in the short-course (2-week) regimen and similarly should not be used in other regimens, unless the organism is methicillin resistant or the patient has penicillin allergy that precludes use of a β-lactam antibiotic.

[k]The additional benefit of an aminoglycoside has not been clearly established. Gentamicin should be used only if the isolate is gentamicin susceptible.

[l]Rifampin should be added in cases of rifampin-susceptible staphylococcal endocarditis in the presence of a prosthetic device; combination therapy is essential to prevent the emergence of rifampin resistance.

[m]If the isolate is gentamicin resistant, another aminoglycoside to which the isolate is sensitive should be used. If resistant to all aminoglycosides, a fluoroquinolone to which the isolate is sensitive should be substituted.

[n]Cefazolin or vancomycin should be used in penicillin-allergic patients. Vancomycin is preferred if immediate-type penicillin hypersensitivity is present.

Adapted from Wilson WR, Karchmer AW, Dajani AS, et al: Antibiotic treatment of adults with infective endocarditis due to streptococci, enterococci, staphylococci and HACEK microorganisms. JAMA 274:1706, 1995. © 1995, American Medical Association.

ing strains of *E. faecalis* that both produce β-lactamase and are highly aminoglycoside resistant; strains of enterococci that exhibit high-level resistance to vancomycin, ampicillin, and aminoglycosides; and gram-negative bacilli, anaerobes, and diphtheroids. In vitro susceptibility testing should be performed for these organisms and the patient treated with the regimen that demonstrates the best bactericidal activity. Bactericidal activity for anaerobic gram-negative bacilli can frequently be achieved with metronidazole; for HACEK organisms, ceftriaxone; for aerobic enteric gram-negative bacilli or *P. aeruginosa*, a cell wall–active agent–aminoglycoside combination or ciprofloxacin; for diphtheroids, a vancomycin-aminoglycoside combination; and for methicillin-resistant coagulase-negative staphylococci causing prosthetic valve endocarditis, a vancomycin-aminoglycoside-rifampin combination.

SURGICAL THERAPY

Surgical replacement of an infected native valve with a prosthetic valve (see Chapter 63) is indicated in the following situations: (1) Increasing or refractory CHF secondary to valvular dysfunction. In patients who are hemodynamically unstable, emergency cardiac valve replacement should not be delayed to allow further antibiotic therapy. Although operative mortality is higher and prosthetic valve endocarditis is more frequent in this situation than when a prosthetic valve is placed in the absence of active infection, the overall outcome is better if the prosthesis is replaced promptly despite active infection, the patient's clinical condition permitting. CHF in infective endocarditis portends a grave prognosis; delay in surgery associated with worsening of CHF increases operative mortality from 6 to 8% in patients with mild or no CHF to 17 to 33% in those with severe CHF. The incidence of reinfection of a newly placed cardiac valvular prosthesis is estimated to be 2 to 3%, far less than the mortality associated with uncontrolled CHF. (2) Multiple clinically significant emboli despite antibiotic therapy for 2 weeks. (3) Infection caused by certain pathogens such as fungi, which rarely respond to medical therapy, high-level ampicillin/aminoglycoside/vancomycin-resistant enterococci, β-lactamase–producing/high-level aminoglycoside–resistant *E. faecalis,* and β-lactam– or quinolone-resistant gram-negative bacilli. Surgical indications for valve ring abscess, which may heal with antimicrobials alone, include extension of infection, development of prosthetic valve dehiscence, heart block or CHF, and persistence of infection despite medical therapy. Patients with valve ring abscess should be monitored for conduction abnormalities, which may require placing a transvenous pacemaker because of the risk of high-grade heart block.

To avoid the complications of prosthetic valve placement (e.g., prosthetic valve endocarditis, bleeding, thromboembolic events, and valve deterioration), new surgical options that have been proposed as an alternative to a prosthetic valve include valve débridement, valvuloplasty, and repair or replacement of the paravalvular structure with a pulmonary root autograft. Prosthetic valve placement in an intravenous drug user is problematic because the prosthetic valve places the patient at continued risk of prosthetic valve endocarditis. Alternatively, for tricuspid valve endocarditis, tricuspid valve resection without prosthetic replacement can be tolerated hemodynamically for extended periods in many of these patients. The surgical indications for prosthetic valve endocarditis are the same as those outlined for native valve endocarditis and include relapse after a course of appropriate antibiotic therapy.

Intrathoracic, intra-abdominal, or peripheral mycotic aneurysms usually require surgical excision. Cerebral aneurysms may heal with medical therapy alone. If symptomatic, cerebral aneurysms should be monitored closely with serial angiography and may require surgery if enlarging or bleeding.

Myocardial revascularization should be performed at the time of elective valve surgery if significant coronary artery disease is present. However, patients who require emergency placement of a prosthetic valve for hemodynamic decompensation secondary to acute endocarditis usually cannot tolerate the dye load necessary for coronary angiography and the additional bypass surgery.

Anticoagulant therapy, although it may impede further enlargement of a vegetation, is relatively contraindicated in endocarditis because of conversion of an unsuspected cerebral infarct into an intracerebral bleed.

SHORTER INPATIENT THERAPY

Shorter courses of antibiotic therapy, oral regimens, and parenteral antibiotic therapy administered at home have been investigated in selected patients as a means of shortening the course of hospitalization. Having a focal infection that would require more than 2 weeks of antimicrobial therapy, prosthetic valve endocarditis, and significant renal or eighth nerve impairment precludes the use of short-course β-lactam–aminoglycoside combination therapy. Absorption of orally administered agents may be unreliable, and oral therapy is generally not recommended. Patients can be selected for parenteral therapy at home by their being at low risk for complications of endocarditis, the most frequent of which are CHF and emboli. In streptococcal endocarditis, heart failure, if not present on admission, rarely initially develops during therapy. Emboli most often occur before or within the first few days of antimicrobial therapy. Before considering outpatient therapy, most patients should initially be evaluated and stabilized in the hospital, although some patients may be managed entirely as outpatients. The standard regimens used to treat penicillin-sensitive streptococci require either continuous infusion of penicillin or frequent intravenous administration. A single daily dose of ceftriaxone is an attractive alternative to penicillin for antibiotic therapy at home. Because of its long half-life and good potency against these streptococci, serum levels of ceftriaxone remain well above the minimal inhibitory and bactericidal concentrations for over 24 hours.

RESPONSE TO THERAPY

Once receiving appropriate antimicrobial therapy, most patients note a sense of well-being, less fatigue, and improved appetite, and their temperature usually falls to normal levels within 2 to 5 days. The size of the vegetation on echocardiography should stabilize or gradually diminish. However, the erythrocyte sedimentation rate, anemia, and renal function may take weeks to months to improve. Circulating immune complexes and related serologic findings, including hypocomplementemia, mixed cryoglobulinemia, and rheumatoid factor, also tend to resolve with effective antibiotic therapy. Blood cultures for streptococci and enterococci should become sterile after 1 to 2 days of appropriate therapy and for *S. aureus,* after 3 to 5 days; however, with vancomycin therapy, blood cultures for *S. aureus* may take 10 to 14 days to become sterile. Blood cultures are obtained daily until sterile. If no organism is isolated from blood but the clinical response to an empirical antimicrobial regimen is good, empirical therapy should be continued in the patient thought to have endocarditis (see Table 326–5). If no organism is isolated and no clinical response is seen to empirical therapy after 1 to 2 weeks, endocarditis caused by a fastidious pathogen, e.g., fungi or anaerobes, or a diagnosis other than endocarditis should be considered. If the pathogen is initially isolated from blood and appropriate antimicrobial therapy started but fever persists or recurs, blood cultures should be repeated to assess persistent or relapsing infection, among other possibilities, which include most commonly pulmonary or systemic embolization (Table 326–9). For non-standard regimens or unusual pathogens, peak serum bactericidal activity may be assayed against the patient's pathogen early in the course of therapy, and if inadequate, the dose of the antibiotic is increased (although not at the cost of toxicity) and the serum retested. Measuring vancomycin or aminoglycoside serum levels may be helpful to ensure adequate but non-toxic antibiotic levels. Blood cultures are repeated 2 and 4 weeks after therapy has

Table 326–9 ■ REASONS FOR INADEQUATE CLINICAL RESPONSE

1. Inadequate therapy: wrong drug, wrong dose
2. Infarcts secondary to emboli
3. Metastatic abscesses of the spleen, kidney, brain, etc., that may require surgical drainage
4. Suppurative thrombophlebitis at site of an IV catheter, with or without superinfecting endocarditis
5. Other superinfections, e.g., *Clostridium difficile* colitis, urinary tract infection
6. Febrile reaction to the antimicrobial agent or another drug
7. Another unrelated febrile illness

Table 326–10 ■ CURE RATES (ANTIMICROBIAL THERAPY +/– SURGERY) (%)

Native Valve Endocarditis	
Non-IVDU	
Viridans streptococci*	>90
Vancomycin, ampicillin, aminoglycoside—	
susceptible enterococci*	75–90
Staphylococcus aureus *	60–75
Fungi	40–50†
IVDU	
S. aureus, left-sided	50
S. aureus, right-sided	95
Prosthetic Valve Endocarditis	
Early onset	12–44
Late onset	47–70

IVDU = intravenous drug user.
*Deaths usually from complications, not failure of antibiotic therapy.
†Antimicrobial therapy plus surgery.

been completed, relapse being most common within 1 month. The relapse organism should be evaluated for the development of antibiotic resistance.

OUTCOMES (Table 326–10)

Factors that affect mortality include the infecting organism (the mortality of endocarditis from fungi and aerobic enteric gram-negative bacilli > staphylococci > enterococci > streptococci), the site of infection (aortic > mitral and left-sided > tricuspid infection), native valve endocarditis versus prosthetic valve endocarditis (early-onset prosthetic valve endocarditis is greater than late-onset prosthetic valve endocarditis is greater than native valve endocarditis), age (higher in the elderly and very young), gender (men > women), and the presence of certain complications such as heart or renal failure, rupture of a mycotic aneurysm, cardiac arrhythmias and conduction abnormalities, and cerebral emboli. Heart failure remains the leading cause of death. However, with increasing use

of prosthetic valve replacement for heart failure, the leading cause of death may shift to neurologic complications caused by embolic episodes or mycotic aneurysms or uncontrolled infection by antibiotic-resistant microorganisms. Following cure of one episode of endocarditis, patients remain at increased risk for reinfection.

PREVENTION

The effect of endocarditis prophylaxis with antimicrobial agents has been estimated to be modest; i.e., fewer than 10% of all cases are preventable by prophylaxis. For example, only about half of cases have recognizable predisposing cardiac lesions, most cases do not follow an invasive procedure, and only about two thirds of cases are due to microorganisms (viridans streptococci and enterococci) against which prophylactic regimens are directed. However, in patients who are known to have a risky cardiac lesion (see Table 326–1) and are to undergo a procedure that is likely to induce bacteremia (see Table 326–3) with organisms having predictable susceptibility to antibiotics with minimal inconvenience, toxicity, and cost, the American Heart Association has made the recommendations shown in Table 326–11. Additional preventive measures are minimizing invasive procedures, avoiding intravascular catheters (a major predisposing event for prosthetic valve endocarditis), aggressively treating focal infections, and maintaining good dental hygiene in patients at increased risk for endocarditis.

Bayer AS, Bolger AF, Taubert KA, et al: Diagnosis and management of infective endocarditis and its complications. Circulation 98:2536, 1998.
Durack DT: Prevention of infective endocarditis. N Engl J Med 332:38, 1995. *Discusses prevention as a complex issue involving diverse aspects of medicine, microbiology, dentistry, surgery, epidemiology, and decision analysis.*
Durack DT. Lukes AS, Bright DK, et al: New criteria for diagnosis of infective endocarditis: Utilization of specific echocardiographic findings. Am J Med 96:200, 1994.
Fowler VO, Li J, Corey R, et al: Role of echocardiography in evaluation of patients with *Staphylococcus aureus* bacteremia: Experience in 103 patients. J Am Clin Oncol 30:1072, 1997.
Kaye D (ed): Infective Endocarditis, 2nd ed. New York, Raven Press, 1992. *This multiauthored text is a thorough, up-to-date review of every aspect of infective endocarditis, written by experts.*
Wilson WR. Steckelberg JM (eds): Infective endocarditis. Infect Dis Clin North Am 7: 1, 1993. *This issue highlights important new developments in pathogenesis, diagnosis, and treatment.*

Table 326–11 ■ PROPHYLACTIC REGIMENS FOR BACTERIAL ENDOCARDITIS

*Dental, Oral, Respiratory Tract, and Esophageal Procedures in Patients at High and Moderate Risk**	
Standard regimen	
Amoxicillin	2.0 g orally 1 hr before procedure
Amoxicillin/penicillin-allergic patients	
Clindamycin	600 mg orally 1 hr before procedure
or	
Cephalexin or cefadroxil†	2.0 g orally 1 hr before procedure
or	
Azithromycin or clarithromycin	500 mg orally 1 hr before procedure
Patients unable to take oral medications	
Ampicillin	IV or IM administration of ampicillin, 2 g within 30 min before procedure
Ampicillin/penicillin-allergic patients unable to take oral medication	
Clindamycin	IV administration of clindamycin, 600 mg within 30 min before procedure
or	
Cefazolin†	IV administration of cefazolin, 1.0 g within 30 min before procedure
Genitourinary/Gastrointestinal (Excluding Esophageal) Procedures in Patients at High Risk‡	
Standard regimen	
Ampicillin, amoxicillin, and gentamicin	IV or IM administration of ampicillin, 2 g plus gentamicin, 1.5 mg/kg (not to exceed 120 mg), within 30 min of starting procedure; 6 hr later, ampicillin, 1.0 g IV/IM, or amoxicillin, 1 g orally
Ampicillin/amoxicillin/penicillin-allergic patients	
Vancomycin and gentamicin	IV administration of vancomycin, 1.0 g over 1–2 hr, plus gentamicin 1.5 mg/kg IV/IM (not to exceed 120 mg); complete infusion or injection within 30 min of starting procedure
Genitourinary/Gastrointestinal (Excluding Esophageal) Procedures in Patients at Moderate Risk	
Standard regimen	
Ampicillin or amoxicillin,	IV or IM administration of ampicillin, 2 g within 30 min of starting procedure, or amoxicillin, 2 g orally 1 hr before procedure
Ampicillin/amoxicillin/penicillin-allergic patients	
Vancomycin	IV administration of vancomycin, 1.0 g over 1–2 hr; complete infusion within 30 min of starting procedure

*Doses in the table are for adults. Pediatric doses are as follows: ampicillin or amoxicillin, 50 mg/kg; cefazolin, 25 mg/kg; cefadroxil or cephalexin, 50 mg/kg; clarithromycin and azithromycin, 15 mg/kg; clindamycin, 20 mg/kg; gentamicin, 1.5 mg/kg; and vancomycin, 20 mg/kg. The total children's dose should not exceed the adult dose.
†Cephalosporins should not be used in individuals with an immediate-type hypersensitivity reaction (urticaria, angioedema, or anaphylaxis) to penicillins.
‡No 2nd dose of vancomycin or gentamicin is recommended.
Adapted from Dajani AS, Taubert KA, Wilson W, et al: Prevention of bacterial endocarditis. Recommendations of the American Heart Association. JAMA 277:1794, 1997.

327 STAPHYLOCOCCAL INFECTIONS

Gordon L. Archer

Staphylococcus aureus has been recognized as one of the most important and lethal human bacterial pathogens since the beginning of this century. Until the antibiotic era, more than 80% of patients growing *S. aureus* from their blood died; most of those dying had been healthy with no underlying disease. Although infections caused by coagulase-positive *S. aureus* were generally known to be potentially lethal, coagulase-negative staphylococci had been dismissed as avirulent skin commensals incapable of causing human disease. However, over the past 20 years, coagulase-negative staphylococcal infections have emerged as one of the major complications of medical progress. They are currently the pathogens most commonly isolated from infections of indwelling foreign devices and are the leading cause of hospital-acquired bacteremias in United States hospitals. This ascendancy of staphylococci as preeminent nosocomial pathogens also has been associated with a major increase in the proportion of these isolates that are resistant to multiple antimicrobial agents. If the trend continues, we may be forced to revisit the serious staphylococcal infections of the preantibiotic era that textbooks had long since relegated to medical history.

BACTERIOLOGY. The name "staphylococcus" means "bunch of grapes" and describes the clusters and clumps of gram-positive cocci seen on Gram stain of both infected material and organisms recovered from culture bottles and agar plates. Staphylococci produce catalase, breaking down hydrogen peroxide to H_2O and O_2; streptococci do not. This is the definitive test for separating the two genera of gram-positive cocci. Staphylococci are non-motile and are facultative anaerobes. The latter characteristic predicts that these organisms should grow equally well in both aerobic and anaerobic media. The coagulase test identifies the exoenzyme produced by *S. aureus* that interacts with a prothrombin-like plasma factor, converting fibrinogen to fibrin and causing plasma to clot. This is the test that traditionally separates the pathogenic species, *S. aureus*, from the numerous non-pathogenic staphylococci, collectively referred to as "coagulase-negative staphylococci." However, in current practice, many clinical microbiology laboratories use rapid tests for identifying *S. aureus* that rely on the clumping of latex beads coated with plasma factors that interact with *S. aureus* cell-surface components rather than coagulase.

S. aureus comprises a homogeneous species, as determined by biochemical testing and nucleic acid analysis, whereas coagulase-negative staphylococci are sufficiently varied to be assigned to numerous species. Coagulase-negative staphylococci are found as normal skin flora on all mammals, and currently, 31 different and distinct species are recognized. Of these, 15 species are found colonizing the cornified squamous epithelium and mucous membranes of humans. Each species has a unique niche on the body, but *S. epidermidis* is the predominant species in terms of numbers and different colonization sites. Because many laboratories report specific species of coagulase-negative staphylococci to clinicians, a list of the most prevalent human pathogenic species is shown in Table 327–1. Because only 60 to 70% of coagulase-negative species identified from specimens processed by the clinical laboratory are *S. epidermidis*, it is clearly improper to refer to coagulase-negative staphylococci as "*S. epidermidis*." However, because no specific pathogenic potential has been recognized for one coagulase-negative staphylococcus versus another, routine species identification of these organisms is useful only for purposes of epidemiology.

EPIDEMIOLOGY. *S. aureus* is carried asymptomatically on the mucous membranes in the anterior nares, nasopharynx, vagina, and/or perianal area in 20 to 40% of normal, healthy adults without underlying diseases. Carriage can be transient, lasting hours to days; intermittent, lasting weeks to months; and recurring or chronic, persisting for months to years despite attempts at eradication. Intact cornified squamous epithelium will not support intermittent or chronic carriage of *S. aureus* for reasons that are not clear but may involve bacteriostatic skin lipids, absence of *S. aureus*–specific receptors, or interference by colonizing coagulase-negative staphylococci. However, transient hand carriage clearly occurs and is an important means of exchange between patients and hospital personnel. Certain conditions have been described, however, that markedly increase skin carriage as well as nasal carriage of *S. aureus*. These include a variety of acute and chronic skin conditions, most prominently burn injuries, atopic dermatitis, eczema, psoriasis, and decubitus ulcers. In addition, needle use by insulin-dependent diabetics and intravenous drug abusers has been associated with increased *S. aureus* carriage; health care workers have been found to have a higher prevalence of nasal colonization than those individuals not involved with patients or hospitals; and patients on chronic hemodialysis, as well as patients with the acquired immunodeficiency syndrome (AIDS), have a higher-than-expected colonization rate.

S. aureus is extremely hardy and can survive drying, extremes of environmental temperature, wide ranges of pH, and high salt. It can therefore survive in the hospital on inanimate objects such as pillows, sheets, and blood pressure cuffs (called fomites) for some time. However, the major reservoir of *S. aureus*, in both hospitals and nature, is humans (see Chapter 315).

In certain cases, *S. aureus* infections result when patients who are carriers infect themselves. This has been shown to be true for most hemodialysis shunt and peritoneal dialysis catheter infections, for infective endocarditis in intravenous drug abusers, for both individuals and families who suffer from recurrent staphyloccal furunculosis, and for sternal wound infections after cardiovascular surgery. Eradicating nasal carriage in patients by using topical mupirocin ointment has been shown to reduce the incidence of shunt infections in hemodialysis patients and recurrent furunculosis.

Coagulase-negative staphylococci colonizing the skin and mucous membranes of hospitalized patients and some hospital personnel have been shown to be more resistant to antimicrobial agents than staphylococci found on the skin of outpatients or hospital personnel not working on inpatient units. The alteration in skin flora is associated with antimicrobial use that selects more resistant organisms on patient skin. This comprises a huge hospital reservoir for multiple-antibiotic–resistant coagulase-negative staphylococci that can be transferred among patients, can be acquired by hospital personnel, and may eventually be inoculated into wounds in association with implanted, indwelling foreign devices.

IMMUNITY AND PATHOGENESIS OF INFECTIONS. *S. aureus* causes disease syndromes by two different mechanisms. The organism can become locally or systemically invasive by producing molecules that thwart host defense mechanisms, or it can elaborate toxins that cause disease without the need for the organism itself to invade tissue (toxinoses).

LOCAL INFECTION. The hallmark of the localized staphylococcal infection is an abscess—a walled-off lesion consisting of central necrosis and liquefaction and containing cellular debris and multiplying bacteria surrounded by a layer of fibrin and intact phagocytic cells. The abscess may be superficial, in skin (furuncle), or deep, in organs (renal carbuncle), as a result of bacteremic dissemination. The factors that result in initial *S. aureus* infections are not clear; normal individuals seem to be fairly resistant to local infection. Intact cornified squamous epithelium is normally a barrier both to colonization and infection by *S. aureus*, and even injecting virulent organisms into the skin will cause infection only if a foreign body (e.g., suture) is also present. Furthermore, most adult serum contains both heat-labile and heat-stable opsonins (complement and specific antibody) that are highly efficient at mediating

Table 327–1 ■ STAPHYLOCOCCAL SPECIES FOUND ON HUMAN SKIN AND MUCOUS MEMBRANES

COAGULASE-POSITIVE	COAGULASE-NEGATIVE	
S. aureus	*S. epidermidis*	*S. cohnii*
	S. saprophyticus	*S. xylosus*
	S. haemolyticus	*S. auricularis*
	S. warneri	*S. simulans*
	S. capitis	*S. schleiferi*
	S. hominis	*S. lugdanensis*
	S. saccharolyticus	*S. caprae*
		S. pasteuri

the phagocytosis and killing of *S. aureus* by neutrophils. Because humoral immunity and opsonophagocytosis are the body's major defense against pyogenic microorganisms such as *S. aureus,* most individuals are well equipped to resist infection. The role of neutrophils and opsonophagocytosis as the primary antistaphylococcal host defense is illustrated by patients with neutrophil defects (see Chapters 171 and 314) who have an increase in *S. aureus* infection. These include defects in intracellular killing (chronic granulomatous disease and Chédiak-Higashi syndrome) and impaired neutrophil chemotaxis and humoral immunity (Job's syndrome). Once the balance is tipped in favor of the organism, *S. aureus* possesses a number of factors that may produce an abscess and promote the organism's survival inside the lesion. Although no single factor has been shown to be the major abscess-forming virulence factor and mutants deficient in each of the factors have been recovered from full-blown infections, there is a general feeling that, because most of these factors differentiate the pathogenic (*S. aureus*) from non-pathogenic (coagulase-negative staphylococci) members of the genus, they probably play some coordinate role in initiating and maintaining infection. Table 327–2 outlines *S. aureus* factors that may contribute to the establishment of local infections.

DISSEMINATED INFECTION. A small percentage of local infections progress to dissemination, where *S. aureus* gains access to the blood. Dissemination is characterized by *bacteremia* and *metastatic infection.* The factors leading to dissemination and the type and appearance of local infections that are more likely to disseminate are not known.

S. aureus produces such enzymes as *staphylokinase* (a fibrinolysin), *hyaluronidase,* and various *proteases* that may enable it to escape the abscess, invade tissue, and eventually enter the blood. Once in the blood, the most lethal immediate consequence is *sepsis* or *septic shock* (see Chapter 96). This syndrome is mediated chiefly by *enterotoxins* and *toxic shock syndrome toxin* (TSST-1), all of which contain similar motifs (superantigens) that enable them to bind to T cells and macrophages, stimulating the production of such sepsis-associated cytokines as interleukin-1, tumor necrosis factor, and interleukin-6. Approximately 60% of *S. aureus* isolates contain a gene for one of the seven serotypes of enterotoxin or TSST-1.

One of the target cells for bacteremic *S. aureus* is the endothelial cell. Organisms adhere to and are internalized by endothelial cells, where, by releasing cytolysins, the bacteria can disrupt the endothelial cell layer and invade underlying tissue. *S. aureus* also can exist inside intact endothelial cells. The ability for the organisms to survive inside phagocytes and endothelial cells may explain their propensity to cause recurrent and refractory bacteremia despite seemingly appropriate therapy.

TOXINOSES. *S. aureus* produces three toxins, or classes of toxin, that produce specific syndromes without the need for the organism itself to invade and disseminate. *Staphylococcal food poisoning* occurs when a preformed, heat-stable *enterotoxin* is ingested and interacts with parasympathetic ganglia in the stomach, producing vomiting. Seven closely related toxin serotypes (A to E, G and H) can all produce the characteristic symptoms. *Staphylococcal*

Table 327–2 ■ *S. AUREUS* FACTORS THAT MAY PROMOTE LOCAL INFECTIONS BY THWARTING HOST DEFENSE

FACTOR	PROPOSED MECHANISMS FOR INTERFERING WITH HOST DEFENSE
Coagulase	Prevents neutrophil access to infection site
Microcapsule	Inhibits phagocytosis
Protein A	Inhibits IgG-mediated opsonization (binds Fc fragment)
Clumping factor (fibrinogen receptor)	Inhibits opsonization (fibrin coating)
Catalase	Interferes with intracellular killing
Proteases, nuclease, lipase, and cytolysins (α, β, and δ)	Liquefaction necrosis and phagocyte dysfunction
Leucocidin and gamma toxin	Neutrophil cytolysis
Fatty acid metabolizing enzyme	Inactivates bactericidal lipids

Table 327–3 ■ INFECTIONS CAUSED BY *S. AUREUS*

Common or Usual Etiologic Pathogen	Less Common Etiologic Pathogen	Uncommon or Rare Etiologic Pathogen
Furuncle or skin abscess	Cellulitis	Community-acquired pneumonia
Bullous impetigo	Hospital-acquired pneumonia	Ascending urinary tract infection
Surgical wound infection	Brain abscess	Meningitis
Hospital-acquired bacteremia	Empyema	Enterocolitis
Acute or right-sided bacterial endocarditis		
Hematogenous osteomyelitis		
Septic arthritis		
Pyomyositis		
Renal carbuncle		
Scalded skin syndrome		
Toxic shock syndrome		
Food-borne gastroenteritis (short incubation)		
Botryomycosis		
Paraspinous or epidural abscess		

scalded skin syndrome results from the production of *exfoliative toxin* by *S. aureus* isolates that colonize or infect the skin of newborns. The characteristic exfoliation of the superficial stratum granulosum layer of the epidermis is due to the action of the toxin on desmosomes that hold the cells of this skin layer together. There are two exfoliating serotypes, A and B. The variety of *toxic shock syndrome* associated with tampon use in young women is due to TSST-1 entering into the blood through the vagina and is produced by *S. aureus* that colonize the mucosa.

DIAGNOSIS. The diagnosis of staphylococcal infections requires that the organism be seen on Gram stain of an infected specimen and be grown on artificial media, preferably in pure culture. Because coagulase-negative staphylococci are the most common contaminants of any culture obtained by crossing skin, it is important that multiple cultures grow the same organism. This is a major reason for drawing blood cultures in pairs from two different sites. Although various tests for serum antibody to *S. aureus* antigens (e.g., teichoic acid antibody) have been evaluated for their ability to differentiate serious, deep-seated infection from trivial infections or self-limited bacteremia, none has proved to have a sensitivity or specificity sufficient to warrant its use as a basis for making clinical decisions.

CLINICAL MANIFESTATIONS: *S. AUREUS* INFECTIONS. SKIN AND SOFT TISSUE INFECTIONS. The most common *S. aureus* infections are *folliculitis* and the *furuncle,* or boil (Table 327–3). These infections involve a single hair follicle or a localized area of the epidermis and dermis. While most *S. aureus* furuncles are without systemic symptoms, those on the face should be treated aggressively because of their potential to migrate directly to the brain by means of the venous circulation. Furuncles can coalesce and spread through deeper skin layers or extend down to and along a fascial plane, causing a much more extensive and serious infection called a carbuncle. Carbuncles are most common over the upper back and back of the neck, where they can form multiple draining sinuses; bacteremia occurs in approximately one fourth of patients. A boil or furuncle also may be called a skin abscess if it becomes large but remains circumscribed, confined to one area, and fluctuant. A non-localized *S. aureus* skin infection is called cellulitis and may resemble the skin infections caused by *Streptococcus pyogenes,* the most common cause of cellulitis (see Chapter 324). *S. aureus* cellulitis also can lead to bacteremia, proving the staphylococcal etiology of some of these infections. *S. aureus* cellulitis is particularly common in individuals with pre-existing chronic skin disease such as stasis dermatitis and diabetic, trophic, or decubitus ulcers. Adults also can develop a form of impetigo called bullous impetigo. The lesions are characterized by erythema with a crusty surface and small or large bullous lesions. The bullae are thought to be the result of the elaboration of exfoliative toxin and are the localized, adult equivalent of the scalded skin syndrome (Ritter's disease) seen in infants.

The most common nosocomial *S. aureus* skin and soft tissue infection is the *wound infection,* in which surgical or catheter exit-site wounds are contaminated with *S. aureus* and become erythematous, draining purulent or serosanguineous fluid. *S. aureus* is the most common and most serious cause of hospital-acquired wound infections, leading to local, deep-wound infections and systemic, metastatic infections due to bacteremia.

Recurrent furunculosis can occur in members of families, usually due to persistent nasal or perineal carriage in family members with autoinoculation of skin due to scratching. The infections are commonly superficial and without systemic symptoms but are painful and annoying. Interruption is not possible until the carrier state is eradicated in all family members. Although most individuals with recurrent furunculosis have normal immune systems, a syndrome called Job's syndrome (see Chapter 171) is recognized in individuals with recurrent *S. aureus* furunculosis. In addition to recurrent furunculosis, patients have high levels of serum IgE, neutrophil chemotactic defects, and a generalized disorder of immunoregulation. Adults with this syndrome usually not only describe a long history of recurrent skin infections since childhood but often also have had recurrent sinopulmonary infections as well.

PLEUROPULMONARY INFECTIONS. *S. aureus* is an uncommon cause of pneumonia in otherwise healthy, unhospitalized adults, accounting for less than 10% of community-acquired pneumonia. However, following influenza A infections, the incidence of *S. aureus* pneumonia markedly increases. Chest radiographs of patients with community-acquired *S. aureus* pneumonia may show abscesses and thin-walled cysts, resembling the pneumatoceles seen in infants.

In contrast to community-acquired pneumonia, *S. aureus* is a prominent cause of nosocomial pneumonia, particularly in intubated patients on mechanical ventilation. Cultures obtained from intubated patients by techniques designed to minimize contamination of specimens by organisms colonizing the upper airway have found *S. aureus* in up to a third of patients. Pneumonia in ventilator-dependent patients is a particularly lethal event, with one fourth to one half of the patients dying as a direct result of their pulmonary infection. There seems to be nothing that distinguishes the radiographic appearance of nosocomial *S. aureus* pneumonia from that of pneumonia due to other nosocomial pathogens. *S. aureus* bacteremia due solely to nosocomial pneumonia also is uncommon.

Septic pulmonary emboli in patients with right-sided *S. aureus* endocarditis (see later) also can present as a primary pneumonia. However, these patients will all have *S. aureus* bacteremia and usually have discrete lesions in multiple lobes, often accompanied by hemoptysis and chest pain.

S. aureus is cultured from the pleural space in up to 15% of adults with empyema, but it is found in pure culture in fewer than 10%. The incidence of *S. aureus* as a cause of empyema seems to have decreased overall in the past 20 years but is still a prominent etiologic pathogen in patients with nosocomial empyema.

ENDOCARDITIS (See also Chapter 326). There are two different and distinct populations who develop endocarditis caused by *S. aureus;* these are compared in Table 327–4. One group consists of

older patients with underlying diseases who develop primarily left-sided endocarditis and have a high mortality rate (20 to 30%). Approximately half will develop heart failure, half will have central nervous system (CNS) manifestations, and 40 to 50% will have had either a skin infection or an intravenous catheter as the presumed portal of entry. Although it is important to realize that patients with left-sided *S. aureus* endocarditis can present acutely, with symptoms compatible with the sepsis syndrome, and that *S. aureus* can infect previously normal valves, the majority of patients will have had more subacute symptoms of fever, malaise, and fatigue for 1 to 2 weeks, and three fourths will have evidence by history or echocardiography of previously damaged or abnormal valves. An increasing proportion of patients in this category infect cardiac valves as a result of a hospital-acquired bacteremia (see later). Patients with nosocomial *S. aureus* endocarditis may be infected with methicillin-resistant staphylococci.

The second population developing *S. aureus* endocarditis consists of those who inject illicit drugs intravenously. These individuals are younger, are healthier, usually have no known valvular heart disease, and have infections of the tricuspid valve in 80 to 90% of cases. The patient is the source of the infecting organism. The major presenting symptoms in these patients are those of septic pulmonary emboli. The chest film typically shows multiple nodular infiltrates in various lobes that often cavitate and occasionally form pneumatoceles. Most of these patients have pure right-sided endocarditis and only rarely will have any peripheral left-sided manifestations. However, a murmur of tricuspid insufficiency is heard in less than half the cases. The mortality rate is extremely low for these patients, usually only 2 to 5%, but recurrence is relatively common, given the individuals' proclivity for continued drug abuse.

BACTEREMIA. *S. aureus* is second only to coagulase-negative staphylococci as a cause of hospital-acquired bacteremia. The usual source of nosocomial bacteremia is intravenous catheters. The consequences of nosocomial bacteremia are usually only fever and malaise, but they can include endocarditis, osteomyelitis, metastatic abscesses in various organs, and death from overwhelming sepsis. Treatment, therefore, is prolonged in order to eradicate the organism from tissues and organs. Bacteremia caused by *S. aureus* is usually high grade, with the organism grown from all blood cultures drawn over a period of time even if there is no endocarditis or infected foreign body present. Furthermore, bacteremia may persist for several days even with appropriate therapy and removal of an infected catheter. This is believed to be due to the organism's ability to survive host phagocytic defense and to be sequestered inside cells.

In contrast to nosocomial *S. aureus* bacteremia, the source of community-acquired bacteremia is often obscure. It may originate from a skin infection, an intravenous injection of illicit drugs, or an infected focus in the heart or at a peripheral site. In all patients with community-acquired *S. aureus* bacteremia, a diligent search should be made for an infected source. If none is found, patients should be treated as if they have endocarditis.

OSTEOMYELITIS (See also Chapter 331). *S. aureus* is the most common cause of acute hematogenous osteomyelitis. Whereas most cases occur in children, adults are also at risk, particularly those who have had documented *S. aureus* bacteremia. Children develop osteomyelitis almost exclusively in long bones, whereas in adults from a third to a half of the cases of hematogenous osteomyelitis are in the lumbar or thoracic vertebrae. Vertebral osteomyelitis results when *S. aureus* initially seeds the intervertebral disk space and then spreads from the disk space to involve contiguous vertebrae. A paraspinous or epidural abscess frequently occurs as an extension of the initial intervertebral focus. Patients present with fever and back pain and may have neurologic symptoms from cord compression. Radiographs typically show narrowing of one or more intervertebral disk spaces with collapse of adjacent vertebrae. A magnetic resonance imaging scan is particularly helpful in defining the extent of vertebral osteomyelitis. Long bones may be involved after hematogenous dissemination of *S. aureus,* but osteomyelitis in these locations is more typically the result of contiguous spread from an infected decubitus, trophic ulcer, or traumatic wound. One of the most common causes of *S. aureus* osteomyelitis of the foot bones is infection of ulcers in diabetics with vascular disease.

Table 327–4 ■ *S. AUREUS* ENDOCARDITIS IN DIFFERENT PATIENT POPULATIONS

PATIENT AND DISEASE CHARACTERISTICS	INTRAVENOUS DRUG ABUSERS	NON–INTRAVENOUS DRUG ABUSERS
Mean age (yr)	30	50
Underlying disease	No	Yes
Portal of *S. aureus* entry	Skin (IV injection)	Skin (infection or IV catheter)
Valves involved	Tricuspid	Mitral, aortic
Pre-existing valve abnormality	No	Yes or no
Presentation	Chest pain, fever hemoptysis	Fever, fatigue, malaise; sepsis (less common)
Peripheral manifestations	Septic pulmonary emboli	Skin manifestations; central nervous system abnormalities; metastatic infection in bone, kidney, and spleen
Heart failure	Rare	Common
Mortality	<5%	20–30%
Treatment duration	2–3 weeks	4–6 weeks

Occasionally, hardware used to repair long bone fractures will become infected with *S. aureus*. These infections are particularly refractory to therapy without removal of the foreign body.

SEPTIC ARTHRITIS (See also Chapter 288). *S. aureus* is a common cause of acute septic arthritis, although spontaneous *S. aureus* septic arthritis in otherwise normal joints is usually seen in children rather than adults. In adults, *S. aureus* septic arthritis typically occurs in joints that previously have been damaged by a chronic inflammatory arthritis or osteoarthritis; that have been violated by needle aspiration, injection, or surgery; or that contain a prosthetic device. Occasionally, an otherwise normal joint will be seeded by the hematogenous route or the joint space will be invaded from a contiguous focus of osteomyelitis. These infections need to be differentiated from such other causes of acute monarticular arthritis in adults as gout and gonococcal infection. In all cases of septic arthritis, arthrocentesis should be performed before beginning therapy so that a specific cultural diagnosis can be made. *S. aureus* pyarthrosis can be present with relatively little systemic toxicity in patients with chronic inflammatory arthritis taking large doses of anti-inflammatory medication; this may be particularly difficult to diagnose. One unique form of *S. aureus* septic arthritis is infection of the sternoclavicular joint usually seen in intravenous drug users or in patients who have had subclavian intravenous catheters.

GENITOURINARY TRACT INFECTIONS. The only important *S. aureus* infections of the genitourinary tract are those that result from hematogenous dissemination. These include microabscesses, renal carbuncles, and perinephric abscesses. The presence of *S. aureus* in the urine, therefore, is either the result of contamination in individuals asymptomatically colonized in the vagina and/or perianal area or an indication that the kidney has been infected during an episode of *S. aureus* bacteremia. The absence of cells in the urine should suggest contamination. However, if *S. aureus* is repeatedly cultured from urine or present in the urine together with pyuria or hematuria, the patient should be evaluated for bacteremia, for a deep focus that might have caused disseminated infection, and for an intrarenal or perinephric abscess. The presence of *S. aureus* in the urine should *never* be assumed to be secondary to an ascending urinary tract infection.

CENTRAL NERVOUS SYSTEM INFECTIONS. Although brain abscess and meningitis can be caused by *S. aureus,* they are relatively rare. Fewer than 10% of cases of meningitis and 20 to 30% of cases of brain abscess are caused by *S. aureus.* They are usually due to metastatic seeding as a result of bacteremia from an identified focus, to direct inoculation after trauma or a neurosurgical procedure, or to infection of an indwelling foreign body, such as a ventricular shunt. The prognosis of patients infected as a result of metastatic seeding is particularly poor, with a mortality rate of 30 to 50%. The one infection associated with the CNS that is uniquely caused by *S. aureus* is a paraspinous or epidural abscess, usually secondary to vertebral osteomyelitis.

PYOMYOSITIS. Infection of the large skeletal muscles is due to *S. aureus* in more than 80% of cases. It is prevalent in tropical countries, giving it the name "tropical pyomyositis," but it is being increasingly described in temperate climates. Patients in tropical countries usually are adults who have no underlying disease and present with fever, pain, and swelling in the involved muscle, but there is often little evidence of local inflammation. Diagnosis is made by needle aspiration of pus. Because eosinophilia is common in patients in tropical countries who have pyomyositis, parasites are believed to have a role in the pathogenesis of this disease. Pyomyositis in temperate climates presents in much the same manner but more often is seen in children or in adults with underlying diseases, particularly those who have AIDS. It is associated with muscle trauma in more than half of patients and more frequently involves more than one non-contiguous muscle group.

TOXINOSES. *Staphylococcal scalded skin syndrome,* also known as Ritter's or Lyell's syndrome, is usually a disease of neonates and is due to the action of the exfoliative toxins A and B. This syndrome results from *S. aureus* colonization or local infection, usually of the umbilical stump, and causes generalized desquamation of the superficial granulosum cell layer of the epidermis. The adult equivalent is bullous impetigo, associated with localized skin involvement, but adult cases of more generalized desquamation have been described. However, it is important to differentiate

Table 327–5 ■ DIFFERENTIATION OF DESQUAMATING SYNDROMES

	STAPHYLOCOCCAL SCALDED SKIN SYNDROME	TOXIC EPIDERMAL NECROLYSIS
Etiology	*S. aureus* exfoliative toxin	Drug hypersensitivity
Pathology	Intraepidermal cleavage plane; no inflammatory cells	Involvement of entire epidermis; infiltration with inflammatory cells
Clinical appearance	Involvement of epidermis only; positive Nikolsky's sign	Involvement of skin, mucous membranes, and multiple organs; negative Nikolsky's sign
Outcome	Low mortality; heals without scarring	High mortality; often heals with scarring

staphylococcal scalded skin syndrome from toxic epidermal necrolysis. Table 327–5 contrasts the two syndromes.

The *toxic shock syndrome* was initially described in young, menstruating women and was associated with tampon use in women vaginally colonized with *S. aureus* that produced TSST-I. However, the number of tampon-associated cases has decreased markedly in recent years. The majority of cases are now secondary to *S. aureus* infections of skin or other sites, and the etiologic toxin is often one of the enterotoxins rather than TSST-I. The criteria for the diagnosis of staphylococcal toxic shock syndrome are shown in Table 327–6. Staphylococcal toxic shock syndrome has a relatively low mortality and is a true toxinosis; bacteremia is rare.

Gastroenteritis or *staphylococcal food poisoning* is due to ingesting preformed staphylococcal enterotoxin. Enterotoxin-producing *S. aureus* are inoculated into food by a colonized or infected food handler. If the food sits at room temperature before being cooked, the organism will multiply and produce toxin. Subsequent cooking will not inactivate the heat-stable toxin, and ingestion will produce symptoms predominantly of vomiting after a short (2 to 8 hours) incubation period.

MISCELLANEOUS INFECTIONS. The older literature describes "botryomycosis," a chronic *S. aureus* infection of skin, lung, or bone that produces granules resembling those seen in actinomycosis, and "enterocolitis," a necrotizing infection of bowel in surgical patients associated with sheets of organisms seen on Gram stain of stool. These infections are rarely seen today.

CLINICAL MANIFESTATIONS: COAGULASE-NEGATIVE STAPHYLOCOCCAL INFECTIONS. The major infections caused by coagulase-negative staphylococci are hospital-acquired and involve indwelling foreign devices. Table 327–7 outlines the characteristics of these infections. In general, coagulase-negative staphylococci are of low virulence, rarely causing metastatic infections, even though they are the most common cause of hospital-acquired bacteremia. Bacteremia is usually the result of intravascular catheter infection. However, coagulase-negative staphylococci can be lethal when they infect prosthetic cardiac valves. They are the most common cause of prosthetic valve endocarditis, presenting in the first year after surgery, presumably inoculated into the area of the sewing ring during valve implantation. Valve dysfunction results from dehiscence or obstruction of the valve orifice, and most patients require surgery for cure. The exception to infections described in Table 327–7 are those caused by *S. saprophyticus.* This organism is second only to *Escherichia coli* as a cause of ascending urinary tract infections in young, sexually active female outpatients, implicated in 15 to 20% of cases in this population. In addition, low

Table 327–6 ■ DIAGNOSTIC CRITERIA FOR STAPHYLOCOCCAL TOXIC SHOCK SYNDROME

1. Fever (usually ≥38.9° C, or 102° F)
2. Rash (diffuse macular erythroderma, sunburn or scarlet fever–like)
3. Desquamation, 1 to 2 weeks after onset of illness, particularly of palms and soles
4. Hypotension (systolic BP <90 mm Hg or orthostatic syncope)
5. Involvement of three or more of the following organ systems: gastrointestinal (nausea and vomiting), muscular (myalgias), mucous membrane (hyperemia), renal, hepatic, hematologic (↓ platelets), central nervous system, or pulmonary (adult respiratory distress syndrome)
6. *S. aureus* infection or mucosal colonization

1. Hospital-acquired
2. Caused by species *S. epidermidis* (70–80%)
3. Resistant to multiple antimicrobial agents (>80% methicillin resistant)
4. Involve indwelling foreign devices (catheters, prosthetic heart valves and joints, vascular grafts)
5. Exhibit a long latent period between device contamination and clinical presentation

Table 327–8 ■ ANTIMICROBIAL AGENTS EFFECTIVE FOR TREATING *S. AUREUS* INFECTIONS

AGENTS	RESISTANCE*	
	Hospital-Acquired	Community-Acquired
Penicillin G	>90	>90
Antistaphylococcal penicillins and cephalosporins	30	S
Erythromycin	40	10
Clindamycin	40	10
Sulfamethoxazole/trimethoprim	20	S
Tetracycline	20	10
Minocycline	S	S
Rifampin	S	S
Gentamicin	30	S
Quinolones	30	S
Vancomycin	S	S

*Numbers are percentage of isolates from patients with hospital-acquired or community-acquired infections resistant to each agent; S = >95% susceptible.

colony counts of this staphylococcal species have been recovered from urine obtained by suprapubic aspiration in some women with the anterior urethral syndrome or symptomatic abacteriuria.

THERAPY. Antimicrobial agents effective for treating *S. aureus* infections are listed in Table 327–8. Treatment of hospital-acquired infections is limited by resistance to many of these agents. Methicillin-resistant isolates are *cross-resistant* to *all β-lactams* (penicillins, cephalosporins, and imipenem) and are usually also resistant to at least three additional classes of antimicrobial agents (multiresistant). However, although only 20 to 30% of nosocomial *S. aureus* isolates are methicillin-resistant, more than 70% of nosocomial coagulase-negative staphylococci are methicillin-resistant and multiresistant. Thus, whereas the treatment of hospital-acquired *S. aureus* infections should be guided by susceptibility testing, infections caused by nosocomial coagulase-negative staphylococci are usually treated with vancomycin. Vancomycin is the only antimicrobial agent to which some isolates of *S. aureus* and coagulase-negative staphylococci are susceptible; and it is, therefore, the mainstay of therapy for infections caused by methicillin-resistant organisms. However, there have been recent reports of a few patients in the United States and Japan who have been infected with *S. aureus* and coagulase-negative staphylococci that have markedly reduced susceptibilities to vancomycin, requiring concentrations of the drug up to eight times that of susceptible isolates for inhibition of bacterial growth to occur. If the appearance of these isolates signals an unfortunate trend toward reduced vancomycin susceptibility among staphylococci, this will have a major impact on chemotherapy.

Treating staphylococcal infections usually consists of administering antimicrobial agents, surgical or catheter drainage of abscesses, and removal of foreign bodies. The duration of therapy is usually 1 to 2 weeks for localized, drained infections not associated with bacteremia or a foreign body. In general, infections can rarely be cured if the foreign material is left in place. Infections requiring more specialized therapeutic decisions are detailed below.

BACTEREMIA AND ENDOCARDITIS. For *S. aureus,* all patients with community-acquired bacteremia who have evidence of a metastatic infection or who have no obvious source for bacteremia should be treated as if they have endocarditis. For intravenous drug abusers with right-sided endocarditis: 2 to 3 weeks of an antistaphylococcal penicillin (nafcillin or oxacillin) or vancomycin, plus gentamicin for the entire treatment period; for left-sided endocarditis: 4 to 6 weeks of an antistaphylococcal penicillin or vancomycin, with gentamicin for the first week. However, in patients with hospital-acquired *S. aureus* bacteremia from a removable focus (usu-

ally an intravascular catheter), the decision becomes more difficult. Those patients whose fever and bacteremia resolve within 3 days after removing the infected focus, those who have no complications or evidence of metastatic infection, and those who have no abnormality of cardiac valves can receive 2 weeks of therapy. All other patients with nosocomial bacteremia who do not meet all the exclusions should be treated as if they have endocarditis (see Chapter 326).

OSTEOMYELITIS. Patients with *S. aureus* osteomyelitis require a minimum of 6 weeks of therapy, with the initial 2 to 4 weeks being parenteral. Therapy for osteomyelitis of long bones often will be unsuccessful if sequestra are left in place.

PREVENTION. Preventing hospital-acquired infections is accomplished by paying attention to tenets of infection control. These include hand washing and regloving between patients and strict adherence to aseptic technique when creating or caring for any kind of wound. Patients undergoing procedures that may result in wound or implanted device infections also should receive prophylactic antibiotics before and during the procedure. Patients with recurrent *S. aureus* infections of skin, catheters, or dialysis shunts should have their nares cultured, and if they are *S. aureus* carriers, they should be treated with topical mupirocin ointment. Chronic carriers resistant to topical *S. aureus* eradication may be given oral rifampin plus sulfamethoxazole/trimethoprim, a fluoroquinolone, or minocycline.

Chambers HF: Methicillin resistance in staphylococci. Molecular and biochemical basis and clinical implications. Clin Microbiol Rev 10:781, 1997. *A good recent review on antistaphylococcal chemotherapy and resistance of staphylococci to the action of therapeutic agents.*

Crossley KB, Archer GL (eds): The Staphylococci in Human Disease. New York, Churchill Livingstone, 1997. *The definitive source for a more detailed discussion of the biology, clinical presentation, and therapy for staphylococcal infections.*

Raad LI, Sabbagh MF: Optimal duration of therapy for catheter-related *Staphylococcus aureus* bacteremia: A study of 55 cases and review. Clin Infect Dis 14:75, 1992. *An excellent study and review of a difficult problem.*

Rupp ME, Archer GL: Coagulase-negative staphylococci: Pathogens of medical progress. Clin Infect Dis 19:231, 1994. *The most recent review of infections caused by coagulase-negative staphylococci.*

BACTERIAL MENINGITIS

328 BACTERIAL MENINGITIS

Morton N. Swartz

Meningitis is an inflammation of the arachnoid, the pia mater, and the intervening cerebrospinal fluid (CSF). The inflammatory process extends throughout the subarachnoid space about the brain and spinal cord and regularly involves the ventricles. Pyogenic meningitis, considered in this chapter, is usually an acute infection

with bacteria that evoke a polymorphonuclear response in the CSF. One of its major forms, that caused by meningococci, is considered in Chapter 329; less acute forms of bacterial meningitis, characterized by a mononuclear cell response in the CSF, are discussed in Chapters 358 and 472.

ETIOLOGY AND INCIDENCE. In the 1970s and 1980s about 20,000 cases of bacterial meningitis occurred annually in the United States. This changed dramatically in the 1990s when the number of cases of community-acquired bacterial meningitis was reduced by 55%. This reduction was the result primarily of the introduction of routine immunization of infants with the *Haemophilus influenzae* type b conjugate vaccines, which effected a 94%

decrease in the number of cases of *H. influenzae* meningitis. As a consequence of *H. influenzae* meningitis having been a disease of infancy and childhood, its virtual elimination raised the median age of persons with bacterial meningitis from 15 months in 1986 to 25 years in 1995. In the 1970s and 1980s, data from the Centers for Disease Control and Prevention indicated that, if all cases were included regardless of the age of patients, *H. influenzae* type b was the most frequent bacterial cause (45%), followed by *Streptococcus pneumoniae* (18%) and *Neisseria meningitidis* (14%); by 1995, *S. pneumoniae* (47%) had become the most common agent, followed by *N. meningitidis* (25%) and group B *Streptococcus* (12%).

The relative frequencies with which the different bacterial species cause community-acquired meningitis are dependent on age (Fig. 328–1). Currently, in the neonatal period group B *Streptococcus* is the leading pathogen (almost 70%) followed by *Escherichia coli*, most commonly possessing the K1 envelope antigen. Thereafter, up through 23 months of age the principal causes are *S. pneumoniae* (45%) and *N. meningitidis* (31%). In persons 2 to 18 years of age, *N. meningitidis* (59%) is the major cause; and in individuals older than 18 years of age *S. pneumoniae* (62%) is the most common cause. *Listeria monocytogenes* accounts for 8% of cases of bacterial meningitis overall but has peak frequencies (about 20%) in the neonatal period and in those 60 years of age and older.

Meningococcal meningitis is the only type that occurs in outbreaks; its relative frequency among the meningitides depends on whether statistics have been gathered in a hyperendemic area or during epidemic or interepidemic periods. In about 10% of patients with pyogenic meningitis, the bacterial cause cannot be defined. Simultaneous mixed meningitis is rare, occurring in the setting of neurosurgical procedures, penetrating head injury, erosion of the skull or vertebrae by adjacent neoplasm, or intraventricular rupture of a cerebral abscess; the isolation of anaerobes should strongly suggest the latter two of these.

Important changes also have occurred in the frequencies of several other types of bacterial meningitis over the past 30 years. Gram-negative bacillary meningitis has doubled in frequency in adults, reflecting more frequent and extensive neurosurgical procedures as well as other nosocomial factors. *L. monocytogenes* has increased 8- to 10-fold as a cause of bacterial meningitis as seen in large urban general hospitals, reflecting the enlarging immunosuppressed population at particular risk. *Listeria* infections appear to be foodborne (dairy products, uncooked vegetables) and involve

particularly organ transplant recipients, patients in hemodialysis units, other patients receiving corticosteroids and cytotoxic drugs, patients with liver disease, pregnant women, and neonates. Meningitis due to coagulase-negative staphylococci, essentially unheard of 30 years ago, now represents about 3% of cases in large urban hospitals. It occurs as a complication of neurosurgical procedures and may present a particular therapeutic problem due to methicillin resistance of many of the involved strains. Rarely, bacterial meningitis complicates invasive neurodiagnostic (e.g., myelographic) and therapeutic spinal puncture and rhizotomy. Whereas in the past those infections were usually due to *Pseudomonas aeruginosa*, other gram-negative bacilli, and *Staphylococcus aureus*, currently, viridans streptococci are the agents most often associated with meningitis complicating diagnostic myelography and percutaneous trigeminal rhizotomy.

In large urban tertiary-care general hospitals, the distribution of bacterial causes of adult meningitis differs from that in smaller community hospitals, where community-acquired disease predominates. For example, at the Massachusetts General Hospital about 40% of cases of bacterial meningitis in adults are of nosocomial origin. In this category, the leading causes are gram-negative bacilli (primarily *E. coli* and *Klebsiella*), accounting for about 40% of nosocomial episodes, and various streptococci, *Staphylococcus aureus*, and coagulase-negative staphylococci, each responsible for 10% of nosocomial cases.

CLINICAL SETTINGS. The clinical setting in which meningitis develops may provide a clue to the specific bacterial cause. Meningococcal disease, including meningitis, may occur sporadically and in cyclic outbreaks. In the past, military recruits were particularly susceptible, but now meningococcal vaccine (polysaccharides of groups A, C, Y, and W135) is employed for their protection. Large urban outbreaks can occur.

Certain predisposing factors are frequently associated with the development of *pneumococcal meningitis*. Acute otitis media (± mastoiditis) occurs in about 20% of adult patients. Pneumonia is present in about 15% of patients with pneumococcal meningitis, a much higher frequency than in meningitis caused by *H. influenzae* or *N. meningitidis*. Acute pneumococcal sinusitis is occasionally the initial focus from which infection spreads to the meninges. A significant head injury (recent or remote) has occurred in about 10% of episodes of pneumococcal meningitis. CSF rhinorrhea (usually caused by a defect or fracture in the cribriform plate) is present in about 5% of patients with pneumococcal meningitis. Meningitis occurring in young children with sickle cell anemia is

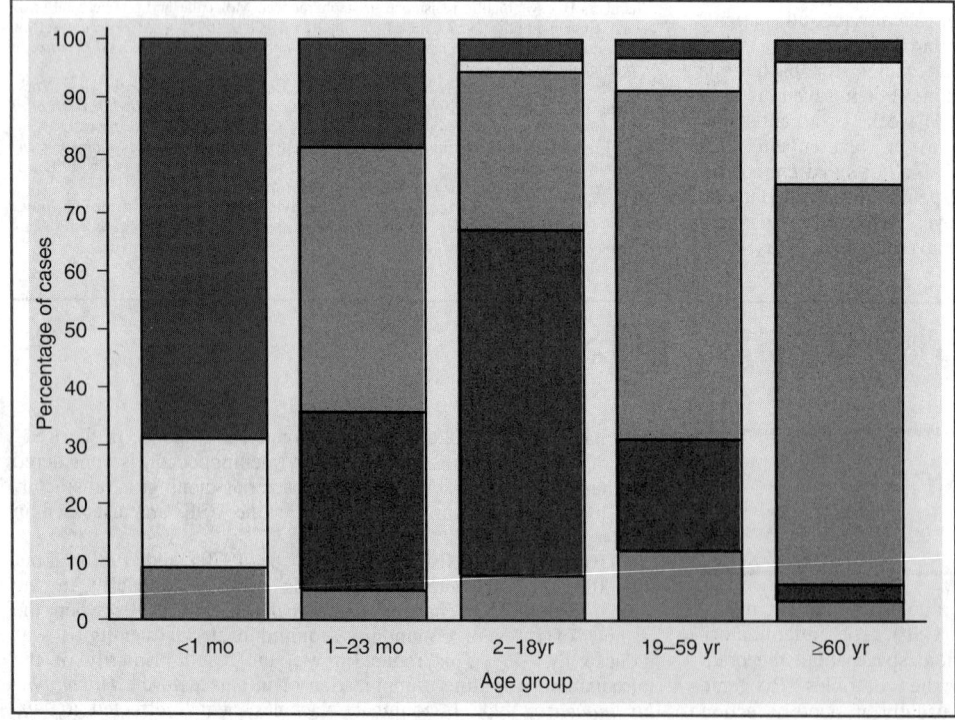

FIGURE 328–1 ■ Pathogenic agents of bacterial meningitis by age group: Dark gray–group B *Streptococcus;* light pink–*Listeria monocytogenes;* pink—*Streptococcus pneumoniae;* red—*Neisseria meningitidis;* light gray—*Haemophilus influenzae*. Meningitis due to *Escherichia coli* or other enteric pathogens among infants younger than 1 month of age is not included in the surveillance data. (From Schuchat A, Robinson K, Wenger JD, et al: Bacterial meningitis in the United States in 1995. N Engl J Med 337:970–976, 1997. Copyright 1997, Massachusetts Medical Society. All rights reserved.)

most likely to be caused by *S. pneumoniae.* A variety of defects in host defenses (primary or acquired immunoglobulin deficiencies, the asplenic state, human immunodeficiency virus infection) may predispose to severe pneumococcal disease, particularly bacteremia and meningitis. Alcoholism is an underlying problem in 10 to 25% of adults with pneumococcal meningitis in urban hospitals.

S. aureus meningitis is seen most commonly as a complication of a neurosurgical procedure, following penetrating skull trauma, or occasionally secondary to staphylococcal bacteremia and endocarditis. Meningitis caused by *gram-negative bacilli* takes one of three forms: neonatal meningitis, meningitis after trauma or neurosurgery, or spontaneous meningitis in adults (e.g., bacteremic *Klebsiella* meningitis in a patient with diabetes mellitus). The most common causes of gram-negative bacillary meningitis in the adult are *E. coli* (about 30%) and *Klebsiella-Enterobacter* (about 40%). The most frequent causes of bacterial meningitis in patients with neoplastic disease are gram-negative bacilli (particularly *Pseudomonas aeruginosa* and *E. coli*), *L. monocytogenes, S. pneumoniae,* and *S. aureus.* Meningitis caused by group A streptococci is uncommon but occasionally occurs after acute otitis media.

In the past, the age-related incidence (children younger than 5 years) of *H. influenzae* type b meningitis has been so striking that the occurrence of this disease in an adult has raised, and should still raise, the question of the presence of an underlying anatomic or immunologic defect, circumventing the usual barrier interposed by serum bactericidal mechanisms.

NEONATAL MENINGITIS. The incidence of meningitis is higher in the first month of life than in any other single month. In the newborn, the group B *Streptococcus* can produce either an "early-onset" (occurring within 8 days of delivery and characterized by a fulminant illness with septicemia, severe respiratory distress, and sometimes meningitis) or a "late-onset" (occurring 10 days to 2 months after delivery and presenting a more insidious, slowly progressive illness that usually includes meningitis) infection. The second leading cause, *E. coli* strains containing K1 capsular antigen, is usually acquired by the neonates from their mothers, who carry the organism in their stool.

The clinical signs in neonatal meningitis suggest sepsis but not necessarily central nervous system (CNS) involvement: fever (in only 60%), jaundice, diarrhea, lethargy, poor feeding or vomiting, respiratory distress (including apnea), seizures, irritability, bulging fontanelle (in only 30%), and nuchal rigidity (15%). Frequently, only by examining the CSF can the presence of meningitis be ruled in or out.

PATHOLOGY. The purulent exudate is distributed widely in the subarachnoid space, is most abundant in the basal cisterns and about the cerebellum initially, but also extends into the sulci over the cerebrum. There is no direct invasion of cerebral tissue by the infecting organism or the inflammatory exudate, but the subjacent brain becomes congested and edematous. The effectiveness of the pial barrier accounts for the fact that cerebral abscess does not complicate bacterial meningitis. Indeed, when these two processes coexist, the sequence usually has been that of an initial abscess subsequently leaking its contents into the ventricular system, producing meningitis. There are two possible exceptions to the aforementioned generalization: (1) neonatal meningitis due to *Citrobacter,* in which the organisms appear to invade the brain after producing a necrotizing vasculitis of small penetrating blood vessels, and (2) *Listeria* rhombencephalitis, a very rare process in which brain stem infection can occur simultaneously with *Listeria* meningitis (or alone). Structures adjacent to the meninges may show a variety of pathologic changes secondary to bacterial meningitis. *Cortical thrombophlebitis* results from venous stasis and adjacent meningeal inflammation. Infarction of cerebral tissue may follow. *Involvement of cortical and pial arteries* with peripheral aneurysm formation and vascular occlusion occurs in bacterial meningitis as well as narrowing (due to spasm and/or arteritis) of the supraclinoid portion of the internal carotid artery at the base of the brain. In one recent prospective study of adults with bacterial meningitis, angiographically documented cerebrovascular involvement was found in 15% (33% in patients with complicated meningitis). Consistent with this has been the relationship of anterior and middle cerebral arteries with markedly increased intracerebral blood flow velocities (an index of stenosis or arterial spasm) on transcranial Doppler ultrasonography to the occurrence of focal cerebral signs. In fulminating cases (particularly meningococcal meningitis),

cerebral edema may be marked even though the pleocytosis is only moderate. Rarely, such patients develop temporal lobe and cerebellar herniation, resulting in compression of the midbrain and medulla. *Damage to cranial nerves* occurs in areas where dense exudate accumulates; the third and sixth cranial nerves are also vulnerable to damage by increased intracranial pressure. *Ventriculitis* probably occurs in most cases of bacterial meningitis; rarely this progresses to the accumulation of pus, *ventricular empyema. Hydrocephalus* can develop during meningitis from obstruction to CSF flow within the ventricular system (obstructive hydrocephalus) or extraventricularly (communicating hydrocephalus). *Subdural effusions* are sterile transudates that develop over the cerebral cortex in about 15% of infants with bacterial meningitis. Rarely such effusions become infected, producing a subdural empyema. In the past, the diagnosis was made almost exclusively in infants, in whom abnormal transillumination or increasing head size can be detected. Now, sterile or infected (showing peripheral contrast medium enhancement) subdural collections can be demonstrated readily by computed tomography (CT) as low-density areas about the cerebrum.

PATHOGENESIS. Bacteria may reach the meninges by several routes: (1) systemic bacteremia, (2) direct ingress from the upper respiratory tract or skin through an anatomic defect (e.g., skull fracture, eroding sequestrum, meningocele), (3) passage intracranially via venules in the nasopharynx, or (4) spread from a contiguous focus of infection (infection of the paranasal sinuses, leakage of a brain abscess). Bacteremic spread to the meninges is probably the most frequent path of infection. However, not all bacteremic organisms have the same likelihood of causing meningitis. Bacteremia with *H. influenzae* and *N. meningitidis* is usually initiated by pharyngeal adhesion and colonization by an infecting strain. Adhesion of such strains, as well as of *S. pneumoniae,* to mucosal surfaces is abetted by their capacity to produce IgA proteases (cleaving this antibody in the hinge region) and thus inactivating this local antibody defense. *N. meningitidis* adhesion to nasopharyngeal cells is effected by fimbriae or pili. In an in vitro nasopharyngeal organ culture these organisms injure ciliated epithelial cells and induce ciliostasis, selectively adhering to non-ciliated epithelial cells. Meningococci invade the nasopharyngeal mucosal cells by means of endocytosis and are transported to the abluminal side in membrane-bound vacuoles. *H. influenzae,* in contrast, invades intercellularly by causing separation of apical tight junctions between columnar epithelial cells. When these meningeal pathogens gain access to the blood stream, their intravascular survival is aided by the presence of polysaccharide capsules that inhibit phagocytosis and confer resistance to complement-mediated bactericidal activity.

After entry into the blood stream, CNS invasion occurs, but the mechanisms by which, and sites at which, this occurs are unclear. A high-grade and sustained bacteremia appears necessary. An important role for specific bacterial adhesion to elements of the blood-brain barrier is likely, as indicated by the preferential binding of fimbriated strains of *E. coli* to the endothelial cell surface of cerebral capillaries and the epithelial cell surface of the choroid plexus and ventricles. Evidence from animal models suggests that CNS invasion sites after bacteremia may develop at foci of non-specific sterile inflammation above the cribriform plate and through the choroid plexus.

Most bacterial species causing meningitis (*H. influenzae* type b, *N. meningitidis, S. pneumoniae, E. coli* K1, group B *Streptococcus*) are antiphagocytic. Whether the capsular polysaccharide confers some special meningeal tropism, possibly through surface receptors, is not known. Although the primary focus initiating the bacteremia is usually in the upper respiratory tract or lung (pneumonia), it may be in the heart (endocarditis) or the gastrointestinal or urinary tracts. Once established in any part of the meninges, infection quickly extends throughout the subarachnoid space. Bacterial replication proceeds relatively unhindered, because CSF levels of complement are low early in meningeal inflammation, resulting in minimal opsonic and bactericidal activity (or none), and because surface phagocytosis of unopsonized organisms is meager in such a fluid environment. A secondary bacteremia may follow meningeal infection and itself contribute to continuing further inoculation of the CSF.

PATHOPHYSIOLOGY. Current experimental evidence suggests

that meningeal inflammation follows bacterial entry and growth in the CSF and that specific bacterial components (e.g., pneumococcal cell walls or lipoteichoic acid, *H. influenzae* lipopolysaccharide) are major elicitors of this response by causing release into the subarachnoid space of various proinflammatory cytokines such as interleukin-1 and tumor necrosis factor from endothelial and meningeal cells, macrophages, and microglia. These cytokines increase adherence and transendothelial movement of neutrophils, as has been shown in endothelial cell monolayers in culture. Cytokines appear to enhance this passage of leukocytes by inducing several families of adhesion molecules that interact with corresponding receptors on leukocytes. The three likely families mediating endothelial-leukocyte adhesion are the (1) immunoglobulin superfamily (e.g., intercellular adhesion molecule-1 and intercellular adhesion molecule-2); (2) integrins (e.g., CD11/CD18 subfamily); and (3) selectins (e.g., endothelial-leukocyte adhesion molecule-1). Cytokines also can act to increase the binding affinity of a leukocyte selectin, leukocyte-adhesion molecule, for its endothelial cell receptor, contributing further to neutrophil trafficking into the subarachnoid space.

Once within the subarachnoid space, neutrophils are further activated to release products such as prostaglandins and toxic oxygen metabolites that increase local vascular permeability and may cause direct neurotoxicity. Evidence of breaching of the blood-brain barrier is found in animal models of meningitis where endothelial intercellular tight junctions are disrupted, where increased pinocytotic vesicles appear in endothelial cells, and where albumin escapes across postcapillary venules into the subarachnoid space.

The foregoing inflammatory changes can contribute to development of increased intracranial pressure and alterations in cerebral blood flow. Cerebral edema is commonly due to increased permeability of the blood-brain barrier (vasogenic) and may be due to cellular swelling in the brain as a result of toxic molecules released by bacteria and neutrophils (cytotoxic); and sometimes increased CSF pressure may result primarily from obstruction to CSF outflow due to inflammation at the level of the arachnoidal villi (interstitial). Cerebral blood flow appears to be increased in the very early stages of meningitis, but subsequently it decreases, substantially in some patients in whom it may be responsible for ensuing neurologic injury. When cerebral perfusion pressure (intracranial pressure minus mean arterial pressure) is markedly reduced, morbidity and mortality of bacterial meningitis is greatest in children in whom these measurements have been made. Localized regions of marked hypoperfusion (attributable to focal vascular inflammation or thrombosis) can occur in patients with normal blood flow. Impairment of autoregulation of cerebral blood flow may be a factor in cerebral edema or ischemia in some patients owing to altered cerebral perfusion pressure.

CLINICAL MANIFESTATIONS. HISTORY. An acute onset of fever, generalized headache, vomiting, and stiff neck are common to many types of meningitis. The majority of patients with pyogenic meningitis of the three common causes have had an antecedent or accompanying upper respiratory tract infection or non-specific febrile illness, acute otitis (or mastoiditis), or pneumonia. Myalgias (particularly in meningococcal disease), backache, and generalized weakness are common symptoms. The illness usually progresses rapidly, with development of confusion, obtundation, and loss of consciousness. Occasionally, the onset may be less acute, with meningeal signs present for several days to a week.

GENERAL PHYSICAL FINDINGS. Evidence of meningeal irritation (drowsiness and decreased mentation, stiff neck, Kernig's and Brudzinski's signs) is usually present. In certain patients, the findings of meningitis may be easily overlooked; infants, obtunded patients, or elderly patients with congestive heart failure or pneumonia may develop meningitis without prominent meningeal signs. Their lethargy should be investigated carefully, and meningeal signs should be sought; if any doubt exists, examination of the CSF is indicated.

The presence of a petechial, purpuric, or ecchymotic rash in a patient with meningeal findings almost always indicates meningococcal infection and requires prompt treatment because of the rapidity with which this infection can progress (see Chapter 329). Rarely, extensive petechial and purpuric lesions occur in meningitis caused by *S. pneumoniae* or *H. influenzae*. Very rarely, skin lesions almost indistinguishable from those of meningococcal bacteremia occur in patients with acute *S. aureus* endocarditis who also have meningeal signs and a pleocytosis (secondary either to staphylococcal meningitis or to embolic cerebral infarction). Usually one or two of the lesions in such a patient are those of purulent purpura; aspiration of material reveals staphylococci on Gram stain. In the summer months, viral aseptic meningitis may produce meningeal signs, macular and petechial skin lesions, and a pleocytosis of several hundred cells, sometimes with neutrophils predominating initially.

NEUROLOGIC FINDINGS AND COMPLICATIONS. Cranial nerve abnormalities, involving principally the third, fourth, sixth, or seventh nerves, occur in 5 to 10% of adults with community-acquired meningitis. These usually disappear shortly after recovery. Persistent sensorineural hearing loss occurs in 10% of children with bacterial meningitis. In another 16% a transient conductive hearing loss develops. The most likely sites of involvement in persistent sensorineural deafness appear to be the inner ear (infection or toxic products possibly spreading from the subarachnoid space along the cochlear aqueduct) and the acoustic nerve. In children, permanent hearing impairment is more common after meningitis due to *S. pneumoniae* than to *H. influenzae* or *N. meningitidis*.

Seizures (focal or generalized) occur in 20 to 30% of patients and may result from readily reversible causes (high fever in infants; penicillin neurotoxicity when large doses are administered intravenously in the presence of renal failure) or, more commonly, from focal cerebral injury. Seizures can occur during the first few days or can appear with associated focal neurologic deficits caused by vascular inflammation some days after the onset of the meningitis (Table 328–1). In adults with seizures accompanying meningitis, *S. pneumoniae* is more commonly the cause, but alcoholism is a confounding factor.

Brain swelling and increased CSF pressure are associated with seizures, third nerve dysfunction, abnormal reflexes, coma, hypertension, and bradycardia. In approximately one fourth of fatal cases of community-acquired meningitis in adults, cerebral edema accompanied by temporal lobe herniation is observed at autopsy.

Papilledema is rare (1%) in bacterial meningitis even with high CSF pressures, probably because the patient is seen early in the process before changes have occurred in the nerve head. Its presence should indicate the possibility of some other associated or independent suppurative intracranial process (subdural empyema, brain abscess). Marked central hyperpnea sometimes occurs in patients with severe bacterial meningitis; CSF acidosis (principally caused by increased lactic acid levels) provides much of the respiratory stimulus.

Focal cerebral signs (principally hemiparesis, dysphasia, visual field defects, and gaze preference) occur in about 25% of adults with community-acquired bacterial meningitis (see Table 328–1).

Table 328–1 ■ CENTRAL NERVOUS SYSTEM FINDINGS IN COMMUNITY-ACQUIRED BACTERIAL MENINGITIS IN ADULTS*

| TIME OF ONSET OF FINDINGS | PERCENTAGE OF EPISODES OF MENINGITIS† | | | | | |
	Hemiparesis	Aphasia	Visual-Field Defect	Gaze Preference	Seizures	Other‡
Early (≤24 hr)	9	6	3	10	15	5
Late (>24 hr)	2	1	0.3	0	8	1
Total†	11	7	3.3	10	23	6

*Based on data of Durand ML, Calderwood SB, Weber DJ, et al: Acute bacterial meningitis in adult: A review of 493 episodes. N Engl J Med 328:21, 1993.
†Total percent of 279 episodes in which individual finding occurred (some episodes involved more than one finding).
‡Other focal findings include nystagmus, diplopia, ataxia, monoparesis, hemianesthesia, and central seventh nerve palsy.

They may develop during early meningitis secondary to occlusive vascular processes or some days later. Also, cerebral blood flow velocity may be decreased in the presence of increased intracranial pressure and lead to temporary or lasting neurologic dysfunction. It is important to distinguish lateralizing findings resulting from postictal changes (Todd's paralysis), which usually persist for no more than several hours.

Prompt treatment of bacterial meningitis usually results in rapid recovery of neurologic function. Persistent or late-onset obtundation and coma without focal findings suggests development of brain swelling, subdural effusion (in the infant), hydrocephalus, loculated ventriculitis, cortical thrombophlebitis, or sagittal sinus thrombosis. The last three are commonly associated with fever and continuing pleocytosis.

Residual neurologic damage remains in 10 to 20% of patients who recover from bacterial meningitis. Developmental delay and speech defects are each observed in about 5% of children. In infants surviving neonatal meningitis, significant sequelae are much more frequent (15 to 50%).

LABORATORY DIAGNOSIS. CEREBROSPINAL FLUID EXAMINATION. Initial CSF pressure is usually moderately elevated (200 to 300 mm H_2O in the adult). Striking elevations (> 450 mm H_2O) occur in occasional patients with acute brain swelling complicating meningitis in the absence of an associated mass lesion.

Gram-Stained Smear. By the time of hospitalization, most patients with pyogenic meningitis have large numbers (at least 10^5/mL) of bacteria in the CSF. Careful examination of the Gram-stained smear of the spun sediment of CSF reveals the etiologic agent in 60 to 80% of cases. In most instances when gram-positive diplococci (or short-chaining cocci) are observed on stained CSF smear, they are pneumococci. In certain clinical settings it is important to distinguish this organism from the relatively penicillin-resistant Enterococcus, an occasional cause of nosocomial meningitis, which would require adding an aminoglycoside to penicillin in treatment. This can be done by identifying pneumococcal polysaccharide in the CSF by latex particle agglutination. Rarely, three species may morphologically mimic Neisseria in the CSF or suggest a mixed infection with short gram-negative rods and meningococci: Acinetobacter baumanii, Moraxella species, and Pasteurella multocida. Culture of the CSF reveals the etiologic agent in 80 to 90% of patients with bacterial meningitis.

Special Immunologic and Serologic Procedures. Rapid antigen disclosure by latex agglutination is available for the detection in CSF of the capsular polysaccharides of common meningeal pathogens (H. influenzae; S. pneumoniae; group B Streptococcus; N. meningitidis serogroups A, C, Y, W 135; and N. meningitidis group B and E. coli K1, which share a common antigen). The sensitivity and specificity of these is highest (over 90%) for H. influenzae. Antigen testing of urine specimens for diagnosis of specific bacterial causes of meningitis or bacteremia has a high rate of false-positive results owing to the presence of cross-reacting species that may be found in urinary tract colonization or infection. Performance of bacterial antigen testing of CSF as routinely practiced is a low yield procedure. Gram-stained smears almost invariably show the causative microorganism when the latex agglutination test is a true positive. Latex agglutination testing may be most useful when the CSF cell count is abnormal, the Gram stain is negative, and blood and CSF cultures are unrevealing at 48 hours (at which time a stored sample of the initial CSF specimen can be tested). Occasionally, when only rare organisms of ambiguous morphology or Gram-staining properties are seen, latex agglutination may be helpful in providing a more specific diagnosis.

Cell Count. The cell count in untreated meningitis usually ranges between 100 and 10,000/mm³, with polymorphonuclear leukocytes predominating initially (≥ 80%) and lymphocytes appearing subsequently. Extremely high cell counts (> 50,000/mm³) may occur rarely in primary bacterial meningitis but also should raise the possibility of intraventricular rupture of a cerebral abscess. Cell counts as low as 10 to 20/mm³ may be observed early in bacterial meningitis (particularly that caused by N. meningitidis and H. influenzae). Occasionally, in granulocytopenic patients or in the elderly with overwhelming pneumococcal meningitis, the CSF may contain very few leukocytes and yet may appear grossly turbid because of the presence of a myriad of organisms. Meningitis caused by several bacterial species (Mycobacterium tuberculosis, Borrelia burgdorferi, Treponema pallidum) characteristically produces a lymphocytic pleocytosis. L. monocytogenes meningitis in infants may produce a primarily lymphocytic response in the CSF; in the adult there is usually a polymorphonuclear response, but rarely lymphocytes predominate.

Glucose. The CSF glucose is reduced to values of 40 mg/dL or less (or <50% of the simultaneous blood level) in 50% of patients with bacterial meningitis; this finding can be very valuable in distinguishing bacterial meningitis from most viral meningitides or parameningeal infections. A normal CSF glucose value does not exclude the diagnosis of bacterial meningitis. The simultaneous blood glucose level should be determined, because patients with diabetes mellitus (or those who are receiving intravenous glucose infusions) have an elevated level of glucose in the CSF, and its significance can be appreciated only on comparison with the simultaneous blood level. However, it may take 90 to 120 minutes for equilibration to occur after major shifts in the level of glucose in the circulation. The hypoglycorrhachia characteristic of pyogenic meningitis appears to be due to interference with normal carrier-facilitated diffusion of glucose and to increased utilization of glucose by host cells.

Protein. The level of protein in the CSF is usually elevated above 100 mg/dL, and the higher values are more commonly observed in pneumococcal meningitis. Extreme elevations, 1000 mg/dL or more, indicate subarachnoid block secondary to the meningitis.

Other Abnormalities in the CSF. Elevated levels of lactic acid occur in pyogenic meningitis. Although lactic dehydrogenase levels are higher in patients with bacterial meningitis than in those with viral infections of the CNS, these alterations are not of help in determining the specific etiologic agent involved. C-reactive protein is increased in about 95% of patients with bacterial meningitis and is not increased in most patients with viral meningitis. However, it does not seem to provide more information than the CSF cell count, is not helpful in diagnosing bacterial meningitis in newborns, and does not provide clues to the bacterial species involved.

OTHER LABORATORY TESTS. Blood and Respiratory Tract Cultures. Bacteremia is demonstrable in about 80% of patients with H. influenzae meningitis, 50% of those with pneumococcal meningitis, and 30 to 40% of those with meningococcal meningitis. Cultures of the upper respiratory tract are not helpful in establishing an etiologic diagnosis. Determining serum creatinine and electrolytes is important in view of the gravity of the illness, the occurrence of specific abnormalities secondary to the meningitis (syndrome of inappropriate secretion of antidiuretic hormone), and problems in therapy in the presence of renal dysfunction (seizures and hyperkalemia with high-dose penicillin therapy). In patients with extensive petechial and purpuric skin lesions, evaluation for coagulopathy is indicated.

RADIOLOGIC STUDIES. In view of the frequency with which pyogenic meningitis is associated with primary foci of infection in the chest, nasal sinuses, or mastoid, radiographs of these areas should be taken at the appropriate time after antimicrobial therapy begins when clinically indicated. CT is not indicated in most patients with bacterial meningitis. If a mass lesion (cerebral abscess, subdural empyema) is suspected by history, clinical setting, or physical findings (papilledema, focal cerebral signs), then CT should be performed. Bacterial meningitis is a medical emergency requiring immediate diagnosis and rapid institution of antimicrobial therapy. Delay in performing a diagnostic lumbar puncture to obtain a CT scan should be avoided except on the basis of findings indicative of a parameningeal collection or other intracranial mass lesions; and in that case it would be important to initiate antimicrobial therapy aimed at meningitis of unknown etiology or brain abscess before performing CT. Changes may be observed on the CT scan during meningitis itself and include cerebral edema and enlargement of the subarachnoid spaces, contrast enhancement of the leptomeninges and the ependyma, or patchy areas of diminished density owing to associated cerebritis and necrosis. Patients with meningitis rarely have significant CT abnormalities in the absence of focal neurologic findings. In the patient with meningitis whose clinical status deteriorates or fails to improve, the CT scan may help demonstrate suspected complications: sterile subdural collections or empyema; ventricular enlargement secondary to communicating or obstructive hydrocephalus; prominent persisting basilar meningitis; extensive areas of cerebral infarction resulting from occlusion of major cerebral arteries, veins, or venous sinuses; or marked ventricular wall enhancement, suggesting ventriculitis or ventricular empyema. Rarely, cerebral hemorrhage, identifiable on CT, may complicate acute bacterial meningitis in adults, occurring much less frequently than thrombotic strokes.

In about 10% of adults with bacterial meningitis, cranial CT findings (mastoid or sinus wall defect, eroding retrobulbar mass, pneumocephalus) are indicative of disruption of the dural barrier.

DIAGNOSIS. Diagnosis of bacterial meningitis is not difficult in a febrile patient with meningeal symptoms and signs developing in the setting of a predisposing illness. The diagnosis may be less obvious in the elderly, obtunded patient with pneumonia or the confused alcoholic patient in impending delirium tremens. Examination of the CSF should be carried out promptly whenever there is any question of meningitis.

Headache, fever, vomiting, stiff neck, and pleocytosis are features of meningeal inflammation and are common to many types of meningitis (e.g., bacterial, fungal, viral) and also to some parameningeal processes. The CSF findings are most helpful in distinguishing among these processes (see Chapter 473). In the patient with meningitis whose CSF does not reveal the etiologic agent on Gram-stained smear, particularly when the CSF glucose is normal and the polymorphonuclear pleocytosis is atypical, certain treatable processes that can mimic bacterial meningitis should be considered in the differential diagnosis:

1. *Parameningeal infections.* The presence of infections (chronic ear or nasal accessory sinus infections, lung abscess) predisposing to brain abscess, epidural (cerebral or spinal) abscess, subdural empyema, or pyogenic venous sinus phlebitis should be sought. Neurologic findings may appear in the course of primary bacterial meningitis, but their presence should alert the physician to the need for close scrutiny for the presence of a space-occupying infectious process in the CNS. Neurologic symptoms or findings antedating the onset of meningeal symptoms should suggest the possibility of a parameningeal infection. The isolation of an anaerobic organism should suggest the possibility of intraventricular leakage of a cerebral abscess.
2. *Bacterial endocarditis.* Bacterial meningitis may occur during bacterial endocarditis caused by pyogenic organisms such as *S. aureus* and enterococci. In subacute bacterial endocarditis, sterile embolic infarctions of the brain may occur and produce meningeal signs and a pleocytosis containing several hundred cells, including polymorphonuclear leukocytes. A history of dental manipulation, fever, and anorexia antedating the meningitis should be sought; careful examination for heart murmurs and peripheral stigmata of endocarditis is indicated.
3. *"Chemical" meningitis.* The clinical and CSF findings (polymorphonuclear pleocytosis and even reduced glucose level) of bacterial meningitis may be produced by chemically induced inflammation. Acute meningitis after a diagnostic lumbar puncture or spinal anesthesia may be due to bacterial or chemical contamination of equipment or anesthetic agent. Chemical meningitis, characterized by a polymorphonuclear pleocytosis, hypoglycorrhachia, and a latent period of 3 to 24 hours, may occur after 1% of metrizamide myelograms. Endogenous chemical meningitis resulting from material from an epidermoid tumor or a craniopharyngioma leaking into the subarachnoid space can produce a polymorphonuclear pleocytosis and hypoglycorrhachia. Birefringent material may be seen on polarizing microscopy of the CSF sediment.

Rarely, a patient develops meningitis characterized by subacute onset and persistent neutrophilic CSF pleocytosis lasting weeks or months without ready bacteriologic diagnosis. The etiologic agent in such cases of *chronic neutrophilic meningitis* has usually been either a fungus (*Aspergillus, Candida, Blastomyces*) or a bacterium such as *Nocardia* or *Actinomyces* species.

NON-NEUROLOGIC COMPLICATIONS. SHOCK. When shock occurs in pyogenic meningitis, it is usually a manifestation of an accompanying intense bacteremia, as in fulminant meningococcemia, rather than of the meningitis itself. Management is guided by the principles of septic shock therapy with appropriate modifications for myocardial failure (see Chapter 329).

COAGULATION DISORDERS. Coagulopathies are frequently associated with the intense bacteremias (usually meningococcal, occasionally pneumococcal) and hypotension, which can accompany meningitis. The changes may be mild, such as thrombocytopenia (with or without prolongation of prothrombin and partial thromboplastin times), or more marked, with clinical evidences of disseminated intravascular coagulation (see Chapter 329).

SEPTIC COMPLICATIONS. Endocarditis. Previously, 5 to 10% of patients with pneumococcal meningitis, particularly those with bacteremia and pneumonia as well, developed acute endocarditis, most commonly on the aortic valve. The incidence is currently much lower, as a result of earlier treatment of the initiating infection. In such patients, febrile relapse and a new murmur may appear shortly after completion of antimicrobial therapy for meningitis.

Pyogenic Arthritis. Septic arthritis may result from the bacteremia associated with meningitis caused by *S. pneumoniae, N. meningitidis,* or *H. influenzae.*

PROLONGED FEVER. With appropriate antimicrobial treatment of meningitis from the three most common bacterial causes, patients become afebrile within 2 to 5 days. Sometimes fever persists beyond this or recurs after an afebrile period. In the patient with persisting headache, obtundation, and cerebral findings, inadequate drug therapy or neurologic sequelae (cortical venous thrombophlebitis, ventriculitis, subdural collections) are important considerations. Re-evaluation of the CSF, particularly Gram-stained smear and culture, is essential under these circumstances. Drug fever may be responsible in the patient who continues to show clinical improvement in all other respects. Metastatic infection (septic arthritis, purulent pericarditis, thoracic empyema, endocarditis) may be the cause of continuing or recurrent fever.

A syndrome consisting of fever, arthritis, and pericarditis 3 to 6 days after initiation of effective antimicrobial therapy of meningococcal meningitis occurs in about 10% of patients (see Chapter 329).

RECURRENT MENINGITIS. Repeated episodes of bacterial meningitis generally indicate a host defect, either in local anatomy or in antibacterial and immunologic defenses (e.g., recurrent *N. meningitidis* infections in patients with congenital or acquired deficiencies of complement, particularly late-acting components). Among episodes of pneumococcal meningitis in adults seen at a large tertiary care general hospital, 11% occurred in patients with recurrent meningitis; but only 0.5% of patients with community-acquired meningitis caused by other microorganisms have had recurrent attacks.

S. pneumoniae is the cause of one third of episodes of community-acquired recurrent meningitis; various streptococci, *H. influenzae,* and *N. meningitidis* are the causes of another one third of episodes. In contrast, in nosocomial recurrent meningitis, gramnegative bacilli and *S. aureus* are the causes of about 60% of episodes. A history of head trauma is much more frequent in patients with recurrent meningitis. Organisms may enter the subarachnoid space directly, through a defect in the cribriform plate (the most common site), in association with the empty sella syndrome, by means of a basilar skull fracture, through an erosive sequestrum of the mastoid, through congenital dermal defects along the craniospinal axis (usually evident before adult life), or as a consequence of penetrating cranial trauma or neurosurgical procedures. The anatomic defect may produce a frank CSF leak (rhinorrhea or, less commonly, otorrhea) or may entrap a vascular cuff of meninges that might subsequently serve as a direct route for organisms to reach the meninges. CSF rhinorrhea may be intermittent, and meningitis may occur months or years after head injury.

Any patient with bacterial meningitis, particularly if meningitis is recurrent, should be evaluated carefully for any congenital or posttraumatic defects. The presence of CSF rhinorrhea should be sought at admission and subsequently (rhinorrhea may clear during active meningitis only to recur when inflammation has resolved). Clinical clues suggesting the presence of a CSF fistula through the cribriform plate, pericranial air sinuses, or temporal bone include (1) salty taste in the throat, (2) positionally dependent rhinorrhea (rhinorrhea only in the lateral recumbent or prone position suggests an otic or sphenoid origin), (3) anosmia (cribriform plate leak), (4) hearing loss or full feeling in the ear, often with a finding of fluid or bubbles behind the tympanic membrane (leakage into the middle ear). Quantitative determination of glucose and chloride content of nasal secretions and detection by protein electrophoresis of a transferrin band unique to CSF can definitively establish the presence of CSF rhinorrhea.

Recurrent pneumococcal meningitis may occur without apparent predisposing circumstances, and cryptic CSF leaks should be sought actively in such patients by CT scanning of the frontal and mastoid regions and by radioisotope techniques. (Radioiodine-labeled albumin is introduced intrathecally, and pledgets of cotton placed in the nares are subsequently examined for the radionuclide. Radioisotopic cisternography has been used successfully.) Intrathecal introduction of fluorescein as a visual tracer (under ultraviolet light) can be employed similarly to detect active leaks. Surgical closure of CSF fistulas should be carried out to prevent further episodes of meningitis. Newer extracranial approaches through the ethmoidal sinuses to repair cribriform plate or sphenoidal sinus dural defects are successful and avoid the higher morbidity associated with craniotomy.

In most patients with CSF otorrhea and rhinorrhea after an acute head injury, the leak ceases in 1 or 2 weeks. *Persistent rhinorrhea for more than 4 to 6 weeks is an indication for surgical repair.* Prolonged administration of penicillin does not prevent pneumococcal meningitis and may encourage infection with more drug-resistant species.

Rarely, recurrent meningitis of non-bacterial cause may mimic bacterial meningitis. *Mollaret's meningitis* consists of repeated febrile episodes of mild meningeal symptomatology, usually without neurologic abnormalities. Initially, large "endothelial" cells may be seen in the CSF along with polymorphonuclear leukocytes, which subsequently are replaced by lymphocytes. *Behçet's syndrome,* characterized by relapsing oral and genital ulcers and ocular lesions (hypopyon), may exhibit a variety of neurologic abnormalities, including recurrent meningitis.

PROGNOSIS. The introduction of antimicrobial agents has converted bacterial meningitis from a disease that was almost always fatal to one that the majority of patients survive without significant neurologic residua. The mortality rate for community-acquired bacterial meningitis in adults varies with the etiologic agent and the clinical circumstances. With current antimicrobial therapy the mortality rate for *H. influenzae* meningitis is below 5% and that for meningococcal meningitis is about 10%. The highest mortality is with pneumococcal meningitis, in which the rate is about 25%. The mortality rate for gram-negative bacillary meningitis, commonly nosocomial in origin, in adults has been 20 to 30%, but it appears to be decreasing in the past 10 to 15 years. The mortality rate for recurrent community-acquired meningitis in adults (about 5%) is strikingly lower than the 20% rate for non-recurrent episodes. Poor prognostic factors include advanced age, presence of other foci of infection, underlying diseases (leukemia, alcoholism), obtundation, seizures within the first 24 hours, and delay in instituting appropriate therapy.

TREATMENT. ANTIMICROBIAL AGENTS. Antimicrobial therapy should be begun promptly in this life-threatening emergency. Treatment should be aimed at the most likely causes based on clinical clues (age of the patient, presence of a petechial or purpuric rash, a recent neurosurgical procedure, CSF rhinorrhea). If the infecting organism is observed on examination of the Gram-stained smear of the CSF sediment, specific therapy is initiated. If the etiologic agent is not seen on smear (and not detected by latex agglutination), treatment of bacterial meningitis of unknown etiology should be carried out (see later).

With the exception of chloramphenicol, the commonly used antimicrobial agents do not readily penetrate the normal blood-brain barrier, but the passage of penicillin and other antimicrobial agents is enhanced in the presence of meningeal inflammation. Antimicrobial drugs should be administered intravenously throughout the treatment period; reducing dosage as the patient improves should be avoided, because normalization of the blood-brain barrier during recovery reduces the CSF levels of drug that are achievable. Bactericidal drugs (penicillin, ampicillin, third-generation cephalosporins) are preferred whenever possible in the treatment of meningitis caused by susceptible bacteria. In animal models of bacterial meningitis, CSF levels of antibiotics at least 10 to 20 times the minimal bactericidal concentration appear to be needed for optimal therapy. Several antimicrobial drugs (first- or second-generation cephalosporins, clindamycin) do not provide effective levels in the CSF and should not be used.

MENINGITIS OF SPECIFIC BACTERIAL CAUSE. The treatment of choice for pneumococcal meningitis in the adult has been penicillin (Table 328–2). For patients allergic to penicillin, chloramphenicol has been a reasonable alternative (see later). However, problems have developed because of the emergence of penicillin resistance in some pneumococcal isolates. Such resistance has arisen as a result of successive stepwise chromosomal mutations in genes for penicillin-binding proteins and is not due to β-lactamase production. Penicillin-resistant isolates are either intermediately resistant (minimal inhibitory concentration [MIC] of 0.1 to 1.0 (μg/mL) or highly resistant (MIC > 1.0 μg/mL). Penicillin-resistant pneumococcal strains have been found worldwide: 44% of isolates in parts of Spain, 45% in regions of South Africa, and almost 60% of isolates in Hungary. In the United States, 20 to 25% of clinical isolates overall are penicillin resistant, with higher percentages being noted in some geographic areas such as Tennessee, Georgia, Maryland, and California and lower percentages in others. In a study of bacterial meningitis in the United States in 1995, 35% of *S. pneumoniae* isolates were penicillin resistant (21% intermediately and 14% highly resistant). Thus, initial treatment decisions for pneumococcal meningitis must take into consideration up-to-date data on penicillin susceptibilities of *S. pneumoniae* isolated in a given region. Antimicrobial susceptibilities should be determined for all pneumococcal isolates from CSF, blood, or sterile body fluids (see Table 328–2). Worrisome has been the recent appearance of pneumococcal strains resistant to third-generation cephalosporins (about 4% of blood and CSF isolates from children). Because commercial MIC panels may not detect resistance to third-generation cephalosporins, it is necessary to determine the MIC to these drugs by means other than using such a panel. If the MIC for cefotaxime or ceftriaxone (<1.0 μg/mL) indicates a susceptible isolate, cefotaxime or ceftriaxone would be the drug of choice. If the isolate is highly penicillin resistant or is resistant to 1.0 μg/mL of ceftriaxone or cefotaxime, alternative therapy (vancomycin with or without rifampin intravenously) is indicated. If the patient has pneumococcal meningitis and comes from an area where highly resistant strains are known to occur, then initial therapy (pending susceptibility testing) with cefotaxime (or ceftriaxone) plus vancomycin intravenously is indicated. Some experts believe that vancomycin should be routinely administered along with a third-generation cephalosporin when *S. pneumoniae* is the suspected agent, regardless of whether highly penicillin-resistant strains have been noted in the region, because of their current widespread dissemination in the United States. When initial adjunctive therapy with dexamethasone is employed (see later) along with vancomycin, it should be borne in mind that vancomycin levels in the CSF may be reduced by the concomitant corticosteroid use.

Although resistance to chloramphenicol is unusual among pneumococcal isolates from the United States, chloramphenicol has shown poor bactericidal activity against penicillin-resistant isolates from children with meningitis in South Africa. The relative chloramphenicol resistance of such strains may not be discerned on usual laboratory testing but is revealed when the minimum bactericidal concentration is determined. In areas where highly penicillin-resistant or chloramphenicol-resistant pneumococci are found, vancomycin replaces chloramphenicol in initial treatment of pneumococcal meningitis in the highly penicillin-allergic patient.

The β-lactam antibiotic meropenem has been studied in the treatment of meningitis due to *S. pneumoniae, N. meningitidis,* and *H. influenzae* in children primarily (but also in adults) and has been found effective. It has the advantage over imipenem of not causing an increased incidence of seizures and not requiring addition of the renal tubular dehydropeptidase inhibitor cilastatin.

Penicillin G or ampicillin intravenously, in the dosage used to treat meningitis due to penicillin-susceptible pneumococci, is used to treat *N. meningitidis* meningitis. Recently, meningococci resistant to penicillin have been isolated occasionally in Spain, South Africa, Canada, and rarely the United States. Most of these isolates have been only intermediately resistant to penicillin (MIC, 0.1 to 1.0 μg/mL), although a rare strain has had high-level resistance due to β-lactamase production. The latter-type strains require the use of third-generation cephalosporins, but "meningitis dosages" of penicillin or ampicillin may provide CSF levels that are sufficient for infections due to some strains of intermediately penicillin-resistant *N. meningitidis.*

Table 328-2 ■ ANTIMICROBIAL THERAPY OF COMMUNITY-ACQUIRED BACTERIAL MENINGITIS OF KNOWN CAUSE*

ORGANISM	PREFERRED THERAPY			ALTERNATIVE THERAPY		
	Antimicrobial	Adults (24-hr Dose)	Children (24-hr Dose)	Antimicrobial	Adults (24-hr Dose)	Children (24-hr Dose)
S. pneumoniae						
Penicillin MIC < 0.1 µg/mL	Penicillin G	24 million units IV, q4h aliquots	300,000 U/kg IV, q4h aliquots	Cefotaxime	12 g IV, q4h aliquots	200 mg/kg IV, q4–6h aliquots
	or			or		
	ampicillin	12 g IV, q4h aliquots	200–400 mg/kg IV, q4h aliquots	ceftriaxone†	4 g IV, q12h aliquots	80–100 mg/kg IV, q12h aliquots
				or		
				vancomycin‡	2 g IV, q8–12h aliquots	50 mg/kg IV, q6h aliquots
				or		
				chloramphenicol		
Penicillin MIC 0.1–1.0 µg/mL	Ceftriaxone†	4 g IV, q12h aliquots	80–100 mg/kg IV, q12h aliquots	Vancomycin‡	4–6 g IV, q6h aliquots	75–100 mg/kg IV, q6h aliquots
	or			or		
	cefotaxime	12 g IV, q4h aliquots	200 mg/kg IV, q4–6h aliquots	meropenem§	2 g IV, q8–12h aliquots	50 mg/kg IV, q6h aliquots
Penicillin MIC > 1.0 µg/mL	Vancomycin‡;¶	2 g IV, q8–12h aliquots	50 mg/kg IV, q6h aliquots	Meropenem§	6 g IV, q8h aliquots	40 mg/kg q8h IV
N. meningitidis	Penicillin G	24 million units IV, q4h aliquots	300,000 U/kg IV, q4h aliquots	Ceftriaxone† or cefotaxime	As above	80–100 mg/kg IV, q12h aliquots / 200 mg/kg IV, q4–6h aliquots
	or			or		
	ampicillin	12 g IV, q4h aliquots	200–400 mg/kg IV, q4h aliquots	chloramphenicol	4–6 g IV, q6h aliquots	75–100 mg/kg IV, q6h aliquots
H. influenzae						
β-Lactamase negative	Ampicillin	12 g IV, q4h aliquots	200–400 mg/kg IV, q4h aliquots	Third-generation cephalosporin** or chloramphenicol as above	Third-generation cephalosporin** or chloramphenicol as above	Third-generation cephalosporin** or chloramphenicol as above
β-Lactamase positive	Ceftriaxone†	4 g IV, q12h aliquots	80–100 mg/kg IV, q12h aliquots	Chloramphenicol as above	6 g IV, q8h aliquots	75–100 mg/kg IV, q6h aliquots
	or					
	cefotaxime	12 g IV, q4h aliquots	200 mg/kg IV, q4–6h aliquots			
L. monocytogenes	Ampicillin ||	12 g IV, q4h aliquots	200–400 mg/kg IV, q4h aliquots	Trimethoprim-sulfamethoxazole	10–20 mg/kg IV,†† q6–8h aliquots	10–20 mg/kg IV,†† q6h aliquots
	or					
	penicillin G ||	24 million units IV, q4h aliquots	300,000 U/kg IV, q4h aliquots			

*Dosages are those for patients with normal renal and hepatic function.
†4 g maximum daily dose.
‡Monitoring of peak and trough serum levels advisable; may need to monitor CSF levels if patient not responding well and if levels are low, may need to increase daily dose temporarily by 0.5–1.0 g in adults or add adjuvant intrathecal vancomycin as in treatment of methicillin-resistant *S. aureus* meningitis (see text).
§Use may be associated with seizures, but much less so than with imipenem.
|| Addition of IV gentamicin to be considered.
¶Addition of rifampin should be considered.
**Ceftriaxone or cefotaxime.
††Dosage based on trimethoprim component of the combination.
Modified from Swartz MN: Acute bacterial meningitis. In Gorbach SL, et al (eds): Infectious Diseases 2nd ed. Philadelphia, WB Saunders, 1998.

At present, 30 to 35% of isolates of *H. influenzae* type b in the United States are β-lactamase producers and ampicillin resistant; cefotaxime is the initial therapy of choice (see Table 328–2). Chloramphenicol combined with ampicillin is an acceptable alternative. If the isolate proves susceptible to ampicillin, the chloramphenicol may be discontinued. Although in areas of Spain more than 50% of isolates are chloramphenicol resistant, less than 1% have been resistant in the United States. Cefuroxime, a second-generation cephalosporin, has been used extensively in the past 10 years, but the third-generation cephalosporins are preferable because of reports indicating slower sterilization of CSF and a higher incidence of sensorineural hearing loss with cefuroxime.

Treatment of adult meningitis caused by methicillin-sensitive *S. aureus* is listed in Table 328–3. For the penicillin-allergic patient, vancomycin is the alternative of choice. Because penetration of vancomycin into the CSF is limited, adjunctive intrathecal (or intraventricular) therapy with vancomycin (without preservative) has occasionally been resorted to when CSF cultures have remained positive after 48 hours of intravenous therapy alone and where CSF levels can be monitored. For adult meningitis due to methicillin-resistant *S. aureus*, intravenous vancomycin (with adjunctive intrathecal vancomycin as needed) is the treatment of choice. In severe or refractory cases, adding another drug (rifampin or gentamicin) for systemic therapy may be warranted.

Cefotaxime (see Table 328–3) is used to treat meningitis known to be due to susceptible gram-negative bacilli (e.g., *E. coli, Klebsiella, Proteus*). It should not be used to treat meningitis due to less susceptible species such as *Pseudomonas aeruginosa* and *Acinetobacter*. Initial treatment (on the basis only of findings on Gram-stained smear of CSF) of adults with gram-negative bacillary meningitis is listed in Table 328–3. After identifying the specific pathogen and determining its drug susceptibilities, alterations in antimicrobial therapy may be indicated. If the organism is *P. aeruginosa*, a third-generation cephalosporin with antipseudomonal activity can be used (see Table 328–3).

BACTERIAL MENINGITIS OF UNKNOWN ETIOLOGY. Initial treatment of meningitis when the etiologic agent cannot be identified on Gram-stained smear of CSF is based on available clinical clues. *In the neonate*, a wide range of gram-positive (group B streptococci, *Listeria*) and gram-negative (*E. coli, Klebsiella, H. influenzae*) organisms may be the cause, indicating the intravenous use of combined therapy with drugs such as ampicillin with gentamicin (or amikacin), or ampicillin with cefotaxime (the combination favored by most pediatric infectious disease specialists), until results of cultures become available. In children, therapy is directed at the three most frequent pathogens: *H. influenzae, S. pneumoniae*, and *N. meningitidis*. The appearance of ampicillin resistance among strains of *H. influenzae* over two decades ago necessitated the shift from single-drug therapy (ampicillin) to a two-drug approach (ampicillin-chloramphenicol) in the treatment of meningitis of unknown cause in this age group, pending results of culture. Now, ceftriaxone (same dosage as for *H. influenzae* meningitis) or cefotaxime is routine therapy used in pediatric centers. *In adults* (Table 328–4), therapy with ampicillin in combination with a third-generation cephalosporin (cefotaxime or ceftriaxone) is employed. This is be-

cause of the role of *L. monocytogenes* (susceptible to ampicillin but not to third-generation cephalosporins) in meningitis of older adults and in previously noted high-risk groups, the emergence of infections due to intermediately penicillin-resistant pneumococci, and the increased frequency of aerobic gram-negative bacilli in nosocomial meningitis and meningitis in immunocompromised patients. In the penicillin-allergic individual, trimethoprim-sulfamethoxazole is a suitable alternative in the treatment of *Listeria* meningitis. In special settings (nosocomial meningitis or presence of endemic highly penicillin-resistant pneumococci) where more resistant species (resistant gram-negative bacilli, *S. aureus*, coagulase-negative staphylococci, or highly penicillin resistant *S. pneumoniae*) are likely to be involved, broader initial therapy (e.g., addition of vancomycin or substitution of ceftazidime for cefotaxime for enhanced coverage of *P. aeruginosa*) may be indicated.

DURATION OF THERAPY. The frequency of CSF examinations depends on the clinical course, but a repeat examination should be done in 24 to 48 hours if there has not been satisfactory improvement, or if the causative microorganism is a more resistant gram-negative bacillus or a highly penicillin- (or cephalosporin-) resistant *S. pneumoniae*.

Routine "end-of-treatment" CSF examination is unnecessary in most patients with the common types of community-acquired bacterial meningitis. Meningococci are rapidly eliminated from the circulation and CSF with appropriate antimicrobial therapy, which should be continued for 5 to 7 days after the patient becomes afebrile. If the patient has responded well, a follow-up lumbar puncture is not necessary. *H. influenzae* meningitis should be treated for 10 days (at least for 7 days after the patient becomes afebrile). Follow-up CSF examination may be omitted in those patients who have responded with rapid clinical resolution of the meningitis. In pneumococcal meningitis, antimicrobial treatment should be continued for 10 to 14 days and follow-up examination of the CSF should be done. More prolonged therapy is indicated with concomitant parameningeal infection. Meningitis due to *L. monocytogenes* should be treated for 14 to 21 days. Treatment of gram-negative bacillary meningitis with parenteral antimicrobials is prolonged, usually for a minimum of 3 weeks (particularly in patients with a recent neurosurgical procedure) to prevent relapse. Repeated examinations of the CSF are necessary both during and at the conclusion of treatment to determine whether bacteriologic cure has been achieved.

OTHER ASPECTS OF TREATMENT. Occasional patients with acute bacterial meningitis develop marked brain swelling (CSF pressure > 450 mm H_2O), which may lead to temporal lobe or cerebellar herniation after lumbar puncture. To decrease the possibility of this complication when the pressure is noted to be this high, only a small amount of CSF should be removed for analysis (the amount present in the manometer) and a 20% solution of mannitol (0.25 to 0.5 g/kg) infused intravenously over 20 to 30 minutes, monitoring (if possible) the decline of CSF pressure to a lower level before the spinal needle is removed. Continued control of increased intracranial pressure, if needed thereafter, may be effected with mannitol,

Table 328–3 ■ THERAPY FOR NOSOCOMIAL MENINGITIS OF KNOWN BACTERIAL CAUSE IN ADULTS

ORGANISM	THERAPY OF CHOICE (24-HR DOSE)*	ALTERNATIVE THERAPY (24-HR DOSE)
Staphylococcus aureus		
Methicillin susceptible	Nafcillin, 10–12 g IV, q4h aliquots; in difficult cases may add rifampin, 600 mg qd IV or PO	Vancomycin, 2 g IV, q8–12h aliquots†
Methicillin-resistant	Vancomycin, 2 g IV, q8–12h aliquots†; in difficult cases may add rifampin as above	
Enterobacteriaceae (susceptible)	Cefotaxime, 12 g IV, q4h aliquots or ceftazidime 6 g IV, q8h aliquots plus aminoglycoside (e.g., gentamicin 5 mg/kg IV, q8h aliquots)‡	Meropenem, 6 g IV, q8h aliquots plus an aminoglycoside IV
Pseudomonas aeruginosa	Ceftazidime, 6 g IV, q6–8h aliquots plus tobramycin, 5 mg/kg, q8h aliquots‡	Meropenem, 6 g IV, q8h aliquots plus tobramycin, 5 mg/kg IV, q8h aliquots‡

*All doses are for adults with normal renal function.

†Monitoring of peak and trough levels advisable; may need to monitor CSF levels if patient not responding well and, if levels are low, may need to increase daily dose temporarily by 0.5–1.0 g or add adjunctive intrathecal vancomycin.

‡If no response to initial therapy, consider adding intrathecal gentamicin (free of preservative), 3–5 mg dose q24h for next few days.

Table 328–4 ■ INITIAL THERAPY FOR COMMUNITY-ACQUIRED PURULENT MENINGITIS OF UNKNOWN CAUSE IN ADULTS

AGE	LIKELY PATHOGENS	PREFERRED DRUG	ALTERNATIVE DRUGS
Immunocompetent			
3 mo through 18 yr	S. pneumoniae, N. meningitidis, H. influenzae	Cefotaxime or ceftriaxone*	*Ampicillin plus chloramphenicol
18–50 yr	S. pneumoniae, N. meningitidis	Cefotaxime or ceftriaxone* ± ampicillin†	Vancomycin plus chloramphenicol
>50 yr	S. pneumoniae, N. meningitidis, L. monocytogenes	Cefotaxime or ceftriaxone* plus ampicillin	Cefotaxime* plus trimethoprim-sulfamethoxazole
Impaired cellular immunity	L. monocytogenes, gram-negative bacilli	Ampicillin plus ceftazidime	Trimethoprim-sulfamethoxozole plus meropenem or chloramphenicol
Cerebrospinal fluid leak, basilar skull fracture	S. pneumoniae, N. meningitidis, H. influenzae, various streptococci	Cefotaxime*	Vancomycin plus chloramphenicol

*When S. pneumoniae is suspected in communities where highly penicillin-resistant or cephalosporin-resistant S. pneumoniae have occurred (or are likely), vancomycin should be added.
†If clinical features suggest L. monocytogenase.

dexamethasone (10 mg intravenously, followed by 4 mg every 6 hours), or both. Brain swelling is about the only established current indication for the adjunctive use of corticosteroids in treating pyogenic meningitis in adults; they should be employed only when the appropriate antimicrobial drugs are administered. In the stuporous patient or one with respiratory insufficiency and markedly increased intracranial pressure, use of a ventilator to reduce the arterial Pco₂ to between 25 and 32 mm Hg is reasonable. Intubation should be carried out with minimal stimulation in the patient with increased intracranial pressure, because tracheal stimulation can produce an appreciable further rise in pressure. Possible adjuncts to facilitate intubation under such circumstances include use of succinylcholine, general anesthesia, or, if hemodynamic instability is present, narcotics. Subsequently, transient increases in intracranial pressure associated with hyperactive airway reflexes can be mitigated by intratracheal instillation of lidocaine before vigorous suctioning. With continued marked and fluctuating elevations of intracranial pressure, use of a continuous intracranial monitoring device may be warranted.

Initial hypovolemia or hypotension, if present, should be treated with fluid and to prevent significantly decreased cerebral blood flow. Over the next 24 to 48 hours in patients in whom inappropriate antidiuretic hormone secretion, sometimes associated with meningitis, is evident and may contribute to further brain swelling, fluid limitation (1200 to 1500 mL or adjusted replacement volumes daily in adults) is appropriate. One study in children with bacterial meningitis suggests that routine fluid restriction does not improve outcome and that the decrease in extracellular water that can ensue may increase the likelihood of a deleterious outcome.

Four prospective, controlled trials in children of the routine use of dexamethasone to reduce the pathophysiologic CNS consequences of the inflammatory response during bacterial meningitis have been performed. Dexamethasone was administered intravenously (either 0.15 mg/kg every 6 hours for 4 days or 0.4 mg/kg every 12 hours for 2 days) either at the time of or 10 to 20 minutes before initiating antimicrobial therapy (third-generation cephalosporin). Corticosteroid use had no effect on mortality but did reduce the incidence of neurologic sequelae (primarily bilateral sensorineural hearing loss). Complicating gastrointestinal bleeding (usually occult) has been observed rarely but merits caution. On the basis of these studies, by 1992 most pediatric infectious disease programs surveyed used dexamethasone in bacterial meningitis of children older than 2 months of age. Most of the children in the studies had H. influenzae meningitis, the most common type at the time, and the results reflect primarily the effects of dexamethasone on this form. Currently, H. influenzae meningitis has been sharply reduced in incidence by the use of protein-conjugate vaccines, but whether dexamethasone will have a similar effect in reducing neurologic sequelae of meningitis due to S. pneumoniae and N. meningitidis in children has not yet been established. Use of adjunctive dexamethasone in cases of severe H. influenzae meningitis in children seems indicated, but whether adjunctive corticosteroid use will have a similar salutary effect in reducing the incidence of sensorineural hearing loss or neurologic sequelae in adults, in whom S. pneumoniae is the leading cause, is not known and awaits results of a multicenter trial. As noted earlier, the presence of markedly

increased intracranial pressure is an indication for adjunctive corticosteroid use in adults (or children) with community-acquired meningitis due to a bacterial species for which bactericidal antimicrobial therapy is employed.

Patients with acute bacterial meningitis should receive constant nursing attention in an intensive-care unit to ensure prompt recognition of seizures and to prevent aspiration. If seizures occur, they should be treated acutely with diazepam (Valium) administered slowly intravenously in a dose of 5 to 10 mg in the adult. Maintenance anticonvulsant therapy can be continued thereafter with intravenous phenytoin (Dilantin) until the medication can be administered orally. Sedation should be avoided because of the danger of respiratory depression and aspiration.

Surgical treatment of an accompanying pyogenic focus such as mastoiditis should be carried out when complete recovery from the meningitis has occurred, but under continuing antibiotic administration. Rarely, the mastoid infection (e.g., Bezold's abscess) is so hyperacute that early drainage may be required after 48 hours or so of antibiotic therapy when the acute meningeal process has subsided somewhat.

Durand ML, Calderwood SB, Weber DJ, et al: Acute bacterial meningitis in adults: A review of 493 episodes. N Engl J Med 328:21, 1993. *A detailed review of an extensive experience in adults between 1962 and 1988 in a large urban general hospital. Community-acquired, nosocomial, and recurrent forms of bacterial meningitis are categorized; the bacteriologic, clinical, CSF, and neurologic findings are well described.*

McIntyre PB, Berkey CS, King SM, et al: Dexamethasone as adjunctive therapy in bacterial meningitis. JAMA 278:925, 1997. *This is a meta-analysis of all randomized clinical trials of adjunctive corticosteroid therapy for bacterial meningitis in children since 1988, confirming a reduction in severe sensorineural hearing loss or neurological sequelae in cases due to H. influenzae type b.*

Odio CM, Faingezicht I, Paris M, et al: The beneficial effects of early dexamethasone administration in infants and children with bacterial meningitis. N Engl J Med 324:1525, 1991. *This study showed that adjuvant dexamethasone treatment resulted in 12 hours in lowered CSF pressures and improved cerebral perfusion pressures and at follow-up, after 15 months, in decreased sensorineural hearing loss or neurologic sequelae.*

Pfister H-W, Feiden W, Einhaupl K-M: Spectrum of complications during bacterial meningitis in adults. Arch Neurol 50:575, 1993. *In this thorough prospective evaluation of 86 adults with bacterial meningitis, neurologic complications (cerebrovascular injury, brain swelling, cerebral herniation, hydrocephalus) are described. This study describes features helpful for identification of these complications and, particularly, their temporal relationships.*

Quagliariello VJ, Scheld WM: Bacterial meningitis: Pathogenesis, pathophysiology, and progress. N Engl J Med 327:864, 1992. *In this insightful and comprehensive review, particular attention is given to the role of bacterial components, cytokines and other mediators, and endothelial and leukocyte adhesins in the generation of the inflammatory response in the subarachnoid space.*

Quagliariello VJ, Scheld WM: Treatment of bacterial meningitis. N Engl J Med 336:708, 1997. *This is a concise but thorough, up-to-date consideration of treatment of bacterial meningitis, including the principles of antimicrobial therapy, empirical management, pathogen-specific therapy, newer drugs for antimicrobial resistant strains, and the role of glucocorticoid therapy.*

Schuchat A, Robinson K, Wenger JD, et al: Bacterial meningitis in the United States in 1995. N Engl J Med 337:970, 1997. *This is the most current summary of the causative agents of community-acquired bacterial meningitis in the United States, with data collected 5 years after H. influenzae type b conjugate vaccines were introduced. This survey documents the change in acute bacterial meningitis from a disease of childhood to one predominantly involving adults.*

Swartz MN, Dodge PR: Bacterial meningitis—A review of selected aspects. N Engl J Med 272:725, 1965. *Detailed account of Massachusetts General Hospital experience. Particularly good on clinical aspects, neurologic complications, and differential diagnosis.*

329 MENINGOCOCCAL INFECTIONS

Michael A. Apicella

Meningococcal infections are a major cause of mortality and morbidity in developed and developing nations. *Neisseria meningitidis* is the causative agent in meningococcal infections. It has become the most common cause of bacterial meningitis in American children since the use of the *Haemophilus influenzae* type b protein-capsular polysaccharide conjugate vaccine in infants dramatically reduced their incidence of meningitis due to this organism. Considerable progress has been made in the management and prevention of infections due to *Neisseria meningitidis* since the organism was first described in 1887. Because the meningococcal vaccine has limited effectiveness in the group at greatest risk to infection, children younger than the age of 2, meningococcal infection is still a major worldwide problem. The devastating nature of systemic meningococcal infection makes it imperative that preventive measures be developed to fully control this disease. In addition, an effective vaccine against meningococcal serogroup B infection has not been developed. Until this goal is realized, it is crucial that the clinician recognize and be able to successfully treat the infection as early as possible in its course to ensure an outcome with minimum mortality and morbidity.

MICROBIOLOGY AND PATHOGENESIS. *Neisseria meningitidis* is a gram-negative diplococcus. Meningococci are considered a fastidious species and media containing appropriate supplementation must be used to ensure reliable growth from clinical samples. The use of selective media such as Thayer-Martin media has allowed isolation of the organism from sites such as the nasopharynx that contain diverse background flora. The organism grows best between 35°, and 37° C in an atmosphere of 5% carbon dioxide. The organism will not grow below 32° C or above 41° C. Laboratory confirmation of the presence of the organism depends on the metabolism of glucose and maltose with the production of acid. Gas is not produced during this metabolic process.

The meningococcus has a very narrow environmental niche. It is a strict human pathogen that has only been isolated from human mucosal surfaces or body fluids. A number of factors contribute to the ability of the organism to colonize and cause infection. The meningococcus has a typical gram-negative cell wall containing lipopolysaccharide or endotoxin, which is the primary toxin of the meningococcus. Meningococci express pili (attachment organelles), which are important in adhesion to nasopharyngeal epithelial cells. Meningococci can express polysaccharide capsules. This is probably the most important virulence factor associated with this species. Thirteen serologically distinct encapsulated forms have been implicated in infection. Immunochemical differences in these capsules are the basis for the principal system used to serogroup encapsulated meningococci. Over 98% of cases are caused by five serogroups: A, B, C, W-135, and Y. Meningococci can be cultured that lack capsular polysaccharides. These are called non-encapsulated strains. Non-encapsulated meningococcal strains are frequently identified in nasopharyngeal cultures during screening in endemic periods. They have not been isolated from body fluids of patients with systemic meningococcal disease. In addition to serogrouping based on capsular antigens, meningococci can also be serotyped based on antigenic differences in their outer membrane proteins and lipopolysaccharides. These serotypes have become important in studies of the epidemiology of infection and in the development of new vaccines.

The molecular pathogenesis of meningococcal infection is now beginning to be understood. Figure 329–1A schematically outlines the process involved in mucosal invasion and Figure 329–1B details the factors associated with the generation of the shock state and disseminated intravascular coagulopathy. The pathogenesis of *N. meningitidis* begins on the nasopharyngeal surface. Colonization of this surface is absolutely necessary for the evolution to systemic infection. The only exceptions are the rare occurrences in which *N. meningitidis* is inoculated parenterally accidentally either in the laboratory or in the clinical setting. Infection of the nasopharynx occurs by inhalation of aerosolized particles containing meningo-

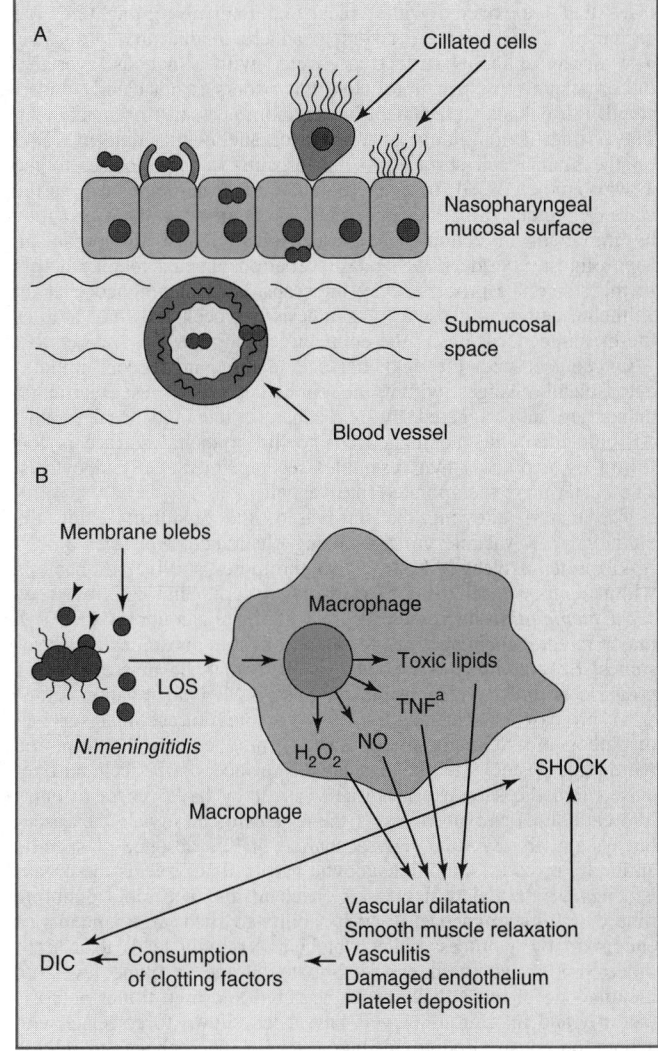

FIGURE 329–1. ■ *A,* A schematic representation of nasopharyngeal invasion by the meningococcus. The process involves attachment to surface of nonciliated cells by meningococcal pili. Short-range attachment factors (meningococcal surface components) are probably involved in the endocytotic engulfment process as microvilli of the nasopharyngeal cell surround the organism. The nonciliated cells through which the organisms transmigrate do not appear to sustain damage. By contrast, the ciliated mucosal cells die and are extruded from the mucosal surface. Meningococcal lipo-oligosaccharide, peptidoglycan, and possibly other toxins are thought to be responsible for this cytolytic activity. Organisms in the submucosal space then have access to entry into capillaries and arterioles and can invade the vascular system. (Data from Stephens DS: Gonococcal and meningococcal pathogenesis as defined by human cell, cell culture, and organ culture assays. Clin Microbiol Rev 2:S104, 1989.) *B,* The rapid doubling time of the meningococcus and its ability to shed large amounts of endotoxin by a process called "blebbing" rapidly lead to a high-grade septic state with shock. Endotoxin (lipo-oligosaccharide, or LOS) interacts with macrophages to release cytokines, vasoactive lipids (prostaglandins), and free radicals such as H_2O_2, O^-, and NO. These substances damage vascular endothelium, resulting in platelet deposition and vasculitis. This leads to vascular disruption and the petechiae and ecchymoses that are frequently seen during meningococcal infection. Clotting factors are consumed, and DIC ensues, which is an ominous consequence of delayed treatment. Occasionally, the intravascular clotting can lead to occlusion of major arterial vessels in the extremities, requiring amputation. The most dire consequence of all these vascular effects is Waterhouse-Friderichsen syndrome, which is multiorgan failure due to shock and hemorrhagic diathesis. (Data from Brandtzaeg P, Ovstebo R, Kierulf P: Compartmentalization of lipopolysaccharide production correlates with clinical presentation in meningococcal disease. J Infect Dis 166:650, 1992.)

cocci. The nasopharynx is a mixed epithelial surface containing ciliated, secretory and non-ciliated, non-secretory cells. There are lymphoid tissues associated with the nasopharynx in the form of adenoidal and tonsillar tissue. These structures have mucosal surfaces that are covered with typical upper airway epithelium. The organism uses adherence factors to adhere to this airway surface. The airway epithelial surface is covered with a mucous layer that the organism must penetrate. How this occurs is not clearly understood. Pili enhance attachment but are not necessary for attachment. The pili act as long-range attachment organelles that bind to CD46 on the human cell surface. As the organisms draws closer to the airway epithelial cell, outer membrane surface proteins such as the class V proteins (opa and opc) play a role in attachment and may be important in defining the tissue specificity of the organism. Lipo-oligosaccharide (LOS) phase variation appears to play a role in the adherence process. Only unencapsulated meningococci enter epithelial cells and capsular biosynthesis has been shown to stop as the meningococcus enters the epithelial cell.

On contact with the epithelial cell, the meningococcus initiates cytoskeletal changes within the epithelial cell. These rearrangements are not triggered by non-adherent meningococcal strains. Attachment of the meningococcus to the epithelial surface is followed by a process that resembles receptor-mediated endocytosis. The bacteria are incorporated into vacuoles.

The factors allowing the survival of the organism within the epithelial cell vacuole are now being elucidated. Neisseria type 2 IgA1 protease cleaves LAMP1 and promotes survival of bacteria within epithelial cells. Infection of human epithelial cells by *Neisseria meningitidis* increases the rate of degradation of LAMP1, a major integral membrane glycoprotein of late endosomes and lysosomes. Several lines of evidence indicate that the neisserial IgA1 protease is directly responsible for this LAMP1 degradation. Thus, IgA1 protease cleavage of LAMP1 promotes intracellular survival of pathogenic Neisseria species. The meningococcus is transported within the vacuole to the basolateral surface of the cell and released into the submucosal space where they have access to entry into capillaries and arterioles. If the organism can invade the vascular system, the capsular polysaccharide, in the absence of specific antibody, provides an antiphagocytic barrier that protects the organism against normal host clearing mechanisms. The rapid doubling time of the meningococcus and its ability to shed large amounts of endotoxin by a process called "blebbing" rapidly leads to a high-grade septic state with shock. Endotoxin and cytokine levels in meningococcal sepsis have been measured and high tumor necrosis factor-α and interferon-γ levels have been shown to correlate with a poor prognosis. Endotoxin interacts with macrophages to release cytokines, vasoactive lipids, and free radicals such as H_2O_2, O^-, and NO. These substances damage vascular endothelium, resulting in platelet deposition and vasculitis. This leads to vascular disruption and the petechiae and ecchymoses that are frequently seen during meningococcal infection. This is responsible for consumption of clotting factors and disseminated intravascular coagulopathies, which are an ominous consequence of delayed treatment. Occasionally, the intravascular clotting can lead to occlusion of major arterial vessels in the extremities, necessitating amputation. The most dire consequence of all of these vascular effects is Waterhouse-Friderichsen syndrome, which is multiorgan failure due to shock and hemorrhagic diathesis.

The propensity of the meningococcus to invade the central nervous system and cause meningitis is poorly understood. The organism probably gains entry through the arachnoid villi. The release of endotoxin and peptidoglycan in the cerebrospinal fluid evokes inflammatory factors that are chemoattractive for polymorphonuclear leukocytes (PMNs). Enzymes released by PMNs intensify the meningeal inflammation, leading to increased cerebrovascular permeability and brain edema.

EPIDEMIOLOGY. *N. meningitidis* can cause endemic and epidemic infection. At the present time, meningococcal infection is endemic in the United States, with approximately 2,500 cases per year reported to the Centers for Disease Control and Prevention. This gives a case rate of approximately 1 in 10^5 total population. The case-fatality rate is approximately 12%. Disease rates in children younger than age 2 are approximately 10 times higher than the overall population. Seasonal variation occurs, with the highest

attack rates in February and March and the lowest in September. The male:female patient ratio is approximately equal. The predominate serogroups causing infection in the United States currently are serogroups B and C.

The epidemic form of meningococcal disease was first described in medical journals in Geneva in 1807, eighty years before the causative organism was identified by Weichselbaum. Before World War II, periodic epidemics of meningococcal infection ravaged American cities. These were caused primarily by the serogroup A meningococcus. With increasing standards of living, these epidemics have abated in this country and infection due to the serogroup A has virtually disappeared.

Large-scale epidemics still occur with a deadly frequency in Africa, parts of Asia, South America, and the countries of the former Soviet Union. These epidemics are most commonly caused by serogroup A meningococcus and occasionally by the serogroup C meningococcus. In an area appropriately named "the meningitis belt," because it crosses the waist of sub-Saharan Africa, epidemics of meningococcal infection occur every 7 to 10 years. The case rate during these epidemics can be as high as 1 in 1000 total population. Case rates in children younger than age 2 can be 1 in 100. In one epidemic in Nairobi, Kenya, which is outside of "meningitis belt," the attack rate was 2.5 cases per 10,000 population. Areas that included Nairobi's largest slums had a particularly high attack rate. This epidemic displayed an unusual age distribution, with high attack rates among the 20- to 29-year olds. The case-fatality rate was approximately 10%. Studies of the genetics of the organism causing this epidemic indicate that it was clonally related to group A strains causing epidemics in other parts of Africa. This suggests that these epidemics are caused by a particularly virulent clone of group A *N. meningitidis*. In the developed nations of Western Europe, epidemics due to serogroup B meningococcus have occurred over the past decade. Norway suffered such an epidemic with case rates of 1 in 10,000 individuals. A high attack rate was seen among teenagers in this epidemic.

The reason for the epidemic spread of the meningococcus is not known. The organism is considered a respiratory pathogen, and spread is most likely by the aerosol route. It is clear that the high attack rates seen in the less well-developed countries is in part due to poverty and the consequences of crowding, poor sanitation, and malnutrition. Factors such as herd immunity and specific virulence factors associated with "epidemic strains" have been implicated as factors in the rapid spread of infection in these situations. From studies of a recent epidemic in central and east Africa, clonal analysis indicated that the epidemic strain had arisen in central Asia almost 7 years before the African epidemic. It had spread through Northern India and Pakistan to Saudi Arabia and then with pilgrims from Mecca to Africa. A number of American pilgrims returning from Mecca at that time were found to have nasopharynx colonization with this epidemic strain.

Predisposition to meningococcal infection has been associated with preceding respiratory tract infection, particularly influenza. In one study of an epidemic limited to American schoolchildren traveling on the same school bus, it was shown that school absenteeism was higher during the 3 weeks before the outbreak than in any time in the preceding 3 years. This suggests a particularly severe outbreak of respiratory illness. The five children who developed meningococcal sepsis all complained of influenza-like symptoms before development of meningococcal disease. Based on serologic analysis, a case-control study revealed that children in this population who complained of respiratory tract symptoms had B/Ann Arbor1/86 influenzae. These data add to evidence suggesting that influenzal respiratory infection predisposes to meningococcal disease.

Epidemic infections in American military recruit camps were a major problem before the introduction of vaccination. Throughout the 19th century, the unique susceptibility of military recruits can be attested to by the clinical descriptions of this infection that can be found in the records of the Crimean and American civil wars. Since introduction of vaccination of all recruits in 1972 with a tetravalent vaccine containing serogroup A, C, Y and W-135 polysaccharides, epidemics have not occurred.

Intimate contacts of cases, including family members, college roommates, and nursery school classmates, are at 100- to 1000-fold increased risk of acquiring meningococcal infection. Such individuals should be told about the increased risk and monitored closely for emergence of co-primary cases (cases that arise within 48 hours of the primary case) and give chemoprophylaxis (see section on treatment later) to prevent secondary cases of infection. Hospital personnel who care for patients with meningococcal disease are not at increased risk of acquisition of infection. Exceptions would include individuals who suffer needle sticks contaminated with body fluids from untreated patients and health care personnel who give mouth-to-mouth resuscitation to individuals with meningococcal infections. It may be wise to manage such individuals with parenteral therapy as cases rather than use chemoprophylaxis. Isolation of patients in hospitals is a common practice. It can be limited to respiratory isolation and terminated 24 hours after institution of appropriate antibiotic therapy.

CLINICAL SYNDROMES. THE CARRIER STATE. There are several different meningococcal infection syndromes. In the early 20th century, the ability to isolate meningococci from the nasopharynx of otherwise healthy individuals led to the concept of asymptomatic carriage of bacterial pathogens. The observation that increased carriage rates coincided with onset of epidemic among military recruits during World War I first linked the relationship of the carrier state to disease. The nasopharyngeal carrier state is considered an active infection because some individuals have symptomatic pharyngitis and develop rises in serologic titers to the infecting organism. It is considered that all cases of acute systemic meningococcal infection are preceded by recent nasopharyngeal colonization. Studies have shown that the carrier state can persist for long periods of time, with about 5% of the population carrying the meningococcus in their nasopharynx during endemic periods. The majority of these isolates are unencapsulated. During epidemics, the carrier rate can rise to over 30% of the population, with the majority of individuals carrying the epidemic strains in their nasopharynx. Generally, most individuals who become carriers are asymptomatic. Evidence exists that the systemic immune system is primed during the period of nasopharyngeal carriage because antibodies to the infecting strains can be shown to evolve concordant with colonization.

In a study of an epidemic among military recruits, it has been shown that nasopharyngeal colonization by the meningococcal strain responsible for the epidemic resulted in a 40% incidence of systemic infection if the person colonized also lacked bactericidal antibodies to the epidemic strain. This study confirmed the role of nasopharyngeal carriage as the source of systemic infection and importance of serum antibody in protection against systemic meningococcal infection.

MENINGITIS AND MENINGOCOCCEMIA. Acute systemic infection can be manifest clinically by three syndromes: meningitis, meningitis with meningococcemia, and meningococcemia without obvious signs of meningitis. Typically, an otherwise healthy patient develops sudden onset of fever, nausea, vomiting, headache, decreased ability to concentrate, and myalgia. The patient will frequently tell the physician that this is the sickest he or she has ever felt. Many have an impending feeling of death. In children, the infection is rare in those younger than age 6 months because of protection from placentally transferred antibodies. Because children younger than age 2 cannot relate many symptoms, sudden onset of fever, leukocytosis, and lethargy become important findings. Initially, the physical examination may be unrevealing, with the exception of an acutely ill patient. The preceding symptoms of pharyngitis that may be associated with nasopharyngeal carriage can lead to a preliminary diagnosis of streptococcal infection. This frequently results in treatment with low-dose penicillin, which has little effect on the emerging meningococcal sepsis. Alternatively, the diagnosis of influenza is assigned to the patient because of complaints of fever, chills, and myalgia. In general, patients with meningococcal infection present considerably sicker than the majority of patients with streptococcal or viral infections. The vital signs will show a low blood pressure with an elevated pulse rate. Diaphoresis is common. In such patients, an intensive search for petechiae should be mounted (Color Plate 8A). A complete examination of the skin with the patient completely undressed is essential. The physical examination should include provocative tests of meningeal irritability, the Kernig and Brudzinski signs. It must be remembered that patients with meningococcemia may not necessarily have meningeal signs, but from 50 to 80% will have petechiae on presentation. An examination of the mucosal surfaces of the soft palate and ocular and palpabral conjunctiva for petechiae must be done.

The infection can progress rapidly. Depending on the presenta-

tion of the patient, a critical situation can occur very quickly. Profound shock with a disseminated intravascular coagulopathy is the most ominous development in these patients. Coagulopathy defined as a partial thromboplastin time of more than 50 seconds or a fibrinogen concentration of more than 150 μg/dl is an excellent predictor of poor prognosis. A number of studies have demonstrated that myocardial dysfunction can occur in meningococcal sepsis. Signs of heart failure including gallop rhythms and congestive heart failure with pulmonary edema are not uncommon. In one large series, 15% of pediatric patients were admitted to intensive-care units because of cardiovascular manifestations. Approximately 25% of patients who died of meningococcal sepsis have evidence of myocarditis. Studies in France of a group of severely ill patients with meningococcal sepsis showed low stroke volume indices (29 mL/m^2) and tachycardia ($>$ 135 beats per minute), a profile suggesting a greater myocardial depression than usually observed in gram-negative sepsis. In infection due to meningococcal serogroup C, pericarditis with tamponade can seriously complicate the course of treatment unless recognized and managed. When disseminated intravascular dissemination occurs, persistent bleeding at intravenous sites and sites of arterial punctures can complicate management of the tamponade.

Neurologic complications include signs of meningeal irritation, an encephalopathic state, and coma. Seizures can occur but are less common than other forms of bacterial meningitis. In general, patients surviving meningococcal central nervous system infection have remarkably few sequelae, but cerebrovascular accidents secondary to intracranial bleeding can lead to paresis. Cases of posterior pituitary insufficiency have been reported in patients recovering from meningococcal infection.

Prognosis can vary depending on the presentation of the patient, the skill and completeness of the physician, and the nature of the facility. At tertiary care hospitals during endemic periods of infection, mortalities as low as 8% have been reported. Patients who present with meningococcemia alone tend to have a higher mortality (up to 20%). During World War II, meningococcal mortality rates using sulfonamides were as low as 2%. Many of these patients were hospitalized and treated as soon as symptoms began. Recent studies in Norway and Africa have supported the concept that early onset of therapy significantly reduces mortality.

LABORATORY DIAGNOSIS. The laboratory diagnosis is based on the isolation of the *N. meningitidis* from blood cultures or cerebrospinal fluid. Blood cultures will be positive in 60 to 80% of untreated patients, whereas cerebrospinal fluid (CSF) cultures will be positive in 50 to 70%. Gram stain analysis of CSF requires a skilled patient observer, but it can provide diagnostic results rapidly. Gram stain of the CSF can be useful as a rapid diagnostic tool especially in patients with meningococcal meningitis. Approximately 50% of these patients will have a positive Gram stain. In cases of meningococcemia without overt meningitis, the CSF Gram stain will be positive in less than 25% of patients. Studies have suggested that Gram stain analysis of punch biopsy or needle aspiration of hemorrhagic skin lesions in meningococcal sepsis without clinical evidence of meningitis can lead to rapid diagnosis. In this study, approximately 70% of such skin lesions were positive. The tinctorial results for punch biopsy specimens were not affected by antibiotics because Gram staining gave positive results up to 45 hours after the start of antibiotic therapy. Cultures of these biopsies or aspirates were also useful diagnostically for as long as 13 hours after the institution of antibiotic therapy. Detection of meningococcal capsular polysaccharide in CSF can also be used as a method for rapid diagnosis. The test is most sensitive for the A and C polysaccharides and considerably less sensitive for serogroup B polysaccharide. In meningococcemia without clinically apparent meningitis, the antigen detection methods can be negative despite profound sepsis. Polymerase chain reaction has been demonstrated as a potentially rapid method for making the diagnosis of CSF infection. Further testing must be done to confirm the specificity and sensitivity of this technique.

TREATMENT OF SYSTEMIC MENINGOCOCCAL INFECTION. In 1933, sulfonamides revolutionized the treatment of meningococcal infection. Before antibiotics, almost all cases resulted in death or profound morbidity with complications. Early administration of appropriate antibiotics is the cornerstone of successful management.

As soon as the practitioner seriously considers the diagnosis of systemic meningococcal infection, institution of therapy must follow within 30 minutes. The patient must be considered a medical emergency. Through organization and documentation of patient management is crucial. Blood cultures should be drawn immediately, an intravenous line established, and penicillin G (chloramphenicol can be used in penicillin-allergic patients) infused over 15 minutes (Table 329–1). There is no evidence that release of endotoxin that may occur after antibiotic administration adversely effects outcome. This should not be a reason to delay onset of therapy. Antibiotic administration should not be delayed while waiting for the spinal tap to be done. If the spinal tap is obtained within 45 minutes of the antibiotics there will be limited reduction in positive CSF cultures and no modification of the CSF cytology or hypoglycorrhachia. In two studies in Great Britain, it has been shown that the administration, before hospitalization, of high-dose penicillin to patients suspected of having meningococcal infection greatly reduced morbidity and mortality.

Patients with meningococcal sepsis frequently have multisystem involvement. If the patient is not at a tertiary care hospital, consideration should be given to transferring the stabilized patient to such a facility. The patient should be cared for in an intensive-care situation with continuous monitoring and careful management of fluids and electrolytes. Because of fluid loss due to fever and the increased vascular permeability, fluids, electrolytes, and colloid should be administered and blood pressure, urine output, and cardiac function monitored. A number of studies indicate that meningococcal sepsis is associated with cardiac failure; thus, attention must be paid to cardiac status during the sepsis and shock state. Treatment of heart failure may be indicated. Vasoactive agents such as dopamine may be necessary to maintain blood pressure and tissue perfusion. Since disseminated intravascular coagulopathies occur frequently, monitoring of clotting parameters such as platelets, fibrin, and fibrin-split products is a crucial part of management. Correction of this problem is a key to survival and reduced morbidity and may require the advice of one skilled in management of bleeding disorders. Studies have shown that the use of fresh frozen plasma may negatively influence outcome in systemic meningococcal. Careful consideration should be give before the administration of such products to these patients. Studies have suggested that exchange transfusion may improve the survival rate among patients with fulminant meningococcal sepsis. The beneficial effect is most likely not based on the elimination of endotoxin. Very promising results have been obtained in patients with meningococcal sepsis using a truncated version of recombinantly produced bactericidal/permeability protein (rBPI). This product is undergoing patient testing and is not available for general use. One of the most serious causes of morbidity in fulminant meningococcal sepsis is skin necrosis and loss of distal digits and limbs. Epidural sympathetic blockade may prove useful in preserving the lower extremities of such patients. Skin necrosis can be managed by debridement, grafting, and nutritional support after the patient's condition has been stabilized.

In the early 1950s, penicillin became the drug of choice for treatment of systemic meningococcal infections. It has remained the cornerstone of therapy since that time. The meningococcus is sensitive to a wide range of antibiotics, including third-generation cephalosporins and quinolones. Ampicillin is equivalent to penicillin G and can be used if there is uncertainty about the etiologic diagnosis at the time that therapy is instituted. Reports from southern Europe (primarily Spain and Greece) of the isolation of penicillin-resistant meningococci could have ominous consequences if epidemics occur due to these organisms. In Spain, the prevalence of *N. meningitidis*

Table 329–1 ■ ANTIBIOTIC MANAGEMENT OF SYSTEMIC MENINGOCOCCAL INFECTION

ANTIBIOTIC	DOSE
Penicillin G	300,000 units/kg/day IV, up to 24 million units/day
Ampicillin	150–200 mg/kg/day IV, up to 12 g/day
Ceftriaxon	2 g/day IV
Chloramphenicol	For use in penicillin-allergic patients, 100 mg/kg day IV, up to 4 g/day

isolates that are moderately susceptible to penicillin and ampicillin has increased to almost 50% of isolates. These strains do not produce β-lactamase. In these strains, the basis of meningococcal resistance to penicillin are alterations in a group of inner membrane enzymes, the penicillin-binding proteins (PBPs), which are responsible for cell wall synthesis. Specifically, alterations in the PBP-2 result in decreased binding affinity of penicillin and ampicillin to these enzymes. Third-generation cephalosporins are usually effective against organisms, which are resistant on this basis. However, careful antibiotic sensitivity testing should be performed to ensure that this is the case because some third-generation cephalosporins may also not bind efficiently to these modified penicillin-binding proteins. Studies have demonstrated that disc diffusion methods can still be used to analyze such strains, although plate dilution methods are preferred. Sulfonamide-resistant meningococci are still common in the United States; hence, sulfonamides should not be used in treatment of acute infections.

COMPLEMENT DEFICIENCY AND MENINGOCOCCAL SEPSIS. Individuals with deficiencies in complement components appear to be uniquely susceptible to meningococcal infection. In properdin-deficient patients, fulminant meningococcal sepsis is a frequent cause of death. Families of such individuals should be investigated for history of sudden septic death in relatives. Such families should be managed closely and undergo vaccination with the tetravalent meningococcal vaccine.

In patients with the late complement component-deficiencies (LCCD), meningococcal infection occurs in older individuals (mean age, 17 years) and tends to be milder (mortality ∼ 2%) and caused by less common serogroups (serogroup Y and W135) then occurs in the general population. LCCD patients respond normally to meningococcal capsular polysaccharide vaccine with the development of antibodies that are functional in both complement-dependent bactericidal assays and opsonophagocytic assays. These patients have a more rapid decline in capsular antibody than that which is seen in normal individuals. These studies suggest that LCCD patients are critically dependent on capsular antibody for protection against meningococcal disease. Vaccination, probably on a recurrent basis, is an important component in the prevention of meningococcal disease in LCCD patients.

OTHER CLINICAL SYNDROMES. CHRONIC MENINGOCOCCEMIA. Chronic meningococcal sepsis, which is indistinguishable from the gonococcal dermatitis-arthritis syndrome, can occur. These patients have typical painful skin lesions usually on the extremities with migratory polyarthritis and tenosynovitis. This form of meningococcal sepsis can persist for weeks if untreated. This syndrome responds promptly to antibiotic therapy.

RESPIRATORY TRACT INFECTION. Pneumonia due to *N. meningitidis* has been reported since the 1930s. In one study of community-acquired infections in Finland, *N. meningitis* was implicated as the etiologic agent in 6%. Epidemic pneumonia due to serogroup Y strains has occurred at a military training center. The patients presented with chills, chest pain, and cough. Rales and fever occurred in almost all patients. Infections in these men were frequently multilobar (40%). The incidence of sepsis associated with these infections is quite low, and the diagnosis is usually made with transtracheal aspirations. There was no mortality in these patients, and all responded well to treatment with penicillin.

MENINGOCOCCAL PERICARDITIS. Pericarditis is usually associated with infections due to *N. meningitidis* serogroup C. It has been associated with meningococcemia and reported as an isolated syndrome. Patients can present with chest pain and signs of tamponade, but relatively asymptomatic disease can occur with detection made by ultrasonography. Treatment with antibiotics and removal of the pericardial fluid usually results in a successful outcome. Pericarditis can occur in patients convalescing from meningococcal sepsis. It should be considered if fever and shortness of breath on minimal exertion occur when the patient is recovering from meningococcal sepsis. Echocardiogram will result in rapid diagnosis of this complication of infection. In convalescent patients, antibiotic therapy should be continued and pericardiocentesis may be indicated. There is no evidence that corticosteroids or anti-inflammatory agents have a role in management.

MENINGOCOCCAL URETHRITIS. Meningococci have been isolated from the urethra and can cause clinical urethritis. In one study of more than 5,000 urethral cultures from homosexual men, the isolation rate was 0.2% compared with 4.7% for *N. gonorrhoeae* among the same population. Eight of these patients had symptomatic urethritis. In the same study, there were no isolates among almost 9,000 urethral cultures from heterosexual males or almost 16,000 cervical cultures. This study strongly suggested that there is an association between orogenital sex and urethral acquisition of the meningococcus. Meningococcal urethritis has been managed successfully with penicillin and/or tetracycline therapy.

CHEMOPROPHYLAXIS. The observation that sulfonamides could clear the nasopharynx carriage of meningococci for weeks after a single day of therapy, led to the concept of chemoprophylaxis for prevention of secondary infection in hyperepidemic situations. During World War II, using carrier rates as a forecaster of epidemics among recruits, military public health officials were able to abort serious epidemics among military trainees. Because of the profligate use of sulfonamides for chemoprophylaxis in the 1950s, the meningococcus developed resistance to these agents; and, in 1963, epidemics were occurring on military bases as the Vietnam military buildup was occurring. These organisms were universally resistant to sulfonamides. This led to intensive research by the U.S. Army on vaccines for disease prevention and new agents for chemoprophylaxis. These studies resulted in an effective anticapsular vaccine in 1970 and the application of minocycline and rifampin for chemoprophylaxis. Eradication of the carrier state in intimate contacts of index cases with chemoprophylaxis is an effective way to prevent secondary cases. The concept behind successful prophylaxis is the use of short-term antibiotic therapy (1 to 2 doses) to achieve long-term (3- to 4-week) eradication of the meningococcus from the nasopharynx. Although physicians realize that prophylaxis is necessary, they fail to appreciate that specific antibiotics must be used for effective management. Penicillin, penicillin derivatives, and first- and second-generation cephalosporins are not effective for prophylaxis because eradication of the meningococcus is not achieved during the short courses of therapy used. Rifampin and ceftriaxone have been shown to be effective agents for prophylaxis (Table 329–2). Quinoline derivatives have also been shown to be effective for chemoprophylaxis.

PREVENTION. The immunologically different meningococcal serogroups were identified in the early 20th century. This observation led to the use of capsular-specific serotherapy for the management of meningococcal infection before the development of effective chemotherapy. The ability of the meningococcal capsular polysaccharides to evoke a protective immune response is the basis for the meningococcal vaccines. An effective tetravalent capsular polysaccharide vaccine (containing A, C, Y and W135 polysaccharide) is available for the prevention of meningococcal infections in individuals older than age 2. Over 100 million doses of this vaccine have been given worldwide with no serious side effects reported. Tetravalent vaccine should be administered to all intimate contacts of index cases at the start of chemoprophylaxis. This vaccine has also been used effectively in the U.S. military and in aborting epidemics caused by serogroup strains represented in the vaccine. A principal drawback of the vaccine is the lack of immunogenicity in children younger than age 2. This has limited widespread application of the current vaccine in countries with recurrent epidemic infections.

Children younger than age 2 respond poorly to polysaccharides for reasons that are not clearly understood. Recent successes in vaccinating young children with *Haemophilus influenzae* polysaccharide conjugated to proteins suggest that a similar strategy might be useful for meningococcal polysaccharides. Such a vaccine is not currently available.

In addition, the lack of an antigen capable of eliciting protection against meningococcal serogroup B infection has limited use of the vaccine. The serogroup B polysaccharide is a poor immunogen even in adults perhaps because it resembles self-antigens. Vaccine development in serogroup B strains has focused on other meningococcal subcapsular surface antigens (proteins and possibly lipopolysaccharide). These vaccines are based on serotypical protein antigens, and the vaccine must be tailored to the serotype of the specific meningococcal strain causing the epidemic. A recent noncapsular serogroup B vaccine has been tested in an epidemic in Brazil, and the results indicate that there was vaccine efficacy in children older than the age of 2.

Apicella MA: *Neisseria meningitidis. In* Mandell GL, Douglas RG, Bennett, JE (eds): Principles and Practices of Infectious Diseases. New York, Churchill Livingstone, 1995, pp 1896–1908. *Complete description of the biology and pathogenesis of* N. meningitidis *infection.*

Control and prevention of meningococcal disease and control and prevention of serogroup C meningococcal diseases: Evaluation and management of suspected outbreaks. MMWR 46:(RR-5) 1–22, 1997. *CDC recommendations for management of meningococcal infections in the community.*

Durand ML, Calderwood SB, Weber DJ, et al: Acute bacterial meningitis in adults. N Engl J Med 328:21–28, 1993. *Recent review of bacterial meningitis in an American hospital.*

Giriorr BP, Quint PA, Barton P, et al: Preliminary evaluation of recombinant amino-terminal fragment of human bactericidal/permeability-increasing protein in children with severe meningococcal sepsis. Lancet 350:1439–1443, 1997. *Study of the use of rBPI to inactivate endotoxin in severely ill patients with meningococcal sepsis.*

Meningococcal disease: Prevention and control strategies for the practice-based physician. Pediatrics 404–412, 1996. *Recommendations from the American Academy of Pediatrics on management of meningococcal infections.*

Schwartz B: Chemoprophylaxis for bacterial infections: Principles of and application to meningococcal infection. Rev Infect Dis 13(Suppl 2):S170–173, 1991. *Review of the concepts and strategies in chemoprophylaxis of meningococcal infection. Studies validate the use of ceftriaxone as an agent for chemoprophylaxis.*

Schwartz B, Moore P, Broome CV: Global epidemiology of meningococcal disease. Clin Rev Microbiol 2:S118–124, 1989. *Review of the international scope of meningococcal infection.*

Table 329–2 ■ CHEMOPROPHYLAXIS AND IMMUNOPROPHYLAXIS FOR PREVENTION OF MENINGOCOCCAL INFECTION

CHEMOPROPHYLAXIS

Antibiotic	Dose
Rifampin	Adults who are not pregnant, 600 mg po q12h for 2 days. Children >1 mo 5mg/kg po, <1 mo 10 mg/kg po q12h for 2 days
Ceftriaxone	Single 250 mg IM dose for adults, single 125 mg IM dose for children <15 years of age
Ciprofloxacin	Adults who are not pregnant, 500 mg as a single PO dose. Limited experience in children <18 and should not be used if other alternatives

Immunoprophylaxis

Monovalent A, monovalent C, bivalent A-C or quadrivalent A, C, Y and W-135 vaccine is administered once by volume according to manufacturer. Amount of polysaccharide delivered is usually 50 µg. Vaccination should be considered on adjunct to antibiotic chemoprophylaxis for household or intimate contacts of meningococcal disease cases when appropriate serogroups are causing disease.

330 INFECTIONS CAUSED BY HAEMOPHILUS SPECIES

Michael S. Simberkoff

DEFINITION. The name *Haemophilus* is derived from the Greek nouns *haima,* meaning "blood," and *philos,* meaning "lover." *Haemophilus* species primarily infect the respiratory tract, skin, or mucous membranes of humans. From these sites, organisms can invade to cause bacteremia, meningitis, epiglottitis, endocarditis, septic arthritis, or cellulitis.

MICROBIOLOGY. The *Haemophilus* species are small, non-motile, aerobic or facultative anaerobic, pleomorphic, gram-negative bacilli. The prototype of this genus, *H. influenzae,* was originally recovered from patients with influenza by Pfeiffer in 1893, and it was considered the cause of that disease for many years. The growth requirements of important *Haemophilus* species are summarized in Table 330–1. Primary isolation of *Haemophilus* species is best accomplished on chocolate agar medium in a CO_2-enriched atmosphere.

INFECTIONS CAUSED BY *H. INFLUENZAE*. GENERAL CONSIDERATIONS AND LABORATORY CHARACTERIZATION. *H. influenzae* is the most important pathogen in this genus. It can be recovered from sites where it colonizes, such as the nasopharynx and upper respiratory tract, and from sites where it causes disease, such as the blood, cerebrospinal fluid (CSF), sputum, pleura, middle ear, female genital tract, and joints (Table 330–2).

H. influenzae consists of encapsulated (typable) and non-encapsu

Table 330–1 ■ GROWTH REQUIREMENTS AND HEMOLYTIC PROPERTIES OF *HAEMOPHILUS* SPECIES

SPECIES	X	V	CO$_2$	HEMOLYSIS
H. influenzae	+	+	–	–
H. influenzae, b. *aegyptius*	+	+	–	–
H. parainfluenzae	–	+	–	–
H. aphrophilus	+*	–	+	–
H. paraphrophilus	–	+	+	–
H. haemolyticus	+	+	–	+
H. parahaemolyticus	–	+	–	+
H. ducreyi	+	–	–	+†

*Hematin needed for primary isolation.
†Delayed hemolysis occurs in 11 to 89% of strains.

lated (non-typable) strains. The former are responsible for most of the invasive infections in children and acute epiglottitis in both children and adults, whereas the latter cause respiratory mucosal infections, including otitis media, sinusitis, exacerbations of chronic bronchitis, and pneumonia; conjunctivitis; female genital tract infections; as well as invasive disease in adults. The capsules of *H. influenzae* consist of polysaccharide antigens. Six capsular serotypes (a through f) exist in the species.

FACTORS AFFECTING VIRULENCE. The capsules of *H. influenzae* are important virulence factors that inhibit opsonization, clearance, and intracellular killing of the organisms. *H. influenzae* type b, formerly the most common cause of meningitis in infancy and childhood worldwide, contains a pentose capsular polysaccharide consisting of polyribosyl-ribitol phosphate (PRP). Other serotypes contain hexose polysaccharides. It is believed that *H. influenzae* type b is more virulent than other serotypes because it is highly resistant to clearance once bacteremia has been initiated.

Fimbriae are important virulence factors that enhance the adherence of *H. influenzae* to mucosal surfaces. Both typable and non-typable *H. influenzae* isolates contain fimbriae. The lipo-oligosaccharides (LOSs) of *H. influenzae* also contribute to their virulence. LOSs appear to play a crucial role in facilitating the survival of *H. influenzae* on mucosal surfaces within the nasopharynx and in initiating invasive disease (blood stream invasion) from these sites.

Outer membrane proteins (OMPs) also serve as virulence factors in *H. influenzae* disease. At least 15 different *H. influenzae* OMPs have been identified. One of these (P2, 39 to 40 kd) functions as a porin, and others are associated with iron binding. Successful scavenging of iron within the human host is crucial for *H. influenzae* to multiply.

HOST DEFENSES. Antibodies have been recognized for decades as an important part of the host defenses against *H. influenzae* diseases. The classic studies of Fothergill and Wright, in 1933, demonstrated that most cases of *H. influenzae* meningitis occurred in children during the ages between their losing passively acquired maternal antibodies and developing active humoral immunity to the organism. It is now recognized that these protective antibodies function primarily to opsonize and facilitate *H. influenzae* clearance rather than to directly kill virulent organisms.

Complement is also an essential component of the host defenses against some *H. influenzae* diseases. Children with congenital deficiencies of C2, C3, and Factor I have an increased incidence of *H. influenzae* infections. Patients who lack a functional spleen or who have undergone splenectomy also are at risk for developing overwhelming infection with *H. influenzae* type b.

PREVALENCE, INCIDENCE, AND EPIDEMIOLOGY. The precise prevalence and incidence of *H. influenzae* infections are unknown. This organism can be detected frequently in the nasopharynx of both children and adults. Between 3 and 5% of infants harbor *H. influenzae* type b in their nasopharynx. Non-typable *H. influenzae* can be detected in the nasopharyngeal culture of more than 70% of young children. Infections, however, occur in only a small fraction of colonized patients. The risk of infection in non-immune household contacts of a patient with invasive *H. influenzae* disease is approximately 600-fold greater than the risk in the age-adjusted general population.

H. influenzae type b was the most common cause of meningitis in young children before effective vaccines were introduced in the 1980s. Vaccination dramatically reduced the incidence of this infection in young children. In a population-based study in Atlanta, over a 1-year period, invasive *H. influenzae* disease occurred in only 5.6 per 100,000 children and 1.7 per 100,000 adults. Forty of the 47 strains associated with invasive disease from adult patients in this study were serotyped. Twenty of these isolates (50%) were *H. influenzae* type b, 19 (47.5%) were non-typable, and 1 (2.5%) was a type f.

Patients with human immunodeficiency virus (HIV) infection are at increased risk for *H. influenzae* infection. Rates of invasive *H. influenzae* infection among men aged 20 to 49 with HIV infection and the acquired immunodeficiency syndrome (AIDS) were 14.6 and 79.2 per 100,000, respectively. The majority of these infections were caused by non-typable *H. influenzae* strains, although in a second study, 10 of 15 bacteremic *H. influenzae* type b infections observed in adults occurred in patients at risk for HIV infection, and AIDS was documented in 7 of these patients.

Other factors also increase the risk of *H. influenzae* infections. These include globulin deficiencies, sickle cell disease, splenectomy, malignancy, pregnancy, CSF leaks, head trauma, alcoholism, and race. Eskimo, Navajo, and Apache children have *H. influenzae* type b infection rates that are significantly greater than those in comparable non-native populations. In addition, day-care attendance, crowding, presence of siblings, previous hospitalizations, and previous otitis media have been shown to increase the risk of *H. influenzae* type b disease in young children, whereas breast feeding decreases this risk.

PATHOGENESIS. *H. influenzae* is spread from person to person. Colonization of an individual depends on the virulence factors described earlier. When *H. influenzae* translocates across damaged epithelial cells, it invades the blood stream. Encapsulated organisms, particularly *H. influenzae* type b, are especially resistant to clearance.

The central nervous system (CNS) is primarily invaded through the choroid plexus. *H. influenzae* and its LOSs initiate an inflammatory process within the subarachnoid that is typical of pyogenic meningitis. This process can be transiently accelerated by using antibiotics that liberate LOSs from organisms if corticosteroids are not administered simultaneously.

CLINICAL SYNDROMES. Meningitis. *H. influenzae* meningitis commonly occurs in children younger than age 5 and in adults with histories of skull trauma or CSF leaks. *H. influenzae* type b strains cause the overwhelming majority of these. A review of 493 episodes of acute bacterial meningitis in adults over a 27-year period showed that 19 cases (4%) were due to *H. influenzae*.

H. influenzae meningitis is clinically indistinguishable from other forms of acute bacterial meningitis. Most patients with *H. influenzae* meningitis have CSF white blood counts of more than 1000/mm³ and hypoglycorrhachia. The CSF Gram stain shows pleomorphic gram-negative bacilli in 60 to 70% of untreated cases. In some patients, however, the bipolar staining may result in a mistaken diagnosis of pneumococcal meningitis. Thus, Gram stain is neither sensitive nor specific for diagnosing *H. influenzae* meningitis.

A diagnosis of *H. influenzae* type b meningitis can be rapidly and reliably established by detecting PRP capsular antigens in CSF. The diagnosis can be established in most cases even when antibiotics have been given before CSF is obtained. Other serotypes (most commonly type f) can cause meningitis in adults.

Table 330–2 ■ SITES OF COLONIZATION AND INFECTIONS BY *H. INFLUENZAE*

SPECIES	NORMAL FLORA	ASSOCIATED DISEASE(S)
H. influenzae	Nasopharynx Upper respiratory tract	Meningitis Epiglottitis Sinusitis Otitis Pneumonia Cellulitis Arthritis Osteomyelitis Obstetric infections Endocarditis
H. influenzae b. *aegyptius*	No	Purulent conjunctivitis Brazilian purpuric fever

Therefore, serologic tests for type b antigen in CSF cannot be relied on to rule out *H. influenzae* meningitis in all cases.

Epiglottitis. *H. influenzae* type b is the most common cause of acute epiglottitis in both children and adults. Epiglottitis is a life-threatening infection in children that usually occurs in patients younger than age 5. The symptoms are fever, drooling, dysphagia, and respiratory distress or stridor, which appear over the course of hours. In adults, fever, sore throat, dysphagia, and odynaphagia occur. Cervical tenderness and lymphadenopathy can be found at all ages. Laryngoscopy demonstrates a swollen, cherry-red epiglottis. However, this procedure should be avoided or undertaken only by experts, because it may precipitate an acute airway obstruction and thus make an emergency tracheotomy necessary. The diagnosis of acute epiglottitis is more safely confirmed by a lateral radiograph of the neck. The patient must be maintained in an upright position during this procedure, however, to avoid additional compromise of the airway. The etiology is usually established by blood culture. Cultures of the pharynx and other mucosal surfaces are less useful because *H. influenzae* may be part of the normal flora. One review suggests that although vaccination has effectively reduced the incidence of this disease in children, it is increasingly observed in adults.

Pneumonia. *H. influenzae* is a common cause of pneumonia in both children and adults. Nosocomial infections, including ventilator-associated pneumonia, also can be caused by these organisms. The clinical features of *H. influenzae* pneumonia include fever, cough, and signs and radiographic findings of lobar consolidation. Parapneumonic effusions or empyema occur commonly in patients with *H. influenzae* pneumonia. Gram-negative bacilli in sputum suggest the diagnosis, but isolation of *H. influenzae* from sputum culture alone is inadequate to prove an etiology because of the high frequency with which this organism colonizes the respiratory tract. A diagnosis can be established by isolating *H. influenzae* from either the blood or pleural fluid.

Tracheobronchitis. Tracheobronchitis is a condition characterized by fever, cough, and purulent sputum that occurs in the absence of radiographic infiltrates suggestive of pneumonia. It frequently occurs in patients with known chronic lung disease. Blood cultures are rarely positive. A combination of pleomorphic gram-negative bacilli predominating in purulent sputum, antibody titers to *H. influenzae* that rise after infection, and the response, at least transiently, to treatment for *H. influenzae* infection strongly suggest this diagnosis.

Sinusitis. *H. influenzae* and *Staplylococcus pneumoniae* are the most frequent bacterial isolates from antral punctures or surgical specimens of patients with acute purulent sinusitis. Most *H. influenzae* isolates are non-typable. Although patients may respond initially to treatment directed against *H. influenzae,* the response is transient if sinus obstruction is not relieved. *H. influenzae* is not an important pathogen in patients with chronic sinusitis.

Otitis Media. *H. influenzae* is the most frequent cause of otitis media in young children. Approximately 90% of the *H. influenzae* isolates obtained by tympanocentesis are non-typable; *H. influenzae* type b causes most of the remaining 10% of infections. Patients with otitis media may present with ear pain or irritability. Drainage can be present. An inflamed, opaque, bulging, or perforated tympanic membrane is usually demonstrated. The etiology can be proven by Gram stain and culture of purulent fluid obtained by tympanocentesis. Otitis caused by *H. influenzae* type b may occur in association with bacteremia and meningitis.

Cellulitis. *H. influenzae* type b is the cause of 5 to 15% of the cases of cellulitis in young children. Most of the infections occur on the face or neck. *H. influenzae* cellulitis is often described as causing a distinctive blue or violaceous discoloration of the skin. However, the fever, erythema, and tenderness observed may not be distinguishable from those from other causes. Diagnosis is established by culture of blood and or tissue aspirates from the involved area.

Bacteremia Without a Primary Focus of Infection. *H. influenzae* causes primary bacteremia in both children and adults. In infants or children, occult meningitis or epiglottitis can be present. A rigorous clinical and laboratory evaluation is essential to avoid missing diagnoses of life-threatening focal infections in these patients. In adults, primary *H. influenzae* type b bacteremia often occurs in patients with underlying diseases such as lymphoma, leukemia, or alcoholism.

Obstetric and Gynecologic Infection. Pregnancy is associated with a significant risk for *H. influenzae* infection. In the Atlanta study, 7 of 47 adult *H. influenzae* invasive infections occurred in pregnant women. Non-typable *H. influenzae* is also an important cause of tubo-ovarian abscess and salpingitis in women.

Pericarditis. *H. influenzae* type b is an important cause of primary bacterial pericarditis in children. It rarely causes this infection in adults; however, pericarditis can occur in association with pneumonia, probably as a result of contiguous spread of the infection.

Endocarditis. *H. influenzae* is a very unusual cause of endocarditis, considering the frequency with which invasive disease occurs. Most infections occur in patients with pre-existing valvular heart disease. Because of its slow initial growth in blood culture media, the diagnosis of this infection may be delayed or missed. Patients with *H. influenzae* endocarditis are at high risk for arterial embolic phenomena.

Septic Arthritis. *H. influenzae* type b is a common cause of septic arthritis in young children; it is rare in adults. *H. influenzae* type b arthritis is clinically indistinguishable from other cause of pyogenic arthritis.

TREATMENT. Third-generation cephalosporins are currently considered to be the treatment of choice for serious *H. influenzae* infections, such as meningitis or epiglottitis. Treatment with ceftriaxone (adult dose: 1 g intravenously every 12 hours) or cefotaxime (adult dose: 2 g intravenously every 8 hours) should be started for patients with proven or suspected *H. influenzae* infection, and this should be continued at least until the full susceptibility data are available.

Ampicillin was considered to be the treatment of choice for all *H. influenzae* infections until the mid 1970s. Since the first reports of ampicillin-resistant *H. influenzae* isolates in 1972, however, this problem has been increasing. At present, 30% of *H. influenzae* type b isolates and 15% of non-typable *H. influenzae* isolates are resistant to ampicillin. The majority contain a plasmid-mediated, R-factor enzyme (TEM-1) β-lactamase, which can be detected rapidly in the laboratory. A small number of isolates, however, have altered penicillin-binding proteins. These proteins bind penicillin and other β-lactam antibiotics poorly. As a consequence, the isolates may be resistant to some cephalosporins, such as cefaclor, cefamandole, and cefuroxime, in addition to ampicillin. Therefore, patients with proven or suspected *H. influenzae* infections should not be treated with ampicillin or with second-generation cephalosporins until susceptibilities to these antibiotics are proven. Chloramphenicol resistance also occurs in *H. influenzae;* resistance is caused by an inactivating enzyme, chloramphenicol acetyl transferase. A small number of *H. influenzae* isolates are resistant to both ampicillin and chloramphenicol.

Amoxicillin can be used for otitis media in children because of the lower prevalence of β-lactamases in non-typable *H. influenzae* isolates. Bactrim is also effective for most isolates. A combination of erythromycin and sulfisoxazole can be used in patients with documented penicillin allergy.

PREVENTION. The first *H. influenzae* type b vaccines were licensed for use in the United States in 1985. These contained purified PRP antigens. However, post-licensing studies of PRP vaccines in the United States showed variable efficacy. The PRP vaccines elicit a type 2, thymus-independent B-cell response, generate few (if any) memory B cells, and fail to stimulate a response in neonates and infants.

Protein-conjugated PRP vaccines were developed to overcome the problem of the lack of immune response in the most susceptible infants and some young children. Several are now licensed for use in infants. At present, protein-conjugated PRP vaccines are recommended for use in all infants over age 2 months, but not earlier than age 6 weeks. Recent studies have shown that protein-conjugated vaccines are effective among diverse populations of infants and societies. True failures after three doses of the protein conjugate PRP vaccines are quite rare.

Antibiotic prophylaxis should be used for unimmunized household or day-care contacts of a patient with invasive *H. influenzae* type b disease. Rifampin is the treatment of choice. It should be given in a dose of 10 mg/kg once daily for 4 days to neonates younger than 1 month, 20 mg/kg (up to a maximum of 600 mg) once daily for 4 days to older children, and 600 mg/day for 4 days to adults.

INFECTIONS CAUSED BY *H. INFLUENZAE, BIOGROUP AE-GYPTIUS* (PURULENT CONJUNCTIVITIS AND BRAZILIAN PURPURIC FEVER). *H. influenzae*, biogroup aegyptius (Koch-Weeks bacillus) causes epidemic purulent conjunctivitis in children. This disease commonly occurs in hot climates or in the summer season. The infection causes conjunctival erythema, edema, mucopurulent exudate, and varying discomfort in the eyes. An unusually virulent clone of *H. influenzae*, biogroup aegyptius, causes an invasive infection called Brazilian purpuric fever, which is characterized by petechial or purpuric skin lesions and vascular collapse, occurring days to weeks after an initial episode of conjunctivitis in infants and children younger than 10 years; this infection is usually fatal.

INFECTIONS CAUSED BY OTHER *HAEMOPHILUS* SPECIES. *H. Parainfluenzae.* *H. parainfluenzae* can be found as part of the normal flora of the mouth and pharynx (Table 330–3). It is a rare cause of meningitis in children and an even rarer cause of meningitis in adults. It may cause dental infections or dental abscesses. Cases of brain abscess, epidural abscess, liver abscess, osteomyelitis, pneumonia, empyema, epiglottitis, peritonitis, septic arthritis, and septicemia caused by this organism have been reported. *H. parainfluenzae* also causes subacute endocarditis, often in young adults. *Haemophilus* species cause approximately 1% of cases of infective endocarditis in non–drug-abusing patients. *H. parainfluenzae* and *H. aphrophilus* (see later) are the species most frequently recovered from these patients. *H. parainfluenzae* forms bulky vegetations on heart valves. Arterial embolization is common in patients with *H. parainfluenzae* endocarditis. Most isolates are sensitive to ampicillin, but some produce β-lactamases. Pending sensitivity reports, patients should be treated with a drug that combines a β-lactam antibiotic and a β-lactamase inhibitor (such as ampicillin sulbactam; adult dose: 3 g intravenously every 6 hours) with ampicillin plus an aminoglycoside or with a third-generation cephalosporin.

H. aphrophilus. *H. aphrophilus* can be found as part of the normal oral flora (see Table 330–3). Like *H. parainfluenzae*, *H. aphrophilus* grows very slowly on primary isolation from blood cultures. It frequently causes bulky vegetations, and arterial emboli are common. *H. aphrophilus* is also a rare cause of brain abscess, periodontal abscess, meningitis, osteomyelitis, and suppurative pulmonary infections. Ampicillin or ampicillin plus an aminoglycoside should be used to treat infections.

H. paraphrophilus. *H. paraphrophilus* can be found as part of the normal flora of the mouth and pharynx (see Table 330–3). *H. paraphrophilus* is a rare cause of endocarditis, and arterial emboli have been observed in 50% of the cases *H. paraphrophilus* endocarditis. It is also a rare cause of brain abscess and liver abscess. Ampicillin is the treatment of choice for this infection.

H. parahaemolyticus. *H. parahaemolyticus* is an important pathogen in domestic animals, causing porcine pleuropneumonia. The organism can be found in the human mouth and pharynx. It is a rare

Table 330–3 ■ SITES OF COLONIZATION AND INFECTIONS BY OTHER *HAEMOPHILUS* SPECIES

SPECIES	NORMAL FLORA	ASSOCIATED DISEASE(S)
H. parainfluenzae	Mouth and pharynx	Endocarditis, brain abscess, liver abscess, pneumonia, epiglottitis, arthritis, osteomyelitis
H. aphrophilus	Mouth	Endocarditis, brain abscess, periodontal abscess, osteomyelitis
H. paraphrophilus	Mouth and pharynx	Endocarditis, brain abscess, liver abscess
H. haemolyticus	Nasopharynx	?
H. parahaemolyticus	Mouth and pharynx	Endocarditis, empyema of gallbladder, ? pharyngitis
H. ducreyi	No	Chancroid

cause of human subacute endocarditis and of empyema of the gallbladder (see Table 330–3). *H. parahaemolyticus* has been isolated from throat cultures of patients with pharyngitis. Animal isolates of *H. parahaemolyticus* are sensitive to tetracycline and sulfa drugs. There is insufficient information about human isolates to permit recommendations for therapy.

H. ducreyi. See Chapter 364.

Adams WG, Keaver KA, Cochi SL, et al: Decline of childhood *Haemophilus Influenzae* type b (Hib) disease in the Hib vaccine era. JAMA 269:221, 1993. *Shows that, in children younger than age 5, there was a 71 to 82% reduction in* H. influenzae *type b meningitis in the year after licensing of the Hib conjugate vaccines in the United States.*

Centers for Disease Control and Prevention: Recommendations for use of the *Haemophilus* b conjugate vaccines and a combined diphtheria, tetanus, pertussis, and *Haemophilus* b vaccine. Recommendations of the Advisory Committee on Immunization Practices (ACIP). MMWR 42(No.RR-13):1, 1993. *Contains recommendations for use of* Haemophilus b *conjugate vaccines for infants beginning at age 2 months (but not earlier than age 6 weeks); also describes the safety, immunogenicity, efficacy, adverse reactions, contraindications, and precautions for vaccine use.*

Durand ML, Calderwood SB, Weber DJ, et al: Acute bacterial meningitis in adults: A review of 493 episodes. N Engl J Med 328:21, 1993. *Summarizes data from a large series of adults with acute bacterial meningitis seen over 27 years.* H. influenzae *caused acute bacterial meningitis in 19 (4%) of the adults. Thirteen of these patients had community-acquired infections and six developed nosocomial* H. influenzae *meningitis after neurosurgery.*

Farley MM, Stephens DS, Brachman PS, et al: Invasive *Haemophilus influenzae* disease in adults. Ann Intern Med 116:806, 1992. *A population-based study showing that 47 cases of invasive* H. influenzae *disease occurred in adults in metropolitan Atlanta from December 1988 through May 1990 (incidence 1.7 per 100,000 adults per year).*

Fothergill LD, Wright J: Influenzal meningitis: The relation of age incidence to the bactericidal power of blood against the causal organism. J Immunol 24:273, 1993. *The classic study showing that* H. influenzae *meningitis occurs in children during the ages between the loss of passively acquired maternal antibodies and the development of active immunity to this organism.*

Mulholland K, Hilton S, Adegloba R, et al: Randomized trial of *Haemophilus influenzae* type-b tetanus protein conjugate for prevention of pneumonia and meningitis in Gambian infants. Lancet 349:1191, 1997. *This study showed that the conjugate vaccine was 95% effective in preventing* Haemophilus influenzae *invasive disease among infants in a developing country.*

OSTEOMYELITIS

331 OSTEOMYELITIS

Barry D. Brause

DEFINITION. Osteomyelitis is an infection by microorganisms that invade bone. Three pathogenetic routes of infection define the major forms of osteomyelitis, with pathogens reaching osseous tissue by (1) hematogenous seeding, (2) contamination accompanying surgical and non-surgical trauma (termed *introduced* infection), or (3) spread from infected contiguous tissue.

ETIOLOGY. Although virtually all microorganisms can infect bone, bacteria are the usual pathogens and staphylococci are the most prominent etiologic agents. *Staphylococcus aureus* causes approximately 60% of hematogenous and introduced infections and is

a principal agent when osseous sepsis spreads by contiguity. *S. epidermidis* has become a major pathogen in bone infections associated with indwelling prosthetic materials, such as joint implants and fracture fixation devices, and is responsible for 30% of these cases. Streptococci, gram-negative bacilli, anaerobes, mycobacteria, and fungi are etiologic agents in a variety of clinical settings (Table 331–1).

INCIDENCE, PREVALENCE, AND EPIDEMIOLOGY. The anatomic location of hematogenous osteomyelitis is age dependent (see Table 331–1). From birth to puberty the long bones of the extremities are the most frequently involved. In adults, blood-borne osteomyelitis generally affects the spine, because vertebrae become more vascular than other skeletal tissue with maturation. Seventy per cent of compound fractures are contaminated, but because of effective débridement and perioperative antibiotic therapy only 2 to 9% develop infection. Osteomyelitis develops by contiguous spread in 30 to 68% of diabetic patients with foot ulcers, and it is notable that

Table 331-1 ■ PREDISPOSITIONS, ANATOMIC SITES, AND PROMINENT PATHOGENS IN FORMS OF OSTEOMYELITIS

FORM OF OSTEOMYELITIS	PREDISPOSING CONDITION	SITE	PROMINENT PATHOGENS
Hematogenous			
Childhood	None	Long bones	*Staphylococcus aureus,* streptococci, *Haemophilus*
	Sickle cell hemoglobinopathy	Multiple	*Salmonella, S. aureus*
Adult	Urinary tract infection or instrumentation	Vertebral	Gram-negative bacilli, streptococci
	Skin infection	Vertebral	*S. aureus,* streptococci
	Respiratory infection	Vertebral	Streptococci, *Mycobacterium tuberculosis*
	Intravenous drug abuse or vascular catheters	Vertebral	Gram-negative bacilli, staphylococci, *Candida*
	Acquired immunodeficiency syndrome	Multiple	Fungi, mycobacteria
Introduced type	Fractures	Fracture site	*S. aureus, S. epidermidis,* gram-negative bacilli
	Prosthetic joint	Prosthesis	*S. epidermidis, S. aureus*
Contiguous spread	Skin ulcer	Foot, leg	Polymicrobial, staphylococci, streptococci, gram-negative bacilli, anaerobes
	Sinusitis	Skull	Streptococci, anaerobes
	Dental abscess	Mandible, maxilla	Streptococci, anaerobes
	Human or animal bites	Hand	Streptococci, anaerobes, *Pasteurella*
	Felon	Finger	*S. aureus*
	Gardening	Hand	*Sporothrix*

more in-hospital days are spent treating foot infections than treating any other complication of diabetes.

PATHOGENESIS. In childhood hematogenous osteomyelitis, the initial infective site is the long bone metaphysis, owing to its large blood flow. In adults, bacteremias seed vertebral bodies preferentially at the more vascular anterior end plates. Osteomyelitis commonly involves two adjacent vertebral bodies and the intervertebral disk space. Infection compromises the nutrient supply to the intervertebral disk, resulting in disk necrosis and disk space narrowing, which is often the earliest sign of vertebral osteomyelitis (Fig. 331–1). Table 331–1 lists examples of clinical conditions that predispose to the development of blood-borne bone infection.

With the introduced form of osteomyelitis, direct septic trauma breaches all protective tissue around the bone, allowing microorganisms into the osseous matrix. The risk of infection is increased further when metallic fixation devices or prosthetic joints are implanted. Indwelling foreign bodies decrease the quantity of bacteria necessary to establish infection in bone and permit pathogens to persist on the surface of the avascular material, often within host or pathogen-derived biofilms, sequestered from circulating immune factors and systemic antibiotics. Osteomyelitis is caused by contiguous extension from infected, adjacent soft tissue when the soft tissue process is sufficiently chronic or uncontrolled (see Table 331–1).

Once infection becomes established in bone, the microorganisms induce local metabolic changes and inflammatory reactions that increase necrosis. As the septic process spreads, local thrombophlebitis develops, further increasing edema and intraosseous pressure, which results in ischemic necrosis of large areas of bone called *sequestra* (Fig. 331–2). When the osseous cortex is breached, subperiosteal abscesses can develop with periosteal inflammation that induces new bone formation in adjacent soft tissue.

CLINICAL MANIFESTATIONS. In the classic presentation of childhood hematogenous osteomyelitis, fever, chills, and malaise are present but are frequently absent in the other forms of bone infection. Localized pain is a characteristic feature of osteomyelitis, with overlying erythema, warmth, and swelling variably observed. Limb motion may be limited if infection is near an articulation,

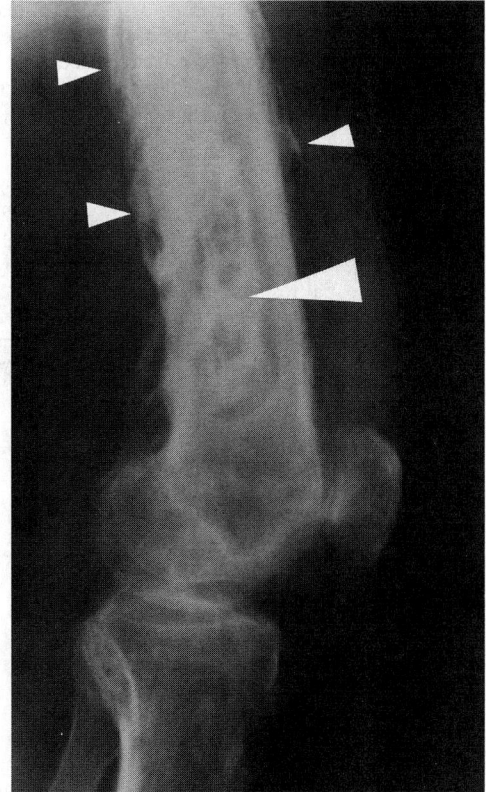

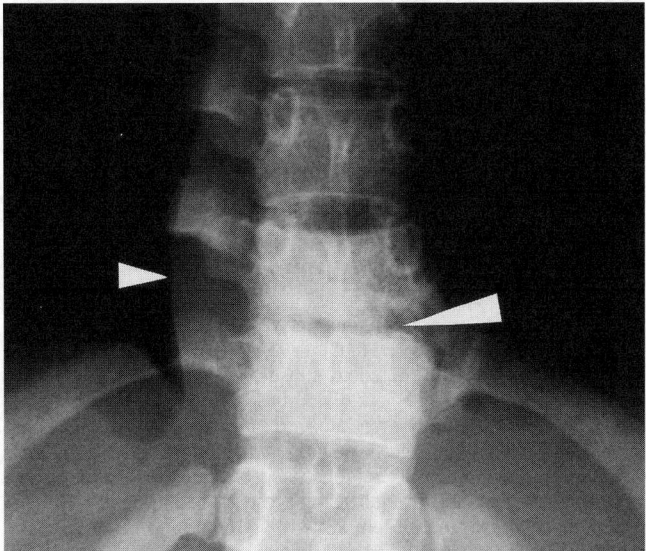

Figure 331–1 ■ Vertebral osteomyelitis. Frontal view of spine illustrates disk space narrowing (large arrowhead) and paraspinal abscess (small arrowhead).

Figure 331–2 ■ Femoral osteomyelitis. Hyperdense central zone is a sequestrum (large arrowhead), and peripheral linear densities are areas of periosteal elevation with periosteal new bone formation (small arrowheads).

and joint effusions can occur but are usually sterile when the epiphyseal cartilage is intact.

Hematogenous vertebral osteomyelitis often presents with back pain, spine tenderness, and low-grade fever after urinary tract instrumentation or infection (30%), skin infection (13%), or respiratory infection (11%). The septic process extending beyond the vertebral column produces suppuration at the particular spinal level of infection such as retropharyngeal abscess, mediastinitis, empyema, subdiaphragmatic and iliopsoas abscesses, as well as meningitis. If paresis, sensory deficits, or bowel or bladder dysfunction develop, spinal epidural abscess—the most feared complication—should be suspected and evaluated immediately. *Mycobacterium tuberculosis* should be considered in relatively indolent infections of vertebrae (as well as at the hip and knee) (see Table 331–1).

Osteomyelitis after trauma or bone surgery is usually associated with persistent or recurrent fevers, increasing pain at the operative site, and poor incisional healing, which is often accompanied by protracted wound drainage or dehiscence. Prosthetic joint infection presents as joint pain (95%), fever (43%), or cutaneous sinus drainage (32%).

Bone involvement by contiguous spread from an overlying chronic ischemic or neuropathic foot ulcer typically occurs in patients with long-standing insulin-dependent diabetes or other vascular disease and involves the metatarsals or the proximal phalanges. It is characterized by local cellulitis with inflammation and necrosis, but pain is only variably found, owing to the frequent presence of sensory neuropathy. Osseous extension is common when the skin ulcer is more than 2 cm² with a depth more than 3 mm or when bone is exposed. Additional examples of osteomyelitis from contiguous spread of infection are listed in Table 331–1.

DIAGNOSIS. Diagnosis requires both confirming the osseous site of involvement and identifying the etiologic microbes. Bone infection must be differentiated from septic arthritis and bursitis, cellulitis and soft tissue abscesses, bone fractures, and neoplasms, as well as bone infarcts seen with sickle cell hemoglobinopathy and Gaucher's disease. Anatomic delineation of bone infection depends largely on radiologic techniques. In hematogenous infection, the earliest osseous changes by radiography are osteopenic or lytic lesions. They require 30 to 50% decalcification to be seen and take 2 to 4 weeks to develop. With further progression, periosteal elevation, thickening, and new bone formation occur, with sequestra and sclerotic changes occurring in chronic infection (see Fig. 331–2). Vertebral osteomyelitis appears initially as disk space narrowing, followed by cortical destruction at the adjacent end plates (see Fig. 331–1). Computed tomography is helpful to identify small osseous alterations and sequestra.

Technetium diphosphonate bone scans, gallium-citrate scans, and indium-labeled leukocyte scintigraphy are far more sensitive than radiography and usually reveal increased radionuclide uptake when symptoms begin. However, these techniques are plagued by inadequate specificity and spatial resolution, so they are not conclusively diagnostic. Inflammatory and degenerative processes in adjacent tissues, recent orthopedic surgery, bone fractures, and neoplasms produce abnormal scans in the absence of osteomyelitis. Magnetic resonance imaging can detect the bone edema of osteomyelitis earlier than radiography; however, differentiation from non-specific reactive marrow edema due to adjacent foci of non-osseous infection and other causes of soft-tissue edema is often not possible. Specificity can be as low as 75%, but magnetic resonance imaging is helpful in identifying paraosseous soft tissue abscesses.

The exact microbial cause of osteomyelitis should be determined, because it is never sufficiently predictable to permit routine presumptive therapy (see Table 331–1). Blood cultures are positive in 25 to 50% of acute childhood hematogenous osteomyelitis but are helpful in less than 10% of the other forms of bone infection. When septic arthritis or soft tissue abscess accompanies the osseous process, arthrocentesis or abscess aspiration cultures can be diagnostic. However, superficial cultures of open wounds or skin ulcers and cultures of cutaneous sinus tracts do not delineate the true bone pathogen(s). In patients with deep chronic skin ulcers from which infection has spread to bone, curettage cultures from the base of the ulcer correlate with osseous tissue 75% of the time. Bone aspirate and biopsy cultures are positive in 70 to 93% of cases and should be sought (percutaneously or by operative débridement) when there is no overlying skin ulcer and the microbiologic diagnosis has not been otherwise established. Specimens for mycobacterial, fungal, and anaerobic cultivation should be considered when routine bacterial cultures are negative.

TREATMENT. Acute osteomyelitis is curable with adequate antimicrobial therapy and surgical débridement when necessary. Parenterally administered antibiotics are usually employed, but oral therapy is also effective when the pathogen is sufficiently susceptible and gastrointestinal absorption is ensured. The exact potency and duration of therapy required to eradicate bone infections are not known. Antibiotics that produce trough serum bactericidal activity at a 1:2 titer have been associated with high cure rates. Treatment should be given for 4 to 6 weeks. Surgery is indicated to drain abscesses, débride necrotic tissues, and remove foreign materials.

PROGNOSIS. Inadequate therapy for acute osteomyelitis results in relapsing infection and progression to chronic osteomyelitis; therefore, definitive treatment of acute infection is obligatory. Because of the presence of gross and microscopic foci of avascular bone, chronic osteomyelitis is not curable except by radical resection (occasionally amputation). Acute exacerbations of these chronic, recurrent infections can be suppressed successfully by débridement of identifiable sequestra followed by protracted courses of parenteral and oral antimicrobial agents.

Brause BD: Infections with prostheses in bones and joints. *In* Mandell GL, Bennett JE, Dolin R (eds): Principles and Practice of Infectious Diseases. New York, Churchill Livingstone, 1994, pp 1051–1055. *Detailed summary of the pathogenesis, microbiology, diagnosis, and treatment of osteomyelitis associated with prosthetic joints.*

Lew DP, Waldvogel FA: Osteomyelitis. N Engl J Med 336:999, 1997. *Detailed description of the pathogenesis, diagnosis, and treatment of osteomyelitis with extensive references.*

Sapico FL, Witte JL, Canawati HN, et al: The infected foot of the diabetic patient: Quantitative microbiology and analysis of clinical features. Rev Infect Dis 6:S171, 1984. *Definitive quantitative microbiology of the correlation between cultures of skin ulcer curettage and bone from amputations in diabetic patients.*

Weinstein M, Stratton C, Hawley HB, et al: Multicenter collaborative evaluation of a standardized serum bactericidal test as a predictor of therapeutic efficacy in acute and chronic osteomyelitis. Am J Med 83:218, 1987. *The best data collection for defining quantitatively effective antibiotic therapy for osteomyelitis.*

WHOOPING COUGH

332 WHOOPING COUGH (PERTUSSIS)

Richard B. Johnston, Jr.

DEFINITION. Whooping cough (pertussis) is a non-invasive, highly communicable bacterial respiratory illness. It occurs at all ages but is most common and most severe in infants and young children. The etiologic agent of the syndrome is usually *Bordetella pertussis*. The descriptive name derives from a distressing, prolonged inspiratory effort that follows paroxysmal coughing. Whooping cough is estimated to cause 500,000 deaths yearly, primarily in infants.

ETIOLOGY. When first isolated, *B. pertussis* is a small, nonmotile, weakly staining, gram-negative coccobacillus, 0.5 to 1.0 μm in length. Capsules can be demonstrated by special procedures, and bipolar metachromatic granules are present. The complex medium containing blood originally employed by Border and Gengou is still used (in modified form) for cultivation. *Primary isolates do not grow on conventional laboratory media.*

An estimated 5 to 10% of clinical whooping cough is caused by *B. parapertussis*. The animal pathogen *B. bronchiseptica* is responsible for a minor percentage of cases. These organisms can be differentiated from *B. pertussis* by growth requirements, enzyme production, and presence of species-specific antigens. It has been suggested that adenoviruses, alone or in concert with *B. pertussis*, and *Chlamydia trachomatis* may play an etiologic role in some cases of whooping cough.

EPIDEMIOLOGY. In non-immune households the attack rate is 80 to 90%. Transmission is by droplet infection. Carriers of *B. pertussis* are found infrequently, but persons previously immunized have been shown during outbreaks of disease to excrete the organism in the absence of clinical symptoms or in the presence of mild or atypical illness.

The mortality rate from whooping cough has fallen since the beginning of the 20th century owing to improved supportive therapy. The incidence of whooping cough, however, did not change until after the 1940s, when immunization of young children became standard practice. In the 1940s, approximately 200,000 cases of pertussis were reported annually in the United States, compared with about 5,000 cases annually in recent years. Most deaths occur in children younger than 1 year of age. The case fatality rate in infants 6 months of age is 1%.

Neither immunization against pertussis nor natural disease provides lifelong protection. In the case of immunization, an attack rate greater than 50% has been reported when the interval after immunization exceeds 12 years. Adolescents and adults represent a large reservoir of susceptibles who can transmit the disease to unimmunized infants, and pertussis is an important cause of persistent cough in adults.

PATHOGENESIS. *B. pertussis* adheres to ciliated epithelial cells of the respiratory tract and multiplies there without invading the tissues. Yet this colonization leads to profound changes in tissues that persist long after the responsible bacteria have been cleared. Such observations suggest that a toxin or toxins from the bacteria play an important part in the pathogenesis of the syndrome. A variety of biologic activities have been demonstrated by injecting *B. pertussis* products into experimental animals. An endotoxin and a heat-labile toxin that can cause tissue necrosis have been identified among these bacterial factors, but the exotoxin *pertussis toxin* (PT) is the best candidate at the moment for a major virulence factor. Immunization with chemically detoxified PT appears to prevent severe whooping cough. PT is believed to be responsible for the characteristic lymphocytosis of whooping cough.

PT is a protein composed of five non-covalently linked subunits (S1–S5). The subunits S2–S5 form a non-toxic unit that binds to the cell membrane; toxicity is mediated by the enzymatically active subunit, S1. Activity of S1 inhibits a subclass of guanosine triphosphate (GTP)-binding proteins (G proteins) that are essential for transmembrane signaling and, thus, certain types of receptor-mediated cell functions.

Adherence of *B. pertussis* to respiratory epithelium is required for the pathogenesis of whooping cough. Adherence appears to involve a bacterial outer membrane protein with a molecular weight of 69 kd, termed *pertactin*. An antigenically similar protein exists on *B. parapertussis* and *B. bronchiseptica*. Injection of this protein into mice or humans elicits agglutinating antibody to *B. pertussis* and protects the mice against lethal *B. pertussis* respiratory challenge. Synthesis of pertactin is controlled by a regulatory gene at the *vir* (virulence) locus, which modulates synthesis of PT and additional factors that may contribute to pathogenesis, including filamentous hemagglutinin.

PATHOLOGY. Lesions caused by *B. pertussis* are found principally in the bronchi and bronchioles, but changes are also seen in the nasopharynx, larynx, and trachea. Masses of bacteria and mucopurulent exudate are intertwined with the cilia of the columnar epithelium. There is necrosis of the midzonal and basilar epithelium with infiltration of polymorphonuclear leukocytes and macrophages. The most frequent findings in the lung are bronchopneumonia, interstitial pneumonitis, and numerous small areas of atelectasis. The brain can show edema and scattered petechiae at autopsy.

CLINICAL MANIFESTATIONS. The incubation period lasts 7 to 14 days (rarely over 2 weeks). It is customary to divide the clinical course into three stages.

CATARRHAL STAGE. Whooping cough begins with symptoms indistinguishable from those of a mild viral upper respiratory tract infection. Sneezing is frequent, conjunctivae are injected, and a

nocturnal cough appears. The temperature may be slightly elevated. Infectivity is greatest at this stage.

PAROXYSMAL STAGE. Seven to 14 days after onset, the cough becomes more frequent, then paroxysmal. In a typical paroxysm there is a series of 5 to 20 short coughs of increasing intensity and then a deep inspiration, making the "whoop." A tenacious mucus plug is usually expelled, and vomiting frequently follows. Paroxysms may occur as often as every half hour and are accompanied by signs of increased venous pressure, including deeply engorged conjunctivae, periorbital edema, petechial hemorrhages, particularly about the forehead, and epistaxis. During the attack, the infant may be cyanotic until the crowing whoop occurs. Between paroxysms, the child usually feels well, although justifiably apprehensive. This phase lasts 2 to 4 weeks.

Physical examination of the chest is often unremarkable except for scattered rhonchi. The chest radiograph sometimes reveals hilar and mediastinal nodal enlargement. The presence of fever should immediately suggest the development of a secondary infectious process.

CONVALESCENT STAGE. Gradually the paroxysms become less frequent and less intense; vomiting ceases, and slow recovery ensues. Convalescence requires 4 to 12 weeks. For many months even a mild, unrelated respiratory infection can induce a return of paroxysmal cough and whoop.

In infants younger than 6 months old, the paroxysms and the whoop are often absent; choking spells and apneic episodes may be the major manifestations. Second attacks of whooping cough as well as disease occurring in previously immunized individuals often present simply as an upper respiratory illness or bronchitis.

COMPLICATIONS. Recurrent vomiting can lead to metabolic alkalosis or malnutrition. Central nervous system changes can result from cerebral anoxia or hemorrhages consequent to the elevated venous pressure. Rarely, cortical degeneration occurs, but the exact pathogenesis of the encephalopathy is unknown. A serous meningitis with lymphocytosis of the cerebrospinal fluid has been described. Pneumothorax and interstitial emphysema are infrequently seen. Secondary bacterial otitis media occurs frequently. The major cause of death in whooping cough is pneumonia, either primary or caused by other bacteria or viruses.

DIAGNOSIS. There is little difficulty in making the clinical diagnosis of whooping cough in a patient who, after a period of coryzal symptoms, develops paroxysmal coughing with a terminal inspiratory whoop. Lymphocytosis often occurs toward the end of the catarrhal stage or early in the spasmodic phase. Characteristically the leukocyte count ranges from 15,000 to 30,000/μL or higher, and 80% of the cells are small lymphocytes. Polymorphonuclear leukocytosis suggests a secondary bacterial complication.

Microbiologic identification of the organisms may be required to make the diagnosis in abortive or mild cases or in young infants or adults. During the early stages, *B. pertussis* can be isolated from approximately 90% of patients. By the third or fourth week, the organism can be recovered in only 50% of cases, and in the convalescent stage it is unusual to obtain a positive culture.

Specimens for culture are best obtained by nasal swab rather than by the cough plate method. A sterile cotton swab wrapped about a flexible copper wire is passed through the nares, and mucus is obtained from the posterior pharynx. *B. pertussis* is readily killed by desiccation, so the specimen should be quickly plated onto fresh medium, to which antibiotic has been added to prevent overgrowth of adventitious organisms.

A fluorescent antibody staining procedure can be applied directly to clinical specimens or organisms grown in culture, but false-positive and false-negative results are relatively common. Probes for *B. pertussis* DNA are available, but their use for diagnosis is uncertain.

Serologic procedures are of little help in diagnosing whooping cough because a rise in titer of most antibodies does not occur until at least the third week of illness. Tests have not been well standardized.

TREATMENT. SUPPORTIVE THERAPY. Young infants, particularly those younger than 6 months of age, should be hospitalized. Supportive measures combined with careful nursing care are of paramount importance. Specific attention must be devoted to the maintenance of proper water and electrolyte balance, adequate nutrition, and sufficient oxygenation. Constant alertness for the presence of secondary infectious complications such as pneumonia is required. Mild cases require only supportive treatment.

ANTIMICROBIAL AGENTS. Specific therapy of severe whooping cough has been disappointing despite the in vitro susceptibility of *B. pertussis* to various antimicrobial agents. Antimicrobial agents given in the catarrhal stage may ameliorate the disease. In the established paroxysmal stage, the organisms can be readily eliminated by antimicrobial agents, but the course of the illness is unaltered. Antibiotics may be justified in order to render the patient non-infectious. Erythromycin is the drug of choice. The daily dose is 40 to 50 mg/kg given in four divided doses. The organism is eliminated after a few days of therapy, but because bacteriologic relapse may occur, treatment should be continued for 14 days. Trimethoprim/sulfamethoxazole (8 mg/kg and 40 mg/kg/day in two doses) is a possible alternative for patients who do not tolerate erythromycin.

PREVENTION. Unfortunately, the diagnosis is usually not made until the end of the catarrhal stage, and by then, spread of the disease has already occurred. Exposed susceptibles should receive erythromycin prophylaxis for 14 days, and close (household, day care, classroom) contacts younger than 7 who have been previously immunized should receive a booster dose of vaccine in addition to erythromycin. Booster doses of vaccine or erythromycin chemoprophylaxis have been used to protect adults, such as hospital staff.

ACTIVE IMMUNIZATION. Women of childbearing age generally do not have significant levels of protective antibody in their sera, and most newborns have received no passive protection. Consequently, active immunization is begun as early as is practicable. At present, it is recommended that the infant receive three injections of pertussis vaccine at 8-week intervals beginning at age 2 months. A fourth injection is given 6 to 12 months after the third dose (15 to 18 months of age), and a booster is given before entering kindergarten. Administration of pertussis vaccine to those older than age 6 has not been recommended as a routine measure, but this practice should probably be reconsidered in view of the improved vaccine and the severity of the disease in some adults.

Whole cell pertussis vaccine consists of inactive *B. pertussis* organisms in suspension with alum-precipitated diphtheria and tetanus toxoids (DTP). The newer acellular pertussis vaccines (DTaP) contain various combinations of the *B. pertussis* products pertussis toxin, pertactin, filamentous hemagglutinin, and fimbrial antigen. In the United States, DTaP is preferred for all doses because of the decreased likelihood of vaccine-associated fever and local reactions.

As previously noted, immunization does not confer lifelong protection. Approximately 80% of those vaccinated within 4 years of exposure are protected, whereas 80 to 90% of a matched unimmunized group with similar exposure contract pertussis. The prophylactic efficacy of pertussis vaccine was clearly demonstrated when epidemics occurred in the United Kingdom in 1977–1979 and 1982 after a 3- to 5-year period during which vaccine acceptance had declined to very low levels. More than 170,000 cases of whooping cough were reported, including 42 deaths, principally among children younger than age 5. Similar outbreaks have followed diminished vaccine utilization in Japan and Sweden.

Reactions at the injection site as well as fever and hyperirritability occur commonly after injection of whole-cell pertussis vaccine. The incidence of postinjection acute encephalopathy is uncertain but apparently rare, and it is not clear whether administering DTP vaccine increases the overall risk in children of chronic nervous system dysfunction. It is clear that the risk of neurologic complications from pertussis immunization is far less than the hazards of whooping cough in the young child. Nevertheless, in infants with a personal history of convulsions or other neurologic disorders, pertussis immunization with either vaccine should be deferred until the condition has stabilized.

Edwards KM, Decker MD, Graham BS, et al: Adult immunization with acellular pertussis vaccine. JAMA 269:53, 1993. *A report of the immunogenicity and safety of the new vaccine in adults.*

Howson CP, Howe CJ, Fineberg HV (eds): Adverse Effects of Pertussis and Rubella Vaccines. Washington, National Academy Press, 1991. *A scientific, fully referenced review by the Institute of Medicine of DTP immunization and possible adverse events.*

Pasternak MS: Pertussis in the 1990's: Diagnosis, treatment and prevention. Curr Clin Top Infect Dis 17:24, 1997. *A thorough discussion of acellular pertussis vaccines.*

Pittman M: The concept of pertussis as a toxin-mediated disease. Pediatr Infect Dis J 3:467, 1984. *A thorough, now classic review of pathogenesis, immunity, and immunization.*

Stratton KR, Howe CJ, Johnston RB Jr (eds): DPT Vaccine and Chronic Nervous System Dysfunction: A New Analysis. Washington, National Academy Press, 1994. *A re-evaluation of this relationship by the Institute of Medicine.*

DIPHTHERIA

333 DIPHTHERIA*

Roland W. Sutter

Diphtheria is an acute infectious disease caused by *Corynebacterium diphtheriae*, a gram-positive bacillus. The organism primarily infects the respiratory tract, where it causes tonsillopharyngitis and/or laryngitis, typically with a pseudomembrane, and the skin, causing a variety of indolent lesions. If the infecting strain produces exotoxin, myocarditis and neuritis may ensue.

ETIOLOGY. *C. diphtheriae* is an aerobic, non-motile, unencapsulated, non-sporulating, pleomorphic gram-positive bacillus. Its name comes from the Greek *korynee* (meaning "club"), describing the shape of the organism on stained smears with one end usually being wider, and *diphtheria* (meaning "leather hide"), for the characteristic adherent membrane. Both non-toxigenic and toxigenic strains exist. Toxigenicity is conferred when a non-toxigenic organism is infected by a β-phage carrying the gene for the toxin (*tox*). *C. diphtheriae* has three biotypes, *gravis*, *mitis*, and *intermedius*, which are distinguished by colonial morphology and varying biochemical and hemolytic reactions. Strains may be distinguished for epidemiologic purposes by molecular techniques. There are a few reports of classic diphtheria, including toxic complications, due to infection with *C. ulcerans*.

EPIDEMIOLOGY. Humans are the only natural reservoir of *C. diphtheriae*, although the organism has been isolated occasionally from a variety of domestic and other animals. Spread occurs in close-contact settings through respiratory droplets or by direct contact with respiratory secretions or skin lesions. The organism survives for weeks and possibly months on environmental surfaces and in dust, and fomite transmission may occur. The majority of nasopharyngeal *C. diphtheriae* infection results in asymptomatic carriers, and approximately one in seven individuals develops clinical disease. However, asymptomatic carriers are important in maintaining transmission.

Diphtheria immunization protects against disease but does not prevent carriage. In the prevaccine era, respiratory disease dominated in temperate climates, with a fall/winter peak in incidence, and most individuals developed natural immunity by the mid-teen years. Cutaneous disease is the predominant form of the disease in tropical countries, but over the past two decades, outbreaks of this form of diphtheria have occurred in the United States and Europe, typically among homeless and alcoholic inner-city adults.

Vaccination with diphtheria toxoid (formalin-treated toxin) was introduced in the 1920s and 1930s. Immunization of children in an era when the majority of older individuals had natural immunity resulted in a dramatic drop in diphtheria incidence and an even more rapid decline in the proportion of toxigenic strains isolated, presumably because the selective advantage of the *tox* gene— promotion of greater replication and spread of the organism—is lost in the immune host. Currently in most Western countries, toxigenic *C. diphtheriae* has been virtually eliminated. In the United States, reported cases fell from 147,991 in 1920, to 15,536 in 1940, to a total of 40 cases from 1980–1993. Since 1988, all

---

*This is a revision and update of the chapter by Iain R. B. Hardy in the 20th edition of this textbook.

culture-confirmed cases have been caused by imported strains. The absence of reported diphtheria cases in the United States in recent years, however, does not indicate that the circulation of toxigenic *C. diphtheriae* has ceased. An investigation in 1996 suggested that *C. diphtheriae* strains may have circulated for more than two decades in a Northern Plains Indian community despite the absence of reported respiratory diphtheria cases.

Vaccine-induced immunity to diphtheria wanes with time, and there is a growing cohort of individuals with no natural diphtheria immunity. Serosurveys indicate that 20 to 60% of adults in industrialized countries have diphtheria antitoxin levels below minimal protective levels. A level of 0.01 IU/mL from an in-vitro neutralization assay, the "gold standard" test, is considered the lower limit of protection. As long as a high proportion of the population remains susceptible, the danger of re-introduction or re-emergence of toxigenic strains exists. Since 1990 there has been a major resurgence of diphtheria in several countries of the former Soviet Union. In Russia, the number of reported cases rose from 593 in 1989 to 39,582 in 1994, with over two thirds of cases occurring among adults. Large-scale mass campaigns with diphtheria toxoid administered to virtually the entire population in the affected new independent states of the former Soviet Union have since led to significant decreases in the incidence of diphtheria, from a peak of 50,449 cases in 1995 to 7,197 cases in 1997, although pre-resurgence levels of control have not been achieved.

PATHOGENESIS. In classic respiratory diphtheria, *C. diphtheriae* colonizes the mucosal surface of the nasopharynx and multiplies locally without blood stream invasion. Released toxin causes local tissue necrosis, and a tough, adherent pseudomembrane forms, composed of a mixture of fibrin, dead cells, and bacteria. The membrane usually begins on the tonsils or posterior pharynx. In more severe cases it spreads, extending progressively over the pharyngeal wall, fauces, soft palate, and into the larynx, which may result in respiratory obstruction. Toxin entering the blood stream causes tissue damage at distant sites, particularly the heart (myocarditis), nerves (demyelination), and kidney (tubular necrosis). Nontoxigenic strains may cause mild local respiratory disease, sometimes including a membrane.

Diphtheria toxin is an extremely potent inhibitor of protein synthesis, with an estimated human lethal dose of 0.1 mg/kg. The extent of toxin absorption varies with site of infection, being much less from skin or nose than from the pharynx.

CLINICAL MANIFESTATIONS. Respiratory Diphtheria. Infection limited to the anterior nares manifests as a chronic serosanguineous or seropurulent discharge without fever or significant toxicity. A whitish membrane may be observed on the septum. The faucial (pharyngeal) form is most common. After an incubation period of 1 to 7 days, the illness begins with a sore throat, malaise, and mild to moderate fever. There is initial mild pharyngeal erythema, usually followed by progressive formation of a whitish tonsillar exudate, which over 24 to 48 hours changes into a grayish membrane that is tightly adherent and bleeds on attempted removal. In more severe cases, the patient appears toxic and the membrane is more extensive. Cervical adenopathy and soft tissue edema may occur, resulting in the typical bull neck appearance and stridor. Laryngeal involvement, which may occur on its own or as a result of membrane extension from the nasopharynx, presents as hoarseness, stridor, and dyspnea.

The likelihood of toxic complications depends primarily on the interval between disease onset and administration of antitoxin. The severity of disease at initial presentation predicts closely the likelihood of severe clinical course, complications, and death. Myocarditis typically occurs in the first or second week after the onset of respiratory symptoms and presents either suddenly or insidiously with signs of low cardiac output and congestive failure. Conduction disturbances, which may occur without other signs of myocarditis, include ST-T wave abnormalities, arrhythmias, and heart block. Neurologic impairment manifests as cranial nerve palsies and peripheral neuritis. Palatal and/or pharyngeal paralysis occurs during the acute phase; peripheral neuritis, symmetrical and predominantly motor, occurs from 2 to 12 weeks after disease onset. Motor deficit may range from minor proximal weakness to complete paralysis. Complete recovery is the rule. In fulminant, sometimes called "hypertoxic," diphtheria, toxic circulatory collapse with hemorrhagic features occurs.

Diphtheria, at the end of the 20th century, remains a serious disease, associated with a high case-fatality rate. In the United States, the diphtheria case-fatality rate has remained virtually unchanged between 5 and 10% over recent decades.

Cutaneous diphtheria lesions are classically indolent, deep, punched-out ulcers, which may have a grayish white membrane. However, the lesions may be indistinguishable from impetigo, or *C. diphtheriae* may infect chronic dermatoses, such as stasis dermatitis. There is frequently co-infection with *Streptococcus pyogenes* and/or *Staphylococcus aureus*. Toxic complications of cutaneous diphtheria are rare.

Uncommonly, *C. diphtheriae,* both toxigenic and non-toxigenic, may cause invasive disease, including endocarditis, osteomyelitis, septic arthritis, and meningitis. Frequently, these patients have predisposing factors such as a prosthetic cardiac valve or underlying immunosuppression.

DIAGNOSIS. The decision to initiate therapy should be made on clinical grounds, because delayed treatment, especially delays in antitoxin administration, is associated with worse outcomes. A high index of suspicion is required. Cultures should be taken from beneath the membrane, from the nasopharynx, and from any suspicious skin lesions. Because special media are required, the laboratory should be alerted to the concern about diphtheria. *C. diphtheriae* is best isolated on selective media that inhibit the growth of other nasopharyngeal organisms; generally one containing potassium tellurite is used. Based on colonial morphology and Gram stain appearance, a presumptive diagnosis may be possible within 18 to 24 hours. Cultures may be negative if the patient received previous antibiotics. Toxigenicity testing should be performed on all *C. diphtheriae* isolates. Because both non-toxigenic and toxigenic strains may be isolated from the same patient, more than one colony should be tested. Traditional methods include guinea pig inoculation and the Elek test, in which the isolate and appropriate controls are streaked on a culture plate in which a filter strip soaked with antitoxin has been embedded; toxin production is confirmed by an immunoprecipitation line in the agar. A recently developed polymerase chain reaction test may allow both detection of the organism and determination of toxigenicity.

The differential diagnosis includes streptococcal and viral tonsillopharyngitis, infectious mononucleosis, Vincent's angina, candidiasis, and acute epiglottitis. A history of travel to a region with endemic diphtheria or of contact with a recent immigrant from such an area increases the possibility of diphtheria, as does a pre-antitoxin treatment serum antitoxin level of less than 0.01 IU/mL.

TREATMENT AND PREVENTION. Treatment goals are to rapidly neutralize toxin, eliminate the infecting organism, provide supportive care, and prevent further transmission. The mainstay of therapy is equine diphtheria antitoxin. Because only unbound toxin can be neutralized, treatment should commence as soon as the diagnosis is suspected, and each day of delay in administration increases the likelihood of a fatal outcome. A single dose is given, ranging in quantity from 20,000 units for localized tonsillar diphtheria up to 100,000 units for extensive disease with severe toxicity. Antitoxin may be given intramuscularly or intravenously; particularly for more severe cases, the intravenous route is preferred. Tests for sensitivity to antitoxin should be performed before administering it and desensitization performed if necessary. Antibiotic therapy, by eliminating the organism, halts toxin production, limits local infection, and prevents transmission. Parenteral penicillin (4 to 6 million units/day) and erythromycin (40 mg/kg/day in four divided doses; maximum, 2 g/day, usually orally if the patient can swallow) are the drugs of choice. General supportive care includes ensuring a secure airway, electrocardiographic monitoring for evidence of myocarditis, treating heart failure and arrhythmias, and preventing secondary complications of neurologic impairment such as aspiration pneumonia. The patient should be in strict isolation until follow-up cultures are negative. Convalescing patients should receive diphtheria toxoid.

The local health department must be notified. Close contacts should be cultured and commenced on prophylactic antibiotics. A positive culture in a contact may confirm the diagnosis if the patient is culture negative. All contacts without full primary immunization and a booster within the preceding 5 years should receive diphtheria toxoid.

Because manufacturers in the United States discontinued diphtheria antitoxin production, no licensed product is available. However, diphtheria antitoxin for the therapeutic purposes can be obtained from the Centers for Disease Control and Prevention, which distributes a European-produced antitoxin (Pasteur Merieux, Lyon, France) under an Investigational New Drug protocol. The antitoxin is comparable to the previous products manufactured in the United States and may be requested by calling 404-639-8255 during working hours or 404-639-2889 at nights or weekends.

Immunization with diphtheria toxoid is the only effective means of primary prevention. The primary series is four doses of diphtheria toxoid (given with tetanus toxoid and pertussis vaccine) at 2, 4, 6, and 12 to 18 months; a preschool booster dose is given at ages 4 to 6 years. Thereafter, Td (tetanus and diphtheria toxoid for adults) boosters should be given as part of the adolescent immunization visit (i.e., between 11 and 13 years of age), followed by doses administered every 10 years.

Centers for Disease Control and Prevention: Toxigenic *Corynebacterium diphtheriae*—Northern plains Indian community, August–October 1996. MMWR Morb Mortal Wkly Rep 46:506–510, 1997. *Evidence for persistence of endemic transmission of C. diphtheriae over two decades in this community in the United States.*

Dixon JMS, Noble WC, Smith GR: Diphtheria; other corynebacterial and coryneform infections. *In* Topley WWC, Parker MT, Collier L, et al (eds): Topley and Wilson's Principles of Bacteriology, 8th ed. Philadelphia, BC Decker, 1990, pp 56–75. *A useful review with especially comprehensive epidemiologic data.*

Farizo KM, Strebel PS, Chen RT, et al: Fatal respiratory disease due to *Corynebacterium diphtheriae:* Case report and review of guidelines for management, investigation, and control. Clin Infect Dis 16:59, 1993. *Includes latest recommendations of the United States Centers for Disease Control and Prevention for case and contact management.*

Harnisch JP, Tronca E, Nolan CM, et al: Diphtheria among alcoholic urban adults: A decade of experience in Seattle. Ann Intern Med 111:71, 1989. *Summary of last major outbreak of diphtheria in the United States.*

Pappenheimer AM: Diphtheria: Studies on the Biology of an Infectious Disease. The Harvey Lectures. New York, Academic Press, 1982, series 76, pp 45–73. *Detailed description of the cellular and molecular biology of diphtheria toxin.*

Peter G (ed): 1997 Red Book: Report of the Committee on Infectious Diseases, 24th ed. Elk Grove Village, IL, American Academy of Pediatrics, 1997, pp 191–195. *Description on public health interventions after detection of a suspected case of diphtheria.*

CLOSTRIDIAL DISEASES

334 CLOSTRIDIAL MYONECROSIS AND OTHER CLOSTRIDIAL DISEASES

Dennis L. Stevens

The genus *Clostridium* encompasses over 60 species of gram-positive anaerobic spore-forming rods that cause a variety of infections in humans and animals by virtue of a myriad of proteinaceous exotoxins (Table 334–1). *C. tetani* and *C. botulinum* manifest specific clinical disease by elaborating single, but highly potent, toxins. Although botulism is usually the result of ingestion of preformed toxin, tetanus requires the bacteria to proliferate at the site of penetrating injury (see Chapters 336 and 337). Frequently, signs of infection are not apparent even with lethal exotoxinemia. In contrast, other strains of clostridia, such as *C. perfringens* and *C. septicum,* cause aggressive necrotizing infections, attributable, in part, to bacterial proteases, phospholipases, and cytotoxins.

MYONECROSIS

TYPES. Clostridial gas gangrene, or myonecrosis, occurs in three different settings. First, and most commonly, traumatic gas gangrene develops after deep, penetrating injury that compromises the blood supply (e.g., knife or gunshot wound, crush injury), creating an anaerobic environment ideal for clostridial proliferation. *C. perfringens* accounts for 80% of such infections. The remaining cases are caused by *C. septicum, C. novyi, C. histolyticum, C. bifermentans,* and *C. fallax.* Other conditions associated with traumatic gas gangrene are bowel and biliary tract surgery, criminal abortion, and retained placenta; prolonged rupture of the membranes; and intrauterine fetal demise or missed abortion in postpartum patients. Second, spontaneous or non-traumatic gas gangrene is most commonly caused by the more aerotolerant *C. septicum.* Lastly, recur-

Table 334–1 ■ CLINICAL DISEASES CAUSED BY CLOSTRIDIA

ORGANISM	CLINICAL DIAGNOSIS	CLINICAL FEATURES	LABORATORY FEATURES	TOXINS
Invasive Infections				
C. perfringens type a	Traumatic gas gangrene	Pain, necrotizing infection, renal impairment, shock	• Renal failure • ↑ CK • Gas in tissues	α toxin θ toxin
C. septicum	Spontaneous gas gangrene	Pain, necrotizing infection, bowel portal	• Renal failure • ↑ CK • Gas in tissues	α toxin
C. sordellii	Malignant edema	No pain, no fever, massive third spacing	• Leukemoid reaction • Hemoconcentration	?
C. tertium	Bacteremia in compromised hosts receiving antibiotics	Bacteremia, shock	• Positive blood cultures	?
Gastrointestinal				
C. perfringens type a	Food poisoning	Nausea, vomiting, watery diarrhea	None	Enterotoxin
C. perfringens type c	Necrotizing enterocolitis	Bloody diarrhea, ruptured bowel	None	β toxin
C. septicum	Neutropenic enterocolitis, "typhlitis"	Right lower quadrant pain, abdominal distention	• Low white blood cell count	Unknown
C. difficile	Pseudomembranous colitis	Water, bloody diarrhea	• Stools positive for organism, toxin, blood and leukocytes	Toxin A Toxin B
Neurologic				
C. tetanii	Tetanus	Spastic paralysis	None	Tetanospasmin
C. botulinum	Botulism	Flaccid paralysis	None	Botulinum toxin (A,B,E,F,G)

CK = creatine phosphokinase.

rent gas gangrene caused by *C. perfringens* has been described in individuals with non-penetrating injuries at sites of previous gas gangrene, where spores of *C. perfringens* remain quiescent in tissue for periods of 10 to 20 years and then germinate when minor trauma provides conditions suitable for growth.

CLINICAL MANIFESTATIONS. The first symptom is usually sudden and severe pain at the site of surgery or trauma. The mean incubation period is less than 24 hours but ranges from 6 to 8 hours to several days, probably depending on the degree of soil contamination or bowel spillage and degree of vascular compromise. The skin may appear pale initially but quickly changes to bronze and then purplish red and becomes tense and exquisitely tender. Bullae develop that may be clear, red, blue, or purple. Gas present in tissue may be obvious by physical examination, soft tissue radiography, or computed tomography. Signs of systemic toxicity develop rapidly, including tachycardia, low-grade fever, and diaphoresis, followed by shock and multiorgan failure. Bacteremia occurs in 15% of patients and is usually associated with brisk hemolysis. Patients have been described with hematocrits of 0% for as long as 24 hours. Complications include jaundice, renal failure, hypotension, and liver necrosis. Renal failure is largely due to hemoglobinuria and myoglobinuria but complicated by acute tubular necrosis after hypotension. Renal tubular cells are likely directly affected by toxins, but this has not been proven.

DIAGNOSIS. Increasing pain at the site of prior injury or surgery, together with signs of systemic toxicity, fever, and gas in the tissue, supports the diagnosis. Definitive diagnosis rests on demonstrating large, gram-variable rods at the injury site. Note that although clostridia stain gram positive when obtained from bacteriologic media, when visualized from infected tissues, they may appear as either gram positive or gram negative. Surgical exploration is essential and demonstrates muscle that does not bleed or contract when stimulated. Grossly, muscle tissue is edematous and may have a reddish blue to black coloration. Usually, necrotizing fasciitis and cutaneous necrosis are also present. Microscopic evaluation of biopsy material invariably demonstrates organisms among degenerating muscle bundles and, characteristically, an absence of acute inflammatory cells.

PATHOGENESIS. The initiating trauma introduces organisms (either vegetative forms or spores) into the deep tissues and produces an anaerobic niche with a sufficiently low redox potential and acid pH for optimal clostridial growth. Necrosis progresses within hours. At the junction of necrotic and normal tissues, no polymorphonuclear leukocytes (PMNs) are present, yet pavementing of PMNs is apparent within capillaries and in small arterioles and postcapillary venules, followed later in the course by leukostasis within larger vessels. Thus, the histopathology of clostridial gas gangrene is completely opposite to that seen in soft tissue infections caused by organisms such as *Staphylococcus aureus,* in which an early luxuriant influx of PMNs localizes the infection without adjacent tissue or vascular destruction.

Studies suggest that θ-toxin and α-toxin, when elaborated in high concentrations at the site of infection, destroy host tissues and inflammatory cells. As the toxin diffuses into surrounding tissues or enters systemic circulation, it promotes dysregulated PMN–endothelial cell adhesive interactions and primes leukocytes for increased respiratory burst activity. These actions lead to vascular leukostasis, endothelial cell injury, and regional tissue hypoxia. Such perfusion deficits expand the anaerobic environment and contribute to the rapidly advancing margins of tissue destruction that are characteristic of clostridial gangrene.

Shock associated with gas gangrene may be attributable, in part, to direct and indirect effects of toxins. α-Toxin directly suppresses myocardial contractility ex vivo and may contribute to profound hypotension by means of a sudden reduction in cardiac output. θ-Toxin contributes indirectly by inducing endogenous mediators that cause relaxation of blood vessel wall tension, such as nitric oxide or the lipid autacoids, prostacyclin, or platelet-activating factor. α-Toxin also induces platelet-activating factor production by endothelial cells and tumor necrosis factor production by monocytes. In experimental studies, reduced vascular tone develops rapidly due to the effects of platelet activating factor and tumor necrosis factor. In response to a precipitous drop in mean arterial pressure, the normal physiologic response is a compensatory increase in cardiac output. Such a response is characteristic of gram-negative sepsis. However, this does not occur in *C. perfringens*–induced shock, owing to the

direct suppression of myocardial contractility by α-toxin. Thus, reduced systemic vascular resistance and declining cardiac output are poor prognostic signs and invariable lead to intractable shock.

TREATMENT. Penicillin, clindamycin, tetracycline, chloramphenicol, metronidazole, and a number of cephalosporins have excellent in vitro activity against *C. perfringens* and other clostridia. No clinical trials have been conducted to compare the efficacy of these agents in humans. Experimental studies in mice suggest that clindamycin has the greatest efficacy and penicillin the least. Slightly greater survival was observed in animals receiving both clindamycin and penicillin; in contrast, antagonism was observed with penicillin plus metronidazole. Resistance of some strains to clindamycin suggests a combination of penicillin and clindamycin is warranted.

Aggressive surgical débridement is mandatory to improve survival and prevent complications. The use of hyperbaric oxygen (HBO) is controversial, although some non-randomized studies have reported excellent results with HBO therapy when it is combined with antibiotics and surgical débridement. Experimental studies demonstrate slight benefit of HBO when combined with penicillin, although survivals were greater with clindamycin alone.

Therapeutic strategies directed against toxin expression in vivo, such as neutralization with specific antitoxin antibody or inhibiting toxin synthesis with antibiotics such as clindamycin, may be valuable adjuncts to traditional antimicrobial regimens. Future strategies may target endogenous proadhesive molecules such that toxin-induced vascular leukostasis and resultant tissue injury are attenuated.

PROGNOSIS. Patients presenting with gas gangrene of an extremity have a better prognosis than those with truncal or intra-abdominal gas gangrene, largely because it is difficult to adequately débride such lesions. HBO could be useful in such patients, yet there are little data on this subject. In addition to truncal gangrene, patients with associated bacteremia and intravascular hemolysis have the greatest likelihood of progressing to shock and death.

PREVENTION. Aggressive débridement of devitalized tissue, as well as rapid repair of compromised vascular supply, greatly reduces the frequency of gas gangrene in contaminated deep wounds. Intramuscular epinephrine, prolonged application of tourniquets, and surgical closure of traumatic, contaminated wounds, particularly those involving fractured bones, should be avoided. Patients with contaminated wounds should receive prophylactic antibiotics.

SPONTANEOUS, NON-TRAUMATIC GAS GANGRENE DUE TO *CLOSTRIDIUM SEPTICUM*

CLINICAL MANIFESTATIONS. The onset of disease is abrupt, often with excruciating pain, although the patient may sense only heaviness or numbness. The first symptom may be confusion or malaise. Extremely rapid progression of gangrene follows. Swelling advances, and blisters appear filled with clear, cloudy, hemorrhagic, or purplish fluid. The skin around such bullae also has a purple hue, perhaps reflecting vascular compromise resulting from bacterial toxins diffusing into surrounding tissues. Histopathology of muscle and connective tissues includes cell lysis and gas formation; inflammatory cells are remarkably absent.

Predisposing factors include colonic carcinoma, diverticulitis, gastrointestinal surgery, leukemia, lymphoproliferative disorders, and either chemotherapy or radiation therapy. Cyclic neutropenia is also associated with spontaneous gas gangrene due to *C. septicum,* and, in such cases, necrotizing enterocolitis, cecitis, or distal ileitis is commonly found. These gastrointestinal pathologic processes permit bacterial access to the blood stream; consequently, the aerotolerant *C. septicum* can become established in normal tissues. Patients surviving bacteremia or spontaneous gangrene due to *C. septicum* should have appropriate diagnostic studies of the gastrointestinal tract to rule out pathology in this area.

DIAGNOSIS. Unlike traumatic gas gangrene, bacteremia precedes cutaneous manifestations by several hours, causing delays in the appropriate diagnosis and, as a consequence, an increase in the mortality rate.

PATHOGENESIS. *C. septicum* produces four toxins—α-toxin (lethal, hemolytic, necrotizing activity); β-toxin (DNase); γ-toxin (hyaluronidase); and δ-toxin (septicolysin, an oxygen-labile hemolysin)—as well as a protease and a neuraminidase. This α-toxin does not possess phospholipase activity and is thus distinct from the α-toxin of *C. perfringens*. Active immunization against α-toxin significantly protects against challenge with viable *C. septicum*. The mechanism by which α-toxin contributes to *C. septicum* pathogenesis is unknown; however, the recent cloning and sequencing of this toxin should facilitate studies in this area.

TREATMENT. Although no comparative human trials have evaluated the efficacy of antibiotics or HBO for treating clinical cases of spontaneous gas gangrene, in vitro data suggests that *C. septicum* is uniformly susceptible to penicillin, tetracycline, erythromycin, clindamycin, chloramphenicol, and metronidazole. The aerotolerance of *C. septicum* may reduce the efficacy of HBO therapy.

PROGNOSIS. The mortality of spontaneous clostridial gangrene ranges from 67 to 100%, with the majority of deaths occurring within 24 hours of onset. Risk factors include underlying malignancy and compromised immune status.

FOOD POISONING (ENTEROTOXEMIA) CAUSED BY *CLOSTRIDIUM PERFRINGENS*

C. perfringens accounts for nearly 20% of all reported cases of food poisoning (see Chapter 125). Ingesting large numbers of vegetative cells from inadequately prepared and stored food leads to multiplication and sporulation in the intestine. When mature spores are released, enterotoxin is liberated into the lumen of the gastrointestinal tract. The alkaline environment of the proximal small intestine and the presence of trypsin (a pancreatic enzyme found in the gut lumen) cause a 2.5-fold increase in biologic activity of enterotoxin. Histologically, enterotoxin causes bleb formation and desquamation of the microvillus tips of the brush border. Physiologically, such cells are incapable of glucose and ion absorption. The net effect is loss of electrolytes and fluid across the brush border, with resultant diarrhea. Other symptoms that manifest 5 to 24 hours after ingesting contaminated food are nausea, vomiting, and abdominal cramping. The definitive diagnosis rests on demonstrating enterotoxin in stool samples. Reliable biologic tests, radioimmunoassays, and an enzyme-linked immunosorbent assay (ELISA) have been developed, although the ELISA is favored, owing to its sensitivity, cost, and quick results.

NECROTIZING ENTERITIS

Neutropenic enterocolitis is a fulminant form of necrotizing enteritis that occurs in neutropenic patients. Neutropenia is often profound and may be related to cyclic neutropenia, leukemia, aplastic anemia, or chemotherapy. Symptoms include abdominal pain, chills, and malaise. Copious watery diarrhea, abdominal distention, and pain localizing to the right lower quadrant develop, followed rapidly by signs of toxicity, such as tachycardia, fever, and delirium. Radiographic examinations may reveal thickening of the wall of the colon or cecum and, in advanced cases, gas in the wall of the colon. Anecdotal reports suggest that computed tomography may be a superior means of diagnosing this condition. Complications include rupture of the bowel, with peritonitis, bacteremia, and death in 100% of cases. Aggressive supportive measures, surgical intervention, and appropriate antibiotics (see previous section on spontaneous gas gangrene) have reduced the mortality to 25%.

Postmortem examinations reveal that among children dying of leukemia, localized infection of the ileocecal region (typhilitis) is extremely common and may have contributed to death in nearly 40%. *C. septicum* is the most common organism isolated from the blood of such patients, and Gram stain and immunofluorescence studies demonstrate that these bacteria invade the bowel wall in most cases.

Other forms of necrotizing enteritis have occurred endemically in New Guinea (pigbel), in epidemic proportion in Germany after World War II (Darmbrand), and sporadically in Africa, Southeast Asia, and the United States. All cases are associated with ingesting meats contaminated with *C. perfringens* type c. Clinical courses vary between abdominal pain, fever, and diarrhea, which resolve spontaneously, to bloody diarrhea, ruptured bowel, and death. β-Toxin from *C. perfringens* type c has been implicated as causing these infections. β-Toxin paralyzes the intestinal villi and causes

friability and necrosis of the bowel wall. Predisposing factors include malnutrition, specifically in those with diets low in protein and rich in trypsin inhibitors such as sweet potato or soy bean. In addition, *Ascaris lumbricoides* is found commonly in such patients, and it, too, secretes a trypsin inhibitor. These protease inhibitors protect β-toxin from intraluminal proteolysis.

Medical management should include aggressive fluid and electrolyte replacement, bowel decompression, and antibiotic treatment with penicillin or chloramphenicol. Surgical resection of necrotic bowel is necessary in 50% of patients, and mortality rates as high as 40% have been described. If peritonitis develops, broader antibiotic coverage may be necessary. Immunization of children in New Guinea with a β-toxoid vaccine has dramatically reduced the incidence of this disease.

CLOSTRIDIUM SORDELLII INFECTION

Patients with *C. sordellii* infection present with unique clinical features, including edema, absence of fever, leukemoid reaction, hemoconcentration, and later shock and multiorgan failure. Often *C. sordellii* infections develop after childbirth or after gynecologic procedures, although some cases involve sites of minor trauma such as lacerations. Unlike *C. perfringens* and *C. septicum* infections, pain may not be a prominent feature. The absence of fever and paucity of signs and symptoms of local infection make early diagnosis difficult. The mechanisms of diffuse capillary leak, massive edema, and hemoconcentration are not well established but clearly are related to elaboration of a potent toxin. Hematocrits of 75 to 80% have been described, and leukocytosis of 50 to 100,000 cells/mm^3 with a left shift is common.

CLOSTRIDIUM TERTIUM INFECTIONS

C. tertium causes bacteremia in compromised hosts who have received long courses of antibiotics, thus explaining the organism's relative resistance to penicillin, cephalosporins, and clindamycin. *C. tertium* is, however, usually quite sensitive to chloramphenicol, vancomycin, and metronidazole. Because this organism can grow aerobically, it may be mistakenly disregarded as a contaminant such as a diphtheroid or bacillus species.

Asmuth DM, Olson RD, Hackett SP, et al: Effects of *Clostridium perfringens* recombinant and crude phospholipase C and ϑ toxin on rabbit hemodynamic parameters. J Infect Dis 172:1317, 1995. *This study demonstrated a profound drop in mean arterial pressure and cardiac output induced by clostridial exotoxins in an awake rabbit model.*

Farnell MB: Neutropenic enterocolitis: A surgical disease? Infect Surg 6:120, 1987. *Describes the clinical presentation of necrotizing lesions of the terminal ileum associated with neutropenic conditions; also describes the evidence that implicates C. septicum as the cause of enterocolitis.*

Stevens DL, Bryant AE, Adams K, et al: Evaluation of hyperbaric oxygen therapy for treatment of experimental *Clostridium perfringens* infection. Clin Infect Dis 17:231, 1993. *This study describes the efficacy of hyperbaric oxygen. In the same issue, editorials describe the pros and cons of hyperbaric oxygen treatment.*

Stevens DL, Musher DM, Watson DA, et al: Spontaneous, nontraumatic gangrene due to *Clostridium septicum*. Rev Infect Dis 12:286, 1990. *A review article concerning clinical features of spontaneous gas gangrene (complete with color plates).*

Stevens DL, Tweten RK, Awad MM, et al: Clostridial gas gangrene: Evidence that α and ϑ toxins differentially modulate the immune response and induce acute tissue necrosis. J Infect Dis 176:189, 1997. *Authors demonstrated that both toxins impede leukocyte infiltration into infected tissues but with differing dynamics.*

335 PSEUDOMEMBRANOUS COLITIS

Robert Fekety

DESCRIPTION. Pseudomembranous colitis (PMC) is a toxin-induced inflammatory process characterized by exudative plaques or pseudomembranes attached to the surface of the inflamed colonic mucosa. The disease is also referred to as "antibiotic-associated colitis" (AAC) because many patients who develop the disease have no grossly visible pseudomembranes, even though biopsy may show microscopically visible pseudomembranes as well as inflammation.

ETIOLOGY. Although most patients with PMC develop it as a complication of antimicrobial therapy or cancer chemotherapy, the disease was recognized in the pre-antibiotic era, when *Staphylococcus aureus* appeared to be the usual cause. Now staphylococci are rarely the cause, and the colitis associated with antimicrobial agents is almost always caused by *Clostridium difficile*. The disease results from the elaboration by this organism in the lumen of the large intestine of two exotoxins, A and B, and it is commonly referred to as *C. difficile*–associated diarrhea (CDAD), especially when the presence of colitis as well as diarrhea has not been proven. For all practical purposes, PMC, AAC, and CDAD are synonyms for a single disease process presenting in different ways to the patient and physician. Toxin A is an enterotoxin because its pronounced effects on the intestinal mucosa of small laboratory animals are more dramatic than its cytotoxic properties. Toxin B, which is called the cytotoxin, is also an enterotoxin for human intestinal epithelial cell cultures. Both exotoxins seem important in the pathogenesis of the disease in humans. Multiplication and toxin production by *C. difficile* within the colonic lumen of humans is promoted by still poorly understood antibiotic-induced alterations in the "colonization resistance" of the normal intestinal flora. *C. difficile*–induced colitis results when there is attachment of toxins A and/or B to the colonic mucosa followed by tissue damage, inflammation, and fluid secretion; invasion of colonic tissues by *C. difficile* is uncommon. About 75% of *C. difficile* isolates produce both toxins; most of the rest do not produce either one. Isolates that do not produce toxins do not cause colitis or diarrhea.

INCIDENCE AND EPIDEMIOLOGY. Although CDAD occurs at all ages, it is surprisingly uncommon in newborns, who often acquire toxigenic *C. difficile* within the first few weeks of life and yet remain well, possibly because the toxins do not bind to the colonic mucosa of most newborns and young infants. CDAD occurs most often in patients in hospitals or nursing homes in association with serious medical and surgical diseases requiring the use of antibiotics. It may occur in healthy persons who have not received antimicrobial agents or cancer chemotherapeutic agents, but this is very uncommon. The frequency of PMC and CDAD is determined in large part by the frequency with which endoscopy and/or laboratory tests to detect the presence of the toxins in diarrheal stools are performed, on the frequency of use of potent antimicrobial agents, on the antibiotic resistance patterns of the prevalent *C. difficile strains,* and on epidemiologic factors favoring transmission of the organism. Nearly all antimicrobial agents have been implicated as factors in the development of PMC and CDAD, but those most frequently implicated are broad-spectrum cephalosporins, ampicillin, clindamycin, and antibiotic combinations. Less frequent are other penicillins, erythromycin, aminoglycosides, tetracyclines, and sulfamethoxazole-trimethoprim. *C. difficile*–induced colitis occurs both sporadically and in clusters or outbreaks in hospitals and chronic care facilities. *C. difficile* can be detected in the stools of 3 to 5% of healthy adults and 20% or more of hospitalized patients without diarrhea, in the environment, and on a variety of inanimate objects in hospitals. *C. difficile* is widely distributed in our environment, including in soil and water. *C. difficile*–associated diarrhea and colitis are especially common in hospitals and nursing homes, where as many as 20 to 30% of patients who have received antibiotics may be asymptomatic carriers and where spread of the organism from patients who are carriers or who have diarrhea can occur. Spread from colonized patients is often the result of transmission by the hands of hospital personnel, although transmission by contact with contaminated objects such as commodes, sinks, and electronic thermometers is also thought to be important.

CLINICAL MANIFESTATIONS. Diarrhea beginning more than 72 hours *after* admission to the hospital is not likely to be caused by other enteropathogens. Although the disease may begin as early as 1 day after antibiotic therapy is started, symptoms usually begin during the first week of treatment. In as many as 20% of patients, diarrhea may not begin until as long as 6 weeks *after* antimicrobials have been discontinued. The most frequent symptoms of CDAD are profuse watery diarrhea, usually without blood or mucus, and cramping abdominal pain. Most patients also have fever (although usually low grade, it may exceed 40° C [104° F]). Leukocytosis is very common, and leukemoid reactions with values as high as 50,000 to 100,000/mm³ occur and should suggest the diagnosis of severe PMC in a patient with diarrhea. In some patients,

marked abdominal tenderness, fever, and leukocytosis are the *only* early clues to PMC, and diarrhea may not begin until several days later; this presentation appears most common in postoperative surgical or obstetric patients and in those who have received opiates for treatment of pain. Other findings include hypoalbuminemia and edema due to protein-losing enteropathy. Mild *C. difficile* diarrhea/colitis is much more common than severe colitis, and many patients simply have annoying watery diarrhea resembling that seen with the so-called benign or simple antibiotic diarrhea thought to be attributable to changes in the normal fecal flora. Complications in severe cases include dehydration, anasarca, electrolyte disturbances, toxic megacolon, and colonic perforation. Unusual manifestations include the development of diarrhea and enterocolitis in infants and very young children with Hirschsprung's disease or with reactive arthritis. The differential diagnosis includes acute and chronic diarrhea caused by other enteric pathogens, an adverse reaction to medications other than antibiotics, idiopathic inflammatory bowel diseases, and intra-abdominal sepsis. Occasionally, *C. difficile* colitis may be complicated afterward by intra-abdominal abscesses or infections at distant sites, such as osteomyelitis.

DIAGNOSIS. The role of the available tests and studies that aid in diagnosis of CDAD is summarized in Table 335–1. Endoscopy is the most rapid way to establish the diagnosis of PMC, but because of expense and discomfort, it is usually reserved for special situations.

Until recently, the "gold standard" laboratory test for establishing the diagnosis of *C. difficile* colitis has been the demonstration in filtrates of diarrheal stools of a cytopathic effect caused by toxin B that is neutralized by specific antitoxin, but this is being replaced by more rapid, simple, and inexpensive enzyme immunoassays for the presence of toxin A and/or B in stools. The specificity of these tests is very high, but it should be noted that their sensitivity ranges from 88 to 96%; that is, false-negative results are not uncommon. Computed tomography may be useful in detecting evidence of PMC, especially in patients presenting with an acute abdominal syndrome without diarrhea; in the early detection of complications of PMC (Figs. 335–1 and 335–2); and in ruling out other conditions.

TREATMENT. Patients with suspect CDAD should have one or more of the various diagnostic tests for the disease (see Table 335–1), but only one stool specimen should be sent for the same test on the same day. Simply discontinuing antimicrobial therapy may result in cessation of mild CDAD within a few days in 15 to 25% of patients. Correction of fluid, electrolyte, protein, and blood losses is of obvious importance.

Patients with severe symptoms should receive prompt specific therapy for colitis. Discontinuation of needed antimicrobial therapy is not essential when specific antibiotic therapy for PMC is given. Opiates and antiperistaltic drugs should be avoided because they may cause intestinal atony, pooling of toxin-laden intestinal contents, and worsening of the illness.

Specific therapy usually is with metronidazole or vancomycin given for 7 to 10 days or longer if the response is slow. The oral route is preferred because the organism multiplies and produces toxins within the intestinal lumen that subsequently attach to mucosa and exert their effects; because the organism rarely invades tissue, it is *not* necessary to obtain good systemic antibacterial activity. Metronidazole, 250 or 500 mg four times per day, is currently preferred over vancomycin for treatment of colitis of mild or moderate severity. Metronidazole may have undesirable side effects in some patients; occasional isolates of *C. difficile* are resistant to metronidazole. Vancomycin is active against virtually all isolates of *C. difficile,* but in the hope of delaying the emergence and spread of vancomycin-resistant staphylococci or streptococci, vancomycin should be reserved for treatment of seriously ill or refractory patients with PMC. Vancomycin, 125 to 500 mg, is usually given orally four times per day for 7 to 14 days; if the patient has impending ileus or is critically ill, the larger dose is preferred. Problems with vancomycin include its relatively high cost, bad taste, and unreliability when given intravenously to treat colitis. Vancomycin given orally is not significantly absorbed systemically in most patients, so systemic side effects are rare when it is given in this way. An alternative treatment for patients with mild CDAD is the use of anion exchange resins such as cholestyramine

Table 335–1 ■ DIAGNOSING *CLOSTRIDIUM DIFFICILE* COLITIS

TEST	COMMENTS
Laboratory Tests on Feces	
Test for fecal leukocytes	A simple screening test but sensitivity only 30 to 50%. Lactoferrin test is probably more reliable. *A positive test rules out benign or simple antibiotic diarrhea.*
Stool culture for *C. difficile*	Results delayed. *Not diagnostic,* because 10 to 25% of patients in hospitals may carry the organism, and only 75% of isolates produce toxins. May be used epidemiologically.
Tests for the presence of fecal toxins	
Cytopathic effect of toxin B in tissue cultures	*"Gold standard,"* but some cell lines are not as sensitive as others, so false-negative results may occur. Time consuming, expensive, and not widely available. Requires antitoxin neutralization for specificity.
Toxin A, B, or AB by ELISA	*Rapid, widely available, relatively inexpensive.* Sensitivity varies and not 100%. If cut point is chosen to minimize false-negative results, false-positive results may be a problem.
Latex agglutination for *C. difficile*	Rapid and inexpensive. *Detects glutamic dehydrogenase* (neither a toxin nor specific for *C. difficile*). Many false-positive and false-negative results.
Radiologic Studies	
Plain film of the abdomen	*Nonspecific* and useful only when colitis is far advanced or complications such as toxic megacolon or perforation are present.
Barium enema	*Nonspecific* findings. May precipitate perforation or megacolon.
Computed tomography	Safe, but expensive, and not highly specific. *Can be useful,* especially when patients present with an acute abdomen without diarrhea. May demonstrate unsuspected pseudomembranous colitis.
Radionuclide scans (indium-labeled white blood cells)	May detect inflammation, but *do not diagnose etiology.*
Procedures	
Flexible sigmoidoscopy	*Most rapid way to make the diagnosis.* Expensive. Misses about 10% of cases (those with only minor or proximal colonic lesions). Biopsy of minor or non-specific lesions increases yield.
Colonoscopy	Rapid and *most sensitive way to make the diagnosis.* Expensive and may be hazardous. Biopsy of minor or non-specific lesions increases yield.

(1 or 2 4-g pouches given orally twice daily for 5 to 10 days) that bind the toxins of C. *difficile*; but these may also bind vancomycin and teicoplanin and other medications. Given by themselves, anion exchange resins may fail in seriously ill patients; furthermore, they may cause obstipation once the diarrhea resolves. Oral bacitracin and teicoplanin have been effective therapeutic alternatives, but bacitracin is not always readily available and teicoplanin is not available in the United States.

Patients who cannot be treated orally or through a nasogastric tube with metronidazole or vancomycin should be given vancomycin in solution (500 mg/500 mL two to four times per day has been used) through a catheter passed to the cecum using a colonoscope, through a long intestinal tube passed from above to the distal ileum, or by means of an ileostomy or colostomy. Therapy with intravenous vancomycin is of no value because little, if any, of the drug gains access to the intestinal lumen when given in this way. Therapy with intravenous metronidazole *may* be a helpful addition in this setting but is *not* reliable by itself. For adults, a loading dose of 15 mg/kg of metronidazole given over 1 hour has been used, followed by 7.5 mg/kg infused over 1 hour every 6 hours. If these measures are not possible or successful, it may be necessary to perform a subtotal colectomy, with postoperative intraluminal administration of the antimicrobial agent or agents.

Relapse or recurrence of colitis within 2 to 8 weeks after discontinuing antibiotic therapy occurs in 15 to 35% of successfully treated patients; whether the patient was treated with vancomycin or metronidazole seems to make no difference. Both of these increase susceptibility to intestinal colonization with *C. difficile*, and both have precipitated attacks of CDAD. Relapses may be caused

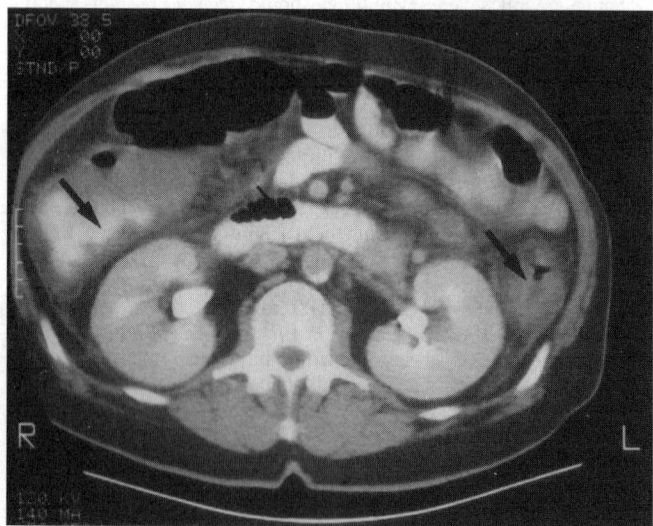

FIGURE 335–1 ■ Computed tomographic scan of abdomen of a neurosurgical patient with postoperative fever and diarrhea. Stools were positive for *C. difficile* cytotoxin. The arrow at left indicates irregularly thickened cecal musosa; the arrow at right indicates luminal narrowing, mucosal thickening, and edema of the descending colon. (From Fekety R: Infectious colitis. *In* Greenfield LJ, et al [eds]: Surgery: Scientific Principles and Practice. Philadelphia, J.B. Lippincott, 1992, p. 1055.)

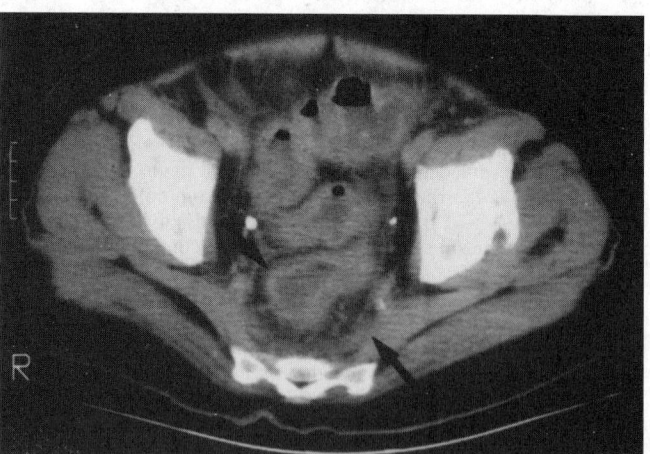

FIGURE 335–2 ■ Computed tomographic scan at another level of the patient with pseudomembranous colitis. The arrow at left points to thickening of the rectal mucosa; the arrow at right indicates edema and inflammation in the perirectal soft tissues. (From Fekety R: Infectious colitis. *In* Greenfield LJ et al [eds]: Surgery: Scientific Principles and Practice. Philadelphia, JB Lippincott, 1992, p 1055.)

GENERAL	OUTBREAK SETTING
Prudent use of antibiotics (narrow spectrum, short courses)	Education about the disease
Washing hands between patients	Emphasize hand washing before and after each patient
Enteric isolation of cases: stool precautions, use of gloves	Use of gloves for handling positive patients
Immunization with *C. difficile* toxoids (future)	Patient (carriers) cohorting
	Treatment of fecal carriers with oral metronidazole, bacitracin, or vancomycin to reduce fecal shedding of *C. difficile*
	Disinfection of unit and fomites to kill spores and vegetative forms with 2% alkaline glutaraldehyde or hypochlorite solutions (1600 ppm)
	Closure of unit (as a last resort)

power of immunotherapy for this disease, and a hint that future progress in prevention may involve active immunization.

by either the initial strain or a newly acquired one. Relapses usually respond well to standard therapy with metronidazole or vancomycin, but neither one is completely reliable in prevention of further relapses. In patients suffering from repeated relapses, attempts have been made in uncontrolled, non-blinded studies to restore the normal fecal flora by giving long courses of intermittent or tapering dosages of oral vancomycin (alone or with rifampin) or metronidazole, live lactobacilli, or mixtures of normal fecal bacteria for various periods of time. Oral administration for 1 month of a live yeast (*Saccharomyces boulardii*) that makes a protease capable of inactivating binding sites on the toxins and/or the mucosa can be an adjunct to treatment with oral vancomycin. Use of *S. boulardii* significantly reduced (by about 50%) the likelihood of further relapses in a double-blind placebo controlled study, but *S. boulardii* is not available in the United States. Encouraging results have been obtained in uncontrolled studies when human immunoglobulin containing IgG against both toxin A and toxin B was given intravenously to young children with immunoglobulin deficiency states who experienced relapses or to adults with severe, prolonged or refractory *C. difficile* colitis.

PREVENTION. The most important preventive measures are enteric isolation precautions, use of gloves and careful hand washing after contact with patients who have the disease or who may be carriers of the organism, elimination of dangerous environmental sources or vectors of the organism, and judicious use or restriction of certain antimicrobial agents (Table 335–2).

Lyerly DM, Neville LM, Evans DT, et al: Multicenter evaluation of the *Clostridium difficile* TOX A/B TEST. J Clin Microbiol 36:184, 1998. *A good discussion of the good and bad things about this most important laboratory aid to the diagnosis of* C. difficile *colitis.*

Fekety R: Guidelines for the diagnosis and management of *Clostridium difficile*-associated diarrhea and colitis. Am J Gastroenterol 92:739,1997. *More details on recommendations and rationales.*

Fekety, R, McFarland LV, Surawicz CM, et al: Recurrent *Clostridium difficile* diarrhea: Characteristics of and risk factors for patients enrolled in a prospective, randomized, double-blinded trial. Clin Infect Dis 24:324, 1997. *Helps identify patients likely to have trouble with recurrences, lists their risk factors, and stresses the importance of avoiding use of antibiotics for minor infections in these patients.*

McFarland LV, Surawicz CM, Greenberg RN, et al: A randomized, placebo-controlled trial of *Saccharomyces boulardii* in combination with standard antibiotics for *Clostridium difficile* disease. JAMA 271:1913, 1994. *Shows the relapse rate was reduced by half with the use of this yeast as an adjunct to specific therapy of patients with multiple relapses.*

Salcedo, J, Keates S, Pothoulakis S, et al: Intravenous immunoglobulin therapy for severe *Clostridium difficile* colitis. Gut 41:366, 1997. *A good discussion of the*

336   BOTULISM

John G. Bartlett

DEFINITION. Botulism is a severe neuroparalytic disease caused by botulinum toxin produced by clostridial species, usually *Clostridium botulinum*. Four categories of disease are recognized: food-borne botulism, infant botulism, wound botulism, and "other."

ETIOLOGY. *C. botulinum* is a gram-positive, spore-forming obligate anaerobe that is widely distributed in nature and frequently found in soil, marine environments, and agricultural products. Each strain produces one of eight antigenically distinct toxins designated A through H. Human disease is caused by types A, B, E, and (rarely) F. These neurotoxins consist of a dichain peptide of approximately 150,000 daltons. The toxin is absorbed from the intestine or produced in an infected wound, and it is disseminated by the systemic circulation and then binds to specific receptors where it blocks acetylcholine release. The result is paralysis reflecting the specific nerves involved, usually expressed as a descending symmetric flaccid paralysis. Botulinum toxin is the most potent poison of humans, with a lethal dose in the systemic circulation estimated to be 10^{-9} mg/kg. Type A botulinum toxin is now available for injection as therapy for ocular muscle disorders such as strabismus and blepharospasm and for dystonias such as torticollis and hemifacial spasm. This toxin is also a candidate for bioterrorism because of its extraordinary potency.

CLINICAL FORMS. The frequency of various forms of human botulism in the United States from 1950 to 1993 is summarized in Table 336–1.

FOOD-BORNE BOTULISM. Food-borne botulism, the most common form of botulism in the world, results from the ingestion of pre-formed toxin in inadequately prepared food. The foods most frequently implicated are home processed. In the United States, an average of 15 "outbreaks" occur annually, and most involve one or two cases. The most frequently implicated source is home canned foods, which usually have a putrefactive odor. Type A is the predominant form in the west and type B predominates in the east. Meat and meat products are more commonly responsible in Europe, and the predominant toxin is type B. In China, the most common vehicle is a vegetable product, and type A toxin predominates. Type E botulism is associated with fish and other marine foods and is most common in Alaska.

WOUND BOTULISM. Wound botulism is a relatively unusual form of botulism that was first described in 1943. Toxin types A and B have been implicated in all cases—a reflection of their presence in soil. Most cases result from traumatic wounds; less frequent causes are surgical wounds and illicit drug abuse. Clinical features are identical to those of food-borne botulism except that the incubation period from the time of injury to the onset of symptoms ranges from 4 to 14 days and gastrointestinal symptoms are few.

Table 336–1 ■ INCIDENCE OF BOTULISM IN THE U.S., 1950–1993

DISEASE FROM	YEARS	TOXIN TYPE**			TOTAL	CASE FATALITY
		A	B	E		
Food-borne	1950–93	436	183	196	1126	17.9%
Wound	1950–93	37	15	0	58	10.3%
Infant	1975–93	575	603	0	1190	1.1%
Other	1978–93	17	6	0	31	29.0%

*Adapted from Hatheway C: *Clostridium botulinum*. *In* Gorbach SL, Bartlett JG, Blacklow NR (eds): Infectious Diseases, 2nd ed. Philadelphia, WB Saunders, 1997, pp 1919–1925.

**Nine cases due to type F and 323 cases with unknown toxin type.

INFANT BOTULISM. Infant botulism was initially described in 1976 and has subsequently become the most frequently recognized form of botulism in the United States. It results from the production of botulinal neurotoxin in the gastrointestinal tract after colonization in children aged 1 to 9 months. The usual source of *C. botulinum* is the soil or, less frequently, honey. Nearly all cases are due to type A or type B. The disease spectrum varies considerably, but the most commonly recognized form is the "floppy baby syndrome." Initial symptoms are lethargy, diminished suck, constipation, weakness, feeble cry, and diminished spontaneous activity with loss of head control. These symptoms are followed by extensive flaccid paralysis. The case fatality rate is only 1%.

UNDETERMINED CLASSIFICATION. Botulism of undetermined classification applies to isolated cases of botulism that have no plausible food or wound source of *C. botulinum*. Some cases are well confirmed on the basis of detection of toxin in serum or stool and isolation of *C. botulinum* from stool. These observations suggest that this form of botulism is due to intestinal colonization rather than ingestion of pre-formed toxin, which makes it analogous to infant botulism.

CLINICAL MANIFESTATIONS. The incubation period is usually 18 to 36 hours but may be as short as 2 hours or as long as 8 days. The incubation period depends to some extent on the inoculum size, so short incubation periods are associated with more severe disease. The bulbar musculature is usually affected first and results in diplopia, dysphonia, dysarthria, and dysphagia. Involvement of the cholinergic autonomic nervous system may result in decreased salivation with dry mouth and sore throat, ileus, or urinary retention. Neurologic evaluation often shows bilateral paresis of the 6th cranial nerves, ptosis, dilated pupils with sluggish reaction, decreased gag reflex, or medial rectus paresis. These symptoms are followed by descending involvement of motor neurons to peripheral muscles, including the muscles of respiration. The most common cause of death is respiratory failure. The spectrum of disease is quite variable; some patients have mild illness whereas others have severe paralysis requiring intensive care with mechanical ventilation. Mentation remains clear, patients are afebrile, and neurologic dysfunction is bilateral, but not necessarily symmetric. In a review of 272 cases of botulism in adults in the United States, the most frequent symptoms were diplopia and blurred vision (90%), dysphagia (76%), generalized weakness (58%), nausea or vomiting (56%), and dysphonia (55%). The most frequent signs in this series were respiratory impairment (73%), specific muscle paresis or paralysis (46%), and ocular muscle impairment (44%). The clinical features of infant botulism are similar to those described above. Findings in over 80% of reported cases include weakness, hypotonia, constipation, failure with oral feeding, diminished gag or suck reflex, respiratory failure, ptosis, and reduced spontaneous movements.

DIAGNOSIS. Standard laboratory tests in cases of suspected food-borne botulism include analysis of serum, stool, gastric contents, and/or food for botulinum toxin and analysis of stool and/or food for *C. botulinum*. With wound botulism, the diagnosis is established by recovery of *C. botulinum* from wound cultures or by detection of the toxin in serum. With both food-borne and wound botulism, failure to detect toxin or recover *C. botulinum* does not exclude the diagnosis. In infants, the recommendation is to test stools for culture and toxin; two negative specimens obtained during the acute phase of disease will generally rule out this diagnosis. The classic test for botulinum toxin is the mouse bioassay using intraperitoneal challenge to demonstrate a lethal toxin that is neutralized by type-specific antitoxin. Alternative antigen assays, including an enzyme-linked immunoassay, have been developed but are not widely available. In general, adult patients with clinical evidence of botulism show demonstrable toxin in sera in one third of cases and toxin in stool in one third of cases, and the organism is recovered from stool in 60%. Because botulism is rare and is a potential public health emergency, diagnostic services of the state health department or Centers for Disease Control and Prevention should be pursued.

Botulism should be suspected in patients with acute flaccid paralysis, especially in the presence of bilateral 6th cranial nerve dysfunction, associated neurologic findings, recent ingestion of possibly contaminated food, and/or typical symptoms in other persons who shared this food. The differential diagnosis includes myasthenia gravis, Guillain-Barré syndrome, tick paralysis, cerebrovascular accident involving branches of the basilar artery, trichinosis, Eaton-Lambert syndrome, hypocalcemia, hypermagnesemia, organophosphate poisoning, atropine poisoning, paralytic poisoning caused by shellfish or puffer fish, and psychiatric syndromes. Electromyography using repetitive stimulation at 40 Hz or greater may prove useful in differentiating botulism from other neurologic syndromes. Electromyography demonstrates a diminished amplitude of muscle action potentials with a single supramaximal stimulus and facilitation of action potentials with paired or repetitive stimuli.

TREATMENT. Respiratory failure is the major risk and patients must be monitored carefully with liberal use of ventilatory support. Toxin may be removed from the gastrointestinal tract with gastric lavage, cathartics, and enemas early in the course of disease. The trivalent antitoxin or type-specific antitoxin for types A, B, or E is usually given to adults. The usual treatment is two vials, one given intravenously and one given intramuscularly. The antitoxin should be given as early as possible. Antitoxin will not reverse paralysis or neutralize toxin bound to nerve endings. The goal is neutralization of unbound toxin in the circulation to prevent further paralysis. The antitoxin is horse serum and is associated with hypersensitivity reactions in about 9%; serum sickness or anaphylaxis develops in occasional patients. Antibiotic treatment is unnecessary except for wound botulism. Infants with botulism should not receive either antibiotics directed against *C. botulinum* or antitoxin because most do extremely well with supportive care alone and it has been suggested that antibiotics may cause toxin release.

PROGNOSIS. The case fatality rate for food-borne botulism was formerly 60 to 70%. Improved management, especially with respiratory support, has reduced the case fatality rate for food-borne botulism in the United States to 6.6% in recent years. The mortality rate with other forms of botulism are summarized in Table 336–1. Patients who survive generally have complete recovery.

PREVENTION. Food-borne botulism is caused by germination of spores in food, with toxin produced by the vegetative forms of *C. botulinum*; the toxin may also be produced in vivo by ingestion of spores and colonization of the gastrointestinal tract. The disease may be prevented by destruction of spores in the original food source, inhibition of germination, or destruction of pre-formed toxin. Specific measures are as follows:

1. Destruction of spores with heat or irradiation. Spores of type A and B may survive boiling for several hours, especially at high altitudes such as in Colorado, where the boiling point may be substantially lower. These spores may be destroyed if kept at 120° C for 30 minutes in pressure cookers. Spores of type E are the most heat labile and are killed with heating at 80° C for 30 minutes.
2. Germination may be inhibited by reducing the pH, refrigerating, freezing, drying, or adding inhibitory substances such as salt, sugar, or sodium nitrate.
3. Inactivation of pre-formed toxin is accomplished by terminal heating for 20 minutes at 80° C or 10 minutes at 90° C.

With regard to infant botulism, honey has been implicated as a vehicle for spores and should not be fed to infants younger than 1 year.

SPECIAL NOTE. Physicians who suspect food-borne botulism or wish to receive botulinal antitoxin should contact their state health department or contact the Centers for Disease Control and Prevention 24-hour hotline at (404) 329-2888.

Chia JK, Clark JB, Ryan CA, et al: Botulism in an adult associated with food-borne intestinal infection with *Clostridium botulinum*. N Engl J Med 315:239, 1986. *The case presented is an example of gastrointestinal colonization by* C. botulinum *with in vivo production of the neurotoxin in an adult.*

Hatheway CL: *Clostridium botulinum. In* Gorbach SL, Bartlett JG, Blacklow NR (eds): Infectious Diseases, 2nd ed. Philadelphia, WB Saunders, 1997, pp 1919–1925. *The author, a noted authority on botulism, reviews the clinical, diagnostic, and therapeutic aspects of this disease.*

Hatheway CL, Ferreira JL: Detection and identification of *Clostridium botulinum* neurotoxins. Adv Exp Med Biol 391:481, 1996. *This is a review of diagnostic tests.*

Montecucco C, Schiavo G: Mechanism of action of tetanus and botulinum neurotoxins. Mol Microbiol 13:1, 1994. *The authors review the similar pathophysiologic mechanisms of neurotoxins produced by Clostridium tetani and* C. botulinum.

Sonnabend OA, Sonnabend WF, Krech U, et al: Continuous microbiological study of 70 sudden and unexpected infant deaths: Toxigenic intestinal *Clostridium botulinum* infection in 9 cases of sudden infant death syndrome. Lancet 2:237, 1985. *The authors review the role of* C. botulinum *in sudden infant death syndrome.*

337 TETANUS

John G. Bartlett

DEFINITION. Tetanus is a neurologic syndrome caused by a neurotoxin elaborated at the site of injury by *Clostridium tetani.*

ETIOLOGY. *C. tetani* is an anaerobic, gram-positive, slender, motile bacillus. The sporulated form has a characteristic drumstick or tennis-racket shape with a terminal spore. The vegetative form produces tetanospasmin, a protein neurotoxin with a molecular weight of approximately 151 kd. Tetanospasmin ranks with botulism toxin as the most potent known microbial toxin; 1 mg is capable of killing 50 to 70 million mice. The vegetative forms of *C. tetani* are highly susceptible to heat, disinfectants, and other adverse environmental conditions, but the spores are highly resistant and can survive in soil for months to years. Killing of spores requires boiling for at least 4 hours or autoclaving for 12 minutes at 121°C.

EPIDEMIOLOGY. *C. tetani* can be found in 20 to 65% of soil samples, the highest yields being in cultivated land and the lowest yields, in virgin soil. The organism can also be found in stool from a variety of animals, house dust, operating rooms, and contaminated heroin. Approximately 10% of humans harbor *C. tetani* in the colon.

Tetanus is most common in warm climates and in highly cultivated rural areas. The greatest problem is in economically deprived countries, owing to poor immunization standards and unhygienic practices. An example is the practice of dressing the umbilical stump with animal dung or "dusting powder," a local dried clay sold for cosmetic purposes, after childbirth by unimmunized mothers. It is estimated that the annual toll from neonatal tetanus in developing countries is 1 million. In the United States, there are 50 to 70 reported cases annually, and almost all occur in unimmunized or inadequately immunized persons. A review of 110 cases of tetanus in 1989–1990 in the United States showed 86 (78%) were associated with an acute injury, 10 (9%) were complications of chronic wounds, and 5 (5%) represented complications of injection drug use. There was one case of neonatal tetanus and 10 (9%) had no recognized portal of entry. The age of these patients was older than 60 years in 58% and younger than 20 years in 6%; this age distribution reflects the impact of waning immunity with aging.

PATHOGENESIS. Clinical tetanus requires a source of the organism, local tissue conditions that promote toxin production, and immunologic naiveté. The usual portals of entry are traumatic wounds, surgical wounds, subcutaneous injection sites, burns, skin ulcers, infected umbilical cords, and otitis media with tympanic membrane perforation. The spores are ubiquitous in the environment, and most cases reflect contamination from exogenous sources, although endogenous infection is conceivable in occasional cases that follow intestinal surgery. Important factors at the site of injury are necrotic tissue, suppuration, and the presence of a foreign body. These are responsible for a reduction in the local oxidation-reduction potential (eH), thus promoting reversion of spores to the vegetative forms that produce tetanospasmin. Tetanospasmin is taken up by the peripheral nerve terminals and carried intra-axonally within membrane-bound vesicles to spinal neurons at a transport rate of approximately 250 mm/day. On reaching the perikarya of the motor neurons the toxin passes to the presynaptic terminals, where it blocks release of neurotransmitters, including glycine, which is the neurotransmitter used by group 1A inhibitory afferent motor neurons. Loss of the inhibitory influence results in unrestrained firing with sustained muscular contraction. The result with spinal cord neurons is rigidity. In severe cases there is also involvement of the sympathetic chain causing autonomic dysfunction. Binding of the toxin is irreversible so that recovery requires generation of new axon terminals.

CLINICAL FEATURES. Forms of tetanus include generalized, localized, cephalic, and neonatal.

Generalized tetanus is the most common, accounting for 85 to 90% of reported cases in the United States. The extent of the associated trauma varies from a rather trivial injury that may be forgotten by the patient to a severe, contaminated crush injury. The usual incubation period is 7 to 21 days, depending largely on the distance of the site of injury from the central nervous system. The "onset period" refers to the time from the first clinical symptoms of tetanus to the first generalized spasm. An incubation period of less than 9 days and an onset period of less than 48 hours appear to be associated with more severe symptomatology. Trismus is the presenting complaint in 75% of cases, so the patient is often initially seen by a dentist or oral surgeon. Other early features include irritability, restlessness, diaphoresis, and dysphagia with hydrophobia and drooling. Sustained trismus may result in a characterisic sardonic smile, or "risus sardonicus," and persistent spasm of the back musculature may cause opisthotonos. These early manifestations reflect involvement of the bulbar muscles and paraspinous muscles, possibly because they are innervated by the shortest axons. Waves of opisthotonos are highly characteristic of the disease. With progression, the extremities become involved in episodes characterized by painful flexion and adduction of the arms, clenched fists, and extension of the legs. Noise or tactile stimuli may precipitate spasms and generalized convulsions, although they occur spontaneously as well. Involvement of the autonomic nervous system may result in severe arrhythmias, oscillation in the blood pressure, profound diaphoresis, hyperthermia, rhabdomyolysis, laryngeal spasm, and urinary retention. In most cases the patient remains lucid. The condition may progress for 2 weeks despite antitoxin therapy because of the time required for intra-axonal toxin transport. Complications include fractures from sustained contractions and convulsions, pulmonary emboli, bacterial infections, and dehydration.

Localized tetanus refers to involvement of the extremity with a contaminated wound and shows considerable variation in severity. In mild cases patients may simply have weakness of the involved extremity, presumably limited by partial immunity. In more severe cases there are intense, painful spasms that usually progress to generalized tetanus. This is a relatively unusual form of tetanus, and the prognosis for survival is excellent.

Cephalic tetanus generally follows a head injury or occurs with *C. tetani* infection of the middle ear. The clinical symptoms consist of isolated or combined dysfunction of the cranial motor nerves, most frequently the seventh cranial nerve. This may remain localized or progress to generalized tetanus. Again, this is a relatively unusual form of tetanus, but the incubation period is only 1 or 2 days, and the prognosis for survival is usually poor.

Tetanus neonatorum refers to generalized tetanus resulting from *C. tetani* infection in neonates. This occurs primarily in underdeveloped countries, where it accounts for up to half of all neonatal deaths. The usual cause is the use of contaminated materials to sever or dress the umbilical cord in newborns of unimmunized mothers. The usual incubation period after birth is 3 to 10 days, and it is sometimes referred to as "the disease of the seventh day," reflecting the average incubation period. The child typically shows irritability, facial grimacing, and severe spasms with touch. The mortality rate exceeds 70%.

DIAGNOSIS. The diagnosis of tetanus is usually made on the basis of clinical observations. The putative agent, *C. tetani,* is infrequently recovered with cultures of the wound. A confirmed history of immunization or a serum antitoxin level of 0.01 unit/dL or higher makes tetanus unlikely, but exceptions are reported. Cerebrospinal fluid analysis is entirely normal, and the electroencephalogram generally shows a sleep pattern. Diagnostic testing is usually not necessary except in cases lacking an identified portal of entry. The differential diagnosis depends on the dominant clinical features and includes oculogyric crisis secondary to phenothiazine toxicity, meningitis, dental abscess, seizure disorder, subarachnoid hemorrhage, hypocalcemic or alkalotic tetany, alcohol withdrawal, and strychnine poisoning. Strychnine also antagonizes glycine, and strychnine poisoning is the only condition that truly mimics tetanus. Strychnine levels in blood and urine establish the diagnosis. Dystonic reactions may resemble tetanus and are distinguished by rapid response to anticholinergic agents.

TREATMENT. Patients with tetanus require intensive care with particular attention to respiratory support, benzodiazepines, autonomic nervous system support, passive and active immunization, surgical débridement, and antibiotics directed against *C. tetani.* There may be clinical progression for about 2 weeks despite antitoxin treatment because of the time required to complete transport of toxin. Disease severity may be reduced by partial immunity so that some patients have mild disease with minimal mortality and others show mortality rates as high as 60% despite expert care.

SUPPORTIVE CARE. It is most important to assess airway function. Many patients will require endotracheal intubation with benzodiazepine sedation and neuromuscular blockade; a tracheostomy should be placed if the endotracheal tube causes spasms. A nasal feeding tube is usually required for nutritional support.

CONTROL OF MUSCLE SPASMS. Benzodiazepines have become the mainstay of therapy to control spasms and provide sedation. The most extensively studied is diazepam given in 5-mg increments; lorazepam or midazolam are equally effective. Tetanus patients may have high tolerance for the sedation effects of these drugs, requiring exceptionally high doses. When tetanus symptoms resolve, the drugs must be tapered over at least 2 weeks to prevent withdrawal reactions. If control of spasms cannot be achieved by benzodiazepines, long-term neuromuscular blockade is performed with vecuronium (6–8 mg/hour).

PASSIVE IMMUNIZATION. Human tetanus immunoglobulin (TIG) should be given as soon as possible to neutralize toxin that has not entered neurons. The usual dose is 500 units intramuscularly. Higher doses or administration intrathecally does not appear to be more effective. An alternative to TIG is pooled intravenous immunoglobulin. Equine tetanus immunoglobulin is equally effective, but the rate of allergic reactions is high, owing to the equine source. This preparation should no longer be used except in underdeveloped countries where cost dictates such medical decisions.

ACTIVE IMMUNIZATION. The standard three-dose schedule of immunization with tetanus toxoid should be given using an injection site separate from that used for immunoglobulin.

ANTIBIOTIC THERAPY. *C. tetani* is susceptible in vitro to penicillins, cephalosporins, imipenem, macrolides, metronidazole, and tetracyclines. Clinical studies favor the use of metronidazole, which should be given in a dose of 2 g/day for 7 to 10 days.

AUTONOMIC NERVOUS SYSTEM DYSFUNCTION. This generally reflects excessive catecholamine release and is usually treated with labetalol (0.25–1.0 mg/min) for blood pressure control. Other treatments for hypertension include morphine by continuous infusion, magnesium sulfate infusion, or an epidural blockade of the renal nerves. Hypotension may require norepinephrine infusion. Bradycardia may require a pacemaker.

SURGERY. Any wounds should be appropriately débrided.

PROGNOSIS. The overall mortality rate for generalized tetanus is 20–25 per cent even in modern medical facilities with extensive resources. Patients with moderate or severe generalized tetanus generally require 3 to 6 weeks for recovery. They may require intensive care during most of this time, but if they survive their recovery is usually complete. The highest mortality rates are at the extremes of age. The most frequent cause of death is pneumonia, but many patients have no obvious findings at autopsy, suggesting that death was directly due to the neurotoxin.

PREVENTION. Nearly all cases of tetanus occur in unimmunized or inadequately immunized individuals. The Immunization Practices Advisory Committee recommends active immunization of infants and children with DPT (diphtheria and tetanus toxoids and pertussis adsorbed) at 2 months, 4 months, 6 months, 15 months, and 4 to 6 years. Tetanus toxoid is a highly effective antigen and protective levels of serum antitoxin in persons who complete the primary series persist for at least 10 years. Td (tetanus and diphtheria toxoids adsorbed for adult use) is recommended every 10 years at mid-decade ages (15 years, 25 years, 35 years, etc.). This is commonly neglected as disclosed by serosurveys showing that 40 per cent of persons over 60 years in the United States lack protective levels of tetanus antitoxin. The recommended primary immunization series for unimmunized persons over 7 years is Td at time 0, 4 to 8 weeks, 6 to 12 months after the second dose, and then every

Table 337–1 ■ GUIDELINES FOR TETANUS PROPHYLAXIS IN WOUND MANAGEMENT

HISTORY OF ADSORBED TETANUS TOXOID	CLEAN AND MINOR WOUNDS		OTHER WOUNDS*	
Number of Doses	Td†	TIG‡	Td†	TIG‡
Unknown or less than three	Yes§	No	Yes†	Yes
Three or more	Yes if over 10 years since last dose	No	Yes if over 5 years since last dose	No

*Included but not limited to wounds contaminated with dirt, feces, soil, saliva, puncture wounds; avulsions; and wounds resulting from missiles, crushing, burns, and frostbite.

†Td: Tetanus and diphtheria toxoids adsorbed. Children younger than 7 should receive DPT (diptheria and tetanus toxoids and pertussis vaccine adsorbed). Too frequent booster doses of tetanus toxoid have been associated with hypersensitivity reactions.

‡TIG: Tetanus immune globulin in a dose of 250 units intramuscularly. The usual prophylactic dose of equine tetanus immune globulin is 1500 to 5000 units intramuscularly. When tetanus toxoid is given concurrently there should be separate syringes and injection sites.

§Unimmunized or incompletely immunized persons (one or two doses of toxoid) should receive complete immunization with Td at time 0, 4–8 weeks later, and 6–12 months later.

10 years. Nearly all states now require DPT immunization for school enrollment. About 95 per cent of tetanus cases in the United States occur in persons who have not received the primary series of tetanus toxoid. Immunized childbearing women confer protection on their infants through transplacental maternal antibody.

Prevention of tetanus after injury requires appropriate wound management, assurance of adequate immunity, and consideration of antibiotic prophylaxis. The aim of surgery is to eliminate necrotic tissue, purulent collections, and foreign bodies that promote the environmental conditions necessary for spore germination. Guidelines for immunoprophylaxis based on immunization status and wound characteristics are summarized in Table 337–1. Passive immunization is recommended only for "tetanus prone" wounds, using TIG for patients with inadequate or unknown primary immunization status. The definition of *tetanus-prone* depends on the interval between injury and treatment, the degree of contamination, the extent of devitalized tissue or foreign bodies within the site of injury, and the depth of the injury. Antimicrobial agents such as penicillin, erythromycin, or metronidazole may be given to inhibit replication of the vegetative forms of *C. tetani*, but immunization and wound cleansing are considered more important.

Armitage P, Clifford R: Prognosis in tetanus: Use of data from therapeutic trials. J Infect Dis 138:1–8, 1978. *Data for 1385 patients with tetanus in India are reviewed to propose a prognostic classification.*

Bizzini B: Tetanus toxin. Microbiol Rev 43:224, 1979. *An extensive discussion of tetanus toxin.*

Bleck TP: *Clostridium tetani. In* Mandell G, Bennett J, Dolin R (eds): Principles and Practice of Infectious Diseases. Philadelphia, WB Saunders, 1995, pp 2173–2178. *The author, a noted tetanus authority, provides an excellent review of the topic, including a detailed treatment plan.*

Faust RA, Vickers OR, Cohn L Jr: Tetanus: 2,449 cases in 68 years at Charity Hospital. J Trauma 16:704–712, 1976. *The authors review a large clinical experience with tetanus in a United States hospital.*

Gergen PJ, McQuillan GM, Kiely M, et al: A population-based serologic survey of immunity to tetanus in the U.S. N Engl J Med 332:761, 1995. *Review of the serologic status of the general population in the United States for tetanus antibodies.*

Griffin JW: Local tetanus. Johns Hopkins Med J 149:84–88, 1981. *A good review of local tetanus and the pathophysiology of tetanospasmin.*

Prevots R, Sutter RW Strebel PM, et al: Tetanus surveillance—United States 1989–1990. MMWR CDC Surveill. Summ 41:1–9 1992. *Review of reported cases of tetanus in the United States for 1989–1990 with information about the type of injury, patient age, clinical type, management, and outcome.*

Schofield F: Selective primary health care: Strategies for control of disease in the developing world XXII. Tetanus: A preventable problem. Rev Infect Dis 8:144, 1986. *The author reviews the tetanus problem in the developing world.*

ANAEROBIC BACTERIA

338 DISEASES CAUSED BY NON–SPORE-FORMING ANAEROBIC BACTERIA

Ellie J. C. Goldstein

Anaerobic bacteria are the predominant indigenous, normal flora of the human body, including the skin and oral, gastrointestinal, and vaginal mucosa (Fig. 338–1; Table 338–1). Although these organisms perform beneficial functions, they are also consummate opportunistic pathogens and can cause serious and lethal infection, often in combination with aerobic bacteria. Their role in disease was first described 100 years ago and has been increasingly appreciated during recent decades. In almost all such infections, anaerobes are mixed with aerobes. Because the flora of these infections is often complex and culture results may be delayed, knowledge of the usual flora at the location of infection is an indispensable guide in selecting and instituting empirical antimicrobial therapy.

TAXONOMY

Anaerobic bacteria range from those that die with very brief exposure to oxygen and are usually isolated only in normal flora studies to those that can survive on the surface of a fresh agar plate even in the presence of atmospheric oxygen (e.g., *Bacteroides fragilis*). Most anaerobes require an environment with a low oxidation-reduction potential (eH gradient), which can be accomplished in association with low pH, tissue destruction, by-products from aerobic bacterial metabolism, or low oxygen content. Although not true anaerobes, some organisms such as microaerophilic streptococci and other capnophilic or hard-to-grow organisms are sometimes lumped together with anaerobes, owing to their fastidious nature. Some genera such as *Lactobacillus* and *Actinomyces* contain both aerobic and anaerobic species.

Table 338–1 ■ LOCATION OF VARIOUS GROUPS OF NON-SPORULATING ANAEROBES AS NORMAL MICROFLORA OF HUMANS

ORGANISM	Skin	Oral/ Respiratory	Gastrointestinal Tract	Genitourinary Tract
Actinomyces		+		
Bacteroides		+	+	
Eubacterium		+	+	
Fusobacterium		+	+	
Lactobacillus			+	+
Peptostreptococcus	+	+	+	+
Porphyromonas		+	+	
Prevotella		+	+	
Propionibacterium	+			
Veillonella		+	+	

Recent taxonomic advances have led to reclassification of many anaerobic species (Table 338–2). The term "*Bacteroides*" will ultimately be reserved for the 10 species of the *Bacteroides fragilis* group. What were previously considered "oral" *Bacteroides* and "pigmented" *Bacteroides* species have been reclassified as *Prevotella*, *Porphyromonas*, and other genera. Those that are capnophilic and not true anaerobes are often more related to *Campylobacter*, *Capnocytophaga*, and other genera. In addition, many new genera and several new species have been created to accommodate pathogens such as *Bilophila wadsworthia*, *Sutterella wadsworthensis*, and *Anaerobiospirillum thomasii*.

VIRULENCE FACTORS

Anaerobic bacteria possess a variety of virulence factors that differ among the species (Table 338–3).

DISEASES

BACTEREMIA. Transient anaerobic bacteremia occurs in approx-

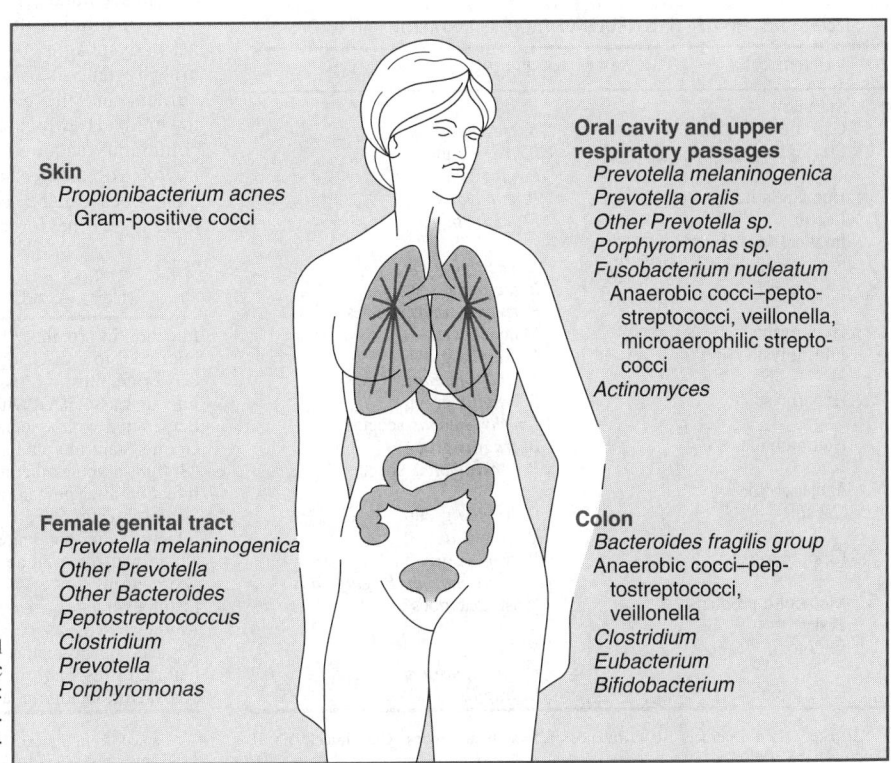

Skin
Propionibacterium acnes
Gram-positive cocci

Oral cavity and upper respiratory passages
Prevotella melaninogenica
Prevotella oralis
Other *Prevotella* sp.
Porphyromonas sp.
Fusobacterium nucleatum
Anaerobic cocci–peptostreptococci, veillonella, microaerophilic streptococci
Actinomyces

Female genital tract
Prevotella melaninogenica
Other *Prevotella*
Other *Bacteroides*
Peptostreptococcus
Clostridium
Prevotella
Porphyromonas

Colon
Bacteroides fragilis group
Anaerobic cocci–peptostreptococci, veillonella
Clostridium
Eubacterium
Bifidobacterium

FIGURE 338–1 ■ Anaerobes as predominant normal microflora of the human body by general anatomic location. (Adapted from Finegold SM, Sutter VL: Diagnosis and Management of Anaerobic Infections. Kalamazoo, MI, Upjohn, 1976. Copyright by Dr. Finegold.)

Table 338–2 ■ TAXONOMY OF ANAEROBIC BACTERIA

CURRENT NAME	SYNONYM/COMMENT
Bacteroides fragilis	
Bacteroides caccae	
Bacteroides distasonis	
Bacteroides merdae	
Bacteroides eggerthii	*B. fragilis* group
Bacteroides stercoris	
Bacteroides ovatus	
Bacteroides thetaiotaomicron	
Bacteroides vulgatus	
Bacteroides uniformis	
Campylobacter gracilis	*Bacteroides gracilis*
Bacteroides ureolyticus	New species
Prevotella bivia	*Bacteroides bivus*
Prevotella buccae	*Bacteroides buccae (ruminicola)*
Prevotella dentalis	New species
Prevotella disiens	*Bacteroides disiens*
Prevotella nigrescens	*P. intermedia*
Prevotella melaninogenica	*Bacteroides melaninogenicus*
Prevotella oralis	*Bacteroides oralis*
Prevotella oris	*Bacteroides oris*
Porphyromonas asacharolytica	*Bacteroides asaccharolyticus*
Porphyromonas gingivalis	*Bacteroides gingivalis*
Porphyromonas salivosa	*Bacteroides salivosus*
Fusobacterium nucleatum sub-species: nucleatum, polymorphum, fusiforme	New subspecies
Fusobacterium necrophorum	
Fusobacterium ulcerans	New species
Anaerobiospirillum thomasii	New species
Bilophila wadsworthia	New species
Sutterella wadsworthensis	New species
Bacteroides forsythus	New species
Bacteroides tectium	New species
Prevotella tannerae	New species
Bacteroides zoogleoformens	New species

imately 85% of patients immediately after dental cleaning or manipulation. More than 220 cases of endocarditis due to anaerobes have been reported and are usually associated with anatomic abnormalities or damaged valves. The majority of anaerobic bacteremias are intermittent and associated with serious intra-abdominal and

Table 338–3 ■ POTENTIAL VIRULENCE FACTORS IN VARIOUS ANAEROBES

FACTOR	SPECIES
Adhesion	
Capsule	*B. fragilis* group
Pili/fimbraie	*B. fragilis* group
	P. gingivalis
Hemagglutinin	*P. gingivalis*
Lectin	*F. nucleatum*
Invasion/Tissue Damage	
Proteases	*F. necrophorum*
	Bacteroides species
	Porphyromonas species
Hemolysins	Many species
Fibrinolysin	*B. fragilis* group
	Porphyromonas species
Heparinase	*B. fragilis* group
	Porphyromonas species
Neuraminidase	*B. fragilis* group
	Porphyromonas species
Antiphagocytic	
Capsule	*B. fragilis* group
	P. gingivalis
Lipopolysaccharide	*B. fragilis* group
	F. necrophorum, P. gingivalis
Metabolic products	Most anaerobes
Toxins	
Endotoxin	*B. fragilis*
	F. necrophorum
Enterotoxin	*B. fragilis*

Adapted from Duerden BI: Virulence factors in anaerobes. Clin Infect Dis 18 (Suppl 4):253, 1994.

Abscesses
Pelvic
Vulvovaginal
Vaginal cuff
Tubo-ovarian
Bartholin's gland
Skene's gland
Endometritis
Myometritis
Parametritis
Pelvic cellulitis
Pelvic thrombophlebitis
Bacterial vaginosis
Salpingitis
Chorioamnionitis
IUD-associated infection
Pelvic actinomycosis
Postabortal sepsis

female genital tract infections. Overall, it has been estimated that 10% of bacteremias are due to anaerobes, and in 80% of those anaerobes are the sole isolates.

HEAD AND NECK. Dental infections, including periodontal disease, gingivitis, acute necrotizing ulcerative gingivitis, localized juvenile periodontitis, adult periodontitis, pericoronitis, endodontitis, dental abscess, and postextraction infection, are associated with a variety of oral anaerobic bacteria.

Peritonsillar abscess is a deep-seated and potentially life-threatening complication of acute tonsillitis. It may extend into the various potential spaces of the neck or even the mediastinum and cause jugular vein thrombosis. Anaerobes may be isolated in more than 50% of such cases, usually in mixed culture with aerobes. Other regional infections include cervicofacial actinomycosis, Ludwig's angina, *Fusobacterium necrophorum* sepsis with metastatic infection (Lemiere's syndrome), and neck space infections. Whereas their acute counterparts are usually infections due to aerobes, chronic sinusitis and chronic otitis media often involve anaerobic bacteria of the normal oral flora.

PULMONARY. Because anaerobic bacteria are the predominant normal flora of the oral cavity and upper respiratory tract and most pneumonias are due to aspiration of indigenous oral flora, it is not surprising that anaerobes are important pulmonary pathogens. They are involved in aspiration pneumonia (both community-acquired and nosocomial), necrotizing pneumonia, empyema, and lung abscess. Aspiration of oral flora may be a result of altered consciousness, dysphagia, or mechanical devices such as intubation. Poor oral hygiene is associated with an increased anaerobic bacterial burden, and the presence of aerobes or tissue necrosis leads to a lowered eH, which in turn facilitates the growth of anaerobes. In community-acquired aspiration pneumonias, anaerobes are involved in 90% of cases, and in many cases may be the sole pathogens. Anaerobes can be isolated in 35% of nosocomial aspiration pneumonias. If one forgets to treat a routine aspiration pneumonia for

Table 338–5 ■ CLUES TO THE PRESENCE OF ANAEROBIC INFECTION

Infection in proximity to a mucous membrane
Foul odor to a discharge or wound
Gas or crepitus in a tissue
Infection associated with necrotic tissue or malignancy
Bacteremia with associated jaundice
Gram's stain morphology consistent with anaerobes
"Sulfur" granules (actinomycosis)
Infection after human or animal bite
Dental infection
Infection after abdominal or pelvic surgery
No growth on routine bacterial culture (especially if Gram's stain shows organisms)
Fistulous tracts
Any abscess
Typical clinical picture of gas gangrene or necrotizing fasciitis
Failure to respond to drugs not active against anaerobes (e.g., sulfamethoxazole/trimethoprim, aminoglycosides, older quinolones)

Adapted from Finegold SM: Anaerobic Bacteria in Human Disease. New York, Academic Press, 1977, p 42.

Table 338-6 ■ SPECIMENS ACCEPTABLE FOR ANAEROBIC CULTURE

Acceptable

Any aspirate: abscess, joint, lung, empyema, suprapubic (urine), brain, myringotomy, percutaneous abdominal, or pelvic
Tissue biopsy
Cellulitis after débridement of superficial debris
Bile
Surgical specimen (not contaminated with normal flora)
Transtracheal aspirate of sputum
Culdocentesis fluid
Antral sinus puncture
Deep gingival pocket

Unacceptable

Sputum
Voided urine
Nasal discharge
Feces/diarrhea
Vaginal discharge
Superficial wounds
Mucous membrane

Table 338-7 ■ GENERAL PRINCIPLES OF THERAPY FOR ANAEROBIC INFECTIONS

Elimination of dead space
Débridement
Drainage
Irrigation
Provide adequate circulation when possible
Remove foreign body
Antimicrobials
    Activity against most likely pathogen(s): location-dependent, normal flora considered
    Absorption, appropriate route of administration
    Penetration into site of infection
    Dosage appropriate for local tissue levels, body mass of patient, renal and liver function
    Duration appropriate for condition
    Susceptibility testing of isolate to guide specific therapy

its anaerobic component, then one must remember the propensity for anaerobes to cause abscess.

Management involves good pulmonary toilet and antimicrobial therapy. Because of the increasing resistance of the "oral *Bacteroides* species" (*Prevotella/Porphyromonas* species), penicillin alone is no longer recommended. Alternatives include penicillin plus metronidazole, β-lactamase inhibitor combinations, second-generation cephalosporins such as cefoxitin and cefotetan, carbapenems, and clindamycin plus penicillin. In choosing coverage, one must also consider the microaerophilic streptococci and the aerobic gram-positive and locally prevalent gram-negative components of the oral flora. Nosocomial aspiration frequently is a mixture of all these components.

INTRA-ABDOMINAL. Because anaerobes outnumber aerobes by 1000:1 in the large intestine, they play an important role in almost all intra-abdominal infections. Most visceral abscesses (e.g., hepatic), chronic cholecystitis, perforated and gangrenous appendicitis, postoperative wound infections and abscesses, diverticulitis, and any infection associated with fecal contamination of the abdominal cavity involve both aerobes and anaerobes. *B. fragilis* group members are especially important pathogens because they are encapsulated and resist phagocytosis, are often resistant to many commonly used antibiotics, and promote abscess formation. They also may be associated with concomitant bacteremia and sepsis.

DIARRHEA. *Anaerobiospirillum thomasii* is a motile gram-negative spiral bacterium with bipolar flagellae. It has been isolated from the feces of asymptomatic dogs and cats and has been transmitted from them to humans. It may also be associated with bacteremia.

Although *B. fragilis* is part of the normal intestinal flora, enterotoxin-producing strains can cause diarrhea in animals and humans and may be associated with bacteremia.

OBSTETRIC-GYNECOLOGIC. Table 338–4 lists the various obstetric-gynecologic diseases that involve anaerobes. Bacterial vaginosis has been linked to a perturbation of the normal anaerobic vaginal flora and accounts for 45% of all cases of vaginitis. It is present in approximately 20% of college women, and up to 45% of women attending sexually transmitted disease clinics. It can be diagnosed by the presence of a foul, gelatinous vaginal discharge, a vaginal pH greater than 4.5, the presence of "clue cells," and a fishy amine odor after 10% KOH is added to vaginal secretions. Bacterial vaginosis has also been associated with premature rupture of membranes, chorioamnionitis, postpartum endometritis, vaginal cuff cellulitis, and postabortal pelvic inflammatory disease. Culture of tubo-ovarian abscess, a complication of chronic pelvic inflammatory disease, grows anaerobes in up to 85% of cases.

SKIN AND SOFT TISSUE. DIABETES. The infected fetid foot is the most frequent infectious cause for diabetics to be hospitalized. The role of anaerobes in more than 50% of these infections is well established. When present, anaerobes are often associated with the more severe cases, especially with vascular insufficiency and tissue necrosis and those that ultimately require amputation. In addition, the presence of fever, long-standing wounds, crepitus, foul odor, abscess, or prior antimicrobial therapy more often involves anaerobes.

BITES. Anaerobes are present in approximately 65% of animal bite wound infections (see Chapter 372), especially those that are more severe or are associated with tissue necrosis or abscess formation. These anaerobes are part of the oral flora of the biting animal. Consequently, the routine bacteriology laboratory may have difficulty in identifying them. Most are penicillin/ampicillin susceptible. Besides anaerobes, *Pasteurella multocida, Staphylococcus intermedius, Staphylococcus aureus,* and streptococci should be considered potential pathogens.

Human bites, both occlusional injuries and clenched fist injuries, tend to be more serious than animal bites. Anaerobes can be isolated from 55% of human bite wounds and are more frequently β-lactamase producing and penicillin resistant. There is also a higher

Table 338-8 ■ ANTIMICROBIAL SUSCEPTIBILITY PATTERNS FOR ANAEROBIC BACTERIA*

BACTERIA	DRUG							
	Penicillin	β-Lactamase†	Cefoxitin	Cefotetan	Imipenem/Meropenem	Trovafloxacin	Clindamycin	Metronidazole
B. fragilis	−	+	+	+	+	+	v	+
B. thetaiotaomicron	−	+	v	v	+	v	v	+
B. fragilis group, other	−	+	v	v	+	+	v	+
Prevotella species	v	+	+	+	+	+	+	+
Fusobacterium nucleatum	v	+	+	+	+	v	+	+
Fusobacterium necrophorum	+	+	+	+	+	v	+	+
Porphyromonas species	+	+	+	+	+	+	+	+
Peptostreptococci	+	+	+	+	+	+	+	v
Propionibacterium acnes	+	+	+	+	+	+	+	−
Veillonella	+	+	+	+	+	+	+	+
Actinomyces	+	+	+	+	+	+	+	−

*Based on a variety of in vitro susceptibility studies from different laboratories and utilizing different techniques.
†β-lactamase inhibitor–β-lactam combination (e.g., ticarcillin/clavulanate, ampicillin/sulbactam, pipericillin/tazobactam).
+ = Susceptible.
− = Resistant.
v = Variable.

frequency of septic arthritis and osteomyelitis associated with human bite wounds. One must consider anaerobes plus *Eikenella corrodens,* streptococci, *S. aureus,* and *Haemophilus* species as potential pathogens when choosing empirical antimicrobial therapy.

GANGRENES. Gangrene indicates necrosis, most often of skin and subcutaneous tissue, and is often rapidly progressive. Several types of "infectious gangrene" have been described and may sometimes be indistinguishable on a clinical basis. These include the following:

1. *Gas gangrene,* which can incidentally involve other anaerobes besides *C. perfringens* and other clostridia.
2. *Progressive bacterial synergistic gangrene* often involves microaerophilic streptococci and peptostreptococci as well as aerobic bacteria such as *S. aureus* and Enterobacteriaceae.
3. *Synergistic necrotizing cellulitis* involves a mixed aerobic and anaerobic bacteria including *B. fragilis* and peptostreptococci. Diabetic patients may be predisposed. The cellulitis is markedly painful, crepitus may be present, and the discharge has a foul odor.
4. *Fournier's gangrene* is a serious infection of the scrotum or perineum that starts with scrotal pain and erythema and rapidly progresses to necrosis and gangrene, which can lead to sloughing of tissue. It is more often seen in diabetics and can be associated with trauma.

PRINCIPLES OF DIAGNOSIS AND THERAPY

Clues as to when one should suspect anaerobic infection are listed in Table 338–5. Obtaining an appropriately collected and acceptable specimen (Table 338–6) must be an active process and specified in the orders.

General principles of therapy are listed in Table 338–7. In general, appropriate antimicrobial therapy coupled with prompt drainage and surgical débridement are essential for therapeutic success. Table 338–8 notes the susceptibility patterns of the various clinically important anaerobes.

Finegold SM, Goldstein EJC (eds): Proceedings of the 1996 Meeting of the Anaerobe Society of the America. Clin Infect Dis 25 (Suppl 1):S77–S295, 1997.
Goldstein EJC, Ueno K (eds): New fluoroquinolones and anaerobic infections. Clin Infect Dis 23 (Suppl 1):1–106, 1996.
Poxton I (ed): Anaerobes 1997: The proceedings of a biennial conference of the Society of Anaerobic Microbiology, July 1997, Cambridge. Rev Med Microbiol 8 (Suppl 1):1–105, 1997.

ENTERIC INFECTIONS

339 INTRODUCTION TO ENTERIC INFECTIONS

Herbert L. DuPont

Enteric infections are second only to respiratory tract infections as common medical problems. In certain populations, enteric infections are hyperendemic: in poorly nourished children living in developing tropical countries where they are significant causes of pediatric mortality, in infants in day-care centers, in residents of custodial institutions for the mentally retarded, in homosexual males, and in those who venture from industrialized to developing regions ("travelers' diarrhea").

In approaching a patient with an enteric infection, epidemiologic (Table 339–1) and clinical features (Table 339–2) are used to determine the proper approach to evaluation and management. One must work through the various considerations to be certain that the proper differential diagnosis and work-up are developed. Recent travel to a mountainous region of North America should raise the possibility of infection by *Giardia lamblia*. Travel to Russia, particularly St. Petersburg, is associated with an increased risk of infection by *Cryptosporidium parvum* and *G. lamblia*. When diarrhea occurs during or after travel to a developing tropical region, a bacterial enteropathogen should be suspected. Infection with *Cyclospora* should be suspected when diarrhea follows travel to Nepal.

A specific food or water vehicle cannot be suspected unless multiple cases of illness with a common exposure occur. In this situation, the incubation period will often help determine the etiologic diagnosis: less than 4 hours in the case of a *Staphylococcus aureus* or *Bacillus cereus* enterotoxin food poisoning or more than 8 hours in the case of intestinal infection. On evaluation of the clinical expression of the illness (see Table 339–2), a tentative diagnosis may be made. In the patient who is receiving an antimicrobial drug, or who has recently completed a course of therapy, and presents with an enteric infection manifested by diarrhea with or without fever and dysenteric disease, *Clostridium difficile* should be suspected. When a person has close contact with an infant or infants attending a day-care center, a number of pathogens found in this setting should be suspected. Finally, the homosexual male with an enteric infection may have acquired it through fecal-oral contamination so common in this setting (and in this case multiple pathogens may be found in stool), through receptive anal intercourse, or when intestinal immunity has become depressed as a result of the acquired immune deficiency syndrome (AIDS).

Enteric infection syndromes may be divided into five groups based on the clinical presentation, including febrile systemic dis-

---

Table 339–1 ■ EPIDEMIOLOGIC FEATURES IMPORTANT IN DETERMINING POTENTIAL CAUSES OF ENTERIC INFECTION

EPIDEMIOLOGIC FEATURE	ETIOLOGIC AGENT TO SUSPECT
Travel to mountainous areas of North America	*Giardia lamblia*
Travel to Russia (especially St. Petersburg)	*Cryptosporidium, G. lamblia*
Travel to Nepal	*Cyclospora*
Travel to the developing tropical/semitropical world from an industrialized region	Enterotoxigenic *Escherichia coli, Shigella, Salmonella* (including *S. typhi*), other bacterial causes, *G. lamblia, Cyclospora,* and *Cryptosporidium*
Presence of associated cases (an outbreak)	Use incubation period and clinical features (see Table 339–2) to determine probable cause
Antibiotic use in the last 2 weeks	*Clostridium difficile*
Contact with day-care centers	Any enteropathogen, often *G. lamblia, Cryptosporidium, Shigella,* or rotavirus
Homosexual male with diarrhea	Any organism spread by fecal-oral route; with proctitis, suspect *Neisseria gonorrhoeae, Chlamydia trachomatis,* herpes simplex or *Treponema pallidium;* with AIDS suspect any agent, especially *Cryptosporidium, Microsporidium, Cyclospora, Salmonella, C. jejuni, C. difficile, Mycobacterium avium-intracellulare,* and cytomegalovirus

Table 339-2 ■ CLINICAL FEATURES OF ENTERIC INFECTION

CLINICAL SYNDROME	ETIOLOGIC AGENTS SUSPECTED	SPECIAL CONSIDERATIONS
Enteric or typhoid fever	*Salmonella typhi, S. enteritidis, Campylobacter, Shigella, Yersinia enterocolitica*	Blood cultures; antibiotics generally needed
Acute watery diarrhea	Any agent may be responsible. Consider: *Vibrio cholerae,* enterotoxigenic *Escherichia coli, Shigella, Salmonella, C. jejuni*	Fluid and electrolyte therapy crucial for recovery in dehydration
Gastroenteritis	Viral agents (rotavirus or small round viruses) or enterotoxin-mediated disease (*Staphylococcus aureus* or *Bacillus cereus*)	In case of an outbreak, incubation period suggests the etiology
Dysentery	*Shigella, C. jejuni, Salmonella,* enterohemorrhagic (0157:H7) or enteroinvasive *E. coli, Aeromonas hydrophilia, Vibrio parahemolyticus, Yersinia enterocolitica, Entamoeba histolytica,* or inflammatory bowel disease	Stool culture and occasionally parasite examination important to determining cause; hemolytic uremic syndrome may complicate diarrheal disease caused by *E. coli* 0157:H7 or *S. dysenteriae* 1
Persistent diarrhea	*Giardia lamblia,* small bowel bacterial overgrowth, bacterial diarrhea, lactase deficiency, Brainerd diarrhea	Stool culture and parasite exam indicated; empirical anti-*Giardia* therapy may be useful; milk should not be consumed; a history of raw milk or untreated (well or surface) water consumption suggests Brainerd diarrhea

ease (enteric fever), acute watery diarrhea (small bowel secretory process), profuse vomiting (gastroenteritis), the passage of many small-volume stools containing blood and mucus (dysenteric disease), and diarrhea lasting longer than 2 weeks (persistent diarrheal disease). Table 339–2 lists the major syndromes along with the expected cause. In the majority of cases of enteric infection, it is not possible to determine the cause of illness on clinical grounds. Laboratory tests are often useful, particularly in the more severe or intensely ill patients, to help establish cause and to develop the proper plan of treatment.

Treatment of diarrhea should be tailored to clinical syndrome. Oral rehydration with fluids and electrolytes is used in acute watery diarrhea and gastroenteritis and in all forms of enteric infection when any degree of dehydration occurs. For enteric fever and dysenteric disease, antimicrobial therapy is indicated. For patients with persistent diarrhea, work-up for cause is indicated before a management plan is developed.

340 TYPHOID FEVER

Thomas Butler

DEFINITION. Typhoid fever is a bacterial disease caused by *Salmonella typhi*. It is characterized by prolonged fever, abdominal pain, diarrhea, delirium, rose spots, and splenomegaly and complicated sometimes by intestinal bleeding and perforation. Enteric fever is synonymous with typhoid fever, which is occasionally caused also by *S. enteritidis* bioserotype paratyphi A or B.

ETIOLOGY. The typhoid bacillus is a motile gram-negative rod in the family Enterobacteriaceae. It possesses a flagellar (H) antigen, a cell wall (O) lipopolysaccharide antigen, and a polysaccharide virulence (Vi) antigen located in the cell capsule. The polysaccharide side chain of the O antigen confers serologic specificity to the organism and is essential in virulence because salmonellae other than *S. typhi* and *S. enteritidis* bioserotype paratyphi A or B do not produce enteric fever in humans.

INCIDENCE AND PREVALENCE. Typhoid fever has been almost eliminated from developed countries because of sewage and water treatment facilities but remains a common disease in developing countries. In 1980, the number of cases occurring yearly was estimated as about 7 million in Asia, over 4 million in Africa, and 0.5 million in Latin America. Outbreaks affecting more than 10,000 persons in Tajikistan were reported in 1996 and 1997. About 500 cases are diagnosed each year in the United States, and over half of these are in recently arrived travelers who contracted their infections abroad.

EPIDEMIOLOGY. Adults and children of all ages and both genders appear equally susceptible to infection. In developing coun-

tries, most cases occur in schoolage children and young adults. Although acquired immunity provides some protection, reinfections have been documented. Typhoid fever occurs during all seasons.

Transmission is by the fecal-oral route through contaminated water or food. The main human sources of infection in the community are asymptomatic fecal carriers and cases during either disease or convalescence. Females and older males are prone to become chronic fecal carriers because underlying cholecystitis enables them to harbor chronic infection in the gallbladder. *S. typhi* is resistant to drying and cooling, thus allowing bacteria to survive prolonged periods in dried sewage, water, food, and ice.

Vi-phage typing of *S. typhi* is a useful epidemiologic tool to trace cases of typhoid fever to a carrier or food source. In endemic situations, multiple phage types are present, and several phage types may be responsible for an epidemic.

PATHOGENESIS AND PATHOLOGY. After *S. typhi* is ingested, the part of the inoculum that survives stomach acid enters the small intestine, where bacteria penetrate the mucosa and enter mononuclear phagocytes of ileal Peyer's patches and mesenteric lymph nodes. Inocula of at least 10^5 bacteria are necessary to initiate disease, and inocula of 10^7 and more cause disease regularly. The incubation period ranges from 8 to 28 days, depending on inoculum size and immune status of the host. Bacteria proliferate in mononuclear phagocytes and spread by way of the blood to the spleen, liver, and bone marrow, where further proliferation in macrophages occurs. The earliest symptoms of fever and chills (Table 340–1) are associated with bacteremia. Inflammatory reactions occur in the spleen, liver, bone marrow, Peyer's patches mainly in the terminal ileum, and skin, consisting of mononuclear cell infiltration, hyperplasia, and focal necrosis. Focal collections of mononuclear leukocytes are called "typhoid nodules." Fever and other constitutional symptoms are probably caused by the release of cytokines, including tumor necrosis factor and interleukin-1, from infected mononuclear phagocytes. Intestinal manifestations are caused by hyperplasia of Peyer's patches with ulcerations of overlying mucosa, resulting in pain, diarrhea, bleeding, or perforation.

CLINICAL MANIFESTATIONS. In the first days of illness, the non-specific symptoms of fever, chills, and headache are mild and in the typical case build up in intensity during the first week, resulting in prostration. The evolution of disease syndromes occurs stepwise over 1 to 3 weeks (see Table 340–1) but may be variable in the time of appearance. The early symptoms of fever, abdominal pain, and prostration tend to persist throughout the illness, which in untreated cases lasts a month or longer. Abdominal pain occurs in more than half of patients and is frequently diffuse or located in the right lower quadrant over the terminal ileum. Diarrhea occurs in about a third of patients and consists of either watery stools or semisolid stools. Melena occurs less commonly. Rose spots occur in more than half of light-skinned individuals but are often not visible in dark-skinned patients. The rash is seen most commonly on the shoulders, thorax, and abdomen and rarely affects the extremities. The lesions are erythematous macules or papules about 1 to 5 mm in diameter that typically blanch with pressure but may become hemorrhagic. Many patients display abnormal behavior or

Table 340–1 ■ EVOLUTION OF TYPICAL SYMPTOMS AND SIGNS OF TYPHOID FEVER

DISEASE PERIOD	SYMPTOMS	SIGNS	PATHOLOGY
First week	Fever, chills gradually increasing and persisting; headache	Abdominal tenderness	Bacteremia
Second week	Rash, abdominal pain, diarrhea or constipation, delirium, prostration	Rose spots, splenomegaly, hepatomegaly	Mononuclear cell vasculitis of skin, hyperplasia of ileal Peyer's patches, typhoid nodules in spleen and liver
Third week	Complications of intestinal bleeding and perforation, shock	Melena, ileus, rigid abdomen, coma	Ulcerations over Peyer's patches, perforation with peritonitis
Fourth week and later	Resolution of symptoms, relapse, weight loss	Reappearance of acute disease, cachexia	Cholecystitis, chronic fecal carriage of bacteria

altered mental status that may be out of proportion to the severity of the systemic illness. Among the common presentations are "toxic" staring, delirium, aphonia, and coma. Seizures are common in children. Patients are rarely jaundiced.

In about 5% of patients, intestinal bleeding or intestinal perforation occurs, usually after the second week of illness. Bleeding occurs from ileal ulcers and may present as melena or bright red blood in stools. Brisk bleeding develops rarely but is an occasional cause of death. Intestinal perforation presents as the sudden onset of more severe abdominal pain, distention, and tenderness. Bowel sounds are diminished, and the abdominal radiograph usually reveals free air. Perforation most often occurs unexpectedly after a few days of treatment when a patient has started to improve. Other complications of typhoid fever include pneumonia, which develops as a superinfection due to other bacteria, myocarditis, acute cholecystitis, and acute meningitis.

Relapses occur in 10 to 20% of patients treated with chloramphenicol. Patients with relapses experience the reappearance of typical symptoms 7 to 14 days after the end of treatment. Relapses tend to be less severe than the initial episode.

DIAGNOSIS. The preferred method of diagnosis is isolation of *S. typhi* from a blood culture, which is positive in most patients during the first 2 weeks of illness. Urine and stool cultures are positive less frequently but should be obtained to increase the diagnostic yield. The bone marrow culture is the most sensitive test, is positive in nearly 90% of cases, and can be used when a bacteriologic diagnosis is crucial or in patients who have been pretreated with antibiotics. The duodenal string test to culture bile has also been used with success in typhoid fever.

The Widal test for agglutinating antibodies against the somatic (O) and flagellar (H) antigens of *S. typhi* is widely used for serodiagnosis. An O agglutinin titer of 1:80 or more or a fourfold rise supports a diagnosis of typhoid fever, whereas the H agglutinins are more often non-specifically elevated by immunization or previous infections with other bacteria. Serodiagnosis is of limited value because false-positive results are often obtained in endemic areas and false-negative results occur in some cases of bacteriologically proven typhoid fever.

Other laboratory findings are anemia of variable severity and a white blood cell count that is normal or decreased with an increased percentage of band forms. Platelets are often diminished, and signs of disseminated intravascular coagulation are present. Liver function tests frequently show elevated levels of aminotransferases and bilirubin. Renal failure is an infrequent complication. In patients with diarrhea, the stool shows fecal leukocytes.

The differential diagnosis depends on infections that are endemic in the area where an individual contracted the infection. For returned travelers from developing countries, the common possibilities are malaria, hepatitis, typhus, amebic liver abscess, shigellosis, non-typhoid salmonellosis, and leptospirosis. In the United States one must consider septicemias originating from the urinary tract, gastrointestinal tract, or gallbladder as well as influenza, infectious mononucleosis, meningococcemia, miliary tuberculosis, and bacterial endocarditis.

TREATMENT. Chloramphenicol has remained the drug of choice since its introduction in 1948 because no other drug has been demonstrated to cause more rapid or consistent improvement of disease. Chloramphenicol is given orally in a dose of 50 to 60 mg/kg/day in four equal portions every 6 hours. After defervescence and clinical improvement the dosage can be reduced

to 30 mg/kg/day to complete a 14-day course. In patients unable to take oral medication, the same dosage should be given intravenously until the patient can take capsules.

Alternative drugs should be considered when *S. typhi* resistant to chloramphenicol is isolated or strongly suspected. Several are nearly equal to chloramphenicol in efficacy. Trimethoprim/sulfamethoxazole is effective in a standard adult dose of 160 mg trimethoprim and 800 mg sulfamethoxazole given orally or intravenously twice a day for 14 days. Other drugs that are effective include ampicillin (intravenously), amoxicillin, cefoperazone, and ceftriaxone. In recent years, most isolates of *S. typhi* from cases in India and Pakistan have shown plasmid-mediated, multidrug resistance to chloramphenicol, ampicillin, and trimethoprim/sulfamethoxazole. These adults can be treated with ciprofloxacin, 500 mg, or ofloxacin, 200 to 400 mg, twice daily for 7 to 14 days, or with other fluoroquinolones. Children with multidrug-resistant infections should receive ceftriaxone or cefixime.

Patients who are dehydrated, anorectic, or suffering from diarrhea should receive intravenous saline with attention to electrolyte and acid-base disturbances. Patients with brisk intestinal bleeding require blood transfusion. Patients with suspected perforation should have an abdominal radiograph to look for free air and peritoneal fluid. Laparotomy should be undertaken as early as possible to suture the perforation.

In some high-risk patients with delirium, coma, or shock, high-dose dexamethasone in addition to antibiotics reduces mortality. The dose should be 3 mg/kg initially, followed by 1 mg/kg every 6 hours for 48 hours. One must be cautious with this therapy because signs and symptoms of perforation are masked by steroids. Antipyretic drugs such as aspirin should be administered with caution because they occasionally markedly reduce blood pressure.

Patients with relapses of typhoid fever should be treated the same as patients with a first attack. Chronic fecal carriers (asymptomatic excretion for a year or longer) should be given high doses of ampicillin or amoxicillin, 100 mg/kg/day, plus probenecid, 30 mg/kg/day for 4 to 6 weeks. Trimethoprim-sulfamethoxazole is also effective. Patients with multidrug-resistant infections can be treated with ciprofloxacin or other quinolones. Patients with gallstones or cholecystitis may require cholecystectomy to eradicate the carrier state. Chloramphenicol neither prevents nor effectively treats the chronic carrier state.

PROGNOSIS. Typhoid fever carried a case-fatality rate of about 12% in the preantibiotic era, which was reduced to about 4% after chloramphenicol became available. Case-fatality rates of more than 10% continue to be reported in developing countries despite availability of antibiotics, whereas developed countries show case-fatality rates of less than 1%. After treatment with chloramphenicol or other effective drug, most patients become afebrile in 4 to 7 days. In the preantibiotic era, about 10% of recovered patients had relapses, and chloramphenicol treatment has not reduced this rate. Intestinal bleeding or perforation occurs in about 5% of patients and may not be prevented by antibiotic treatment. Thus, bleeding or perforation is occasionally detected after patients have defervesced during treatment. One to 3 percent of patients become chronic fecal carriers after recovery.

PREVENTION. Travelers to developing countries should avoid consuming untreated water, drinks served with ice, peeled fruits, and other food that is not served hot. American international travelers face an overall risk of developing typhoid fever of fewer than 1 case in 10,000 trips, but travelers to high-risk countries like India and Pakistan have a probability of about 4 in 10,000 trips of getting typhoid fever. Travelers wishing immune protection should receive either typhoid vaccine live oral Ty21a given as one capsule every other day for a total of four capsules or typhoid Vi polysaccharide vaccine given as a single intramuscular injection, with booster doses given every 2 years if needed. These vaccines give only partial protection, and thus vaccinated persons should still exercise dietary precautions. The traditional method of controlling typhoid is to follow stool cultures of convalescent cases and report positive cultures to the health department. The health department investigates non-imported typhoid cases to identify possible food sources or contact with a chronic carrier.

Engels EA, Falagos ME, Lau J, et al: Typhoid fever vaccines: A meta-analysis of studies of efficacy and toxicity. BMJ 316:110, 1998. *Review of field trials of three different vaccines concluded that whole cell vaccines were most effective but the live oral Ty21a and Vi polysaccharide vaccines were less toxic.*

Keuter M, Dharmana E, Gasem MH, et al: Patterns of proinflammatory cytokines and inhibitors during typhoid fever. J Infect Dis 169:1306, 1994. *In Indonesian patients, tumor necrosis factor and interleukins 6 and 8 were modestly elevated, but anti-inflammatory molecules, including receptors for tumor necrosis factor and interleukin-1 receptor antagonist, were more prominent.*

Mirza SH, Beeching NJ, Hart CA: Multi-drug resistant typhoid: A global problem. J Med Microbiol 44:317, 1996. *In China, India, and Pakistan, large numbers of cases of infection caused by* Salmonella typhi *resistant to ampicillin, chloramphenicol, and trimethoprim/sulfamethoxazole have emerged. Resistance is mediated by a 120-Md plasmid in H1 incompatibility group.*

Smith MD, Duong NM, Hoa NTT, et al: Comparison of ofloxacin and ceftriaxone for short-course treatment of enteric fever. Antimicrob Agents Chemother 38:1716, 1994. *In Vietnam, a short course of ofloxacin for 5 days was more effective than a 3-day course of ceftriaxone.*

Zenilman JM: Typhoid fever. JAMA 278:847, 1997. *A case report of an unimmunized pregnant patient who recently returned from India is presented. Prevention of infection by the live oral Ty21a vaccine or the Vi polysaccharide vaccine for travelers is advised.*

341 *SALMONELLA* INFECTIONS OTHER THAN TYPHOID FEVER

Donald Kaye

DEFINITION. *Salmonella,* a genus of the family Enterobacteriaceae, can cause an asymptomatic intestinal carrier state or clinical disease in both humans and animals. In humans, the most common clinical manifestation is enterocolitis, with diarrhea as the major symptom. Some patients develop bacteremia without gastrointestinal manifestations. Localization from bacteremia may result in osteomyelitis, a mycotic aneurysm, or other localized infection. *S. typhi,* a pathogen of humans only, causes enteric fever. Enteric fever produced by *S. typhi* is called typhoid fever, whereas enteric fever caused by other salmonellae is named paratyphoid fever.

An asymptomatic intestinal carrier state of variable duration may follow inapparent or symptomatic infection. Most carriers are transient carriers. A chronic carrier state, defined as lasting more than 1 year, is usually permanent and is most often related to persistent infection in the gallbladder. With the exception of *S. typhi,* in which a human carrier is always implicated, most *Salmonella* infections are acquired from food products derived from infected animals (e.g., eggs, poultry, meat, milk).

ETIOLOGY. Salmonellae are motile, gram-negative, non–spore-forming bacilli. They are differentiated from other Enterobacteriaceae by biochemical tests. They ferment glucose, maltose, and mannitol but not lactose or sucrose. Almost all salmonellae produce acid and gas with fermentation. Exceptions to the rules that are helpful in identification are the following: *S. typhi* does not produce gas, and *S. gallinarum-pullorum* is non-motile. As another confounding exception, lactose-fermenting strains of salmonellae have been isolated.

Salmonellae can be differentiated into over 2000 serotypes (serovars) by their somatic (O) antigens, which are composed of lipopolysaccharides and are part of the cell wall, and their flagellar (H) antigens. There are five serogroups based on O antigens, A through E. Each serovar is commonly referred to as a separate species and is so indicated in this chapter. In this system, some of the important serovars and their groups are *S. typhi* (group D), *S. choleraesuis* (group C$_1$), *S. typhimurium* (group B), and *S. enteritidis* (group D).

S. enteritidis and *S. typhimurium* are the most common causes of human disease and together represent almost 50% of human isolates. Other common isolates are *S. heidelberg, S. hadar, S. newport, S. agona, S. montevideo, S. oranienburg, S. meunchen,* and *S. thompson.* In recent years, *S. enteritidis* outbreaks related to eggs have been increasing.

EPIDEMIOLOGY. *S. typhi, S. paratyphi A, S. schottmuelleri (S. paratyphi B), S. hirschfeldii (S. paratyphi C),* and *S. sendai* are either solely or almost always pathogens in humans only, and human-to-human transmission is important.

The remaining serovars of salmonellae are widely spread in the animal kingdom, and salmonellae have been isolated from virtually all species, including birds, poultry, mammals, reptiles, amphibians, and insects. *Salmonella* infection in humans usually occurs from ingesting contaminated animal food products, most often eggs, poultry, and meat. Eggs usually become contaminated from feces on the surface of the egg, with small cracks allowing entry into the egg. However, infection of the ovary allows primary incorporation of salmonellae into the egg. Meat and poultry become widely contaminated at the slaughterhouse with salmonellae spread from carcass to carcass, usually on the surface. *S. choleraesuis* is associated with pig products and *S. dublin* with cattle and consumption of unpasteurized milk from cattle. Salmonellae may survive cooking at relatively low temperatures in the center of eggs or turkeys, or food may be contaminated after cooking from kitchen utensils or from the hands of food preparers who handle raw food. Multiplication of organisms can then occur if food is not refrigerated. In 1994, an estimated 224,000 persons in the United States developed *S. enteritidis* gastroenteritis from contamination of bulk ice cream made by one manufacturer. This was related to transport of pasteurized ice cream base in containers previously used for transport of non-pasteurized liquid eggs.

Salmonella infections have been acquired after contamination of food or water with feces of pet turtles, chicks, ducks, birds, dogs, cats, and many other species. These pets become infected from their food.

Salmonella infection also can be acquired by eating food or, less commonly, drinking water contaminated by a human carrier who has not washed his or her hands adequately. Infection has been spread by the fecal-oral route in children, by contaminated enema and fiberoptic instruments, by diagnostic and therapeutic preparations made from animal or insect products (e.g., pancreatic extract, carmine dye) and from intentional contamination of restaurant salad bars. Homosexual men are prone to fecal-oral infection.

Outbreaks of salmonellosis occur in institutionalized patients, who are probably more prone to develop *Salmonella* infections for three reasons. First, there are more underlying diseases that decrease host defense mechanisms against salmonellae such as disorders of gastric acidity and intestinal motility; second, use of antimicrobial agents reduces the normal, protective intestinal flora; and third, institutional food prepared in bulk is more likely to be contaminated than individually prepared meals. Outbreaks in nurseries and in the elderly in nursing homes have the highest mortality rates (i.e., >5%). Diabetes may be an additional risk factor for *Salmonella* infection.

Most cases of *Salmonella* infection occurring in the United States are sporadic rather than related to outbreaks. However, when an infection occurs in a family, other members of the household also tend to have positive stool cultures. About 40,000 cases of culture-confirmed *Salmonella* infection have been reported annually to the Centers for Disease Control and Prevention in recent years, a marked increase over the past 30 years. However, this undoubtedly represents only a fraction of actual cases. It has been estimated that 2 to 4 million cases actually occur each year. A disproportionate number of infections occur in July through October, probably related to the warm weather. *Salmonella* infections are most common in infants and in children younger than 5 years of age.

Salmonellae have become increasingly resistant to antibiotics, usually by acquiring resistance transfer factors. It is believed that much of the resistance has been related to widespread use of antimicrobial agents in farm animals. A multidrug-resistant strain of

S. typhimurium (definitive type 104 [DT 104]) has emerged as an important cause of infection in the United Kingdom, with very recent outbreaks reported in the United States.

PATHOGENESIS. After ingestion of organisms, the determinants of whether or not infection results, as well as the severity of infection, are the dose and virulence of the *Salmonella* strain and the status of host defense mechanisms. Large inocula such as 10^7 bacteria are usually required to produce clinical infection in the normal host. Smaller inocula are more likely to result in no infection or to produce a transient intestinal carrier state. Gastric acid serves as a host defense mechanism by killing many of the ingested organisms, and intestinal motility is also probably a host defense mechanism. In the absence or decrease of gastric acidity (as in the elderly, after gastrectomy, vagotomy, or gastroenterostomy, with H_2-receptor antagonists, and with antacids) and with decreased intestinal motility (as with antimotility drugs), much smaller inocula can produce infection and the infection tends to be more severe.

Administration of antimicrobial agents before ingestion of salmonellae can markedly reduce the size of inoculum needed to produce infection, presumably by reducing the protective bowel flora.

Although any *Salmonella* serotype can produce any of the *Salmonella* syndromes (transient asymptomatic carrier state, enterocolitis, bacteremia, enteric fever, and chronic carrier state), each serotype tends to produce certain syndromes much more often than others. For example, *S. anatum* usually causes asymptomatic intestinal infection, whereas *S. typhimurium* usually causes enterocolitis. *S. choleraesuis* is more likely to produce bacteremia (often with metastatic infection) than asymptomatic infection or enterocolitis, and some serotypes such as *S. typhi* are most likely to cause enteric fever as well as the chronic carrier state. Fortunately, most *Salmonella* serotypes are of relatively low pathogenicity for humans; and, therefore, although food products are commonly contaminated, large outbreaks occur only when more virulent serotypes are involved.

To produce infection, invasion must occur across the mucosa of the intestine. When the organisms reach the lamina propria, an influx of polymorphonuclear leukocytes serves as a defense mechanism to prevent invasion of lymphatics. Certain serotypes seem more able than others to invade lymphatics and subsequently produce bacteremia. For example, *S. dublin*, which has been isolated from unpasteurized milk, commonly produces bacteremia after intestinal infection. Both the small intestine and colon are involved in the inflammatory process. The diarrhea in *Salmonella* enterocolitis results from the inflammation. In addition, watery stools may occur, apparently the result of secretion of water and electrolytes by small intestinal epithelial cells in response to an enterotoxin secreted by some of the *Salmonella* strains or in response to tissue mediators of inflammation.

Patients with diseases that impair host defense mechanisms seem to have an increased frequency of severe *Salmonella* infection. For many years, a striking association has been recognized between diseases producing hemolysis and *Salmonella* bacteremia. Specifically, *Salmonella* bacteremia is common in patients with sickle cell disorders, malaria, and bartonellosis. In fact, because of the frequency of *Salmonella* bacteremia in sickle cell diseases and the underlying bone disease in these patients to which salmonellae localize, these organisms are the most common cause of osteomyelitis in patients with sickle cell disorders. Prolonged *Salmonella* bacteremia occurs in patients with hepatosplenic schistosomiasis, probably related to localization on and in the intravascular schistosomes. Patients with lymphoma and leukemia also are more prone to develop *Salmonella* bacteremia. Prolonged and recurrent refractory *Salmonella* bacteremia has been observed in patients with the acquired immunodeficiency syndrome (AIDS).

CLINICAL SYNDROMES. Asymptomatic Intestinal Carrier State. The asymptomatic intestinal carrier state may result from inapparent infection, which is the most common form of *Salmonella* infection, or may follow clinical disease (convalescent carrier). The carrier state is usually self-limited to several weeks to months, with the incidence of positive stool cultures rapidly decreasing. By 1 year, far less than 1% still have positive stools. The major exception is with *S. typhi*: about 3% of those infected excrete the organism for life. A patient who has had *Salmonella* in the stool for 1 year (chronic carrier) is likely to become a lifelong carrier. Patients with *Schistosoma haematobium* infections are predisposed to become chronic urinary carriers of *Salmonella*.

Enterocolitis. After an incubation period, which is usually 12 to 48 hours, the illness starts suddenly with crampy abdominal pain and diarrhea. A chill is common. Although occasional patients have nausea and vomit once or twice, vomiting is not persistent. The diarrhea may be watery and of large volume or small volume. The stools may contain mucus and occasionally blood. Polymorphonuclear leukocytes are present in the stool. Diarrhea may be mild or may be severe with up to 20 to 30 stools a day. Fever is present in most patients, whose temperature may reach 40° C (104° F) or higher. The abdomen is tender to palpation. Transient bacteremia may occur and is most likely in infants, the elderly, and patients with impaired host defense mechanisms.

Symptoms usually improve over a period of days, with fever lasting no more than 2 to 3 days and diarrhea no more than 5 to 7 days. However, these symptoms may occasionally persist for up to 14 days. More severe disease is seen with malnutrition, inflammatory bowel disease, and AIDS. Reactive arthritis may follow enterocolitis in up to 7% of cases. It is especially frequent in those with the HLA-B27 phenotype.

Enteric Fever. Paratyphoid fever is an enteric fever syndrome identical to typhoid fever but produced by a serotype other than *S. typhi* (most often *S. paratyphi A, S. schottmuelleri,* or *S. hirschfeldii*). On occasion, it may immediately follow classic enterocolitis caused by the same organism. The syndrome, characterized by prolonged sustained fever, relative bradycardia, splenomegaly, rose spots, and leukopenia, is described in Chapter 340. Enteric fever produced by serotypes of *Salmonella* other than *S. typhi* is usually milder than typhoid fever, and the chronic carrier state follows less commonly than after typhoid fever.

Bacteremia. Patients with the syndrome of *Salmonella* bacteremia usually complain of fever and chills for a period of days to weeks. Gastrointestinal symptoms are unusual, but in some patients the syndrome of *Salmonella* bacteremia follows classic enterocolitis. Other symptoms are non-specific, such as malaise, anorexia, and weight loss. Metastatic infection of bones, joints, mycotic aneurysm (particularly of the abdominal aorta), meninges (mainly in infants), pericardium, pleural space, lungs, heart valves, cysts, uterine myomas, malignancies, and other sites is common, and symptoms may be related to the site of metastatic infection. Stool cultures are usually negative for *Salmonella*, but blood cultures are positive.

Although any *Salmonella* serotype can produce the syndrome of bacteremia, *S. choleraesuis* is most likely to cause this syndrome; over 50% of *S. choleraesuis* infections are bacteremic.

Salmonella bacteremia occurs with increased frequency in infants and the elderly and in patients with diseases associated with hemolysis (such as sickle cell diseases, malaria, and bartonellosis), with lymphoma, with leukemia, and perhaps with systemic lupus erythematosus. Localization to bone is common in patients with sickle cell diseases.

Prolonged *Salmonella* bacteremia lasting for months occurs in patients with hepatosplenic schistosomiasis. Patients with AIDS develop recurrent, relapsing *Salmonella* bacteremia that is difficult to cure with antibiotics.

DIAGNOSIS. The diagnosis of *Salmonella* infection is made by isolating the organism from the stool in enterocolitis, from the blood in bacteremia, from blood and stool in enteric fever, and from the local site in localized infection. Serologic studies are of little clinical value in *Salmonella* infections other than typhoid fever, but they may be of use in epidemiologic studies. A stained smear of the stool usually demonstrates polymorphonuclear leukocytes in patients with *Salmonella* enterocolitis.

The differential diagnosis of *Salmonella* enterocolitis includes all causes of acute diarrhea, including invasive bacteria such as *Campylobacter jejuni, Shigella* species, invasive *Escherichia coli, Yersinia enterocolitica,* and *Vibrio parahaemolyticus;* toxigenic bacteria such as *V. cholerae,* enterotoxigenic *E. coli, E. coli 0157:H7, S. aureus, Bacillus cereus, Clostridium perfringens,* and *C. difficile;* viruses; and protozoa such as *Entamoeba histolytica, Giardia lamblia,* and *Cryptosporidium* species. Invasive bacterial causes of diarrhea, *E. coli 0157:H7,* and *C. difficile* infection are also associated with polymorphonuclear leukocytes in the stool, whereas bacterial toxigenic causes (other than *C. difficile* and *E. coli 0157: H7*), viruses, and protozoa generally are not. The bacterial toxigenic causes of diarrhea other than *C. difficile* and *E. coli* 0157:H7 do not produce fever.

Stool culture is definitive for the diagnosis of *Salmonella* enterocolitis; but by the time the results of the stool culture are available, most patients are recovering.

The differential diagnosis of *Salmonella* bacteremia includes all acute infectious and non-infectious causes of fever, including bacteremia caused by other organisms.

The differential diagnosis of enteric fever is the same as discussed in Chapter 340.

TREATMENT. Enterocolitis. The primary approach to treatment of *Salmonella* enterocolitis is fluid and electrolyte replacement. Drugs with antiperistaltic effects such as loperamide or diphenoxylate with atropine can relieve cramps but should be used sparingly because they can prolong the diarrhea.

Salmonella enterocolitis is self-limited. Furthermore, there has been a reluctance to treat *Salmonella* enterocolitis because antibiotic therapy has been reported to have no effect on the clinical course and, in some studies, to prolong the period of time salmonellae are excreted in the stool. In addition, most patients are improving by the time that salmonellae or other bacterial pathogens are isolated from the stool. However, infants, the elderly, and those with sickle cell disease, lymphoma, leukemia, or other serious underlying diseases who are severely ill and may have bacteremia may benefit from antimicrobial therapy.

The fluoroquinolones are active against virtually all bacterial pathogens that cause diarrhea except for *C. difficile*, and it is reasonable to use them empirically in the early therapy of adults with severe diarrhea of presumed bacterial etiology. It is also reasonable to use them for patients with known *Salmonella* enterocolitis who are suspected of being bacteremic. Ciprofloxacin, 500 mg every 12 hours orally or 400 mg every 12 hours intravenously for 3 to 5 days, has been widely used.

Other agents, such as amoxicillin (1 g every 6 hours orally), ampicillin (1 to 2 g IV every 6 hours), trimethoprim-sulfamethoxazole (one double-strength tablet every 12 hours orally), and trimethoprim-sulfamethoxazole (10 mg/kg/day IV of the trimethoprim component) have also been widely used in severely ill adults. However, many strains of *Salmonella* are now resistant to these agents.

Bacteremia and Enteric Fever. The agents of choice to treat these disorders are the third-generation cephalosporins, such as ceftriaxone, cefotaxime, and ceftizoxime, or the fluoroquinolones, such as ciprofloxacin and ofloxacin. Typical doses are ceftriaxone, 1 g every 12 hours intramuscularly or intravenously, and ciprofloxacin, 400 mg every 12 hours intravenously. After response, therapy can be changed to oral ciprofloxacin, 500 mg every 12 hours, or oral cefixime, 400 mg every 12 hours. When the salmonellae are known to be susceptible, ampicillin or trimethoprim-sulfamethoxazole can be used in the doses described in the section on enterocolitis. Chloramphenicol, 50 mg/kg/day in four equally divided doses orally or intravenously, is an alternative regimen.

Therapy is continued for 7 to 14 days for enteric fever and bacteremia without localization of organisms and for much longer periods of time with localization to bone, aneurysms, heart valves, and various other sites. Surgical drainage or removal of foreign bodies or resection of an aneurysm is often necessary to cure localized infection.

Curing schistosomiasis in patients with *Salmonella* bacteremia may cure the bacteremia. Patients with AIDS tend to relapse repeatedly after treatment courses for *Salmonella* bacteremia. Long-term suppressive therapy has been recommended by some.

Carriers. Chronic carriers (i.e., over 1 year) of salmonellae other than *S. typhi* are rare. Stools of convalescent carriers spontaneously become negative over a period of weeks to months, and no therapy should be given. The rare chronic carrier of non–*S. typhi* serotypes (usually infected with *S. paratyphi A, S. schottmuelleri*, or *S. hirschfeldii*) may be treated with 4 to 6 g of ampicillin plus 2 g of probenecid orally each day in four divided doses for 6 weeks. The fluoroquinolones are probably equally effective. Patients who experience relapse usually have gallbladder disease (most often calculi) and will not be cured with antimicrobial therapy. Cholecystectomy plus antimicrobial therapy may cure these patients, but it is doubtful that the carrier state per se is a sufficient indication for cholecystectomy.

PROGNOSIS. Mortality in *Salmonella* enterocolitis is rare; infants and the elderly are at greatest risk, with death occurring from dehydration and electrolyte imbalance. Mortality from *Salmonella* bacteremia or enteric fever is not uncommon and is most likely to occur in the very young and the very old. *S. choleraesuis* bacteremia has the highest mortality rate of any *Salmonella* serotype, as high as 20 to 30% if untreated.

PREVENTION. *Salmonella* infection is best prevented by properly managing the water supply and sewage disposal, cooking and refrigerating foods made from animal products, pasteurizing milk and milk products, and hand washing before preparing foods and after handling animals and uncooked animal products. Despite these precautions, because of the widespread presence of salmonellae in the animal kingdom, it is unlikely that the frequency of *Salmonella* infections will be significantly diminished.

There is no vaccine for any infection with salmonellae other than that for infection with *S. typhi*.

Centers for Disease Control and Prevention: Multidrug-resistant *Salmonella* serotype typhimurium—United States, 1996. MMWR Morbid Mortal Wkly Rep 46:308–310, 1997. *A report of an outbreak of multidrug-resistant Salmonella typhimurium infection in the United States caused by definitive type 104 (DT104), a strain that has been an increasing cause of infection in the United Kingdom.*
Centers for Disease Control and Prevention: Outbreaks of *Salmonella* serotype enteritidis infection associated with consumption of raw shell eggs—United States, 1994–1995. MMWR Morbid Mortal Wkly Rep 45:737–742, 1996. *A description of the increasing importance of Salmonella enteritidis as a cause of infection associated with consumption of eggs.*
Gruenewald R, Blum S, Chan J: Relationship between human immunodeficiency virus infection and salmonellosis in 20- to 59-year-old residents of New York City. Clin Infect Dis 18:358–363, 1994. *A report of the strong association between Salmonella infection and AIDS.*
Hennessy TW, Hedberg CW, Slutsker L, et al: A national outbreak of salmonella enteritidis infections from ice cream. N Engl J Med 334:1281–1286, 1996. *A description of a major outbreak of Salmonella enteritidis infection from ice cream caused by transport of pasteurized ice cream base in containers previously used for transport of non-pasteurized liquid eggs.*
Mahon BE, Ponka A, Hall WN, et al: An international outbreak of *Salmonella* infections caused by alfalfa sprouts grown from contaminated seeds. J Infect Dis 175:876–882, 1997. *A description of a Salmonella outbreak caused by alfalfa sprouts grown from contaminated seeds.*
Torok TJ, Tauxe RV, Wise RP, et al: A large community outbreak of salmonellosis caused by intentional contamination of restaurant salad bars. JAMA 278:389–395, 1997. *A description of a large outbreak of Salmonella infection related to intentional contamination of restaurant salad bars.*

342 SHIGELLOSIS

Thomas Butler

DEFINITION. Shigellosis is an acute bacterial infection caused by the genus *Shigella* resulting in colitis affecting predominantly the rectosigmoid colon. "Bacillary dysentery" is synonymous with shigellosis. The disease is characterized by diarrhea, dysentery, fever, abdominal pain, and tenesmus. Shigellosis is usually limited to a few days. Early treatment with antimicrobial drugs results in more rapid recovery.

ETIOLOGY. Shigellae are non-motile gram-negative bacilli belonging to the family Enterobacteriaceae. Four species of shigellae are recognized on the basis of antigenic and biochemical properties: *S. dysenteriae* (group A), *S. flexneri* (group B), *S. boydii* (group C), and *S. sonnei* (group D). Among these species there are over 40 serotypes, each of which is designated by the species name followed by a specific Arabic number. *S. dysenteriae* 1 is called the "Shiga bacillus" and causes epidemics with higher mortality than other serotypes. With the exception of *S. flexneri* 6, they do not ferment lactose.

Serotypes are determined by the O polysaccharide side chain of the lipopolysaccharide (endotoxin) in the cell wall. Endotoxin is detectable in the blood of severely ill patients and may be responsible for the complication of the hemolytic-uremic syndrome. To be virulent, shigellae must be able to invade epithelial cells, as tested in the laboratory by keratoconjunctivitis in the guinea pig (Sereney test) or HeLa cell invasion. Bacterial invasion of cells is genetically governed by three chromosomal regions and a 140-Md plasmid.

Shiga toxin is produced by *S. dysenteriae* 1 and in lesser amounts by other serotypes. It inhibits protein synthesis and has enterotoxic activity in animal models, but its role in human disease is uncertain.

INCIDENCE AND PREVALENCE. In the United States there were more than 14,000 cases reported in 1996 with species distribution of 73% *S. sonnei*, 19% *S. flexneri*, 2% *S. boydii*, and 1% *S. dysenteriae*. Most cases were in young children, women of childbearing age, and low-income minority residents; and a large proportion occurred in population groups living in homes for the mentally ill or in nursing homes. A large outbreak in 1987 in Tennessee affected more than 1000 persons camping under unsanitary conditions at a mass gathering.

Worldwide, most cases of shigellosis occur in children of developing countries, where *S. flexneri* is the predominant species. In 1994, an epidemic in Rwandan refugees caused an estimated 30,000 deaths.

EPIDEMIOLOGY. Shigellosis is transmitted by the fecal-oral route. Crowded living conditions, low standards of personal hygiene, poor water supply, and inadequate sewage facilities all contribute to an increased risk of infection. Transmission most often occurs by close person-to-person contact through contaminated hands. During clinical illness and for up to 6 weeks after recovery, organisms are excreted in the feces. Although the organisms are sensitive to desiccation, they may survive several months in food or water, which are occasional vehicles of transmission.

Children between 1 and 4 years old have the greatest risk of developing shigellosis. Inhabitants of custodial institutions, such as homes for retarded children, are at highest risk. Intrafamilial spread follows often when the initial case has occurred in a preschool child. In young adults, the incidence is higher in women than in men, which probably reflects closer contact of women with children. The male homosexual population in the United States is at increased risk for shigellosis, which is one of the causes of the "gay bowel syndrome."

Humans and higher primates are the only known natural reservoirs of shigellosis. Transmission shows variable seasonal patterns in different regions. In the United States, the peak incidence is in late summer and early autumn.

PATHOGENESIS AND PATHOLOGY. Because the microorganisms are relatively resistant to acid, shigellae pass the gastric barrier more readily than other enteric pathogens. In volunteer studies, as few as 200 ingested bacilli regularly initiate disease in 25% of healthy adults. This contrasts strikingly to the much larger numbers of typhoid or cholera bacilli required to produce disease in normal individuals. During the incubation period (usually 12 to 72 hours), the organisms traverse the small bowel, penetrate colonic epithelial cells, and multiply intracellularly. An acute inflammatory response ensues in the colonic mucosa attended by prodromal symptoms (Table 342–1). Epithelial cells containing bacteria are lysed, resulting in superficial ulcerations and shedding of shigella organisms into stools. The mucosa is friable and covered with a layer of polymorphonuclear leukocytes. Biopsy specimens show ulcers and crypt abscesses. Initially, the inflammation is confined to the rectosigmoid colon but after about 4 days of illness may advance to involve the proximal colon and sometimes even the terminal ileum; a pseudomembranous type of colitis may develop. Levels of proinflammatory cytokines are elevated in stool and plasma and correlate with disease severity. Diarrhea results because of impaired absorption of water and electrolytes by the inflamed colon.

Although the colonic inflammation is superficial, bacteremia occurs occasionally, especially in *S. dysenteriae* 1 infections. Susceptibility of organisms to serum complement–mediated bacteriolysis may explain the infrequency of bacteremia and disseminated infection. Colonic perforation is a rare complication during toxic megacolon. Children with severe colitis due to *S. dysenteriae* 1 are prone to develop the hemolytic-uremic syndrome. In this complication, fibrin thrombi are deposited in the renal glomeruli, causing cortical necrosis and fragmentation of red cells.

CLINICAL MANIFESTATIONS. Most patients with shigellosis begin their illness with a non-specific prodrome (see Table 342–1). The height of the temperature varies, and children may have febrile convulsions. The initial intestinal symptoms soon follow as cramps, loose stools, and watery diarrhea, which usually precede the onset of dysentery by 1 or more days. The average fecal output is about 600 g/day for adults. The dysentery consists typically of flecks and small clots of bright red blood and mucus in stools that are small in volume. Frequency of passage is often as high as 20 to 40 times a day, with excruciating rectal pain and tenesmus during defecation. Some patients develop rectal prolapse during severe straining. The amount of blood in stools varies widely but usually is small because of the superficial colonic ulcerations. Abdominal tenderness is often most marked in the left lower quadrant over the sigmoid colon but also may be generalized. The fever is likely to abate after a few days of dysentery, making afebrile bloody diarrhea an occasional clinical presentation. After 1 to 2 weeks of untreated disease, spontaneous improvement occurs in most patients. Some patients with mild disease develop only watery diarrhea without dysentery.

Complications include dehydration, which can cause death, especially in children and the elderly. *Shigella* septicemia occurs mainly in malnourished children with *S. dysenteriae* 1 infections. The leukemoid reaction and hemolytic-uremic syndrome may develop in children late in the course after antimicrobial treatment when the dysentery has started to improve. Neurologic manifestations can be striking and include delirium, seizures, and nuchal rigidity.

The important postdysenteric syndromes are arthritis and Reiter's triad of arthritis, urethritis, and conjunctivitis (see Chapter 287). These are non-suppurative phenomena that occur in the absence of viable *Shigella* organisms 1 to 3 weeks after resolution of dysentery.

DIAGNOSIS. Shigellosis should be considered in any patient with acute onset of fever and diarrhea. Examination of the stool is essential. Blood and pus are grossly apparent in severe bacillary dysentery; even in milder forms of the disease, microscopic examination of the stool often reveals numerous leukocytes and erythrocytes. The fecal leukocyte examination should be performed with a portion of liquid stool, preferably containing mucus. A drop of stool is placed on a microscopic slide, mixed thoroughly with two drops of methylene blue, and overlaid with a coverslip. The presence of abundant polymorphonuclear leukocytes helps distinguish shigellosis from diarrheal syndromes caused by viruses and enterotoxigenic bacteria. The fecal leukocyte examination is not helpful in distinguishing shigellosis from diarrheal illnesses caused by

Table 342–1 ■ EVOLUTION OF CLINICAL SYNDROMES IN SHIGELLOSIS

STAGE	TIME OF APPEARANCE AFTER ONSET OF ILLNESS	SYMPTOMS AND SIGNS	PATHOLOGY
Prodrome	Earliest	Fever, chills, myalgias, anorexia, nausea, vomiting	None or early colitis
Non-specific diarrhea	0–3 days	Abdominal cramps, loose stools, watery diarrhea	Rectosigmoid colitis with superficial ulceration, fecal leukocytes
Dysentery	1–8 days	Frequent passage of blood and mucus, tenesmus, rectal prolapse, abdominal tenderness	Colitis extending sometimes to proximal colon, crypt abscesses, inflammation in lamina propria
Complications	3–10 days	Dehydration, seizures, septicemia, leukemoid reaction, hemolytic-uremic syndrome, ileus, peritonitis	Severe colitis, terminal ileitis, endotoxemia, intravascular coagulation, toxic megacolon, colonic perforation
Postdysenteric syndromes	1–3 weeks	Arthritis, Reiter's syndrome	Reactive inflammation in HLA-B27 haplotype

other invasive enteric pathogens (non-typhoidal *Salmonella, Campylobacter,* and *Yersinia*). Amebic dysentery is excluded by the absence of trophozoites on a microscopic examination of fresh stool under a coverslip. The peripheral white cell count is of little diagnostic value, because it may range from less than 3000 to more than 30,000/mm³. Sigmoidoscopic examination reveals diffuse erythema with a mucopurulent layer and friable areas of mucosa with shallow ulcers 3 to 7 mm in diameter.

Definitive diagnosis depends on isolating shigellae by selective media. A rectal swab, a swab of a colonic ulcer obtained by sigmoidoscopic examination, or a freshly passed stool specimen should be inoculated immediately on culture plates or into carrying media. Because isolation rates of shigellae from freshly passed stools of patients with shigellosis may be as low as 67%, culturing for 3 successive days is recommended. Stool cultures are generally positive within 24 hours after onset of symptoms and may remain positive for several weeks in the absence of antimicrobial therapy. Appropriate culture media include blood, desoxycholate, and *Salmonella-Shigella* (S-S) agars. Selected colonies should be diagnosed by agglutination with polyvalent *Shigella* antisera. S-S agar is inhibitory for *S. dysenteriae* 1.

Definitive bacteriologic diagnosis becomes critically important for distinguishing the more severe and prolonged cases of shigellosis from ulcerative colitis, with which it may be confused both clinically and on sigmoidoscopic examination. Patients with shigellosis have been subjected to colectomy because of a mistaken diagnosis of ulcerative colitis; a positive culture should prevent such a misadventure.

TREATMENT. Appropriate antimicrobial therapy instituted early may decrease the duration of symptoms by 50% and decrease the duration of excretion of shigellae (an important epidemiologic factor) by a far greater percentage. Because of the increasing frequency of plasmid-mediated antimicrobial resistance to *Shigella* infections, surveillance of drug susceptibility in an endemic area is important. In adults, ciprofloxacin given orally in a dose of 500 mg twice daily for 5 days or 1 g as a single dose is the treatment of choice when the susceptibility of a strain is unknown. In children, treatment should be trimethoprim-sulfamethoxazole, ampicillin, or azithromycin, depending on susceptibilities of *Shigella* in a given location.

Fluid losses in shigellosis are qualitatively similar to those in other infectious diarrheal diseases, and the patient should be treated with appropriate intravenous or oral electrolyte repletion fluids in quantities adequate to correct clinical signs of saline depletion. The requirement for fluids is generally small, but fluid repletion is lifesaving in exceptional cases.

Agents that decrease intestinal motility should not be used. Such preparations as diphenoxylate and paregoric may exacerbate symptoms, presumably by retarding intestinal clearance of the microorganisms. There is no convincing evidence that pectin- or bismuth-containing preparations are helpful.

PROGNOSIS. The mortality rate in untreated shigellosis depends on the infectious strain and ranges from 10 to 30% in certain outbreaks caused by *S. dysenteriae* 1 to less than 1% in most *S. sonnei* infections. Even with infection caused by *S. dysenteriae* 1, mortality rates should approach zero if appropriate fluid replacement and antimicrobial therapy are initiated early.

About 2% of patients may develop arthritis or Reiter's syndrome weeks or months after recovery from shigellosis.

PREVENTION. Individuals excreting shigellae should be excluded from all phases of food handling until negative cultures have been obtained from three successive stool specimens collected after completion of antimicrobial therapy. In institutional outbreaks, strict and early isolation of infected individuals is mandatory. Targeted antimicrobial chemoprophylaxis has been disappointing. The most important control measure is rigorous hand washing with soap and water by all individuals involved in handling of food or changing diapers. Reporting of shigellosis cases to health authorities should be mandatory.

For the traveler to countries with major *Shigella* problems, no chemoprophylactic agent is an adequate substitute for good personal hygiene and avoiding contaminated food and water. A variety of vaccines has been developed and tested, but no vaccine is now commercially available.

Bogaerts J, Verhaegen J, Munyabikali JP, et al: Antimicrobial resistance and serotypes of *Shigella* isolates in Kigali, Rwanda (1983–1993): Increasing frequency of multiple resistance. Diagn Microbiol Infect Dis 28:165, 1997. *Emergence of multidrug resistance, including resistance to nalidixic acid in S. dysenteriae 1, in infected refugees posed threats to effective therapy.*

Khan WA, Seas C, Dhar U, et al: Treatment of shigellosis: V. Comparison of azithromycin and ciprofloxacin. Ann Intern Med 126:697, 1997. *Azithromycin and ciprofloxacin were equally effective against multiresistant infections in Bangladesh.*

Kolavic SA, Kimura A, Simons SL, et al: An outbreak of *Shigella dysenteriae* type 2 among laboratory workers due to intentional food contamination. JAMA 278:396, 1997. *In Texas, 12 laboratory personnel became ill after ingesting muffins and doughnuts that had been deliberately contaminated by an unusual laboratory stocked strain. Pulsed-field gel electrophoresis of isolated strains confirmed the likely source of the outbreak.*

Raqib R, Wretlind B, Andersson J, et al: Cytokine secretion in acute shigellosis is correlated to disease activity and directed more to stool than to plasma. J Infect Dis 171:376, 1995. *Proinflammatory cytokine levels were elevated in stool and plasma during acute disease, whereas interferon-γ was below normal levels.*

Tauxe RV, Puhr ND, Wells JG, et al: Antimicrobial resistance of *Shigella* isolates in the USA: The importance to international travelers. J Infect Dis 162:1107, 1990. *In the United States, resistance of Shigella isolates to trimethoprim-sulfamethoxazole occurred in 4% of domestically acquired cases and 20% of travel-related cases.*

Wharton M, Spiegel RA, Horan JM, et al: A large outbreak of antibiotic-resistant shigellosis at a mass gathering. J Infect Dis 162:1324, 1990. *Poor sanitation at a camp site in Tennessee led to an attack rate of more than 50% in several thousand attendees; disease was caused by multiresistant S. sonnei.*

343 *CAMPYLOBACTER* ENTERITIS

Richard L. Guerrant

Enteric infection with a member of the genus *Campylobacter* usually results in an inflammatory, occasionally bloody diarrhea or dysentery syndrome in industrialized, temperate areas. *Campylobacter jejuni* is often the most commonly recognized cause of community-acquired inflammatory enteritis. The diarrhea also may be watery, especially in developing, tropical areas. An enterocolitis or protocolitis syndrome similar to that seen with *C. jejuni* is also seen in homosexual males with several "*Campylobacter*-like organisms," that are now being classified as *Helicobacter* species such as *H. cinaedi, H. fennelliae* and others. Like *C. jejuni*, these *Campylobacter*-like organisms may cause life-threatening bacteremic infections in patients with the acquired immunodeficiency syndrome. The other major *Campylobacter* species that infects humans is *C. fetus*, a relatively uncommon cause of bacteremia and occasional intravascular infection in immunocompromised hosts. *Helicobacter pylori* (the cause of gastritis and peptic ulcers) was once called *Campylobacter pylori*, but is now reclassified.

ETIOLOGY. *Campylobacter* (meaning "curved rod") is a curved or spiral, motile, non–spore-forming, gram-negative rod measuring 1.5 by 3.5 μm that is distinguished from Enterobacteriaceae by its inability to ferment or oxidize carbohydrates. It was once called a "vibrio," but is now recognized as a separate genus on the basis of its distinctive DNA content. It is both oxidase and catalase positive and is a microaerophilic organism that requires reduced oxygen (5 to 10%) and increased carbon dioxide (3 to 10%). The organism does not grow at either aerobic or strictly anaerobic conditions. Perhaps reflecting its avian reservoir, *C. jejuni* also requires an increased temperature to 42° C for optimal growth. *C. jejuni* is distinguished from *C. fetus* by its higher growth temperatures, cephalothin resistance, and nalidixic acid sensitivity. As shown in Table 343–1, the additional *Campylobacter* species that infect humans include *C. lari*, a thermophilic organism commonly found in healthy sea gulls that has been reported in children with mild recurrent diarrhea and in an elderly patient with sepsis and terminal multiple myeloma. The weak or non–catalase-producing *C. upsaliensis* may cause diarrhea or bacteremia, and *C. hyointestinalis*, like *C. fetus*, causes occasional bacteremia in compromised hosts. These organisms are also inhibited by cephalothin that is in some selective culture media. Like *C. fetus*, the *Campylobacter*-like organisms (*H. cinaedi, H. fennelliae*, others) do not grow at 42° C or in the presence of cephalosporin antibiotics (present in some selective media for *C. jejuni*) and may require several days to grow on microaerophilic subcultures on blood agar. *C. jejuni* is further subdivided into over 90 serotypes on the basis of heat-stable somatic

Table 343–1 ■ HUMAN *CAMPYLOBACTER* INFECTIONS

SPECIES	GROWTH TEMPERATURE	RESERVOIR	CLINICAL MANIFESTATIONS
C. jejuni/coli	37–42° C	Poultry, mammals	Common cause of dysentery/diarrhea
C. fetus (sub. sp. *fetus*, old sub sp. *intestinalis*)	25–37° C	Cattle, sheep	Uncommon, bacteremia; intravascular infections in debilitated hosts
C. laridis	30–42° C	Sea gulls	Uncommon, childhood diarrhea, one case of sepsis
C. upsaliensis	37–42° C	Dogs	Occasional diarrhea
C. hyointestinalis	37° C	Swine	Occasional bacteremia in compromised hosts
"*Campylobacter*-like organisms": (including *Helicobacter cinaedi, H. fennelliae*)	37° C	?	Proctocolitis, rarely sepsis, in homosexual males

lipopolysaccharide O antigens or some 112 heat-labile flagellar and cellular antigens or even additional subtypes based on phage restriction DNA or ribosomal RNA digests, all markers that are helpful in tracing the epidemiology of this common enteric pathogen.

EPIDEMIOLOGY. Although the frequency of other *Campylobacter* infections is either low or unclear. *C. jejuni* infections are extremely common throughout the world. In many studies, the frequency of *Campylobacter* enteritis exceeds that of *Salmonella* or *Shigella* infections, and it has been estimated that as many as 2 million *Campylobacter* enteritis cases occur annually in the United States. The reservoirs of *C. jejuni/coli* include a wide range of mammalian species. Between 30 and 100% of chickens, turkeys, and water fowl may be infected asymptomatically in their intestinal tracts, and commercially prepared poultry in supermarkets can often be shown to be culture positive. In addition, swine, cattle, sheep, horses, and even household pets and rodents may carry *C. jejuni, C. coli*, or *C. fetus*. Dogs and cats are more likely to be infected with *C. upsaliensis*. Enteric symptoms may be found, particularly in puppies, kittens, calves, or lambs, which may have diarrhea when infected. Furthermore, the organisms survive days to weeks in fresh or salt water and in milk and are killed most effectively by pasteurization, chlorination, drying, or freezing.

The transmission of *Campylobacter* infections is likely via the fecal-oral route. Fecal-oral spread may occur by contact among animals, those practicing oral-anal sex, and those in day-care centers. Secondary transmission is relatively infrequent, and the infectious dose appears to vary from 500 to over 1 million organisms. The majority of infections are probably acquired by ingesting contaminated food, water, or milk vehicles. Many cases and outbreaks are associated with ingesting inadequately cooked poultry, unpasteurized milk, inadequately treated water, and even cake icing, salads, beef, and clams.

The majority of those infected in well-described outbreaks are symptomatic. Asymptomatic infection appears to be relatively infrequent in temperate climates and in adults. An exception is among young children in certain tropical developing areas such as Bangladesh, where as many as 39% of children younger than age 2 years may be infected asymptomatically (Table 343–2). These frequent asymptomatic infections in tropical areas raise important questions about possible strain differences in virulence, host susceptibility, and protective immunity against disease that might be acquired very early in developing areas.

Throughout the world, *Campylobacter* infections appear to predominate during the warmer or wet season. As with diarrheal illnesses in general, the highest age-specific attack rate is in young

children. However, the greatest proportion of positive fecal cultures occurs in older children and young adults. The latter contributes a small peak in the age-specific attack rates during the "second weaning," when young adults leave home and lack experience with cooking poultry and other products. There is little, if any, sexual predominance of recognized *C. jejuni* infections.

PATHOGENESIS AND PATHOLOGY. *C. jejuni* and *C. coli* are reasonably susceptible to gastric acidity. However, the reported variation in infectious dose suggests considerable host or strain variability. After an incubation period of 1 to 7 (median 4) days, symptoms of the enteric infection begin. *C. jejuni* organisms are attracted toward mucus and fucose in bile, and the flagellae may be important in both chemotaxis and adherence to epithelial cells or mucus. Adherence also may involve lipopolysaccharide or other outer membrane components. Several laboratories around the world have documented the production by *C. jejuni* of a cholera-like, heat-labile enterotoxin that binds to ganglioside and is neutralized by anticholera toxin antiserum. However, the genetic code and role of this toxin in disease remain elusive. Studies from Mexico have shown that antitoxic immunity develops after infection, often with watery diarrhea, suggesting that this toxin is significant in those infections.

However, more characteristic in temperate areas is a diffuse, often bloody exudative enteritis involving the ileum and colon. These pathologic changes may include non-specific crypt abscesses that on colonoscopy and histopathology may mimic the changes seen with inflammatory bowel disease. Such invasive pathology is also seen in rabbit, chick, mouse, dog, and monkey models of infection. Although *C. jejuni* is negative in the Sereny test for guinea pig conjunctivitis, some have reported the production of cytotoxins by certain strains of *C. jejuni* that may be involved in the pathogenesis of the invasive colitis. The relative infrequency of blood-stream invasion by *C. jejuni*, compared with *C. fetus*, likely relates to the relative serum sensitivity of most *C. jejuni* strains and to the rapid development of bactericidal antibody with infection in normal individuals. Volunteer studies suggest that effective immunity develops to rechallenge with the homologous strain, and animal studies suggest that protective immunity may be transferred in immune milk to suckling offspring. Additional evidence of effective immunity comes with the decreasing illness/infection ratio among children in endemic areas as well as among regular consumers of raw milk.

Once patients are infected, they shed 10^7 to 10^9 organisms per gram of stool for a median duration of 2 to 3 weeks, if not treated with effective antibiotics. Although some may continue to excrete the organism for 2 to 3 months, chronic asymptomatic intestinal carriage is rare.

CLINICAL MANIFESTATIONS. As noted in Table 343–1, the major recognized disease with human *Campylobacter* infections is the characteristic diarrheal illness seen with *C. jejuni* or *C. coli* infections. Although asymptomatic infections and watery, non-inflammatory diarrhea are seen with *C. jejuni* infections in tropical, developing areas as shown in Table 343–2, *C. jejuni* is characteristically associated with an inflammatory, febrile enteritis in industrialized countries throughout the world. After an incubation period of 1 to 7 days, a brief prodrome of fever, headache, and myalgias lasting for 12 to 24 hours is promptly followed in a case of *C. jejuni* enteritis in a child or young adult with the symptoms of acute enteritis. These characteristically include crampy abdominal pain, fever to 39 or 40° C, and diarrhea with up to 10 or more

Table 343–2 ■ CLINICAL PRESENTATIONS OF *CAMPYLOBACTER JEJUNI* INFECTION

	INDUSTRIALIZED COUNTRIES	DEVELOPING COUNTRIES
Percent of all diarrhea with *C. jejuni*	5–13	2–35
Percent of *C. jejuni* diarrhea with:		
Fecal polymorphonuclear leukocytes	78–93	22–46
Blood in stool	60–65	5–17
Asymptomatic infection rates (%)	<2	0–39*

*Depending on age—39% if younger than 2 years old.

loose, often bloody bowel movements per day. Occasionally, the abdominal pain may predominate as an appendicitis-like syndrome, with mesenteric adenitis or terminal ileitis being the predominant pathology. On physical examination, the abdomen is diffusely tender and may mimic appendicitis. Although the acute febrile enteritis is usually self-limited to 5 to 7 days, 10 to 20% of cases may last longer than 1 week and 5 to 20% of untreated cases may relapse with a similar illness.

Complications, particularly if antimotility agents are used, include toxic megacolon, pseudomembranous colitis, and colonic hemorrhage. In addition, hemolytic-uremic syndrome, postinfectious polyneuritis, or Guillain-Barré syndrome may follow *C. jejuni* enteritis. Some suggest that *C. jejuni* (especially O type 19) may be a major recognized predisposing cause of Guillain-Barré syndrome. As in many inflammatory colitis syndromes, reactive arthritis and full-blown Reiter's syndrome may follow weeks after *Campylobacter* enteritis. Bacteremia may occur relatively rarely (usually <2% of cases), particularly in the very young or the elderly, in whom meningitis, endocarditis, cholecystitis, urinary tract infections, and pancreatitis have been described. In patients with hypogammaglobulinemia or human immunodeficiency virus infection, *C. jejuni* infections are more often bacteremic and may be prolonged or severe despite appropriate antimicrobial therapy.

In striking contrast to *C. jejuni,* the slow-growing *C. fetus* is primarily an uncommon cause of bacteremia, often in immunocompromised hosts. Although *C. fetus* would be missed on most routine stool cultures for *C. jejuni,* studies with filtration methods suggest that it is a relatively infrequent cause of diarrhea. Instead, *C. fetus* tends to cause intravascular, meningeal, or localized infec-

tions such as arthritis, cellulitis, abscesses, cholecystitis, and urinary, placental, or pleural infections, often in elderly or debilitated hosts. As it does in animals, *C. fetus* may cause stillbirth or septic abortions more often than generally recognized in humans. *C. fetus* infections are often recognized only by astute clinical microbiology technicians who methodically examine or subculture cultured specimens of blood or other body fluids after 1 week in the laboratory. The clinical course of *C. fetus* bacteremia is often related to its recognition and appropriate treatment as well as to the underlying disease.

DIAGNOSIS. The diagnosis of *Campylobacter* infections is related to a careful history for exposure or characteristic clinical syndromes, direct stool examination, and selective culture methods. *C. jejuni* enteritis should be suspected in anyone presenting with a febrile enteritis, especially if there is a history of recent ingestion of inadequately cooked poultry, unpasteurized milk, or untreated water. As suggested in Figure 343–1, such a history should prompt obtaining a fecal specimen in a cup if at all possible and direct microscopic examination using methylene blue or Gram stain for leukocytes or a test for fecal lactoferrin as well as gross and/or occult blood. In many industrialized areas, the presence of blood or fecal leukocytes or lactoferrin with fever strongly suggests the presence of a cultivable enteric pathogen such as *C. jejuni, Salmonella,* or *Shigella,* with *C. jejuni* being most common. Additional immediate clues to *C. jejuni* infection may be seen on dark-field or phase microscopy for characteristic darting motility or on a carbolfuchsin Gram stain of stool for characteristic curved rods or sea

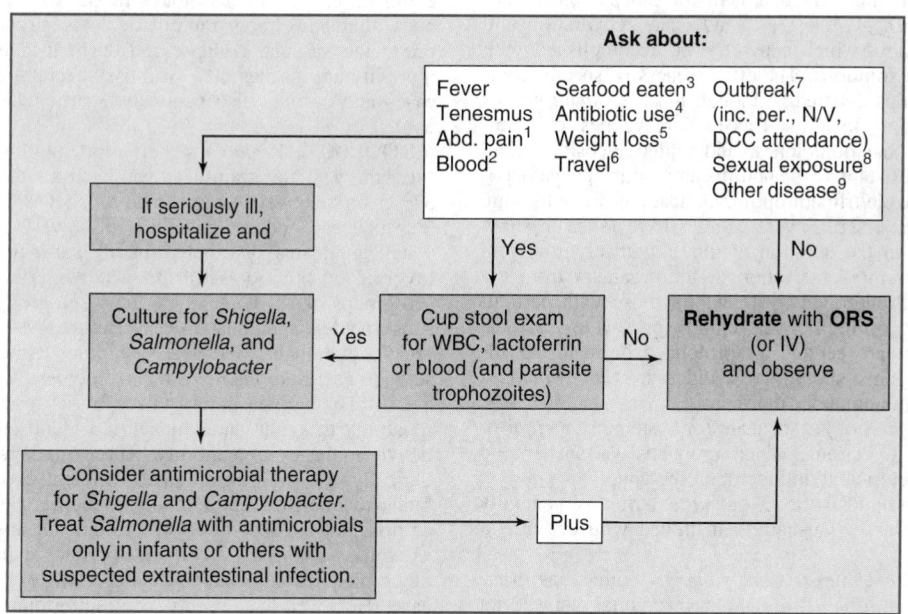

FIGURE 343–1 ■ Approach to the diagnosis and management of acute infectious diarrhea.

1. If unexplained abdominal pain and fever persist or suggest an appendicitis-like syndrome, culture for *Yersinia enterocolitica.*
2. Bloody diarrhea, especially if without fecal leukocytes, suggests enterohemorrhagic (*Shiga* toxin-producing) *E. coli* 0157 or amebiasis (where leukocytes are destroyed by the parasite).
3. Ingestion of inadequately cooked seafood should prompt consideration of *Vibrio* infections or Norwalk-like viruses.
4. Associated antibiotics should be stopped if possible and cytotoxigenic *C. difficile* considered.
5. Persistence (>10 days) with weight loss should prompt consideration of giardiasis or cryptosporidiosis.
6. Travel to tropical areas increases the chance of enterotoxigenic *E. coli* as well as viral (ex. Norwalk-like or rotaviral), parasitic (ex. *Giardia, Entamoeba, Strongyloides, Cryptosporidium*), and, if fecal leukocytes are present, invasive bacterial pathogens as noted in the algorithm.
7. Outbreaks should prompt consideration of *S. aureus, B. cereus, Anisakis* (incubation period <6 hours), *C. perfringens,* ETEC, *Vibrio, Salmonella, Campylobacter, Shigella* or EIEC infection. If unexplained, consider saving *E. coli* for LT, ST, invasiveness, adherence testing, and serotyping, and save stool for rotavirus and stool + paired sera for Norwalk-like virus testing.
8. Sigmoidoscopy in symptomatic homosexual males should distinguish procititis in the distal 15 cm only (caused by herpesvirus, gonococcal, chlamydial, or syphilitic infection) from colitis (*Campylobacter, Shigella, C. difficile,* or chlamydial [LGV serotypes] infections) or noninflammatory diarrhea (due to giardiasis).
9. Immunocompromised hosts should have a wide range of viral (ex. CMV, HSV, coxsackie, rotavirus), bacterial (ex. *Salmonella, Mycobacterium avium-intracellular, Listeria*), fungal (ex. *Candida*), and parasitic (ex. *Cryptosporidium, Strongyloides, Entamoeba,* and *Giardia*) agents considered.

(Adapted from Guerrant RL, Shields DS, Thorson SM, et al.: Evaluation and diagnosis of acute infectious diarrhea. Am J Med 78:91, 1985; Guerrant RL, Bobak DA: Bacterial and protozoal gastroenteritis. N Engl J Med 325:327, 1991; and Choi SW, Park CH, Silva TMJ, Zaenker EI, Guerrant RL. To culture or not to culture: Fecal lactoferrin screening for inflammatory diarrhea. J Clin Microbiol 34:928–932, 1996.)

gull morphology. However, dark-field and Gram stains, although reasonably specific with trained observers, are each only 50 to 66% sensitive. Patients with febrile enteritis, particularly with blood and leukocytes in the stool, should have cultured done for *C. jejuni.*

Additional differential diagnostic possibilities for febrile inflammatory enteritis include *Salmonella* and *Shigella* infections, for which one should seek a history of an outbreak or contact exposure (such as in day-care centers or among homosexual males, respectively). If the patient has recently taken antibiotics, *C. difficile* colitis or *Salmonella* enteritis should be considered. Recent ingestion of raw seafood should prompt investigation for *Vibrio* infection that may present as either inflammatory or non-inflammatory diarrhea. A history of sick pet exposure, persisting abdominal pain, or unexplained inflammatory diarrhea also should prompt consideration of *Yersinia enterocolitica* infections, and travel exposure to tropical areas or residence in an institution where careful hygiene is difficult should prompt an examination of stool and possibly rectal biopsy specimens for *Entamoeba histolytica* (which often destroys fecal leukocytes). Another frequent diagnosis that is considered, especially if *Campylobacter* enteritis has relapsed once or twice, is inflammatory bowel disease. However, it is imperative that anyone who is being considered for that diagnosis have treatable causes such as *Campylobacter* enteritis or amebiasis excluded by appropriate cultures or stains, because treatment with corticosteroids may worsen *Campylobacter* or amebic enteritis, with potentially devastating consequences. Additional non-infectious causes of bloody diarrhea with abdominal pain include intussusception and vascular insufficiency.

THERAPY. The most important treatment for *Campylobacter* enteritis, as with all diarrheal illnesses, is adequate rehydration and maintenance fluid therapy, which can often be accomplished with oral glucose-electrolyte solutions. The effectiveness of specific antimicrobial therapy remains debated. Although most *C. jejuni* strains are sensitive to erythromycin as well as to tetracyclines, chloramphenicol, clindamycin, the quinolones, and aminoglycosides, they are characteristically resistant to penicillin, ampicillin, cephalosporins, and sulfamethoxazole/trimethroprim. Indications for antibiotic treatment remain controversial. Several studies have failed to show a significant reduction in the duration of illness with erythromycin treatment despite its prompt eradication of the organism from the stool. Some reserve antimicrobial treatment for those with particularly severe symptoms of high fever, bloody or severe diarrhea, young children in day-care centers, or prolonged or relapsing illnesses. Antimotility agents should be avoided in *Campylobacter* enteritis, as with any inflammatory diarrhea.

Oral erythromycin may not be adequate for systemic *C. jejuni* or *C. fetus* endovascular infections, which probably warrant 2 to 4 weeks of parenteral bactericidal antimicrobial therapy.

PROGNOSIS. The prognosis of *C. jejuni* enteritis is generally quite good, and the disease is usually self-limited with or without specific therapy.

PREVENTION. Because most *Campylobacter* infections arise from fecal contamination, often from animal reservoirs, many if not most *Campylobacter* infections are potentially preventable by education. The most common recognized vehicles of spread are inadequately cooked food, unpasteurized milk, and inadequately treated water. Consequently, thoroughly cooking meat and poultry, careful hand washing after preparing food, pasteurizing milk, and adequately chlorinating drinking water should greatly reduce the frequency of *Campylobacter* infections. Parents should be warned that sick pet kittens or puppies may harbor potential human pathogens such as *C. jejuni* and keep them away from small children and practice careful hygienic measures in their care.

Allos BM, Lastovica AJ, Blaser MJ: Atypical campylobacters and related microorganisms. *In* Blaser MJ, Smith PD, Ravdin JI, et al (eds): Infections of the Gastrointestinal Tract. New York, Raven Press, 1995, pp 849–865. *Excellent overview of C. fetus, upsaliensis, lari, H. cinaedi, H. fennelliae and related campylobacters.*

Guerrant RL, Lahita RG, Winn WC, et al: Campylobacteriosis in man. Pathogenic mechanisms and review of 91 bloodstream infections. Am J Med 65:584, 1978. *Review of both C. fetus and C. jejuni infections and their presentations as bacteremic illnesses.*

Guerrant RL, Bobak DA: Bacterial and protozoal gastroenteritis. N Engl J Med 325: 327, 1991. *Update on epidemiology and pathogenesis as well as a practical clinical approach to diagnosis and management of bacterial and other causes of diarrhea.*

Hoge CW, Gambel JM, Srijan A, et al: Trends in antibiotic resistance among diarrheal pathogens isolated in Thailand over 15 years. Clin Infect Dis 26:341–345, 1998. *Important report of the alarming increase of ciprofloxacin resistance among* Campylobacter *species from zero before 1991 to 84% in 1995 (with concomitant resistance to the new macrolide azithromycin in 15%).*

Nachamkin I, Blazer MJ, Tompkins LS: *Campylobacter jejuni:* Current Status and Future Trends. Washington, DC, ASM, 1992. *An excellent compendium of multiauthored chapters on epidemiology, microbiology, clinical manifestations, pathogenesis, immunity and therapy of* Campylobacter *infections.*

Skirrow MB, Blaser MJ: *Campylobacter jejuni.* In Blaser MJ, Smith PD, Ravdin JI, et al (eds): Infections of the Gastrointestinal Tract, New York, Raven Press, 1995, pp 825–848. *Good review of cultivation methods, epidemiology, pathogenesis and clinical presentations of* C. jejuni *infections.*

Tee W, Mijch A: *Campylobacter jejuni* bacteremia in HIV-infected and non–HIV-infected patients: Comparison of clinical features and review. Clin Infect Dis 26:91–96, 1998. *Excellent review of increased risk of* C. jejuni, *bacteremia in AIDS, with extraintestinal involvement such as pneumonitis or cellulitis.*

Walker RI, Caldwell MB, Lee EC, et al: Pathophysiology of *Campylobacter* enteritis. Microbiol Rev 50:81, 1986. *Excellent review of the virulence traits, pathogenic mechanisms, and animal models of* C. jejuni *infections.*

344 CHOLERA

William B. Greenough, III

DEFINITION. Cholera is an epidemic, acute watery diarrheal disease caused by *Vibrio cholerae,* serogroups 01 and 0139, that occurs both sporadically and as large outbreaks. Fluid loss may be extreme, exceeding 1 L/hour. In such cases, loss of solute-rich body fluids in stools rapidly depletes circulating plasma volume, producing vascular collapse and death in hours. Without treatment, mortality approaches 60% of those severely affected; however, mild cases and carriers also occur and participate in the spread of disease.

ETIOLOGY. *V. cholerae* are short, slightly curved, rapidly motile, uniflagellate gram-negative bacteria that grow aerobically at 37° C on relatively simple media. They are currently classified as Vibrionaceae and are members of a very large group of surface water organisms distributed in all parts of the world, especially favoring brackish or salt-fresh water interfaces. There are many O serogroups of *V. cholerae,* but only serogroups 01 and 0139 Bengal cause epidemic human disease. Before 1992, two major serotypes, Ogawa and Inaba, and a less common Hikojima variant were observed. There are also two main biotypes, "classical" and "El Tor." The El Tor biotype is recognized by its resistance to polymyxin B, its ability to agglutinate chicken red blood cells, and its characteristic vibriophage susceptibility. These markers are of use epidemiologically. *V. cholerae* produces a potent exotoxin (choleragen) that binds to intestinal epithelium, producing a chloride ion–driven secretion and malabsorption of sodium ion and water. Other vibrios, as well as *Escherichia coli,* can produce exotoxins but do not have other biologic characteristics that lead to spreading epidemic disease. However, an entirely new serogroup (0139 Bengal) is currently responsible for major epidemics.

EPIDEMIOLOGY. Cholera is thought to be a disease of antiquity, with clear written descriptions dating before 500 B.C. The present global spread (seventh pandemic) has been due to an El Tor biotype first recognized in 1911 at the El Tor quarantine station in the Persian Gulf. Epidemics due to this organism first appeared in the Celebes in the 1930s, spreading westward through Southeast Asia and reaching the Mediterranean and Africa in the 1970s. However, in the Ganges delta, epidemics of classic *V. cholerae* were replaced by El Tor late in the 1960s. There have been small but regular outbreaks of cholera in the United States in the Mississippi delta regions since 1973. The El Tor strains isolated have not been the same as the global epidemic strain. In 1991, *V. cholerae* 01 El Tor caused explosive outbreaks of cholera in Peru and have subsequently spread throughout Latin America (Fig. 344–1). The newly arisen *V. cholerae* 0139 Bengal is now spreading globally. *V. cholerae* serogroups 01 and 0139 can be identified by gene amplification or immunofluorescent methods in many surface waters and are often associated with phytoplankton.

MODE OF SPREAD. During epidemics, cholera is mainly water-

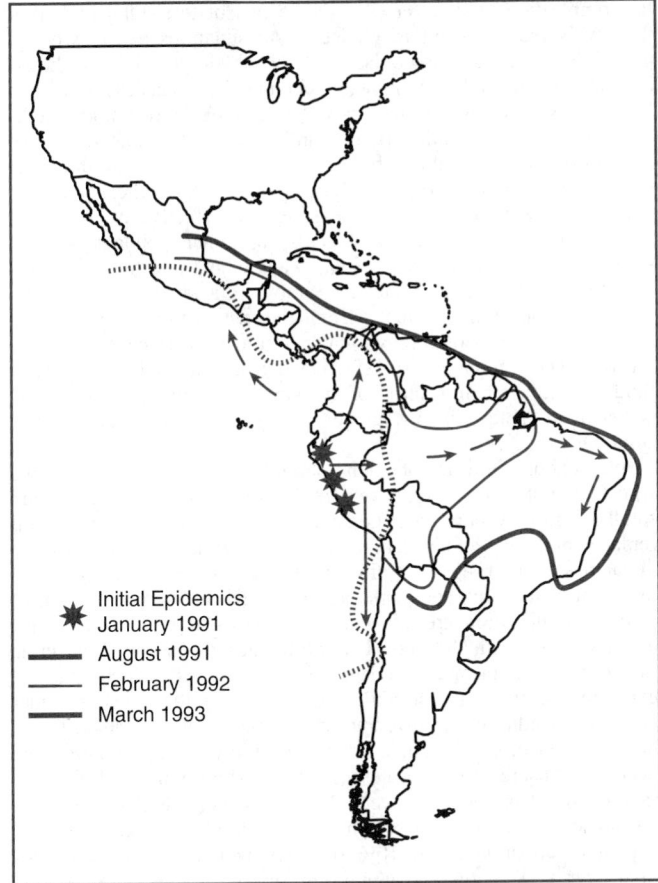

FIGURE 344–1 ■ Geographic extent of the Latin American epidemic over time. Lines represent the advancing front of the epidemic at different times. By March 1993, all Latin American countries except Uruguay had reported cholera, and no cases had been reported from the Caribbean.

Initial Epidemics
★ January 1991
━━━ August 1991
──── February 1992
▬▬▬ March 1993

borne. Large numbers of vibrios enter water sources from the voluminous liquid stools that soak clothing and linens and contaminate the environment. The setting for epidemics is often extreme poverty with lack of safe water. However, an outbreak in Portugal affected the most careful travelers who used only bottled water, which unfortunately had been supplied from a spring contaminated with *V. cholerae*. Occasionally, contaminated foods spread disease. Most often raw or undercooked shellfish or fresh vegetables washed with contaminated water are responsible. These played an important role in the recent Latin American epidemics. There is a high risk of secondary spread in families or institutions in which water and food are shared. Contamination of household food and water sources is the rule. It is easy to understand how this occurs when an adult patient may produce 30 to 50 L of stool in 2 to 3 days and is usually too weak to use a commode or toilet. Mild cases and convalescent carriers probably spread the disease between communities. True long-term carries are rare enough to be reportable. During interepidemic periods *V. Cholerae* lurks in many brackish surface waters in an unculturable form that can be detected by specific gene amplification methods.

SUSCEPTIBILITY TO CHOLERA. In areas where cholera occurs each year, children younger than 5 have the highest rates. Rates of older children and adults are lower because of local intestinal immunity, which decreases risk; but these older individuals make up a larger part of the population, and many patients present when older than age 5. Breastfed infants rarely get cholera because they receive protection from antibodies in their mother's milk. When cholera attacks a population that has not experienced it for many years, as was true during the present pandemic in the Philippines and Africa, all ages are attacked equally, but morbidity and mortality are greatest among the very young and very old. Individuals with low gastric acid production, or those who are on acid-suppressing medications or who have had gastrectomies, are especially

vulnerable, because *V. cholerae* is quite sensitive to acid. Cholera tends to attack persons of blood group O more frequently and with greater severity, whereas individuals with AB blood group have less severe disease. People with a safe, piped water supply and effective disinfected waste disposal are at least risk regardless of host susceptibility.

PATHOGENESIS. After *V. cholerae* is ingested, vomiting and diarrhea may begin as early as 12 hours or not appear for more than a week. Illness occurs when viable organisms reach the duodenum and jejunum where alkaline pH, nutrients, and bile salts favor rapid multiplication. Actively motile vibrios penetrate mucous layers and attach to the brush border of the intestinal epithelium, where they secrete a potent exotoxin. This toxin is a protein of 84,000 daltons consisting of five B subunits that bind irreversibly to a specific chemical receptor on the cell surfaces (GM_1-ganglioside). The toxic moiety or A subunit is linked to the B aggregate and gains entry once binding has occurred. Adenosine diphosphate ribosylates the α-subunit of G protein, producing increased adenylate cyclase activity and consequent raised cyclic adenosine monophosphate levels in the enterocytes or any other affected cells. The most visible result in the small intestine is the profuse watery diarrhea resulting from abolition at the villous tips of the normal absorption of sodium ion and with it anions and water, and stimulation of crypt cells to secrete chloride, drawing with them cations and water from the blood stream into the gut lumen. The resulting solute-rich stream originating in the duodenum and jejunum is profuse, eliciting vomiting as it progresses cephalad and diarrhea as it flushes from small intestine through the colon. The fluid lost in cholera is a slightly fishy-smelling, non-fecal, whitish, mucous-flecked liquid ("rice water stool"). There is no cellular damage and no inflammation or loss of plasma proteins or formed elements of the blood into the gut lumen. There is also increased secretion of hepatic and pancreatic fluids, prostaglandins, and other intestinal hormones. All signs and symptoms of cholera derive from the fluid losses, which approach in composition an ultrafiltrate of plasma enriched in potassium and bicarbonate (Table 344–1). There is no evidence for systemic effects by cholera toxin itself, because *V. cholerae* does not invade the body, nor is the toxin absorbed. It exerts all its effects topically by adhering to the intestinal lining and producing toxin that is bound at cell surfaces. Cells at the intestinal surface other than epithelial cells are also affected by the toxin and may contribute to symptoms by release of cytokines and neural signals.

CLINICAL MANIFESTATIONS. Cholera can reduce a perfectly healthy, robust adult to shock and death in 4 to 6 hours. More usually, death ensues in 18 or more hours. In rare instances, "cholera sicca" shock and death occur before diarrhea appears, the voluminous secretions pooling in distended loops of bowel and not escaping as either diarrhea or vomiting. Despite the capacity of cholera to cause severe illness, many of the infected patients have only a mild diarrhea indistinguishable from that of ordinary gastroenteritis. In epidemics, many of those infected have either no symptoms or very mild illness.

Without fluid replacement, cholera patients have signs of severe volume depletion—sunken eyes, poor skin turgor, hoarse voice, extreme thirst, faint heart sounds, weak or absent peripheral pulses, and severe muscle cramps. Patients are oriented but appear apa-

Table 344–1 ■ **TYPICAL CHEMICAL VALUES IN STOOL AND PLASMA FROM PATIENTS WITH SEVERE CHOLERA**

	STOOL	PLASMA	
		Untreated	Treated†
Sodium*	138 (105)	141	142
Chloride*	102 (90)	107	106
Potassium*	18 (25)	4.5	3.6
Bicarbonate*	45 (30)	9	21
Arterial pH	—	7.21	7.43
Plasma specific gravity	—	1.040	1.026

*Milliequivalents per liter. Stool values in parentheses are for children younger than 10 years old.
†Four hours after water and electrolyte replacement.

thetic except for thirst. If patients survive and have not received adequate hydration, a "reactive" phase occurs with fever secondary to sepsis and pneumonia. Pulmonary edema can ensue with even modest fluid replacement due to prolonged severe acidosis.

In children, unconsciousness and/or convulsions may signal hypoglycemia. Initial laboratory values from depleted cholera patients (see Table 344–1) reflect the loss of isotonic fluid without larger molecules such as albumen. This results in increased concentrations of plasma proteins and blood cells. Loss of bicarbonate leads to acidosis with a low arterial pH and bicarbonate. Potassium depletion, which may be severe, is not reflected by low plasma values until acidosis has been corrected.

DIAGNOSIS. Cholera should be considered in any patient with acute watery diarrhea. Travel to or residence in a cholera-endemic area should raise the index of suspicion. In clusters of acute watery diarrhea, particularly where sanitation is poor, it is especially important to recognize cholera early to permit advance actions to prevent deaths of large numbers of people.

Treatment does not depend on an etiologic diagnosis. Fluid replacement should be started without delay as soon as any watery diarrhea begins. After initiating treatment, stool should be examined directly for red and white blood cells. Except in mixed infections with invasive organisms, which do occur in cholera outbreaks, fecal red and white cells are not a feature of cholera. If phase or dark-field microscopy is available, the characteristic darting motility of vibrios can be recognized in fresh wet preparations. To be certain that these motile bacteria are *V. cholerae,* serogroups 01 and 0139 antisera can be applied to wet preparations, immobilizing the organisms in a rapid and specific diagnostic test. For greater sensitivity of this test, a stool sample or rectal swab can be incubated in an enrichment medium for vibrios, such as alkaline peptone water, for 12 to 18 hours. Stool culture is best done on a selective medium, because colonies of *V. cholerae* may be overgrown or are easily missed on standard enteric media. A simple method uses thiosulfate citrate-bile salt-sucrose (TCBS) agar, which is very stable and selective for vibrios. Opaque flat yellow colonies form on TCBS agar in 18 hours at 37° C. Confirmation of serogroup and serotype can be done by direct slide agglutination with specific antisera that are available commercially, including against the new 0139 Bengal strain. Biotyping requires more elaborate procedures, but resistance to polymyxin B is a quick way to recognize the El Tor biotype. There is also a kit based on a monoclonal antibody against *V. Cholerae* 01 lipopolysaccharide called a SMART test availabe for rapid diagnosis.

Although the first line of immune defense is local at the intestinal epithelium, circulating antibodies occur to the specific O antigens. Testing for these is of use only as an epidemiologic tool to judge prevalence of disease in a specific population.

TREATMENT. Early and complete replacement of fluid loss averts death and all complications. Advanced oral hydration solutions based on rice or other starchy foods hydrate efficiently and reduce diarrhea and vomiting substantially (30 to 50%), as compared with intravenous treatment or glucose-based oral rehydration solutions. In all except the most severe cases, oral rehydration therapy is sufficient to treat cholera, especially if started as soon as diarrhea begins. All varieties of watery diarrhea lose fluid of similar composition, which varies with the rate of loss. Oral hydration therapy is the treatment of choice in all situations except when a patient is in shock or is comatose. Oral rehydration therapy should be used in hospitals, at home, or in the field, because it entails fewer risks, is much less expensive, does not require trained medical personnel for administration, and is effective. The discovery that absorption of sodium by co-transport pathways in intestinal mucosa is spared during cholera and other diarrheal diseases opened the way for safe, inexpensive, and effective oral replacement solutions. Glucose, amino acids, and small peptides, are absorbed by separate co-transport pathways of the intestine and carry with them sodium ions. Water and anions follow down the osmotic and electochemical gradients from the gut lumen to the blood stream. Originally, oral rehydration solutions were based only on glucose. These remain very effective but do not diminish diarrheal fluid losses. The composition of available oral rehydration solutions is listed in Table 344–2, together with some standard intravenous solutions.

Intravenous fluid replacement should be reserved for patients who have not received early oral replacement and are in shock and for those rapidly purging patients who exceed the capacity of oral replacement. In a cholera epidemic it is essential that all individuals at risk be thoroughly familiar with oral rehydration therapy and use it early to minimize deaths and the need for intravenous fluids. Thirst and urination are adequate guides to oral replacement therapy even in small children. This eliminates the need for accurate intake and output measurements and weighings, which even in excellent hospitals are difficult and are out of the question under epidemic conditions. Intravenous replacement for patients who are depleted and in shock should be given rapidly through a large-bore needle to ensure infusion rates of 50 to 100 mL/min until a strong radial pulse has been achieved. Remaining fluid deficits may then be replaced less rapidly over 2 hours. The fluid deficit in a severely depleted patient is about 10% of body weight (for a 50-kg patient—5 L). As soon as patients are strong enough to drink, oral rehydration therapy should begin, preferably with a rice- or other cereal-based solution of the proper solute composition. If this is done adequately, no further intravenous fluids are needed. In semicomatose patients who are unable to cooperate, nasogastric intubation permits adequate enteral replacement. For both intravenous and oral solutions the composition is crucial and should be within a range to properly replace losses of solutes and water (see Table 344–2). Many drinks ordinarily given to diarrhea patients are not adequate, although they may complement oral rehydration therapy. Vomiting is not a contraindication for oral rehydration therapy. However, fluids of high osmolarity should be avoided.

If a commercial preparation of oral rehydration salts is not available, a home solution can be prepared. The safest and most effective of these is a thick but drinkable suspension prepared from rice or other suitable ground starchy foods. If precooked products are available, these are very convenient but not essential. To a pint of water with cereal thickly suspended, a half-level teaspoon (one three-finger pinch of salt) is added and the mixture cooked only long enough to soften the ground cereal powder. The mixture should be used within 6 hours and may be taken warm or cold. This mixture lacks potassium, which can be made up with potassium-rich foods. If hydration is well maintained, the kidney will

Table 344–2 ■ CHOLERA AND ACUTE DIARRHEA TREATMENT SOLUTIONS (ORAL AND INTRAVENOUS)

	SUBSTRATE (g/L)	Na⁺	K⁺ (millimoles/L)	BASE*	Cl⁻	OSMOLALITY
Oral						
WHO/UNICEF	20 (glucose)	90	20	30	80	330
Pedialyte	25 (glucose)	45	20	30	65	300
Rice solution	80 (rice)	90	20	30	80	240
Infalyte	30 (rice digest)	50	25	34	45	200
Ceralyte†	40 (rice digest)	90	20	30	65	235
Intravenous						
Dhaka solution	0	134	13	48 (bicarbonate)	99	294
Ringer's‡	0	130	4	28 (lactate)	109	271

*Citrate is generally used but bicarbonate is equally effective, and lactate or acetate are used in intravenous solutions.
†Available as dried powder in packets.
‡Also contains calcium, 3.0 mEq per liter.

compensate for stool bicarbonate loss. In cholera it may be necessary to drink a great deal of fluid every hour The patient must be offered sips every few minutes to minimize overloading the stomach and consequent vomiting. This is labor intensive but does not require medical skills. Especially in epidemics, family members and friends are the backbone of a successful treatment program.

In treating either children or adults, fluid therapy should be guided by thirst, observations on the circulation, urine output, and presence of edema or rales at the lung bases. Feeding is important and should be initiated immediately. Breast feeding is especially useful in affected infants, although few breast-fed babies contract cholera except in non-endemic areas where maternal milk lacks protective antibodies. Feeding should be with appetizing foods rich in complex carbohydrates and proteins and culturally adapted to the taste of the patient.

Adjunctive antibiotic therapy may be indicated. This varies with the epidemic strain, but tetracyclines and macrolides have been effective when resistance is not present. However, resistance is common and must be monitored to avoid wasting high-cost antimicrobial agents that are ineffective. Antibiotic prophylaxis has not been useful and encourages the emergence of resistant strains.

PREVENTION. Safe water supplies and appropriate disposal of human waste prevent spread of cholera but may not be achievable under conditions of poverty. Rapid loss of large volumes require the use of special beds (cholera cots) or fecal conduits that avoid widespread dissemination into surrounding areas. *V. cholerae* is a fragile organism and cannot withstand drying, mild oxidation, or acid conditions. Thus a variety of disinfectants are effective for soiled articles. Bleaching powder is frequently used. Hand washing with soap before food handling is important. Patients suspected to have cholera should be reported to state health authorities by telephone or facsimile machine because of epidemic risks.

The available injected cholera vaccine is not useful, but there are effective killed bacterial and toxoid oral vaccines as well as very promising genetically altered live vaccines. At present, a single dose of live oral cholera vaccine strain CVD 103-HgR is licensed in many countries and is available in Europe under the trade name Orachol and in Canada as Mutachol. This is a vaccine that can be administered in a liquid formulation with Ty 21a oral typhoid vaccine and gives protection beginning in 8 days. The oral killed vaccine is available in Sweden and has been extensively field tested for safety and efficacy.

Barua D, Greenough WB III: Cholera. New York, Plenum Scientific Publishing Co., 1992. *A broad review of all aspects of cholera.*

Islam MS, Drason BS, Albert MS, et al: Toxigenic *Vibrio cholerae* in the environment: A minireview Trop Dis Bull 94:R1–R11, 1987.

Sanchez JL, Taylor DN: Cholera. Lancet 349:1825–1830, 1997. *An excellent summary of recent knowledge of microbiology, epidemiology, ecology, treatment, and prevention of cholera, including risk to travelers and in The Western hemisphere.*

Wachsmuth IK, Blake PA. Olsvik O: *Vibrio cholerae* and Cholera: Molecular and Global Perspectives. Washington. ASM Press, 1994. *Comprehensive, current review on new epidemic strains, epidemiology, and microbiology of cholera.*

Weber JT, Levine WC, Hopkins DP, Tauxe RV: Cholera in the United States 1965–1991: Risks at home and abroad. Arch Intern Med 184:55, 1994. *Summary of risks of cholera in the United States.*

Addressing emerging infectious disease threats: Preventive strategy for the U.S. MMWR 43:1, 1994. *Emphasizes risks of emerging infectious diseases, including* V. cholerae *0139 Bengal.*

345   ENTERIC *ESCHERICHIA COLI* INFECTIONS

Richard L. Guerrant

Escherichia coli is the predominant aerobic, coliform species in the normal colon. However, *E. coli* also can be an enteric pathogen and cause intestinal disease, usually diarrhea. Diarrhea caused by *E. coli* may be watery, inflammatory, or bloody, depending on which genetic codes for virulence traits the organism happens to possess. Consequently, diarrheogenic *E. coli* must be defined more specifically according to its virulence traits. Specific virulence traits determine the type of disease the organism causes, such as enterotoxi-

genic, enteroinvasive, enterohemorrhagic, enteropathogenic, or enteroadherent *E. coli* diarrhea. Each of these categories is being further resolved by the type of enterotoxin (such as the cholera-like, heat-labile toxin, LT, or the heat-stable toxin, ST) or adherence (such as localized and effacing, aggregative, or diffuse) it causes. Taken separately, organisms such as enterotoxigenic *E. coli* constitute major bacterial causes of diarrhea morbidity and mortality on a global scale, particularly among children in tropical, developing areas and in travelers. Taken together, the varied types of *E. coli* diarrhea not only constitute the major category of bacterial enteric pathogens but also illustrate the wide array of ways that enteric pathogens can cause disease.

As noted in Table 345–1, at least three different types of *E. coli* enterotoxins may cause intestinal secretion (ETEC), others are enteroinvasive (EIEC), still others cause foodborne hemorrhagic colitis (EHEC) and produce the Shiga-like toxin (EHEC), whereas the classically recognized enteropathogenic *E. coli* (EPEC) serotypes are neither enterotoxigenic nor invasive but attach and efface the epithelium. Still additional types of enteroadherent *E. coli* exhibit aggregating (EAggEC) or diffuse adherence (DAEC) traits and may be associated with prolonged diarrhea among children in tropical, developing areas and in patients with the acquired immunodeficiency syndrome (AIDS).

ETIOLOGY. *E. coli* is a small, catalase-positive, oxidase-negative, gram-negative bacillus in the family Enterobacteriaceae. It characteristically reduces nitrates, ferments glucose and usually lactose, and is either motile (with peritrichate flagella) or non-motile. It gives a positive methyl red reaction and negative reactions with Voges-Proskauer, urease, phenylalanine deaminase, and citrate agents. *E. coli* constitutes the predominant facultative gram-negative bacillus in the intestinal tract of humans and other mammals. As with other gram-negative organisms, the lipopolysaccharide cell wall contains lipid A and 2-keto-3-deoxyoctanate (KDO), a core glycolipid that has been used to develop vaccines that provide cross-protection against systemic infections with other gram-negative organisms. Smooth (S) forms of *E. coli* have O-specific carbohydrate chains attached to this core glycolipid to provide 169 O serogroups as well as at least 60 heat-labile protein flagellar (H) antigens by which strains are currently serotyped. Historically, some 80 variably heat-labile capsular (K) antigens also have been described (L, B, and A), not to mention the more recently appreciated numerous adherence, enterotoxin, cytotoxin, and invasiveness factors that may be gained or lost by a particular serotype, because they are characteristically encoded on transmissible genetic elements such as plasmids or bacteriophages. Consequently, this common inhabitant of the normal human intestinal tract becomes a pathogen when it houses one or more specific traits contributing to its colonization and virulence in the intestinal tract. Other traits such as O and H serogroup also may be important for certain enteropathogenic and enteroinvasive organisms. For reasons that remain obscure, only a few O serogroups tend to predominate in the normal human colon (O groups 1, 2, 4, 6, 7, 8, 18, 25, 45, 75, and 81) whereas others noted in Table 345–1 tend (albeit not absolutely) to be associated with specific virulence traits and thus different types of pathogenesis in the intestine. The O antigens of invasive *E. coli* often cross-react with various *Shigella* species, suggesting further that, in addition to the 140-Md plasmid, serotype also has a role in pathogenesis.

EPIDEMIOLOGY. Enteric *E. coli* infections are essentially acquired by the fecal-oral route, reflecting primarily a human reservoir for most recognized types of *E. coli* enteropathogens. Enterotoxigenic *E. coli* is also an important veterinary pathogen, especially in calves and piglets. However, the attachment traits of animal strains are different from those that infect humans and likely substantially influence their epidemiology.

The infectious doses of enterotoxigenic, enteroinvasive and enteroaggregative *E. coli* have been determined in volunteers to be 10^6 to 10^{10}, numbers that usually require multiplication in contaminated food or water vehicles for their transmission. Heavy contamination with enterotoxigenic *E. coli* has been documented in foods prepared in homes, restaurants, and at street vendors as well as in drinking water in many tropical areas, and contaminated water and foods likely represent the major sources of their acquisition, primarily in the warm or wet season. In the United States, major

Table 345–1 ■ DIFFERENT TYPES OF ENTERIC *E. COLI* INFECTIONS

TYPE	MECHANISM	PREDOMINANT O SEROGROUPS	GENETIC CODE	DETECTION	CLINICAL SYNDROMES
Enterotoxigenic E. coli (ETEC)					
1. Cholera-like, heat-labile toxin (LT)	Activates intestinal adenylate cyclase	6, 8, 11, 15, 20, 25, 27, 63, 80, 85, 139	Plasmid	ELISA, RIA, PIH, CHO, Y1 cells, 18-h loops, gene probe	Watery diarrhea, travelers' diarrhea
2. Heat-stable toxin (STa: STh or STp)	Activates intestinal guanylate cyclase	12, 78, 115, 148, 149, 153, 155, 166, 167	Plasmid (transposon)	ELISA, RIA, suckling mice, 6-h loops, gene probes	Watery diarrhea, travelers' diarrhea
3. Heat-stable toxin (STb)	?; Not cyclic adenosine or guanosine monophosphate		Plasmid	Piglet loops, gene probe	?
Enteroinvasive E. coli					
4. Enteroinvasive E. coli	Cell invasion and spread	11, 28ac, 29, 124, 136, 144, 147, 152, 164, 167	Plasmid (140 Md, pWR110)	Sereny test, gene probe, (lys⁻, NM, oft, lactose⁻)	Inflammatory dysentery
Enterohemorrhagic E. coli					
5. Enterohemorrhagic (EHEC)	Shiga-like toxin(s) (SLT) and adhesin fimbriae	26, 39, 113, 121, 128, 139, 145, 157, occ 55, 111	Phage(s) & adhesin plasmid(s)	ELISA for SLT, serotype, HeLa, Vero cells, sorbitol, agar, SLT or eae gene probes	Bloody non-inflammatory diarrhea; hemolytic-uremic syndrome
Enteropathogenic E. coli					
6. Focal attaching and effacing (EPEC)	Attach, then efface the mucosa	55, 111, 119, 125, 126, 127, 128, 142, 158,	Plasmid (60 Md, pMAR2) + chromosomal (*esp, eae, and tir*)	Serotype, focal HEp2 adhesion, gene probes for EAF or eae	Infantile diarrhea
Enteroadherent E. coli					
7. Enteroaggregating E. coli (EAggEC)	Colonize ? toxins (EAST, EALT)	3, 15, 44, 51, 77, 78, 91	Plasmid	HEp2 cell adherence; AA probe	Persistent diarrhea
8. Diffusely adherent E. coli (DAEC)	Colonize (F 1845 fimbriate adhesin)	75 (F 1845), 15 (57-1), ? (189)	Chromosomal/plasmid	HEp2 cell adherence; DA gene probe	Persistent diarrhea in children > 18 mo old

outbreaks of water- or food-borne *E. coli* diarrhea of different types have been documented in the past 10 to 15 years. A large waterborne outbreak of diarrhea at a popular national park was found to be caused by enterotoxigenic *E. coli* (ETEC), and a widespread outbreak of enteroinvasive *E. coli* (EIEC) enteritis was traced to consumption of French Camembert cheese. More recently, bloody, non-inflammatory diarrhea has been increasingly associated with enterohemorrhagic *E. coli* (EHEC) (0157 and others) from eating hamburgers from large distributors or several fast-food chains, or from ingestion of contaminated unpasteurized apple juice or seed sprouts such as raddish or alfalfa sprouts. EHEC infections are especially alarming because they are increasing in frequency and may cause hemolytic-uremic syndrome, which can be fatal despite antimicrobial therapy. Occasional nosocomial outbreaks of enterotoxigenic *E. coli* and enteropathogenic *E. coli* serotypes (EPEC) also have occurred in hospitalized infants in the United States and other industrialized countries.

As with most diarrheal illnesses, the highest age-specific attack rates of enterotoxigenic *E. coli* infections are in young children, especially at the time of weaning, when enterotoxigenic *E. coli* account for 15 to 50% of illnesses. Like immunologically inexperienced young children, the traveler visiting tropical areas has a 30 to 50% chance of acquiring travelers' diarrhea over a 2- to 3-week stay unless untreated water or ice and uncooked foods such as salads are strictly avoided. The most commonly recognized pathogen associated with travelers' diarrhea around most tropical areas of the world is enterotoxigenic *E. coli* that produces either the STa, LT, or both enterotoxins (see Chapter 346).

Of potential immunologic significance is the continued occurrence of symptomatic infections with *E. coli* that produce the less immunogenic STa in adult residents of tropical or other areas endemic for enterotoxigenic *E. coli* infections. In contrast, adult residents in endemic areas often carry LT-producing *E. coli* asymptomatically, suggesting that they may be protected from symptoms, if not from colonization.

Limited data on invasive *E. coli* suggest that the infectious doses are relatively high. As with enterotoxigenic *E. coli* infections, such

large numbers have been readily spread in food with high attack rates. Enteropathogenic *E. coli* have been recognized primarily in urban areas, especially among hospitalized infants in their first year of life, with apparent cross-infection in hospital nurseries. Although sporadic cases still occur, nosocomial outbreaks of EPEC diarrhea during the summer appear to have become less common and less severe in industrialized countries in the last few decades. Enteroaggregative *E. coli* increasingly appear to be important causes of persistent diarrhea and malnutrition, especially in children in tropical areas and in patients with AIDS.

PATHOGENESIS AND PATHOLOGY. The pathogenesis of enteric *E. coli* infections begins with the ingestion of the organism in contaminated food or water, which then faces the normal gastric acid barrier. Both enterotoxigenic *E. coli* and enteroinvasive *E. coli* appear to be sensitive to gastric acid; neutralization by gastric acid reduces the infectious dose by 100- to 1000-fold. This is followed by an incubation period of 2 to 7 days, during which colonization of the involved part of the intestinal tract and toxin production, invasion or other disruption of cell function take place. Best characterized is the colonization by enterotoxigenic *E. coli* in the upper small bowel, which involves one of at least five major colonization factor antigen groups (which are fimbriate or fibrillar protein structures on the surface of the organism). The colonization fimbriae bind the organism to cell surface receptors in the upper small bowel where the enterotoxin is delivered to reduce normal absorption and cause net electrolyte and water secretion. The heat-labile toxin (LT) with a molecular weight of about 86,000 has a binding and active subunit that, like choleratoxin, binds to a monosialoganglioside (Gm1) receptor. Also like choleratoxin, the active subunit adenosine diphosphate ribosylates the regulatory subunit of adenylate cyclase to activate adenylate cyclase. The consequently increased chloride secretion and reduced sodium absorption combine to cause net isotonic electrolyte loss that must be replaced to prevent severe dehydration and hypotension and its potential consequences. Other strains produce the heat-stable toxin (STa), a much smaller molecule of 18 to 19 amino acids (molecular weight less than 2000), which activates intestinal particulate guanylate cyclase.

Like cyclic adenosine monophosphate, the cyclic guanosine monophosphate thus formed also causes net secretion. A third type of *E. coli* enterotoxin (STb) causes secretion in porcine intestine without activating adenylate or guanylate cyclase; STb has no known role in human disease. Similarly, the roles of enterotoxins such as LTII, EAST, EIET, and others seen in ETEC, EAggEC, and EIEC, respectively, are unclear at present. Both the colonization traits and enterotoxin production are encoded on transmissible plasmids. Besides the complications of dehydration, the only significant pathologic change is depletion of mucus from intestinal goblet cells.

Other *E. coli*, often of certain serogroups noted in Table 345–1, have the capacity, analogous to *Shigella*, to invade and multiply in epithelial cells, cause conjunctivitis in guinea pigs (Sereny test), and cause inflammatory colitis and dysenteric or bloody diarrhea. As seen with shigellosis, a striking inflammatory response is seen, with sheets of polymorphonuclear leukocytes in the stool. The colon shows patchy, acute inflammation in the mucosa and submucosa with focal denuding of the surface epithelium but usually without deeper invasion or systemic spread. While epithelial cell invasiveness in both enteroinvasive *E. coli* and *Shigella* appears to be encoded on a large 120- to 140-Md plasmid, several chromosomal determinants, including the O antigen, are crucial for full invasive virulence.

Classically recognized enteropathogenic *E. coli* serotypes often fail to produce known enterotoxins or to be invasive. Nevertheless, they are well-established causes of infantile diarrhea and exhibit a remarkable array of chromosomal and plasmid-encoded traits that orchestrate their initial attachment and subsequent effacement of the brush border epithelium. The majority of classically recognized EPEC serotypes such as O55 and O111 exhibit both plasmid-encoded localized adherence to epithelial cells and chromosomally mediated attachment and effacement of the microvilli. There is also villus atrophy, mucosal thinning, inflammation in the lamina propria, and variable crypt cell hyperplasia. These morphologic changes are associated with a reduction in the mucosal brush border enzymes and may contribute to the impaired absorptive function and diarrhea.

Enterohemorrhagic *E. coli,* most notably serotype 0157:H7 but also serogroups 026, 39, and others, are associated with foodborne outbreaks of bloody, non-inflammatory diarrhea and with the hemolytic-uremic syndrome. These organisms produce Shiga-like toxins that may be responsible for the characteristic colonic mucosal and hemorrhage, as well as the complication of hemolytic-uremic syndrome. Sigmoidoscopy usually reveals only moderately hyperemic mucosa, and barium enema may reveal a thumbprint pattern of submucosal edema in the ascending and transverse colon. Some patients have superficial ulceration with mild neutrophil infiltration in the edematous submucosa. The mechanisms by which EAggEC (which adhere in an aggregative pattern to the mucosa and produce heat-stable and heat-labile "toxins"), DAEC, or colonization alone may cause diarrhea remain unclear at present.

CLINICAL MANIFESTATIONS. The most common clinical manifestation of enteric *E. coli* infections is the watery diarrhea that characterizes enterotoxigenic *E. coli* infections, particularly in young children and travelers to tropical or developing areas. This may range from mild to severe, cholera-like diarrhea that may be life threatening, especially in small children and elderly patients, who are particularly prone to suffer the most severe consequences of dehydration, undernutrition, and electrolyte imbalance (especially hypokalemia and acidosis).

The incubation period (2 to 7 days) varies with the size of the inoculum. Characteristic symptoms include malaise, abdominal cramping, anorexia, and watery diarrhea, occasionally associated with nausea, vomiting, or low-grade fever. The illness is usually self-limited to 1 to 5 days and rarely extends beyond 10 days or 2 weeks. Infections with *E. coli* that produce both ST and LT or ST alone may be more severe than those with only LT-producing *E. coli*. The persistence of impaired mucosal absorptive capacity for 1 to 3 weeks may further compound the cycle of malnutrition that complicates diarrheal illnesses in children in developing, tropical areas.

Infection with EIEC is characterized by inflammatory colitis, often with abdominal pain, high fever, tenesmus, and bloody or dysenteric diarrhea essentially like that seen with *Shigella*, to which this organism is closely related. The incubation period is usually 1 to 3 days with the duration usually self-limited to 7 to 10 days.

Outbreaks of EPEC infections in newborn nurseries have ranged from mild transient diarrhea to severe and rapidly fatal diarrheal illnesses, especially in premature or otherwise compromised infants. The more severe illnesses appear to have been more common in industrialized countries before 1950. However, more recent outbreaks and sporadic cases are well documented.

Hemorrhagic colitis associated with the Shiga-like toxin producing *E. coli* (EHEC) 0157:H7, 026:H11, and others is characterized by grossly bloody diarrhea often with remarkably little fever or inflammatory exudate in the stool. Although the diarrheal illnesses have been self-limited, a significant number of children and adults have subsequently developed a potentially fatal hemolytic-uremic syndrome or thrombotic thrombocytopenic purpura. Outbreaks of hemorrhagic colitis due to EHEC in nursing homes or other institutions may be quite severe and more common than previously appreciated. The incubation period in two outbreaks has been 3 to 4 days (range, 1 to 7 days), and the illness is characteristically self-limited to 5 to 12 days (mean 7.8).

Enteroaggregative *E. coli* have been associated with persistent diarrhea and malnutrition in children in developing area and in patients with AIDS. Diffusely adherent *E. coli* have also been associated with diarrhea in children older than 18 months of age.

DIAGNOSIS. With the exception of enterohemorrhagic *E. coli* (EHEC), which should be sought by enzyme-linked immunosorbent assay (ELISA), or other testing for the Shiga-like toxin (SLT) and for sorbitol-negative EHEC 0157:H7 in all patients with bloody diarrhea, definitive etiologic diagnosis of *E. coli* diarrhea requires the documentation of a specific virulence trait, such as enterotoxin, invasiveness, enteroadherence, or serotype, which requires specialized immunologic, tissue culture, animal bioassay, or gene probes that are usually available only in research and reference laboratories. Except for EHEC, such tests are rarely cost effective or clinically indicated, except in outbreak or research situations. Fortunately, a likely diagnosis often can be suspected by the clinical and epidemiologic setting. For example, self-limited, non-inflammatory diarrhea in tropical, developing areas is most likely due to enterotoxigenic *E. coli*, rotaviruses (young children), or Norwalk-like viruses (older children and adults). Non-inflammatory diarrhea in winter months in temperate areas in older children or younger adults is more likely to be due to Norwalk-like viruses. Specific tests for the respective virulence traits of different types of *E. coli* are noted in Table 345–1. One should also consider *Vibrio* infections in areas endemic for cholera or in any coastal area where inadequately cooked seafood may be eaten. If non-inflammatory diarrhea persists, especially with weight loss, one also should consider *Giardia lamblia* or *Cryptosporidium* infection. In outbreaks of food poisoning, *S. aureus, Clostridium perfringens,* and *Bacillus cereus* should be considered.

Inflammatory colitis with high fever, tenesmus, and leukocytes, mucus, and blood in the stool may well be due to enteroinvasive *E. coli* but should prompt a stool culture for more common invasive pathogens such as *Campylobacter jejuni, Shigella,* and *Salmonella* or even *Clostridium difficile, Yersinia enterocolitica,* or non-cholera *Vibrio* (see Chapter 343). On the other hand, bloody diarrhea without high fever and few, if any, fecal leukocytes (or minimal or no fecal lactoferrin elevations) should prompt consideration of the Shiga-like toxin producing enterohemorrhagic *E. coli* (EHEC) such as strain O157:H7. This organism is often suspected as a sorbitol-negative *E. coli,* which may require further study for serotype or Shiga-like toxin production.

THERAPY. As with all diarrheal illnesses, the primary treatment is replacement and maintenance of water and electrolytes. Losses of water and electrolytes may be particularly severe and even life threatening with enterotoxigenic *E. coli* and can usually be replaced with a simple oral rehydration solution that uses the intact, sodium-coupled glucose, and/or amino acid absorption to replace fluid losses, as described in Chapter 344. This oral rehydration solution should be given ad libitum with free water and, in breast-fed infants, continued breast feeding and early refeeding should be done to compensate for the nutritional losses.

Because most *E. coli* diarrhea is self-limited, the role of antimicrobial agents is debated and remains of secondary importance to rehydration. In areas where the enterotoxigenic *E. coli* remains sensitive, early initiation of sulfamethoxazole/trimthoprim, tetracycline, or a quinolone antibiotic may reduce a 3- to 5-day illness to a 1- to 2-day illness if the agent is started with the first loose stool in travelers to endemic, tropical areas (see Chapter 346). The use of antimotility agents should be tempered by the potential added risk of worsening or prolonging inflammatory diarrheas and by their lack of effectiveness in reducing fluid loss even though abdominal cramping and overt diarrhea may be temporarily reduced. Because of the potential severity of the disease in infants, some pediatricians use neomycin, 100 mg/kg/day orally, divided into three or four daily doses for 5 days, for documented enteropathogenic *E. coli* infections in neonates. Bismuth subsalicylate may reduce symptoms in travelers' diarrhea but should be used with caution to avoid toxic doses of salicylate. A number of pharmacologic agents enhance absorption or reduce secretion with experimental diarrhea but remain inadequately studied or too toxic for recommended use to date.

The role of antimicrobial agents in treating EHEC infections or in preventing serious complications remains controversial. The treatment of hemolytic-uremic syndrome requires careful supportive care and may require plasma exchange as well.

PROGNOSIS. The overall prognosis in *E. coli* diarrheas of the various types noted, if fully and adequately treated, is generally excellent. However, the impact of *E. coli* and other common diarrheas on mortality and morbidity (particularly with repeated infections compounding malnutrition in young children) remains one of the major health problems on a global scale; this problem may actually be worsening in some transitional areas. The potentially serious complication of hemolytic-uremic syndrome may follow EHEC infection.

PREVENTION. The prevention of many *E. coli* enteric infections is ultimately related to basic economic development and adequate sanitary facilities and wide availability of sufficient quality and quantity of water. In the interim, especially in areas where adequate water supplies and sanitary facilities are not available, such measures as breast feeding for at least 6 to 12 months and hygienic measures like hand washing should reduce the likelihood of acquiring *E. coli* enteric infections. Travelers to developing or tropical areas should avoid drinking untreated or unboiled water or ice and should avoid eating uncooked fruits or vegetables that may have been "freshened" with highly contaminated water. Although a number of antimicrobial agents have been documented to be effective over short periods of time when taken prophylactically, their effectiveness is sharply limited by the rapidly emerging resistance to antimicrobial drugs as well as by the potential side effects of their indiscriminate, widespread use. For example, tetracycline resistance among enterotoxigenic *E. coli* is common, and combined sulfamethoxazole/trimethoprim resistance is rapidly emerging around the world. Finally, currently developing toxoid or colonization factor vaccines hold considerable promise for the prevention of enterotoxigenic *E. coli* diarrhea. EHEC infections can be largely prevented by adequately cooking beef, especially hamburgers, and by careful hand washing and other hygienic measures in day-care centers and nursing homes.

Bhan MK, Raj P, Levine MM, et al: Enteroaggregative *Escherichia coli* associated with persistent diarrhea in a cohort of rural children in India. J Infect Dis 159:1060, 1989. *A first report of a clinical role for new types of enteroadherent* E. coli.

Carter AO, Borczyk AA, Carlson AK, et al: A severe outbreak of *E. coli* O157:H7 associated hemorrhagic colitis in a nursing home. N Engl J Med 317:1496, 1987. *A a common source outbreak with secondary probable person-to-person spread of this cause of bloody diarrhea and hemolytic-uremic syndrome in the institutionalized elderly.*

Griffin PM: *Escherichia coli* O157-H7 and other enterohemorrhagic *E. coli. In* Blaser MJ, Smith PA, Raudin JI, et al (eds): Infection of the Gastrointestinal Tract. New York, Raven Press, 1995, pp 739–761. *Excellent review of the increasing problem of enterohemorrhagic* E. coli *infections and complications, often associated with rare hamburger and other foods and also seen in day-care centers and institutions.*

Guerrant RL, Kirchhoff LV, Shields DS, et al: Prospective study of diarrheal illnesses in northeastern Brazil: Patterns of disease, nutritional impact, etiologies and risk factors. J Infect Dis 148:986, 1983. *A detailed study of endemic diarrhea in a tropical area, including seasonality, risk after weaning, and nutritional impact, as well as relationship of enterotoxigenic* E. coli *to other pathogens.*

Guerrant RL, Steiner TS, Lima AAM, Bobac DA: How intestinal bacteria cause disease. J Infect Dis 179:S331–S337, 1999. *Overview of ways that intestinal bacteria disrupt mucosal function using the different types of* E. coli *as the paradigm.*

Guerrant RL, Thielman NM: Types of Escherichia coli enteropathogens. *In* Blaser MJ, Smith PD, Ravdin JI, et al (eds): Infection of The Gastrointestinal Tract. New York, Raven Press, 1995, pp 687–690. *Concise overview of 6 to 10 types of* E. coli *pathogenesis with update on new clinical and pathogenic studies of different types of* E. coli *pathogens.*

Levine MM: *Escherichia coli* that cause diarrhea: Enterotoxigenic, enteropathogenic,

enterohemorrhagic, and enteroadherent. J Infect Dis 155:377, 1989. *A good overview of major pathogenic mechanisms of* E. coli *diarrhea.*

Nataro JP Kaper JB: Diarrheagenic *Escherichia coli.* Clin Microbiol Rev 11:142–201, 1998. *Excellent overview of recent advances regarding the pathogenesis of diarrheagenic* E. coli *infections.*

NIH Consensus Development Conference on Traveler's Diarrhea. JAMA 253:2700, 1985. *A balanced critical appraisal of the epidemiology, etiologies, presentation, and treatment of travelers' diarrhea.*

Steiner TS, Lima AAM, Nataro JP, Guerrant RL: Enteroaggregative *Escherichia coli* produce intestinal inflammation and growth impairment and cause interleukin-8 release from intestinal epithelial cells. J Infect Dis 177:88–96, 1998. *First report of emerging enteroaggregative* E. coli *causing inflammation and malnutrition as well as diarrhea in children in the tropics.*

346 THE DIARRHEA OF TRAVELERS

R. Bradley Sack

Travelers from the developed world who visit the developing world are highly susceptible to an acute infectious diarrheal illness known as "travelers' diarrhea," or by more colorful names that fit the locale in which the travelers find themselves incapacitated. The primary etiologic agents of this syndrome are the same as those that cause endemic diarrheal illness, primarily in children, throughout the areas of the world in which sanitation is less than optimal. Travelers (see Chapter 316) from sanitized, developed countries are, in a sense, immunologically naive "children" who are suddenly transported to an endemic area of infection, where they are highly susceptible to the local pathogens. Other than during a common-source outbreak of diarrheal disease (e.g., a gross fecal contamination of a water supply), the attack rates among travelers are the highest known in any identifiable population. Twenty-five to 50 per cent of travelers will experience a diarrheal illness during their first 3 weeks of stay in a developing country; this will decrease markedly thereafter as immunity develops.

By way of contrast, travelers from developing countries who visit other developing countries usually have a considerably lower attack rate, owing to their prior exposure and subsequent immunity to these organisms. As expected, these same visitors who visit the developed world do not develop the illness.

ETIOLOGY. Multiple studies have described the causes of this syndrome throughout the world, and it is clear that enterotoxigenic *Escherichia coli* is the most common pathogen. Other bacteria, viruses, and protozoa are also involved, but with lesser frequency (Table 346–1). In certain localities and in certain seasons, the prevalence of *Campylobacter* or *Salmonella* may be particularly high. Even now, a considerable proportion of episodes (20 to 30%) cannot be diagnosed microbiologically, and new etiologic organisms continue to be discovered. Contrary to "popular" notions, relatively few cases of travelers' diarrhea are caused by *Entamoeba histolytica* or *Giardia lamblia.*

PATHOGENESIS AND CLINICAL PICTURE. The clinical syndrome of travelers' diarrhea is typically that of a non-febrile, secretory, watery diarrhea that is produced by the enterotoxins of bacte-

Table 346–1 ■ ETIOLOGIC AGENTS OF TRAVELERS' DIARRHEA

AGENT	PERCENTAGE
Enterotoxigenic *Escherichia coli*	30–70
Shigella	5–10
*Salmonella**	<5
*Campylobacter**	<5
Enteroaggregative *E. coli*	5–10
Rotavirus	<5
Giardia lamblia	<5
Entamoeba histolytica	<3
Cryptosporidium	<5
Cyclospora*	<1
Others†	<1
Unknown agents	20–30

*May be higher in certain geographic areas.
†Includes Shiga toxin–producing *E. coli*, *Vibrio cholerae*, non-cholera vibrios, other viruses.

ria, particularly *E. coli* (see Chapter 345). The watery diarrhea usually lasts 2 to 4 days and, when most severe, may result in 15 to 20 evacuations per day, with significant water and electrolyte loss, leading to clinical signs of dehydration. The vast majority of illnesses are much milder, however, consisting of only three to five diarrheal stools per day, and are important primarily because they limit the activities of the traveler. Episodes due to invasive bacteria, such as *Shigella* or *Campylobacter*, may be dysentery-like, with abdominal pain, fever, and blood in the stool (see Chapter 342).

Nearly all episodes are self-limited, but a few (<3%) may become persistent and require evaluation after the return home. Some of these prolonged episodes may be due to infection with *E. histolytica, Giardia lamblia,* or *Cyclospora,* an intracellular coccidian most recently found in the developing world.

TRANSMISSION. Transmission of the enteric pathogens occurs almost exclusively through fecally contaminated food and water. Of highest risk to the traveler are foods that are not cooked or peeled, foods obtained from roadside vendors, or foods kept unrefrigerated for long periods of time.

PREVENTION. Because the modes of transmission are known, prudent attention to the ingestion of uncontaminated food and water should entirely prevent the disease. This has been shown in the military or on board cruise ships, where all food is hygienically prepared and packaged. For the usual traveler, however, food must be obtained from local sources and contamination cannot be entirely prevented. Even the "best" hotels in the developing world may have unsanitary kitchens, and "first class" travelers are therefore not exempt.

Many studies have now shown that a number of drugs can prevent 80 to 90% of diarrheal episodes when taken regularly during short-term travel (<3 weeks). Medication is begun on the day before reaching the locale and discontinued on the day after leaving. The antimicrobial agents that have been well studied are shown in Table 346–2. Doxycycline, which was the earliest antimicrobial agent shown to be effective, is no longer recommended because of a marked increase in antibiotic resistance of enterotoxigenic *E. coli*. Because the antibacterial spectrum of the fluoroquinolones includes *Campylobacter*, these drugs provide the broadest spectrum of antibacterial coverage against the disease. A non-antimicrobial drug, bismuth subsalicylate (BSS), taken four times a day, also has given a significant but lesser degree (approximately 60%) of protection. Other antimicrobial agents also have been used successfully (i.e., erythromycin, mecillinam, trimethoprim) but have not been tested as extensively.

Drugs that have been tested and found to be of little or no benefit include neomycin, streptotriad, hydroxyquinolines, and *Lactobacillus* preparations.

TREATMENT. Treatment is best carried out by the patient, who must be able to recognize when to take the medication. Instructions for therapy should be given by the traveler's physician, who must be familiar with the disease. One aim of self-treatment is to avoid consultation by the traveler with local practitioners who may provide less than adequate advice and medications. Treatment includes specific fluid replacement when indicated, specific antimicrobial therapy directed against the most likely causative agents, and, if necessary, symptomatic therapy directed at relieving the frequency of stooling and abdominal cramps.

Fluids may be replaced by increasing the amount of liquids ingested, such as soup and fruit juices, if the diarrhea is mild. For more severe diarrhea, an oral glucose (or rice-based) electrolyte solution, which has been developed to treat all dehydrating diar-

rheas regardless of etiologic agent or age of the patient, should be taken. This solution is available commercially in packets; the traveler can carry and use them as required by mixing the contents with appropriate volumes of potable water.

In many controlled studies, a short course (1 to 3 days) of appropriate antimicrobial agents has been shown to significantly shorten the disease to 12 to 24 hours. The most widely used drugs (see Table 346–2) are also the ones that have been shown to be effective in prevention. In addition, some of the newer fluoroquinolones (e.g., ofloxacin, fleroxacin) and aztreonam have been shown to be equally effective.

Symptomatic therapy with antimotility agents, such as loperamide, may be useful for travelers who need to participate in certain vital events during which the need to evacuate frequently would be embarrassing and particularly inconvenient, such as during long bus rides or while giving lectures. The combination of loperamide with an effective antimicrobial agent has been shown to resolve the illness more quickly than would the antimicrobial agent alone.

BSS also has been shown to give significant but less striking symptomatic improvement, although the exact mechanism of action is unknown. Kaolin-pectin preparations are of no significant effect in treatment.

When to give antimicrobial agents prophylactically and when to rely on early patient-initiated treatment is subject to differing opinions. The decisions should be based on the following considerations. It is known that all persons who travel to developing countries, regardless of whether they are taking antimicrobial agents, have an alteration in their microbial gut flora, which includes acquiring antibiotic-resistant bacteria. Antimicriobial agents are widely available without prescription in most developing countries and are used widely; therefore, the contribution of tourists taking antibiotics to the local microbial ecology is probably negligible. The real concern of giving antimicrobial agents prophylactically is side effects. Although adverse effects are known to be infrequent, some travelers will experience them. Contraindications include known allergies, pregnancy, and age. Therefore, the following suggestions are made when considering prophylaxis: Travelers should be on short-term visits (<3 weeks), they should request the use of antimicrobial agents, and they should be able to understand and accept the risk of possible side effects. Certain travelers with medical illnesses, for whom an episode of diarrhea would be particularly deleterious, also may be given special consideration for prophylaxis. The more widely recommended strategy is to have the traveler carry the medicines and self-administer them on recognition of the onset of illness.

The problem of travelers' diarrhea will continue until the general sanitation of the developing world approaches that of industrialized countries or until effective vaccines against the major diarrheal pathogens become available. (Vaccines against both enterotoxigenic *E. coli* and *Shigella* are being field-tested.) However, this common syndrome will need to be addressed for some time. Fortunately, this can now be done rationally and effectively based on our knowledge of causes and modes of transmission.

DuPont HL, Ericsson CD: Prevention and treatment of travelers' diarrhea. N Engl J Med 328:1821, 1993. *A review of the problem with an extensive discussion of management options.*

Traveler's diarrhea: Recent advances. Chemotherapy 41 (Suppl 1):1–82, 1995. *A review of all aspects of the problem of traveler's diarrhea, including a list of all trials of prophylaxis and treatment of traveler's diarrhea.*

Table 346–2 ■ PREVENTION AND TREATMENT OF TRAVELERS' DIARRHEA WITH ANTIMICROBIAL AGENTS

	PREVENTION*	TREATMENT†	
ANTIMICROBIAL	Daily Dose (mg)	Dose (mg)	Duration‡ (days)
Norfloxacin	400	400 bid	3
Ciprofloxacin	500	500 bid	3
Trimethoprim/sulfamethoxazole	160/800	160–800 bid	3

*For periods up to 3 weeks.
†Loperamide given along with antimicrobial agents has given further improvement.
‡Some studies have shown larger doses given as only a single dose to be effective.

347 EXTRAINTESTINAL INFECTIONS CAUSED BY ENTERIC BACTERIA

Elizabeth J. Ziegler

Bacteria constitute over half the dry weight of stool. *Bacteroides* species far outnumber other genera, at 10^{12} organisms per gram. Other anaerobes such as fusobacteria, clostridia, and peptostreptococci also are abundant. Among the facultative bacteria, members of the family Enterobacteriaceae predominate, at about 10^9 organisms per gram. Pseudomonads, enterococci, other non-hemolytic streptococci, and yeasts are present as well.

These bacteria that normally inhabit the human gastrointestinal tract perform important functions beneficial to the host. *Bacteroides fragilis,* clostridia, and enterococci deconjugate bile acids for participation in fat metabolism. Some intestinal bacteria synthesize menaquinone, or vitamin K, a cofactor for blood coagulation. Normal gut flora discourage colonization of the bowel with primary pathogens and overgrowth of bacteria usually present in small numbers. Colonization resistance is not understood completely, but it must involve bacteriocins, regulation of local oxidation-reduction potential, competition for receptors, and balance of nutrients as well as unknown factors. Breakdown of colonization resistance is illustrated by the increase in susceptibility of antibiotic-treated animals to *Salmonella* and by the emergence of fecal *Pseudomonas aeruginosa* and *Candida* in patients receiving antimicrobial agents.

PATHOGENESIS OF INFECTIONS

Enteric bacteria are not primary pathogens but cause disease when they escape from their usual gastrointestinal habitat. Direct penetration of the bowel wall by surgical, traumatic, or spontaneous rupture spills fecal contents into the peritoneal cavity and into open wounds. Gut bacteria on the perineal skin gain access to the urinary tract and proliferate there, especially when the flushing action of urine flow is disrupted by mechanical obstruction or neurologic dysfunction. When the biliary tract is obstructed by gallstones or tumor, the upper small bowel, which normally is sterile, becomes colonized with facultative bacteria (*Escherichia coli,* klebsiella, enterococci) or, less often, with bacteroides and clostridia, which then infect the gallbladder and bile ducts. Intestinal flora can be introduced into the respiratory tract from contaminated skin or the environment; they proliferate there under the influence of antibiotics and in the presence of underlying pulmonary disease and tracheal instrumentation. Penetrating foreign bodies, such as intravenous catheters and intraventricular cerebral pressure monitors, become colonized by gut flora on the skin and in respiratory secretions and then induce infection in adjacent tissues. In burns, destruction of the skin barrier, the rich culture medium of oozing tissue fluid, and a shift of surface flora by application of local and systemic antibacterial agents result in local necrotizing infection of the burn wound with gut flora and frequent secondary gram-negative bacteremia.

In the absence of mechanical and surface abnormalities, such as those outlined earlier, systemic resistance to enteric bacteria is very strong. The mainstay of this resistance is the polymorphonuclear neutrophil, destruction or malfunction of which leads almost inevitably to blood stream invasion by bowel bacteria. Serum complement must be protective against invasion of some organisms, because very few gram-negative bacilli isolated from blood are sensitive to complement-mediated bacteriolysis, whereas many enteric rods in feces are susceptible. Microbial factors are important, too. Although anaerobes predominate over facultative bacteria and aerobes in the gut, these anaerobes rarely cause bacteremia or metastatic infection even in neutropenia. The presence of certain bacterial polysaccharide capsules (e.g., *E. coli* K1) or production of large amounts of capsule (e.g., by *Klebsiella pneumoniae* in hyperglycemic or glycosuric diabetics) predisposes to systemic invasion by these organisms.

Infections with enteric bacteria have increased dramatically during the past four decades. The reasons should be apparent from the foregoing discussion. Advances in surgical and intensive care, trauma and burn management, blood transfusion, antimicrobial and cancer chemotherapy, transplantation, and immunosuppression all create opportunities for these infections. The average lifespan has lengthened, so that those receiving medical attention carry the added risks of advanced age. Many extraintestinal infections with enteric bacteria now arise in the hospital, and they exact a high toll in mortality and increased hospital costs. Furthermore, they jeopardize the success of the advanced treatments we have worked so hard to develop. Therefore, physicians should understand the pathogenesis of each infection so that they can effect a cure and prevent recurrence if possible.

SPECIFIC INFECTIONS WITH ENTERIC BACTERIA

The diagnosis and management of each of the following gram-negative infections are discussed in depth in the appropriate section elsewhere in this textbook. A few points are emphasized here.

PERITONITIS (See Chapter 142). It can be difficult to recover bacteria from patients with spontaneous bacterial peritonitis; large volumes of fluid should be submitted for culture. Patients undergoing chronic peritoneal dialysis frequently develop peritonitis. If the same organism is isolated from repeated episodes and especially if it is an enteric rod or *Pseudomonas,* infection of the subcutaneous catheter tunnel should be suspected. A radiolabeled white blood cell scan can be helpful in detecting such infections so that the infected catheter can be removed.

PYELONEPHRITIS (See Chapter 111). Urinary tract infections localized to the bladder or kidneys can have important implications for therapy. Symptoms may be misleading, selective ureteral catheterization carries considerable risk, and examination of urine for antibody-coated bacteria is not practical in most laboratories. A simple culture technique (Fairley test) can differentiate between upper and lower urinary tract infections in difficult cases in which parenteral antibiotics would be required for kidney infection. In brief, the test employs a newly placed three-way bladder catheter through which a combination antibiotic and enzyme mixture (fibrinolysin and DNase) is instilled for 30 minutes to sterilize the bladder. Neomycin (32 mg/200 mL saline) is used for most organisms; polymyxin B (160,000 units/200 mL saline) can be used for *Pseudomonas* and amphotericin B (20 mg/200 mL 5% dextrose in water) for yeast. Bladder instillation is followed by a large-volume sterile water wash. Then the catheter is clamped, and three 10-minute specimens are collected. Increasing bacterial counts after the wash point to pyelonephritis. If infection is limited to the bladder, this procedure can cure it. The test is unreliable in patients with low urinary output, and it should not be performed in those with neutropenia.

PROSTATITIS (See Chapter 118). Most antibiotics available for treating infections with enteric bacilli do not penetrate the prostate well. For this reason, chronic prostatitis rarely is cured. However, the role of chronic prostatitis as a nidus of recurrent acute urinary tract infection in males can be curbed by low levels of suppressive antibiotics in bladder urine, achieved by a single tablet of an oral antibiotic given daily.

MENINGITIS (See Chapter 328). Enteric rods, especially *E. coli* and *Klebsiella,* are a frequent cause of neonatal meningitis. In adults, meningitis with enteric bacilli is exceedingly rare except in cases of head trauma or neurosurgery. Bacteria may be infrequent and difficult to see on stained smears of spinal or ventricular fluid. Treatment with a third-generation cephalosporin that penetrates the blood-brain barrier at high dose may be sufficient, but infections with organisms resistant to such drugs may require chloramphenicol or a combination of intravenous and intrathecal aminoglycosides. Infected foreign bodies must be removed.

PNEUMONIA (See Chapters 82 and 322). Seeing gram-negative rods in respiratory secretions or growing them from the secretions does not necessarily imply pneumonia. Susceptible patients often have severe acute or chronic lung disease with abnormal chest radiographs. Many are on respirators with inflammation around endotracheal tubes and have abnormal gram-negative nasopharyngeal flora. Evidence of increasing infiltrates, fever, increasing leukocytosis, and/or worsening respiratory function should be sought before the diagnosis of gram-negative pneumonia is made in such cases.

INFECTIONS OF INTRAVENOUS CATHETERS. Critically ill patients may have limited numbers of sites for placing intravenous catheters. If catheter infection is suspected, it may be impractical or impossible to remove all the lines. Comparing simultaneous quantitative blood cultures drawn through each catheter and from one peripheral vein can identify the infected site and preserve the uninfected catheters in place.

INFECTIONS IN NEUTROPENIA (See Chapter 314). The most common bowel infection in neutropenia is perirectal abscess. Inflammation may be modest, but patients complain of severe pain.

Examination can cause bacteremia. Surgical drainage may not be required unless neutropenia resolves and fluctuance develops. A less common but much more serious condition is typhlitis, an infection of the cecum associated with gas in the bowel wall, peritonitis, perforation, and bacteremia. This condition can be fatal within hours. Surgical resection has been helpful in a few cases, but surgical mortality is very high. Aggressive antibiotic therapy should be directed against *E. coli* and *P. aeruginosa,* the most common etiologic agents.

Necrotic skin lesions can accompany gram-negative bacteremia in neutropenic patients. These lesions, called ecthyma gangrenosum, are seen most frequently in *Pseudomonas* bacteremia. Cases have been reported with other gram-negative rods and with *Candida* and *Aspergillus* septicemia as well. The lesions can be scraped to search for the organism on smear. If nothing is seen, a punch biopsy for culture and histologic section can be done safely even in severe thrombocytopenia. In fungemia, the histologic section may be the only premortem specimen from which a diagnosis is obtained.

GRAM-NEGATIVE BACTEREMIA

(See Chapter 96). Gram-negative bacteria gain access to the blood stream from foci of tissue infection or, when host resistance is depressed, from sites of heavy colonization and minor trauma. Although bacteremia creates the opportunity for metastatic infections, a more immediate and serious consequence is septic shock. Mortality varies with the severity and nature of underlying disease, the source of bacteremia, the causative organisms, and the incidence of serious sequelae. In comparable groups, shock is somewhat more frequent in gram-negative bacteremia than in gram-positive bacteremia or fungemia. However, gram-negative bacteremia is distinguished from the other septicemias by the fact that very small numbers of circulating bacteria are associated with hypotension. Figure 347–1 is a schematic representation of the complex relationship between sepsis, bacteremia, hypotension, and endotoxemia in gram-negative infection. Septic shock also may result from non-enteric gram-positive bacteremic or non-bacteremic infections.

For therapeutic purposes, the diagnosis of gram-negative bacteremia cannot await the results of blood cultures but must be made on clinical grounds alone. The clinical setting is very helpful. A diagnosis of gram-negative bacteremia should be considered when sudden deterioration occurs in patients with focal infections usually caused by gram-negative bacteria (e.g., pyelonephritis, cholecystitis), in patients with significant focal infections from which gram-negative bacteria already have been isolated, and in patients with compromise in host defenses (e.g., neutropenia, burn injury), rendering them susceptible to their own bacterial flora. Neutropenic patients rarely have physical signs to localize the source of their bacteremia, but careful conversation often reveals a history of minor trauma, slight pain, or diarrhea. Gram-negative bacteremia and endotoxin infusion both cause transient neutropenia followed by neutrophilic leukocytosis. Large "toxic" vacuoles are seen. The first leukocyte count often is obtained after the leukopenic phase, but patients recovering from chemotherapy may have limited leukocyte reserves and thus exhibit only an apparent reversal of marrow recovery. Isolated thrombocytopenia or full-blown disseminated intravascular coagulopathy is not diagnostic of gram-negative bacteremia but, if present, is good supporting evidence. Arterial blood gas determinations may reveal unexplained hypoxemia without overt pulmonary disease, followed by metabolic acidosis.

TREATMENT. The correct choice of antibiotics is crucial to successful treatment of gram-negative bacteremia. When inappropriate drugs are used or the doses are too low, outcome is poor. It is never wise to give a single antibiotic to a patient at the onset of a bacteremic episode, even if the diagnosis and etiology seem certain. Many other infections can mimic gram-negative bacteremia. Sometimes more than one bacterial species is involved. In neutropenia, the outcome of *Pseudomonas* bacteremia is much better if more than one effective antibiotic is used. The choice of empirical antibiotics should be made on the basis of the site of the focal infection

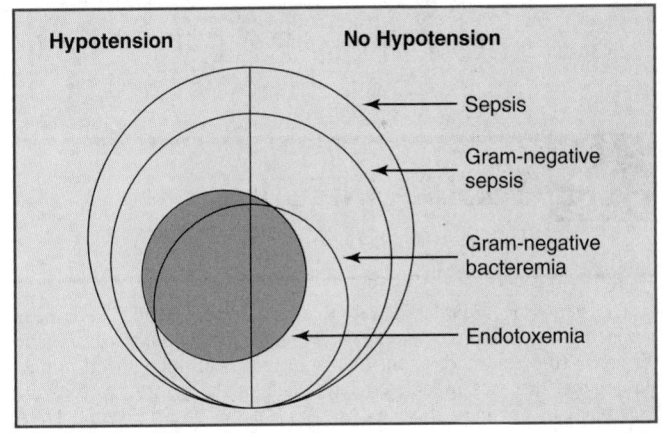

FIGURE 347–1 ■ Schematic representation of etiologies of the sepsis syndrome. (Courtesy of Craig R. Smith.)

(or infections) present, the known antimicrobial sensitivities of previous isolates from the patient or from recent nosocomial infections in the hospital, and the patient's underlying diseases. Choice of antibiotics has become increasingly difficult because of the recent explosion of antibiotic resistance caused mainly by emergence of organisms exhibiting several new types of β-lactamase–mediated resistance. In most patients the best regimen seems to be a combination of an aminoglycoside with a third-generation β-lactam. An antistaphylococcal drug should be added if *S. aureus* infection is possible. If bowel perforation or infarction has occurred, *Bacteroides fragilis* must be covered. If *Clostridium perfringens* is suspected to be part of a mixed infection, concomitant high-dose penicillin should be used. (*C. perfringens* decolorizes easily in the Gram's stain and may be distinguishable from gram-negative rods only by its boxlike rectangular shape.) A common mistake in use of aminoglycosides is to tailor the initial regimen to the first renal function tests. If azotemia is acute and attributable to poor perfusion, initial low doses will give inadequate levels as soon as hypotension is reversed. Renal toxicity from these drugs rarely occurs early; it is far more important to treat infection effectively in the first 24 hours than to avoid short-term aminoglycoside toxicity.

Gram-negative bacteremia cannot be cured without eradicating the source of bacteremia. In cases of infection associated with ureteral or biliary obstruction, bacteremia and shock may persist in the face of adequate antibiotics until the obstruction is relieved. All likely sites of infection should be cultured, if possible, before antibiotics are given. However, antibiotic treatment should not be delayed for this reason. Wound cultures often remain positive after blood and urine have been sterilized. Physicians should not be content until they have found a satisfactory explanation for bacteremia. New fever or clinical deterioration can signal a new infection in a susceptible patient, the emergence of resistant bacteria, spread of the original focal infection, inadequate antibiotic levels, or a drug reaction. Such an episode requires complete re-evaluation with physical examination and repeat cultures.

Pitout JDD, Sanders CC, Sanders WE Jr: Antimicrobial resistance with focus on β-lactam resistance in gram-negative bacilli. Am J Med 103:51, 1997. *A concise, readable overview of the most difficult current issues in treatment of extraintestinal infections with enteric bacteria.*

Quartin AA, Schein RMH, Kett DH, Peduzzi PN: Magnitude and duration of the effect of sepsis on survival. JAMA 277:1058, 1997. *A large study of 1,505 septic patients and 91,830 uninfected controls, done by the VA Systemic Sepsis Cooperative Studies Group, illustrating the considerable impact of a septic episode on survival even after other disease factors are considered.*

Svanborg C: Bacterial virulence in urinary tract infection. Infect Dis Clin North Am 11:513, 1997. *A succinct well-referenced review of bacterial factors important in the development of urinary tract infections.*

OTHER BACTERIAL INFECTIONS

348 *YERSINIA* INFECTIONS

J. Glenn Morris, Jr.

The genus *Yersinia* contains at least 10 species that have been isolated from humans. *Y. enterocolitica, Y. pseudotuberculosis,* and *Y. pestis* (the causative agent of plague) are well-recognized human pathogens; diseases associated with each of these three species are described in detail in this chapter. Within the past 15 years, DNA hybridization and other studies have resulted in the delineation of seven additional "*Y. enterocolitica*—like" species: *Y. frederiksenii, Y. kristensenii, Y. intermedia, Y. aldovae, Y. mollaretii* (formerly biogroup 3A of *Y. enterocolitica*), *Y. bercovieri* (formerly biogroup 3B of *Y. enterocolitica*), and *Y. rhodei.* These seven species carry antigens that in some instances are identical to those of *Y. enterocolitica* strains (allowing strains to be serotyped with *Y. enterocolitica* typing sera) and may be identified as *Y. enterocolitica* in some laboratory identification systems. It remains controversial as to whether these species do, indeed, cause human illness.

YERSINIA ENTEROCOLITICA

DEFINITION. *Y. enterocolitica* is an enteric pathogen that can cause gastroenteritis, mesenteric adenitis and ileitis ("pseudoappendicitis"), and sepsis. Infection may also trigger a variety of autoimmune phenomena, including reactive arthritis.

Y. enterocolitica is a gram-negative bacillus within the family Enterobacteriaceae; when first identified, it was designated *Pasteurella X.*

DISTRIBUTION AND EPIDEMIOLOGY. *Y. enterocolitica* is widely distributed in the environment (especially in cooler, temperate regions) and frequently colonizes wild and domestic animals. The organism is a common pharyngeal commensal in swine, with potentially pathogenic strains isolated from 25 to 90% of pork tongues after slaughter. Fifty-eight per cent of *Y. enterocolitica* infections in Belgium (which has one of the highest rates of *Y. enterocolitica* disease in the world) have been attributed to eating raw pork; in the United States, illness has been associated with home preparation of chitterlings. *Y. enterocolitica* outbreaks have also been linked with milk, in which the organism grows at refrigerator temperatures. *Y. enterocolitica* may be introduced into a household by pets or by symptomatic or asymptomatic human carriers. Once the organism is present within a household, infants and young children appear to be at greatest risk for infection.

In parts of Canada and western Europe, *Y. enterocolitica* rivals *Salmonella* and surpasses *Shigella* as a cause of acute diarrheal disease. In the United States, isolation rates from diarrheal stool samples are somewhat lower, generally between 5 and 30% of those for *Salmonella.* Isolation rates tend to be much lower in tropical areas. In one study in Bangladesh, *Y. enterocolitica* was isolated from only 0.06% of diarrheal stool samples from children younger than age 7; this very low rate may reflect both the decreased frequency of environmental isolation outside of cold areas and the dietary restrictions limiting pork consumption in Moslem countries.

PATHOGENESIS. *Y. enterocolitica* is an intracellular pathogen. It invades and survives within macrophages and may persist and grow within lymph nodes and other lymphoid tissue for extended periods. It can also produce one or more protein enterotoxins, which may be responsible for or contribute to the diarrheal disease caused by the organism. Autoimmune phenomena occurring after *Y. enterocolitica* infections appear to be due to cross-reactivity between host and bacterial antigens; several putative target antigens are under active investigation, including bacterial antigens that may cross-react with the HLA-B27 antigen.

Human illness is most commonly associated with *Y. enterocolitica* strains in serogroups (O:3, O:5,27, O:8, O:9, and others) and biogroups (1B, 2, 3, 4), which carry a virulence plasmid and share certain virulence characteristics, including the ability to invade epithelial cells.

CLINICAL AND LABORATORY FEATURES. The most common clinical manifestation of *Y. enterocolitica* infection is diarrhea, frequently accompanied by abdominal pain and fever; vomiting occurs in 20 to 40% of cases. Diarrhea is mild to moderate in severity and may last 1 to 2 weeks. As many as 10 to 20% of patients are reported to have bloody diarrhea. The limited available data suggest that leukocytosis is common.

Abdominal pain may be quite severe, mimicking appendicitis, and may occur in the absence of diarrhea. This has resulted in several outbreaks of "pseudoappendicitis" associated with transmission of *Y. enterocolitica* in a common food item.

Y. enterocolitica can cause pharyngitis (8% of *Y. enterocolitica* cases identified in one large, multistate outbreak), hepatic and splenic abscesses, peritonitis, and septicemia. Sepsis has been closely linked with iron overload states (and the administration of deferoxamine, used in treating iron overload) and with the presence of underlying conditions such as cirrhosis, chronic renal failure, diabetes, and immunosuppression. *Y. enterocolitica* sepsis has been reported in association with transfusion of red blood cell units contaminated with the organism, with 21 such cases reported in the United States between 1985 and 1996. Very young infants (<3 months) with intestinal *Y. enterocolitica* infections appear to have an increased susceptibility to septicemia; these infants may or may not be febrile and may have protein-losing enteropathy and failure to thrive.

Infection with *Y. enterocolitica* can trigger myriad autoimmune processes, most notably erythema nodosum and a reactive polyarthritis. Arthritis generally occurs within 1 to 2 weeks of onset of gastrointestinal symptoms, usually in HLA-B27–positive patients. Viable organisms cannot be cultured from involved joints; however, *Yersinia* antigens have been identified in synovial fluid cells and peripheral blood mononuclear cells. *Y. enterocolitica* infections have also been implicated in the development of Reiter's syndrome, carditis, glomerulonephritis, Graves' disease, and Hashimoto's thyroiditis.

DIAGNOSIS. Diagnosis is based on isolation of the organism from stool, blood, or other clinical specimen.

Although not generally available in the United States, serologic diagnosis of *Y. enterocolitica* infections is widely used in Europe.

TREATMENT. Available data do not indicate that antimicrobial therapy is efficacious in cases of uncomplicated *Y. enterocolitica* enteritis, but it is indicated in systemic disease or focal extraintestinal infection. *Y. enterocolitica* strains are susceptible in vitro to aminoglycosides, chloramphenicol, tetracycline, trimethoprim-sulfamethoxazole, third-generation cephalosporins, and quinolones; isolates are resistant to penicillins and first-generation cephalosporins. Data suggest that fluoroquinolones may be the drug of choice for extraintestinal *Y. enterocolitica* infections, in combination with a third-generation cephalosporin or an aminoglycoside in severe cases.

PROGNOSIS. Most cases of *Y. enterocolitica* enteritis are self-limited, and recovery is complete. Mortality rates among persons with *Y. enterocolitica* sepsis were originally reported to exceed 50%. In more recent studies, with aggressive antimicrobial therapy and supportive care, mortality has been approximately 7.5%. Arthritis may persist for a period of months (mean of 3.2 months in one study), with mild residual symptoms occurring in 50% of patients; 1 to 2% develop chronic arthritis.

YERSINIA PSEUDOTUBERCULOSIS

Y. pseudotuberculosis is most commonly recognized as a cause of mesenteric adenitis. Cases of enteritis in children have been reported from Japan (Izumi fever), and septicemia is seen in patients who have underlying liver disease or immunosuppression. The organism is widely distributed in the environment (including water from wells and mountain springs in endemic areas) and is carried by wild and domestic animals. Secondary immunologic complications, such as erythema nodosum, arthritis, and renal insufficiency, have also been observed; in one recent Korean study, 14% of affected children had acute renal failure.

YERSINIA PESTIS (PLAGUE)

DEFINITION. *Y. pestis* is the etiologic agent for plague. The most common clinical form is bubonic plague, or acute regional lymphadenitis; septicemic and pneumonic forms also occur. Epidemics of plague have had a major impact on human history. Whereas cases today are confined largely to isolated endemic foci, recent outbreaks in Madagascar, India, Peru, and East Africa highlight the continued potential for human transmission. The 1994 plague outbreak in India also highlights the profound psychological impact that the diagnosis of plague can have on a community, with the early reports of pneumonic plague cases in Surat resulting in over 600,000 of the estimated population of 2 million fleeing the city.

DISTRIBUTION AND EPIDEMIOLOGY. Among rodent populations, plague is spread by transmission from rodents to fleas and back to rodents (sylvatic plague). Soil can also be contaminated by infected dead fleas and rodents; rodents coming from non-infected areas can become infected when they dig burrows in previously infected areas. This cycle may be relatively stable (enzootic) or may result in periodic epidemics (epizootics) in susceptible rodent populations. Humans are an accidental host in this natural cycle, with cases occurring when infected fleas bite people, or after direct contact or skin inoculation with body fluids of an infected animal (including wild carnivores, rabbits, and cats and dogs). Direct, person-to-person transmission occurs only in the setting of pneumonic plague.

In the United States, plague is found west of the 100th meridian, which runs from North Dakota to Texas. Animals most commonly involved have included ground squirrels, rock squirrels, and prairie dogs. From 1947 through 1996, a total of 390 cases of plague were reported to the Centers for Disease Control and Prevention. Approximately one third of recent cases have occurred in Native Americans; this is presumably a function of lifestyle, which may involve herding animals, assisted by dogs, in enzootic areas. Since 1977, there have been 18 U.S. cases in which cats were implicated as the probable source of infection; it is possible that some of these cases represented pneumonic transmission of the organism from the cat to the affected human.

CLINICAL AND LABORATORY FEATURES. Plague presents most commonly as an acute regional lymphadenitis, or bubonic plague. Symptoms generally occur after an incubation period of 2 to 6 days. Illness is marked by the sudden onset of fever, chills, weakness, and headache. Then, or shortly thereafter, patients note an intensely painful swelling in one region of lymph nodes, usually the groin, axilla, or neck. This swelling, or bubo, is typically oval, varying from 1 to 10 cm in length; the overlying skin is elevated and warm and may appear stretched or erythematous. The bubo itself is firm, extremely tender to palpation, and non-fluctuant. Patients with bubonic plague usually do not have skin lesions. However, in studies in Vietnam, about one fourth of patients had pustules, vesicles, eschars, or papules near the bubo or in areas drained by the affected nodes; these were presumed to represent sites of flea bite inoculations.

In the absence of therapy, disease progresses rapidly to a septicemic phase, with marked toxicity, prostration, and shock. The white blood cell count is elevated, and evidence of disseminated intravascular coagulation may appear. Purpura may be seen, associated with vasculitis and thrombosis. Some patients do not develop a bubo and progress directly to septicemia (septicemic plague). Diagnosis in these cases may be particularly difficult, because initial symptoms are relatively non-specific (fever, headache, sore throat, malaise, myalgia, nausea, diarrhea, vomiting).

One of the feared complications of plague is plague pneumonia. Secondary pneumonia results from hematogenous spread of *Y. pestis* to the lung. Patients develop cough and chest pain and may have hemoptysis. Radiographically, there is patchy bronchopneumonia or confluent consolidation. Sputum is purulent and contains the etiologic organism. Plague pneumonia is highly contagious by airborne transmission; persons inhaling the organism, from either an infected person or an animal, are susceptible to infection (primary plague pneumonia). Plague meningitis is a rarer complication; it typically occurs more than a week after inadequately treated bubonic plague but may be seen as a primary manifestation, without associated lymphadenopathy.

DIAGNOSIS. Plague can be diagnosed by isolating *Y. pestis* from blood, from an aspirate of a bubo, or from sputum. A presumptive diagnosis can be made in the appropriate clinical setting by demonstrating (by Gram stain or fluorescent antibody) characteristic organisms in sputum or in an aspirate of the bubo. In the absence of culture results, infection can be diagnosed by serology.

TREATMENT AND PROGNOSIS. In the absence of therapy, plague has an estimated mortality of more than 50%; untreated primary septicemic or pneumonic plague is invariably fatal. Fatality rates of up to 22% continue to be reported in the United States, owing primarily to delays in initiation of appropriate therapy. Because of this, therapy should be started immediately if the diagnosis of plague is suspected.

Streptomycin was the first drug to be shown to have activity against plague, and, in the absence of controlled trials with other agents, it remains the drug of choice. Chloramphenicol and tetracycline are thought to be acceptable alternative therapies. Recent animal studies suggest that other aminoglycosides and the fluoroquinolones (ciprofloxacin, ofloxacin) may also be effective. Penicillin and first-generation cephalosporins are not effective, are associated with a high mortality, and should not be used. There has now been one report from Madagascar of isolation of a *Y. pestis* strain resistant to multiple "first line" antibiotics (including streptomycin, chloramphenicol, tetracycline, and sulfonamides), emphasizing the need for routine testing of antimicrobial susceptibility of isolates. Aggressive supportive care is essential for patients in shock or with disseminated intravascular coagulation.

PREVENTION. All suspected plague cases should be reported immediately to local health authorities. Patients with bubonic plague (with no cough and a normal chest radiograph) should be placed on drainage secretion precautions; if any evidence of pneumonic involvement is present, patients should be placed in strict isolation with precautions against airborne spread of the organism. Isolation should be maintained for a minimum of 3 days after starting appropriate antimicrobial therapy. Clinical samples must be carefully handled to minimize the risk of skin contact or aerosolization of the organism. Close contacts of suspected or confirmed plague pneumonia cases (including medical personnel) should be provided with chemoprophylaxis with tetracycline or sulfonamides.

Persons living in endemic areas should be advised to protect themselves against rodents and fleas; this includes measures designed to reduce rodent populations near homes and application of insecticides, as necessary, to control flea populations. Veterinarians should be aware of the potential risk of transmission from infected cats. A formalin-killed vaccine, plague vaccine, is commercially available. Its use is recommended for persons traveling to epidemic areas, for individuals who must live and work in close contact with wild rodents, and for laboratory workers who must handle *Y. pestis* cultures. New, subunit vaccines for plague are also under active development.

Bottone EJ: *Yersinia enterocolitica*: The charisma continues. Clin Microbiol Rev 10: 257–276, 1997. *A comprehensive review of the microbiology, pathogenesis, and epidemiology of Y. enterocolitica and Y. enterocolitica–like species.*

Crook LD, Tempest B: Plague: A clinical review of 27 cases. Arch Intern Med 152: 1253, 1992. *A description of 27 plague cases seen at the Gallup, New Mexico, Indian Medical Center between 1965 and 1989; 19 patients had bubonic plague and 8 had septicemic plague.*

Perry RD, Fetherston JD: *Yersinia pestis*—etiologic agent of plague. Clin Microbiol Rev 10:35–66, 1997. *A comprehensive review of the microbiology, pathogenesis, and epidemiology of plague.*

349 TULAREMIA

Richard B. Hornick

DEFINITION. Tularemia is a rare infectious disease caused by a small gram-negative pleomorphic rod, *Francisella tularensis*. This organism is acquired from an animal reservoir, frequently cottontail rabbits, by direct contact with diseased animal tissues, the bite of an infected tick or deer fly, ingestion of contaminated food or water, and inhalation of aerosolized bacteria. Clinical manifestations usually include a cutaneous ulcer with enlargement of regional lymph nodes. Rarely, a pneumonitis results from inhalation of *F. tularensis* or secondary spread from the skin ulcer and lymph nodes. Confirmation of the diagnosis by cultural technique is not advocated because of the high contagion risk to personnel handling this organism. The therapeutic response to effective antibiotic therapy is rapid.

The typhoidal form of tularemia was first described in Japan in 1818. A clear description of the organism occurred in 1906 when McCoy uncovered a "plaguelike" disease among ground squirrels in Tulare County, California. In Japan, tularemia may be referred to as Ohara's disease or Yato-byo (wild hare disease).

ETIOLOGY, SPECIFIC LABORATORY DIAGNOSIS, AND EPIDEMIOLOGY. *F. tularensis* is a small gram-negative pleomorphic rod-shaped bacterium. Organisms are not seen in smears of infected tissue unless special staining techniques are used. Fluorescent antibody conjugate staining and modified Dieterle staining are the best methods. All tularemia strains are serologically identical, but there are biochemical and virulence differences for mammals that have allowed differentiation of two strains. These are called Jellison A and B; the former, found only in North America, is lethal for domestic rabbits (*Oryctolagus*) and causes severe disease in humans. The unique biochemical capabilities of this strain (e.g., it ferments glycerol and contains citrulline ureidase) do not explain its increased virulence. Strain B lacks these biochemical features, is not lethal for cottontails, causes milder disease in humans, usually is isolated from rodents or from water, and is distributed over Europe, Asia, and North America. Reasons for the differences in virulence are unknown.

CULTURE METHODS. The direct isolation of *F. tularensis* from blood (rarely), pus from ulcers or buboes, sputum, or pharyngeal or gastric aspirations in a patient with pneumonitis can be achieved by two methods. This is a class 4 organism requiring an effective hood or an adequate isolation laboratory to prevent human disease or epizootics. The two methods for isolation are intraperitoneal inoculation of guinea pigs and direct plating of a specimen onto glucose cysteine blood agar, cystine heart agar, or eugon agar. The colonies are small on these media; they appear in 48 to 72 hours of incubation at 37° C. The polymerase chain reaction has been used to expedite the identification of *F. tularensis* in patients with ulceroglandular disease. This test reduces the chance of laboratory-acquired disease. As few as one to five viable organisms will cause the death of guinea pigs in 5 to 10 days. Appropriate facilities are needed to prevent spread of the disease to other animals.

SEROLOGIC DIAGNOSIS. The measurement of serum agglutinating antibodies is a useful and safer method of diagnosing tularemia. Titers begin to rise in 7 to 10 days and peak in 3 to 4 weeks. Paired serum specimens obtained 2 weeks apart and demonstrating a fourfold or greater rise are diagnostic of tularemia. However, a single specimen with a titer of 1:160 or greater in a patient thought to have tularemia on clinical grounds is diagnostic. Antibiotic therapy does not appear to dampen the antibody response. Titers remain elevated for 6 to 8 months and then decline in the subsequent 1 to 1.5 years to low or undetectable levels. There is a cross-reaction with *Brucella* antigen during the early phase of the antibody response. The *Brucella* titer falls off faster than, and is never so high as, the tularemia titer (see Chapter 356).

SKIN TESTING. A skin test antigen has proved to be reliable for diagnostic and epidemiologic purposes. A positive test result, similar in appearance to a tuberculin test response, is present during the first week of illness, frequently before the agglutinins are detectable, and remains positive for years. There is no known cross-reacting skin test antigen. The antigen is derived from *F. tularensis* by ether extraction; however, it is not commonly available. It can be obtained from the Centers for Disease Control and Prevention (CDC) in Atlanta. In 10% of patients, the skin test antigen may boost pre-existing agglutinating antibody titers. Skin test reactivity can be shown to be associated with sensitized lymphocytes.

EPIDEMIOLOGY. Tularemia is a sporadic disease; humans acquire it when bitten by an infected tick or deer fly or when handling an infected animal. In the process of dressing a rabbit or skinning a muskrat, the hands may become contaminated with infected blood, subcutaneous abscesses, or liver and spleen that contain millions of organisms. The act of eviscerating the animal can create an aerosol that can be inhaled. Contaminated water or food is the least likely method of acquiring tularemia. Many carnivores such as dogs, cats, bull snakes, and others may feed on diseased rabbits, resulting in contamination of the teeth and saliva. These animals are relatively resistant to tularemia. Contact with the teeth of a pet dog or cat has resulted in ulceroglandular tularemia. Studies in volunteers have quantified the susceptibility of humans to infection and disease and the virulence of *F. tularensis* for humans. As few as 50 type A organisms injected subcutaneously cause ulceroglandular disease. Pneumonic tularemia can be induced by a similar inoculum size if the aerosolized and inhaled particles are small (<5 μm). Type B organisms require an inoculum about 1000 times larger to induce ulceroglandular or respiratory disease in humans.

The incidence of tularemia is low: 96 cases were reported in 1994, the last year that tularemia was included in the CDC's list of notifiable diseases. The peak incidence was in 1939, when almost 2300 cases were reported. Laws passed at that time prohibited the sale of wild rabbits, especially cottontails, and this legislation plus increased public awareness of the danger of handling sick or dying wild animals has contributed to the decline. Most cases occur in the Midwest, but the disease is not restricted to any one geographic location in the United States. Cottontail rabbits in urban and suburban areas provide the reservoir from which tularemia can occur. Epizootics among these or other animals can cause epidemics in humans. Tularemia has been reported only north of the 30th parallel. The cottontail is not found in Europe; various rodents such as voles, muskrats, and hares carry *F. tularensis* (Jellison B type) in that part of the world. Diseased jackrabbits, found west of the Mississippi River, may be an important source of contamination of ticks and deer flies.

In the summer months, most cases of tularemia are caused by tick or deer fly bites. Ulceroglandular disease begins with an ulcer at the site of the bite (e.g., groin, axilla, or scalp). In the fall during hunting season, sporadic cases, usually ulceroglandular, occur among hunters and trappers. In Scandinavia, epidemics have occurred in winter when farmers handling stored hay contaminated by diseased voles inhaled *F. tularensis* and developed pneumonic tularemia.

MECHANISMS OF INFECTION AND PATHOLOGY. The most common form of tularemia results from *F. tularensis* penetrating the skin. This penetration may be through hair follicles or minute areas of trauma. Subsequent disease develops in 2 to 6 days, depending on the number of bacteria and their virulence. The organisms multiply in the dermis and induce a marked inflammatory process consisting primarily of mononuclear cells with a perivascular distribution. This process produces an erythematous tender papule. The inflamed area continues to swell until the induced ischemia causes the skin to ulcerate. The base of the ulcer becomes black and depressed and the edges sharply demarcated. At the time of penetration, some organisms may be phagocytized and transported in the lymph to regional nodes. There is no clinically apparent lymphangitis. The nodes enlarge and become painful when caseation occurs. Histologic sections reveal geographic necrosis and disruption of the capsule. Fluctuation of the node is a late and rare event. It may then rupture. The necrotic, purulent, painful lymph node is termed a *bubo*. Healing of a bubo takes months even with appropriate antibiotic treatment. Aspiration of an unruptured node may lead to an indolent draining sinus tract. *F. tularensis* may remain in the necrotic tissue and purulent drainage for many weeks. The ulcer heals slowly and usually leaves a depigmented, rounded area in the skin.

Oculoglandular tularemia may occur when the conjunctival sac is infected from an ulcer or contaminated finger. Small yellowish granulomatous lesions develop on the palpebral conjunctivae, accompanied by enlargement of the preauricular lymph nodes. In untreated patients the cornea may perforate.

Inhaled small particle aerosols (<5 μm in diameter) containing *F. tularensis* (usually type A) are ultimately deposited in the terminal bronchioles and alveoli, although infection of the trachea and large bronchi also occurs. A peribronchial inflammation develops, with infiltration by neutrophils and mononuclear cells. This produces necrosis of alveolar walls and results in localized pneumonitis. In humans, small areas of pneumonitis represent the most common findings on chest roentgenograms. Often these are ill defined and difficult to interpret. Lobar consolidation or lung abscesses, infrequent in humans, represent extensive spread and necrosis. Mediastinal and peritracheal lymph nodes enlarge and may be apparent on chest films. They may be partially responsible, along with the bronchitis, for the substernal burning common with tularemic pneumonia. The incubation period for this form of tularemia varies inversely with the size and virulence of the inhaled inoculum. After an inoculum of 10 to 50 organisms, disease appears in about 4 to 7 days in volunteers.

Typhoidal tularemia follows systemic spread of *F. tularensis* from the oropharynx and probably the gastrointestinal tract when a huge inoculum is swallowed. Enlargement of cervical lymph nodes, and presumably nodes in the mesentery, occurs. This latter process causes abdominal pain and is associated with an ileus. This is the most unusual form of tularemia in this country.

CLINICAL MANIFESTATIONS. Disease initiated by a tick bite is manifested by an ulcer at the site or adjacent to it. The tick defecates after feeding, and the infected feces may be scratched into the epidermis. Usually the lesion is in the inguinal, axillary, or scalp skin. If contact with tularemia organisms results from handling an infected animal, an ulcerative lesion evolves in the skin of the hands, frequently around a fingernail. This lesion may be so trivial that it is ignored by the patient. The ulcer is depressed into the dermis, has sharply demarcated edges, and gradually develops a black base. Initially, the lesion produces a thick, yellowish exudate. Regional lymph nodes enlarge and are tender to palpation. Fever and chills are common. The temperature curve is usually remittent or continuous in character. Without antibiotic therapy, most patients remain febrile for several weeks, the ulcer heals slowly over weeks to months, and the enlarged lymph nodes persist for months. Untreated patients may occasionally develop a secondary necrotizing pneumonia as a consequence of bacteremia, causing acute illness.

Primary tularemia pneumonia involves the sudden development of substernal burning and a non-productive paroxysmal cough associated with fever and chills. Headache, myalgia, photophobia, malaise, and prostration are common. The temperature elevates quickly to 39.4 to 40° C and remains at that level (continuous fever curve) until antibiotic treatment is given. Sixty to 70 per cent of patients survive without specific therapy, and in these a slow defervescence occurs over several months. Radiographs of the lungs may reveal ill-defined, scattered oval areas of infiltration, with enlarged peritracheal lymph nodes. Pleural effusions, lobar consolidation, and lung abscess are other manifestations of this form of tularemia. Cervical lymph nodes are palpable and tender.

DIAGNOSIS AND DIFFERENTIAL DIAGNOSIS. The diagnosis of ulceroglandular tularemia is made on the basis of the clinical manifestations and serologic studies. Paired serum specimens collected over a 2- to 3-week period are required to demonstrate a fourfold rise in titer. A baseline agglutinin titer of 1:160 in a patient with a history of an indolent ulcer for 2 or more weeks is diagnostic of tularemia. Culture of an ulcer and blood should be performed only if the hospital laboratory has appropriate protective isolation hoods. Patients with sporotrichosis or *Mycobacterium marinum* infections may have ulcers suggestive of tularemia but are usually afebrile. Enlarged lymph nodes extending centripetally as a beaded chain are a characteristic finding in sporotrichosis. Lesions of the fingers infected with staphylococci or β-streptococci usually produce more pus and may be associated with lymphangitis. *Bacillus anthracis* can produce an ulcer (anthrax) with black-based, sharply demarcated edges similar to that initiated by *F. tularensis*. A careful history and serologic data help in the differential diagnosis. In patients in whom any form of tularemia is suspected, the skin test antigen is helpful. The test result is usually positive before agglutinating antibodies develop.

Tularemia pneumonia must be differentiated from the more common bacterial, viral, and mycoplasmal pneumonias. The history and the presence of ulceroglandular disease are helpful. Skin testing and serologic studies are diagnostic. The chest radiographs may yield suggestive findings consisting of ill-defined, small, oval, multiple infiltrates but is not diagnostic.

Patients infected with *F. tularensis* usually have a normal leukocyte count with an elevated sedimentation rate. The white blood cell count is elevated when a bubo or a lung abscess is present.

COMPLICATIONS. Pericarditis and meningitis are rare events that usually occur in patients who have been misdiagnosed and

have received inappropriate treatment. Pericarditis results from direct extension of the infection from the purulent, necrotic mediastinal lymph nodes or the involved lung. Constrictive pericarditis has been reported. Meningitis develops rarely, represents a seeding of the meninges during bacteremia, and is characterized by a lymphocytic pleocytosis in the cerebrospinal fluid.

TREATMENT. Patients with all forms of tularemia respond to the antibiotics streptomycin, gentamicin, tetracycline, and chloramphenicol. The aminoglycoside antibiotics are recommended; they produce a prompt cure of patients with the most severe form of tularemia. Patients with pneumonitis are afebrile within 24 to 48 hours and do not relapse. Ulcers and tender lymph nodes heal in 7 to 10 days. Gentamicin, 5 mg/kg/day in divided doses, is given for 10 days. Streptomycin was the principal drug for treating tularemia before gentamicin; 1 g is given every 12 hours for 10 days. Treatment with tetracycline or chloramphenicol may produce an equally rapid response, but relapses occur in 15 to 20% of the patients. These drugs are not recommended unless gentamicin and streptomycin are contraindicated. Doses of 3 to 4 g of tetracycline or 3 g of chloramphenicol daily for 10 days can be used. Naturally acquired resistance to any of these antibiotics has not been found. Ceftriaxone has excellent in vitro inhibitory activity but in one study failed to cure eight pediatric patients. In vitro studies also indicate the potential antibacterial effect of the quinolones. However, no systematic in vivo testing has been reported.

Patients with ulceroglandular tularemia respond well to these antibiotics. Fluctuant lymph nodes should not be aspirated until the patient has finished the course of the antibiotic treatment. Isolation of patients with any form of tularemia is not required; there is no evidence of person-to-person spread.

PROGNOSIS. The mortality for untreated ulceroglandular disease is about 5%. Patients infected with type B strains and untreated probably have a mortality less than 1%. Many cases probably go undiagnosed, because the disease is mild and self-limiting. Treatment with antibiotics prevents death and promotes healing in a week to 10 days.

The mortality for pneumonic tularemia in the preantibiotic period was 30 to 40%. Treatment with streptomycin or tetracycline has lowered this figure to less than 1%. Healing occurs without residual lung damage or deficits in pulmonary function.

PREVENTION. Patients who recover from tularemia have a high degree of resistance to reinfection. If *F. tularensis* is reintroduced into the skin, a positive skin test reaction ensues without ulceration. Resistance to pulmonary disease may be associated with sensitized lymphocytes and alveolar macrophages.

A live attenuated strain of *F. tularensis* has been prepared as a vaccine. This can be administered by the acupuncture route, and it produces excellent immunity. The vaccine can be obtained from the Commander, U.S. Army Medical Research Institute of Infectious Diseases, Frederick, Maryland 21701. Its use is limited to persons considered at high risk, such as selected laboratory workers, forest rangers, game wardens, and perhaps others known to be exposed during an outbreak. The vaccine works by stimulating cellular immune mechanisms. Circulating agglutinins are not associated with resistance to disease.

Ancuta P, Pedron T, Girard R, et al: Inability of the *Francisella tularensis* lipopolysaccharide to mimic or to antagonize the induction of cell activation by endotoxins. Infect Immun 64:2041–2046, 1996. *The LPS of* F. tularensis *is atypical; when the organism is phagocytized by monocytes in vitro, the LPS does not induce NO and thus the organism avoids this antimicrobial activity and persists intracellularly.*

Capellan J, Fong IW: Tularemia from a cat bite: Case report and review of feline-associated tularemia. Clin Infect Dis 16:472, 1993. *Summarizes literature reports of patients acquiring tularemia from cats. Offers advice on management of cat bite wounds not healing with penicillin therapy.*

Enderlin G. Morales L, Jacobs RF, Cross JT: Streptomycin and alternative agents for the treatment of tularemia: Review of the literature. Clin Infect Dis 19:42, 1994. *Compares in vitro with in vivo results. A good guide to current therapy.*

Evans ME, Gregory DW, Schaffner W, et al: Tularemia: A 30-year experience with 88 cases. Medicine 64:251, 1985. *An excellent summary of the clinical presentations of* F. tularensis *disease.*

Penn RL, Kinasewitz GT: Factors associated with a poor outcome in tularemia. Arch Intern Med 147:265, 1987. *A retrospective study of the factors leading to poor outcomes. One significant factor was delay in diagnosis and treatment.*

Sjostedt A, Eriksson U, Berglund L, Tarnvik A: Detection of *Francisella tularensis* in ulcers of patients with tularemia by PCR. J Clin Microbiol 35:1045–1048, 1997. *As in other infections the PCR is more sensitive than culturing the organism. The PCR has been very effective in animal models in identifying the organism in blood as well as splenic tissue.*

350 ANTHRAX

Jonas A. Shulman

DEFINITION. Anthrax is a zoonotic disease caused by *Bacillus anthracis,* a large gram-positive, spore-forming bacillus transmitted to humans by contact with infected animals or contaminated animal products. Other names for anthrax include woolsorter's disease, Siberian ulcer, malignant pustule, charbon, malignant edema, and ragsorter's disease. In 1877, Koch described *B. anthracis* as one of the first microbes identified as a cause of a specific disease, thereby making anthrax the prototype for Koch's postulates and the first disease to satisfy them. Anthrax has all but disappeared from North America, Western Europe, and Australia since being nearly eradicated in livestock after extensive veterinary programs, including vaccination. The disease is still prevalent in many developing countries, however, especially Asia, Africa, and Central America, where livestock are only marginally subjected to veterinary control and where environmental conditions are favorable for an animal-to-soil-to-animal cycle.

Anthrax occurs primarily in herbivorous animals, especially cattle, goats, and sheep, but many other animals, including pigs, buffalo, and elephants, have also been infected. Cattle are particularly susceptible to the systemic form of anthrax, which clinically progresses to death in 24 to 48 hours. The large numbers of organisms found in infected cattle may contaminate not only the animal but also its products and environs, thereby allowing infection to occur in animals more resistant to anthrax, such as humans.

The primary forms of anthrax in humans are cutaneous, inhalation, gastrointestinal, and oropharyngeal. Septicemia and meningitis may occur from any of these primary foci. By far the most common form of the disease in the United States is the cutaneous lesion, which accounts for more than 95% of clinical cases. Inhalation anthrax has occurred only rarely in the United States in the past 25 years, and gastrointestinal anthrax has never been reported in this country.

ETIOLOGY. *B. anthracis* is a large gram-positive, non-motile, spore-forming bacillus (1 to 1.3 × 3 to 8 μm). Although spores of *B. anthracis* do not form in living tissue, they are induced by aerobic conditions in the external environment and may persist for years in the soil, in animal products, or in an appropriate industrial setting. The organism grows well aerobically on ordinary laboratory media at 35° to 37° C. The colonies produced are especially sticky (positive tenacity test, positive string of pearls test) and have a tendency to stand up in stalagmite fashion when lifted with a bacteriologic loop. The Gray-white colonies are non-hemolytic, rough, and flat, with many comma-shaped outgrowths on blood agar. Microscopic examination of organisms growing on artificial media shows long, parallel chains of organisms frequently described as having a rather characteristic "boxcar" appearance. Spores are oval and occur either centrally or paracentrally but cause no swelling of the bacillus. Material from fresh lesions contains single or short chains of two or three bacilli, which may appear encapsulated, the ends of which are slightly rounded.

Anthrax organisms can be differentiated from the saprophytic *Bacillus* species by fluorescent antibody staining, lysis with a specific γ bacteriophage, and virulence for mice, guinea pigs, and rabbits. Parenteral inoculation into these species results in death in 1 to 3 days.

INCIDENCE AND PREVALENCE. *B. anthracis* is a soil organism that has worldwide distribution. Animal anthrax is endemic in some areas of Asia, Africa, and Latin America, especially in rural regions that have inadequate animal vaccination programs and inadequate animal husbandry. These areas are more likely to have a number of human cases as well. Certain areas within the United States and other parts of the world may provide a particularly favorable environment for large numbers of resistant spores to survive in the soil for many years. In fact, a number of epizootics related to focal regions of heavily contaminated soil have occurred.

Because no reliable reporting of anthrax exists, and in many

instances the diagnosis may never be made, the actual worldwide incidence of anthrax is not known. Estimates in the past have ranged between 20,000 and 100,000 human cases per year, but these figures have more recently been estimated at 2,000 to 20,000 cases per annum. In the United States, approximately one case of human anthrax per year was reported between 1970 and 1985, but only three cases have been documented since 1984. Reports of human anthrax have been especially frequent in Turkey, Pakistan, Iran, Haiti, and several Asian and African countries. There are probably many parts of the world with significant endemic problems but from which data are not available.

The potential for large outbreaks in animals and humans continues to exist, especially when economic or political upheaval is present. One of the largest epidemics of anthrax was reported in Zimbabwe between 1978 and 1980, when nearly 10,000 human cases of cutaneous anthrax and a few cases of gastrointestinal anthrax occurred, resulting in approximately 100 deaths. This outbreak was related to an extensive epizootic infection in cattle. Another major outbreak of anthrax occurred in Siberia in 1979. It was initially thought by some to be related to inhalation, perhaps relative to the explosion of a germ-warfare facility, but more recently the route of infection has been identified as the ingestion and handling of infected "black market" meat. The source of anthrax in the cattle in this epidemic appeared to be a single 29-ton lot of bone meal used as animal feed that likely was made from the bones of animals that had died of anthrax the previous year.

Very rare cases of inhalation anthrax have developed in workers exposed to aerosolized anthrax spores generated during the processing of contaminated materials such as woolens, hides, or bone meal, and even more rarely in people who have simply been in the vicinity of a wool-processing mill or tannery but who were not directly involved in the processing of the product. Cases have even been reported in home weavers, such as those using contaminated goat yarn, or in individuals working with contaminated bone meal fertilizer.

In the United States, the average annual occurrence has diminished. From 1977 to 1988, the number of cases was only 0.8, as opposed to 127 cases reported to occur annually between 1916 and 1925. The case fatality rate of the 221 U.S. cases of cutaneous anthrax from 1955 to 1986 was approximately 5.0% (11 of 221), whereas the case fatality rate was 82% in the patients with inhalation anthrax (9 of 11). The overall mortality rate in these 232 American cases of anthrax was 8.6%.

EPIDEMIOLOGY. Cases of anthrax are classified generally as either agricultural or industrial. Most of the agricultural cases of human anthrax result from direct contact with contaminated discharges from infected animals. Occasional human cases have been transmitted by bites of flies that have fed on the carcasses of animals dead of anthrax. Others have been caused by ingestion of poorly cooked or raw infected meat. Industrial cases usually result from contact with anthrax spores contaminating animal products, such as goat hair, wool, hides, and animal bones, especially those imported from areas of high endemicity. Transmission usually occurs during the processing of these animal products, either by direct contact with the contaminated raw material or by indirect contact with a contaminated environment; rarely, transmission may occur from airborne particles produced during the manufacturing process. Because the *B. anthracis* spores can survive for long periods, a wide variety of unusual products have been associated with human infection, such as imported bongo drums made with goat skins, shaving brushes, various leather or woolen blankets, and ivory piano keys. Laboratory-acquired infections have been reported; however, human-to-human transmission of anthrax is not thought to occur.

Most cases of anthrax in the United States are sporadic, but occasional epidemics have been reported. In 1957, the largest and most serious of these occurred in New Hampshire, where nine employees of a textile mill acquired anthrax while processing a batch of contaminated goat hair imported from Asia. This outbreak included four cutaneous cases and five inhalation cases, with four fatalities reported in the latter group.

PATHOGENESIS. The virulence of *B. anthracis* is determined by both a plasmid-mediated group of exotoxins (plasmid pX01) and another plasmid-mediated antiphagocytic polydiglutamic acid capsule (plasmid pX02). Three toxic proteins (exotoxins) have been identified and cloned, including a protective antigen (PA), an edema factor (EF), and a lethal factor (LF). A combination of two of these proteins (PA and EF) has been demonstrated to decrease polymorphonuclear neutrophil function, suggesting that this is one of the ways that host susceptibility to infection with *B. anthracis* may be increased.

Furthermore, a combination of PA and EF causes local edema, whereas the combination of PA and LF may cause death in as little as 60 minutes. None of these three toxins, when administered alone, has any biologic effect in experimental animals. Protective antigen is able to bind to cell-surface receptors, in turn enabling them to be used by both EF and LF to reach the cytoplasm. Recently, EF has been found to be related to its ability to increase cyclic AMP. EF, in fact, is a calmodulin-dependent adenylate cyclase, and it is likely that the edema is produced through this mechanism.

As noted, virulent strains of *B. anthracis* contain two large plasmids, pX01 and pX02, both of which are necessary for virulence. Strains that contain only one of these plasmids are totally avirulent.

In cutaneous anthrax, the organism is introduced either through a wound or by means of infected animal fibers that disrupt the skin. The organism is not known to penetrate intact skin. Once in the subcutaneous tissue, the anthrax spore is thought to germinate, multiply, and produce both its exotoxin and the antiphagocytic capsular material. The toxins are capable of provoking a marked edematous response and tissue necrosis with a paucity of neutrophil invasion. Phagocytosis of the organisms by local macrophages occurs, and these bacilli are then spread to regional lymph nodes, where further production of toxins produces a hemorrhagic, necrotic, and edematous lymphadenitis. Bacilli may enter the circulation, at times producing meningitis, pneumonia, and systemic toxicity.

Inhalation anthrax is fortunately a very uncommon clinical presentation of anthrax, as it is associated with close to 100% mortality. In the United States, inhalation anthrax is now essentially obsolete, with only two cases reported during the past 25 years; however, this is still a cause of significant disease in many parts of the world. A major current concern is the possibility of the use of *B. anthracis* as a biologic weapon for the production of the inhalation form of anthrax. Inhalation anthrax, commonly known as woolsorter's disease, occurs not as a result of direct contact with infected animals but rather by inhalation of an aerosol of spores in particle sizes less than 5 μm. These aerosols usually occur during processing of contaminated material. In humans, spores are inhaled, reach the alveoli, and may then eventually be phagocytized by macrophages and carried by these cells to the mediastinal lymph nodes. Germination, growth, and toxin formation at this site can produce severe, massive hemorrhagic lymphadenitis and mediastinitis. *B. anthracis* may also directly affect the pulmonary capillary endothelium, causing thrombosis and respiratory failure. Pleural effusion is common. Anthrax is not thought to cause primary pneumonia, but secondary bacterial pneumonia may complicate inhalation anthrax. *B. anthracis* may also enter the bloodstream from this site, with the evolution of intense bacteremia. The number of organisms per milliliter of blood may be so great that in some instances the organism may be seen on smears of the peripheral blood. Hemorrhagic meningitis may ensue. Respiratory failure, shock, and pulmonary edema are frequent causes of death.

Ingestion of markedly contaminated, poorly cooked meat may result in either the oropharyngeal or the gastrointestinal form of infection. When oropharyngeal anthrax occurs, there is localized swelling of the pharynx, sometimes causing tracheal obstruction, and marked cervical adenopathy with overlying brawny edema. Similarly, the organism may reach the small and large intestines and cause a gastrointestinal syndrome. In this case, the spores that are deposited in the submucosa of the intestinal tract may germinate, multiply, and produce toxin, again resulting in marked edema, hemorrhage, and necrosis. Regional mesenteric lymphadenopathy is common, and findings associated with the syndrome include fever, vomiting, abdominal pain and distention, massive bloody diarrhea, mesenteric adenitis, hemorrhagic ascites, and septicemia. Gastrointestinal anthrax is a very severe form of the disease, has a high mortality rate (25 to 75%), and is rarely diagnosed during life except in the setting of an epidemic.

Although antimicrobial agents may rapidly eradicate the organism, the persistence of the toxin that has been produced may result in continued development of the disease process until the toxin is

metabolized. Thus, although the mortality rate may be diminished by appropriate antibiotic therapy, especially in the cutaneous form of the disease, the clinical process may continue to progress even after the institution of antimicrobial therapy. Antitoxins have been tried by some in the past, but such antitoxins are not currently available.

CLINICAL MANIFESTATIONS. Cutaneous anthrax is the most common form of the disease in humans, accounting for more than 95% of cases. After an incubation period of 1 to 7 days, the infection generally begins with a small, somewhat pruritic papule at the site of an abrasion, which over the next several days develops into a vesicle containing serosanguineous fluid teeming with organisms. The lesion generally occurs on the upper extremities, especially the arms and hands, or on the face, neck, or other areas that are likely to be exposed to the contaminated animal product or infected soil. As the lesion progresses, ulceration occurs, with formation of a necrotic ulcer base frequently surrounded by smaller vesicles. The characteristic black eschar evolves over several weeks to a size of several centimeters, gradually separating and leaving a scar. This black eschar accounts for the name *anthrax,* which comes from the Greek word for coal. The edema is frequently nonpitting, gelatinous, and brawny and is very striking. It may be quite extensive, spreading over a wide area in severe cases. With involvement near the eye, periorbital swelling may be especially intense. The edema may be so dramatic that hypotension occurs in part because of the loss of intravascular volume as fluid enters the subcutaneous tissues. This edema, in combination with the vesicle progressing to the necrotic black eschar, forms the lesion that is highly characteristic of anthrax. Despite the dramatic appearance of the lesion, it is frequently painless.

In association with the localized cutaneous lesion, most patients have minimal constitutional findings, such as fever, malaise, myalgias, and headaches. In those with extensive edema, the systemic symptoms may be more severe. Localized lymphadenopathy may occur at times and may be complicated by bacteremia and even meningitis. Death is rare if appropriate antimicrobial therapy is instituted; in untreated cases of cutaneous anthrax, however, the mortality rate remains about 25%.

Bacterial adenitis due to staphylococci and streptococci, tularemia, plague, orf, cat-scratch disease, localized herpes, and ecthyma gangrenosum are diagnostic considerations, and lesions seen in these diseases may be confused with those of anthrax. The diagnosis of cutaneous anthrax will rarely be missed if the disease is considered in any patient who has had exposure to an appropriate animal or animal product and who develops a painless ulcer surrounded by small vesicles, along with marked edema and eschar formation. Gram stains of the vesicular fluid and lesion usually readily demonstrate the characteristic gram-positive bacilli, as the organisms are present in large numbers in these lesions and are readily isolated by culture. Informing the bacteriology laboratory of the possibility of the diagnosis of anthrax is important to prevent the organism from being discarded as merely a probable contaminant of *Bacillus* species, which is frequently not fully characterized. At times, secondary bacterial infection may occur in these ulcers. Rarely, more than one lesion may be present, resulting from coprimary infections.

Inhalation anthrax is very rare, usually fatal, and extremely difficult to diagnose. The incubation period in this syndrome is generally 1 to 6 days, and the illness is generally biphasic in its presentation. Initially, a brief, non-specific "influenza-like" illness occurs, manifested by fever, fatigue, myalgias, malaise, a non-productive cough, and at times some chest discomfort. Few physical findings are noted at this time; however, within several days after a short period of clinical improvement, the patient becomes much more ill. This second phase is manifested by severe dyspnea, cyanosis, hypoxia, hemoptysis, stridor, chest pain, and diaphoresis. Physical examination may reveal some crepitant rales and evidence of pleural effusions. Fever, tachycardia, and trachypnea are common. Some subcutaneous brawny edema of the chest wall and neck may be noted. The chest radiograph in these patients shows a rather distinctive clinical finding, namely, a widened mediastinum without a definite infiltrate. Bacteremia, shock, and meningitis are frequently present, and death generally follows within 1 to 2 days of the onset of the respiratory distress. The mortality rate is 80 to 100%, even with appropriate therapy.

Inhalation anthrax should be considered in patients with appropriate exposure to an animal product, as in a weaver using imported goat hair or a textile mill worker. It must also be considered in the setting of potential germ warfare or biologic terrorism. The most important clue is the presence of an appropriate epidemiologic history in a patient developing severe respiratory distress and a rapidly enlarging mediastinum.

Gastrointestinal anthrax is a rare disease. It has an incubation period of 2 to 5 days, although there are some cases in which a more prolonged incubation period has been postulated. The diagnosis is rarely suspected before death except in areas where anthrax is highly endemic and in which multiple human cases are occurring. The symptoms include severe abdominal pain, hematemesis, melena, rapid onset of ascites, and, at times, marked diarrhea. Paracentesis may reveal hemorrhagic ascites, and sometimes these cases may simulate an "acute" or "surgical abdomen." The disease usually progresses to bacteremia, toxemia, shock, and eventually death in many patients. No cases of intestinal anthrax have been reported in the United States.

Oropharyngeal anthrax presents as severe sore throat with neck swelling, adenopathy, dysphagia, and at times tracheal compression and dyspnea. Cervical and submandibular lymphadenopathy is common. Again, bacteremia and its complications may ensue.

Meningitis is a relatively rare complication of any of the forms of anthrax and almost never is found without a primary focus of infection. It is frequently hemorrhagic and most often fatal.

DIAGNOSIS. The clinician who elicits a careful epidemiologic history and who has a high index of suspicion of anthrax will not have problems establishing the diagnosis in cutaneous anthrax and will even be alert to the rarer and more difficult to recognize cases of inhalation, gastrointestinal, or oropharyngeal anthrax.

Inhalation anthrax is rarely suspected before death and only if an epidemiologic history of aerosol exposure is obtained or if an epidemic is recognized. The major finding in the clinical evaluation, other than epidemiologic history, is the presence of a widened mediastinum or, at times, hemorrhagic pleural effusions or associated hemorrhagic meningitis. Ordinarily, Gram stains of sputum and cultures do not demonstrate *B. anthracis*. These patients frequently do develop bacteremia, however, and in these cases the organism can be readily isolated and sometimes seen on stains of the peripheral blood.

A number of serologic tests are available to diagnose anthrax retrospectively, but many of these very ill patients die so quickly that the initial serologic studies may not be especially helpful to the clinician. In some cases, however, serology has been a helpful diagnostic tool, especially when prior antibiotics have eradicated the bacteria before cultures or smears were obtained. Current serologic tests considered valuable include an enzyme-linked immunosorbent assay (ELISA), which detects antibodies to the capsular antigen, and an electrophoretic immunotransblot test, which detects antibodies to the PA exotoxin. Both of these serologic tests are quite sensitive and specific enough to be useful, but the test for antibody to the PA exotoxin may be more specific.

TREATMENT. Penicillin G is the drug of choice for treatment of anthrax. Only a few isolates of *B. anthracis* have been identified as resistant to penicillin G. In cutaneous anthrax, cultures of the infected blisters have become negative for the organism within 5 hours of the patient's receiving 2 million units of penicillin G. As previously mentioned, however, the presence of the toxin may persist, and the cutaneous lesion frequently goes through its various phases of evolution, even though the organism has been eradicated and the mortality rate reduced.

For cutaneous anthrax, intravenous penicillin G is given, 4 million units every 6 hours for several days, followed by a 7- to 10-day course of oral penicillin G. In patients with severe, overwhelming edema, corticosteroids have been thought by some to be helpful, although no controlled studies of their use have been performed. Severe neck swelling may require intubation or tracheostomy. In patients who are allergic to penicillin, effective alternatives include ciprofloxacin, tetracycline, streptomycin, erythromycin, and chloramphenicol. No local surgery should be performed on these patients, because no pus requiring drainage is usually present

and excision of the lesion has been reported to increase the risk of organism spread. The lesion should be covered with a sterile dressing. No definite cases have been reported of spread of anthrax from human to human.

In inhalation, gastrointestinal, or oropharyngeal anthrax or in anthrax meningitis, high dosages of intravenous penicillin G, in the range of 24 million units/day, or intravenous ciprofloxacin 500 mg every 8 to 12 hours, are recommended, along with excellent supportive care for the problems of hypotension and respiratory distress. Some suggest that ciprofloxacin should be selected as the initial drug of choice for inhalation anthrax until susceptibility test results are available. When the patient is hospitalized, good infection control practices are required. Soiled dressings must be incinerated or autoclaved.

PROGNOSIS. Inhalation anthrax is considered to be fatal in 80 to 100% of cases, and gastrointestinal anthrax has a case fatality rate of 25 to 75%. The case fatality rate for cutaneous anthrax is 20 to 25% without treatment but generally is less than 1% with appropriate treatment.

PREVENTION. Control of anthrax in animals is essential to control of the disease in humans. All cases of anthrax (animal as well as human) should be reported to the state health department or the appropriate veterinary agency. Live avirulent animal vaccines are effective and may help control anthrax in endemic areas. Animals dead of anthrax should be cremated or buried, and care must be taken at autopsy to avoid additional environmental contamination by infected blood and tissues. Human anthrax can be partially prevented by proper disposal of the infected animals. In addition, formaldehyde has been used successfully to decontaminate raw wool and hair. A cell-free filtrate vaccine has been shown to protect humans from anthrax and is available from the Michigan State Department of Health. This vaccine should be offered to workers likely to be exposed to contaminated animal products in high-risk industries.

The United States military has decided to vaccinate more than 2 million members of the armed forces against anthrax in view of the threat of biologic warfare or terrorism. Even wider use of an anthrax vaccine may be necessary in the future. A protective antibody response does not develop until 7 days after the second dose of vaccine. The vaccine is well tolerated and has been shown to be highly effective in rhesus monkeys after a lethal aerosol challenge. It is given at 0, 2, and 4 weeks and at 6, 12, and 18 months. An annual booster is required to maintain immunity. For emergency use after aerosol exposure to anthrax, the vaccine should be given promptly and again 2 weeks later. In addition after exposure oral doxycycline, 100 mg twice daily, or ciprofloxacin, 500 mg twice daily, should be given for at least 30 days.

Newer vaccines are being evaluated, such as a PA toxoid vaccine and a PA-producing live vaccine. In the former Soviet Union, in addition to the chemical vaccine, a live anthrax spore vaccine has been widely used for prophylaxis against anthrax in both humans and animals.

Because none of the currently available vaccines is ideal, efforts at developing better agents are a major area of research. Among the newer approaches for anthrax vaccine development for human use are (1) combination of the PA with adjuvants derived from the BCG strain or killed cells of *Bordetella pertussis* and (2) PA cloned into a *Bacillus subtilis* as a recombinant vaccine that does not contain the *B. anthracis* genome.

Good personal hygiene, as well as the use of protective clothing and respirators when contaminated aerosols are likely to be encountered, may also prove to be helpful preventive measures. Gastrointestinal anthrax can be prevented by proper cooking of meat and by avoiding ingestion of potentially contaminated meat. Care must be taken by the laboratory personnel working with *B. anthracis*, because cases of anthrax have been acquired in this setting.

Anthrax vaccine. Med Lett 40:52, 1998. *Good discussion of currently available vaccine and primary prevention as well as prevention after exposure.*

Farrar E: Anthrax: Virulence and vaccines. Ann Intern Med 121:379, 1994. *Excellent editorial outlining newer molecular biologic features of* B. anthracis *and the role of virulence factors in pathogenesis of the disease produced; also highlights new approaches to vaccine development.*

Harrison LH, Ezzell JW, Abshire TG, et al: Evaluation of serologic tests for diagnosis of anthrax after an outbreak of cutaneous anthrax in Paraguay. J Infect Dis 160:706, 1989. *Serologic methods for diagnosis and detection of immunity.*

Ivins BE, Welkos SL: Recent advances in the development of an improved human anthrax vaccine. Eur J Epidemiol 4:12, 1988. *An approach to vaccines for anthrax.*

Ivins BE, Welkos SL, Little SF, et al: Immunization against anthrax with *Bacillus* anthracis protective antigen combined with adjuvants. Infect Immun 60:662, 1992. *Discusses the protective efficacy of immunization against anthrax with B. anthracis protective antigen combined with different adjuvants.*

Knudson GB: Treatment of anthrax in man: History and current concepts. Milit Med 151:71, 1986. *Reviews history of anthrax with emphasis on treatment.*

Shlyakov EN, Rubenstein E: Human live anthrax vaccine in the former USSR. Vaccine 12:727, 1994. *Describes the history of the development and use of the Soviet live spore human anthrax vaccine.*

351 DISEASES CAUSED BY PSEUDOMONADS

Stephen C. Schimpff

PSEUDOMONADS. Pseudomonads are gram-negative aerobic bacilli that prefer moist environments and are relatively non-invasive yet can cause serious and often fatal infection when the host defense mechanism is damaged or deficient. Each species is different in its pathogenic properties, each causes somewhat different types of infection, and each invades as a result of different host defense defects; but with each pseudomonad, the environmental source is usually water, moist soil, or a contaminated medical device, infusion, or injection.

Pseudomonads are divided into five major groups based on RNA homology (Table 351–1). Most human infections are caused by members of groups I, II, and V. For purposes of discussion, this chapter considers *Pseudomonas pseudomallei* (the cause of melioidosis), *Pseudomonas mallei* (the cause of glanders), *Pseudomonas aeruginosa* (which principally causes bacteremia, endocarditis, pneumonia, keratitis, and urinary tract infections), and *Pseudomonas cepacia, Pseudomonas pickettii,* and *Xanthomonas (Pseudomonas) maltophilia* (which cause bacteremia, pseudobacteremia, endocarditis, and urinary tract infections). Many of the pseudomonads have been reclassified based on genetic characteristics. *Pseudomonas maltophilia* (RNA group I) became *Xanthomonas maltophilia* over a decade ago and now is known as *Stenotrophomonas maltophilia;* and, recently, the RNA group II organisms became *Burkholderia mallei, pseudomallei, cepacia,* and *pickettii,* respectively. For convenience, both nomenclatures are used here.

PSEUDOMONAS (BURKHOLDERIA) PSEUDOMALLEI. This organism causes melioidosis, which is often characterized as a glanders-like infectious disease. It was first described in Rangoon among debilitated morphine addicts. The term *melioidosis* means "a similarity to distemper of asses." Despite the clinical resemblance to glanders, it has a totally different epidemiology. Melioidosis occurs in animals and humans in endemic areas of southeast Asia and northern Australia and has now been recognized to occur in epidemic-like form in specific areas, given the combination of the environment (an appropriate rainy season with water-covered rice paddies) and a susceptible host (abraded skin in barefoot farmers who have a high prevalence of diabetes mellitus, renal disease, or both). Melioidosis has been detected in a few patients in India (who had not traveled to known endemic areas) and occasionally in Central and South America. The organism also has been isolated in multiple areas of southern and coastal China.

P. (B.) pseudomallei is a gram-negative, motile, aerobic bacillus that is small and may grow in filamentous chains. Staining with methylene blue or Wright's stain shows a bipolar "safety pin" pattern. *P. pseudomallei* has a characteristic wrinkling appearance of the colonies on agar if held long enough. The organism, like most pseudomonads, can be isolated from soil and water and particularly streams, rice paddies, and ponds of the endemic areas and on plants, including commonly consumed vegetables. Most human infection probably occurs through skin abrasions. In endemic areas, the organism is easy to culture from soil samples of flooded rice paddies and is still detectable during dry seasons from deep soil samples that are moist. However, laboratory animals have been found to become infected by the respiratory route, so inhalation may be a possible human route of acquisition, which would explain the occurrence of primary pneumonia. Both this pathogen and *P. (B.) mallei* have a polysaccharide biopolymer capsule that adversely affects phagocytosis.

At the conclusion of U. S. involvement in the Vietnam War, 343 cases were reported, with 36 deaths; however, serologic surveys suggest that either mild or inapparent infection may be fairly common, with positive serologies found in 1 to 2% of healthy, non-wounded Army troops returning to the United States. This would suggest that as many as 225,000 military personnel may have had subclinical infection with *P. (B.) pseudomallei.* The importance of this observation is that recrudescence of disease, usually as cavitary pneumonia, has been observed many years after primary infection.

In addition to inapparent infection or asymptomatic pulmonary infection, the frequently observed forms of melioidosis are an acute, localized, suppurative soft tissue infection, an acute pulmonary infection, and an acute septicemic presentation. The localized infections are probably related to skin abrasion, with development of a nodule with secondary lymphangitis and regional lymphadenitis. An apparent primary pulmonary infection ranges from bronchitis to necrotizing pneumonia. The patient with pneumonia usually has high fever and signs and symptoms of consolidation, ordinarily in an upper lobe. It is an acute pyogenic process, frequently leading to early cavitation and giving a pulmonary appearance consistent with tuberculosis. Progression to bacteremia is rare. In Singapore, *P. (B.) pseudomallei* is the cause of a small but important percentage of the severe community-acquired pneumonia cases that require hospitalization.

Patients with the acute septic form characteristically present with a short history of fever and no clinical evidence of focal infection, although skin abrasion is the presumed site of origin. Most are profoundly ill, with signs of sepsis, such as tachypnea or Kussmaul's breathing, and occasional evidence of septic shock. Clinical and radiologic evidence frequently demonstrates progression to diffuse bilateral and patchy pulmonary infiltrate, which progresses to abscess and cavity formation if the patient survives. Subcutaneous abscesses are relatively uncommon but can occur at multiple sites. Liver abscess, usually multiple, is not uncommon and is accompanied in more than 50% by multiple splenic abscesses, a combination unlikely for most other causes of liver abscess.

The diagnosis should be considered in any patient living in an endemic area who has a febrile illness and especially one occupationally at risk and, perhaps, at further risk of sepsis because of diabetes or renal disease. The diagnosis is highly suggested in such an individual with a rapidly progressive, extensive pulmonary process if subcutaneous lesions are present or in one whose condition progresses to a cavitary form indistinguishable from tuberculosis. Although frequently negative, a Gram stain of pulmonary or abscess exudate may show small gram-negative bacilli and methylene blue staining shows the characteristic bipolar "safety pin." The organism grows on standard media and is usually detected in blood cultures within 48 hours. Efforts are underway to create rapid

Table 351–1 ■ CLASSIFICATION OF PSEUDOMONADS THAT HAVE BEEN ISOLATED FROM CLINICAL SPECIMENS

GROUP/SUBGROUP	GENUS AND SPECIES
RNA group I	
Fluorescent group	P. aeruginosa
	P. fluorescens
	P. putida
Non-fluorescent group	P. stutzeri
	P. alcaligenes
	P. pseudoalcaligenes
RNA group II	P. (Burkholderia) mallei
	P. (Burkholderia) pseudomallei
	P. (Burkholderia) cepacia
	P. (Burkholderia) pickettii
RNA group III	P. acidovorans
	P. testosteroni
RNA group IV	P. diminuta
	P. vesicularis
RNA group V	Xanthomonas (Stenotrophomonas) maltophilia

From Sanford JP: *Pseudomonas* species (including melioidosis and glanders). *In* Mandell GL, Dolin R, Bennett JE (eds): Principles and Practice of Infectious Diseases, 4th ed. New York, Churchill Livingstone, 1995, pp 2003–2009. Modified to recognize new nomenclatures of RNA groups II and V.

immunoassays to detect antigen in urine or antibody in serum or to identify the organism in specimens or early cultures.

In northeast Thailand, a report from a hospital serving a population of nearly 2 million rural rice farming families determined that about 20% of all community-acquired bacteremias were caused by *P. (B.) pseudomallei* and that during the rainy season, when the paddy fields are under water (from June to September), *P. (B.) pseudomallei* was the single most common organism isolated from blood culture, representing nearly one half of all documented cases of community-acquired bacteremia in the month of August (Fig. 351–1). An interesting observation was the higher than expected frequency of both diabetes mellitus and renal calculi in patients with sepsis who are from this region, where both diabetes and calculi are common.

Pulmonary and septic disease have a very high mortality and, hence, when suspected, should be treated aggressively with intravenous ceftazidime (imipenem or piperacillin as acceptable substitutes). Treatment needs to be prolonged, including intravenous therapy for 2 to 4 weeks, followed by oral therapy (perhaps amoxicillin-clavulanic acid) for 6 months or longer to prevent recrudescence.

The prognosis for patients with localized disease should be excellent with appropriate therapy. However, those with the septicemic form are often gravely ill at the time of admission, and the mortality rate, even with current therapy, is about 40%. Patients with the highest mortality include those who are hypothermic, azotemic, or unable to produce a leukocytosis. Prompt early therapy with ceftazidime has now been found to reduce the mortality by 50% when historically compared with combination therapy with chloramphenicol, doxycycline, and cotrimoxazole as used before 1987. Relapses are common, perhaps 25% overall, with clinical severity and initial therapy the crucial risk factors (Fig. 351–2). Long-term oral treatment with amoxicillin–clavulanic acid appears logical to reduce relapses, since recurrence carries a high mortality rate.

PSEUDOMONAS (BURKHOLDERIA) MALLEI. P. (B.) mallei can cause an infection in horses, mules, and donkeys that occasionally has been transmitted to humans. The name "glanders" comes from the prominent pulmonary involvement, although the infection can, instead, be characterized by subcutaneous ulcerative lesions or lymphatic thickening with nodules (known as farcy).

Glanders was never a common human infection, and with the

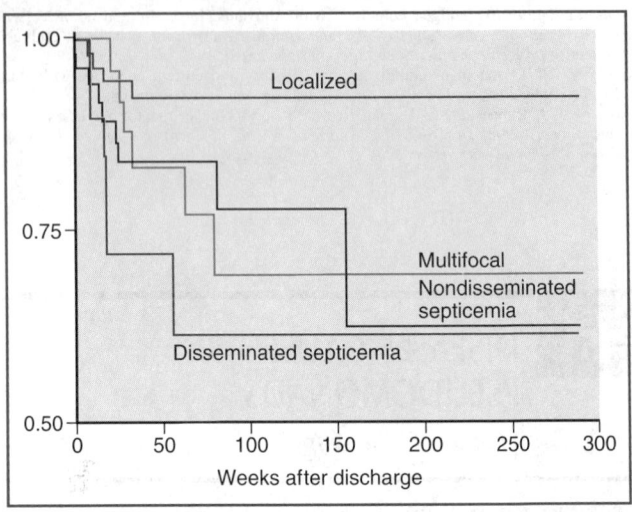

FIGURE 351–2 ■ Relapse-free probability in survivors of acute melioidosis stratified by clinical severity on first admission. (From Chaowagul, W, Suputtamongkol Y, Dance DAB, et al: Relapse in melioidosis: Incidence and risk factors. J Infect Dis 168:1181, 1993.)

decline in the use of horses for day-to-day activities and with improved sanitation, glanders has become a very rare disease. Apparently, there have been no naturally acquired infections in the United States since 1938, although the occasional case occurs in other countries. Glanders was used as a form of biologic warfare in World War I with deliberate infection of animals near the front lines.

Like melioidosis, glanders tends to occur as an acute localized suppurative infection, an acute pulmonary infection, an acute septicemic infection, or a chronic suppurative infection. An abraded area of skin may lead to a local nodule with acute lymphangitis. Inoculation into an abraded mucous membrane can lead to extensive ulcerating granulomatous lesions. These forms of infection seem to have an incubation period of 1 to 5 days; in contrast, after inhalation, a primary pneumonia tends to develop 10 to 14 days later. Symptoms are relatively non-specific and include fever, occasional rigors, malaise, fatigue, and headache. Examination findings depend on the form of infection. Leukocytosis is common. Chest radiographs of the acute pulmonary form usually show densities consistent with early lung abscess; however, lobar or bronchopneumonia-type infiltrates are common. Chronic suppurative disease involves multiple subcutaneous and intramuscular abscesses, especially on the extremities, with lymphatic involvement and, in many, a nasal discharge with or without ulceration.

The organism is usually difficult to find in exudates but when seen with a Gram stain or methylene blue appears similar to *P. (B.) pseudomallei*. It is reasonably easy to cultivate.

The treatment of glanders is uncertain because of its rarity, hence the inability to carry out clinical trials. A reasonable recommendation is to initiate therapy with regimens found effective for melioidosis, recognizing that the acute septicemic form has been uniformly fatal and suggesting that full dosage of intravenous combinations of agents be given initially.

PSEUDOMONAS AERUGINOSA. The name *aeruginosa* comes from the fluorescent blue-green pigment pyocyanin produced by many, but not all, strains. Like other pseudomonads, *P. aeruginosa* grows well in multiple moist settings with limited nutrients. Found in soil, in water, and on plants, it also can be a normal commensal in animals and humans. Colonization in humans usually takes place in moist areas, such as the perineum, auditory canal, axillae, and the lower alimentary canal. It is commonly found in faucet aerators, sink traps, ice machines, and kitchen settings in the hospital; it can become a particular problem when it contaminates medications or medical devices with a moist environment, such as ventilators, endoscopes, or pressure monitors. It can withstand many disinfectants and is resistant to a broad variety of antimicrobial agents. In the non-hospital setting, infections have been related to growth in swimming pools, contact lens solutions, and hot tubs.

Infection with *P. aeruginosa* has become, to a large degree, a by-product of medical advances in technology. In the 20 years

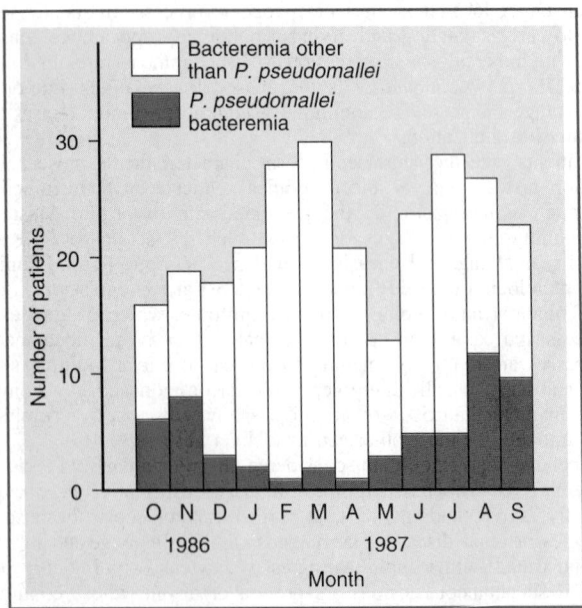

FIGURE 351–1 ■ Number of persons with community-acquired bacteremia caused by *P. (B.) pseudomallei* and other organisms in northeast Thailand from October 1986 to September 1987. (From Chaowagul W, White NJ, Dance DAB, et al: Melioidosis: A major cause of community-acquired septicemia in northeastern Thailand. J Infect Dis 159:890, 1989; by permission of the University of Chicago Press, 1989.)

before 1960 at the Johns Hopkins Hospital, only 91 cases of *P. aeruginosa* bacteremia occurred. In recent years, *P. aeruginosa* has been the fourth most common cause of primary nosocomial gram-negative bacteremia and the fourth most frequently isolated nosocomial pathogen, causing about 10% of all hospital-acquired infections nationwide.

The most common infections caused by *P. aeruginosa* include nosocomial bacteremia, nosocomial pneumonia, nosocomial urinary tract infection, surgical wound infection, endocarditis related to intravenous drug abuse or placement of artificial heart valves, respiratory tract infection associated with cystic fibrosis, external otitis (including "malignant" external otitis), corneal keratitis, uncommon occurrences of spinal osteomyelitis in heroin addicts (see Chapter 331), and rare cases of meningitis or brain abscess. A common origin of bacteremia in the granulocytopenic patient is infection along the alimentary canal, especially perianal cellulitis, colonic lesions, and, occasionally, pharyngitis or esophagitis. Finally, extensive burns are commonly colonized by *P. aeruginosa,* with progression to sepsis and death.

P. aeruginosa almost never causes infection in the absence of (1) damage to a normal host defense mechanism (e.g., cancer chemotherapy–induced mucosal damage to the alimentary canal, granulocytopenia, or extensive third-degree burns); (2) deficiency or alteration in a defense mechanism (e.g., the progressive respiratory tract changes of cystic fibrosis); or (3) bypass of a normal defense mechanism (e.g., respiratory assist device directly inoculating organisms into the bronchial tree while concurrently limiting or damaging the mucociliary mechanism, or insertion of an indwelling urinary catheter, circumventing the normal bladder clearance mechanism). Thus, infections with *P. aeruginosa* are seen most commonly in patients with a chronic urinary catheter; those neutropenic from disease, chemotherapy, or both; those with cystic fibrosis; those with extensive thermal injuries; those in the intensive-care unit who are subjected to any number of invasive procedures; those with head trauma, allowing entry either directly or by means of a pressure monitoring device; those with artificial heart valves or damaged endocardium from contaminants in illicit drugs; and those who have had extensive surgery, particularly when there is consequent need for open drainage. Pulmonary infection late in the course of the acquired immunodeficiency syndrome may present as an acute infection or as an indolent, frequently recurrent infection mimicking that seen with cystic fibrosis.

Pollack has pointed out three distinct stages of *Pseudomonas* infection: stage I—bacterial attachment and colonization; stage II—local invasion; and stage III—blood stream dissemination and systemic disease. Stage I is a prerequisite to stage II, which, in turn, is a prerequisite to stage III, although obviously not all colonized individuals have local invasion and not all those with local invasion progress to dissemination or systemic disease. The three stages relate to the fact that this organism is both invasive and toxigenic. Colonization in a normal person is relatively uncommon at most sites, although, over time, a fair proportion of the population will have transient colonization of the colon. However, hospitalized patients have a much higher frequency of colonization, related in part to changes in host defenses, as discussed earlier, and partly to the frequency of hospital reservoirs of this organism. In addition, broad-spectrum antimicrobial therapy suppresses other normal microbial flora, especially along the alimentary canal. This suppression reduces the body's normal mechanism of colonization resistance so that an organism such as *P. aeruginosa* or other species resistant to the antibiotics used can more readily colonize multiple locations in high concentration. Additional specific factors further predispose to colonization by *P. aeruginosa.* These include the presence of pili for attachment, flagella for motility, and exoproducts, especially proteinases. Also involved is the secretory protease-induced loss of fibronectin from epithelial cells during serious illness (among patients hospitalized or not), which in turn allows the pili or fimbriae to adhere to the oral, pharyngeal, and respiratory epithelium. Thus, the illness determinants of protease production are major modulators of the oral flora. This colonization in turn can be accentuated by local damage caused by an endotracheal tube, by viral infection (such as influenza), by thermal injury, or by cancer chemotherapy and is exacerbated by antibiotics. *P. aeruginosa,* in some settings, can help protect itself from defense mechanisms by producing a glycocalyx, a carbohydrate produced by many bacteria, which, by surrounding the cell and anchoring it to epithelial cells

or invasive devices such as an intravascular or urinary catheter, protects the bacterium from antibody, complement, and polymorphonuclear leukocytes or macrophages.

After colonization, *P. aeruginosa* can invade in the appropriate setting through the effect of extracellular enzymes (toxins). These include elastase, alkaline protease, cytotoxin, and hemolysins. Elastase and protease have been demonstrated to cause necrotizing lesions in the skin, lung, and cornea, along with small vessel necrotizing lesions, which cause the characteristic skin finding known as ecthyma gangrenosum. It is this combination of local necrosis and blood vessel destruction that is the essence of the initial invasive characteristic of *P. aeruginosa.* Cytotoxin damages granulocytes and may be involved in initial adult respiratory distress syndrome. Hemolysins are cytotoxic as well, thus augmenting tissue invasion.

The third stage of *Pseudomonas* infection, dissemination and systemic disease, is due, in the first case, to these same extracellular enzymes and, in the second case, to *Pseudomonas* liposaccharide (endotoxin) and exotoxin A. As with other septicemias caused by gram-negative bacilli, endotoxin is thought to be a critical factor in the activation of the clotting, fibrinolytic, kinin, and complement systems, along with the production of prostaglandins and leukotrienes, the release of β-endorphins, and the release of cytokines, including tumor necrosis factor. By some interaction of many or all of these factors come fever, shock, disseminated intravascular coagulation (which is relatively uncommon with *Pseudomonas* bacteremia), and the adult respiratory distress syndrome. The other factor, exotoxin A, is similar to diphtheria toxin in that it inhibits protein synthesis. It causes local necrosis and encourages bacterial dissemination to the systemic circulation and, in itself, has been shown to produce shock in animal models.

Pseudomonas bacteremia occurs most commonly in cancer patients who are receiving intensive chemotherapy that produces granulocytopenia, in patients with extensive third-degree burns, and, occasionally, in patients with immunoglobulin or hypocomplementemia states. It is also a common cause of bacteremia in the patient with urinary catheterization. Sepsis in burn patients arises from the thermally damaged skin. Bacteremia in neutropenic patients arises principally from the lower intestinal tract and occasionally from primary pneumonia. Granulocytopenic patients frequently become colonized, and nearly all colonized patients will develop bacteremia if profound (<100 cells/μL) granulocytopenia persists for more than a few days. Ecthyma gangrenosum, usually a sign of fairly advanced systemic infection, is not pathognomonic but is most frequently associated with *P. aeruginosa* bacteremia. These skin lesions at first are small and indurated and then rapidly enlarge, become necrotic, and may ulcerate. Bacteria, on histologic section, are seen to be invading small arteries and veins, with remarkably minimal evidence of inflammation. A histologically similar lesion can be found in the lungs as a secondary consequence of bacteremia. The mortality of *Pseudomonas* sepsis is high, with the underlying status of the patient's host defenses and the promptness of instituting empirical antibiotic therapy being the two critical factors affecting survival. The presence of septic shock, the evidence of septic metastases, or both when antibiotics are started are usually considered adverse prognostic signs but, in reality, represent another measure of late institution of therapy.

The standard approach to suspected gram-negative sepsis, including that caused by *P. aeruginosa,* is a combination using an antipseudomonal β-lactam (penicillin or cephalosporin) with an aminoglycoside. Imipenem and perhaps the antipseudomonal quinolones—again, in combination with an aminoglycoside—are also effective. Although in some cases, such as in the febrile neutropenic patient, monotherapy has been recommended with agents such as ceftazidime or imipenem, a two-drug regimen is advised for initial empirical therapy of the patient with suspected *P. aeruginosa* sepsis. Studies suggest that survival is improved when two antibiotics to which the organism is susceptible are given immediately and that survival is further improved if the two agents prove to be synergistic in activity. For example, in a study of 200 episodes of *P. aeruginosa* bacteremia, most not neutropenic, combination therapy yielded a mortality of 27%, whereas monotherapy mortality was 47%. Finally, imipenem therapy is being increasingly recognized as a predisposition to multiresistant *P. aeruginosa*, especially among organ transplant patients.

Respiratory tract infections (see Chapter 321) can take the form of a primary pneumonia, a secondary pneumonia due to bacteremia, or a chronic infection with intermittent exacerbations. Primary pneumonia occurs almost exclusively in hospitalized patients whose oropharynx or tracheobronchial tree is colonized by *P. aeruginosa*, the latter as a result of intubation. Frequently, *Pseudomonas* pneumonia occurs in the setting of additional pulmonary damage, such as blunt trauma, substantial atelectasis, or hemothorax. Atelectasis appears to be a key contributing pathogenic factor. Early, aggressive physiotherapy for the chest sometimes clears what appears to be a pneumonia but, in fact, is atelectasis that has resulted in fever, purulent sputum production, and a positive chest radiograph. However, once actual pneumonia has begun, the prognosis is poor and early empirical therapy is crucial.

The pneumonia that follows bacteremia is usually fulminant, with multiple areas of hemorrhage around small and medium-sized pulmonary arteries and lesions caused by necrosis of the small muscular arteries and veins in a fashion similar to ecthyma gangrenosum. Survival is limited even with prompt, aggressive therapy.

Chronic *Pseudomonas* respiratory tract infections are largely limited to patients with cystic fibrosis (see Chapter 76), with the frequency of this infection increasing with age so that, ultimately, almost all patients will have significant *Pseudomonas* pulmonary infection. The age differential is probably related to the progressive development of airway obstruction, a crucial factor in development of *Pseudomonas* infection. This chronic infection is associated with chronic cough, nutritional losses, and progressive loss of pulmonary function. The standard treatment has been an antipseudomonal penicillin plus an aminoglycoside. The development of resistance is common, so therapy must be based on susceptibility patterns. Ceftazidime, imipenem, or a quinolone also may be considered. Acute exacerbations may be reduced or even prevented with intermittent therapy a number of times each year, irrespective of whether the infection is currently quiescent.

OTHER PSEUDOMONADS. *PSEUDOMONAS (BURKHOLDERIA) CEPACIA*. This species of *Pseudomonas* can grow as well in distilled water as it can in trypticase soy broth; it is resistant to many of the commonly used hospital disinfectants; it can use penicillin as a carbon source; and it is resistant to many of the commonly used antimicrobials. Its virulence properties are not understood.

Community-acquired infections are rare. However, certain hosts are at substantially increased risk. Endocarditis has occurred among intravenous drug abusers; skin infections related to extensive burns have occurred; a necrotizing, occasionally recurrent pneumonia has occurred among patients with the phagocytic dysfunction of chronic granulomatous disease; and an emerging problem for cystic fibrosis patients has been a relentless, often fulminating pneumonia caused by *P. (B.) cepacia*. Indeed, after *P. aeruginosa*, *P. (B.) cepacia* has

become the second leading cause of chronic progressive lung infection among cystic fibrosis patients in whom it causes major pulmonary deterioriation.

Nosocomial infections and pseudoinfections are considered together because of a common origin and because it can be difficult to distinguish between the two. The source of hospital *P. (B.) cepacia* is usually a moist or water-based reservoir, which, given the technologic advances of medicine, suggests that *P. (B.) cepacia* has the potential to become a not infrequent cause of infection and pseudoinfection in the high-technology or intensive-care setting. *P. (B.) cepacia* has been found to cause pneumonitis, endocarditis, wound infections, and urinary tract infections, along with primary bacteremia. The origins of iatrogenic bacteremia can be conveniently divided into those related to contaminated solutions, injectables, and medical devices. Among the contaminated solutions implicated in bacteremia or pseudobacteremia have been multidose albuterol used with ventilators, disinfectant solutions, heparinized flushing solutions, distilled water, topical anesthetics, and intravenous infusates, including human serum albumin and cryoprecipitate. Contaminated injectables have included saline, methylprednisolone, and fentanyl. The implicated devices all include a moist environment where the organism can multiply; pressure monitoring devices, respiratory assist devices, peritoneal dialysis machines, reusable hemodialysis coils, and blood gas analyzers have been documented as point sources. Dental equipment contamination may be one source of colonization among cystic fibrosis patients.

Figure 351–3 shows an epidemic of *P. (B.) cepacia* bacteremia among patients at the Clinical Center of the National Institutes of Health. The figure indicates *that P. (B.) cepacia*–positive blood cultures were uncommon in the years preceding this outbreak and that the majority during the epidemic occurred within the medical intensive-care unit. A blood gas analyzer in an adjoining laboratory was found to be contaminated, and this served as the point source for this series of bacteremias. Although some were apparently pseudobacteremias (i.e., the blood culture became positive owing to contamination by skin or other sources), others were true bacteremias with significant morbidity. Indeed, among those highly compromised patients, many with cancer and significant immune suppression, the mortality resulting from the *P. (B.) cepacia* infection itself was 38%. Respiratory colonization in an appropriately predisposed host can progress to pneumonia, as evidenced by 14 of 37 patients with colonization and hematologic malignancies who developed pneumonia during an 18-month outbreak. In another outbreak of 14 bacteremias among cancer patients, all had central venous lines flushed with a contaminated heparin solution.

P. (B.) cepacia is resistant to many of the commonly used broad-spectrum antibiotics but is usually susceptible to trimethoprim-sulfamethoxazole and ceftazidime.

***PSEUDOMONAS (BURKHOLDERIA) PICKETTII*.** This is an uncommon cause of infection. In the past 30 years, 49 cases of bacteremia were reported. Thirty-eight of the 49 were caused by contaminated

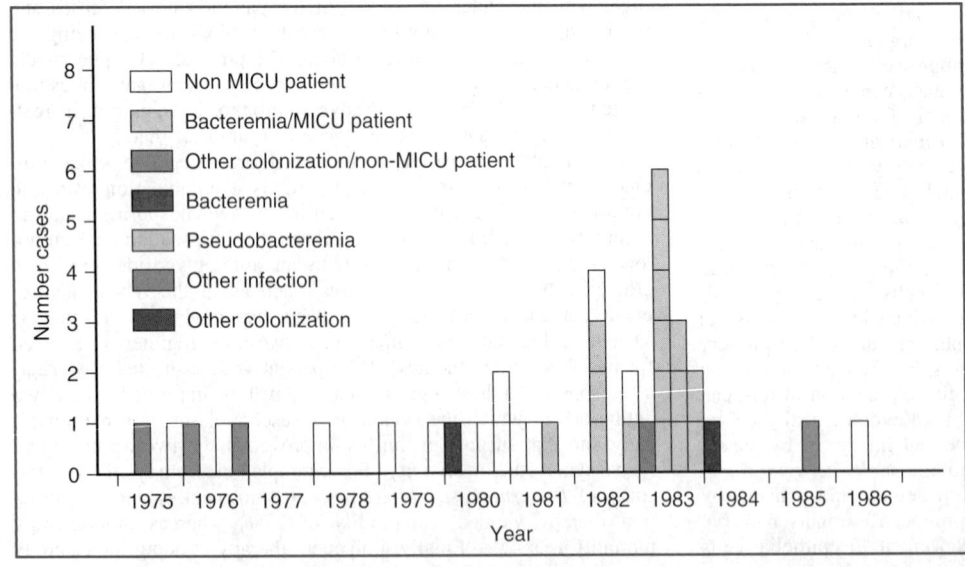

FIGURE 351–3 ■ An epidemic of *Pseudomonas (Burkholderia) cepacia* bacteremia among patients at the Clinical Center of the National Institutes of Health. Note that the epidemic in 1982–1983 within the medical intensive-care unit was caused by a contaminated nearby blood gas analyzer. (From Henderson DK, Baptiste R, Parillo J, et al: Indolent epidemic of *Pseudomonas [Burkholderia] cepacia* bacteremia and pseudobacteremia in an intensive care unit traced to a contaminated blood gas analyzer. Am J Med 84: 75, 1988. With permission from Excerpta Medica, Inc.)

injected solutions; 7 more were related to contaminated ventilators or dialysis equipment. Four patients had bacteremia related to indwelling intravenous catheters; all were treated at one institution over a 2-year period. *P. (B.) pickettii* is usually resistant to aminoglycosides but susceptible to cephalosporins and antipseudomonal penicillins.

XANTHOMONAS MALTOPHILIA (STENOTROPHOMONAS OR PSEUDOMONAS MALTOPHILIA).

X. (Stenotrophomonas) maltophilia is atypical of the other pseudomonads in that the oxidase test is negative or equivocal. It is probably a fairly common commensal and a part of the transient flora, especially of hospitalized patients. In hospitals it is not infrequently found in moist or wet settings. The organism is resistant to most of the first- and second-generation cephalosporins, semisynthetic penicillins, and aminoglycosides, although it has variable susceptibility to the antipseudomonal penicillins. It is generally susceptible to many of the third-generation cephalosporins, trimethoprim-sulfamethoxazole, and rifampin. Synergy has been noted with trimethoprim-sulfamethoxazole plus carbenicillin and with the triple regimen of trimethoprim-sulfamethoxazole plus carbenicillin and rifampin.

X. (S.) maltophilia is an uncommon cause of a wide spectrum of diseases that, in general, are less severe than infections caused by other gram-negative bacilli in similar locations. The most common types of infection are pneumonia, endocarditis, urinary tract infection, and iatrogenic bacteremia or pseudobacteremia. Cholangitis and meningitis have been reported but are quite unusual, and wounds, although a common site for *X. (S.) maltophilia* isolation, are rarely infected by this organism. Pneumonias tend to occur in debilitated patients with prior antibiotic therapy in a nosocomial setting, but they are very uncommon, and the organism should be questioned as causative in the absence of a pure culture by means of bronchoscopy, thoracentesis, or blood. Endocarditis in the community occurs among intravenous drug abusers and in the hospital as a complication of open-heart surgery, usually among those with abnormal valves. Traumatized victims, especially with contaminated wounds, develop serious infections in association with ventilatory assist and broad-spectrum antimicrobial agents. *X. (S.) maltophilia* is being increasingly recognized as a cause of serious infection (pneumonia, bacteremia, and urinary tract and wound infection) among transplant patients and cancer patients who are granulocytopenic and have received broad-spectrum antibiotics, especially imipenem.

X. (S.) maltophilia bacteriuria is found occasionally in patients with indwelling long-term catheters; however, only rarely has the organism been shown to cause clinical infection. When infection has occurred, it has usually been in association with significant instrumentation, genitourinary surgery, or both. The morbidity has tended to be low, and therapy, especially with trimethoprim-sulfamethoxazole, has frequently been effective.

Iatrogenic bacteremia and pseudobacteremia caused by this organism have been reported often. In one epidemic of 25 patients with positive blood cultures, it was determined that these cases were pseudobacteremias due to contaminated blood collection tubes. In another setting, eight children were found to have bacteremia after open-heart surgery, apparently as a result of contamination of the monitoring transducers in the intensive-care unit. *X. (S.) maltophilia* has been found to contaminate the deionized water used for diluting disinfectants, and the organism can even survive in the diluted disinfectant. It is important to emphasize that not all of these bacteremias have been "pseudobacteremias"; for example, two fatal cases of endocarditis have been noted as a result of bacteremia caused by a contaminated device or solution. Permanent indwelling vascular catheters are a major source of bacteremias; imipenem therapy is an important predisposing factor.

Bodey GP, Jadeja L, Elting L: *Pseudomonas* bacteremia: Retrospective analysis of 410 episodes. Arch Intern Med 145:1621, 1985. *A review of* P. aeruginosa *bacteremia.*

Chaowagul W, Suputtamongkol Y, Dance DAB, et al: Relapse in melioidosis: Incidence and risk factors. J Infect Dis 168:1181, 1993. *A 23% relapse rate was related to initial infection severity and therapy.*

Hamill RJ, Houston ED, Georghiou PR, et al: An outbreak of *Burkholderia* (formerly *Pseudomonas*) *cepacia* respiratory tract colonization and infection associated with nebulized albuterol therapy. Ann Intern Med 122:762, 1995. *The intensive-care unit can be a dangerous place.*

Henderson DK, Baptiste R, Parillo J, et al: Indolent epidemic of *Pseudomonas cepacia* bacteremia and pseudobacteremia in an intensive care unit traced to a contaminated blood gas analyzer. Am J Med 84:75, 1988. *A nice review of bacteremia and pseudobacteremia due to* P. cepacia.

Hilf M, Yu VL, Sharp J, et al: Antibiotic therapy for Pseudomonas aeruginosa bactere-mia: Outcome correlations in a prospective study of 200 patients. Am J Med 87:540, 1989. *A critical evaluation of antimicrobial therapy for* P. aeruginosa *bacteremia suggesting an advantage for combination therapy.*

Marshall WF, Keating MR, Anhalt JP, Steckelberg JM: *Xanthomonas maltophilia:* An emerging nosocomial pathogen. Mayo Clin Proc 64:1097, 1989. *A thorough review.*

Pollack M: *Pseudomonas aeruginosa. In* Mandell GL, Bennett JE, Dolin R (eds): Principles and Practice of Infectious Diseases, 4th ed. New York, Churchill Livingstone, 1995, pp 1980–2003. *A very thorough discussion of the microbiology, epidemiology, pathogenic factors, and clinical syndromes of* P. aeruginosa.

Raveh D, Simhon A, Gimmon Z, et al: Infections caused by *Pseudomonas pickettii* in association with permanent indwelling intravenous devices: Four cases and a review. Clin Infect Dis 17:877, 1993. *A review of the few reported cases of bacteremia by this organism.*

Sanford JP: Pseudomonas species (including melioidosis and glanders). *In* Mandell GL, Bennett JE, Dolin R (eds): Principles and Practice of Infectious Diseases, 4th ed. New York, Churchill Livingstone, 1995, pp 2003–2009. *Broad discussion of melioidosis and glanders by an expert in infections of importance to the U.S. military.*

Spencer RC: The emergence of epidemic, multiple-antibiotic-resistant *Stenotrophomonas (Xanthomonas) maltophilia* and *Burkholderia (Pseudomonas) cepacia.* J Hosp Infect 30(S):453, 1995. *Antibiotic pressure is leading to increased frequency of infection.*

Troillet N, Samore MH, Carmeli Y: Imipenem-resistant *Pseudomonas aeruginosa:* Risk factors and antibiotic susceptibility patterns. Clin Infect Dis 25:1094, 1997. *Discussion of resistance patterns and epidemiology.*

White NJ, Dance DAB, Chaowagul W, et al: Halving of mortality of severe melioidosis by ceftazidime. Lancet 2:697, 1988. *Ceftazidime has had a major impact on mortality.*

352 LISTERIOSIS

Alan M. Stamm

DEFINITION. Listeriosis is an infectious disease caused by the bacterium *Listeria monocytogenes.* The majority of afflicted patients are immunocompromised and present with meningoencephalitis.

ETIOLOGY. *L. monocytogenes* is a gram-positive bacillus but may stain unevenly and/or appear coccoid. It is facultatively anaerobic, non-spore forming, and β-hemolytic on blood agar. It grows optimally at 35 to 37° C, grows less well at temperatures as low as 4° C, and exhibits tumbling motility at 20 to 25° C.

Although at least 16 serotypes of *L. monocytogenes* are identified, each of the types 1/2a, 1/2b, and 4b accounts for about 30% of human disease in the United States. These serotypes are uniformly distributed throughout this country. Six other species of *Listeria* exist, but they are rarely pathogenic for humans.

EPIDEMIOLOGY. *L. monocytogenes* is distributed widely in nature throughout the world. It is recovered from water, soil, decaying vegetation, silage, sewage, insects, crustaceans, fish, birds, and wild and domestic mammals. Sporadic as well as epizootic disease, manifest as meningitis, encephalitis, or spontaneous abortion, occurs in sheep, cattle, and goats. Asymptomatic human intestinal carriage is present in 1 to 5% of normal adults and in 10 to 20% of case contacts.

Neonates and the elderly have the highest attack rates of listeriosis. The genders are equally represented. The incidence of disease is not significantly different across the United States or from one continent to another. Consistent seasonal patterns are noted, with disease occurring most commonly in domestic animals in late winter to early spring and in humans in late summer to early fall. However, the correlation between the number and location of animal cases and human cases is poor in any one region.

Epidemiologic investigations of outbreaks of listeriosis have demonstrated their frequent foodborne etiology. Manure from infected sheep was used to fertilize cabbage plants in the Maritime Provinces of Canada; 41 cases of human disease in 1980–1981 were linked to the ingestion of cole slaw prepared from these cabbages. Milk from cows was pasteurized but nonetheless implicated in 49 cases of listeriosis in Massachusetts in 1983; whether the microorganism survived pasteurization or contaminated the product afterward remains controversial. A large epidemic occurred in southern California in 1985; 142 cases were associated with the consumption of soft, Mexican-style cheese made with unpasteurized milk. Similarly, an outbreak of 122 cases in Switzerland during 1983–1987 was attributed to a soft cheese. A doubling in the incidence of listeriosis in the United Kingdom between 1985 and 1989 was linked with paté produced by a single manufacturer. Epidemics in France in 1992 and 1993 involving 279 and 39 individuals, respectively, were both propagated by ready-to-eat pork products. Consumption of contaminated commercial pasteurized chocolate milk at a cow show in Illinois in 1994 resulted in 45 cases of gastroenteritis due to *L. monocytogenes*. During periods of increased disease activity, the organism causing an epidemic is differentiated from that causing sporadic disease by serotyping, electrophoretic enzyme typing, ribotyping, or DNA fingerprinting.

Further evidence for foodborne acquisition of *L monocytogenes* is provided by recent microbiologic investigations. The microorganism has been identified as a fairly common contaminant of raw and pasteurized milk; ice cream; soft cheese; raw beef, pork, and lamb; ready-to-eat meat products, including salami, sausages, paté, and hot dogs; retail poultry; cooked shrimp and crab; raw vegetables such as cabbage, cucumbers, potatoes, and radishes; and packaged salads. Although commercial food production methods may effectively kill the microorganism, products may become contaminated during subsequent processing and packaging before leaving the production facility.

PATHOGENESIS. Most adults with listeriosis have impaired cell-mediated immunity caused by cytotoxic chemotherapy for malignancy, immunosuppressive therapy for organ transplantation, or pregnancy. Both helper and suppressor T cells are centrally involved, whereas immunoglobulin and complement play lesser roles as opsonins. The gastrointestinal tract is the usual portal of entry. Bacteria are taken up from the lumen by endocytosis of epithelial cells covering intestinal villi. The inoculum required to cause disease may depend on the immunologic health and gastric acidity of the host as well as the virulence characteristics of the microorganism.

Dissemination occurs via simple bacteremia and/or circulation of infected monocytes. *L monocytogenes* is a facultative intracellular parasite capable of multiplying within the non-immune monocyte-macrophage. Listeriolysin O, a hemolysin structurally similar to streptolysin O, is an important virulence factor in this process. Phagocytosis of the bacterium stimulates its production; it binds to cholesterol in cell membranes, leading to their disruption. This allows the microorganism to escape from phagolysosomes but to persist and multiply within the cytoplasm. *Listeria* migrate to the periphery, create protrusions of the outer membrane, and are ingested by adjacent cells. Thus, the microorganism spreads directly from cell to cell avoiding the extracellular environment.

CLINICAL MANIFESTATIONS. The incubation period varies from hours to weeks. Recognition of *L. monocytogenes* as a foodborne pathogen has led to the discovery that listeriosis may present as 1 to 2 days of fever, diarrhea, and crampy abdominal pain. However, the traditional spectrum of the disease is meningitis in 50 to 60% of cases; bacteremia without evident localized disease in 25 to 30%; parenchymal disease of the central nervous system (CNS), with or without meningitis, in 10%; and endocarditis in 5%. Infrequent manifestations due to hematogenous dissemination include anterior uveitis, endophthalmitis, cervical lymphadenitis, pneumonia, empyema, myocarditis, pericarditis, peritonitis, hepatitis, liver abscess, cholecystitis, mycotic aneurysm, osteomyelitis, and arthritis.

L. monocytogenes is the cause in about 1% of cases of acute bacterial meningitis. However, among patients with cancer, it is responsible for more than one fifth of episodes. Conversely, among patients with *Listeria* meningitis, 25% have a malignancy; 25% are transplant recipients; 20% have another underlying disorder, such as diabetes mellitus or cirrhosis, or are receiving glucocorticosteroids; and 30% have no predisposing condition. Two thirds of patients experience a fairly sudden onset of symptoms, but one third note an insidious progression over several days. No features distinguish *Listeria* meningitis. High fever is almost always reported. Headache, meningismus, and a decreased level of consciousness are present in more than one half of patients. Focal neurologic deficits and seizures are found in about one fourth. Most patients have 100 to 10,000 white blood cells/mm³ of cerebrospinal fluid (CSF), with two thirds of them being polymorphonuclear cells. The CSF glu-

cose level is less than 50 mg/dL in one half of cases, and the protein level is usually 50 to 300 mg/dL. The Gram stain of CSF is interpreted as revealing gram-positive bacilli in only 25% of cases. Cultures of blood are positive in 60%. The differential diagnosis includes disease due to *Streptococcus pneumoniae,* a gram-negative bacillus, or *Cryptococcus neoformans.*

Parenchymal disease of the CNS is associated with clinical and CSF findings of meningitis in only 50% of cases. Anatomically, the spectrum of disease includes diffuse and localized cerebritis, brain stem meningoencephalitis (rhombencephalitis), and macroscopic abscess formation in the brain or spine. All patients are febrile; other common symptoms and signs are decreased consciousness in two thirds of patients, headache and hemiparesis in one half, and seizures and cranial nerve palsies in one third. *Listeria* rhombencephalitis merits special mention. Eighty per cent of reported victims have been previously healthy. The illness has a biphasic course: a 3- to 10-day prodrome of fever, headache, and vomiting is terminated by the abrupt onset of asymmetrical palsies of cranial nerves V, VI, VII, IX, and/or X, cerebellar signs, paresis, hypesthesia and respiratory failure. In patients without concurrent meningitis, the analysis of CSF is usually normal or reveals only a mild pleocytosis and increased protein; Gram stain and culture are positive in a minority. Blood cultures are positive in most patients with parenchymal CNS disease. The differential diagnosis includes tuberculosis, toxoplasmosis, nocardiosis, mycoses, and stroke.

Bacteremia without evident localized disease (primary bacteremia) occurs in patients with hematologic malignancies (33% of cases), organ transplant recipients (25%), pregnant women (13%), and individuals suffering from alcoholism or cirrhosis (11%). *Listeria* bacteremia has no distinguishing features. Up to one fourth have premonitory gastrointestinal symptoms: nausea, vomiting, abdominal pain, and/or diarrhea.

Endocarditis occurs not in immunocompromised hosts but usually in those with underlying valvular heart disease. The aortic valve is involved in two thirds of cases and the mitral valve in one third, and prosthetic valve disease is well described. The onset of illness is subacute, with a median duration of symptoms before hospitalization of 5 weeks. Fever is cited in 75% of reported cases, a new or changing murmur in 40%, splenomegaly in 35%, and hepatomegaly, CNS emboli, and pulmonary emboli each in 25%.

One third of all cases of listeriosis are associated with pregnancy. Most commonly, in the third trimester, the mother develops a "flu-like" illness with fever, sore throat, myalgias, crampy abdominal pain, and diarrhea. After 3 to 7 days, premature labor or abortion ensues. Transplacental transmission of disease becomes clinically evident in the newborn within hours of delivery; this severe septicemic illness is known as "granulomatosis infantiseptica." Babies also may acquire infection in the birth canal or nosocomially in the nursery; at a mean of 14 days of life, disease presents as anorexia, fever, or meningismus. *L. monocytogenes* is the third most common cause of neonatal sepsis and meningitis after *Escherichia coli* and group B streptococci.

The complete spectrum of listeriosis is seen among patients with acquired immunodeficiency syndrome (AIDS). Chemoprophylaxis of pneumocystosis with trimethoprim/sulfamethoxazole may prevent listeriosis.

DIAGNOSIS. The microbiologic diagnosis of listeriosis is established by culture of blood, CSF, or tissue. In cases of granulomatosis infantiseptica, meconium, amniotic fluid, and lochia are cultured. Initial growth in the laboratory may be slow and require several days. Unwary technicians may misinterpret these gram-positive bacilli as diphtheroids and label them contaminants.

TREATMENT. Ampicillin is the antimicrobial agent of choice for listeriosis. Although no comparative trials have been conducted, it has an established record of efficacy and can be administered safely even during pregnancy and infancy. The standard dosage in patients with meningitis is 200 mg/kg/day in six divided doses given intravenously. The duration of therapy necessary for consistent cure is 3 weeks. Seriously ill and immunocompromised patients are treated with ampicillin plus gentamicin; the latter drug is administered intravenously in doses sufficient to yield peak serum concentrations of 5 to 8 μg/mL and predictable CSF concentrations of 1 to 2 μg/mL. Most in vitro studies and animal model trials suggest that these two drugs act synergistically against *L. monocytogenes.*

Trimethoprim/sulfamethoxazole is the preferred therapy for patients allergic to penicillins. The combination is bactericidal at achievable serum and CSF concentrations. Experience to date suggests an initial dosage of 160 mg of trimethoprim plus 800 mg of sulfamethoxazole given intravenously every 6 to 12 hours in adults with normal renal function. A review of 22 cases from Vandoeuvre, France, suggests that the combination of ampicillin plus trimethoprim/sulfamethoxazole may be even more efficacious than ampicillin plus gentamicin.

The inordinate number of treatment failures and relapses among patients treated with cephalosporins or chloramphenicol indicates that these agents are not to be used. Newer β-lactams, including imipenem, are not as active as ampicillin against *L. monocytogenes*. The quinolones do not appear to be sufficiently active at achievable concentrations to be useful clinically. There has been no significant change in the antimicrobial susceptibility profile of *L. monocytogenes* over the past 25 years.

PROGNOSIS. The overall mortality rate of *Listeria* meningitis is 30%, being higher in patients with cancer, hypoglycorrhachia, or bacteremia and lower in previously healthy individuals. Parenchymal CNS disease and endocarditis are fatal in 50% of cases.

PREVENTION. Individuals at increased risk should avoid raw milk, wash raw vegetables carefully, and cook meats thoroughly. In the hospital, patients with listeriosis should be isolated from immunocompromised hosts.

Dalton CB, Austin CC, Sobel J, et al: An outbreak of gastroenteritis and fever due to *Listeria monocytogenes* in milk. N Engl J Med 336:100, 1997. *A detailed description of a recent outbreak illustrating the methods and tools of investigation.*
Lorber B: Listeriosis. Clin Infect Dis 24:1, 1997. *A comprehensive clinical review by an authority on the disease.*
Southwick FS, Purich DL: Intracellular pathogenesis of listeriosis. N Engl J Med 334:770, 1996. *An elegant discussion of the interaction of* Listeria *and man with many clinical correlations.*

353 ERYSIPELOID

Annette C. Reboli

DEFINITION. *Erysipelothrix rhusiopathiae* causes three well-defined patterns of human infection: (1) erysipeloid, a cellulitis of the fingers and hands (also known as whale finger or pork finger), which is the most common manifestation of infection with *E. rhusiopathiae*; (2) a diffuse cutaneous form; and (3) a bacteremic form, with or without cutaneous involvement, usually complicated by endocarditis. The term *erysipeloid* refers to cutaneous infection caused by *E. rhusiopathiae* and should not be confused with erysipelas, which is a superficial cellulitis due to streptococci or staphylococci.

ETIOLOGY. *E. rhusiopathiae* is a thin, pleomorphic, non-sporulating, microaerophilic, gram-positive rod. It may be confused with other gram-positive bacillary organisms, in particular *Listeria monocytogenes* and *Corynebacterium* species. It can be differentiated from *L. monocytogenes* by its lack of motility, lack of catalase and coagulase production, and resistance to neomycin. Most strains of *E. rhusiopathiae* produce hydrogen sulfide on triple sugar iron agar slants, a feature that distinguishes *E. rhusiopathiae* from *L. monocytogenes* and from corynebacteria. Because α-hemolysis may be seen after 48 hours of incubation of *E. rhusiopathiae*, confusion with streptococci also may occur.

EPIDEMIOLOGY. *E. rhusiopathiae* is found worldwide as a commensal or a pathogen in a variety of animals, including swine, sheep, cattle, horses, dogs, and rodents; fowl, including chickens, ducks, turkeys, and parrots; and flies, ticks, mites, and lice. The greatest commercial impact of *E. rhusiopathiae* infection is due to disease in swine, but infection of sheep and poultry is also important economically. Although the organism colonizes the mucoid surface slime of fish, it does not appear to cause disease in these animals. Environmental surfaces in contact with infected animals or their products are potential sources of *E. rhusiopathiae*. It can persist for prolonged periods in contaminated soil. Although *E. rhusiopathiae* is resistant to smoking, salting, and pickling, it is killed within 15 minutes by heating to 55° C.

Infection in humans is usually the result of contact with infected animals or their products. Persons at greatest risk for infection include fishermen, fishmongers, butchers, slaughterhouse workers, and veterinarians. The organism gains entry through cuts and abrasions on the skin. The seasonal incidence of erysipeloid parallels that of swine erysipelas and is highest in the summer and early fall.

CLINICAL MANIFESTATIONS. Because of its mode of acquisition (contact with infected animals or their products with organisms inoculating abrasions on the skin), lesions are usually confined to the fingers and hands. A well-defined, slightly elevated, violaceous lesion, accompanied by a very painful, throbbing, burning, or itching sensation, develops within 2 to 7 days of traumatic dermal inoculation. The infected area is swollen. Vesicles may be present, but suppuration is absent. The lesion spreads slowly to other fingers but rarely involves the fingertips or the skin above the wrist. As the lesion spreads peripherally, the central area clears. Systemic signs and symptoms are rare. There may be sterile arthritis of an adjacent joint. Regional lymphadenopathy or lymphadenitis occurs in about 20% of cases, and low-grade fevers occur in approximately 10%. Because *E. rhusiopathiae* is located only in deeper parts of the skin in cases of erysipeloid, biopsy of the entire thickness of the dermis from the edge of the lesion yields maximum recovery of the organism. *E. rhusiopathiae* grows on routine laboratory media. Lesions usually resolve within 3 weeks without treatment. Relapse occurs in 1% of cases.

The diffuse cutaneous form is rare. The cutaneous lesion progresses proximally from the site of inoculation or appears at remote areas. The patients often have fever and arthralgias, but blood cultures are usually negative.

Systemic infection with *Erysipelothrix* is uncommon. Approximately 60 cases of bacteremia have been reported; 90% of the patients had endocarditis. All but two cases involved native valves. In 60% of cases, infection developed on apparently normal heart valves. One third of patients had an antecedent or concurrent skin lesion of erysipeloid. Clinical manifestations of endocarditis due to *E. rhusiopathiae* and other microorganisms are similar. *E. rhusiopathiae* endocarditis correlates highly with occupation, exhibits a tropism for the aortic valve, affects more males than females, and is associated with a high mortality. Very few cases of systemic infection have occurred in immunocompromised hosts, although one third had a history of ethanol abuse. There has been a suggestion that bacteremia due to *E. rhusiopathiae* without endocarditis occurs more frequently than was previously believed and that bacteremia may be occurring with increased frequency in immunocompromised patients while endocarditis usually occurs in immunocompetent patients. Routine blood culture techniques are adequate for growth and isolation of the organism in suspected cases of bacteremia or endocarditis. Focal infections including brain abscess, osteomyelitis, and chronic arthritis have been reported.

TREATMENT. Most isolates of *E. rhusiopathiae* are susceptible to penicillin, cephalosporins, imipenem, clindamycin, ciprofloxacin, and ofloxacin. Some resistance has been observed with erythromycin, tetracycline, and chloramphenicol. *E. rhusiopathiae* is resistant to vancomycin, aminoglycosides, trimethoprim/sulfamethoxazole, and sulfonamides. Penicillin G is the treatment of choice. Uncomplicated cutaneous lesions usually respond well to a 5- to 7-day course of oral penicillin. Treatment hastens healing, although relapse may still occur. Bacteremia should be treated with intravenous penicillin; cases of endocarditis should be treated with 12 to 20 million units of penicillin G daily for 4 to 6 weeks. Cephalosporins are an alternative for the penicillin-allergic patient. Use of quinolones, in particular, ofloxacin or ciprofloxacin, may be considered in *Erysipelothrix* infections when the patient is allergic to β-lactams. Valve replacement may be necessary in patients with endocarditis.

Barnett JH, Estes SA, Wirman JA, et al: Erysipeloid. J Am Acad Dermatol 9:116, 1983. *A complete review of the clinical and pathologic features of Erysipelothrix infections and their treatment.*
Gorby GL, Peacock JE: Erysipelothrix rhusiopathiae endocarditis: Microbiologic, epidemiologic, and clinical features of an occupational disease. Rev Infect Dis 10:317, 1988. *Compares and contrasts cases of E. rhusiopathiae endocarditis and endocarditis caused by other organisms.*
Reboli AC, Farrar WE: Erysipelothrix rhusiopathiae: An occupational pathogen. Clin Microbiol Rev 4:354, 1989. *Reviews epidemiology, clinical features, and bacteriology.*
Venditti M, Gelfusa V, Tarasi A, et al: Antimicrobial susceptibilities of Erysipelothrix rhusiopathiae. Antimicrob Agents Chemother 34:2038, 1990. *In vitro susceptibility data on 10 isolates of E. rhusiopathiae to 16 antimicrobial agents.*

354 ACTINOMYCOSIS

Ward E. Bullock

DEFINITION. Actinomycosis is a chronic bacterial infection that induces both a suppurative and a granulomatous inflammatory response. It spreads contiguously through anatomic barriers and frequently forms external sinuses, from which may extrude "sulfur granules" that are characteristic but not pathognomonic. The most common clinical forms are cervicofacial, thoracic, abdominal, and, in females, genital.

ETIOLOGY. Members of the genus *Actinomyces* are prokaryotes with cell walls that contain both muramic acid and diaminopimelic acid. Unlike the cell walls of fungi, the cell walls of these organisms do not contain sterols and are insensitive to polyene antibiotics. *Actinomyces israelii* is the species most often recovered from human cases of actinomycosis. However, *A. naeslundii, A. odontolyticus, A. viscosus, A. meyeri,* and a related genus, *Arachnia propionica,* cause identical clinical infections and bear close resemblance in primary culture. *Actinomyces bovis* produces "lumpy jaw" in cattle but is not a human pathogen. These gram-positive bacteria are filamentous (0.5 to 1.0 mm in diameter) with branching and are non–acid fast, with a tendency to break up into coccobacilli. They require anaerobic to microaerophilic conditions for growth, which is quite slow; it usually takes 3 to 10 or more days before these organisms can be macroscopically detected in culture.

EPIDEMIOLOGY. Actinomycosis is observed throughout the world, and its prevalence is unrelated to climate, occupation, race, or age. The disease has been reported more commonly in men than in women (3:1). However, since the recognition of pelvic actinomycosis in association with the use of intrauterine devices (IUDs) for contraception, the male prevalence ratio may be decreasing. The number of cases of actinomycosis reported annually to the Centers for Disease Control and Prevention is fewer than 100. These infections are not easily recognized by clinicians, and the organisms are fastidious; therefore, it is likely that the true incidence is substantially greater. Although many animal species are susceptible to actinomycosis, infection is neither transmissible from animal to human nor transmissible from person to person. *Actinomyces* species are part of the indigenous microbiota colonizing the teeth and oral cavity. They also may be found in the tonsillar crypts of asymptomatic individuals, in the fecal flora, and within the female reproductive tract.

PATHOGENESIS AND PATHOLOGY. *Actinomyces* species maintain their niche within the microbial community of the mouth by adherence to oral surfaces, especially to dental plaque, a thin film of salivary proteins and glycoproteins that coats the enamel surface. Adherence is achieved by complex protein-protein stereochemical interactions and by lectin-carbohydrate interactions, the latter of which also mediate cellular coaggregation of oral *Actinomyces* with the *Streptococcus milleri,* group *S. sanguis,* and other mouth flora. This propensity for coaggregation may explain, in part, why actinomycotic infections often are polymicrobial, with "associate" mouth flora frequently isolated from cervicofacial, thoracic, and central nervous system (CNS) abscesses. The "associate" flora may play a synergistic role in infection by maintaining the low oxygen tension necessary for *Actinomyces* growth. To cause disease, these organisms must be introduced into tissue through a break in the mucous membrane resulting from dental infections and manipulations or from aspiration of infected dental debris. They may enter the abdominal cavity by perforation of the lower gastrointestinal tract or by ascending infection of the genital tract in women.

Actinomycotic infection evokes a combination of suppurative and granulomatous inflammatory responses accompanied by intense fibrosis. Plasma cells and multinucleated giant cells often are observed within lesions, as may be large macrophages with foamy cytoplasm around purulent centers. The infection spreads through fascial planes and ultimately may produce draining sinus tracts, especially in infections of the pelvis and abdomen. Sulfur granules within lesions and sinus drainage are a typical feature but not always present. These granules are gritty aggregates of organisms measuring 1 to 2 mm in diameter; the centers have a basophilic staining property, with eosinophilic rays terminating in pear-shaped "clubs" on the surface. They contain calcium phosphate, probably as a result of phosphatase activity of both the host and the organisms.

CLINICAL MANIFESTATIONS. Cervicofacial actinomycosis comprises 50 to 60% of reported cases. Infection is usually observed in a setting of poor oral hygiene with tooth decay, periodontal disease, or gingivitis, in which mucosal integrity is disrupted by dental manipulations or other injury. The infection generally evolves as a chronic or subacute soft tissue swelling or mass involving the submandibular or paramandibular region. The swelling may have a ligneous consistency caused by tissue fibrosis. More rapidly developing lesions often simulate pyogenic infections. Trismus may be present, and advanced lesions may discharge odorless pus containing "sulfur granules" through one or more sinuses. Fever, pain, and leukocytosis may be present. The infection can extend to the tongue, salivary glands, pharynx, and larynx. Bone (most commonly the mandible) may be invaded from the adjacent soft tissue. Cervical spine or cranial bone infection may lead to subdural empyema and invasion of the CNS. The differential diagnosis includes tuberculosis (scrofula), fungal infections, nocardiosis, suppurative infections by other organisms, and neoplasms.

Thoracic actinomycosis comprises 15 to 30% of the disease spectrum and usually results from aspiration of infective material from the oropharynx. Less commonly, thoracic infection may be introduced by esophageal perforation, by extension into the mediastinum from the neck, or by spread from an abdominal site; hematogenous spread to the lung is rare. Pulmonary actinomycosis commonly spreads from an early pneumonic focus across lung fissures to involve the pleura and the chest wall, with eventual fistula formation and drainage containing sulfur granules (Fig. 354–1). Granules rarely are present in the sputum. The incidence of this complication, as well as the destruction of thoracic vertebrae and adjacent ribs, has declined in the antibiotic era.

The complaints of patients with thoracic actinomycosis are non-specific. The most common are a productive cough, dyspnea, weight loss, fever, and chest pain. Anemia, mild leukocytosis, and an elevated sedimentation rate are relatively common. There often is a history of underlying lung disease, and patients rarely present in an early stage of infection. The pulmonary lesions may resemble tuberculosis, especially when cavity formation occurs, and blastomycosis, which may destroy ribs posteriorly but rarely form sinuses. Nocardiosis, bronchogenic carcinoma, and lymphoma can also mimic thoracic actinomycosis.

ABDOMINAL-PELVIC ACTINOMYCOSIS. Actinomycosis of the abdomen and pelvis is a chronic, localized inflammatory process that often is preceded weeks or months by surgery for acute appendicitis with perforation or for perforated colonic diverticulitis or by emergency surgery on the lower intestinal tract after trauma. Occasionally, abdominal actinomycosis may manifest without identifiable predisposing factors. The ileocecal region is involved most frequently, with the formation of a mass lesion. The infection extends slowly to contiguous organs, especially the liver, and may involve retroperitoneal tissues, the spine, or the abdominal wall. Persistent draining sinuses may form, and those involving the perianal region can simulate Crohn's disease or tuberculosis. The extensive fibrosis of actinomycotic lesions, presenting to the examiner as a mass, often suggests tumor. A frequent finding on computed tomography (CT) is an infiltrative mass with dense, inhomogeneous contrast medium enhancement. Constitutional symptoms and signs are non-specific; the most common are fever, weight loss, nausea, vomiting, and pain.

An association has been recognized between long-term use of IUDs and actinomycosis of the genital tract. Manifestations of infection may range from a chronic vaginal discharge to pelvic inflammatory disease with tubo-ovarian abscesses or pseudomalignant masses. No association exists between actinomycotic infection and the type of IUD used. Accurate data on the prevalence and incidence of infection among IUD users are sparse, because cytologic criteria and fluorescent antibody staining techniques are the principal means of detecting *Actinomyces* in vaginal smears and other genital tract specimens. Anaerobic cultures of the female genital tract generally are unsuccessful.

It is generally agreed that *Actinomyces* species may be part of the indigenous genital tract flora of females and that demonstrating their presence by morphologic criteria and fluorescent antibody stains does not predict disease. However, colonization of the endo-

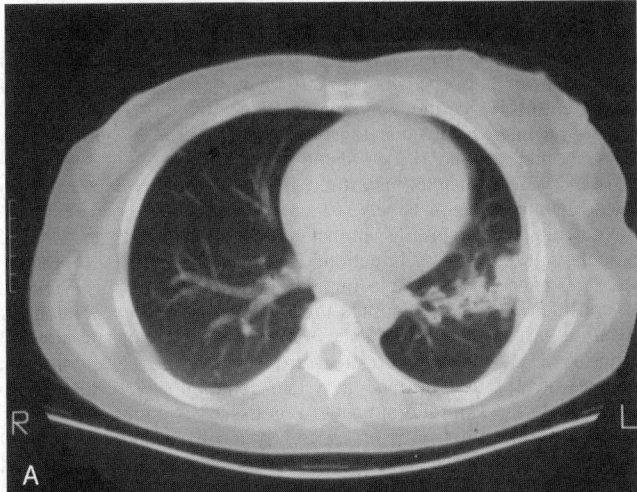

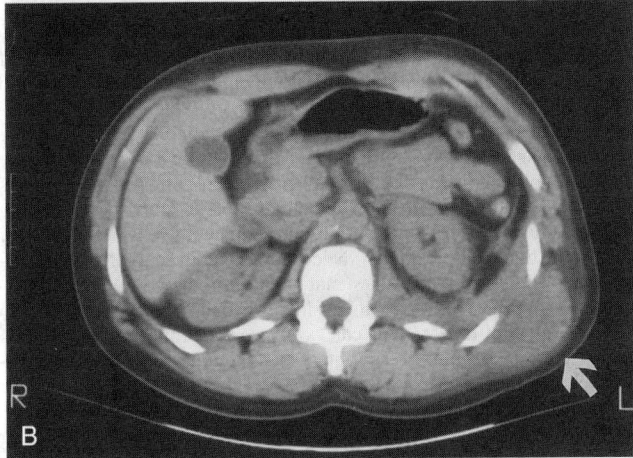

FIGURE 354–1 ■ Thoracic computed tomographic scan of a 43-year-old woman with pulmonary actinomycosis. There is consolidation of the lung with pleural thickening adjacent to the parenchymal disease (*A*). Abscess extended into the left breast and inferiorly to the costophrenic sulcus, to the retroperitoneum, and into the lateral abdominal wall (*B*) (arrow).

metrium appears to require the presence of an IUD. Although many cases of genital-pelvic actinomycosis associated with IUD use have been reported, the actual incidence of disease appears to be low relative to the millions of women who use IUDs.

CNS and disseminated actinomycosis are very uncommon. Most infections of the CNS manifest as single or multiple encapsulated brain abscesses that appear as ring enhancing lesions on computed tomography with intravenous contrast material and are indistinguishable from those caused by other organisms. Most actinomycotic infections of the CNS are thought to be seeded hematogenously from a distant primary site; however, direct extension of cervicofacial disease is well recognized. Sinus formation is not a characteristic of CNS disease. The rare meningitis caused by *Actinomyces* is chronic and basilar in location, and the pleocytosis usually is lymphocytic. Thus, it may be misdiagnosed as tuberculous meningitis.

Unlike *Nocardia* species (see Chapter 355), *Actinomyces* species usually are not opportunistic in the immunocompromised host. Few systemic actinomycotic infections have been reported among patients with the acquired immunodeficiency syndrome.

DIAGNOSIS. Crucial to the diagnosis is a high index of suspicion communicated to the microbiology diagnostic laboratory, along with material from draining sinuses, from deep needle aspiration, or from biopsy specimens. Anaerobic culture is required, and no selective media are available to restrict overgrowth of the slow-growing *Actinomyces* by associated microflora. The presence, in pus or tissue specimens of non–acid-fast, gram-positive organisms with filamentous branching is very suggestive of the diagnosis. The characteristic morphology of "sulfur granules" and the presence of gram-positive organisms within are helpful. However, the granules must be distinguished from similar structures that are sometimes

produced in infections and that are caused by *Nocardia, Monosporium, Cephalosporium, Staphylococcus* (botryomycosis), and others. *Actinomyces* and *Arachnia* generally can be differentiated from other gram-positive anaerobes by means of growth rate (slow), by catalase production (negative, except *A. viscosus*), and by gas-liquid chromatographic detection of acetic, lactic, and succinic acids produced in peptone-yeast-glucose broth. Direct fluorescent antibody conjugates can be used to detect *Actinomyces* in clinical material or culture but are not readily available to clinical microbiology laboratories. There are no reliable serologic tests or skin tests.

TREATMENT. Penicillin G is the drug of choice for treating an infection caused by any of the *Actinomyces*. It is given in high dosage over a prolonged period, because the infection has a tendency to recur, presumably because antibiotic penetration to areas of fibrosis and necrosis and into "sulfur granules" may be poor. Most deep-seated infections can be expected to respond to intravenous penicillin G, 10 to 20 million units/day given for 2 to 6 weeks, followed by an oral phenoxypenicillin in a dosage of 2 to 4 g/day. A few additional weeks of oral penicillin therapy may suffice for uncomplicated cervicofacial disease; complicated cases and extensive pulmonary or abdominal disease may require treatment for 12 to 18 months. Little evidence exists of acquired resistance to penicillin G by *Actinomyces* during prolonged therapy. Radical excision of large sinus tracts should be considered in some cases. Alternative first-line antibiotics for treating *Actinomyces* infections include tetracycline, erythromycin, and clindamycin. First-generation cephalosporins, ceftriaxone, and imipenem also have been employed successfully. Antifungal drugs are not active against these organisms. In vitro antibiotic sensitivity testing of *Actinomyces* is difficult, and the results may not be predictive of antibiotic activity in vivo.

The need to use combination antibiotic therapy to attack microorganisms that are isolated in association with *Actinomyces* has not been established. The generally good results obtained with penicillin G alone over nearly three decades indicate that monotherapy is effective in most cases. In complicated infections of the lower abdomen, where anaerobic gram-negative organisms, among others, may be the "associates," combination antibiotic therapy is appropriate. Surgical treatment may be necessary if extensive necrotic tissue or fistulas are present, if malignancy cannot be excluded, and if large abscesses cannot be drained by percutaneous aspiration.

The presence of organisms presumed to be *Actinomyces* on a Papanicolaou smear, obtained from an asymptomatic female with or without an IUD in place, is not an indication for therapy. When patients experience well-defined IUD-related symptoms and Papanicolaou smears demonstrate *Actinomyces* by specific fluorescent-labeled antibody, the IUD should be removed. Antibiotic administration for a 2-week period may be indicated. More serious infections require prolonged therapy as recommended previously.

PROGNOSIS. The advent of antibiotics has greatly improved the prognosis for all forms of actinomycosis. At present, cure rates are high and neither deformity nor death is common.

Bennhoff DF: Actinomycosis: Diagnostic and therapeutic considerations and a review of 32 cases. Laryngoscope 94:1198, 1984. *A general review.*

Fiorino AS: Intrauterine contraceptive device–associated actinomycotic abscess and *Actinomyces* detection on cervical smear. Obstet Gynecol 87:142, 1996.

Ha HK, Lee HJ, Kim H, et al: Abdominal actinomycosis: CT findings in 10 patients. AJR Am J Roentgenol 161:791, 1993. *A helpful summary.*

Richtsmeier WJ, Johns ME: Actinomycosis of the head and neck. CRC Crit Rev Clin Lab Sci 11:175, 1979. *An excellent review, with an emphasis on infection of the head and neck.*

Smego RA Jr: Actinomycosis of the central nervous system. Rev Infect Dis 9:855, 1987. *A good review of 70 cases of CNS actinomycosis.*

355 NOCARDIOSIS

Ward E. Bullock

DEFINITION. Nocardiosis is a subacute or chronic bacterial infection that evokes a suppurative response. The most common sites of primary infection are, first, the lung and then the skin, from which bacteria may disseminate hematogenously to the central nervous system (CNS) and other tissues. The infection often pursues a more acute and aggressive course in immunosuppressed patients.

ETIOLOGY. The nocardiae are gram-positive, aerobic actinomycetes, many of which are weakly acid fast in tissue or on initial isolation. They reproduce by filamentous branching, with fragmentation into bacillary and coccoid forms. *Nocardia* species are distributed widely in nature and commonly are found in soil, grasses, and rotting vegetation. Members of the *N. asteroides* complex, a heterogeneous group of organisms, are the most frequent cause of nocardiosis in humans. Other species that produce pulmonary and/or disseminated infection include *N. farcinica, N. nova, N. otitidiscaviarum, N. transvalensis, and N. brasiliensis. N. brasiliensis* is the most common cause of actinomycetoma in Latin and South America.

INCIDENCE AND PREVALENCE. A 1976 survey estimated the incidence of nocardiosis in the United States to be 500 to 1000 new cases per year. At present, the incidence undoubtedly is higher as a consequence of an ever expanding population of people who are immunosuppressed iatrogenically or by underlying diseases. Nocardiosis has been reported worldwide in all ages and races and is two to three times more common in men than in women. No occupational related risks have been found.

EPIDEMIOLOGY. The majority of infections caused by *N. asteroides* occur in patients with impaired cell-mediated immunity. However, the organism is capable of infecting apparently normal persons. Nocardiosis presumably is acquired by inhaling airborne bacteria, since the primary site of infection is the lung in the majority of cases. Other mammals can be infected, but no well-established evidence exists for animal-to-person transmission or for person-to-person transmission. Occasional clusters of nocardial infection have been reported among immunosuppressed hospital patients, suggesting possible nosocomial acquisition. *N. asteroides* has been recovered from the sputum, skin, and other body regions of patients who do not have apparent disease. Nevertheless, repeated isolation of *Nocardia* species from any immunocompromised person should be considered evidence of infection rather than colonization, and treatment should be initiated. Nocardiosis can manifest as a primary cutaneous infection (especially *N. brasiliensis*) after inoculation through local injury and may disseminate to other organs.

PATHOGENESIS AND PATHOLOGY. The typical nocardial lesion within the lung and other tissues is one of liquefactive necrosis with abscess formation. Polymorphonuclear leukocytes predominate in association with varying proportions of macrophages and lymphocytes. Granuloma formation is infrequent, and in contrast to actinomycotic lesions, fibrosis is rare. Confluent daughter abscesses are common. Sulfur granules are not present in visceral lesions, as they are in actinomycosis. However, they may be seen in nocardial lesions of the skin.

That cell-mediated immunity plays a major role in host defense against nocardiosis is suggested by the fact that immunocompromised patients are prone to this infection. The importance of antigen-specific T lymphocyte immune function is illustrated by the increased susceptibility of athymic nude mice to *Nocardia* infection and by the capacity of T lymphocytes from rabbits immunized with *N. asteroides* to augment phagocytosis and growth inhibition of these organisms by macrophages. Neutrophils exhibit poor nocardicidal activity in vitro but may inhibit growth of organisms during an early phase of infection before maturation of cellular immune responses.

N. asteroides may counter host defenses by inhibiting the phagolysosome fusion that enables phagocytic cells to kill ingested bacteria, by producing superoxide dismutase and catalase, and by blocking the acidification of parasitized phagolysosomes.

CLINICAL MANIFESTATIONS. Pulmonary infection is the most frequent manifestation of nocardiosis (about 75% of the reported cases). The clinical manifestations are non-specific and include fever, productive cough, dyspnea, pleuritic pain, and weight loss. The range of pulmonary involvement extends from transient or inapparent infection to confluent bronchopneumonia with complete consolidation. Radiographic examination of the chest may reveal one or more of the following: nodules, fluffy infiltrates, multiple abscess formation with cavitation in 20 to 50% of cases, bulging fissures,

masses, and empyema. Hilar involvement and calcification are infrequent. Nocardia can disseminate to other organs from pulmonary lesions, especially in patients who are immunosuppressed after solid organ or allogeneic bone marrow transplantation and in individuals with the acquired immunodeficiency syndrome (AIDS). Patients who have received extensive x-irradiation and chemotherapy for malignancies and those treated with high doses of corticosteroids also are prone to metastatic infection, and evidence thereof should be sought aggressively.

Nocardial organisms disseminate to the CNS in 20 to 40% of patients with pulmonary infection. Therefore, computed tomography (CT) or magnetic resonance imaging scanning of the head should be considered. Typical findings are brain abscesses, either singular or multiple, that "ring enhance" after administration of contrast material. Headache and focal neurologic findings are common, whereas meningitis is infrequent. Other common sites of dissemination include the skin and subcutaneous tissues, kidneys, eyes, liver, and lymph nodes. In cases of apparently localized nocardial lesions of skin, it is important to distinguish between the possibilities of primary inoculation and hematogenous dissemination to the skin from another site.

DIAGNOSIS. The clinical and radiographic findings in pulmonary nocardiosis are non-specific and may be mistaken for a variety of other bacterial infections of the lung, including actinomycosis and tuberculosis, as well as fungal infections and malignancies. Alertness to the possibility of nocardiosis can expedite the diagnostic work-up, especially in immunosuppressed patients, in whom the disease may coexist with other opportunistic infections. Cultures and stains should be done on specimens of sputum, pleural fluid, and bronchial lavage fluid and on percutaneous lung aspirates or open-lung biopsy specimens. Needle biopsy of cerebral mass lesions should be considered strongly in immunocompromised patients who have pulmonary nocardiosis because of the multiplicity of infections and tumors that can present in a similar manner.

Skin lesions should be aspirated if fluctuant or biopsied. Specimens should be submitted for culture and the smear preparations or histologic sections examined for organisms. Nocardiosis often can be diagnosed with confidence by direct examination of sputum or purulent material. The presence of gram-positive, filamentous branching rods that stain unevenly with crystal violet to give a beaded appearance is highly suggestive of either *Actinomyces* or *Nocardia*. *Nocardia* species are not visible in tissue specimens stained by hematoxylin and eosin or by the periodic acid–Schiff procedure. They can be visualized by a tissue Gram stain or after slight overstaining by the Gomori methenamine silver method. If the organisms are acid fast on a modified Ziehl-Neelsen stain, the probability of *Nocardia* is high. However, lack of acid-fast staining does not exclude *Nocardia*.

Nocardia species are not fastidious and grow aerobically, although slowly, on routinely used media. Characteristic heaped, waxy colonies, often colored tan, orange, or gray that produce a musty odor, may be seen after 3 to 14 days of culture. Longer times may be required. Thus, the microbiology laboratory should be advised of possible nocardiosis to ensure that selective media are employed to limit overgrowth by microbial contaminants (particularly in sputum samples) and that plates are held for at least 14 days. Several simple tests can assist in the presumptive identification of nocardial species and differentiation from other aerobic actinomycetes and from rapidly growing mycobacteria. These include tests for the decomposition of casein, xanthine, hypoxanthine, and tyrosine and the ability to grow in the presence of lysozyme. Most clinical laboratories should rely on reference facilities for definitive taxonomic designations.

TREATMENT. The sulfonamides are equally efficacious and are first-line agents for treatment, as is the combination of trimethoprim/sulfamethoxazole (TMP/SMX). The dosage of sulfadiazine is 6 to 10 g/day given in three to six divided doses, with adjustment as needed to achieve peak serum levels of 12 to 15 mg/dL. Dosing schedules of TMP/SMX range from 160 mg/800 mg to 320 mg/1600 mg every 6 or 8 hours. These antimicrobial agents penetrate well into the CNS and other body compartments. A high percentage of *Nocardia* isolates are sensitive to sulfonamides and to TMP-SMX by in vitro testing. Techniques for in vitro sensitivity testing with *Nocardia* have not been standardized, in part because of technical difficulties created by slow growth in culture and problems in obtaining a homogeneous suspension of cells for standardization of the inoculum. Thus, the results of in vitro tests may not predict in vivo efficacy and should be interpreted with caution.

Not all patients respond to sulfonamide or TMP/SMX therapy. Development of resistance to the sulfonamides during therapy has been documented, and metastatic lesions can appear during the course of apparently successful treatment. Hypersensitivity reactions, nephrotoxicity, or hematopoietic toxicity induced by these drugs may force discontinuation of treatment, especially in solid organ and bone marrow transplant recipients given cyclosporine and in patients with AIDS. The alternative antibiotics that have proved to be most efficacious, both in vitro and clinically, are imipenem, amikacin, and minocycline. Ceftriaxone, cefuroxime, and cefotaxime display in vitro activity against many, but by no means all, clinical isolates of the *Nocardia* species. Isolates of *N. otitidiscaviarum* are usually resistant to sulfamethoxazole as are most *N. farcinica* to cefotaxime and many *N. brasiliensis* to imipenem. Therefore, despite problems inherent in testing the sensitivity of Nocardiae to antibiotics, these studies should be performed to assist in the choice of long-term antibiotic therapy. Some studies in vitro and a few in experimental animal models indicate that imipenem plus amikacin and certain other antibiotic combinations can exert synergistic activity against *Nocardia*. As yet, no good clinical evidence exists that combination antibiotic regimens are superior to single-agent therapy.

Prolonged treatment is necessary because relapse of nocardiosis is common. In patients with intact host defenses, treatment should be continued for at least 6 weeks after clinical recovery. In those who have AIDS or who are otherwise immunocompromised, treatment should be continued for a year or more. As a rule, it is necessary to perform surgical drainage of brain abscesses, empyema, and subcutaneous abscesses. Patients with cerebral nocardiosis or other deep abscesses are best monitored by serial CT. If patients are receiving immunosuppressive drugs, the dosage should be reduced if at all possible.

PROGNOSIS. The prognosis for clinical cure of nocardiosis is influenced by (1) the rapidity of diagnosis, (2) the location of the infection, (3) pre-existing impairment of cellular immunity from underlying disease or drug therapy, and (4) the aggressiveness of the patient's management. Mortality rates range from near zero in patients with isolated skin lesions to more than 40% in cases of CNS involvement. The overall mortality rate in patients with pulmonary disease is in the range of 15 to 30%, including those who are immunocompromised.

Arduino RC, Johnson PC, Miranda AG: Nocardiosis in renal transplant recipients undergoing immunosuppression with cyclosporine. Clin Infect Dis 16:505, 1993. *A review of nocardiosis in renal transplant patients.*

Mamelak AN, Obana WG, Flaherty JF, Rosenblum ML: Nocardial brain abscess: Treatment strategies and factors influencing outcome. Neurosurgery 35:622, 1994. *An excellent analysis of 131 cases.*

Palmer DL, Harvey RL, Wheeler JK: Diagnostic and therapeutic considerations in *Nocardia asteroides* infection. Medicine 53:391, 1974. *A comprehensive literature review of 243 cases of nocardiosis (including 13 patients in the authors' own experience).*

Uttamchandani RB, Daikos GL, Reyes RR, et al: Nocardiosis in 30 patients with advanced human immunodeficiency virus infection: Clinical features and outcome. Clin Infect Dis 18:348, 1994. *A current discussion of nocardial infection in AIDS patients.*

356 BRUCELLOSIS

Robert A. Salata

DEFINITION. Bacteria of the genus *Brucella* cause disease with protean manifestations. Infection is transmitted to humans from animals as a consequence of occupational exposure or ingestion of contaminated milk products. Despite the attempt to institute effective control measures, brucellosis remains a significant health and economic burden in many countries.

ETIOLOGY. Brucellae are slow-growing, small, aerobic, non-motile, non-encapsulated, non–spore-forming, gram-negative coccobacilli. *B. abortus, B. suis, B. melitensis,* and *B. canis* are known to infect humans and are typed on the basis of biochemical, metabolic, and immunologic criteria. There are differences in virulence among these four species. *B. abortus,* with a reservoir in cattle, usually is associated with mild to moderate sporadic disease; sup-

purative or disabling complications are rare. *B. suis* infection, resulting from swine contact, is often associated with destructive, suppurative lesions and may have a prolonged course. *B. melitensis,* with a reservoir in sheep and goats, may cause severe, acute disease and disabling complications. *B. canis,* spread to humans from infected dogs, causes disease with an insidious onset, frequent relapse, and a chronic course that is indistinguishable from infection related to *B. abortus.*

EPIDEMIOLOGY. Over 500,000 cases of brucellosis are reported yearly to the World Health Organization from 100 countries. *B. melitensis* infection, distributed primarily in the Mediterranean region (particularly Spain and Greece), Latin America, the Arabian gulf and the Indian subcontinent, accounts for the majority of cases. *B. abortus* infection occurs worldwide but has been effectively eradicated in several European countries, Japan, and Israel. *B. suis* occurs mainly in the midwestern United States, South America, and Southeast Asia, whereas *B. canis* infection is most common in North and South America, Japan, and Central Europe. Identification of the *Brucella* species recovered in humans can provide clues to the likely source of infection.

In association with effective control programs in animals, human brucellosis has decrease dramatically in the United States, from over 6000 cases in 1947 to fewer than 200 cases per year since 1980. States reporting the greatest number of cases include Texas, California, Virginia, and Florida. In North America, brucellosis occurs mainly in spring and summer and is most common in men, usually related to occupational exposure.

Brucella infection in the United States most frequently occurs in high-risk groups, including slaughterhouse workers, farmers and dairymen, veterinarians, travelers to endemic areas, and laboratory workers handling the organisms. More than one half of reported cases occur in the meat-processing industry, particularly in the kill areas, where infection is spread through abraded or lacerated skin and the conjunctiva, possibly by aerosolization, and rarely by ingestion of infected tissue. Many cases of *B. abortus* infection in veterinarians have accidentally occurred from the strain 19 vaccine used to immunize cattle. *B. melitensis* infection, transmitted through the ingestion of goat's milk cheese, has been seen in U.S. travelers to and immigrants from Mexico. Brucellosis contracted abroad may not become symptomatic until the patient returns to the United States.

Brucellosis in children accounts for only 3 to 10% of all reported cases worldwide, is common in endemic areas (may account for 20 to 25% of cases), and is often a mild, self-limited process. Infection occurs most frequently in school-age children and in familial outbreaks; no convincing evidence exists to associate *Brucella* infection with abortion in humans.

PATHOGENESIS AND IMMUNITY. After penetrating the epithelial cells of human skin, conjunctiva, pharynx, or lung, *Brucella* organisms initially induce an exuberant polymorphonuclear neutrophil response in the submucosa. After ingestion of organisms by neutrophils and tissue macrophages, spread to regional lymph nodes occurs. If host defenses within the lymph nodes are overwhelmed, bacteremia follows. The usual incubation period between infection and bacteremia is 1½ to 3 weeks. Bacteremia is accompanied by phagocytosis of free *Brucella* organisms by neutrophils and localization of bacteria primarily to the spleen, liver, and bone marrow, with the formation of granulomas.

If the inoculum is large and the patient receives no treatment, large granulomas may form, suppurate, and serve as a source of persistent bacteremia with the potential for multiorgan spread. The primary virulence factor of *Brucella* appears to be cell wall lipopolysaccharide.

Both virulent and attenuated strains of *Brucella* are readily phagocytized by neutrophils after opsonization with normal human serum. Whole bacteria and extracts of *Brucella* species may inhibit neutrophil oxidative burst activity and degranulation. Intracellular killing of ingested bacteria has been demonstrated with *B. abortus* but not *B. melitensis;* this may explain differences in pathogenicity between these species.

Humoral factors may be important in the host defense against *Brucella.* Even in the absence of specific agglutinating antibody, normal human serum is bactericidal for *Brucella* organisms; *B. abortus* is more susceptible to serum lysis than is *B. melitensis.*

The intracellular location of the organism may provide a means for the bacteria to escape the lethal effects of serum. Specific serum agglutinating antibody has opsonic activity but does not correlate with the development of protective immunity.

A role for mononuclear phagocytes and cell-mediated immunity in brucellosis has been demonstrated. Protection against *Brucella* infection in animals is associated with preceding infection with *Listeria monocytogenes* or *Mycobacterium tuberculosis,* both of which stimulate cell-mediated immune mechanisms. Skin testing with *Brucella* proteins elicits a typical delayed hypersensitivity response in infected individuals. Macrophages, activated with cytokines (e.g., interferon-γ and tumor necrosis factor-α), kill *Brucella* in vitro. In some cases of chronic brucellosis, depressed proliferative responses to classic T-cell mitogens or to *Brucella* antigen occur.

CLINICAL MANIFESTATIONS. Clinically, human brucellosis may be conveniently divided into subclinical illness, acute/subacute disease, localized disease and complications, relapsing infection, and chronic disease (Table 356–1).

SUBCLINICAL ILLNESS. Deleted only by serologic testing, asymptomatic or clinically unrecognized human brucellosis often occurs in high-risk groups, including slaughterhouse workers, farmers, and veterinarians. More than 50% of abattoir workers and up to 33% of veterinarians have high anti-*Brucella* antibody titers but no history of recognized clinical infection. Children in endemic areas frequently have subclinical illness.

ACUTE AND SUBACUTE DISEASE. After an incubation period of several weeks or months, acute brucellosis may occur as a mild, transient illness (with *B. abortus* or *B. canis*) or as an explosive, toxic illness with the potential for multiple complications (with *B. melitensis*). Approximately 50% of patients have an abrupt onset over days, whereas the remainder have an insidious onset over weeks. Symptoms in brucellosis are protean and non-specific. More than 90% of patients experience malaise, chills, sweats, fatigue, and weakness. More than 50% of patients have myalgias, anorexia, and weight loss. Fewer patients complain of arthralgias, cough, testicular pain, dysuria, ocular pain, or visual blurring. Likewise, few localizing physical signs are apparent. Fever, often greater than 39.4° C (103° F), occurs in 95%. An undulating or intermittent fever pattern is unusual. A relative pulse-temperature deficit may occur. Splenomegaly is present in 10 to 15%, lymphadenopathy occurs in up to 14% (axillary, cervical, and supraclavicular locations are most frequent, related to hand-wound or oropharyngeal routes of infection); hepatomegaly is less frequent. Other laboratory findings in acute or subacute disease may include mild anemia, lymphopenia or neutropenia (especially with bacteremia), lymphocytosis, thrombocytopenia, or (rarely) pancytopenia. The majority of infected individuals recover completely without sequelae if the diagnosis is appropriately made and prompt therapy is initiated.

LOCALIZED DISEASE AND COMPLICATIONS. *Brucella* organisms may localize in almost any organ, most commonly in bone, joints, central nervous system (CNS), heart, lung, spleen, testes, liver, gallbladder, kidney, prostate, and skin. Localized disease may occur simultaneously at multiple sites. Localized complications most often appear in association with a more chronic course of illness, although complications may occur with acute disease due to *B. melitensis* or *B. suis*. In the United States, localized disease is most frequently related to *B. suis*.

RELAPSING INFECTION. Up to 10% of patients with brucellosis relapse after antimicrobial therapy. This probably results from the intracellular location of the organisms, which protects the bacteria from certain antibiotics and host defense mechanisms. Relapses occur most frequently within months after initial infection but may occur as long as 2 years after apparently successful treatment. Relapsing infection is difficult to distinguish from reinfection in high-risk groups with continued exposure. Recent studies have shown that relapses are associated with inappropriate or insufficient antimicrobial therapy, positive blood cultures on initial presentation, and an acute onset of disease.

CHRONIC DISEASE. Disease with a duration of more than 1 year has been called chronic brucellosis. A majority of patients classified as having chronic brucellosis really have persistent disease caused by inadequate treatment of the initial episode, or they have focal disease in bone, liver, or spleen. About 20% of patients diagnosed as having chronic brucellosis complain of persistent fatigue, malaise, and depression; in many aspects this condition resembles the chronic fatigue syndrome. These symptoms frequently are not associated with clinical, microbiologic, or serologic evidence of active infection.

DIAGNOSIS. Many more common illnesses mimic the clinical presentation of brucellosis. The most conclusive means of establishing the diagnosis of brucellosis is by positive cultures from normally sterile body fluids or tissues. Isolation of the organism can be enhanced by use of special media. The culture of *Brucella* organisms is potentially hazardous to laboratory personnel. Therefore, most cases of brucellosis are diagnosed by serologic testing.

In acute brucellosis, positive blood cultures are obtained in 10 to 30% of cases (as high as 85% with *B. melitensis*). Blood culture positivity decreases with increasing duration of illness. With *B. melitensis* infection, bone marrow cultures are of higher yield than are blood cultures. Blood cultures processed in radiometric detection or isolator systems may yield positive cultures in less than 10 days. With localized brucellosis (e.g., lymph nodes, spleen, liver, or skeletal system), cultures of purulent material or tissues usually yield *Brucella* organisms. Culture of cerebrospinal fluid is positive in 45% of patients with meningitis. Antibody against *Brucella* may be demonstrated in cerebrospinal fluid by enzyme-linked immunosorbent assay (ELISA).

Most patients mount significant serologic responses to *Brucella* infections. The most frequently used test is the standard tube agglutination (STA) test, measuring antibody to *B. abortus* antigen. A

Table 356–1 ■ CLINICAL CLASSIFICATION OF HUMAN BRUCELLOSIS

	DURATION OF SYMPTOMS BEFORE DIAGNOSIS	MAJOR SYMPTOMS AND SIGNS	DIAGNOSIS	COMMENTS
Subclinical		Asymptomatic	Positive (low titer) serology, negative cultures	Occurs in abattoir workers, farmers, and veterinarians
Acute and subacute	Up to 2–3 mo and 3 mo to 1 yr	Malaise, chills, sweats, fatigue, headache, anorexia, arthralgias, fever, splenomegaly, lymphadenopathy, hepatomegaly	Positive serology, positive blood or bone marrow cultures	Presentation can be mild, self-limited (*B. abortus*), or fulminant with severe complications (*B. melitensis*)
Localized	Occurs with acute or chronic untreated disease	Related to involved organs	Positive serology, positive cultures in specific tissues	Bone/joint, genitourinary, hepatosplenic involvement most common
Relapsing	2–3 mo after initial episode	Same as acute illness but may have higher fever, more fatigue, weakness, chills, and sweats	Positive serology, positive cultures	May be extremely difficult to distinguish relapse from reinfection
Chronic	Longer than 1 yr	Non-specific presentation but neuropsychiatric symptoms and low-grade fever most common	Low titer or negative serology, cultures negative	Most controversial classification; localized disease may be associated

Table 356–2 ■ **TREATMENT FOR BRUCELLOSIS**

	TREATMENT	COMMENTS
Acute		
With no endocarditis or CNS involvement	Doxycycline (200 mg/day) plus rifampin (600 to 900 mg/day) for 6 weeks	Treatment of choice by World Health Organization Widely used; low rate of relapse; intramuscular administration of streptomycin may be difficult
	or	
	Tetracycline (2 g/day) for 6 weeks plus streptomycin (1 g/day) or gentamicin for 3 weeks. *Alternative agents:* chloramphenicol, fluoroquinolones, trimethoprim/sulfamethoxazole, imipenem	Combination therapy still preferred
In children	Trimethoprim/sulfamethoxazole	
CNS	Third-generation cephalosporin with rifampin	
Localized	Surgically drain abscesses plus antimicrobial therapy for 6 or more weeks	
Brucella endocarditis	Bactericidal drugs; early valve replacement may be necessary	Possible aortic valve destruction and/or major arterial emboli

fourfold or greater rise in titer to 1:160 or higher is considered significant. A presumptive case is one in which the agglutination titer is positive ($\geq$ 1:160) in single or serial specimens, with symptoms consistent with brucellosis. By 3 weeks of illness, more than 97% of patients demonstrate serologic evidence of infection. This test equally detects antibodies to *B. abortus, B. suis,* and *B. melitensis* but not to *B. canis.* Serologic confirmation of *B. canis* infection requires *B. canis* or *B. ovis* antigen. Despite adequate antibiotic treatment, significant STA titers can persist for up to 2 years in 5 to 7% of cases. Because the STA titer may remain elevated, it is not useful in differentiating relapsing infection from other febrile illnesses in patients with past *Brucella* infections. Individuals with subclinical infection may demonstrate significant STA titers. In chronic localized brucellosis, STA titers may appear absent or low owing to a prozone phenomenon. This prozone effect appears to be related to the presence of immunoglobulin G (IgG) or immunoglobulin A (IgA) blocking antibodies; it can be eliminated if dilutions are carried out to at least 1:1280. False-positive STA titers due to immunologic cross-reactivity have been associated with *Brucella* skin testing, cholera vaccination, or infections due to *Vibrio cholerae, Francisella tularensis,* or *Yersinia enterocolitica.*

Immunoglobulin M (IgM) is the major agglutinating antibody formed in the first few weeks after infection with *Brucella* organisms. Thereafter, IgG levels also rise. The STA test measures both IgM and IgG. With prompt and adequate therapy, IgG antibody levels usually become undetectable after 6 to 12 months. If therapy is given, those patients who develop persistent *Brucella* infection usually maintain elevated IgG agglutinins. In the absence of rising STA titers, a single elevated 2-ME *Brucella* agglutination titer ($\geq$ 1:160) suggests either current or recent infection. Certain newer antibody tests, including an ELISA and radioimmunoassay, are more sensitive than the STA; these methods are becoming more widely employed.

TREATMENT. Antibiotic treatment of *Brucella* infections is complicated by a number of complex issues, including the requirement for antibiotics that penetrate intracellularly, for prolonged therapy to prevent relapse, and for bactericidal antibiotics in treating CNS infection and endocarditis, as well as the lack of controlled, randomized, double-blind studies comparing different antimicrobial regimens. Debate is still considerable regarding which antibiotic regimens are clearly superior. Current recommendations are given in Table 356–2.

PROGNOSIS. Brucellosis appropriately treated within the first month of symptom onset is curable. Acute brucellosis often produces severe weakness and fatigue, and patients are frequently unable to work for up to 2 months. Immunity to reinfection follows initial *Brucella* infection in the majority of individuals. With early antimicrobial therapy, cases of chronic brucellosis or localized disease and complications are rare. Of patients who die of brucellosis, 84% have endocarditis involving a previously abnormal aortic valve, often associated with severe congestive heart failure.

PREVENTION. The control of human brucellosis relates directly to prevention programs in domestic animals and avoiding unpasteurized milk and milk products. In slaughterhouses, important means of prevention include careful wound dressing, protective glasses and clothing, prohibition of raw meat ingestion, and the use of previously infected (immune) individuals in high-risk areas.

Akova M, Uzun O, Akalin E, et al: Quinolones in the treatment of human brucellosis: Comparative trial of ofloxacin-rifampin versus doxycycline-rifampin. Antimicrob Agents Chemother 37:1831, 1993. *The quinolone-rifampin combination was as effective as doxycycline plus rifampin regardless of the complications of the disease.*

Ariza J, Pujol M, Valverde J, et al: Brucella sacroiliitis: Findings in 63 episodes and current relevance. Clin Infect Dis 16:761, 1993. *Epidemiologic, clinical, diagnostic, and treatment aspects of sacroiliitis reviewed over a 15-year period in Spain suggest that a mild disease exists with a good outcome similar to uncomplicated brucellosis.*

Hall WH: Modern chemotherapy for brucellosis in humans. Rev Infect Dis 12:1060, 1990. *A comprehensive analysis of the world's literature related to therapy of brucellosis that stresses that prolonged combined chemotherapy in conjunction with surgery, where indicated, is the key to successful treatment.*

357 DISEASE CAUSED BY BARTONELLA SPECIES

David A. Relman ■ *Craig Hoesley* ■ *C. Glenn Cobbs*

The genus *Bartonella* includes 11 species, but only 4 (*B. henselae, B. quintana, B. bacilliformis,* and *B. elizabethae*) are known to be pathogenic in humans. Three major pathologic varieties of disease are attributed to *Bartonella* infection: (1) vasculoproliferative disease, (2) endovascular disease with primary bacteremia, and (3) granulomatous disease. Examples of vasculoproliferative disease include bacillary angiomatosis and peliosis caused by *B. henselae* or *B. quintana* (formerly members of the *Rochalimaea* genus), and verruga peruana, which is a manifestation of chronic *B. bacilliformis* infection. The cutaneous lesions of bacillary angiomatosis and Kaposi's sarcoma share a similar gross appearance. Bacteremia may occur during any form of bartonellosis; however, it is convenient to consider separately the specific disorders of the endovascular compartment in which bacteremia is a dominant feature: trench fever (caused by *B. quintana*), infective endocarditis, and Oroya fever (caused by *B. bacilliformis*). *B. henselae* also causes the granulomatous disorder known as cat-scratch disease, which primarily affects lymph nodes but can sometimes cause systemic complications.

The state of host immune system integrity plays an important role in determining which of these disparate forms of pathology become manifest during *Bartonella* infection. For example, *B. henselae* usually causes bacillary angiomatosis in immunocompromised individuals and cat-scratch disease in immunocompetent hosts. Genetic differences between *Bartonella* species or strains may also account for differences in pathogenicity and host response. *B. quintana* and *B. henselae* are equally likely to cause cutaneous lesions of bacillary angiomatosis, but *B. quintana* is more likely to induce subcutaneous or osseous lesions whereas *B. henselae* is almost exclusively implicated in disease of the liver, spleen, and lymph nodes.

ETIOLOGY. VASCULOPROLIFERATIVE DISEASE. Bacillary angiomatosis (epithelioid angiomatosis) was first described in 1983 in a person infected with human immunodeficiency virus (HIV). It was not until 1990 that a visualized but uncultivated bacillus was identified from tissues affected by this disease using molecular methods. In a serendipitous development, the same organism was cultivated for the first time in that same year; it was subsequently named *Rochalimaea henselae*. The close evolutionary relationships between this organism, *R. quintana*, and *Bartonella bacilliformis* led to the reclassification of all of these species within the *Bartonella* genus in 1993 (Fig. 357–1). *B. henselae* and *B. quintana* have each been cultivated directly from and detected in tissues affected by bacillary angiomatosis, as well as a variant form of pathology, bacillary peliosis. *B. henselae* is responsible for cases of bacillary angiomatosis-peliosis associated with cat exposure, and *B. quintana* infection is associated with low income, homelessness, and exposure to lice.

Classic bartonellosis (*B. bacilliformis* infection; Carrión's disease) is an insect-borne disorder characterized by two well-defined clinical stages: Oroya fever and verruga peruana, the second of which is associated with vascular proliferative lesions. The common bacterial cause of the two stages was established in 1885 by Daniel Carrion, a Peruvian medical student, when he developed acute hemolytic anemia (Oroya fever) 39 days after self-inoculation with material from a verruga lesion. In 1909, Barton named the causative agent *Bartonella bacilliformis*.

BACTEREMIC DISEASE. Trench fever was described as a specific clinical entity during World War I when more than 1 million military personnel were affected by this disorder. Trench fever has also been called 5-day or quintan fever, shinbone fever, shank fever, and His-Werner disease and has primarily been recognized during war-related epidemics. The etiologic agent was initially considered to be a member of the *Rickettsia* genus, but in 1961 the organism was isolated from infected lice and human blood and assigned to the genus *Rochalimaea* as *R. quintana*. In 1964, Koch's postulates were fulfilled when trench fever was experimentally induced in human volunteers after inoculation with *R. quintana* organisms from patients with trench fever. The agent was renamed *B. quintana* in 1993. *B. quintana*, *B. henselae*, and *B. elizabethae* have all been associated with endocarditis in humans.

GRANULOMATOUS DISEASE. In 1983, small pleomorphic weakly gram-negative but strongly argyrophilic bacilli were first described in cat-scratch disease tissues. An organism subsequently cultivated from such tissues in a small number of cases, *Afipia felis*, was suspected to be the causative agent, but this suspicion could not be confirmed. Instead, beginning in 1992, data have increasingly supported a causative role for *B. henselae* in the vast majority of cases. Eighty-four to 88 per cent of patients who meet traditional diagnostic criteria for cat-scratch disease (see later) demonstrate a significant elevation of serum IgG antibodies directed against *B. henselae*, whereas approximately 20% of asymptomatic cat owners and 3 to 4% of the general population have elevated titers. In addition, *B. henselae* DNA and antigens can be detected in tissues from these patients with the polymerase chain reaction (PCR) and in situ immunohistochemistry. *B. henselae* has also been cultivated from blood and tissues of patients with cat-scratch disease. However, Koch's postulates have not been fulfilled for this organism. In addition, there may be a role for other species such as *B. clarridgeiae* in a minority of cat-scratch disease cases.

B. henselae is a slightly curved, small (0.5 × 1 to 2 μm), self-aggregating, gram-negative bacillus that is capable of twitching motility. Optimal growth occurs on enriched media supplemented with 5% sheep or rabbit blood, at 35° C in a 5 to 10% CO_2-humified atmosphere. Colonies become visible after 9 to 21 days of primary culture (two different morphologies) and after 3 to 5 days on subsequent laboratory passage. *B. quintana* grows under similar conditions, especially after co-cultivation with endothelial cell monolayers. *B. bacilliformis* grows preferentially at 25 to 30° C. Species identification requires specific antisera, cellular fatty acid analysis, or DNA polymorphism or sequence analysis.

EPIDEMIOLOGY. VASCULOPROLIFERATIVE DISEASE. Cats and other felids are reservoirs for *B. henselae* in many regions of the world. In one study, 41% of cats were bacteremic with this organism. Bacteremia is more common in cats that are younger than 1 year of age, free ranging, and seropositive. It is asymptomatic and may persist for the lifetime of the animal. Thus, it is not surprising that cat ownership and cat bites or scratches are the strongest risk factors for *B. henselae*–associated bacillary angiomatosis. Cat fleas transmit this species among cats, but their role in transmission to humans is less clear. *B. quintana* has not been detected in cats, and cat exposure is uncommon among patients with *B. quintana*–associated bacillary angiomatosis. Humans appear to be the sole reservoir of *B. quintana;* and the human body louse, *Pediculus humanus*, serves as the transmission vector. The microorganism has been found in saliva, feces, and material regurgitated by lice. Direct human-to-human transmission has not been demonstrated. Risk factors for *B. quintana*–associated disease include homelessness, low

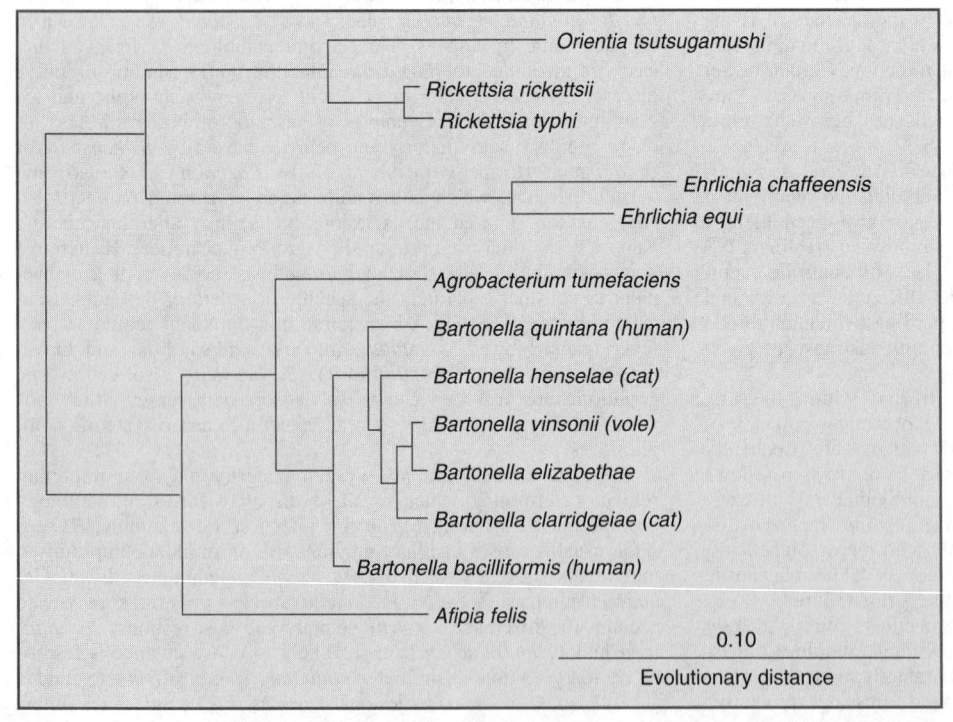

FIGURE 357–1 ■ Phylogenetic relationships among some of the α-proteobacteria, including the four *Bartonella* species pathogenic for humans, based on small subunit ribosomal RNA sequence analysis. Many of these organisms are endosymbiotic and may have evolved in close association with insects or plants. The primary reservoirs for the *Bartonella* species are indicated in parentheses after their names. (The reservoir for *B. elizabethae* is unknown.)

economic status, and louse infestation. Approximately 90% of patients with bacillary angiomatosis-peliosis are co-infected with the human immunodeficiency virus or are immunocompromised by another mechanism.

B. bacilliformis infection is restricted to the habitat of its principal vector, the sandfly, *Phlebotomus verrucarum.* The sandfly breeds and transmits the infection in river valleys of the Andes Mountains at altitudes between 2500 and 9000 feet. Humans are the only known reservoir of the microorganism. Convalescent individuals may have low-grade bacteremia for months to years after infection, and *B. bacilliformis* may be recovered from 5 to 10% of apparently healthy persons in an endemic area. These carriers represent the greatest epidemiologic threat.

BACTEREMIC DISEASE. Trench fever and *B. quintana* have a worldwide distribution; disease occurs sporadically in endemic sites, such as eastern Europe, Russia, and Mexico. Epidemic disease was described during World Wars I and II in Europe. In the 1990s, temporal and geographic clusters of endemic disease were recognized for the first time among urban homeless populations in the United States and western Europe. In one study, 20% of attendees at an inner-city clinic in Seattle had elevated antibody titers to *B. quintana.* Poor hygiene, alcoholism, and crowding characterize settings for the emergence of trench fever.

Bartonella species account for approximately 3% of all cases of infective endocarditis and a significant portion of "culture-negative" endocarditis cases in both immunocompetent and immunocompromised hosts. *B. henselae* has been incriminated in 5% of cases of fever of unknown origin in children.

GRANULOMATOUS DISEASE. Cat-scratch disease affects approximately 22,000 persons in the United States per year. The highest incidence of the disease occurs in the 5- through 14-year-old age group and in the South, where cat fleas are most prevalent and *B. henselae* infection of cats is most common. The disease usually occurs in the summer and autumn. A history of cat scratch or bite is elicited in approximately 75% of patients. Fewer than 5% of cases of cat-scratch disease belong to a family cluster; however, small clusters of disease with neurologic complication have been noted.

PATHOLOGY AND PATHOGENESIS. VASCULOPROLIFERATIVE DISEASE. The lesions of bacillary angiomatosis assume diverse macroscopic appearances, including an erythematous, polypoid or papular, cutaneous or mucosal pattern; deeply erythematous and indurated dermal plaques; and subcutaneous or visceral nodules. In all of these lesions, a distinctive lobular proliferation of capillaries is seen within a fibrous stroma. Hematoxylin and eosin staining reveals granular amphophilic material in the interstitium between vessels. This material corresponds to clumps of extracellular bacteria, as viewed with the Warthin-Starry silver stain or with electron microscopy. Bacillary peliosis is a histologic variant form of bacillary angiomatosis that is characterized by blood-filled cystic spaces, fibromyxoid stroma, and inflammatory cells; it is almost always associated with *B. henselae* and occurs most often within the liver and spleen. The pathogenesis of bacillary angiomatosis includes early blood-borne dissemination of organisms throughout the body. The bartonellae attach readily to and may enter erythrocytes; persistence within the intravascular compartment suggests bacterial mechanisms for avoidance of opsonization and host phagocytosis.

After inoculation by the sandfly, *B. bacilliformis* invades erythrocytes and endothelial cells. Most untreated patients who survive the acute hemolytic anemia go on to develop the chronic cutaneous lesions of verruga peruana. These hemangiomatous nodules consist of proliferating small vessels infiltrated by lymphocytes and macrophages. Verrugas may also occur in the viscera, bone, and central nervous system.

BACTEREMIC DISEASE. The pathology and pathogenesis of trench fever are not well characterized. In contrast to the angioproliferation seen with bacillary angiomatosis, biopsy specimens of skin lesions from patients with trench fever reveal perivascular lymphocytic infiltration; bacteria are not seen within vascular endothelial cells. *Bartonella* endocarditis usually occurs in persons with preexisting valvular (most often aortic valve) disease and leads to further valve destruction. Electron microscopy reveals intracellular and extracellular clusters of bacteria in valve tissue. In Oroya fever, erythrocyte parasitization results in increased fragility of red blood cells and increased phagocytosis by the reticuloendothelial system. In severe cases, as many as 90% of the circulating erythrocytes

may be parasitized. Peripheral blood smears reveal a normochromic macrocytosis and striking polychromasia, Howell-Jolly bodies, Cabot's rings, and nucleated erythrocytes. The Coombs test and other assays for red cell agglutinins and hemolysins are usually negative. Cells of the reticuloendothelial system may contain intracellular organisms, presumably as a result of erythrophagocytosis. Reactive hyperplasia of lymphatic tissue is common.

GRANULOMATOUS DISEASE. Histologic changes in lymph nodes evolve over a period of months in patients with cat-scratch disease. Follicular hyperplasia and hypertrophy, sinus histiocytosis, and B-cell proliferation are followed by granuloma formation and later by neutrophilic infiltration with central or stellate necrosis and surrounding palisades of histiocytes. Microabscesses are common. Bacilli are best visualized with the Warthin-Starry silver impregnation stain early in the course of the disease. It remains possible that bacterial strain–associated characteristics, as well as host factors, help to determine whether granulomatous or angioproliferative responses result from infection.

CLINICAL MANIFESTATIONS. VASCULOPROLIFERATIVE DISEASE. Bacillary angiomatosis is most often associated with tender cutaneous or subcutaneous lesions. Mucosal lesions are also common. These lesions may be solitary or multiple, red, purple, or flesh-colored dome-shaped papules, nodules, polypoid tumors, or plaques. With age the lesions may ulcerate, form a crust, or develop a collarette of scale. Subcutaneous lesions sometimes erode underlying bone. In an undetermined percentage of cases, visceral bacillary angiomatosis-peliosis occurs, sometimes in the absence of cutaneous disease. Visceral involvement may be asymptomatic or, as in disseminated cutaneous disease, may be associated with fever, chills, malaise, and anorexia. Liver, spleen, and internal lymph nodes appear to be the most frequent sites of extracutaneous disease. Biliary obstruction has resulted from external compression of periportal lymph nodes. Other sites affected by bacillary angiomatosis include bone marrow, lung, and brain.

Verruga peruana develops after a latent period of weeks to months following the resolution of acute *B. bacilliformis* infection in untreated patients. This disorder is characterized by 1- to 2-cm hemangiomatous nodules that typically evolve over a period of 1 to 2 months in crops on exposed skin, but also on mucous membranes and within internal organs. The lesions are usually non-tender and may vary morphologically, appearing sometimes as ulcers or as secondarily infected pustules. The verrugas may persist for months to years in untreated patients.

BACTEREMIC DISEASE. The incubation period for trench fever ranges from 4 to 35 days. In human volunteers the average duration was 22 days. Clinical manifestations vary from a febrile illness of 4 to 5 days' duration in some patients to a severe illness with prolonged fever in others. In the classic descriptions of more severe disease, infected persons experience three to five febrile paroxysms each lasting approximately 5 days (quintan or 5-day fever). A syndrome of continuous fever lasting 2 to 6 weeks has also been noted. In addition to fever and chills, symptoms of trench fever include malaise, anorexia, night sweats, headache with retro-orbital pain, and severe bone pain in the neck, back, and lower extremities, especially the tibia (shinbone fever). Conjunctival injection, hepatosplenomegaly, mild to moderate leukocytosis, and an erythematous maculopapular truncal rash occur in the majority of patients. Symptoms and signs are typically most severe during the initial febrile period. Subsequent attacks are milder, with the exception of persistent, severe bone pain. Irregular episodes of remission and late relapses have been reported. Specific antibodies to *B. quintana* appear within several weeks of primary infection, but they are not fully protective, because reinfection has been documented within 3 to 6 months of the initial illness.

The clinical manifestations of *Bartonella* endocarditis are similar to those of more typical forms of infective endocarditis. In a retrospective analysis of 22 patients, the majority presented with fever with a temperature greater than 38° C and approximately 40% manifested embolic phenomena. Echocardiography revealed a valvular vegetation in 86% of patients. Approximately 90% required valve surgery despite antibiotic therapy; the mortality rate was close to 30%. *B. henselae, B. quintana,* and *B. elizabethae* have all been reported to cause infective endocarditis.

Signs of sepsis or localized (granulomatous or angioproliferative) disease are uncommon in cases of *B. henselae* or *B. quintana* bacteremia. Fever, headache, myalgias, and arthralgias may persist or recur over a period of weeks to months despite therapy. In some cases, *B. henselae* bacteremia has been associated with a lymphocytic meningitis.

Within 2 to 6 weeks after the bite of an infected sandfly, the non-immune host develops Oroya fever. It is characterized by the insidious onset of myalgias and low-grade fever, followed by high fever, headache, and painful muscles and joints. Tender lymphadenopathy is common; splenomegaly is rare. Erythrocyte counts decrease rapidly within a few days and many fall as low as 1 million/mm³. In some patients there is a febrile crisis, followed by rapid resolution of symptoms and signs, increased erythropoiesis, and gradual reduction of fever. Recurrence of fever after initial improvement suggests secondary infection. Salmonellosis is an especially important complication of acute *B. bacilliformis*–associated disease in South America and may reflect transient immunosuppression. In addition, malaria, amebiasis, and tuberculosis also appear to be more common in these patients. Mortality in untreated Oroya fever approaches 50% as a result of both acute hemolytic anemia and secondary infections. After resolution of the febrile hemolytic anemia, immunity develops; relapses or reinfections are unusual.

GRANULOMATOUS DISEASE. After an incubation period of 3 to 10 days, an erythematous papule develops at the inoculation site in more than half of those later diagnosed with cat-scratch disease. These lesions may form a crust or become pustular; they resolve spontaneously in 1 to 3 weeks. Within a few weeks of inoculation, regional lymphadenopathy becomes apparent; usually a lymph node in the axillary or neck regions is found to be enlarged and tender (Table 357–1). Low-grade fever, malaise, anorexia, and nausea each occur in a minority of patients. In a typical case of cat-scratch disease, lymph nodes remain enlarged for at least 2 to 4 months. Infrequently, inoculation of the eye results in a granulomatous lesion of the conjunctiva and in preauricular adenopathy, a condition known as the oculoglandular syndrome of Parinaud (affecting 4 to 6% of cat-scratch disease patients).

Severe or systemic, non-neurologic manifestations are reported in 2% of cat-scratch disease patients. These include persistent fever, weight loss, splenomegaly, diffuse papular rash, erythema nodosum, pleuritis, splenic abscess, central lymphadenopathy, osteolytic lesions, hepatitis, and thrombocytopenic purpura. An additional 2% of cat-scratch disease patients develop neurologic complications. Encephalopathy or encephalitis are most common and are manifest by seizures and confusion; other presentations include radiculitis, meningitis, cranial neuritis, neuroretinitis, and cerebral arteritis. Neurologic complications occur 2 to 3 weeks after onset of the initial illness. Spontaneous, complete resolution is the rule in these cases.

DIAGNOSIS. VASCULOPROLIFERATIVE DISEASE. The diagnosis of both bacillary angiomatosis and cat-scratch disease rests on tissue examination and serologic tests in a compatible clinical setting. Histology typical of bacillary angiomatosis in hematoxylin and eosin–stained tissue is suggestive of the diagnosis. Warthin-Starry stains will usually confirm this diagnosis (i.e., revealing clumps of small, pleomorphic bacilli). Commercial laboratories, as well as the Centers for Disease Control and Prevention, offer an immunofluorescent or enzyme-linked immunosorbent assay for serum IgG antibodies directed against *B. henselae*, *B. quintana*, and *B. elizabe-*

Table 357–1 ■ **SELECTED CLINICAL FEATURES OF CLASSIC CAT-SCRATCH DISEASE**

FEATURE	% OF CASES
Site of lymphadenopathy	
Axilla	25–52
Neck	26–39
Groin	7–18
Elbow	2–13
Preauricular region	5–7
Single node involvement	43–85
Lymphadenopathy only	48–51
Fever	31–48
Splenomegaly	11–12
Hospitalization	9–17

Table 357–2 ■ **TREATMENT SUGGESTIONS**

Severe Cat-Scratch Disease*	
Doxycycline, plus	100 mg bid
rifampin	300 mg bid
or ciprofloxacin	500 mg bid
or azithromycin	500 mg qd × 1 d, then 250 mg qd × 4 d
Bacillary Angiomatosis-Peliosis or Bartonella Bacteremia†	
Erythromycin or	250–500 mg qid
doxycycline	100 mg bid
plus rifampin (severe disease)	300 mg bid
Azithromycin	500 mg qd × 1 d, then 250 mg/d

*Therapy with doxycycline plus rifampin or ciprofloxacin should be continued for at least 14 days.

†Treat patients with bacillary angiomatosis-peliosis for at least 3 to 4 months, patients with *Bartonella* bacteremia for 2 to 4 weeks, and patients with *Bartonella* endocarditis for at least 6 weeks.

thae. Most assays cannot distinguish reliably among humoral responses to each of these species. Cultivation of *Bartonella* species and detection of specific genetic sequences by PCR or antigens by immunohistochemical methods are more specialized procedures and are not available at most clinical microbiology laboratories. Kaposi's sarcoma is the most important entity confused with bacillary angiomatosis. Visual detection of bacilli distinguishes the latter from the former. Lytic bone lesions in an HIV-infected individual should raise the possibility of bacillary angiomatosis.

BACTEREMIC DISEASE. *Bartonella* species are slow-growing and fastidious, but they can be cultivated on blood-enriched media or in the presence of endothelial cells (see earlier). Formation of colonies on an agar surface directly from an infected clinical specimen may require more than 21 days of incubation and subculturing on freshly prepared media. Acridine orange staining procedures and lysis centrifugation culture methods enhance the detection and recovery, respectively, of *Bartonella* species from blood specimens. Serologic methods may aid in the diagnosis of *Bartonella* bacteremic disease. The serologic cross-reactivity of *Chlamydia* and *Bartonella* species may present a diagnostic problem because both groups of microorganisms must be considered in cases of culture-negative endocarditis. PCR assays have also proven successful in detecting *Bartonella* species on resected heart valve tissue.

The differential diagnosis of trench fever includes epidemic (louse-borne) typhus, which occurs under similar demographic circumstances and shares the same vector (*P. humanus*) as trench fever, endemic (murine) typhus, ehrlichiosis, Q fever, Rocky Mountain spotted fever, relapsing fever, Lyme disease, malaria, and plague. Local disease endemicity or history of body louse infestation should raise the clinical suspicion of trench fever.

The diagnosis of Oroya fever is made by examining a peripheral blood smear. Bacilli may be seen within red blood cells as single organisms or in pairs or clusters. With Giemsa staining, the bacilli appear as 0.3- to 1.5-μm pleomorphic red-purple rods.

GRANULOMATOUS DISEASE. Cat-scratch disease is diagnosed most often by examination of Warthin-Starry silver-stained tissue or by using serologic methods. The differential diagnosis for localized cat-scratch disease may include pyogenic lymphadenitis, mycobacterial infection, tularemia, brucellosis, lymphogranuloma venereum, syphilis, fungal disease, toxoplasmosis, and Epstein-Barr virus or cytomegalovirus infection.

TREATMENT. There are few data from prospective randomized studies from which to choose an antimicrobial regimen for *Bartonella*-associated disease. Retrospective or empirical clinical observations offer the primary basis for the suggested approaches in Table 357–2. Corticosteroids are not recommended for any of these diseases.

VASCULOPROLIFERATIVE DISEASE. All forms of *Bartonella*-associated vasculoproliferative disease warrant antimicrobial treatment. *Bartonella* species are susceptible in vitro to β-lactams, gentamicin, tetracyclines, chloramphenicol, and macrolides; however, clinical experience in the treatment of patients with bacillary angiomatosis-peliosis does not support all of these laboratory findings. In particular, there are well-documented instances of clinical failure with β-lactam agents. Based on empirical observations, the treatment of choice for bacillary angiomatosis-peliosis is either erythromycin, 500 mg every 6 hours, or doxycycline, 100 mg every 12 hours. Azithromycin is an alternative. Patients who are severely ill or unable to absorb oral medications should be treated with intravenous formulations. Rifampin should be added to the regimen for patients in the former category. Because disease relapse is otherwise so common in these immunocompromised hosts, patients should be treated for at least 3 months. Verruga lesions do not respond consistently to antimicrobial agents and sometimes require surgical resection.

BACTEREMIC DISEASE. *Bartonella* bacteremia also warrants antimicrobial treatment, despite the fact that some immunocompetent hosts with *B. quintana* bacteremia will clear their infection spontaneously. The same drugs and doses listed earlier for treatment of bacillary angiomatosis-peliosis are recommended for primary bacteremias. All patients should be evaluated for endocarditis. Treatment should be administered for at least 6 weeks and for 2 to 4 weeks in patients with and without endocarditis, respectively. Rifampin should be added to the regimen for treatment of endocarditis. Close monitoring of hemodynamics is essential because historically the majority of endocarditis patients have ultimately required valve repair or replacement, perhaps related to delay in diagnosis in many instances. Patients with trench fever usually respond rapidly to antibiotic therapy with resolution of fever and other symptoms within 1 to 2 days. Relapses in treated patients have been well described.

In patients with Oroya fever, clinical observations suggest that penicillin, chloramphenicol, tetracycline, and streptomycin are effective. Chloramphenicol at a dose of 2 to 4 g/day for 7 or more days is the therapy of choice because of the frequent association of *Salmonella* infection in endemic regions. After the institution of therapy, fever generally disappears within 2 to 3 days, although blood smears may remain positive for some time.

GRANULOMATOUS DISEASE. Most patients with cat-scratch disease do not require more than symptomatic support. A fluctuant or suppurative lymph node may benefit from needle aspiration. Antibiotic therapy should be reserved for immunocompromised individuals or those with evidence of severe or systemic disease. It remains unclear what constitutes the most useful agents in this setting. Doxycycline plus rifampin is probably effective, as is probably ciprofloxacin. One published randomized placebo-controlled study suggests that a 5-day course of azithromycin speeds resolution of cat-scratch lymphadenopathy.

Anderson BE, Neuman MA: *Bartonella* spp. as emerging human pathogens. Clin Microbiol Rev 10:203, 1997. *Useful review of the biology of the bartonellae. Emphasizes diagnostic approaches.*

Bass JW, Freitas BC, Freitas AD, et al: Prospective randomized double blind placebo-controlled evaluation of azithromycin for treatment of cat-scratch disease. Pediatr Infect Dis J 17:447, 1998. *First published prospective randomized study of treatment for cat-scratch disease. Suggests that azithromycin might speed resolution of disease in some cases.*

Koehler JE, Glaser CA, Tappero JW: *Rochalimaea henselae* infection: A new zoonosis with the domestic cat as reservoir. JAMA 271:531, 1994. *The first definitive demonstration that B. henselae bacteremia is common in asymptomatic domestic cats! Even though cat fleas were implicated, the mechanism(s) of B. henselae transmission from the cat reservoir to humans is believed to be direct inoculation.*

Koehler JE, Sanchez MA, Garrido CS, et al: Molecular epidemiology of *Bartonella* infections in patients with bacillary angiomatosis-peliosis. N Engl J Med 337:1876, 1997. *Defines the different epidemiologic settings for B. henselae and B. quintana–associated disease.*

Relman DA, Loutit JS, Schmidt TM, et al: The agent of bacillary angiomatosis: An approach to the identification of uncultured pathogens. N Engl J Med 323:1573, 1990. *Describes the first clinical application of a molecular approach for identifying previously uncharacterized fastidious or uncultivated microbial pathogens directly from infected host tissue. The results of this study suggested a close relationship between the agent(s) of bacillary angiomatosis and the Rochalimaea/Bartonella genus.*

Spach DH, Kanter AS, Dougherty MJ, et al: *Bartonella (Rochalimaea) quintana* bacteremia in inner-city patients with chronic alcoholism. N Engl J Med 332:424, 1995. *The first description of urban trench fever in the United States. These unexpected findings occurred after the institution of a more sensitive blood culture protocol at a major public hospital in Seattle.*

DISEASES DUE TO MYCOBACTERIA

358 TUBERCULOSIS

Michael D. Iseman

DEFINITION. Tuberculosis is an infectious disease caused by *Mycobacterium tuberculosis.* Characteristic features include a generally prolonged latency period between initial infection and overt disease, prominent pulmonary disease (although other organs can be involved), and a granulomatous response associated with intense tissue inflammation and damage.

ETIOLOGIC AGENT. Mycobacteria are small, rod-shaped, aerobic, non–spore-forming bacilli. In the genus *Mycobacterium,* there is a group of organisms so closely related that they are referred to as "the tuberculosis complex": *M. tuberculosis, M. bovis, M. africanum,* and *M. microti.* However, given the singular epidemiologic, clinical, public health, and therapeutic considerations associated with *M. tuberculosis,* the term *tuberculosis* should be reserved exclusively for infection or disease caused by this organism. Disease caused by other organisms of this genus should be referred to as "mycobacteriosis due to *M. x*" and not "atypical tuberculosis" or "tuberculosis due to . . ." (see also Chapter 359).

The mycobacteria are primarily soil or environmental organisms. However, *M. tuberculosis* has become so adapted to the human body that it has no natural reservoirs in nature other than infected/diseased persons. Although disease due to strain identified as *M. tuberculosis* has been reported rarely in primates, elephants, and other mammals, the presumption is that the animals acquired the infection from humans.

Mycobacterial cell walls contain high concentrations of lipids or waxes, making them resistant to standard staining techniques. They can be induced to take up a dye such as carbol fuchsin by alkalinity or by heating; and once so colored, they are resistant to the potent decolorizing agent acid-alcohol, hence the reference to "acid-fast" bacilli.

M. tuberculosis and most of the other mycobacteria grow quite slowly; their doubling time in most media is approximately 18 hours. Readily discernible colonies typically do not appear on solid media for 3 to 5 weeks; because of this, culture confirmation, speciation, and drug susceptibility testing have proven clinically problematic.

M. tuberculosis is an obligate aerobe and a facultative intracellular parasite. Tissues attacked are characterized by high regional oxygen tension. The ability to invade and spread throughout the human body has largely to do with the capacity of tubercle bacilli to survive and proliferate within mononuclear phagocytes.

TRANSMISSION. Infection is spread almost exclusively by aerosolization of contaminated respiratory secretions. Patients with *cavitary* lung disease are particularly infectious because their sputum usually contains 1 to 100 million bacilli/mL, and they cough frequently.

However, the intact skin and respiratory mucous membranes of normal exposed individuals are quite resistant to invasion. For infection to occur, bacilli must be delivered to the distal air spaces of the lung, the alveoli, where they are not subject to bronchial mucociliary clearance. Once deposited in alveoli, bacilli are adapted to promote uptake by alveolar macrophages, which—depending on innate, genetically determined properties—may be more or less permissive to bacillary proliferation (see later).

To reach the alveoli, which lie at the end of a ramifying system of progressively smaller airways, the bacilli must be suspended in very fine units that behave as the air itself and not as particles with significant mass. These units are the dehydrated residuals of the tinier particles generated by high-velocity exhalational maneuvers; cough-inducing procedures such as bronchoscopy or endotracheal intubation are particularly likely to generate infectious aerosols. These droplet nuclei are calculated to be 1 to 5 μm in diameter, may remain suspended in room air for many hours, and when inhaled can traverse the airways to reach the alveoli.

Although patients with cavitary tuberculosis expectorate massive numbers of bacilli, the probability of generating *infectious* particles is relatively low. Household contacts of patients with extensive pulmonary disease who have had productive coughs for weeks or months before diagnosis have, on average, less than a 50% chance of being infected. Hence the usual case of pulmonary tuberculosis is of a low order of infectiousness compared with an airborne disease such as measles. However, infrequent cases demonstrate extremely high rates of transmission; specific factors in these instances have not been clearly elucidated.

The preponderance of transmission occurs as described earlier but other mechanisms of transmission have been identified. Aerosols generated by débridement or by dressing changes of skin or soft tissue abscesses due to *M. tuberculosis* have been shown to be highly infectious. Also, tissue agitation associated with autopsies and direct inoculation into soft tissues from contaminated instruments or bone fragments also have been reported. Fomites do not play a significant role in transmission.

PATHOGENESIS AND IMMUNITY. The natural history and various clinical syndromes of tuberculosis are intimately related to the hosts' defenses. Tubercle bacilli do not elaborate classic endo- or exotoxins; rather, the inflammatory illness and tissue destruction are mediated by products elaborated by the host during the "immune" response to the infection (see Part XX).

When an immunologically naive alveolar macrophage engulfs a tubercle bacillus, it initially provides a nurturing environment within its phagosome in which the bacilli survive and replicate. However, the infected macrophage releases substances that attract T lymphocytes; the macrophages then present antigens from the phagocytized bacilli to these lymphocytes, initiating a series of committed immune effector cells. The lymphocytes, in turn, elaborate cytokines that "activate" the macrophages, enhancing their antimicrobial capacity. Thus is set in motion an elaborate, delicately balanced struggle between the host and the parasite.

Among "normal" adult persons, the host initially prevails in more than 95% of cases. However, this initial encounter typically extends over a few weeks to several months during which the bacillary population has proliferated massively and undergone variable degrees of dissemination. Tissues that are seeded during this bacillemia, such as the apices of the lungs, the kidneys, bones, meninges, or other extrapulmonary sites, are potential foci for subsequent "reactivation" tuberculosis. Through complex interactions involving mononuclear phagocytes and various T-cell subsets, host defenses are enhanced. This results in more competent macrophages capable of inhibiting the intracellular replication of mycobacteria. Also, disruption of permissive macrophages that support bacillary multiplication occurs in order that more competent macrophages may engulf and limit the growth of the mycobacteria. These phenomena are broadly referred to as "cell-mediated immunity" (CMI) and "delayed-type hypersensitivity" (DTH), respectively. DTH is associated clinically with the development of the tuberculin reaction, an indurated response 48 to 72 hours after the intradermal injection of tuberculosis protein antigens (such as purified protein derivative, or PPD). Skin test reactivity typically develops 4 to 6 weeks after infection, although intervals up to 20 weeks have been noted.

As these defenses gain momentum, involution of the numerous disseminated granulomatous foci in the lungs, lymph nodes, and scattered sites occurs. Typically, all that remains to overtly mark this encounter is the tuberculin skin test reactivity. In a minority of cases, a small single residual of the primary infection appears in the lung parenchyma (the Ghon focus); occasionally, this is accompanied by calcifications of the ipsilateral hilar nodes. Some patients also develop fibronodular shadowing in one or both lung apices ("Simon foci"); these presumably are the residua of subclinical disease at these sites.

The majority of cases occur due to late reactivation of the vestigial lesions of this primary infection, either in the lungs or in extrapulmonary sites. Rapid progression to overt disease occurs in a minority of newly infected persons who cannot mount sufficient immune responses. Groups at high risk include infants through age 4, the infirm elderly, and immunocompromised subjects, including those with human immunodeficiency virus (HIV) infection or acquired immunodeficiency syndrome (AIDS), organ transplant recipients, and those with other immunosuppressive illnesses or chemotherapy.

EPIDEMIOLOGY. Globally, tuberculosis is now the leading infectious cause of morbidity and mortality. However, in the more industrialized nations, the disease has retreated from the general

populations, afflicting selected groups. Recognition of these high-risk groups is vital in terms of diagnosis, prevention, and control programs.

GLOBAL. The World Health Organization (WHO) estimates that approximately one third of the world's population is latently infected with *M. tuberculosis.* From this pool, 8 to 10 million new active cases emerge per year; WHO estimates that roughly 50% of these are communicable forms of pulmonary disease. Regions in the world where the infection and disease are most prevalent include the Pacific Rim nations (excluding Japan), Southeast Asia, Indo-Asia, sub-Saharan Africa, and Latin America. Because of delayed, inadequate, or unavailable therapy, 2 to 3 million persons die annually; indeed, WHO estimates that 26% of preventable deaths in the developing nations are attributable to tuberculosis.

UNITED STATES. The United States has a considerably lower prevalence of infection; recent Centers for Disease Control and Prevention (CDC) estimates suggest that only 4 to 6% of the population—10 to 15 million persons—harbor latent infections. Case rates in the United States had fallen consistently from 1953 to 1984; however, from 1985 to 1992 there was a substantial upsurge resulting in more than 75,000 surplus cases in this period (Fig. 358–1). Elements feeding this rise included HIV, immigration, and—critically—deterioration of the public health infrastructure in America's larger cities. In response to this pattern, treatment programs were strengthened and measures were taken to reduce nosocomial transmission; from 1992 to 1997 case rates dropped substantially, with an all-time low of 19,851 cases in 1997. This represents a 26% reduction from 1992; case rates fell from 10.5 to 7.4 per 100,000 per year in this period. Notable is the fact that in 1997 six states (California, New York, Texas, Florida, Illinois, and New Jersey) contributed 57% of the national case load.

U.S. morbidity entails remarkable disparities according to race, age, and national origins. Among non-white Americans, it is largely a disease of young adults, with the peak incidence between ages 25 and 44 years; by contrast, the peak age among whites is 70 years and older, due presumably to latent early infections (Fig. 358–2). In 1996, 71% of U.S. tuberculosis cases occurred among minorities.

Immigration has contributed significantly to the upturn in morbidity. In 1997, roughly 39% of cases occurred among foreign-born persons (up from 20% in 1985). Major sources of these cases include Mexico, the Philippines, Southeast Asia, the Caribbean, and Latin America, the bulk occurring within 5 years of arrival in the United States. This rising percentage reflects both declining case rates among the indigenous population and relatively high rates among immigrants. In 1997, case rates for foreign-born persons were five-fold higher than in U.S.-born persons.

HIV INFECTION/AIDS (See Part XXIII). HIV infection and AIDS have contributed to the rising case rates of tuberculosis through three broad pathways: (1) Individuals with latent tuberculosis infection who acquired HIV infection are at much greater risk of reactivation as their immune capacity diminishes; (2) persons with HIV infection or AIDS may well be at higher risk of acquiring new

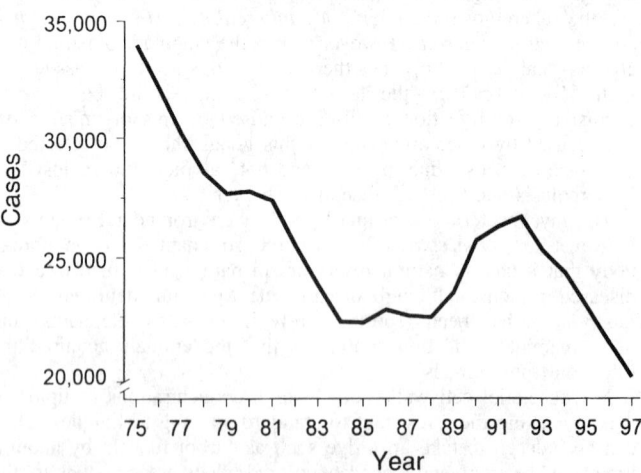

FIGURE 358–1 ■ Reported tuberculosis cases in the United States, 1975–1997.

Year	Cases	Case Rate (per 100,000)
1993	25,287	9.8
1994	24,361	9.4
1995	22,860	8.7
1996	21,337	8.0
1997	19,851	7.4

FIGURE 358-2 ▪ Tuberculosis morbidity in the United States, 1993–1997.

infections with tuberculosis, due probably to both biologic factors (they may be more prone to become infected on exposure due to impaired defenses) and situational factors (they are more likely to be exposed due to time spent in high-risk, congregate environments); and (3) young adults with HIV infection and active tuberculosis transmit tuberculosis to people with whom they reside.

In the United States, the upsurge in tuberculosis from 1985 to the present has been clearly linked to the HIV epidemic, although full quantification of the association is not possible due to incomplete serologic testing.

CLINICAL PRESENTATIONS. Because the primary pulmonary infection results in bacillemic dissemination, tuberculosis commonly entails disease in extrathoracic as well as pulmonary or pleural sites. As a generalization, hosts with more competent immunity tend to have disease limited to their lungs or other single sites, whereas those with less robust defenses experience multifocal or disseminated disease.

NORMAL ADULTS. Overall, excluding the influence of HIV infection, about 85% of adults present with pulmonary parenchymal disease, 15% with disease at extrapulmonary sites, and approximately 4% with simultaneously active disease at intrathoracic and extrathoracic locations.

Two important comments should be made about clinical tuberculosis in normal adults: (1) The tuberculin skin test (TST) will be falsely negative in 20 to 25% at the time of diagnosis, and (2) although most complain of feeling "feverish," a substantial proportion do not have fever when measured. Thus, a clinician should not be diverted from considering the diagnosis by non-reactive TSTs or lack of fever in patients with other typical features of tuberculosis.

Pulmonary Disease. Classic symptoms include the following: cough is nearly universal; typically, it is initially dry but then progresses with increasing volumes of purulent secretions and the variable appearance of blood streaking or gross hemoptysis. Feverishness is common as the disease advances; actual temperatures range from subnormal to extreme elevations. Sweating, including drenching night sweats, is quite typical. Other common complaints include malaise, fatigue, weight loss, non-pleuritic chest pain, and dyspnea.

Signs may be quite limited until the disease is in advanced stages. Fever with peaks as high as 40 to 41°C, typically occurring in the evening, is seen among patients with disease of various forms and extent. Localized rales are early findings; coarse rhonchi evolve as secretions become more voluminous and tenacious; signs of lung consolidation are rarely heard. Wheezing and/or regionally diminished breath sounds may be heard in cases with peri- or endobronchial airway compression.

The chest radiograph is central to the diagnosis. Upper lung zone fibronodular shadowing involving one or both apices is seen in the majority of cases. As these lesions advance, they enlarge and become fluffy or softly marginated; coalescence occurs, and cavitation devolves as intense local inflammation produces necrosis and sloughing of lung tissue. The most common sites involved in reactivation adult tuberculosis are, in descending order, the posterior and apical segments of the right upper lobe, the apical-posterior segment of the left upper lobe, and the superior segments of the lower lobes. Lower zone disease is the presenting appearance in less than 15% of HIV-negative adults; it is seen somewhat more commonly in diabetics and patients with prominent peribronchial and endobronchial involvement. Pleural effusions are uncommon in adults with reactivation-type pulmonary disease.

Sputum smears and cultures are the most specific components of diagnosis. Some contemporary laboratories still use the classic acid-fast stains (Ziehl-Neelsen or Kinyoun); however, most use a modi-fied acid-fast method, the fluorochrome technique, which relies on the uptake and acid-fast retention of auramine-O, a dye that fluoresces when excited by ultraviolet light. With the fluorochrome technique, the tubercle bacillus is more easily discernible (bright yellow contrasted to an inky black background) than the older methods (red on a blue and white background); hence the fluorochrome system is visually more sensitive. Microscopic acid-fast bacilli (AFB) found in respiratory secretions associated with suitable clinical, epidemiologic, and radiographic findings highly suggests tuberculosis. However, microscopy is not specific, because other pathogenic or saprophytic mycobacteria may be found in sputum. The test is not very sensitive; the likelihood of positive smears depends heavily on the extent of pulmonary involvement. With readily visible cavities and no prior treatment, it would be rare to have negative sputum microscopy. However, with non-cavitary fibronodular or miliary patterns on chest films, negative microscopy is common. Overall, 50 to 60% of patients with active pulmonary tuberculosis yield AFB smear-positive sputum. Cultures are the gold standard for diagnosis; however, current methods typically entail 3 to 6 weeks to cultivate and identify species. More rapid cultivation and identification techniques that use liquid media and/or radiometric, molecular biologic, or chromatographic methods have reduced the required time substantially. Nucleic acid amplification techniques potentially offer 1- to 2-day diagnosis but have not been approved for sputum AFB smear-negative specimens. The diagnosis is occasionally made on the basis of symptoms, radiographic findings, and response to empirical therapy *without* culture confirmation. Because of the rising prevalence of resistance to standard drugs, susceptibility testing on all initial *M. tuberculosis* isolates is recommended.

As noted earlier, the TST will be falsely negative in 20 to 25% of HIV-negative adults with pulmonary tuberculosis. Testing with other delayed-type hypersensitivity antigens may help identify persons who are broadly anergic; however, selective anergy to tuberculin occurs.

Extrapulmonary Tuberculosis (XPTB). XPTB occurs in roughly one sixth of HIV-negative adults in the United States with active disease. The most common sites and relevant features are displayed in Table 358–1 (see also Part XXIII).

Clinically, it should be noted that the severe wasting seen with advanced pulmonary diseases—consumption—is rarely seen with XPTB. Feverishness occurs with more extensive disease, prominently including miliary, pleural, and genitourinary disease.

Diagnosis is problematic in most forms of XPTB due to the relative paucity of bacilli. Histopathology of involved tissues typically shows giant cell granulomas with caseating necrosis and few, if any, demonstrable AFB. Analysis of mesothelial effusions (pleural, peritoneal, or pericardial) characteristically reveals a lymphocyte-rich exudate with low concentrations of glucose; however, the *initial* inflammatory responses in these spaces may be polymorphonuclear (PMN) leukocyte predominant. Cerebrospinal fluid (CSF) in meningitis begins with a modest leukocytosis, shifting from PMN to lymphocyte dominance; leukocyte counts typically range from 50 to 300 cells/mL. The CSF protein concentration is typically moderately elevated. Glucose levels are progressively depressed in relation to the degree of leukocytosis. Because of the scarcity of AFB in the CSF, the polymerase chain reaction test may be useful in establishing the diagnosis, although the test is not yet approved for this indication.

TUBERCULOSIS IN PERSONS WITH HIV INFECTION/AIDS. Early in the course of HIV infection, the clinical manifestations of tuberculosis are quite similar to those in normal hosts. However, with the progressive reduction in the T-lymphocyte population, the following major changes ensue: (1) a steady reduction in the proportion who react significantly to tuberculin skin testing, reaching a nadir of 10 to 20% reactors among those with advanced AIDS; (2) substantially greater extrapulmonary involvement, reaching 60 to 80% prevalence of XPTB including exotic presentations such as diffuse lymphadenitis, cutaneous disease, or an acute syndrome mindful of gram-negative sepsis among those with CD4 counts less than 50; and (3) changing patterns of disease on chest radiography, evolving from classic upper zone fibronodular, cavitary disease to lower zone, nondescript pneumonic patterns, infrequent cavity for-

Table 358–1 ■ COMMON FORMS OF EXTRAPULMONARY TUBERCULOSIS IN PATIENTS WITHOUT HIV INFECTION

ORGAN SYSTEM	RELATIVELY HIGH-RISK GROUPS	COMMON CLINICAL MANIFESTATIONS	DIAGNOSIS	MANAGEMENT
Lymphatic	Youngsters and young adults; F > M, Asian and Indian females high-risk	Unilateral, cervical; painless; sinus tracts late	Excisional biopsy with culture; PPD usually positive	May respond slowly to medication; rarely may require excision
Pleural	Young adults with primary infection; older adults with reactivation disease	May be acute or indolent; severe pleurisy or asymptomatic	Lymphatic exudate; AFB smear usually negative; biopsy with culture gives best yield	Usually responds well to medication; do not drain with tube thoracostomy
Genitourinary	Rare in young; more frequent among females, foreign born, and Native Americans	May involve kidneys, ureters, bladder, testes, epididymis, uterus, fallopian tubes	Culture urine; biopsy and culture masses and uterine scrapings	Usually responds well to medication; beware of early or late obstructive uropathy
Bone/joint	More common in elderly, although seen in all ages	Lumbar and low dorsal spine common in older; high dorsal in young; weight-bearing bones/joints	Needle biopsy and aspirate for spinal lesions; synovial biopsy and culture for joints	Débride and stabilize spine; try to avoid fusing joints
Disseminated	Most frequent in very young or old; blacks and Native Americans	Chest film abnormalities may lag; progressive fever and inanition; PPD negative in 50%	Smears and cultures of involved fluids, organs, and mesothelia; smear and culture urine	Early therapy vital; corticosteroids of uncertain value
Meninges/CNS	Most common among infants/children with XPTB; higher risk for Hispanics, blacks, and Native Americans	Three stages; early fever, headache, and malaise; later confusion, obtundation, seizures, and coma	Lumbar puncture: ↑ protein and cells; ↓ glucose, ↑ pressure; smears rarely positive; special tests (see text)	Prognosis related to stage; corticosteroids indicated in most cases; drugs must penetrate CNS
Peritoneal/gastrointestinal	Increases with age; higher risk among minorities	Mainly mesothelial but ileal involvement may resemble Crohn's; abdominal swelling and vague pain common	Laparoscopic biopsy ideal; smear and culture ascites; stool cultures may be useful	Beware of adhesions and obstruction; corticosteroids may be useful
Pericardial	Rare in children; more common in blacks	Acute pain rare; cough, dyspnea, and vague discomfort	Widened cardiac silhouette; left pleural effusion; ECG low voltage and chronic ST/T wave changes; ↓ heart sounds, rubs rare	Corticosteroids ↓ effusion, improve performance; may reduce late adhesive complications; pericardiectomy for tamponade

Note: Among persons without HIV infection, roughly 16% of tuberculosis presents as extrapulmonary involvement. Lymphatic and pleural disease are the most common forms.

mation, interstitial or miliary shadowing, very prominent hilar or paratracheal adenopathy, and substantial pleural effusions.

TREATMENT. One unique aspect to the care of tuberculosis patients merits emphasis before discussing specific therapy: Because of the hazard of casual, airborne transmission of infection and of the potentially morbid or lethal consequences for the recipients, there is a singular public health mandate that *persons with communicable tuberculosis must either be treated or quarantined.* U.S. public health policy throughout the 20th century has empowered governmental representatives to quarantine patients with potentially lethal infectious diseases. In the case of tuberculosis, modern chemotherapy has, in effect, become "chemical quarantine"; thus, non-adherence to treatment may be seen as breaching this quarantine. Because of the consequences of inadequate or incomplete treatment, directly observed therapy (DOT) to prevent non-compliance is being employed increasingly (see the section on non-adherence later).

INDICATIONS FOR COMMENCING TREATMENT. Because it usually takes 3 to 8 weeks to culture and identify species, treatment for most patients is initiated before a "definitive" diagnosis is established, based rather on an amalgam of historical, epidemiologic, radiographic, tissue or fluid analysis, and microscopic findings. Beginning empirical therapy for patients with potentially rapid, life-threatening conditions such as central nervous system (CNS) or miliary disease usually entails a low threshold of suspicion; however, care should be taken to obtain optimal diagnostic specimens before commencing medication, lest the chemotherapy suppress growth from paucibacillary material.

THE PRINCIPLES OF MULTIDRUG TREATMENT. Patients with active tuberculosis should receive multiple agents both to prevent the emergence of drug-resistant mutants and to accelerate the bacterial clearance. Of these, the former is more crucial, because the emergence of a substantial population of drug-resistant bacilli may significantly and permanently compromise the treatment outcome.

Biologically, tubercle bacilli have the well-documented capacity to undergo spontaneous mutations that confer resistance to the various antituberculosis medications. These mutations occur at predictable frequencies, usually in the range of 1 in 10^5 to 10^8 replications, and are unlinked, resulting in resistance to only one drug or drug category. In patients with cavitary tuberculosis, the population of bacilli is so numerous that small numbers of mycobacteria exist that are resistant to each of the standard medications. However, because the mutations are unlinked, there is an extremely low probability of spontaneous resistance to two or more drugs by a single microbe; for example, the isoniazid-resistant mutants would be killed by rifampin (RIF) and the rifampin-resistant mutants killed by isoniazid (INH). Thus, early in treatment when the mycobacterial burden is greatest, it is vital that *at least* two effective agents be employed.

If patients are non-adherent, that is, stop one of their medications unbeknownst to their clinician, the unopposed mutants are allowed to proliferate, resulting in treatment failures or relapses associated with acquired drug resistance. When this happens serially, multidrug resistance is created. Such organisms can be transmitted then to other persons, giving rise to initial drug-resistant tuberculosis.

In addition to combating drug resistance, multidrug regimens can shorten the required duration of treatment through unique contributions by the various agents. A regimen of INH and ethambutol (EMB) requires 18 months to cure the typical case of pulmonary tuberculosis; adding RIF to INH reduces the duration to 9 months; and when an initial 2-month phase of pyrazinamide (PZA) is added to INH and RIF, cure occurs in 6 months.

CHOICE OF REGIMEN. Because of concern over the rising prevalence of drug resistance, recent CDC recommendations advocate a four-drug regimen for most cases of known or suspected tuberculosis (Table 358–2). INH and RIF are the central agents of any regimen based on their superior bactericidal activity and low toxicity. PZA has special utility in promoting rapid, early reduction in bacillary burden; in drug-susceptible cases, PZA need be given only for the initial 2 months to produce this effect. EMB is useful primarily to protect against the emergence of drug resistance in cases with unknown initial susceptibility patterns and large mycobacterial burdens; EMB may be terminated if susceptibility is reported or be continued throughout the duration of treatment if resistance is noted (see later). Streptomycin (SM), a parenteral agent, has found a diminishing role in modern therapy due to problems with regularly administering intramuscular injections; however, for patients with very extensive tuberculosis, SM may accelerate initial bactericidal activity. Dosage and toxicity for these agents are displayed in Table 358–3.

Does every patient need to receive such a four-drug regimen? In actual practice, clinicians should review every proven or suspected case and consider individual modifications or exemptions of this standard program. For example, (1) an elderly patient with known remote exposure to tuberculosis in the prechemotherapy era, with no recent contacts and no history of tuberculosis medical treatment, might reasonably be started on a three-drug (INH, RIF, EMB) or even two-drug (INH, RIF) regimen because of the very low likelihood of drug resistance; and (2) an injection drug-using 35-year-old HIV-positive man from the Bronx who has been previously hospitalized in this community might receive initial seven-drug treatment because of the risk of disease due to nosocomial acquisition of one of the multidrug-resistant tuberculosis strains prevalent in the New York City area.

Common factors that might influence the initial choice of drugs are included in Table 358–4. Additional considerations in selecting therapy are noted below.

AIDS. (SEE PART XXIII). The most salient particular issue in patients with AIDS and tuberculosis is to ensure adequate absorption of the antituberculosis medications. Due to a variety of AIDS-associated enteropathies, there is a risk of grossly reduced serum drug concentrations, which can result in treatment failure and po-

Table 358–2 ■ RECOMMENDED REGIMEN OPTIONS FOR TUBERCULOSIS, UNITED STATES

REGIMEN	MEDICATIONS	TOTAL DURATION	COMMENTS
ATS/CDC (as modified by ACET)	INH and RIF daily for 6 mo PZA and SM or EMB daily for 2 mo	6 mo	Add SM or EMB in areas/patients at risk for initial drug resistance. Stop PZA, EMB, or SM after 2 mo if strain susceptible; continue or modify regimen if resistance present.
Denver	INH, RIF, PZA, and SM daily for 2 wk; then twice weekly for 6 wk. Follow with INH and RIF twice weekly for 18 wk	6 mo	Stop PZA and SM at 8 wk if strain is susceptible; continue through 6 mo if there is initial INH resistance. May substitute EMB for SM. 24 weeks of twice-weekly therapy facilitates directly observed therapy.
Hong Kong	INH, RIF, PZA, and SM or EMB thrice weekly for 6 mo (may stop PZA, SM, or EMB after 2 mo)	6 mo	All-intermittent. If strain is susceptible, may stop PZA and SM or EMB after 2 mo. If there is INH resistance, stop INH and add the fourth drug (EMB or SM).
Arkansas	INH and RIF daily for 1 mo; then INH and RIF twice weekly for 8 mo	9 mo	This regimen should only be employed in populations with a very low prevalence of drug resistance. Initial therapy probably should include a third drug until drug susceptibility is reported.

Note: Currently, the Advisory Council for the Elimination of Tuberculosis of the CDC advocates initial four-drug therapy for cases in communities with a background prevalence of initial drug resistance of 4% or greater. If susceptibility has been demonstrated or if resistance is deemed very unlikely, initial three-drug regimens may be used. INH = isoniazid; RIF = rifampin; PZA = pyrazinamide; SM = streptomycin; EMB = ethambutol.

Table 358–3 ■ DOSAGE, TOXICITY, AND SPECIAL CONSIDERATIONS FOR STANDARD ANTITUBERCULOSIS MEDICATIONS

DRUG	DAILY	USUAL ADULT DOSE THRICE WEEKLY ‖ TWICE WEEKLY	TOXICITY	SPECIAL CONSIDERATIONS	COMMENTS
Isoniazid (INH)	300 mg PO	600 ‖ 900 mg	Hepatitis, neuritis, mood/cognition, lupus reaction	Pregnancy: safe Liver disease: caution Renal impairment: ↓ dose if severe	Monitor liver function tests monthly in most patients; clinically significant interactions with phenytoin and antifungal agents (azols)
Rifampin (RIF)	600 mg PO 450 mg in persons <50 kg body weight	600 ‖ (same)	Hepatitis, thrombopenia, nephritis, flu syndrome	Pregnancy: acceptable Liver disease: caution Renal impairment: safe	Key: multiple, profound drug interactions possible (see later); turns urine and fluids red
Pyrazinamide (PZA)	25–30 mg/kg PO	30–35 mg/kg ‖ (same)	Hepatitis, arthralgias and arthritis secondary to hyperuricemia, gastrointestinal distress, rash	Pregnancy: unknown (avoid) Liver disease: caution Renal impairment: caution	Urate levels always rise; do not treat or stop PZA unless unmanageable gout develops
Ethambutol (EMB)	15 mg/kg PO	35 mg/kg ‖ 50 mg/kg	Optic neuritis	Pregnancy: safe Liver disease: safe Renal impairment: ↓ dose/frequency	Monitor visual acuity and color vision regularly
Streptomycin (SM)	12–15 mg/kg IM	15 mg/kg ‖ (same)	Vestibular and auditory, cation depletion	Pregnancy: high-risk (avoid) Liver disease: safe Renal impairment: ↓ dose/frequency	Reduce dose and/or frequency in case of renal impairment

Note: Rifampin drug interactions have been reported with anti-retroviral agents including protease inhibitors and non-nucleoside reverse transcriptase inhibitors, oral contraceptives, anticoagulants, methadone, corticosteroids, estrogen replacement, calcium channel blockers, β-blockers, cyclosporine, antifungal agents (azols), phenytoin, theophylline, sulfonylureas, haloperidol, and others (see *Physicians' Desk Reference*).

Table 358-4 ■ HIGH-RISK CANDIDATES FOR IPT

Candidates for preventive chemotherapy—persons at high risk for tuberculosis. Various persons with latent tuberculosis infection are at relatively great risk of developing active disease. The degree of tuberculin skin test reactivity to identify such persons varies based on epidemiologic and biologic factors. The recommended duration of therapy is 6 months for most candidates but 12 months for HIV-infected persons or patients with upper-zone fibronodular shadows on chest film.

High-Risk Groups

Certain groups within the infected population are at greater risk than others and should receive high priority for preventive therapy. *In the United States, persons with any of the following six risk factors should be considered candidates for preventive therapy, regardless of age, if they have not previously been treated:*

1. Persons with human immunodeficiency virus (HIV) infection (≥ 5 mm) and persons with risk factors for HIV infection whose HIV infection status is unknown but who are suspected of having HIV infection.
2. Close contacts of persons with newly diagnosed infectious tuberculosis (≥ 5 mm). In addition, tuberculin-negative (< 5 mm) children and adolescents who have been close contacts of infectious persons within the past 3 months are candidates for preventive therapy until a repeat tuberculin skin test is done 12 weeks after contact with the infectious source.
3. Recent converters, as indicated by a tuberculin skin test (≥ 10 mm increase within a 2-year period for those < 35 years old; ≥ 15 mm increase for those ≥ 35 years of age).
4. Persons with abnormal chest radiographs that show fibrotic lesions likely to represent old healed tuberculosis (≥ 5 mm).
5. Intravenous drug users known to be HIV seronegative (≥ 10 mm).
6. Persons with medical conditions that have been reported to increase the risk of tuberculosis (≥ 10 mm).

In addition, in the absence of any of the above risk factors, persons younger than 35 years of age in the following high-incidence groups are appropriate candidates for preventive therapy if their reaction to a tuberculin skin test is ≥ 10 mm:

1. Foreign-born persons from high-prevalence countries.
2. Medically underserved low-income populations, including high-risk racial or ethnic minority populations, especially blacks, Hispanics, and Native Americans.
3. Residents of facilities for long-term care (e.g., correctional institutions, nursing homes, and mental institutions).

In addition to these groups, public health officials should be alert for other high-risk populations in their communities. For example, through a review of cases reported in the community over several years, health officials may use geographic or sociodemographic factors to identify groups that should be targeted for intervention. Screening and preventive therapy programs should be initiated and promoted within these populations based on an analysis of cases and infection in the community. To the extent possible, members of high-risk groups and their health-care providers should be involved in the design, implementation, and evaluation of these programs. Staff of facilities in which an individual with disease would pose a risk to large numbers of susceptible persons (e.g., correctional institutions, nursing homes, mental institutions, other health-care facilities, schools, and child-care facilities) may also be considered for preventive therapy if their tuberculin reaction is ≥ 10 mm induration.

From screening for tuberculosis and tuberculous infection in high-risk populations and the use of preventive therapy for tuberculous infection in the United States. Recommendation of the Advisory Committee for the Elimination of Tuberculosis. MMWR 39(No. RR-8):7, 1990.

tentially promote acquired drug resistance. Almost unique to persons with AIDS is rifampin monoresistance. Direct determination of drug levels at some time early in treatment is the ideal means for addressing this issue. If this is not feasible, very close monitoring of responses to treatment and use of high-range drug dosing may be appropriate. Also, because of the polypharmacy typically used with AIDS, special attention should be given to the potential impact of RIF-induced hepatic catabolism of other medications (see Table 358-4). The most critical current aspect of drug-drug interaction is the effect of rifampin on the bioavailability of anti-retroviral agents, including protease inhibitors and non-nucleoside reverse transcriptase inhibitors. Rifampin, by accelerating the hepatic degradation of these drugs, may lower their bioavailability to the extent of lost efficacy and acquired viral resistance to these agents. Various options have been suggested to deal with this situation. They range from delaying anti-retroviral therapy until tuberculosis treatment is completed, using rifampin for only 2 months, substituting rifabutine (which induces the cytochrome P450 pathways less

than does rifampin), or using a non-rifamycin regimen. Such cases should probably be decided on an individual basis after specialized consultation.

CNS DISEASE. Smaller un-ionized molecules such as INH and PZA cross the blood-brain barrier well, even in the absence of gross inflammation. RIF crosses less well, although therapeutic effects are seen. EMB CSF levels are significantly lower than those in serum, and its use in meningitis is less well established. SM and the other aminoglycoside antibiotics are large, complex, and ionically charged molecules; they cross the barrier very poorly, even in the presence of inflammation.

COMBATING NON-ADHERENCE WITH DIRECTLY OBSERVED INTERMITTENT CHEMOTHERAPY. Treatment given intermittently, thrice or twice weekly, is generally comparable in efficacy with daily treatment. These intermittent schedules make it practical that patients either come to treatment centers or have visits by outreach workers at home or in shelters, schools, or work sites to observe ingestion or actually administer medications. Most reported regimens have begun with a daily phase of therapy and switched to an intermittent schedule after 1 or 2 months. However, effective treatment can either entail a brief (2-week) initial daily phase *or* be intermittent (thrice weekly) throughout. Not all patients need to receive directly observed therapy; some can be trusted to self-administer their drugs. However, it is extremely difficult to predict those who are likely to be compliant, and careful attention should be given to patient education and ongoing monitoring of medication-taking behavior for all patients. If non-adherence is demonstrated or reasonably anticipated (on the basis of risk factors such as homelessness, substance abuse, personality or thought disorders, language or cultural barriers), supervised treatment will benefit patients, their future contacts, and ultimately the community at large. Directly observed therapy may be the only feasible means of stemming the rising prevalence of tuberculosis in general and multidrug-resistant tuberculosis in particular in certain communities and populations.

COMMON CLINICIAN ERRORS IN RELATION TO ACQUIRED DRUG RESISTANCE. Among the more common errors that contribute to the evolution of multidrug resistance are failure to recognize and cope with non-adherence in a timely manner, failure to identify an individual at high risk for pre-existing drug resistance resulting in use of an inadequate initial regimen, and adding a single drug to a failing regimen.

MONITORING FOR AND COPING WITH DRUG TOXICITY. In the general population about a 5% incidence of significant reactions requiring transient or permanent discontinuation of one or more drugs is seen in a typical three- or four-drug regimen. Common drug toxicities are listed in Table 358-4. Vague gastrointestinal complaints are relatively common in association with all the first-line oral drugs. However, with coaching and encouragement, most patients can be induced to tolerate these drugs. Caution should be taken that patients, in an effort to diminish gastrointestinal intolerance, do not take their oral medications directly with meals, antacids, or H_2 blockers, any of which may substantially reduce absorption of certain of these agents. Regular monitoring of liver chemistries is indicated for all patients receiving multidrug therapy; monthly surveillance is common. In addition, patient education regarding the typical symptoms of hepatitis and regular reminders may be of major importance in preventing serious liver injury. When patients experience serious hepatitis, all potentially hepatotoxic drugs should be held until liver chemistries and symptoms normalize; then the drugs can be reintroduced one at a time at 3- to 4-day intervals, monitoring liver function tests and symptoms to identify the offending agent. Elderly patients receiving SM or other aminoglycosides should have baseline and periodic audiometry; in addition, surveillance of vestibular function is required. For younger patients who are receiving only 2 months of SM, objective testing is generally not indicated.

DURATION OF TREATMENT AND POST-TREATMENT SURVEILLANCE. Currently, a 6-month regimen consisting of INH and RIF supplemented by an initial 2-month phase of PZA is regarded as sufficient and curative for the vast majority of cases caused by drug-susceptible strains. If these three agents cannot be used, the duration of treatment may be prolonged (see Table 358-3). Other situations in which therapy may be extended beyond 6 months include the following:

HIV infection/AIDS: although no well-controlled studies have demonstrated the superiority of longer therapy, some clinicians fear that impaired immunity will place these patients at higher risk of relapse.

Far-advanced, cavitary lung disease with delayed clinical response or sputum conversion: about 95% of patients will become culture negative by 3 months of treatment; for those who remain positive longer than this, treatment for 3 months *after* conversion is recommended.

Irregular, interrupted therapy: if patients fail to attend 10% or more of DOT encounters or are otherwise deemed to have been significantly non-adherent to their treatment, extended treatment is prudent.

Miliary or meningeal cases: due both to the concern that such patients may be less competent hosts and the implications of disease recurrence, therapy may be extended to 9 to 12 months.

A low and unavoidable risk of relapse exists after treatment; for the regimens described earlier in usual populations, the probability is less than 5%. The majority of such recurrences occur within 2 years and are usually associated with the same drug susceptibility profile as pretreatment. Current guidelines do not compel post-treatment surveillance. Rather, patients should be instructed to return after treatment when there are changes in their clinical status; suitable tests including sputa, chest radiographs, or other studies should be obtained if symptoms or signs appear.

INDICATIONS FOR CORTICOSTEROID THERAPY. Corticosteroids may be used to reduce acute inflammation and limit delayed fibrotic complications. Acute reductions in inflammation with significant benefits in outcome have been demonstrated in meningitis and pericarditis cases treated with corticosteroids. Prednisone, at 1 mg/kg, is usual. Less well proven are the benefits of such therapy in pleural, peritoneal, miliary, or extensive pulmonary disease, although salutary effects may occur in individual cases. Whereas high-dose corticosteroids may impair immune responses, there is no evidence that they adversely affect the outcome of treatment when given for 4 to 8 weeks to patients who are receiving adequate chemotherapy.

Adrenal insufficiency due to tuberculous destruction is uncommon in this era. However, among patients with marginal cortisol production, RIF may precipitate hypocortisolism by accelerating catabolism of endogenous steroids.

DRUG-RESISTANT TUBERCULOSIS. In a 1991 CDC survey, the national prevalence of resistance to one or more drugs was 14.2%. Resistance to INH was noted most commonly: 8.2% of new cases and 21.5% of recurrent cases. Resistance to INH and RIF was noted in 3.5% of strains studied; cases with resistance to INH and RIF, with or without resistance to other drugs, are referred to as "multidrug-resistant tuberculosis" (MDR-TB). This report indicated that the regional patterns of resistance varied widely, and it is incumbent on clinicians to consider this when choosing empirical therapy. For example, in New York City, resistance to INH and RIF was found in 12.9% of isolates. Owing to a variety of factors, the prevalence of MDR-TB has diminished substantially, including in New York City, over the past decade. The particular importance of MDR-TB is that, in the absence of INH and RIF, the period required for treatment is doubled, the probability of cure drops substantially, and the ability to provide effective preventive therapy for infected contacts is sorely compromised.

Risk markers for the likelihood of drug resistance include prior treatment for tuberculosis, close contact to such persons, and time spent in communities/countries with known high prevalence, such as the Dominican Republic, Bolivia, India, Latvia, Lithuania, or Estonia. Cases proven or suspected to involve MDR-TB should be referred with alacrity to specialty facilities for expedited laboratory studies and individualized management.

CONTACT INVESTIGATION. It is vital that clinicians realize that their responsibilities are not complete when they have established the diagnosis and initiated chemotherapy for their patient. Tuberculosis is a reportable disease in all U.S. communities and states; clinicians are obligated to promptly notify public health authorities of all cases of proven or suspected tuberculosis. Contact investigation of the home, workplace, school, or other congregate facilities may well reveal other active cases or newly infected persons who are at substantial risk for tuberculosis. Priority must be given to investigations in which infants or AIDS patients have been exposed owing to their compressed incubation periods for potentially lethal forms of tuberculosis. Preventive chemotherapy of infected contacts is a highly efficient means of curtailing tuberculosis morbidity (see later).

PREVENTION OF TUBERCULOSIS. Multiple modalities are involved with the efforts to control tuberculosis. In the United States over the past 30 years, INH preventive chemotherapy (IPT) has been relied upon. For the remainder of the world, vaccination with bacille Calmette-Guérin (BCG) has been the central element. The relative merits and limitations of these methods are discussed next.

ISONIAZID PREVENTIVE THERAPY: PRINCIPLES AND EFFICACY. Because most U.S. tuberculosis cases arise from endogenous reactivation of latent infection acquired remotely in time, authorities reasoned that chemotherapy given to persons harboring such infections might be an efficient prevention strategy. In a series of randomized, placebo-controlled studies, IPT demonstrated 75% reduction of morbidity in the year of treatment and 54% protection in the post-treatment years; even higher rates of protection were shown in a large trial in Eastern Europe, ranging from 70 to 90% with 6- and 12-month IPT, respectively.

INDICATIONS FOR IPT. The focus of IPT recommendations is on persons who are deemed to be at relatively higher risk for experiencing reactivation. Specific groups or conditions that are regarded at high risk and to be candidates for IPT are noted in Table 358–4.

In most instances, the TST is the central modality to identify latent infection. Interpretation of the TST, however, is influenced by circumstances. Thus, in some instances, IPT would be recommended despite non-reactivity, whereas in other cases 15 mm or more of induration is required for significance.

SPECIAL CONSIDERATIONS IN PREVENTIVE THERAPY. HIV infection is the most potent risk factor for endogenous reactivation. Hence, persons with positive HIV serology or strong epidemiologic or clinical markers for HIV risk should be assigned very high priority for IPT. In addition to protecting the individual patient from tuberculosis, IPT may extend survival by ameliorating the accelerated progression of HIV infection seen with active tuberculosis *and* could prevent transmission to other very vulnerable HIV-infected persons (e.g., in shared health care, social, or residential facilities).

Persons exposed to and presumed infected by resistant strains of *M. tuberculosis* pose problems for preventive therapy. If the strain from the source case is resistant only to INH, RIF likely would be a highly effective substitute. However, if the source-case strain is resistant to both INH and RIF, there are no really promising alternatives. For very high-risk persons (such as AIDS patients) exposed to an MDR-TB case, preventive therapy with a fluoroquinolone such as levofloxacin and EMB may be indicated but should be undertaken only after expert consultation.

MONITORING FOR COMPLIANCE AND TOXICITY. Patients receiving preventive chemotherapy should be seen periodically to both promote adherence to the treatment and survey for signs or symptoms of drug toxicity. Intermittent, directly observed preventive therapy is not widely feasible; however, it may be applicable in selected circumstances such as prisoners, especially with HIV infection, or recently infected infants or children in households where reliable treatment is unlikely.

The major toxicity of INH is hepatitis, which may prove fatal if therapy is continued into the period of symptoms and gross chemical derangements. Therefore, it is important that initial education alert the patient and/or responsible family members to the early manifestations of liver injury (anorexia, nausea, malaise, loss of taste for cigarettes, dark urine) with instructions to stop the INH and report promptly for evaluation. Also, patients should have monthly communication with a health care worker, directly if possible but by telephone as an alternative, to inquire regarding their health and to reiterate the education. Biochemical monitoring of liver chemistries is indicated for persons 35 years of age or older, owing to the age-related risk of hepatitis, and should be obtained at baseline and monthly intervals. Innocent increases in the transaminase levels three- to fourfold over baseline without symptoms are noted among up to 20% of persons on IPT; this is not an indication to discontinue the drug but to maintain close surveillance. However, liver chemistries elevated to higher levels or those associated with symptoms should result in discontinuation of the INH. The decision to rechallenge with this drug or to use an alternative agent should be made after expert consultation.

VACCINATION WITH BCG. BCG is a live vaccine prepared from an attenuated strain of *M. bovis*. It has been used widely around the world, but its efficacy and utility are debated. The performance of various strains of BCG, given to different populations over time, has ranged from 80% protection to detrimental effects (more tuberculosis in those receiving the vaccine). A recent meta-analysis of published BCG studies indicated that vaccinations offered an overall 50% protective effect, with higher levels of protection against meningeal or disseminated tuberculosis. This study revealed that the efficacy of BCG diminished at sites near the equator. Although the calculated protection in this meta-analysis reached statistical significance, no explanation was offered for the failure to show efficacy in two large, recently conducted trials.

In addition, because BCG is presumed to work by conferring tuberculoimmunity to those *not* previously infected, it is not appropriate for widespread use in the United States, where most cases arise among those already infected with *M. tuberculosis*. Some have called for BCG vaccinations for health care workers at high risk for tuberculosis infection. However, given the disputable protection afforded by the vaccines and the loss of utility of the TST (due to reactivity induced by BCG) as a tool to mark recent infection and to qualify for preventive chemotherapy—which *has* proven efficacy—this seems to be a dubious proposition.

LIMITING NOSOCOMIAL TRANSMISSION. Substantial microepidemics of tuberculosis have been documented recently in various institutions, including hospitals, clinics, residential facilities, and prisons. To prevent institutional transmission, the CDC has advocated a three-tiered system: administrative measures, environmental programs, and personal respiratory protection. These measures are being employed by Occupational Safety and Health Administration (OSHA) as criteria to assess institutional tuberculosis control programs. *Administrative measures* include educational programs to alert staff on how to recognize and isolate possible active cases early. Also, staff tuberculin skin testing is required to assess the risks of intrainstitutional transmission. *Engineering or environmental programs* are intended to effectively isolate proven or suspected cases by placing them in negative-pressure rooms and diluting the air in the patients' environment through six or more air changes per hour, with the options of decontamination via the adjunctive use of HEPA filtration or ultraviolet germicidal irradiation. *Personal respiratory protection* entails respirators or masks that theoretically can filter out the infectious "droplet nuclei." Presently a NIOSH category N95 personal respiratory device meets federal guidelines. The optimal role for personal respirators is controversial. Perhaps the most suitable role would be to protect health care workers who have unavoidable exposure to smear-positive cases during cough-inducing procedures such as bronchoscopy or intubation. Use in other circumstances depends on source case and environmental factors. The regulations regarding mandated use of these devices are under review. For considerations of both public health concerns and regulatory oversight, all institutions that might be involved with caring for tuberculosis patients should have an active program to limit the hazard of nosocomial transmission to health care workers and other patients or clients.

American Thoracic Society: Treatment of tuberculosis and tuberculosis infection in adults and children. Am J Respir Crit Care Med 149:1359, 1994. *Most recent guidelines for treatment and prevention in adults, children, and infants. Excellent overview of contemporary issues.*

Bloch AB, Cauthen GM, Onorato IM, et al: Nationwide survey of drug-resistant tuberculosis in the United States. JAMA 271:665, 1994. *A careful delineation of the patterns, frequencies, and special risk factors for drug resistance in the United States in the 1990s. Helpful in selecting empirical drug regimens and preventive chemotherapy.*

Cantwell MF, Snider DE Jr, Cauthen GM, et al: Epidemiology of tuberculosis in the United States, 1985–1992. JAMA 272:535, 1994. *Recent trends in demographics and special risk factors. Helps quantify the impacts of HIV infection and immigration upon case rates; also targets high-risk groups for screening, case detection, and prevention.*

Iseman MD: Treatment of multidrug-resistant tuberculosis. N Engl J Med 329:784, 1993. *Reviews recent epidemiology, management, and prevention of multidrug-resistant tuberculosis; discusses use of second-line medications and resectional surgery.*

359 OTHER MYCOBACTERIOSES

Laurel C. Preheim

MICROBIOLOGY. Among the mycobacteria, *M. tuberculosis*, *M. bovis*, and *M. leprae* have caused most human infections. In the 1950s, however, Timpe and Runyon established that other mycobacteria could cause disease in humans and classified these organisms based on pigment production, growth rate, and colonial characteristics. Photochromogens (group I) grow slowly on culture media (>7 days). Their colonies change from a buff shade to bright yellow or orange after exposure to light. Scotochromogens (group II) also grow slowly but demonstrate pigmented colonies when incubated in the dark or the light. Group III mycobacteria grow slowly and lack pigment in the dark or light. Rapid growers (group IV) also lack pigment, but they grow in culture within 3 to 5 days. Collectively, these four groups have been called the "atypical mycobacteria," non-tuberculous mycobacteria (NTM), mycobacteria other than tubercle bacilli (MOTT), or "potentially pathogenic environmental mycobacteria" (PPEM).

EPIDEMIOLOGY. The rate of isolation of NTM is increasing and has surpassed that for *M. tuberculosis* in some areas. Ubiquitous in nature, many have been isolated from ground or tap water, soil, house dust, domestic and wild animals, and birds. Despite their wide distribution, some species are more common in certain geographic locations. Most infections, including those that are hospital acquired, result from inhalation or direct inoculation from environmental sources. Ingestion may be the source of infection for children with NTM cervical adenopathy and for patients with the acquired immunodeficiency syndrome (AIDS) whose disseminated infection may begin in the gastrointestinal tract. Because person-to-person transmission is extremely rare, infected patients do not require isolation.

PATHOPHYSIOLOGY. The pathogenic potential for human disease varies among NTM. As a group, these organisms are less virulent for humans than *M. tuberculosis* and may colonize body surfaces or secretions without causing disease. Tissue invasion is most likely to occur in individuals with predisposing conditions associated with impaired local or systemic host defenses. In general, disease is slowly progressive and histopathologic findings resemble those seen in tuberculosis.

DIAGNOSIS. The steps taken to diagnose tuberculosis generally apply to NTM infections. Standardized, specific skin test antigens for NTM, however, are unavailable. In addition, colonization of asymptomatic individuals and environmental contamination of specimens can yield positive cultures in the absence of clinical disease. NTM disease can be considered present in patients with a cavitary infiltrate on chest radiogram when (1) two or more sputum specimens (or sputum and a bronchial washing) are smear-positive for acid-fast bacilli and/or yield moderate to heavy growth on culture and (2) other reasonable causes for the disease process have been excluded (e.g., fungal disease, tuberculosis, malignancy). An additional criterion, failure of the sputum cultures to convert to negative with either bronchial hygiene or 2 weeks of specific mycobacterial drug therapy, is applied in the presence of a non-cavitary infiltrate not known to be due to another disease.

The diagnosis is also established if transbronchial, percutaneous, or open-lung biopsy tissue reveals mycobacterial histopathologic changes and yields the organism. Extrapulmonary or disseminated disease is confirmed by isolation of the organism from normally sterile body fluids, closed sites, or lesions and when environmental contamination of specimens is excluded. Radiometric culture systems, DNA probes, and polymerase chain reaction assays have increased the speed and accuracy of laboratory diagnosis of pulmonary and extrapulmonary infections.

CLINICAL DISEASE. NTM cause a broad spectrum of diseases (Table 359–1). The following discussion includes infections caused by selected species most likely to be encountered in clinical settings. Therapeutic approaches continue to evolve and therefore remain controversial. Most conventional antituberculous agents have

Table 359–1 ■ NON-TUBERCULOUS MYCOBACTERIAL DISEASES AND ETIOLOGIC SPECIES

CLINICAL DISEASE	ETIOLOGIC SPECIES (RUNYAN GROUP)*	
	Common	Less Common
Pulmonary	M. avium complex (III) M. kansasii (I) M. abscessus (IV) M. xenopi (II)	M. simiae (I) M. szulgai (II) M. malmoense (III) M. fortuitum (IV) M. chelonei (IV)
Lymphadenitis	M. avium complex (III) M. scrofulaceum (II)	M. fortuitum (IV) M. chelonei (IV) M. abscessus (IV) M. kansasii (I)
Cutaneous	M. marinum (I) M. fortuitum (IV) M. chelonei (IV) M. abscessus (IV) M. ulcerans (III)	M. avium complex (III) M. kansasii (I) M. terrae (III) M. smegmatis (IV) M. haemophilum (III)
Disseminated	M. avium complex (III) M. kansasii (I) M. chelonei (IV) M. abscessus (IV) M. haemophilum (III)	M. fortuitum (IV) M. xenopi (II) M. simiae (I) M. gordonae (II) M. terrae complex (III) M. neoarum (II) M. celatum (III) M. genavense (?III)

*I = photochromogen; II = scotochromogen; III = nonpigmented; IV = rapid grower.

little or no activity against the majority of these organisms. Many treatment regimens contain new agents or older antimicrobial agents newly found to have activity against mycobacteria. Therapeutic decisions must weigh all potential drug toxicities and interactions as well as the results of susceptibility testing.

MYCOBACTERIUM AVIUM-INTRACELLULARE. *M. avium* and *M. intracellulare* are closely related and commonly grouped as *M. avium-intracellulare* (MAI) or *M. avium* complex (MAC). Distributed worldwide, they rank first among NTM isolates in the United States. MAI causes about 80% of NTM lymphadenitis cases. *M. scrofulaceum* is responsible for most of the rest. Excisional therapy without chemotherapy is curative in about 95% of cervical adenopathy cases. Pulmonary infection usually occurs in individuals with underlying lung disease and generally follows an indolent or slowly progressive course. Differentiation between colonization and true infection may be difficult initially. Extrapulmonary or disseminated disease, infrequently seen in immunocompetent patients, occurs in up to 40% of individuals with AIDS. It usually affects patients with advanced human immunodeficiency virus infection. Therefore, prophylaxis with clarithromycin (500 mg twice daily) or azithromycin (1200 mg once weekly) is recommended for patients with CD4+ T-lymphocyte counts less than 50 cells/μL. Suggestive symptoms of disseminated MAI include fever, weight loss, anorexia, abdominal pain, and diarrhea. Findings may include hepatosplenomegaly and generalized lymphadenopathy, including mediastinal adenopathy. Diagnosis of disseminated disease is commonly made by culture of the organism from blood, bone marrow, stool, or tissue biopsy.

Newer regimens for MAI infections are based on trials involving patients with AIDS who received treatment for disseminated disease. These guidelines can be applied to patients with or without AIDS who have either pulmonary or disseminated infections. Treatment regimens should include at least two agents. Every regimen should contain either azithromycin (600 mg once daily) or clarithromycin (500 mg twice daily). Many experts prefer ethambutol (15 mg/kg once daily) as the second drug. One or more of the following may be added as second, third, or fourth agents: rifabutin (300 mg/day), ciprofloxacin (750 mg twice daily), ofloxacin (400 mg twice daily) and, in some situations, amikacin (7.5–15 mg/kg/day). Isoniazid and pyrazinamide are not effective. No specific regimen has emerged as being superior for pulmonary or disseminated disease, and the optimal duration of therapy remains unknown. Immunocompetent patients probably should receive a minimum of 18 to 24 months of therapy. Therapy should continue for the lifetime of patients with AIDS if clinical and microbiologic improvement is observed.

MYCOBACTERIUM KANSASII. *M. kansasii,* the most important photochromogen, often appears beaded or cross-barred on acid-fast stain. It ranks second among NTM in causing human infections. Most disease occurs in midwest and southern United States. Pulmonary infection resembling tuberculosis is the usual clinical presentation. Although adult white men are most commonly affected, infection can occur in individuals of any age, sex, or race. Extrapulmonary disease can involve any organ system, and risks of dissemination are increased in immunocompromised patients.

Standard treatment of pulmonary disease is isoniazid (300 mg/day), rifampin (600 mg/day), and ethambutol (15 mg/kg/day) for 18 months. In patients who are unable to tolerate isoniazid, rifampin, and ethambutol with or without streptomycin for the first 3 months is an alternative regimen. These treatment regimens apply to patients with pulmonary or extrapulmonary infection and have been used with some success in individuals with AIDS. The optimal agents or duration of therapy for disseminated disease in patients with AIDS is unknown. Alternative agents such as clarithromycin (500 mg twice daily) or trimethoprim/sulfamethoxazole (160/800 mg twice or thrice daily), amikacin, ofloxacin, or sparfloxacin may be effective against *M. kansasii* strains that are resistant to first-line antimicrobial agents.

RAPIDLY GROWING MYCOBACTERIA. Rapidly growing mycobacteria are acid-fast rods that resemble diphtheroids on Gram's stain. Growth is rapid on subculture to solid media (<7 days), but primary isolation from clinical specimens may require 2 to 30 days. Unlike other mycobacteria, they grow well on most routine laboratory media. Sporadic, community-acquired infections have been reported from most areas of the United States. The spectrum of diseases ranges from localized to disseminated, with cutaneous involvement being most common. Most infections are acquired by inoculation after accidental trauma, surgery, or injection. Nosocomial epidemics or clusters have been reported in numerous settings, including augmentation mammaplasty, hemodialysis, plastic surgery, long-term venous catheters, cardiac surgery, and jet injector use.

These NTM are highly resistant to conventional antituberculous drugs but may be sensitive to traditional or newer antibiotics. Susceptibility testing of individual isolates is important because resistance patterns vary by and within species subgroups. The newer macrolides, clarithromycin and azithromycin, are highly effective against most strains of rapidly growing mycobacteria. They may be successful as monotherapy for minor infections. Extensive disease, however, often requires combination therapy. *M. fortuitum* and *M. peregrinum* are usually also susceptible to amikacin, fluoroquinolones, sulfonamides, cefoxitin, and imipenem and occasionally to doxycycline. *M. abscessus* is generally also susceptible to amikacin, imipenem, and cefoxitin. In contrast, *M. chelonei* is most likely to be susceptible to tobramycin or imipenem. In addition to the new macrolides, therapeutic options for *M. mucogenicum* may include trimethoprim/sulfamethoxazole, tetracyclines, fluoroquinolones, amikacin, imipenem, or cefoxitin.

Treatment duration should be a minimum of 3 months for serious disease and 6 months for bone infections. Any regimen should include surgical débridement of infected wounds or excision of infected foreign bodies.

OTHER NON-TUBERCULOUS MYCOBACTERIA. *M. marinum* cutaneous infections commonly follow aquatic-related inoculation. Papules on an extremity, especially on the elbows, knees, and dorsum of feet and hands, may progress to shallow ulceration and scar formation. Therapeutic approaches have included simple observation for minor lesions, surgical excision, and the use of antimicrobial agents. Acceptable regimens include doxycycline (100 mg twice daily), trimethoprim/sulfamethoxazole (160/800 mg twice daily), or rifampin (600 mg/day) plus ethambutol (15 mg/kg/day) for a minimum of 3 months. Recent studies indicate clarithromycin (500 mg twice daily) may be effective as a single agent.

M. gordonae, a scotochromogen, is also known as the "tap water bacillus." This organism has been associated with nosocomial pseudo-outbreaks, and its isolation is commonly due to environmental contamination of a clinical specimen. *M. gordonae* has been reported to cause pulmonary or disseminated infections in patients with AIDS.

M. xenopi, M. malmoense, M. szulgai, M. simiae, M. haemophilum, M. terrae, M. neoarum, M. celatum, and *M. genavense* are being reported with increasing frequency as causes of pulmonary or disseminated infections in Europe, England, Canada, and the United States. Patients with AIDS appear particularly prone to disseminated disease. Initial therapy for these infections should consist of isoniazid, rifampin, ethambutol, with or without streptomycin or amikacin pending results of antimicrobial susceptibility testing. Optimal duration of therapy is unknown, but at least 18 to 24 months is recommended.

A growing number of uncommon NTM, including *M. shimoidei, M. branderi, M. asiaticum, M. gastri, M. phlei, M. thermoresistible, M. flavescens,* and *M. intermedium,* are being implicated as rare causes of pulmonary, extrapulmonary, or disseminated infections. The clinical significance of these NTM is likely to increase among patients with AIDS or other immunocompromising conditions.

American Thoracic Society: Diagnosis and treatment of disease caused by nontuberculous mycobacteria. Am Rev Respir Dis 142:940, 1990. *Benchmark guidelines for the diagnosis and therapy of NTM.*

Falkinham JO III: Epidemiology of infection by nontuberculous mycobacteria. Clin Microbiol Rev 9:177, 1996. *An excellent, very comprehensive review that includes 571 references.*

Preheim LC: Other nontuberculous mycobacteria and *Mycobacterium bovis. In* Schlossberg D, (ed): Tuberculosis and Nontuberculous Mycobacterial Infections, 4th ed. Philadelphia, WB Saunders, 1999. *This chapter contains additional information on less common NTM.*

360 LEPROSY (HANSEN'S DISEASE)

Gilla Kaplan

DEFINITION. Leprosy is a bacterial disease of great chronicity and low infectivity that occurs worldwide. The primary host is the human, in whom the causative agent *Mycobacterium leprae* accumulates largely in the skin and peripheral nerves, leading to a variety of cutaneous lesions and loss of nerve conduction. Serious disfigurement and loss of digits may result and represent the stigmata of this biblical disease. The clinical manifestations are largely governed by the ability of the host to mount a cell-mediated immune (CMI) response to the organism and its antigens. Patients unable to generate an immune response develop widely distributed skin lesions of the lepromatous state and allow unrestricted growth of bacilli. In contrast, a moderate to vigorous immune response leads to reduced numbers of bacteria in localized cutaneous lesions of the tuberculoid state. In addition to these polar states, there are intermediate forms that demonstrate gradations in reactivity. Spontaneous modulation of the disease toward more polar forms can occur and may lead to tissue damage through humoral (immune complex) and cellular (CMI) mechanisms. Multiple-drug therapy promptly reduces viable organisms and transmissibility but must be maintained for at least 6 months for the disappearance of skin lesions and a reduction in bacterial load.

TRANSMISSION. Little detailed information is available about how the bacillus is transmitted from one individual to another. This deficit in our understanding is related to the long incubation period (6 months–10 years) and the absence of adequate information about the life of the organism in the environment. Other than in humans, the disease has been discovered in feral armadillos studied in Louisiana and Texas. These animals contain large numbers of acid-fast bacilli in parenchymatous organs, which by DNA hybridization and restriction fragment length polymorphism (RFLP) analysis techniques are identical to bacilli obtained from humans. The sooty mangabey, a New World monkey, can become infected naturally in the wild or when injected with human bacilli. In both armadillos and monkeys it takes 18 to 24 months for the injected bacilli to reach high numbers. These infections are quite unlike the spectrum of human disease.

How the localized lesions of tuberculoid leprosy and the generalized cutaneous distribution of lepromatous disease develop is unclear. Direct inoculation through trauma and puncture wounds might lead to an initial focus with bacilli. The initial route of infection may be through the respiratory or gastrointestinal tract. Whatever the source and route of infection at some point during the infection in lepromatous leprosy patients, hematogenous spread occurs with wide seeding of the body.

The incidence of the disease within a household containing an infected tuberculoid or lepromatous index patient may be four to eight times that of the general population. Lepromatous patients with lesions in the nasal mucosa discharge large numbers of organisms. Bacilli recovered from dry nasal discharges retain some viability for up to 7 to 10 days, with somewhat greater viability under conditions of higher humidity. Transmission of the disease from an untreated, infected mother to an infant is not uncommon and should always be considered. Nevertheless, accumulated clinical wisdom indicates that disease transmission takes place only after years of exposure. Little likelihood of transmission is present in a ward or hospital setting, and patients are now cared for on an ambulatory basis with a minimum of precautions.

SUSCEPTIBILITY. Leprosy occurs worldwide and in individuals of all ages. It appears more frequently in young adults, but this may be related to a parental index case and the long period of incubation. A number of studies suggest, but do not prove, that the overall susceptibility to leprosy may be controlled by immune response genes including major histocompatibility complex (MHC) class II antigens. Early analysis of the disease incidence and susceptibility in identical twins has not been conclusive. More recent studies suggest that the type of leprosy rather than overall disease susceptibility may be controlled by human leukocyte antigen determinants and other genes regulating the immune response. Environmental factors such as nutrition and coincident microbial and parasitic infections may also contribute to susceptibility.

The acquired immunodeficiency syndrome (AIDS) pandemic has been associated with a rise in the incidence of other mycobacterial diseases. This association has not yet been observed in leprosy.

EPIDEMIOLOGY. The worldwide number of leprosy cases has been reported by the World Health Organization to be about 1.2 million in 1997. In many countries, valid statistics are not available, and the incidence in outlying, rural areas is poorly documented. The highest prevalence rates are in Asia and Africa, followed by Central and South America and Oceania. The highest rates do not usually exceed 55 per 1000 but may be as high as 200 per 1000 in selected villages. With effective chemotherapy and advanced diagnostic and public health methods the worldwide prevalence is dropping. However, the incidence does not appear to be changing and the number of new cases detected worldwide each year is about 500,000.

The majority of leprosy cases are found in tropical areas. Socioeconomic condition, availability of health care, and body exposure to the environment may all contribute to this. However, the disease also occurs in the colder climates of Tibet, Nepal, Korea, and Siberia. In previous centuries, the disease occurred more commonly in Scandinavia and those countries bordering the North Sea. Small numbers (300 to 500 per year) of cases currently occur in the United States. The majority of these are in immigrant groups from Asia and South America, although occasional cases are seen in the southern states and those bordering Mexico.

The nature of the disease varies considerably with geographic distribution. In African and Asian countries there is a predominance of tuberculoid leprosy, and 20% or fewer of the cases are of the lepromatous type. In contrast, larger numbers of lepromatous cases are reported in Brazil and Venezuela. Early infection and/or sensitization with cross-reacting antigens of other mycobacteria have been considered as an explanation for the variation in type of leprosy with which an individual presents.

ETIOLOGIC AGENT. *M. leprae,* discovered by Hansen in 1873, is the causative agent of human leprosy. No evidence of strain variation has been noted by DNA-DNA hybridization or RFLP. The organism is acid-alcohol fast when stained by the Ziehl-Neelsen method. *M. leprae* is an obligate intracellular parasite and has never been cultivated extracellularly in laboratory media. It is a resident of the phagolysosomes of macrophages, Schwann cells, and endothelial cells. *M. leprae* is classified as a mycobacterium and contains mycolic acid, arabinogalactan, and phenolic glycolipid in the cell wall. The latter molecule is the only *M. leprae*–specific component. Recently, a major effort to identify the more than 300 proteins of *M. leprae* has resulted in the detection of proteins preferentially found in either the cytosol, the bacterial membrane, and the cell wall. How these components contribute to the pathogenicity and immunogenecity of *M. leprae* infection in humans remains to be elucidated.

The absence of a culture system for *M. leprae* has complicated any investigations of the physiology and pathogenicity of the organism. However, the armadillo has been used to grow large numbers of the mycobacteria. Eighteen to 24 months after inoculation, 10^9 bacilli per gram can be purified from liver and spleen and serve as a source for genetic, chemical, and antigenic analysis. The *M. leprae* genome has now been almost fully sequenced, providing many new insights into the physiology of the organism. Many of the metabolic activities of *M. leprae* appear to be low compared with other mycobacteria. *M. leprae* lacks catalase activity, and de novo purine biosynthesis appears to be missing. *M. leprae* replicates very slowly within host cells and has a doubling time of approximately 13 days. It prefers ambient temperatures below 37° C and grows selectively in cooler portions of the body such as skin, testes, and nasal mucosa.

Determining bacillary viability and resistance to chemotherapeutic agents depends on slow bacillary growth in the foot pads of mice—a bioassay taking about 12 months. Accelerated growth occurs in the athymic nude mouse but still requires 6 or more months. These properties impose severe restrictions on determination of viability and antibiotic sensitivity. Use of polymerase chain reaction–based technology, in which selected DNA sequences are amplified a millionfold, may facilitate more efficient analyses of these properties.

IMMUNOLOGIC CONSIDERATION. A specific immunologic defect occurs in patients with lepromatous leprosy. This is expressed as a selective unresponsiveness of T cells to *M. leprae* and is evident in skin test (Mitsuda) anergy and the in vitro lymphocyte transformation test for *M. leprae* antigens (Table 360–1). In contrast, T cells from patients with the tuberculoid form of the disease respond normally to *M. leprae* antigens. In neither form of the disease are there abnormalities in humoral immunity. The association between cell-mediated cutaneous responses, T-cell accumulation in lesions, and the number of *M. leprae* in the tissues is shown in Table 360–1. These parameters are inversely related. In the absence of *M. leprae*–specific T-cell reactivity, TH1 type cytokine production is depressed or absent and tissue macrophages fail to be activated to an antimicrobial state. Thus, bacilli taken up by macrophages of the skin of lepromatous leprosy patients are able to multiply intracellularly, leading to multibacillary vacuoles. Normally (as in tuberculoid leprosy patients), macrophage activation occurs largely through the local release of interferon-gamma (IFN-γ), a lymphokine that enhances the production of toxic oxygen intermediates in these cells. In these patients, the bacilli are largely destroyed and only small numbers survive to perpetuate the cell-mediated immune reactions.

Lepromatous patients, although unresponsive to *M. leprae* antigen, develop adequate reactions to other antigens to which they have been sensitized, including skin test antigens such as purified protein derivative (PPD), mumps, *Candida,* trichophytin, and tetanus toxoid.

CLINICAL DIAGNOSIS. Patients with leprosy are first seen and followed by dermatologists because the anesthetic cutaneous lesions are often the presenting complaint. The range in immune response to *M. leprae* is reflected clinically by a wide variation of skin lesions and peripheral nerve involvement. In this section we review the characteristics of the major polar and borderline forms.

POLAR TUBERCULOID LEPROSY (TT). This form presents as one to a few asymmetrical plaques or macules defined by a sharp, raised border. In dark-skinned patients, the lesions are often centrally hypopigmented with a more erythematous border. The central area is scaly, lacks hair, and is anesthetic. Nerves leading to the ear, elbow, and knee may be palpably enlarged. Almost any area of the skin may be affected except for the warmer regions of the scalp, axilla, and perineum. The disease is stable.

BORDERLINE TUBERCULOID AND BORDERLINE LEPROMATOUS LEPROSY (BT AND BL). As the body burden of bacilli increases, in association with a partial reduction in immunity, the number, distribution, and nature of the cutaneous lesions increase in complexity. The skin exhibits a polymorphic array of macular, erythematous, hypopigmented lesions involving the trunk, extremities, and face. These vary randomly in number and distribution. Larger nerve trunks are infiltrated with a granulomatous reaction, leading to nerve damage resulting in footdrop, flexion contractions of the digits, and corneal abrasions. The anesthesia of hands and feet and the resulting damage from burns, trauma, and secondary infection leads to loss of digits, plantar ulcerations, and blindness. These widely dispersed lesions suggest hematogenous spread and a cell-mediated reaction that is not capable of controlling bacillary growth. Disease is unstable and may evolve toward the polar forms. Reactional states are common.

LEPROMATOUS LEPROSY (LL). Here there is little or no CMI, and tremendous numbers of organisms are dispersed throughout the skin. Again, the lesions are pleomorphic but often are less "angry" or erythematous than in borderline disease. Macules, papules, and nodules may cover wide areas of the trunk and extremities, and lesion distribution is often symmetrical. Almost any area of affected or "normal"-looking skin contains bacilli. Often there are no obvious lesions, but the skin looks shiny and "full," as the dermis is expanded with macrophages containing bacilli. This is particularly prominent on the ears, eyebrows, and face, giving rise to an appearance called "leonine facies." Eyebrow loss is frequent; a saddle nose deformity may result from cartilage destruction; gynecomastia from reduced testosterone levels secondary to testicular damage may be present; and blindness and iridocyclitis, laryngeal stenosis, loss of incisor teeth, and loss of digits may occur. Nerve damage in lepromatous leprosy is more slowly progressive but is eventually severe and diffuse and leads to a sensory polyneuropathy. Rigid, swollen nerves are palpable in many locations. Disease is stable. The deformities associated with long-term untreated lepromatous leprosy are the stigmata that result in the ostracism of the leper from his or her community and necessitate custodial care. However, today patients undergoing chemotherapy often remain members of their households.

REACTIONAL STATES. ERYTHEMA NODOSUM LEPROSUM (ENL). Patients with BL and LL disease maintain high levels of circulating anti–*M. leprae* antibodies as well as high antigen levels. After effective chemotherapy, a prompt and extensive kill of bacilli takes place and large amounts of soluble antigens are liberated extracellularly. More than 30% of such patients develop ENL and present with painful subcutaneous erythematous nodules that arise diffusely and may eventually lead to necrosis and suppuration. These symptoms, accompanied by fever and malaise, can continue for months, are extremely debilitating, and are often accompanied by acute inflammation of the eyes, testes, nerves, lymph nodes, and joints. Some patients develop glomerulonephritis with the deposition of complement and immune complexes in the glomeruli. Enhanced production of the cytokine tumor necrosis factor alpha (TNF-α) has been associated with ENL. This serious complication requires prompt diagnosis and therapy.

REVERSAL REACTION. This reactional state also may occur after chemotherapy but differs from ENL in that acceleration or decrease

Table 360–1 ■ IMMUNOLOGIC FEATURES OF LEPROSY PATIENTS

	TUBERCULOID	BORDERLINE TUBERCULOID	MID-BORDERLINE	BORDERLINE LEPROMATOUS	LEPROMATOUS
Acid-fast bacilli in skin lesions	–	–/+	+	+++	+++
Lepromin (Mitsuda) reaction	+++	+++	–	–	–
Lymphocyte transformation test	95%	40%	10%	1–2%	1–2%
Anti–*M. leprae* antibodies	–/+	–/++	++	+++	+++
CD4+/CD8+ T-cell ratio in lesions	1.35	1.11	NT	0.48	0.20

of the local cell-mediated reaction is observed, accompanied by widespread erythema and induration of pre-existing lesions as well as systemic symptoms (e.g., pyrexia). The onset of this state is slower than that of ENL (weeks to months), and it may persist for many months if not properly treated. Rapid progression of pre-existing peripheral nerve damage may take place. Irreversible changes in nerve conduction should be considered a medical emergency and treated accordingly.

Both of these reactions as well as progressive nerve damage can occur or recur even after completion of the course of therapy and bacteriologic cure.

LABORATORY DIAGNOSIS. In addition to clinical manifestations, the primary method for diagnosing leprosy is by identification of acid-fast bacilli in the skin. The slit smear technique is used throughout the world. Skin is incised with a scalpel, squeezing the area to maintain a bloodless field. The edges of the slit are scraped with the edge of the scalpel, smeared on a slide, fixed, and stained by the Ziehl-Neelsen method. A microscopic logarithmic score (1+ to 6+; 5+ equals 100 to 1000 acid-fast bacilli per high-power field) is used to quantitate the bacterial load. Usually six sites on the ear lobes, elbow, knee, and a lesion are prepared. This simple method, when skillfully applied, is as sensitive as any other diagnostic procedure.

A more definitive estimate of bacillary numbers in the skin comes from biopsy material. A logarithmic score is made by counting the number of bacilli in high-power fields. This ranges from 1+ to 6+ and is a useful index in following the response of patients to therapy in terms of bacillary numbers and histopathologic classification. (Bacterial index: 0—no bacilli in 100 microscopic fields [×100]; 1+ = 1 to 10 bacilli in 100 fields; 2+ = 1 to 10 bacilli in 10 fields; 3+ = 1 to 10 bacilli per field; 4+ = 10 to 100 bacilli per field; 5+ = 100 to 1000 bacilli per field; and 6+ = 1000s per field.)

A skin test may be used that distinguishes the immunologically reactive (tuberculoid) and non-reactive (lepromatous) poles of the disease. A crude antigen consisting of heat-killed bacilli prepared from infected armadillos is injected and induces local induration and the formation of granulomas in 3 to 4 weeks in most tuberculoid patients. Patients with lepromatous leprosy fail to react to the antigen and may remain unresponsive long after effective chemotherapy.

Serologic tests are useful in assaying the level of anti–*M. leprae* antibodies in multibacillary lepromatous but not in the paucibacillary tuberculoid patients. However, the many cross-reactive antigenic epitopes shared with other mycobacteria complicate interpretation and differential diagnosis. Enzyme-linked immunosorbent assay (ELISA), which recognizes antibodies against the carbohydrate moieties of the phenolic glycolipids, the only molecule that is *M. leprae* specific, is positive in patients with lepromatous but not tuberculoid disease and declines after chemotherapy is initiated. Patients with lepromatous leprosy have a polyclonal hypergammaglobulinemia, as well as acute-phase reactants such as C-reactive protein and immune complexes in the circulation. Ten per cent of patients give false-positive tests for syphilis, and 30% have cryoglobulinemia.

HISTOPATHOLOGY AND IMMUNOPATHOLOGY. Microscopic analysis of tissue plays a primary role in diagnosing and classifying the various clinical forms of leprosy and uses the standardized classification described by Ridley and Jopling. Five groups have been defined spanning the spectrum from polar tuberculoid (TT) to polar lepromatous (LL) and include borderline (BB) as well as borderline tuberculoid (BT) and borderline lepromatous (BL). Our discussion focuses on the polar forms, and the details pertaining to the intermediate manifestations can be found in more specialized texts.

LESIONS OF THE SKIN. Tuberculoid Leprosy. Microscopic examination of hematoxylin and eosin–stained sections of biopsy specimens obtained from a TT macular plaque reveals heavy infiltration of the dermis by mononuclear leukocytes organized in well-developed granulomas. These contain large numbers of lymphocytes scattered between and surrounding other components of the granulomatous response, including macrophage-derived epithelioid cells and Langerhans-type multinucleated giant cells (Fig. 360–1). Occasional plasma cells but few granulocytes are found. Antigen-presenting Langerhans' cells are found within the dermal infiltrate in significant numbers. Staining with monoclonal antibodies shows

that the majority of lymphocytes are T cells and that the CD4+ "helper type" phenotype predominates over CD8+ "suppressor cytotoxic" cells.

The epidermis overlying the dermal infiltrate is thickened (two-fold to three-fold), and individual keratinocytes are enlarged. The keratinocytes display large amounts of MHC class II determinants on their surface. This is a response to the local production of IFN-γ in the dermis and is accompanied by the expression of other IFN-γ–induced molecules by keratinocytes and other cell types.

Acid-fast staining of sections reveals an occasional bacillus or bacillary remnants within macrophages. BT lesions are similar except that acid-fast bacilli are more readily seen.

Lepromatous Leprosy. In contrast to TT lesions, the lepromatous lesion contains only small numbers of lymphocytes, predominantly of the CD8+ phenotype, scattered through a background of loosely organized dermal macrophages and collagen (Fig. 360–2). The macrophages often have a pale, foamy cytoplasm and may contain large clumps of *M. leprae* called "globi" (Fig. 360–3). By electron microscopy, these organisms are seen to reside within large cytoplasmic vacuoles, embedded in a lucent matrix that contains phenolic glycolipid. Remnants of the osmiophilic bacilli are present along with structurally intact organisms (Fig. 360–3B). A gram of skin may contain 10^9 bacilli. Langerhans' cells are rarely seen in the

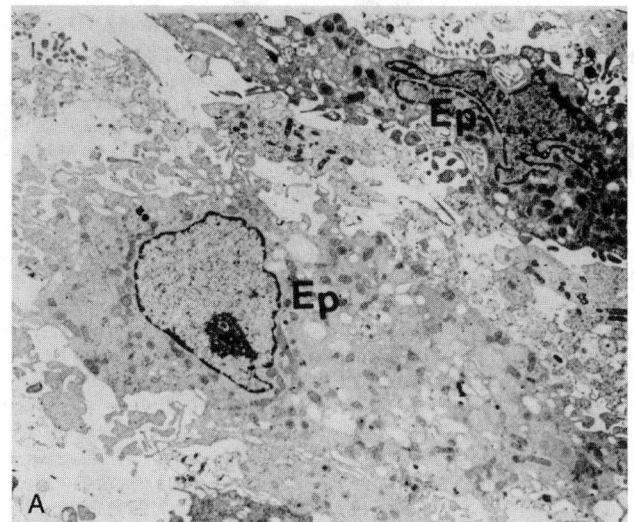

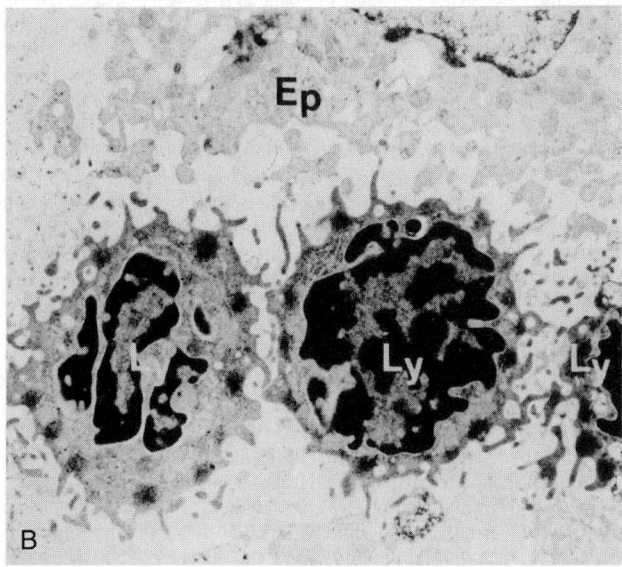

FIGURE 360–1 ■ Transmission electron photomicrographs of cutaneous granulomas from a patient with tuberculoid leprosy. *A,* The granuloma contains large epithelioid cells (Ep) with multiple cytoplasmic organelles (×4500). *B,* Three T lymphocytes (Ly) and an epithelioid cell are observed (×9000).

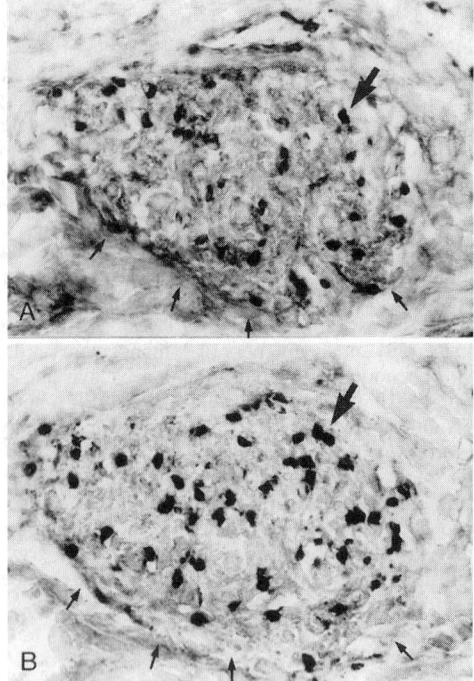

FIGURE 360–2 ■ Lepromatous leprosy—cutaneous lesion. Frozen serial sections stained with Leu 3 (anti-CD4–helper T-cell subset) *(A)* and with Leu 2 (anti-CD8–suppressor/cytotoxic T-cell subset) *(B)*. The inflammatory infiltrates *(small arrows)* contain few T cells. Cells of the CD4+ subset *(large arrow in A)* are less numerous than those of the CD8+ subset *(large arrow in B)*. Immunoperoxidase, counterstained with hematoxylin (×200).

dermis; the overlying epidermis is thin and atrophic and fails to show surface MHC class II antigens.

The loose bacilli-rich infiltrates of LL are present in almost every area of the skin, and individual infected macrophages may be observed surrounded by collagen bundles.

LESIONS OF PERIPHERAL NERVE. Tuberculoid Leprosy. The paucibacillary granulomatous response is associated with significant destruction of peripheral nerve fascicles and late in the disease may lead to caseous necrosis of nerve trunks. Large numbers of T cells and mononuclear phagocytes breach the perineurium and lead to destruction of Schwann cells and axons alike. By the time the skin lesion is apparent, nerve damage and sensory loss have occurred. The mechanism of the nerve damage in TT is unclear but is related to CMI and the granulomatous response.

Lepromatous Leprosy. Many bacilli are observed within Schwann cells and macrophages surrounding and within the perineural sheath in the majority of subcutaneously placed nerve trunks (Fig. 360–4). Nerve damage is relatively slow as compared with a TT but more extensive and insidious. Few, if any, lymphocytes are part of the nerve lesion. Schwann cells are capable of taking up *M. leprae* and serve as permissive hosts for their replication (see Fig. 360–4).

OTHER ORGANS. Lepromatous lesions can be seen in the lymph nodes, liver, spleen, bone marrow, endocrine organs, and eye. These contain bacilli-infected macrophages but are not considered to be an important site of infection. Patients with untreated multibacillary disease can have a constant bacteremia of 10^5 acid-fast bacilli per milliliter, all of which are present within monocytes. The total body burden of *M. leprae* can reach 10^{12}.

LESIONS OF REACTIONAL STATES. Erythema Nodosum Leprosum. Examination of the skin nodules of ENL shows extensive mixed leukocyte infiltration of neutrophils and mononuclear cells and tissue necrosis. Immune complexes are evident, and there is a panvasculitis of dermal arteries and veins. These are all hallmarks of an extensive acute inflammatory response resulting in tissue damage. TNF-α and other monocyte cytokine-induced cell surface antigens can be demonstrated.

Reversal Reactions. Patients with BT, BB, or BL leprosy, who are partially responsive to *M. leprae* antigens, occasionally undergo an

upgrading reaction after several months of therapy. This differs from ENL in the migration of a predominantly T-cell infiltrate into pre-existing affected sites. Many of the T cells are of the helper phenotype and are secreting lymphokines into their environment. T-cell migration into skin lesions is associated with mononuclear phagocyte differentiation into organized granuloma and is often associated with the rapid progression of peripheral nerve damage. This enhancement of CMI leads to limited bacillary destruction. A downgrading or reduction in CMI also may occur. Such reactions may continue for weeks or months and are associated with severe morbidity leading to serious sequelae.

PATHOGENESIS. Recovery from infections with obligate intracellular parasites such as *M. leprae* requires the host to mount an effective CMI response. Antigen-presenting cells must recognize and cluster with appropriate T cells, leading to T-cell stimulation, differentiation, and replication. T helper cells synthesize and secrete a variety of hormone-like lymphokines, which enhance the microbicidal activity of monocytes and macrophages as well as stimulate other cells in the environment (e.g., keratinocytes, endothelial cells, and fibroblasts). This leads to the development of T cells, which are antigen specific and MHC class II or class I restricted. Along with natural killer and lymphokine-activated killer cells, they serve as potent specific and non-specific cytotoxic effector cells.

In lepromatous leprosy, in the absence of local lymphokine production, bacilli multiply in macrophages that have the capacity

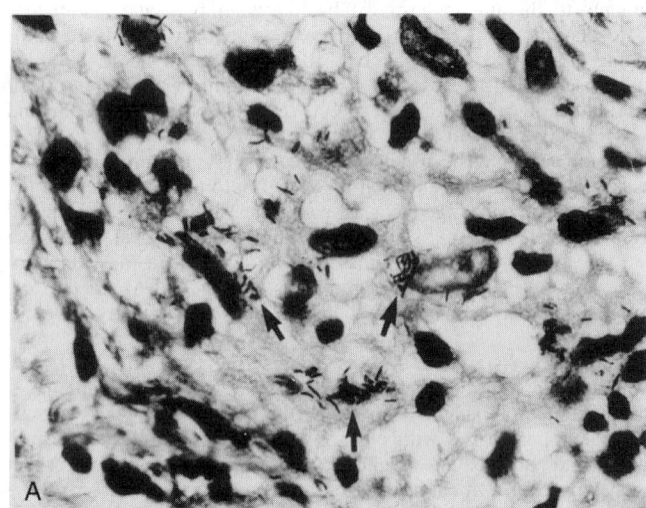

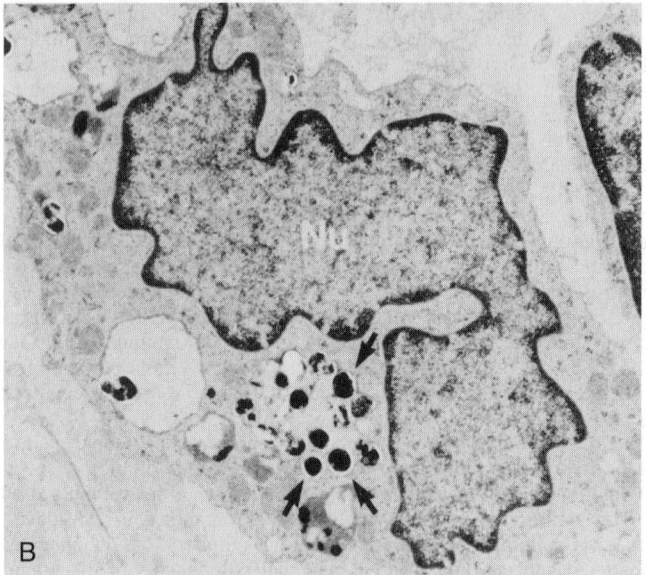

FIGURE 360–3 ■ Lepromatous leprosy—cutaneous lesions. Acid-fast staining of histologic section *(A)* and transmission electron photomicrograph *(B)* of *M. leprae*–parasitized foamy macrophages *(arrows)*. The phagocytes have large nuclei and many light and electron lucent vacuoles containing darkly staining bacteria *(A, ×500; B, ×9000)*. Nu = nucleus.

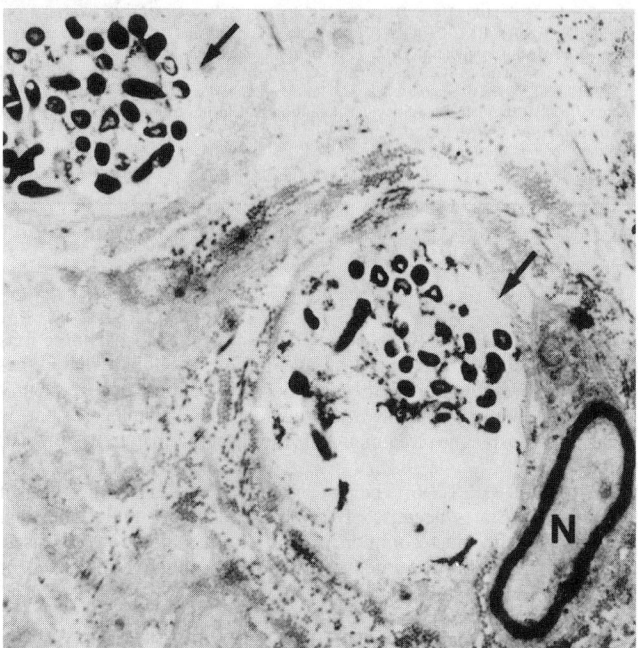

FIGURE 360–4 ■ Transmission electron micrograph of an infiltrated peripheral nerve of a cutaneous lesion from a lepromatous leprosy patient. The myelinated neuron (N) and two *M. leprae*–infected Schwann cells *(arrows)* are observed (×9000).

neither to kill the organism nor to be activated by lymphokines. To modify this fertile intracellular culture environment, the host must destroy the heavily parasitized macrophage, liberating its contents into the extracellular milieu. Here, newly emigrated monocytes ingest, kill, and degrade *M. leprae* with the help of a lymphokine stimulus. This is the situation that occurs in the tuberculoid form of the disease and is lacking in the lepromatous state.

RECOMMENDED TREATMENT SCHEDULES. The most commonly used drug in the therapy for leprosy is 4,4′-diaminodiphenylsulfone (dapsone, DDS). Because of the widespread emergence of dapsone-resistant strains of *M. leprae,* all patients now receive multidrug therapy. The components and schedules vary depending on the presence of dapsone-sensitive strains and the part of the world in which the patient resides. In the United States, the following recently modified regimens are employed:

1. *Paucibacillary disease of the TT and BT categories*
   a. Dapsone-sensitive *M. leprae:* dapsone is given in a daily dose of 100 mg and rifampin at a daily dose of 600 mg for 1 year.
   b. Dapsone-resistant *M. leprae:* clofazimine at a daily dose of 50 to 100 mg is substituted for dapsone.
2. *Multibacillary disease of the BB, BL, and LL categories*
   a. Dapsone-sensitive or dapsone-resistant *M. leprae:* dapsone is given in a dose of 100 mg/day, rifampin is given in a dose of 600 mg/day, and clofazimine is given in a dose of 50 mg/day for 2 years.

To evaluate the dapsone sensitivity, the mouse foot pad assay must be used; this procedure is available only in specialized facilities.

A modified schedule for third world country control programs was issued by the World Health Organization (WHO) in 1982 and is based on practical consideration, including the availability of slit smear facilities and financial constraints:

1. *Paucibacillary disease—a bacillary index of 0 at all six skin sites.* Dapsone is given daily at a dose of 100 mg, unsupervised. Rifampin is given at a dose of 600 mg once a month, supervised. Treatment is given for 6 months and is then discontinued.
2. *Multibacillary disease—a bacillary index of 1+ or more at any one of six skin sites.* Dapsone is given daily at 100 mg with clofazimine 50 mg daily, unsupervised. Rifampin 600 mg and clofazimine 300 mg are given once monthly, supervised. This therapy is continued for 2 years.

The WHO schedule for intermittent rifampin therapy is based in part on its expense and on clinical and laboratory trials. It should be noted, however, that many leprologists use rifampin at 450 to 600 mg/day for 2 to 3 years. Relapses under the WHO schedule are infrequent.

Rifampin is the most rapidly effective bactericidal agent and kills the majority of *M. leprae* within 2 to 3 weeks. This is evident by mouse foot pad assays. Resistance to rifampin is well known in the therapy of *M. tuberculosis* and is now becoming evident with *M. leprae.*

Therapy with clofazimine, a phenazine derivative, has certain unpleasant side effects based on its lipophilicity. The compound is a red-purple dye taken up and concentrated by macrophages of the skin, causing increased skin pigmentation. This is distressing to certain light-skinned patients. Clofazimine is also deposited in the small intestine, where at high concentrations it causes segmental thickening associated with crampy pain and diarrhea. If clofazimine is unacceptable to patients, the physician should consider substitution with 100 mg/day of minocycline or 400 mg/day of ofloxacin.

THERAPY OF REACTIONS. ERYTHEMA NODOSUM LEPROSUM. The acute onset of ENL may be mild enough to require only salicylates or other cyclooxygenase inhibitors. With severe episodes, high doses of corticosteroids (prednisone, 60 to 80 mg/day) are necessary and should be tapered off as soon as feasible. However, exacerbations occur frequently, and repeated dosing is necessary. A particularly useful drug in severe ENL is thalidomide, a selective inhibitor of TNF-α. It is given initially at 200 mg twice a day and then tapered to levels of 50 to 100 mg/day. Thalidomide is a potent teratogen and should be assiduously avoided if pregnancy is possible. Clofazimine also has been found useful in ENL but requires 4 to 6 weeks to achieve therapeutic effects. ENL in some patients responds poorly to thalidomide, and prednisone and/or clofazimine are employed.

REVERSAL REACTIONS. The chronicity and potential nerve damage of this cell-mediated reaction require high-dose corticosteroids and careful evaluation of peripheral nerve condition. Thalidomide is not used in this condition, but clofazimine along with corticosteroids allows the more rapid withdrawal of prednisone.

OTHER COMPLICATIONS. A number of surgical procedures are available at specialized leprosy hospitals to help correct footdrop, hand deformities, madarosis, and lagophthalmos. Plastic surgical procedures can replace nasal septa and help close large plantar ulcerations. On occasion, patients with gynecomastia request the removal of glandular tissue.

The presence of a cold abscess of a peripheral nerve with sudden increase in pain and functional loss requires immediate decompression by surgical drainage.

IMMUNOMODULATION. Recombinant lymphokines that can enhance the microbicidal properties of macrophages and stimulate the expression of CMI may find a place in the care of leprosy patients. Preliminary studies with the T-cell mitogen interleukin-2 (IL-2) have already been carried out in patients with lepromatous leprosy. The intradermal injection of IL-2 leads to a local cell-mediated reaction associated with induration, the destruction of parasitized macrophages, and a marked reduction in the bacillary load. Trials with more prolonged administration have demonstrated that a systemic response can be achieved.

PROGNOSIS. Tuberculoid leprosy is usually self-limited and responds well to chemotherapy. Nerve damage is, however, irreversible. In lepromatous disease, prolonged courses of multiple drugs arrest the progression of the illness when compliance is good. It is the ability of the public health infrastructure to monitor compliance that is central to effective therapy. Recurrences due to poor maintenance therapy are not infrequent.

PREVENTION AND PROPHYLAXIS. Education of the general public plays an important role in sensitizing individuals to the nature of leprosy and the ability to cure the illness with medication. Once a case has been identified in a household, careful physical examination of all contacts with the biopsy of suspicious lesions should be carried out. The threat of contagion is much higher in children younger than age 16. In this adolescent category, the prophylactic use of dapsone should be considered.

Vaccine trials have been carried out sponsored by WHO. These have employed bacille Calmette-Guérin (BCG) vaccine with and without heat-killed *M. leprae* or other mycobacteria in highly endemic areas of Africa, Asia, and India. There is evidence that BCG vaccination alone may reduce the incidence of disease.

Cohn ZA, Kaplan G: Leprosy, cell-mediated immunity and recombinant lymphokines.

J Infect Dis 163:1195, 1991. *Discussion of the regulation of CMI with cytokines.*
Guinto RS, Abalos RM, Cellona RV, Fajardo TT: An Atlas of Leprosy. Sasakawa Memorial Health Foundation, 1983. *Excellent pictorial atlas of diagnostic signs.*
Hastings RC, Franzblau SG: Chemotherapy of leprosy. Annu Rev Pharmacol Toxicol 28:231, 1988. *Current update of therapy and complications thereof.*
Pessolani MCV, Brennan PJ. Molecular definition and identification of new proteins of *Mycobacterium leprae.* Infect Immun 64:5425, 1996. *Up-to-date discussion of* M. leprae *proteins and their properties.*

SEXUALLY TRANSMITTED DISEASES

361 INTRODUCTION TO SEXUALLY TRANSMITTED DISEASES AND COMMON SYNDROMES

P. Frederick Sparling

Sexually transmitted diseases (STDs) are a diverse group of infections, caused by biologically dissimilar microbial agents, that are grouped together because of certain common clinical and epidemiologic features. Advent of the acquired immunodeficiency syndrome (AIDS) has heightened public awareness of the importance of STDs and the dangers of unsafe sexual practices. New knowledge has accumulated rapidly about old diseases; for instance, it is now clear that cervical carcinoma is a complication of certain human papillomavirus (genital wart virus) infections. Some relatively less severe infections, such as chlamydial ones, are known to be alarmingly prevalent in young persons. In this chapter certain common features of some of these infections are discussed, as well as the differential diagnosis and management of several of the common syndromes of genital infections.

DEFINITIONS. Those infectious agents that are frequently transmitted by sexual contact, and for which sexual transmission is epidemiologically important, are considered STDs. In some cases, such as gonorrhea and genital herpes simplex virus infection, sexual transmission is the only important mode of transmission, at least between adults. In others, such as the hepatitis viruses, giardiasis, shigellosis, and amebiasis, there are also important non-sexual means of acquiring infection. Table 361–1 lists the important infectious agents commonly transmitted sexually, as well as their known or probable disease syndromes. "Sexual" includes the full range of heterosexual or homosexual behavior, including genital, oral-genital, oral-anal, and genital-anal contact.

EPIDEMIOLOGIC CONSIDERATIONS. Sexually transmitted infections are prevalent in many segments of society but, for obvious reasons, are most prevalent in the groups with the most promiscuous sexual activity. It is not sexual activity per se but the number and type of different sexual partners that determine the risk of acquiring STDs. The highest rates of gonorrhea are found in the young (15 to 30) and unmarried and in groups of low educational and socioeconomic status. Rates of gonococcal infection may be 50-fold higher in young, single inner-city persons than in married middle- to upper-middle-class persons. Rates of syphilis and gonorrhea are much higher in African Americans than other ethnic groups and in the rural Southeast and inner cities, presumably because of linkage of socioeconomic and behavioral factors. Decisions regarding the cost-effectiveness of screening for STDs should be governed by these considerations; screening is most effective in high-risk groups.

Multiple infections are frequent in patients with sexually transmitted infection. In venereal disease clinics, about 20% of men with gonorrhea also have urethral chlamydial infection and 30 to 50% of women with gonorrhea also have cervical chlamydial infection. The frequent coexistence of multiple sexually acquired infections probably reflects the multiplicity of sexual partners among the subject patients.

Control of sexually transmitted infections is complicated by the frequent lack of significant symptoms. The majority of gonococcal and chlamydial infections in women probably are associated with few symptoms. From 10 to 50% of urethral gonococcal infections in men are oligosymptomatic or asymptomatic. Chlamydial infections are more common than gonococcal infections and frequently are asymptomatic. One of the crucial issues in management is proper diagnosis and treatment of the asymptomatically infected partner.

INCIDENCE OF STDS. The true incidence of STDs is not known in the United States because of serious problems of underreporting. Gonorrhea is the most common of the reported infectious diseases, with more than 500,000 infections reported annually. Incidence of

Table 361–1 ■ **SEXUALLY TRANSMITTED AGENTS AND THEIR SYNDROMES***

MICROORGANISM	SYNDROMES
Bacteria	
Neisseria gonorrhoeae	Urethritis, cervicitis, bartholinitis, proctitis, pharyngitis, salpingitis, epididymitis, conjunctivitis, perihepatitis, arthritis, dermatitis, endocarditis, meningitis, amniotic infection syndrome
Mobiluncus species and *Gardnerella vaginalis*	Bacterial vaginosis
Treponema pallidum	Syphilis (multiple clinical syndromes)
Haemophilus ducreyi	Chancroid
Calymmatobacterium granulomatis	Granuloma inguinale
Shigella species	Enteritis in homosexual men
Campylobacter species	Enteritis in homosexual men
Group B *Streptococcus*	Neonatal sepsis and meningitis
Chlamydiae	
Chlamydia trachomatis	Nongonococcal urethritis, purulent hypertrophic cervicitis, epididymitis, salpingitis, conjunctivitis, trachoma, pneumonia, perihepatitis, lymphogranuloma venereum, Reiter's syndrome
Mycoplasmas	
Ureaplasma urealyticum	Nongonococcal urethritis, ? premature rupture of membranes and abortion
Mycoplasma hominis	Postpartum fever, pelvic inflammatory disease
Viruses	
Herpes simplex virus (HSV)	Genital herpes, proctitis, meningitis, disseminated infection in neonates
Hepatitis A virus	Hepatitis in homosexual men
Hepatitis B virus	Hepatitis, periarteritis nodosa, hepatoma; especially prevalent in homosexual men
Cytomegalovirus	Congenital infection (birth defects, infant mortality, mental deficiency, hearing loss), mononucleosis syndrome
Human papillomavirus (HPV)	Condyloma acuminatum, cervical and perianal
Molluscum contagiosum virus	Molluscum contagiosum
Human immunodeficiency virus (HIV)	Acquired immunodeficiency syndrome (AIDS) and related illnesses
Protozoa	
Trichomonas vaginalis	Trichomonal vaginitis, occasional urethritis
Entamoeba histolytica	Enteritis in homosexual men
Giardia lamblia	Enteritis in homosexual men
Fungi	
Candida albicans	Vaginitis, balanitis
Ectoparasites	
Phthirus pubis	Pubic lice infestation
Sarcoptes scabiei	Scabies

*The relative importance of sexual transmission in the epidemiology of several of these agents remains to be defined; these include group B streptococci, hepatitis A virus, cytomegalovirus, *Candida albicans*, and others.

gonorrhea and syphilis has declined significantly in the last decade of the 20th century, even in the United States, which lagged the rest of the industrialized Western nations in this regard. Although genital chlamydial infections generally are not reported, their prevalence certainly exceeds that of gonorrhea. Herpes simplex virus (HSV) and human papillomavirus infections also are more prevalent than gonorrhea. The relative incidence of STDs is quite variable in different areas of the world. For instance, chancroid is currently uncommon in the United States but is about as common as gonorrhea in certain areas of the Far East and Africa.

COMMON SYNDROMES. URETHRITIS IN MALES. Urethritis in males is a very common syndrome. It is ordinarily classified as either gonococcal or non-gonococcal urethritis (NGU), depending on whether the presence of gonococci can be demonstrated by Gram stain or culture. In STD clinics, the prevalence of gonococcal and non-gonococcal urethritis is similar, but NGU is considerably more common in private practice and in college infirmaries. Several studies of asymptomatic sexually active young persons found an incidence of up to 15% of genital chlamydial infection.

A large number of studies have established *Chlamydia trachomatis* as a cause of approximately 40% of cases of NGU. Case-control studies have provided evidence that suggests *Ureaplasma urealyticum* (formerly T-strain *Mycoplasma*) is a significant factor in chlamydia-negative NGU. In addition, urethral inoculation of volunteers with pure cultures of *U. urealyticum* produced rather typical NGU. In practice, however, it is difficult to define the importance of *Ureaplasma* infection in patients with urethritis, because colonization of these organisms occurs in up to 70% of asymptomatic sexually active persons. A small proportion of cases of NGU in men is due to *Trichomonas vaginalis*, HSV, or *Mycoplasma genitalium* infection.

Diagnosis of urethritis requires demonstration of an inflammatory urethral exudate. A discharge may not be evident if the patient has recently voided, and patients preferably should be examined several hours after their last urination. The discharge may be present only in the morning, before urination. Demonstration of discharge often requires urethral "milking" and may require insertion of a small calcium alginate or similar swab into the anterior urethra, with examination of a direct Gram-stained smear of the swab for leukocytes. Presence of an average of at least five polymorphonuclear leukocytes per high-power (100×) field suggests the diagnosis of urethritis.

The patient should be questioned for past history of urethritis and for symptoms suggestive of systemic diseases such as Reiter's syndrome or disseminated gonococcal infection. Examination should be made for signs of conjunctivitis, arthritis, dermatitis, and epididymitis. Prostatitis is rarely present unless there are symptoms of perineal, suprapubic, or rectal discomfort; and rectal examination is not routinely indicated. Rectal examination and urine culture are indicated in men with dysuria but without signs of anterior urethral discharge.

Laboratory studies are ordinarily limited to a Gram stain of urethral exudate. Demonstration of typical gram-negative diplococci, many of which are inside neutrophils, establishes the diagnosis of gonococcal urethritis. A Gram stain is positive in at least 90% of men with symptomatic culture-proven urethral gonorrhea. In occasional patients, especially those with an equivocal Gram stain, it may be necessary to culture the anterior urethra or freshly voided urine sediment for gonococci. This is particularly important in asymptomatic male contacts of patients with disseminated gonococcal infection or gonococcal salpingitis, because a Gram stain of urethral contents is positive in only about 60% of men with asymptomatic urethral gonorrhea.

Diagnosis of NGU usually is made by exclusion of gonorrhea. Immunoassays and a DNA hybridization test for *Chlamydia* are widely available and have sensitivities of 70 to 80% and specificities of more than 90%. Ligase chain reaction (LCR) tests for presence of gonococcal or chlamydial DNA are becoming widely available and are highly specific as well as extremely sensitive. LCR on urine is as sensitive as purulent genital secretions. Cost limits the use of LCR in some settings. Culture is not as sensitive as LCR for diagnosis of genital *Chlamydia*. There is no serologic test that is clinically useful. Tests for *Ureaplasma* are not readily available and rarely are indicated. Examination of a saline suspension of urethral exudate occasionally may reveal motile trichomonads in patients with recurrent urethritis who fail to respond to appropriate therapy. A serologic test for syphilis should be obtained, but the diagnostic yield is low.

Management is outlined in Figure 361–1 and is discussed further in gonococcal infections. Sexual partners of men with gonococcal or non-gonococcal urethritis should be treated to prevent both reinfection of the patient and development of complications in the partners.

The syndrome of *postgonococcal urethritis* (persistence or recrudescence of urethritis after administration of therapy that has eradicated gonococcal infection) is usually due to concomitant urethral chlamydial infection that was not eradicated by the original treatment. Accordingly, oral doxycycline, a macrolide such as azithromycin, or other agents effective against *Chlamydia* should be used in conjunction with ceftriaxone therapy for gonorrhea.

GENITAL ULCER SYNDROME. Genital skin lesions may be either ulcerative or non-ulcerative. In patients seen in a venereal disease clinic, the most common sexually transmitted non-ulcerative genital lesions are due to scabies, genital warts, molluscum contagiosum, or *Candida* species, but differential diagnosis includes a long list of dermatologic conditions.

The most common cause of ulcerative genital lesions in patients in the United States is HSV, but differential diagnosis includes syphilis, chancroid, lymphogranuloma venereum, granuloma inguinale, and trauma. Chancroid, lymphogranuloma venereum, and granuloma inguinale are rare. The most important distinction is among syphilis, genital herpes, and chancroid. Sometimes the appearance

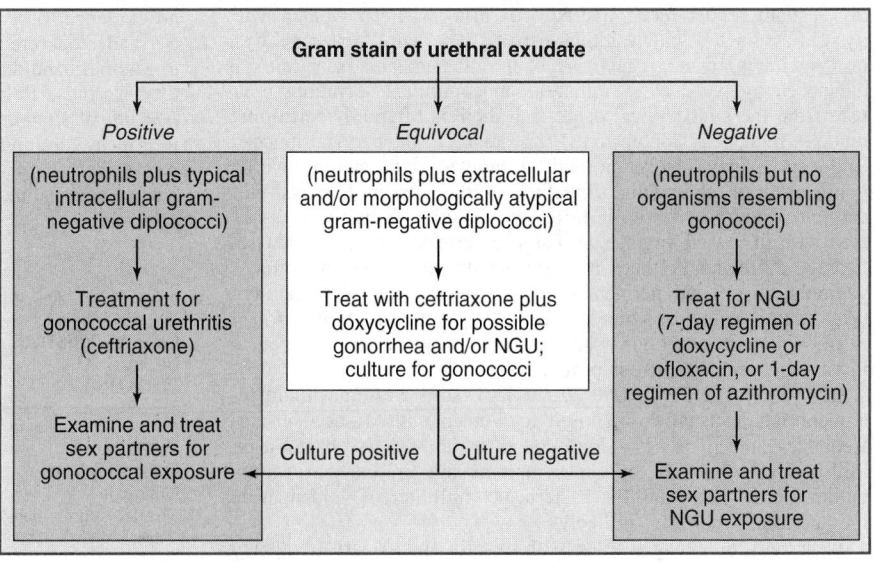

FIGURE 361–1 ■ Management of male patients with urethritis.

is virtually diagnostic: grouped, painful, superficial vesicles are nearly diagnostic of herpes, whereas a single, clean-based, non-painful ulcer with indurated margins suggests primary syphilis. About 60% of penile syphilitic chancres have this classic appearance. Painful ulcers suggest herpes or chancroid. Genital herpes may occur as a single ulcer, particularly in patients with recurrent herpes, and syphilis may occur with multiple ulcers. Secondarily infected lesions of primary syphilis may be painful.

It is a useful rule to obtain a serologic test for syphilis on all patients with genital ulcers and, if the initial serologic findings are negative and if the diagnosis remains uncertain, to obtain a second serologic examination about 2 weeks later. A darkfield examination for syphilis should also be done, and it should be repeated twice on successive days if syphilis is seriously suspected and the initial examination is negative. A multiplex polymerase chain reaction–based test is being developed that will distinguish syphilis, HSV, and chancroid in ulcer secretions.

Infection by HSV may be efficiently diagnosed by viral culture. Giemsa's or Wright's stain of cells scraped from the base of a vesicle may reveal multinucleate giant cells (Tzanck's test), but this test is particularly insensitive in herpetic lesions that have become ulcerated. Serologic tests for herpesvirus are not helpful in management but may indicate persons with latent infection.

Chancroid was epidemic in certain cities in the United States but now is most likely to be seen in travelers returning from Africa or Asia, where chancroid is common. Attempts should be made to isolate the causative agent, *Haemophilus ducreyi;* selective culture media are an improvement over previously available methods. No serologic tests are available.

Therapy clearly depends on the correct diagnosis. Topical antibiotics are never indicated. Initial genital herpes (first infection) is best treated with oral administration of acyclovir or its derivatives (valacyclovir, famcyclovir). Therapy for chancroid is with ciprofloxacin, azithromycin, erythromycin, or ceftriaxone. Occasional empirical trials of oral ciprofloxacin, azithromycin, or erythromycin are warranted in patients with persistent genital ulcers not readily attributable to herpesvirus or syphilis, but repeated attempts to isolate *H. ducreyi* should be made in such instances. It is not possible to arrive at an unequivocal diagnosis of the cause of genital ulcers in all patients.

LOWER GENITAL TRACT INFECTIONS IN WOMEN. Infections of the female genitourinary tract produce a variety of syndromes, often with overlapping symptoms (dysuria, vaginal discharge, vulvar irritation). These infections are very common, relatively poorly understood by most physicians, sometimes difficult to treat, and often frustrating for both doctor and patient. However, the various syndromes usually can be distinguished on relatively simple clinical and laboratory grounds, and a precise microbial cause often can be established.

It is most helpful first to determine the primary anatomic site of infection: urethra or bladder, endocervix, or vagina. This can sometimes be accomplished by history; women with urinary tract infection usually experience "internal" dysuria, whereas women with dysuria associated with vaginitis usually experience "external" dysuria, owing to passage of urine over inflamed labia. Cervicitis is diagnosed by physical examination; mucopurulent secretions emanate from the endocervical canal, and there is often a hypertrophic, mucoid, reddened "cobblestone" appearance to the cervical mucosa. The cervix may appear normal in women with culture-positive gonococcal or chlamydial infection of the cervix. Patients with cervicitis may also have urethritis or vaginitis. Vaginitis is associated with increased vaginal discharge of several types, as discussed later, and frequently there are associated signs and symptoms of vaginal, vulvar, and perineal irritation (dyspareunia, external dysuria, itching, pain). In patients with lower genitourinary infection, it is important to determine whether the upper genitourinary tract is involved (pyelonephritis, salpingitis).

THE URETHRAL SYNDROME. Bacterial cystitis with or without pyelonephritis is usually diagnosed in women with dysuria, urinary frequency, and pyuria if colony counts are at least 10^5 bacteria per milliliter of urine. If similar symptoms are present but routine cultures grow less than 10^4 bacteria per milliliter of voided urine, the "urethral syndrome" is likely.

In a study of young women with dysuria and urinary frequency,

and who did not have vaginitis or active herpes simplex infection, 43% had the urethral syndrome (urethritis). Among women with urethritis, 25% had positive urethral cultures for *C. trachomatis.* Gonococci also were shown to cause this syndrome. Thus, women as well as men may have urethritis caused by gonococci and chlamydiae.

Patients with symptoms of UTI who do not have bacteriuria should have urethral and cervical cultures for *Neisseria gonorrhoeae.* If these cultures are also negative, a therapeutic trial may be made with a tetracycline, azithromycin, or ofloxacin. LCR tests for gonococci or *Chlamydia* in voided urine are useful.

VAGINITIS. In a large study of women in a primary care clinic who had lower genitourinary complaints, vaginitis was more than five times as common as urinary tract infections. In this and similar studies, there were three predominant types of vaginitis: yeast infection *(Candida albicans)*, Trichomonas *(T. vaginalis)* infection, and bacterial vaginosis (BV) caused by organisms other than *Candida* and *T. vaginalis.* The incidence of these types of vaginitis varies in different patient populations, but, in general, *Candida* and BV are more common than *T. vaginalis* vaginitis.

Symptoms of vaginitis include increased volume of vaginal discharge, which is often abnormally yellow or green and may be malodorous. Vaginal and vulvar itching may be troublesome, especially in *Candida* infection. There may be vaginal tenderness and pain, dyspareunia, or dysuria.

The most common sign of vaginitis is an increased vaginal discharge. In *T. vaginalis* infections, there is often a profuse and frothy discharge. A curdlike, white discharge is common in *Candida* infections, and many patients with BV have an adherent, often gray, and frequently malodorous discharge. Microscopic examination shows many polymorphonuclear leukocytes (PMNs) in the discharge in all but BV. Speculum examination may show signs of endocervicitis as well, with purulent discharge issuing from the cervical os. In occasional patients, no objective signs of vaginal inflammation are found despite the presence of troublesome symptoms (Table 361–2).

Candida Vaginitis. Most vaginal yeast infections are due to *C. albicans.* The discharge in *Candida* vaginitis is not malodorous. Diagnosis is usually made by visualizing yeasts or pseudohyphae by microscopic examination of vaginal secretions suspended in normal saline or 10% potassium hydroxide (KOH). Microscopic examination is less sensitive than culture. However, many asymptomatic women have positive vaginal cultures for *C. albicans,* and therefore microscopy is preferred initially to culture. Culture for *Candida* may be helpful in women with discharge of normal acidity (pH < 4.5) and negative microscopy.

Therapy for *Candida* vaginitis is with one of the imidazole compounds (e.g., clotrimazole, miconazole, butoconazole, or terconazole) once each night for 1 to 14 days intravaginally or with an oral azole agent (ketoconazole, fluconazole, or itraconazole) for 1 to 5 days. A single oral dose of 150 mg of fluconazole appears to be as effective as other therapies. No convincing evidence exists that attempts to eradicate yeast from the gastrointestinal tract significantly affect rates of cure or relapse of *Candida* vaginitis. There is no evidence to warrant therapy of sexual partners. Attempts should be made to correct ancillary conditions that increase susceptibility to vaginal candidiasis: antibiotic therapy, diabetes, or oral anovulatory steroids. Relapse is a significant problem in some patients. Antifungal suppression therapy may be warranted in some women. Regimens that appear useful include oral fluconazole, 100 mg once weekly, or vaginal clotrimzole, 500 mg suppositories once weekly. No therapy is indicated for asymptomatic vaginal carriers of *C. albicans.*

Table 361–2 ■ DIFFERENTIAL DIAGNOSIS OF VAGINITIS

CHARACTERISTICS OF VAGINAL DISCHARGE	C. ALBICANS VAGINITIS	T. VAGINALIS VAGINITIS	BACTERIAL VAGINOSIS
pH	4.5	>5.0	>5.0
White curd	Usually	No	No
Odor with KOH	No	Yes	Yes
Clue cells	No	No	Usually
Motile trichomonads	No	Usually	No
Yeast cells	Yes	No	No

T. vaginalis Vaginitis. Diagnosis is made ordinarily by visualizing motile trichomonads in a normal saline suspension of vaginal secretions. The saline suspension should be examined promptly. Culture is more sensitive, but about 70% of culture-positive cases are detected by microscopy. Addition of a drop of 10% KOH to vaginal secretions often results in liberation of a detectable fishlike odor, attributed to release of volatile amines. The pH of vaginal secretions is usually more than 5.0 In these latter two respects, *T. vaginalis* vaginitis is similar to BV. Secretions contain many polymorphonuclear PMNs in *Trichomonas* vaginitis but few in BV.

Therapy for trichomoniasis is with one of the nitroimidazoles, either metronidazole or newer compounds such as tinidazole. A single 2-g oral dose of metronidazole is as effective as multiple-day regimens. Metronidazole should be used with caution in pregnancy because of unsubstantiated concerns about teratogenicity. Because more than one third of male sexual partners of women with trichomoniasis are asymptomatic urethral carriers of *T. vaginalis,* the male partners should also be treated with a single 2-g dose of metronidazole.

Although *T. vaginalis* can be transmitted sexually, it probably is transmitted by other means as well. This conclusion is based on prevalence studies that show one peak in young, sexually active women and a second peak in older women who have no other evidence for sexually transmitted infection.

Bacterial Vaginosis. BV is the most common cause of vaginitis in women of childbearing age. This syndrome is probably due to mixed infection by *Gardnerella vaginalis* and anaerobic bacteria, including the curved or comma-shaped rods now known as *Mobiluncus* species. *G. vaginalis* is a small, gram-variable coccobacillus that can be grown on partially selective enriched media. Among women with abnormal vaginal discharge who do not have yeast infection or trichomoniasis, more than 90% grow *G. vaginalis,* but normal women may have *G. vaginalis* as well. There usually are increased numbers of anaerobic vaginal bacteria and decreased numbers of hydrogen peroxide–producing vaginal lactobacilli. The pathophysiology of this syndrome is still under investigation.

Diagnosis of BV is by exclusion of trichomoniasis, candidiasis, and purulent cervicitis. Abnormal cells termed *clue cells* are often seen in a wet mount or Gram's stain of vaginal secretions in normal saline; these are stippled, granular-appearing vaginal epithelial cells that contain large numbers of adherent *G. vaginalis.* Few PMNs are present. Addition of a drop of 10% KOH usually results in production of an unpleasant fishy odor. The pH of the vaginal secretions is nearly always more than 5.0.

Optimal therapy is being investigated. Metronidazole has only borderline activity in vitro against *G. vaginalis,* but in a dose of 500 mg by mouth twice daily for 7 days it is effective in eradicating both *G. vaginalis* and the symptoms of vaginitis in at least 90% of women. Single-dose therapy results in increased rates of relapse. This suggests that the principal cause of this syndrome is an anaerobe, because metronidazole is principally effective against anaerobes. Clindamycin (300 mg orally twice daily for 7 days) also is effective, as is topical therapy with either metronidazole or clindamycin. More than 90% of male partners are urethral carriers of *G. vaginalis.* However, treatment of male partners does not seem to affect the recurrence rate in women.

Mixed Vaginitis. In 2 to 16% of patients, vaginitis may be due to polymicrobial infection with two or three organisms. Such mixed infection may account for some instances of treatment failure. Particular care should be given to identification of all causative organisms in patients who have recurrent or relapsing vaginitis.

CERVICITIS. Two organisms are recognized as probable causes of mucopurulent endocervicitis: *N. gonorrhoeae* and *C. trachomatis.* Women who are sexual partners of men with *Chlamydia*-positive NGU have a much higher rate of isolation of chlamydiae from the cervix than do women who are partners of men with *Chlamydia*-negative NGU, and they also have significantly higher rates of mucopurulent cervicitis. HSV can also cause cervicitis, especially in primary infection. However, the clinical appearance in herpetic cervicitis is different, with cervical vesicles and ulcers rather than mucopurulent cervicitis.

True cervicitis should not be confused with cervical ectopy, which is merely the appearance of endocervical columnar epithelium on the exposed, visible exocervix. This results in a red-appearing cervix and may result in increased production of a mucoid vaginal discharge but does not require therapy.

Diagnosis of mucopurulent endocervicitis requires visualization of purulent discharge from the cervical os. There often is a roughened cobblestone appearance to the cervix. Gram stain is about 60% sensitive and more than 90% specific for gonorrhea if typical intracellular gonococci are seen, but cultures or other specific tests, especially LCR for *N. gonorrhoeae* should be taken. Tissue culture for isolation of *C. trachomatis* is rarely employed, having been replaced either by antigen detection or by molecular tests, especially LCR. First-voided urine is a convenient source of material for diagnostic LCR for either gonococci or chlamydia. Cytologic methods are not sufficiently sensitive to warrant widespread use.

Antibiotic therapy appears to result in clinical improvement in mucopurulent cervicitis. Patients with negative cultures for the gonococcus should be treated with doxycycline (100 mg twice daily for 7 days); alternatives are oral azithromycin in a single dose of 1 g or oral ofloxacin in a dose of 300 mg twice daily for 7 days. No other form of cervicitis has been shown to respond to antimicrobial therapy.

UPPER GENITAL TRACT DISEASE IN WOMEN: SALPINGITIS. Full coverage of this important topic is precluded by space considerations. This is a very important clinical problem, resulting in considerable morbidity in the estimated 250,000 to 500,000 women who are affected yearly in the United States.

Etiology. The gonococcus accounts for 20 to 50% of cases in the United States, particularly among women with relatively severe and first-episode salpingitis. Fifteen to 20 per cent of women with gonococcal cervicitis probably subsequently develop salpingitis. Genital chlamydial infections also are a significant cause of salpingitis. Salpingitis due to genital chlamydial infections may be mild, and patients may not seek medical care. Nevertheless, complications may follow, particularly tubal scarring and infertility. BV may predispose to salpingitis (as well as preterm delivery), and douching may be an additional risk factor for salpingitis. Many cases of salpingitis are caused by mixed infection with microaerophilic streptococci and enteric bacilli, often including *Bacteroides* species. These polymicrobial infections appear to be more common in recurrent attacks of salpingitis.

Diagnosis. Clinical diagnosis of salpingitis is inexact. Perhaps only 20% of patients have the classic syndrome of lower abdominal pain and tenderness, cervical tenderness, fever, leukocytosis, and elevated sedimentation rate. The most common findings are lower abdominal tenderness, which is usually bilateral, and adnexal and cervical tenderness. Patients with gonococcal salpingitis are more likely to have fever and more commonly have onset near the menses, whereas patients with non-gonococcal salpingitis more commonly have adnexal masses. Laparoscopy is invasive but provides definitive evidence and also allows cultures to be taken from the fimbriated end of the fallopian tubes. In current practice, vaginal ultrasonography and computed tomography help to define the cause of pelvic pain syndromes.

Complications. Complications are primarily infertility and ectopic pregnancy. Rates of involuntary infertility are about 15% after one attack of salpingitis and about 75% after three or more attacks. Total hysterectomy may eventually be necessitated by symptoms of chronic salpingitis.

Therapy. Initial therapy for outpatients may include cefoxitin, 2 g intramuscularly, along with probenecid, 1 g orally, followed by doxycycline, 100 mg orally twice daily for 10 to 14 days. An alternative regimen for penicillin-allergic patients is ofloxacin, 400 mg orally twice daily for 14 days, plus either clindamycin, 450 mg orally four times daily, or metronidazole, 500 mg orally twice daily for 14 days. There are no controlled data on efficacy of various regimens used for hospitalized patients. Current recommendations call for doxycycline, 100 mg twice daily, plus cefoxitin, 2 g intravenously four times daily; or clindamycin, 900 mg intravenously three times daily, plus gentamicin, 1.5 mg/kg three times daily. After discharge, either doxycycline (100 mg orally twice daily) or clindamycin (450 mg orally four times daily) should be given to complete 10 to 14 days of therapy. Patients should usually be hospitalized if they are very ill, are pregnant, or have significant adnexal masses; if previous therapy failed; or if the differential diagnosis includes a surgical emergency such as appendicitis or ectopic pregnancy.

Prevention. Sexual partners of women with gonococcal or chlamydial salpingitis must be identified, examined, and treated to prevent subsequent reinfection of the patient. Many of the infected male partners of women with salpingitis are asymptomatic. Effective community programs to detect and treat asymptomatic genital gonococcal and chlamydia infections reduce the incidence of pelvic inflammatory disease.

Marrazzo JM, White CL, Krekeler B, et al: Community-based urine screening for Chlamydia trachomatis with a ligase chain reaction assay. Ann Intern Med 127:796, 1997. One of many papers that proves the use of this simple but not cheap test.
McCormack WM: Pelvic inflammatory disease. N Engl J Med 330:115, 1994. A concise, still timely overview.
Shcoles D, Stergachis A, Heidrich FE, et al: Prevention of pelvic inflammatory disease by screening for cervical chlamydia infection. N Engl J Med 334:1362, 1996. A randomized controlled trial in an HMO setting that showed that a strategy to screen certain high-risk women was effective in reducting rates of PID.
Sobel JD: Vaginitis. N Engl J Med 337:1896, 1997. An excellent concise general review.

362 GONOCOCCAL INFECTIONS

P. Frederick Sparling

Neisseria gonorrhoeae is a common sexually transmitted organism that causes anterior urethritis in males and endocervicitis and urethritis in females. Other types of primary infection include pharyngitis, proctitis, conjunctivitis, and vulvovaginitis; the last-named occurs principally in prepubescent females. Complications may occur by direct extension of infection, including epididymitis, prostatitis, Bartholin gland abscess, salpingitis, and perihepatitis. Bacteremia may occur, with production of characteristic cutaneous lesions, arthritis, and tenosynovitis; rare complications include endocarditis and meningitis. Conjunctival infection formerly was a common cause of blindness in neonates.

Gonorrhea is the most common reportable infectious disease in the United States, with nearly 400,000 reported cases in 1995. The true incidence is probably twice as high. Incidence has declined dramatically in much of the industrialized west in recent years and now is decreasing in the United States as well.

EPIDEMIOLOGY. The only natural hosts for *N. gonorrhoeae* are humans. The organism normally resides on the columnar epithelium of mucosal surfaces and is usually transmitted by intimate sexual contact. The incidence of gonorrhea varies greatly in different groups. As many as 5% of persons in high-risk populations may be infected at any time. Highest incidence is found in young (15 to 30) single persons of low socioeconomic and educational status, probably because these factors correlate positively with sexual promiscuity. Incidence is highest in inner cities and in the rural Southeast and in African Americans. The common factor in each instance is low socioeconomic status.

The risk of acquiring infection depends on the type of contact with an infected person. Sixty to 80 percent of females in contact with a male with urethral gonorrhea develop gonococcal cervicitis. By contrast, it is estimated that only 20 to 30% of males having sex with an infected female develop gonorrhea. This difference may be due to exposure of females to a larger inoculum of gonococci. A person having oral sex with a male with gonococcal urethritis has considerable risk of acquiring pharyngeal gonorrhea. Transmission of infection by oral contact with the genitalia of an infected female is rare. Infection is apparently efficiently spread by penile-rectal contact.

Gonococci die rapidly on drying, and transmission by fomites is rare. Epidemics were reported in prepubertal females living in proximity in orphanages, but such episodes are now very uncommon.

Control of gonorrhea is difficult because of the frequency of asymptomatic infection. Perhaps 50% of infections in females are asymptomatic or only minimally symptomatic, and at least 10% of incident infections in males are asymptomatic. Prevalence studies commonly show that up to 50% of infected men have too few symptoms to seek medical care.

In past years there was considerable emphasis on case finding by endocervical culture in young, sexually active females. The merit of this strategy depends on the prevalence of infection in the community and the lifestyle of the patient. A more cost-effective method for finding infected patients is to obtain a culture in patients about 6 weeks after treatment for gonorrhea; as many as 15 to 20% of such cases are culture positive, usually because of reinfection.

THE ORGANISM. *N. gonorrhoeae* is a gram-negative, aerobic diplococcus. Many strains require 3 to 10% CO_2 for optimal growth. They are highly autolytic and die rapidly when outside their normal human environment. They are sensitive to fatty acids and grow best on media with added starch to inhibit fatty acids present in agar. Several partially selective media are available; most employ antibiotics to inhibit growth of other microorganisms.

Presumptive identification in vitro is made by colonial morphology, Gram stain, and a positive oxidase test. Differentiation from the closely related meningococcus and the various non-pathogenic *Neisseria* is ordinarily by patterns of utilization of various simple carbohydrates; gonococci use glucose but not maltose or sucrose.

Gonococci are highly variable and occur in a number of different colonial forms. Small colonial types are piliated and more virulent in humans than the larger, non-piliated variants. Variation is also found in certain outer membrane proteins. Gonococci undergo rapid variation in the antigenic type of pilus expressed, which probably contributes to prolonged infections without treatment and to the ability of persons to acquire repeat infections after treatment. The importance of surface components of the gonococcus in the pathogenesis of infection is under intense investigation.

Gonococci can be serotyped on the basis of antigenic differences in outer membrane proteins. These tests are not routinely available.

PATHOGENESIS. Surface pili undoubtedly help to attach the bacteria to the mucosal surface. Typical urethral infections result in moderately severe inflammation, probably due to release of toxic lipopolysaccharide from gonococci and to production of chemotactic factors that attract neutrophilic leukocytes. Certain strains can cause asymptomatic urethral infection for reasons not completely understood. These strains are usually penicillin sensitive, resistant to the bactericidal effects of normal human serum, and particularly likely to cause bacteremia and septic arthritis.

In the preantibiotic era, symptoms usually persisted for 2 to 3 months before host defenses finally eradicated the infection. Host defenses include serum opsonic and bactericidal antibodies, as well as local (mucosal) antibodies of the IgG and IgA classes. All gonococci produce an enzyme, IgA protease, that cleaves the major class of secretory IgA, perhaps contributing to persistence of local gonococcal infections.

Serum bactericidal antibodies are undoubtedly important in preventing bacteremic infection. The best evidence for this has been provided by patients who suffer from homozygous deficiency of one of the complement components C6, C7, C8, or C9. This results in deficiency of serum bactericidal activity but no alteration of serum opsonic activity. Such individuals are particularly prone to recurrent bacteremic gonococcal infection or to recurrent meningococcal meningitis or meningococcemia.

CLINICAL PATTERNS OF DISEASE. GONORRHEA IN MALES. Gonococcal urethritis in males ("the clap" or "the strain") is characterized by a yellowish, purulent urethral discharge and dysuria. The usual incubation period is 2 to 6 days. The discharge in gonorrhea is slightly more copious and purulent than in non-gonococcal urethritis. Symptoms are probably produced by 90% of infections, although asymptomatic infections do occur and may persist for many months. Males with asymptomatic infection do not seek treatment, whereas those with symptomatic infection are usually promptly treated and cured. This is the probable explanation for prevalence studies that show that up to 50% of infected males are asymptomatic. Asymptomatic infection in males and females is of great epidemiologic importance, because such carriers may continue to spread infection to new sexual partners for months if the infection is not properly diagnosed and treated.

Complications of gonococcal urethritis in males are now rare. Urethral stricture was formerly a common complication but was probably due in part to the use of caustic treatment regimens. Epididymitis and prostatitis, relatively common complications in the past, are seen only occasionally today. The principal complication is disseminated gonococcal infection, which is estimated to

DIAGNOSIS	TREATMENT
Uncomplicated genital, rectal, or pharyngeal infection of men and women	Ceftriaxone, 125 mg IM once, plus doxycycline, 100 mg PO twice daily for 7 days *or* Cefixime, 400 mg PO once, plus doxycycline, 100 mg PO twice daily for 7 days *or* Ciprofloxacin, 500 mg PO once, plus doxycycline, 100 mg PO twice daily for 7 days *or* Ofloxacin, 400 mg PO once, plus doxycycline, 100 mg PO twice daily for 7 days
Gonorrhea in pregnancy	Ceftriaxone, 125 mg IM once, plus erythromycin base, 500 mg PO 4 times daily for 7 days *or* Spectinomycin, 2 g IM, plus erythromycin (as in ceftriaxone regimen)
Salpingitis—outpatient	Cefoxitin, 2 g IM, plus doxycycline, 100 mg PO twice daily for 10–14 days *or* Ofloxacin, 400 mg PO twice daily for 14 days, plus either clindamycin, 450 mg PO 4 times daily or metronidazole, 500 mg PO twice daily for 14 days
Salpingitis—inpatient	Doxycycline, 100 mg IV twice daily, plus cefoxitin, 2 g IV 4 times daily until improved, followed by doxycycline, 100 mg PO twice daily to complete 14 days of therapy; alternative regimens include clindamycin plus an aminoglycoside
Disseminated gonococcal infection	Ceftriaxone, 1 g IM every 24 hours *or* Spectinomycin 2 g IM every 12 hours (see text)

affect about 1% of persons with gonorrhea. This entity is discussed later. The differential diagnosis of gonococcal urethritis is discussed in Chapter 361.

Gonococcal infections of the pharynx and rectum are common problems in homosexual males. Most patients with pharyngeal infection are asymptomatic, but occasional patients have exudative pharyngitis with cervical adenopathy. Gonococcal infection of the rectum causes a wide spectrum of symptoms, ranging from no symptoms to severe proctitis with tenesmus and bloody, mucopurulent discharge. Although rectal cultures are also positive in approximately 40% of females with cervical gonorrhea, symptoms of proctitis in females are unusual. This has suggested that the trauma of rectal intercourse may contribute to the proctitis observed in males. Sigmoidoscopy may be indicated to exclude ulcerative colitis, Crohn's colitis, rectal lacerations, or other infections such as shigellosis, amebiasis, or syphilis, all of which are common in male homosexuals.

Gonococcal epididymitis is usually unilateral. Both *Chlamydia trachomatis* and the gonococcus are significant causes of epididymitis in men younger than 35, whereas coliform bacteria are the usual cause in older males. The differential diagnosis includes trauma, tumor, and torsion of the testis, suggested by sudden onset and elevation of the testis. If there is question of testicular torsion, consultation with a urologist is necessary. In epididymitis there is often a urethral exudate, which should be cultured for gonococci and other bacteria. Treatment of gonococcal epididymitis includes scrotal elevation and 7 to 10 days of appropriate antibiotics (Table 362–1).

GONORRHEA IN FEMALES. In incidence studies, approximately one half of women infected with the gonococcus are asymptomatic or have so few symptoms that they do not seek medical care. The most commonly involved site is the endocervix (80 to 90%), followed by the urethra (80%), rectum (40%), and pharynx (10 to 20%). Most pharyngeal, urethral, and rectal infections cause few or no symptoms. Cervical infection may result in vaginal discharge or abnormal menstrual bleeding. Neither of these symptoms is specific for gonococcal infection. Gonococcal urethritis may mimic cystitis caused by enteric bacilli, although standard urine cultures are negative because gonococci do not grow on culture media ordinarily used to diagnose urinary tract infection. Culture methods are discussed later under Laboratory Diagnosis. The differential diagnosis of cervicitis, vaginitis, and the urethral syndrome is discussed in Chapter 361.

The most important complication of gonorrhea is salpingitis. The less precise term *pelvic inflammatory disease* (PID) is often used synonymously. Although many other organisms can cause a similar syndrome, the gonococcus accounts for about half of the cases of PID in the United States. About 15% of women with gonococcal cervicitis develop PID, often in proximity to a menstrual period. Symptoms usually include abdominal pain, and often there is fever. Physical examination usually discloses cervical motion tenderness and bilateral adnexal tenderness; in a small proportion of cases the disease may be unilateral, causing confusion with appendicitis or ectopic pregnancy. There may be signs of generalized peritonitis. Laboratory studies often show elevation of the white blood cell count and sedimentation rate. The diagnosis of PID is inexact, as shown by laparoscopic examination; many cases of PID are missed if undue reliance is placed on presence of fever or elevation of white blood cell count or sedimentation rate.

Although PID is uncommon in pregnancy, it may be particularly severe, and pregnant patients with PID should probably be hospitalized. The incidence of gonococcal PID is increased about threefold in women using an intrauterine device (IUD) for contraception.

A single attack of gonococcal PID seems to increase twofold the risk of developing another with subsequent gonococcal cervicitis. About half of the male sexual partners of women with gonococcal PID are infected, and half of these infections are asymptomatic. Failure to diagnose cases and treat properly the male partners exposes the patient to the risk of further attacks of PID. After the patient has been effectively treated, it often is wise to refer her and her sexual partners to a public health clinic for follow-up.

The major complication of gonococcal PID is tubal scarring and infertility. The incidence of involuntary infertility is estimated as 15% after one attack of PID and about 50% after three attacks. The incidence of ectopic pregnancy is increased from 7- to 10-fold in women with previous salpingitis, with resultant increased fetal and maternal mortality. Treatment is indicated in Table 362–1.

Gonococci may spread upward to the liver, causing perihepatitis (Fitz-Hugh-Curtis syndrome). This syndrome is more common in women but rarely occurs in men with gonococcal bacteremia. Gonococcal perihepatitis causes tenderness and pain in the region of the liver, mimicking acute cholecystitis. However, it resolves promptly with appropriate antibiotic therapy. Peritoneoscopy may be indicated rarely for diagnostic purposes; "violin-string" adhesions between the liver capsule and the peritoneum are seen.

GONORRHEA IN CHILDREN. Infants born to a mother with cervicovaginal gonorrhea may develop gonococcal conjunctivitis, although routine use of prophylactic 1% silver nitrate eye drops (or, in some hospitals, topical erythromycin or tetracycline) has markedly reduced the incidence of this problem. Neonates may also acquire pharyngeal, respiratory, or rectal infection and may develop gonococcal sepsis. Older children up to 1 year of age usually acquire conjunctival or vaginal infection by accidental contamination from an adult, whereas from 1 year to puberty most childhood gonorrhea is the result of purposeful sexual abuse by an adult.

GONOCOCCAL BACTEREMIA. Approximately 1% of adults with gonorrhea develop the syndrome of gonococcal bacteremia, dermatitis, and arthritis, or disseminated gonococcal infection (DGI). In most series, the majority of patients with DGI are women. The regional incidence of DGI probably varies because of geographic differences in prevalence of the usually antibiotic-sensitive, serum-bactericidal-resistant strains of *N. gonorrhoeae* that cause this syndrome. The severity of the syndrome is variable, from a slowly evolving mild illness with little or no fever, mild arthralgias, and few skin lesions to a fulminant illness with high temperature and prostration. Most episodes of DGI are relatively mild in comparison with meningococcemia.

Many patients with DGI have no local symptoms of gonococcal infection. Initial manifestations are usually migratory asymmetrical polyarthralgias and skin lesions that are often accompanied by fever. Many patients have tenosynovitis, typically involving the flexor tendon sheaths of the wrist or the Achilles tendon (colloquially known as "lover's heels"). Skin lesions are few in number (<30 usually), are acral in distribution (fingers, toes, extremities), and may be painful before they are visible. The individual lesions may be papules, pustules, or bullae on an erythematous base; less commonly seen are petechiae or necrotic lesions. The rash is not pathognomonic but is sufficiently typical that it should strongly suggest DGI when seen in young patients with polyarthralgia. Blood cultures are often positive at this stage, and circulating immune complexes may be present. Gram stain of the skin lesions is positive in only about 5% of patients, but gonococcal antigens can be detected in these lesions in about two thirds of patients by use of immunofluorescent-labeled antigonococcal antibody.

The early stage of gonococcemia may subside spontaneously or may merge indistinctly after about 1 week into a second stage of septic arthritis. Skin lesions have usually disappeared by this time, and blood cultures are nearly always negative. Septic arthritis may occur without preceding skin lesions or polyarthralgia. One large joint (elbow, wrist, hip, knee, ankle) is usually involved, although some series report involvement of two joints in a significant minority of patients. On infrequent occasions, symmetrical involvement of the fingers may mimic acute rheumatoid arthritis. Physical examination typically discloses a swollen, warm joint with evident intra-articular fluid. Aspiration of the joint often reveals marked neutrophilic leukocytosis (50,000 to 100,000 leukocytes/mm³ millimeter), although early in the development of the septic joint the synovial leukocyte count may be much lower. Cultures of joint fluid are often positive if the leukocyte count is 80,000/mm³ or more but are often negative when leukocyte counts are 20,000/mm³ or less.

Other complications of gonococcal bacteremia include mild hepatitis, myocarditis, the Fitz-Hugh-Curtis syndrome, meningitis, and endocarditis. In the preantibiotic era, gonococcal infection accounted for up to 10% of all endocarditis, but it is now rare. Gonococcal endocarditis is often a rapidly progressive infection with severe valvular damage; it should be suspected in patients with a new murmur, severe prostrating illness, severe myocarditis, or evidence of renal failure, or in the presence of stigmas of peripheral embolization.

The differential diagnosis of the gonococcal bacteremia arthritis syndrome includes Reiter's syndrome, rheumatic fever, rheumatoid arthritis, systemic lupus erythematosus, other infectious or postinfectious arthritis, subacute bacterial endocarditis, meningococcemia, and viral hepatitis. In young males, Reiter's syndrome is the principal consideration. Conjunctivitis is rarely seen in gonococcemia but is common in Reiter's syndrome. In the absence of typical skin lesions, DGI may not be suspected until culture results are known.

Diagnosis of DGI is secure when gonococci are recovered from the blood, skin lesions, or synovial fluid. The diagnosis of DGI is probably correct in patients in whom the only positive cultures are from local mucosal surfaces but in whom there are both typical skin lesions and a prompt response to antigonococcal therapy.

LABORATORY DIAGNOSIS. Gram stain of urethral exudate in symptomatic males has a sensitivity of 90 to 98% and a specificity of 95 to 98%. Accordingly, urethral cultures are not ordinarily indicated in untreated symptomatic males. Since the sensitivity of the Gram stain is only about 60% in asymptomatic male urethral infection, cultures of the anterior urethra or fresh urine sediment are recommended when epidemiologic evidence suggests possible asymptomatic urethral infection. Gram stain of the endocervix is 50 to 60% sensitive and 82 to 97% specific in women with positive cervical cultures for N. gonorrhoeae. Care must be taken to avoid mistaking normal endocervical flora and neutrophils for gonorrhea; only smears showing several neutrophils with multiple, typical intracellular gram-negative diplococci should be read as presumptively positive for gonorrhea. Cultures for N. gonorrhoeae should be obtained in all women, even if the Gram stain appears positive. Non-culture tests are supplanting culture in some circumstances. Urine-based ligase chain reaction is highly sensitive and specific,

and avoids speculum examination. It is more expensive than culture, however, and does not allow sensitivity testing.

Cultures should be plated immediately if possible onto chocolate agar or chocolate agar containing selective antibiotics (e.g., modified Thayer-Martin medium [MTM]). Holding media such as Amies' or Stuart's transport media may be used if necessary, but viability of gonococci drops after 12 to 24 hours in such media. In infected women, a single endocervical culture on modified Thayer-Martin medium is 80 to 90% sensitive, as judged by yields obtained with multiple cultures from multiple sites. In 3 to 5% of women the only positive culture is at the pharyngeal, urethral, or rectal site. The yield from these sites is too low to warrant routine pharyngeal, urethral, or rectal cultures. Urethral cultures are indicated in women with the urethral syndrome. Both cervical and rectal cultures should be obtained as part of the test of cure in women after treatment, because inclusion of the rectal culture increases the diagnostic yield of treatment failures by as much as 50%. Pharyngeal cultures should be obtained from patients with symptomatic pharyngitis or from persons exposed by fellatio to infected males. Patients with possible DGI should have culture samples taken from all possible mucosal sites (pharynx, urethra, cervix, rectum), as well as blood and synovial fluid.

Cultures of the cervix should be taken under direct visualization during speculum examination, using a cotton-tipped swab. Lubricant jellies may be deleterious to gonococci and should be avoided. Cultures of the anterior urethra of males should be obtained with calcium alginate swabs or a sterile wire loop. Immediate culture of first-voided urine is also useful.

Positive cultures from the pharynx or rectum should be carefully evaluated by the microbiology laboratory to avoid confusion between gonococci and meningococci. Meningococci are more common than gonococci in throat cultures. No serologic test available is sufficiently sensitive and specific to merit use for screening or diagnostic purposes.

TREATMENT. Gonococci frequently have chromosomal mutations that result in relative resistance to penicillin, tetracycline, and other antibiotics. Strains with chromosomally mediated resistance (CMRNG strains) have become prevalent in certain areas of the United States and are more common in parts of Asia. These strains do not respond to penicillin but do respond to spectinomycin or ceftriaxone. About 10% of all gonococci in the United States now are CMRNG.

Gonococci that carry a β-lactamase (penicillinase) plasmid emerged in the Far East and elsewhere in 1975 and have spread to much of the world. Penicillinase-producing gonococci (PPNG) account for 30 to 50% of all gonorrhea in certain cities in Africa and the Far East but are less common in the United States. The incidence of PPNG is about 10% in the United States but varies in different locales. The gonococcal plasmids are similar to penicillinase plasmids found in Haemophilus species. PPNG are resistant to clinically attainable doses of penicillins but are sensitive to spectinomycin and to certain cephalosporins (cefuroxime, cefoxitin, ceftriaxone). PPNG are known to cause DGI and salpingitis.

Plasmid-encoded tetracycline resistance, Tcr, also is a problem. These strains do not respond to tetracycline but do respond to spectinomycin or ceftriaxone and may respond to penicillin. Incidence of Tcr gonococci is increasing and is 5 to 15% in various U.S. cities. Recently, gonococci with clinically significant levels of resistance to fluoroquinolones have emerged in several areas of the world, including the United States.

The antibiotic regimens recommended for gonorrhea in the United States are summarized in Table 362–1. Ceftriaxone has replaced penicillin and ampicillin, because of the prevalence of CMRNG and Pcr strains. Tetracyclines no longer are acceptable therapy for gonorrhea because of the prevalence of Tcr strains. Because gonococcal infections commonly are associated with genital chlamydial infection, most authorities now recommend a 7-day course of a tetracycline (usually doxycycline) for all patients with gonorrhea as follow-up to initial ceftriaxone therapy. A single dose of 1 g of azithromycin orally is as effective for chlamydia as the 7-day regimen of doxycycline.

Each of the recommended regimens is highly effective for genital gonorrhea. In patients who do not respond, isolates can be tested for production of penicillinase, and spectinomycin should be used for re-treatment. However, most apparent failures are really reinfections. Some studies show that 15% of patients are reinfected within 6 weeks of successful therapy. On this basis, many authorities recommend that recultures should be obtained 6 weeks after treatment.

In the absence of an effective vaccine, control of this disease depends on proper diagnosis and treatment of patients' sexual contacts. If patients are given simple instructions, many bring their contacts to the physician for examination. There are sound epidemiologic reasons for treating contacts immediately. Local health departments are not utilized sufficiently for help in examination and treatment of contacts.

Treatment of salpingitis (PID) has not been studied adequately (see Table 362–1). Most authorities recommend removal of IUDs in women with PID. It is crucial to examine and treat all sexual partners of women with gonococcal PID.

Therapy for gonococcal arthritis is ordinarily highly successful with each of the recommended regimens (see Table 362–1). Failure to improve in 3 days suggests that the patient does not have DGI. Septic joints should be aspirated, both to make the initial diagnosis and to remove inflammatory exudate. Open drainage is rarely indicated, except in infection of the hip in childhood. Repeat closed aspiration may be necessary if joint fluid rapidly reaccumulates, but most patients require only one or a few joint aspirations. Antibiotics should not be injected into the joint space. Most patients with DGI should be hospitalized initially, but outpatient therapy may be used to conclude a 7-day course of treatment. Oral therapy may be used initially in carefully selected, compliant patients with a definite diagnosis and only mild infection. Antibiotics for oral use in this situation include cefixime, 400 mg twice daily, or ciprofloxacin, 500 mg twice daily. Therapy should be continued for 7 days.

Gonococcal conjunctivitis should be treated by immediate saline irrigation and intravenous ceftriaxone.

PREVENTION. Although vaccines are under intense study, an effective gonococcal vaccine is still only a hope. Condoms prevent most infection. Certain contraceptive foams have antigonococcal activity but are of unproven efficacy clinically.

Cohen MS, Sparling PF: Mucosal infection with *Neisseria gonorrhoeae:* Bacterial adaptation and mucosal defenses. J Clin Invest 89:1699, 1992. *A review of pathogenesis with emphasis on interactions with the host.*
Handsfield HH, Sparling PF: *Neisseria gonorrhoeae. In* Mandell GF, Bennett JE, Dolin R (eds): Principles and Practice of Infectious Diseases, 4th ed. New York, Churchill Livingstone, 1995, pp 1909–1926. *Highly referenced overview of pathogenesis, epidemiology, clinical presentation, diagnosis, and treatment.*
Kilmars PH, Knapp JS, Xia M, et al: Intercity spread of gonococci with decreased susceptibility to fluoroquinolones: A unique focus in the United States. J Infect Dis 177:677, 1998. *"The days for fluoroquinolone use for gonorrhea may be nearing the end."*
Smith KR, Ching S, Lee H, et al: Evaluation of ligase chain reaction for use with urine for identification of *Neisseria gonorrhoeae* in females attending a sexually transmitted disease clinic. J Clin Microbiol 33:455, 1995. *"One of many papers showing the urine-based LCR tests are simple, sensitive, and specific."*
Sparling PF, Cohen MS, Wyrick PB, Elkins C: Vaccines for bacterial sexually transmitted infections: A realistic goal? Proc Natl Acad Sci USA 91:2456, 1994. *Discussion of immunobiology of gonorrhea and prospects for a vaccine.*

363 GRANULOMA INGUINALE (DONOVANOSIS)
Edward W. Hook III

Granuloma inguinale, also known as donovanosis, is a slowly progressive ulcerative disease involving principally the skin and subcutaneous tissues of the genital, inguinal, and anal regions. It is primarily transmitted sexually but probably can be transmitted by non-sexual contact as well. Multiple sexual contacts with an infected partner seem necessary for transmission of infection. The disease is uncommon in the United States, with fewer than 100 recorded cases annually. It is quite common, however, in certain other areas of the world, especially Papua New Guinea.

ETIOLOGY. The causative organism is *Calymmatobacterium granulomatis,* a gram-negative bacterium immunologically related to certain *Klebsiella* strains. Current evidence suggests that *C. granulomatis* is not a member of the *Klebsiella-Enterobacter-Serra-tia* family; its exact taxonomic status is uncertain. The organism can be grown in yolk sacs, but only with great difficulty on artificial medium. It is apparently a facultative intracellular parasite because in infected lesions it is found primarily in histiocytes or other mononuclear cells.

CLINICAL MANIFESTATIONS. The initial lesion usually appears as a subcutaneous nodule that erodes through the surface and develops into a beefy, elevated granulomatous lesion. This usually is painless and unassociated with systemic symptoms. Secondary bacterial infection may cause a necrotic painful ulcerative lesion that may be rapidly destructive. A cicatricial form may also occur with a depigmented elevated area of keloid-like scar containing scattered islands of granulomatous tissue. Lesions in the genital area are commonly associated with pseudobuboes in the inguinal region; these swellings are usually not due to involvement of the inguinal lymph nodes but rather to granulomatous involvement of the subcutaneous tissues. Metastatic infection of bones or other viscera is occasionally seen. Clinical experience suggests that secondary carcinomas may be a complication of granuloma inguinale.

DIFFERENTIAL DIAGNOSIS. The differential diagnosis includes tumor, lymphogranuloma venereum, chancroid, syphilis, and other ulcerative granulomatous diseases. Chancroid is usually differentiated by its irregular undermined borders, which are not seen in the usual cases of granuloma inguinale. Darkfield examination and serologic tests should help to distinguish syphilis. Biopsy lesions may be necessary to distinguish granuloma inguinale from certain tumors.

DIAGNOSIS. Diagnosis is made by demonstrating intracellular "Donovan bodies" in histiocytes or other mononuclear cells from lesion scrapings or biopsies. Wright's stain and Giemsa's stain of fresh impression smears or unfixed biopsies usually demonstrate the bacilli relatively easily, although multiple biopsies may be necessary in chronic cases. Culture is not practical at present. A serologic test has been devised but is not clinically available. Histologic examination of biopsy specimens shows mononuclear cells with some infiltration by polymorphonuclear leukocytes but no giant cells.

TREATMENT. Recommended treatment consists of trimethoprim/sulfamethoxazole, one double-strength tablet twice daily, or doxycycline, 100 mg twice daily, for at least 3 weeks. Other regimens that have proved effective include ampicillin, chloramphenicol, and gentamicin. Limited experience suggests that lincomycin may be used successfully. Patients should be followed for at least several weeks after treatment is discontinued because of the possibility of relapse. Although the risk of communicability appears to be low, sexual contacts should also be examined; at present, treatment of contacts is not indicated in the absence of clinically evident disease.

PREVENTION. No effective prevention is known.

Kuberski T: Granuloma inguinale (donovanosis). Sex Transm Dis 7:29, 1980. *An excellent short review.*
Rosen T, Tschen JA, Ramsdell W, et al: Granuloma inguinale. J Am Acad Dermatol 11:433, 1984. *An American epidemic of this relatively rare disease is described.*

364 CHANCROID
Edward W. Hook III

Chancroid is a sexually transmitted infection caused by the gram-negative bacillus *Haemophilus ducreyi.*

EPIDEMIOLOGY. Worldwide, chancroid is considerably more common than syphilis, and in parts of Africa and in Southeast Asia it is nearly as great a problem as gonorrhea. In the United States it is an uncommon disease. In the mid 1980s, chancroid rates increased more than five-fold, peaking at 4986 cases in 1987. Since then, rates have steadily declined to 243 cases in 1997. In North America there are strong epidemiologic links between chancroid and both prostitution and illegal drug use. Although all genital ulcer diseases are associated with increased risk for human immunodeficiency virus (HIV) acquisition, the association is particularly strong for chancroid. The majority of reported cases occur in males. An outbreak in Greenland was exceptional in that about 40% of cases were noted in women. It is quite likely that there has been significant underdiagnosis of chancroid in women in the past.

CLINICAL MANIFESTATIONS. The usual incubation period is 2 to 5 days but it may be up to 14 days. In the Greenland outbreak the incubation period averaged nearly 2 weeks in women. The clinical manifestations of chancroid are quite variable. Classically, the initial manifestation is an inflammatory macule that then becomes a vesicle-pustule and finally a sharply circumscribed, somewhat ragged, and undermined painful ulcer. The base is moist and may be covered with a grayish necrotic exudate. Removal of the exudate reveals purulent granulation tissue. There is usually surrounding cutaneous erythema. Lesions typically are single but may be multiple, possibly owing to autoinoculation of nearby tissues. There are rarely systemic symptoms. Inguinal adenopathy is noted in one half of patients, approximately two thirds of whom have unilateral adenopathy. Lesions are usually noted on the penile shaft or glans. In women, lesions may occur on the cervix, vagina, vulva, or perianal area. Lesions may occasionally occur primarily on or spread to the abdomen, thigh, breast, fingers, or lips. Intraoral lesions are uncommon.

There are reports of a transient genital ulcer, followed by significant inguinal adenopathy. This may be difficult to distinguish from lymphogranuloma venereum. Other uncommon clinical variants include the *phagedenic type* of ulcer with secondary superinfection and rapid tissue destruction; *giant chancroid,* which is characterized by a very large single ulcer; *serpiginous ulcer,* which is characterized by rapidly spreading, indolent, shallow ulcers on the groin or the thigh; and a *follicular* type with multiple small ulcers in a perifollicular distribution.

DIFFERENTIAL DIAGNOSIS. The differential diagnosis includes syphilis, herpes genitalis, lymphogranuloma venereum, traumatic ulcers, and granuloma inguinale. Of these, the most commonly confused are syphilis and genital herpes. Multiple infections are relatively common. Outpatients with suspected chancroid should have a serologic test for syphilis and preferably a darkfield examination as well.

DIAGNOSIS. The diagnosis of chancroid is most often made on the basis of the clinical appearance of the lesions plus either morphologic demonstration of typical organisms in the lesions or demonstration of *H. ducreyi* by culture or polymerase chain reaction (PCR) assays. PCR assays for chancroid diagnosis have been developed and found to be more sensitive than culture but are not currently commercially available. Culture is the preferred method in non-research settings, but selective culture media are often not available. Under optimal conditions, positive cultures can be obtained in more than 80% of cases. Best culture results seem to be obtained with supplemented chocolate agar media containing 3 μg/mL of vancomycin and incubated at 33° C. Necrotic debris should be removed from the ulcer with physiologic saline. The base and edges of the ulcer should be swabbed with a cotton-tipped swab and inoculated directly onto the culture plate if possible; swabs may be put into Amies transport medium if culture plates are not immediately available. Smears obtained from the undermined edges should be gently rolled onto a slide. *H. ducreyi* is a small gram-negative bacillus with rounded ends that typically forms chains or parallel aggregates in lesions. Typical organisms are seen in 50 to 80% of cases. Organisms may also be obtained by aspirating inguinal nodes. Nodes should be aspirated by placing the needle through normal skin to avoid formation of fistulous tracts. Nodes should not be incised. There is no commercially available serologic test for chancroid.

TREATMENT. The drug of choice is a single intramuscular dose of ceftriaxone, 250 mg. A single 1-g dose of azithromycin, given orally, is highly effective. Erythromycin, 500 mg orally four times daily for 7 days, is also usually curative. Another effective agent is ciprofloxacin, 500 mg orally twice daily for 3 days. Ampicillin should not be used because some strains of *H. ducreyi* produce a typical TEM-type β-lactamase and are quite ampicillin resistant. Interestingly, the plasmids containing the gene for production of β-lactamase are very closely related to the penicillinase plasmids present in *H. influenzae* and *Neisseria gonorrhoeae.* Tetracycline resistance is common. Serologic testing for HIV is recommended for all patients treated for possible chancroid. All regular sexual partners should be examined and epidemiologically treated with a similar regimen.

PREVENTION. No vaccine is available. Use of a condom is presumably helpful. There are no data regarding efficacy of antibiotic prophylaxis.

Blackmore CA, Limpakarnjanarat K, Rigau-Perez JG, et al: An outbreak of chancroid in Orange County, California: Descriptive epidemiology and disease-control measures. J Infect Dis 151:840, 1985. *A very large continental U.S. outbreak is described. Sulfa and tetracycline resistance was common, but erythromycin and cotrimoxazole were effective.*

Centers for Disease Control and Prevention: 1998 Guidelines for treatment of sexually transmitted diseases. MMWR 47(RR-1):18–20, 1998. *Current treatment and management recommendations for chancroid.*

Telzak EE, Chaisson MA, Bevier PJ, et al: HIV-1 seroconversion in patients with and without genital ulcer disease. Ann Intern Med 119:1181, 1993. *In this study of heterosexual men attending New York City STD clinics, a diagnosis of chancroid was associated with a more than three-fold increased likelihood of HIV acquisition.*

365 SYPHILIS

Edward W. Hook III

DEFINITION. Syphilis is a chronic infectious disease caused by the bacterium *Treponema pallidum.* It is usually acquired by sexual contact with another infected individual. Syphilis is remarkable among infectious diseases in its large variety of clinical presentations. It progresses, if untreated, through primary, secondary, and tertiary stages. The early stages (primary and secondary) are infectious. Spontaneous healing of early lesions occurs, followed by a long latent period. In about 30% of untreated patients, late disease of the heart, central nervous system (CNS), or other organs ultimately develops. At one time this disease was called "the great imitator." Although the disease is less common now than previously, it remains a great challenge to the clinician because of its protean manifestations and is of great interest to biologists as well because of the long and tenuous balance between the host and the invading spirochete.

ETIOLOGY. The cause of syphilis was discovered in 1905 by Schaudinn and Hoffman when they visualized spirochetal organisms in early infectious lesions. The causative agent of syphilis, *T. pallidum,* is closely related to other pathogenic spirochetes, including those causing yaws (*T. pallidum* subspecies *pertenue*) and pinta (*T. carateum*).

T. pallidum is a thin, helical bacterium approximately 0.15 μm wide and 6 to 50 μm long. Ordinarily there are 6 to 14 spirals. The organism is tapered on either end. It is too thin to be seen by ordinary Gram stain but can be visualized in wet mounts by darkfield microscopy (see later) or by silver stains or fluorescent antibody methods.

Studies have described several unusual characteristics of the *T. pallidum* outer membrane that may provide clues to the pathogenesis of syphilis. Unlike most bacteria having protein-rich outer membranes, the outer membrane of *T. pallidum* appears to be predominantly made up of phospholipids with few surface-exposed proteins. It has been hypothesized that because of this structure syphilis can progress despite a brisk antibody response (to non–surface-exposed, internal antigens). Between the outer membrane and the peptidoglycan cell wall are six axial fibrils. The axial fibrils are attached three at each end and overlap in the center of the organism. They are structurally and biochemically similar to flagella and are in part responsible for the motility of the organism.

It is possible to culture *T. pallidum* in vitro, but sustained in vitro cultivation is not yet possible and yields are very low. Culture is of limited use in research but of no use in clinical practice. *T. pallidum* can be maintained by serial passage in rabbits without loss of virulence. Only a few strains have been isolated in rabbits and carefully studied, and little evidence is available regarding the genetic diversity of the organism. All studied isolates have been susceptible to penicillin and are similar antigenically. Immunity to the homologous strain develops after prolonged untreated infection in rabbits. The only known natural hosts for *T. pallidum* are humans and certain monkeys and higher apes.

PATHOGENESIS AND HOST RESPONSE. *T. pallidum* may penetrate through normal mucosal membranes and also through minor abrasions of epithelial surfaces. In experimental rabbit syphilis, spirochetes can be found in the lymphatic system within 30 minutes of inoculation and are found in blood shortly thereafter. There have been occasional instances in humans of transfusion syphilis resulting from use of blood from a donor who was in the incubation stage of the disease. Therefore, it seems clear that syphilis is a systemic disease from the onset in humans as well. However, the first lesions appear at the site of primary inoculation, presumably because of the large numbers of treponemes implanted at this site. In laboratory animals, there is an inverse relationship between numbers of treponemes inoculated and time required for development of the primary cutaneous lesion. The minimal number of treponemes required to establish infection is not known but may be as low as one treponeme. Multiplication of organisms is very slow, with a division time in rabbits of approximately 33 hours. Similarly, slow growth of treponemes in humans probably accounts in part for the protracted nature of the illness and for the relatively long incubation period.

T. pallidum is not known to produce any toxins. Treponemes are capable of specific attachment to host cells, but it is not known whether attachment results in damage to host cells. Most treponemes are found in intercellular spaces, but occasional treponemes can be seen within phagocytic cells. However, there is no evidence for prolonged intracellular survival of treponemes.

The primary pathologic lesion of syphilis is a focal endarteritis. There is an increase in adventitial cells, endothelial proliferation, and presence of an inflammatory cuff around affected vessels. Lymphocytes, plasma cells, and monocytes predominate in the inflammatory lesion, and in some cases polymorphonuclear cells are seen as well. The vessel lumen is frequently obliterated. With healing there is considerable fibrosis. Treponemes may be seen in most early lesions of syphilis and in some of the late lesions such as the meningoencephalitis of general paresis.

Granulomatous reaction is also frequent in secondary syphilis and in late syphilis. The granuloma is histologically non-specific, and cases of syphilis have been incorrectly diagnosed as sarcoidosis or other granulomatous diseases. Human inoculation studies suggest that the pathogenesis of the gumma, which is a granulomatous lesion, involves hypersensitivity to small numbers of virulent treponemes introduced into a previously sensitized host.

Intracutaneous inoculation of patients with syphilis in various stages with partially purified antigens of *T. pallidum* showed that delayed cellular hypersensitivity developed only in late secondary syphilis but was uniformly present in latent syphilis. There may be temporary hyporesponsiveness of lymphocytes from patients with primary and secondary syphilis to treponemal antigens. It is possible but not proved that the unusual waxing and waning of lesions in early syphilis depend on the balance between development of effective cellular immunity and suppression of thymus-derived lymphocyte function.

The host also responds to infection with production of numerous antibodies, and in some instances circulating immune complexes may be formed. The nephrotic syndrome has been recognized occasionally in secondary syphilis, and renal biopsy specimens from such cases have shown membranous glomerulonephritis characterized by focal subepithelial basement membrane deposits. The deposits contain both IgG and C3 and also treponemal antibody.

Antibodies useful in diagnosis are discussed under Serologic Tests, later.

EPIDEMIOLOGY. Syphilis, with the exception of congenital syphilis, is acquired almost exclusively by intimate contact with the infectious lesions of primary or secondary syphilis (chancre, mucous patches, condylomata lata). This is usually through sexual intercourse, including anogenital and orogenital intercourse. Health care workers have sometimes been infected during unsuspecting examination of patients with infectious lesions. Infection by contact with fomites is extremely uncommon.

Syphilis is most common in large cities and in young, sexually active individuals. The highest rate in both men and women occurs at ages 25 to 29, somewhat older than for gonorrhea and chlamydial infection. In 1997, 2324 (75%) of 3115 U.S. counties reported

no cases of primary or secondary syphilis and 31 (1%) of counties accounted for about 50% of all reported infections. The disease is most prevalent in the Southeast.

Syphilis spares no class, race, or group but is more prevalent in the United States among the poorly educated and economically deprived than among more prosperous groups. In 1997, U.S. syphilis rates were 44-fold greater among African-Americans than among non-Hispanic whites (22 vs. 0.5 per 100,000 population). Increased numbers of different sexual partners and perhaps indiscriminate choice of partner increase the risk of acquiring sexually transmitted disease. Patients with primary and secondary syphilis name on the average nearly three different sexual contacts within the previous 90 days. A traditional cornerstone of syphilis control has been epidemiologic investigation and treatment of sexual contacts of patients with primary or secondary lesions, and of patients with early latent disease. More recently, as syphilis has been associated with drug use and anonymous sex, epidemiologic investigations have become less efficacious.

In the 1970s and 1980s, male homosexuals accounted for an increasing proportion of the total cases of infectious syphilis. The ratio of male:female cases of primary and secondary syphilis in the United States rose from 1.6:1.0 in 1965 to 2.5:1.0 in 1975 and to about 3:1 in the mid 1980s. Similar trends were noted in other countries. From 1986 to 1990, U.S. syphilis rates nearly doubled to reach 50,578 cases in 1990. This epidemic disproportionately affected non-white heterosexual men and women and occurred contemporaneously with an epidemic of crack cocaine use. Many cases were related to the exchange of sex for drugs or money to buy drugs. After 1990, syphilis rates again declined; and in 1997 there were 8550 cases of primary and secondary syphilis reported, the lowest number since 1959. The epidemic of the late 1980s is likely to have also contributed to the spread of human immunodeficiency virus (HIV) infection (see Syphilis-HIV Interactions, later) and to dramatic increases in congenital syphilis.

The annual incidence of syphilis has generally declined worldwide for approximately 100 years with the exception of periods of extensive war. With the introduction of penicillin there was a rapid decline in primary and secondary syphilis after World War II, to annual rates of approximately 4 cases per 100,000 in 1957. This resulted in declining federal expenditure for syphilis control, however, and there was a subsequent resurgence in infectious primary and secondary syphilis in the United States, reaching peaks of more than 12 cases per 100,000 several times in the period 1965–1983. Because many cases of syphilis are not reported, the true incidence is much higher.

Reported deaths from syphilis declined from 2434 in 1965 to 200 in 1976. Infant deaths from syphilis fell by 98 to 99% by 1980 but rose sharply in 1988–1990. Patients with clinically manifest late syphilis, particularly those with gummas, are becoming less common, perhaps as a result of the effectiveness of penicillin therapy for early syphilis. However, surveys indicate that there still are significant numbers of patients with untreated cardiovascular and neurologic syphilis, especially among older age groups. There is suggestive evidence that neurosyphilis may be presenting with atypical clinical manifestations and therefore may not be easily recognized.

NATURAL COURSE OF UNTREATED SYPHILIS. The incubation period from time of exposure to development of the primary lesion at the place of initial inoculation of treponemes averages approximately 21 days but ranges from 10 to 90 days. A painless papule develops and soon breaks down to form a clean-based ulcer, the chancre, with raised, indurated margins. The chancre persists for 2 to 6 weeks and then heals spontaneously. Several weeks later the patient characteristically develops a secondary stage characterized by low-grade fever, headache, malaise, generalized lymphadenopathy, and a mucocutaneous rash. There may be involvement of visceral organs. The secondary eruption may occur while the primary chancre is still healing or several months after the disappearance of the chancre. The secondary lesions heal spontaneously within 2 to 6 weeks, and the infection then enters latency. Over 20% of untreated patients will later develop relapsing lesions similar to those of the secondary stage; rarely, the relapse takes the form of recurrence of the primary chancre. About one third of untreated patients eventually develop late destructive tertiary lesions involving one or more of the eyes, central nervous system, heart, or other organs, including skin. These may occur at any time from a few years to as late as 25 years after infection.

The incidence of late complications of untreated syphilis is unknown but seems less than noted previously. Cases of gumma are at present so rare as to be reportable.

CLINICAL MANIFESTATIONS. PRIMARY SYPHILIS. The typical lesion of primary syphilis, the chancre, is a painless, clean-based, indurated ulcer. The chancre starts as a papule, but then superficial erosion occurs, resulting in the typical ulcer. The borders of the ulcer are raised, firm, and indurated. Occasionally, secondary infections change the appearance, resulting in a painful lesion. Most chancres are single, but multiple ulcers are sometimes seen, particularly when skin folds are opposed ("kissing chancres"). The untreated chancre heals in several weeks, leaving a faint scar. The chancre is usually associated with regional adenopathy, which may be either unilateral or bilateral. The regional nodes are movable, discrete, and rubbery. If the chancre occurs in the cervix or in the rectum, the affected regional iliac nodes are not palpable (Fig. 365–1).

Chancres may occur at any site of potential inoculation by direct contact. The majority of chancres occur at anogenital locations. Chancres may also be seen in the pharynx, on the tongue, around the lips, on the fingers, on the nipples, or in diverse other areas. The morphology depends in part on the area of the body in which they occur and also on the host immune response. Chancres in previously infected individuals may be small and may remain papular. Chancres of the finger may appear more erosive and may be quite painful.

The *differential diagnosis* of a genital ulcer should include genital herpes. Classically, herpetic ulcers are multiple, painful, superficial, and, if seen early, vesicular. However, atypical presentations may be indistinguishable from a syphilitic chancre. Genital herpes is orders of magnitude more common than syphilis. Thus, genital herpes is now the most common cause of a "typical chancre" in North America. Herpetic ulcers, unlike syphilitic ulcers, may yield positive findings on Tzanck's test—multinucleated giant cells in the base of the ulcer. The ulcers of chancroid are usually painful, often multiple, and frequently exudative and non-indurated. Lymphogranuloma venereum may produce a small papular lesion asso-

ciated with a regional adenopathy. Other conditions that must be distinguished include granuloma inguinale, drug eruptions, carcinoma, superficial fungal infections, traumatic lesions, and lichen planus. Final distinction in most cases is made on the basis of darkfield examination, which is positive only in syphilis.

SECONDARY SYPHILIS. Four to 8 weeks after the appearance of the primary chancre, patients typically develop lesions of secondary syphilis. They may complain of malaise, fever, headache, sore throat, and other systemic symptoms. Most patients have generalized lymphadenopathy, including the epitrochlear nodes. Approximately 30% of patients have evidence of the healing chancre, although many patients, including male homosexuals and women, give no history of a primary lesion.

At least 80% of patients with secondary syphilis have cutaneous lesions or lesions of the mucocutaneous junctions at some point in their illness. The diagnosis is usually first suspected on the basis of the cutaneous eruption. The rash is often minimally symptomatic, however, and many patients with late syphilis do not recall either primary or secondary lesions. The rashes are quite varied in their appearance but have certain characteristic features. The lesions are usually widespread, are symmetric in distribution, and often are pink, coppery, or dusky red (particularly the earliest macular lesions). They usually are non-pruritic, although occasional exceptions have been noted, and are almost never vesicular or bullous in adults. They are indurated except for the very earliest macular lesions and frequently have a superficial scale (papulosquamous lesions). They tend to be polymorphic and rounded, and on healing they may leave residual pigmentation or depigmentation. The lesions may be quite faint and difficult to visualize, particularly on dark-skinned individuals.

The earliest pink macular lesions are frequently seen on the margins of the ribs or the sides of the trunk, with later spread to the rest of the body. The face is often spared except around the mouth. Subsequently, a papular rash appears, which is usually generalized but is quite marked on the palms and soles. These rashes frequently are associated with a superficial scale and may be hyperpigmented. When the rash occurs on the face, it may be pustular, resembling acne vulgaris. On occasion, the scale may be so great as to resemble psoriasis. Deep nodular lesions may cause confusion. Ulceration may occur, producing lesions resembling ecthyma. In malnourished or debilitated patients, extensive destructive ulcerative lesions with a heaped-up crust may occur, the so-called rupial

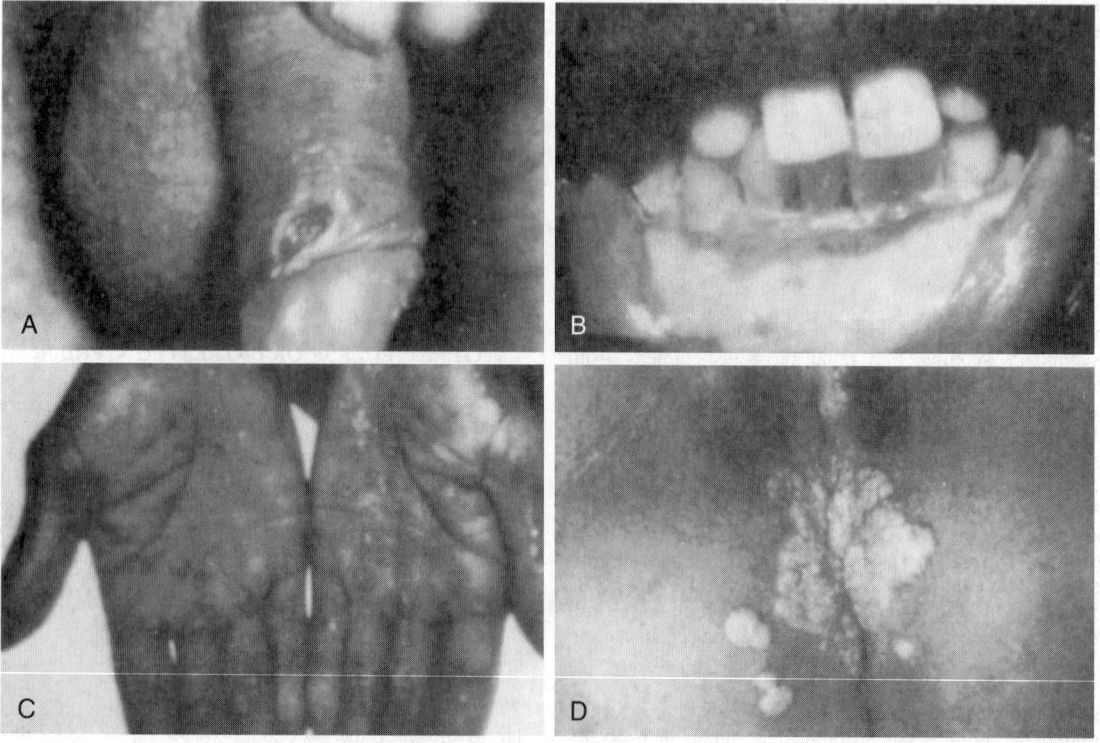

FIGURE 365–1 ■ *A,* Primary syphilis, chancre. *B,* Secondary syphilis, mucous patch. *C,* Secondary syphilis, papulosquamous rash. *D,* Secondary syphilis, condylomata lata.

lesion. Lesions around the hair follicles may result in patchy alopecia of the beard or of the scalp.

Ringed or annular lesions may occur, especially around the face, particularly on black individuals. Lesions at the angle of the mouth or the corner of the nose may have a central linear erosion (the so-called split papule).

In warm, moist areas such as the perineum, large, pale, flat-topped papules may coalesce to form condylomata lata. These may also be seen in the axilla and rarely in a generalized form. They are extremely infectious. They are not to be confused with the common venereal warts (condylomata acuminata), which are small, often multiple, and more sharply raised than condylomata lata.

Other lesions of the mucous membranes are common. The palate and pharynx may be inflamed. Approximately 30% of secondary syphilis patients develop the so-called mucous patch. This is a slightly raised oval area covered by a grayish-white membrane, which when raised reveals a pink base that does not bleed. These may be seen on the genitalia, in the mouth, or on the tongue and, like condylomata lata, are highly infectious.

Other manifestations of secondary syphilis include hepatitis, which has been reported in up to 10% of patients in some series. Jaundice is rare, but an elevated alkaline phosphatase level is common. Liver biopsy reveals small areas of focal necrosis and mononuclear infiltrate or periportal vasculitis. Spirochetes can often be visualized with silver stains. Periostitis with widespread lytic lesions of bone has been reported occasionally; bone scanning appears to be a sensitive test for early syphilitic osteitis. An immune complex type of nephropathy with transient nephrotic syndrome has been rarely documented. There may be iritis or an anterior uveitis. From 10 to 30% of patients have pleocytosis in the cerebrospinal fluid (CSF), but symptomatic meningitis is seen in less than 1% of patients. Symptomatic gastritis may be present.

Differential diagnosis of secondary syphilis includes a large number of diseases. The cutaneous eruptions may be mimicked by pityriasis rosea, which can be differentiated by the occurrence of lesions along lines of skin cleavage and frequently by the presence of a herald patch. Drug eruptions, acute febrile exanthems, psoriasis, lichen planus, scabies, and other diseases must also be considered in some cases. The mucous patch may superficially resemble oral candidiasis (thrush). Infectious mononucleosis may appear very similar to secondary syphilis, with sore throat, generalized adenopathy, hepatitis, and a generalized rash. Infectious hepatitis may also cause confusion. A high index of suspicion is required to make the diagnosis of syphilis in some cases. Unfortunately, even classic cases with widespread, hyperpigmented, papulosquamous lesions involving the palms and the soles are not infrequently misdiagnosed today. Fortunately, if the serologic tests for syphilis are obtained, they are positive in 99% of patients. The condylomata lata and mucous patches contain large numbers of treponemes on darkfield examination. Aspiration of lymph nodes may occasionally reveal motile *T. pallidum*.

RELAPSING SYPHILIS. After resolution of primary or secondary syphilis skin lesions, 20 to 30% of patients experience cutaneous recurrences. Recurrent lesions may be fewer or more firmly indurated than initial lesions and, like typical lesions of primary or secondary syphilis, are infectious for exposed sexual partners.

LATENT SYPHILIS. By definition, latent syphilis is that stage in which there are no clinical signs of syphilis and the CSF is normal. Latency begins with the passing of the first attack of secondary syphilis and may last for a lifetime thereafter. It is usually detected by reactive serologic tests for syphilis. The test must be shown to be reactive on more than one occasion to rule out technical errors. Diseases known to cause occasional false-positive non-treponemal test reactions for syphilis, such as systemic lupus erythematosus, must be excluded. In addition, congenital syphilis must be excluded before the diagnosis of latent syphilis can be made. Patients may or may not have a history of earlier primary or secondary syphilis, although such history is obviously helpful in making a firm diagnosis of latent syphilis.

Latency has been divided into two stages: early and late latency. Evidence suggests that most infectious relapses occur in the first year, and epidemiologic evidence shows that the most infectious spread of syphilis occurs during the first year of infection. Therefore, early latency in the United States is defined as the first year after the resolution of primary or secondary lesions or as a newly reactive serologic test for syphilis in an otherwise asymptomatic individual who has had a negative serologic test within the preceding year. Late latent syphilis is ordinarily not infectious except for the case of the pregnant woman, who may transmit infection to her fetus after many years.

LATE SYPHILIS. Late, or tertiary, syphilis is the destructive stage of the disease and can be crippling. Late syphilitic complications are still important medical problems, but newly recognized cases of late syphilis have been declining steadily in the United States since World War II. Although the incidence of late syphilis is unknown, the prevalence of various types of late syphilis has been approximated (Table 365–1).

Late syphilis is usually very slowly progressive, although certain neurologic syndromes may have sudden onset owing to endarteritis and thrombosis in the CNS. Late syphilis is non-infectious. Any organ of the body may be involved, but three main types of disease may be distinguished: late benign (gummatous), cardiovascular, and neurosyphilis.

Late Benign Syphilis. Late benign syphilis, or gumma, was the most common complication of late syphilis in the Oslo Study of untreated patients (1891–1951). In the penicillin era gummas are rare. They typically develop from 1 to 10 years after the initial infection and may involve any part of the body. Although they may be very destructive, they respond rapidly to treatment and therefore are relatively benign. Histologically, the gumma is a granuloma. The histologic findings are non-specific and may be associated with central necrosis surrounded by epithelioid and fibroblastic cells and occasionally giant cells. There is sometimes vasculitis. *T. pallidum* is ordinarily not demonstrable by silver stains but can sometimes be recovered by inoculation of rabbits.

Gummas may be solitary or multiple. They are usually asymmetric and are often grouped. They may start as a superficial nodule or as a deeper lesion that breaks down to form punched-out ulcers. They are ordinarily indolent, slowly progressive, and indurated on palpation. There often is central healing with an atrophic scar surrounded by hyperpigmented borders. Cutaneous gummas may resemble other chronic granulomatous ulcerative lesions caused by tuberculosis, sarcoidosis, leprosy, and other deep fungal infections. Precise histologic diagnosis may not be possible. However, the syphilitic gumma is the only such lesion to heal dramatically with penicillin therapy. Another form of gumma is papulosquamous and may mimic psoriasis.

Gummas may also involve deep visceral organs, of which the most common are the respiratory tract, the gastrointestinal tract, and bones. In earlier centuries, gummas of the nose and palate commonly resulted in septal perforations and disfiguring facial lesions. Gummas may also involve the larynx or the pulmonary parenchyma. Gumma of the stomach may masquerade as carcinoma of the stomach or lymphoma. Gummas of the liver were once the most common form of visceral syphilis, presenting often with hepatosplenomegaly and anemia, occasionally with fever and jaundice. Skeletal gummas typically produce lesions in the long bones, skull, and clavicle. A characteristic symptom is nocturnal pain. Radiologic abnormalities, when present, include periostitis and either lytic or sclerotic destructive osteitis.

Cardiovascular Syphilis. The primary cardiovascular complications

Table 365–1 ■ NEWLY DIAGNOSED TERTIARY SYPHILIS IN 105 PATIENTS IN DENMARK, 1961–1970

TYPE OF TERTIARY SYPHILIS	NO. OBSERVED*
Neurosyphilis	72
Asymptomatic	45
Tabes dorsalis	11
General paresis	13
Meningovascular	1
Optic atrophy	2
Cardiovascular syphilis	44
Aortic insufficiency	16
Aortic aneurysm	13
Uncomplicated aortitis†	15
Late benign syphilis (gumma)	4

*Some patients had more than one form of late syphilis.
†Autopsy diagnoses only.

of syphilis are aortic insufficiency and aortic aneurysm, usually of the ascending aorta. Less commonly, other large arteries may be involved, and rarely involvement of the coronary ostia results in coronary insufficiency. These complications in all cases are due to obliterative endarteritis of the vasa vasorum with resultant damage to the intima and media of the great vessels. This results in dilatation of the ascending aorta and eventually in stretching of the ring of the aortic valve, producing aortic insufficiency. The valve cusps remain normal. Death may eventually result from congestive heart failure. There has been some success with placing prosthetic heart valves in patients with syphilitic aortic insufficiency. Aneurysms occasionally present as a pulsating mass bulging through the anterior chest wall. Syphilitic aortitis may involve the descending aorta, but this is almost always proximal to the renal arteries, unlike atherosclerotic aneurysms, which typically involve the descending aorta below the renal arteries.

The disease usually begins within 5 to 10 years after initial infection but may not become clinically manifest until 20 to 30 years after infection. Cardiovascular syphilis is thought to be more common in men than in women and possibly in blacks than in whites. Cardiovascular syphilis does not occur after congenital infection—a phenomenon that remains unexplained.

Asymptomatic aortitis is best diagnosed by visualizing linear calcifications in the wall of the ascending aorta by radiography. The signs of syphilitic aortic insufficiency are the same as for aortic insufficiency of other causes. In aortic insufficiency resulting from dilatation of the aortic ring, the decrescendo murmur is often loudest along the *right* sternal margin. Syphilitic aneurysms may be fusiform but are more typically saccular and do not lead to aortic dissection. Ten to 25 per cent of patients with cardiovascular syphilis have coexistent neurosyphilis.

At present, syphilis is a relatively more common cause of aortic insufficiency among the elderly than among younger patients; this is due to the progressively decreasing incidence of new cases of late cardiovascular syphilis.

Neurosyphilis. Neurosyphilis may be divided into four groups: asymptomatic, meningovascular, tabes dorsalis, and general paresis. These are more fully described in Chapter 474. Division is not absolute, and overlap between syndromes is typical. Current cases of neurosyphilis are more likely than heretofore to be variants of the classic syndromes, possibly as a result of use of antimicrobial agents for other diseases.

Asymptomatic Neurosyphilis. Asymptomatic neurosyphilis is diagnosed when there are CSF abnormalities (pleocytosis, protein elevation, or a reactive Venereal Disease Research Laboratories [VDRL] test; see Serologic Tests and Table 365–2) in a syphilis patient in the absence of signs and symptoms of neurologic disease. Although numerous other processes may cause CSF pleocytosis or protein elevations, false-positive VDRL test results are very rare in CSF in the absence of a traumatic tap. The CSF usually shows an increased total protein and a lymphocytic pleocytosis. If the CSF is normal 2 or more years after the initial infection, the patient is not likely to develop a positive CSF finding later. Although up to 50% of patients with untreated secondary syphilis have an abnormal CSF, recommended therapy with 2.4 million units of intramuscular benzathine penicillin apparently prevents progression to late symptomatic neurosyphilis. Because of this, routine lumbar punctures for examining CSF are not indicated in early syphilis unless the patient is known to have HIV infection. Unfortunately, it has become common practice to avoid lumbar punctures in later stages of syphilis as well. Instead, patients are treated with doses of penicillin thought to be effective for neurosyphilis, if present. As a result, there are few data on the present frequency and course of asymptomatic neurosyphilis.

Some laboratories perform a fluorescent treponemal antibody absorption (FTA-ABS) test (see Serologic Tests and Table 365–2) on CSF. Interest in tests such as this has been prompted by good evidence that patients with untreated neurosyphilis may have a non-reactive CSF-VDRL. Reports were published of positive FTA-ABS test results in the CSF of patients with otherwise normal CSF in whom there were clinical signs and symptoms compatible with neurosyphilis. However, the CSF FTA-ABS test has not been standardized, and some evidence exists that reactive CSF test results are caused by passive transfer of serum antibody into CSF. At present, although a non-reactive CSF FTA-ABS may be useful to rule out the diagnosis, no diagnosis of asymptomatic (or symptomatic) neurosyphilis should be based solely on the CSF FTA-ABS test (see Serologic Tests and Table 365–2).

Meningovascular Syphilis. An acute to subacute aseptic meningitis may occur at any time after the primary stage but usually within the first year of infection. It frequently involves the base of the brain and may result in unilateral or bilateral cranial nerve palsies. In about 10% of cases, the onset of meningitis coincides with the rash of secondary syphilis. The CSF shows a lymphocytic pleocytosis with increased protein and usually normal glucose concentration. The CSF-VDRL is nearly always reactive. Rarely, CSF glucose concentration is decreased. This syndrome can mimic tuberculous or fungal meningitis or non-purulent meningitis of various causes.

In other patients, the meningeal involvement may be less prominent but there is sufficient endarteritis and perivascular inflammation to result in cerebrovascular thrombosis and infarction. This usually occurs 5 to 10 years after the initial infection and is more common in males. There often is associated aseptic meningitis as well. Most cerebrovascular accidents are not due to syphilitic arteritis even in patients with a reactive serologic test for syphilis. However, syphilis should be considered as the cause in young patients with a history of syphilis and without other causes for cerebrovascular accidents.

Tabes Dorsalis. Tabes dorsalis is a slowly progressive degenerative disease involving the posterior columns and posterior roots of the spinal cord, resulting in progressive loss of peripheral reflexes, impairment of vibration and position sense, and progressive ataxia. There may be chronic destructive changes in the large joints of the affected limbs in far-advanced cases (Charcot's joints). Incontinence of the bladder and impotence are common. Sudden and severe painful crises of uncertain cause are a characteristic part of the syndrome. These most typically involve the lower extremities but may occur at any site. Not infrequently, severe, sharp abdominal pains lead to exploratory surgery. These attacks may be triggered by exposure to cold or other stresses or may arise with no obvious precipitating cause.

Optic atrophy is seen in 20% of cases. The pupils are abnormal in 90% of cases: they are bilaterally small and fail to constrict further in response to light but do constrict normally to accommodation (Argyll Robertson pupils).

The cause of tabes dorsalis is unclear. Spirochetes cannot be demonstrated in the posterior column or dorsal root.

Onset of the disease is usually delayed, first being noted often 20 to 30 years after initial infection. It is thought to be more common in whites and in men. Typical cases of patients presenting with lightning pains, ataxia, Argyll Robertson pupils, absent deep tendon reflexes, and loss of posterior column function are easy to diagnose. Atypical cases may be more troublesome, particularly because the VDRL test result in the serum is normal in as many as 30 to 40% of patients and 10 to 20% of patients (even before the advent of penicillin) have normal CSF-VDRL results as well. The FTA-ABS test in serum is nearly always reactive.

Treatment is unsatisfactory. Penicillin usually arrests progression but does not reverse the symptoms. Carbamazepine in doses of 400

Table 365–2 ■ SEROLOGIC TESTS FOR SYPHILIS

TYPE	USE
Nontreponemal (anticardiolipin) antibodies:	
VDRL (slide flocculation)	Screening, quantitation, after response to treatment
RPR (circle-card) (agglutination)	Screening
Specific treponemal antibodies:	
FTA-ABS (immunofluorescence with absorbed serum)	Confirmatory, diagnostic, not for routine screening
MHA-TP (microhemagglutination)	Similar to FTA-ABS but can be quantified and automated

VDRL = Venereal Disease Research Laboratories test; RPR = rapid plasma reagin test; FTA-ABS = fluorescent treponemal antibody absorption test; MHA-TP = microhemagglutination assay for *Treponema pallidum.*

to 800 mg/day has been reported to effectively treat the lightning pains.

Tabes dorsalis is now thought to be uncommon, although a survey of newly diagnosed late syphilis in Denmark in the decade 1961–1970 showed that in approximately 10% of all persons with late syphilis and 40% of all persons with clinical neurosyphilis there was evidence of tabes dorsalis.

General Paresis. This form of neurosyphilis is a chronic meningoencephalitis resulting in gradually progressive loss of cortical function. It typically occurs 10 to 20 years after the initial infection. Pathologically, there is a perivascular and meningeal chronic inflammatory reaction with thickening of the meninges, a granular ependymitis, degeneration of the cortical parenchyma, and abundant spirochetes in the tissues.

The most devastating effect of general paresis is on the mind. With effective penicillin therapy this disease has become much less common; in the United States, first admissions to mental hospitals because of syphilitic psychosis declined from 7694 in 1940 to 154 in 1968, the last year for which definite figures are available.

In its early stages, general paresis results in non-specific symptoms such as irritability, fatigability, headaches, forgetfulness, and personality changes. Later, there is impaired memory, defective judgment, lack of insight, confusion, and often depression or marked elation. The patients may be delusional, and seizures are sometimes seen. There may also be loss of other cortical functions, including paralysis or aphasia.

Physical signs are primarily those of the altered mental status. Cranial nerve palsies are uncommon. Optic atrophy is rare. The complete Argyll Robertson pupil is also uncommon, but irregular or otherwise abnormal pupils are not infrequent. Peripheral reflexes are often somewhat increased.

The CSF is nearly always abnormal, with lymphocytic pleocytosis and increased total protein. The VDRL is usually reactive in both CSF and serum. The disease responds well to penicillin therapy if administered early, although as many as a third of treated patients may develop progressive neurologic decline in later years. Fever therapy induced with malaria was formerly an effective adjunct to treatment with arsenicals but has now been abandoned.

Even though classic general paresis is now infrequent, it remains reasonable to suspect syphilis as the cause of undiagnosed neurologic illness.

Syphilis HIV Interactions. Syphilis and HIV infection interact on multiple levels. Thus, clinicians evaluating patients with newly diagnosed syphilis should consider whether coexistent HIV infection is present and how the two diseases might be interacting. Conversely, clinicians seeing patients with newly diagnosed HIV should be attuned to the possible existence of previously undiagnosed syphilis.

Syphilis, like other genital ulcer diseases, is associated with a three- to fivefold increased risk for HIV acquisition. Presumably, genital ulcers act as portals of entry through which HIV may more readily infect exposed individuals. In individuals with HIV infection who acquire syphilis, the natural history of the infection may be modified. HIV-infected syphilis patients are more likely to present with secondary syphilis than are non–HIV-infected patients. In addition, HIV-infected secondary syphilis patients are more likely to have coexistent chancres than are HIV-negative secondary syphilis patients, suggesting that either the healing of chancres is delayed or the appearance of secondary manifestations is accelerated in the presence of HIV co-infection.

Several reports have suggested that neurosyphilis may be more common in patients with HIV infection; however, no large or carefully controlled studies document this association. In HIV-infected syphilis patients in whom therapy fails, neurosyphilis may be a more common presenting feature than in patients without HIV infection.

Most experts agree that failure of treatment using currently recommended regimens for syphilis therapy is more common in patients with coexistent HIV infection. The magnitude of this increase, however, is small; and, as a result, alternate treatment regimens are not currently recommended. Rather, closer follow-up is suggested to permit early detection of treatment failure and to help prevent disease progression or transmission of infection to others.

CONGENITAL SYPHILIS. Congenital syphilis results from transplacental hematogenous spread of syphilis from the mother to the fetus. The incidence of congenital syphilis diagnoses in the United States fell below 1000 per year for the first time in 1975, and fewer than 500 cases occurred per year until 1988, when the epidemic of syphilis in adults led to similar epidemic increases in congenital infections. From 1990 through 1993 more than 3000 new cases of congenital syphilis have been reported each year. Each case of congenital syphilis represents a tragedy that could have been prevented by better case reporting and by proper prenatal care. A VDRL should be obtained in all expectant mothers at the beginning and near the end of pregnancy.

Spirochetes can be found in abortuses of as little as 9 to 10 weeks' gestation. The risk of fetal infection is greatest in the early stages of untreated maternal syphilis and declines slowly thereafter, but the mother may infect her fetus during at least the first 5 years of her infection. Adequate treatment of the mother before the 16th week usually prevents manifest clinical illness in the neonate. Later treatment may not prevent late sequelae of the disease in the child. Untreated maternal infection may result in stillbirth, neonatal death, prematurity, or syndromes of early or late congenital syphilis among surviving infants.

Manifestations of early congenital syphilis are often seen in the perinatal period but may not develop until the infant has been discharged from the hospital. The disease resembles secondary syphilis of the adult except that the rash may be vesicular or bullous, which is extremely rare in adults. There often is rhinitis, hepatosplenomegaly, hemolytic anemia, jaundice, and pseudoparalysis (immobility of one or more extremities) resulting from painful osteochondritis. There may be thrombocytopenia and leukocytosis. The early stages of congenital syphilis must be differentiated from rubella, cytomegalovirus infection, toxoplasmosis, bacterial sepsis, and other diseases.

Late congenital syphilis is defined as congenital syphilis of more than 2 years' duration. The disease may remain latent with no manifest late damage. Cardiovascular alterations have not been observed in congenital syphilis. Neurologic manifestations are common, and there may be eighth cranial nerve deafness and interstitial keratitis. The latter occurs in more than 10% of patients but may not be apparent until the 10th year of life or later. Periostitis may result in prominent frontal bones, depression of the bridge of the nose (saddle nose), poor development of the maxilla, and anterior bowing of the tibias (saber shins). There may be late-onset arthritis of the knees (Clutton's joints). The permanent dentition may show characteristic abnormalities known as Hutchinson's teeth; the upper central incisors are widely spaced, centrally notched, and tapered in the manner of a screwdriver. The molars may show multiple poorly developed cusps (mulberry molars). Some of the late manifestations such as interstitial keratitis and Clutton's joints may be due to hypersensitivity responses and are benefited by corticosteroids in some cases.

DIAGNOSIS. DARKFIELD EXAMINATION. The most definitive means of making a diagnosis is finding spirochetes of typical morphology and motility in lesions of early acquired or congenital syphilis. The darkfield examination is often positive in primary syphilis and in the moist mucosal lesions of secondary and congenital syphilis. It may occasionally be positive in aspirates of lymph nodes in secondary syphilis. Problems arise, however, because of false-negative results in primary syphilis owing to application by the patient of soaps or other toxic compounds to the lesions. A single negative result is therefore insufficient to exclude syphilis. Optimally, patients with suspicious lesions but with an initially negative darkfield examination should be instructed to avoid washing the lesion and to return daily for two successive examinations. In practice, however, for high-risk individuals (drug users, homosexually active men), it may be more appropriate to treat patients with suspicious lesions presumptively after obtaining serologic tests. Confusion may also arise because of the presence of spirochetes that are morphologically indistinguishable from *T. pallidum* in the mouth, particularly around the gingival margins. For lesions in these areas, diagnosis often depends on clinical appearance, history, and serologic testing.

To perform the darkfield examination, the surface of the suspected ulcerative lesion should be cleaned with saline solution and gauze without producing bleeding. The presence of red cells in the specimen makes it difficult to visualize small numbers of *T. palli-*

dum. Squeezing of the lesion (with gloves on) may help produce serous fluid, which is picked up on a glass slide, covered with a coverslip, and examined with the darkfield microscope. Living *T. pallidum* organisms demonstrate gradual motion to and fro, rotational movement around the long axis, and rather sudden 90-degree bending near the center of the organism. Because most physicians do not have the proper equipment and are not familiar with the techniques of darkfield microscopy, the public health authorities can be called for assistance.

T. pallidum may also be demonstrated in biopsy or pathologic specimens by fluorescent antibody stains or by silver stains.

SEROLOGIC TESTS. Two basic types of serologic tests for humoral antibody are widely used to diagnose infection with *T. pallidum:* (1) non-treponemal tests that detect antibodies reactive with diphosphatidylglycerol (cardiolipin), which is a normal component of many tissues, and (2) specific treponemal antibodies. Non-specific antibodies against cardiolipin were formerly designated *reagin,* a term that should be discarded to avoid confusion with another "reagin," IgE. The kinds of tests used in syphilis are summarized in Table 365–2.

Non-treponemal Tests. Anticardiolipin antibodies were first discovered by Wassermann in 1907, using extracts of congenitally syphilitic livers as the antigen for a complement fixation test. Subsequently, it was shown that normal livers contained the same antigen as do many other tissues; the antigen for this class of test is now extracted from beef heart. As yet there is no convincing explanation for why patients infected with *T. pallidum* develop increasing titers of antibody against a normal tissue component.

The Wassermann test has now been replaced by related tests. The standard test in use today to detect anticardiolipin antibody is the VDRL test, which is an easily quantified slide flocculation test. Many similar tests, including the rapid plasma reagin (RPR) test and the unheated serum reagin (USR) test, are frequently used for screening for syphilis.

The VDRL and related tests are simple, well-standardized, and inexpensive and the screening tests of choice. The VDRL is readily quantified and, for that reason, is the test of choice for following the response of patients to treatment. Because the VDRL detects antibody against a normal tissue component, it may be falsely positive in a significant number of conditions. The relative proportion of patients with a false-positive VDRL depends on the prevalence of syphilis in the community; the lower the prevalence of syphilis, the higher the proportion of reactive VDRL tests that are due to non-syphilitic causes.

The VDRL test begins to turn positive within 1 week after the onset of the chancre. In a large series of patients with primary syphilis, approximately two thirds have had a positive VDRL test result. Obviously, then, a non-reactive VDRL test does not exclude primary syphilis, particularly if the lesion is less than 1 week old. The VDRL test is positive in 99% of patients with secondary syphilis, the only exceptions being patients with such high titers of antibody that they are in antibody excess; dilution of the serum then paradoxically results in conversion of a negative test to positive. In patients with coexistent HIV infection, the serologic responses to syphilis may be modified. In large groups of syphilis patients, non-treponemal test titers tend to be higher than for comparison groups of patients without HIV infection. In contrast, however, there are also case reports of patients with advanced HIV infection in whom development of a serologic response was delayed or absent and infection could be diagnosed only by biopsy of typical lesions. For most patients with HIV infection, however, serologic tests for syphilis remain useful for diagnosis and management. VDRL reactivity tends to diminish in later stages of the disease, and only about 70% of patients with cardiovascular or neurosyphilis have a positive VDRL test result.

The *quantitative titer* of the VDRL test is somewhat useful in diagnosis and quite useful in following therapeutic response. The titer is reported as the highest dilution that gives a positive response. Most patients with secondary syphilis have titers of at least 1:16. Most patients with false-positive VDRL tests have titers of less than 1:8. No single titer is in itself diagnostic. Significant rises (fourfold or greater) in paired sera, however, are strongly indicative of acute syphilis.

Treponemal Tests. There are many varieties of specific treponemal

antibody tests. The most widely used is the FTA-ABS test. Patient serum is absorbed with extracts of non-pathogenic cultivable treponemes to remove cross-reacting group treponemal antibody. Agglutination of red blood cells to which *T. pallidum* antigens have been fixed is the basis of the microhemagglutination assay for *T. pallidum* (MHA-TP).

The precise nature of the antigens involved in these tests is not known. Characterization of the antigens of *T. pallidum* has been greatly hindered by inability to grow the organism in cell-free culture. Recent success in cloning *T. pallidum* antigens into *Escherichia coli* may circumvent this problem. Antibodies reactive in the various tests are found in all major immunoglobulin classes (IgG, IgM, IgA). A modification of the FTA-ABS test has been developed using fluorescein-labeled anti–human IgM (IgM FTA-ABS). The IgM FTA-ABS test is of some use in the diagnosis of early congenital syphilis but is of no use in distinguishing acute disease from old infections in adults.

The FTA-ABS test is best used as a confirmatory test. It is somewhat more difficult to perform than the VDRL test and cannot be easily quantified. It is sensitive and has a high degree of specificity, being reactive in only approximately 1% of normal individuals. It is reactive in 85% of patients with primary syphilis, 99% with secondary syphilis, and at least 95% with late syphilis. It may therefore be the only test positive in patients with cardiovascular or neurologic syphilis. In late syphilis the FTA-ABS test often remains reactive for life despite adequate therapy. It (as well as the MHA-TP) is positive in other treponemal diseases, such as pinta, yaws, and endemic syphilis (formerly bejel) (see Chapter 366).

The FTA-ABS test is reported in terms of relative brilliance of fluorescence, from borderline to 4+. Borderline reactivity has the same meaning as non-reactive for clinical purposes. Most laboratories report 1+ positive tests as reactive, but some studies have shown that such tests may be difficult to reproduce. Occasional laboratories therefore report as positive only tests with 2+ or greater reactivity. In patients lacking historical or clinical evidence of syphilis but with a reactive FTA-ABS test, one should repeat the FTA-ABS test. Use of another treponemal test such as the MHA-TP may be helpful in problem cases.

The MHA-TP test is less sensitive than either the VDRL or the FTA-ABS test in primary syphilis. Its sensitivity and specificity otherwise are nearly identical to those of the FTA-ABS test, being reactive in nearly all patients with secondary syphilis and in more than 95% of patients with late syphilis. The reactivity of serologic tests for syphilis in various stages of disease is shown in Table 365–3.

FALSE-POSITIVE SEROLOGIC TEST RESULTS FOR SYPHILIS. The VDRL or RPR test may be reactive in a variety of diseases other than syphilis. A false-positive result is defined as a reproducible positive test in a patient with no clinical or historical evidence of syphilis and whose serum FTA-ABS or MHA-TP test is negative.

Acute (<6 months) false-positive VDRL test results occur with low frequency in atypical pneumonia, malaria, and other bacterial or viral infections and may occur after smallpox or other vaccinations as well. Chronic false-positive VDRL tests (lasting > 6 months) are relatively common in autoimmune disorders such as SLE, in parenteral drug users, in HIV infection, in leprosy, and in aged persons. From 8 to 20% of patients with SLE have been reported as having a false-positive VDRL test, and the false-positive result may develop many years before the onset of other manifestations of the disease. A chronic false-positive VDRL test in females aged 20 or younger carries a significant risk of future development of SLE, thyroiditis, or other autoimmune disorders, and such patients should be followed carefully for a considerable period of time. As many as one third of parenteral drug users have a false-positive VDRL test. More than 1% of patients aged 70 and 10% of patients over age 80 have a low-titer false-positive VDRL

Table 365–3 ■ **FREQUENCY OF POSITIVE SEROLOGIC TESTS IN UNTREATED SYPHILIS**

STAGE	VDRL (%)	FTA-ABS (%)	MHA-TP (%)
Primary	70	85	50–60
Secondary	99	100	100
Latent or late	70	98	98

test. Most false-positive VDRL tests have a titer of less than 1:8, although occasional patients with lymphoma and other diseases have been described with very high-titer false-positive VDRL tests.

A reactive FTA-ABS result is usually indicative of recent or past syphilis. However, there is an increased incidence of false-positive FTA-ABS results in SLE and in other chronic inflammatory diseases associated with hyperglobulinemia, including rheumatoid arthritis, biliary cirrhosis, and others.

Occasionally, one encounters reproducible positive FTA-ABS results in patients with no clinical or historical evidence of syphilis and in whom there is no evidence of diseases associated with false-positive FTA-ABS results. It may be wise to obtain CSF for examination of total protein, cells, and VDRL reactivity to rule out neurosyphilis. If in doubt and if the patient is not allergic to penicillin, it is often wisest to treat such patients for possible syphilis.

IgM FTA-ABS TEST FOR CONGENITAL SYPHILIS. Mothers with a reactive VDRL or FTA-ABS are delivered of infants with a reactive VDRL and FTA-ABS because of passive transfer of the IgG antibodies reactive in these tests. Because many infants with congenital syphilis are clinically normal at birth but develop serious symptomatic disease some weeks later, it is important to determine whether a newborn with a reactive VDRL or FTA-ABS test has passively transferred maternal antibody or is actively infected. Because maternal IgM antibodies are not passively transferred to the fetus, an IgM FTA-ABS test has been developed to detect syphilis in the newborn. Unfortunately there is approximately a 35% incidence of false-negative IgM FTA-ABS test results in delayed-onset congenital syphilis. There also is a false-positive rate of approximately 10%. For these reasons the IgM FTA-ABS test is of limited use for diagnosing neonatal syphilis.

If the mother has been adequately treated for syphilis during pregnancy and the infant is clinically normal at birth, one may elect to follow the infant carefully by serial examination and VDRL titers. If the reactive VDRL in the infant is due to passively transferred maternal antibody, the titer of reactivity falls markedly in the first 2 months of life. A rising titer indicates active disease and the need for treatment. Many physicians are unwilling to risk failure of proper follow-up of VDRL-positive but clinically normal neonates and instead administer effective therapy immediately. The risk of penicillin allergy in neonates is very low.

TREATMENT. *T. pallidum* is highly susceptible to penicillin, being inhibited by less than 0.01 mg of penicillin G. Because treponemes divide slowly and because penicillin acts only on dividing cells, it is necessary to maintain serum levels of penicillin for many days. Studies in animals and in humans show that more therapy is required as the length of infection increases. Current recommendations for treatment of syphilis are summarized in Table 365–4.

EARLY (<1 YEAR) INFECTIOUS SYPHILIS. Early syphilis may be treated with a single injection of 2.4 million units of benzathine penicillin G, which provides low but effective serum levels for more than 2 weeks. Extensive studies in the 1940s and 1950s with regimens that provided similar serum levels and duration of therapy showed that approximately 95% of patients were cured by such treatment. Some of the remaining 5% who had clinical or serologic evidence of relapse may actually have been reinfected. It is not necessary to examine the CSF at this stage because penicillin prevents development of later neurosyphilis. Motile treponemes disappear from primary lesions in 24 hours following treatment.

A single injection of 2.4 million units of aqueous procaine penicillin, which provides relatively high serum levels for a brief period, is ineffective in established early syphilis but is curative if the disease is still in the incubating stage. The ceftriaxone regimen currently useful for gonorrhea probably is curative for incubating syphilis, but data are few, and careful follow-up is indicated if there is reason to suspect exposure to syphilis in a patient treated for gonorrhea with ceftriaxone. The incidence of incubating syphilis in gonorrhea patients is 2% or more in several series.

For patients allergic to penicillin, doxycycline, 100 mg twice daily for 14 days, is recommended. Particularly careful follow-up is necessary in patients treated with drugs other than penicillin, because patients may not be fully compliant with these prolonged courses of oral therapy and these regimens have been less fully evaluated clinically. Ceftriaxone, 2 g intramuscularly daily for 10 days, may be effective but has not been well studied. Chloramphenicol is of equivocal efficacy and for this reason, as well as because of the risk of toxicity, should not be used. Spectinomycin and quinolone antibiotics have essentially no effect on syphilis. Erythromycin is of questionable efficacy.

SYPHILIS OF MORE THAN 1 YEAR'S DURATION. Larger doses of penicillin are needed for neurosyphilis (see Chapter 474) than for syphilis of less than 1 year's duration. In general, patients with general paresis respond better to treatment than do patients with tabes dorsalis, although patients with paresis should be expected to show residual effects of the infection. This is particularly true in advanced cases. Meningovascular syphilis usually responds well, except for residual damage resulting from ischemic infarcts. Published studies show that a total of 6.0 to 9.0 million units of penicillin G results in a satisfactory clinical response in approximately 90% of patients with neurosyphilis, in the absence of HIV infection.

Benzathine penicillin regimens have received relatively little study in neurosyphilis but were previously recommended. However, there are reports of patients who have failed standard benzathine penicillin therapy for neurosyphilis but who responded to intensive intravenous therapy that provided high serum levels of penicillin. Benzathine penicillin does not provide measurable levels of penicillin in the CSF or aqueous humor of the eye. There are anecdotal

---

Table 365–4 ■ PENICILLIN TREATMENT PRACTICE IN SYPHILIS AS RECOMMENDED BY UNITED STATES PUBLIC HEALTH SERVICE

INDICATIONS FOR SYPHILIS THERAPY†	DOSAGE AND ADMINISTRATION*	
	Benzathine Penicillin G	Aqueous Benzyl Penicillin G or Procaine Penicillin G
Primary, secondary, and early latent syphilis (<1 year); epidemiologic treatment	Total of 2.4 million units; single IM dose of two injections of 1.2 million units in one session	Total of 4.8 million units IM in doses of 600,000 units daily for 8 consecutive days
Late latent (>1 year) or when CSF was not examined in "latency"; cardiovascular syphilis, late benign (cutaneous, osseous, visceral gumma)	Total of 7.2 million units IM in doses of 2.4 million units at 7-day intervals, over 21 days	Total of 9 million units IM in doses of 600,000 units daily over 15 days
Symptomatic or asymptomatic neurosyphilis	2 to 4 million units of aqueous (crystalline) penicillin G IV every 4 hours for at least 10 days	2 to 4 million units procaine penicillin IM daily and probenecid, 500 mg orally four times daily for 10–14 days
Congenital		
Infants	CSF normal: Total of 500,000 units/kg IM in a single or divided dose at one session	CSF abnormal: Total of 50,000 units/kg IM per day for 10 consecutive days‡
Older children	CSF normal: Same as for early congenital syphilis, up to 2.4 million units	CSF abnormal: 200,000–300,000 units/kg/d IV aqueous crystalline penicillin for 10–14 days

CSF = cerebrospinal fluid
*Individual doses can be divided for injection in each buttock to minimize discomfort.
†In *pregnancy,* treatment is dependent on the stage of syphilis.
‡For aqueous penicillin, give in two divided IV doses per day; for procaine penicillin, give as one daily dose IM.

reports of increased treatment failures in patients with concomitant HIV infection. Therefore, there is considerable rationale to treatment with intravenous penicillin G (20 million units/day for at least 10 days). Therapy for neurosyphilis not infrequently results in increased CSF pleocytosis for 7 to 10 days after starting treatment and may transiently convert a normal CSF to abnormal.

Limited evidence suggests that treating latent syphilis with 7.2 million units total dose of benzathine penicillin (administered as three successive weekly injections of 2.4 million units) is curative even if the patient has asymptomatic neurosyphilis. However, because of the possible lack of the efficacy of benzathine penicillin in some patients with CNS syphilis, it is preferable to examine CSF in all patients with latent syphilis to exclude asymptomatic neurosyphilis. This is particularly important in HIV-positive patients. Alternatively, a lumbar puncture may be performed at the conclusion of the follow-up period (2 years); if the CSF is normal, the patient can be reassured that neurosyphilis will not develop.

There is no evidence that therapy with antimicrobial drugs is clinically beneficial to patients with cardiovascular syphilis. Nevertheless, treatment of cardiovascular syphilis is recommended to prevent further progression of disease and because approximately 15% of patients with cardiovascular syphilis have associated neurosyphilis.

There is no evidence regarding the efficacy of other antimicrobial agents in the treatment of later syphilis. Therefore, if patients are allergic to penicillin, it is mandatory that the CSF be examined before therapy is undertaken. Either tetracycline or doxycycline taken for 4 weeks is probably effective.

SYPHILIS IN PREGNANCY. All pregnant women should be examined with a VDRL or RPR test during pregnancy; if they are at high risk for syphilis, a second test should be obtained before delivery. Because of the risk to the fetus, evaluation and treatment of the VDRL-positive patient should be done as rapidly as possible, particularly for patients first seen in the later stages of pregnancy. If a confirmatory FTA-ABS is positive and the patient has not been treated, penicillin should be administered in doses appropriate for early or late syphilis, as outlined earlier. Penicillin-allergic patients should not be treated with tetracycline or erythromycin because of toxicity (tetracycline) or lack of efficacy (erythromycin). Penicillin desensitization may be considered but also carries risks. For patients who are VDRL positive but FTA-ABS negative and who have no clinical signs of syphilis, treatment may be withheld. In such patients a quantitative VDRL test and another FTA-ABS test should be repeated in 4 weeks. If the VDRL titer has risen by fourfold or more, or if clinical signs of syphilis have developed, the patient should be treated. If after repeat examination the diagnosis remains equivocal, the patient should be treated to prevent possible disease in the neonate. After treatment, a quantitative VDRL titer should be followed monthly; if it rises fourfold, the patient should be treated a second time.

CONGENITAL SYPHILIS. Proper treatment of the mother usually prevents active congenital syphilis in the neonate. However, infected infants may be clinically normal at birth, and the infant may be seronegative if the mother's infection was acquired late in pregnancy. The infant should be treated at birth if the mother has received no or inadequate treatment, or has been treated with drugs other than penicillin; if the mother has not yet responded to possibly effective therapy; or if the infant cannot be carefully followed up for several months after birth. The CSF should be examined before the infant is treated. If the CSF is normal, treatment may be with a single injection of 50,000 U/kg of benzathine penicillin G. If the CSF is abnormal, treatment should be with aqueous penicillin G, 50,000 U/kg intramuscularly or intravenously daily, given twice daily, for a minimum of 10 days. Alternatively, a single daily intramuscular injection of procaine penicillin G, 50,000 U/kg, may be given for 10 days. These recommendations are based on the failure of benzathine penicillin to provide adequate treponemicidal levels in CSF and on evidence that aqueous or procaine penicillin does provide adequate CSF levels of penicillin. Many experts believe that all syphilis in infected infants should be treated with either procaine or aqueous penicillin to ensure adequate CSF levels. Tetracycline should not be used to treat children younger than age 8. Antimicrobial agents other than penicillin are not recommended for treating congenital syphilis.

FOLLOW-UP EXAMINATIONS. All HIV-seronegative patients with early syphilis or congenital syphilis should return for quantitative VDRL titers and clinical examination 6 and 12 months after treatment. Treatment failure is somewhat more common in patients with HIV infection; and although more aggressive therapy is usually not required, more aggressive follow-up is suggested. Serologic tests should be repeated at 1, 2, 3, 6, 9, and 12 months. Patients with late latent syphilis should be examined also at 24 months after therapy; if CSF was not examined before therapy, a lumbar puncture should be done before discharge to rule out inadequately treated asymptomatic neurosyphilis.

In about 85% of patients with early (primary, secondary, or early latent) syphilis, quantitative VDRL titers become non-reactive in 12 to 24 months after therapy. Prolonged reactive VDRL test results are associated with higher initial VDRL titers, prolonged infection, more advanced stage (primary < secondary < early latent), or repeated infection. In a small percentage of patients with early syphilis, the VDRL remains reactive in low titer for long periods. Chronic low-titer VDRL reactivity after therapy is much more common in late syphilis and should not be viewed with alarm. The FTA-ABS test may remain positive for years, despite adequate therapy. A fourfold or greater rise of VDRL titer after therapy is sufficient evidence for re-treatment. Patients with treated early syphilis are fully susceptible to reinfection, and many clinical and serologic relapses after therapy are probably reinfections. As such, they represent failures of proper epidemiologic case finding and of preventive therapy of the patient's sexual contacts.

Patients with neurosyphilis should be followed with serologic tests for at least 3 years and with repeat examination of CSF at 6-month intervals. The CSF pleocytosis is the first abnormality to disappear, but cell counts may not be normal for 1 to 2 years. The elevated CSF protein level falls more slowly, followed by the positive CSF-VDRL test, which may take years to become negative. It is not known whether high-dose intravenous penicillin therapy accelerates the return of CSF to normal. Rising CSF cell counts, protein, and VDRL titer obtained at follow-up are an indication for re-treatment.

EPIDEMIOLOGIC INVESTIGATION AND TREATMENT. All patients with syphilis should be reported to public health authorities. In the absence of an effective vaccine, control of syphilis depends on finding and treating persons with infectious lesions of primary and secondary syphilis before they can further transmit the disease and on finding and treating persons with incubating syphilis before they develop infectious lesions. All patients with early syphilis (<1 year) should be carefully interviewed by qualified persons to determine the nature of their recent sex contacts. Approximately 16% of the named recent contacts of patients with early syphilis are found to have active untreated syphilis on examination, and a similar proportion of individuals named as suspects or associates also have active syphilis.

Most authorities, particularly in the United States, recommend treating sexual contacts of patients with early syphilis even if the contacts are clinically and serologically normal on examination. This is justifiable, because 30% of clinically normal individuals named as contacts of persons with infectious lesions of syphilis within the previous 30 days go on to develop syphilis if untreated. In general, preventive treatment is given to all sexual contacts of the past 90 days, although nearly all cases of syphilis in contacts develop within 60 days of exposure.

JARISCH-HERXHEIMER REACTIONS. Up to 60% of patients with early syphilis, and a significant proportion of patients with later stages of syphilis, experience a transient febrile reaction after therapy for syphilis. This usually occurs in the first few hours after therapy, peaks at 6 to 8 hours, and disappears within 12 to 24 hours of therapy. Temperature elevation is usually low grade, and there is often associated myalgia, headache, and malaise. The skin lesions of secondary syphilis are often exacerbated during the Herxheimer reaction, and cutaneous lesions that were not visible may become visible. It is usually of no clinical significance and may be treated with salicylates in most cases. In patients with syphilis of the coronary ostia or of the optic nerve, there is a theoretical risk that local inflammation coincident with the Herxheimer reaction could precipitate serious damage. This is the subject of much discussion in the old literature, but there is little current evidence that "local Herxheimer reactions" constitute a significant risk to the patient. Corticosteroids have been used to prevent adverse effects of the Herxheimer reaction, but there is no evidence that they are clinically beneficial (other than reducing fever) or necessary. Institution of treatment with small doses of penicillin does not prevent the Herxheimer reaction.

The pathogenesis of the Herxheimer reaction is unclear. It may be due to liberation of antigens from the spirochetes. There is evidence that the complement cascade (see Chapter 271) is activated, including transient consumption of C3, C4, C6, and C7, and of transient decrease in treponemal antibodies coincident with the Herxheimer reaction. There is also evidence for endotoxemia, obtained by positive limulus amebocyte gelatin tests, at the time of the Herxheimer reaction, although *T. pallidum* does not contain biologically active endotoxin. These seemingly contradictory observations could be explained if the reaction resulted in release of endogenous endotoxin from the gut.

PERSISTENCE OF TREPONEMES AFTER TREATMENT. Studies in humans and in rabbits have shown that spiral forms may be visualized by silver stains in lymph nodes after effective treatment. Living virulent treponemes have occasionally been recovered by rabbit inoculation from lymph nodes, CSF, or ocular fluids after effective treatment has been given. These documented cases of treponemal persistence are very rare, however. At present there is little reason to worry about persistence of virulent treponemes after therapy with penicillin, with the possible exception of CNS syphilis, which needs further evaluation. No evidence exists for selection of penicillin-resistant mutants of *T. pallidum*.

PROSPECTS FOR PREVENTION. Solid immunity develops in rabbits after prolonged infection with virulent *T. pallidum*. It has not yet been possible to transfer immunity passively in laboratory animals by either immune serum or immune lymphocytes alone, suggesting that both cellular and humoral systems are necessary for immunity. Rabbits have been effectively immunized with multiple injections of treponemes that have been rendered avirulent by irradiation or by exposure to cold. However, a very large number of injections and a large mass of treponemes are necessary to effect immunity in the laboratory animal. For this reason and because *T. pallidum* cannot yet be grown in a virulent state in cell-free medium, there is no immediate prospect for a vaccine. However, significant immunity does develop in humans after prolonged infection. For the present, control depends entirely on clinical awareness on the part of physicians, adequate reporting to public health authorities, and vigorous application of epidemiologic investigation and preventive treatment of sexual contacts.

Cox DL, Chang P, McDowell A, Radolf JD: The outer membrane, not a coat of host proteins, limits the antigenicity of virulent *Treponema pallidum*. Infect Immun 60: 1076, 1992. *New data regarding the causative agent of syphilis and the reasons humoral antibody does not control or prevent infection.*
Holmes KK, Märdh P-A, Sparling PF, et al: Sexually Transmitted Diseases, 2nd ed. New York, McGraw-Hill, 1990. *The definitive text on sexually transmitted diseases.*
Hook EW III, Marra CM: Acquired syphilis in adults. N Engl J Med 326:1060, 1992. *A review of syphilis in the 1990s, including syphilis-HIV interactions.*
Magnuson HJ, Thomas EW, Olansky S, et al: Inoculation syphilis in human volunteers. Medicine 35:33, 1956. *A classic paper reporting results of a study in which prison volunteers were inoculated with virulent* T. pallidum. *Immunity to inoculation syphilis was observed only in individuals who had congenital or late syphilis.*
Rolfs RT, Joesoef MR, Hendershot EF, et al: A randomized trial of enhanced therapy for early syphilis in patients with and without human immunodeficiency virus infection. N Engl J Med 1997;337:307–314.

SPIROCHETAL DISEASES OTHER THAN SYPHILIS

366 NON-SYPHILITIC TREPONEMATOSES

Edward W. Hook III

DEFINITION. The non-syphilitic treponematoses (yaws, endemic syphilis [previously known as bejel], and pinta) are the spirochetal diseases caused by *Treponema pallidum* subspecies (yaws and endemic syphilis) or a closely related organism, *T. carateum* (pinta). Like syphilis the non-syphilitic treponematoses are usually transmitted through direct contact with an infectious cutaneous or mucosal lesion. The natural history of the non-syphilitic treponematoses is likewise similar to syphilis. Primary nodular or ulcerative lesions typically develop at sites of inoculation after an incubation period of several weeks. Untreated primary lesions serve as a source for local spread through scratching or for hematogenous dissemination, which gives rise to the secondary stage of infection characterized by development of widespread manifestations involving skin, lymph nodes, and bone or cartilage. Without therapy the primary and secondary manifestations of infections resolve and the infection becomes latent, although periodic recurrent secondary manifestations may occur for several years. Persons with long-standing untreated infections are at risk for late sequelae, which may include bony deformity, destruction of nasal cartilage, or chronic skin changes.

Unlike syphilis, the non-syphilitic treponematoses are primarily diseases of children, are not congenitally transmitted across the placenta, and do not invade the central nervous system. Treatment with benzathine penicillin G is effective, and the World Health Organization (WHO) has carried out extensive treatment campaigns in endemic areas.

ETIOLOGY. Yaws is caused by *Treponema pallidum* subspecies *pertenue*; pinta is caused by *T. carateum*; and endemic syphilis is caused by *T. pallidum* subspecies *endemicum*. The *T. pallidum* subspecies causing non-syphilitic treponematoses is closely related to *T. pallidum* subspecies *pallidum*, which causes venereal syphilis; there is a high degree of DNA homology, and they share unique, pathogen-restricted antigens. Like *T. pallidum*, these treponemes are spirochetal bacteria with helical structures and measure about 0.2 μm in diameter and 10 μm in length. They are visible by darkfield microscopy but cannot be cultivated for prolonged periods in vitro.

DISTRIBUTION AND EPIDEMIOLOGY. Yaws is prevalent in rural areas of tropical Africa, the Americas, Southeast Asia, and Oceania. The highest incidence is in children between ages 2 and 5 years. Endemic syphilis occurs in Africa, in Eastern Mediterranean countries, on the Arabian peninsula, in Central Asia, and in Australia. It is most prevalent in arid regions. Pinta occurs in rural areas of tropical Central and South America and affects mostly older children and adolescents. Humans are the only known carriers of the non-syphilitic treponematoses. The spirochete enters the skin only after it is broken, as by a scratch or insect bite. Transmission is believed to occur by contacting the skin directly or indirectly by contaminated hands or fomites and is facilitated by conditions of poor personal hygiene and crowding.

CLINICAL FEATURES. Yaws produces a skin papule at the inoculation site after an incubation period of 3 to 4 weeks. The most common sites are the legs and buttocks. The papule enlarges, ulcerates, and develops a serous crust from which treponemes can be recovered. Regional lymphadenitis may accompany the papule, which will heal spontaneously within 6 months. A generalized secondary rash will occur before or after the initial lesion heals, and these rashes are also papular and often covered with brown crusts. Relapsing crops of lesions can occur. Papillomas may result, and the plantar surfaces of the feet are involved with hyperkeratotic lesions. Periostitis of long bones leads to tender bones, and fever may be present. Relapsing lesions may occur over several years, resulting in chronic ulcerations and destructive gummatous lesions affecting the skin and bones.

Endemic syphilis produces patches on the mucous membranes of the oral cavity and pharynx and can cause split papules at the mucocutaneous junction of the oral angles. Anal, genital, and other intertriginous skin areas can be affected by lesions that resemble secondary syphilis. Regional lymphadenitis is common, and generalized rashes are rare. Healing of these early lesions is followed by latency manifested by seropositivity or by late lesions that resemble tertiary syphilis. These include nodular ulcers of skin, deformities of bones, and ulcerative lesions that can perforate the palate.

Pinta starts similarly as a cutaneous papule with regional lymphadenitis that is followed by a generalized maculopapular eruption. One to 3 years after healing of the initial lesion, large hyperpigmented macules that are brown or blue develop and subsequently lose their pigment and become white. The time required for lesions to pass through these stages varies, so that the same patient may have coexisting areas of increased pigment and loss of pigment.

DIAGNOSIS. By darkfield microscopy, the causative spirochetes from early skin lesions can be observed directly. Spirochetes have been demonstrated also in lymph node aspirates. There is no specific test for any of the non-syphilitic treponematoses. Serologic tests for syphilis detect cross-reacting antibodies in these diseases. The Venereal Disease Research Laboratories test, the serologic test for syphilis, and the fluorescent treponemal antibody absorption test each give positive results if serum is obtained at least 2 weeks after the lesions initially appear.

TREATMENT AND PROGNOSIS. Long-acting benzathine penicillin G given as 1.2 million units intramuscularly is the preferred treatment for patients with early lesions. For patients with late manifestations, this therapy should be repeated twice at approximately 7-day intervals. The early lesions heal rapidly, and most seropositive cases convert to seronegative status. Late destructive lesions take longer to show improvement.

PREVENTION. The prevalence of these diseases was reduced in the 1950s by mass treatment campaigns using penicillin. The World Health Organization treated about 53 million cases of yaws and 350,000 cases of pinta in the 1950s with good results. These campaigns, however, were not adequate to eradicate the disease, and in recent years the prevalence of yaws has again increased. It has been suggested that reduction in transmission requires improvements in the sanitation and economic standards of people living in endemic areas.

Koff AB, Rosen T: Nonvenereal treponematoses: Yaws, endemic syphilis, and pinta. J Am Acad Dermatol 29:519, 1993. *With worldwide travel there is a need to consider diagnosis of non-venereal treponematoses in appropriate clinical and historical situations.*

Vorst FA: Clinical diagnosis and changing manifestations of treponemal infection. Rev Infect Dis 7(Suppl 2):S327, 1985. *This paper shows that yaws in populations after mass treatment with penicillin assumes attenuated forms characterized by shorter duration of papillomas and lower antibody titers.*

367 RELAPSING FEVER

William A. Petri, Jr.

DEFINITION. Relapsing fever is a spirochetal infection with bacteria of the genus *Borrelia*. There are two modes of transmission: epidemic louse-borne and endemic tick-borne relapsing fever.

ETIOLOGY. *Borrelia* are spirochetes that measure 0.5 μm in diameter and 5 to 40 μm in length. They are aerophilic and require long-chain fatty acids for growth. Louse-borne relapsing fever is caused by *B. recurrentis*. Tick-borne relapsing fever organisms are named after their tick vector and include the closely related species *B. duttonii* (Old World) and *B. hermsii*, *B. turicatae*, and *B. parkeri* (North America).

EPIDEMIOLOGY. Louse-borne epidemic relapsing fever is carried from person to person by the human body louse. There is no animal reservoir. The spirochete lives in the hemolymph, and infection is transmitted to humans when the louse is crushed. Epidemics have occurred at wartime when breakdown in sanitation favors transmission of body lice. Louse-borne disease remains endemic in Ethiopia, Somalia, and the Sudan.

Tick-borne endemic relapsing fever is carried by *Ornithodoros* ticks, which become infected by feeding on wild rodents. In the United States, relapsing fever is limited to mountainous areas of the West at altitudes of 1500 to 8000 feet where the tick vector *O.*

hermsii resides in forests of ponderosa pine and Douglas fir. A key diagnostic clue has been a history of sleeping in rodent-infested rustic cabins in western national parks.

PATHOLOGY AND PATHOGENESIS. *Borrelia* infection begins in the skin at the site of the louse or tick bite and is followed by rapid dissemination of the spirochetes through the blood stream. Spirochetes are visible on Wright's stained peripheral blood smears during the initial febrile episode and during each relapse in most patients. Clearance of spirochetes from the blood is associated with the production of serotype-specific immune sera; anti-*Borrelia* antibodies have been shown in animal models to be the major mechanism of immune clearance of infection.

Relapses are associated with antigenic variation in the variable major proteins (VMPs), which are the abundant outer-membrane proteins of the spirochete that carry the serotype-specific epitopes. Antigenic variation is the consequence of recombination events occurring between VMP genes at silent and expression sites on linear plasmids.

CLINICAL FEATURES. An abrupt onset of fever to 38.5 to 40° C (>39° C in most patients), headache, myalgias, and shaking chills characterize the onset of illness. Cough, nausea and vomiting, and fatigue are less frequent complaints. Signs include fever, tachycardia, lethargy or confusion, conjunctival injection, and epistaxis. Hepatosplenomegaly, jaundice, and often a truncal petechial rash are common signs in louse-borne relapsing fever. Untreated louse-borne disease lasts 6 days, and relapses occur once after an afebrile period of 9 days. Tick-borne relapsing fever lasts about 4 days without antibiotic treatment and an average of two relapses occur after a 10-day afebrile period.

Relapsing fever in pregnancy results in miscarriage in one third of patients. Neonatal infection presents in both the tick- and louse-borne forms with jaundice, hepatosplenomegaly, and often sepsis and hemorrhage. Fever and hepatosplenomegaly are also common signs in children.

LABORATORY FEATURES. Spirochetes can be demonstrated in the Wright's stained peripheral blood smear of most patients. The white blood cell count is usually normal, but platelet counts less than 50,000/mm³ occur in up to 90% of cases of louse-borne disease. Prothrombin and partial thromboplastin times are often prolonged. In louse-borne disease, elevations in hepatic enzymes and blood urea nitrogen are common. The degree of spirochetemia is often 10⁵ organisms.

DIAGNOSIS. Spirochetes can be demonstrated on peripheral blood smears taken during the febrile episodes in 70% of patients. With an average incubation period of 1 week, relapsing fever is often diagnosed in a non-endemic area after the individual has returned from a stay in the Rocky Mountains. Only a few patients will remember tick exposure, because *O. hermsii* is a night feeder and only remains attached for 15 minutes. Culture of the organism requires a special medium and is not practical in a clinical laboratory setting. Because the number of organisms in blood is extremely high, the diagnosis is most often made by direct visualization of the organism on a blood smear.

PROGNOSIS. Epidemics of louse-borne relapsing fever have been reported, with mortalities approaching 40%. With antibiotic treatment, mortality is less than 5% in all recent series, with complete recovery expected. Autopsies of patients with louse-borne disease have documented intracranial hemorrhage, brain edema, bronchopneumonia, hepatic necrosis, and splenic infarcts.

THERAPY AND PREVENTION. A single 500-mg dose of tetracycline may be as effective as longer treatments in clearing spirochetemia of louse-borne disease, although many physicians still treat with 500 mg tetracycline every 6 hours for 5 to 10 days. Erythromycin is also effective and should be used in children younger than age 7 (in whom tetracyclines can stain the permanent teeth). Penicillin treatment has been reported to clear the spirochetemia more slowly than tetracycline.

The Jarisch-Herxheimer reaction (typically characterized by a rise in body temperature of 1° C, rigors, a slight fall followed by a rise in blood pressure, and transient leukopenia) occurs 2 to 3 hours after treatment in many patients with louse-borne disease, less commonly in tick-born disease, and should be anticipated and managed supportively. Deaths due to shock from the Jarisch-Herxheimer reaction occur rarely. The Jarisch-Herxheimer reaction has been associated with accelerated phagocytosis of spirochetes by neutrophils and transient elevations of tumor necrosis factor, interleukin-6, and interleukin-8.

Barbour AG: Antigenic variation of a relapsing fever *Borrelia* species. Annu Rev Microbiol 44:155, 1990. *Immunology and molecular biology of antigenic variation are reviewed.*

Common source outbreak of relapsing fever—California. MMWR 39:579, 1990. *Six individuals who had at different times spent the night in the same cabin at Big Bear Lake in California all developed relapsing fever with sudden onset of high fever, severe headache, prostration, nausea, and vomiting. Inhabited ground squirrel burrows were found under the cabin.*

Seboxa T, Rahlenbeck SI: Treatment of louse-borne relapsing fever with low dose penicillin or tetracycline: A clinical trial. Scand J Infect Dis 27:29, 1995. *Low-dose penicillin treatment (100,000 IU IM) had a higher relapse rate than tetracycline (250 mg PO) but a lower incidence of Jarisch-Herxheimer-like reaction (JHR). Because mortality is linked to severe JHR, the authors recommend treatment with low-dose penicillin and not tetracycline.*

368 LYME DISEASE

Stephen E. Malawista

Lyme disease is a tick-borne inflammatory disorder caused by the spirochete *Borrelia burgdorferi*. Its clinical hallmark is an early expanding skin lesion, *erythema migrans* (EM; previously called *erythema chronicum migrans*), which may be followed weeks to months later by neurologic, cardiac, or joint abnormalities. Symptoms may refer to any one of these four systems alone or in combination. All stages of Lyme disease may respond to antibiotics, but treatment of early disease is the most successful. Although cases of the illness are concentrated in certain endemic areas, foci of Lyme disease are widely distributed within the United States, Europe, and Asia.

"Lyme arthritis" was recognized in November 1975 because of unusual geographic clustering of children with inflammatory arthropathy in the region of Lyme, Connecticut. It soon became clear that this was a multisystem disorder (Lyme disease) occurring at any age, in both sexes, and often preceded by a characteristic expanding skin lesion, EM. In Europe EM had been associated with the bite of the sheep tick, *Ixodes ricinus*, and with tick-borne meningopolyneuritis. In the Lyme region, a closely related deer tick, *I. scapularis* (thought until recently to represent a new species, called *I. dammini*), was implicated as the principal disease vector on epidemiologic grounds. In 1982, Burgdorfer and associates isolated a spirochete, now called *B. burgdorferi*, from *I. scapularis* and linked it serologically to patients with Lyme disease. It was soon recovered from patient specimens.

DISTRIBUTION AND EPIDEMIOLOGY. Lyme disease is widespread. In the United States there are three distinct foci: the Northeast from Southern Maine to Maryland, the upper Midwest, and the West in northern California. Over 90% of reported cases come from eight states: Connecticut, Maryland, Massachusetts, New Jersey, New York, Pennsylvania, Minnesota, and Wisconsin. However, the illness has been reported in 48 states, as well as across Europe and Asia. The earliest known cases in the United States occurred on Cape Cod in 1962 and in Lyme, Connecticut, in 1965; annual cases now number more than 10,000. Disease can occur at any age and in either gender. Onset of illness is generally between May 1 and November 30, with the peak in June and July.

Lyme disease accounts for over 90% of reported vector-borne infectious diseases in the United States. Its primary vectors are tiny ixodid ticks. Major foci of disease correspond to the distribution of *I. scapularis* (Northeast, Midwest), *I. pacificus* (West), *I. ricinus* (Europe), and *I. persulcatus* (Eurasia, Asia). In one U.S. study 31% of 314 patients recalled a tick bite at the skin site where EM developed days to weeks later. The six ticks that were saved were invariably nymphal *I. scapularis*, whose peak questing period is May through July; the nymphal stage is primarily responsible for transmission of disease. Preferred hosts for *I. scapularis* nymphs are white-footed mice and, for adults, white-tailed deer, in whose fur they mate. A less successful transmission cycle involving the dusky footed woodrat has been described in California.

The rising incidence of Lyme disease in recent years in the United States may be explained by multiple factors, including an increase in the numbers of ixodid ticks, the outward migration of residential areas into previously rural woodlands (habitats favored by ixodid ticks and their hosts), an exploding deer population, and increased recognition.

In areas endemic for Lyme disease, the prevalence of *B. burgdorferi* in nymphal *I. scapularis* ranges from about 20 to more than 60% (cf. *I. pacificus*, 1 to 2%). The organism has been isolated, or specific antibody found, in blood and tissues of a wide variety of large and small animals, including domestic dogs and birds. Indiscriminate feeding on a variety of animals by immature *I. scapularis* may favor the spread of infection.

PATHOGENESIS. Recovery of *B. burgdorferi* is straightforward from the tick but difficult from patients—except from EM lesions, where the clinical diagnosis is usually obvious—in part because of a relative paucity of organisms in specimens of tissue and fluids from the latter. Nevertheless, rare positive cultures are reported at all stages of the illness—from blood (early), secondary annular lesions, meningitic cerebrospinal fluid (CSF), heart, joint fluid, ligament, and even a late skin lesion, *acrodermatitis chronica atrophicans*, that had been present for 10 years. Spirochetes have been identified by silver stain or by immunofluorescence in some histologic sections of EM and rarely of secondary annular lesions, synovium, brain, eye, heart, striated muscle, ligament, liver, spleen, kidney, and bone marrow.

From these data, combined with clinical (see later) and epidemiologic features of Lyme disease, the following pathogenetic sequence is likely. *B. burgdorferi* is transmitted to the skin of the host via the tick vector but only, in general, after at least 48 hours of engorgement. Within 3 to 32 days, the organism migrates outward in the skin, and EM spreads in lymph (regional adenopathy), or disseminates in blood to organs (e.g., central nervous system [CNS], joints, heart, and presumably liver and spleen) or other skin sites (secondary annular lesions; see later). Maternal-fetal transmission is distinctly uncommon. Although organisms are hard to find in later stages of Lyme disease, it is entirely possible that persistent live spirochetes or their undegraded antigens are driving the illness throughout its course. Evidence for this interpretation includes the responsiveness of many patients to antibiotics, the rare sightings of spirochetes in affected tissues, the variable recovery from affected tissues and fluids of spirochetal DNA amplified by the polymerase chain reaction (PCR), and an expansion of the antibody response to additional spirochetal antigens over time. If live spirochetes are invariably present, it is not yet clear how they occasionally remain out of harm's way in the face of both antibiotic therapy and the body's usual phagocytic and other immune clearance mechanisms. Autoimmune mechanisms have been proposed, but not proven, in the propagation of chronic Lyme arthritis.

In the clinical laboratory characteristic immune abnormalities are found. At disease onset (EM), almost all patients have evidence of circulating immune complexes. At that time, the findings of elevated serum immunoglobulin M (IgM) levels and cryoglobulins containing IgM predict subsequent nervous system, heart, or joint involvement; that is, early humoral findings have prognostic significance. These abnormalities tend to persist during neurologic or cardiac involvement. Later in the illness, when arthritis is present, serum IgM levels are more often normal. By then, immune complexes are usually lacking in serum but are present uniformly in joint fluid, where their titers correlate positively with the local concentration of polymorphonuclear leukocytes. Mononuclear cells from peripheral blood increase their antigen-specific proliferative response as the disease progresses, but the greatest reactivity to antigen is seen in cells from inflamed joints. Adjacent to that joint fluid, on biopsy a proliferative synovium is seen, often replete with lymphocytes and plasma cells that are presumably capable of producing immunoglobulin locally. Thus, an initially disseminated, immune-mediated inflammatory disorder becomes in some patients localized and propagated in joints.

Although *B. burgdorferi* seem not to destroy tissue directly, they non-specifically activate monocytes, macrophages, synovial lining cells, natural killer cells, B cells, and complement, resulting in the elaboration of a host of proinflammatory materials. These spirochetes adhere to extracellular matrix proteins, to endothelial cells (and penetrate endothelial monolayers), and to neural glycolipid.

They can induce the production of cross-reactive antibodies and of specific immune B and T lymphocytes that may be associated histologically with endarteritic microvascular occlusive changes (e.g., in nervous tissue, hearts, joints), but it is not clear that these phenomena persist in the absence of live spirochetes.

In addition to factors related to the pathogenicity of specific isolates of *B. burgdorferi,* immunogenetic makeup may play a role in whether infected individuals can rid themselves of spirochetes, their antigens, or their effects. Patients with treatment-resistant chronic arthritis have been reported to have an increased frequency of the B-cell alloantigen HLA DR4.

CLINICAL CHARACTERISTICS. Lyme disease is conveniently divided into three clinical stages, but the stages may overlap, most patients do not exhibit all of them, and in fact seroconversion can occur in asymptomatic individuals. The illness usually begins with EM and associated symptoms (stage 1), sometimes followed weeks to months later by neurologic or cardiac abnormalities (stage 2) and weeks to years later by arthritis (stage 3). Chronic neurologic and skin involvement also may occur years after onset.

EARLY MANIFESTATIONS. EM, the unique clinical marker for Lyme disease, is recognized in 90% or more of patients. It begins as a red macule or papule at the site where the tick vector, usually long gone, had engorged. As the area of redness expands to 15 cm or so (range, 3 to 68 cm), there is usually partial central clearing (see Color Plate 8*B*). The outer borders are red, generally flat, and without scaling. The centers are occasionally red and indurated, even vesicular or necrotic. Variations may occur—multiple rings, for example. The thigh, groin, and axilla are particularly common sites. The lesion is warm to touch, but not often sore, and is easily missed if out of sight. Routine histologic findings are non-specific: a heavy dermal infiltrate of mononuclear cells, without epidermal change except at the site of the tick bite.

Within days of onset of EM, one fourth or less of U.S. patients develop multiple annular secondary lesions (more did so in the initial study; Table 368–1). These lesions, from which spirochetes have been cultured, represent clear evidence of dissemination. They resemble EM itself but are generally smaller, migrate less, and lack indurated centers. Individual lesions may come and go, and their borders sometimes merge. Other occasional skin lesions are noted in Table 368–1. In addition, benign lymphocytoma cutis has been reported in Europe. EM and secondary lesions fade in 3 to 4 weeks (range, 1 day to 14 months). They may recur.

Skin involvement is often accompanied by musculoskeletal flu-like symptoms—malaise and fatigue, headache, fever and chills. myalgia, and arthralgia (Table 368–2). Even without EM, this syndrome in summer, in an endemic area for Lyme disease, is grounds for treatment. Some patients have evidence of meningeal irritation or mild encephalopathy—for example, episodic attacks of excruciating headache and neck pain, stiffness, or pressure—but

Table 368–1 ■ EARLY SIGNS OF LYME DISEASE IN A STUDY OF 314 PATIENTS

SIGNS	NO. OF PATIENTS (%)
Erythema migrans	314 (100)*
Multiple annular lesions	150 (48)
Lymphadenopathy	
Regional	128 (41)
Generalized	63 (20)
Pain on neck flexion	52 (17)
Malar rash	41 (13)
Erythematous throat	38 (12)
Conjunctivitis	35 (11)
Right upper quadrant tenderness	24 (8)
Splenomegaly	18 (6)
Hepatomegaly	16 (5)
Muscle tenderness	12 (4)
Periorbital edema	10 (3)
Evanescent skin lesions	8 (3)
Abdominal tenderness	6 (2)
Testicular swelling	2 (1)

*Erythema migrans was required for inclusion in this study.
From Steere AC, et al: The early clinical manifestations of Lyme disease. Ann Intern Med 99:76. © 1983, Massachusetts Medical Society. All rights reserved.

Table 368–2 ■ EARLY SYMPTOMS OF LYME DISEASE IN A STUDY OF 314 PATIENTS

SYMPTOMS	NO. OF PATIENTS (%)
Malaise, fatigue, and lethargy	251 (80)
Headache	200 (64)
Fever and chills	185 (59)
Stiff neck	151 (48)
Arthralgias	150 (48)
Myalgias	135 (43)
Backache	81 (26)
Anorexia	73 (23)
Sore throat	53 (17)
Nausea	53 (17)
Dysesthesia	35 (11)
Vomiting	32 (10)
Abdominal pain	24 (8)
Photophobia	19 (6)
Hand stiffness	16 (5)
Dizziness	15 (5)
Cough	15 (5)
Chest pain	12 (4)
Ear pain	12 (4)
Diarrhea	6 (2)

From Steere AC, Bartenhagen NH, Craft JE, et al: The early clinical manifestations of Lyme disease. Ann Intern Med 99:76, 1983.

typically lasting only for hours at this stage of the illness and without CSF pleocytosis or objective neurologic deficit. Except for fatigue and lethargy, which are often constant, the early signs and symptoms are typically intermittent and changing. For example, a patient may have meningitic attacks for several days, a few days of improvement, and then the onset of migratory musculoskeletal pain. This last may involve joints (generally without swelling), tendons, bursa, muscle, and bone. The pain tends to affect only one or two sites at a time and to last a few hours to several days in a given location. The various associated symptoms may occur several days before EM (or without it) and last for months (especially fatigue and lethargy) after the skin lesions have disappeared.

LATER MANIFESTATIONS. Neurologic Involvement. Within several weeks to months of the onset of illness, about 15% of patients develop frank neurologic abnormalities, including meningitis, encephalitis, chorea, cranial neuritis (including bilateral facial palsy), motor and sensory radiculoneuritis, or mononeuritis multiplex, in various combinations. The usual pattern is fluctuating meningoencephalitis with superimposed cranial nerve (particularly facial) palsy and peripheral radiculoneuropathy, but Bell's-like palsy may occur *alone.* By now, patients with meningitic symptoms have a lymphocytic pleocytosis (about 100 cells/mm³) in CSF and sometimes diffuse slowing on electroencephalogram. However, the neck is rarely stiff except on extreme flexion; Kernig's and Brudzinski's signs are absent. Neurologic abnormalities typically last for months but usually resolve completely (late neurologic complications are noted later).

Cardiac Involvement. Also within weeks to months of onset, about 8% of patients develop cardiac involvement. The most common abnormality is fluctuating degrees of atrioventricular block (first-degree, Wenckebach, or complete heart block). Some patients have evidence of more diffuse cardiac involvement, including electrocardiographic changes compatible with acute myopericarditis, radionuclide evidence of mild left ventricular dysfunction, or, rarely, cardiomegaly. None has had heart murmurs. Cardiac involvement is usually brief (3 days to 6 weeks), but it may recur.

Arthritis. From weeks to as long as 2 years after the onset of illness, about 60% of patients develop frank arthritis, usually characterized by intermittent attacks of asymmetric joint swelling and pain primarily in large joints, especially the knee, one or two joints at a time. Affected knees are commonly more swollen than painful, often hot, rarely red; Baker's cysts may form and rupture early. However, both large and small joints may be affected, and a few patients have had symmetrical polyarthritis. Attacks of arthritis, which generally last from weeks to months, typically recur for several years, decreasing in frequency with time. Fatigue is common with active joint involvement, but fever or other systemic symptoms at this stage are unusual. Joint fluid white blood cell counts vary from 500 to 110,000 cells/mm³, with an average of about 25,000 cells/mm³, mostly polymorphonuclear leukocytes. Total protein ranges from 3 to 8 g/dL. The C3 and C4 levels are generally greater than one-third, and glucose levels usually greater than two-thirds, that of serum. Rheumatoid factor and antinuclear antibody are absent.

In about 10% of patients with arthritis, involvement in large joints may become chronic, with pannus formation and erosion of cartilage and bone. Synovial biopsy findings may mimic those of rheumatoid arthritis: surface deposits of fibrin, villous hypertrophy, vascular proliferation, and a heavy infiltration of mononuclear cells. In addition, there may be an obliterative endarteritis and (rarely) demonstrable spirochetes. As noted earlier, *B. burgdorferi* stimulates mononuclear cells to produce cytokines (e.g., interleukin-1, tumor necrosis factor-α, interleukin-6), and elevated concentrations of inflammatory cytokines have been found in synovial fluid. In one patient with chronic Lyme arthritis, synovium grown in tissue culture produced large amounts of collagenase and prostaglandin E_2. Thus, in Lyme disease the joint fluid cell counts, the immune reactants (except for rheumatoid factor), the synovial histology, the amounts of synovial enzymes released, and the resulting destruction of cartilage and bone may be similar to those in rheumatoid arthritis.

Other late findings (years) associated with this infection include a chronic skin lesion—*acrodermatitis chronica atrophicans*—well known in Europe but still rare in the United States. One sees violaceous infiltrated plaques or nodules, especially on extensor surfaces, that eventually become atrophic. Uncommon late chronic neurologic disease includes transverse myelitis, diffuse sensory axonal neuropathy, and demyelinating lesions of the CNS. Mild memory impairment, subtle mood changes, and chronic fatigue states may also occur.

LABORATORY TEST RESULTS. The diagnosis of Lyme disease is based on recognizing clinical features of the illness in a patient with a history of possible exposure to the causative organism. Culture of *B. burgdorferi* from patients is definitive but has rarely been successful except from skin biopsy specimens. The organism can be isolated from blood in a significant minority of patients with systemic manifestations of early disease (it grows very slowly). Special tissue staining techniques generally have a low yield and are not readily available. Determination of specific antibody titers, usually performed by enzyme-linked immunosorbent assay (ELISA), is currently the most helpful additional diagnostic test for Lyme disease. In serum, specific IgM antibody titers against *B. burgdorferi* usually reach a peak between the third and sixth weeks after the onset of disease; specific immunoglobulin G (IgG) antibody titers rise more slowly and are generally highest months later when arthritis is present (Fig. 368–1). Individuals with untreated Lyme disease of more than 6 weeks' duration can be expected to have elevated levels of specific antibodies. However, the tests employed are not standardized, and results from different commercial laboratories may vary, especially for borderline elevations. The vast majority of individuals with established Lyme arthritis have elevated specific IgG titers. This finding makes antibody titers against *B. burgdorferi* particularly useful in differentiating Lyme disease from other rheumatic syndromes, especially when EM is missed, forgotten, or absent. This antibody cross-reacts with other spirochetes, including *Treponema pallidum,* but patients with Lyme disease do not have positive VDRL test results. Western blots are important when false-positive ELISAs are suspected.

Another test of diagnostic interest uses the PCR to detect spirochetal DNA in host material. Although this powerful tool is notorious for false-positive results when not performed under the most stringent conditions, it shows great promise, particularly in Lyme arthritis, in which synovial fluid from the large majority of untreated patients appears to be positive.

The most common non-specific laboratory abnormalities, particularly early in the illness, are a high erythrocyte sedimentation rate, an elevated serum IgM level, or increased serum levels of aspartate transaminase (AST). The enzyme levels generally return to normal within several weeks. Patients may be mildly anemic early in the illness and occasionally have elevated white blood cell counts with shifts to the left in the differential count. A few patients have had

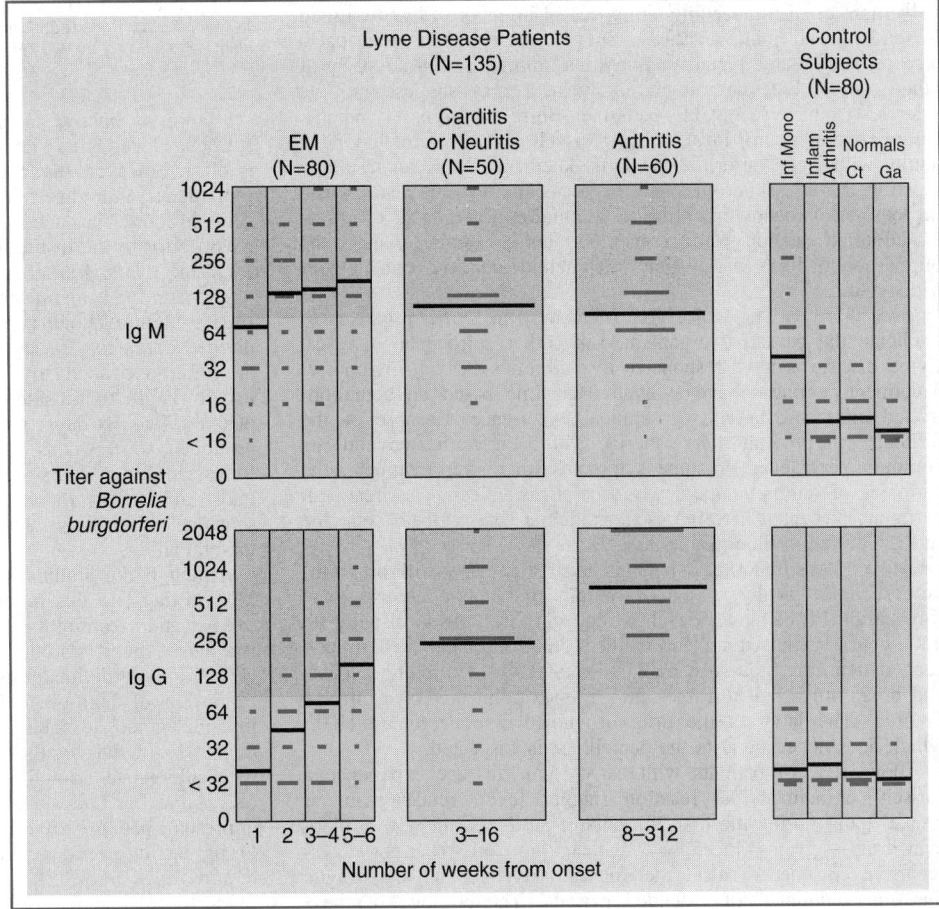

FIGURE 368–1 ■ Antibody titers against *Borrelia burgdorferi* are shown in serum samples from 135 patients with different clinical manifestations of Lyme disease, and from 80 control subjects with infectious mononucleosis, inflammatory arthritis, or no disease (titers determined by indirect immunofluorescence). The black bar shows the geometric mean titer for each group; the pink shaded areas indicate the range of values generally observed in control subjects. Note that all patients with Lyme arthritis have elevated IgG antibody titers. (Adapted from Steere AC, Grodzicki RL, Kornblatt AN, et al: The spirochetal etiology of Lyme disease. N Engl J Med 308:733–740, 1983. Copyright 1983 Massachusetts Medical Society.)

microscopic hematuria, sometimes with mild proteinuria (dipstick); values for creatinine and blood urea nitrogen have been normal. Throughout the illness, serum C3 and C4 levels are generally normal or elevated. Rheumatoid factor and antinuclear antibodies are usually absent.

DIFFERENTIAL DIAGNOSIS. EM is the unique herald lesion of Lyme disease. When present in its classic form, there is little else that might be confused with it. However, some patients are not aware of having had EM and in others, its appearance is not always characteristic. Secondary lesions might suggest *erythema multiforme,* but blistering, mucosal lesions, and involvement of the palms and soles are not features of Lyme disease. Malar rash may suggest systemic lupus erythematosus, an urticarial rash, hepatitis B infection, or serum sickness. Evanescent blotches and circles may resemble *erythema marginatum,* but those of Lyme disease do not expand.

Early musculoskeletal flulike symptoms may be misinterpreted, especially when EM is absent or missed or is not the first manifestation. In patients with particularly severe constitutional symptoms, consider possible concomitant infection with two other illnesses whose causative agents are transmitted by the same tick: the ricketsial-like disorder, human granulocytic ehrlichiosis (HGE; watch for leukopenia, thrombocytopenia, elevated transaminases, occasional inclusions in granulocytes) (see Chapter 371) or the malaria-like disorder, babesiosis (occasional inclusions in erythrocytes) (see Chapter 429).

Severe headache and stiff neck may resemble aseptic meningitis, abdominal symptoms, hepatitis, and generalized tender lymphadenopathy and splenomegaly, infectious mononucleosis. As in the last infection, fatigue in Lyme disease may be a major and persistent complaint. However, initial presentations of an isolated chronic fatigue syndrome or of fibromyalgia-like complaints (diffuse aching, trigger points, sleep disturbance) are not characteristic of Lyme disease.

In later stages, Lyme disease may mimic other immune-mediated disorders. Like rheumatic fever, Lyme disease may be associated with sore throat followed by migratory polyarthritis (more often, polyarthralgias) and carditis, but without evidence of valvular involvement or of a preceding streptococcal infection. Migratory pain in tendons and joints may also suggest disseminated gonococcal disease. An isolated facial weakness may mimic Bell's-like palsy of other causes. Late neurologic involvement may suggest multiple sclerosis (transverse myelitis), Guillain-Barré syndrome (symmetrical peripheral neuropathy), primary psychosis, or brain tumor. In adults with Lyme arthritis, the large knee effusions can resemble those in Reiter's syndrome, and the occasional symmetrical polyarthritis, that of rheumatoid arthritis. In children, the attacks of arthritis, although generally shorter, may be identical to those seen in the oligoarticular form of juvenile rheumatoid arthritis, but without iridocyclitis.

TREATMENT. The major goal of therapy in Lyme disease is to eradicate the causative organism. Like other spirochetal diseases, Lyme disease is most responsive to antibiotics early in its course. Treatment regimens have evolved over time based on both controlled clinical data and on clinical experience. Because of the difficulty in proving that bacteria have been eradicated and the common persistence of some symptoms long after treatment, the endpoint of antibiotic therapy is not always clear. The treatment regimens presented here represent guidelines that will no doubt be further refined in time (Table 368–3).

EARLY LYME DISEASE. If patients are treated early with oral antibiotics, EM typically resolves promptly, and major later sequelae (myocarditis, meningoencephalitis, or recurrent arthritis) usually do not occur. Prompt treatment is therefore important, even though such patients may be susceptible to reinfection. Antibiotic choices and doses are listed in Table 368–3, amoxicillin or doxycycline is favored. The latter is the drug of choice if concomitant HGE, which does not respond to the penicillins, is suspected.

About 10% of patients with early Lyme disease experience a Jarisch-Herxheimer–like reaction (higher fever, redder rash, or greater pain) during the first 24 hours of antibiotic therapy. Whichever drug is given, 30 to 50% of patients have brief (hours to days) recurrent episodes of headache, musculoskeletal pain, and fatigue that may continue for extended periods. The etiology of these

Table 368–3 ■ RECOMMENDATIONS FOR ANTIBIOTIC TREATMENT OF LYME DISEASE*

Early Lyme Disease†
Amoxicillin, 500 mg three times daily for 21 days‡
Doxycycline, 100 mg twice daily for 21 days
Cefuroxime axetil, 500 mg twice daily for 21 days
Azithromycin, 500 mg daily for 7 days§
  (less effective than other regimens)

Neurologic Manifestations
Bell's-like palsy (no other neurologic abnormalities)
  Oarl regimens of doxycycline or amoxicillin for 21–28 days ‖
Meningitis (with or without radiculoneuropathy or encephalitis) ‖
  Ceftriaxone, 2 g daily for 14–28 days
  Penicillin G, 20 million units daily for 14–28 days
  Doxycycline, 100 mg twice daily (oral or intravenous) for 21–28 days¶

Arthritis**
Amoxicillin, 500 mg three times daily for 30–60 days
Doxycycline, 100 mg twice daily for 30–60 days
Ceftriaxone, 2 g daily for 30 days
Penicillin G, 20 million units daily for 30 days

Carditis
Ceftriaxone, 2 g daily for 14–28 days
Penicillin G, 20 million units daily for 14–28 days
Doxycycline, 100 mg orally twice daily for 30 days††
Amoxicillin, 500 mg three times daily for 30 days††

Pregnancy
Localized early disease
  Amoxicillin, 500 mg three times daily for 21 days
Any manifestation of disseminated disease
  Penicillin G, 20 million units daily for 14–28 days
Asymptomatic seropositivity
  No treatment necessary

*These are guidelines, to be modified by new findings and to be applied always with close attention to the clinical context of individual patients.
†Without neurologic, cardiac, or joint involvement. For early Lyme disease limited to single EM lesion, 10 days may suffice.
‡Some experts advise addition of probenecid 500 mg three times daily.
§Experience with this agent is limited; optimal duration of therapy is unclear.
‖ Optimal duration of therapy has not been established. There are no controlled trials of therapy longer than 4 weeks for any manifestation of Lyme disease.
¶No published experience in the United States.
**An oral regimen should be selected only if there is no neurologic involvement.
††Oral regimens have been reserved for mild carditis limited to first-degree heart block with PR ≤ .30 sec and normal ventricular function.
Adapted from Rahn DW, Malawista SE: Treatment of Lyme disease (special article). *In* Mandell GL, Bone RC, Cline MJ, et al (eds): 1994 Year Book of Medicine. St. Louis, Mosby–Year Book, 1994.

symptoms is unclear at present; they may result from undegraded spirochetal antigen(s) rather than persistence of live spirochetes. It is clear, however, that the risk of delayed resolution is greatest in individuals with disseminated manifestations of disease (multiple skin lesions, headache, fever, lymphadenopathy, or Bell's-like palsy) prior to the institution of antibiotics.

LATER LYME DISEASE. For Lyme meningitis, with or without other neurologic manifestations (cranial neuropathy or radiculoneuropathy), intravenous penicillin G, 20 million units a day in six divided doses for 10 days, is effective therapy; in practice, courses are often extended to 3 to 4 weeks. Headache and stiff neck usually begin to subside by the second day of therapy and disappear by 7 to 10 days; motor deficits and radicular pain frequently require 7 to 8 weeks for complete recovery but do not require longer antibiotic courses. For Bell's-like palsy alone, oral regimens may suffice, but these patients may be at higher risk of later sequelae than are individuals with early disease without neurologic dissemination.

Although not studied systematically, carditis also responds rapidly (in days) to this regimen. Recovery from carditis was the rule even in the preantibiotic era, but untreated patients are at high risk for later manifestations of Lyme disease. Prednisone, 40 to 60 mg/day in divided doses, has, in the past, seemed to hasten resolution of high-grade heart block, but one should hesitate to institute glucocorticoids during antibiotic administration because they may impede eradication of infecting organisms. For patients with allergy to penicillin, doxycycline, 100 mg twice a day, is reasonable but unevaluated. If second- or third-degree heart block is present, patients should be admitted to hospital for cardiac monitoring and intravenous antibiotics; temporary pacing is occasionally required for complete heart block.

In clinical practice, ceftriaxone (2 g daily for 14 to 21 days) has largely replaced penicillin for the therapy of disseminated Lyme disease. Arguments in favor of this practice are a once-daily administration schedule that is amenable to outpatient intravenous antibiotic programs and improved penetration of the CSF in comparison with penicillin. However, in a recent study, 3 weeks of oral doxycycline was equally effective for acute disseminated disease excluding meningitis. Penicillin and cefotaxime have been found equally effective for the treatment of acute neurologic Lyme disease (meningitis or radiculitis) in a group of patients studied in Germany. Ceftriaxone also appeared responsible for the complete recovery of six of nine unusual Austrian patients with dilated cardiomyopathy attributed to Lyme disease.

LATE LYME DISEASE. Lyme arthritis has been successfully treated with both oral and parenteral antibiotics, but failures occur with any regimen chosen. Unless CNS involvement coexists, first-line treatment with 1 or 2 months of doxycycline, 100 mg twice a day, or amoxicillin 500 mg three times a day, is recommended. The large majority of patients respond, although complete response can be delayed as long as 3 months or more after therapy is completed, and some patients may develop neurologic disease later. During treatment, the affected joint should be kept at rest and effusions drained by needle aspiration as for any infected joint. In patients who fail one or more courses of antibiotics, arthroscopic synovectomy can result in a long-term response and perhaps cure. Even without antibiotic or surgical treatment, persistent Lyme arthritis tends to resolve within several years.

Optimal therapy for the later neurologic complications of Lyme disease is also not yet clear, but 28 days of intravenous ceftriaxone or penicillin (see Table 368–3) are recommended. The frequency of subtle chronic encephalopathy and peripheral neuropathy is debated at present. These entities, when suspected, should be carefully documented through neurologic, neuropsychological, and electrophysiologic testing before aggressive or prolonged antibiotic therapy is instituted. Although some current thinking favors longer periods of the highest tolerated oral doses of amoxicillin (with probenecid), doxycycline, or even intravenous antibiotics in difficult cases, there is no controlled experience with courses of antibiotics longer than 1 month for any manifestation of Lyme disease. The infiltrative lesions of *acrodermatitis chronica atrophicans* are usually cured by 30 days of penicillin V, 1 g three times a day, or of doxycycline, 100 mg twice a day.

PREGNANCY. Because the spirochetes that cause relapsing fever and syphilis can cross the placenta, there has been concern regarding this possibility in Lyme disease. Maternal-fetal transmission of *B. burgdorferi* resulting in either neonatal death or stillbirth has been reported in rare instances in which symptomatic early Lyme disease occurred early in pregnancy and was either untreated or inadequately treated. In follow-up studies conducted by the Centers for Disease Control and Prevention, maternal Lyme disease was not directly implicated as a cause of fetal malformations. There have been no cases of fetal infection occurring when currently recommended antibiotic regimens for Lyme disease have been used during pregnancy. A lower threshold for initiating therapy for suspected Lyme disease in pregnancy is understandable, but women acquiring the illness during pregnancy should be reassured that the vast majority of infants born to women in these circumstances have been entirely well.

TICK BITES. A final treatment issue regards the advisability of administering antibiotics prophylactically to individuals sustaining ixodid tick bites in endemic areas. Studies completed to date have not supported this common practice. Because nymphal ixodid ticks must, in general, feed for at least 48 hours before transmitting spirochetes, ticks removed before this time are unlikely to have transmitted *B. burgdorferi* even if infected. Tick bite sites should be observed for development of EM and patients cautioned regarding the common associated symptoms of early Lyme disease. A watched tick bite allows for very early treatment of EM in the small minority of patients in whom it will develop, and this is the stage of disease most amenable to therapy.

VACCINATION. Two vaccines against Lyme disease, both based on one of the outer surface proteins (OspA) of *B. burgdorferi*, appear to be safe and effective; one of them is available as of this writing. Their mechanism of action is unique: spirochetes are killed in the midgut of the tick by the antibody-laden blood meal before they ever reach the host.

Bockenstedt LK, Malawista SE: Lyme Disease. *In* Rich RR (ed): Clinical Immunology. St. Louis, Mosby–Year Book, 1995. *An expanded version of this chapter with extensive references.*

Dattwyler RJ, Luft BJ, Kunkel MJ, et al: Ceftriaxone compared with doxycycline for the treatment of acute disseminated Lyme disease. N Engl J Med 337:289, 1997. *Oral doxycycline for 3 weeks and intravenous ceftriaxone for 2 weeks were both excellent in preventing late manifestations of disease in patients with acute disseminated disease (i.e., multiple EM lesions or other definite organ involvement excluding meningitis). Oral therapy has fewer adverse drug-related effects and is much less expensive.*

Malawista SE, Steere AC, Hardin JA: Lyme disease: A unique human model for an infectious etiology of rheumatic disease. Yale J Biol Med 57:473, 1984. *The larger significance of Lyme disease, a disorder that is infectious in origin but inflammatory or "rheumatic" in expression.*

Rahn DW, Malawista SE: Treatment of Lyme disease (special article). *In* Mandell GL, Bone RC, Cline MJ, et al. (eds): 1994 Year Book of Medicine. St. Louis, Mosby–Year Book, 1994. *Evolution of recommendations for therapy, based on published studies, practical considerations, and clinical experience.*

Sigal LH: Pitfalls in the diagnosis and management of Lyme disease. Arthritis Rheum 41:195, 1998. *An insightful analysis of fact, assertion, and rumor.*

Sigal LH, Zahradnik JM, Lavin P, et al: A vaccine consisting of recombinant *Borrelia burgdorferi* outer-surface protein A to prevent Lyme disease. N Engl J Med 339:216, 1998. *One of two double-blind placebo-controlled phase 3 vaccine studies, published back-to-back (~10,000 subjects in each), showing safety and efficacy in the prevention of Lyme disease.*

Steere AC, Malawista SE, Snydman DR, et al: Lyme arthritis: An epidemic of oligoarticular arthritis in children and adults in three Connecticut communities. Arthritis Rheum 20:7, 1977. *The first description of a new nosologic entity, recognized because it clusters geographically; rheumatoid arthritis does not.*

369 LEPTOSPIROSIS

William A. Petri, Jr.

DEFINITION. Leptospirosis is a spirochetal infection with bacteria of the genus *Leptospira*. The severe icteric form of infection is called Weil's disease, after the investigator who in 1886 described four men with an acute but self-limited infectious illness characterized by fever, jaundice, nephritis, and hepatomegaly and a biphasic course, with fever recurring 1 to 7 days into convalescence.

ETIOLOGY. There are two species of *Leptospira*: *L. interrogans*, which is pathogenic in humans and animals, and *L. biflexa*, which is free-living. *L. interrogans* is divided into more than 200 serovars grouped into 19 serogroups based on shared major agglutinins. Virulence does not in general correlate with serovars, although serovar classifications can be useful epidemiologically to identify common-source outbreaks. *Leptospira* are motile spirochetes 6 to 20 μm in length and 0.1 to 0.2 μm in diameter that are obligate aerobes with unique nutritional requirements for long-chain fatty acids.

EPIDEMIOLOGY. Leptospirosis is one of the most common, widespread, and underdiagnosed infections transmitted from animals to humans. *L. interrogans* can survive for months in the proximal convoluted tubules of the kidney in asymptomatically infected animals and upon excretion in urine survives in the environment for as long as 6 months. The optimal temperature for growth is 28 to 32° C, with slightly alkaline water ideal for growth and survival. Herbivores with alkaline urines, such as pigs, shed higher numbers of organisms than animals with acidic urine, such as dogs. The most common source of exposure in the United States is dogs, followed by livestock, rodents, and other wild animals. Humans become infected through recreational (e.g., windsurfing, kayaking, swimming) or occupational exposure to animal urine or urine-contaminated water and soil. Epidemics in developing countries are associated with exposure to flood waters during rainy season. Occupations with the greatest documented risks include New Zealand dairy farmers (incidence of 1.1 infections per 10 person-years), Glasgow sewer workers (3.7 infections per 10 person-years), and U.S. Army soldiers undergoing jungle warfare training in Panama (4.1 infections per 10 person-years). Approximately 15% of veterinarians and abattoir workers have serologic evidence of infection. Leptospirosis is up to 10 times more frequent in rural than in urban dwellers and three times more frequent in men, with a peak incidence in men at ages 30 to 39.

PATHOLOGY AND PATHOGENESIS. *Leptospira* penetrate intact mucous membranes and abraded skin and disseminate widely through the blood stream. In the first week to 10 days of illness, spirochetes can be cultured with special media from blood and cerebrospinal fluid (CSF). Leptospirosis is an infectious vasculitis, with damage to capillary endothelial cells responsible for the major clinical manifestations of disease, including renal tubular and hepatic dysfunction, myocarditis, and pulmonary hemorrhage. Intravascular to extravascular fluid shifts secondary to endothelial damage lead to hypovolemia, which complicates renal dysfunction and can lead to shock. Fatal cases are associated with widespread hemorrhage of mucosal, skin, and serosal surfaces. Examination of the kidneys from autopsies has revealed ischemic damage, including epithelial cell necrosis in the distal convoluted tubules and the ascending loop of Henle, and interstitial nephritis but only rarely glomerular damage. Liver pathology includes disorganization of liver cell plates, marked variation in the size and shape of parenchymal cells, mitotic figures, and evidence of cholestasis but not necrosis. Muscle biopsies have demonstrated focal necrotic changes with a mild mononuclear infiltrate. Only rarely is the spirochete visualized in the infected tissue. Hemorrhagic myocarditis has been observed frequently in autopsies. The secondary "immune" phase of leptospirosis is associated with the clearance of the organism from blood and CSF and the appearance of agglutinating anti-*Leptospira* antibodies.

CLINICAL FEATURES. Symptoms develop 7 to 12 days after exposure. Most patients have an abrupt onset of a self-limited 4- to 7-day anicteric illness characterized by the sudden onset of fever, mild to severe headache, myalgias, chills, cough, chest pain, neck stiffness, and/or prostration. An estimated 10% of patients will present with jaundice, hemorrhage, renal failure, and/or neurologic dysfunction (Weil's disease). Signs of leptospirosis include fever of 38 to 40° C (97 to 100% of patients), conjunctival suffusion (40 to 100%), hepatomegaly (80% of icteric cases), splenomegaly (15 to 25%), diffuse abdominal tenderness (5 to 30%), muscle tenderness (40 to 80%), meningeal signs (12 to 40%), disturbances in sensorium (50% of icteric cases), jaundice (10%), and a truncal rash that can be macular, urticarial, or purpuric (7 to 9%). Pretibial, raised, 1- to 5-cm erythematous lesions are seen characteristically in a form of leptospirosis called "Fort Bragg fever."

Classically, leptospirosis has been considered a biphasic illness, although many patients with mild disease will not have symptoms of the secondary "immune" phase of illness, and patients with very severe disease will have a relentless progression from onset of illness to jaundice, renal failure, hemorrhage, hypotension, and coma. Overall, about half the patients with leptospirosis will have a relapse. Typically 1 week after the initial fever resolves, fever, headache, and meningeal signs return. This immune phase of the illness can last several days to a month. A late complication is anterior uveitis, which may be seen in 10% of patients during and months to years after convalescence. Leptospirosis in pregnancy is associated with spontaneous abortion; children born with congenitally acquired leptospirosis have not been described to have congenital anomalies and have been treated successfully with antibiotics.

LABORATORY FEATURES. *Leptospira* can be cultured with special media from blood and CSF early in the illness, but incubation of the cultures for 5 to 6 weeks at 28 to 30° C is often required. Mild proteinuria is seen in most patients and may be accompanied by pyuria, casts, and microscopic hematuria. In patients with renal failure, the blood urea nitrogen level rarely exceeds 100 mg/dL and the creatinine concentration is usually less than 8 mg/dL. Liver function test results are usually abnormal only in icteric patients, where twofold to threefold elevations in aminotransferases and alkaline phosphatase are observed (lower than the elevations commonly seen in acute viral hepatitis), and a predominantly conjugated bilirubinemia is seen. Myositis with elevated serum creatine phosphokinase (MM band) occurs in about half of patients. Thrombocytopenia (usually $\geq 50,000/\mu L$), anemia, and leukocytosis are commonly seen. Thrombocytopenia is seen most commonly in patients with renal failure. CSF examination shows a pleocytosis (<500 cells/mm^3) with an early neutrophilic and late mononuclear cell predominance, a normal glucose level, and mildly elevated protein level (50 to 110 mg/dL). Chest radiographs were abnormal

in the majority of patients in one study, with small nodular densities showing a tendency to consolidate. First-degree atrioventricular block and changes consistent with acute pericarditis have been documented in one third of patients.

DIAGNOSIS. The presentation of the illness in anicteric cases is non-specific. It is important to search for an exposure history to animal urine in a patient with a flu-like illness, respiratory illness, aseptic meningitis, acute hepatitis, acute renal failure, pericarditis, atrioventricular block, or anterior uveitis. In some developing countries, leptospirosis is more common than hepatitis A as a cause of acute hepatitis. Useful means to distinguish icteric leptospirosis from acute viral hepatitis include the prominent myalgias, conjunctival suffusion, elevated serum creatine phosphokinase, and the only twofold to threefold elevations in aminotransferases seen in leptospirosis. The diagnosis is usually made retrospectively by a fourfold rise in agglutinating antibody titer. The microscopic agglutination test (MAT) detects serum antibodies against the 21 most common serovars of *Leptospira*. The MAT is the most reliable test and is available from the Centers for Disease Control and Prevention. Agglutinins characteristically appear within the first 1 to 2 weeks of illness and peak at 3 to 4 weeks. It is possible to grow the organism from blood and CSF collected during the first week of illness, but it may take 4 to 6 weeks for the cultures to be positive because the organism is so slow growing.

PROGNOSIS. Case fatality rates for leptospirosis are less than 1% in studies in which aggressive surveillance has been conducted (increasing the proportion of mild cases). The illness is usually self-limited. Liver and renal dysfunction are for the most part reversible, with return to normal function over 1 to 2 months. The mortality rate for icteric disease has been reported in different studies to be 2.4 to 11.3%, with deaths occurring secondary to renal failure, gastrointestinal and pulmonary hemorrhage, and the adult respiratory distress syndrome.

THERAPY AND PREVENTION. Antibiotic treatment is most beneficial when started within 4 days of illness; unfortunately, the diagnosis of leptospirosis is rarely made this rapidly. Doxycycline, 100 mg orally twice a day for 7 days, started within 48 hours of illness, decreased the duration of illness by 2 days in one study; penicillin at a dose of 2.4 to 3.6 million units per day also has been successful early treatment. A beneficial effect of antibiotic therapy later in disease course has not been uniformly seen. While a randomized, double-blinded trial of penicillin treatment (1.5 million units intravenously every 6 hours for 7 days) started on average 9 days into illness showed a decrease in fever duration from 11.6 to 4.7 days and in elevated serum creatinine level from 8.3 to 2.7 days, a second randomized trial of penicillin in patients with icteric leptospirosis and a median duration of illness of 1 week demonstrated no beneficial effect. Jarish-Herxheimer reactions (fever, rigors, hypotension, and tachycardia) rarely occur on initiation of antibiotic therapy. Supportive care and treatment of the hypotension, renal failure (including rehydration and dialysis), and hemorrhage, which can complicate leptospirosis, are crucial for a good outcome.

Immunization of animals is not necessarily effective at preventing human disease, because leptospiruria can still occur in immunized animals. Because asymptomatically infected wild animals can chronically excrete large numbers of spirochetes in their urine, controlling environmental sources of leptospirosis is difficult if not impossible. Occupationally exposed individuals (abattoir workers, veterinarians) should wear protective clothing to prevent exposure of skin and mucous membranes to potentially infected urine. Bodies of water associated with recreational exposures to leptospirosis may need to be placed off limits. Doxycycline, 200 mg orally once a week, has been 95% effective at preventing leptospirosis in U.S. troops undergoing training in the jungle warfare school in Panama and has a place in the short-term prevention of the disease in high-risk settings. No licensed vaccine is available in the United States for humans.

Regina C, Abdulkader RM: Acute renal failure in leptospirosis. Renal Failure 19:191, 1997. *Renal failure occurs in 15 to 69% of cases of leptospirosis and is characteristically non-oliguric and normokalemic or hypokalemic. Jaundice is present in almost all cases, and the many patients respond to rehydration.*

Vinetz JM, Glass GE, Flexner, CE et al: Sporadic urban leptospirosis. Ann Intern Med 125:794, 1996. *Three patients developed leptospirosis after percutaneous exposure to rat urine in Baltimore alleys.*

Zaki SR, Shieh WJ, Epidemic Working Group at the Ministry of Health in Nicaragua: Leptospirosis associated with outbreak of acute febrile illness and pulmonary haemorrhage, Nicaragua, 1995. Lancet 347:535, 1996. *After widespread flooding in Nicaragua an epidemic of leptospirosis affecting approximately 2000 people was associated with pulmonary hemorrhage.*

370 DISEASES CAUSED BY CHLAMYDIAE

Robert C. Brunham

Chlamydiae are obligate intracellular bacteria whose extreme biosynthetic defects in intermediate metabolism and energy generation cause them to be absolutely dependent on a host cell to grow and replicate. They are among the most common of all human infectious agents and produce much disability although little mortality.

CHLAMYDIAE AS ORGANISMS

Chlamydiae are a unique monophyletic bacterial phylum as defined by 16S rDNA sequences with an extremely ancient origin within the bacterial domain and are composed of four species (Table 370–1).

The chlamydial bacterial cell has a gram-negative cell wall structure consisting of an outer membrane and an inner cytoplasmic membrane. However, no peptidoglycan layer is found within the periplasmic space separating these two layers. The outer membrane is protein-rich, composed of a single major outer membrane protein (MOMP 40 kd) and two minor outer membrane proteins (60 and 12.5 kd). All three proteins are extraordinarily rich in the amino acid cysteine, and intermolecular and intramolecular disulfide bonding produces a supramolecular protein complex that confers structural rigidity on the bacterial cell analogous to the role played by peptidoglycan in other bacteria. Within *Chlamydia trachomatis*, MOMP variation determines the serologic types that characterize the individual serovars. As with other gram-negative bacteria, the chlamydial outer membrane also contains lipopolysaccharide (LPS). Chlamydial LPS is a rough type without O-saccharides and is composed of a trisaccharide of 3-deoxy-D-manno-octulosonic acid (KDO). Although the core KDO sequences are shared by LPS from many other gram-negative bacteria, the chlamydial LPS is unique because two of the three KDOs are bonded through a 2.8 instead of a 2.4 linkage. Thus, antibodies to chlamydial LPS are specific. Because all four species of chlamydiae share the same LPS structure, antibodies to chlamydial LPS are genus specific.

Chlamydiae share a common and distinctive growth cycle. Figure 370–1 shows the distinctive developmental cycle typical for all chlamydiae. The size of the chlamydial genome is small at 1042 kilobases, containing 894 protein coding genes. Most strains of chlamydiae also contain a 7-kilobase cryptic plasmid; some strains contain a 4 kilobase phage. Chlamydiae absolutely depend on host cells to obtain nutrients from the extracellular environment and convert them into forms they can use. In comparison with other bacteria, chlamydiae are virtually unique in being able to transport phosphorylated compounds found in the host cell cytoplasm, and this undoubtedly represents their premiere adaptation to the intracellular environment. Despite sharing many characteristics in cell architecture and in the developmental cycle, chlamydiae are surprisingly diverse at the DNA level. By DNA-DNA homology, the chlamydial species share less than 33% homology. Within each species, DNA-DNA homology varies between 14 and 95%.

CHLAMYDIAE AS PATHOGENS

Immune Responses

Depending on the species of chlamydiae, macrophage or non-macrophage host cells support the organisms' replication. Macrophages appear to be the principal target cell for *C. psittaci* and *C. trachomatis* lymphogranuloma venereum (LGV) biovars. Columnar epithelial cells found in mucous membranes are the usual host cells for trachoma biovar and for *C. pneumoniae* replication. Host cell trophism correlates with the type of inflammation elicited by chlamydiae. LGV biovar and *C. psittaci,* which infect macrophages, produce granulomatous inflammation characteristic of delayed hypersensitivity reactions. Trachoma biovar, which infects epithelial cells, produces neutrophilic exudate during acute infection and submucosal mononuclear infiltration with lymphoid follicle formation during later stages of infection.

Chlamydiae elicit both humoral and cellular immune responses. *C. trachomatis* elicits secretory IgA and circulatory IgM and IgG antibodies. Serum antibodies commonly recognize the chlamydial LPS as detected in the complement-fixation assay. *C. trachomatis* infection also elicits antibodies to the MOMP detected by the microimmunofluorescence assay. Women with reproductive sequelae such as tubal infertility or ectopic pregnancy due to *C. trachomatis* infection often have antibody responses to the heat shock protein 60 of chlamydiae.

Because chlamydiae produce intracellular infection, T cell–mediated immune responses are prominent. Both CD4 and CD8 T-cell responses occur. CD4 TH1 activation with interferon-gamma (IFN-γ) secretion correlates with immunity and CD4 TH2 activation correlates with persistent infection. CD8 T-cell responses are difficult to detect and their role in resistance is unclear.

PATHOGENESIS AND MECHANISM OF HOST INJURY

Most animal model studies of chlamydial infection demonstrate an acute self-limited course. However, case reports of human LGV biovar and *C. psittaci* infections that last 10 to 20 years and observations from a longitudinal follow-up study of untreated cervical *C. trachomatis* infection showing that infection can last 15 months or more suggest that chlamydiae also can produce chronic persistent infection. Chronic persistent infection or repeated episodes of acute infection appear to elicit the immune mechanisms that cause host injury. Infection of a previously exposed host results in an accelerated and intensified inflammatory response, and tissue destruction appears to be directly correlated with the intensity of inflammation. This is best elucidated for *C. trachomatis* ocular infection. Inflammatory and scarring (cicatricial) trachoma are diseases of reinfection, and the more intense the inflammatory response, the more prominent is the late fibrotic response. Thus, the mechanism for host injury with *C. trachomatis* infection is thought to be mediated by cellular immune responses.

CHLAMYDIAL DISEASES

Table 370–2 lists the most frequent chlamydial diseases.

Chlamydia trachomatis

The major diseases caused by *C. trachomatis* are trachoma produced by serovars A, B, Ba, and C, sexually and perinatally transmitted diseases caused by serovars D through K, and sexually transmitted lymphogranuloma venereum caused by serovars L₁, L₂, and L₃. Trachoma and lymphogranuloma venereum are essentially restricted to developing areas of the world, whereas sexually and perinatally transmitted chlamydial infections are distributed globally. Trachoma and sexually/perinatally transmitted chlamydial infections are restricted to the mucosal surfaces of the body, and lymphogranuloma venereum causes systemic infection, principally of the lymphoid system.

Table 370–1 ■ CLASSIFICATION OF BIOLOGIC VARIANTS (BIOVARS) AND SEROLOGIC VARIANTS (SEROVARS) OF THE GENUS *CHLAMYDIA*

	BIOVAR	SEROVAR
C. trachomatis	Trachoma	12
	Lymphogranuloma venereum	3
	Mouse pneumonitis	1
C. pneumoniae	TWAR	1
C. psittaci	Birds, mammals	Unknown, multiple
C. pecorum	Ruminants	Unknown, multiple

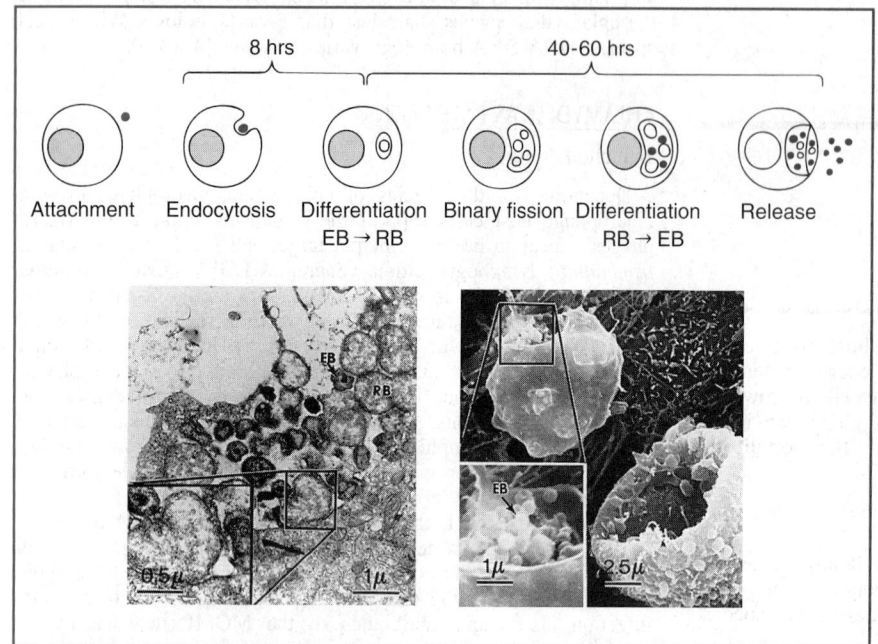

8 hrs   40-60 hrs

Attachment   Endocytosis   Differentiation   Binary fission   Differentiation   Release
                              EB → RB   RB → EB

FIGURE 370–1 ■ The top panel schematically shows the developmental cycle common to all chlamydiae. The red circles represent elementary bodies (EBs) and the open circles represent reticulate bodies (RBs). Chlamydiae infect eukaryotic cells through multiple attachment mechanisms, best understood for *C. trachomatis*. A trimolecular complex with a secreted heparan sulfate–like glycosaminogin synthesized by *C. trachomatis* acts as a bridge between ligands on the chlamydial EB and the eukaryotic cell surface. Different mechanisms exist among different chlamydial species and may explain their distinct trophism. After attachment, EBs enter the cell within a membrane-bound vacuole that remains unfused with lysosomes. EBs reorganize into RBs and asynchronously replicate 8 to 12 times with a doubling time of 2 to 3 hours. At the conclusion of the growth cycle, RB's differentiate back to EBs, and each inclusion yields 100 to 1000 new infectious EBs. The bottom left-hand panel is a transmission electron micrograph at 40 hours after infection showing the large RBs and the smaller EBs, which have a condensed nucleoid structure within their cytoplasm. The bottom right-hand panel is a scanning electron micrograph at 60 hours after infection showing a membrane-bound vacuole containing many EBs and apparently exiting from an infected HeLa cell.

TRACHOMA. EPIDEMIOLOGY. Trachoma is a distinctive ocular disease from infection by specific serovars of *C. trachomatis*. An estimated 150 million people worldwide are afflicted with trachoma, most of whom are young children. Trachoma is especially common in poor areas of sub-Saharan Africa. Trachoma is a major public health problem because 1 to 5% of infected individuals later develop scarring, which deforms the eyelid, causes inward turning of the eyelashes (entropion), and results in corneal abrasion (trichiasis). Corneal damage results in blindness. Trachoma is the most common preventable cause of blindness; an estimated 6 million people are blind as a result of trachoma. Most of these individuals are middle-aged and elderly adults. Active trachoma often first occurs within the first 1 to 2 years of life but after the first month. Recurrences of active disease are common during childhood and spontaneously cease by age 10 to 15. Among children, the frequency of face washing, access to water, sharing a sleeping room with an affected individual, and intensity of eye-seeking fly exposure are important risk factors for trachoma. Active trachoma also can occur in adults, especially in mothers caring for young children with active disease. Trichiasis is related to repeated intense trachoma episodes in childhood, is more common in women than in men, and preferentially occurs in families.

The *C. trachomatis* serovars that produce trachoma are spread by direct contact with contaminated fomites such as washcloths or eye-seeking flies. Perinatal exposure to *C. trachomatis* from maternal genital tract infection is not important in transmitting trachoma.

CLINICAL FEATURES. Trachoma is a chronic follicular conjunctivitis that causes macroscopically visible lymphoid follicles to form in the submucosa. These are especially apparent along the upper tarsal plate. The bulbar conjunctiva is minimally involved. Limited mucoid ocular discharge occurs; preauricular lymphadenopathy is rare and, if present, suggests other diagnoses such as adenovirus infection. The cornea may be involved with superficial vascularization and lymphocytic infiltration (pannus). Epidemic bacterial conjunctivitis due to *Haemophilus influenzae* can supervene on trachoma and cause a marked purulent conjunctivitis involving the bulbar conjunctiva. Bacterial conjunctivitis worsens the trachoma inflammatory damage. Tarsal conjunctival scarring deforms the eyelid structure and produces entropion and trichiasis in adulthood. Eventually, the corneal epithelium is eroded, and bacterial keratitis occurs. The cornea subsequently heals with opacification, resulting in blindness.

DIAGNOSIS. Trachoma is most often a clinical diagnosis and is made if two of the following findings are observed: lymphoid follicles along the upper tarsal plate, lymphoid follicles (or Herbert's pits) along the corneal limbus, linear conjunctival scarring, and corneal pannus. Because most cases of trachoma occur in remote areas of the developing world without access to laboratory testing, most cases are diagnosed clinically. When laboratories are available, isolating *C. trachomatis* in cell culture provides definitive proof of the diagnosis. Culture is most often positive in young children with active disease and is rarely positive in adults with late scarring disease. Even in young children with active disease, culture is positive in only one third to one half of cases. Nonculture tests such as the direct immunofluorescent detection of elementary bodies (EBs) with monoclonal antibody or detecting chlamydial antigen by enzyme-linked immunosorbent assay (ELISA) are more frequently positive than are cultures. Detecting chlamydial DNA by the polymerase chain reaction (PCR) is the most sensitive diagnostic test, with about 70 to 80% of children

Table 370–2 ■ MAJOR DISEASES CAUSED BY *CHLAMYDIA* AND CARDINAL EPIDEMIOLOGIC FEATURES

	DISEASE	HOST RESERVOIR	TRANSMISSION ROUTE	EPIDEMIOLOGIC PERIODICITY
C. trachomatis	Trachoma	Children	Fomites/flies	Endemic
	Urethritis/cervicitis	Sexually active teenagers and adults	Direct sexual contact	
	Epididymitis/salpingitis	Sexually active teenagers and adults	Direct sexual contact	
	Lymphogranuloma venereum	Sexually active teenagers and adults	Direct sexual contact	
	Inclusion conjunctivitis	Infected pregnant mothers	Direct perinatal contact	
	Infant pneumonia			
C. psittaci	Atypical pneumonia	Birds	Aerosol	Epidemic
	Culture-negative endocarditis			
C. pneumoniae	Bronchitis	Humans	Respiratory droplet	Epidemic and endemic
	Atypical pneumonia			

with active trachoma testing positive. Few adults with late cicatricial disease are found to have positive tests for chlamydial EBs, antigen, or DNA.

TREATMENT AND PREVENTION. Active trachoma in children can be treated with the topical ocular application of tetracycline or erythromycin ointment for 21 to 60 days. Because extraocular *C. trachomatis* infection of the nasopharynx and gastrointestinal tract is relatively common during childhood trachoma, oral antibiotics such as erythromycin may be preferred. Single-dose oral azithromycin (20 mg/kg) seems as effective as 6 weeks of topical tetracycline. Trichiasis can be alleviated by depilation.

The prevalence of trachoma in a community responds dramatically to socioeconomic development. Mass chemotherapy for young school-aged children has a temporary impact on trachoma prevalence. Control of fly exposure also assists in trachoma control. No vaccine is available.

SEXUALLY AND PERINATALLY TRANSMITTED CHLAMYDIAL INFECTIONS. EPIDEMIOLOGY. Currently, *C. trachomatis* is the most prevalent sexually transmitted bacterial infection in the United States. More than 4 million chlamydial infections occur annually, and prevalence rates are highest (>10%) among sexually active adolescent females. Prevalence is higher in inner-city areas among lower socioeconomic status individuals and among minority ethnic groups such as African-Americans in the United States and Native Americans in Canada. Importantly, although prevalence rates are higher in these subgroups, with few exceptions, prevalences are 5% or more irrespective of geographic region, urban location, or ethnicity. In the United States, the direct and indirect costs of chlamydial disease exceed $2.4 billion annually. From a global perspective, sexually transmitted chlamydial infections are a major cause of total disease burden and morbidity because of effects on the reproductive health of women and because they facilitate the transmission of human immunodeficiency virus.

CLINICAL FEATURES. Urethritis. *C. trachomatis* causes 30 to 40% of cases of non-gonococcal urethritis (NGU) in men, and an estimated 40 to 60% of urethral chlamydial infections are symptomatic with NGU. NGU is characterized by complaints of mild urethral discharge, urethral discomfort, and mild dysuria. On examination, a mild to moderate clear or cloudy urethral exudate can be detected. Often this is best observed in the morning before voiding. Sometimes, urethral discharge is apparent only on "milking" the urethra from the base of the penis to the glans. Gram stain of urethral exudate demonstrates 5 or more polymorphonuclear leukocytes per 1000× field and no gram-negative intracellular diplococci. Asymptomatic urethral infection is common with *C. trachomatis* infection and can be recognized by the urinary leukocyte esterase test on unspun first-void urine.

C. trachomatis urethral infection also occurs in women, in whom it produces the acute urethral syndrome. In such cases, the individual complains of dysuria, and pyuria (≥5 white blood cells per 1000× field) is found on urinalysis, but culture for uropathogens is negative. Urinary frequency and urgency are usually absent. Mild urethral exudate may be observed during pelvic examination when the urethra is compressed against the pubic ramus.

Epididymitis. In some men with urethral chlamydial infection (an estimated 1 to 3%), infection spreads from the urethra to the epididymis. This results in unilateral testicular pain, scrotal erythema and tenderness, or swelling over the epididymis. Epididymitis associated with urethritis is most commonly due to *C. trachomatis* or *Neisseria gonorrhoeae* (see Chapter 362). Among men younger than 35 years of age, *C. trachomatis* is the principal cause of epididymitis. Among men older than 35 years of age, complicated urinary tract infection with uropathogens is more commonly the cause of epididymitis.

Reiter's Syndrome. Reactive arthritis can complicate chlamydial infection (see Chapter 287). About 50% of men with non-diarrheal Reiter's syndrome have urethral *C. trachomatis* infection. It is estimated that approximately 1% of men with chlamydial urethritis develop Reiter's syndrome.

Mucopurulent Cervicitis. Mucopurulent cervicitis in women is the clinical counterpart of NGU in men. As with NGU, *C. trachomatis* causes 40 to 50% of cases of mucopurulent cervicitis. Twenty to fifty per cent of women with cervical chlamydial infection have mucopurulent cervicitis. Women with mucopurulent cervicitis may complain of mucoid vaginal discharge. Unless concurrent infection with other pathogens is present, the vaginal discharge lacks odor,

and vulvar pruritus does not occur. Mucopurulent cervicitis is best recognized during vaginal speculum examination with the cervix fully exposed and well illuminated. There is a yellow or cloudy mucoid discharge from the cervix, although the color may be better appreciated on the tip of a cotton swab than in situ. Gram stain of endocervical mucus shows more than 10 polymorphonuclear leukocytes per 1000× field. Often, a red area of columnar epithelium is visible on the face of the cervix (ectopy). The area is erythematous, is edematous, and bleeds easily when touched with a cotton-tipped swab.

Endometritis and Salpingitis. *C. trachomatis* infection can spread from the cervix to the endometrium to produce endometritis and to the fallopian tubes to produce salpingitis. Spread occurs in 10 to 40% of women with cervical chlamydial infection. If *C. trachomatis* spreads to the endometrium after therapeutic or postvaginal delivery, it can produce late onset postpartum or postabortal endometritis. More commonly, chlamydial infection spreads spontaneously to the upper reproductive tract. Although endometritis and salpingitis can occur subclinically, clinically patent disease includes the following features: subacute onset of low abdominal pain during menses or during the first 2 weeks of the menstrual cycle, pain on sexual intercourse (dyspareunia), and prolonged menses or intermenstrual vaginal bleeding. Fever is not a common feature of *C. trachomatis* endometritis or salpingitis.

Infant Inclusion Conjunctivitis and Pneumonia. Perinatally transmitted *C. trachomatis* infection is an important health problem for infants. Approximately, two of three infants perinatally exposed to *C. trachomatis* acquire infection. Clinically patent disease occurs in about 75% of infected infants, and 25% are subclinically infected. Inclusion conjunctivitis of the newborn develops in one in three exposed infants and a distinctive pneumonia syndrome in about one in six. Because 5 to 20% of pregnant women in the United States have *C. trachomatis* cervical infection, the morbidity due to perinatally transmitted chlamydial infection is substantial.

The distinctive pneumonia syndrome has a subacute onset in infants between ages 1 and 4 months. The natural history of illness is protracted, and, importantly, fever is absent. The cardinal clinical characteristic is a distinctive staccato cough reminiscent of pertussis but without the whoop or post-tussive vomiting. Hematologic examination consistently shows eosinophilia and hypergammaglobulinemia.

Lymphogranuloma Venereum. LGV is the result of sexually transmitted infection with *C. trachomatis* serovars L_1, L_2, or L_3. This is a systemic infection that involves lymphoid tissue. LGV is most common in sub-Saharan Africa, although accurate statistics are lacking. LGV is rare in the United States, with a few hundred cases reported annually.

The *C. trachomatis* serovars that produce LGV are much more invasive than are other *C. trachomatis* serovars. Similar to diseases due to other *C. trachomatis* serovars, LGV produces acute disease and late fibrotic complications. Among heterosexuals, primary LGV infection produces an evanescent and rarely observed genital ulcer 2 to 3 weeks after exposure. The ulcer spontaneously heals, and 2 to 4 weeks later painful bilateral inguinal lymphadenopathy develops, often associated with signs of systemic infection such as fever, headache, arthralgias, leukocytosis, and hypergammaglobulinemia. In the absence of treatment, LGV spontaneously heals, sometimes leaving lymphatic scarring. Late fibrotic complications of LGV include genital elephantiasis, strictures, and fistulas of the penis, urethra, and rectum.

In women and homosexual men, rectal infection with *C. trachomatis* L_1, L_2, or L_3 strains produces a severe febrile proctocolitis illness. Patients complain of frequent painful defecation (tenesmus) with urgency and, less commonly, mucopurulent bloody discharge in stool. Biopsy of rectal mucosa shows submucosal granulomas, crypt abscesses, and diffuse mononuclear cell inflammation. The clinical, endoscopic, and histopathologic findings can mimic Crohn's disease of the rectum.

LABORATORY DIAGNOSIS. Empirical treatment for *C. trachomatis* infection should be initiated when a specific chlamydial syndrome is recognized. However, definitive diagnosis of *C. trachomatis* infection depends on laboratory identification of the organism. Laboratory diagnosis confirms the clinical diagnosis, assists in managing contacts of infected cases, and detects asymptomatic but infectious individuals. Screening women for *C. trachomatis* has been demonstrated to reduce the incidence of acute salpingitis.

The gold standard for diagnosing *C. trachomatis* infection is isolating the organism in cell culture. The development of culture-independent technologies to identify *C. trachomatis* infection was an important advancement. Culture-independent tests detect (1) *C. trachomatis* EBs in mucosal exudate by fluorescent labeled monoclonal antibody, (2) antigen (mainly lipopolysaccharide) in extracted mucosal exudate by ELISA, (3) plasmid DNA by direct probing, and (4) chlamydial DNA by PCR amplification. The relative sensitivity of these tests is as follows: cell culture or PCR (capable of detecting a single EB) > LPS antigen detection by ELISA (lower limit of detection approximately 10^3 EBs) > chromosomal or plasmid DNA probe detection (lower limit of detection about 10^3 to 10^4 EBs). Because many chlamydial infections such as NGU, salpingitis, and trachoma are characterized by low numbers of organisms, amplification-based tests are preferred. At present, the higher costs of these tests will limit their widespread use, and antigen-based or probe-based tests remain the most commonly used tests. Interpreting a positive ELISA test for chlamydia antigen can be difficult in situations in which the prevalence of *C. trachomatis* is low (<5%) because such tests typically have false-positive rates of 1 to 3%. For example, when an antigen-ELISA has a specificity of 98%, has a sensitivity of 80%, and is used to screen 1000 individuals from a high-risk population with a *C. trachomatis* prevalence of 15%, the predictive value of a positive test is 88%. When the same test is used to screen 1000 individuals from a low-risk population with a *C. trachomatis* prevalence of 2%, the predictive value of positive tests falls to 44%. Clinicians should verify positive antigen-ELISA tests with a second *C. trachomatis* diagnostic test based on a different method if the risk of false-positive tests results in adverse medical, social, or psychological consequences.

Serology is infrequently used to diagnose *C. trachomatis* infection except in two circumstances: Specific *C. trachomatis* IgM antibody at a titer of 1:32 or more is useful to diagnose the infant pneumonia syndrome, and a complement-fixation antibody titer of 1:64 or more suggests LGV.

TREATMENT. *C. trachomatis* is uniformally susceptible to tetracyclines, macrolides, and sulfonamides. Recent data also suggest that selected quinolones (ofloxacin) are useful to treat *C. trachomatis* infection.

The recommended treatment for uncomplicated *C. trachomatis* urethritis and mucopurulent cervicitis is doxycycline (100 mg orally twice daily for 7 days) or azithromycin (1 g orally in a single dose), although azithromycin is substantially more expensive than doxycycline. Alternate treatment regimens include erythromycin base (500 mg orally four times a day for 7 days), or ofloxacin (300 mg orally twice daily for 7 days). *C. trachomatis* epididymitis and endometritis/salpingitis should be treated for 10 to 14 days. LGV should be treated for 3 weeks.

Sexual partners and parents of infants infected with *C. trachomatis* should be evaluated, tested, and empirically treated. Sexual contacts within the preceding 30 to 60 days should be seen.

Chlamydia pneumoniae

In 1986, a new chlamydial pathogen was recognized—*C. pneumoniae*—which causes respiratory illness. Although initially confused with *C. psittaci*, *C. pneumoniae* is a separate species with less than 10% DNA homology with the other three chlamydial species. Pneumonia and bronchitis are the most frequently identified illnesses caused by *C. pneumoniae*. Recent evidence suggests that *C. pneumoniae* may cause atherosclerosis.

EPIDEMIOLOGY. More than 50% of adults in the United States and from other developed countries are seropositive. Most seroconversion occurs during childhood with rates of 6 to 9% per year for the age group 5 to 14. Many seroconversions occur subclinically. *C. pneumoniae* causes both endemic and epidemic atypical pneumonia syndromes. In Seattle, the average annual endemic incidence of *C. pneumoniae* pneumonia was 1.2 per 1000 population. Approximately 10% of pneumonia illnesses were attributed to *C. pneumoniae*. Periods of increased incidence were observed at 3- to 4-year cycles. The bacteria also produces epidemics of atypical pneumonia in closed populations such as military recruits, univer-

sity students, and the institutionalized elderly. Case-to-case transmission appears to involve respiratory droplet spread with an average case-to-case interval of 1 month. Both diseased and asymptomatically infected individuals transmit infection.

CLINICAL FEATURES. Even though most acute infections occur in children, most *C. pneumoniae* disease occurs in adults, especially the elderly. It causes an afebrile, usually relative mild pneumonia. Extrapulmonary findings are not prominent. Non-productive cough with sore throat and hoarseness are characteristic. The time from onset of illness to clinic presentation is long. On auscultation, localized crackles are often heard. Chest radiography shows a pneumonitis, most often evident as a single subsegmental lesion. Hematologic studies show a normal leukocyte count but a high erythrocyte sedimentation rate.

C. pneumoniae also causes bronchitis and sinusitis. Bronchitis is often subacute in onset, lasting several days or weeks. Some patients with the bronchitis illness unexpectedly have pneumonia on radiography. Sinusitis is often demonstrated by sinus percussion tenderness. Isolated pharyngitis is rarely attributable to *C. pneumoniae* infection, but when pharyngitis, sinusitis, and bronchitis are observed in association with pneumonia, *C. pneumoniae* is a likely cause.

LABORATORY DIAGNOSIS. Serology, isolation, and non-culture detection are the primary methods for laboratory diagnosis of *C. pneumoniae* infection. The indirect microimmunofluorescent test for *C. pneumoniae* antibodies remains the best method for laboratory diagnosis. Isolating *C. pneumoniae* in cell culture (HL cell line) is successful in 50 to 75% cases of serologically confirmed infections but is technically demanding. PCR of *C. pneumoniae*–specific DNA is about 25% more sensitive than culture and likely will become the diagnostic test of choice. At present, no effective diagnostic method for *C. pneumoniae* is commercially available.

TREATMENT. *C. pneumoniae* is susceptible to tetracycline and macrolides but not sulfonamides. Antimicrobial therapy of *C. pneumoniae* infection can be difficult, and clinical response is not dramatic. Recommended treatment includes tetracycline or erythromycin base 500 mg orally four times a day for 10 to 14 days.

ASSOCIATION WITH ATHEROSCLEROSIS. Four lines of evidence suggest that *C. pneumoniae* may cause atherosclerosis and plaque instability. Seroepidemiologic studies have shown a constant excess prevalance of *C. pneumoniae* antibodies among atherosclerosis cases, compared with controls. *C. pneumoniae* has been isolated from atherosclerotic plaques on several occasions and has been identified in plaques by non-culture tests in over 50% of cases. *C. pneumoniae* infection in a rabbit model causes atherosclerosis. Two intervention trials have shown that antibiotic treatment substantially reduced coronary events among individuals presenting with ischemic heart disease. Additional large-scale antibiotic intervention trials are underway.

Chlamydia psittaci

EPIDEMIOLOGY. Strangely, *C. psittaci* is the least common but the only reportable chlamydial infection. This is so because it produces common-source outbreaks of serious disease often related to infected imported birds. *C. psittaci* is a heterogeneous chlamydial species that naturally infects a variety of non-human mammals and birds. *C. psittaci* strains appear to be host-specific, and most human psittacosis infections are linked to bird and not mammal exposure. One hundred to 200 cases of psittacosis are reported annually in the United States with no apparent periodicity. The annual incidence has been stable for the past 15 years. Psittacine birds (parrots, parakeets, budgerigars) are most commonly implicated as source contacts, although human cases have been traced to contact with pigeons, ducks, turkeys, chickens, and other birds. Among infected birds, *C. psittaci* is present in nasal and cloacal secretions, guano, and feathers. Psittacosis in birds is a mild illness manifested by ruffled feathers and anorexia. Recovered and asymptomatically infected birds can shed the organism for months.

Transmission to humans is by the aerosol route to the respiratory tract. The infectious inoculum is likely very small, and brief contact with a contaminated environment can result in transmission. Person-to-person spread of *C. psittaci* rarely occurs.

CLINICAL FEATURES. Psittacosis is a systemic infection of the reticuloendothelial system and of the interstitium and alveoli of the lung by *C. psittaci*. Seven to 14 days after aerosol exposure, an abrupt febrile illness begins with shaking chills and a fever as high as 40° C. Headache, myalgias, and arthralgias can be disabling. Cough appears early in the illness but is usually non-productive. Auscultation may be normal or show bilateral crackles. Chest radiograph shows single or multiple localized bronchopneumonic patches. Clinically, psittacosis can resemble legionnaires' disease. In distinction to *C. pneumoniae* pneumonia, psittacosis is more severe with high fever and absent or minimal upper respiratory complaints.

Extrapulmonary findings are usual with psittacosis, and myalgias can mislead the clinician to suspect meningitis or pyelonephritis. Fulminant psittacosis can produce meningoencephalitis, hepatitis, and a faint macular rash (Horder's spots) resembling the rose spots of typhoid fever. Like typhoid fever, psittacosis may cause abdominal pain, diarrhea, constipation, and splenomegaly. Occasional patients, especially with underlying valvular heart disease, develop endocarditis, and *C. psittaci* is a recognized, if rare, cause of culture-negative endocarditis. Untreated psittacosis can be fatal, but most patients recover slowly after an illness lasting 10 to 21 days.

LABORATORY DIAGNOSIS. The diagnosis can be established by isolating the organism in cell culture or by serology. Because laboratory-acquired *C. psittaci* infections are well documented, cell culture isolation is discouraged, and serology is the preferred test method. If culture is attempted, it is essential to contain the specimen in a biosafety cabinet for processing. Blood and respiratory secretions can be used to isolate the organism during acute disease. Psittacosis is most readily diagnosed by demonstrating a rising titer of complement-fixing antibody in the serum. Acute and 3- to 6-week convalescent sera should be tested.

TREATMENT. *C. psittaci* is susceptible to tetracyclines and macrolides but resistant to sulfonamides. Tetracycline has had the greatest clinical use. Psittacosis is the most gratifying of all chlamydial diseases to treat. Defervescence and marked symptomatic relief of systemic signs occur within 24 to 48 hours after starting tetracycline 500 mg four times a day. Treatment should be continued for 10 to 14 days.

PREVENTION. Epidemic psittacosis is a preventable disease by quarantining and giving all imported psittacine birds tetracycline. Preventing psittacosis acquired from non-psittacine birds is more problematic and will remain a continuing source for human infection. No vaccine is commercially available.

Danesh J, Collins R, Peto R: Chronic infections and coronary heart disease: Is there a link? Lancet 350:430, 1997. *A meta analysis of the role of C. pneumoniae in atherosclerosis concludes that the hypothesis remains plausible but unproven.*

Gurfinkel E, Bozovich G, Daroca A, et al, for the ROXIS Study Group: Randomised trial of roxithromycin in non–Q-wave coronary syndromes: ROXIS pilot study. Lancet 350:404, 1997. *A randomized intervention trial demonstrated that treatment with an antibiotic active against* C. pneumoniae *reduced subsequent coronary events by over 70%.*

Hackstadt T, Fischer ER, Scidmore MA, et al: Origins and functions of the chlamydial inclusion. Trends Microbiol 5:288, 1997. *A comprehensive review of the unique cell biology of chlamydiae.*

Scholes D, Stergachis A, Heidrich FE, et al: Prevention of pelvic inflammatory disease by screening for cervical chlamydial infection. N Engl J Med 334:1362, 1996. *A randomized clinical trial establishes that screening for cervical chlamydial infection reduced the risk of pelvic inflammatory disease by 56%.*

Stephens RS, Kalman S, Lammel C, et al. Genome sequence of an obligate intracellular pathogen of humans: Chlamydia trachomatis. Science 282–754, 1998. *The first publication of the entire genetic blueprint for a chlamydiae.*

371 RICKETTSIAL DISEASES

Richard B. Hornick

The rickettsiae are small obligate intracellular, gram-negative pathogens. They do not have a symbiotic relationship with human host cells, and therefore cause metabolic derangements that result in cell death. Infections with the typhus and spotted fever groups of rickettsiae involve endothelial cells. This host-pathogen interaction results in a perivasculitis. Q fever induces granulomas in the liver plus interstitial pneumonia. Ehrlichiosis is a relatively new human disease, and two species have been identified: the first, *Ehrlichia chaffeensis* invades human monocytes, and the other is identical to strains known to cause disease in dogs and horses—thus *E. equi/phagocytophilia*—and invades granulocytes. These diseases are called human monocytic ehrlichiosis (HME) and human granulocytic ehrlichiosis (HGE). Both are characterized by fever with leukopenia and thrombocytopenia.

Each of the rickettsiae is transmitted to humans by ticks, mites, lice, fleas, or aerosols originating from animal products (placentas, Q fever) or from feces of the aforementioned insects. In the United States, there are relatively few cases of rickettsial infections. Rocky Mountain spotted fever (RMSF) is the most prevalent, with 600 to 700 cases having been reported annually since 1985. Fewer cases of Q fever and murine typhus are identified each year. Certain other rickettsial infections are major public health problems in developing countries but are not found in the United States (e.g., scrub typhus). The potential for tourists to return to the United States with an emerging rickettsial infection is increasing. Because of the rarity of rickettsial infections in this country, diagnosis may be delayed. Delays in diagnosing these illnesses can adversely affect the potential for recovery.

In this chapter Tables 371–1 through 371–3 are included that summarize (1) the epidemiologic features of rickettsial infections; (2) the host cells involved in the pathogenesis of the clinical manifestations of the disease; and (3) those clinical features that will assist in differentiating the various forms of rickettsial infections. Additional details on the major rickettsial infections that occur in the United States or that represent potential threats to persons traveling abroad are found under separate sections in this chapter.

THE TYPHUS GROUP

This group of conditions includes three established clinical and epidemiologic entities: epidemic louse-borne typhus fever, the oldest disease known to be caused by rickettsiae; Brill-Zinsser disease, a classic example of reactivation of a latent infection; and flea-borne murine typhus. The first two conditions are induced by *Rickettsia prowazekii*, a pathogen transferred from person to person by the bite of body lice. Persons who have recovered from epidemic typhus have persistent rickettsiae in various host cells, presumably in the reticuloendothelial cells; stresses that cause a defect in the suppressive lymphocytes will, years later, permit these rickettsiae to be reactivated, resulting in a mild typhus-like illness, called Brill-Zinsser disease. In 1975, *R. prowazekii* was isolated from flying squirrels in the southeastern United States. A number of persons acquired typhus fever from squirrels living in their attics and probably harboring infected fleas or lice or both.

Flea-borne murine typhus, caused by *R. typhi*, is a mild form of typhus fever occurring in the U.S. and elsewhere. It is transmitted by fleas from rodents. *R. canada* is a tick-borne (mouse-rabbit reservoirs), rickettsial organism, formerly classified with the typhus group. It is distinct from the typhus, as well as the spotted fever group. Whether it is a significant human pathogen requires more study. It has been implicated by serologic means as the cause of acute febrile cerebrovasculitis in one patient.

Epidemic Louse-Borne Typhus

Synonyms include classic, historic, and European typhus; jail, war, camp, and ship fever; *Flichfieber* (German); *typhus exanthematique* (French); and *tifus exantematico* and *tabardillo* (Spanish). Many of these names indicate the location of the outbreaks—military and concentration camps, crowded ships with poor and starved immigrants, outbreaks in persons living in occupied countries during wartime, and so forth. Each implies crowded, unsanitary living conditions where bathing and laundry facilities are inadequate. These conditions allow for body lice to breed and propagate.

DEFINITION. Classic typhus fever is manifested by the sudden onset of headache, fever, rash, and an altered mental state. (Typhus is derived from the Greek word meaning cloudy or misty. Applied to typhus, it describes the obtunded, lethargic state of mind.) *R. prowazekii* is transmitted by human body lice (*Pediculus humanus humanus*).

ETIOLOGY. *R. prowazekii* is a small obligate intracellular, gram-negative bacillus. In cells it stains red when exposed to Gimenez's

Table 371–1 ■ SUMMARY OF SOME EPIDEMIOLOGIC FEATURES OF SELECTED RICKETTSIAL DISEASES OF HUMANS

DISEASE	ORAGNISM	ARTHROPOD VECTOR	RESERVOIR/ MAMMALIAN HOST	USUAL MODE OF TRANSMISSION TO HUMANS	COMMON OCCUPATIONAL OR ENVIRONMENTAL ASSOCIATION	GEOGRAPHIC DISTRIBUTION
Typhus group						
Murine typhus	*Rickettsia mooseri* (*R. typhi*)	Flea	Rodents	Infected flea feces into broken skin or aerosol to mucous membranes	Rat-infected premises (shops, warehouses, grain elevators)	Scattered foci, worldwide
Epidemic typhus	*R. prowazekii*	Body louse	Humans*	Infected crushed louse or feces into broken skin or aerosol to mucous membranes	Louse-infected human population with louse transfer	Worldwide
Brill-Zinsser disease	*R. prowazekii*	Recrudescence months to years after primary attack of louse-borne typhus			Unknown; stress	Worldwide
Spotted fever group (selected examples)						
Rocky Mountain spotted fever	*R. rickettsii*	Dog, wood ticks	Ticks/small mammas	Tick bite, mechanical transfer to mucous membranes, ?airborne	Tick-infested terrain, houses, dogs	Western hemisphere
Boutonneuse fever	*R. conorii*	Ixodid ticks	Ticks/rodents, dogs	Tick bite	Tick-infested terrain, houses, dogs	Mediterranean littoral, Africa, ?Indian subcontinent
Rickettsialpox	*R. akari*	Mouse mite	Mite/mice	Mouse mite bite	Unique mouse- and mite-infested premises (incinerators)	United States, former USSR, Korea, Central Africa
Scrub typhus						
Tsutsugamushi disease	*O. tsutsugamushi* (multiple serotypes)	Chigger	Chigger/?rodents	Chigger bite	Chigger-infested terrain; secondary scrub, grass airfields, golf courses	Asia, Australia, New Guinea, Pacific Islands
Q fever	*Coxiella burnetii*	?Ticks	Ticks/mammals	Inhalation of dried airborne infective material; ?tick bite	Domestic animals or products, dairies, lambing pens, slaughterhouses	Worldwide
Ehrlichiosis						
Human monocytic ehrlichiosis (HME)	*Ehrlichia chaffeensis*	Ticks	?Dogs	Tick bite	Tick-infected areas	At least 30 states in United States, Europe, and Africa
Human granulocytic ehrlichiosis (HGE)	*E. phagocytophilia/E. equi* group	Ticks/Ixodid	Ticks/Mammals	Tick bite	Tick-infested areas	At least 11 U.S. states and Europe

*Recent isolations of putative *R. prowazekii* from flying squirrels in the eastern United States have not been evaluated as reservoirs for human infection. Previous claims of involvement of domestic animals are now largely discounted.

stain. Viable rickettsiae stimulate the endothelial cell to act like a phagocyte to engulf the rickettsiae in a phagosome and internalize it. If rickettsiae do not break out of the phagosome promptly they begin to disintegrate, perhaps owing to enzymatic activities. The rickettsiae have an enzyme, phospholipase A, that enables them to lyse the phagosome wall and to multiply freely in the cytoplasm.

R. prowazekii escape from the cell by destroying it. The necrotic cell stimulates an inflammatory response that leads to the vasculitis and subsequent clotting abnormalities.

TRANSMISSION AND EPIDEMIOLOGY. The unique feature of infection with *R. prowazekii* is that no animal reservoir has been implicated, at least until its isolation from the flying squirrel (*Glau-*

371–2 ■ RICKETTSIA TARGET CELL RELATIONSHIPS AND PATHOLOGIC LESIONS OF HUMAN RICKETTSIOSES

DISEASE	TARGET CELL	HOST-CELL ASSOCIATION	BASIC LESION
Typhus group	Endothelial	Free intracytoplasmic	Vasculitis
Scrub typhus	Endothelial	Free intracytoplasmic	Vasculitis
Spotted fever group	Endothelial	Free intracytoplasmic and intranuclear	Vasculitis
Ehrlichiosis	Neutrophils/monocytes	Intracytoplasmic inclusion body (morulae)	Leukopenia, thrombocytopenia liver cell damage
Q fever	Reticuloendothelial	Intracytoplasmic vacuole	Granulomas

Adapted from Stickland (ed): Hunter's Tropical Medicine. Philadelphia, WB Saunders, 1984.

Table 371-3 ■ SOME CLINICAL FEATURES OF SELECTED RICKETTSIAL DISEASES

DISEASE	USUAL INCUBATION PERIOD (DAYS)	ESCHAR	RASH			USUAL DURATION OF DISEASE (DAYS)	USUAL SEVERITY*	FEVER AFTER CHEMOTHERAPY (HOURS)
			Onset, Day of Disease	Distribution	Type			
Typhus group								
Murine typhus	12 (8–16)	None	5–7	Trunk → extremities	Macular, maculopapular	12 (8–16)	Moderate	48–72
Epidemic typhus	12 (10–14)	None	5–7	Trunk → extremities	Macular, maculopapular	14 (10–18)	Severe	48–72
Brill-Zinsser Disease		None		Trunk → extremities	Macular	7–11	Relatively mild	48–72
Spotted Fever Group								
Rocky Mountain spotted fever	7 (13–12)	None	3–5	Extremities → trunk, face	Macular, maculopapular, petechial	16 (10–20)	Severe†	72
Boutonneuse fever	5–7	Often present	3–4	Trunk, soles, extremities, face, palms	Macular, maculopapular, petechial	10 (7–14)	Moderate	24–48
Rickettsialpox	?9–17	Often present	1–3	Trunk → face, extremities	Papulovesicular	7 (3–11)	Relatively mild	
Ehrlichiosis	7–21	None	?Rare	Unknown	Petechial	7 (3–19)	Moderate	72
Scrub typhus (tsutsugamushi disease)	1–12 (9–18)	Often present	4–6	Trunk → extremities	Macular, maculopapular	7 (3–11)	Relatively mild	
Q fever	10–19	None	None			(2–21)	Relatively mild‡	48 (occasionally slow)

*Severity can vary greatly.
†Untreated disease.
‡Occasionally subacute or chronic infections occur (e.g., hepatitis, endocarditis).

comys volans). It is still uncertain how significant the flying squirrel will be in amplifying the incidence of this disease. Very few, if any, cases of classic typhus occur each year in the United States (Centers for Disease Control and Prevention [CDC] does not have an active surveillance for it). Fifteen cases were reported in 1980 and 1981, all in persons having contact with flying squirrels.

Classic typhus is a disease of humans. An individual with rickettsemia can infect body lice. The lice acquire the organisms in their blood meal. These ectoparasites may then find another person to whom they transmit the rickettsiae via infected feces. Body lice do not survive the ingestion of rickettsiae. The organisms multiply in the gut of the louse, destroy the epithelial cells, and the louse dies (usually in 1 to 3 weeks). However, during the period of infetion, the louse passes feces heavily laden with rickettsiae. Either the human host scratches the site of the bite and thereby self-inoculates the rickettsiae, or the feces and rickettsiae contaminate minute apertures in the epidermis, allowing the organisms to find cells in which to multiply. Dried, contaminated feces can also become airborne (e.g., by shaking out clothing loaded with lice and feces and thereby creating an infectious aerosol). When inhaled, the rickettsiae can penetrate the mucosal cells and enter endothelial cells. Laboratory accidents frequently generate aerosols that induce infection in technicians. Nurses and other medical personnel are at risk for inhaling airborne particles when they remove the clothing from a patient.

When the body louse obtains a blood meal containing antibody-coated rickettsiae, the louse may modify the infectivity of the rickettsiae-antibody combination by partially digesting the antibody coating of the organism in its gut. This digestion destroys the Fc portion of the antibody that would have permitted attachment to macrophages. The rickettsia is then free of the inhibiting action of the antibody when it infects the next person.

The louse does not transmit *R. prowazekii* transovarially to offspring and is not an amplifier for further propagation. Patients who recover from classic typhus have the opportunity to develop Brill-Zinsser disease and at that time have rickettsemia and are able again to infect body lice. However, this happens rarely, for few cases of Brill-Zinsser disease have been detected among the many hundreds of thousands of soldiers who acquired typhus in World War II; one estimate suggested a rate of 10 per 100,000 cases of primary typhus. More cases may be recognized as the geriatric population continues to increase. This group will have significant illness, surgical procedures, and chemotherapy that could cause reactivation of the latent rickettsiae.

Typhus fever remains a threat to persons living under unsanitary and deprived circumstances. As long as there are persons who are latent reservoirs for *R. prowazekii,* an epidemic can erupt. One country with persistent typhus is Ethiopia. There, prolonged drought, poverty, and malnutrition contribute to the perpetuation of the disease.

PATHOLOGY. The rickettsiae invade only endothelial cells, as described in the section on RMSF. This leads to vasculitis, with differing pathologic changes in various organs. There is no eschar in this disease. The rash appears to have its origin in the leakage of blood and fluid from the damaged capillaries. The damage to the endothelial cells results in cell death, and at these sites platelet-fibrin thrombi form, platelet-active substances are released, and vaso-constriction and occlusion of small vessels occur. These changes can lead to infarcts in various organs, edema of tissue, leakage of inflammatory cells around small blood vessels ("typhus nodules" of the brain, for instance), stimulation of clotting mechanisms, and the development of shock. Almost all organs are involved in patients with untreated disease. The inflammatory exudate consists of mononuclear cells, plasma cells, histiocytes, and polymorphonuclear leukocytes. Gangrene of skin and limbs occurs in the presence of extensive thrombotic activity.

CLINICAL MANIFESTATIONS AND COURSE. The incubation period averages about 7 days but can range from 6 to 15 days. The onset is abrupt with intense headache, chills, fever, and myalgia. There is back or leg pain—presumably due to the muscle damage secondary to the vasculitis. Bites of lice may cause pruritus, and persons infested with lice may have numerous scratches in the skin. Sometimes the skin has a yellow-gold hue because of frequent lice bites. The headache is described as the "worst ever," and the pain is unremitting unless treated with narcotic analgesics. The temperature rises quickly during the first 2 days and persists for about 2 weeks, maintaining a continuous fever pattern if not altered by antibiotics or antipyretic medications. During the first week, there is a bradycardia relative to the temperature elevations of 39° to 41° C. Conjunctivae are injected, and photophobia is present. Deafness, tinnitus, and sometimes vertigo are prominent features. The patient appears to be in a toxic state, with a flushed face, obtundation, and profound weakness. There may be a cough, but no rales are apparent on auscultation of the lungs. The pharyngeal mucous lining is dry and inflamed.

The rash, characteristic of the typhus group, appears on the fourth to seventh day of disease. The lesions appear first on the trunk and axillary folds (areas of skin stress) and spread to the extremities but spare the palms and soles of the feet. The lesions are reddish-pink macules that fade on pressure. With treatment or in mild cases, the rash disappears within several days. In untreated patients, it can spread and coalesce, leading to gangrene of portions of the skin, especially over regions of bony prominences. In 5 to 10% of patients, the rash may not be present.

These and other manifestations occur because of the initial unchecked multiplication and spread of the rickettsiae, involving ever-enlarging segments of the endothelial surface. The resulting damage to the organs evolves because of the compromised circulation and the associated acute inflammatory responses. Whether rickettsial toxin or endotoxin contributes to the pathologic changes is still debated. Whatever processes are involved, certain organs are regularly involved: the skin, heart, kidneys, and skeletal muscle. In patients with severe disease, hypotension and renal failure portend a fatal outcome.

The altered mental status that occurs as the disease progresses (in untreated patients) is striking. The patient may progress from stupor to coma. The stupor may be interrupted by brief periods of delirium. Patients may have to be restrained to protect them from trauma. At this stage, lymphocytic pleocytosis of the cerebrospinal fluid (CSF) may be present. Despite the seriousness of the patient's condition, complete recovery can ensue. Cranial nerve lesions are common. There are also temporary mental aberrations.

Patients who have acquired typhus fever in the United States from flying squirrels have had signs and symptoms of the classic disease. The rash was noted in 8 of 15, and it was evanescent. Significant central nervous system involvement was reported in five patients; two had coma and three had confusion or delirium.

Death in untreated patients occurs between the 9th and 18th days. Recovery from the disease begins with a rapid lysis of fever after about 2 weeks of disease. When the fever disappears, mental function returns quickly. Recovery of a sense of well-being is protracted, owing to the need to counter the stresses of prolonged negative nitrogen balance, inanition, and loss of muscle mass.

Brill-Zinsser disease is manifested in a manner similar to classic typhus. All signs and symptoms are milder, presumably because the host has well-developed immune mechanisms that can regain control in a short time. Serologic studies in these patients demonstrate immunoglobulin G (IgG) rather than immunoglobulin M (IgM) antibodies. Occasionally, patients with unrecognized Brill-Zinsser disease die. An underlying disease or procedure may permit activation of the latent rickettsiae, and this combination can culminate in death. Reactivation has been noted after surgical procedures and the use of immunosuppressive drugs. In experimental animals that have recovered from the primary disease, isolation of rickettsiae at a future date is facilitated by steroid administration.

PROGNOSIS. The fatality rate in untreated groups of patients with classic typhus is 10 to 60%. Children usually have a mild illness with minimal risk of death. Patients older than age 60 have the highest mortality rate. Recovery is the rule with appropriate antibiotic treatment.

TREATMENT. *R. prowazekii* responds well to tetracycline and chloramphenicol antibiotics. Doxycycline, 200 mg as a single oral dose, is the treatment of choice. Tetracycline, 25 mg/kg/day in four doses, or chloramphenicol 50 mg/kg/day in four doses, is an effective alternative. Therapy should be continued for 2 to 3 days after the fever has defervesced. Most patients are afebrile within 48 to 72 hours and improve quickly from the debilitating headache or mental aberrations or both. Relapses occur in persons who are

treated early, on day 1 or 2 of illness. Such patients do not develop the required immune mechanisms to contain the proliferation of the residual rickettsiae. Furthermore, these antibiotics are rickettsiostatic and do not eradicate all of these intracellular parasites even when specific immune mechanisms are introduced. Recovery from disease without antibiotics also allows rickettsiae to remain in cells, later to be activated and cause Brill-Zinsser disease. In the severely ill patient, fluid therapy and proper nutrition are mandatory. Fortunately, antibiotic therapy has simplified the need for supportive care.

PREVENTION AND CONTROL. To prevent and control the spread of classic typhus, the body lice (and feces) associated with patients and their clothes must be destroyed. The clothing should be carefully placed in plastic bags and sealed and carefully removed only in the area where they are to be treated. Clothes that can sustain boiling are boiled, and the rest should be subjected to steam and dry heat. It is also possible to kill the lice (also the eggs present in seams and elsewhere—these eggs will hatch in a week) with insecticides. Lice now are generally resistant to 10% DDT (chlorophenothane) and 1% lindane dust. Malathion (1%) and 2% temefos (Abate) are effective in most areas. These dusts are applied to the fully clothed individual. This approach controls the acute outbreaks of disease when applied to all persons in the community. Long-time use of insecticides is not effective because resistance develops, because long-term compliance is difficult, and because the insecticides may adversely affect the ecology of the region. Control requires improvement of sanitary conditions and standards of living as well as health education.

Health personnel treating patients with classic typhus are at risk for acquiring the disease from lice picked up from the patients or their clothing. There is no risk of direct human-to-human transfer of the rickettsiae other than by aerosolized, dried, contaminated feces. Once the patient has been deloused, no isolation barriers are required.

No vaccine is available for preventing classic typhus.

Travelers to endemic areas are rarely at risk unless, for example, they work in camps for displaced persons or carry out relief work that brings them in contact with persons with lice. Decontaminating the clothing overnight with insecticides or wearing insect repellent-treated clothes provides some protection. Prophylactic doxycycline has been effective when given weekly to prevent scrub typhus and would be expected to be effective in preventing *R. prowazekii* infections. This drug should be used only for short periods, 2 to 4 weeks. It is important under these circumstances to monitor the temperature for 2 weeks at least, as the drug may have masked the initial infection and delayed the onset of symptoms. Re-treatment with doxycycline at the onset of the fever is curative.

Murine Thypus

DEFINITION. Murine typhus, a milder form of classic typhus, is caused by *Rickettsia typhi* and is transmitted from rodents to humans by means of the rat flea (*Xenopsylla cheopis*). A closely related new pathogen, ELB agent or *Rickettsia felis,* is isolated from cat fleas. It infects the tissues of opossums and can cause a clinical syndrome similar to murine typhus. Very few patients are infected by these organisms in the United States.

ETIOLOGY. *R. typhi* is a small gram-negative obligate intracellular pathogen. Like *R. prowazekii,* it can penetrate into endothelial cells by induced phagocytosis. Its disease potential resides in its ability to multiply in these cells, destroy them, and initiate a vasculitis. *R. typhi* is catalogued with the typhus group because it shares common antigens with *R. prowazekii* and *R. canada*. In addition, there is cross-immunity between *R. prowazekii* and *R. typhi* induced by infections. Despite these similarities, it is clear from DNA homology studies that the two are not closely related.

TRANSMISSION AND EPIDEMIOLOGY. *R. typhi* causes disease worldwide. Wherever there are large rodent populations, there is the potential for outbreaks. The rat as well as free ranging cats, dogs, and opossums serve as reservoirs of this disease. *Rattus rattus* and *Rattus norvegicus* are two species of rats that can sustain the *R. typhi,* serve as a source of rickettsiae for the rat flea, and have no obvious illness from carrying this human pathogen. The rat flea disseminates the infection not through its bite but by placing contaminated feces on the skin. These may be rubbed or scratched into the skin; they can be carried to the conjunctival sac or mucous membranes on the fingers, where the rickettsiae can invade; or they can be aerosolized after drying and cause infection if inhaled. In the flea, the rickettsiae multiply in the enterocytes in the gut, do not kill the flea, and continue to be shed in the feces for the life of the flea. Transovarial transmission of *R. typhi* occurs in the oriental rat flea.

Murine typhus is no longer a reportable disease to the CDC. The last report was in 1993 when 25 cases were noted. In the previous 10 years, the number ranged from 28 to 67 annually, with Texas and California having the highest numbers. Cases are probably under-reported. A dramatic drop occurred in the number of reported cases after the mid 1940s. In 1944 there were over 5400 cases. By 1954 there were 163. This decline was due to intensive efforts at rodent control. Most of the cases occur in the warmer months, when rat fleas are plentiful.

PATHOLOGY. Descriptions of the pathologic lesions in this disease are few because of the rarity of fatal cases. Because the rickettsiae are known to invade endothelial cells, the pathologic consequences should mimic those seen in other rickettsial infections. The reasons for the differences in virulence of these rickettsiae and the varying severity of illnesses produced are unknown.

CLINICAL MANIFESTATIONS AND COURSE. Headache, fever, and myalgia are the principal symptoms and signs. These appear after an incubation period of 1 to 2 weeks. A faint macular-papular pink-colored rash appears in about 80% of patients after 4 to 5 days of illness. It may be difficult to see in poor light. When present, it may be visible for 4 to 8 days before it gradually fades.

Rarely are there any significant complications of this infection, but because it is an infection of the endothelial cells, a vasculitis can cause widespread organ derangement. The patients, especially if older, are debilitated when not treated. They may remain febrile, with a temperature of 39 to 40° C for 2 weeks. This metabolic stress necessitates prolonged convalescence. Antibiotic therapy brings about a prompt recovery.

DIAGNOSIS. This disease has no distinguishing characteristics during the early days of symptoms. The rash appearing on the fourth or fifth day should alert the physician to the possibility of a rickettsial infection. The history of a possible exposure to areas where rats are known to exist (e.g., grain elevators, port facilities, and farm buildings) provides useful information. Flea bites, if seen early, are discrete and may have a central hemorrhagic punctum. The location and grouping of flea bites are important diagnostic features. They occur in covered parts of the body, in irregular groups of several to a dozen or more, in the region of the belt, shoulders, and hips, or on the legs.

Differentiating this disease from RMSF may be difficult. The rash of RMSF usually begins on the wrists and palms and on the soles of the feet and then extends to the skin of the thorax and abdomen. In murine typhus the lesions are on the skin of the chest and abdomen and rarely on the extremities. The history of a tick bite or exposure provides evidence for a clinical diagnosis of RMSF.

Serologic studies confirm the rickettsial infection. Weil-Felix OX-19 reaction is positive in most patients who have not received antibiotic treatment. This test, however, does not distinguish murine typhus from the spotted fever group of infections. The indirect immunofluorescent test can be used to identify *R. typhi* infections. However, because of the common antigens shared with *R. prowazekii*, the serum requires cross-absorption with special antigens from these two rickettsia strains. Isolating the organism is possible but should be done only in special laboratories where containment facilities are available.

PROGNOSIS AND TREATMENT. The mortality rate is less than 5% in untreated patients. Appropriate antibiotic treatment results in prompt cure, and the mortality rate is reduced almost to zero. Two deaths were reported between 1982 and 1991.

Tetracycline and chloramphenicol are effective for treating this rickettsial infection. A 5- to 7-day course of either is effective. The usual dosage of 25 mg/kg of tetracycline per day in four doses or chloramphenicol, 50 mg/kg/day in four doses, effects a prompt cure. The organisms are sensitive to these antibiotics. No resistant strains have been identified. Relapses do occur when antibiotics are administered early in the course of the illness. Re-treatment with the antibiotic of choice provides prompt response.

PREVENTION AND CONTROL. There is no vaccine to prevent this disease. Control of rats has been shown to be very effective.

When rat control programs are instituted, appropriate insecticides should be simultaneously used to prevent the fleas from seeking humans for feeding as the rat population is decreased.

ROCKY MOUNTAIN SPOTTED FEVER

SYNONYMS AND DEFINITION. RMSF is also known as *fiebre manchada* (Mexico), *fiebre petequial* (Colombia), and *febre maculosa* or São Paulo typhus (Brazil).

It is a sometimes fatal systemic infection manifested by fever, severe headache, rash, and other organ disease caused by the vasculitis induced by *Rickettsia rickettsii*. The organism is usually transmitted to humans from animal reservoirs by a tick bite.

ETIOLOGY. *R. rickettsii* organisms are small gram-negative coccobacillary bacteria that can grow only inside eukaryotic host cells. They cannot be isolated on cell-free culture media. In human infections the rickettsiae invade and multiply within endothelial cells of arteries and veins. Different strains of *R. rickettsii* vary in virulence in human as well as animal hosts. Mortality rates appear to be higher in Montana than on the Eastern seaboard. Attempts to correlate virulence with structural components in the polysaccharide portion of the cell wall have been unsuccessful.

DISTRIBUTION AND INCIDENCE. This disease was named for the geographic site of its original discovery; the causative agent was named for the discoverer, Howard T. Ricketts. By the 1940s the disease had become more common on the East Coast than in the West. The incidence rose sharply beginning in 1971 and peaked in 1981 at 0.53 per 100,000 population in the United States. In 1996 831 cases were reported, reversing a previous downward trend. (Fig. 371–1). Reasons for these fluctuations are unknown.

Serologic surveys in children and adults in North Carolina, the state with the highest number of reported cases, demonstrate that subclinical infections occur. Almost 20% of the children had OX-19 agglutination titers in the diagnostic range, and a smaller number had positive indirect fluorescent antibody titers, a more specific test. None of these children was previously diagnosed as having had RMSF.

TRANSMISSION AND EPIDEMIOLOGY. Ninety per cent of reported cases occur between April 1 and September 30, with two thirds in May, June, and July. Children and young adults account for about 40% of cases. Ninety per cent of patients give a history of a tick bite or attachment or of having been in a tick-infested area 14 days before onset of illness. Infected ticks are found in urban as well as rural areas. A park in New York City was the source of ticks that transmitted *R. rickettsii* to four children, one of whom died.

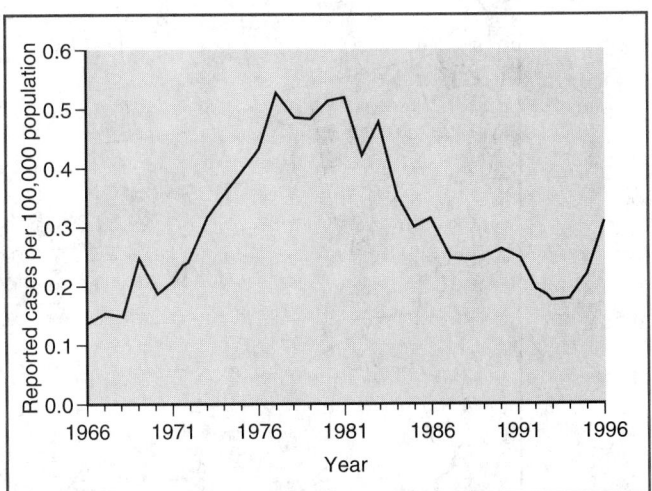

FIGURE 371–1 ■ ROCKY MOUNTAIN SPOTTED FEVER (RMSF)—by year, United States, 1966–1996. Increases in reported cases of Rocky Mountain spotted fever may reflect heightened awareness and surveillance for emerging tick-borne diseases (e.g., ehrlichiosis). Biological factors (e.g., increases in tick populations resulting from favorable environmental conditions) also could be involved in this resurgence.

RMSF occurs in humans when an infected tick bites and injects *R. rickettsii* into the skin. Probably fewer than 10 organisms injected intradermally are sufficient to induce disease.

Several species of ticks are commonly involved in transmission of disease: *Dermacentor andersoni,* the wood tick, in the Rocky Mountain states; *D. variabilis,* the dog tick, in the East and Oklahoma; *Amblyomma americanum* in Texas and Oklahoma; and *Rhipicephalus sanguineus* in Texas and Mexico. These ticks feed on small mammals such as ground squirrels and rabbits as well as on larger animals such as bear and deer. Dogs serve as a reservoir to infect ticks and then other animals or humans. Figure 371–2 shows the distribution of cases of RMSF by state in the United States in 1992.

Laboratory-acquired infections have occurred in persons exposed to droplets from accidental generation of aerosols from solutions of the organism. However, even in circumstances conducive to airborne transmission, person-to-person transmission does not occur. RMSF can also be acquired by the transfusion of contaminated blood.

PATHOLOGY. The basis of the pathologic changes in this disease, as in other rickettsial infections, is the inflammatory response stimulated by the irreparable damage of the endothelial cells. *R. rickettsia* invade these cells and multiply in the cytoplasm; they may penetrate the nucleus, and they penetrate into adjacent cells. This infectious process results in changes in the endoplasmic reticulum, the outer nuclear membrane, and the plasma membrane. Such changes are probably due to oxidant-mediated injury. In addition, studies using infected cultured human umbilical vein endothelial cells have demonstrated induced production of tissue factor (TF), an essential cofactor for Factor VII in the coagulation pathways. Also, plasminogen activator inhibitor 1 production is increased; these and other substances (e.g., platelet factors) can contribute to the development of thrombosis. In patients dying within 3 to 5 days of onset of disease, significant coagulation abnormalities are present. Microinfarcts result from occlusions of small vessels, and edema and hemorrhages occur secondary to increased permeability of the vasculature. Such lesions can be found in the heart, kidneys, adrenals, lungs, brain, skin, spleen, and subcutaneous tissues.

The rash is thought to result from the vasculitis and the associated permeability changes. Petechial lesions are caused by microhemorrhages secondary to the vasculitis and thrombocytopenia.

Patients with glucose-6-phosphate dehydrogenase (G6PD) deficiency appear to be prone to severe infections caused by *R. rickettsii* and other rickettsial agents. These patients have severe hemolytic reactions and significant thrombotic lesions in the glomeruli, resulting in oliguria.

CLINICAL MANIFESTATIONS. The incubation period of naturally acquired disease has a range of 2 to 14 days with an average of 7 days. The onset of disease in the typical case is sudden, with a severe headache, often retrobulbar in location, chills, fever, myalgia, malaise, nausea and vomiting, conjunctival injection, and photophobia. Tenderness may be present in large muscle groups. The duration of fever in untreated cases is about 2 weeks, but recovery from the debilitating effects of the disease requires several additional weeks.

Rash appears in 80 to 90% of patients—usually on the third or fourth day of fever, rarely after 5 or more days. It consists of pink macules, 2 to 5 mm, often noted first around the wrists and ankles. Lesions then spread to arms, chest, face, feet, and abdomen. Rarely does the rash involve the mucous membranes. Initially, these lesions blanch with pressure, but after 2 to 3 days they become fixed and turn dark red or purple and then slowly disappear during convalescence. The latter lesions represent microhemorrhages. Lesions on the palms and soles of the feet, in conjunction with the rash elsewhere, and petechial lesions in the skin folds of the axillae and around the ankles, constitute the classic distribution of the rash. Biopsy of the rash reveals perivascular round cell infiltration. Staining of the specimens of skin with fluorescent tagged antibodies to *R. rickettsii* shows the intracellular organisms.

In patients with unrecognized and inappropriately treated disease, the rash coalesces as the spread of the infectious process involves additional and larger vessels. This can result in large ischemic and gangrenous lesions. Especially susceptible is the skin of the tip of the nose, earlobes, digits, and scrotum. Involvement of the cooler portions of the body may reflect the optimal temperature for growth of *R. rickettsii* (32° C). Thrombosis of larger arteries can cause gangrene of a limb or hemiplegia. Patients with untreated disease may die of myocarditis and pulmonary edema.

The reported incidence of pulmonary abnormalities varies from 10 to 40% in large series of patients. Respiratory symptoms and signs as part of this illness have not been emphasized sufficiently.

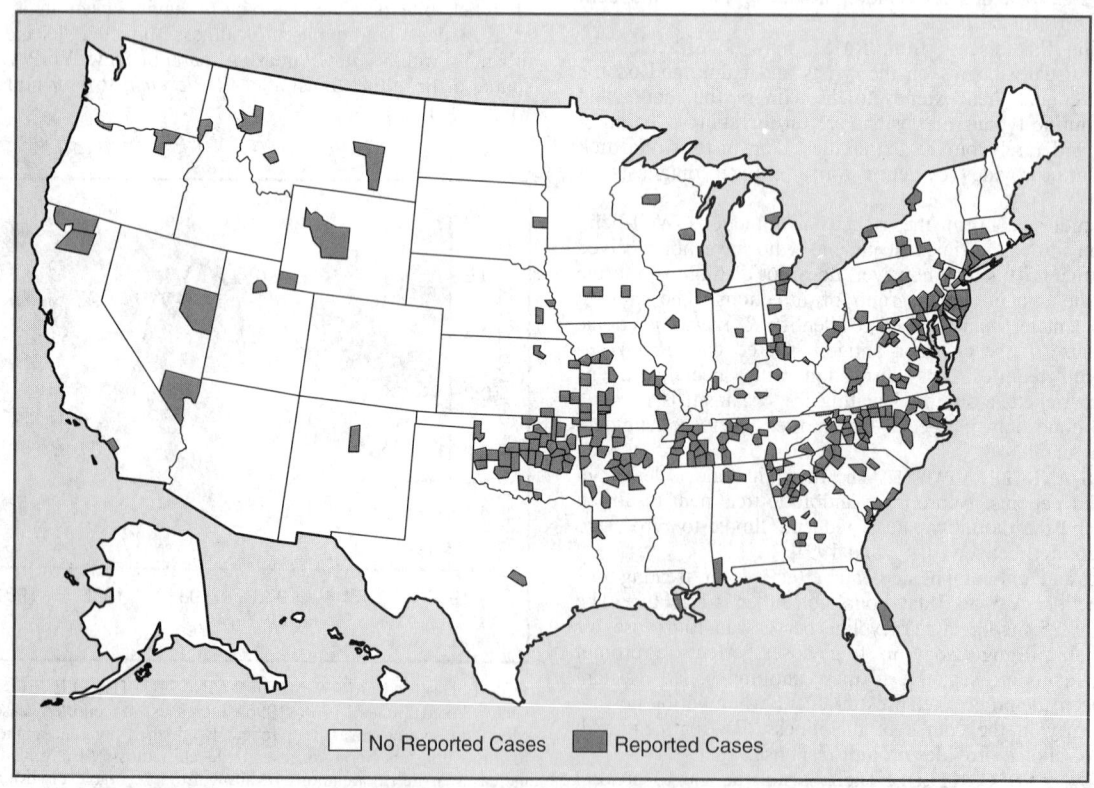

No Reported Cases   Reported Cases

FIGURE 371–2 ■ United States counties reporting cases of Rocky Mountain spotted fever, 1992.

In fact, after the spleen, the heaviest concentrations of rickettsiae can be demonstrated by fluorescent antibody staining in the endothelial cells of the pulmonary vasculature.

Edema of the brain and ring hemorrhages may cause delirium and stupor and ultimately lead to death. Fortunately, even though microinfarcts are probably common insults to the central nervous system during the acute disease, few patients, if appropriately treated, sustain permanent neurologic sequelae. Neuroimaging studies demonstrated infarctions, edema, meningeal enhancement, and prominent perivascular spaces in 4 of 44 computed tomographic scans and 4 of 6 magnetic resonance imaging studies. A magnetic resonance image of the spine was abnormal. However, clinical symptoms present in these patients returned to baseline in 67%. Ninety-three per cent of those with normal neuroimaging had complete resolution of their symptoms. One patient has been reported with the Guillain-Barré syndrome associated with RMSF.

DIAGNOSIS. The diagnosis of RMSF is difficult in the patient presenting with non-specific complaints such as sudden onset of fever, headache, myalgia, and malaise. A history of travel, camping, or outdoor recreational activities where tick exposure could occur and of recent tick bites is an especially important part of any work-up of a febrile patient during the warmer months. The patient complains of a severe headache, photophobia, and pain when moving the eyes. There is no meningismus. Lumbar puncture usually reveals normal CSF. Patients with stupor or coma may demonstrate elevated CSF protein and a few mononuclear cells. The presence of a faint, pink-colored rash on wrists and ankles should raise a suspicion of RMSF. The information that the rash appeared after the fever helps make the diagnosis.

A search for an attached tick should concentrate on the scalp and groin. Hard body ticks such as *D. andersoni* tend to remain attached for long periods. The finding of an engorged tick should settle the clinical diagnosis. There usually is no ulceration or scar from the tick bite.

Most patients have thrombocytopenia but not significant clotting abnormalities. In severe cases, disseminated intravascular coagulopathy (DIC) occurs with hypofibrinogenemia and prolonged prothrombin and partial thromboplastin times. Other laboratory studies are not helpful in making a diagnosis. The white blood cell count is usually normal.

RMSF is confirmed by immunofluorescence staining of tissue specimens and by serologic analyses. The detection by immunofluorescence of rickettsiae in tissues, such as skin or rash biopsies, is the one test that can provide the most rapid (4 to 6 hours) and early (day 3 to 4) diagnosis. The state health department should be contacted about the availability of this test.

Serologic tests do not provide rapid diagnostic confirmation. The Weil-Felix reaction uses the polysaccharide antigens of three *Proteus* strains (OX-19, OX-2, and OX-K) to agglutinate antibodies produced by a rickettsial infection. Serum specimens from patients with RMSF agglutinate OX-19 and OX-2 but not OX-K. The peak titer occurs at 2 to 3 weeks and then falls rapidly. Antibiotic treatment blunts the antibody response. The test is inexpensive; and with a fourfold or greater increase in titer of OX-19 or OX-2, or both, in paired specimens (drawn 2 weeks apart), confirmation is obtained. Indirect immunofluorescent antibody (IFA) testing is the most specific and sensitive serologic test available. It has replaced the complement fixation test and, in many laboratories, the Weil-Felix reaction. The IFA is now used in epidemiologic surveys because of the persistence of these antibodies compared with the short-lived antibodies demonstrated in the Weil-Felix reaction. A diagnostic rise (fourfold or greater) in titer also takes 2 to 3 weeks.

Differentiation of this disease from other infections is difficult without the history of a tick bite or the information about the fever preceding the rash. In children measles and atypical measles (in those who received killed vaccine) can mimic the early phase of RMSF illness. The location and type of lesions making up the rash, the presence of Koplik's spots, and a history of measles-like illness in close associates should permit a differentiation. Meningococcemia with meningitis usually produces petechiae or purpura, or both, in the patient earlier in the course of the disease than expected in all but rare patients with RMSF. Furthermore, the CSF indicates the septic nature of the meningitis caused by the meningococci.

PROGNOSIS. RMSF is a serious infectious disease that involves endothelial cells throughout the host. Prompt antibiotic therapy is necessary to assist cellular immune mechanisms to eliminate the pathogen. In some patients, the pathologic processes spread rapidly and cause irreversible damage, and death ensues within 3 to 5 days (fulminant disease). Certain risk factors correlate with severe diseases: presence of G6PD/A−, time of onset of specific antibiotic therapy, and old age. Patients with the classic form of RMSF who are untreated have a prolonged febrile illness lasting 2 to 3 weeks with many complications. The mortality rate in such patients is 20 to 30%, with the highest rate occurring in the elderly. Antibiotic treatment has lowered the mortality rate to 3%. Mortality rates increase when treatment is delayed. For patients in whom therapy is started within 4 days of onset of symptoms, death is three times less likely than for those who were treated at 5 or more days. Patients older than age 40 have a higher mortality risk than children and young adults. This is a serious disease requiring that patients be hospitalized and carefully monitored to detect changes in pulmonary findings and evidence of hypotension, oliguria, myocarditis, or increasing intracranial pressure.

TREATMENT. Prompt initiation of tetracycline or chloramphenicol therapy is mandatory to ensure optimal chances for recovery. Tetracycline (25 to 50 mg/kg/day), doxycycline (100 mg every 12 hours in adults), and chloramphenicol (50 mg/kg/day) are the drugs of choice. Usually the fever abates in 2 to 3 days, and concurrently a sense of well-being is restored. Antibiotic treatment can be discontinued 2 to 3 days thereafter. No instances of strains resistant to the tetracyclines or chloramphenicol have been reported. The third-generation cephalosporins or the aminoglycoside antibiotics have not been evaluated in RMSF. Evaluation of four aminoquinolone antibiotics in various infected tissue culture cell lines has revealed antibacterial activity equal to that of tetracyclines. Clinical evaluations are not available. Relapses after tetracycline or chloramphenicol treatment are uncommon.

PREVENTION AND CONTROL. Immunity to reinfection after recovery from RMSF appears to be complete. No naturally acquired second cases have been reported. There is no effective vaccine.

The best method for preventing disease is to avoid contact with ticks. Ticks are brushed off grass onto clothes or skin. Ticks usually remain stationary until the host is quiet. They then seek warm, dark areas and migrate to the groin or the scalp, where they can grasp hair shafts while inserting their mouth parts into the skin. Small barbs on each side of the mouth make it difficult to withdraw the whole tick from the skin while it is feeding; the mouth parts may remain embedded. Ticks should be searched for at the end of each day spent in tick-infested country and removed with forceps or tweezers. A drop of acetone or a lighted match brought close to the tick may ensure that the tick withdraws its mouth parts. The tick should not be removed with exposed fingers because a tick crushed between the fingers may induce disease. Prophylactic antibiotics are not indicated for persons with known tick bites. They should be advised concerning the usual incubation period and urged to watch for development of fever or headache. Oral temperature should be recorded twice a day for 2 weeks. On elevation, medical attention should be obtained promptly. Therapy begun before the onset of fever could result in a prolongation of the incubation period.

OTHER TICK-BORNE RICKETTSIOSES

DEFINITIONS. Mediterranean spotted fever (MSF), also known as North African tick typhus, Kenya tick-bite fever, Indian tick typhus, and boutonneuse fever, is caused by *Rickettsia conorii*. A second disease, called North Asian tick-borne rickettsiosis, is induced by *R. siberica*. A third tick-borne rickettsial infection, called Queensland tick typhus, is caused by *R. australis*. The disease produced by these agents consists of headache, fever, rash, myalgia, and malaise. The rickettsiae induce disease by invading endothelial cells and producing a vasculitis. Outcome is usually favorable. The illnesses are mild compared with RMSF. One other difference is the usual presence of a depressed black ulcer—the site of the tick bite. This is the *tache noire,* or eschar, and has been likened to a cigarette burn.

ETIOLOGY, DISTRIBUTION, AND EPIDEMIOLOGY. MSF occurs in countries bordering the Mediterranean Sea, but also in the

Middle East, India, and Pakistan. Several species of ticks are involved. The brown dog tick. *Rhipicephalus sanguineus,* is the main vector, but ticks common to wild animals transmit *Rickettsia conorii* in African countries. Italian epidemiologists have demonstrated a dramatic increase in the incidence of this disease in Italy, Spain, and Israel. The assumption is that the suburbanization of cities and towns resulted in increased opportunities for humans to contact ticks.

The distribution of *R. siberica* extends from European Russia through Siberia to the Soviet Far East and south into the Indo-Pakistan subcontinent. Several species of hard, or ixodid, body ticks appear to be the vectors: *Haemaphysalis concinna, Dermacentor sylvarum,* and *D. nuttallii.* Transovarian transmission occurs in these three naturally infected ticks.

Queensland tick typhus is one of several rickettsial infections found in Australia. The *R. australis* is carried by the tick *Ixodes holocyclus,* and marsupial animals are among known animal reservoirs.

PATHOLOGY. These three rickettsiae are very similar to *R. rickettsii.* There is more than 90% homology by DNA hybridization between the latter strain and *R. conorii.* All share group-specific antigens but have species-specific antigens as well that allow for their identification. These strains invade endothelial cells and cause cell death, resulting in a vasculitis (see earlier). Each of these three strains produces an eschar at the site of the tick bite.

SYMPTOMS, LABORATORY FINDINGS, AND DIAGNOSIS. The onset of disease caused by each of these three rickettsiae is sudden and characterized by fever, headache, malaise, myalgia, and conjunctival injection. These symptoms and signs appear 5 to 7 days after the tick bite. The eschar is the distinguishing sign that confirms the diagnosis. It should be looked for in the scalp, axillae, and groin area, regions of the body favored by ticks. Because of the necrotic nature of the eschar, lymph nodes draining the region of the eschar are enlarged. The lesion has been appropriately likened to a cigarette burn, 2 to 5 mm in diameter with a black center and a raised, erythematous rim. The lesion is only mildly tender.

As with RMSF, a generalized rash appears on the fourth to fifth day, including the palms and soles of the feet. The faint pink macular-papular lesions represent small hemorrhages into the skin. The duration of the disease is about 2 weeks. Death is unusual.

The Weil-Felix reaction demonstrates agglutinating antibodies to OX-19 antigen in most patients; these appear in the second to third week of disease. The microimmunofluorescence test for antibodies to *R. conorii* is the serologic test of choice, if available.

A skin biopsy stained with immunofluorescent antibody stain is the most rapid and earliest diagnostic procedure. This is indicated only when the diagnosis of spotted fever is suspected and an eschar is not present.

TREATMENT AND PROPHYLAXIS. Excellent outcomes are reported in patients receiving 200 mg of doxycycline every 12 hours for two doses. Tetracycline, chloramphenicol, and rifamycin can be used. Defervescence occurs over 2 days.

Tick bites should be avoided. Travelers into wild game country of Africa should check their clothes and skin carefully for ticks. Tourists traveling to southern European countries should search for ticks if they go hiking through suburban and rural areas during the spring and summer months.

Recovery from these rickettsial infections imparts solid immunity. In experimental animals *R. conorii* is relatively avirulent compared with most strains of *R. rickettsii.* However, animals recovered from infections with the former strain are protected against challenge with virulent *R. rickettsii.* This protection is mediated by T lymphocytes that recognize antigens on other species of rickettsial agents of the spotted fever group.

HUMAN EHRLICHIOSIS (SPOTLESS ROCKY MOUNTAIN SPOTTED FEVER). The first reported case of infection with a species of *Ehrlichia* in the United States occurred in 1986. A patient was found to have intracytoplasmic inclusions (morula) in monocytes and subsequently had an antibody rise to *E. canis.* This organism is known to cause severe pancytopenia in dogs. It is one of four species known to infect animals—*E. canis, E. equi, E. risticii,* and *E. phagocytophilia.* An additional species, *E. sennetsu,* was isolated from a patient in Japan in 1954, who had an infectious mononucleosis–like syndrome. This strain has not been iden-

tified outside the Far East. In the United States since 1986, many investigators tried to isolate *E. canis* or a similar strain from patients with clinical and serologic evidence of ehrlichiosis. In 1990, the first isolation was made on a continuous cell line of canine macrophage cells using blood drawn from a patient with a 3-day history of fever, headache, pharyngitis, nausea, and vomiting. This isolate was named *E. chaffeensis* because the patient was an Army reservist stationed at Ft. Chaffee, Arkansas. This strain is different from but closely related to *E. canis* and is now used as the antigen for serologic studies. Patients suspected of having ehrlichiosis, but with no antibodies when tested with *E. canis,* do have antibodies to this human isolate. The organism can be stained in circulating monocytes, thus the disease is called human monocytic ehrlichiosis (HME). The organisms are found in the cytoplasm as a clump (0.2 to 1.5 μm) enclosed in a membrane; this mass is the morula (mulberry-like). These organisms have been found in *D. variabilis* ticks, one of the same tick species that transmits *R. rickettsii.* Most cases have been identified in Oklahoma, Missouri, and Arkansas—states in which RMSF is common.

In 1994 another *Ehrlichia* species was associated with human disease. Infection with this agent was confirmed in 12 patients in Wisconsin and Minnesota by serologic studies (IFA and/or polymerase chain reaction [PCR]). Two of the patients died of infection. This strain was cultured in 1996 in a human promyelocyte leukemia cell line. It is different from *E. chaffeensis,* as demonstrated by various serologic studies, and is closely related to the *E. equi/E. phagocytophilia* group. *Ixodes scapularis (Ixodes dammini)* ticks are the common vectors for human granulocytic ehrlichiosis (HGE). These ticks also transmit *Borrelia burgdorferi* and *Babesia microti.* Coinfection in patients with two of these three agents have been demonstrated. Serologic studies of serum samples from small mammals (mice, voles, shrews, and chipmunks) confirm the source for colonization of ticks. The unique feature of infection with this strain is the location of the morulae. They are found in granulocytes in the circulation and in the bone marrow, hence the name.

The clinical symptoms of both forms of ehrlichiosis are similar and can be difficult to distinguish from those found in patients with RMSF. Fever, chills, myalgias, headaches are common. Nausea, vomiting, and asthenia add to the patient's discomfort. The physical examination usually is non-revealing. Rash has been reported in about 20% of patients with HME but not in those with HGE. The rash has been described with a variety of lesions—macular or papular or both, petechial or erythematous. It is seen most frequently on the thorax, legs, and arms. The rash appears after the onset of symptoms; the median day of onset was 5 days in a series of 212 patients. Striking laboratory values are leukopenia, thrombocytopenia, and abnormal results of liver function tests. The alanine aminotransferase (ALT) and aspartate aminotransferase (AST) values peak at the end of the first week of illness. The platelet count drops to its lowest level at about the same time. The leukocyte count falls quicker, within the first 3 to 5 days of disease. The presence of the morula in lymphocytes and monocytes (HME) and in granulocytes (HGE) is a significant laboratory diagnostic clue. This finding needs to be identified by skilled observers.

The severity of the clinical illnesses ranges from mild to fatal. Patients with HGE may develop postinfectious peripheral neuropathy (e.g., brachial plexopathy). Severe central nervous system disease can occur with both strains. Serologic evidence exists to indicate that more infections with *E. chaffeensis* are asymptomatic than those requiring medical attention. The PCR assay is now available at the CDC for precise diagnosis; when widely available it will provide a rapid diagnostic test.

Elderly patients are most prone to acquire the disease and to have the most severe illnesses. In the few patients who have died, the diagnosis was usually made late in the course of the disease. Therefore, there was a delay in onset of specific therapy, and frequently life-threatening complications were seen with severe infections (e.g., renal failure, meningitis, coma, DIC). The rapid appearance of pancytopenia in the sick patients has been postulated to be due to bone marrow hypoplasia, but more recent investigations point to sequestration or destruction of various blood elements (the hemophagocytic syndrome) as the most likely explanation.

The diagnosis of ehrlichiosis is based on epidemiologic information regarding possible tick exposure in areas where the tick-borne diseases are present, plus the aforementioned clinical and laboratory features. This febrile illness needs to be differentiated from Colorado tick fever and Lyme disease (see Chapter 368). The geographic location of the patient helps determine the possibility of Colorado tick fever. Differential features of Lyme disease include the classic erythema migrans lesion and the usual lack of leukopenia and thrombocytopenia. In the small percentage of patients with a rash more typical of RMSF, a mistaken diagnosis of RMSF is possible. Confusion with *R. rickettsii* disease is not a serious clinical management problem if the patient is treated with a tetracycline antibiotic or chloramphenicol. Failure to consider either disease and administer appropriate therapy can lead to serious consequences for the patient. Prompt antibiotic treatment needs repeated emphasis because delay is associated with the poorest prognosis.

Treatment of patients infected with either of the known strains of *Ehrlichia* requires doxycycline (100 mg every 12 hours for the first day and 100 mg once daily for at least 3 days after the fever abates). Tetracycline (500 mg once daily) can also be used. With early therapy the febrile course is short. Ciprofloxacin, ofloxacin, and trovafloxacin were bactericidal against HGE in tissue culture systems. They and rifampin may be useful when tetracycline cannot be used. Heparin therapy is not recommended because the pancytopenia disappears promptly as the disease is brought under control with antibiotics.

RICKETTSIALPOX

DEFINITION. Rickettsialpox is a rare mite-borne infectious disease caused by *Rickettsia akari*. This mild, self-limited illness consists of headache, fever, an eschar at the site of the mite bite, and a papulovesicular rash.

ETIOLOGY. *R. akari* is classified with the spotted fever group of rickettsiae. It is a small, gram-negative, coccobacillus-shaped, obligate intracellular organism.

DISTRIBUTION AND INCIDENCE. Rickettsialpox was first described in 1946. In the subsequent few years, more than 500 cases were diagnosed, primarily in New York City. Since the early 1950s, only one outbreak has occurred, again in New York City. The disease is virtually unknown throughout the rest of the United States.

TRANSMISSION AND EPIDEMIOLOGY. The original description included *R. akari* isolated from persons with the disease, from mites *(Allodermanyssus sanguineus)* that feed on rodents, and from house mice *(Mus musculus)*. Engorged mites were occasionally found on the mice; attachment was usually around the rump. The mites remain in the nest, where access to mice is readily available. Human intrusion into this animal-ectoparasite cycle can result in an infected mite's biting and inducing disease. The ecologic range of *A. sanguineus* covers most of the United States, and mice are ubiquitous animals. Thus the elements for potential epidemics exist. Isolated cases may develop from unusual exposure to mice, as in persons working in landfills or in homeless persons sleeping in abandoned buildings.

Rickettsialpox is fairly common in some urban areas of Ukraine, where rats appear to be the animal reservoir. In Korea, small field mice are infected.

PATHOLOGY. The known pathologic changes are limited to the skin, because this is a non-fatal infection. Histologic examination of the eschar (site of mite bite) reveals intense inflammation with necrosis. Other findings are similar to those in RMSF: thrombosis and necrosis of capillaries, edema, and a monocytic perivascular infiltrate. The characteristic rash in this disease is papulovesicular. The lesions contain fluid that may yield *R. akari* on culture.

CLINICAL MANIFESTATIONS AND COURSE. The bite of the mite is not painful and goes unnoticed. This site undergoes a localized inflammatory reaction over the next week to 10 days. During this time the edema and cellular components of the reaction create a slowly enlarging, firm, erythematous papule, which may reach 1 to 1.5 cm in diameter. The involved skin separates gradually, creating a vesicle that finally breaks down to form an ulcer. The base of the ulcer is usually black and is surrounded by a rim of erythematous skin. This progression occurs over 3 to 7 days, at the end of which there is the sudden onset of fever, chills, sweats, headache, backache, and malaise. The lymph nodes draining the area of the eschar enlarge but are non-tender. These symptoms and signs may be present for a week if no specific antibiotic treatment is administered.

As with other members of the spotted fever group, a rash appears after 2 to 3 days of illness. Initially the lesions are maculopapular, few in number, and distributed mostly on the trunk and abdomen, rarely involving the palms or soles. The lesions evolve quickly and uniformly into vesicular lesions; the vesicle appears to sit on top of an erythematous papule. These lesions persist for about a week; the fluid in the vesicle is slowly absorbed, and a scab forms, which leaves a brownish discoloration in the skin after it falls off. This gradually clears without leaving a scar. There is no significant internal organ involvement.

DIAGNOSIS. The diagnosis is made by clinical observation; the unique lesions of the rash, the presence of the eschar, and a history that suggests contact with rodents in the past 2 weeks provide sufficient evidence to make the diagnosis. Serologic studies confirm the diagnosis; complement-fixing antibody titers have been the standard, but indirect immunofluorescent antibodies are more specific, when available. Confusion exists regarding whether the Weil-Felix reaction can be used to diagnose rickettsialpox. In about 10% of patients in small series, significant titer rises to OX-19 and OX-2 have been observed. The test lacks sensitivity for confirming the diagnosis. The organism can be isolated from the vesicular fluid or from clotted blood specimens. These materials must be injected into animals or embryonated eggs. Laboratory tests are of no diagnostic help, although leukopenia is common.

The rash may be confused with the lesions of chickenpox, but no eschar is present in chickenpox (see Chapter 383). In addition, the lesions of chickenpox are usually in various stages of maturity, whereas the character of those in rickettsialpox is more uniform. Finally, the vesicle of rickettsialpox appears to sit on a papule, whereas those of chickenpox lack such a base.

PROGNOSIS AND TREATMENT. Rickettsialpox is a benign illness, and recovery occurs without therapy.

Treatment with tetracycline or doxycycline shortens the febrile period and hastens recovery. Antibiotic treatment need only be administered for 3 to 4 days to ensure a cure. No relapse will occur.

PREVENTION AND CONTROL. Rickettsialpox is a zoonosis involving a common house pest, the mouse. Control of this reservoir through elimination of mouse harborages and use of residual acaricides to walls adjacent to mice-infested areas should control mite populations. There is no available vaccine.

SCRUB TYPHUS

DEFINITION. Scrub typhus is an acute febrile illness caused by *Orientia tsutsugamushi* (formerly *Rickettsia*) from the Japanese: *tsutsuga,* "dangerous"; *mushi,* "bug"). This rickettsia is inoculated into humans during the bite by a chigger. The site of the bite develops into an eschar.

ETIOLOGY. *O. tsutsugamushi* is a small gram-negative, obligate intracellular organism. Unlike other rickettsial infections, infection with *O. tsutsugamushi* does not induce solid protection against additional bouts of scrub typhus. This results from the variable antigenic compositions of the strains.

This is the only rickettsia whose polysaccharides bear an antigenic relationship to *Proteus* OX-K. This *Proteus* strain is used in serologic tests to confirm scrub typhus.

DISTRIBUTION. This disease occurs almost exclusively in the large triangular region extending from the northern islands of Japan southwest to Australia and southeast to the South Pacific Islands. This region contains the larval form of mites that are both vector and reservoir of rickettsiae.

TRANSMISSION AND EPIDEMIOLOGY. *O. tsutsugamushi* is transmitted to humans by the bite of the larva of trombiculid mites (chiggers). Chiggers are the only stage in the life cycle of these mites *(Leptotrombidium deliensis* and others) that can feed on humans. Chiggers are almost microscopic, often brilliantly colored (red bugs). The chiggers feed on rats and other small rodents. The word "scrub" was applied because of the type of vegetation—transitional between forests and clearings—that maintains the chigger-mammal relationship. But other regions (e.g., semiarid, sandy beaches) also support rodents and mites. Humans encounter scrub typhus when they enter such areas to build roads, to clear fields or forests, or on military expeditions. Circumscribed regions are highly endemic, a reflection of the lack of mobility of the chiggers and their rodent hosts. Mites transmit the rickettsiae to their offspring through the ova. Therefore, they can serve as vector and reservoir of the etiologic agent.

This disease has been called river or flood fever because of the increased incidence during the rainy seasons. Chiggers and mites proliferate in warm, wet environments.

PATHOLOGY. *O. tsutsugamushi* invades endothelial cells to produce a vasculitis. The serious pathologic manifestations in untreated patients are predominantly myocarditis, meningoencephalitis, and pneumonitis. Coagulopathy develops but is less severe than in RMSF or typhus.

The site of the chigger bite develops into a papular lesion that ulcerates to form an eschar. This is associated with regional and later generalized lymphadenopathy.

CLINICAL MANIFESTATIONS AND COURSE. The incubation period for development of the primary papular lesion ranges from 6 to 18 days. This lesion can occur anywhere on the body. It enlarges, undergoes central necrosis, and crusts to form the eschar. As the eschar matures, the patient has the sudden onset of headache, fever, chills, and malaise. Over the next several days, these symptoms increase in severity with further elevation of the temperature. The patient, if untreated, may become stuporous as meningoencephalitis develops. Signs of cardiac dysfunction, including minor electrocardiographic abnormalities such as first-degree heart block and inverted T waves, can appear. The rash of scrub typhus appears at the end of the first week of disease. This is a faint, pink maculopapular rash appearing first on the trunk and spreading to the extremities.

Physical findings late in the first week of illness include generalized lymphadenopathy and palpable spleen and occasionally liver. Pulmonary findings are often absent despite radiographic evidence of interstitial pneumonia. In those patients with myocarditis, there may be a gallop rhythm, poor-quality heart sounds, and systolic murmurs.

Various cranial nerve deficits have been noted in untreated patients. Deafness, dysarthria, and dysphagia may occur but are usually transient, although deafness can last for several months.

All of 87 (non-immune) soldiers in Vietnam who developed scrub typhus had fever and headache, 46% had an eschar, and 35% had a rash. Eighty-five per cent had generalized lymph node enlargement. It is not surprising that many were misdiagnosed as having infectious mononucleosis.

Laboratory studies reveal leukopenia early in the disease with subsequent increase of white blood cell counts to normal levels. Coagulopathies can be demonstrated, but only rare patients develop the disseminated intravascular clotting syndrome. Liver enzyme values may be elevated, indicating hepatocellular damage. Proteinuria is common.

Patients with untreated disease remain febrile for about 2 weeks and have a long convalescence of 4 to 6 weeks thereafter.

DIAGNOSIS. The variable presentations in this disease make the clinical diagnosis difficult. The eschar and rash should suggest a rickettsial infection, but these may be found in fewer than one half of patients. Furthermore, the eschar and rash may suggest other rickettsial infections, such as tick-borne typhus. The endemic foci of scrub typhus and whether the patient has traveled or worked in such areas constitute important epidemiologic information. A therapeutic trial of tetracycline or chloramphenicol is indicated in patients in whom the diagnosis of scrub typhus is suspected. Defervescence should occur within 24 hours.

The specific serologic test is the detection of significant increases (greater than fourfold) of IFAs in paired serum specimens obtained 2 weeks apart. The *Proteus* OX-K antigen test is readily available and inexpensive, so that it is frequently employed in endemic areas. About 50% of patients have diagnostic titers. In Malaya, the sensitivity and specificity of both tests were found to be about the same, but their usefulness was enhanced when they were used concurrently.

O. tsutsugamushi can be isolated from a patient's blood by inoculating it, intraperitoneally, into white mice. The rickettsiae can be demonstrated in the tissues of the mice.

PROGNOSIS AND TREATMENT. Without treatment, the mortality rate ranges from 0 to 30% depending on virulence and resistance factors; with treatment, survival is the expected outcome. Second or third attacks of scrub typhus, caused by different serotypes, usually result in a mild illness, usually with no eschar or rash.

Persistence of *O. tsutsugamushi* in lymph node tissues has been demonstrated 1 year after recovery. This finding raises the possibility of disease reactivating during immunosuppression.

Tetracycline, doxycycline, and chloramphenicol are all effective. The drug should be continued for at least 2 days after the patient has become afebrile.

PREVENTION AND CONTROL. Vaccines were developed and tested during and after World War II. Some were effective against homologous strains. However, no single antigen has been identified that induces protection against all of the antigenically diverse strains of *O. tsutsugamushi*. In military populations in endemic areas, weekly doses of doxycycline protect against scrub typhus.

Avoidance of chigger attachment can be accomplished by insect repellents applied to the skin and by use of protective clothing impregnated with benzyl benzoate. Diethyltoluamide preparations such as OFF and DEET are also effective if sprayed on clothing and exposed skin but are removed rapidly by water. Applying this chemical to socks is especially important in preventing chigger bites.

Q FEVER

DEFINITION. Q fever is a systemic infection caused by inhaling small numbers of *Coxiella burnetii*. Domestic animals and pets are the usual sources of infection for humans. This highly infectious rickettsial agent induces mild febrile illness, occasionally associated with pneumonitis, but in a few patients causes chronic hepatitis and life-threatening endocarditis.

ETIOLOGY. *C. burnetii* is unique among the rickettsiae in the following ways: It is not transmitted to humans by arthropod vectors; rather, it is readily disseminated by aerosols. No rash ensues despite the similarity of the infection of endothelial cells (vasculitis) to that with *Rickettsia rickettsii*. The organism resides uniquely inside the phagolysosome in the cytoplasm of the infected cell. *C. burnetii* does not have cross-reacting antigens with *Proteus vulgaris*, and therefore antibodies developed during infection do not agglutinate in the Weil-Felix test. These rickettsiae are resistant to destruction by environmental stresses (e.g., sunlight, humidity).

Isolation of *C. burnetii* from pulmonary secretions, liver biopsy specimens, and surgical cardiac valve specimens is possible but not recommended unless appropriate laboratory facilities are available. This is a highly infectious agent that can readily cause laboratory-acquired infections. These materials are injected into eggs and/or guinea pigs. In the latter, the production of agglutinating antibodies confirms the presence of the organism. *C. burnetii* can exist in two phases. Phase I organisms are usually associated with chronic, severe clinical illnesses, such as endocarditis. Phase II organisms evolve (through the loss of monosaccharide and polysaccharide chains of the lipopolysaccharide surface antigens) after multiple transfers in eggs. Antibodies to phase II organisms are predominant in most patients with Q fever. However, patients with endocarditis have higher titers of antibodies to phase I organisms, specifically IgA and IgG; the latter two types of antibodies are diagnostic for this entity.

Virulence factors associated with *C. burnetii* include three plasmids. These appear to be specific for acute versus chronic disease; they control the production of proteins that may be involved in the infectious processes. The lipopolysaccharide antigen is another virulence factor. The antigen in strains causing chronic disease is different from that in strains involved in acute disease. The organism may resist destruction inside the phagolysosome by producing large quantities of acid phosphatase, which inhibits the superoxide production of the host cell, thereby avoiding lysis. In addition, its ability to survive in the acid milieu of the phagolysosome provides an environment that impairs the efficacy of most antibiotics. Raising the pH in tissue culture systems results in increased antibiotic efficacy. These virulence factors can enable *C. burnetii* to establish chronic infections.

EPIDEMIOLOGY. Human disease is acquired by inhaling aerosols containing *C. burnetii*. The organisms are disseminated from infected ruminants and pets (cats). The placentas from these animals contain huge concentrations of rickettsiae. During delivery of the placenta, aerosols are generated that may be wind borne to contaminate soil, clothing, and the wool or fur of other animals or may be transmitted hundreds of yards to susceptible persons. Trucks carrying sheep appear to disseminate organisms to persons passed on the streets. Sheep regularly transported to research laboratories through hallways in a medical center caused an epidemic that persisted for 6 months. Organisms are also found in amniotic fluid, feces, and the mammary glands and milk of sheep and cows. The ability of *C. burnetii* to form sporelike structures that resist environmental destruction allows these organisms to cause disease long after the initial contamination occurs and at sites distant from the original source.

The animals are infected by ticks. There are ticks that transmit the organisms among wild animals, such as the kangaroo in Australia. Spread to domestic animals occurs when the two populations of animals intermingle. Ticks have not been implicated in the transmission from animals to humans. Q fever is a mild and inapparent infection in animals. It may be responsible for placental deficiencies that lead to stillbirth of kittens and lambs. *C. burnetii* attach to the head of the sperm from infected mice. Males can infect female mice by sexual contact. Whether this occurs in humans is unknown.

Various volunteer studies, designed to evaluate vaccine effectiveness, have demonstrated that very few organisms, probably fewer than 10, are sufficient to induce disease. For this reason, as well as the ability to survive in most environments, *C. burnetii* is a hazardous organism with which to work. In one laboratory 21 of 50 cases diagnosed over a 15-year period occurred in persons working in laboratories (or offices) not directly involved in Q fever research. Presumably, these persons were infected by widely disseminated aerosols from laboratory accidents or from contaminated clothing of workers socializing outside their laboratory. Despite the infectious nature of the organism and its presence in sputum, human-to-human transmission does not occur and respiratory isolation for infected patients is not needed.

In the United States and Canada, *C. burnetii* (and antibodies) has been found in milk from numerous herds of cattle. Despite this evidence, documented cases of Q fever occurring after unpasteurized milk from such cows was ingested have not been identified. The ingestion of 10^5 organisms by mouth by volunteers failed to induce disease. If disease occurs, it could originate from aerosols created in the act of pouring the milk into a glass.

The incubation period varies indirectly with inoculum size. Large doses result in disease at about 7 days. Most persons develop symptoms at 13 to 18 days.

PATHOLOGY. Knowledge of the pathologic changes is greatest for the more severe form of this disease. For example, microscopic examinations of liver biopsies and autopsy material from patients dying of chronic hepatitis and from heart valves infected with *C. burnetii* are available. Patients with pneumonitis usually have a mild illness so tissue specimens are scarce. Animal studies have provided complementary pathohistologic data.

HEPATITIS. Granulomas with fatty necrosis are typical microscopic findings. These granulomas are doughnut-shaped. While they are common in Q fever, they also are seen in patients with tuberculosis. Fatty metamorphosis is also seen. Patients with mild forms of Q fever may have elevated liver enzyme values indicative of minimal liver cell damage.

SUBACUTE AND CHRONIC ENDOCARDITIS. This is a life-threatening disease because it is difficult to eradicate the infection. These patients may have large vegetations on the aortic valve and less likely on the mitral valve. They have negative blood cultures and frequently have a history of a febrile illness with or without pneumonitis months previously. The vegetations have a histologic picture similar to that in other forms of endocarditis, an avascular collection of fibrin and platelets. These patients also have enlarged livers and spleens, plus signs of vasculitis associated with endocarditis (e.g., splinter hemorrhages, Roth spots, and petechiae).

PNEUMONITIS. In the few autopsies performed, consolidation similar to that of other bacterial pneumonias was the gross finding. The microscopic examination revealed an exudate loaded with his-

tocytes and no polymorphonuclear leukocytes. This inflammatory response is compatible with a non-bacterial process. The histologic features have been described as those of a severe intra-alveolar, focally necrotizing, hemorrhagic pneumonia with associated necrotizing bronchitis and bronchiolitis.

The portal of entry of *C. burnetii* is the respiratory tract; small particles less than 3 to 5 μm in diameter can reach the terminal bronchioles. The pneumonia does not appear until the third or fourth day of fever. In a mouse model, the rickettsiae enter pneumatocytes, histocytes, and fibroblasts. The self-limiting nature of this infection is probably related to the destruction of the organisms in the macrophages. However, *C. burnetii* can persist for 2 months inside those cells. Some of the macrophages can be damaged by *C. burnetii*, leading to an inflammatory response. Cellular immune mechanisms attack these damaged cells. Numerous factors are involved in the pathogenesis of pneumonia—the number and virulence of the rickettsiae, particle size, and the functional status of the macrophages and parenchymal cells of the lung.

CLINICAL MANIFESTATIONS. The onset of Q fever is very abrupt; the manifestations are not specific. The patient develops a high fever that is associated with headache, chills, myalgia, and malaise. This flulike syndrome differs from influenza disease because of the height of the temperature, frequently 39.4° to 40° C. The fever also persists for 10 to 14 days. No rash occurs. Retroorbital pain, common in other rickettsial infections, is reported by 10 to 15% of patients.

Patients may have a dry, non-productive cough indicative of the bronchiolitis and the minimal pneumonitis produced by the invading *C. burnetii*. Physical findings of consolidated lung are lacking early in the course of the pneumonia. There may be decreased breath sounds, but rales are unlikely until the lesions start to resolve. The chest films reveal patchy infiltrates that frequently are multiple round, segmental opacities. These are discrete lesions. Larger areas of the lung may show consolidation, and linear atelectatic lesions occur in about half the patients with pneumonia. Resolution of the lesions is slow. The incidence of pneumonitis varies from 4 to 97% in series of cases reported from the United States (28%), Australia (4 to 75%), and Switzerland (97%). The reasons for these variations are unknown.

Most patients (85%) with Q fever have hepatic involvement as measured by abnormal liver cell enzymes. Hepatomegaly is noted in about 65% of patients, but few patients (10%) have liver tenderness. Jaundice is unlikely (about 5% of cases) unless chronic hepatitis ensues, a very rare manifestation. Liver biopsy specimens have demonstrated, by direct immunofluorescent studies, rickettsia residing in hepatic cells. Q fever may account for a few cases of acute hepatitis. Patients with a strong exposure history should be evaluated for infection by *C. burnetii*.

The clinical manifestations of Q fever endocarditis are characteristic of those associated with the syndrome of endocarditis (e.g., splenomegaly, splinter hemorrhages, and heart murmurs). Few cases of *C. burnetii*–induced valvular infections are seen in the United States; small series are reported from countries in which Q fever is more common. Evidence of endocarditis in a patient occurs years after the acute infections. The lack of positive cultures contributes to a delay in diagnosis. The diagnosis is made by serologic means, demonstrating high (> 1:800 for IgG and > 1:50 for IgA) or rising titers of phase I antibodies by indirect immunofluorescence. The level of phase I antibodies exceeding those for phase II antibodies is indicative of chronic Q fever, whether it is endocarditis or a localized infection of bone, vascular prosthesis, aneurysm, liver, or joint. Phase II antibodies indicate a recent exposure or an acute infection.

PROGNOSIS. The key to diagnosing Q fever in a patient with a debilitating febrile illness is obtaining a history of contact with sheep, cattle, goats, or cats or the skins or wool from these animals. This history should be compelling enough to initiate antibiotic treatment and to obtain acute and convalescent serum for serologic studies. These latter studies are the practical and definitive diagnostic aids. Phase II antibodies (complement fixing [CF] or IFA) are present in two thirds of patients at the end of 2 weeks of illness and in 90% at 1 month. Phase I antibodies, if present, are found in titers lower than phase II antibodies. IFA is more sensitive than CF in detecting early antibody formation (IgM) and also in demonstrating persistence of antibody at 1 year or longer. The presence of phase I antibodies in excess of phase II, and specifically phase I IgA, is diagnostic of Q fever endocarditis.

The non-specific clinical manifestations of early symptoms and signs of Q fever (e.g., headache, fever, myalgia) suggest numerous infectious diseases. Influenza infections are seasonal, the temperature is less than that in Q fever, and liver function tests are normal. The white blood cell count is not helpful, because it is normal in both infections. Other diseases such as typhoid fever and brucellosis can be diagnosed by bacterial cultures. Viral hepatitis can be mistaken for Q fever. Appropriate serologic studies and liver biopsy provide diagnostic evidence. In those patients with pneumonitis, the differential diagnosis includes viral or mycoplasmal causes, tularemia, psittacosis, and *Legionella pneumophila*. Serologic and culture results identify these organisms.

TREATMENT AND PROGNOSIS. *C. burnetii* is known to be susceptible to a number of antibiotics. Sensitivity studies have been conducted in eggs, guinea pigs, and acute and chronically infected tissue culture cells. Tetracycline and doxycycline or chloramphenicol have been effective in vitro as well as in clinical studies. Early institution of tetracycline (within 3 days of onset) reduces the febrile course by half. Tetracycline, 500 mg four times a day, or doxycycline, 100 mg twice a day, should be continued for at least 1 week after the patient becomes afebrile (usually 2 to 3 days). The prognosis with such therapy is excellent, with no mortality expected. Those patients who receive no antibiotics also do well, with a recovery rate of more than 99%. If a febrile relapse occurs, retreatment with the same antibiotic is effective.

The recommended treatment of patients with Q fever endocarditis is not settled. Doxycycline and a quinolone have been somewhat effective, but cures have not been achieved even after 2 years of continuous therapy. The mortality rate remains high (24%). The location of the organism in an acid environment inside the phagolysosome interferes with the activity of antibiotics. Experimental studies designed to alkalize the fluid helped to eradicate the organisms in phagocytes. The combination of doxycycline and chloroquine in these studies was most effective and may be useful in patients with chronic Q fever. Surgical resection of infected valves is usually required because the large vegetations cause hemodynamic deficiencies in cardiac function.

PREVENTION. There is no commercially available vaccine for Q fever. Experimental vaccines using either phase I or phase II organisms have been effective in preventing disease in volunteers and in several field trials. For those persons at high risk, such as researchers working with sheep, veterinarians, or exposed laboratory workers, vaccine can be obtained under an investigational new drug application.

Focusing on controlling disease in the workplace is more effective than attempting to control the disease in animals. Three recommended measures include knowing the serologic status of the employees, not permitting pregnant women or persons with valvular heart disease to be in the high-risk jobs, and confining the research on sheep to a building dedicated solely to that purpose. Vaccination of employees should also be attempted.

Bakken JS, Dumler JS, Chen S. et al: Human granulocytic ehrlichiosis in the upper midwest United States. JAMA 272:212, 1994. *The first report on a new disease entity caused by another species of* Ehrlichia.

Brouqui P, Dupont HT, Drancourt M, et al: Chronic Q fever: Ninety-two cases from France, including 27 cases without endocarditis. Arch Intern Med 153:642, 1993. *An excellent review of chronic Q fever.*

Conlon PJ. Procop GW, Fowler V, et al: Predictors of prognosis and risk of acute renal failure in patients with Rocky Mountain spotted fever. Am J Med 101:621–626, 1997.

Dalton MJ, Clarke MJ, Holman RC, et al: National surveillance for Rocky Mountain spotted fever, 1981–1982: Epidemiologic summary and evaluation of risk factors for fatal outcome. Am J Trop Med Hyg 52:405, 1995.

Everett ED, Evans KA, Henry B, et al: Human ehrlichiosis in adults after tick exposure. Ann Intern Med 120:730, 1994. *Presents data on 30 patients diagnosed and followed by this group.*

Fishbein DB, Dawson JE, Robinson LE: Human ehrlichiosis in the United States, 1985 to 1990. Ann Intern Med 120:736, 1994. *This report follows Everett et al. and is the usual excellent CDC review of 237 cases garnered by a laboratory surveillance.*

Yeaman MR, Roman MJ, Baca OG: Antibiotic susceptibilities of two *Coxiella burnetii* isolates implicated in distinct clinical syndromes. Antimicrob Agents Chemother 33: 2053, 1989. *A new method to evaluate sensitivities of Q fever isolates to antibiotics.*

372 ZOONOSES

Stuart Levin

Zoonoses are most simply defined as human infections derived from animals. Approximately 200 different infectious agents, many of them rare, cause disease in humans and fulfill the definition of zoonoses. There are more than 40 million dogs in the United States, and man's best friend has been targeted as facilitating the transmission of more than 50 infectious agents while being credited with more than 1 million bite injuries each year in the United States. There are more than 30 million cats in the United States and more than 40 infectious diseases have been transmitted by this creature. Almost all arthropod transmitted infectious agents in the United States are due to either ticks or mosquitos, with ticks being the more common villain and Lyme disease being the most common arthropod-transmitted infectious disease in the United States.

The risk of developing a zoonosis is increased by direct animal contact, outdoor activities, exposure to and inhalation of infectious air particles, insect bites, contact with previously infected human blood products, and contact with and ingestion of infectious agents transmitted by animal-contaminated water and insufficiently cooked meat, eggs, dairy products, fish, and shellfish. Raw shellfish are the garbage filters of the ocean and can transmit at least 25 different infectious or toxic illnesses to humans. In addition, the farmer, pet owner, hunter, laboratory researcher, and cave explorer, among others, is at higher risk than the general population to develop a zoonosis. Infective agents transmitted by these routes from animal sources essentially include members of all microbial classes: viruses, bacteria, fungi, and parasites. Immunocompromised hosts such as splenectomized patients, transplant patients, patients with the acquired immunodeficiency syndrome, as well as pregnant women and their fetuses are at high risk of developing clinical disease when exposed to these various infectious agents. New emerging infectious diseases seem inevitable because of increased interest in xenotransplantation, global warming trends, human intrusion in previously underexplored or never-explored sites, and an increasing threat of biological terrorism or warfare. Preventive measures to decrease infection in the compromised host include utilizing routine pet care immunization, neutering pets, using caution when handling pet fomites, and avoiding ingestion of undercooked meat, fish, and eggs.

Massive warming changes and man's entry into previously unaccessible geographic areas both increase the potential to encounter previously described infectious diseases on a more frequent basis and new emerging pathogens.

Non–animal-associated environmental- or travel-related infectious diseases can be confused with zoonoses. The vast majority of clinical diseases caused by *Legionella pneumophila, Plasmodium falciparum, Entamoeba histolytica, Giardia lamblia, Pseudomonas pseudomallei, Chromobacterium violaceum, Aeromonas hydrophila, Francisella philomiragia,* and airborne fungi such as *Blastomyces dermatitides, Coccidioides immitis,* and *Histoplasma capsulatum* are acquired through environmental exposure and are only rarely related to animal hosts. One exception is *Sporotrichosis schenckii,* which generally is considered an environment-acquired pathogen from vegetation injuries. This fungus has been associated with the zoonotic transmission from draining cutaneous ulcers of cats to owners and animal handlers. Histoplasmosis has been acquired by explorers (spelunkers) in caves contaminated by bat guano.

Unfortunately, some descriptive disease titles can be misleading to clinicians and thus can interfere with correctly considering the possible diagnosis. The transmission of tick-borne Rocky Mountain Spotted Fever actually occurs more commonly in the southeastern United States than in the Rocky Mountains and has even been acquired in the middle of New York City. Vegetarians and other strict non–pork-eating persons have been seriously infected with the pig tapeworm *Taenia solium* as a result of fecal contamination of food from unsuspected infected human sources. Human influenza A is not typically considered a zoonosis; however, inter-species spread of swine, avian, and human influenza viruses can occur in unique geographic areas, such as southern China, where dense

Table 372–1 ■ RESPIRATORY TRACT ZOONOSES

DISEASE	MICROORGANISM	CLINICAL SYNDROME AND DIAGNOSTIC TOOL	RESERVOIR AND/OR VECTOR
Psittacosis*	Chlamydia psittaci	Pneumonia, often severe; serology	Aerosols from parrots, ducks, turkeys
Q-Fever	Coxiella burnetii	Pneumonia, hepatitis or myocarditis; serology	Airborne from soil contaminated by sheep, goats, and cats, particularly if parturient
Tularemia	Francisella tularensis	Cutaneous ulcer and regional node, pneumonia and hilar node; pleural	Rabbit contact (winter) and tick bites
Plague	Yersinia pestis	Inguinal nodes, bubonic plague (10% will develop basilar pneumonia); hilar node enlargement; serology Gram's stain of node aspirate	Fleas from prairie dogs, rock squirrels, rats, cats
Hantavirus syndrome	Hantavirus	Upper respiratory to lower respiratory to adult respiratory distress syndrome to death; serology	Deer mouse formites: urine, feces, saliva
Rhodococcus pneumonia	Rhodococcus equi	Pneumonia, often cavitates, in patients with acquired immunodeficiency syndrome and other immunosuppressed patients; sputum culture	Horse manure, soil
Mycoplasma arginini pneumonia	Mycoplasma arginini	Pneumonia, sepsis neutropenia	Sheep, goats special culture
Foot and mouth disease	Aphthovirus	Non-specific upper respiratory tract infection, oral vesicles; serology	Cloven-footed mammals
Bordetella bronchoseptica		Pneumonia, bronchitis, Whooping cough	Dogs
Histoplasmosis	Histoplasma capsulatum	Pneumonia or fever of unknown origin	Bats

Note: See Table of Contents and Index for more detailed discussion of each disease.
*Occurs in more than 1000 animal species.

Table 372–2 ■ CENTRAL NERVOUS SYSTEM (CNS) INFECTION: ZOONOSES

DISEASE	ORGANISM	CLINICAL SYNDROME AND DIAGNOSIS	RESERVOIR
Listeriosis	Listeria monocytogenes	Purulent meningitis during pregnancy and in neonate; immunosuppression; culture	Unpasteurized cheese and other dairy products; cattle; goats
Leptospirosis	Leptospira interrogans	Aseptic meningitis, hepatorenal syndrome; serology, culture	Asymptomatic dogs, cattle, water source common
Herpes B encephalitis	Herpes simiae	Diffuse, progressive encephalitis; culture	Macaca monkey bites or scratches
Lyme disease	Borrelia burgdorferi	Lymphocytic meningitis, motor-sensory neuropathy, facial palsy; serology	Reservoir acquired from tick bites, mouse
Lymphocytic choriomeningitis	Lymphocytic choriomeningitis virus	Lymphocytic meningitis occasionally with pneumonia; serology	Inhalation of mouse secretions, urine, feces, saliva
Mosquito-borne encephalitis—USA	Eastern, Western equine encephalitis; St. Louis, California encephalitis	Diffuse encephalitis; least severe: California encephalitis; most severe: Eastern equine encephalitis; serology	Mosquito-borne from horses, birds
Rabies encephalitis	Rabies virus	Almost always fatal; encephalitis;	Bites from dogs, skunks, bats, raccoons, foxes
Toxoplasmosis	Toxoplasma gondii	CNS, multiple brain masses, AIDS patient; CNS scan, serology, biopsy	Cat feces or ingestion of undercooked lamb or pork
Cerebral cysticercosis	Taenia solium	Epilepsy, CNS cysts, eosinophilic meningitis, hydrocephalus; scan, serology	Fecal-oral; contamination of food; with tapeworm eggs
New varient: Creutzfeldt-Jakob disease	Prion (proteinaceous infectious particle)	Dementia, ataxia, and myoclonus	Beef from cattle fed scraps from contaminated sheep carcasses

Note: See Table of Contents and Index for more detailed discussion of each disease.

Table 372–3 ■ RASHES: ZOONOSES

DISEASE	MICROORGANISM	CLINICAL INFORMATION AND DIAGNOSIS	RESERVOIR AND/OR VECTOR
Ehrlichiosis	Ehrlichia chaffeensis (monocytic)	Macular rash (one third of patients), central distribution; in south central United States; culture, serology	Tick bite
Leptospirosis	Leptospira interrogans	Central macular rash in 20%, with occasional enanthem; serology, culture	Urine-contaminated water, dogs, cattle
Lyme disease	Borrelia burgdorferi	Primary lesion is erythema chronicum migrans; 40% have multiple lesions; serology/culture	Mouse reservoir—tick bite
Rocky Mountain spotted fever	Rickettsia rickettsii	Acral or peripheral distribution of macular papular to hemorrhagic rash to gangrenous lesions; serology/biopsy of skin	Tick bite
Typhus (endemic)	Rickettsia prowazeckii	Central distribution, macular rash (can be hemorrhagic); serology	Flying squirrel fleas or fomites
Scabies	Sarcoptes scabiei	Pruritic macules on trunk; skin burrow	Dogs—close contact. Up to one third of asymptomatic dogs have mite infection.
Flea bite dermatitis	Pulex irritans	Pruritic papules, urticarial vesicles; fleas found on pets or in the environment	Fleas on dogs
Cat-scratch disease	Bartonella species	Bacillary angiomatosis, peliosis hepatitis, cervical adenopathy, subacute bacterial endocarditis and fever of unknown origin; culture, serology, silver stain biopsy	Cat scratch or bite

Note: See Table of Contents and Index for more detailed discussion of each disease.

Table 372-4 ■ HIGHLY FATAL ZOONOSES

DISEASE	FATALITY RATE (%)
Creutzfeldt-Jakob disease (new variant)	100
Rabies	100
Anthrax pneumonia	100
Herpes simiae*	50–75
Ebola virus	70
Eastern equine encephalitis	50–70
Hantavirus pulmonary syndrome—US†	60
Yellow fever‡	20–50
Lassa fever‡	15–25
Plague*	50–80
Rocky Mountain spotted fever*	20–60
East African sleeping sickness*	20–30
Anthrax*—cutaneous	20
Tularemia	10–15
Visceral leishmaniasis*	5–25
Louse-borne relapsing fever*	5–40

Note: See Table of Contents and Index for more detailed discussion of each disease.
*Fatality rate if untreated.
†If jaundiced.
‡Case mortality of hospitalized patients.

concentrations of ducks, pigs, and people cohabit. Viral incubation of the three influenza species in the pig with reassortment of antigens and subsequent spread to humans of virulent "new" influenza strains can lead to influenza pandemics that in sheer number (billions) surpass any past epidemics of smallpox or plague.

Leprosy, a human-to-human-transmitted illness of biblical notoriety, is endemic in at least three animal species, including the armadillo. This animal has rarely been implicated in the transmission of this disease to humans in the United States.

Despite the large number of zoonoses described, clinicians evaluating an individual patient usually need consider only a limited number of historical details to arrive at an appropriate differential diagnosis:

1. Questions regarding direct contact with animals or animal products, animal bites, arthropod exposures, and food ingestion may offer clues to the correct etiology.
2. Consideration must be given to a patient's travel history, because a number of zoonoses are quite limited in their geographic distribution.
3. Details about occupational and recreational high-risk activities must be ascertained.
4. The patient's clinical presentation (course and organ involvement) is used to focus simultaneously on the most likely cause and disease considerations. Tables 372–1 through 372–5 take advantage of this "syndrome" approach. Additional lists of zoonotic agents can be generated for the differential diagnoses of arthritis, jaundice, diarrhea, sepsis and shock, renal failure, fever of unknown origin, and endocarditis.

Cook GC: Canine-associated zoonoses: An unacceptable hazard to human health. Q J Med 70:5126, 1989.
Eastaugh J, Shepherd S: Infectious and toxic syndromes from fish and shellfish consumption. Arch Intern Med 149:1735, 1989.
Glaser CA, Angulo FJ, Rooney JA: Animal-associated opportunistic infections among persons infected with the human immunodeficiency virus. Clin Infect Dis 18:14, 1994.
Maquire JH, Keystone JS: Parasitic diseases. Infect Dis Clin North Am 7:467–738, 1993. *All of these sources are interesting descriptions of the syndromes and disease categories mentioned in the chapter.*
Weinberg AN, Weber DJ: Animal associated human infections. Infect Dis Clin North Am 5:1–181, 1991.

Table 372-5 ■ NEWLY CHARACTERIZED ZOONOSES

DISEASE	INFECTIOUS AGENT	CLINICAL INFORMATION	VECTOR
Ehrlichiosis monocytic	*Ehrlichia chaffeensis*	Fever, myalgia, leukopenia	Tick bite
Ehrlichiosis granulocytic	(HGE) Human Granulocytic Ehrlichia	Fever, myalgia, leukopenia	Tick bite
Cat-scratch disease	*Bartonella species*	Cervical lymphadenopathy in normal hosts and cutaneous and hepatic angiomatosis in AIDS patients	Cat scratch or bite
Hemorrhagic diarrhea	Enterohemorrhagic *Escherichia coli* 0157-H7 (other species)	Rectal bleeding, dysentery, hemolytic uremic syndrome	Contaminated, undercooked meat
Hantavirus pulmonary syndrome (HPV)	Hantavirus–sin nombre	Adult respiratory distress syndrome	Fomites of rodents
Cryptosporidum diarrhea	*Cryptosporidium parvum* (?)	Diarrhea	Contaminated water
Dysentery	*Campylobacter jejuni*	Dysentery, Reiter's syndrome, Guillian-Barré syndrome	Contaminated chicken
Pyogenic skin ulcer	*Capnocytophaga Canimorsus*	Sepsis, skin infection	Dog bites

Note: See Table of Contents and Index for more detailed discussion of each disease.

■ VIRAL DISEASES

373 INTRODUCTION TO VIRAL DISEASES

R. Gordon Douglas, Jr.

Viruses are among the simplest and smallest of all forms of life. They are obligate intracellular parasites that require host cell structural and metabolic components for replication. They infect bacteria as well as plants and animals. More than 400 distinct viruses infect humans. They produce diseases ranging from subclinical infections and mild, self-limited, localized infections to common systemic infections and overwhelming, highly lethal infections such as meningoencephalitis or hemorrhagic fever with shock.

CHARACTERISTICS OF VIRUSES. Essentially, virus particles, or "virions," consist of nucleic acid enclosed in a protein coat. They lack metabolic activity and do not possess ribosomes or most enzymes necessary for replication. In addition, some possess a lipid envelope. Both the lipid and the protein coats protect the nucleic acid from enzymatic degradation. The nucleic acid may be either deoxyribonucleic acid (DNA) or ribonucleic acid (RNA). It may code for only a few or, in some cases, several hundred proteins. The protein coat, or "capsid," consists of repeating, identical subunits called "capsomeres." The capsid and nucleic acid together are called the "nucleocapsid." The smallest (parvoviruses) are only 18 nm in diameter; some poxviruses may be as large as 450 nm.

PLATE 9   INFECTIOUS AND PROTOZOAN DISEASES

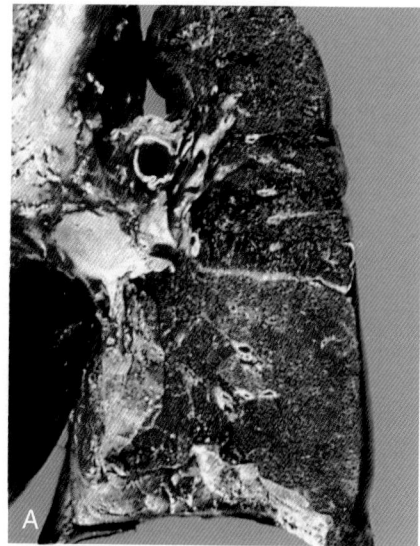

A, Autopsy specimen shows lobar consolidation (gray and red hepatization) of the left lower lobe due to *Streptococcus pneumoniae*. Note the absence of abscess formation and the presence of dense consolidation extending from the hilum to the pleural surface.

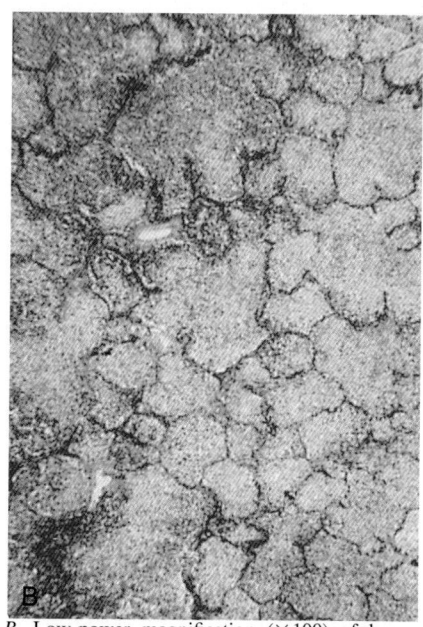

B, Low-power magnification (×100) of hematoxylin and eosin (H & E) stain of tissue section from left lower lobe of pneumonia shown in A. Note intact alveolar walls and alveoli filled with edema and thick cellular exudate.

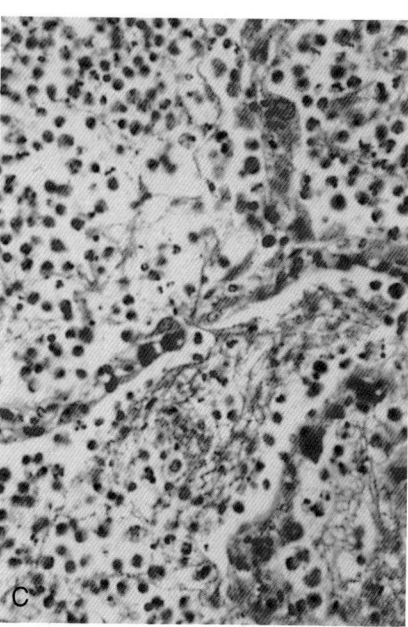

C, Higher magnification (×500) H & E stain depicted in B. Note heavy infiltrate of polymorphonuclear cells and intact alveolar walls.

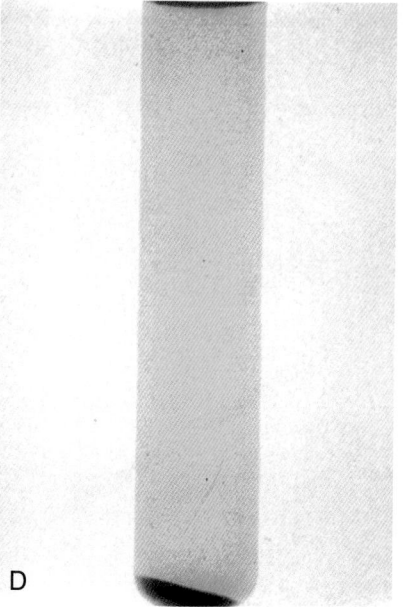

D, Fluid removed from the pleural space in a patient with early pneumococcal pneumonia and pleural effusion. The fluid may be serous, serosanguineous, green, or thick and white.

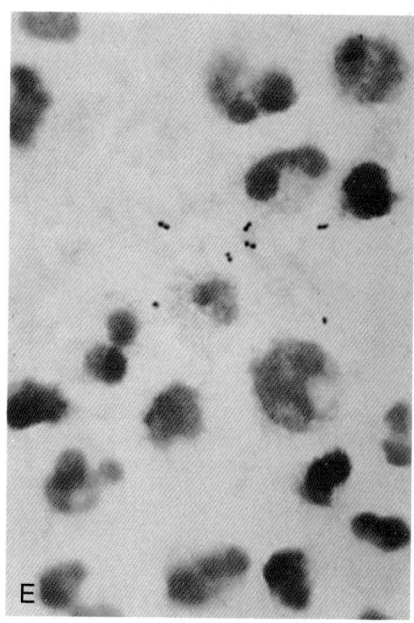

E, Gram stain of pleural fluid shown in D, revealing the presence of polymorphonuclear cells and typical gram-positive diplococci in pairs, consistent with pneumococci.

F, Cutaneous leishmaniasis due to *Leishmania braziliensis.* (From Jeronimo SMB, Pearson RD: Subcell Biochem 18:1,1992.)

G, Brazilian patient with mucosal leishmaniasis due to *Leishmania braziliensis.* Note the destructive lesions involving the nose, nasal septum, and lips. (From Pearson RD, et al.: Rev Infect Dis 5:907, 1983.)

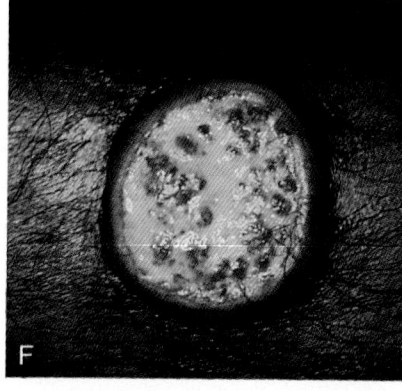

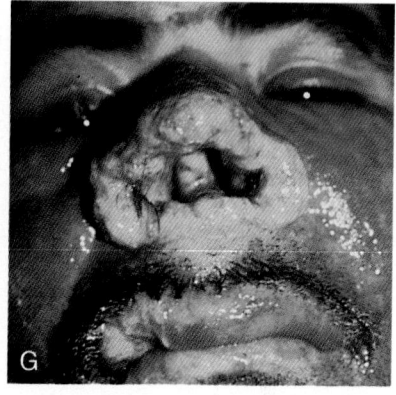

PLATE 9 INFECTIOUS AND PROTOZOAN DISEASES *Continued*

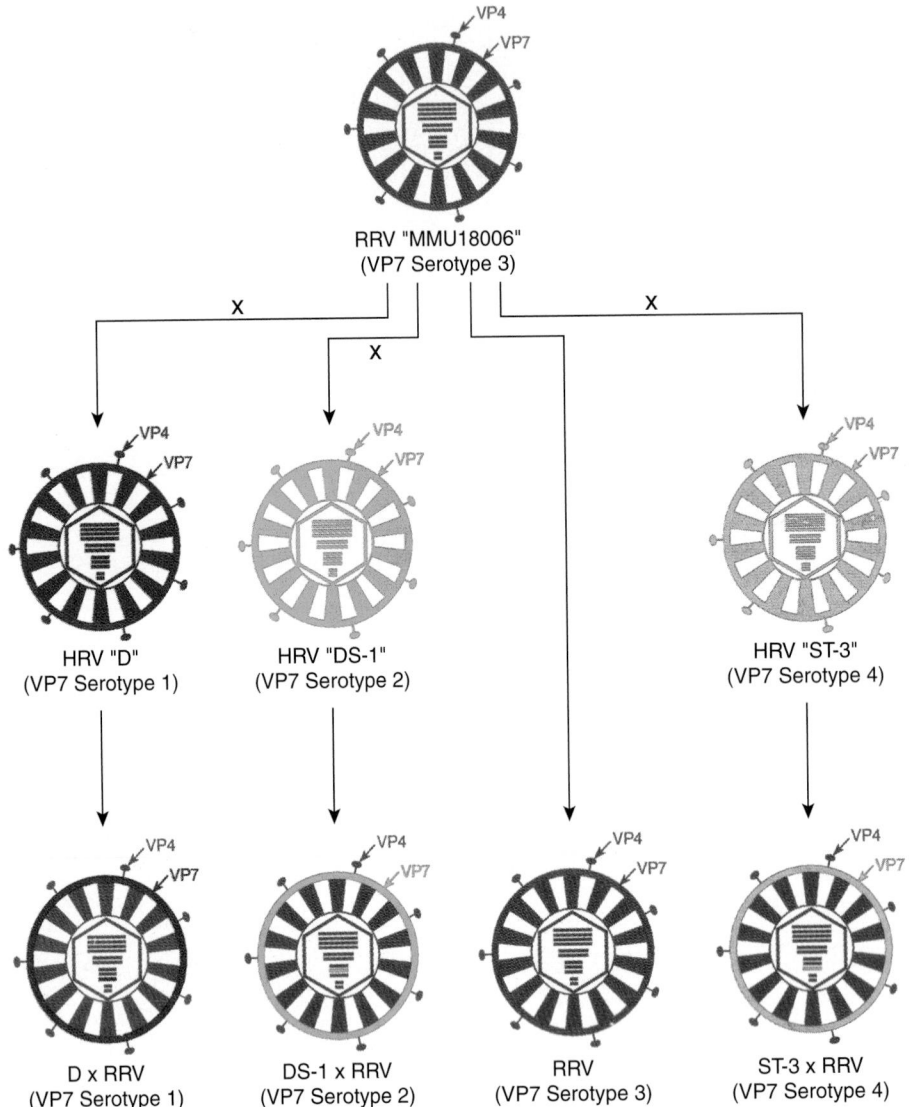

H, Production of a rhesus rotavirus (RRV), human rotavirus (HRV) ×RRV reassortant, quadrivalent vaccine with VP7 serotype 1, 2, 3, and 4 specificity. (From Kapikian AZ, Hoshino Y, Chanock RM, Perez-Schael I: Efficacy of a quadrivalent rhesus rotavirus-based human rotavirus vaccine aimed at preventing severe diarrhea in infants and young children. J Infect Dis 174(suppl1):S65–S72, 1996.)

PLATE 10 INFECTIOUS AND PROTOZOAN DISEASES AND HIV

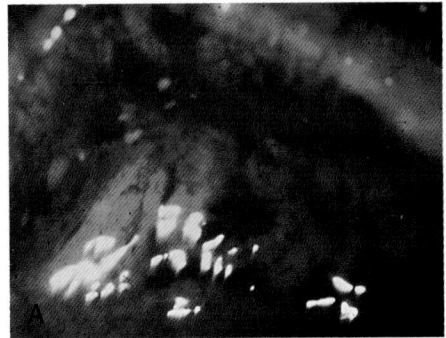

A, Conjunctival petechiae.

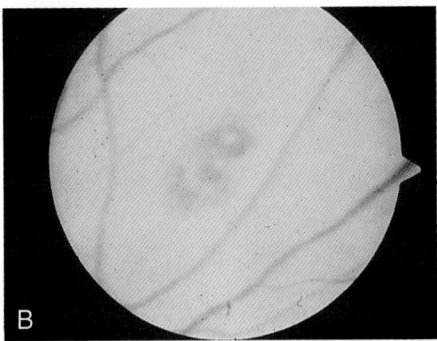

B, Roth's spots on retina.

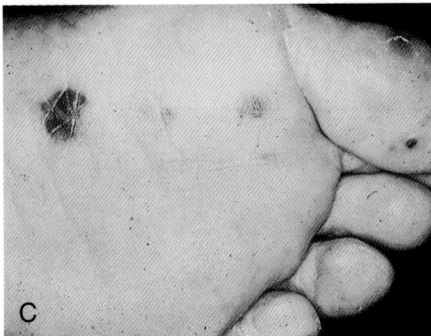

C, Janeway lesion: painless hemorrhagic macule on sole. (From Korzeniowski O, Kaye D: Infective endocarditis. *In* Braunwald E [ed]: Heart Disease, 4th ed. Philadelphia, WB Saunders, 1992.)

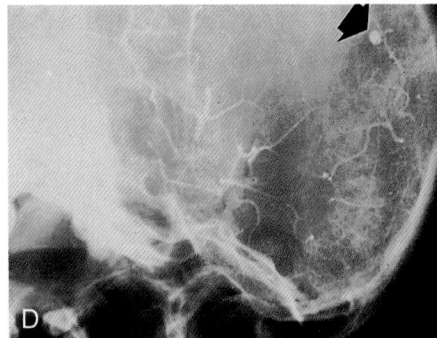

D, Cerebral angiogram illustrating a mycotic aneurysm (arrow). (From Kaye D [ed]: Infective Endocarditis. Baltimore, University Park Press, 1976.)

H, Section of liver from a patient with zidovudine-induced steatosis. The hepatocytes are swollen with lipid vacuoles (mixed macrovesicular and microvesicular steatosis). A necrotic hepatocyte is seen at the center of the field (H & E, ×400). (Courtesy of Dr. D. Kleiner.)

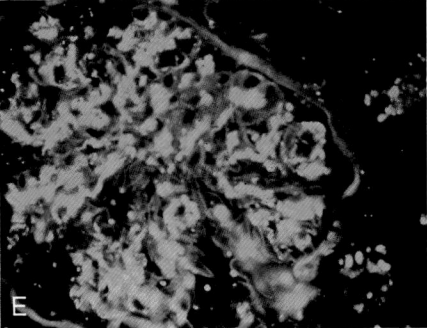

E, Fluorescent immunoglobulin staining of a glomerulus in a patient with glomerulonephritis. (From Kaye D [ed]: Infective Endocarditis. Baltimore, University Park Press, 1976.)

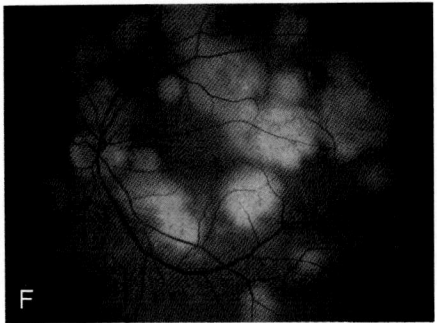

F, Photomicrograph of the indirect funduscopic examination of the left eye of a 35-year-old AIDS patient who was receiving aerosolized pentamidine for secondary prophylaxis of *Pneumocystis* pneumonia. There is extensive choroidal exudation but, unlike CMV retinitis, there is sparing of the retina and minimal hemorrhage. (From Rao NA, Zimmermann PL, Boyer D, et al.: A clinical, histopathologic, and electron microscopic study of *Pneumocystis carinii* choroiditis. Am J Ophthalmol 107:218, 1989.)

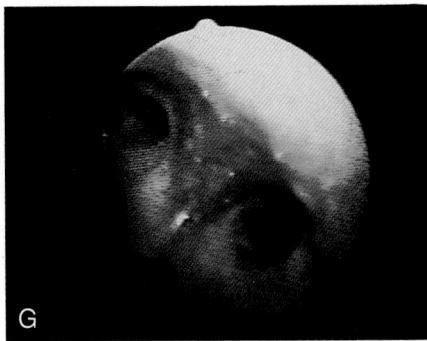

G, Bronchoscopic view of a typical endobronchial Kaposi's sarcoma lesion. The lesion is macular and bright red and straddles a carina. These lesions are sufficiently distinctive to be diagnostic of Kaposi's sarcoma.

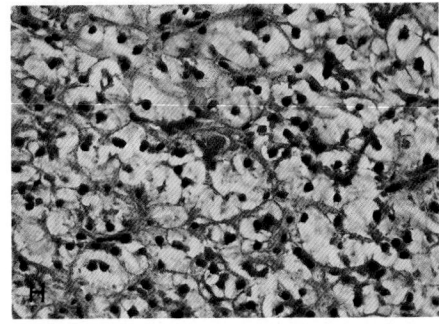

PLATE 11 HIV AND ASSOCIATED DISORDERS

A to *E* show dermatologic abnormalities in AIDS.

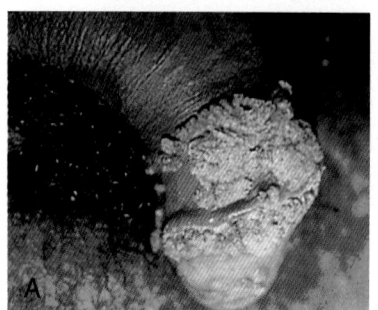

A, Prominent condyloma surrounding the corona and shaft of the penis.

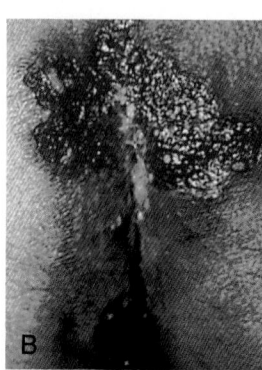

B, Chronic ulcerative herpetic infection is commonly seen in the intergluteal fold.

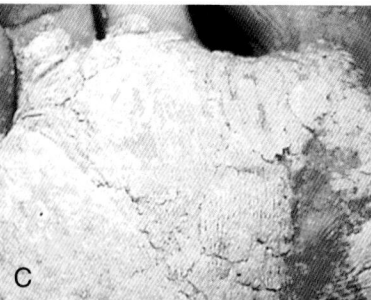

C, Marked hyperkeratosis characterizes keratoderma blennorrhagicum of Reiter's syndrome in HIV-seropositive patients.

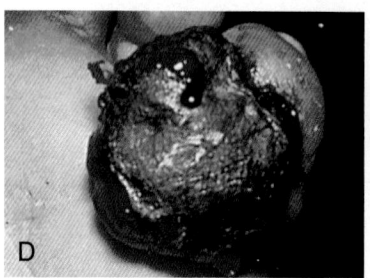
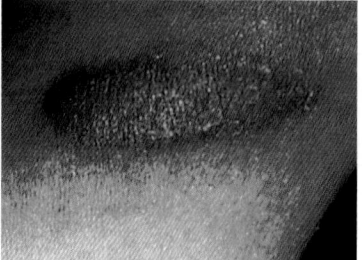

D, Left, An exophytic tumor of Kaposi's sarcoma on the sole. *Right,* Lesion demonstrating the linear configuration frequently noted in Kaposi's sarcoma of the skin in patients with AIDS.

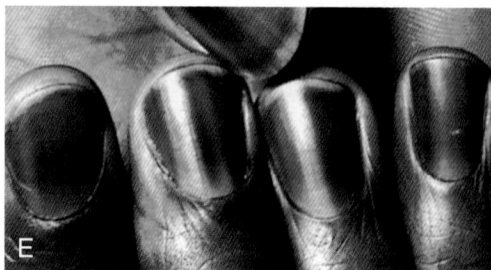

E, Bluish discoloration of the nail plates developed during treatment with AZT.

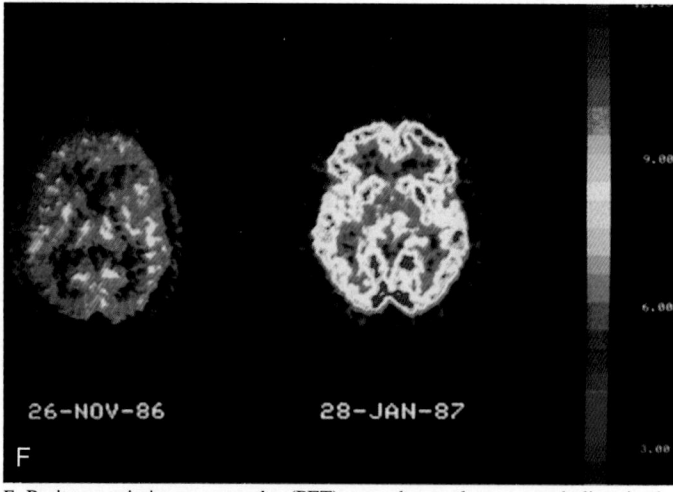

F, Positron emission tomography (PET) scan shows glucose metabolism in the brain of a patient with AIDS dementia before *(left)* and during *(right)* therapy with AZT. This patient had marked improvement of cognitive function associated with a relative normalization of glucose metabolism in the brain. (Reproduced with permission from Brunetti A, Berg G, Di Chiro G, et al.: Reversal of brain metabolic abnormalities following treatment of AIDS dementia complex with 39-azido-29, 39-dideoxythymidine [AZT, zidovudine]: A PET-FDG study. J Nucl Med 30:581–590, 1989.)

PLATE 11   HIV AND ASSOCIATED DISORDERS *Continued*

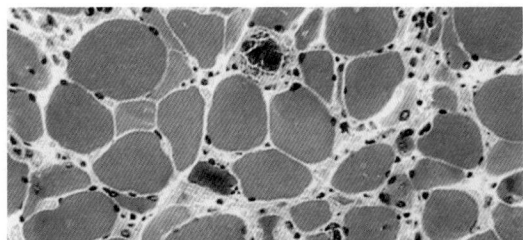

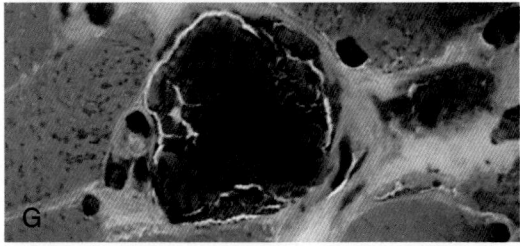

G, Pathologic findings in a patient with AZT-induced myopathy. *Top,* Destructive changes with variation in fiber size and a "ragged-red" fiber. Inflammatory changes can be seen in both AZT-induced myopathy and the myopathy of HIV infection. However, ragged-red fibers are seen only in patients receiving AZT. Transverse section, stained with the modified Gomori trichrome stain (×320). *Bottom,* Detail showing a ragged-red fiber (×900). (Courtesy of Dr. M. C. Dalakos.)

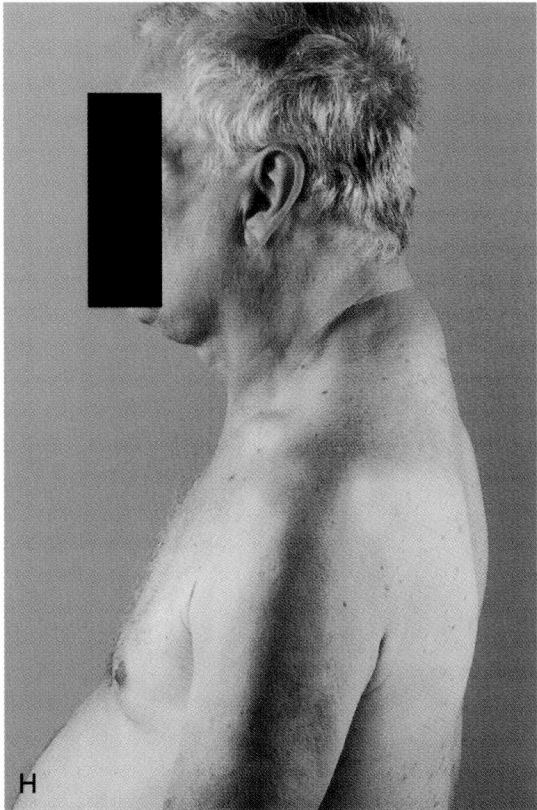

H, Abnormal fat distribution in an HIV-infected patient being treated with an HIV-protease inhibitor. Note the cervical fat pad in a "buffalo hump" distribution and increased intra-abdominal fat deposits. (Courtesy of Drs. Kirk Miller and Henry Masur.)

PLATE 12 SKIN DISEASES

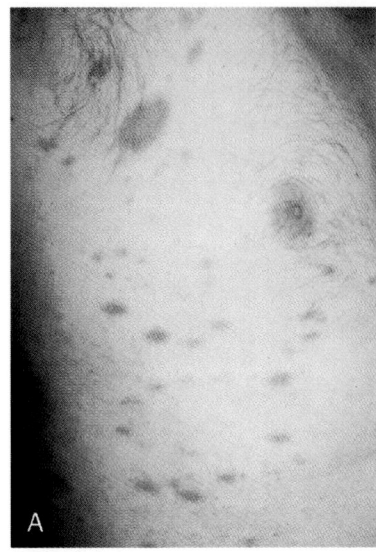

A, Pityriasis rosea.

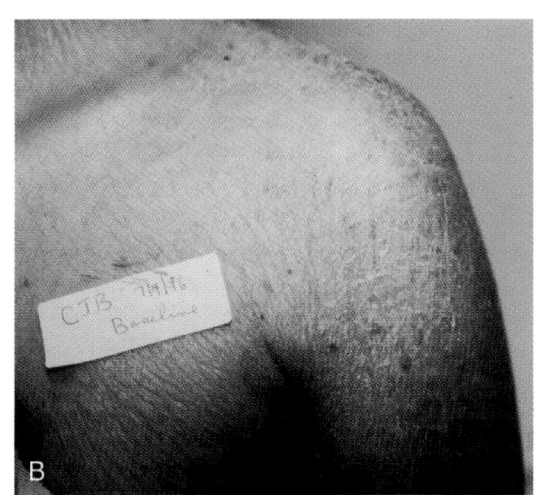

B, Ichthyosis.

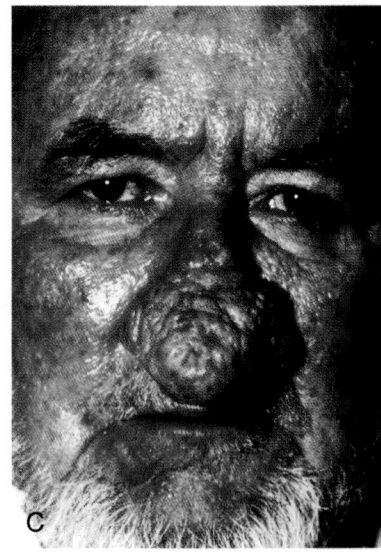

C, Rhinophyma.

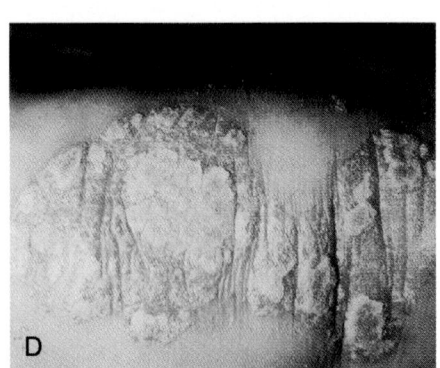

D, Psoriasis.

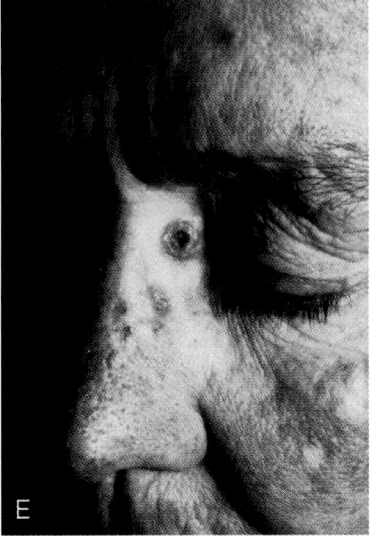

E, Basal cell cancer.

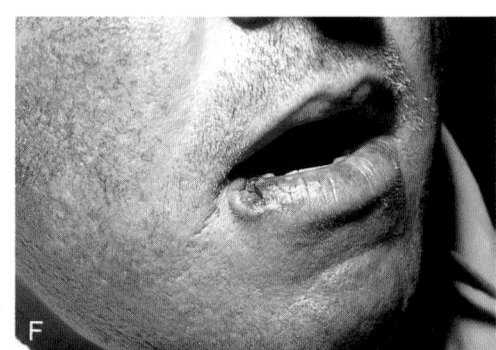

F, Squamous cell cancer. Firm nodule with eroded surface on the lower lip.

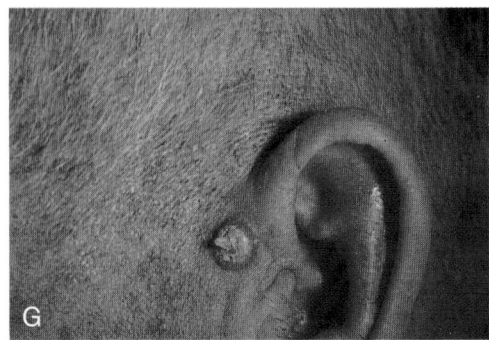

G, Cutaneous horn. Keratotic horn evolving from red nodule at base. These commonly are squamous cell cancers.

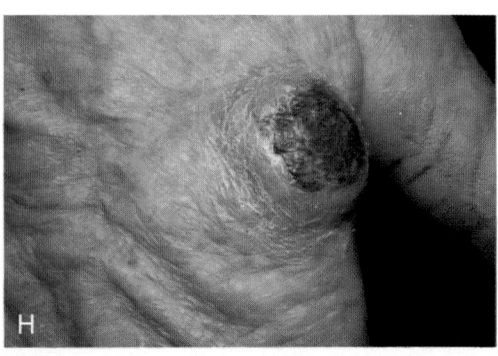

H, Keratoacanthoma. Large nodular lesion with central keratotic crater.

PLATE 13   SKIN DISEASES

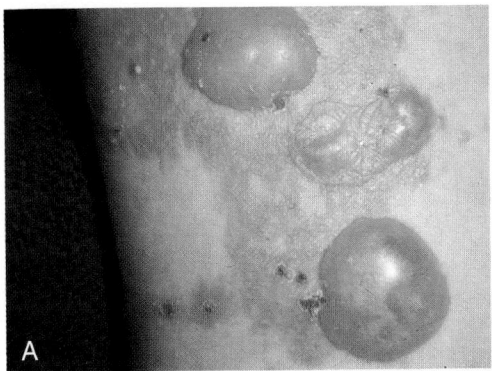

A, Bullous pemphigoid. Tense subepidermal bullae on an erythematous base.

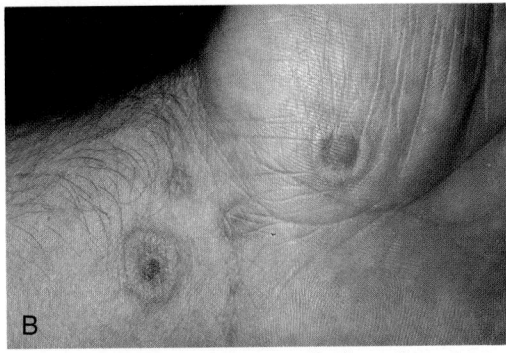

B, Erythema multiforme. Target or "bull's-eye" annular lesions with central vesicles and bullae.

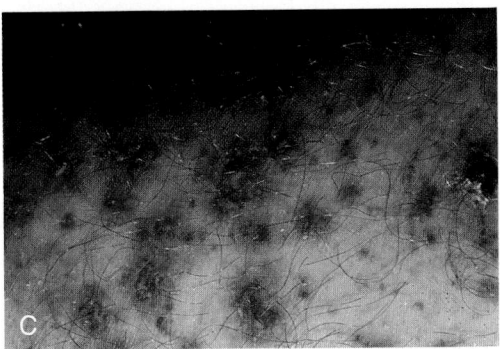

C, Palpable purpura. Leukocytoclastic vasculitis commonly causes raised purpuric and ulcerated lesions on legs.

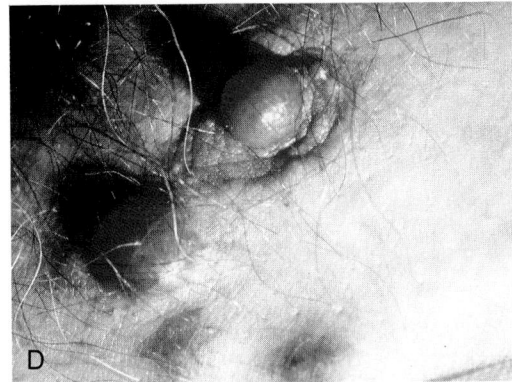

D, Skin metastases. Firm, hard, red nodules.

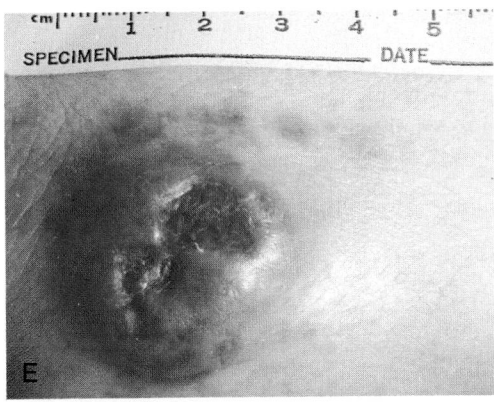

E, Mycosis fungoides, tumor stage.

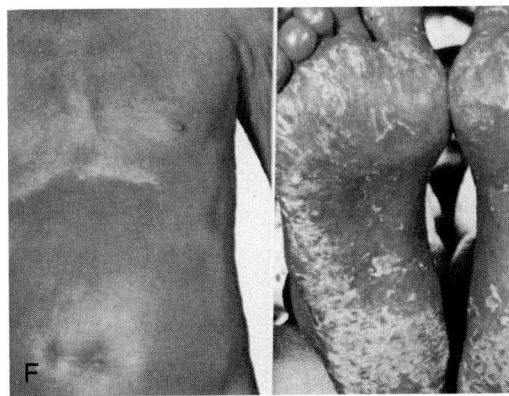

F, Sézary syndrome, exfoliative dermatitis stage.

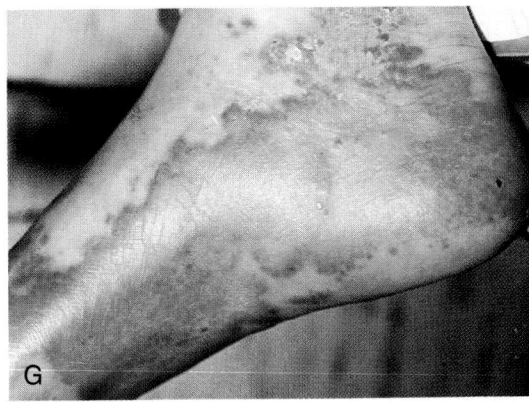

G, Classic Kaposi's sarcoma.

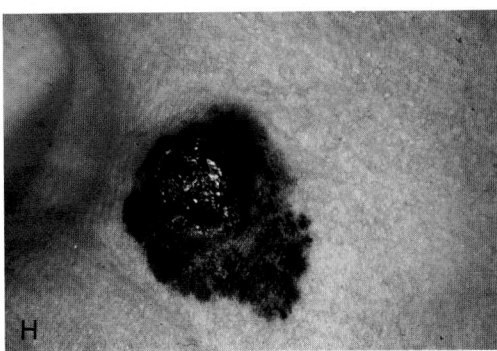

H, Malignant melanoma. Darkly pigmented, nodular lesion with irregular outline, irregular shades of dark pigmentation, and irregular surface configuration.

PLATE 14 SKIN DISEASES

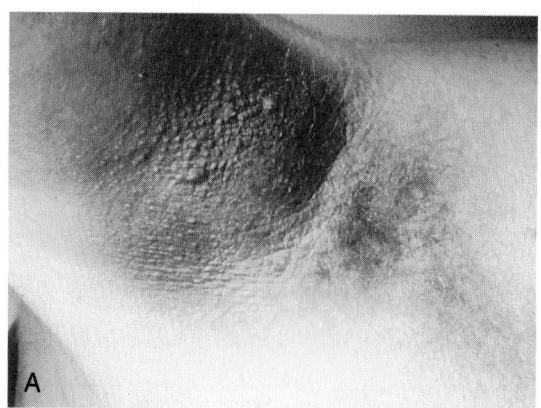

A, Acanthosis nigrans. Axillary lesion.

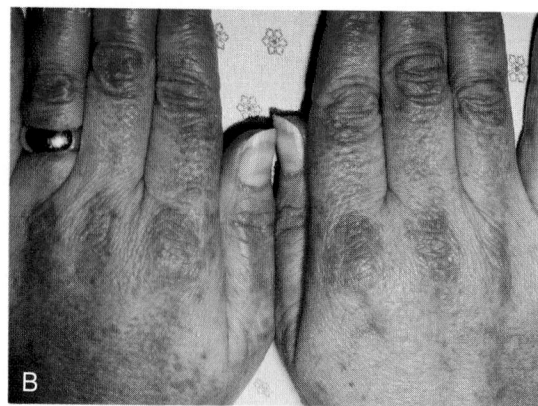

B, Dermatomyositis. Gottron's papules over the knuckles.

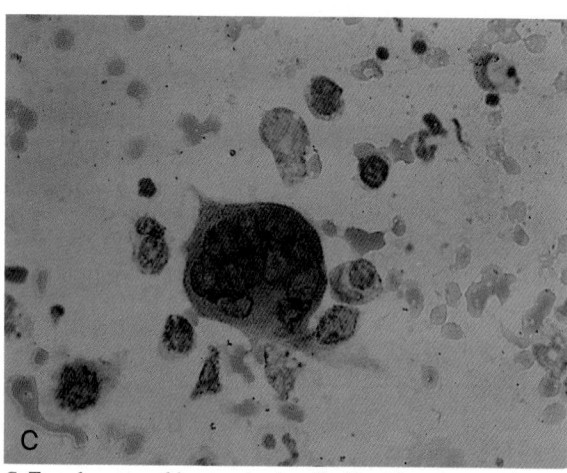

C, Tzanck smear of herpes simplex. Positive Tzanck smear is seen as multinucleated giant cell.

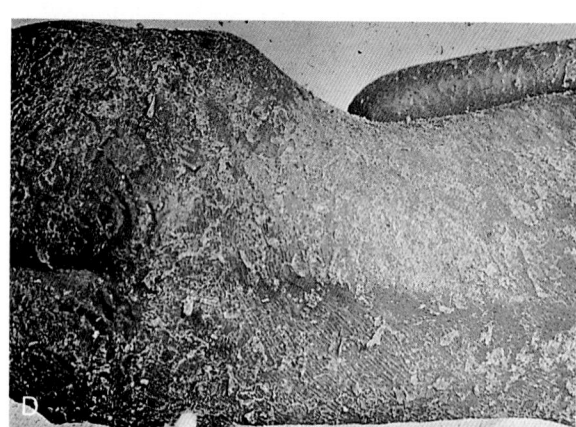

D, Exfoliative erythroderma. Diffuse inflammatory reaction of the entire skin with thickening, lichenification, redness, and scaling.

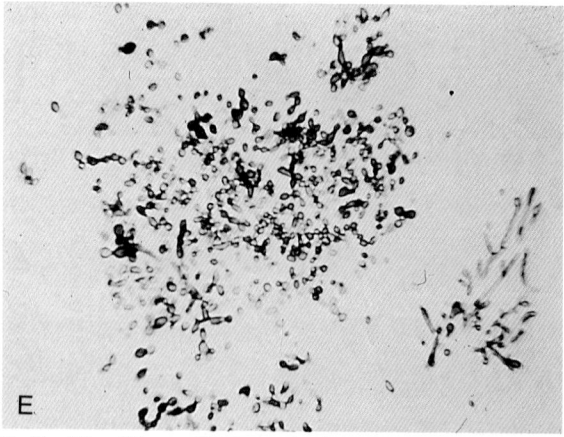

E, Candida albicans. KOH examination of candidal skin lesion. Short, stubby hyphae and budding yeast elements.

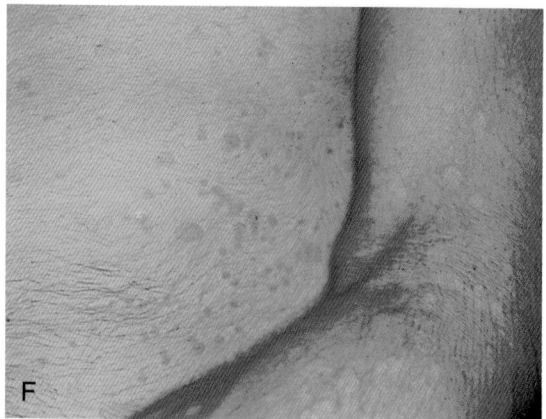

F, Tinea versicolor. Discrete areas of red-brown scaling lesions on the trunk.

PLATE 15   SKIN DISEASES

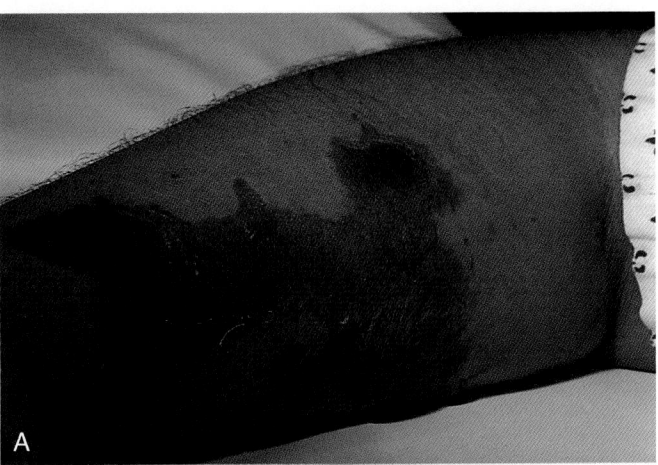

A, *Macule:* flat circumscribed color change. This is a purpuric area of skin in a patient with purpura fulminans.

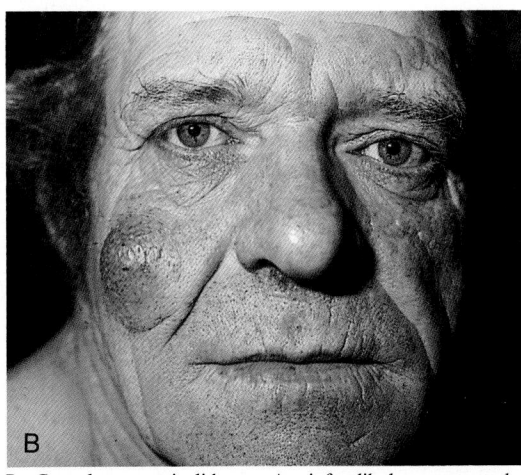

B, *Cyst:* large semisolid sac. An infundibular cyst on the right cheek. Note that this is a smooth round, nodular lesion.

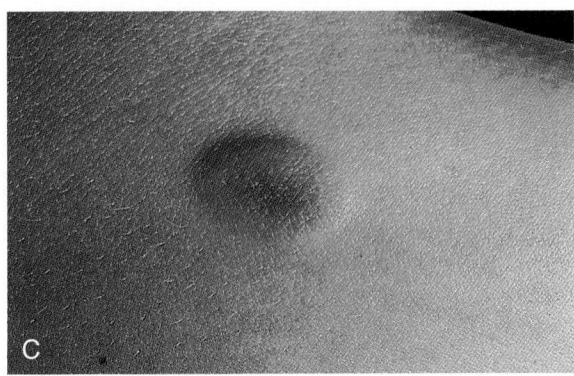

C, *Papule:* a solid elevation of 1 cm or less. This is a papule of granuloma annulare.

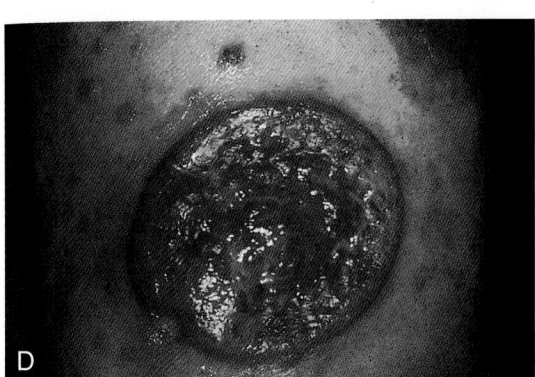

D, *Plaque:* a raised, circumscribed, flat-topped lesion. A typical mycosis fungoides–eroded plaque.

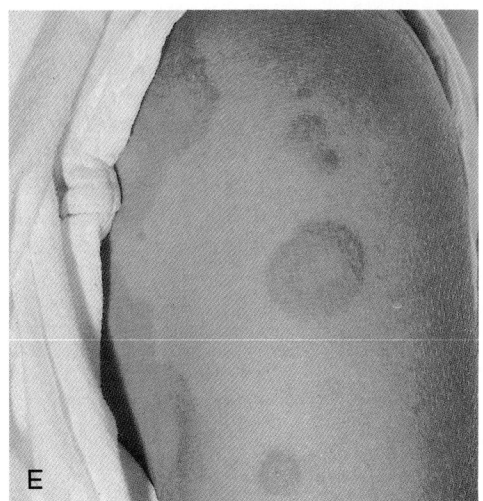

E, *Wheal:* erythematous edematous plaque that is evanescent. This is an urticarial lesion due to penicillin.

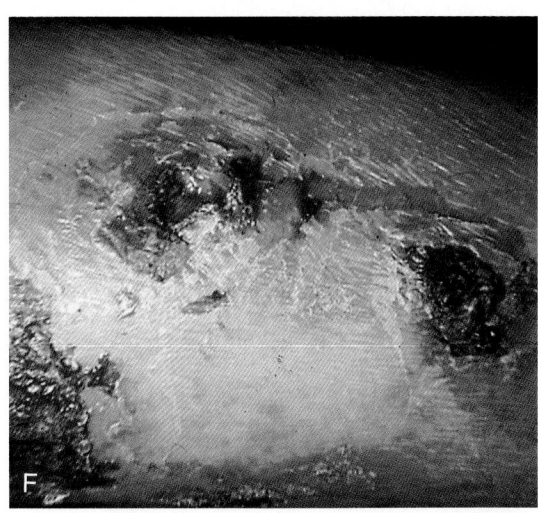

F, *Erosion:* superficial denudation of epidermis. Ecthyma, a superficial staphylococcal infection.

PLATE 16   SKIN DISEASES

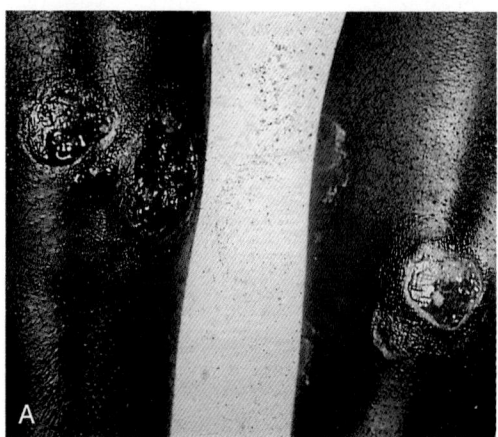

A, Ulcer: deep defect in the skin extending to the dermis. These ulcers are secondary to ischemia due to sickle cell anemia.

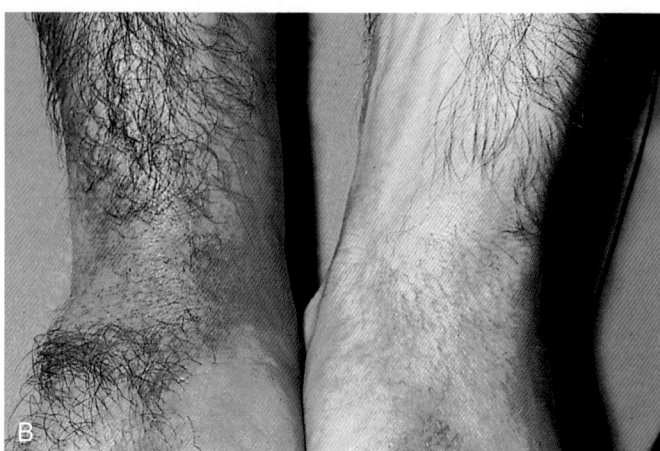

B, Atrophy: loss of epidermal or dermal substance with thinning of skin. Here the atrophy is due to scleroderma. Note loss of hair follicles and shiny atrophic areas of skin.

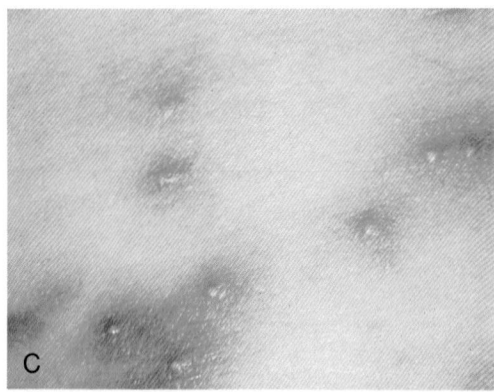

C, Pustule: fluid-filled sac filled with neutrophils. This patient had hot tub dermatitis due to *Pseudomonas* infection.

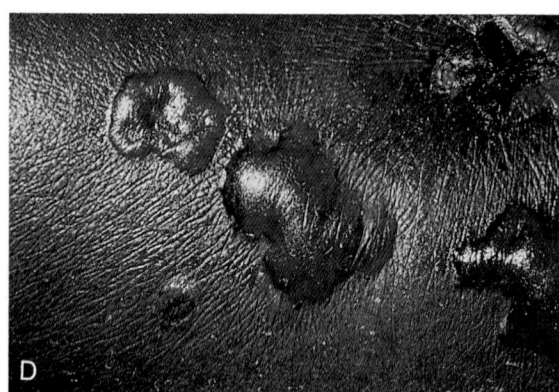

D, Bullae: fluid-filled lesions 0.5 cm or larger. Bullous impetigo.

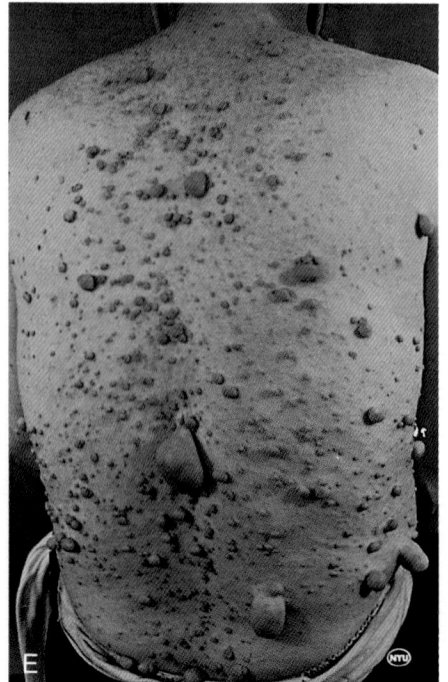

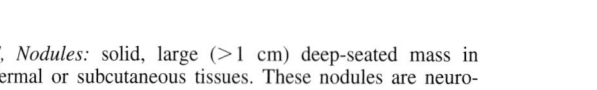

F, Scar: an area of replacement fibrosis of the dermis or subcutaneous tissue. These scars are healed diabetic ulcers.

E, Nodules: solid, large (>1 cm) deep-seated mass in dermal or subcutaneous tissues. These nodules are neurofibromas in a patient with neurofibromatosis.

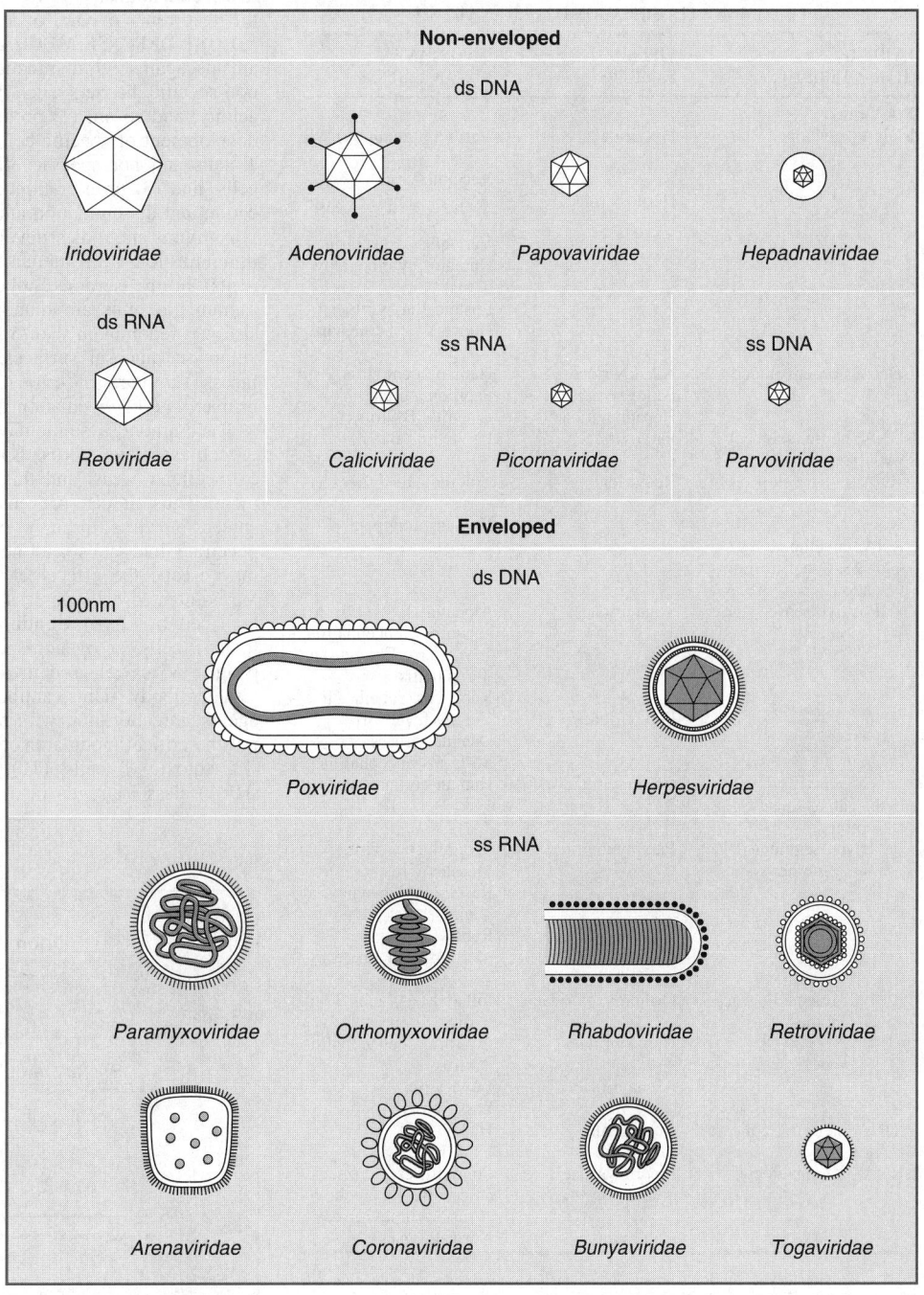

FIGURE 373–1 ■ Structure and relative size of human virus families. (Modified from Matthews REF: Classification and nomenclature of viruses. Intervirology 12:158, 1979.)

There are two major types of structures of virus particles. In the first type, capsomeres are arranged as a regular polyhedron with 20 triangular faces and 12 corners. Such a virus exhibits icosahedral symmetry. Many non-enveloped viruses are of this type. Other viruses exhibit helical symmetry in which a helix is formed of ribonucleoprotein and nucleic acid. Helical viruses are always enveloped, whereas icosahedral viruses may be enveloped or non-enveloped. The envelope is derived from host cell membranes and modified by insertion of one or more spikelike glycoproteins. These and other proteins on the surface of enveloped or non-enveloped viruses are important for two reasons: they provide specific interaction with receptors on host cells, and they serve as the major antigens of the virus.

Figure 373–1 demonstrates schematically the marked variety in size, shape, and structure of human viruses. In addition, there is great diversity in the structure of the viral genome: either RNA or DNA may be single stranded or double stranded. The genome may be linear or circular and may exist as single or multiple segments.

Viruses are classified by the International Committee on Taxonomy of Viruses according to the scheme presented in Table 373–1. The following order of virion characteristics is used: nucleic acid type, presence or absence of envelope, genome replication strategy, positive- or negative-sense genome, and genome segmentation.

Because virus structure varies and genomes are complex, mechanisms of replication are diverse. Following a random collision between a virus particle and a cell surface, attachment occurs by binding of a surface protein of a virus to a host cell virus receptor. The nature of the viral attachment protein has been identified for a number of viruses. Penetration of the plasma membrane of the cell occurs by endocytosis, a process similar to receptor-mediated endocytosis of non-viral ligands, or by non-endocytic pathways such as direct translocation across the plasma membrane. After acidification of the endosome, the viral membrane fuses with that of the vesicle, releasing the nucleocapsid. After uncoating of the viral nucleic acid, macromolecular synthesis of nucleic acid and protein occurs. The strategy for genome replication depends on the type of nucleic acid. Assembly of virus components then occurs, with release of mature viruses by budding, in the case of enveloped viruses, or by

Table 373–1 ■ CLASSIFICATION OF HUMAN VIRUSES

DIVIDING CHARACTERISTICS	VIRUS FAMILIES	IMPORTANT HUMAN VIRUSES
DNA Viruses		
dsDNA, enveloped	Poxviridae	Variola (smallpox) virus
		Vaccinia virus
	Herpesviridae	Herpes simplex virus types 1 and 2
		Varicella-zoster virus
		Human cytomegalovirus
		Epstein-Barr virus
		Human herpesvirus type G
dsDNA, non-enveloped	Adenoviridae	Human adenovirus
	Papovaviridae	Papillomavirus
	Hepadnaviridae	Hepatitis B virus
ssDNA, non-enveloped	Parvoviridae	Parvovirus B19
RNA Viruses		
dsRNA, nonenveloped	Reoviridae	Colorado tick fever virus
		Human rotaviruses
ssRNA, enveloped		
No DNA step in replication		
Positive-sense genome	Togaviridae	Alphavirus: Eastern equine encephalitis, Western Equine encephalitis
		Rubivirus: rubella virus
	Flaviviridae	Yellow fever virus
		Dengue viruses
		St. Louis encephalitis
	Coronaviridae	Human coronaviruses
Negative-sense genome		
Non-segmented genome	Paramyxoviridae	Parainfluenza virus
		Measles virus
		Respiratory syncytial virus
	Rhabdoviridae	Rabies virus
	Filoviridae	Marburg and Ebola viruses
Segmented genome	Orthomyxoviridae	Influenza A and B virus
	Bunyaviridae	California encephalitis virus
	Arenaviridae	LCM virus
		Lassa virus
DNA step in replication	Retroviridae	HTLV, I, II
		HIV, I, II
ssRNA, non-enveloped	Picornaviridae	Polioviruses, coxsackieviruses, echoviruses, rhinoviruses
	Caliciviridae	Norwalk virus

LCM = lymphocytic choriomeningitis; ss = single stranded; ds = double stranded; HTLV = human T-cell lymphotropic virus; HIV = human immunodeficiency virus.
From Murphy FA, Kinsbury DW: Virus taxonomy. *In* Fields BN, Knipe DM (eds): Fields Virology, 2nd ed. New York, Raven Press, 1990.

lysis of the cell, in the case of some non-enveloped viruses. Such released virions are infectious for other cells.

Viruses cause cell injury by a number of mechanisms: directly by lysis resulting from viral replication, by lysis induced by antiviral antibody and complement, or by cell-mediated immune mechanisms recognizing infected host cells. As virus infection spreads and sufficient numbers of cells are injured, disease results. Viral infection may be limited to the initial site of infection or may spread through the lymphatic, blood, or nervous system to distal sites. A role for viral toxins has never been established, and such enzymes as are virus coded have a role in viral replication but not directly in cellular injury, and they do not affect host tissues at distant sites. However, products of inflammation released from sites of cell injury and circulating interferon and other lymphokines contribute to the signs and symptoms of viral infection.

In addition to lytic effects on cells, viral infection may transform cells so that they proliferate continuously and, in vertebrates, mammals, and humans, may produce tumors, sometimes as a result of the occurrence of viral oncogenes in such viruses.

HOST DEFENSE MECHANISMS. Three main host defense mechanisms against viral infections have been described in addition to non-specific barriers such as skin, respiratory epithelium, gastric acidity, and so on: (1) production of specific antiviral antibody, (2) development of specific cell-mediated immunity involving cytotoxic T cells and non-specific effector cells such as natural killer (NK) cells, and (3) proliferation of macrophages that restrict virus replication and dissemination and also destroy infected cells.

Antiviral antibodies develop in response to viral infection and to immunization with attenuated or inactivated virus or viral components. In the serum, antibodies of all classes and subclasses of immunoglobulins are found; in addition, secretory antibodies consisting predominantly of immunoglobulin A (IgA) molecules develop on mucosal surfaces in response to infection of their surfaces. They are of critical importance in diseases in which the primary site of inoculation is a mucosal surface.

The immune system may interact with extracellular (free) virus or cell-associated virus. Specific antibody inactivates (neutralizes) extracellular virus, and this activity may be enhanced by complement. Thus, it can prevent initial infection or restrict cell-to-cell spread of virus through extracellular fluids. It cannot, however, penetrate into cells and neutralize intracellular virus. Thus, virus may escape the effects of antibody by direct cell-to-cell transfer. Virus-infected cells possess viral antigens on their surface and may be lysed by specific antibody and complement, by specific cytotoxic T cells, or by non-specific cells such as NK cells or macrophages. Virus released in the process may be neutralized by antiviral antibody. Thus, antibody may play a key role in protection against infection but, with the exception of enteroviral infection, is not the critical modulator of active viral infection.

Cytotoxic T cells (Tc), which are human leukocyte antigen (HLA) class I antigen restricted, also develop in response to infec-

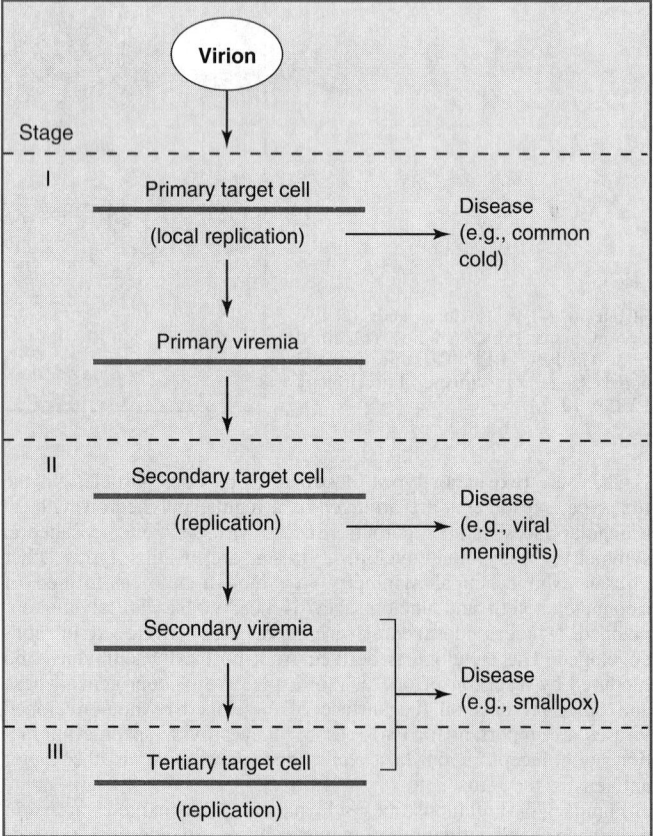

FIGURE 373–2 ■ Stages of viral pathogenesis. Initial invasion may involve only primary target cells or may lead to secondary or tertiary target cell invasion, which results in the characteristic disease. (Courtesy of ED Kilbourne.)

tion or immunization (see Chapter 270). They are important in limiting the growth of certain viruses in the infected host.

NK cells are another important host defense mechanism against viral infections. NK cells lyse virus-infected cells directly and produce cytokines that impede viral replication and enhance antiviral immune responses. They are not HLA class restricted. During early stages of viral infection.

Virus-induced interferons and cytokines have important roles in protection against virus infection through their ability to prevent viral replication and by means of their regulatory function in the immune system. Selected interferons (IFN-α, IFN-γ, IFN-β), tumor necrosis factor, and interleukin-1 have all been shown to contribute to antiviral defenses, but the specific contributions varied by infection. Interferon and cytokines also may account, in part, for some of the systemic signs, and symptoms that accompany viral infections.

MECHANISMS OF PATHOGENESIS. Infection is initiated, often when one or a very few virus particles are deposited in the respiratory, gastrointestinal, or genitourinary tract or are injected percutaneously or pass transplacentally. As shown in Figure 373–2, human viral infections may be classified according to mechanisms of pathogenesis. Many infections are limited to cells at the portal of entry, and dissemination does not occur. Conjunctivitis due to ade-

novirus type 8 and common colds due to rhinoviruses are examples of this type of pathogenesis.

Other virus infections spread hematogenously to distal sites. Infection at the primary site may or may not result in symptoms, but viral replication in the distal site usually results in the characteristic illness associated with such a virus infection. Enteroviruses such as coxsackievirus infect the gastrointestinal tract as their primary site, and this infection is usually clinically silent but produces a primary viremia, following which encephalitis, meningitis, or other central nervous system disease may occur as these tissues are infected. Other viruses reach target organs through nerves: rabies, varicella-zoster virus, and herpes simplex virus.

In other infections, viral replication in the secondary site produces a viremia that results in replication in still other sites. Such was the case with smallpox and may be the case with measles. Rash may be a manifestation of either primary or secondary viremia.

Many virus infections have clinical characteristics that permit diagnosis: measles, mumps, chickenpox, and poliomyelitis. However, many others do not, and many syndromes have multiple causes as is shown in Table 373–2. In fact, as many as 200

Table 373–2 ■ VIRUSES COMMONLY ASSOCIATED WITH DIFFERENT SYNDROMES

DISEASE CATEGORY	COMMON ASSOCIATED VIRUS	DISEASE CATEGORY	COMMON ASSOCIATED VIRUS
Respiratory Tract		**Gastrointestinal Tract**	
Upper respiratory tract infection (including common cold and pharyngitis)	Rhinoviruses	Gastroenteritis	Rotavirus
	Coronaviruses		Norwalk-like agents
	Parainfluenza 1–3		Adenovirus
	Influenza A, B	Hepatitis	Hepatitis A
	Herpes simplex		Hepatitis B
	Adenoviruses		Hepatitis C
	Echoviruses		Hepatitis D
	Coxsackieviruses		Hepatitis E
	Epstein-Barr virus		Epstein-Barr virus
	Respiratory synctial		Cytomegalovirus
Croup	Parainfluenza 1–3		
	Influenza A, B	**Skin**	
	Respiratory syncytial	Maculopapular rash	Measles
Bronchiolitis	Respiratory syncytial		Rubella
	Parainfluenza 1–3		Parvovirus B19
Pneumonia (adults)	Influenza A		Echoviruses
Pneumonia (children)	Respiratory syncytial		Coxsackievirus A16
	Parainfluenza 1–3		Enterovirus 71
	Influenza A	Hemorrhagic rash	Herpesvirus G
Central Nervous System			Alphavirus
Aseptic meningitis	Mumps		Bunyavirus
	Coxsackievirus B1–5		Flaviviruses
	Coxsackievirus A9	Localized lesions	Herpes simplex
	Echovirus 4, 6, 9, 11, 14, 18, 30, 31		Human papillomavirus 1, 2, 4, 41
Paralysis	Poliovirus 1–3		Molluscum contagiosum
Encephalitis	Human immunodeficiency virus I	**Neonatal**	
	Alphaviruses	Teratogenic effects	Rubella
	Flaviviruses		Cytomegalovirus
	Bunyaviruses	Disseminated disease	Coxsackievirus B1–5
	Herpes simplex 1		Echoviruses
	Enterovirus 71		Hepatitis B
	Mumps		Parvovirus B19
			Cytomegalovirus
Genitourinary Tract			Herpes simplex
Vulvovaginitis, cervicitis	Herpes simplex 2	Lower respiratory disease	Respiratory syncytial
Penile and vulvar lesions	Herpes simplex 2		Influenza
	Molluscum contagiosum	Enteritis	Rotavirus
	Human papillomavirus 6, 10, 11, 40–45, 51	**Other**	
Acute hemorrhagic cystitis	Adenovirus 11	Arthritis	Rubella
Ocular			Parvovirus B19
Conjunctivitis	Adenovirus 3, 4, 7, 8, 19		Hepatitis B
	Herpes simplex	Myositis	Togaviruses
	Varicella-zoster		Influenza B
	Measles	Carditis	Coxsackievirus B
Acute hemorrhagic conjunctivitis	Enterovirus 70	Parotitis, pancreatitis, and orchitis	Mumps
	Coxsackievirus A24		
Immune System			
Acquired immunodeficiency syndrome	Human immunodeficiency virus I		

Modified from Manegus MA, Douglas RG Jr: Viruses, rickettsiae, chlamydiae, and mycoplasmas. *In* Mandell GL, Douglas RG Jr, Bennett JE (eds): Principles and Practice of Infectious Diseases, 3rd ed. New York, Churchill Livingstone, 1990.

serologically distinct viruses may cause the common cold and related disorders. In the case of some syndromes—for example, ambulatory pneumonia—the etiology may be shared with other infectious organisms: *Mycoplasma pneumoniae, Chlamydia pneumoniae,* and *Legionella pneumophila.* Others, however, are exclusively viral in etiology.

PREVENTION AND CONTROL. Recent advances in antiviral chemotherapy have produced a number of specific antiviral agents that are available and effective for prophylaxis or treatment, or both, of certain viral diseases. For many other viral infections, however, no specific therapy exists. Proper use of antiviral agents may require specific viral diagnosis. Fortunately, in the case of herpes zoster, the diagnosis can usually be made clinically, and in influenza, the diagnosis can often be made on clinical and epidemiologic grounds; however, for many infections, laboratory diagnosis is required.

Vaccines are available for a number of viral infections, and many have greatly affected morbidity and mortality due to specific infections. Antibodies induced by vaccination may block initiation of infection in a primary site, as in the case in influenza. Others, such as inactivated poliomyelitis vaccine, are designed to prevent primary viremia after initial infection has occurred. Live attenuated viruses induce cell-mediated as well as humoral immune response.

Fields BN, Knipe DM (eds): Fields Virology, 2nd ed. New York. Raven Press, 1990. *Excellent definitive textbook of basic virology.*
Tyler UL, Fields BN: Introduction to viruses and viral diseases. *In* Mandell GL, Bennett JE, Dolin R (eds): Principles and Practice of Infectious Diseases, 4th ed. New York, John Wiley & Sons, 1995. *Excellent detailed review of virus structure, virus-cell interactions, virus-host interactions, and virus transmission.*

374 ANTIVIRAL THERAPY (NON-AIDS)
Richard J. Whitley

Advances in the chemotherapy of viral diseases are increasingly common. Nevertheless, in the United States, only a few antiviral agents of proven clinical value are available and for a limited number of indications. The problems associated with the development of antiviral agents can be summarized as follows: (1) viruses are obligate intracellular parasites that use biochemical pathways of the infected host cell, so it is difficult to achieve clinically useful antiviral activity without also adversely affecting host cell metabolism; (2) early diagnosis of viral infection is crucial for effective antiviral therapy, yet by the time symptoms appear, several cycles of viral multiplication may have occurred and replication has begun to wane; (3) precise diagnosis is difficult for many viral infections because of the lack of specificity of symptoms; and (4) because many of the disease syndromes caused by viruses are common, relatively benign, and self-limiting, the therapeutic index (ratio of efficacy to toxicity) must be extremely high for therapy to be acceptable.

As with all infectious diseases, the effectiveness of therapy is related to host defenses. Not only is the incidence of reactivation of certain viral diseases high in the immunocompromised host, but these infections also are often much more severe. These patients require high doses of antiviral agents for long periods of time and have a high morbidity and mortality with currently approved antiviral therapy.

ANTIVIRALS FOR HERPESVIRUS INFECTIONS

Acyclovir

MECHANISM OF ACTION. Acyclovir is an acyclic analogue of guanosine. Virus-specified thymidine kinase phosphorylates acyclovir to its monophosphate derivative, an event that does not occur in uninfected cells to a significant extent. Acyclovir is then further phosphorylated by cellular enzymes to its triphosphate derivative. Acyclovir triphosphate binds viral DNA polymerase, acting as a DNA chain terminator. Because acyclovir is taken up selectively by virus-infected cells, the concentration of acyclovir triphosphate is 40 to 100 times higher in infected than in uninfected cells. Furthermore, viral DNA polymerase exhibits a 10- to 30-fold greater affinity for acyclovir triphosphate than does cellular DNA polymerases. The higher concentration in infected cells plus the affinity for viral polymerases results in the very low toxicity of acyclovir for normal host cells. Although Epstein-Barr virus (EBV) and cytomegalovirus (CMV) do not have virus-specific thymidine kinases, acyclovir does have minimal activity against these viruses.

LICENSED USES. Acyclovir is available in ointment, capsule, and intravenous formulations. In the topical form, acyclovir is licensed for managing primary herpes genitalis in both immunocompetent and immunocompromised hosts as well as in limited, non–life-threatening mucocutaneous herpes simplex virus (HSV) infections in immunocompromised hosts. It is less active topically than when delivered by other routes, and its use by this route should be discouraged.

Oral acyclovir is indicated in the management of most cases of primary or initial genital herpes in all patient populations and as suppressive therapy in normal hosts with frequently recurrent genital herpes (six or more recurrences a year). Oral acyclovir is also used as prophylaxis and treatment in immunocompromised patients with a history of HSV infections (e.g., herpes labialis or genital herpes). High-dose oral acyclovir (i.e., 800 mg five times per day) has been approved for use in immunocompetent patients with localized herpes zoster.

Intravenous acyclovir is indicated in severe initial herpes genitalis of immunocompetent patients and in the treatment of some initial and recurrent mucocutaneous infections in immunocompromised patients, as well as in the treatment of herpes simplex encephalitis (HSE). Intravenous acyclovir is approved for treatment of varicella-zoster virus (VZV) infections in immunocompromised hosts.

TOXICITY. Acyclovir has an excellent safety profile and is well tolerated. The major adverse effect of acyclovir is that it alters renal function. High-dose bolus injection of acyclovir can cause crystallization in renal tubules and subsequent acute tubular necrosis or simply a reversible elevation of serum creatinine. Dehydration, pre-existing renal insufficiency, and higher doses of acyclovir are risk factors for renal toxicity. Dosage alterations are required with renal impairment (Table 374–1). In addition, there have been a few brief reports suggesting central nervous system (CNS) toxicity after intravenous administration of acyclovir. Oral acyclovir has not been associated with renal toxicity, even when given in high doses (800 mg five times a day).

Because acyclovir is a nucleoside analogue that can be incorporated into both viral and host-cell DNA, it has been studied extensively for its potential as a carcinogen, teratogen, and mutagen. There is no significant evidence that acyclovir is a carcinogen in humans, and animal studies indicate that acyclovir is not a significant teratogen in clinically used doses. Acyclovir is not a significant mutagen in vitro but seems to be able to induce chromosomal events as does caffeine. Because of the many possible indications for acyclovir during pregnancy, as well as the likelihood of frequent first-trimester exposures to drug before pregnancy is established, it is extremely important to define its risk. The safety of acyclovir in pregnancy, therefore, has not been unequivocally established. Because acyclovir crosses the placenta and can concentrate in amniotic fluid, there is valid concern about the potential for renal toxicity in the fetus.

RESISTANCE TO ACYCLOVIR. Resistance to acyclovir develops through mutations in one of two HSV genes, namely, those speci-

Table 374–1 ■ DOSAGE ADJUSTMENTS FOR INTRAVENOUS ACYCLOVIR IN PATIENTS WITH IMPAIRED RENAL FUNCTION

CREATININE CLEARANCE (ML/MIN/1.73 M^2)	PERCENTAGE OF STANDARD DOSE	DOSING INTERVAL (HOURS)
>50	100	8
25–50	100	12
10–25	100	24
0–10*	50	24

*Administered after hemodialysis.

fying viral thymidine kinase (TK) or DNA polymerase. Clinical isolates resistant to acyclovir are almost uniformly deficient in TK. Until recently, such resistance has been rare; all such mutants had reduced neurovirulence and did not readily establish latency. However, acyclovir-resistant HSV mutants are being reported more frequently in the immunocompromised patient population and in one normal host. These mutants are deficient in viral TK and sensitive to vidarabine and foscarnet, drugs that do not require viral TK for activation. Some isolates are fully neurovirulent and able to establish latency in a murine model. With the growing population of immunocompromised patients (due to both human immunodeficiency virus [HIV] infection and therapeutic immunosuppression) who suffer from frequent and severe herpesvirus infections, it is expected that acyclovir resistance will become more prevalent.

Valaciclovir

MECHANISM OF ACTION. Valaciclovir is the L-valyl ester of acyclovir that, after oral administration, is cleaved in the gastrointestinal tract and liver by an enzyme identified as valaciclovir hydrolase. The end product is acyclovir and the natural amino acid L-valine. The mechanism of action and disposition of acyclovir are described previously.

LICENSED USES. Valaciclovir is licensed for the treatment of primary, recurrent, and suppressive therapy of genital HSV infections. In comparative studies, valaciclovir is as effective as treatment with acyclovir; however, dosing frequency can be decreased in many patients to once daily (Table 374–2).

Valaciclovir is also licensed for the treatment of herpes zoster in the immunocompetent host (see Table 374–2). In a clinical trial that directly compared valaciclovir and acyclovir therapy, valaciclovir significantly accelerated the resolution of zoster-associated pain and therefore is the medication of preference. A dosing interval of three times a day provides an advantage over acyclovir.

TOXICITY. In general, valaciclovir is well tolerated because it is metabolized to acyclovir. However, in HIV-infected individuals who were exposed to high doses of valaciclovir for prolonged periods of time, a thrombotic thrombocytopenic purpuric syndrome was reported. On detailed analysis, other concomitantly administered drugs were associated with greater risk ratios for this syndrome.

Valaciclovir is under investigation for suppression of reactivation of CMV infections in transplant recipients.

Penciclovir/Famciclovir

MECHANISM OF ACTION. Penciclovir is another nucleoside analogue in which the base, guanine, is normal but the sugar moiety has a structural modification. The structural similarities to acyclovir is apparent; however, there is no oxygen atom in acyclic sugar moiety, although an OH group exists in the position equivalent to that of the 3′ OH group in the normal nucleoside, guanosine. Like acyclovir, penciclovir is converted to its monophosphate by herpes simplex virus or varicella-zoster virus thymidine kinase. Penciclovir triphosphate inhibits viral DNA polymerase, but it is not a DNA chain terminator; therefore, there is potential for internal incorporation of penciclovir residues into viral DNA and further DNA elongation. The initial conversion of penciclovir to its monophosphate is more efficient than the phosphorylation of acyclovir; however, the penciclovir triphosphate formed in infected cells is less active than acyclovir triphosphate as an inhibitor of HSV and VZV DNA polymerase.

The triphosphate of penciclovir has a significantly longer intracellular half life than acyclovir triphosphate. The full implication of this observation remains to be elucidated. The oral bioavailability of penciclovir is poor (< 5 %).

Famciclovir is the diacetyl ester of penciclovir. When administered orally, the compound undergoes a two-step modification to penciclovir. Penciclovir, then, behaves as noted earlier.

LICENSED USES. Famciclovir is licensed for the treatment of primary, recurrent, and suppressive therapy of genital HSV infections (see Table 374–2). In addition, famciclovir has been shown to be equivalent to acyclovir for suppression of HSV reactivation in immunocompromised hosts.

Famciclovir is also licensed for the treatment of herpes zoster in the normal host (see Table 374–2).

Penciclovir is only licensed in its topical formulation (Denavir) for the treatment of herpes simplex labialis.

TOXICITY. Famciclovir and penciclovir (applied topically) have excellent safety profiles and are well tolerated. The most commonly reported adverse events are headache, nausea, and diarrhea; however, these event rates have occurred at no greater frequency than either background or concomitant acyclovir administration. The long-term toxicity of penciclovir has not been well established, although carcinogenicity in animal models has been demonstrated. The relevance of this latter finding is unknown.

Ganciclovir

MECHANISM OF ACTION. Ganciclovir, also known as DHPG, is an acyclic nucleoside analogue of acyclovir that has increased in vitro activity against all herpesviruses as compared with acyclovir, including an 8 to 20 times greater antiviral activity against CMV. Like acyclovir, the activity of ganciclovir in HSV-infected cells depends on phosphorylation by virus-specific TK. Also like acyclovir, ganciclovir monophosphate is further converted to its di- and triphosphate derivatives by cellular kinases. In cells infected by HSV-1 or HSV-2, the triphosphate (DHPG-TP) competitively inhibits the incorporation of guanosine-TP into viral DNA and terminates chain synthesis. The mode of action of ganciclovir against CMV and EBV (which do not produce virus-specific TK) is not entirely known, but it has been suggested that these viruses may induce a cellular TK or viral kinase that efficiently promotes the obligatory initial phosphorylation of ganciclovir to its monophosphate.

LICENSED USES. Ganciclovir has been licensed by the U.S. Food and Drug Administration for treating CMV retinitis and life-threatening CMV diseases in acquired immunodeficiency syndrome (AIDS) and other immunocompromised patients.

TOXICITY. The most important side effects of ganciclovir are neutropenia and thrombocytopenia. Neutropenia occurs in approximately 35% of patients and is usually (but not always) reversible with dose adjustment or discontinuation. Thrombocytopenia occurs in about 20% of patients. Numerous other side effects possibly related to ganciclovir, such as nausea, vomiting, dizziness, and headache, are usually not of clinical significance. Agents with significant myelotoxicity, such as antimetabolites or alkylating agents, cannot be used concomitantly with ganciclovir. Zidovudine (azidothymidine or [AZT]) may be used cautiously in low doses in patients receiving ganciclovir, but hematologic parameters must be monitored closely.

Ganciclovir also has significant gonadal toxicity in animal screening systems, most notably as a potent inhibitor of spermatogenesis. As an agent affecting DNA synthesis, ganciclovir has carcinogenic potential.

CLINICAL USE. Ganciclovir has been the most widely tested drug for the treatment of CMV infections. There is support for clinical benefit in immunocompromised patients with CMV retinitis and gastrointestinal infection. Benefit is suggested but has been less dramatic for CMV pneumonia in AIDS patients and organ transplant recipients. Ganciclovir has effectively suppressed the reactivation of CMV infections in organ transplant recipients.

Cidofovir

MECHANISM OF ACTION. Cidofovir (hydroxyphosphonylmethoxycytosine) is unlike nucleoside analogues. Cidofovir does not require specific conversion to the monophosphate derivative to initiate its inhibitory effects. Although the mechanism of action has not been completely elucidated, the essential target is virus-specific DNA polymerase. Cidofovir has an additionally important feature, namely, a very prolonged tissue half-life. In humans, a dose of once weekly for induction and biweekly thereafter for maintenance has been established for the treatment of cytomegalovirus retinitis in patients with AIDS.

LICENSED USES. Cidofovir is only licensed for the treatment of CMV retinitis in patients with AIDS (Table 374–2). Cidofovir provides an alternative to ganciclovir or foscarnet therapy for retinitis in this patient population.

TOXICITY. Cidofovir is directly associated with nephrotoxicity. In the presence of proteinuria or elevated serum levels of creati-

Table 374–2 ■ INDICATIONS FOR THE USE OF AVAILABLE ANTIVIRAL AGENTS

INDICATION	ANTIVIRAL AGENT	ROUTE	DOSE	COMMENTS
Respiratory syncytial virus infection (infants)	Ribavirin	Aerosol	Diluted in sterile water to a concentration of 20 mg/mL, then delivered via aerosol for 12–18 hr/d for 3–7 days	Only for infants at high risk
Life- or sight-threatening cytomegalovirus (CMV) infections in immunocompromised hosts	Ganciclovir	IV	5.0 mg/kg q12h × 14 days	Maintenance therapy for 5.0 mg/kg/d recommended for AIDS patients. Leukopenia is a frequent complication; in bone marrow transplant patients with CMV pneumonia, CMV immune globulin may be a useful adjunct
	Foscarnet	IV		
	Cidofovir	IV	5 mg once weekly × 3	Induction therapy
		IV	5 mg biweekly	Maintenance
Condyloma acuminatum	Interferon-α	Intralesional	1.0 million units injected into the base of each lesion, up to 3 times per week for 3 weeks	Flu-type symptoms may occur with administrations
Influenza A infection	Amantadine	Oral	Adults: 100–200 mg/d for 5–7 days Children ≤ 9 years: 4.4–8.8 mg/kg/d for 5–7 days not to exceed 150 mg/d	Normal person >65 years should receive 100 mg/day
Prophylaxis against influenza A virus infection	Amantadine	Oral	Adults: 100–200 mg/d Children ≤ 9 years: 4.4–8.8 mg/kg/d (not to exceed 150 mg/d)	Continued for the duration of the epidemic or for 2 weeks in conjunction with influenza vaccination (until vaccine-induced immunity develops); normal persons >65 years should receive 100 mg/d
	Rimantadine	Oral	100 mg PO bid × season	
Herpes simplex virus (HSV) encephalitis	Acyclovir	IV	10 mg/kg (1-hour infusion) every 8 hours for 10–14 days	Morbidity and mortality are significantly lower in patients treated with acyclovir than with vidarabine
Neonatal herpes	Acyclovir	IV	10 mg/kg (1 hour infusion) every 8 hours for 10 days	Efficacy of vidarabine is established; vidarabine and acyclovir show equal efficacy
Mucocutaneous HSV in immunocompromised hosts	Acyclovir or	IV	5.0 mg/kg (1 hour infusion) every 8 hours for 7 days	Choice of topical, oral, or intravenous preparation depends on clinical severity and setting; topical acyclovir is appropriate only when it can be applied to all lesions; it does not affect untreated lesions or systemic symptoms
	Acyclovir	Oral	400 mg 3–5 times/d for 10 days	
	Acyclovir Valaciclovir		Oral 500 mg bid	10 days
	Famciclovir	Oral	500 mg tid	10 days
Prophylaxis against mucocutaneous HSV during intense immunosuppression	Acyclovir or	Oral	200 mg 3–4 times/day	Oral therapy most convenient; lesions recur when therapy stops
	Acyclovir	IV	5 mg/kg/q 8 hr	Lesions recur when therapy stops
Treatment of initial genital HSV infections	Acyclovir or	Oral	200 mg 5 times/d for 10 days or 400 mg tid × 10 day	Drug of choice in most clinical settings; treatment has no effect on subsequent recurrence rates
	Acyclovir	IV	5 mg/kg (1 hour infusion) every 8 hours for 5–7 days	For patients requiring hospitalization or with neurologic or other visceral complications
	Valaciclovir	Oral	1 g bid	5–10 days
	Famciclovir	Oral	250 mg tid	5–10 days
Recurrent genital herpes	Acyclovir	Oral	400 mg tid/d for 5 days	No effect on subsequent recurrence rates; efficacy greater if used early in attack
	Valaciclovir	Oral	500 mg bid or 1 g qd	5–7 days
	Famciclovir	Oral	250 mg tid	5–7 days
Prophylaxis against frequently recurring genital herpes	Acyclovir	Oral	200 mg 3–5 times/d	Occasional "breaking through" attacks and/or asymptomatic virus shedding during treatment; re-evaluation every 6 months recommended
	Valaciclovir	Oral	500 mg bid or 1 g/d	
	Famciclovir	Oral	250 mg tid	
Treatment of HSV keratitis	Trifluorothymidine or	Topical	One drop of 0.1% ophthalmic solution every 2 hours while awake (up to 9 drops/d)	3% acyclovir ointment (ophthalmic) is equal or superior to idoxuridine, vidarabine, and trifluridine for treatment of HSV keratitis but is not available in the United States
	Vidarabine or	Topical	One-half-inch ribbon of 3% ophthalmic ointment 5 times/d	
	Idoxuridine	Topical	One-half-inch ribbon of 0.5% ophthalmic ointment 5 times/d	
Localized herpes zoster in immunocompetent hosts	Acyclovir or Famciclovir or Valaciclovir	Oral	800 mg 5 times/d for 7–10 days 250 mg tid × 5–7 days 1 gram tid × 5–7 days	Shortens time to lesion healing, but not shown to decrease the incidence of postherapetic neuralgia

Table 374–2 ▪ INDICATIONS FOR THE USE OF AVAILABLE ANTIVIRAL AGENTS *Continued*

INDICATION	ANTIVIRAL AGENT	ROUTE	DOSE	COMMENTS
Chickenpox in immunocompromised hosts	Acyclovir	IV	500 mgM^2 (1-hour infusion) every 8 hours for 7 days	In the absence of comparative data, acyclovir is preferred because of its ease of administration and lower toxicity
	or	IV		
Treatment of severe localized or disseminated herpes zoster in immunocompromised hosts	Acyclovir or	IV	500 mg/M^2 of 12.4 mg/kg (1-hour infusion) every 8 hours for 5–7 days	Comparative trials in severe localized and disseminated herpes zoster are underway; pending results, acyclovir is preferred because of its ease of administration and lower toxicity
	Valaciclovir	Oral	1 g tid	7–10 days
	Famciclovir	Oral	500 mg tid	7–10 days
Chronic hepatitis B	Interferon-α	SQ	10 × 10^6 units tiw for 16 weeks or 5 × 10^6 units daily for 16 weeks	Patients must have compensated liver disease
Chronic hepatitis C	Interferon-α	SQ	3 × 10^6 units tiw for 24 weeks	Must have compensated liver disease

nine, significant risk of renal failure exists. As a consequence, pretreatment hydration and concomitant administration with probenecid are mandatory before the use of this medication.

Idoxuridine and Trifluorothymidine

Idoxuridine and trifluorothymidine are analogues of thymidine. When administered systemically, these nucleosides are phosphorylated by both viral and cellular TK to active triphosphorylate derivatives that inhibit both viral and cellular DNA synthesis. The result is antiviral activity but also sufficient host cytotoxicity to prevent the systemic use of these drugs. Toxicity of these compounds is not significant, however, when applied topically to the eye in the treatment of HSV keratitis. Both idoxuridine and trifluorothymidine, as well as vidarabine, ophthalmic ointments are effective and licensed for such treatment. Acyclovir as an ophthalmic preparation also appears to be effective but is not yet licensed. Trifluorothymidine appears to be the most efficacious of these compounds. Although these agents are not of proven value in the treatment of stromal keratitis and uveitis, trifluorothymidine is more likely to penetrate the cornea. Some forms of stromal keratitis and uveitis are thought to be caused by immune mechanisms and thus would not respond to antiviral drugs. The ophthalmic preparations of idoxuridine, vidarabine, and trifluorothymidine may cause local irritation, photophobia, edema of the eyelids and cornea, punctual occlusion, and superficial punctate keratopathy.

Vidarabine

Vidarabine has been shown to be effective when administered parenterally for HSE, neonatal herpes, and VZV infections in the immunocompromised host. Because of a lower therapeutic index than acyclovir, it is only available as an ophthalmic preparation for therapy of HSV keratitis.

Foscarnet

Foscarnet, a pyrophosphate analogue of phosphonoacetic acid, has potent in vitro and in vivo activity against herpesviruses. Foscarnet inhibits the DNA polymerase of all human herpesviruses by blocking the pyrophosphate binding site and preventing chain elongation. Unlike acyclovir, which requires activation by a virus-specific TK, foscarnet acts directly on the virus DNA polymerase. TK-deficient, acyclovir-resistant herpesviruses remain sensitive to foscarnet.

Foscarnet was recently approved for the treatment of CMV retinitis in HIV-infected patients. Data collected from the Soka clinical trial indicate the equal effectiveness of foscarnet and ganciclovir therapy for retinitis in this population. However, use of foscarnet in combination with zidovidine resulted in enhanced survival. These findings remain to be confirmed in a larger study population. Foscarnet has been used for induction therapy of retinitis as well as when ganciclovir is not tolerated. However, administration of foscarnet is not without toxicity. Renal toxicity has been documented as well as hypocalcemia and altered levels of serum magnesium. Foscarnet's lack of bone marrow toxicity offers an advantage over ganciclovir. Additionally, foscarnet also has been used to treat acyclovir-resistant herpes simplex genital disease.

ANTIVIRALS FOR RESPIRATORY VIRAL INFECTIONS

It is difficult to overestimate the impact of respiratory viral illnesses on human health. Almost 90% of the population experiences one of these illnesses each year, resulting in a staggering number of days lost from work and school, as well as significant potential for serious morbidity and even death. Nonetheless, because these conditions in most patient populations are self-limited and rarely fatal, the requirements for new drugs are stringent: an extreme degree of safety, moderate to high effectiveness, ease of administration, and low cost. Accordingly, only two such antiviral agents are approved for use in the United States, each with fairly limited indications. Because of the number of developmental programs identifying new antiviral agents for treatment of respiratory viruses, it seems likely that an expanded armamentarium will be forthcoming.

Amantadine and Rimantadine

MECHANISM OF ACTION. Amantadine and rimantadine have a narrow spectrum of activity and at concentrations achievable in humans are useful only against influenza A infections. Although amantadine was the first antiviral agent to be approved in the United States, its mechanism of action is not yet completely understood. Influenza A viruses differ in their susceptibility to amantadine, and the drug may have different actions depending on the concentration and virus strain. Early studies indicated that amantadine acted by preventing the penetration and/or uncoating the virus. More recently, low concentrations of the drug were shown to inhibit virus assembly by interacting with hemagglutinin; high concentrations appear to inhibit an early stage of the infection involving fusion between the virus envelope and the membrane of secondary lysosomes. Rimantidine has a similar mechanism of action.

LICENSED USES. As antiviral agents, amantadine and rimantidine are licensed for both the chemoprophylaxis and the treatment of influenza A infections. Both drugs can be used for any unimmunized member of the general population who wishes to avoid influenza A, but prophylaxis is especially recommended to control presumed influenza outbreaks in institutions housing high-risk persons. High-risk individuals include adults and children with chronic disorders of the cardiovascular or pulmonary systems requiring regular follow-up or hospitalization during the preceding year, as well as nursing homes and other chronic-care facilities residents. In these instances, drugs should be administered to all residents of the institution, whether or not they received influenza vaccination the previous fall. To reduce spread of virus and to minimize disruption of patient care, it is also recommended that amantadine prophylaxis be offered to unvaccinated staff who care for high-risk patients. Amantadine prophylaxis is also recommended in the following situations:

1. As an adjunct to late immunization of high-risk individuals.

Amantadine does not interfere with antibody response to the vaccine.

2. For persons who have not been immunized and who care for high-risk persons in home settings, both to reduce spread of virus and to allow persons to maintain care for high-risk persons in the home setting.
3. For immunodeficient persons, who may be expected to have a poor antibody response to vaccine.
4. For persons for whom influenza vaccine is contraindicated (e.g., for persons hypersensitive to egg protein).

Both drugs are also indicated in the treatment of uncomplicated respiratory illness caused by influenza A. Studies have shown a beneficial effect on the signs and symptoms of acute influenza, as well as a significant reduction in quantity of virus in respiratory secretions. Because of the short duration of disease, amantadine must be administered within 48 hours of symptom onset to show benefit. The effect of amantadine on the prevention of complications in high-risk groups is under evaluation.

Rimantadine is a structural analogue of amantadine, with the same spectrum of activity, mechanism of action, and clinical indications. Rimantadine is somewhat more effective than amantadine against influenza type A viruses at equal concentrations. Absorption of rimantadine is delayed when compared with amantadine, and, furthermore, equivalent doses of rimantadine produce lower plasma levels than does amantadine. The lower plasma levels may explain the lower incidence of side effects at similar doses. Rimantadine has similar CNS side effects even though, unlike amantadine, this drug does not affect CNS catecholamine release and is not effective in the treatment of Parkinson's disease. The efficacy of rimantadine in both the prophylaxis and treatment of influenza A infections is similar to that of amantadine. There has been a recent report of rimantadine-resistant strains of influenza isolated from patients treated for acute influenza A.

TOXICITY. Amantadine is reported to cause side effects in 5 to 10% of healthy young adults taking the standard adult dose of 200 mg/day. These side effects are usually mild, cease soon after amantadine is discontinued, and often disappear even with continued use of the drug. CNS side effects are most common and include difficulty in thinking, confusion, lightheadedness, hallucinations, anxiety, and insomnia. Activities requiring mental alertness (e.g., driving) should be avoided until it is reasonable to assume that these symptoms will not occur. More severe adverse effects (e.g., mental depression and psychosis) are usually associated with doses exceeding 200 mg daily. About 5% of patients complain of nausea, vomiting, or anorexia. Older individuals are more likely to experience side effects. Rimantidine appears to be somewhat better tolerated.

Patients with renal disease should receive doses based on their creatinine clearance (Table 374–3). Doses for older people and children are usually lower as well. Persons with an active seizure disorder may be at increased risk for seizures when amantadine is given at standard doses.

Ribavirin

MECHANISM OF ACTION. Ribavirin is a nucleoside analogue whose mechanisms of action are poorly understood and probably not the same for all viruses; however, its ability to alter nucleotide pools and the packaging of mRNA appears to be important. This process is not totally virus specific, but there is a certain selectivity in that infected cells produce more mRNA than non-infected cells. The capacity of viral mRNA to support protein synthesis is markedly reduced by ribavirin. High concentrations also inhibit cellular protein synthesis.

LICENSED USES. The development of a mechanism to deliver ribavirin by means of a small-particle aerosol greatly enhanced the potential usefulness of this drug for respiratory viral infections. At this time ribavirin is licensed for the treatment, by aerosol administration, of carefully selected hospitalized infants and young children with severe lower respiratory tract infections caused by respiratory syncytial virus (RSV). The vast majority of infants and children with RSV infection have disease that is mild and self-limited and do not require ribavirin.

Of note, ribavirin is also undergoing evaluation for the treatment of chronic hepatitis C when co-administered with interferon.

TOXICITY AND CLINICAL PROBLEMS. No adverse effect has been clearly attributable to aerosol therapy with ribavirin, although reports of adverse effects during or after therapy in infants with RSV have included bronchospasm, pulmonary function test changes, pneumothorax in ventilated patients, apnea, cardiac arrest, hypotension, and concomitant digitalis toxicity. Precipitation of drug within the ventilatory apparatus of patients on mechanical ventilation can be a serious problem. When proper precautions are taken, such as frequent changes in ventilator tubing, safe delivery of ribavirin to ventilated patients can be accomplished. Reticulocytosis, rash, and conjunctivitis have been associated with the use of ribavirin aerosol. Although there are no pertinent human data, ribavirin has been found to be teratogenic and mutagenic in nearly all species in which it has been tested. This drug is therefore contraindicated in women who are or may become pregnant. Some concern has been expressed about the risk to persons in the room with infants being treated with ribavirin aerosol, particularly females of childbearing age. Although this risk seems to be minimal with limited exposure, awareness and caution are warranted.

FUTURE ANTIVIRAL AGENTS

Advances in molecular virology continue to define those sites of viral replication that may be vulnerable to attack without harm to the host cell. Further characterization of the viral DNA polymerase, required for replication but not used by the host cell, is a major research focus. In addition, classes of compounds, many of them nucleoside analogues, are being systematically evaluated to identify more efficacious and less toxic antiviral agents. A description of some of the most promising drugs follows.

Zanamivir

Zanamivir is a novel sialic acid analogue inhibitor of the neuraminidases of influenza A and B. The design of the molecule was based on the characterization of crystallographic structure of influenza viral neuraminidase that has been shown to be essential for viral replication in vitro. This viral enzyme cleaves terminal sialic acid residues from cellular and viral glycoproteins and glycolipids to allow release of virus from infected cells, preventing vital aggregation and possibly preventing binding and inactivation by respiratory mucous. Zanamivir is a highly specific and potent inhibitor of influenza viral neuraminidase with little activity against mammalian or bacterial neuraminidase. It is inhibitory for a range of influenza A and B viruses in cell culture and in explants of human respiratory epithelium.

Zanamivir is under evaluation for topical administration to prevent and treat influenza infections. In experimentally infected healthy individuals, intranasal zanamivir administration beginning 4 hours before viral inoculation was highly protective against infection with febrile illness, after intranasal challenge with influenza virus. In naturally occurring infection, adults with uncomplicated illness of less than 48 hours in duration, zanamivir therapy accelerated resolution of disease significantly. No evidence of toxicity was reported in these studies. Currently, the compound is undergoing extensive phase III evaluation in anticipation of licensure. Of note, the oral bioavailability of zanamivir is poor, and, as a consequence, the compound can only be delivered topically to mucosal surfaces.

Gilead Sciences has also identified a neuraminidase inhibitor, GS

Table 374–3 ■ DOSAGE ADJUSTMENT FOR ORAL AMANTADINE IN PATIENTS WITH IMPAIRED RENAL FUNCTION

CREATININE CLEARANCE (ML/MIN/1.73 M²)	SUGGESTED ORAL MAINTENANCE REGIMEN AFTER 200 MG (100 MG BID) ON THE FIRST DAY
≥80	100 mg bid
60–80	100 mg bid alternating with 100 mg daily
40–60	100 mg daily
30–40	200 mg (100 mg bid) twice weekly
20–30	100 mg three times each week
10–20	200 mg (100 mg bid) alternating with 100 mg every 7 days
<10	100 mg every 7 days

4104, which is undergoing extensive phase II evaluation worldwide. This compound differs from zanamivir only in terms of administration. GS 4104 can be administered orally. In similar challenge studies, it was efficacious for both prevention and treatment of influenza infections.

Lamivudine

Lamivudine (2'-deoxy-3'-thiacytidine [3TC]) is a nucleoside analogue that is an inhibitor of reverse transcriptase. Its activity in the treatment of individuals with HIV infection is described elsewhere. However, of note, lamivudine has activity in treatment of chronic hepatitis B virus infections. It is undergoing extensive evaluation as monotherapy and combination therapy in the treatment of chronic hepatitis B.

INTERFERONS

HISTORY AND INTRODUCTION. Interferons (IFN) are glycoprotein cytokines (intracellular messengers) with a complex array of immunomodulating, antineoplastic, and antiviral properties. The name *interferon* was derived from landmark experiments by Isaacs and Lindemann in 1957 demonstrating the existence of a biologic substance that "interfered" with viral replication in infected cells. Interferons are currently classified as α, β, or γ, with natural sources of these classes, in general, being leukocytes, fibroblasts, and lymphocytes, respectively. Each type of IFN can now be produced through recombinant DNA technology. The complexity of the response to IFN, including the variability of dose response, duration of therapy, and combination with other treatments, creates enormous challenges to determine appropriate clinical scenarios in which IFN might be a worthwhile therapeutic agent.

MECHANISM OF ACTION. Binding of IFN to the intact cell membrane is the first step in establishing an antiviral effect. IFN binds to specific cell surface receptors; IFN-γ appears to have a different receptor from either IFN-α or β, which may explain the purported synergistic antiviral and antitumor effects sometimes observed when IFN-γ is given with either of the other two IFN species.

A prevalent view of IFN action is that after binding there is synthesis of new cellular RNAs and proteins that mediate the antiviral effect. The antiviral state is not fully expressed until these primed cells are infected with virus. In addition to their antiviral effect, IFNs have a number of other biologic activities, including inhibition of cell proliferation and enhancement of the cytotoxic activities of lymphocytes, the expression of cell surface antigens, and the phagocytic and tumoricidal activities of macrophages. These properties may play an important role in the in vivo antiviral and antitumor effects of the IFNs.

LICENSED USES. Although promising for a number of viral infections and HIV-associated conditions, the only licensed use of IFN as an antiviral agent is its intralesional administration in the treatment of condyloma acuminatum, or genital warts, which are caused by human papillomaviruses, and therapy for chronic hepatitis B and C. Only IFN-α is licensed.

TOXICITY AND CLINICAL PROBLEMS. Side effects are frequent with IFN administration and are usually dose limiting. Influenza-like symptoms (i.e., fever, chills, headache, and malaise) commonly occur, but these symptoms usually become less severe with repeated treatments. At doses used in the treatment of condyloma acuminatum, these side effects rarely cause termination of treatment and may be reduced in severity by pretreatment with acetaminophen. For local treatment (intralesional injection), pain at the injection site does not differ significantly from that in placebo-treated patients and is short lived. Leukopenia is the most common hematologic abnormality, occurring in up to 26% of patients treated for condyloma. Leukopenia is usually modest, not clinically relevant, and reversible when therapy is discontinued. Increased alanine aminotransferase levels also may occur, as well as nausea, vomiting, and diarrhea.

At higher doses of IFN, neurotoxicity is encountered, as manifested by personality changes, confusion, loss of attention, disorientation, and paranoid ideation. Early studies with IFN-γ show similar side effects as treatment with IFN-α and IFN-β but with the additional side effects of dose-limiting hypotension and a marked increase in triglyceride levels.

CLINICAL TRIALS. IFN has potential use against virtually all

viral infections. Its ultimate utility depends on a number of factors, including the acceptability of side effects, cost, and the availability of other antiviral agents. Of the many viral infections in which IFN has been tested, treatment of condyloma acuminatum, chronic hepatitis B, chronic hepatitis C, and recurrent respiratory papillomatosis and prophylaxis of rhinovirus and coronavirus upper respiratory tract infection have been promising.

CONDYLOMA ACUMINATUM. Several large controlled trials have demonstrated the clinical benefit of IFN-α therapy for condyloma acuminatum. These studies have demonstrated clearance rates of treated lesions from 36 to 62%. Up to one third of lesions treated with IFN recur. Much research remains to be done to examine the effects of different routes of administration, prolonged therapy, repeated courses of treatment, and combined treatment with other therapeutic modalities (i.e., cryotherapy podophyllin, and laser ablation).

RESPIRATORY PAPILLOMATOSIS. Recurrent respiratory papillomatosis is a disease in which squamous papillomata relentlessly recur within the larynx and trachea of both children and young adults. Standard management consists of careful microendoscopic excision, usually with a CO_2 laser. In recent years, there have been numerous case reports and uncontrolled studies supporting benefit from IFN as an adjunct to surgery. Results of placebo-controlled trials have suggested benefit.

HEPATITIS. The inhibitory effect of human leukocyte IFN-α on hepatitis B virus (HBV) replication was first reported more than 10 years ago. Treatment with IFN-α in chronic hepatitis B subsequently has been investigated in several large, randomized, controlled trials. The earlier studies were encouraging, but the response rate was low at approximately 30%.

In an attempt to enhance the efficacy of antiviral therapy, combinations of IFN with other agents also have been studied. Vidarabine and acyclovir have been used in such studies with little success. It has been observed, however, that a short course of corticosteroids before treatment with IFN-α results in "immunologic rebound" after prednisone withdrawal. This phenomenon, which seems to be directed at virus-infected hepatocytes, is characterized by an acute hepatitis-like elevation of serum aminotransferases and a transient decline in levels of HBV DNA polymerase and HBV DNA. A large multicenter trial comparing patients randomly assigned to receive one of two doses of IFN-α versus prednisone followed by IFN-α or no treatment recently showed that a 4-month treatment regimen of subcutaneous IFN-α in a dose of 5 million units daily resulted in a complete response (loss of serum HBeAg and HBV DNA) in nearly 40% of patients and that re-activation of infection within 6 months after treatment was no greater than 2%. The beneficial effect of pretreatment with a tapering dose of prednisone was limited to patients with low baseline levels of alanine aminotransferase (<100 units/L). The best predictor of response in this study was the HBV DNA level before treatment, with approximately half of the patients having levels less than 100 pg/mL experiencing a complete response. Long-term follow-up studies are required to determine the duration of antiviral effect and the impact on survival.

The efficacy of IFN for treating chronic hepatitis C (non-A, non-B hepatitis) has been established. The first large, randomized, placebo-controlled study of IFN-α therapy in patients with chronic hepatitis C showed that the serum alanine aminotransferase levels declined to normal in 38% of patients treated with 3 million units of IFN-α for 6 months, compared with 4% of untreated patients. However, only 52% of the patients who initially responded to treatment remained in remission during 6 months of follow-up.

RESPIRATORY INFECTIONS. The upper respiratory tract infection known as the "common cold" has a multitude of possible viral causes (see Chapter 375). It has been demonstrated that nasal spray or drops of IFN-α provide prophylaxis against the common cold caused by rhinovirus or coronavirus infection. Although clinical benefit was demonstrated in these studies, administration of IFN-α for 2 to 3 weeks led to hemorrhage of nasal mucosa.

IMMUNOGLOBULIN THERAPY

Efficacy has been established for prophylactic immunoglobulin administration for several viral infections, but the use of immunoglobulin alone for therapy for established disease has not been proven unequivocally beneficial for any viral infection. Benefit has been shown for the administration of intravenous immunoglobulin or CMV hyperimmune globulin when combined with ganciclovir in the treatment of CMV pneumonia in bone marrow transplant recipients. Survival was increased to 52 to 79%, which is significantly better than that of historical controls treated with either agent alone. Currently active areas of research include the efficacy of CMV hyperimmune globulin for prevention and treatment of disease in bone marrow, kidney, and heart transplant patients, and that of CMV monoclonal antibody, in the treatment of established CMV disease in AIDS patients.

Although relatively few antiviral drugs are licensed for use at this time, there is significant interest in the development of antiviral compounds. Table 327–3 summarizes the use of currently available antivirals for indications other than therapy of HIV infections. Systematic approaches have revealed a number of promising new drugs and biologic agents in various stages of evaluation. A better understanding of the molecular biology of virus replication and pathogenesis should elucidate agents with enhanced virus-specific activity.

Balfour HH Jr: Antiviral drugs (review). N Engl J Med 340:1255, 1999. *Excellent, up-to-the-minute reviews of cervical therapeutic modalities.*

Buhles WC, Mastre BJ, Tinker AJ, et al: Ganciclovir treatment of life- or sight-threatening cytomegalovirus infection: Experience in 314 immunocompromised patients. Rev Infect Dis 10:495, 1988. *Describes the clinical efficacy of ganciclovir when used to treat infections of the retina, gastrointestinal tract, and lungs.*

Couch R: Respiratory diseases. *In* Galasso G, Whitley R, Merigan T (eds): Antiviral Agents and Viral Diseases of Man, 3rd ed. New York, Raven Press, 1990, pp 327–372. *This chapter contains a summary of the published work regarding the efficacy and toxicity of amantadine, rimantadine, and ribavirin for influenza and respiratory syncytial virus infections.*

Davis GL, Esteban-Mur R, Rustgi V, et al: Interferon alfa-2b alone or in combination with ribavirin for the treatment of relapse of chronic hepatitis C. International Hepatitis Interventional Therapy Group. N Engl J Med 339:1493, 1998. *Demonstrates progress in treatment of HCV.*

Dorsky DI, Crumpacker CS: Drugs five years later: Acyclovir. Ann Intern Med 107:859, 1987. *A detailed analysis of the chemistry, antiviral activity, and clinical efficacy of acyclovir.*

Hirsch MS, Kaplan JC: Antiviral Agents. *In* Fields BN, Knipe DM (eds): Virology, 2nd ed. New York, Raven Press, 1990, pp 441–468. *A comprehensive text that includes a detailed analysis of antiviral therapy.*

Martin DF, Kuppermann BD, Wolitz RA, et al: Oral ganciclovir for patients with cytomegalovirus retinitis treated with ganciclovir implant. Roche Ganciclovir Study Group. N Engl J Med 340:1109, 1999. *Demonstrates a new approach to chronic therapy for viral diseases.*

Perillo RP, Schiff ER, Davis GL, et al: A randomized, controlled trial of interferon alfa-2b alone and after prednisone withdrawal for the treatment of chronic hepatitis B. N Engl J Med 323:295, 1990. *A multicenter study of combination therapy for chronic hepatitis B.*

Reichman RC, Oakes D, Bonnez W, et al: Treatment of condyloma acuminatum with three different interferons administered intralesionally. Ann Intern Med 108:675, 1988. *Intralesional injections of three different interferon preparations were found to be efficacious in the treatment of condyloma acuminatum.*

VIRAL INFECTIONS OF THE RESPIRATORY TRACT

375 THE COMMON COLD

J. Owen Hendley

DEFINITION. The common cold, also known as an upper respiratory infection (URI) or acute coryza, is an acute, self-limited illness caused by a virus. Nasal symptoms including rhinorrhea and nasal obstruction are invariably present; sore/scratchy throat and/or cough may be present. Many myths surround the source of the virus causing colds. There are no normal viral flora of the respiratory tract in humans (two possible exceptions are human herpesvirus type 6 in saliva and adenovirus, which can be recovered from adenoid tissue of otherwise healthy children by co-cultivation with susceptible cells). In sharp contrast, luxuriant normal bacterial flora occur in the upper respiratory tract and mouth. Because viruses are not part of normal flora, the viruses that cause colds are not present in the host ready to be activated because "resistance" has been lowered by chilling, loss of sleep, or bad diet. Instead, the virus must be *passed* from another human to produce the cold.

ETIOLOGY. Colds are common because the viruses with few serotypes reinfect many times, and the viruses that infect an individual only once have multiple serotypes (Table 375–1). Rhinoviruses (*rhino* = "nose") cause at least 50% of colds in adults, and coronaviruses (*corona* = "crown") are responsible for 10 to 15%. Each of the other virus groups listed in Table 375–1 cause less than 5% of colds. Adults are susceptible to respiratory syncytial virus (RSV) and parainfluenza virus, but the illness in adults is usually a cold rather than the more severe involvement seen in infants. Some of the viruses that cause colds are characteristically associated with other syndromes. Influenza viruses cause febrile respiratory disease with lower tract involvement, adenoviruses cause pharyngoconjunctival fever or acute undifferentiated febrile illness, echoviruses and other enteroviruses are an important cause of aseptic meningitis, and coxsackievirus A causes herpangina.

EPIDEMIOLOGY AND TRANSMISSION. Colds are the most frequent disease of humans and the single most common cause of absenteeism from school and work. Frequency of colds varies with age. Even before widespread day-care attendance, colds were particularly common in children younger than age 6. In the Cleveland family study in the 1950s, infants younger than age 1 had an average of 6.7 colds per year, 1- to 5-year olds had 7.4 to 8.3 colds per year, and teenagers averaged about 4.5 colds per year. Mothers reported 4.5 colds and fathers 3.5 colds per year. The wider exposure to other preschoolers in day care has increased the frequency of colds in children younger than 6 even more. The number of colds in adults may increase for several years because of exposure to young children, which highlights the fact that children commonly introduce new viruses to their families. At least with rhinovirus, the home setting is the primary site for viral transmission. Coworkers in an insurance company office with simultaneous rhinovirus colds usually were infected with different serotypes of virus, but each worker's serotype was found in his or her family contacts.

In temperate climates, colds are epidemic in the winter months (Fig. 375–1). The epidemic starts with a sharp rise in frequency in September after children have returned to school; the incidence then remains at an almost constant level until spring. This epidemic curve is produced by successive waves of different viruses moving through the community. Although rhinovirus infections occur year-round, the epidemic is initiated by a sharp rise of rhinovirus infections in early fall. Parainfluenza viruses move through in October and November, followed by RSV and coronaviruses in winter

Table 375-1 ■ IMMUNITY TO COMMON COLD VIRUSES

a. Solid immunity not produced by infection (repeated infection with same serotype usual)	
Virus	**No. of Serotypes**
Respiratory syncytial virus	1
Parainfluenza virus	4
Coronavirus	4

b. Immunity produced by infection (reinfection with same serotype uncommon)	
Virus	**No. of Serotypes**
Rhinovirus	>100
Adenovirus	≥33
Influenza	3 (type A subtypes change)
Echovirus	31
Coxsackievirus	
Group A	23
Group B	6

From Hendley JO: Immunology of viral colds. *In* Veldman JE, McCabe BF, Huizing EH, Mygind N (eds.): Immunobiology, Autoimmunity, Transplantation in Otorhinolaryngology. Amsterdam, Kugler Publications, 1985, pp 257–260.

MONTH

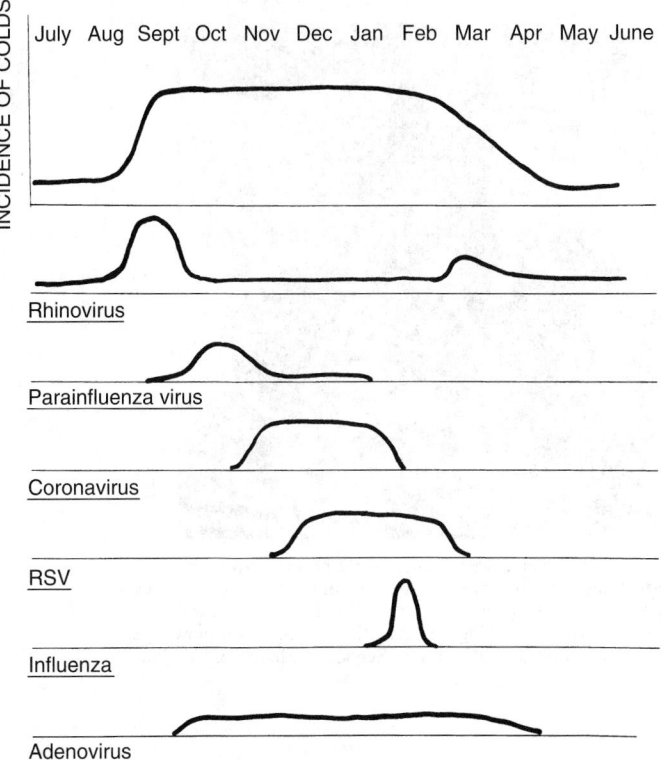

FIGURE 375–1 ▪ Schematic diagram of the incidence of colds and frequency of the causative viruses.

months. Influenza viruses appear later in winter, then rhinovirus has a resurgence in spring. Summer colds are usually caused by rhinovirus or one of the enteroviruses. The wave of each virus moving through is not sharp, and many times two or three viruses may be overlapping. Adenovirus and parainfluenza virus type 3 contribute to the burden of illness throughout the epidemic.

Determinants of this yearly epidemic of colds are not established but certainly include human behavior, with more virus transmitted by higher indoor contact in colder months. Another determinant might be attributes of the viruses. Enveloped viruses, including RSV, parainfluenza virus, influenza virus, and coronavirus, may survive outside the host for longer periods in winter when the relative humidity of indoor (but not outdoor) air is very low.

Transmission of viruses causing colds could occur by one or more of three mechanisms: (1) small-particle (<5 μ in diameter) aerosol in which virus may be suspended in air for an hour and infect by inhalation, (2) large-particle (>10 μ in diameter) airborne droplets that travel less than 1 m and infect by landing on a mucosal surface such as conjunctiva or nasal mucosa, and (3) direct transfer of virus in secretions via hand contact from a person with a cold to a well person, who inoculates the virus onto his or her own conjunctival or nasal mucosa. Oral inoculation of rhinovirus or RSV does not result in infection, presumably because the stratified squamous epithelium of the mouth and oropharynx is not susceptible. The transmission route under natural conditions in the home has not been definitely established for any of the viruses. However, the importance of spread of colds in the home favors direct contact and/or large-droplet spread as being most likely. Influenza virus clearly can be transmitted by small-particle aerosol in some circumstances.

PATHOGENESIS. It had been assumed until recently that the symptoms of colds were produced by a viral cytopathic effect destroying the nasal mucosa. However, one recent study found that the histologic appearance of the nasal mucosa in biopsy specimens taken during natural colds could not be distinguished from that of biopsy specimens taken 2 weeks after illness except for an increased number of polymorphonuclear leukocytes (PMNs) during illness. The unexpected infiltration of PMNs in the nose in uncomplicated colds was confirmed in another study; the number of PMNs in nasal secretions increased coincidently when symptoms

appeared in experimentally induced rhinovirus colds. Rhinovirus and coronavirus, in contrast to influenza virus and adenovirus, were not found to be destructive of nasal epithelium in organ cultures in vitro. Because mucosal damage by the virus during colds does not adequately explain the symptoms, the hypothesis that the viral infection of the nose triggers a cascade of inflammatory mediators that results in the symptoms is being explored. Initial support for this hypothesis was provided in volunteers with experimentally induced rhinovirus colds. Kinins (primarily bradykinin) and PMNs appeared in nasal secretions of infected volunteers at the time that they became ill, and their presence paralleled cold symptoms. More recent work has suggested that viral infection of individual epithelial cells in the mucosa of the nose and nasopharynx can lead to elaboration of cytokines that effect the symptomatic illness and influx of PMNs. Infected cells have been shown to elaborate interleukin (IL)-8, which is a chemoattractant for PMNs. Increased levels of IL-1β, IL-6, and IL-8 have been detected in nasal secretions during colds. Whether the release of proinflammatory cytokines from the host cells induced by the viral infection can be interrupted has not been ascertained. However, the concept that it might be possible to ablate cold symptoms by blocking the mediators of the host response without having to kill the virus is exciting.

CLINICAL MANIFESTATIONS. The clinical manifestations of colds, which are familiar to all, are predominately subjective. In adults, rhinorrhea, nasal obstruction, and scratchy/sore throat are usually noted. The rhinorrhea is usually clear early in illness and may become white or yellow-green. Some malaise and non-productive cough are common; sneezing is noted in some colds. Other common symptoms include sinus fullness and a "nasal" quality to the voice. Hoarseness is sometimes present. Objective findings in an adult with a cold are usually minimal. The nasal mucosa may be red but not to a degree that differs from normal. Mild erythema of the pharynx and redness around the external nares from nose blowing may be noted. Fever ($>38°$ C) is uncommon in a cold in an adult; the presence of fever would suggest influenza or a bacterial complication of the cold. The symptoms of the cold usually abate in 5 to 7 days.

Colds in infants and children may be associated with more objective signs than in adults. In addition to rhinorrhea and nasal obstruction, moderate enlargement of the anterior cervical lymph nodes is frequent. Fever during the first 2 to 3 days of a cold in young children is not unusual, even when the child's parent or older sibling does not have an elevated temperature during the cold due to the same virus. In contrast to in adults, the usual duration of cold symptoms in children is 10 to 14 days.

DIAGNOSIS. Self-diagnosis of a cold by the patient is usually accurate. Laboratory tests including white blood cell count and differential are not helpful. Sloughed ciliated cells may be present, and PMNs would be expected in nasal secretions during viral colds. The differential diagnosis of a cold includes an intranasal foreign body in a child and allergic or vasomotor rhinitis in adults and children. Examination of the nose should exclude a foreign body; the chronicity of symptoms with allergic or vasomotor rhinitis should differentiate these conditions from an acute cold.

Etiologic (virologic) diagnosis of a cold can be attempted by inoculation of a sample of nasal secretions into tissue cell cultures, but this is rarely needed or useful. Rhinovirus can be grown in human embryonic lung fibroblast cultures. Coronavirus infections have been diagnosed by serologic titer rise because coronaviruses cannot be detected accurately in cell culture. Assays using polymerase chain reaction for detection of rhinovirus and coronavirus have been developed that will facilitate diagnosis of these infections. Influenza and parainfluenza viruses can be grown in primary rhesus monkey kidney cell culture, and adenoviruses will grow in human embryonic kidney cells. RSV antigen in nasal secretions can be reliably detected with commercially available rapid tests. In addition, a new test for detection of the nucleoprotein of influenza virus A appears to be useful as a rapid screen for this virus.

TREATMENT. Given the self-limited nature of colds, any treatment should be completely safe. Antibiotics have no place in therapy for uncomplicated colds, because they neither hasten nor delay recovery from the cold, nor do they reduce the frequency of bacterial complications.

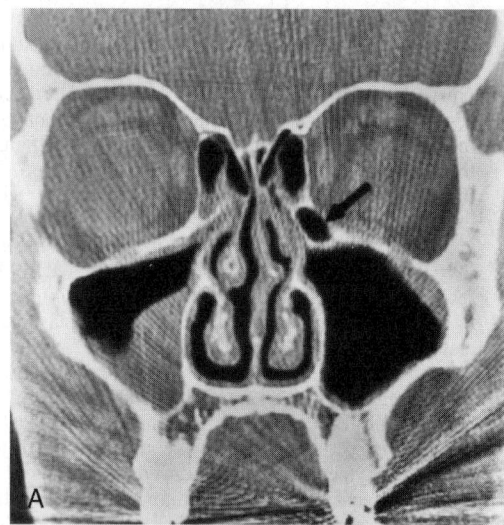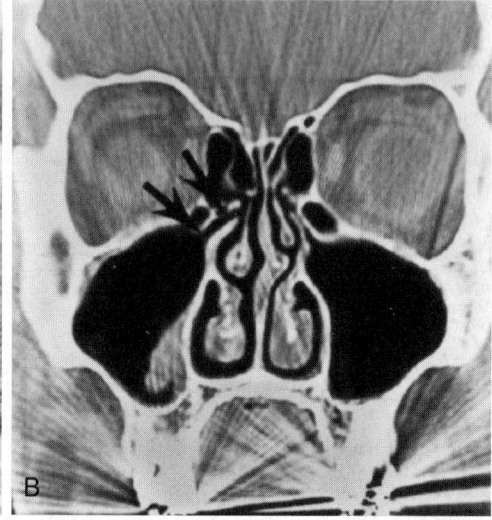

FIGURE 375-2 ■ Sinus CT scan of adult during symptomatic cold *(left panel)* and 2 weeks later *(right panel).* Arrow in the left panel denotes an infraorbital air cell (Haller cell). Bilateral abnormalities were observed in the ethmoid and maxillary sinuses during the cold, with an air-fluid interface in the right maxillary sinus. Two weeks later, all abnormalities had cleared except for a residual density in the right maxillary sinus. The infundibulum *(two arrows)* draining the maxillary antrum was now open. (Courtesy of Dr. Jack M. Gwaltney, Jr., Department of Internal Medicine, University of Virginia School of Medicine, Charlottesville, Virginia).

Because the subjective symptoms of a cold disappear in 7 days without intervention, a variety of actually ineffective treatments have been reported to be effective due to inadequate blinding of placebo recipients. One example of this phenomenon was a study of large doses of vitamin C to prevent colds, in which many placebo recipients dropped out of the study because they could tell by tasting the medication that they were not receiving the vitamin C. Another example was the use of zinc gluconate lozenges as an antiviral treatment for colds. In the blinded trial, the only appropriate placebo that could be found to match the noxious taste of the zinc was denatonium benzoate, which is so bitter that it has been painted on the thumbs of children to discourage them from thumb-sucking.

No antiviral agents are currently available for treating colds. Individual symptoms may be treated. Malaise may be relieved by analgesics (e.g., aspirin, acetaminophen, ibuprofen). Nasal congestion may be relieved by decongestants by mouth (pseudoephedrine, 60 mg, three times a day) or by topical application (oxymetazoline 0.05%, two sprays to each nostril twice daily). Oral first-generation antihistamines (e.g., brompheniramine, chlorpheniramine, clemastine) may provide modest relief of sneezing and rhinorrhea in colds.

COMPLICATIONS. Secondary bacterial infection may complicate viral colds. The most common is bacterial suppurative otitis media, which occurs in some 5% of colds in preschool-aged children. Otitis media may be heralded by a secondary fever with associated ear pain. Bacterial sinusitis is estimated to occur in 0.5% of colds, primarily in adults. Sinusitis would be suggested by the presence of fever and/or facial pain (see Chapter 515). Bacterial pneumonia is thought to complicate colds, but it is very uncommon.

Clinical differentiation between primary viral and secondary bacterial infection of the respiratory tract is a challenge, because respiratory viruses may involve the middle ear or paranasal sinuses in the absence of bacterial infection. Tympanocentesis or maxillary sinus puncture provides definitive information on viral versus bacterial infection, but these are too invasive for routine use. Coronal computed tomography (CT) is an accurate non-invasive method for imaging the paranasal sinuses. Recent work using CT has demonstrated that abnormalities in the sinuses may occur in colds not complicated by secondary bacterial infection. Coronal CT in 27 (87%) of 31 young adults during uncomplicated colds had abnormalities in one or more sinuses (Fig. 375-2). In 11 (79%) of the 14 subjects who had repeat scans 2 weeks later, the abnormalities had cleared or were markedly improved without antibiotic therapy.

An important complication of viral colds occurs in adults and children with underlying reactive airways disease or asthma. Wheezing occurs in 30 to 50% of episodes of viral colds in prospective studies of patients with asthma. Colds in these patients produce a large burden of illness, because up to 50% of asthma exacerbations in children and up to 20% of exacerbations in adults have been associated with an identified virus.

PREVENTION. Vaccine(s) to prevent common colds are unlikely to be useful given the multiplicity of immunotypes of some of the viruses and the lack of solid immunity to reinfection with the other viruses (see Table 375-1). Prophylaxis with topical interferon applied intranasally for 5 days after one family member appears with a cold has been shown to be moderately effective in preventing other family members from acquiring a cold, particularly colds due to rhinovirus. The practicality of this preventive approach may be argued, particularly in view of the fact that prolonged use of intranasal interferon is complicated by alteration or damage of the nasal mucosa.

Probably the only practical, albeit imperfect, means of preventing colds available is to prevent virus from reaching the nasal or conjunctival mucosa by way of one's own hands. If transmission occurs by inhalation of airborne small particles or by adherence of large droplets to a mucosal surface, infection is inevitable for those who enjoy contact with other humans. However, if transmission occurs by self-inoculation with virus on contaminated fingertips, the simple measure of ridding the fingers of viable virus before touching one's eye or nose might be helpful. The virus can be removed physically by rinsing the hands. Applying a virucide to the hands might be another approach.

Arruda E, Pitkaranta A, Witek TJ Jr, et al: Frequency and natural history of rhinovirus infections in adults during autumn. J Clin Microbiol 35:2864, 1997. *Use of PCR in addition to cell culture demonstrated that 80% of colds in the fall were caused by rhinovirus.*

Gwaltney JM Jr, Phillips CD, Miller RD, et al: Computed tomographic study of the common cold. N Engl J Med 330:25, 1994. *Sinus CT during naturally acquired common colds demonstrated that one or more of the sinuses was abnormal in more than 80% of subjects. Most abnormalities had cleared on repeat scan after the cold was over.*

Hendley JO: Epidemiology, pathogenesis, and treatment of the common cold. Semin Pediatr Infect Dis 9:50, 1998. *Review of differences in colds in children versus adults and of recent work on pathogenesis of symptoms.*

Pattemore PK, Johnston SL, Bardin PG: Viruses as precipitants of asthma symptoms: I. Epidemiology. Clin Exp Allergy 22:325, 1992. *Review of evidence incriminating viral respiratory infections as common precipitants of wheezing. Rhinovirus and RSV were most commonly associated with episodes of wheezing, but all respiratory viruses have been found.*

Winther B. Gwaltney JM, Hendley JO: Respiratory virus infection of monolayer cultures of human nasal epithelial cells. Am Rev Respir Dis 141:839, 1990. *Growth of rhinovirus and coronavirus in nasal epithelial cells produced no visible destruction of the epithelial layer, whereas influenza and adenovirus produced obvious disruption.*

376   VIRAL PHARYNGITIS, LARYNGITIS, CROUP, AND BRONCHITIS

Maurice A. Mufson

DEFINITION. Viral infections that localize to the upper and middle respiratory passages produce an acute inflammatory response and, depending on the anatomic site involved, evoke the clinical manifestations of pharyngitis, laryngitis, croup (laryngotracheobronchitis), and bronchitis. These infections do not ordinarily involve the pulmonary alveoli. Pharyngitis, laryngitis, and bronchitis can occur in persons of any age. Croup occurs exclusively in children and mainly during the second year of life. Usually these illnesses begin abruptly with predominant upper respiratory tract signs and symptoms and limited systemic findings. Mainly uncomplicated illnesses, they abate after 5 to 10 days.

ETIOLOGY. The viral pathogens of the respiratory tract that cause pharyngitis, laryngitis, croup, and bronchitis include members of the myxoviruses (influenza, parainfluenza, and respiratory syncytial viruses), adenoviruses, coronaviruses, picornaviruses (rhinoviruses and enteroviruses), and herpesviruses (Table 376–1). However, they differ in their propensity to cause these illnesses (Table 376–2). An etiologic diagnosis requires either isolation of virus or detection of viral antigen or demonstration of a rise in antibody during convalescence. Such diagnostic studies infrequently need to be done in advance of beginning treatment.

Pharyngitis also can occur as part of systemic viral illnesses associated with *Epstein-Barr virus* (see Chapter 387) or *cytomegalovirus* (see Chapter 386) infection, and laryngitis and bronchitis can occur in *measles virus* infection (see Chapter 381). When coryza represents the main feature of an upper respiratory infection, the term *common cold* (see Chapter 375) prevails. When influenza virus is the infecting virus, the designation *influenza* describes an acute respiratory tract infection with fever and systemic features (see Chapter 379).

INCIDENCE AND PREVALENCE. Most children and adults experience three to five viral infections of the upper respiratory tract each year. In infants and children, croup is a serious illness that peaks in the second year of life, as high as 47 cases per 1000 children per year, and by age 4 to 5 it declines to under 15 cases per 1000 children per year.

EPIDEMIOLOGY. Viral pharyngitis, laryngitis croup, and bronchitis occur during all months of the year, in parallel with the occurrence of individual viruses. Respiratory syncytial virus, influenza A and B viruses, and parainfluenza virus type 1 occur in epidemics, mainly in the late fall, winter, and spring (see Table 376–3). The other viral pathogens occur endemically or sporadically. Virus infections of the respiratory tract spread mainly by direct person-to-person contact, and less commonly by infectious aerosols and fomites.

CLINICAL MANIFESTATIONS. VIRAL PHARYNGITIS. Acute viral pharyngitis is characterized by a scratchy and sore throat, but pain on swallowing is not a prominent or constant feature. Dysphagia occurs infrequently in viral pharyngitis. Cough is not a feature of acute viral pharyngitis. Pharyngeal erythema and enlarged tender lymph nodes may be the only physical findings. Fever and malaise often accompany influenza and adenovirus infections; they infrequently occur with the other respiratory virus infections. Adenovirus pharyngitis may be associated with conjunctivitis. Exudative tonsillitis occurs in adenovirus infections, infectious mononucleosis associated with Epstein-Barr virus infection, herpetic pharyngitis (with or without vesicles or small ulcers), as well as streptococcal pharyngitis. Bronchospasm occurs as a feature of herpes tracheobronchitis in elderly persons.

VIRAL LARYNGITIS. In acute viral laryngitis, hoarseness predominates, associated with difficulty in talking, pain on clearing respiratory secretions, and often fever, depending on the infecting virus. Cough and pharyngitis may be present. The larynx appears erythematous and edematous, and the regional lymph nodes show slight enlargement and tenderness. Wheezes may be audible on auscultation.

VIRAL CROUP. The clinical picture of croup characteristically includes inspiratory stridor, hoarseness, and a brassy cough. This distinctive triad of symptoms reflects the acute and intense edema and mucoid exudative secretions of the larynx and associated obstruction of the subglottic portion of the upper airway. These symptoms develop acutely, accompanied by fever, cough, tachypnea, and wheezing. Retractions of the chest wall occur. Hemoptysis does not occur. Rhonchi, rales, or wheezes, alone or in combination, may be audible on auscultation of the lungs. Radiographic examination of the neck can demonstrate subglottic narrowing, and views of the chest can show hyperinflation of the lungs. In the uncomplicated case, the findings resolve in several days, but some children develop respiratory failure and pneumonia. Children who experience multiple episodes of croup may as an adolescent or adult manifest bronchial hyperreactivity and peripheral airways obstruction.

Table 376–1 ■ **VIRUSES THAT CAUSE PHARYNGITIS, LARYNGITIS, CROUP, AND BRONCHITIS**

VIRUS	SEROTYPE
Influenza	Types A, B,
Parainfluenza	Types 1, 2, 3
Respiratory syncytial	Subgroups A, B1, B2
Adenovirus	Types 1, 2, 3, 4, 5, 6, 7 (also others)
Coronavirus	Types 229E, OC43 (also others)
Rhinovirus	Most or all of more than 100 serotypes
Enterovirus	At least some of more than 75 serotypes
Herpes simplex	Type 1

Table 376–2 ■ **RELATIVE IMPORTANCE OF VIRUSES CAUSING PHARYNGITIS, LARYNGITIS, CROUP, AND BRONCHITIS**

VIRUS	OCCURRENCE IN INDICATED ILLNESS*			
	Pharyngitis	Laryngitis	Croup	Bronchitis
Influenza A	++++	++++	+	++++
B	++	++		++
Parainfluenza 1	++	++	++++	++
2	+	+	+++	+
3	++	++	++++	++
Respiratory syncytial	+		+	+++
Adenovirus	++++	++		++
Coronavirus	+	+		+++
Rhinovirus	+	+		+
Enterovirus	+			
Herpes simplex	+		+	+

*Graded from minimal (+) to major (++++) importance; blank means unlikely occurrence; and ± means rare occurrence.

Table 376–3 ■ **EPIDEMIOLOGY OF VIRUSES THAT CAUSE PHARYNGITIS, LARYNGITIS, CROUP, AND BRONCHITIS**

EPIDEMIC	ENDEMIC	SPORADIC
Parainfluenza 1*	Parainfluenza 3	Parainfluenza 2
Influenza A†	Adenovirus	Herpes simplex
Influenza B	Coronavirus	
Respiratory syncytial‡	Rhinovirus	
	Enterovirus	

*Alternate years, usually.
†Epidemic and pandemic.
‡Annual epidemics.

Table 376–4 ■ ANTIVIRAL DRUG THERAPY OF VIRUSES THAT CAUSE PHARYNGITIS, LARYNGITIS, CROUP, AND BRONCHITIS

VIRUS	DRUG	DOSE (DURATION)	ROUTE
Influenza A	Amantadine*	200 mg daily (7–10 days)	Oral
	Rimantidine*	200 mg daily‡ (7–10 days)	Oral
Respiratory syncytial	Ribavirin	20 mg/mL solution (administered over 12–18 hours for 3–7 days)	Aerosol
Herpes simplex†	Acyclovir	8 mg/kg q8h (7–10 days)	IV

*More commonly used for prophylaxis at same daily dose over longer periods of time until the virus leaves the community.

†Herpes simplex tracheobronchitis treated with intravenous acyclovir.

‡In patients with hepatic dysfunction or renal failure and elderly nursing home residents, the dose for treatment and for prophylaxis is 100 mg/day.

VIRAL BRONCHITIS. In acute viral bronchitis, cough, with or without sputum production, and fever are the main features. The sputum is slightly mucoid or watery and white. Other symptoms and signs include hoarseness, non-pleuritic substernal chest pain, malaise, rhonchi, and rales. The chest roentgenogram may show increased intensity of the vascular pattern, but not pulmonary infiltrates. Acute bronchitis associated with influenza or coronavirus infection occurs often as an exacerbation of chronic bronchitis. Persons with chronic respiratory disease suffer more severe exacerbations.

TREATMENT AND PROGNOSIS. Viral pharyngitis, laryngitis, and bronchitis are self-limited illnesses and not severe, except for herpes tracheobronchitis infections. The symptoms of these illnesses should be treated with analgesics, fluids, and rest. Persistent cough can be treated with suppressant preparations. Antibiotics are not indicated. Secondary bacterial infection complicates mainly influenza virus infection; it should be treated with antibiotics. In pharyngitis, pharyngeal pain or dysphagia should be treated with analgesics and fluids.

Less serious cases of croup can be managed by having the child rest in bed at home and use a room vaporizer. Children with severe croup require hospitalization, supportive treatment, and constant monitoring for the development of respiratory distress. If hypoxemia develops, oxygen therapy is essential; hypoxemia requiring oxygen can develop even before cyanosis becomes evident. Subglottic edema may be reduced by the administration of racemic epinephrine. Some children with moderately severe croup may show reduced severity of their illness within 24 hours after a single intramuscular injection of dexamethasone (0.6 mg/kg). Antiviral drug therapy is available for influenza A, respiratory syncytial, and herpes simplex viruses (Table 376–4). Ribavirin lessens the severity of serious respiratory syncytial virus infection in the infant and child. Herpes tracheobronchitis responds to treatment with acyclovir. Influenza virus vaccine must be administered to persons in high-risk groups (unless contraindicated) to diminish the chance of infection.

Cruz MN, Stewart G, Rosenberg N: Use of dexamethasone in the outpatient management of acute laryngotracheitis. Pediatrics 96:220, 1995. *In most children with moderately severe croup, a single intramuscular injection of dexamethasone reduces severity within 24 hours.*

Mancao MY, Sindel LJ, Richardson PH, Silver FM: Herpetic croup: Two case reports and a review of the literature. Acta Paediatr 85:118, 1996. *Herpesvirus is an infrequent cause of croup.*

Marx A, Torok TJ, Holman RC, et al: Pediatric hospitalizations for croup (laryngotracheobronchitis): Biennial increases associated with human parainfluenza virus 1 epidemics. J Infect Dis 176:1423, 1997. *Major epidemics of parainfluenza 1 virus occur in alternate (odd-numbered) years and are associated with croup illnesses.*

Mufson MA, Åkerlind-Stopner B, Örvell C, et al: A single season epidemic with respiratory syncytial virus subgroup B2 during 10 epidemic years, 1978 to 1988. J Clin Microbiol 29:162, 1991. *Annual winter-spring epidemics of respiratory syncytial virus. Subgroup A predominated. One third to one half of infections were limited to the upper respiratory tract.*

Wiselka MJ, Kent J, Cookson JB, Nicholson KG: Impact of respiratory virus infection in patients with chronic chest disease. Epidemiol Infect 111:337, 1993. *Adults with chronic chest disease suffer worse symptoms due to virus infections of the respiratory tract.*

377 RESPIRATORY SYNCYTIAL VIRUS

Edward E. Walsh

DEFINITION. Respiratory syncytial virus (RSV) causes yearly outbreaks of illness during the fall, winter, and early spring. Since its discovery in 1957, RSV has been found to be the single most important cause of bronchiolitis and pneumonia in young infants and is a common cause of upper respiratory illness in older children and young adults. In addition, RSV is a cause of serious respiratory infection in the elderly, adults with underlying cardiopulmonary disease, and those who are severely immunocompromised.

ETIOLOGY. RSV is an enveloped virus of the family Paramyxoviridae, genus *Pneumovirus*. The single-stranded negative-polarity RNA encodes 10 proteins, of which 8 are found in purified virions. Three transmembrane glycoproteins (G, attachment protein; F, fusion protein; SH protein) protrude from a lipid bilayer encompassing three nucleocapsid proteins (N, P, polymerase) complexed with the genome. Two additional proteins (M, M2) are associated with the viral envelope. Neutralizing antibodies are directed at F and G glycoproteins, whereas F, N, and M2 are targets for cytotoxic T cells. Two major virus groups (A and B), each with four to five subgroups, are distinguishable by antigenically divergent G proteins.

EPIDEMIOLOGY. Similar to influenza, worldwide RSV outbreaks occur annually. In the United States, epidemics generally begin in the southern states in late fall, move steadily north, and peak in February and March in colder climates. RSV causes approximately 90,000 hospitalizations and accounts for 60% of bronchiolitis and 25% of pneumonia cases in infants in the United States. In the first year of life, over half of all infants become infected, with the remainder infected the following year. Family studies suggest that schoolchildren introduce RSV into the home with subsequent spread to parents and younger siblings, with infection rates of 43% and 62%, respectively. Like rhinovirus (see Chapter 375), RSV is transmitted principally by direct contact with large-particle fomites from respiratory secretions, in contrast to the primary mode of spread of influenza virus, aerosolization.

Approximately 0.5% of infected infants require hospitalization, but underlying prematurity, congenital cardiac abnormalities, bronchopulmonary dysplasia, and immunosuppression significantly increase the risk of serious disease. Hospitalization is most frequent between the ages of 1 to 6 months, with a median age of 2 months. Maternally derived antibody appears to protect in the first month of life when serious lower respiratory symptoms are infrequent, but this benefit is rather brief. Reinfection occurs frequently throughout life, although illness is less severe and hospitalization infrequent, except for those with underlying cardiac or pulmonary conditions.

Although often not considered in adults, RSV infection in certain populations may be severe. RSV has been identified as a relatively common cause of community-acquired pneumonia in adults, ranking third behind pneumococcus and influenza in one large study. Elderly persons appear to be at highest risk, and nosocomial outbreaks in nursing homes are common. In addition, RSV infection has been associated with about 10% of hospitalizations for cardiopulmonary deterioration in the winter among community-dwelling elderly. RSV infection in severely immunocompromised adults, such as bone marrow transplant recipients and those with acute leukemia undergoing cytotoxic chemotherapy, often results in very high morbidity and mortality.

Both RSV groups usually co-circulate during outbreaks, although group A strains usually dominate and are associated with more severe disease in hospitalized infants. Evidence suggests that strain variation alone does not solely account for reinfections. Partial immunity to RSV develops over time, as indicated by the resistance to both infection and illness. Experimental studies suggest that immunopathologic mechanisms, principally mediated by T helper cells, and their cytokines, contribute to disease manifestations.

CLINICAL MANIFESTATIONS. After an incubation period of 3 days, previously uninfected infants develop upper respiratory symptoms. Conjunctival injection, mucopurulent nasal discharge, cough, and low-grade fever (38° C) are typical and indistinguishable from other respiratory infections. Otitis media occurs commonly, generally in association with bacteria. After several days, lower respiratory tract symptoms develop in 25 to 50% of infants. Cough, wheezing, increased respiratory rate, accessory muscle use, intercostal retractions, and cyanosis are seen as the disease progresses. Expiratory wheezes, rhonchi, and fine rales are the most common findings on lung examination. Sudden apnea may develop in the youngest infants. Mortality for otherwise healthy children is about 1% in hospitalized infants but can reach 37% in infants with cardiac disorders. Hyperinflation and diffuse interstitial pneumonitis are the most frequent radiographic findings. Infiltrates are usually diffuse, but consolidation is seen in up to one fourth.

Virus is shed from respiratory secretions for 7 to 10 days, although immunocompromised infants (i.e., those with human immunodeficiency virus infection) may excrete virus for a month or longer. Interestingly, clinical symptoms may not correlate with prolonged shedding. Co-infection with other respiratoy viruses is not uncommon but is not clinically discernible. Should bacterial superinfection develop, with *Streptococcus pneumoniae* and *Haemophilus influenzae* the most frequent organisms isolated, treatment with antibiotics is indicated. Long-term sequelae of lower respiratory tract infection include development of childhood asthma, although the precise contributions of RSV infection and allergic predisposition are unknown.

Normal adults typically manifest nasal discharge, pharyngitis, and low-grade fever, and virus is shed for an average of 3 days. Elderly persons with RSV infection may develop cough, dyspnea, fever, wheezing, and, in some cases, respiratory failure. Adults most at risk of severe infection are the frail elderly, those with underlying chronic obstructive pulmonary disease or congestive heart failure, and those with severe immunocompromise. Attack rates are variable in nosocomial outbreaks in nursing homes, averaging 10 to 15%. Rales and wheezes are evident in one third of patients, and radiographically confirmed pneumonia is noted in approximately 10%. Symptoms are similar among community-dwelling elderly, and infection can lead to exacerbation of underlying congestive heart failure or chronic bronchitis.

RSV infection has been documented in up to 10% of bone marrow transplant recipients and those with acute leukemia during the winter months. The illness begins with upper respiratory symptoms but frequently spreads to the lower respiratory tract. If RSV infection occurs before marrow engraftment, pneumonia will develop in half with an attendant mortality of 90%. Notably, this is somewhat higher than the mortality with influenza virus pneumonia in this population. Chest radiographs demonstrate diffuse interstitial and alveolar infiltrates. A useful clinical clue to the presence of RSV is the almost universal presence of radiographically proven sinusitis. The presence of upper respiratory tract symptoms distinguishes this illness from cytomegalovirus pneumonia.

DIAGNOSIS. In the pediatric setting, a presumptive diagnosis is suggested by typical symptoms occurring during the epidemic season. In adults, the diagnosis is often never considered. Because the clinical picture of RSV is indistinguishable from illness caused by other infectious agents of respiratory disease, laboratory confirmation of RSV infection is required, especially if antiviral therapy is contemplated. In infants, RSV is readily grown from respiratory secretions on HEp-2, human diploid fibroblast, and HELA cell lines. The sensitivity of viral culture is about 75%. Rapid diagnostic tests rely on detecting viral antigen or RNA in respiratory secretions. Immunofluorescence (IF) is a widely used test and has a sensitivity of about 80%, whereas commercial enzyme immunoassay (EIA) is less sensitive and less specific than IF. Serologic diagnosis can be made but is not useful in immediate management. Reverse transcription-polymerase chain reaction (RT-PCR) is more sensitive than culture but is not comercially available. In normal adults, diagnostic tests, with the exception of serology, are significantly less sensitive: approximately 50% for virus culture and 10% or less for IF and EIA antigen detection. In immunocompromised adults, detection of RSV antigen in throat swabs by EIA is only 15% sensitive, but it is 90% sensitive when bronchoalveolar lavage specimens are used.

THERAPY AND PREVENTION. Therapy for hospitalized infants includes hydration, oxygen, bronchodilators, and specific antiviral medication. Severely ill infants are commonly dehydrated and require intravenous fluid. Supplemental oxygen, administered as a humidified mist, should be given to all infants with hypoxia. The value of bronchodilators for the treatment of wheezing is controversial, because most studies have not demonstrated clear benefit, but a trial of inhaled bronchodilators is probably indicated. Specific antiviral therapy is currently limited to inhaled ribavirin (1-β-D-ribafuranosyl-1,2,4-triazole-3-carboxamide), a nucleoside analogue with activity against several RNA viruses. Ribavirin is administered via aerosol, typically for 4 hours three times a day for 3 to 5 days, although longer therapy has been used. High-dose, short-duration (2 hours three times daily) treatment is considered equivalent. Some placebo-controlled clinical trials demonstrate more rapid resolution of respiratory symptoms and hypoxia. The majority of infants do not require therapy, but ribavirin treatment may be indicated for infants at high risk of serious disease and those who are severely ill. Although short- or long-term toxicity of ribavirin has not been recognized, hospital personnel and family members of patients should minimize exposure to the drug and pregnant health care workers should avoid exposure altogether. Inhaled ribavirin has also been used in treatment of immunocompromised adults with RSV pneumonia. Although results from controlled trials are not available, anecdotal data suggest benefit, but only if therapy is begun before respiratory failure develops. Finally, intravenous high-titer RSV immunoglobulin or humanized monoclonal antibody has demonstrated benefit when administered prophylactically to high-risk infants with underlying cardiopulmonary disease or prematurity. Immunoglobulin, in combination with inhaled ribavirin, has been used in treatment of RSV pneumonia in immunosuppressed adults.

Adherance to standard infection-control principles (e.g., gloves, gowns, and frequent hand washing) can substantially reduce nosocomial spread. A vaccine for prevention of RSV is not available, although both inactivated purified subunit and live attenuated vaccines are in clinical trials.

Committee on Infectious Diseases: Reassessment of the indications for ribavirin therapy in respiratory syncytial virus infections. Pediatrics 97:137–140, 1996. *Recommendations by clinical virology experts on appropriate use of aerosolized ribavirin in infants.*

Dowell SF, Anderson LJ, Gary HE, et al: Respiratory syncytial virus is an important cause of community-acquired lower respiratory infection among hospitalized adults. J Infect Dis 174:456–462, 1996. *Clinical epidemiology of RSV as a cause of community-acquired pneumonia in adults.*

Englund JA, Piedra, PA, Whimbey E: Prevention and treatment of respiratory syncytial virus and parainfluenza viruses in immunocompromised patients. Am J Med 104:61–70, 1997. *Review of studies describing RSV infection and treatment in immunocompromised adults.*

Falsey AR, Cunningham CK, Barker WH, et al: Respiratory syncytial virus and influenza A infections in the hospitalized elderly. J Infect Dis 172:389–394, 1995. *Prospective description of RSV and influenza virus infection in elderly hospitalized with cardiopulmonary deterioration.*

Falsey AR, Treanor JJ, Betts RF, Walsh EE: Viral respiratory infection in the institutionalized elderly: Clinical and epidemiologic findings. J Am Geriatr Soc 40:115, 1992. *This prospective study of respiratory illness in a long-term care facility describes clinical features of RSV infection in the elderly with comparison with other viral pathogens.*

378 PARAINFLUENZA VIRAL DISEASE

Edward E. Walsh

DEFINITION. Parainfluenza viruses are important causes of a wide spectrum of respiratory illness in infants and young children, producing syndromes ranging from the common cold and otitis media to severe croup, bronchiolitis, and pneumonia. In older children and adults, illness is usually limited to the upper respiratory tract, although immunocompromised individuals may develop fatal respiratory failure.

ETIOLOGY. The parainfluenza viruses are enveloped single-stranded non-segmented RNA viruses and belong to the family Paramyxoviridae, which also includes measles, mumps, and respiratory syncytial viruses (RSV). The genome encodes for six structural proteins, of which the hemagglutinin-neuraminidase (HN) and fusion proteins (F) are exposed on the bilayered lipid envelope that

Table 378–1 ■ PARAINFLUENZA PATTERNS

TYPE	MANIFESTATION	SEASON	COMMENTS
1	Epidemic croup	Fall of odd-number years	Since 1970
2	Epidemic croup	Fall or early winter	Less predictable than type 1; less widespread
3	Epidemic bronchitis and pneumonia	Late winter, early spring	Recently epidemic; often following influenza season; low levels of virus year-round
4	Unknown	?	Mild illness; frequently unrecognized

surrounds a helical nucleocapsid-RNA complex. The two surface proteins, which mediate attachment and penetration of the virus into susceptible mammalian cells, have retained antigenic stability for more than 30 years.

There are four serotypes of human parainfluenza viruses, types 1 through 4, with two subgroups (A and B) of type 4 virus. In addition, numerous animal strains of parainfluenza viruses exist, including shipping fever virus of cattle and Newcastle disease virus of chickens, important causes of lost income for the livestock industry. These viruses do not cause human illness.

EPIDEMIOLOGY. The parainfluenza viruses are ubiquitous and have worldwide geographic distribution. Spread principally by large-particle fomites and close person-to-person contact, each of the four serotypes displays somewhat different epidemiologic features.

Over the years, parainfluenza virus activity has displayed both endemic and epidemic patterns (Table 378–1). Primary infection with parainfluenza viruses begins soon after birth, with each serotype favoring different age groups and distinct clinical syndromes. Significant overlap exists in this regard, thus precluding specific diagnosis based on clinical and epidemiologic grounds. Among the parainfluenza viruses, type 3 infects infants first, with more than 50% showing serologic evidence of infection in the first year of life. Parainfluenza virus type 3 is second only to RSV as a cause of bronchiolitis and pneumonia in this youngest age group. Parainfluenza virus type 1, which exhibits characteristic epidemiology with biennial outbreaks in the fall of odd-numbered years, and type 2 infections occur later in childhood between ages 2 through 6. The peak incidence of infection with parainfluenza virus 1, manifested principally as croup, occurs between ages 1 and 2. The lower infection rate with parainfluenza type 1 and 2 viruses in very young infants suggests that maternally derived antibody is protective, in contrast to parainfluenza virus type 3 infection, in which maternal antibody has only limited benefit. After primary infection, a relatively brief period of immunity against homotypic reinfection develops; however, the fact that reinfections are common later in childhood highlights the lack of durable immunity.

CLINICAL MANIFESTATIONS. Illness associated with primary parainfluenza virus infection varies by age and the virus serotype, although substantial overlap occurs. Underlying medical conditions, such as cardiopulmonary or immune disorders, also will influence the severity of disease. In general, parainfluenza virus types 1 and 2 are associated with croup whereas parainfluenza virus type 3 causes bronchiolitis and pneumonia. Other causes of croup include influenza A and RSV.

Infection typically starts with upper respiratory signs and symptoms, notably coryza, rhinorrhea, pharyngitis without cervical adenopathy, and low-grade fever. In 15%, signs of lower respiratory tract disease develop. If croup evolves, the child manifests a raspy, barking cough with notable inspiratory stridor, dyspnea, and respiratory distress. These latter symptoms, which may be spasmodic, are due to subglottic inflammation and edema. Typically, in mild to moderate illness symptoms last 3 to 5 days but may be quite unpredictable and result in sudden respiratory failure. In hospitalized infants, hypoxia is universal, and hypercarbia is present in half. In severe stridor, differentiation from epiglottis due to *Haemophilus influenzae* type b (see Chapter 330) may be suggested by lateral neck radiography, which can show subglottic edema and narrowing, in contrast to epiglottic swelling. Although also a cause of croup, parainfluenza virus type 3 more commonly causes disease indistinguishable from RSV: tracheobronchitis, bronchiolitis, and pneumonia. Cough, rales, and wheezing associated with hypoxia and air trapping on radiography are common.

Reinfection with the parainfluenza viruses is less severe and typically causes cold symptoms in normal children and adults. However, similar to the situation with RSV, some adults may develop severe disease. Nursing home outbreaks with a high incidence of pneumonia have been reported, and parainfluenza viruses have been implicated in severe pneumonia in immunocompromised children and adults. In a report of more than 1000 bone marrow transplant recipients, 61 parainfluenza virus infections were documented; of these patients 44% developed pneumonia and 27% died, with most having had preceding upper respiratory symptoms. This latter finding is clinically useful in distinguishing parainfluenza virus pneumonia from cytomegalovirus pneumonia in this group. Many of the parainfluenza infections in immunosuppressed persons are acquired nosocomially. Similar to RSV infection, the most severe illnesses and 90% of the deaths due to parainfluenza virus pneumonia occur in the first 100 days after transplantation when lymphopenia is most pronounced. Fever, cough, shortness of breath, and sputum production are the most common symptoms, whereas bilateral pulmonary infiltrates are the most common radiographic finding.

DIAGNOSIS. Although the clinician may suspect parainfluenza virus based on clinical and epidemiologic grounds, specific diagnosis requires isolating the virus or detecting viral antigen in respiratory secretions. Monkey kidney or human embryonic kidney cell cultures are optimal for virus recovery, generally in 5 to 10 days, with the exception of type 4 virus, which requires up to 3 weeks in culture. Indirect immunofluorescent tests are also available for rapid antigen detection and, although specific, are less sensitive than culture. Diagnosis of parainfluenza infection in adults may be more difficult than in children, but virus can usually be recovered from the nasal or pharyngeal secretions of bone marrow transplant recipients with pneumonia and also generally from bronchoalveolar specimens in this group.

THERAPY AND PREVENTION. Specific antiviral treatment for parainfluenza virus is currently unavailable. Aerosolized ribavirin, approved for use in RSV infection, has in vitro activity against the parainfluenza viruses. Uncontrolled studies of ribavirin therapy of immunocompromised children and adults with severe parainfluenza virus pneumonia suggest possible benefit when administered at a dose of 20 mg/mL for 12 to 20 hours per day for 7 to 14 days.

Treatment of croup in children, under usual circumstances, includes mist and supplemental oxygen. Aerosolized bronchodilators (racemic epinephrine) have definite but only transient benefit, whereas corticosteroid use is controversial. Antibiotics are indicated only when bacterial superinfection is documented, an uncommon occurrence. Immunization to prevent parainfluenza virus infection with live attenuated vaccines is under study.

Lewis, VA, Champlin R, Englund J, et al: Respiratory disease due to parainfluenza virus in adult bone marrow transplant recipients. Clin Infect Dis 23:1033–1037, 1996. *Clinical description of parainfluenza viurs infections in bone marrow transplant patients.*

Marx A, Torok TJ, Holman RC, et al: Pediatric hospitalizations for croup (laryngotracheobronchitis): Biennial increases associated with human parainfluenza virus 1 epidemics. J Infect Dis 176:1423–1427, 1997. *Describes the epidemiology and associated clinical illness of parainfluenza virus infections in the United States from 1979 to 1993.*

Reed G, Jewett PH, Thompson J, et al: Epidemiology and clinical impact of parainfluenza virus infections in otherwise healthy infants and young children < 5 years old. J Infect Dis 175:807–813, 1997. *This report describes the epidemiology and clinical characteristics of parainfluenza virus infection among outpatient infants and children during a 20-year period at a single center.*

379 INFLUENZA

Frederick G. Hayden

Influenza is an acute febrile respiratory illness that occurs in annual outbreaks of varying severity. The causative virus infects the respiratory tract, is highly contagious, and typically produces prominent systemic symptoms early in the illness. Influenza virus infection can produce various clinical syndromes in adults, including common colds, pharyngitis, tracheobronchitis, and pneumonia. Conversely, infections with other respiratory viruses, such as respiratory syncytial virus or adenovirus, may produce influenzal illness. Influenza A viruses can cause worldwide epidemics (pandemics) and have done so four times this century (Table 379–1). The pandemic of 1918–1919 caused at least 500,000 deaths in the United States and over 20 million worldwide. Influenza epidemics are associated with enormous morbidity, economic loss, and often substantial mortality. Each epidemic causes on average over 20,000 deaths and about 150,000 hospitalizations in the United States.

ETIOLOGY. Influenza viruses belong to the family Orthomyxoviridae and are divided into three types (A, B, and C) distinguished by the antigenicity of their internal and external proteins (Table 379–2). The virion (Fig. 379–1) is a medium-sized enveloped pleomorphic particle covered with two types of surface glycoprotein spikes, the hemagglutinin (H or HA) and neuraminidase (N or NA). The envelope is composed of a lipid bilayer overlying the matrix (M1) protein that surrounds the segmented viral genome. The genome comprises eight segments of single-stranded RNA. Influenza C viruses have seven segments and only a single surface glycoprotein. Whereas influenza B and C viruses are human pathogens, influenza A viruses infect diverse animal species, including birds, horses, swine, and marine mammals. Influenza A viruses are further classified into subtypes based on their HA and NA glycoproteins. Each strain within a subtype is identified by site, sample number, and year of isolation. Three hemagglutinins (H1, H2, and H3) and two neuraminidases (N1 and N2) have been recognized in human influenza A viruses. In addition, in 1997 an avian H5N1 subtype virus caused a cluster of severe illnesses in humans in Hong Kong, and cases of avian H9N2 subtype virus infection have been recently documented in humans.

EPIDEMIOLOGY. ANTIGENIC VARIATION. Influenza viruses are unique among the respiratory viruses with regard to their extent of antigenic variation, epidemic behavior, and association with excess mortality during community outbreaks. The changing antigenicity of the surface glycoproteins accounts in part for the continuing epidemics of influenza in humans. Antibody to the HA neutralizes viral infectivity and thus is the major determinant of immunity. Anti-NA antibody limits viral replication and therefore the severity of infection. Variation involves either relatively minor (antigenic drift) or major (antigenic shift) changes in antigenicity. Significant antigenic variation is much less frequent with influenza B than with influenza A and may not occur with influenza C.

Antigenic drift refers to small changes that occur frequently (every year or every few years) within an influenza A or B virus. For example, the original H3N2 variant, A/Aichi/68, has undergone successive drifts resulting in epidemic strains that include the recent circulation of A/Sydney/5/97-like viruses. Antigenic drift re-

sults from an accumulation of point mutations in the RNA segment coding for the HA that cause amino acid substitutions in at least one of five antigenic sites on the HA. Immunologic selection favors the new variant over the old for transmission because of the less frequent presence of antibody in the population to the new virus.

Antigenic shift results from the appearance of an influenza A virus with HA or with HA and NA glycoproteins new to humans or possible reappearance of virus after decades of absence. Because of the lack of immunity to the new strain within the human population, a virulent new strain can cause pandemic disease (see Table 379–1). Infection by one subtype does not provide cross-protection against another. The origin of new pandemic strains and the basis for their apparent recirculation remain incompletely defined. Reassortment of gene segments may occur when two influenza viruses simultaneously infect a single cell. At least 15 HA and 9 NA subtypes exist in animal influenza A viruses, particularly aquatic birds, and these serve as the reservoir or new genes for human pandemic strains. Although avian influenza viruses generally do not cause infections directly in humans, bird to human transmission of an avian H5N1 subtype virus has been documented. Spread from swine and other animals to humans rarely occurs.

EPIDEMIC OR INTERPANDEMIC INFLUENZA. An "epidemic" is an outbreak of influenza confined to one geographic location. In a given community, epidemics of influenza A virus infection have a characteristic pattern. They usually begin rather abruptly, reach a sharp peak in 2 or 3 weeks, and last 6 to 10 weeks. Increased numbers of school children with febrile respiratory illness are often the first indication of influenza in a community. This is soon followed by illnesses among adults and about a week later by increased hospital admissions of patients with influenza-related complications. Hospitalization rates in high-risk persons increase two- to fivefold during major epidemics (Table 379–3). School and employment absenteeism increases, as does mortality from pneumonia and influenza, especially in older persons (see Table 379–3). The latter finding is a highly specific indicator of influenza activity.

Epidemics occur almost exclusively during the winter months in temperate areas but influenza activity may continue year-round in the tropics. Regional differences in the time of occurrence of influenza outbreaks are common, and major outbreaks may occur in some communities or regions whereas others are experiencing no activity whatsoever. During epidemics, the overall attack rates typically average 10 to 20%. Attack rates of 40 to 50% are not uncommon in closed populations, including hospital and nursing homes, and in certain highly susceptible age groups. In recent years it has been recognized that two different strains within a single subtype, two different influenza A subtypes (H1N1 and H3N2), or both influenza A and B viruses may co-circulate. In addition, simultaneous outbreaks of influenza A and respiratory syncytial viruses have been found. Strains circulating at the end of one season's epidemic are likely to be responsible for the next season's outbreak (the so-called herald wave phenomenon). Furthermore, other than the association of influenza outbreaks with colder seasons, the factors are unknown that allow an epidemic to develop or those responsible for the tapering off of an epidemic, when only some susceptible persons have been infected.

Pneumonia and influenza (P + I)-related deaths fluctuate annually, with peaks in the winter months. When such P + I deaths

Table 379-1 ■ ANTIGENIC SUBTYPES OF INFLUENZA A VIRUS ASSOCIATED WITH PANDEMIC INFLUENZA

YEAR	INTERVAL (YEARS)	DESIGNATION	EXTENT OF ANTIGENIC CHANGE IN INDICATED SURFACE PROTEIN*	SEVERITY OF PANDEMIC
1889	?	H2N2	?	Severe
1900	11	H3N8?	H+++N?	Moderate
1918	18	H1N1†	H+++N+++	Very severe
1957	39	H2N2	H+++N+++	Severe
1968	11	H3N2	H+++N−	Moderate‡
1977	9	H1N1	H+++N+++	Mild§

*Compared with antecedant or co-circulating virus: + = minor change; ++ = moderate change; +++ = major change; − = no change.
†Formerly designated as H0N1 (swine virus prototype) or Hsw1N1.
‡Population had some immunity to the N2 neuraminidase.
§Most of population immune due to prior infection with earlier circulating antigenically identical virus.

Table 379-2 ■ INFLUENZA VIRUS PROTEINS

DESIGNATION	LOCATION (APPROXIMATE NO. PER VIRION)	FUNCTION	OTHER
Hemagglutinin (HA)	Surface (500)	Cell attachment and penetration; fusion activity	Subtype- and strain-specific antigens
Neuraminidase (NA)	Surface (100)	Virus release; enzymatic activity	Subtype- and strain-specific antigens; site of action of zanamivir, GS4071
Membrane or M1 matrix	Internal (3000)	Major structural envelope protein; virus assembly	Type-specific antigen
M2	Surface (20–60)	Virus uncoating and assembly; ion channel	Site of action of amantadine/rimantadine
Nucleoprotein (NP)	Internal (1000)	Associated with RNA and polymerase proteins	Type-specific antigen
Polymerases (PB1, PB2, PA)	Internal (30–60)	RNA replication and transcription	Probable site of action of ribavirin
NS1	Nonstructural (infected cells)	Regulation of virus replication	Interferon antagonist
NEP	Internal (130–200)	Nuclear export factor	Formerly NS2

Adapted from Lamb RA, King RM: Orthomyxoviridae. *In* Fields BN, Knipe DM, Howley PM (eds): Fields Virology, 3rd ed. Philadelphia, Lippincott–Raven, 1996, p 1355.

exceed the predicted number, this is due to influenza A or occasionally to influenza B virus or respiratory syncytial virus activity. Although mortality is greatest during pandemics, substantial total mortality occurs with epidemics. Over 85% of P + I deaths occur among persons aged 65 and older (see Table 379–3). Other cardiopulmonary and chronic diseases also show increased mortality after influenza epidemics.

PANDEMIC INFLUENZA. Pandemics of influenza A result from the emergence of a new virus capable of sustained person-to-person transmission and to which the population contains no or limited immunity. The virus spreads worldwide and infects persons of all ages (see Table 379–1). The pandemics of 1957, 1968, and 1977 all began in mainland China, and Southeast Asia has been postulated to be the epicenter for such strains. The interval between pandemics is variable and unpredictable. The most severe pandemics have resulted when there were major antigenic alterations in both the major surface antigens. Furthermore, it appears that virulence is a virus-coded function that also varies among strains. The intrinsic virulence of recent H1N1 viruses appears to be milder than that of H3N2 viruses. After one or more waves of pandemic influenza, the level of immunity in the population increases. Repeated epidemics caused by strains showing antigenic drift within the subtype occur in subsequent years. After 10 to 40 years of circulation of variants within this given subtype, the population's immunity to all variants within the subtype is very high, and the conditions for the emergence of a new virus are favorable.

PATHOGENESIS AND PATHOLOGY. Influenza virus infection is transmitted from person to person by virus-containing respiratory secretions. Small-particle aerosols appear most important, but transmission by other routes, including fomites, may be possible. Virtually all cells lining the respiratory tract can support viral replication. Once the virus initiates infection of the respiratory tract epithelium, successive cycles of viral replication infect large numbers of cells and result in destruction of ciliated epithelium. The incubation period averages 2 days and varies from 1 to 4 days. The quantity of virus in respiratory tract specimens correlates with severity of illness, which suggests that a major mechanism in producing illness is virally mediated cell death. Elevations of proinflammatory cytokines like interferon-α, interleukin-6, and tumor necrosis factor-α occur in blood and respiratory secretions and may contribute to systemic symptoms and fever. The duration of viral shedding depends on age and generally lasts for 3 to 5 days in adults and often into the second week in children. Viremia or extrapulmonary dissemination is rarely found.

Nasal and bronchial biopsy specimens from persons with uncomplicated influenza reveal desquamation of the ciliated columnar epithelium. Individual cells show shrinkage, pyknotic nuclei, and loss of cilia. In addition, the lungs in fatal influenza show extensive hemorrhage, hyaline membrane formation, and paucity of polymorphonuclear (PMN) cell infiltration. Secondary bacterial infections develop as a result of altered bacterial flora, damage to bronchial epithelium with depressed mucociliary clearance, decreased PMN and alveolar macrophage functions, and/or alveolar fluid.

Neutralizing, hemagglutination-inhibiting (HAI), antineuraminidase, complement-fixing, enzyme-linked immunosorbent assay (ELISA), and immunofluorescent antibodies begin to develop in the sera of persons with primary influenza virus infection during the second week after infection and reach a peak by 4 weeks. Secretory antibodies develop in the respiratory tract after influenza infection and consist predominantly of IgA antibodies that reach peak titers in 14 days. Cell-mediated immune responses also occur. Immunity

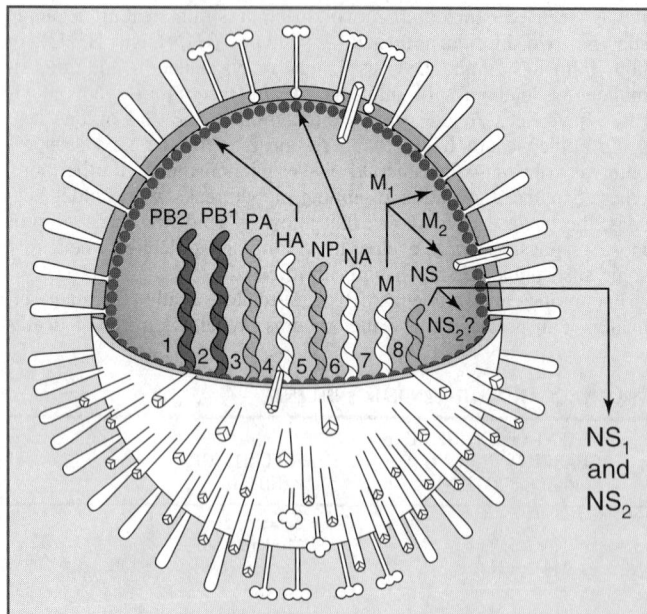

FIGURE 379–1 ■ Diagram of influenza virus structure. Eight segments of viral RNA are contained within the envelope and matrix (M1) shell. Each codes for one or two proteins that form the virus or regulate its intracellular replication. The presumed functions of each are listed in Table 379–2. (Courtesy of Dr. Robert G. Webster.)

Table 379-3 ■ AGE-SPECIFIC RATES FOR ILLNESS AND MORTALITY DURING URBAN INFLUENZA EPIDEMICS

AGE (YEARS)	PHYSICIAN VISITS PER 100	ARD HOSPITALIZATIONS PER 10,000	P + I MORTALITY PER 100,000
<5	28	43	3
5–14	14	5	1
15–44	10	8	1
45–54	9	13	10
55–64	10	21	10
≥65	—	73	104

ARD = acute respiratory disease; P + I = pneumonia and influenza; — = not stated.

Adapted from Glezen WP: Anatomy of an urban influenza epidemic. *In* Hannoun C, Kendal AP, Klenk HD, et al (eds): Options for the Control of Influenza II. Amsterdam, Elsevier Science, 1993, p 12.

to influenza appears to be subtype-specific and durable. Protection against illness is generally associated with serum HAI titers of 1:40 or greater, serum-neutralizing antibody titers of 1:8 or greater, or nasal neutralizing antibody titers of 1:4 or greater.

CLINICAL FINDINGS. INFLUENZA SYNDROME. The abrupt onset of feverishness, chilliness, or frank rigors, headache, myalgia, and malaise is characteristic of influenza. Systemic symptoms predominate initially, and prostration occurs in more severe cases. Usually myalgia or headaches are the most troublesome early symptoms, and their severity is related to the level of fever. Arthralgia is common, and less often ocular symptoms, photophobia, tearing, burning, and pain on moving the eyes are helpful diagnostically. Respiratory symptoms, particularly dry cough and nasal discharge, are usually also present at the onset but are overshadowed by the systemic symptoms. Nasal obstruction, hoarseness, and sore throat are also common. As systemic illness diminishes, respiratory complaints and findings become more apparent. Cough is the most frequent and troublesome and may be accompanied by substernal discomfort or burning. Cough, lassitude, and malaise may persist for several weeks before full recovery.

Fever is the most important initial physical finding. The temperature usually rises rapidly to a peak of 38 to 40° C within 12 hours of onset, concurrently with systemic symptoms. Fever is usually continuous but may be intermittent, especially if antipyretics are administered. As fever subsides, the systemic symptoms diminish. Typically, the duration of fever is 3 days, but it may last from 1 to 5 or more days. Uncommonly, a biphasic fever course occurs. Early in the course of illness, the patient appears toxic, the face is flushed, and the skin is hot and moist. The eyes are watery and reddened. Clear nasal discharge is common. The mucosa of the nose and throat are hyperemic, but exudate is not observed. Small, tender cervical lymph nodes are often present. Transient scattered rhonchi or localized areas of rales are found in less than 20% of cases.

The pattern of illness just described occurs with any strain of influenza A or B virus. Illness is more frequent and severe in smokers, and attack rates are higher in children than in adults. Maximum temperatures are higher in children, cervical adenopathy may be more frequent, and gastrointestinal symptoms of nausea, emesis, or abdominal pain more common. Women experience increased complications of influenza during the second and third trimesters of pregnancy. Symptoms may be protracted for some human immunodeficiency virus (HIV)–infected persons and they are also at higher risk of complications. Older adults (≥ 60 years) experience muscle aches, sore throat, and headache less often but have higher rates of pulmonary complications. Influenza C virus generally causes only sporadic upper respiratory tract illness.

RESPIRATORY COMPLICATIONS. Three kinds of pneumonic syndromes have been described: primary influenza viral pneumonia, secondary bacterial pneumonia, and mixed viral and bacterial pneumonia. Influenza A and B virus infections may be associated with other respiratory tract complications, including exacerbations of chronic bronchitis, asthma, or cystic fibrosis; croup and bronchiolitis in young children; and otitis media, sinusitis, and rarely parotitis or bacterial tracheitis. Apparently uncomplicated influenza is often accompanied by abnormal tracheobronchial clearance, airway hyperactivity, and small airways dysfunction lasting weeks. A syndrome mimicking pulmonary embolism with transiently altered perfusion scans also has been described.

Primary influenza vital pneumonia occurs predominantly among persons with underlying pulmonary and cardiac disorders, pregnancy, or immunodeficiency states, although up to 40% of reported cases have no recognized underlying disease. Following a typical onset of influenza, there is rapid progression of fever, cough, dyspnea, and cyanosis. Physical examination and chest radiographs reveal bilateral findings consistent with the adult respiratory distress syndrome. Blood gas studies show marked hypoxia. Gram's stain of the sputum may show abundant PMNs but scant bacterial flora. Sputum maybe bloody. Viral cultures of sputum or tracheal aspirates yield high titers of influenza virus. Antibiotics are not helpful, and the value of antiviral therapy is uncertain.

Bacterial superinfection is often clinically distinguishable from primary viral pneumonia. The patients are most often elderly or have chronic pulmonary, cardiac, metabolic, or other diseases. After a typical influenza illness, a period of improvement lasting from 1 to 4 days may occur. Recrudescence of fever is associated with

symptoms and signs of bacterial pneumonia, such as cough, sputum production, and a localized area of consolidation apparent on physical and chest radiographic examination. Gram stain and culture of sputum most often reveal *Streptococcus pneumoniae, Staphylococcus aureus,* or *Haemophilus influenzae* (see relevant chapters for specific bacterial diseases). Such patients usually respond to specific antibiotic therapy, although staphylococcal infections may be particularly virulent and cause destructive pulmonary lesions. Invasive aspergillosis occurs rarely after influenza.

In addition, during an outbreak of influenza, many less distinct cases are observed that do not clearly fit into either of these categories. These patients may have viral tracheobronchitis, milder forms of localized viral pneumonia, or mixed viral and bacterial infection. Many respond to antibiotics. Such cases are more likely to be confused with a pneumonia due to *Mycoplasma pneumoniae* than to that produced by other bacterial infection. Immunocompromised hosts including transplant recipients and acute leukemia patients undergoing chemotherapy have high rates of pneumonia and mortality after influenza.

NON-PULMONIC COMPLICATIONS. Reye's syndrome is a well-recognized hepatic and central nervous system (CNS) complication of influenza A and B virus infections, typically in children and rarely in adults (see Chapter 481). Toxic shock syndrome due to respiratory tract infection with toxin-bearing *S. aureus* has been reported. Outbreaks of meningococcal infections have been associated with both influenza A and B virus infections. Myositis with tender leg muscles and elevated serum creatine kinase levels may develop uncommonly, more often in children. Disseminated intravascular coagulation (DIC) develops rarely, as does renal failure related to DIC or myoglobinuria. Myocarditis or pericarditis has been described rarely. Aseptic meningitis, myelitis, encephalopathy associated with acute illness, and postinfluenzal encephalitis also occur.

DIAGNOSIS. In an individual case, influenza often cannot be distinguished from infection with a number of other viruses (and occasionally streptococcal pharyngitis) that produce headache, muscle aches, fever, and/or cough. In summer, enteroviruses produce a similar clinical picture, and the acute manifestations of many other infections, including those of respiratory syncytial viruses, parainfluenza viruses, and adenoviruses, may mimic influenza. On the other hand, when public health authorities report an epidemic of influenza A and B virus infection in a given community and a patient is seen with typical illness, it is highly likely that these symptoms are caused by an influenza virus infection.

Influenza virus is readily isolated from throat or nasal specimens, sputum, or tracheal secretion specimens in the first 2 or 3 days of illness. Usually infectivity is detected within 48 to 72 hours in cell cultures. Immunofluorescence testing of respiratory cells or of inoculated cell cultures (shell vials) can reduce time to detection. Commercially available enzyme immunoassays or neuraminidase detection-based assay can document influenza virus infection rapidly but may have limited sensitivity in adults. Serologic methods are less useful clinically because they require a convalescent serum obtained 14 to 21 days after the onset of infection.

TREATMENT. Oral rimantadine or amantadine therapy shortens the duration of fever and of systemic and respiratory symptoms in uncomplicated influenza A by 1 to 2 days and speeds functional recovery. The possible effectiveness of these drugs in treating pulmonary complications of influenza is unknown. The usual dosage is 100 mg twice daily for 5 days. A daily dose of 100 mg should be used in older adults. Rimantadine has a lower risk of the CNS side effects that occur with amantadine. Amantadine is excreted unchanged in the urine, so dose adjustments are needed for those with renal impairment. These agents are ineffective for influenza B infections. Treated persons sometimes transmit drug-resistant virus to close contacts. Inhaled zanamivir (10 mg twice daily) and oral GS4104 (75 mg twice daily), investigational neuraminidase inhibitors active against influenza A and B viruses, are also effective in treating acute influenza.

Other symptomatic measures include antipyretics and cough suppressants. Many authorities recommend that aspirin not be used, especially for children younger than age 16, because of its association with Reye's syndrome.

Influenza viral pneumonia in its severe form requires intensive

Table 379–4 ▪ TARGET GROUPS FOR INFLUENZA IMMUNIZATION

Groups at Increased Risk of Complications

Persons aged 65 and older

Residents of nursing homes and other chronic care facilities

Patients with chronic pulmonary (including asthma) or cardiac disorder

Patients with chronic metabolic disease (including diabetes), renal dysfunction, hemoglobinopathies, or immunosuppression

Children and teens receiving long-term aspirin

Pregnant women who will be in second or third trimester during influenza season

Groups in Contact with High-Risk Persons

Physicians, nurses, and other health care providers

Employees of nursing homes and chronic care facilities

Providers of home care to high-risk persons

Household members (including children) of high-risk persons

Other Groups

Providers of essential community services (e.g., police, fire)

International travelers

Students, dormitory residents

Anyone wishing to reduce risk of influenza

Adapted from Advisory Committee on Immunization Practices, Centers for Disease Control and Prevention. MMWR 47(No. RR-6):1–26, 1998.

respiratory monitoring and support. Oral amantadine or rimantadine, intravenous ribavirin, aerosolized ribavirin, and nebulized zanamivir have been used with uncertain benefit. Secondary bacterial pneumonia should be treated with appropriate antibiotics. When studies of the sputum do not clearly indicate an infecting bacterium, antibiotics that are effective against the likely pathogens, including *S. aureus,* should be used.

PREVENTION. The mainstay of prevention is using inactivated influenza virus vaccines. These vaccines provide 60 to 90% protection against influenzal illness when vaccine matches the epidemic strain. Immunogenicity and hence protection rates are often lower in the elderly, particularly in infirm nursing home residents, and immunosuppressed patients, including those with advanced HIV infection or receiving chemotherapy. In the ambulatory and institutionalized elderly, immunization is 50 to 60% effective in preventing hospitalization and pneumonia and reduces mortality. Immunization also appears cost effective in working adults. The antigenic composition is reviewed annually so that the vaccine contains the most recently circulating strains, usually one or more subtypes of influenza A and an influenza B virus. Between 1 and 2% of immunized adults have fever and less than 10% have systemic symptoms peaking at 8 to 12 hours after vaccination, but 25% or more may have mild local reactions at the site of injection. Persons with malignant disease should receive vaccine between chemotherapy courses.

The priority groups for vaccine include those at highest risk for influenza complications and their immediate contacts (Table 379–4), although vaccine can be safely administered to anyone trying to avoid influenza. Vaccine should be given each year in the fall before the influenza season. The vaccine is contraindicated in persons with chicken egg anaphylactic hypersensitivity. Rarely reported and unproven complications of inactivated vaccine include Guillain-Barré syndrome, systemic vasculitis syndrome, and theophylline or warfarin toxicities. Intranasal cold-adapted attenuated vaccines are highly protective in young children and are currently being studied in adults.

Rimantadine and amantadine are 70 to 90% effective in preventing influenza A illness and can be used to supplement vaccine programs. Persons who are not vaccinated in the fall should be placed on prophylaxis when an outbreak occurs or throughout the influenza season for the highest-risk group. If vaccine is available, persons may be vaccinated simultaneously and drug therapy stopped after 14 days. Alternatively, if vaccine is not available, administration may be continued for duration of the outbreak. When given to patients and staff alike, these drugs may be helpful in managing nosocomial outbreaks. Postexposure prophylaxis in households is also effective. The neuraminidase inhibitors, inhaled zanamivir and oral GS4104, are also effective for chemoprophylaxis. Hospitalized patients should be placed in respiratory isolation.

Advisory Committee on Immunization Practices, Centers for Disease Control and Prevention: Prevention and control of influenza: MMWR 47(No. RR-6):1–26, 1998.

Recommendations for influenza immunization and antiviral use that are updated on an annual basis.

Brown LE, Hampson AW, Webster RG (eds): Options for Control of Influenza III. Amsterdam, Elsevier Science, 1996, pp 1–860. *Compilation of review articles and papers from an international conference covering recent developments in influenza, including newer antivirals and vaccines.*

Hayden FG, Aoki FY: Amantadine, rimantadine, and related agents. *In* Yu VL, Merigan TC, White NJ, Barriere S (eds): Antimicrobial Chemotherapy. Baltimore, Williams & Wilkins, 1999, pp 1344–1365. *Detailed review of antiviral properties, pharmacology, and chemical use of these drugs.*

Nicholson KG, Webster RG, Hay AJ (eds): Textbook of Influenza. Malden, MA, Blackwell Science, 1998, p 578. *Multi-authored, authoritative text covering all aspects of influenza virus infections.*

Subbaroo K, Klimov A, Katz J, et al: Characterization of an avian influenza A (H5N1) virus isolated from a child with a fatal respiratory illness. Science 279:393–396, 1998. *First detailed report of an avian H5N1 subtype infection in humans.*

380 ADENOVIRUS DISEASES

John J. Treanor

VIROLOGY

The adenoviruses are found in a variety of animal species, including humans, simians, horses, pigs, goats, and dogs. These viruses have been the subject of intense investigation for many years because of their ability to undergo latency and to induce tumors in experimental animals; consequently, the molecular biology of the adenoviruses is among the most completely known of all viruses. However, despite much effort in this regard, there is no well-documented association between adenoviruses and any human tumor.

The virus is non-enveloped, with a double-stranded DNA genome. The human adenoviruses are grouped into six subgenera (A–F) based on differences in genome content, pattern of hemagglutination, and ability to cause tumors in experimental animals. In addition, at least 47 distinct serotypes are defined based on neutralization tests. Specific disease syndromes or hosts are often associated with specific adenovirus serotypes (Table 380–1).

CLINICAL FEATURES

DISEASE IN NORMAL HOSTS. The adenoviruses can infect and cause disease in a variety of human epithelial tissues, including those of the eye, respiratory tract, gastrointestinal tract, and urinary

Table 380–1 ▪ ADENOVIRUS SEROTYPES AND ASSOCIATED SYNDROMES

HOST AND DISEASE CATEGORY	EPIDEMIOLOGIC FEATURES	ASSOCIATED ADENOVIRUS SEROTYPES
Immunocompetent Hosts		
Pharyngoconjunctival fever	Epidemics in schools, families, and the military, associated with swimming pools	3, 7
Epidemic keratoconjunctivitis	Sporadic epidemics in schools, families, and industrial sites; may cause nosocomial outbreaks; more common in fall and winter	8, 19, 37
Endemic upper respiratory disease	Seen predominantly in children, in families, and day-care settings	1, 2, 5
Acute respiratory disease of military recruits		3, 4, 7, 14, 21
Acute hemorrhagic cystitis	Male predominance	7, 11, 21, 35
Gastroenteritis	Predominant in children <2 yr	40, 41
Immunocompromised Hosts		
Transplantation		7, 11, 31, 34, 35
Acquired immunodeficiency syndrome		Multiple, 35, 42–47

bladder. Most infections in immunologically competent individuals are subclinical. Virus may be shed for months after infection from either the gastrointestinal or respiratory tract. Adenoviruses appear to utilize multiple mechanisms to circumvent the host immune response, including inhibition of the antiviral effects of interferons, down-regulation of the expression of human leukocyte antigen molecules on the surface of infected cells, and antagonism of the effects of tumor necrosis factor-α.

EYE DISEASE. Pharyngoconjunctival Fever (see Chapter 376). The syndrome of pharyngoconjunctival fever (PCF) is seen predominantly in children and is characterized by bilateral conjunctivitis accompanied by mild pharyngitis without exudate. Fever, myalgias, and malaise also may be present. The eyes are itchy but not painful, with a boggy, hyperemic conjunctiva, and watery discharge. Occasionally, the syndrome may be complicated by punctate keratitis.

PCF is highly contagious (see Table 380–1) and can be spread by contact with the eyes and mouth for 8 to 10 days after the onset of symptoms. The incubation period is 5 to 8 days. The illness is self limited, with a duration of from a few days to as long as 3 weeks. There is no specific therapy.

Epidemic Keratoconjunctivitis. In contrast to PCF, epidemic keratoconjunctivitis (EKC) presents as unilateral disease in the majority of cases and is generally not accompanied by sore throat, fever, or systemic symptoms. The patient may complain of a mild foreign body sensation with watery tearing but is not in significant discomfort. Physical findings include a swollen eyelid, conjunctival hyperemia with edema and chemosis, and tender preauricular adenopathy. Keratitis eventually develops in about 80% of patients and is usually noted on about the eighth day of illness with the onset of pain, photophobia, lacrimation, and blepharospasm. Visual acuity also may be temporarily reduced during the height of illness. Subepithelial corneal infiltrates can be detected in about one third of patients and may take weeks or months to resolve.

Many EKC outbreaks (see Table 380–1) have been attributed to contamination of ophthalmologic equipment, such as tonometers, and sterilization of such equipment between patients and other infection control procedures are critical in terminating nosocomial outbreaks.

RESPIRATORY DISEASE. Upper Respiratory Tract Illness (see Chapter 376). Acute pharyngitis is the most common respiratory syndrome attributed to the adenoviruses. Adenoviruses can cause an exudative tonsillitis similar to that caused by group A streptococci. In children, common associated syndromes include otitis media, coryza, and undifferentiated fever. Overall, adenoviruses are associated with about 7% of acute febrile illnesses in children, with a peak age of incidence between 6 months and 2 years. High secondary attack rates are seen in families or in the day-care setting.

Lower Respiratory Tract Illness. Adenoviruses have been implicated as causing approximately 10% of childhood pneumonias. Clinical features are nondescript, and chest radiographs are similar to those in other forms of viral pneumonia, with the exception that hilar adenopathy is more common in children with adenoviral pneumonia than with other forms of viral pneumonia. Mixed bacterial/viral pneumonia is often present and may be suggested by elevations in band forms in peripheral blood.

Military recruits generally present with the atypical pneumonia syndrome (see Table 380–1), and illness clinically resembles that due to *Mycoplasma pneumoniae*. Although the illness is typically mild, more severe disseminated infections and deaths have been reported. Multiple radiographic patterns are noted; there may be large pleural effusions. Prodromal symptoms of upper respiratory tract infection are reported by most patients, and pharyngitis is often found on presentation. Bacterial superinfection, particularly with *Neisseria meningitidis,* may occur. The disease is classically seen in military recruits and appears to be associated with the special conditions of fatigue and crowding found in military barracks. Outbreaks have also recently been reported among young adults in psychiatric hospitals. However, this syndrome does not commonly occur in similarly crowded situations such as college dormitories.

Because adenoviruses rarely cause pneumonia in otherwise healthy adults (Fig. 380–1) but are frequently shed asymptomatically, isolation of adenovirus from stool or respiratory secretions in normal adults with pulmonary infiltrates should be interpreted with caution.

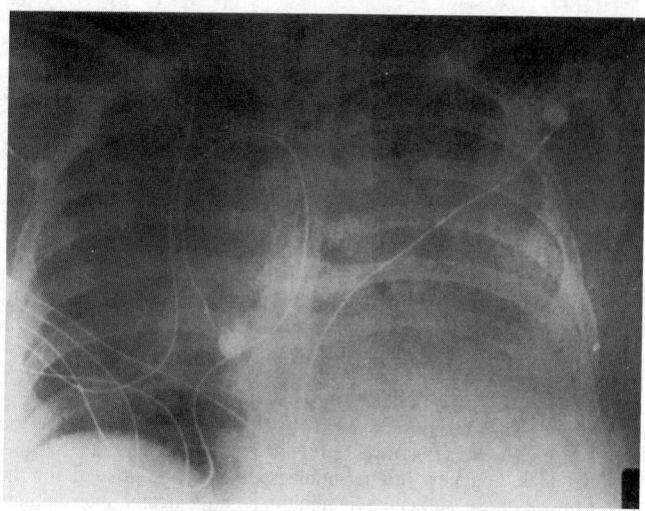

FIGURE 380–1 ▪ Portable upright chest film of a previously healthy 36-year-old woman with adenovirus pneumonia, showing consolidation of the left lower lobe and lingula as well as left-sided pleural effusion. (From Klinger JR, Sanchez MP, Curtin LA, et al: Multiple cases of life-threatening adenovirus pneumonia in a mental health care center. Am J Respir Crit Care Med 157:645–649, 1998. Used with permission.)

URINARY DISEASE. Hemorrhagic Cystitis. Acute hemorrhagic cystitis (AHC) may be caused by adenoviruses (see Table 380–1). The patient complains of gross hematuria and dysuria. The presentation may be confused with glomerulonephritis, but laboratory tests of renal function remain normal, and fever and hypertension do not occur. AHC is generally self-limited.

GASTROINTESTINAL DISEASE. Gastroenteritis (see Chapter 390). Although multiple adenovirus serotypes may be shed in the stool, only the so-called enteric adenoviruses (i.e., types 40 and 41) have been convincingly associated with acute gastroenteritis. These adenovirus types belong to the newly created group F and differ from other adenoviruses in being highly restricted in their ability to replicate in conventional cell culture.

Gastroenteritis due to enteric adenovirus is a disease predominantly of children younger than age 2. Clinical features include watery diarrhea and vomiting similar to those seen with infection with group A rotavirus. In contrast to gastroenteritis due to the rotaviruses and astroviruses, adenoviral gastroenteritis shows no significant seasonal variability. The frequency of illness is about 5 to 10% of that caused by rotavirus in the same age group. Adenoviruses are rarely causes of acute gastroenteritis in adults.

OTHER SYNDROMES ASSOCIATED WITH ADENOVIRUSES IN IMMUNOCOMPETENT HOSTS. Adenoviruses are often isolated in cases of pertussis-like syndrome, but there is no evidence that adenoviruses by themselves are important causes of whooping cough. A toxic shock–like presentation of disseminated adenovirus infection in a normal host has been reported. Adenoviruses have occasionally been isolated from cerebrospinal fluid in immunocompetent individuals with meningitis or meningoencephalitis. These viruses also have been implicated in sudden infant death syndrome (SIDS). Adenoviruses may be detected in mesenteric lymph nodes at the time of surgery for intussusception, and it is postulated that viral infection causes an acute mesenteric lymphadenitis that then leads to the development of this condition.

DISEASE IN IMMUNOCOMPROMISED HOSTS. Transplantation. Adenoviruses are causes of morbidity and mortality in immunocompromised patients, particularly after transplantation. In contrast to infection in normal hosts, infection in immunocompromised subjects tends to be disseminated, with virus isolated from multiple body sites, including lung, liver, and gastrointestinal tract, and in urine. In addition, the spectrum of serotypes includes both those found in immunocompetent individuals and a markedly increased frequency of higher-numbered serotypes found rarely in immunologically normal subjects (see Table 380–1). The source of infection may be reactivation of latent virus; nosocomial infection has also been documented.

Adenoviruses may cause hemorrhagic cystitis in bone marrow

transplant recipients, which may be confused with that due to cyclophosphamide. Differentiation between these two possibilities is generally made by virus culture and by the timing of cystitis in relationship to drug administration. Individuals with cystitis may develop pneumonia, hepatic necrosis, gastroenteritis, and encephalitis. The case-fatality rate of disseminated infection can be as high as 60%. Disseminated disease after liver transplantation can be seen and frequently leads to loss of the transplanted liver. However, this does not appear to preclude successful transplant of a new liver if one is available. Adenovirus disease in renal transplant recipients is generally not as severe as that seen in other transplants. Hemorrhagic cystitis is the most commonly seen problem, with pneumonia seen more rarely.

AIDS. Adenoviruses also have been isolated frequently from the stool and urine of individuals with the acquired immunodeficiency syndrome (AIDS), particularly those with relatively low CD4 lymphocyte counts. The most remarkable aspect of this situation is the isolation of a wide variety of serotypes in these patients (see Table 380–1), including new, higher-numbered serotypes isolated for the first time in these subjects. In addition, antigenically intermediate types have been isolated that possibly reflect recombination events made possible by prolonged virus replication in these hosts.

Because adenoviruses are almost always isolated in these patients in conjunction with multiple other opportunistic pathogens, it is difficult to ascribe specific clinical syndromes to them. Described associations include pneumonia, meningoencephalitis, hepatitis, gastroenteritis, and colitis. Adenoviruses have been detected in the large bowel of such patients in association with chronic diarrhea, but generally these have not been the enteric adenoviruses most commonly associated with gastroenteritis in immunologically normal hosts.

DIAGNOSIS

Virus can be isolated efficiently from conjunctival swabs, respiratory secretions, urine, or stool in primary cells of human epithelial origin, such as human embryonic kidney cells. However, diagnosis is complicated by the prolonged time required for isolation. Other means of directly detecting viral antigen or nucleic acid in clinical specimens are therefore widely used, including enzyme immunoassays, immunofluoresecence tests, and polymerase chain reaction techniques. In addition, the time required to detect virus in cell culture can be shortened to as little as 2 days by applying centrifugation culture systems coupled with detection of early virus replication in culture using immunofluorescent or other means.

TREATMENT AND PREVENTION

THERAPY. CONJUNCTIVITIS. Therapy is generally supportive Corticosteriods should be avoided in mild cases of conjunctivitis, because symptoms will usually recur when these agents are discontinued. In more severe cases of keratitis, mild topical corticosteroids may be used with cycloplegics as needed for iritis. Topical antibiotics may be administered to prevent bacterial superinfection.

SYSTEMIC INFECTIONS. There is no antiviral therapy that has been proven to be effective in any systemic adenoviral syndrome. A number of antiviral compounds including gancyclovir and cidofovir (HPMPC) are active against common adenovirus serotypes in vitro, and there have been uncontrolled anecdotal reports of successful treatment of AHC in immunocompromised hosts with intravenous ribavirin, a broad-spectrum antiviral drug.

VACCINATION. Live adenovirus vaccines have been developed for serotypes 4 and 7. These vaccines are administered orally in enteric-coated capsules and bypass the respiratory tract to replicate asymptomatically in the intestine. They have been shown to provide effective serotype-specific protection against adenovirus respiratory disease in high-risk military recruits, but these vaccines have not been used in civilian populations because of the plethora of additional serotypes causing severe disease in this population.

Because relatively large portions of the adenovirus genome can be replaced without affecting viral viability, adenoviruses have received considerable attention in constructing recombinant vaccines for other infectious diseases, such as hepatitis B, and as a vector for the delivery of gene therapy.

Baum SG: Adenovirus. *In* Mandell G, Dolin R, Bennett J (eds): Principles and Practice of Infectious Diseases, 4th ed. New York, Churchill-Livingstone, 1995. pp 70–75. *Readily accessible, detailed review of the clinical significance of the human adenoviruses.*

Hierholzer JD: Adenoviruses in the immunocompromised host. Clin Microbiol Rev 5: 262, 1992. *A complete description of reported cases of adenovirus infection in individuals with primary and secondary immunodeficiencies, including AIDS.*

Shenk T: Adenoviridae: The viruses and their replication. *In* Fields BN, Knipe DM, Howley PM (eds): Virology, 3rd ed. Philadelphia, Lippincott–Raven, 1996, pp 2111–2148. *Detailed description of the molecular biology of adenovirus replication.*

EXANTHEMS AND MUMPS

381 MEASLES

Philip A. Brunell

DEFINITION. Measles is an acute, highly contagious disease characterized by fever, coryza, cough, conjunctivitis, and both an enanthem and an exanthem.

ETIOLOGY. The virus is an enveloped, negative-stranded RNA paramyxovirus (genus Morbillivirus) measuring 120 to 250 mm in diameter, similar to other members of the Paramyxovirus family but lacking neuraminidase. Its single antigenic serotype has been remarkably stable throughout the world for many years; however, sequencing has revealed geographic strain differences. The virus contains six major polypeptides, which are responsible for a number of structural and functional properties, including hemagglutination (of primate erythrocytes), hemolysis, cell fusion, and others. Isolation of virus from clinical specimens is most successful with primary kidney cell cultures of human or simian origin, but newer cell lines may be equally sensitive.

EPIDEMIOLOGY. With the introduction of routine immunization against measles in the United States in 1963, the incidence of the disease fell by about 99%. Smaller outbreaks have occurred at increasing intervals in 1971, 1976, and 1986. A somewhat larger outbreak appeared in 1989. Before the advent of measles vaccine, almost every child got measles, most before entering school. In developing countries, where measles in the very young is common, it is estimated that there are from 1 to 2 million deaths annually worldwide. As a result of eradication efforts the number of cases globally has fallen, particularly in Latin America.

During the 1989–1990 epidemic in the United States, the highest attack rates were in infants, followed by preschool children. The largest number of measles deaths in over a decade, 89, was reported in 1990. About 30% occurred in those older than age 20 years, many in those who were immunocompromised. Almost all the remaining deaths occurred in those younger than age 5 years, most of whom were unimmunized and otherwise normal. During the past few years, however, the reported cases of measles have been at an all-time low and indigious transmission may have been interrupted at times. Most isolated strains appear to be of foreign origin.

COMMUNICABILITY. Measles is one of the most highly contagious infections. Almost all unprotected household contacts are infected. Demonstration of virus in nasopharyngeal secretions during the prodromal, pre-eruptive phase and in the first days of rash is in accord with epidemiologic evidence of contagiousness. Close physical proximity or direct person-to-person respiratory droplet contact is the usual requisite for infection, although airborne transmission has been documented.

IMMUNITY. An unmodified attack of measles is followed by lifelong immunity. Passively transferred maternal antibody protects the young infant during the early months of life.

PATHOLOGY AND PHYSIOLOGIC RESPONSES. Pathologic changes in fatal measles usually represent the compound effect of viral and secondary bacterial infection. Pneumonia is almost invariably present; it is most frequently interstitial. More representative are changes of the uncomplicated viral diseases within the tonsillar, nasopharyngeal, and appendiceal tissue removed during the prodrome. These changes consist of round cell infiltration and the presence of multinucleated giant cells. Giant cells also are observed in tissue cultures infected with measles virus. The skin and mucous membranes contain perivascular round cell infiltrates with congestion and edema. Koplik's spots are inflammatory lesions of the submucous glands with similar microscopic features.

Simultaneous with the onset of rash, measles-specific antibodies are detectable in serum. Leukopenia is observed on the first day of rash mainly due to a decrease in lymphocytes; subsequently, granulocytopenia ensues as well. Measles virus replicates in lymphoid tissues (spleen, thymus, lymph nodes) and can be isolated from monocytes and other mononuclear cells during acute infection. The virus is propagable in suspension of leukocytes in vitro.

IMMUNOSUPPRESSIVE EFFECTS OF MEASLES. It has long been known that cell-mediated immunity is impaired during measles. There is transient suppression of the tuberculin reaction (observed also with measles vaccines); improvement in eczema and allergic asthma and the induction of remissions in nephrosis have been described. In severe disease, the magnitude of depression of the total lymphocytes has been positively correlated with a lessened chance of recovery.

CLINICAL MANIFESTATIONS. After an incubation period that averages 11 days, measles becomes clinically manifest with symptoms of fever, malaise, myalgia, and headache. Within hours, *ocular symptoms* of photophobia and conjunctival injection occur. The palpebral and, to a lesser extent, the bulbar conjunctivae are involved. There is usually no exudate. Sneezing, coughing, and nasal discharge occur almost simultaneously. Less commonly, hoarseness and aphonia may reflect laryngeal involvement. In this prodromal stage of 1 to 4 days' duration, tiny white spots on the buccal mucosa may herald the appearance of rash. The white lesions described by Koplik characteristically occur lateral to the molar teeth and typically are mounted on a bluish red areola of injected mucosa, superimposed on a diffuse red background. They generally appear a day or so before the rash and disappear within 2 days after its appearance. They constitute a pathognomonic diagnostic sign. The enanthem may involve other mucous membranes such as the palpebral conjunctiva and vaginal lining.

The *rash* of measles follows the prodromal symptoms by 2 to 4 days, occasionally as late as 7 days. It first appears behind the ears or on the face and neck as a blotchy erythema, spreads downward to cover the trunk, and finally is manifest on the extremities. The hands and feet may escape involvement. Initially, the eruption consists of discrete red macules that blanch with pressure. Subsequently, these lesions become papular, tend to coalesce, and may develop a red, non-blanching component. In adults, the rash generally is more extensive, with a greater tendency to become confluent and slightly raised and redder than in children. This is particularly true on the face. The rash fades in the order of its appearance; its disappearance about 5 days after onset may be attended by a fine, powdery desquamation that spares the hands and feet. In adults, malaise may continue for 1 to 2 weeks.

The *fever* of measles may persist for about 6 days and frequently reaches 40 or 41° C. Throughout the febrile period, productive cough and auscultatory evidence of bronchitis may be evident. These manifestations may persist after defervescence, and cough is often the last symptom to disappear. Bronchopulmonary symptomatology is an integral part of the primary viral infection; roentgenographic evidence of pulmonary involvement is frequently seen in the uncomplicated disease in the absence of leukocytosis and obvious bacterial infection. Generalized lymphadenopathy accompanies the acute febrile illness and may persist for several weeks thereafter. Nausea and, less commonly, emesis appear to be more common in adults and are often accompanied by slightly elevated serum aminotransferase levels.

COMPLICATIONS. The persistence or recurrence of fever and development of leukocytosis are presumptive evidence of the common bacterial sequela of otitis media or pneumonia. Transtracheal aspirates in patients with pneumonia have yielded a variety of bacterial organisms.

Laryngitis of sufficient severity to embarrass respiration has been observed. Keratoconjunctivitis is part of the acute phase. Electrocardiographic abnormalities may be found. Severe measles has been described in pregnant women with hepatitis and pneumonia, the latter sometimes fatal. Premature labor has resulted in prematurity and stillbirths.

ENCEPHALOMYELITIS. A rare (0.1%) but serious consequence of measles is a demyelinating encephalomyelitis that may appear from 1 to 14 days after the onset of rash. This complication is associated with recurrence of fever and headache, vomiting, and stiff neck. Stupor and convulsions usually follow. Death ensues in about 10% of patients; more than half of survivors suffer permanent residuals of varying severity. Abnormal electroencephalograms were recorded in about half of children with measles without clinical signs of encephalitis.

Infection of brain cells results in an incomplete viral replicative cycle with production of defective virions lacking the matrix (M) measles virus protein. Studies of patients with acute measles encephalomyelitis and those with late-onset subacute sclerosing panencephalitis show high titers in serum and cerebrospinal fluid of antibodies to all the measles virus proteins except M.

Other late sequelae of measles are thrombocytopenic purpura and exacerbation or activation of pre-existing pulmonary tuberculosis. The late complication of subacute sclerosing panencephalitis is discussed in Chapter 479.4.

GIANT-CELL PNEUMONIA. In patients who are immunocompromised (e.g., those with the acquired immunodeficiency syndrome [AIDS]), measles virus may induce an interstitial pneumonia characterized by giant cells and intracellular inclusion bodies that is often fatal. This also has been reported in a human immunodeficiency virus (HIV)–positive vaccine recipient.

MEASLES MODIFIED BY ADMINISTERING ANTIBODIES. Attenuation of the natural disease by antibody prophylaxis may result in an illness of lessened severity comparable with the milder infection as seen in infants with illness modified by maternally acquired antibody. Fever alone may be observed, but some degree of exanthem is usually apparent. Koplik's spots may not appear. In general, the course is truncated and relatively uncomplicated. Lasting immunity is uncertain. Later routine immunization of these individuals is probably indicated.

ATYPICAL MEASLES. From 1963 to 1967, two types of measles vaccine, one live attenuated and the other inactivated or "killed," were available in the United States. The live attenuated vaccine has been the sole product licensed and used in this country since 1967. A severe illness was reported in killed vaccine recipients after exposure to natural measles. These patients had high fever, pneumonia with pleural effusion, obtundation, and an unusual rash. The exanthem was hemorrhagic and was most marked on the extremities. In some instances, vesicular, macular, or maculopapular phases have been observed. The rash is sometimes accompanied by edema of hands and feet. Concomitantly, these patients' sera revealed extraordinarily high liters of measles-specific antibodies.

Subsequent investigations showed that patients who had received inactivated measles vaccines failed to develop antibodies to the fusion (F) protein of the virus. Lack of antibodies to the cell fusion factor is believed to have permitted these patients to support measles infection. Thus the atypical measles syndrome is believed to be due to an anamnestic antibody response in the face of an abundance of measles antigens.

In addition to the rash and pulmonary findings, these patients may have elevated liver enzymes, disseminated intravascular coagulation, and marked myalgia. Nodular pulmonary changes have persisted in some patients. Some cases of pneumonia are reported to have occurred in the absence of rash. Initial diagnoses on presentation have included Rocky Mountain spotted fever and meningococcemia because of the similarities of rash and toxicity. Because inactivated vaccines were available only from 1963 through 1967, the past recipients are now adults. This atypical measles syndrome is of increasing importance to the internist. Atypical measles has been reported in some patients who received live vaccine alone or after killed vaccine. Recipients of killed vaccine who later received live vaccine may have severe local and systemic reactions to reimmunization.

DIAGNOSIS. The diagnosis should be suspected during an epi-

Table 381–1 ■ A GUIDE TO THE DIFFERENTIAL DIAGNOSIS OF MEASLES

	CONJUNCTIVITIS	RHINITIS	SORE THROAT	ENANTHEM	LEUKOCYTOSIS	SPECIFIC LABORATORY TESTS AVAILABLE
Measles	++	++	0	+	0	+
Rubella	0	±	±	0	0	+
Exanthem subitum	0	±	0	0	0	+
Enterovirus infection	0	±	±	0	0	+
Adenovirus infection	+	+	+	0	0	+
Scarlet fever	±	±	++	0	+	+
Infectious mononucleosis	0	0	++	±	±	+
Drug rash	0	0	0	0	0	0

0 Not usually present; no test available.
± Variable in occurrence.
+ Present: test available (virus or bacterial culture, serology).
++ Present and severe.

demic or after history of exposure or of foreign travel. Before the appearance of rash, the diagnosis may be difficult unless Koplik's spots are present. Finding an uncomfortable patient in a darkened room who has conjunctivitis, coryza, and cough should make one suspect measles. The rash in adults may be more violaceous, confluent, slightly raised, and more extensive than in children. A history of having received measles vaccine does not preclude the diagnosis, because most individuals with measles of school age or older have had the vaccine.

Differential diagnosis (Table 381–1) includes consideration of rubella, scarlet fever, infectious mononucleosis, secondary syphilis, drug eruptions, toxic shock syndrome, and Kawasaki's disease. Of value in excluding these possibilities are the milder course, post-auricular nodes, and pinker rash of rubella; the sore throat, eventual desquamation, strawberry tongue, and leukocytosis of scarlet fever; and serologic tests for infectious mononucleosis. Fever, enanthem, and catarrh are uncommon with the cutaneous manifestations of drug hypersensitivity. Erythema infectiosum is usually an afebrile illness with rash on the cheeks, arms, and legs. There is no prodrome or accompanying respiratory tract involvement. Kawasaki's disease is rare in adults.

SPECIFIC DIAGNOSIS. Virus isolation is technically difficult. Increase in specific antibody may be detected as early as the first or second day of rash. Generally acute and convalescent sera are required. Demonstration of measles IgM is available in some laboratories.

Presumptive diagnosis may be made if giant cells are detected in stained smears of nasal exudate in the pre-eruptive period.

PROGNOSIS. Uncomplicated measles is rarely fatal, and complete recovery is the rule. Fatalities are almost always the result of pneumonia, occurring in adults or children younger than age 1. Congestive cardiac failure is a common cause of death in patients older than age 50 years. The prognosis is particularly poor in patients with AIDS or other immunocompromised patients (see Chapter 407).

Antimicrobial drugs effective against the usual secondary invaders have reduced the case fatality rate of measles sharply. They have proved effective in therapy of bacterial complications but not in prophylaxis.

Encephalitis occurs as frequently in mild as in severe measles (i.e., about 1 in 1000 cases); subacute sclerosing panencephalitis occurs about 7 years after measles and has essentially disappeared with widespread vaccine use.

TREATMENT. There is no specific antiviral therapy for measles with demonstrated efficacy, although ribavirin has been used in some cases.

SYMPTOMATIC THERAPY. In the absence of complications, bed rest is the essence of treatment in this self-limited disease. Codeine sulfate may be useful to ameliorate headache and myalgia and is effective for cough. Analgesics and antipyretics may be useful. Fluids should be encouraged. Bright light is not an ocular hazard, but photophobia may require darkening the patient's room.

ANTIMICROBIAL PROPHYLAXIS. The course of uncomplicated measles is not influenced by antimicrobial drugs, and their use during the acute illness has resulted in no decrease of secondary bacterial complications (otitis, sinusitis, pneumonia). Instead, the

same rates of complications (10–15%) have been observed, but with organisms resistant to the antibiotics used during the viral illness. If careful observation of the patient is possible, rational therapy is based on promptly recognizing and defining the cause of complications, followed by starting the appropriate antimicrobial drug in proper dosage.

PREVENTION. VACCINATION. A highly effective vaccine available for preventing measles is derived from the Edmonston strain of virus isolated originally in the laboratory of Dr. John Enders. This live virus vaccine produces immunity by infection. A second dose now is recommended routinely. In children older than age 1, seroconversion after vaccination in recent years is 98 to 99%. Measles vaccine usually is given as a single preparation as measles, mumps, and rubella (MMR) vaccine. Failure of measles immunization was much more common before 1980. The reasons for this are unclear. It may be due to poor recall or faulty documentation of immunization, age of immunization, use of immune globulin with the vaccine, receipt of killed rather than live vaccine, or the type of live vaccine.

Vaccine recommendations vary depending on the measles experience in the community (see Chapter 15). The first dose is now recommended at age 12 months as MMR. During epidemics, it may be given as monovalent measles vaccine to infants as young as 6 months of age. In the latter case, it should be repeated in combination with mumps and rubella (MMR) after the first birthday. A second routine dose of MMR at school entry is recommended. All entering college students and beginning health care workers born after 1956 should show evidence of measles immunity (e.g., positive serologic test, physician-documented measles, or receipt of two doses of measles vaccine or preferably MMR). The immune status of those contemplating foreign travel should be reviewed. A large number of military personnel have been reimmunized without significant side effects. Measles vaccine may be given at the same time as other live or killed vaccines.

Contraindications to live virus vaccine include pregnancy, immunodeficiency, leukemia, other systemic malignant diseases, active tuberculosis, and administration of resistance-depressing drugs such as corticosteroids and antimetabolites. Measles immunization of HIV-infected children is recommended with the caveat to avoid severly immunocompromised individuals.

Annunziato D, Kaplan MH, Hall WW, et al: Atypical measles syndrome: Pathologic and serologic findings. Pediatrics 70:203, 1982. *Excellent clinical description and explanation of a syndrome now seen in young adults.*

Atmar RL, Englund JA, Hammill H: Complications of measles during pregnancy. Clin Infect Dis 14:217, 1992. *A review of the complications and the treatment of measles in pregnancy.*

Centers for Disease Control and Prevention: Measles prevention: Recommendations of the Immunization Practices Advisory Committee (ACIP). MMWR 38:1, 1989. *Everything you want to know about the use of measles vaccine.*

Gilad M: Measles in adults: A prospective study of 291 consecutive cases. BMJ 295:1313, 1987. *A brief summary of findings in a large number of adults.*

Gremillion DH, Crawford GE: Measles pneumonia in young adults. Am J Med 71:539, 1981. *A large series of cases of measles pneumonia in young adults and other features of measles in this group.*

Gustafson TL, Brunell PA, Lievens AW, et al: Measles outbreak in a "fully-immunized" secondary school population. N Engl J Med 316:771, 1987. *School outbreaks are described in a presumably well-immunized population.*

Measles Evaluation: Recommendations from a meeting co-sponsored by the World Health Organization, the Pan American Health Organization and CDC. MMWR

46(No. RR-1), 1997. *A progress report and recommendations for the worldwide eradication of measles.*

Panum PL: Observations Made During the Epidemic of Measles on the Faroe Islands, New York, Delta Omega Society, 1940. *A classic clinical epidemiologic description of measles introduced into an isolated population with disease among all susceptibles born since the previous epidemic 65 years earlier.*

382 RUBELLA (GERMAN MEASLES)

Philip A. Brunell

DEFINITION. Rubella is an acute, usually benign infectious disease characterized by a 3-day rash, generalized lymphadenopathy, and minimal or no prodromal symptoms. Since 1941, it has been known to cause congenital malformations when infection occurs during the early months of pregnancy.

ETIOLOGY. Rubella is a small, spherical, enveloped virus containing single-stranded RNA of positive polarity. Structural proteins include two envelope glycoproteins and a nucleocapsid protein. The virus is classified as a togavirus, genus *rubivirus*. It multiplies slowly in a variety of primary cell culture systems and in some continuous cell lines in most systems without detectable cytopathic effects.

EPIDEMIOLOGY. Before rubella vaccines were available, the disease was worldwide in distribution, produced major epidemics at 6- to 9-year intervals, and was recognized mainly in school-age children; it also produced outbreaks in settings such as military recruit bases and college campuses where large numbers of susceptible young adults gathered in relatively crowded conditions. Since licensure in 1969 of the vaccine in the United States, there has been strikingly altered epidemiology. There has been no major epidemic since 1964–1965. In other nations, where rubella vaccine has not been widely used, the epidemiology has remained unchanged. Because the disease may be quite non-specific clinically, with nearly one third of adults undergoing infection without rash, epidemiologic reporting tends to underestimate its prevalence. Since 1966, congenital rubella has been a reportable disease. It is probable that rubella is spread by the respiratory route and by close and sustained personal contact. The incubation period in experimentally infected individuals was found to be 12 to 19 days, with most cases occurring 14 to 15 days after exposure. Although virus was isolated as early as 7 days before and as late as 21 days after onset of rash, infectivity probably is greatest throughout the period of prodromal symptoms and for as long as 7 days after the appearance of rash. Infants with congenitally acquired infection may excrete virus in respiratory secretions and in urine for months after birth and are contagious during this time. In hospital environments, especially in nurseries, the newborn with congenital rubella had been a source of nosocomial infection of personnel involved in his or her care.

Immunity is lifelong after initial infection. Authenticated second attacks are exceedingly rare and require serologic documentation because of the non-specific nature of the clinical syndrome. Subclinical reinfection demonstrated by increase in IgG serum antibody has been documented. Such reinfections are not associated with viremia and thus pose little threat to pregnant women. IgM response has been used to distinguish primary infection from reinfection. Immunity that follows artificial immunization with live virus vaccine is apparently of equal duration even though the antibody titers induced may be somewhat lower.

PATHOLOGY. Death from postnatal rubella is usually due to encephalitis. Thus, most autopsies describe only the brain findings. Since 1962, it has been possible to investigate the pathogenesis and to correlate clinical findings with virologic events. After initial invasion of the upper respiratory tract, virus spreads to local lymphoid tissue, where it multiplies and initiates a viremia of approximately 7 days' duration. Respiratory tract shedding of virus and the viremia rise to peak levels until the onset of rash, at which time the latter becomes undetectable, whereas respiratory secretions contain diminishing quantities of virus over the succeeding 5 to 15 days. Specific serum antibodies can be demonstrated with the onset of rash, and circulating immune complexes are detectable soon thereafter.

CONGENITAL RUBELLA. Necropsies of fetal and neonatal victims of intrauterine infection have shown a variety of embryonal defects related to developmental arrest involving all three germ layers.

The virus establishes chronic persistent infection of many tissues, with resultant intrauterine growth retardation. Delayed and disordered organogenesis produces embryopathic structural defects of the eye, brain, heart, and large arteries; continued viral infection during the fetal and postnatal period causes organ and tissue damage (e.g., hepatitis, nephritis, myocarditis, pneumonia, osteitis, meningitis, cochlear degeneration, and pancreatitis with the development of diabetes).

CLINICAL MANIFESTATIONS. POSTNATALLY ACQUIRED RUBELLA. Twelve to 19 days after exposure, the onset of rubella is manifested by the appearance of a rash with mild accompanying constitutional symptoms of malaise and occasionally mild sore throat. Enlargement of the postauricular and suboccipital nodes generally appears about a week before the rash. Moderate fever may accompany or precede the rash. Generalized peripheral lymphadenopathy and, more rarely, splenomegaly may occur.

The exanthem of rubella is usually apparent within 24 hours of the first symptoms as a faint macular erythema that first involves the face and neck. Characterized by its brevity and evanescence, it spreads rapidly to the trunk and extremities, sometimes leaving one site even as it appears at the next. The pink macules that constitute the rash blanch with pressure and rarely stain the skin. Rubella virus has been isolated from the skin lesions as well as from uninvolved sites. The truncal rash may coalesce, but the lesions on the extremities remain discrete. The eruption usually vanishes by the third day. Rubella may occur without rash. In the absence of an epidemic and of serologic or virologic confirmation, the clinical diagnosis of rubella is not reliable.

COMPLICATIONS. Recovery is almost always prompt and uneventful. In contrast to measles, secondary bacterial infections are not encountered in rubella. Transient polyarthralgia and polyarthritis are more common among adolescents and adults with rubella, particularly females. They appear 3 or more days after onset of rash and may last 5 to 10 days. The knees and joints of the hands and wrists are most often involved. Surveys during urban epidemics have revealed rates of 5 to 15% in males and 10 to 35% in females.

Thrombocytopenia, when sought by serial platelet counts, is common but rarely of clinical consequence. A meningoencephalitis of short duration may occur 1 to 6 days after the appearance of rash. Its incidence is estimated at 1 in 5000 cases, and it is fatal in approximately 20% of those afflicted. Rubella encephalopathy is not associated with demyelinization, in contrast to other postviral encephalitides. Survivors may have electroencephalographic abnormalities, but intellectual function seems to be preserved.

CONGENITAL RUBELLA. Congenital transplacental infection of the fetus occurs as a consequence of maternal infection, usually in the first 4 months of pregnancy. Virus is demonstrable in placental and fetal tissues obtained by therapeutic abortion at that time. If pregnancy is not interrupted, fetal infection persists, and on delivery of the infant, virus is recoverable from the throat, urine, conjunctivae, bone marrow, and cerebrospinal fluid of the living infant and from most organs at autopsy. From 20 to 80% of infants born to mothers infected in the first trimester of pregnancy have stigmata of infection readily recognizable in the first year of life. These include cardiac lesions and eye defects (e.g., cataracts, glaucoma, retinitis, microphthalmia). Most infants in whom virus is detectable do not have evidence of disease at birth or may simply have intrauterine growth retardation. In others, more severe disease occurs. Most prominent of these manifestations is thrombocytopenic purpura, which disappears soon after birth. Hepatosplenomegaly with active hepatitis may persist for months. Other involvement includes interstitial pneumonia, meningoencephalitis, hearing loss of varying extent, and lesions of the long bones. Recently, a progressive panencephilitis simulating subacute sclerosing panencephalitis has been observed in the second decade after congenital infection. The long-term sequelae for infants with congenital rubella include psychomotor retardation, hearing loss, retinopathy, and diabetes.

A striking finding has been the persistence of virus in the pharynx, urine, and cerebrospinal fluid for as long as 1 year after birth in 7% of infants. Infective virus was found in a congenital cataract after 3 years. This evidence of continuing viral synthesis occurs coincidentally with circulating antibody. The character of the antibody changes during the first months from maternal IgG to IgM, indicating a primary response of the infant to the persisting viral antigen. Studies of older infants and children with stigmata of congenital rubella show them to be free of demonstrable virus and to possess the IgG immunoglobulins that characteristically persist after other viral infections.

DIAGNOSIS. Rubella may be diagnosed clinically with assurance only during an epidemic. Distinction from measles may be made on the basis of fainter, non-staining rash, the milder course, and the minimal or absent systemic complaints. Sore throat is a more prominent complaint in scarlet fever; the course of infectious mononucleosis is often more protracted, and splenomegaly is more frequent than in rubella. Specific diagnosis of rubella is made by isolating the virus in any of several cell culture systems or by demonstrating a rise by latex agglutination, hemagglutination inhibition, enzyme-linked immunosorbent assay, or complement fixation.

PROGNOSIS. Complete recovery from postnatally acquired rubella is almost invariable. The rare deaths attributable to rubella follow the infrequent complication of meningoencephalitis. Infection in pregnancy constitutes a grave hazard to the fetus but not to the mother.

TREATMENT. There is no specific antiviral therapy. Few patients suffer discomfort severe enough to warrant symptomatic medication. Headache and myalgia or arthritis may be controlled by analgesics.

PREVENTION. PASSIVE IMMUNIZATION. Administration of gamma globulin to the pregnant woman may only mask her symptoms of infection and not protect the fetus from viral invasions. Thus its use may only obscure the picture and confound decision about the need to terminate the pregnancy.

ACTIVE IMMUNIZATION. Rubella may be prevented in children and adults by parenteral attenuated live virus vaccines produced in cell cultures. Seroconversion rates after immunization are at least 98% with the current RA 27/3 vaccine. Joint symptoms are less common than with the older HPV 7-DE strain, occurring in about 2.5% of adults. Arthritis occurs 13 to 19 days after immunization and lasts 2 to 11 days. The fingers are most often affected, with the wrists and knees less commonly involved. Arthralgias generally begin 10 to 25 days after vaccination and last 1 to 9 days. Joint symptoms are less common in men than in women. In children, vaccination is attended by little or no reaction. Although rubella vaccine allegedly has been the cause of chronic arthritis, evidence has been accumulating that there is no etiologic relationship.

It was initially recommended in the United States that immunization be carried out principally in childhood. There now is a more aggressive attempt to immunize those remaining susceptible women and adolescent girls. Current policy recommends vaccinating all such persons who have no history of previous rubella immunizations. Postpartum immunization of those found to be seronegative during pregnancy is encouraged. Although occasionally vaccine virus has been transmitted to the newborn by breast milk, this has proven to be of little consequence. Only non-pregnant individuals should be immunized, and contraception, when appropriate, should be carried out for at least 3 months after vaccination. Inadvertent administration of vaccine to pregnant women has occasionally resulted in attenuated vaccine viruses infection of the fetus. In more than 500 such cases studied, no infant has been observed with congenital malformations as a result. The frequency of fetal infection with the RA 27/3 vaccine currently used is less than with the previous rubella vaccine. Use of vaccine in the United States prevented a large epidemic of rubella expected in the early 1970s and has reduced the reported annual occurrence from more than 50,000 cases annually, with epidemic peaks of 200,000 to 500,000, to an all-time low in 1995 of 128 cases. A slight increase in cases of rubella accompanied by cases of congenital rubella syndrome occurred in 1990.

Centers for Disease Control and Prevention: Rubella and congenital rubella syndrome—United States. MMWR 38:173, 1989. *A summary report of progress in rubella "eradication" in the United States.*

Gregg NM: Congenital cataract following German measles in the mother. Trans Ophthal Soc Aust 3:35, 1941. *The original "classic" report associating rubella in pregnancy with congenital malformations.*

Sherman FE, Michaels RH, Kenny FM: Acute encephalopathy (encephalitis) complicating rubella. JAMA 192:675, 1965. *A clinical, pathologic, and epidemiologic study of rubella encephalitis.*

Townsend JJ, Stroop WG, Baringer JR, et al: Neuropathology of progressive rubella panencephalitis after childhood rubella. Neurology 32:185, 1982. *A review of the clinical and neuropathologic findings.*

Weibel RE, Vilarejos VM, Klein EB, et al: Clinical and laboratory studies of live attenuated RA 27/3 and HPV 77-DE rubella virus vaccines (40931). Proc Soc Exp Biol Med 165:44, 1980. *A description of the clinical and serologic response to rubella vaccine.*

383 VARICELLA (CHICKENPOX, SHINGLES) (See also Chapter 477)

Philip A. Brunell

DEFINITION. Varicella, or chickenpox, is an acute communicable disease characterized by a generalized vesicular rash. Because it is highly contagious, most individuals contract it in childhood. Herpes zoster, due to reactivation of varicella-zoster virus (VZV), is a dermatomal cutaneous eruption.

ETIOLOGY. Varicella is caused by VZV, which is a member of the alpha Herpesviridae subfamily. It has the characteristic structure of a herpesvirus with an envelope, a tegument, a capsid, and a core of double-stranded DNA. The DNA is organized with terminal and internal repeats flanking unique short and long segments containing about 125,000 base pairs coding for approximately 70 genes. There are at least six glycoproteins. Its thymidine kinase has been a target for antiviral agents. There is some diversity in the restriction enzyme patterns among wild isolates; there is only a single serotype. Although the human is the only known natural host, a closely related virus has been identified in a simian species.

EPIDEMIOLOGY. Varicella is a highly contagious disease. After continuing household exposure, as would occur in a family, almost all susceptibles are infected. The subclinical attack rate is believed to be no more than 4%. The results of non-household exposure are less predictable. Chickenpox may be most contagious the day before the onset of rash. The period of contagiousness lasts for no more than 5 days after the appearance of the first lesion. Children may return to school at this time or earlier if the lesions are crusted. The incubation period is usually about 14 days. Ninety-nine per cent of the cases occur 10 to 20 days after exposure. The disease is known to be spread by direct contact. Airborne spread also has been demonstrated, most notably in hospitals.

Nosocomial spread of varicella has been well documented. This has occurred room to room by airborne spread as well as between patients and staff. Adults with herpes zoster who are hospitalized are less likely to cause secondary cases of chickenpox among adult contacts than among children. The reason is that hospitalized children are more likely to be susceptible to chickenpox than hospitalized adults. Strict isolation is recommended for hospitalized patients with varicella and for children or immunocompromised adults with herpes zoster. Adults with localized herpes zoster require less stringent isolation procedures.

Most cases of chickenpox occur in childhood. Most children contract chickenpox either in day-care situations or shortly after they enter school. Fewer than 2% of the cases occur after the second decade. Less than 10% of hospital workers with a negative history are seronegative. Almost all individuals with a positive history are seropositive. A single attack of chickenpox usually confers lifetime immunity.

There appears to be more efficient transmission of disease in temperate than in tropical climates. The reason for this is uncertain but may be due to temperature rather than urbanization. Varicella occurs most commonly during the late winter and spring months, the peak being about in March. Sporadic cases occur into the early summer and start in late fall.

Varicella is more common than other childhood diseases during the early months of life. In this situation the disease is generally mild. Maternal antibody transferred across the placenta may not be as effective in protecting infants against this disease as are antibodies against other viruses. However, nursery outbreaks have been rare. Children who develop varicella during the early months of life or are exposed in utero have a greater risk of developing herpes zoster in childhood.

PATHOGENESIS. Replication of virus is believed to occur initially in the epithelial cells of the mucosa of the upper respiratory tract. Because VZV produces a disseminated rash, one can assume that blood stream distribution must have occurred. Virus can be isolated from white blood cells from 5 days before to 2 days after the appearance of rash. After clinical recovery, the virus infection continues in the absence of clinical symptoms in a latent phase. During this time, DNA and some species of messenger RNA (mRNA) can be demonstrated in neurons in dorsal root ganglia. The segmental distribution of herpes zoster (see Chapter 477.3), which usually occurs decades after the initial VZV infection, is consistent with a dorsal root ganglion site for the latent virus. In uncomplicated chickenpox, rises in serum aminotransferase levels have been demonstrated. This suggests that there is visceral involvement in the normal course of this disease.

The vesicular lesions of varicella contain a predominance of polymorphonuclear leukocytes even during the early phase of vesicle formation. Multinuclear giant cells are occasionally found in the base of the lesions, often containing eosinophilic intranuclear inclusions. Large amounts of virus can be demonstrated in vesicular fluid by electron microscopy and virus can be isolated.

Postmortem descriptions of patients with varicella have usually involved immunocompromised subjects. In these cases, inflammatory changes are usually found in multiple organs, including the lung, liver, spleen, and skin, together with anoxic changes in the brain. Similar involvement is found in the newborn. Focal areas of necrosis and intranuclear eosinophilic inclusions in mononuclear cells are common. Changes in otherwise normal individuals usually include myocardial and pulmonary lesions. On microscopic examination, the brain has demonstrated edema with some lymphocyte cuffing around the cerebral vessels.

CLINICAL MANIFESTATIONS. Varicella is characterized by a generalized eruption that is centripetal in distribution; erythematous macules, papules, vesicles, and scabbed lesions may be present at the same time. The vesicles are superficial, with varying amounts of erythema at their bases. Adults tend to have considerably more erythema than children. During the early phase of the eruption, lesions are found on the face, scalp, and trunk. Often lesions can be detected in the scalp before their appearance on the skin by running the fingers through the hair. Later, new lesions appear on the extremities. By this time, the earlier lesions have dried and crusted. Excoriations are common, attesting to the pruritic nature of the lesions. Mucous membranes of the conjunctiva and oropharynx are more frequently involved in adults than in children. New lesions continue to appear over a 3- or 4-day period, after which the rate of their appearance decelerates markedly.

There is a striking variation in the extent of systemic symptoms associated with varicella. Most children have a mild illness with few systemic complaints and an average maximal temperature of about 38.3° C. It is more common for adults to have considerable malaise, muscle ache, arthralgia, and headache. These may precede the first skin lesions by 24 to 48 hours.

In the immunocompromised subject, the disease often is very severe. Approximately 30% of children with leukemia or lymphoma who get varicella and receive no prophylaxis or treatment develop "progressive varicella." Vesicles continue to erupt into the second week of illness, accompanied by high fever. Lesions tend to be deep seated rather than superficial. Toward the end of the first week and the beginning of the second week, the lesions are more common on the extremities than on the trunk. Indeed, the distribution and appearance may resemble those with smallpox. Visceral involvement occurs in about 30% of these patients. The lung, liver, pancreas, and brain may be involved. Death occurs in about 9% of immunocompromised patients who develop varicella. The death usually is due to pulmonary involvement. Patients with human immunodeficiency virus infections may have recurrent attacks of varicella in the absence of exposure or a persistent eruption that may continue for months, this latter usually in severely immunocompromised patients.

Varicella in pregnant women is believed to be more serious than in non-gravid females; fatalities have been reported. The rate of fetal wastage is not increased. About 1% of infants born to mothers who have had varicella early in pregnancy, however, have been found at birth to have "varicella embryopathy." The infants are born with cerebral damage and a variety of ocular findings, and characteristically they have a scarred, atrophic limb. The children are generally small for gestational age and may have other abnormalities as well. When mothers develop chickenpox within a few days of delivery, "varicella of the newborn" may occur. If the onset of varicella is between 5 and 10 days after birth, it is associated with a higher risk of serious disease and even death.

Bacterial infections of the skin are the most common complication of chickenpox in childhood. The frequency of invasive streptococcal superinfection has increased in recent years. The rate of complications is much higher in adults than in children. Although fewer than 2% of the reported cases occur after the second decade, almost 35% of the deaths occur in this group. A disproportionate rate of hospitalization also is found in adults. The major complications of varicella in adults are encephalitis and pneumonia.

Approximately 1 in 400 adults with chickenpox are hospitalized for pneumonia. In a prospective study, however, it was found that only 6% of young adults with chickenpox had respiratory symptoms, whereas 16% had roentgenographic evidence of pulmonary involvement.

Infection produces a diffuse interstitial type of pneumonia with hypoxia resulting from poor diffusion of gases. Diffuse calcification of the lung parenchyma may be found years after recovery.

Encephalitis in childhood is most commonly manifested by a cerebellitis, which usually occurs at the end of the first week or during the second week after onset of rash. This complication is almost always self-limited. In contrast, an acute form of encephalitis usually occurring soon after the onset of rash often has a fulminating course: it is characterized by severe brain swelling. When Reye's syndrome was prevalent, as many as 20% of cases were preceded by chickenpox. A variety of other neurologic complications, including optic neuritis, transverse myelitis, and Guillain-Barré syndrome, may be associated with chickenpox. Hemorrhagic complications of chickenpox include thrombocytopenic purpura and purpura fulminans. Nephritis, myocarditis, hepatitis and arthritis also have been described.

DIAGNOSIS. There is usually little difficulty in recognizing typical forms of chickenpox, particularly if there has been a history of exposure. The diagnosis may be more difficult in immunocompromised hosts, because they may have features of progressive varicella with visceral involvement. Modified cases of chickenpox may occur after passive or active immunization. These cases may require laboratory confirmation. The most common sources of confusion are insect bites, generalized herpes in the immunocompromised host, rickettsialpox, or "hand, foot, and mouth disease" caused by an enterovirus. The differentiation of disseminated herpes zoster from chickenpox may be difficult. The former usually has dermatomal involvement initially. Generalization usually does not occur until 3 to 5 days after onset of the zosteriform rash. In severely immunocompromised patients (e.g., bone marrow recipients), generalization may occur earlier and the clinical differentiation may be difficult.

Fluorescence microscopy is a rapid and accurate method of confirming the diagnosis from vesicular scrapings. Virus can usually be isolated during the first 3 or 4 days of lesions. The virus is quite labile; it must be stored at −70° C if cultures cannot be inoculated immediately. My preference is to collect vesicular fluid in unheparinized capillary tubes and put the specimen directly into human embryonic lung fibroblasts at the bedside. Specimens from throat, urine, or stool are of little value for isolation of virus. Polymerase chain reaction can be used to demonstrate the presence of virus in vesicular fluid and throat swabs.

Serologic confirmation of diagnosis can be made using a variety of techniques. The enzyme-linked immunosorbent assay (ELISA) or, the latex agglutination assay are the most generally available. The laboratory director should be consulted regarding appropriate time of collection of specimens as well as interpretation of data.

Determining the immune status of contacts can be done with the ELISA or latex agglutination test. Because complement-fixing antibody is lost rapidly after infection, it cannot be used for determining susceptibility. Fluorescence antibody testing using fixed cells sometimes yields false-positive results. A number of laboratories have developed tests for VZV immunoglobulin M (IgM). It was hoped that these might differentiate varicella from herpes zoster in cases in which this was unclear. Unfortunately, these tests have not been very useful, because VZV IgM is present in the sera of many patients with acute herpes zoster.

TREATMENT. Major therapeutic objectives are the prevention of superinfection and relief of pruritus. The latter can be accomplished frequently by application of calamine lotion. Occasionally this does not suffice, and a systemic antipruritic agent such as trimeprazine may be necessary. It is advisable to trim and file nails to reduce the damage from scratching. Bacterial superinfection can best be prevented by encouraging daily bathing with an antibacterial soap. Following this with a colloidal starch bath also may be useful for relieving pruritus.

Relief of systemic symptoms may require additional medication such as acetaminophen, although this may increase pruritus. Salicylates are contraindicated, since there is an association between their use and development of Reye's syndrome in children. Special care should be taken to be certain that over-the-counter medications containing salicylates are avoided. Necrotizing fasciitis due to group A *Streptococcus* has been associated with the use of ibuprofen.

Some patients, particularly those who are immunocompromised, may require antiviral therapy. Intravenous acyclovir has been shown to be effective in immunocompromised children with varicella. A dose of 500 mg/m² repeated every 8 hours has been used. VZV is generally less sensitive to acyclovir than herpes simplex. For this reason, larger doses are probably required. Studies on the use of oral acyclovir in the treatment of varicella have demonstrated some efficacy. Newer drugs (e.g., valacyclovir and famciclovir) have been effective in treating zoster with less-frequent dosing. Patients who are sick enough to require antiviral therapy probably should be treated with parenteral rather than oral medication.

Patients on high doses of corticosteroids or other immunosuppressive drugs who have been exposed to chickenpox are at high risk of developing progressive varicella. Corticosteroids appear to be most deleterious when given during the incubation period. They have been used in the treatment of pneumonia after the eruption has occurred without any obvious deleterious effects.

PREVENTION. Live attenuated varicella vaccine is recommended for all children aged 1 through 12 years and for certain adults. A single dose is recommended for children and two doses at least 2 months apart are given to adults. Most adults, including those with a positive history, are immune to varicella. Immunization of child care or institution workers, those traveling abroad, the military, and postpartum women is highly desirable. Immunization during pregnancy should be avoided but if it occurs it should be reported by calling 1-800-986-8999. Immunity of health care workers should be ensured.

The vaccine is quite safe and effective. Breakthrough cases generally are mild. Some vaccinees have developed a rash after immunization and may spread vaccine virus to contacts. Caution is advised when immunizing those who may come in contact with pregnant women or immunocompromised individuals. The latter should not be immunized.

Increased immunization of health care workers and increased use of the vaccine in the general population would be expected to decrease the risk of nosocomial infection. However, cases occurring after exposure to zoster will continue to be a problem. Some immunized staff may develop varicella and have the potential to infect others. Patients who develop varicella should have strict isolation precautions in a negative pressure room if possible. Those who are susceptible and cannot be discharged should be isolated from the 10th to the 20th day after exposure. Screening for susceptibility with the latex agglutination test may be useful in cohorting patients. This test is not as reliable for predicting protection of vaccinees. Some susceptible persons, especially those who are immunocompromised, should be passively immunized with varicella-zoster immune globulin (VZIG). Consideration should be given to administration of acyclovir orally from the seventh day after expo-

sure for 7 days. This was found to be effective in preventing disease in exposed children.

Immune serum globulin does not prevent varicella. Massive doses are required to produce measurable modification. If prevention or modification is indicated, VZIG should be given. Candidates are those who (1) are susceptible, (2) are at high risk of developing complicated varicella, and (3) have had a significant exposure to the disease. Any individuals fulfilling the first two criteria who have had a household exposure should receive prophylaxis. It is often difficult to judge the degree of intimacy in other types of exposure. Reference to guidelines published by the Academy of Pediatrics or Centers for Disease Control and Prevention may be helpful.

Patients considered at high risk are (1) those who are immunocompromised by virtue of either disease or immunosuppressive therapy, (2) infants born to mothers who have had varicella less than 5 days before or 2 days after delivery, (3) certain premature infants, (4) bone marrow transplant recipients regardless of susceptibility, and (5) certain adults.

A history of varicella is usually reliable in both adults and children. Children who have a negative history are usually susceptible. Serologic testing of adults who have a negative history is useful if it does not delay administration of VZIG. VZIG should be given as soon as possible after exposure and has not been shown to be effective if delayed more than 96 hours.

Brunell PA: Varicella in pregnancy, the fetus and the newborn: Problems in management. J Infect Dis 166:542, 1992. *A comprehensive review of varicella in pregnancy.*

Brunell PA: Varicella vaccine—where are we? Pediatrics 78:721, 1986. *A symposium on the epidemiology, cost burden, and complications of varicella and on varicella vaccine.*

Brunell PA: Varicella-zoster virus. *In* Rose NR, Friedman H, Fahey JL (eds): Manual of Clinical Laboratory Immunity, 4th ed. Washington, DC, American Society for Microbiology, 1992, pp 560–562. *A review of serologic tests for varicella-zoster antibody.*

First International Conference on Varicella. J Infect Dis 166(Suppl 1):SI, 1992. *A comprehensive review of basic and clinical information.*

Prevention of varicella: Recommendation of the Advisory Committee on Immunization Practice (ACIP). MMWR 45 (No. RR-11), 1996. *Everything you need to know about varicella vaccine.*

Srugo I, Israele V, Wittek, AE, et al: Clinical manifestations of varicella-zoster virus infections in human immunodeficiency virus-infected children. Am J Dis Child 147: 742, 1993. *A description of the various manifestations of VZV infection in HIV-infected children.*

Varicella-zoster infections. Report of the Committee on Infectious Diseases, 24th ed. Evanston, IL, American Academy of Pediatrics, 1997, pp 510–517. *A useful guide to management of patients exposed to varicella, including control of nosocomial infection.*

384 MUMPS

John W. Gnann, Jr.

Mumps is an acute systemic viral infection that occurs most commonly in children, is usually self-limited, and is clinically characterized by non-suppurative parotitis.

VIROLOGY. Mumps virus is a member of the Paramyxovirus family. Mumps virions are pleomorphic, roughly spherical, enveloped particles with an average diameter of 200 nm. Glycoprotein spikes project from the surface of the envelope, which encloses a helical nucleocapsid composed of nucleoproteins and linear, nonsegmented, single-stranded, negative-sense RNA. Humans are the only natural hosts for mumps virus, although infection can be induced experimentally in a variety of mammalian species. In vitro, mumps virus can be cultured in many mammalian cell lines and in embryonated hens' eggs.

EPIDEMIOLOGY. In unvaccinated urban populations, mumps is a disease of school-aged children (5 to 9 years), and more than 90% will have mumps antibodies by age 15 years. Before the mumps vaccine was released in the United States in 1967, mumps was an endemic disease with a seasonal peak of activity occurring between January and May. Mumps epidemics occurred at 2- to 5-year intervals. The largest number of cases reported in the United

States was in 1941, when the incidence of mumps was 250 cases per 100,000 population. In 1968, when the mumps vaccine was first entering clinical use, the incidence of mumps was 76 cases per 100,000 population. In 1985, only 2982 cases of mumps were reported, an incidence of 1.1 per 100,000 population, representing a 98% decline from the number of cases reported in 1967. Between 1985 and 1987, the incidence of mumps in the United States increased fivefold to 5.2 cases per 100,000 population. More than one third of the cases reported between 1985 and 1989 occurred in adolescents and young adults, reflecting the slow acceptance of universal mumps vaccination during the 1970s. Epidemiologic studies of mumps epidemics in high schools, colleges, and military units during the 1980s demonstrated that outbreaks were due principally to failure to vaccinate. Renewed emphasis on vaccination resulted in a further decline in the annual incidence of mumps. More recent studies have attributed smaller mumps outbreaks in the 1990s to primary vaccine failure and possibly to waning vaccine-induced immunity. In 1996, the Centers for Disease Control and Prevention reported only 751 cases of mumps in the United States, the lowest annual total ever recorded.

PATHOGENESIS. Mumps is highly contagious and can be transmitted experimentally by inoculation of virus onto the nasal or buccal mucosa, suggesting that most natural infections result from droplet spread of upper respiratory secretions. The average incubation period for mumps is 18 days. Primary viral replication takes place in epithelial cells of the upper respiratory tract, followed by spread of virus to regional lymph nodes and subsequent viremia and systemic dissemination. Virus can be isolated from saliva for 5 to 7 days before and up to 9 days after the onset of clinical symptoms, meaning that an infected individual is potentially able to transmit mumps for a period of about 2 weeks. An estimated 30% of mumps infections in children are subclinical or associated only with non-specific upper respiratory infection symptoms.

CLINICAL MANIFESTATIONS. PAROTITIS. Mumps usually begins with a short prodromal phase of low-grade fever, malaise, headache, and anorexia. Young children may complain initially of ear pain. Patients then develop the characteristic parotid tenderness and enlargement, which lifts the earlobe forward and obscures the angle of the mandible. The parotid glands are involved most commonly, although other salivary glands occasionally may be enlarged. Parotitis initially may be unilateral, with swelling of the contralateral parotid gland occurring 2 to 3 days later; bilateral parotitis eventually develops in 70% of patients with symptomatic salivary gland involvement. Painful parotid gland enlargement progresses over about 3 days, followed by defervescence and resolution of parotid pain and swelling within about 7 days. Long-term sequelae of mumps parotitis are uncommon.

ASEPTIC MENINGITIS. Symptomatic meningitis occurs in 15% of cases and is the second most common manifestation of mumps. About 50% of patients with mumps parotitis have cerebrospinal fluid (CSF) pleocytosis, although many have no signs or symptoms of meningitis. Signs and symptoms of meningeal irritation (headache, neck stiffness, vomiting, and lethargy) plus high fever usually develop 4 to 5 days after the onset of parotitis, although the meningitis may occasionally precede the parotitis. Indeed, 40 to 50% of all cases of documented mumps meningitis occur in patients who never develop clinical parotitis. For unexplained reasons, symptomatic central nervous system (CNS) involvement with mumps is two to three times more common in males than in females. Examination of the CSF usually reveals normal opening pressure and a mononuclear cell pleocytosis with an average cell count of 450/mm³. A polymorphonuclear leukocyte predominance may be seen in some patients early during the course of mumps meningitis. The CSF protein is usually normal or mildly elevated (<100 mg/dL). Hypoglycorrhachia, which is not usually seen in viral meningitis, may be present in 10 to 30% of patients with mumps meningitis. Mumps virus can be recovered from CSF. Whereas the symptoms of mumps meningitis usually resolve within 7 to 10 days, the CSF abnormalities may persist for up to 5 weeks. Mumps meningitis is usually benign, and significant neurologic complications are rare.

ENCEPHALITIS. The spectrum of mumps-induced CNS disease ranges from mild "aseptic" meningitis (which is common) to severe encephalitis (which is rare). Some cases of encephalitis develop concurrently with the parotitis and are thought to result from direct extension of viral infection from the choroid plexus ependyma into parenchymal neurons. Other cases of mumps encephalitis occur 1 to 2 weeks after the onset of parotitis and may represent a demyelinating postinfectious encephalitis. Clinical findings in mumps encephalitis include obtundation (and less commonly delirium), generalized seizures, and high fever. Other neurologic findings can include focal seizures, aphasia, paresis, and involuntary movements. Recovery from mumps encephalitis is usually complete, although complications such as aqueductal stenosis with hydrocephalus, seizure disorders, and psychomotor retardation have been reported. The overall mortality from mumps encephalitis is 0.5 to 2.3%.

ORCHITIS. Epididymo-orchitis is rare in boys with mumps but occurs in 15 to 35% of postpubertal men with mumps. Orchitis is most often unilateral (bilateral involvement occurs in 17 to 38% of cases) and results from replication of mumps virus in seminiferous tubules with resulting lymphocytic infiltration and edema. Orchitis typically develops within 1 week of the onset of parotitis, although orchitis (like mumps meningitis) can develop before or even in the absence of parotitis. Mumps orchitis is characterized by marked testicular swelling and severe pain, accompanied by fever, nausea, and headache. The pain and swelling resolve within 5 to 7 days, although residual testicular tenderness can persist for weeks. Testicular atrophy may follow orchitis in 35 to 50% of cases, but sterility is an uncommon complication even among men with bilateral orchitis.

OTHER MANIFESTATIONS. Mumps can cause inflammation of other glandular tissues, including pancreatitis and thyroiditis. Oophoritis and mastitis have been reported in postpubertal women with mumps. Transient renal function abnormalities are common in mumps, and virus can be isolated readily from urine; significant renal damage is rare, however. Other infrequent manifestations of mumps include sensorineural deafness (either transient or permanent), arthritis, myocarditis, and thrombocytopenia. Maternal mumps infection during the first trimester of pregnancy results in an increased frequency of spontaneous abortions, but no clear association between congenital malformations and maternal mumps has been demonstrated.

IMMUNE RESPONSE. Transient IgM antibody responses are detected early in the course of mumps infection, followed by the appearance of IgG antibody and cytotoxic T lymphocytes. Mumps-specific IgG can be detected during the first week of acute infection, peaks at 3 to 4 weeks, and persists for decades. Lifelong immunity follows natural infection. Patients who report more than one episode of mumps probably had parotitis due to another cause.

A variety of serologic tests are available to determine susceptibility to mumps. The neutralizing antibody assay has been considered the "gold standard" test but is technically demanding. The hemagglutination inhibition assay is simple to perform but less specific due to cross-reactivity with other paramyxoviruses. Detection of complement-fixing antibodies against "V" (hemagglutinin-neuraminidase) and "S" (nucleocapsid) antigens previously has been the routine method for determining immune status but has been replaced by a sensitive and specific enzyme-linked immunosorbent assay. The mumps skin test is not a reliable indicator of immune status.

DIAGNOSIS. The diagnosis of mumps is usually made on the basis of clinical findings in a child who presents with fever and parotitis, particularly if the individual is known to be susceptible and has been exposed to mumps during the preceding 2 to 3 weeks. However, an atypical clinical presentation (e.g., meningitis or orchitis without parotitis) will require laboratory confirmation. Culturing for mumps virus is definitive but not universally available. Testing of acute and convalescent sera should demonstrate a diagnostic fourfold rise in mumps antibody titer. Alternatively, finding mumps IgM antibody provides good evidence of recent infection. About 30% of patients will have an elevated serum amylase level that may be due to parotitis or pancreatitis.

The differential diagnosis of parotitis includes infections caused by other viruses such as influenza A, parainfluenza virus, coxsackievirus, lymphocytic choriomeningitis virus, or bacteria such as *Staphylococcus aureus*. Parotid gland enlargement also can be associated with Sjögren's syndrome, sarcoidosis, amyloidosis, thiazide ingestion, iodine sensitivity, tumor, or salivary duct obstruction. A careful examination should distinguish parotitis from lymphadenopathy.

THERAPY. Management of the patient with mumps consists of conservative measures to provide symptomatic relief and to ensure adequate hydration and nutrition. Treatment of orchitis includes bed rest, scrotal support, analgesics, and ice packs. Patients with significant CNS involvement will require hospitalization for observation and supportive care. There is currently no established role for antiviral drugs, corticosteroids, or passive immunotherapy.

PREVENTION. The cornerstone of mumps prevention is active immunization using the live attenuated mumps vaccine. In the United States, mumps vaccine is administered in combination with the measles and rubella vaccines (MMR) to children at age 12 to 15 months and produces protective antibody levels in more than 95% of recipients. A second dose of MMR is recommended for children at age 4 to 6 years. The mumps vaccine is also indicated for susceptible adults.

The "Jeryl-Lynn" strain of attenuated mumps virus used in the United States since 1967 is a very well-tolerated vaccine, although rare instances of fever, parotitis, and possibly aseptic meningitis have been reported after immunization. In 1988 and 1989, however, an increased frequency of cases of vaccine-related mumps meningitis was recognized in Canada and Japan. These cases occurred after administration of an MMR vaccine that contained the Urabe AM-9 mumps virus, and in several cases, the vaccine virus was isolated from CSF and positively identified by nucleotide sequencing. This problem has not been recognized in the United States, where the Jeryl-Lynn mumps vaccine continues to be used.

Questions regarding prevention often arise when an individual with no history of mumps (typically an adult male) is exposed to a patient with active mumps. The immune status of the exposed individual can be determined by serologic testing, although this may involve some delay. The vast majority of adults born in the United States before 1957 have been naturally infected and are therefore immune. Mumps vaccine can be safely administered to an individual of unknown immune status, although vaccine given to a susceptible individual after exposure to mumps may not provide protection.

Centers for Disease Control and Prevention: Measles, mumps, and rubella—vaccine use and strategies for measles, rubella, and congenital rubella syndrome elimination and mumps control: Recommendations of the Advisory Committee for Immunization Practices (ACIP). MMWR 47(RR-08):1, 1998. *Current recommendations for mumps vaccination.*

Centers for Disease Control and Prevention: Mumps surveillance—United States, 1988–1993. MMWR 44(SS-3):1, 1995. *Epidemiology of mumps in the United States over the past decade.*

THE HERPES GROUP OF VIRUSES

385 HERPES SIMPLEX VIRUS INFECTIONS

Richard J. Whitley

Herpes simplex virus (HSV), a member of the family Herpesviridae, has been implicated in human infections since descriptions of cutaneous spreading lesions in ancient Greek times. Scholars of Greek civilization define the word *herpes* to mean "to creep or crawl," in reference to the spreading nature of the observed skin lesions. More recently, infection has been defined by the spectrum of illnesses caused by HSV. In 1968, well-defined antigenic and biologic differences were demonstrated between herpes simplex virus type 1 (HSV-1) and herpes simplex virus type 2 (HSV-2). HSV-1 was more frequently associated with non-genital infection and HSV-2 with genital disease. Further study has revealed that, of all the herpesviruses, HSV-1 and HSV-2 are the most closely related, with approximately 60% genomic homology. These two viruses can be distinguished most reliably by DNA restriction enzyme analyses; however, differences in antigen expression and biologic properties also serve as methods for differentiation.

STRUCTURE. Membership in the family Herpesviridae is based on the structure of the virion (Fig. 385–1). HSV contains double-stranded DNA at the central core, has a molecular weight of approximately 100 million, and encodes at least 80 polypeptides. The DNA core is surrounded by a capsid that consists of 162 capsomers, arranged in icosapentahedral symmetry. The capsid is 100 to 110 nm in diameter. Tightly adherent to the capsid is the tegument, consisting of amorphous material. Loosely surrounding the capsid

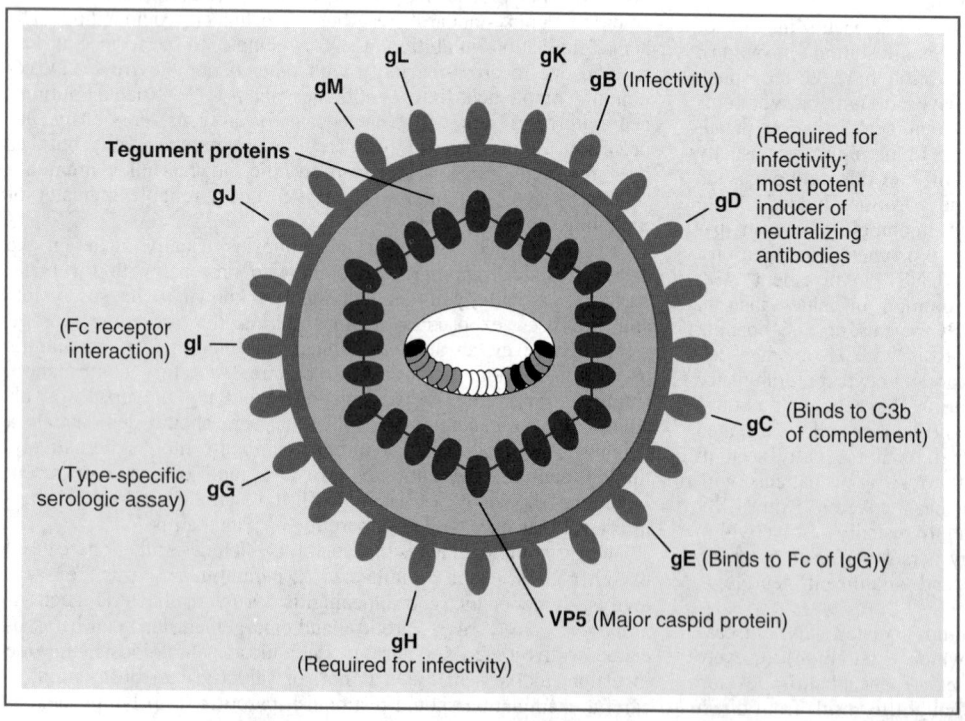

FIGURE 385–1 ■ Schematic diagram of the HSV virion.

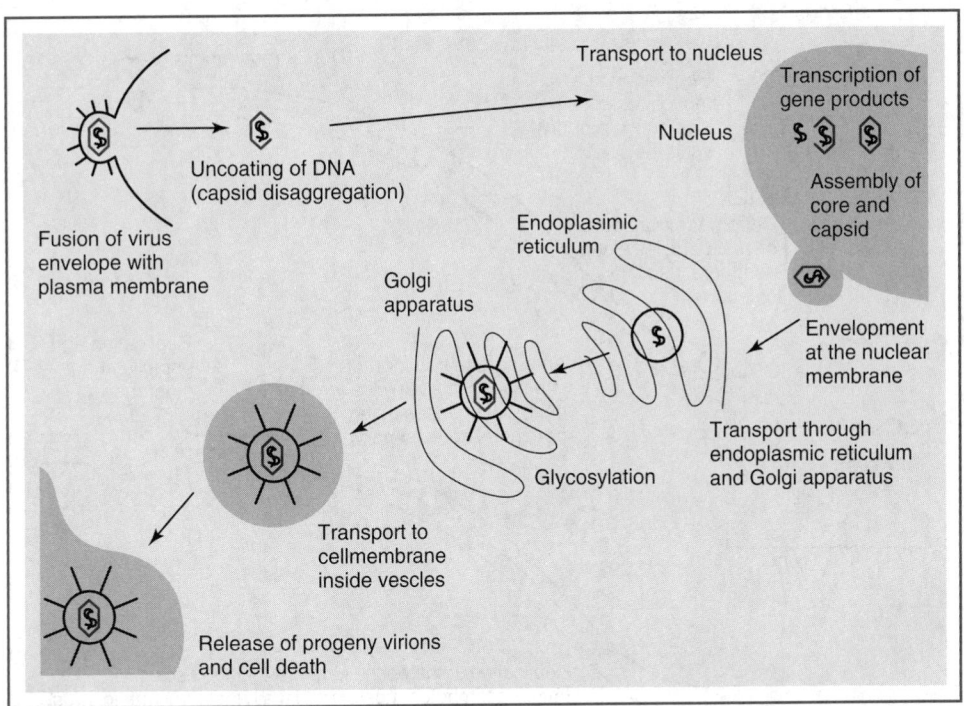

Transport to nucleus

Transcription of gene products

Nucleus

$ $ $

Uncoating of DNA (capsid disaggregation)

Assembly of core and capsid

Endoplasimic reticulum

Fusion of virus envelope with plasma membrane

Golgi apparatus

Envelopment at the nuclear membrane

Glycosylation

Transport through endoplasmic reticulum and Golgi apparatus

Transport to cellmembrane inside vescles

Release of progeny virions and cell death

FIGURE 385–2 ■ Schematic diagram of HSV replication.

and tegument is a lipid bilayer envelope derived from host cell membranes. The envelope consists of polyamines, lipids, and glycoproteins. These glycoproteins confer distinctive properties to the virus and provide unique antigens to which the host is capable of responding. Notably, glycoprotein G (gG) provides antigenic specificity to HSV and therefore results in an antibody response that allows for the distinction between HSV-1 (gG-1) and HSV-2 (gG-2).

A unique feature of HSV DNA is its genomic sequence arrangement. The genome consists of two components, L (long) and S (short), each of which contains unique sequences that can invert on themselves, leading to four isomers. Viral DNA extracted from virions of infected cells consists of four equimolar populations, differing only with respect to the relative orientation of the two unique components. Biologic relevance of this phenomenon is unknown.

REPLICATION. Replication of HSV is a multistep process (Fig. 385–2). After the onset of infection, DNA is uncoated and transported to the nucleus of the host cell. This is followed by transcription of immediate-early genes, which encode for the regulatory proteins, and is followed by the expression of proteins encoded by early and then late genes. These proteins include enzymes necessary for viral replication and structural proteins.

Assembly of the viral core and capsid takes place within the nucleus. Envelopment at the nuclear membrane and transport out of the nucleus occur through the endoplasmic reticulum and the Golgi apparatus. Glycosylation of the viral membrane occurs in the Golgi. Mature virions are transported to the outer membrane of the host cell inside vesicles. Release of progeny virus is accompanied by cell death. Replication for all herpesviruses is considered inefficient, with a high ratio of non-infectious to infectious viral particles.

PATHOGENESIS AND LATENCY. A critical factor for transmission of HSV, regardless of virus type, is intimate contact between a person who is shedding virus and a susceptible host. With inoculation onto the skin or mucous membrane, HSV replicates in epithelial cells; the incubation period is 4 to 6 days (Fig. 385–3). As replication continues, cell lysis and local inflammation ensue, resulting in characteristic vesicles on an erythematous base. Regional lymphatics and lymph nodes become involved with the draining of infected secretions from the area of viral replication. Viremia and visceral dissemination may develop depending on the immunologic competence of the host. In all hosts, the virus generally ascends peripheral sensory nerves to reach the dorsal root ganglia. Replica-

tion of HSV within neural tissue is followed by spread of the virus to other mucosal and skin surfaces by means of the peripheral sensory nerves. Virus replicates further in epithelial cells, reproducing the lesions of the initial infection, until infection is contained through host immunity.

The histopathologic changes induced by HSV replication are similar for both primary and recurrent infection. Changes induced by viral infection include ballooning of infected cells and the appearance of condensed chromatin within the nuclei of cells, followed by subsequent degeneration of the cellular nuclei. Cells lose intact plasma membranes and form multinucleated giant cells. They also may demonstrate the intranuclear inclusion bodies known as Cowdry type A bodies, which are suggestive but not diagnostic of HSV infection. With cell lysis, a clear vesicular fluid containing large quantities of virus forms between the epidermis and dermal layer. The dermis reveals an intense inflammatory response, more so with primary infection than with recurrent disease. As healing progresses, the clear vesicular fluid becomes pustular with the recruitment of inflammatory cells. The pustule then forms a scab, with scarring being uncommon.

The vascular changes in the area of infection include perivascular cuffing and hemorrhagic necrosis. These changes are particularly prominent when organs other than skin are involved, as is the case with herpes simplex encephalitis or disseminated neonatal HSV infection. Local lymphatics can show evidence of infection with intrusion of inflammatory cells due to the draining of infected secretions from the area of viral replication. As host defenses are mounted, an influx of mononuclear cells can be detected in infected tissue.

A unique characteristic of the herpesviruses is their ability to establish latent infection, persist in an apparently inactive state for varying amounts of time, and then be reactivated (Fig. 385–4). The latent viral genome may be either extrachromosomal or integrated into host-cell DNA.

Latency is established when HSV reaches the dorsal root ganglia after retrograde transmission through sensory nerve pathways. Latent virus may be reactivated and enter a replicative cycle at any point in time. The reactivation of latent virus is a well-recognized biologic phenomenon but not one that is understood from a molecular standpoint. Stimuli that have been observed to be associated with the reactivation of latent HSV have included stress, menstruation, and exposure to ultraviolet light. Precisely how these factors interact at the level of the ganglia remains to be defined. Reactiva-

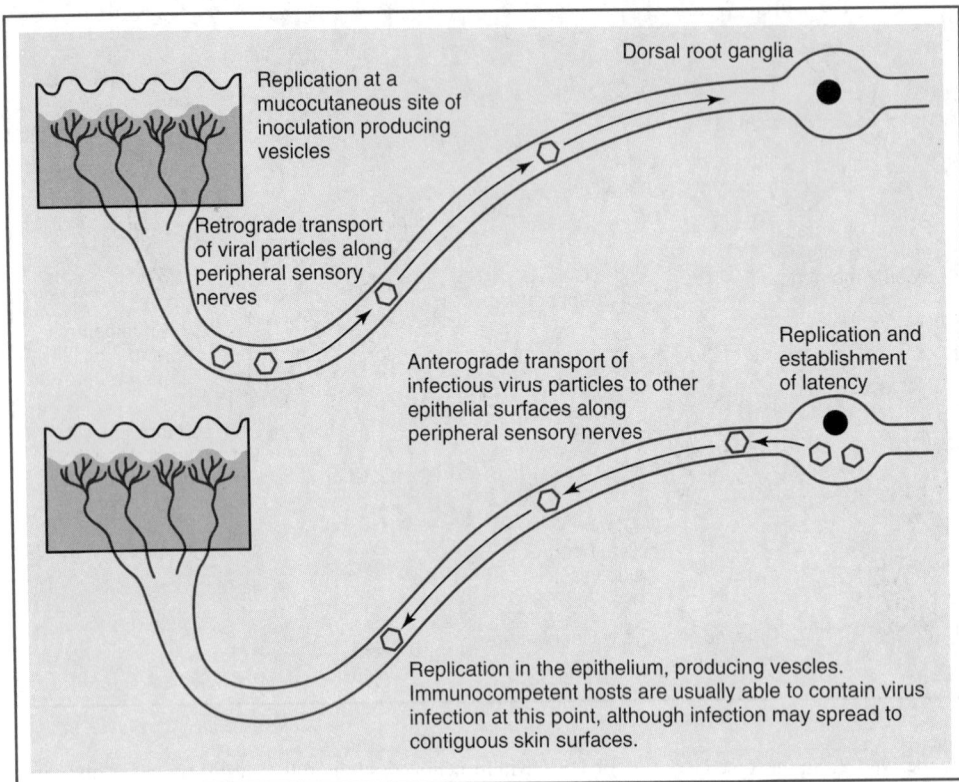

Dorsal root ganglia

Replication at a mucocutaneous site of inoculation producing vesicles

Retrograde transport of viral particles along peripheral sensory nerves

Anterograde transport of infectious virus particles to other epithelial surfaces along peripheral sensory nerves

Replication and establishment of latency

Replication in the epithelium, producing vescles. Immunocompetent hosts are usually able to contain virus infection at this point, although infection may spread to contiguous skin surfaces.

FIGURE 385–3 ■ Schematic diagram of primary HSV infection.

tion may be clinically asymptomatic, or it may produce life-threatening disease.

DIAGNOSIS. The definitive diagnosis of HSV infection requires isolation of virus. Swabs of clinical specimens or other body fluids can be inoculated into susceptible cell lines and observed for the development of characteristic cytopathic effects. This technique is very useful for the diagnosis of HSV-1 and HSV-2 infection because of the short replicative cycles.

In the absence of diagnostic virology facilities, cytologic examination of cells scraped from a clinical lesion may be useful in making a presumptive diagnosis of HSV infection. Material obtained from scraping the base of a lesion should be smeared on a glass slide and promptly fixed in cold ethanol. The slide can be stained according to the methods of Papanicolaou, Giemsa, or Wright. The presence of intranuclear inclusions and multinucleated giant cells is indicative, but not diagnostic, of HSV infection. This method has a sensitivity of only 60 to 70% and should not be the sole diagnostic method used.

Additional diagnostic techniques of clinical utility include in situ and dot-blot hybridization and DNA amplification by polymerase

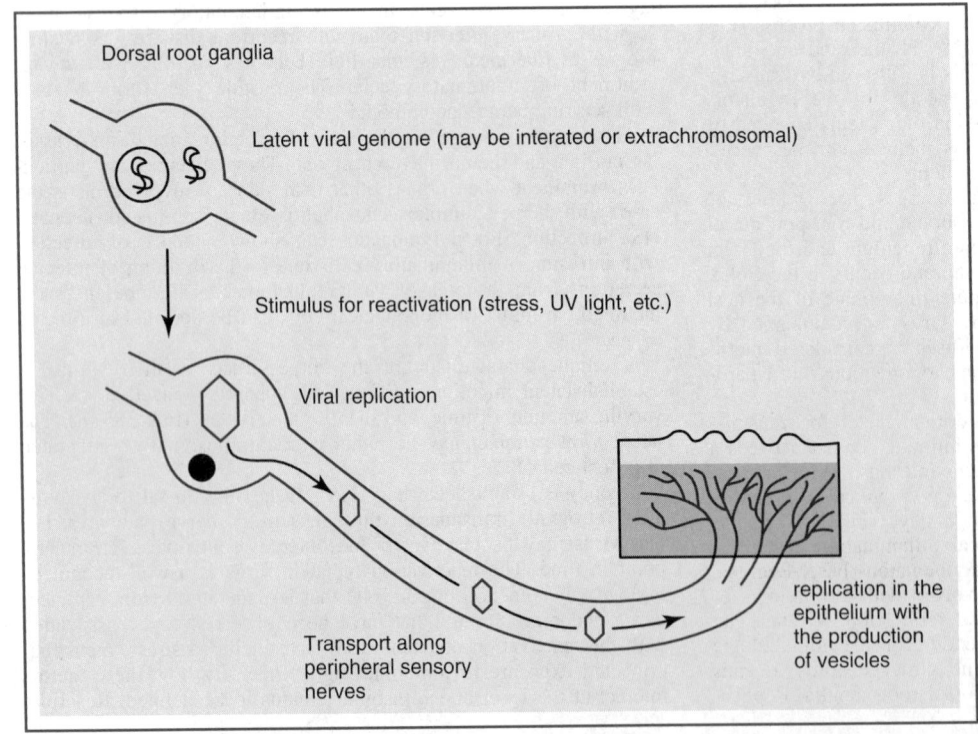

Dorsal root ganglia

Latent viral genome (may be interated or extrachromosomal)

Stimulus for reactivation (stress, UV light, etc.)

Viral replication

Transport along peripheral sensory nerves

replication in the epithelium with the production of vesicles

FIGURE 385–4 ■ Schematic diagram of HSV latency and reactivation.

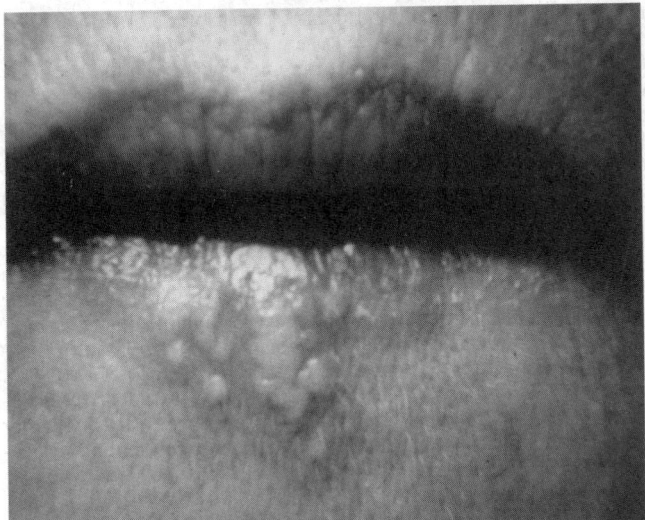

FIGURE 385-5 ■ Herpes simplex labialis.

chain reaction (PCR). DNA amplification is particularly useful in assessing cerebrospinal fluid (CSF) specimens for evidence of HSV infection.

In addition to new tests for virus gene products and viral DNA, improved serologic assays are also becoming available. However, these tests are useful only for making a diagnosis in retrospect.

CLINICAL MANIFESTATIONS. MUCOCUTANEOUS INFECTIONS. Gingivostomatitis. Gingivostomatitis (usually caused by HSV-1) occurs most frequently in children younger than age 5. Illness is characterized by fever, sore throat, pharyngeal edema, and erythema, followed by the development of vesicular or ulcerative lesions on the oral and pharyngeal mucosa. Recurrent HSV-1 infections of the oropharynx are most frequently manifest as herpes simplex labialis (cold sores) and usually appear on the vermilion border of the lip (Fig. 385-5). Intraoral lesions as a manifestation of recurrent disease are uncommon.

Genital Herpes. Genital herpes is most frequently caused by HSV-2. Primary infection in women usually involves the vulva, vagina, and cervix. In men, initial infection is most often associated with lesions on the glans penis, prepuce, or penile shaft. In individuals of either gender, primary disease is associated with fever, malaise, anorexia, and bilateral inguinal adenopathy. Women frequently have dysuria and urinary retention due to urethral involvement. As many as 10% of individuals develop an aseptic meningitis with primary infection. Sacral radiculomyelitis may occur in both men and women, resulting in neuralgias, urinary retention, or obstipation. The complete healing of primary infection may take several weeks. It has been recognized that the first episode of genital infection is less severe in individuals who have had previous HSV-1 infections at other sites. Antibodies to HSV-1 appear to ameliorate the expression of HSV-2 clinical disease.

Recurrent genital infections in either men or women can be particularly distressing. The frequency of recurrence varies significantly from one individual to another. Of note, viral DNA can be detected by PCR in genital secretions at a greater frequency than symptomatic recurrences. It has been estimated that one third have virtually no or few recurrences, one third have approximately three recurrences per year, and another third have more than three per year. Seroepidemiologic studies have found that between 25 and 65% of individuals in the United States in 1988 had antibodies to HSV-2 and that seroprevalence is correlated with the number of sexual partners.

Herpetic Keratitis. Herpes simplex keratitis is usually caused by HSV-1 and is accompanied by conjunctivitis in many cases. It is considered the most common infectious cause of blindness in the United States. The characteristic lesions of HSV keratoconjunctivitis are dendritic ulcers best detected by fluorescein staining. Deep stromal involvement also has been reported and may result in visual impairment.

Other Cutaneous Manifestations. HSV infections can occur at any skin site. Common among health care workers are lesions on

abraded skin or the fingers, known as herpetic whitlows. Similarly, wrestlers, because of physical contact, may develop disseminated cutaneous lesions known as herpes gladiatorum.

NEONATAL HERPES SIMPLEX VIRUS INFECTION. Neonatal HSV infection is estimated to occur in approximately 1 in 3500 deliveries in the United States each year. Approximately 70% of cases are caused by HSV-2 and usually result from contact of the fetus with infected maternal genital secretions at the time of delivery. Manifestations of neonatal HSV infection can be divided into three categories: (1) skin, eye, and mouth disease; (2) encephalitis; and (3) disseminated infection. As the name implies, skin, eye, and mouth disease consists of cutaneous lesions and does not involve other organ systems. Involvement of the central nervous system may occur with encephalitis or disseminated infection and generally results in a diffuse encephalitis. The CSF formula characteristically reveals an elevated protein and a mononuclear pleocytosis. Disseminated infection involves multiple organ systems and can produce disseminated intravascular coagulation, hemorrhagic pneumonitis, encephalitis, and cutaneous lesions. Diagnosis can be particularly difficult in the absence of skin lesions, which occurs in as many as 36% of cases. The mortality rate for each disease classification varies from zero for skin, eye, and mouth disease to 15% for encephalitis and 60% for neonates with disseminated infection, even with appropriate antiviral treatment. In addition to the high mortality associated with these infections, morbidity is significant in that children with encephalitis or disseminated disease develop normally in only 40% of cases, even with appropriate antiviral therapy.

HERPES SIMPLEX ENCEPHALITIS. Herpes simplex encephalitis is characterized by hemorrhagic necrosis of the temporal lobe. Disease begins unilaterally, spreads to the contralateral temporal lobe, and is characterized by hemorrhagic necrosis (Fig. 385-6). It is the most common cause of focal, sporadic encephalitis in the United States today and occurs in approximately 1 in 150,000 individuals. Most cases are caused by HSV-1. The actual pathogenesis of herpes simplex encephalitis requires further clarification, although it has been speculated that primary or recurrent virus can reach the temporal lobe by ascending neural pathways, such as the trigeminal tracts or the olfactory nerves.

Clinical manifestations of herpes simplex encephalitis include headache, fever, altered consciousness, and abnormalities of speech and behavior, findings characteristic of temporal lobe involvement. Focal seizures also may occur. The CSF formula for these patients is variable but usually consists of a pleocytosis with both polymorphonuclear leukocytes and monocytes present. The protein concentration is characteristically elevated, and glucose is usually normal. Diagnosis can be achieved by PCR evaluation of CSF in experi-

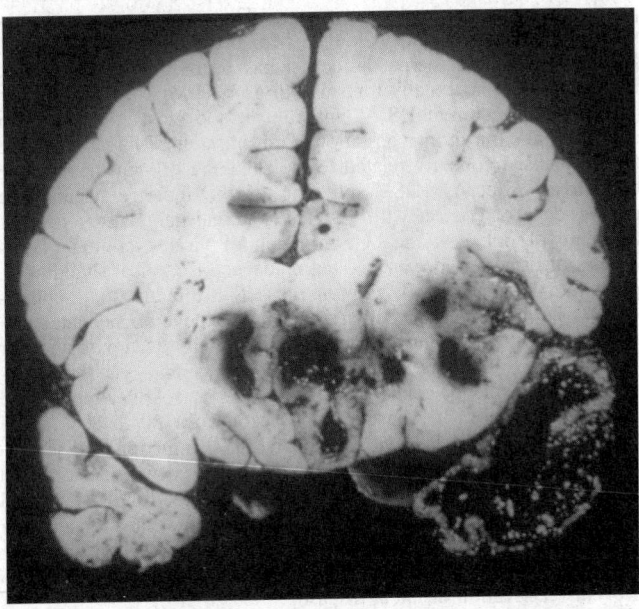

FIGURE 385-6 ■ Hemorrhagic necrosis in herpes simplex encephalitis.

enced laboratories. The mortality and morbidity are high, even with appropriate antiviral therapy. At present, the mortality rate is approximately 30% 1 year after treatment. In addition, approximately 50% of survivors have moderate or severe neurologic impairment.

HERPES SIMPLEX VIRUS INFECTIONS IN THE IMMUNOCOMPROMISED HOST. HSV infections in the immunocompromised host, including patients with the acquired immunodeficiency syndrome (AIDS), are usually due to reactivation of latent infection and are clinically more severe, may be progressive, and require a longer time to heal. Manifestations of HSV infections in this patient population include pneumonitis, esophagitis, hepatitis, colitis, and disseminated cutaneous disease. Individuals suffering from human immunodeficiency virus (HIV) infection may have extensive perineal or orofacial ulcerations. HSV infections are also noted to be of increased severity in individuals with extensive burns.

EPIDEMIOLOGY. HSV infections are distributed worldwide and have been reported in both developed and underdeveloped countries. Animal vectors for human HSV infections have not been described, and there is no seasonal variation in the incidence of HSV infections. The virus is transmitted from infected to susceptible individuals during close personal contact, and virus must come in contact with mucosal surfaces or abraded skin for infection to be initiated. Because approximately one third of the world's population has recurrent HSV infections, and because infection is rarely fatal, a large reservoir of HSV exists in the community.

Although HSV-1 and HSV-2 are usually transmitted by different routes and involve different areas of the body, there is a great deal of overlap between the epidemiology and clinical manifestations of infections caused by these viruses. The mouth and lips are clearly the most common sites of HSV-1 infection. Primary HSV-1 infection in the young child is usually asymptomatic but may be manifest as gingivostomatitis. Primary infection in young adults has been associated with pharyngitis and sometimes a mononucleosis-like syndrome. Seroprevalence studies have demonstrated that acquisition of HSV-1 infection is related to socioeconomic factors. Antibodies, which indicate past infection, are found early in life among individuals of lower socioeconomic groups. This presumably is a consequence of crowded living conditions that provide a greater opportunity for direct contact with infected individuals. As many as 75 to 90% of individuals from lower socioeconomic populations develop antibodies by the end of the first decade of life. In contrast, only 30 to 40% of persons in middle and upper socioeconomic groups are seropositive by the middle of the second decade of life.

Because infections with HSV-2 are usually acquired through sexual contact, antibodies to this virus are rarely found until the onset of sexual activity. There is a progressive increase in infection rates with HSV-2 in all populations beginning in adolescence. As with HSV-1 infections, the rate of acquisition of HSV-2 infection appears related to socioeconomic factors. The number of sexual contacts is also an important risk factor for the acquisition of HSV-2. Importantly, genital herpes infection has been found to be a risk factor for another sexually transmitted virus, HIV.

Localized, recurrent HSV-2 infection is the most common form of HSV infection during gestation. Transmission of infection to the fetus is most frequently related to the shedding of virus at the time of delivery. Because HSV infection of the fetus is usually the consequence of contact with infected maternal genital secretions at the time of delivery, the determination of viral excretion at this time is of utmost importance. The incidence of cervical shedding in pregnant women with asymptomatic HSV infection is approximately 1%. Interestingly, most infants who develop neonatal disease are born to women who are completely asymptomatic for genital HSV infections at the time of delivery and who have neither a past history of genital herpes nor a sexual partner reporting a genital vesicular rash. These women account for 60 to 80% of all women whose children develop neonatal HSV infection.

PREVENTION. At present, there are no licensed vaccines directed against HSV. However, experimental vaccines for HSV-1 and HSV-2 are being evaluated. Acyclovir, valaciclovir, and famciclovir are being given to recipients of solid organ and bone marrow transplants in the immediate post-transplant period in an effort to prevent reactivation of latent disease.

TREATMENT. Infections caused by HSV-1 and HSV-2 are amenable to therapy with antiviral drugs (see Chapter 374). Both vidarabine and acyclovir have proved useful for managing specific infections caused by these viruses. At present, acyclovir is the treatment of choice for mucocutaneous HSV infections in the immunocompromised host, herpes simplex encephalitis, and neonatal HSV infections. Intravenous administration is preferred for therapy for life-threatening disease. Intravenous acyclovir is also recommended for clinically severe initial genital herpes in the immunocompetent host. This includes patients with complications such as urinary retention or aseptic meningitis, and they should receive 5 mg/kg every 8 hours for 5 to 7 days. Caution must be exercised when acyclovir is used intravenously because it may crystallize in the renal tubules when given too rapidly or to dehydrated patients.

Immunocompromised individuals with mucocutaneous HSV infections that are not life threatening may be given oral acyclovir. Oral acyclovir is also useful in treating initial genital herpes. Recurrent episodes, however, are not as responsive to acyclovir. For individuals who experience severe or frequent recurrences of genital herpes, a "suppressive" regimen of acyclovir in doses of 600 to 800 mg/day may be useful. The efficacy of acyclovir for primary or recurrent oropharyngeal HSV in the immunocompetent host has not been well established.

Brown ZA, Selke S, Zeh J, et al: The acquisition of herpes simplex virus during pregnancy. N Engl J Med 337:509–515, 1997.
Fleming DT, McQuillan GM, Johnson RE, et al: N Engl J Med 1105–1111.
Roizman B: Herpesviridae. In Fields BN, Knipe DM, Howley PM, et al (eds): Fields Virology, 3rd ed. Philadelphia, Lippincott-Raven, 1996, pp 2221–2230.
Roizman B: New viral footprints in Kaposi's sarcoma (editorial). N Engl J Med 332: 1227, 1995. *Discusses the discovery of human herpesvirus 8 by a novel technique and that the virus' footprints were found in cells affected by Kaposi's sarcoma.*
Straus SE: Clinical and biological differences between recurrent herpes simplex virus and varicella-zoster virus infections. JAMA 262:3455, 1989. *A concise article that emphasizes the distinctions between recurrent herpes simplex virus infections, and recurrent varicella-zoster infections.*
Wald A, Zeh J, Selke S, et al: Virologic characteristics of subclinical and symptomatic genital herpes infections. N Engl J Med 333:770–775, 1995.
Wald A, Zeh J, Barnum G, et al: Suppression of subclinical shedding of herpes simplex virus type 2 with acyclovir. Ann Intern Med 124:8–15, 1996.
Whitley RJ: Herpes simplex virus. In Fields BN, Knipe DM, Howley PM, et al (eds): Fields Virology, 3rd ed. Philadelphia, Lippincott-Raven, 1996, pp 2297–2342.
Whitley RJ, Kimberlin DW, Roizman B: Herpes simplex viruses. Clin Infect Dis 26: 541–553, 1998.

386 INFECTIONS ASSOCIATED WITH HUMAN CYTOMEGALOVIRUS

William J. Britt

Human cytomegalovirus (HCMV) is the largest and most structurally complex human herpesvirus. Its linear double-stranded DNA genome consists of 250,000 base pairs that can potentially encode over 200 different proteins. Two different types of infections have been defined: primary and recurrent. Recurrent infection may follow reactivation of previous infection or reinfection by a superinfecting viral strain. Host immunity is thought to be protective, because clinical evidence of infection rarely develops in the immunocompetent host. Abnormalities in immune responses caused by immunosuppressive drugs after allotransplantation, retroviral infections in patients with human immunodeficiency virus (HIV), or developmental immune dysfunction in the fetus predispose these unique populations to HCMV-induced disease.

EPIDEMIOLOGY. HCMV circulates within the population, and there is no evidence of epidemics or seasonal dependence. In most underdeveloped countries, HCMV is acquired early in childhood, likely as a result of either breast feeding or secondary to crowded living conditions. Seropositivity reaches nearly 100% in these populations before childbearing age. In contrast, the seroprevalence in the United States is dependent on age and socioeconomic status. By childbearing age, the seroprevalence often exceeds 90% in lower socioeconomic groups. In individuals in higher socioeconomic groups, approximately 50% are seropositive by early adulthood.

Several routes of virus transmission have been documented, including transmission after sexual contact. Previous studies have documented large amounts of virus within semen and cervical secretions. Epidemiologic studies have demonstrated a correlation between a history of sexually transmitted disease with HCMV seropositivity. Transmission from young children represents another important source of HCMV infection. Careful epidemiologic studies within child care centers demonstrated virus transmission between young children, as well as transmission to adult caretakers and susceptible parents. The importance of children as a major source of virus can be appreciated if one considers that approximately 1% of all infants are born with HCMV infection (congenital) and that 30 to 70% of breast-fed infants of seropositive mothers will become infected. Because these infants often excrete large amounts of virus in their saliva and urine for months to years after infection, they provide an important reservoir of infectious HCMV.

Major sources of virus exposure among hospitalized patients include blood products and transplanted organs. Transfusion-acquired HCMV infection, before routine serologic screening of donor blood products, occurred at a consistent rate of approximately 2.5% per unit of whole blood. Numerous studies have demonstrated that leukocytes present within various blood products were responsible for the majority of transfusion-acquired HCMV infections. Measures that reduce leukocyte contamination within blood products or, alternatively, screening blood donors and matching HCMV serologic status of donor and recipient have reduced the incidence of transfusion-associated HCMV infection. Nosocomial transmission of HCMV to health workers is uncommon, even in personnel caring for patients excreting large amounts of HCMV, such as congenitally infected infants.

PATHOLOGY. Although HCMV can be consistently propagated in vitro only in human fibroblast cells, it can be isolated from a myriad of organs and cell types from infected humans. HCMV has been demonstrated in the endothelium of the vasculature, epithelium of almost every organ (including endocrine and exocrine organs), and neuronal cells of the central nervous system (CNS). Pathologic findings range from extensive tissue destruction to isolated cytomegalic cells. The histologic appearance of the typical cytomegalic cell consists of an enlarged cell with scant to reduced cytoplasm containing a large nucleus with prominent nucleoli and intranuclear inclusions.

PATHOGENESIS. Cellular-, antibody-, and cytokine-mediated immune responses have been proposed to limit HCMV infection in vivo, although in most cases direct evidence is lacking. A number of studies in bone marrow and solid organ allograft recipients have provided a strong correlation between the depression of HCMV-specific T-lymphocyte responses and susceptibility to HCMV-associated infection and, more importantly, clinical disease. These responses have included both major histocompatibility (MHC) class II–restricted CD4+ T lymphocytes and class I–restricted CD8+ cytotoxic T lymphocytes. Findings from several laboratories have suggested that a limited number of virion structural proteins (pp65 and pp150) are major targets of protective cellular immune responses. Several studies have documented that passively transferred antiviral antibodies failed to prevent HCMV infection in susceptible patients but modulated clinical disease associated with HCMV infection. The importance of natural killer cell responses and cytokines to the course of HCMV infection is unknown.

As yet, poorly defined non-lytic effects of the virus may contribute to disease syndromes associated with HCMV infection. Clinical syndromes of bacterial and fungal infections after HCMV infection in allograft recipients are consistent with an immunomodulatory activity of the virus; however, specific mechanisms accounting for this immunosuppressive activity of HCMV remain inadequately defined.

CLINICAL ASPECTS OF HCMV INFECTION. Although infection in the immunocompetent host rarely results in clinically apparent disease, infrequently, normal hosts will exhibit a mononucleosis-like syndrome. Approximately 8% of cases of infectious mononucleosis may be caused by HCMV. Clinically, this infection is indistinguishable from mononucleosis caused by Epstein-Barr virus, with the exception that it is heterophile negative. Non-specific constitutional symptoms predominate, including malaise, decreased appetite, and low-grade fever. Laboratory abnormalities include atypical lymphocytosis, chemical hepatitis and cholestasis and, less frequently, thrombocytopenia. Similar but often exaggerated findings have been associated with transfusion-acquired HCMV, including the previously described postperfusion syndrome that followed cardiopulmonary bypass.

Congenital HCMV infection (present at birth) is common, occurring in approximately 1% of all live births in the United States. Some 10% of these will suffer signs and symptoms of cytomegalic inclusion disease, which include petechiae, hepatosplenomegaly, jaundice, and microcephaly. Thrombocytopenia, cholestasis, and evidence of hepatocellular damage are consistent laboratory findings. Although almost all end-organ disease is self-limited, CNS damage associated with congenital HCMV infection is permanent and can result in significant developmental delays, seizure activity, gross neurologic impairment, and, most frequently, hearing loss. Subclinical congenital HCMV infection is less commonly associated with permanent CNS sequelae; however, between 8 and 15% of infants with subclinical infection may exhibit evidence of CNS damage, such as sensorineural hearing loss. Both forms of congenital HCMV infection result in chronic virus excretion, which may persist for years, thus providing an important source of HCMV exposure in the community.

HCMV infection after allograft transplantation is the most common infection in the post-transplant period. An estimated 50 to 100% of seropositive renal transplant recipients will excrete HCMV after transplantation. Although the vast majority of patients will not exhibit evidence of invasive HCMV infection, HCMV is a major cause of disease in heart, heart-lung, liver, and bone marrow transplant recipients. In the latter setting, HCMV pneumonia has been the leading infection-related cause of death, with mortality rates approaching 50 to 60%. Sources of HCMV infection in the allograft recipient include (1) reactivated infection in the HCMV-seropositive recipient, (2) exogenous blood products given in the post-transplant period, and (3) most commonly, from the transplanted organ obtained from an HCMV-seropositive donor. The highest risk for infection and disease is observed in the HCMV-seronegative recipient of an allograft from a HCMV-seropositive allograft donor (see Chapter 314). Other factors associated with clinically significant HCMV infections in solid organ allograft recipients include the use of cadaveric grafts, leukocyte-containing blood products, and immunosuppressive agents that deplete T lymphocytes such as antithymocyte globulin or anti-CD8 monoclonal antibodies. Very recent reports have indicated that the HCMV viral burden in transplant recipients is most predictive of invasive disease, irrespective of donor-recipient status. In bone marrow allograft recipients, the severity of HCMV infection often parallels the development of graft-versus-host disease.

Clinical evidence of HCMV infection usually develops 4 to 6 weeks after transplantation and can present as a variety of end-organ diseases such as pneumonitis or hepatitis and more commonly as a syndrome similar to HCMV mononucleosis, which can include fever, leukopenia, thrombocytopenia, and hepatitis. Virus can be isolated from the urine in almost all infected patients and from the blood in a subset of patients. This latter finding may presage the development of invasive multiorgan disease. Potentially fatal invasive infections include pneumonitis, severe gastrointestinal ulcerative disease with perforation, and life-threatening hepatitis. HCMV pneumonitis most commonly presents insidiously as a diffuse interstitial pneumonia that progresses in the absence of specific therapy. Acute allograft loss may accompany HCMV disease either as a direct result of graft involvement, as seen in hepatic transplants, or secondary to the reduction in immunosuppression that may be necessary during treatment of invasive HCMV disease. Long-term allograft survival also appears to be reduced as a result of HCMV infection. In cardiac allografts this has been proposed to result from virus-associated acceleration of coronary artery atherosclerosis of the allograft, whereas in hepatic allografts it has been suggested that HCMV causes increased expression of MHC antigens resulting in enhanced immunologic recognition of the graft.

HCMV has been a major cause of morbidity and mortality in patients with acquired immunodeficiency syndrome (AIDS) (see Part XXIII). Because of the importance of sexual transmission in the spread of HCMV in adult populations, it is not surprising that the rate of HCMV seropositivity approaches 100% in populations at high risk for HIV infection. Thus, endogenous virus and frequent sexual exposure to reinfecting viral strains are likely sources of

HCMV in these populations. The importance of HCMV co-infection to progression of AIDS remains controversial even though in vitro findings have suggested a potential role of HCMV in enhanced replication of HIV. Risk factors for the development of invasive HCMV disease in this population include a CD4+ lymphocyte count of less than 50/mm³. In the recent past, the development of invasive HCMV disease was a grave prognostic sign, because overall survival was significantly shortened in patients with documented HCMV end-organ disease.

Invasive HCMV infections in patients with AIDS have included end-organ disease in almost all organ systems, with three systems being more frequently involved: the CNS, gastrointestinal system, and pulmonary system. HCMV infection of the CNS, although uncommon in allograft recipients, is more frequently seen in HIV-infected patients. Encephalopathies, both diffuse and focal, as well as myelopathies and neuropathies, have been ascribed to HCMV. The most common and important disease associated with HCMV in this population is retinitis. Before the introduction of newer antiretroviral agents, it was estimated that between 8 and 25% of long-lived patients with AIDS developed this invasive HCMV infection. Gastrointestinal involvement includes both colitis and esophagitis and less frequently gastritis. Clinical and laboratory evidence of HCMV colitis is often found in association with other gastrointestinal pathogens, thus raising questions about the importance of HCMV as a primary pathogen. Likewise, most investigations do not view HCMV as a significant cause of pneumonitis in AIDS patients. With the advent of highly active antiretroviral therapy, the incidence of invasive HCMV disease has decreased significantly in patients with AIDS. Immune restoration/reconstitution has been proposed as mechanism(s) for the declining rate of invasive HCMV disease in this population, and resolution of disease and clearance of viral DNA from the plasma has been correlated with increased numbers of CD4+ lymphocytes.

DIAGNOSIS. The diagnosis of HCMV has conventionally relied on isolating the virus from urine, saliva, blood, or biopsy specimens obtained from patients exhibiting symptoms compatible with HCMV infection. Adaptation of immunocytochemistry and centrifugation-enhanced culture techniques has shortened the time required to identify HCMV in clinical specimens to less than 24 hours. There is no convenient method to distinguish acute, invasive infection from peripheral shedding after reactivation of a pre-existing infection. In the transplant and AIDS population, this has prompted diagnostic approaches for measuring viral burden, including HCMV blood cultures, cultures from biopsy specimens, and quantitative polymerase chain reaction (PCR) assays, all of which more closely correlate with invasive disease as compared with qualitative assays of viruria.

Serologic determination of HCMV is valuable when both IgG and IgM virus-specific antibodies are measured but usually only in normal hosts. Measurement of IgG alone is of limited value because of the high seroprevalence of HCMV in the population and the persistence of antibody responses to the virus. Although HCMV-specific IgM antibodies persist for up to 4 months in most normal individuals, their predictive value in the diagnosis of invasive infection in immunocompromised hosts is often limited because of their low positive and negative predictive value of invasive disease.

Newer methods of diagnosis include the PCR using several different body fluids as well as biopsy material as a source of template. PCR has been used successfully to detect viremia and plasma HCMV DNA. Quantifying PCR results has defined a threshold of viral burden that is associated with a high likelihood of development of invasive disease. Similarly, a semiquantitative assay of viral burden that utilizes a monoclonal antibody to detect virus-encoded protein in polymorphonuclear leukocytes, the antigenemia assay, appears predictive of invasive disease in allograft recipients and patients with AIDS. This assay is less sensitive than PCR but has a similar predictive value for invasive disease when compared with quantitative PCR and is technically more straightforward.

THERAPY. Until recently, effective antiviral therapy was not available for HCMV infection. Two agents, ganciclovir and foscarnet, have been shown to be virostatic in vitro and in vivo. Clinical trials have documented efficacy of these agents in treating invasive HCMV disease in both transplant and AIDS patients. Both have

significant toxicity, which often precludes their long-term administration. Ganciclovir causes dose-limiting hematopoietic toxicity, often resulting in clinically significant neutropenia. Foscarnet has significant nephrotoxicity, which limits its use in patients with azotemia. In addition, long-term therapy in immunocompromised patients has resulted in the development of viral resistance to both agents. Local therapy for HCMV retinitis has included intraocular injection of cidofovir and antisense oligonucleotides. Both therapies are well tolerated and lack systemic toxicity.

Perhaps the most beneficial use of these agents has been as prophylaxis in the immediate transplant period. Both foscarnet and ganciclovir have been used successfully to reduce the incidence of HCMV disease in the post-transplant period in both solid organ and bone marrow transplant recipients. More recent protocols include the use of quantitative assays of viral burden and so-called preemptive therapy in those patients at risk for developing invasive disease. This approach is not only more cost-effective but will also limit the development of resistance by reducing the indiscriminate use of these agents.

Immunoprophylaxis of HCMV infection has included passive transfer of antibody and limited clinical trials of a live-virus vaccine. The use of intravenous immunoglobulin containing anti-HCMV antibodies remains controversial, although clinical trials in solid organ allograft recipients has provided evidence of its efficacy. Its use in bone marrow transplantation is contentious, but accumulating evidence suggests that any beneficial effects may result from poorly understood immunomodulatory properties that influence the severity of GVHD. Active immunization with a replicating HCMV virus as a means of inducing protective immunity has been attempted on a limited scale in renal transplant recipients. The results of this trial remain controversial, although there was some evidence suggesting that protective immunity was induced by the vaccine virus.

Britt WJ, Alford CA: Cytomegalovirus. *In* Fields BN, Knipe DM, Howley PM, et al: (eds): Fields Virology, 3rd ed. Philadelphia, Lippincott–Raven, 1996, pp 2493–2523. *Discussion of biology and clinical syndromes associated with HCMV.*

Cope AV, Sabin C, Burroughs A, et al: Interrelationsips among quantity of human cytomegalovirus (HCMV) DNA in blood, donor-recipient serostatus, and administration of methylprednisolone as risk factors for HCMV disease following liver transplantation. J Infect Dis 176:1484, 1997. *A very complete study of the relationship between virus load and disease in solid organ allograft recipients. This paper also demonstrates that viral load is predictive of disease development, independent of donor:recipient serologic matching.*

Hoover DR, Peng Y, Saah A, et al: Occurrence of cytomegalovirus retinitis after human immunodeficiency virus immunosuppression. Arch Ophthalmol 114:821, 1996. *More recent study of HCMV retinitis in HIV-infected patients.*

Pass RF, Britt WJ, Stagno S: Cytomegalovirus. *In* Lennette EH, Lennette DA, Lennette ET (eds): Diagnostic Procedures for Viral, Rickettsial and Chlamydial Infections, 7th ed. Washington, APHA, 1994. *Discussion of commonly used methodologies for diagnosing HCMV.*

Seu P, Winston DJ, Holt CD, et al: Long-term ganciclovir prophylaxis for successful prevention of primary cytomegalovirus (CMV) disease in CMV-seronegative liver transplant recipients with CMV-seropositive donors. Transplantation 64:1614, 1997. *This report describes the efficacy of ganciclovir prophylaxis in liver allograft recipients.*

387 INFECTIOUS MONONUCLEOSIS: EPSTEIN-BARR VIRUS INFECTION

Elliott D. Kieff

DEFINITION. Infectious mononucleosis is a clinical syndrome characterized by malaise, headache, fever, pharyngitis, pharyngeal lymphatic hyperplasia, lymphadenopathy, atypical lymphocytosis, heterophile antibody, and mild transient hepatitis. The syndrome occurs most commonly in adolescents and young adults.

ETIOLOGY. Primary Epstein-Barr virus (EBV) infection is the cause of almost all typical infectious mononucleosis syndromes. EBV is a herpesvirus. In vitro, it infects only human B lymphocytes. Virus infection of B lymphocytes in vitro results in lymphocyte proliferation and immunoglobulin secretion. EBV usually remains latent in the infected B lymphocytes and can be induced to replicate in these cells using a variety of chemicals.

EPIDEMIOLOGY. The usual mode of EBV infection is by direct contact of saliva from a previously infected person with the oropharyngeal epithelium of a non-immune person. Infection in infancy commonly results from eating food premasticated by an infected mother, whereas infection in adolescence or as an adult is usually from salivary transfer during kissing. Virus survival in expectorated saliva is probably brief, because infection does not usually spread to susceptible roommates. Spread among young children sharing toys has not been studied.

After oropharyngeal inoculation with infected saliva, the virus replicates in oropharyngeal epithelial cells. Although the amount of virus in saliva is highest during primary infection and for months thereafter, virus replication in the oropharynx occurs intermittently for many years, possibly for life. In the course of primary oropharyngeal infection, EBV infects tonsillar and peripheral blood B lymphocytes. Virus persists indefinitely in a small fraction of the peripheral blood B lymphocytes. Transfusion of whole blood, bone marrow, blood fractions, or tissue containing viable B lymphocytes to susceptible (non-immune) persons can result in symptomatic primary infection. After bone marrow transplantation, the donor's virus may predominate in the recipient and may emerge as the dominant virus in the oropharynx of the recipient, indicating that a bone marrow or blood cell such as B lymphocytes are a site of persistent latent infection and the source of virus for continuing infection of the epithelium. EBV has also been found in salivary gland secretions and in cervical secretions, indicating that latently infected B lymphocytes can transmit virus to other epithelial tissues.

Previously infected normal persons are immune to the development of infectious mononucleosis. In less industrialized societies or among lower socioeconomic groups in industrialized societies, most children experience primary infection in the first decade of life. Among middle and higher socioeconomic groups, primary infection usually occurs as a consequence of adolescent or postadolescent kissing. More than 90% of adults in all human populations have serologic evidence of previous primary EBV infection and are carriers of the virus. Although EBV infection is limited to humans, each Old World primate species is endemically infected with a related virus characteristic of that species. New World primates are free of EBV-related viruses and can be experimentally infected. Experimental infection of some species with a sufficient EBV inoculum results in acute fatal lymphoproliferation.

CLINICAL MANIFESTATIONS. The syndrome of infectious mononucleosis was a distinctive clinical entity for at least 40 years before the discovery of its etiologic agent. After a 2- to 5-week incubation period, most infected non-immune adolescents and young adults develop malaise, headache, fever, pharyngitis, and lymphadenopathy lasting from 1 to several weeks. Temperatures may reach 40° C. Tonsillar or cervical lymph nodes may be quite enlarged, painful, and tender. Laboratory findings include relative or absolute lymphocytosis and a high titer of antibody to horse or ox red blood cells, referred to as a heterophile antibody. Up to 40% of the peripheral lymphocytes are atypical large cells with unusually abundant cytoplasm and a large pale pleomorphic nucleus. Other common manifestations are listed in Table 387–1. Malaise or weakness may recur over several months. Rashes are significantly more common in patients with primary EBV infection receiving penicillin or ampicillin treatment than in untreated patients or patients with other diseases who are treated with penicillin. Almost all normal people completely recover from acute infectious mononucleosis within 3 to 4 months. Persistent systemic, hematologic, neurologic, or cardiac abnormalities are rare.

Outside of the adolescent and young adult populations, primary EBV infection frequently does not result in the full infectious mononucleosis syndrome. In younger children, fever and pharyngitis from primary EBV infection may be clinically indistinguishable from upper respiratory tract infections caused by other viruses, mycoplasma, or streptococci. At any age cerebritis, neuritis, pneumonitis, hepatitis, carditis, autoimmune hemolytic anemia, or thrombocytopenia may be the predominant clinical manifestation. Atypical lymphocytosis or heterophile antibody may be less prominent or absent.

Severe, progressive, and sometimes fatal primary EBV infections occur in children in X-linked lymphoproliferative disease (Duncan's syndrome). Non-X-linked, sporadic cases also occur. Although these children have no obvious pre-existing immune deficiency,

Table 387–1 ■ CLINICAL MANIFESTATIONS OF INFECTIOUS MONONUCLEOSIS

Common Manifestations
Splenomegaly (50%)
Vomiting (20%)
Hepatitis (20–50%)
Jaundice (5%)
Palatal petechiae
Rash (4%)
Albuminuria (10%)
Less Frequent Manifestations (0.5–1%)
Cough
Pneumonitis
Neck stiffness
Aseptic meningitis
Cerebritis
Cerebellar dysfunction
Mononeuritis or polyneuritis
Transverse myelitis
Guillain-Barré syndrome
Uveitis
Subcapsular splenic hemorrhage or rupture
Myocarditis
Pericarditis
Cardiac conduction abnormalities
Nephrotic syndrome
Renal dysfunction
Diarrhea
Hemolytic anemia with anti-i antibody
Thrombocytopenia
Agranulocytosis
Pancytopenia
Hemophagocytic syndrome

primary EBV infection leads to massive lymphoproliferation, fever, anemia, hepatitis, or fulminant hepatic necrosis. The proliferating B lymphocytes are EBV-infected cells that express EBV-latent-infection–associated proteins. The early proliferation is polyclonal. Fulminant hepatic failure is a frequent cause of death. Recovery may be accompanied by persistent anemia, hypogammaglobulinemia, or pancytopenia. Oligoclonal or uniclonal EBV-infected B lymphomas may occur during the primary infection or after recovery. Similar illnesses with polyclonal lymphoproliferative disease occur in other immunosuppressed patients with primary EBV infection. Administration of high-dose cyclosporine as part of immunosuppressive regimens for heart, lung, liver, or bone marrow transplantation has been associated with severe EBV infection and polyclonal lymphoproliferative disease. The lymphoproliferative process may involve cervical, abdominal, or gastrointestinal lymphatics. Moreover, children with human immunodeficiency virus (HIV) infection are also at risk for severe EBV infection and lymphoproliferative disease (see Chapter 416), and EBV-infected lymphocytes are a frequent cause of the central nervous system lymphomas that occur in the acquired immunodeficiency syndrome (AIDS) or organ transplant recipients. In AIDS patients, replicating EBV has also been found in hairy leukoplakia of the tongue, a proliferative epithelial lesion.

Very rare cases of chronic progressive primary EBV infection in otherwise normal young adults have been well documented. These few patients have had severe acute mononucleosis that persists with clinical manifestations that include lymphadenopathy or visceral organ involvement and abnormally high antibody titers to EBV replicative cycle antigens. These titers are characteristically 10- to 100-fold higher than those in normal persons after primary EBV infection. Some patients have lacked antibody to EBV nuclear antigens. Most patients eventually recover without specific treatment. In one patient, acyclovir treatment produced clinical remission.

Persistent active EBV infection has been proposed to be the cause of a more common chronic mononucleosis or *chronic fatigue syndrome.* This syndrome is characterized by recurrent episodes of malaise and weakness, sometimes accompanied by myalgias, arthralgias, pharyngitis, lymphadenitis, or mild fever. The persistent lack of significant objective clinical or laboratory abnormalities distinguishes most patients with this poorly defined syndrome from those with documentable infectious, autoimmune, oncologic, metabolic, or neurologic diseases that can also occur with chronic fatigue. EBV-specific antibody titers in most patients with the chronic fatigue syndrome do not differ significantly from those of normal infected adults (see later). Thus, there is little to support the initial hypothesis that EBV is a frequent cause of this syndrome.

Latent EBV infection is also associated with B lymphomas in immunosuppressed patients, with Burkitt-type lymphoma in African children, with some of the sporadic Burkitt-type lymphomas that occur in developed societies, with about 50% of cases of Hodgkin's disease, with some T-cell lymphomas in adolescents or young adults, and with anaplastic nasopharyngeal carcinoma. A substantial fraction of B lymphomas occurring in immunocompromised patients have EBV DNA in the tumor cells. In B lymphomas in which the virus is latent in all of the tumor cells, the virus probably provides an initial, and in some cases an ongoing, stimulus for cell proliferation. Malignant conversion in many late postinfection lymphomas requires at least one additional factor, because these cells frequently also have a chromosome translocation that enhances c-myc oncogene expression. In a prospective study of African children, a correlation was noted between children with higher EBV antibody responses in the years after primary infection and tumor occurrence, suggesting that the extent of EBV replication is an important parameter in tumor induction.

In the last few years, considerable evidence has been amassed that EBV is an etiologic agent in Hodgkin's disease (see Chapter 180). EBV DNA is present in about 50% of Hodgkin's disease, with the highest incidence of EBV positivity being in younger patients, in Hispanic patients, and in patients with the mixed cellularity form of Hodgkin's disease. When present, EBV DNA is in all of the Hodgkin's disease "tumor" cells, and the cells are uniclonal with regard to EBV infection, indicating that infection did not occur after the onset of Hodgkin's disease.

EBV infection is also associated with anaplastic nasopharyngeal carcinomas. In retrospective and prospective clinical studies, high levels of IgA antibody to EBV antigens have been closely associated with anaplastic nasopharyngeal carcinoma. EBV has been uniformly found in each of the tumor cells of anaplastic nasopharyngeal carcinoma. The uniclonality of the virus genomes in these tumor cells indicates that the tumors arise in a single virus-infected cell. The virus is therefore likely to be necessary for this oncogenic conversion. Chinese and some North African and Canadian and U.S. Native American populations have a high incidence of nasopharyngeal carcinoma. Among peoples of Southern Chinese extraction, anaplastic nasopharyngeal carcinomas are the most common or second most common malignant growth. Genetic factors are therefore likely to be important determinants of tumor incidence. Other factors in the pathogenesis of nasopharyngeal carcinoma have not been defined.

PATHOLOGY AND PATHOGENESIS. EBV first infects pharyngeal epithelial cells and then spreads to subepithelial circulating B lymphocytes. The virus carries a gene similar to the human interleukin-10 gene, and the expression of this protein partially blocks the initial interferon, natural killer (NK), and T-cytotoxic responses. Infection may be confined to epithelial and B-lymphocyte tissues, because only these cells have EBV receptors. The EBV receptor is also the receptor for the C3d fragment of complement. Tonsils and regional and systemic lymph nodes enlarge because of follicular hyperplasia, owing in part to virus-infected B lymphocytes and infiltration of sinuses and paracortex with reactive, atypical T lymphocytes. Loss of normal architecture and the presence of Reed-Sternberg-like cells may make EBV infection difficult to distinguish from Hodgkin's disease. Similar changes occur in the spleen. In patients with significant hepatitis, hepatic lobules or portal areas may be infiltrated with mononuclear cells. The bone marrow is usually unaffected. Early in the illness, up to 1 or 2% of the circulating leukocytes may be EBV-infected B lymphocytes. The predominant atypical lymphocytes in the peripheral blood, however, are reactive NK cells and T cells. EBV-infected B lymphocytes can be detected by their expression of EBV nuclear proteins (EBNAs) and latent infection membrane proteins or by their ability to proliferate continuously in vitro or in severe combined immunodeficiency (SCID) mice, a property that normal B lymphocytes lack. EBV infection of B lymphocytes stimulates both B-cell proliferation and Ig secretion, particularly IgM. The heterophile antibody

may be the direct product of EBV-infected B lymphocytes, or it may be produced as a result of lymphokines produced by EBV-infected or reactive lymphocytes.

Lymphoproliferation following EBV infection of normal B lymphocytes in vitro is associated with the expression of six EBV nuclear proteins or EBNAs, two EBV integral membrane proteins or latent infection membrane proteins (LMPs), and two small RNAs. The same repertoire of genes is expressed in the peripheral B lymphocytes in acute infectious mononucleosis and in EBV-associated lymphoproliferative disease. The EBV-encoded nuclear proteins are transactivators of virus and cell gene expression. The virus LMP1 gene encodes the primary transforming protein of the virus. This protein is characteristically expressed in EBV-associated lymphoproliferative disease, in EBV-associated Hodgkin's disease, and in early nasopharyngeal carcinomas. The *LMP2* gene encodes a protein that prevents reactivation of virus lytic infection in response to usual B-cell activators. In normal patients with primary EBV infection, the acute, non-B-lymphocyte response to EBV infection is multifunctional. Some T lymphocytes suppress both B-lymphocyte proliferation and Ig secretion. Other peripheral blood T lymphocytes and NK cells from patients with infectious mononucleosis are cytotoxic to autologous EBV-infected B cells. Most cytotoxic T lymphocytes are largely CD8+ and recognize EBNA or LMP epitopes in the context of class I histocompatibility molecules. Other T lymphocytes may augment the T- and B-lymphocyte immune responses. Two EBV types are endemic in humans. These two types differ in their EBNA proteins and in their ability to transform B lymphocytes in vitro. Some cytotoxic T-lymphocyte clones are specific for EBNA proteins. Some of these EBNA-specific cytotoxic T lymphocytes recognize only the EBNA protein of one virus type.

After the patient recovers from acute infectious mononucleosis, the proportion of circulating B lymphocytes infected with EBV is 1 in 10^5 to 10^6. Most of these lymphocytes express only the EBNA 1 protein, which is not usually recognized by immune cytotoxic T lymphocytes. These latently infected B lymphocytes are likely to be the site of virus persistence, since long-term suppression of virus replication in the oropharynx with antiviral chemotherapy does not decrease the number of circulating EBV-infected B lymphocytes; and after cessation of treatment, the virus rapidly returns to the oropharyngeal epithelium. Also after bone marrow transplantation, the donor's rather than the recipient's virus may persist in the oropharynx of the recipient. Long after primary EBV infection, T lymphocytes, which can suppress or kill HLA-related EBV-infected cells that express EBNAs or LMPs, continue to circulate in the peripheral blood. Cyclosporine administration for organ transplantation indirectly inhibits the EBV-specific T-lymphocyte immune response, thereby enabling EBV-infected B lymphocytes to overgrow in transplantation recipients receiving high doses of cyclosporine and other immunosuppressive drugs. In this patient group, EBV-associated lymphoproliferative diseases are a significant, albeit unusual, problem.

DIAGNOSIS. In normal adolescents the diagnosis of acute infectious mononucleosis can usually be made on clinical grounds and confirmed by the laboratory findings of atypical lymphocytosis and heterophile antibody to ox or horse erythrocytes. Bacterial throat culture should be obtained in patients with significant pharyngitis to exclude concomitant β-hemolytic streptococcal infection. The rapid heterophile tests are more than 95% sensitive and more than 95% specific in an adolescent or young adult population. Titers are substantially diminished by 3 months after primary infection and undetectable by 6 months. In patients with absence of or equivocal heterophile antibodies, EBV-specific serologic testing should be done. The differential diagnosis may include streptococcal or gonococcal pharyngitis; cytomegalovirus, hepatitis virus A or B, HIV, HHV6, adenovirus, or *Toxoplasma* infection; leukemia; lymphoma; and Hodgkin's disease. Most heterophile-negative infectious mononucleosis with pharyngitis is also caused by EBV. In the absence of pharyngitis, however, cytomegalovirus, *Toxoplasma* hepatitis virus, or HIV infections are likely causes of heterophile-negative or low-titer heterophile-positive infectious mononucleosis. In some patient populations, acute HIV infection is a significant cause of typical or atypical infectious mononucleosis syndromes. HIV antigen or nucleotide sequence-specific detection may be necessary to

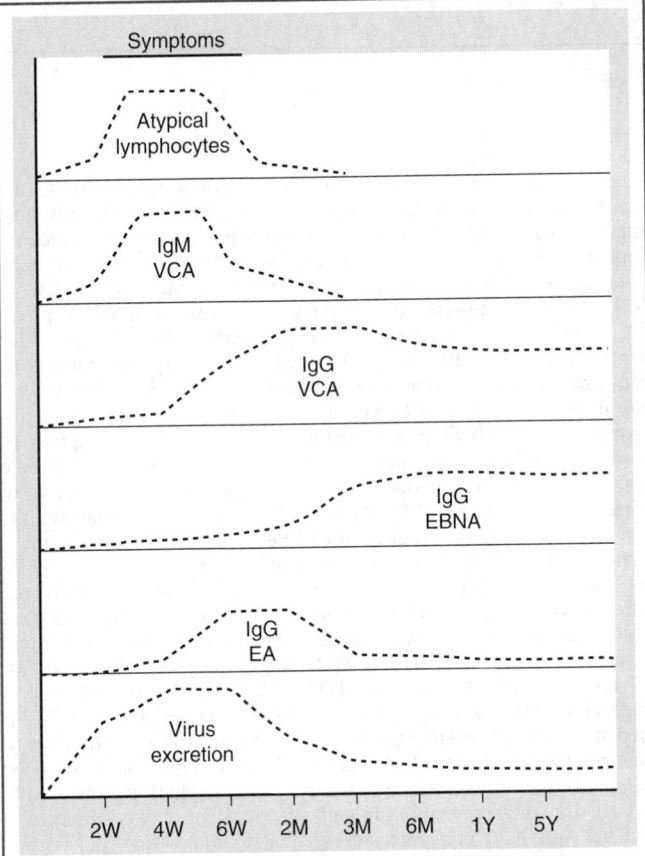

Symptoms

Atypical lymphocytes

IgM VCA

IgG VCA

IgG EBNA

IgG EA

Virus excretion

2W 4W 6W 2M 3M 6M 1Y 5Y

FIGURE 387–1 ■ The usual incubation period after EBV infection is 10 days to 2 weeks. By the time headache, malaise, and fever develop there are usually a few atypical lymphocytes and the monospot or heterophile test may be slightly positive. By 4 weeks, symptoms, monospot test, atypical lymphocytosis, and IgM antibody against EBV viral capsid antigen (VCA) are usually at their maximum. They may persist for another 2 to 3 weeks. IgG anti-EBV early antigen (EA) and anti-VCA are frequently detectable at 4 weeks but reach their maximum at 6 to 8 weeks. Anti-EBV nuclear protein (EBNA) IgG is usually not detectable until symptoms begin to resolve. Malaise may persist for 8 to 12 weeks. By 3 months, patients are usually fully recovered. IgG anti-VCA and EBNA titers persist at a high level for many years thereafter. EBV infection in normal humans is persistent but asymptomatic.

diagnose HIV infection early in the illness. Later, seroconversion may establish the diagnosis.

Specific serologic testing for EBV infection involves determining antibody titers to latently infected (anti-EBNA), early replication cycle (anti-EA), or late replication cycle (anti-VCA) viral proteins (Fig. 387–1). This is usually done by indirect immunofluorescence microscopy or by enzyme-linked immunoassay. Infection titers are listed in Table 387–2. Those rare patients with chronically progressive EBV infection tend to have abnormally high titers of antibodies to some or many EBV antigens. On the other hand, serologic diagnosis may be misleading in immunosuppressed patients, including children with X-linked immunodeficiency. These infected children may have high or low antibody titers. EBV serologic studies

Table 387–2 ■ ANTIBODY TESTS FOR EPSTEIN-BARR VIRUS

	TITERS
Acute Primary Infection	
IgM EA and VCA	High
IgG VCA and EBNA	Low
Recovering From Primary Infection	
IgM EA or VCA	Lower
IgG VCA	Rising
EBNA	Low
After Several Months	
IgM EA and VCA	Low or normal
IgG VCA and EBNA	Persist at high for several years

are helpful in following patients with anaplastic nasopharyngeal carcinoma or in screening for early detection of this malignant disease in high-risk populations. Patients at risk for primary anaplastic nasopharyngeal carcinoma or for recurrences have high IgG or IgA EA antibody titers.

TREATMENT. No treatment is necessary for most EBV infections. Rest during the period of acute symptoms and slow return to normal activity are commonly advised, although the therapeutic efficacy of this regimen has not been firmly established. Patients with splenomegaly should restrict their involvement in sports to avoid traumatic rupture. Acetaminophen or aspirin may be used to reduce temperature and pharyngeal pain in most patients who have normal or only slightly abnormal liver function. Very brief courses of glucocorticoid treatment (e.g., 60 mg prednisone per day for 4 days followed by rapidly decreasing doses) have been effective in shrinking obstructing tonsils, probably by ameliorating an overactive T-cell response. Autoimmune hemolytic anemia, granulocytopenia, and thrombocytopenia usually respond to longer courses of glucocorticoid therapy. The use of glucocorticoids for other manifestations of EBV infection is less certain to be beneficial. Glucocorticoids have no antiviral activity and are contraindicated in most herpesvirus infections. A few patients with severe hemorrhagic thrombocytopenia refractory to glucocorticoids have responded to intravenous immunoglobulin. Early plasmapheresis is indicated in patients with Guillain-Barré syndrome. Acyclovir and its derivatives have activity against EBV in vitro and in vivo but are not approved for use against EBV. These drugs should not be used in normal patients with EBV infections because they do not affect the length or severity of illness. Acyclovir can be used for AIDS patients with oral hairy leukoplakia or for patients with well-documented chronically progressive EBV infection. Acyclovir has not affected the outcome of EBV-associated lymphoproliferative syndromes in immunosuppressed patients. Partial restoration of immune function by lowering immune suppression has been beneficial. In one patient with X-linked lymphoproliferative disease recombinant interferon-γ produced rapid clinical remission.

Ernberg I, Andersson J: Acyclovir efficiently inhibits oropharyngeal excretion of Epstein-Barr virus in patients with acute infectious mononucleosis. J Gen Virol 67: 2267, 1986. *Effect of acycloguanosine on EBV infection.*

Kieff E: Epstein-Barr virus and its replication. *In* Fields B, Knipe D, Howley PM, et al (ed): Fields Virology, 3rd ed. Philadelphia, Lippincott–Raven, 1996. *Review of the biochemistry of Epstein-Barr virus and its effect on lymphocytes.*

Liebowitz D: Epstein-Barr virus—an old dog with new tricks (editorial). N Engl J Med 332:55, 1995.

Rickinson A, Kieff E: Epstein-Barr virus: Biology, pathogenesis and medical aspects. *In* Fields B, Knipe D, Howley PM, et al (eds): Virology, 3rd ed. Philadelphia, Lippincott–Raven, 1996. *Review of EBV-associated diseases.*

RETROVIRUSES

388 RETROVIRUSES OTHER THAN HIV

William A. Blattner

The discovery of human T-lymphotropic virus type I (HTLV-I) in the late 1970s culminated a search for a human retrovirus dating back to the turn of the century and began a new age of medical virology. It resulted in discoveries that linked human retroviruses to diverse lymphoreticular and chronic degenerative conditions and to the discovery in 1983 of the human immunodeficiency virus (HIV), a lente-retrovirus, the cause of the acquired immunodeficiency syndrome (AIDS) (see Part XXIII). These discoveries had scientific roots in the search for human cancer viruses in the early decades of this century; they were propelled by studies of mammalian cancer-causing retroviruses and the delineation of a replication cycle involving reverse transcriptase, which catalyzes the creation of a proviral DNA copy from a viral RNA template that is integrated into the cell genome resulting in lifelong infection. This chapter focuses on the virologic, epidemiologic, and clinical correlates of the HTLV class of viruses; it reviews the distribution of HTLV-I and HTLV-II and presents the known and possible disease associations and summarizes treatment approaches. Part XXII provides a comprehensive review of HIV and AIDS, and Chapter 179 reviews cancer chemotherapy for patients with aggressive T-cell lymphomas and leukemia.

VIROLOGY

HTLV-I and HTLV-II are single-stranded RNA viruses containing a diploid genome that replicates through a DNA intermediary able to integrate into the host cell genome as a provirus. The integration process is essential to the ability of this class of virus to cause lifelong infection, evade immune clearance, and produce diseases of long latency such as leukemia and lymphoma. Morphologically, HTLV-I is approximately 100 nm in diameter with a thin electron-dense outer envelope and an electron-dense, roughly spherical core. The genomic structure of HTLV-I is shown in Figure 388–1. The long terminal repeats (LTR) at the 5′ and 3′ ends of the genome contain regulatory elements that control virus expression and virion production, particularly binding sites for the major regulatory elements of HTLV *tax* and *rex*. Retroviral structural genes generally code for large overlapping polyproteins that are later processed into functional peptide products by virally encoded protease and cellular proteases. The encoding genes of the virus are

gag (group-specific antigen), *pol* (polymerase/integrase/protease), *env* (envelope), and a series of regulatory genes, *tax* and *rex,* that regulate virus expression. The *gag* proteins function as structural proteins of the matrix, capsid, and nucleocapsid. The *pol* gene encodes for several enzymes-reverse transcriptase (involved in RNA to DNA transcription), endonuclease (ribonuclease-H), protease (overlapping *gag* and *pol*), and integrase, which functions for viral integration. The *env* gene encodes the major components of the viral coat: the surface glycoprotein of 46,000 MW (gp46) and the transmembrane 21,000 MW (gp21). The regulatory region, pX, expresses *tax,* which is responsible for enhanced transcription of viral and cellular gene products; it has been postulated to play a crucial role in leukemogenesis. *Rex* (regulator of expression of virion proteins for HTLV) modulates, in a complex manner, the pattern of viral RNA production and the transport of virion components in the production of virus particles.

The initial step in the life cycle of HTLV is attachment of the virus envelope glycoprotein to an unknown cell surface receptor. Data suggest that postattachment interactions between virus and target cell result in preferential infection of CD4 T-helper cells for HTLV-I and of CD8 cells for HTLV-II. After uptake and uncoating, viral RNA is transcribed by *reverse transcriptase,* an RNA-dependent DNA polymerase complexed to the RNA in the core of the virus particle, into double-stranded DNA. This double-stranded viral DNA is integrated into the host cell nucleus by the virally encoded integrase, resulting in cell infection that may be lifelong.

The viral LTR elements are essential to integration and regulation of viral genome expression. They form the sites for covalent attachment of the provirus to cellular DNA and contain important regulatory elements such as the U3 region where viral *tax* exerts its up-regulatory effects through interactions with the AFT/CREB family of DNA-binding proteins whose active complexes are enhanced by a stabilizing effect of *tax*. The virus may remain "hidden" (unexpressed, not replicated) in cells for long periods. This may contribute to the long interval (sometimes many years to decades) between the time of infection and disease.

Factors that control viral replication (viral regulatory genes, cell stimulation, and possibly co-infections) may also be cofactors in disease progression. When the DNA provirus is expressed (transcribed by a cellular RNA polymerase), viral genomic and messenger RNA and subsequently viral proteins are made by the cell. These assemble at the cell membrane to be packaged and released (budding). During the budding process the envelope incorporates the cell's lipid bilayer, producing an infectious virion of about 100 nm.

HTLV-I and HTLV-II are routinely detected through blood bank screening assays that use whole HTLV-I virus lysates. Recently these assays were shown to be insensitive to HTLV-II detection, so newer test kits with enhanced HTLV-II sensitivity through addition of HTLV-II antigens have been developed and current U.S. Food and Drug Administration guidelines require detection of both HTLV virus types. Confirmation of positives is done by Western blotting. The current generation of assays uses whole virus lysates and recombinant viral antigens; these increase sensitivity and the ability to distinguish HTLV-I from HTLV-II. Polymerase chain reaction is another technique useful in research settings for detecting and distinguishing virus type and, more recently, in quantifying cell-associated virus as a marker in disease.

DISTRIBUTION OF HTLV

The source of human retroviruses is not known. Primate retroviruses called simian T-lymphotropic virus (STLV) have been isolated from several primate species in Africa and Asia; these viruses share significant homology with human HTLV-I and raise the possibility of enzootic transmission to humans. How HTLV has spread among various human populations is not known; it appears to represent an ancient virus that has followed the migrations of vari-

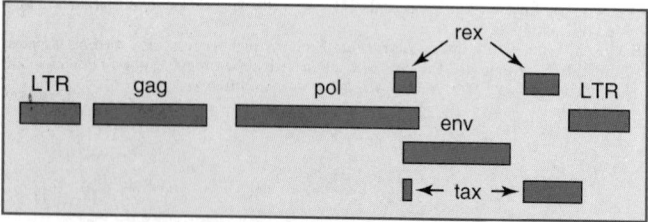

FIGURE 388–1 ■ Genomic structure of human T-lymphotropic viruses. LTR = long terminal repeat, which is organized into three regions: U5, R, and U3, which house the polyadenylation site; and the *rev* = response element and the transactivating response element, which are involved in controlling virus expression. *gag* = group specific antigen, whose products form the skeleton of the virion (matrix, capsid, nucleocapsid, nucleic acid binding protein); *pol* = gene for reverse transcriptase, integrase, and protease; *env* = envelope gene; *tax* = transactivator gene; *rex* = viral regulatory gene involved in promoting genomic RNA production. (Courtesy of Dr. Robert C. Gallo.)

Table 388–1 ■ TRANSMISSION OF HTLV-I AND II

MODES OF TRANSMISSION	HTLV-I	HTLV-II
Mother to infant		
Transplacental	Yes	Not known
Breast milk	Yes	Probable
Sexual		
Male to female	Yes	Yes
Female to male	Yes	Yes
Male to male	Yes	Not known
Parenteral		
Blood transfusion	Yes	Yes
Intravenous drug use	Yes	Yes
	Co-factors	
Elevated virus load		
Mother to infant	Yes	Not known
Heterosexual	Yes	Not known
Ulcerative genital lesions	Yes	Not known
Cellular transfusion products	Yes	Yes
Sharing of "works"	Yes	Yes

ous human populations. So far, five major molecular subtypes of HTLV-I have been identified: the Cosmopolitan (widespread all over the world), Japanese, West African, Central African and Melanesian (Papua New Guinea, Melanesia, and Australian aborigine) subtypes. HTLV-I clusters are found in southern Japan, among Melanesian peoples in Papua New Guinea and northern Australia, throughout Western and Equatorial Africa, and among persons of African descent in the Caribbean and South America. The virus from Melanesia differs molecularly from the Japanese and African strains by 5 to 10%, the result of the independent evolution of the virus in these populations separated for tens of thousands of years. A concentration of HTLV-I in northeastern Iran may have resulted from the cross-cultural migrations occurring along the trade routes from the Far East to the Middle East and Europe. HTLV-II is found among Native American peoples throughout North, Central, and South America. An Asian focus was recently reported in remote areas of Mongolia, among people who share genetic links with Native American populations whose ancestors emigrated from this region during the Ice Age. HTLV-II has also been detected in Africa, originally among pygmies in Equatorial Africa but more recently in some areas of West Africa. Infections in Europe occur among injection drug users who may have acquired the virus from contact with U.S. drug users.

Table 388–1 summarizes the routes, cofactors, and viral characteristics associated with HTLV-I transmission; the basic modes of transmission for HTLV-I and HIV-1 are similar.

SEXUAL TRANSMISSION. A sexual transmission of HTLV-I from male to female and female to male as well as from male to male has been documented. HTLV-I transmission is cell associated and appears to be at least an order of magnitude less infectious than HIV-1. Coincidental infection with other sexually transmitted diseases, particularly those associated with ulcerative genital lesions in males and inflammatory lesions in women, amplify the risk of transmission. For HTLV-I, elevated antibody titer, which appears to correlate with elevated virus load, is linked to heightened transmission. In viral endemic regions there is a characteristic age-dependent rise in HTLV-I seroprevalence. This increase first becomes evident in the adolescent years; it is steeper in women than in men and continues in women after age 40, whereas rates in men plateau around age 40. This pattern reflects more efficient male-to-female transmission. For HTLV-II the pattern differs; here, the rates for both genders are equal. This finding suggests that there may be differences between the two viruses in the kinetics of transmission.

PERINATAL TRANSMISSION. The second major route of transmission is from mother to child. For HTLV-I, breast feeding is more efficient than in utero or perinatal transmission. For example, whereas 20% of breast-fed infants on average seroconvert to HTLV-I, only 1 to 2% of bottle-fed infants of HTLV-I–positive mothers become infected. In this regard, HTLV-I differs significantly from HIV-1; in utero and perinatal transmission accounts for virtually all HIV-1 transmission in the West, where breast-feeding is discouraged. The rate of breast milk–associated HIV-1 transmission is estimated to be approximately 15%. HTLV-II has been detected in breast milk, but mother to child transmission by this route has not been documented.

TRANSFUSION AND INJECTION DRUG USE. The third major route of transmission is parenteral, through either transfusion or injection drug use. Surveys of blood donors in the United States document that more than half of the HTLV infections are due to HTLV-II. Among injection drug users the vast majority of infections are due to HTLV-II; it is projected that HTLV-II is more efficiently transmitted by this route than is HTLV-I.

Prospective studies of transfusion transmission indicate that both HTLV-I and HTLV-II are transmitted in association with cellular components. This is in sharp contrast to HIV-1, which is transmitted by cells, plasma, or plasma products. Approximately one half of the recipients of HTLV-I– and HTLV-II–positive blood seroconvert; the percentage for HIV-1 is more than 95%.

The only documented illness linked to HTLV-I or HTLV-II transfusion transmission is the HTLV-associated demyelinating neurologic syndrome described later. Leukemia has not been associated with transfusion of HTLV-positive blood. Among U.S. blood donors who are confirmed HTLV positive (slightly less than half are HTLV-I and the others are HTLV-II), the major risk factors are intravenous drug use, birthplace in a viral endemic area, or sexual contact with a person with this profile.

Co-infection with HTLV-I and HIV-1 appears to increase the progression to AIDS through unexplained mechanisms, possibly related to the cell-proliferative effects of HTLV-I on HIV-1–infected T cells. Such a relationship has not been shown for HTLV-II. Other modes of transmission involving "casual contact," mosquito transmission, and so on are not a source of infection. Health care and laboratory workers who experience a needle stick, skin, or mucous membrane exposure in the absence of protective barriers have little or no risk for infection with a single case of such infection documented after exposure to a "microtransfusion" from a syringe.

HTLV-ASSOCIATED DISEASES

Adult T-Cell Leukemia/Lymphoma (ATL)

HTLV-I-associated diseases are listed in Table 388–2. The most common malignancy caused by HTLV-I is ATL, a form of peripheral T-cell lymphoma often with spread in the peripheral blood. The subtypes of ATL (acute, chronic, smoldering, and lymphoma-type) have different clinical features and prognosis (Fig. 388–2). These tumors represent high-grade lymphomas, usually of large, medium, and/or pleiotropic morphology and advanced clinical stage, and are associated with a poor prognosis.

The incidence of ATL is approximately 1 per 1000 carriers per year, and thus the number of cases varies by the underlying prevalence of infection. Worldwide among the 3 to 4 million infected persons worldwide there are approximately 2500 to 3000 cases per year. In the United States, with a low prevalence of infection it is estimated that there are approximately 30 cases per year. In HTLV-I endemic areas such as southern Japan and the Caribbean Islands, ATL accounts for half or more of adult lymphoid malignancies. The chance of an infected individual developing a malignancy over a lifetime is approximately 5%; studies of mothers of ATL cases emphasizes that early life exposure is associated with the greatest risk for subsequent disease.

The age group of cases ranges from adolescence to a peak in middle-aged (40s in the Caribbean and 50s in Japan) adults. The diagnosis should be considered in an adult with mature T-cell lymphoma and hypercalcemia and/or cutaneous involvement, particularly if the individual is from a known risk group or endemic region. The diagnosis is established by testing serum for HTLV-I antibodies. Occasionally, cases are antibody negative but provirus is detectable in the blood or in biopsy specimens.

The acute form of ATL (Figs. 388–2 and 388–3) is characterized by an aggressive mature T-cell lymphoma whose clinical course is often associated with high white blood cell count, hypercalcemia, and cutaneous involvement. Other cases resemble T-prolymphocytic leukemia and are called chronic ATL. Smoldering ATL may clinically resemble mycosis fungoides/Sézary syndrome, with cutaneous involvement presenting as erythema or as infiltrative plaques or tumors. Sometimes a long prodrome of signs (e.g., cutaneous rashes) and symptoms (e.g., fevers) are noted before

Table 388–2 ■ HTLV-ASSOCIATED DISEASES

DIAGNOSIS	NATURE OF SYNDROME	STRENGTH OF ASSOCIATION
HTLV I–Associated Diseases		
Adult T-cell leukemia/lymphoma	Aggressive lymphoproliferative malignancy of mature T lymphocytes	Strong
B-cell chronic lymphocytic leukemia	Tumor-associated immunoglobulin reacts to HTLV antigen	2 cases reported
Tropical spastic paraparesis (TSP) HTLV-associated myelopathy (HAM)	Chronic progressive demyelinating syndrome of long motor tracks of spinal cord	Strong
Polymyositis	Degenerative inflammatory syndrome of skeletal muscles	Probable
Infective dermatitis	Chronic generalized eczema of skin in children; potential for preleukemia and immunodeficiency	Strong
Uveitis	Inflammatory infiltration of the uvea of the eye	Strong
HTLV-associated arthritis	Large joint polyarthropathy; rheumatoid factor positive with HTLV-I positive cells infiltrating the synovia	Probable
Immune deficiency	Anecdotal reports of AIDS-like illness in HTLV-I positives; subclinical (e.g., decreased PPD response) or clinical (e.g., poor response to therapy for symptomatic strongyloidiasis)	Possible
Miscellaneous clinical conditions	Case reports or case series of Sjögren's syndrome, interstitial pneumonitis, small cell lung cancer with monoclonal HTLV-I integration, and invasive cervical cancer	Uncertain
HTLV II–Associated Diseases		
T-hairy cell/large granulocytic leukemia	Case reports of T-cell/NK-cell malignancy with either monoclonal or polyclonal integration	Possible
HTLV-associated myelopathy	Case reports of TSP HAM in association with HTLV-II. In some cases ataxic form of neurologic involvement is reported	Probable
Miscellaneous clinical conditions	Case reports or case series of HTLV-II linked to mycosis fungoides, asthma, glomerular nephritis, pulmonary disease	Uncertain

transformation to an acute, rapidly fatal form of disease occurs. In addition to differences in clinical presentation, the different forms of ATL—acute, chronic and smoldering—have distinctive morphologic features, as shown Figure 388–3. A particularly distinctive morphology are the so-called flower cells shown in Figure 388–3b, which represent a sine qua non of HTLV-I–associated leukemia. Interestingly, cells with this morphology are also seen in healthy carriers. Sometimes ATL presents as a T-cell non-Hodgkin's lymphoma with many of the signs and symptoms of acute ATL such as hypercalcemia and monoclonal integration of HTLV-I proviral DNA in the tumor cells but without the characteristic peripheral blood involvement of acute ATL. Patients with acute and lymphoma-type ATL have a poor prognosis, especially when hypercalcemia is present and death within 6 months of diagnosis is common. The cause of death is usually an explosive growth of tumor cells, hypercalcemia, and various opportunistic infections, including *Pneumocystis carinii* pneumonia and other infections observed in AIDS patients.

THERAPY. ATL has proven refractory to most conventional and experimental chemotherapeutic regimens (Fig. 388–4). In general,

smoldering ATL is the least aggressive form. The chronic type has a relatively poor prognosis, with death occurring within a few years of diagnosis. Patients with chronic and smoldering ATL receive no therapy, or they are treated with prednisone with or without cyclophosphamide. The more indolent forms of ATL have a high rate of complicating infections resulting from the immunosuppressive effects of aggressive therapy. Acute and lymphoma-type ATLs are aggressive high-grade lymphomas with a generally poor prognosis, although approximately 15% of cases do respond to multidrug regimens with prolonged remission. Conventional combination chemotherapy, such as CHOP, VEPA, MACOP-B, and PROMACE, achieve response rates of more than 50% with clinical remission rates of approximately 20%, but relapses within 6 months are almost universal owing to resistance and to presence of residual disease (see Fig. 388–4). Approaches to therapy intensification, such as use of granulocyte colony-stimulating factor and stem cell rescue, may provide additional benefit, but data are preliminary. Unfavorable prognosis is associated with poor performance status at diagnosis, age older than 40, extensive disease, hypercalcemia, and high serum LDH level. Relapses in long-term survivors often occur in the central nervous system and prove refractory to subsequent therapy. Experimental approaches under investigation include topoisomerase inhibitors, monoclonal antibodies, and interferon and zidovudine. The topoisomerase inhibitors have promising effects in early phase trials. Monoclonal antibodies against interleukin (IL)-2 α-chain and interferon conjugated or not to toxins selectively target leukemic cells with long-term survival in some patients but with 50% relapse at 5 months. Zidovudine and interferon-α induce responses (66%) in cases, but overall survival is poor. Future approaches will focus on combining conventional and novel approaches to sustain longer-term responses.

A possible association was reported between HTLV-I and some cases of B-cell chronic lymphocytic leukemia. In these cases, chronic stimulation of B-cell proliferation by viral antigens coupled with virus-induced impairment of CD4 cell function resulted in malignant transformation in B cells with HTLV-I–specific cell surface antibodies.

Tropical Spastic Paraparesis/HTLV-I–Associated Myelopathy (TSP/HAM)

HTLV-I is linked to a neurologic syndrome known as TSP/HAM. This disease is characterized by a chronic, slowly progressive development of spastic paraparesis resulting from the demyelination of the long motor neurons of the spinal cord. Symptoms often begin with a stiff gait, progressing (usually slowly) to in-

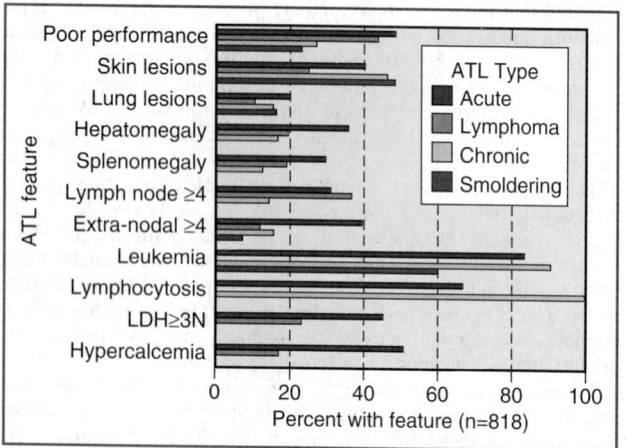

FIGURE 388–2 ■ Features of adult T-cell lymphoma/leukemia in Japan. A combination of clinical and laboratory features is involved in defining the various subtypes of ATL (see text for details). (From Blattner W: Human T-cell lymphotropic viruses and cancer causation. *In* Devita VT, Hellman S, Rosenberg SA [eds]: Cancer Prevention, Update. Philadelphia, JB Lippincott, 1993, p 1.)

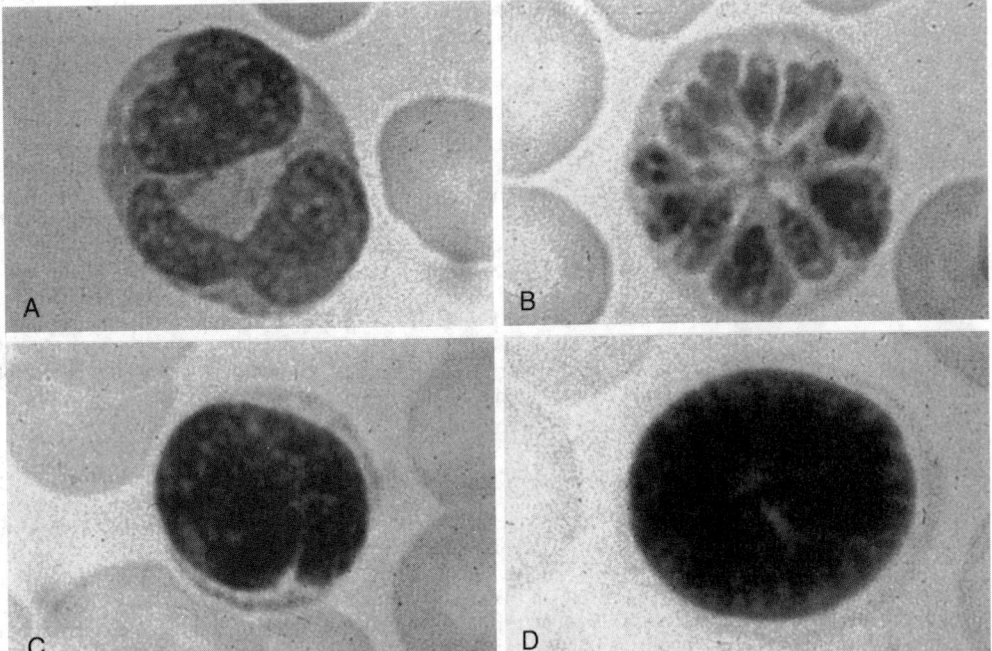

FIGURE 388-3 ■ Photomicrographs demonstrating the morphologic features of leukemic cells observed in different subtypes of ATL. Panel *A* and *B* display the polylobulated morphology of the acute type, with the highly characteristic "flower cell" shown in panel *B*. Panel *C* is a typical cleaved cell seen in the chronic type. Panel *D* displays the typical morphology of smoldering ATL. (Photographs courtesy of K. Yamaguchi and K. Takatsuki.)

creasing spasticity and weakness, with incontinence and impotence developing later in the course of the illness. Sometimes ataxia develops. In some cases, isolated lesions of the CNS are detected on a nuclear magnetic resonance scan. This syndrome differs from classic multiple sclerosis because of its generally slow, progressive course and the absence of a waxing and waning symptomatology and the primary neurologic defect of demyelination of the long motor neurons. However, some cases are acutely progressive; such cases are sometimes associated with the transfusion of HTLV-I–positive blood.

The incidence of disease is approximately half of the rate for ATL. The diagnosis is suspected in unexplained CNS disease with loss of pyramidal tract functions and is confirmed by testing sera for HTLV-I antibodies. Treatment with corticosteroids and immunosuppressive therapies benefit some patients, ranging between 30 and 50% in one series, particularly those with rapidly progressive disease; danazol, and androgenic steroid, improves urinary and fecal incontinence but does not affect the underlying neurologic deficit. Recently, pentoxifylline was reported in an uncontrolled trial to have favorable effects on clinical symptoms and on subclinical immunologic perturbations. Based on the association between the IL-2 complex and the immune activation in TSP/HAM, a humanized anti–IL-2 receptor antibody was used in treatment of seven cases and resulted in a reduction of viral load confirmed by polymerase chain reaction, with clinical stabilization in six cases and clinical improvement in 1 case.

TSP/HAM is the prototype for a series of immune-mediated syndromes characterized by high virus load, significant immune activation, and an indirect pathogenic mechanism produced by virally induced perturbations in immune function. Examples of these conditions include polymyositis of the skeletal muscle, uveitis of the eye, a large joint arthritis, and Sjögren's syndrome. Additional oncogenic effects are suggested by a Japanese case of small cell lung cancer with monoclonal HTLV integration and association with invasive cervical cancer. HTLV-I has also been linked to immunosuppression through clinical and laboratory observations of Japanese patients with AIDS-like illnesses associated with HTLV-I (in the absence of underlying malignancy), perturbations in skin test reactivity, and the finding that parasitic infestations (e.g., strongyloidiasis) are refractory to conventional treatments. The infective dermatitis syndrome first reported in Jamaica represents the first childhood HTLV-I syndrome. In children and adults with this syndrome, patients develop refractory bacterial infections with saprophytic skin organisms that respond to antibiotic therapy but relapse when therapy is stopped. It is hypothesized that these symptoms result from immunosuppressive effects of HTLV-I. Long-term fol-

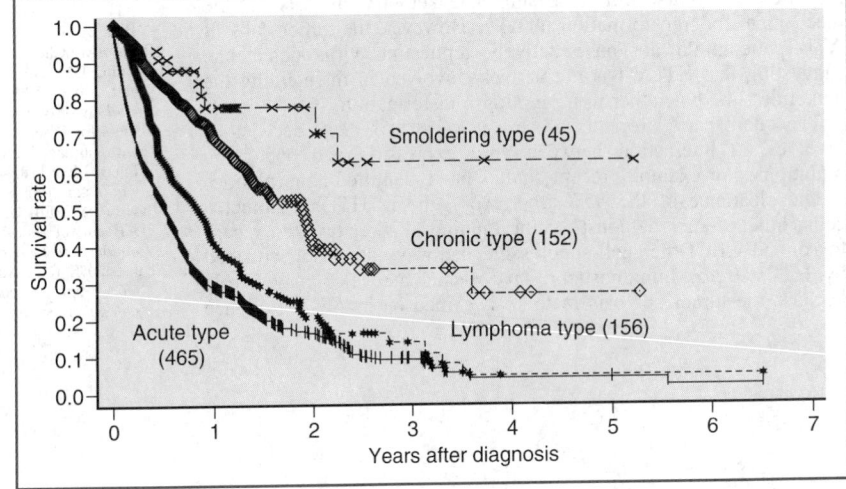

FIGURE 388-4 ■ Survival by ATL subtype after polychemotherapy in Japan. Poorest survival is observed in patients with acute and lymphoma-type ATL. (From Tsukasaki K, Ikeda S, Murata K, et al: Characteristics of chemotherapy-induced clinical remission in long survivors with aggressive adult T-cell leukemia/lymphoma. Leuk Res 17:157, 1993.)

low-up of some patients has documented the subsequent development of ATL and TSP/HAM in patients originally diagnosed with infective dermatitis.

HTLV-II Infection

At this time, HTLV-II continues to be an "orphan" virus with no true disease association. Although HTLV-II was originally isolated from a patient with hairy T-cell leukemia that on reanalysis was thought to represent large granulocytic cell leukemia, a malignancy with a natural killer cell phenotype, there has been no consistent evidence of an association of HTLV-II with this or any lymphoid malignancy.

More than a dozen TSP/HAM cases associated with HTLV-II have been reported. In some instances the clinical pattern had features of the ataxic form, but most had the more typical spastic paraparesis. Preliminary data suggest this syndrome is infrequent compared with its occurrence in HTLV-I carriers.

HTLV PATHOGENESIS

A great deal has been learned about the pathogenesis of HTLV-I–associated leukemia. Early in infection, HTLV-I infects only a small number of T cells and probably the monocyte/macrophage. The DNA provirus randomly integrates into the DNA of infected cells. Although HTLV-I may exist as a latent virus, the virus genes promote cell proliferation by direct and indirect mechanisms, including various lymphokine and cell regulatory pathways. In particular, *tax* directly binds to essential elements of the NF-κB pathway, which plays a central role in controlling cellular transcription and immune activation pathways. In this way, Tax promotes the expression of additional activated target cells and thereby amplifies virus spread. For example, when lymphocytes from HTLV-I–infected normal persons are placed in tissue culture, they undergo spontaneous (in the absence of exogenous antigens or mitogens) lymphocyte proliferation. Early in the infection phase, host immune responses to the virus are activated, producing viral antibodies and cytotoxic T cells targeted at viral antigens. In some cases, persons with documented exposure (e.g., via blood transfusion) do not seroconvert and develop cell-mediated immune responses that presumably clear virus infection. Some healthy carriers develop T-cell polyclonal and oligoclonal proliferations that can later progress to malignancy or may disappear spontaneously. Morphologically distinct "flower cells," (see Fig. 388–3*B*) representing T cells with deeply lobulated nuclei resembling ATL leukemic cells, are seen on peripheral blood smears of healthy carriers but do not presage risk for subsequent disease. In ATL, the HTLV-I provirus is found integrated in the DNA of the leukemic cells in a clonal fashion with one (or occasionally two) copy of the provirus integrated in the same chromosomal location in each cell. This would indicate that ATL is tumor derived from a single transformed cell that sprouted from a virus infection before transformation and clonal expansion rather than afterward as a passenger virus. Tumors from different patients have proviral integration in different locations. This indicates that *cis*-activation of a nearby cellular gene by the LTR of the virus, as occurs with some animal leukemia viruses, is not the mechanism for transformation in ATL. However, the tumor cells of ATL patients do not have actively replicating virus detectable, suggesting that HTLV-I is not actively involved in maintaining the leukemic state but rather in promoting transformation.

The latent period for this process is years to several decades; it involves an interaction between viral expression and oncogenic mutations. For example, recent studies have identified abnormalities in the clearance of the *p53* suppressor gene in HTLV-I–infected cells; other studies demonstrate the binding of viral tax to a receptor on NF-kB. Other cell-suppressive pathways are also perturbed by HTLV-I *tax*. Immunosuppressive events may also play a role because the tumor necrosis factor-β is turned on in ATL. Evidence is growing that, at some stage, transformation involves the expression of the Tax protein encoded by the *px* gene of HTLV-I. Because the tax protein induces expression of cellular genes critical for T-cell proliferation, including IL-2 and its receptor (IL-2R), an autocrine mechanism may be involved, particularly in the first steps of leukemogenesis, which involves polyclonal expansions of T cells. For malignancy to develop, additional genetic changes most probably take place (e.g., cytogenetic changes, oncogene alterations). Because tax gene expression is detectable in tumor samples, even in some cases of antibody-negative ATL, this viral gene may be crucial in oncogenesis. However, the *tax* gene is not widely expressed in the tumor cells.

TSP/HAM occurs with a latency from infection to disease of months to years, which contrasts to the years-to-decades incubation for ATL. Current data suggest an indirect mechanism of pathogenesis involving immune-mediated responses that appear to cause local damage in the myelin sheath of the long motor neuron.

PREVENTION

A major issue confronting practicing physicians is what to tell patients identified as HTLV positive based on blood bank screening. First and foremost, they must emphasize that disease complications related to HTLV-I are rare and that for HTLV-II no specific disease has been verified. Second, it should be emphasized that the viruses are not easily transmitted. Third, the patient should be clearly counseled concerning the distinction between the HTLV and the HIV viruses because the greatest fear the patient may have is that he or she has the "AIDS virus." Recently, guidelines for prevention and counseling have been developed for HTLV-I and HTLV-II by a Centers for Disease Control and Prevention Working Group:

1. Blood for donation should be screened before transfusion, and positive donors should be deferred from donating.
2. HTLV-I/II–positive mothers should be discouraged from breast feeding when practicable to prevent mother-to-infant transmission (except in particular settings, such as in the tropics, where diarrheal disease in non–breast-fed infants presents a high risk for morbidity and mortality).
3. Condoms should be used by discordant couples, but, given the relatively low frequency of sexual transmission per sexual encounter, couples who desire a pregnancy could time unprotected sexual intercourse to coincide with periods of maximal fertility. (Such decisions require careful discussion between physician and patient; there are no absolute guidelines in this area.)

Vaccines containing whole virus and recombinant HTLV-I envelope antigens have successfully prevented HTLV-I infection in monkeys and in a rabbit model; it is uncertain whether a vaccine for HTLV-I or HTLV-II will ever be implemented for humans. For example, in Japan, epidemiologic data show that new infections are declining because of changing socioeconomic and lifestyle factors, whereas in developing countries rates as high as 1 to 1.5% per year are reported in sexually active populations. It is unclear whether the disease burden associated with these viruses warrants a vaccine.

Blattner W, Pombo de Oliveira M: Human T lymphotropic viruses: HTLV-I and HTLV-II. *In* Broder S, Merigan T, Bolognasi D (eds): Textbook of AIDS Medicine. 1998. *A clinically oriented review of HTLV-I and HTLV-II and related diseases.*

Cann AM, Chen ISY: Human T-cell leukemia virus types I and II. *In* Fields BN, Knipe DM, Howley PM, et al (eds): Fields Virology, 3rd ed. Philadelphia, Lippincott–Raven, 1996. *A through review of the molecular pathogenesis of HTLV-I in the etiology of associated diseases.*

Centers for Disease Control and Prevention: Guidelines for counseling persons infected with human T-lymphotropic virus type I (HTLV-I) and type II (HTLV-II). Ann Intern Med 118:448, 1993. *Presents important information to clinicians confronted with counseling persons referred with HTLV infection.*

Pawson R, Mufti G, Pagliuca A: Management of adult T-cell leukemia/lymphoma. Br J Haematol 100:453, 1998. *Provides a comprehensive summary of current treatment options and management strategies.*

Takatsuki K (ed): Adult T-cell Leukemia. Oxford, Oxford Press, 1994. *Comprehensive monograph on human T-cell leukemia virus including chapters on virology, immunology, epidemiology, clinical features, and management.*

ENTERIC VIRAL INFECTIONS

389   ENTEROVIRUSES

Michael N. Oxman

Enteroviruses, so named because they generally infect the alimentary tract and are shed in the feces, cause a variety of diseases in humans and lower animals. They comprise one of the five major subgroups, or genera, of the Picornavirus (*pico,* small; *rna,* ribonucleic acid) family. The other Picornavirus genera are: *rhinoviruses,* which inhabit the upper respiratory tract and include the principal recognized etiologic agents of the common cold (see Chapter 375); *cardioviruses,* recovered chiefly from rodents and only very rarely implicated in human disease; *aphthoviruses,* named for the vesicular lesions that they produce in cloven-footed animals; and *hepatovirus,* a newly designated genus with human hepatitis A virus as its only currently recognized member.

Enteroviruses are differentiated from rhinoviruses primarily by their resistance to acid; they are fully infectious at pH 3 or even lower. Consequently, enteroviruses that have undergone limited replication in the oropharynx survive passage through the stomach and implant in the lower intestinal tract, where they undergo more extensive multiplication. In contrast, rhinoviruses are acid labile; they begin to lose infectivity at pH 6 and are completely inactivated at pH 3. They are further distinguished from enteroviruses by their lower optimal temperature of replication (33° C versus 37° C for enteroviruses) and higher buoyant density in cesium chloride. Because rhinoviruses inhabit the nasopharynx, they have no obvious need for acid stability, and preferential replication at lower than body temperature probably reflects their adaptation to the cooler nasal passages.

Hepatitis A virus was originally classified as an enterovirus and designated enterovirus 72. However, it is more resistant to inactivation by heat than enteroviruses, and its genome has relatively little nucleotide sequence homology with members of the enterovirus genus. Furthermore, in contrast to enteroviruses, hepatitis A virus does not cause a rapid shut-off of host cell protein synthesis, and the infected cells are not lysed. Because of these important differences, hepatitis A virus has been accorded its own genus, Hepatovirus, within the Picornavirus family. Hepatitis A virus is discussed in Chapter 149.

Within the enterovirus genus, species are distinguished immunologically by the ability of specific antisera to neutralize only the homotypic virus. There are now 67 recognized human enterovirus species (serotypes or immunotypes), as well as numerous enteroviruses of lower animals. Humans appear to be the only natural host for the human enteroviruses, and, in general, the enteroviruses of lower animals are not natural pathogens for humans.

Historically, human enteroviruses have been subclassified into *polioviruses,* group A and group B *coxsackieviruses,* and *echoviruses* on the basis of antigenic relationship differences in host range, and type of disease produced (Table 389–1). By 1969, 67 species (serotypes) of human enteroviruses had been identified and classified according to these criteria, although reclassification and redundancy have reduced this number to 63. The distinguishing characteristics of these enterovirus subgroups are outlined here.

POLIOVIRUSES. The first human enteroviruses to be recognized, polioviruses produce characteristic lesions when inoculated into the central nervous system (CNS) of primates. Clinical isolates replicate only in primates and in primate cell cultures (see Chapter 476). There are three poliovirus serotypes.

COXSACKIEVIRUSES. In contrast to polioviruses, coxsackieviruses produce paralysis and death when inoculated into suckling mice. This property was responsible for their detection and differentiation from polioviruses when they were first recovered in 1948 from the feces of two children in the village of Coxsackie, New York, who were suffering from a poliomyelitis-like paralytic illness. With the isolation of additional serotypes, it was recognized that when inoculated into suckling mice, some coxsackieviruses, designated group A coxsackieviruses, produced generalized myositis of skeletal muscles that resulted in flaccid paralysis, whereas others, designated group B coxsackieviruses, produced only focal myositis but caused an encephalitis that resulted in spastic paralysis and a generalized infection that involved the myocardium, brown fat, pancreas, and other organs. Moreover, group B coxsackieviruses could be readily propagated in primate cell cultures, whereas group A coxsackieviruses grew poorly or not at all. Twenty-three group A and six group B coxsackievirus serotypes have been identified.

ECHOVIRUSES. The use of the cell culture techniques developed by Enders and colleagues led to the recovery, from the feces of healthy children, of additional enteroviruses that produced cytopathic effects in primate cell cultures but failed to produce disease in suckling mice or in the CNS of primates. These agents, initially considered "orphan" viruses because they were unrelated to any disease, were called echoviruses (enteric cytopathic human orphan). Echoviruses have now been associated with a variety of diseases, and 31 serotypes have been identified. Most echoviruses are readily propagated in primate cell cultures.

SIMPLIFIED TAXONOMIC SCHEME. The detailed comparison of enterovirus genomes supports the validity of this classification scheme. Different serotypes within the same human enterovirus subgroup (e.g., group B coxsackieviruses) generally have 30 to 50% of their nucleotide sequences in common, whereas serotypes from different subgroups generally share less than 20% of their nucleotide sequences. About 5% of the nucleotide sequences are conserved among all human enteroviruses.

Table 389–1 ■ CLASSIFICATION OF HUMAN ENTEROVIRUSES*

ENTEROVIRUS GROUP	NUMBER OF SEROTYPES	NUMERICAL DESIGNATION	GROWTH IN PRIMATE CELL CULTURE	PATHOGENICITY FOR SUCKLING MICE	PATHOGENICITY FOR MONKEYS
Poliovirus	3	1–3	+	–	+
Coxsackievirus, group A	23	A1–22, A24†	+/–‡	+	–§
Coxsackievirus, group B	6	B1–6	+	+	–
Echovirus	31	1–9, 11–27, 29–34¶	+	–	–
Enterovirus	4	68–71**	+	Variable††	Variable‡‡

*Many enterovirus strains have been isolated that do not conform to these criteria.
†Coxsackievirus A23 has been reclassified as echovirus 9.
‡Except for a few serotypes (e.g., A7, A9, A16), primary isolates of group A coxsackieviruses grow poorly or not at all in cell culture; virus isolation requires inoculation of suckling mice.
§Coxsackievirus A7 is neurovirulent in monkeys.
¶Echovirus 10 has been reclassified as reovirus type 1; echovirus 28 has been reclassified as rhinovirus 1A.
**Hepatitis A virus, formally classified as human enterovirus 72, is now classified as a member of the Hepatovirus genus.
††Enteroviruses 70 and 71 are pathogenic for suckling mice.
‡‡Enteroviruses 70 and 71 are neurovirulent in monkeys.

Over the years, however, an increasing number of enterovirus isolates were identified that could not be subclassified unambiguously by these criteria (e.g., viruses serologically related to known echoviruses but with a host range characteristic of coxsackieviruses). Consequently it was agreed in 1970 that newly recognized human enteroviruses would be classified simply as enteroviruses and numbered sequentially, beginning with enterovirus 68. To avoid confusion with the older literature, the original classification (poliovirus, group A and group B coxsackievirus, and echovirus) has been retained for the first 63 serotypes. Since adoption of this simplified taxonomic scheme, four new human enteroviruses, enteroviruses 68 to 71, have been recognized.

ENTEROVIRUSES 68 TO 71. Enterovirus 68 was initially isolated from the throat of an infant with bronchiolitis and pneumonia. Few isolates have since been reported, and the agent is little studied. Enterovirus 69 was recovered from the feces of an asymptomatic child, and this serotype has not yet been associated with disease. Enterovirus 70 is the principal cause of acute hemorrhagic conjunctivitis, a disease first recognized in 1969, which has subsequently affected tens of millions of persons throughout the world. Enterovirus 70 has an unusually broad host range; it causes meningoencephalitis in humans and in experimentally infected monkeys, and it infects both primate and non-primate cell cultures. Genome analysis and serologic surveys raise the possibility that enterovirus 70 may be a zoonotic enterovirus that has recently extended its host range to include humans. Enterovirus 71, first recognized as the cause of an outbreak of aseptic meningitis and encephalitis in California between 1969 and 1972, is neurovirulent in monkeys and produces a myositis in suckling mice that is typical of that produced by group A coxsackieviruses. Enterovirus 71 has been recovered throughout the world in association with a variety of clinical manifestations and many fatal infections. These have included respiratory infections, aseptic meningitis, hand-foot-and-mouth disease, maculopapular exanthems, and encephalitis. In addition, enterovirus 71 has been responsible for epidemics of acute paralytic disease indistinguishable from poliomyelitis.

The discovery of the enteroviruses, as well as the origins of modern virology, were closely associated with efforts to control poliomyelitis. Poliovirus type 1 is the prototype for the enterovirus genus and for the Picornavirus family. It is one of the most extensively studied and thoroughly characterized agents of disease. Although a number of non-polio enteroviruses have also been well characterized and the genomes of many have been cloned and sequenced, much of our present understanding of enterovirus structure, replication, genetics, pathogenesis, and immunology is derived from studies carried out with wild type and vaccine strains of poliovirus.

The enteroviruses have many features in common, and they are discussed here as a group before considering the special features of individual members. Because polioviruses are the subject of Chapter 476 this discussion will be limited to the non-polio enteroviruses.

PHYSICAL AND BIOCHEMICAL CHARACTERISTICS OF ENTEROVIRUSES

The enteroviruses share with all picornaviruses certain important physical and biochemical characteristics: They are small, spherical, non-enveloped viruses approximately 30 nm in diameter. Their genome consists of a linear, single-stranded, unsegmented molecule of RNA with a molecular weight of about 2.6×10^6 daltons (approximately 7500 nucleotides) which has the same polarity as messenger RNA; that is, it is plus (+) stranded and is thus infectious. In fact, purified enterovirus RNA can initiate the synthesis of complete infectious virions in vitro in cell-free extracts from susceptible cells. The viral genome has a small virus-encoded polypeptide (VPg) covalently bound to its 5′ end and a poly (A) tail at its 3′ end. It contains a single-open reading frame of about 6620 nucleotides flanked by 5′ (740–750 nucleotides) and 3′ (70–90 nucleotides) non-translated regions. These non-translated regions are highly conserved among enteroviruses and are involved in the regulation of viral RNA translation and replication. The viral genome is tightly packed within an icosahedral protein shell or *capsid*

composed of 60 identical subunits or *protomers,* each of which has a molecular mass of 90,000 to 100,000 daltons and is itself composed of four non-identical virus-encoded polypeptides (VP1, VP2, VP3, and VP4). VP1, VP2, and VP3 are exposed on the virion surface, whereas VP4 lies buried in association with the RNA core. Like all picornaviruses, enteroviruses exhibit a unique pattern of replication in which the viral genome binds directly to host cell ribosomes at a site in the 5′ nontranslated region and is translated into a single giant *polyprotein* of about 250,000 daltons. This polyprotein is then cleaved by endogenous viral proteinases into the individual viral structural and non-structural proteins.

Enteroviruses are stable over a wide range of pH (pH 3 to 10) and retain infectivity for days at room temperature, weeks at refrigerator temperature, and indefinitely when frozen at −20° C or lower. They are readily inactivated at temperatures above 50° C, but this inactivation is inhibited by molar magnesium chloride, which greatly enhances the stability of enteroviruses at all environmental temperatures. Thus, magnesium chloride is widely used as a stabilizer for oral poliovirus vaccines.

Enteroviruses are resistant to proteolytic enzymes and to inactivation by organic solvents, deoxycholate, and various detergents that destroy lipid-containing enveloped viruses such as herpes viruses, orthomyxoviruses, and paramyxoviruses. Enteroviruses are inactivated by formaldehyde, chlorination, and ultraviolet light but are protected from inactivation by dissolved organic matter, the formation of virus aggregates, and adsorption to particulate matter. Consequently, enteroviruses may survive secondary sewage treatment and chlorination as generally practiced and are abundant in urban sewage and treated waste water. The agricultural use of treated sewage and recycled waste water may thus contaminate food and water supplies. Because sewage treatment that destroys fecal coliform bacteria does not eliminate enteroviruses, the use of fecal coliform counts to assess the sanitary quality of water is inadequate with respect to its potential for transmission of enteroviral diseases. Enteroviruses are often detectable in samples of recreational water judged acceptable on the basis of fecal coliform counts. Although person-to-person (fecal-oral) spread is the dominant mode of transmission, and water-borne outbreaks of enterovirus infection have rarely been documented, the hazard associated with the discharge of virus-laden sewage into coastal waters is demonstrated by the occurrence of shellfish-associated outbreaks of hepatitis A. Clams, mussels, and oysters are filter-feeders that concentrate virus and function as passive virus carriers. Most of the enteroviruses in sewage are associated with suspended solids, and virus adsorbed to sediment remains infectious for long periods in the marine environment. The reintroduction of specific enteroviruses into coastal populations when marine sediments are disturbed by storms, dredging, and so on, might explain the sudden occurrence of epidemics as well as the reappearance of certain enterovirus serotypes after years of absence from the human population.

EPIDEMIOLOGY

Human enteroviruses are worldwide in distributions, and humans are their only known reservoir. The prevalence of enterovirus infection varies markedly with season and climate, and with the age and socioeconomic status of the population studied. In tropical and semitropical regions, enterovirus infections are frequent throughout the year. In temperate climates, the incidence of infection is markedly increased in the summer and early fall; in Europe and North America 80 to 90% of enterovirus isolates are recovered from June through October, with peak recovery in August. Even within the United States, climatic and socioeconomic factors affect the prevalence of enterovirus infections. Enterovirus isolation rates from young children are twofold to threefold higher in southern than in northern cities, and threefold to sixfold higher in lower than in middle and upper socioeconomic districts. In developed countries, usually only one to three enterovirus serotypes are highly prevalent in a given community each year, with different serotypes prevalent in different years, and isolation rates in young children rarely exceed 10%. In developing countries with poor sanitation, a greater number of enterovirus serotypes circulate simultaneously, and isolation rates in children are regularly more than 75%, with many fecal specimens yielding three or more enterovirus serotypes.

Some enteroviruses appear to be endemic, being isolated at low frequency in the same locality each year, whereas others produce local or regional epidemics and then disappear, only to return again years later. Occasionally an enterovirus will spread worldwide, infecting tens of millions of persons and producing pandemic disease. This pattern was observed with echovirus 9 in the late 1950s and with enterovirus 70, which caused a pandemic of acute hemorrhagic conjunctivitis beginning in 1969.

With the elimination of wild-type polioviruses by immunization, non-polio enteroviruses now account for virtually all of the 10 to 30 million symptomatic enterovirus infections observed annually in the United States. Although the predominant serotype varies from year to year, certain serotypes are regularly among those most commonly detected, and the 10 most frequently detected serotypes account for 60 to 80% of all isolates identified. In recent years in the United States, these have included echoviruses 6, 7, 9, 11, and 30, and coxsackieviruses A9 and B2, B3, B4, and B5.

Enteroviruses exhibit a high rate of mutation during replication in the human gastrointestinal tract, and this can lead to the appearance of antigenic varients, as well as virus strains with altered tissue tropism and virulence. Such mutations are readily detected within days after administration of attenuated poliovirus vaccines to normal children. They have also been observed in a number of non-polio enteroviruses. Recently isolated strains of several coxsackieviruses, echoviruses, and enterovirus 70 have been found to differ in many epitopes from the corresponding prototype strains isolated more than a decade earlier, a pattern of "antigenic drift" not unlike that seen with influenza viruses. In addition, recombination between the genomes of different enterovirus serotypes can be observed in multiply infected individuals (e.g., in young children in developing countries) and in recipients of trivalent oral poliovirus vaccines. Antigenic changes and alterations in cell tropism produced by mutation and recombination may help to account for the ability of individual enterovirus serotypes to persist in nature and to cause a variety of clinical syndromes.

Transmission of human enteroviruses is chiefly by the fecal-oral route directly from person to person or through fomites; spread by respiratory secretions plays a lesser role. After infection by most serotypes, virus can be recovered from the oropharynx and intestine of both symptomatic and asymptomatic individuals, but virus is shed in greater amounts and for a longer period (a month or more) in the feces.

Young children have the highest rates of infection, and enteroviruses are most efficiently disseminated by infected children younger than 2 years of age. Spread is from child to child, and then within family groups, and is facilitated by crowding and poor hygiene. Secondary attack rates of approximately 90% for polioviruses, 75% for coxsackieviruses, and 50% for echoviruses are observed in families. Middle-class parents with children in day-care centers are at particular risk. Reared in circumstances that minimized their childhood exposure, they are likely to be susceptible to infection by many of the enteroviruses brought home from day-care centers by their asymptomatically infected toddlers.

Although the epidemiology of most enteroviruses is similar, patterns of infection with some serotypes are distinctive. Enterovirus 70 and coxsackievirus A24, etiologic agents of acute hemorrhagic conjunctivitis, are transmitted by direct inoculation of the conjunctivae by fingers and fomites contaminated with infected tears. Replication of these viruses in the alimentary tract, if it occurs at all, is limited. Coxsackievirus A21 is shed primarily from the upper respiratory tract, where it produces a rhinovirus-like illness. It is transmitted by respiratory secretions.

The incubation period for illnesses caused by enteroviruses may vary from less than 1 day to more than 3 weeks, but it is generally 2 to 7 days. It is shortest when symptoms are the direct result of virus replication at the portal of entry (e.g., acute hemorrhagic conjunctivitis caused by enterovirus 70 or coxsackievirus 24) and longest when they reflect tissue injury that involves immunopathology in target organs infected following viremia (e.g., some forms of coxsackievirus myocarditis).

PATHOGENESIS OF ENTEROVIRUS INFECTIONS

The pathogenesis of enterovirus infections is understood best for polioviruses, which have been extensively studied in experimentally infected primates and in humans infected with attenuated vaccine

strains. The pathogenesis of most non-polio enterovirus infections appears to be similar, except for the principal target organs affected.

After ingestion of fecally contaminated material, virus implants in susceptible tissues of the pharynx and distal small intestine. Whereas some replication occurs in the pharynx, the primary site of infection is the distal small intestine; virus traverses the intestinal lining cells without causing detectable cytopathology and reaches Peyer's patches in the lamina propria where significant replication occurs. Within a day or two virus spreads to regional lymph nodes, and on about the third day small quantities escape into the blood stream (the "minor viremia") and are disseminated throughout the reticuloendothelial system and to other receptor-bearing target tissues. In most cases, infection is contained at this stage by host defense mechanisms with no further progression, resulting in *asymptomatic infection*. In a minority of infected persons, replication continues in reticuloendothelial tissues producing, by about the fifth day, heavy sustained viremia (the "major viremia") that coincides with the "minor illness" of poliovirus infection (see Chapter 476) and with the "non-specific febrile illness" caused by other human enteroviruses.

The major viremia disseminates large amounts of virus to target organs, such as the spinal cord, brain, meninges, heart, and skin, where further virus replication results in inflammatory lesions and cell necrosis. In most such patients, host defense mechanisms quickly terminate the major viremia and halt virus replication in target organs; only rarely is virus replication in target organs extensive enough to be clinically manifest. Although other host defense mechanisms (e.g., macrophages, natural killer [NK] cells, interferon production) are doubtless involved, neutralizing antibodies play a major role in terminating viremia and limiting enterovirus multiplication in target tissues. Serotype-specific neutralizing antibodies may be detected in the serum within 4 or 5 days of the infection, and they generally persist for life. Evidence for the critical role of antibodies in terminating infection is provided by the occurrence of chronic persistent enterovirus infections in agammaglobulinemic children. Host defenses do not, however, terminate virus replication in the intestine, and fecal shedding continues for weeks after both symptomatic and asymptomatic enterovirus infections. Reinfection (i.e., virus excretion by a person with pre-existing homotypic antibodies) is relatively uncommon. When it occurs, infection is confined to the alimentary tract and is not associated with illness, and the duration of virus shedding is markedly reduced.

The clinical syndrome(s) caused by a given enterovirus reflect the particular target organs and tissues that it infects (i.e., its *cell tropism*). All of the determinants of cell tropism have not been elucidated, but a major factor is the presence on the cell surface of specific *receptor* molecules to which the virus attaches. Different groups of enteroviruses utilize different receptors, many of which are encoded by genes on human chromosome 19. A number of distinct receptors, each shared by multiple enterovirus serotypes, have been identified. The receptor used by all three polioviruses (PVR) and a receptor used by a subset of group A coxsackieviruses and by the majority of human rhinoviruses (ICAM-1) are both members of the immunoglobulin superfamily. A receptor used by a subset of the echoviruses (VLA-2) and another used by coxsackievirus A9 are members of the integrin family. Decay-accelerating factor (DAF), a surface glycoprotein that protects cells from complement-mediated lysis, is used as a receptor by another group of echoviruses and by enterovirus 70. All six group B coxsackieviruses share the same receptor, a 46-kd cell surface glycoprotein that is also utilized as a receptor by several human adenoviruses.

These enterovirus receptors bind to specific sites on the floor of a canyon at the junction of capsid proteins VP1 and VP3. This binding is followed by a conformational change in the enterovirus capsid that leads to the entry of the viral RNA into the cell cytoplasm. Neutralizing antibodies bind to sites on the canyon wall, blocking entry of the receptor into the canyon.

CLINICAL MANIFESTATIONS OF ENTEROVIRUS INFECTIONS

The majority of non-polio enterovirus infections (50 to 80%) are asymptomatic. Most symptomatic infections consist of *undifferen-*

Table 389–2 ■ CLINICAL MANIFESTATIONS OF NON-POLIO ENTEROVIRUS INFECTIONS*

CLINICAL SYNDROME	GROUP A COXSACKIEVIRUSES†	GROUP B COXSACKIEVIRUSES	ECHOVIRUSES	ENTEROVIRUSES
Asymptomatic infection	All serotypes	All serotypes	All serotypes	All serotypes
Undifferentiated febrile illness ("summer grippe") with or without respiratory symptoms	All serotypes	All serotypes	All serotypes	68, 70, 71
Aseptic meningitis	1, 2, 3, 4, 5, 6, 7, 8, 9, 10, 11, 14, 16, 17, 18, 22, 24	1, 2, 3, 4, 5, 6	1, 2, 3, 4, 5, 6, 7, 8, 9, 10, 11, 12, 14, 16, 17, 18, 19, 20, 21, 22, 23, 25, 30, 31, 33	70, 71
Encephalitis	2, 4, 5, 6, 7, 9, 10, 16	1, 2, 3, 4, 5	2, 3, 4, 6, 7, 9, 11, 14, 17, 18, 19, 22, 25, 30, 33	70, 71
Paralytic disease (poliomyelitis-like)	4, 5, 6, 7, 9, 10, 11, 14, 16, 21	1, 2, 3, 4, 5, 6	1, 2, 4, 6, 7, 9, 11, 14, 16, 17, 18, 19, 30	70, 71
Myopericarditis	1, 2, 4, 5, 7, 8, 9, 14, 16	1, 2, 3, 4, 5, 6	1, 2, 3, 4, 6, 7, 8, 9, 11, 14, 16, 17, 19, 22, 25, 30	
Pleurodynia	1, 2, 4, 6, 9, 10, 16	1, 2, 3, 4, 5, 6	1, 2, 3, 6, 7, 8, 9, 11, 12, 14, 16, 19, 23, 25, 30	
Herpangina	1, 2, 3, 4, 5, 6, 7, 8, 9, 10, 16, 22	1, 2, 3, 4, 5	6, 9, 11, 16, 17, 22, 25	
Hand-foot-and-mouth disease	4, 5, 7, 9, 10, 16	2, 5		71
Exanthems	2, 4, 5, 6, 7, 9, 10, 16	1, 2, 3, 4, 5	2, 4, 5, 6, 9, 11, 16, 18, 25	71
Common cold	2, 10, 21, 24	1, 2, 3, 4, 5	2, 4, 8, 9, 11, 20, 25	
Lower respiratory tract infections (broncheolitis, pneumonia)	7, 9, 16	1, 2, 3, 4, 5	4, 8, 9, 11, 12, 14, 19, 20, 21, 25, 30	68, 71
Acute hemorrhagic conjunctivitis‡	24			70
Generalized disease of the newborn	3, 9, 16	1, 2, 3, 4, 5	3, 4, 6, 7, 9, 11, 12, 14, 17, 18, 19, 20, 21, 22, 30	

*A great many enterovirus serotypes have been implicated in most of these syndromes, at least in sporadic cases. The serotypes listed are those that have been clearly and/or frequently implicated. Serotypes with the strongest association are underlined.

†Because isolation of many of the group A coxsackieviruses requires suckling mouse inoculation, they are likely to be underreported as causes of illness.

‡Conjunctivitis without hemorrhage is frequently seen in association with other manifestations in patients infected with many group A and group B coxsackieviruses and echoviruses, especially coxsackieviruses A9, A16, and B1–5 and echoviruses 2, 7, 9, 11, 16, and 30.

tiated febrile illnesses ("summer grippe"), often accompanied by upper respiratory symptoms. These are generally mild and last only a few days. This syndrome is totally non-specific; it can be caused by virtually any enterovirus serotype, as well as by members of a number of other virus families (e.g., adenoviruses, paramyxoviruses, orthomyxoviruses). The so-called characteristic enterovirus syndromes, such as aseptic meningitis, hand-foot-and-mouth disease, and pleurodynia, are, in fact, unusual manifestations of enterovirus infection. They represent the very small tip of a very large iceberg.

Some clinical syndromes are highly associated with certain enterovirus serotypes or subgroups (e.g., hand-foot-and-mouth disease with coxsackievirus A16, myopericarditis with group B coxsackieviruses), but even these associations are not specific. The same syndrome may also be caused by a number of other enterovirus serotypes. Conversely, a single enterovirus serotype may cause several different syndromes, even within the same outbreak (Table 389–2). The more important syndromes are discussed next.

CENTRAL NERVOUS SYSTEM SYNDROMES

ASEPTIC MENINGITIS. Aseptic meningitis is the most common significant illness caused by non-polio enteroviruses, and these viruses are responsible for more than 80% of the cases of aseptic meningitis in which an etiologic agent is identified. Almost every enterovirus serotype has been implicated, but those most frequently associated include coxsackieviruses A2, A4, A7, A9, A10, and B1-5, echoviruses 3, 4, 6, 9, 11, 14, 16, 17, 18, 19, 25, 30, and 33, and enteroviruses 70 and 71, all of which have been responsible for outbreaks as well as sporadic cases. Although attack rates are generally highest in children, cases also occur in adults, especially during larger outbreaks. Initial symptoms, which are typical of the undifferentiated febrile illness (e.g., fever, headache, malaise, myalgias, and sore throat), are followed, usually within a day, by signs

and symptoms of meningitis, including a more severe headache that is often retrobulbar, photophobia, meningismus, stiffness of the neck and back, and nausea and vomiting, especially in children. The illness is sometimes biphasic like poliomyelitis. The cerebrospinal fluid (CSF) is clear and under slightly increased pressure. The total cell count, which can vary from less than 10/mm³ to more than 3000/mm³, averages 50 to 500/mm³. Initially, neutrophils may predominate (although they rarely exceed 90%), but they are quickly replaced by mononuclear cells. The glucose concentration is usually normal, although levels less than 40 mg/dL are occasionally observed. The protein concentration is normal or slightly elevated, but rarely exceeds 100 mg/dL. Fever and signs of meningeal inflammation subside in 3 to 7 days, although pleocytosis may persist for an additional week or more. The great majority of children and adults recover fully without sequelae. However, enteroviral meningitis during the first year of life may, in up to 10% of affected infants, result in permanent neurologic damage, as evidenced by paresis, reduced head circumference, spasticity, and impaired intellectual function.

In some cases, especially those caused by echoviruses and enterovirus 71, meningitis may be accompanied by a rash, which, if petechial, may raise the spectre of meningococcemia. It is frequently necessary to distinguish enteroviral meningitis from partially treated bacterial meningitis. In bacterial meningitis, even when treated with appropriate antibiotics, the polymorphonuclear pleocytosis is usually more persistent, the protein concentration higher, and the glucose concentration lower. Aseptic meningitis may be caused by a number of other infectious and non-infectious agents, including mumps virus, arthropod-borne viruses, lymphocytic choriomeningitis virus (LCM), human immunodeficiency virus (HIV), herpes simplex virus, Lyme borreliosis, and leptospirosis. Differential diagnosis is aided by the distinct epidemiologic features and characteristic signs and symptoms of these other diseases.

PARALYTIC DISEASE. Paralytic disease may occur in the course of many non-polio enterovirus infections. It is similar, but generally less severe, than that caused by polioviruses. Muscle weakness is far more common than frank paralysis, and recovery is usually complete, although occasional patients suffer cranial nerve palsies or severe, sometimes fatal, bulbar involvement. Frequently implicated serotypes include coxsackieviruses A7, A9, and B2-5, echoviruses 2, 4, 6, 9, 11, and 30, and enteroviruses 70 and 71. In contrast to paralytic poliomyelitis, which in the prevaccine era occurred in epidemics, cases of paralysis associated with non-polio enteroviruses are generally sporadic. However, several non-polio enteroviruses produce paralytic disease with sufficient frequency to cause local outbreaks and epidemics. A variant of coxsackievirus A7 has caused outbreaks, as well as numerous sporadic cases of paralytic disease. In fact, coxsackievirus A7 was once thought to be a fourth serotype of poliovirus. Paralytic disease resembling poliomyelitis, with a significant incidence of residual paralysis and muscle atrophy, has been observed in patients with acute hemorrhagic conjunctivitis caused by enterovirus 70. Enterovirus 71 has caused outbreaks and epidemics of cutaneous and CNS disease in temperate regions around the world since its initial isolation in California in 1969. These have included epidemics of poliomyelitis-like paralytic disease with residual flaccid paralysis, encephalitis, and significant mortality.

ENCEPHALITIS. Encephalitis is a well-recognized but uncommon manifestation of enterovirus infection. Thus, despite their prevalence, enteroviruses account for only 10 to 20% of the cases of encephalitis in the United States of proven viral etiology. The most frequently implicated serotypes include coxsackieviruses A9, B2, and B5, echoviruses 4, 6, 9, 11, and 30, and enterovirus 71. In most cases, encephalitis complicates the course of aseptic meningitis; parenchymal involvement is indicated by the onset of confusion, coma, abnormalities of motor function, hemiparesis, vasomotor instability, cranial nerve palsies, cerebellar ataxia, and focal or generalized seizures, singly or in various combinations. Cerebral involvement is usually generalized, but focal encephalitis does occur and may be clinically indistinguishable from herpes simplex encephalitis. In fact, in one series, enteroviruses were demonstrated by brain biopsy in 13% of patients suspected of having herpes simplex encephalitis. Recovery from enteroviral encephalitis is usually complete, although neurologic sequelae and deaths do occur, especially in young infants and during enterovirus 71 epidemics.

OTHER REPORTED NEUROLOGIC COMPLICATIONS. Other neurologic complications, including Guillain-Barré syndrome, transverse myelitis, Reye's syndrome, and cerebellar ataxia, have been reported in patients with enterovirus infections. However, no clear epidemiologic or etiologic linkage to enteroviruses has been established. Given the high prevalence of asymptomatic enterovirus infections, these associations may be only coincidental.

EPIDEMIC PLEURODYNIA (BORNHOLM DISEASE)

Epidemic pleurodynia is an acute febrile viral illness characterized by the sudden onset of intense paroxysmal lower thoracic or abdominal pain. Synonyms include Bornholm disease, devil's grip, epidemic myalgia, epidemic benign dry pleurisy, and Sylvest's disease. The name, pleurodynia (pleura, side; odyne, pain) reflects the characteristic intercostal location of the pain and does not connote disease of the pleura. Pleurodynia is usually an epidemic disease, but sporadic cases do occur.

ETIOLOGY. The enteroviral etiology of epidemic pleurodynia was established in 1949. Group B coxsackieviruses, especially B3 and B5, are the principal cause. Other viruses associated with epidemic disease include echoviruses 1 and 6. Sporadic cases have also been associated with these viruses, as well as with many other enteroviruses, including coxsackieviruses A1, A2, A4, A6, A9, A10, and A16 and echoviruses 2, 3, 7, 8, 9, 11, 12, 14, 16, 19, 23, 25, and 30.

EPIDEMIOLOGY. Epidemics of pleurodynia have been recognized in Scandinavian countries for more than two centuries, but the disease was little known elsewhere until 1933, when the Danish physician Ejnar Sylvest described an epidemic on Bornholm, a Danish island in the Baltic Sea. Since then, epidemics and sporadic cases have been recognized in many parts of the world. As with other enteroviral infections, the majority of illnesses occur in summer and early fall. However, in contrast to the annual outbreaks of

enteroviral aseptic meningitis, epidemics of pleurodynia are much less frequent, generally occurring at intervals of 10 to 20 years.

Transmission is primarily from person to person, and multiple family members may be attacked almost simultaneously or in rapid succession at intervals of 2 to 5 days. In epidemics, disease is observed in children and adults of both genders. Although the peak age of incidence is somewhat older than with other enterovirus syndromes, the majority of cases occur in persons younger than 30 years of age. The incubation period is generally 2 to 5 days.

PATHOGENESIS. Pleurodynia is a disease of skeletal muscle, not of the pleura or peritoneum. As in most enteroviral diseases, infection is initiated in the alimentary tract. Skeletal muscle is probably most often infected during the primary (minor) viremia, although it may be infected later, during the major viremia in the minority of patients in whom pleurodynia is preceded by a prodromal illness. Host immune responses terminate viremia and halt virus replication in the tissues, but they also contribute to the severity of local inflammation. Histopathologic data in humans are lacking because of the benign nature of the disease, but studies in murine models of coxsackievirus infection suggest that the myositis results from a combination of direct virus-induced cytolysis and immunopathology mediated by sensitized T lymphocytes.

CLINICAL MANIFESTATIONS. Pleurodynia is characterized by the abrupt onset of fever and sharp, paroxysmal pain over the lower ribs or upper abdomen. In about 25% of patients, this is preceded by a 1- or 2-day prodrome of headache, malaise, anorexia, sore throat, and diffuse myalgia. The pain varies in intensity, but is often severe. It is accentuated, sometimes elicited, by deep breathing, coughing, and movement. The pain of pleurodynia has been described as catching (a "stitch" in the side), stabbing, knifelike, lancinating, crushing, or vise-like. In adults, the pain is primarily in muscles of the thorax, especially the intercostals. In children, abdominal muscles are more often involved. Occasionally it may involve muscles in the neck or limbs. The pain is often unilateral and is generally experienced in only one or two locations. Muscle tenderness and, occasionally, swelling can be detected at the site of pain, and characteristic paroxysms of pain can often be elicited by pressure on the affected muscles. Pleural friction rubs are uncommon, and peritonitis has generally not been observed in patients who have come to laparotomy. The level of creatine kinase in the serum may be elevated, reflecting injury to striated muscle. Other laboratory values are usually normal, although there may be mild leukopenia in some patients.

During paroxysms of severe pain, the patient lies still in bed, sweating profusely and appearing acutely ill and apprehensive. Respiration, limited by pain, is shallow, rapid, and grunting, suggesting pneumonia or pleural inflammation. A temperature of 38° C to 40° C is present at the onset of pain, reaches its peak during the episode, and resolves between paroxysms. Multiple paroxysms of pain occur, each lasting from a few minutes to several hours. The initial paroxysm is usually the most severe, and patients frequently appear relatively well between paroxysms.

The acute illness generally lasts for 2 to 6 days, with a range of 12 hours to 3 weeks. The disease is often biphasic; the initial pain and fever resolve and the patient is asymptomatic for a day or more, and then the pain and fever recur, frequently at the same site. Rarely, patients will have several recurrences over a period of several weeks or will have a late recurrence after being symptom free for a month or more.

DIFFERENTIAL DIAGNOSIS. The most useful distinguishing feature of pleurodynia is the intermittent paroxysmal character of the pain. Epidemiologic information, such as the occurrence of similar illnesses in family members or in the community, may also suggest the diagnosis. Nevertheless, depending upon the location of the pain, pleurodynia may be confused with any of a number of more serious diseases. When the pain is thoracic, these include pneumonia, pulmonary infarction, rib fracture, costochondritis, and myocardial infarction. The absence of physical and roentgenographic evidence of fracture, costochondritis, or pulmonary parenchymal disease, lack of sputum production, absence of leukocytosis, and normal electrocardiogram help to exclude these diagnoses. When the pain is abdominal, it can be difficult to differentiate pleurodynia from serious causes of acute abdominal pain, such as peritonitis, cholecystitis, appendicitis, perforated peptic ulcer, and acute intestinal obstruction. Thus, during epidemics of pleurodynia, it is common to have as many children with the disease admitted to surgical wards as to medical wards, and in one epidemic 9 of 49 of these children underwent laparotomy with normal findings before the nature of their disease was recognized. The absence of signs of peritonitis and the normal white blood cell count are helpful in excluding these diagnoses, as are normal ultrasound and roentgenographic studies. Pleurodynia may also be confused with the pain of pre-eruptive herpes zoster, herniated intervertebral disk, and renal colic. However, the pain of pre-eruptive herpes zoster is usually more constant, and the localization of pain and tenderness to the affected muscle, normal roentgenographic and neurologic examinations (except perhaps for a local area of hyperesthesia over the affected muscle), and the absence of hematuria help to exclude the other two diagnoses.

TREATMENT AND PROGNOSIS. Treatment of pleurodynia is symptomatic. Episodes of pain can usually be controlled with salicylates or other mild analgesics, but opiate analgesics are recommended for severe pain once serious intra-abdominal processes have been excluded. Heat applied to affected muscles may also be useful. Despite the tendency of the disease to relapse, patients with epidemic pleurodynia eventually recover completely. Occasionally, convalescence may be prolonged, with malaise or asthenia persisting for several months. Complications, which reflect dissemination of virus to other tissues, are relatively uncommon. When they do occur, they generally become apparent within several days after the onset of the disease. Aseptic meningitis is observed in approximately 5% of cases, and orchitis in a similar proportion of postpubertal males. Pericarditis and myocarditis are rare complications of epidemic pleurodynia.

MYOCARDITIS AND PERICARDITIS CAUSED BY ENTEROVIRUSES

Myocarditis and pericarditis have long been known to occur in association with epidemic viral diseases, including measles, mumps, rubella, varicella, influenza, poliomyelitis, and pleurodynia. Because many of these diseases have been controlled with vaccines, enteroviruses have emerged as the major recognized infectious cause of myocarditis and pericarditis in North America and Western Europe. The pathogenesis, clinical manifestations, and outcome of enteroviral infections of the heart vary markedly, depending on properties of the virus and characteristics of the host, especially age. Neonatal infections frequently result in severe myocarditis, widespread involvement of other organs, and high mortality, whereas in older children and adults, pericarditis often predominates and the disease is generally benign and self-limited. In fact, it appears that the clinical manifestations are generally so subtle that cardiac involvement during enteroviral infections is often unrecognized. However, idiopathic dilated cardiomyopathy may, in many cases, be a late sequela of both recognized and unrecognized enteroviral myocarditis.

ETIOLOGY. The evidence linking specific enteroviruses with myocarditis or pericarditis varies markedly. Proof of causation requires isolation of virus from, or demonstration of viral proteins or nucleic acids in, the myocardium, pericardium, or pericardial fluid. Except in neonatal myopericarditis, virus is rarely isolated from cardiac tissue or pericardial fluid, and detection of viral proteins has been difficult, primarily because lack of specificity has led to false-positive results. However, increasing use of endomyocardial biopsy and application of new techniques such as in situ hybridization and, especially, polymerase chain reaction (PCR) for detection and amplification of enteroviral nucleic acid has substantially improved our ability to establish the etiology in cases of myocarditis and pericarditis. Although these techniques are only now becoming widely available, their limited application has already demonstrated the presence of enteroviral RNA in 20 to 30% of myocardial specimens from patients with acute myocarditis. In most instances, however, the association of a particular enterovirus with myocarditis or pericarditis is based only on isolation of virus from noncardiac sources (e.g., feces) and/or serologic evidence of recent or concurrent enterovirus infection. These associations may often be coincidental rather than causal.

Coxsackieviruses B1 through B6, A4, and A16 and echoviruses 9, 11, and 22 have been proven to cause myopericarditis in children and adults. Coxsackieviruses A1, A2, A5, A8, A9, and A14 and echoviruses 1, 2, 3, 4, 6, 7, 8, 14, 16, 19, 25, and 30 have also been implicated. The group B coxsackieviruses are the most common etiologic agents of myocarditis and pericarditis. They appear to account for approximately 50% of sporadic cases of acute myocarditis and for virtually all cases that have occurred in epidemics. Group B coxsackieviruses also appear to account for 30% or more of sporadic cases of acute non-bacterial pericarditis.

EPIDEMIOLOGY. Enteroviral myocarditis and pericarditis occur most frequently in the summer and early fall. Idiopathic myopericarditis also peaks during this period of maximum enteroviral prevalence; this is consistent with the notion that most cases of idiopathic myopericarditis are caused by enteroviruses.

The incidence of myopericarditis during enteroviral infections depends on the virus and characteristics of the host, especially age. Myopericarditis has been the predominant manifestation in only about 3% of group B coxsackievirus infections. However, 5 to 10% of infected adults and children older than 9 who have sought medical care during coxsackievirus B5 epidemics have been found to have evidence of acute myopericarditis. The incidence of myocarditis and disseminated disease during group B coxsackievirus infection is very high during the neonatal period. It drops to a minimum (e.g., ≥ 1% of symptomatic coxsackievirus B5 infections) in children 1 to 9 years of age and then increases again in older children and adults. Thus, despite the higher frequency of enterovirus infections in younger children, enteroviral myopericarditis is primarily a disease of adolescents and young adults. At least two thirds of the cases occur in males, and the risk of cardiac involvement also appears to be increased during pregnancy and immediately post partum. Enterovirus transmission associated with myocarditis and pericarditis is the same as that of enteroviruses in general: it is primarily fecal-oral.

PATHOGENESIS. When enteroviral infections involve the heart they almost always cause an inflammatory response in both the myocardium (myocarditis) and the pericardium (pericarditis). Although one or the other usually predominates, the term myopericarditis best describes the pathologic process. The hallmark of enteroviral myopericarditis is injury to myocytes with an adjacent inflammatory infiltrate. Cardiac myosites, which bear a receptor utilized by all 6 group B coxsackieviruses, are infected and lysed. The acute process may resolve completely or progress. Healing and progression are reflected by the development of interstitial fibrosis and loss of myocytes. Enteroviral pericarditis is almost always accompanied by focal subepicardial myocarditis, which has these same pathologic characteristics.

In neonatal enteroviral myopericarditis, the relatively short incubation period, the widely disseminated infection, and the presence of high titers of virus in the heart and other organs indicate that the primary pathogenic mechanism is direct cytolytic virus infection of the tissues involved. In myopericarditis in older children and adults, the longer incubation period, the presence of virus-specific antibodies and T lymphocytes at clinical presentation, the low frequency of virus isolation from the heart and pericardial fluid, and the later occurrence of relapses all suggest that immunopathologic mechanisms are involved. Patients with myocarditis have also been found to have cytotoxic T lymphocytes that react with normal cardiac myocytes, as well as high titers of antimyocyte antibodies.

Idiopathic dilated cardiomyopathy (IDC; see Chapter 64) may in many instances represent the end stage of an immunologically mediated disease initiated by an episode of enteroviral myocarditis. This notion is supported by the development of chronic cardiomyopathy in approximately 10% of patients observed long-term after group B coxsackievirus myocarditis and by the demonstration of progressive fibrosis in such patients by serial endomyocardial biopsies. It is also supported by the demonstration of molecular mimicry of cardiac antigens by group B coxsackievirus epitopes. The question of whether enteroviruses persist in IDC and contribute directly to the chronic inflammatory process has yet to be answered. The failure to isolate enteroviruses from myocardial biopsy specimens, as well as the failure of several groups to detect enteroviral RNA with extremely sensitive nested PCR assays in cardiac tissue obtained from cases of end-stage IDC at the time of heart transplantation, suggest that enteroviruses do not persist after acute myocarditis. However, there are also reports of the detection of enteroviral RNA in cardiac tissue from patients with IDC by in situ hybridization and PCR assays, and thus the question of enteroviral persistence in IDC is still unresolved.

CLINICAL MANIFESTATIONS. Although the term *myopericarditis* best describes the pathologic process observed in enteroviral infections of the heart, *myocarditis* or *pericarditis* usually predominates, and the two syndromes are sufficiently distinct in clinical presentation and pathophysiology to warrant separate consideration. They are discussed in detail in Chapters 64 and 65.

NEONATAL MYOCARDITIS. Most severe neonatal enterovirus infections begin during the first week of life; the infant's mother has frequently been infected shortly before delivery and has transmitted the virus transplacentally or by contact during or soon after delivery without also transferring virus-specific neutralizing antibodies. However, the disease can be present at birth or may occur at any time during the first 3 months of life after a 2- to 8-day incubation period. It is usually a manifestation of generalized enteroviral disease of the newborn.

MYOCARDITIS AND PERICARDITIS IN OLDER CHILDREN AND ADULTS. In contrast to the neonate, enteroviral infections of the heart in older children and adults often present clinically as pericarditis rather than myocarditis, although the myocardium is almost always involved to some degree. Approximately 60% of older children and adults with symptomatic group B coxsackievirus-associated heart disease have a clinical diagnosis of pericarditis; approximately 40% have a clinical diagnosis of myocarditis. More than two thirds of the patients are male. See Chapters 64 and 65 for clinical features of myocarditis and pericarditis.

TREATMENT AND PROGNOSIS. Specific antiviral chemotherapy is not yet available for enterovirus infections, and treatment of neonatal myocarditis is supportive. Infants with neonatal myocarditis are unlikely to have received transplacental antibodies to the causative virus from their mothers. Thus it seems reasonable to administer human immune serum globulin, which contains high titers of neutralizing antibodies to a number of enterovirus serotypes, in an attempt to terminate viremia and limit further virus replication in infected tissues. This approach is supported by anecdotal experience, but results of randomized clinical trials involving adequate numbers of patients are not available.

Treatment of enteroviral myopericarditis in older children and adults is primarily supportive. It should include control of pain with analgesics; careful monitoring for arrhythmias, heart failure, and hemodynamic compromise; and prompt treatment of these complications if they arise. Bed rest is an important component of therapy because of clear evidence in mice with coxsackievirus B3 myocarditis that exercise markedly increases the extent of myocardial necrosis and mortality during the acute phase of the disease. Adequate oxygenation should be assured and fluid overload avoided and promptly treated if it develops. In severe cases cardiac assist devices may be lifesaving.

Corticosteroids should not be administered to patients with suspected enteroviral myocarditis or pericarditis. Their use during the acute phase of viral myocarditis has been associated with rapid clinical deterioration.

Clinical trials are underway to assess the efficacy of a class of antienteroviral drugs (capsid binding inhibitors, WIN compounds) that bind within a hydrophobic pocket under the floor of the receptor-binding canyon in the enterovirus capsid. This binding inhibits virus replication by blocking receptor attachment and/or virus penetration and uncoating. If effective, these antiviral drugs would be recommended for the early treatment of neonatal enteroviral infections and acute myopericarditis in children and adults.

The majority of children and adults with enteroviral myopericarditis recover without obvious sequelae. Acute mortality is low (0 to 5%), and deaths occur as a result of arrhythmias or congestive heart failure in patients with myocarditis; cardiac tamponade is extremely rare in enteroviral pericarditis.

Approximately 20% of patients experience one or more episodes of recurrent myopericarditis within 1 year of their initial illness and persistent electrocardiographic (ECG) abnormalities are observed in 10 to 20% of patients. Cardiomegaly persists in 5 to 10% of patients, and long-term follow-up suggests that 10% or more may develop chronic cardiomyopathy. Constrictive pericarditis rarely occurs following enteroviral pericarditis.

INSULIN DEPENDENT DIABETES MELLITUS

Epidemiologic evidence suggests a role for enteroviruses, especially group B coxsackieviruses, in the etiology of insulin-dependent diabetes mellitus (IDDM) (see Chapter 242). A number of serologic studies have found evidence of a higher frequency of coxsackievirus B infection in children with new-onset IDDM than in matched controls, and maternal enterovirus infections during pregnancy have been associated with the subsequent development of IDDM in offspring during early childhood. Moreover, enteroviral RNA has been identified by PCR in children with new-onset IDDM. Studies in mouse models suggest several potential mechanisms by which enteroviruses might be involved in the genesis of IDDM. Enteroviruses could initiate IDDM directly by infecting and destroying pancreatic β cells. Enteroviral infection could also initiate autoimmune responses to pancreatic β cells in genetically susceptible individuals, either as a consequence of direct cytolytic infection or by molecular mimicry. For example, there are homologous domains on coxsackievirus B protein 2C and a pancreatic β cell autoantigen, glutamic acid decarboxylase (GAD_{65}), that induce cross-reactive humoral and cellular immune responses. Alternatively, enterovirus infection could accelerate an already ongoing process of immunologically mediated β cell damage or precipitate the symptom of IDDM when the majority of β cells have already been destroyed. These mechanisms are not mutually exclusive, and their relative importance may vary depending on the properties of the inciting enterovirus and the age and genetic susceptibility of the host.

MUCOCUTANEOUS SYNDROMES CAUSED BY ENTEROVIRUSES

Enteroviruses are the leading cause of exanthematous disease in the United States and most other developed countries. Almost all enteroviruses can cause maculopapular eruptions, and most serotypes are occasionally responsible for petechial or papulovesicular exanthems and enanthems, as well. Moreover, a given enterovirus may cause more than one pattern of mucocutaneous disease, even within a single infected household. Consequently, except for hand-foot-and-mouth disease, which is usually caused by coxsackievirus A16 or enterovirus 71, there are no clinical or epidemiologic characteristics of any given enteroviral rash that point to a specific enterovirus as its cause.

EPIDEMIOLOGY. The epidemiology of enteroviral exanthems and enanthems is the epidemiology of enteroviral infections in general. The vast majority occur during the summer and early fall. The incidence of enanthems and exanthems in infected persons varies among different enteroviruses and even among different strains of the same enterovirus. For example, enanthems and exanthems are often seen in more than 50% of infected children during outbreaks of infection caused by echovirus 9 or coxsackievirus A16 but are rare during outbreaks caused by echovirus 6 or coxsackievirus A7. Host factors, especially age, are also important; infants and young children are more likely to develop mucocutaneous lesions, whereas other manifestations of enterovirus infection, such as aseptic meningitis, are more likely to develop in older children and adults. Thus, during outbreaks of echovirus 9 infection, rash is often seen in the majority of infected children younger than 5 years of age, but in less than 5% of infected adults, and it is not uncommon when evaluating an adult with aseptic meningitis and no rash to find that a child in the same household is convalescing from an illness characterized by a maculopapular rash. Enteroviral exanthems and enanthems occur in outbreaks and as sporadic cases. Asymptomatic infections are common and are often the source of virus for symptomatic infections. Attack rates are highest in young children, who frequently introduce the virus into households where several members may become infected simultaneously or sequentially, with an incubation period of 3 to 10 days.

PATHOGENESIS. Enteroviral lesions in the oropharyngeal mucosa and skin are manifestations of a systemic virus infection. They result from the secondary infection of endothelial cells of small vessels in the underlying lamina propria and dermis, which occurs during the viremia that regularly follows enteroviral infection and replication in the alimentary tract. Their pathogenesis thus resembles that of the mucocutaneous lesions of measles, rubella, and varicella and contrasts to the pathogenesis of the lesions of acute herpetic gingivostomatitis, human papillomavirus infections (warts), and acute hemorrhagic conjunctivitis, which are the direct result of exogenous virus infection and replication in epithelial cells at the portal of entry.

The obligatory occurrence of alimentary tract replication and viremia before mucocutaneous lesions develop explains the 3- to 10-day incubation period and the frequent occurrence of prodromal signs and symptoms. Moreover, the simultaneous dissemination of virus to a number of target organs explains the concurrent appearance of other manifestations of enterovirus infection, such as aseptic meningitis and myopericarditis.

CLINICAL MANIFESTATIONS. ENANTHEMS. The oropharyngeal mucosa is involved to some degree during most symptomatic enteroviral infections. This is usually manifest by mild pharyngitis and mucosal erythema, but it may also result in a variety of enanthems. These may consist of macules, papules, vesicles, petechiae, or ulcers, and they may occur alone or in association with exanthems and other manifestations of systemic enteroviral infection. They are often transient and frequently unrecognized, but they occasionally lead to diagnostic confusion, for example, when they resemble Koplik's spots and accompany a morbilliform exanthem in a child infected by echovirus 9. Two enanthems are sufficiently unique to warrant separate description.

Herpangina. Herpangina (*herpes,* vesicular eruption, *angina,* inflammation of the throat) is a syndrome characterized by sudden onset of fever, sore throat, pain on swallowing, and a vesicular enanthem of the posterior pharynx. It is seen primarily in children between ages 3 and 10. The disease begins abruptly, after a 3- to 10-day incubation period, with temperature ranging from 38° to 41° C, sore throat, and pain on swallowing. There may also be anorexia, vomiting, and abdominal pain. Fever tends to be greater in younger children, who may suffer febrile convulsions; older children and adults frequently complain of headache and myalgia. On examination there is pharyngeal erythema but little or no tonsillar exudate. The characteristic lesions are discrete 1- to 2-mm vesicles and ulcers surrounded by 1- to 5-mm zones of erythema. Lesions are few, averaging 4 to 5 per patient, with a range of 1 or 2 to 20. They occur most frequently on the anterior tonsillar pillars, the posterior edge of the soft palate, and the uvula, and less frequently on the tonsils, the posterior pharyngeal wall, and the posterior buccal mucosa. They begin as small papules, progress to vesicles, and ulcerate within 24 hours. The shallow ulcers, which are moderately painful, may enlarge over the next day or two to a diameter of 3 to 4 mm. Symptoms generally disappear in 3 or 4 days, but the ulcers may persist for up to a week. Most cases are mild and resolve without complications, but herpangina is occasionally associated with exanthems, aseptic meningitis, or other serious manifestations of systemic enterovirus infection.

Outbreaks of herpangina are common during the summer, and sporadic cases are also observed. Group A coxsackieviruses (A1-6, A8, A10, and A22) account for the majority of outbreaks, but outbreaks have also been caused by other enteroviruses, including coxsackievirus B1 and echoviruses 16 and 25. In addition, these viruses, as well as coxsackieviruses A7, A9, A16 and B2-5, and echoviruses 6, 9, 11, 17 and 22, have been isolated from sporadic cases.

Acute Lymphonodular Pharyngitis. Acute lymphonodular pharyngitis is a variant of herpangina that has been described in children infected with coxsackievirus A10. The lesions have the same distribution as typical cases of herpangina, but instead of evolving into vesicles and ulcers, they remain papular and are infiltrated with lymphocytes to form 2- to 3-mm gray-white nodules surrounded by narrow zones of erythema. The disease is otherwise indistinguishable from herpangina.

Hand-Foot-and-Mouth Disease. Hand-foot-and-mouth disease (vesicular stomatitis with exanthem) is a mild enteroviral disease characterized by a vesicular eruption in the mouth and over the extremities. It occurs most frequently in children younger than age 5. After an incubation period of 3 to 6 days, the disease begins with mild fever ranging from 38° to 39° C, anorexia, malaise, and, often, a sore mouth. Within 1 or 2 days vesicular lesions appear in the oral cavity, most frequently on the anterior buccal mucosa and the

tongue, but also on the labial mucosa, gingivae, and hard palate. In the majority of preschool children, but in only about 10% of infected adults, the oral lesions are accompanied by vesicular skin lesions, most often on the dorsal or lateral surfaces of the hands and feet and on the fingers and toes, but not infrequently on the palms and soles. Less often, lesions occur on the buttocks or more proximally on the extremities, and rarely on the genitalia. They are generally 3 to 7 mm in diameter and surrounded by a narrow zone of erythema. They range from 2 or 3 to 30 or more and consist of subepidermal vesicles containing a mixed inflammatory infiltrate of lymphocytes, monocytes, and neutrophils and are accompanied by acantholysis and cellular degeneration in the overlying epidermis. Hand-foot-and-mouth disease is caused most frequently by coxsackievirus A16, less frequently by enterovirus 71 and coxsackieviruses A5, A9, and A10, and occasionally by coxsackieviruses A4, A7, B2, and B5. Outbreaks and sporadic cases occur primarily in the summer and early fall. It may be accompanied by more serious manifestations, especially when caused by enterovirus 71.

EXANTHEMS. Enterovirus exanthems themselves are benign, but they are clinically important for at least three reasons: (1) They constitute direct evidence of enterovirus dissemination and thus provide a clue to the presence and the etiology of coexistent disease referable to other infected target organs, such as the heart and the CNS; (2) they represent the "tip of the iceberg" of enterovirus infection in the community; and (3) they are often confused with other infectious exanthems, some of which have more serious consequences, require specific control measures, or are amenable to specific anti-infective therapy. Because enteroviral rashes are not sufficiently distinctive to permit an etiologic diagnosis to be made on clinical grounds, laboratory diagnosis is required. However, the problem of confusing enteroviral rashes with other infectious exanthems can be approached by comparing the enterovirus rashes to the non-enterovirus rashes that they resemble.

The most common cutaneous manifestation of enterovirus infection is an erythematous maculopapular rash that appears together with fever and other manifestations of systemic infection. This is also a common manifestation of infection by a variety of other organisms, but it is more often caused by enteroviruses. Only certain enteroviruses (e.g., echovirus 9) cause this syndrome with high frequency, but almost all can produce it at least occasionally. The rash begins on the face and quickly spreads to the neck, trunk, and extremities. It consists of 1- to 3-mm erythematous macules and papules that may be discrete (*rubelliform,* resembling rubella) or confluent (*morbilliform,* resembling measles). It usually lasts for 2 to 5 days and does not itch or desquamate. Enteroviral exanthems are generally not accompanied by significant posterior cervical, suboccipital, or postauricular lymphadenopathy, but there are many exceptions. For example, posterior cervical and suboccipital lymphadenopathy similar to that seen in rubella has been observed in many children with exanthems caused by coxsackievirus A9.

Enteroviral rashes are sometimes petechial and occasionally purpuric. While this pattern is seen most frequently in echovirus 9 and coxsackievirus A9 infections, it is observed occasionally with many other enterovirus serotypes.

Vesicular exanthems are most often seen as a component of hand-foot-and-mouth disease (see earlier), but several enteroviruses, including echovirus 11 and coxsackievirus A9, may cause vesicular exanthems without an associated enanthem. The lesions resemble those caused by varicella-zoster and herpes simplex viruses. In contrast to varicella, however, vesicular rashes caused by enteroviruses are usually peripheral in distribution and consist of relatively few lesions that heal without crusting. When they are not associated with hand-foot-and-mouth disease, vesicular lesions caused by enteroviruses are often confused with insect bites or poison ivy. Echovirus 11 and several coxsackievirus serotypes have been associated with skin lesions resembling papular urticaria, lesions that usually result from insect bites.

Enteroviral rashes are generally accompanied by fever; they develop at or within 1 or 2 days of its onset. In some cases, however, the rash does not develop until the fever subsides, a pattern resembling that of *roseola infantum* (exanthem subitem), a benign sporadic disease of infants 6 to 24 months old now known to be caused by human herpesvirus 6. These roseola-like enterovirus infections are typified by the "Boston exanthem," caused by echovirus 16 and first described during an epidemic in Boston in 1951. It is characterized by fever (to 38° to 39° C) lasting 2 to 4 days, followed by defervescence and then by the appearance of a salmon-pink maculopapular rash on the face and upper chest. The rash resolves in 1 to 5 days without sequelae. Frequently, multiple cases occur sequentially in households; the illness is mild in children and more severe in adults, who often develop high fever and aseptic meningitis without rash. In addition to echovirus 16, a number of other enterovirus serotypes have occasionally been associated with roseola-like illnesses.

DIFFERENTIAL DIAGNOSIS. Herpangina is most often confused with bacterial pharyngitis or tonsillitis, or with pharyngitis caused by other viruses. Other considerations include hand-foot-and-mouth disease, primary herpes simplex virus infections, particularly acute herpetic pharyngotonsillitis, and herpes zoster involving the palate.

The vesicular lesions of hand-foot-and-mouth disease resemble those caused by herpes simplex and varicella-zoster viruses. Patients with primary herpetic gingivostomatitis usually have more toxicity, cervical lymphadenopathy, and more prominent gingivitis. Their cutaneous lesions are usually perioral but may occasionally involve a finger that has been in the mouth. Recurrent herpes simplex (herpes labialis) usually involves the vermilion border of the lip or the adjacent skin, is rarely accompanied by lesions on the hands or feet, often has a neuralgic prodome, and frequently has a history of recurrent episodes. The cutaneous lesions of varicella are generally more extensive and are centrally distributed, sparing the palms and soles. Oral lesions are far less prominent in varicella, and its prevalence in winter and spring further distinguish it from hand-foot-and-mouth disease. Aphthous stomatitis is distinguished from hand-foot-and-mouth disease by the absence of fever and other signs of systemic illness, the absence of cutaneous lesions, and often by a history of recurrence.

Maculopapular exanthems caused by enteroviruses are distinguished from measles and rubella by their summertime occurrence, the usual absence of posterior cervical, suboccipital, and postauricular lymphadenopathy, and their relatively short incubation period. The absence of significant coryza and conjunctivitis further distinguishes the typical enteroviral exanthems from measles. In addition, the probability of measles and rubella is markedly reduced in persons with a well-documented history of adequate immunization.

When enteroviral rashes are maculopapular they may be confused with drug reactions; when they are petechial they may be confused with bacterial or rickettsial rashes. When enteroviral rashes are petechial or purpuric it is impossible to rule out meningococcemia on clinical grounds alone, and when the rash is associated with aseptic meningitis (as is often the case in echovirus 9 and coxsackievirus A9 infections), it is clinically indistinguishable from meningococcal meningitis. Laboratory investigation is required, even during proven outbreaks of enteroviral disease, because concurrent enteroviral and meningococcal infections can occur.

TREATMENT AND PROGNOSIS. Enteroviral enanthems and exanthems are benign self-limited illnesses that require only symptomatic therapy for headache and sore throat. When illness mimics meningococcemia or meningococcal meningitis, antimicrobial chemotherapy should be initiated until bacterial infection is ruled out by appropriate cultures and antigen-detection assays.

RESPIRATORY TRACT DISEASE CAUSED BY ENTEROVIRUSES

A number of enteroviruses have been associated with mild upper respiratory tract illness in children and adults, especially coxsackieviruses A21, A24, and B1 through B5 and echoviruses 9 and 11, as well as 2, 4, 8, 20, and 25. Many of the enteroviruses, most notably coxsackievirus A21, produce illness that resembles the common cold, except for a higher incidence of fever. In contrast to most other enteroviruses, coxsackievirus A21 is shed primarily from the upper respiratory tract, rather than in feces. Enteroviruses have also been associated with lower respiratory tract illnesses in infants and children, although rarely in adults. These include tracheitis, bronchitis, croup, bronchiolitis, and pneumonia. Frequently implicated serotypes include coxsackieviruses A7, A9, A16, and B1 through B5; echoviruses 4, 8, 9, 11, 12, 14, 19, 20, 21, 25, and 30; and enterovirus 68. In addition, respiratory tract symptoms frequently accompany the undifferentiated febrile illnesses (summer grippe) caused by most enteroviruses. Surveillance data indicate that enteroviruses account for 2 to 10% of viral respiratory disease and that 10 to 15% of symptomatic enterovirus infections are asso-

ciated with respiratory symptoms. The respiratory illnesses caused by enteroviruses are clinically indistinguishable from similar illnesses caused by viruses more commonly considered to be respiratory tract pathogens, such as rhinoviruses, influenza viruses, parainfluenza viruses, respiratory syncytial virus, and adenoviruses. However, infections with these viruses occur most frequently during the winter, whereas enterovirus infections occur primarily in the summer and early fall. Viral respiratory tract infections are discussed in Chapters 375 through 380.

ACUTE HEMORRHAGIC CONJUNCTIVITIS

Acute hemorrhagic conjunctivitis (AHC) is an acute, highly contagious, self-limited disease of the eye characterized by sudden onset of pain, photophobia, conjunctivitis, swelling of the eyelids, and prominent subconjunctival hemorrhages. Since its first appearance in 1969, AHC has occurred in explosive epidemics throughout the world. The disease was initially nicknamed Apollo 11 disease because its appearance in Ghana coincided with the Apollo 11 moon landing.

ETIOLOGY. Enterovirus 70, a new enterovirus isolated from patients during the initial pandemic of AHC that began in Ghana in 1969, has been responsible for tens of millions of cases that have occurred in widespread epidemics during the past 25 years. A variant of coxsackievirus A24, which first appeared at about the same time as enterovirus 70, has been responsible for hundreds of thousands of cases of the disease that have occurred in a number of more circumscribed epidemics during the same period. Both viruses have been involved concurrently in some epidemics. To date, coxsackievirus A24 has been responsible for fewer cases of epidemic conjunctivitis than enterovirus 70, and it does not cause subconjunctival hemorrhages in as high a proportion of patients. Nucleic acid hybridization and serologic studies have shown that the two viruses are genetically and antigenically unrelated.

Enterovirus 70 is a most unusual enterovirus. In addition to being a naturally occurring temperature-sensitive virus that causes disease at its portal of entry and is not transmitted by the fecal-oral route, it has an exceptionally broad host range. Oligonucleotide mapping of a series of epidemic strains suggests that they all evolved from a hypothetical ancestor strain that did not exist before 1967. Serologic studies have reinforced the notion that enterovirus 70 has only recently emerged as a human pathogen; neutralizing antibodies to enterovirus 70 have generally not been found in human sera collected before 1969, even sera from elderly persons. Neutralizing antibodies to enterovirus 70 have been detected in animal sera from Japan and West Africa collected before 1969, indicating that enterovirus 70 or a very similar virus was circulating in animals before the first appearance of AHC in humans. These observations suggest that enterovirus 70 may represent a zoonotic picornavirus that extended its host range to humans, perhaps as a consequence of recombination with poliovirus type 3.

EPIDEMIOLOGY. Although mild conjunctivitis may occur as a minor manifestation of infection by many enteroviruses, especially in children, its occurrence as the major clinical manifestation of enterovirus infection was not observed until 1969, when explosive epidemics of AHC occurred in Ghana and almost simultaneously in Indonesia. Over the next 2 years the disease assumed pandemic proportions, with large epidemics occurring in many areas of Africa, Southeast Asia, the Far East, India, and Japan, and involving tens of millions of people. A number of smaller outbreaks also occurred in Europe. Scattered epidemics of AHC continued to occur in these same areas during the remainder of the decade, and the recurrence of epidemics in the same geographic areas suggests that immunity to AHC may be short-lived.

AHC is a highly contagious disease. In contrast to most enteroviral infections, it is transmitted by direct inoculation of the conjunctivae with virus-contaminated fingers or fomites (i.e., transmission is eye to finger or fomite to eye). Enterovirus 70 and the coxsackievirus A24 variant are both naturally occurring temperature-sensitive viruses that replicate optimally at 33° to 35° C, the temperature of the conjunctivae. There appears to be little or no virus replication in the alimentary tract. Virus is abundant in the conjunctivae and in the ocular exudate, from which it can be readily isolated early in infection. During epidemics, all age groups are affected; attack rates of clinical illness are highest in young adults, but infection rates are highest in children younger than 10 years of age, many of whom experience mild or inapparent infections. Infection rates are also substantially higher among the poor than in middle and upper socioeconomic groups. School-age children are most likely to introduce infection into households, where secondary attack rates are often more than 50%.

PATHOGENESIS. In contrast to other enteroviral infections, AHC is transmitted by direct inoculation of the conjunctivae with virus on contaminated fingers or fomites (e.g., ophthalmologic instruments, shared towels). Disease results from local virus replication at the portal of entry; prior replication in the alimentary tract and viremia are not required to disseminate virus to ocular tissues. This explains the unusually short incubation period, generally lasting 24 hours or less (range, 12 to 72 hours).

The major complication of AHC is poliomyelitis-like flaccid paralysis, which occurs in a very small proportion of patients with AHC caused by enterovirus 70 but apparently not at all in patients with AHC caused by coxsackievirus A24. The pathogenesis of this AHC-associated paralytic disease is not clear, but infections and destruction of motor neurons appears to reflect axonal rather than viremic spread of enterovirus 70 to the CNS.

CLINICAL MANIFESTATIONS. AHC begins with the sudden onset of eye pain and foreign body sensation, lacrimation, photophobia, blurred vision, and bulbar conjunctivitis. Signs and symptoms rapidly increase in severity with the development of palpebral conjunctivitis, conjunctival edema, swelling of the eyelids, subconjunctival hemorrhages in the bulbar conjunctivae, and a serous or seromucoid ocular discharge containing large numbers of polymorphonuclear leukocytes. The subconjunctival hemorrhages, which are the hallmark of the disease, range from discrete petechiae to confluent hemorrhages that occupy virtually the entire bulbar conjunctiva. They are present, usually within 24 hours of onset, in 70 to 90% of patients with AHC caused by enterovirus 70, but are much less frequent in AHC caused by coxsackievirus A24. AHC often begins unilaterally, but it rapidly spreads to the other eye. Signs and symptoms peak within 24 to 36 hours of onset, by which time most patients have also developed hypertrophy of palpebral follicles and papillae, preauricular lymphadenopathy, and punctate epithelial keratitis with tiny corneal erosions that are often seen only by slit-lamp examination after fluorescein staining. Clinical improvement usually begins by the second or third day, and recovery is generally complete without sequelae within 7 to 10 days. Constitutional symptoms, including headache, low-grade fever, and malaise, occur in a minority of patients.

Poliomyelitis-like motor paralysis occurs as a rare complication of AHC caused by enterovirus 70, but not in AHC caused by coxsackievirus A24. It occurs predominantly in adult males. The neurologic disease generally does not begin until 2 to 5 weeks after AHC (range, 5 to 60 days or more), and thus its relationship to the conjunctivitis is often overlooked by physicians as well as by the patients themselves. Radicular pain and paresthesia, usually accompanied by headache, fever, and malaise, are followed in 1 to 3 days by acute asymmetrical areflexic paresis or paralysis of one or more limbs. Proximal muscles are usually affected more than distal muscles and lower limbs more than upper limbs. Bulbar involvement, as evidenced by paralysis of one or more cranial nerves, is observed in one third or more of affected patients. The CSF is characterized by mononuclear pleocytosis and elevated protein concentration. Permanent paralysis and muscular atrophy occur in approximately 25% of affected patients. More than 200 cases have been reported to date, and the long interval between AHC and paralysis almost certainly accentuates underreporting. Nevertheless, in view of the many tens of millions of cases of AHC that have occurred since 1969, the incidence of this neurologic complication is probably less than 1 in 10,000 cases of AHC.

DIFFERENTIAL DIAGNOSIS. During major epidemics, AHC is unlikely to be confused with other eye infections. However, small outbreaks and sporadic cases may be mistaken for adenovirus infections, either acute follicular conjunctivitis or the more severe epidemic keratoconjunctivitis.

A variety of non-infectious conditions can produce the signs and symptoms of conjunctivitis.

TREATMENT AND PROGNOSIS. AHC almost always resolves spontaneously without sequelae, and treatment is symptomatic. Topical application of antihistamine/decongestant eye drops and cold compresses may be used to reduce discomfort. Corticosteroids, a component of many topical ophthalmic preparations, are contraindicated. Transmission of AHC can be prevented by careful handwashing, avoidance of contaminated washcloths and towels, and sterilization of all ophthalmologic instruments. These practices should be routine in eye clinics.

CHRONIC MENINGOENCEPHALITIS IN AGAMMAGLOBULINEMIC PATIENTS. Enteroviruses, primarily echoviruses, have been responsible for a syndrome of chronic meningoencephalitis in patients with inherited or acquired defects in B lymphocyte function, most often children with X-linked agammaglobulinemia. The majority of these patients also have a dermatomyositis-like syndrome, and many have chronic hepatitis. Surprisingly, despite the presence in their CSF of abundant virus, an increased number of lymphocytes, and elevated protein concentration, these patients generally exhibit few if any clinical signs of meningitis. Enteroviruses have been recovered from many sites in addition to the CSF, including cardiac and skeletal muscle. However, the pathogenesis remains to be elucidated. Some of these patients have improved after treatment with immune serum globulin containing high titers of neutralizing antibody to the responsible virus.

DIAGNOSIS

The enteroviral etiology of a disease may be suspected on clinical and epidemiologic grounds, but the multiplicity of agents capable of causing most clinical syndromes makes it impossible to establish a specific etiologic diagnosis on the basis of such information alone. Virus isolation from the site of pathology (e.g., CSF in aseptic meningitis; brain biopsy in encephalitis; myocardial tissue and pericardial fluid in myopericarditis; vesicle fluid in hand-foot-and-mouth disease; eye swabs or tears in acute hemorrhagic conjunctivitis) has been the "gold standard" of enteroviral diagnosis. Isolation of an enterovirus from the nasopharynx or feces is less definitive, because isolation of an enterovirus from these sites may be due to an intercurrent asymptomatic enterovirus infection or prolonged virus shedding from an earlier enterovirus infection and be etiologically unrelated to the observed illness.

The recent development and commercialization of methods for the detection and identification of enterovirus RNA that employ reverse transcription and amplification by polymerase chain reaction (RT-PCR) makes it possible to provide an accurate diagnosis of enterovirus infection in less than a day with a sensitivity substantial greater than virus isolation and a specificity of 100%.

Serologic testing has a very limited role in the diagnosis of enteroviral infections because of the great diversity of serotypes and the lack of a common antigen.

TREATMENT AND PREVENTION

Specific antiviral chemotherapy and chemoprophylaxis are not yet available for enterovirus infections. Treatment is symptomatic and, in severe disease, supportive. Corticosteroids, which have a deleterious effect on coxsackievirus-infected mice, should not be administered during acute enterovirus infections. Strenuous exercise and intramuscular injections, both of which may precipitate paralysis of the involved muscles during poliovirus and enterovirus 70 infections, should also be avoided during the acute, presumably viremic, phase of symptomatic enterovirus infections. Intravenous immunoglobulin (IVIG), which contains high titers of neutralizing antibodies to many enteroviruses, appears to have been useful in some agammaglobulinemic patients with chronic enteroviral meningoencephalitis. IVIG may also have a role in the treatment of enteroviral infections in other patients with severely compromised B lymphocyte function. Infants with generalized neonatal enterovirus infections are unlikely to have received transplacental antibodies to the causative virus from their mothers. Consequently it would seem reasonable to administer IVIG to such infants in an attempt to terminate their viremia and limit virus replication in infected tissues. Prophylactic IVIG should also be considered for patients with severely compromised B lymphocyte function, including bone marrow transplant recipients. Several promising inhibitors of enterovirus replication are undergoing clinical evaluation. They belong to a class of antienterovirus drugs known as capsid binding inhibitors or WIN compounds that bind within a hydrophobic pocket under the floor of the receptor-binding canyon in the enterovirus capsid. If proven effective, these drugs would be useful for the treatment of serious enteroviral diseases provided that treatment can be initiated early.

Live attenuated and inactivated poliovirus vaccines have been remarkably successful in preventing paralytic poliomyelitis (see Chapter 476). However, the large number of non-polio enterovirus serotypes, and the benign nature of most non-polio enterovirus infections, have precluded the development of vaccines for these agents. Pre-exposure administration of immune serum globulin reduces the risk of paralytic poliomyelitis. Because immune serum globulin also contains neutralizing antibodies to many non-polio enteroviruses, it would probably prevent many non-polio enteroviral diseases as well. This approach has proven effective for pre-exposure and postexposure prophylaxis of hepatitis A and probably reduces the frequency of severe enteroviral infections in agammaglobulinemic patients receiving replacement therapy. However, the benign nature of most enterovirus infections, the fact that exposures are rarely recognized (most result from contact with an asymptomatically infected person), and the relatively short half-life of exogenous immune serum globulin make this approach to prevention impractical in most situations. Nursery outbreaks of severe enteroviral disease provide an exception. The administration of IVIG to all infants in the nursery offers protection to those infants without transplancentally acquired neutralizing antibody who have not yet been infected.

Bergelson JM, Cunningham JA, Droguett G, et al: Isolation of a common receptor for coxsackie B viruses and adenoviruses 2 and 5. Science 275:1320–1323, 1997. *Isolation and characterization of the receptor for coxsackie B viruses and adenoviruses.*

Graves PM, Norris JM, Pallansch MA, et al: The role of enteroviral infections in the development of IDDM. Diabetes 46:161–168, 1997. *A critical review of the evidence linking enterovirus infections with IDDM.*

Melnick JL: Poliovirus and the other enteroviruses. *In* Evans AS, Kaslow RA (eds): Viral infections of Humans, Epidemiology and Control, 4th ed. New York, Plenum Medical Book Company, 1997, pp 583–663. *Authoritative review with emphasis on epidemiology and an extensive bibliography.*

Modlin JF: Coxsackieviruses, echoviruses, and newer enteroviruses. *In* Mandell GL, et al (eds): Principles and Practice of Infectious Diseases, 5th ed. New York, Churchill Livingstone, 1999. *Extensive review of epidemiology and clinical manifestations of non-polio enterovirus infections with excellent bibliography.*

Rotbart HA: Enteroviruses. *In* Richman DD, Whitley RJ, Hayden FG (eds): Clinical Virology. New York, Churchill Livingstone, 1997, pp 997–1023. *Authoritative review of all aspects of enterovirus infections by the leader in the application of PCR technology to enteroviral diagnosis.*

Rotbart HA (ed): Human Enterovirus Infections. Washington, DC, American Society for Microbiology, 1995, pp 1–445. *Comprehensive coverage of all aspects of enterovirus infection and disease, including diagnosis and therapy, with chapters by experts in the field.*

Rueckert RR: Picornaviridae and their replication. *In* Fields BN, et al (eds): Fields Virology, 3rd ed. New York, Lippincott-Raven Publishers, 1996. *Detailed summary of current knowledge of picornavirus structure, replication, and virus-cell interactions.*

Savoia MC, Oxman MN: Myocarditis and pericarditis. *In* Mandell GL, et al (eds): Principles and Practice of Infectious Diseases, 5th ed. New York, Churchill Livingstone, 1999. *Well-referenced review of etiology, pathogenesis, clinical manifestations, and diagnosis of myocarditis and pericarditis.*

390 VIRAL GASTROENTERITIS

Albert Z. Kapikian

DEFINITION

Viral gastroenteritis (acute infectious nonbacterial gastroenteritis, epidemic diarrhea, winter vomiting disease, sporadic infantile gastroenteritis) is a common acute infectious disease of all age groups, characterized by vomiting or watery diarrhea, or both, that may be accompanied by fever, nausea, anorexia, and malaise. It ranges from a mild, self-limited illness of short duration to life-threatening dehydration, especially in infants and young children.

The importance of this disease in a developed country was high-lighted in the Cleveland Family Study, in which infectious gastroenteritis, presumably nonbacterial, was the second most common disease experience, accounting for 16% of approximately 25,000 illnesses in a period of almost 10 years, averaging 1.5 episodes per person per year, an incidence that was remarkably similar in two family studies carried out 20 to 30 years later. In developing countries the impact of diarrheal illnesses is staggering: in the under-5-year age group, in Africa, Asia (excluding China), and Latin America, revised estimates indicate that 1 billion episodes of diarrheal illness and 3.3 million diarrhea-associated deaths occur annually, with an incidence of 2.6 episodes per child per year. In addition, diarrheal illness has been ranked first or second (to lower respiratory tract illnesses) among infectious diseases in incidence and mortality in these developing areas.

Despite major discoveries in bacteriology and parasitology in the past century, the etiology of most acute diarrheal illnesses remained elusive for many years. In the 1940s and 1950s, oral administration of bacteria-free stool filtrates from patients with acute diarrhea induced illness in volunteers, but the suspected viral etiologic agent could not be identified. In 1972, Kapikian and colleagues, employing immune electron microscopy (IEM), discovered the first virus-like particles that could be implicated as an important cause of acute gastroenteritis, in a stool suspension derived from a gastroenteritis outbreak in Norwalk, Ohio. In 1973, Bishop and associates, using electron microscopy (EM), discovered rotavirus particles in duodenal biopsies from infants and young children hospitalized with acute gastroenteritis. Rotaviruses have emerged as the major known cause of severe diarrhea of infants and young children worldwide.

ETIOLOGY (Table 390–1)

NORWALK VIRUS GROUP. The 27 nm Norwalk virus is the prototype strain of a group of fastidious, nonenveloped 27- to 40-nm particles usually named after the geographic location of the gastroenteritis outbreak from which they were first derived. They share these common characteristics: (1) they are detected in feces of patients with gastroenteritis; (2) they lack a distinctive morphologic appearance by EM; (3) they have not been grown in cell culture; (4) they possess a positive sense single-stranded RNA genome; (5) they have a buoyant density of 1:33 to 1:41 g/cm² in cesium chloride; (6) they possess a single primary virion-associated protein with a molecular weight of approximately 60,000. The Norwalk virus group includes at least four serotypes: Norwalk, Hawaii, Snow Mountain, and Taunton viruses, but a unified serotyping system is not yet available. Related viruses include the Montgomery County (MC), Southampton, Lorsdale, Desert Shield, Toronto (formerly minireovirus), Otofuke, and other small roundstructured viruses (SRSVs). Although lacking the distinctive cuplike surface indentations of the "classical" caliciviruses (calix = cup in Latin), the Norwalk virus group is now classified in a separate genus in the family Caliciviridae. Previously, other noncultivatable human enteric viruses, which were associated with gastroenteritis in children or with outbreaks in the elderly, were considered to be "classical" caliciviruses morphologically. These "classical" caliciviruses (provisionally named the "Sapporo-like" caliciviruses) have recently been classified into a genus in the Caliciviridae, that is distinct from the Norwalk virus group.

ROTAVIRUS. Rotaviruses are classified as a genus in the family Reoviridae and are etiologic agents of diarrhea in humans and in numerous animal and a few avian species. They are 70 nm in diameter, nonenveloped, and possess a distinctive double-layered capsid which surrounds a third layer, the core, that contains the genome consisting of 11 segments of double-stranded RNA (Fig. 390–1). The name rotavirus (rota = wheel) was adopted because the sharply defined circular outline of the outer capsid was reminiscent of the rim of a wheel placed on short spokes radiating from a wide hub. The virions have a density of 1.36 g/cm² in cesium chloride. Rotaviruses possess three important antigenic specificities—group, subgroup, and serotype—which are mediated by different proteins: group specificity prominently by VP6 and subgroup by VP6 alone (encoded by RNA segment 6). Serotype specificity has been defined by VP7, a glycoprotein that is one of the two

Table 390–1 ■ VIRUSES ASSOCIATED WITH ACUTE GASTROENTERITIS IN HUMANS

VIRUS	SIZE (nm)	EPIDEMIOLOGY	IMPORTANT AS A CAUSE OF HOSPITALIZATION
Rotavirus			
Group A	70	Single most important cause (viral or bacterial) of endemic severe diarrheal illness in infants and young children worldwide (in cooler months in temperate climates)	Yes
Group B	70	Outbreaks of diarrheal illness in adults and children in China	No
Group C	70	Sporadic cases and occasional outbreaks of diarrheal illness in children	No
Enteric adenovirus	70–80	Second most important viral agent of endemic diarrheal illness of infants and young children worldwide	Yes
Norwalk virus group of caliciviruses	27–32	Important cause of outbreaks of vomiting and diarrheal illness in older children and adults in families, communities, and institutions; frequently associated with ingestion of food	No
"Sapporo-like" caliciviruses ("classical")	28–40	Sporadic cases and occasional outbreaks of diarrheal illness in infants, young children, and the elderly	No
Astroviruses	28	Sporadic cases and occasional outbreaks of diarrheal illness in infants, young children, and the elderly	No

Adapted from Kapikian AZ: Viral gastroenteritis. JAMA 269:627, 1993.

major neutralization antigens located on the outer capsid (encoded by RNA segment 7, 8, or 9). The other outer capsid protein VP4, which is encoded by RNA segment 4 and which protrudes from the smooth outer surface as a series of 60 short spikes of about 12 nm in length, also induces neutralizing antibodies. VP4 is the hemagglutinin in certain strains. Antibodies to both VP4 and VP7 are associated with protection against rotavirus illness. There are ten human rotavirus serotypes as defined by VP7 (also designated as "G" [for glycoprotein] serotypes), of which only four (numbers 1, 2, 3, or 4) are of epidemiologic importance worldwide, although recently G5 and G9 serotypes have appeared in selected settings. Many human and animal rotavirus strains share VP7 serotype specificity. Most animal and human rotaviruses share the common group antigen and are thus classified as group A rotaviruses, and these are further divided into subgroups. A serotyping scheme based on neutralization of VP4 (also designated "P" [for protease sensitive]) has been developed. The VP4 genotype of various strains has also been described, based on sequence analysis and/or nucleic acid hybridization of VP4. The human rotaviruses have only relatively recently been grown efficiently in cell culture. Several human and animal rotavirus strains have been discovered that do not share the common group antigen and are classified as non–group A rotaviruses (groups B to G). In this chapter, when the term *rotavirus* is used, it is meant to describe only those rotaviruses belonging to group A, unless specified otherwise.

OTHER AGENTS. Other viral agents have been associated with gastroenteritis and include enteric adenoviruses belonging to types 40 and 41 (70 to 80 nm in diameter); astroviruses (28 to 30 nm); small, round viruses other than the Norwalk virus group (20 to 30 nm); putative coronavirus-like particles (100 to 150 nm); the pleomorphic, fringed toroviruses (100 to 140 nm); 35 nm "picobirnaviruses"; and a pestivirus antigen. The role of these viruses as etiologic agents of severe infantile diarrhea appears to be minor, with the exception of the enteric adenoviruses, which are associated with approximately 3 to 10% of the diarrheal illnesses of infants and young children requiring hospitalization. In addition, the role of these other agents in epidemic viral gastroenteritis appears to be minor. Additional systematic studies are needed to assess the role of these other agents in gastroenteritis. It should be noted that about one third to one half of gastroenteritis episodes in developed countries have yet to be associated with an etiologic agent.

EPIDEMIOLOGY

NORWALK VIRUS GROUP. The Norwalk group of viruses comprises major etiologic agents of acute nonbacterial gastroenteritis, which typically occurs as a sharp outbreak affecting adults, school-age children, and family contacts. The location or source of contamination responsible for these outbreaks includes various settings such as schools, camps and recreational areas, nursing homes, swimming facilities, cruise ships, and restaurants. For example, the

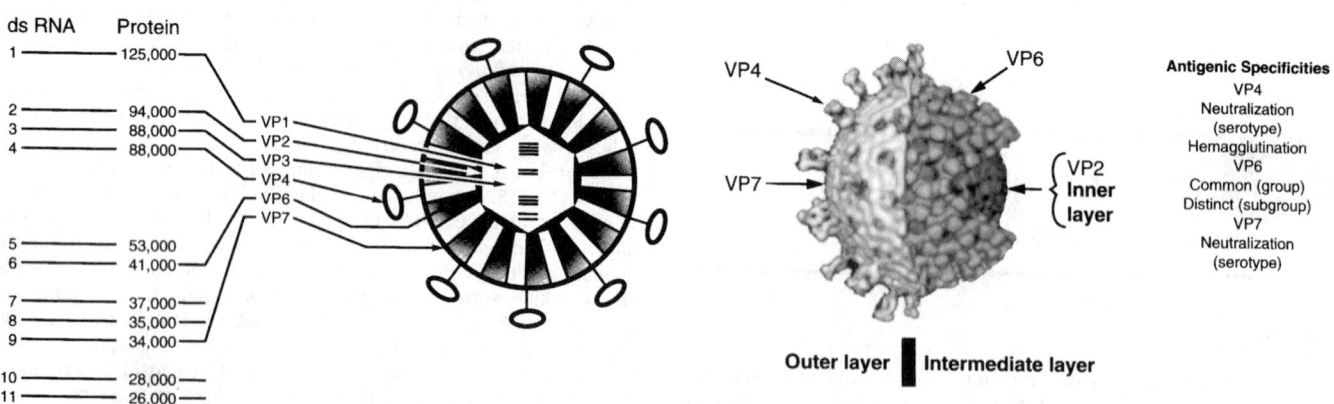

FIGURE 390–1 ■ *Left.* Schematic representation of the rotavirus double-shelled particle. *Right.* Surface representations of the three-dimensional structures of the outer layer of the complete particle (left) and a particle (right) in which the outer layer and a small triangular portion of the intermediate layer have been removed, exposing the inner layer. (Figure on *left* modified from Kapikian AZ, Chanock RM. Rotaviruses. *In* Fields BN. et al. [eds]: Fields Virology, 3rd ed. Philadelphia, Lippincott-Raven Publishers, 1996; three-dimensional figure on *right* courtesy of B.V.V. Prasad.) (From Kapikian AZ: Overview of viral gastroenteritis. *In* Chiba S, Estes MK, Nakata S, Calisher CH [eds]: Viral gastroenteritis. Arch Virol 12(suppl):7–19, 1996.)

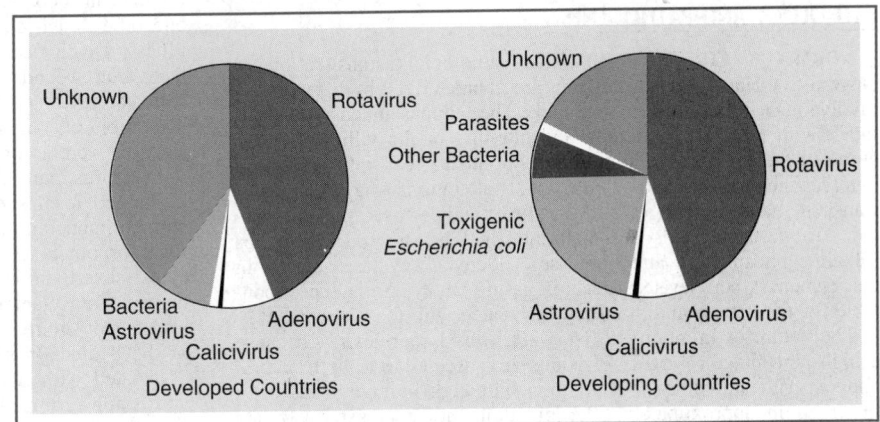

FIGURE 390-2 ■ An estimate of the role of etiologic agents in severe diarrheal illnesses requiring hospitalization of infants and young children in developed countries (*left*) and in developing countries (*right*). (From Kapikian AZ: Viral gastroenteritis. JAMA 269:627, 1993.)

Norwalk virus was derived from an outbreak in an elementary school in Norwalk, Ohio, in which 50% of the students and teachers developed gastroenteritis within a 2-day period. Norwalk virus has been linked with 42% of 74 nonbacterial gastroenteritis outbreaks investigated from 1976 to 1980 and approximately 10% of all acute gastroenteritis outbreaks. In the United States, antibody to the Norwalk virus is acquired gradually in childhood and somewhat more rapidly in the adult years, so that by age 50 years at least 50% of individuals have serum antibody. In developing countries, infants and young children acquire Norwalk antibody at an earlier age, and the virus is associated with mild gastroenteritis in this age group. Although young children do undergo infection with the Norwalk virus, the contribution of this group of agents to the etiology of severe diarrhea in this young age group appears to be quite low or infrequent.

Norwalk virus is most likely transmitted via the fecal-oral route; however, it has also been detected in vomitus. Although sporadic cases attributed to person-to-person transmission may occur, the explosive nature of outbreaks associated with the Norwalk virus group often suggests a common source of infection, such as water or food. Common-source outbreaks have been attributed to contamination of community and noncommunity public water systems, stored water on cruise ships, or recreational swimming water and to ingestion of various foods, such as tainted oysters, lettuce, potato salad, cole slaw, or cake frosting. Secondary person-to-person transmission to contacts is relatively common. The incubation period ranges from 10 to 51 hours, with a mean of 24 hours, and symptoms usually last 24 to 60 hours. Norwalk virus outbreaks occur throughout the year without a peak season.

Norwalk virus infections have been detected in individuals with travelers' diarrhea. However, this agent is not considered to be an important cause of this disease.

The Norwalk virus or related agents have recently been shown to be important agents of acute gastroenteritis in military personnel deployed to different parts of the world. The "classical" caliciviruses have been associated primarily with pediatric gastroenteritis that characteristically is not severe enough to require hospitalization.

ROTAVIRUS. Rotaviruses are the major known etiologic agents of severe diarrhea in infants and young children in most areas of the world and are usually associated with sporadic or endemic infantile gastroenteritis, which differs from epidemic viral gastroenteritis associated with the Norwalk virus group in the following characteristics: (1) it usually does not occur in sharp outbreaks; (2) it can cause severe diarrheal illness in infants and young children; (3) it does not usually cause illness in adults; and (4) the attack rate among family contacts of index cases is low, although subclinical infections occur frequently in contacts. In addition, in contrast to Norwalk virus infections, about 90% of infants and young children in both developed and developing countries experience a rotavirus infection (as determined from antibody prevalence) by 3 years of age.

The most compelling evidence for the importance of rotaviruses in severe infantile gastroenteritis has emerged from numerous cross-sectional studies in developed and developing countries. In developed countries, including the United Slates, rotaviruses are associated with approximately 35 to 52% of acute diarrheal illness requiring hospitalization of infants and young children. It is estimated that annually in the United States in infants and young children under 5 years of age, rotaviruses are responsible for 2.7 million episodes of diarrheal illness, 410,000 visits to a physician, 160,000 emergency room visits, 50,000 hospitalizations, and 20 deaths. The contribution of other enteric pathogens is consistently relatively minor. A similar pattern is also usually observed in developing countries, where rotaviruses are the most frequently detected pathogens in children younger than 2 years who have severe gastroenteritis; however, bacterial agents also play an important role in such areas. It is estimated that in developing countries 873,000 infants and young children under age 5 years die from rotavirus diarrhea each year. It should be noted that in developing countries during longitudinal studies in a community setting where all diarrheal episodes are monitored, the incidence of rotavirus diarrhea is lower than that of diarrhea caused by various other pathogens, but characteristically dehydration is more often associated with rotavirus disease than with illness caused by other agents.

In temperate climates, rotavirus gastroenteritis has a characteristic seasonal occurrence during the cooler months of the year with peak prevalence in the winter months. In tropical countries it occurs throughout the year, with less pronounced peaks. Rotavirus diarrhea occurs most frequently in children between age 6 months and 24 months. Infants younger than 6 months have the next highest frequency, although in certain studies the highest frequency is observed in this age group. The low frequency of clinical illness in neonates who undergo rotavirus infection is an unusual paradox that has not been explained, although the protective role of maternal antibodies is considered to be of prime importance. Rotavirus gastroenteritis occurs infrequently in adults, but subclinical infections are common.

Rotaviruses are likely transmitted by the fecal-oral route, although respiratory transmission remains a possibility, because there is such a rapid acquisition of serum antibody during the first 2 years of life regardless of hygienic conditions. Nosocomial rotavirus infections occur frequently. The incubation period of rotavirus illness is approximately 2 to 4 days. There are ten recognized group A human rotavirus serotypes of which those numbered 1 to 4 appear to be consistently clinically important. Group B rotavirus has been responsible for widespread outbreaks of gastroenteritis in adults in China, and a relatively small number of group C rotaviruses have been recovered from individuals with gastroenteritis in various countries. With the exception of the group B rotaviruses in China, the role of the non–group A rotaviruses in other regions of the world appears to be relatively minor at this time.

Rotavirus infections have been observed in individuals with travelers' diarrhea. However, rotaviruses are not considered to be an important cause of this illness.

An estimate of the role of rotaviruses and other microbial agents in the etiology of severe diarrhea of infants and young children is shown in Figure 390-2. In addition, a summary of key findings regarding the epidemiology and importance of various viruses associated with acute gastroenteritis is shown in Table 390-1.

PATHOLOGY AND PATHOGENESIS

NORWALK VIRUS GROUP. Histopathologic lesions following Norwalk or Hawaii virus infection are characterized by a reversible involvement of the upper jejunum. The jejunal mucosa remains intact with marked broadening and blunting of the villi and shortening of the microvilli, along with mononuclear cell infiltration and cytoplasmic vacuolization. Functional alterations may include a transient malabsorption of fat, D-xylose, and lactose and a significant decrease in levels of small intestinal brush border enzymes (alkaline phosphatase and trehalase). Adenylate cyclase activity in the jejunum is not elevated. Delay in gastric emptying may be responsible for the nausea and vomiting associated with these agents.

The nature of immunity to Norwalk virus is perplexing, because a high percentage ($\sim$ 50%) of adults are susceptible to both natural and experimental illness. In addition, although immunity has been observed in approximately 50% of adults, it appears to correlate inversely with the level of serum or local jejunal antibody.

ROTAVIRUS. The major histopathologic lesions are characterized by reversible involvement of the proximal small intestine. The mucosa remains intact, with shortening of the villi, mononuclear cell infiltration in the lamina propria, distended cisternae of the endoplasmic reticulum, mitochondrial swelling, and sparse, irregular microvilli. Functional alterations may include impaired D-xylose absorption and depressed levels of disaccharidases (maltase, sucrase, and lactase). A nonstructural protein NSP4 with enterotoxin activity (encoded by gene 10) has recently been shown to induce diarrhea in a mouse model by its effect on calcium regulation. Its role in humans awaits further study.

The mechanism of immunity to human rotaviruses is not clear. Although significant levels of serum antibodies correlate with resistance to illness, the role of local intestinal immunity has not been evaluated as extensively. Animal studies indicate that antibody in the small intestine is the major determinant of resistance to illness. A high rate of subclinical infection in neonates is well documented and may be related to passively acquired maternal antibody, host factors, or naturally attenuated rotaviruses that are able to persist in newborn nurseries.

CLINICAL MANIFESTATIONS

NORWALK VIRUS GROUP. Clinical characteristics of illness induced by the Norwalk group of viruses include nausea, vomiting, diarrhea, anorexia, or abdominal discomfort, or any combination. Accompanying clinical manifestations may also include myalgias, low-grade fever, headache, and chills. In children, vomiting occurs more often than diarrhea, whereas in adults the opposite is observed. The onset of illness may be abrupt, marked by vomiting, diarrhea, or both. The illness is usually mild and lasts about 24 to 60 hours. However, severe gastroenteritis has been observed in middle-aged patients and has contributed to the death of elderly, debilitated individuals. The stools are characteristically loose and watery; blood, mucus, and leukocytes are not typically present. A transient decrease in the T, B, and null cell lymphocyte subpopulations has been observed. The role of Norwalk virus in the etiology of gastroenteritis in human immunodeficiency virus (HIV)-positive individuals appears to be similar to that observed in non-HIV infected controls.

ROTAVIRUS. Rotavirus infection can produce a variety of responses in infants and young children, ranging from subclinical infection and mild diarrhea to a severe and occasionally fatal dehydrating illness. Clinical characteristics include vomiting, diarrhea, abdominal discomfort, or fever, or any combination. Fever and vomiting often develop before the diarrhea. Accompanying clinical manifestations may include dehydration, irritability, and pharyngeal or tympanic membrane erythema. In hospitalized patients, the mean duration of confinement is 4 days, with a range of 2 to 14 days. The stools are characteristically loose and watery and only infrequently contain blood or leukocytes.

Although rotaviruses can cause severe or fatal dehydrating illnesses in developing countries, deaths have also been documented in developed countries. In a study in Canada, rotavirus gastroenteritis was implicated in the deaths of 21 children 4 to 30 months old (mean, 11 months) over a period of about 5 years. Twenty children

were dead or moribund on arrival at hospital, and one child was infected nosocomially. With the exception of the latter patient and one other, each child was considered healthy prior to the rotaviral illness. Death occurred within 1 to 3 days of onset of symptoms. Dehydration and electrolyte imbalance leading to cardiac arrest were believed to be the major cause of death in 16 patients; aspiration of vomitus was the cause of death in 3 patients; and seizures were a contributing factor in the remaining 2 patients.

Rotavirus can also induce chronic symptomatic diarrhea with prolonged fecal shedding of the virus and antigenemia in patients with primary immunodeficiency diseases. Infections with rotaviruses or other viral and bacterial enteric pathogens may be especially severe in individuals who are immunosuppressed for bone marrow transplantation. In one study, 8 of 78 such patients (average age of entire group, 20.5 years) shed rotavirus in stools and 5 of the 8 died. In addition, nosocomial rotavirus infection has been associated with severe diarrhea in adult renal transplant recipients; and a non–group A rotavirus was associated with severe gastroenteritis in an 8-year-old bone marrow transplant patient. Rotavirus infections have also been persistent and severe in children with severe combined immunodeficiency. Rotavirus infections have also been associated with necrotizing enterocolitis and hemorrhagic gastroenteritis in neonates.

Outbreaks of rotavirus gastroenteritis have occurred in elderly individuals in nursing homes with several fatalities.

Rotaviruses do not appear to have an important role as etiologic agents of acute diarrhea in HIV-positive adults.

DIAGNOSIS

NORWALK VIRUS GROUP. Because a specific diagnosis of infection with this group cannot be made by clinical observation, the diagnosis must be made in the laboratory and relies on detection of virus in the stool or a serologic response to a viral-specific antigen. These tests include IEM (for the entire group) and by enzyme-linked immunosorbent assay (ELISA) when stool is available for antigen. Recent molecular biologic advances (notably the cloning and sequencing of Norwalk and related viruses and expression of their capsids in baculovirus, which resulted in a ready source of recombinant virus-like particles) have led to a proliferation of diagnostic assays such as PCR-based and ELISA procedures for research use. By IEM for the Norwalk virus, shedding is maximal at or shortly after onset of illness and minimal at 72 hours following onset. However, by PCR the peak of virus shedding in volunteers was 25 to 72 hours after challenge, with virus detection for at least 7 days. The characteristic absence of fecal leukocytes in Norwalk infection may be helpful for differentiation from *Shigella* or *Salmonella* enteritis.

Although a specific clinical diagnosis of infection with Norwalk virus cannot be made in the individual patient, a tentative diagnosis of infection can be made during an outbreak if certain criteria are met: (1) bacterial or parasitic pathogens are not detected; (2) vomiting is present in at least 50% of cases; (3) incubation period is 24 to 48 hours; and (4) mean or median duration of illness is 12 to 60 hours.

ROTAVIRUS. The clinical manifestations of rotavirus gastroenteritis are not distinctive enough to enable diagnosis. Thus, diagnosis requires either detection of the virus or demonstration of a significant serologic response to rotavirus in paired acute and convalescent sera. The epidemiologic pattern relating to the age of the patient, the temporal occurrence of illness, and the signs and symptoms of illness, however, may suggest the diagnosis. In addition, the usual absence of fecal leukocytes in rotavirus diarrhea may help in early differentiation from *Shigella* or *Salmonella* enteritis.

By conventional assays such as EM and ELISA, stools obtained from the first to fourth day of illness are optimal for detecting rotavirus, but virus shedding may continue up to 21 days. Virus is characteristically present in stools during the early phase of diarrhea, but diarrhea may continue for 2 to 3 days after virus shedding has ceased. However, by a recently developed PCR-based assay, the duration of virus shedding ranged from 4 to 57 days after onset of diarrhea, with 30% of the children shedding virus for 25 ot 57 days.

More than 25 assays have been developed to detect rotavirus in stools. The most rapid method is still direct EM because in negatively stained preparations these agents have a distinctive morphologic appearance and are present in large amounts. The non–group A rotaviruses, which do not share the common group antigen, can also be detected by EM. However, an electron microscope may not be readily available, and its use may be impractical when evaluating a large number of specimens. Thus, other rapid and highly effective methods for virus detection have been developed, including ELISA, counterimmunoelectroosmophoresis (CIEOP), radioimmunoassay (RIA), reverse passive hemagglutination assay (RPHA), latex agglutination (LA), RNA electrophoresis (electropherotyping), dot hybridization, and recently PCR. Commercial kits are now available for the ELISA, and LA, assays. A popular method is the confirmatory ELISA because it is simple to perform, is sensitive, does not require specialized equipment, and has a negative serum antibody control for detecting nonspecific reactions. An ELISA using monoclonal anti-VP7 antibody is also available. The non–group A rotaviruses cannot be detected by these assays, because they lack the common group antigen; however, an ELISA for group B and group C rotaviruses has been developed. Diagnosis of group A rotavirus infection by growth in cell cultures is not practical. Serotyping by ELISA or PCR remains a research tool.

There are many methods for measuring a serologic response to rotavirus infection, including IEM, complement fixation (CF), immunofluorescence, immune adherence hemagglutination assay, ELISA, neutralization, hemagglutination-inhibition (HI), inhibition of RPHA, and a competition solid-phase immunoassay that measures epitope-specific immune responses to individual rotavirus serotypes. Complement fixation is an efficient assay for detecting a serologic response to rotavirus in patients age 6 to 24 months but is not as effective in adults or infants younger than 6 months.

Detection of rotavirus or demonstration of a serologic response does not necessarily establish an etiologic association with the patient's illness, especially in newborns and adults, who frequently undergo subclinical infection.

TREATMENT

NORWALK VIRUS GROUP. Because the Norwalk group of viruses characteristically causes mild, self-limited gastroenteritis, replacement of fluid and electrolyte loss with orally administered isotonic fluids is usually sufficient. However, if severe vomiting or diarrhea occurs, parenteral fluid replacement may be necessary. Oral administration of bismuth subsalicylate significantly reduces the severity of abdominal cramps, with a decrease in the median duration of gastrointestinal symptoms from 20 hours to 14 hours. However, the number, weight, and water content of stools and the level of virus excretion are not affected significantly. The American Academy of Pediatrics did not recommend the use of bismuth subsalicylate for treatment of acute diarrhea of infants and young children because of concerns about toxic effects.

ROTAVIRUS. Because rotavirus gastroenteritis may lead to severe dehydration in infants and young children, the early replacement of fluids and electrolytes is essential. Intravenous fluids have been used effectively in treating dehydration. However, in many parts of the world where such treatment is not feasible, efforts have been made to evaluate the effectiveness of an oral rehydration salts (ORS) solution. In a double-blind study comparing ORS with intravenous fluids in children with rotavirus gastroenteritis, ORS solution containing either glucose (20 g/L) or sucrose (40 g/L) plus electrolytes was found to be as effective as intravenous therapy for rehydration. Glucose electrolyte solutions are recommended for optimal results. The recommended World Health Organization (WHO) ORS solution is made by adding the following to 1 L of water: sodium chloride, 3.5 g; trisodium citrate, dihydrate, 2.9 g; potassium chloride, 1.5 g; and glucose, anhydrous, 20 g. Sodium bicarbonate, 2.5 g, may be substituted for the trisodium citrate, dihydrate. The efficacy of oral glucose-electrolyte solutions that contained either 90 mmol of sodium per liter (as in the WHO formula above) or 50 mmol of sodium per liter, plus additional electrolytes, was examined in well-nourished ambulatory or hospitalized children with mild or moderate dehydrating diarrheal illnesses of varied etiology (including rotavirus but excluding cholera), and each was found to be safe and effective. After the initial calculated fluid deficit is corrected by the ORS, water or fluids without added electrolytes, such as breast milk or some other form of low-solute feeding, should be given orally in addition to the ORS solution, to replace both continued diarrheal fluid and electrolyte losses and to provide normal daily fluid requirements. If oral rehydration fails to correct the fluid and electrolyte loss or if the patient is severely dehydrated or in a state of shock or near shock, or has depressed consciousness (see below), intravenous therapy must be given immediately.

In recent studies, rice-based ORS solutions were also found to be effective in rehydrating infants and young children hospitalized with mild to moderate dehydration caused by diarrhea associated with various pathogens, including rotavirus. Both glucose-based or rice-based ORS solutions were effective in rehydration and maintenance therapy. Oral rehydration therapy should not be given to infants and younger children with depressed consciousness because of the possibility of fluid aspiration.

With regard to antidiarrheal compounds for treatment of acute diarrhea of infants and young children, the American Academy of Pediatrics did not recommend the use of loperamide, anticholinergic agents, bismuth subsalicylate, adsorbents or lactobacillus-containing compounds; in addition, they stated that the use of opiates as well as opiate and atropine combination drugs for the treatment of acute diarrhea in infants and young children was contraindicated.

In a limited study, chronic rotavirus illness in immunodeficient children has been treated effectively by oral feeding of pooled human milk that contained rotavirus antibody. Oral administration of preparations containing rotavirus antibody has produced conflicting results regarding their efficacy for treatment of normal children during episodes of rotavirus gastroenteritis.

PREVENTION

NORWALK VIRUS GROUP. There are no specific methods for preventing illness by the Norwalk virus group. However, because of the extremely infectious nature of these agents, careful handwashing and proper disposal of contaminated material should minimize transmission. In addition, hygienic preparation of food and measures to decrease contamination of drinking water or swimming facilities should limit the frequency of Norwalk virus outbreaks. Active immunization against this group of viruses is not yet feasible.

ROTAVIRUS. Epidemiologic studies indicate the global need for a rotavirus vaccine to prevent rotavirus diarrhea in the first 2 years of life, when illness is most severe. Recent efforts have focused on developing a live, attenuated oral vaccine that is effective against all serotypes. A promising initial strategy involved the "Jennerian" approach, in which a related rotavirus from a nonhuman host (a bovine or rhesus rotavirus strain) was used as the immunizing agent. Efficacy trials of several such candidate rotavirus vaccines gave variable results and it soon became apparent that these vaccines did not induce satisfactory heterotypic immunity in infants not primed by previous rotavirus infection. The rhesus rotavirus vaccine (a VP7 serotype 3 strain) induced protection against rotavirus diarrhea in the 1- to 4-month age group in a study in which VP7 serotype 3 was predominant, but it failed in other studies to protect unprimed infants against illnesses caused by other than serotype 3 rotaviruses. Thus, the Jennerian approach was modified with the goal being a quadrivalent vaccine composed of rhesus rotavirus (serotype 3) and three reassortant rotaviruses each containing 10 rhesus rotavirus genes and a single human rotavirus gene that encodes VP7 serotype 1, 2, or 4 specificity (Fig. 390–3; Color Plate 9H). Field trials of the quadrivalent vaccine in infants and young children have shown that three oral doses of live, attenuated quadrivalent (or tetravalent) rotavirus vaccine is highly effective in preventing severe rotavirus diarrhea, achieving an efficacy of 80% in a U.S. multicenter trial (100% against dehydration), 91% in Finland (97% against dehydration and 100% against hospitalization), 88% in Venezuela (75% against dehydration) and 69% in Native Americans (too few cases of dehydration to evaluate). Efficacy against any rotavirus diarrhea ranged from 48 to 68%, which is consistent with the goal of the rotavirus vaccine to prevent severe (but not any) rotavirus diarrhea, because reinfections also occur commonly following natural rotavirus infection. In these trials, up to 29% of vaccinees developed a characteristically low-grade transient fever of 38.1°C or greater (rectal) within 5 days of the first dose of vaccine. Furthermore, in June 1998, the U.S. Advisory Committee on Immunization Practices recommended rou-

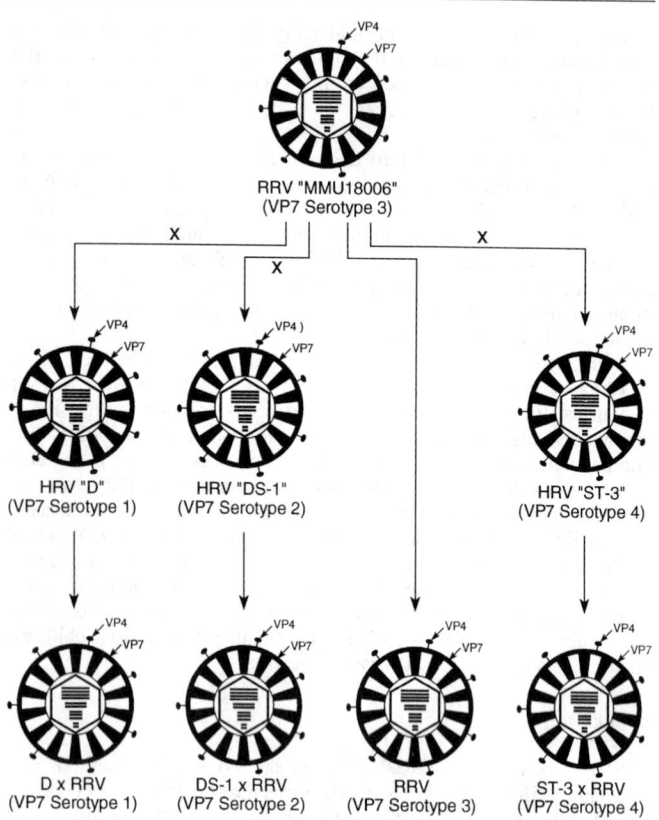

FIGURE 390-3 ■ Production of a rhesus rotavirus (RRV), human rotavirus (HRV) × RRV reassortant, quadrivalent vaccine with VP7 serotype 1, 2, 3, and 4 specificity. (From Kapikian AZ, Hoshino Y, Chanock RM, Pérez-Schael I: Efficacy of a quadrivalent rhesus rotavirus-based human rotavirus vaccine aimed at preventing severe diarrhea in infants and young children. J Infect Dis 174[suppl1]:S65–S72, 1996.)

tine immunization with three oral doses at 2, 4, and 6 months of age. Subsequently, in August 1998, this quadrivalent rotavirus vaccine (RotaShield) was licensed by the U.S. Food and Drug Administration for the immunization of infants at 2, 4, and 6 months of age. Later, in November 1998, the American Academy of Pediatrics recommended this vaccine for infants at 2, 4, and 6 months of age. More recently, in May 1999, the European Commission issued marketing authorization for the rotavirus vaccine (RotaShield). This approval covers all 15 member countries of the European Community, including Austria, Belgium, Denmark, Finland, France, Ireland, Italy, Luxembourg, Germany, Greece, the Netherlands, Portugal, Spain, Sweden, and the United Kingdom.

Breast milk is generally considered to confer some degree of protection against clinically significant rotavirus diarrhea during infancy. The prophylactic oral administration of human serum globulin containing rotavirus antibody to low-birth-weight neonates provides significant protection against rotavirus diarrhea. In addition, passive oral immunization of infants and young children with bovine colostrum that contained antibodies to human rotavirus was effective in preventing rotavirus illness when compared with a control group.

American Academy of Pediatrics Committee on Infectious Diseases: Prevention of rotavirus disease: Guidelines for use of rotavirus vaccine. Pediatrics 102:1483–1491, 1998. *An up-to-date overview of the epidemiology, clinical characteristics, immunology, treatment, and prevention of rotavirus with special emphasis on their recommendations for use of the newly licensed rotavirus vaccine. Contains key references.*

Barnes GL, Uren E, Stevens KB, Bishop RF: Etiology of acute gastroenteritis in hospitalized children in Melbourne, Australia, from April 1980 to March 1993. J Clin Microbiol 36:133–138, 1998. *A comprehensive 13-year survey of infants and children admitted to the hospital with acute gastroenteritis. The importance of rotavirus is clearly shown.*

Chiba S, Estes MK, Nakata S, Calisher CH (eds): Viral gastroenteritis. Arch Virol 12(suppl):1–311, 1996. *A comprehensive volume presenting the proceedings of an international symposium. It encompasses the major advances in etiology, molecular biology, epidemiology, and prevention of viral gastroenteritis.*

Kapikian AZ, Estes MK, Chanock RM: Norwalk group of viruses. In Fields BN, et al (eds): Virology, 3rd ed. Philadelphia, Lippincott-Raven, 1996, pp. 783–810. *A detailed review of the Norwalk group of viruses from a virologic, epidemiologic, and clinical point of view, 277 references.*

Kapikian AZ, Chanock RM: Rotaviruses, In Fields BN, et al (eds): Virology, 3rd ed. Philadelphia, Lippincott-Raven, 1996, pp 1657–1708. *A detailed review of rotaviruses from a virologic, epidemiologic, and clinical point of view (993 references).*

Provisional Committee on Quality Improvement, Subcommittee on Acute Gastroenteritis: Practice parameter: The management of acute gastroenteritis in young children. Pediatrics 97: 424–433, 1996. *A comprehensive examination of issues in the management of acute gastroenteritis from the American Academy of Pediatrics. Important reading for the clinician.*

HEMORRHAGIC FEVER VIRUSES

391 INTRODUCTION TO HEMORRHAGIC FEVER VIRUSES

Robert E. Shope

The viral hemorrhagic fevers encompass syndromes that vary from febrile hemorrhagic disease with capillary fragility to acute severe shock leading rapidly to death. The causative agents include arthropod-borne and rodent-associated viruses. The rodent-associated viruses do not require an arthropod vector but are transmitted directly to vertebrates by aerosol spread or contact with infected excreta or body secretions of the rodent. The reservoir and natural mode of transmission for the African hemorrhagic fever viruses, Marburg and Ebola, are not known.

At least 18 viruses cause human hemorrhagic fevers (see Table 391–1). They are in the families Flaviviridae, Bunyaviridae, Arenaviridae, and Filoviridae. All contain RNA, and nearly all are zoonoses.

The hemorrhagic fevers form a special group of diseases characterized by viral replication in lymphoid cells, followed by fever and myalgia and leading to hemorrhagic manifestations and hypovolemic shock. The basic physiologic defect in most is capillary leakage. In some, such as yellow fever, hepatocellular damage is prominent. In others, such as hantavirus disease, renal or pulmonary lesions are striking. The mortality rates may be high, and the pathogenesis is poorly understood. Disseminated intravascular coag-

ulopathy (DIC) is a feature in some cases, but probably not all. Antigen-antibody complexes may lead to release of mediators of shock in some cases, and direct effects of viral replication on capillary permeability in some have not been ruled out. It is important to understand the pathogenetic mechanism to manage these infections, but our knowledge is sparse at present.

Control can be achieved by interrupting the cycle of infection, including peridomestic rodent control (Bolivian hemorrhagic fever) and, for arboviruses, vaccination of reservoir animals (Rift Valley fever), vector control, and education on methods to avoid the vector (dengue) or rodent reservoir (hantavirus pulmonary syndrome). Vaccines are available or are under development for some of the agents, such as Rift Valley fever, yellow fever, dengue, and Junin viruses. For others such as Lassa virus, we now have an antiviral drug, and for still another (Junin) pre-exposure and postexposure protection is afforded by human immune plasma.

391.1 Yellow Fever

DEFINITION. Yellow fever is an acute viral disease caused by infection with yellow fever virus. The disease is exemplary of the viral hemorrhagic fevers described in the following sections (see Table 391–1). The infection is often subclinical, but it may lead to disease whose severity varies from mild and self-limited to fulminant with a fatal outcome. Classic yellow fever is characterized by sudden onset, moderately high fever, nausea, bradycardia, prostration, vomiting of altered blood, jaundice, oliguria, and albuminuria. Natural cycles of the infection occur periodically in mosquitoes and

Table 391–1 ■ CLINICAL PARAMETERS OF VIRAL HEMORRHAGIC FEVERS

DISEASE	VIRAL AGENT	INCUBATION PERIOD (DAYS)	CLINICAL SYNDROMES					CASE-FATALITY RATE (%)
			Hemorrhage	Hepatitis	Encephalitis	Nephropathy	ARDS*	
Yellow fever	Yellow fever	3–6	Major	Major	Absent	Moderate	Absent	2–20
Dengue hemorrhagic fever	Dengue 1–4	5–8	Moderate	Moderate	Absent	Absent	Absent	2–10
Rift Valley fever	Rift Valley fever	3–6	Major	Major	Moderate	Absent	Absent	0.2–10
Crimean-Congo hemorrhagic fever	Crimean-Congo hemorrhagic fever	2–9	Major	Major	Minor	Absent	Absent	30–50
Kyasanur Forest disease	Kyasanur Forest disease	3–8	Minor	Minor	Moderate	Absent	Absent	5–10
Omsk hemorrhagic fever	Omsk hemorrhagic fever	3–8	Minor	Minor	Moderate	Absent	Absent	0.4–2.5
Hemorrhagic fever with renal syndrome	Hantaan, Puumala, Dobrava, Seoul	2–42	Moderate	Rare	Minor	Major	Major	2–5
Hantavirus pulmonary syndrome	Sin Nombre	12–16	Minor	Minor	Absent	Minor	Major	40–50
Venezuelan hemorrhagic fever	Guanarito	7–14	Moderate	Rare	Rare	Minor	Absent	33
Brazilian hemorrhagic fever	Sabiá	8–12	Major	Minor	Minor	Minor	Absent	33
Argentine hemorrhagic fever	Junin	10–14	Minor	Rare	Moderate	Minor	Absent	10–20
Bolivian hemorrhagic fever	Machupo	7–14	Moderate	Rare	Moderate	Minor	Absent	15–30
Lassa fever	Lassa	3–16	Minor	Major	Minor	Minor	Absent	15
African hemorrhagic fever	Marburg	3–9	Major	Major	Minor	Absent	Absent	20–30
African hemorrhagic fever	Ebola	3–18	Major	Major	Minor	Absent	Absent	53–88

*Adult respiratory distress syndrome.

primates of tropical South America as far north as Panama and in tropical west, central, and east Africa.

ETIOLOGY. Yellow fever virus is in the genus *Flavivirus* of the family Flaviviridae. Members of the family are single-stranded, negative-sense RNA viruses, spherical and approximately 40 nm in diameter. Particles form in the cytoplasm in close association with endoplasmic reticulum. They contain a lipid envelope and replicate in both arthropod and vertebrate cells. Other members of the Flaviviridae, including dengue, West Nile, and St. Louis encephalitis, cross-react with yellow fever virus in serologic tests and may confound the diagnosis. Minor antigenic differences exist between strains of yellow fever virus from Africa and South America, and among strains from different regions of Africa; however, the 17D yellow fever vaccine protects against all strains. The virus can be isolated in mosquitoes, arthropod, and vertebrate tissue cultures; baby mice; and several monkey species. Rhesus monkeys regularly succumb following experimental inoculation, and their disease mimics severe human disease.

EPIDEMIOLOGY. Two epidemiologic types of yellow fever are distinguished: the urban and the sylvan (jungle) forms. Urban yellow fever is transmitted by *Aedes aegypti* mosquitoes from person to person, whereas sylvan yellow fever is maintained in a forest cycle of monkeys and forest-canopy mosquitoes; humans are infected when they enter the forest or when infected monkeys exit to establish transmission in mosquitoes at the forest fringe. The two types do not differ clinically.

A. aegypti is a domiciliary mosquito that breeds in abandoned tires, jars, cans, water-storage containers, roof catchments, and drains in and around houses. Urban yellow fever was a major killer until the early 1900s, when mosquito control in Havana, Rio de Janeiro, Guayaquil, and other large urban centers eliminated the disease. The last recorded urban case in the Americas was in Trinidad in 1954. *A. aegypti* continues to be prevalent in African cities, and *A. aegypti*–transmitted outbreaks still occur there. Major epidemics were recorded in Ethiopia, 1960–1962; Nigeria, 1969; Senegal, 1965 and 1979; Gambia, 1978; Ghana and Burkina Faso, 1983; and Kenya, 1993. In 1986, an epidemic involving at least 3000 persons occurred in Nigeria, in Benue and Cross River States, and it extended into Oyo and Niger States in 1987. An estimated 39,000 cases, with 8400 deaths, were recorded.

Yellow fever virus in Africa is transmitted by *A. aegypti* not only in the cities but also in semirural areas. In addition, some African epidemics are maintained by other *Aedes* species, such as *A. bromeliae* and the tree hole–breeding *A. africanus, A. luteocephalus,* and *A. furcifer-taylori,* which transmit the virus in savannah and the transition forest-savannah zones of west Africa.

Sylvan yellow fever was recognized initially in Brazil in 1932. After urban yellow fever had been controlled in the Americas, sporadic cases continued to occur in persons exposed to mosquitoes in the jungles of South America and Africa. This sylvan form is maintained in tropical America by *Haemagogus* mosquitoes and forest primates, and sometimes by other sylvan animals. Evidence favors the hypothesis that the virus moves through the forest, cycling in one place until the monkeys are immune, then dying out and moving to areas where susceptible monkeys live. People entering the forest are at risk. Sylvan yellow fever extends periodically outside the enzootic zone into forests such as those in Panama and Central America. The virus can be maintained over dry periods by transovarial transmission in mosquitoes, although it remains to be shown whether maintenance in mosquito eggs is more than a temporary mechanism.

The sylvan cycle in Africa is more complicated than in the Americas; in tropical Africa, the virus cycles between *A. africanus* and monkeys. Another African mosquito, *A. bromeliae,* which feeds on both humans and monkeys, serves in some areas as a link between primates in the deep forest and people in the African villages.

A. aegypti was once carried on sailing ships between tropical ports and into temperate-zone cities. Modern oceangoing ships no longer harbor mosquito-breeding sites, but the mosquito continues to travel by small boats, airplanes, and cars, and especially in the form of dried eggs transported by used tires. Cities such as Rio de

Janeiro, which were once freed of the mosquito, are now reinfested, as are most tropical Latin American cities. Dengue fever, which is also spread by *A. aegypti*, reappeared in Rio de Janeiro in 1986 and subsequently spread widely. To control the mosquito again in the Americas will be difficult because of insecticide resistance, population growth, and the high price of labor and materials. Jungle yellow fever continues to cycle, reappearing in the same locale every 5 to 40 years. The scene is thus set again for emergence of the virus from the jungle to reinitiate the urban cycle in the Americas.

A. aegypti is easily identified. It has white thoracic scales in the shape of a lyre and black legs with white bands. Mosquitoes that have fed on a viremic vertebrate become infective after an extrinsic incubation period of 9 to 30 days, the shorter periods correlating with higher ambient temperatures. This extrinsic incubation period in the mosquito accounts for the delay from the first human infection in an urban outbreak to subsequent clusters of infection.

Yellow fever is not found in Asia, although large areas harbor *A. aegypti* that are capable of transmitting the virus, should it be introduced. India and other Asian nations require vaccination of travelers from yellow fever-endemic regions.

All age groups and races are susceptible. However, sylvan yellow fever is found almost always in young males because they are the individuals who venture into the forest. Immunity following vaccination or infection is long-lasting. During an epidemic, the population at risk may therefore be limited to age groups not covered by prior immunization or those born since a prior outbreak. There is also some evidence that persons may be protected by antibody to heterologous flaviviruses.

During the 24-year period from 1965 to 1988, 3324 cases of yellow fever were reported in the Americas and 7701 in Africa. The numbers of cases are greatly underestimated; as of 1998, the World Health Organization (WHO) estimates that 200,000 yellow fever cases and 30,000 deaths occur annually. Case-fatality rates are usually about 20%, but they are higher in some epidemics. Ratios of apparent to inapparent infection, estimated at 1:10, may vary greatly.

PATHOLOGY AND PATHOGENESIS. The lesions of yellow fever involve primarily the liver, heart, kidneys, and lymphoid tissues. Grossly, the skin is icteric, and there may be multiple hemorrhages or petechiae of the skin, mucous membranes, and multiple organs. The liver is normal in size, icteric, and fatty. The heart is soft and flabby, and the kidneys are swollen and a pink-gray color. Small peritoneal and pleural effusions are sometimes observed.

Histologic findings are often characteristic in patients who die before the ninth day of illness, but the lesions are not always pathognomonic. The most striking lesion is the eosinophilic degeneration and coagulation of hepatocytes (Councilman's bodies). Hepatocyte destruction is most marked in the midzone of the lobule, with relative sparing of the central vein and portal areas. Intranuclear eosinophilic granular inclusions or enlarged nucleoli (Torres bodies) are also described. Both microvacuolar and multivacuolar fatty changes are prominent, especially after the first week of illness. Inflammation is uncommon, and the reticulum framework is unaffected, probably accounting for the absence of postnecrotic fibrosis in convalescence and the regeneration of hepatocytes in recovered patients. The kidneys show cloudy swelling of tubular epithelium leading to acute tubular necrosis. The glomeruli are not obviously affected, but special stains indicate Schiff-positive alterations in the basal membranes, and proteinaceous material accumulates in the capsular spaces and lumina of the proximal tubules. The myocardium is characterized by granular or fatty infiltration of muscle fibers and of the atrioventricular (AV) conduction system and cloudy swelling and degeneration of myocytes without inflammation. Large monocytes replace lymphocytic cells in the splenic follicles and lymph nodes. Encephalitis is rare, although petechial hemorrhage in the brain stem and cerebral edema are observed.

Knowledge of the pathogenesis of yellow fever is sparse. Yellow fever cases occur in remote areas, and pathophysiologic studies of yellow fever patients are usually done with only rudimentary laboratory facilities. The virus replicates in the hepatocytes and myocytes, and it is presumed that lesions in these target cells are a direct effect of the virus. Jaundice and prolonged prothrombin time can be explained by hepatocellular damage; bradycardia and arrhythmias are explained by myocyte and AV node perturbation. The etiology of renal tubular necrosis is not clear, but it may be secondary to hepatic changes. Some, but not all, fatal cases are associated with thrombocytopenia; increased prothrombin, partial thromboplastin, and thrombin times; diminished factor VIII and fibrinogen levels; and the presence of fibrin split products. The bleeding in these cases may be secondary to DIC, but this is not generally accepted by all investigators. Hypoglycemia, metabolic acidosis, and hyperkalemia characterize the terminal stage and are probably the result of multiple organ-system failure.

CLINICAL MANIFESTATIONS. Severe yellow fever is a fulminant febrile illness with 50% or greater mortality. A great deal of variation occurs, however; most cases are mild with a better prognosis, and only about 10 to 20% are in the severe category. The intrinsic incubation period is 3 to 6 days, and in exceptional cases as long as 10 days.

The clinical syndrome is classified as very mild, mild, moderately severe, or malignant. Patients with very mild cases have fever and headache and recover in 48 hours or less. Those with mild cases have sudden fever and headache with nausea, sometimes bleeding of the gums or epistaxis, bradycardia, or albuminuria. These patients recover in 2 or 3 days. Those with moderately severe cases have more marked manifestations of bleeding, definite bradycardia in relation to the fever, nausea and vomiting, jaundice, and striking albuminuria. The illness may be aborted after 3 to 4 days or serious hemorrhagic manifestations may develop, such as black vomit, melena, and metrorrhagia. Moderately severe yellow fever may last 1 week or even longer.

Classic yellow fever is characterized as malignant and is divided into three periods: infection, remission, and intoxication. The period of infection involves sudden onset of fever and headache, with initial rapid pulse, but by day 2, the pulse slows despite continued fever (Faget's sign). Headache, backache, and muscle pain may be severe, blood oozes from the gums, and other signs of bleeding become prominent. The face is flushed, the tongue is reddened (strawberry tongue), and the conjunctivae are injected; the patient is irritable, unable to sleep, and frequently constipated. The temperature is often 40°C or higher. On the third day of illness, nausea, vomiting of coffee-ground material, and notable albuminuria are characteristic. The bleeding is usually gastric, not lower intestinal, in origin. In the period of remission, often on day 4, the patient feels better, the fever drops, and headache and nausea subside. Remission lasts a few hours to 2 days. It is followed by the period of intoxication in which the classic signs of fever, epigastric tenderness with vomiting of altered blood, nosebleeds, and albuminuria leading to oliguria or anuria occur. Dehydration may predispose to suppurative parotitis; the lungs are usually normal, but bacterial pneumonia may complicate the disease. Intoxication lasts from 3 days up to 2 weeks and may be accompanied by heart failure with drop in blood pressure, hiccup, coma, and death. Sometimes the patient is lucid until the end.

The clinical syndrome may be predominantly one of hepatic, renal, or cardiac failure. Meningoencephalitis has also been recorded. Death usually occurs between the seventh and the tenth day of illness. Patients who survive generally recover completely, although the convalescence may be prolonged, and late death from cardiac failure or arrhythmias is a rare complication.

CLINICAL LABORATORY FINDINGS. Early in the course of disease, the following may be present: leukopenia with relative neutropenia (but sometimes with normal or elevated leukocyte count), decreased prothrombin time, and elevation of serum bilirubin level. After the third day of illness, full-blown yellow fever is associated with abnormalities referable to the liver, kidneys, and heart. The total and conjugated bilirubin concentration values are elevated and rise together. The mean bilirubin value is 9 to 10 mg/dL, but it averages 15 to 20 mg/dL in severe cases, and may be much higher. Prothrombin and partial thromboplastin times are increased, and platelets, blood glucose, and clotting factors II, V, VII, IX, and X are decreased. Alkaline phosphatase levels are normal. Aminotransferase levels are of prognostic value; serum aspartate aminotransferase and alanine aminotransferase levels are consistently elevated in jaundiced patients.

Albuminuria usually appears on the fourth day, reaching levels of 3 to 5 mg/L (much higher in severe cases). Blood urea averages 109 mg/dL, and creatinine averages 5.9 mg/dL in fatal cases; the averages are much lower in nonfatal yellow fever. The urine may

contain bile and casts. Electrocardiogram abnormalities are sometimes present, including abnormal ST-T waves and prolonged PR and QT intervals. The cerebrospinal fluid (CSF) is under increased pressure and may contain increased protein with normal cell counts.

DIAGNOSIS. Diagnosis can be made by histopathologic examination of the liver, by isolation of yellow fever virus from blood during life and from liver and other tissues post mortem, by demonstration of specific nucleic acid, or by serologic tests. Yellow fever should be suspected in any febrile patient from endemic zones of Africa and the Americas and in areas of high *A. aegypti* prevalence where yellow fever may be introduced. Postmortem diagnosis by examination of liver taken by a viscerotome was successfully used in South America routinely for many years, and postmortem immunohistochemistry of liver is sensitive and relatively specific. Liver biopsy should not be attempted because of the danger of uncontrolled bleeding.

Yellow fever virus can be isolated from serum and blood during the first 4 days of fever by inoculation intracerebrally into baby mice or onto mammalian or mosquito cell cultures. Mice are observed for death; the virus causes cytopathic effect in Vero cells and is detected by immunofluorescence tests in mosquito cells 3 to 6 days after inoculation. The most rapid methods of diagnosis are identification of RNA by reverse transcription-polymerase chain reaction (RT-PCR) and detection of antigen in acute-phase blood by the antigen-capture enzyme-linked immunosorbent assay (ELISA). The tests can be completed in a few hours, although detection of antigen by ELISA is less sensitive than virus isolation.

Serologic diagnosis is made by demonstrating immunoglobulin M (IgM) by the antibody-capture ELISA. Because IgM is relatively specific and is detectable in high titer for only a short time after infection, this technique is reliable using a single convalescent serum specimen. Alternatively, tests of sera collected during the acute and convalescent phases are diagnostic if they show a fourfold or greater rise (or fall) of yellow fever antibody. The neutralization test is highly specific, but the complement fixation, hemagglutination-inhibition, and ELISA are usually used because they are quicker and lend themselves to field laboratory use. The laboratory must also rule out cross-reacting antibody by related viruses such as dengue. A radiolabeled RNA probe was able to detect yellow fever RNA in fixed human liver that had been stored for more than 20 years.

DIFFERENTIAL DIAGNOSIS. The mild form of yellow fever is not clinically distinguishable from other tropical fevers. Severe yellow fever simulates viral hepatitis, including hepatitis D; other hemorrhagic fevers; leptospirosis; rickettsial fevers; malignant malaria; and drug- and toxin-related conditions.

PROGNOSIS. Two to 20% of patients with clinically evident yellow fever die, although as many as 50% of severely ill patients die. It is not clear whether these patients would survive if they received the most modern supportive treatment, because most cases are treated in primitive clinics in Africa and South America. Patients who enter the period of intoxication have a guarded prognosis, especially if they develop anuria, high levels of albuminemia and bilirubinemia, a prothrombin time prolonged beyond 25% of normal, a rapid and weak pulse, uncontrolled bleeding, persistent hiccup, delirium, hypotension, or coma.

TREATMENT. Treatment consists of complete bedrest, fluid and blood replacement, and supportive care, including monitoring of vital signs. Analgesics and antiemetics may be useful, but aspirin is contraindicated because it may exacerbate bleeding. Patients are placed under bed nets to prevent possible mosquito transmission to other patients and to hospital personnel. Malaria and bacterial complications should be treated if diagnosed. Electrolyte imbalance should be corrected. Dialysis has not been used in cases of renal tubular damage, but on theoretical ground, it may benefit patients with renal failure. If DIC is evident by laboratory tests, heparin may be used cautiously, although experience to date is insufficient to predict its efficacy. Interferon and other antiviral substances have not been tried in patients with yellow fever.

PREVENTION AND CONTROL. Yellow fever can be prevented by inoculation of 17D attenuated vaccine. This vaccine is safe and induces antibody that persists at least 10 years in more than 90%

of vaccinees, usually for life. The vaccine is produced in eggs and should not be given to persons with egg allergies. Travelers should be vaccinated at least 10 days before arrival in yellow fever-endemic areas. Because the presence of yellow fever often goes undetected and unreported in tropical Africa and South America, the vaccine should be given to travelers whether or not there is known active transmission. Human immunodeficiency virus (HIV) infection is not a contraindication to vaccination. Unless the risk of exposure to yellow fever is great, vaccine is not recommended during pregnancy; however, it is not known to have caused fetal damage. In an epidemic, mosquito control measures and personal protection with repellents are recommended until vaccine can be obtained. An urban epidemic may represent an international emergency and should trigger immediate public health measures, both locally and abroad.

391.2 Hemorrhagic Fever Caused by Dengue Viruses

DEFINITION. Dengue hemorrhagic fever (DHF) is an acute febrile illness characterized by decreased platelet counts and hemoconcentration in patients infected with any one of the four serotypes of dengue virus. The disease affects children primarily and adults occasionally. Capillary permeability and coagulation defects lead to hemorrhagic manifestations and, in the more severe cases, to hypovolemic shock (dengue shock syndrome), with death in 40 to 50% of untreated shock syndrome patients. The disease has been endoepidemic in Southeast Asia since 1953 and is increasing in prevalence. It was restricted to Asia and the Pacific until 1981, when epidemic DHF appeared in Cuba; between 1981 and mid-1998, 54,248 DHF cases were reported from 25 tropical American countries.

ETIOLOGY. DHF is caused by infection with dengue viruses, but it is not yet established why hemorrhagic fever develops in one patient and classic dengue fever develops in another. Initially, it was hypothesized that strains of dengue virus that caused DHF were more virulent than others; this may still be true, but overwhelming evidence indicates that infection is enhanced and disease is more severe when the host has been sensitized by a prior dengue infection of different serotype.

EPIDEMIOLOGY. The epidemiology of DHF is that described for dengue fever with some added features. Epidemics of DHF are limited to Southeast Asia, the Pacific Islands, and, since 1981, the Caribbean and South America. It is estimated that fewer than 7% of individuals with dengue develop DHF. The attack rate in Thailand is highest in children, with a minor peak in infants, when maternal antibody is waning, and a major peak at ages 4 to 12 years, when second dengue infections are most common; adults as well as children develop DHF in some outbreaks, such as those in Cuba in 1981 and 1997. Well-nourished children in Southeast Asia appeared to be at higher risk than the undernourished, and blacks in the 1981 Cuban epidemic had milder illness than whites; well-controlled studies are needed to substantiate these observations.

PATHOLOGY. Post mortem, focal hemorrhages, vascular congestion, and edema are evident in multiple organs. The spleen and lymphoid tissues show marked lymphocytolysis and phagocytosis of lymphocytes, primarily in the T-cell–dependent zones. Proliferation of lymphoblasts and young plasma cells is also noted. Monocytic and lymphocytic non-necrotizing perivascular infiltration is found in skin lesions, resembling an antibody-dependent Arthus reaction.

PATHOGENESIS. Dengue virus infects the macrophages, lymphocytes, and endothelial cells. On rare occasions, DHF occurs in primary dengue, indicating that direct infection of these cells with the virus can lead to the syndrome; however, the vast majority of cases consist of secondary infections. In these cases, the anamnestic antibody response is rapid, with formation of antigen-antibody complexes. Experimentally, formation of complexes enhances infectivity of the virus for monocytes through attachment of complexes at the Fc receptor site and entry of virus into the cell. Between

0.05 and 0.1% of monocytes in the peripheral blood can be visualized carrying dengue antigen. The replication of dengue virus in the monocyte is postulated to be the effector pathway leading to vascular permeability. Monocyte infection is presumably responsible for the observed complement activation and consumption via the classic and perhaps the alternate pathway. This process may result in formation of C3a and C5a, which are anaphylatoxins, or some other as yet unknown mediator of vascular permeability may be activated. Another effector pathway leads to coagulation defects, including thrombocytopenia and abnormal clotting. The entire process is rapid. It may evolve in a few hours to shock and death or, if managed effectively, to complete recovery. Although the pathogenesis is not understood, the pathophysiologic events are known and can be treated rationally.

CLINICAL MANIFESTATIONS. DHF usually starts with sudden onset of high fever and the signs and symptoms of dengue fever, which include facial flush, anorexia, headache, nausea, and pains in the muscles and joints. Hepatic tenderness, epigastric or generalized abdominal pain, and sore throat are frequent. The liver is usually palpable in children, and the spleen is characteristically prominent on radiographs. A high temperature continues for 2 days to a week. A positive tourniquet test result, easy bruising, and fine petechiae on the face, soft palate, and extremities indicate a hemorrhagic disorder. Sometimes gum bleeding and epistaxis are noted. The majority of cases are moderately severe or mild, and the patients recover after lysis of fever. The lysis may be associated with sweating, coolness of extremities, and transient lowering of blood pressure.

More severe cases are associated with shock. The fall in blood pressure occurs suddenly on the third to the seventh day of illness and is accompanied by cool, blotchy skin, circumoral cyanosis, and tachycardia. The patient becomes restless and may complain of acute abdominal pain. The pulse pressure drops to 20 mm Hg or less, and in severe cases, blood pressure and pulse may not be detectable. Uncorrected shock may lead to metabolic acidosis and severe bleeding from the gastrointestinal tract and other sites. Death or recovery usually occurs in 12 to 24 hours. Surviving patients do not usually have sequelae. The white blood cell count is normal or slightly elevated, with lymphocytosis and atypical lymphocytes commonly seen. Hemoconcentration and elevated serum aspartate aminotransferase and blood urea nitrogen levels are noted.

DIAGNOSIS. The laboratory diagnosis is that of dengue fever (see Chapter 392); RT-PCR provides the possibility of rapid diagnosis. DHF with shock syndrome is a medical emergency, and therefore early clinical diagnosis is essential. DHF presents with (1) acute onset of fever, which is high, continuous, and lasts 2 days or more; (2) positive tourniquet test result, with spontaneous petechiae or ecchymoses; bleeding from gums or nose; hematemesis or melena; (3) hepatomegaly, observed in more than 90% of pediatric Asian patients; (4) hypotension with cold, clammy skin, restlessness, and pulse pressure less than 20 mm Hg; (5) thrombocytopenia; (6) hematocrit increased 20% over the convalescent value; and (7) radiographic or ultrasound evidence of pleural and peritoneal effusion. Fever, hemorrhagic phenomena, thrombocytopenia, and hemoconcentration are the hallmarks of DHF, and, with hypotension or narrow pulse pressure, of dengue shock syndrome (DSS). Hepatoencephalopathy sometimes develops as a late manifestation. Bacterial endotoxic shock and meningococcemia can mimic DHF/DSS.

TREATMENT. No specific treatment has been established. The object of therapy is to maintain hydration, to combat acidosis, and to correct coagulation abnormalities. Salicylates may contribute to bleeding and acidosis, and they are contraindicated. Paracetamol may be used. Steroids should not be used. Hematocrit should be determined frequently, at least daily, to measure the degree of plasma loss and the need for intravenous fluids. Fluid should be started at 20 mL/kg of body weight. One-third to one-half of fluid should be physiologic saline, and the remainder should be 5% glucose in water. If acidosis is present, one quarter of fluid should be 0.167 mol/L of sodium bicarbonate. In shock cases, one should use Ringer's lactate solution, 5% glucose in physiologic saline, 5% glucose in one-half physiologic saline, 5% glucose in one-half Ringer's solution, or 5% glucose in one-third physiologic saline (depending on degree of dehydration and age). One should monitor for signs of cardiac failure during rapid fluid administration.

In case of shock, one should administer fluid rapidly and under pressure if necessary. Plasma or another volume expander should be given if shock persists and the vital signs and hematocrit should be followed. The hematocrit should decline with fluid therapy, which is continued until the hematocrit is less than 40%, urine output is adequate, and the appetite returns. If levels of electrolytes and blood gases indicate acidosis, sodium bicarbonate should be administered. Heparin for intravascular coagulopathy (prolonged prothrombin and partial thromboplastin times) is usually not needed, but it may be used cautiously in refractory cases. Chloral hydrate should be given for sedation, oxygen should be administered for shock, and blood should be administered as needed.

PROGNOSIS. Case fatality from DHF is 2 to 10%; deaths occur in patients with shock. Most patients survive when treated early by experienced health-care workers. Recovery is rapid and without sequelae.

PREVENTION. Prevention is as described for dengue fever (see Chapter 392).

391.3   Tick-Borne Flavivirus Diseases: Kyasanur Forest Disease and Omsk Hemorrhagic Fever

DEFINITION. Kyasanur Forest disease (KFD) of India and Omsk hemorrhagic fever (OHF) of western Siberia are tick-transmitted flavivirus fevers characterized by hemorrhage or encephalitis. Some patients manifest both syndromes.

ETIOLOGY. KFD and OHF viruses belong to the tick-borne complex of flaviviruses, which also encompasses the closely related viruses of central European tick-borne encephalitis, Russian spring-summer encephalitis, and Powassan encephalitis of North America and Asia.

EPIDEMIOLOGY. KFD was originally limited to the forests of Shimoga District of Karnataka State, India, but since its discovery in 1957 it has spread in an unpredictable fashion to three other neighboring forested districts. The largest outbreak occurred during 1982–1983 in a new focus in Nidle Forest. Many tick species are involved in transmission, especially nymphal *Haemaphysalis spinigera.* Small terrestrial mammals, as well as birds and bats, are infected in nature. When the forest is felled for plantations, the ecology is upset. Cattle brought in to graze at the forest fringe are not infected but serve as hosts that greatly increase the numbers of ticks. Infected ticks feed on black-faced langur monkeys and South Indian bonnet macaques, which become viremic, serve as amplifiers of infection, and often die. At the same time, epidemics occur in persons with forest occupations. People are infected incidentally and do not form part of the transmission cycle.

OHF occurs in the forest-steppe areas of the lake region of western Siberia. Epidemics of as many as 600 cases were recorded in the 1940s, but in recent years the disease has become uncommon. Numbers of cases peak in May and again in August and September. The virus is transmitted by *Dermacentor pictus* ticks and is maintained in small-mammal populations. Muskrats, which were introduced for hunting in the 1920s, are susceptible and apparently transmit OHF virus to other muskrats and to hunters by direct contact. Lake water contaminated by dead muskrats is said to be responsible for water-borne disease. Both KFD and OHF are transmitted transovarially and trans-stadially in ticks.

CLINICAL MANIFESTATIONS AND PATHOLOGY. The incubation period is 3 to 8 days. Onset is sudden, with temperature up to 40°C, headache, papulovesicular lesions of the soft palate, myalgia, and prostration lasting 1 to 2 weeks. In more severe cases, nasal, enteric, uterine, or pulmonary hemorrhage may be evident. Leukopenia, thrombocytopenia, and albuminuria are found. Some patients have a diphasic course, with a more severe illness and meningoencephalitis after a 1- or 2-week afebrile period. The second phase is characterized by fever, severe headache, meningismus, mental disturbances, and tremors. Hemorrhagic manifestations or pneumonia may also be prominent in the second phase. The case fatality rate of KFD is 5 to 10%; that of OHF is 0.4 to 2.5%. There are no sequelae. Infections in laboratory workers are common but are usually mild. Histopathologic findings are minor in comparison to the gravity of the clinical disease. Findings include extravasation of red blood cells, edema, and thrombi in the small vessels.

DIAGNOSIS AND TREATMENT. Diagnosis is by isolation of virus from the blood during the first 10 days of illness and by demonstration of antibody rise or presence of specific immunoglobulin M (IgM) during convalescence. There is no specific treatment, but fluid and electrolyte balance should be maintained and blood transfused if needed. Analgesics other than aspirin may be indicated.

PREVENTION. Tick repellents, protective clothing, and spraying of forest tracts with acaricides are the only measures available for prevention.

391.4   Crimean-Congo Hemorrhagic Fever

DEFINITION. Crimean-Congo hemorrhagic fever (CCHF) is an acute febrile hemorrhagic tick-borne disease of Asia, Europe, and Africa. Mortality is high and hospital-based outbreaks are common.

ETIOLOGY. The disease is caused by CCHF virus of the *Nairovirus* genus, family Bunyaviridae. The virus kills baby mice and replicates in CER cells and several other cell culture systems.

EPIDEMIOLOGY. CCHF virus is transmitted in nature principally by hard ticks of the genus *Hyalomma,* but also by ticks in the genera *Rhipicephalus, Boophilus,* and *Amblyomma.* Virus is maintained by transovarial and trans-stadial passage in the tick and is amplified by hares and possibly hedgehogs, sheep, and cattle. Giraffe, rhinoceros, eland, buffalo, kudu, zebra, and dogs in southern Africa have antibody to CCHF virus.

The virus or its antibody is found in the distribution of *Hyalomma* ticks. Foci occur in the former Soviet Union, the Balkan nations, Iraq, Iran, Pakistan, Afghanistan, western China, the Middle East, and most of sub-Saharan Africa, including South Africa. Outbreaks occur among military personnel, campers, and in persons tending sheep and cattle. Medical workers are at high risk because of frequent spread in hospitals from infected human blood and tissue.

CLINICAL MANIFESTATIONS. The incubation period is usually between 2 and 9 days. Onset is sudden, with severe headache, fever, chills, myalgia (especially in the back and legs), sore throat, abdominal pain, nausea, vomiting, diarrhea, photophobia, and conjunctival injection. The fever is constant but may be remitting. The patient is often confused or aggressive, with a marked mood change. Leukopenia and thrombocytopenia are usually observed. On days 3 to 6, hemorrhagic manifestations and a petechial rash on the trunk, limbs, and oral cavity appear. Epistaxis, hematemesis, melena, and uterine bleeding may be severe and require transfusion. The liver is sometimes enlarged and tender. In severe cases, hepatorenal failure or multiple organ system failure leads to death, usually on days 6 to 14 of illness. Death may also result from blood loss, cerebral hemorrhage, dehydration after diarrhea, or pulmonary edema. Patients recover gradually, starting on day 10 when the rash fades. Asthenia may last for a month or more. Recovery is usually complete, although neuritis may persist for months. Liver function tests are abnormal, especially the aspartate aminotransferase, and serum bilirubin levels are often elevated late in the illness. Abnormal prothrombin, activated partial thromboplastin, and thrombin times, as well as increased fibrin degradation products, are indicative of DIC.

DIAGNOSIS. Virus is easily isolated during the first 8 days of illness. Antibodies are detectable by immunofluorescence and enzyme-linked immunosorbent assay (ELISA) in surviving patients. Specific immunoglobulin M (IgM) and immunoglobulin G (IgG) are present by days 7 to 9 of illness.

TREATMENT AND PROGNOSIS. Patients suspected of having CCHF should be housed in an isolation facility with needle and blood precautions. Health-care personnel who work with them should use respirators and protective clothing. Treatment is supportive, including monitoring and correcting fluid and electrolyte imbalance and treating DIC. The vital signs and hematocrit should be tested frequently, and blood should be replaced by transfusion. Case-fatality rates range from 30 to 50%.

PREVENTION. Protection from tick bites and care in handling blood and tissue of sick sheep and cattle are the only preventive measures available in the case of exposure in natural foci.

391.5 Hemorrhagic Diseases Caused by Arenaviruses (Argentine, Bolivian, Venezuelan, and Brazilian Hemorrhagic Fevers and Lassa Fever)

DEFINITION. Argentine, Bolivian, Venezuelan, and Brazilian hemorrhagic fevers and Lassa fever are acute febrile diseases characterized by hemorrhagic diatheses, marked myalgia, and, in severe cases, shock. Case-fatality rates are between 5 and 33%.

ETIOLOGY. The diseases are caused by the viruses Junin (Argentina), Machupo (Bolivia), Guanarito (Venezuela), Sabiá (Brazil), and Lassa (West Africa) of the family Arenaviridae.

EPIDEMIOLOGY. The reservoirs are rodents that excrete virus in urine and possibly other body fluids. The viruses involved with various rodents are: Junin virus, *Calomys musculinus, C. laucha,* and *Akodon arenicola;* Machupo virus, *C. callosus;* Guanarito virus, *Zygodontomys brevicauda;* Sabiá virus, not known; and Lassa virus, *Mastomys natalensis.* People are believed to be infected by inhaling or eating contaminated excreta or by passage of virus through abraded skin or mucous membranes. In Argentina, exposure to Junin virus is primarily in workers harvesting corn in Cordoba and Buenos Aires provinces in the north. In Bolivia, domestic and peridomestic exposure to Machupo virus occurs in Beni province, and in Venezuela, exposure occurs to Guanarito virus in agricultural settings in Portugesa and Barinas states. The site of exposure to Sabiá virus in São Paulo State, Brazil, is not known. Lassa virus is endemic in west and central Africa, especially in Liberia, Sierra Leone, and parts of Nigeria, where it is transmitted in and around homes that have an abundance of its host, *M. natalensis.*

Argentine hemorrhagic fever epidemics involving hundreds of farm workers were recorded annually until vaccination was carried out starting in 1988. Bolivian hemorrhagic fever epidemics were common in the 1960s, but after institution of rodent control measures, the disease was not reported after 1974 until it reappeared in 1994. Lassa fever was recognized first in 1969 in a nosocomial outbreak in Nigeria. Several other nosocomial outbreaks were subsequently diagnosed, but studies in Sierra Leone established the basic endemic nature of the disease. In the eastern province, 8 to 52% of the population have antibody, and the annual seroconversion rate in susceptible subjects ranges between 5 and 22%. It is estimated that 5 to 14% of all fevers are Lassa virus infections and that Lassa fever accounts for 10 to 16% of the adult hospital admissions.

PATHOGENESIS AND PATHOLOGY. The diseases are characterized by multiple organ impairment, yet specific lesions are absent. The prominent findings are focal diapedesis and capillary hemorrhage, but inflammation is minimal. Focal areas of liver necrosis in Lassa fever are not sufficient to account for the profound shock and death. It is postulated that the virus infects cells of the reticuloendothelial system, including the B and T cells. It causes temporary inhibition of immune cell function, leading to prolonged and high-titered viremia. It is not known whether subsequent capillary damage and parenchymal edema are direct or indirect effects of the virus.

CLINICAL MANIFESTATIONS. The five diseases have many similarities. The incubation period of Lassa fever is 3 to 16 days; of Argentine hemorrhagic fever, 10 to 14 days; and of Bolivian hemorrhagic fever, 7 to 14 days. Onset is insidious, initially with fever, chills, malaise, asthenia, headache, retro-ocular pain, anorexia, nausea, vomiting, and muscle pain (especially at the costovertebral angle in the South American forms and the legs in Lassa fever). Fever, between 39 and 40.5°C, is nonremitting. Sore throat is not prominent in the Argentine, Venezuelan, and Bolivian dis-

eases, but purulent pharyngitis and aphthous ulcers are common in Lassa fever.

Signs include conjunctivitis; facial edema; enanthem with pharyngeal vesicles; exanthem of the face, neck, and upper thorax; tenderness of thighs; laterocervical and other polyadenopathy; and petechiae (especially in the axillae). No jaundice or hepatosplenomegaly is present. Leukopenia, thrombocytopenia, and albuminuria with casts are characteristic.

Late in the first week of illness, the signs and symptoms become more pronounced. Signs of dehydration, decreased blood pressure, and relative bradycardia are prominent. Hemorrhage from the gums, nose, stomach, intestines, uterus, and urinary tract indicates a severe hemorrhagic diathesis. Bleeding was observed commonly in the South American forms, but in only 17% of Lassa fever cases. Blood loss is not massive enough to account for the shock. The acute phase usually lasts 7 to 15 days. Death is the result of uremia or hypovolemic shock, usually in the second week of illness. Recovery is heralded by lysis of fever; there is usually a prolonged convalescence marked by periods of sweating, flush, and postural hypotension, but patients suffer no permanent non-neurologic sequelae.

Neurologic signs are prominent in Bolivian hemorrhagic fever; nearly 50% of patients have an intention tremor of the tongue and hands at about the fifth day of illness, and in 25%, symptoms progress to more serious encephalopathy with delirium and convulsions. The CSF is normal in these patients. A similar syndrome is occasionally seen in Lassa fever, and about 5% of patients develop unilateral or bilateral eighth cranial nerve damage, which may be permanent. Other transient complications are loss of hair and Beau's lines of the nails.

Most patients have leukopenia with depression of both lymphocytes and neutrophils; however, some Lassa fever patients have markedly elevated white blood cell counts. Thrombocytopenia is present during the first week of illness.

DIAGNOSIS. The diagnosis can be made definitively only with laboratory tests. Fever, muscle pain, and diminished white blood cell count in the endemic areas should alert the physician to the diagnosis. RT-PCR is used to detect and identify specific RNA. Virus can be isolated in Vero cells from blood, CSF, and throat washings during life and from most tissues at necropsy. Virus is recoverable even in the presence of antibody. Isolation of virus from Bolivian hemorrhagic fever cases is more difficult than from the Argentine or West African form. Virus isolation should be attempted only in laboratories with high biosecurity containment equipment because of the risk of infection of laboratory workers. Serologic diagnosis is made by the immunofluorescence test. Immunoglobulin G is present in 53% of Lassa fever patients on admission to hospital, and IgM is present in 67%. The IgM test is useful for early and rapid diagnosis.

TREATMENT. Supportive therapy, including attention to electrolyte and fluid balance, is essential. Hematocrit and urine protein measurements aid in detection of hypovolemic shock. Plasma expanders are effective if used early, but may precipitate pulmonary edema late in the clinical course.

Specific Junin virus-immune human plasma given during the first 8 days of Argentine hemorrhagic fever reduced the case-fatality rate from 16 to 1%. A neurologic illness was observed about 3 weeks after the acute attack in some patients receiving this therapy. Most of these patients recovered completely.

Ribavirin given to Lassa fever patients early in the illness significantly reduced mortality. The drug was administered intravenously, 60 mg/kg/day for the first 4 days, and then orally, 30 mg/kg/day for 6 days more. Immune plasma was not effective in Lassa fever patients in controlled trials.

PROGNOSIS. In Lassa fever, bleeding manifestations, high levels of circulating virus in the blood, and elevated aspartate aminotransferase levels in serum are predictive of death. There are no such predictors for the South American arenavirus hemorrhagic fevers. Shock or abnormal neurologic findings indicate a poor prognosis.

PREVENTION AND CONTROL. Environmental sanitation, including rodent-proofing of homes, and proper storage of grains and other foods to diminish rodent populations, are the only community-control measures now available. A live attenuated vaccine for Junin virus has proved efficacious in Argentina. Barrier nursing, with use of gloves and gowns, should be instituted in suspected cases of arenaviral hemorrhagic fevers. Blood and other tissue are infective and should be decontaminated.

391.6 African Hemorrhagic Fever (Marburg-Ebola Disease)

DEFINITION. African hemorrhagic fever is an acute, often fatal, hemorrhagic disease. Fever, rash, hemorrhage, hepatic and pancreatic inflammation, and prostration are hallmarks of the illness.

ETIOLOGY. The disease is caused by Marburg and Ebola viruses of the family Filoviridae. The two viruses are distinct antigenically but are of very similar morphology.

EPIDEMIOLOGY. African hemorrhagic fever caused by Marburg virus was described in 1967 in Germany and Yugoslavia, where workers in vaccine manufacturing facilities sickened and died after they were exposed to infected tissue of African green monkeys from Uganda. Where the monkeys became infected is not known, although Marburg virus is indigenous to Africa. (Additional isolated cases in South Africa and Kenya have been recorded.) Ebola virus epidemics in Sudan and Zaire in 1976 were traced to contact with infected patients and, in Zaire, to spread by needle. The disease recurred in Sudan in 1979, and there was an isolated case in Kenya in 1980. The outbreak in Kikwit, Zaire, in 1995 involved 315 cases, and a single case in Ivory Coast followed exposure of a Swiss ethologist during necropsy of a naturally infected chimpanzee in 1994. (The ethologist recovered.) In 1996, an Ebola outbreak in Gabon involved 54 cases and 41 deaths. A physician infected in Gabon flew to South Africa and fatally infected a nurse there. The source of the outbreaks is unknown, and the natural history remains a mystery. A third filovirus, most closely related to Ebola virus, was isolated in 1989 from sick cynomolgus monkeys recently imported to the United States from the Philippines. Animal handlers in the United States experienced seroconversion to the virus without associated illness.

PATHOLOGY. African hemorrhagic fever is a systemic disease with multiple organ involvement, most prominently the lymphatic system, testes, ovaries, and liver. Liver cell necrosis with eosinophilic inclusions, unlike that in yellow fever, is random and focal. Fibrin deposits are found in the renal glomeruli, consistent with DIC. There is edema and diffuse inflammation in the brain.

CLINICAL MANIFESTATIONS. The incubation period is 3 to 9 days for Marburg virus infection and 3 to 18 days for Ebola virus. Onset is abrupt, with severe headache, backache, muscle pains, and, sometimes, abdominal pain. At this stage, the disease is not readily differentiated from malaria, typhoid fever, and other bacterial, rickettsial, or viral illnesses. On about the third day, nausea, vomiting, and profuse watery diarrhea with mucus and blood commence. Diarrhea may continue for several days. A maculopapular rash appears on the trunk and spreads to the rest of the body. On day 4 or 5, the patient's status becomes critical, with high, unremitting fever and an altered mental state, including confusion, aggression, or lethargy. Spontaneous bleeding from injection sites is seen as are hematemesis, melena, hemoptysis, and, in pregnant patients, abortion, often with massive blood loss. Renal failure may be a terminal event. Death occurs from day 8 to 17, often on day 8 or 9. Recovery is marked by fatigue, anorexia, weight loss, hair loss, and, sometimes, psychological problems.

The pathophysiology is characterized by leukopenia, thrombocytopenia, increased prothrombin time, and other abnormalities in the liver function tests; increased serum amylase; proteinuria; and electrocardiographic changes indicative of myocardial disease. DIC has been documented in some cases.

DIAGNOSIS. Antigen is detected in acute-phase blood by antigen-capture ELISA. Alternatively, virus is isolated from acute-phase blood, liver, and other organs by inoculation into guinea pigs or cell culture. Antibody is detected by the immunofluorescence and ELISA during the second week of illness.

TREATMENT AND PROGNOSIS. No specific treatment is available. Supportive therapy consists of maintenance of fluid and electrolyte balance and administration of blood, platelets, or fresh frozen plasma to control bleeding. Peritoneal dialysis for renal failure and heparin for DIC have been recommended, but their value in

African hemorrhagic fever has not been established. Convalescent blood transfusion appeared to be beneficial in an uncontrolled study in Kikwit, Zaire. The presence of bleeding indicates a poor prognosis. The case-fatality rate under relatively sophisticated hospital conditions in Marburg, Germany, was 22% in 1967, and under Third World conditions in Zaire it was 90% in 1976 and 78% in 1995.

PREVENTION. Control activities are not carried out because the natural reservoir is unknown. Nosocomial spread can be minimized by barrier nursing and handling of blood and tissue in isolator laboratory units with proper decontamination.

391.7 Hemorrhagic Fever with Renal Syndrome

DEFINITION. Hemorrhagic fever with renal syndrome (HFRS) is a disease of Europe and Asia characterized by fevers, capillary dilatation, leakage of blood leading to hemorrhagic manifestations, and, in severe cases, shock and renal tubular disease.

ETIOLOGY. HFRS is caused by any one of several closely related viruses of the genus *Hantavirus*, family Bunyaviridae. The prototype is Hantaan virus, originally isolated from *Apodemus agrarius* field mice in the endemic region of Korea.

EPIDEMIOLOGY. The virus is transmitted from rodents. *A. agrarius* in Korea and other parts of Asia, *Clethrionomys glareolus* in Finland and west of the Ural Mountains, and *Rattus rattus* and *R. norvegicus* in cities of Japan, Korea, and Belgium serve as reservoirs. The rodent excretes virus in urine, saliva, and feces for weeks, and sometimes for months, after infection. Transmission is presumably by respiratory spread or direct contact with fomites contaminated by rodent excreta. Persons at risk include soldiers in field operations, campers, farmers, woodsmen, and, especially in the winter, family groups in houses that harbor field rodents seeking shelter from the cold. Outbreaks have also occurred in laboratories housing field rodents or laboratory rats that carry the virus as an inapparent infection. Nosocomial infections have not been reported.

PATHOLOGY. Patients who die of shock in the early stages demonstrate retroperitoneal gelatinous edema. Macroscopic hemorrhages are seen in the pituitary and right atrium. The renal medulla is congested and hyperemic, and patients who die later in the course of the disease have marked renal tubular necrosis. Petechial hemorrhages found in the skin and in multiple organs indicate widespread capillary fragility.

CLINICAL MANIFESTATIONS AND PATHOLOGIC PHYSIOLOGY. The incubation period ranges from 2 to 42 days but is usually about 2 weeks. Eighty per cent of cases are mild (demonstrating only fever, facial flush, backache, and muscle ache) or moderate (fever plus proteinuria, and petechial hemorrhages). The remaining 20% are severe. They progress through five characteristic phases: febrile, hypotensive, oliguric, diuretic, and convalescent. The febrile phase lasts about 5 days, during which fever, facial flush, conjunctival injection, and backache precede the appearance of petechial hemorrhages and albuminuria. In the hypotensive phase, the temperature returns to baseline, and the patient manifests nausea, vomiting, abdominal pain, and about 3 days of capillary leakage with a rising hematocrit, heavy proteinuria, leukocytosis, thrombocytopenia, and decreased renal clearance. This is followed for about 4 days by the oliguric phase, when extravascular fluid is resorbed, leading to relative hypervolemia, hypertension, metabolic acidosis, and, sometimes, pulmonary edema and/or acute renal failure. The diuretic phase is accompanied by return of renal clearance to normal, but with marked electrolyte and fluid imbalance, which may lead to death if it is not adequately managed. The convalescent phase may last 1 to 3 months, with slowly recovering renal function. The clinical diagnosis may be reliable during an outbreak with classic severe cases but not with mild infections; serologic confirmation is obtained by immunofluorescence, ELISA, and neutralization tests, which become positive at the end of the first week of illness. Antibody titers peak at 2 weeks and antibody lasts for many years.

TREATMENT AND PROGNOSIS. Management includes careful monitoring of electrolytes and fluid intake and output with correction, especially during the oliguric and diuretic phases. Plasma expanders can be used for shock, and hemodialysis can be undertaken in cases of renal failure with hyperkalemia. Ribavirin improves survival if given within 5 days of onset. The case-fatality rate in Korea is about 5% with hospital management; the disease in northern Europe is milder with a more favorable prognosis.

PREVENTION. Rodent control should be practiced where feasible, especially in urban settings.

391.8 Hantavirus Pulmonary Syndrome

DEFINITION. Hantavirus pulmonary syndrome (HPS) is a disease of North and South America first recognized in the Four Corners region of New Mexico in 1993 and characterized by fever, muscle pain, and gastrointestinal symptoms, progressing to acute respiratory failure and shock. Case-fatality approaches 50%.

ETIOLOGY. HPS is caused by any one of several closely related viruses of the genus *Hantavirus*, family Bunyaviridae. The prototype is Sin Nombre virus, originally characterized from human lung by RT-PCR analysis of its RNA.

EPIDEMIOLOGY. The viruses are transmitted from Cricetid rodent excreta, presumably by inhalation and percutaneous contamination. *Peromyscus maniculatus* (Sin Nombre virus) in New Mexico and neighboring states, *Peromyscus leucopus* (New York virus) in New York, *Oryzomys palustris* (Bayou virus) in Texas and Louisiana, and *Sigmodon hispidus* (Black Creek Canal virus) in Florida serve as reservoirs of different but related viruses in North America. Transmission, seasonality, and risk factors are very similar to those of hantaviruses in Europe and Asia. No person-to-person transmission has been documented in North America. Patients range in age from 12 to 69 years, with a median age of 35 years. The disease has not been recognized in young children. Fifty-four per cent of patients are male and 62% are white. Subclinical infections are rare.

HPS was first recognized in South America in 1995. Disease in Argentina and Chile caused by Andes virus resembled that in North America, except that person-to-person transmission was documented for the first time, and disease was recognized in children. As in North America, HPS is caused by genetically different hantaviruses, each with a different rodent reservoir.

PATHOLOGY. Pleural effusions and lung edema are found at autopsy. Microscopically, alveolar edema and pulmonary interstitial infiltrates of T cells and macrophages are evident in the absence of necrosis. Splenomegaly may be present, but lymph nodes and other organs appear grossly normal. Infiltrates of atypical mononuclear cells are found in the spleen, liver, and lymph nodes. The hemorrhage, retroperitoneal effusions, and kidney lesions of hemorrhagic fever with renal syndrome (HFRS) are usually absent.

CLINICAL MANIFESTATIONS AND PATHOLOGIC PHYSIOLOGY. A prodrome of fever and myalgia, sometimes with abdominal pain, nausea, vomiting, and dizziness, lasts 3 to 6 days. A cardiopulmonary phase follows in which the patient has fever, cough, dyspnea, hypoxia, noncardiogenic pulmonary edema, and shock. Surviving patients recover completely, usually within a week after onset of respiratory signs, although fever may continue. The partial thromboplastin and prothrombin times are prolonged, and thrombocytopenia and hemoconcentration are common, as are increased levels of aspartate aminotransferase and serum lactate dehydrogenase. Leukocytosis, atypical lymphocytes, and immature granulocytes are noted in the peripheral blood. Metabolic acidosis develops in severe cases. Signs of renal involvement in Sin Nombre virus infections are minimal; however, Bayou and other New World hantaviruses may cause renal insufficiency and elevated creatine kinase levels. Viral antigen has been found in capillary endothelium of several organs. Diagnosis depends on demonstration of specific antibodies by immunofluorescence, ELISA, and Western blot. IgM detected with hantavirus antigens is usually present on admission to the hospital. RT-PCR and immunohistochemistry of lung or other tissues have also been used for diagnosis.

TREATMENT AND PROGNOSIS. Management includes adequate oxygenation and monitoring of hemodynamic status. Mechanical ventilation may be needed. Invasive monitoring is required in hypotensive patients and will guide therapy with pressors and/or inotropic agents. Crystalloids are recommended instead of colloids for volume replacement because of the increased pulmonary capillary permeability. Overhydration should be avoided. Ribavirin efficacy in HPS is not established, but it is available for intravenous administration to HPS patients under an investigational protocol.

Breman JG, van der Groen G, Peters CJ, Heymann D: International colloquium on Ebola virus research: Summary report. J Infect Dis 176:1058, 1997. *Insightful review of Ebola disease and research.*

Butler JC, Peters CJ: Hantaviruses and hantavirus pulmonary syndrome. Clin Infect Dis 19:387, 1994. *State-of-the-art clinical review of hantavirus pulmonary syndrome.*

de Manzione N, Salas RA, Paredes H, et al: Venezuelan hemorrhagic fever: Clinical and epidemiological studies of 165 cases. Clin Infect Dis 26:308, 1998. *Clinical and epidemiological description of Venezuelan hemorrhagic fever.*

Preston R: The Hot Zone. New York, Random House, 1994. *Historical novel dealing with Marburg-Ebola disease.*

Proceedings of the International Symposium on Hemostatic Impairment Associated with Hemorrhagic Fever Viruses, May 26–28, 1987.

Rev Infect Dis 11(suppl 4):5669–5896, 1989. *A comprehensive compilation of reviews of the viral hemorrhagic fevers, including DHF, Crimean-Congo hemorrhagic fever, arenaviral hemorrhagic fevers, African hemorrhagic fevers, and HFRS.*

Schmaljohn C, Hjelle B: Hantaviruses: A global disease problem. Emerg Infect Dis 3:95, 1997. *Current review that includes South American hantavirus pulmonary syndrome.*

Swanepoel R, Shepherd AJ, Leman PA, et al: Epidemiologic and clinical features of Crimean Congo hemorrhagic fever in Southern Africa. Am J Trop Med Hyg 36:120, 1987. *Clinical description and review of CCHF literature.*

WHO Expert Committee Report: Viral Haemorrhagic Fevers, WHO Tech Rep Series No. 721. Geneva, WHO, 1985. *Excellent review of hemorrhagic fevers by an international group of experts with detailed guide to management of patients, investigation of outbreaks, and vector control.*

World Health Organization: Dengue Haemorrhagic fever: Diagnosis, Treatment and Control, 2nd ed. Geneva, World Health Organization, 1997. *A comprehensive manual for the physician faced with management of patients with DHF.*

392 OTHER ARTHROPOD-BORNE VIRUSES

R. Gordon Douglas, Jr.

Arthropod-borne viruses (arboviruses) are transmitted by an arthropod to a vertebrate host, either a human or a lower animal. During an incubation period, the viruses replicate in the arthropod, which may be a mosquito, tick, phlebotomus sandfly, or culicoid midge. The viruses are transmitted by bite to the vertebrate, which becomes viremic and then can infect another biting arthropod. Some arboviruses also are transmitted vertically through the egg of the arthropod and may be maintained this way between seasons.

There are nearly 500 arthropod-borne viruses, and at least 100 of these infect humans. Most fit into five families—Togaviridae, Flaviviridae, Bunyaviridae, Rhabdoviridae, and Reoviridae. Within each family are one or more genera, each usually corresponding to an antigenic group.

Most infections are inapparent. The remainder are associated with one or more of five major syndromes: (1) undifferentiated fever, (2) fever with rash and/or arthritis, (3) pulmonary disease, (4) encephalitis, and (5) hemorrhagic fever.

This chapter describes several of the more important arboviruses known to infect people. Table 392–1 lists some that cause fever, rash, or polyarthritis in humans; those that cause encephalitis in humans are listed in Table 392–2.

The diseases described here are nearly all "zoonoses" (i.e., illnesses caused by viruses transmitted from animals to humans). They are more prevalent in the tropics and subtropics and are usually focal because of ecologic restrictions on their transmission. Diagnosis depends on a careful history encompassing exposure to vertebrate animals and arthropod vectors, age, season, and travel, including geographic site of exposure. The physician must have a high index of suspicion. Fevers are often diagnosed erroneously as malaria; indeed, in malaria-endemic regions, the patient frequently has malaria concomitantly with an arboviral infection.

Table 392–1 ■ ARTHROPOD-BORNE VIRUSES THAT CAUSE FEVER, RASH, OR POLYARTHRITIS

FAMILY (GENUS) VIRUS	HUMAN DISEASE	DISTRIBUTION	VECTOR
Togaviridae (Alphavirus)			
Mayaro	Fever, arthritis, rash	South America	Mosquito
Ross River	Arthritis, rash, sometimes fever	Australia, South Pacific	Mosquito
Chikungunya	Fever, arthritis, hemorrhagic fever	Africa, Asia, Philippines	Mosquito
O'nyong-nyong	Fever, arthritis, rash	Africa	Mosquito
Sindbis	Arthritis, rash, sometimes fever	Africa, Europe, Australia	Mosquito
Flaviviridae (Flavivirus)			
Dengue (4 types)	Fever, rash, hemorrhagic fever	Worldwide (tropics)	Mosquito
Yellow fever	Fever, hemorrhagic fever	Tropical Americas, Africa	Mosquito
West Nile	Fever, rash, hepatitis, encephalitis	Asia, Europe, Africa	Mosquito
Bunyaviridae (Bunyavirus)			
Oxopouche	Fever	Brazil, Panama	Midge
Bunyaviridae (Phlebovirus)			
Sandfly fever viruses	Fever	Asia, Africa, tropical Americas	Sand fly, mosquito
Rift Valley fever	Fever, hemorrhagic fever, encephalitis, retinitis	Africa	Mosquito
Bunyaviridae (Hantavirus)			
Sin Nombre, others	Pulmonary disease	Americas	Rodent
Reoviridae (Coltivirus)			
Colorado tick fever	Fever	Western U.S.	Tick

Note: Shown are the most important of more than 100 arboviruses that infect humns.

Table 392–2 ■ ARTHROPOD-BORNE VIRUSES THAT CAUSE ACUTE CENTRAL NERVOUS SYSTEM INFECTION AND ENCEPHALITIS

VIRUS BY GROUP	MODE OF TRANSMISSION	GEOGRAPHIC DISTRIBUTION	DISEASE IN DOMESTIC LIVESTOCK
Viruses Principally Associated with the Encephalitis Syndrome; Epidemic and Endemic			
Togaviridae, alphavirus			
Eastern equine encephalitis	Mosquito	Eastern North America, Caribbean, South America	Equines, penned pheasants
Western equine encephalitis	Mosquito	Western North America, South America	Equines
Venezuelan equine encephalitis	Mosquito, possibly other	Florida, Central and South America	Equines
Flaviviridae, flavivirus			
St. Louis encephalitis	Mosquito	North America, Caribbean, Central and South America	None
Japanese encephalitis	Mosquito	East and Southeast Asia, India	Equines, swine
Rocio encephalitis	Mosquito	Brazil	None
Murray Valley encephalitis	Mosquito	Australia	(Equines)*
Tick-bone encephalitides			
Russian spring-summer and Central European encephalitis	Tick, ingestion of milk	Europe, former U.S.S.R.	None
Louping ill	Tick	British Isles	Sheep, equines, cows
Powassan	Tick	North America	None
Bunyaviridae, California subgroup			
California encephalitis, LaCrosse, Jamestown Canyon, snowshoe hare	Mosquito	North America, China, former U.S.S.R.	None
Viruses Principally Associated with Other Syndromes, but Occasionally Causing Encephalitis; Epidemic and Endemic			
Togaviridae, alphavirus			
Sindbis (febrile illness with rash)	Mosquito	Africa, Europe	None
Semliki Forest (febrile illness)	Mosquito	Africa, Southeast Asia	(Equines)*
Flaviviridae, flavivirus			
West Nile (febrile illness with rash)	Mosquito	Africa, Middle East	(Equines)*
Kyasanur Forest disease†	Tick	India	None
Omsk hemorrhagic fever†	Tick	Central Asia	None
Bunyaviridae, phlebovirus			
Rift Valley fever (febrile illness, hemorrhagic fever, retinitis)	Mosquito, direct contact	Africa	Sheep, cows, goats
Crimean hemorrhagic fever†—Congo	Tick	Eastern Europe, former U.S.S.R., Africa	None
Reoviridae, orbivirus			
Colorado tick fever (febrile illness)	Tick	Western North America	None
Rare and Sporadic Infections Associated with Encephalitis			
Flaviviridae, flavivirus			
Ilheus‡	Mosquito	South America	None
Negishi	Tick	Japan, China	None
Langat†	Tick	Asia	None
Orthomyxovirus			
Thogoto	Tick	Africa	None

*Disease rare or suspected but not well documented.
†Tick-borne hemorrhagic fevers.
‡Encephalitis recorded in laboratory infections or experimental infections of cancer patients only; significance in naturally acquired infections unknown.

Laboratory confirmation of infection is essential. The virus may be isolated from acute phase serum or whole blood in laboratory animals or in tissue culture. Neutralization, complement-fixation, hemagglutination-inhibition, fluorescent antibody, and enzyme-linked immunosorbent assays (ELISA) tests of acute and 3-week convalescent sera also produced the correct diagnosis. Antigen detection and IgM-capture ELISA often permit diagnosis on initial presentation and at least within a week of illness onset in most cases.

Treatment is symptomatic and may include bed rest, antipyretics, and analgesics. Ribavirin has shown some activity against certain viruses, but controlled clinical trials have not been done.

Control can be achieved by interrupting the cycle, including vaccination of reservoir animals, vector control, and education on vector avoidance. Vaccines are available in the United States for yellow fever and Japanese encephalitis. They are under development for other infections such as Rift Valley fever, Venezuelan encephalitis, and dengue.

FEVER AND RASH SYNDROMES

COLORADO TICK FEVER. Colorado tick fever (CTF) is an acute, benign tick-transmitted viral infection that occurs throughout the Rocky Mountain area. It is characterized by headache, myalgia, a biphasic febrile course lasting about 1 week, and leukopenia.

ETIOLOGY. CTF virus is an RNA virus in the coltivirus genus of the Reoviridae family; it is unrelated to other major arbovirus groups. The hard-shelled wood tick, *Dermacentor andersoni,* transmits the virus to humans by bite. Human cases are limited to the combined geographic distribution of the tick vector and the major mammalian rodent reservoirs, ground squirrels and chipmunks.

EPIDEMIOLOGY. Exposure usually occurs during the spring and summer in mountainous terrain and high plains between 4000 and 10,000 feet. Cases occur at lower altitudes during April and May and at higher altitudes during June and July, presumably because ticks emerge later at higher altitudes. Most patients find attached ticks, but others may have seen ticks on their body or clothing. Postexposure travel during the incubation period or accidental transportation of infected adult ticks in clothing or bedding may result in cases outside the endemic area.

CTF virus has been recovered from up to 14% of *D. andersoni* collected in endemic areas. The virus overwinters in hibernating nymphal and adult ticks and in infected hibernating rodent hosts. Infected nymphal ticks feed on ground squirrels and chipmunks in the spring, and because viremia in the rodent reservoirs lasts for weeks or months, a cycle involving larval and nymphal ticks and their rodent hosts evolves. Humans are accidental hosts; disease in humans results from the bite of an adult tick.

INCIDENCE AND PREVALENCE. The disease has been reported from most states in the Rocky Mountain area and from western Canadian provinces. The several hundred cases diagnosed annually in the endemic area probably represent only a fraction of the total. Mild or wholly subclinical infections probably occur.

The virus has been isolated from other species of ticks and from numerous species of small mammals, suggesting that the disease may occur over a wider geographic area than is currently appreciated.

PATHOGENESIS. There is no unusual local reaction to the tick bite. The virus replicates in hematopoietic stem cells, and symptoms begin 3 to 6 days after tick exposure. Viremia can be demonstrated at onset of fever and in red blood cells long after the virus has vanished from serum and neutralizing antibody has appeared. Transfusion-transmitted CTF has been documented.

Fatal cases are rare. Occasional patients have clinical evidence of central nervous system (CNS) or meningeal involvement, and CTF virus has been recovered from cerebrospinal fluid (CSF).

CLINICAL MANIFESTATIONS. The disease begins abruptly, with chills, fever of 38 to 40°C, myalgia (especially in the back and legs), headache, retro-orbital pain, and photophobia. Malaise and nausea may occur, but vomiting is uncommon. Physical findings during the first 2 to 3 days of illness are nonspecific. The patient may be flushed with conjunctival and pharyngeal erythema. Mild splenomegaly is sometimes present. Up to 12% of patients suffer rashes, commonly macular or macropapular and distributed over the entire body, sometimes petechial and involving primarily the extremities. Tachycardia is in proportion to the temperature elevation.

In approximately one half of cases, a distinctly biphasic illness occurs, the so-called saddleback fever. Symptoms and fever abate after 2 to 3 days, and the patient feels relatively well for 1 or 2 days, after which fever, headache, and back pain return abruptly, often more intensely than in the first phase. The second phase lasts 2 to 4 days and then subsides, leaving the patient with weakness and lassitude that disappear during the succeeding week or two. A prolonged convalescence of 3 weeks or more may ensue in patients older than 30 years. Some patients do not exhibit the typical biphasic course, experiencing only one bout of fever, three phases of fever, or a single protracted febrile illness lasting 5 to 8 days.

Children are most susceptible to CNS involvement. Findings may include aseptic meningitis with nuchal rigidity and mononuclear pleocytosis or encephalitis with a depressed sensorium or stupor. Hemorrhagic manifestations have been described in a few children with encephalitis.

Laboratory findings very early in the illness are generally not helpful, but leukopenia usually is present by the third day and becomes even more pronounced during the second phase, reaching levels as low as 1000/mm^3. The most striking decrease is in the granulocyte series, with relative lymphocytosis, and accompanying thrombocytopenia is often present. Atypical, vacuolated lymphocytes are often observed. Bone marrow examination reveals a maturation arrest in the granulocyte series.

DIAGNOSIS. CTF should be suspected in any person with a history of tick exposure in the endemic area 3 to 7 days before the onset of a febrile illness. Findings during the first phase, however, cannot be differentiated from many other acute febrile illnesses. A brief symptom-free interval followed by a second febrile illness should strongly suggest CTF.

Isolation of the virus from serum or whole blood, via inoculation of suckling mice, confirms the diagnosis. Direct immunofluorescent staining of virus in the patient's erythrocytes may provide more rapid identification. A diagnostic rise in antibody titers can be detected by indirect immunofluorescence or by neutralization test; an ELISA is also available.

The differential diagnosis can be troublesome, inasmuch as Rocky Mountain spotted fever (see Chapter 371) is transmitted in the tick fever endemic area by the same vector, *D. andersoni.* Paradoxically, Rocky Mountain spotted fever is abating in the state of Colorado; CTF now outnumbers it by at least 20-fold. Nevertheless, differential diagnosis may be impossible early in the course of disease, before the characteristic rash of Rocky Mountain spotted fever appears. A relatively symptom-free interval after 2 or 3 days would be most unusual in Rocky Mountain spotted fever and strongly favors the diagnosis of CTF.

TREATMENT AND PROGNOSIS. Therapy is entirely supportive. The disease is almost invariably benign, and the prognosis is excellent. Severe illness, complicated by CNS involvement, is seen infrequently and only in children.

PREVENTION. The most effective means of preventing CTF is for people outdoors in endemic areas during the spring and summer months to wear protective clothing or use tick repellents, together with frequent body inspection and prompt tick removal. Transfusion-associated disease can be prevented by excluding convalescent donors for a minimum of 6 months.

DENGUE. Dengue is an acute arbovirus infection that presents chiefly with fever, malaise, lymphadenopathy, and rash. Epidemics occur worldwide over large areas of the tropics and subtropics, including the Pacific Basin, Southeast Asia, and Africa. Outbreaks recurred in the Caribbean, including Puerto Rico and the U.S. Virgin Islands, in 1969. A small number of cases (40 to 80) are imported each year into the United States. Indigenous infections were recognized in the continental United States in 1980, but they have not recurred recently.

Dengue viruses are members of the Flaviviridae family. Single-stranded nonsegmented RNA viruses, they occur in four distinct serogroups, types I through 4.

EPIDEMIOLOGY. Dengue virus is transmitted from person to person primarily by *Aedes aegypti* mosquitoes, although other species of *Aedes* are involved in Asia and the Pacific. *A. aegypti* is peridomestic, biting humans readily or even preferentially. A single mosquito can infect a number of people. Small collections of water in backyard litter, especially tires, are favored breeding sites. *A. aegypti* has reappeared along the U.S. Gulf Coast; hence, the threat of dengue reemerging in the United States is real.

Dengue viruses multiply in the midgut epithelium and salivary glands of mosquitoes without producing pathologic changes. Mosquitoes remain infectious for life.

Zoonotic cycles of dengue virus transmission involving monkeys and forest *Aedes* species occur in Malaysia and West Africa. The mechanism for maintaining the virus between epidemics has not been defined, but vertical transmission in *Aedes* has been documented experimentally.

Nonimmune individuals are uniformly susceptible, and susceptibility is not influenced by age. During outbreaks, attack rates in nonimmune individuals may be high; in Puerto Rico and the U.S. Virgin Islands, the overall rate of clinical disease was 20%, with infection rates as determined by serologic surveys as high as 79%. Immunity against homotypic reinfection is complete and probably lifelong, but cross-protection between different serotypes lasts for less than 3 months.

CLINICAL FEATURES AND TREATMENT. Dengue virus infection is often inapparent. When disease occurs, three overlapping clinical forms are recognized: classic dengue, a mild to moderate febrile illness; dengue hemorrhagic fever (DHF), a severe form; and the dengue shock syndrome (DSS). Classic dengue (breakbone fever) occurs primarily in nonimmune individuals, often nonindigenous children and adults. Disease begins abruptly after a 2- to 7-day incubation with severe splitting headache, retro-orbital pain, backache (especially in the lumbar area), leg pain, and arthralgia. Most patients complain of pain on moving their eyes. True rigors are common during the illness but usually do not herald the onset. Other common symptoms include insomnia, nausea, anorexia with taste aberrations, cutaneous hyperesthesia, and generalized weakness. Mild rhinopharyngitis occurs in one fourth of patients. Examination reveals relative bradycardia, scleral injection (30 to 90%), tenderness on pressure on the ocular globes, and pharyngeal injection. A transient macular rash may appear on the first or second day. Within 2 to 3 days after onset, the temperature may decrease to nearly normal and other symptoms subside. Remission in this biphasic illness typically lasts 2 days. Fever then returns, as may other symptoms, although they are generally less severe. On the third to fifth day (with the second phase), a more definite maculopapular rash usually appears on the trunk and then spreads to the arms and legs while sparing the palms and soles. The rash is often characterized by 2- to 5-mm "islands of white in a sea of red." The rash is accompanied in some cases by complaints of burning in the palms and soles. On resolution, the rash may desquamate. Concurrently, generalized nontender lymphadenopathy, typically including posterior cervical, epitrochlear, and inguinal chains, develops. The biphasic febrile course is considered characteristic but often is not encountered. The entire illness lasts 5 to 7 days and terminates abruptly. Complaints of fatigue and depression for an additional several weeks are common.

In addition to the classic syndrome, a mild illness characterized by fever, anorexia, headache, myalgia, and evanescent rashes sometimes occurs and is usually not associated with lymphadenopathy. At onset in both classic and mild dengue, leukocyte counts may be normal or low; however, by the third to fifth day leukocyte counts are decreased (<5000/mm³ with granulocytopenia). Thrombocytopenia (<100,000/mm³) also may be a feature. Urinalysis may show moderate albuminuria.

A history of travel to dengue-endemic areas and occurrence of other cases in a community are important reminders to include dengue in the differential diagnosis. Specific diagnosis depends on virus isolation or serologic tests. Viremia can be detected for the initial 3 to 5 days with dengue types 1, 2, and 3 by inoculation of mosquito tissue cell cultures. Viral titers in patients with dengue 4 are considerably lower than in patients with types 1, 2, and 3, making viral isolation less common. Of serologic tests, neutralization is most specific. IgM antibodies indicate recent dengue infection but do not provide a type-specific diagnosis and cross-react with other flavivirus antibodies, including those following immunization with yellow fever vaccine.

Treatment is entirely symptomatic. In the absence of DHF or DSS, mortality is nil. Preventing epidemics relies principally on reducing or eradicating *A. aegypti* by eliminating breeding sites and using larvacides. Ultra-low-volume aerial spraying of organophos-

phate insecticides (malathion) to reduce the population of adult female mosquitoes has been successful in emergency control of epidemics.

WEST NILE FEVER. Like dengue, West Nile fever is a mosquito-transmitted, acute, self-limited illness that presents chiefly with fever, malaise, lymphadenopathy, and rash. A flavivirus, West Nile fever viral strains from Africa, Europe, the former U.S.S.R., and the Middle East are antigenically distinct from strains isolated in India and the Far East.

Virus transmission involves mosquitoes and wild birds, with mammals, including humans, as incidental end-stage hosts. The mosquito vector species varies: *Culex univittatus*, *C. pipiens*, and *C. molestus* in the Middle East and Africa, *Mansonia metallicus* in Uganda, and *C. tritaeniorhynchus* in Asia. In endemic areas, human infections are extremely common, with over 60% of young adults having antibodies; this suggests a high prevalence of inapparent or undifferentiated febrile illness in children. There is no gender predominance.

CLINICAL FEATURES. Following an incubation period of 1 to 6 days, the onset is usually abrupt without prodromal symptoms. The temperature rises quickly to 38.3 to 40°C, with rigors in one third of patients. Symptoms include drowsiness, severe frontal headache, ocular pain, myalgia, and pain in the abdomen and back. A small number of patients have dryness of the throat, anorexia, and nausea. Cough is common. Examination shows facial flushing, conjunctival injection, and coating of the tongue. The predominant finding is generalized lymphadenopathy. Nodes are of moderate size and nontender and usually include the occipital, axillary, and inguinal chains. The spleen and liver are occasionally slightly enlarged. The temperature curve may be biphasic. In half of patients, a pale roseolar maculopapular rash, predominantly on the trunk and upper arms, appears from the second to fifth day. It may be evanescent (several hours) or persist until defervescence; and it does not desquamate. Vesicular lesions may occur but are rare. The illness is self-limited and lasts 3 to 5 days in 80% of patients.

Infection also may result in aseptic meningitis or meningoencephalitis, especially in the elderly. CSF examinations may reveal a lymphocytic pleocytosis with some increase in protein concentration. Other rare complications include myocarditis, pancreatitis, and hepatitis. Convalescence is often prolonged, lasting several weeks with prominent symptoms of fatigue. Lymph node enlargement requires several months to regress. Laboratory findings include leukopenia (<4000/mm³ in one-third of patients).

Clinically, West Nile fever resembles dengue. West Nile virus can be isolated from the blood of three fourths of patients on the first day, with viremia persisting but decreasing over 5 days. Serologic diagnosis is possible using a number of tests; however, cross-reactions with other flaviviruses complicate interpretation.

Treatment is symptomatic. Ribavirin has activity against West Nile fever virus, but since the disease is self-limited and almost never fatal, its use does not seem indicated.

PHLEBOTOMUS FEVER. Phlebotomus (sandfly, pappataci, or 3-day) fever is an acute, relatively mild, self-limited infection transmitted by *Phlebotomus* flies.

The sandfly fever group of viruses are enveloped, single-stranded, trisegmented RNA viruses belonging to the phlebovirus genus of the Bunyaviridae family. There are at least five immunologically distinct phleboviruses (Naples, Sicilian, Punto Toro, Chagres, and Candiru). The principal vector of Phlebotomus fever viruses in the Mediterranean, Middle East, and northwest India is *Phlebotomus paptasii*, which breeds in dry sandy areas and feeds in early evening. In Central America, *Lutzomyia*, a forest-dwelling species, is the primary culprit. Although undefined, sandfly fever viruses presumably are maintained in a vector-host wildlife cycle between epidemics. During epidemics, humans may act as the major host. Transovarial transmission probably serves as an alternative mechanism for virus perpetuation. Sandflies are small (2 to 3 mm), which enables them to penetrate screens and mosquito netting. There is no pain or itching after the bite; hence, only about 1% of patients remember being bitten.

CLINICAL FEATURES AND TREATMENT. After an incubation period of 2 to 6 days, symptoms develop abruptly in more than 90% of patients. Temperatures rise to 37.8 to 40.1°C. Headache is nearly always present and often is accompanied by pain on ocular movement and retro-orbital pain. Myalgia is common and may be localized, for example, to the abdomen; if to the chest, it resembles pleurodynia. Other symptoms include vomiting, photophobia, alteration or loss of taste, and arthralgia. Conjunctival injection is seen in one-third of patients. With severe illness, mild papilledema has been seen. Small vesicles occur on the palate. Malcular or urticarial rashes may erupt. The spleen is rarely palpable, and lymphadenopathy is absent. Pulse is proportional to the temperature on the first day, followed by relative bradycardia. Fever persists for 2 to 4 days in most patients and gradually decreases. Weakness and feelings of depression are common during convalescence. Second attacks occur 2 to 12 weeks after the first in 15% of cases. Aseptic meningitis may develop. CSF findings include pleocytosis (average cell counts of 90/mm³ with either mononuclear or neutrophilic leukocytes). Laboratory findings include leukopenia (<5000/mm³) in 90% of patients. The leukopenia may not occur until the third day. Lymphopenia with an increase in band neutrophils early in the illness is followed by a relative lymphocytosis (40 to 65%). Urinalyses are usually normal.

Diagnosis is made on the basis of clinical and epidemiologic findings. Sandfly fever viruses replicate and produce plaques in Vero cell cultures. Serologic tests are not available.

Treatment is symptomatic. No fatalities have been reported.

RIFT VALLEY FEVER. Rift Valley fever (RVF) is an acute disease principally of livestock—sheep, goats, cattle, and camels—caused by the mosquito-transmitted RVF virus. The virus is an enveloped, single-stranded, trisegmented RNA virus belonging to the phlebovirus genus and the Bunyaviridae family. The virus multiplies readily in most common cell cultures, is cytopathic, and forms plaques.

RVF virus can be transmitted by a number of mosquito species; in Egypt, *Culex pipiens,* in South Africa, *C. theileri,* and in East Africa, *Aedes* species are the major vectors. Epizootics in large domestic animals have been associated with particularly wet rainy seasons and high mosquito density. In cattle and sheep, most pregnant ewes and cows abort, and mortality in newborn lambs is > 90%. A wildlife-mosquito cycle during interepizootic periods has been postulated but not confirmed. Transovarial vertical transmission is an alternative. During an epizootic, disease occurs first in animals and then in humans. Direct transmission to humans by contact with blood or tissues of infected animals may be more frequent than mosquito transmission. Laboratory-acquired infections presumably due to aerosols are common. In addition to eastern and southern Africa, RVF virus has been isolated in western Africa. Zinga virus, a cause of sporadic human disease in central Africa, is a strain of RVF virus.

CLINICAL FEATURES. After an incubation period of 3 to 6 days, illness begins with an abrupt onset, malaise, occasionally rigors, headache, myalgia, and backache. The temperature rises rapidly to 38.3 to 40°C. Later complaints include anorexia, loss of taste, photophobia, and epigastric pain. Findings may include facial flushing and conjunctival injection. Biphasic fever, with the initial elevation lasting 2 to 3 days, followed by remission and then a second febrile period, is common. Fever generally lasts a total of about 1 week. Convalescence is usually rapid. Normally a benign illness with almost no fatalities, rare cases with severe complications—meningoencephalitis, retinopathy, or hepatic or hemorrhagic manifestations—have resulted in death. Encephalitis with intense headache, confusion, and stupor may appear as the acute infection subsides. The CSF shows a lymphocytic pleocytosis with normal CSF glucose values. Ocular complications including visual loss occur 2 to 7 days after the onset. Findings on ophthalmoscopic examination include macular edema, cotton-wool exudates on the macula, hemorrhages, retinitis, and vascular occlusion. One-half of such patients have some permanent loss of visual acuity. Hepatic and hemorrhagic manifestations may develop during the acute illness. Deaths from massive hepatic necrosis occur 7 to 10 days after onset. Hemorrhagic manifestations include epistaxis, hematemesis, melena, and intracranial hemorrhage. The fatality ratio in severely ill patients exceeds 50%. Laboratory findings include initial normal to increased total leukocyte counts initially, followed by leukopenia with granulocytopenia but an increase in band forms. Thrombocytopenia and clotting defects occur.

DIAGNOSIS. Isolating virus from blood by inoculating mice con-

firms the diagnosis. Three fourths of patients are viremic at the onset of illness. Neutralizing antibodies appear as early as 4 days.

TREATMENT AND PREVENTION. Treatment is symptomatic. In patients with hemorrhagic manifestations, transfusion of platelets and fresh frozen plasma may be beneficial. Ribavirin has been partially protective in experimentally infected animals. Thus, one might consider administering ribavirin (2.0-g loading dose IV, then 1.0 g IV every 6 hours for 4 days, then 0.5 g IV every 8 hours for 6 days) to patients with severe disease. Because the virus can be spread by contact with blood and tissues, and humans show high levels of viremia, blood and needle precautions are essential.

POLYARTHRITIS. Fever, rash, and polyarthritis are caused by at least six viruses belonging to the alphavirus genus of the Togaviridae family. This group of single-stranded RNA viruses shares antigenic determinants and is transmitted by mosquitoes to vertebrate hosts.

CHIKUNGUNYA VIRUS. EPIDEMIOLOGY. Chikungunya virus (CK) is of major importance in Africa and Asia. CK virus is transmitted by *Aedes* mosquitoes in Africa; in the tropical forests of the continent, the mosquitoes belong to the subgenera *Stegomyia* and *Diceromyia.* Nonhuman primates—monkeys or baboons—serve as primary hosts, with transmission occurring mostly in the rainy season. Human involvement is largely secondary. *A. aegypti* also functions as a vector in villages and urban areas, where humans may serve as the vertebrate host. In sub-Saharan Africa, except in the dry areas and below 18 degrees latitude, antibody prevalence surveys range from 20% to > 90%. In Asia, transmission is primarily human to human via *A. aegypti.* CK virus is present in India, Southeast Asia, and the Philippines. Seroprevalence rates of 31% were observed in Bangkok. The potential exists for CK virus transmission outside the current distribution, i.e., Central and South America, as well as the southern United States.

CLINICAL FEATURES. The incubation period is usually 2 to 3 days but may be as long as 12 days. The onset is usually abrupt, with temperatures rising to 38.3 to 40°C, often accompanied by rigors and incapacitating arthralgia. The arthralgias are polyarticular and migratory, involving predominantly the small joints of the hands, wrists, ankles, and toes. Pain is increased with motion and worse in the morning. Joint swelling is common, but effusions are not. The arthralgia is associated with generalized myalgia. Other symptoms include headache, photophobia, sore throat, anorexia, and vomiting. Flushing of the face and neck occur at onset. Other signs include conjunctival injection and lymphadenopathy. A macropapular rash, usually involving the trunk and limbs, typically occurs on the second to fifth day. The rash lasts 1 to 5 days and may just fade or may desquamate. On the second or third day, the fever may remit for 1 to 2 days and then recur. However, the biphasic course is not as striking as that seen with dengue. Laboratory findings may include leukopenia with relative lymphocytosis, although leukocyte counts are usually normal. Mild thrombocytopenia may develop. The joint symptoms may persist for long periods, only one-third of individuals being asymptomatic within a few weeks. About 5% of patients have persistent joint pain, stiffness, and recurrent effusions. Persistence may be more common in HLA-B27–positive patients. In African children, disease is milder, with arthralgia being less prominent. In Asia, CK virus is responsible for a hemorrhagic fever syndrome closely resembling dengue hemorrhagic fever or the DSS. Other features may include encephalitis and myocarditis.

DIAGNOSIS AND TREATMENT. CK virus disease should be suspected clinically given the appropriate epidemiologic history and the triad of fever, acute arthralgia/arthritis, and rash. Most patients are viremic during the first 48 hours. Hemagglutination inhibition (HI) (III) antibodies appear by the fifth to seventh day. Treatment is symptomatic.

O'NYONG-NYONG VIRUS. The name *o'nyong-nyong* (in the language spoken in the Ugandan province of Acholi) means "weakening of the joints." Epidemics have occurred in Uganda and Kenya. *Anopheles funnestus* and *A. anogambiae* mosquitoes are o'nyong-nyong (ON) virus vectors.

Clinical features are similar to those of CK disease. The incubation period may be somewhat longer, at least 8 days. Fever is less prominent, exceeding 38.3°C only in one third of patients. Rash occurs in 60 to 70%. In contrast to CK virus disease, generalized lymphadenopathy is a common feature, and there appears to be less residual arthropathy. Diagnosis is based on virus isolation or seroconversion by HI assays, but cross-reactions with CK virus make interpretation difficult.

MAYARO VIRUS. Mayaro virus (MYV) has been associated with epidemics of acute polyarthritis in Brazil and Bolivia.

MYV exists in the forested areas of Central and South America with annual infection rates of 10 to 60% and a 2:1 male predominance. The vectors for MYV are *Haemagogus* mosquitoes. The virus causes high-level viremia in marmosets and other primates.

CLINICAL FEATURES. After a 1-week incubation period, illness begins abruptly with fever, chills, severe frontal headache, myalgia, and dizziness. Arthralgia (which in some cases precedes the fever) is uniform, very prominent, and occasionally incapacitating, striking small joints, wrists, fingers, ankles, and toes. Temperatures usually exceed 40°C. Other initial symptoms (less than one-third of patients) include nausea, vomiting, and diarrhea. Initial clinical features include occasional conjunctival suffusion, inguinal lymphadenopathy (one-half of patients), and joint swelling (one-quarter of patients). About the fifth day, maculopapular rash develops over the chest, back, arms, and legs. Rash appears in 90% of children and one-half of adults and lasts about 3 days. The clinical course of MYV is usually 3 to 5 days except for the arthralgia, which may persist for several months. Laboratory findings include leukopenia (as low as 2500/mm³). Urinalyses revealed albuminuria (2+) in one fourth of patients. Some patients showed increases in AST levels. Occasional fatalities have been reported.

DIAGNOSIS. Diagnosis is confirmed by virus isolation. MYV-specific IgM responses have been observed.

ROSS RIVER VIRUS. Ross River (RR) virus outbreaks occur almost entirely between December and June. RR virus infection exists in Australia, New Guinea, the Solomon Islands, Fiji, and the Samoan, Cook, and some Melanesian islands. The natural vector-reservoir relationships have not been well established. *Culex annulirostris* is probably the major vector, although other species of mosquitoes may be involved. Several mammalian species, especially the New Holland mouse and wallabies, are important hosts in Australia. In the Pacific outbreak, *Aedes vigilax* also may have been an important vector, and human-mosquito-human transmission was likely. Infection rates are equal at all ages and in both genders, but clinical disease rates are 4% in patients under age 20 years and 42% in those older than 20 years. The clinical attack rate of males to females is 1:1.7.

CLINICAL FEATURES. In Australia, incubation is 7 to 9 days, whereas in the Pacific the incubation period is shorter. At onset, the illness is characterized by headache, myalgia, nausea, and vomiting, and occasionally tenderness of the palms and soles. Initially, fever may be absent or minimal (highest 38°C). About one-half of patients experience arthritis involving mainly the small joints, wrists, and ankles. Knee involvement also is common. The joint swelling and paresthesias may precede a rash by 1 to 15 days. In the other half of patients, the rash precedes the arthralgia. The rash, which is usually maculopapular, appears on the cheeks and forehead, occasionally spreads to the trunk, or may be restricted to extremities. The rash may be pruritic. Vesicles occur rarely. Tender lymphadenopathy occurs in one-fifth of patients. Recovery is slow, only one-half being able to return to work by 1 month and 10% still having joint symptoms at 3 months. Laboratory findings are not striking; leukocyte counts are normal or minimally decreased. The erythrocyte sedimentation rate is increased acutely but normalizes over several weeks, even with continued joint symptoms. Antinuclear antibody and rheumatoid factor tests are negative. Synovial fluid changes are not striking: cell counts of 1000 to 60,000, predominantly mononuclear, normal viscosity. Urinalyses are normal, although recently RR virus has been associated with segmental sclerosing glomerulonephritis.

The diagnosis is usually based on clinical features. In Australia patients seldom have viremia on presentation, whereas in the Pacific outbreak viremia was readily detected. HI antibodies appear early. Treatment is symptomatic.

SINDBIS VIRUS (OKELBO DISEASE, POGOSTA DISEASE, KARELIAN FEVER). Sindbis virus has caused disease in Egypt, elsewhere in Africa, in Europe, and in Australia. In the former U.S.S.R. it is known as "Karelian fever," in Sweden as "Okelbo disease," and in Finland as "Pogosta disease." *C. univittatus* is the principal vector, and birds are the major hosts. Human infection is common where birds and *Culex* mosquitoes are in close proximity. Human antibody rates are commonly 20 to 30% in the Nile Valley of Egypt. Because Sindbis and West Nile fever virus share the same transmission cycles, Sindbis transmission often parallels that of West Nile fever virus. In northern Europe, symptomatic disease appears in late summer between 60 and 65 degrees of north latitude, usually affecting adults with forest occupations. The virus has been isolated from *Culiseta, Aedes,* and *Culex* mosquitoes. The host has not been identified.

CLINICAL FEATURES AND TREATMENT. The incubation period for Sindbis has not been defined. The illness more closely resembles Ross River virus disease than chikungunya or o'nyong-nyong disease. Clinically, fever is low grade and is accompanied by malaise, myalgia, rash, and arthralgia in wrists, ankles, knees, and elbows. Periarticular involvement and tendinitis are common. The rash begins on the trunk as scattered macules and spreads to the extremities, palms, and soles. The rash may precede or follow the joint symptoms by 1 to 2 days. Unlike that caused by other alphaviruses, the rash frequently becomes vesicular, especially on the feet and hands. The rash fades within a week. In Europe, persistence of joint complaints is a common feature. In Sweden, more than 20% of patients had joint symptoms longer than 1 month after onset.

Antibodies can be detected by HI tests within 7 to 10 days of onset. Treatment is symptomatic.

PULMONARY SYNDROMES

HANTAVIRUS PULMONARY SYNDROME. Hantavirus pulmonary syndrome (HPS) is a Pan-American zoonosis. No arthropod is involved. HPS results from infection with New World hantaviruses (Sin Nombre, Bayou, Black Creek Canal, and New York-1 viruses), members of the Bunyaviridae family, a group of large, enveloped, negative-sense RNA viruses with tripartite genomes. Other hantaviruses cause hemorrhagic fever (see Chapter 391). Hantaviruses are maintained by a single rodent reservoir species belonging to the subfamily sigmodontinae (*Peromyseus maniculatus* [deer mouse], *P. leucopas* [white-footed mouse], *Sigmodon hispidis* [cotton rat], and *Oryzomys palustris* [rice rat]). Humans are infected by exposure to aerosols of secretions and excretions from infected rodents. Approximately 400 cases have occurred throughout the Americas.

PATHOLOGY. The lungs of patients dying from HPS show interstitial infiltration of T lymphocytes and alveolar pulmonary edema without marked necrosis or polymorphonuclear leukocyte infiltration. The major abnormality is thought to be an increase in vascular permeability via an immunopathologic mechanism.

CLINICAL FEATURES. The disease begins abruptly with fever and myalgia, often accompanied by gastrointestinal symptoms and headache; it is indistinguishable from other nonspecific acute febrile illnesses such as influenza. Examination is unrevealing except for fever, tachycardia, and tachypnea. The respiratory symptoms begin after 4 to 5 days. The patient first notes cough and dyspnea, but acute pulmonary edema and hypotension develop rapidly in most patients. The case-fatality rate is 40 to 60%.

Laboratory abnormalities include elevated hematocrit, marked leukocytosis (median count 26,000/mm³) with shift to the left, abnormal lymphocytes on smear, thrombocytopenia, prolonged prothrombin and partial thromboplastin times, and mildly elevated alananine transaminase (ALT) and lactate dehydrogenase (LDH) levels. The severe renal abnormalities seen in hemorrhagic fever with renal syndrome (HFRS) (see Chapter 103) characteristic of other hantavirus infections, are not seen, although mild elevations of serum creatinine and proteinuria have been observed. Blood gases reveal marked hypoxia of adult respiratory distress syndrome (ARDS).

DIAGNOSIS. HPS should be considered when an otherwise healthy adult develops an ARDS-like picture without any of the known causes of ARDS. The diagnosis can be confirmed serologically: Virtually all patients will have specific IgM and IgG antibodies detectable by ELISA on admission to hospital. Virus recovery from clinical specimens is difficult. Polymerase chain reaction and immunohistochemical staining can detect virus in tissue.

TREATMENT AND PREVENTION. Intravenous ribavirin has been used to treat HPS in patients, but its efficacy has not been established. Nonspecific treatment of ARDS, shock, and other complications may be helpful.

Avoiding contact with rodent urine and feces and rodent control in the home form the basis of HPS prevention.

ARTHROPOD-BORNE VIRAL ENCEPHALITIDES

Arboviral encephalitis is a significant health problem in Europe, the former U.S.S.R., parts of Asia, and Central and South America, but not Africa. The disease is of particular concern in the Americas not only because of its multiple etiologic agents and widespread occurrence but also because of its concurrent affliction of domestic animals and humans and its potential for epidemic spread.

The most important arthropod-borne viruses that cause encephalitis are shown in Table 392-2. Only a small fraction of persons infected with these viruses experience severe CNS manifestations, and human infection is most often subclinical (Table 392-3). The ratio of inapparent to clinically overt infections is a distinctive, age-dependent quality of each disease. The neurologic disease usually begins after a variable period of nonspecific, systemic symptoms and may take the form of aseptic meningitis, meningoencephalitis, or encephalitis. These syndromes are not distinguishable on clinical grounds alone from similar syndromes caused by other infectious agents.

PATHOLOGY AND PATHOGENESIS. Two pathologic processes are common to the arboviral encephalitides: (1) neuronal and glial damage mediated by intracellular viral infection and (2) migration of immunologically active cells into the perivascular space and brain parenchyma. Endothelial cell swelling and proliferation, destruction of myelin sheaths in deep white matter areas, and vasculitis are present in some arboviral encephalitides.

After a bite by an infected arthropod, viral replication occurs in local tissues and in regional lymph nodes. Viremia, which seeds extraneural tissues, occurs and persists depending on the extent of replication in extraneural sites, the rate of viral clearance by the reticuloendothelial system, and the appearance of humoral antibodies. Sites of extraneural infection vary from virus to virus. Many alphavirus and flaviviruses involve striated muscle and vascular endothelium, whereas Venezuelan encephalitis virus is associated with myeloid and lymphoid tissue invasion. During this viremia, the neural parenchyma may be invaded, but the mode of penetration of virus across the blood-brain barrier is not completely understood. Possible mechanisms include passive movement of virus across vascular membranes and virus replication in cerebral capillary endothelial cells. Factors that increase vascular permeability promote neuroinvasion. In experimental animals infected with some flaviviruses, virus enters the CNS via the olfactory neuroepithelium.

The immature brain is more susceptible to damage by western equine, Venezuelan equine, and California encephalitis viruses (see Table 392-3). St. Louis encephalitis principally affects the elderly, whereas Japanese encephalitis and eastern equine encephalitis have a bimodal incidence, striking both children and elderly persons. In endemic areas, immunity accumulated with increasing age may reduce the incidence of disease in older persons for some viruses; however, the reasons for increased severity of illness with other viruses remain unknown.

DIFFERENTIAL DIAGNOSIS. The most important consideration in diagnosis is to differentiate arthropod-borne viral encephalitis from acute CNS infection due to treatable organisms. The early prodro-

mata resemble influenza, dengue, or other influenza-like illnesses. Bacterial meningitis (especially early or partially treated), infective bacterial endocarditis, brain abscess, subdural empyema, and cerebral thrombophlebitis may mimic viral encephalitis, and CSF changes are sometimes similar. Other infections that occasionally cause meningoencephalitis resembling arthropod-borne viral encephalitis include tuberculosis, cryptococcosis, histoplasmosis, coccidioidomycosis, Rocky Mountain spotted fever, leptospirosis, falciparum malaria, trichinosis, *Naseglleria* meningitis, typhoid fever, Lyme disease, and *Mycoplasma* pneumonia.

Acute meningoencephalitis may result from infections with other viruses, including herpesviruses, human immunodeficiency virus (HIV), mumps virus, enteroviruses, lymphocytic choriomeningitis virus, rabies, influenza, and the exanthematous viral infections of childhood. Exposure history, presence of an outbreak of similar disease in the community, and summer-fall occurrence are principal clues to an arboviral etiology. Enteroviruses also cause summer-fall outbreaks, but the predominant syndrome is aseptic meningitis, and the occurrence of rash or pleurodynia is a helpful clue. Herpes simplex encephalitis presents an important diagnostic challenge, because chemotherapy is available. The presence of localizing neurologic signs, localizing findings on computed tomography (CT) or magnetic resonance imaging (MRI) scans, or brain biopsy may help distinguish herpes simplex encephalitis from that due to arthropod-borne viral encephalitides.

Noninfectious diseases of the CNS such as *cerebrovascular accident* may be confused with viral encephalitis. For example, St. Louis encephalitis, a disease of the elderly, has been misdiagnosed as a stroke. Subarachnoid hemorrhage produces meningismus, fever, headache, and neurologic signs that mimic an infectious etiology. *Metabolic encephalopathies* may present features suggesting infectious encephalitis. *Neoplastic* or *granulomatous diseases* involving the CNS and a variety of diseases of uncertain etiology (cat scratch disease, Behçet's disease, Reye's syndrome, acute multiple sclerosis, and systemic lupus erythematosus) must be considered in the differential diagnosis as well.

WESTERN EQUINE ENCEPHALITIS (WEE). ETIOLOGIC AGENT. WEE virus is a member of the alphavirus genus of the Togaviridae family.

EPIDEMIOLOGY. Incidence and Prevalence. Since 1987, very few (0 to 2) cases of WEE have been reported in the United States in the area from the Mississippi River west to the Rocky Mountains. Mixed outbreaks of WEE and St Louis encephalitis are common. Epidemics occur in early or midsummer and may follow heavy snow melt or flooding, conditions favorable for breeding of mosquitoes. Cases of encephalitis in equines often precede the appearance of human disease. The illness principally affects residents of rural communities, and the incidence is higher in males than in females. WEE is most severe in infants and young children. The case-fatality rate is between 3 and 5%. The ratio of inapparent to apparent infection is also age-dependent, ranging from about 1:1 in infants under age 1 year, to 58:1 in children aged 1 to 4 years, to over 1000:1 in persons over age 14 years.

WEE virus also occurs in South America. Equine epizootics in Argentina have been associated with human cases.

Transmission. WEE virus circulates between wild birds and *C. tarsalis* mosquitoes. *C. tarsalis* is responsible for infection of humans and equines, which develop low or undetectable viremia and do not perpetuate the chain of transmission. In temperate areas, transmission ceases during the winter months.

Table 392-3 ■ DIFFERING FEATURES OF ARTHROPOD-BORNE ENCEPHALITIDES IMPORTANT IN THE UNITED STATES

	WESTERN EQUINE ENCEPHALITIS	EASTERN EQUINE ENCEPHALITIS	VENEZUELAN EQUINE ENCEPHALITIS	ST LOUIS ENCEPHALITIS	CALIFORNIA ENCEPHALITIS
Incidence	0–2/year, mostly infants and children	10/year	Rare in U.S.; mostly children	0–2000/year, mostly adults	10–50/year, mostly children
Time of year	Early or midsummer	Late summer, early fall	Summer	Mid- to late summer	July–September
Case-fatality	3–5% in children	50–70%, highest in children <15 yr and adults >55 yr	35% in children; <10% in older persons	9% overall; 0% <20 yr, 30% >65 yr	<1%
Residual damage	33% in infants	30–50%, especially in children	Frequent in children	Frequent in elderly	Probably rare
Cerebrospinal fluid	<500 cells	500–2000 cells PMNs*	<500 cells	<500 cells	<500 cells

*Polymorphonuclear leukocytes.

CLINICAL FEATURES AND PATHOLOGY. The disease usually begins with an influenza-like illness consisting of fever, headache, malaise, and myalgia lasting 1 to 4 days. Somnolence, lethargy, photophobia, vomiting, and neck stiffness may follow; neurologic involvement may rapidly progress to stupor, coma, and convulsions. Paresis, cranial nerve deficits, tremors, and abnormal reflexes may be present. In fatal cases, patients die 1 to 2 days after coma develops. Survivors generally experience a sudden and rapid recovery. However, about one third of surviving infants suffer retardation, cerebellar damage, choreoathetosis, and spastic paralysis. Children with protracted illnesses who develop convulsions during the acute stage are more likely to suffer long-term neurologic impairment. Adults may have a prolonged convalescent syndrome, but objective residua are rare. Congenital infections are documented and result in severe and progressive neurologic deterioration.

Leukocytosis and shift to the left are common. The CSF contains <500 white cells/mm (at first polymorphonuclear, then mononuclear) and elevated protein concentration (usually 90 to 110 mg/dL).

Pathologic examination of the brains of infants reveals massive neuroparenchymal destruction; children dying months or years after the acute insult often have large cystic lesions in many areas of the brain. In older children and adults, acute WEE is characterized by focal necrosis and perivascular cuffing, predominantly in the basal ganglia and thalamic nuclei but also in deep cerebral white matter.

DIAGNOSIS. Viral isolation from blood or CSF is almost never successful. Diagnosis is achieved by demonstrating a rise in HI, fluorescent, complement-fixing (CF), ELISA, or neutralizing-antibody titers in appropriately timed (10 to 14 days apart) paired sera. IgM antibodies demonstrated in serum or CSF by ELISA provides a presumptive diagnosis.

TREATMENT. There is no specific therapy for WEE. Supportive care is essential and may reduce mortality. Control of high fever, cerebral edema, convulsions, fluid and electrolyte imbalances, and airways is critical.

PREVENTION AND CONTROL. An experimental formalin-inactivated vaccine grown in chick embryo cell cultures has been used to protect laboratory workers but is not indicated for others. In threatened or ongoing epidemics, residents should be advised to use protective clothing, insect repellents, and window screens and to restrict outdoor activity in the early morning, late afternoon, and evening (times of greatest mosquito activity). Public health measures include spraying insecticides aimed at the adult *C. tarsalis* vector.

EASTERN EQUINE ENCEPHALITIS (EEE). ETIOLOGIC AGENT. EEE virus is a member of the Togaviridae family, alphavirus genus.

EPIDEMIOLOGY. Incidence and Prevalence. The disease in humans is relatively rare, with fewer than 10 cases occurring each year in the Gulf Coast and Atlantic states, usually associated with a predominantly equine epizootic involving 100 to 300 animals. Outbreaks usually occur during the late summer and early fall. The occurrence of equine cases or outbreaks of fatal encephalitis in penned exotic birds (pheasants, chukar partridges) precedes the appearance of human cases by several weeks or more. Epizootics of EEE have been reported in the Caribbean (Hispaniola) and South America.

Despite the small size of EEE epidemics, the severity is high. The case-fatality rate is 50 to 70%. Incidence and mortality are highest in children under age 15 years and in persons over 55 years, with no gender predilection.

Transmission. In temperate areas, EEE virus circulates between wild birds and *C. melanura* mosquitoes in freshwater swamp habitat. Equine epizootics and associated human cases result from extension of the transmission cycle to involve *Aedes* and *Coquillettidia* mosquitoes, which feed on horses and humans.

CLINICAL FEATURES AND PATHOLOGY. The disease is more acute and rapidly progressive than the other arboviral encephalitides. Onset is abrupt, with high fever, vomiting, and somnolence. Stupor, coma, myoclonus, and generalized convulsions appear within 24 to 48 hours. Autonomic disturbances (sialorrhea) may be prominent, and respiratory difficulty and cyanosis are frequent. In children, facial, periorbital, or generalized edema may be present. Death usually occurs during the first week; in surviving patients, recovery begins during the second week and may progress rapidly. Good functional recovery is associated with a long prodromal course and absence of coma. Residual damage, found in 30 to 50% of the patients, is often severe, especially in children, and is characterized by retardation, spastic paralyses, and atrophy of brain sustance.

A striking peripheral leukocytosis and shift to the left are frequent findings in patients with EEE. Examination of the CSF reveals 500 to 2000 white cells/mm³ (predominantly polymorphonuclear). As the total cell count falls, polymorphonuclear cells persist as a significant fraction. Red blood cells may be present, the protein is elevated, and glucose is normal.

In contrast to St Louis encephalitis and WEE, the brain is grossly edematous and congested, and the inflammatory response is predominantly polymorphonuclear. The areas most affected are basal ganglia, thalamus, hippocampus, and frontal and occipital cortex. Focal vasculitis, endothelial cell swelling, intravenous and arteriolar thrombus formation, demyelination, necrosis, neuronolysis, and neuronophagia are prominent.

SPECIFIC DIAGNOSIS. Isolating the virus from blood and CSF is rarely successful. Serologic diagnosis by demonstrating a rise in antibody titer using appropriately timed paired sera is the most practical and available test. Because of the rapid course of the clinical disease, sera should be obtained at 2- to 3-day intervals during the acute phase of illness.

TREATMENT, PREVENTION, AND CONTROL. Treatment is supportive (see previous discussion of WEE). An experimental formalin-inactivated chick embryo cell culture vaccine is used to protect laboratory and field workers. Reduction of mosquito populations by appropriate use of insecticides may be effective in threatened or established outbreaks.

VENEZUELAN EQUINE ENCEPHALITIS (VEE). ETIOLOGY. The causative agent of VEE is a member of the Togaviridae family and alphavirus genus. Six antigenic subtypes (I to VI) and multiple antigenic variants of subtypes I and III are recognized by serologic tests. Subtypes IAB and IC are responsible for epidemics involving humans and equines. In Florida, subtype II is enzootic and produces sporadic human disease.

EPIDEMIOLOGY. Incidence and Prevalence. Before 1973, large equine epizootics occurred at 5- to 10-year intervals in Venezuela, Colombia, Ecuador, and Peru, involving many thousands of animals and incurring mortality rates as high as 40%. Associated human morbidity also was great (up to 32,000 clinical cases). No outbreaks of equine or human disease have been recognized in more than 15 years.

The predominant syndrome is a self-limited influenza-like illness; only about 4% of infected persons, principally children under age 15 years develop encephalitis. Subclinical infections are rare. The case-fatality rate in children up to 5 years old with encephalitis is approximately 35%, but in older persons it is less than 10%. Laboratory infections are common in unvaccinated persons working with the virus or infected animals.

Transmission. A large variety of mosquito vectors, including species of the genera *Aedes, Psorophora,* and *Mansonia,* transmit subtypes IAB and IC during epizootic epidemics. Equines are the principal viremic hosts. Virus may be present in pharyngeal excretions of human patients; contact or aerosol person-to-person spread, although possible, is not epidemiologically important.

The other members of the VEE viral complex, including subtype II in Florida, have enzootic transmission cycles involving *Culex (Melanoconion)* species mosquitoes and small forest rodents and marsupials. Human disease is sporadic and relatively uncommon.

CLINICAL FEATURES AND PATHOLOGY. After an incubation period of 2 to 5 days, there is sudden onset of fever, chills, malaise, and headache, followed by myalgias, nausea, vomiting, and occasionally diarrhea. Physical examination reveals fever, tachycardia, conjunctival injection, and, in some cases, nonexudative pharyngitis. The acute illness generally subsides in 4 to 6 days, and convalescent symptoms may last up to 3 weeks. A biphasic course has sometimes been noted; acute symptoms reappear after a brief remission, within a week after the initial onset.

Some patients exhibit evidence of mild CNS involvement (photophobia, somnolence, confusion) during the typical influenza-like illness. When it occurs, severe encephalitis is characterized by meningeal signs, convulsions, tremor, stupor, coma, spastic paralysis, abnormal reflexes, cranial nerve palsies, and central respiratory failure. Residual neurologic damage occurs in severe cases. Infections of pregnant women acquired during the first and second trimesters may result in fetal encephalitis and death.

The peripheral leukocyte count is often low, with decrease in both lymphocytes and neutrophils, or normal, with a relative lymphopenia. In patients with CNS signs the CSF contains up to 500 cells/mm³ predominantly lymphocytes. The serum LDH and glutamic-oxaloacetic transaminase levels may be elevated.

Pathologic changes in the CNS include edema, congestion, meningeal and perivascular inflammation, intracerebral hemorrhages, neuronal degeneration, and vasculitis. In addition, hepatocellular degeneration and necrosis, widespread lymphoid depletion and follicular necrosis, and interstitial pneumonitis are frequent findings. In the congenitally infected fetus, there are massive and widespread necrosis of brain tissue, hemorrhages, and resorption of brain material, resulting in hydranencephaly.

DIAGNOSIS. In contrast to the other arthropod-borne encephalitides, VEE virus can be isolated from the blood or from throat swabs or washings during the first 3 or 4 days of illness. Serodiagnosis is usually more practical and is achieved by testing appropriately timed paired sera by HI, CF, ELISA, neutralization, or IgM immunoassay.

TREATMENT, PREVENTION, AND CONTROL. No specific therapy is available, and treatment of encephalitis cases is supportive. An experimental live, attenuated vaccine made from subtype IAB is used for adult laboratory personnel. It provides solid immunity to subtype IAB and its closest relative (IC) but incomplete protection against infection with other heterologous VEE viruses. Epidemics and epizootics can be prevented by effective vaccination of equines. Spraying insecticides to reduce adult (infective) mosquito populations is the only means of immediate control in the face of an ongoing epidemic. Individual protection against mosquitoes also is advised.

ST. LOUIS ENCEPHALITIS (SLEn). ETIOLOGY. St Louis encephalitis virus, a member of the family Flaviviridae, shares close antigenic relationships with Japanese encephalitis, Murray Valley encephalitis, and West Nile viruses and is related to yellow fever and dengue viruses. Strains associated with *C. pipiens*–borne epidemics in the eastern United States are distinct from endemic strains transmitted by *C. tarsalis* in the western states.

EPIDEMIOLOGY. Incidence and Prevalence. The virus is present in all parts of the Western Hemisphere, but epidemics occur only in North America and some Caribbean islands. During epidemic years, the virus has been responsible for up to 80% of all reported cases of encephalitis of known etiology in the United States. Epidemics of up to 2000 cases have taken place, the last in 1990, mainly in urban-suburban localities of the Ohio-Mississippi River basin, in eastern and central Texas, and Florida. Small outbreaks also have occurred in the western United States. Epidemics usually transpire between July and September but may arise later in the year in warm areas such as Florida. Prior exposure and immunity to dengue may provide a degree of cross-protection against clinical SLEn.

The overall case-fatality rate is approximately 9%. Mortality is negligible in persons under age 20 years but rises steeply after age 55 years to approximately 30% in patients over age 65 years. The inapparent to apparent infection ratio is 800:1 in children up to age 9 years, 400:1 in persons aged 10 to 49 years, and 85:1 in persons older than 60 years.

Transmission. In most of the eastern United States, SLEn virus circulates between wild birds and *C. pipiens* mosquitoes, which breed in polluted water. In Florida and in parts of the Caribbean, *C. nigripalpus* is the principal vector. The cycle in the western United States also involves wild birds, but the vector is *C. tarsalis,* the vector of WEE. Because of the similar ecology of SLEn and WEE viruses in the west, mixed outbreaks occur, mostly in rural, agricultural areas.

Above-average summer temperatures and conditions such as deficient rainfall, which create stagnant pools suitable for *C. pipiens* breeding, are associated with epidemics in the eastern United States. SLEn in the western states is favored by warm spring temperatures, heavy snow melt, and flooding.

CLINICAL FEATURES AND PATHOLOGY. Three clinical syndromes are recognized: febrile headache, aseptic meningitis, and encephali-

tis. After an incubation period of 4 to 21 days, there is a variable period of nonspecific symptoms, including fever (38 to 41°C), headache, malaise, drowsiness, myalgia, and sore throat. This may be followed by the acute or subacute onset of meningeal or encephalitic signs or both. Nausea, vomiting, and photophobia are common. Neurologic abnormalities occur in up to 25% of patients. Extrapyramidal abnormalities (tremor of tongue, face, and limbs) and an altered state of consciousness are the most significant findings. Others include altered sensorium, meningismus, cranial nerve deficits (particularly nerve VII), abnormal reflexes, tremors, myoclonic twitching, nystagmus, and ataxia. Motor abnormalities are infrequent and sensory changes extremely uncommon. Convulsions occur in 10% of patients and are a poor prognostic sign, as is a persistent high temperature of 40 to 41°C. Signs of markedly increased intracranial pressure are very unusual. Guillain-Barré syndrome has occasionally been associated with SLEn, both as an acute presentation and during the convalescent period. Approximately half the patients with fatal outcome succumb during the first week and 80% within 2 weeks after onset.

In uncomplicated cases of SLEn, moderate peripheral neutrophilic leukocytosis and shift to the left are noted. CSF pressure is elevated, protein mildly elevated, and sugar normal. Pleocytosis up to 500 cells/mm³ is present. Polymorphonuclear cells predominate early, the change to lymphocytes occurring within several days. Serum creatinine phosphokinase, glutamic-oxaloacetic transaminase, and serum aldolase levels are frequently elevated. The electroencephalogram typically shows amorphous delta wave activity and diffuse generalized slowing, most prominently in the frontal and temporal regions, but brain scans are normal. Inappropriate secretion of antidiuretic hormone is present in one-third of patients.

Genitourinary tract symptoms (urgency, frequency, incontinence, and retention), microscopic hematuria, pyuria, and proteinuria, and elevated blood urea nitrogen are frequent. SLEn viral antigen in cells of the urinary sediment has been detected by fluorescent techniques and virus-like particles in urine by immunoelectronmicroscopy.

A convalescent syndrome characterized by weakness, fatigue, nervousness, tremulousness, sleeplessness, irritability, depression, difficulty in concentrating, and headaches occurs in 30 to 50% of older persons and clears in 80% of these within 3 years.

Pathologic changes in fatal cases are limited to microscopic findings. Leptomeningitis is characterized by lymphocytic inflammation. Parenchymal changes consist of lymphocytic perivascular cuffing, cellular nodule formation, and neuronal degeneration.

DIAGNOSIS. SLEn virus is rarely isolated from blood or CSF obtained during the acute phase of illness. Serologic diagnosis is achieved by demonstrating changing antibody titers; the HI, fluorescent, ELISA, and neutralizing tests demonstrate antibody within the first week after onset, and titers rise during the ensuing 2 weeks. CF antibodies appear 10 to 20 days after onset. Rapid, early diagnosis is possible by detecting IgM antibodies by ELISA in serum and CSF. Serologic cross-reactions may occur in persons with prior exposures to dengue and other related flaviviruses.

TREATMENT, PREVENTION, AND CONTROL. Treatment is supportive. No vaccine is available for SLEn. Surveillance of viral activity in vectors and avian hosts is used to define the risk of human infection and initiate vector control efforts. In an established outbreak, avoiding mosquito bites and spraying to reduce infected adult mosquitoes are the only effective means of control.

CALIFORNIA ENCEPHALITIS. ETIOLOGY. At least four members of the California serogroup of the Bunyaviridae family (Bunyavirus genus)—LaCrosse, California encephalitis, Jamestown Canyon, and snowshoe hare virus—cause encephalitis. California encephalitis virus occurs in the western United States (California, New Mexico, Utah, Texas) and has been implicated in only three human cases. In contrast, LaCrosse virus, distributed more widely in the eastern half of the United States and southern Canada, is a major human pathogen. Recently, Jamestown Canyon and snowshoe hare viruses have been implicated in sporadic human encephalitis cases in the north central United States and Canada. California serogroup viruses have been implicated in human disease in the People's Republic of China and the former U.S.S.R.

EPIDEMIOLOGY. Incidence and Prevalence. California encephalitis occurs as an endemic rather than an epidemic disease, with individual or small clusters of cases scattered across the affected areas. Ten to 50 cases are reported each year, generally occurring between July and September, with peak incidence in August. The virus primarily affects persons younger than 15 living in rural and suburban areas characterized by deciduous hardwood forests. It is most prevalent in the north central states, where it is responsible for as many as 20% of cases of acute CNS infection in children. Focal "hot spots" (communities, even backyards) of recurrent summertime viral activity are recognized. The case-fatality rate is less than 1%. The inapparent/apparent infection ratio has been estimated variably at between 26:1 and 157:1.

Transmission. The vector of LaCrosse virus is *A. triseriatus,* which breeds both in forest tree holes and in peridomestic artificial containers. The vector also serves as a reservoir of LaCrosse virus. Wild rodents (squirrels, chipmunks) contribute to a cycle of transmission as viremic hosts. Humans acquire the disease by being bitten by an infected mosquito.

A. communis, A. stimulans, A. triseriatus, and possibly anopheline mosquitoes are involved in transmitting Jamestown Canyon virus, and deer are the principal vertebrate hosts.

CLINICAL FEATURES. The clinical spectrum of California virus infection includes nonspecific febrile illness, aseptic meningitis, and meningoencephalitis. The disease begins with fever, headache, sore throat, and gastrointestinal symptoms, with appearance of the neurologic disorder within 1 to 3 days. In mild cases, CNS signs appear on the third day after onset and subside within 7 to 8 days. In the more severe form, neurologic signs appear within 24 to 48 hours of onset, usually in the form of generalized seizures and altered consciousness, and are more prolonged. Papilledema or abnormal optic disc margins have been noted. Encephalitis may be quite severe in the acute stage, but the disease is almost always self-limited, and death is extremely rare. The question of permanent sequelae is unsettled. Many researchers believe LaCrosse virus infection is responsible for residual psychological problems, emotional lability, hyperkinesis, infantilism, compulsive behavior, and auditory and visual perceptual problems. Cases of hemiparesis and persistent seizure disorders have been reported.

The peripheral white cell count is elevated, with a predominance of polymorphonuclear cells and a shift to the left. The CSF contains up to 500 lymphocytes/mm^3, normal or mildly elevated protein, and normal glucose concentrations. The electroencephalogram reveals generalized slowing in the delta and theta range, indicating diffuse cortical dysfunction. Focal delta wave activity related to cortical destruction or focal seizures is also a common finding.

Histopathologic features in the CNS are qualitatively similar to those of other viral encephalitides; however, absence of inflammatory lesions in cerebellum, medulla, and spinal cord has been postulated to be a distinguishing feature of LaCrosse infection.

DIAGNOSIS. The virus cannot be recovered from blood or CSF obtained during the acute phase. Diagnosis is best achieved by tests for antibody in paired acute and convalescent sera using counterimmunoelectrophoresis, HI, CF, fluorescent, ELISA, and neutralization tests. The most practical, sensitive, and reliable methods are the HI test using the LaCrosse viral antigen and IgM antibody capture ELISA.

TREATMENT, PREVENTION, AND CONTROL. Treatment is supportive. There is no vaccine for California encephalitis. Vector control methods are of uncertain usefulness in this disease. In defined "hot spots" of recurrent viral activity, efforts to eliminate breeding sites for *A. triseriatus* should be made. Parents should protect children by limiting exposure and using mosquito repellents.

JAPANESE ENCEPHALITIS (JE). ETIOLOGY AND EPIDEMIOLOGY. Incidence and Prevalence. JE virus is a member of the Flaviviridae family. It causes epizootics of clinical encephalitis in equines. The disease occurs throughout Asia, including Japan, the Korean peninsula, Taiwan, the People's Republic of China, Okinawa, Vietnam, the Philippines, Burma, Malaysia, Bangladesh, east and south India, Sri Lanka, Thailand, and Indonesia. More than 30,000 causes occur annually. JE is a summertime disease in temperate areas but occurs sporadically year-round in the tropics. Epidemics have been most frequent at the northern fringe of the tropical zone. JE is predominantly a rural disease, and the incidence in males is often higher than in females. In hyperendemic areas, over 70% of adult populations surveyed have antibodies, and children under age 15 years principally are affected by the disease. In areas without a high prevalence of background immunity (e.g., northern India), however, all age groups are affected. In Japan where schoolchildren have been protected by vaccination cam-

paigns targeted at this age group, occurrence of encephalitis in the elderly has become prominent. The inapparent/apparent infection ratio is over 500:1 in children and decreases with age; in Korea, the ratio among American servicemen was estimated at 25:1. The case-fatality rate probably is about 25%, but rates of 50% or more have been reported, which may reflect underrecognition of nonfatal cases.

Transmission. The natural cycle involves *Culex* mosquito vectors and wild birds and swine. Humans and equines are incidental hosts.

CLINICAL FEATURES AND PATHOLOGY. Manifestations of JE include febrile headache, aseptic meningitis, and meningoencephalitis. Onset is abrupt, with fever, headache, and gastrointestinal symptoms. Meningeal irritation develops within 24 hours and is followed on the second or third day by the appearance of irritability, impaired consciousness, convulsions (especially in children), muscular rigidity, masklike facies, ataxia, coarse tremor, involuntary movements, cranial nerve deficits, paresis, hyperactive deep tendon reflexes, and pathologic reflexes. Weight loss and dehydration are often striking findings. In mild cases, fever subsides after the first week and neurologic signs resolve by the end of the second week after onset. In severe cases, hyperpyrexia, progressive neurologic dysfunction, and coma result in death, usually between the seventh and tenth days. About 25% of patients undergo a prolonged recovery, often leaving permanent sequelae. Cardiorespiratory complications are frequent during the acute stage in these patients. A poor prognosis is associated with protracted high fever, frequent or prolonged seizures, high protein content in the CSF, Babinski's sign, and early appearance of respiratory depression. Fetal death and abortion due to transplacental JE infection have been reported.

The occurrence of sequelae correlates with severity of the acute stage of illness. Young children are most susceptible, and sequelae such as mental impairment, emotional lability, choreoathetosis, tremor, parkinsonism, autonomic disturbances, motor paralysis, and pathopsychologic syndromes (including schizophrenia) have been reported in up to 75% of patients.

A moderate peripheral leukocytosis and neutrophilia occur early in the disease. Pleocytosis, protein elevation, and normal glucose in the CSF are usual findings.

Neuropathologic changes and distribution of lesions are similar to those described for St Louis encephalitis (see earlier discussion of SLEn).

DIAGNOSIS. Isolating JE virus from blood is uncommon; virus may be recovered from the CSF of about one-third of patients who progress to a fatal outcome but rarely from patients who live. HI and neutralizing antibodies appear during the first and CF antibodies during the second week after onset. Cross-reactions with other flaviviruses make serodiagnosis difficult. Specific IgM antibodies in serum or CSF are detectable by immunoassays in over three fourths of patients at the time of hospital admission.

TREATMENT, PREVENTION, AND CONTROL. Treatment is supportive (see WEE). Uncontrolled trials of intrathecal interferon suggest a beneficial effect but require confirmation. Inactivated, partially purified mouse brain vaccines produced in Japan are safe and effective in preschool- and school-aged children. Recently licensed for use in the United States, a vaccine produced in Japan is available to U.S. citizens traveling to high-risk areas. Information should be sought from state health departments or the Centers for Disease Control and Prevention. Because three doses of the inactivated vaccine are used and approximately 1 month is required to confer protection, vaccination is not a practical measure in the face of an ongoing epidemic. Reduction of vector mosquito populations by applying insecticides may help to abort outbreaks. Immunization of swine is an ancillary control strategy.

MURRAY VALLEY ENCEPHALITIS AND ROCIO ENCEPHALITIS. Murray Valley encephalitis and Rocio encephalitis are similar to JE in pathogenesis and clinical features and are caused by closely related flaviviruses. Murray Valley encephalitis has occurred in small epidemics in the Murray and Darling River valleys of Victoria and New South Wales, Australia. The virus is endemic in northern Australia and New Guinea, where it is maintained in a bird-mosquito cycle. Rocio encephalitis has caused epidemics of 1000 cases in Saam Paulo State, Brazil.

TICK-BORNE ENCEPHALITIS. ETIOLOGIC AGENTS. A complex of six antigenically related tick-borne flaviviruses cause encephalitis: Powassan, tick-borne encephalitis (TBE), louping ill, Kyasanur Forest disease (KFD), Omsk hemorrhagic fever (OHF), and Langat viruses. The predominant syndrome in KFD and OHF is hemorrhagic fever (see Chapter 391.3), but meningoencephalitis may be a component of the disease spectrum. Two subtypes of TBE virus (Central European encephalitis and Russian spring-summer encephalitis) are distinguished by special serologic tests, are ecologically distinct, and differ in virulence for humans. Powassan and louping ill viruses are rare causes of encephalitis in North America and the British Isles, respectively. These viruses are serologically easily distinguished from mosquito-borne flaviviruses but induce cross-reactions within the complex.

Tick-Borne Encephalitis (TBE). TBE occurs in Europe (including Eastern Europe and Ukraine), southern Scandinavia, and far eastern Russia during summer months, corresponding to peak tick vector populations. Several hundred to 2000 cases are reported annually, with morbidity rates of up to 20 per 100,000 inhabitants. Inapparent infections are common. Adults over age 20 years are mainly affected, and persons frequenting wooded areas that are heavily tick-infested are at highest risk. In Europe, the disease is relatively mild (case-fatality rate 1 to 2%), but in the Far East, it is severe (20 to 25%).

In Europe, the vector of TBE is *Ixodes ricinus*, and in the Far East, *I. persulcatus*. The tick vector also serves as a reservoir of the virus. Larval ticks parasitize small rodents, which serve as amplifying viremic hosts during the spring and summer. Large vertebrates (goats, sheep, cattle) are hosts for nymphal and adult ticks. Outbreaks have occurred in families or groups of individuals ingesting unpasteurized milk or cheese from goats or sheep.

TBE in Europe typically (but not invariably) has a biphasic course, beginning 7 to 14 days after exposure with an influenza-like illness lasting 1 week, followed by a period of clinical remission for several days and then abrupt onset of aseptic meningitis or meningoencephalitis. The latter is usually benign, although severe paralytic illness, myelitis, myeloradiculitis, and bulbar forms may occur. Convalescence is often prolonged, and residual paralysis may follow in severe cases. In the Far East, TBE begins suddenly with fever, headache, and gastrointestinal symptoms, followed rapidly by appearance of depressed sensorium, coma, convulsions, and paralysis. Bulbar paralysis and cervical myelitis are frequent findings. In fatal cases, death occurs in the first week after onset. Survivors have a high incidence of residual paralyses, especially lower motor neuron paralysis of upper extremities or shoulder girdle. Aseptic meningitis and milder forms of encephalitis also occur.

Chronic forms of TBE have been described, with active clinical and pathologic abnormalities a year or more after onset.

In TBE, virus isolation from blood is also possible during the early phase of illness. Serologic diagnosis is achieved by the HI, CF, N, or ELISA techniques.

Treatment is supportive (see WEE).

In eastern Europe and the former U.S.S.R., TBE vaccines are used in high-risk groups (forestry and agricultural workers, military personnel). In Austria, immunization of the general population has resulted in a marked decline in incidence. Avoiding tick exposure by wearing protective clothing and using repellents may be recommended in areas of high TBE activity.

Louping Ill Encephalitis. Louping ill causes encephalitis in sheep (rarely in cattle, horses, and swine) in Scotland and in northern England and Ireland. Sporadic human cases have been recognized. Louping ill virus is maintained in nature by *I. ricinus* ticks and a variety of hosts, including small mammals, ground-dwelling birds (grouse), and probably sheep. The clinical features of louping ill resemble the European form of TBE.

Powassan Virus Encephalitis. Powassan virus encephalitis has been documented in a small number of cases in the northeastern United States and eastern Canada, with a case-fatality rate of 50%. The virus is not associated with animal disease. The transmission cycle of Powassan virus involves *I. cookei, I. marxi* (and possibly other tick species), and mammals, particular rodents and carnivores. Powassan encephalitis is characterized by fever and nonspecific symptoms, followed by encephalitic signs, which are frequently severe. Residual paralysis may occur. Peripheral blood and CSF changes are similar to those described in other forms of flaviviral encephalitis.

Khan AS, Khabbaz RF, Armstrong LR, et al: Hantavirus pulmonary syndrome: The first 100 U.S. cases. J Infect Dis 173:1297–1303, 1996. *Detailed description of the disease.*

Markoff L: Alphaviruses. *In* Mandell G, Bennett J, Dolin R (eds.): Principles and Practice of Infectious Diseases, 4th ed. New York, Churchill-Livingstone, 1995. *Clear description of alphaviruses and important syndromes including fever, polyarthritis, and encephalitis in a well-referenced, easily accessible source.*

Peters CJ, Johnson KM: Bunyaviridae: California encephalitis viruses, Hantavirus, and other Bunyaviridae. *In* Mandell G, Bennett J, Dolin R (eds.): Principles and Practice of Infectious Diseases, 4th ed. New York, Churchill-Livingstone, 1995. *An up-to-date, well-referenced review of important Bunyaviruses and their infections in humans.*

Rigou-Perez JG, Gubler DJ, Vorndam AV, Clark GE: Dengue in travelers from the United States, 1986–1994. J Travel Med 4:65–71, 1997. *An alert to the possibility of dengue in patients in the United States.*

Spach DH, Liles WC, Campbell GL, et al: Tick-borne diseases in the United States. N Engl J Med 329:936, 1993. *Reviews advances in understanding these diseases, especially their microbiology, epidemiology, diagnosis, and treatment; 145 references.*

■ THE MYCOSES

393 INTRODUCTION TO THE MYCOSES

William E. Dismukes

Fungi are classified as eukaryotic microorganisms, in contrast to bacteria, which are considered prokaryotic. Eukaryotes, such as fungi, possess a discrete nuclear membrane and a nucleus that contains several chromosomes, whereas prokaryotes have no nucleus or nuclear membrane and possess only a single chromosome. Fungi also differ from bacteria in the ability of the former to reproduce sexually or asexually. Most fungi reproduce by asexual spore formation. When sexual mating of two closely related species, e.g., *Cryptococcus neoformans,* serotypes A and D, takes place, the "perfect state" (*Filobasidiella neoformans* var *neoformans*) is produced. Fungi for which a perfect state has not been identified are referred to as fungi imperfecti (e.g., *Candida albicans* and *Coccidioides immitis*). The cell walls of fungi are rigid, usually composed of chitin, glucan, and mannoproteins, another feature that distinguishes fungi from bacteria. In addition, the cytoplasmic membrane of fungi contains sterols, principally ergosterol, which are the target sites of action for the major classes of antifungal drugs.

The terms "fungal diseases" and "mycoses" are used interchangeably. Fungal infections that involve only the skin and its appendages are referred to as cutaneous or superficial mycoses (e.g., ringworm of the scalp or groin and tinea versicolor). By contrast, fungal infections that are acquired primarily by inhalation and spread via lymphohematogenous dissemination to involve one or more organs, such as the lungs, skin, liver, spleen, and central nervous system, are referred to as systemic mycoses (Table 393–1). Candidiasis is a mycosis that may cause superficial disease (e.g., intertrigo, oral thrush, and vaginitis) or deep organ disease (e.g., candidemia and disseminated candidiasis).

Fungi causing systemic disease may also be classified by the morphologic or structural form of the organism. For example, *Aspergillus* species and zygomycetes (*Mucor* and *Rhizopus* species) are molds that grow as a hyphal structural form both in the laboratory (and nature) and in humans. By contrast, other fungi are

Table 393–1 ■ COMMON SYSTEM MYCOSES

DISEASE	CAUSATIVE FUNGUS
Aspergillosis	*Aspergillus* species
Zygomycosis (mucormycosis)	*Mucor* and *Rhizopus* species
Candidiasis	*Candida* species
Cryptococcosis	*Cryptococcus neoformans*
Blastomycosis	*Blastomyces dermatitidis*
Coccidioidomycosis	*Coccidioides immitis*
Histoplasmosis	*Histoplasma capsulatum*
Paracoccidioidomycosis	*Paracoccidioides brasiliensis*
Sporotrichosis	*Sporothrix schenckii*

dimorphic (i.e., they have the ability to transform morphologically into either a mold or a yeast form, depending on the environmental conditions). *Blastomyces dermatitidis, Coccidioides immitis, Histoplasma capsulatum, Paracoccidioides brasiliensis,* and *Sporothrix schenckii* exist as hyphal or filamentous forms in nature, but as yeasts (*B. dermatitidis, H. capsulatum, P. brasiliensis, S. schenckii*) or endosporulating spherules (*C. immitis*) in humans. *Cryptococcus neoformans* is a true yeast, growing as the same spherical form in both nature and humans. (For information on the many other fungal organisms that have been increasingly recognized as causes of human disease see Kwon-Chung and Bennett: Medical Mycology.)

The epidemiologic features of the major systemic mycoses are summarized in the individual chapters that follow. Soil and other environmental niches are the natural reservoirs for most of the causative organisms. Infections of humans primarily result from inhaling aerosolized spores (respiratory route of transmission). Exceptions include sporotrichosis, for which most cases are acquired via cutaneous inoculation, and candidiasis, which results either from an endogenous site of colonization such as the oropharynx, skin, or vagina, or from person-to-person contact. The other systemic mycoses are not transmitted routinely from human to human. The natural habitat of several fungal pathogens is limited to specific geographic areas. Consequently, persons living in these areas are at highest risk of acquiring infection. The diseases caused by such organisms are referred to as endemic mycoses and include blastomycosis, coccidioidomycosis, histoplasmosis, and paracoccidioidomycosis. These diseases typically are associated with asymptomatic or mild pulmonary infection that heals spontaneously. Progressive pulmonary infection or spread to extrapulmonary sites occurs less frequently.

Some fungal organisms are considered opportunistic pathogens and are especially prone to cause disease in the setting of altered host defense (Table 393–2). Common predisposing conditions or factors include interruptions in anatomic barriers (burns and endotracheal tubes) or indwelling foreign bodies (arterial or central venous catheters, urinary catheters, and prosthetic heart valves or joints); granulocyte dysfunction secondary to hematologic malignancies (leukemia) or cytotoxic chemotherapy; and depressed cell-mediated immunity associated with organ transplantation, acquired immunodeficiency syndrome (AIDS), or immunosuppressive therapy, such as corticosteroids and azathioprine. Other conditions that may predispose to systemic mycoses include diabetic ketoacidosis (rhinocerebral mucormycosis) and intravenous drug abuse (*Candida* endocarditis and basal ganglia mucormycosis).

Culture for fungus and histopathologic studies using special stains of infected body fluids (sputum, blood, urine, and cerebrospinal fluid [CSF]) and tissue (skin, lung, liver, bone marrow, and

Table 393–2 ■ ALTERED HOST DEFENSE AND OPPORTUNISTIC FUNGAL DISEASE

ALTERATION IN HOST DEFENSE	OPPORTUNISTIC FUNGAL DISEASE
Interruption of mechanical barriers or indwelling foreign bodies	Candidiasis (invasive)
Granulocyte dysfunction (quantitative or qualitative)	Aspergillosis
	Candidiasis
	Zygomycosis
Depressed cell-mediated immunity	Aspergillosis
	Candidiasis (mucosal)
	Coccidioidomycosis
	Cryptococcosis
	Histoplasmosis

lymph nodes) are the mainstays of diagnosis of the mycoses. If fungal disease is suspected, the microbiology laboratory should be alerted to use appropriate culture media. For example, the likelihood of recovering fungi in blood cultures is enhanced by using one of the new highly sensitive systems such as lysis centrifugation, biphasic media, or automated nonradiometric methods. Skin testing with fungal antigens has no place in the diagnosis of individual infections, although skin tests may be useful indicators of prior infection in epidemiologic studies of prevalence. Although most serologic tests for mycoses have limited value in diagnosis because of either low sensitivity and specificity or poor standardization of assay reagents and methods, there are exceptions. A positive latex agglutination test for cryptococcal antigen in CSF or serum is a highly reliable indicator of cryptococcal disease; similarly, a positive titer for complement-fixing antibody in serum or CSF is a reliable marker of coccidioidal disease. Widely available serologic tests that are both sensitive and specific would be very useful in the diagnosis of invasive aspergillosis and candidiasis.

Table 393–3 shows the currently available classes of antifungal drugs, with examples of each class and their mechanisms of action. Although amphotericin B remains the standard of therapy for many systemic fungal diseases, especially serious life-threatening infections in immunocompromised patients, this drug has two principal disadvantages: it must be administered intravenously and it is associated with a high toxicity profile, including azotemia, hypokalemia, and bone marrow suppression, especially anemia. Three lipid formulations of amphotericin B, either encapsulated in liposomes or complexed with lipids, have recently been licensed in the United States: liposomal amphotericin B (AmBisome), colloidal dispersion of amphotericin B (Amphotec), and amphotericin B lipid complex (Abelcet). These new lipid formulations offer advantages over conventional amphotericin B (Fungizone), including less toxicity (especially nephrotoxicity), increased tropism for reticuloendothelial organs, and increased dosing of active drug. However, the high cost of these new formulations is a serious concern. Although the indications for these drugs as first-line therapy remain controversial, most authorities agree that they should be used in patients with serious invasive fungal disease (such as aspergillosis), who are refractory to or intolerant of conventional amphotericin B. In addition, data indicate that AmBisome is effective and well tolerated as empirical therapy for presumed fungal infection in neutropenic patients with persistent fever. Owing to their exciting potential, most tertiary hospitals have added one of these new lipid formulations to their formulary.

Since the late 1970s, progress in antifungal therapy has also been made with regard to antifungal azoles. Miconazole, the first of this class of drugs and a parenteral formulation, is highly toxic and therefore is of limited usefulness. The licensing of three orally administered azoles, ketoconazole (imidazole) in 1981, fluconazole (triazole) in 1990, and itraconazole (triazole) in 1992, represented a major breakthrough. Fluconazole possesses several pharmacologic advantages over ketoconazole and itraconazole, including availability as either an oral or parenteral formulation, significant urinary excretion of active drug, and excellent penetration into CSF (60 to 80% of plasma concentration). In addition, the two triazoles, fluconazole and itraconazole, are better tolerated and less toxic than

Table 393–3 ■ CURRENTLY AVAILABLE DRUGS FOR THERAPY OF SYSTEMIC MYCOSES BY CLASS AND MECHANISM OF ACTION

CLASS OF ANTIFUNGAL DRUG WITH EXAMPLES	MECHANISM OF ACTION

Polyene
  Nystatin
  Amphotercin B
	Binds irreversibly to ergosterol, resulting in increased permeability of cell membrane with leakage of intracellular contents

Azole
  Clotrimazole
  Miconazole
  Ketoconazole
  Fluconazole
  Itraconazole
	Blocks synthesis of ergosterol via inhibition of cytochrome P-450 dependent enzyme, 14α-demethylase

Substituted pyrimidine Flucytosine	Inhibits both DNA and protein synthesis

ketoconazole and are not associated with clinically significant suppression of endogenous steroid synthesis in humans, as is ketoconazole. The azole antifungal agents are capable of interacting with many co-administered drugs, leading to either decreased plasma concentration of the azole or increased plasma concentration of the co-administered drug, often with harmful clinical consequences. Therefore, awareness of potentially interacting drugs is essential when prescribing antifungal azoles. Several promising broad-spectrum triazole drugs, including voriconazole and SCH 56592 with enhanced in vitro and in animal in vivo activity against *Aspergillus* species and fluconazole-resistant *Candida* species, are under development.

The only other antifungal drug currently approved for treating systemic mycoses is flucytosine, an oral preparation, which is often used in combination with amphotericin B to provide a synergistic effect against *C. neoformans* and *Candida* species and is sometimes used alone as therapy for chromomycosis. Unfortunately, flucytosine is potentially toxic to the bone marrow and liver; in addition, its use, especially as a single agent, may be associated with rapid emergence of resistant organisms.

Gallis HA, Drew RH, Pickard WW: Amphotericin B: 30 years of clinical experience. Rev Infect Dis 12:308, 1990. *A practical review of the pharmacology, clinical uses, and adverse effects of amphotericin B, the most important intravenous antifungal agent (190 references).*

Heimenz JW, Walsh TJ: Lipid formulations of amphotericin B: Recent progress and future directions. Clin Infect Dis: 22(suppl 2):S133, 1996. *An important comparative review of the three recently available lipid formulations, amphotericin B lipid complex, amphotericin B colloidal dispersion, and liposomal amphotericin B, focusing on pharmacology, in vivo animal and human studies, and potential indications (83 references).*

Hoesley C, Dismukes WE: Overview of oral azole drugs as systemic antifungal therapy. Semin Resp Crit Care Med 18:301, 1997. *An up-to-date review of the pharmacology, resistance, adverse effects, drug interactions, and treatment and prophylactic indications of the available azole drugs (99 references).*

Kwon-Chung KJ, Bennett JE (eds): Medical Mycology. Philadelphia, Lea & Febiger, 1992. *An exhaustive, well-illustrated text that considers all fungal pathogens and their diseases, including the common and uncommon.*

394 HISTOPLASMOSIS

William E. Dismukes

DEFINITION. Histoplasmosis, the most common endemic systemic mycosis in the United States, is associated with a variety of clinical syndromes, the most frequent of which is an asymptomatic or self-limited influenza-like respiratory infection. Less frequently, histoplasmosis manifests as chronic cavitary pulmonary disease, progressive disseminated disease involving multiple organs, or immune-mediated disease of the mediastinum or eye.

HISTOPLASMOSIS

Causative fungus	*Histoplasma capsulatum*
Primary geographic distribution	Worldwide; endemic in North and South Central United States
Primary route of acquisition	Respiratory (inhalation of spores)
Principal sites of disease	Lungs, lymph nodes, liver, spleen, bone marrow, adrenal glands, gastrointestinal tract
Opportunistic infection in compromised hosts	Frequent, especially in AIDS patients
Drug of choice for most patients	Itraconazole
Alternative therapy	Amphotericin B, ketoconazole, or fluconazole

ETIOLOGY. *Histoplasma capsulatum* is the imperfect state of a dimorphic fungus that grows as a mycelial form at temperatures below 35° C in the laboratory and in soil, its natural habitat, and as a yeast form at 37° C and in infected hosts. The perfect state is *Ajellomyces capsulatus.* The mycelial form bears two types of infectious spores, macroconidia and microconidia, both of which are readily airborne, but the smaller microconidia (2 to 6 μm versus 8 to 14 μm) more easily reach alveoli or small bronchioles on inhalation. The oval yeast cells (2 to 4 μm) reproduce by single narrow-based buds, are unencapsulated, and are usually found within macrophages in viable tissue. A variant strain, *H. capsulatum* var *duboisii,* which is found solely in Central Africa, is characterized by a larger yeast form (7 to 15 μm).

EPIDEMIOLOGY. Results of skin test surveys using histoplasmin antigen indicate that histoplasmosis is worldwide in distribution, with greatest prevalence in tropical and temperate zones. The disease is endemic in the South Central and North Central United States, especially along the Mississippi, Tennessee, Missouri, Ohio, and St Lawrence river basins. A high prevalence has also been noted in selected areas of the eastern United States. In these endemic areas, more than 80% of persons are infected by age 20 years. *H. capsulatum* can be readily recovered from soil, especially that enriched by bird and bat guano. Because of high body temperatures, birds are not infected, whereas bats are. Soil contaminated by chicken, pigeon, blackbird, or starling droppings and areas frequented by bats, such as caves, hollow trees, old buildings, and attics, are frequently identified sources of outbreaks. The disturbance of soil or sites by wind, bulldozing, demolition, or other construction-related activities may greatly increase the number of airborne spores and result in exposure of both nearby and distantly located persons. Although *H. capsulatum* is more prevalent in bird- or bat-related microenvironments, aerosolized microconidia are commonly present as "air pollutants" in endemic areas and may account for the majority of sporadic infections.

Pulmonary infection does not convey protective immunity; consequently, reinfection may occur. Person-to-person transmission of histoplasmosis is not known to occur. Although age, sex, and race do not significantly affect susceptibility to infection, middle-aged white men with pre-existing chronic obstructive pulmonary disease (COPD) appear to be at highest risk of developing chronic pulmonary histoplasmosis. Over recent years, *H. capsulatum* has emerged as an opportunistic fungal pathogen, especially in hosts with altered cellular immunity secondary to organ transplantation, corticosteroid or cytotoxic drug therapy, or infection with human immunodeficiency virus (HIV). In some endemic areas, disseminated histoplasmosis is the most common acquired immunodeficiency syndrome (AIDS)-defining opportunistic infection.

PATHOGENESIS AND PATHOLOGY. Aerosolized microconidia of *H. capsulatum,* after being inhaled into the lungs, undergo transformation into yeast forms at body temperature and are promptly phagocytized by macrophages. In non-immune persons, macrophages are initially unable to kill the yeasts, which multiply intracellularly.

These infected macrophages migrate to the mediastinal lymph nodes and to other organs of the mononuclear phagocyte system (reticuloendothelial system) such as the spleen. Recent evidence indicates that L3T4$^+$ cells are a critical determinant of an effective host response to *H. capsulatum*. In normal hosts, once antigen-specific cellular immunity becomes established, infection is usually contained by a sequence of events including a vasculitic response, granuloma formation with caseation necrosis, enlargement of regional lymph nodes followed by fibrosis, and, ultimately, calcification. In contrast, in persons with impaired cell-mediated immunity, the mononuclear phagocyte system is unable to contain the infection, and viable *H. capsulatum* organisms disseminate widely to macrophage-rich tissues, including liver, spleen, visceral lymph nodes, and bone marrow. In these individuals, because normal reaction of host tissue to parasitized macrophages is either minimal or absent, infection goes unchecked, and progressive disseminated disease ensues. The pathogenesis of mediastinal fibrosis and ocular histoplasmosis, two uncommon but clinically significant complications of infection with *H. capsulatum,* is presumed to be immune mediated, at least in part. Mediastinal fibrosis appears to develop in hypersensitive persons with a large antigen load in caseous mediastinal nodes. Exuberant fibrous encapsulation of nodes and adjacent tissues may lead to bronchial or vascular occlusion or erosion.

In histopathologic specimens stained with periodic acid-Schiff (PAS), Giemsa's, or Gomori's methenamine silver (GMS), the characteristic ovoid yeast forms of *H. capsulatum,* surrounded by a clear space resembling a capsule (but actually due to fixation artifact), are generally found in macrophages. Organisms are more difficult to visualize in tissue stained with hematoxylin-eosin. The likelihood of identifying organisms in tissue sections is directly related to the effectiveness of cellular immunity in a given host. In immune individuals with an intact host defense, fungi are rare, granuloma formation is well developed, and extent of disease is limited. By contrast, in compromised hosts with impaired cellular immunity, macrophages, including those in peripheral blood, are filled with intracellular yeasts, granulomas are poorly developed or absent, and disease is extensive.

CLINICAL MANIFESTATIONS. Pulmonary disease in histoplasmosis is conveniently classified into acute and chronic forms. Acute disease, which results from primary infection, most often resolves spontaneously over 3 to 6 weeks but may be associated with early and late complications.

ACUTE PULMONARY INFECTION. The vast majority of primary infections with *H. capsulatum* are either asymptomatic or associated with a flu-like illness, manifested by fever, chills, headache, nonproductive cough, pleuritic or substernal chest pain, malaise, and myalgia. The incubation period and severity of illness are directly related to the inoculum of inhaled spores and the prior immune status of the individual. In non-immune persons with a heavy exposure, respiratory symptoms tend to be more severe and progressive and include severe dyspnea. A normal chest radiograph is most common, but abnormalities range from one or two patchy infiltrates, with or without mediastinal and hilar adenopathy, to diffuse interstitial or miliary opacities, which frequently heal in a pattern of "buckshot" calcifications. Pleural effusion and cavitation are uncommon. Extrapulmonary symptoms and signs, including arthralgia, erythema nodosum, and erythema multiforme, may be present, especially in young women. Early and late complications of acute or primary pulmonary infection may result from vigorous host reactions causing enlarged mediastinal or hilar nodes and exuberant encapsulating fibrosis, which in turn lead to compression or erosion of adjacent mediastinal structures. These rare complications include acute pericarditis; tracheal, bronchial, or esophageal obstruction; esophageal diverticuli; bronchoesophageal fistula; broncholithiasis (secondary to erosion of a calcification into a bronchus); mediastinal granuloma; mediastinal fibrosis or fibrosing mediastinitis; and enlarging histoplasmoma (usually located in the peripheral lung parenchyma and recognized by concentric laminations of calcium). Mediastinal granuloma, which tends to develop more often in the right paratracheal area, is more circumscribed, smaller in size, and associated with fewer sequelae than is mediastinal fibrosis. Both entities are recognized causes of superior vena cava syndrome.

CHRONIC PULMONARY INFECTION. Chronic pulmonary histoplasmosis often resembles pulmonary tuberculosis in symptomatology and radiographic manifestations, although the course of this type of histoplasmosis tends to be milder and more indolent than that of tuberculosis. The pathogenesis and course of chronic pulmonary histoplasmosis are highly complex; pathologic studies indicate two basic lesions. An interstitial pneumonitis is characteristic of the early lesion, whereas the chronic lesion is manifested by organization of diseased tissue, with prominence of giant cells and progressive cavitation. In the thicker-walled cavities, infection is persistent, with continuing necrosis, leading to progressive cavity enlargement (marching cavity) at the expense of the surrounding lung parenchyma. In general, the symptoms and roentgenographic findings reflect the two types or stages of disease, namely, pneumonitis and progressive cavitation. Although symptoms overlap, they tend to be more abrupt in onset, with more severe constitutional symptoms, such as fever, night sweats, and malaise, in the pneumonitis stage; hemoptysis and progressive dyspnea are more typical of the cavitation stage. In 80% of cases, the pneumonitis stage tends to resolve spontaneously over 2 to 3 months, with a small fibrotic residuum, whereas the cavitation stage, especially that associated with thick-walled cavities, tends to be relentlessly progressive, leading to destruction and diminution of lung parenchyma, fibrosis, and, eventually, respiratory insufficiency.

DISSEMINATED HISTOPLASMOSIS. This less common form of histoplasmosis (about 10% of cases) develops primarily in persons with defective host immunity, including infants with immature immune systems; compromised hosts, such as corticosteroid-treated organ recipients and HIV-infected persons; and individuals with either no measurable defect or a highly selective defect, such as the failure of host lymphocytes to undergo in vitro blast transformation on exposure to *H. capsulatum* antigen. The severity of the symptoms and signs of disseminated disease and the attendant histopathologic findings in a given patient mirror the level of immunocompetence of the individual. For example, in patients with the mildest and most chronic forms of disseminated disease, well-developed tuberculoid granulomas, typical of the response in normal hosts, can be found in reticuloendothelial tissues. In contrast, in patients with overwhelming multiorgan histoplasmosis superimposed on a severely immunocompromising condition, such as AIDS, the host response is suboptimal, with the pathologic findings consisting of large numbers of diffusely scattered macrophages filled with yeast forms and minimal or no granuloma formation.

Fever, chills, and other nonspecific constitutional symptoms, including malaise and weight loss, predominate. On initial presentation, many patients satisfy criteria for fever of unknown origin. Enlargement of liver and spleen is common; less frequently, peripheral lymphadenopathy is present. Mucous membrane ulceration, especially of the oropharynx, occurs in about 25 to 75% of patients with subacute disease and should alert the physician to the possibility of histoplasmosis. Laboratory clues may include pancytopenia (anemia, leukopenia, and thrombocytopenia) as evidence of impaired bone marrow function or replacement of the marrow, elevated alkaline phosphatase level, elevated erythrocyte sedimentation rate, and electrolyte abnormalities suggestive of adrenal insufficiency. In some patients, adrenal hypofunction may not be clinically manifest until years later. Chest radiographs may be normal or show findings suggestive of earlier primary infection or of interstitial pneumonitis consistent with hematogenous spread of infection. Unusual syndromes, including cardiac involvement with culture-negative endocarditis associated with large emboli, gastrointestinal involvement with bleeding secondary to mucosal ulceration, or central nervous system (CNS) involvement with chronic lymphocytic meningitis, occasionally dominate the clinical course. Cutaneous lesions, manifested by diffusely scattered papulonodules on an erythematous base, and CNS disease are more likely in HIV-positive persons. In some AIDS patients, disseminated histoplasmosis represents reactivation of dormant foci, as evidenced by the development of symptoms and signs during a period of residence in a nonendemic area, years after having lived in an endemic region.

OCULAR HISTOPLASMOSIS. Vision loss associated with the triad of punched-out choroidal lesions or "spots," macular neovascular membranes, and peripapillary atrophy or scarring, in the absence of inflammatory changes in the vitreous or anterior chamber, has been labeled *presumed ocular histoplasmosis syndrome* (POHS). Although no direct relationship to active ongoing infection with *H. capsulatum* has been established, POHS is believed to represent a localized hypersensitivity response to *Histoplasma* antigen. In almost all instances, the syndrome occurs in young adults with no evidence of pulmonary or disseminated histoplasmosis. Antifungal therapy, either systemic or intraocular, is not indicated. Laser photocoagulation appears to be the most beneficial therapeutic modality to prevent or reduce vision impairment.

DIAGNOSIS. The diagnostic approach varies in part with the clinical syndrome under consideration. Special features or presentations that should raise suspicion of histoplasmosis include atypical pneumonia syndrome that occurs in a resident of an endemic area, right paratracheal adenopathy, superior vena cava syndrome secondary to adenopathy or a mediastinal mass, an oral ulcer resembling carcinoma, chronic progressive upper lobe cavitation associated with negative sputum smears and cultures for tuberculosis, sarcoid-like illness, adrenal insufficiency, "buckshot" calcifications in the lungs or spleen, and persistent unexplained fever in an HIV-infected person. In most instances, diagnosis should be based on demonstrated *H. capsulatum* by culture or by histopathologic study of involved organs. The histoplasmin skin test, although important in epidemiologic studies, is not recommended for diagnostic purposes, owing to the high positivity rate among persons residing in endemic areas. In addition, the skin test may falsely elevate titers of serum antibodies.

For patients with suspected pulmonary histoplasmosis, detection of serum antibody to *H. capsulatum* by complement fixation is the most widely used serologic test. Although a titer of 1:32 or more or a fourfold rise in titer provides presumptive evidence of active infection, a negative or lower titer does not exclude histoplasmosis. Similarly, titers do not parallel disease activity, correlate with response to therapy, or predict outcome. Testing of serum by immunodiffusion to detect precipitin bands to M and H antigens appears to be a more specific but less sensitive serologic method than complement fixation. All antibody tests are associated with frequent false-positive reactions to *Histoplasma* antigens among patients with tuberculosis and other fungal diseases, especially blastomycosis and coccidioidomycosis. However, detection of *H. capsulatum* polysaccharide antigen in body fluids, such as serum and urine, by radioimmunoassay (Histoplasmosis Reference Laboratory, Indiana University) is a relatively sensitive and specific marker, especially for patients with disseminated histoplasmosis. Antigen levels fall with treatment; consequently, this test is useful for both diagnosing and evaluating response to therapy.

The diagnosis of primary pulmonary histoplasmosis should be suspected on the basis of clinical, radiographic, and epidemiologic clues (e.g., an acute febrile respiratory illness accompanied by scattered patchy infiltrates and hilar adenopathy in an individual with high risk of exposure to *Histoplasma* spores). An elevated complement fixation titer and/or precipitin bands in serum provide presumptive evidence. Whereas sputum cultures are rarely positive (only 10 to 20%) in primary pulmonary disease, the likelihood of positive sputum cultures is significantly higher in chronic pulmonary histoplasmosis. Among patients with chronic disease, about 60% with marching thick-walled cavities have positive cultures, and a significant percentage of these also have positive smears of stained sputum. Although serologic tests for antibody are only moderately helpful (positive results in only 50% of cases), an elevated complement fixation titer in a patient with characteristic radiographic findings provides strong supportive evidence. Definitive diagnosis of chronic pulmonary histoplasmosis must be based on a positive sputum culture or smear or on histopathologic studies and special stains of lung tissue obtained by bronchoscopy.

The diagnosis of disseminated histoplasmosis depends on either demonstrating intracellular yeast forms by histopathologic study or a positive culture of blood, bone marrow, lymph node, skin or mucous membrane, liver, lung, or other involved site. A Wright-stained smear of peripheral blood is positive in more than 50% of acute or subacute cases. A computed tomographic scan of the abdomen and retroperitoneal area may detect hepatosplenomegaly, adrenal masses, and retroperitoneal adenopathy. Serum and urine should be examined for *H. capsulatum* antigen by radioimmunoassay. The cerebrospinal fluid of patients with chronic unexplained culture-negative lymphocytic meningitis should be tested for antigen and antibodies to *H. capsulatum*.

TREATMENT. For most patients with primary pulmonary histoplasmosis, no antifungal therapy is necessary. For those with severe or progressive primary infection, short-course intravenous amphotericin B (around 1000 mg total dose), oral ketoconazole (400 mg daily for 3 to 6 months), or oral itraconazole (200 to 400 mg daily for 3 to 6 months) is recommended, although none of these regimens has been prospectively evaluated in this setting. The treatment of chronic pulmonary histoplasmosis is even less standardized, in large part owing to the relative difficulty in clinically and radiologically distinguishing the pneumonitic and cavitary stages of disease. Although the early pneumonitic form of chronic pulmonary disease has been reported to resolve spontaneously in 80% of cases, rest and inactivity clearly promote healing. Traditionally, antifungal therapy has been advocated only for patients with progressive or marching cavitary disease, manifested by persistent or enlarging, thick-walled (>2 mm) cavities. Amphotericin B (total dose, 2.0 to 2.5 g), ketoconazole (400 mg daily for at least 6 months), or itraconazole (200 to 400 mg daily for 6 to 9 months) is effective therapy. Liberalizing criteria for treatment in patients

with chronic pulmonary disease may have merit. Rather than reserving therapy only for patients with advanced cavitary disease, some authorities suggest that oral ketoconazole or itraconazole may be indicated for all patients with chronic pulmonary disease, regardless of the stage. Although itraconazole is better tolerated and less toxic, ketoconazole is less expensive.

In contrast to the somewhat controversial guidelines regarding therapy of pulmonary histoplasmosis, there is no question that all patients with disseminated histoplasmosis should be treated. For patients with severe life-threatening disease, immunocompromised hosts such as organ transplant recipients or corticosteroid-treated patients, and the rare patients with CNS or cardiac histoplasmosis, amphotericin B (total dose, 2.0 to 2.5 g) is the drug of choice. Itraconazole (200 to 400 mg daily for 6 to 12 months) is an effective alternative in immunocompetent patients with mild to moderate disease. Experience during the past decade with disseminated histoplasmosis in AIDS patients indicates that an aggressive approach to treatment is necessary in an attempt to prevent relapse. For AIDS patients with moderate to severe or life-threatening disease, intensive "induction" primary therapy with intravenous amphotericin B (total dose, 1.0 to 2.0 g) should be used to gain control of disease and reduce the organism load. For AIDS patients with milder disease, itraconazole (200 mg twice daily for 10 to 12 weeks) is highly effective primary therapy; fluconazole (400 to 800 mg daily) may be an effective alternative. The role of itraconazole or fluconazole in central nervous system histoplasmosis has not been clearly defined. The approach of initiating therapy with intravenous amphotericin B and completing it with an oral agent may prove applicable to selected non-AIDS patients with either chronic pulmonary or disseminated histoplasmosis. Regardless of which primary therapy regimen is used, lifelong maintenance or suppressive therapy is required to prevent relapse of histoplasmosis in patients with AIDS. Itraconazole (200 to 400 mg daily) is the regimen of choice. In patients who cannot take itraconazole because of intolerance or drug interaction, fluconazole (400 mg daily) can be used. Ketoconazole is inadequate for primary or maintenance therapy in patients with AIDS. A recent placebo-controlled trial has shown that itraconazole, 200 mg daily, can markedly reduce the occurrence of histoplasmosis in HIV-infected persons with CD4 counts less than 100/mm³, living in the endemic area. Accordingly, for this high-risk group, prophylactic therapy with itraconazole should be considered.

The management of mediastinal fibrosis presumed secondary to *H. capsulatum* infection is largely unsatisfactory, as evidenced by progressive morbidity in many patients and a mortality rate of at least 30%. Antifungal chemotherapy is generally not recommended. In selected cases, surgical extirpation may be beneficial in alleviating entrapment or obstructive syndromes.

PROGNOSIS. Although primary pulmonary histoplasmosis may be associated with acute or chronic intrathoracic complications, this form of disease is usually self-limited. In contrast, chronic cavitary pulmonary histoplasmosis is usually progressive, and even if treated, may result in respiratory insufficiency and death. Disseminated histoplasmosis is variable in its severity and course, depending on the immune status of the host. Although a single course of therapy may be curative in some patients with disseminated histoplasmosis, long-term maintenance therapy to prevent relapse is required in others, especially patients with AIDS.

Dismukes WE, Bradsher RW Jr, Cloud GC, et al: Itraconazole therapy for blastomycosis and histoplasmosis. Am J Med 93:489, 1992. *In a prospective, non-randomized open trial among 35 patients with non–life-threatening, non-meningeal histoplasmosis treated for 2 or more months with itraconazole, the success rate was 86%. Only one of these patients had AIDS as an underlying disease.*

Wheat LJ, Connolly-Stringfield PA, Baker RL, et al: Disseminated histoplasmosis in the acquired immune deficiency syndrome: Clinical findings, diagnosis and treatment, and review of the literature. Medicine 69:361, 1990. *An informative review of disseminated histoplasmosis, a common opportunistic disease among AIDS patients living in or with a history of exposure to the endemic area.*

Wheat J, Hafner R, Korzun AH, et al: Itraconazole treatment of disseminated histoplasmosis in patients with the acquired immunodeficiency syndrome. Am J Med 98: 336, 1995. *Itraconazole is highly effective therapy for mild disseminated histoplasmosis in AIDS patients. Patients with moderate to severe disease should be managed with induction-therapy amphotericin B followed by consolidation therapy with itraconazole.*

395 COCCIDIOIDOMYCOSIS

John N. Galgiani

DEFINITION. Coccidioidomycosis is a systemic fungal infection due to *Coccidioides immitis,* endemic to some deserts of the Western Hemisphere.

COCCIDIOIDOMYCOSIS

Causative fungus	*Coccidioides immitis*
Primary geographic distribution	Lower Sonoran deserts of the Western Hemisphere, including parts of Arizona, California, New Mexico, west Texas, and parts of Central and South America
Primary route of acquisition	Respiratory (inhalation of arthroconidia)
Principal site of disease	Lungs most common; spread to skin, bones, meninges, and other viscera, uncommon but serious
Opportunistic infection in compromised hosts	Diffuse pneumonia and widespread infections common in patients with T-lymphocyte defects or during high-dose corticosteroid therapy
Drug of choice for most patients	No antifungal is required for uncomplicated pneumonia; fluconazole or itraconazole for progressive forms of infection
Alternative therapy	Amphotericin B (especially with diffuse pneumonia or rapidly progressive infections); ketoconazole

ETIOLOGY. *C. immitis* is a dimorphic fungus that is classified as an ascomycete by ribosomal gene homology. In its vegetative state, mycelia with true septations mature to produce arthroconidia, single cells approximately 2 to 5 mm in size. After infection, an arthroconidium enlarges to as much as 75 mm in diameter as a spherule, undergoing internal septation to produce scores of endospores. When spherules rupture, packets of endospores are released, and these produce more spherules in infected tissue or revert to mycelia if removed from the body.

EPIDEMIOLOGY. *C. immitis* can be recovered from the soil of the low deserts of Arizona; the Central Valley of California; parts of other states, including New Mexico and Texas; and parts of Central and South America. Endemic regions follow the climatologic Sonoran life zone, which is characterized by modest rainfall, mild winters, and low humidity. Mycelia bloom beneath the surface during periods of rain, and arthroconidia develop as the earth dries. Rates of infection are highest during dry months and are accentuated when soil is disturbed by windstorms or construction equipment. Exposure to contaminated bales of cotton or other fomites can result in infection beyond the endemic regions, but this is rare. Person-to-person transmission of pulmonary infection has not been reported, and isolation precautions are unnecessary.

INCIDENCE AND PREVALENCE. In general, the annual risk of infection within the most strongly endemic areas is 3% and results in approximately 100,000 new infections. With unusually intense exposure, such as at archeology sites or during military maneuvers within endemic regions, infections can develop in the majority of persons exposed for only a matter of days. More than 60% of new infections are likely to occur in Arizona because of the rapid growth of populations in the Phoenix and Tucson areas.

PATHOGENESIS AND PATHOLOGY. Inhaling an arthroconidium to the level of the terminal bronchiole initiates virtually all coccidioidal infections. Fungal proliferation engenders both granulomatous inflammation, which is associated with intact spherules, and acute inflammation including eosinophils, which is associated with spherule rupture. Focal pneumonia is often associated with ipsilateral hilar adenopathy, and, less frequently, infection enlarges peritracheal, supraclavicular, and cervical nodes. Lesions occurring elsewhere are the result of hematogenous dissemination and most become apparent within 2 years of the initial infection. Although progressive dissemination results from fewer than 1% of infections, as many as 8% of persons with self-limited infection manifest asymptomatic chorioretinal scars, suggesting that subclinical hematogenous spread may be frequent. Within weeks after infection, durable T-cell immunity normally arrests fungal proliferation, allowing inflammation to resolve and preventing reinfection in the future. However, control of the infection may occur without sterilizing lesions, and reactivation of dormant infection or second infections is possible in patients whose cell-mediated immunity becomes deficient.

CLINICAL MANIFESTATIONS. At least two of every three infections are detected only by finding dermal hypersensitivity to coccidioidal antigens. Those who become ill usually experience self-limited pulmonary syndromes. However, a minority of patients develop complications or progressive forms of infection that display a broad variety of manifestations and pose difficult problems in management for the clinician.

PRIMARY PULMONARY INFECTIONS. Symptoms develop within 5 to 21 days after exposure. Fever, weight loss, fatigue, a dry cough, and pleuritic chest pain are common but not specific complaints. Arthralgia of multiple joints without significant effusions is also frequent and is referred to as "desert rheumatism." Occasionally skin manifestations develop, including a short-lived non-pruritic maculopapular rash, *erythema multiforme,* or *erythema nodosum.* These arthritic and dermatologic manifestations are mediated by circulating immune complexes or other immunologic phenomena rather than fungal dissemination. Radiographs of the chest may show no abnormalities or may demonstrate pulmonary infiltrates, either segmental or lobar. Hilar adenopathy is often a distinctive finding. Peripneumonic pleural effusions may occur and usually resolve without intervention, although cultures of pleural biopsies usually yield *C. immitis.* Eosinophilia is frequently a prominent finding in differential leukocyte counts of peripheral blood, and the erythrocyte sedimentation rate is usually elevated. Symptoms may persist for several weeks before improvement is clearly under way, and the illness, especially lassitude, may persist for months.

The primary pulmonary process produces a variety of sequelae. The most frequent is the development of a pulmonary nodule (Fig. 395–1), typically measuring 1 to 4 cm and lying within 5 cm of the hilus. Despite their harmless nature, coccidioidal nodules may engender concern because of their similarity to a malignant mass. For this reason, management usually requires percutaneous needle aspiration or resection. Another consequence of pulmonary coccidioidomycosis is cavitation of the infiltrate, which occurs in approximately 5% of cases of pneumonia. Most cavities are solitary and thin walled, residing in an upper lobe close to the pleura. Occasionally they produce pain, hemoptysis, or adjacent infiltrates. Cavities may acquire mycetomas either from *C. immitis* itself or some other colonizing mould. Infrequently a cavity ruptures, forming a pyopneumothorax. This usually is the first symptom of coccidioidal infection and typically occurs in otherwise healthy young males. An air-fluid level in the pleural space, detectable by roentgenography, often helps differentiate this problem from a spontaneous pneumothorax. Surgical resection of the cavity is the preferred treatment for this complication. The least common pulmonary complication is persistent fibrocavitary infection that progresses from involvement of lobes to involvement of both lungs.

EXTRAPULMONARY DISSEMINATION. Coccidioidomycosis in immunosuppressed patients, such as organ recipients, those with AIDS or lymphoma, or women during their third trimester of pregnancy, usually results in dissemination beyond the lungs. However, disseminated infection also occurs in some patients who have no underlying disease and do not manifest heightened susceptibility to other infections. The most common locations for disseminated lesions are skin (cutaneous papules or subcutaneous abscesses); joints (especially the knee); bones, including vertebrae; and the basilar meninges. Such infections may produce one or many lesions and

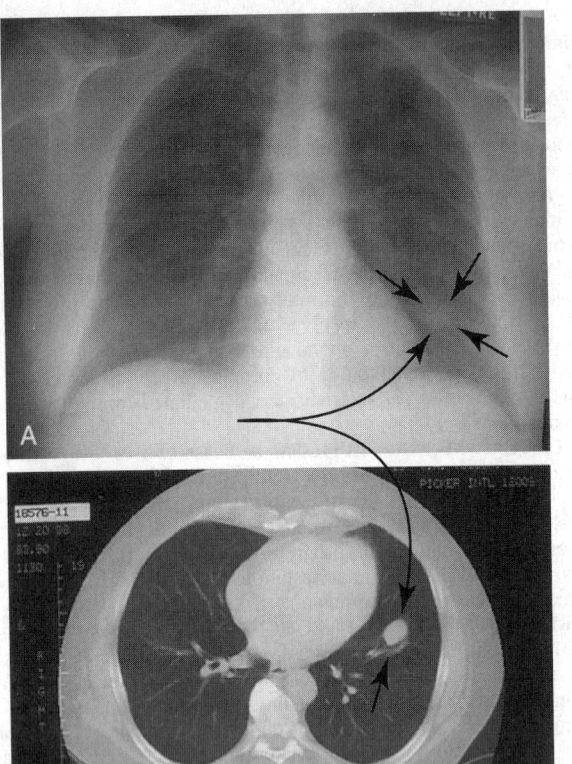

FIGURE 395-1 ▪ *A*, Benign nodule due to coccidioidomycosis. *B*, Computed tomographic image of the nodule shown in *A*.

frequently are subacute or chronic in their presentation. In broadly immunosuppressed patients, coccidioidal infections may be more fulminant, with fungemia detectable with blood cultures and diffuse reticulonodular embolic pulmonary infiltrates. Although the kidneys and the urinary bladder are rarely involved, *C. immitis* may be recovered from concentrated specimens of urine, because of either transient fungemia or focal dissemination to the prostate. In contrast to histoplasmosis, the gastrointestinal tract is rarely involved in coccidioidomycosis.

DIAGNOSIS. The diagnosis is firmly established by recovering *C. immitis* from clinical specimens. On direct examination of respiratory specimens or tissue, spherules can be seen as large structures with refractile walls and internal organization; these are also seen on hematoxylin-eosin, silver, or periodic acid–Schiff stains of histologic preparations. The Gram stain does not detect spherules. In culture, mycelial growth is often evident within the first week of incubation, and DNA probing with commercially available kits allows rapid species identification. Recovery of *C. immitis* may be difficult in patients who have only scant respiratory secretions asso-

ciated with the initial pneumonia and from the cerebrospinal fluid (CSF) of patients with meningitis.

A presumptive diagnosis of coccidioidal infection is often based on detecting specific antibodies in serum. Within the first weeks of initial infections, a precipitin-type antibody is detected, usually by immunodiffusion techniques. Later, complement-fixing (CF)–type antibodies usually appear. When reported quantitatively, CF antibodies generally are found to be highest in the most extensive infections and to decrease in concentration in patients whose infections are controlled. An important means of diagnosing coccidioidal meningitis is by detection of CF antibodies in the CSF, along with other abnormalities, such as leukocytosis, elevated protein concentration, or low glucose concentration.

TREATMENT. The role of antifungal therapy for primary uncomplicated infections is controversial because clinical trials have not been performed to determine if treatment either shortens the course of symptoms or diminishes the chances of complications. However, the value of treatment is clear for patients with progressive illness. Because many coccidioidal infections are chronic in nature, treatment with oral azole antifungal agents, such as ketoconazole, fluconazole, and itraconazole, is often used for initial therapy. Doses of these azoles are 400 mg/day or higher and treatment is usually continued for a year or more. Responses with these agents are satisfactory in approximately two-thirds of patients. Fluconazole is effective therapy for coccidioidal meningitis and has greatly reduced the number of patients treated with intrathecal amphotericin B. Unfortunately, cessation of azole therapy, especially of therapy for coccidioidal meningitis, often is followed by recurrence of symptoms. Therefore, many patients may need protracted or even life-long therapy to maintain control of disease activity. Amphotericin B remains a rational choice in cases in which treatment with azole antifungals has failed. Daily doses range from 0.4 to 1.0 mg/kg and cumulative therapy ranges from 0.5 to 3.0 g. Occasionally, in a patient in whom disease progression is rapid, amphotericin B may produce a more rapid therapeutic response and therefore is preferred initial therapy. Delivery of amphotericin B in liposomes or lipid complexes is being explored as a means of reducing its well-recognized toxic effects. In addition to selection of antifungal agents, surgical removal of necrotic tissue is often essential to control the damage from specific lesions.

PROGNOSIS. After resolution of the initial infection, most patients maintain life-long immunity, and infections after reexposure are rare. However, cessation of symptoms is often accomplished without eradicating *C. immitis* completely, and recurrence of the original infection up to many years after the original episode is a well-recognized risk of intercurrent profound immunosuppression. For patients in whom the initial infection cannot be resolved, the disease typically follows a protracted course. Although infection is more often debilitating than fatal, fulminant respiratory failure can occur and, if untreated, coccidioidal meningitis is nearly always fatal within 2 years.

McNeil MM, Ampel NM: Opportunistic coccidioidomycosis in patients infected with human immunodeficiency virus: Prevention issues and priorities. Clin Infect Dis 21 (suppl 1): S111, 1995. *An important finding from this study is that 46% of all coccidioidal infections in patients with AIDS occurred outside of the endemic regions, indicating the increased importance of this disease as a national problem.*

Galgiani JN: Coccidioidomycosis: A regional disease of national importance. Ann Intern Med 130:293, 1999. *Emphasis on the primary care aspects of valley fever.*

Galgiani JN, Ampel NM, Catanzaro A, et al: Treatment guidelines for coccidioidomycosis. Clin Infect Dis, in press. *Consensus statement regarding current therapy of coccidioidomycosis.*

Pappagianis D, Zimmer BL: Serology of coccidioidomycosis. Clin Microbiol Rev 3: 247, 1990. *Comprehensive review of diagnostic tests for coccidioidomycosis.*

Stevens DA: Current concepts: Coccidioidomycosis. N Engl J Med 332:1077, 1995. *Review of coccidioidomycosis with more detailed discussion of its pathogenesis.*

396 BLASTOMYCOSIS

William E. Dismukes

DEFINITION. Blastomycosis (North American blastomycosis, Gilchrist's disease) is an endemic systemic mycosis that occurs primarily in non-compromised hosts. As with the other important endemic mycoses, such as coccidioidomycosis and histoplasmosis, infection follows inhalation of the aerosolized spore form of the fungus. Clinical disease most commonly involves the lungs, skin, skeletal system, and male genitourinary tract.

BLASTOMYCOSIS	
Causative fungus	*Blastomyces dermatitidis*
Primary geographic distribution	Endemic in North and South Central United States
Primary route of acquisition	Respiratory (inhalation of spores)
Principal sites of disease	Lungs, skin, bone, joints, prostate
Opportunistic infection in compromised hosts	Infrequent
Drug of choice for most patients	Itraconazole
Alternative therapy	Amphotericin B, ketoconazole, or fluconazole

ETIOLOGY. *Blastomyces dermatitidis,* the imperfect or asexual state of *Ajellomyces dermatitidis,* is a dimorphic fungus, growing as a mycelial form in the environment and in the laboratory at room temperature and as a yeast form in mammalian tissue and in the laboratory at 37° C. The yeast cells, which are identical in vitro and in vivo in tissue and fluid specimens, vary from 8 to 15 μm in diameter, have a thick, highly refractile cell wall, and reproduce by single broad-based buds. In the laboratory, growth of *B. dermatitidis* is somewhat slow; white, mold colonies may not appear for 1 to 3 weeks.

EPIDEMIOLOGY. Because no highly sensitive and specific skin test or serologic marker is currently available, the epidemiology of blastomycosis is less well understood than that of coccidioidomycosis and histoplasmosis. The prevalence of subclinical blastomycosis is largely unknown and the incidence of clinically manifest blastomycosis appears to be lower than the incidence of clinical disease associated with the two other endemic mycoses. During 1985–1996 in Wisconsin, the mean annual incidence of clinical blastomycosis was 1.4 cases per 100,000 persons. Isolated cases of blastomycosis have been reported worldwide, including Africa and Central and South America; however, the disease is concentrated or endemic in the South and North Central United States, especially in areas bordering the Mississippi and Ohio river basins, and the Great Lakes. In these endemic areas, infection occurs both sporadically and epidemically; small point-source outbreaks of blastomycosis have been associated with recreational or occupational activities in wooded areas along waterways. Current evidence indicates that *B. dermatitidis* exists in warm, moist soil enriched by organic debris, including decaying vegetation or wood. It is not surprising, therefore, that persons with occupational or avocational exposure to soil and the outdoors appear to be at highest risk of acquiring infection. Data from point-source outbreaks indicate that the median incubation period from exposure to infection is about 43 days, with a range of 3 weeks to 3 months. Animals, especially dogs and horses, are also susceptible to infection, which may progress to clinical disease. Among humans, clinical illness is most common among middle-aged men. Although *B. dermatitidis,* in contrast to the other dimorphic fungi, is a relatively uncommon opportunistic pathogen, studies over the past decade indicate that blastomycosis is being increasingly observed in immunocompromised hosts, e.g., corticosteroid- and cytotoxic drug-treated patients, organ transplant recipients, and patients with acquired immunodeficiency syndrome (AIDS). This observation suggests that reactivation blastomycosis may be more common than previously suspected.

PATHOGENESIS AND PATHOLOGY. Humans and animals, for the most part, acquire infection by inhaling aerosolized conidia that convert to the yeast form in the lungs at body temperature. Percutaneous inoculation of *B. dermatitidis* has been documented rarely, as a result of either a laboratory accident or a dog bite. The clinical manifestations of disease at body sites other than lung (and rarely skin) result from the hematogenous spread of organisms.

T-cell–mediated immunity appears to be the most important arm of host defense against *B. dermatitidis.* In vivo and in vitro studies indicate that macrophages, stimulated by lymphokines, are more effective in inhibiting or killing this yeast than are granulocytes. A growth-inhibiting or protective role of humoral immunity in blastomycosis has not been established. The organism's large size and thick cell wall, which consists of chitin, glucan, and structural proteins, likely contribute to its ability to resist host cell mechanisms during the early inflammatory response. Host-pathogen interactions appear to be modulated by WI-1 and α-1,3-glucan, two surface antigens of the yeast form of *B. dermatitidis.* The typical histopathologic picture of pulmonary blastomycosis and other non-mucocutaneous sites of disease consists of noncaseating granulomas as well as clusters of neutrophils. By contrast, cutaneous and mucous membrane lesions are characterized by pseudoepitheliomatous hyperplasia with microabscesses.

CLINICAL MANIFESTATIONS. In general, blastomycosis is a chronic indolent systemic fungal disease associated with a variety of pulmonary and extrapulmonary manifestations. Among the latter, cutaneous disease predominates, occurring in about 40 to 80% of cases. Multiple organ involvement occurs in approximately 50 to 60% of cases. Extrapulmonary disease may occur in the absence of clinical or radiologic evidence of lung disease.

PULMONARY. Most primary infections are believed to be either asymptomatic or unrecognized as being due to *B. dermatitidis* on the basis of nonspecific flu-like symptoms. In patients with proven acute pulmonary blastomycosis, the radiologic findings usually consist of infiltrative or nodular air space opacities, most often in the lower lobes. By contrast, chronic pulmonary blastomycosis, which is found in about 75% of cases, usually manifests as a chronic pneumonia syndrome, characterized by productive cough, pleuritic chest pain, dyspnea, weight loss, and low-grade fever. Although the disease has no distinguishing radiologic characteristics, consolidation, one or more fibronodular infiltrates, or mass lesions (with or without cavitation) are common, often mimicking the findings in other granulomatous diseases or lung cancer. Although hilar adenopathy and pleural effusions occur, they are uncommon. Patients with overwhelming pulmonary blastomycosis may develop diffuse, bilateral, interstitial alveolar infiltrates on the chest radiograph and clinical evidence of acute respiratory distress syndrome.

SKIN. The cutaneous lesions, which often prompt the patient with blastomycosis to seek medical evaluation initially, are of two general types, verrucous and ulcerative; both types tend to occur more commonly on exposed parts. The verrucous lesions, which begin as papulopustules, are more characteristic; these progress slowly over weeks to months to become crusted, heaped-up, and warty in appearance, often with a reddish-black or violaceous hue, an area of central healing and scarring, and a well-circumscribed outer border. Microabscesses, manifested by black dots on the surface, are typically located at the periphery of verrucous lesions; removing the crusted eschar often reveals purulent material in which the yeast form of the organism can be demonstrated by wet preparation. Ulcerative lesions overlying a bed of friable red granulation tissue are less common. Occasionally, mucosal ulcerations may be found in the mouth, nose, or larynx, mimicking the mucocutaneous lesions of histoplasmosis.

OTHER. After lung and skin disease, bone and joint involvement is next most common and is seen in up to 25% of cases. Osteolytic lesions, with or without sclerotic margins, are typically located in long bones and vertebrae. Often, patients with bone disease present as a result of overlying chronic draining sinuses or contiguous soft tissue lesions rather than bone pain. Septic arthritis, which is much less common than osteomyelitis, is frequently secondary to contiguous extension. Up to one third of men with blastomycosis have genitourinary tract disease, manifested most commonly by prostatic enlargement with obstructive symptoms and less frequently by epididymitis. Central nervous system (CNS) disease in the form of either granulomatous meningitis or a mass lesion (intracerebral blastomycoma) occurs in about 5% of cases. Clinically apparent blastomycotic involvement of other organs (e.g., gastrointestinal tract, liver, spleen, adrenals, and kidneys) is unusual, except in patients with fulminant disseminated disease.

DIAGNOSIS. As is true for all systemic mycotic diseases, the definitive diagnosis of blastomycosis requires a positive fungal culture from clinical specimens. A presumptive diagnosis may be based on the finding of characteristic yeast forms in a wet preparation of sputum, pus, or other body fluid or in a histopathologic section of tissue (e.g., skin, lung, bone, or prostate). *B. dermatitidis* in wet preparations of fluid specimens mixed with 10% potassium hydroxide appears as a broad-based single budding yeast, and in fixed-tissue specimens stained with hematoxylin-eosin or periodic acid-Schiff (PAS) reagents it appears as single or budding yeast cells with a doubly refractile cell wall. Because a presumptive clinical diagnosis based on "characteristic" skin lesions or radiologic findings is associated with an unacceptably high error rate, obtaining fluids or tissue from involved sites for culture and histopathologic study is mandatory in the evaluation of all patients with suspected blastomycosis. Moreover, documented cutaneous and/or pulmonary disease should signal the possibility of bone or genitourinary disease and lead to appropriate diagnostic studies, such as bone scan and prostate examination and massage. As a diagnostic test, the blastomycin skin test lacks sensitivity and specificity and should not be used. Similarly, the complement fixation assay for serum antibody is highly cross-reactive and of no diagnostic value. Recent studies suggest that immunodiffusion, enzyme immunoassay, or radioimmunoassay tests for antibody to the A antigen of *B. dermatitidis* or antibody to other more purified antigens (e.g., WI-1, a 120 kDa surface protein) are better serologic markers of disease. Similarly, recent developments with DNA probes and exoantigen technology for rapid identification of yeast colonies in cultured specimens are promising.

TREATMENT. At present, three drugs, amphotericin B, ketoconazole, and itraconazole, are approved for the treatment of blastomycosis. Although intravenous amphotericin B has been traditionally considered the drug of choice for all forms of disease, studies and experience gained over recent years indicate that the oral azoles, ketoconazole and itraconazole, are highly effective, especially in patients with chronic indolent disease and non-involvement of the CNS. Ketoconazole should be initiated at a dosage of 400 mg/day, advanced by 200-mg increments at monthly intervals, up to a maximum of 800 mg/day in patients with progressive disease, and continued for a minimum of 6 months. Itraconazole in a dose of 200 to 400 mg/day for 6 months or longer is even more effective than ketoconazole (90 to 95% success rate versus 80%) and associated with less toxicity. Accordingly, itraconazole is considered the drug of choice for most patients with blastomycosis. Fluconazole, at usual therapeutic doses of 200 to 400 mg/day, is not as effective as ketoconazole or itraconazole. Higher doses of fluconazole, which are associated with higher costs and increased potential for toxicity, appear necessary for cure. Amphotericin B, a total dose of 1.5 to 2.5 g, should be reserved for patients with overwhelming life-threatening or CNS disease, rare patients who are immunocompromised, and those in whom oral azole therapy has failed. In selected situations, some investigators advocate an induction course of amphotericin B (total dose, approximately 500 mg) for a rapid fungicidal effect to gain control of disease, followed by maintenance or "consolidation" therapy with itraconazole for 3 to 6 months. Although controversy exists about whether or not to treat patients with acute pulmonary blastomycosis who are identified as part of point-source outbreaks, available data suggest that most such patients do not require therapy. However, careful long-term follow-up of untreated patients is important to monitor for evidence of disease activity.

PROGNOSIS. In contrast to the past, now most patients with blastomycosis are identified and treated before the development of overwhelming or fatal disease. Antifungal therapy with either amphotericin B or itraconazole in normal hosts is associated with a cure rate of about 90% and relapse rate of less than 10%.

Bradsher RW: Histoplasmosis and blastomycosis. Clin Infect Dis 22 (suppl 2): S102, 1996. *An informative review of the epidemiology, clinical manifestations, diagnosis, and treatment of two important endemic mycoses.*

Brown LR, Swensen SJ, Van Scoy RE, et al: Roentgenologic features of pulmonary blastomycosis. Mayo Clin Proc 66:29, 1991. *A well-illustrated description of the varied radiographic findings in pulmonary blastomycosis. Consolidation and mass patterns are most common, whereas hilar adenopathy and pleural effusion are rare.*

Klein BS, Vergeront JM, Davis JP: Epidemiologic aspects of blastomycosis, the enigmatic systemic mycosis. Semin Respir Infect 1:29, 1986. *A valuable review that focuses on seven point-source epidemics and the ecologic niche of the organism.*

Meyer KC, McManus EJ, Maki DG: Overwhelming pulmonary blastomycosis associated with the adult respiratory distress syndrome. N Engl J Med 329:1231, 1993. *Overwhelming infection with B. dermatitidis can cause diffuse pneumonitis and the adult respiratory distress syndrome, even in immunocompetent hosts.*

Pappas PG, Threlkeld MG, Bedsole GD, et al: Blastomycosis in immunocompromised patients. Medicine 72:311, 1993. *This review documents the increasing occurrence of blastomycosis in compromised hosts, including corticosteroid-treated and oncologic patients, organ transplant recipients, pregnant patients, or those with AIDS, and describes the clinical manifestations and treatment approaches in these high-risk groups.*

397 PARACOCCIDIOIDOMYCOSIS

William E. Dismukes

DEFINITION. Paracoccidioidomycosis is a chronic granulomatous disease that typically involves the lungs, skin, mucous membranes, and lymph nodes, and is limited to an endemic area extending from Mexico south to Argentina.

PARACOCCIDIOIDOMYCOSIS	
Causative fungus	*Paracoccidioides brasiliensis*
Primary geographic distribution	Endemic in Mexico, Central America and parts of South America
Primary route of acquisition	Respiratory (inhalation of spores)
Principal sites of disease	Lungs, mucous membranes, skin, lymph nodes, liver, and spleen
Opportunistic infection in compromised hosts	Infrequent
Drug of choice for most patients	Itraconazole
Alternative therapy	Sulfonamide, amphotericin B, or ketoconazole

ETIOLOGY. The causative agent, *Paracoccidioides brasiliensis*, is a dimorphic fungus that grows as a mycelial form in nature and in the laboratory and as an oval or round yeast form in host tissues or at 37° C. Histopathologic identification of characteristic multiple budding or "pilot wheel," thick-walled yeast cells, 10 to 40 μm in diameter, provides presumptive evidence of disease. Because the organism grows slowly on primary isolation in the laboratory, fungal cultures should be held for at least 4 weeks before being discarded.

EPIDEMIOLOGY. Most cases occur in persons living in or with a history of prior exposure to southern Mexico, Central America, or South America; in selected countries such as Brazil, paracoccidioidomycosis is the most common systemic mycosis. Owing to the long period of latency, overt disease may develop in persons many years after they have left the endemic region. Infection is acquired by inhaling spores. Neither human-to-human transmission nor common-source outbreaks have been documented, although cases tend to concentrate around humid forests. The majority of cases occur in adult males, especially those who labor in the outdoors, so-called agriculturists. The preponderance of cases in men may also be related to the observation that estrogens inhibit the mycelium-to-yeast transformation of the organism. Although cases have been reported in compromised hosts, in general, paracoccidioidomycosis is not considered an opportunistic fungal disease. However, paracoccidioidomycosis has been reported in patients with acquired immunodeficiency syndrome (AIDS) living in endemic areas of Latin America.

PATHOGENESIS AND PATHOLOGY. After inhaling spores, infection may remain confined to the lungs or may spread by lymphohematogenous dissemination to multiple organs. The host pathologic response caused by *P. brasiliensis* is similar to that caused by tissue invasion with *Blastomyces dermatitidis* and *Coccidioides immitis* (i.e., both granulomas and suppuration may develop). The type of tissue pathology and the spectrum of clinical disease are in large part dictated by the integrity of the cell-mediated defenses of the host.

CLINICAL MANIFESTATIONS. Pulmonary paracoccidioidomycosis may be asymptomatic or may result in symptomatic acute or chronic disease. Whereas the acute form of pulmonary paracoccidioidomycosis is usually non-specific and indistinguishable from other influenza-like illnesses, the clinical and radiographic features of the chronic form often resemble those of chronic pulmonary coccidioidomycosis. Any or all lobes may be infected, but the upper lobes tend to be less frequently involved. In addition, cavities, if present, are usually small (so-called microcavities). The juvenile form of paracoccidioidomycosis represents about 5% of all cases, occurs in persons younger than 30 years, and is characterized by acute onset, extrapulmonary disease often manifested by lymphadenopathy and hepatosplenomegaly, and a poor prognosis. The chronic form, adult type, accounting for about 90% of cases, occurs in older adults as an indolent illness, manifested by oropharyngeal and laryngeal mucous membrane ulcers; verrucous, ulcerative, or nodular skin lesions, often on the face or mucocutaneous borders; and enlarged or necrotic, draining lymph nodes, especially in the cervical region; pulmonary disease also occurs in the majority of patients. Other sites of less frequent involvement are the gastrointestinal tract, adrenal glands, testes, epididymis, and skeletal system. Central nervous system and eye disease secondary to *P. brasiliensis* are rare. Paracoccidioidomycosis heals by fibrosis; consequently, residual fibrotic sequelae in the affected organs, despite therapy, may be incapacitating, especially in patients with pulmonary disease.

DIAGNOSIS. Demonstration of the characteristic "pilot wheel," multiple-budding *P. brasiliensis* yeast cells by wet mounts or potassium hydroxide preparations of sputum, pus, or other body fluids, or by special fungal stains of biopsy or cell-block specimens, provides presumptive evidence of paracoccidioidomycosis. A positive culture of body fluid or tissue specimens is diagnostic. Two serologic tests, immunodiffusion and complement fixation, are commonly utilized. Precipitin bands appear early in the course of active infection and may persist for years, even after successful therapy. Complement-fixing antibodies appear later and are more useful in evaluating response to treatment. Both tests have high specificity. Alternative serologic tests, including enzyme-linked immunosorbent assay (ELISA) and counter-immunoelectrophoresis (CIE), as well as newer ones for detecting various glycoprotein antigens and antibodies to these antigens are under investigation. Skin tests have no role in diagnosis.

TREATMENT. In the past, oral sulfonamides were the mainstay of therapy, in large part owing to low cost; however, sulfonamides have two major drawbacks, namely, a high rate of relapse even after prolonged suppression therapy and a high frequency of adverse reactions, especially rashes. Intravenous amphotericin B is effective therapy and is usually used for more severe forms of paracoccidioidomycosis, such as pulmonary or disseminated multiorgan disease, and for more refractory cases. Follow-up chronic suppression therapy with sulfonamides is recommended. Oral antifungal azole drugs represent a significant advance in the treatment of this disease. Ketoconazole, an imidazole, is highly effective in both in vivo animal models and humans. Cure is usually achieved with dosages of 200 to 400 mg/day, given for at least 1 year. Itraconazole, a triazole, in a dose of 100 mg/day for 6 to 12 months, is as effective as ketoconazole and better tolerated; as a result, authorities now consider itraconazole the drug of choice for paracoccidioidomycosis. Experience in this disease with fluconazole, the other available oral triazole, has been limited. Because of the tropism of *P. brasiliensis* for the adrenal glands and the possibility of adrenal insufficiency during active disease or even after therapy is discontinued, periodic tests of adrenal function are recommended.

PROGNOSIS. Untreated disseminated paracoccidioidomycosis is generally fatal. As a rule, the more common indolent forms of adult disease, usually associated with reactivation, are amenable to

prolonged therapy, given over months to years. Unfortunately, clinically significant fibrotic sequelae often persist despite therapy.

Brummer E, Castaneda E, Restrepo A: Paracoccidioidomycosis: An update. Clin Microbiol Rev 6:89, 1993. *A comprehensive review of the disease, focusing on the causative agent, epidemiology, pathogenesis, diagnosis, and therapy, with 329 references.*

Goldani LZ, Sugar AM: Paracoccidioidomycosis and AIDS: An overview. Clin Infect Dis 21:1275, 1995. *This review focuses on clinical manifestations, diagnosis, and therapy of paracoccidioidomycosis in 27 patients with advanced AIDS who were not receiving trimethoprim-sulfamethoxazole prophylaxis (41 references).*

Naranjo MS, Trujillo M, Munera MI, et al: Treatment of paracoccidioidomycosis with itraconazole. J Med Vet Mycol 28:67, 1990. *Forty-five of 47 patients had the chronic form of disease. Itraconazole, 100 mg/day, given for a mean duration of 6 months, was highly effective, as measured by radiographic and cultural responses, falling serologic titers, and improvement in clinical severity scores.*

398 CRYPTOCOCCOSIS

William E. Dismukes

DEFINITION. Cryptococcosis is a systemic mycosis that most often involves the lungs and central nervous system (CNS) and, less frequently, the blood, skin, skeletal system, and prostate gland. *Cryptococcus neoformans,* the causative organism, is the most common agent of fungal meningitis, and since the onset of the acquired immunodeficiency syndrome (AIDS) epidemic in the early 1980s, it has been increasingly recognized as an opportunistic fungal pathogen.

CRYPTOCOCCOSIS	
Causative fungus	*Cryptococcus neoformans*
Primary geographic distribution	Worldwide
Primary route of acquisition	Respiratory (inhalation of spores)
Principal sites of disease	Lungs, CNS, blood, skin, bone, joints, prostate
Opportunistic infection in compromised hosts	Frequent, especially in corticosteroid-treated and AIDS patients
Drug of choice in most patients	Amphotericin B (with or without flucytosine) or fluconazole
Alternative therapy	Itraconazole

ETIOLOGY. *C. neoformans* is a yeast-like round or oval fungus, 5 to 10 μm in diameter, that is surrounded by a polysaccharide capsule and that reproduces by budding. Characteristics used to distinguish the genus *Cryptococcus* from other yeasts include a lack of pseudohyphae, assimilation of carbohydrate and nitrate, and production of phenyloxidase, melanin, and urease. There are two varieties of *C. neoformans:* var *neoformans* and var *gattii,* and four different serotypes, A, B, C, and D (based on the antigenic specificity of the capsule). In the laboratory, *C. neoformans* var *neoformans* (serotypes A and D) grows at 37° C on niger seed agar as smooth brown colonies within a few days after inoculation. By contrast, *C. neoformans* var *gattii* (serotypes B and C) grows more slowly, and nonpathogenic *Cryptococcus* species grow poorly or not at all at 37° C. Color reactions on canavanine-glycine-bromthymol blue (CGB) agar are also used to determine varietal status. Nomenclature of the perfect or sexual states is based on mating properties. For example, strains of serotypes A and D, which include the majority of clinical isolates, can be mated to produce the perfect state (*Filobasidiella neoformans* var *neoformans*).

EPIDEMIOLOGY. Cryptococcosis is worldwide in distribution. *C. neoformans* var *neoformans* is found in soil and other environmental areas, especially those contaminated by pigeon droppings; pigeons themselves are not infected. Although less is known about the ecologic niche of *C. neoformans* var *gattii,* this organism has been isolated from bark, wood, and leaves of river red gum (*Eucalyptus calmaldulensis*) trees in tropical and subtropical regions, areas of the world in which this variety of *C. neoformans* is endemic (southeast Asia and parts of Africa and Australia). Although humans and animals acquire infection after inhaling aerosolized spores, clusters of cases or mini-outbreaks of cryptococcosis rarely occur. Only two unusual cases of presumed person-to-person transmission of cryptococcosis have been observed. No obvious age, sex, or occupational predilection exists. Immunosuppression related to altered T-cell function is the most common predisposing factor: examples include corticosteroid therapy, lymphoproliferative malignancies, sarcoidosis (even in the absence of corticosteroid therapy), human immunodeficiency virus (HIV) infection, organ transplantation, and, perhaps, diabetes mellitus. The association of cryptococcosis and organ transplantation probably relates in large part to immunosuppression with corticosteroids. Cyclosporine, at least in a murine model, inhibits growth of *C. neoformans.* Among patients with AIDS in the United States, the incidence of cryptococcosis has been estimated to be between 5 and 10%. However, recent data from New York City showing the annual prevalence to be between 6.1 and 8.5% argue that the true cumulative risk for cryptococcosis among HIV-infected persons in the United States is underestimated. In Africa and other developing areas, the incidence of cryptococcosis in AIDS patients approaches 30%. Although cryptococcosis occurs most frequently in immunosuppressed hosts, in some countries, about 20 to 30% of patients with the disease have no apparent underlying condition or predisposing factor (except for unexplained CD4 cytopenia in some).

PATHOGENESIS AND PATHOLOGY. After aerosolized spores are inhaled, most infections begin with an asymptomatic pulmonary focus. In individuals with normal host defense, cryptococci remain localized in the lungs and are eventually eliminated. By contrast, in immunocompromised individuals, there is hematogenous spread to extrapulmonary organs. Phagocytosis of cryptococci by neutrophils and monocyte-derived macrophages appears to be mediated in part by complement and several proinflammatory cytokines including interferon-γ, tissue necrosis factor, various interleukins, including IL-8 and IL-12, and GM-CSF. In addition, nonphagocytic effector cells, such as natural killer cells and CD4$^+$ and CD8$^+$ T lymphocytes, kill *C. neoformans* by both oxidative and nonoxidative mechanisms. Cryptococcal polysaccharide is a major virulence factor and may be immunosuppressive, inhibit phagocytosis, limit production of nitric oxide (an inhibitor of cryptococcal cells), and interfere with antigen presentation processes. Paradoxically, cryptococcal polysaccharide has also been shown to activate the alternative complement pathway. Other cryptococcal virulence factors include soluble constituents of the capsule (glucuronoxylomannan, galactoxylomannan, and mannoprotein), melanin, and mannitol. Although immunity in large part depends on functioning, sensitized T-cells, and an intact cell-mediated arm of host defense, anticryptococcal antibody and complement appear to be critical components of some of the cellular mechanisms.

Patients with defective or altered T-cell immunity, such as those with HIV infection, are highly susceptible to infection with *C. neoformans* and progressive disease. The occurrence of cryptococcosis in AIDS patients is highly associated with CD4 counts of less than 50 cells/mm³. The preferential involvement of *C. neoformans* for the CNS is explained, in part, by the absence of complement and soluble anticryptococcal factors (present in normal serum) in normal cerebrospinal fluid (CSF), as well as a decreased to absent inflammatory response to cryptococci in brain tissue. As a result, well-formed granulomas are generally absent in histopathologic sections of infected tissue. The characteristic lesion in cryptococcal meningoencephalitis consists of cystic clusters of fungi; the meninges, basal ganglia, and the cortical gray matter are the sites of heaviest involvement. In other organs such as the lung, the inflammatory response varies in intensity from minimal to heavy and consists of an array of cells, including organism-containing macrophages, giant cells, plasma cells, and lymphocytes. No necrosis is present, and tissue is usually displaced by multiplying organisms. Yeast-like cryptococci with characteristic narrow-based buds stain

poorly with hematoxylin-eosin but are easily visualized with Gomori's methenamine silver (GMS) or periodic acid-Schiff (PAS) stains. Mucicarmine stain further aids identification by giving a rose color to the polysaccharide capsule.

CLINICAL MANIFESTATIONS. PULMONARY CRYPTOCOCCOSIS. The pattern of pulmonary cryptococcal infection is highly variable, ranging from the extremes of saprophytic airway colonization without clinical or radiographic evidence of disease to full-blown acute respiratory distress syndrome in compromised hosts, such as AIDS patients. More typically, radiographic findings include either patchy pneumonitis or solitary or multiple small nodules in asymptomatic persons or those with mild to moderate symptoms (e.g., fever, malaise, cough, scant sputum, pleuritic pain, or, rarely, hemoptysis). Although tumor-like masses mimicking carcinoma are not uncommon, cavitation and pleural effusions are less likely. The course of pulmonary cryptococcosis is also variable. In patients with normal host defenses, spontaneous regression of both clinical and radiographic manifestations is the rule, although chronic stable infection is known to occur. In contrast, pulmonary cryptococcosis in immunocompromised patients is more likely to progress and therefore requires antifungal therapy. Pulmonary disease may occur in the absence of extrapulmonary cryptococcosis, and, conversely, extrapulmonary disease such as meningitis may develop in the absence of apparent lung involvement.

CENTRAL NERVOUS SYSTEM CRYPTOCOCCOSIS. Meningitis, usually subacute or chronic in nature, is the most common manifestation of CNS cryptococcosis. Complications include hydrocephalus, increased intracranial pressure associated with cerebral edema and resistance to CSF outflow in the absence of hydrocephalus, encephalitis, involvement of the optic pathways, brain-stem vasculitis, and mass lesions (cryptococcomas) of the brain parenchyma or spinal cord. The clinical presentation and course of cryptococcal meningitis vary greatly, related in part to the underlying condition and immune status of the host. In "normal" hosts, the onset is often insidious, whereas in compromised hosts, such as HIV-infected or corticosteroid-treated patients, the onset tends to be more acute and the course more rapidly progressive. The most common symptoms are headache and alteration in mental status (e.g., confusion, lethargy, obtundation or coma, and personality change). Nausea and vomiting are frequent; fever and stiff neck are less common. Ocular symptoms, such as blurred vision, photophobia, vision loss, and diplopia are secondary to perineuritic adhesive arachnoiditis, papilledema, optic nerve neuritis, chorioretinitis, or retinovitreal abscess, and are present in about 25% of patients. Other manifestations include hearing deficits, seizures, ataxia, and aphasia. Dementia is important to recognize as a potential sequela because it may be curable. Cryptococcomas, which are uncommon, can rarely be seen in the absence of meningeal disease. The mortality rate varies from 5 to 25%; most deaths occur in the first few weeks of illness.

MISCELLANEOUS. After the lungs and CNS, the next most commonly involved organs in patients with disseminated cryptococcosis are the skin and skeletal system. Cutaneous manifestations occur in 10 to 15% of cases and usually take the form of papules, pustules, nodules, ulcers, or draining sinuses. Typically, cellulitis with prominent erythema and induration is seen in corticosteroid-treated transplant recipients, and umbilicated papules resembling molluscum contagiosum are observed in AIDS patients. Oral mucosal chancres have been reported rarely. Osteomyelitis is more common than septic arthritis. Less commonly involved sites of cryptococcal disease include pericardium, myocardium, muscle, liver, peritoneum, adrenal glands, kidneys, and prostate gland. Infections of these organs are being increasingly identified in AIDS patients. For example, the prostate has been reported to be a sanctuary of residual infection in this population group.

DIAGNOSIS. As with other systemic mycoses, the definitive diagnosis of cryptococcosis depends on demonstrating the characteristic yeast-like organism with its surrounding capsule in tissue or fluid obtained from involved sites, together with cultural confirmation. In addition, in patients with suspected cryptococcosis, the latex agglutination test to detect cryptococcal polysaccharide antigen in serum and CSF is an extremely important adjunct to diagnosis, unlike the situation for most other fungal disease, in which serologic tests lack specificity and sensitivity. Cryptococcal antigen is found in CSF in more than 90% and in serum in about 75% of patients with meningitis, especially if serial specimens are examined over time. Sensitivity of the test is even higher in AIDS patients, and titers are especially high. In patients with extraneural cryptococcal disease, antigen is detected in only 25 to 50% of cases. Proper controls are necessary to eliminate rheumatoid factor, which may give rise to a false-positive result. Serum of patients with disseminated infection caused by *Trichosporon beigelii* may also test positive for cryptococcal antigen. False-negative tests for cryptococcal antigen may be due to low numbers of cryptococcal organisms invading tissue or in CSF, unencapsulated or poorly encapsulated strains, or a prozone phenomenon. Tests for cryptococcal antibody are not useful for diagnosis.

Pulmonary cryptococcosis is difficult to diagnose in most cases without obtaining lung tissue via bronchoscopy, open lung biopsy, or thorascopy. Wet preparations of sputum are only occasionally helpful, and sputum cultures are positive for *C. neoformans* in only 20% of cases. In patients with pleural effusions, fluid tested for cryptococcal antigen may be positive, thereby obviating a more invasive procedure. In every patient with established pulmonary cryptococcosis, a lumbar puncture should be performed, whether or not CNS disease is apparent. Blood cultures and tissue for culture and histopathologic study of any other suspected sites of involvement (e.g., skin or bone) should also be obtained.

The diagnosis of cryptococcal meningitis is easier to establish than the diagnosis of cryptococcal pulmonary disease. Once the diagnosis of meningitis is considered, a lumbar puncture should be performed. Most patients, except for those with AIDS (see below), have significant CSF abnormalities, including elevated opening pressure, depressed glucose levels (hypoglycorrhachia), elevated protein levels, and lymphocytic pleocytosis. The India ink preparation of centrifuged CSF to detect budding yeast cells and surrounding capsule is positive in 50 to 75% of cases; because the incidence of false-positive smears is high, confirmation of findings by culture is imperative. Culturing of centrifuged sediment of large volumes (5 to 10 mL) of CSF obtained by repeated lumbar punctures is associated with a positive culture rate of 90 to 95%. In AIDS patients, the CSF formula is often normal or only minimally abnormal, owing to a diminished or absent inflammatory response. Yet in most cases, opening pressures are elevated, cultures are positive, cryptococcal antigen titers are high, and India ink preparations reveal organisms. The chest roentgenogram may or may not be abnormal. Blood should be cultured and tested for antigen in all patients. In addition, computed tomographic scans (CT) or magnetic resonance imaging (MRI) of the head is indicated in most patients, especially those with coma, suspected hydrocephalus, focal neurologic findings, seizures, or clinical deterioration after initial improvement.

TREATMENT. Approaches to therapy of cryptococcosis vary according to site of involvement and underlying host status. Whereas all patients with CNS cryptococcosis or other forms of extrapulmonary disease require treatment, some cases of pulmonary cryptococcosis alone in the "normal" host resolve without antifungal therapy. By contrast, other patients with pulmonary cryptococcosis, including patients with AIDS and other immunocompromising conditions, those with accompanying extrapulmonary disease, and those with progressive disease require antifungal therapy. Although specific guidelines are poorly defined, the two commonly used drugs are amphotericin B (total dose, 1.0 to 2.0 g) and fluconazole (400 mg daily for 3 to 6 months). Fluconazole should be reserved for patients with mild to moderate forms of cryptococcal lung disease. As a rule, therapy should be continued until clinical, radiographic, and mycologic resolution of disease is evident. Surgical resection may be an important adjunct to drug therapy in patients with extensive lobar consolidation and large mass lesions.

The therapy of cryptococcal meningitis has been more extensively studied than the therapy of any other systemic fungal disease. Data indicate that (1) all patients require treatment; (2) several treatment regimens, including oral azole drugs, may be used; (3) a combination of amphotericin B and flucytosine is the regimen of choice, especially for patients with moderate to severe disease including complications such as obtundation, coma, blindness, cranial nerve palsies, and hydrocephalus; (4) regardless of regimen, 5 to 25% of patients die of the disease; and (5) treatment considerations are somewhat different for AIDS patients with cryptococcal meningitis (see below). Although the standard regimen in non-

AIDS patients is combination amphotericin B (0.5 to 1.0 mg/kg/day) and flucytosine (100 mg/kg/day) for 4 to 6 weeks, both the daily dose and total dose should be individualized, balancing the risks of toxicities of the drugs and the potential benefits of synergy and increased efficacy. Both renal function and serum flucytosine levels should be closely monitored, and flucytosine doses should be adjusted to maintain serum concentrations in the range of 50 to 100 mg/mL. Potential toxic effects of flucytosine include bone marrow suppression, hepatitis, diarrhea, and rash. Although experience with fluconazole (400 mg daily for 10 weeks) in non-AIDS cryptococcal meningitis is limited, this drug may be an effective alternative therapy. A second alternative regimen for non-AIDS patients is induction therapy followed by consolidation therapy (see Therapy in Patients with AIDS, item 4). Intrathecal therapy with amphotericin B is rarely used nowadays, usually reserved for patients who experience relapse or whose disease is refractory to prolonged courses of high-dose intravenous amphotericin B. After completion of primary therapy in selected non-AIDS patients with persistent T-cell dysfunction (e.g., renal transplant recipients receiving immunosuppressive therapy), some authorities recommend prolonged maintenance therapy with fluconazole, 200 mg daily, to prevent relapse.

THERAPY IN PATIENTS WITH AIDS. Because cryptococcal meningitis in AIDS patients may be highly refractory and associated with a relapse rate of 50% if therapy is stopped, both aggressive primary therapy and long-term maintenance therapy are required.

PRIMARY THERAPY. Several alternative treatment regimens may be used.

1. Combination amphotericin and flucytosine may be given for the entire period of primary therapy. However, this regimen is not commonly employed, as some AIDS patients may not tolerate flucytosine because of a high incidence of drug-induced cytopenia, often superimposed on pre-existing bone-marrow suppression secondary to antibacterial and antiviral drugs, cytotoxic chemotherapy, and opportunistic infectious diseases. In addition, flucytosine for prolonged duration should not be used unless serum levels can be monitored. In such situations, amphotericin B may be used alone.

2. Azole therapy alone is effective in highly selected patients (e.g., those with mild disease and normal mental status at time of diagnosis). Fluconazole is favored over itraconazole, another triazole, in cryptococcal meningitis because of fluconazole's water solubility, minimal protein binding, and good to excellent penetration into CSF (60 to 80% of serum concentration). In addition, an intravenous formulation of fluconazole is available. A major disadvantage of fluconazole and itraconazole is their less rapid sterilization of CSF than with amphotericin B.

3. The novel combination of two oral drugs, flucytosine and fluconazole, has been studied in both animal models and, to a lesser extent, in patients with AIDS-associated cryptococcal meningitis. However, because of unacceptable toxicity of flucytosine administered over a prolonged period, this regimen cannot be recommended over more established treatments.

4. Results obtained from a recent, large (381 patients) multicenter clinical trial argue that induction therapy with combination amphotericin (0.7 mg/kg/day) and flucytosine (100 mg/kg/day) for 2 weeks followed by consolidation therapy with fluconazole (400 mg/day) for 8 weeks is now the preferred treatment regimen for AIDS-associated cryptococcal meningitis. This unique regimen was extremely well tolerated and resulted in an increased rate of sterilization of CSF and decreased mortality as compared with regimens used in previous studies. Overall, mortality was 5.5% in the first 2 weeks and 3.9% over the next 8 weeks. In this study, flucytosine given for only 2 weeks was associated with minimum toxicity and combined with amphotericin B was more effective in sterilizing CSF than amphotericin B alone. Other studies have utilized an even higher dose of amphotericin B, 1.0 mg/kg/day, with similar success. Consequently, amphotericin B (0.7 to 1.0 mg/kg/day) in combination with flucytosine (100 mg/kg/day) is recommended over amphotericin B alone for induction therapy of AIDS-associated cryptococcal meningitis. Itraconazole (400 mg/day) may be a suitable

alternative for patients unable to take fluconazole during consolidation therapy.

5. Recent data indicate that passive antibody in the form of murine or humanized monoclonal antibodies has the potential to enhance cellular immunity; trials are ongoing.

Chemotherapy alone is not adequate treatment for all patients. Ventricular shunting of CSF should be performed in obtunded or comatose patients with hydrocephalus demonstrated by imaging studies. Among patients with no overt hydrocephalus but abnormal or worsening mental status and elevated intracranial pressure, an aggressive management approach is mandatory (frequent lumbar punctures to cautiously lower CSF pressure, placement of a lumbar drain, or ventriculostomy with pressure monitoring and placement of ventriculoperitoneal shunt if indicated). Mechanical measures to reduce intracranial pressure are more effective than medical measures, such as high-dose dexamethasone or mannitol.

MAINTENANCE THERAPY. Once primary therapy has sterilized the CSF (i.e., converted the fungal culture from positive to negative), maintenance therapy in AIDS patients should be initiated. Fluconazole (200 mg daily) is more effective in preventing relapse than amphotericin (1 mg/kg weekly) and much better tolerated, resulting in better patient compliance. Fluconazole is also more effective than itraconazole. Chronic suppressive therapy must be continued for life.

PROGNOSIS. Pretreatment prognostic factors that adversely affect outcome in patients with cryptococcal meningitis include any underlying condition predisposing to T-cell dysfunction (e.g., HIV infection/AIDS, corticosteroid or other immunosuppressive therapy, or organ transplantation); absence of headache as a presenting symptom; altered mental status as evidenced by obtundation, stupor, or coma; positive extraneural cultures for *C. neoformans;* CSF white cell count less than 20/mm³; and high cryptococcal antigen serum and CSF titers. Among these factors, T-cell dysfunction and abnormal mental status appear to be most important. A rise in CSF antigen during maintenance therapy is associated with relapse; by contrast, other abnormalities of CSF such as hypoglycorrhachia, elevated protein, or positive India ink preparation may persist for months after therapy has been discontinued and do not appear to correlate with relapse.

PREVENTION. Because an environmental source of infection cannot be determined in the vast majority of patients who develop cryptococcal disease, attempts at eliminating *C. neoformans* from soil or other habitats are not feasible or practical. With the availability of effective and safe oral antifungal drugs, such as fluconazole and itraconazole, use of these as prophylactic agents in high-risk groups such as HIV-infected persons has been evaluated. Data indicate that oral fluconazole, 200 mg daily, in patients with CD4 counts of less than 200 cells/mm³, is effective in reducing the frequency of systemic fungal disease, especially cryptococcosis, but it does not prolong survival. Consequently, use of fluconazole to prevent cryptococcosis in patients with advanced AIDS is not routinely recommended.

Levitz SM: The ecology of *Cryptococcus neoformans* and the epidemiology of cryptococcosis. Rev Infect Dis 13:1163, 1991. *Reviews of the two varieties of* C. neoformans (*var.* neoformans *and var.* gattii) *with emphasis on their distribution in nature and the epidemiologic characteristics of infected patients.*

Mitchell TG, Perfect JR: Cryptococcosis in the era of AIDS—100 years after the discovery of *Cryptococcus neoformans.* Clin Microbiol Rev 8:515, 1995. *A comprehensive review of the disease, including the virulence factors and biology of the organism, pathogenesis and host defenses, clinical manifestations, laboratory diagnosis, and treatment (529 references).*

Powderly WG: Cryptococcal meningitis and AIDS. Clin Infect Dis 17:837, 1993. *Focuses on clinical and laboratory features as well as different treatment options, including primary therapy for acute disease and maintenance therapy to prevent relapse.*

Powderly WG, Saag MS, Cloud GA, et al: A controlled trial of fluconazole or amphotericin B to prevent relapse of cryptococcal meningitis in patients with the acquired immunodeficiency syndrome. N Engl J Med 326:793, 1992. *The definitive trial showing that daily fluconazole is superior to weekly intravenous amphotericin B as maintenance preventive therapy in AIDS-associated cryptococcosis.*

Van der Horst CM, Saag MS, Cloud GA, et al: Treatment of cryptococcal meningitis associated with the acquired immunodeficiency syndrome. N Engl J Med 337:15, 1997. *Results of this large, double-blind, multicenter trial indicate that the combination of higher-dose amphotericin B and flucytosine is associated with an increased rate of sterilization of cerebrospinal fluid and decreased mortality at 2 weeks as compared with regimens used in previous studies.*

399 SPOROTRICHOSIS
William E. Dismukes

DEFINITION. Sporotrichosis is a chronic mycotic disease that typically involves skin, subcutaneous tissue, and regional lymphatics as a result of cutaneous inoculation of *Sporothrix schenckii.* Extracutaneous disease, secondary to either lymphohematogenous dissemination or inhalation of organisms, is rare.

SPOROTRICHOSIS	
Causative fungus	*Sporothrix schenckii*
Primary geographic distribution	Worldwide, mainly in temperate and tropical areas
Primary route of acquisition	Cutaneous inoculation
Principal sites of disease	Skin, lymphatics; less commonly, lungs and joints
Opportunistic infection in compromised hosts	Infrequent
Drug of choice for most patients	Itraconazole
Alternative therapy	Cutaneous disease: saturated solution potassium iodide, fluconazole, or surgery Extracutaneous disease: amphotericin B

ETIOLOGY. *S. schenckii* is a dimorphic fungus that grows in nature and in the laboratory at 30° C on Sabouraud's agar as a white mold, which, with time, becomes brownish black. In tissue and at 37° C, the organism exists as yeastlike cells, which appear as round, spherical, or cigar-shaped budding forms, 2 to 6 μm in size.

EPIDEMIOLOGY. Sporotrichosis is worldwide in distribution. *S. schenckii* appears to be ubiquitous in soil and in both living and decaying vegetation. Although the organism does not appear to infect plants, it may infect animals, especially cats and dogs, as well as humans, especially those who frequently handle or come in contact with mulch, sphagnum moss, hay, timber, and thorny bushes. Consequently, sporotrichosis is considered an occupational disease of certain groups, including farmers, tree nursery or forestry workers, gardeners, florists, landscapers, and carpenters. In 1988, the largest known epidemic of sporotrichosis in the United States occurred among 84 forestry workers exposed to sphagnum moss obtained from a single source. Transmission almost always results from the percutaneous inoculation of organisms. In the majority of patients with extracutaneous disease, the route of acquisition is unclear. Rarely, pulmonary sporotrichosis may result from inhalation of aerosolized conidia. Although person-to-person transmission is not known to occur, transmission from animals, especially cats and squirrels, to humans has been documented. The number of cases of cutaneous disease in males and females is similar; sex and age appear to play less of a role than does environmental exposure. By contrast, extracutaneous sporotrichosis is more common in males. As a rule, *S. schenckii* is not considered an opportunistic fungal pathogen, although sporotrichosis in compromised hosts is being recognized increasingly. For example, cases have been observed in a few patients with acquired immunodeficiency syndrome (AIDS).

PATHOGENESIS AND PATHOLOGY. Cutaneous inoculation may follow either inapparent or obvious penetrating trauma. In the majority of patients, clinical disease does not extend beyond the site of inoculation or the draining lymphatics. Localized disease may persist for years, and cell-mediated immunity appears to be responsible for preventing or limiting the spread to extracutaneous sites. Conversely, multiorgan disease involving skin and distant sites, such as lungs, bones, and joints, is more common in immunosuppressed hosts.

The basic histopathologic pattern in cutaneous sporotrichosis is a combination of suppuration and granulomas, often accompanied by pseudoepitheliomatous hyperplasia. This pattern is not diagnostic, as it may also be seen in malignancy as well as other fungal diseases, such as blastomycosis, coccidioidomycosis, and chromomycosis. Because the yeastlike cells, typical of *S. schenckii,* are uncommonly identified in tissue sections, cultural confirmation is usually necessary for diagnosis. The finding of large asteroid bodies (radiate eosinophilic material surrounding fungal yeast cells) provides presumptive evidence of sporotrichosis.

CLINICAL MANIFESTATIONS. Two distinctive clinical forms of cutaneous and extracutaneous disease, which differ in management and prognosis, are seen.

CUTANEOUS. This form of sporotrichosis can be further divided into two types: plaque (or fixed) and lymphocutaneous. Plaque sporotrichosis, which is less common, consists of a single ulcerative or nodular lesion at the site of primary inoculation, usually on an exposed extremity or the face. The lesion begins as a small painless red papule, which gradually enlarges and finally ulcerates (sporotrichotic chancre). A violaceous hue and intermittent serosanguineous drainage are characteristic. Lymphocutaneous sporotrichosis, which is the more typical type and is found in about 75% of cases, represents an extension of the primary lesion. Subcutaneous nontender nodular lesions appear proximally along thickened lymphatics over days to weeks, and they occasionally ulcerate. Lymph nodes are rarely enlarged. Similarly, constitutional symptoms, such as fever and chills, are usually absent. This type of sporotrichosis, which usually remains confined to the primary site and its regional lymphatics, may wax and wane over years if untreated. Lymphohematogenous spread to distant organs is uncommon.

EXTRACUTANEOUS. The pathogenesis of the majority of cases of extracutaneous sporotrichosis is uncertain because most cases are not accompanied by clinically apparent cutaneous disease. The skeletal system is the most commonly involved extracutaneous organ. Although indolent monoarticular arthritis of the knees, ankles, wrists, and elbows is most frequent, osteomyelitis (especially of the tibia), tenosynovitis, and carpal tunnel syndrome have been reported. Multiarticular arthritis is more likely in compromised hosts with widespread hematogenous spread to multiple organs. Pulmonary sporotrichosis is far less common than osteoarticular disease. Fewer than 100 cases of pulmonary disease have been reported. This form of insidious infection occurs primarily in older male alcoholics and mimics reactivation tuberculosis. Thin-walled cavitary lesions in a single upper lobe are characteristic; bilateral fibrocavitary disease may be seen occasionally. Extrapulmonary spread of disease is uncommon. Ocular sporotrichosis results from traumatic inoculation of the conjunctiva or cornea; endophthalmitis is unusual. Chronic lymphocytic meningitis may be a complication of sporotrichosis, even in the absence of obvious extraneural disease. In any patient with chronic meningitis of unknown origin, cerebrospinal fluid (CSF) should be tested for antibody to *S. schenckii.* Meningeal sporotrichosis has been reported in at least two patients with AIDS.

DIAGNOSIS. As a rule, the diagnosis of sporotrichosis must be based on cultural demonstration of the organism in tissue or fluid obtained from involved sites (e.g., skin, subcutaneous nodule, joint, bone, or lung). Histopathologic findings are usually non-specific, and the characteristic yeastlike cells are often not identified by special stains, such as Gomori's methenamine silver or periodic acid-Schiff. Direct immunofluorescence, if available, may be helpful. Although testing of serum or CSF by latex agglutination or enzyme immunoassay for antibody to *S. schenckii* may be useful, especially in patients suspected of having extracutaneous disease, positive low-level antibody titers may be observed in normal persons. No skin test is commercially available.

TREATMENT. Itraconazole, in a dosage of 100 to 400 mg/day, has replaced saturated solution of potassium iodide (SSKI) as conventional therapy for cutaneous sporotrichosis. Itraconazole, which should be administered for 3 to 6 months, is more effective than the other two oral azoles, ketoconazole and fluconazole, and is easier to administer and better tolerated than SSKI. Oral SSKI is begun at a dosage of 5 drops, three times a day, and increased dropwise (3 to 5 drops/day) up to a maximum of 120 drops/day or until the development of iodine toxicity (manifested by rash, lacrimation, parotid swelling, or nonspecific gastrointestinal symptoms). Iodide therapy should be continued for at least 1 month after clinical resolution of the disease. For patients in developing countries, SSKI may be preferred over itraconazole or other azoles because of cheaper cost. Terbinafine, an oral allylamine antifungal drug, has promise as an alternative therapy for cutaneous sporotrichosis. For patients who are intolerant of their drugs or who are pregnant, prolonged daily use of local hyperthermia is an effective alternative treatment for lymphocutaneous disease.

Itraconazole, 200 to 600 mg/day for 12 months or longer, is moderately effective in treating extracutaneous sporotrichosis, especially osteoarticular disease. Amphotericin B should be reserved for patients with cutaneous or extracutaneous disease in whom azole or iodide therapy has failed and as therapy in immunocompromised patients with severe, life-threatening, widely disseminated sporotrichosis, and/or meningeal sporotrichosis. In patients with disseminated or meningeal disease, consideration may be given to switching to itraconazole after a successful induction course of amphotericin B. Cure rates may be improved in selected patients with bone and joint disease or single-cavity pulmonary disease by surgical resection of synovial tissue, bone, or lung, as an adjunct to antifungal therapy.

PROGNOSIS. Although untreated cutaneous sporotrichosis may remit and relapse for years, and rarely disseminate, treatment is recommended, as the likelihood of cure with itraconazole or iodide therapy is high. In contrast, extracutaneous disease, especially pulmonary and disseminated disease, is often refractory to therapy including itraconazole, amphotericin B, and surgery, and is associated with significant morbidity and mortality.

Dixon DM, Salkin IF, Duncan RA, et al: Isolation and characterization of *Sporothrix schenckii* from clinical and environmental sources associated with the largest U.S. epidemic of sporotrichosis. J Clin Microbiol 29:6, 1991. *A detailed microbiologic analysis of 21 clinical and 69 environmental isolates of* S. schenckii *associated with this sporotrichosis outbreak (84 cases).*

Kauffman CA: Old and new therapies for sporotrichosis. Clin Infect Dis 21:981, 1995. *A concise review and helpful discussion of the currently recommended treatment regimen for all clinical forms of sporotrichosis (63 references).*

Winn RE, Anderson J, Piper J: Systemic sporotrichosis treated with itraconazole. Clin Infect Dis 7:210, 1993. *A report of six cases of extracutaneous sporotrichosis, three with bone and joint disease and three with disseminated disease, successfully treated with itraconazole. One patient suffered relapse.*

400 CANDIDIASIS

William E. Dismukes

DEFINITION. *Candida* species can cause a variety of clinical syndromes that are generically termed candidiasis and are usually categorized by site of involvement. Broadly speaking, the two most common syndromes are mucocutaneous candidiasis (e.g., oropharyngeal disease or thrush, esophagitis, and vaginitis) and invasive or deep-organ candidiasis (e.g., candidemia, chronic disseminated or hepatosplenic disease, endocarditis, and endophthalmitis). In most patients, candidiasis is an opportunistic disease.

CANDIDIASIS

Causative fungus	*Candida* species (*C. albicans* most common)
Primary geographic distribution	Worldwide; part of normal flora of humans and in environment
Primary route of acquisition	Endogenous; person-to-person
Principal sites of disease	Mucous membranes (oropharynx, vagina), skin, esophagus, blood, liver, spleen, kidneys, eyes, heart
Opportunistic infection in compromised hosts	Frequent; e.g., mucosal disease in patients with AIDS and deep-organ disease in patients with granulocytopenia
Drug(s) of choice for most patients	Mucosal disease: topical or oral azole drug (clotrimazole or fluconazole) Deep-organ disease: amphotericin B or fluconazole
Alternative therapy for deep-organ disease	Amphotericin B plus flucytosine

ETIOLOGY. Among more than 190 recognized species of *Candida, C. albicans* is the most commonly identified pathogen in humans. Other clinically important species include *C. tropicalis, C. parapsilosis, C. glabrata, C. krusei, C. pseudotropicalis, C. lusitaniae,* and *C. guilliermondi. Candida* organisms share two morphologic features: small, spherical yeast forms (4 to 6 μm), which reproduce by budding; and pseudohyphae (pseudomycelia), which are chains of elongated yeasts separated by constrictions. In body fluids or tissue, both budding cells and fragments of pseudohyphae may be visualized. Identification and speciation in the microbiology laboratory are based on both morphologic characteristics and results of metabolic tests. The ability of *C. albicans* to produce germ tubes allows presumptive identification. CHROM-agar *Candida,* which is a chromogenic medium, is useful for identifying multiple yeast species in a single specimen (e.g., urine or blood) and for more rapidly identifying non–*C. albicans* species.

EPIDEMIOLOGY. Candidiasis occurs worldwide. *C. albicans* is part of the normal human flora of the mouth, gastrointestinal tract, and vagina; it normally lives in balance with other microorganisms in the body; and, in most individuals, it exists as a saprophytic colonizer or commensal. When this balance is upset by certain drugs (e.g., broad-spectrum antibiotics or corticosteroids) or conditions (e.g., diabetes mellitus or human immunodeficiency virus [HIV] infection), endogenous *C. albicans* may become a pathogen and cause either mucocutaneous or deep-organ disease. *C. albicans* may also be recovered from soil, hospital environments, food, and other substrates. In contrast to *C. albicans,* the non–*C. albicans* species that are pathogenic for humans less frequently colonize the skin, gastrointestinal tract, or vagina of normal individuals. These species more often reside in the environment and on inanimate objects and thus reach the body from exogenous sources; consequently, they are generally regarded as opportunistic fungal pathogens. Unlike other fungi, *Candida* species may be transmitted from person to person (e.g., between sexual partners, by hands of medical personnel, and during birth, from colonized vagina to neonatal oropharynx).

Candidiasis, both mucocutaneous and deep forms, has emerged as the most common opportunistic fungal disease, owing to the progressively increasing use of antibiotics (both prophylactic and therapeutic) and immunosuppressive and cytotoxic drugs; indwelling foreign bodies, including prosthetic heart valves, prosthetic joints, and intravascular monitoring devices; venous, arterial, urinary, and peritoneal catheters; and organ transplantation. In addition, the acquired immunodeficiency syndrome (AIDS) epidemic has been highly contributory.

PATHOGENESIS AND PATHOLOGY. Several components of the host defense system are important in protecting against infection with *Candida* species. An intact integumentary barrier, including skin and mucous membranes, prevents invasion of normally colonizing organisms, which possess adherence properties as yet not fully understood. Disruption or loss of normal barriers as a consequence of percutaneous catheters, endotracheal tubes, severe burns, or abdominal surgery is a common predisposing factor, especially to deep invasive or disseminated disease. Polymorphonuclear leukocytes and monocytes are the major cellular defenses against *Candida* species; both oxidant-dependent and -independent effector mechanisms are necessary for killing of organisms. Although less well defined, tissue macrophages, lymphocytes and cell-mediated immunity also play a role. Predisposing abnormalities of host defense include T-cell dysfunction, associated with mucocutaneous disease (oropharyngeal or esophageal candidiasis in HIV-infected persons) as well as chronic mucocutaneous candidiasis, and granulocytopenia secondary to underlying disease or therapy, associated with deep disease (candidemia or invasive candidiasis). In cutaneous candidiasis, histopathologic evidence of chronic dermatitis with yeasts confined to the stratum corneum is characteristic. By contrast, microabscesses interspersed in normal tissue are the characteristic pathologic finding in visceral candidiasis. Neutrophils appear initially, followed by histiocytes and giant cells and, in some cases, a readily apparent granulomatous response. In severely immunocompromised patients, the inflammatory response may be minimal or absent. Both yeasts and pseudohyphae can usually be visualized by special stains, such as periodic acid-Schiff or Gomori's methenamine silver.

CLINICAL MANIFESTATIONS. MUCOCUTANEOUS INFECTIONS. Thrush or oropharyngeal candidiasis is manifested by creamy white, curdlike, exudative patches on the tongue, buccal mucosa, palate, or other oral mucosal surfaces. These patches are actually pseudomembranes, which, on removal, may leave a raw, bleeding, painful surface. Poorly fitting dentures may be a predisposing factor, and areas of erythema may be the only marker of disease. Cheilosis, an inflammatory reaction at the corners of the mouth, and atrophic changes, either acute or chronic, are less common presentations of oropharyngeal disease. Esophagitis, which may occur as an extension of thrush or may occur in the absence of thrush in up to one-third of patients, is manifested typically by odynophagia, dysphagia, or substernal chest pain and uncommonly by bleeding. Thrush or esophagitis, occurring in the absence of any known predisposing condition, should raise the suspicion of HIV infection. Gastrointestinal candidiasis involving the mucosa of the stomach and small and large bowel is most common in patients with cancer and is an important source of disseminated infection.

Intertrigo, a cutaneous *Candida* infection involving warm, moist surfaces, such as the axillae, gluteal and inframammary folds, and groin, may be variable in appearance but is usually manifested as well-marginated, erythematous, exudative patches surrounded by satellite vesicles or pustules. Paronychia, a painful, tense, reddened swelling at the base of the nail or along the sides, is commonly caused by *Candida* species, especially in diabetics and persons whose hands are chronically immersed in water. Although *Candida* species may cause onychomycosis, this chronic deforming infection of the nails is most frequently due to one of the genera of superficial dermatophytes, such as *Trichophyton* or *Epidermophyton.* Vulvovaginitis, the most common *Candida* mucocutaneous infection in women, especially in association with pregnancy, oral contraceptives, antibiotic therapy, diabetes, and HIV infection, is typically caused by *C. albicans* and is characterized by thick, creamy vaginal discharge, erythematous labia, and intense pruritus. Balanitis in males, often acquired through sexual intercourse, is manifested by superficial vesicles and exudative patches, usually on the glans penis. *Candida* cystitis, which at cystoscopy resembles oral thrush, is most often a complication of an indwelling bladder catheter. Chronic mucocutaneous candidiasis, a rare condition manifested by a heterogeneous group of persistent, often disfiguring *Candida* infections involving skin, mucous membranes, hair, and nails, occurs primarily in persons with altered T-cell function or an endocrinopathy (e.g., hypoparathyroidism or hypoadrenalism).

DEEP-ORGAN CANDIDIASIS. Numerous diagnostic categories or labels for serious or deep *Candida* infection exist, including candidemia, disseminated candidiasis, systemic candidiasis, invasive candidiasis, visceral candidiasis, and terms indicating involvement of specific organs, such as hepatosplenic candidiasis and ocular candidiasis. Here, discussion focuses on two major categories: (1) candidemia, which may or may not be associated with visceral organ involvement; and (2) chronic disseminated candidiasis, which implies systemic multiorgan disease and encompasses other subgroups, such as visceral, invasive, and hepatosplenic disease.

Candidemia. Candidemia, which is defined as one or more positive blood cultures for *Candida* species, may occur in the presence or absence of clinical manifestations (e.g., fever or skin lesions) and is often preceded by *Candida* colonization or infection at a site other than the bloodstream. The incidence of candidemia has risen dramatically over recent years in association with the increased number of compromised hosts (e.g., patients with cancer or burns, patients in intensive care units, and organ transplant recipients) managed by aggressive interventions, including empirical broad-spectrum antibiotics, cytotoxic chemotherapy, hemodialysis, and most important, intravenous and intra-arterial catheters, as well as other intravascular devices. In many hospitals, *Candida* species have become one of the three to five most common causes of bloodstream infections. Previously, "transient candidemia" was used to imply short duration (<24 hours) of fungemia and to indicate either clearing of the candidemia on removal of an infected intravascular catheter or a benign condition not requiring antifungal therapy. Current data strongly argue against this concept and suggest that catheter removal alone is insufficient, even in the noncompromised patient, to prevent metastatic hematogenous dissemination to visceral organs.

Although *C. albicans* is the most common species identified in blood, recent studies indicate that candidemia is increasingly caused by non–*C. albicans* species, especially *C. tropicalis*, *C. parapsilosis*, and *C. glabrata*. Candidemia developing in patients already receiving antifungal therapy is more likely caused by non–*C. albicans* species, often associated with resistance to fluconazole, the most widely used azole drug. The frequency of non–*C. albicans* species as causes of fungemia varies widely from institution to institution, in part due to differing practices of empirical antibacterial therapy and antifungal prophylaxis as well as to differing subsets of patients with cancer and other causes of immunosuppression. For example, *C. tropicalis* and *C. krusei* are more likely in oncology patients, whereas *C. albicans* is significantly more common in non-oncology patients.

Catheters of various types are the most important portals of entry, accounting for more than half of episodes of candidemia. In the majority of cases, removing or changing catheters, either peripheral or central, is necessary to eradicate candidemia, especially persistent candidemia. Other portals of entry are the gastrointestinal tract, especially in patients with granulocytopenia, and surgical wounds. The urinary and respiratory tracts, although frequently colonized by *Candida* species, are less common sources of bloodstream infection. The mortality rate of candidemia caused by all species is high, ranging from 40 to 60%. Mortality is significantly associated with a high Acute Physiology and Chronic Health Evaluation (APACHE) II score, a rapidly fatal underlying disease, and sustained candidemia. The mortality rate in catheter-associated candidemia is lower than in candidemia related to other sources.

The frequency with which candidemia results in localized single-organ disease (e.g., ocular candidiasis) or widespread disseminated multiorgan disease is uncertain. Premortem diagnosis of invasive or disseminated candidiasis must be based on histopathologic demonstration of tissue invasion by *Candida* organisms. Because blood cultures are negative in about 50% of patients with disseminated candidiasis and there are no other reliable markers, such as serologic tests, disseminated *Candida* disease may not be suspected and appropriate invasive diagnostic procedures may not be performed. Autopsy series indicate that disseminated disease involving kidneys, liver, spleen, brain, myocardium, and eyes is most likely in patients with some rapidly fatal underlying disease, such as leukemia complicated by neutropenia, and is least likely in patients with candidemia in the setting of non-oncologic disease, especially when the bloodstream infection is catheter-related. In addition, patients whose candidemia is treated are less likely to develop disseminated disease.

Cutaneous Lesions of Disseminated Candidiasis. Papulopustules or macronodules on an erythematous base, usually widely distributed over the trunk and extremities, are the hallmark lesions associated with persistent candidemia. Hemorrhagic bullae have also been reported.

Ocular Candidiasis. This form of localized candidiasis may result

from either hematogenous spread or direct inoculation (e.g., after cataract extraction or intraocular lens implantation). Any eye structure may be infected; endophthalmitis is the most fulminant manifestation and may result in blindness. Single or multiple fluffy, white, cotton ball–like chorioretinal lesions, often extending into the vitreous, are characteristic. These lesions can be easily recognized on funduscopic examination and should be repeatedly looked for in all patients with known candidemia.

Renal Candidiasis. Infection of the kidneys may be secondary to ascending extension from the bladder (*Candida* cystitis), resulting in papillary necrosis, calyceal invasion, or formation of a fungus ball in the ureter or renal pelvis. More commonly, renal candidiasis is secondary to hematogenous spread in patients with either documented or undocumented candidemia, which results in pyelonephritis with diffuse cortical and medullary abscesses. The triad of candidemia, candiduria, and *Candida* organisms within casts in urinary sediment provides presumptive evidence of upper urinary tract involvement.

Hepatosplenic Candidiasis. This visceral form of deep infection occurs most commonly in patients with hematologic malignancies, especially leukemia, who are in remission after prolonged chemotherapy-induced neutropenia. Gastrointestinal candidiasis complicated by portal fungemia is the source in most patients; documented candidemia or evidence of disease in other organs is usually absent. Persistent unexplained fever, right upper quadrant tenderness and pain, elevated alkaline phosphatase levels, and multiple scattered "bull's-eye" lesions in the liver and spleen, demonstrated by abdominal ultrasonographic examination or computed tomography (CT), are features. Diagnosis is established by characteristic histopathologic findings on liver biopsy.

Pulmonary Candidiasis. Whereas colonization by yeasts of the tracheobronchial tree is common in seriously ill, debilitated patients who are receiving mechanical ventilation intensive care units, bona fide pneumonia caused by *Candida* species is rare. Diagnosis should be based on histopathologic evidence of yeast invasion of lung parenchyma.

Cardiac Candidiasis. Disseminated candidiasis is complicated frequently by *Candida* myocarditis (>50% of cases) and occasionally by *Candida* pericarditis. *Candida* is the most common cause of fungal endocarditis and should be suspected in the setting of indwelling cardiac prostheses, intravenous drug abuse, and prolonged use of central venous catheters for chemotherapy, hyperalimentation, or hemodynamic monitoring. Because fungal valvular vegetations are large and friable, major embolic events involving the central nervous system (CNS), coronary arteries, and large peripheral arteries are common.

Central Nervous System Candidiasis. Meningitis and intracerebral microabscesses and macroabscesses frequently complicate disseminated candidiasis and often are a complication of active intravenous drug abuse or ventricular shunt infection. Cerebrospinal fluid pleocytosis (most often lymphocytic), hypoglycorrhachia, and elevated protein levels are typical; yeast organisms can be identified by wet preparation, Gram's stains, or culture in fewer than half of cases.

Musculoskeletal Candidiasis. Manifestations include myositis (abscess) in neutropenic patients and costochondritis, arthritis, and osteomyelitis (special predilection for vertebrae and intervertebral disks) in intravenous drug users. All of these complications may develop in any patient with disseminated candidiasis, whatever the setting or source.

DIAGNOSIS. Mucocutaneous lesions are diagnosed on the basis of clinical appearance and by examination of potassium hydroxide wet mounts or Gram-stained smears of lesion material obtained by scraping or swabbing. Masses of spherical budding yeast forms and pseudohyphae are characteristic. Patients suspected of having *Candida* esophagitis should undergo not only endoscopy and brushing, but also biopsy, in an attempt to histopathologically demonstrate mucosal invasion of *Candida* organisms. Esophagitis caused by either herpes simplex virus or cytomegalovirus may mimic the symptoms and appearance of *Candida* esophagitis; infection in a single patient caused by more than one microorganism is not unusual. Blood cultures in patients with suspected candidemia or disseminated candidiasis should be performed using one of the new highly sensitive systems including lysis centrifugation, biphasic media, or automated non-radiometric methods (e.g., BACTEC, BacT/

Alert, or ESP). Two sets of blood cultures on 2 consecutive days should be obtained. Data gathered over the past decade indicate that a single positive blood culture for *Candida* species should be assumed to represent clinically significant candidemia that merits antifungal therapy. The finding of heavy growth of *Candida* species in cultures of sputum, tracheal aspirate, wounds, or urine may increase the likelihood of bloodstream invasion but does not prove that dissemination has occurred. Because blood cultures may be negative in as many as 50% of patients with disseminated candidiasis, diagnosis must often depend on the results of histopathologic study and fungal cultures of tissue obtained by biopsy. Diagnostic procedures that should be considered include CT of the head, thorax, and abdomen; echocardiography; thoracentesis; arthrocentesis; lumbar puncture; and biopsy of skin, liver, kidney, myocardium, bone, muscle, or lung. Although quantitative or semiquantitative cultures of selected tissue specimens have been advocated as useful predictors of disseminated disease, no correlative data support this concept. Skin testing with *Candida* antigen may be useful in assessing for anergy but has no role in diagnosing candidiasis. Although much effort has been devoted to the development of reliable, simple, sensitive, and specific serologic assays for detecting serum antibodies to *Candida*, circulating *Candida* antigen (e.g., cell wall mannan or cytoplasmic enolase), or a metabolite, controversy persists about the value of these serodiagnostic procedures. Because false-positive and false-negative results are common, the decision to initiate treatment cannot be based on results of serologic tests alone. Genotypic typing methods, including electrophoretic karyotyping, DNA probes, restriction endonuclease analysis of genomic DNA, restriction fragment–length polymorphism, and random amplified polymorphic DNA, are sensitive means of discriminating strains of *Candida* species and greatly facilitate the epidemiologic investigation and control of *Candida* species as nosocomial pathogens.

TREATMENT. In non-AIDS patients with mucocutaneous infections, any one of several topical preparations, including nystatin or various azole drugs, provides effective therapy. Nystatin suspension and clotrimazole troches appear to be equal in efficacy as therapy for oral thrush, but clotrimazole is better tolerated. Although the clinical manifestations of *Candida* vulvovaginitis are usually eliminated by local topical therapy administered for 3 to 7 days, the disease tends to recur frequently in some patients. Newer approaches to acute vulvovaginitis use single-dose therapy (e.g., clotrimazole, 500 mg vaginal tablet; miconazole, 1200 mg vaginal suppository; or oral fluconazole, 150 mg oral tablet). In refractory cases, prolonged therapy with a topical agent or an orally absorbed azole, provided that pregnancy has been excluded, may be beneficial. Oral ketoconazole or fluconazole is the treatment of choice for chronic mucocutaneous candidiasis and must be continued indefinitely to avoid relapse. In contrast, AIDS patients with mucocutaneous forms of candidiasis respond less rapidly than other patient groups and often have incomplete clearance of exudative patches. Nystatin suspension appears to be less effective than either clotrimazole troches or an oral azole drug in AIDS patients with oropharyngeal or esophageal candidiasis. Fluconazole (tablet or liquid suspension) and itraconazole (oral cyclodextrin solution) are more effective than ketoconazole. Recent clinical microbiologic and epidemiologic data indicate an emerging problem of resistance to fluconazole among AIDS patients with oral thrush who have low CD4 cell counts and a history of prolonged exposure to fluconazole therapy. Although cross-resistance may develop to itraconazole, the oral solution of this triazole is an effective therapeutic alternative in many patients with fluconazole-resistant disease. In refractory cases associated with severe disease and/or fluconazole-resistance, low-dose amphotericin B can be used.

Consensus guidelines are emerging regarding therapy of serious *Candida* disease (e.g., candidemia or disseminated candidiasis). First, in most patients with catheter-related candidemia, the catheter, if still present, should be removed or changed. Consideration should be given to attempting to eradicate candidemia before changing a surgically implanted catheter. Second, in patients with suppurative peripheral thrombophlebitis, surgical segmental venous resection is necessary. Third, because of the high risk of metastatic complications of candidemia, such as endophthalmitis, osteomyelitis, arthritis, nephritis, myocarditis, and cerebritis, all patients with candidemia, even non-neutropenic hosts, deserve a course of antifungal chemotherapy. For patients with candidemia, both amphotericin B and fluconazole are effective in selected populations. For example, in non-neutropenic patients with catheter-associated candidemia, initial therapy with fluconazole, 400 to 800 mg/day for 14 days (initial intravenous therapy followed by oral therapy), is commonly utilized. By contrast, amphotericin B, 0.5 to 1.0 mg/kg/day for 7 to 14 days, should usually be given to compromised hosts, especially those with granulocytopenia, patients with persistent candidemia (whatever the cause), and patients who are clinically unstable or have septic shock syndrome due to *Candida* species. In these types of patients, several options are available: one of the newly licensed lipid formulations of amphotericin B, flucytosine (100 mg/kg/day) in combination with amphotericin B, fluconazole alone (400 to 800 mg/day), or fluconazole in combination with amphotericin B. Until additional guidelines are forthcoming from ongoing prospective studies, the decisions regarding which drugs to use and at what dosages must be based on the host defense status of the patient, underlying conditions, predisposing factors, results of serial blood cultures, and physical examinations for complications of candidemia, and causative *Candida* species. Non–*C. albicans* species vary in susceptibility to fluconazole; *C. krusei* is intrinsically resistant, and *C. glabrata* may be relatively resistant.

Patients with documented disseminated disease, manifested as either localized deep disease (e.g., hepatosplenic candidiasis, CNS candidiasis, renal candidiasis, or *Candida* endocarditis) or multiorgan disease, should be treated with amphotericin B (total dose, 2.0 to 3.0 g), often in combination with flucytosine (100 mg/kg/day). Fluconazole may be used in the therapy of most patients with hepatosplenic candidiasis, either as primary therapy or consolidation therapy after an initial course of amphotericin B, with or without flucytosine. Valve replacement is a necessary adjunct to chemotherapy in most patients with *Candida* endocarditis.

Candida cystitis, in contrast to renal candidiasis, can be cured by removing the bladder catheter in the majority of cases. Therapeutic options available for managing candiduria that is persistent after catheter removal or in diabetic patients include oral flucytosine, 75 to 100 mg/kg/day for 7 to 14 days, or oral fluconazole, 100 to 200 mg/day for 7 to 14 days. Although both of these antifungal agents are excreted by the kidneys, fluconazole is preferred because it is less toxic. Eradication of candiduria in patients whose condition justifies a persistent indwelling catheter is difficult and is rarely necessary, because asymptomatic candiduria rarely leads to significant complications such as ureteral obstruction or candidemia.

Therapy for *Candida* peritonitis, which most often is a complication of continuous ambulatory peritoneal dialysis (CAPD) and is less often associated with perforation of the gastrointestinal tract and/or intra-abdominal surgery, is less straightforward. Ideally, in patients with CAPD peritonitis, the catheter should be discontinued, and either oral fluconazole or intravenous amphotericin B should be administered until clinical symptoms and signs resolve and cultures become negative. Usually, therapy is initiated with fluconazole. For patients in whom the catheter must be maintained, instilling either amphotericin B or fluconazole in the dialysate fluid may be successful.

Managing ocular candidiasis requires close cooperation with an ophthalmologist experienced in eye infections. For most cases of uncomplicated endophthalmitis, fluconazole is preferred as initial therapy. For patients with progressive or complicated disease, intravenous amphotericin B, with or without flucytosine, plus partial vitrectomy to remove vitreous abscesses is required. Findings at vitrectomy may also be used to confirm the diagnosis and monitor efficacy. The practice of administering intravitreal amphotericin B is controversial.

PREVENTION. Given the increasing incidence of nosocomial candidemia and its potential severity, awareness of the problem and measures aimed at prevention assume increasing importance. The frequency and duration of use of intravascular catheters and monitoring devices should be reduced. Special attention should be paid to long-term surgically implantable access devices for chemotherapy or other purposes. Similarly, the frequency, breadth, and duration of courses of antibiotics should be reduced. Antifungal drugs are commonly used in seriously ill hospitalized patients, especially those with granulocytopenia, to prevent *Candida* infection. Although fluconazole, the drug most commonly used, appears to be more beneficial in bone marrow transplant recipients than in patients with acute leukemia, prolongation of survival has not been shown consistently. Moreover, widespread or injudicious use of oral azoles in prophylaxis does not offer protection against natively resistant pathogenic fungi (*Aspergillus* species, Mucorales, *Fusarium* species, *C. krusei*, and *C. glabrata*), and it may increase the likelihood of emergence of resistant organisms and not be cost-effective.

Edwards JE Jr, Bodey GP, Bowden RA, et al: International Conference for the Development of a Consensus on the Management and Prevention of Severe Candidal Infections. Clin Infect Dis 25:43, 1997. *A useful commentary by a team of experts on prevention and treatment strategies for the various* Candida *syndromes, including the roles of amphotericin B (conventional and lipid formulations) and the azoles.*

Nguyen MH, Peacock JE Jr, Morris AJ, et al: The changing face of candidemia: Emergence of non-*Candida albicans* species and antifungal resistance. Am J Med 100:716, 1996. *In four tertiary care medical centers over a 3.5 year study period (1990–1994), non-*C. albicans *species, especially* T. glabrata, C *tropicalis, and* C. parapsilosis, *emerged as frequent causes of fungemia. Candidemia developing during antifungal therapy was more frequently caused by non-*C. albicans *species, and these species were more likely to be resistant to fluconazole.*

Rex JH, Rinaldi MG, Pfaller MA: Resistance of *Candida* species to fluconazole. Antimicrob Agents Chemother 39:1 1995. *A nice review of this emerging problem, with emphasis on risk factors, especially in AIDS patients, and management options in patients with fluconazole-resistant* Candida *disease.*

Slavin MA, Osborne B, Adams R, et al: Efficacy and safety of fluconazole prophylaxis for fungal infections after marrow transplantation: A prospective, randomized, double-blind study. J Infect Dis 171:1545, 1995. *This and an earlier placebo-controlled trial (Goodman JL, et al: N Engl J Med 326:845, 1992) in bone-marrow transplant recipients showed that fluconazole decreased the incidence of disseminated deep-organ fungal infection, but only the Slavin trial showed that fluconazole improved survival.*

401 ASPERGILLOSIS

David A. Stevens

DEFINITION

Aspergillosis refers to infection with any of the species of the genus *Aspergillus*. These are in mold form in the environment, on artificial media, and when invading tissues.

ASPERGILLOSIS

Causative fungus	*Aspergillus* species: *A. fumigatus, A. flavus, A. niger, A. terreus*
Primary geographic distribution	Ubiquitous: human habitat, soil, water, air
Primary route of acquisition	Inhaling spores
Principal site of disease	Lung
Opportunistic infection in compromised hosts	Invasive form, pulmonary
Drug of choice for most patients	Amphotericin, itraconazole
Alternative therapy	None

ETIOLOGY AND EPIDEMIOLOGY

Aspergilli are ubiquitous in the environment and have been isolated with ease from soil and air, and even swimming pools and saunas. They are associated with decaying matter and may grow in temperatures of 40 to 50°C, e.g., self-heating organic compost. The ease with which they are isolated from composting materials, silos, and the cooling canals of nuclear power plants has been an environmental and industrial concern. They are easily isolated from houses, particularly from basements, crawl spaces, bedding, humidifiers, ventilation ducts, potted plants, wicker or straw material, and house dust; in surveys they have been found in, for example, condiments, pasta, and marijuana samples. This pervasiveness

should not make it surprising that they are sometimes found in normal expectorated sputa. They are important pathogens of insects (of economic importance to beekeepers) and birds, both domesticated and wild, and cause abortion in cattle. As they grow, they produce toxins, such as aflatoxin—one of the most potent carcinogens known—which contaminates the food chain, posing a risk to animals and humans. Their threat to hospitalized patients has been revealed in outbreaks of infection, particularly pulmonary infection in compromised hosts, associated with building renovation and new construction. The suspected vector has been unfiltered air, as from inlets contaminated with bird excreta and fireproofing materials.

The most common species infecting humans are *A. fumigatus, A. flavus, A. niger,* and *A. terreus.* Some are speciated by the clinical laboratory only with difficulty, and they may be reported only as "*Aspergillus* species." In tissues they may be seen as septate hyphae, dichotomously branched (resembling the divergence of fingers from one another), and they may produce their characteristic conidia in tissues or artificial media, which is one way to differentiate them. If the septation can be seen, they can be differentiated from the zygomycetes; they may be confused with *Pseudallescheria boydii,* however, unless the characteristic terminal spores of the latter are seen.

Aspergillosis generally results from airborne conidia and is not contagious.

SYNDROMES

The main forms of clinical aspergillosis are shown in Table 401–1.

The *invasive* form of the disease is generally a problem of immunocompromised hosts (see Chapter 314), and more aggressive immunosuppression and anticancer therapy are the most important factors contributing to the rise of *Aspergillus* infections. Series have reported an incidence as high as 41% in those with acute leukemia at autopsy, and in 89% of these cases it played a significant role in the death of the patient. In 97%, pulmonary involvement was present, and in 25%, the infection was disseminated widely to various organs. Similarly, in a group of heart transplant patients, the incidence of infection was 28%. This is also a problem in diabetics and patients with the neutrophil defect of chronic granulomatous disease. Diagnosis is difficult because aspergilli frequently are contaminants in sputum and even in other cultures during handling. In patients with leukemia, there is particularly an association with relapses of the malignancy, and usually three or four of the following factors are present: leukopenia, glucocorticoid therapy, cytotoxic chemotherapy, and broad-spectrum antibacterials. The classic picture is that of fever and pulmonary infiltrates or nodules, especially progressing to a cavity (usually when granulocytopenia is reversed), or wedge-shaped densities resembling infarcts. The pulmonary pathology in all these entities is that of hemorrhagic infarction and pneumonia. Pulmonary emboli are common because of the organism's tendency to invade blood vessel walls. These processes often combine to produce a "target lesion" pathologically, consisting of a necrotic center surrounded by a ring of hemorrhage. The sputum culture is positive in only 8 to 34% of cases, and obtaining tissue is necessary to make the diagnosis. Prospective culturing of the nose of granulocytopenic patients has been of some value, because a positive nasal culture (and particularly the presence of nasal *Aspergillus* lesions) has led to the early diagnosis of concurrent pulmonary or sinus disease. However, negative nasal cultures are common in pulmonary aspergillosis.

Targets of *disseminated disease* include the central nervous system, where abscesses are characteristic. The cerebrospinal fluid (CSF) glucose level is normal, and cultures of the CSF are nega-

Table 401–1 ■ ASPERGILLOSIS SYNDROMES

Invasive disease	Asthma
Aspergilloma (fungus ball)	Invasive airways disease
Superficial bronchial disease	Bronchocentric granulomatosis
Extrinsic allergic alveolitis	Pleural disease
Mixed forms	Local disease
Allergic bronchopulmonary disease	Endocarditis

tive. Mycelia invading blood vessels may produce a microangiopathic hemolytic anemia. Dissemination can result in Budd-Chiari syndrome, myocardial infarction, gastrointestinal disease, or skin lesions. Esophageal ulcers may produce gastrointestinal bleeding. Abscesses are common in the kidney, liver, and myocardium.

Endocarditis is associated with cardiac surgery, particularly prostheses, or intravenous drug abuse. Major arterial emboli occur in 83% of patients, and neurologic presentations are common. Only 8% have positive blood cultures, and this positivity usually is delayed 14 to 20 days, contributing to the poor record of diagnosis ante mortem, which is usually made on histologic examination of an embolus. Overall survival is about 5%, and these individuals have had valve replacement. The disease should be suspected in any post-cardiac surgery patient who presents with endocarditis or emboli and negative blood cultures.

The typical picture of an aspergilloma is a fungus ball (matted hyphae and debris) in a cavity in an upper lobe (Fig. 401–1). This has been reported as a complication in as many as 11% of old tuberculous cavities. The patients present with cough (87%), hemoptysis (81%), dyspnea (61%), weight loss (61%), fatigue (61%), chest pain (31%), or fever (25%). The sputum culture is positive in most. Total immunoglobulin G (IgG) and immunoglobulin A (IgA) levels are elevated. Invasion of the parenchyma is rare.

Pleural disease is associated with tuberculosis and bronchopleural fistulas. It may occur after surgery or spontaneously.

Allergic bronchopulmonary aspergillosis is usually seen superimposed on a background of chronic asthma or cystic fibrosis. It is characterized by episodic airway obstruction, fever, eosinophilia, mucous plugs, positive sputum cultures, and the presence of grossly visible brown flecks in the sputum (hyphae), transient infiltrates and parallel "tram-line" or ring markings on chest radiographs, proximal bronchiectasis, upper lobe contraction, and elevated levels of total immunoglobulin E (IgE), especially when the patient is symptomatic. It is more common in agricultural areas and in the winter, presumably representing an association with stored agricultural products (especially moldy hay) and spore production. The eosinophilia is present in blood, sputum, and the lung on biopsy. The mucous plugs contain mycelia, and the plugs may be the cause of the infiltrates, with collapse and inflammation occurring peripherally, or inflammatory edema may be responsible. The parallel or ring markings are caused by thickened ectatic bronchi, and the upper lobe changes are a result of progressive apical fibrosis. The infiltrates may be nonsegmental and transient, with a clinical presentation of "eosinophilic pneumonia" and asthma, with eosinophils in blood and sputum; alternatively, they may be segmental, associated with the blocking of bronchi by plugs, and asthma and eosinophilia may be absent. A biphasic skin test response may assist in the diagnosis. A scratch test with *Aspergillus* antigens produces an immediate wheal and flare reaction, mediated by IgE and blocked by antihistamines, but not by corticosteroids. An intracutaneous test with the antigens produces a later (6 to 8 hours) reaction, mediated by IgG antibody and complement and blocked by steroids. Similarly, bronchial challenge with the antigens can produce a biphasic response. Immediate, short-lived

wheezing may result, reproducing the asthmatic symptoms and associated with increased airways resistance; this can be blocked by β-blockers, antihistamines, and cromolyn, but not by steroids. There may be a later (2 to 6 hours) reaction, of two types. One is increased airways resistance, as described. The other is a restrictive defect occurring peripherally, which may be associated with influenza-like symptoms, fever, leukocytosis, and infiltrates. These reactions are associated with IgG precipitins and are believed to account for some transient infiltrates.

Extrinsic allergic alveolitis is an unusual form of *Aspergillus* lung disease and has been most associated with *A. clavatus* in malt workers. The patients develop a hypersensitivity pneumonitis with dyspnea and fever 4 hours after exposure. Diffuse micronodular infiltrates may be present at the time of symptoms. The patients have IgG precipitins and cell-mediated immune reactions against *Aspergillus* antigens, and granulomas are present on biopsy. Eosinophilia is not a feature. The scratch test is negative, although an intradermal test produces a reaction in 4 hours, with immunoglobulins and complement present on biopsy. Bronchial challenge produces a reaction in 4 hours, with systemic symptoms and a restrictive defect but without airway resistance. The entity can progress to irreversible fibrosis. The same pathophysiology may be involved in episodes following massive inhalation of spores, usually in farm environments. Symptoms are present within 24 hours, and granulomas are found on biopsy.

Superficial bronchial disease, an acute or chronic bronchitis with brown-flecked sputum, *extrinsic asthma* due to airborne conidia, and *bronchocentric granulomatosis,* peribronchial destructive disease with wheezing or fever and weight loss, are other important pulmonary diseases. The aspergilloma, allergic, alveolitis, and superficial forms rarely progress to invasive disease. However, more *invasive airway disease* with ulcerative, pseudomembranous, or plaquelike tracheobronchitis occurs, particularly in immunocompromised hosts, and may presage parenchymal invasion. *Chronic necrotizing pulmonary aspergillosis* is a poorly defined entity that usually occurs in patients with underlying lung disease, often with features of invasive disease and aspergilloma.

Examples of *locally invasive disease* abound and are usually severe. These include invasion of burn wounds, keratitis, external otitis (particularly in the tropics), focal rhinitis (particularly in immunosuppressed and/or granulocytopenic hosts), sinusitis (in these hosts or following dental procedures) and osteomyelitis or endophthalmitis (after fungemia, trauma, or surgery). Cutaneous ulcers have been associated with the use of adhesive tape. Bloodborne disease in addicts can produce foci of dissemination that are similar to those associated with the invasive pulmonary form of the disease. A noninvasive form of sinus disease has a predominantly allergic component and eosinophilia. It is responsive to drainage and corticosteroids.

DIAGNOSIS

Some of the modalities of diagnosis have been mentioned in connection with specific syndromes. Antibody to *Aspergillus* has been detected by a variety of techniques and with a variety of antigen preparations. Data from the more commonly reported techniques suggest a high degree of sensitivity in allergic disease or aspergillomas, but generally a low sensitivity in invasive disease. Because the frequency of false-positive reactions, even in the presence of other mycoses, is low, a positive test in invasive disease may be useful. IgE and IgG antibody specific to *Aspergillus* antigens is another serodiagnostic adjunct in allergic disease. Detection of antigenemia and of antigen in bronchoalveolar lavage fluid also is promising in diagnosis of invasive disease. The problem with all serodiagnostic modalities is the lack of a generally available, standardized technique. The physician should know the background data for the laboratory to which the specimens may be sent, i.e., the sensitivity and specificity of the assay in the various syndromes. Serial antibody testing in groups of patients predisposed to aspergillomas (i.e., those with lung cavities), to endocarditis (cardiac surgery patients), or to invasive disease may increase the utility of otherwise problematic serodiagnostic methods.

In severe disease, an aggressive, invasive approach, as well as making a tissue diagnosis early in the illness, appears to be a key to survival. In the appropriate clinical setting, such as an immuno-

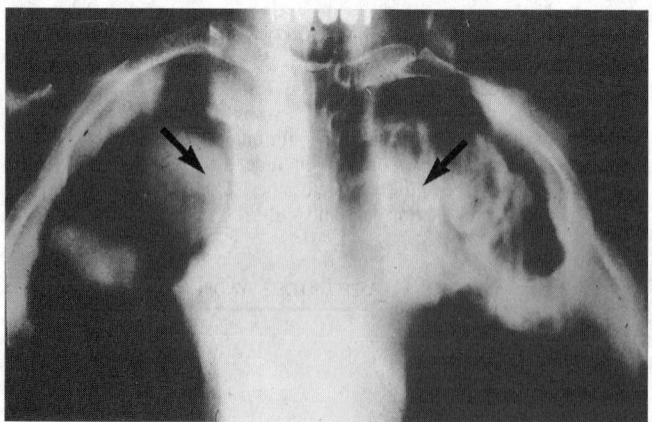

FIGURE 401–1. ■ Tomogram of pulmonary aspergillomas.

compromised host with fever and a pulmonary infiltrate, repeated isolation of the same species in culture, and particularly a bronchial lavage or other endobronchial culture, correlates with invasive disease; sometimes even a single sputum culture (especially with heavy growth) may have to be the stimulus for therapy if invasive procedures cannot be done. Negative cultures do not rule out invasive disease. Blood cultures are rarely helpful. Computed tomographic (CT) scanning of the chest done at the earliest suspicion of this diagnosis initially may reveal a lesion with peripheral haziness ("halo sign") or, later, a lesion with an air crescent, which are highly predictive of this diagnosis. These are radiographic correlates of edema or hemorrhage, and infarction, related to the organism's vasculotropism.

THERAPY AND PREVENTION

In invasive disease, prompt, aggressive chemotherapy has produced superior survival statistics at some institutions, although recovery from neutropenia is a necessary accompaniment of recovery in almost every success. The role of granulocyte transfusions or colony-stimulating factors is unclear. In endocarditis, in addition to prompt, aggressive chemotherapy, valve replacement appears necessary. Locally invasive disease in other sites also requires systemic or local chemotherapy, particularly intravitreal therapy or nephrostomy irrigation in renal disease. Surgical excision has an important role in the invasion of bone, burn wounds, epidural abscesses, vitreal disease, sinus disease of noncompromised hosts, and removal of catheters for peritonitis and of silk sutures in bronchial stump (postpneumonectomy) aspergillosis. It may have a function in invasive pulmonary disease for which chemotherapy has failed or where disease impinges on major vascular structures.

In cases involving aspergilloma, there is evidence that patients with fever, cough, weight loss, malaise, and hemoptysis have an element of allergy, which can be demonstrated by bronchial challenge or the presence of specific IgG and IgE. These patients symptomatically improve if given glucocorticoids. Intravenous amphotericin B therapy of patients with aspergilloma produces results no better than those with routine pulmonary toilet. Intracavitary antifungals, instilled through a catheter, are an heroic form of therapy that has been attempted in some patients. The role of surgery in this entity is controversial. Seven to 15% of mycetomas undergo spontaneous lysis. The overall operative mortality aggregated from several series is 7%, but may be as high as 14% in some large series. The frequency of various operative complications is 22%, aggregated from several series, with a range of 7 to 60%. Furthermore, new aspergillomas have later developed after surgical successes. On the other hand, in various series, 18 to 26% of patients with adequate follow-up treated without surgery died of disease complications, usually hemoptysis, whereas 50% have shown significant improvement symptomatically and radiographically. If any consensus exists, it is that surgical resection has a role in recurrent, significant hemoptysis. An alternative temporary therapy, particularly for the nonsurgical patient, is selective bronchial arterial embolization to the bleeding vessel.

In pleural disease, locally instilling nystatin, amphotericin, or miconazole has succeeded. In allergic disease, measures that have *not* worked include hyposensitization, avoidance of sites in the environment, and aerosolized corticosteroids. Cromolyn is inadequate in most patients. Aerosolized antifungals have produced remissions but do not prevent recurrences. Treating the clinical disease is more complicated than the effects of drug blockade demonstrable in challenge tests. The continuous use of systemic glucocorticoids can prevent the infiltrates and some accompanying symptoms. Intermittent use of glucocorticoids or raising the dose in patients on chronic therapy can produce rapid resolution of marked symptomatic episodes. The long-term beneficial effects of glucocorticoids are less clear; they are not so useful in arresting dyspnea or wheezing in the long term, and they do not prevent the development of the accompanying bronchiectasis. A recent randomized study using oral itraconazole indicated amelioration of disease and a steroid-sparing effect. The proper approach to extrinsic alveolitis is to avoid the stimulus.

For those entities in which systemic chemotherapy is indicated, most clinical experience has been with amphotericin B in deoxycholate. Its track record is generally poor in invasive or disseminated disease in compromised hosts (especially so in those with cerebral or hepatic disease or in bone marrow transplant patients). In the compromised host, it should be used aggressively, with prompt progression to a full therapeutic dose, which should be ≥ 1 mg per kilogram per day, if tolerated. Prophylactic therapy may have a role in patients who have survived invasive disease and will become neutropenic again. Rifampin almost always potentiates the activity of amphotericin in vitro against aspergilli, whereas results with flucytosine are unpredictable. Moreover, animal models have shown an enhanced effect of combinations of these drugs over that with amphotericin alone. Clinical data to support combination therapy are limited, but given the poor record of amphotericin alone in invasive disease, combination therapy appears a logical avenue to explore, particularly if synergy in vitro can be demonstrated. Of the azole drugs, itraconazole as sole therapy has produced similar response rates in invasive disease and is an alternative if the patient is reliable, can be shown to absorb the drug adequately (by monitoring serum concentrations), and is not receiving other drugs that interact with itraconazole. A new oral solution in cyclodextrin lessens absorption problems. Lipid-complexed amphotericin B given in higher doses than deoxycholate amphotericin has also produced similar response rates in historical comparisons and is less nephrotoxic (but more expensive). Comparative clinical trials are needed to assess all alternative forms of systemic therapy. Therapy should be continued after lesions are resolving, cultures are negative, and reversible underlying predispositions have abated.

Prophylaxis of susceptible patients, such as immunocompromised hosts, using intranasal, inhaled, or systemic antifungals, or allergic patients, using inhaled or systemic antifungals, is an approach to avoid disease and the need for therapy. Reducing airborne spores, such as by filtering hospital air and restricting contaminated materials (e.g., potted plants), is believed to be a worthwhile effort for patients who will be transiently immunosuppressed or neutropenic.

Andride VT: *Aspergillus* infections: Problems in diagnosis and treatment. Inf Agents Dis 5:47,1996. *Recent review with emphasis on antigen detection.*

Denning DW, Stevens DA: The treatment of invasive aspergillosis. Rev Infect Dis 12: 1147, 1990. *Reviews and tabulates data from more than 2000 published cases in 497 articles to give a current picture of therapeutic results.*

402 *Pneumocystis Carinii* PNEUMONIA

Judith E. Feinberg ■ *Fred R. Sattler*

Pneumocystis carinii pneumonia remains the most frequent case-defining infection in acquired immunodeficiency syndrome (AIDS), despite an almost 50% decrease in the number of first episodes (see Chapter 412) recently reported to the Centers for Disease Control and Prevention (CDC). A large number of second or third episodes also occur annually in AIDS patients, although these are less well reported.

Moderate to severe episodes cause appreciable morbidity, and even with effective therapy, up to 20% of cases are fatal. For mild episodes, the fatality rate is less than 5%, but the diagnosis can be challenging as signs and symptoms may mimic community-acquired bacterial infections and the presentation may be atypical in patients receiving prophylaxis. It is, therefore, imperative that episodes be detected when alteration of gas exchange is mild and lung damage minimal if hospitalization and mortality are to be minimized. Clinicians caring for human immunodeficiency virus (HIV)-infected patients must be aware of various manifestations of *P. carinii* infection so that therapy can be initiated as early as possible.

ETIOLOGY. *P. carinii* is a eukaryotic microbe with morphologic features similar to those of protozoa. Lack of growth on fungal culture media and response to anti-protozoan agents have also supported the notion that it is a protozoan. However, *P. carinii* has an affinity for fungal stains, is ultrastructurally similar to fungi, and is phylogenetically closely related to the Ascomycetes yeasts by molecular analysis of its 16S ribosomal RNA and mitochondrial DNA. The base pair sequence of its mitochondrial DNA contains genes of NDH dehydrogenase subunits and cytochrome oxidase subunits, which show 60% homology with fungi but only 20% with protozoa. Finally, the dihydrofolate reductase (DHFR) of *P. carinii,* like that of fungi, is a single enzyme with lower molecular weight than the dual thymidylate synthetase–DHFR enzyme found in protozoa.

This is not a purely academic issue. Although *P. carinii* does not respond to antifungal drugs such as amphotericin or azoles, β-glucan synthesis in the cyst wall is inhibited by newer antifungal agents, such as echinocandins and papulocandins. These agents are active against both the cyst and trophozoite forms in experimental infections, whereas traditional anti-*Pneumocystis* therapies affect only the trophozoite. Novel therapeutic approaches that affect both stages of the life cycle are therefore being developed in an attempt to improve response rates.

EPIDEMIOLOGY AND TRANSMISSION. Within the first few years of life, nearly all children have serologic evidence of exposure to *P. carinii.* Thus, the most accepted hypothesis for pathogenesis has been that *P. carinii* remains latent in the lung with active disease due to reactivation during severe immune depression. Yet, few data support chronic carriage, because the organism is neither detected in lung sections at autopsy of previously healthy individuals nor by polymerase chain reaction (PCR) in bronchoalveolar lavage fluid of immunocompetent adults.

P. carinii may be found incidentally in lungs of immunocompromised patients, and genetic sequences have been detected in the absence of histologic evidence of infection. Case clusters and familial spread have been reported, and in one natural history study of HIV-infected patients, upper respiratory infections peaked in winter months followed by *P. carinii* pneumonia 4 months later, suggesting that *P. carinii* may have been acquired by prior exposure to infected aerosols when community respiratory infections were common. These data suggest that *P. carinii* may be acquired by person-to-person spread.

PATHOGENESIS AND PATHOPHYSIOLOGY. In cortisone-treated rats, inhaled *P. carinii* adheres to type 1 alveolar cells through fibronectin. After several weeks, small clusters of *P. carinii* can be detected in alveolar spaces. Later, air sacs become filled with organisms, indicating that replication is slow, but proliferation is extensive. Two morphologic forms are readily detected. The majority are small pleomorphic trophozoites. A more mature, larger, thick-walled cyst containing up to eight intracystic bodies is less common. Histology typically shows foamy alveolar exudates consisting of degenerative *P. carinii* cell membranes, surfactant, host proteins, and a modest number of alveolar macrophages. As infection progresses, septal hypertrophy occurs, and interstitial edema is evident. Mononuclear cells accumulate and similar abnormalities occur in humans.

These abnormalities result in increased alveolar-capillary permeability, which is associated with physiologic alterations: impaired gas exchange and decreased membrane diffusing capacity, compliance, total lung capacity, and vital capacity. Soon after anti-*Pneumocystis* therapy begins, lung function is further impaired by an inflammatory response, as evidenced by a rapid decline in oxygenation that reaches its nadir after 3 to 4 days. This inflammatory reaction appears to be mediated by tumor necrosis factor-α (TNF-α) and interleukin-1, -6, and -8 released by alveolar macrophages. TNF-α is modulated by the β-glucan component of the cell wall, providing further evidence that *P. carinii* is a fungus.

RISK FOR INFECTION. In the rat model, depletion of T lymphocytes is the critical determinant in the development of *P. carinii* pneumonia. In humans, *Pneumocystis* occurs in association with lymphoreticular malignancy, certain congenital immune disorders, solid organ transplantation (recipients), and therapy with cyclosporine or corticosteroids, which have in common variable defects in T-cell function. In patients with HIV, the risk of developing *P. carinii* pneumonia is related to a decrease in T lymphocytes with CD4 surface phenotype. The median CD4 count is typically 50 to 70 at the time of a first episode. That *P. carinii* pneumonia may occur with transient declines in CD4 counts to less than 100 during primary HIV infection suggests it is the absolute number of CD4 cells and not the stage of HIV infection that is important in determining risk for infection. Although more than 90% of episodes

occur at total counts less than 200, *P. carinii* pneumonia may occur at higher counts in individuals whose CD4 cells are declining rapidly and those with thrush and unexplained fever ($\geq$100° F for $\geq$2 weeks).

HISTOPATHOLOGY. Microscopy of lung tissue from AIDS patients with *P. carinii* pneumonia shows a prominent eosinophilic, foamy, intra-alveolar exudate; proliferation of type II pneumocytes; but only mild interstitial inflammation. Detection of *P. carinii* requires special stains. The cysts are uniformly 5 to 7 mm and collapse easily, which gives them a helmet or banana shape. Trophozoites are smaller, measuring 1 to 4 mm, and, unlike the cysts, are pleomorphic.

Diffuse alveolar damage is commonly found. Interstitial fibrosis is present in approximately 6% and intraluminal fibrosis in almost 40% of cases; fibrosis appears to be related to the severity of the inflammatory response and duration of therapy. In contrast, acute exudative alveolar damage is unusual, and hyaline membranes have been detected in fewer than 5% of lung biopsies, but they may occasionally be so prominent that they obscure the typical eosinophilic alveolar material. Other less common histologic abnormalities include pneumatoceles and cavities, granulomas, lymphocytic interstitial infiltrates, microcalcifications, vasculitis, and alveolar proteinosis. In patients with cavitation and pneumothorax, *P. carinii* invades the interstitium, and unlike typical cases, greater proportions of trophozoites are present.

CLINICAL MANIFESTATIONS. Early recognition and treatment are imperative. Figure 402–1 shows that the risk of a fatal outcome increases progressively for patients whose room air arterial oxygen partial pressure (PaO$_2$) values are less than 75 and alveolar-arterial oxygen differences (A − aDO$_2$) are 35 mm Hg or more at presenta-

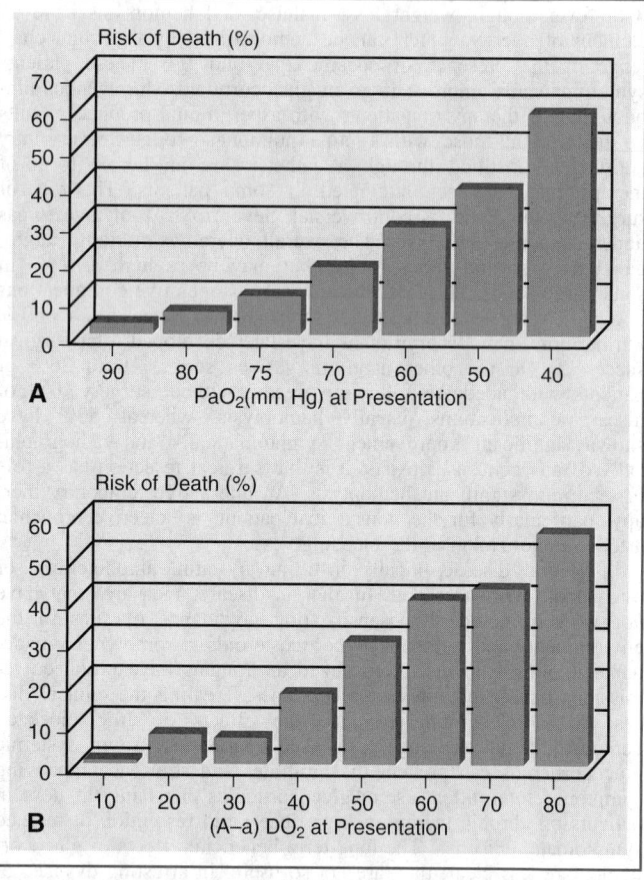

FIGURE 402–1 ■ *A,* Risk of death, according to the partial pressure (PaO$_2$) of oxygen on room air at time of admission to the hospital for patients receiving conventional therapies without adjunctive corticosteroids. *B,* Risk of death, according to alveolar-arterial oxygen difference (A − aDO$_2$) on room air at time of admission to the hospital for patients receiving conventional therapies without adjunctive corticosteroids. (Adapted from the U.S. Public Health Service Consensus Statement on the Use of Corticosteroids as Adjunctive Therapy for *Pneumocystis* Pneumonia in the Acquired Immunodeficiency Syndrome.)

tion. Clinicians must therefore be familiar with both the typical manifestations and the unusual presentations of *P. carinii* pneumonia.

TYPICAL PRESENTATIONS. The onset of *P. carinii* pneumonia in AIDS patients is usually insidious. The cardinal manifestation is a hacking, typically nonproductive cough that may have been present for weeks. Retrosternal chest tightness, intensified by coughing and inspiration, is also common. Fever occurs in 80 to 90%. Dyspnea occurs later, when oxygenation is moderately to severely impaired. In contrast, *P. carinii* pneumonia in HIV-seronegative patients is typically acute in onset, with high fever and chest x-ray abnormalities.

Physical findings are often limited and nonspecific. No tachypnea is usually present with mild episodes, whereas respiratory distress and use of accessory respiratory muscles may be seen in severe episodes. Auscultation of the lungs is frequently normal because rales occur in only 30 to 40% of cases and are usually a late finding, indicating greater severity. Occasionally patients have wheezing or overt bronchospasm. In one report, 84% of patients had peak expiratory flow rates (PEFR) less than 80% of predicted, with 54% of these responding to bronchodilator therapy, compared to those without *Pneumocystis,* of whom only 23% had low PEFR, and 3% had a response to bronchodilator therapy.

Physical findings outside the lung may be helpful. Oral thrush is a nearly universal finding in patients not taking antifungals. Facial seborrheic dermatitis is also common. Generalized adenopathy with lymph nodes larger than 1 cm is rare because patients with *P. carinii* generally have severe immunodeficiency with hypoplastic lymph nodes.

In one study of 2526 men and 544 women, women were more likely to be hospitalized for their first episode of *P. carinii* pneumonia, were less likely to be white, and were more likely to die in the hospital. These differences in clinical course suggest that *P. carinii* pneumonia has been less frequently diagnosed early in HIV-infected women.

ATYPICAL PRESENTATIONS. Pneumothorax and Cavitation. Pneumothoraces that may be associated with refractory bronchopleural fistulas and chronic lung cavitation are an increasingly frequent presentation and may occur in up to 10% of episodes. Pneumothoraces occurred spontaneously in 20 (2%) of 1030 patients with AIDS at one medical center; 50 to 95% of episodes are associated with active *P. carinii* pneumonia. Thus, HIV-positive patients with spontaneous pneumothorax should undergo work-up and treatment for *P. carinii* pneumonia along with lung re-expansion.

Lung destruction and cavitation may appear as solitary thin-walled cavities, regional honeycombing, blebs, or bullae; these findings are often bilateral, and they usually occur in the upper lobes and precede the development of pneumothorax. Although cavitation and pneumothorax were initially associated with aerosol pentamidine prophylaxis, these complications may occur in the absence of aerosol therapy, in non-smokers, and in first episodes, as well as in patients with prior bronchoscopy or mechanical ventilation and barotrauma.

Fever of Unknown Origin. In some AIDS patients, *P. carinii* pneumonia may present as an occult febrile illness, with few or no respiratory symptoms. Non-specific complaints of high fever, night sweats, fatigue, and malaise are prominent. Other etiologies of fever of unknown origin in this population, such as occult sinusitis, cytomegalovirus retinitis, disseminated *Mycobacterium avium* infection and endocarditis, must be excluded, and oxygen desaturation with exercise and histologic evidence of *P. carinii* should be sought.

Extrapulmonary *P. carinii* Infection. Infection with *P. carinii* may occur outside the lung in 0.5 to 3.0% of patients with *P. carinii* pneumonia. At the time at which extrapulmonary *Pneumocystis* infection is diagnosed, more than 50% of patients have concurrent *P. carinii* pneumonia. Nucleotide sequences of the *P. carinii* DHFR gene have been detected by PCR in blood of 5 of 11 patients with acute *P. carinii* pneumonia, which suggests that hematogenous dissemination occurs.

Clinical presentations have included external auditory polyps, mastoiditis, choroiditis, cutaneous lesions or digital necrosis secondary to vasculitis, small bowel obstruction, ascites with gross nodules in the stomach and duodenum, hepatic or splenic infiltration, hilar or mediastinal lymphadenopathy, thyroiditis, thymic involvement, and cytopenia due to bone marrow infection. At au-

topsy, disseminated infection has been documented in other organs, including abdominal lymph nodes, pancreas, gastric mucosa, adrenal glands, myocardium, kidneys, and central nervous system. Lymph nodes, liver, spleen, and bone marrow are the most commonly affected organs.

Histology of affected organs show foci of eosinophilic frothy exudates, and special stains reveal *P. carinii.* Unlike the lung, these lesions are often calcified (punctate or rimlike) and show vasculitis with frank invasion of vessel walls.

Nonspecific complaints of fever and sweats predominate. Two extrapulmonary sites are associated with specific symptoms or signs. Thyroid involvement may present with neck pain, hyperthyroidism or hypothyroidism, and goiter, which may be multinodular or a solitary neck mass. The thyroid is usually "cold" on ^{125}I scanning, and the diagnosis is made by fine-needle aspiration. Choroiditis appears as slightly elevated, yellow-white plaques, and it is generally limited to the choroid without involvement of retinal vessels (unlike cytomegalovirus retinitis) or evidence of intraocular inflammation. Identification of typical choroidal lesions may provide the first clue of disseminated infection. Although the lung is involved in nearly 90% of cases, choroiditis may be the only evidence of extrapulmonary disease.

Extensive extrapulmonary infection portends a poor prognosis, frequently associated with organ failure and death, but involvement of a single extrapulmonary site often responds favorably to anti-*Pneumocystis* therapy.

LABORATORY ABNORMALITIES. PULMONARY FUNCTION TESTS. Hypoxemia is the most useful marker of *Pneumocystis* pneumonia and is highly predictive of outcome. At presentation, PaO_2 less than 80 mm Hg or A − aDO_2 greater than 15 on room air occurs in more than 80% of episodes.

In patients with normal or nearly normal PaO_2 A − aDO_2, and chest radiographs, graded exercise testing results in increases in the A − aDO_2, and oxygen desaturation can be readily demonstrated with pulse oximetry. The carbon monoxide diffusing capacity (DL_{CO}) is also a sensitive but nonspecific marker. Despite the lack of specificity, DL_{CO} values greater than 80% make *Pneumocystis* unlikely (i.e., negative predictive values are >98%). In AIDS patients with asthma who have cough and hypoxemia, results of DL_{CO} should be normal when hypoxemia is due solely to bronchospasm.

RADIOGRAPHIC PROCEDURES. Routine Radiology. Routine chest radiographs typically show interstitial infiltrates, beginning in perihilar areas and spreading to the lower and finally upper lung fields in a butterfly pattern. The apices are usually spared. Alveolar patterns with air bronchograms may be superimposed on the interstitial process in more advanced infection, although alveolar infiltrates may be the initial presentation in up to 10% of cases. Because *P. carinii* pneumonia is so common, the range of radiographic findings is wide. In 10 to 30% of cases the radiograph is atypical, with asymmetrical or predominantly upper lobe infiltration, especially in patients receiving aerosol pentamidine prophylaxis. Other atypical abnormalities include cysts, pneumatoceles, cavitation, "honeycombing," pneumothorax, adenopathy (with or without calcifications), pleural effusions, abscesses, lobar or segmental consolidation, solitary parenchymal nodules, or postobstructive infiltration secondary to endobronchial nodules. In one series of 100 patients with *P. carinii* pneumonia, cysts were documented in 34%, and of these, 32 had multiple cysts measuring 1.0 to 5.0 cm that occurred predominantly in the upper lobes. Cysts resolved partially or completely in most cases with specific therapy for *Pneumocystis* infection, but 12 (35%) of the 34 patients developed pneumothoraces compared with only 2 of 30 patients without cysts. These cystic cavitary lesions may mimic those of tuberculosis (Fig. 402–2). Normal chest radiographs at presentation may be seen in 10 to 20% of patients with documented *Pneumocystis* infection.

Computed Tomography. Computed tomographic (CT) scans typically show fine, diffuse alveolar consolidation with bronchial wall thickening, even when chest radiographs are normal, and less often show regional consolidation or cystic air spaces. Low-attenuation lesions and calcifications of lymph nodes, spleen, liver, and kidneys may be present in patients with extrapulmonary involvement. CT is primarily valuable in patients who have normal chest radiographs or unsuspected extrapulmonary *Pneumocystis* infection.

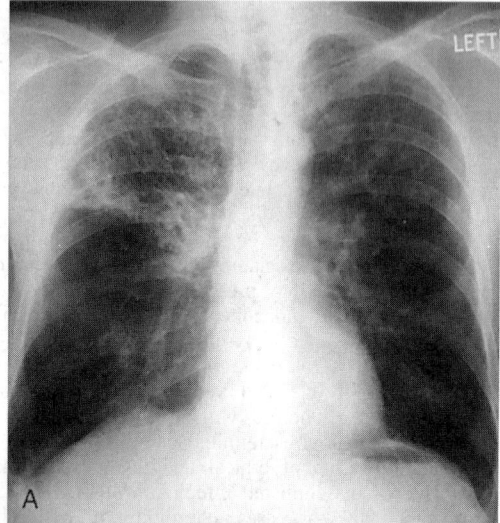

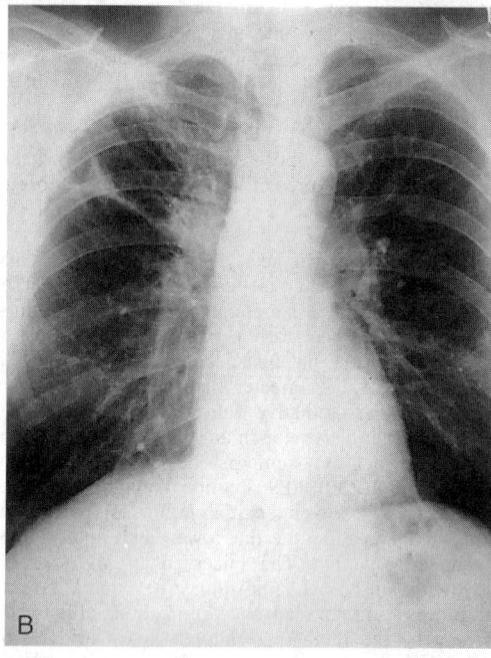

FIGURE 402–2 ■ *A*, This chest radiograph was obtained from a 42-year-old homosexual man who presented with a 14-month history of chronic cough, dyspnea with minimal exertion, and 25-lb weight loss. He was treated for 8 weeks with four standard antituberculous drugs plus intravenous amikacin, but cultures for *Mycobacterium tuberculosis* remained negative. A repeat induced sputum at that time showed large numbers of *P. carinii*. *B*, Chest radiographs from the same patient after a 3-week course of therapy with oral trimethoprim-sulfamethoxazole (15 mg/kg/day of the trimethoprim component). At the completion of therapy, cough and dyspnea had completely subsided.

Nuclear Imaging. Nuclear imaging may be of ancillary value in some cases, such as in patients with chronic lung disease, abnormal radiographs, and worsening respiratory symptoms. Gallium 67 accumulates in activated macrophages through transferrin receptors in areas of lung inflammation, but pulmonary uptake is not specific for *Pneumocystis*. Specificity is improved when scans are reported as positive only if gallium uptake in lung equals or exceeds uptake in liver; images are read at 48 to 72 hours after injection.

LACTATE DEHYDROGENASE. Serum lactate dehydrogenase (LDH) level is more elevated in patients with *Pneumocystis* pneumonia than in matched patients with other pulmonary complications of HIV. Although serum levels of LDH are not highly specific, the sensitivity was greater than 90% in one study of patients with dyspnea and *Pneumocystis* when values exceeded 220 IU/L. However, LDH values greater than 500 IU/L at presentation are associated with an increased risk for a fatal outcome. Equally important, serial tests gradually improve in survivors.

CD4 CELL COUNTS. Typically counts are less than 100 cells/mm³, and more than 90% of patients have values of less than 200 cells/mm³ when *Pneumocystis* pneumonia is diagnosed.

DIAGNOSIS. BRONCHOALVEOLAR LAVAGE. Bronchoalveolar lavage (BAL) is the cornerstone of diagnosis and consistently has a sensitivity of 86 to 96%. The diagnostic yield is lower—only 62%—for patients who have received aerosol pentamidine and who have predominantly upper lobe disease. Several approaches may increase the yield for such patients. Bilateral BAL yields a diagnosis in 94%, compared with 84% in patients who have previously undergone BAL on one side. Because severalfold more organisms may be recovered from upper than from lower lobes, sampling involved sites is likely to increase the yield.

TRANSBRONCHIAL BIOPSY. The yield from transbronchial biopsy approaches BAL if tissue is obtained without crush artifact and contains at least 25 alveoli. If both BAL and transbronchial biopsies are obtained, the diagnostic sensitivity approaches 100%. The risk of pneumothorax makes BAL more attractive.

SPUTUM INDUCTION. Pulmonary secretions may be obtained by ultrasonic nebulization of hypertonic saline. If these specimens are treated with mucolytic agents to solubilize oral debris prior to centrifugation, cytostaining procedures have resulted in diagnostic yields of 15 to 90%. Fluorescent staining with monoclonal antibodies for *P. carinii* generally produces the highest yields. Because the sensitivity is variable and yields greater than 80% have been consistently achieved in only a few centers, a negative induced sputum does not exclude the diagnosis.

IDENTIFICATION OF *P. CARINII.* Cyst Wall Stains. The standard staining procedure for identifying *P. carinii* in clinical specimens has used Gomori's methenamine silver because the sensitivity is generally greater than 95%. Toluidine blue O also stains the cyst, is more rapid, and is comparably reliable.

Noncyst Wall Stains. Wright-Giemsa and Diff-Quik stains are commonly used; they stain trophozoites, nuclei of cysts, and intermediate forms, and they can be completed within 30 minutes. However, organisms may be missed in 10 to 15% of cases. Papanicolaou silver stains the nonspecific foam surrounding large clusters of *P. carinii*, but organisms are not readily identified. The methodology is quick and useful for screening.

Immunochemical Stains. Immunofluorescent staining with monoclonal antibody results in yields greater than 90% for BAL specimens and appears to be more sensitive for sputum samples than silver or Wright-Giemsa stains.

Molecular Identification. Oligonucleotide probes and PCR are promising methodologies that may increase the diagnostic yield in identifying *P. carinii*, especially in induced sputum specimens.

TREATMENT. INITIATING THERAPY. The key to successful treatment is prompt suspicion of the diagnosis and early initiation of therapy when episodes are mild. Because sputum induction and bronchoscopies are generally not done after hours, and results of special stains may not be immediately available, patients with typical clinical features of *Pneumocystis* pneumonia and moderate-to-severe hypoxemia should be treated empirically. This does not impair the ability to make a diagnosis, as large numbers of *P. carinii* are detectable in lung tissue and secretions for weeks after therapy is begun.

SEVERE EPISODES. Parenteral Therapy. Initial therapy should be given parenterally for patients with moderate-to-severe impairment in oxygen exchange, namely PaO₂ less than 70 mm Hg or A − aDO₂ greater than 35 (Table 402–1). Drugs with high oral bioavailability, such as trimethoprim-sulfamethoxazole, may be erratically absorbed from the gut in subjects with severe hypoxemia. In addition, AIDS patients may have enteropathy and malabsorption even in the absence of diarrhea; consequently, drug concentrations may be subtherapeutic.

Trimethoprim-Sulfamethoxazole. The antifolate combination of trimethoprim-sulfamethoxazole is the gold standard for severe episodes (see Chapters 412 and 418). Three recent prospective, double-blind studies, each involving more than 300 patients, confirmed that trimethoprim-sulfamethoxazole was more effective than trimetrexate, atovaquone, or aerosolized pentamidine in AIDS patients

Table 402–1 ■ ESTABLISHED THERAPIES FOR INITIAL TREATMENT OF *Pneumocystis carinii* PNEUMONIA

Intravenous therapy

1. Trimethoprim-sulfamethoxazole	5 mg/kg of trimethoprim component every 6–8 hr
2. Pentamidine*	4 mg/kg, once daily
3. Trimetrexate plus leucovorin	For patients <50 kg: 1.5 mg/kg trimetrexate once daily plus leucovorin, 0.5 mg/kg IV or PO every 6 hr
	For patients 50–80 kg: 1.2 mg/kg trimetrexate daily plus leucovorin, 0.5/kg IV or PO every 6 hr
	For patients >80 kg: 1.0 mg/kg trimetrexate daily plus leucovorin, 0.8 mg/kg IV or PO every 6 hr
	Continue leucovorin for 72 hr after last dose of trimetrexate
4. Clindamycin plus primaquine base (oral)†	600–900 mg every 8 hr plus 15–30 mg PO, once daily

Oral therapy

1. Trimethoprim-sulfamethoxazole	2 double-strength tablets tid
2. Trimethoprim plus dapsone	4–5 mg/kg tid plus 100 mg once daily
3. Clindamycin plus primaquine base†	450–600 mg tid or qid plus 15–30 mg once daily
4. Atovaquone‡	750 mg tid

Aerosol therapy

1. Pentamidine	600 mg daily via Respirgard II§

*Intramuscular therapy may cause sterile abscesses and should be avoided.
†The combination is not advisable in situations in which absorption may be impaired (severe hypoxemia, vomiting, diarrhea, ileus, malabsorption) because clindamycin alone has no activity against *P. carinii.*
‡Must be given with fatty food because serum concentrations are 2- or 3-fold lower when drug is administered on an empty stomach.
§Administered at 50 psi and 8 L/minute of oxygen.

with *Pneumocystis.* Although no comparably rigorous studies have compared trimethoprim-sulfamethoxazole with parenteral pentamidine, trimethoprim-sulfamethoxazole is associated with less serious toxic effects.

The most frequent potentially serious toxic effect with trimethoprim-sulfamethoxazole is neutropenia (Table 402–2). Because this reaction is dose-dependent, a lower dose (15 mg/kg/day of trimethoprim) is now preferred. Several controlled trials have indicated

Table 402–2 ■ TOXICITIES ASSOCIATED WITH STANDARD THERAPIES FOR *Pneumocystis carinii* PNEUMONIA

DRUG	FREQUENT CAUSES OF DRUG MORBIDITY	INFREQUENT CAUSES OF MORBIDITY
Trimethoprim-sulfamethoxazole	Fever Morbilliform rash Nausea and vomiting Neutropenia* Thrombocytopenia† Anemia‡	Stevens-Johnson syndrome Exfoliative dermatitis Diarrhea Liver test abnormalities Elevated serum creatinine Hyperkalemia Hyponatremia Renal impairment Hallucinations or agitation
Parenteral pentamidine	Fever Morbilliform rash Nausea and vomiting Renal impairment Hypoglycemia Hypotension Pancreatitis	Hypocalcemia Ventricular tachycardia/fibrillation Torsades de pointes Neutropenia Thrombocytopenia Liver test abnormalities Ketoacidosis and diabetes Hypomagnesemia Myoglobinuria Hematuria
Trimetrexate plus leucovorin	Fever Neutropenia	Liver test abnormalities Morbilliform rash Thrombocytopenia Mucositis
Dapsone	Fever Morbilliform rash Nausea and vomiting	Methemoglobinemia Hemolytic anemia Sulfone syndrome
Clindamycin	Fever Morbilliform rash Diarrhea	Liver test abnormalities *Clostridium difficile* colitis
Primaquine	Nausea Abdominal distress Neutropenia	Methemoglobinemia Hemolytic anemia Hypertension Arrhythmias
Atovaquone	Rash	Fever Nausea and vomiting Liver test abnormalities
Aerosolized pentamidine	Cough Bronchospasm Metallic taste	Contact dermatitis Morbilliform rash Hypoglycemia Pancreatitis Renal impairment

*Reduced to <1000 cells/μL.
†Reduced to <50,000 cells/μL.
‡>2 g/dL decline.

that this dose results in survival rates greater than or equal to 88% for severe episodes, suggesting that it does not compromise outcome.

Parenteral Pentamidine. Parenteral pentamidine is also highly effective. As with trimethoprim-sulfamethoxazole, toxic reactions are common (see Table 402–2). In one study in which patients received a minimum of 14 days of therapy, nephrotoxicity (>1 mg/L rise in serum creatinine) occurred in 64% of patients, hypotension in 27%, and hypoglycemia in 21%. Impaired renal function and hypoglycemia are dose-dependent and more likely to be seen after 2 weeks of therapy or a total dosage of more than 4 g. Hypotension generally occurs during or shortly after intravenous infusion and may last several hours, although low blood pressures may persist for several months.

Hypoglycemia is the most treacherous reaction and occurs in 10 to 20% of AIDS patients treated with pentamidine; this results from sudden increases in serum insulin caused by lysis of pancreatic β cells. Because of the prolonged binding of pentamidine to tissue, precipitous hypoglycemia may occur after the drug is discontinued, with fatal reactions occurring up to 2 weeks after the last dose. When hypoglycemia is detected, pentamidine should be discontinued and patients should be monitored closely with daily capillary glucose measurements for several weeks.

Trimetrexate. Trimetrexate (NeuTrexin) is a powerful antifolate drug that binds to the DHFR of *P. carinii* nearly 1500 times more avidly than does trimethoprim, and it is concentrated in *P. carinii*. Leucovorin (folinic acid) must be co-administered to protect against bone marrow toxicity. In a comparative study, trimetrexate was effective but inferior to trimethoprim-sulfamethoxazole for moderate-to-severe episodes. Treatment-limiting toxicity, particularly critical neutropenia, thrombocytopenia, and anemia, occurred significantly more often with trimethoprim-sulfamethoxazole than with trimetrexate.

Adjunctive Corticosteroids. The major breakthrough in the search for more effective therapies for *Pneumocystis* has been the irrefutable evidence that mortality for severe episodes can be reduced nearly twofold by use of corticosteroids within 72 hours after beginning specific anti-*Pneumocystis* therapy (Table 402–3). With adjunctive corticosteroids, oxygen desaturation occurs less often, and fewer patients require mechanical ventilation. Serious adverse consequences are uncommon, perhaps because the course is limited (21 days) and the tapering period is rapid; an increase in mucocutaneous herpes infections was seen in the largest study. However, adjunctive corticosteroids could be deleterious if given with empirical anti-*Pneumocystis* therapy for patients who actually have pulmonary fungal infection or tuberculosis, because these patients may show initial improvement, which could thereby delay diagnosis and specific antimicrobial therapy. Corticosteroids can also aggravate and accelerate the progression of cutaneous and pulmonary Kaposi's sarcoma.

Salvage Therapy. Once respiratory failure has developed, prognosis is poor. Parenteral trimethoprim-sulfamethoxazole, pentamidine, trimetrexate, and clindamycin-primaquine have all been evaluated for salvage in uncontrolled studies and appear to provide limited benefit. Little reason has been put forward to favor any of these,

and no data are available to support the use of multiple concurrent therapies.

MILD EPISODE. For mild episodes (PaO$_2$ > 70 mm Hg or A − aDO$_2$ <35), management should focus on tolerable oral agents that can be used in an ambulatory setting, because mortality rates are low (see Table 402–1). Trimethoprim-sulfamethoxazole is inexpensive and can be conveniently given orally, but it causes substantial toxic effects.

Trimethoprim-Dapsone. Trimethoprim-dapsone, like trimethoprim-sulfamethoxazole, results in sequential blockade of folate synthesis in *P. carinii*. Dapsone, a sulfone, binds to dihydropteroate synthetase twofold more avidly than sulfamethoxazole. Treatment-limiting neutropenia and transaminase elevations occur less frequently than with trimethoprim-sulfamethoxazole.

Clindamycin-Primaquine. Clindamycin and the antimalarial drug primaquine together have excellent activity against *P. carinii* in a limited cell culture system and in the murine model, but neither agent alone is effective, and the mechanism of action is unclear. The combination has been effective for *Pneumocystis* as initial therapy, with response rates in the range of 90% regardless of whether clindamycin is given intravenously or orally and whether the dose of primaquine base is 15 or 30 mg/day. Controlled trials have not established whether trimethoprim-dapsone or clindamycin-primaquine are as effective as trimethoprim-sulfamethoxazole. In a comparative study of these three oral regimens for mild to moderate disease, the frequency of treatment-limiting toxicity effects was not significantly different among the arms of the study, although the specific types of adverse effects were not evenly distributed. Clindamycin-primaquine was the most common cause of severe rash and anemia, whereas trimethoprim-sulfamethoxazole more frequently caused hepatitis, and trimethoprim-dapsone caused nausea and vomiting. Awareness of the potential problems with each of these regimens permits better matching of *Pneumocystis* therapy to the patient's clinical status at diagnosis. The U.S. Public Health Service has not recommended adjunctive corticosteroids for mild episodes because mortality is very low. However, a recent study indicated that there is less desaturation, better exercise tolerance, and a quicker return of elevated LDH levels to baseline with adjunctive corticosteroids in episodes of mild to moderate severity.

Atovaquone. Atovaquone (Mepron) is an oral hydroxynapthoquinone originally developed as an antimalarial, and it is well-tolerated. The drug inhibits mitochondrial electron transport necessary for the biosynthesis of pyrimidines in protozoa, but its mode of action against *P. carinii* is unknown. In a comparative study of atovaquone for 322 patients with mild to moderate (A − aDO$_2$ <45) *Pneumocystis* pneumonia, failures due to inadequate therapeutic response occurred in 31% of patients receiving atovaquone and in 16% receiving trimethoprim-sulfamethoxazole (P = 0.002). Mortality was also imbalanced, with one death in the trimethoprim-sulfamethoxazole group and 11 in the atovaquone arm. Patients in whom atovaquone failed were more likely to have low plasma concentrations (<15 mg/mm) and diarrhea. Atovaquone must be given with fatty food, because blood levels are twofold to threefold lower when it is taken on an empty stomach.

OUTCOME AND PROGNOSIS. Clinical parameters at presentation that are associated with an increased risk for fatal outcome include an elevated serum LDH of more than > 500 IU/dL, PaO$_2$ < 70 mm Hg or A − aDO$_2$ > 35, BAL neutrophils greater than 5%, and low triiodothyronine (T$_3$) and reverse = T$_3$ hormone concentrations.

CHANGING THERAPY. It can be difficult to know when therapy is failing in a specific patient. Persistence of fever or lack of improvement on chest radiographs is common, especially during the first several days of treatment. Unchanged or progressive infiltrates frequently occur even in patients who show an ultimate response. Oxygenation reaches its nadir 3 to 4 days after beginning treatment. A sustained respiratory rate greater than 35/minute or absolute increase in room air A − aDO$_2$ >20 above baseline have proven to be reproducible end points for failure in clinical trials. These signs provide objective justification for changing therapy and for evaluating other possible complications in the lung. It is important to remember that another concurrent pulmonary diagnosis exists in up to 15% of AIDS patients with *Pneumocystis* pneumonia.

SUPPORTIVE CARE. Evidence suggests that the degree of alveolar damage is the most important determinant of outcome. Thus, as

Table 402–3 ■ ADJUNCTIVE CORTICOSTEROIDS* FOR PATIENTS WITH *Pneumocystis carinii* PNEUMONIA AND A − aDO$_2$ ≥ 35 mm Hg OR PaO$_2$ ≤ 70 mm Hg

DRUG	DOSE	TREATMENT DAYS
Oral		
Prednisone	40 mg bid	1–5
	40 mg once daily	6–10
	20 mg once daily	11–21
Intravenous		
Methylprednisolone	30 mg bid	1–5
	30 mg once daily	6–10
	15 mg once daily	11–21

*Efficacy established only when adjunctive corticosteroids are initiated within 72 hours of starting specific treatment for *P. carinii*.

Table 402–4 ■ PROPHYLACTIC THERAPIES FOR PREVENTION OF *Pneumocystis carinii* PNEUMONIA

DRUG	DOSE OR REGIMEN	ALTERNATE DOSE OR REGIMEN
Antifolate regimens		
Trimethoprim-sulfamethoxazole	1 double-strength tablet daily	1 double-strength tablet 3 times weekly
		1 single-strength tablet daily
Dapsone	100 mg tablet daily	50 mg tablet once or twice daily
Dapsone-pyrimethamine	50 mg tablet dapsone daily	None
	50 mg tablet pyrimethamine weekly	
Aerosolized pentamidine	300 mg monthly by Respirgard II jet nebulizer	None established
Other regimens		
Atovaquone	1500 mg once daily	None
Primaquine-clindamycin	Unknown	None

*Patients receiving therapy for toxoplasmosis are unlikely to need additional prophylaxis for *Pneumocystis* because pyrimethamine-sulfadiazine has been used successfully to treat *Pneumocystis* pneumonia, and the alternative combination of pyrimethamine-clindamycin is similar to the regimen of primaquine-clindamycin, which is also an effective treatment for *Pneumocystis*.

with adult respiratory distress syndrome (ARDS), which has similar histologic features to severe *Pneumocystis infection,* supportive care is crucial for severely ill patients. Continuous positive airway pressure by face mask improves oxygenation in patients with tachypnea, and refractory desaturation with standard masks and may mitigate the need for mechanical ventilation.

MECHANICAL VENTILATION AND INTENSIVE CARE UNIT CARE. Mortality for AIDS patients on mechanical ventilators in intensive care units (ICU) has ranged from 30 to 50% in recent reports, supporting the value of aggressive measures in selected patients. Low albumin level, arterial pH less than 7.35, or need for positive end expiratory pressure greater than 10 cm H_2O after 96 hours in the intensive care unit portend a severalfold greater risk for a fatal outcome. Thus, patients with better nutritional status and those who have less severe alveolar damage and a normal pH may benefit most from ventilatory support.

PROPHYLAXIS. The U.S. Public Health Service recommends prophylaxis for pneumocystis in patients at high risk (Table 402–4). Those at highest risk include (1) patients with prior *Pneumocystis infection,* (2) those with fewer than 200 CD4 cells, and (3) patients with thrush and a fever greater than 100° F for at least 2 weeks; a prior AIDS-defining illness may also increase the risk of *Pneumocystis* infection. Trimethoprim-sulfamethoxazole is currently the most effective form of prophylaxis. In several studies, the relative hazard of developing *Pneumocystis* was approximately three to four times less with trimethoprim-sulfamethoxazole than with aerosolized pentamidine. In controlled trials, dapsone has been comparable to aerosolized pentamidine, but somewhat inferior to trimethoprim-sulfamethoxazole. When combined with pyrimethamine (usually 50 mg given once weekly), this approach is also effective in preventing toxoplasmosis. Atovaquone and dapsone appear equally useful in the sulfa-intolerant patient.

Bozzette SA, Sattler FR, Chui J, et al: A controlled trial of early adjunctive treatment with corticosteroids for *Pneumocystis carinii* pneumonia in the acquired immunodeficiency syndrome. N Engl J Med 323:1451, 1990. *A pivotal study demonstrating that adjunctive corticosteroids reduce mortality for patients with severe* Pneumocystis.

Hardy DW, Feinberg J, Finkelstein DM, et al: A controlled trial of trimethoprim-sulfamethoxazole or aerosolized pentamidine for secondary prophylaxis of *Pneumocystis carinii* pneumonia in patients with the acquired immunodeficiency syndrome: AIDS Clinical Trials Group Protocol 021. N Engl J Med 327:1842, 1992. *Results demonstrate the superiority of trimethoprim-sulfamethoxazole compared with aerosolized pentamidine for preventing* Pneumocystis *in AIDS patients with a prior episode of* Pneumocystis *infection.*

Safrin S, Finkelstein DM, Feinberg J, et al: Comparison of three regimens for treatment of mild to moderate *Pneumocystis carinii* pneumonia in patients with AIDS: A double-blind, randomized trial of oral trimethoprim-sulfamethoxazole, dapsone-trimethoprim, and clindamycin-primaquine. Ann Intern Med 124:792–802, 1996. *Equivalent rates of treatment-limiting toxicity were seen for all three regimens, although specific types of toxicity were different for each therapy.*

Sattler FR, Frame P, Davis R, et al: Trimetrexate with leucovorin versus trimethoprim-sulfamethoxazole for moderate to severe episodes of *Pneumocystis carinii* pneumonia in patients with AIDS: A prospective, controlled multicenter investigation of the AIDS Clinical Trials Protocol 029/031. J Infect Dis 170:165, 1994. *Results established the relative effectiveness and tolerability of trimetrexate for moderate to severe* P. carinii *pneumonia.*

Toma E, Fournier S, Dumont M, et al: Clindamycin-primaquine versus trimethoprim-sulfamethoxazole as primary therapy for *Pneumocystis carinii* pneumonia in AIDS: A randomized, double blind pilot trial. Clin Infect Dis 17:178, 1993. *Results confirm prior reports of the incidence of adverse effects with these treatment regimens and*

suggest that clindamycin-primaquine is highly effective as initial therapy for P. carinii *pneumonia.*

403

MUCORMYCOSIS

Sandy F. S. Chun and David A. Stevens

DEFINITION

Mucormycosis is generally an acute and rapidly developing fungal infection caused by fungi of the class Zygomycetes. In healthy hosts, these organisms seldom cause infection. However, in debilitated or immunosuppressed hosts, they produce a fulminant opportunistic infection, resulting in marked tissue destruction. Several predisposing conditions have been identified. The infection is most commonly associated with the acidotic patient, especially those in diabetic ketoacidosis. Prolonged treatment with antibiotics, corticosteroids, and cytotoxic drugs and, most recently, the use of deferoxamine in the dialysis patient have also been associated, as have severe malnutrition, hematologic malignancies, and extensive burns.

MUCORMYCOSIS

Causative fungus	The order Mucorales; *Rhizopus, Mucor* species most common
Primary geographic distribution	Ubiquitous: air, bread, fruit, vegetables, soil, manure
Primary route of acquisition	Inhaling spores
Principal sites of disease	Rhinocerebral, pulmonary, cutaneous, gastrointestinal, disseminated, central nervous system (CNS)
Opportunistic infection in compromised hosts	Pulmonary, rhinocerebral
Drug of choice for most patients	Amphotericin B
Alternative therapy	Amphotericin combined with rifampin, azoles, flucytosine

THE PATHOGENS

The pathogenic zygomycetes are largely in the order Mucorales, which is related to the term for this infection, mucormycosis. Zygomycosis has also been used to refer to the disease caused by organisms of the class, but that term would include diseases due to fungi of the order Entomophthorales. The latter diseases usually are different from those caused by the Mucorales (largely superficial infections) and are rare in North America. Phycomycosis is another older term in the literature describing the same infections. The Mucorales are morphologically distinct. Their hyphae are non-septated, broad, and variable in size and shape. Furthermore, the branching of the hyphae is usually irregular and at right angles. Species of the genera *Rhizopus* and *Mucor* are the common pathogens of this group. Other genera, including *Absidia, Cunninghamella, Rhizomucor,* and *Apophysomyces,* have also been reported to cause disease. These fungi cannot be differentiated histopathologically. Further speciation requires culturing the pathogen and characterizing the isolates by their morphologic and physiologic features.

EPIDEMIOLOGY

The Mucorales are ubiquitous saprophytic fungi and are abundant in nature. They have been recovered from bread, fruits, vegetables, soil, and manure. These fungi have been isolated from the nose, stool, and sputum of healthy individuals. Despite their widespread distribution, they cause disease infrequently. Fortunately, even in the severely immunocompromised hosts, mucormycosis remains a rare opportunistic infection. The disease is not contagious.

PATHOGENESIS AND PATHOLOGY

Currently, there is no unifying concept of the pathogenesis of mucormycosis. In diseases of the airways (sinus, lung), the infection is presumed to originate from inhaled spores, although the lung may also be involved secondary to bloodstream invasion. Diabetic patients appear to be more frequently colonized. Whereas normal human serum can inhibit their growth, serum obtained from patients with diabetic ketoacidosis is not inhibitory and may even promote fungal growth. Undefined defects of macrophages and neutrophils contribute to the loss of immunity against this infection in the susceptible host. Corticosteroids weaken normal inhibitors of spore germination in tissue. Unlike most pathogenic fungi, these can grow in the absence of oxygen.

Invasion, thrombosis, and necrosis are the characteristic findings in this disease. Once the fungal spores have germinated at the site of infection, the hyphal elements are very aggressive and tend to invade blood vessels, nerves, lymphatics, and tissues. The infarction leads to further tissue hypoxia and acidosis, resulting in a vicious circle enhancing rapid growth and infection. The paucity of a granulomatous reaction is quite characteristic. The fungal hyphae sometimes have little or no inflammation around them.

CLINICAL MANIFESTATIONS

Mucormycosis can be manifested as at least six distinct clinical entities, dependent on the types of predisposing factors of the patient and the portal of entry of the organism (Table 403–1).

Rhinocerebral mucormycosis is the most common presentation, accounting for more than 75% of the cases in the literature. It frequently affects the poorly controlled diabetic patient who is also in ketoacidosis. It has also been reported in patients with hematologic malignancies who have been neutropenic for an extended period and who have received broad-spectrum antibacterial drugs or immunosuppressive therapy, in other acidotic patients, and in those with azotemia. This is one of the most rapidly fatal fungal diseases if left undiagnosed. Hyphae invade the paranasal sinuses and palate from the oronasal cavity. From the sinuses, especially the ethmoid sinus, the infection spreads to involve the retro-orbital region or the CNS. Epistaxis, severe unilateral headache, alteration in mental status, and eye symptoms such as lacrimation, irritation, or periorbital anesthesia are common symptoms. Examination of the nose may reveal the classic black necrotic turbinates (too often mistaken for dried blood) or even nasal septum perforation. However, at the early stage of infection, the nasal mucosa may appear only inflamed and friable. Facial cellulitis and palatal necrosis may be seen. The early eye findings include mild proptosis, periorbital edema, decreased visual acuity, or lid swelling. In more advanced orbital involvement, exophthalmos, complete ophthalmoplegia, conjunctival hemorrhage, blindness, fixed and dilated pupil, and corneal anesthesia may be found. These conditions result from fungal invasion of the roof of the orbit, affecting the nerves (third, fourth, and sixth cranial nerves and the ophthalmic branch of the fifth cranial nerve), muscles, and orbital vessels, a condition also known as the "orbital apex syndrome." The infection can spread through the superior orbital fissure or the cribriform plate to involve the brain. Cavernous sinus thrombosis is a frequent complication usually resulting from hematogenous spread from the ophthalmic veins.

This spread results in additional cranial nerve involvement outside the orbital apex, specifically the trigeminal nerve ganglion and the root of the facial nerve, leading to ipsilateral paresthesia of the face or peripheral facial palsy. Internal carotid artery thrombosis, from retrograde spread from the ophthalmic artery or invasion from the cavernous sinus, is another late complication, leading to cerebral infarction. The middle ear may be involved via the blood, cerebrospinal fluid (CSF), or eustachian tube.

The radiographic manifestations are nonspecific. Plain roentgenograms of the sinuses and orbits may reveal nodular thickening of the mucosa of multiple sinuses, usually without air-fluid levels, or spotty destruction of the bone through the walls of the sinuses or into the orbit. Computed tomography (CT) or magnetic resonance imaging (MRI) is useful in better defining the bone destruction and soft tissue involvement, which could be important in guiding subsequent surgical intervention. The CSF findings are usually nonspecific and often normal even in the presence of CNS involvement. The common findings are pleocytosis, with about 50% polymorphonuclear cells and slight protein elevation; hypoglycorrhachia is rare. Smear and culture of CSF are usually negative for fungus even in cases with documented meningeal involvement. Several infectious diseases can present a similar picture. Black necrotic lesions may also be seen with invasive aspergillosis and with infections by *Pseudomonas aeruginosa* or *Pseudallescheria boydii.* The only definitive method of differentiating between these possibilities is by examination of tissue. Cavernous sinus thrombosis due to *Staphylococcus aureus,* as well as rhinoscleroma, aggressive orbital tumor, midline granuloma, and other fungal infections, can mimic the disease as well.

Pulmonary mucormycosis occurs most frequently in patients with hematologic malignancies being treated with antibacterial drugs or immunosuppressive therapy. The presentation usually is acute, and the patients are often profoundly ill, with variable complaints of cough, fever, and sputum production. There is no specific lobar predilection. Pulmonary vascular thrombosis and infarction are universal findings. No pathognomonic clinical or radiographic findings exist. Sputum culture usually is negative. In fact, ante mortem diagnosis is seldom made because of the acuteness of the illness, the lack of consideration of the diagnosis, and the need for tissue to establish the diagnosis.

Invasive pulmonary aspergillosis or other mycoses, or nocardiosis, other bacterial infections, such as *Pseudomonas* infection, malignant invasion, hemorrhage, or pulmonary embolism and infarction may mimic the presentation of pulmonary mucormycosis.

Cutaneous mucormycosis is rare and is primarily a nosocomial infection in burn and blunt trauma victims. Local infection has resulted from using contaminated elastic bandages. The involved area is erythematous and painful, with varying degrees of central necrosis that can progress to gangrenous cellulitis. Cutaneous infection can also occur as a result of dissemination from another site of involvement. Skin and subcutaneous infection in diabetics can occur.

Gastrointestinal mucormycosis is the rarest form of infection. It is seen primarily in patients suffering from intrinsic abnormalities of the gastrointestinal tract or severe malnutrition. The infection is thought to arise from fungi entering the body with food. Any part of the gastrointestinal tract is susceptible to infection, with the stomach, terminal ileum, and colon being the most common sites. Wall invasion, ischemic infarction, and ulceration are characteristic. The diagnosis is frequently made at autopsy.

Table 403–1 ■ CLINICAL MANIFESTATIONS OF MUCORMYCOSIS

Rhinocerebral	Gastrointestinal
Pulmonary	Widely disseminated
Cutaneous	Central nervous system

Disseminated mucormycosis is defined as infection occurring in two or more noncontiguous organ systems. The distant sites are infected by bloodstream invasion from a local site. Although any organ can be affected, the lungs and CNS are the two common sites. The outcome of this infection is almost invariably fatal.

Isolated CNS mucormycosis results from hematogenous spread and is seen primarily in intravenous drug addicts.

DIAGNOSIS

The diagnosis of any form of mucormycosis is dependent on direct and histologic examinations of scrapings and biopsies of necrotic material. In contrast to most fungi, these organisms are readily seen in hematoxylin and eosin-stained tissue. The Gomori methenamine silver stain usually is adequate, but some special fungus stains, such as periodic acid–Schiff, do not demonstrate the organism well. However, a more rapid but preliminary diagnosis can sometimes be made by demonstrating hyphal elements after potassium hydroxide digestion of fresh tissue scraping. The alkali digests some of the tissue debris, but not the fungus, and makes identifying the fungi easier. Swabs of discharge or abnormal tissue are not adequate and can give erroneous information. Fungal cultures are occasionally positive, but a negative culture result does not exclude the diagnosis nor make it less likely. Teasing rather than homogenization of the tissue may increase the yield of cultures. The media used for culturing these fungi should not contain cycloheximide. At present, no skin tests or serologic methods are adequate for diagnosing mucormycosis. Blood cultures are not helpful.

THERAPY

The hallmarks of successful outcome in this aggressive infection rely on early diagnosis by invasive procedures, immediate correction of the underlying predisposing condition, aggressive surgical débridement, and early systemic amphotericin therapy. Amphotericin B is the only drug with proven clinical efficacy, and a high therapeutic dosage (such as 1.0 to 1.5 mg per kilogram per day, if tolerated) should be achieved as soon as possible. This may be reduced to alternate-day dosing once the patient is stabilized. Typically, a cumulative dose of 2 to 5 grams may be needed to achieve cure. Lipid-complexed amphotericin could enable continued aggressive therapy in the nephrotoxic patient. Although local irrigation of infected sites with amphotericin is an unproven adjunct, given the difficulties in perfusion of infected areas because of the tendency to thrombosis, this measure seems logical. Similarly, potentiation of amphotericin with other drugs (such as rifampin, azoles, flucytosine) is of unproven benefit, but given the poor results with conventional therapy, this should be considered if susceptibility testing can be done in vitro with the patient's isolate to show synergy and exclude antagonism. The newer orally administered azole derivates have no proven activity alone against these fungi. Improvement of survival may necessitate repeated major surgical débridement of necrotic tissue, resulting in significant disfiguring. Hyperbaric oxygen therapy may be of some value in deterring progression. Colony-stimulating factors could accelerate neutrophil return in neutropenic patients. If the patient survives, major reconstructive surgery may be needed.

PROGNOSIS

Mucormycosis remains a disease with guarded prognosis. It is difficult to ascertain accurately the effectiveness of any therapeutic approach because the disease is relatively rare and there is a general bias toward reporting cases only if therapy is effective. With the introduction of amphotericin B in 1961, it is generally accepted that the survival rate significantly improved. Rhinocerebral mucormycosis is the most common form of infection and is thought to have an overall mortality rate of about 50%. Patients who develop hemiplegia, facial necrosis, or nasal deformity have a higher mortality. Pulmonary or disseminated mucormycosis frequently escapes ante mortem diagnosis, and only a handful of patients have been reported to recover from these. Superficial infections, particularly in immunocompetent patients, can be successfully treated with débridement and antifungal therapy. Deeper cutaneous infections of

the extremities usually require amputation, and when the head or trunk is involved, the condition is commonly fatal.

At this time, the most aggressive approach we can take toward this lethal disease is rapid diagnosis and immediate institution of surgical débridement plus systemic and local chemotherapy.

Boelaert JR: Mucormycosis (zygomycosis). Is there news for the clinician? J. Infect 28 (suppl 1):1, 1994. *An update reviewing increased risk with deferoxamine therapy, and utility of MRI and CT scans of sinus and brain in guiding response to therapy and débridement surgery.*

Sugar AM: Mucormycosis. Clin Infect Dis 14 (suppl 1):S126, 1992. *A review of all forms of the disease.*

Yohai RA, Bullock JD, Aziz AA, Markert RJ: Survival factors in rhino-orbital-cerebral mucormycosis. Surv Ophthal 39:3, 1994. *Comprehensive review of 208 cases in the literature since 1970. Factors are identified that help determine prognosis. Standard treatment is discussed, as well as data on hyperbaric oxygen.*

404 MYCETOMA

Michael S. Saag

DEFINITION

Mycetoma is a chronic, localized, subcutaneous infection characterized by draining sinus tracts that frequently discharge purulent material containing granules. The disease most often affects the lower extremities, with the majority of cases involving the foot. Originally described in the mid-1800's, the disease was initially referred to as "Madura foot," named after the region in India where it was first identified. Although still referred to as maduromycosis, the preferred name and the term used most often to describe the disorder is mycetoma.

EUMYCETOMA	
Primary geographic distribution	*P. boydii* (U.S.; N. America)
	L. senegalensis (W. Africa)
	M. grisea (S. America)
	M. mycetomatis (Worldwide; Saudi Arabia)
Primary sites of disease	Lower extremities; hands (direct inoculation)
Drug of choice	Itraconazole (as an adjunct to surgical débridement)
Alternative therapy	Ketoconazole
	Amphotericin B (resistant cases)

ACTINOMYCETOMA	
Primary geographic distribution	*A. madurae* (U.S.)
	S. somaliensis (Africa)
	A. pelletieri (S. America)
	N. brasiliensis (Mexico)
Primary sites of disease	Lower extremities; hands (direct inoculation)
Drug of choice	Trimethoprim/ sulfamethoxazole (as adjunct to surgery)
Alternative therapy	Dapsone
	Streptomycin

ETIOLOGY

More than 20 species of fungi and bacteria have been implicated as etiologic agents of mycetoma. Approximately 40% of cases are

Table 404-1 ■ CAUSATIVE ORGANISMS OF MYCETOMA AND THE CHARACTERISTIC PIGMENT OF THEIR ASSOCIATED GRANULES

EUMYCETOMA	ACTINOMYCETOMA
White to yellow grains	
Pseudallescheria boydii	*Nocardia brasiliensis*
Acremonium species	*Nocardia asteroides*
Trichophyton species	*Nocardia cavae* (tiny grains)
Microsporum species	*Actinomadura madurae* (large grains)
Fusarium species	
Aspergillus nidulans	
Yellow to brown grains	
Neotestudina (Zophia) rosatii	*Streptomyces somaliensis*
Black grains	
Madurella mycetomatis	*Streptomyces paraguayensis*
Madurella grisea	
Exophiala jeanselmei	
Leptosphaeria senegalensis	
Leptosphaeria thompkinsii	
Red to pink grains	
	Actinomadura pelletieri

due to true fungi (eumycetoma), and 60% are caused by aerobic actinomycetes (actinomycetoma). The organisms are distributed throughout the world, and the predominant organisms responsible for disease are subject to regional variation. Etiologic agents of eumycetoma and actinomycetoma may be presumptively identified based on the characteristic pigment of their granules. A listing of the predominant causative organisms is given in Table 404–1.

EPIDEMIOLOGY

Mycetomas have been reported from all over the world but are endemic in tropical regions of Africa, India, Central and South America, and the Far East. The geographic distribution of the disease is more related to rainfall than any other climatic factor. Most of the etiologic agents have been cultured from the soil in endemic areas, and occasionally organisms have been identified on plant thorns, which may be responsible for intradermal inoculation. *Pseudallescheria boydii* is the most common cause of mycetoma in the United States and is readily isolated from the soil in the United States and Canada. *Nocardia brasiliensis* and *Actinomadura madurae* are the most frequently isolated organisms in Central America, South America, and the Caribbean.

The majority of cases occur in males, many of whom are field laborers or herdsmen who have long-term trauma to their feet while in wet or swampy soil. Although the disease afflicts people of all ages, most cases are reported in young adults. Person-to-person transmission is not believed to occur, and the disease is unrelated to animal contact.

PATHOGENESIS AND PATHOLOGY

In contrast to systemic mycoses, which usually are established via the respiratory route, mycetomas are initiated through direct inoculation of the organism into the skin or mucosal surface, frequently as a consequence of trauma. Although the foot is the most common site of infection, direct inoculation of organisms into the hand, back, neck, and back of the head can occur in individuals who carry loads contaminated with soil.

The precise mechanism of pathogenesis remains unknown. Once inoculated, the organism induces a subacute to chronic suppurative inflammatory response that is primarily neutrophilic in nature but that may be associated with a granulomatous reaction. Over time, localized necrosis, fibrosis, abscess formation and, frequently, bone and joint disease ensue. Deep sinuses with fistulas commonly develop and present as draining sinus tracts on the skin surface. The purulent drainage from those tracts often contains grains or granules, which consist of the causative organism embedded in a host-derived, proteinaceous matrix. The size, character, and color of the granules suggest the underlying etiologic agent (see Table 404–1).

The inflammatory process usually extends along fascial planes and may result in substantial regional destruction of deep tissues and bone. Distal spread of disease via the lymphatics or the bloodstream may occur but is distinctly uncommon.

CLINICAL MANIFESTATIONS

Most cases of mycetoma present late in the course of a long-standing, chronic inflammatory disease. The initial lesion appears as a small, painless nodule several weeks to months after primary inoculation. The patient generally cannot recall a precipitating event or specific traumatic incident. The lesions slowly extend into deep tissues, and the resultant lymphatic obstruction, fibrosis, and tissue thickening give the foot a shortened, raised appearance. Skin nodules may break down, yielding granulomatous tissue with serosanguineous to purulent discharge. Later in the course of disease, sinus tracts begin to appear, through which the characteristic fungal granules are expelled onto the skin surface. The sinus tracts spontaneously heal, only to be replaced by new tracts at nearby sites. Eumycetomas tend to be more circumscribed, remain localized, and progress more slowly than actinomycetomas, which have less well-defined margins, merge with surrounding tissue, and progress more rapidly. The lesions tend to remain painless until deep bone involvement occurs, although many patients may complain of a deep itching sensation during active disease progression. Systemic involvement is rare, and patients feel remarkably well even in the presence of advanced localized disease.

DIAGNOSIS

The definitive diagnosis of mycetoma depends on culture of the causative organism from tissue specimens. The disease is suspected in the appropriate clinical setting, especially when grains are identified in the purulent discharge. Examination of the grains can establish a differential diagnosis of eumycetoma or actinomycetoma based on the presence of characteristic broad (fungal) or narrow (actinomycete) filaments. The characteristics of the granules, when combined with geographic and epidemiologic information, can yield a presumptive identification of the specific organism. However, cultural data are required for confirmation. Serologic tests are not routinely available.

TREATMENT

The response to therapy is dependent on the underlying etiologic agent. Eumycetomas are unresponsive to antimicrobial therapy, although partial responses to amphotericin B, liposomal amphotericin B, miconazole, ketoconazole, itraconazole, and thiabendazole have been reported. Fortunately, eumycetomas tend to be well circumscribed, yielding ready access to surgical approaches. If the lesion is not removed in its entirety and residual disease is present, relapse is inevitable.

Actinomycetomas are more responsive to antimicrobial therapy. Regimens consisting of high-dose penicillin (10 to 12 million units per day), sulfadiazine (3 to 10 grams per day), or minocycline (150 mg twice daily) have been reported to have some effect. The most successful regimens consist of trimethoprim-sulfamethoxazole (160 mg of trimethoprim and 800 mg of sulfamethoxazole given twice daily), combined with either streptomycin (1 to 3 grams per day for 3 weeks) or rifampin (600 mg per day for 3 to 4 months); or dapsone (100 mg twice daily) combined with streptomycin (1 gram per day for 1 month, given intramuscularly). The dapsone regimen often is preferred, owing to its low cost. Amoxicillin-clavulanic acid therapy has been successful in some cases which were unresponsive to conventional therapy. The duration of therapy with either the trimethoprim-sulfamethoxazole or the dapsone regimen is usually 9 months, depending on response.

PROGNOSIS

If the disease is diagnosed early, the prognosis for mycetoma is good. Unfortunately, many cases are not identified until late in the course of disease, when response to therapy is limited, and amputation may be required. When disease is located on the back, neck, trunk, or abdomen, very little therapeutic intervention can be offered. The prognosis for survival is quite good; however, the quality of life may be dramatically lessened.

Fincher RM, Fisher JF, Lovell RD, et al.: Infection due to the fungus acremonium (cephalosporium). Medicine 70:398, 1991. *Case report and review of the literature of this saprophytic organism that may cause disease in humans, especially immunocompromised hosts.*

Mahgoub ES: Medical management of mycetoma. Bull WHO 54:303, 1976. *Summarizes general principles of diagnosis and management.*

McGinnis MR: Mycetoma. Dermatol Clin 14:97–104, 1996. *An overview of mycetoma and the 31 fungal species known to cause this disorder.*

Smego RA Jr, Gallis HA: The clinical spectrum of *Nocardia brasiliensis* infection in the United States. Rev Infect Dis 6:164, 1984. *An important review of the pathogenesis, diagnosis, and therapy of the most common cause of mycetoma worldwide.*

Welsh O, Salinas MC, Rodriguez MA: Treatment of Eumycetoma and Actinomycetoma. Current Topics in Medical Mycology 6:47–71, 1995. *A thorough review (105 references) of the approach to treatment of mycetoma, including the use of newer triazole therapies.*

405 DEMATIACEOUS FUNGAL INFECTIONS

Michael S. Saag

DEFINITION

The term "dematiaceous" is applied to fungi that produce an intrinsic characteristic pigment. Diseases caused by dematiaceous fungi are divided into two groups: chromomycosis (chromoblastomycosis) and phaeohyphomycosis.

ETIOLOGY

Chromomycosis is caused by several species of related fungi, most notably *Fonsecaea, Phialophora, Cladosporium,* and *Acrotheca* species. These agents are brown-pigmented saprophytes commonly found in soil and wood. The microscopic appearance, which is virtually identical for all of the causative agents, consists of thick-walled, dark brown bodies ("sclerotic cells" or "copper pennies"), single or clustered. Sclerotic cells represent an intermediate form between yeasts and hyphae and multiply by horizontal and vertical separation, not by budding.

Phaeohyphomycosis may be caused by several organisms, frequently referred to as "black" fungi. They differ from the agents of chromomycosis in their clinical appearance and the absence of sclerotic cells. The black fungi usually exist in tissues as yeast-like cells (solitary or in small chains), as septated hyphae (branched or unbranched), or as a combination of yeast and hyphae. The hyphal forms are frequently confused with *Aspergillus* species but may be distinguished by using the Fontana-Masson staining procedure (a melanin-specific stain) or via in vitro culture. The most common agents of phaeohyphomycosis identified in humans include species in the following genera: *Curvularia, Bipolaris, Exserohilum, Alternaria, Mycocentrospora, Pyrenochaeta, Trichomaris, Wangiella, Xylohypha,* and *Exophiala.*

EPIDEMIOLOGY AND PATHOGENESIS

The organisms causing chromomycosis and phaeohyphomycosis are worldwide in distribution. Chromomycosis occurs predominantly in young males and usually is inoculated into the skin via thorns, splinters, and other penetrating wounds. The disease is more prevalent in rural populations, especially among those with suboptimal nutritional status and personal hygiene. Chromomycosis appears to be endemic in certain areas, such as Madagascar and Costa Rica.

Phaeohyphomycosis is becoming an important disease among immunocompromised hosts. Despite the ubiquity of black fungi in the environment, disease due to these organisms had in the past been sporadic. More recently, however, clusters of cases have been reported from major medical centers as opportunistic infections in transplant recipients, especially bone marrow transplant patients.

CLINICAL MANIFESTATIONS

Chromomycosis initially manifests as a wart-like papule that slowly enlarges into a verruciform plaque. The lesions may progress to ulceration with or without an exudate. Over time, the lesions become dry and crusted with a raised border, which may be serpiginous. Large plaques frequently develop central scarring. Occasionally, the lesions become pedunculated and acquire a cauliflower-like appearance. Systemic spread to distal sites is distinctly uncommon, although spread through autoinoculation or via lymphatic drainage may occur. Rarely, widespread disseminated disease to the pancreas, liver, bowel, lymph nodes, meninges, and brain is noted.

Phaeohyphomycosis may occur as a wide spectrum of clinical disease. Superficial phaeohyphomycosis is the most benign and is found in the stratum corneum or around the hair shaft. Tinea nigra and black piedra are examples of this disorder. More invasive skin disease involving nonliving layers of keratinized epithelium include the dermatomycoses and onychomycoses. Mycotic keratitis may result in extensive corneal damage and subsequent blindness. Subcutaneous disease usually results from direct inoculation of fungi through intact skin. Cystic lesions with well-defined walls and central abscess formation, occasionally surrounding a foreign body such as a splinter, are characteristic.

Invasive phaeohyphomycosis is a potentially life-threatening disease that occurs predominantly in immunocompromised hosts. Localized invasive disease frequently occurs in the paranasal sinuses, lower respiratory tract, and bone. Disease due to *Cladosporium, Curvularia, Bipolaris, Xylohypha,* and *Exserohilum* species is especially prone to invade the central nervous system.

DIAGNOSIS

The diagnosis of chromomycosis and phaeohyphomycosis is made by histopathologic examination of tissue biopsy specimens or KOH (10%) preparations. The brown sclerotic cells of chromomycosis are readily identified, and special stains are not usually required. Phaeohyphomycosis is best diagnosed using the Fontana-Masson technique, which distinguishes organisms producing melanin from *Aspergillus* species. Cultures are required to identify the specific genera causing chromomycosis and phaeohyphomycosis. All cultures should be held for at least 8 weeks, because some of the organisms grow slowly. No serologic or skin tests are available.

TREATMENT

Surgical excision, when feasible, is the most effective mode of therapy for subcutaneous or deeply invasive disease. Unfortunately, unless lesions are diagnosed and treated early, the rate of relapse is high. Systemic antifungal therapy with amphotericin B often is used; however, the results are generally disappointing. Flucytosine (5-FC; 150 mg per kilogram per day) has been used on an investigational basis in patients with chromomycosis, with some success (16 of 23 patients cured); however, resistance developed in several treated patients. The response to therapy of phaeohyphomycosis is highly dependent on the causative organism. Many black fungi are resistant to 5-FC, and amphotericin B therapy yields variable results. Newer triazole antifungal agents, such as fluconazole and itraconazole, show some promise as effective agents.

Adam RD, Paquin ML, Petersen EA, et al.: Phaeohyphomycosis caused by the fungal genera *Bipolaris* and *Exserohilum*. Medicine 65:203, 1986. *These fungi have been previously misclassified as* Helminthosporium *or* Drechslera *species, but the latter fungi appear not to produce human disease. This paper serves as an excellent review.*

Bayles MA: Chromomycosis. Current Topics in Medical Mycology 6:221, 1995. *A thorough review of infections caused by dematiaceous fungi (98 references).*

Bennett JE, Bonner H, Jennings AE, et al.: Chronic meningitis caused by *Cladospor-*

ium trichoides. Am J Clin Pathol 59:398, 1973. *Comprehensive review of cerebral infection with dematiaceous fungi.*

McGinnis MR: Chromoblastomycosis and phaeohyphomycosis: New concepts, diagnosis and mycology. J Am Acad Dermatol 8:1, 1983. *Clear-cut exposition of clinical and mycologic criteria for these diagnoses. A very important review.*

Rex JH, Walsh TJ, Anaissie EJ: Fungal infections in iatrogenically compromised hosts. Adv Intern Med 43:321, 1998. *An up-to-date review of systemic fungal diseases that occur in immunocompromised patients (290 references).*

Sudduth EJ, Crumbley AJ III, Farrar WE: *Phaeohyphomycosis due to Exophiala* species: Clinical spectrum of disease in humans. Clin Inf Dis 15:639, 1992. *An indepth review of infections due to* Exophiala. *Case report and review of the literature.*

PART XXIII

HIV AND THE ACQUIRED IMMUNODEFICIENCY SYNDROME

406 INTRODUCTION TO HIV AND ASSOCIATED DISORDERS

Gerald L. Mandell

The acquired immunodeficiency syndrome (AIDS), caused by the diabolically unique human immunodeficiency virus (HIV-1), has profoundly changed contemporary society and medical practice. The chapters in this part enable the physician to understand the virus and its effects on humans. In addition, there is an extensive discussion of involvement of various organ systems, both by the virus itself and by opportunistic infections. The management of patients with HIV infection is presented in detail.

In 1981, the first cluster of cases of what we now call AIDS was recognized and reported. Nearly all of the early identified cases were in young homosexual men, but it was quickly learned that HIV infection could be transmitted by heterosexual contact and by blood transfer from infected to noninfected individuals.

After an initial flurry of fearful reactions by health care workers who believed that they were at a very significant risk for acquiring HIV infection, the facts are somewhat reassuring and protective procedures have been established. It is clear that the greatest risk to health care workers is needle stick (or other sharp) transmittal of blood from infected patients to health care workers, with an infection rate of about 3 per 1000: Universal precautions were established on the premise that blood and body fluids from all patients should be considered potentially infectious. Recent data indicate that antiretroviral therapy reduces the risk of infection after accidental inoculation with HIV. Medical students and house officers training in many of our large medical centers are now just as likely to see patients with *Pneumocystis carinii* pneumonia as patients with pneumococcal pneumonia. The possibility of HIV infection must be considered in patients with a broad array of presenting symptoms because of the protean manifestations of this disease and its accompanying opportunistic infections and malignancies.

In the United States and other countries, governmental agencies have reacted to the HIV infection pandemic. New civil rights and public health legislation has been passed. The potential penalty for acquiring a sexually transmitted disease has now escalated to death. Despite this, countries around the world have been relatively slow to realize that the rules of the game for sexual contact have changed. We cannot wait for a vaccine to wipe out HIV infection. Educational efforts to reduce the spread of this disease have been supported by nearly all medical and public health groups, but have been opposed by other factions on religious or moral grounds. The process for drug testing, development, and approval has been altered. Activist groups have caused re-examination of some of the processes and regulations regarding approval of new therapies. This has resulted in "fast tracks" for certain agents. The concept of "surrogate markers" for disease progression has emerged. In a disease where time from infection to death is about 10 years, the use of survival measurements to determine efficacy of therapy would be impossibly slow. Therefore, surrogate markers such as CD4 counts and viral load are widely considered appropriate.

Despite more than a decade of significant progress related to understanding the molecular biology of the virus and details of pathogenesis of the disease, neither a cure nor an effective vaccine is in sight. However, modern therapy is very effective in those patients who are compliant and who can tolerate multiple drug regimens.

Study of patients who have resisted acquiring infection despite multiple exposures, and those who have had slow or no progression of their HIV infections, has uncovered the importance of chemokine receptors for viral entrance into cells. There is exciting potential to exploit this knowledge for new strategies of treatment and prevention.

All practicing physicians must know the basics of AIDS pathogenesis, disease presentation, and principles of management in order to effectively care for patients in the present era.

407 IMMUNOLOGY RELATED TO AIDS

Bruce D. Walker

The clinical consequences of human immunodeficiency virus (HIV) infection are due to the ability of this retrovirus to disarm the host immune system, a process that occurs by virtue of the fact that the primary target for the virus is the helper-inducer subset of lymphocytes. This lymphocyte subset, defined by its surface expression of the CD4 molecule, acts as the pivotal orchestrator of a myriad of immune functions. HIV-i infection can therefore be considered a disease of the immune system, characterized by the progressive loss of CD4-positive (CD4+) lymphocytes (Table 407–1), with ultimately fatal consequences for the infected host.

Despite this immunosuppression induced by HIV, a number of specific immunologic defenses against the virus are generated in infected individuals and may contribute to the long, asymptomatic phase that follows infection by keeping the virus at least partially contained. The potential significance of such responses is also underscored by the recent demonstration in animal AIDS models that a state of vaccine-induced protective immunity can be achieved against retroviruses related to HIV, and by the identification of infected persons who maintain control of HIV-1 viremia without

Table 407–1 ■ POTENTIAL CAUSES OF CD4+ CELL DEPLETION

1. Direct toxic consequences of infection
2. Syncytia formation
3. Innocent bystander destruction of cells with adsorbed gp120
4. Impaired regeneration of the peripheral T cell compartment
5. Autoimmune destruction
6. Superantigens
7. Apoptosis

drug therapy. An understanding of the immunology related to HIV provides insight not only into the clinical sequelae of infection, but also into the prospects for development of an effective vaccine against HIV.

HIV-INDUCED IMMUNOSUPPRESSION

An understanding of HIV life cycle (see Chapter 408 and Fig. 407–1) is necessary to appreciate the induction of immunosuppression. The hallmark of HIV-1 infection is progressive depletion of the CD4 helper-inducer subset of lymphocytes. Because of the central role of these cells in immunologic functioning, the clinical disease manifestations of immunosuppression and susceptibility to opportunistic infections and neoplasms are not surprising. The immunologic deficits associated with HIV-1 infection are widespread and involve numerous interdependent effector arms of the immune system, including both cellular and humoral elements.

Direct Immunosuppressive Properties of Viral Products

Protein products of a number of retroviruses have been shown to have direct immunosuppressive properties independent of viral infection. A synthetic peptide corresponding to a highly conserved region in the HIV-1 envelope gp41 transmembrane protein has been demonstrated in vitro to inhibit lymphocyte proliferative responses to mitogenic or antigenic stimuli. This region is analogous to a highly conserved immunosuppressive protein of human T-lymphotrophic virus I (HTLV-I), and similar inhibitory transmembrane proteins have been identified in other animal retroviral infections, such as feline leukemia virus (FeLV). Whether such a phenomenon contributes to the global immunosuppression seen in HIV-infected individuals has not been determined, but the possibility that HIV-1 proteins may be immunosuppressive has raised concerns about inclusion of such sequences in potential HIV vaccine candidates.

T Lymphocyte Abnormalities

Lymphocyte abnormalities associated with HIV-1 infection can be classified as both quantitative and qualitative. Qualitative deficiencies become apparent soon after infection and before CD4 depletion is evident, and may be related to virus-related functional defects in the helper-inducer subset of lymphocytes. Studies using purified subpopulations of lymphocytes from AIDS patients have demonstrated a selective defect in soluble antigen (e.g., tetanus toxoid) recognition, although these cells are still able to respond to mitogen (e.g., phytohemagglutinin). In other words, the weapon is loaded, but only mitogens and not antigens cause the trigger to be pulled. These studies also indicate that the central defect is lack of helper cell function, rather than an overabundance of suppressor cell activity. Other lymphocyte abnormalities observed with HIV-1 infection include decreased lymphokine production, decreased expression of interleukin-2 (IL-2) receptors, decreased alloreactivity, and decreased ability to provide help to B cells. The functional T lymphocyte abnormalities are also likely to contribute to the loss of delayed-type hypersensitivity reactions that become more prevalent as disease progresses.

The quantitative abnormality of T lymphocytes is the result of progressive depletion of the CD4+ helper T lymphocyte population (Table 407–1), which begins soon after primary infection. This downhill trend continues until the normal levels of 800 to 1200 CD4 cells per cubic millimeter drop below 50 cells per cubic millimeter and often lower than 10 cells per cubic millimeter in the later stages of disease. CD4 cell depletion cannot be attributed solely to direct cytotoxic effects of virus infection, because only a minority of helper cells are actually infected, even in later stages of illness. Other factors potentially contributing CD4 depletion include (1) syncytia formation, in which a single infected cell fuses via its surface gp120 with the CD4 molecule on uninfected cells, forming multinucleated giant cells; (2) "innocent bystander" destruction of uninfected CD4 cells that have bound free gp 120 to the CD4 molecule, rendering them susceptible to immune attack; (3) HIV-1 infection of stem cells or HIV–1-induced thymic depletion, resulting in decreased helper cell production; (4) autoimmune mechanisms, whereby cross-reactive antibodies or cellular immune responses to the virus result in killing of uninfected CD4 cells; (5) superantigen effects, in which a viral protein would be hypothesized to lead to stimulation and ultimately depletion of CD4 lymphocytes bearing a specific T cell receptor; and (6) apoptosis, whereby virus or viral products would induce programmed cell death (PCD). Whatever the mechanisms of the CD4 cell depletion, the resultant consequence to immune function is so profound that total CD4 number is an important prognosticator of disease progression. The risk of certain opportunistic infections increases significantly when the total CD4 cell number is lower than 200 per cubic millimeter, which is why routine prophylaxis against *Pneumocystis carinii* pneumonia (PCP) is instituted at this stage. At levels below 50 to 100 cells per cubic millimeter, the risk for other complications, such as disseminated mycobacterium avium or cytomegalovirus (CMV) infections, increases dramatically.

Lymphocytes also represent a very important reservoir of persistent infection. It is estimated that approximately one million CD4 lymphocytes in an infected person contain stably integrated provirus that is in a latent state but fully capable of replication when the cell is activated. Because these cells do not make viral proteins until they are activated, they are hidden from immune attack and are not susceptible to current antiviral drugs, and thus represent a substantial hurdle for ultimate eradication of the virus.

B Lymphocyte Abnormalities

As with T lymphocyte abnormalities in HIV-1 infection, the B lymphocyte abnormalities are both quantitative and qualitative. Most characteristic, particularly in the early stages of infection, is intense polyclonal activation of B cells, evidenced clinically by elevated levels of immunoglobulins G and A, the presence of

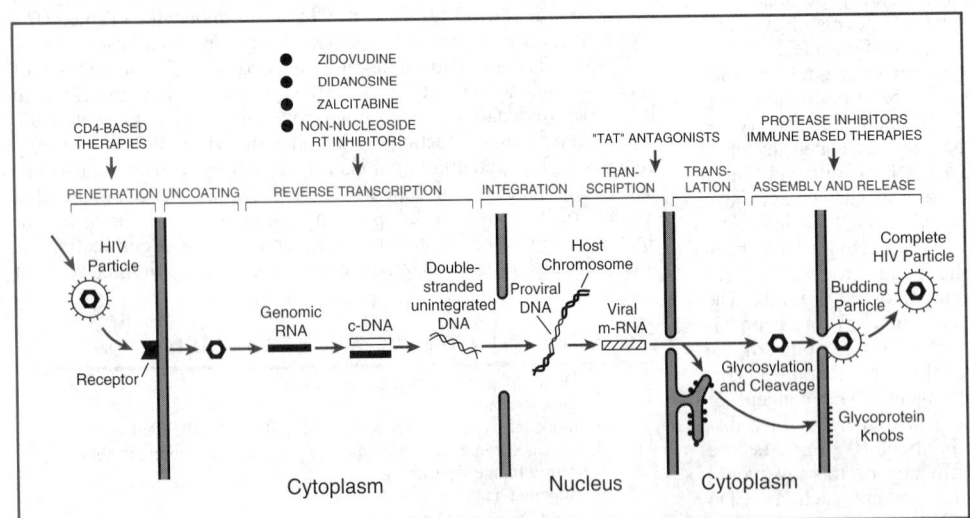

FIGURE 407–1 ■ The life cycle of HIV. The target sites for antiretroviral agents are shown. (Reprinted with permission from Johnson VA, Hirsch MS: *In* AIDS Clinical Review. New York, Marcel Dekker, 1990, p 238.)

circulating immune complexes, and an increased number of peripheral blood B lymphocytes that secrete immunoglobulin spontaneously. These B cell abnormalities are unlikely to be a direct consequence of HIV-1 infection of B cells. Whereas B cells can express low levels of CD4 and have been infected in vitro, there are no conclusive data indicating that these cells became infected in vivo. Rather, the virus itself or viral proteins appear to directly interact with and stimulate uninfected cells. Other potential contributors to this polyclonal activation include concurrent viral infections. For example, CMV and Epstein-Barr virus (EBV) infection occur with greatly increased frequency in HIV–1-infected individuals and can lead to B cell hyperactivity.

Functional abnormalities of B cells consist particularly of impaired antibody responses to antigenic stimuli, and impaired T cell helper function also may contribute to this problem. These impaired antibody responses may account for the increase in pyogenic infections seen in advanced HIV-1 infection. In addition, decreased antibody responsiveness to vaccination against viruses such as influenza A and hepatitis B is also characteristic of late-stage HIV infection.

Monocyte/Macrophage Abnormalities

It has been clearly demonstrated that HIV-1 also infects cells of the monocyte/macrophage lineage, which express CD4 as well as the coreceptor molecule CCR5. Infection and high-level replication of HIV-1 have also been demonstrated in monocyte/macrophage progenitor cells of normal bone marrow and may contribute to the pancytopenia seen with HIV infection. Unlike CD4 lymphocytes, however, macrophages appear to be relatively resistant to the cytopathic effects of HIV infection and may therefore constitute a persistent reservoir of infection. Macrophages may also play an important role in viral dissemination within the infected individual, in particular carrying virus across the blood-brain barrier to the central nervous system (CNS).

At least in part as a consequence of HIV infection, a number of monocyte/macrophage abnormalities have been detected in HIV-seropositive persons. The ability of monocyte/macrophages to act as antigen-presenting cells is impaired, particularly in later stages of illness. Some defects in these cells in AIDS patients may be a consequence of chronic in vivo activation, such as increased IL-2 receptor expression, IL-1 secretion, and increased chemotactic ligand receptor expression. The reasons for this chronic activation likely are multifactorial and may relate to exposure to viral proteins or lymphokines or to direct effects of HIV infection. These abnormalities may have immunopathogenic consequences, because defects in the ability to present antigens ultimately could impair the ability to sustain an immune response against HIV-1 or other pathogens.

In the brain, cells of the macrophage lineage appear to be the major cell type infected with HIV-1 and directly or indirectly may contribute to the CNS dysfunction observed in this disease. In the lung, infected alveolar macrophages may stimulate HIV–1-specific immune responses, the byproducts of which have been postulated to contribute to the observed alveolitis. Deficient CD4 T helper cell function also indirectly may contribute to the observed defects in monocyte/macrophages, because a minority of monocyte/macrophages appear to be actually productively infected in vivo.

Natural Killer Cell Abnormalities

Natural killer (NK) cells are thought to be an important component of immunosurveillance against virus-infected cells, allogeneic cells, and tumor cells. NK cells typically are large granular lymphocytes that recognize foreign antigens on cells, resulting in activation of lytic machinery. NK cells are phenotypically and numerically normal in AIDS patients, but they are functionally defective. This may relate in part to an observed defect in the trigger mechanism necessary to deliver the lethal blow to a target cell. In addition, defective lymphokine production in HIV–1-infected persons may also contribute to NK cell dysfunction. However, adding IL-2 to these cells in vitro only partially restores NK function.

Autoimmune Abnormalities

Autoimmune phenomena are also part of the immunologic derangement in HIV-1 infection and may also contribute to the disease manifestations seen clinically. When sensitive assays are used, circulating immune complexes can be detected in the majority of HIV-infected individuals. These may help to explain the occurrence of HIV–1-related arthralgias, myalgias, renal disease, and vasculitis.

VIRUS-SPECIFIC HOST IMMUNE RESPONSES (TABLE 407–2)

The initial phase of HIV-1 infection is characterized by high-level viremia, associated with the ability to detect the viral core protein p24 in the serum. However, soon after infection the level of viremia and p24 antigenemia rapidly decrease (see Fig. 407–6). A long period of relatively asymptomatic infection ensues, suggesting that virus-specific immune responses may play a role in limiting viral replication and thereby disease progression. With the AIDS epidemic now entering its third decade, identification of the precise protective components of anti-HIV immunity remains an elusive goal, although significant progress has been made.

Neutralizing Antibodies

HIV infection induces B lymphocytes to produce antibodies directed against viral proteins, and some of these antibodies are capable of neutralizing the virus. Antibody responses are typically observed 1 to 3 months after primary infection, although longer periods before antibody responses develop have been documented in rare instances. Neutralizing antibodies directly neutralize free virus at a stage before the virus has entered the cell and become uncoated. In a number of viral infections, neutralizing antibody induced by immunization correlates with protection from subsequent viral infection. HIV-1 infection results in the production of HIV-specific antibodies directed at a number of viral proteins, and some of these antibodies demonstrate neutralizing activity. The primary target of neutralizing antibodies is the envelope glycoprotein, in particular a loop structure within a relatively hypervariable region of the gp120 glycoprotein termed the principal neutralizing domain or V3 loop, as well as epitopes in the region involved in CD4 binding that recognize conformationally determined regions that are composed of discontinuous segments brought together in the tertiary structure of the envelope protein.

Neutralizing antibodies have been demonstrated to be present at all stages of HIV-1 infection, and although titers are generally lower in later stages of illness, attempts to correlate neutralizing antibody titers with disease progression have yielded conflicting results. Detailed studies in primary HIV-1 infection have demonstrated that antibodies capable of neutralizing the infecting strain of virus appear after clearance of the primary viremia, suggesting that other immune mechanisms may be important in the early control of viremia. In addition, it has been demonstrated that antibodies from infected persons at a given point in time tend to be poorly able to neutralize the infecting strain of virus, but much better at neutralizing laboratory strains of virus. Although a number of animal studies have shown that neutralizing antibodies can confer protection against viral challenge, this protection has been largely in highly idealized situations in which maximal titers were induced just prior to challenge and a low inoculum of virus was given intravenously. Whether induction of neutralizing antibodies alone would be able to confer protection against naturally acquired infection is not known, but it will be important for vaccine candidates to be able to induce these responses.

The ability of HIV-specific neutralizing antibodies to confer protection may be impaired in part by the high degree of antigenic variation exhibited by HIV. This antigenic variation is particularly pronounced in the envelope region of the virus, and virus variants may emerge within an infected individual that are neutralization resistant. This also has significant implications for vaccine design, because neutralizing antibodies generated in response to a single

Table 407–2 ▪ HIV-SPECIFIC IMMUNE RESPONSES

1. Neutralizing antibodies
2. Antibody-dependent cellular cytotoxicity
3. Cytotoxic T cells
4. Cellular proliferative responses

immunizing strain of virus are likely to neutralize only very closely related viruses, a phenomenon known as type specificity. New studies suggest that antibodies directed at the fusion complex of gp41 may be particularly able to neutralize widely divergent viruses, which offers encouragement that induction of more effective neutralizing antibodies may be a realistic goal.

Antibodies constitute the first line of defense at mucosal surfaces, in the form of secretory IgA. Such secretory antibodies have been found in blood, saliva, and other body fluids of persons infected with HIV, but their potential role as a protective immune response in HIV-1 infection remains undetermined.

Antibody-Dependent Cellular Cytotoxicity (ADCC)

Another mechanism the immune system can use to limit the spread of infection is ADCC, which involves both cellular and humoral components. ADCC is a process whereby virus-specific antibodies bind directly to viral proteins expressed on the surface of infected cells, thereby sensitizing these cells for lysis by cells that bind to the exposed Fc portion of the antibody. The cells mediating this response are typically NK cells, which express the CD16 Fc receptor for IgG. Antibodies that can mediate ADCC have been identified in the majority of HIV-infected individuals; these are present soon after seroconversion and are maintained throughout the disease course. It has been postulated that ADCC may limit cell-cell spread of virus by providing an early cytotoxic host defense. ADCC may correlate with better clinical stage in children born to infected mothers, and ADCC titers have been shown to be higher in early stages of infection in some studies. However, the contribution of this immune response to protection from disease progression remains unclear.

Cytotoxic T Lymphocytes (CTL)

Cytotoxic T lymphocytes have been demonstrated to be one of the protective host defenses generated in response to a number of viral infections. CTL can kill virus-infected cells by recognizing viral protein fragments on the infected cell surface, where these proteins form a trimolecular complex with a surface HLA molecule and $\beta 2$ microglobulin. CTL recognition of this complex leads to lysis and elimination of the infected cell.

Although the hallmark of HIV-1 infection is the development of profound immunosuppression, extremely vigorous HIV-1-specific CTL responses have been detected in the peripheral blood of infected individuals. These responses are directed not only against the major viral structural proteins, but also against the reverse transcriptase protein and regulatory proteins such as *vif* and *nef*. These responses appear to be mediated predominantly by CD8+ lymphocytes, which recognize processed HIV proteins on the surface of infected cells in conjunction with HLA class I (A,B,C) molecules.

A protective role for CTL has been demonstrated in numerous experimental models of viral infection, and emerging data indicate an antiviral role for CTL in HIV-1 infection. High levels of HIV-1-specific CTL are detected in acute infection, and their appearance correlates with initial control of viremia. There is at least indirect evidence to suggest that the CTL response might indeed retard disease progression. For example, CD8+ lymphocytes from HIV-infected individuals can inhibit HIV replication in autologous CD4 lymphocytes in vitro. Similar inhibitory CD8 cells have also been identified in simian immunodeficiency virus (SIV)-infected macaque monkeys, and in vivo depletion of these cells leads to dramatic increases in viremia. Recent studies of adoptively transferred CTL clones indicate that these cells migrate to infected cells in vivo. Other indirect evidence that CTL may be important in retarding disease progression stems from studies quantifying HIV-specific CTL in infected persons. As clinical disease progresses, CTL numbers decline, which could help to explain the observed increase in viremia observed in later stages of illness. More recently, new techniques that allow for direct visualization of CTL by flow cytometry indicate that there is a negative correlation between CTL responses and viral load. The detection of vigorous HIV-1-specific CTL responses in long-term nonprogressors who control viremia is further evidence for a protective role of these cells.

Cellular Proliferative Responses

T cell immunity to viral pathogens consists not only of cytotoxic T lymphocytes, but also helper T cell proliferation and cytokine production in specific responses to viral antigens. This CD4+ proliferative response generally is triggered by recognition of viral antigen in association with class II (HLA-D) molecules on the surface of antigen-presenting cells. Cross-sectional data indicate a negative association between viral load and T helper cell responses to the Gag protein, providing supportive evidence for a critical role of T helper cells in controlling viremia. Strong helper cell responses are associated with strong CTL responses, and it is likely that the antiviral effect of T helper cells is mediated through enhancing effects on CTL responses. The majority of infected persons lack strong HIV-1-specific T helper cell responses, but persons with acute HIV-1 infection who are treated with potent antiviral therapy before seroconversion all develop strong Gag-specific T helper cell responses. This observation has led to the hypothesis that a significant proportion of HIV-1-specific T helper cells are lost in the earliest stages of infection as they become activated, perhaps because HIV preferentially infects activated CD4 cells.

IMMUNOTHERAPY FOR HIV INFECTION (TABLE 407-3)

Recent studies in persons with long-term non-progressing infection suggest that the immune response to HIV may be of sufficient magnitude, in rare cases, to successfully contain the virus and prevent the development of disease. This observation has led to more focused attempts to reconstitute effective immunity in infected persons. Encouraging data showing that potent antiviral therapy can augment production of naïve CD4 cells, and may augment thymic function, provide further encouragement for these approaches.

A number of approaches for immune-based therapy are being investigated. Passive immunotherapy with immunoglobulins as well as HIV-1-specific gamma globulins and monoclonal antibodies may have direct antiviral effects, but efficacy may be limited because of lack of broad cross reactivity of antibody responses. Cytokines may serve to regulate immune responses as well as HIV-1 expression. Trials of intermittent IL-2 infusion are under way, as are trials of IL-12 therapy. Some in vitro studies have shown that IL-12 can restore some HIV-1-specific cell-mediated immune responses. Adoptive cellular therapy with autologous cloned HIV-1-specific CTL as well as polyclonal populations of CD8 cells are under way, and although efficacy has not yet been determined, the early data indicate that this approach seems to be safe and that infused CTL home to infected cells. Trials of adoptive therapy with autologous uninfected CD4 cells to correct the CD4 cell deficit are being planned.

PROSPECTS FOR VACCINE DEVELOPMENT (TABLE 407-4)

Ultimate global control of the HIV epidemic will likely require a vaccine that can elicit protective immunity. Although efforts to define the components of productive immunity in infected persons have been unsuccessful thus far, recent data from animal models of retrovirus infection indicate that a state of protective immunity may be an attainable goal. When immunized with an attenuated, *nef*-deleted SIV, rhesus macaques were found to be protected when subsequently challenged with wild-type pathogenic SIV. Not only were the animals protected from low-dose challenge, but they were also protected from high-dose challenge. Although the precise

Table 407-3 ■ IMMUNE-BASED INTERVENTIONS FOR HIV INFECTION

Passive immunity
Immunoglobulins
Monoclonal antibodies
Thymic hormones
Cytokine treatment
Interleukin-2
Tumor necrosis factor
Interferons
Interleukin-12
Adoptive cellular therapy
Therapeutic vaccination

Table 407–4 ■ POTENTIAL HIV-1 VACCINES IN CLINICAL TRIALS

1. Soluble protein/peptides
   gp160
   p24
   p17
   gp120
   V3 loop peptides
2. Recombinant live vaccines
   Vaccinia–HIV-1 gp160
   Canarypox gp160
3. Retroviral vectors
4. Pseudovirion vaccines
5. Whole inactivated HIV
6. DNA vaccines
7. Combination vaccines

mechanism whereby these animals were protected has not been determined, these results indicate that protective immunity may be an achievable goal for HIV-1 infection.

Despite these promising results in the SIV model of HIV-1 infection, a number of potential obstacles exist to the development of an effective AIDS vaccine (Table 407–5). Foremost among these is the genetic diversity of the viral genome. Most of this diversity occurs in the envelope gene, with as much as 20% divergence in nucleotide sequence among field isolates. Even within a single individual, multiple divergent strains of virus have been identified, reflecting an extremely high intrinsic mutation rate for the virus. The implications of such diversity for vaccine development are profound, because the virus acts as a moving target for any immune response that is generated. Another obstacle to be overcome is the type specificity of immune responses generated to candidate vaccines, because immune responses generated by an immunogen representing a single field isolate are unlikely to cross react with all field isolates. In addition, although some of the protein-based HIV-1 vaccine candidates have induced reasonably strong neutralizing antibodies when tested against laboratory strains of virus, these antibodies have been much less effective in neutralizing field isolates of HIV-1.

Once candidate immunogens are identified, animal testing for efficacy would be ideal, but may be difficult for a number of reasons. Although chimpanzees become infected with HIV-1, they do not generally develop disease. Rhesus macaques develop an immunodeficiency disease similar to AIDS when infected with SIV, but cannot be infected with HIV, are expensive to maintain, and are in limited supply. The potential utility of immunodeficient mice reconstituted with human fetal tissues, providing them with a "human" immune system, remains to be demonstrated. The biggest obstacle will be demonstration of efficacy, which will require large field trials in a population showing a high enough incidence of new infection that statistically significant data can be generated in a reasonable period. Demonstration of efficacy in one population may not translate to other populations. For example, protection of persons infected by sexual exposure will not necessarily imply that such a vaccine would protect intravenous drug abusers as well, who may be exposed to a higher initial inoculum of virus. As with HIV-infected persons, the potential for discrimination against vaccines due to positive serology will have to be addressed.

Although these obstacles exist, a number of clinical trials are already under way with a variety of vaccine candidates. These include soluble Gag or envelope proteins; recombinant vaccine virus containing the HIV-1 envelope gene; pseudovirion vaccines that resemble whole HIV particles but are modified to exclude the viral genome or render it harmless; retroviral vectors; and whole killed virus vaccines. A number of these approaches also are being evaluated as potential therapeutic vaccines in an attempt to improve the host immune response to the virus. Combinations of some of these

approaches also are under investigation, and appear to be the most promising. In subjects immunized with vaccinia–HIV-1 GP 160, dramatic increases in HIV-1 envelope antibodies were observed when vaccinees were boosted with recombinant gp 160 protein. Other approaches in various stages of development include use of recombinant vaccinia viruses. Modified vaccinia Ankara (MVA) looks particularly immunogenic. Given the potential importance of inducing mucosal immune responses, there also is interest in attenuated salmonella-HIV recombinants, which may be more effective at inducing mucosal immunity.

Autran B, Carcelain G, Li TS, et al: Positive effects of combined antiretroviral therapy on CD4+ T cell homeostasis and function in advanced HIV disease [see comments]. Science 277:112–116, 1997. *Treatment of persons with prolonged highly active antiretroviral therapy leads to the progressive generation of naïve CD4 lymphocytes. The possibility that these cells might be reeducated offers hope for immunotherapy and immune reconstitution.*

Brodie SJ, Lewinsohn DA, Patterson BK, et al: In vivo migration and function of transferred HIV–1-specific cytotoxic T cells. Nature Medicine 5:34, 1999. *This is the best demonstration that adoptively transferred CTL are able to home to sites of viral replication, indicating an antiviral role for these cells.*

Douek DC, McFarland RD, Keiser PH, et al: Changes in thymic function with age and during the treatment of HIV infection. Nature 396:690, 1998. *This study shows that the thymus continues to remain functional well into adult life, and that thymic production of naive cells is increased in persons treated with highly active antiviral therapy.*

Kahn JO, Walker BD: Acute human immunodeficiency virus type 1 infection. N Engl J Med 339:33–39, 1998. *A review of HIV pathogenesis in the early stages of infection.*

LaCasse RA, Follis KE, Trahey M, et al: Fusion-competent vaccines: Broad neutralization of primary isolates of HIV. Science 283:357–362, 1999. *This study shows that broadly cross-reactive neutralizing antibodies can be generated with an immunogen consisting of the fusion complex of the envelope glycoprotein.*

Letvin NL: Progress in the development of an HIV-1 vaccine. Science 280:1875–1880, 1998. *An excellent review article regarding the current state of vaccine development for HIV, and the problems being encountered.*

Ogg GS, Jin X, Bonhoeffer S, et al: Quantitation of HIV-1 specific cytotoxic T lymphocytes and plasma load of viral RNA. Science 279:2103–2106, 1998. *This study demonstrates that there is a negative correlation between CTL and viral load in HIV infection, and introduces a novel technology that allows for direct visualization of CTL by flow cytometry.*

Rosenberg ES, Billingsley JM, Caliendo AM, et al: Vigorous HIV–1-specific CD4+ T cell responses correlate with control of viremia. Science 278:1447, 1997. *This study demonstrates that virus-specific T helper cells are a critical host defense mechanism, and that early treatment of acute HIV infection results in the generation of these responses.*

Schmitz JE, Kuroda MJ, Santra S, et al: Control of viremia in simian immunodeficiency virus infection by CD8+ lymphocytes. Science 283:857–860, 1999. *Depletion of Cd8 cells and CTL leads to a dramatic increase in viral load in an animal model of AIDS virus infection. These data indicate that CTL are critical to maintaining the viral set point in chronic infection.*

---

408 BIOLOGY OF HUMAN IMMUNODEFICIENCY VIRUSES

George M. Shaw

DISCOVERY OF HUMAN IMMUNODEFICIENCY VIRUSES

The identification of HIV-1 as the causative agent of acquired immunodeficiency syndrome (AIDS) just 3 years after the clinical syndrome initially was described represents a remarkable scientific achievement that had its roots in earlier discoveries of animal and human retroviruses (see Chapter 388). The selective loss of CD4+ helper T lymphocytes in patients with the disease implicated an agent with T-lymphocyte cell tropism. As expected for an etiologic agent, HIV-1 was shown to be uniformly present in subjects with AIDS and to reproduce the hallmark of disease, destruction of T lymphocytes, in tissue culture.

GENERAL BIOLOGIC PROPERTIES OF HIV-1

Soon after its discovery, HIV-1 was shown to be biologically, structurally, and genetically distinct from human T-lymphotrophic virus I (HTLV-I) and HTLV-II and more like members of the

---

Table 407–5 ■ POTENTIAL OBSTACLES TO HIV VACCINE DEVELOPMENT

1. Genomic diversity of the viral genome
2. Type specificity of immune responses
3. Potential generation of enhancing antibodies
4. Lack of animal models of HIV infection and AIDS
5. Field trials to demonstrate efficacy
6. Idemnification of vaccinees from discrimination

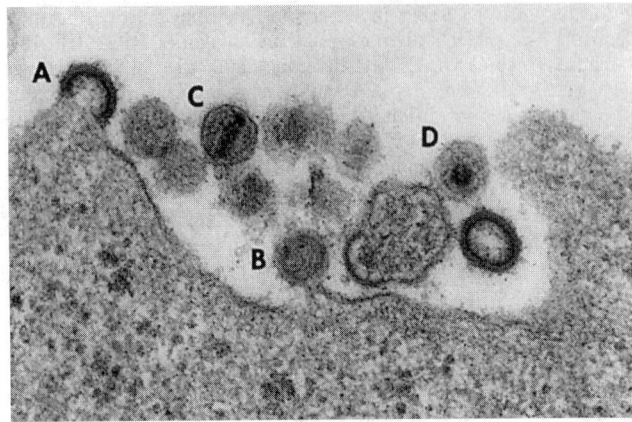

FIGURE 408–1 ■ Transmission electron micrograph of HIV-1. Virions are shown at all stages of morphogenesis: early (*A*) and late (*B*) budding forms and cell-free mature virions (*C* and *D*) with condensed central cores. The diameter of virions is approximately 110 nm.

lentivirus subfamily of retroviruses (see Chapter 388). Unlike the leukemia viruses, which lead to immortalization of lymphocytes in vitro and in vivo, HIV-1 exhibits pronounced cytopathic properties for lymphocytes, causing syncytia formation and cell death. Morphologically, HIV-1 differs from HTLV-I and other type C oncogenic retroviruses in exhibiting a dense, cylindrical core surrounded by a lipid envelope typical of lentiviruses (Fig. 408–1).

The structural organization of HIV-1 is shown diagrammatically in Figure 408–2. Like all retroviruses, HIV-1 is a single-stranded plus-sense RNA virus. The RNA-dependent DNA polymerase, or reverse transcriptase, is packaged within the virion core and is responsible for replicating the single-stranded RNA genome through a double-stranded DNA intermediate, which in turn serves as the precursor molecule for proviral integration within the host cell genome. The major structural core proteins of HIV-1 are the p24 capsid protein and the p18 matrix protein, as shown. Surrounding the viral core protein structures is a bilayered lipid envelope that is derived from the outer limiting membrane of the host cell as the virus buds from the cell surface during replication. Studding this outer viral membrane are the envelope glycoproteins, gp120

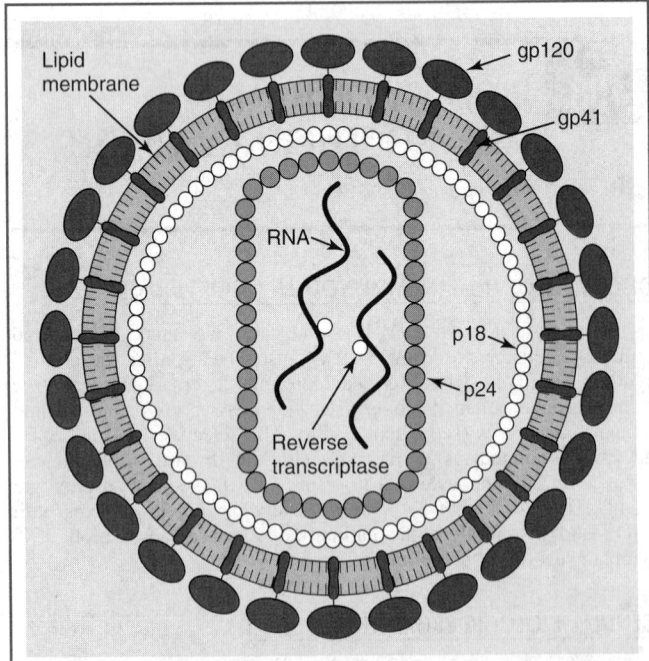

FIGURE 408–2 ■ Structure of HIV-1. (Adapted from RC Gallo. Copyright © 1987 by Scientific American, Inc., and George V. Kelvin. All rights reserved.)

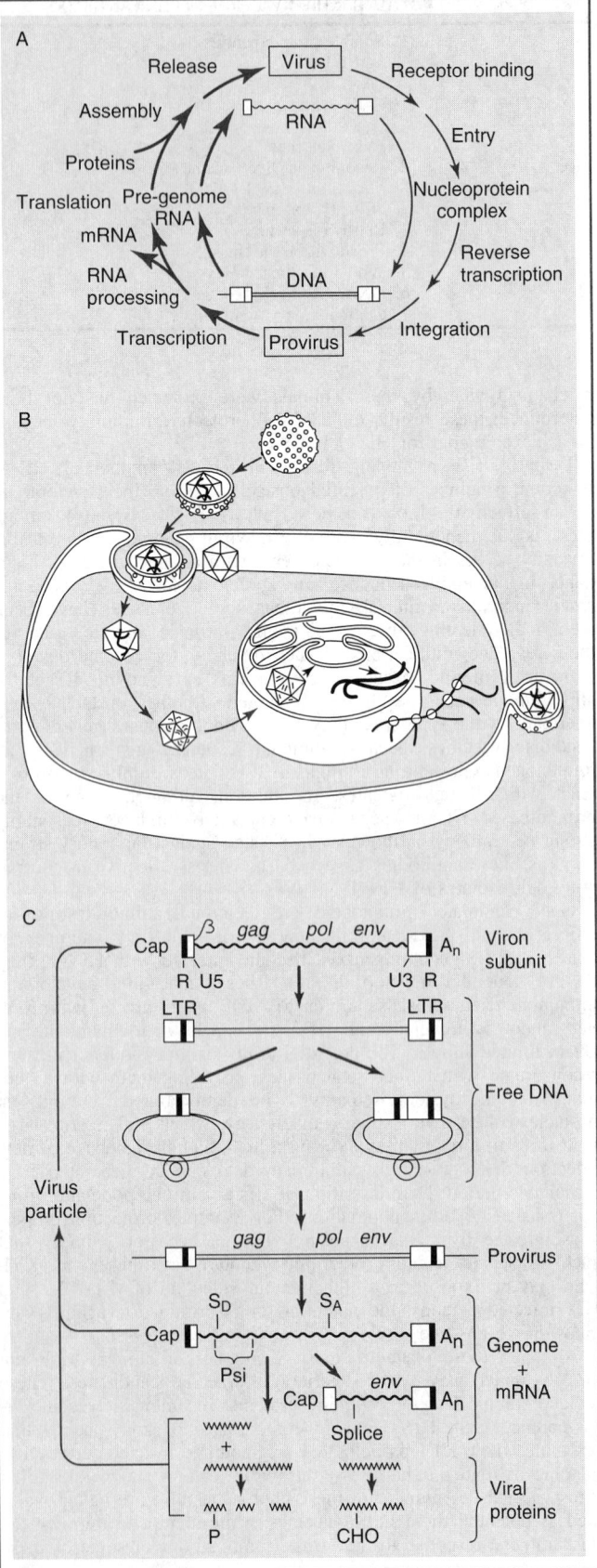

FIGURE 408–3 ■ Different representations of the HIV-1 life cycle. *A,* Thick arrows denote amplification of viral products that may occur in the latter half of the replication cycle. *B,* A pictorial overview of the virus life cycle outlined in *A. C,* A detailed illustration of the major transformations of retroviral genetic information during the life cycle. Cap denotes the 5' methyl-G-nucleotide, A_n the poly (A) tract, and S_D and S_A the splice donor and acceptor sites. Psi denotes the viral packaging signal sequence, P a phosphorylation site, and CHO a glycosylation site. (Reprinted with permission from Varmus H, Brown P: Retroviruses. *In* Berg DE, Howe MM [eds]: Mobile DNA. Washington, DC, American Society for Microbiology, 1989, p 53.)

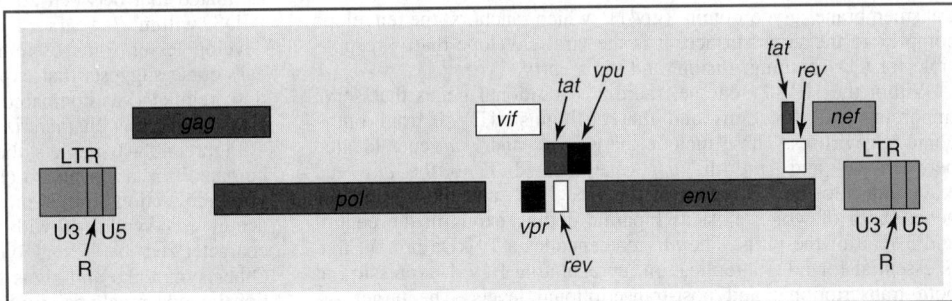

FIGURE 408-4 ■ Genomic organization of HIV-1.

and gp41, which are encoded by viral-specific genes and are responsible for cell attachment and entry.

The lifecycle of HIV-1 is shown diagrammatically in Figure 408-3. Features of this lifecycle distinguish retroviruses from all other viruses. The cell-free virion first attaches to the target cell through a specific interaction between the viral envelope and the host cell membrane. The specificity of this interaction between virus and cell has been shown to be due to a high-affinity specific interaction between the viral gp120 envelope glycoprotein and the target cell-associated CD4 molecule. Following virus adsorption, the viral and cellular membranes fuse, resulting in internalization of the nucleoprotein viral complex. Reverse transcription catalyzed by the viral reverse transcriptase generates a double-stranded DNA copy of the viral RNA within the nucleoprotein complex, and this migrates to the nucleus where covalent integration of viral DNA into the host chromosomes leads to formation of the provirus. Subsequent expression of viral DNA is controlled by a combination of viral and host cellular proteins that interact with viral DNA and RNA regulatory elements. Transcribed viral mRNA is translated into viral proteins, and new virions are assembled at the cell surface where genomic-length viral RNA, reverse transcriptase, structural and regulatory proteins, and envelope glycoproteins are assembled. Because the HIV-1 provirus is covalently integrated within the host cell chromosome, it represents a stable component of the host genome and is replicated and transmitted to daughter cells in synchrony with cellular DNA. Relevant to subsequent discussions of viral pathogenesis, the integrated provirus is thus permanently incorporated into the host cell genome and may remain transcriptionally latent or may exhibit high levels of gene expression with explosive production of progeny virus.

MOLECULAR STRUCTURE AND FUNCTION OF HIV-1

The genomic organization of HIV-1 is shown diagrammatically in Figure 408-4. The HIV-1 genome, like other retroviral genomes, is diploid, consisting of two identical viral RNA molecules assembled in a hydrogen-bonded 70S complex. These genomic subunits are plus strands of viral RNA in that they have the same chemical polarity as the mRNA from which viral products are translated. Like eukaryotic mRNAs, the genomic viral RNA con-

tains a 5′ methylated-G nucleotide, a poly(A) tract of 100 to 200 nucleotides at its 3′ end, and a number of methylated(A) residues. Host cell–derived tRNA incorporated within the virion is base paired over a stretch of 18 nucleotides to the primer binding site of the genomic viral RNA near its 5′ terminus and serves to prime the synthesis of minus-strand DNA during the initial stages of viral replication following infection.

The HIV-1 genome is bounded by long terminal repeat (LTR) elements and contains genes encoding structural and enzymatic proteins (*gag, pol,* and *env*) found in all other replication-competent retroviruses. In addition to these, however, HIV-1 contains genes encoding other viral functions unique to this family of viruses that are responsible for their biologic behavior. The LTR sequences of HIV-1 direct and regulate expression of the viral genome (Fig. 408-5).

The *gag* gene encodes a precursor protein of 55 kilodaltons (p 55), which is cleaved into four smaller products with the linear order NH$_2$-p18-p24-p9-p7-COOH. These proteins constitute the core protein structure of the virus and also subserve nucleic acid and lipid membrane binding functions. The *gag* proteins of HIV-1, like those of other retroviruses, are synthesized as a polyprotein precursor that subsequently is cleaved during the viral maturation process. This facilitates the assembly of the different components of the virus core structure into a three-dimensional configuration that, when cleaved by a specific virus-derived protease, acquires the specialized functions characteristic of the mature virion. The polymerase gene products are translated from the same genomic RNA message as the *gag* proteins but in a different, overlapping reading frame as a result of ribosomal frame shifting. The *pol* gene encodes three proteins that are cleaved from a larger precursor polypeptide. These genes include NH$_2$-protease(p13)-reverse transcriptase (p66/p51)-integrase(p31)-COOH. The HIV-1 protease plays a critical role in virus biology, acting specifically to cleave *gag* and *pol* precursor polypeptides into functionally active proteins. The reverse transcriptase of HIV-1 is a magnesium-requiring, RNA-dependent DNA polymerase responsible for replicating the RNA viral genome. The integrase protein is required for proviral integration into the host cell genome. The envelope gene *(env)* encodes a glycosolated polypeptide precursor (gp160) that is processed to form the exterior envelope glycoprotein (gp120) and the

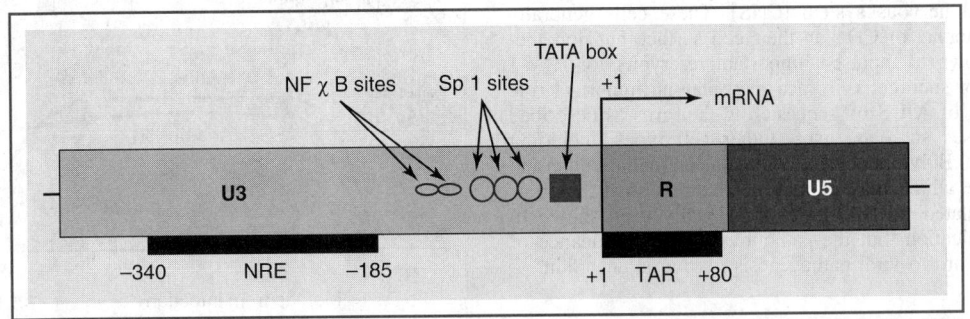

FIGURE 408-5 ■ Regulatory regions in the long terminal repeat (LTR) of HIV-1. Deletion mutant studies of the LTR have identified at least five regions for gene expression, including the TATA box and promotor where RNA polymerase binds and transcription is initiated (+1); a negative regulatory element (NRE) located between nucleotides −340 and −185, deletion of which increases the level of gene expression directed by the viral LTR; enhancer elements (NRκB and Sp 1) located between nucleotides −137 and −17; and a *trans*-acting responsive region (TAR) located between nucleotides +1 and +80 which represents the putative binding region for regulatory factors responsible for *tat*-mediated transcriptional activation.

transmembrane glycoprotein (gp41), which anchors the envelope complex to the virus surface. It is the viral envelope that is responsible for CD4 binding, fusion, and virus entry.

Within the HIV-1 genome, there are additional genes that serve important viral functions and that distinguish HIV-1 from oncogenic retroviruses. These include the *vif, vpr,* and *vpu* genes located between *pol* and *env;* the *nef* gene located 3' to the *env* and extending into the U3 region of the viral LTR; and the *tat* and *rev* genes, both of which exist as bipartite coding exons in the central and 3' end of the virus. The *tat* gene encodes a 14-kDa protein that is essential for HIV-1 replication, upregulating HIV-1 expression at both transcriptional and post-transcriptional levels. The target sequence for *tat*-mediated upregulation of HIV-1 expression is the *trans*-acting responsive region (TAR) of the LTR, which apparently interacts with cellular factors induced by *tat* because the *tat* protein itself has not been shown to bind and activate TAR directly. The *rev* gene is also absolutely required for HIV-1 replication, facilitating transport of unspliced viral mRNA from the nucleus to cytoplasm. In the absence of *rev* genes, *gag* and *env* mRNA, transcripts are multiply spliced such that *gag* and *env* proteins are not made. The *vif* gene encodes a protein product of 23 kDa, which is required for the production of virions that are fully infectious. The mechanisms of *vif* action are currently unknown. The *vpr* gene encodes a protein of 15 kDa which is involved in transport of the viral preintegration complex (see Fig. 408–3) to the nucleus. The *vpu* gene encodes a 16-kDa protein that is involved in virus assembly and release. The *nef* gene encodes a 27-kDa protein that decreases CD4 expression in virally infected cells, and by this or other means, accentuates viral pathogenesis in vivo.

In summary, HIV-1 encodes the usual structural and enzymatic proteins typical of other replication-competent retroviruses, including *gag, pol,* and *env,* but in addition it encodes a group of at least six regulatory or auxiliary proteins (*vif, vpr, vpu, tat, rev,* and *nef*) whose activities are critically important in regulating the lifecycle and pathogenesis of the virus.

CELL TROPISM

The hallmark of AIDS is a selective depletion of CD4+ helper-inducer lymphocytes. This defect is believed to result largely from the selective tropism of HIV-1 for this population of cells based on the high affinity of the viral gp120 envelope protein for the CD4 molecule (km = 4×10^{-0}M). CD4 normally serves as a ligand for MHC II (major histocompatibility complex type II) interaction, but in HIV-1 infection it is used as the primary receptor molecule for HIV-1 targeting. This has been shown conclusively by studies demonstrating (1) direct complexing of gp120 and CD4 during viral infection; (2) viral attachment and infection inhibited by anti-CD4 monoclonal antibodies that prevent gp120 binding; (3) the ability of recombinant CD4 to confer susceptibility to HIV-1 infection to transfected human cells that normally do not express CD4 (e.g., HeLa cells).

A variety of cell types other than helper-inducer lymphocytes are known to express CD4 on their surface and are capable of replicating HIV-1. These include blood monocytes, tissue macrophages, Langerhans cells in skin, and microglial and multinucleated giant cells in the central nervous system (CNS). These cells generally express smaller amounts of CD4 on their cell surface but nonetheless have been shown to represent important reservoirs for HIV-1 in vivo. Infection of such cells, in fact, may play an important role in the pathogenesis of AIDS by sequestering the virus as described for other lentiviruses such as visna. Other cell types, including neurons, glial cells, B lymphocytes, colorectal epithelial cells, and myeloid precursors, which may or may not express small amounts of CD4 or CD4-related mRNA, have occasionally been shown to support HIV-1 replication, but the pathophysiologic significance of such findings in regard to viral pathogenesis in vivo is uncertain.

VIRAL PATHOGENESIS

Retroviral diseases are typically characterized by restricted viral gene expression, latency, and lifelong persistence of virus in the face of substantial host immune responses. From cohort studies of individuals infected with HIV-1 at known points in time, it is estimated that between 26 and 36% of infected individuals develop AIDS within 7 years of infection and that an additional 40% develop lesser signs of immune dysfunction. This protracted clinical course suggests that expression of the HIV-1 genome in vivo is downregulated as compared to in vitro infection of lymphocytes by HIV-1, which is characterized by explosive lytic viral infection.

Figure 408–6 depicts the natural history of HIV-1 infection of humans in relationship to clinical symptoms, immune function, and viral replication. Initial infection with HIV-1 frequently causes an acute viral syndrome with protean manifestations most frequently characterized by fever, lymphadenopathy, pharyngitis, and rash. Other symptoms and signs that may occur with acute HIV-1 infection include myalgias and arthalgias, leukopenia, thrombocytopenia, nausea, diarrhea, headache, and encephalopathy. During this primary phase of infection, symptoms are accompanied by high-level HIV-1 plasma viremia, with peak titers reaching 10^7 virions per milliliter. Viremia is also accompanied by high levels of circulating HIV-1 p24 antigen, only part of which is virion-associated, the remainder circulating alone or complexed with immunoglobulin. Studies of individuals who have become infected with HIV-1 at defined points in time have shown that there is a relatively prolonged "window" period ranging from 2 weeks to 6 months during which patients remain antibody-negative. During this time, they may or may not have symptoms of acute infection prompting medical attention. Generally, such patients become p24 antigenemic in the few days or weeks immediately preceding seroconversion. Subsequently, antibodies to viral core and envelope proteins appear coincident with resolution of clinical symptoms. An important recent finding regarding HIV-1 pathogenesis is that viral replication is only partially controlled in the months and years following infection and seroconversion. That is, the initial high levels of virus produced in lymphoid tissues and circulating in plasma in titers of 10^6 to 10^7 virions per milliliter decrease only to levels of 10^3 to 10^5 virions per milliliter. This indicates that even during the clinically quiescent stages of infection substantial viral replication ensues, leading to progressive CD4 cell destruction. This serves as the rationale for clinical studies examining the utility of antiviral therapy earlier in the disease process.

The protracted clinical course of HIV-1 infection raises clinically relevant questions regarding viral pathogenesis: What are the mechanisms responsible for CD4+ cell loss in vivo? What are the viral and host interactions that underlie the chronicity of HIV-1 infection? The precise biologic mechanisms responsible for the cytopathic effects of HIV-1 in vivo are not known. Molecularly cloned HIV-1 proviral DNA, transfected into human cells, has been shown in cell culture experiments to contain all necessary information to generate infectious and cytopathic virus. Thus, there is no question that HIV-1 alone has the potential for direct cytopathic activity against CD4+ lymphocytes in vitro and in vivo. Expression of

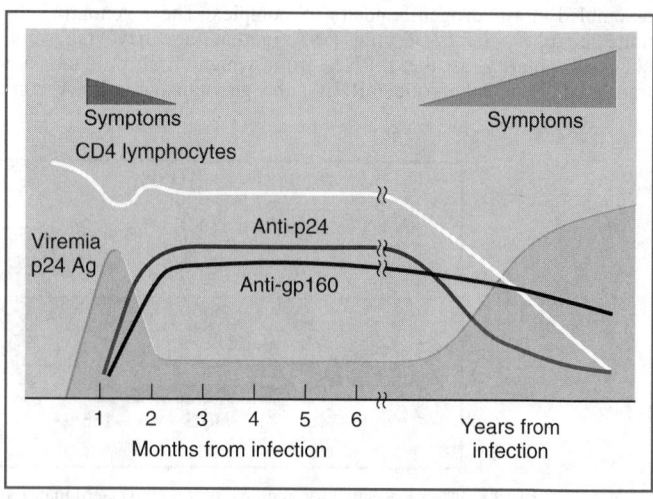

FIGURE 408–6 ■ Natural history model for HIV-1 infection. Viremia denotes cell-free infectious virus in plasma, p24 Ag denotes circulating viral p24 antigen in plasma, and anti-p24 and anti-gp 160 correspond to antibodies to viral core and envelope proteins.

only the HIV-1 envelope on lymphocytes is sufficient for inducing fusion of cells with normal uninfected CD4+ bystander cells, suggesting that syncytium formation mediated by gp120-CD4 interaction may also contribute to cell loss in vivo. However, other mechanisms of CD4 cell loss may also be operative. Cell-free HIV-1 gp120 envelope protein has been shown to adsorb to CD4+ cells and could serve as an effective antigen for mediating antibody-dependent cell-mediated cytotoxicity, and when processed by antigen-presenting cells, to constitute a target for direct T-cell cytotoxicity. The relative importance of these processes to CD4 cell loss in vivo remains to be determined. Similarly, in the CNS of infected individuals, wherein the predominant cell types infected with HIV-1 are cells of the monocyte/macrophage lineage, additional mechanisms of cytopathology are likely involved. Possibilities include the elaboration of cytotoxic factors from infected cells and interference with neurotropic factors both leading to the clinically recognized AIDS dementia complex.

Viral and host factors responsible for the partial downregulation of HIV-1 replication following initial infection are also largely unknown. A strong humoral and cellular immune response to HIV-1 has been documented on the basis of ELISA, immunoblot, and radioimmunoprecipitation assays of patient sera and cell-mediated cytotoxicity to target cells displaying viral antigens. Neutralizing antibodies, antibody-dependent cell-mediated cytotoxicity, antibody-dependent complement-mediated cytotoxicity, MHC-restricted virus-specific cytotoxic T-lymphocyte-mediated cytotoxicity, and NK cell-mediated cytotoxicity have all been found to have activity against HIV-1 in vitro and may play an important role in the downmodulation of viral replication. However, the relative efficacy of the various immune effector arms and the changes that occur with time which eventually allow uncontrolled viral replication are unknown.

An additional component of the viral-host interaction of potentially great clinical importance is the regeneration capacity of the immune system. Recent studies of the clinical effects of novel, potent inhibitors of HIV-1 reverse transcriptase and protease genes indicate that patients with even severely depressed CD4 lymphocyte counts can experience substantial increases in such cells. Such responses have been of limited duration, however, owing to the development of viral resistance to these drugs. Yet they illustrate the potential benefits that may accrue if more effective antivirals are developed.

Genetic variability is a hallmark of HIV-1. The variability of the HIV-1 genome is characteristic of retroviruses in general because reverse transcription of viral RNA into proviral DNA and transcription of proviral DNA into genomic viral RNA are not subject to cellular proofreading mechanisms. The rate of nucleotide misincorporation by the viral reverse transcriptase is of the order of 10^{-4} per nucleotide per replication cycle. Because the HIV-1 genome is 10^4 nucleotides in length, this high rate of nucleotide misincorporation means that virtually no two viruses are identical and that HIV-1 isolates must, by definition, be described in terms of a "quasispecies" composed of populations highly related by distinct viral genomes. Direct nucleotide sequence analysis of uncultured, virally infected human tissues using polymerase chain reaction amplification has confirmed these findings. The clinical importance of HIV-1 variability is still not fully understood. However, it is clear that viral resistance to reverse transcription inhibitors and protease inhibitors commonly develops and limits the effectiveness of these agents. Antigenic properties of the virus may also vary, thereby limiting the effectiveness of the immune response. Moreover, genetic variability leads to biologic changes in the virus over time, frequently resulting in the accumulation of virus strains with pronounced syncytium-including (SI) phenotypes in late stages of infection. Such a switch from non-SI to SI virus strains in vivo carries a worsened clinical prognosis.

HUMAN IMMUNODEFICIENCY VIRUS TYPE 2

Following the discovery of HIV-1 as the cause of epidemic AIDS in the United States, Europe, and Asia, patients in West Africa with AIDS-like symptoms were identified whose sera reacted more strongly with an immunodeficiency virus (SIV_{MAC}) isolated from captive rhesus macaques in US primate centers than with HIV-1. The identification of patients with serologic reactivity

for SIV_{MAC} raised the possibility that certain African human and simian populations could be infected with immunodeficiency viruses related to but distinct from HIV-1. An extensive survey of African primate species for such viruses led to the identification of distinct SIV viruses in African green monkeys (SIV_{AGM}), mandrills (SIV_{MND}), sooty mangabeys (SIV_{SM}), and chimpanzees (SIV_{CPZ}) (Fig. 408–7). West African patients with AIDS-like symptoms and healthy individuals at risk for AIDS were identified who were infected with a virus closely related to SIV_{SM}. This virus was isolated, molecularly cloned and characterized, and shown to represent a second major class of human immunodeficiency viruses termed HIV-2. Although originally limited geographically to West Africa, HIV-2 has now been identified in patients in Europe, the United States, South America, and India. HIV-2 is approximately 40 to 50% similar to HIV-1 in overall nucleotide sequence homology. There are two major differences in the genomic organization of HIV-1 and HIV-2. The *vpu* gene of HIV-1 is not present in HIV-2, and HIV-2 contains an additional gene, *vpx*, in a central region that is not present in HIV-1. Although the function of *vpx* is not entirely clear, it is packaged in the viral particle, like *vpr*, and it may have a similar function related to nuclear transport or processing of the viral preintegration complex. Antigenically, HIV-2 and HIV-1 are distinct, with greatest cross reactivity in structural proteins and least in envelope proteins. Currently licensed ELISA tests to detect HIV-1 infection generally include HIV-2 antigens. However, confirmation requires specific testing by Western immunoblot using HIV-2–specific proteins as antigen. Like HIV-1, HIV-

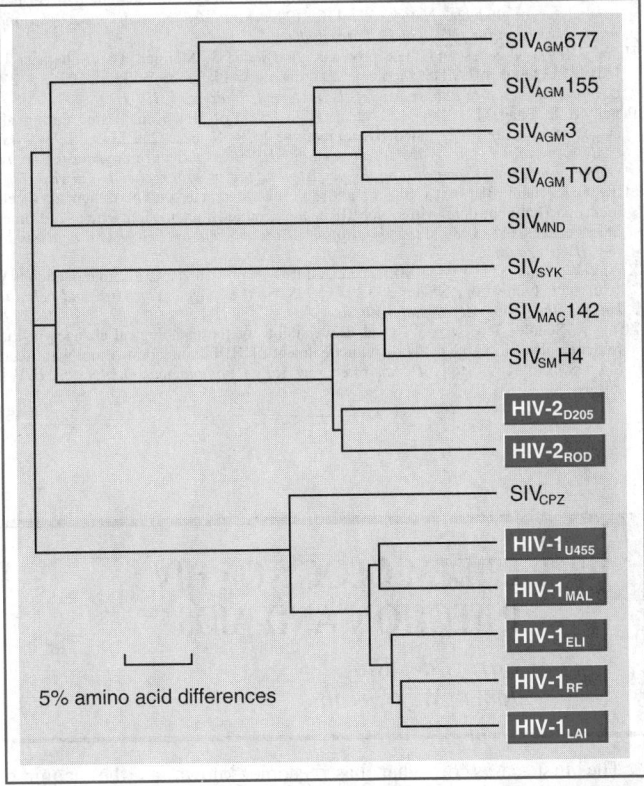

FIGURE 408–7 ■ Phylogenetic relationships among primate lentiviruses, inferred from *pol* protein sequences. Independent isolates of SIV obtained from African green monkeys (AGM), mandrill (MND), Sykes' (SYK), rhesus macaque (MAC), sooty mangabey (SM), and chimpanzee (CPZ) are depicted along with representative isolates of HIV-1 and HIV-2 (boxed). The horizontal branch lengths are drawn to scale and can be used to determine the percentage difference in *pol* protein sequences between the different virus strains. The figure shows five major and roughly equidistant phylogenetic lineages of viruses (SIV_{AGM}; SIV_{MND}; SIV_{SYK}; SIV_{MAC}/SIV_{SM}/HIV-2; and SIV_{CPZ}/HIV-1). HIV-1 and HIV-2 appear as members of larger viral lineages composed of both simian- and human-derived viruses. Such relationships are indicative of cross-species transmission. (Adapted with permission from Hahn BH: Viral genes and their products. *In* Broder S, Merigan TC, Bolognesi D [eds]: Textbook of AIDS Medicine. Baltimore, Williams & Wilkins, 1994, p 21.)

2 selectively infects CD4+ cells. Although HIV-2 can cause profound immunodeficiency and an AIDS syndrome indistinguishable from that caused by HIV-1, evidence suggests that HIV-2 may in general be less virulent than HIV-1 and cause disease over a more prolonged period of time.

The discovery of two distinct types of human immunodeficiency viruses (HIV-1 and HIV-2) having closely related counterparts in African primates (SIV_{CPZ} chimpanzees and SIV_{SM} in wild-caught sooty mangabeys, respectively), along with epidemiologic findings revealing Africa as the geographic source of all human and SIVs, suggest cross-species (zoonotic) infection for the origin of HIV-1 and HIV-2. This conclusion is strengthened by a molecular phylogenetic analysis of the genomes of all known primate lentiviruses (Fig. 408–7). This figure indicates that HIV-1 and HIV-2 are members of a much larger group of lentiviruses that infect a number of different primate species in the wild. It is apparent that the closest phylogenetic relative of HIV-1 is SIV_{CPZ}, and for HIV-2, is SIV_{SM}. Nevertheless, it is premature to conclude that the chimpanzee and sooty mangabey are the proximal hosts for the human viruses because other primate species in Africa remain to be evaluated and could also serve as natural reservoirs. Such studies are fundamentally important to the elucidation of the origin of the current AIDS epidemic, the molecular basis for the pathogenicity of HIVs and SIVs in natural and unnatural host species, and an explanation for the relatively recent appearance of AIDS as an epidemic.

Gallo RC, Salahuddin SZ, Popovic M, et al: Frequent detection and isolation of cytopathic retroviruses (HTLV-III) from patients with AIDS and at risk for AIDS. Science 224:500, 1984. *Initial report conclusively identifying HIV-1 as the etiologic agent responsible for AIDS.*
Gao F, Bailer E, Robertson DL, et al: Origin of HIV-1 in the chimpanzee Pan troglodyter troglodyter. Nature 397:436, 1999. *First definition of the origin and primary revision for HIV-1 in P. T. troglodytes.*
Hahn BH: Viral genes and their products. *In* Broder S, Merigan TC, Bolognesi D (eds.): Textbook of AIDS Medicine. Baltimore, Williams & Wilkins, 1994, p 21. *Comprehensive up-to-date review of the molecular biology of HIV-1.*
Piatak M Jr, Saag MS, Yang LC, et al: High levels of HIV-1 in plasma during all stages of infection determined by competitive PCR. Science 259:1749, 1993. *First study to accurately and systematically quantify HIV-1 in plasma throughout the entire course of infection, demonstrating the persistent nature of viral replication in vivo.*
Shaw GM, Hahn BH, Arya SK, et al: Molecular characterization of human T-cell leukemia (lymphotropic) virus type III in the acquired immunodeficiency syndrome. Science 226:1165, 1984. *First description of the molecular cloning and analysis of the HIV-1 provirus.*
Xiping W, Sajal KG, Taylor ME, et al: Viral dynamics in human immunodeficiency virus type 1 infection. Nature 373:117, 1995. *First description of viral and cellular kinetics underlying HIV-1 pathogenesis.*
Zhang Z, Schuler T, Covert W, et al: Reversibility of the pathological changes in the follicular dendritic cell network with treatment of HIV-1 infection. Proc Natl Acad Sci USA 96:5169, 1999. *Demonstrates reversal of pathological changes in HIV-1 disease.*

409 EPIDEMIOLOGY OF HIV INFECTION AND AIDS

Carlos del Rio
James W. Curran

The first cases of what has become known as the acquired immunodeficiency syndrome (AIDS) were reported in mid-1981 from Los Angeles, California. One month following these five reports of *Pneumocystis carinii* pneumonia (PCP) in young homosexual men, 26 cases of Kaposi's sarcoma (KS) in homosexual men in New York and California and additional cases of PCP and other opportunistic infections were reported. Reports of cases in the United States continued to rise, and soon the occurrence of PCP, KS, or other serious opportunistic infections in a person with unexplained immune dysfunction became known as AIDS. In retrospect, sporadic cases may have occurred in the United States, Europe, or Africa as much as three decades earlier, but the worldwide epidemic was not apparent until the 1980s.

The initial occurrence of AIDS in homosexual men and injecting drug users (IDUs) suggested by 1982 that a transmissible agent

was the likely cause. The transmissible agent hypothesis gained credence by early 1983 with the documented occurrence of AIDS in persons with hemophilia and in recipients of blood transfusions. Within a year, the retrovirus, now termed human immunodeficiency virus (HIV), was isolated and shown to be the cause of AIDS.

Recent data support the theory that the HIV virus originated in Africa. Blood obtained in 1959 from an adult Bantu man in the Democratic Republic of Congo represents the oldest known HIV-1 virus infection.

HIV INFECTION AND AIDS IN THE UNITED STATES

Through December of 1997, the United Nations AIDS Programme (UNAIDS) and the World Health Organization (WHO) estimate that over 30 million people are living with HIV infection worldwide, with the overwhelming majority living in developing countries and most not knowing that they are infected. Since 1981 and through November of 1997 more than 1.7 million cases of AIDS have been reported from 197 countries. More than 35% of these were reported from the United States, reflecting the relatively high incidence of the syndrome here and a well-established, national active surveillance system. All 50 states require that AIDS be reported to state health departments and subsequently without names to the Centers for Disease Control and Prevention (CDC). The surveillance case definition for AIDS initially was developed before its cause was known, but was revised following the development of diagnostic tests for HIV infection and the widespread use of CD4 lymphocyte monitoring in clinical management of persons with HIV disease. The current definition provides a consistent method to monitor trends of serious HIV-associated morbidity and mortality (Tables 409–1 and 409–2). Patients infected with HIV exhibit a spectrum of manifestations ranging from no symptoms to AIDS. Systems have been developed to classify these manifestations in children and adults. Twenty-seven states also require reporting of all HIV infections. Because of the changing nature of the disease and due to the fact that currently available drugs may prevent the patient from developing an advanced immunodeficiency, there is a renewed interest in adding HIV infection to AIDS case reporting nationwide. However, different issues, such as confidentiality, have prevented this from being implemented uniformly throughout the United States.

INDICENCE AND TRENDS OF AIDS IN THE UNITED STATES

By December 1997, 641,086 cases of AIDS in adults and children had been reported to the CDC; and >390,000 were reported to have died, including >80% of those diagnosed before 1990. In 1996, for the first time in the epidemic, the number of persons diagnosed with an AIDS opportunistic infection as well as the number of deaths among persons with AIDS declined. The recently available antiretroviral treatments as well as the success of a variety of preventive interventions are credited with these declines. The rates of reported AIDS cases vary substantially by age, gender, race-ethnicity, and geographic region, emphasizing that the epi-

Table 409–1 ■ **1993 REVISED CLASSIFICATION SYSTEM FOR HIV INFECTION AND EXPANDED AIDS SURVEILLANCE CASE DEFINITION FOR ADOLESCENTS AND ADULTS***

	CLINICAL CATEGORIES		
$CD4^+$ T-cell categories	(A) Asymptomatic, acute (primary) HIV or PGL†	(B) Symptomatic, not (A) or (C) conditions	(C) AIDS-indicator conditions
(1) ≥500/μL	A1	B1	C1
(2) 200–449/μL	A2	B2	C2
(3) <200/μ AIDS-indicator T-cell count	A3	B3	C3

*Shaded areas indicate conditions included in the 1993 AIDS surveillance case definition for adolescents and adults. Clinical conditions in C are listed in Table 409–2.

†PGL = persistent generalized lymphadenopathy.

Bacterial infections, multiple or recurrent*
Candidiasis of bronchi, trachea, or lungs
Candidiasis, esophageal
Cervical cancer, invasive†
Coccidioidomycosis, disseminated or extrapulmonary
Cryptococcosis, extrapulmonary
Cryptosporidiosis, chronic intestinal (>1 month duration)
Cytomegalovirus disease (other than liver, spleen, or nodes)
Cytomegalovirus retinitis (with loss of vision)
Encephalopathy, HIV-related
Herpes simplex, chronic ulcer(s) (>1 month duration); or bronchitis, pneumonitis, or esophagitis
Histoplasmosis, disseminated or extrapulmonary
Isosporiasis, chronic intestinal (>1 month duration)
Kaposi's sarcoma
Lymphoid interstitial pneumonia and/or pulmonary lymphoid hyperplasia*
Lymphoma, Burkitt's (or equivalent term)
Lymphoma, immunoblastic (or equivalent term)
Lymphoma, primary, of brain
Mycobacterium avium complex or *M. kansasii,* disseminated or extrapulmonary
Mycobacterium tuberculosis, any site (pulmonary† or extrapulmonary)
Mycobacterium, other species or unidentified species, disseminated or extrapulmonary
Pneumocystis carinii pneumonia
Pneumonia, recurrent†
Progressive multifocal leukoencephalopathy
Salmonella septicemia, recurrent
Toxoplasmosis of brain
Wasting syndrome due to HIV

*Children <13 years old.
†Added in the 1993 expansion of the AIDS surveillance case definition for adolescents and adults.

demic in the United States (as well as in the world) is not one epidemic but the product of "hundreds of epidemics" of varying intensity. Figure 409–1 depicts 1997 case rates by gender throughout the United States, highlighting these substantial geographic disparities.

Among AIDS cases reported in 1997, 35% of those in adults were homosexual or bisexual men and 24% were IDUs. Heterosexual contact was responsible for 7% of cases among men and 38% of cases among women; it is estimated that heterosexual sex has now surpassed injecting drug use as the major risk factor for HIV infection among women. However, sex with an IDU was identified as the risk factor in 27% of cases of heterosexually acquired AIDS in 1997 and, thus, the heterosexual epidemic in the United States remains closely linked to drug use. Less than 1% of AIDS cases notified in 1997 have hemophilia or other coagulation disorders; 1% of cases were associated with transfusion of blood, blood components, or tissue transplantation. Most transfusion-associated AIDS cases in the United States received the infected blood prior to 1985, when HIV antibody screening of all blood and plasma donations was instituted; however, 37 adults and 2 children have developed AIDS after receiving blood that was screened negative for HIV antibodies, and 13 adults have developed AIDS after receiving tissue, organs, or artificial insemination from HIV-infected donors. Four of the 13 received these from a donor who was negative for HIV antibodies at the time of donation. The proportion of AIDS cases initially reported without risk information has increased in recent years, especially among women. However, after investigation, most of these cases are reclassified within the usual risk categories.

By December 1997, a total of 8086 cases of AIDS had been reported in children younger than age 13 years, with 58% reported to have died. Most pediatric AIDS cases are the result of perinatal transmission of HIV infection. However, as a consequence of implementation in 1994 of the results of the ACTG 076 trial—the U.S./France multicenter study that proved that zidovudine given to the HIV-infected mother could reduce by 66% the risk that the infant also will become infected—there has been a dramatic reduction in the number of perinatally acquired HIV/AIDS cases. In the United States, the number of infants under 1 year of age diagnosed with AIDS decreased from 905 cases in 1992 to 516 cases in 1996.

AIDS has disproportionately affected black and Hispanic minor-

ity populations in the United States. In 1997, 45% of reported adult/adolescent cases (40% of reported cases among men and 61% among women) and 62% of pediatric cases were black. That same year, 21% of adult/adolescent and 23% of pediatric cases were among Hispanics. In contrast, blacks and Hispanics are estimated to account for 11% and 9% of the U.S. population, respectively.

In 1997, AIDS rates were approximately 20 and 7 times higher for black and Hispanic women than for white women. The rates for black and Hispanic men were 7 and 3 times higher than for white men. Racial disparities in pediatric AIDS rates reflect those in women (Table 409–3). HIV infection and AIDS cases continue to increase more rapidly in those racial-ethnic minority populations, particularly in association with injecting drug use and heterosexual transmission.

Because AIDS related deaths have declined markedly, the prevalence of HIV/AIDS has actually increased in the United States. The CDC estimates that approximately 250,000 people are living with AIDS, of which 40% are white, non-Hispanic; 38% are black; and 20% are Hispanic.

HIV infection has had a large impact on mortality in young adults in the United States. By 1992, HIV infection had become the leading cause of death in men in the 25- to 44-year-old age group and the fourth leading cause of death in women in that age group in the United States. The number of deaths due to HIV/AIDS peaked in the United States in 1995 with 50,700—three quarters of which was in the 25- to 44-year-old age group. In 1996, the number of AIDS-related deaths declined 23% to 39,200 (Fig. 409–2); however, this decline has been more marked among whites (33%) than among blacks or Hispanics (13% and 20%, respectively). AIDS is now the second leading cause of death among people between the ages of 25 and 44 years, following unintentional injuries.

PREVALENCE AND INCIDENCE OF HIV INFECTION IN THE UNITED STATES

Trends in reported AIDS cases do not provide a complete picture of the prevalence of the public health problem that HIV infection poses for a population group, community, or nation, because HIV infection per se precedes the clinical diagnosis of AIDS by many years. In some groups, reported AIDS continues to increase after HIV infection has declined. For example, despite very dramatic declines in HIV incidence associated with blood and plasma transfusions after 1985, when antibody screening of blood donations was instituted in the United States, reported cases of AIDS associated with transfusions and in persons with hemophilia continued to increase through the end of the decade. Conversely, reported AIDS case rates may underestimate greatly the future impact of HIV infection, especially in communities or populations more recently affected by the epidemic. Most notable are the emerging HIV infection epidemics in Thailand, India, Viet Nam, and other areas of Asia, where few cases of AIDS have reached the clinical horizon. For this reason, AIDS surveillance must be accompanied by carefully conducted HIV serosurveys to accurately monitor the public health problem.

Estimates of the prevalence of HIV infection in the United States by the U.S. Public Health Service (USPHS) in 1997 are between 750,000 and 900,000. In addition, it is estimated that approximately 0.6% of men and 0.1% of women are infected; however, the prevalence is much higher for blacks, where 2% of men and 0.6% of women are estimated to be infected. These estimates were based on both available HIV seroprevalence data and on statistical models using AIDS surveillance data and information on the natural history of infection.

National data on HIV prevalence have been directly measured from HIV testing of first-time blood donors, military recruit applicants, job corps applicants, and surveys of antibody status of newborn infants. The prevalence of HIV infection in both military recruit applicants and blood donors grossly underestimates true HIV prevalence rates because homosexual men, IDUs, and persons with hemophilia are discouraged from applying for military service and actively deferred from donating blood.

The highest HIV prevalence rates detected have been among

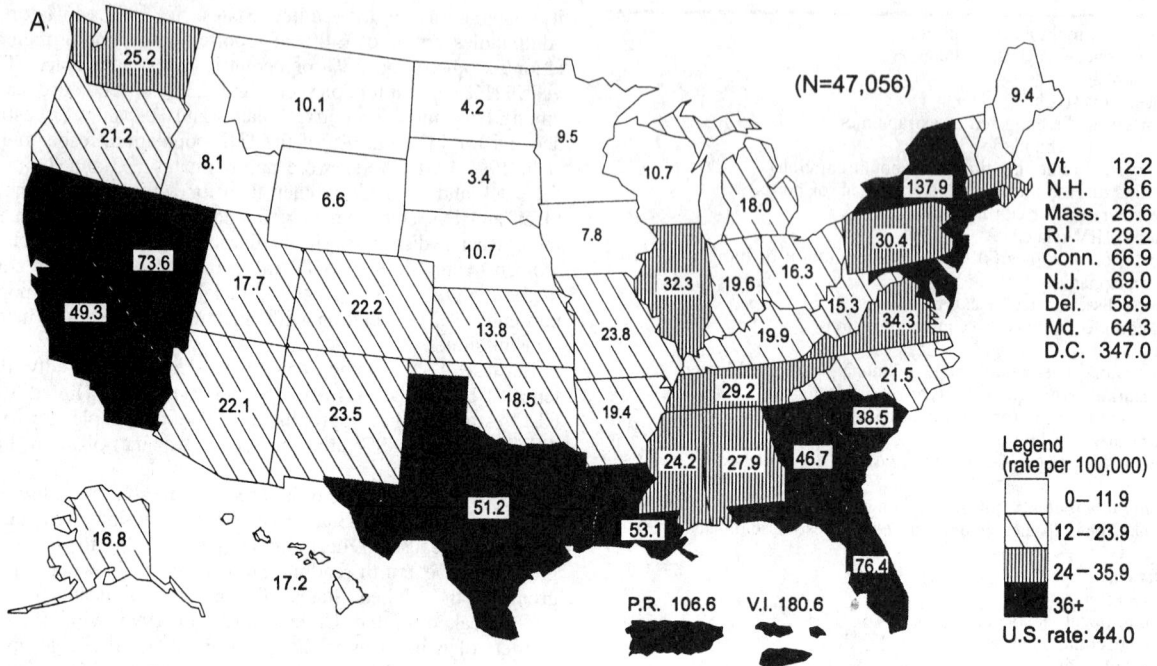

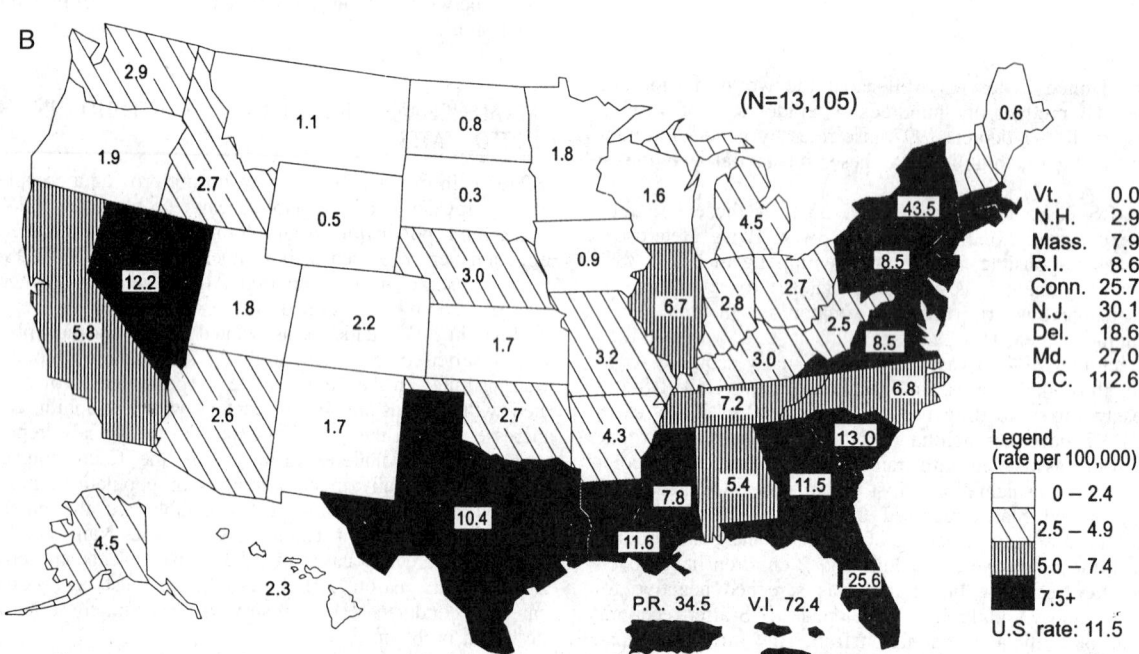

FIGURE 409–1 ■ Adult/adolescent AIDS annual rates per 100,000 population, for cases reported in 1997 in the United States for *(A)* males and *(B)* females. (Source: Centers for Disease Control and Prevention: *HIVAIDS Surveillance Report,* 9 [No. 2]:23, 1997.)

homosexual or bisexual men, IDUs, and persons with hemophilia who received untreated factor concentrates. Prevalence rates in these groups ranged widely in studies—homosexual/bisexual men, 10 to 70%; IDUs, 1 to 50%; and persons with hemophilia, 15 to 90%. Because most surveys in homosexual men and IDUs were conducted among persons seeking medical care for sexually transmitted diseases (STDs) or treatment for drug abuse, the data may not be completely representative of these populations. HIV prevalence rates in persons with hemophilia A and B were directly related to the amount of clotting factor received prior to 1985. HIV seroprevalence rates among female prostitutes varied widely, from 0 to >50%, with the differences largely attributed to the extent of

injecting drug use in the population surveyed and the HIV prevalence among IDUs in the community at that time. HIV prevalence rates among male prostitutes parallel rates in homosexual and bisexual men seen in STD clinics in the same communities.

Standardized HIV serosurveys conducted in STD clinics among heterosexual men and women who do not inject drugs showed a median seroprevalence of 0.9% for men and 0.6% for women in 1992. Among adolescents, as with other STDs, HIV infection rates were higher in women than in men. The close association of clinical tuberculosis with HIV infection is apparent from surveys in tuberculosis clinics, in which HIV seroprevalence had a median rate of 10% by 1990.

Table 409–3 ■ NUMBER AND RATES (PER 100,000) OF AIDS CASES BY RACE/ETHNICITY—UNITED STATES, REPORTED IN 1997

	ADULTS/ADOLESCENTS						Children <13 years		Total	
	Males		Females		Total					
RACE/ETHNICITY	No.	Rate	No.	Rate	No.	Rate	No.	Rate	No.	Rate
White, not Hispanic	17,649	22.5	2,485	3.0	20,134	12.4	63	0.2	20,197	10.4
Black, not Hispanic	18,903	163.4	7,880	58.8	26,783	107.2	292	4.0	27,075	83.7
Hispanic	9,778	78.5	2,578	21.5	12,356	50.6	110	1.3	12,466	37.7
Asian/Pacific Islander	381	10.2	64	1.5	445	5.6	3	0.1	448	4.5
American Indian/Alaska Native	168	23.0	36	4.7	204	13.6	2	0.4	206	10.4
Total*	47,056	44.0	13,105	11.5	60,161	27.3	473	0.9	60,634	22.3

*Totals include 242 persons whose race/ethnicity is unknown.
(Source: Center for Disease Control and Prevention: HIV/AIDS Surveillance Report, 9 [No. 21]: 17, 1997.)

HIV seroprevalence rates in childbearing women have been measured by blinded testing of residual blood samples collected on filter paper from newborns for routine metabolic screening such as for phenylketonuria. Based on data from 35 states, approximately 7000 births occurred in HIV-infected women annually in 1991–1992, for an annual rate of 1.7 per 1000 childbearing women nationwide. At a perinatal transmission rate of 20 to 30%, 1400 to 2100 infants were infected with HIV perinatally in the United States in 1992. Seroprevalence rates varied widely among states, from <1 per 1000 to >1 to 3% in northeastern urban areas. The survey results in New York State (HIV prevalence of 0.67% statewide and >1.4% in New York City in childbearing women in 1989) resulted in a state policy that encourages HIV counseling of all women of childbearing age and offers counseling and HIV testing to women contemplating pregnancy or already pregnant. Seroprevalence approached or exceeded 0.5% in New Jersey, Maryland, Florida, Puerto Rico, the District of Columbia, and New York by 1992. Nationwide, these blinded surveys were discontinued in 1995.

Because incident HIV infections seldom cause persons to seek medical care, direct measurement of HIV incidence is very difficult in most populations. Using a combination of approaches, the USPHS estimated that 55,000 new HIV infections occurred in adults and adolescents in 1996. HIV incidence estimates must be refined to measure the growth of the epidemic, as well as the effectiveness of prevention efforts.

MODES OF HIV TRANSMISSION

HIV is transmitted primarily through sexual contact, parenteral exposure to blood or blood products, and perinatally from infected mothers to their infants.

Sexual Transmission

The predominant mode of HIV transmission throughout the world is sexual contact. The risk of acquiring HIV infection during a single sexual contact depends on several factors. Most important, of course, is the likelihood that the contact is with an HIV-infected partner. Because the prevalence of HIV varies widely between populations within countries as well as between countries, the rates of sexual transmission also vary. Other factors affecting the efficiency of sexual transmission include the type of sexual practice; the infectivity of the source partner; coexisting sexually transmitted infections in either partner, particularly those causing genital ulceration; and consistency of condom use. HIV transmission has been attributed to vaginal, anal and, less frequently, oral intercourse.

In epidemiologic studies among homosexual men, the risk of

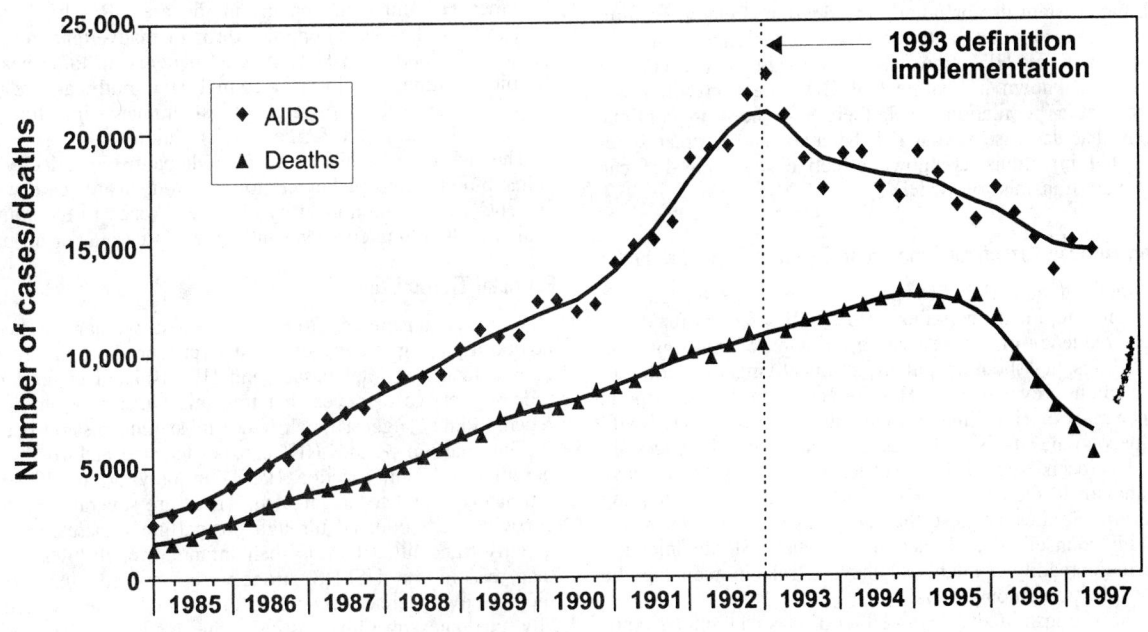

FIGURE 409–2 ■ Estimated incidence of AIDS and deaths of persons with AIDS, adjusted for delays in reporting, by quarter-year of diagnosis/death, United States, January 1985 through June 1997. (Source: Centers for Disease Control and Prevention: *HIV/ AIDS Surveillance Report*, 9 [No. 2]: 1997.)

HIV acquisition increases with the number of sexual partners, the frequency of receptive anal intercourse, and practices associated with rectal trauma such as receptive "fisting" and anal douching. No sexual activity potentially involving the exchange of semen or blood, however, should be considered without risk. The relative efficiency of HIV transmission through various sexual practices was difficult to estimate precisely because most HIV-infected homosexual men in epidemiologic studies had engaged in multiple practices. Although the frequency of female-to-female transmission would seem to be quite low, such HIV infections associated with traumatic sexual practices have been reported. Most cases of HIV infection reported among bisexual women and lesbians are attributed to injecting drug use or heterosexual contact.

Most heterosexual transmission of HIV occurs during vaginal intercourse, although some studies suggest that receptive anal intercourse increases the risk of HIV transmission from an infected man to a woman. Some infected persons may be more efficient transmitters than others, perhaps owing to differences in viral strains or other factors. Transmission efficiency is inversely related to the immunologic status of the infected partner. In studies conducted among spouses and other steady sexual partners of HIV-infected persons, male-to-female, female-to-male, and male-to-male sexual transmission of HIV increased as the index partner's T-helper lymphocyte numbers declined. These findings are not surprising, because the quantity of HIV in blood and semen increases as the disease progresses and the immune system weakens. Several studies have documented that infections such as *Haemophilus ducreyi, Treponema pallidum,* herpes simplex virus, and other pathogens causing genital or anal ulcers facilitate acquisition or transmission of HIV through sexual contact, most likely by disrupting the genital or anal skin and mucous membranes. Undoubtedly, the higher rates of untreated genital ulcer disease contribute to the high rates of sexual transmission of HIV observed in some areas of the developing world. Several investigators have reported increased risks of HIV acquisition for women with cervical infections with *Neisseria gonorrhoeae* or *Chlamydia trachomatis* or with cervical ectopy. To the extent that coexisting sexually transmitted infections increase the rate of HIV transmission, populations throughout the world with higher rates of these infections are at higher risk of HIV infection. Conversely, preventing and treating other sexually transmitted infections should have a beneficial effect on preventing HIV transmission. Cohort studies of couples discordant for HIV infection clearly indicate that consistent condom use reduces heterosexual as well as homosexual HIV transmission by ≥90% compared with inconsistent use or nonuse of condoms. Finally, preliminary studies suggest that antiretrovirals may reduce but not eliminate the risk of HIV transmission through sexual contact. However, it is unknown if treatment of HIV infection will lower infectiousness at a population level, there is a need to continue interventions that decrease sexual risk behavior and to treat sexually transmitted infections as known effective strategies that can lower the sexual transmission of HIV.

Transmission Through Parenteral Exposure to Blood or Blood Products

HIV is transmitted to IDUs by parenteral exposure to contaminated injection equipment, including needles. Risk factors for infection include frequency of needle sharing, duration of injecting drug use, use of drugs in "shooting galleries," and living in a community with a high prevalence of HIV infection in IDUs. Among IDUs, higher rates of HIV infection have also been associated with lower socioeconomic status, homelessness, and minority race-ethnicity. As has been true of homosexual men, many IDUs have changed behavior to reduce their HIV risk, particularly by reducing needle sharing. Studies suggest that drug abuse treatment, street outreach with counseling, and measures to make sterile injection equipment more readily available all have a role in reducing the risk of HIV infection among IDUs.

HIV has been transmitted by whole blood, plasma, cellular components, and clotting factors, but not by other products produced in the United States from blood. No HIV transmission has been linked to receipt of immune serum globulin, hepatitis B immune globulin, Rh₀ (O) immune globulin, or hepatitis B vaccine. The latter products have been produced by fractionation and other processes that remove and inactivate HIV. Conversely, receipt of whole blood, packed cells, or plasma from an HIV-infected donor has been shown to transmit HIV virtually 100% of the time. It has been estimated that >12,000 living persons in the United States were infected with HIV through blood transfusions, as were several thousand additional persons with hemophilia from infected clotting factor concentrates between 1978 and 1985. In the United States and most industrialized countries, screening of all donated blood and plasma for HIV, donor deferral procedures, and heat treatment of clotting factor concentrates have minimized the risk of HIV transmission through transfusions. The exceptions occur largely in donors very recently infected who have yet to develop detectable antibody. This so-called window period is estimated to average 6 to 8 weeks after infection. The rate of HIV transmission from such HIV-seronegative donors was estimated to range from 1 in 36,000 to 1 in 225,000 units transfused in the United States, with even lower estimates in recent years. Because HIV transmission has been reported in recipients of organs, tissues, and semen from HIV-infected donors, the USPHS recommends that potential donors be screened for HIV antibody and that organ, tissue, and semen of those who test positive not be used for transplantation or insemination.

Transmission in the Health Care Environment

Exposure to HIV-infected blood poses a definite risk for HIV infection for health care, laboratory, and home health care workers. Large prospective collaborative studies have found the risk of seroconversion following needle stick or other parenteral exposures to the blood of HIV-infected persons to be approximately 0.3%. In addition, there are a few well-documented, published reports of infections in health care workers following mucous membrane or extensive skin exposures. Such transmission can occur, but the risk is much lower than following parenteral exposures. The use of zidovudine after occupational exposures (needle stick injuries) has been shown to decrease the risk of HIV seroconversion among exposed health care workers. The USPHS has recently recommended the use of combination antiretroviral chemoprophylaxis, including a protease inhibitor, after high-risk percutaneous exposures.

Transmission of HIV infection from an infected dentist to six patients and the transmission from a surgeon to a patient remain the only documented transmissions of HIV to patients from health care workers. These patients had no other confirmed exposure to HIV and each was infected with an HIV strain nearly identical genetically to that of the health care worker and dissimilar to that of other HIV-infected persons in the area. Rarely, HIV infection transmission has been reported through inadvertent intravenous injection of blood from HIV-infected patients in home health care or hospital settings. Major nosocomial HIV outbreaks resulted from improper sterilization or reuse of contaminated injection equipment in Romania and in the former Soviet Union.

The risk of transmission of HIV, hepatitis B and C viruses, and other blood borne pathogens to and from health care workers and patients can be minimized by close adherence to recommendations, which include universal precautions when caring for all patients.

Perinatal Transmission

HIV is transmitted from an infected woman to her fetus or newborn during pregnancy or delivery or through breast-feeding. HIV detected in fetal tissues and HIV isolated in cord blood provide suggestive evidence that transmission can occur in utero, but recent studies suggest much if not most transmission occurs during the intrapartum period. HIV can be detected at birth by culture or polymerase chain reaction (PCR) in only 30 to 50% of infants ultimately found to be infected. There are several reports of mothers who were infected through postpartum transfusions and subsequently transmitted HIV to their infants through breast-feeding. For that reason, the USPHS strongly recommends that HIV-positive mothers avoid breast-feeding in the United States, where nutritionally adequate and safe substitutes are available. The rate of perinatal transmission in published studies varies from 13 to >40%, with higher rates associated with advanced maternal HIV disease or increased viral load and reduced CD4 count, higher rates of breast-feeding, and the presence of chorioamnionitis with more than 4 hours of rupture of membranes. In an important randomized, placebo-controlled trial (ACTG 076), zidovudine administered to asymptomatic HIV-infected pregnant women with CD4 counts >200 per cubic millimeter reduced perinatal transmission by two thirds. The regimen was initiated after the thirteenth week of gestation and accompanied by intravenous zidovudine during parturition and 6 weeks of therapy to the newborn. Based on these data, the USPHS issued guidelines on use of zidovudine during pregnancy to reduce perinatal transmission of HIV infection. The implementation of such recommendations has lead to a 43% reduction in perinatally acquired HIV infection between 1992 and 1996 in the United States. In 1997, less than 500 cases of pediatric AIDS were reported in the United States.

Other Modes of Transmission

Throughout the world, the above routes of transmission have accounted for the overwhelming majority of HIV infections, but there has been considerable concern about other theoretical modes of transmission, especially through "casual" contact with HIV-infected persons, exposure to saliva or aerosols, or insect vectors. More than 700 nonsexual household contacts of adults or children with HIV infection have been evaluated in prospective studies. In thousands of person-years of close contact, including sharing bathroom and kitchen facilities, and frequent personal interactions including kissing and hugging, no transmission other than sexual or perinatal has occurred. HIV has been isolated from saliva but less frequently than in blood, and at least two definite cases of HIV transmission through kissing have been reported in the United States. In addition, a case report of HIV transmission between siblings suggested a bite as the possible route of transmission, although the precise mode of transmission in this case was unclear because seroconversion was not documented and the bite did not break the skin or result in bleeding. Because saliva can contain other pathogenic organisms, appropriate precautions for health care and dental workers remain important, including universal precautions if gross contamination with blood is present. Aerosols have not been reported to transmit blood-borne pathogens such as HIV or hepatitis B in health care or other settings. Extensive laboratory and epidemiologic studies of hepatitis B have failed to detect HBsAg in respirable particles in air samples in dental operatories or dialysis units during procedures on infected patients when aerosols were generated. Because the concentration of HBsAg in body fluids is much higher than that of HIV, it is unlikely that HIV would be detected. Extensive laboratory studies have failed to demonstrate replication of HIV in insects that were fed high concentrations of HIV or injected with HIV-contaminated blood. Epidemiologic studies in the United States, Haiti, and Central Africa show no evidence of insect-borne HIV transmission.

The possibility of previously unrecognized modes of HIV transmission cannot be entirely excluded, but they are likely to be rare, if found.

AIDS AND HIV INFECTION OUTSIDE THE UNITED STATES

Within 3 years after the syndrome was recognized in the United States, cases of AIDS were reported from every continent. By November of 1997, more than 1.7 million cases had been reported from 197 countries to WHO (Table 409–4). WHO also estimates that >60 milion people would be infected with HIV by the end of century. AIDS case reporting from developing countries is much less complete than in industrialized countries and, because the developing world is most heavily affected by HIV/AIDS, WHO esti-

mates that the number of reported AIDS cases worldwide are less than 15% of the total estimated number of AIDS cases that have occurred throughout the epidemic. Extensive HIV serosurveys in Africa, South and Central America, and parts of Asia provide evidence that AIDS case reports greatly underestimate the magnitude of the HIV problem in many countries in these regions.

Modes of transmission of HIV are similar throughout the world, but the relative frequency varies considerably between countries and regions. In North America, Europe, Australia, New Zealand, and some areas of South America, the majority of HIV infections first occurred in homosexual men and IDUs; heterosexual and perinatal transmission initially resulted mostly from transmission from IDUs and their partners. In most countries in Africa and some in the Caribbean and Central America, most HIV infections have occurred through heterosexual transmission. HIV seroprevalence rates are highest in urban prostitutes and sexually active young adults. High rates of infection in young women translate into a substantial amount of perinatal transmission. In some areas of Africa, pediatric HIV infection has significantly increased already high infant mortality rates. In many developing countries, transfusion of HIV-infected blood remains a substantial problem because of inadequate blood banking and serologic testing capacity. Reuse of nonsterile needles and syringes and other medical practices have caused major HIV outbreaks in the former Soviet Union and Romania. In Asian countries such as Thailand and India, emergence of HIV infection as a major public health problem began in IDUs and prostitutes, but rapidly spread more widely through heterosexual transmission to other young adult populations. India is now the country believed to have the highest number of HIV-infected persons, with an estimated 2 to 5 million people currently infected. In Eastern Europe and the newly independent states of the former Soviet Union, HIV infections are rapidly increasing, primarily in association with injecting drug use. In yet other countries, primarily in the Middle East, Asia, and the Pacific region, HIV has not yet been recognized as an important public health problem. The future course of HIV in these countries may depend on their ability to anticipate and respond to the problem; it can be approximately predicted by the extent and pattern of sexually transmitted and transfusion-associated infections and the extent of injecting drug use that currently exists in each country.

A second human immunodeficiency virus, HIV type 2 (HIV-2), was first described in asymptomatic West Africans with AIDS in 1986. HIV-2 infection remains most prevalent in West Africa, although well-documented cases have been reported from Western Europe, Canada, Brazil, the United States, and Central Africa. HIV-2 is generally less virulent than HIV-1. The average viral titer usually is lower, perhaps explaining the lower rates of sexual and perinatal transmission and the slower rate of disease progression in persons infected with HIV-2 than HIV-1. HIV-1 and HIV-2 are closely related; tests for antibody for one virus often cross react with those for the other. For example, licensed enzyme immunoassays for detecting HIV-1 find HIV-2 antibody in 60 to 90% of infected patients. In the United States, combined HIV-1/HIV-2 assays are used to test donated blood. As of 1994, HIV-2 infection remained rare in the United States, with nearly all cases detected in persons from West Africa.

Recently, additional HIV variants, classified together as subtype O, were reported from Cameroon. The antibody response elicited by group O strains is not consistently detected by enzyme immunoassay (EIA) kits commercially available in Europe and the United States. In 1996, a patient with HIV-1 group O infection was diagnosed in California, which reinforces the need for strong international collaboration in maintaining surveillance for variants of HIV and other emerging infections.

Table 409–4 ■ CASES OF AIDS REPORTED TO WHO AS OF NOVEMBER 20, 1997

CONTINENT	NUMBER OF CASES	NUMBER OF COUNTRIES REPORTING CASES
Africa	617,463	54
Americas	839,189	45
Asia	74,431	42
Europe	197,374	40
Oceania	8,501	16
Total	1,736,958	197

(Source: WHO Weekly Epidemiological Record 72;357; 1997)

Goedert JJ, Eyster EE, Biggar RJ, et al: Heterosexual transmission of HIV: Association with severe depletion of T-helper lymphocytes in men with hemophilia. AIDS Res Hum Retroviruses 3:355, 1988. Holmberg SD, Horsburgh CR, Ward JW, et al: Biologic factors in the sexual transmission of human immunodeficiency virus. J Infect Dis 160:116, 1989. Ellerbrock TV, Lieb S, Harrington PE, et al: Heterosexual transmitted human immunodeficiency virus infection among pregnant women in a rural Florida community. N Engl J Med 327:1704, 1992. De Vincenzi I, et al: A longitudinal study of human immunodeficiency virus transmission by heterosexual partners. N Engl J Med 331:341, 1994. Connor EM, Sperling RS, Gelber R, et al: Reduction of maternal-infant transmission of human immunodeficiency virus type 1 with zidovudine treatment. N Engl J Med 331:1173, 1994. CDC: Perinatally acquired HIV/AIDS—United States, 1997. MMWR 46:1086, 1997. CDC/USPHS Task

Force Recommendations for the Use of Antiretroviral Drugs in Pregnant Women Infected with Human Immunodeficiency Virus-1 for Maternal Health and for Reducing Perinatal HIV-1 Transmission in the U.S. MMWR 47 (RR-2):1, 1998. *These summarize available information on factors related to heterosexual transmission of HIV and prevention of perinatal transmission.*

Mann JM, Tarantola DJM (eds): AIDS in the World II Global Dimensions, Social Roots and Responses. New York: Oxford University Press, 1996. *This volume summarizes and updates what is known about HIV infection and prevention activities throughout the world.*

1993 Revised classification system for HIV infection and expanded surveillance, case definition for AIDS among adolescents and adults. MMWR 41(RR-17):1, 1992. Redfield RR, Wright DC, Tramont EA: The Walter Reed staging classification for HTLV-IIILAV infection. N Engl J Med 314:131, 1986. *These are the most widely used classification systems in the United States.*

Update: Trends in AIDS incidence, deaths, and prevalence—United States, 1996. JAMA 277:874, 1997. CDC: AIDS among racial/ethnic minorities—United States, 1993. MMWR 43:644, 1993. Denning PH, et al: Recent trends in the HIV epidemic in adolescent and young adult gay and bisexual men. JAIDS 16:374, 1997. Karon JM, et al: Prevalence of HIV infection in the United States, 1984 to 1992. JAMA 276:126, 1996. McQuillan GM, et al: Update on the seroepidemiology of human immunodeficiency virus in the United States household population: NHANES III, 1988–1994. JAIDS 14:355, 1997. Weainstock HS, et al: Trends in HIV seroprevalence among persons attending sexually transmitted disease clinics in the United States, 1988–1992. JAIDS 9:514, 1995. Pub Health Rep 105:113, 1990. National serosurveillance summary, Volume 3—Centers for Disease Control and Prevention, HIVNCID11-913036; Gwinn M, Pappaioanou M, George JR, et al: Prevalence of HIV infection in childbearing women in the United States. JAMA 265:1704, 1991. *These articles summarize recent methods and data on HIV seroprevalence in the United States.*

Update: Universal precautions for prevention of transmission of HIV, hepatitis B virus, and other bloodborne pathogens in health care setting. MMWR 37:337, 1988. Public Health Service Guidelines for the Management of Health-Care Worker Exposures to HIV and Recommendations for Postexposure Prophylaxis. MMWR 47 (RR-7):1, 1998. Recommendations for preventing transmission of human immunodeficiency virus and hepatitis B virus to patients during exposure-prone invasive procedures. MMWR 40(RR-8):1, 1991. *These documents summarize data on transmission of HIV in the health care setting and list recommended precautions.*

410 PREVENTION OF HIV INFECTION

Michael S. Saag

Prevention of HIV infection requires a thorough understanding of the modes of viral transmission, the populations at risk, and the established guidelines to avoid high-risk exposures. HIV has been identified in virtually every body fluid and tissue, including blood, semen, vaginal secretions, saliva, tears, breast milk, cerebrospinal fluid, amniotic fluid, urine, and fluid obtained from bronchoalveolar lavage. In most instances, the virus resides in lymphocytes present within body fluids; therefore, any fluid that contains lymphocytes could be implicated theoretically in the spread of the virus. Nonetheless, no cases of HIV transmission have been documented through any body fluids except blood and fluids grossly contaminated with blood, semen, vaginal secretions, and, rarely, breast milk. HIV has been transmitted through transplanted organs, including kidney, liver, heart, pancreas, and bone.

MODES OF HIV TRANSMISSION AND PREVENTION

Sexual Transmission

HIV infection is a sexually transmitted disease (STD). Like other STDs, HIV spreads bidirectionally and appears to be transmitted from male to female and female to male with greater efficiency (up to three-fold) from male to female. Although the majority of sexually transmitted cases reported in the United States occur via male homosexual activity, heterosexual transmission is one of the fastest growing modes of transmission reported in the United States and is the primary mode of disease acquisition in many African countries, where male-to-female prevalence ratios are approximately 1.1:1.

Certain cofactors are associated with an increased risk of acquiring HIV infection. Among homosexual men, receptive anal intercourse and contact with a large number of different sexual partners are the most important risk factors. Activities that may lead to damage of the rectal mucosa, such as rectal douching, manual penetration of the rectum ("fisting"), and concomitant ulcerative

STDs, increase the likelihood of disease acquisition. Insertive rectal intercourse, fellatio, and ingestion of semen are associated with HIV transmission to a lesser degree. The likelihood of heterosexual acquired disease increases with a higher number of sexual partners, contact with intravenous drug users (IVDUs), prostitution, sexual practices that damage vaginal or rectal mucosa, and a previous history of other STDs. Female-to-female transmission has been reported via orogenital contact.

Prevention

Abstinence is the only absolute way of preventing sexual acquisition of HIV infection. Persons who have been engaged in a mutually monogamous relationship since the mid-1970s are at extremely low risk of acquiring disease; however, the assurance that both partners have remained "faithful" is sometimes difficult to confirm. For the majority of sexually active individuals it should be assumed that their partner is seropositive until demonstrated otherwise. Verbal claims of seronegativity should be viewed with skepticism. When a couple, heterosexual or homosexual, is establishing a long-term relationship, it may be recommended that they undergo serologic testing to determine their HIV status. However, the decision to be tested should be of mutual consent and viewed in the context that exposures outside the relationship may lead to seropositivity in the future.

In situations in which a decision to engage in sexual activity has been made and the HIV status of the partner is unknown or in doubt, safe sexual practices ("safe sex") should be implemented (Table 410–1). Mutual masturbation is considered "safe," assuming it is nontraumatic and not followed by ingestion of body fluids such as semen or vaginal secretions. Transmission of HIV has never been documented to occur through saliva; however, no group of patients has ever been studied who engage in deep "French" kissing as their sole means of sexual activity. Because HIV exists in saliva, albeit in very low titers, deep French kissing cannot be considered absolutely safe even though the likelihood of HIV transmission is extremely low. Condom use is the most effective means of preventing HIV infection among individuals who engage in oral, vaginal, or anal intercourse. To be effective, however, the condom should be made of latex and must be used properly. Natural skin condoms have been shown to leak in laboratory studies, whereas latex condoms maintain their integrity and are more durable. Nonoxynol-9, a spermicide with some antiviral activity, enhances the protective effects of condoms and should be used in conjunction with condoms either as a spermicidal jelly or impregnated into the latex condom itself. Petroleum-based lubricants enhance the likelihood of latex condom rupture and should be avoided. If needed, water-based lubricants such as K-Y Jelly should be used.

Both partners should be knowledgeable about the correct use of condoms. Discussions regarding condom use should occur before the need arises, and ideally, condom placement should be practiced in advance. A new condom should be used for each act of intercourse and each condom should be used only one time. Even under the best of circumstances, a 5 to 15% failure rate has been noted among couples using condoms as their sole means of contraception, and HIV transmission has been reported in discordant couples using condoms. Condom ineffectiveness most often is due to improper placement, falling off during intercourse, and rupture. Therefore, although condom use during intercourse is considered "safer" sex, it is not absolutely safe.

Table 410–1 ■ SAFE AND UNSAFE SEXUAL PRACTICES IN ORDER OF "SURENESS" OF SAFETY

Safe
Abstinence
Monogamous relationship with confirmed seronegative partner
Manual sex (manual masturbation)
Kissing
Intercourse with latex condom (used in combination with nonoxynol-9)
Unsafe
Intercourse with "natural skin" condom
Intercourse with latex condom lubricated with petroleum-based lubricants
Unprotected orogenital sex
Unprotected vaginal intercourse
Unprotected anal intercourse

HIV Transmission in Intravenous Drug Users

The primary mode of HIV transmission in IVDUs is sharing of contaminated needles and syringes. Sharing of injection paraphernalia ("works") is commonplace among IVDUs and is reinforced by the cultural economic and legal environment in the IVDU community. The risk of HIV transmission is highest among IVDUs who share needles and use drugs that are injected more often, such as cocaine. HIV is frequently transmitted from IVDUs to their sexual partners through both heterosexual and homosexual activity, and ultimately, the virus may be transmitted to their children via perinatal exposure. Many cases of heterosexual transmission, including transmission from prostitutes, are associated with intravenous drug use.

Prevention

The primary mode of preventing HIV transmission in IVDUs is to prevent the use of intravenous drugs in the first place. Education programs that are culturally sensitive and geared to young audiences have the best chance of preventing drug use. Access to treatment centers is the best approach for those individuals already using IV drugs. For those IVDUs who do not wish to seek treatment or who are unable to gain access to treatment, the most effective way to prevent HIV infection is to avoid sharing needles and works. Where works are in short supply, needles and syringes should be cleaned after each use, preferably with readily accessible virucidal cleansers such as chlorine bleach (diluted 1:100). Some communities have adopted programs that provide free needles and syringes for IVDUs. Voluntary HIV testing and outreach programs that rigorously maintain confidentiality can be effective in reducing transmission to sexual partners of IVDUs. In order to be effective, antibody testing should be combined with intensive pretest and post-test counseling.

The efficacy of many community programs is limited, however, by cultural barriers, including lack of trust, fear of prosecution, misconceptions regarding the prevalence of HIV infection within the local drug-using population, and the use of ineffective language in delivering anti-HIV messages by program staff. When combined with the relative paucity of IV drug treatment resources, HIV education among IVDUs which ultimately results in behavioral changes represents the most challenging HIV prevention goal.

Transmission of HIV Through Blood Products

HIV has been transmitted via transfusion of single-donor blood and blood products, including whole blood, fresh frozen plasma, packed red blood cells, cryoprecipitate, clotting factors, and platelets. Prior to May 1985, when the Red Cross began testing the blood supply for evidence of HIV antibodies, an estimated 10,000 to 12,000 individuals received blood products from HIV-infected donors. Most recipients develop infection after transfusion with HIV-tainted blood products, and recent data suggest that the time to development of advanced disease is shorter among transfusion recipients than among those who acquired their disease via sexual contact.

Since 1985, the rate of HIV transmission through transfusion has dropped precipitously. The current estimated rate of transmission is 1 in 40,000 to 1 in 200,000 units of blood, depending on the prevalence of HIV infection in the community where the blood was collected. Pooled plasma components often require 2000 to 30,000 donors per lot and represent a higher potential risk of transmission than single-donor blood products if the pooled product is not treated to eliminate infectious virus.

Prevention

Aggressive efforts by the American Red Cross have greatly reduced the risk of HIV transmission via transfusion in the United States. Voluntary self-deferral of donors at risk for HIV acquisition in the community was initiated in 1983. The effectiveness of self-deferral is limited, however, by social pressures. Some high-risk individuals view blood donation as a means of being tested for HIV and provide erroneous screening information in order to receive free, confidential evaluation of their HIV status. Other at-risk individuals may be coerced to participate in blood donation drives at work. Potentially infected donors may feel uncomfortable excusing themselves from donation and provide false information on screening in order to avoid possible disclosure of a high-risk life-style to their coworkers. Self-deferral programs are most effective when free, voluntary testing centers are readily available elsewhere in the community and when blood drives encourage potential donors to come to donation centers by themselves and not in groups.

The institution of HIV antibody testing of donated blood and blood products in 1985 has had the most dramatic effect on lowering the incidence of transfusion-related transmission. When combined with voluntary self-deferral, the blood supply has become relatively free of HIV. Heat inactivation processes for cryoprecipitate and clotting factor concentrates have virtually eliminated transmission of HIV through use of these products. Other products, such as immune globulin preparations and hepatitis B vaccines, are produced via methods that inactivate HIV and have never been associated with transmission of HIV.

Transmission of HIV to Health Care Workers

Transmission of HIV in the health care delivery setting has been the subject of intense investigation throughout the course of the epidemic. The percentage of health care workers with AIDS who have "no identified risk" for HIV infection has remained low (< 10%) and has not increased over time, despite the dramatic increase in the number of AIDS cases and concomitant exposure of health care workers to patients with HIV disease. More importantly, detailed studies examining the risk of specific exposures, such as needle stick injuries and mucous membrane exposures, have demonstrated very low risk of disease acquisition in the workplace. More than 3628 health care workers have been examined prospectively in carefully designed surveillance studies at 10 high-incidence medical centers. The overall risk of seroconversion after a percutaneous needle stick from a known HIV-positive source is 0.25% per exposure. Although mucous membrane exposures to HIV-positive blood have resulted in seroconversion in at least three health care workers, prospective studies of over 900 splash exposures have failed to identify any seroconverters, implying that the risk of infection is even lower after mucous membrane exposure than through percutaneous needle stick. To date, no transmission has occurred after exposure to body fluids other than blood or fluids heavily contaminated with blood. Therefore, although the potential for HIV transmission to health care providers clearly exists, the risk of infection is inherently low and can be further minimized by following routine precautions to prevent transmission.

Prevention

In August 1987, the Centers for Disease Control and Prevention (CDC) published guidelines designed to minimize health care worker exposure to blood and body fluids which may be infected with blood-borne pathogens, such as HIV. These guidelines remain the principal mode of HIV prevention among health care workers today. These so-called universal precautions are based on the premise that any patient may be infected with blood-borne infectious agents and it may be difficult, if not impossible, to differentiate those with infection from their uninfected counterparts. Thus all specimens containing blood or blood-tinged fluids obtained from *any* patient should be considered hazardous and handled as such (Table 410–2).

Handwashing is the cornerstone of universal precautions, as it is with all infection-control practices. Gloves should be worn when spillage of blood or body fluids is likely. Gloves should *never* be washed and should be changed after soiling or after gross contamination, with handwashing immediately after the gloves are removed. Gowns, protective eyewear, and masks usually are not needed except in circumstances in which splattering or splashing of blood-containing fluids is likely to occur. Masks should always be worn in situations in which eyewear is required. Reusable equipment should be cleansed of visible organic material, placed in an impervious bag, and returned to central supply for decontamination. Although heat is the single best decontamination method, chemical agents that possess mycobactericidal activity are effective against both hepatitis B and HIV and are acceptable alternatives when heat inactivation is impractical. Blood spills should be cleaned with appropriate caution. After placing gloves and other appropriate barrier precautions, excess blood should be removed with absorbent materials (e.g., paper towels), the area then cleaned with soap and

Table 410–2 ■ SUMMARY OF UNIVERSAL PRECAUTIONS

Specimens, including blood, blood products, and body fluids, obtained from all patients should be considered hazardous and potentially infected with transmissible agents.

Handwashing should be performed before and after patient contact; after removing gloves; and immediately if hands are grossly contaminated with blood.

Gloves should be worn when hands are likely to come in contact with blood or body fluids.

Gowns, protective eyewear, and masks should be worn when splashing, splattering, or aerosolization of blood or body fluids is likely to occur.

Sharp objects ("sharps") should be handled with great care and disposed of in impervious receptacles.

Needles should never be manipulated, bent, broken, or recapped.

Blood spills should be handled via initial absorption of spill with disposable towels, cleaning area with soap and water, followed by disinfecting area with 1:10 solution of household bleach.

Contaminated reusable equipment should be decontaminated using heat sterilization, or when heat is impractical, using a mycobactericidal cleanser.

Pocket masks or mechanical ventilation devices should be available in areas where cardiopulmonary resuscitation procedures are likely.

Health care workers with open lesions or weeping dermatitis should avoid direct patient contact and should not handle contaminated equipment.

Private rooms are not required for routine care; select circumstances, however, such as the presence of concomitant transmissible opportunistic disease, may warrant respiratory, enteric, or contact isolation.

water, and the area disinfected with a 1:10 solution of sodium hypochlorite (household bleach) and water. Health care workers with denuded skin, open lesions, or active dermatitis should avoid direct patient contact and should not process contaminated equipment or materials. Private rooms generally are not required for patients known to be HIV infected unless a concomitant opportunistic disease is present which requires respiratory, enteric, or contact isolation. Food service should be provided as usual on reusable dishware.

Because *all* blood and body fluids should be handled as potentially hazardous and *all* patients presumed to be infected, it makes little sense to identify infected patients or their specimens with "blood and body fluid" labels. The use of such labels on *known* infected patients implies that unlabeled specimens or specimens from patients of unknown status are less hazardous and may be handled with less care. Indeed, studies have shown that more than half of the specimens containing antibodies to either HbsAg or HIV went to the laboratory unlabeled. The handling of sharp instruments ("sharps") represents the greatest risk of HIV transmission to health care workers. Although sharp injuries cannot be entirely eliminated, the number of exposures can be reduced substantially by adhering to guidelines put forth in universal precautions. Before a sharp instrument is used, thought should be given regarding where the instrument will be disposed after use. Impervious containers should be readily available in all patient care areas and identified by the health care worker *prior to* "sharp" utilization. The containers should be checked frequently and should not be allowed to overfill. Used needles should never be manipulated, bent, broken, or recapped. Recapping of needles is the single most common activity that results in needle stick injuries.

Despite their logical basis and relative ease of implementation, universal precautions have not been used routinely by many health care providers. Recent studies have shown that > 50% of health care workers engage in inadequate infection control practices, even in high-impact AIDS centers, and up to 40% of the needle stick exposures were judged to be preventable. Although lack of adequate education may partly explain these findings, implementation of infection control practices has been generally poor historically. Between 200 and 400 health care workers die each year as a result of hepatitis B infection acquired on the job. The use of universal precautions helps minimize the transmission of many transmissible diseases in addition to HIV.

Even in the best of circumstances, accidental mucous membrane and percutaneous exposures to blood from HIV-infected patients do occur. Each institution and health care facility should adopt procedures for managing these exposures based on guidelines published by the CDC (recently updated; MMWR 47(RR-7): 1–28, 1998).

The essential elements of management following needle stick or mucous membrane exposure include defining the type of exposure, appropriately evaluating the donor (patient) and recipient (health care worker) at the time of exposure, and follow-up of the health care worker for at least 1 year after exposure.

Proposed definitions of the types of exposure are summarized in Table 410–3. Health care workers with any kind of parenteral exposure should be counseled and evaluated for possible acquisition of HIV and receive routine prophylaxis against hepatitis B. The source patient (donor) should be evaluated for HIV infection; if the donor's HIV status is unknown, the donor should be informed about the incident and encouraged to allow voluntary, confidential screening of his/her blood for HIV and hepatitis B antibody. If the patient refuses or cannot give consent, he/she should be considered to be infected. In cases where exposure to HIV is documented or presumed to have occurred, the health care worker should be evaluated serologically for the presence of HIV as soon as possible after the exposure (baseline) and again at 6 weeks, 12 weeks, 24 weeks, and 1 year after the exposure to determine whether HIV transmission has occurred. The health care worker should report any acute illnesses that occur during the follow-up period, especially during the first 6 to 12 weeks after exposure. Exposed workers should follow the recommended guidelines for preventing HIV transmission, including using safe sexual practices; refraining from blood, semen, and organ donation; and avoiding breast feeding. If the source patient is seronegative for HIV and has no clinical manifestations of HIV disease, no further follow-up of the exposed health care workers is necessary, although some workers prefer follow-up for their own peace of mind. Serologic testing should be made available to all health care workers who are concerned about potential on the job exposure.

The use of chemoprophylaxis following parenteral exposure to HIV is now routinely recommended for all health care workers

Table 410–3 ■ DEFINITIONS OF EXPOSURES TO BLOOD AND BODY FLUIDS FROM HIV-INFECTED PATIENTS

	CHEMOPROPHYLAXIS
Massive parenteral exposure	
Transfusion of blood	Recommended
High-inoculum injection of blood (>1 mL) or laboratory materials containing high viral titers	
Definite parenteral exposure	
Deep intramuscular injury with a needle contaminated with blood or a body fluid	Recommended
Small volume injection of blood or body fluid (<1 mL)	
Laceration caused by instrument contaminated with blood or body fluids	
Laceration inoculated with blood, body fluids, or virus samples (research materials)	
Possible parenteral exposure	
Subcutaneous or superficial injury with an instrument or needle contaminated with blood or body fluids	Available
Injury with a contaminated instrument or needle which does not cause visible bleeding	
Previous wound or skin lesion contaminated with blood or body fluids	
Mucous membrane exposure to blood or body fluids	
Doubtful parenteral exposure	
Subcutaneous injury by instrument or needle contaminated with noninfectious fluids†	Discouraged
Contamination of a wound, previous skin lesion, or mucous membrane with noninfectious fluids	
Intact skin visibly contaminated with blood	

*Dual nucleoside therapy (e.g., zidovudine plus lamivudine), usually with a potent protease inhibitor or non-nucleoside reverse transcriptase inhibitor (NNRTI); see text.

†Body fluids considered to be potentially infectious include blood, blood products, cerebrospinal fluid, amniotic fluid, menstrual discharge, inflammatory exudates, pleural fluid, peritoneal fluid, pericardial fluid, and any fluid visibly contaminated with blood. All other fluids are considered noninfectious.

who experience a massive or definite parenteral exposure. Many clinicians favor using prophylactic antiretroviral therapy after possible parenteral exposures, although this practice remains controversial. The firm recommendation to administer routine chemoprophylaxis in cases of massive or definite exposure is based on increasing evidence of the beneficial protective effects from its use in both animal and human studies. In some animal models of retroviral infection, zidovudine (ZDV), when given early after inoculation, modifies the course of disease. Very recent reports from the CDC indicate an 80% reduction in anticipated transmission rates of HIV to parenterally exposed health care workers who had received ZDV prophylaxis. With the introduction of more potent antiretroviral therapy, even more reduction in HIV transmission in the health care worker setting is anticipated. Therefore, in most medical centers, multidrug chemoprophylaxis has become a standard of practice. The CDC recommends use of at least a dual nucleoside regimen (e.g., zidovudine with lamivudine), with or without the addition of a third agent, usually a potent protease inhibitor or a non-nucleoside reverse transcriptase inhibitor. Health care workers with doubtful parenteral or nonparenteral exposures generally should not take chemoprophylaxis. The optimal timing and dosage of chemoprophylaxis are unknown; however, animal studies suggest that higher doses given as soon as possible after exposure have the best chance of being effective. Therefore, most centers that offer chemoprophylaxis to their employees have established mechanisms whereby the health care worker can be evaluated and the drugs administered within 2 to 4 hours after the exposure. Standard doses of the antiretroviral agents are administered for 4 to 6 weeks.

Transmission from Infected Health Care Workers to their Patients

In July 1990, the first case of possible transmission of HIV from an infected health care worker (dentist) to his patients was reported. Six patients are believed to have acquired infection from the dentist based on the absence of other risk factors among the patients and the high degree of homology between the viruses isolated from the dentist and those isolated from the patients. Although each patient underwent an invasive procedure in the dental office, the precise mode of transmission remains unknown.

Based on the known transmission of other blood-borne pathogens from health care providers to their patients (e.g., hepatitis B), it was anticipated that HIV may also be transmitted in this fashion. Remarkably, despite the prolonged duration of the epidemic, the dentist described above remains the only documented case of transmission to patients in the health care setting. Several "look-back" studies of over 4000 patients who underwent invasive surgical procedures performed by HIV-infected physicians have failed to identify any additional cases of nosocomial transmission. Therefore, the risk of transmission from infected health care workers to patients is thought to be very low (between 1 in 42,000 and 1 in 420,000). Routine use of universal precautions should minimize the risk of transmission from HIV-infected patients to health care providers and vice versa.

VACCINE DEVELOPMENT

Education is the only means of HIV prevention currently available. Over the past few years significant efforts have been directed toward the development of an effective vaccine against HIV. Although substantial progress has been achieved, several obstacles still remain. Despite enormous advances in understanding the immunopathogenesis of HIV infection, the precise mechanism of protective immunity remains unknown. Without such knowledge, it is difficult to develop vaccines that are assured of targeting the appropriate arm of the immune system that confers long-term protective immunity. Another obstacle is the lack of correlation of data from animal models to the potential protective effects of vaccines in humans. Therefore, even if an effective vaccine were available, it would take years of human testing to demonstrate its effectiveness. Moreover, once a candidate vaccine is in human trials, the relatively low rate of HIV transmission and, in some cases, the difficulty in determining whether HIV infection has actually occurred will complicate the evaluation process. Despite the enormous progress made in vaccine development over the last few years, it will take several more years before protective efficacy can be estab-

lished. Even if an effective vaccine is established, education will remain the primary mode of HIV prevention, owing to the difficulty in knowing how long the protective immune effect will last. Never before has so much been known about an epidemic during the time it was occurring. The challenge is to disseminate the knowledge to populations at risk in language they can understand and, ultimately, to modify activities so that the risk of transmission is minimized.

Bell DM: Occupational risk of human immunodeficiency virus infection in healthcare workers: An overview. Am J Med 102 (Suppl 5B), 9–15, 1997. *A thorough overview of risks of HIV transmission. Part of a dedicated supplement to the American Journal of Medicine on this subject.*

Centers for Disease Control: Recommendations for prevention of HIV transmission in health-care settings. MMWR 36(Suppl 2):1S, 1987. *Original description of universal precautions. Critical reading for all health care providers.*

Centers for Disease Control: Update: Investigations of persons treated by HIV-infected health-care workers—United States. MMWR 42:329, 1993. *Summary of look-back studies that examine the status of patients who received care from HIV-infected health care workers.*

Centers for Disease Control: Public Health Service guidelines for the management of health care worker exposures to HIV and recommendations for postexposure prophylaxis. MMWR 47(RR-7):1–26, 1998. *A comprehensive summary of guidelines for management of HCW exposure to HIV. A "must" for employee health and infection control counselor. Extensive reference list.*

Gerberding JL: Is antiretroviral treatment after percutaneous HIV exposure justified? Ann Intern Med 118:979, 1993. *Succinct overview of current thinking on postexposure prophylaxis. Cites key references.*

Lo B, Steinbrook R: Health care workers infected with the human immunodeficiency virus: The next steps. JAMA 267:1100, 1992. *Thoughtful review of the medical, epidemiologic, and ethical issues surrounding the practice of HIV-infected health care providers.*

411 NEUROLOGIC COMPLICATIONS OF HIV-1 INFECTION

Richard W. Price

The neurologic complications of HIV-1 infection are both common and varied. Indeed, only rarely do the central and peripheral nervous systems of HIV-infected patients remain unaffected through the course of untreated disease. Because each of the individual neurologic disorders is discussed in more detail elsewhere in this volume, the major purpose of this chapter is to provide an overview and a general guide to diagnosis and management.

Although the major susceptibility to neurologic complications occurs in the late phase of HIV-1 infection, at the time when immunosuppression leads to a marked increase in vulnerability to a host of conditions, patients may also manifest certain neurologic afflictions early in infection. Because the neurologic complications of early and late HIV-1 infection differ, they are considered separately. Indeed, because of these stage-related differences in susceptibility, when approaching diagnosis in HIV-infected patients it is important to characterize their "background" systemic HIV-1 infection, either clinically with respect to the presence or absence of previous opportunistic infections indicating compromised immunity or by assessment of surrogate markers, particularly the blood CD4+ lymphocyte count. Emerging data suggest that susceptibility to late neurologic complications can be delayed or reversed by highly active antiretroviral therapy (HAART), sustaining the value of the CD4+ count in predicting disease vulnerability.

EARLY HIV-1 INFECTION

Although less common than in the late stages of HIV-1 infection, the nervous system may also be afflicted earlier, indeed as early as the stage of primary infection and seroconversion. Thus, individual reports have described examples of focal or diffuse encephalopathy, ataxia, myelopathy, and meningitis presenting within the context of HIV-1 seroconversion. These conditions appear to evolve acutely or subacutely, to pursue a monophasic course, and to be followed by good recovery. Peripheral nervous system disorders, including mononeuropathy involving cranial or segmental nerves, brachial plexopathy, and polyneuropathy, have also been reported during this phase. At times these peripheral and central nervous system (CNS) disorders occur together.

Subsequently, during the "clinically latent" phase of infection, several neurologic conditions have been reported. Among these is the Guillain-Barré syndrome and its more protracted counterpart, chronic idiopathic demyelinating polyneuropathy (CIDP), both of which are clinically indistinguishable from demyelinating polyneu-ropathies affecting non–HIV-1-infected individuals, except for higher cerebrospinal fluid (CSF) cell counts and perhaps a poorer prognosis. Response to treatment with corticosteroids, plasma ex-change, and intravenous immunoglobulin has been noted, support-ing an autoimmune pathogenesis. Because of the potential hazards of corticosteroids, plasma exchange and immunoglobulin are the preferred therapies. Isolated cases of a multiple sclerosis–like de-myelinating CNS disease have also been reported in this stage of HIV-1 infection, but this appears to be rare.

An additional important aspect of HIV-1 infection, with both diagnostic and pathogenetic implications, is the early development of CSF abnormalities, which relate to early *asymptomatic HIV-1 infection of the CNS* soon after initial systemic infection. Prospec-tive studies have reported that the majority of asymptomatic HIV-1-infected individuals exhibit mild CSF changes, including eleva-tions in the cell count and protein and immunoglobulin levels as well as evidence of local "intra-blood-brain barrier" synthesis of anti-HIV-1 antibody. Additionally, in a substantial number of asymptomatic patients HIV-1 can be detected in the CSF using nucleic acid amplification techniques. These findings have not been shown to have an adverse prognostic significance for the subject; indeed, it is clear that patients with such abnormalities can continue to function without symptoms or signs of neurologic impairment. These "background" abnormalities may confound CSF analysis.

LATE HIV-1 INFECTION

The evolving, and eventually severe, impairment of immune de-fenses caused by HIV-1 renders the nervous system highly vulnera-ble to a broad spectrum of disorders. The following overview emphasizes general principles of pathogenesis and approach to di-agnosis.

Pathophysiology

A number of pathophysiologic processes may lead to neurologic dysfunction in the late phase of HIV-1 infection (Table 411–1). These include conditions that distinguish the AIDS patient from other groups, such as *opportunistic infections, opportunistic neo-*

Table 411–1 ■ PATHOPHYSIOLOGIC CLASSIFICATION OF SOME COMMON NEUROLOGIC COMPLICATIONS OF LATE HIV-1 INFECTION

UNDERLYING PROCESS	EXAMPLES
Opportunistic infections	Cerebral toxoplasmosis
	Cryptococcal meningitis
	Progressive multifocal leukoenceph-alopathy
	Cytomegalovirus encephalitis, poly-radiculitis
Opportunistic neoplasms	Primary central nervous system lym-phoma
	Metastatic lymphoma
Conditions possibly related to HIV-1 itself	AIDS dementia complex
	Aseptic meningitis
	Predominantly sensory polyneuropa-thy
Metabolic and vascular complica-tions of systemic disease	Hypoxic, sepsis-related encephalop-athies
	Stroke (nonbacterial thrombotic en-docarditis, coagulopathies)
Toxic reactions	Dideoxyinosine, dideoxycytidine neu-ropathies
	AZT myopathy
Functional (psychiatric) disorders	Anxiety disorders
	Psychotic depression

plasms, and several conditions that appear to relate to more *direct effects of HIV-1* itself. AIDS patients are also susceptible to the neurologic conditions that affect other acute and chronically ill populations, including metabolic brain disease resulting from sys-temic organ dysfunction, stroke related to nonbacterial thrombotic endocarditis or coagulopathies, toxic effects of medications, and primary psychiatric disturbances. Here we focus on those disorders that particularly distinguish AIDS patients.

Opportunistic Nervous System Infections

As with other organ systems, the spectrum of opportunistic in-fections of the nervous system results from the intrinsic vulnerabili-ties of the tissue (fertile soil) and the pattern of immunosuppres-sion, in this case circumscribed impairment of T-cell/macrophage defenses. The patient's long-term history of exposure to particular organisms is also important because most of the opportunistic in-fections result from reactivation of latent infections rather than from new encounters with pathogens. An important implication of the pre-eminence of reactivated infection relates to serologic test-ing, which is most useful for assessing prior exposure to an organ-ism and hence susceptibility to clinically important reactivation, but not for defining active infection. For example, patients with cere-bral toxoplasmosis nearly always exhibit antecedent positive *Toxo-plasma gondii* blood serology, and therefore a negative serum IgG antibody titer militates against this diagnosis. On the other hand, these serum antibody titers most often do not rise before or during the course of disease, and therefore a fourfold increase cannot be relied upon to establish disease activity. Moreover, as long as immunosuppression persists and therapy still cannot eliminate latent infection, suppressive antibiotic therapy must be maintained for the remainder of the patient's life. Prophylaxis also influences vulnera-bility to some infections and therefore their diagnostic probability. Thus, whether or not a patient is taking trimethoprim-sulfamethox-azole affects the likelihood of cerebral toxoplasmosis.

The reason for the intrinsic vulnerability of the nervous system to certain infections (e.g., *T. gondii*) and not others (e.g., *Pneumo-cystis carinii*) in many cases remains uncertain. However, in some instances susceptibility relates to the capacity of local cells to support intracellular replication. Thus, the virus causing progressive multi-focal leukoencephalopathy (PML), JC virus, causes a produc-tive and lytic infection of oligodendrocytes and hence leads to spreading infection and demyelination as the processes of these myelin-producing cells disappear. In the case of HIV-1, productive infection appears to involve monocyte-derived macrophages and local microglial cells.

The circumscribed nature of the immunologic defect in AIDS determines the range of opportunistic infections, which therefore differs somewhat from that of other immunosuppressed states. For example, AIDS patients are particularly susceptible to cerebral tox-oplasmosis but, unlike patients with organ transplants, are much less likely to develop cerebral *Candida* or *Aspergillus* infections. For this reason, AIDS patients present a unique set of disease probabilities.

Opportunistic Neoplasms

The major consideration in this category is primary brain lym-phoma. These B-cell lymphomas arise in the CNS, usually are multicentric (at least microscopically), and rarely metastasize sys-temically. Characteristically, they develop late in HIV-1 infection when blood CD4+ lymphocytes are low, i.e., in the same setting as major opportunistic infections. Indeed, the tumor cells are nearly always positive for Epstein-Barr virus (EBV), which likely plays an important role in their genesis. Recently, this association has been exploited diagnostically using PCR DNA amplification to detect EBV sequences in CSF. Radiation therapy usually results in tumor regression, and some patients do well, although more generally the prognosis is poor, principally because other complications develop; the role of chemotherapy is uncertain, but aggressive treatment is often not possible because of reduced bone marrow reserves. Sys-temic lymphoma can also spread to the CNS, although usually to the leptomeninges rather than brain parenchyma. Although Kaposi's sarcoma has been reported to metastasize to brain, this is exceed-ingly rare.

Effects of HIV-1 on the Nervous System

Several disorders have been suggested to relate in a more direct or fundamental way to HIV-1 infection. These include the AIDS dementia complex, aseptic meningitis, and perhaps predominantly sensory neuropathy. Although considerable uncertainty still exists regarding their pathogenesis, the uniqueness of these conditions in HIV-1-infected compared with other immunosuppressed patients, as well as more direct evidence of virus infection in some patients with the AIDS dementia complex, lends support to this contention.

Diagnosis: Neuroanatomic Approach

As with other neurologic disease, diagnosis in AIDS patients begins with localization of symptoms and signs and hence involves neuroanatomic classification (Table 411–2).

Meningitis and Headache

Several disorders may involve the leptomeninges in patients with advanced HIV-1 disease. The most important of these is infection by *Cryptococcus neoformans* (see Ch. 398). This condition may present subacutely with headache, nausea, vomiting, and confusion, just as in non-AIDS patients. However, importantly, in some patients initial symptoms can be remarkably mild, with only low-grade headache or fever. Likewise, the CSF findings may be bland, with few or no cells and little or no perturbation in either glucose

Table 411–2 ■ NEUROANATOMIC CLASSIFICATION OF THE LATE COMPLICATIONS OF HIV-1 INFECTION

Meningitis and headache
  Cryptococcal meningitis
  Aseptic meningitis (HIV-1)
  Idiopathic, "HIV-1–related" headache
  Tuberculous meningitis (*Mycobacterium tuberculosis*)
  Syphilitic meningitis
  Lymphomatous meningitis (metastatic)
Diffuse brain diseases
  With preservation of consciousness
    AIDS dementia complex
  With concomitant depression of arousal
    Metabolic encephalopathies (alone or as an exacerbating influence)
    Toxoplasmosis ("encephalitic" form)
    Cytomegalovirus encephalitis
    Herpes encephalitis
Focal brain diseases
  Subacute
    Cerebral toxoplasmosis
    Primary CNS lymphoma
    Progressive multifocal leukoencephalopathy
    Tuberculous brain abscess (*M. tuberculosis*)
    Cryptococcoma
    Varicella-zoster virus encephalitis
    Herpes encephalitis
  Acute
    Vascular disorders (VZV vasculitis)
Myelopathies
  Subacute/chronic, progressive and "diffuse"
    Vacuolar myelopathy
    HTLV-1–associated myelopathy
  Acute/subacute and segmental
    Transverse myelitis
      Varicella-zoster virus (herpes zoster)
      Spinal epidural or intradural lymphoma
    With polyradiculopathy
      Cytomegalovirus
Peripheral neuropathies
  Polyneuropathies
    HIV-1-related distal sensory polyneuropathy
    Nucleoside toxic neuropathies
    Autonomic neuropathy
    CD8 cell neuropathy associated with diffuse infiltrative lymphocytosis syndrome
  Focal neuropathies and radiculopathies
    CMV polyradiculopathy
    Mononeuritis multiplex
      CMV-related malignant type
      Early, benign vasculopathic form
    Mononeuropathy associated with aseptic meningitis
    Neuropathy related to lymphomatous meningitis or epidural compression
Myopathies
  Inflammatory
  Noninflammatory
  Zidovudine toxic myopathy

or protein levels. For this reason the clinician should have a low threshold for lumbar puncture and should routinely examine CSF for *Cryptococcus* (India ink stain, cryptococcal antigen determination, culture). Initial treatment is usually gratifying, although continued chronic therapy is required.

The syndrome of aseptic meningitis, presumably relating to direct HIV-1 infection of the leptomeninges, may complicate advanced HIV-1 infection but most often develops in the period of transition to AIDS. Both acute and chronic forms are accompanied by headache and meningeal symptoms, whereas signs of meningeal irritation are more characteristic of the acute group. Cranial nerve palsies affecting the seventh and, less often, the fifth and eighth nerves may complicate the course. The CSF shows a modest mononuclear pleocytosis, usually with normal glucose and mildly elevated protein. The presumption that this condition is due to direct HIV-1 infection of the meninges derives from the fact that the virus can be identified in the CSF and no other cause has been found. The syndrome itself is characteristically benign but may imply a poor prognosis in relation to impending progression to AIDS. The efficacy of antiretroviral or other therapies in this disorder has not been studied.

Other, less common meningeal disorders (including meningeal lymphoma, tuberculous meningitis, meningovascular syphilis) resemble their counterparts in the non-AIDS patient. A number of other conditions may present with symptoms resembling meningitis; for example, parenchymal brain diseases such as toxoplasmosis and primary CNS lymphoma may initially manifest with headache as an important symptom. More common, however, is the development of headache of uncertain cause. Although not well understood, this headache is not rare in late HIV-1 infection and at times can be a severe, debilitating problem. In some patients this headache may relate to systemic infection but in others the explanation is elusive and for this reason has been referred to as *HIV headache*.

Predominantly Focal Brain Disorders

In approaching diagnosis of parenchymal brain disease, it is useful to separate the conditions that cause predominantly focal symptoms and signs from those producing more generalized brain dysfunction. Patients in the former group present with hemiparesis, aphasia, apraxia, hemisensory abnormalities, visual field loss, and the like, as a result of focal macroscopic lesions in cortical or subcortical brain regions. The most important of the focal brain diseases are cerebral toxoplasmosis, primary CNS lymphoma and PML. Although the incidence of each of these has declined with widespread use of HAART, toxoplasmosis, which was once the most common of the three, has decreased disproportionately related to trimethoprim-sulfamethoxazole prophylaxis. Less common are a miscellany of other infections and cerebrovascular disorders.

Although the three major focal disorders all characteristically have a subacute onset and may be clinically indistinguishable, they tend to have somewhat different temporal profiles (Table 411–3). Thus, cerebral toxoplasmosis typically progresses most rapidly (over a few days) and PML evolves most slowly (over a few weeks), with primary CNS lymphoma somewhere in between. Each may cause similar neurologic deficits, but there are often differences in the associated findings. Thus, toxoplasmosis commonly presents with a combination of focal deficit and generalized encephalopathy with confusion or clouding of consciousness; fever and headache may also be present. This contrasts with PML in which focal neurologic deficits are unaccompanied by either diffuse brain dysfunction or evidence of a systemic toxic state. CNS lymphoma, when accompanied by significant mass effect or when deep in the frontal or periventricular region, may cause more global mental dysfunction, but, again, these patients are usually afebrile without constitutional symptoms or signs.

Once the focal nature of the patient's symptoms and signs is recognized, neuroimaging, including computed tomography (CT) or preferably magnetic resonance imaging (MRI), is critical both to confirm the presence of macroscopic focal disease and to determine the nature of the abnormalities (Table 411–3). Multiple lesions involving the cortex or deep brain nuclei (thalamus, basal ganglia) surrounded by edema strongly favor cerebral toxoplasmosis. In most cases *Toxoplasma* abscesses exhibit ringlike contrast enhancement. Cerebral lymphoma may produce a similar neuroimaging appearance, although the lesions of lymphoma are usually less

Table 411-3 ■ COMPARATIVE CLINICAL AND RADIOLOGIC FEATURES OF CEREBRAL TOXOPLASMOSIS, PRIMARY CNS LYMPHOMA, AND PROGRESSIVE MULTIFOCAL LEUKOENCEPHALOPATHY

	CLINICAL ONSET			NEURORADIOLOGIC FEATURES		
	Temporal Profile	Level of Alertness	Fever	Number of Lesions	Type of Lesions	Location of Lesions
Cerebral toxoplasmosis	Days	Reduced	Common	Multiple	Spherical, ring-enhancing	Basal ganglia, cortex
Primary CNS lymphoma	Days to weeks	Variable	Absent	One or few	Irregular, weakly enhancing	Periventricular white matter
Progressive multifocal leuko-encephalopathy	Weeks	Preserved	Absent	Multiple	Nonenhancing, no mass effect	White matter

numerous (one or two definable lesions), commonly exhibit more diffuse or less clear-cut contrast enhancement, and are more often located in the white matter adjacent to the ventricles. Spread beneath the ependymal lining or across the corpus callosum is also characteristic. PML characteristically involves the white matter, most often adjacent to the cortex, and is without mass effect or contrast enhancement.

The approach to diagnosis of focal brain lesions has evolved in the last few years related to appreciation of their neuroimaging characteristics and the value of toxoplasma serology along with the advent of CSF PCR in diagnosis. The first step in patients with focal neurologic symptoms and signs involves neuroimaging. Where mass lesions are present, the next step usually is distinguishing primary brain lymphoma from toxoplasmosis. If the blood toxoplasma serology is negative and the MRI shows lesions characteristic of lymphoma, then either EBV DNA sequences should be sought in CSF or brain biopsy undertaken without delay so that therapy can begin quickly. If the brain lesions appear more characteristic of toxoplasmosis and the serology is negative, then a trial of antitoxoplasma therapy is undertaken with expectation of clinical improvement within several days and neuroimaging improvement within 1 to 2 weeks. Unless herniation threatens, corticosteroids should be avoided because their effect on lymphoma and brain edema can obscure the more specific influence of antitoxoplasma treatment. Lack of improvement or suspicion of another diagnosis should signal the need for brain biopsy or other diagnostic measures. PML can usually be identified by the combination of steadily progressive focal neurologic dysfunction and the characteristic white matter lesions on MRI. Where further confirmation is needed, either CSF PCR for JC virus or brain biopsy can be used.

Other focal CNS disorders are uncommon but include some treatable lesions. This includes cryptococcal invasion of brain which nearly always develops in the setting of meningitis. Varicella-zoster virus (VZV) can cause both a demyelinating focal disease resembling PML and a cerebral vasculitis and cytomegalovirus (CMV) may rarely cause macroscopic lesions accompanied by focal clinical deficit. Herpes simplex viruses have also been reported to cause focal deficits. All of these evolve subacutely, as do the more common opportunistic problems. Acutely evolving neurologic deficits may follow seizures (Todd's palsy) or ischemic events.

Predominantly Nonfocal Brain Disorders

The disorders presenting with more general or diffuse brain dysfunction and without focal features can be further divided into those in which consciousness remains fully preserved and those accompanied by a concomitant decrease in alertness. Most important among the former is the AIDS dementia complex, a clinical syndrome characterized by cognitive, motor, and, at times, behavioral dysfunction.

Both the incidence and severity of the AIDS dementia complex increase with advancing immunosuppression. Although thought to relate to an effect of HIV-1 brain infection, the mechanisms linking this infection to neurologic dysfunction are uncertain. Most speculation centers on the activation of cytokines and related endogenous neurotoxins. Its early, mild form is usually characterized by impaired concentration and attention along with reduced mental agility, resulting in complaints of forgetfulness and slowness in performing complex mental tasks. In those who progress to more severe involvement, cognitive dysfunction worsens and involves other domains, and motor dysfunction becomes clinically manifest

with gait unsteadiness and difficulty with rapid, fine movements of the hands. Personality change with apathy, lack of initiative, or, at times, hyperactivity and agitation may be part of the syndrome. In its most severe form, global dementia, paraplegia, and virtual mutism may evolve with resultant incapacity. Although it is in part a diagnosis of exclusion, the symptoms and signs of the AIDS dementia complex are sufficiently distinct to allow bedside diagnosis in most patients on the basis of their stereotypy. Neuroimaging characteristically reveals cerebral atrophy, and MRI may additionally demonstrate increased signal in white matter or basal ganglia. Several studies have shown that zidovudine (AZT) can prevent and partially reverse the signs and symptoms of the AIDS dementia complex. This precedent suggests that combination HAART might be even more effective in this regard, although evidence for this is only beginning to be reported anecdotally or in case series.

In the AIDS dementia complex there is relative preservation of alertness in relation to cognitive loss. This contrasts with most metabolic encephalopathies developing as sequelae of the systemic diseases suffered by AIDS patients; for example, hypoxia and sepsis are characteristically accompanied by a degree of lethargy and confusion which parallels the decline in cognition. Likewise, CNS-active drugs often cloud mentation and alertness together. Although such metabolic and toxic disorders may present alone, they may also have an exacerbating or unmasking influence on the AIDS dementia complex, resulting in a mixture of the two conditions. HIV-1-infected patients may also be more sensitive to neuroleptics and thereby manifest parkinsonian or other movement disorders as side effects at seemingly low doses.

Brain infections may also produce diffuse brain dysfunction. Most important is CMV, which can be difficult to diagnose. Clinical features that raise suspicion include clouded consciousness, ataxia and nystagmus or seizures, whereas MRI findings of contrast enhancement or increased attenuation of the ventricular ependyma also support this diagnosis. CSF PCR detection of CMV sequences provides diagnostic confirmation in this setting. Although CNS toxoplasmosis characteristically causes focal neurologic symptoms and signs, in some patients generalized encephalopathy predominates. Similarly, CNS lymphoma may infiltrate deep structures and impair cognition and motor function without prominent focal symptoms or signs. Herpes simplex virus types 1 and 2 may also cause subacute nonfocal encephalitis.

Myelopathies

The most common spinal cord affliction in AIDS patients is the pathologically defined vacuolar myelopathy, which has been included within the broader clinical designation of the AIDS dementia complex because it is usually accompanied by evidence of concomitant brain dysfunction. The disorder is generally of subacute or gradual onset and progression with painless gait disturbance characterized by ataxia and spasticity. Bladder and bowel difficulty usually follow deterioration of gait, and sensory symptoms and signs are less prominent than gait dysfunction unless there is concomitant neuropathy. Patients do not manifest a distinct sensory or motor "level" as in transverse myelopathies but rather distal loss of large-fiber modalities accompanied by increased deep tendon reflexes (again, in the absence of neuropathy) and Babinski signs. The efficacy of antiretroviral therapy in this subgroup of AIDS dementia complex patients is uncertain, but personal experience suggests that some respond.

Infections by two other retroviruses, human T-lymphotropic viruses types one and two (HTLV-I and HTLV-II), can also cause similar myelopathies and coexist in the same population at risk for HIV-1 or even co-infect the same patient. Diagnosis of these infections is established by serology, and other than the overlap in epidemiology related to sexual or intravenous inoculation, they do not appear to interact in causing CNS disease. HTLV-I/II myelopathy may be aided by detection of antiviral IgG antibodies in the CSF. MRI is not helpful in distinguishing these from vacuolar myelopathy and usually is negative. In fact, MRI is most useful in detecting and characterizing the segmental myelopathies listed in Table 411–2.

Peripheral Neuropathies

HIV-1 infection can be complicated by several neuropathies, including both polyneuropathies and focal neuropathies (Table 411–2). The most common of these, sometimes called HIV-related distal sensory polyneuropathy, is a distal, predominantly sensory polyneuropathy that manifests in late HIV-1 infection. In this axonal neuropathy, sensory symptoms exceed both sensory and motor dysfunction and severity ranges from asymptomatic increase in sensory thresholds to paresthesias and numbness to severe neuropathic pain. The latter begins with distal burning of the toes or bottoms of the feet and may ascend subacutely or more indolently to the ankles or beyond. Although associated with HIV-1 infection, like the AIDS dementia complex, its pathogenesis is unknown and is speculated to relate to cytokine-mediated injury. Unlike the CNS disease, however, antiretroviral therapy does not appear to reverse the condition. Rather, treatment is directed at relief of pain, using tricyclic antidepressants, gabapentin or, when necessary, narcotic analgesics.

A second and clinically very similar sensory polyneuropathy is caused by some of the nucleoside antiretroviral drugs, including zalcitabine, didanosine, and stavudine. Clinical differentiation of this dose-related neuropathy from HIV-related polyneuropathy is difficult and relies on temporal linking of onset with drug therapy or its alleviation, after a delay of several weeks, when the drug is stopped. Electromyography or other laboratory studies are not helpful in separating these conditions.

Among the focal neuropathies, CMV causes an uncommon but severe polyradiculopathy that usually begins with pain, weakness and sensory loss in the lumbosacral roots and progresses over days in ascending fashion to affect thoracic and cervical roots. The CSF usually has a characteristic polymorphonuclear cell-predominant pleocytosis. Rapid institution of treatment is paramount in halting its progression which may otherwise be fatal. CMV can also cause a severe mononeuritis multiplex, often involving proximal nerves. This occurs in the setting of low CD4+ lymphocyte counts and also mandates rapid treatment, even without laboratory proof of its cause. It should be distinguished from a more benign and limited mononeuritis multiplex that can occur with higher CD4 counts and likely has an immunopathologic basis.

Myopathies

Several types of myopathy may complicate HIV-1 infection. Both inflammatory and noninflammatory myopathies have been described, ranging in severity from asymptomatic creatine kinase elevation to severe proximal weakness. Patients with inflammatory, polymyositis-like illnesses have improved with corticosteroid therapy.

Zidovudine can also cause proximal weakness and loss of muscle mass. This toxic myopathy appears to develop only after prolonged use of the antiretroviral and perhaps relates to the drug's effect on mitochondria; muscle biopsy may reveal excessive or abnormal mitochondria. Discontinuing the drug usually results in clinical improvement.

Baumbartner JE, Rachlin JR, Beckstead JH, et al: Primary central nervous system lymphomas: Natural history and response to radiation therapy in 55 patients with acquired immunodeficiency syndrome. J Neurosurg 73:206, 1990. *Describes an extensive experience with primary CNS lymphoma in AIDS.*

Berger JR, Levy RM: AIDS and the Nervous System, 2nd ed. Philadelphia, Lippincott-Raven, 1997. *A multi-authored book with a number of useful chapters and extensive primary source references.*

Berger J, Lorraine P, Lanska D, Whiteman M: Progressive multifocal leukoencephalopathy in patients with HIV infection. J Neuro Virol 4:59, 1998. *A review of experience with PML in AIDS.*

Gendelman HE, Lipton SA, Epstein L, Swindells S: The Neurology of AIDS. New York: Chapman & Hall, 1998. *Another useful book, though focused heavily on the interactions of HIV-1 with the nervous system.*

Navia BA, Jordon BD, Price RW: The AIDS dementia complex. J. Clinical features,

Ann Neurol 19517, 1986. *Report characterizing the clinical features of the AIDS dementia complex.*

Price RW: Management of the neurological complications of HIV-1 and AIDS. *In* Sande MA, Volberding PA (eds). The Medical Management of AIDS, 5th ed. Philadelphia, W.B. Saunders, 1997, pp 197–216. *A review chapter that extends this section.*

Zuger A, Louie E, Holzman RS, et al: Cryptococcal disease in patients with the acquired immunodeficiency syndrome: Diagnostic features and outcome of treatment. Ann Intern Med 104:234, 1986. *Describes the clinical features of cryptococcal meningitis in AIDS.*

412 PULMONARY MANIFESTATIONS OF HIV INFECTION

Philip C. Hopewell

Lung disease, specifically *Pneumocystis carinii* pneumonia (PCP), was the first recognized mode of expression of infection with the human immunodeficiency virus (HIV). Since the original clusters of cases of PCP were reported in 1981, the respiratory system has continued to be a common site of involvement in persons infected with HIV. Although pulmonary disorders are more frequent among persons who have advanced immunosuppression, meeting the current surveillance definitions for the acquired immunodeficiency syndrome (AIDS), lung diseases also occur with an increased frequency in individuals with HIV infection who have lesser degrees of immunosuppression. This chapter describes the relative frequency and spectrum of lung diseases that occur among persons infected with HIV and focuses on the approach to evaluating symptoms that originate from the respiratory tract in this unique group of patients.

EFFECTS OF HIV ON RESPIRATORY TRACT DEFENSES

The hallmark of the effect of HIV infection on host immune response is a progressive reduction in the number of circulating CD4+ lymphocytes or "T-helper" cells (see Chapter 407 and 408). The CD4+ lymphocyte plays a central role in orchestrating both cellular and humoral immune responses. Consequently, as HIV disease becomes progressively more severe, the ability of the host to ward off or contain infecting organisms becomes more and more limited. Many of the immune defects that have been described in HIV-infected persons can be attributed simply to a reduction in numbers of CD4+ lymphocytes. However, HIV infection also induces functional defects in these cells: Circulating CD4+ lymphocytes fail to proliferate in response to antigens that have been encountered previously. This loss of memory may account for failure to continue to contain infections, such as with *Mycobacterium tuberculosis* or *P. carinii*, and for the inability to prevent reinfection, as may occur with *M. tuberculosis*. Reductions in production of interleukin-2 (IL-2) and interferon-γ by CD4+ lymphocytes from HIV-infected persons have also been demonstrated. These cytokines are responsible for stimulating clonal proliferation of specifically activated alveolar macrophages and lymphocytes. Defects in production of IL-2 and interferon-γ are detectable early in the course of HIV infection and account for a functional decrease in immune response out of proportion to reduced numbers of circulating CD4+ lymphocytes (see Chapter 407).

Alveolar macrophages from persons with HIV infection have reduced chemotactic ability, but the ability to phagocytose and kill ingested organisms is thought to be normal. Alveolar macrophages express CD4 surface antigens and thus can be infected with HIV, yet they remain viable. It has been postulated that these cells can serve as reservoirs in which HIV may be sequestered. The protected virions may then infect other cells. It has also been demonstrated that cytokines, especially tumor necrosis factor-α and IL-3, stimulated by opportunistic infections such as tuberculosis, result in upregulation of HIV production within macrophages. Given these findings, the alveolar macrophage may play roles in protecting both

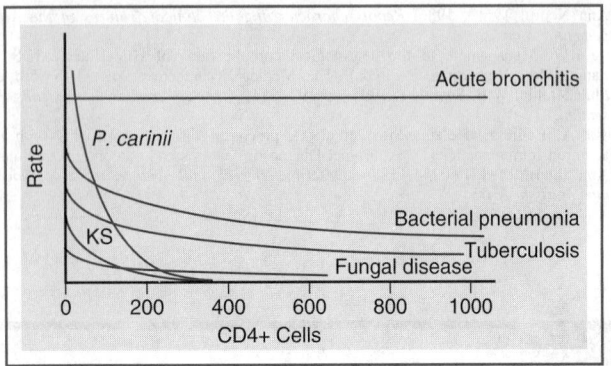

FIGURE 412-1 ■ The relative frequency and spectrum of lung diseases change as the CD4+ lymphocyte count declines. This graph presents a conceptual depiction of these changes. The x-axis could also be equated with time following acquisition of HIV infection.

the host and the virus and may contribute to accelerated HIV disease in the presence of opportunistic infections.

CORRELATION OF RESPIRATORY TRACT DISORDERS WITH STAGE OF HIV DISEASE

The conceptual relationship between the frequency and spectrum of lung diseases and CD4+ lymphocyte count is shown in Figure 412-1. The data that support this concept have been derived from a large, national, multicenter investigation, The Pulmonary Complications of HIV Infection Study (PCHIS). The cohort that formed the basis for this study generally mirrored the characteristics of the known HIV-infected persons in the United States (that is, reported AIDS cases), had a broad range of severity of immune compromise (47% of the cohort had CD4+ lymphocyte counts > 400 cells per microliter at the time of enrollment), and were followed for a median of 53 months.

Table 412-1 shows the diseases and their rates per 100 person-years of observation in the PCHIS. Because an HIV-negative control group made up of subjects from the two largest HIV transmission categories (homosexual/bisexual men and injecting drug users [IDUs]) was included, it was demonstrated that acute bronchitis, a disorder not usually regarded as opportunistic, is significantly more common among HIV-infected persons. It should be noted that because there were no study centers in areas in which histoplasmosis and coccidioidomycosis are endemic, there were few instances of these relatively common fungal infections of the lung noted in the cohort. This observation raises an important point: the spectrum of HIV-associated lung diseases varies with geographic location as well as with severity of immune compromise and the demographic (including transmission category) make-up of the HIV-infected population in any given medical center or geographic area.

Table 412-1 ■ CUMULATIVE FREQUENCY OF DISEASES WITH RESPIRATORY TRACT INVOLVEMENT IN A COHORT OF PERSONS WITH HIV INFECTION (INCLUDES MULTIPLE EPISODES PER PERSON)

DIAGNOSIS	EPISODES PER 100 PERSON-YEARS
Acute bronchitis	9.72
Pneumocystis carinii pneumonia	5.65
Bacterial pneumonia	5.63
Nontuberculous mycobacterial diseases	0.74
Interstitial lung disease	0.60
Pulmonary tuberculosis	0.58
Cytomegalovirus	0.42
Kaposi's sarcoma	0.33
Lymphoma	0.19
Cryptococcosis	0.16

RELATIONSHIP OF RESPIRATORY TRACT DISEASES TO CD4+ LYMPHOCYTE COUNT, DEMOGRAPHIC CHARACTERISTICS, AND TRANSMISSION CATEGORY

PCP is the most common lung disease in persons with CD4+ counts < 200 cells per microliter. However, in the PCHIS, 11 (6%) cases of PCP occurred in persons with CD4+ lymphocyte counts > 200 cells per microliter. The patients with higher counts were marked by having other HIV-associated symptoms or findings such as fever, unintentional weight loss, oral thrush, and lymphadenopathy. Other lung diseases that usually occur only in persons with advanced HIV infection include fungal infections, pulmonary Kaposi's sarcoma (KS), lymphoma, and nontuberculous mycobacterial infections. In the case of *Mycobacterium avium* complex, it is difficult to determine if the organism is actually causing lung disease or is simply colonizing the airways. Thus, the frequency of *M. avium* complex lung disease is difficult to establish. The same difficulty applies to determining the frequency of cytomegalovirus (CMV) pulmonary disease.

It is not yet known if the increase in CD4+ count that occurs with combination antiretroviral therapy is associated with a reduction in risk of opportunistic infections or a change in their relative frequency.

Both demographic characteristics and HIV transmission category bear some relationship to the frequency of various lung diseases. Bacterial pneumonia tends to be more common among IDUs (with or without HIV infection) than in the other HIV transmission categories. Presumably, this relates, at least in part, to the effects of opiates on ventilation, cough, and ability to protect the airway. Tuberculosis is also more common in IDUs. Injection drug use had been shown to be a risk factor for tuberculosis prior to the HIV epidemic, so the finding of an increased amount of tuberculosis among drug users with HIV infection is not surprising.

Data from the PCHIS have shown that whites have a higher rate of PCP than blacks. Although the basis for this is unknown, the finding is consistent with the observation that PCP is rare in Africa. It has generally been assumed that the rarity of *P. carinii* in Africa is related to the organism being less common in the environment. However, the finding of a racial difference in risk suggests that genetic factors may play a role in predisposing whites to or protecting blacks from the disease.

CLINICAL FEATURES OF HIV-ASSOCIATED DISORDERS OF THE RESPIRATORY TRACT

Disorders Not Necessarily Associated with Severe Immune Suppression

Bronchitis

Acute bronchitis in the PCHIS was defined by the presence of cough with sputum production for at least 48 hours and a chest film that showed either no or stable parenchymal infiltrations occurring in a study subject who did not develop an identified pulmonary infection. Evaluations to attempt to determine the microbial cause of the bronchitis were not performed in the PCHIS. It was the general impression of the investigators that the illness tended to be self-limited but recurrent. Not surprisingly, bronchitis was more common among cigarette smokers.

Airways disease may be recognized on plain chest films by the presence of peribronchial thickening (Fig. 412-2A) and is more clearly seen on computed tomographic (CT) scans, especially thin-section scans (Fig. 412-2B). In addition, bronchiectasis may also occur without a recognized antecedent lung infection (Fig. 412-3). Bronchiectasis may also be a sequela of bacterial lung infection or, occasionally, PCP.

Although in the PCHIS cohort the episodes of acute bronchitis were neither associated with nor portended any other significant pulmonary diseases, the disorder may be problematic in that the symptoms may be mistaken as an indication for further, often invasive, evaluations. In general, however, bronchitis is recognizable by the absence of parenchymal infiltrations on chest films and, thus, when the constellation of symptoms and findings described previously is noted, one should, generally, simply observe the patient, with or without antimicrobial therapy, and not undertake further evaluations.

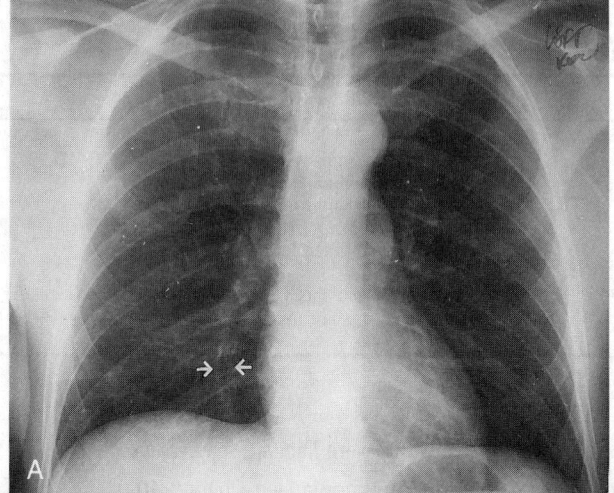

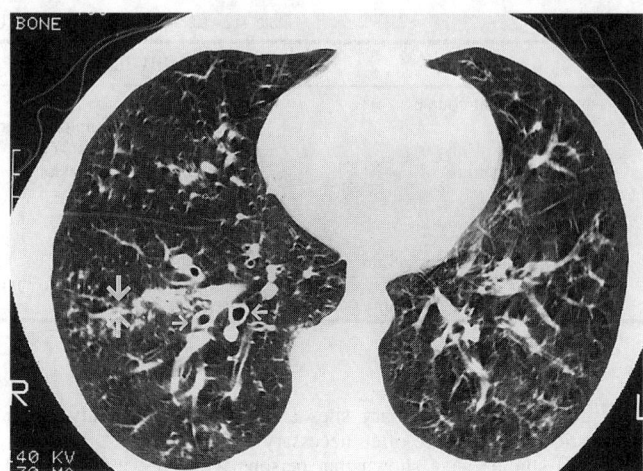

FIGURE 412–3 ■ High-resolution CT scan of the chest of the patient whose films are shown in Figure 365–2. The scan is at a lower level and shows dilated airways with thickened walls indicative of bronchiectasis (*horizontal arrows*) and areas of mucus plugging and infiltration (*vertical arrows*). (Courtesy of Dr. James Gruden, Department of Radiology, San Francisco General Hospital.)

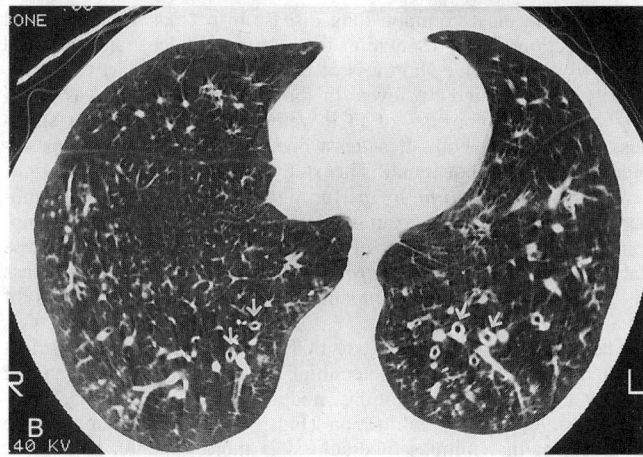

FIGURE 412–2 ■ Bronchitis in HIV infection. *A,* A frontal view chest radiograph showing peribronchial thickening, right lower lung zone (*arrows*) consistent with bronchitis. *B,* A high-resolution CT scan of the chest showing bilateral peribronchial thickening (*arrows*) consistent with bronchitis. (Courtesy of Dr. James Gruden, Department of Radiology, San Francisco General Hospital.)

Bacterial Pneumonia (see related chapter for each infection in Part XXII)

As shown in Table 412–1, bacterial pneumonia occurred at a rate of 5.63 episodes per 100 person-years of observation in the PCHIS cohort. Bacterial pneumonia was defined as the presence of cough that was productive of purulent sputum, an area of parenchymal infiltration on chest film, and a response to antimicrobial therapy. A specific causative agent was identified in 35% of cases, a proportion that is consistent with the results of studies of the etiology of community-acquired pneumonia in persons without HIV infection.

Of the episodes for which the cause was established, *Streptococcus pneumoniae* accounted for 67% and *Haemophilus influenzae* 15%. These two agents have been generally ranked first and second in most reports of bacterial pneumonia in persons with HIV infection. In most reports, *Staphylococcus aureus* has been the third most common agent and seems to be especially common among persons with pulmonary KS. A long list of other bacterial pathogens has also been described as causing pneumonia in the setting of HIV infection (Table 412–2).

Bacterial pneumonia, especially pneumococcal pneumonia, commonly tends to be associated with bacteremia and, occasionally, sepsis syndrome. Other than the high frequency of bacteremia, the mode of clinical presentation of bacterial pneumonia does not differ in persons with and without HIV infection. Pneumonias caused by *S. pneumoniae* and *H. influenzae* tend to present as an acute illness of short duration characterized by fever, chills, and productive cough. Lobar consolidation is the most common finding on chest radiographs, and pleural fluid may be present.

The diagnostic evaluation should include sputum Gram stain and culture, Gram stain and culture of pleural fluid if present, and blood cultures. Antimicrobial therapy should be guided by the usual principles for treating infectious disorders. The response to therapy should be prompt and comparable to the response of non-immunocompromised patients. Clinicians should have a low threshold for initiating further diagnostic evaluations if the response is not prompt or is incomplete or there is worsening after an initial response. In a retrospective review of pneumococcal pneumonia in patients with HIV infection, all patients who failed to respond to usual antimicrobial therapy had superimposed PCP.

Another feature of HIV-associated bacterial pneumonia is the tendency for recurrence. This may be related to the failure to generate protective antibodies to infecting organism or to bronchiectasis.

Tuberculosis

Because *M. tuberculosis* is a very pathogenic organism, little or no immune compromise is needed for tuberculosis to develop. For this reason, tuberculosis tends to occur earlier in the course of HIV disease than diseases caused by less pathogenic organisms. The degree of immunosuppression present in a given patient has an important influence on the clinical features of tuberculosis in the presence of HIV infection, as described in Table 412–3. Persons with HIV infection and relatively well-preserved immune function tend to have "typical" features of tuberculosis, whereas tuberculosis that occurs among persons with advanced HIV disease commonly involves extrapulmonary sites and has diffuse lung infiltration with no cavitation and hilar and mediastinal adenopathy (Fig. 412–4). In terms of symptoms, tuberculosis may present as an acute illness or as a more indolent progressive process. When the lungs are involved, sputum smears and cultures are as likely to be positive in persons with HIV infection as in non–HIV-infected patients. How-

Table 412–2 ■ **REPORTED CAUSES OF BACTERIAL PNEUMONIA IN PERSONS WITH HIV INFECTION**

Streptococcus pneumoniae
Haemophilus influenzae
Staphylococcus aureus
Nonpneumococcal streptococci
Pseudomonas aeruginosa
Moraxella catarrhalis
Rhodococcus equi
Neisseria meningitidis
Legionella species
Nocardia species
Actinomyces species

Table 412–3 ■ FEATURES OF TUBERCULOSIS IN PATIENTS WITH HIV INFECTION

	EARLY IN HIV DISEASE	LATE IN HIV DISEASE
Clinical course	More indolent	More acute
	Fewer systemic symptoms/signs	Systemic symptoms/signs may predominate
Sites of disease	Predominantly pulmonary	Predominantly extrapulmonary and disseminated
Chest film	Upper lobe cavitary lesions	Diffuse or lower lobe infiltration
		Adenopathy
		Occasionally normal when lungs involved
Tuberculin test	Usually positive	Usually negative
Sputum smear/culture	Usually positive	Usually positive in patients with pulmonary disease
Infectiousness	Infectious when lungs are involved	Infectious when lungs are involved
Response to therapy	Excellent	Excellent

ever, because extrapulmonary sites are involved commonly, other diagnostic specimens are often necessary (Table 412–4).

Several studies have shown that persons with HIV infection and tuberculosis respond well to antituberculous therapy. In a series of patients, those who failed to respond to standard antituberculous therapy or who responded and then worsened had another superimposed disease, often PCP.

Nonspecific and Lymphoid Interstitial Pneumonitis

In the PCHIS cohort, undiagnosed "interstitial disease" occurred at a rate of 0.60 cases per 100 person-years. It is not known, however, if these cases met the diagnostic criteria for either nonspecific interstitial pneumonitis (NIP) or lymphoid interstitial pneumonitis (LIP). LIP, although common in children with HIV infection, is thought to be rare in adults; thus, most of the cases in the PCHIS cohort were probably NIP. The cause of these conditions is not known, but it is speculated that they represent a response to the HIV itself. NIP tends to be self-limited in most instances and to resolve without therapy. LIP is more persistent and/or progressive but in some instances has seemed to respond to corticosteroids.

The diagnosis of both NIP and LIP can be made only by biopsy. Although transbronchial biopsy tissue usually is not sufficient to provide a definitive diagnosis, findings that are consistent with NIP in the absence of any other identified diagnosis is sufficient to infer a diagnosis of NIP. Because of the apparent benign course of the disease and the lack of any therapeutic modalities, invasive tests to establish a diagnosis of NIP are not warranted.

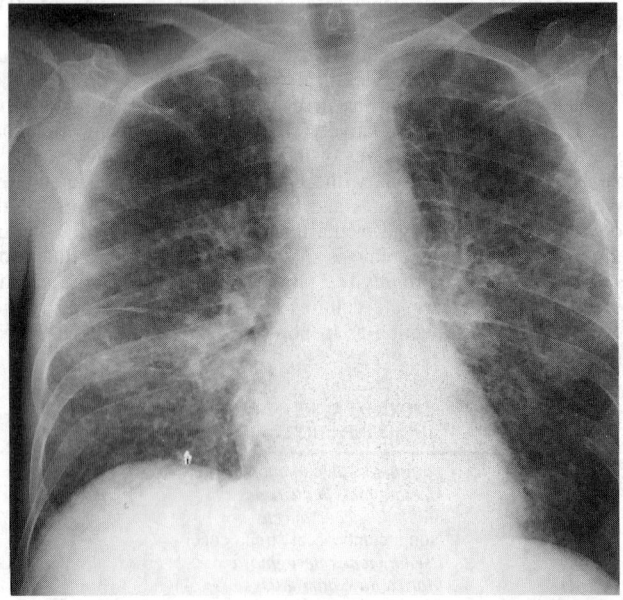

FIGURE 412–4 ■ Frontal view chest radiograph showing diffuse pulmonary parenchymal infiltration and bilateral hilar and right paratracheal adenopathy. The patient had acid-fast bacilli seen on microscopic examination of his sputum, and *Mycobacterium tuberculosis* was isolated from sputum and blood. (Courtesy of Dr. James Gruden, Department of Radiology, San Francisco Hospital.)

Disorders Associated with Severe Immune Suppression

Pneumocystis carinii Pneumonia (see Chapter 402)

PCP is the most common lung disease in persons with advanced HIV infection. The presentation tends to be indolent, characterized by slowly progressive shortness of breath and nonproductive cough, usually accompanied by fever. In the PCHIS cohort, it was noted that virtually all episodes of PCP were marked by cough or shortness of breath, or both. If at least one of these symptoms was not present, PCP was not found. This study also examined the utility of screening for *P. carinii* by performing chest radiographs, pulmonary function tests, and examination of induced sputum on asymptomatic subjects. No cases of PCP were found. Based on these data, an evaluation for *P. carinii* should not be undertaken unless an HIV-infected person complains of cough and/or shortness of breath.

The radiographic findings of PCP are extremely varied. Most frequently there is diffuse "interstitial" infiltration, but there may be any manner of focal infiltrations, nodules or cavitary lesions, pneumatoceles, or miliary infiltration (Fig. 412–5). Focal upper lobe involvement that mimics tuberculosis is more common in persons who have been given aerosol pentamidine as prophylaxis against PCP. Pneumatoceles and spontaneous pneumothorax may occur with first episodes of PCP but are more common with subsequent episodes.

Commonly, the response to antipneumocystis therapy is slow, and radiographic abnormalities and gas exchange may worsen during the first 4 to 6 days of treatment. Co-administration of corticosteroids may minimize this initial worsening. Generally, particularly if the diagnosis has been established by bronchoscopy, most clinicians who repeat bronchoscopy early in the course of therapy find that it does not yield any additional diagnoses. However, worsening later in the course may be associated with a second, superimposed disease.

Nontuberculous Mycobacterial Disease (see Chapter 359)

Soon after AIDS was initially described, it was recognized that a group of closely related mycobacteria collectively named *Mycobac-*

Table 412–4 ■ RESULTS OF MICROSCOPIC EXAMINATION AND MYCOBACTERIAL CULTURES IN PATIENTS WITH ADVANCED HIV INFECTION AND TUBERCULOSIS

	NO. POSITIVE/NO. TESTED (%)	
SPECIMEN	Acid-fast Smear	Culture
Sputum	43/69 (62)	64/69 (93)
Bronchoalveolar lavage	9/44 (20)	39/44 (89)
Transbronchial lung biopsy	1/10 (10)	7/10 (70)
Blood	—	15/46 (33)
Lymph node	21/44 (48)	39/43 (91)
Bone marrow	4/22 (18)	13/21 (62)
Cerebrospinal fluid	—	4/21 (19)
Urine	—	12/17 (71)
Other*	5/31 (16)	24/32 (75)

*Includes pleural fluid/biopsy; pericardial fluid/biopsy, stool, liver biopsy, abscess drainage, peritoneal fluid, bone biopsy.

Data from Small PM, Schecter GF, Goodman PF, et al: Treatment of tuberculosis in patients with advanced human immunodeficiency virus infection. N Engl J Med 324: 289, 1991.

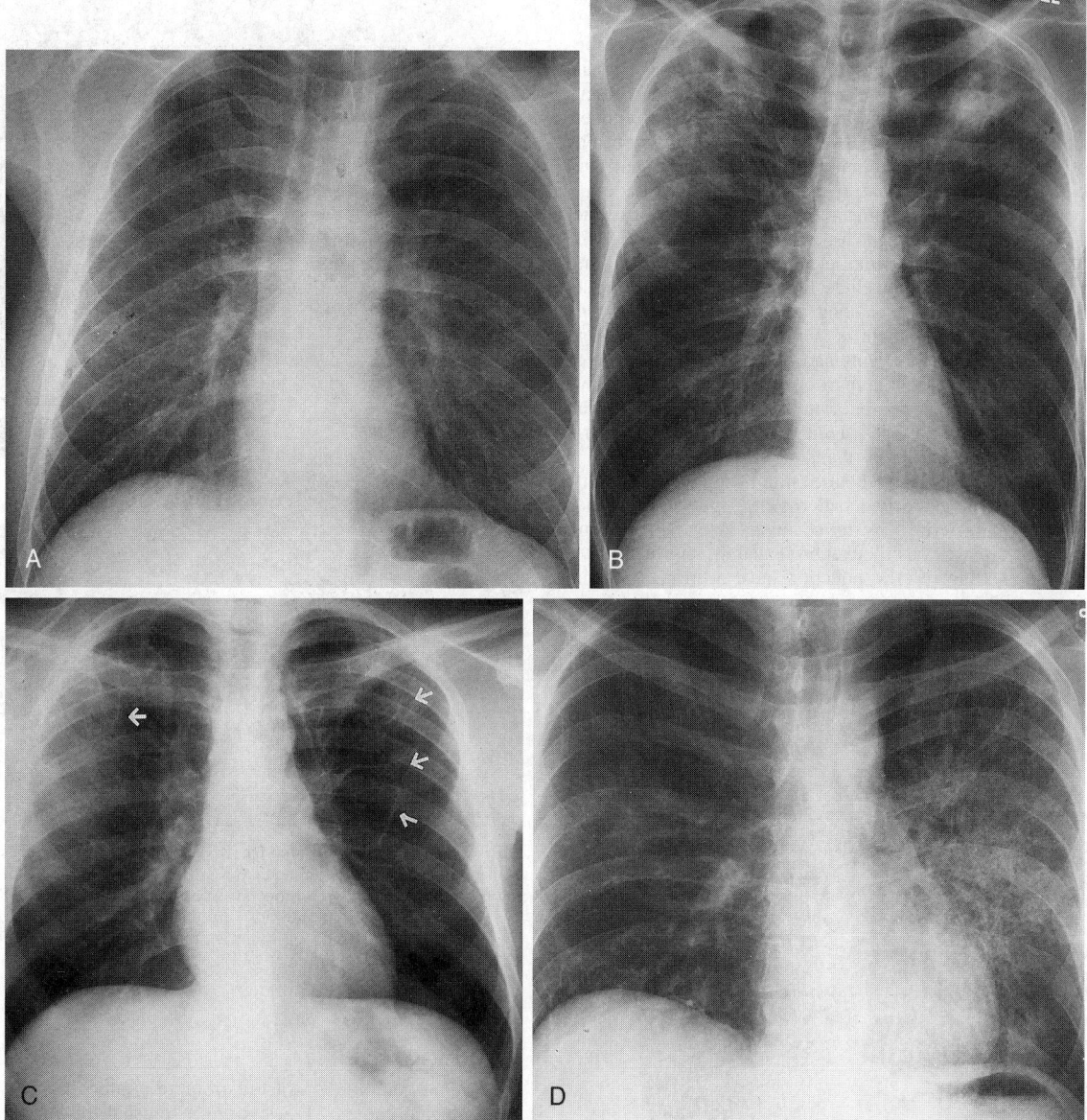

FIGURE 412–5 ■ Radiographic findings of *Pneumocystis carinii* pneumonia (PCP). *A,* A frontal view chest radiograph showing diffuse hazy infiltration caused by early PCP. *B,* A frontal view chest radiograph with bilateral upper lobe infiltrations. *C,* A frontal view chest radiograph showing multiple bilateral thin-walled pneumatoceles *(arrows). D,* A frontal view chest radiograph with unilateral left-sided infiltration. (Courtesy of Dr. James Gruden, Department of Radiology, San Francisco General Hospital.)

terium avium complex was a common cause of disseminated infection in patients with the syndrome. Although *M. avium* complex organisms are commonly isolated from respiratory tract specimens in persons with advanced HIV infection, actual lung disease is unusual. Occasionally, however, the organism may cause focal lung disease. Endobronchial lesions may be seen on bronchoscopy, and on biopsy these lesions may contain granulomas, a histologic feature that is unusual in other organs involved in disseminated *M. avium* disease. Colonization of the lungs may precede and be a marker for subsequent disseminated *M. avium* infection. Disseminated *M. avium* complex disease occurs late in the course of HIV disease, usually when the CD4 + lymphocyte count is < 50 cells per microliter. Fever, weight loss, diarrhea, and abdominal pain are common symptoms. Pulmonary involvement is usually indicated by cough. Because it is difficult to distinguish between colonization and infection, the radiographic features of *M. avium* pulmonary disease are not well-defined. As noted above, focal infiltration may occur. Rarely, there may be diffuse lung involvement with an interstitial pattern on chest films. However, in the presence of a diffusely abnormal chest film, *M. avium* complex should not be accepted as the cause until other diseases have been excluded.

Among the nontuberculous mycobacteria, *M. kansasii* is a distant second to *M. avium* complex as a cause of disease in HIV-infected persons; although its frequency seems to be increasing. As with *M. avium* complex, *M. kansasii* infections tend to be disseminated in persons with HIV infection. However, when *M. kansasii* is isolated from a respiratory tract specimen, it is more likely to be a cause of lung disease than is *M. avium* complex. As with most lung infections, *M. kansasii* usually presents with fever, cough, and, subsequently, shortness of breath. *M. kansasii* is probably more likely to cause diffuse infiltration on chest film than *M. avium* complex (see Chapter 359).

Fungal Infections (see Chapters 393 to 402)

Both histoplasmosis and coccidioidomycosis are common HIV-associated infections in the areas in which the causative organisms are endemic and are seen sporadically outside of the endemic regions. The presenting clinical features of both histoplasmosis and coccidioidomycosis are nonspecific and variable. Histoplasmosis is commonly a protracted, febrile, wasting illness. Both infections are usually disseminated, with respiratory symptoms and abnormal chest films reported in varying proportions. Both histoplasmosis and coccidioidomycosis can present with an acute sepsis syndrome including acute respiratory failure.

Chest radiographs are abnormal in the majority of patients, especially those who have respiratory symptoms. With histoplasmosis, the most common pattern is diffuse infiltration that is either reticulonodular or "alveolar." Coccidioidomycosis is associated with either localized or scattered nodular lesions or diffuse infiltration. For histoplasmosis, the diagnosis is commonly established by stain and culture of bone marrow, buffy coat, or blood. With coccidioidomycosis involving the lungs, specimens from the respiratory tract usually serve to establish the diagnosis.

Cryptococcosis is not limited to an endemic area. The presenting complaints are nonspecific and include fever, weight loss, fatigue, and headache, often present for a long period prior to diagnosis. Most often pulmonary involvement is silent, although in one large retrospective review, 31% of patients had respiratory complaints at the time of presentation. The findings on chest radiographs have been varied. Focal and diffuse infiltration, localized or scattered nodules, some of which may be cavitary, pleural effusions, and hilar adenopathy all have been described.

Aspergillosis has been diagnosed in a small number of patients with HIV infection. There are two patterns of *Aspergillus* pulmonary disease, one characterized by tissue invasion and the second largely an airway disease, obstructive bronchial aspergillosis. Reported risks in the setting of HIV infection have been neutropenia, use of corticosteroids, marijuana smoking, and use of broad-spectrum antimicrobial agents. Fever and cough that is sometimes productive of bronchial casts are the usual presenting complaints. The radiographic findings include focal infiltration, cavitary lesions, and pleura-based densities (Fig. 412–6). Atelectasis and airway filling patterns may be seen with obstructive bronchial aspergillosis.

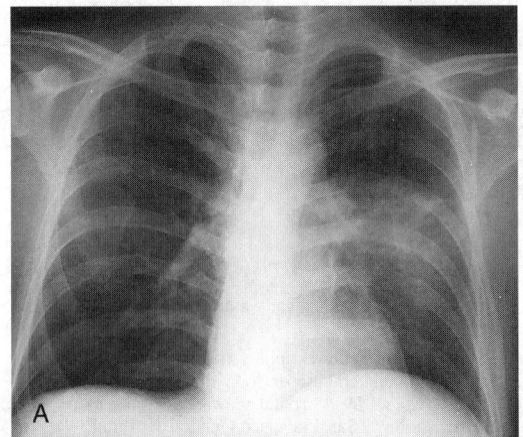

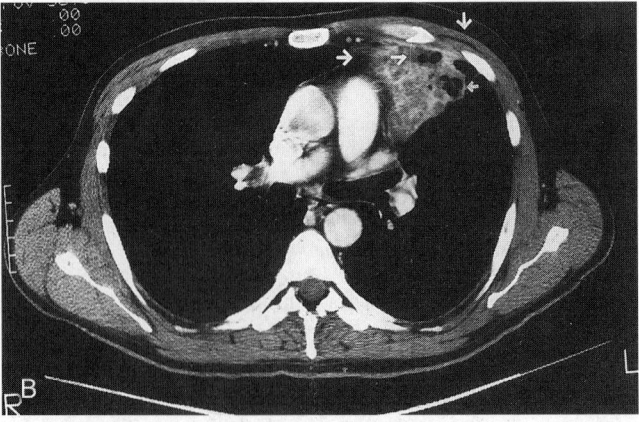

FIGURE 412–6 ■ Invasive aspergillosis in an HIV-infected man. *A,* A frontal view chest radiograph showing infiltration in the right mid-lung zone. *B,* A CT scan of the chest at the level of the infiltration. The scan shows areas of necrosis *(horizontal arrows)* and probable chest wall invasion *(vertical arrow)*. (Courtesy of Dr. James Gruden, Department of Radiology, San Francisco General Hospital.)

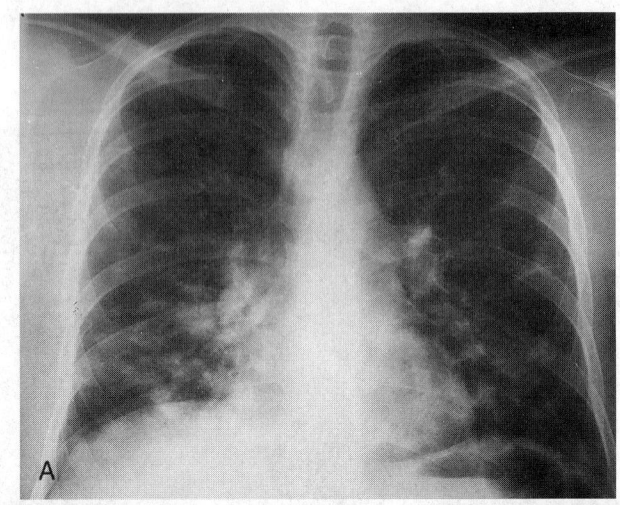

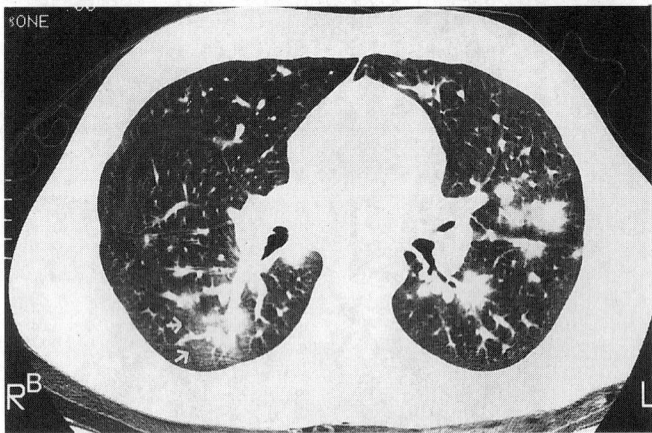

FIGURE 412–7 ■ Kaposi's sarcoma (KS). *A,* A frontal view chest radiograph with typical findings of pulmonary KS. *B,* A high-resolution CT scan of the lower chest. Masslike peribronchovascular lesions typical of KS are seen. The lesions on the right side are surrounded by areas of fainter infiltration *(arrows),* a so-called halo sign that is highly suggestive of KS. (Courtesy of Dr. James Gruden, Department of Radiology, San Francisco General Hospital.)

Cytomegalovirus

CMV is commonly isolated from respiratory tract specimens in HIV-infected patients. However, it is unusual for lung disease to be attributable to this agent even when specific cytomegalic cells are seen on biopsy specimens. Thus, the diagnosis of CMV pneumonia can be made only when the virus is isolated in culture, specific histopathologic changes are seen on biopsy, and no other diagnosis is established. Because it is difficult to determine if CMV is the cause of lung disease in a given patient, the radiographic features of CMV pneumonia are not well-defined. In general, however, it is thought to cause diffuse infiltration that is not distinguishable from the pattern caused by many other organisms and by nonspecific interstitial pneumonitis.

Neoplastic Diseases

In the PCHIS cohort, KS involving the lungs occurred at a rate of 0.33 cases per 100 person-years of observation (14 [13%] pulmonary cases of 105 total cases), and pulmonary involvement with lymphoma occurred at a rate of 0.19 cases per 100 person-years. However, among persons with advanced HIV disease, pulmonary KS has been diagnosed in 8 to 14% of patients being evaluated for respiratory symptoms, in 21 to 49% of patients with respiratory symptoms and mucocutaneous lesions, and in 47 to 75% of patients with known KS undergoing autopsy. It is likely that the reported frequency of KS is less than actually occurs because the lung involvement may be clinically silent.

The diagnosis of pulmonary KS is nearly always established by the appearance of lesions on bronchoscopy. Typically, endobronchial KS is seen as flat, red or purple submucosal lesions that are similar in appearance to submucosal hemorrhages induced by bronchoscope trauma (see Color Plate 10*G*). The lesions may be found in any location, from vocal cords to peripheral airways, and tend to favor airway bifurcations. Because of their submucosal location, the lesions are difficult to biopsy; however, the findings are sufficiently characteristic in appearance to enable a high degree of diagnostic certainty. In a few instances, pulmonary parenchymal KS has been diagnosed by transbronchial or open biopsy in persons with no endobronchial lesions seen.

The chest radiographs of patients who had pulmonary KS without coexisting infection showed lesions that were predominantly central and consisted mainly of bronchial wall thickening and nodules (Fig. 412–7). Kerley B lines and pleural effusions were noted in 71 and 52%, respectively. Hilar or mediastinal adenopathy was present in 15%.

Non-Hodgkin's lymphoma is the second most frequent malignancy involving the lungs in patients with HIV infection. The frequency of pulmonary involvement in reported series is 0 to 25%. The presentation, even in patients who have pulmonary involvement, is generally dominated by systemic symptoms. The most common chest radiographic findings are patchy parenchymal infiltrates, nodules, and solitary masses. Intrathoracic adenopathy has been reported in a minority of cases. The diagnosis can be established by transbronchial biopsy, needle aspiration biopsy, or thoracoscopic or open biopsy.

AN INTEGRATED APPROACH TO DIAGNOSIS

Although the differential diagnosis of lung disease in a person with HIV infection is quite broad, the probabilities of the various diagnoses can be reduced in a given patient by knowing the patient's symptoms, HIV transmission category, and CD4+ lymphocyte count and further refined by the findings on the chest film. A general approach to the diagnostic evaluation in patients with a CD4+ lymphocyte count of ≤ 300 cells per microliter is shown in Figure 412–8.

The first step in the diagnostic evaluation is to define the patient's symptoms, especially whether or not the patient has cough and/or shortness of breath. If cough is present, it is important to ascertain if it is productive of purulent sputum. It is very uncommon for patients with PCP to have purulent sputum. Moreover, depending on the stain used, the presence of purulent debris in respiratory tract specimens makes it difficult to detect *P. carinii* in smears of sputum or bronchoalveolar lavage (BAL) fluid. As noted previously, acute bronchitis and bacterial pneumonia are relatively more frequent among persons with higher CD4+ lymphocyte cell counts. Additionally, IDUs have higher rates of bacterial pneumonia and tuberculosis than persons in other HIV transmission categories. Also as noted, the differential diagnosis varies somewhat with the geographic area, with histoplasmosis and coccidioidomycosis being common in their respective endemic areas.

As in all patients with significant respiratory symptoms, radiographic examination of the chest is usually the first test performed. If the chest film shows no abnormalities in a patient with purulent sputum, the likely diagnosis is bronchitis. Patients with a diagnosis of bronchitis should be followed to be certain that the symptoms resolve and, if there is no resolution or worsening, further evaluation should be undertaken. It must be kept in mind that both tuberculosis and PCP may present with normal chest films.

Patients who have normal chest films and a nonproductive cough may also have bronchitis, but if the CD4+ lymphocyte count is < 300 cells per microliter, *P. carinii* should be considered. In this circumstance, pulmonary function testing with measurement of the diffusing capacity for carbon monoxide (DLCO) should be performed. If the DLCO is < 75% of the predicted normal value, further evaluation directed toward detecting *P. carinii* should be undertaken. An alternative approach is to replace measurement of the DLCO with thin-section CT scanning, using a limited number of images to reduce cost. This approach has the potential advantage of being able to distinguish among PCP, emphysema and vascular obliteration caused by foreign particle embolization from intravenous drug use (Fig. 412–9).

If the chest film is abnormal, the next step depends on the type of abnormality. Focal infiltration, especially consolidation, in a patient with purulent sputum is most consistent with a diagnosis of bacterial pneumonia or tuberculosis (see Fig. 412–8). Sputum

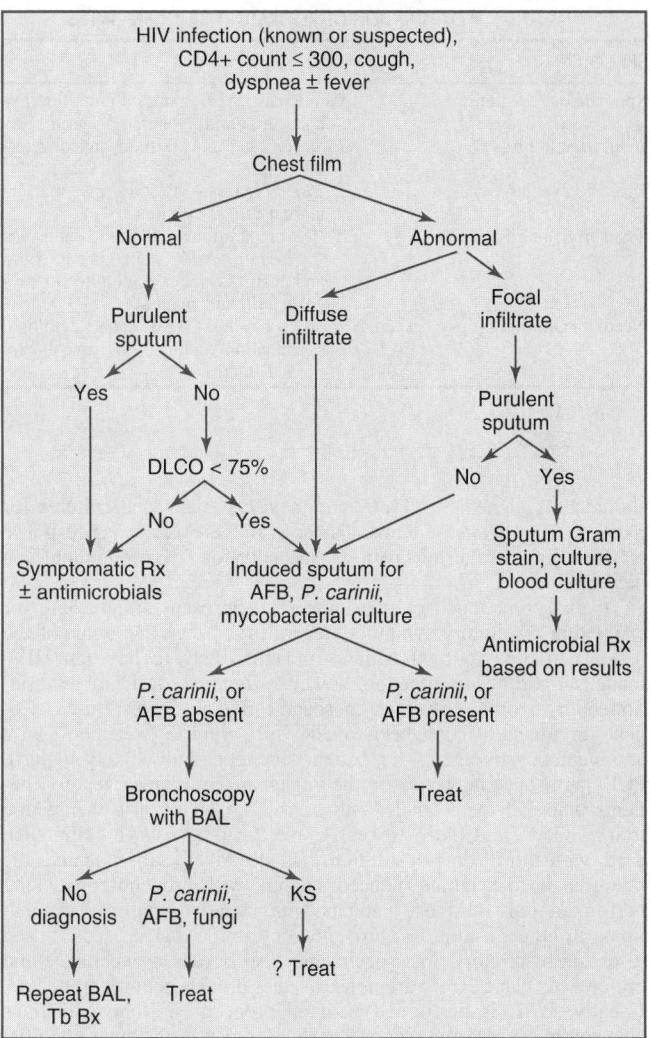

FIGURE 412–8 ■ Algorithm of the diagnostic approach to patients who are known or suspected of having HIV infection resulting in significant immunocompromise. < 300 CD4+ lymphocytes per microliter. DLCO = Pulmonary diffusing capacity for carbon monoxide; AFB = acid-fast bacilli; BAL = bronchoalveolar lavage; Tb Bx = transbronchial lung biopsy.

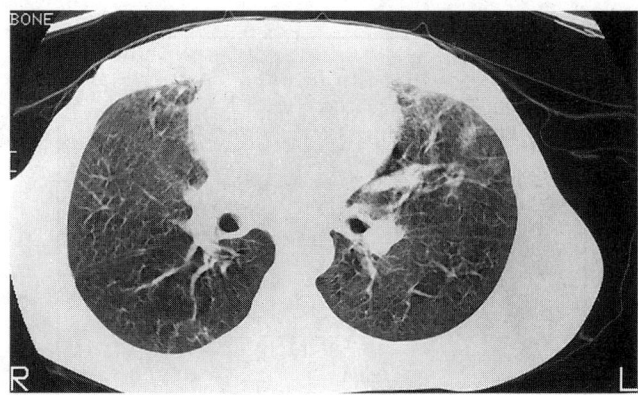

FIGURE 412–9 ■ High-resolution CT scan of the chest of a patient who complained of shortness of breath but whose plain chest film was normal. The scan shows patchy "ground-glass" infiltration in the anterior portions of both lungs. The patient was found to have *P. carinii* in an induced sputum sample. The findings noted in the scan are typical of early *P. carinii* pneumonia. (Courtesy of Dr. James Gruden, Department of Radiology, San Francisco General Hospital.)

Table 412–5 ■ EXAMINATION OF RESPIRATORY TRACT SPECIMENS

SPECIMEN	TEST
Spontaneous sputum	Gram stain, AFB stain, cultures for mycobacteria and pyogenic bacteria
Induced sputum	*P. carinii* stain, AFB stain, mycobacterial culture
Bronchoalveolar lavage fluid	*P. carinii* stain, AFB stain, mycobacterial and fungal cultures
Transbronchial biopsy tissue	Touch preparations and tissue stains for *P. carinii*, AFB stain, hematoxylin and eosin tissue stain, culture for mycobacteria and fungi
Needle aspiration biopsy tissue	*P. carinii* stain, AFB stain, cytologic examination, cultures for mycobacteria and fungi

AFB = Acid-fast bacilli.

should be obtained for Gram stain, acid-fast stain, and cultures for pyogenic organisms and mycobacteria. If there is a poor response or worsening, further evaluation, especially for *P. carinii*, should be performed.

To this point much of the diagnostic approach is applicable for evaluating respiratory symptoms regardless of the HIV status of the patient. In the group of patients thought likely to have an HIV-related opportunistic infection, however, there is considerable variation both in philosophy and in specific diagnostic tests used. Cogent arguments have been made for empiric treatment with antipneumocystis agents for patients thought highly likely to have PCP, with specific tests for the organism being reserved for patients who fail to respond. With or without an empiric therapeutic trial, when it is decided to seek a specific diagnosis, the approach used varies. In some institutions, as described subsequently, the first step is to examine induced sputum, with bronchoscopy being performed only in those patients with negative sputum examinations. In other institutions, bronchoscopy is the first procedure used to obtain respiratory tract specimens. Also based on experience and preference, there are variations in the bronchoscopic procedure. Usually, BAL is performed with all procedures. Many clinicians also routinely perform a transbronchial biopsy at the time of initial bronchoscopy, whereas others perform biopsies on a case-by-case basis, and others do so only if the BAL does not provide a diagnosis (and perhaps not even then).

If there is diffuse or focal infiltration in a person with a nonproductive cough, generally the evaluation should be directed toward opportunistic organisms. In many institutions the next diagnostic step is to induce sputum by having the patient inhale a hypertonic (3%) saline mist generated by an ultrasonic nebulizer. Careful attention to the details of selecting patients and inducing, processing,

and examining the sputum specimens is essential to obtain good results.

Diagnosis of mycobacterial disease and fungal infections can also be established by examining induced sputum. However, in HIV-infected patients, because of the high frequency of oral candidiasis, fungal cultures are frequently overgrown with *Candida* species.

Because the negative predictive value of a negative examination of induced sputum for *P. carinii* is in the range of 60%, patients having a negative sputum examination generally should undergo bronchoscopy with BAL unless another diagnosis has been established or the procedure is contraindicated. At San Francisco General Hospital, *P. carinii* infection, either alone or with another diagnosis, was found in 32% of bronchoscopic examinations in patients who had a negative sputum examination. KS was found in 15%, nontuberculous mycobacteria in 25%, *M. tuberculosis* in 5%, and fungal pathogens in 4%. In addition, nearly all of the pathogens were found by BAL, and only rarely did transbronchial biopsy provide additional information.

In patients whose chest films show focal or isolated nodular or mass lesions, needle aspiration biopsy, if the lesion is accessible, is an efficient diagnostic approach, and in some instances fluoroscopically guided transbronchial biopsy should be attempted. Enlarged intrathoracic lymph nodes may also be approached via needle aspiration biopsy, either through the bronchoscope (Wang needle) or via a transthoracic approach. The tests that should be performed on the various sorts of specimens described above are listed in Table 412–5.

PREVENTING LUNG DISEASES IN PERSONS WITH HIV INFECTION

Much of the improved survival for patients with HIV infection in recent years owes to the prevention of PCP. Hence, the use of antipneumocystis agents such as trimethoprim-sulfamethoxazole, dapsone, pentamidine aerosol, and atovaquone for persons with HIV infection and CD4+ lymphocyte counts < 200 cells per microliter is a high-priority intervention. This is described in more detail in Chapter 402.

Preventive interventions for tuberculosis also should be accorded a high priority. All HIV-infected persons should receive a tuberculin skin test, and, if the test is positive (≥ 5 mm induration), isoniazid preventive therapy should be given regardless of the CD4 + lymphocyte count. Isoniazid should also be given to all HIV-infected persons who have been exposed to a person with infectious tuberculosis regardless of the tuberculin test result. The use of isoniazid preventive therapy for nonexposed persons who are defined as anergic has not been shown to be of benefit. A combination of rifampin and pyrazinamide given for 2 months has also been shown to be effective in preventing tuberculosis in persons with HIV infection who have a positive tuberculin skin test.

It is not established whether pneumococcal vaccine reduces the rate of pneumococcal disease in persons with HIV infection. However, because of the low likelihood of adverse reactions to the vaccine, any benefit would not be offset by risk. Data from the PCHIS cohort suggest that trimethoprim-sulfamethoxazole as antipneumocystis prophylaxis decreases the frequency of pneumococcal disease, thus providing an additional benefit for this preventive intervention.

Finally, it has been shown that prophylactic administration of newer macrolide agents (clarithromycin, azithromycin) reduces the frequency of *M. avium* complex disease by approximately 70%. Current recommendations are that macrolide prophylaxis be given to persons with HIV infection and CD4+ counts of < 100 cells per microliter. Although less effective than the macrolides, rifabetin may also be used to prevent *M. avium* complex disease. Persons who are candidates for rifabutin should be carefully evaluated for tuberculosis. Rifabutin administered to a person who has undiagnosed tuberculosis would quickly result in resistance of *M. tuberculosis* to rifabutin *and* rifampin, a major antituberculosis drug. The relationship of preventive interventions to CD4+ lymphocyte count is summarized in Figure 412–10.

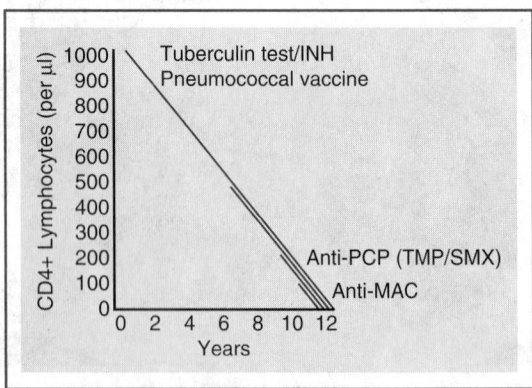

FIGURE 412–10 ■ Schematic representation of the use of preventive interventions in persons with HIV infection. The timing of the interventions is based on the CD4+ lymphocyte count and the risk of the common HIV-associated lung infections. INH = Isoniazid; PCP = *P. carinii* pneumonia; TMP-SMX = trimethoprim-sulfamethoxazole; MAC = *Mycobacterium avium* complex.

Chin DP: *Mycobacterium avium* complex and other nontuberculous mycobacteria in patients with HIV. Semin Respir Infect 8:124, 1993. *Describes the epidemiology, clinical presentation, diagnosis, and management of the nontuberculous mycobacterial diseases with a focus on* M. avium *complex.*

Hopewell PC: Tuberculosis in persons with human immunodeficiency virus infection:

Clinical and public health aspects. Semin Resp Crit Care Med 18:471, 1997. *Describes the overall impact of HIV infection on all aspects of tuberculosis.*

Irwin DH, Kaplan LD: Pulmonary manifestations of acquired immunodeficiency syndrome malignancies. Semin Respir Infect 8:139, 1993. *Describes the clinical features and management of pulmonary Kaposi's sarcoma and non-Hodgkin's lymphoma.*

Stansell JD: Pulmonary fungal infections in HIV infected persons. Semin Respir Infect 8:116, 1993. *Reviews the epidemiology, clinical features, diagnosis, and management of the fungal infections that involve the lungs in patients with HIV infection.*

Stancell JD, Huang L: *Pneumocystis carinii* pneumonia: *In* Sande MA, Volberding PA (eds.): The Medical Management of AIDS, 5th ed. Philadelphia, WB Saunders, 1997, p 275. *A comprehensive review of the epidemiology, pathogenesis, clinical features, diagnosis, and treatment of PCP.*

Wallace JM, Hansen NI, Lavange L, et al: Respiratory disease trends in the pulmonary complications of HIV infection study cohort. Am J Respir Crit Care Med 155:72, 1997. *Describes the frequency and spectrum of lung diseases after 50 months of follow-up in a cohort of HIV-infected persons from the major transmission categories. Included are subjects who have little apparent immunosuppression.*

413 GASTROINTESTINAL MANIFESTATIONS OF AIDS

John G. Bartlett

The gastrointestinal tract is an especially common site for clinical expression of human immunodeficiency virus (HIV) infection and is an important factor in morbidity from opportunistic infections in late-stage disease, as well as gastrointestinal complications from antiretroviral agents or other drugs. Nearly all opportunistic infections occur when the CD4 count is less than 200/mm³, and almost all seem to respond well to immune reconstitution when achieved with antiretroviral therapy.

ORAL LESIONS. Oral candidiasis ("thrush") is encountered at some time in 80 to 90% of all patients with advanced stages of HIV infection. The usual finding is white patches that show yeast forms and pseudohyphae on KOH preparation. Thrush is often asymptomatic, and treatment in such cases is unnecessary. Common symptoms include mouth pain, dysphagia, and taste change. The diagnosis is usually made by visual appearance. Treatment consists of topical agents (nystatin, clotrimazole troches, or amphotericin B), oral therapy with azoles or amphotericin B, or in severe refractory cases, intravenous amphotericin. Relapse rates are high, so continuous therapy with topical agents or azoles is often necessary.

Oral hairy leukoplakia is characterized by white patches consisting of white fibrillar projections that are usually located on the tongue and are often confused with thrush. Oral hairy leukoplakia is usually asymptomatic, but occasional patients complain of pain or voice changes; symptomatic patients usually respond to treatment with acyclovir. Herpes simplex virus (HSV) often causes painful oral lesions that have the typical appearance of vesicles on an erythematous base and break down to form ulcers. Herpetic oral lesions are common in the general population, but they tend to be more severe and prolonged in patients with advanced HIV infection. The usual treatment is acyclovir, famciclovir, or valacyclovir given orally; severe cases may require intravenous acyclovir or, for

acyclovir-resistant strains, foscarnet given parenterally. The major source of confusion is aphthous ulcers of unknown etiology, which seem to respond best to thalidomide or to corticosteroids given topically or systemically. Patients with Kaposi's sarcoma often have involvement of the oral cavity, most frequently with typical purplish raised lesions on the palate, although any site in the oral cavity may be involved. Most are asymptomatic; symptomatic lesions generally respond to irradiation, laser treatments, or vinblastine injections. Periodontal disease is relatively common, with either gingivitis or periodontitis. Treatment consists of topical chlorhexidine (Peridex) or systemically administered metronidazole.

ESOPHAGITIS. Dysphagia or odynophagia generally indicates an esophageal lesion. The most common cause is candidiasis, and most such patients also have thrush. Patients with odynophagia in late-stage HIV infection are usually treated empirically with fluconazole. Alternative causes of esophagitis include herpes simplex, cytomegalovirus (CMV), or aphthous ulcers (Table 413–1). Endoscopy is recommended for patients with atypical symptoms and those who fail to respond to fluconazole. Occasional cases are due to fluconazole-resistant *Candida* spp. and require intravenous amphotericin B. Ulcerative esophagitis is usually due to CMV or aphthous ulceration; HSV esophagitis is unusual. Herpes simplex may be treated with acyclovir, CMV responds to ganciclovir, and aphthous ulcers are optimally treated with systemic corticosteroids or thalidomide.

GASTRIC LESIONS. Patients with acquired immunodeficiency syndrome (AIDS) often have gastric achlorhydria; less common gastric lesions are Kaposi's sarcoma and opportunistic infections. Gastric intolerance to medications is common, especially with zidovudine, ritonavir, didanosine, indinavir, saquinavir, macrolides, trimethoprim-sulfamethoxazole, and pentamidine. Symptoms include nausea, vomiting, anorexia, and epigastric pain and usually resolve promptly when use of the implicated drug is discontinued.

SMALL BOWEL AND COLON LESIONS. Acute and/or chronic diarrhea is a frequent complication and may be due to medications, opportunistic infections, or common causes seen in the general population such as viral gastroenteritis or irritable bowel syndrome. The antiretroviral agent that most commonly causes diarrhea is nelfinavir. Treatment with bacterial agents may be complicated by *Clostridium difficile*–associated diarrhea or colitis, but the frequency and severity do not appear to be increased by immunosuppression per se.

DIAGNOSTIC EVALUATION. The approach to patients with HIV infection and diarrhea requires knowledge of four factors: medication history, CD4 count, a distinction between acute and chronic diarrhea, and emphasis on features that distinguish between colitis and enteritis. Regarding the latter, patients with colitis usually have cramps, fever, fecal leukocytes, and small-volume "fraction" stools. Enteritis is characterized by large-volume watery stools without fecal leukocytes or cramps and often without fever.

The most common microbial causes of acute diarrhea in HIV-infected patients are *Salmonella* spp., *C. difficile*, and enteric viruses. Common opportunistic pathogens that cause chronic diarrhea in late-stage HIV include cryptosporidia, microsporidia, CMV, and *Mycobacterium avium* (Table 413–2). The diagnostic evaluation begins with a review of medications and discontinuation of treatment with suspected agents. Many patients with other forms of

Table 413–1 ■ ESOPHAGEAL COMPLICATIONS OF HIV INFECTION

AGENT	FREQUENCY* (%)	CD4 COUNT (mm³)	CLINICAL FEATURES	DIAGNOSIS	TREATMENT
Candida	50–70	<200	Odynophagia, thrush, diffuse pain, usually afebrile	Usually treated empirically. Endoscopy shows plaques	Fluconazole
Cytomegalovirus (CMV)	10–20	<50	Odynophagia, focal pain, usually febrile	Biopsy of ulcer to show CMV inclusions	Ganciclovir
Herpes simplex virus (HSV)	2–5	<200	Odynophagia, oral HSV lesions common, usually afebrile	Biopsy of ulcer to show HSV inclusions	Acyclovir
Idiopathic	10–20	<300	Odynophagia, focal pain, usually afebrile	Negative biopsy of ulcer	Prednisone or thalidomide

*Approximate frequency in HIV-infected patients with odynophagia.

Table 413–2 ■ AGENTS OF ACUTE AND CHRONIC DIARRHEA

AGENT	FREQUENCY* (%)	CD4 COUNT	CLINICAL FEATURES	DIAGNOSIS	TREATMENT
Acute Diarrhea					
Salmonella	5–15	Any	Watery diarrhea, fever	Stool and blood culture	Fluoroquinolone
Clostridium difficile	10–15	Any	Cramps, watery diarrhea, fever	Stool toxin assay	Metronidazole
Enteric viruses	15–30	Any	Watery diarrhea, usually afebrile	None	Symptomatic
Idiopathic	25–40	Any	Variable	Negative culture, O&P exam, and *C. difficile* toxin	Symptomatic
Chronic Diarrhea					
Cryptosporidium	10–30	<100	Watery diarrhea, fever variable, may be devastating fluid losses	Stool O&P with AFB	Paromomycin ± azithromycin
Microsporida	15–30	<100	Watery diarrhea, afebrile	Stool trichrome stain	Albendazole (*Enterocytozoon intestinalis*)
Isospora	1–3	<100	Watery diarrhea	Stool O&P	TMP-SMX
Mycobacterium avium	10–20	<50	Watery diarrhea, fever, wasting	Blood culture	Clarithromycin + ethambutol
Cytomegalovirus	15–40	<50	Watery or bloody diarrhea; fever, fecal WBCs	Colon biopsy	Ganciclovir
Idiopathic	20–30	Any	Watery diarrhea	Negative culture, O&P, *C. difficile* toxin, endoscopy	Symptomatic

*Frequency among HIV-infected patients with acute or chronic diarrhea.
O&P = ova and parasites; AFB = acid-fast bacillus; TMP-SMX = trimethoprim-sulfamethoxazole; WBCs = white blood cells.

diarrhea respond to symptomatic therapy, so diagnostic studies for infectious causes are usually restricted to patients with severe symptoms, symptoms suggesting colitis, or chronic diarrhea. Standard tests include stool for culture, ova and parasite examination, including acid-fast bacillus stain, and *C. difficile* toxin. Endoscopy is recommended for undiagnosed cases with symptoms that are severe or persist. Patients with diarrhea should have a diet of frequent small-volume feedings, bland food, and avoidance of fat, caffeine, milk, and milk products. Antiperistaltic agents such as loperamide are often given for symptomatic relief.

Cryptosporidia tend to cause intermittent diarrhea that persists for months and may be responsible for severe fluid losses, dehydration, and electrolyte abnormalities. Small bowel biopsies show villous atrophy, crypt hyperplasia, and intraepithelial lymphocytes with typical schizonts that appear to be adherent to the brush border. Functional tests show D-xylose malabsorption, and stools show no fecal leukocytes. The usual diagnostic test is a stool examination for oocysts that appear like yeast but are easily detected with modified acid-fast stains. Complications include papillary stenosis with obstruction of the common bile duct. The usual treatment of cryptosporidial diarrhea is supportive care and paromomycin with or without azithromycin, but the response is variable and temporary. The best response is achieved with immune reconstitution.

Microsporidia are a group of small unicellular parasites; the two pathogens in AIDS patients are *Enterocytozoon bieneusi*, which accounts for about 80% of cases, and *Enterocytozoon intestinalis*. The organism can be detected in stool with a trichrome stain. Histopathologic changes are similar to those noted with cryptosporidiosis except for the unique morphologic features and location of the organism within the cytoplasm of the enterocyte. Treatment with albendazole is effective in the majority of cases caused by *E. intestinalis*; *E. bieneusi* is usually refractory to antimicrobials and responds best to immune reconstitution.

M. avium may cause pathologic changes in the small bowel that appear identical to those of Whipple's disease, with foamy macrophages distended by vesicles containing periodic acid–Schiff–positive material in the lamina propria. However, unlike Whipple's disease, the putative agents in the macrophage are acid fast and do not cross-react with antibacterial typing sera. The diagnosis is usually made with blood cultures for mycobacteria. *M. avium* generally responds to treatment with clarithromycin plus ethambutol.

CMV commonly causes disseminated infection in the late stages of HIV infection at any level of the gastrointestinal tract, including the mouth, esophagus, stomach, small bowel, colon, and perirectal region. The most common infection is a diffuse colitis with superficial ulcerations. Common symptoms ascribed to this infection include fever, diarrhea, abdominal pain, and bloody stools. Less common is a solitary ulcer, toxic megacolon, or intestinal perforation. CMV is the most common opportunistic pathogen in late-stage AIDS that causes colitis; the major alternative diagnostic consideration is *C. difficile*–associated colitis. The diagnosis of CMV is generally established by demonstrating typical viral inclusions in intestinal biopsies, but the role of this organism as a cause of symptomatic disease is sometimes controversial even when seen. A large number of inclusion bodies per square millimeter of tissue and the presence of high-grade inflammation or typical CMV vasculitis are possibly important correlates in interpretation. Ganciclovir or foscarnet is effective therapy, but patients may require continuous treatment to prevent relapse.

Isospora belli is another enteric pathogen that is found with increased frequency in patients with advanced stages of HIV infection. It is a protozoan parasite that may cause symptoms similar to those described for cryptosporidiosis. The diagnosis is established by recognition of large acid-fast oocysts (20 to 30 × 10 to 20 μm) in stool. This organism responds well to treatment with trimethoprim-sulfamethoxazole, although the relapse rate is high, so long-term maintenance treatment is often necessary.

Tumors of the gastrointestinal tract associated with HIV infection include Kaposi's sarcoma, non-Hodgkin's lymphoma, cloacogenic carcinoma of the rectum, and squamous cell carcinoma of the rectum and anus. The most common of these is Kaposi's sarcoma, which has been found in gut tissue at autopsy in 40 to 50% of persons with typical cutaneous lesions. Endoscopy typically shows raised red nodules, but histologic confirmation is difficult owing to the depth of pathologic changes. The great majority are asymptomatic; less common manifestations include diarrhea, subacute intestinal obstruction, protein-losing enteropathy, and rectal ulcer. The lymphomas associated with HIV infection are usually high-grade B-cell lymphomas that are extranodal in origin. The gastrointestinal tract is affected in up to 20%, and any site may be involved from the oral cavity to the rectum.

AIDS ENTEROPATHY. Endoscopy in patients with advanced AIDS often shows morphologic changes in the small bowel in the absence of evidence of a superimposed opportunistic infection. Characteristic features are villous blunting, a reduced villus-crypt ratio, and an inappropriately low number of mitotic figures. In the absence of an enteric pathogen, the findings are sometimes referred to as "AIDS enteropathy." Studies of gastrointestinal function in the presence of AIDS enteropathy usually show malabsorption with abnormal D-xylose and ^{14}C-glycerol-tripalmitin absorption tests. The cause of these changes is not known, but the major considerations include direct invasion by HIV, an opportunistic infection that has not been detected, or a consequence of immune suppression.

MALNUTRITION AND WASTING. The average patient with late-stage AIDS loses 15 to 20% of baseline weight. Protein-calorie malnutrition is a common and important sequela that may accelerate progressive immunosuppression. Factors contributing to malnutrition include a hypermetabolic state associated with chronic infection (especially with fever), oral lesions causing pain, esophageal lesions resulting in dysphagia, reduced taste sensation, depression, HIV-associated subcortical dementia, gastrointestinal side effects of medications, and AIDS enteropathy. Many patients lose weight with sequential opportunistic infections that is not regained during asymptomatic intervals. Therapy for wasting depends on the severity, cause, patient gender, and response. Immune reconstitution with antiretroviral therapy has been associated with remarkable weight gain. Prevention of opportunistic infections is an important factor in stabilizing weight. A number of pharmacologic agents are in common use, with variable responses in terms of the amount and the quality of the weight gained (fat versus muscle). The most commonly used agents for wasting are appetite stimulants (megestrol acetate, dronabinol), anabolic steroids (oxandrolone, nandrolone), testosterone, or thalidomide.

HEPATOBILIARY DISEASE. The prevalence of markers for hepatitis B (hepatitis B surface antigen [HBsAg], antibody to HBsAg, or antibody to hepatitis B core antigen) is 35 to 80% in AIDS patients, which is a reflection of their prevalence among homosexual men, intravenous drug abusers, and hemophiliacs. HBsAg is found in 5 to 10%. Hepatitis C antibody indicates chronic infection in most patients and is found in up to 90% of injection drug users. The seroprevalence of hepatitis C virus is low in other HIV risk categories. Chronic hepatitis B or C virus infection does not appear to notably alter the course of HIV infection, although HIV may accelerate the course of chronic hepatitis C. Other viral causes of hepatitis include herpes simplex virus and CMV. Granulomatous hepatitis is most often due to *M. avium*; less common are histoplasmosis, cryptococcosis, and tuberculosis. Hepatotoxic drugs commonly taken by HIV-infected patients include protease inhibitors, azoles, sulfonamides, isoniazid, and rifampin. Cholestasis secondary to papillary stenosis and sclerosing cholangitis are most often due to *Cryptosporidium*, Microsporida, or CMV or are idiopathic.

CONDITIONS NECESSITATING ABDOMINAL SURGERY. The most common clinical syndromes in persons with HIV infection that require abdominal surgery are peritonitis associated with perforation secondary to CMV infection, lymphoma of the gut (most frequently manifested as involvement of the terminal ileum by obstruction or bleeding), Kaposi's sarcoma, and *M. avium* infection involving the retroperitoneal lymph nodes or spleen. Patients with AIDS cholangiopathy usually respond to endoscopic retrograde cholangiopancreatography, but the benefit is usually temporary. The experience with abdominal surgery indicates that patients with HIV infection tolerate surgical procedures well and do not have an unusually high incidence of postoperative complications.

Greenson JK, Belitsos PC, Yardley JH, et al: AIDS enteropathy: Occult infections and duodenal mucosal alterations in chronic diarrhea. Ann Intern Med 114:366, 1991. *The authors review histopathologic changes and etiologic agents of AIDS patients with chronic diarrhea.*

Johanson JF, Sonnenberg A: Efficient management of diarrhea in the acquired immunodeficiency syndrome (AIDS). Ann Intern Med 112:942, 1990. *Review of the efficacy and cost-effectiveness of various strategies for evaluating diarrhea in AIDS patients suggests that endoscopy and other costly tests are infrequently warranted.*

Kotler DP, Clayton F, Scholes JV, Orenstein JM: Small intestinal injury and parasitic diseases in AIDS. Ann Intern Med 113:444, 1990. *The authors review histopathologic findings, including electron microscopy, in AIDS patients with cryptosporidiosis and microsporidiosis.*

Laughon BE, Druckman DA, Vernon A, et al: Prevalence of enteric pathogens in homosexual men with and without acquired immunodeficiency syndrome. Gastroenterology 94:984, 1988. *This is an exhaustive study of stool to detect bacterial, viral, fungal, and parasitic pathogens in homosexual men without AIDS, with AIDS, and with proctitis or diarrhea.*

Sharpstone D, Gazzard B: Gastrointestinal manifestations of HIV infection. Lancet 348:379, 1996. *The authors review the clinical features of gastrointestinal complications of HIV infection, including esophageal disease, diarrhea, and wasting.*

Soave R, Johnson WD Jr: Cryptosporidium and Isospora belli infections. J Infect Dis 157:225, 1988. *The authors review* Cryptosporidium *and* Isospora *with particular attention to their role in AIDS patients.*

Weinert M, Grimes RM, Lynch DP: Oral manifestations of HIV infection. Ann Intern Med 125:485, 1996. *The authors provide guidelines for recognizing, diagnosing, and managing oral complications of HIV infection.*

414 CUTANEOUS SIGNS OF AIDS
Neal S. Penneys

Cutaneous signs and symptoms associated with acquired immunodeficiency syndrome (AIDS) increase in frequency and severity as the disease advances. However, infection by human immunodeficiency virus (HIV) may produce a transient macular roseola–like eruption. As HIV infection progresses, infectious processes and neoplastic disease are most often seen. Patients also may have symptoms such as pruritus without visible skin lesions.

Cutaneous infections are a common feature of AIDS. Superficial infections such as dermatophytosis, candidiasis, and scabies may be extensive and have altered appearances. Superficial fungal infections may coexist with other pathogens such as herpesvirus or cytomegalovirus to produce unusual complex cutaneous infections.

Cutaneous viral infections also may have unpredictable presentations. Molluscum contagiosum occurs commonly and is persistent; lesions may become quite large. Human papillomavirus–induced lesions may occur, ranging from persistent verrucae to severe anogenital condyloma (see Color Plate 11*A*). Molluscum contagiosum and human papillomavirus lesions frequently occur in cosmetically sensitive areas. Locally destructive treatments such as curettage and cryotherapy are effective, but lesions almost always recur or new lesions develop, particularly as CD4 counts decrease.

Herpes zoster may be a reliable sign of the presence or progression of HIV infection in an otherwise asymptomatic person. With the diminishing immune response, the usually self-limited herpetic infections become chronic and fail to heal (see Color Plate 11*B*). Chronic herpetic lesions may not have the characteristic morphologic characteristics of acute lesions in immunocompetent individuals. Both herpes simplex and herpes zoster viruses may produce disseminated skin lesions in HIV-infected individuals. The diagnosis of herpetic infections can be made by morphologic features of the clinical lesion, examination of a Tzanck preparation (Wright's stain of a scraping taken from the base of a lesion), skin biopsy, or viral culture and/or molecular diagnostic methods. For chronic or recurrent herpetic infection and for long-term suppression, oral antiviral therapy is helpful.

Unusual primary and disseminated infections occur in the skin in the context of HIV infection. Mucosal and cutaneous lesions of histoplasmosis, cryptococcosis, and other systemic fungal disorders can be signs of disseminated infection in AIDS patients. Mycobacterial infections produced by *M. tuberculosis, M. avium-intracellulare, M. haemophilum,* and others affect the skin in patients with AIDS. A long list of unusual or unique infections has been observed, including disseminated amebiasis, *Trichosporon beigelei,* sporotrichosis, *Strongyloides* infection, alternariosis, and superficial pheohyphomycosis. A new entity, bacillary angiomatosis caused by *Bartonella henselae/quintana,* produces vascular proliferations in the skin as well as in other sites. Reiter's syndrome, with typical cutaneous findings, is found with increased frequency in patients with AIDS (see Color Plate 11*C*). It is safe to predict that unusual presentations of disseminated infectious diseases will continue to be described in the skin of AIDS patients.

Mucous membranes are commonly affected by infectious processes in patients with HIV infection. Oral candidiasis may be present and is one harbinger of the progression of HIV infection. Human papillomavirus and herpesvirus can produce lesions in the oral cavity. Oral hairy leukoplakia, a mixed infectious process, produces a characteristic "hairy" appearance to the sides of the tongue. Severe necrotizing gingivitis and recurrent oral ulcers are common. Lastly, disseminated infectious disease and malignant lymphoma can affect the mucous membranes.

The most common neoplasm in the context of AIDS is Kaposi's sarcoma (see Color Plate 11*D*) a proliferation now associated with the presence of human herpesvirus 8. In AIDS, however, Kaposi's lesions may be solitary or disseminated; vary in color from light tan to deep purple; vary in appearance from macules to tumor nodules; or be arranged in a follicular, zosteriform, or linear pattern; they are generally atypical when compared with the lesions of

Kaposi's sarcoma occurring in non-HIV-infected individuals. Kaposi's sarcoma found in AIDS patients frequently affects the mucosae. Other malignant tumors have an increased incidence in the setting of HIV infection, including squamous cell carcinoma and a variety of lymphomas, and all may have cutaneous involvement.

A number of poorly classified eruptions occur in AIDS patients. Best known is seborrheic dermatitis, which occurs in the usual locations but can be persistent and difficult to treat. Patients with AIDS also may have persistent pruritic eruptions, annular eruptions that resemble granuloma annulare, folliculitis, vasculitis, alopecia areata, vitiligo, porphyria cutanea tarda, eosinophilic folliculitis, and others. Certain well-characterized dermatoses such as psoriasis and atopic dermatitis appear to be worsened by the presence of HIV infection. Many AIDS patients receive a panoply of therapeutic agents that in turn produce a spectrum of cutaneous reactions including certain recognizable reactions, such as discolored nails from azidothymidine therapy (see Color Plate 11E).

Penneys NS: Skin Manifestations of AIDS, 2nd ed. London, Martin Dunitz, 1995. *This reference is the easiest way to see the most common skin changes associated with HIV infection; has primary references.*

415 OPHTHALMOLOGIC MANIFESTATIONS OF AIDS

Mark A. Jacobson, M.D.

Infectious or noninfectious ocular disorders, some of which may lead to severe visual impairment, have been reported in 40 to 90% of patients with acquired immunodeficiency syndrome (AIDS) referred for formal ophthalmoscopy. In prospective observational cohort studies conducted prior to the clinical availability of the new, more potent generation of antiretroviral agents for the treatment of human immunodeficiency virus (HIV) disease, the incidence of cytomegalovirus (CMV) retinitis (the most common ophthalmologic complication of AIDS) was reported to be in the range of 20 to 40% in patients with an AIDS diagnosis. In the first 18 months since potent HIV protease inhibitors became widely available in the United States and Europe, the incidence of new CMV retinitis diagnoses decreased markedly. How sustained this decrease will be is unknown, but if new antiretroviral treatment strategies ultimately lead to extensive HIV cross resistance to these agents, the incidence of CMV retinitis may again increase.

The differential diagnosis of HIV-associated ocular disease is best considered by its anatomic location.

DISEASES OF THE CHOROID, RETINA, AND VITREOUS

Retinal Microvascular Disease

The most common ophthalmologic complication observed in patients with HIV infection is retinal microvascular disease, which usually manifests as asymptomatic cotton-wool spots or small retinal hemorrhages. Cotton-wool spots have been reported in up to half of patients with advanced HIV disease. Histopathologically, these lesions represent areas of retinal ischemia. Both immune complex deposition and direct HIV retinal infection have been implicated in the pathogenesis of cotton-wool spot lesions. On funduscopic examination, they typically appear as white spots with feathered edges on the surface of the retina. A common location is near major posterior retinal vessels, and these lesions can have small associated retinal hemorrhages. It may be difficult to differentiate between cotton-wool spots and early lesions of CMV retinitis, which can have a very similar appearance. Sometimes the distinction can be made only by serial ophthalmoscopic examination. Cotton-wool spots remain stationary or resolve, whereas the lesion of CMV retinitis increases in size. Because cotton-wool spots virtu-

ally never cause symptomatic loss of vision and often spontaneously resolve, no treatment is indicated.

Small retinal hemorrhages and other microvascular abnormalities have been reported in up to 40% of patients with AIDS. These lesions also are asymptomatic, except in the rare case where perifoveal involvement may result in visual blurring.

Cytomegalovirus Retinitis

CMV retinitis is the most common sight-threatening ocular opportunistic infection in patients with AIDS. It usually occurs only in patients with a history of an absolute CD4+ (T helper) lymphocyte count <50 cells/μL. The typical appearance is a white, cottage cheese–like retinal exudate, often associated with hemorrhage and frequently located adjacent to major retinal vessels. In tissue sections, full-thickness retinal necrosis and swollen retinal cells containing intranuclear and intracytoplasmic inclusions are observed.

Patients with CMV retinitis typically present with complaints of painless visual impairment—either "floaters," blurred vision, decreased visual acuity, or visual field defects—almost always affecting one eye more than the other. Several studies of untreated CMV retinitis have demonstrated a natural history of progressive retinal destruction caused by new retinal lesions or increasing size of previous lesions usually evident within weeks by serial ophthalmoscopy.

CMV retinitis is diagnosed primarily by its typical clinical appearance. The differential diagnosis includes cotton-wool spots, retinal hemorrhages, choroidal granulomas, acute retinal necrosis syndrome, and toxoplasmic and syphilitic retinitis. Because differentiating between these entities may be difficult, and the therapy of CMV retinitis is expensive, time-consuming, and toxic, the diagnosis of CMV retinitis must be confirmed by an experienced ophthalmologist. Because of poor specificity and sensitivity, CMV cultures of blood or urine are not clinically useful diagnostic tests. However, recent studies of more sensitive techniques of detecting CMV viremia (e.g., CMV DNA amplification by polymerase chain reaction [PCR] or staining peripheral blood leukocytes for CMV antigen) appear to have better predictive value for identifying patients at high risk for developing CMV retinitis. It is not yet clear whether these more sensitive tests have clinical utility in screening.

The current treatment options for CMV retinitis include chronic intravenous treatment with ganciclovir or foscarnet, initial therapy with intravenous ganciclovir followed by chronic oral ganciclovir therapy, intermittent intravenous therapy with cidofovir, or surgical placement of an intraocular device that releases ganciclovir intravitreally for 6 to 8 months combined with chronic oral ganciclovir (Table 415–1). Ganciclovir is a nucleoside analogue prodrug that is preferentially phosphorylated within CMV-infected cells to an active drug, ganciclovir triphosphate, which inhibits CMV replication. Foscarnet is a pyrophosphate analogue that does not require phosphorylation for its anti-CMV activity. Cidofovir is a very potent

Table 415–1 ■ THERAPY FOR CYTOMEGALOVIRUS (CMV) RETINITIS

Ganciclovir: Induction therapy: 5 mg/kg IV q 12 hr × 14 d
    Chronic maintenance therapy: 5–6 mg/kg IV qd or 5d/wk, or 1 g PO tid
    Intraocular device: must replace after 6 to 8 months
  Efficacy: intraocular device >IV >PO
  Adverse effects: systemic therapy can cause granulocytopenia, thrombocytopenia, azoospermia. Intraocular device placement can be complicated by retinal detachment, bleeding, or endophthalmitis. High risk of contralateral or extraocular CMV disease with intraocular device as sole therapy; should have PO ganciclovir co-administered.

Foscarnet: Induction therapy: 90 mg/kg IV q 12 hr × 14 d
    Chronic maintenance therapy: 90–120 mg/kg IV qd
  Efficacy: equivalent to IV ganciclovir
  Adverse effects: nephrotoxicity, ionized hypocalcemia (seizure or arrhythmia with overdose), hypomagnesemia, hypophosphatemia, hypocalcemia, hypokalemia, genital ulcers, nephrogenic diabetes insipidus

Cidofovir: Induction therapy: 5 mg/kg IV q week × 2
    Chronic maintenance therapy: 5 mg/kg IV q 2 weeks
    Concomitant saline hydration and oral probenecid must be coadministered to decrease risk of nephrotoxicity.
  Efficacy: has not been compared to other anti-CMV treatments.
  Adverse effects: nephrotoxicity, neutropenia, probenecid-induced hypersensitivity reaction or nausea, neuropathy, anterior uveitis, hypotony

anti-CMV nucleotide analogue that does not require phosphorylation by CMV-encoded enzymes. In the absence of marked immune reconstitution, therapy must be given indefinitely to minimize further irreversible visual impairment. Both ganciclovir- and foscarnet-resistant strains of CMV have emerged and have been associated with therapeutic failure. In such cases, use of these agents in combination or of cidofovir may be effective in controlling retinitis progression.

Because atrophy occurs in areas of active CMV retinitis, patients are susceptible to rhegmatogenous retinal detachment (resulting from a scar in a thinned portion of the retina) even when active retinitis has been controlled with antiviral therapy. For such patients, surgical reattachment by removal of the vitreous and injection of silicone oil can be temporarily effective in restoring functional vision.

Toxoplasmic Chorioretinitis (Table 415–2)

Toxoplasmic chorioretinitis is rare compared to CMV retinitis, but may complicate up to 20% of cases of AIDS-associated toxoplasmic encephalitis. Unlike toxoplasmic retinitis in immunocompetent individuals, which typically results from reactivation of congenitally acquired cysts latent in the retina, AIDS-associated toxoplasmic chorioretinitis does not appear to originate in pre-existing retinochoroidal scars, but from dissemination of organisms from nonocular sites of disease. Necrotizing retinal lesions are often bilateral and multifocal, and (as in CMV retinitis) may result in rhegmatogenous retinal detachment. Vitreous inflammation and anterior uveitis are more common and associated hemorrhage less common than in CMV retinitis. Because nearly all cases of toxoplasmic chorioretinitis are associated with toxoplasmic encephalitis, a computed tomographic (CT) or magnetic resonance (MR) scan of the brain should be done whenever this diagnosis is considered. Specific antiparasitic therapy (pyramethamine and sulfadiazine, or pyramethamine and clindamycin, in the same doses used to treat toxoplasmic encephalitis) usually is effective in preventing further retinal necrosis, but chronic maintenance therapy must be continued indefinitely to prevent relapse.

Acute Retinal Necrosis Syndrome

Widespread, often bilateral, necrotizing retinitis caused by herpes simplex or varicella-zoster virus is now a well-characterized, although rare, AIDS-associated condition. Unlike CMV retinitis, this disease often is associated with ocular pain and concomittant keratitis or iritis. Many individuals have had recent or concurrent trigeminal zoster or orolabial herpes simplex infection, and evidence of concurrent viral meningoencephalitis may be present. On funduscopic examination, widespread, pale or gray, peripheral retinal lesions are noted. Although intravenous acyclovir is effective in preventing further retinal necrosis, subsequent retinal detachment is a frequent, sight-threatening complication.

Progressive Outer Retinal Necrosis Syndrome

Progressive outer retinal necrosis is a recently described clinical variant of varicella-zoster retinitis occurring in patients with CD4+ lymphocyte counts less than 100 cells/μL and characterized by multifocal, deep retinal lesions that rapidly progress to confluence. Less inflammatory cell response is observed in this condition than in acute retinal necrosis. The clinical response to available antiviral therapies is poor.

Other Causes of Chorioretinitis and Vitritis

Cases of syphilitic retinitis have been reported in individuals with AIDS, AIDS-related complex (ARC) and asymptomatic HIV infection. There is no characteristic ophthalmologic appearance, but nearly all reported cases have had markedly positive serologic tests for active syphilis and dermatologic or central nervous system (CNS) manifestations of secondary syphilis. Generally, response to intravenous penicillin therapy has been good. Disseminated pneumocystosis (associated with use of inhaled pentamidine prophylaxis against *Pneumocystis carinii* pneumonia), *Mycobacterium tuberculosis,* and *Mycobacterium avium* complex infection with choroidal infiltrates have been described, but these lesions generally have not been sight-threatening. Rare cases of indolently progressive retinitis have been attributed to endogenous bacterial infection on the basis of retinal histopathology and response to broad-spectrum antibiotics. Also, vitritis (i.e., endophthalmitis) due to disseminated candidiasis may occur in parenteral drug users who are HIV infected or AIDS patients with indwelling central venous catheters.

OPTIC NEUROPATHY

Opportunistic infectious diseases affecting the optic nerve of patients with ARC or AIDS may result in visual impairment or blindness. The most common cause of optic neuropathy is CMV infection. When CMV retinitis involves the optic disc, swelling of the optic nerve head (papillitis) leads to decreased visual acuity. This may occur in the presence or absence of other areas of retinitis and may affect the intraorbital optic nerve (optic neuritis) or retrobulbar nerve (retrobulbar neuritis). The acute retinal necrosis syndrome caused by herpes simplex or varicella zoster virus infection may cause papillitis; syphilis may cause papillitis, optic neuritis, or retrobulbar neuritis in patients at any stage of HIV disease. The most serious ocular complication of crytococcal meningitis is an arachnoiditis that compresses the retrobulbar optic nerve, occasionally causing blindness. The cause of optic neuropathy usually can be established by seeking the other characteristic features of the specific infection. However, specific antimicrobial therapy for the cause of optic neuropathy often fails to improve vision once significant visual loss has occurred.

ANTERIOR UVEITIS

Severe anterior uveitis is uncommon in patients with HIV disease, but when such cases occur, syphilis or varicella-zoster virus infection are the most common causes. Mild, asymptomatic anterior uveitis commonly is observed in patients with CMV retinitis, but inflammation severe enough to cause symptoms is extremely rare (with the exception of patients receiving cidofovir therapy, which can cause severe, persistant uveitis). Occasional cases of toxoplasmic anterior uveitis also have been reported.

KERATITIS

Inflammatory disease of cornea (keratitis) is most frequently caused by varicella zoster or herpes simplex virus, and the clinical features usually make diagnosis relatively simple. Patients with advanced HIV disease who develop this complication may require

Table 415–2 ■ DIAGNOSTIC FEATURES OF IMPORTANT CAUSES OF HIV-ASSOCIATED RETINITIS

FEATURE	CYTOMEGALOVIRUS	ACUTE RETINAL NECROSIS (VZV, HSV)	TOXOPLASMOSIS	SYPHILIS
Ocular symptoms	Floaters, visual field defect or decreased visual acuity	Same	Same	Same
	Painless	Pain common	± Photophobia	± Photophobia
Associated clinical findings	AIDS	Orolabial herpes, trigeminal zoster	AIDS, encephalitis	Rash, hearing loss
Typical retinal lesion	Cottage-cheese exudate with hemorrhage	Confluent, gray or pale retina	White or yellow exudate	Variable
Typical retinal location	Adjacent to major vessel	Peripheral	Multifocal	Focal or posterior
Risk of retinal detachment	+++	++++	++	+
Serology, culture	Not helpful	Viral culture of skin lesion	*T. gondii* IgG titer	VDRL, FTA-ABS

Modified from Culbertson WW: Infection of the retina in AIDS. Int Ophthalmol Clin 29:108, 1989.

intravenous acyclovir therapy in addition to topical trifluridine. Microsporida infection has also been reported to cause keratitis in HIV-infected patients.

DISEASES OF THE CONJUNCTIVA AND ADNEXA

Kaposi's sarcoma (KS) has a predilection to involve ocular structures. Conjunctival Kaposi's lesions appear as bright red subepithelial nodules, and small lesions may be mistaken for subconjunctival hemorrhages. Periorbital edema may be caused by lymphangitic KS, even in the absence of apparent ocular or cutaneous lesions. Most ocular lesions respond to local irradiation.

Nonspecific, nonprurulent conjunctivitis that often is self-limited has been reported in up to 10% of AIDS patients. Topical steroid and sulfa therapy may be beneficial for this condition. Other rare causes of conjunctivitis include syphilis and molluscum contagiosum infection. Orbital KS or Burkitt's lymphoma may present with ptosis and diplopia.

de Smet MD, Nussenblatt RB: Ocular manifestation of AIDS. JAMA 266:3019, 1991. *Detailed review, with references, of non-CMV ocular complications of AIDS.*
Jacobson MA: Treatment of cytomegalovirus retinitis in patients with the acquired immunodeficiency syndrome. N Engl J Med 337:105, 1997. *Reviews and compares advantages and disadvantages of available treatments for CMV retinitis.*
Margolis TP, Lowder CY, Holland GN, et al: Varicella-zoster virus retinitis in patients with the acquired immunodeficiency syndrome. Am J Ophthal 112:119, 1991. *Detailed description of unique clinical characteristics of varicella-zoster virus retinitis.*

416 HEMATOLOGY/ONCOLOGY IN AIDS

David T. Scadden ■ *Jerome E. Groopman*

A signature abnormality of human immunodeficiency virus (HIV) infection is the decline in the number of CD4 lymphocytes over time. However, other cytopenias also are seen in advanced disease, with anemia reported in 60%, thrombocytopenia in 40%, and neutropenia in 50% of patients with acquired immunodeficiency syndrome (AIDS). These cytopenias occur in conjunction with progressive deterioration of immune function and are less common in the earlier stages of HIV infection or in patients responding to antiretroviral medications. Thrombocytopenia is the exception and may constitute a manifestation of HIV infection during the asymptomatic phases. Multiple contributing factors frequently are operative in the cytopenia in advanced HIV infection, including direct and indirect effects of HIV; opportunistic infections; neoplasms; and toxic antiretroviral, antimicrobial, or antitumor chemotherapy. Evaluation of patients with low blood counts should focus on infectious processes and attendant myelotoxic effects of therapy. In addition to the usual laboratory approaches to cytopenia based on impaired production, excess consumption, and/or sequestration, a number of other diagnostic studies should be considered. These include blood isolator cultures for fungi and mycobacteria, and serum assessment for cytomegalovirus (CMV) antigen or IgM antibody to parvovirus.

Although the utility of bone marrow aspirate and biopsy in an HIV-infected patient with low blood counts has been debated, morphologic changes such as giant pronormoblasts in parvovirus infection and special stains for mycobacteria and fungi may hasten identification of a reversible cause of myelosuppression. Marrow sampling is not more sensitive, however, than routine microbiologic tests in diagnosing these abnormalities.

Morphologic abnormalities of myeloid and erythroid lineages often are present in the bone marrow of patients with HIV disease in the absence of infection or neoplasm. These changes are nonspecific and include hypercellularity, dysplasia with frequent megaloblastosis, lymphoid aggregates, and increased plasma cells and reticulin. The pathogenetic mechanisms for these morphologic abnormalities and the associated impaired hematopoiesis are not well

defined. Laboratory studies of hematopoiesis in HIV infection have yielded variable and differing results. The bulk of evidence suggests that HIV does not directly infect early progenitors but may alter the proliferative capacity of progenitors by two possible mechanisms: (1) induction of inhibitory factors in the marrow microenvironment, or (2) interaction with the progenitor cell surface and induction of cell death (apoptosis) without infecting stem cells.

THROMBOCYTOPENIA (SEE CH. 184)

Thrombocytopenia may be a presenting laboratory finding in an otherwise asymptomatic HIV-infected person. HIV infection should be considered in the differential diagnosis of thrombocytopenia, and the history should include questions regarding risk factors for infection. Clinically asymptomatic but thrombocytopenic HIV-infected patients have a similar rate of progression to AIDS as asymptomatic HIV-seropositive persons without thrombocytopenia. Thrombocytopenia is not a criterion for more advanced HIV disease according to the staging system developed by the Centers for Disease Control and Prevention (CDC). Multiple causes need to be considered in evaluating thrombocytopenia in HIV infection. Immune-mediated destruction and ineffective hematopoiesis are generally both operative. In addition, cases of AIDS with apparent hemolytic-uremic syndrome or thrombotic thrombocytopenic purpura have been described, but are rare. Isolated thrombocytopenia is most often clinically similar to classic autoimmune thrombocytopenic purpura (ITP). Bone marrow examination reveals an increased number of megakaryocytes, and there are elevated levels of bound immunoglobulin on the platelet surface. However, distinct from ITP, the immunoglobulin is generally immune complexes often involving anti-HIV antibodies, and splenomegaly is common. Detection of antibody on platelet surfaces does not correlate with thrombocytopenia, possibly because reticuloendothelial cell dysfunction often occurs in AIDS and may reduce platelet clearance. In addition to peripheral destruction of platelets, reduced production appears to be common in HIV disease. Even in patients with an ITP-like presentation, production is reduced. This mechanism predominates in patients with thrombocytopenia in the setting of AIDS.

The thrombocytopenia in HIV-infected patients has similar sequelae to classic immune thrombocytopenia, yet special attention to the issue of thrombocytopenia should be given in HIV-infected hemophiliacs. Complications from thrombocytopenia may be more severe in hemophiliacs, so therapy should be considered at a higher platelet count than in HIV-infected patients without other coagulation defects. An important observation has been the improvement in platelet count due to treatment with zidovudine (AZT) in HIV-infected patients with significant thrombocytopenia, regardless of risk group. Nearly two thirds of such patients may respond to AZT therapy and increase their platelet counts (mean, threefold increase) within 12 weeks of initiating treatment. There are a number of anecdotal reports of responses to other antiretroviral agents as well, should AZT be an unacceptable option. If there is no response to AZT, then several treatment modalities may be considered, including corticosteroids, interferon-α, splenectomy, danazol; for rapid temporary reversal of severe thrombocytopenia, intravenous gamma globulin and anti-RhD preparations have been shown to be quite active.

Theoretical risk of steroid use exists in an HIV-infected individual, including exacerbation of fungal infection, Kaposi's sarcoma (KS), and the replicative activity of HIV itself. Nonetheless, most patients have tolerated corticosteroids for short intervals. Their long-term use in HIV-associated thrombocytopenia cannot be recommended.

ANEMIA

Anemia increases in incidence in HIV-infected patients as their degree of immune dysfunction worsens. The anemia is usually normochromic and normocytic with iron studies that are either normal or indicative of chronic disease. Occasionally the vitamin B_{12} level is decreased, but true vitamin B_{12} deficiency is uncommon; rather, transcobalamin transport may be altered and therapy with the vitamin does not lead to improved erythropoiesis. Should a low vitamin B₁₂ level be found, then a true deficiency needs to be ruled out by a Schilling test and other studies (see Ch. 163).

The Coombs' test (antiglobulin) may be positive in the majority of patients with AIDS and in about a third of asymptomatic HIV-infected individuals. Although anti-i or other specific antibodies may occur, nonspecific binding of antiphospholipid antibodies or immune complexes to erythrocytes is more common. Immune-mediated hemolysis is unusual in HIV-infected patients as a cause of anemia.

Impaired erythropoiesis accounts for anemia in most HIV-infected individuals. Serum erythropoietin levels are often low for the degree of anemia in the patient without renal abnormalities and is of unclear origin. Parvovirus infection has been reported in HIV-infected patients and may result in red cell aplasia. Gamma globulin therapy has been reported to reverse this unusual cause of severe anemia.

AZT is associated with both dose-related and idiosyncratic suppression of erythropoiesis, whereas other antiretroviral drugs generally are not associated with anemia. Macrocytic changes occur in the erythrocytes with AZT therapy. The mechanism of impaired erythropoiesis due to the drug appears to be impairment of DNA synthesis in developing progenitors.

Recombinant erythropoietin therapy may decrease the transfusion requirement and increase the hemoglobin in anemic AIDS patients on AZT. The response to recombinant erythropoietin treatment is most clearly seen in patients with pretreatment serum erythropoietin levels below 500 mU per milliliter. Some anemic AIDS patients receiving AZT have developed red cell aplasia that does not improve with recombinant erythropoietin therapy.

NEUTROPENIA

Neutropenia occurs in the HIV-infected patient in concert with decreases in other cell counts with progressive deterioration of the immune system. In addition to neutropenia, neutrophil dysfunction has been reported in AIDS. The extent to which neutrophil defects, particularly of microbial killing, contribute to host immune impairment is unknown.

Neutropenia is most commonly caused by myelosuppressive therapy in AIDS patients. AZT treatment is at times limited by neutropenia, although other antiretrovirals do not seem to cause this problem. Other therapies, including trimethoprim-sulfamethoxazole for *Pneumocystis carinii* pneumonia, pyrimethamine-sulfadiazine for central nervous system (CNS) toxoplasmosis, acyclovir for disseminated herpes simplex or herpes zoster, and most prominently ganciclovir for CMV retinitis may be myelotoxic and result in neutropenia.

HEMATOPOIETIC GROWTH FACTORS

Suppression of leukocyte or erythrocyte production can be a limiting factor in treating HIV infection or its complications. This problem has become less limiting with newer antiretroviral therapies and better control of HIV-1. However, for those patients who do develop severe cytopenia, hematopoietic growth factors are useful in raising cell counts. It is clear that in most patients with anemia due to HIV infection and or concomitant AZT therapy, with baseline serum erythropoietin concentrations <500 mU per milliliter, recombinant erythropoietin increases the hemoglobin and reduces the transfusion requirement. Use of the myeloid growth factors, granulocyte colony-stimulating factor (G-CSF) or granulocyte macrophage colony-stimulating factor (GM-CSF) to ameliorate leukopenia due to HIV infection and or therapy with AZT, interferon-α, ganciclovir, or cancer chemotherapy has also been successful. Use of G-CSF has recently been shown to modestly reduce bacterial infection rates in HIV-infected individuals with neutrophil counts between 750 and 1000/mm³.

The major issue in the safety profile of the myeloid growth factors relates to their potential effects on replication of HIV. In vitro data indicate that HIV replication is stimulated by GM-CSF but not G-CSF. The data conflict as to whether this phenomenon occurs in vivo, but there are data that indicate that GM-CSF combined with AZT does not result in any increase in HIV-1 viral load.

Recent trials have indicated that the lymphopoietic cytokine in-

terleukin-2 (IL-2) may be used to enhance lymphoid cell numbers, particularly CD4-positive T lymphocytes. Intermittent use of this cytokine has been shown to raise CD4 counts with tolerable toxicity in patients whose baseline CD4 count is greater than 200 cells/mm³. Use of concurrent antiretroviral therapy is necessary to prevent enhanced virus replication. Whether this cytokine results in any clinical benefit remains controversial, and this approach should still be regarded as experimental pending data on clinical outcomes.

Neoplasms that occur with increased frequency in the setting of HIV disease are KS, B-cell lymphoma, and squamous cell neoplasia of the anogenital region. Smaller, but statistically meaningful increases have also been noted in Hodgkin's disease, leiomyosarcoma (in children only), seminoma, and plasmacytoma. Clinical management of AIDS-associated neoplasia must balance therapy directed at HIV-1 and opportunistic infections, as well as the tumors.

KAPOSI'S SARCOMA (See Chapters 178, 190, and 414)

Kaposi's sarcoma is the most frequent neoplastic manifestation of HIV infection and is one of the CDC criteria that define an HIV-infected individual as having AIDS. AIDS-associated KS more frequently is seen among homosexual or bisexual men with HIV than in other HIV transmission risk groups. This epidemiologic observation led to a search for a second transmissible factor, which resulted in the identification of a new member of the gamma herpesvirus family, Kaposi's sarcoma herpesvirus (KSHV) or human herpesvirus 8 (HHV-8). This virus has now been associated not just with KS, but also with a subset of B-cell lymphomas (discussed below), Castleman's disease and, perhaps, multiple myeloma. The epidemiologic data indicate that exposure to this virus is more common in promiscuous homosexual men and in populations with higher frequencies of "classic" or "endemic" KS not associated with HIV-1. It is found in KS tissue regardless of the epidemiologic background, but the mechanism by which the virus participates in tumor development is unclear. There are a number of KSHV genes with human homologues that suggest possible direct effects of the virus (cyclin D, bcl-2 or activated G-protein coupled receptor homologues) or effects at a distance (interleukin-6, chemokine and Ox-2 homologues). Hypotheses for how this virus is oncogenic are wide ranging and the mechanisms involved may be quite distinct from other tumor viruses. The nature of the immunologic response to KSHV remains ill defined, but clearly plays an important role in the control of KSHV-related tumors. KS in the setting of organ transplant often regresses with reduction of immunosuppressive medication. Similarly, in AIDS, patients treated with potent antiretroviral drug combinations have both a markedly reduced incidence of KS and often have pre-existing KS regress.

Histopathologically, KS lesions are a mixture of different cell types. Endothelial cells are quite present within the KS lesions, as is a prominent spindle-cell proliferation surrounded by extravasated erythrocytes and macrophages. The cell of origin of the neoplasm is still debated, as is the clonality of the disease. There are some patients who have multiple independent clones of tumor, whereas a subset of patients appear to have metastatic lesions derived from a single clone. In general, however, aggressive treatment of the original lesion has not had substantial impact on the ultimate development of other lesions.

KS often is a cutaneous nonblanching red macule. As lesions increase in size, they often have surrounding ecchymoses and acquire more of a violet hue. At times, the lesions may become nodular and, with advanced disease, the lesions may become confluent with large plaques developing, particularly on the legs. There is no orderly pattern of tumor progression, and presentation may be with lesions at multiple sites. The rate of growth of the primary lesions, as well as the appearance of new lesions, is quite variable. The lesions may occur on any cutaneous site and on mucous membranes. Lymphatic involvement is not unusual, and KS may present as lymphadenopathy. Visceral involvement, particularly of the trachea, lungs, and gastrointestinal tract, occurs commonly and may be seen in the absence of cutaneous disease. The most striking morbidity associated with KS is that of lymph node involvement and consequent lymphedema involving the lower extremities, groin,

Table 416–1 ■ TREATMENT OF KAPOSI'S SARCOMA

Chemotherapy single agent	Liposomal doxorubicin	20 mg/m² IV every 3 weeks
	Liposomal daunorubicin	40 mg/m² IV every 2 weeks
	Paclitaxel	100 mg/m² IV every 2 weeks
Combined therapy	Bleomycin/vincristine	Bleomycin 15 U IV
		Vincristine 2 mg IV every 2–3 weeks
	Doxorubicin-bleomycin-vincristine	Doxorubicin 20 mg/m²
		Bleomycin 15 μm² IV
		Vincristine 2 mg IV every 3 weeks

and head and neck. Extensive parenchymal or pleural involvement of the lung may result in life-threatening respiratory compromise.

The diagnosis of KS is relatively straightforward in HIV-infected individuals presenting with an erythematous or violaceous cutaneous or mucosal lesion. However, bacillary angiomatosis caused by *Rochalimaea* species (see Ch. 357) may result in similar lesions. This process, which is treatable with antibiotics, should be excluded by Warthin-Starry staining of biopsy material. Following diagnosis, an assessment should be made of the distribution of the lesions. The presence of visceral disease does not necessarily correlate with poor response of lesions to therapy, so that an extensive evaluation for gastrointestinal or lymphadenopathic KS is not indicated unless there are specific symptoms referable to such involvement.

In patients with symptomatic visceral disease, lesions associated with edema, or rapidly evolving extensive cutaneous disease, chemotherapy can often provide symptomatic relief (Table 416–1). The most active chemotherapeutic drugs appear to be paclitaxel, liposomal anthracyclines, or combinations of vincristine/bleomycin or doxorubicin/vincristine/bleomycin. Liposomal doxorubicin or liposomal daunorubicin have been shown to be active with reduced toxicity compared with standard agents and often are used as a first-line approach. For those patients who fail liposomal agents (common after 10 weeks), low-dose paclitaxel has been shown to be highly active, desirable, and well tolerated. Response to chemotherapy usually occurs within the first few weeks of treatment. Unfortunately, the lesions regrow when the chemotherapy is stopped, so treatment is generally chronic.

Patients with KS who do not have rapidly progressive disease and therefore do not require immediate intervention may be treated with several other approaches. The most important among these is aggressive antiretroviral therapy. Regression of KS is common among patients treated with combinations of antiretroviral drugs occurring 2 to 4 months after control of viremia has been achieved. For those patients whose KS persists despite antiretrovirals, options include observation, single-agent interferon-α, local radiation, intralesional chemotherapy, local cryotherapy, or combinations of these. Selecting the optimal therapeutic approach involves determining the clinical status of the patient, particularly using the staging classification (Table 416–2), as well as lifestyle issues. Patients who are categorized as "good risk" by the TIS staging system are also good candidates for response to interferon-α, but toxicity is common. A number of agents currently in clinical trial appear to have potential for this patient group. Among these are thalidomide, 9-*cis* retinoic acid, and angiogenesis inhibitors.

NON-HODGKIN'S LYMPHOMA

B-cell lymphoma frequently occurs in immunosuppressed individuals. Genetic disorders of the immune system such as Wiskott-Aldrich syndrome, as well as immunosuppressive therapy used in organ transplantation, are associated with malignant transformation of B cells and an oligoclonal or monoclonal lymphoma. Non-Hodgkin's B-cell lymphoma is a frequent manifestation of HIV infection, occurring in 4 to 10% of the affected population. The relative risk of lymphoma in HIV-infected individuals compared with matched uninfected controls is 60- to 100-fold. The incidence of B-cell lymphoma in this population appears stable despite the introduction of potent antiretroviral therapy and may increase as survival lengthens and control of opportunistic infections improves.

Causative factors operative in the development of lymphoma in AIDS are likely to be multiple (see Ch. 145). HIV provides a permissive environment in which lymphoma develops. Lymphoma in this setting may be regarded as an opportunistic neoplasm and is considered an AIDS-defining illness. Proliferative signals to B cells, whether from dysfunctional T cells, aberrant cytokine production, or infections (such as Epstein-Barr virus or HIV-1 itself), may induce polyclonal expansion of the B-cell population (see Ch. 387). This expanded population may provide targets for genetic abnormalities that lead to malignant transformation and emergence of several dominant clones. The oligoclonal populations of malignant B cells seen in some HIV-infected individuals with lymphoma support such a model. Ultimately, a single malignant clone may emerge, leading to a monoclonal neoplasm. The chromosomal abnormalities frequently seen in B-cell lymphoma involve translocation of loci encoding the immunoglobulin genes with the *c-myc* oncogene. Over 75% of AIDS-related lymphomas manifest alterations in at least one proto-oncogene, and a large fraction also have alterations in at least one tumor-suppressor gene. Genetic evidence of Epstein-Barr virus is found in about one half of B-cell lymphomas in AIDS patients and virtually all primary CNS lymphomas in AIDS. A number of interacting factors are likely to be important in the pathogenesis of lymphoma in those patients with HIV infection united by the disorganization of immune function induced by HIV. Recently, KSHV or HHV-8 infection has been associated with a distinct subset of B-cell lymphomas that presents with body cavity effusions. These aggressive lymphomas also frequently have genomic material from Epstein-Barr virus.

Clinically, B-cell lymphoma in AIDS patients tends to be of high-grade histologic pattern and follows an aggressive clinical course. Small, noncleaved or large cell histologies account for

Table 416–2 ■ KAPOSI'S SARCOMA (KS): RECOMMENDED STAGING CLASSIFICATION

	GOOD RISK (0) (ALL OF THE FOLLOWING)	POOR RISK (1) (ANY OF THE FOLLOWING)
Tumor (T)	Confined to skin and/or lymph nodes and/or minimal oral disease*	Tumor-associated edema or ulceration, extensive oral KS, gastrointestinal KS or KS in other non-nodal viscera
Immune system (I)	CD4 cells ≥200 μL	CD4 cells <200/μL
Systemic illness (S)	No history of OI† or thrush	History of OI and/or thrush, "B" symptoms present
	No "B" symptoms‡	
	Performance status ≥70 (Karnofsky)	Performance status <70
		Other HIV-related illness (e.g., neurologic disease, lymphoma)

*Minimal oral disease is non-nodular KS confined to the palate.
†OI = opportunistic infection.
‡"B" symptoms are unexplained fever, night sweats, >10% involuntary weight loss, or diarrhea persisting more than 2 weeks.
Modified from Krown SE, Metroka C, Wernz J: Kaposi's sarcoma in the acquired immune deficiency syndrome: A proposal for uniform evaluation, response, and staging criteria. J Clin Oncol 7:1201–1207, 1989.

nearly all lymphomas in this setting. The low-grade lymphomas are uncommon and may represent background rather than a neoplasm directly associated with immunosuppression. Rarely, B-cell acute lymphoblastic leukemia or T-cell neoplasms have been reported.

Most patients have extranodular disease involving the gastrointestinal tract, CNS, liver, soft tissues, or bone marrow. In one large series, nearly 80% of all patients diagnosed with B-cell lymphoma in AIDS had extra-nodal involvement. Lymphoma strictly confined to lymph nodes is uncommon. Gastrointestinal lymphoma may occur anywhere from the esophagus to the anus. Primary CNS lymphoma is usually immunoblastic in histologic type (see Ch. 411). Such patients generally have solitary mass lesions in the parenchyma of the brain, whereas CNS involvement in conjunction with systemic lymphoma is more often meningeal in location. All AIDS patients diagnosed with systemic non-Hodgkin's lymphoma should undergo careful CNS assessment with computed tomographic (CT) scan or magnetic resonance imaging (MRI) scan, as well as lumbar puncture with cytology.

Most AIDS patients with B-cell lymphoma are classified as having stage III (involving both sides of the diaphragm without visceral involvement) or stage IV (visceral involvement). Systemic "B" symptoms are frequent, but fever should not be immediately ascribed to lymphoma in AIDS patients, and secondary infectious causes need to be ruled out. Staging of patients should follow the approach used in other settings of non-Hodgkin's lymphoma, with particular attention to the gastrointestinal tract, bone marrow, and CNS.

The major differential diagnosis to be considered with primary CNS lymphoma is *Toxoplasma gondii* infection or progressive multifocal leukoencephalopathy (PML) (see Ch. 411). PML usually can be distinguished from CNS lymphoma by its lack of enhancement with gadolinium on MRI. CNS lesions due to lymphoma may be isodense or hypodense and contrast-enhancing on CT scan, and enhance on MRI, thereby resembling toxoplasmosis. Nonetheless, toxoplasmosis usually presents with multiple lesions throughout the neuraxis, whereas primary CNS lymphoma tends to be a single lesion located in a paraventricular site. Accessible lesions should be biopsied to distinguish between lymphoma and toxoplasmosis; lesions difficult to approach surgically may be empirically treated with antitoxoplasmal therapy for a limited time, generally 1 to 2 weeks. If no response is seen, lymphoma becomes more likely. Alternatively, cerebrospinal fluid analysis for Epstein-Barr virus DNA compared with SPECT scanning may help distinguish abscess from non-Hodgkin's lymphoma. Treatment for primary CNS lymphoma is radiation therapy and steroids, with taper of the steroids as rapidly as tolerated. Approaches are currently in clinical trial for those patients who relapse with reasonable underlying immune function and performance status.

The treatment of AIDS-related B-cell lymphoma pivots on a balance between the poor prognosis of the neoplasm and the limited tolerance of aggressive chemotherapy in this patient population. Both opportunistic infection and bone marrow suppression often limit the delivery of high doses of chemotherapy on schedule. Patients with prior AIDS-defining illness, particularly a history of opportunistic infection, have a poor prognosis compared with patients who present with lymphoma as their initial manifestation of AIDS. Similarly, more severely immunocompromised patients with low CD4 cell numbers have a poor outcome and are less tolerant of chemotherapy than are those patients with more intact immune function.

Among "good prognosis" patients with relatively intact immune function and/or those presenting with lymphoma as their AIDS manifestation, aggressive therapy with combination regimens is indicated. The regimen of cyclophosphamide, doxorubicin, vincristine, and prednisone ("CHOP") is most often used, although infusional regimens with etoposide, doxorubicin, and cyclophophamide also have reported good results. Hematopoietic growth factors to ameliorate cytopenias generally are needed. Antiretroviral therapy generally can be sustained, but systematic pharmacokinetic studies are lacking and significant drug-drug interactions may occur. We have noted no undue toxicity when using indinavir, 3TC, and d4T in conjunction with CHOP. For those patients who do not have CNS involvement at the time of presentation, prophylactic therapy to the CNS often is given to prevent CNS relapse. This may be particularly important for patients with small, noncleaved cell histology or bone marrow, or testicular or Waldeyer's ring involve-ment. The response rate in patients undergoing systemic chemotherapy is on the order of 50%, but the long-term survival rate is still poor owing to frequent relapse and intervening infections. The potential for eradication of the non-Hodgkin's lymphoma is real and should be pursued in select patients. Fifty per cent of patients achieve a complete remission and have a median survival of 18 months or longer. For those failing initial therapy, no clear second-line approach has been defined. Patients with this disorder should be treated in clinical trial settings whenever possible.

Patients with poor prognosis based on severe immune suppression and/or complicating opportunistic infections pose a particularly complex treatment dilemma. Some patients have opted for palliative therapy with corticosteroids because intensive chemotherapy may lead to further immune compromise and infection. Yet lymphoma is generally rapidly growing and fatal in patients who are not aggressively treated. Thus, the clinician needs to pursue therapy in such patients only with an informed discussion of the risks and benefits of treatment, honestly emphasizing the poor prognosis with or without chemotherapy.

Other Malignancies

The incidence of Hodgkin's disease has been estimated to be up to 18-fold greater in HIV-infected individuals compared to the HIV-seronegative population. In patients with HIV infection and Hodgkin's disease, the clinical presentation usually includes B-symptoms (fever, night sweats, anorexia, and weight loss), stage III or IV disease, and extranodular disease. The histopathology is often the mixed cellularity or lymphocyte-depleted types. Furthermore, HIV-infected individuals with Hodgkin's disease appear to tolerate chemotherapy less well and may have a higher incidence of tumor relapse than do those without HIV infection.

Hodgkin's disease therapy among HIV-infected patients should be according to guidelines for non–HIV-positive individuals (see Ch. 314). The major difference is to incorporate prophylaxis against opportunistic infections, particularly *P. carinii* pneumonia, to be particularly alert to infectious complications during therapy, and to integrate growth factor support given the frequent cytopenias in HIV-infected hosts. We generally continue antiretroviral therapy, but drug interactions are possible and poorly defined at present.

Anal cancer and, to a lesser extent, cervical cancer occur with a higher incidence in HIV-infected patients. This is due to the high prevalence of papillomavirus infection in groups at risk for HIV (see Ch. 361) and the dysplasia associated with it. Frequent careful cervical examinations including colposcopy are indicated in HIV-infected women to detect early malignant change. Ongoing surveillance programs of HIV-infected individuals using Papanicolaou smears on cells from the transitional zone of the anus and cervix should provide important data as to the increased incidence and optimal surveillance programs for these cancers in this population. Invasive cancer of the uterine cervix has recently been added as an AIDS-defining illness in women infected with HIV.

Although anecdotal reports abound of other malignancies in HIV-infected individuals, it is unclear whether these occur above that of the background prevalence in the general population. Nonetheless, consideration should be given to the significance of the HIV infection in clinical management. These patients have a propensity to develop opportunistic infections when starting chemotherapy or radiation therapy and, in general, have fared poorly because of these infectious complications.

Ballem PJ, Belzberg A, Devine DV, et al: Kinetic studies of the mechanism of thrombocytopenia in patients with human immunodeficiency virus infection. N Engl J Med 327:1779, 1992. *A study on thrombocytopenia in HIV disease.*

Goedert JJ, Cote TR, Virgo P, et al: Spectrum of AIDS-associated malignant disorders. Lancet 351:1833, 1998. *An excellent summary of the epidemiology of AIDS-related cancers.*

Karcher DS, Alkan S: Human herpesvirus-8–associated body cavity-based lymphoma in human immunodeficiency virus-infected patients: A unique B-cell neoplasm. Hum Pathol 28:801, 1997. *Description of a recently recognized lymphoma due to a novel herpes virus.*

Lee FC, Mitsuyasu RT: Chemotherapy of AIDS-related Kaposi's sarcoma. Hematol/Oncol Clin North Am 10:1051, 1996. *A review of treatments for Kaposi's sarcoma.*

Luft BJ, Hafner R, Korzun AH, et al: Toxoplasmic encephalitis in patients with the acquired immunodeficiency syndrome. N Engl J Med 329:995, 1993. *A discussion of outcomes from anti-toxoplasmosis treatment of CNS lesions in patients with AIDS.*

Palefsky JM: Anal human papilloma virus infection and anal cancer in HIV-positive individuals: An emerging problem. AIDS 8:283, 1994.

Roizman B: New viral footprints in Kaposi's sarcoma [editorial]. N Engl J Med 332: 1227, 1995. *Discusses the discovery of herpesvirus 8 and the presence of the virus in cells affected by Kaposi's sarcoma.*

Straus DJ: Human immunodeficiency virus–associated lymphomas. Med Clin North Am 81:495, 1997. *A review of AIDS-related lymphoma with an excellent bibliography.*

417 RENAL, CARDIAC, ENDOCRINE, AND RHEUMATOLOGIC MANIFESTATIONS OF HIV INFECTION

Michael S. Saag

Infection with the human immunodeficiency virus type I (HIV) is a multisystem disease. Manifestations of pulmonary, gastrointestinal, neurologic, hematologic, and oncologic disease are well described in the literature, owing mainly to their high prevalence and often dramatic modes of presentation. In contrast, HIV-related renal, cardiac, endocrine, and rheumatologic diseases are more insidious in presentation. As overall survival of HIV-infected individuals continues to improve and therapeutic regimens become more sophisticated, clinicians will undoubtedly encounter disorders of the latter organ systems with increasing frequency.

RENAL DISEASE

Renal disease associated with HIV infection may present as fluid-electrolyte and acid-base abnormalities, acute renal failure, coincidental renal disorders, or a glomerulopathy directly related to underlying HIV infection, the so-called HIV-associated nephropathy (HIVAN). Originally observed in patients with AIDS and referred to as AIDS-associated nephropathy, recent studies have described the characteristic renal changes of HIVAN in both asymptomatic HIV-infected individuals and those with early symptomatic HIV disease, thereby broadening the definition to include all HIV-infected patients. With the advent of the potent protease inhibitor indinavir, renal stones have been reported with increasing frequency. Up to 4% of indinauir recipients experience flank pain, with or without hematuria, while on therapy. Crystallization of drug in the renal collecting system leads to development of "sludge," or frank stones, resulting in renal colic.

Fluid, Electrolyte, and Acid-Base Disorders

Fluid-electrolyte disorders are common in patients with advanced HIV infection. Hyponatremia is noted in up to 40% of hospitalized AIDS patients and occurs in the setting of both hypovolemia and euvolemia. Hypovolemia, most often due to gastrointestinal fluid losses, is the most common cause of hyponatremia among this group of patients. The syndrome of inappropriate antidiuretic hormone release (SIADH) is responsible for the majority of cases of euvolemic hyponatremia and is most often due to underlying *Pneumocystis carinii* infection, malignancy, or central nervous system (CNS) disease. The presence of hyponatremia is associated with increased morbidity and mortality, especially in conjunction with certain opportunistic infections, such as cryptococcosis.

Adrenal insufficiency is a less frequent cause of hyponatremia. Although abnormalities of the adrenal glands are frequently reported at autopsy, overt adrenal insufficiency occurs in <5% of patients. The typical findings of hyponatremia, hyperkalemia, non–anion gap metabolic acidosis, hypovolemia, renal salt wasting, and mild renal insufficiency are usually present in some combination.

Drugs are an important cause of fluid and electrolyte disorders in HIV-infected patients and can mimic the abnormalities associated with adrenal dysfunction. Hyperkalemia and non–anion gap metabolic acidosis have been noted in patients receiving parenteral pentamidine. Amphotericin B is associated with hypokalemia, hypomagnesia, renal tubular acidosis, and renal insufficiency. Foscarnet therapy is associated with decreased levels of ionized calcium and, on occasion, renal insufficiency. Nucleotide analogs, such as cidofovir and adefovir, are associated with renal insufficiency and electrolyte disorders. A Fanconi-like proximal renal tubule disorder (see Chapter 109), characterized by hypophosphatemia and creatinine elevation, has been observed frequently in patients receiving adefovir; the incidence of this disorder increases dramatically after 24 weeks of adefovir therapy. Chemotherapeutic agents used to treat AIDS-associated malignancies may lead to fluid and electrolyte disturbances through direct nephrotoxicity or gastrointestinal losses associated with prolonged vomiting or diarrhea.

Acute Renal Failure

As with most chronic illnesses, acute renal dysfunction may develop as a complication in the management of HIV-infected patients. Prerenal azotemia often results from hypovolemia secondary to poor fluid intake, increased gastrointestinal losses, or both. Acute tubular necrosis can be ischemic in origin, usually secondary to hypotension or sepsis, or due to nephrotoxic agents. Acute interstitial nephritis is another complication associated with drugs used to treat HIV-related diseases. A listing of agents with nephrotoxic potential commonly used in HIV-infected patients is presented in Table 417–1.

Opportunistic infections, invasion of renal parenchyma with lymphoma or Kaposi's sarcoma, and amyloidosis, which occurs as a complication of subcutaneous narcotic abuse, all may result in interstitial nephritis. Other renal lesions, such as hepatitis B–induced membranous glomerulonephritis, IgA nephropathy, acute glomerulonephritis secondary to bacterial infection, direct infection of the renal parenchyma with cytomegalovirus (CMV), fungi, or mycobacteria, and the hemolytic-uremic syndrome have all been associated with renal dysfunction in HIV-infected individuals. The diagnosis and management of acute renal failure are no different in HIV-infected patients than in their uninfected counterparts (see Chapter 103).

HIV-Associated Nephropathy

Definition

HIVAN was first established as a unique clinical entity in 1984. Originally called AIDS-associated nephropathy (AAN), many investigators questioned whether AAN was indeed a unique manifestation of AIDS or simply represented heroin-associated nephropathy (HAN) occurring in intravenous drug users (IVDUs) who also happened to be infected with HIV. Although the lesions and clinical manifestations of HAN are similar to those of AAN, further studies have established clear distinctions between the two entities. Of note, AAN occurs in individuals, including children, who have never used intravenous drugs. Indeed, nearly half of the cases presenting with the manifestations of AAN have early (asymptomatic or minimally symptomatic) HIV disease. Therefore, HIVAN has replaced AAN as the most appropriate name for this entity.

Epidemiology

The first cases of HIVAN were described in major urban centers, such as New York and Miami, which also had many IVDUs among their HIV patient population. In contrast, centers whose HIV population consisted primarily of Caucasian homosexual and

Table 417–1 ■ DRUGS WITH NEPHROTOXIC POTENTIAL COMMONLY USED IN THE TREATMENT OF HIV-RELATED DISEASE

Acyclovir	Nonsteroidal anti-inflammatory agents
Aminoglycosides	Penicillins
Amphotericin B	Pentamidine
Aspirin	Phenytoin
Cephalosporins	Rifabutin
Cimetidine	Rifampin
Cis-platinum	Spiramycin
Dapsone	Sulfonamides
Ethambutol	Tetracyclines
Foscarnet	Thiazides
Ganciclovir	Trimethoprim

bisexual men, such as San Francisco and the National Institutes of Health, were not observing the renal changes of HIVAN in their patients, thereby implying that HIVAN was a manifestation of HAN. More recent epidemiologic data indicate that 50% of patients with HIVAN are IVDUs, with the remaining cases occurring in homosexual and bisexual men, immigrants from Haiti, women who have acquired HIV from heterosexual contacts, and children born to infected mothers, many of whom did not use intravenous drugs.

Over 90% of patients with HIVAN are black. No explanation regarding the high prevalence of cases among blacks has been established, although many investigators have speculated that cofactors such as superimposed infection(s) or specific immune response genes may be responsible.

Pathology and Pathogenesis

Focal and segmental glomerulosclerosis (FSGS) is the characteristic renal lesion identified in patients with HIVAN, occurring in 80 to 90% of patients. On gross inspection, the kidneys usually are enlarged and the cortical surface is smooth, even in advanced uremia. Microscopic examination of early lesions reveals diffuse mesangial hyperplasia with minimal glomerular sclerosis over time. A variable number of glomeruli develop segmental sclerosis characterized by hyperplastic visceral epithelial cells with coarse cytoplasmic vacuoles, collapsed capillary walls or capillaries obliterated by protein deposits (hyalinosis), and foam cells (lipid-filled monocytes) in the lumina (Fig. 417–1). Bowman spaces are usually dilated and tubular damage is universal. Microcystic dilation of tubules is a unique feature of HIVAN not reported in the FSGS of HAN (Fig. 417–2). Interstitial changes consisting of mild edema with scattered mononuclear cells are usually evident in HIVAN kidneys but not nearly to the degree noted in HAN. Similarly, although interstitial fibrosis may be present in advanced HIVAN disease, it is not nearly as prominent as the marked interstitial fibrosis noted in HAN disease.

The etiology of HIVAN remains unknown; however, many investigators suspect that an infectious agent perhaps HIV itself, is responsible. Ultrastructural studies have demonstrated tuboloreticular structures in vascular endothelium as well as in circulating and tissue lymphocytes. Other findings, such as a large number of nuclear bodies existing as budding forms in renal and lymphoid tissues, have been interpreted by some investigators to suggest a viral etiology. In situ hybridization studies have demonstrated proviral HIV DNA in renal tubular and glomerular epithelial cells, implicating HIV as the causative agent. However, the predominance of HIVAN in blacks and the relative paucity of cases among Caucasian homosexual men suggest that other factors not yet identified must play a role in the pathogenesis of HIVAN.

Clinical Manifestations

HIVAN is characterized by the development of proteinuria, nephrotic syndrome, and rapidly progressive irreversible azotemia. The proteinuria is typically heavy and presents as an early manifestation. Untreated, the time to the development of end-stage renal

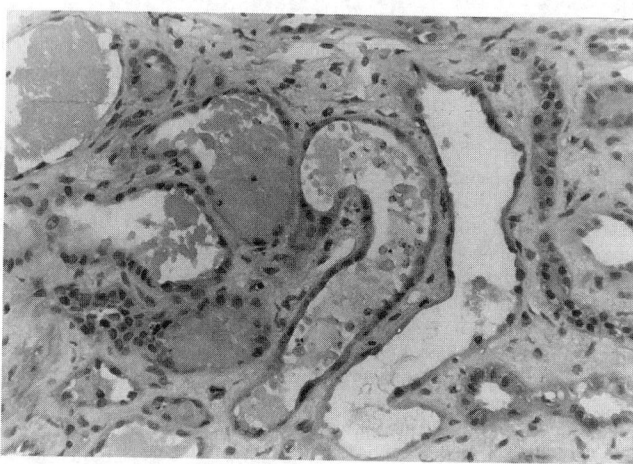

FIGURE 417–2 ■ Dilated degenerated tubules demonstrating flattened epithelium and loss of nuclei and containing proteinaceous casts from a patient with HIV-associated nephropathy. (Hematoxylin-eosin; magnification ×200. Courtesy of Dr. William L. Clapp.)

disease (ESRD) from the initial diagnosis of proteinuria is 4 to 16 weeks in patients with HIVAN, compared to 20 to 40 months among patients with HAN. Another clinical distinction between HIVAN and HAN is the relative absence of significant hypertension among patients with HIVAN. Accelerated hypertension is a hallmark of HAN. Peripheral edema and anasarca are conspicuously absent in a large number of HIVAN patients with high-grade proteinuria and hypoalbuminemia.

Nephropathy has been documented in patients months to years before the onset of clinical symptoms of early symptomatic HIV disease or AIDS. HIVAN is being reported with increasing frequency among HIV-infected children and appears to be independent of the risk factors for HIV infection in their mothers. It is anticipated that the incidence of HIVAN will continue to grow and should be considered as a diagnostic possibility in any HIV-infected patient who presents with unexplained proteinuria regardless of the stage of disease.

Diagnosis

Quantitative measurement of the amount of protein excreted in the urine along with estimation of the creatinine clearance via a 24-hour urine collection should be performed early in the course of evaluation. Other reversible causes of renal insufficiency such as bacterial infection, crystalluria, and obstructive uropathy should be ruled out using urine culture, urinalysis, and ultrasonography. The kidneys are enlarged early in HIVAN and remain enlarged throughout the course of disease. Since a variety of other renal lesions, such as membranous nephropathy related to hepatitis B, membranoproliferative disease, and immune complex–related glomerular damage, may also present as nephrotic syndrome in HIV-infected patients, renal biopsy should be encouraged. The presence of the typical features of FSGS with tubular involvement as described above establishes the diagnosis of HIVAN when renal tissue is obtained.

Treatment

Improved outcome, including reversal of renal insufficiency and marked reduction in proteinuria, has been reported with a number of interventions. The use of highly active antiretroviral therapy, usually consisting of a regimen containing a potent protein inhibitor, in combination with other modalities (e.g., conticosteroids or ACE-inhibitor therapy) is the cornerstone of therapy. Corticosteroids (60 mg prednisone daily over 2 to 6 weeks) have been shown to partially reverse the progressive azotemia and prevent the need for dialysis in a subgroup of patients. Several uncontrolled studies have demonstrated benefit of ACE-inhibitors, either captopril or fosinopril, in the treatment of biopsy-proven HIVAN. Outcomes were better among those receiving ACE-inhibitors along with potent antiretroviral therapy.

Nutritional support in the form of high-protein, high-calorie diets

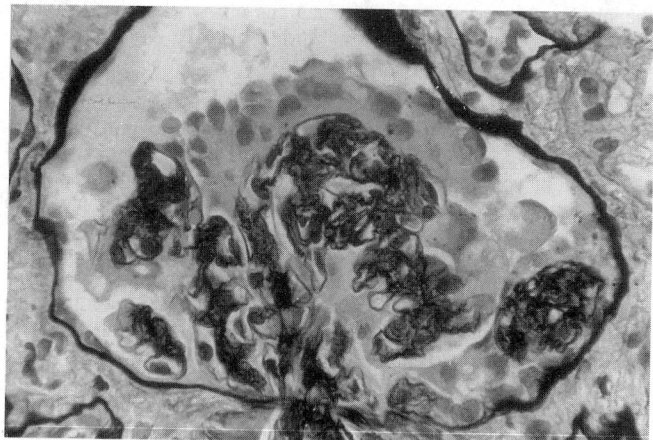

FIGURE 417–1 ■ Glomerulus from a patient with HIV-associated nephropathy demonstrating global collapse of the glomerular capillaries, increased mesangial sclerosis, and a proliferative "cap" of visceral epithelial cells. (Silver methenamine: magnification ×400. Courtesy of Dr. William L. Clapp.)

along with appropriate dosage adjustments of nephrotoxic drugs is crucial. Hemodialysis is of marginal benefit in prolonging survival of patients with advanced HIV disease once they have reached end-stage renal disease. Among patients with AIDS, hemodialysis provides significant prolongation of life. Patients who are asymptomatic or have early symptomatic HIV disease survive longer, with some patients living >6 years on chronic hemodialysis. Peritoneal dialysis should be considered in patients who are suitable candidates. Chronic ambulatory peritoneal dialysis (CAPD) may offer several advantages over hemodialysis, including avoiding leukopenia caused by the hemodialysis membranes, fewer problems with anemia, and theoretical advantages of less stimulation of HIV-infected T lymphocytes via membrane-induced cytokine release. A potential disadvantage of CAPD is the higher incidence of peritonitis. Renal transplantation is not considered a viable option in HIV-infected patients owing to the intensive immunosuppressive regimens required to prevent rejection. In some patients with advanced HIV infection or AIDS who develop HIVAN it may be appropriate to withhold dialysis support because of the generally poor prognosis. As always, such decisions should be individualized, taking into account the wishes of the patient, the family, and significant others.

CARDIAC DISEASE

A wide variety of cardiac abnormalities have been reported in HIV-infected patients, including ventricular dysfunction myocarditis, pericarditis, endocarditis, and arrhythmias. Most often, cardiac involvement is clinically silent and is noted as an incidental finding at autopsy. When clinical symptoms are present, however, disease manifestations can be debilitating, and, in many cases, life threatening. Unlike HIV-associated renal disease, no specific cardiac syndrome or disease state has been described.

Epidemiology

Cardiac abnormalities have been observed in 25 to 75% of HIV-infected patients studied at autopsy. Myocardial disease is noted most frequently, occurring in >90% of subjects with cardiac findings. Pericardial disease, often with adjacent myocardial involvement, is observed in >20% of cases with cardiac abnormalities. Endocarditis is evident histologically in 3 to 5% of cases reported in autopsy series. No characteristic epidemiologic factor, such as age, gender, race, or means of acquiring HIV infection, has been identified which predisposes patients to cardiac disease. Although cardiac abnormalities are observed more frequently in AIDS patients, up to 30% of patients with early symptomatic HIV disease are noted to have abnormal findings on echocardiograms and electrocardiograms.

Pathology and Pathogenesis

HIV-related heart disease may result from metastatic extension of a concomitant opportunistic infection or malignancy but most often is seen as lymphocytic infiltration of the myocardium or as an unspecified myocarditis. The mechanism responsible for the myocarditis remains unknown, although many investigators believe that HIV itself may be directly responsible. Other viruses, such as CMV, may be responsible for the development of myocarditis, although the typical "owl's eye" inclusion bodies are rarely seen in patients with HIV-associated cardiomyopathy. Additional mechanisms, such as postviral myocarditis or catecholamine-induced myocarditis, have been postulated, but little evidence exists to support their role.

A broad range of opportunistic infections and malignant diseases has been described in cardiac tissue examined at autopsy. Among the infectious disorders, fungal and viral pathogens are identified most often, followed by bacterial and protozoal infections (Table 417–2). Although the invading pathogen is frequently diagnosed at another primary site antemortem, cardiac involvement is rarely (<2%) identified before autopsy. This is largely due to the clinically silent nature of cardiac disease in HIV infection and a low index of suspicion by clinicians. Kaposi's sarcoma and metastatic lymphoma are the most common neoplastic diseases reported that invade the heart. Primary cardiac lymphoma has been reported rarely.

Table 417–2 ■ INFECTIOUS CAUSES OF CARDIAC DISEASE IN HIV-INFECTED PATIENTS

Bacteria
   Bacteria (endocarditis)
   Mycobacterium tuberculosis
   Mycobacterium avium-intracellulare
   Nocardia asteroides
   Actinomyces
Fungi
   Cryptococcus neoformans
   Histoplasma capsulatum
   Coccidioides immitis
   Candida species
   Aspergillus species
Viruses
   Cytomegalovirus
   Herpes simplex virus
   Human immunodeficiency virus
Protozoa
   Toxoplasma gondii
   Pneumocystis carinii

Pericardial disease is almost invariably associated with adjacent myocardial involvement. Pericarditis is usually nonspecific in origin, but when an etiologic process is identified, Kaposi's sarcoma or a pathogen, such as *Mycobacterium tuberculosis* or *Cryptococcus neoformans,* is responsible most often. Drugs used to treat HIV-associated disorders, such as doxorubicin for Kaposi's sarcoma, may cause myocardial damage. Other toxins, vitamin deficiencies, or metabolic abnormalities (e.g., hypothyroidism) may also result in myocardial dysfunction or pericardial disease.

Endocardial disease has been described in up to 3% of cases studied at autopsy and usually presents as either nonbacterial thrombotic (marantic) endocarditis or healed bacterial endocarditis. The precise etiology of marantic endocarditis is unknown, but it has been reported in other long-term wasting illnesses and malignant diseases. Vegetations are usually located on the mitral valve, although lesions on the tricuspid valve have been noted in up to 29% of AIDS patients with this disorder. Significant embolization to the spleen and brain was noted in >50% of patients with marantic endocarditis studied at autopsy. Bacterial endocarditis is reported rarely in AIDS patients. Healed lesions from previous bouts of bacterial endocarditis have been reported in autopsy series but are of little clinical significance.

Clinical Findings

Most cardiac disease in HIV-infected patients is clinically silent. When symptoms are present they usually consist of the ordinary findings noted in non-HIV-infected patients with myocarditis or pericarditis, such as fever, dyspnea, chest pain, fatigue, cough, and orthopnea. Hepatomegaly and jugular venous distention are the most common signs noted on physical examination, followed by rales, systolic murmurs, and the presence of an S3 gallop. Signs of advanced pericardial disease with impending tamponade are among the most common clinical manifestations observed in patients who present with clinical symptoms of cardiac disease.

Diagnosis

Demonstrated cardiomegaly on a chest roentgenogram is an important marker of underlying cardiac disease in HIV-infected patients. Right ventricular enlargement is usually the result of pulmonary artery hypertension, which in AIDS patients is often due to severe or recurrent opportunistic pneumonia. Left ventricular or biventricular enlargement is a characteristic finding of congestive cardiomyopathy due to any cause. Echocardiography is a more sensitive and specific noninvasive test that is used to assess the degree of ventricular dysfunction and to characterize the extent of pericardial effusion, if present. Several series have demonstrated echocardiographic abnormalities in up to 50% of HIV-infected patients who had no cardiac symptoms at the time of study. Ventricular enlargement, pericardial effusion, and ventricular hypokinesis were the abnormalities noted most frequently. In view of the overall silent nature of cardiac disease, the high likelihood that infiltrative processes will be evident and diagnosed at another site, and the often limited therapeutic options available for treating cardiac disease in HIV-infected patients, routine echocardiography should be discouraged in those without cardiac symptoms. The experience with endomyocardial biopsies in HIV-infected patients is quite limited; however, in those individuals who show signs of cardiac disease and have not had a specific diagnosis established, endomyocardial biopsy is a viable option for a definitive diagnosis.

Treatment

Supportive treatment consisting of diuretic therapy, reducing preload and afterload when appropriate, and correcting cardiac arrhythmias is the obvious initial approach to treating myocardial disease. Pericardial disease requires careful volume management with avoidance of aggressive diuresis or preload reduction. In the case of pericardial tamponade, surgical intervention is warranted. When the underlying etiology of the cardiac disease is known, appropriate therapy directed at the specific infectious agent or malignancy is indicated.

ENDOCRINE DISORDERS

Endocrine dysfunction has not been prominent in HIV infection. Nonetheless, all glands of the endocrine system may be infiltrated with opportunistic infections or malignancies or may be affected by drugs used to treat HIV-related disorders. More recently, hyperlipidemia and lipodystrophy have been associated with the use of highly active antiretroviral therapy, especially with certain protease inhibitors. The specific etiology of these disorder remains unclear. The subtle presentations of endocrine diseases create difficult diagnostic challenges.

Adrenal Gland Dysfunction

The adrenal gland is the endocrine gland most commonly affected in AIDS patients examined at autopsy, although clinical evidence of adrenal insufficiency is observed in <8% of AIDS patients. Widespread lipid depletion and varying degrees of adrenal necrosis are the most prevalent pathologic findings in postmortem examinations. Adrenal invasion by CMV is noted in up to 50% of patients with adrenal pathology. *Mycobacterium avium* complex, Kaposi's sarcoma, *C. neoformans,* and *Histoplasma capsulatum* involve the adrenal glands in 5 to 12% of cases. Drug therapy, with agents such as ketoconazole (adrenal dysfunction) or rifampin (increased clearance of cortisol) may also result in adrenal insufficiency. Fatigue, anorexia, nausea, vomiting, orthostatic hypotension, and hyponatremia are symptoms frequently noted in many HIV-infected patients; however, only a few with these symptoms are actually adrenal insufficient when evaluated using standard laboratory criteria.

Basal 8 A.M. plasma cortisol levels are usually higher in patients with advanced HIV disease than in asymptomatic patients and uninfected healthy controls. However, other ACTH-dependent steroids, such as desoxycorticosterone (DOC), compound B, and 18-hydroxy-DOC, are not elevated and show a blunted response to corticotropin (ACTH) stimulation, implying subnormal adrenal reserves. Patients who fail to achieve plasma cortisol levels >20 μg per deciliter 60 minutes after ACTH stimulation should be considered to have, or be at high risk of developing, adrenal insufficiency. Plasma ACTH levels are frequently normal or subnormal even when plasma cortisol levels are depressed, suggesting that adrenal insufficiency in some HIV-infected patients is due to a primary pituitary or CNS disorder. Treatment of adrenal insufficiency in HIV-infected patients is the same as in other individuals with abnormal adrenal function (see Chapter 240).

Hypogonadism

The most common abnormality of endocrine function noted clinically is hypogonadism. Decreased libido occurs in over one half of male patients with AIDS, and impotence, usually associated with low serum testosterone levels, is reported in up to 30% of AIDS patients. Serum gonadotropin levels may be below normal or inappropriately within normal limits in hypogonadal men with AIDS. When pituitary responsiveness to gonadotropin-releasing hormone is assessed in these hypogonadotropic males, normal release of luteinizing hormone (LH) and follicle-stimulating hormone (FSH) has been observed, suggesting a hypothalamic basis for the central hypogonadotropism. Other studies have demonstrated appropriately elevated levels of LH and FSH in hypogonadal men, implying primary testicular dysfunction. Drugs, such as ketoconazole, ganciclovir, and acyclovir have been associated with low testosterone levels or decreased spermatogenesis. Chronic use of megesterol acetate is invariably associated with suppression of testosterone levels in men. Studies of gonadal function in women are limited, although menstrual irregularities are common in women with advanced HIV disease.

Thyroid Disease

Thyroid function remains remarkably normal throughout the course of HIV disease. Low levels of thyroxine (T$_4$), triiodothyronine (T$_3$), and free-thyroxine index (FTI) in the setting of low concentrations of thyrotropin (TSH), the so-called euthyroid sick syndrome, is remarkably uncommon among ambulatory HIV-infected patients. Decreased levels of T$_3$ resin uptake and elevated levels of T$_4$-binding globulin are frequently noted in ambulatory patients with advanced disease; however, concentration of T$_3$ and T$_4$ are most often within normal limits. Invasive disease due to CMV, *P. carinii, C. neoformans,* Kaposi's sarcoma, and lymphoma have all been described in the thyroid. Remarkably, even patients with infiltrating opportunistic diseases of the thyroid gland usually remain euthyroid throughout the course of their disease. Nonetheless, despite the relative infrequency of clinical disease, hypothyroidism represents a potentially reversible cause of fatigue, malaise, altered mental status, and "failure to thrive" in HIV-Infected individuals and should be routinely evaluated.

Less common causes of hypothyroidism in HIV-infected patients include adverse effects of medications. Ketoconazole has been associated with primary hypothyroidism on rare occasions. In addition, drugs that are strong inducers of hepatic microsomal enzymes, such as rifampin, may lead to increased clearance of T$_4$.

Metabolic Abnormalities

Hyponatremia is the most common electrolyte disturbance noted in HIV-infected individuals (see discussion in renal section). Disorders of carbohydrate metabolism have been reported in association with direct pancreatic invasion by opportunistic processes and with drug therapy. Pancreatic lesions caused by CMV, toxoplasmosis, Kaposi's sarcoma, and lymphoma are noted in up to 35% of cases at autopsy. Yet the development of type I diabetes mellitus has been reported in only a few instances. Hypoglycemia is the most common alteration in glucose metabolism. Direct toxic effects of drugs may induce premature release of insulin by β cells, resulting in hypoglycemic episodes that may be severe and prolonged. Pentamidine isothionate is the most common cause of hypoglycemia, occurring in 4 to 33% of treated patients. Renal insufficiency is a predisposing factor in the development of pentamidine-induced hypoglycemia. Although most hypoglycemic episodes result from parenteral administration of pentamidine, several cases have been reported in patients receiving aerosolized drug.

Disorders of calcium metabolism are relatively uncommon but do occur. Hypercalcemia is associated with HIV-related leukemia and lymphoma. Hypocalcemia usually is the result of drug therapy with agents, such as amphotericin B and foscarnet, which induce magnesium wasting and decrease levels of ionized calcium, respectively. CMV has been observed in parathyroid tissue, however, CMV-induced hypoparathyroidism is extremely rare.

Hyperlipidemia is noted commonly in HIV-infected patients. Isolated elevation of triglycerides is reported in up to 50% of patients with either asymptomatic HIV disease or AIDS. Although hypertriglyceridemia is routinely noted among patients with HIV wasting syndrome, no relationship has been noted between the serum triglyceride level and the degree of wasting. Elevation of cachectin (tumor necrosis factor), inhibition of lipoprotein lipase, and decreased clearance of circulating lipoproteins have all been proposed as potential mechanisms of hypertriglyceridemia, but no clear association of any of these factors has been established.

In the era of highly active antiretroviral therapy (HAART), patients receiving protease inhibitor therapy have been noted to have elevated plasma triglyceride and cholesterol levels. Initial reports identified ritonavir as the most likely cause of these metabolic abnormalities, but more recently, indinavir, nelfinavir, and saquinavir have also been implicated. Sporadic reports of nonprotease inhibitor-containing regimens causing this syndrome have also appeared. In addition to hyperlipidemia, glucose intolerance and frank diabetes mellitus have been associated with HAART regimens. Insulin resistance appears to play a role in the development of this entry, but the precise mechanism remains unclear. To complete the syndrome, abnormalities in body fat distribution have been observed in some individuals on HAART regimens. Loss of peripheral body fat in the extremities and excess accumulation of fat in the abdominal region (so-called "protease paunch") and breasts have been reported, to some degree, in up to 80% of patient on HAART; severe manifestations are observed in 10% of patients. Dorsocervical fat pad enlargement (buffalo hump) among HAART recipients has been reported in 55 patients in the published literature. These patients have normal cortisol levels and varying degrees of hypertriglyceridemia or lipodystrophy. No specific therapeutic approaches for this syndrome have been elucidated. In severe cases, the HAART regimen must be modified.

RHEUMATOLOGIC DISEASE

Rheumatologic manifestations of HIV disease are being recognized with increased frequency. Musculoskeletal complaints are reported in 33 to 75% of HIV-infected patients and may present as a variety of rheumatologic disorders (Table 417–3). The severity of disease ranges from intermittent arthralgias to debilitating arthritis and vasculitis. An array of autoimmune antibodies, including antinuclear, antiplatelet, antilymphocyte, antigranulocyte, and antiphospholipid (anticardiolipin and lupus anticoagulant) antibodies are associated with HIV infection along with circulating immune complexes, rheumatoid factor, and cryoglobulins. Despite the presence of these antibodies in some patients, the precise mechanisms by which the rheumatologic abnormalities develop have not been elucidated and most likely are different for each particular disorder.

Arthralgias

Arthralgia is a common manifestation of acute HIV seroconversion, in addition to fever, myalgia, headache, sore throat, abdominal cramps, and lymphadenopathy. Generalized arthralgias are reported in up to one third of HIV-infected patients with minimally symptomatic disease. Some patients develop arthralgias and myalgias when zidovudine therapy is initiated; however, these symptoms are usually self-limited and abate within 4 to 6 weeks after starting treatment. The "painful articular syndrome" is characterized by severe articular pain of 2 to 24 hours' duration. Although uncommon, this disorder is quite incapacitating and usually unresponsive to oral nonsteroidal anti-inflammatory agents (NSAIDs) or narcotic analgesics. Its etiology remains unknown. With the exception of the painful articular syndrome, most of the arthralgias associated with HIV disease are treated with nonsteroidal agents.

Myopathies

Polymyositis-like illnesses, characterized by myalgias, proximal muscle weakness, and wasting, have been reported in several HIV-infected patients and have been the initial HIV-defining presentation in a few. The findings of creatinine phosphokinase (CPK) elevation (>5 times normal) and abnormal electromyography are indistinguishable from idiopathic polymyositis. Muscle biopsies reveal necrosis, fibrosis, and inflammation, but usually to a lesser extent than is noted in non–HIV-infected individuals. The presence of nemaline rods, often noted in muscle biopsies of older adults with myositis, suggests the likelihood of underlying HIV infection when noted in biopsy specimens obtained from younger adults, especially in the absence of inflammation.

Although virus-like particles have been demonstrated rarely in synovial tissue and HIV p24 antigen has been noted in the cytoplasm of degenerating muscle cells, no specific viral etiology has been determined. All attempts to culture HIV-1 from muscle tissue of patients with myositis have been unsuccessful.

Patients receiving long-term zidovudine therapy may develop myositis characterized by muscle weakness, elevated CPK levels, myalgias, and evidence of myopathy with a paucity of inflammatory cells on biopsy. Zidovudine-associated myositis usually responds to drug discontinuation and may recur on rechallenge. No definitive therapy exists for HIV-associated polymyositis, although corticosteroid therapy has been successful in reversing symptoms in some patients. If corticosteroid therapy is contemplated, the potential risks of superimposing immunosuppressive therapy on an immunocompromised host must be considered.

Reiter's Syndrome (see also Chapter 287)

Reiter's syndrome is noted in up to 10% of HIV-infected patients who develop arthritis, and an additional 10 to 20% of patients are classified as having "reactive arthritis" because they lack the nonarticular features of Reiter's. Severe, persistent oligoarticular arthritis associated with urethritis, conjunctivitis, painless oral ulcerations, keratoderma blennorrhagicum, or circinate balanitis are the hallmarks of Reiter's disease in both HIV-infected and noninfected individuals. Clinical manifestations of Reiter's syndrome may precede or occur at the time of the initial diagnosis of HIV infection but most often follow the onset of immunodeficiency. HLA-B27 positivity is noted in 65 to 75% of HIV-infected patients with Reiter's syndrome. However, studies of African HIV patients with Reiter's disease or reactive arthritis revealed no increased incidence of HLA-B27, suggesting involvement of other gene markers in this group. *Shigella, Campylobacter, Ureaplasma,* and other bacterial species associated with the development of reactive arthropathies are rarely described in HIV patients with Reiter's syndrome. However, underlying concomitant sexually transmitted disease(s) may prove to be an important etiologic factor.

Treatment options for HIV patients with Reiter's disease are quite limited. Responses to NSAIDs are minimal, and more potent immunosuppressive agents, such as methotrexate and azathioprine, frequently lead to opportunistic diseases and Kaposi's sarcoma shortly after initiation of therapy.

Table 417–3 ■ RHEUMATOLOGIC DISEASES ASSOCIATED WITH HIV INFECTION

Autoimmune phenomena
  Anticardiolipin antibodies
  Antigranulocyte antibodies
  Antilymphocyte antibodies
  Antinuclear antibodies
  Antiplatelet antibodies
  Circulating immune complexes
  Cryoglobulins
  Rheumatoid factor
Dermatologic
  Dermatomyositis
  Malar flush
  Psoriasis
Joint disease
  Arthralgias
  Arthritis
  Enthesopathies
  HIV-associated arthritis
  "Painful articular syndrome"
  Psoriatic arthritis
  Reactive arthropathy
  Reiter's disease
  Septic arthritis
  Systemic lupus erythematosus (lupus-like syndrome)
Myopathies
  Infectious (septic) myositis
  Myalgias
    Idiopathic
    Zidovudine-associated
  Necrotizing, noninflammatory myopathy
  Nemaline rod polymyositis
  Polymyositis
  Pyomyositis
Sjögren's syndrome
  Sicca complex
Vasculitis
  Central nervous system angiitis
  Eosinophilic vasculitis
  Henoch-Schönlein purpura
  Hypersensitivity (drug-induced)
  Leukocytoclastic vasculitis
  Polyarteritis nodosa
  Unspecified vasculitis

Sjögren's Syndrome (see also Chapter 291)

Xerophthalmia and xerostomia, the characteristic symptoms of Sjögren's syndrome (SS), have been reported with increasing frequency in AIDS patients. Features that closely resemble idiopathic SS, including sicca symptoms, a positive Schirmer test, abnormal salivary gland emptying, and abnormal salivary gland biopsies, have been reported in HIV-infected patients. As a result, it has been suggested that AIDS be an exclusionary disease for the diagnosis of idiopathic SS. The predominance of male patients, the absence of anti-Ro/SS-A and anti-La/SS-B antibodies, the absence of a well-defined connective tissue disease, the presence of HLA-DR52 and DR5 alleles instead of the characteristic A1, B8, DR3, DR2, and DQ1/DQ2 antigens, and a predominance of CD8+ lymphocytes instead of CD4+ cells infiltrating salivary tissue are the characteristic features of AIDS-associated SS, which differs from classic idiopathic SS. Treatment is primarily symptomatic.

Septic Arthritis

Joint space infection is remarkably uncommon in HIV-infected patients. Sporadic case reports have been published of septic arthritis due to fungal pathogens, such as *C. neoformans, H. capsulatum,* and *S. schenkii,* mycobacteria, and routine pyogenic organisms. The approach to diagnosis and treatment of septic arthritis is the same for HIV-infected patients as non–HIV-infected individuals.

HIV-Associated Arthropathy

A relatively uncommon arthritis has been described in patients with moderately advanced HIV disease who demonstrate no other signs of any recognizable rheumatologic disease. The so-called HIV-associated arthropathy (HIVAA) presents as a mono- of pauciarticular arthritis. The arthritis is usually severe, affects primarily the knees and ankles, and lasts from 1 week to 6 months. No extra-articular manifestations have been noted. The synovial fluid is noninflammatory in nature, although a mild synovitis consisting of a chronic mononuclear cell infiltrate is noted on biopsy. Rheumatoid factor, antinuclear antibodies, anti-DNA antibodies, and antibodies against RNP, Sm, Ro/SS-A, and La/SS-B are negative. No predominant HLA pattern has been described. NSAIDs are of some benefit, but some patients require intra-articular steroid injections.

Vasculitis (see also Chapter 292)

Several varieties of vasculitis have been reported in association with HIV infection. Necrotizing vasculitis of the polyarteritis nodosa type is reported most commonly and presents as a peripheral sensory or sensorimotor neuropathy. The vasculitis involves the medium-sized vessels of the nerves, skin, and muscle. None of the reported patients with HIV-related PAN were hepatitis B surface antigen positive. Primary angiitis of the CNS has been noted in two patients, one of whom had persistent varicella-zoster virus infection. Lymphomatoid granulomatosis has also been reported in HIV-infected patients. Henoch-Schönlein purpura has been reported rarely; however, no distinct etiology has been elucidated. Drug-induced hypersensitivity vasculitis, usually presenting as cutaneous disease, has been reported associated with penicillin, trimethoprim-sulfamethoxazole, amitriptyline, and griseofulvin. Recently, several cases of uveitis have been reported with rifabutin therapy, especially when this drug is administered with fluconazole and clarithromycin.

It is unclear whether HIV-associated vasculitis is the result of direct HIV invasion of the vessels, an immunologic reaction to an underlying viral infection, or a response to an opportunistic viral pathogen that invades vascular tissue. As with other serious rheumatologic manifestations of HIV disease, treatment options are limited by the underlying immunodeficiency of the host.

Buskila D, Gladman D: Musculoskeletal manifestations of infection with human immunodeficiency virus. Rev Infect Dis 12:223, 1990. *Extensively referenced review of the musculoskeletal complaints associated with HIV disease.*

Carr A, Samaras K, Chisholm DJ, et al: Pathogenesis of HIV-1 protease inhibitor-associated peripheral lipodystrophy, hyperlipidemia, and insulin resistance. Lancet 351:1881, 1998. *A comprehensive report describing the newly recognized lipodystrophy syndrome associated with therapy, including proposed mechanism for its occurrence.*

Etzel JV, Brocavich JM, Torre M: Endocrine complications associated with human immunodeficiency virus infection. Clin Pharm 11:705, 1992. *A practical, easy-to-read overview of the endocrine abnormality seen in HIV-infected patients.*

Fernández SM, Cardenal A, Balsa A: Rheumatic manifestations in 556 patients with human immunodeficiency virus infection. Semin Arthritis Rheum 21:30, 1991. *One of the largest published reports on the rheumatological manifestations of HIV infection. Numerous tables, charts, and figures.*

Gherardi R, Belec L, Mhiri C, et al: The spectrum of vasculitis in human immunodeficiency virus-infected patients. Arthritis Rheum 36:1164, 1993. *A thorough review of an uncommon yet diverse complication of HIV disease.*

Herskowitz A, Vlahov D, Willoughby S, et al: Prevalence and incidence of left ventricular dysfunction in patients with human immunodeficiency virus infection. Am J Cardiol 71:955, 1993. *A study of 98 patients followed at Johns Hopkins Hospital Clinics who were evaluated for left ventricular dysfunction. Includes patients referred to the cardiology service as well as asymptomatic "controls."*

Kaul S, Fishbein MC, Siegel RJ: Cardiac manifestations of acquired immune deficiency syndrome: A 1991 update. Am Heart J 122:535, 1991. *Overview of the cardiac manifestations of HIV disease. Special focus on cardiomyopathy.*

Marks JB: Endocrine manifestations of human immunodeficiency virus (HIV) infection. Am J Med Sci 302:110, 1991. *A review of the pathologic and clinical reports in the literature regarding endocrinopathies in AIDS patients.*

Rao TKS: Human immunodeficiency virus (HIV) associated nephropathy. Annu Rev Med 42:391, 1991. *Succinct review of the renal complications of HIV disease, with special focus on the HIV-associated nephropathy.*

Smith MC, Austen JT, Casey JT, et al: Prednisone improves renal function and preteinuria in HIV associated nephropathy. Am J Med 101:41, 1996. *A case series of successful outcomes using steroid therapy for HIVAN.*

418 TREATMENT OF HIV INFECTION AND AIDS

Robert Yarchoan ■ Samuel Broder

Since the identification of the acquired immunodeficiency syndrome (AIDS) as a new entity in 1981, dramatic changes have occurred in therapy for this disease and its related disorders. In 1984, therapy was either entirely supportive or directed at a bewildering array of infectious and oncologic complications. The identification of human immunodeficiency virus (HIV) as the causative agent of AIDS and the elucidation of its life cycle have enabled the development of specific antiretroviral therapy, and such therapy is now recognized as being the cornerstone of treatment for HIV infection and AIDS. Substantial advances have been made over the past several years. At least 13 antiretroviral drugs are now approved belonging to three major classes: nucleoside reverse transcriptase inhibitors (NRTIs), non-nucleoside reverse transcriptase inhibitors (NNRTIs), and protease inhibitors (PIs) (Table 418–1). It has also been shown that these drugs are particularly effective if used in combination regimens that effectively suppress HIV replication. The physician treating HIV-infected patients thus has a wide array of active regimens to chose from; and although none is curative, the use of these drug regimens has substantially improved the outlook for HIV-infected patients. At the same time, however, these recent developments have increased the complexity of therapy, and it has been shown that the experience of physicians in treating AIDS has a direct bearing on their patients' survival. It is thus essential that physicians setting out to treat HIV-infected individuals have a good understanding of the issues involved. In this chapter, the principles underlying the therapy for HIV infection, the drugs used, the approaches now being used, and the limitations of these approaches are discussed. It should be noted, however, that this is an extremely rapidly moving field and that physicians treating HIV-infected patients should make a particular effort to stay informed of new developments.

PRINCIPLES AND GOALS FOR THE TREATMENT OF HIV INFECTION

For some time after the discovery of HIV, the technology for measuring virus was relatively insensitive and it appeared that the degree of T-cell destruction was much greater than could be accounted for by the level of HIV replication. In the past several years, sensitive assays to measure HIV RNA in plasma have been developed. Studies of viral dynamics utilizing these assays have revealed that HIV-infected patients often have extremely high rates

Table 418-1 ■ NAMES AND USUAL ADULT ORAL DOSES OF ANTI-HIV DRUGS

DRUG	DOSAGE
Nucleoside Reverse Transcriptase Inhibitors	
Zidovudine (AZT)	200 mg three times daily or 300 mg twice daily*
Didanosine (ddI)	>60 kg: 200 mg twice daily (tablets) between meals†
	<60 kg: 125 mg twice daily (tablets) between meals†
Zalcitabine (ddC)	0.75 mg three times daily
Stavudine (d4T)	>60 kg: 40 mg twice daily
	<60 mg: 30 mg twice daily
Lamivudine (3TC)	>50 kg: 150 mg twice daily*
	<50 kg: 2 mg/kg twice daily
Abacavir	300 mg twice daily
Non-Nucleoside Reverse Transcriptase Inhibitors	
Nevirapine	200 mg/d for 14 days, then 200 mg twice daily
Delavirdine	400 mg three times daily (in water as slurry)
Efavirenz	600 mg once daily at nighttime
Protease Inhibitors	
Indinavir	800 mg q8h between meals or with low-fat meal
Ritonavir	600 mg q12h with food if possible
Saquinavir	
Hard-gel capsule	600 mg three times daily with large meal
Soft-gel capsule	1200 mg three times daily with large meal
Nelfinavir	750 mg three times daily with food or light snack

*Zudovudine is also available in a combined capsule with lamivudine.
†For the buffered powder formulation of didanosine, the doses are 250 mg twice daily for patients > 60 kg and 167 mg twice daily for patients < 60 kg.

of viral production of 10^9 to 10^{10} or more virions per day. There is now an appreciation that in the absence of effective therapy for HIV, nearly all HIV-infected individuals have active HIV replication that leads to immune system damage and progression to AIDS. Also, a number of studies have shown that the plasma HIV RNA levels are a good measure of the level of HIV replication and are good predictors of subsequent CD4 decline and clinical deterioration. In particular, high viral loads are associated with a substantially higher rate of future disease progression (and CD4), and regimens that effectively suppress the viral loads are associated with better outcomes. CD4 counts provide a measure of the present status of the immune system and the current risk of developing opportunistic complications. These two parameters can thus be used together to assess the disease status of patients and as a guide for treatment decisions.

It is now generally accepted that a goal of anti-HIV therapy should ideally be to completely inhibit HIV replication in a patient to the extent possible. This concept was recently articulated by a panel convened by the National Institutes of Health to define the principles of therapy for HIV infection. Suppression of viral replication will stop the process of HIV-induced immune destruction and permit some reconstitution of the immune system to occur. As is described later, one of the most exciting recent advances in AIDS therapy was the finding that combinations of a PI with two NRTIs could suppress HIV replication in many patients to the point where HIV RNA could not be detected in the plasma for many months, even with highly sensitive assays.

Because of the ability of proviral HIV to integrate into host cells in a latent form, an absence of plasma viral RNA does not indicate that patients have been cured or rendered free of HIV, or even that all HIV replication in the body has been stopped. It has been hypothesized that with sufficiently prolonged effective therapy all the HIV-infected cells might eventually die. However, it has recently been shown that long-lived memory T cells can act as a reservoir for HIV, indicating that anti-HIV therapy would have to be maintained for years for these cells to die out. This goal may become even more elusive as we learn more about other potential reservoirs (such as the central nervous system). At the same time, there is now some interest in strategies to activate such cells to produce HIV so they can be eliminated, either through a viral-induced cytopathic effect or through immunologic destruction. Also, if sufficient immune reconstitution can be attained, it may be possible to substantially control HIV replication for long periods of time, possibly with long-term or intermittent anti-HIV therapy.

Thus, in the future it may be conceivable to attain long-term survival of HIV-infected patients even without complete eradication of their disease.

HIV has an extremely high mutation rate (approximately one mutation for every one to three genomes copied), and resistant strains can emerge to any of the available drugs. Resistance to reverse transcriptase inhibitors is associated with amino acid substitutions in the reverse transcriptase, whereas resistance to PIs is associated with amino acid substitutions in HIV protease. For some of the available drugs (e.g., lamivudine or nevirapine), a single mutation in the *pol* gene encoding reverse transcriptase can confer high-level (100-fold to over 1000-fold) resistance. By contrast, resistance to certain other drugs is of a lesser extent or requires the development of several mutations. There is evidence that because of the high replication rate of HIV and the high mutation rate, patients generally harbor viruses resistant to antiviral drugs even before antiretroviral therapy is initiated. Under the selective pressure of anti-HIV therapy, resistant strains can then rapidly predominate. In patients given monotherapy with lamivudine or nevirapine, for example, clinically significant outgrowth of resistant strains can occur within 4 weeks of the initiation of therapy. In fact, the emergence of HIV resistance is perhaps the most challenging obstacle to the development of prolonged effective anti-HIV therapy, and it is of utmost importance to choose and manage antiretroviral therapy in individual patients in a way to forestall the development of resistance.

It has recently been shown that the emergence of resistant strains can be substantially delayed or even prevented by highly potent combination regimens that suppress HIV replication to undetectable levels. This was initially shown in a study in which patients received a PI (indinavir), two NRTIs (zidovudine plus didanosine), or the three drugs together. During a 24-week period, patients on the triple-drug combination had significantly fewer mutations conferring resistance either to the PI or the NRTI than the respective arms in which patients received just the PI or the NRTI. Thus, regimens that effectively suppress HIV replication (at least below the limits of detection of plasma HIV RNA) can forestall or prevent the emergence of resistant strains. This provides a strong rationale for achieving and maintaining complete HIV suppression whenever possible. Indeed, drugs such as nevirapine whose activity in other settings may be limited by the rapid emergence of resistance may be of greater value when used in regimens that achieve complete HIV suppression.

DRUGS USED IN THE TREATMENT OF HIV INFECTION

Before going on to discuss specific recommendations for therapy, it is of value to review the drugs that are presently available for the treatment of HIV. As noted earlier, these drugs fall into three broad categories: NRTIs, NNRTIs, and PIs (see Table 418–1). NRTIs and NNRTIs target reverse transcriptase and thus prevent the formation of the DNA provirus. These drugs thus inhibit early steps in HIV infection but do not prevent the production of infectious virions by cells already infected. PIs target HIV protease and prevent the production of mature HIV virions by cells that are already infected. Combination regimens that use both reverse transcriptase inhibitors and PIs thus have the advantage of simultaneously targeting both early and late steps in HIV replication.

Nucleoside Reverse Transcriptase Inhibitors

The first drugs to be developed and approved for the treatment of HIV infection were members of a class of compounds called dideoxynucleosides, special analogues of nucleosides that have a sugar and a purine or pyrimidine base (Fig. 418–1). Included in this class of drugs are zidovudine (formerly azidothymidine [AZT]), didanosine (ddI), zalcitabine (ddC), stavudine (d4T), lamivudine (3TC), and abacavir. In these drugs, the 3'-hydroxy (-OH) group in the sugar is replaced by another group that does not form phosphodiester linkages. These drugs are not active in themselves but must be phosphorylated in target cells to form active 5'-triphosphate moieties. In this form, they block reverse transcription and thus inhibit the formation of a (double-stranded) DNA proviral copy of the viral RNA. The activation of dideoxynucleosides, called anabolic phosphorylation, involves a series of host-cell enzymes (kinases) that usually serve to phosphorylate physiologic

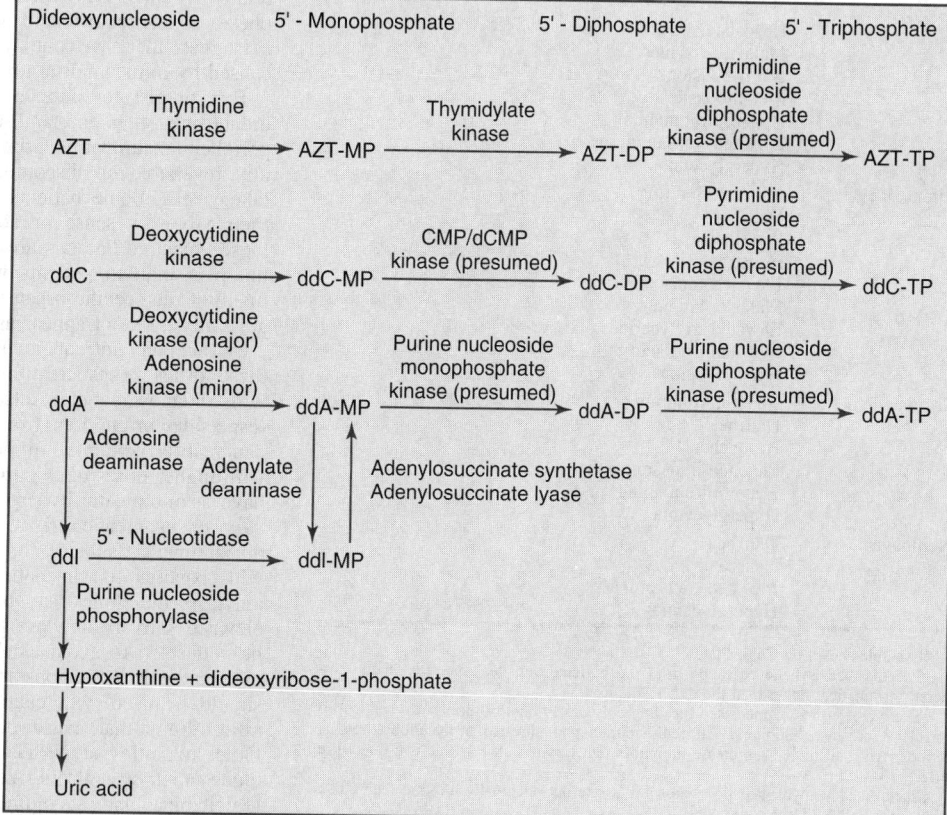

FIGURE 418–1 ■ Structures of thymidine and five nucleoside reverse transcriptase inhibitors (NRTI). Zidovudine and stavudine are analogues of thymidine with substitutions of the 3′-hydroxy (OH⁻) group.

deoxynucleosides (Fig. 418–2). For many purposes, each drug in this broad family is unique. Even a one-atom shift in the sugar or the base of the parent compound can radically change activity and toxicity. Also, there are substantial differences in the rates at which various human cells phosphorylate these compounds and in their enzymatic pathways, and these differences may be important in their antiretroviral activity and differing toxicity profiles (Table 418–2). For example, thymidine kinase, the enzyme responsible for the initial step in the phosphorylation of thymidine analogues such as zidovudine or stavudine, is a cell-cycle dependent enzyme. As a result, the activity of these drugs is relatively greater in replicating

lymphocytes or cytokine-stimulated monocytes than in resting cells of the same lineage. By contrast, the activity of didanosine, zalcitabine, or lamivudine is not substantially affected by the state of activation of the cells. Therefore, these two groups of drugs can preferentially target different cell populations, and combination regimens combining a member of each group can be especially effective.

As triphosphates, the dideoxynucleosides are believed to inhibit reverse transcriptase in two ways: (1) as DNA chain terminators and (2) as competitive inhibitors for the binding of physiologic deoxynucleoside-5′-triphosphates to relevant sites within reverse

FIGURE 418–2 ■ Activation pathways for zidovudine (AZT), zalcitabine (ddC), and didanosine (ddI) to the active triphosphate moieties in human cells. Also shown is dideoxyadenosine (ddA), an experimental drug closely related to ddI. MP = 5′-monophosphate; DP = 5′-diphosphate; TP = 5′-triphosphate.

Table 418–2 ■ PRINCIPAL TOXICITIES OF ANTI-HIV DRUGS

DRUG	SIDE EFFECTS
Nucleoside Reverse Transcriptase Inhibitors§	
Zidovudine	Anemia, neutropenia
	Malaise, fever, fatigue
	Headaches
	Myositis, myalgias
	Nausea, vomiting
	Insomnia
	Bluish nail pigmentation*
Didanosine	Sporadic pancreatitis
	Peripheral neuropathy
	Nausea, diarrhea†
	Sporadic hepatitis
	Insomnia, irritability
	Retinal depigmentation (in children)
	Diabetes mellitus
Zalcitabine	Peripheral neuropathy
	Aphthous ulcers
	Esophageal ulceration
	Rash
	Sporadic pancreatitis
Stavudine	Peripheral neuropathy
	Elevated transaminases
	Anemia
	Arthralgias
	Sporadic pancreatitis
Lamivudine	Sporadic pancreatitis (more in children)
	Peripheral neuropathy
	Anemia, neutropenia
Abacavir	Hypersensitivity reaction (fever, rash, nausea, vomiting)
Non-Nucleoside Reverse Transcriptase Inhibitors	
Nevirapine	Rashes (can be severe)
	Elevated transaminase levels
	Hepatitis
Delavirdine	Rashes (can be severe)
	Headaches
Efavirenz	Rashes (can be severe)
	Elevated transaminase levels
	Central nervous system symptoms
Protease Inhibitors	
Indinavir‡	Nephrolithiasis
	Nausea
	Headache
	Malaise, dizziness
	Blurred vision
	Metallic taste
	Hyperbilirubinemia
	Elevated transaminases
	Hyperglycemia
Ritonavir‡	Nausea, vomiting
	Diarrhea
	Paresthesias
	Hepatitis
	Elevated transaminases
	Malaise, fatigue
	Elevated triglycerides
	Elevated uric acid
	Hyperglycemia
Saquinavir‡	Nausea, vomiting
	Diarrhea
	Headaches
	Elevated transaminases
	Hyperbilirubinemia
	Hyperglycemia
Nelfinavir‡	Diarrhea
	Nausea
	Elevated transaminases
	Hyperglycemia

*Example shown on Color Plate E.

†The diarrhea is believed to be from the buffered vehicle, especially in the powdered formulation, rather than the didanosine itself.

‡There are reports of increased bleeding episodes in hemophiliacs who were receiving HIV protease inhibitors. Fat redistribution and elevated triglyceride levels are reported with all the HIV protease inhibitors, but it is not clear if this is a direct drug effect.

§Lactic acidosis with hepatic steatosis is a rare but potentially life-threatening complication of all NRTIs.

transcriptase. Reverse transcriptase, but not mammalian DNA polymerase-α, preferentially uses dideoxynucleoside-5'-triphosphates in place of the respective physiologic deoxynucleoside-5'-triphosphates, and this is an important basis for their selective antiretroviral activity. Human mitochondrial DNA polymerase-γ is also relatively sensitive to inhibition by these drugs as 5'-triphosphates and this may be an important basis for clinical toxicities including myopathy and rare cases of hepatic steatosis in patients receiving dideoxynucleoside therapy.

The first NRTI to be developed clinically was zidovudine. Clinical trials of zidovudine conducted during 1985 and 1986 convincingly showed that the drug was effective at reducing morbidity and mortality in patients with advanced HIV infection. Patients receiving zidovudine were noted to have increased numbers of CD4 cells, improved immunologic function, and clinical improvement. However, if zidovudine is used as a single drug, these benefits are usually transient, lasting from 3 to 6 months in patients with advanced AIDS to a year or longer in patients with earlier disease. It is now appreciated that this drug, like other NRTIs given as single agents, generally induces only a moderate decline in the viral load of HIV (a decrease to about a third to a tenth of the starting value, or of 0.5 to 1.0 $\log_{10}$ viral particles/mL). Also, the clinical activity of zidovudine as a single agent, like that of other anti-HIV drugs, is limited by the emergence of viral resistance. As described earlier, the development of resistance can be substantially delayed by the use of highly active combination regimens combining two NRTIs with a PI.

There are some important differences among the NRTIs that physicians should be aware of as they build combination regimens. As noted earlier, different enzymes catalyze the intracellular phosphorylation of these agents; and in part because of this, they have different toxicity profiles (see Table 418–2). The most frequent dose-limiting toxicity of zidovudine is bone marrow suppression, especially macrocytic anemia. Patients starting on this drug often experience malaise, nausea, and headaches. Also, patients receiving zidovudine for several months sometimes develop myositis associated with "ragged-red" fibers on biopsy (see Color Plate 11G). Occasional HIV-infected patients receiving zidovudine alone or in combination with other dideoxynucleosides have been reported to develop a poorly understood syndrome involving severe macrovesicular hepatic steatosis (a condition related to Reye's syndrome) and lactic acidosis (see Color Plate 10H). A high proportion of these patients have died of this complication. Most of these patients had relatively early HIV infection and were well nourished or even obese. A disproportionate number were female. There is evidence to suggest that this condition, like zidovudine-induced myositis, is caused by mitochondrial toxicity.

By contrast to zidovudine, a principal toxicity of zalcitabine, didanosine, stavudine, and, to a lesser extent, lamivudine is painful peripheral neuropathy, primarily involving the feet. This is generally reversible on discontinuing the drug, but the resolution can take weeks. Some patients with this condition have a decrease in their vibratory sense or ability to discriminate temperatures, but these objective findings are generally less pronounced in relation to the pain than in patients with HIV-induced neuropathy. As with many of the specific organ toxicities induced by NRTIs, neuropathy generally does not appear until after at least 10 weeks of therapy.

A relatively infrequent but serious toxicity seen with several of these drugs is pancreatitis. This complication is best associated with didanosine but is also reported with the use of lamivudine (especially in children), zalcitabine, or stavudine. The incidence of pancreatitis is higher in patients with more advanced disease or with higher doses of the drugs. Some patients receiving these drugs have asymptomatic hyperamylasemia, which may be of either salivary or pancreatic origin. Although it is prudent to temporarily discontinue didanosine (or the other drugs whose use is associated with pancreatitis) in patients with elevated levels of pancreatic amylase, the drugs may be continued in patients who have only elevated salivary amylase levels. Patients taking didanosine should be counseled to avoid alcohol, and this drug should be avoided in patients with a previous history of pancreatitis. Also, these drugs should be used with caution or stopped if patients are receiving other drugs that cause pancreatitis (e.g., systemic pentamidine). Other toxicities of NRTIs that physicians should be aware of include aphthous ulcers (zalcitabine), arthralgias (stavudine), rash (zalcitabine and stavudine), and diabetes mellitus (didanosine).

About 2 to 5% of patients receiving abacavir develop a hypersensitivity reaction with rash, fever, nausea, and vomiting. The drug should be stopped in such patients and they should not be rechallenged.

All of the NRTIs can be given orally and most have good absorption (60 to 86%) when taken by mouth. However, didanosine is unstable in the acid environment of the stomach, and for this reason it is formulated with buffers as either a tablet or powder. In these forms, it has an oral bioavailability of 30 to 40%. It should be noted that the buffers used with didanosine sometimes cause diarrhea and can interfere with the absorption of drugs such as delavirdine or indinavir that require a low stomach pH. If didanosine is used together with either of these drugs, they should be spaced at least an hour (delavirdine) or 2 hours (indinavir) apart. With the exception of lamivudine, the serum half-life of the NRTI is generally short, on the order of 1 to 1.6 hours. However, the intracellular half-life of most of these compounds is somewhat longer, and for this reason they can be effective when given two to three times daily. In this regard, the intracellular half-life of the active moiety of didanosine is quite long (25 to 40 hours), and this compound is active even when administered twice or even once daily. Efforts are now underway to develop a formulation of didanosine for once-daily dosing. Zidovudine penetrates well into the central nervous system; and of all the dideoxynucleosides, this has the best documented activity in patients with HIV-induced cognitive impairment (see Color Plate 11F). Stavudine can also penetrate reasonably well. However, non–thymidine-based NRTIs have better in vitro activity in resting cells, and there is evidence that some (such as didanosine) can have activity in the brain.

The requirement for NRTIs to undergo intracellular phosphorylation can also lead to drug interactions. There is evidence that the 5′-triphosphate of zidovudine interferes with the phosphorylation of stavudine, and these two drugs should not be used together. As noted earlier, there is evidence that thymidine-based and non–thymidine-based NRTIs preferentially target different cell populations, and there are thus advantages to combination regimens that use one drug from each class.

Resistance to most dideoxynucleosides develops relatively slowly, and this is one reason that they are important components of combination regimens. Strains resistant to zidovudine generally have two or more mutations in the gene encoding reverse transcriptase. Of these, substitution of tyrosine (or phenylalanine) for threonine at codon 215 appears to be the most important. High-level (over 100-fold) resistance can develop to zidovudine; however, because it requires several mutations, it generally emerges only after several months or more of therapy. Resistance to most of the other NRTIs can develop with a single mutation; however, the level of resistance attained is generally small (on the order of 10-fold or so) and in part for that reason it also emerges relatively slowly.

A notable exception to this pattern is lamivudine. A single base substitution of valine for methionine at codon 184 can induce high-level (1000-fold or more) resistance to this drug, and clinical resistance can emerge within 2 to 4 weeks in patients receiving lamivudine as a single agent. If one examines the sugar ring of lamivudine, one notices that it is flipped with respect to physiologic nucleosides (and the other NRTI), and it is possible that this structural difference facilitates the development of resistance. Interestingly, the mutation at codon 184 that confers resistance to lamivudine also partially reverses resistance to zidovudine in HIV strains with a mutation at codon 215, and in part for this reason the combination of zidovudine and lamivudine is associated with long-term activity. A similar pattern of antagonistic resistance occurs with zidovudine and the mutation at codon 74 that is induced by didanosine, and this combination is also associated with long-term activity. Up to 15% of patients who have received long-term sequential or combination treatment with NRTI have been observed to develop a unique pattern of broad HIV resistance to this class of drugs associated with a substitution of methionine for glutamine at codon 151 along with several other mutations. Because of the importance of NRTI in combination regimens, such patients have very limited treatment options at present. However, two NRTIs under development, lodenosine (F-ddA) and adefovir dipivoxil, have some activity against these strains of HIV and may prove to be useful in these patients. Lodenosine is a fluorinated analogue of didanosine that has a unique resistance pattern and, because of the

fluorine substitution, is resistant to acid degradation. It may be suitable for once-daily dosing. Adefovir dipivoxil is now available under an expanded access program; the principal toxicities associated with this drug are proximal renal tubular dysfunction, nausea, and elevated liver function tests. Other NRTIs currently under development include PMPA and FTC. PMPA is a phosphorylated nucleotide phosphate that can thus bypass the initial phosphorylation step. This drug has been shown to be very active against simian immunodeficiency virus.

Non-Nucleoside Reverse Transcriptase Inhibitors

Starting in the early 1990s, a number of structurally unrelated non-nucleoside compounds were discovered to be potent non-competitive inhibitors of HIV reverse transcriptase. These compounds share the property of having highly specific activity against HIV-1 but not against HIV-2 or other retroviruses. These compounds bind to a deep pocket in reverse transcriptase and disrupt the catalytic site of the enzyme. Three NNRTIs, nevirapine, delavirdine, and efavirenz, are presently approved, and several others are in various stages of development.

The biggest drawback to this class of drugs is that high-level resistance can emerge within 2 to 4 weeks in patients receiving these compounds as single drugs. This resistance is associated with one or more mutations in reverse transcriptase. There is some evidence that the development of this resistance is slowed somewhat and that more sustained activity of these compounds can be obtained if they are used in potent combination drug regimens in which the viral load is suppressed to undetectable levels. This finding has increased the interest somewhat in this class of drugs, and several others are now in clinical development, including HBY097, MKC-442, and calanolide A. However, there is a substantial degree of cross-resistance among the NNRTI, and patients who become resistant to one may not respond to others in the future. This point underscores the importance of using anti-HIV drugs in a manner that reduces the development of resistance.

Nevirapine, delavirdine, and efavirenz are all metabolized by the cytochrome P-450 system. However, whereas nevirapine induces the P-450 system, delavirdine acts as an inhibitor of P-450 CYP3A and can thus suppress the metabolism of PIs such as saquinavir. This may make delavirdine attractive to use in combination with PIs. Efavirenz is a mixed inducer/inhibitor of cytochrome P-450 and can have mixed effects on these drugs. The principal toxicity of these drugs is a rash, which can on occasion progress to Stevens-Johnson syndrome. Other toxicities include headache, fatigue, and elevated hepatic transaminase levels. Efavirenz can also cause central nervous system symptoms.

Protease Inhibitors

The second enzyme of HIV to be successfully targeted was the viral aspartyl protease. HIV produces the structural proteins of the viral core, as well as the integral viral enzymes, as Gag and Gag-Pol polyproteins that subsequently must be cleaved by the HIV protease. This cleavage is essential to the production of mature virions; and if HIV protease is inhibited, the virions produced are not infectious. The three-dimensional structure of HIV protease has been elucidated, and this information, as well as previous studies elucidating its target sequence, permitted the rational development of inhibitors of this enzyme. Unlike the reverse transcriptase inhibitors, PIs block the production of infectious virions by chronically infected cells. PIs can thus suppress viral production by macrophages and other cells that can produce virus over relatively long periods of time.

Although HIV protease was an attractive target, a number of obstacles had to be overcome to develop clinically useful inhibitors. Many of the initial candidate compounds were highly potent in vitro but had poor bioavailability and relatively short plasma half-lives. In addition, the compounds are quite complex and difficult to synthesize. Nonetheless, by March 1997, four HIV PIs had been approved and several others are presently in clinical development. The PIs developed to date fall into several broad structural categories. Saquinavir and indinavir are peptide-based inhibitors with substitutions in the dipeptidic cleavage site. Ritonavir is a twofold (C_2) symmetrical inhibitor, designed to take advantage of the symmetry of the protease active site. Finally, nelfinavir is a non-peptidic inhibitor. All of these are highly selective for viral protease and have little or no activity against human proteases.

Used alone, PIs can induce substantial decreases in the HIV viral load of 100-fold (2 $\log_{10}$) or more. However, their usefulness as single agents is limited by the relatively rapid development of resistance, often within 3 months if used alone. This resistance is associated with the emergence of HIV strains with mutations at key sites in the HIV protease gene. Usually two or more mutations are required for high-level resistance to emerge. Cross-resistance among these drugs is frequently found, but because the resistance generally involves several mutations, the issue of cross-resistance in this class of compounds is a complex one. It is worth noting that there is no cross-resistance between PIs and either NRTIs or NNRTIs. As noted earlier, the development of resistance to PIs can be substantially slowed or even prevented by their use in highly potent combinations with NRTIs, and they should generally only be used in such combinations.

The first PI to be developed was saquinavir. Although this drug was found to be active and reasonably well tolerated, its usefulness was somewhat limited by its poor oral bioavailability, which is 4% when given with food and less in the fasting state. However, when saquinavir is given with an inhibitor of cytochrome P-450 (such as ritonavir), the area under the time-plasma concentration curve is substantially increased. When used in this manner, saquinavir has quite effective anti-HIV activity. The other approved PIs are better absorbed by mouth, although each must be taken in a defined way with relation to food. The serum half-life of these drugs ranges from 1 to 2 hours (saquinavir) to as much as 3½ to 5 hours (nelfinavir). One potential drawback to this class of drugs is that in general they penetrate but poorly into the central nervous system.

All of the presently available PIs are metabolized by the cyto-chrome P-450 system, and all of them inhibit cytochrome P-450 (particularly 3A4) to various degrees. Because of this, a large number of drug interactions occur with this class of drugs, some of which can be quite serious or even fatal. Ritonavir is a potent inhibitor of cytochrome P-450, and thus has a greater potential than the other available PIs for affecting the metabolism of other drugs. Even so, all the members of this class of drugs can cause drug interactions, and they can be quite complex to use, especially in sick patients who may require a number of other drugs. Some drugs that are recommended to be avoided with one or more of the PIs are listed in Table 418–3. In addition, a number of drug interactions may require adjusting the dose levels. It is beyond the scope of this chapter to list all the drug interactions involving the HIV PIs, and physicians prescribing any of these drugs should pay particular attention to the information on drug interactions found in the package inserts and in pharmaceutical reference works such as that published by the American Hospital Formulary Service.

The toxicity profile of the PI is generally different from that of the NRTI. All the members of this class of drugs can cause gastrointestinal intolerance, ranging from nausea to diarrhea. Ritonavir and saquinavir can cause elevated hepatic transaminase levels, and some cases of hepatitis have been observed in patients on ritonavir. Indinavir can cause a clinically inconsequential elevation of the indirect bilirubin level. The most frequent dose-limiting toxicity seen with indinavir is nephrolithiasis with drug crystals, and it is important to keep patients receiving this drug well hydrated. There have also been reports of increased bleeding episodes in hemophiliac patients receiving PIs, and diabetes mellitus has also been reported to occur in patients receiving these drugs. Also, a number of patients who have been on combination therapy that included a PI have developed a form of lipodystrophy. These patients characteristically have wasting of the face and limbs along with adipose tissue accumulations in the abdomen and the back of the neck, the

Table 418–3 ■ SELECTED DRUGS THAT SHOULD NOT BE USED WITH PROTEASE INHIBITORS*

Note: Based on theoretical considerations of pharmacokinetic interactions, the following should not be used with the noted protease inhibitors. This table is not intended as an exhaustive list, and physicians should consult the package inserts and more complete pharmacology reference works when using protease inhibitors with other drugs.

DRUG CATEGORY	INDINAVIR	RITONAVIR	SAQUINAVIR	NELFINAVIR
Analgesics		Meperidine Piroxicam Propoxyphene		
Cardiac		Amiodrone Encainide Flecainide Propafenone Quinidine		
Antimycobacterial	Rifampin	Rifabutin†	Rifampin Rifabutin	Rifampin
Calcium channel blocker		Bepridil		
Antihistamine	Astemizole Terfenadine	Astemizole Terfenadine	Astemizole Terfenadine	Astemizole Terfenadine
Gastrointestinal	Cisapride	Cisapride	Cisapride	Cisapride
Antidepressant		Bupropion		
Neuroleptic		Clozapine Pimozide		
Psychotropic	Midazolam Triazolam	Midazolam Triazolam Clorazepate Diazepam Estazolam Flurazepam Zolpidem	Midazolam Triazolam	Midazolam Triazolam
Ergot alkaloids	Ergotamines D.H.E. 45	Ergotamines D.H.E. 45	Ergotamines D.H.E. 45	Ergotamines D.H.E. 45

*Based on recommendations of the panel convened by the Department of Health and Human Services and the Henry J. Kaiser Family Foundation.
†The combination of ritonavir and rifabutin is generally not recommended. If they must be used together, however, the dose of rifabutin should be reduced to one fourth of its standard dose.

latter giving a "buffalo hump" appearance. The pathogenesis of this condition is not clear at present and there is some evidence to suggest that it may result from the substantial suppression of HIV in advanced patients rather than from a direct drug toxicity.

A substantial body of knowledge has been accumulated about the three-dimensional structure of the HIV protease, about its interactions with its peptide substrate and available PIs, and on the patterns of mutations that develop. Some of this information had been used to develop the present drugs, and new generations of PIs are being developed using sophisticated computer modeling techniques along with iterative rounds of synthesis and in vitro testing to optimize desirable properties. Some PIs now in clinical testing include VX-478, a non–peptide-based PI that may penetrate better into the central nervous system than some other members of this class; 141W94 (amprenavir), a highly active C_2 symmetry-based inhibitor; PNU-140690; and DMP-450. Amprenavir is now available under an expanded access program.

GENERAL RECOMMENDATIONS FOR THE TREATMENT OF HIV INFECTION

The substantial recent developments in AIDS therapy and in our ability to monitor viral dynamics have led to a major shift in the thinking about HIV therapy. Several panels have convened to reconsider the best treatment strategies for HIV infection in the face of these developments. Some of the panels making recommendations have included one convened by the Department of Health and Human Services (DHHS) and the Henry J. Kaiser Family Foundation, a USA Panel convened by the International AIDS Society, and one convened by the British HIV Association. Because of the rapid development of new therapies and in the ability to monitor the viral load, the recommendations have been based to a large degree on the principles of therapy articulated earlier and on small or short-term clinical trials with laboratory end points. It will probably be years before randomized trials with clinical end points are conducted to evaluate many of these recommendations, and in a number of cases these trials may never be undertaken.

Although there are some differences between the recommendations made by these panels, overall they were quite similar. The recommendations articulated here apply to adults and adolescents infected with HIV and are largely derived from those of the DHHS-Kaiser panel. It is anticipated that these recommendations will evolve over the next several years, and physicians treating HIV-infected patients are strongly urged to keep alert for such changes. Updated recommendations from the DHHS-Kaiser group are to be posted by the AIDS Treatment Information Services Website at Internet Uniform Resource Location *http://www.hivatis.org.*

Once it is established that a patient has HIV infection, the two most useful tests for guiding therapy are the plasma HIV RNA level (viral load) and the CD4+ T-cell count. Both of these tests should be performed at the time of diagnosis. The viral load should subsequently be performed every 3 to 4 months, whereas the CD4 count should be measured every 3 to 6 months. Plasma RNA levels can be acutely affected by immune stimulation, and for this reason they should generally not be measured within 4 weeks after successful treatment of intercurrent infections, resolution of symptomatic illnesses, or immunizations. Also, there are some differences in the assays used to measure viral RNA; the viral load assessments obtained with branched DNA technology are generally about one half of the magnitude of those obtained with reverse transcriptase polymerase chain reaction (RT-PCR) technology. For this reason, one assay type should ideally be used throughout in following a given patient. Guidelines given here will be keyed to the results of RT-PCR assays. Ideally, decisions of when to institute therapy should be made based on two measurements of CD4 count and viral load, except in those patients with advanced disease, in whom the dangers of a delay in treatment associated in repeating the test may outweigh the advantages. Other evaluations that should be undertaken in patients before initiating therapy include a complete history and physical examination, a complete blood cell count, and a chemistry profile. Also, if not already performed, a VDRL, a tuberculin skin test, *Toxoplasma* IgG serology, a gynecologic examination with a Papanicolaou smear, and other clinically appropriate tests should be obtained.

Considerations for Initiating Antiretroviral Therapy

The decision to undertake antiretroviral therapy in patients is an important one and should only be made in the setting of careful patient counseling and education (see Chapter 419). It has clearly been shown that antiretroviral therapy can benefit patients with advanced HIV infection and immunosuppression, and such patients should generally be treated. The decision to treat asymptomatic patients with established HIV infection, however, should be individualized based on a careful consideration of the patient's disease status and the likelihood of compliance with therapy. Therapy of such patients is based on the principle that continued viral replication is always harmful. In this context, the potential benefits of preventing disease progression by initiating therapy must be weighed against the risks of drug toxicities, the inconvenience of the treatment regimens, and the risk of selecting for resistant strains of virus. Non-compliance with drug regimens can create periods of time during which there is incomplete HIV suppression and hasten the emergence of resistant strains, thus both thwarting the effectiveness of the present regimen and reducing future therapeutic options. Thus, an important factor in the decision to initiate antiretroviral therapy is the likelihood of patient adherence to the prescribed regimen after counseling and education.

There are two general approaches to initiating therapy in asymptomatic patients with established HIV infection. The more aggressive approach is heavily based on the principles of therapy discussed earlier and involves offering therapy to all patients with less than 500 CD4+ cells/mm^3 or with 20,000 HIV virions/mL (by RT-PCR). The more conservative approach would observe patients with 350 to 500 CD4+ cells/mm^3 and less than 20,000 virions/mL. Although there is currently a move toward the more aggressive strategy, it is worth remembering that in every case the patient should make the final decision on the acceptance of therapy after discussion of the issues concerning his or her own clinical situation. The DHHS-Kaiser panel recommended that for patients with over 500 CD4+ cells/mm^3 and less than 20,000 virions/mL, observation alone is reasonable to consider. They noted, however, that some experts would treat such patients. It is worth noting that these recommendations are based largely on the principles of therapy presented earlier. Over the years, the recommendations of when to begin therapy for HIV have fluctuated back and forth, and a prior trend to treat most patients with fewer than 500 CD4+ cells/mm^3 with zidovudine was subsequently modified by the results of a large randomized study (the Concorde trial) showing that such early zidovudine monotherapy did not yield an improvement in survival. The present recommendations are backed by a substantially greater understanding of disease pathogenesis and involve more potent regimens, but they may again be modified as the field evolves.

A number of patients experience an acute retroviral syndrome at the time of their HIV infection (see Chapter 408). The symptoms of this syndrome often include fever, sweats, lymphadenopathy, pharyngitis, and myalgias. Physicians should be alert for the possibility of HIV infection in such patients and obtain appropriate laboratory tests, including plasma HIV RNA. Treating such patients has the potential of decreasing the spread of HIV through the body, reducing the viral load in the asymptomatic period after the acute infection, and potentially reducing the rate of viral mutation. With this in mind, it is generally recommended that patients with acute HIV infection be offered antiretroviral therapy. Some experts also recommend treating patients in whom seroconversion has been documented to have occurred within the past 6 months. In either case, it is recommended that antiretroviral therapy be utilized for at least 1 year, and some experts would continue the therapy indefinitely.

Regimens for Initial Antiretroviral Therapy

The goal of therapy should be to suppress HIV replication to undetectable levels. This will provide the greatest protection against further immune destruction and permit some degree of immune reconstitution to occur. To accomplish this, potent regimens should be used with each drug given at full dose if possible. This is particularly important when instituting therapy for the first time. The initial therapy provides the single best opportunity to achieve a

Preferred regimens include one drug or combination from the left column plus one of the nucleoside reverse transcriptase inhibitor combinations in the right column

NON-NRTI		NRTI COMBINATIONS
Indinavir or Nelfinavir or Ritonavir or Saquinavir-soft gel or Ritonavir plus saquinavir (soft or hard gel) or Efavirenz	*plus*	Zidovudine plus didanosine or Stavudine plus didanosine or Zidovudine plus zalcitabine or Zidovudine plus lamivudine or Stavudine plus lamivudine

Note: Listings in each column are in random order, not priority order.
*Based on recommendations of the panel convened by the Department of Health and Human Services and the Henry J. Kaiser Family Foundation.

prolonged suppression of HIV replication, at least below the limits of detection, and thus a delay in (or even prevention of) the emergence of resistant strains. As noted earlier, there is substantial cross-resistance among drugs within each of the classes, and for this reason it is much harder to achieve effective HIV suppression once resistance has emerged to this first regimen. It is thus essential that the initial regimen used be one that is very likely to yield complete suppression and that patient compliance is maximized by the patient wholeheartedly undertaking the therapy after careful education and counseling.

At present, the preferred regimens for this initial therapy generally involve the use of two NRTIs and either a potent single PI or efavirenz (Table 418–4). In general, one of the NRTIs should be thymidine-based, while the other should not be thymidine-based. However, the combination of stavudine and zalcitabine, both of which can cause peripheral neuropathy, is not recommended (Table 418–5). The role of abacavir for initial therapy is expected to be considered in the near future. With regard to the PIs, all are considered preferred except for the current hard-capsule formulation of saquinavir (because of its relatively poor absorption and low plasma levels). However, the combination of saquinavir and ritonavir is acceptable in the initial regimen. Alternative regimens that can be considered acceptable but are generally considered less desirable include two NRTIs along with either nevirapine or delavirdine.

The International AIDS Society USA panel suggested that use of two NRTIs was also acceptable as a first-line regimen, especially in asymptomatic patients with a relatively lower risk of progression. However, although such a regimen can provide clinical benefit, a randomized trial with clinical end points has since shown better short-term results with a three-drug regimen and there is now a movement away from this approach. Another concern with the use of only two NRTIs as initial therapy is that sustained viral suppression is generally not achieved and thus resistance is not optimally suppressed. The choice of therapy in patients with more advanced HIV disease can be complicated by the potential for drug interactions with their other medications and their greater susceptibility to certain toxicities (such as bone marrow suppression). A particular problem in this regard is the effects of PIs and NNRTIs on the cytochrome P-450 pathway. For this reason, antiretroviral therapy should be initiated in any patient only after a careful drug history is obtained (including over-the-counter and alternative medicines), and patients on antiretroviral therapy should be carefully instructed not to change any medications without discussing the change with their physician or other health care provider.

Patients should be carefully instructed to take their antiretroviral therapy as instructed once it is initiated. Suboptimal doses, omitting

one of the drugs in a regimen, or missed doses all can lead to suboptimal viral suppression and increase the likelihood of resistance emerging. There is a misconception that once antiretroviral therapy is started, it can never be stopped or resistance will emerge. Actually, if all the drugs are stopped simultaneously, there is no longer evolutionary pressure for resistance to develop, and in fact, this is the preferred strategy if one or two of the drugs need to be stopped for any extended period of time.

Changing Antiretroviral Therapy

There are three main reasons to consider changes in antiretroviral therapy: (1) for drug toxicity or incompatibilities, (2) for regimens that are believed to be suboptimal, and (3) for a failure to achieve adequate suppression or a rebound in viral load after a period of complete suppression. In the case of patients who need to change therapy because of toxicity to a particular drug, it is acceptable to substitute an appropriate alternative drug of the same class. However, for patients who have virologic drug failure, it is desirable to change at least two and preferably three new drugs whenever possible to maximize the likelihood that complete suppression will again be attained. Before changes in regimen are undertaken, however, it is important to assess compliance with the regimen and determine if poor compliance is the principal reason for failure.

The viral load should be measured immediately before initiating antiretroviral therapy, at 4 to 8 weeks after the initiation of therapy, and then every 3 to 4 months. In most patients, a potent regimen will result in a decrease of 0.5 to 0.75 $\log_{10}$ viral load by week 4 and 1 $\log_{10}$ by week 8. Plasma HIV RNA should be undetectable using the most sensitive assay available by months 4 to 6 after therapy is initiated. A failure to meet any of those standards suggests that the therapy is not working optimally and consideration should be given to a change in regimen. Other factors that suggest that the regimen should be changed include the re-emergence of detectable plasma HIV RNA (especially if over 5000 copies/mL) after suppression to undetectable levels; a significant (threefold or greater) increase in the viral load not explained by intercurrent infections; or a persistent decline in the CD4 count. When the decision to change therapy is based on viral load determination, it is preferable to have a second confirmatory viral load test. Many experts believe that patients receiving therapy with only two NRTIs should have a change in therapy (rather than simply adding a PI), even if their virus is undetectable, because of their likelihood of subsequent virologic failure. Finally, clinical deterioration (such as the development of a new opportunistic infection) may prompt a reconsideration of the therapy. However, such an event may merely represent the prior immune compromise of the patient and thus may not necessitate a change in antiretroviral therapy.

In patients who have been on one or two NRTIs alone, physicians can consider switching therapy to two new NRTIs along with a potent PI (or with ritonavir and saquinavir), a new NRTI along with an NNRTI and a potent PI, or even two PIs along with an NNRTI. In patients who have been on a three-drug regimen with two NRTIs and a PI, the choice of a second-line salvage regimen depends in part on the initial PI used. It is generally desirable to select a new regimen with two new NRTIs and either a new PI, a combination of a new PI and an NNRTI, or even two new PIs (usually saquinavir plus either ritonavir or nelfinavir). It is usually

Table 418–5 ■ NUCLEOSIDE COMBINATIONS THAT ARE GENERALLY NOT RECOMMENDED

REGIMEN	REASON FOR NOT USING
Stavudine plus zidovudine	Antagonistic intracellular phosphorylation
Zalcitabine plus didanosine	Overlapping toxicity (neuropathy)
Zalcitabine plus stavudine	Overlapping toxicity (neuropathy)
Zalcitabine plus lamivudine	Little data; potential for cross-resistance

best to avoid switching from ritonavir to indinavir or vice versa in the new regimen or from indinavir to nelfinavir because of the high level of cross-resistance. Similarly, it is best to avoid changing among nevirapine, delavirdine, and etavirenz. For certain patients, one or more drugs newly licensed or available on expanded access programs may also be worth considering after the physician has studied the agents. Experience with some of these regimens, or with other four-or-more drug regimens that some physicians are using, is limited, and there remains the real possibility of unexpected interactions and results. Genotypic analysis of HIV resistance mutations may help select regimens in certain patients. However, the value of this approach in various settings remains to be fully established. There are also limited data on the value of re-starting drugs to which patients have become resistant. There is some evidence that non-resistant viral strains can gradually predominate when a drug to which a patient's HIV has become resistant is stopped. However, many copies of the resistant virus can remain in proviral form and resistant virus can very rapidly re-emerge when the drug is restarted.

Many patients have but limited options for new regimens of desired potency, and in some cases it may be rational to continue suboptimal therapy if partial viral suppression is obtained. Because of the limitations imposed by patterns of resistance, intolerance, or toxicity, some regimens that would be deemed suboptimal for initial therapy may be quite appropriate as second-or third-line regimens, especially in patients with late-stage disease. Indeed, it may be rational to withhold therapy altogether for some patients with no viable treatment options.

The experience of many physicians is that once viral strains become resistant to an initial therapy, the success of subsequently administered therapies is rather limited. Even if suppression of the viral load to undetectable levels is attained, it is often relatively short lived. This is one reason why it is so important that the initial regimen be carefully chosen and followed. Many physicians currently have a very low threshold for sequentially changing regimens in the face of persistent viral replication. A real danger of this approach is that even with 13 approved drugs, patients can rapidly use up their therapeutic options. Any regimen or change in regimen must be undertaken with attention to the effect that this decision will have on subsequent therapeutic options. In patients in whom one or more antiretroviral regimens have failed, treatment can be very challenging, and it is important for both the physician and the patient to have a realistic expectation of what can be accomplished. When possible, it is recommended that the decisions to change therapy and the design of new regimens be undertaken with the assistance of a clinician who is experienced in the care of HIV-infected patients.

Treatment of the Pregnant HIV-Infected Patient

Although a complete discussion of the therapy for the pregnant HIV-infected patient is beyond the scope of this chapter, it is worth highlighting several important issues. First, it is generally accepted that women should receive optimal therapy for their HIV whether or not they are pregnant. At the same time, consideration has to be given to the potential effects of the drugs used on the fetus as well as the effects on the perinatal transmission of HIV. HIV can be transmitted from the mother to the child in utero, at the time of birth, or through breast-feeding. Breast-feeding should thus be avoided in such patients. Moreover, it has been shown quite clearly in a randomized, double-blind clinical trial that the risk of perinatal HIV transmission can be substantially reduced by the administration of zidovudine orally to the mother after the first 14 weeks of gestation, intravenously during the intrapartum period, and to the newborn during the first 6 weeks of life. This has only been shown with zidovudine, and for this reason zidovudine should be included in the treatment regimen of the mother whenever possible and the intrapartum and neonatal zidovudine components of this treatment regimen should be administered to reduce the risk of perinatal transmission.

With regard to the treatment of the mother, zidovudine is the only drug that has been extensively studied in pregnancy, and there are only limited data on the pharmacokinetics and safety of the other agents. Many of the drugs now used for the treatment of HIV turn up positive on at least one of the in vitro and animal screening tests for the effects of drugs on the fetus, and even zidovudine has

been shown to induce tumors in mice exposed to very high doses in utero. Even so, there is at least some experience in the use of these drugs in pregnancy, and most members of the DHHS-Kaiser panel recommended continuing or (for mothers who were not on therapy) initiating optimal therapy regardless of the gestational age of the fetus. With regard to the PI, there are some theoretical concerns regarding the use of indinavir late in pregnancy. The hyperbilirubinemia and the renal stones that can be associated with the use of this drug could be particularly problematic in newborns if substantial transplacental passage of this agent occurs; and for this reason, this drug might best be avoided just before the time of delivery. Health care providers who treat HIV-infected pregnant women are strongly encouraged to report cases of perinatal exposure to these drugs to the Antiretroviral Pregnancy Registry, which is a collaborative project of the National Institutes of Health, the Centers for Disease Control and Prevention, and staff from various pharmaceutical manufacturers.

IMMUNE RECONSTITUTION AND OTHER APPROACHES

We are just beginning to learn about the immune reconstitution attained when HIV-infected patients attain substantial viral suppression with highly active antiretroviral therapy (see Chapter 407). For the first few months of therapy, patients have a relatively rapid increase in their CD4+ cell population that can be to a large extent explained by an expansion of their pre-existing memory CD4 cells. However, such patients have also been observed to have a gradual increase in their naive (CD45RA+) CD4+ T-cell population. This can occur even in patients who begin with very low CD4 counts. This finding raises the possibility that such patients may be able to at least partially reconstitute their immune system, have an increase in the number of naive T cells, and recover some of their T-cell immune defect. At the same time, physicians should realize that such patients still can retain substantial gaps in their immune repertoire. In particular, they can still develop opportunistic infections even when their CD4 counts have risen to levels that are infrequently associated with such infections. However, there is some evidence to suggest that partial reconstitution of the immune repertoire and ability to defend against such infections can occur and this will be an important area for research in the next several years.

The demonstration that HIV replication can be effectively suppressed with antiretroviral therapy has also renewed interest in more direct approaches to immune reconstitution. Even before the development of highly active three-drug regimens, it was shown that intermittent administration of interleukin-2 could induce an increase in the peripheral CD4 count in HIV-infected patients who began with over 200 CD4 cells/mm^3. A theoretical concern of this approach is that interleukin-2 can stimulate HIV replication. However, this effect appears to be minor and with the present highly active regimens can be easily controlled. It remains to be shown whether this increase in CD4 cells is accompanied by a functional improvement in the immune system, and a large-scale international trial is in progress to assess this point.

A variety of other approaches for immunoreconstitution in HIV infection are either under consideration or actively in clinical trial, including interleukin-12, a combination of interleukin-2 and interleukin-12, and interleukin-15. Also, there is some renewed interest in boosting the specific immune response to HIV through therapeutic vaccination. Ultimately, the aim of all such approaches is to achieve a reconstituted immune system that can also suppress the replication of HIV. Even if complete eradication of the virus is not possible, long-term control of HIV may be feasible and permit a prolonged survival.

At the same time, the available approved drugs permit only a limited number of three-drug regimens to be sequentially used in a given patient, and there remains an urgent need for new effective therapies. We have discussed some of the NRTIs, the NNRTIs, and the PIs under development. There also continues to be a substantial interest in developing drugs that act at new viral targets. Such agents, used in combination with the presently available drugs, may enable even more complete and sustained viral suppression to be attained. It was known for some time that one cellular receptor for HIV was CD4. It has recently been shown that certain chemokine receptors act as a co-receptor for HIV. The most important of these are CCR5 for monocytotropic strains and CXCR4 for T-tropic strains. Moreover, individuals with a homozygous deletion in the CCR5 receptor have been shown to be naturally resistant to becoming infected with HIV. Agents that block the binding of HIV to these receptors have been identified, and one such agent, T-20, has been shown to have clinical activity in early trials. It is possible that other strategies including gene therapy might also be able to take advantage of this finding.

Another target of interest is HIV integrase, which catalyzes the insertion of the HIV provirus into the target cell DNA. There is an effort underway to identify specific inhibitors for this enzyme. Another novel target is the HIV-1 nucleocapsid protein zinc fingers. These are structural components necessary for both acute infection and virion assembly. Their protein sequence is very highly conserved, and it has been hypothesized that they might be relatively resistant to mutation. Several inhibitors have been identified, and at least two are now in clinical trial.

Substantial advances have been made in AIDS therapy over the past several years. The development of highly active combination regimens of NRTIs and PIs has represented a substantial advance. Patients on these regimens have had substantial increases in their CD4 counts, fewer opportunistic infections, and prolonged survival. These advances have also resulted in a substantial drop in the death rate from AIDS starting in about 1996. In addition, the widespread use of zidovudine in the peripartum period has resulted in a marked drop in the incidence of vertically acquired HIV infection.

At the same time, the available regimens are quite expensive and require taking many pills daily in a complex schedule. This is an impediment for patient compliance. There is a need for simpler effective drug regimens, ideally involving once-daily dosing. We do not know how long the viral suppression attained with potent three-drug therapies will last when these regimens are used as initial therapy. Also, as we have seen, once patients fail their initial regimen, further therapeutic regimens are generally not as effective. Complete eradication of HIV remains an elusive goal, because memory T cells can serve as a long-lived reservoir for HIV, and it is quite possible that other reservoir sites (such as the brain) will be identified. For these reasons, it is important that we not get lulled into a false sense of security but rather use this period to redouble our efforts to develop long-lasting effective therapies for this disorder.

Carpenter CCJ, Fischl MA, Hammer SM, et al: Antiretroviral therapy for HIV infection in 1997: Updated recommendations of the International AIDS Society—USA Panel. JAMA 277:1962–1969, 1997. *Describes one recent set of therapeutic recommendations.*

De Clercq E: Toward improved anti-HIV chemotherapy: Therapeutic strategies for intervention with HIV infections. J Med Chem 38:2491–2517, 1995. *Review of the medicinal chemistry of anti-HIV drugs.*

Deeks SG, Smith M, Holodniy M, Kahn JO: HIV-1 protease inhibitors: A review for clinicians. JAMA 277:145–153, 1997. *Clinical overview of HIV protease inhibitors.*

Delta Coordinating Committee: DELTA: A randomized double-blind controlled trial comparing combinations of zidovudine plus didanosine or zalcitabine with zidovudine monotherapy in individuals with HIV infection. Lancet 348:293–291, 1996. *A second trial examining combination NRTI therapy.*

Department of Health and Human Services Panel on Clinical Practices for Treatment of HIV Infection. Guidelines for the use of antiretroviral agents in HIV-infected adults and adolescents. November 5, 1997. ⟨http://www.cdcac.org⟩ or ⟨http://www.hivatis.org⟩. *Provides guidelines for HIV therapy.*

Eron JJ, Benoit SL, Jemsek J, et al: Treatment with lamivudine, zidovudine, or both in HIV-positive patients with 200 to 500 CD4+ cells per cubic millimeter. N Engl J Med 333:1662–1669, 1996. *Results of a clinical trial utilizing zidovudine and lamivudine.*

Flexner C: HIV-protease inhibitors. N Engl J Med 338:1281–1292, 1998. *General review of protease inhibitors.*

Hammer S, Katzenstein D, Hughes M, et al: A trial comparing nucleoside monotherapy with combination therapy in HIV-infected adults with CD4 cell counts from 200 to 500 per cubic millimeter. N Engl J Med 335:1081–1090, 1996. *Results of a clinical trial showing the superiority of combination therapy over zidovudine monotherapy.*

Hammer SM, Squires KE, Hughes MD, et al: A controlled trial of two nucleoside analogues plus indinavir in persons with human immunodeficiency virus infection and CD4 cell counts of 200 per cubic millimeter or less. AIDS Clinical Trials Group 320 Study Team. N Engl J Med 337:725–733, 1997. *Results of a clinical trial showing the superiority of three-drug combination therapy involving a protease inhibitor over two-NRTI therapy.*

Roberts NA, Craig JC, Sheldon J: Resistance and cross-resistance with saquinavir and other HIV protease inhibitors: Theory and practice. AIDS 12:453–460, 1998. *Article describing patterns of PI resistance and how they can influence therapeutic decisions.*

419 MANAGEMENT AND COUNSELING FOR PERSONS WITH HIV INFECTION

John A. Bartlett

Treatment advances in human immunodeficiency virus (HIV) disease have dramatically changed the management of chronically infected persons. Advances in three areas have contributed to these successes: (1) an improved understanding of the dynamic nature of HIV replication and its implications for treatment, (2) the technology to measure HIV RNA levels with an understanding of their correlation with prognosis in untreated and treated persons, and (3) the availability of an expanding number of antiretroviral agents with increased potency. These advances have resulted in profound virologic suppression in treated patients with an associated improvement in clinical outcomes and survival. However, despite these treatment advances, significant gaps remain in our understanding of the strategies needed to guide treatment initiation, and when to change a failing regimen. Coincident with these treatment advances, persons with HIV infection in the United States are increasingly impoverished, more likely to abuse drugs, and have less access to health care. The use of complex antiretroviral regimens has created a scheduling challenge for many patients, and the success of therapy is absolutely dependent on patient adherence. Therefore, health care providers must carefully assess the resources and commitment of persons beginning antiretroviral therapy, design a highly potent and convenient regimen for individual patients, optimize adherence through patient preparation and education, and continually reassess the entire process in a patient on treatment. Significant questions remain unanswered regarding the durability of successful antiretroviral therapy, the potential infectivity of persons on treatment, and the optimal management of treatment failure. These uncertainties may make counseling difficult because individual patients may experience emotional extremes in periods of treatment successes and failures.

CLINICAL EVALUATION OF THE PATIENT

The clinical approach to the HIV-infected patient should be guided by several important principles. First, it is important to establish the degree of immunosuppression in every patient through the history and physical examination and the measurement of absolute CD4+ lymphocyte count. Second, an individual's risk of disease progression can be assessed through the measurement of plasma HIV RNA levels. Third, past histories of sexually transmitted diseases (STDs), positive purified protein derivative (PPD) testing or exposure to tuberculosis, and places of residence may be very useful in predicting complications of HIV infection. Finally, the sharing of pertinent medical information with patients may improve the quality of personal observations that they report to the physician in subsequent visits. Such educational efforts may result in greater adherence to medications and may also improve the physician's ability to establish early diagnoses, provide effective outpatient treatment, and communicate regarding treatment options and risk reduction. Information regarding the stage of HIV disease, and thus the degree of immunosuppression, provides important insight into predicting clinical complications and guiding therapeutic decisions. Such a clinical approach will allow the physician to optimize the chronic management and counseling of HIV-infected persons.

THE INITIAL EVALUATION (Table 419–1). The initial evaluation of an HIV-infected person should begin with a careful history of past evaluations for HIV infection. Previous history of risk behaviors, mononucleosis-like symptoms that could represent acute HIV infection, and previous HIV testing may all offer insight into a patient's duration of HIV infection. Previous plasma HIV RNA levels, CD4+ lymphocyte counts, history of acquired immunodeficiency syndrome (AIDS) indicator conditions, and other clinical manifestations are important historical factors. The physician must

History
How long has the patient been HIV infected?
What complications of HIV have occurred?
What past evaluations has the patient undergone?
What past treatment has the patient received?
Any past history of sexually transmitted diseases?
Past history of positive purified protein derivative (PPD) test or exposure to tuberculosis?
Medications and allergies?
Substance abuse?
Residential history?
Physical Examination
Laboratory Evaluation
Complete blood cell count
Chemistries including liver enzymes and serum creatinine
Plasma HIV RNA level
Absolute CD4+ lymphocyte count and CD4+ lymphocyte percentage
Syphilis and *Toxoplasma* serologies
PPD Testing
Immunizations
Pneumococcal vaccine
Influenza vaccine
Hepatitis B vaccine if non-immune

also elicit a medical history, especially a history of STDs (syphilis, herpes simplex, hepatitis B and C, genital or perianal warts, and cervical dysplasia are important examples), past PPD testing or exposure to tuberculosis, substance abuse, and medication allergies. On physical examination, particular attention should be focused on the skin (severe seborrhea, molluscum contagiosum, chronic herpetic ulcerations, and Kaposi's sarcoma all suggest progressive HIV infection), lymph nodes (generalized lymphadenopathy usually correlates with earlier HIV infection and involution may signal progression of disease), oropharynx (candidiasis, oral hairy leukoplakia, and Kaposi's sarcoma indicate progression), genitalia (severe warts, recurrent vaginal candidiasis, frequently recurrent or severe herpetic ulcerations, cervical dysplasia, and Kaposi's sarcoma suggest progression), and central nervous system (neurocognitive and memory deficits suggest progression to AIDS dementia). The initial laboratory examination should include a complete blood cell count with differential; routine chemistries including liver enzymes and serum creatinine, plasma HIV RNA level, absolute CD4+ lymphocyte count, and CD4+ lymphocyte percentage; and syphilis and *Toxoplasma* serologies. Patients should also undergo 5-TU PPD testing; a positive response in an HIV-infected patient is defined as induration of 5 mm or more. All HIV-infected patients should receive the pneumococcal pneumonia vaccine due to their increased risk of pneumococcal infections. The hepatitis B vaccine may be given to previously uninfected patients, and the influenza vaccine may be given yearly.

Once the initial evaluation is complete, the physician should be able to establish a Centers for Disease Control and Prevention (CDC) classification (Fig. 419–1) and assess the patient's risk of disease progression. In addition, potential co-infections with *Treponema pallidum* or *Mycobacterium tuberculosis* should be recognized and treated for personal and public health benefits. Finally, counseling may result in the reduction of risk behaviors through education and the identification and treatment of substance abuse.

STRATEGIC DECISIONS

With improving longevity for HIV-infected persons receiving antiretroviral treatment, but also acknowledging the finite durability of each regimen and a limited number of regimens, the optimal strategy for the use of antiretroviral therapy is crucial to maximize clinical benefit. Significant unanswered questions include the optimal initiation of antiretroviral therapy and the timing of a switch from a failing regimen to a secondary one.

TREATMENT INITIATION. Most clinicians follow HIV-infected persons not receiving antiretroviral treatment every 3 to 6 months with a careful history and physical examination and monitoring of plasma HIV RNA levels and absolute CD4+ cell counts. In asymptomatic HIV-infected persons the potential benefits of antiretroviral therapy should outweigh their imposition, toxicities, and cost. Many asymptomatic HIV-infected persons may be at low risk for clinical progression of disease due to host and virologic factors. Therefore, antiretroviral therapy should ideally be offered to those patients at greatest risk of clinical progression. Before considering treatment initiation, it is prudent to repeat plasma HIV RNA levels and absolute CD4+ cell counts because of potential variability. The risk of disease progression is related to a patient's symptoms, plasma HIV RNA level, and absolute CD4+ cell number. Therapy is strongly recommended for all symptomatic patients. The optimal levels of plasma HIV RNA and absolute CD4+ cells to guide the initiation of therapy are not known, but most clinicians recommend therapy at conservative thresholds of more than 20,000 copies HIV RNA/mL or CD4+ cells less than 300/mm^3.

Critical to the success of treatment interventions is a patient who is prepared and committed to beginning therapy. Therefore, decisions on treatment initiation must be highly individualized. Many clinicians never initiate treatment for a patient during his or her first visit; rather, they evaluate and educate the patient during several visits. Physicians must recognize the essential role of strict adherence to antiretroviral regimens and optimize circumstances such as patient education, emotional support, substance abuse rehabilitation, and the resources to obtain a continuing supply of medications. Studies of adherence have demonstrated that socioeconomic status, race/ethnicity, gender, and educational level do not predict successful adherence; therefore, physicians should not preclude treatment based on these factors.

With an expanding number of available antiretroviral drugs, clinicians can tailor regimens based on potency, convenience, predicted toxicities, and drug interactions. The importance of convenience and its relationship to adherence should not be underestimated. Significant issues may include dosing schedules, pill burden, food interactions, drug interactions, and toxicities. Clinicians should take a careful history regarding daily activities including employment and meals and project alternative medication schedules in discussions with their patients. When an initial regimen has been chosen, many clinicians will have patients return in 1 to 4 weeks to reinforce adherence and assess possible toxicities. Continuing attention to adherence at the time of all follow-up visits may assist in achieving long-term treatment success.

TREATMENT FAILURE. Successful antiretroviral therapy appears to achieve profound suppression of HIV replication, but the reservoir of chronically infected cells may not diminish over time.

	A	B	C
	Asymptomatic or PGL	Early symptomatic HIV disease	AIDS indicator conditions
1 CD4 > 500/mm^3	A1	B1	C1
2 CD4 > 200–499/mm^3	A2	B2	C2
3 CD4 > 200/mm^3	A3	B3	C3

FIGURE 419–1 ■ CDC classification system for HIV infection. The shaded areas (classes A3, B3, C1-3) meet the CDC definition of AIDS. PGL = Progressive generalized lymphadenopathy.

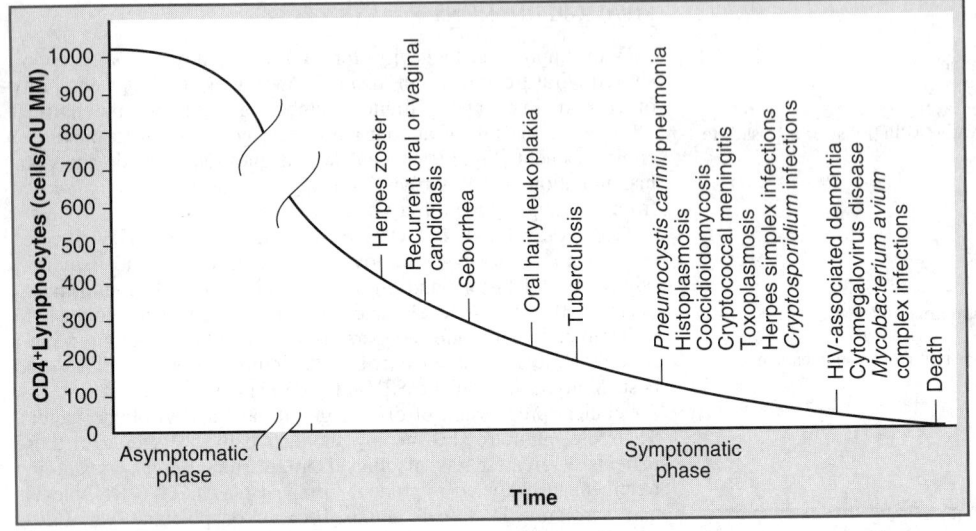

FIGURE 419–2 ■ Complications of HIV disease as related to lymphocyte count.

As a result, compromise in chronic suppression leads to reactivation of HIV from this reservoir and recurrence in plasma viremia. The reasons for treatment failure may include diverse factors such as adherence, individualized pharmacokinetic responses, drug interactions, and antiretroviral resistance.

Most clinicians follow plasma HIV RNA levels every 3 months in patients on stable, fully suppressive antiretroviral regimens. Such intensive monitoring of plasma HIV RNA levels is associated with greater suppression of virus over time. Currently, there is no consensus definition of treatment failure based on plasma HIV RNA levels. Increasing levels may indicate antiretroviral resistance, and the prolonged administration of a failing drug regimen can result in the accumulation of multiple resistance mutations with greater potential for cross-resistance. Conversely, modest increases in plasma HIV RNA levels do not appear to correlate with rapid falls in absolute CD4+ cell counts or immediately worsening clinical outcomes. Therefore, a balance must be reached when considering the discontinuation of an initial antiretroviral regimen and the substitution of a secondary one. Pending the elucidation of factors influencing the optimal timing for treatment changes, most clinicians follow individual patients closely to ascertain the rapidity of their virus recurrence and change medications accordingly.

When choosing a secondary treatment regimen, the new combination should include at least two new drugs predicted not to have cross-resistance with agents from previous regimens. The inclusion of at least two new drugs clearly offers better virologic results than the addition of a single new agent. At the present time, resistance patterns can only be predicted based on a past treatment history. However, studies to correlate genotypic and/or phenotypic resistance patterns with subsequent virologic responses may yield improved opportunities for laboratory-based assessments. It is important to recognize that the virologic success of secondary treatment regimens is compromised relative to the virologic success of initial treatment regimens.

EVALUATION OF THE FEBRILE PATIENT. Fever is a common physical finding among patients with HIV infection, and the potential causes are many. Fever may indicate a self-limited viral upper respiratory tract infection in a patient with early HIV infection or the presence of *Pneumocystis carinii* pneumonia (PCP) in a patient with progressive HIV infection. Differentiating the clinical manifestations of the two infections may be difficult for the physician; therefore, the physician should use any available information on HIV staging for the patient. In this context, the absolute CD4+ lymphocyte count may be an extremely useful guide in assessing the likelihood of opportunistic infections. If the absolute CD4+ lymphocyte count is more than 200/mm³, the likelihood of PCP or other opportunistic infections is significantly decreased. Thus, the absolute CD4+ lymphocyte count may guide the most appropriate diagnostic considerations. Of note, the uncommon patient may present with an opportunistic infection at absolute CD4+ lymphocyte counts of more than 200/mm³; therefore, it is imperative to reconsider such diagnoses if the fever persists.

COMPLICATIONS OF HIV INFECTION

As HIV infection progresses, it creates increasing immunosuppression, resulting in a predisposition to complicating opportunistic infections and neoplasms. The pattern of these complications can be predicted by following a patient's absolute CD4+ lymphocyte count (Fig. 419–2). On the basis of these correlations between absolute CD4+ lymphocytes and the predicted complications of HIV infection, clinicians can anticipate an increased risk of certain opportunistic infections in an individual patient, which may lead to an earlier diagnosis or the use of antimicrobial prophylaxis to prevent specific opportunistic infections. Successful prophylaxis has been identified against PCP, toxoplasmic encephalitis, disseminated *Mycobacterium avium* complex (MAC) infection, cryptococcal meningitis, and cytomegalovirus (CMV) disease (Table 419–2).

Table 419–2 ■ PROPHYLAXIS OF OPPORTUNISTIC INFECTIONS

INFECTION	AVAILABLE AGENTS	COMMENTS
Pneumocystis carinii pneumonia	SMX-TMP Dapsone Atovaquone Aerosolized pentamidine	SMX-TMP most effective and least expensive but potentially toxic
Mycobacterium avium complex (MAC)	Rifabutin Azithromycin Clarithromycin	Delay in disseminated MAC infection; potential pharmacokinetic interactions with protease inhibitors and zidovudine; resistant isolates possible
Toxoplasmic encephalitis	SMX-TMP Dapsone-pyrimethamine	
Cryptococcal meningitis	Fluconazole	Delay in deep fungal infections but costly; resistant isolates possible
Cytomegalovirus	Oral ganciclovir	Delay in CMV disease but costly

SMX-TMP = Sulfamethoxazole-trimethoprim.

Persons at highest risk for PCP include those recovering from their first episode (secondary prophylaxis, 1-year risk of recurrence without prophylaxis 60%), those with absolute CD4+ lymphocytes less than or equal to 200/mm³ (primary prophylaxis, 1-year risk of PCP ≥ 18%), those with CD4+ lymphocyte percentages less than 20%, and those with a non-PCP AIDS indicator condition (both primary prophylaxis). Sulfamethoxazole/trimethoprim (SMX-TMP) is the most successful prophylaxis against PCP. In patients intolerant of SMX-TMP, desensitization may be undertaken or dapsone, atovaquone, or aerosolized pentamidine may be used. SMX-TMP and dapsone-pyrimethamine can also be given to prevent toxoplasmic encephalitis among patients who are seropositive for previous infection with *Toxoplasma gondii*.

Clarithromycin, azithromycin, or rifabutin can delay disseminated MAC infection. These drugs are prescribed for patients at highest risk, usually those with absolute CD4+ lymphocytes less than 100/mm³. Fluconazole has also demonstrated efficacy in delaying invasive fungal infections in patients with absolute CD4+ lymphocytes less than 200/mm³. Oral ganciclovir has also successfully delayed the onset of CMV disease in seropositive HIV-infected patients. The widespread use of these prophylaxes must include consideration of their potential drug interactions, the potential for drug resistance, and cost effectiveness.

PCP was once the most common AIDS indicator condition, but HIV-associated wasting, disseminated MAC infection, and CMV disease are now more common clinical manifestations. Overall, the incidence of opportunistic infections has declined with the use of potent antiretroviral combinations. Undoubtedly, the future complications of progressive HIV infection will continue to evolve as improved antiretroviral therapies and prophylactic strategies against additional opportunistic infections are identified and as survival lengthens for persons with AIDS.

When patients do develop opportunistic infections, clinicians should attempt to establish a diagnosis and initiate treatment as soon as possible. Early diagnosis results in an improved prognosis for most opportunistic infections, and with early diagnosis many patients may receive outpatient therapy. Successful outpatient therapy frequently results in greater patient satisfaction and lower health care costs.

COUNSELING

Counseling HIV-infected patients can present great challenges to their physicians. Many HIV-infected persons enter the physician-patient relationship with significant emotional distress and numerous complicating circumstances. These complicating circumstances can include issues of sexual orientation and sexuality, the need for risk reduction, substance abuse, societal discrimination, and increasing poverty as the epidemic evolves in the United States. The physician must enter this relationship prepared to address these issues with knowledge and compassion and without becoming judgmental about their content.

A crucial component involved in counseling HIV-infected persons is education concerning HIV disease, its transmission, and its potential treatments. This process should continue for the duration of the physician-patient relationship; and given the extensive knowledge base of many persons with HIV infection, there may be a mutual exchange of important information. The best medical interventions will not succeed unless HIV-infected persons have been carefully counseled regarding their potential benefits, costs, and acquisition. A well-informed patient can be a strong ally in

tackling difficult therapeutic decisions, and many therapeutic decisions are currently not straightforward, such as the optimal time to initiate antiretroviral therapy. A well-informed patient will be more adherent with prescribed medications and may better recognize the early manifestations of HIV-related clinical complications and potential drug toxicities. Finally, a well-informed patient can constructively guide decisions regarding advance directives for his or her care if HIV disease progresses.

Education regarding the transmission of HIV and alterations in risk behavior is another important goal of counseling. Efforts to encourage behavioral changes resulting in temporarily decreased HIV transmission have succeeded in homosexual men in San Francisco, although recent evidence suggests an increasing number of new infections, especially among young individuals. Intensive efforts to decrease HIV transmission have also succeeded in smaller populations of injecting drug users and high-risk heterosexuals. All patients should be well informed regarding safer sex precautions and the avoidance of needle sharing. This information must be presented in language appropriate to the culture of the patient. Significant behavioral changes are frequently not accomplished during a single visit, and enduring change requires ongoing re-education and support from the physician.

Treating substance abuse is crucial in decreasing the risk of HIV transmission through needle sharing and sexual contact and in avoiding the medical and psychological consequences of continued substance abuse. Physicians must advocate for their patients in seeking access to frequently inadequate and overwhelmed drug treatment programs. Physicians also must acknowledge the high recidivism rates associated with substance abuse and continue to treat their recidivous patients firmly and without judgment. Finally, physicians should reinforce positively those recovering addicts who have succeeded in treatment and struggle to avoid relapse on a daily basis.

The clinical course of persons with HIV infection is frequently complicated by significant anxiety and depression. Pharmacologic measures may prove useful in their management, although physicians should be cautious about the potential for drug interactions with protease inhibitors. In the circumstance of late-stage HIV infection complicated by HIV encephalopathy and depression, ritalin may be of benefit. Physicians should identify AIDS service organizations in their community that may provide support services such as patient education, case management, transportation, shelter, food, medications, or support groups to their clients. Formal psychiatric referral may also be necessary in individual patients. Patients may experience depression throughout the course of HIV infection—in early infection, during successful treatment, and in disease progression. Past coping strategies may be useful in such instances. A careful history may provide assistance in identifying these strategies.

Bartlett JG: Medical Management of HIV Infection. Glenview, IL, Physicians and Scientists Publishing Co, 1997. *A review for health care professionals describing the medical management of HIV-infected persons.*

Carpenter CJ, Fischl MA, Hammer SM, et al: Antiretroviral therapy for HIV infection in 1997: Updated recommendations of the International AIDS Society—USA Panel. JAMA 227:1962–1969, 1997. *A review of the continually evolving recommendations for antiretroviral therapy.*

Kitahata MM, Koepsell TD, Deyo RA, et al: Physician's experience with acquired immunodeficiency syndrome as a factor in patient survival. N Engl J Med 334:701–706, 1996. *Increased experience of physicians in treating AIDS improves survival.*

Royce RA, Sena A, Cates W, Cohen MS: Sexual transmission of HIV. N Engl J Med 336:1072–1078, 1997. *A review of the factors affecting the sexual transmission of HIV, the predominant mechanism of continuing spread.*

PART XXIV

DISEASES OF PROTOZOA AND METAZOA

420 INTRODUCTION TO PROTOZOAN AND HELMINTHIC DISEASES

Keith A. Joiner

Interactions between micro-organisms and their hosts can be classified as mutualistic, commensalistic, parasitic. Only in a parasitic relationship does the organism flourish at the expense of host fitness. By this definition, all human pathogens are parasites. By convention, however, the term parasitic infection is used to describe infestations with protozoans and helminths. These two categories of organisms are typically (although not always) distinguished from other human pathogens by having complex lifecycles, often involving sequential developmental stages in different hosts or in a free-living state, by causing chronic infections, and by expression of highly evolved immune evasion mechanisms.

There are several essential distinctions between protozoan and metazoan (helminthic) pathogens and the infections they cause. Protozoa are unicellular, are typically microscopic in size, and replicate within their mammalian host. Hence, disease from protozoans can result even when the initial parasite inoculum to which the host is exposed is small, and the time of exposure is short. In contrast, helminths are generally macroscopic, multicellular organisms that do not multiply within their mammalian hosts. Helminthic disease typically requires repeated exposure to infective forms in order to increase the organism burden to a level sufficient to cause disease. This usually necessitates prolonged residence in the endemic area. Sexual reproduction does occur in the host, but the eggs or larvae that are generated must be passed from the host into the environment in order for development of a stage infective for humans to occur.

THE BIOLOGY OF PARASITES

Molecular Parasitology

The field of molecular parasitology has undergone revolutionary advances in the last decade. Many fundamental new paradigms in eukaryotic molecular and cellular biology, such as trans-splicing of mRNA and anchoring of membrane proteins by glycosylphosphatidylinositol anchors, were first revealed in parasites. DNA for either endogenous or foreign genes can now be introduced into most pathogenic protozoan parasites, and gene function can be further assessed after gene knockout in leishmania, trypanosomes, plasmodia, and toxoplasma. Reverse genetics can be used to identify genes that encode critical parasite functions. This has stimulated the interest of the scientific community at large, and induced investigators from other fields to begin working in parasite systems. The nucleotide sequence of entire parasite genomes will be available by early in the next century. The hope, still largely unrealized, is that these tools will lead to the identification of new diagnostic methods, new targets for chemotherapy, and new candidates for successful vaccine development.

Immunity and Vaccine Development

Protozoa and helminths exhibit elaborate strategies for evading the host response, which contributes to their chronicity and latency. Antigenic variation, in which the major antigen on the microbial surface undergoes periodic and spontaneous switching, thereby precluding effective antibody-mediated clearance by the host, was first described in *Trypanosoma brucei*. This phenomenon is now known to occur in some form or another with many other pathogenic protozoans, including plasmodia, giardia, and *T. cruzi*. The relevance of the observation that immunologic effector functions could be divided into two categories based on lymphokine expression by CD4 cells (the Th1/Th2 paradigm) was first demonstrated with *Leishmania major,* and is now commonly recognized with a wide variety of parasitic diseases. Parasites have proved instrumental in defining effector mechanisms of host resistance that are critical for effective vaccine development, although disappointingly, after decades of research there is still no commercially available vaccine for any parasitic infection of man.

EPIDEMIOLOGY

The magnitude of parasitic infections worldwide is staggering. One billion individuals are infected with ascariasis or trichuriasis, and 600 million are infected with malaria and either schistosomiasis or filariasis.

One of the most important recent changes in the epidemiology of protozoal diseases is the association of selected infections with HIV (see Part XXIII). Some infections, such as *Toxoplasma* and *Cryptosporidia,* occur to an equal extent in the developed and the underdeveloped world. In contrast, more than 90% of the 30 million individuals infected with HIV live in tropical and subtropical countries where malaria, leishmaniasis, and trypanosomiasis are endemic. Although malaria incidence and severity are surprisingly unaltered by HIV, the risk of developing visceral leishmaniasis is increased by as much as 500-fold, and the resultant disease is more severe and difficult to treat. HIV-infected individuals with chronic *T. cruzi* infection have an increased incidence of central nervous system disease.

DIAGNOSIS AND THERAPY

Probably nowhere else in clinical medicine is the question "Where have you been?" more important than in the diagnosis of parasitic and helminthic disease. A precise accounting of the places visited in chronological order, and extent of rural travel and exposure to water and vegetation, is essential. The answer to these questions then leads the clinician to a consideration of the geographic distribution and the major modes of clinical presentation of various parasitic diseases (see Chapter 316). Adjunctive laboratory data, most notably peripheral blood eosinophilia, may provide an additional clue to the presence of infection with a tissue-invasive helminth.

There are a limited number of effective agents for protozoal and helminthic infections. Fortunately, most parasites remain susceptible to the limited armamentarium of available agents. The situation is decidedly different with malaria, where chloroquine resistance is now worldwide.

CDC: Health Information for International Travel 1996–1997. Atlanta, DHHS, 1997.

Web site: www.cdc.gov/travel/yellowbk. *A review of the recommendations for pro-phylaxis and vaccination for international travel by destination. Frequently updated.*

Drugs for parasitic infections. Med. Lett. Drugs 40:1, 1998. *Review of drugs for parasitic infections, providing dose, adverse reactions, and alternative agents. Published and updated annually.*

Pearce EJ, Scott PA, Sher A: Immune regulation in parasitic infection and disease. *In* Fundamental Immunology. WE Paul (ed). New York, Raven Press, 1998. *A detailed review of the immune response to parasitic infection, and of the current status of vaccine development.*

Wilson ME: A Worldwide Guide to Infections: Diseases, Distribution, Diagnosis. New York, Oxford University Press, 1991. *A description of the manifestations and diagnosis of diseases worldwide, grouped by geographic distribution.*

■ PROTOZOAN DISEASES

421 MALARIA

Donald J. Krogstad

Malaria is characterized by recurrent fever and chills associated with the synchronous lysis of parasitized red blood cells. Its name is derived from the belief of the ancient Romans that malaria was due to the bad air of the marshes surrounding Rome.

ETIOLOGY

Malaria is produced by intraerythrocytic parasites of the genus *Plasmodium.* Four plasmodia produce malaria in humans: *Plasmodium falciparum, P. vivax, P. ovale,* and *P. malariae.* The severity and characteristic manifestations of malaria are governed by the infecting species, the magnitude of the parasitemia, the metabolic effects of the parasite, and the cytokines released as a result of the infection.

INCIDENCE, PREVALENCE, AND RESURGENCE

Incidence

Although precise data are difficult to obtain, malaria is one of the most common infectious diseases. At least 200 to 300 million cases of malaria occur each year, with 1 to 2 million deaths. Most deaths are due to *P. falciparum* infection and occur among children less than 5 years old in sub-Saharan Africa. One of the major unanswered questions about malaria is how plasmodia produce repetitive infections without stimulating an effective (protective) immune response.

Prevalence

The prevalence of malaria varies widely; it may reach 70 to 80% or more among children in hyperendemic areas during the transmission season. Thus its impact on the health of the developing world is enormous.

Resurgence

The major factors responsible for the resurgence of malaria are drug resistances: (1) the widespread resistance of the anopheline vector to economical insecticides such as chlorophenothane (DDT), and (2) the increasing prevalence of chloroquine resistance in *P. falciparum,* which is now established in South America, Southeast Asia, and Africa.

LIFE CYCLE AND EPIDEMIOLOGY

Life Cycle

The life cycle can be viewed as beginning with the synchronous asexual replication of the erythrocytic stage of the parasite (Fig. 421–1). During the asexual erythrocytic cycle, the parasites mature

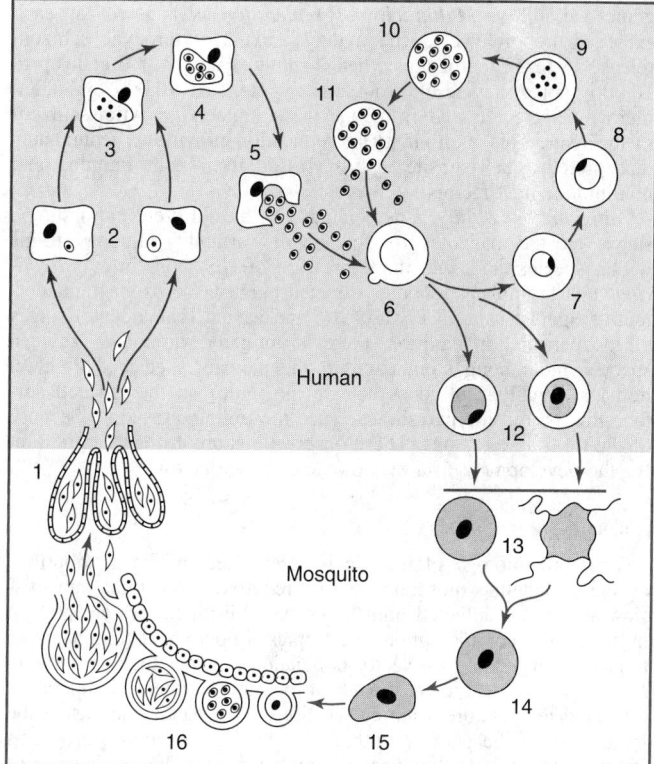

FIGURE 421–1 ■ Life cycle of the malaria parasite. The upper and lower halves of the diagram indicate the human and anopheline mosquito parts of the cycle, respectively. Sporozoites from the salivary gland of a female *Anopheles* mosquito are injected under the skin (1). They then travel through the bloodstream to the liver (2) and mature within hepatocytes to tissue *schizonts* (4). Up to 30,000 parasites are then released into the bloodstream as *merozoites* (5) and produce symptomatic injection as they invade and destroy red blood cells. However, some parasites remain dormant in the liver as *hypnozoites (2, dashed lines from 1 to 3).* These are the parasites that cause relapsing malaria (in *P. vivax* or *P. ovale* infection). Once within the bloodstream, merozoites (5) invade red cells (6) and mature to the *ring* (7,8), *trophozoite* (9), and *schizont* (10) asexual stages. Schizonts lyse their host red cells as they mature and release the next generation of merozoites (11), which invade previously uninfected red cells. Within the red cell some parasites differentiate to sexual forms (male and female *gametocytes*) (12). When taken up by a female *Anopheles* mosquito, the gametocytes mature to *male* and *female gametes,* which produce *zygotes* (14). The zygote invades the gut of the mosquito (15) and develops into an *oocyst* (16). Mature oocysts produce *sporozoites,* which migrate to the salivary gland of the mosquito (1) and repeat the cycle. The dashed line between 12 and 13 indicates that absence of the mosquito vector prevents natural transmission via this cycle. Infection by the injection of contaminated blood bypasses this constraint and permits transmission among intravenous drug addicts or to recipients of blood transfusions. (Reproduced with permission from Krogstad DJ: Blood and tissue protozoa. *In* Schaechter M, Medoff G, Eisenstein BI [eds.]: Mechanisms of Microbial Diseases. 2nd ed © 1993, p 600, the Williams & Wilkins Company, Baltimore.)

from rings to trophozoites to schizonts, which ultimately rupture the red cell and release merozoites that enter uninfected red cells via receptors such as Duffy factor in *P. vivax;* the cycle is then repeated. In contrast, some erythrocytic parasites mature to sexual forms (gametocytes) that are ingested by the female anopheline mosquito. Within the mosquito intermediate host, male and female gametocytes mature to gametes, fuse to form an ookinete that matures to a zygote and ultimately produces the sporozoites that are infectious for humans. When an infected mosquito bites a human, sporozoites travel via the bloodstream to the liver, where they enter hepatocytes and mature to tissue schizonts, which release merozoites that are infectious for red cells and produce the asexual erythrocytic cycle. Two of the four species that infect humans (*P. vivax* and *P. ovale*) produce dormant (hypnozoite) forms in the liver, which may mature 2 to 11 months or more after the initial infection and thus produce relapsing malaria.

Two characteristics of the life cycle are essential for the long-term survival of the parasite: multiplicity of replication and antigenic variability. *Multiplicity of replication* is apparent at each stage of the life cycle. The mature asexual erythrocytic schizont releases 8 to 32 merozoites when it ruptures its host red cell; up to 10,000 sporozoites result from one zygote; and 10,000 to 30,000 merozoites are released from one tissue (exoerythrocytic) schizont in the liver. This multiplicity of replication provides a redundancy that protects the parasite against losses from both immune and nonimmune host factors.

Antigenic variability is associated with the different morphologic stages in the parasite lifecycle, with variability among strains within species, and with the expression of *var* genes in *P. falciparum.* For example, antibodies directed against sporozoites are ineffective against asexual erythrocytic and sexual (gametocyte) stages of the parasite. In addition, there is antigenic variability between species and among strains within the parasite species that infect humans. Finally, *var* genes encode molecules on the red cell surface that permit the parasite to evade the immune response because of their variable regions. These observations are critically important for the development of a malaria vaccine (see below).

Epidemiology

The epidemiology of malaria is determined by the distributions of the anopheline mosquito vectors required for natural transmission and of the infected human reservoir. Both factors are present in endemic areas throughout the tropics. Important determinants of transmission include the vector population (vectors such as *Anopheles gambiae* in Africa are thought to be more efficient), temperature (elevated temperatures shorten the life of the vector and hasten the maturation of the parasite within the vector), and control programs (which reduce both the vector population and the prevalence of human infection).

Competent mosquito vectors are present in the United States (*A. albimanus* in the east, *A. freeborni* in the west). Although transmission in the United States is limited by the absence of infected humans, natural mosquito-borne transmission can and does occur with the importation of infected humans (e.g., the return of soldiers after their exposure in endemic areas). Mosquito-borne transmission (*introduced malaria*) occurred in the United States after World War II, the Korean War, the Vietnam War, and the arrival of refugees from Southeast Asia.

PATHOGENESIS

Species-Dependent Factors

Malaria is a multifactorial disease that can be explained in part, but not completely, by the magnitude of the parasitemia. *P. falciparum* is the most lethal parasite because it can invade red cells of any age and can thus produce unrestricted parasitemias involving 10^6 or more parasitized red cells per cubic millimeter of blood ($\geq 20\%$ of circulating red cells). Conversely, *P. vivax* and *P. ovale,* which invade only young red cells, are limited to parasitemias $\leq 25,000$ per cubic millimeter, and *P. malariae,* which invades only older red cells, is limited to parasitemias $\leq 10,000$ per cubic millimeter.

The Host Immune Response

Because millions of people experience repetitive episodes of malaria throughout their lives in the tropics, the immune response to natural infection is inadequate by definition. Thus the term *semi-immune* is used for residents of endemic areas who are at reduced risk of severe or complicated malaria but are reinfected regularly. The reasons for the inadequate host immune response are only partially clear and are likely to be central to developing a successful vaccine. For example, most exposed persons make antibodies directed against the repetitive epitope or epitopes on the surface of the sporozoite, and antibodies to asexual stages have been shown to reduce the magnitude of the parasitemia in children. However, cell-mediated immune responses may be essential for effective immunity. Factors potentially responsible for the poor cell-mediated responses to sporozoite antigen include (1) host immune restriction related to HLA haplotype, and (2) the dependence of cellular responses on hypervariable regions downstream from the coding region.

Peripheral Sequestration of Parasitized Red Cells

With maturation, red cells containing *P. falciparum* parasites develop knobs that contain histidine-rich proteins. In vivo, these knobs adhere to endothelial cells in the peripheral microvasculature via receptors such as thrombospondin, intercellular adhesion molecule 1, or CD36. This phenomenon has at least two consequences: (1) It enhances the microvascular obstruction and pathology produced by the parasite, and (2) it removes mature *P. falciparum* parasites from the circulation, so that only early asexual erythrocytic stages, such as rings, are seen on peripheral blood smears.

Cytokines in the Pathogenesis of Malaria

Recent studies suggest that cytokine release in malaria is a central factor in the pathogenesis of severe disease. Cytokines that have been shown to be important include tumor necrosis factor-α (TNF-α). Serum levels of TNF-α are elevated in severe *P. falciparum* infection and correlate with complications such as cerebral malaria and death, although a direct cause-and-effect relationship has not been established. Interferon-γ (IFN-γ) has antiparasitic activity against the exoerythrocytic stages of the parasite in the liver.

PATHOLOGY

The pathology of severe malaria is that of a microvascular disease involving the brain, lung, and kidney. Post-mortem examination in fatal *P. falciparum* infection demonstrates parasitized red cells in the capillaries and venules of the brain and other affected organs. In severe cases, acute tubular necrosis may be present, and the liver, spleen, and other sites in the reticuloendothelial system may be filled with dark malarial pigment from the phagocytosis of parasitized red cells. This predominantly microvascular pathology is consistent with the importance of sequestration and cytokine release in the pathogenesis of severe *P. falciparum* malaria (see above). By contrast, the other malarias that infect humans produce lower parasitemias, do not sequester, and are rarely fatal.

CLINICAL MANIFESTATIONS

Fever and Chills

Most patients with malaria have recurrent fever and chills (at 48-hour intervals for *P. vivax* and *P. ovale* and at 72-hour intervals for *P. malariae*). By contrast, patients with *P. falciparum* infection typically have irregular fever and chills and rarely present with a regular 48-hour cycle of symptoms despite the 48-hour cycle of the parasite.

Coma

Coma (cerebral malaria) is the most feared complication of *P. falciparum* infection and has a substantial fatality rate. Although it has been attributed to the blockage of capillaries with parasitized red cells, both hypoglycemia and the effects of cytokines such as TNF-α are important factors. Hypoglycemia in *P. falciparum* malaria may have at least three causes: (1) insulin released from the pancreatic β cell by quinine or quinidine during treatment, (2) glucose consumption by the massive numbers of parasites present in the patient, and (3) liver glycogen depletion in persons who have not eaten for several days before seeking medical care because they were ill with malaria. Hypoglycemia is particularly important to consider because it is treatable. Although the effects of TNF-α undoubtedly contribute to cerebral malaria, it is difficult to separate them from the magnitude of the parasitemia because the concentration of TNF-α and the magnitude of the parasitemia correlate with each other.

Renal Failure

Patients with massive parasitemias may have dark urine from the free hemoglobin produced by hemolysis (black-water fever) and may later develop renal failure. In most instances, the patients recover uneventfully; however, acute renal failure may occur with a time course similar to that of other causes of acute tubular necrosis.

Pulmonary Edema

This complication also occurs in patients with high *P. falciparum* parasitemias ($\geq 5\%$ of circulating red cells). Hemodynamic measurements indicate that this is a noncardiogenic form of pulmonary edema with normal pulmonary arterial and capillary pressures. These findings and the association with high TNF-α levels suggest that the pathogenesis of pulmonary edema may be similar in malaria and bacterial septicemia.

Gastrointestinal Manifestations

Diarrhea is common among children with *P. falciparum* infection. Although the pathogenesis of this complication is unclear, postmortem studies of children with diarrhea have revealed parasitized red cells in the microvasculature of the intestine.

DIAGNOSIS

Giemsa-Stained Thick and Thin Smears

The most direct way to diagnose malaria is to examine Giemsa-stained thick or thin smears using oil immersion magnification ($\times 1000$). Giemsa stain is preferable to Wright's stain, especially for persons with *P. vivax* or *P. ovale* infection, because the Schüffner's dots characteristic of those infections are often not visible with Wright's stain. Thick smears are more sensitive than thin smears because the red cells have been lysed. As a result, approximately 10 times as much blood can be examined per field and thus per unit of time. However, because the red cells have been lysed, it is not possible to determine the effect of the parasite on red cell size or the position of the parasite within the red cell on a thick smear (Table 421–1). Therefore, persons without previous experience in reading thick smears should consider using thin smears to identify the infecting parasite or parasites. A common mistake is to require characteristic gametocytes for a diagnosis of *P. falciparum* infection. Because gametocytes require longer to develop than asexual parasites (7 to 10 versus 2 days), they are usually not present in the peripheral blood when nonimmune tourists or expatriates first become symptomatic. Conversely, gametocytes are frequently present in the blood of semi-immune residents of endemic areas with few or no symptoms or asexual parasites. A second common mistake is to assume that the patient can have only one parasite species: Approximately 5% of persons with malaria have infections with more than one parasite species.

Antigen Detection

Testing for parasite antigen (histidine rich protein 2—ParaSight F) is a potential alternative to microscopy for the diagnosis of *P. falciparum* infections, especially in non-endemic areas where skilled microscopists are rare. Potential disadvantages of this approach include negatives with *P. vivax, P. ovale,* and *P. malariae* infections, and some false-negatives with *P. falciparum* infections from spontaneous deletion of the *hrp2* gene.

Fluorescent Staining with Acridine Orange (QBC)

Because parasitized red cells are less dense, they are found at the top of the red cell layer after centrifugation. Although parasites of all species stain with acridine orange and can be visualized with

Table 421–1 ■ MALARIA PARASITES THAT INFECT HUMANS

	PARASITEMIA (per μl blood)	COMPLICATIONS
P. falciparum	$\geq 10^6$	Coma (cerebral malaria) Hypoglycemia Pulmonary edema, renal failure Anemia
P. vivax	$\leq 25,000$	Late (2–3 mo) splenic rupture
P. ovale	$\leq 25,000$	—
P. malariae	$\leq 10,000$	Immune complex nephrotic syndrome

MORPHOLOGY			
	Red Blood Cell Size	Schüffner's Dots	Stages
P. falciparum	No RBC enlargement	Absent	Rings, occasionally gametocytes
P. vivax	Enlarged host RBC	Present	All forms
P. ovale	Enlarged host RBC	Present	All forms
P. malariae	No RBC enlargement	Absent	All forms

	RELAPSE FROM HYPNOZOITES	ANTIMALARIAL RESISTANCE
P. falciparum	No	Chloroquine, meftoquine, pyrimethamine-sulfadoxine, plus partial resistance to quinine and quinidine
P. vivax	Yes	Chloroquine
P. ovale	Yes	None known
P. malariae	No	None known

RBC = red blood cells

fluorescence microscopy, a number of investigators have had difficulty distinguishing among species with this technique.

DNA Probes and PCR

Both DNA probes and PCR may achieve the sensitivity of a thick smear. However, problems have included the need for nonisotopic methods (probes), and the requirement for expensive equipment (thermocycler) and reagents for PCR. For these reasons, neither method is routinely used in malaria-endemic areas.

Serology (Antibody Testing)

Testing for antibodies to plasmodia is of limited value. In endemic areas, most persons have antibody titers from previous infections whether they have been infected recently or not. In addition, 3 to 4 weeks may be required to develop a diagnostic rise in antibody titer, whereas the decision to treat should be made in the first few hours of evaluation. However, serology may be of value retrospectively in nonimmune persons (expatriate tourists) who have been treated empirically for malaria without a microscopic diagnosis. For example, a high titer of antibodies against *P. vivax* suggests that the patient has had a recent *P. vivax* infection and should receive primaquine if it has not been given previously (see the section on treatment, below).

PREVENTION

Exposed nonimmune persons may prevent malaria by taking antimalarials prospectively (chemoprophylaxis); by using insect repellents and otherwise reducing contact with the anopheline vector; and possibly, in the future, by a malaria vaccine (immunoprophylaxis).

Chemoprophylaxis

Drugs used for chemoprophylaxis must be safe because they are given to healthy persons for long periods. Several have been chosen for their long serum half-lives so that they can be given infrequently. On the basis of these criteria, chloroquine is an excellent drug for chemoprophylaxis in areas without chloroquine-resistant *P. falciparum* (Table 421–2). It is the only chemoprophylactic agent known to be safe for pregnant women and does not produce retinal toxicity at the doses used for antimalarial chemoprophylaxis. Unfortunately, chloroquine-resistant strains of *P. falciparum* are now established in Southeast Asia, South America, and Africa. For areas with chloroquine-resistant *P. falciparum,* mefloquine is now the recommended chemoprophylactic agent, although resistance to mefloquine is developing in Southeast Asia. Doxycycline is an alternative, with the advantage that it also reduces the frequency of traveler's diarrhea. The disadvantages of doxycycline include the need to take it daily, photosensitivity reactions, and vaginitis. Because of hypersensitivity reactions to pyrimethamine-sulfadoxine (Fansidar) and both agranulocytosis and hepatitis with amodiaquine, neither of these agents is recommended for chemoprophylaxis.

Vector Control

Because of widespread drug resistance in *P. falciparum,* increasing emphasis has been placed on reducing exposure to the anopheline vector, especially in areas with intense transmission such as Africa. Strategies that are successful and should be considered include DEET-containing insect repellents and pyrethrin (insecticide)–impregnated bed nets. DDT is no longer effective in most regions of the world because of widespread resistance.

Immunoprophylaxis—Development of a Malaria Vaccine

Although a malaria vaccine is not available, it is hoped that this goal will ultimately be achievable. Because the three major parasite stages in humans are antigenically distinct, a successful vaccine will likely need to contain at least three parasite antigens (sporozoite, merozoite, and gametocyte). However, a vaccine need not be 100% effective to be valuable. For example, a vaccine that required boosting could be quite effective for residents of endemic areas because of repetitive exposure to natural infection. In addition, a vaccine that limited the magnitude of the parasitemia could have a marked effect on survival even if it had no effect on the incidence of infection, because severe morbidity and death are associated with high parasitemias.

TREATMENT

Successful treatment of patients with malaria depends primarily on effective antimalarial drugs. However, it also depends on ancillary measures as diverse as the infusion of glucose and dialysis. Monitoring of the blood glucose level is important because hypoglycemia is a common cause of coma and because both quinine and quinidine stimulate the release of insulin directly from the pancreatic β cell. Steroids are contraindicated in cerebral malaria because they prolong the duration of coma.

The treatment of chloroquine-susceptible malaria (*P. vivax, P. ovale,* or *P. malariae* malaria and chloroquine-susceptible *P. falciparum* malaria) is satisfactory (Table 421–3) because chloroquine is a safe and effective antimalarial. Patients with chloroquine-resistant *P. vivax* have recently been treated successfully with either mefloquine or halofantrine. However, the treatment of chloroquine-resistant *P. falciparum* infection is unsatisfactory. Patients able to tolerate oral medications may be treated with mefloquine alone in areas without mefloquine resistance. In areas with mefloquine resistance, treatments include halofantrine alone, quinine plus pyri-

Table 421–2 ■ CHEMOPROPHYLAXIS OF MALARIA*

For Areas without Chloroquine-Resistant *Plasmodium falciparum*:

Chloroquine phosphate (Aralen)	500 mg/wk (300 mg chloroquine base) during exposure and for 4 wk after leaving the endemic area

For Areas with Chloroquine-Resistant *Plasmodium falciparum*:

Mefloquine (Lariam)	250 mg/wk during exposure and for 4 wk after leaving the endemic area
Doxycycline	100 mg/d during exposure and for 4 wk after leaving the endemic area

Alternatives for areas with chloroquine-resistant *P. falciparum* include proguanil (200 mg/day) plus weekly chloroquine, although this regimen has not been approved by the FDA and breakthroughs occur with some frequency in areas with chloroquine-resistant *P. falciparum.* Updated information on malaria chemoprophylaxis may be obtained from the CDC Hot Line and Web Sites at 404-223-4559, 404-332-4565, and *www.cdc.gov,* respectively.

Table 421–3 ■ TREATMENT OF MALARIA

Table 421–3 ■ TREATMENT OF MALARIA

***P. vivax, P. ovale, P. malariae,* and Chloroquine-Susceptible *P. falciparum*:**

For patients able to take oral medications:

PO chloroquine:	10 mg/kg = 600-mg base, followed by an additional 300-mg base after 6 hr and 300-mg base again on days 2 and 3

For patients unable to take oral medications:

IM chloroquine:	2.5 mg/kg IM q 4 hr or 3.5 mg/kg q 6 hr (total dose not to exceed 25 mg/kg base)
IV chloroquine:	10 mg/kg base over 4 hr, followed by 5 mg/kg base q 12 hr (given in a 2-hr infusion; total dose not to exceed 25 mg/kg base)

Chloroquine-Resistant *P. vivax*:

PO mefloquine:	750 mg (15 mg per kg) as a single dose
OR	
PO halofantrine:	500 mg q 8 hours × 3 over 24 hours for a total dose of 1500 mg

Chloroquine-Resistant *P. falciparum*:

For patients able to take oral medications:

PO mefloquine*:	750 mg (684-mg base) as a single oral dose, followed by 500 mg in 6–8 hours
OR	
PO halofantrine:	500 mg q 6 hours × 3 doses and repeat in 1 week
OR	
PO quinine:	650 mg quinine sulfate q 8 hours × 3 days, plus
plus Pyrimethamine-sulfadoxine:	3 tables (1500 mg sulfadoxine, 75 mg pyrimethamine) as a single dose
or Doxycyline (Vibramycin):	100 mg 2 id × 7 days
or Clindamycin:	900 mg 3 id × 5 days
OR Atovaquone:	1000 mg q day × 3 days
plus Proguanil (Malarone):	400 mg 1 day × 3 days
or Doxycyline:	100 mg 2 id × 3 days

For patients unable to tolerate oral medications:

IV quinidine:	6.25 mg base/kg (10 mg gluconate salt/kg, maximum of 600 mg salt) over 1–2 hours, followed by 0.0125 mg/kg base (0.02 mg gluconate salt)/min until parasitemia is <1% or patient tolerates oral medications
OR IV quinine:	16.7 mg/kg base (20 mg dihydrochloride salt) loading dose over 4 hours, followed by 8.3 mg base/kg over 2–4 hours q 8 hours until patient tolerates oral medications
OR IM quinine:	8.3 mg base/kg (10 mg dihydrochloride salt) q 8 hours (maximum of 1500-mg base [1800 mg salt] per day)
OR IM artemether:	4 mg/kg initially, followed by 2 mg/kg every 8 hours for ≥72 hours

For Multiply resistant *P. falciparum*:

PR artesunate:	200 mg PR at 0, 4, 8, 12, 24, 36, 48 and 60 hours for a total PR dose of 1600 mg, or 100 mg Artesunate PO × 1, followed by 50 mg PO q 12 hours × 5 days for a total of 600 mg
plus PO mefloquine:	650 mg at 72 hours, plus 500 mg at 84 hours

To Prevent Relapse in *P. vivax* or *P. ovale* Infection:

PO primaquine:	15 mg primaquine base (26.3 mg salt) per day × 14 days

To Prevent Relapse in *P. vivax* or *P. ovale* Infection:

PO primaquine:‡	15 mg primaquine base (26.3 mg primaquine phosphate) daily × 14 days

*For areas without mefloquine resistance.
†Not yet available in the United States.
‡To prevent potentially severe hemolysis, patients should be tested for glucose-6-phosphate dehydrogenase deficiency prior to treatment with primaquine.

methamine-sulfadoxine, docycycline or clindamycin, or atovaquone plus proguanil or doxycycline (Table 421–3). For patients who cannot tolerate oral medications, potential strategies include IV quinidine, IV quinine, IM quinine, and IM artemether (which is reported to be effective without detectable neurologic toxicity, although it has not yet been approved by the FDA). The general principle of parenteral treatment is to stabilize patients until they can tolerate oral medications. In addition, oral regimens are now available for multiply resistant *P. falciparum.*

Patients with *P. vivax* or *P. ovale* infection should be tested for glucose-6-phosphate dehydrogenase deficiency before treatment with primaquine, which is used to eradicate persistent hypnozoites in the liver in order to prevent relapse.

PROGNOSIS

Virtually all patients with *P. vivax, P. ovale,* or *P. malariae* infection respond well to chloroquine and make an uneventful recovery. The chloroquine-resistant strains of *P. vivax* reported from Indonesia have thus far responded to treatment with either mefloquine or halofantrine. For patients with *P. falciparum* infection, the quantitative parasite count is the best predictor of the outcome. Patients with ≥5% parasitemia (≥250,000 parasites per microliter of blood) are at increased risk of severe and complicated malaria, including death. In addition to standard antimalarial treatment directed at the parasite (outlined above), such patients may require glucose for hypoglycemia, treatment of acidosis, dialysis for renal failure and respiratory support. The role of exchange transfusion is controversial, in part because there have been no controlled clinical trials. Finally, it should be clear that oral treatment (including nasogastric) treatment may be successful even in patients with severe or cerebral malaria.

Curtis CF: Impregnated bednets, malaria control and child mortality. Trop Med Intl Hlth 1:137, 1996. *Summary of recent bednet research, which suggests that their efficacy may decrease with increasing intensity of transmission.*
De D, Krogstad FM, Cogswell FB, Krogstad DJ: Aminoquinolines that circumvent resistance in *P. falciparum in vitro.* Am J Trop Med Hyg 55:579, 1996. *Alteration of the side chain produces 4-aminoquinolines active against chloroquine- and mefloquine-resistant P. falciparum.*
Horuk R, Chitnis CE, Darbonne WC, et al: A receptor for the malarial parasite *Plasmodium vivax:* The erythrocyte chemokine receptor. Science 261:1182, 1993. *Receptors for parasite entry into the red cell are part of the chemokine superfamily.*
Stoute JA, Sloui M, Heppner DG, et al: A preliminary evaluation of a recombinant circumsporozoite protein vaccine against *Plasmodium falciparum* malaria: RTS,S Malaria Vaccine Evaluation Group. N Engl J Med 336:86, 1997. *Promising preliminary results with a vaccine based on circumsporozoite protein.*
Su XZ, Heatwole VM, Wertheimer SP, et al: The large diverse gene family *var* encodes proteins involved in cytoadherence and antigenic variation of *Plasmodium falciparum*-infected erythrocytes. Cell 82:89, 1995. *This paper and others in the same issue describe the identification of molecules on the red cell surface that mediate cytoadherence to the microvascular endothelium.*
Su X-Z, Kirkman LA, Fujioka H, Wellems TE: Complex polymorphisms in a ~330 kDa protein are linked to chloroquine-resistant *Plasmodium falciparum* in Southeast Asia and Africa. Cell 91:591, 1997. *This recently identified molecule may be responsible for chloroquine resistance in P. falciparum.*

422 AFRICAN TRYPANOSOMIASIS (SLEEPING SICKNESS)

Thomas C. Quinn

DEFINITION

Known widely as sleeping sickness, African trypanosomiasis is an acute and chronic disease caused by *Trypanosoma brucei.* The parasites are transmitted to humans through the bite of tsetse flies located in 36 countries of Africa between 15 degrees north and 15 degrees south latitude. In humans, there are two distinct forms of the disease, East African trypanosomiasis caused by *T. brucei rhodesiense* and West African trypanosomiasis caused by *T. brucei gambiense.* Although there is some clinical overlap, East African trypanosomiasis primarily causes an acute febrile illness with myo-

carditis and meningoencephalitis that is rapidly fatal if not treated, whereas West African trypanosomiasis is characterized as a chronic debilitating disease with mental deterioration and physical wasting (Table 422–1). A closely related variant, *T. brucei brucei,* is non-infectious for humans, but causes a chronic wasting illness in cattle, called nagana, which has a considerable indirect effect on human nutrition in sub-Saharan Africa.

ETIOLOGY AND LIFECYCLE

Trypanosomes are motile hemoflagellates with a single undulating membrane that passes along the length of the parasite, terminating in an anterior flagellum (see Color Plate 8E). Located anteriorly is a kinetoplast, an organelle containing topologically interlocked circular DNA molecules and mitochondria. In the peripheral blood of humans, trypanosomes vary in length from 10 to 40 μm. Both short stumpy and long slender forms can be present in a patient at the same time. The different variants of *T. brucei* cannot be distinguished morphologically but can be identified by differences in pathogenicity for certain animals, as well as in biochemical requirements, electrophoretic pattern of component enzymes, and DNA hybridization.

T. brucei is transmitted by the tsetse fly *Glossina,* within which it undergoes several developmental changes. When biting an infected host, trypanosomes are ingested and within the insect midgut rapidly differentiate into procyclic forms with loss of their dense surface coat, composed of variant surface glycoprotein. After 2 to 3 weeks of multiplication within the midgut the procyclic trypanosomes migrate to the insect's salivary glands, where they change morphologically into epimastigotes. These forms further undergo multiplication and ultimately differentiate into metacyclic trypanosomes that are coated with characteristic variant surface glycoprotein and are infectious to mammalian hosts. When a new host is bitten by the tsetse fly, the trypanosomes present in the salivary glands are injected into the connective tissue and blood. Within the human host they divide by binary fission and undergo antigen variation, a process by which they continually change their variable surface glycoproteins (VSG) and evade the immune system of the host. With the bite of another tsetse fly, ingestion of the parasite occurs, and the life cycle of the organism is completed (Fig. 422–1). Mechanical transmission can theoretically also occur via blood transfusion or by interrupted biting of a tsetse fly feeding on an infectious person and directly thereafter biting an uninfected individual.

EPIDEMIOLOGY

It is estimated that African trypanosomiasis infects more than 40,000 Africans annually and that approximately 50 million people live at risk of acquiring trypanosomiasis because of the presence of the disease and its vector. Within recent years, there has been a resurgence in African trypanosomiasis, particularly in central African countries, due to decreased surveillance, prophylaxis, and treatment as a consequence of war and civil unrest. In some areas the prevalence of African trypanosomiasis has increased tenfold over the past decade. Approximately 4 million square miles in Africa remain unpopulated because of the presence of *T. brucei brucei* infection, which results in the loss of domestic and wild animals, including cattle, waterbuck, bushbuck, and buffalo.

T. b. gambiense occurs primarily in the west and central regions of sub-Saharan Africa. Although it primarily infects humans, there may be animal reservoirs, such as pigs, dogs, and sheep. Gambian sleeping sickness is spread mainly by three species of tsetse fly, *Glossina palpalis, G. tachinoides,* and *G. fuscipes.* Distribution of these flies includes shaded areas along rivers and streams, where the conditions of temperature, darkness, and moisture are optimum.

T. b. rhodesiense differs from *T. b. gambiense* in that it is primarily a parasite of wild game, with humans serving only as occasional hosts. The geographic distribution of *T. b. rhodesiense* is primarily East Africa from Ethiopia and eastern Uganda south to Zambia and Botswana. Rhodesian sleeping sickness is spread by tsetse flies of the *G. morsitans* group, including *G. pallidipes* and *G. swynnertoni.* These flies can survive in the open savanna, and

Table 422-1 ■ A COMPARISON OF GAMBIAN AND RHODESIAN SLEEPING SICKNESS

	GAMBIAN (WEST AFRICAN)	RHODESIAN (EAST AFRICAN)
Etiologic agent	*Trypanosoma brucei gambiense*	*Trypanosoma brucei rhodesiense*
Vector	*Glossina palpalis or tachinoides* (riverine tsetse)	*Glossina morsitans* (savanna tsetse)
Distribution	West and Central Africa	East Africa
Reservoir	Humans (domestic animals)	Wild game
Course of infection	Slow (months—years)	Rapid (<1 yr)
Clinical features		
Lymphadenopathy	++ (Winterbottom's sign)	±
Myocarditis, heart failure	–	++
Neurologic symptoms	++	+
Disseminated intravascular coagulation	–	+
Parasitemia	Low	High

Rhodesian sleeping sickness usually occurs among individuals visiting or traveling through an endemic area. Consequently, hunters, fishermen, and tourists are at risk, exposing themselves to vectors that usually feed on wild animals.

Imported African trypanosomiasis is a rare disease. Most cases were due to *T. b. rhodesiense* acquired by Americans who had been on safari in East Africa for a very brief period. Nearly all of these cases were initially misdiagnosed because of the unfamiliarity of United States physicians with this disease. With an increase in international travel, 20,000 Americans are now estimated to visit endemic areas yearly, and approximately 10,000 aliens enter the United States each year from countries in Africa where the infection is endemic.

PATHOGENESIS AND PATHOLOGY

Following the bite of the tsetse fly, trypanosomes accumulate in the connective tissue, where they multiply to produce a local chancre (trypanoma). The organisms subsequently spread through the lymphatics, resulting in enlargement of lymph nodes secondary to reactive plasma cell and macrophage infiltration. The trypanosomes eventually disseminate to the circulatory system, where the parasitemia usually remains at low intensity and the organisms multiply by binary fission. Systemic African trypanosomiasis without central nervous system (CNS) involvement is generally referred to as stage I disease.

The host immune response plays an integral role in the pathogenesis of African sleeping sickness, although the exact nature of the immunopathogenic reactions has not been clearly defined. Trypanosomes survive by periodically altering their surface antigenic coat, avoiding successful eradication by the host. Any single parasite may contain some 1000 genes for VSG which can be activated in a variety of ways and selected by the host-antibody response. Consequently trypanosomes occur in the peripheral blood of infected individuals in waves, with each parasite wave consisting of a serologically distinct organism.

Tissue damage is induced by either toxin production or immune complex reaction with release of proteolytic enzymes. Immune complexes consisting of variant antigens of the organism and complement-fixing antibodies have been demonstrated in both the circulation and the target organs of infected patients. The production of autoantibodies is a prominent feature, and they are frequently directed against antigen components of red cells, brain, and heart. Thus the host-parasite interaction can result in generalized febrile episodes, lymphadenopathy, and myocardial and pericardial inflammation, along with anemia, thrombocytopenia, disseminated intravascular coagulation, and renal disease primarily during the acute stage of the disease.

Stage II of human African trypanosomiasis involves invasion of the CNS, which occurs during the period of circulatory dissemination when trypanosomes localize in the small vessels of the CNS. Pathologic changes in the CNS are most prominent in chronic cases of Gambian sleeping sickness. The meninges are thickened and infiltrated with lymphocytes, plasma cells, and morular cells. Morular cells are modified plasma cells (up to 20 mm in diameter) with large granular inclusions that have been shown to consist of immunoglobulin. These cells may play an important role in the local production of immunoglobulin M (IgM) in the cerebrospinal fluid (CSF). Edema, hemorrhages, and granulomatous lesions are frequently present, along with thrombosis as a result of endarteritis and with neuronal degeneration.

African trypanosomes appear to induce a state of B cell polyclonal activation caused either by interference with host T cell control of antibody production or by a B cell mitogen released by the parasite. Polyclonal hypergammaglobulinemia, with very high levels of IgM, is commonly seen. High levels of nonspecific heterophile antibody, rheumatoid factor, and autoantibodies are also produced. In patients with late-stage *T. b. gambiense*, circulating levels of tumor necrosis factor-α and interleukin-10 are markedly elevated, which decline following effective treatment.

CLINICAL FEATURES

The signs and symptoms of sleeping sickness differ according to the infecting organism (Table 422–1). Rhodesian sleeping sickness, due to *T. b. rhodesiense,* causes a rapid progressive disease often resulting in cardiac failure and acute neurologic manifestations. Gambian sleeping sickness, caused by *T. b. gambiense,* is typically a more chronic illness with primarily neurologic features. However, this difference is not absolute; in some cases Gambian sleeping sickness can progress rapidly, and occasionally Rhodesian sleeping sickness may follow a more chronic course.

Gambian Sleeping Sickness

Within several days following the bite by an infected tsetse fly, a trypanosomal nodule or chancre develops, typically on the exposed parts of the body. Within a week the lesion becomes a hard, painful nodule surrounded by erythema and swelling, which persists for 1 to 2 weeks. After this incubation period, clinical features develop after systemic, lymphatic, and circulatory invasion of the trypanosomes. Fever, headache, dizziness, and weakness occur in the majority of these patients. Febrile episodes may last 1 to 6 days, alternating with afebrile periods. Lymphadenopathy with prominent supraclavicular and posterior cervical enlargement is seen in > 80% of infected individuals. Known as Winterbottom's sign, these enlarged lymph nodes are usually discrete, rubbery, and painless. Moderate splenomegaly may occur, and urticaria and erythematous rashes have also been observed. Electrocardiograms are often abnormal, but clinical signs of heart disease are unusual.

Six months to several years after symptoms first appear, the clinical features of this early hemolymphatic stage progress to a late meningoencephalitic stage. Behavioral and personality changes are often the first signs of CNS involvement. Later, more florid psychological changes may occur, with hallucinations and delusions. Reversion of sleep rhythm is characteristic, with drowsiness during the day, a feature from which the disease derives its name. Other nervous symptoms include tremor, most characteristically of the face and lips, and hyperesthesia, causing some patients to avoid common practices such as closing (Kerandel's sign) or locking doors (key sign). Without treatment, the patient's level of consciousness progressively deteriorates until there is lapse into stupor. Alterations in thermoregulation may lead to hypothermia or hyperthermia, and progressive neurologic alterations lead to convulsions, chorea, and athetosis. Adrenal insufficiency, hypothyroidism, and hypogonadism are frequently observed, and pituitary function tests suggest an unusual combined central (hypothalamic/pituitary) and peripheral defect in hormone secretion. The CSF shows an increase in cells and protein, much of which is IgM. Free immunoglobulin light chains may be present. Most of the cells are lymphocytes, but a few are plasma cells and morula cells. Trypanosomes may also be evident within the CSF.

Rhodesian Sleeping Sickness

This disease is more acute than Gambian sleeping sickness, and symptoms usually occur a few days after the victim has been bitten by the tsetse fly. Alternating periods of high fever, malaise, and headache, followed by several days of well-being, are often misinterpreted as acute malaria infection. Lymphadenopathy is not prominent in this variety of the disease, and Winterbottom's sign is usually absent. Tachycardia with arrhythmias and extrasystoles is common. Anemia, thrombocytopenia, and disseminated intravascular coagulation are usually evident within the first several weeks of infection. Liver enzyme values are often elevated, and electrocardiograms are abnormal, usually reflecting underlying myocarditis. Neurologic features are similar to those described for Gambian sleeping sickness, but they occur much earlier and with more rapid deterioration. Without treatment the disease may result in death within a matter of weeks to months, without clear distinction into an early and late phase, as described for Gambian trypanosomias.

DIAGNOSIS

Although a presumptive diagnosis of trypanosomiasis is based on clinical suspicion, history of travel to areas where this disease is endemic, and tsetse fly exposure, confirmation of the diagnosis is based solely on the demonstration of trypanosomes. These organisms may be found in the blood (see Color Plate 10*E*), bone marrow, centrifuged CSF, lymph node aspirates, and scrapings from the chancre. Giemsa or Wright's stain of the buffy coat of centrifuged heparinized blood makes identification easier because the trypanosomes are often concentrated in the buffy coat. In one technique, referred to as the quantitative buffy coat (QBC), 60 μL of blood obtained by a fingerprick is drawn up in a glass hematocrit tube precoated with acridine orange and anticoagulate. Following centrifugation, the buffy coat can be examined and trypanosomes fluoresce greenish yellow, remain motile, and are easily identified. In patients with Gambian sleeping sickness, in which trypanosomes are found less frequently in the blood, concentration methods such as anion exchange chromatography, diethylaminoe-

thyl (DEAE) filtration, culture, or animal inoculation should be used.

All patients should have a lumbar puncture prior to and following therapy to determine whether CNS involvement is present. Documentation of CNS involvement is imperative because suramin, drug effective against the hemolymphatic stage of *T. brucei*, does not penetrate the spinal fluid. CNS disease is manifested by pleocytosis (>5 PMNs/mL) and elevation of spinal fluid total protein and IgM levels. Trypanosomes can be found in most patients, provided that the CSF is examined immediately after collection and that clean glassware is used. For those patients in whom trypanosomes cannot be found, measuring the CSF IgM is often of great diagnostic help. A high CSF IgM value and a modest increase in total protein are almost pathognomonic of sleeping sickness.

Several immunodiagnostic tests have been developed for African trypanosomiasis, including an indirect hemagglutination test, indirect fluorescent antibody test, and enzyme-linked immunosorbent assay (ELISA), which are useful for epidemiologic surveys. A card agglutination trypanosome test (CATT) with prefixed trypanosomes is frequently used for rapid serodiagnosis. Although very sensitive, CATT may remain positive for several years after successful treatment, thereby decreasing its ability to differentiate between acute infection and a previous, treated infection.

TREATMENT

Suramin* is the drug of choice for the early hemolymphatic stage of both *T. b. gambiense* and *T. b. rhodesiense* infections before CNS invasion has occurred. Suramin does not cross the blood-brain barrier in increased amounts, and it does not cure the disease once CNS invasion has occurred. The dose is 20 mg per kilogram of body weight given intravenously up to a maximum single dose of 1 gram. Suramin is freshly prepared as a 10% aqueous solution. Intramuscular injection is not advised because of local irritation and pain. Suramin binds to plasma proteins and may persist in the circulation at low concentrations for as long as 3 months. A test dose of 200 mg is given initially; if no adverse side effects are noted, then full doses of the drug may be given on days 1, 3, 7, 14, and 21. A single course for an adult is usually 5 grams; it should not exceed 7 grams.

Suramin is a toxic drug that may result in idiosyncratic reactions in some individuals (1 in 20,000). The drug is excreted entirely by the kidneys; renal damage may result because the drug is deposited in the renal tubules. The urine should be examined before administering each dose of suramin, and if proteinuria or casts are present, treatment should be stopped. Other side effects include a papular eruption, photophobia, arthralgias, peripheral neuritis, fever, and agranulocytosis.

Pentamidine isethionate* is an alternative drug for treating early hemolymphatic African trypanosomiasis, but it is much less active against *T. rhodesiense* than is suramin. The dose is 4 mg per kilogram of body weight; it is given every other day by intramuscular injection for a total of 10 injections. Pentamidine is also ineffective for treating CNS trypanosomiasis.

The arsenical melarsoprol* (Mel B) is the treatment of choice for both Gambian and Rhodesian sleeping sickness once involvement of the CNS has occurred. The drug is given in three courses of 3 days each. The recommended dosage is 2.0 to 3.6 mg per kilogram per day given intravenously in three divided doses for 3 days, followed 1 week later by 3.6 mg per kilogram per day in three divided doses for 3 days. This latter course is then repeated 10 to 21 days later. Melarsoprol is a highly toxic drug and should be administered with great care. If signs of arsenical toxicity occur, the drug should be discontinued.

The most important side effects involve the CNS. A reactive encephalopathy, probably due to release of trypanosomal antigens, may occur early in the course of treatment, and its incidence has been reported to be as high as 18%. It may develop very rapidly or insidiously, and its mortality is about 50%. Clinical indications of reactive encephalopathy include high fever, headache, tremor, seizures, and finally coma. It has been suggested that corticosteroids

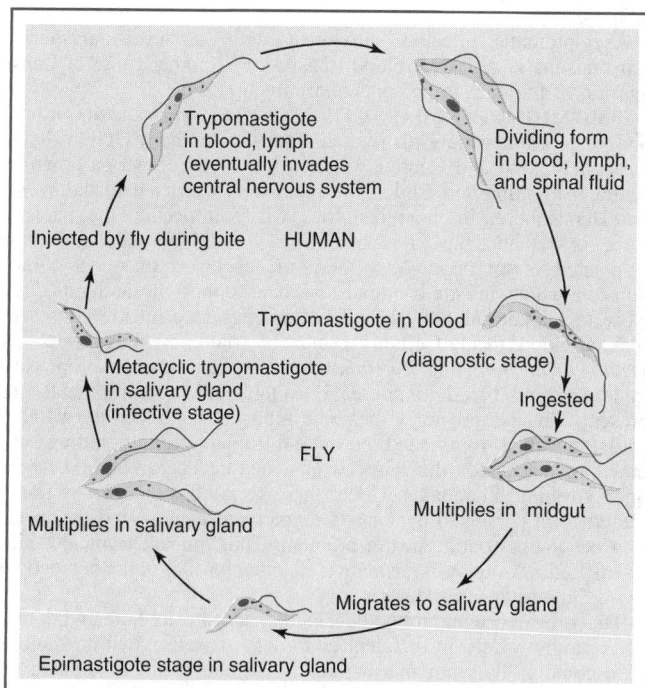

FIGURE 422–1 ■ Life cycle of *Trypanosoma (Trypanozoon) brucei, T. (T.) b. gambiense,* and *T. (T.) b. rhodesiense.*

*Available from the Centers for Disease Control and Prevention, Atlanta, GA.

protect patients from melarsoprol encephalopathy, but this assertion has not been clearly documented. An alternative drug for both systemic and CNS involvement includes difluoromethylornithine (eflornithine, DFMO), a specific, irreversible inhibitor of orboxylase. In one large trial of 207 patients with late-stage *T. b. gambiense* sleeping sickness, eflornithine was highly effective in successful treatment of both hemolymphatic and CNS stages of infection. Eflornithine dramatically reduced symptoms and rapidly cleared parasites from blood and CSF, even in those patients who had relapsed after melarsoprol therapy. The recommended dosage is 400 mg per kilogram per day given intravenously in four divided doses for 2 weeks, followed by 300 mg per kilogram per day given orally in four doses for 30 days. Frequent side effects include diarrhea and anemia. Unfortunately, its efficacy in *T. b. rhodesiense* has been quite variable, and its cost and long duration of therapy have limited its usefulness in the field. In addition, immunocompromised patients such as those with HIV infection do not respond to treatment as effectively with any of the above agents because a normal immune response is necessary for a cure. Regular follow-up with clinical examination of a lumbar puncture is necessary for all patients for at least a year after treatment.

PROGNOSIS

Untreated African sleeping sickness is almost invariably fatal. Many patients with early Gambian sleeping sickness may remain relatively well for months to years without treatment, but once CNS involvement has occurred, death is inevitable unless treatment is given. Death frequently results from pneumonia in Gambian sleeping sickness and from heart failure in Rhodesian sleeping sickness. Treatment with suramin in the early phase of sleeping sickness results in a cure rate of >90%. A few patients may subsequently develop CNS involvement and require further treatment. Mel B achieves a parasitologic cure in at least 90% of cases of advanced disease, and many patients may recover completely. Unfortunately, some patients are left with irreversible neurologic damage. Approximately 5% of patients may die during the course of Mel B therapy.

CONTROL AND PROPHYLAXIS

Measures to prevent and control African trypanosomiasis can be instituted at three different levels: surveillance and treatment, chemoprophylaxis, and vector control. Surveillance with treatment is necessary to reduce the human reservoir of infection, particularly in areas where epidemics have occurred in the past. Pentamidine has been successfully used as a chemoprophylactic in Gambian sleeping sickness following mass screening and treatment of seropositive and trypanosomal positive individuals regardless of symptoms. Pentamidine is given as a single intramuscular injection of 4 mg per kilogram every 3 to 6 months. However, the drug is generally not recommended for mass use, and it appears to be ineffective against Rhodesian trypanosomiasis.

Vector control requires destruction of tsetse fly habitats by selective clearing of vegetation and spraying with insecticides, which are effective only temporarily. Because of the wide range of the tsetse fly, these vector control measures are not economically feasible except when it is necessary to break transmission in epidemics. For individual protection, avoidance of contact with infected tsetse flies is best achieved by the use of repellents and protective clothing.

A vaccine is not currently available because of the occurrence of antigenic variation. However, the potential for development of a vaccine has increased with the progress in cultivation of *T. brucei* in vitro and analysis of the chemical structure of its variant antigens.

Doua F, Miezan TW, Sanon Singaro JR, et al: The efficacy of pentamidine in the treatment of early-late stage *Trypanosoma brucei gambiense* trypanosomiasis. Am J Trop Med Hyg 55:586, 1996. *This paper describes the treatment of 58 patients infected with* Trypanosoma brucei gambiense *with pentamidine with a cure rate of 94%, which was comparable to treatment with melarsoprol or eflornithine.*

Ekwanzala M, Pepin J, Khonde N, et al: In the heart of darkness: Sleeping sickness in Zaire. Lancet 48:1427, 1996. *An excellent report demonstrating the resurgence of African trypanosomiasis in central Africa as a result of the deterioration in surveillance, prophylaxis, and treatment of trypanosomiasis due to the consequences of war, civil strife, and movement of refugee populations.*

Pepin J, Milord F, Khonde AN, et al: Risk factors for encephalopathy and mortality during melarsoprol treatment of *T.b. gambiense* sleeping sickness. Trans Royal Soc Trop Med Hyg 89:92, 1995. *This paper reviews the incidence of and risk factors for drug-induced encephalopathy and mortality during treatment with melarsoprol of 1083 patients with* T. b. gambiense *sleeping sickness between 1983 and 1990.*

423 AMERICAN TRYPANOSOMIASIS (CHAGAS' DISEASE)

Franklin A. Neva

DEFINITION. Chagas' disease, resulting from infection with the protozoan parasite *Trypanosoma cruzi,* is named after the Brazilian physician Carlos Chagas, who discovered the parasite. Distinction should be made between infection by the parasite (i.e., positive serologic result only) and presence of clinical disease. Chronic disease manifestations develop years after initial infection in the form of chronic cardiomyopathy with conduction defects or with dysfunction of the esophagus or colon (mega syndromes).

LIFE CYCLE OF THE CAUSATIVE AGENT. The causative agent, *T. cruzi,* is usually transmitted as a zoonosis. Various species of blood-sucking reduviid bugs become infected when they take a blood-meal from animals or humans who have circulating parasites, trypomastigotes, in the blood. The ingested parasites transform into epimastogotes and multiply in the midgut of the insect vector, where they later transform once again into metacyclic trypomastigotes in the hindgut of the bug. When the infected bug takes a subsequent blood meal, it frequently defecates during or after feeding, so that the infective metacyclic forms are deposited on the skin. Transmission to a second vertebrate host occurs when the feeding puncture site or a mucous membrane is inadvertently contaminated with infective bug feces. The parasites can penetrate a variety of host cell types, within which they transform into intracellular amastigote forms. In contrast to certain other intracellular organisms, amastigotes of *T. cruzi* are not enclosed in phagolysosomes. They multiply in the cytoplasm, elongate, transform into motile trypomastigotes, and rupture out of the cells. Liberated organisms penetrate new cells or are carried into the blood stream to initiate further cycles of multiplication, preferentially in muscle cells, or are ingested by new vectors to maintain the cycle (Fig. 423–1).

Asymptomatic infected individuals with low-level parasitemia can transmit *T. cruzi* via blood transfusion. Another route of transmission of the parasite is congenital infection.

EPIDEMIOLOGIC CHARACTERISTICS. *T. cruzi* and its arthropod vectors are widely distributed from the southern United States through Mexico and Central America into South America down to central Argentina and Chile. The parasite is restricted to the Western Hemisphere. In most countries where it occurs, the parasite cycle is sylvatic; i.e., it takes place in wild animals and their associated vector bugs. A peridomestic cycle occurs under conditions in which infected animals, such as opossums and rats, live close to human habitations, and vector bugs may invade houses to seek a blood meal. Certain species of triatomine bugs, such as *Triatoma infestans* and *Rhodnius prolixus,* have a great propensity to invade and breed in houses if suitable microenvironments are present. Cracks and holes in adobe mud huts or in crude wooden walls, thatched roofs, and household rubble provide hiding and breeding places for the bugs, which venture out at night to feed upon sleeping inhabitants. Under these conditions *T. cruzi* is transmitted from person to person—a domiciliary cycle—and the infection becomes a public health problem. Thus, human trypanosomiasis in Latin America is primarily an infection of rural poor people living in substandard housing.

The prevalence of antibodies to the parasite in human populations varies widely in different countries, as well as within regions of a country. It is not unusual for up to half of all inhabitants in selected villages to be antibody-positive. But, since 1984 the overall prevalence of seropositivity in Brazil, for example, has decreased greatly from about 4 per cent to less than 0.5 per cent.

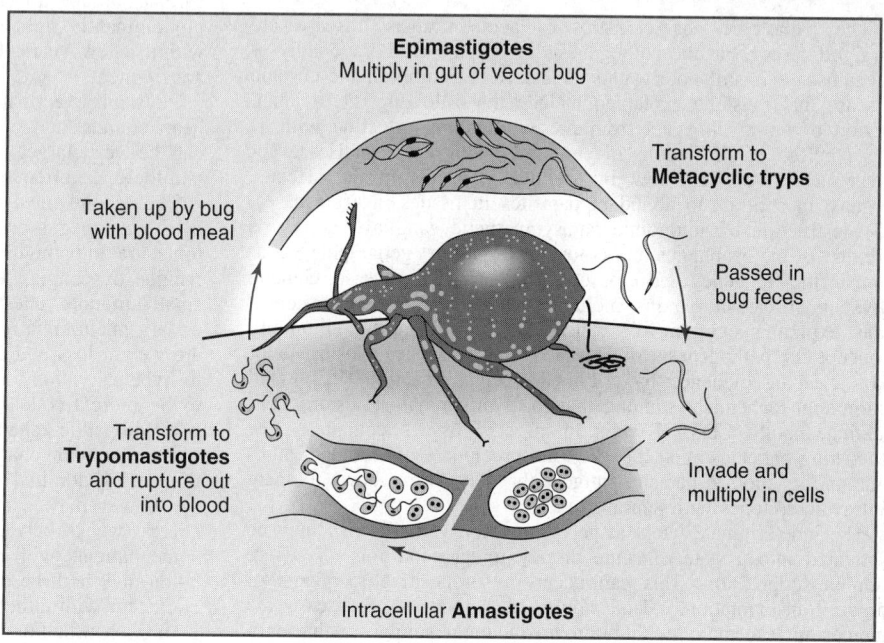

Epimastigotes
Multiply in gut of vector bug

Transform to
Metacyclic tryps

Taken up by bug
with blood meal

Passed in
bug feces

Transform to
Trypomastigotes
and rupture out
into blood

Invade and
multiply in cells

Intracellular **Amastigotes**

FIGURE 423–1 ■ Life cycle of *Trypanosoma cruzi.*

Countries with the highest incidence of both infection and disease due to *T. cruzi* include Brazil, Argentina, Chile, Bolivia, and Venezuela. It is estimated that in all of the Americas a total of 15 million people are infected. In many Latin American countries, positive serologic findings for *T. cruzi* constitute a social stigma; a lower socioeconomic background is implied, and employers are reluctant to hire someone who may later have chronic Chagas' disease.

Considerable geographic variation exists in both the prevalence and the type of chronic disease manifestations. In Brazil, for example, cardiomyopathy and megadisease are common, and often a patient has both types of involvement. However, chagasic megaesophagus and megacolon are virtually unknown in Venezuela, Colombia, and Panama, whereas cardiomyopathy is relatively high, moderate, and low in prevalence, respectively. In general, the frequency of cardiac disease in Central America and Mexico in seropositive persons is low, even though rates of seropositivity may be substantial. Also in these countries heart disease tends to develop later in life than in Brazil, Bolivia, or Argentina.

The situation regarding Chagas' disease in the United States is interesting because only four autochthonous acute cases have been recognized despite the presence of *T. cruzi* in vector bugs as well as in animal reservoirs. The lack of transmission of *T. cruzi* to humans in this country is probably due to preference of the vectors for sylvatic habitats and their tendency to defecate late after feeding. Yet in some areas of the West, bites from aggressive and abundant reduviid bugs can be a source of annoyance to, and allergic reactions in, suburbanites and outdoorspeople. Because of increased Hispanic immigration in recent years, sporadic cases of chronic Chagas' disease are encountered in the United States.

PATHOLOGIC FEATURES AND PATHOGENESIS. A local inflammatory lesion called a *chagoma* may develop at the site of entry of the parasite. Histologically, the chagoma shows mononuclear cell infiltration, interstitial edema, and intracellular aggregates of amastigotes in cells of the subcutaneous tissue and muscle. Biopsy specimens from enlarged lymph nodes show hyperplasia, and amastigotes may be present in reticular cells. Skeletal muscle tissue from muscle biopsy specimens has shown organisms and focal inflammation. In acute cases that have a fatal outcome there is invariably myocarditis with an enlarged heart. Microscopically, degeneration of cardiac muscle fibers and prominent but patchy areas of inflammation with nests of amastigotes in the muscles are observed. The brain and meninges may also be parasitized in acute Chagas' disease. Virtually all organs and cell types can be invaded by *T. cruzi.*

The organs primarily affected in *chronic Chagas' disease* are the heart and hollow viscera, especially the esophagus and colon. Sur-

prisingly, the intracellular *T. cruzi* usually cannot be found in the affected organs, or a few may be demonstrable after protracted search of many tissue sections. The heart in those patients with chronic disease who die suddenly, presumably of ventricular arrhythmias or heart block, may be normal in size or only moderately enlarged. Other patients with chronic chagasic cardiomyopathy experience cardiomegaly and die of intractable failure. The hearts are both hypertrophied and dilated, with thinning, especially at the apex to form a characteristic apical aneurysm. Mural thrombi, with subsequent embolization of the lungs and peripheral organs, are frequently seen. The coronary arteries are generally normal.

Microscopic findings in the heart are not specific, consisting of focal mononuclear cell infiltrates, hypertrophy of cardiac fibers with patchy areas of necrosis, variable fibrosis, and edema. The components of the conduction system of the heart most often involved by inflammatory changes are the sinoatrial and atrioventricular nodes, as well as the right branch and left anterior branches of the bundle of His. Andrade's detailed studies of these pathologic changes, indicated that they correlated well with electrocardiographic (ECG) changes during life, but were diffusely scattered without specific localization to the conducting system.

When either the esophagus or the colon is affected in chronic Chagas' disease, the gross appearance is of dilatation and hypertrophy of the affected organ. The microscopic pathologic changes are disappointingly similar to those in the heart, again with no or very few organisms. However, myenteric ganglion cells are strikingly reduced in number. This type of parasympathetic denervation may also be found in other hollow viscera, such as duodenum, ureters, or biliary tree.

The significant pathologic characteristic of *congenital Chagas' disease* is chronic placentitis, with inflammatory changes and focal necrosis in the chorionic villi. Amastigotes of *T. cruzi* are present in the lesions. The presence of lesions and organisms in the placenta may be associated with abortion, stillbirth, or acute disease in the fetus. However, pregnancy may result in a normal fetus, even though placental lesions are present.

Individuals with antibodies to *T. cruzi,* but without evidence of clinical disease are considered to represent the *indeterminate* form. Some of these patient maintain a low-level parasitemia demonstrable only with very sensitive techniques. So, one point of view is that indeterminate cases have a smouldering disease process that will become evident later. However, there are no tests that can predict whether or when evidence of chronic disease will develop. Even in those areas where chronic disease is common, one half or more of those with positive serologic findings will die of causes other than Chagas' disease. In countries of lower endemicity the risk of chronic disease is correspondingly less.

The pathologic characteristics of acute Chagas' disease are straightforward, but the pathogenesis of chronic cardiomyopathy or megadisease is still poorly understood. Key features of the chronic disease that must be explained include the following: (1) a latent period of up to 20 years from presumed initial infection with *T. cruzi* before manifestations of cardiomyopathy or megadisease appear; (2) no or very few intracellular parasites in the affected organs, in contrast to abundant parasites in tissues in acute cases; (3) destruction of autonomic parasympathetic ganglia (Auerbach's plexus) of the esophagus and colon; and (4) great geographic variation in the frequency and type of chronic Chagas' disease. Genetic diversity in parasite strains, including variation in animal virulence, may explain geographic differences in disease. The autoimmunity concept for pathogenesis of chronic disease has been losing favor to increasing evidence by polymerase chain reaction (PCR) and immunohistochemical staining that focal inflammatory lesions containing mainly CD8+ T cells in affected tissues contain a few persisting parasites. Yet, this does not preclude a concomitant autoimmune reaction to parasite antigens that have been shown to share antigenic epitopes with neural tissues.

The indeterminate latent stage of infection with *T. cruzi* may be activated into a state of acute disease under conditions of severe immunosuppression. This can occur in seropositive recipients of organ transplantation. Also, reports of activation of disease are increasing, especially with brain involvement similar to that produced by *Toxoplasma* sp., in patients with acquired immunodeficiency syndrome (AIDS) who also have latent *T. cruzi* infection.

CLINICAL PRESENTATION. In endemic areas, first exposure to *T. cruzi* generally is subclinical and unnoticed. When those initially exposed do have clinical manifestations, the disease is an acute systemic infection. Chronic Chagas' disease, in contrast, evolves as a later sequela with specific organ involvement and no systemic features.

ACUTE CHAGAS' DISEASE. Although acute Chagas' disease is most commonly seen in children in endemic areas, it can occur at any age, depending upon epidemiologic circumstances. The incubation period under natural conditions cannot be established accurately but is probably at least a week. A local area of erythema and induration (chagoma) may develop in the skin at the site of parasite entry. When infection takes place via the conjunctival route, as it frequently does, the local periorbital swelling is referred to as Romaña's sign. The chagoma is often accompanied by regional adenopathy and persists for several weeks. Other signs of acute Chagas' disease include fever, generalized lymphadenopathy, hepatosplenomegaly, and transient skin rashes.

Myocarditis, accompanied by tachycardia and non-specific ECG changes, can occur in the acute stage. Meningoencephalitis is another serious complication, particularly in very young patients. The fact that trypanosomes may be found in the spinal fluid of some acute cases who show no obvious meningeal signs helps explain the frequent involvement of the brain in latent infections activated by HIV/AIDS. Fatal outcome in acute Chagas' disease is rare, but when it does occur, it is due to myocarditis and congestive failure or to meningoencephalitis.

Signs and symptoms of acute disease gradually subside within a few weeks to several months even without treatment. Trypanosomes, which have been demonstrable by direct microscopy in the peripheral blood during the acute phase, become more difficult to find and then disappear. The patient then enters the *indeterminate phase*. This state of apparent complete recovery with positive serologic findings may continue indefinitely without further evidence of disease or sequelae. However, a variable proportion of indeterminate cases, years to a decade or more later, will develop signs and symptoms of chronic Chagas' disease. Except for epidemiologic experience from a particular geographic region, there are no laboratory or clinical indicators to predict the likelihood of future chronic disease.

CHRONIC CHAGAS' DISEASE. Cardiac signs and symptoms are the most common manifestations of chronic disease and are likely to begin with palpitations, dizziness, precordial discomfort, and even syncope. These reflect a variety of arrhythmias, including ventricular extrasystoles, bouts of tachycardia, and various degrees of heart block. Sudden death due to ventricular tachycardia in an otherwise healthy young adult is not unusual. Symptoms due to arrhythmias

may be present for a long time before cardiomegaly or evidence of cardiac failure appears. When congestive failure develops, it is predominantly right sided and is likely to lead to a fatal outcome within a few years. Peripheral emboli to the brain or other organs are frequent.

Physical examination reveals only an irregular pulse, distant heart sounds, and perhaps a gallop rhythm. With failure, the heart can be very large, functional regurgitant murmurs may be heard, and there are often congestive hepatomegaly and peripheral edema.

The second most common chronic manifestation is megadisease of the esophagus or colon, most frequently the former. The symptoms are indistinguishable from those of idiopathic achalasia and include dysphagia, feeling of fullness after eating or drinking only small amounts, chest pain, and regurgitation. Aspiration with secondary pneumonia is a common complication in advanced cases, as are weight loss and cachexia. Salivary gland hypertrophy secondary to hypersalivation is sometimes seen. Esophageal cancer is reported to be more frequent in patients with chagasic megaesophagus, as with idiopathic achalasia.

Patients with chagasic megacolon suffer from chronic constipation and abdominal pain. Volvulus, obstruction, and perforation of the bowel may occur. An astonishing history of an interval of several weeks between bowel movements has been obtained from some patients with severe megacolon. Megaesophagus and megacolon may both be present in the same patient, and cardiomyopathy can occur with either form of megadisease.

DIAGNOSIS. For both acute and chronic Chagas' disease, a history of possible exposure to *T. cruzi* should be sought. Usual tourist travel to endemic areas is not likely to provide sufficient exposure to infected vectors. Blood transfusion from a chronically infected donor can be a source of infection.

For *acute Chagas' disease* direct microscopic examination of anticoagulated blood or a buffy coat preparation for motile trypanosomes is the most important procedure. Organisms are more difficult to find on stained thin or thick blood films, but the morphologic features of organisms seen on direct microscopy should be confirmed in a stained preparation. Red cells may be lysed, using 0.083% NH_4Cl to concentrate parasites by centrifugation. If parasites cannot be found in the peripheral blood and acute disease is still suspected, blood can be cultured on Novy, MacNeal, and Nicolle's medium (NNN) or other suitable media. Inoculation of mice with the patient's blood may sometimes result in recovery of the parasite. Biopsy of an enlarged lymph node or of skeletal muscle for culture and/or histologic examination is another possibility.

A time-honored, labor-intensive, but very sensitive technique for recovering trypanosomes from the blood is a procedure referred to as *xenodiagnosis*. It is basically a form of blood culture using the insect vector, by allowing up to 40 normal, laboratory-reared reduviid bugs to feed directly upon the patient or on the patient's blood through a membrane. Circulating parasites ingested by the bugs multiply in the gut and can be detected when the intestinal contents are examined 30 days later. PCR detection of *T. cruzi* DNA will likely replace other methods in terms of sensitivity and convenience.

Serologic testing is generally not needed to diagnose acute disease. Parasite-specific immunoglobulin M (IgM) antibodies detected by immunofluorescence or direct agglutination do not become positive until 20 to 40 days after the onset of symptoms. In certain situations this delayed antibody response permits the demonstration of seroconversion. Other laboratory tests often show non-specific changes, such as a lymphocytic leukocytosis, elevated sedimentation rate, or transient ECG abnormalities. Reversible cardiomegaly and even pericardial effusion may occur.

The diagnosis of *chronic Chagas' disease* requires demonstration of antibodies to *T. cruzi* in the presence of the characteristic cardiac abnormalities and/or megadisease. Thus, except for the positive serologic findings, the diagnosis relies heavily upon clinical judgment in excluding other causes of heart disease or gastrointestinal dysfunction. A positive xenodiagnosis or PCR reaction is strongly supportive, but not in itself diagnostic of chronic disease, since patients in the indeterminate phase may have low-level parasitemia. A variety of assays for specific antibody are available, and generally the results of different tests are comparable. However, there are cross-reactions in some tests with sera from patients with leishmaniasis or syphilis, for example. Therefore, in individual

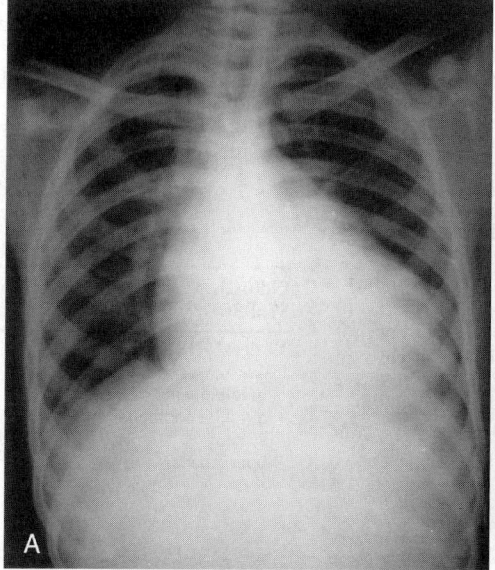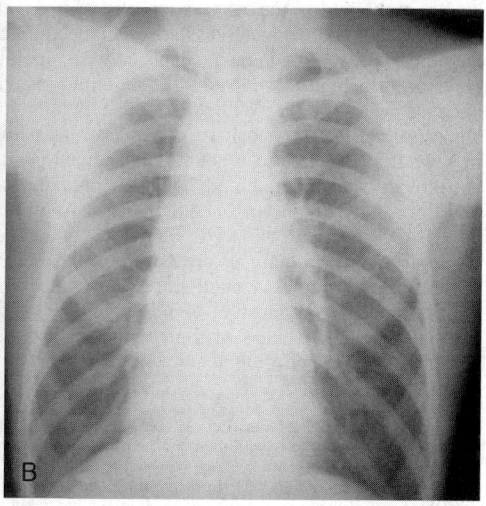

FIGURE 423-2 ■ *A*. Cardiac silhouette in a patient with chronic chagasic cardiomyopathy and heart failure. *B*. Chest radiograph showing a widened mediastinum due to a greatly dilated megaesophagus of chronic Chagas' disease.

cases it may be helpful to confirm the presence of antibody to specific antigens of *T. cruzi* with more sophisticated tests, such as immunoblots.

Symptomatic heart involvement in the chronic disease is manifested by characteristic ECG abnormalities, often without cardiomegaly. The most common of these is complete right bundle branch block. Other frequent ECG findings are left anterior hemiblock, ventricular extrasystoles, and even complete heart block. If heart failure is present, the findings of radiographs and echocardiograms will show generalized cardiomegaly with a reduced ejection fraction (Fig. 423–2).

Chagasic megaesophagus in the early stages shows only delayed emptying and minimal dilatation on studies after a barium swallow. With more advanced disease, retention of swallowed material and esophageal dilatation are progressively increased. Manometric studies show spasm of the esophageal sphincter and uncoordinated peristaltic movements. Endoscopy should be performed to rule out malignant disease. However, all of these findings are indistinguishable from these of idiopathic achalasia. Barium enema with air contrast shows the dilated colon with impaired peristalsis, but other causes of colonic obstruction must be ruled out.

DIFFERENTIAL DIAGNOSIS. When acute Chagas' disease is symptomatic and severe, it can resemble a variety of acute systemic infections. Romaña's sign must be distinguished from other causes of unilateral orbital edema, such as the reaction to an insect bite, trauma, or orbital cellulitis.

Congenital infections are virtually indistinguishable from congenital toxoplasmosis, cytomegalic inclusion disease, and syphilis.

Various cardiomyopathies, such as postpartum, alcoholic, and endomyocardial fibrosis, can resemble chronic Chagas' heart disease. Routine endomyocardial biopsy is of limited diagnostic value. However, a substantial yield of PCR-positive biopsy specimens have been reported when the procedure is guided by imaging techniques to sites of myocardial inflammation. The characteristic heart murmurs of rheumatic valvular disease are helpful in differentiating this entity from chagasic cardiomyopathy. The value of positive serologic findings for *T. cruzi* in the differential diagnosis of both heart disease and megadisease will depend upon the background prevalence of antibodies in the general population.

TREATMENT. Two drugs with reasonable antitrypanosomal activity are currently in use for treating Chagas' disease. One of these is a nitrofuran derivative, nifurtimox*, which has been extensively evaluated. Nifurtimox is the only drug available in the United States for treating Chagas' disease; it is used in a dose of 8 to 10 mg/kg/day. The second drug, benznidazole, is a nitroimidazole derivative that appears to be equal to nifurtimox in efficacy,

*An investigational drug that must be obtained from the Centers for Disease Control and Prevention Drug Service (404-639-3670).

although there is less experience with its use. The exact mechanism of antitrypanosomal action of both of these drugs is not known.

There is now considerable evidence that if patients with acute Chagas' disease are treated with either nifurtimox or benznidazole, the extent of disease and parasitemia usually are reduced. But more important, in many patients treated in the acute phase antibodies to *T. cruzi* never develop or do so only transiently. From this observation, plus the fact that xenodiagnosis in such treated patients often has negative findings, it is assumed that parasites can be eliminated and the patient cured if treated in the acute stage. However, nifurtimox is not uniformly effective in producing these results, and parasite strains from certain geographic areas (Brazil) appear to be less responsive to treatment than do strains from other countries (Argentina and Chile).

The frequency of side effects from both nifurtimox and benznidazole is high; because they are administered for 60 to 90 days, drug toxicity is a serious problem. The most common adverse effect with nifurtimox is gastrointestinal intolerance, with anorexia, nausea, vomiting, and abdominal pain. Neurologic symptoms include restlessness, insomnia, disorientation, paresthesias, polyneuritis, and even seizures. Skin rashes can also occur. Peripheral neuropathy and bone marrow suppression have been reported with benznidazole. These side effects subside when the dosage of the drugs is reduced or treatment is stopped.

Since these drugs have shown effectiveness in treatment of acute Chagas' disease, some Latin American physicians are also treating chronic and indeterminate cases. There is no evidence that the established pathologic changes of chronic Chagas' disease can be reversed by nifurtimox or benznidazole therapy. The question of whether drug treatment in the indeterminate case, i.e., the asymptomatic patient with positive serologic findings, would prevent development of later chronic disease is controversial. Some data suggest that low-level parasitemia, as assessed by xenodiagnosis, can be reduced or eliminated after treatment with antitrypanosomal drugs, including allopurinol. But such studies require critical confirmation to establish their ultimate influence on the development of chronic disease, as well as risk versus benefit evaluation.

The treatment of patients with established chronic heart disease is supportive. Patients with frequent ventricular premature beats can benefit from antiarrhythmic drugs such as amiodarone. Cardiac pacemakers will prolong survival of those with complete heart block. The congestive failure of chagasic cardiomyopathy is disappointingly refractory to the usual cardiotropic drugs.

More options are open for managing and treating megadisease. In the early stages of megaesophagus, pneumatic dilation of the sphincter is probably more effective than bougienage. For more advanced cases, various surgical procedures involving myotomy of the sphincter or partial resection are necessary. Early stages of megacolon can be managed by manipulating diet and using laxatives and occasional enemas. Sometimes an aperistaltic section of the colon can be resected in more severe cases.

PREVENTION. Chagas' disease could be eliminated as a serious health problem for the rural poor of Latin America by adequate housing and education. But stark socioeconomic realities dictate another approach to control. This consists mainly of the use of residual insecticides directed at domiciliary vectors, and sprayed once or twice a year. With this measure, plus screening in blood banks to exclude seropositive donors, the transmission of *T. cruzi* in several south American countries has been greatly reduced.

Serologic testing in blood banks to prevent use of seropositive donors is carried out in endemic areas. Another precaution is to add 1:4000 gentian violet to blood 24 hours before use to kill trypanosomes that may be present. With the recent occurrence of several transfusion-associated cases of acute Chagas' disease in North America, the question of serologic screening of blood donors has been raised for areas of the country with large Latin American populations. The development of vaccines is still in the research stage.

De Lourdes Higuchi M, Martins Reis M, DeMarchi Aiello V, et al: Association of an increase in CD8+ T cells with the presence of *T. cruzi* antigens in chronic, human, chagasic myocarditis. Am J Trop Med Hyg 56:485, 1997. *One of the papers supporting the concept that persisting parasites and parasite antigens that provoke a CD8+ T-cell response are important factors in chronic disease.*

Kirchhoff LV: American trypanosomiasis (Chagas' disease): A tropical disease now in the United States. N Engl J Med 329:639, 1993. *A concise "Current Concepts" review of the subject, including potential problems for blood banks and health care providers dealing with immigrant populations.*

Rocha A, deMeneses ACO, daSilva AM, et al: Pathology of patients with Chagas' disease and acquired immunodeficiency syndrome. Am J Trop Med Hyg 50:261, 1994. *A review of 23 patients, 20 of whom had severe, multifocal meningoencephalitis; Chagas' disease was activated by AIDS.*

Viotti R, Vigliano C, Armenti H, et al: Treatment of chronic Chagas disease with benznidazole: Clinical and serologic evolution of patients with long-term follow up. Am Heart J 127:151,1994. *A study that indicates that treatment of indeterminate cases can prevent development of chronic disease: an important contribution if it can be confirmed by others.*

424 LEISHMANIASIS

Richard D. Pearson
Anastacio de Queiroz Sousa

Leishmaniasis comprises a spectrum of clinical disease produced by *Leishmania* species. They are endemic in scattered areas on every continent except Australia and Antarctica. *Leishmania* spp. reside within mononuclear phagocytes in humans and other mammals. Transmission requires an infected animal or human reservoir, a competent sandfly vector, and a susceptible host. The clinical manifestations of infection vary as a function of parasites' pathogenicity, which differs among *Leishmania* species, and the genetically defined cell-mediated immune responses of the human host. Some leishmanial infections are asymptomatic and self-resolving. Others are limited to the skin, resulting in cutaneous leishmaniasis, or affect the mucosa of the nose, mouth, or oral pharynx, resulting in mucosal leishmaniasis. In visceral leishmaniasis parasites disseminate to mononuclear phagocytes throughout the reticuloendothelial system.

An estimated 350 million people worldwide live in areas where there is a risk of infection. The incidence of cutaneous disease is estimated to be 1.0 to 1.5 million cases a year, and the incidence of visceral leishmaniasis is estimated to be 500,000 cases per year. Major epidemics of visceral leishmaniasis have occurred in eastern India and Bangladesh, among refugees in the Sudan, and in urban areas of northeastern Brazil. Visceral leishmaniasis has emerged as an important opportunistic infection among persons with human immunodeficiency virus (HIV) infection in Southern Europe. Cutaneous leishmaniasis poses a substantial risk for settlers, residents, military personnel, and expatriates working or traveling in endemic areas. Mucosal leishmaniasis is an important problem in Brazil and other Latin American countries.

CLASSIFICATION AND LIFE CYCLE

The *Leishmania* species that produce human disease, their geographic locations, and the clinical syndromes that they produce are summarized in Table 424–1. Although there are slight ultrastructural differences, they cannot be used to differentiate one *Leishmania* species from another. Isoenzyme analysis is used at World Health Organization reference laboratories for speciation. Species-specific monoclonal antibodies and DNA probes are also available.

Table 424–1 ■ GEOGRAPHIC DISTRIBUTION AND CLINICAL SYNDROMES CAUSED BY *LEISHMANIA* SPECIES

CLINICAL SYNDROMES	LEISHMANIA SPECIES	LOCATION
Visceral leishmaniasis		
Kala-azar: generalized involvement of the reticuloendothelial system (spleen, bone marrow, liver, etc.)	*L. donovani*	Indian subcontinent, North and East China, Pakistan, Nepal
	L. infantum	Middle East, Mediterranean littoral, Balkans, Central and Southwest Asia, North and northwestern China, North and sub-Saharan Africa
	L. donovani (archibaldi)	Sudan, Kenya, Ethiopia
	Leishmania species	Kenya, Ethiopia, Somalia
	L. chagasi	Latin America
	L. amazonensis	Brazil (Bahia State)
	L. tropica	Israel, India, and "viscerotropic" disease in Saudi Arabia (U.S. troops)
Post–kala-azar dermal leishmaniasis	*L. donovani*	Indian subcontinent
	Leishmania species	Kenya, Ethiopia, Somalia
Old World cutaneous leishmaniasis		
Single or limited number of skin lesions	*L. major*	Middle East, Northwest China, Northwest India, Pakistan, Africa
	L. tropica	Mediterranean littoral, Middle East, western Asiatic area, Indian subcontinent, Kenya
	L. aethiopica	Ethiopian highlands, Kenya, Yemen
	L. infantum	Mediterranean basin
	L. donovani (archibaldi)	Sudan, East Africa
	Leishmania species	Kenya, Ethiopia, Somalia
Diffuse cutaneous leishmaniasis	*L. aethiopica*	Ethiopian highlands, Kenya, Yemen
New World cutaneous leishmaniasis		
Single or limited number of skin lesions	*L. mexicana* (chiclero ulcer)	Central America, Mexico, Texas
	L. amazonensis	Amazon basin including Brazil and neighboring countries
	L. braziliensis	Multiple areas of Central and South America
	L. guyanensis (forest yaws)	Guyana, Surinam, northern Amazon basin
	L. peruviana (uta)	Peru (western Andes), Argentinean highlands
	L. panamensis	Panama, Costa Rica, Colombia
	L. pifanoi	Venezuela
	L. garnhami	Venezuela
	L. venezuelensis	Venezuela
	L. chagasi	Central and South America
Diffuse cutaneous leishmaniasis	*L. amazonensis*	Amazon basin, neighboring areas, Bahia and other states in Brazil
	L. pifanoi	Venezuela
	L. mexicana	Mexico, Central America
	Leishmania species	Dominican Republic
Mucosal leishmaniasis	*L. braziliensis* (Espundia)	Multiple areas in Latin America

Adapted from Pearson RD, Sousa AQ: Clinical spectrum of leishmaniosis. Clin Infect Dis 22:1, 1996. Data from Lainson R, Shaw JJ: Evolution, classification and geographic distribution. *In* Peters W, Killick-Kendrick R (eds.): The Leishmaniases in Biology and Medicine, vol. 1. University of Chicago, publisher.

Polymerase chain reaction (PCR)–based assays are being developed and may emerge as the method of choice for diagnosis and speciation in the future. Refinement of the current classification system is also likely.

The life cycle is depicted in Figure 424–1. In humans and other mammals leishmania organisms are found within mononuclear phagocytes as intracellular amastigotes that are oval or round in shape and 2 to 3 μm in diameter. They have a relatively large, eccentrically placed nucleus; an internalized flagellum; and a rod-shaped specialized mitochondrial structure, the kinetoplast. Amastigotes are adapted to mammalian temperature and multiply in the acid environment of phagolysosomes in macrophages.

Female sandflies, *Lutzomyia* species in Latin America and *Phlebotomus* species in the rest of the world, serve as vectors. Some are peridomestic and live in rubble and debris near houses or farm buildings; others thrive in thick vegetation in forest areas. Sandflies are modified pool feeders. They ingest amastigote-containing macrophages when they take a blood meal. Rodents, dogs, or occasion-

ally other animals serve as reservoirs for some *Leishmania* species, and humans are the reservoir for others.

Leishmania convert to flagellated, extracellular promastigotes in the gut of the sandfly. Promastigotes are 15 to 26 μm in length and 2 to 3 μm in width. They multiply at ambient temperatures of 22° C to 26° C. They differentiate through multiple steps to become infectious metacyclic promastigotes that migrate to the proboscis and are inoculated when the sandfly attempts to take its next blood meal. Promastigotes are ingested by macrophages in the skin and convert to amastigotes within them. Sandfly saliva contains a factor(s) that enhances promastigote infectivity.

IMMUNOLOGIC CHARACTERISTICS

The outcome of leishmanial infection depends on genetically determined cell-mediated immune responses. Antileishmanial anti-

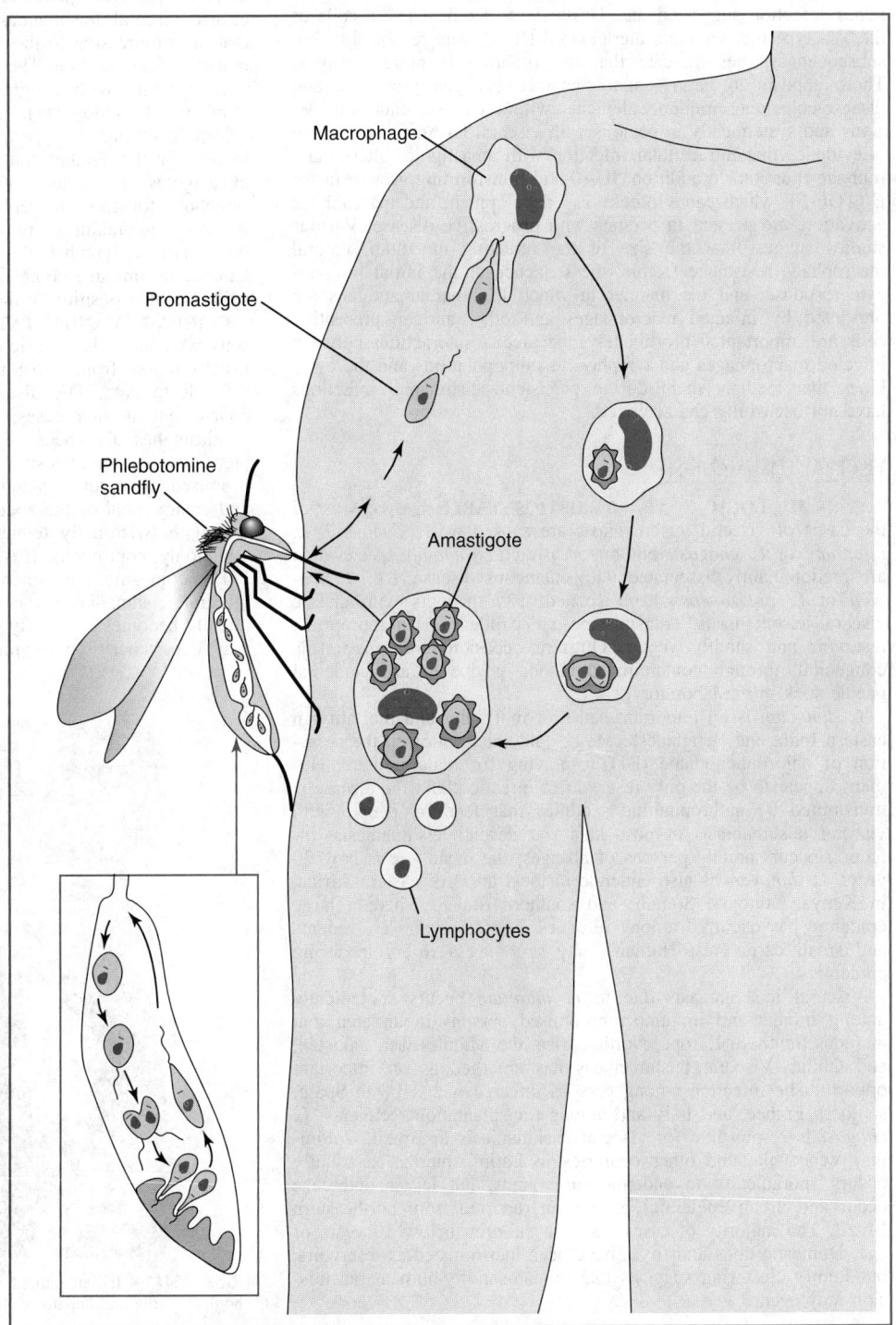

FIGURE 424–1 ■ Life cycle of leishmania. Humans serve as the reservoir for *L. donovani* in India as depicted here. In most settings leishmaniasis is a zoonosis with rodents or canines as reservoirs.

bodies are produced, but they are not protective. Animal models and humans with leishmaniasis have been extensively studied in an attempt to identify the cell populations and cytokines involved. There is evidence for both protective and disease-enhancing responses. Resolution of infection and protection against reinfection correlate with the expansion of CD4 T cells of the T helper 1 T_H1 type (see Chapter 270) that secrete interferon γ and interleukin 2 (IL-2) in response to leishmanial antigens. Interferon γ or direct contact with leishmania-specific CD4 T cells activates macrophages to inhibit and kill intracellular parasites. L-arginine-dependent production of nitric oxide following induction of nitric oxide synthase appears to be the dominant effector mechanism. Interleukin 12 (IL-12) and tumor necrosis factor-α (TNF-α) play important roles in the initiation and maintenance of protective immune responses.

Data from animal models and humans suggest that the development of protective immune responses is inhibited locally in chronic skin lesions and systemically in persons with progressive visceral leishmaniasis. Early studies in a murine model of visceralizing *L. major* infection suggested that *Leishmania*-specific CD4 T cells of the T_H2 type that secreted interleukin 4 (IL-4) were responsible, but subsequent studies indicate that the situation is more complex. There appears to be a tenuous balance between protective and disease-enhancing immune elements within chronic cutaneous lesions and systemically in persons with visceral leishmaniasis. There is evidence that intracellular infection with amastigotes alters macrophage function. In addition, IL-10 and transforming growth factor β (TGF-β), which can suppress T_H1 development and macrophage activation, are present in persons with progressive disease. Various studies suggest that the size of the infecting inoculum, natural macrophage resistance factors, the sequence of the initial lymphocyte response, and the manner in which leishmanial antigens are presented by infected macrophages and other antigen presenting cells are important. Unfortunately, the precise interactions between infected macrophages and lymphocyte subpopulations and the cytokines that mediate them during persistent leishmanial infections have not been fully characterized.

VISCERAL LEISHMANIASIS

EPIDEMIOLOGIC CHARACTERISTICS (TABLE 424–1). Most of the cases of visceral leishmaniasis are caused by *L. donovani, L. infantum,* or *L. chagast,* but on occasion *Leishmania* species that are predominantly associated with cutaneous disease, e.g., *L. tropica* or *L. amazonensis,* are isolated from patients with classic visceral leishmaniasis. Transmission is dependent on an appropriate reservoir and sandfly vector. On rare occasions transmission is congenital, through contaminated blood, or due to an accidental needle stick in the laboratory.

L. donovani is an important cause of morbidity and mortality in eastern India and Bangladesh. Major epidemics followed the cessation of chlorophenothane (DDT) spraying for malaria there. Humans appear to be the only reservoir of infection, and the disease is transmitted by anthropophilic sandflies that feed on people with visceral leishmaniasis or post–kala-azar dermal leishmaniasis. Infection occurs among persons of all ages; the mean age is now 20 years. *L. donovani* is also endemic in focal areas of eastern Africa, in Kenya, Ethiopia, Somali, and southern Sudan, where a large epidemic has occurred among refugees. The reservoirs are rodents and small carnivores. Humans may serve as a reservoir during epidemics.

Visceral leishmaniasis due to *L. infantum* occurs sporadically among infants and immunocompromised persons in an area that includes Southern Europe, North Africa, the Middle East, Pakistan, and China. Visceral leishmaniasis has emerged as an important opportunistic infection among persons infected with HIV in Spain, southern France, and Italy and among transplantation recipients. *L. chagasi* is responsible for visceral leishmaniasis in Brazil, Colombia, Venezuela, and other countries in Latin America. It usually occurs sporadically in endemic rural areas, but larger outbreaks occur and urban epidemics have been reported from northeastern Brazil. The majority of cases occur in children below 10 years of age. Domestic dogs and foxes have been incriminated as reservoirs, but family clustering suggests that human-sandfly-human transmission may occur.

In addition, a small group of American troops who were in Saudi Arabia during the Persian Gulf War in 1991 experienced a viscerotropic syndrome due to *L. tropica,* a species that is usually associated with cutaneous disease. They presented with visceral dissemination but lacked many of the manifestations of classical progressive visceral leishmaniasis.

PATHOPHYSIOLOGIC CHARACTERISTICS. Infection with *L. donovani* and related organisms is acquired when promastigotes are inoculated by sandflies into an exposed area of skin. The parasites convert to amastigotes and multiply within mononuclear phagocytes. Although a cutaneous nodule or ulcer may develop, most patients are unaware of the site of primary inoculation. Amastigotes subsequently disseminate via regional lymphatics and the vascular system to mononuclear phagocytes throughout the reticuloendothelial system. The majority of infections are asymptomatic and resolve spontaneously. A minority progress to classic, full-blown visceral leishmaniasis, known in many areas as kala-azar. A subset of children infected with *L. chagasi* in Brazil has been reported to have a prolonged course with minimal symptoms; in some the infection resolves spontaneously whereas in others it progresses to classic visceral leishmaniasis. The ratio of *L. chagasi* infections that are progressive to those that resolve spontaneously is approximately 1:6 in children. The ratio is lower among adults.

In patients with progressive visceral leishmaniasis, increased numbers of mononuclear phagocytes are found in the liver and spleen, resulting in hypertrophy. In the liver there is a dramatic increase in the number and size of Kupffer's cells, many filled with amastigotes. The spleen often is massively enlarged, and splenic lymphoid follicles are replaced by parasitized mononuclear cells. Amastigote-containing mononuclear phagocytes are found in the bone marrow, lymph nodes, skin, intestinal tract, and other organs. Circulating immune complexes are common, and there is histologic evidence of deposition in the kidney, but renal failure is rare.

CLINICAL MANIFESTATIONS. The incubation period for persons who have the classic clinical syndrome is quite variable but usually ranges from 2 to 8 months. The onset is often insidious and difficult to date. The disease usually has a subacute or chronic course, but in some cases, there is an abrupt onset. Visceral leishmaniasis has also been reported in former residents of endemic areas, years after exposure, when they have become immunocompromised. Symptoms include fever, malaise, anorexia, weight loss, and enlargement of the abdomen. Fever may be intermittent, remittent with twice-daily temperature spikes to 38 to 40° C, or less commonly, continuous. It is usually well tolerated.

Hepatomegaly and splenomegaly are hallmarks of progressive visceral leishmaniasis; the spleen is firm and non-tender and frequently becomes massively enlarged (Fig. 424–2). Patients in India may experience hyperpigmentation, which led to the name *kala-*

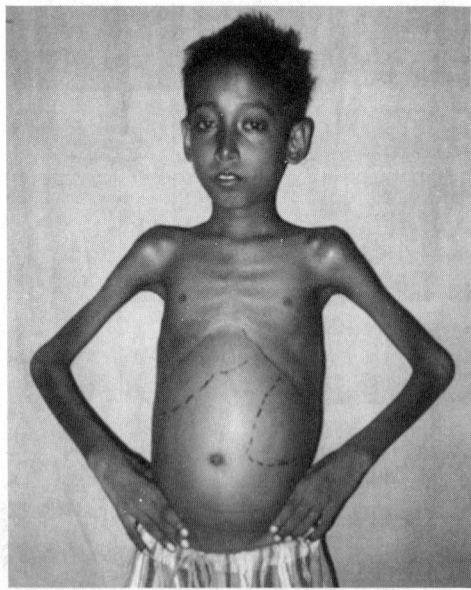

FIGURE 424–2 ■ Indian patient with kala-azar. Note wasting of thorax and shoulder girdle and hepatosplenomegaly as outlined.

azar, meaning "black fever" in Hindi. Jaundice is occasionally present. Late in visceral leishmaniasis patients may have epistaxis, gingival bleeding, and petechiae on their extremities. They may have edema and ascites due to hypoalbuminemia.

On laboratory examination, anemia, thrombocytopenia, neutropenia, and hypergammaglobulinemia are common findings. The anemia is usually normocytic and normochromic unless complicated by blood loss. The white blood count may be as low as 1000 per cubic millimeter; eosinopenia is common. Platelet numbers are also decreased. The erythrocyte sedimentation rate is elevated. The levels of gamma globulin are markedly increased, at times in the range of 9 to 10 grams per deciliter. This is a result of polyclonal B-cell activation. Circulating immune complexes and rheumatoid factors are present in the majority of patients. Levels of liver enzymes and bilirubin are elevated in some.

Untreated persons with visceral leishmaniasis typically have a progressive, downhill course over several months. Severe cachexia may develop. Patients with advanced visceral leishmaniasis evidence neutropenia as well as anergy to multiple T-cell antigens. Bacterial pneumonia, measles, dysentery, tuberculosis, gangrenous stomatitis, and other secondary infections are common and frequently lead to death. The death rate in developing areas approaches 10% even with appropriate antileishmanial chemotherapy.

VISCERAL LEISHMANIASIS IN PERSONS WITH HIV. The majority of persons with visceral leishmaniasis and concurrent HIV infection present in the classic manner, but splenomegaly may be absent, and atypical presentations with involvement of the lungs, pleura, oral mucosa, esophagus, stomach, small intestine, or skin may occur. Several patients have presented with aplastic anemia. Asymptomatic leishmanial infections have also been reported.

VISCEROTROPIC LEISHMANIASIS. In the *L. tropica*–related "viscerotropic" syndrome observed in American military personnel who served in Operation Desert Storm, symptoms included chronic low-grade fever, malaise, fatigue, and, in some instances, diarrhea. The troops did not experience massive splenomegaly or the progressive wasting associated with classic visceral leishmaniasis.

POST–KALA-AZAR DERMAL LEISHMANIASIS. A small percentage of persons in India and Africa who are treated for visceral leishmaniasis develop post–kala-azar dermal leishmaniasis after the other manifestations of disease have resolved. In Africa the lesions appear shortly after treatment and persist for several months. In India they appear up to 2 years after treatment and persist for months to as long as 20 years. The skin lesions vary from hyperpigmented macules to frank nodules and contain *L. donovani* amastigotes. They are frequently found on the face, trunk, and extremities and may be confused with leprosy.

DIAGNOSIS. A presumptive diagnosis of visceral leishmaniasis is easily made by the classic clinical presentation in an endemic area. The diagnosis may be delayed or missed in an immigrant or traveler returning to a nonendemic country, particularly if the person has concurrent HIV infection and lacks splenomegaly. The diagnosis is confirmed by identifying *Leishmania* species amastigotes in tissue or by growing promastigotes in culture. Splenic aspiration results in a diagnosis in 96 to 98% of cases. It is relatively safe when performed by an experienced physician, but significant hemorrhage can occur, particularly in patients with clotting abnormalities. Bone marrow aspiration for examination and culture results in a diagnosis in more than half of the cases. Alternative sites for aspiration and/or biopsy include the liver and lymph nodes if they are enlarged, or culture of the buffy coat. PCR-based assays applied to blood, bone marrow, or other samples appear promising, but they are not yet widely available. In patients with concurrent HIV infections amastigotes are frequently identified in unexpected sites such as bronchoalveolar lavage fluid, pleural effusions, or biopsy specimens of lesions in the oral pharynx, larynx, stomach, or intestine.

Antileishmanial antibodies are present in high titer in immunocompetent patients with visceral leishmaniasis. They can be measured by enzyme-linked immunosorbent assays (ELISAs), indirect immunofluorescence assays, direct agglutination tests, or several alternative assays. Persons with advanced HIV and those with viscerotropic *L. tropica* infections frequently have low or undetectable levels of antileishmanial antibodies. The leishmanin skin test, also known as the Montenegro test, yields negative findings in persons with visceral leishmaniasis, but the result becomes positive in the majority of those who undergo successful chemotherapy and in those with self-revolving infections. The antigen preparation is not approved for use in the United States.

CUTANEOUS AND MUCOSAL LEISHMANIASIS

EPIDEMIOLOGIC CHARACTERISTICS (SEE TABLE 424–1). *Leishmania* species produce a spectrum of cutaneous disease. Most common are chronic, localized, ulcerative lesions, often referred to as "oriental sores" (see Color Plate 9F). In the Americas cutaneous leishmaniasis is caused by *L. mexicana, L. amazonensis, L. braziliensis, L. panamensis, L. guyanensis, L. peruviana,* and several other species including *L. chagasi*. Except for *L. peruviana* and *L. chagasi,* which infect dogs and other canines, the reservoirs are forest rodents. The vectors are ground dwelling or arboreal sandflies. Humans become infected when they live in or enter endemic forested areas for work, recreation, or military activities. *L. mexicana* is found in focal areas extending from Texas to Argentina. *L. braziliensis* is endemic throughout Latin America and produces mucosal disease in a small subset of those infected.

Most cases of cutaneous leishmaniasis outside Latin America are caused by three *Leishmania* species. *L. major* is an important problem among settlers, visitors, and troops in endemic rural areas of the Middle East, Central Asia, and North Africa. Rodents are the principal reservoir. *L. tropica* is usually found in urban areas of the Middle East, the Mediterranean littoral, India, Pakistan, and Central Asia. The reservoirs are dogs and humans. *L. aethiopica* is endemic in Ethiopia, Kenya, and southwest Africa, where hyrax are reservoirs. On occasion *L. donovani* or *L. infantum* causes cutaneous lesions.

PATHOPHYSIOLOGIC CHARACTERISTICS. A cutaneous lesion develops at the site where promastigotes are inoculated by sandflies. Amastigote-infected macrophages are the predominant histologic finding early in infection. Over time, a granulomatous response develops with increasing numbers of lymphocytes, decreasing numbers of parasites, and necrosis of the skin resulting in ulceration. Peripheral blood mononuclear cells from persons with typical cutaneous leishmaniasis proliferate and produce interferon γ in response to leishmanial antigens in vitro, and patients evidence delayed-type hypersensitivity responses in vivo. In the lesion there seems to be a stalemate between protective and suppressive elements of the immune response. Eventually T_H1 cells dominate and the lesion heals, leaving an atrophic scar.

The spectrum of cutaneous leishmaniasis includes several variants. On one extreme is diffuse cutaneous leishmaniasis, a relatively infrequent, anergic condition characterized by disseminated nodular skin lesions composed of large numbers of amastigote-infected macrophages. These lesions do not ulcerate, protective T_H1 responses do not develop, and the syndrome persists indefinitely. On the other extreme are the chronic, destructive, granulomatous lesions observed in patients with mucosal leishmaniasis. Amastigotes are usually scant. There is evidence of a vigorous T_H1-like response, but the lesions persist. The clinical spectrum of cutaneous leishmaniasis is similar to that of leprosy, but there are differences at the pathophysiologic level.

CLINICAL MANIFESTATIONS. CUTANEOUS LEISHMANIASIS. Cutaneous leishmaniasis may involve single or multiple lesions. They are relatively heterogeneous and vary as a function of the infecting *Leishmania* species and the host's immune response. They are usually found on exposed areas of the skin. A typical lesion starts as an erythematous papule at the site where promastigotes are inoculated by a sandfly, slowly increases in size, becomes a nodule, and eventually ulcerates. "Wet" lesions are covered with exudate and have raised borders (see Color Plate 9G). They are frequently associated with superficial, secondary bacterial or fungal infections. Other lesions are "dry" with a central crust. Satellite lesions may be found at or near the edges of the primary site of infection.

Cutaneous lesions persist for months and in some cases years before they spontaneously heal, leaving flat, hypopigmented, atrophic scars. On occasion cutaneous leishmaniasis may appear nodular, suggesting skin cancer, or involve local lymphatics, mimicking sporotrichosis. Secondary bacterial or fungal infections may complicate lesions. Disseminated cutaneous leishmaniasis has been reported in a few persons. Some were apparently immunocompetent; others had the acquired immunodeficiency syndrome (AIDS).

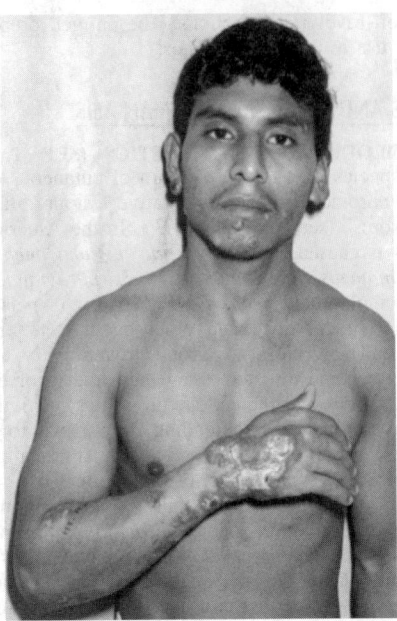

FIGURE 424–3 ■ Patient with diffuse cutaneous leishmaniasis of 5 years' duration. Note nonulcerative lesions of chin, ear lobes, right arm, and hand.

It was once thought that cutaneous leishmaniasis was confined to the skin, but recent observations in Brazil indicate that *L. braziliensis* can cause regional lymphadenopathy, fever, and other constitutional symptoms before the primary cutaneous lesion becomes apparent. These findings resolve as the skin ulcer develops. Splenomegaly occurs in some patients. It is thought that *L. braziliensis* may disseminate to distant mucosal sites during this early phase of infection.

DIFFUSE CUTANEOUS LEISHMANIASIS. Diffuse cutaneous leishmaniasis is a rare anergic variant. It starts as a localized papule that does not ulcerate, and satellite lesions develop as amastigotes disseminate in the skin (Fig. 424–3). Multiple cutaneous nodules develop on the face and extremities. The disease progresses slowly and may persist for decades.

LEISHMANIASIS RECIDIVA. Leishmaniasis recidiva, typically associated with *L. tropica* infection in the Middle East, is a chronic syndrome with skin lesions on the face or exposed extremities that enlarge slowly, tend to heal in the center, and persist for many years. Biopsy findings of the lesions reveal chronic inflammatory changes; amastigotes are sparse.

MUCOSAL LEISHMANIASIS (ESPUNDIA). A small percentage of persons with *L. braziliensis* infection in Latin America develop mucosal lesions of the nose, mouth, pharynx, or larynx months to years after the primary skin ulcer heals (see Color Plate 9*G*). The disease typically begins with nasal inflammation and stuffiness, followed by ulceration of the mucosa. The lesions are characterized by a chronic granulomatous response. There is destruction of the mucosa and eventually of the underlying cartilage of the nasal septum or palate. Mucosal involvement is also occasionally observed in persons with visceral leishmaniasis, particularly those with concurrent human immunodeficiency virus (HIV) infection or post–kala-azar dermal leishmaniasis, and those who have leishmaniasis recidiva with contiguous extension. The differential diagnosis of American mucosal leishmaniasis includes paracoccidioidomycosis, histoplasmosis, tertiary syphilis, tertiary yaws, sarcoidosis, Wegener's granulomatosis, angiocentric T-cell lymphoma, rhinoscleroma, and basal cell carcinoma.

DIAGNOSIS. The diagnosis of cutaneous leishmaniasis should be considered in any person with a chronic, localized skin lesion who has been exposed in an endemic area. It is confirmed by identifying amastigotes in tissue or by growing promastigotes in culture. A punch biopsy and aspirate should be obtained from the margin of the lesion after it has been meticulously cleaned. Touch preparations are stained with a Wright-Giemsa preparation. The remaining tissue should be divided and used for culture and histopathologic analysis. Species-specific PCR-based diagnostic assays are under development. Antileishmanial antibodies may be detectable in the serum of some patients with cutaneous leishmaniasis, but the titers are usually low. The leishmanin skin test result is positive in persons with simple cutaneous leishmaniasis, leishmaniasis recidiva, and mucosal leishmaniasis, but the test yields no reaction in patients with diffuse cutaneous leishmaniasis.

Parasites are often scant in mucosal lesions due to *L. braziliensis*. A positive leishmanin skin test, presence of antileishmanial antibodies, history of exposure in an endemic area, and evidence of a healed cutaneous lesion allow for a presumptive diagnosis.

TREATMENT

VISCERAL LEISHMANIASIS. Pentavalent antimonials, stibogluconate sodium (Pentostam) and meglumine antimoniate (Glucantime), have been the mainstays of therapy for visceral leishmaniasis. They are still used in many countries, but therapeutic failures are increasingly recognized in some areas, and they are associated with important untoward effects. Amphotericin B and pentamidine have been effective, but toxic alternatives. Recent reports indicate that short-course therapy with liposomal amphotericin B or lipid-complexed amphotericin B is effective and generally well tolerated. Liposome-encapsulated amphotericin B recently became the first drug licensed for the treatment of visceral leishmaniasis in the United States. It is likely to emerge as the treatment of choice.

Stibogluconate sodium is available in the United States through the Centers for Disease Control and Prevention (CDC) Drug Service. It is also used in Europe, Africa, and India. Meglumine antimoniate is available in Latin America, France, and francophone countries in Africa.

Stibogluconate sodium and meglumine antimoniate are administered on the basis of their pentavalent antimony content. When properly manufactured and stored, they appear to be of comparable efficacy and toxicity. The recommended treatment course of pentavalent antimony is 20 mg/kg body weight/day for 20 to 28 days. A prolonged course is frequently used in patients who do not respond to the initial course of therapy.

Chemical pancreatitis is common in patients receiving pentavalent antimonials. Other side effects include pain at the injection site when the drug is given intramuscularly, arthralgias, myalgias, nausea, vomiting, liver enzyme abnormalities, leukopenia, and ST-T wave changes indicated by electrocardiography. Cardiac toxicity and sudden death have occurred in patients who received more than the recommended dose.

Amphotericin B and pentamidine are alternative drugs, but both have important side effects (see Chapter 393). Amphotericin B (0.5 to 1.0 mg/kg daily or every other day for up to 8 weeks) has been used successfully to treat patients with visceral leishmaniasis. Lipid-encapsulated amphotericin B, 3.0 mg/kg body weight/day on days 1 through 5, 14, and 21 for immunocompetent persons, is also effective and is much better tolerated. A higher dose and longer duration are recommended for immunocompromised patients. Lipid-associated amphotericin is theoretically attractive because the drug is delivered to macrophages, the sanctuary of leishmania. Recombinant interferon γ with pentavalent antimony has proved effective in the treatment of patients with visceral leishmaniasis when antimony therapy alone failed. Failures have been reported when interferon γ was used as a single agent.

Unfortunately, some patients relapse after therapy with pentavalent antimony or other drugs, most within the first few months. Relapses are particularly common in patients with AIDS, and secondary prophylaxis with pentavalent antimony or an alternative regimen should be considered for them.

CUTANEOUS LEISHMANIASIS. Cutaneous lesions that are large or located in cosmetically important sites and those that are caused by *L. braziliensis* or other *Leishmania* species associated with mucosal disease should be treated. Small, inconspicuous, or healing lesions caused by *Leishmania* species that are not associated with mucosal disease can be followed expectantly. Pentavalent antimonials, stibogluconate sodium and meglumine antimoniate, effectively treat cutaneous leishmaniasis in many situations, but, as described, they are frequently associated with toxicity and clinical failures occur. They are common in persons infected with *L. aethiopica*. Full doses of 20 mg/kg body weight/day are recommended for 20 days; lower doses may favor the development of antimony resistance. Cutaneous lesions heal slowly during antimony therapy.

A number of other drugs and therapeutic approaches, including immunotherapy with killed promastigotes and bacille Calmette-Guérin (BCG), or local treatment of lesions, have been studied. A topical formulation of paromomycin sulfate, methylbenzethonium chloride, and white paraffin has been used successfully against *L. major*. The injection of pentavalent antimony into cutaneous lesions is effective in some patients. Oral itraconazole or ketoconazole has been effective in some persons infected with *L. mexicana*, but failures have been common in those with *L. braziliensis*.

Therapeutic failures and relapses are common among persons with diffuse cutaneous leishmaniasis or mucosal leishmaniasis who are treated with pentavalent antimony. Amphotericin B and pentamidine are effective, but toxic alternatives for those who experience failure or relapse. Lipid-encapsulated amphotericin B has not been evaluated in these conditions. Recombinant interferon γ administered with pentavalent antimony has been used effectively in a limited number of persons with diffuse cutaneous leishmaniasis.

PROPHYLAXIS

The transmission of *Leishmania* species depends on the presence of appropriate vectors and reservoirs. Large-scale control programs have been attempted in areas where dogs are the apparent reservoir, but their efficacy is debated. Residual insecticide spraying has been used successfully to limit disease where transmission is due to peridomestic sandflies, but it is seldom employed now because of emerging insect resistance and environmental concerns. Personal protective measures using insect repellents containing N,N-diethyl-methyltoluamide (DEET) applied to the skin and wearing permethrin-impregnated clothing reduce the frequency of sandfly bites and transmission. Fine mesh netting provides protection at night. Unfortunately, these measures are often not available for residents of endemic areas, and no vaccine is available.

Herwaldt BL, Stokes SL, Juranek DD: American cutaneous leishmaniasis in U.S. travelers. Ann Intern Med 118:779, 1993. *Cutaneous leishmaniasis is occasionally contracted by U.S. travelers in endemic areas. This is a summary of their exposures and the delay that frequently occurs in diagnosis. Recommendations are made for prevention and management.*

Magill AJ, Grögl M, Gasser RA Jr, et al: Visceral infection caused by *Leishmania tropica* in veterans of Operation Desert Storm. N Engl J Med 328:1383, 1993. *Some Operation Desert Storm soldiers experienced a viscerotropic syndrome with L. tropica, which resulted in a temporary ban on blood and organ donations from all those involved in the operation.*

Pearson RD, Sousa AQ: Clinical spectrum of leishmaniasis. Clin Infect Dis 22:1, 1996. *The epidemiologic characteristics, clinical manifestations, diagnosis, and treatment of leishmaniasis are reviewed.*

Reed SG, Scott P: T-cell and cytokine responses in leishmaniasis. Curr Opin Immunol 5:524, 1993. *Excellent review of the immunologic characteristics of leismaniasis.*

Zijlstra EE, el-Hassan AM, Ismael A: Endemic kala-azar in eastern Sudan: Post-kala-azar dermal leishmaniasis. Am J Trop Med Hyg 52:299, 1995. *Visceral leishmaniasis is endemic in the Sudan, and a major epidemic has occurred there among refugees.*

425 TOXOPLASMOSIS

Oliver Liesenfeld ■ *Jack S. Remington*

DEFINITION. *Toxoplasma gondii* is a protozoan parasite that is ubiquitous in nature and infects a variety of mammals and birds throughout the world. The *acute acquired* infection in humans is usually asymptomatic. However, clinical and/or pathologic evidence of disease (toxoplasmosis) may occur, particularly in the immunocompromised patient, the congenitally infected fetus and child, and those in whom chorioretinitis develops during the acute acquired infection. Infection is characterized by two stages: acute (recently acquired) and chronic (latent). For information on congenital toxoplasmosis, the reader is referred to Remington and Klein (1995).

LIFE CYCLE. There are three forms of the parasite: the tachyzoite, which is the asexual invasive form; the tissue cyst (containing bradyzoites), which persists in tissues of infected hosts during the chronic phase of the infection; and the oocyst (containing sporozo-

ites), which is produced during the sexual cycle in the intestine of members of the cat family (the definitive host). The extraintestinal asexual cycle is present in all incidental hosts and in cats. After ingestion of tissue cysts or oocysts, bradyzoites or sporozoites, respectively, are released into the intestinal lumen, where they invade surrounding cells, become tachyzoites, and disseminate throughout the body via the blood. The *tachyzoite* has a crescent shape, measures approximately 3 by 7 μm, requires an intracellular habitat for survival, and can infect all mammalian cells. Continued multiplication ultimately results in destruction of the host cell and release of tachyzoites, which can then infect other cells. Tachyzoites are found in tissues during the acute stage of the infection or during reactivation of the chronic infection. Freezing and thawing, desiccation, and gastric secretions kill tachyzoites. Development of immunity is associated with disappearance of tachyzoites and formation of tissue cysts. Tissue cysts measure from 10 to 200 μm in diameter, may contain up to several thousand bradyzoites, can be found in all organs, and are most readily observed in the central nervous system (CNS) and myocardial, skeletal, and smooth muscle. In humans, they appear to persist for life. Unlike tachyzoites, bradyzoites released from tissue cysts are relatively resistant to the digestive process of the gastrointestinal tract. The enteroepithelial sexual cycle results in the formation of oocysts in the cat's intestine. *Oocysts* containing sporozoites measure 10 to 12 μm in diameter, are excreted in the feces 3 to 34 days after the cat becomes infected, and continue to be excreted for 7 to 20 days, after which excretion rarely recurs. They become infectious only after they are excreted and sporulation occurs; the duration of this process depends on environmental conditions but usually is 2 to 5 days. They may remain infectious in the environment for more than 1 year. Thus, transmission is primarily by the oral route through ingestion of raw or undercooked meat containing *T. gondii* cysts or through accidental ingestion of food or water contaminated with oocysts.

Virulence in laboratory mice, isoenzyme pattern analysis, and restriction-fragment length polymorphisms have been used to differentiate virulent and avirulent strains of *T. gondii*. *T. gondii* strains can be divided into three clonal lineages, designated I, II, and III. Whereas most strains isolated from acquired immunodeficiency syndrome (AIDS) patients are type III, type I strains are commonly found in cases of congenital disease.

EPIDEMIOLOGIC CHARACTERISTICS. In the United States, there is no significant difference in prevalence of antibodies to *T. gondii* between men and women. Depending on geographic locale and population group, 3 to 67% of adults have serologic evidence of infection. In other parts of the world, including tropical countries and some areas of Western Europe, up to 75% of adults are seropositive. Transmission to humans occurs by ingestion of tissue cysts or oocysts, the transplacental route, blood product transfusion, solid organ transplantation (kidney, heart, or liver from a seropositive donor into a seronegative recipient), and laboratory accident. Epidemics of toxoplasmosis due to eating of undercooked meat or exposure to oocysts (e.g., in contaminated water) have occurred. In 1995, an epidemic occurred in Victoria, British Columbia, Canada, in which more than 100 persons became infected. The outbreak was attributed to a contaminated water supply. In the United States, transmission by eating undercooked or raw meat containing tissue cysts or vegetables or other food products contaminated with oocysts appears more common than transmission by contact with cat feces, but further data are needed to verify this hypothesis. Commercial cuts of pork and lamb (but rarely beef) may contain tissue cysts that remain infectious unless the meat is frozen to −20° C or heated throughout to 66° C.

The incidence of congenital toxoplasmosis in the United States has been estimated to be from 1 in 1000 to 1 in 8000 live births. Transplacental infection resulting in congenital infection can occur in immunocompetent pregnant women with recently acquired *T. gondii* infection and in immunocompromised pregnant women with reactivation of their chronic infection. Frequency of transmission to the fetus likely depends on maternal parasitemia, maturity of placenta, and competency of the maternal immune response to *T. gondii*. Congenital transmission has been shown to vary considerably, depending on the time during gestation the mother acquired her infection (Table 425-1). Approximately 85% of infants with congenital infection appear normal at birth. However, if untreated,

Table 425–1 ■ INCIDENCE OF CONGENITAL *Toxoplasma gondii* INFECTION ACCORDING TO GESTATIONAL AGE AT TIME OF INFECTION OF THE MOTHER

WEEKS OF GESTATION*	NO. OF INFECTED FETUSES/ TOTAL NO. OF FETUSES (%)
0–2	0/100 (0)
3–6	6/384 (1.6)
7–10	9/503 (1.8)
11–14	37/511 (7.2)
15–18	49/392 (13)
19–22	44/237 (19)
23–26	30/116 (26)
27–30	7/32 (22)
31–34	4/6 (67)
Unknown	8/351
Total	194/2632 (7.4)

*Patients were treated with spiramycin.

Reprinted, by permission, from the New England Journal of Medicine 331, 695–699, 1994.

as many as 85% of these children will later have signs and symptoms of the disease, in most cases chorioretinitis or delays in development. Maternal infection acquired around the time of conception and within the first 2 weeks of gestation usually does not result in transmission. Maternal infection acquired weeks or a few months prior to gestation rarely has been reported to result in fetal infection. The earlier the transmission to the fetus, the more severe the outcome. Toxoplasmic encephalitis (TE) in AIDS patients (and in Hodgkin's disease patients and bone marrow transplantation recipients) in the United States is almost always due to reactivation of a chronic infection. Therefore, the incidence of this disease is proportional to the prevalence of *T. gondii* antibodies (latent infection) in a given population and the stage of human immunodeficiency virus (HIV) infection in the respective patients (usually CD4 count < 200/μL). In the United States, *T. gondii* seroprevalence in HIV-infected individuals varies from 10 to 45%. It is estimated that 20 to 47% of HIV-infected, *T. gondii*–seropositive patients ultimately develop TE if they are not receiving appropriate prophylaxis.

PATHOGENESIS. After infection by the oral route, tachyzoites disseminate from the gastrointestinal tract and can invade virtually any cell or tissue, where they proliferate, infect adjoining cells, and produce necrotic foci surrounded by inflammation. In immunocompromised individuals, acute infection may result in severe damage to multiple organs. Both cell-mediated immunity and humoral immunity play a crucial role in resistance against *T. gondii*. Immune mechanisms that contribute to control of the acute infection and termination of continued tissue destruction by the proliferating parasite include activation of the cytokine system, especially the T-helper 1–(T_H1)-type response. *T. gondii* infection triggers production of the immunoglobulins IgG, IgM, IgA, and IgE antibodies against multiple *T. gondii* proteins. Activation of the monocyte/macrophage system after phagocytosis of parasites leads to death of the parasite. In addition, $\alpha\beta$ T cells are activated and sensitized CD4 and CD8+ T cells are cytotoxic for *T. gondii*–infected cells. Both up-regulatory (e.g., γ interferon [IFN-γ]; tumor necrosis factor α [TNF-α]) and down-regulatory (e.g., interleukin 10 [IL-10], transforming growth factor [TGF]) cytokines affect the response; IFN-γ plays the pivotal role in this immunity. Despite a normal immune response, tissue cysts form in multiple organs. Although disruption of cysts or "leakage" of bradyzoites from cysts appears to occur in normal hosts without causing disease, this can result in life-threatening disease in immunocompromised patients. Immunocompetent children or adults with congenital *T. gondii* infection can have a localized reactivation that usually manifests clinically as recurrent retinochoroiditis.

In murine models of the disease, genetic susceptibility to infection has been reported. Recently, the first evidence for genetic regulation of susceptibility to toxoplasmic encephalitis in AIDS patients has been reported; human leukocyte antigen DQ3 (HLA-DQ3) appeared to be a genetic marker of susceptibility, whereas HLA-DQ1 was found to be a genetic marker of resistance to development of TE.

PATHOLOGIC CHARACTERISTICS. Pathologic changes vary, depending on the immune status of the individual. Histologic preparations of tissues of normal individuals rarely reveal the presence of tissue cysts; when present, they are without a surrounding inflammatory response. The exception occurs in immunocompetent adults suffering toxoplasmic retinochoroiditis, who may have tachyzoites, necrosis, and mononuclear cell infiltrates in their retina and choroid.

Histopathologic changes of toxoplasmic lymphadenitis in immunocompetent patients consist of a distinctive and usually diagnostic triad of reactive follicular hyperplasia, irregular clusters of epithelioid histiocytes that encroach on and blur the margins of germinal centers, and focal distension of sinuses with monocytoid cells. These findings reflect an immune response to infection rather than the presence of the organism, which is rarely observed.

Tissues of immunocompromised patients with toxoplasmosis exhibit, in addition to tissue cysts, foci of intracellular tachyzoite proliferation with resultant cell death, tissue necrosis, and inflammation. The inflammatory response can occur in multiple tissues and consists of lymphocytes, plasma cells, mononuclear phagocytes, and few neutrophils. This occurs most commonly in the brain, lung, heart, and gastrointestinal tract but has also been observed in the liver, spleen, pancreas, kidney, seminiferous tubules, prostate, adrenals, bone marrow, and skeletal muscle. The most frequently clinically apparent site of involvement in these patients is the central nervous system (CNS), which may have acute focal or diffuse meningoencephalitis with necrosis, microglial nodules, and perivascular mononuclear inflammation. These lesions are usually multiple and diffuse in distribution. Tachyzoites and tissue cysts are usually found at the periphery of necrotic areas. TE has a predilection for the subcortical area of the cerebral hemispheres, basal ganglia, cerebellum, and brain stem. Some patients have a diffuse form of TE with widespread microglial nodules without abscess formation that involves the gray matter of the cerebrum, cerebellum, and brain stem. Spinal cord involvement can occur and mimic tumor. Pulmonary involvement is second in frequency only to TE in AIDS patients and is characterized by interstitial or necrotizing pneumonitis and/or areas of consolidation.

CLINICAL MANIFESTATIONS. ACUTE INFECTION IN IMMUNOCOMPETENT PATIENTS. *T. gondii* infection is symptomatic in only approximately 10% of immunocompetent individuals. In these patients, toxoplasmosis most often presents as lymphadenopathy. Although any or all lymph node groups may be involved, cervical lymphadenopathy is most common; nodes are usually discrete, nontender, non-suppurative, and asymptomatic. However, some patients may experience fever, myalgias, arthralgias, fatigue, headache, visual disturbances (due to chorioretinitis), sore throat, maculopapular rash, urticaria, hepatosplenomegaly, small numbers (<10%) of atypical lymphocytes, and rarely myocarditis. Involvement of retroperitoneal or mesenteric nodes may be associated with abdominal pain. Toxoplasmic lymphadenopathy is a self-limited disease, although fatigue and/or lymphadenopathy may persist or recur for months. Clinical illness due to reinfection from an exogenous source has not been reported.

OCULAR TOXOPLASMOSIS IN IMMUNOCOMPETENT PATIENTS. *T. gondii* infection has been reported to be responsible for approximately 35% of retinochoroiditis in older children and adults in the United States. Uncommonly individuals with recently acquired infection experience ocular involvement, but this manifestation is increasingly being recognized. In 19% of patients with *T. gondii* infection or toxoplasmosis chorioretinitis developed during a recent outbreak of toxoplasmosis in Canada; such cases have serologic test results indicating acute toxoplasmosis infection. *T. gondii* retinochoroiditis usually presents as a late manifestation of congenital infection. These latter patients are usually asymptomatic until adolescence or adulthood. Reactivation is uncommon after age 40; adults diagnosed as having toxoplasmic chorioretinitis should be studied serologically to define whether the chorioretinitis is due to a recently acquired infection. Patients may have blurred vision, scotoma, pain, photophobia, or epiphora. Macular involvement may impair central vision. Systemic symptoms usually do not accompany ocular involvement. Ophthalmologic examination reveals multiple yellow-white, cotton-like patches with indistinct margins, located in small clusters in the posterior pole. Flareup of congenitally acquired chorioretinitis is often associated with scarred lesions juxtaposed to the fresh lesion. Chorioretinitis in the context of congenital infection is often bilateral, whereas retinochoroiditis in patients with recently acquired infection is typically unilateral. Retinochoroiditis may be part of a syndrome of panuveitis; isolated anterior uveitis has not been associated with *T. gondii*. Lesions may heal spontaneously, in which case they become atrophic with whitish gray plaques with distinct margins surrounded by areas of black choroidal pigment. Lesions at different stages of development may occur simultaneously. Multiple relapses may occur and may result in glaucoma and loss of vision.

TOXOPLASMOSIS IN IMMUNOCOMPROMISED PATIENTS. Toxoplasmosis in the immunocompromised patient in most cases is the result of reactivation of the latent infection. Numerous conditions that compromise the immune system have been associated with toxoplasmosis, with the highest frequencies in patients with AIDS, Hodgkin's disease or other lymphoma, and in other patients who are on high-dose corticosteroids and/or other immunosuppressive agents for treatment of malignancies, collagen-vascular disorders, or prevention of organ transplant rejection. In patients with these conditions, toxoplasmosis may also be due to exogenous acquisition of infection, especially in seronegative recipients of organ transplants from seropositive donors. If untreated, toxoplasmosis in immunocompromised patients is often rapidly progressive and fatal. Clinical manifestations most commonly occur secondary to involvement of the central nervous system (CNS), lungs, eyes, and heart. In 30 to 50% of HIV-infected toxoplasma-seropositive individuals TE will develop if they are not receiving appropriate prophylaxis. TE is the most common manifestation and along with lymphoma is the most frequent cause of intracerebral mass lesions in patients with AIDS (see Chapter 411). As a result of multifocal involvement of the CNS, clinical findings vary widely; they include alterations in mental status, seizures, motor weakness, cranial nerve disorders, sensory abnormalities, cerebellar signs, meningismus, movement disorders, and neuropsychiatric manifestations; typically, TE is characterized by focal neurologic abnormalities of subacute onset, frequently accompanied by non-focal signs and symptoms such as headache, altered mental status, and fever. The most common focal neurologic sign is motor weakness, but patients may also experience cranial nerve abnormalities, cognitive disorders, speech disturbances, visual field defects, sensory disturbances, cerebellar signs, focal seizures, and movement disorders. Meningeal signs may be present. Analysis of cerebrospinal fluid (CSF) may detect slight mononuclear pleocytosis, increased protein level, and normal glucose level. Although radiologic findings are not pathognomonic, the presence of multiple focal lesions in AIDS patients strongly favors the diagnosis of TE, whereas the presence of a single lesion makes TE less likely and lymphoma more likely. Results of computed tomographic (CT) scans usually show multiple bilateral cerebral lesions, which tend to be located at the corticomedullary junction and the basal ganglia. These lesions are generally hypodense and show ring enhancement after intravenous contrast. CT scans tend to underestimate the number of lesions and may show a single lesion when magnetic resonance imaging (MRI) reveals two or more lesions. Thus, because MRI is more sensitive for detecting the lesions of TE, it is the preferred radiologic method for patients with suspected TE and is of particular importance in patients with only a single lesion indicated on CT. The differential diagnosis of TE includes CNS lymphoma, progressive multifocal leukoencephalopathy, and infections due to other pathogens, including viruses, fungi, and bacteria.

Toxoplasmic pneumonitis may develop in the absence of extrapulmonary disease and is associated with a high mortality rate (e.g., 35%) even when treated. Its clinical and radiologic features are non-specific and may mimic those of *Pneumocystis carinii* pneumonia. Patients experience fever, dyspnea, and non-productive cough, and the chest radiograph finding usually shows bilateral interstitial infiltrates. Disseminated toxoplasmosis in AIDS patients has been reported to present a picture of septic shock and adult respiratory distress syndrome (ARDS). Although ocular toxoplasmosis is infrequent in patients with AIDS, it is still the second most common cause of retinal infection in these individuals (see Chapter 415). Toxoplasmic chorioretinitis in AIDS patients is characterized by yellow-white areas of retinitis with fluffy borders. It should be distinguished from ocular involvement due to cytomegalovirus, syphilis, herpes simplex, varicella zoster, *P. carinii*, lymphoma, and fungi. When compared to those of cytomegalovirus (CMV) retinitis, lesions of toxoplasmic chorioretinitis usually occur at the posterior pole, are more fluffy and edematous, have ill-defined margins, and are non-hemorrhagic. Clinical manifestations secondary to cardiac involvement occur but are unusual. In non-AIDS immunocompromised patients, congestive heart failure, arrhythmias, and pericarditis have been noted. Toxoplasmic myocarditis can mimic heart transplant rejection.

DIAGNOSIS. Toxoplasmosis can be diagnosed by isolation of the organism, polymerase chain reaction (PCR), demonstration of tachyzoites in tissues or body fluids by histologic or cytologic analysis, and serologic testing. Whereas direct demonstration of the parasite is often used for diagnosis of the infection in immunocompromised patients, serologic analysis is most commonly used for diagnosis in immunocompetent patients. Serologic tests for detection of *Toxoplasma* immunoglobulin G (IgG) and IgM antibodies are most commonly used for diagnosis of *T. gondii* infection and toxoplasmosis in the immunocompetent patient. Many commercial serologic testing kits to detect *T. gondii* IgM antibodies are not adequate and give unacceptable numbers of false-positive and/or false-negative results. Only the most commonly used tests are discussed here. IgG antibodies can be detected with the Sabin-Feldman dye test (considered the gold standard), indirect fluorescent antibody (IFA), agglutination, or enzyme-linked immunosorbent assay (ELISA) test. IgG antibodies measured by the dye test and IFA test usually appear 1 to 2 weeks after infection, peak in 6 to 8 weeks, and gradually decline thereafter; low titers usually persist for life. The agglutination test is a sensitive and inexpensive method to screen for IgG antibodies.

Detection of IgM antibodies is frequently useful when attempting to diagnose the acute infection. IgM antibodies are demonstrable as early as 5 days after infection and usually decrease after a few weeks or months. However, since IgM antibodies may persist for 1 year or longer after infection, a positive IgM antibody titer finding does not necessarily mean that the patient has recently been infected. The greatest value of an IgM antibody test lies in determining whether an otherwise normal individual has *not* recently been infected. A negative IgM serologic test result in immunocompetent patients virtually rules out recently acquired infection unless sera are tested so early that an antibody response has not yet developed or is not yet detectable. Correct interpretation of serologic test results is of utmost importance for diagnosis of infection in pregnant women, who may choose abortion when informed of a positive IgM test result. For example, a negative IgM test result late in gestation may reflect either that the patient had not recently acquired the infection or that IgM antibodies, due to *T. gondii* infection acquired early in pregnancy, may have disappeared by that time. Appropriate diagnosis and interpretation of results in pregnant women often require that a panel of tests be performed and evaluated in a reference laboratory to assist in discriminating between recent and more distant infection. Recent results of confirmatory testing in a reference laboratory revealed that recently acquired infections had occurred in only 40% of those women who had positive results in tests for IgM antibodies in commercial laboratories; 17% of these women had their pregnancy terminated when informed of the results. In that study, communication of the results and their correct interpretation by an expert in *Toxoplasma* serologic characteristics decreased the rate of unnecessary abortions by 50% among those women with positive IgM *Toxoplasma* antibody test results by commercial laboratories.

A definitive serologic diagnosis of acute infection requires the demonstration of seroconversion (from seronegative to seropositive). Recent infection is likely when serial specimens obtained at least 3 weeks apart and tested in parallel show a significant rise in IgG antibody titers, and when IgM, IgA, or IgE antibody titers are present in conjunction with an "acute" pattern in an avidity test result.

Serologic testing in HIV-infected patients is mainly useful in identifying those at risk for development of toxoplasmosis and in assisting the physician faced with the problem of diagnosing the cause of CNS lesions in such individuals. Therefore, all HIV-positive patients should be tested for the presence of IgG antibodies. In addition, in AIDS patients with CD4 counts < 200/μL high IgG *Toxoplasma* antibody titers are associated with a greater likelihood of development of TE. Serologic tests findings may be misleading in chronically infected patients who receive heart or other organ transplant, because these patients can show rising titers of IgG and IgM antibodies without clinical evidence of active *T. gondii* infection. Definitive diagnosis of toxoplasmosis in immunodeficient patients ultimately relies on histologic studies, isolation of the parasite, and/or identification of *T. gondii* DNA in body fluids or tissues. However, a presumptive diagnosis of TE in AIDS patients can be made when a compatible clinical presentation, multiple ring-enhancing lesions on CT or MRI scan results, and IgG *Toxoplasma* antibodies are present. HIV-infected patients who have a single lesion on the MRI scan result, are seronegative for *T. gondii* antibodies, or are not responding to specific treatment should be considered for brain biopsy.

Isolation of *T. gondii* is accomplished by inoculating blood, CSF, bronchoalveolar lavage (BAL) fluid, vitreous fluid, amniotic fluid, or tissue specimens into mice or cell culture. Mouse inoculation is more sensitive but less rapid than cell culture. Positive results obtained in isolation studies from tissue samples do not necessarily indicate acute infection since a positive result may be due to the presence of bradyzoites (cysts), indicating latent infection.

Polymerase chain reaction (PCR) has been used successfully on CSF, amniotic fluid, samples from BAL, and blood to diagnose toxoplasmosis. The sensitivity of PCR on cerebrospinal fluid ranges from 11 to 77%; PCR on blood has been successfully used primarily in patients with disseminated disease due to *T. gondii*. PCR on amniotic fluid has been successfully used for the diagnosis of fetal infection at 18 weeks of gestation. Because of its greater sensitivity and specificity, which approach approximately 100%, rapid performance, and safety, PCR on amniotic fluid should replace conventional prenatal diagnostic techniques, including fetal blood sampling, when feasible. Routine histologic and cytologic staining may not allow tachyzoites to be identified in tissue sections. An immunohistochemical method (e.g., immunoperoxidase staining) should be used to confirm their presence. The presence of multiple cysts in tissue sections near an area of inflammation and necrosis is highly suggestive of active infection. The characteristic lymph node histologic findings are in most cases sufficient to make the diagnosis of toxoplasmic lymphadenitis.

TREATMENT. The need for and duration of therapy depend on the clinical manifestations of toxoplasmosis and the immune status of the patient. The drug combination pyrimethamine and sulfadiazine is considered the regimen of choice and is synergistic against tachyzoites. It is not active against the tissue cyst form. In adults, a loading dose of 200 mg of pyrimethamine is administered orally in two divided doses on the first day. Thereafter, patients receive 25 to 100 mg/day orally; the dosage depends on the severity of the disease and the immunologic status of the patient (see later). Sulfadiazine is administered as a loading dose of 75 mg/kg (up to 4 g) orally, followed by a daily dose of 100 mg/kg (up to 6 g) divided into two doses. Other sulfonamides have less activity against *T. gondii*. Treatment is usually continued for 1 to 2 weeks after resolution of signs or symptoms of the infection in other than the most severely immunocompromised patients such as those with AIDS (see later). Thereafter careful follow-up observation is indicated. Because pyrimethamine is a folate antagonist, the most common side effect is dose-related bone marrow suppression. Patients receiving pyrimethamine should thus be placed on an oral dose of 5 to 20 mg/day of folinic acid (not folic acid) and have complete blood cell and platelet counts measured twice weekly. Patients receiving sulfonamides should maintain high urinary flow to prevent crystal-induced nephrotoxicity. Other important side effects of sulfonamides are fever, rash, leukopenia, and hepatitis.

ACUTE INFECTION IN IMMUNOCOMPETENT PATIENTS. Patients with toxoplasmic lymphadenitis do not require antimicrobial therapy unless symptoms are severe and persistent. Infections acquired after a blood transfusion or laboratory accident may be severe and therefore should be treated. Patients with toxoplasmic retinochorioiditis may be treated with pyrimethamine & sulfadiazine (P + S). The recommended dose of pyrimethamine in these cases is 50 mg/day as a single dose. Clindamycin, either alone or in combination with pyrimethamine or sulfadiazine, has also been effective. Systemic corticosteroids are added to the regimen when the chorioretinitis involves the macula, optic nerve head, or papillomacular bundle.

ACUTE INFECTION IN PREGNANT WOMEN. Spiramycin at a dose of 3 g/day (obtained from the Food and Drug Administration; phone [301] 827-2335) has been stated to reduce the incidence of fetal infection by about 60%. If prenatal diagnosis reveals infection in the fetus, the pregnant patient should receive pyrimethamine and sulfadiazine in order to treat the fetus. Because of potential teratogenicity, pyrimethamine should not be administered in the first trimester. If necessary, sulfadiazine may be used, but its efficacy when used alone for this purpose has not been studied.

TOXOPLASMOSIS IN IMMUNOCOMPROMISED PATIENTS. Immunodeficient patients with toxoplasmosis or with serologic evidence of an acute *T. gondii* infection should be treated. Chronic asymptomatic infection does not require treatment. In non-AIDS immunodeficient patients, therapy is usually administered until 4 to 6 weeks after all clinical evidence of toxoplasmosis resolves. Treatment is usually based on the presumptive diagnosis of TE. Treatment of toxoplasmosis in AIDS patients has two phases: acute stage therapy and maintenance treatment. Acute therapy should be administered for at least 3 weeks; 6 weeks is recommended in

Table 425–2 ■ GUIDELINES FOR ACUTE AND MAINTENANCE THERAPY OF TOXOPLASMIC ENCEPHALITIS IN AIDS PATIENTS

	ACUTE THERAPY	MAINTENANCE THERAPY*
Suggested regimens		
Pyrimethamine	Oral 200 mg loading dose, then 50 to 75 mg q.d.	25 to 50 mg q.d.
plus		
Folinic acid (leucovorin)	Oral, IV, or IM 10 to 20 mg q.d. (up to 50 mg q.d.)	10 to 20 mg q.d.
plus one of the following		
Sulfadiazine or	Oral 1 to 1.5 g q 6 hr	0.5 to 1.0 g p.o. q.i.d.
Clindamycin	Oral or IV 600 mg q 6 hr (up to IV 1200 mg q 6 hr)	450–600 mg q 6 hr
Pyrimethamine-sulfadoxine (Fansidar)	No adequate data	1 tablet b.i.w.
Alternative regimens†		
Trimethoprim-sulfamethoxazole	Oral or IV, 5 mg (trimethoprim component)/kg q 6 hr	No adequate data
Pyrimethamine	No adequate data	50 mg q.d.
plus		
Folinic acid		10 to 20 mg q.d.
Pyrimethamine and folinic acid	As in suggested regimens	As in suggested regimens
plus one of the following		
Clarithromycin or	Oral 1 g q 12 hr	1 g q 12 hr
Azithromycin or	Oral 1200 to 1500 mg q.d.	1200 to 1500 mg q.d.
Atovaquone or	Oral 750 mg q 6 hr	750 mg q 6 hr
Dapsone	Oral 100 mg q.d.	100 mg b.i.w.

*Drugs administered orally.
†Data inadequate for definitive recommendation.
Adapted from Liesenfeld O, Wong SY, Remington JS: Toxoplasmosis in the setting of AIDS. *In* Merigan TC Jr, Bartlett JG, Bolognesi D (eds): Textbook of AIDS Medicine. Baltimore, Williams & Wilkins, pp 225–259, 1999.

Table 425-3 ■ PRIMARY PROPHYLAXIS FOR TOXOPLASMOSIS IN AIDS PATIENTS*

For the *T. gondii*–seropositive HIV-infected individual†	
Trimethoprim-sulfamethoxazole	1 DS tab q.d.
	2 DS tab b.i.w.
Pyrimethamine-dapsone	Pyrimethamine, 50 mg once a week, plus dapsone, 50 mg q.d.
	Pyrimethamine, 25 mg b.i.w., plus dapsone, 100 mg b.i.w.
	Pyrimethamine, 75 mg once a week, plus dapsone, 200 mg once a week
Pyrimethamine-sulfadoxine (Fansidar)	3 tablets every 2 weeks
	1 tablet b.i.w.
For prevention of congenital transmission of *T. gondii* in seropositive, HIV-infected pregnant women‡	
Spiramycin	1 g q 8 hr

AIDS = acquired immunodeficiency syndrome; HIV = human immunodeficiency syndrome; DS = double strength.

*Drugs are administered orally.

†These regimens have been reported to be effective for primary prophylaxis of toxoplasmic encephalitis in AIDS patients.

‡Although at present no data are available on the efficacy of prophylaxis against congential transmission in this group of patients, we consider it prudent to recommend spiramycin because preliminary studies suggest that the transmission rate for congenital toxoplasmosis in these women is remarkably and significantly higher than in non-HIV-infected, *T. gondii*-seropositive women.

Adapted from Liesenfeld O, Wong SY, Remington JS: Toxoplasmosis in the setting of AIDS. *In* Merigan TC Jr, Bartlett JG, Bolognesi D (eds): Textbook of AIDS Medicine. Baltimore, Williams & Wilkins, 1999, pp 225–259.

patients with severe illness or no significant clinical and/or neuroradiologic response. P + S and pyrimethamine plus clindamycin (P + C) have been used with comparable results (Table 425-2). Most patients respond to these regimens, and neurologic improvement usually occurs within the first 7 days. Brain biopsy should be considered if clinical improvement does not occur during the first 10 days of treatment or if deterioration occurs during the first 7 days. Brain biopsy should also be considered at initial presentation in AIDS patients who are seronegative for IgG antibodies to *T. gondii* and those compliant with primary prophylaxis against toxoplasmosis who have focal lesions indicated by neuroimaging study results (see Prevention). Many AIDS patients do not tolerate one or the other regimen because of rash (P + S), rash and diarrhea (P + C), or bone marrow suppression (P + S, P + C). Short courses of corticosteroids can be administered to treat cerebral edema and intracranial hypertension. The mortality rate in treated patients ranges from approximately 1 to 25%. Because most AIDS patients relapse when treatment is discontinued, maintenance therapy is necessary. The optimal regimen has not been identified. Usually the same drugs used for acute therapy are continued but at lower doses (Table 425-2). For patients who do not tolerate any of these regimens for acute stage or maintenance therapy, alternatives listed in Table 425-3 can be tried in combination with pyrimethamine.

PREVENTION. Preventing the infection is particularly important for seronegative immunocompromised patients and pregnant women. Since the infection is acquired primarily via the oral route—through ingestion of either undercooked meat or food contaminated with oocysts—it is in most cases preventable. Therefore, it is the responsibility of the physician to instruct patients on how to prevent infection. Recommendations include eating meat only if it is well cooked throughout, washing hands after touching raw meat, washing fruits and vegetables, and avoiding contact with cat feces. To attempt to prevent congenital toxoplasmosis, routine serologic screening of pregnant women has been performed in order to identify fetuses at risk of becoming infected. Mandatory screening programs have been successfully implemented in France and Austria. If serologic testing should be chosen, the serologic status of pregnant women should be evaluated no later than the 10th or 12th week of gestation. Those who are seronegative should be retested at the 20th to 22nd week and then again near term. Administering spiramycin to acutely infected pregnant women (see section on treatment) appears to reduce the incidence of congenital infection by approximately 60%. In Massachusetts, a secondary screening program consisting of screening of all newborns for IgM antibodies has been implemented because of the lack of feasibility of screening all pregnant women. Compared to initial clinical examination, neonatal screening showed a dramatically higher sensitivity for di-

agnosis of congenital infection. However, detection of IgM antibodies in newborns is only 25–75% sensitive; thus, this program will have missed a significant number of subclinically infected infants or infants infected in the late third trimester. Furthermore, a secondary prevention program does not allow for prenatal diagnosis and subsequent treatment of the fetus.

It seems prudent to avoid transfusions of blood products from a seropositive donor to a seronegative immunocompromised patient when feasible. If possible, seronegative recipients should receive transplanted organs from seronegative donors. If that is not feasible, seronegative patients who receive organs from seropositive donors should be treated with pyrimethamine, 25 mg/day for 6 weeks.

For primary prophylaxis in *T. gondii*–seropositive HIV-infected patients with a CD4 count < 200 cells/μL, administering either trimethoprim-sulfamethoxazole, pyrimethamine-dapsone, or pyrimethamine-sulfadoxine (Fansidar) is indicated to prevent development of toxoplasmosis (Table 425-3). Secondary prophylaxis (maintenance therapy) in AIDS patients has proved effective in prevention of relapse of TE (Table 425-2).

Bowie WR, King AS, Werker D, et al: Outbreak of toxoplasmosis associated with municipal drinking water. Lancet 350:173, 1997. *Report on epidemiologic, clinical, and serologic features of a unique outbreak of toxoplasmosis attributed to drinking water contaminated with oocysts.*

Hohlfeld P, Daffos F, Costa J-M, et al: Prenatal diagnosis of congenital toxoplasmosis with a polymerase-chain-reaction test on amniotic fluid. N Engl J Med 331:695, 1994. *Definitive study reporting the greater sensitivity of PCR on amniotic fluid than of conventional prenatal diagnostic methods for the diagnosis of congenital infection with Toxoplasma gondii.*

Liesenfeld O, Wong SY, Remington JS: Toxoplasmosis in the setting of AIDS. *In* Broder S, Merigan TC, Bolognesi D (eds): Textbook of AIDS Medicine, 2nd ed. Baltimore, Williams & Wilkins, 1998. *A comprehensive overview of the clinical presentation, diagnosis, management, and prevention of toxoplasmosis in AIDS patients.*

Montoya JG, Remington JS: Studies on the serodiagnosis of toxoplasmic lymphadenitis. Clin Infect Dis 20:781, 1995. *An overview of the value of conventional and newer serologic tests for the diagnosis of toxoplasmic lymphadenitis.*

Montoya JG, Remington JS: Toxoplasmic chorioretinitis in the setting of acute acquired toxoplasmosis. Clin Infect Dis 23:277, 1996. *A unique report on clinical and serologic findings in adults with acute toxoplasmic chorioretinitis in the setting of acute post-natally acquired toxoplasmosis.*

Remington JS, McLeod R, Desmonts G: Toxoplasmosis. *In* Remington JS, Klein KO (eds): Infectious Diseases of the Fetus and Newborn Infant, 4th ed. Philadelphia, WB Saunders, 1995, p 140. *A comprehensive discussion of congenital toxoplasmosis and the diagnosis and management of acute* T. gondii *infection during pregnancy.*

426 CRYPTOSPORIDIOSIS

Beth D. Kirkpatrick ■ *Cynthia L. Sears*

Cryptosporidiosis is a leading cause of endemic and epidemic diarrheal disease worldwide. *Cryptosporidium parvum*, the agent of human cryptosporidiosis, is an intestinal protozoan parasite of the phylum Apicomplex, related to *Toxoplasma* and *Cyclospora* species.

C. parvum was first described by Tyzzer in 1912, in the intestinal tract of mice. Human disease was recognized in 1976 and attracted interest in the early 1980s, when it was identified as a cause of chronic diarrhea in patients with acquired immunodeficiency syndrome (AIDS). Cryptosporidiosis came to public attention in 1993 as a result of the Milwaukee *C. parvum* outbreak, which affected 403,000 people: the largest recorded diarrheal disease outbreak from a public water supply in U.S. history. Recognition of the impact of *C. parvum* infections on public health has led to its classification as an "emerging infectious disease" in the landmark 1992 Institute of Medicine Report, Emerging Infections: Microbial Threats to Health in the United States.

EPIDEMIOLOGIC CHARACTERISTICS

Transmission of *C. parvum* is fecal-oral, via the ingestion of oocysts, which are shed in very high numbers in the feces of many mammals, including humans. For example, AIDS patients with symptomatic cryptosporidiosis may shed up to 1.2 billion oocysts per day. Originally cryptosporidiosis was thought to be predominantly a zoonosis; it is now clear that the primary mode of transmission of *C. parvum* is person-to-person contact or contaminated water. Transmission from environmental sources, food, and animals also occurs. Recent data, based on genotyping studies, suggest that distinct species termed "human-adapted" and "animal-adapted" exist; both cause human disease.

The oocysts of *C. parvum* are ubiquitous and highly infectious. Thick-walled cysts survive well in the environment and are extremely resistant to sterilizing agents, including iodine and chlorine. In the United States, it is estimated that 80% of surface water and 26% of treated drinking water contain *C. parvum* oocysts. Studies of human volunteers have demonstrated that clinical disease may result from ingestion of less than 10 to 500 oocysts, depending on the *C. parvum* strain. As a result of the high infectivity, secondary transmission occurs, ranging from 5% if an adult is the index case to 20% if a child is the index case. Thus, the secondary transmission rate of *C. parvum* parallels that of other highly infectious enteric organisms, such as *Shigella* sp.

Waterborne outbreaks of cryptosporidiosis have highlighted its epidemic potential. Attack rates during epidemics of cryptosporidiosis are as high as 62%. In addition to the magnitude of the 1993 Milwaukee outbreak, a notable 1994 Las Vegas outbreak occurred with a state-of-the-art water filtration system without signs of malfunction, indicating that current water treatment regulations do not prevent *C. parvum* water contamination. Swimming pools and lakes have been the source of waterborne outbreaks at recreational sites. Food-borne outbreaks, which result from fecal contamination of food, are infrequently recognized. In 1993, 160 cases of cryptosporidiosis resulted from contamination of unpasteurized apple cider by cattle feces. Multiple outbreaks also have been reported as a result of direct person-to-person transmission, in day care settings and through nosocomial spread. Inapparent fecal contamination of objects has also caused nosocomial disease, including one outbreak from a contaminated ice machine on a psychiatric ward. Because of the technical difficulty of identifying oocysts in stool specimens, false outbreaks have also been reported.

C. parvum is responsible for endemic diarrheal disease in the normal host, both domestically and abroad. Prevalence of infection varies greatly from industrialized to developing countries. In immunocompetent adults in industrialized nations, the prevalence of *C. parvum* in stool is approximately 2–6% and seroprevalence, 17–32%. In less developed countries, however, cryptosporidiosis is primarily a disease of childhood; for example, in Brazil, over 95% of children are seropositive by 5 years. Populations at increased risk of exposure and infection include veterinary workers, caregivers of infected patients, and day care workers. In addition, cryptosporidiosis is a cause of acute and persistent traveler's diarrhea. In immunocompromised patients, particularly those with primary T-cell defects, infection is typically much more serious than in the normal host. In patients with AIDS, *C. parvum* may be the cause of up to 14–24% of cases of chronic diarrhea.

LIFE CYCLE, PATHOGENESIS, AND IMMUNOLOGIC CHARACTERISTICS

C. parvum has a complex life cycle, which it completes in a single host (monoxenous). After oocysts are ingested, excystation occurs in the upper small intestine after contact with gastric acid and proteolytic enzymes. Four crescentic sporozoites per oocyst are released. Sporozoites penetrate the brush border membrane of the enterocyte to reside in a distinctive intracellular but extracytoplasmic position. Sporozoites develop into trophozoites intracellularly and divide asexually to form a schizont with four to eight merozoites, which are released by rupture of the enterocyte. Some merozoites invade adjacent cells, expanding the infection asexually. Others form sexual stages in host cells to produce male and female gametocytes, which result in oocyst formation. It appears that 80% of oocysts are thick-walled and excreted into the environment, whereas 20% are thin-walled and capable of initiating cycles of autoinfection. Autoinfection expands and augments infection and, if

uncontrolled by host defenses, is presumed to cause persistent disease in immunocompromised hosts. Furthermore, the intracellular position of *C. parvum* may protect the organism from host immune defenses.

All structures contiguous to the intestine that are lined with polarized epithelial cells are at risk of infection. Infection is typically concentrated in the small bowel with lesser colonic involvement. The biliary and pancreatic tracts and, rarely, the respiratory tree may also be infected. Intestinal infection results in villous atrophy and crypt hyperplasia, causing a malabsorptive and/or a secretory diarrhea. Combined small and large bowel infection correlates with the severity of clinical disease in AIDS patients. A variable inflammatory infiltrate of neutrophils and/or mononuclear cells is found in the lamina propria.

Piglet studies of the pathophysiologic characteristics of *C. parvum* infection indicate that impaired glucose-stimulated sodium and water absorption in the jejunum and ileum contributes to the occurrence of malabsorptive diarrhea. Cholera-like (20 liters) stool losses in some AIDS patients infected with *C. parvum* have prompted the search for a possible enterotoxin. Although no specific toxin has been found, animal models show a net increase in chloride secretion, mediated by prostaglandin E_2, which may be responsible, in part, for secretory diarrhea. The secretory response may be further augmented by epithelial cell secretion of proinflammatory cytokines. Disruption of the intestinal epithelial barrier as a result of impairment of tight junctions by *C. parvum* infection also increases membrane permeability to the back-diffusion of water and ions into the gut lumen.

The specific immune response to *C. parvum* in humans is poorly understood. Severe cryptosporidiosis is found in patients with either cellular or humoral immune defects, and both arms of the immune response are thought necessary to control infection. In humans, specific serum antibodies (immunoglobulin G [IgG], IgM, and IgA) and intestinal secretory IgA (sIgA) are found in response to infection but have not been shown to be protective. Epidemiologic data suggest that maternal antibodies may be an important defense; breast-fed children appear to have less *C. parvum* infection before 6 months of age. Studies of cell-mediated immune responses have demonstrated a role for systemic and intraepithelial CD4+ T-helper cells and interferon γ, but not CD8+ cytotoxic T cells or natural killer cells, in prevention of and recovery from disease. However, high levels of interferon γ are not helpful in controlling infection in AIDS patients. Interleukin-12 protects against infection in a mouse model.

CLINICAL FINDINGS

Clinical manifestations of infection vary with age and immune status. Diarrhea is the predominant symptom in all groups. In otherwise healthy adults, the incubation period is 2–14 days, followed by the onset of non-inflammatory (watery and non-bloody) diarrhea, which may be copious, as seen in other infectious diarrheal diseases. Diarrhea is frequently associated with abdominal cramping, nausea, flatulence, and vomiting. Symptoms are usually self-limited, with recovery in 10–14 days. Recurrent diarrhea after 1–2 days of apparent recovery is not uncommon. Fever and other systemic signs of infection are infrequent, but weight loss may be prominent. In the Milwaukee outbreak, approximately 75% of otherwise healthy people with diarrhea lost weight, a median of 10 pounds. Infection with *C. parvum* may also be asymptomatic.

In developing nations, cryptosporidiosis is predominantly a childhood disease and is recognized as a major cause of persistent diarrhea in these populations. As found in Peru and Brazil, children less than 1 year of age appear to be at greater risk for persistent diarrhea and may suffer enhanced morbidity as a result of other enteric infections and growth stunting after *C. parvum* infection.

In the immunocompromised host, the severity and duration of infection are directly related to the type and degree of immunosuppression. Disease is more likely to become fulminant, persistent, and life-threatening. Excessive fluid and electrolyte losses with malabsorption can cause progressive weight loss, dehydration, and malnutrition. Although most data are from patients with AIDS, severe, chronic cryptosporidiosis has been found in almost all immunocompromised populations, including patients with common variable immunodeficiency, hematologic malignancies, and hypogammaglobulinemia, and in those having chemotherapy or using steroids. The majority of these have primary T-cell defects. Reversal of the immune compromise often results in rapid cessation of symptoms of cryptosporidiosis.

In AIDS patients with chronic diarrhea, intestinal cryptosporidiosis has been considered an AIDS-defining illness since 1983 (see Chapter 413). Up to 30% of this group may also have a second intestinal coinfection. Uncontrolled persistent diarrhea is directly related to CD4 count; patients with CD4 levels over 180 mm³ are able to recover from *C. parvum* infection, whereas patients with lower CD4 counts often have persistent diarrhea with an associated poor survival of approximately 6 months. In this population, the disease fits one of four patterns: cholera-like (31%), chronic diarrhea (37%), relapsing (14%), or resolved (17%). Acalculous cholecystitis and, less frequently, sclerosing cholangitis are found in 10–15% of AIDS patients with cryptosporidiosis, causing symptoms of fever, right upper quadrant pain, and nausea. Pancreatitis and respiratory tract involvement have also been reported, although the clinical significance of the latter is unknown. The use of highly active antiretroviral therapy (HAART) (see Chapter 418) has dramatically decreased clinically apparent cryptosporidiosis in patients with AIDS. Resolution of established cryptosporidial diarrhea in AIDS patients has been shown after initiation of effective HAART therapy.

DIAGNOSIS AND DIFFERENTIAL

C. parvum infection is diagnosed by stool examination. The classic acid-fast stain of the stool with modified Ziehl-Nielsen stain demonstrates bright pink 4- to 6-μm oocysts. Sensitivity is diminished with formed stool but is increased by techniques to concentrate oocysts. Direct immunofluoresence with monoclonal antibodies to the oocyst wall and a specific *C. parvum* enzyme-linked immunosorbent assay (ELISA) are reported to be more sensitive than stool examination. Cysts must be differentiated from yeast and the oocysts of *Cyclospora* sp., which are 8–10 μm and, unlike those of *C. parvum,* glow with ultraviolet (UV) light. Serologic methods are not useful in diagnosis of acute disease. Diagnostic polymerase chain reaction (PCR) techniques are under development. Rarely, intestinal biopsy is necessary for diagnosis. Histologic samples are stained by hemoxylin and eosin and demonstrate *C. parvum* life cycle stages in the brush border of intestinal epithelial cells.

Other laboratory findings are non-specific. Signs of malabsorption may be found by measuring serum B_{12} level, stool fat, or *d*-xylose absorption. In biliary disease, the alkaline phosphate, γ-glutamyl transferase (GGT), and bilirubin levels may be increased; levels of transaminases are usually normal. Ultrasound and computed tomography (CT) scan may show dilatation of the biliary ducts. Endoscopic retrograde cholangiopancreatography (ERCP) to obtain bile or tissue is the most sensitive method of diagnosing biliary disease.

Acute diarrhea with *C. parvum* has no distinguishing features, and the differential diagnosis varies with the patient population and the clinical setting. In patients with AIDS and persistent diarrhea, other parasitic infections such as those caused by *Microsporidia, Isospora,* and *Cyclospora* spp. should be considered, as well as cytomegalovirus and *Mycobacterium avium-intercellulare* (MAI) infections. Cryptosporidiosis should be included in the differential diagnosis of persistent diarrhea in all hosts (particularly in children of developing nations, travelers, and immunocompromised populations) and as a cause of any epidemic of diarrheal disease.

TREATMENT AND PREVENTION

The cornerstone of therapy is fluid replacement, and in immunocompromised patients, an attempt to reverse the immunodeficiency. MAI chemoprophylaxis with rifampin and the macrolide clarithromycin in AIDS patients is protective against the development of cryptosporidiosis. There is no clearly demonstrated successful drug therapy once infection is established; therapeutic data have been limited to studies in AIDS patients. The non-absorbable aminoglycoside paromomycin, in case reports, has temporarily decreased oocyst excretion and stool frequency in infected AIDS patients. However, in a controlled clinical trial (ACTG 192), paromomycin

treatment of cryptosporidiosis in patients with advanced AIDS yielded no clinical benefit. Case reports (but no controlled studies) suggest that treatment of AIDS patients with Nitazoxanide, an antiparasitic agent, may lead to clinical improvement. Passive transfer of antibody via hyperimmune bovine colostrum has had limited success in diminishing symptoms in AIDS patients with cryptosporidiosis. Future rational drug development for cryptosporidiosis will be enhanced by the growing knowledge of basic parasite biology.

Eliminating exposure to *C. parvum* oocysts is the cornerstone of preventing infection. Avoidance of contact with human and animal feces in water and food and via sexual practices is essential for all hosts, but particularly immunocompromised patients. Contact with newborn animals and patients with diarrhea should be minimized and hand washing emphasized. The difficulty of eliminating *C. parvum* from public drinking water remains an important public health problem. In outbreak settings, drinking water can be considered safe when boiled for 1 minute at sea level or if purified with ozone or an absolute <1-μm filter or by reverse osmosis. Filters should meet the National Sanitation Foundation standard #53 criteria for "cyst removal." Since recommendations of sources differ, bottled water should not be assumed to be free of oocysts. The risk of acquiring cryptosporidiosis in tap water in non-outbreak settings is unknown. No special tap water precautions are currently recommended for human immunodeficiency virus (HIV) and immunocompromised patients.

Clark DP, Sears CL: The pathogenesis of cryptosporidiosis. Parasitology Today 12(6): 222, 1996. *A detailed review of the pathogenesis of* C. parvum *infection.*

Goodgame RW: Understanding intestinal spore forming protozoa: Cryptosporidia, microsporidia, isospora and cyclospora. Ann Intern Med 124:429, 1996. *An excellent review, comprehensively referenced.*

Guerrant, RL: Cryptosporidiosis: An emerging highly infectious threat. Emerg Infect Dis 3(1):51, 1997. *An up-to-date synopsis, with an emphasis on prevalence and the public health impact of outbreaks.*

427 GIARDIASIS
Cynthia L. Sears

ETIOLOGY. *Giardia lamblia* (also known as *G. intestinalis, G. duodenalis*) is the most common human protozoan enteric pathogen worldwide and causes both endemic and epidemic diarrheal illnesses. However, the parasite is also often carried asymptomatically by humans. Discovered in 1681, it is now recognized to be among the most primitive eukaryotes known and to have a simple life cycle alternating between trophozoite and cyst stages. The pear-shaped flagellated trophozoites (10–20 μm long × 5–15 μm wide) contain four nuclei and resemble a "face" microscopically. Trophozoites proliferate in the small bowel and may be identified in the liquid stools of symptomatic patients. Encystation in the ileum yields the infective cyst stage (12 μm long × 7–10 μm wide), which is identified in the formed stools of asymptomatic carriers as well as in the liquid stools of symptomatic patients. The oval cysts are resistant to chlorine and can survive in water for up to 3 months. These features facilitate spread of infection and make this parasite one of the most frequently identified waterborne pathogens in the United States. Importantly, the parasite is quite genetically heterogeneous, and some strains appear more biologically fit than others, a factor potentially important in disease pathogenesis. Recent work indicates that *G. lamblia* undergoes surface antigenic variation most likely stimulated by the host immune response. Sequential presentation of differing surface antigens to elude the host immune response increases the parasite's chances of a successful reinfection and/or development of a persistent initial infection.

EPIDEMIOLOGY. Transmission of *G. lamblia* infection occurs either directly person-to-person or indirectly by ingestion of contaminated water or, less often, food. Person-to-person fecal-oral transmission and small-scale water contamination results in endemic infection, whereas epidemic disease is recognized when food or large-scale drinking water contamination occurs. The infection is transmitted by ingestion of as few as 10 to 100 *G. lamblia* cysts. Persons of all age groups are susceptible to this infection. In the developing world, infection is nearly universal by age 5 yet recurrent infections are not uncommon, indicating that the primary immune response to infection is incompletely protective. In the United States, infection is usually sporadic, with certain groups of individuals at higher risk including children (particularly those attending day-care centers), male homosexuals engaging in oral-anal sexual behavior, campers and hikers (from ingestion of untreated surface water), and international travelers. A notable association of travel to Russia (particularly St. Petersburg) with acquisition of *G. lamblia* infection is amply documented. Although both T and B cell–mediated immune mechanisms appear necessary to eradicate infection, only immunocompromised patients with hypogammaglobulinemia (e.g., common variable immunodeficiency, X-linked hypogammaglobulinemia) are at increased risk of prolonged, sometimes intractable, infections. *G. lamblia* does not exhibit enhanced virulence in patients with human immunodeficiency virus infection. Similar to other enteric infections, achlorhydria or hypochlorhydria enhances the likelihood of infection. Although humans are the main reservoir of *G. lamblia* infection, genetically indistinguishable species infect humans, beavers, guinea pigs, cats, and dogs, strongly suggesting that *G. lamblia* infection is a zoonosis. Surface water (such as streams) contaminated with cysts excreted by beavers has been linked to human infection.

PATHOGENESIS. *G. lamblia* is strictly a small bowel non-invasive enteric pathogen. Infection is initiated by the ingestion of the cyst form of the parasite, which releases two trophozoites in the alkaline conditions of the upper small bowel. The low concentration of bile salts and the anaerobic conditions in this intestinal region stimulate trophozoite multiplication. Trophozoites firmly attach by means of a ventral surface disc-shaped sucker to the small bowel mucosa, aided initially by a surface lectin and, subsequently, by contractile parasitic proteins and the negative pressure created by the parasite's beating flagella. Attachment is most often patchy and imprints the mucosa, creating localized microvillus damage. In some patients, these events culminate in onset of symptoms after an incubation period of 6 to 15 days. As trophozoites migrate distally in the small bowel, the higher bile concentrations in the ileum stimulate encystation, resulting in the excretion of the environmentally resistant cyst form of the parasite.

The histopathologic response to *G. lamblia* infection varies and imperfectly correlates with the clinical findings. In asymptomatic patients, no abnormalities may be identified on histopathologic examination of a small bowel biopsy by light microscopy yet electron microscopy often reveals evidence of ultrastructural changes in the microvilli. In contrast, biopsies of symptomatic patients may, but do not always, reveal villous atrophy and crypt hyperplasia with an inflammatory lamina propria infiltrate consisting of polymorphonuclear leukocytes, plasma cells, and lymphocytes. Lymphoid nodular hyperplasia has been associated with both giardiasis and/or hypogammaglobulinemia.

One of the unresolved puzzles is how *G. lamblia* causes a broad spectrum of disease ranging from asymptomatic infection to acute and sometimes chronic diarrhea. Two major postulates accounting for disease variability exist. First, *G. lamblia* strains may vary in virulence, as suggested by experimental animal and human infections. However, specific virulence traits of the parasite have yet to be identified. Second, the host response, particularly the mucosal immune response, to the parasite may vary. Although both the variable histopathology and clinical course of giardiasis support this hypothesis, it is also possible that this variability is driven by strain-dependent *G. lamblia* virulence. Clarification of the host-parasite relationship will require the ability to characterize the infecting strain by molecular approaches and correlate these results with the clinical disease observed.

The mechanisms by which *G. lamblia* results in diarrhea appear to be multifactorial. First, documented disaccharidase deficiencies and the ultrastructural and histopathologic changes observed in association with some *G. lamblia* infections are consistent with the clinical observation of malabsorption in infected patients. Experimental animal infections also reveal impaired glucose and amino acid–dependent sodium absorption and, in some instances, net chloride secretion. Second, the patchy distribution of *G. lamblia*

infection (in contrast to the large surface area of the small bowel) and the absence of overt abnormalities in gut architecture in some symptomatic individuals have suggested that the parasite may secrete a factor (e.g., an enterotoxin) that alters intestinal transport. Only limited experimental data support this hypothesis at present. Third, the nature of the mucosal immune response is likely to contribute to intestinal secretion, given that particular cytokines released by host inflammatory cells in the lamina propria are known to stimulate chloride secretion by intestinal epithelial cells.

CLINICAL DISEASE. Giardiasis presents in one of three clinical forms: (1) asymptomatic carrier state (accounting for up to one half of infections); (2) acute, self-limited diarrheal illnesses; and (3) chronic diarrhea associated with malabsorption and, in young children in the developing world, growth retardation. Forty to 50 per cent of infected persons develop acute diarrhea. Symptomatic patients experience anorexia and nausea combined with, most characteristically, explosive, watery, foul-smelling diarrhea with increased passage of gas. Only low-grade fever occurs. Fecal leukocytes and blood are not present and even mucus in the stool is rare. Nevertheless, the diarrheal illness caused by *G. lamblia* is indistinguishable from that caused by other small bowel enteric pathogens. In some, the infection or diarrhea may clear spontaneously. Experimental studies suggest intestinal secretory IgA and helper T lymphocytes (CD4) contribute to infection resolution. Alternatively, more indolent, non-dehydrating, intermittent diarrhea persists. This may result in malabsorption potentially manifested by foul-smelling oily stools that float. Weight loss may be prominent. Twenty to 40 per cent of patients with diarrhea and *G. lamblia* infection experience lactose intolerance, which may last for several weeks after successful therapy. Rare associations with *G. lamblia* infection include urticaria, cholecystitis, pancreatitis, arthritis, retinal arteritis, and iridocyclitis. The white blood cell count is normal in *G. lamblia* infection.

DIAGNOSIS. Demonstration of the cysts or, more rarely, trophozoites of *G. lamblia* in fecal specimens is most often essential for diagnosis. However, diagnosis can be elusive because (1) cyst excretion in this infection is erratic and (2) symptoms may begin before the organism is detectable in stool. Although standard recommendations are to examine three stools from separate days (typically within a 10-day time frame), examination of two concentrated stools using a trichrome stain or a more sensitive direct immunofluorescence assay generally yields the diagnosis in 90% of infected individuals. Direct visualization of cysts can be complemented by newer enzyme-linked immunosorbent assay (ELISA) techniques that detect giardial antigens in stool with high sensitivity and specificity (>95%). Limited data suggest that detection of *G. lamblia* approaches 100% with a single examination if an ELISA is added to the standard stained smear of a stool concentrate. Although use of an "Enterotest" (gelatin capsule-string test) and/or endoscopy will improve detection of trophozoites in the upper small bowel, these examinations are rarely necessary for patient management.

THERAPY. Three major drugs are used for the therapy of giardiasis based on clinical experience. Treatment failures may occur with any of these standard therapies consistent with in vivo and in vitro data, suggesting that strain-dependent drug resistance not only exists but also may be induced during therapy. The nitroimidazoles, metronidazole and tinidazole (not available in the United States), are most often the drugs of choice and are more than 90% efficacious. Notable side effects include a metallic taste as well as gastrointestinal and allergic adverse reactions. Quinacrine (mepacrine), the second major drug used in therapy, appears to be about equal in efficacy to the nitroimidazoles but is no longer available in the United States. This drug may precipitate a toxic psychosis in adults and may aggravate certain skin disorders. Lastly, furazolidone (approximately 80% effective) is often used in children, in part, owing to its availability as a suspension. Furazolidone may precipitate hemolysis in patients with glucose-6-phosphate deficiency. Each of these medications inhibits aldehyde dehydrogenase and, thus, may precipitate a disulfiram-like reaction if taken with alcohol. None of these therapeutic alternatives is clearly safe in pregnancy; therefore, the poorly absorbed oral aminoglycoside paromomycin has been suggested for use in this clinical situation. It is unknown if dual drug therapy offers benefit in recalcitrant infections. Limited clinical data suggest that the anthelminthic albendazole has antigiardial activity.

PREVENTION. Because *G. lamblia* is a zoonosis transmitted by environmentally resistant cysts and does not stimulate complete protective immunity, prevention of infection requires public health measures to ensure the availability of clean water and education to promote excellent personal hygiene to interrupt the infection cycle. Boiling of water for 1 minute or treatment with 2 to 4 drops of household bleach or 0.5 mL of 2% tincture of iodine per liter for at least 60 minutes (overnight if the water is cold) before drinking renders the parasite non-infective. The antigenic variability of *G. lamblia* combined with the presently ill-defined correlates of protective immunity greatly hinder vaccine development for this infection.

Farthing MJG: Giardiasis. Gastroenterol Clin North Am 25:493–515, 1996. *This article provides a comprehensive overview of the epidemiology, mechanisms of disease, and clinical illnesses resulting from G. lamblia infection.*

Nash TE, Herrington DA, Losonsky GA, Levine MM: Experimental human infections with *Giardia lamblia*. J Infect Dis 156:974–984, 1987. *The human studies in this report illustrate the natural history and variability of G. lamblia infections.*

Steiner TS, Thielman NM, Guerrant RL: Protozoal agents: What are the dangers for the public water supply? Annu Rev Med 48:329–340, 1997. *This summary highlights the public health threat and importance of G. lamblia and Cryptosporidium parvum in waterborne enteric disease.*

428 AMEBIASIS

Jonathan I. Ravdin

Human amebiasis is due to infection with the enteric protozoan *Entamoeba histolytica*. This parasite infects 1% of the world's population, with the disease burden highest in poor, developing areas. To manage patients with amebiasis appropriately, physicians must know the biology of the organism, risk factors for infection, mechanisms of disease, pathogenesis and host immunity, the presenting manifestations of the invasive syndrome, the correct diagnostic approach, alternative therapeutic drug regimens, and strategies for preventing infection.

BIOLOGY OF *E. HISTOLYTICA* AND EPIDEMIOLOGY. Infection results from ingestion of the excreted acid-resistant cysts in fecally contaminated water or food. Excystation occurs in the small bowel, leading to colonization of the colon with trophozoites. Transmission of infection may also result from direct fecal-oral contact because of poor hygiene or anal-oral sexual practices. Epidemiologic and molecular biology studies indicate that there are two distinct species, the pathogenic *E. histolytica* and the non-pathogenic *E. dispar*. Infection with the latter is much more common but does not result in systemic invasive disease or a humoral immune response. Approximately 10% of those with *E. histolytica* infection present clinically with invasive amebiasis, although all manifest a serum anti-amebic antibody response. The relative frequency of *E. histolytica* and *E. dispar* infection varies, depending on geographic area. Regions of the world with a high incidence of invasive amebiasis include Mexico, parts of South America, West and South Africa, the Indian subcontinent, the Middle East, and Southeast Asia. High-risk groups in the United States include sexually promiscuous male homosexuals, the institutionalized mentally challenged population, and travelers or emigrants (especially Mexican-Americans) from areas of high prevalence. Groups that experience an increased severity of invasive amebiasis, when infected, are the very young (younger than age 2 years), pregnant women, malnourished individuals, and patients receiving corticosteroids.

PATHOGENESIS AND HOST IMMUNITY. *E. histolytica* trophozoites cause disease by sequentially adhering to colonic mucins, disrupting mucosal barriers with proteolytic enzymes, and contact-dependent lysis of host cells, including responding inflammatory cells. Trophozoite adherence to colonic mucins is mediated by a galactose-binding surface lectin; attachment by this lectin is the first step in the amebic lysis of human cells. Intestinal infection with *E. dispar* usually clears within 8 to 12 months without evidence of a systemic immune response. Cure of invasive amebiasis is associated with resistance to recurrent disease and immunity for a year or more to asymptomatic intestinal infection. Protective immunity is apparently mediated by development of a serum anti-

body and an amebicidal cell-mediated immune response with lymphokine-activated macrophages and a CD8 subset of cytotoxic lymphocytes serving as effector cells. Acute amebiasis is associated with the occurrence of antigen-specific suppression of cell-mediated responses to *E. histolytica*, facilitating parasite survival in tissues. The mucosal secretory IgA antiamebic antibody response that develops after *E. histolytica* infection has a protective role against recurrent intestinal infection.

CLINICAL DISEASE SYNDROMES. The disease syndromes caused by *E. histolytica* are summarized in Table 428–1. It is unknown whether health is impaired by asymptomatic infection with *E. histolytica*. Occasionally, infected patients present with non-specific gastrointestinal complaints, such as bloating and cramps, without evidence of invasive colitis. Amebic rectocolitis is characterized by the subacute onset of bloody diarrhea over days, abdominal tenderness, and weight loss. Fever occurs in only one third of cases. Fulminant colitis with perforation is uncommon; patients are in a toxic state, are acutely ill, and have a rigid, tender abdomen. Toxic megacolon is an unusual complication that is associated with the inappropriate use of corticosteroids when amebic colitis is mistaken for idiopathic inflammatory bowel disease. Chronic non-dysenteric amebic colitis can manifest with years of intermittent bloody diarrhea, a syndrome symptomatically indistinguishable from ulcerative colitis. Ameboma is a rare, segmental form of chronic amebic colitis commonly found in the cecum and ascending colon; it presents as a tender abdominal mass and can be confused with colonic carcinoma.

Extraintestinal disease consists mainly of amebic liver abscess, which can occur up to 5 months after the onset of intestinal infection. The presentation may be acute with fewer than 10 days of high fever and marked right upper quadrant tenderness. Alternatively, with more than 10 days of symptoms, fever is less frequent and pain and weight loss predominate. Fewer than a third of patients have concurrent diarrhea. Extension of an amebic liver abscess into the peritoneum or pericardium is a very acute clinical presentation that is more likely with a left lobe abscess. Disease can extend to the pleura, causing empyema, or, less likely, disseminate hematogenously to the lung and brain.

DIFFERENTIAL DIAGNOSIS AND WORK-UP. Algorithms for the diagnosis of amebic colitis and liver abscess are provided in Figures 428–1 and 428–2, respectively. The differential diagnosis of acute amebic colitis includes infection due to *Shigella*, *Campylobacter*, *Salmonella*, *Yersinia*, and invasive *Escherichia coli* species or *Clostridium difficile* toxin–mediated disease. Amebiasis is one cause of inflammatory colitis in which fecal leukocytes may be absent, owing to the ability of trophozoites to lyse human neutrophils. Recently, several research groups succeeded in correctly diagnosing *E. histolytica* and *E. dispar* intestinal infections by directly detecting amebic antigen in feces and serum. Although these diagnostic tests are commercially available, in current clinical practice the diagnosis of intestinal amebiasis still rests on the morphologic identification of trophozoites in fecal specimens. At least three stool samples are necessary to reach a 90% yield; samples

Table 428–1 ■ CLINICAL SYNDROMES ASSOCIATED WITH *E. HISTOLYTICA* INFECTION

Intestinal Disease
Asymptomatic infection
Acute rectocolitis (dysentery)
Fulminant colitis with perforation
Toxic megacolon
Chronic nondysenteric colitis
Ameboma
Extraintestinal Disease
Liver abscess
Liver abscess complicated by:
   Peritonitis
   Empyema
   Pericarditis
Lung abscess
Brain abscess
Genitourinary disease

From Mandell GL, Douglas RG Jr, Bennett JE (eds): Principles and Practices of Infectious Diseases, 3rd ed. New York, Churchill Livingstone, 1989.

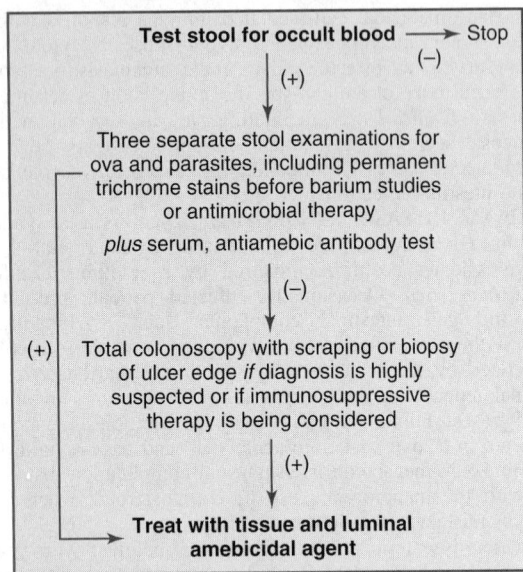

FIGURE 428–1 ■ Diagnostic evaluation for acute amebic rectocolitis in a patient with suggestive epidemiology and clinical manifestations. (From Kass EH, Platt R [eds]: Current Therapy in Infectious Disease—3. Philadelphia, BC Decker, 1990.)

should be refrigerated or placed in fixative if they cannot be processed immediately. Laboratories in the United States frequently falsely identify fecal leukocytes as trophozoites; careful study with skilled microscopy is necessary. Serology for antiamebic antibodies is positive in more than 90% of patients with amebic colitis having at least 1 week of symptoms and is very helpful in making a correct diagnosis. Interpretation of results can be difficult in highly endemic areas, where up to 25% of the population is seropositive owing to the persistence of serum antibodies for years after asymptomatic E. histolytica infection. Endoscopy with biopsies of the ulcer edge is diagnostic in 90% of cases; this is helpful for a rapid diagnosis and to differentiate amebiasis from idiopathic inflammatory bowel disease.

The key study for diagnosing amebic liver abscess is abdominal ultrasonography, a rapid, non-invasive procedure that differentiates biliary tract disease from a non-homogeneous cavitary defect in the liver. The differential diagnosis can then be narrowed to amebic liver abscess, pyogenic bacterial abscess, echinococcal cyst, and hepatoma. Attention to epidemiologic risk factors and detecting serum antiamebic antibodies are usually sufficient to establish the diagnosis, with the caveat that serology may be negative in patients with fewer than 7 days of symptoms. However, if there is sufficient risk for a bacterial abscess and a serologic study is not immediately available, then a "skinny-needle" aspiration, guided by ultrasonography or computed tomography, can be performed. This procedure with culture will diagnose and assist in therapy of a bacterial abscess; aspiration of an amebic abscess yields a yellow proteinaceous fluid often without white blood cells or amebas. The trophozoites are found in tissue at the periphery of the liver lesion.

THERAPY. Regimens for treating amebiasis are summarized in Table 428–2. Therapy for invasive amebiasis requires a tissue-active agent followed by a drug effective in the bowel lumen. In pregnant women, the use of non-absorbable agents (paromomycin) or the judicious use of metronidazole is advisable. Therapy for asymptomatic intestinal infection with E. dispar is not indicated; however, it is advisable for asymptomatic E. histolytica infection in which serology for serum antiamebic antibodies should be positive. Careful follow-up stool examinations are necessary, because all available agents are not always effective in eradicating intestinal infection. Patients with amebic liver abscess respond gradually to therapy, with decreased pain and fever over 3 to 5 days. A small minority do not respond at all within 3 days or have a very large abscess that appears close to rupture; needle aspiration is indicated in such patients. After aspiration, continued therapy with metronidazole should be adequate. Studies have revealed a high incidence of intestinal infection by culture in patients with amebic liver abscess. To avoid a recurrence of disease, therapy must include a luminal cysticidal agent.

PREVENTION. E. histolytica infection can be prevented by the availability of clean water, adequate sanitation, and avoidance of sexual practices or living conditions that facilitate direct fecal-oral contamination. Boiling is the only reliable way of killing cysts; halide solutions are not reliable. In endemic areas, uncooked foods such as salads and vegetables should be avoided. No vaccine or acceptable form of chemoprophylaxis is available; however, current research on the pathogenesis of amebiasis and the host immune response has led to the production of multiple, recombinant E. histolytica antigens that are effective as subunit vaccines in experimental models of amebic liver abscess.

AMEBIC MENINGOENCEPHALITIS. Amebic meningoencephalitis is a rare clinical syndrome caused by the free-living amebas Naegleria fowleri and Acanthamoeba species. N. fowleri causes a primary amebic meningoencephalitis (PAM), whereas Acanthamoeba produces a subacute granulomatous amebic encephalitis (GAE).

N. fowleri in trophozoite or flagellate form grows best at high temperatures (46° C); encystment occurs at low temperatures. Acanthamoeba species, which have a trophozoite and cyst form, grow at normal ambient temperatures (25 to 35° C). PAM is a highly infrequent disease despite the massive exposure of populations to warm fresh water. GAE is usually restricted to immunosuppressed populations, such as those with AIDS or those with organ transplants. N. fowleri enters the central nervous system (CNS) by penetrating the nasal mucosa and cribriform plate and is highly cytolytic. GAE probably results from hematogenous dissemination and can be distinguished from PAM by the presence of cysts in tissue.

PAM is characterized by the abrupt onset of headache, fever, and meningismus, with rapid development of focal neurologic findings, including olfactory loss. CT demonstrates non-specific edema. A neutrophilic cerebrospinal fluid (CSF) pleocytosis is frequently associated with increased CSF protein and hypoglycorrhachia. A negative CSF Gram stain result, India ink preparation, culture for bacteria, and cryptococcal antigen study in a patient with acute

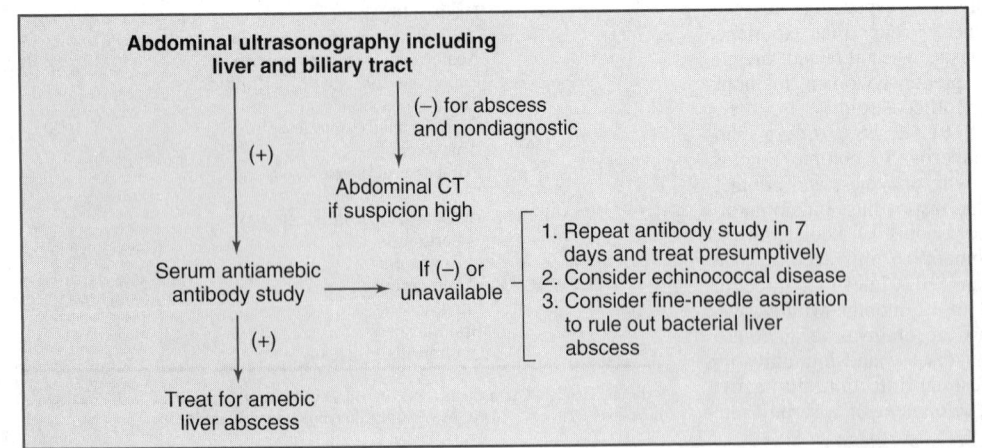

FIGURE 428–2 ■ Diagnostic evaluation for amebic liver abscess in a patient with suggestive epidemiology and clinical manifestations. (From Kass EH, Platt R [eds]: Current Therapy in Infectious Disease—3. Philadelphia, BC Decker, 1990.)

Table 428-2 ■ THERAPEUTIC REGIMENS FOR TREATMENT OF AMEBIASIS*

Cyst Passers

Diloxanide furoate, 500 mg twice daily × 10 days, or
Paromomycin, 30 mg/kg/d in three divided doses × 5–10 days, or
Tetracycline, 250 mg four times a day × 10 days, then diiodohydroxyquin, 650 three times a day × 20 days

Invasive Rectocolitis

Metronidazole, 750 mg three times a day × 5–10 days
or 2.4 g/d × 2–3 days
or 50 mg/kg × 1 dose
  plus diloxanide furoate or paromomycin or if metronidazole not tolerated
Dehydroemetine, 1–1.5 mg/kg/d × 5 days plus diloxanide furoate or paromomycin

Liver Abscess

Metronidazole, 750 mg three times a day × 5–10 days or 2.4 g/d × 1–2 days plus diloxanide furoate or paromomycin or if metronidazole not tolerated
Dehydroemetine, 1–1.5 mg/kg/d × 5 days plus diloxanide furoate or paromomycin

*All dosages are for oral administration except dehydroemetine, which is given intramuscularly; metronidazole can be used intravenously.

Adapted with permission from Mandell GL, Douglas RG Jr, Bennett JE (eds): Principles and Practices of Infectious Diseases, 3rd ed. New York, Churchill Livingstone, 1989.

meningitis who has a history of exposure to fresh water suggests the need to examine the CSF for motile trophozoites (10 to 30 mm), a finding that is diagnostic. Polymerase chain reaction and DNA probes specific for *N. fowleri* have been developed but are not yet clinically appropriate. In contrast, GAE manifests subacutely over weeks with focal CNS signs, headache, fever, and depressed mental status and is often complicated by seizures. The presence of *Acanthamoeba* organisms in a nodular or ulcerative skin lesion is helpful; study of the CSF usually reveals a nonspecific lymphocytosis with abnormally elevated protein levels. A brain biopsy is necessary to differentiate GAE from toxoplasmosis, pyogenic brain abscess, and other causes of focal CNS disease.

There is no treatment known to be efficacious for PAM or GAE. Treatment with systemic and intrathecal amphotericin B, which is effective in a mouse model, resulted in survival in two patients with PAM. *Acanthamoeba* organisms are usually susceptible in vitro to ketoconazole, miconazole, 5-flucytosine, and pentamidine. After determination of susceptibility of the patient's isolate in vitro, these agents and amphotericin B can be considered. These are rare disorders, and the risk of PAM from diving or water skiing in warm fresh water cannot be quantified. Other opportunistic infections are much more frequent than those caused by *Acanthamoeba* in immunosuppressed patients.

Barnett ND, Kaplan AM, Hopkin RJ, et al: Primary amoebic meningoencephalitis with *Naegleria fowleri:* Clinical review. Pediatr Neurol 15:230–234, 1996. *An excellent up-to-date review on PAM.*

Clark, CG: *Entamoeba dispar,* an organism reborn. Trans R Soc Trop Med Hyg 92: 361–364, 1998. *A excellent review of the biology of* E. dispar.

Huston CD, Petri WA Jr: Host-pathogen interaction in amebiasis and progress in vaccine development. Eur J Clin Microbiol Infect Dis 17:601–614, 1998. *An up-to-date review of pathogenesis and immunity in amebiasis.*

Katzenstein D, Rickerson V, Braude A: New concepts of amebic liver abscess derived from hepatic imaging, serodiagnosis, and hepatic enzymes in 67 consecutive cases in San Diego. Medicine 61:237, 1982. *Excellent clinical study of amebic liver abscess.*

Kidney DD, Kim SH: CNS infections with free-living amebas: Neuroimaging findings. Am J Roentgen 171:809–812, 1998. *Up-to-date discussion of neuroimaging findings with CT and MR in PAM and GAE.*

Stanley SL, JR: *Progress towards development of a vaccine for amebiasis.* Clin Microbiol Rev 10:637–649, 1997. *A recent review of the progress and future promise for development of an amebiasis vaccine.*

429 OTHER PROTOZOAN DISEASES

Richard D. Pearson

CYCLOSPORIASIS

Cyclospora cayetanensis has emerged as an important cause of gastroenteritis throughout the world among residents of developing

areas, including Peru, Nepal, Mexico, and Caribbean countries. It has also been reported among international travelers and among North Americans who ingested raspberries imported from Guatemala. *C. cayetanensis* is acquired through contaminated food and water and lives within enterocytes in the small bowel. It produces watery diarrhea, flatulence, fatigue, and abdominal pain. Symptoms may be prolonged and associated with substantial weight loss, particularly in persons with acquired immunodeficiency syndrome (AIDS).

The diagnosis is usually made by identifying cyclospora in stool samples. They can be stained with modified acid-fast preparations and appear fluorescent in stool specimens examined by ultraviolet microscopy. *C. cayetanensis* responds to treatment with trimethoprim, 160 mg, and sulfamethoxazole, 800 mg, b.i.d. for 7 days. Chronic suppressive therapy may be necessary in patients with human immunodeficiency virus (HIV).

Herwaldt BL, Ackers ML: An outbreak in 1996 of cyclosporiasis associated with imported raspberries: The Cyclospora Working Group. N Engl J Med 336:1548, 1997. *The paper summarizes a large outbreak of cyclosporiasis in the United States caused by imported raspberries.*

Soave R: *Cyclospora:* An overview. Clin Infect Dis 23:429, 1996. *This is an excellent review of the epidemiologic characteristics, clinical manifestations, and treatment of cyclosporiasis.*

OTHER ENTERIC PROTOZOANS

A number of other protozoa can cause enteric disease (Table 429–1). They are acquired by ingesting contaminated food or water. Some reside in the lumen of the bowel; others invade and multiply within enterocytes. Enteric protozoan pathogens should be considered in the differential diagnosis of patients with persistent diarrhea and abdominal symptoms, particularly those who have a history of recent international travel or who are infected with HIV.

The diagnosis is typically made by identifying parasites in the stool. Microscopic examination should be performed by experts because fecal debris may be confused with protozoa. Pathogenic protozoa must also be differentiated from non-pathogens such as *Entamoeba coli, Endolimax nana, Iodamoeba butschlii, Pentatrichomonas hominis,* and *Chilomastix mesnili.* Polymerase chain reaction–(PCR)-based diagnostic assays are under development. Therapy includes rehydration and administration of the appropriate antiprotozoal drug (Table 429–1).

Drugs for parasitic diseases. Med Lett Drugs Ther 40:1, 1998. *Consensus recommendations for the treatment of parasitic diseases are provided in tables. Key articles are referenced.*

Goodgame RW: Understanding intestinal spore-forming protozoa: Crytosporidia, microsporidia, isospora, and cyclospora. Ann Intern Med 124:429, 1996. *Excellent review of several emerging enteric pathogens.*

BABESIOSIS

Babesiosis is a tick-borne malaria-like disease. It is caused by *Babesia* species that infect erythrocytes. They are important pathogens of animals around the world and occasionally infect people. Most human infections in North America are caused by *B. microti,* which is found in zoonotic areas of coastal New England including the barrier islands of Nantucket, Martha's Vineyard, Long Island, Block Island, and Shelter Island; the upper Midwest, particularly Wisconsin; and occasionally elsewhere. Sporadic human cases due to *Babesia* WA1 strain have been reported from Washington and northern California. *B. divergens* is responsible for most of the European cases.

In the northeastern United States the major reservoir is the white-footed mouse, *Peromyscus leucopus,* but other rodents are involved. The vector is the deer tick, *Ixodes scapularis,* the same tick that transmits *Borrelia burgdorferi,* the cause of Lyme disease (see Chapter 368) and human granulocytic ehrlichiosis. Concurrent cases of Lyme disease and babesiosis have been reported. *Babesia* organisms are transmitted to humans by the nymph stage of the tick, which is 1 to 2 mm in length and easily missed, or less commonly by adults, which are somewhat larger. Blood transfusions have also been implicated in a few cases. *B. divergens* is transmitted by *Ixodes ricinus* in Europe.

In immunocompetent persons *Babesia* infections are usually asymptomatic or mild and self-limited, but they can be severe, particularly in asplenic persons, the elderly, or the immunocompro-

Table 429–1 ■ OTHER ENTERIC PROTOZOA

ORGANISM	EPIDEMIOLOGY	MANIFESTATIONS	THERAPY*
Balantidium coli	Primarily an infection of animals, especially pigs, but also affects humans	Asymptomatic or mild and self-resolving; a few cases are more severe with abdominal pain, blood, and mucus in the stool	Tetracycline (500 mg q.i.d. for 10 days) *Alternative:* Metronidazole (750 mg t.i.d. for 5 days) *or* Iodoquinol (650 mg t.i.d. for 20 days)
Blastocystis hominis	Probably worldwide, including North America; often found concomitantly with *Giardia lamblia*	Pathogenicity is debated	The need for treatment is debated, but efficacy has been reported with Metronidazole (750 mg t.i.d. for 10 days) *or* Iodoquinol (650 mg t.i.d. for 20 days)
Cyclospora cayetanensis	Distribution appears to be worldwide; associated with imported raspberries from Guatemala	Can produce severe, watery diarrhea and fatigue lasting weeks and prolonged disease in those with AIDS	Trimethoprim, 160 mg and Sulfamethoxazole, 800 mg b.i.d. for 7 days; suppressive therapy may be necessary in persons with AIDS
Dientamoeba fragilis	Worldwide distribution; frequently found concomitantly with the pinworm *Enterobius vermicularis*	Most asymptomatic; diarrhea reported	Iodoquinol (650 mg t.i.d. for 20 days) *or* Paromomycin (25–30 mg/kg body weight/d in 3 doses for 7 days) *or* Tetracycline (500 mg q.i.d. for 10 days)
Entamoeba polecki	Most cases reported from Papua New Guinea, but probably worldwide distribution; primarily found in pigs and monkeys; human infections are rare	Most asymptomatic; some have symptoms similar to those of *Entamoeba histolytica* colitis	Metronidazole (750 mg t.i.d. for 10 days)
Isospora belli	Worldwide distribution, most prevalent in Latin America and Africa	Self-limited diarrhea in immunocompetent residents and travelers, but persistent, severe diarrhea in patients with AIDS	Trimethoprim 160 mg plus sulfamethoxazole 800 mg q.i.d. for 10 days then b.i.d. for 3 weeks; suppressive therapy may be necessary in persons with AIDS
Microspordia (*Enterocytozoon bieneusi* and *Encephalitozoon* [*Septata*] *intestinalis*)	Apparent worldwide distribution	AIDS patients with persistent diarrhea and wasting; rare cases in immunocompetent persons	Uncertain: abendazole 400 mg b.i.d.; suppressive therapy may be necessary in persons with AIDS
Sarcocystis species	Common pathogens of animals; rare in humans; acquired by ingesting contaminated beef or pork	Nausea, vomiting, abdominal pain, and diarrhea; eosinophilic necrotizing enteritis has been reported	No specific therapy

*Recommendations based on drugs for parasitic infections. Med Lett Drugs Ther 40:1, 1998. The dosages and durations are for adults.

mised, including those with AIDS. The incubation period varies from 1 to 6 weeks with tick transmission and up to 9 weeks with blood transfusion. The majority of those infected by ticks are unaware of the bite. Symptomatic patients experience irregular fever, sweats, chills, myalgia, fatigue, headache, and other constitutional symptoms. Unlike in malaria, there is no periodicity to the disease. Fever is frequently the only abnormality found on physical examination, but hepatomegaly or splenomegaly may be present. Erythema migrans may be observed in persons with concurrent *B. burgdorferi* infection.

There is evidence of hemolytic anemia of varying severity. The white blood count may be normal or decreased and the platelet count low. Levels of liver enzymes and bilirubin are often elevated. Severe cases may be associated with gross hemaglobinuria, jaundice, pancytopenia, hemophagocytosis, or the acute respiratory distress syndrome. Parasitemia persists from a few weeks to several months in untreated persons. In Europe *B. divergens* has been associated with severe disease and death; most of the patients are asplenic.

Babesiosis is diagnosed by identifying intraerythrocytic parasites in Giemsa-stained blood smears. They must be differentiated from malaria. In some cases dividing babesia make up four daughter cells that appear as the characteristic "Maltese cross." In contrast to organisms that cause malaria *Babesia* species do not form pigmented granules. Blood smear results may be negative in patients with low parasitemia. Antibodies can be detected by an indirect immunofluorescent assay that is specific for *B. microti*, but the test does not differentiate persons with prior exposure from those with acute infection. Inoculation of Syrian hamsters and PCR-based assays have been used to diagnose cases of *B. microti* in which parasites are not seen in blood smears.

Most cases of babesiosis in North America occur in immunocompetent persons and resolve spontaneously. In adult patients who have symptoms, particularly those who are asplenic, elderly, or

immunocompromised, babesiosis is treated with clindamycin 1.2 g b.i.d. (parenterally) or 600 mg t.i.d. (orally) administered concurrently with quinine sulfate 650 mg t.i.d. (orally) for 7 days. Exchange transfusions have been used in patients with high levels of parasitemia and severe disease. Therapy should be initiated early in persons infected with *B. divergens* in Europe because rapidly increasing parasitemia can result in massive hemolysis, renal failure, and death. Azithromycin and atovaquone have been shown to have activity against *Babesia* species in animal models.

Boustani MR, Gelfand JA: Babesiosis. Clin Infect Dis 22:611, 1996. *The life cycle, epidemiologic characteristics, clinical manifestations, and therapy of human babesiosis are reviewed in detail.*

TRICHOMONIASIS

Trichomonas vaginalis is among the most prevalent of all pathogenic protozoa. The organism is oval, approximately 10 by 15 μm wide, and has four free flagella at its anterior pole and a fifth in an undulating membrane that runs along the cell. *T. vaginalis* is usually spread by sexual contact. The highest incidences of disease are among women with multiple sexual partners and those with other sexually transmitted diseases (see Chapter 361). It can also be passed from infected mothers to their newborn daughters, but it is seldom symptomatic in girls before menarche. *T. vaginalis* is able to survive for some time in moist environments, and non-venereal transmission can occur.

As many as half of the *T. vaginalis* infections in women are asymptomatic. The remainder are associated with vaginal discharge, vulvovaginal irritation, dyspareunia, or dysuria. The discharge tends to be watery and copious, but in some cases it is thick and may be yellow or green. Patients may notice an odor, but that is more common with bacterial vaginosis. On pelvic examination there is usually inflammation of the vaginal walls. Punctate hemorrhages on the exocervix, causing the classic "strawberry cervix," are uncommonly found on gross inspection, but they are observed in approximately half of infected women if colposcopy is performed. The pH of the vaginal contents is typically elevated above the normal level of 4.5, as it is in bacterial vaginosis.

Most men with *T. vaginalis* are asymptomatic, but the organism is isolated on occasion from men with symptoms of urethritis who have negative findings for *Neisseria gonorrhoeae* and *Chlamydia trachomatis* (see Chapter 370). Urethral discharge is usually scant in such cases. On rare occasions *T. vaginalis* can cause epididymitis; produce superficial penile ulcerations, which are usually located under the prepuce; or involve the prostate.

Diagnosis of trichomonas vaginitis is usually made by identifying the parasite in vaginal discharge. The trophozoites have a twitching movement with active flagella. They are seen in wet mounts of vaginal secretions in approximately 60% of infected women. Polymorphonuclear leukocytes are usually present. Culture is the most sensitive method of diagnosis, and commercial kits are now available. In men a wet mount of material from a platinum loop scraping of the anterior urethra reveals the organism in approximately half of the cases. Prostatic massage prior to collecting urine for trichomonas culture is the most sensitive diagnostic approach. Sero-diagnostic studies lack sensitivity and specificity.

Metronidazole is the treatment of choice; a single dose of 2 g is effective. Sexual partners should be treated concurrently to prevent reinfection. Metronidazole, 250 mg three times a day for 7 days, is an alternative. Single-dose therapy ensures patient compliance, but the higher dose can produce nausea and a metallic taste. Metronidazole also has a disulfiram-like effect, and patients consuming it with alcohol may experience severe nausea, vomiting, and flushing. The use of metronidazole is relatively contraindicated during pregnancy. Treatment failures with metronidazole are encountered. Some are due to reinfection, others to poor compliance, but a subset is apparently due to metronidazole resistance. In such cases high doses of metronidazole have been administered for longer periods. Tinidazole, which is not licensed for use in the United States, is also effective for trichomoniasis when administered as a single 2-g dose.

duBouchet L, Spence MR, Rein MF, et al: Multicenter comparison of clotrimazole vaginal tablets, oral metronidazole, and vaginal suppositories containing sulfanilamide, aminacrine hydrochloride, and allantoin in the treatment of symptomatic trichomoniasis. Sex Transm Dis 24:156, 1997. *A comparative study demonstrating that oral metronidazole is more effective than topical preparations for the treatment of vaginal trichomoniasis.*

Krieger JN, Jenny C, Verdon M, et al: Clinical manifestations of trichomoniasis in men. Ann Intern Med 118:844, 1993. *Summarizes the clinical manifestations of trichomoniasis in men.*

Rein MF: *Trichomonas vaginalis. In* Mandell GL, Bennett JE, Dolin R: Principles and Practice of Infectious Diseases, 4th ed. New York, Churchill Livingstone, 1995, p 2493. *The epidemiologic characteristics, diagnosis, and treatment of trichomoniasis are reviewed.*

HELMINTHIC DISEASES

430   CESTODE INFECTIONS

Charles H. King

The eight cestode species that most commonly cause human infection are listed in Table 430–1. Although this class of parasites is often referred to, collectively, as "tapeworms," not all cestode parasites develop into tapeworms in the human host. The key to understanding the rather broad spectrum of cestode-associated illness is to recall that these parasites divide their life cycle between two or more different animal hosts, termed *intermediate* and *definitive* hosts. The intermediate host harbors the immature parasite as a tissue cyst, whereas the subsequent definitive host harbors the mature parasite as a tapeworm. For a given cestode species, humans may serve as *either* intermediate or definitive hosts.

The *intermediate* host is typically an insect or herbivorous (omnivorous) vertebrate that ingests parasite eggs in fecally contaminated food or water. The cestode eggs hatch into invasive oncospheres in this primary host's intestinal tract, then migrate into the host viscera or muscles to develop into immature cystic forms, called cysticerci or cysticercoids (for Cyclophyllidea cestodes such as *Taenia* and *Hymenolepis*), or procercoid and plerocercoid larvae (for Pseudophyllidea cestodes such as *Diphyllobothrium*). Humans become intermediate hosts for cestode species by ingesting parasite eggs in food or water, as in echinococcosis, or rarely by direct transfer of plerocercoid larvae from animal tissues, as in sparganosis.

The *definitive* host for a cestode species is a carnivorous or omnivorous mammal that acquires infection by consuming larval cysts in the uncooked tissues of an intermediate host. Upon exposure to stomach acid and bile salts in the digestive tract, the larvae excyst and develop into mature tapeworms within the intestinal lumen. Adult tapeworms contain two sections: a *scolex* (or head) used to adhere to the wall of the intestine and a *strobila*, or tapelike chain of developing segments called proglottides. The hermaphroditic proglottides produce large numbers of fertile, infectious parasite eggs that reach the environment either free or enclosed within parasite segments in the host's feces. Carnivorous humans become definitive hosts by ingesting cyst-infested meat of intermediate hosts (e.g., fish, pork, or beef), after which the cysts develop into intraluminal, intestinal tapeworms.

We are strictly definitive hosts for the cestodes *D. latum* (the "fish" tapeworm) and *T. saginata* (the "beef" tapeworm). These adult tapeworms do not enter the tissues of the human body and cause only minimal clinical symptoms. In contrast, we are solely

Table 430–1 ■ COMMON HUMAN CESTODE INFECTIONS

SPECIES	STAGE FOUND IN HUMANS	COMMON NAME	PATHOLOGY	THERAPY
Diphyllobothrium latum	Adult	Fish tapeworm	Pernicious anemia	Niclosamide Praziquantel
Hymenolepis nana	Adult	Dwarf tapeworm	Rarely symptomatic	Niclosamide Praziquantel
Taenia saginata	Adult	Beef tapeworm	Rarely symptomatic	
Taenia solium	Adult	Pork tapeworm	Rarely symptomatic	Niclosamide Praziquantel
	Larva	Cysticercosis	Brain and tissue cysts	Albendazole Praziquantel Surgery
Echinococcus granulosus	Larva	Hydatid cyst disease	Solitary tissue cysts	Surgery Albendazole
Echinococcus multilocularis	Larva	Alveolar cyst disease	Multilocular cysts	Surgery Albendazole
Taenia multiceps	Larva	Bladderworm, coenurosis	Brain and eye cysts	Surgery
Spirometra mansonoides	Larva	Sparganosis	Subcutaneous larvae	Surgery

intermediate hosts for *Echinococcus granulosus* (hydatid cyst disease), *Echinococcus multilocularis* (alveolar cyst disease), *T. multiceps* (coenurosis), and *Spirometra* species. In the human body, these parasites develop as larval cysts and cause significant symptomatic tissue damage.

There are two exceptions to this rule. First, patients with *Taenia solium* infection may be infected with larval cysts (cysticercosis), adult tapeworms ("pork" tapeworm), or both. Second, in the case of the dwarf tapeworm, *Hymenolepis nana*, complete egg-to-tapeworm development can take place within a single human host. *H. nana* can thus be transmitted directly from person to person, and internal autoinfection may substantially increase the tapeworm burden of an infected individual. For all other cestode infections, increases in parasite burden occur only by means of continued exposure to egg-contaminated or larvae-infested foods and water.

INTESTINAL CESTODE (TAPEWORM) INFECTIONS

Diphyllobothrium Latum

D. latum tapeworms are the largest parasites that infect humans, ranging up to 10 meters in length. Infection is acquired by ingestion of parasite cysts in the tissues of smoked or uncooked freshwater fish (e.g., as sushi, sashimi, or ceviche). Tapeworms develop to maturity within 3 to 6 weeks after exposure and may survive for up to 20 years. Infection is prevalent (up to 2% of local residents) in many parts of the world; endemic foci are found in lake or delta regions of Scandinavia, the former Soviet Union, Japan, Europe, Chile, and North America. Contamination of fresh-water bodies by raw sewage increases the risk for *D. latum* infection, but stable transmission may also occur owing to local infection of alternate definitive hosts, such as foxes, wolves, minks, and bears.

CLINICAL MANIFESTATIONS. For most patients, *D. latum* infection produces few, if any, symptoms. These are typically limited to nonspecific complaints of weakness, dizziness, craving for salt, diarrhea, and intermittent abdominal discomfort. Occasional patients may experience vomiting, severe abdominal pain, and weight loss. In cases of multiple infection, biliary or intestinal obstruction may occur. One to 2% of patients with *D. latum* infection develop significant vitamin B_{12} deficiency, resulting in megaloblastic anemia and/or neurologic disease. Folate deficiency may also occur. Vitamin B_{12} deficiency is a product of extensive vitamin uptake by the worm as well as worm-induced interference with gastrointestinal uptake by the host (despite normal gastric acidity and intrinsic factor production). Vitamin B_{12} deficiency is most common among older patients and is more likely to occur in patients with low dietary intake of vitamins, multiple tapeworms, or a tapeworm in the proximal jejunum. In the debilitated host, nervous system complications can be quite extensive and can range from peripheral neuropathy to the syndrome of severe combined degeneration (see Chapter 489).

DIAGNOSIS. The diagnosis of *D. latum* infection is made by stool examination for characteristic operculated eggs that are 65 by 45 μm. Recovery of proglottides is infrequent owing to segment degeneration during intestinal transit.

TREATMENT. Treatment is with niclosamide or praziquantel, as summarized in Table 430–2. Severe vitamin B_{12} deficiency can be rapidly treated by parenteral vitamin injections.

PREVENTION. Fish tapeworm infection is prevented by avoiding consumption of raw, smoked, or salted fish from endemic areas. Parasite cysts may be killed by cooking (above 56°C for 5 minutes) or by freezing ($-$ 20°C for 24 hours).

Hymenolepis Nana

H. nana, or dwarf tapeworm, is found frequently in warm, dry climates and is prevalent in Southern and Eastern Europe, Asia, Africa, Central and South America, and Australia. It is the only human tapeworm that does not require an intermediate host. In the small intestine, hatching eggs release oncospheres that penetrate the villi of the mucosa. Four to 5 days later, the developed cysticercoid ruptures out of the villus, and a parasite scolex attaches to the lining of the ileum, maturing in 10 to 12 days. Mature worms are small, measuring 25 to 40 mm long by 1 mm wide. Autoinfection can occur internally, i.e., within the small bowel, or externally, via the fecal-oral route, resulting in heavy infection. With time, however, a regulatory immunity to infection may develop, so that *H. nana* infection can be spontaneously cleared. Intensive infection is more common in institutionalized, malnourished, or immunodeficient individuals.

CLINICAL MANIFESTATIONS. The clinical manifestations of *H. nana* vary with intensity and may include diarrhea, anorexia, abdominal pain, and pallor. A statistical association with phlyctenular keratoconjunctivitis has been observed and has been tentatively ascribed to the immune response to infection.

DIAGNOSIS. The diagnosis of *H. nana* infection is made by examining stool for eggs 30 to 47 μm that have a characteristic double membrane. Proglottides are usually not seen in the stool.

TREATMENT. Treatment is with niclosamide or praziquantel, as outlined in Table 430–2. Compared with the treatment of other tapeworm infections, longer courses of niclosamide and higher doses of praziquantel are recommended for the therapy of *H. nana* infection because of the relative resistance of larval cysticercoids to drug therapy. Because of the potential for late emergence of worms from viable cysticercoids remaining in the ileum, heavily infected individuals should be retested for infection and retreated 10 to 14 days after initial therapy.

PREVENTION. Because *H. nana* is easily transmitted from person to person, sanitation and hand washing are essential to control this parasite. Mass chemotherapy may also be used to suppress endemic transmission, particularly within closed institutions.

Taenia Saginata

T. saginata, or beef tapeworm, is widespread in cattle-breeding areas of the world. Endemic foci (defined as prevalence >10%) are found in the southern Russian republics, in the Near East, and in central and eastern Africa. Infection is less common in other parts of the world but is found at prevalence rates of 0.1 to 5% in Europe, Southeast Asia, and South America. Infection is acquired by consuming cysticerci in the muscle tissue of infected cattle. The consumption of dishes such as steak tartare, "bleu" or rare steak,

Table 430–2 ■ **THERAPY FOR INTESTINAL CESTODE (TAPEWORM) INFECTION**

	NICLOSAMIDE	PRAZIQUANTEL
Dosage Adults Children >34 kg Children 11–34 kg	2 grams (4 tablets) 1.5 grams (3 tablets) 1 gram (2 tablets)	10–12 mg/kg for all age groups (25 mg/kg for *H. nana*)
Administration	For most tapeworm species, taken as a single dose; tablets must be thoroughly chewed before swallowing to obtain complete therapeutic effect; a 7-day course of drugs used for *H. nana,* with reduced pediatric doses on days 2–7	Taken as a single dose for all species; may repeat after 7 days for heavy *H. nana* infections.
Side effects	Nausea, vomiting, abdominal pain, diarrhea, drowsiness, dizziness, headache, pruritus	Mild but frequent, including dizziness, myalgias, nausea, vomiting, diarrhea, abdominal pain
Pregnancy	No known mutagenic effects; considered safe if indicated; because of risk of cysticercosis by autoinfection in T. solium tapeworm infection, therapy should not be delayed	

and undercooked shish kebabs is associated with infection in North American travelers to endemic areas.

CLINICAL MANIFESTATIONS. *T. saginata* infection may cause nonspecific complaints of weakness and mild abdominal discomfort in a minority (one third) of patients. Because *T. saginata* proglottides are motile, they may cause acute abdominal symptoms by migrating into and obstructing the appendix or the pancreatic and biliary ducts. A psychologically distressing feature of infection (and often the first symptom reported by the patient) occurs when motile proglottides migrate out of the anus onto skin or clothing or when they are observed moving in the feces.

DIAGNOSIS. The diagnosis of taeniasis is most readily established by stool examination and perianal inspection for parasite proglottides and eggs. It is not possible, however, to distinguish *T. saginata* eggs from those of *T. solium* morphologically, and the definitive diagnosis of *T. saginata* infection requires pathologic examination of proglottid features or DNA hybridization studies. In practice, because patients with *T. solium* are at risk for self-infection with cysticercosis (see below), and because medical therapy for taeniasis is both safe and highly effective, treatment of an undetermined *Taenia* species infection should not be delayed pending speciation of the infecting tapeworm.

TREATMENT. Treatment of beef tapeworm infection is with praziquantel or niclosamide, as outlined in Table 430–2. Both medications are highly effective in eliminating infection, and no special preparation or purgation is required. After therapy, the parasite scolex is digested within the gastrointestinal tract before it is passed in the feces. Although with the highly effective medications currently in use one no longer needs to collect the scolex to be assured that the parasite head has been expelled, digestive destruction of the head limits the ability to establish a species-specific clinical diagnosis for individual *Taenia* infections.

PREVENTION. *T. saginata* infection is prevented by avoiding foods containing undercooked or raw beef. As for the fish tapeworm, cooking to 56°C for 5 minutes or freezing at −20°C for 7 to 10 days destroys the infective larvae.

Taenia Solium

T. solium, also known as pork tapeworm, causes human infection in two different forms. Individuals who consume undercooked pork containing intermediate parasite cysts develop intestinal *T. solium* tapeworms. Individuals who consume parasite eggs may develop intermediate parasite cysts within the tissues of the body. (This condition, called *cysticercosis*, is described in more detail in the section on tissue cestode infections.) Autoinfection, most likely via the fecal-oral route, is possible, and a single patient may harbor both adult tapeworm and tissue cysticerci. *T. solium* infection is prevalent in Mexico, Central and South America, Africa, the Cape Verde Islands, southern Europe, Southeast Asia, and the Philippines. Most infections seen in the United States and Canada are found in immigrants from these endemic foci.

CLINICAL MANIFESTATIONS. *T. solium* tapeworms are relatively short (3 meters) but may survive for several decades once established in the human jejunum. Generally, tapeworm infections with *T. solium* produce minimal or no symptoms, being limited to mild, nonspecific abdominal complaints. Unlike *T. saginata* proglottides, the segments of *T. solium* are nonmotile and are unlikely to cause obstruction.

DIAGNOSIS. The diagnosis of intestinal infection with *T. solium* tapeworm is made by examining the stool for eggs and proglottides. Because the eggs are morphologically indistinguishable from those of *T. saginata*, study of the proglottid or head of the tapeworms is required for species identification. Stool samples and proglottides should be handled with care because of the risk of acquiring cysticercosis by accidental ingestion of *T. solium* eggs.

TREATMENT. *T. solium* tapeworm infection is treated with either niclosamide or praziquantel, as outlined in Table 430–2. Once diagnosis is established, therapy should be instituted as soon as possible because of the risk of autoinfection with cysticercosis. Therapy of concurrent cysticercosis is substantially longer and more intensive than that for intestinal infection and is described in detail in the section on tissue cestode infections.

Other Intestinal Cestodes

Other tapeworms that occasionally infect humans include the dog tapeworm *Dipylidium caninum* and the rodent tapeworm *Hymenolepis diminuta*. These are most common in children and are acquired

by inadvertently ingesting the intermediate larval forms of these parasites in the bodies of fleas or other insects. Usually, *D. caninum* and *H. diminuta* infections produce minimal symptoms. Diagnosis is established by stool examination, and infections are readily treated with standard doses of niclosamide or praziquantel.

TISSUE CESTODE (CYST) INFECTION

Echinococcosis

Human echinococcosis causes significant morbidity and mortality in livestock-raising regions in all parts of the world. The causative agents of "hydatid" and "alveolar" cyst disease in humans are the intermediate larval forms of the tapeworms *Echinococcus granulosus* and *E. multilocularis,* respectively.

Like other cestodes, *Echinococcus* tapeworms have both intermediate and definitive hosts. For *Echinococcus* species, dogs and other canines are the definitive hosts. Tapeworm-infected animals pass eggs in their feces, which contaminate the local environment. Contamination of grazing areas and foodstuffs results in egg ingestion by intermediate hosts, e.g., humans, sheep, goats, camels, and horses for *E. granulosus* and mice or other small rodents for *E. multilocularis*. Life-cycle transmission is completed when the definitive carnivore host consumes meat or offal of the intermediate host that contains hydatid or alveolar cysts. Protoscolices within the cysts mature in the lumen of the canine gut to become adult, egg-bearing tapeworms. Because the cysts of *Echinococcus* contain a germinal layer that can produce multiple internal "daughter" cysts by asexual budding, an individual dog may develop infection with dozens of tapeworms after consuming a single large cyst. Once the tapeworms mature, a heavily infected dog may contaminate 10 or more hectares of ground with infectious eggs in a week.

In most areas of the world, burial practices make humans a "dead-end" host for *Echinococcus;* i.e., human infection does not perpetuate transmission in the local ecosystem. Nevertheless, the "inadvertent" hydatid cyst disease caused by *E. granulosus* and the more aggressive alveolar cyst disease caused by *E. multilocularis* are severe or even fatal illnesses for a significant minority of infected individuals.

EPIDEMIOLOGY. *E. granulosus* is common in livestock-raising areas of both developed and developing countries. Sheep- and goat-herding populations that keep dogs as pets or work animals are at highest risk for hydatid cyst disease. Until recently, hydatid disease was common in Australia, New Zealand, Argentina, Chile, Ireland, Scotland, the Basque country, the Mediterranean basin, and throughout middle Europe. Currently, the area with the highest prevalence in the world is the Turkana and Samburu regions of northwestern Kenya, where domestic and feral transmission of *E. granulosus* is perpetuated among nomadic farmers by poor hygienic practices. Occasional hydatid disease transmission is also found in central Asia, Mexico, the United States, and South America.

Alveolar cyst disease due to *E. multilocularis* is usually transmitted by wild animals, e.g., foxes and bush dogs, and is found in the arctic regions of the United States, Canada, and the former Soviet Union, as well as in rural areas of Europe and Turkey.

CLINICAL MANIFESTATIONS. Human disease caused by *Echinococcus* species results from bloodborne invasion of the liver (50 to 70% of patients), lungs (20 to 30%), or other organs by developing parasite oncospheres. As these mature, they grow within tissues by concentric enlargement *(E. granulosus)* or by extension through adjacent host tissues *(E. multilocularis)*. At any given time, most infected individuals are asymptomatic, and it may take 5 to 20 years for a cyst to grow to sufficient size (3 to 15 cm) to cause symptoms. When present, symptoms and findings refer to the anatomic site of involvement and derive from local inflammation, secondary bacterial infection, obstruction, or local mass effect. In hydatid cyst disease, the growing cyst becomes surrounded by a fibrous capsule formed by host immune reaction. Within this primary unilocular cyst, multiple daughter cysts, each containing an infective protoscolex, develop by asexual budding of the germinal layer. In alveolar cyst disease, the parasite cyst is not well separated from surrounding tissues, and lateral budding and malignancy-like growth (including distant metastasis of daughter cysts) may occur.

Patients with symptomatic hydatid liver cysts may complain of abdominal discomfort or mass in the right upper quadrant. Cyst leakage into the peritoneal cavity or pleural space may be associated with fever, urticaria, or a severe anaphylactoid reaction. Invasion of the biliary system often leads to the passage of daughter cysts into the common bile duct, with clinical and chemical evidence of intermittent obstruction resembling choledocholithiasis. Individuals with symptomatic hydatid involvement of the lungs present with cough, hemoptysis, and pleurisy. Spontaneous rupture of the cyst may lead to intrathoracic spread or to evacuation of daughter cysts via the bronchus. At either lung or liver sites, bacterial superinfection may cause an acute presentation with symptoms of sepsis. Hydatid involvement of the brain is marked by slow-onset mass effect, hydrocephalus and, often, seizures. Cysts of the bone frequently fail to form a discrete capsule but rather cause local erosion of the cortex, resulting in pathologic fracture.

Symptomatic alveolar cyst disease most frequently refers to liver involvement and manifests as vague, mild upper quadrant and epigastric pain. Signs of hepatomegaly or obstructive jaundice may be present. Occasionally, metastatic lesions in the lung or brain are the first to cause symptoms by local inflammation or mass effect.

DIAGNOSIS. Laboratory evaluation may show marked eosinophilia, but this finding is inconstant (30% prevalence). In hydatid cyst disease, radiographic and ultrasonographic studies typically show characteristic large, avascular cysts containing internal structures consistent with daughter cysts. Detection of mural calcification strongly favors the diagnosis of hydatid cyst. The differential diagnosis includes hemangioma, metastatic carcinoma, and remote bacterial or amebic liver abscess. Confirmatory evidence of infection may be obtained by serology (sensitivity of 60 to 90%, depending on the test used). Serologic testing is available commercially or from the Centers for Disease Control and Prevention (CDC), Atlanta, GA (through local state health departments). Until recently, it has not been recommended to perform closed aspiration on the cyst for diagnosis, as cyst leakage has the potential to initiate a severe allergic reaction and may result in the metastatic spread of daughter cysts. However, recent clinical series have reported successful computed tomography (CT)-guided thin-needle aspiration of hydatid cysts for diagnosis. This procedure, when followed by immediate instillation of ethanol to kill viable protoscoleces, was associated with minimal side effects and was followed by apparent regression of cysts on CT scans.

With alveolar cyst disease due to *E. multilocularis,* the organism's appearance on radiographic and sonographic imaging often mimics that of hepatic carcinoma. A definitive diagnosis may require either angiography or open biopsy at surgery. Precautions must be taken to prevent metastatic dissemination of daughter cysts at the time of surgery.

TREATMENT. Stable, asymptomatic, calcified cysts do not require specific therapy but should be monitored by serial imaging over several years to ensure a benign resolution. When technically feasible, expanding, symptomatic, or infected cysts are best removed in toto at surgery, with care taken to isolate and kill the cyst (with hypertonic saline [25 to 30 grams per deciliter] or other cidal agents [such as ethanol]) prior to excision, to avoid secondary spread of parasite cysts. Controversy has developed over the practice of intraoperative instillation of cidal agents, as some patients have developed sclerosing cholangitis as a late complication of surgery. Perioperative drug therapy alone may prevent spread of daughter cysts at the time of surgery. Iodophor and formalin instillation should be avoided. Surgical resection should include careful closure of biliary and enteric fistulas and extensive postoperative drainage of the cyst bed to prevent fluid accumulation and secondary bacterial infection. Alveolar cyst disease may require wide resection, i.e., total lobectomy of liver or lung organ or even transplantation, to remove all cyst material.

In many cases, symptomatic echinococcal cysts are not amenable to resection. In such cases, oral drug therapy with the anthelminthics, either long-term mebendazole (40 mg per kilogram of body weight per day in three divided doses for 6 to 12 months) or albendazole (400 mg twice a day for one to eight periods of 28 days each, separated by drug-free rest intervals of 14 to 28 days), has been recommended for cure or palliation. Cure rates, particularly for difficult cases with recurrent or extrahepatic/extrapulmonary cysts, have been low (<33%), although a majority of patients show some improvement. Because the efficacy of drug therapy is

limited, a combined medical-surgical approach should be formulated for each patient.

Cysticercosis

Cysticercosis represents human tissue infection with the intermediate cyst forms of the pork tapeworm *T. solium.* Cysticercosis is acquired by ingestion of *T. solium* eggs in contaminated foods. Infection prevalence is approximately 1 to 10% in endemic areas of Latin America, India, Asia, Indonesia, and parts of Africa. Because of its potentially life-threatening complications, cysticercosis has greater clinical significance than does intestinal *T. solium* tapeworm infection, particularly if cyst disease involves the CNS, the eyes, the heart, or other vital organs.

CLINICAL MANIFESTATIONS. Clinical manifestations depend on the location and number of infecting cysts. Cysticerci are bladder-like, fluid-filled cysts containing an invaginated protoscolex. They are often surrounded by a dense fibrous capsule of host origin. In infected humans, cysticerci are usually multiple, 0.5 to 2 cm in size, and distributed widely throughout the body. Many patients have minimal, if any, symptoms of infection. However, symptomatic *neurocysticercosis* (i.e., cerebral cysticercosis, eye or spinal cord involvement) requires medical attention. This syndrome has an estimated mortality rate of up to 50%, and any neurologic, cognitive, or personality disorder in an individual from an endemic area should be considered a possible manifestation of undiagnosed neurocysticercosis. Diagnosis of this condition has been facilitated by CT scanning and magnetic resonance imaging (MRI), both of which are highly sensitive in detecting central nervous system (CNS) cysticerci. Patients with CNS involvement have an average of 10 cysts distributed throughout the brain and spinal cord. These cysts may be in different stages of development, with symptoms commonly arising when older cysts begin to die, lose osmoregulation, and release antigenic material to provoke significant host inflammatory response.

In practice, neurocysticercosis may be divided into six discrete syndromes for management. In the *acute invasive* stage of cysticercosis, immediately after infection, the patient may experience fevers, headache, and myalgias associated with significant peripheral eosinophilia. Heavy infection at this stage may result in a clinical picture of "cysticercal encephalitis" associated with coma and rapid deterioration. This presentation should be treated aggressively with antiparasitic agents and anti-inflammatory drugs. After cysticerci become established, *parenchymal CNS cysticercosis* (50% of cases) is associated with seizures, intellectual impairment, and personality changes. Compression due to swelling or inflammation around the cysts may result in focal deficits, signs of cerebral edema, and/or hydrocephalus. Seizures may be focal (jacksonian), referring to the specific cortical locus of involvement, or may be generalized. *Subarachnoid cysticercosis* (30% of cases) is frequently associated with obstruction of cerebrospinal fluid (CSF) flow. Intracranial hypertension may manifest as vomiting, headache, and visual disturbances. Sensorial changes may include apathy, amnesia, dementia, hallucination, and emotional disturbance. Like other forms of basilar meningitis, pericysticercal inflammation at the base of the brain may cause obstruction or vasculitis of the cerebral arteries, leading to intermittent ischemia or stroke. *Intraventricular cysticercosis* (15% of cases) is, because of its location, the most difficult to diagnose and treat. Symptomatic cysts are most frequent in the fourth ventricle, where they cause outflow obstruction and increased intracranial pressure without localizing signs. An aggressive variant of ventricular neurocysticercosis, called racemose cysticercosis, frequently involves the basal cisterns. This form of cysticercosis has been noted most often in young women and involves multiple, rapidly spreading cysts in the cerebrum and around the base of the brain. Whereas symptoms due to isolated cysts may remit, racemose cysticercosis usually has a progressive, deteriorating course if therapy is not given. Those with *spinal cysticercosis* may present with cord compression, radiculopathy, transverse myelitis, or signs of meningitis, depending on the location of involvement. *Ocular cysticercosis* is a distinct syndrome that manifests as eye pain, scotomata, and decreasing vision due to iridocyclitis, clouding of the vitreous, and retinal inflammation or detachment.

DIAGNOSIS. A definitive diagnosis of cysticercosis requires examination of biopsy material obtained from a tissue cyst. However, a presumptive diagnosis may be made on the basis of a history of residence in an endemic area, the presence of characteristic radiographic findings on plain films (calcified cysts in soft tissues) or scans (multiple, low-density, enhanced, and unenhanced lesions on CT or MRI), and suggestive laboratory findings. Infection with *T. solium* tapeworm is present in about 25% of neurocysticercosis cases. In neurocysticercosis, examining the CSF may show hypoglycorrhachia, elevated total protein levels, and lymphocytic and eosinophilic pleocytosis (5 to 500 cells per microliter). Serum and CSF enzyme-linked immunosorbent assay and Western blot testing for specific immunoglobulin M (IgM) and IgG anticysticercal antibodies have a sensitivity of 75 to 100%. These tests are available through commercial laboratories or from the CDC (samples should be sent through state health departments). It should be noted, however, that antiparasite antibodies may persist long after infection, and a positive IgG serology merely indicates prior *Taenia* exposure, not necessarily active disease. The differential diagnosis of neurocysticercosis includes tumor, hydatid cyst disease, vasculitis, and chronic fungal and mycobacterial infection.

TREATMENT. Given the high prevalence of cysticercosis in some areas of the world, it is evident that most cysticerci do not cause significant symptoms. For *symptomatic* cysts outside the CNS, the optimal therapy is surgical removal, as this ensures complete elimination of the cyst. In the case of symptomatic neurocysticercosis, which carries an associated mortality of up to 50%, therapy is definitely indicated, but surgery may be risky or technically unfeasible. An alternative approach to controlling some forms of neurocysticercosis has been demonstrated in recent clinical studies. Drug therapy with either praziquantel (50 mg per kilogram per day in three divided doses for 14 to 30 days) or albendazole (15 mg per kilogram per day for 30 days) has been associated with alleviation of symptoms and regression of cyst size and number in patients with viable (nonenhancing) cysts in the cerebral parenchyma. However, drug therapy has provided only limited improvement in patients with arachnoiditis and no improvement in patients with intraventricular cysts. For these latter presentations, the treatment of choice remains surgery and/or palliation with shunting, anticonvulsants, and anti-inflammatory agents. It should be noted that in about 20% of treated cases, starting drug therapy is associated with a severely symptomatic, increased inflammatory response at the site of the cyst. This inflammation may be controlled with corticosteroids, but corticosteroids are not recommended for routine use in all patients, as they may significantly alter the pharmacokinetics of the anthelminthics used to treat infection. Follow-up tomographic scanning should be repeated 3 months after therapy is stopped to ensure adequate response. If necessary, a repeat course of drug therapy with the alternate agent may be given to improve response. Because parasite-induced ocular inflammation does not respond well to systemic anti-inflammatory agents, patients with cysticercosis of the eye (20% of cases of neurocysticercosis) should not receive drug therapy until the eye disease has been controlled surgically.

Coenurosis

A different, but more rare, form of tissue cysticercosis may be caused by larval stages of the dog tapeworms *T. multiceps* and *T. serialis*. Lesions tend to be solitary and are distinguished pathologically from *T. solium* cysticerci on biopsy. Ocular involvement is common, and surgical resection is currently the only effective mode of therapy.

Sparganosis

Sparganosis is a tissue cestode infection caused by the plerocercoid larval stages of *Spirometra*, species tapeworms of cats and other carnivores. Humans may become infected by ingesting infected water fleas *(Cyclops),* by ingesting uncooked meat from infected animals (reptiles, birds, or mammals), or by cutaneous exposure (e.g., via traditional skin or eye poultices) to uncooked, infected meat. Usually, the larva encysts within the intestinal submucosa or skin. In some cases, however, parasites may invade the eye or CNS and cause significant inflammatory pathology at the site of encystment. Occasionally, proliferation into surrounding tissues occurs by lateral budding of the parasite (termed *sparganum proliferum*). The treatment of choice for sparganosis is ethanol injection and/or surgical removal, as limited experience with medical anthelminthic therapy has shown no beneficial effect.

Ammann RW, Eckert J: Cestodes: Echinococcus. Gastroenterol Clin North Am 25:655, 1996. *A comprehensive review of* E. granulosus *and* E. multilocularis *infection with discussion of current therapeutic controversies.*
Schantz PM: Tapeworms (cestodiasis). Gastroenterol Clin North Am 25:637, 1996. *Concise summary of tapeworm biology and infections in humans by a leading expert.*
White AC: Neurocysticercosis: A major cause of neurological disease worldwide. Clin Infect Dis 24:101, 1997. *A "state of the art" article discussing the different presentations of CNS cysticercosis and their management.*
WHO: Guidelines for treatment of cystic and alveolar echinococcosis in humans. Bull WHO 74:231, 1996.

431 SCHISTOSOMIASIS (BILHARZIASIS)

Edgar M. Carvalho ▪ *Aldo A. M. Lima*

DEFINITIONS. Schistosomiasis is one of the most important parasitic diseases of the humans. It is estimated that over 200 million people are currently infected worldwide, mainly in rural agricultural and peri-urban areas. Schistosomiasis may cause a severe degree of morbidity and pathologic changes that if left undiagnosed and untreated may result in major disability or mortality.

EPIDEMIOLOGY. There are five major species of *Schistosoma* affecting humans: *S. mansoni, S. haematobium, S. japonicum, S. intercalatum,* and *S. mekongi.* Other species that occasionally infect humans include *S. bovis, S. mathei,* and some avian schistosomes. These species differ not only biologically from one another but also in their geographic distribution and in the type of disease they produce. *S. mansoni* is spread less widely in Africa than *S. haematobium,* occurring intensely in the Nile delta north of Cairo and in one belt across Africa south of the Sahara from Mali to Ethiopia and in another belt south to Mozambique. It is also present in Madagascar and Angola. In the Western Hemisphere it is established in Brazil, Venezuela, Surinam, Puerto Rico, Antigua, Dominican Republic, Guadeloupe, Martinique, Montserrat, Nevis, and St. Lucia. *S. japonicum* is confined to the Far East. It is highly endemic in the Yangtze river valley of Central China. There are numerous foci in the Philippines and small foci in Indonesia. Transmission to humans has probably ceased in Japan. *S. mekongi* has been discovered in the Mekong river valley between Laos and Thailand.

The endemicity of schistosomiasis depends on the urban disposal of urine (*S. haematobium*) and feces (*S. mansoni, S. japonicum, S. intercalatum, S. mekongi*), the presence of suitable snail hosts, and human exposure to cercariae. The freshwater snail intermediate hosts are *Biomphalaria* in Africa and *Biomphalaria glabrata (Australorbis)* and *Tropicarbis* in South America and the West Indies. In some cases, the endemicity of schistosomiasis may be maintained by animal reservoirs. This is the case with *S. japonicum,* which infects dogs and cows. Rodents, monkeys, and baboons have been found infected in nature, but the role of these animals as reservoirs does not seem to be epidemiologically important.

ETIOLOGY AND LIFE CYCLE (Fig. 431–1). The schistosomes are digenetic parasitic trematodes. Although they are morphologically distinctive, the species of *Schistosoma* that infect humans share some common factors. The large male (0.6–2.2 cm × 2–4 mm) has a ventral gynecophoric canal in which the female (1.2–2.6 cm × 1–2 mm) is held during copulation. Adult worms live in the mesenteric veins (*S. mansoni, S. japonicum, S. mekongi,* and *S. intercalatum*) or in the venous plexus around the lower ends of the ureters and the urinary bladder (*S. haematobium*). At these sites they start their sexual reproduction by releasing eggs. Once deposited in the host, eggs may stay in the mesenteric vein, be trapped in the intestines, escape to intestinal lumen, and migrate by portal blood to the liver (*S. mansoni, S. japonicum*). Eggs of *S. haematobium* may be trapped in the intestines and bladder and may escape to the intestinal or bladder lumen. After exposition by feces or urine in fresh water the eggs hatch and release ciliated motile

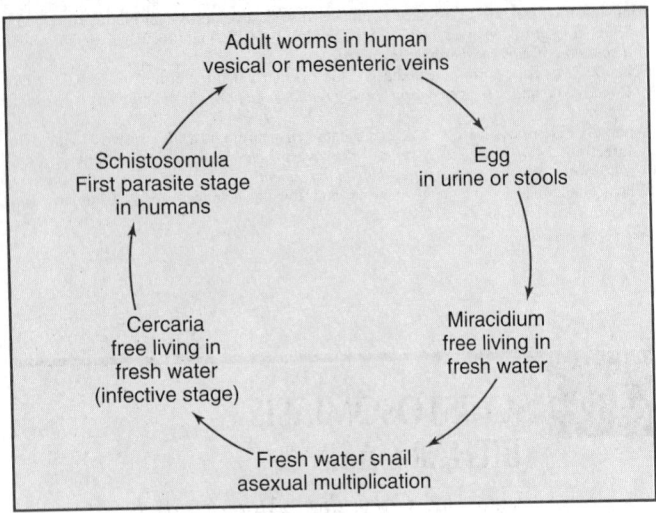

FIGURE 431–1 ■ Schistosome life cycle.

miracidia that penetrate in the snail intermediate host. After asexual multiplication in the snail, the development of cercariae, the infective forms for humans, takes 4 to 7 weeks. After leaving the snails, the cercariae can survive in fresh water for almost 72 hours. During penetration in the skin of the human host, the cercariae lose their tails and change into schistosomula. The schistosomula migrate to the lungs and, in about 6 weeks, mature to adult worms and descend to their final habitat. Viable eggs can be seen in the excretions 5 to 9 weeks after cercarial penetration. The mean lifespan of the worms range from 5 to 10 years.

PATHOGENESIS AND CLINICAL MANIFESTATIONS (Table 431–1). Clinical manifestations of schistosomiasis are divided in schistosome dermatitis, acute schistosomiasis, and chronic schistosomiasis. Schistosome dermatitis or swimmer's itch is seen mainly when avian cercariae penetrate the skin and are destroyed. Although this manifestation is not common in human schistosomiasis, recognition of this clinical entity is gradually expanding. Schistosome dermatitis is a sensitization phenomena, because it occurs in previously exposed persons. The cercariae are destroyed in the epithelial layers of the skin. They evoke an acute inflammatory response with edema, early infiltration of neutrophils and lymphocytes, and later invasion of eosinophils. Clinically, a pruritic papular rash occurs within 24 hours after penetration of cercariae reaching maximal intensity in 2 to 3 days.

The pathogenesis of human schistosomiasis is mainly related with egg deposition and liberation of antigens of adult worms and eggs. Acute schistosomiasis, also called Katayama fever, occurs more often with *S. japonicum,* but it is also observed in heavy infection by *S. mansoni.* One of the main reasons why acute schistosomiasis is more likely to be associated with *S. japonicum* than

other species is that *S. japonicum* female worms produce about 2000 to 3000 eggs per day. This is nearly 10 times the egg output of the female *S. mansoni.* It has been speculated that the acute schistosomiasis may represent an immune complex–mediated disease, although the leukocytosis and prominent eosinophilia indicate that immediate hypersensitivity and inflammatory response to egg antigens are important. Acute disease is more frequently observed in individuals living outside the endemic areas of schistosomiasis. It is possible that modulation of the immune response by antigens or idiotypes transferred from mother to child may explain the low frequency of this manifestation in subjects living in endemic areas. Acute schistosomiasis occurs with the beginning of oviposition, usually 20 to 50 days after primary exposure. The disease is characterized by fever, chills, hepatosplenomegaly, lymphadenopathy, weight loss, headache, and cough. Leukocytosis with eosinophilia is the main laboratory finding. Most symptoms and signs disappear within a few weeks, but death may occur.

In chronic schistosomiasis, tissue injury is mediated by egg-induced granulomas and subsequent appearance of fibrosis. Because the habitat of *S. mansoni, S. japonicum, S. mekongi,* and *S. intercalatum* worms is the mesenteric blood vessels, the intestines are involved primarily and egg embolism results in secondary involvement of the liver. Abdominal pain, irregular bowel movements, and blood in the stool are the main symptoms of intestinal involvement. Colonic polyposis may occur, especially in Egypt.

Hepatosplenic involvement is the most important cause of morbidity in *S. mansoni* and *S. japonicum* infections. Patients may remain asymptomatic until the manifestation of hepatic fibrosis and portal hypertension. Hepatic fibrosis is due to a granulomatous reaction to *Schistosoma* eggs that were carried to the liver. Hepatic fibrosis in *S. mansoni* infection has been associated with intensity of infection, genetic background, and immunologic response. Although the severity of infection is clearly linked with liver disease, the immune response, collagen deposition, and genetic factors potentiate disease in some individuals with only moderate infections, or inhibit disease in others with heavy infections. Both Th1 and Th2 cytokines are involved in the granulomatosus response, but granuloma growth and maintenance is largely associated with Th2 cytokines, down-regulated by interleukin-12. Additionally, eosinophils constitute approximately 50% of the cells in the granuloma. Recently, an association between HLA class II allele DQ B1*0201 and a greater chance for hepatosplenism has been demonstrated.

Enzymes and antigens released from eggs sensitize the host lymphocytes, which migrate to areas of egg deposition and recruit other cell types, such as macrophages, eosinophils, and fibroblasts. The size of these granulomas and the resulting fibrosis lead to most of the chronic fibro-obstructive lesions in schistosomiasis. In the liver, the granulomas result in perisinusoidal obstruction of portal blood flow, portal hypertension, splenomegaly, esophageal varices, and portosystemic collateral circulation. Liver cell perfusion is not reduced; consequently, liver function test results remain normal for a long time. Hematemesis from bleeding esophageal or gastric varices may occur. In such cases, anemia and decreasing levels of serum albumin are observed. A few patients have a severe hepatosplenic disease with decompensated liver disease. Jaundice, ascites,

Table 431–1 ■ DIAGNOSIS OF SCHISTOSOMIASIS

SCHISTOSOME	EGGS	DIAGNOSIS
S. haematobium	Mainly found in urine but may be found in stools or rectal biopsy Eggs: 143 × 50 μm; spindle shaped: rounded anterior, conical posterior, tapering to a terminal delicate spine	Obtain urine sample at midday (when eggs are excreted); more than one sample may be needed Examine urine directly or by filtering 10 mL urine through Nuclepore membrane Rectal biopsy in suspected cases with normal urine Serologic testing to diagnose early or light infection
S. mansoni	Eggs: 155 × 66 μm; oval with lateral, long spine	Examine stool for eggs Use Kato thick smear method for quantification purposes Rectal biopsy or serologic testing to diagnose stool-negative cases, particularly in lightly infected patients
S. japonicum	Found in stool; eggs: 89 × 67 μm; oval or rounded with lateral, short, sometimes curved spine	Examine stool for eggs Kato thick smear (for quantitative assessment) Rectal biopsy for those with light infections, especially with less common manifestation (i.e., cerebral schistosmiasis)
S. mekongi	Found in stool; eggs: 60 × 32 μm; smaller than eggs of *S. japonicum*	Examine stool for eggs
S. intercalatum	Found in stool; eggs: 180 × 65 μm; terminal spine	Examine stool for eggs

and liver failure are then observed. Association of *S. mansoni* or *S. japonicum* infection with hepatitis B virus may cause high morbidity and mortality. Concomitant infection by *Salmonella* species and, less extensively, gram-negative bacteria with *S. mansoni* or *S. haematobium* leads to a picture of prolonged fever, hepatosplenomegaly, and mild leukocytosis with eosinophilia. Other complications associated with hepatosplenic schistosomiasis include pulmonary hypertension, glomerulonephritis, infantilism, and hypersplenism. In adult hospitalized patients with *S. japonicum* infection, cerebral schistosomiasis occurs in 1.7 to 4.3%. It may occur as early as 6 weeks after infection, and the most frequent sign is focal jacksonian epilepsy. Signs and symptoms of generalized encephalitis may occasionally be found. In *S. mansoni* infection, nervous system involvement is rare and characterized mainly by transverse myelitis.

In *S. haematobium* infection, the main system involved is the urinary tract. The acute granulomatous response to parasite eggs in the early stages causes urinary tract disease, such as urethral ulceration and bladder polyposis. In chronic disease, usually in older patients, granulomas at the lower end of the ureters impede urinary flow and cause hydroureter and hydronephrosis. Bladder fibrosis and calcification are also seen in this phase. Up to 50 to 70% of infected individuals have hematuria, dysuria, or frequency. Urine examination reveals proteinuria and hematuria. Radiologic findings include hydronephrosis, hydroureter, ureteric stricture, dilatation or distortion, ureteric calcification, ureterolithiasis, calcified bladder, polyps, reduction in bladder capacity, irregular contraction of the bladder wall, or dilated bladder due to bladder neck fibrosis. An increased incidence of squamous cell carcinoma of the bladder has been reported in endemic areas of *S. haematobium* infection, but the mechanism of carcinogenesis is unknown. *S. haematobium* eggs have occasionally been found in the lungs with subsequent focal pulmonary arteritis and pulmonary hypertension.

In schistosome-infected populations, intensity of infection increases during the first two decades of life, as children accumulate worms, and then declines. The susceptibility of younger children to infection is even more evident when intensities of reinfection are studied after the elimination of existing worms by chemotherapy. Although there is a decrease in exposure with age, the lower intensities of infection in older individuals are due in part to an acquired resistance. Both Th1 (interferon [IFN]-γ) and Th2 type of immune response, mediated by IgE, may participate in resistance to reinfection. In the *S. haematobium*–infected population, IgE increases progressively with age and IgE antibodies directed against adult worm antigens are associated with subsequent low intensities of reinfection. Similar associations between high IgE levels or IgE:IgG$_4$ ratio and resistance to reinfection have been found among Brazilian and Kenyan subjects exposed to *S. mansoni*. Evidence that a Th1 type immune response may also be involved in the protection against *S. mansoni* comes from the immunologic studies in subjects that are highly exposed to contaminated water but have negative stool examinations. In these subjects there are higher IFN-γ production in response to *S. mansoni* membrane extract. The existence of a major co-dominant gene, called *SM1*, controlling the intensity of infection by *S. mansoni* has been demonstrated. The localization of *SM1* on chromosome 5q31-q33, close to several genes involved in the regulation of immune response, including *CSF1R* (colony-stimulating factor-1 receptor), *GM-CSF* (granulocyte-macrophage colony-stimulating factor), *IL-3, IL-4, IL-5, IL-13, IRF1* (immune regulatory factor-1), and a locus regulating IgE levels, indicates that genetic factors are probably critical to susceptibility and resistance to schistosome infection.

DIAGNOSIS (See Table 431–1). A definitive diagnosis of schistosomiasis can be made only by finding schistosome eggs in feces, urine, a biopsy specimen, usually from the rectum. The history of contact with contaminated water and clinical manifestations are important steps in establishing the diagnosis. Because schistosome eggs may be few in number, concentration by sedimentation should be employed. All eggs from the feces, urine, or tissues should be examined under high power to determine their viability by the activity of the cilia of the excretory flame cell of the enclosed miracidium. Dead eggs may persist for a long time after successful therapy or natural death of the worms. The presence of only dead eggs should not necessarily require treatment. Because intensity of infection is associated with morbidity, quantitative techniques are recommended. For *S. mansoni* and *S. japonicum* the Kato thick smear method is used. Rectal biopsy may be used for those with light infection. In patients with chronic *S. mansoni* and *S. japonicum* infection and liver disease, diagnosis is sometimes made by the documentation of eggs in liver specimens. Ultrasonography allows determination of the degree of liver fibrosis. Diagnosis of *S. mekongi* and *S. intercalatum* infections is performed by examining the stool for eggs.

Urine examination for *S. haematobium* eggs can be performed by direct or concentration methods. Samples should be obtained at midday when excretion of the eggs is maximal. Rectal biopsy may be done in patients with light infection and negative urine results. Once *S. haematobium* infection is diagnosed, assessment of urinary tract pathology by ultrasonography is recommended. Because of an increased incidence of carcinoma of the bladder, cancer surveillance should be performed in patients with *S. haematobium* infection.

Several serologic tests with detection of IgM, IgG and IgA antibodies to *Schistosoma* antigens are available. Serologic tests are important in the diagnosis of acute infection because the symptoms are not specific and the finding of eggs in the stool may be due to a chronic infection. High levels of IgA anti-egg antigen and IgM and IgG antibodies to Keyhole limpet hemocyanin (KLH) are predominantly observed during the acute phase. The KLH from the murine mollusk *Megathura crenulata* shares carbohydrate epitopes with the surface of schistosomula.

Quantification of circulating antigens in serum and urine has been shown to be an alternative for the diagnosis of schistosome infection. However, the sensitivity of the method decreases in cases of light infection (i.e., less than 100 eggs per gram of feces). This test has also been used to monitor efficacy of schistosome chemotherapy. Significant decrease in antigen levels or negativation of the test is observed as early as 10 days after therapy.

MANAGEMENT. Chemotherapy is by far the major tool for the control and cure of schistosomiasis. Three compounds are currently in use—metrifonate, oxamniquine, and praziquantel—and all three are included in the World Health Organization's list of essential drugs. Praziquantel, a pyrazinoisoquinoline derivative, is the drug of choice for the treatment of schistosomiasis for four reasons: (1) high efficacy against all schistosome species and against cestodes, (2) lack of serious short-term and long-term side effects, (3) administration as a single oral dose, and (4) competitive cost.

The standard recommended treatment consists of a single dose of 40 mg/kg for *S. mansoni, S. hematobium,* and *S. intercalatum* infection. In *S. japonicum* infection, a total dose of 60 mg/kg is recommended, split in two or three doses in a single day. *S. mekongi* may require two treatments at 60 mg/kg of body weight. Using these dosages, recorded cure rates are 75 to 85% for *S. hematobium,* 63 to 85% for *S. mansoni,* 80 to 90% for *S. japonicum,* 89% for *S. intercalatum,* and 60 to 80% for double infections with *S. mansoni* and *S. hematobium.*

Praziquantel is well tolerated and effective in patients of all ages and in different clinical forms of schistosomiasis, including advanced hepatosplenic cases (*S. mansoni*), cerebral schistosomiasis (*S. japonicum*), and neurologic syndromes (*S. mansoni* and *S. hematobium*), possibly in association with corticosteroids.

The effects of praziquantel on schistosomes can be summarized under three headings: (1) muscular contraction; (2) tegumental damage (vacuolization and blebbing); and (3) metabolic alterations (decreased glucose uptake, lactate excretion, and glycogen content). The praziquantel activity is also dependent on the immune system. Several studies have reported that praziquantel induces the exposure of worm surface antigens that may function as targets to immune responses.

The most common side effects observed on praziquantel or oxamniquine administration are related to the gastrointestinal tract: abdominal pain and/or discomfort, nausea, vomiting, anorexia, and diarrhea. These symptoms can be observed in up to 50% of patients but are usually well tolerated. Other side effects are related to the central nervous system (headache, dizziness, drowsiness) and the skin (pruritus, eruptions) or may be non-specific (fever, fatigue). Toxicity is very low in animal studies with praziquantel, and, at present, no genotoxic risk is reported. In general, the cumulated experience from a huge number of studies permits the conclusion that praziquantel is an extremely well-tolerated drug, requiring minimal medical supervision and, thus, particularly suitable for mass chemotherapy programs.

Although the reduction of the intensity of infection and morbidity has been documented with mass chemotherapy, provision for clean water, use of molluscicide, and adequate sanitation should be combined to control the disease.

Cioli D, Pica-Mattoccia L, Archer S: Antischistosomal drugs: Past, present...and future? Pharmacol Ther 68:35–85, 1995. *Detailed and up-to-date description of antischistosomal drugs, including history, chemistry, pharmacokinetics, clinical use, side effects and toxicity, and mode of action of metrifonate, oxamniquine, praziquantel, and other future drugs.*

Marquet S, Abel L, Hillaire D, et al: Genetic localization of a locus controlling the intensity of infection by *Schistosoma mansoni* on chromosome 5q31-q33. Nature Genet. 14:181, 1996.

Mwatha JK, Kimani G, et al: High levels of tNF, soluble tNF receptors, soluble ICAM-1 and IFNγ, but low levels of IL-5, are associated with hepatosplenic disease in human *Schistosomiasis mansoni*. J. Immunol 160:1992, 1998.

Prata A: *Schistosomiasis mansoni* in Brazil. *In* Mahmoud AAF (ed): Clinical Tropical Medicine and Communicable Diseases, Vol 2, Schistosomiasis. London, Bailliere Tindall, 1987, pp 349–369. *A review of clinical features as seen in an endemic area, with emphasis on diagnostic methods.*

Waine GJ, McManus DP: Schistosomiasis vaccine development. Curr Picture Bioassays 19:435, 1997. *A general review about epidemiologic and immunologic aspects of schistosomiasis with focus on immunologic protective mechanisms and antigens candidates for vaccine development.*

World Health Organization: The Control of Schistosomiasis. Technical Report Series 728, pp 1–86. Geneva, World Health Organization, 1993. *Description of the epidemiology, morbidity, and methods of control of schistosomiasis. This report also includes a summary of control programs in endemic areas and outline for strategy of morbidity control.*

432 LIVER, INTESTINAL, AND LUNG FLUKE INFECTIONS

Adel A.F. Mahmoud

Parasitic flukes belong to the phylum Platyhelminthes. These organisms are dorsoventrally flattened and are typically bilaterally symmetrical. With the exception of the schistosomes, all flat worms of clinical significance are hermaphroditic. Morphologically the body of adult worms is leaf shaped and possesses two prominent suckers, one located anteriorly and the other ventrally. These are attachment organs that help anchor adult worms in their habitat within the organs of the definitive host. During the typical life cycle of a flat worm, the organism utilizes two, three, or more hosts; one is the definitive host and the others are intermediate hosts. Flukes challenge the protective mechanisms of the definitive hosts because of their size, complex anatomic and antigenic structure, and remarkable abilities to evade expulsion. Clinically relevant flukes are usually grouped according to the main location of adult worms in the definitive host. These include liver, intestinal, and lung flukes (Table 432–1). Blood flukes or schistomes are discussed in Chapter 431.

Approximately 50 million individuals are infected worldwide with liver, intestinal, or lung flukes (Table 432–2); the liver flukes

Table 432–2 ■ GEOGRAPHIC DISTRIBUTION OF FLUKES

FLUKE	DISTRIBUTION
Liver	
Opisthorchis viverrini	Thailand, Laos, Cambodia
O. felineus	Russia, Eastern and Central Europe
Clonorchis sinesis	China, Japan, Korea, Taiwan, Vietnam, Hong Kong (imported fish from China)
Fasciola hepatica	United States, Europe, Africa, Asia
F. gigantica	less common: Africa, Asia, Hawaii
Dicrocoelium sp.	Europe, Africa, Asia, North America
Intestinal	
Fasciolopsis sp.	Taiwan, Thailand, Bangladesh, India, plus other Asian and Western countries
Echinostoma sp.	Indonesia, Philippines, Thailand, Taiwan
Heterophyes heterophyes	Egypt, Iran, Far East, Southeast Asia
Metagonimus yokogawai	China, Japan, Kora, Taiwan
Gastrodiscoides hominis	India, Southeast Asia, Russia
Lung	
Paragonimus sp.	Asia, West Africa, Central and South America

Clonorchis sinensis, Opisthorchis felineus, and *O. viverrini* are the most prevalent. Liver, intestinal, and lung flukes are similar morphologically, but vary in size from 1 mm to 7 cm. The pattern of life cycle of these flukes is similar. Eggs are passed in the feces or sputum of infected individuals. Eggs hatch in the aquatic outside environment, releasing miracidia that seek specific snail intermediate hosts, where they undergo several asexual multiplication steps, resulting finally in the release of cercariae. This stage is free living but of limited lifespan; it has to encyst on vegetation or in the tissues of fish or crabs, where it changes into the metacercarial stage, which is infective to humans. Human acquisition of infection depends on ingestion of metacercaria in raw or improperly cooked aquatic plants or animals. Diagnosis of a specific tissue fluke is a significant clinical challenge: Knowing the geographic distribution of infection, the specific symptoms and signs, and the proper identification of eggs in feces or sputum samples is necessary. Recently the specificity and sensitivity of serologic tests have progressed to being helpful in diagnosis with a certain degree of confidence.

LIVER FLUKES

Several species of liver flukes are capable of inducing significant morbidity and mortality in humans. Opisthorchiasis and clonorchiasis are the most common of these infections.

Opisthorchiasis

Human infection is caused by *O. viverrini* or *O. felineus,* parasitic flukes of cats, dogs, and other fish-eating mammals. Human infection is acquired by ingestion of metacercariae found in the second intermediate host (cyprinoid fish, carp). The metacercariae excyst in the duodenum and migrate through the ampulla of Vater to reach their final habitat in the bile ducts. The incidence of *O. viverrini* in northeastern Thailand (Table 432–2) has recently been increasing, reaching 90% of the population in specific foci.

Table 432–1 ■ MAJOR LIVER, INTESTINAL, AND LUNG FLUKE INFECTIONS IN HUMANS

INFECTION	CAUSATIVE ORGANISMS	SECOND INTERMEDIATE HOST	SIZE OF ADULT FLUKE (mm)	FINAL HABITAT IN HUMANS	SIZE OF EGGS (μm)
Opisthorchiasis	*O. viverrini* *O. felineus*	Cyprinoid fish	5–10 × 1–2	Distal bile ducts, gallbladder	28 × 16 Operculated
Clonorchiasis	*C. sinensis*	Carp fish	10–24 × 3–5	Bile and pancreatic ducts	29 × 16 Operculated
Fascioliasis	*F. hepatica* *F. gigantica*	Aquatic vegetation or water	20–30 × 13 75 × 20	Large biliary ducts	140 × 75 Inconspicuous operculum 175 × 80
Fasciolopsiasis	*F. buski*	Aquatic plants	50–75 × 8–20	Small intestine	135 × 35 Small operculum
Paragonimiasis	*P. westermani*	Freshwater and brackish water crabs	7–16 × 4–8	Lungs, brain, or abdominal organs	100 × 60 Operculated

PATHOGENESIS AND CLINICAL FEATURES. Adult flukes inhabit the distal bile ducts and may occasionally be seen in the gallbladder. The majority of infected individuals are asymptomatic. Lesions have been demonstrated in the biliary system, varying from hyperplasia of ductal epithelium to obstruction and bile retention. There is significant correlation between intensity of infection and severity of observed lesions.

Most infected individuals are asymptomatic; infection is diagnosed when the characteristic eggs are found during routine fecal examination. Since very few controlled studies have been performed on infected and uninfected populations of endemic areas, the specificity of symptoms and signs is questionable. Symptomatic infections are associated with right upper quadrant discomfort, dyspepsia, and change in bowel habits. Generalized symptoms such as decrease of appetite and weight loss have also been observed. In severe cases, relapsing cholangitis and cholecystitis may occur. An association between *O. viverrini* and cholangiocarcinoma, gallstones, and obstructive jaundice has been reported. Liver enlargement is demonstrated in most symptomatic individuals along with imaging evidence for biliary tree disease.

Infection with *O. felineus* has a characteristic clinical course. In its acute phase (2 to 3 weeks after infection), the clinical features include irregular fever, lymphadenopathy, myalgia, and eosinophilia. In chronic infections, symptoms and signs of biliary disease resemble those of *O. viverrini* infection; however, the worms may also be found in the pancreatic duct, causing manifestations related to this organ.

Clonorchiasis

C. sinensis is also frequently referred to as the Chinese or oriental liver fluke. Carnivorous animals such as dogs, cats, and rats are probably the reservoir hosts in nature. Human infection is acquired by ingestion of the second intermediate host, a freshwater carp of the family Cyprinidae. In endemic areas (Table 432–2), many species of this family have been found to be parasitized with *C. sinensis* metacercariae. Clonorchiasis is also seen in many countries, including the United States among immigrants from endemic areas. Importation of *C. sinensis* is a risk in the international food trade.

PATHOGENESIS AND CLINICAL FEATURES. The life cycle, pathologic features, and clinical manifestations of clonorchiasis are similar to those of opisthorchiasis. Adult flukes reside in the medium-sized and small bile ducts. They may also be found in the gallbladder, common bile duct, and pancreatic duct. In early infection the pathologic features consist of edema and epithelial desquamation in bile ducts associated with an inflammatory response. Later, metaplasia and glandular proliferation occur with dilatation and thickening of bile ducts. The final pathologic insult is related to marked periductal fibrosis. The specificity of symptoms due to clonorchiasis such as anorexia, epigastric pain, or diarrhea has been questioned in studies performed on immigrants to the United States from the Far East. In chronic infection as seen in endemic areas, the association with cholangitis, gallstones, and cholangiocarcinoma has been reported repeatedly. Sonography or computed tomography (CT) demonstrates the pathologic changes in the liver: flukes within dilated bile ducts and periductal changes.

Fascioliasis

Human infection with the zoonotic flukes *Fasciola hepatica* and *F. gigantica* is acquired by ingestion of metacercariae that are attached to various aquatic plants or through drinking of water contaminated with the infective stage of the organisms. The natural hosts of fascioliasis include sheep, goats, cattle, and horses; endemic regions are listed in Table 432–2. Once the infective metacercariae are consumed they excyst in the duodenum, penetrate its wall, and travel via the peritoneal cavity to enter the liver through its capsule. The organisms migrate into the liver parenchyma to reach their final habitat in large bile ducts.

PATHOGENESIS AND CLINICAL FEATURES. Human fascioliasis is usually associated with mild clinical features. The resulting syndromes may be conveniently divided into the *acute migratory phase,* while the organisms are finding their way through the peritoneal cavity to the liver capsule and parenchyma, and the *established phase,* which is associated with the mature flukes' taking

residence in the bile ducts. The acute phase is marked with fever, right upper quadrant or epigastric pain, and eosinophilia. The clinical presentation may last 4 to 8 weeks after ingestion of metacercariae and is usually self-limited. It has to be noted that stool examination during this phase usually yields negative findings for parasite eggs. During the established phase, most infected individuals are asymptomatic. Some may complain of abdominal pain and dyspepsia. Hepatomegaly and jaundice may be noted, as well as significant peripheral blood eosinophilia. Borderline changes in liver function test results have also been reported. CT of the liver may help in demonstrating hepatic lesions, including the nodular or the more characteristic linear hypodense tracks, particularly if they are located subcapsularly. In the *biliary stage,* ultrasonography may demonstrate the adult flukes in the bile ducts or gallbladder.

Dicroceliasis

Human infection with *Dicrocoelium dendriticum* or *D. hospes* is rare (Table 432–2). Dicroceliasis is a zoonosis in sheep, goats, deer, and other herbivores. Its life cycle is similar to that of other liver flukes except that metacercariae encyst in ants, the second intermediate host. Humans are infected via eating melacercariae-containing ants. Most cases of dicroceliasis are asymptomatic. In those with heavy infection, vague abdominal complaints—vomiting, diarrhea or constipation, and biliary colic—have been observed.

INTESTINAL FLUKES

Human infection with 1 of more than 50 species of intestinal trematodes has been reported from the Far East, Middle East, and North Africa. Clinically significant disease may be encountered in infection with only few species, as outlined later.

Fasciolopsiasis

The giant intestinal fluke *Fasciolopsis buski* inhabits the small intestine of pigs. The life cycle of the helminth is similar to that of *Fasciola hepatica*. Humans are infected by ingestion of raw stems, leaves, and pods of aquatic plants with encysted metacercariae. The geographic distribution is listed in Table 432–2. Endemicity depends on close contact among water plants, pigs, and populations that consume raw aquatic plants.

F. buski attach to the mucosa of small intestine, particularly the duodenum and jejunum. Most infected individuals are asymptomatic. The site of attachment, however, becomes ulcerated and a local inflammatory response follows. In heavy infection, intestinal obstruction and protein-losing enteropathy have been reported. With heavy infection, abdominal pain and diarrhea may be observed along with edema and anasarca caused by hypoalbuminemia.

Echinostomiasis

Humans can be infected with any of several genera of the family Echinostomatidae (Table 432–2). The common species are *Echinostoma ilocanum*, *E. malayaman*, and *E. revolutum*. Adult flukes are parasites of the small intestine of birds and mammals. Humans are occasionally infected after eating undercooked *pila*, other fish, and tadpoles. Mature adult worms attach to intestinal mucosa, causing ulceration and subsequent inflammatory response. Little morbidity has been reported in association with echinostomiasis. High-intensity infection may be associated with abdominal pain and diarrhea.

Heterophyiasis

Heterophyes heterophyes infects not only humans but also cats, dogs, and other fish-eating mammals. Infection is acquired by ingestion of the fish second intermediate host, which contains the fluke metacercariae. The common fish hosts include mullet and minnow and the brackish water fish *Mugil capito*. They are usually consumed either raw or salted. Metacercariae can live in salted fish for approximately 1 week. Adult *H. heterophyes* attach to the mucosa of jejunum and upper ileum, producing shallow ulcers and mild inflammatory response. Symptomatic patients complain of gastroenterocolitis with diarrhea and tenesmus. Stools characteristically contain abundant mucus and occasionally blood.

OTHER INTESTINAL FLUKES

Several other species may cause disease limited to defined geographic areas (Table 432–2). The *Metagonimus yokogawai* life cycle and the associated disease syndromes are similar to those in *H. heterophyes* infection, but *M. yokogawai* may invade the mucosa of small intestine, resulting in ulceration and granuloma formation. Another intestinal fluke, *Gastrodiscoides hominis* (Table 432–2), has its final habitat in humans in the cecum. Clinically it is believed to produce mucous diarrhea.

Lung Flukes: "Paragonimiasis"

Human infection by species of *Paragonimus* may cause considerable pulmonary or extrapulmonary morbidity in several endemic areas (Table 432–2). *Paragonimus* infection exists in nature in humans and carnivores. There are at least 10 species of *Paragonimus* known to cause human disease; of these *P. westermani* is most common. Infection is acquired by ingestion of metacercariae encysted in freshwater and brackish water crabs or crayfish (raw or undercooked). Infection may also be transmitted to humans through contaminated utensils used to prepare crabs or crayfish. Rarely, consumption of wild boar meat may result in transmission of immature flukes to humans, in whom they complete their development into adult worms.

PATHOGENESIS AND CLINICAL FEATURES. Disease in infected humans is related to migration of young flukes from the gastrointestinal tract to their final habitat (early or acute stage) and more characteristically results when adult worms become established in the lungs or at extrapulmonary sites (late or chronic stage).

Acute paragonimiasis occurs during the 3-week period following infection. It passes unnoticed in most infected individuals. Symptoms include diarrhea, abdominal pain, fever, and malaise associated with cough, dyspnea, and night sweats. Pulmonary paragonimiasis results from invasion of the host lungs and establishment of adult worms in cysts or abscess cavities. The lung parenchyma demonstrates hemorrhage and an inflammatory response of predominantly eosinophils. Worm cysts are 1 to 2 cm in diameter and usually contain one or two worms. Pathologic changes in the remaining lung tissues may result in bronchopneumonia, bronchiectasis, fibrosis, and pleural thickening. The established pulmonary stage of paragonimiasis results usually in mild chronic cough with production of mucoid rusty-brown sputum. Hemoptysis that may be severe and life-threatening occurs rarely. Microscopic examination of sputum demonstrates necrotic tissue and parasite eggs. Results of physical examination of patients with pulmonary paragonimiasis are usually within normal limits. Chest radiography findings may be normal in 10 to 20% of cases. Typical changes in the lungs include pathway infiltrate and ring shadow with a crescent-shaped "corona." Cystic and nodular lesions are also commonly seen. Furthermore, pleural lesions, including effusion, pneumothorax, and thickening, may be encountered in approximately two thirds of infected individuals. Other imaging methods, e.g., CT, may define better the pulmonary abnormalities, including worm migration tracks.

Extrapulmonary paragonimiasis occurs either because maturing flukes migrate to tissues other than the lungs, or adult flukes migrate from the lungs to other tissues. It is believed that extrapulmonary paragonimiasis may be mainly due to *Paragonimus* flukes other than *P. westermani*. The tissues most commonly affected are the brain, abdominal organs, and skin. In cerebral paragonimiasis, the clinical presentation may be acute or chronic. Acute cerebral paragonimiasis presents as fever, headache, visual disturbances, paralysis, and generalized or focal convulsions. Evidence for an intracranial inflammatory process may be demonstrated as papilledema, high cerebrospinal fluid pressure, and eosinophilic pleocytosis. Chronic cerebral paragonimiasis is characterized by space-occupying lesions that cause epilepsy or paralysis. Abdominal or cutaneous paragonimiasis results from invasion of liver, spleen, or skin by maturing or adult flukes. This results in space-occupying lesions, abscesses, or migratory swellings.

MANAGEMENT OF LIVER, INTESTINAL, AND LUNG FLUKE INFECTIONS

Diagnosis of human infection with liver, intestinal, or lung flukes requires knowledge of the geographic distribution of these infections, a high degree of clinical correlation of mainly non-specific symptoms and signs with history of possible exposure, and peripheral blood eosinophilia. Definitive diagnosis is established by finding the characteristically shaped fluke eggs in fecal samples or sputum. In general, the sensitivity of fecal or sputum examination is enhanced by examining two or three separate specimens. Seroimmunodiagnostic tests are available for fascioliasis and paragonimiasis. They are particularly helpful in early infection, in which parasitologic diagnosis usually yields negative results.

Chemotherapy for fluke infections has become a more effective management strategy with the introduction of praziquantel. This orally administered 1-day antihelminth results in cure rates of 70 to 90% and an even more remarkable decrease in egg counts. Its administration is associated with few side effects. The recommended dose of praziquantel is 75 mg/kg body weight divided into three doses and given in 1 day. A 2-day course of praziquantel is necessary for treatment of paragonimiasis. For fascioliasis the drug of choice is bithionol given orally as 30 to 50 mg/kg every other day for 10 to 15 doses.

Prevention of infection with any of these parasitic trematodes depends on proper medical advice given to individuals traveling or planning to reside in endemic areas (see Chapter 316). Avoidance of ingestion of suspect intermediate hosts and the proper washing, cooking, or preservation methods of such food items constitute the most effective strategy. Engaging in some of the local dietary habits in endemic areas is to be discouraged. Water for drinking must be properly purified to prevent the possible transmission of *F. hepatica*. Control of parasitic trematodes in endemic areas is a much more complex challenge. It involves changing long-established cultural, dietary, and sanitary habits. With the availability of a safe broad-spectrum antihelminth (praziquantel), chemotherapy may play a significant role in controlling infection and disease. As a long-term strategy, vaccines and socioeconomic development will be needed.

Drugs for Parasitic Infections. Med Lett Drugs Ther 40:1, 1998. *Yearly update of drugs of choice and alternatives.*

Harinasuta T, Bunnag D: Liver, lung and intestinal trematodiasis. *In* Warren KS, Mahmoud AAF (eds): Tropical and Geographical Medicine, 2nd ed. New York, McGraw-Hill, 1990, pp 473–489. *An authoritative description of the causative agents, clinical syndromes, and management strategies.*

Im JG, Whang HY, Kim WS, et al: Pleuropulmonary paragonimiasis: Radiologic findings in 71 patients. AJR 159:39, 1992. *Retrospective evaluation of 71 individuals with evidence of pleuropulmonary paragonimiasis. Report details frequency of specific radiographic and CT findings.*

King CH: Liver, lung and intestinal trematodiasis. *In* Mahmoud AAF (ed): Tropical and Geographical Medicine. 2nd ed. Companion Handbook. New York, McGraw-Hill, 1993, pp 149–154. *Summary of the salient clinical features and diagnostic and therapeutic approaches to tissue fluke infection.*

Lim JH: Radiologic findings of clonorchiasis. AJR 155:1001, 1990. *Detailed description of the epidemiologic and parasitologic characteristics of clonorchiasis as well as the sonographic and CT findings based on examining a large group of infected individuals.*

433 NEMATODE INFECTIONS

James W. Kazura

Nematodes (phylum Nematoda), or roundworms, include a vast number of species of free-living and parasitic helminths. These multicellular organisms differ from unicellular bacteria and protozoa in that they have organ systems with specialized nervous, muscular, gastrointestinal, and reproductive functions. Parasitic nematodes vary in length from several millimeters to approximately 2 meters. They have four larval stages and adult worms of both sexes. With the exception of *Strongyloides* sp. and a few other helminths of medical importance, larvae are produced after mating of sexually mature adult worms, which by themselves are incapable of multiplying in the mammalian host. The inability of adult worms to replicate has important implications for the propensity of this class of organism to establish an infection and cause disease. Unlike the situation pertaining to bacterial, viral, or protozoan infections, casual or limited exposure to infective stages of parasitic helminths generally does not result in patent infection or pathologic manifestations. Repeated or intense exposure to a large number of infective larvae is required for infection to be established and disease to develop.

Nematode infections are endemic in both temperate and tropical climates. They are transmitted either by the fecal–oral route or by inoculation of infective larvae into the skin, primarily by blood-feeding intermediate insect vectors. The prevalence of infection is greatest in circumstances conducive to the development and transmission of infective forms of the parasites, i.e., overcrowded, perennially warm geographic areas with poor sanitation, such as in many developing countries of Africa, Asia, and Latin America and economically poor areas of North America and Europe.

The epidemiologic characteristics of human nematode (as well as trematode and cestode) infections have several unique features. The infection in an endemic area has a negative binomial distribution; i.e., the majority of individuals have low parasite burdens and a small number harbor relatively high burdens. Persons in the latter group are important from an epidemiologic perspective in that they contribute most substantially to transmission and are most likely to experience pathologic manifestations. This characteristic implies that transmission in an endemic area may be decreased or interrupted by reduction of the parasite burden in a small proportion of the population. In addition, because total worm load correlates directly with the propensity to development of disease, treatment of lightly infected persons may not be indicated or may be unnecessary, especially if the available chemotherapy has major side effects.

Nematode infections of medical importance may be broadly classified into those in which the route of infection, larval migration, and disease manifestations are primarily gastrointestinal and those that affect other tissues. The former group includes hookworms (*Ancylostoma duodenale, Necator americanus*), the roundworm *Ascaris lumbricoides*, the pinworm *Enterobius vermicularis*, and the whipworm *Trichuris trichiuria*. Animal intestinal nematodes such as *Trichostrongylus* and *Anisakis* species also occasionally infect and cause disease in humans. *Trichinella spiralis, Strongyloides stercoralis*, and *Angiostrongylus cantonensis* infect humans by the oral route, but disease manifestations are due primarily to migration in other tissues. Tissue-invasive nematodes include lymphatic filariae (*Wuchereria bancrofti, Brugia malayi*, and *B. timori*), skin-dwelling *Onchocerca volvulus* and *Loa loa*, and the guinea worm *Dracunculus medinensis*.

Anderson RM, May RM: Helminthic infections of humans: Mathematical models, population dynamics, and control. Adv Parasitol 24:1, 1985. *An excellent discussion of the relationship of the biologic characteristics of parasitic helminthic infections to their epidemiologic features and control strategies.*

INTESTINAL NEMATODES

Intestinal nematode infections include hookworm disease, ascariasis, enterobiasis, trichuriasis, and rarely animal nematodiases. They are prevalent in temperate and tropical areas of the world, especially those with overcrowding and poor sanitation. Intestinal nematode infections cause little morbidity in most cases and are easily treated with mebendazole. The adverse impact of chronic infection on growth of children in developing countries is substantial.

Hookworm Disease

CAUSATIVE AND EPIDEMIOLOGIC CHARACTERISTICS. The major hookworms that infect humans are *Ancylostoma duodenale* and *Necator americanus. A. ceylanicum* infection is less common and occurs primarily in the South Pacific. Animal hookworms such as *A. braziliense* and *Uncinaria stenocephala* do not undergo full development in incidentally exposed humans. Infection occurs when exposed skin maintains contact for several minutes with soil contaminated with parasite eggs containing viable larvae. Larvae penetrate the skin and subsequently migrate to and mature in the lungs. The parasites then break into the air spaces, ascend the trachea, and are swallowed. Adult worms mature in the upper small intestine and attach to the mucosa. Female worms release more than 10,000 eggs per day, which are passed in the stools and deposited in the soil. The pre-patent period (duration of time between infection and passing of eggs in the feces) is 40 to 105 days. Adult hookworms have a lifespan of 2 to 5 years.

Hookworms infect over 1 billion persons worldwide. The highest prevalence of infection (80 to 100%) occurs in tropical and less developed countries, where environmental and socioeconomic conditions are especially favorable to transmission. These include warm, moist soil; lack of public sewage disposal systems; and the habit of walking barefoot. The higher prevalence of hookworm infection in children than in adults results from more frequent exposure of skin to larvae in soil. Acquired resistance is minimal or does not appear to develop as a consequence of previous infection.

PATHOGENESIS AND CLINICAL MANIFESTATIONS. Hookworm disease is due primarily to gastrointestinal blood loss and attendant iron deficiency anemia. The latter correlates directly with the total worm burden. Adult worms attached to the mucosa of the upper small intestine digest ingested blood as well as cause focal bleeding. *A. duodenale* is estimated to cause a blood loss of 0.3 mL/day/worm; *N. americanus* induces loss of approximately 0.03 mL/day. Light infections (feces with <400 eggs/g) do not cause blood loss sufficient to induce iron deficiency. Nutritional deficiencies secondary to coexisting conditions that result in low iron stores (e.g., malabsorption or insufficient dietary intake in children and multiparous women) contribute significantly to morbidity. Hypoproteinemia has been reported in children with hookworm disease in less developed countries. This complication is most likely due to coexisting malnutrition rather than gastrointestinal disease caused by hookworm infestation per se. Abdominal signs or symptoms are not caused by hookworm infection.

Pruritus at the site of larval skin penetration ("ground itch") occurs occasionally. In the case of primary exposure, local itching and erythematous papules lasting 1 week develop. More intense pruritus, vesiculation, and edema of 2 to 3 weeks' duration may occur after repeated exposure to infective larvae. Hookworm larvae migrating through the lungs rarely cause pulmonary symptoms.

DIAGNOSIS. Hookworm infection is diagnosed by identification of the characteristic round eggs containing convoluted larvae. Direct smears of freshly passed stool using the Kato or other techniques are satisfactory for the diagnosis of moderately to heavily infected cases (> 400 eggs/g).

TREATMENT AND PREVENTION. Mebendazole is the treatment of choice (Table 433–1). The ideal method for preventing hookworm infection is improvement of hygienic conditions. Use of footwear, especially by children, is currently the only practical means of preventing infection.

Table 433–1 ■ TREATMENT FOR INTESTINAL NEMATODES

NEMATODE	TREATMENT
Hookworm	Mebendazole, 100 mg orally b.i.d. for 3 days. Do not give to pregnant women; iron supplementation (if warranted by anemia and complicating illnesses)
Ascaris	Mebendazole, 100 mg orally b.i.d. for 3 days. Children with heavy infections, biliary tract obstruction: piperazine, 50–75 mg/kg body weight for 2 days
Enterobius	Pyrantel pamoate, 11 mg/kg once, with a repeated dose 2 weeks later; maximum single dose, 1 g. Several treatments may be required (every 3–4 months) if exposure continues (i.e., in institutional setting)
Trichuris	Mebendazole, at same dosage as for ascariasis
Other animal nematodes	
Trichostrongylus	Pyrantel pamoate, 11 mg/kg once; maximum dose of 1 g
Anisakis	Thiabendazole, 25 mg/kg b.i.d. for 3 days if surgery is not required
Capillaria	Mebendazole, 200 mg b.i.d. for 20 days. Alternative: albendazole, 400 mg/d for 10 days. Supportive care: replacement of fluid and electrolytes, high-protein diet
Gnathostoma	For subcutaneous lesions: surgical removal. For CNS infection: albendazole, 400 mg b.i.d. for 21 days.

Ascariasis

CAUSATIVE AND EPIDEMIOLOGIC CHARACTERISTICS. *Ascaris lumbricoides* are roundworms 2 to 3 cm in length that reside in the lumen of the jejunum and in the midileum. Infection occurs by the oral route when soil containing embryonated eggs is ingested. Larvae are released from eggs in the small intestine, penetrate the gut, and migrate to the liver and then lungs via the blood or lymphatic circulation. Following maturation in the lungs over a 4-week period, the parasites ascend the respiratory tract and are swallowed. Adult worms reach sexual maturity (i.e., female worms release eggs that are detectable in feces) approximately 60 days after infection.

Ascariasis affects approximately one quarter of the world's population and is likely the most prevalent helminthiasis of humans. Infection is common in Africa, Asia, and Latin America, especially in areas of high population density and unhygienic conditions. The use of human feces as fertilizer, defecation in soil, and hand-to-mouth contact with contaminated soil are major factors that contribute to the spread of *Ascaris*. The ability of *Ascaris* eggs to remain viable in harsh environmental conditions (embryonated eggs remain infectious after exposure to freezing temperatures and desiccation for several weeks) also facilitates transmission.

PATHOGENESIS AND CLINICAL MANIFESTATIONS. Disease caused by *A. lumbricoides* is infrequent and generally correlates with the intensity of infection. The majority of infected individuals are asymptomatic.

Symptomatic cases can be divided into two broad categories, which are based on the phase of infection and site of abnormality in the pulmonary or gastrointestinal tract. Pulmonary disease is caused by the migration of larvae in the small vessels of the lung and their subsequent rupture into alveoli. Tissue damage is thought to be due to the host immune response, which includes production of immunoglobulin E (IgE) and eosinophilia. Transient pulmonary infiltrates, fever, cough, dyspnea, and eosinophilia lasting 1 to several weeks are the major clinical manifestations. This complex of symptoms and signs is frequently seasonal and coincidental with environmental changes that favor development of infective-stage larvae in eggs (e.g., spring rains that follow cold and dry periods). Intestinal signs and symptoms are due either to obstruction caused by the presence of an exceptionally large number of parasites in the small intestine or to migration of adult worms to unusual sites, such as the biliary tree or pancreatic duct. Intestinal obstruction almost always occurs in children <6 years old. The onset is sudden and characterized by colicky abdominal pain and vomiting. Heavily infected children are also prone to biliary disease or pancreatitis secondary to *Ascaris* lodging in the ducts draining these organs. A malabsorption syndrome characterized by steatorrhea and low vitamin A levels has been reported in Latin American children with ascariasis.

DIAGNOSIS. Intestinal infection is diagnosed by the presence of the typical oval, thick-shelled *Ascaris* eggs in thick smears of fecal specimens. The existence of adult worms in pancreatic or biliary ducts should be suspected in children who have high egg outputs in conjunction with jaundice or pancreatitis. Pulmonary ascariasis cannot be diagnosed on the basis of identification of ova in feces because adult worms have not yet matured and reached the intestinal tract. Biopsy examination of the lung is unlikely to demonstrate larvae and is not recommended.

TREATMENT AND PREVENTION. Treatment for uncomplicated intestinal ascariasis is listed in Table 433–1. Treatment causes neuromuscular paralysis of the worms and expulsion of intact helminths. No specific treatment is recommended for pulmonary ascariasis because the condition is self-limited.

The major means of preventing *Ascaris* infection is improvement of hygienic and socioeconomic conditions. Mass chemotherapy successfully reduces worm loads but requires frequent treatment.

Enterobiasis

Enterobius vermicularis or pinworm infection is cosmopolitan in its distribution. It is common in overcrowded settings and spreads rapidly in conditions in which person-to-person contact is frequent, such as in institutions for children.

Infection occurs by the fecal–oral route. Embryonated eggs carried on the fingernails, bed clothing, or bedding are ingested and hatch in the upper small intestine. Larvae develop in the large bowel into adult worms 2 to 5 mm long. Female worms migrate nightly out of the rectum and deposit large numbers of ova (11,000 per worm) in the perianal and perineal areas. Larvae in the deposited eggs become infective within several hours of exposure to ambient oxygen. Infectivity is usually maintained for 1 to 2 days.

The vast majority of pinworm infections are asymptomatic or associated with perianal pruritus and consequent sleep deprivation. *E. vermicularis* is a rare cause of appendicitis and, when the adult worms follow an aberrant path of migration, vulvovaginitis, urethritis, or peritonitis.

The diagnosis of pinworm infection is easily made by identifying ova on a piece of cellophane tape applied to the perirectal area in the morning. *E. vermicularis* eggs are oval and slightly flattened on one side. It is unusual to find eggs in feces or adult worms in the perianal area. Repeated examinations may be necessary.

Treatment (Table 433–1) is mebendazole given to affected individuals as well as close associates, such as family members. Although personal cleanliness is recommended as a means of limiting transmission, there is no clear-cut demonstration that it prevents infection.

Trichuriasis

Trichuris trichiuria or whipworm infection is similar to pinworm infection in that it is limited to the gastrointestinal tract and does not have a tissue migratory phase. Eggs containing infective larvae mature in warm, moist soil over a 2-week period. Ingested eggs hatch in the small bowel and subsequently develop in epithelial cells of the cecum and ascending colon into adult worms that are 40 mm in length. The body of the parasite protrudes into the colonic lumen. Its anterior portion has a whiplike shape.

As is the case with most intestinal nematode infections, trichuriasis is most common in overcrowded areas with poor sanitation. The estimated prevalence worldwide is 800 million, with approximately 2 million cases in the southern United States. Children are more frequently infected than adults and also more likely to have higher worm burdens.

Adults with trichuriasis are usually asymptomatic. In children with heavy infections (>10,000 eggs/g of feces), a syndrome of dysentery, growth retardation, and rectal prolapse has been described. The pathologic manifestations include infiltrates of eosinophils and neutrophils accompanied by epithelial denudation. Complicating diseases such as shigellosis and amebiasis may contribute to this condition in children.

Whipworm infection is diagnosed by identification of football-shaped eggs in direct smears of fecal specimens. Mebendazole at the same dosage indicated for ascariasis listed in Table 433–1 is satisfactory treatment.

Other Animal Nematodiases

Humans may serve as paratenic hosts for several nematodes that ordinarily parasitize the intestine of other mammals. These helminths are incapable of completing their life cycle in humans and display aberrant migration patterns in both intestinal and non-intestinal tissues.

Several species of the genus *Trichostrongylus* infect both humans and domestic ruminants. The infection is found widely in the Middle and Far East and Australia. Ova are passed in the stool of ruminants and hatch in the soil. Humans are incidentally infected when larvae are ingested with leafy vegetables. The adult worms live in the intestines and suck small amounts of blood; heavy infections result in anemia. Diagnosis is made by identifying ova, which resemble those of hookworm, in the stool. Treatment is listed in Table 433–1.

Anisakis is an intestinal nematode of marine mammals. Several species of saltwater fish are intermediate hosts. Human infection occurs when raw fish is eaten. The larvae of both *Anisakis* and *Phocanemia decipiens* have been implicated. Most cases have been reported in Japan or Western Europe, particularly Scandinavia. The larvae invade the wall of the small intestine or stomach, causing pain and, rarely, intestinal obstruction or perforation. Gastric anisakiasis can be diagnosed endoscopically and treated by removal of the worms. Intestinal anisakiasis often resembles acute conditions that require surgery leading to laparotomy. Thiabendazole treatment is listed in Table 433–1. Infection is prevented by cooking or freezing fish prior to eating.

Capillaria philippinensis infection has been reported from the Philippines and Thailand. This nematode is thought to parasitize birds, with fish and crustaceans serving as intermediate hosts. Humans are infected by eating the raw intermediate hosts. The ingested larvae mature and live in the crypts of the small intestine, where they reproduce. The result is often a heavy infection; up to 40,000 adult worms have been recovered at one autopsy. The clinical syndrome includes severe malabsorption and protein-losing enteropathy. The diagnosis is made by finding eggs or larvae in the stool; an intradermal test is also available. The treatment of choice is mebendazole (Table 433–1).

Gnathostoma spinigerum is an intestinal nematode of dogs and cats; fish are intermediate hosts. The infection is endemic in rodents in the Far East and Thailand. Human infection has also been reported in South America. Infective larvae are ingested by humans in raw or undercooked fish. The larvae do not complete their life cycle in humans but migrate through the body. The most frequent site is subcutaneous tissues, where larvae are found in eosinophilic granulomas. A few weeks after infection, pruritic or painful subcutaneous nodules and swellings appear. These may be migratory and develop into abscesses. In central nervous system (CNS) gnathostomiasis, hemorrhagic tracts may be found in the brain. Fever, vomiting, and abdominal pain occur a few days after larvae are ingested. Paralysis of the extremities, encephalitis, and subarachnoid hemorrhage have been reported. Eye involvement with uveitis and orbital cellulitis represents a third variety.

Peripheral eosinophilia is usual in cutaneous gnathostomiasis; the diagnosis may be established by biopsy. In CNS infection, blood eosinophilia is an inconstant feature, but eosinophils are present in the cerebrospinal fluid (CSF), as in the case of angiostrongyliasis. Treatments are listed in Table 433–1. The infection may be prevented by thorough cooking of fish.

Several nematodes that ordinarily parasitize the intestine of monkeys occasionally infect humans. *Oesophagostomum* has been reported from Africa, Asia, and Brazil; it is responsible for the formation of granulomas in the intestinal wall. *Ternides deminutus* is sometimes found in the human colon in Africa and Asia; a heavy infection may cause anemia. *Physaloptera mordens,* also reported from Africa, may attach itself to the esophagus, stomach, or small intestine of humans. The definitive host of *Lagochilascaris minor* is unknown. About 30 human cases have been reported from Central and South America, usually with worms invading the soft tissues of the neck, throat, and sinuses.

Drugs for parasitic infections. Med Lett 40:1, 1998.

Khuroo MS, Zargar SA, Mahajan R: Sonographic appearances in biliary ascariasis. Gastroenterology 93:267, 1987. *A discussion of the ultrasound appearance of this unusual but clinically important aspect of ascariasis.*

Smith JW, Wootten R: Anisakis and anisakiasis. Adv Parasitol 16:93, 1978. *An exceptionally complete review.*

TOXOCARIASIS

DEFINITION. Visceral larva migrans (VLM) and ocular larva migrans (OLM) are caused by ingestion and subsequent development and migration of embryonated eggs of the canine roundworm *Toxocara canis.* Roundworms of cats *(T. cati)* and raccoons *(Baylisascaris procyonis)* also rarely cause VLM.

CAUSES. In its normal canine host, *T. canis* follow a route of migration similar to that described for *Ascaris;* i.e., ingested larvae penetrate the small intestine, migrate to the lungs, are reswallowed, and develop into adult worms in the small intestine; the adult worms lodge there and release eggs that are passed in the feces. When embryonated *T. canis* eggs are ingested by humans, larvae also migrate throughout the body (lung, liver, brain, muscles, and occasionally eyes) but fail to complete development to the adult stage. Tissue necrosis secondary to penetrating larvae and associated host inflammatory reactions, such as eosinophil-rich granulomas, are the underlying cause of disease.

EPIDEMIOLOGIC CHARACTERISTICS. Toxocariasis is endemic in both temperate and tropical areas of the world. The vast majority of symptomatic cases occur in young children. This age group is most likely to be infected by virtue of frequent and intimate handling of dogs (especially newborn puppies that may be hyperinfected), playing in areas where dogs and cats defecate (e.g., public sandboxes), and the habit of geophagia. The potential of exposure to embryonated eggs is high in that *T. canis* infection is common in dogs (a 20% infection rate in dogs in the United States).

CLINICAL MANIFESTATIONS. The vast majority of children who ingest *T. canis* eggs are asymptomatic. VLM is the most common clinically defined entity attributable to *T. canis.* It is most frequent in children younger than 5 (there are no published series of adults with VLM) and is characterized by fever <39° C; pulmonary symptoms, including wheezing and cough; and, less frequently, pain in the right upper quadrant. These symptoms have a gradual onset and resolve over 4 to 8 weeks. Physical signs include wheezing and hepatomegaly in about one quarter of cases. Larvae less commonly migrate to the brain and heart and cause focal neurologic defects and heart failure.

OLM has an incidence approximately one tenth that of VLM and affects children older than 8 to 10 years. Visual disturbances due to VLM are not distinguishable from other causes of focal intraretinal granulomas or space-occupying lesions, such as tuberculosis and retinoblastoma. *T. canis* larvae may migrate intraretinally and produce transient and recurrent impairment of vision.

DIAGNOSIS AND TREATMENT. VLM is diagnosed on the basis of suspicion of ingestion of *T. canis* eggs in a child with the symptoms described. Eosinophilia, elevated erythrocyte sedimentation rate, and generalized hypergammaglobulinemia are also consistent with the diagnosis. Biopsy to document the presence of larvae is insensitive and not recommended. An enzyme-linked immunosorbent assay (ELISA) for measuring anti-*Toxocara* antibodies is helpful if elevated levels of immunoglobulin M (IgM) antibodies and a rise in titer between acute and convalescent phases are documented. Most cases of VLM are not life-threatening and are self-limited. Treatment is therefore not required. In persons with severe pulmonary, cardiac, or neurologic involvement and high-grade eosinophilia (>10,000/mm^3 of blood), diethylcarbamazine, 6 mg/kg/day in three doses for 7 to 10 days, and corticosteroids may be used to reduce symptoms and shorten the course of the illness. No controlled studies, however, demonstrate the efficacy of chemotherapy.

OLM represents a diagnostic dilemma in that it must be distinguished from intraretinal neoplasms and infections. Expert ophthalmologic consultation is necessary. Computed tomography and fluorescein angiography are helpful in diagnosis. Elevated anti-*Toxocara* antibody titers in aqueous fluid relative to serum values are consistent with OLM. It is unclear whether anthelmintics are useful for the treatment of OLM.

VLM and OLM may be prevented by periodic deworming of dogs, especially puppies, and limiting of their defecation in public places.

Glickman LT, Schantz PM, Cypess RH: Epidemiologic characteristics and clinical findings in patients with serologically proven toxocariasis. Trans R Soc Trop Med Hyg 73:254, 1979. *An excellent description of the major clinical manifestations of toxocariasis.*

CUTANEOUS LARVA MIGRANS

Animal hookworms, most frequently the dog parasite *Ancylostoma braziliense* and less commonly *Uncinaria stenocephala* and *Bunostomum phlebotomum,* are the major causative agents of cutaneous larva migrans, or creeping eruption. *Ancylostoma duodenale, Necator americanus,* and *Strongyloides stercoralis* may produce a similar syndrome during the phase of infection that involves penetration of the skin.

The disease occurs when skin comes into direct and prolonged contact with hookworm larvae contained in the feces of dogs, cats, or humans. Moist areas visited by animals, such as vegetation near beaches and exposed soil covered by porches, are common sites in which humans may be infected. Cutaneous larva migrans in the United States is most prevalent in southern coastal regions.

Clinical manifestations result from penetration and migration of larvae in the epidermal-dermal junction of the skin. Within several hours of contact with exposed skin, the patient notes pruritus and raised erythematous serpiginous lesions. The lesions migrate approximately 1 cm/day and evolve into bullae. Multiple lesions may appear if large areas of the body have been exposed, as in sunbathing.

Creeping eruption may be treated by topical application of thiabendazole oral suspension. This may be prepared by trituration of a 500-mg tablet in 5 g of petroleum jelly. If untreated, cutaneous larva migrans is self-limited; signs and symptoms resolve in several weeks to 2 months.

ANGIOSTRONGYLIASIS

Angiostrongylus cantonensis is a cause of eosinophilic meningitis in Asia and the South Pacific. Small numbers of cases have also been reported in Cuba and Africa. *Angiostrongylus costaricensis* is a rare cause of gastrointestinal bleeding. The nematode is limited in its distribution to Central and South America. Humans are infected with these rodent (primarily rat) nematodes after ingesting poorly cooked or raw intermediate mollusk hosts, such as snails, slugs, and prawns. Fresh vegetables may also be contaminated with infective larvae and serve as a vehicle of infection.

In the case of *A. cantonensis* infection, ingested infective larvae penetrate the gut wall and migrate to small vessels of the meninges and, less commonly, the spinal cord and eye. An intense local inflammatory reaction ensues within 1 week. Fever, meningismus, and headache develop in association with eosinophilic pleocytosis of the CSF. Strabismus, paresthesias, and vomiting have been observed in a minority of cases. Diagnosis is based on a history of ingesting potentially contaminated foodstuffs and the presence of eosinophils in CSF. Larvae are usually not found in CSF. Other infectious causes of eosinophilic meningitis include *Trichinella spiralis*, *Taenia solium*, *Toxocara canis*, *Gnathostoma spinigerum*, and *Paragonimus westermani*. Symptomatic *A. cantonensis* infection resolves over a 2-week period. The value of anthelmintic therapy or corticosteroids has not been established.

A. costaricensis larvae penetrate the mucosa of the terminal ileum, appendix, and ascending colon. The larvae subsequently develop into adult worms in the local lymphatics and mesenteric arterioles. Eggs released by the female worms elicit multiple eosinophil-rich granulomatous reactions that cause edematous, thickened bowel and necrosis (secondary to mesenteric blood vessel obstruction). Clinical presentations typically include right-sided abdominal pain, vomiting, and fever. Abnormal laboratory findings include leukocytosis with eosinophilia. Parasite larvae and eggs are not present in stools. A palpable mass secondary to granulomatous lesions may be present and cause intestinal obstruction. Less frequently, gastrointestinal bleeding is the principal manifestation. Treatment is surgical. There is no demonstrated benefit of specific anthelmintic chemotherapy.

Koo J, Pien F, Kliks M: *Angiostrongylus (Parastrongylus) eosinophilic meningitis*. Rev Infect Dis 10:1155, 1988. *An excellent discussion of the biologic features of the helminth and the clinical manifestations of human infection.*

TRICHINOSIS

DEFINITION. Infection by *Trichinella spiralis* occurs when infective larvae are eaten in undercooked pork or other meats. The majority of infected individuals are asymptomatic. Clinical manifestations in heavily infected persons include diarrhea, myalgias, fever, and, less commonly, myocarditis and neurologic disease. Trichinosis occurs in all areas of the world, including the Arctic and temperate regions. The incidence of trichinosis in the United States has decreased markedly over the past several decades.

CAUSE. Infection is initiated by ingesting infective larvae encysted in striated muscle. Excystment occurs in the acid-pepsin environment of the stomach, and parasites develop into sexually mature adult worms in the upper to middle small intestine of the human host. Completion of the enteric phase of the parasite life cycle takes about 1 week, with adult worms remaining viable and productive of larval offspring for an additional 3 to 5 weeks. The systemic phase commences 1 week after infection, when larvae released by female worms migrate through blood vessels and lymphatics and invade multiple organ systems. Mature third-stage larvae develop in host-derived nurse cells in striated skeletal and cardiac muscle, where they become encysted and remain viable for years. As is the case with most helminthiases, the severity of symptoms is related to the total parasite load. Because adult worms are incapable of reproducing themselves, the number of infective

larvae ingested is the most important determinant of worm load (i.e., number of larvae that invade muscle and other tissues).

EPIDEMIOLOGIC CHARACTERISTICS. *T. spiralis* infection is enzootic in omnivorous and carnivorous animal populations, including rats, bears, and aquatic mammals of the Arctic. The nematode is introduced into domestic animals such as pigs and horses by feeding them garbage containing carcasses of these animals, most commonly rats. Human infection usually occurs in two settings: first, when undercooked or smoked pork products or beef contaminated with nematodes is eaten, and second, when flesh of poorly cooked wild game, such as bear or boar meat, is ingested. An important source of infection in Alaskan and Canadian Arctic native populations is uncooked walrus meat.

The annual incidence of human trichinosis in the United States has decreased markedly over the past 50 years. This decline is primarily due to a decrease in the number of cases related to ingestion of commercial pork products. Recent cases in the United States occur in point-source outbreaks associated with eating game or non-commercial pork products.

PATHOGENESIS AND CLINICAL MANIFESTATIONS. Tissue-invasive *T. spiralis* larvae elicit an eosinophilic granulomatous reaction that may result in significant end-organ tissue damage and dysfunction. Skeletal muscle is the most frequent site involved. Myocardial damage, pulmonary infiltration, and focal neurologic damage secondary to invasion by larvae are seen in only the most heavily infected persons. The systemic phase of infection usually occurs 2 to 3 weeks after ingestion of infective larvae and may last for 2 months. Clinical manifestations typically include myalgias (especially of the gastrocnemius and masseter), periorbital edema, and fever. Myocardial damage may manifest as heart failure or dysrhythmias.

The enteric phase of infection may cause gastrointestinal signs and symptoms, such as diarrhea and abdominal cramps. These typically occur within 1 week of eating contaminated meat and last less than 2 weeks. Reports from the Canadian Arctic suggest that the *T. spiralis* larvae that infect walrus meat may cause diarrhea of 1 to 3 months' duration.

DIAGNOSIS. A diagnosis of trichinosis should be considered in individuals with generalized myalgias and eosinophilia (>600 eosinophils/mm^3). Serologic testing for *T. spiralis* antibodies is available at the Centers for Disease Control and Prevention. Elevation of the level of IgM antibodies or a more than four-fold rise in titer between acute and convalescent phases of infection is helpful in diagnosis. The levels of creatine phosphate kinase and of serum immunoglobulins and the erythrocyte sedimentation rate are also increased for several weeks after infection. Muscle biopsy (e.g., of the gastrocnemius) may demonstrate larvae, although their absence does not exclude the diagnosis.

TREATMENT AND PREVENTION. If patients present at a time when adult parasites are in the intestine (i.e., during the initial 1 to 2 weeks after infection, when gastrointestinal symptoms are prominent), mebendazole is recommended at a dosage of 200 to 400 mg/ three times per day for 3 days, followed by 400 to 500 mg three times per day for 10 days. It is not clear whether larvae in muscle are killed by this drug, and treatment is primarily symptomatic with antipyretics and analgesics. Although there are too few recent cases to establish a possible beneficial effect of corticosteroids, they may be useful to diminish the severity of inflammation when signs of myocarditis, neurologic disease (e.g., seizures, focal weakness), or pulmonary insufficiency develop. *T. spiralis* infection is prevented by killing larvae in meat products. This is achieved by heating until no trace of pink flesh remains. Freezing, smoking, or exposure to microwaves does not reliably kill the helminth.

Bailey TM, Schantz PM: Trends in the incidence and transmission patterns of trichinosis in humans in the United States: Comparisons of the periods 1975–1981 and 1982–1986. Rev Infect Dis 12:5, 1990. *A comprehensive review of the epidemiologic characteristics of trichinosis.*

MacLean JD, Viallet J, Law C, et al: Trichinosis in the Canadian Arctic: Report of five outbreaks and a new clinical syndrome. J Infect Dis 160:513, 1989. *Excellent description of severe gastrointestinal manifestations of* T. spiralis *in a population in which the prevalence of trichinosis is among the highest in the world.*

STRONGYLOIDIASIS

DEFINITION. *Strongyloides stercoralis* infection is endemic in warm climates worldwide, including the southern United States. In immunologically normal individuals, infection is usually asymptomatic or causes gastrointestinal dysfunction, manifest as abdominal pain, bloating, or bleeding. In persons who have deficient cell-mediated immunity an autoinfective and hyperinfective life cycle of the nematode that markedly increases the total worm load can develop. Life-threatening acute pulmonary disease and organ dysfunction due to dissemination of larvae to aberrant sites such as the brain, pancreas, and kidneys may result in immunocompromise in the host.

CAUSE. *S. stercoralis* infection occurs when skin contacts free-living filariform larvae in the soil. After penetrating the skin, the parasite embolizes to the small vessels of the lungs via the venous circulation. Rhabditiform larvae then break into the alveolar spaces, ascend the respiratory tree, and are swallowed. Further development to adult worms occurs in the duodenum and upper jejunum, where egg-laying parasites live in the mucosa and submucosa. Rhabditiform larvae are released from eggs and are passed from the body in stools. Infective filariform larvae develop in the soil by two alternative means, either directly by transformation from rhabditiform larvae or indirectly from free-living intermediate forms.

Several unusual features of the life cycle of *S. stercoralis* are crucial to understanding how this parasitic nematode causes life-threatening disease. First, unlike the vast majority of human helminthic parasites, adult worms reproduce parthogenetically in the gastrointestinal tract. The total worm burden in the host may therefore be greatly increased in the absence of repeated exposure to infective larvae in the environment. Second, rhabditiform larvae may develop into infective filariform larvae in the gastrointestinal tract as well as after passage in feces. Occurrence of the former process in immunocompromised hosts allows autoinfection, whereby larvae pass directly through the bowel (internal autoinfection) or perianal skin (external autoinfection) to reinitiate migration and development in the lungs. When this event is frequent, a hyperinfection syndrome ensues. Disseminated strongyloidiasis entails a condition of hyperinfection in which the organisms also migrate to and cause pathologic disorders in organs not usually traversed by larvae, such as the central nervous system (CNS).

EPIDEMIOLOGIC CHARACTERISTICS. *S. stercoralis* infection is endemic in Africa, Asia, Latin America, and areas of Eastern and Southern Europe. Prevalence rates based on stools examined for rhabditiform larvae vary from more than 40% in areas of sub-Saharan Africa to 1 to 7% in rural Eastern Europe. In the United States, the infection is endemic in rural Appalachia and other parts of the South. Prevalences range from 0.4 to 3% in the United States. Refugees from Asia have a higher prevalence of infection than do indigenous Americans. Surveys of homosexual men indicate a frequency of infection of 3.9%. It is likely that most studies of prevalence underestimate infection because they are based on examination of a single stool specimen, which is less sensitive than multiple examinations performed over days or weeks.

Strongyloidiasis is especially common in overcrowded situations in which sanitation and personal hygiene are poor, such as in institutions for retarded children and POW camps. An unusually high frequency of *S. stercoralis* infection has also been reported in persons with asymptomatic human T-cell lymphotropic virus (HTLV) type I infection.

PATHOGENESIS. Adult worms and larvae penetrating the upper small bowel cause an enteritis characterized histopathologically by eosinophil and mononuclear cell infiltration of the lamina propria. Edema and mucosal atrophy are found on gross examination. Ulcerative lesions with hemorrhages are present in the most severe cases. Filariform larvae in the lungs elicit an inflammatory response in the alveoli consisting of mononuclear cells and eosinophils. In hyperinfection syndrome, these may coalesce and result in alveolar hemorrhage.

Autoinfection leading to exceptionally high worm loads (hyperinfection) and disseminated strongyloidiasis occur in persons with deficient cell-mediated immunity. Groups at risk include persons who are chronically taking corticosteroids, renal transplanation recipients, patients with Hodgkin's disease and other lymphomas, and leukemic patients. Because *S. stercoralis* may persist and remain asymptomatic for decades after exposure, it is important to keep in mind that a change in immune status may convert a previously asymptomatic infection to hyperinfection. In this regard, there is a suspected association between acquired immunodeficiency syndrome (AIDS) and disseminated strongyloidiasis.

CLINICAL MANIFESTATIONS. More than 50% of immunocompetent infected persons are asymptomatic. The frequency of clinical manifestations among infected immunocompromised subjects is not known.

Signs and symptoms of *S. stercoralis* infection are attributable to the presence of adult worms in the upper gastrointestinal tract and larval invasion and attendant host pathologic responses in the lung, skin, and aberrant sites of migration, such as the brain, eyes, pancreas, and kidney. Immunocompetent individuals rarely have signs or symptoms attributable to larval migration outside the gut.

Gastrointestinal disease usually manifests as abdominal bloating, vague epigastric pain, and diarrhea with nausea. Symptoms are exacerbated by eating. Hematochezia and melena occur in <20% of subjects with intestinal strongyloidiasis. Major causes of morbidity related to *S. stercoralis* infection of the intestine are paralytic ileus, small bowel obstruction, and a malabsorption syndrome.

Pulmonary signs and symptoms in immunocompromised persons with hyperinfection syndrome are similar to those seen in the adult respiratory distress syndrome, i.e., acute onset of dyspnea, productive cough, and hemoptysis. These are accompanied by fever, tachypnea, hypoxemia, and respiratory alkalosis. *Strongyloides* larvae may also invade the CNS, pancreas, and eye and cause signs and symptoms attributable to tissue destruction in these sites.

Dermatologic manifestations include self-limited creeping eruption and, more commonly, larva currens. The latter is due to migration of filariform larvae produced by a process of external autoinfection as described above. The larvae elicit serpiginous erythematous papules and occasionally urticaria around the buttocks, upper thigh, and lower abdomen. Larva currens has been noted among former prisoners of war in the South Pacific.

DIAGNOSIS. The unequivocal diagnosis of *S. stercoralis* infection depends on identifying larvae in host tissues or gastrointestinal and pulmonary secretions. The existence of filariform larvae in stools implies an active autoinfection.

Intestinal strongyloidiasis is most easily diagnosed by identification of parasites in direct smears of freshly passed stools. Rhabditiform larvae are 225 to 380 μm in length. Repeated examinations and concentration of stools increase the sensitivity of this method from approximately 25 to 80%. Examination of fluid obtained by duodenal aspiration or passage of a swallowed string into the upper small bowel may also be used if stool examination findings are negative. Serologic tests are sensitive but not generally available. The differential diagnosis of intestinal *S. stercoralis* infection includes sprue, peptic ulcer, regional enteritis, and ulcerative colitis.

Hyperinfection syndrome and disseminated strongyloidiasis are diagnosed by identification of filariform larvae (500 to 600 μm long) in gastrointestinal secretions, as described, or in pulmonary tissues, secretions, or washings, such as those obtained by bronchoalveolar lavage or in sputum. Larvae have also been recovered from CSF peritoneal washings, kidneys, urine, skin, and brains of immunocompromised persons.

Accompanying abnormalities in laboratory results frequently include eosinophilia. However, eosinophilia may not develop in immunocompromised hosts. Lack of eosinophilia is therefore not helpful in excluding strongyloidiasis in the differential diagnosis. The differential diagnosis of hyperinfection and disseminated strongyloidiasis includes overwhelming bacterial or fungal sepsis.

COMPLICATIONS. Disseminated strongyloidiasis is frequently accompanied by fungal or bacterial sepsis. Gram-negative enterococcal and polymicrobial septicemia has been observed. These infections likely result from translocation of gut organisms by migrating larvae.

TREATMENT. Uncomplicated intestinal strongyloidiasis should be treated with ivermectin (200 μg/kg/day for 2 days). Parasitologic cure rates are >90%. Thiabendazole (50 mg/kg/day in two divided doses) should be given to immunocompromised patients with hyperinfection syndrome (i.e., pulmonary disease) or disseminated disease. The drug should be continued for a minimum of 5 to 7 days, although 1 to 2 weeks may be required if organ dysfunction and larval recovery persist. Symptomatic improvement and absence of larvae in gastrointestinal secretions or other sites are indicative of cure. Corticosteroids and other immunosuppressive agents should be discontinued when possible.

PREVENTION. Infection is preventable by avoiding skin contact with contaminated soil. Immunocompromised patients in endemic areas should be advised to avoid walking barefoot. Persons residing in endemic areas who are to become immunosuppressed (e.g., for renal transplantation) should have their stools examined three times for the presence of larvae, and they should be treated if the examination result is positive. Because infected individuals may be incorrectly categorized as uninfected by this test, it is suggested by some authorities that prophylactic thiabendazole (25 mg/kg body weight/day for 2 days) be given in the month preceding iatrogenic immunosuppression. Positive serologic findings for *S. stercoralis* are also an indication for thiabendazole administration prior to immunosuppression.

Cook GC: *Strongyloides stercoralis* hyperinfection syndrome: How often is it missed? Q J Med 64:625, 1987. *Discusses in detail the differential diagnosis and pitfalls in diagnosis of strongyloidiasis in the immunocompromised host.*

Lessnav K-D, Can S, Talavera W: Disseminated *Strongyloides stercoralis* in human immunodeficiency virus–infected patients: Treatment failure and a review of the literature. Chest 104:119. *A discussion of the difficulties in diagnosis in AIDS patients.*

Mahmoud AA: Strongyloidiasis. Clin Inf Dis 23:949, 1996. *A general review of diagnosis and treatment.*

Robinson PD, Lindo JF, Neva FA, et al: Immunoepidemiologic studies of *Strongyloides stercoralis* and human T lymphotropic virus type I infection in Jamaica. Infect Dis 169:692, 1994. *Describes the association between HTLV-I infection and strongyloidiasis.*

434 FILARIASIS

David O. Freedman

INTRODUCTION

The filariases are a group of arthropod borne parasitic diseases of humans caused by thread-like nematodes that in their mature adult stage reside in the lymphatics or in connective tissue. Eight filarial species infect humans (see Table 434–1): *Wuchereria bancrofti, Brugia malayi, Brugia timori, Onchocerca volvulus, Loa loa, Mansonella streptocerca, Mansonella perstans,* and *Mansonella ozzardi.* Three species, *W. bancrofti, B. malayi,* and *O. volvulus,* which infect approximately 150 million individuals, are responsible for the majority of human filarial disease in the world. Loiasis, however, is a relatively common affliction of returned travelers and expatriates.

Infection of the human host begins with the bite of an infected arthropod vector (see Table 434–1). Infective larvae are deposited into the skin or blood of a new host, where at least 3–12 months is required for the development of the mature adult female capable of producing larvae called *microfilariae.* To complete the life cycle, microfilariae, which either circulate in the blood or migrate through the skin, are ingested by another arthropod vector to develop into new infective larvae ready to be passed to the next human host in a blood meal. Generally, infection is only established with repeated

and prolonged exposure to infective larvae. After successful infection, no multiplication of the adult worms occurs in the human host. Because adult worms live for 5–15 years, these are chronic diseases. Microfilariae live for approximately 5–15 months. The long asymptomatic incubation period significantly lessens the chance the relevant travel history will be elicited in an individual who has the non-specific symptoms that occur with many of the filarial infections.

Disease expression varies. The adult parasite itself may provoke chronic inflammatory reactions in tissues; whereas in other filariases reaction to microfilariae migrating through tissue may incite the abnormality observed. Newly exposed individuals characteristically have manifestations of acute symptoms that are exaggerated when compared to those of chronically infected natives of the endemic area.

Definitive diagnosis of any of the filarial infections is generally dependent upon the parasitologic demonstration of 170 to 300-μm-long by 5- to 9-μm-wide microfilariae in blood or in skin snips. The presence or absence of a sheath, the arrangement of the nuclei in the tail, and the tissue of origin are usually sufficient to differentiate the species. Diagnostic blood sampling must be timed during the day to account for the periodicity of every filarial parasite that is epidemiologically possible in the particular patient. Available serologic methods utilize crude heterologous antigen preparations. A positive result is not species-specific and individuals resident in endemic areas will have antibodies whether they are currently infected or not. A positive result may be helpful in individuals infected with filarial parasites who are originally from non-endemic areas and were presumably seronegative initially.

Diethylcarbamazine (DEC) and ivermectin are the backbone of antifilarial treatment. DEC has substantial adulticidal effects against *L. loa* and the lymphatic filariases. Curative efforts with repeated courses of adulticidal therapy are more important in those non-endemic individuals who will not be subsequently re-exposed to the parasite. DEC is microfilaricidal to all species of human filaria except *M. ozzardi* and *M. perstans.* Ivermectin is not an adulticide and is microfilaricidal to *O. volvulus, W. bancrofti, Brugia* sp., *L. loa, M. ozzardi,* and *M. streptocerca.* Suppression of microfilaremia may vary from weeks to months. Treatment regimens will differ according to whether the ultimate aim is treatment and cure of an individual patient or widespread single-dose community based interruption of transmission by suppression of microfilariae available to vectors. Albendazole has significant antifilarial activity but lack of data precludes its use as first-line therapy of individual patients at present.

LYMPHATIC FILARIASIS

CAUSE. *Wuchereria bancrofti, Brugia malayi,* and *Brugia timori* adults are thread-like worms that are convoluted in lymph nodes but have been shown by ultrasound to be extended into afferent lymph vessels. The females, which are about twice the size (80–100 mm in length and 0.2–0.3 mm in width) of the males, produce microfilariae that circulate in the peripheral blood until ingestion by mosquito intermediate hosts. After a 1- to 3-week incubation, mosquitoes take a second blood meal and infective larvae penetrate the skin at the puncture wound. An additional 4–12 months elapses for development into mature adults in the lymphatics of the new host.

Table 434–1 ■ THE COMMON FILARIAL PARASITES OF HUMANS

SPECIES	DISTRIBUTION	VECTOR	PRIMARY PATHOLOGY	MICROFILARIAE Primary Location	Periodicity	Presence of Sheath
Wuchereria bancrofti	Tropics worldwide	Mosquitoes	Lymphatic, pulmonary	Blood, hydrocele fluid	Nocturnal, subperiodic	+
Brugia malayi	Southeast Asia, West Pacific	Mosquitoes	Lymphatic, pulmonary	Blood	Nocturnal, subperiodic	+
Brugia timori	Indonesia	Mosquitoes	Lymphatic	Blood	Nocturnal	+
Onchocerca volvulus	Africa, Central and South America	Black fly	Skin, eye, lymphatic	Skin, eye	None or minimal	−
Loa loa	Africa	Deer fly	Allergic	Blood	Diurnal	+
Mansonella perstans	Africa, South America	Midge	? Allergic	Blood	None	−
Mansonella streptocerca	Africa	Midge	Skin	Skin	None	−
Mansonella ozzardi	Central and South America	Midge	Vague	Blood	None	−

PREVALENCE AND EPIDEMIOLOGIC CHARACTERISTICS.

An estimated 120 million people are affected by lymphatic filariasis—90% with bancroftian and 10% with brugian filariasis. Humans are the only definitive host for *W. bancrofti,* which has no animal reservoir. *W. bancrofti* is found in 76 countries throughout the tropics and subtropics, encompassing areas of South America, the Caribbean, Africa, Asia, and the South Pacific. Two forms of the parasite are distinguished by the periodicity of their circulating microfilariae. Nocturnally periodic forms of the parasite, found in most endemic areas, have microfilariae detectable in blood primarily at night, peaking between 10:00 P.M. and 2:00 A.M. Subperiodic bancroftian filariasis is found only in the Pacific islands, with microfilariae circulating at all hours but with peak levels in the late afternoon. The natural vectors are *Culex quinquefasciatus* in urban settings and usually anopheline or aedean mosquitoes in rural areas.

Brugia malayi is restricted to an area of Asla from India in the west to Korea in the northeast. Foci also exist in Indonesia, Vietnam, Malaysia, China, and the Philippines. Two forms of *B. malayi* are distinguished. The nocturnally periodic form, which has no animal reservoir, is transmitted by *Mansonia* and *Anopheles* species in India, Sulawesi, Vietnam, and China. The nocturnally subperiodic form is transmitted by *Mansonia* species and co-exists with periodic forms in Malaysia and Indonesia. Subperiodic *B. malayi* can produce a natural infection of cats. *B. timori,* transmitted by anophelines, has been described from only two Indonesian islands.

PATHOLOGIC FEATURES.

Microfilariae in blood are not associated with any disorder. The mature adult lymphatic dwelling parasite induces a parasite-specific local inflammatory reaction with both cell-mediated and humoral components leading to hypertrophy of the vessel walls. The worm itself does not seem to cause blockage of the vessel. Endothelial and connective tissue proliferation leads to vessel dilatatation and intraluminal polyposis that diminish normal lymphatic function. The resulting lymphedema is reversible in its early stages. Worm death leads to necrosis and granulomatous reaction with infiltration of plasma cells, eosinophils, and giant cells. Over time fibrosis and obstruction of lymph flow within the lumen lead to irreversible elephantiasis of the affected part. Though some recanalization and collateralization of lymph vessels take place, lymphatic function remains compromised.

At least two other components play clear-cut roles at differing stages of disease. First, mechanical damage to lymph vessels due to the whip-like action of the constantly motile adult worms and toxic effects of parasite excretory secretory products are important early in the clinically asymptomatic non-inflammatory stage of infection. Second, at an uncertain point during the clinical evolution of the lymphatic insufficiency, repeated limb bacterial infections in previously damaged vessels may become superimposed on other processes. The relative contribution to disease evolution of each of the components and the degree of interindividual variability are incompletely defined at present.

Until recently, entirely asymptomatic individuals with microfilaremia but no overt clinical manifestations of filarial infection had been thought to have infection but not disease. Imaging of the lymphatic system with both ultrasound and radionuclide lymphoscintigraphy as well as biopsy of affected tissue have now demonstrated that lymphatic structural and functional abnormalities are often far advanced even before overt lymphatic insufficiency is manifest clinically.

CLINICAL MANIFESTATIONS.

The common clinical outcomes of lymphatic filariasis are asymptomatic microfilaremia, acute episodic adenolymphangitis (also called "filarial fever"), and chronic lymphatic obstruction. Clinically asymptomatic microfilaremia is the most common outcome of lymphatic filariasis. These individuals, however, almost uniformly have underlying lymphatic damage with impaired lymphatic function. Microscopic hematuria and low-grade proteinuria are common but of uncertain clinical significance.

Acute attacks of retrograde adenolymphangitis, accompanied by fever, chills, and malaise, lasting 3–15 days each, can occur up to 10 times per year and are often presenting manifestations of progressive filarial disease. Patients usually give a clear history of pain, erythema, and tenderness in the affected lymph node region for hours or a day prior to onset of the lymphangitis. Some individuals may have only one or a few attacks in a lifetime. Adenolymphangitis most often affects the groin, and in males the lymphatics of the genitalia, leading to funiculitis, orchitis, and epididymitis, but essentially any lymph node group and any body part may be involved. Patients with filarial fevers may be microfilaremic but often are not.

After months to years of acute episodes ranging from very insidious to severe, transient then chronic obstructive disease due to lymphatic insufficiency develops. Pitting edema progresses to brawny edema, and thickening of subcutaneous tissue and hyperkeratosis develop. Fissuring of the skin develops along with nodular and papillomatous hyperplasia. Bacterial superinfection of limbs with such loss of integrity of skin surfaces manifests as a typical cellulitis type of presentation with a warm edematous extremity and anterograde lymphangitis. In many areas the most common chronic manifestation is hydrocele, and scrotal lymphedema is seen in more advanced cases. That many patients give no history of earlier acute attacks emphasizes the need for disrobing of all male patients in order to carry out a genital examination. Females may occasionally have lymphedema of the vulva. If retroperitoneal lymphatics are obstructed, the rupture of renal lymphatics leads to the development of intermittent chyluria. In endemic areas, the prevalence of chronic manifestations increases with age. Patients with chronic disease may be microfilaremic but most often are not. Attacks of acute adenolymphangitis often continue even in those with far advanced disease.

Newly exposed individuals (e.g., long-term visitors, military personnel, migrants) characteristically have manifestations of typical acute inflammatory symptoms with more rapid progression to chronic or irreversible abnormality than do those born in the endemic area. Prolonged severe episodes of adenolymphangitis often with genital involvement may lead to the relatively rapid development of lymphedema and elephantiasis within 6–12 months of arrival. Disease abates quickly with removal of the patient from the endemic area. These individuals are uniformly amicrofilaremic.

Brugian filariasis differs in several respects from bancroftian filariasis. In *B. malayi* infection only the lower leg is affected, whereas in *W. bancrofti* infection, the thigh as well as the lower leg are involved. In brugian filariasis, infected superficial nodes, usually inguinal, may suppurate and form sterile abscesses that heal with a characteristic scar. In general, brugian filariasis is more clinically dramatic. Insidious onset of chronic lymphedema, as may occur in bancroftian filariasis, is uncommon. Urogenital disease and chyluria do not occur.

DIAGNOSIS.

Definitive diagnosis often depends on the parasitologic demonstration of the 250- to 320-μm-long microfilariae in blood. Diagnostic sampling must take into account the periodicity of the microfilariae in the area of exposure. A Giemsa-stained thick blood smear, performed as for the diagnosis of malaria, will detect heavily infected individuals but is relatively insensitive. Parasites may be concentrated by passage through a polycarbonate membrane filter (3-μm pore size) or by centrifugation at 1 mL of anticoagulated blood in a conical tube with 9 mL of 2% formalin. The filter itself or the sediment is then stained and examined. Microfilariae of *W. bancrofti* have occasionally been found in urine but are usually not present in chyluric patients. Only an experienced pathologist can identify the sections of adult worms that are found incidentally in specimens of diverse human body tissues. Lymph node biopsy is not indicated in suspected filariasis unless neoplasia is also a diagnostic concern.

Serologic measurement of antifilarial antibodies is often not useful because existing assays cannot distinguish among the eight human filarial parasites. The assays cannot distinguish actively infected patients from those previously infected, and those merely exposed but not infected may also have positive findings. Cross-reactivity occurs with other helminth infections. A rapid card test assay sensitive enough to detect circulating *W. bancrofti*–specific antigen liberated by adult worms (and present in the blood both day and night) has dramatically advanced the serologic approach to diagnosing filariasis. The card test is commercially available but is not U.S. Food and Drug Administration (FDA)-approved.

Ultrasound techniques have been used to visualize rapidly moving ("dancing") adult worms in the dilated scrotal lymphatics of infected men. Such findings are pathognomonic of filarial parasites, but the technique is less sensitive than other modalities. Abnormalities detected by lymphoscintigraphy are not specific for filarial disease.

Bacterial infection, thrombophlebitis, or trauma may be mistaken for acute filarial adenolymphangitis. Filarial lymphangitis is retrograde, a characteristic that helps differentiate it from bacterial lymphangitis. In cases of orchitis and epididymitis, the sexually transmitted diseases must be considered. Chronic lymphedema may be caused by malignancy, post-operative changes, congenital malformations, as well as renal or cardiac failure. Physical examination cannot distinguish a filarial from a non-filarial cause of lymphedema or elephantiasis. A foreign body reaction to silica dust introduced into traumatized legs accounts for elephantiasis in some parts of the world. Patients with filarial lymphedema are often amicrofilaremic; therefore, so diagnosis depends on the clinical history, the epidemiologic features, as well as the physical examination result and may be supported by a positive serologic or antigen assay result.

TREATMENT. Individual patients, whether symptomatic or asymptomatic, with lymphatic filariasis should be treated with diethylcarbamazine (DEC) 6 mg/kg/day in three divided doses for 2–3 weeks. DEC is FDA-approved but at present only available through the Centers for Disease Control (CDC) Drug Service (404-639-3670). Side effects are due to dying parasites, not to direct drug toxicity, and are directly proportional to the number of circulating microfilariae. They include fever, chills, headache, dizziness, nausea, vomiting, and arthralgias, all usually occurring in the first 24 to 36 hours and then subsiding even with continued therapy. In highly parasitemic persons, one can initiate treatment with single doses of 50–100 mg of DEC on the first 2 days or pre-medicate the patients with steroids. Some patients may experience adenolymphangitis due to dying adult worms. A single dose of DEC is microfilaricidal so is used in control programs where the aim is to break transmission by suppression of microfilariae available to vectors. In individual patients who will not be returning to endemic areas, adulticidal therapy, which requires a prolonged course of DEC, is necessary. If the patient remains microfilaremic, at least two repeat courses at several-month intervals should be considered. Patients with lymphedema or elephantiasis should receive low-dose DEC daily for at least a year in an attempt to determine whether any reversible component of the chronic disease is present. Limb elevation, massage, use of elastic stockings, and prevention of superficial bacterial and fungal infection through meticulous hygiene are important in the care of a lymphedematous extremity. Suspected bacterial superinfection should receive antibiotic therapy. In preliminary trials, albendazole has adulticidal and microfilaricidal activity in lymphatic filariasis, but appropriate dosing regimens for the treatment of individual patients have yet to be developed.

Single doses of DEC, ivermectin, or albendazole either alone or in combination are effectively microfilaricidal for periods of up to a year. These regimens are well tolerated and therefore are ideally suited for mass treatment as part of control programs.

PROGNOSIS. Though the psychosocial morbidity associated with this deforming disease is profound, there is little mortality associated with lymphatic filariasis. It is likely that some but not all untreated asymptomatic microfilaremic individuals become symptomatic, but factors determining such clinical changes are unknown. The determinants of which patients with chronic manifestations have a component that is reversible with therapy are not defined. Disease should not progress in those removed from an endemic area and adequately treated.

PREVENTION. DEC has some value as a prophylactic agent in humans in a dose of 10 mg/kg on 2 consecutive days each month. Yearly mass treatment with a single dose of DEC significantly reduces the prevalence of infection within a community. DEC-supplemented table salt can reduce the number of blood-borne microfilariae in the community to levels so low that transmission is interrupted. Vector control in endemic areas has proved difficult but bed net programs may have some efficacy.

TROPICAL EOSINOPHILIA

Tropical pulmonary eosinophilia (TPE) is a syndrome that develops in a small percentage of individuals infected with lymphatic filarial parasites. The characteristic patient is a male (4:1 male to female ratio) in his teens or 20s who is a resident of India, Pakistan, Sri Lanka, Brazil, or Southeast Asia. Characteristic clinical findings include paroxysmal cough and wheezing that occurs almost exclusively at night, weight loss, low-grade fever, adenopathy, and extreme blood eosinophilia. Chest radiograph results generally show diffusely increased bronchovascular markings or mottled opacities in middle and lower lung fields. Both restrictive and obstructive abnormalities are found through pulmonary function tests. Total serum immunoglobulin E (IgE) level as well as antifilarial antibody levels are both extremely elevated.

TPE is thought to occur as a result of unusually rapid immune-mediated clearance of blood microfilariae with trapping in the lung. The pulmonary symptoms result from allergic (IgE-mediated) and inflammatory reactions to the cleared parasites (*W. bancrofti* or *B. malayi*). Several reports have described microfilariae or their degenerating remnants in lung biopsy specimens and eosinophils are present in bronchial lavage fluid. Untreated disease can progress to interstitial fibrosis.

Differential diagnosis of TPE includes asthma, Löffler's syndrome (which can be due to migrating larval forms of other helminths), allergic bronchopulmonary aspergillosis, Churg-Strauss syndrome or other systemic vasculitides, chronic eosinophilic pneumonia, and idiopathic hypereosinophilic syndrome. Diagnosis of TPE is usually confirmed by the coexistence of nocturnal wheezing, very high antifilarial titers, and rapid initial response to DEC therapy in a patient with the right geographic exposure. DEC at 6 mg/kg/day for 14–21 days is the treatment of choice. Ivermectin is not useful for TPE. Symptoms typically respond within a week but may relapse even after an interval of years in 25%, necessitating re-treatment.

ONCHOCERCIASIS (RIVER BLINDNESS)

CAUSE. Transmission of *Onchocerca volvulus* is via the bites of black flies (*Simulium* species) that ingest microfilariae from the skin of an infected person. After development in the vector, infective larvae are transmitted to a new human host. Over a period of several months, the larvae develop into adult worms that are coiled within fibrotic subcutaneous nodules. Nine to 18 months after infection, each mature female worm begins to produce up to 2000 microfilariae per day, which migrate primarily through the skin and ocular tissues.

Adult female worms are 23 to 70 cm in length, whereas the males are 3 to 6 cm long. Microfilariae are unsheathed and 200 to 300 μm long and 6 to 9 μm wide. The average lifespan of the adult worm is 8 to 10 years and that of the microfilariae, 13 to 14 months. Two distinct strains or biotypes of *O. volvulus* are present in West Africa. The blinding or savanna strain is associated with the development of ocular disorders, whereas the non-blinding or forest strain is generally not associated with ocular disease.

PREVALENCE AND EPIDEMIOLOGIC FEATURES. Onchocerciasis is endemic in 34 countries, 27 in equatorial Africa in a broad belt extending from the Atlantic coast to the Red Sea, and more focally in 6 Latin American (Guatemala, Mexico, Venezuela, Brazil, Colombia, and Ecuador) countries, and in the Arabian peninsula (Yemen and Saudi Arabia). Current estimates are that approximately 18 million people are infected, 270,000 of whom are blind and another 500,000 of whom have severe visual disability. Over 99% of the cases occur in sub-Saharan Africa, almost half in Nigeria and Zaire. Because the black flies depend on well-oxygenated, fast flowing waterways for egg-laying and reproduction, both the vectors and the disease are concentrated around streams and rivers, often in the most fertile farming areas.

O. volvulus–induced blindness is associated with a life expectancy that is decreased by at least 10 years over that of non-blinded individuals in the same area. However, more than the blinding disease, which affects only a small proportion of those infected, the pervasiveness of the chronic skin lesions and intense pruritus caused by onchodermatitis make it a leading cause of morbidity in infected areas.

PATHOLOGIC CHARACTERISTICS AND PATHOGENESIS. Onchocerciasis predominantly affects the skin, the eyes, and the lymph nodes. The inflammatory reaction is elicited by the microfilariae and not the adult worms, whose encapsulation seems to protect them from the immune response. Tissue damage results primarily from the host response to the secretion of toxic products by granulocytes, particularly granular proteins from eosinophils that adhere to microfilariae. The pathogenesis of sclerosing keratitis, the major cause of blindness, is due to a parasite antigen–specific, lymphocytic inflammatory reaction to dying intraocular microfilariae that appears dependent on TH_2 cytokines. With time neovascularization and scarring of the cornea lead to loss of transparency and to blindness. Ongoing low-grade inflammation in the skin eventually leads to loss of elastic fibers and atrophy. Chronic inflammatory changes and fibrosis are seen in lymph nodes.

CLINICAL MANIFESTATIONS. DERMATITIS. The pruritus of onchocerciasis is often intractable and unresponsive to antipruritus medication. In heavily infected endemic individuals scratching and excoriation to the point of bleeding, and even suicide, occur. Episodes of localized rash, erythema, and angioedema may be superimposed on the ongoing dermatologic manifestations at essentially any stage of disease. The five categories used to classify onchodermatitis are not mutually exclusive in a given patient, and the clinical findings are not necessarily specific for onchodermatitis: (1) acute papular onchodermatitis—small pruritic papules that may be scattered on limbs, shoulders, and trunk, lesions may progress to become vesicular or pustular; (2) chronic papular onchodermatitis—papules, which are often flat-topped, that are larger but more variable in size and height than in the acute papular eruption, lesions are less pruritic than in the acute eruption; (3) lichenified dermatitis (also called Sowda)—an intensely pruritic eruption limited to one limb, usually the leg, consisting of hyperpigmented papules and plaques with accompanying edema of the entire limb; (4) atrophy—premature atrophy, which is due to degeneration of one or more of the structural elements of the skin, pruritus is uncommon and fine wrinkles will appear on skin after pushing along the surface with one finger, and loss of elasticity can be demonstrated by slow return to position of skin pinched between two fingers; (5) depigmentation—areas of complete depigmentation over the anterior shin with islands of normally pigmented skin, also called "leopard skin." In short-term residents of endemic areas an evanescent acute papular dermatitis is almost always the sole manifestation of infection.

EYE. Involvement of all tissues of the eye has been described. Inflammation due to microfilariae of *O. volvulus* as they migrate through the eye initially presents as a punctate keratitis or as snowflake corneal opacities. Free microfilariae may be visible by slit lamp examination in the anterior chamber or aqueous humor but are rarely found in infected short-term visitors, who are typically very lightly infected. Longstanding infection with savanna strain *O. volvulus* leads to sclerosing keratitis characterized by a fibrovascular pannus. Iridocyclitis with flare and cells in the anterior chamber leads to development of synechiae, raised intraocular pressure, and secondary glaucoma. Chorioretinitis and chorioretinal atrophy are the common manifestations of posterior ocular disease. Optic neuritis and optic atrophy occur in savannah regions. Infected short-term visitors do not have ocular involvement.

SUBCUTANEOUS NODULES. Asymptomatic 0.5- to 3.0-cm subcutaneous onchocercomata occurring most often over bony prominences are freely movable encapsulated nodules that contain coiled masses of adult worms. In Latin America, the nodules are often located on the head and upper body, whereas in Africa the nodules are most often over the hips and lower limbs. Over 80% of nodules are nonpalpable and in the lightly infected expatriates are rarely detectable.

LYMPHADENOPATHY. Lymphadenopathy is frequently found in inguinal and femoral areas. When it occurs in inguinofemoral nodes in a sling of stretched out atrophic abdominal skin, the so-called hanging groin results. Lymph nodes are non-tender and fibrotic.

DIAGNOSIS. Definitive diagnosis is dependent on the demonstration of motile microfilariae in superficial bloodless skin snips. This type of skin biopsy employs either a razor blade to slice a thin piece of skin that has been tented up with a needle or a corneoscleral biopsy instrument to obtain 1 to 2 mg of skin bloodlessly. Six snips, one from over each scapula, iliac crest, and lateral aspect of each calf, are incubated with saline solution in microplate wells and examined microscopically. Deep punch biopsy of the skin is not necessary and multiple skin snips will have a higher yield than one random traumatic deep biopsy. When available, polymerase chain reaction (PCR) amplification of parasite DNA directly from skin snips is far more sensitive than direct visualization. Blood contamination of a skin snip may cause one of the blood-borne microfilaria to escape into the specimen. If the patient has been in an area endemic for *Mansonella streptocerca* it is then necessary to fix the skin and to stain the microfilariae for identification. In well-equipped clinical settings, biopsy or ultrasound demonstration of adult parasites in any nodules that are present can be diagnostic. Elevated titers of antifilarial antibodies may support the diagnosis of onchocerciasis but should not be used alone. The total eosinophil count is unhelpful diagnostically as it is often but inconstantly elevated in onchocerciasis.

Scabies, insect bites, hypersensitivity reactions, miliaria rubra, and atopic or contact dermatitis enter the differential diagnosis of acute pruritic disease. In expatriates, Calabar swellings (see the discussion of loiasis), clinically similar episodes of localized rash and mild angioedema, can mimic onchodermatitis. Tuberculoid leprosy, streptocercosis, and excema should be considered if there are chronic skin changes. Dermatomycoses, previous trauma, and yaws can also cause hypopigmented skin lesions. The posterior eye lesions are not at all specific for onchocerciasis.

TREATMENT. No available non-toxic agent is able to kill the long-lived adult worms of *O. volvulus*. Repeated microfilaricidal therapy with ivermectin 150 μg/kg in a single dose every 6 to 12 months is effective in ameliorating symptoms. For unclear reasons, pruritus in lightly infected expatriates may be refractory to 6-monthly therapy and many clinicians find it necessary to treat more aggressively for the first 2 years or so. Appropriate duration of therapy in those without further exposure is not known but probably should be offered for at least 10 years. In *L. loa* co-infected individuals with high circulating microfilaremia, ivermectin therapy may precipitate a toxic encephalopathy. In areas endemic for loiasis, high microfilaremia should be ruled out prior to ivermectin administration for onchocerciasis. Because of frequent unacceptable reactions to dying microfilariae, ranging from urticaria and angioedema to hypotension and death, DEC should no longer ever be used for microfilaricidal treatment of onchocerciasis. Suramin (available from the CDC drug service) is adulticidal but because of toxicity and even potentially life-threatening effects should be used only in extreme situations. Surgical removal of palpable nodules in order to reduce the microfilarial load and the ensuing disorder has been successful in some areas. Nodulectomy is appropriate for cosmetic reasons but cannot be expected to cure infection because most nodules are impalpable.

PROGNOSIS. Ivermectin is effective in reversing existing early skin and ocular abnormalities but must be given repeatedly because adult parasites begin producing microfilariae again with time. The atrophic skin changes, sclerosing keratitis, and established lesions in the posterior segment of the eye are not helped by therapy.

PREVENTION. There are no effective vaccines or chemoprophylactic drugs. For expatriates or others with sufficient resources, personal mosquito protection using repellents is likely of benefit. The Onchocerciasis Control Program has been ongoing in West Africa since 1974 and involves vector control in 11 countries and 50,000 km of rivers. It is estimated that 30 million people have been protected from infection, 10 million children have been born into areas that are free of disease transmission, and blindness has in 125,000 to 200,000 others been prevented. Building a sustainable infrastructure for the mass community-based distribution of the microfilaricide ivermectin has now become the primary global control strategy. Annual mass treatment of an affected community with ivermectin, which is available free through a remarkable donation program of Merck & Co., Inc., should break the transmission cycle within 10–15 years by eliminating microfilariae available to vectors from the skin of infected individuals. There is no non-human reservoir of *O. volvulus*.

LOIASIS

CAUSE AND EPIDEMIOLOGIC CHARACTERISTICS. *Loa loa*, the African eye worm, is restricted to the rain forest area of Central and West Africa. Prevalence and endemicity are imprecisely defined, but loiasis appears to be most prevalent in Gabon, Cameroon, Congo, Nigeria, and the Central African Republic. Adult parasites (females, 50–70 mm long; males, 25–35 mm long) live a constantly migratory existence in subcutaneous tissues. Microfilariae are blood-borne with a diurnal periodicity peaking between noon and 4:00 P.M. Tabanid flies of *Chrysops* sp. are the vector. In temporary residents, a shorter period of exposure appears necessary in order to acquire infection when compared to that of other filarial parasites.

PATHOLOGIC FEATURES. The pathogenesis of the angioedematous reaction that occurs in response to the adult worm is poorly understood. The extremely elevated serum IgE level and eosinophilia seen in newly infected individuals prone to Calabar swellings indicate a hypersensitivity reaction to adult worms or worm products.

CLINICAL MANIFESTATIONS. More so than with the other filarial infections clinical manifestations are much exaggerated in short-term residents or visitors to endemic areas when compared to those of natives. Non-endemic persons, who are usually amicrofilaremic, have severe allergic symptoms with frequent and incapacitating Calabar swellings, pruritus, and urticaria. Calabar swellings are localized areas of evanescent erythema and angioedema (up to 5 to 10 cm in diameter) that occur primarily on the extremities and last 1 to 3 days. The subcutaneous adults, which are large enough to be visible, only rarely migrate across the conjunctiva. Among endemic individuals, infection is most often asymptomatic with microfilaremia and a much lower incidence of Calabar swellings and allergic manifestations. Eye worm occurs in up to 50% of these individuals. In chronically infected individuals nephropathy and cardiomyopathy occur very rarely.

DIAGNOSIS. Definitive diagnosis is dependent on the demonstration of characteristic sheated microfilariae on afternoon blood film. Non-endemic individuals are usually amicrofilaremic so that diagnosis often cannot be made parasitologically and must be based on the characteristic history, clinical presentation, blood eosinophilia, and elevated antifilarial antibody titers. *O. volvulus, M. perstans, M. ozzardi,* and *M. streptocerca* all cause overlapping syndromes and must, if epidemiologically possible, be ruled out by a complete search for microfilariae in blood and skin. Occasionally an adult *L. loa* is excised while crawling across the conjunctiva or under the skin. Definitive diagnosis sometimes occurs after initiation of DEC therapy and subcutaneous biopsy of a swelling developing at the site of a dying adult worm.

TREATMENT AND PROGNOSIS. DEC (6–10 mg/kg/day for 21 days) has both microfilaricidal and adulticidal effect. Decisions about retreatment should be based on clinical resolution, and multiple courses of DEC may be required before signs and symptoms completely resolve. One course of therapy will cure about half those infected, and a second course will cure half of the remaining infected individuals. Eosinophilia and antifilarial titers resolve slowly even with effective therapy so should not be closely followed as a test of cure. However, an antifilarial titer or an eosinophilia that is increasing or unchanged after 6 months should prompt suspicion of failure of treatment given up until that time.

In patients with any microfilaremia, DEC therapy should be initiated with low doses of drug (50 mg/day) on the first few days and pre-treatment with corticosteroids should be considered. With microfilaremia greater than a few hundred microfilariae per milliliter of blood DEC-induced inflammatory reactions to dying microfilariae may progress to encephalopathy and death. If available, apheresis to remove circulating microfilariae can be performed prior to initiating DEC therapy in these individuals. If this latter option is not available for highly microfilaremic individuals, limited data support the use of albendazole (200 mg twice a day for 21 days) as it appears to be moderately adulticidal without effect on the microfilariae. Ivermectin is microfilaricidal but has no adulticidal effect and may cause toxic encephalopathy in highly microfilaremic individuals. If epidemiologically appropriate, onchocerciasis must be carefully ruled out before the initiation of DEC therapy for loiasis in order to prevent toxicity due to dying *O. volvulus* microfilariae.

PREVENTION. DEC is effective in preventing loiasis when taken in prophylactic doses of 300 mg/week.

DRACUNCULIASIS

Dracunculiasis, or guinea worm disease, caused by the helminth *Dracunculus medinensis,* is close to eradication. A global effort reduced incidence from 3.2 million cases in 1986 to 152,000 cases in 1996, of which 78% were in Sudan. The infection has essentially been eradicated from the Indian subcontinent and remains in only 16 countries of sub-Saharan Africa.

Transmission to humans is through drinking water contaminated with tiny crustaceans called *copepods* that carry larval forms of the parasite. A year or so later adult female worms up to 1 m long emerge through the skin, usually of the lower leg or foot. Transmission is perpetuated when the female releases thousands of larvae into the water if the human host immerses that part of the body in a source of drinking water. Emergence of the worm is accompanied by a painful blister that ruptures and ulcerates. Fever and allergic symptoms including wheezing and urticaria often precede rupture of the blister. Affected persons may be incapacitated for weeks or months often coinciding with major planting or harvesting seasons. Secondary bacterial infection of the ulcer with abscess formation is common.

Emerging worms can be extracted by winding of a few more centimeters on a stick each day. Chemotherapy is ineffective. Worms may be removed surgically. Prevention is achieved through the provision of safe drinking water.

OTHER FILARIASES

PERSTANS FILARIASIS. *Mansonella perstans* infection occurs commonly throughout Central Africa and in northeast South America but exact numbers are unknown. The blood-borne microfilariae circulate without periodicity and adults reside in serous body cavities (pleural, peritoneal, and pericardial) and in the mesenteric, perirenal, and retroperitoneal tissues. Most individuals are asymptomatic or at most mildly symptomatic, but a distribution that overlaps with several other human filarids has hampered definition of distinct clinical features. Reported manifestations include transient angioedematous swellings, pruritus, fever, headache, arthralgias, abdominal pain, and neurologic syndromes. Pericarditis and hepatitis have been reported. Eosinophilia and elevated antifilarial antibody titers are often present. No reliable therapy exists. DEC and ivermectin are clearly ineffective. Some success with albendazole (two 400-mg/day doses) or mebendazole (two 100-mg/day doses) for at least 1 month has been reported.

STREPTOCERCIASIS. *Mansonella streptocerca,* transmitted by midges, has been thought to be restricted to the tropical forest zone of Africa from Ghana to Zaire but has recently been described as far east as Uganda. The adult worms are subcutaneous, and the microfilariae, which have characteristic hooked tails, are found in the skin, most often on the upper body. Ocular involvement does not occur. Infection is usually asymptomatic, but pruritus and acute or chronic papular dermatitis similar to that of onchodermatitis can be found on the trunk and upper extremities of up to 24% of those infected. Inguinal adenopathy is common. In areas of epidemiologic overlap skin snips must be stained to differentiate *M. streptocerca* from *O. volvulus*. Both adult worms and microfilariae are killed by DEC 6 mg/kg/day for 2 weeks. Ivermectin 150 μg/kg in a single dose is microfilaricidal.

***Mansonella Ozzardi* INFECTION.** *M. ozzardi* is found only in Central and South America and certain islands of the Caribbean. The blood-borne microfilariae circulate without periodicity and the location of adults is unclear. Adult worms have been recovered only twice, both times from the peritoneal cavity. Although it is generally considered non-pathogenic, articular pain, headache, fever, pulmonary symptoms, adenopathy, hepatomegaly, and pruritic skin eruptions are reported. Ivermectin 150 μg/kg in a single dose appears to suppress microfilaremia reliably for at least several months but is not likely adulticidal. DEC is ineffective.

ZOONOTIC FILARIAL INFECTIONS. Uncommonly, several animal filariae, including *Dirofilaria immitis* and *D. repens* in dogs, as well as *D. tenuis* in raccoons, can infect humans. Distribution is worldwide and found in non-tropical as well as tropical climates. The parasites die in the larval stages before reaching maturity and cause few symptoms. Localization is to the lungs in *D. immitis* infection (appearing as coin lesions) or to the subcutaneous tissues and lymph nodes in the other *Dirofilaria* species. Subcutaneous lesions may be migratory. Zoonotic *Brugia* sp. infection localizes to lymph nodes. Eosinophilia and positive antifilarial antibody titers are unusual. Surgical removal of lesions is diagnostic and curative. Chemotherapy is uniformly ineffective.

Boussinesq M, Gardon J: Prevalences *of Loa loa* microfilaremia throughout the area endemic for the infection. Ann Trop Med Parasitol 91:573, 1997. *Extensive graphical material on infection prevalence down to the village level.*

Burnham G: Onchocerciasis. Lancet 351:1341, 1998. *Concise review of clinical, parasitologic, and epidemiologic aspects of onchocerciasis with very up-to-date references.*

Fischer P, Bamuhiiga J, Buttner DW: Occurrence and diagnosis of *Mansonella streptocerca* in Uganda. Acta Tropica 63:43, 1997. *First large clinical study of an underinvestigated infection in over 25 years.*

Michael E, Bundy DAP, Grenfell BT: Re-assessing the global prevalence and distribution of lymphatic filariasis. Parasitology 112:409, 1996. *Most comprehensive review of infection prevalence ever done, extensively referenced.*

435 ARTHROPODS AND LEECHES

David Schlossberg

Arthropods are bilaterally symmetrical invertebrates with an exoskeleton, segmented bodies, and jointed appendages. In the phylum Arthropoda, six classes are important sources of disease in humans: Arachnida, Pentastomida, Chilopoda, Diplopoda, Crustacea, and Insecta. Table 435–1 lists these classes and their members are discussed in this chapter.

Arthropods cause disease in humans directly and indirectly. They bite, sting, envenomate, and evoke hypersensitivity reactions; they also serve as vectors for infectious pathogens. Arthropods are thus the link between humans and age-old scourges like plague, typhus, and malaria.

Infections spread by arthropod vectors are listed in Table 435–2. They are each described in greater detail elsewhere in this text and will not be reviewed further here.

SCABIES

Mites are small arachnids, about the size of a grain of sand. They have a single apparent body region, with a fused cephalothorax and abdomen. The best-known mite, *Sarcoptes scabei,* is the cause of scabies. It has a worldwide distribution and is associated with war, poverty, malnutrition, and sexual promiscuity. Although it causes dramatic skin manifestations, the scabies mite is not a vector for other infectious diseases.

Scabies is spread by skin to skin contact, for example, shaking hands, sharing a bed, and having sexual relations. It is also spread by fomites, since the mite is able to survive for 2 to 3 days away from human skin and may infect clothing, towels, and bed linen. Activated by warmth, the mite burrows under the skin to the bottom of the stratum corneum in 2.5 minutes. The female moves at a rate of 2 to 3 mm/day and lays eggs as she tunnels. The male (seldom seen, because it is smaller than the female and dies a day or two after copulation) makes side chambers or branches in the

Table 435–1 ■ MEDICALLY IMPORTANT ARTHROPODS

1. Arachnida (four pairs of legs)
   A. Acari—mites, ticks
   B. Araneida—spiders
   C. Scorpionida
2. Pentostomida—tongue worms
3. Chilopoda—centipedes
4. Diplopoda—millipedes
5. Crustacea
   A. Copepoda—cyclops, diptomus
   B. Decapoda—shrimp, lobster, crayfish, crab
6. Insecta (three pairs of legs)
   A. Anoplura—lice
   B. Coleoptera—beetles
   C. Diptera—flies (mosquitoes, black flies, midges, horse flies, deer flies, greenheads, tsetse flies, stable flies, sand flies, houseflies, bluebottle flies, cockroaches; myiasis)
   D. Hemiptera—bed bugs, cone-nose bugs
   E. Hymenoptera—ants, bees, wasps
   F. Lepidoptera—moths, caterpillars
   G. Siphonoptera—fleas

Table 435–2 ■ ARTHROPOD VECTORS OF INFECTION

Mites	Western equine encephalitis,* St. Louis encephalitis,* murine typhus,* rickettsialpox*
Ticks	Colorado tick fever,* Powasson encephalitis,* Crimean-Congo hemorrhagic fever, Central European encephalitides, Rocky Mountain spotted fever,* Q fever,* fièvre boutonneuse, Asian tick typhus, Queensland tick typhus, ehrlichiosis,* relapsing fever,* Lyme disease,* babesiosis,* tularemia*
Crustaceans	Dracunculosis, nematode and cestode infestation, paragonimiasis
Lice	Typhus,* trench fever, relapsing fever*
Mosquitoes	Malaria, filariasis, viral encephalitis,* dengue,* yellow fever
Deer flies	Loiasis, tularemia*
Black flies	Onchocerciasis
Tsetse flies	Trypanosomiasis
Sand flies	Leishmaniasis, bartonellosis, sand fly fever
Cone-nose bugs	Chagas' disease
Fleas	Plague,* murine typhus,* ?*Bartonella henselae,* Rickettsia felis,* Dypilidium caninum,* Hymenolepis diminuta*

*Can be acquired in the United States.

female's burrows. Thus, burrows contain mites, fecal pellets, and eggs. In 2 to 3 days a larva is born; eventually it molts through nymphal stages to an adult. This cycles takes 10 to 17 days. During the female's lifespan of 4 to 5 weeks, she will lay a total of 40 to 50 eggs.

Typical lesions are small papules over the female mite with wavy or linear burrows indicating her path. Typical locations of lesions are the interdigital webs, wrist folds, elbows, axillae, feet, thigh, nipples in women, genitalia, buttocks, and beltline. Crusted, excoriated, pruritic papules on the penis or buttock are almost pathognomonic for scabies. Infants may have involvement of head, neck, palms, and soles, areas typically spared in the adult, although geriatric and immunosuppressed adults (for example, acquired immunodeficiency syndrome [AIDS] patients) may also have head and neck involvement.

These lesions cause severe itching, especially at night. A generalized rash may occur separate from the burrows. Other secondary local phenomena include urticaria, eczematous plaques, excoriation, and impetigo. Superimposed streptococcal infection occasionally results in post-streptococcal glomerulonephritis.

Many of the clinical phenomena result from sensitization. Thus, the incubation period for the initial infection is from 2 weeks to 2 months, since time is required for this sensitization. With subsequent infection, however, itching may begin in 1 to 4 days. During the prolonged incubation period patients may be entirely asymptomatic even though they can transmit the disease. A clue to the presence of scabies is the appearance of typical lesions in multiple family members.

In elderly and immunosuppressed patients the skin reaction may be muted, with pruritus but minimal inflammation. Thus, outbreaks in nursing homes and early disease in AIDS patients may go undetected. Scabies may also be asymptomatic (*scabies incognito*) in patients receiving topical or systemic corticosteroids. Diagnosis is made by applying washable ink or tetracycline (which fluoresces under a Wood's light) to an area of suspected involvement. When the area is washed off, remaining ink or tetracycline may indicate the presence of burrows. For microscopic diagnosis, mineral oil may be applied to a scalpel blade and allowed to flow onto a burrow or papule, which is then scraped gently (until pinpoint bleeding occurs). Then the oil and tissue mixture may be microscopically examined for mites, eggs, or fecal pellets.

Scabies may take other forms. Nodular scabies forms red brown papules and nodules in the groin, axillae, and genitalia. Histopathologically, these lesions may mimic Hodgkin's disease because of multinucleated cells that resemble Reed-Sternberg cells. Bullous scabies is seen in infants and children and mimics bullous impetigo and pemphigus. In the adult, vesicular scabetic lesions mimic dermatitis herpetiformis, especially when in a sacral and gluteal location. The mites that cause scabies in animals (mange) are transmissible to humans after direct contact with horses, dogs, and other infested species. These mites are unable to propagate in humans, although they may cause papules or vesicles. *Norwegian* or crusted scabies is seen in patients with altered cell-mediated immunity or in the elderly. It occurs as local or generalized dermatitis with scaling and crusting. When the extremities are involved there may be heavy involvement of the nails. Itching is often minimal. In this disease, thousands of mites are present, as opposed to 3 to 50 in normal scabies. Thus, it is extremely contagious. Diagnosis is relatively easy since there are so many mites, and scrapings should demonstrate their presence. This form of scabies may be complicated by bacteremia.

The treatment of choice is permethrin (Elimite). This cream is applied from the neck to the feet and washed off 8 to 14 hours later. One application is usually adequate. In infants, scalp, temple, and forehead are included. Crotamiton or Eurax is also effective. It is applied from the neck down and repeated in 24 hours. Then the patient bathes and washes off the crotamiton 48 hours later. Again, in infants it is applied to the entire body. Lindane had been the mainstay of treatment for years, but it is limited in application as a result of toxicity; excessive absorption of lindane may result in central nervous system (CNS) toxicity. Thus, it should not be used in individuals who have Norwegian scabies, premature infants, young children, pregnant or nursing mothers, or patients with a history of seizure disorder. In treating Norwegian scabies the patient should take a bath first and apply lotion and repeat after 12 hours. It should again be repeated in a week, and an additional scraping should be done afterward in case additional therapy is necessary. Recently, ivermectin has been given orally in the treatment of scabies. It is especially helpful in Norwegian scabies since it is difficult to penetrate the crust of Norwegian scabies with topical agents. Although, ivermectin is not approved for treatment of scabies in the United States, it has been found effective in a single oral dose of 200 μg/kg. Nodular scabies may be treated by intralesional steroids. Antiscabetic medication is not effective in nodular scabies since there are no mites at this stage of the disease. Fortunately, its natural history is resolution with time. In all of the therapies discussed it is important to follow the manufacturer's instructions. Also, patients should trim their nails and scrub under their nails with a toothbrush that is then discarded. Close contacts and family members who have had skin-to-skin contact should also be treated without waiting for lesions to appear. It is not necessary to clean furniture or carpets, but bed covers, pillow cases, sheets, outer clothes, and underwear if used in the previous 48 hours should be put in a hot water cycle or dry cleaned.

After one course of treatment scabies is no longer contagious. In the hospital, patients should have contact isolation for 24 hours after the start of therapy. Clothes and linens should be placed in plastic laundry bags and handled only by personnel wearing gloves. Particular care should be taken for patients with Norwegian scabies since it is highly contagious, and these patients should be isolated.

After therapy for scabies pruritus may persist for 1 to 2 weeks. Most of the time this does not indicate treatment failure. Symptomatic therapy with antipruritics is indicated.

OTHER MITES

Mites other than scabies generally do not cause permanent infestation. Most of them can bite and produce pruritic or allergic reactions. However, since their involvement with humans is transitory, treatment is symptomatic and involves elimination of the mite from a pet or the local environment. Topical therapy with corticosteroids and oral antihistamines is useful.

The follicle mite (*Demodex*) is an elongated worm-like mite that occurs on the face, living in hair follicles or sebaceous glands. It rarely causes discomfort or needs therapy. Dust mites do not bite, but exposure to them may result in rhinitis, asthma, and childhood eczema. Infestation with these organisms requires treating the house by cleaning carpets, mattresses, and blankets and by minimizing household humidity. Fowl mites infest humans in association with birds such as pigeons, and they are capable of biting and may cause a local dermatitis. Some of them are occasionally important vectors. For example, the fowl mite *Ornithonyssus sylviarum* can

transmit the western equine encephalitis virus, and the viruses of St. Louis encephalitis and western equine encephalitis have been isolated from the chicken mite *Dermanyssus gallinae.*

A variety of food mites, e.g., *Pyemotes ventricosus,* are associated with cheeses, cereals, sugar, flour, grain, dried vegetable products, eggs, and other foodstuffs. These mites penetrate the superficial epithelium and cause a papulovesicular or urticarial eruption. Occasionally exposure to them results in fever, diarrhea, and anorexia. More commonly, it causes a chronic dermatitis; it has been held responsible for "grocer's itch," "copra itch," "dried fruit dermatitis," and "vanillism" (in those who work with vanilla pods). When inhaled, some of the food mites cause pulmonary infiltrates and peripheral eosinophilia, called *acariasis.*

The best known of the non-scabies mites is the harvest mite, chigger, or "red bug." These are *Trombicula* species and are the bane of picnickers and campers. They are bright orange to red and attach where clothing fits snugly, especially at the ankles, groin, and waist. They do not burrow but feed at a sweat pore or the base of a hair follicle for several days. It is the larva stage, not the adult, that attacks humans. Chigger larvae are tiny, about 0.2 mm long, in contrast to the 1-mm adults. The initial reaction to their bite is itching within 3 to 6 hours. Some patients experience a papular, urticarial, or vesicular rash, occasionally with fever and adenopathy. Treatment is a warm soapy bath or shower plus antipruritic lotions; topical corticosteroids or anesthetic ointments are also used. These mites are the vector for *Rickettsia tsutsugamushi* (scrub typhus) in Central and Eastern Asia.

An important mite associated with rats is *Ornithonyssus bacoti,* a vector of murine or endemic typhus (*Rickettsia typhi*). Another medically important vector is *Liponyssoides sanguineus,* the mouse mite, which transmits rickettsialpox (*Rickettsia akari*) to humans. This mite is capable of biting and is seen on rats and other rodents as well as mice. Cheyletiellid mites are parasites of dogs, cats, rabbits, and other small mammals and are the cause of "walking dandruff" in these animals. They do not burrow, but live on the keratin layer of the epidermis, producing a mange-like dermatitis in the animal. Humans, often pet owners, experience transient pruritus and a rash, typically papulovesicles on the flexor side of the arms, breasts, or abdomen. Cure in humans follows treatment of the pet.

The straw itch mite is also capable of biting; it is acquired by handling grain or sleeping on straw mattresses. The clover mite, associated with ivy, grass, clover, and fruit trees, may infest humans but does not bite.

TICKS

Like mites, ticks have a single disk-shaped body region with a fused cephalothorax and abdomen. They are larger than mites, about the size of a pea. However, after feeding, engorged ticks may appear much larger. Conversely, the larvae of some species may be extremely small, resembling a sesame seed. Ticks are divided into soft and hard varieties based on a dorsal plate, or scutum. Most infections transmitted to humans are from hard ticks.

Ticks cause disease in a variety of ways: They transmit microorganisms that cause infection; they cause toxic and hypersensitivity reactions to their salivary secretions; and they directly inject toxin into a human host.

Most tick bites occur in the spring and summer. The bites are usually not painful or even symptomatic. Local swelling and erythema may result, and occasionally blistering or ecchymosis follows, sometimes followed by necrosis and ulceration. In some cases a chronic granulomatous reaction may develop and persist for years.

Ticks do not fly, jump, or swim. They "quest" for host animals by waiting on low-lying vegetation and waving their legs or moving around on the plant, responding to nearby vibrations or carbon dioxide. Once they contact their host they move around to find a suitable location, often for 1 to 2 hours, before actually attaching to feed.

Ticks need time to transmit disease. For example, to transmit Rocky Mountain spotted fever, the tick has to feed for at least 8 to 14 hours before rickettsiae are released from salivary glands. For Lyme disease, the tick needs at least 24 hours of feeding and possibly 72 hours to transmit disease efficiently. Thus, a tick removed while it is still wandering in search of a location for feeding or before it has had an adequate chance to feed is not likely to have spread disease to its human host.

Tick paralysis is not an infection but an intoxication. Worldwide, 50 species of ticks cause paralysis in humans or animals. In North America there are six species that have been identified, including the species that also cause Lyme disease, tularemia, Rocky Mountain spotted fever, ehrlichiosis, Colorado tick fever, and babesiosis. Thus, it is possible to acquire both infection and tick paralysis simultaneously. The paralysis begins 5 to 7 days after attachment of the tick. It occurs most frequently in small girls. The child becomes irritable and lethargic and leg weakness, which may progress to complete paralysis, develops. The weakness can ascend and cause bulbar paralysis. Cranial nerve involvement includes the face and extraocular muscles. Eventually, respiratory paralysis supervenes and death may occur. The patient remains afebrile. Characteristic features of this disease are its symmetry, the flaccid nature of the paralysis, normal pupils, intact sensory examination findings, clear sensorium, preservation of sphincter tone, lack of fever, and normal cerebrospinal fluid. Unusual presentations can be extremely misleading and have included unilateral Bell's palsy, ataxia, chorea, and localized weakness of one arm or leg. These unilateral localized presentations are attributed to the nearby location of the tick. Thus, facial weakness has resulted from a paralytic tick in the ipsilateral ear. The differential diagnosis for tick paralysis is extensive, and tick paralysis has been misdiagnosed as Guillain-Barré syndrome, botulism, poliomyelitis, spinal cord compression, myasthenia gravis, and transverse myelitis. It is important to consider tick paralysis in a susceptible host; without removal the process may be fatal, but after the tick is removed most patients improve within a few hours.

Tick removal has acquired an elaborate folklore. The safest and most efficient method is to grab the tick at the skin surface with tweezers or blunt forceps. The tick is then pulled steadily and gently out of the skin. None of the mouthparts should be left in the skin. The tick itself should be incinerated and the site disinfected. The best ways to prevent tick attachment are to keep pant legs tucked in boots or socks and to use an effective repellent.

SPIDERS

Spider bites cause secondary infection, allergic reactions, and envenomation. Approximately 50 species bite humans but only 4 cause severe disease in the United States: the widow (*Latrodectus*), the brown recluse (*Loxosceles*), the hobo spider or aggressive house spider (*Tegenaria*), and the yellow sac spider (*Cheiracanthium*), a greenish-gray garden dweller that is the most common domestic spider in many areas of the United States. Bites from other spiders may be painful but are not dangerous. Therefore, it is important for a bite victim to take the spider for identification.

Local treatment requires washing the area, applying cold compresses, and administering tetanus prophylaxis. The brown recluse, or *Loxosceles*, is the best known cause of necrotic arachnidism in the United States. Those spiders have a 2- to 4-cm leg span. There is a violin-shaped marking from the eyes to the abdomen, with the base pointing forward. The brown recluse is not aggressive but hides in clothing and in the bathroom, attic, and closets. It bites only when threatened. Bites are painless until 3 to 8 hours afterward; then the lesion ranges from a local urticarial reaction to full-thickness skin necrosis. Redness, swelling, and tenderness develop; slough, ulceration, and scabbing may follow. Some lesions show central blistering with ecchymosis surrounded by blanched skin, which in turn is surrounded by erythema. This is called the "red, white, and blue sign." The lesion tends to extend downward gravitationally, "to flow downhill." Systemic reactions include fever, arthralgias, maculopapular rash, nausea, and vomiting. Treatment includes antibiotics, which help prevent abscess formation and secondary infection; elevation; and ice packs. Some advocate use of dapsone for its leukocyte-inhibiting qualities. The use of antivenin is controversial. Surgical excision is avoided early in the course; if used at all, excision should be postponed until later in the course, when the venom is less likely to impair wound healing. Some advocate corticosteroid administration for systemic symptoms. Eventually, many patients require extensive plastic surgical repair.

The hobo spider and yellow sac spider cause necrotic arachnidism similar to the envenomation seen after brown recluse bites. Hobo spider bites may be complicated by severe headaches and aplastic anemia.

The widow spider, also known as the hourglass, shoe-button, or po-ko-moo spider, injects a neurotoxin (α-latrotoxin) into its victims. This toxin results in acetylcholine depletion at neuromuscular junctions. The bite causes pain at the bite site, which then spreads to local and regional muscle groups as a dull aching and sometimes numbness. This is followed by sweating, nausea, tremor, myalgias, muscle spasm, board-like abdomen, chest pain, paralysis, bradycardia, seizures, and rarely death. Fortunately, fewer than 1% of bites are fatal.

The female spider (males do not bite humans) has a leg span of 3 to 4 cm. There is a red-orange hourglass on the ventral side of the abdomen; however, some species have red markings on the dorsal side, and in some the hourglass is incomplete, appearing more like hatch marks. The wound should be cleaned and ice packs applied. Systemic therapy is undertaken with intravenous calcium gluconate, muscle relaxants, and tetanus toxoid. Antivenin is given if the the envenomation is severe.

SCORPIONS

In the United States the only dangerous species of scorpions is *Centruroides exilicauda,* found in Arizona and New Mexico. Otherwise, scorpion bites in the United States are not serious unless patients have a severe allergic reaction to them.

Scorpions inject a neurotoxic venom when they sting. The sting produces local swelling, pain, and numbness. Systemic signs may be neurologic (coma, tremor, paralysis of respiratory muscles, seizures), cardiac (hypertension, arrhythmias, pulmonary edema), and pancreatic (scorpion bite is a common cause of pancreatitis in Brazil). Death may ensue within hours.

Therapy of bites includes ice packs and antihistamines. Some advocate applying a tourniquet and removing the venom from the wound by suction. Antivenin use is controversial. It has been suggested that patients receive non-opiate analgesics, since opiates may have a synergistic effect with the venom of some scorpions.

TONGUE WORM (PENTASTOMIASIS)

Pentastomiasis is human infection by two genera of Pentastomids, *Armillifer* and *Linguatula.* These worm-like arthropods are found principally in Asia and Africa and reside in the respiratory tract of birds, reptiles, dogs, and other mammals. Animals such as sheep or goats may also serve as intermediate hosts to the parasite, and when humans eat uncooked viscera or lymph nodes of these animals, gastric juices liberate the nymphs, which are encapsulated in the viscera, and they ascend the esophagus and anchor themselves in the upper respiratory tract. This produces severe inflammation with violent coughing and occasionally asphyxiation. This syndrome is known as "halzoun" or "marrara" syndrome, referring to suffocation. Other symptoms include hemoptysis, sneezing, lacrimation, aural pruritus, coryza, facial edema, and vomiting.

Visceral infection is acquired by ingesting eggs in water contaminated with the sputum of animals harboring the pentastome in their upper respiratory tract. These eggs then hatch and develop into larvae that spread hematogenously through the body. This infection is usually asymptomatic and is discovered incidentally by the pathologist or radiologist as comma-shaped pleural or peritoneal calcifications. However, fatal infections do occur rarely.

CENTIPEDES AND MILLIPEDES

Chilopods (centipedes) and diplopods (millipedes) are elongated multisegmented arthropods. The centipede or "hundred legger" has one pair of legs per segment and is a carnivore. Its bite produces a painful wound, and the larger species seen in the tropics and subtropics are also capable of secreting a venom through their claws while holding their victim. The site of this envenomation may become ulcerated and necrotic, and patients may experience nausea, vomiting, and headache. Secondary infection is not uncommon. The wounds should be washed and cool compresses applied; antibiotics should be given for secondary infection, and some patients have required administration of corticosteroids and local injection of anesthetic for the extreme pain.

The millipede or "thousand legger" has two pairs of legs per body segment. This arthropod is a vegetarian and does not bite or sting. However, some tropical species emit a toxic fluid from glands on each segment when they are threatened. This fluid may cause local skin discoloration and burning, with the formation of blisters. If the eyes are contaminated a conjunctivitis or keratitis results, rarely causing blindness. Some species are able to squirt these secretions as far as 80 cm. Treatment includes washing the involved area of skin, and some advocate the application of solvents such as ether or alcohol to help remove the toxic fluid. If the eyes are involved, they should be irrigated copiously with water.

CRUSTACEANS

The crustaceans may function as intermediate hosts of parasites that infect humans. Copepods are tiny aquatic arthropods that may be intermediate hosts of the guinea worm *Dracunculus medinensis,* the nematode *Gnathostoma spinigerum,* and the cestodes *Spirometra mansonoides* and *Diphyllobothrium latum.* The decapods include shrimp, lobster, crab, prawn, and crayfish. Land crabs and freshwater prawns may be host to the rat lungworm *Angiostrongylus* sp.; the lung fluke *Paragonimus westermani* is an occasional parasite of freshwater crabs and crayfish.

LICE

Lice are small (2–4 mm) dorsoventrally flattened wingless insects that have mouthparts modified for piercing and sucking blood. They are parasites exclusively of humans and are seen in three varieties: (1) *Pediculus humanus* var *capitis* (head louse), (2) *Pediculus humanus* var *humanus* (body louse), and (3) *Phthirus pubis* (crab louse).

The head louse ("motorized dandruff") is transmitted by direct contact or by fomites such as combs, hats, and bedding. It is seen under circumstances of crowding and poor hygiene and is particularly common among schoolchildren, the elderly, and the senile. The organisms live for approximately 1 month on the scalp but are able to live only a few days (as long as a week) if removed from the warmth and blood meals available on the scalp.

Infestation of scalp hairs produces severe itching and occasionally secondary pyogenic infection and cervical lymphadenopathy. The head lice favor hair in the back of the head. Lice may be visible crawling on hair shafts and they may move quite rapidly, approximately 23 cm/minute. However, they are few in number, i.e., less than 10, and it is much easier to identify the nits, the gray-white glistening oval eggs, 0.6 to 0.8 mm, that the lice attach to the base of scalp hairs. These nits are cemented securely to the hair shafts and are difficult to remove. They fluoresce under ultraviolet light (for example, Wood's light), facilitating diagnosis, especially when large numbers of patients are screened.

Patients should be treated with 1% permethrin (Nix), which is also ovicidal. It is available over the counter. The patient should shampoo, rinse, and dry the hair; then apply it to the hair and scalp. After 10 minutes it is rinsed off. Repetition in 1 week is necessary only if lice are again seen. As a result of growing resistance, there may be treatment failure with 1% permethrin, in which case 5% permethrin (Elimite) or a single oral dose of ivermectin (200 µg/kg) can be tried. When the patient is treated, all infested family members should be treated simultaneously. Combing the nits reduces the number of viable ova and decreases the chance of relapse and treatment failure. Clothing that had contact with the patient's head should be washed and dried in a dryer or dry cleaned.

Body lice ("cooties") look like head lice but are slightly larger. However, they have different clinical behavior. Body lice are seen in cold climates (because of heavy clothing) and under conditions of crowding and poor sanitation. They are most common in jails and crowded tenements and among military personnel. Unlike head lice, body lice are infrequent among affluent members of our society.

Lice and eggs are found in the seams of clothing, and very few lice are seen on the body of patients. The lice favor clothing fibers, especially wool, and live in the clothing, visiting the body only to feed. Clinically, the major manifestation is itching. Small red spots are produced, especially on the back and under the arm. Ultimately, excoriations, urticaria, pigmentary changes, and secondary infection may occur. "Vagabonds' disease" refers to the hyperpigmentation and thickening of the skin seen in chronic untreated infestation. Body lice are also a vector for serious diseases of humanity, including typhus (*Rickettsia prowazekii*), trench fever (*Bartonella quintana*), and relapsing fever (*Borrelia recurrentis*).

Treatment of body lice requires only improved hygiene and cleaned clothing in mild cases. Heat kills both ova and lice in clothing. In severe cases and in epidemics, topical pediculocidal agents may be used.

Crab lice are transmitted predominantly by sexual contact, clothes, or infected hairs. During coitus both adult lice and nits are transmitted on broken hairs. Less frequently they are transmitted by toilet seats or bedding. Although typically found on pubic hair, crab lice occasionally infect other short hairs of the body, including eyebrows, eyelashes, the edge of the scalp, moustache, and axilla.

Symptoms may not begin for 30 days after infection. On close inspection, nits are visible, and the louse may be seen clinging to one or two hairs. Also evident in these infestations are dried serous fluid, blood, and louse feces. The combination of louse saliva and blood produces a blue-gray macule known as *macula caerulea.* The crab louse dies after 24 to 48 hours off the host.

Treatment is similar to that for pediculosis capitis. It is also important to clean bedding and clothing, which should be washed in hot water. Treatment failure often results from not treating other involved areas of the body. Infestation of the eyelid can be treated with petrolatum occlusions, yellow oxide of mercury ointment, or mechanical removal of nits. Sexual partners and intimate contacts should be treated when they have evidence of lice. One third of patients with pubic lice have other sexually transmitted diseases, including human immunodeficiency virus (HIV) infection, and should be screened for them. Children with pubic lice infestation in facial hair or eyes should be evaluated for the possibility of sexual abuse.

Symptomatic treatment of pruritus in all types of lice infestation consists of antihistamines, and, in some cases, topical corticosteroids may be applied to affected areas for additional symptomatic relief.

BEETLES

Of the 250,000 species of beetles, some are injurious to humans. The most common beetle injury is not from a bite or sting but from the formation of blisters. The best known blister beetle is *Lypta vesicatoria,* the Spanish fly. This beetle fills its breathing tube with air and closes its breathing pores to elevate body pressure. This forces the toxin cantharidin out through its leg joints. On human skin, cantharidin forms blisters within hours. Some of the blistering may evolve to ulceration and secondary infection. Clues to this cause of blisters are the presence of multiple blisters in the same stage of development and the lack of an accompanying rash. Sometimes the blisters form a line, reflecting the path of the beetle as it crossed the skin. When ingested, cantharidin causes nausea and abdominal pain. Cantharidin has been prepared commercially and used as a diuretic, aphrodisiac, and rubefacient. Other beetles, for example, the carpet beetle, cause a papulovesicular dermatitis. Treatment of these beetle-related skin injuries is soap and water and wet compresses. Occasionally, topical or systemic corticosteroids are used.

FLIES

The order Diptera contains the true flies, which transmit more disease than any other arthropod order. Prominent among the flies is the mosquito, a slender delicate insect that is a vector for disease throughout the world. *Anopheles* sp. mosquitoes transmit malaria and filariasis; *Aedes* sp. mosquitoes transmit viral encephalitis, dengue, yellow fever, and filariasis; and the *Culex* sp. mosquitoes transmit encephalitis and filariasis. In addition to functioning as vectors, mosquito bites per se are irritating. The female mosquito lacerates human skin with her jaws and inserts a blood tube. Her salivary secretions contain an anticoagulant and cause local inflammation, pruritus, and urticaria. Mosquitoes prefer blacks to whites, young to old, warmth, strong scents, bright colors, and carbon dioxide, which is an effective attractant when humans and animals are grouped. Mosquito bites may be prevented by netting, protective clothing, and repellents.

Black flies (buffalo gnats) are bloodsucking flies that are small (2 to 3 mm) and humpbacked. This fly injects an anesthetic compound into the wound so that the initial bite is not painful. However, subsequently the bitten area becomes pruritic, red, and swollen. Black flies transmit onchocerciasis in the tropics. Biting midges (punkies, gnats, no seeums, flying teeth) are tiny (1 to 1.5 mm). They cause immediate pain and erythema and eventually papulovesicles, with a nodular reaction that may last for months. These flies are small enough to pass through screens. Tabanid flies are large and colorful and include the horse flies, deer flies, and greenheads. They cause painful bites that often bleed because of the relatively large size of the fly and its blade-like mouthparts. Only the Chrysops (deer fly) is a vector of human disease in this group; it transmits loiasis in Africa and tularemia in the United States.

The Muscidae include *Glossina* sp. (tsetse flies), the vector of trypanosomiasis, and *stomoxys* sp. (stable flies, storm flies, stinging flies, dog flies). The stomoxys is slightly larger than the common housefly, and its resemblance has misled some patients into thinking they were bitten by a housefly (which does not bite). The Phlebotomid sand flies cause a painful bite and also transmit leishmania, *Bartonella bacilliformis*, and sandfly fever, a non-fatal viral disease. The bites of all of these flies are treated symptomatically, by cleaning with soap and water, treating secondary infection with antibiotics, and applying soothing topical ointments or corticosteroids. Non-biting flies such as houseflies, flesh flies, and blowflies (bluebottle flies) can transmit disease, particularly that caused by gastrointestinal pathogens, by acting as mechanical vectors. They are also occasional causes of myiasis (see later). Eye gnats do not bite but may transmit bacterial conjunctivitis and yaws.

Other than biting and acting as vectors of disease, flies may affect humans by causing myiasis, infestation of the skin or a body orifice with fly larvae. A well-known example is the botfly found in the American tropics, which glues its eggs to a bloodsucking fly like the mosquito; when the mosquito bites humans, the larvae leave the mosquito, hatch, and penetrate the skin of their new host. A similar form of myiasis is caused by the tumbu or mango fly in Africa, which lays its eggs on the ground or on soiled clothing. Upon direct contact with humans, the larvae then penetrate the skin. The screw worm lays its eggs at the edge of wounds and may infect nose, eyes, ears, and other body orifices. This larva often travels through tissues. Sarcophagid flies deposit their living larvae on the hosts. Some larvae migrate in tortuous channels and produce a type of larva migrans (hypoderma). Other flies that feed on decaying tissue occasionally cause myiasis in humans; the larvae enter living tissue after feeding on necrotic wounds. Although usually confined to the skin or superficial wounds, myiasis can involve the genitourinary tract and the intestine; the larvae are usually passed spontaneously, although uretheral involvement sometimes requires cystoscopy. Areas of cutaneous myiasis are frequently misdiagnosed as pyogenic infection, and this diagnosis should be kept in mind for a "boil" that is refractory to medical therapy if a patient has visited an endemic area. Treatment for the cutaneous form requires mechanical removal with tweezers or by excision; this may be facilitated by covering the embedded larvae with petrolatum or strips of raw bacon fat, both of which encourage them to move upward, where they are grasped more easily.

Cockroaches are an important pest. They are able to consume any human or animal food, dead plant or animal material, leather, glue, fabrics, grease, hair, wallpaper, and book bindings. They may function as mechanical vectors of pathogens and are sometimes intermediate hosts of helminths. Cockroaches can bite, but these bites are not particularly painful. Their glandular secretions can cause asthma when ingested, and cockroaches may be an important cause of asthma in children, in which group sensitization to cockroach allergens is commonly demonstrable.

HEMIPTERA—BUGS

Hemiptera are the "true" bugs, comprising bed bugs, cone-nose bugs, and wheel bugs. Bed bugs are 5-mm-long, flat, oval insects that resemble large ticks or small cockroaches. The most common species in temperate climates is *Cimex*. Bed bugs are not an important vector of disease, but their bites cause inflammation and occasionally hemorrhagic bullae. They are nocturnal feeders with a distinct odor and are capable of hiding successfully in the seams of mattresses, in couches, behind loose wallpaper, and under baseboards.

The cone-nose bugs are members of the Reduviid family. They are 1 to 3 cm long and can fly. The best known of these are the assassin bug (so named because it kills other insects) and the "kissing" bug (because it often bites around the lips and face). The kissing bug may transmit Chagas' disease, caused by *Trypanosoma cruzi*. Although some species of Reduviid bugs produce painful bites that occasionally ulcerate and resemble necrotic arachnidism, the vectors of Chagas' disease produce painless bites. The bug defecates after eating, and it is the human host who scratches the trypanosomes into the skin. Although some species of cone-nose bugs are found throughout the United States, those that transmit Chagas' disease are found in Mexico, Central and South America, and only rarely in the U.S. Southwest.

The bites of all these bugs are treated symptomatically, with topical antipruritic ointments and corticosteroids when needed, antihistamines for allergic reactions, and antibiotics for secondary infections.

HYMENOPTERA

The Hymenoptera include bees, wasps, hornets, and ants. These insects have an ovipositor, designed to deposit eggs; however, the ovipositor has been modified to a stinging apparatus that injects venom, causing severe local inflammation and sometimes hypersensitivity. The familar honeybee is yellow and black striped and has an ovipositor that is barbed; thus, after the honeybee stings, the stinger and venom sacs are left in its victim and the bee dies. During stinging, the honeybee releases pheromones that attract other bees to attack. "Killer" bees are africanized honeybees imported to South America to improve honey production. However, multiple swarms escaped from experimental colonies, and they have spread northward to Central America and the southern United States. The sting of the killer bee is not more toxic or allergenic than that of the domesticated honeybee, but the killer bee is more aggressive; it attacks with less provocation and exhibits massive stinging behavior in defense of the colony. In fact, up to 50% of the bees in a killer bee colony are guard bees that respond to perceived threats. The bumble bee is not as aggressive as the honeybee but otherwise exhibits similar behavior. Wasps include yellowjackets, hornets, and paper wasps. The yellowjackets are usually 1.5 to 2 cm in length and are attracted to sweet products, soda, meats, and so on. They have familar black bands and produce a large honeycombed nest with a paper envelope. Hornets are larger than yellowjackets, 2.5 to 3.5 cm., and are brown, orange, and red. Paper wasps are the same size as yellowjackets but may be black, brown, red, or yellow. Their nest is a single open comb of gray paper, usually attached to a building or tree.

Of the 15 species of ants capable of stinging humans, 8 are found in the United States. The imported fire ants are the most troublesome; found in the southeastern states, they both bite and sting. They attach to the skin with their jaws and then pivot around their head, stinging multiple times. The harvester ant, found in the western and southeastern states, stings its victim, and, like that of the honeybee, its stinger may be torn off after envenomation. Velvet ants (wooly ants, cow killers, mutillid wasps) look like ants but are in actuality wingless female wasps. They are red, orange, or yellow and achieve a size of 0.75 to 2.5 cm. Found in the western and southeastern states, they are capable of a painful sting.

The Hymenoptera produce both local and systemic reactions. The local reaction is an area of inflammation that involves the immediate area of the sting, appears within 2 to 3 minutes, and abates within hours. Fire ant stings often develop into pustules, and lymphangitis may complicate harvester ant bites. Patients who have extensive local reactions have a slightly increased risk for future anaphylaxis. Local reactions themselves are not life-threatening except for instances of multiple stings (50 to 100 or more), which may be fatal as a result of toxicity as opposed to hypersensitivity. The effects of multiple stings suggest excessive histamine release; thus, antihistamines may be appropriate in this setting. Otherwise, local reactions are treated with ice, elevation, local analgesics, corticosteroid creams, and lotions such as calamine. If a stinging apparatus remains in the skin, it should be removed. Systemic anaphylactic reactions are treated with epinephrine, corticosteroids, and antihistamines (see Chapter 275). Patients with severe Hymenoptera allergies should consider venom immunotherapy (see Chapter 276).

LEPIDOPTERA

Lepidoptera cause dermatologic and systemic disease through the hairs of caterpillars and moths. The caterpillars of several moth and butterfly families secrete venom from a gland at the base of specialized hairs or from cells lining the lower part of sharp spines. These hairs and spines can be both irritating and allergenic when touched. An immediate burning sensation develops, followed by swelling, numbness, urticaria, extreme pain referred to regional lymph nodes, and, rarely, headache, nausea, paralysis, and seizures. In the United States, the most bothersome varieties are the caterpillars of the IO, brown-tail, saddleback, and gypsy moths, and the puss caterpillar. The puss caterpillar is a particular problem in the southern United States; it does not look like a caterpillar, but rather like a teardrop-shaped tuft of yellow cotton. Some caterpillars, for example, the gypsy moth larvae, do not sting, but contact with their hair causes dermatitis, which has occurred in outbreak form in the northeastern United States. Some moths have scales or hairs that become airborne and cause urticaria, skin irritation, upper respiratory symptoms, and conjunctivitis. When occurring in great numbers, such airborne spread has caused epidemics both on land or on board ship. Treatment of caterpillar stings includes repeated stripping of the sting site with cellophane or adhesive tape to remove spines, in addition to local application of ice, antihistamines, calamine lotion, and corticosteroids; zinc oxide and lime water have been found helpful as well. Some advocate use of Meperidol, codeine, or intravenous calcium gluconate for pain in view of the poor analgesic effect of aspirin for these lesions. Systemic symptoms are treated with epinephrine, antihistamines, and corticosteroids.

FLEAS

Fleas are small brown wingless insects that are flattened laterally. Both human and animal (cat, dog, bird, rat, etc.) species may bite humans. Animal fleas can live for months without a host. If humans are available and their natural host is still not accessible, they will bite. Their ability to jump several inches increases humans' vulnerability. Flea bites produce a punctate hemorrhagic area initially, followed by a maculopapular pruritic dermatitis; typically the papules are linear or clustered. The dermatitis may be more severe in previously sensitized patients. Most fleas feed on humans only transiently, but the chigoe flea (jigger, nigua, chica, pico, pique, suthi) *Tunga penetrans* burrows into the dermis, lays her eggs, and remains embedded in the skin. The chigoe is found in tropical America, Africa, the Near East, and India; lesions are most commonly seen between the toes and under the toenails. If it is found within the first 48 hours a sterile needle removes the flea; later, surgical removal is usually necessary.

The term "sand flea" is used loosely by the lay public to indicate chigoes, cat fleas, dog fleas, human fleas, and tiny crustaceans found in seaweed along coastal beaches.

Other than the minor discomfort of bites or the focal persistence of the chigoe, fleas are vectors. The rat flea *Xenopsylla cheopis* is the most efficient vector of plague (*Yersinia pestis*) and murine typhus (*Rickettsia typhi*). In the southwestern United States a natural reservoir of plague exists among wild rodents, especially ground squirrels; domestic pets may then carry these infected fleas to their owner's home. Recent observations associate *Bartonella henselae* (which causes cat scratch disease, bacillary angiomatosis, and peliosis hepatis) with exposure to flea-infested cats. A newly described rickettsial agent, *Rickettsia felis,* is maintained in cat fleas by transovarian passage and uses the opossum as a reservoir host. It has caused a murine-typhus-like illness in humans. Fleas may also act as mechanical vectors for numerous bacterial and viral infections by contaminated windborne feces that reach humans' mucous membranes. In addition, several flea species act as intermediate hosts of the dog tapeworm *Dypilidium caninum* and the rat tapeworm *Hymenolepis diminuta,* infecting humans when fleas are accidentally ingested.

DELUSORY PARASITOSIS

The psychiatric disorder delusory parasitosis can torture both patient and physician. Typically, patients are elderly white women who have seen many physicians and now present the physician with a container or small bag containing the suspected "bugs." Often they claim that these bugs are in their vagina or rectum and emerge at night. Some patients have skin lesions from excoriation. After excluding true parasitosis and somatic disease, physicians should refer patients for psychiatric evaluation. Some patients have responded to therapy with pimozide or haloperidol.

LEECHES

Leeches are members of the phylum Annelida, class Hirudinea. They are segmented worms found in fresh water and salt water and on land. The aquatic leeches are found in temperate and tropical climates. They attach to their swimming or wading hosts to acquire a blood meal. The bite of salt water leeches is painful, whereas the attachment of the freshwater variety may be asymptomatic. Smaller leeches may invade the upper respiratory or gastrointestinal tract, eye, nose, vagina, urethra, and anus.

Bites of leeches often bleed freely after the leech has stopped feeding, because the leech injects hirudin, an anticoagulant that inhibits thrombin. Other allergens the leech introduces may elicit anaphylaxis or a local hypersensitivity response, including bullae, urticaria, or necrotic ulceration.

In the Far East, land leeches attach themselves to travelers in tropical forests, often crawling between boot and sock and feeding by penetrating the material of the sock. Treatment is removal, often facilitated by local anesthetic, salt solutions, alcohol, vinegar, or a lighted match. No mouthparts should be left behind. The wound is then cleaned and disinfected; residual bleeding can be stemmed by a styptic pencil. Leeches have been used in plastic surgery to reduce vascular congestion in tissue flaps. They have also been applied to sites of cutaneous ischemia in patients with purpura fulminans.

Other marine annelids related to the leech can bite or envenomate. The bloodworm, used as fish bait in North America, causes a painful bite that takes days to resolve. The bristle worm, found in Asia and the Gulf of Mexico and California, has chitinous spines filled with venom. A sting from one of these spines causes pain, rash, swelling, and occasionally skin necrosis. It is important to remove the spines in addition to applying topical soothing creams and ice.

Fitzpatrick TB, Eisen AZ, Wolff K, et al: Dermatology and General Medicine, 4th ed. New York, McGraw-Hill, 1993. *Clinically oriented discussion of the ectoparasitic dermatoses, with striking photographs of lesions and organisms.*

Goddard J: Physician's Guide to Arthropods of Medical Importance, 2nd ed. Boca Raton, FL, CRC Press, 1996. *A thorough compendium of the biologic characteristics, classification, and behavior of medically important anthropods.*

Neva FA, Brown HW: Basic Clinic Parasitology, 6th ed. Norwalk, CT, Appleton & Lange, 1994. *A helpful reference, particularly for the life cycles, epidemiologic characteristics, and pathogenesis of arthropod-borne disease.*

436   VENOMOUS SNAKE BITES*

Rodney D. Adam ■ John B. Sullivan

EPIDEMIOLOGIC CHARACTERISTICS

In the United States, approximately 5000 snake bites are reported to poison control centers per year, of which one third to one half are caused by poisonous snakes. Approximately 20% of bites from venomous snakes result in no envenomation, and another 30 to 40% result in relatively mild envenomation. Seven deaths were reported from 1984 to 1996, all occurring from rattlesnakes; however, it should be noted that reporting of poisonous snake bites is not required and these figures may substantially underestimate the true numbers. In many parts of the world, deaths are more common than in the United States, both because of poor access to medical care and because of the presence of snakes with more lethal venom (e.g., Russell's viper in southern Asia and lance-headed vipers in Brazil).

The poisonous snakes of major medical importance are from two families, Viperidae and Elapidae (Table 436–1). The Viperidae include the subfamilies Viperinae (true vipers and adders) and Crotalinae (pit vipers). Crotalinae (rattlesnakes, water moccasins or cottonmouths, copperheads) and Elapidae (coral snakes) are found in the United States. Most of the bite injuries sustained within the United States are caused by rattlesnakes or by copperheads. Most bite victims are male (75 to 90%) and most bites occur in the extremities (two thirds upper and one third lower extremities). The great majority of bites occur during the months of April through October with a peak occurring in June through September. On the basis of data from the 1950s, the southeastern states have the highest frequency of snake bites, followed by Arizona and New Mexico. Whether the increased urbanization of many of these areas has significantly changed the frequency is unknown. Frequently, alcohol intoxication and/or intentional handling of the snake is an accompanying risk factor.

The pit vipers are identified by a small depression between the eyes and nostrils. This pit is a heat sensing organ, which detects minute changes in temperature and allows the snake to locate its mammalian victim. The pit viper has fangs that are folded against the upper jaw while the snake is at rest. When the snake strikes, the fangs rotate down and forward, allowing penetration as deep as 8 to 20 mm. Other characteristics that distinguish pit vipers from non-venomous snakes include a triangular head, which is distinct from the remainder of the body; an elliptical (rather than round) eye; and a single row of ventral scales (rather than a double row). In addition, a rattle is found on the tail of the rattlesnakes. However, not all strikes are preceded by a rattle, and snakes too young to have a well-developed rattle may still be venomous.

Coral snakes are found in the southern and western states, typically on dry ground near rivers or lakes. The eastern coral snake is found in the southeastern states, extending as far west as west Texas; the western coral snake is found in Arizona and New Mexico. The coral snakes found in the United States have red bands circling the body that are bordered by yellow or white, whereas the similar appearing non-venomous snakes have red bands bordered by black. Their fangs are short and permanently erect. Envenomation occurs through chewing movements. The eastern coral snake is the more dangerous of the two and the only coral snake for which antivenin is available. Coral snakes are generally nocturnal and shy; only 1% of reported snake bites are caused by coral snakes.

PIT VIPERS (CROTALINAE)

PATHOGENESIS. The pathogenesis of bite injuries caused by venomous snakes is related to the action of the various components of the venom as well as the degree of envenomation. The relative makeup of the venom varies, not only by genus and species, but

Table 436–1 ■ MAJOR VENOMOUS SNAKES OF THE WORLD

CLASSIFICATION*	GEOGRAPHIC LOCATION
Viperidae	
Viperinae (true vipers and adders)	
Viper (*Vipera, Daboia*)	
Adder (*Bitis, Echis*)	
Crotalinae (pit vipers)	
Asian pit viper (*Calloselasma, Agkistrodon, Trimeresurus*)	Asia
Lance-headed viper (*Bothrops*)	South America
Moccasin and copperhead (*Agkistrodon*)	North America
Rattlesnake (*Crotalus, Sistrurus*)	Americas
Elapidae	
Cobra (*Naja*)	Africa and Asia
African mamba (*Dendroaspis*)	Africa
Asian krait (*Bungarus*)	Asia
Asian coral snake (*Calliophis, Maticora*)	Asia
American coral snake (*Micrurus*)	Americas

*The Colubridae (e.g., African boomsland, twig snake), Hydrophiidae (sea snake), and Atractaspididae (burrowing asp) are venomous snakes of lesser medical importance.

also with the individual snake. Pit viper venom contains proteases that lead to tissue necrosis. Hyaluronidase cleaves acid mucopolysaccharides, decreasing the viscosity of connective tissue and allowing the venom to spread. Phospholipase A2, which hydrolyzes an ester bond of lecithin, releases lysolecithin, which in turn releases histamine from mast cells. Phospholipase A2 also damages erythrocytes and muscle fibers. L-amino acid oxidase causes tissue destruction. Thrombin-like enzymes and amino acid esterases act as defibrinating anticoagulants. Other enzymes with less well-defined roles in pathogenesis include collagenase, nucleases, and arginine ester hydrolase.

The cardiovascular effects of pit viper bites result primarily from the hypovolemia that is caused by increased vascular permeability and vasodilation. Tachycardia, weakness, and hypotension are commonly found in cases of moderate to severe envenomation. Hemoconcentration may be found early in the course.

Platelet aggregation may be induced by the tissue damage at the site of the injury or may be directly induced by the snake venom. Coagulopathy may result from the thrombin-like enzyme, which clots fibrinogen, resulting in a decrease in fibrinogen level and increase in fibrin degradation products. Elevated prothrombin time and partial thromboplastin time may be seen, but when bleeding occurs, it is usually not life-threatening. Burring of the erythrocytes may result from the membrane effects of the venom; anemia occurs as a result of decreased red blood cell survival.

The neuromuscular effects of pit viper envenomation are generally overshadowed by the local effects. However, the subset of Mojave rattlesnakes (*Crotalus scutulatus scutulatus*) producing venom A typically has greater neurotoxicity than other rattlesnakes. The blockade at the pre-synaptic site of the neuromuscular junction can result in weakness and paralysis. In contrast, bites from the venom B–producing Mojave rattlesnakes result in relatively greater local tissue injury and less neurotoxicity.

CLINICAL MANIFESTATIONS (TABLE 436–2). The most common clinical manifestation of the bite of a pit viper consists of edema and pain at the location of the bite, beginning as early as 10 minutes after the bite. Mild envenomation is characterized by local edema (1 to 5 inches in diameter) and pain without systemic symptoms or signs. With moderate envenomation, local findings are more extensive: edema of 6 to 12 inches in diameter in addition to ecchymosis and tender regional lymphadenopathy. Systemic findings of moderate envenomation include weakness or dizziness, sweating, nausea or vomiting, and paresthesias of the scalp and tips of the extremities. Severe envenomation may result in necrosis, usually in the cutaneous and subcutaneous levels. More rarely, the venom may be injected into the muscle layer, resulting in myonecrosis. The systemic effects of severe envenomation include tachycardia and hypotension, tachypnea, hypothermia, muscle fasciculations, and occasionally clinically significant bleeding from the gingivae or gastrointestinal or genitourinary tract.

LABORATORY FINDINGS. Most of the significant laboratory

---

*This chapter is revised and updated from the chapter by Jay Sanford in the 20th edition. Dr. Sanford is remembered for his life and numerous contributions to medicine.

Table 436–2 ■ MANIFESTATIONS OF PIT VIPER ENVENOMATION

LOCAL	(PERCENTAGE)	SYSTEMIC	(PERCENTAGE)	ABNORMAL RESULTS*	(PERCENTAGE)
Fang mark	100	Weakness or dizziness	10–80	Thrombocytopenia	18–42
Swelling	74–98	Nausea and vomiting	31–70	Elevated PTT	48
Pain	60–81	Fasciculations	8–41	Elevated PT	12–15
Paresthesia	48–73			Decreased fibrinogen	17–35
Discoloration	27–69			Increased FDP	39–54
Bullae	6–15				
Necrosis	4–27				

*PTT = partial thromboplastin time; PT = prothrombin time; FDP = fibrin degradation product.
The data were compiled from Russell FE: Snake venom poisoning in the United States. Annu Rev Med 31:247, 1980, reproduced, with permission, from the Annual Review of Medicine, volume 31, © 1980, by Annual Reviews Inc.; Plowman DM, Reynolds TL, Joyce SM: Poisonous snakebite in Utah. West J Med 163:547, 1995; Sullivan JB Jr, Wingert WA, Norris RL: North American venomous reptile bites. *In* PS Auerbach (ed): Wilderness Medicine, 3rd ed. St. Louis, Mosby, 1995, pp 680–709.

findings involve coagulation and hematologic abnormalities. Hemoconcentration may be found at presentation; anemia is commonly seen later as a result of increased red blood cell (RBC) fragility. Increased platelet consumption may result in thrombocytopenia.

CORAL SNAKES (ELAPIDAE)

The bite wound of the coral snake usually resembles scratch marks and is somewhat painful, but there is little or no edema. The onset of systemic manifestations is usually delayed for 1 to 6 hours. Paresthesias around the bite may occur within several hours. Systemic symptoms may include weakness, apprehension, giddiness, nausea, vomiting, excess salivation, and even a sense of euphoria. Bulbar and cranial nerve paralysis may develop with ptosis, diplopia, pupillary dilatation, excess salivation, dysphagia, dysphonia, and respiratory failure. Paralysis may last 6 to 14 days, and muscular strength may not be fully regained for 6 to 8 weeks.

TREATMENT

PRE-HOSPITAL TREATMENT. The major goal of pre-hospital treatment is to provide rapid and safe transport to a hospital with the resources to care for snake bites (see Table 436–3). If at all possible, this should include restraining the patient to minimize muscular activity. With neurotoxic venoms, absorption may result in respiratory arrest, for which resuscitation is essential. Respiratory paralysis may develop within 15 minutes of cobra bites. Accurate identification of the snake is useful, but not always possible. A snake should not be handled, because of the risk of incurring another bite injury. Even a dead snake must be handled with care, since the head of an apparently dead snake can deliver a venomous bite after being severed. The potential value of incision and suction is lower than the risk, and they should not be done. However, the site of the bite should be wiped. Negative pressure suction devices may remove up to 30% of venom if used in the first few minutes after envenomation. The affected part should be immobilized and the patient should be promptly transported to the nearest medical treatment facility.

The affected area should not be placed in ice. A tourniquet should not be placed. Cryotherapy and tourniquets increase the likelihood of local tissue damage and the potential need for amputation. Compressive bandages have commonly been recommended, but there are no data supporting their use for pit viper bites and they should not be used.

HOSPITAL TREATMENT. Determine whether the bite was inflicted by a pit viper or a coral snake and whether envenomation has occurred. The state or regional poison control center can be a valuable source of information regarding assessment and treatment of the patient. Among the different species of rattlesnakes, there are differences in the likelihood of severe envenomation, but there are enough differences among bite injuries that the major determinant of the required therapy is the clinical assessment of envenomation. The degree of envenomation should be graded as none, mild, moderate, or severe (Table 436–4), remembering that the envenomation grade may worsen during the first few hours after the bite. Therapy includes administration of intravenous fluids and monitoring of vital signs and electrocardiographic and coagulation status in an intensive care unit. In addition, antivenin is used for rattlesnake bites with moderate to severe envenomation. Two antivenins are available: a polyvalent preparation for North American pit vipers and another for eastern coral snakes. The currently available antivenins are horse serum products, which entail high risk for anaphylactic reactions during administration (3 to 54%) and later serum sickness (nearly 100% with high doses). Preparations of antivenin using F(ab) fragments appear to have good efficacy and substantially reduced toxicity but have not been approved by the Food and Drug Administration at the time of publication. The bites of water moccasins, copperheads, and western coral snakes can be managed without antivenin.

For moderate envenomation, 10 to 15 ampules of the Wyeth antivenin should be diluted into 500 mL of a crystalloid fluid such as normal saline solution and infused over 30 minutes to 2 hours. Skin sensitivity tests are unreliable in predicting early reactions to antivenin and should not be used. Immediate reactions should be watched for closely with epinephrine available before the infusion is started. When bronchospasm, hypotension, or angioedema occurs, the infusion should be halted and 0.5 mL or 1:1000 epinephrine given intramuscularly in addition to H_1 and H_2 receptor blocking antihistamines, such as diphenhydramine and cimetidine. This is usually effective and allows the antivenin to be restarted. A

Table 436–3 ■ PRE-HOSPITAL TREATMENT

DO	DON'T
Minimize muscular activity	Perform incision and suction of bite wound
Immobilize affected part	Allow "dead" snake to bite care-givers or patient
Wipe bite site	Apply tourniquet or occlude arterial blood supply
Identify snake if it can be done safely	Place affected part in ice
Transport immediately to nearest medical treatment facility	Give patient alcohol
Observe respiratory status; resuscitate if necessary	

Table 436–4 ■ DEGREES OF ENVENOMATION AFTER A PIT VIPER BITE

GRADE	CLINICAL CHARACTERISTICS*
None	Minimal pain and no significant swelling
Minimal	Local swelling of less than 15 cm from bite wound No systemic manifestations
Moderate	Local swelling of 15–30 cm Systemic signs or symptoms
Severe	Local swelling of greater than 30 cm Severe systemic signs and symptoms, including coagulation abnormalities

*By definition, fang marks are present for all levels. This classification system is satisfactory in most cases. A more precise classification system can be found in Dart RC, Hurlbut KM, Garcia R, Boren J: Validation of a severity score for the assessment of crotalid snakebite. Ann Emerg Med 27:321, 1996.

history of immediate reaction to horse serum is a relative contraindication to the use of antivenin, but antivenin should be considered for severe envenomation. A reaction can frequently be attenuated or prevented by pre-treatment with diphenhydramine, cimetidine, epinephrine, and possibly corticosteroids.

If the amount of antivenin is adequate, swelling will not progress and paresthesias will decrease. If progression occurs, the dose should be repeated. For severe envenomation, 30 vials may be required. In one series, the average dose required for adults with severe bites was 16 vials. Antivenin neutralizes both the local and the systemic effects of the venom.

For coral snake bites, the neuromuscular manifestations, including respiratory failure, are more prominent than the local signs and may be delayed by several hours or longer. Even in the absence of symptoms, patients should be observed in the hospital for 1 to 2 days because the onset of symptoms may be delayed and insidious. If symptoms or signs of envenomation develop within the first several hours after the bite of an eastern coral snake, 3 to 5 vials of antivenin should be given intravenously. A coral snake bite victim for whom antivenin was unavailable has been successfully treated with neostigmine, which has been shown to be effective for cobra bites (see later). Therefore, neostigmine treatment can be considered if neurotoxicity develops and antivenin is unavailable or has not worked.

Results of bacteriologic cultures of rattlesnake venom and fangs show growth from over 90% of specimens, including enterobacteriaceae, *Pseudomonas* sp., and *Clostridium perfringens.* Abscesses occurred after about 8% of pit viper (*Bothrops*) bites in a South American study. The organisms causing abscesses include enterobacteriaceae, group D streptococci, and *Bacteroides* sp. A randomized study of antibiotic prophylaxis (gentamicin and chloramphenicol) actually showed a higher incidence of abscess formation in patients who received antibiotics. Therefore, antibiotics should be administered if infection occurs but should not necessarily be given prophylactically.

For severely envenomated patients, supportive measures include stabilization of the cardiovascular, respiratory, and renal systems. Glucocorticoids have been recommended, but a controlled trial of prednisone therapy was effective for neither local nor systemic effects of poisoning. The only legitimate role for glucocorticoids is in treatment or possibly prevention of early antivenin reactions and in treatment of serum sickness. Despite the hypofibrinogenemia and increase in fibrin degradation products, heparin is not of benefit. Decompressive fasciotomy should not be used for most patients with snake bites. It may be considered if compartmental pressures are greater than 30 mm Hg and arterial blood supply is compromised.

PROGNOSIS. If adequate antivenin has been administered, the mortality rate is low. If cryotherapy and tourniquets have been avoided, amputation or serious deformities are uncommon. After approximately 1 to 2 weeks, the majority of patients given moderate to high amounts of antivenin will experience serum sickness, consisting of maculopapular rash, urticaria, fever, malaise, and arthralgia. An antihistamine in addition to oral prednisone (2 mg/kg/day for 1 week and tapered over the second week) can be used for treatment of the serum sickness.

When a pit viper bite occurs during pregnancy, high maternal (10%) and fetal (43%) mortality rates have been reported; however, these figures are likely subject to reporting bias of cases with more severe envenomation.

BITES CAUSED BY SNAKES NOT FOUND IN THE UNITED STATES

VIPER (VIPERIDAE) BITES. Bites by Russell's viper are the leading cause of fatal snake bite in Pakistan, India, Bangladesh, Sri Lanka, Myanmar, and Thailand. They are an occupational hazard of rice farmers. Up to 70% of the protein content of the venom is phospholipase A2, which can induce hemolysis, rhabdomyolysis, pre-synaptic neurotoxicity, and shock. Geographic variation in clinical manifestations is striking. The most common systemic signs are those of neurotoxicity: external ophthalmoplegia, ptosis, difficulty in opening the mouth (pseudotrismus), and inability to protrude the tongue. Symptoms include drowsiness, headache, vomiting, and abdominal pain. Incoagulability of blood commonly leads

to spontaneous hemorrhage, often massive. Generalized muscle tenderness, myoglobinuria, and oliguria are also common. In some countries, viper bite envenomation is the most common cause of acute renal failure. Management requires intensive supportive therapy and specific antivenin. Antivenin is most effective when administered within 4 hours; 400 to 500 mL is often required. Adequate doses restore blood coagulability but do not reverse shock, nephrotoxicity, or myotoxic signs. Causes of death include shock; pituitary, intracranial, and gastrointestinal hemorrhage; and tubular or renal cortical necrosis. Individuals who recover often show clinical or laboratory evidence of hypopituitarism.

COBRA (ELAPIDAE) BITES. Coral snake bites are almost invariably painful. Local necrosis is often preceded by bullae, which may not develop for 2 to 4 days after the bite. Neurotoxic symptoms may appear as early as 3 minutes after a bite, and respiratory paralysis may occur within 15 minutes. The neurotoxic effects can usually be reversed by edrophonium chloride. If neurotoxic signs appear, an edrophonium test should be done: atropine sulfate (0.6 mg) given by slow intravenous infusion, followed by edrophonium chloride (10 mg) intravenously over 2 minutes. If improvement occurs, neostigmine methylsulfate should be administered (beginning with 25 μg/kg/hour) by continuous infusion. The effectiveness of cobra antivenin is inconsistent. Maintaining adequate ventilation is essential. In survivors, neurotoxic manifestations usually resolve within 1 week.

Dart RC, Hurlbut KM, Garcia R, Boren J: Validation of a severity score for the assessment of crotalid snakebite. Ann Emerg Med 27:321, 1996. *A useful method for assessing the degree of envenomation from a pit viper bite.*

Dart RC, Seifert SA, Carroll L, et al: Affinity-purified, mixed monospecific crotalid antivenom ovine Fab for the treatment of crotalid venom poisoning. Ann Emerg Med 30:33, 1997. *Results obtained with an F(ab) fragment antivenin. Serum sickness did not occur.*

Holstege CP, Miller MB, Wermuth M, et al: Crotalid snake envenomation. Crit Care Clin 13:889, 1997. *A well-written and extensive review of crotalid snake bites in the United States, dealing primarily with rattlesnake bites.*

Meier J, White J (eds): Handbook of Clinical Toxicology of Animal Venoms and Poisons. Boca Raton, FL, CRC Press, 1995. *Extensive well-referenced monograph, which covers venomous snakes from throughout the world.*

Warrell DA: Venomous bites and stings in the tropical world. Med J Aust 159:773, 1993. *A review of bites caused by poisonous snakes found in the tropics.*

437 VENOMS AND POISONS FROM MARINE ORGANISMS

Jay W. Fox

It is generally accepted that the term *envenomation* implies penetration by an organism for delivery of a venom containing one or more toxins. In contrast, poisons are toxins that are acquired from the environment by mechanisms such as absorption, inhalation, and ingestion. In the marine environment, both forms of intoxication occur, with effects ranging from mild irritation and discomfort to death. Previously, most clinically relevant intoxications were envenomations from marine organisms primarily found in tropical and subtropical waters. In recent times, however, severe outbreaks of poisoning from ingesting marine organisms containing toxins have occurred. This is likely due to increased microorganism growth in coastal waters as a result of eutrophication. Encroachment on the marine environment for recreation, living space, and food sources may be expected to increase the frequency of adverse encounters with venomous and poisonous marine organisms. In this chapter, the marine organisms responsible for the majority of clinically significant intoxications are discussed, with emphasis on the pharmacologic and symptomatic properties of the toxins. Table 437–1 is a list of names of venomous and poisonous marine organisms that can produce severe intoxication or death and includes whether antivenin is available. The sites of action of some marine neurotoxins are depicted in Figure 437–1.

VENOMOUS MARINE ORGANISMS

Venomous marine organisms deliver their venoms by biting and stinging (see Table 437–1). Envenomation involves penetration of the skin. Thus, consideration must be given to the potential of infection by microorganisms, especially in situations involving deep puncture wounds and bites, as well as to the treatment of the toxicologic effects of the venom.

SEA SNAKES. Sea snakes are members of the family Hydrophiidae and are generally found in tropical and subtropical waters. Sea snakes are very common in the coastal waters of Thailand, Indonesia, the Persian Gulf, Australia, and India. With regard to the Americas, one species of sea snake, *Pelaramis platurus*, the yellow-bellied sea snake, is found in the Pacific coastal waters of Central America. These snakes are very capable swimmers but do not come ashore and are relatively immobile on land. They inject their venom with two small maxillary fangs (2 to 4 mm) containing ducts connected to venom glands located posterior and ventral to the maxillary bone. The relatively short aspect of the fangs prevents effective envenomation through most protective clothing such as dive suits. In the case of human envenomation, if the subject reacts by violent retraction the fangs are often dislodged from the maxillary bone of the snake and may remain in the site.

Because of the nature of the venom and the size of the fangs, the sea snake bite itself is generally not painful. One or two small prick marks are present at the envenomation site, as occasionally are additional marks from the other teeth in the snake's mouth. The primary toxin in sea snake venom is a postsynaptic peptide neurotoxin that functions by blocking the acetylcholine receptor at neuromuscular junctions (see Fig. 437–1). The symptoms of sea snake envenomation are mainly neurologic and typically appear within 30 minutes to 2 hours after the bite. Ptosis, dysphagia, and non-rigid paralysis occur. In severe cases, respiratory failure may occur and respiratory intervention may be necessary.

MOLLUSKS. BLUE-RINGED OCTOPUS. The blue-ringed and spotted octopuses (*Hapalochlaena maculosa* and *H. lunulata*), found in Australian waters, inject their venom by a relatively painless bite producing two small puncture wounds. Hemorrhage at the site may occur. The major toxic component in the venom is tetrodotoxin, a postsynaptic neurotoxin that causes perioral and intraoral paresthesias, dysphagia, nausea, ataxia, aphonia, flaccid muscular paralysis, and respiratory distress or failure. Fatal envenomations have occurred.

CONE SHELLS. Cone shell venoms are injected into victims through a hollow, harpoon-like tooth. The venom is primarily neurotoxic, causing paresthesias, hypotension, and respiratory impairment/failure. Three types of neurotoxins have been identified in cone shell venoms: ω-conotoxin, α-conotoxin, and μ-conotoxins, all of which are short polypeptides. The ω-conotoxins block depolarization-induced calcium uptake through N-type presynaptic channels (see Fig. 437–1). The bite is very painful and may be followed by such systemic symptoms as dysphagia, aphonia, pruritus, blurred vision, syncope, muscular paralysis, and respiratory and cardiac failure. In cases of severe envenomation, preparation for cardiovascular and respiratory support should be made. Rare cases of coagulopathies have been noted. Fatal envenomations have occurred.

WEEVERFISH/SCORPIONFISH/STONEFISH/LIONFISH. Weeverfish are of the Trachinidae family whereas the scorpionfish, stonefish, and lionfish all belong to the family Scorpaenidae. Members of the Scorpaenidae family are mostly found in tropic and subtropic waters. Weeverfish occur in European and African waters. All of these fish sting by using dorsal spines. Additionally, anal spines of the Scorpaenidae fish and opercular spines of the Trachinidae fish can also deliver venom. The spines are encased in an integumentary sheath that is torn when the spine punctures the victim's skin. Venom glands are located at the base of the spine.

Few details are known regarding the biochemistry and pharmacology of the toxins in weeverfish venom. The sting of the weeverfish is extremely painful and may produce systemic effects such as aphonia, fever, chills, dyspnea, cyanosis, nausea, syncope, hypotension, and arrhythmias. The wound is edematous, erythematous, and ecchymotic. Bacterial infection is typical, and gangrene has been known to develop in severe cases of infection. The venom may be somewhat heat labile, and soaking in tolerably hot water may relieve some pain as well as attenuate the effects of the venom. Death from a weeverfish sting is rare.

Scorpionfish (*Scorpanena*) are primarily found in tropical and subtropical waters and the Mediterranean. The stings of these fishes have been described to be very similar to those of the weeverfish. Lionfish (*Pterois*) dwell in tropical waters; their stings generally are the most severe of all of the fish stings and occasionally cause death. Because the venom is heat labile, soaking in hot water is recommended. The stonefish (*Synanceja*) group is found throughout the India-Pacific area, China, Australia, and the Indian Ocean and is considered to be the most venomous fish. Symptoms are similar to those from the stings of members of the other groups. Similar, high-molecular-weight toxins, verrucotoxin from *S. verrucosa*, stonustoxin from *S. horrida*, and cytolysin from *S. trachynis* have recently been isolated and characterized. These are multimeric, heat-labile protein toxins composed of α- and β-subunits and are the toxins that are primarily responsible for many of the symptoms associated with the sting from these fish. Soaking of the wound site

Table 437–1 ■ SIGNIFICANT VENOMOUS AND POISONOUS MARINE ORGANISMS

ORGANISM	TYPE OF ENVENOMATION (POISONING)	PRIMARY TOXINS	ANTIVENOM AVAILABLE
Sea snakes (Hydrophiidae)	Bite	Post-synaptic neurotoxin	Yes
Blue-ringed octopus (Octopodidae)	Bite	Post-synaptic neurotoxin (tetrodotoxin)	No
Cone shell (Conidae)	Bite	Pre- and post-synaptic neurotoxins	No
Box jellyfish (*Chironex fleckeri, Chiropsolmus quadrigatus*)	Sting	Hemolysins, proteinases, cardiotoxin necrotoxins	Yes
Portuguese man-o-war (*Physalia physalis*)	Sting	Hemolysins, proteinases, cardiotoxin necrotoxins	No; may be a need
Sea nettles (*Chrysaora quinquecirrha; Cyanea capillata*)	Sting	Hemolysins, proteinases, cardiotoxin necrotoxins	No; generally no need
Sea anemone (*Anemonia sulcata*)	Sting	Neurotoxins	No; generally no need
Scorpionfish (Scorpaenidae)	Sting puncture	Hemolysins, necrotoxins ?	Yes
Lionfish (Scorpaenidae)	Sting puncture	Hemolysins, necrotoxins ?	No
Stonefish (Scorpaenidae)	Sting puncture	Hemolysins, necrotoxins ?	Yes
Weeverfish (Trachinidae)	Sting puncture	Hemolysins, necrotoxins ?	No
Stingrays (Rajiformes)	Sting puncture	?	No
Dinoflagellates		Ciguatera poisoning, ciguatoxins, maitotoxin (neurotoxins)	
Gambierdiscus toxicus	Poisonous (found in fish)		
Ptychodiscus brevis	Poisonous (found in shellfish)	Neurotoxic shellfish poisoning, neurotoxins	
Gonyaulax species	Poisonous (found in shellfish)	Paralytic shellfish poisoning	
Pyrodinium species	Poisonous (found in shellfish)	Saxitoxin, neosaxitoxin and gonyautoxin	
Jania species	Poisonous (found in shellfish)	Okadaic acid (phosphatase inhibitors)	
Pufferfish (Tetraodontiformes)	Poisonous	Tetrodotoxin (neurotoxin)	No
Porcupinefish (Tetraodontiformes)	Poisonous	Tetrodotoxin (neurotoxin)	
Sunfish (*Mola* species)	Poisonous	Tetrodotoxin (neurotoxin)	

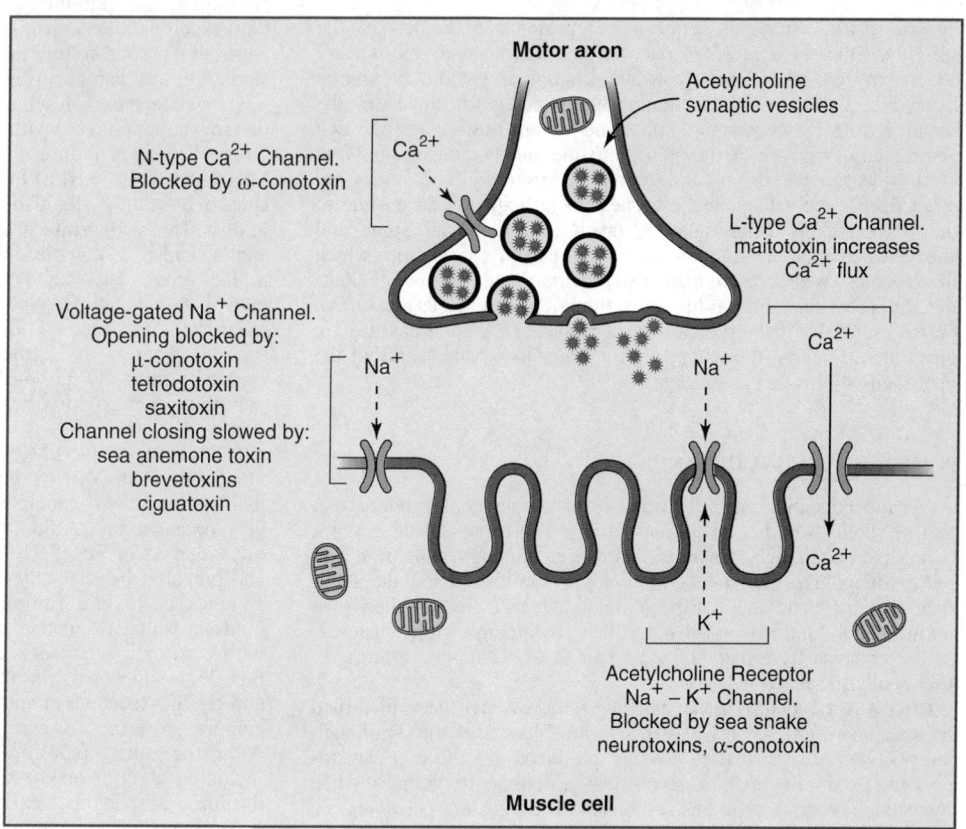

FIGURE 437–1 ■ Schematic representation of a motor axon synapse and the sites of action of various marine neurotoxins.

in hot water (45° C) is recommended. In cases of severe blistering, the blisters should be excised to flush residual active venom from the blister fluid to ameliorate dermal necrosis. As with all fish stings, care should be taken to ensure that no broken portions of the spines remain in the wound; vigilance against bacterial infections should be observed.

COELENTERATES. JELLYFISH AND ANEMONES. These organisms belong to the Cnidaria phylum, thus named because of their venomous organelles, cnidae. The cnidae found in jellyfish and anemones (termed *nematocysts* and *spirocysts,* respectively) are located on exposed tentacles. On tactile stimulation the tentacles send forth a tethered projectile to deliver venom through the dermis. As the victim's surrounding musculature contracts, the venom is disseminated. The toxins contained in the venom from these organisms have not been fully documented. Hemolysins, DNAses, and histamine releasers have been identified in some venoms. Several peptide toxins have been characterized from the sea anemone, *Anemonia sulcata,* which act similarly to α-scorpion toxins by inactivating the sodium channel. Stings by jellyfish and anemones typically produce immediate pain at the site of envenomation, followed by erythematous, urticarial lesions. Anaphylaxis is not common in most situations unless previous sensitization has occurred. Depending on the severity of the sting, wheals and whiplike patterns at the sites of envenomation may appear within a few minutes or be delayed by several hours, followed in some cases by dermal necrosis. Recurrence of eruptions days after the envenomation has been reported. Systemic reactions may include muscle spasms and cramps, vomiting, nausea, diarrhea, diaphoresis, and, in rare cases, cardiorespiratory failure. Verapamil will eliminate cardiac arrhythmia but will not ameliorate respiratory depression. Unfired nematocysts on tentacles adhering to the skin may be neutralized by either vinegar or baking soda depending on the species of jellyfish. Vinegar seems to be most useful for the Portuguese man-of-war (*Physalia physalis*) and Australian blue bottle (*P. utriculus*) stings, whereas baking soda appears more efficacious for sea nettle (*Chrysaora quinquecirrha*) stings. Box jellyfish (*Chironex fleckeri*) found in Australian waters are perhaps the most venomous jellyfish, producing very severe stings that may cause death from hypotension, muscular and respiratory paralysis, and, ultimately, cardiac arrest.

Treatment of box jellyfish stings must include consideration of the option of respiratory support and administration of an antivenin.

SPONGES. Some sponges colonized by coelenterates elaborate toxins that can produce either a pruritic allergenic dermatitis or an irritant dermatitis. These toxins are delivered by the sharp spicules present in the sponges, which when handled penetrate the dermis. The toxins can cause the typical sponge diver's disease, characterized by local burning and itching, which in severe cases may be accompanied by soft tissue edema and purulent vesiculation. Serious illness is rare.

CORALS. Fire coral (*Millepora alcicornis*) is found in shallow tropical waters. Stings are a common consequence of brushing or rubbing against the coral. Envenomation produces a burning or stinging sensation followed by severe pruritus. Edematous wheals may occur but generally dissipate over the course of several days. The site of envenomation should be soaked in dilute acetic acid or isopropanol to relieve pain.

BRISTLEWORMS. Bristleworms (Annelida) are segmented invertebrates found in tropical Pacific waters and the Gulf of Mexico. The bristles present on the segments of the organism are capable of penetrating the skin and producing a severely painful envenomation with pruritus and burning that may persist for several days. Local paresthesia is likely and may linger for weeks. Treatment is symptomatic, with consideration of possible tetanus infection. Little is known regarding the chemistry of bristleworm venoms.

SEA URCHINS. Of the echinoderms, sea urchins and sea stars are responsible for most stings to humans. The venom is delivered by the long spines and pedicellariae protruding from the sea urchin body. The spines are covered at the tips with a venom sac that is broken when it penetrates the skin. The pedicellariae, present on some species of sea urchins, are pincer-like appendages carrying venom glands. The toxins of sea urchin venoms are not well characterized. Stings can produce pain, hemorrhage, aphonia, paresthesias, paralysis, hypotension, nausea, syncope, and respiratory distress. Immersion in hot water helps inactivate heat-labile toxins in the venoms. Attached pedicellariae and embedded spines must be removed to prevent additional envenomation.

STINGRAYS. Stingrays (order Rajiformes) are found in most seas but are predominant in the Indo-Pacific area. Venom is delivered by stings from spines (one or more) present on the tail of the stingray. Stingray spines are retroserrated on the margins and are covered by an integumentary sheath. Venomous glandular tissue is located at the base of the spines. On puncture of the skin, the sheath is torn by the serrated spine and venom flows along the two ventrolateral grooves of the spine into the surrounding tissue. One of the identified toxins in the venom is serotonin. The spines are often deeply embedded in the tissue and difficult to extract due to the retroserration. Care must be taken to remove all spine and sheath fragments. A sting produces severe pain and edema, which in extreme cases is accompanied by hemorrhage, syncope, vomiting, hypotension, and cardiac arrhythmia. In rare cases death can occur, especially if the pericardial, peritoneal, or pleural cavities are penetrated. Soaking the wound in hot water inactivates some of the heat-labile toxins in the venom.

POISONOUS MARINE ORGANISMS

Marine poisoning nearly always results from consumption of a fish or shellfish harboring various toxins. The causes of three types of marine poisoning are fish or shellfish containing toxins produced by dinoflagellates (ciguatera, neurotoxic shellfish, paralytic shellfish, and diarrhetic shellfish poisoning); fish that produce their own toxin (Tetraodontiformes fish); and fish containing significant levels of bacteria that have metabolized histidine to histamine, resulting in pseudoallergic reactions.

CIGUATERA POISONING. Ciguatera toxins have been identified in more than 400 species of fish. During blooms of the dinoflagellate *Gambierdiscus toxicus,* toxins produced by these organisms concentrate in the fish to levels that are toxic to humans when ingested. The primary toxins responsible for ciguatera poisoning are ciguatoxin(s), which are cyclic polyethers and act as excitatory agents by binding to sodium channels. Maitotoxin, from the same dinoflagellate, is a water-soluble polyether and acts by enhancing calcium entry through L-type calcium channels. Symptoms of ciguatera poisoning generally appear within 2 to 12 hours after ingestion of contaminated fish. Gastrointestinal symptoms including diarrhea, abdominal pain, nausea, and vomiting appear first, followed by neurologic and cardiovascular symptoms. Neurologic symptoms include aphonia, dental dysesthesias, fatigue, tremor, ataxia, pruritus, extremity and perioral dysesthesia, vertigo, headache, myalgias, arthralgias, temperature reversal, and hyporeflexia. Cardiovascular symptoms, such as bradycardia and hypotension, occur least often. There is no specific treatment for ciguatera poisoning; supportive, symptom-based therapy is indicated. Death from ciguatera poisoning has occurred but is rare.

NEUROTOXIC SHELLFISH POISONING (NSP). NSP is caused by eating shellfish that contain brevetoxins produced by the dinoflagellate *Ptychodiscus brevis.* Brevetoxins are cyclic polyethers that function similarly to the ciguatoxins. Gastrointestinal and neurologic symptoms of intoxication appear within 3 hours after toxic shellfish is eaten and are similar to those of ciguatera poisoning. Treatment is supportive. No deaths have been reported for NSP.

PARALYTIC SHELLFISH POISONING (PSP). PSP is significantly more severe than NSP and predominantly involves neurologic symptoms with less pronounced gastrointestinal symptoms such as nausea, vomiting, and diarrhea. The toxins responsible for PSP are from the dinoflagellate genera *Gonyaulax, Pyrodinium,* and *Jania* and are harbored in a variety of shellfish. The primary PSP toxins—saxitoxin, neosaxitoxin, and gonyautoxin—are heterocyclic compounds that block nerve and muscle action potentials by binding to sodium channels. The site of binding overlaps with tetrodotoxin, resulting in paralysis. Symptoms appear soon after consump-

tion of contaminated shellfish (minutes to hours) beginning with circumoral and extremity paresthesias. Additional neurologic symptoms, such as ataxia, arthria, dysphagia, dysmetria, diaphoresis, and tachycardia, soon follow the initial paresthesias. Respiratory depression or failure can occur and may result in death, usually within 12 hours of the onset of symptoms. As with other shellfish poisoning, therapy is supportive, with close attention given to potential respiratory distress or failure.

DIARRHETIC SHELLFISH POISONING (DSP). DSP is also caused by eating shellfish that are contaminated by dinoflagellate toxins. The two primary toxins associated with DSP are okadaic acid(s) and pectenotoxins. Okadaic acid is a polyether derivative of a 38 carbon fatty acid. It functions as an inhibitor of protein phosphatase-1 and -2A and causes smooth and cardiac muscle contraction. Symptoms of DSP begin with abdominal cramps and nausea and progress to diarrhea. Additional, delayed symptoms occurring approximately 35 hours after ingestion may appear and include vomiting, vertigo, diarrhea, cramps, and headache. Treatment is supportive.

TETRAODONTIFORMES (PUFFERFISH, PORCUPINEFISH, AND SUNFISH) POISONING. Pufferfish (also called blowfish, balloonfish, and toadfish), porcupinefish, and sunfish *(Mola* species*)* have a very potent toxin, tetrodotoxin, present in their liver, gonads, intestines, and skin. The flesh of the fish (fugu) is a delicacy in Japan and prepared by specially trained chefs to avoid serving significant amounts of toxins. Tetrodotoxin is a heterocyclic compound that binds at voltage-sensitive sodium channels (at an overlapping site with saxitoxin) to block sodium passage, preventing nerve and muscle action potentials, thus resulting in paralysis. Symptoms occur rapidly (several minutes to several hours) beginning with circumoral paresthesias and progressing to widespread paresthesias. After the initial paresthesias, additional symptoms soon follow, including ataxia, weakness, aphonia, diaphoresis, excess salivation, dyspnea, dysphagia, weakness, and respiratory distress or failure. Gastrointestinal symptoms include nausea, vomiting, and diarrhea. Coagulopathologies have been reported in association with tetrodotoxin intoxication. Respiratory intervention is crucial in light of the potential for complete flaccid paralysis. Without respiratory assistance, death is not unusual in cases of severe intoxication.

SCOMBROID FISH POISONING. Scombroid poisoning is a pseudoallergic fish poisoning caused by consumption of certain types of fish that have been improperly stored, including the scombroid fish (tuna, mackerel, wahoo, bonito, albacore, skipjack) and non-scombroid fish (mahi-mahi, amberjack, sardines, and herring). The poisoning results from high levels of histamine and saurine present in the fish because of bacterial catabolism of histidine. Presentation of symptoms from intoxication is rapid (within minutes to hours), beginning with a flushing of the skin, oral paresthesias, pruritus, urticaria, nausea, vomiting, diarrhea, vertigo, headache, bronchospasm, dysphagia, tachycardia, and hypotension. Therapy should follow a course for allergic reaction and anaphylaxis. Symptoms usually resolve in several hours.

Adams ME: Neurotoxins. Trends Neurosci 17(4 Suppl):151–155, 1994. *This issue is a concise tabulation of neurotoxins, their biological sources, and pharmacological activities.*

Auerbach PS: Marine envenomations. N Engl J Med 325:486, 1991. *A thorough guide to the types of marine envenomations and symptoms that they cause.*

Burnett JW: Human injuries following jellyfish stings. Md Med J 41:509, 1992. *This article describes the mechanism of jellyfish stings and therapy.*

Gwee MCE: A review of stonefish venoms and toxins. Pharmacol Ther 64:509–528, 1994. *This is a review article that describes the biological, clinical and biochemical properties of stonefish venom and envenomation.*

Hall S, Strichartz G (eds): Marine Toxins: Origin, Structure and Molecular Pharmacology. Washington, DC, American Chemical Society, 1990. *This is a collection of papers on marine toxins with particular emphasis on experimental pharmacology.*

Miller DM (ed): Ciguatera Seafood Toxins. Boca Raton, FL, CRC Press, 1991. *A compilation of information on the toxicology of ciguatoxin poisoning.*

Tu AT (ed): Handbook of Natural Toxins, Vol 3, Marine Toxins and Venoms. New York, Marcel Dekker, 1988. *This volume discusses many types of marine toxins as well as provides a section on treatment.*

PART XXV

NEUROLOGY

■ EVALUATION OF THE PATIENT

438 APPROACH TO THE PATIENT
Robert C. Griggs

The symptoms of nervous system diseases are a part of everyday experience for most normal people. Slips of the tongue, headaches, backache and other pains, dizziness, light-headedness, numbness, muscle twitches, jerks, cramps, and tremors all occur in totally healthy persons. Mood swings with feelings of elation and depression, paranoia, and displays of temper are equally a part of the behavior of completely normal people. The rapid increase in information about neurologic diseases coupled with the intense interest of people in all walks of life in medical matters has focused public attention on both common and rare neurologic conditions.

Most older people are concerned that they or their spouse have or are developing Alzheimer's disease or stroke or both. The almost ubiquitous tremor of the elderly prompts concern about Parkinson's disease. Many younger patients are concerned about multiple sclerosis or brain tumor, and few normal people lack one or more symptoms suggesting the diagnosis of a serious neurologic disease. For most of these and other common diagnoses, imaging and other tests are typically normal when symptoms first appear and should not be obtained to reassure the patient or physician. Moreover, the widespread availability of neurodiagnostic imaging and electrophysiologic, biochemical, and genetic testing has detected "abnormalities" in many young and most elderly persons. In evaluating a patient's symptoms, it is imperative that a clinical diagnosis be reached without reference to a neurodiagnostic laboratory finding. Patients with disorders such as headache, anxiety, or depression usually do not have abnormal laboratory studies. Abnormalities that are noted on various neurodiagnostic studies are often incidental findings whose treatment may be justified and necessary but will not improve the patient's symptoms. Abnormalities detected incidentally that do not have signs or symptoms may, as for disorders such as hypertension, require aggressive evaluation and treatment, but in general, the adage that it is difficult to improve the asymptomatic patient should be kept in mind. Thus, in elderly patients, few imaging or electrophysiologic studies are interpreted as "normal" but in the absence of specific complaints consistent with the findings, treatment and even further evaluation should reflect an estimate of the specificity and sensitivity of the test, as well as the likelihood that the patient will require and benefit from treatment. It is a good rule-of-thumb that one should never obtain (or refer to the result of) a neurodiagnostic procedure without a specific diagnosis or at least a differential diagnosis in mind.

It is important to allow the patient to describe any symptoms in his or her own words. Direct questions are often necessary to fully characterize the patient's problem, but suggested terms or descriptors for symptoms are frequently grasped by the patient unfamiliar with medical terminology and then parroted to subsequent interviewers. The patient's terms should always be used when recording symptoms. Terms such as *lameness, weakness, numbness, heaviness, cramps,* and *tiredness* may each mean pain, weakness, or alteration of sensation to some patients.

439 THE NEUROLOGIC HISTORY
Ralph F. Józefowicz

The neurologic history is the most important component of neurologic diagnosis. A careful history frequently determines the cause and allows one to begin localizing the lesion(s), aiding in the determination whether the disease is diffuse or focal. Symptoms of acute onset suggest a vascular cause or seizure; symptoms that are subacute in onset suggest a mass lesion such as a tumor or abscess; symptoms that have a waxing and waning course with exacerbations and remissions suggest a demyelinating cause; symptoms that are chronic and progressive suggest a degenerative disorder.

The history is often the only way of diagnosing neurologic illnesses that typically have normal or non-focal findings on neurologic examination. These illnesses include many seizure disorders, narcolepsy, migraine and most other headache syndromes, the various causes of dizziness, and most types of dementia. The neurologic history may often provide the first clues that a symptom is psychological in origin. The following are points to consider when obtaining a neurologic history:

- **Carefully identify the chief complaint or major problem.** Not only is the chief complaint important in providing the first clue to the physician as to the differential diagnosis, it is also the reason why the patient is seeking medical advice and treatment. If the chief complaint is not properly identified and addressed, the proper diagnosis may be missed and an inappropriate diagnostic work-up may be undertaken. Establishing a diagnosis that does not incorporate the chief complaint frequently focuses attention on a coincidental process irrelevant to the patient's concerns.

- **Listen carefully to the patient for as long as is necessary.** A good rule of thumb is to listen initially for at least 5 minutes without interrupting the patient. The patient often volunteers the most important information at the start of the history. During this time, the examiner can also assess mental status, including speech, language, fund of knowledge, and affect, and observe the patient for facial asymmetry, abnormalities of ocular movements, and an increase or a paucity of spontaneous movements as seen with movement disorders.

- **Steer the patient away from discussions of previous diagnostic test results and of the opinions of previous caregivers.** Abnormal results of laboratory studies may be incidental to the patient's primary problem or may simply represent a normal variant.

- **Take a careful medical history, medication history, psychiatric history, family history, and social and occupational history.** Many neurologic illnesses are complications of underlying medical disorders or are due to adverse effects of drugs. For example, parkinsonism is a frequent complication of use of metoclopramide and most neuroleptic agents. A large number of neurologic disorders are hereditary, and a positive family history may establish the diagnosis in many instances. Occupation plays a major role in various neurologic disorders such as carpal tunnel syndrome (in computer keyboard operators), and peripheral neuropathy (caused by exposure to lead or other toxins).

- **Interview surrogate historians.** Patients with dementia or altered mental status are usually unable to provide exact details of the history, and a family member may provide key details needed to make an accurate diagnosis. This is especially true for patients with dementia and certain right hemispheric lesions with various agnosias (lack of awareness of disease) that may interfere with their ability to provide a cogent history. Surrogate historians also provide missing historical details for patients with episodic loss of consciousness, such as syncope and epilepsy.

- **Summarize the history for the patient.** Summarizing the history is an effective way to ensure that all details were covered sufficiently to make a tentative diagnosis. Summarizing will also allow the physician to fill in historical gaps that may not have been apparent when the history was initially taken. In addition, the patient or surrogate may correct any historical misinformation at this time.

- **End by asking the patient what he or she thinks is wrong.** This allows the physician to evaluate the patient's concerns about and insight into the condition. Some patients have a specific diagnosis in mind that spurs them to seek medical attention. Multiple sclerosis, amyotrophic lateral sclerosis, Alzheimer's disease, and brain tumors are diseases that patients often suspect may be the cause of their neurologic symptoms.

440 CLINICAL DIAGNOSIS AND NEUROLOGIC EXAMINATION

Robert C. Griggs

CLINICAL DIAGNOSIS

In neurologic diagnosis, the history usually indicates the nature of the disease or the diagnosis, whereas the neurologic examination localizes it and quantitates its severity. For many diseases the history is almost the only avenue to explore. Examples of such disorders include headaches, seizures, developmental disorders, memory disorders, and behavioral diseases. In arriving at a diagnosis, the following points are useful. Consider the entire medical history of the patient. Early-life events or long-standing processes such as head or spine trauma, unilateral hearing or visual loss, poor prowess in sports, poor performance in school, spinal curvature, or bone anomalies are easily overlooked but may point to the underlying disease process.

Consider the tempo and duration of symptoms. Have the symptoms been progressive without remission, or have there been plateaus or periods of return to normal? Cerebral mass lesions (tumor, subdural) tend to have a progressive but fluctuating course; seizures and migraine, an episodic course; strokes, an abrupt, ictal onset with worsening for 3–5 days followed by partial or complete recovery.

Ask yourself, Can one disease account for all of the symptoms and signs? Formulate a diagnostic opinion in anatomic terms. Is the history suggestive of a single (e.g., stroke or tumor) *focus* or of multiple sites of nervous system involvement (e.g., multiple sclerosis)? Or is the process a disease of a *system:* B$_{12}$ deficiency, myopathy, or polyneuropathy?

Two common situations provide special challenges to the diagnostic skills of a physician:

PHYSICAL ABUSE AS A CAUSE OF NEUROLOGIC SYMPTOMS. Traumatic injury inflicted by family members or other close contact with patients is usually difficult to detect by medical history and examination. Physically battered babies, abused children, battered women, and traumatized seniors are often unable or un-

willing to complain of this cause or contribution to symptoms. The only method to prevent overlooking this frequent cause of common problems is systematic consideration of the possibility in every patient and awareness of the (often subtle) signs that suggest physical trauma: ecchymoses or fractures (often attributed to a logical cause), denial of expected symptoms, failure to keep appointments, and unexplained intensification of neurologic symptoms (headache, dizziness, ringing in the ears, blackouts).

ALCOHOLISM AND DRUG ABUSE. A host of neurologic disorders can be the result of the intentional ingestion of toxins. Patients do not give an accurate account of their use of these agents. Consequently, physical signs and laboratory screening test results that give evidence of drug-related hepatic and other metabolic abnormalities (see the discussion of alcoholism) may point to a major underlying problem.

ACUTE NEUROLOGIC DISORDERS REQUIRING IMMEDIATE DIAGNOSIS AND TREATMENT. Most neurologic diagnoses are arrived at by a careful, thorough history and an appropriately complete examination. However, the tempo of illness and the availability of lifesaving treatment, that is only effective if administered within minutes of first evaluating a patient dictates rapid action in several specific circumstances. *Coma, repetitive seizures, acute stroke, suspected meningitis and encephalitis, head and spine trauma, and acute spinal cord compression* are each considered in chapters that follow. In each, diagnosis by clinical and laboratory assessment and urgent treatment must be instituted as soon as ventilation and cardiac status are stabilized.

NEUROLOGIC EXAMINATION

The neurologic examination is always tailored to the clinical setting of the patient. The complete neurologic examination of the child is much different from that of an elderly adult, and the examination of a patient with specific complaints will focus on findings pertinent to that patient. Thus, more detailed testing of cognition is indicated in patients with behavioral or memory disturbance and more detailed testing of sensation should be performed in patients with complaints of pain, numbness, or weakness.

However, many tests of neurologic function are routinely indicated in all patients because they provide a baseline for future examination and because they are so frequently helpful in detecting unsuspected neurologic disease in apparently normal persons or in patients whose symptoms initially suggest disease outside the nervous system. It is particularly important to perform all routine tests in patients with abnormalities in one sphere of neurologic dysfunction; otherwise, erroneous localization of a lesion or disease process is likely. It is essential for a physician to have extensive experience in the routine assessment of normal persons, in order to recognize and quantitate deviations from the normal.

THE GENERAL EXAMINATION. Specific neurologic symptoms or signs should prompt attention to the assessment of general findings. Head circumference should be measured in patients with central nervous system or spinal cord disease (normally 55 ± 5 cm in adults). Head enlargement is occasionally a normal, often hereditary, variant but should suggest a long-standing anomaly of the brain or spinal cord. The skin should be inspected for café au lait maculas, adenoma sebaceum, vascular malformations, lipomas, neurofibromas, and other lesions (see Chapter 456). Neck range of motion, straight leg raising, and spinal curvature (scoliosis) should be assessed. Carotid auscultation for bruits is indicated in all older adults; carotid palpation is seldom informative. In patients with bladder, bowel, or leg symptoms, rectal sphincter examination for tone and ability to contract voluntarily is usually indicated. Limitation of joint range of motion or painless swelling of joints is often a sign of an unsuspected neurologic lesion.

THE NEUROLOGIC EXAMINATION. The various aspects of the detailed neurologic examination are considered in specific symptom and disease sections noted later. The five major divisions of the examination should be assessed in all patients. During a careful medical history the mental status is often adequately assessed: level of consciousness, orientation, memory, language function, affect, and judgment. If abnormal, more detailed testing is needed. Cranial nerve function that should be tested in all patients includes visual acuity (with and without correction); optic fundi; visual fields; pupils (size and reactivity to direct and consensual light); ocular motility; jaw, facial, palatal, neck, and tongue movement; and hearing.

Motor system examination (also see Chapters 505 to 511) is essential in all patients because incipient weakness is usually overlooked by the patient. Muscle tone (flaccid, spastic, or rigid), muscle size (atrophy or hypertrophy), and muscle strength can be assessed rapidly. Muscle strength testing should always assess specific functional activities including the ability to walk on heel and toe; sit up from a supine position; rise from a deep knee bend or deep chair; lift the arms over the head; and make a tight fist. Gait, stance, and coordination are assessed. The patient should be observed for tremor, fasciculations, and other abnormal movements and the muscles inspected for fasciculations.

Sensory testing (see Chapters 497 to 504) need not be detailed unless there are sensory symptoms. However, vibration perception in the toes as well as the normality of perception of pain, temperature, and light touch in the hands and feet should be assessed.

Muscle stretch reflexes and plantar responses should always be assessed, evaluating right/left symmetry and disparity between proximal or distal reflexes or arm versus leg reflexes. Biceps, triceps, brachioradialis, quadriceps, and ankle reflexes should be quantitated 1–4 (4 = clonus; 3 = spread; 2 = brisk; 1 = hypoactive).

THE COMATOSE PATIENT. The rapid examination required for a patient with an altered state of consciousness is much different from that of an alert, aware individual. The approach is detailed in Chapter 445. Many aspects of the neurologic examination cannot be tested: cognitive function; subtleties of sensory perception; specific motor functions; coordination; gait; stance. Moreover, the muscle stretch reflexes are likely to fluctuate from one moment to the next and minor asymmetries are much less significant than in an awake patient. Instead, attention should focus on the examination of (1) level of consciousness, (2) respiratory pattern, (3) eyelid position and eye movements, (4) pupils, (5) corneal reflexes, (6) optic fundi, (7) motor responses. Particular elements of the general examination must also be assessed quickly: evidence of cranial and spine trauma, tenderness of the skull to percussion, nuchal rigidity (but not in patients with head or neck trauma), evidence of physical abuse.

441 NEUROGENETICS

Robert C. Griggs

The molecular characterization of neurologic diseases has had a major impact on the laboratory diagnosis of neurologic disorders, has changed disease classification, and has begun to explain disease mechanisms and to facilitate the development of treatment. Whereas neurologic diseases are not unique in this regard, the impact has been arguably greater for nervous system diseases than for any other system. Three specific discoveries have made it necessary to make major changes in textbooks:

1. Diseases once considered to be single clinical and pathologic entities have proved to be multiple diseases caused by two or more different genes. Examples include Alzheimer's disease (8 or more genes), amyotrophic lateral sclerosis (5 or more genes), and limb girdle muscular dystrophy (14 or more genes).
2. There are many different mutations in single genes. These allelic variants may have widely differing severity of disease. Examples include Friedreich's ataxia, once considered invariably severe and uniformly life-threatening in late childhood and early adulthood. Whereas most mutations in the Friedreich's ataxia gene produce this phenotype, certain mutations produce a much less severe phenotype.
3. Many "different" diseases are caused by an abnormality of a single gene. Examples include the periodic paralyses in which at least five diseases can be caused by mutations in different portions of the α-subunit of the sodium channel.

Thus, neurologic disease classification is changing rapidly. Even more changes will occur as soon as the molecular cause of diseases

once given eponyms or characterized by their clinical symptoms and signs or pathology are defined. The following "new" categories of disease are rapidly being identified: channelopathies, trinucleotide repeat diseases, structural protein defects, enzymopathies, and mitochondriopathies. There will undoubtedly be others.

With the recognition that the majority of neurologic diseases are either caused or predisposed to by genetic factors, the family history is an important but emotionally charged and potentially distressing part of the patient's history. Alzheimer's disease, epilepsy, Tourette's syndrome, and other common diseases are often denied on family history and, if present, imply a considerable risk to the patient or the patient's offspring. Previous diagnostic evaluations of relatives were often inadequate or the results misunderstood. Absence of a family history of a disease is seldom an argument against considering that the patient may have an hereditary condition. Two specific features of neurologic disorders are important to consider in obtaining a family pedigree. *Anticipation*, the worsening of a disease with successive generations, is a feature of the trinucleotide repeat diseases. Many *mitochondrial* genetic diseases are transmitted only from mothers to their male and female offspring.

442 NEUROLOGIC DIAGNOSTIC PROCEDURES

Ralph F. Józefowicz

LUMBAR PUNCTURE

Sampling of cerebrospinal fluid (CSF) via lumbar puncture is crucial for accurate diagnosis of meningeal infections and carcinomatosis. CSF analysis is also helpful in evaluating patients with central or peripheral nervous system demyelinating disorders and with intracranial hemorrhage, particularly when imaging studies are inconclusive.

The CSF formula often provides an important clue as to the pathologic process involved. An elevated WBC count is seen with infections and other inflammatory diseases, as well as with carcinomatosis. The WBC differential cell count may point to a specific class of pathogen: polymorphonuclear leukocytes suggest a bacterial process, whereas mononuclear cells suggest a viral, fungal, or immunologic cause. The CSF glucose concentration is typically reduced in bacterial and fungal infections, as well as with certain viral infections (e.g., mumps virus) and with sarcoidosis. The CSF protein concentration is elevated in a variety of disorders, including most infections and demyelinating neuropathies. Table 442–1 lists characteristic CSF formulas for several neurologic conditions.

A lumbar puncture should not be performed in patients who have obstructive, non-communicating hydrocephalus or a focal CNS mass lesion causing raised intracranial pressure, because reducing the CSF pressure acutely in these settings via lumbar puncture may result in cerebral or cerebellar herniation. Lumbar puncture may be safely performed in patients with *communicating* hydrocephalus, such as with idiopathic intracranial hypertension (pseudotumor cerebri), and it may even be an effective treatment for selected patients with this condition.

ELECTROENCEPHALOGRAPHY

Electroencephalography (EEG) is the recording and measurement of scalp electrical potentials to evaluate baseline brain functioning and paroxysmal brain electrical activity suggestive of a seizure disorder.

An EEG is performed by securing 20 electrodes to the scalp at predetermined locations, based on an international system that uses standardized percentages of the head circumference, the "10–20 system." Each electrode is labeled using a letter and a number, the

Table 442–1 ▪ CHARACTERISTIC CSF FORMULAS

	TURBIDITY AND COLOR	OPENING PRESSURE	WBC (Cells/mm³)	DIFFERENTIAL CELLS	RBC COUNT	PROTEIN	GLUCOSE
Normal	Clear, colorless	70–180 mm H₂O	0–5	Mononuclear	0	<60 mg/dL	>2/3 serum
Bacterial meningitis	Cloudy, straw-colored	↑	↑↑	PMNs	0	↑↑	↓
Viral meningitis	Clear or cloudy, colorless	↑	↑	Lymphocytes	0	↑	Normal
Fungal and tuberculous meningitis	Cloudy, straw-colored	↑	↑	Lymphocytes	0	↑↑	↓↓
Viral encephalitis	Clear or cloudy, straw-colored	Normal to ↑	↑	Lymphocytes	0 (herpes ↑)	Normal to ↑	Normal
Subarachnoid hemorrhage	Cloudy, pink	↑	↑	PMNs and lymphocytes	↑↑	↑	Normal (early) ↓ (late)
Guillain-Barré syndrome	Clear, yellow	Normal to ↑	0–5	Mononuclear	0	↑	Normal

letter identifying the skull region (Fp = frontopolar, F = frontal, P = parietal, T = temporal, O = occipital, V = vertex) and the number identifying the specific location, with odd numbers representing the left-sided electrodes and even numbers the right-sided electrodes. These electrodes are then connected in various combinations of pairs to generate voltage potential differences, and the potentials are recorded on a chart recorder.

To delineate the spatial distribution of the changing electric field for an EEG, orderly arrangement of electrode pairs are used, and each specific arrangement is known as a *montage*. Montages are generally of two types: *referential*, in which each electrode is connected to a single reference electrode, such as the ear; and *bipolar*, in which electrodes are connected sequentially to one another, forming a chain. A standard EEG generally records about 30 minutes of brain activity, both in the awake state and in the first two stages of sleep. Various activating procedures are used during the recording of an EEG, including hyperventilation and photic stimulation. These activating procedures may precipitate seizure discharges in some patients with seizure disorders, increasing the sensitivity of the test.

The amplitudes of scalp electrical potentials are quite low, averaging 30 to 100 μV; they represent a summation of excitatory postsynaptic potentials (EPSPs) and inhibitory postsynaptic potentials (IPSPs) that are largely generated by the pyramidal cells in layer four of the cerebral cortex, which behave as electric dipoles. Action potentials are of too brief a duration to have an effect on the EEG.

The EEG is analyzed with respect to symmetry between each hemisphere, wave frequency and amplitude, and the presence of spikes (20 to 70 msec) and sharp waves (70 to 200 msec) that may

Table 442–2 ▪ EEG ABNORMALITIES

EEG ABNORMALITY	CLINICAL CORRELATE
Background Rhythm Abnormalities	
Generalized slowing	Most metabolic encephalopathies
Triphasic waves	Hepatic and renal encephalopathies
Focal slowing	Large mass lesions (tumor, large stroke)
Electrocerebral inactivity with lack of response to all stimuli	Brain death
Paroxysmal Abnormalities	
3 Hz spike and wave, augmented by hyperventilation	Absence epilepsy
3–4 Hz spike and wave in light sleep or with photic stimulation	Primary generalized epilepsy
Central to midtemporal spikes	Benign Rolandic epilepsy
Anterior temporal spikes or sharp waves	Simple or complex partial seizures of mesial temporal origin
Hypsarrhythmia (high-voltage chaotic slowing with multifocal spikes)	Infantile spasms (West syndrome)
Burst suppression	Severe anoxic brain injury, barbiturate coma

indicate a seizure focus. EEG frequencies are divided into four categories as follows:

Delta: <4 Hz
Theta: 4 to 7 Hz
Alpha: 8 to 13 Hz
Beta: >13 Hz

The normal waking EEG in a patient with eyes closed contains rhythms of alpha frequency in the occipital leads and beta frequency in the frontal leads. Normal sleep causes a generalized slowing of the EEG frequencies and an increase in amplitude in each stage of sleep, such that stage 4 sleep consists of greater than 50% large-amplitude delta rhythms.

EEG abnormalities are of two types: abnormalities in background rhythm and abnormalities of a paroxysmal nature. Some of the more common EEG abnormalities are noted in Table 442–2 and Figure 442–1.

The major usefulness of EEG is for diagnosis and categorization of a seizure disorder. It is important to realize that EEGs are neither highly sensitive nor completely specific for diagnosing seizures. Because seizures are paroxysmal events, it is not unusual for an EEG to be normal, or only minimally abnormal, in a patient with epilepsy if it is recorded during an interictal phase (the time period between seizures). In fact, only about 50% of patients with seizures show epileptiform activity on the first EEG. Repeating the EEG with provocative maneuvers, such as sleep deprivation, hyperventilation, and photic stimulation, may increase this percentage to 90%. Conversely, about 1% of adults and 3.5% of children who are neurologically normal and who never had a seizure will have epileptiform activity on an EEG.

The EEG may provide clues in the diagnosis of certain neurologic conditions, including viral encephalitis, slow virus infections, and some forms of coma. In each of these situations, the EEG can have specific patterns that suggest a specific neurologic diagnosis. In herpes simplex encephalitis, periodic lateralizing epileptiform discharges (PLEDs) emanating from the temporal lobes are frequently present. Triphasic slow waves are the hallmark of hepatic encephalopathy. Creutzfeldt-Jakob disease is characterized by the presence of bilateral synchronous repetitive sharp waves. The EEG is also helpful in confirming brain death when an apnea test cannot be performed because of cardiac instability.

In the past, the EEG was often used for localizing neurologic lesions such as stroke, brain tumor, or abscess. With the advent of neuroimaging, EEG is almost never used for these purposes.

NERVE CONDUCTION STUDY

A nerve conduction study (NCS) is the recording and measurement of the compound nerve and muscle action potentials elicited in response to an electrical stimulus.

To perform a motor NCS, a surface (active) electrode is placed over the belly of a distal muscle that is innervated by the nerve in question. A reference electrode is placed distally over a joint. The nerve is then supramaximally stimulated at a predetermined dis-

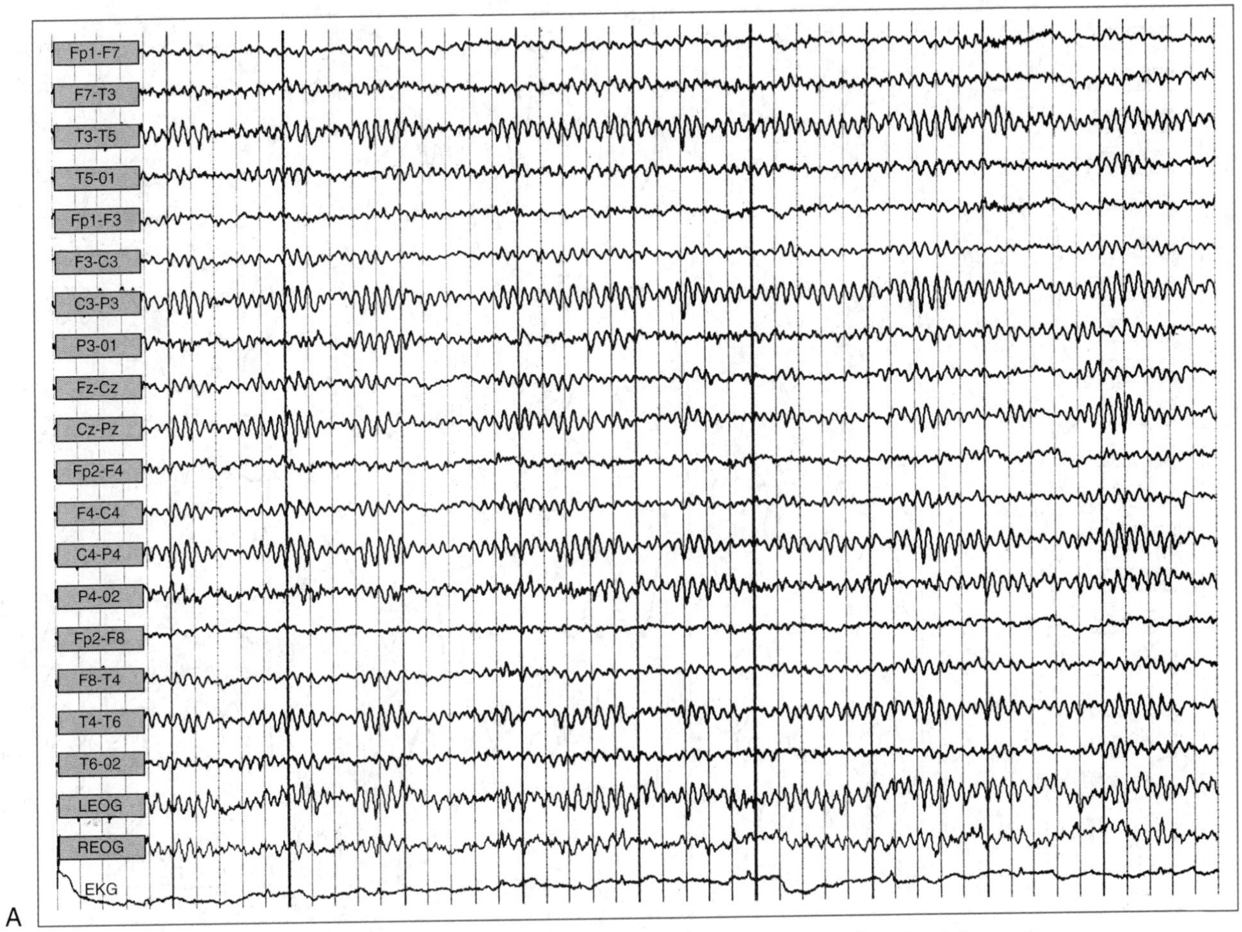

A

FIGURE 442–1 ■ Normal and abnormal EEGs. *A*, The EEG of a normal awake adult.

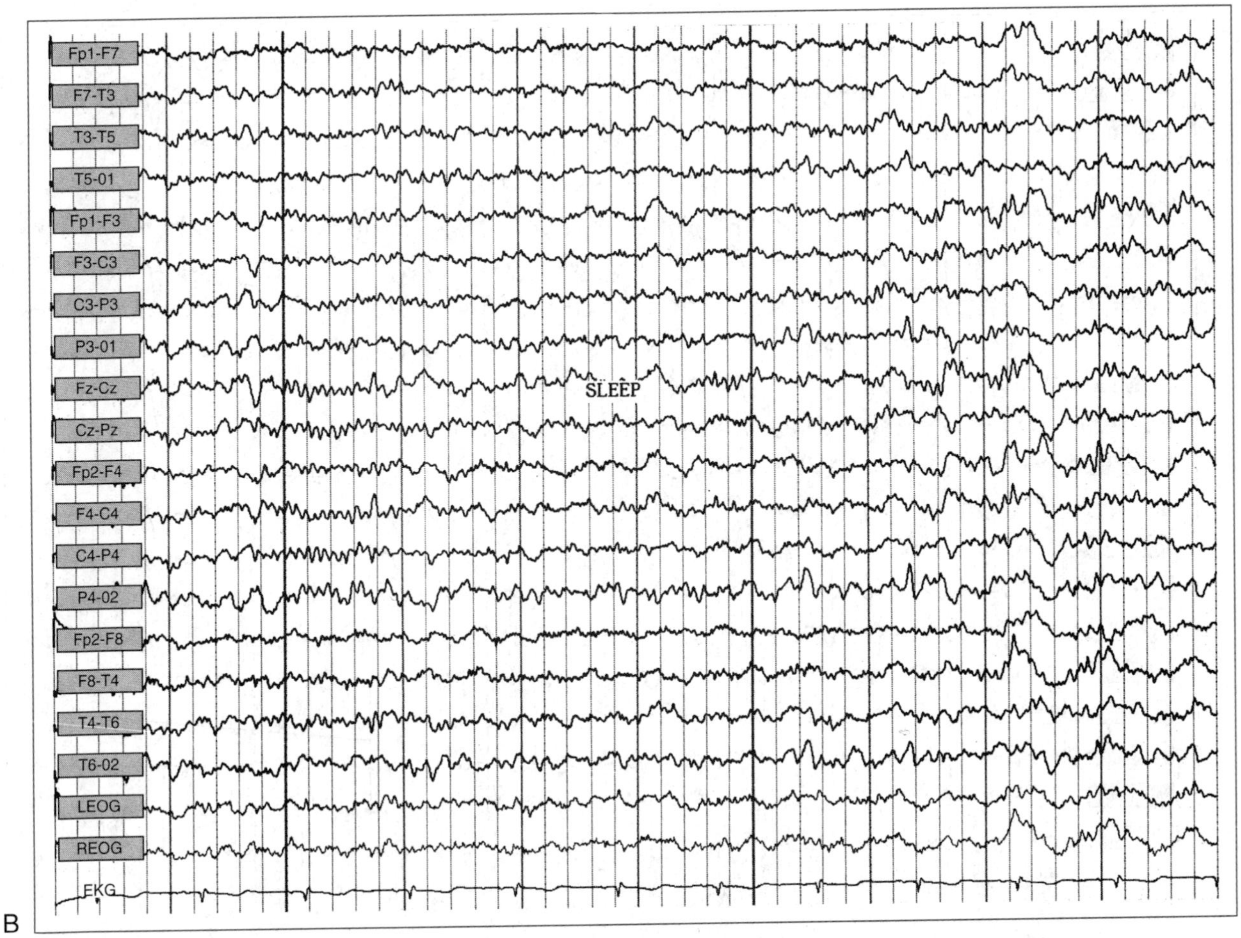

B

FIGURE 442–1 ■ *Continued. B*, Stage 2 sleep in a normal adult, demonstrating sleep spindles and K complexes.

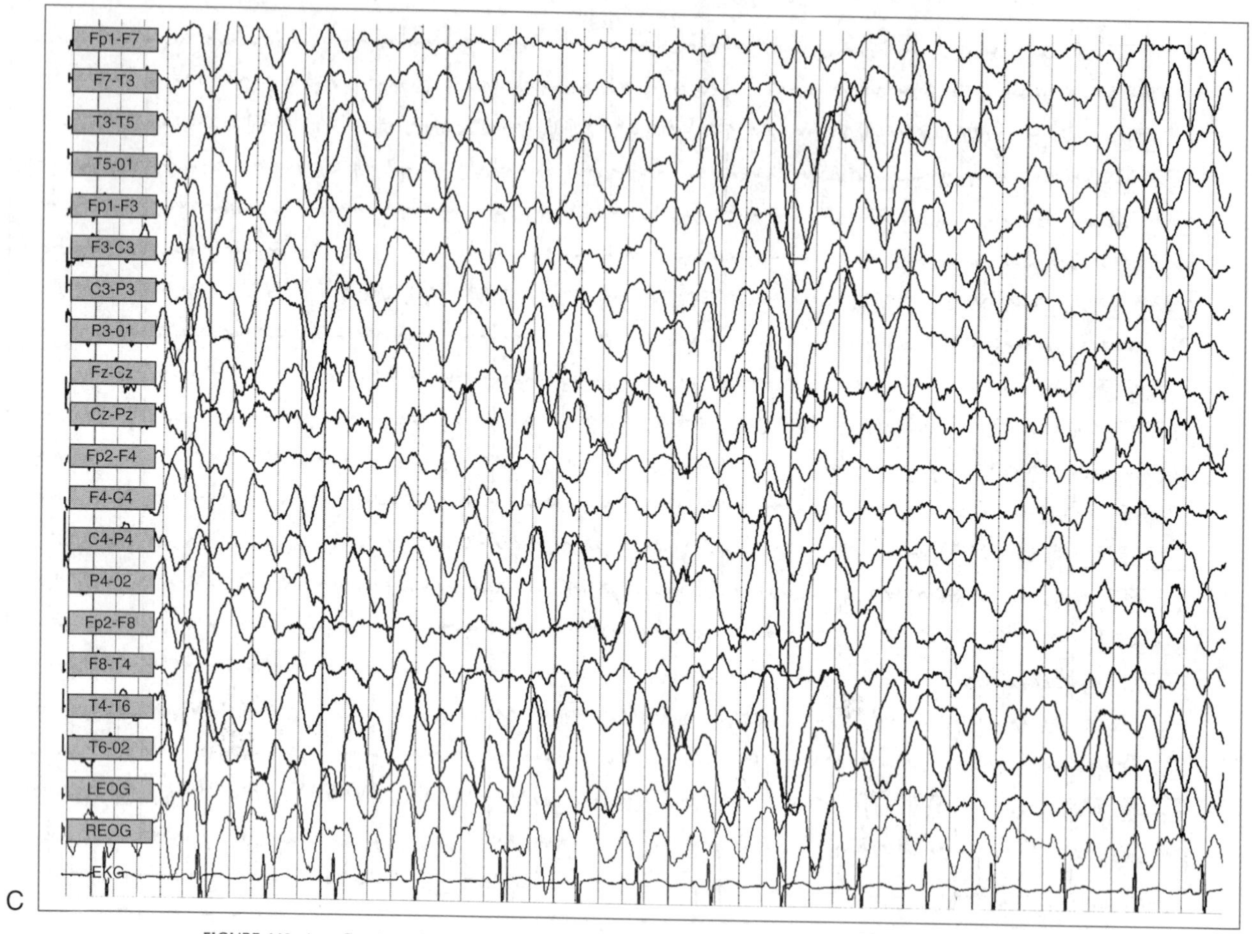

C

FIGURE 442–1 ■ *Continued. C,* Diffuse encephalopathy, with high-voltage, polymorphic delta waves.

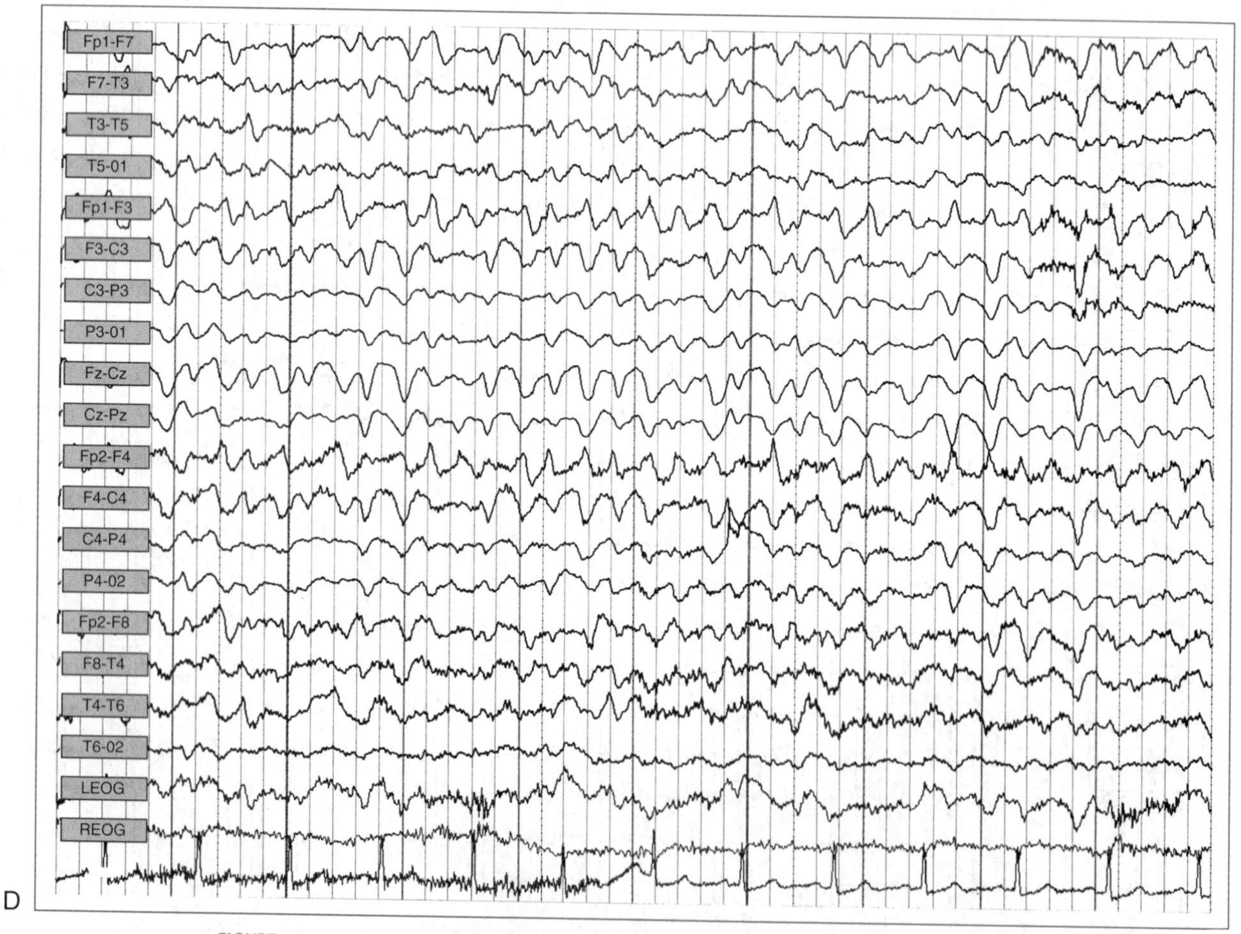

D

FIGURE 442–1 ■ *Continued. D,* Triphasic slow waves, a pattern seen in hepatic encephalopathy.

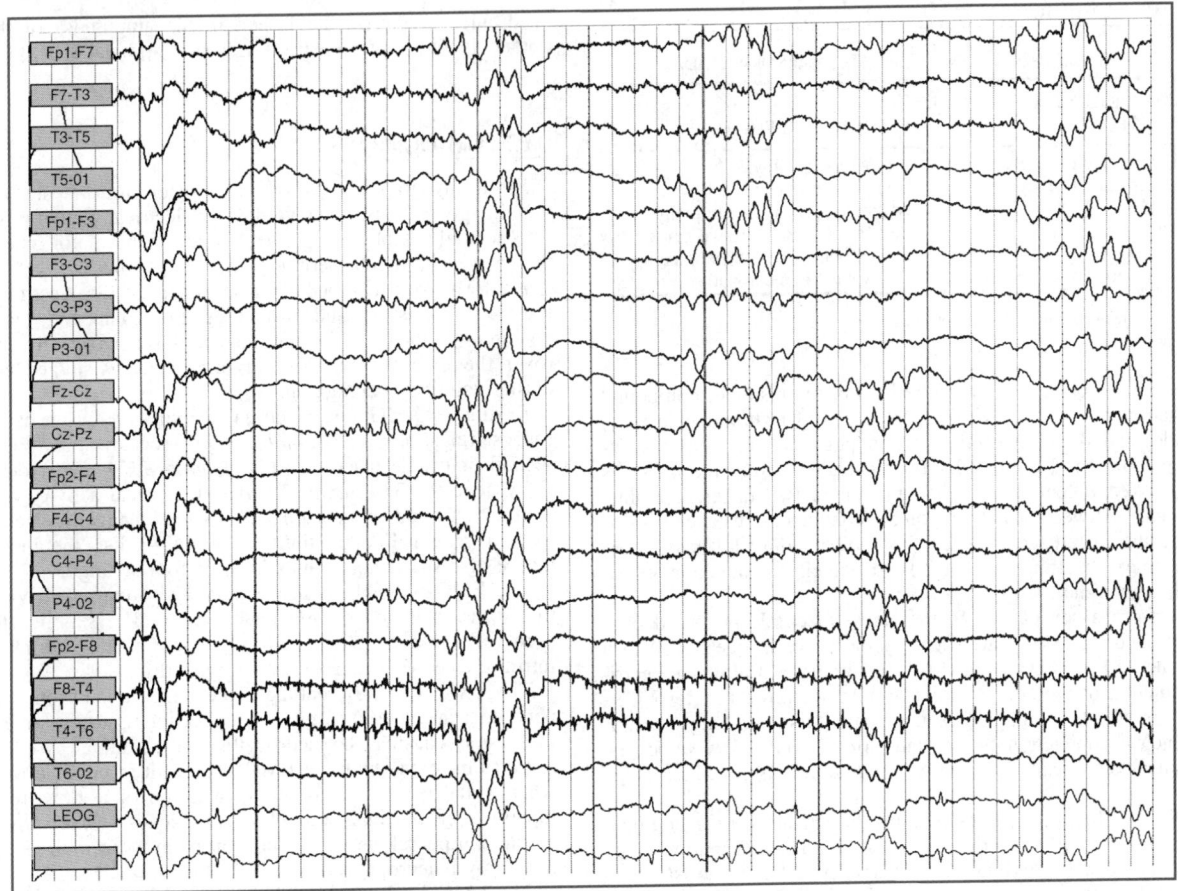

E

FIGURE 442-1 ■ *Continued. E,* Burst-suppression, a pattern seen in severe cerebral dysfunction.

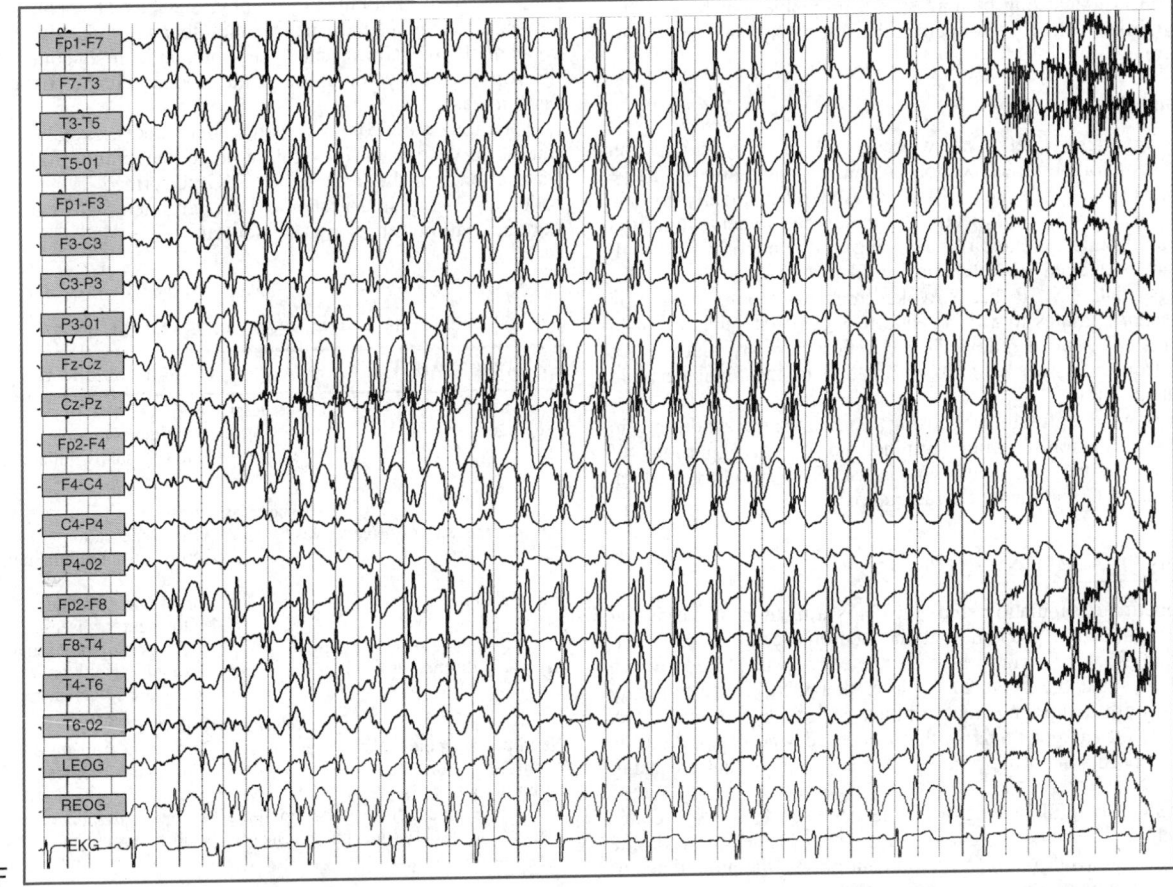

F

FIGURE 442-1 ■ *Continued. F,* A 3 Hz spike and wave activity, a pattern seen in absence epilepsy. In each record, channels 1 through 8 and 11 through 18 represent left- and right-sided bipolar electrode placements, respectively. Channels 9 and 10 represent midline bipolar electrode placements, and channels 19 and 20 represent the left and right electro-oculograms (eye movements). Each major horizontal division represents 1 second.

Table 442–3 ■ NERVE CONDUCTION STUDY ABNORMALITIES

NERVE CONDUCTION STUDY ABNORMALITY	CLINICAL CORRELATE
Reduced amplitude of CMAP	Axonal neuropathy
Prolonged terminal latency	Demyelinating neuropathy
	Distal compressive neuropathy
Conduction block	Severe focal compressive neuropathy
	Severe demyelinating neuropathy
Slowed conduction velocity	Demyelinating neuropathy

CMAP = compound muscle action potential.

tance proximal to the active electrode, and the resultant compound motor action potential (CMAP) is recorded. The terminal latency, amplitude, and duration of the evoked potential are measured directly, and the conduction velocity is calculated from the latencies of the evoked potentials with stimulation at two different points: the distance between the two points (conduction distance) is divided by the difference between the corresponding latencies (conduction time), resulting in a calculated velocity (conduction velocity = distance/time).

To perform a sensory NCS, the active electrode is placed over that portion of the skin innervated by the nerve in question, and a sensory nerve action potential (SNAP) is recorded following electrical stimulation of the nerve, similar to that noted for a motor NCS.

NCS abnormalities include reduced amplitudes, prolonged terminal latencies, conduction block, and slowed conduction velocities. The clinical significance of these abnormalities is noted in Table 442–3.

An NCS is helpful in documenting the existence of a neuropathy, quantifying its severity, and noting its distribution (i.e., whether it is distal, proximal, or diffuse). In addition, the NCS can provide information on the modality involved (i.e., motor versus sensory) and can give clues about the underlying pathologic process, whether the lesion is axonal or demyelinating. An NCS is also helpful in diagnosing compressive neuropathies, such as carpal tunnel syndrome, ulnar palsy, peroneal nerve palsy, and tarsal tunnel syndrome.

F Wave and H Reflex

The F wave and H reflex are ways of looking at the conduction characteristics for proximal portions of nerves, including the nerve roots. The F wave is a late CMAP evoked intermittently from a muscle by a *supramaximal* electrical stimulus to the nerve, and it is due to antidromic activation (backfiring) of α-motor neurons. F waves can be elicited from practically all distal motor nerves. The H reflex is a late CMAP that is evoked regularly from a muscle by a *submaximal* stimulus to a nerve, and it is due to stimulation of Ia afferent fibers (a spinal reflex). The H reflex can only routinely be obtained from calf muscles with stimulation of the tibial nerve in the popliteal fossa.

F waves are helpful in diagnosing Guillain-Barré syndrome, in which demyelination is often confined to proximal portions of nerves early in the course of the disease. The H reflex is often absent in patients with acute S1 radiculopathy.

REPETITIVE STIMULATION STUDY

The repetitive stimulation study (RSS) is a method of measuring electrical conduction properties at the neuromuscular junction. To perform an RSS, a surface recording electrode is placed over a muscle belly, and the nerve innervating that muscle is electrically stimulated with a supramaximal stimulus at a certain frequency. A series of electrical potentials is then recorded whose amplitude is roughly proportional to the number of muscle fibers that are being activated.

The RSS is helpful in diagnosing neuromuscular junction disorders, such as myasthenia gravis and the myasthenic syndrome (Lambert-Eaton syndrome). In myasthenia gravis, the amplitudes of the evoked potentials become progressively smaller with repetitive stimulation in clinically involved muscles. Clinically uninvolved muscles often do not demonstrate this decrement. In the myasthenic

syndrome, an *increment* is seen in the amplitudes of the evoked potentials with rapid repetitive electrical stimulation.

ELECTROMYOGRAPHY

Electromyography (EMG) is the recording and study of insertional, spontaneous, and voluntary electrical activity of muscle. This test allows physiologic evaluation of the motor unit, including the anterior horn cell, peripheral nerve, and muscle.

An EMG is performed by inserting a needle electrode into the muscle in question and evaluating the compound motor action potentials both visually (on the oscilloscope screen) and aurally (over the loudspeaker). Muscles are typically studied at rest and during voluntary contraction.

During an EMG, the electrical activity of muscle is studied in four settings: (1) *insertional activity* (occurring within the first second of needle insertion); (2) *spontaneous activity* (electrical activity at rest); (3) *voluntary activity* (electrical activity with muscle contraction); and (4) *recruitment pattern* (change in electrical activity with maximal contraction). Table 442–4 lists the clinical significance of EMG abnormalities in these four settings.

The EMG is helpful when evaluating patients with weakness, in that it can help to determine whether weakness is due to anterior horn cell disease, nerve root disease, peripheral neuropathy, or an intrinsic disease of muscle itself (myopathy).

The EMG can differentiate acute denervation from chronic denervation, and may thus give an indication as to the time course of the lesion causing the neuropathy. In addition, based on which muscles have an abnormal EMG pattern, it is possible to determine whether the neuropathy is due to a lesion of a nerve root (radiculopathy), the brachial or lumbosacral plexus (plexopathy), an individual peripheral nerve (mononeuropathy), or multiple peripheral nerves (polyneuropathy).

The EMG is also helpful in differentiating active (inflammatory) myopathies from chronic myopathies. The active myopathies include dermatomyositis, polymyositis, inclusion body myositis, and some forms of muscular dystrophy, such as Duchenne dystrophy. The chronic myopathies include the other muscular dystrophies, the congenital myopathies, and some metabolic myopathies. Myotonic dystrophy and myotonia congenita produce characteristic myotonic discharges.

It is important to note that it may take several weeks for a muscle to develop EMG signs of acute denervation following nerve transection. For this reason, an EMG performed in the acute setting following nerve injury should be interpreted with caution, and it may need to be repeated at a later date.

Table 442–4 ■ EMG ABNORMALITIES

EMG ABNORMALITY	CLINICAL CORRELATE
Insertional Activity	
Prolonged	Acute denervation
	Active (usually inflammatory) myopathy
Spontaneous Activity	
Fibrillations and positive waves	Acute denervation
	Active (usually inflammatory) myopathy
Fasciculations	Chronic neuropathies
	Motor neuron disease (rare fasciculations may be normal)
Myotonic discharges	Myotonic disorders
	Acid maltase deficiency
Voluntary Activity	
Neuropathic potentials: large-amplitude, long-duration, polyphasic potentials	Chronic neuropathies and anterior horn cell diseases
Myopathic potentials: small-amplitude, short-duration, polyphasic potentials	Chronic myopathies Neuromuscular junction disorders
Recruitment	
Reduced	Chronic neuropathies
Rapid	Chronic myopathies

EVOKED POTENTIALS

Evoked potentials are ways of measuring conduction velocities for sensory pathways in the central nervous system by means of computerized averaging techniques. Three types of evoked potentials are routinely performed: visual, brain-stem auditory, and somatosensory.

Pattern Reversal Visual Evoked Responses

The pattern reversal visual evoked response (PVER) measures conduction velocities for central visual pathways, in particular the optic nerves. To perform this test, EEG electrodes are placed over the occipital regions of the scalp and the patient is asked to look at the center of a black-and-white checkerboard screen with one eye patched for 3 minutes. The color of the checks alternates about twice per second, a process known as pattern reversal. The scalp potentials elicited by the pattern reversal are then recorded and signal-averaged by a computer. This signal averaging cancels the random EEG activity and differentially amplifies the evoked potential. A single waveform (P 100) is recorded for each eye, and the amplitude and latency are measured. The normal latency for the P 100 waveform is approximately 100 msec. A prolonged P 100 latency in one eye implies slowed conduction velocity in the optic nerve and suggests demyelination of that nerve.

PVER testing is helpful when multiple sclerosis is suspected clinically and it is necessary to document the presence of a second demyelinating lesion in the CNS that may not be clinically evident (Fig. 442–2).

Brain Stem Auditory Evoked Responses

The brain stem auditory evoked response (BAER) measures conduction velocities for central auditory pathways in the brain stem. EEG electrodes are placed over the posterior scalp, and a series of clicks at a frequency of 5 Hz are delivered to each ear separately for 3 minutes. The scalp potentials elicited by the clicks are then recorded and signal-averaged by a computer. This signal averaging cancels the random EEG activity and differentially amplifies the evoked potential. A series of five waves is recorded for each ear, and each wave corresponds to a different point in the central auditory pathway as noted in Table 442–5. The wave latencies for the right and left ears are compared, and a delay in any of the latencies suggests a lesion at that point in the central brain stem auditory pathway. BAER testing is helpful in diagnosing acoustic schwannoma. In patients with this lesion, only wave I is present, indicating a lesion in the distal acoustic nerve.

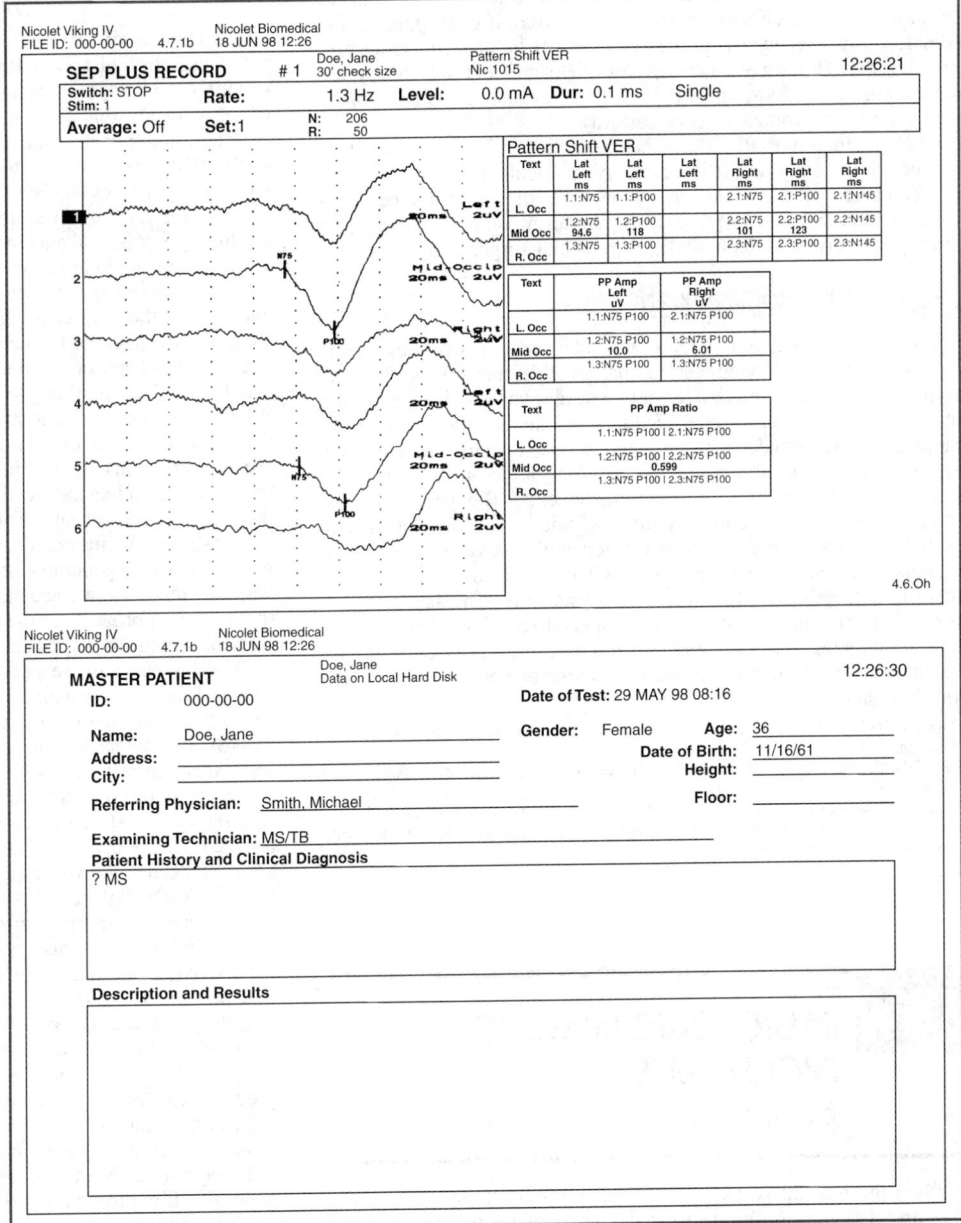

FIGURE 442–2 ■ Abnormal PVER in a patient with multiple sclerosis, demonstrating a prolonged P 100–wave latency with left eye stimulation, and suggesting a conduction defect in the left optic nerve. The top three channels represent right eye stimulation and the bottom three channels represent left eye stimulation. Each horizontal division represents 20 msec.

Table 442–5 ■ BAER WAVE GENERATORS

WAVE	LOCATION
I	Auditory nerve
II	Cochlear nucleus
III	Superior olivary nucleus
IV	Lateral lemniscus
V	Inferior colliculus

Somatosensory Evoked Responses

The somatosensory evoked response (SER) measures conduction velocities for central somatosensory pathways in the posterior columns of the spinal cord, brain stem, thalamus, and primary sensory cortex in the parietal lobes. To perform the SER, recording electrodes are placed over Erb's point (for medial nerve stimulation), popliteal fossa, and lumbar spine (for peroneal or tibial nerve stimulation), as well as over the posterior and lateral regions of the scalp. A series of electrical shocks at a frequency of 5 Hz are delivered to the median nerve (for an upper-extremity SER) or to the peroneal or tibial nerves (for a lower-extremity SER) for 3 minutes. The scalp potentials elicited by the electrical shocks are then recorded and signal-averaged by a computer. This signal averaging cancels the random EEG activity and differentially amplifies the evoked potential. A series of waves is recorded for each nerve stimulated, with each wave corresponding to a different point in the somatosensory pathways in the spinal cord, brain stem, and cerebral cortex. The wave latencies for the right and left limbs are compared, and a delay in any of the latencies suggests a lesion at that point in the somatosensory pathways.

SER testing, like PVER, is helpful when multiple sclerosis is suspected clinically and it is necessary to document the presence of a second demyelinating lesion in the CNS that may not be clinically evident. SER is also useful in monitoring spinal cord function intraoperatively in patients undergoing spinal surgery.

ELECTRONYSTAGMOGRAPHY (ENG)

Electronystagmography (ENG) accurately records eye movements and nystagmus following certain provocative maneuvers. To perform this test, disk electrodes are placed over the bridge of the nose and lateral to each outer canthus, and the electrical leads from these disks are connected to an oscilloscope. Because the cornea is electropositive and the retina is electronegative, these electrodes will accurately record lateral eye movements. The patient is first observed for spontaneous nystagmus with the eyes open and closed, and then for nystagmus evoked with lateral gaze, for nystagmus induced by hot and cold air instilled in the outer ears (caloric-induced), and for positional nystagmus. The latter is performed by rotating the patient in a specialized chair. Spontaneous nystagmus suggests a vestibular pathologic lesion, as does an imbalance in the nystagmus evoked by these maneuvers in the right and left ears.

Chiappa KH: Evoked Potentials in Clinical Medicine, 3rd ed. Philadelphia, Lippincott-Raven, 1997.
Daly DD, Pedley TA: Current Practice of Clinical Neurophysiology. New York, Raven Press, 1990.
Misulis KE: Spehlmann's Evoked Potential Primer. Boston, Butterworth-Heinemann, 1994.
Preston D, Shapiro B: Electromyography and Neuromuscular Disorders. Boston, Butterworth-Heinemann, 1998.

443 RADIOLOGIC IMAGING PROCEDURES

Robert I. Grossman

Over the past 20 years, medical imaging has rapidly evolved into its current pivotal position in the diagnosis of neurologic disorders.

With computed tomography (CT) and magnetic resonance imaging (MRI), the clinician can noninvasively identify most areas of the brain and spine that are responsible for the signs and symptoms that have brought the patient to seek medical attention. Conventional angiography is still often employed in the work-up of vascular causes of neurologic disease. Although less commonly performed, myelography is utilized in certain cases particularly where MRI is contraindicated. Ultrasound, magnetic resonance spectroscopy (MRS), positron emission tomography (PET), and single photon emission computed tomography (SPECT) have specific applications in the diagnosis of neurologic disease. For the physician to understand how to intelligently employ these imaging techniques requires understanding of the specificity and limitations of each modality. Although the cost of procedures is extremely important in the decisions about the work-up of neurologic problems, this chapter will only focus on what is generally considered to be the best modality to answer specific neurologic questions. In general, choosing the best test is the most cost-effective approach. Furthermore, the assumption is that most of the imaging modalities discussed in this chapter are readily available.

Table 443–1 indicates the strengths and weaknesses of commonly used imaging modalities. Table 443–2 is a basic algorithm for the work-up of frequently encountered neurologic problems.

CONTRAST AGENTS AND THE BLOOD-BRAIN BARRIER (BBB)

The concept of the BBB dates back to the 19th century when the noted bacteriologist Paul Ehrlich observed that dyes injected intravenously stained all organs of an animal except the brain. The BBB is responsible for the lack of significant enhancement in the normal brain parenchyma following contrast injection. Alterations of the BBB result in contrast enhancement in the brain parenchyma and leptomeninges. This is a nonspecific phenomenon. Any alteration of the BBB such as inflammation, infection, or neoplasm can produce contrast enhancement. Factors determining the degree of enhancement include the intravascular concentration of contrast, the interval between injection and imaging, the delivery of the contrast material to the region of the brain, the permeability of the lesion area, and the volume of the accumulation space.

Contrast agents or radionuclide tracers that cross an altered BBB can be used as markers to detect central nervous system lesions. Whether or not a patient should have a contrast enhanced image is determined by the differential diagnosis. Table 443–3 lists those clinical situations in which contrast is recommended and those in which an unenhanced scan may suffice. As with any algorithm there are many caveats. For example, no contrast is necessary to demonstrate an intraparenchymal hemorrhage. However, an enhanced study is generally necessary to determine if the hemorrhage was the result of a metastasis. Table 443–3 should be viewed as the initial approach to the imaging examination based upon the particular neurologic presentation.

Other issues with respect to the use of intravenous contrast are centered on the particular imaging modality. For CT, the debate focuses on the use of low-osmolar (generally nonionic—more expensive but safer) versus high-osmolar (ionic—less expensive but less safe) contrast agents. There are data to suggest that the number of severe contrast reactions (hypotensive shock, pulmonary edema, respiratory arrest, cardiac arrest, or convulsions) is substantially reduced (from 157 to 126 per 100,000) by using low-osmolar contrast agents; however, there appears to be no reduction in the risk of death (0.9 per 100,000 uses). Both high- and low-osmolar contrast agents are thus extremely safe. An additional consideration is that iodinated agents (both ionic and nonionic) are potentially nephrotoxic, particularly in patients with diseases or clinical states that predispose to kidney injury such as multiple myeloma, severe diabetes, dehydration, recent aminoglycoside exposure, anuria, hepatorenal syndrome, serum creatinine > 3 mg/dL, and administration of glucophage. The best approach is to use MRI in any patient predisposed to contrast nephropathy.

Specific indications for nonionic contrast agents include previous adverse reaction to an ionic agent, asthma, cardiac problems including congestive heart failure and pulmonary hypertension, severe general debilitation, and patient request.

The incidence of reaction is much lower with MRI contrast

Table 443–1 ■ STRENGTHS AND WEAKNESSES OF IMAGING MODALITIES

MODALITY	STRENGTHS	WEAKNESSES
Magnetic resonance imaging (MRI)	1. Noninvasive 2. No radiation 3. Multiplanar 4. Extremely sensitive 5. Soft tissue resolution 6. Safe contrast agent	1. Not as sensitive as CT for detection of subarachnoid hemorrhage and calcification. 2. Need cooperative patient 3. Time consuming
Magnetic resonance angiography (MRA)	1. Noninvasive 2. Very good screening tool for both extra and intracranial vascular disease 3. Readily repeatable 4. Safe 5. May be performed without contrast	1. Cooperative patient 2. Technically demanding 3. Can miss extracranial tandem lesions 4. May overestimate the degree of vascular stenosis 5. Cannot image distal vessels optimally without contrast 6. May miss small lesions such as aneurysms <3 mm
Proton magnetic resonance spectroscopy (MRS)	1. Localization of seizure focus 2. May be useful in helping to diagnose and classify dementias, such as Alzheimer's disease 3. May be useful in evaluation of brain tumors 4. May be useful for distinguishing radiation necrosis from recurrent tumor	1. Specificity of the technique has yet to be determined 2. Not fully available 3. Need particular expertise 4. Low resolution 5. Time consuming
Ultrasound	1. Fast 2. Easy to use 3. Can be performed at the bedside	1. Does not assess the vertebral arteries 2. Less sensitive and specific than MRA 3. Cannot visualize vessels in the upper neck and cranial base 4. Can misdiagnose high-grade lesions as occlusions Does not provide images of vessels
Transcranial Doppler (TCD)	1. Fast 2. Easy to use 3. Assesses vascular velocities quantitatively 4. Can assess cerebral vasospasm	
Computed tomography (CT)	1. Fast 2. Can easily detect acute intraparenchymal/subarachnoid hemorrhage and calcification 3. Easy to monitor patients 4. Excellent for studying bones and bone lesions	1. Less sensitive to parenchymal lesions than MR 2. Potential for significant contrast reaction
Conventional angiography	Best imaging modality for vascular diagnosis including aneurysms, vascular malformations, and vasculitis	1. Invasive 2. Small but significant risk of stroke and other complications 3. Significant expertise needed to perform procedure 4. Can be lengthy
Computed tomographic angiography	Less artifact than conventional angiography	1. Injection of intravenous iodine 2. Need to process data off line 3. Can only be performed once per session because of contrast injection
Conventional myelography	1. Good images of nerve roots and small osteophytic lesions 2. Accurate for bony stenosis 3. Can detect block of cerebrospinal fluid	1. Invasive with small risk of complications from lumbar puncture and installation of contrast 2. Does not image intramedullary lesions well 3. Has poor soft tissue resolution 4. Difficulty in imaging conus
CT myelography	Excellent for imaging nerve roots and detecting root compression from degenerative processes	Same as 1 and 2 above
Positron-emission tomography (PET)	1. Sensitive for diffuse brain pathologic processes 2. Can study diseases of the basal ganglia including Parkinson's disease and multisystem atrophy 3. Cerebral blood flow/volume 4. Functional imaging	1. Requires a cyclotron to generate radioisotopes with a short half-life 2. Lower resolution than MR/CT
Single photon emission tomography (SPECT)	1. Epilepsy 2. Sensitive to diffuse brain pathologic processes 3. Easier to implement than PET	Lower resolution than MR/CT

agents. MRI, barring any contraindications, is generally the modality of choice when a contrast-enhanced examination of the central nervous system is indicated. It usually requires a small dose (between 10 and 20 mL) and is not associated with contrast-induced nephropathy. The rate of severe anaphylactoid contrast reactions with gadolinium agents is reported to be between 0.0003 and 0.01%.

IMAGING TECHNIQUES

Magnetic Resonance Imaging (MRI)

ECHO PLANAR IMAGING (EPI). This is the fastest imaging technique available, acquiring entire images in less than 50 milliseconds. EPI has the ability to produce motion frozen "snapshots" of function such as in the heart and lung and can also be used to

Table 443–2 ■ IMAGING METHODOLOGIES FOR NEUROLOGIC PROBLEMS

NEUROLOGIC PROBLEM/DISORDER	IMAGING METHODOLOGY	COMMENT
Nonlocalized symptoms	MRI without and with contrast	Once a physician decides that an imaging study is warranted, MRI is the most sensitive modality for initial imaging
Suspected subarachnoid hemorrhage	CT without contrast	Best imaging method to detect subarachnoid hemorrhage
Suspected intracranial aneurysm (high probability, e.g, acute 3rd nerve palsy)	Conventional angiography	Definitive
Familial history of aneurysm or predisposing condition, e.g, polycystic kidney disease	MRA	Nonvasive and excellent at detecting aneurysms
Suspected stroke	CT	CT is fast and can detect whether or not there is an intraparenchymal hemorrhage or ischemic infarction
	Diffusion-weighted MRI	Fast and extremely sensitive for the diagnosis of acute stroke
Suspected neoplasm	MRI without and with contrast	Most sensitive imaging test
Suspected multiple sclerosis	MRI without and with contrast	Most sensitive imaging test
Suspected infection/inflammation	MRI without and with contrast	Most sensitive imaging test
Dementia work-up	MRI without contrast (rarely is contrast helpful)	The first test should be MRI to detect any lesion such as a frontal meningioma that might be responsible for dementia syndrome. Normal pressure hydrocephalus and multiinfarct dementia can also be easily demonstrated. PET and SPECT scanning may also be helpful
Seizures/epilepsy	MRI without and with contrast	The first test should be MRI to detect any lesion that is the seizure source. Other useful techniques may be SPECT, PET, and MRS
Head trauma	Acute-CT, MRI is additionally useful as well as for follow-up	CT is the fastest method to asses head trauma. MRI is more sensitive and specific for detecting diffuse axonal injury
Intrinsic spinal cord lesion	MRI without and with contrast	Most sensitive imaging modality for detection of spinal cord disease
Extradural spinal process	MRI without and with contrast and CT myelogram	For nonneoplastic disease, MRI without contrast is all that is required. CT myelogram is particularly useful for cervical spine degenerative disease.

study diffusion and perfusion as well as perform task-induced functional images of the brain. The rapidity of EPI imaging is also useful in uncooperative patients and in children. EPI images are not yet as high quality as spin echo or FSE images.

FLUID-ATTENUATED INVERSION RECOVERY (FLAIR) IMAGING. FLAIR is a pulse sequence that yields heavily T2 weighted images in which cerebrospinal fluid (CSF) is nulled (dark). FLAIR images have the ability to increase the conspicuity of lesions that are at the interface between brain (bright) and CSF (dark). With conventional spin echo or FSE images, cortical/subcortical or periventricular lesions are generally difficult to visualize because of the lack of contrast between high-intensity cortex and high-intensity CSF, whereas on FLAIR images such high-intensity lesions would be highlighted against the juxtaposed dark CSF.

DIFFUSION-WEIGHTED IMAGING. Diffusion of molecules implies a random process of molecular displacements caused by thermal agitation (Brownian motion). Random displacement of the molecules (i.e., diffusion) in the imaging voxel leads to echo attenuation. The phenomenon has been interpreted as follows: cellular swelling secondary to breakdown of the sodium-potassium pump

reduces the extracellular space. Since the dominant contribution to diffusion arises from extracellular water molecules, diffusion will become restricted with a net reduction in the diffusion coefficient. This results in an increase in the signal of diffusion-weighted images (i.e., less echo attenuation) and a very bright region seen on the image. Conversely, if apparent diffusion coefficient (ADC) maps are displayed, reduced diffusivity will show up as a zone of lower intensity. ADC maps are particularly helpful in situations where there are abnormalities in which the tissue has increased water content (e.g., an old infarct). This will produce an area of brightness (but not very bright) on the diffusion-weighted image that is termed "T2 shine-through." The ADC map, however, will correctly separate the acute lesion (lower intensity) from the old infarct (higher intensity).

The observation that the diffusivity is reduced in cerebral ischemia and stroke gave diffusion-weighted MRI a major impetus. It can detect cerebral ischemia within minutes of its onset in contrast to conventional MRI, which is not abnormal until a few hours after a cerebral infarction. Based upon diffusion characteristics, one can differentiate acute versus chronic infarction. This is sometimes dif-

Table 443–3 ■ INDICATIONS FOR UNENHANCED AND ENHANCED IMAGING (CT/MRI) IN DISEASES OF THE BRAIN AND SPINE

UNENHANCED IMAGES	ENHANCED
Hemorrhagic event	Infection
Ischemic event	Inflammation
Congenital anomaly	Neoplasia—either primary or metastatic
Head trauma	Process thought to involve the leptomeninges, nerve roots
Neurodegenerative disease	Seizures
Degenerative disease of the spine (not operated)	Intrinsic spinal cord lesions or suspected lesions in the subarachnoid space
Spinal cord trauma	Extradural spinal cord lesions from primary neoplastic or metastatic lesions
	Postoperative spine to separate scar from recurrent disk

ficult on standard T2-weighted or FLAIR images, since both acute and chronic infarction will be high intensity on both studies. Diffusion-weighted imaging is a rapid pulse sequence (either EPI or FSE) with a total imaging time of usually less than 2 minutes that demonstrates the presence of acute infarction (very bright) on MRI.

PERFUSION IMAGING. Perfusion imaging differs from diffusion imaging in that its aim is to characterize microscopic flow at the capillary level. Conventional radiologic techniques including catheter angiography, positron emission tomography (PET), and single photon emission computed tomography (SPECT) have been used for estimation of tissue perfusion, but MRI perfusion imaging may have higher spatial resolution and is of minimal invasiveness. Techniques include the use of either exogenous contrast agents (gadolinium) or magnetic labeling (spin tagging) of arterial water. There is some evidence that subtraction of perfusion from diffusion images can demonstrate an area of ischemic brain that is at risk for infarction following stroke (ischemic penumbra). In the near future, perfusion imaging may be used in combination with diffusion imaging to develop an algorithm for acute stroke treatment. In such a scenario, the larger the difference between the perfusion and diffusional abnormalities, the greater the need for acute intervention with thrombolytic agents. If there is no perfusional abnormality, or it is equal to the diffusional lesion, infarction has occurred and the probability that thrombolysis will be effective is low. At the present time, perfusion imaging is still undergoing study with more data needed before such an algorithm is validated and implemented.

BLOOD OXYGEN LEVEL DEPENDENCE (BOLD) EFFECT AND FUNCTIONAL IMAGING. The magnetic properties of blood can be exploited to produce contrast. This approach has recently been applied to the visualization of those regions of the brain involved in task activation such as sensory and motor cortices or the visual cortex. Intravascular deoxyhemoglobin is paramagnetic, hence susceptibility-induced gradients between the intra- and extracellular compartments cause spin dephasing and signal loss in a gradient echo sequence. Replacement of deoxyhemoglobin by oxyhemoglobin during increased blood flow, induced by task activation, lowers the extent of these gradients, thus causing a slight increase in signal intensity. Subtracting one data set from the other (one obtained with, the other without a stimulus) results in a difference image highlighting the zone of altered tissue oxygenation. Since the magnitude of the effect scales with field strength, operation at field strengths of 3 to 4 Tesla has been shown to offer substantial advantages. This effect is the basis of functional MRI (FMRI), which is being used to localize brain function in the study of neurologic disease as well as to study normal brain function. Examples of its application include identification of discrete motor and speech areas of the brain. FMRI is useful prior to surgical treatment of tumors or vascular malformations located in or near these eloquent regions of the brain.

INDICATIONS AND LIMITATIONS OF MRI. MRI is at present the most commonly used imaging modality for the central nervous system. Its power lies in the ability to produce multiplanar images of high resolution with considerable sensitivity to pathologic abnormalities. With few exceptions, it can answer most questions about the brain and spine that a clinician may pose. The exceptions to MRI as a first study are discussed below.

1. Rule out subarachnoid hemorrhage. In this clinical circumstance, the patient typically presents with "the worst headache of my life." Noncontrast CT is the fastest, most sensitive and specific imaging modality to demonstrate subarachnoid hemorrhage. The presence of subarachnoid blood on CT obviates the need for lumbar puncture in most patients with symptoms/signs consistent with this diagnosis. The next study following a positive CT is an angiogram, which is performed to find the cause of the bleeding. What should the clinician do in the face of a negative CT? This finding does not preclude subarachnoid hemorrhage. Situations in which this would occur include hemorrhage from a vascular lesion of the spinal cord, if the CT is performed very early with only a small amount of blood being present at the time of imaging, or if the subarachnoid blood disappears rapidly before imaging is performed. CT can be negative in approximately 2 to 5% of cases with definite subarachnoid hemorrhage. If there is clinical suspicion of subarachnoid hemorrhage and a negative CT, the next step is a lumbar puncture. Delayed lumbar puncture (12 hours) can detect xanthochromic blood pigments (formed after lysis of red blood cells) and distinguish true subarachnoid hemorrhage from a bloody traumatic lumbar puncture.

2. Detection of calcification. CT is more sensitive and specific with respect to calcification. This can be important in distinguishing certain lesions such as craniopharyngioma, retinoblastoma, chondrosarcoma, Sturge-Weber syndrome, toxoplasmosis, and tuberous sclerosis whose lesions have a strong tendency to calcify. In cases where the detection of calcium is important, noncontrast CT is necessary.

3. Questions of bony cortical abnormalities. Although MRI easily detects the fat in bone marrow, the cortex of bone is seen as a signal void. Thus, subtle cortical fractures are relatively easy to miss. After skull trauma, displaced shards of bone or cranial penetration by foreign matter may be difficult to visualize with MRI. In the setting of acute cranial/facial trauma, CT is useful to detect facial/skull fractures.

4. CT is also the first study in other clinical situations including acute head trauma or facial trauma, sinusitis, temporal bone problems such as inflammatory or congenital lesions, and the immediate postoperative craniotomy patient.

5. In situations where MRI cannot be performed. There are many circumstances in which MRI is relatively or absolutely contraindicated. These include patients with pacemakers, non-MRI-compatible vascular clips, and metallic implants or foreign bodies in the eyes. Agitated or uncooperative patients require sedation for MRI; such sedation may be contraindicated. With respect to specific appliances, it is best to check with the manufacturer regarding MRI compatibility. There are many instances in which there are questions regarding orbital metallic foreign bodies. Here anterior-posterior plain skull films can determine if there are metallic fragments that preclude MRI examination.

Magnetic Resonance Angiography (MRA)

MRA has great inherent appeal and is rapidly replacing conventional angiography. Conventional neuroangiography is an invasive procedure with a very low but significant morbidity and mortality. There are two different techniques used to generate MRA—time-of-flight (TOF) and phase contrast (PC) angiography. Once the imaging data are gathered, they may be processed by a number of display techniques. The one most commonly employed is termed maximal intensity projection (MIP), which finds the brightest pixels along a ray and projects them along any viewing angle. MIP is fast and insensitive to low-level variations in background intensity.

TOF. The principle is that protons not immediately exposed to an RF pulse (unsaturated spins) flow into the imaging volume and have higher signal than the partially saturated stationary tissue (which has lost signal secondary to the RF pulse). This is a T1 effect and has also been termed "flow related enhancement." The images can be acquired as individual slices (2D) acquisition or as a volume (3D) acquisition. In either case, flowing blood will appear bright. The 2D TOF techniques are very sensitive to slow or moderate flow (since flow-related enhancement is maximized), whereas 3D techniques are better than 2D MRA for rapid flow and have higher resolution.

PC. The principle of PC involves using bipolar flow-sensitizing gradients of opposite polarity to tag-moving spins, which are then identified as a result of their position change at the time of each gradient application. The operator chooses the flow velocities that the angiogram will be sensitive to, termed the VENC, which varies in neuroradiology from 30 cm/sec for arterial flow to 15 cm/sec for venous flow. Complex subtraction of data from the two acquisitions (one of which inverts the polarity of the bipolar gradient) will cancel all phase shifts except those due to flow. This technique provides excellent background suppression to differentiate flow from other causes of T1 shortening such as methemoglobin or fat. This technique is less often implemented but is useful in cases of suspected venous thrombosis to differentiate between flow and thrombus. In TOF images, both thrombus containing methemoglobin and flow can be bright whereas only flow will have signal on PC images.

CONTRAST-ENHANCED MRA (cMRA). A new and potentially important improvement in MRA has been the use of paramagnetic contrast enhancement in association with 3D TOF imaging. The procedure generally requires very fast pulse sequences combined with software that can time the intravenously administered bolus of contrast. This method has many advantages over the noncontrast approach. The use of paramagnetic vascular enhancement abolishes the signal loss secondary to spin saturation from slow flow or in-plane flow. The result is a high resolution image of the extra- or intracranial vessels including the aortic arch. Timing is critical, as enhancement of veins confounds the ability to demonstrate arterial anatomy. This methodology may be useful to exclude aneurysm or other vascular malformations and study the carotid bifurcation as well as the aortic arch. cMRA may also be able to delineate the exact location of large vessel intracranial vascular occlusions from embolic disease, the presence of intracranial stenosis, and the narrowing of vessels from vasculitis.

INDICATIONS AND LIMITATIONS OF MRA. MRA is the best noninvasive technique for evaluating the extracranial vasculature for the presence of a hemodynamically significant lesion of the carotid arteries, dissection of the vertebral and carotid arteries, extracranial traumatic fistula, extracranial vasculitis such as giant cell arteritis, or congenital abnormalities of the vessels such as fibromuscular disease. Intracranial MRA is used to detect aneurysms particularly in those cases where there is a relatively low probability of occurrence. This includes asymptomatic relatives of patients with aneurysms and patients with headache where concern is raised about aneurysm. Table 443–4 lists disorders that have been associated with aneurysm in which MRA could play a screening role. Other situations where MRA could provide information is in the follow-up of unruptured aneurysms, and in cases where a diagnosis is important but treatment or conventional angiography is contraindicated, or in the follow-up of treated aneurysm. Additional indications for MRA include the work-up of intracranial vasculitis, stroke, venous occlusive disease, congenital AVMs, vascular compression syndromes, and definition of the blood supply to vascular neoplasms. However, conventional angiography remains the definitive diagnostic modality for the diagnosis of intracranial aneurysm including those patients presenting with acute third nerve palsy. Small aneurysms, particularly less than 3 mm in diameter, can be missed by MRA.

The limitations of extracranial MRA include a tendency to overestimate stenosis, particularly if 2D TOF methods are used. It is also difficult to detect tandem lesions with MRA. Ulcerations in atheromas are poorly seen. If blood flow is very slow, MRA may falsely suggest occlusion in a vessel that has a high-grade stenosis. This distinction is important because surgery is often performed for stenosis but not indicated for total vascular occlusion. MRA requires that patients be cooperative, since motion degrades the images. In the case of carotid stenosis, only performing the extracra-

Table 443–4 ■ DISORDERS ASSOCIATED WITH INTRACRANIAL ANEURYSMS*

Autosomal dominant polycystic kidney disease (10% of asymptomatic patients)
Ehlers-Danlos syndrome type IV
Marfan's syndrome
Neurofibromatosis type 1
Fibromuscular dysplasia
Moya moya disease
Coarctation of the aorta
Takayasu's disease
Collagen vascular disease
Pseudoxanthoma elasticum
α-Glucosidase deficiency
α₁-Antitrypsin deficiency
Alkaptonuria
Anderson-Fabry disease
Homocystinuria
Familial idiopathic nonarteriosclerotic cerebral calcification syndrome
Hereditary hemorrhagic telangiectasia
Noonan's syndrome
Tuberous sclerosis
Werner's syndrome
3M syndrome

*Schievink WI, Schaid DJ, Rogers HM, et al: On the inheritance of intracranial aneurysms. (Review.) *Stroke* 25(10):2028–2037, 1994.

nial MRA can preclude diagnosis of additional vascular lesions such as an aneurysm or AVM in the brain. Additionally, patients with a history of transient ischemic attacks or recent neurologic deficits may have unrecognized embolic occlusions, which are difficult to detect with intracranial MRA because of poor visualization of the distal vessels. Surgery in such cases can be associated with hemorrhagic complications.

MRA images, particularly of distal intracranial vessels, are often difficult to interpret. Vasculitis and other diseases of distal vessels require careful examination of all images, preferably after the image is segmented so that each vessel can be viewed independently without overlap of other vessels. In comparison with CT angiography (see below), MRA generally involves no or low doses of contrast agents and no radiation; MRA can be repeated multiple times (if no contrast is used) during the same examination, and has a larger field of view that commonly includes the origin of the posterior inferior cerebellar artery.

Magnetic Resonance Spectroscopy (MRS)

MRS, currently primarily proton MRS, offers the potential ability to identify chemical compounds within the central nervous system. It is being increasingly applied to the study of brain diseases, including brain neoplasms, Alzheimer's disease, HIV infection, epilepsy, and multiple sclerosis. The proton MRI spectrum is characterized by at least three peaks representing the compounds creatine (CR), which is associated with cellular energy metabolism, choline (CHO), associated with cell membranes, and N-acetyl aspartate (NAA), which is considered to be a marker of neuronal integrity. Lactate is not detectable in the MRS of normal brain but may be seen with inflammation and infarction. Other peaks may be found in proton spectra, particularly those acquired at short echo times, and these include inositol, the methyl group of lipids, and peaks associated with GABA, glutamate, and glutamine. The appearance of the latter peaks in the adult MRI spectrum may be associated with pathologic conditions. MRI spectra are acquired using primarily one of two volume localization techniques: point-resolved spectroscopy (PRESS) and stimulated echo acquisition mode (STEAM). Spectroscopic images of metabolites may also be acquired using methods that are hybrids of conventional spectroscopy and imaging techniques. Analysis is carried out to obtain either relative metabolite measurements (peak area ratios) or absolute metabolite concentrations with the use of a variety of techniques. Decreased NAA has been associated with neuronal loss, and this finding can be useful in the localization of temporal lobe epilepsy and for the diagnosis of HIV encephalopathy. Increased CHO levels may indicate myelin breakdown, inflammation, or neoplasia and have the potential to detect abnormal membrane metabolism. MRS is a rapidly expanding technique with a promise of increasing the diagnostic specificity of MRI. It also may provide a surrogate marker for monitoring treatment trials for neoplasia or multiple sclerosis.

Computed Tomography (CT)

CT employs a highly collimated x-ray beam that passes through the patient and is differentially absorbed by tissue. The photons are detected and imaged, and contrast is dependent upon the differential absorption of the photons by the tissue being studied. The scale [in *Hounsfield units* (HU)] for CT absorption ranges from +1000 to −1000 with zero being water and −300 to −1000 representing fat. White matter and gray matter are in the 30 to 50 HU range, hematomas 50 to 80 HU, and calcification 150 HU. These values can vary somewhat with different manufacturers' equipment. In axial CT, each revolution of the gantry around the patient produces one data set or slice. The patient is then incremented in the scanner, and another slice is produced. The latest CT technology employs the x-ray tube rotating continually (helical CT) as the table moves through the x-ray scan field allowing a continuous volume of transaxial data to be rapidly acquired. In this situation, the term "pitch" is used to specify the distance the table moves in millimeters for every rotation of the tube. "Pitch factor" is the pitch divided by the slice thickness. This is a unitless term. A continuous set of volume data is produced that provides the ability to perform rapid imaging (scan times of less than 1 second per slice) and slice thickness of 1 millimeter. The x-ray dose to the patient is generally less than 3 rads (to the imaged volume).

INDICATIONS AND LIMITATIONS. CT is a fast alternative to

MRI for imaging of the brain. It is not quite as sensitive for parenchymal and leptomeningeal processes, particularly white matter lesions such as seen in multiple sclerosis, but is better for detecting subarachnoid hemorrhage, calcification, and cortical bone abnormalities. CT is used in patients in whom MRI is contraindicated (e.g., metallic foreign body, pacemaker).

Computed Tomographic Angiography (CTA)

CTA is emerging as an alternative to MRA for imaging both the extracranial and intracranial blood vessels. It requires the placement of a small catheter usually in the antecubital vein with injection of approximately 75 mL of iodinated contrast material. After a short delay following contrast injection, imaging commences and a 3D data set acquired. Computer post-processing is necessary for MIP images and to exclude the bony base of the skull structures. CTA is fast and noninvasive but does require the injection of intravenous iodinated contrast. It is probably as good as MRA at detecting aneurysms 3 mm or larger (i.e., those having the greatest likelihood of rupture). CTA is (1) fast (less than 32 seconds); (2) less motion-sensitive than MRI; (3) without the flow-related effects seen in MRA; (4) can easily visualize slow flow or turbulent flow in aneurysms (particularly large aneurysms); (5) involves no MRI compatibility problems with intubated patients or aneurysm clips; and (6) can present a multiplanar view of the vascular anatomy from any perspective. It can also detect calcification in the neck of an aneurysm, provide bony surgical landmarks, and detect intraluminal thrombus, all of which may be useful for planning treatment.

The limitations of CTA include (1) risks of intravenous iodinated contrast injection; (2) the length of time for postprocessing of data (45 or more minutes); (3) exposure to radiation; (4) vessels at the base of the skull may be obscured by enhancement in the cavernous sinus or bone at the base of the skull; (5) in subarachnoid hemorrhage, the high density of blood can obscure the bleeding aneurysm; (6) the acquisition volume (usually less than 4 cm) can miss the take-off of the posterior inferior cerebellar arteries unless specifically directed to this area (MRA may have similar problems); (7) aneurysm clips in the postoperative patient produce artifacts that may obscure anatomic detail (MRA has similar problems); (8) calcifications in the walls of the vessels, in the anterior clinoid processes, and other areas can produce artifacts; (9) there is only one opportunity to perform the study as opposed to MRA, which can be repeated; and (10) the 3D reconstruction process is operator-dependent. At present, CTA is employed as a screening tool, mostly to rapidly show aneurysms in symptomatic patients and to screen asymptomatic patients at risk for cerebral aneurysms.

Conventional Angiography

Arterial catheter angiography is the definitive imaging modality for vascular lesions of the brain and great vessels of the neck. In most cases, the catheter is passed via the femoral artery selectively into the great vessels of the neck and their branches. In many institutions, images are performed by digital subtraction as opposed to conventional film-screen methods, which, in combination with low osmolar contrast and currently employed catheters, are safe and produce high-quality images of vascular structures. The incidence of all complications for femoral artery catherizations is approximately 8.5% with the range of permanent complications (the most significant of which is stroke) from 0.1% to 0.33%, a 2.6% incidence of transient complications, and a 4.9% incidence of local complications.

Interest in the detection of extracranial occlusive carotid artery disease has been accelerated because of the reported results in two recent large trials for the treatment of symptomatic and asymptomatic patients. The North American Symptomatic Carotid Endarterectomy Trial (NASCET) and Asymptomatic Carotid Atherosclerosis Study (ACAS) confirmed the benefit of carotid endarterectomy in patients with high-grade carotid stenosis (>60%). Hemodynamically significant narrowing occurs when the diameter of the vessel is decreased by 50 to 60%.

One issue with respect to carotid stenosis is the method of measurement. In the NASCET study, the per cent stenosis was measured as:

1—the diameter of lumen at the point of the maximal stenosis divided by the diameter of the lumen of the normal artery distal to the stenosis × 100%

while in the European Carotid Surgery Trial, the per cent stenosis was measured as:

1—the diameter of lumen at the point of the maximal stenosis divided by the estimated "true" lumen diameter at the point of stenosis

Both methods have their strengths and weakness. The former method may underestimate stenosis when the distal lumen narrows as a result of the severe proximal stenosis that limits volume flow. The latter method has problems because the observer must extrapolate what is thought to be the true lumen.

Depending upon the beliefs of surgeons and physicians caring for the particular patient, extracranial occlusive vascular disease may be worked-up solely with noninvasive imaging techniques including ultrasound and MRA, or noninvasive imaging may be followed by catheter angiography. In ambiguous or problematic cases, catheter angiography is usually performed.

Conventional angiography is routinely employed for the diagnosis of aneurysm, arteriovenous malformation, and vasculitis. Careful technique is required to make the diagnosis. Each vessel must be scrutinized separately. In patients in which aneurysm has to be ruled out, all intracranial vessels must be injected. Injection of one vertebral with excellent reflux down the other may be adequate, but care must be taken to identify the contralateral posterior inferior cerebellar artery origin as well as to ascertain whether or not there is visualization of that entire vessel. Depending upon the age of the patients and the amount of atherosclerosis, the catheter tip can be placed in the common or internal carotid artery.

In cases of subarachnoid hemorrhage (the majority of which are the result of rupture of intracranial aneurysms), the clinician must ascertain whether or not there is an aneurysm, and, if there is not, what other process can explain the presence of subarachnoid hemorrhage. Identification of the aneurysm is critical. Rebleeding occurs in approximately 20% of patients within 2 weeks of initial hemorrhage, in 30% by 1 month, and in 40% by 6 months. Rebleeding is associated with a mortality in excess of 40%, mandating a meticulous search for an aneurysm. In the absence of finding an aneurysm or intracerebral vascular malformation it is important to (1) assess the extracranial vessels for a dural malformation; (2) consider spinal angiography to rule out a spinal malformation as a source of the subarachnoid hemorrhage; (3) ascertain whether the patient has vasculitis; (4) perform external carotid angiography to search for a dural malformation which can rarely produce subarachnoid hemorrhage; and (5) repeat the study in 1 to 2 weeks. If an aneurysm is found, it must be determined if it is the source of the bleed and if there exist any other lesions associated with the aneurysm such as arterial spasm, extracranial occlusive vascular disease, vasculitis, AVM, etc.

Carotid Ultrasound/Transcranial Doppler

Ultrasound scanning uses sound waves to image structures or measure the velocity and direction of blood flow. In infants, it provides a rapid global assessment of the brain and is used for the detection of germinal matrix or other intraparenchymal hemorrhage, extracerebral collections, congenital abnormalities including hydrocephalus, Dandy Walker cysts, agenesis of the corpus callosum, anencephaly, holoprosencephaly, and other malformations. It has been used in utero to detect hydrocephalus, anencephaly, and spinal cord abnormalities including spina bifida and meningomyelocele in patients with elevated α-fetoprotein levels. Intraoperative ultrasonography is used to localize lesions in the brain and the spine and is also used as a guide for ventricular shunt placement.

Color-coded Doppler ultrasound can depict the residual lumen of the extracranial carotid artery more accurately than conventional duplex Doppler. However, the results from color-coded Doppler ultrasound examination can be influenced by the skills and bias of the operator. Problems include distinguishing high-grade stenosis from occlusion, calcified plaques interfering with visualization of the vascular lumen, inability to show lesions of the carotid near the skull base, difficulty with tandem lesions, and inability to image the origins of the carotid or the vertebral arteries. In the NASCET study, Doppler measurements were 59.3% sensitive and 80.4% specific for the detection of stenosis greater than 70%. A battery of ultrasonic noninvasive carotid studies including indirect tests monitoring the superficial and deep orbital circulations and direct studies using imaging and function have been advocated to increase the accuracy particularly in significant vascular disease.

Transcranial Doppler ultrasound is a noninvasive means used to evaluate the basal cerebral arteries through the infratemporal fossa. It evaluates the flow velocity spectrum of the cerebral vessels and can provide information regarding the direction of flow, the patency of vessels, focal narrowing from atherosclerotic disease or spasm, and cerebrovascular reactivity. It can determine adequacy of middle cerebral artery flow in patients with carotid stenosis and evidence of embolus within the proximal middle cerebral artery. It is very useful in the detection of cerebrovascular spasm following subarachnoid hemorrhage or after surgery, and can rapidly assess the results of intracranial angioplasty or papaverine infusions to treat vasospasm.

Nuclear Medicine Techniques: Positron Emission Tomography (PET) and Single-Photon Emission Computed Tomography (SPECT)

Nuclear medicine methodology uses a variety of radioactive substances that can be localized by a crystal scintillation device (gamma camera). PET employs positron-emitting isotopes that are manufactured in a cyclotron while SPECT uses an iodinated radiotracer, technetium 99m, or other radiotracers. These have been advocated for diagnosis of a wide variety of neurologic diseases. They are most useful in diagnosing disorders that do not possess easily identifiable anatomic correlates or are associated with diffuse disease throughout the brain. These techniques image function predominantly and anatomy to a lesser degree. In nuclear medicine, thallium imaging is at present being advocated to distinguish lymphoma (hot) from toxoplasmosis (not hot) in AIDS. Indium can be instilled into the subarachnoid space to aid in detecting and localizing cerebrospinal fluid leaks from surgery, trauma, or congenital abnormalities. It has also been used to aid in the diagnosis of normal pressure hydrocephalus.

Both PET and SPECT have been used to aid in making the diagnosis of Alzheimer's disease. The finding that has been emphasized is hypoperfusion in the temporal-parietal regions. There is a great deal of variability with respect to results, with the reported sensitivity of SPECT ranging from 64 to 96% while in severely demented patients the sensitivity has been reported as 95% or greater. FDG PET studies have revealed that the cerebral metabolic rate of glucose (CMRGLc) was decreased 20 to 30% in Alzheimer's disease when compared with normal healthy controls. Technetium-99m hexamethylpropyleneamine oxime (99mTc-HMOAO) SPECT and FDG PET have been also applied to study other degenerative dementias including Pick disease and Creutzfeldt-Jacob disease. CT and MRI are often normal, even with advanced disease, and when abnormal are quite nonspecific, revealing only atrophy. It has been reported that altered metabolic activity that can be detected by either PET or SPECT precedes neuronal loss and may even occur before electrical cortical changes.

These modalities have been applied to lateralizing temporal lobe epilepsy. Ictal SPECT is both sensitive and specific but is dependent upon the temporal relationship of the ictus and study. For the best information, interictal and ictal SPECT should be compared using computer-assisted techniques. PET is also very sensitive but is not widely available. Recent reports suggest that proton MRI spectroscopy is more sensitive than PET for lateralizing temporal lobe seizures.

Early work with [18F] 2-fluoro-2-D-deoxyglucose (FDG) PET suggested that it might be possible to differentiate recurrent tumor from radiation necrosis. Recent reports indicate that the ability of FDG PET to differentiate the two lesions is limited with both false-positive and false-negative results producing low sensitivity and specificity.

PET/SPECT have also been used to diagnose movement disorders such as Parkinson's disease and Huntington's disease. The results of these studies are controversial.

SPINE IMAGING

MRI is generally the best modality for imaging the spinal cord and the spaces surrounding it. The approach for intramedullary (within the spinal cord) and extramedullary intradural lesions should consist of multiplanar images including T2 and post-contrast pulse sequences. The diagnosis of spinal cord compression from extradural metastatic lesions, trauma, or osteoporotic compression is also best performed by the same imaging approach.

Although plain films and CT of the spine are usually the first study ordered in suspected spinal trauma, MRI is the best method for studying those cases in which the spinal cord may have sustained injury. It can detect both intrinsic damage to the spinal cord and extrinsic compression from bone and disk fragments as well as ligamentous injury. CT with multiplanar reconstruction is used in addition to plain cervical spine films to identify difficult anatomic regions not well visualized by plain films including C1–C2, C6–C7, and C7–T1.

MRI is the first approach for presumed vascular lesions of the spinal cord including small dural malformations that result in venous hypertension. However, the definitive study for vascular lesions of the spinal cord is spinal angiography. This technique must be performed in a meticulous fashion to precisely demonstrate the exact vascular supply to the lesion.

Thoracic and lumbar degenerative disk disease is also easily imaged with axial and sagittal T1 and T2 weighted MRI sequences. Contrast is necessary only in the postoperative patient with persistent problems ("failed back") to separate scar, which usually enhances, from recurrent or residual disk, which usually does not avidly enhance. Although MRI is generally the most efficient method to study cervical spine degenerative disease, it may not be the most sensitive. CT myelography provides the best images of degenerative spine lesions such as small osteophytes impinging upon nerve roots. The disadvantages are the need for intrathecal contrast injection and the use of x-rays.

Multiplanar MRI is also excellent for studying lesions that affect the peripheral nerves including the brachial plexus.

Plain Films

Plain skull films are rarely, if ever, indicated and should never be ordered as the primary imaging study. They provide little useful unambiguous information. When imaging is indicated, a CT or MRI examination should be ordered. If paranasal sinus studies are needed, CT performed in the coronal planes is the study of choice. Plain films of the spine are also less informative than MRI or CT; however, they aid in triage for acute spinal cord trauma by assessment of bony fractures and dislocations. Passive flexion-extension plain films provide some measure of the stability following cervical spine injury, although MRI imaging can precisely demonstrate the ligamentous injury.

Interventional Neuroradiology

Although the techniques used in this area of special interest are beyond the scope of this chapter, it is important to understand that there is a broad spectrum of neurologic vascular diseases that may be amenable to treatment by endovascular surgery. These techniques enable temporary occlusions of vessels to determine if the patient can tolerate removal of vessels that are encased by tumor. This is particularly useful in head and neck tumors. One early and important application of endovascular intervention is the occlusion of carotid-cavernous sinus fistula by detachable balloons. This technique generally preserves the parent vessel and taponades the fistulous tract.

This alternative to conventional surgery is being used to occlude intracranial aneurysms by packing them with tiny balls of wire (coiling) via an endovascular catheter. Many varieties of vascular malformations in the brain and spinal cord may be occluded using an endovascular approach with occlusive agents or detachable balloons. Vascular tumors such as meningiomas may be treated by preoperative embolization to decrease intraoperative blood loss. Intracranial vascular spasm following subarachnoid hemorrhage may be reduced by balloon dilatation of the involved vessels or local infusion of papaverine. Intra- and extracranial arterial stenosis may be dilated with a balloon catheter and a vascular stent then positioned in the vessel to prevent restenosis. Vascular stenting has also been used in vascular dissection and in the treatment of pseudoaneurysm. Such endovascular therapies are rapidly evolving. Their use relative to traditional approaches is under intensive study.

Atlas SW: Magnetic Resonance Imaging of the Brain and Spine, 2nd ed. Philadelphia, Lippincott–Raven, 1996.
Grossman RI, Yousem DM: Neuroradiology, The Requisites. St. Louis, Mosby–Year Book, 1994.
Osborn AG: Diagnostic Neuroradiology. St. Louis, Mosby–Year Book, 1994.

■ DISORDERS OF CEREBRAL FUNCTION

444 COMA AND DISORDERS OF AROUSAL

Roger P. Simon

Coma is a sleep-like state from which the patient cannot be aroused. It is sleep-like in that the eyes are closed and remain closed in the face of vigorous stimulation. A poorly responsive state in which the eyes are open and an agitated confused state or delirium do not constitute coma but may represent early stages of the same disease processes and should be investigated in the same manner.

Consciousness requires an intact and functioning brain stem reticular activating system and its cortical projections. The reticular formation begins in the midpons and ascends through the dorsal midbrain to synapse in the thalamus for its thalamocortical connections. Knowledge of this anatomic substrate provides the short list of regions to be investigated while searching for a structural cause of coma; a brain stem or bihemispheric dysfunction must satisfy these anatomic requirements or it is not the cause of the patient's unconsciousness. In addition to structural lesions, meningeal inflammation, metabolic encephalopathy, or seizure satisfies the anatomic requirements and completes the differential diagnosis of the patient in coma.

PATHOPHYSIOLOGIC CHARACTERISTICS

MENINGEAL IRRITATION. Meningeal irritation caused by infection or blood in the subarachnoid space is among the most important early considerations in coma evaluation as it is treatable and (especially with purulent meningitis) may not be diagnosed by computed tomography (CT) scans (see Table 444–1). The mechanism by which inflammatory processes in the subarachnoid space result in unconsciousness is incompletely understood. A combination of the release of humoral factors, including interleukin 1, tumor necrosis factor, and arachidonic acid metabolites (promoting blood-brain barrier permeability); vasogenic cerebral edema; altered cerebral blood flow; and perhaps an increase in neurotoxic excitatory amino acid neurotransmitters may all be causative. Later, vasculitis and thrombosis of meningeal veins result in a diffuse cortical and white matter necrosis.

HEMISPHERIC MASS LESIONS. Hemispheric mass lesions result in coma either by expanding across the midline laterally to compromise both cerebral hemispheres or by impinging on the brain stem to compress the rostral reticular formation. These processes have been referred to as *lateral herniation* (lateral movement of the brain) and *transtentorial herniation* (vertical movement of hemispheric content across the cerebellar tentorium, which separates the hemispheric compartment from the brain stem and posterior fossa). Although horizontal or vertical movement of the brain in isolation may occur to produce coma, a combination of these processes is the most common cause. At the bedside, however, clinical signs of an expanding hemispheric mass evolve in a level-by-level rostral-caudal manner (Figure 444–1). Hemispheric lesions of adequate size to produce coma are readily seen on CT scan.

BRAIN STEM MASS LESIONS. Brain stem mass lesions produce coma by directly compromising the reticular formation. As the pathways for lateral eye movements (the pontine gaze center, medial longitudinal fasciculus, and oculomotor—third nerve—nucleus) traverse the reticular activating system, impairment of reflex eye movements is often the critical element in diagnosis. A comatose patient without impairment of reflex lateral eye movements does not have a mass lesion compromising brain stem structures in the posterior fossa. CT scanning is not able to detect some lesions in this region. This aspect of the examination is therefore critical to rapid diagnosis. Posterior fossa lesions may compromise cortical function by upward herniation across the cerebellar tentorium or by blocking of cerebral spinal fluid flow from the lateral ventricles, resulting in the dangerous state of non-communicating hydrocephalus.

METABOLIC ABNORMALITIES. Metabolic abnormalities characterize syndromes caused by the presence of *exogenous toxins* (drugs) or *endogenous toxins* (organ system failure), resulting in diffuse dysfunction of the nervous system without localized signs such as hemiparesis or unilateral pupillary dilatation. A diagnosis of "metabolic encephalopathy" indicates that the examiner has found no focal anatomic features in examination or neuroimaging study results to explain coma but does not state that a specific metabolic cause, such as hypernatremia, has been established. Such global impairment of function is particularly typical of endogenoustoxins. Drugs have a predilection for affecting the reticular formation in the brain stem and producing paralysis of reflex eye movement on examination.

SEIZURES. Generalized seizures produce diffuse abnormal electrical discharges throughout the reticular formation and cortex, thus satisfying the anatomic criteria for coma. In the late stages of status epilepticus motor movements may be subtle even though seizure activity is continuing throughout the brain. Once seizures stop, the abnormal electrical activity is followed by a state of electrical inhibition, which may be prolonged. This so-called post-ictal state produces coma and if the inciting seizures are not witnessed can also be a cause of unexplained coma.

DIAGNOSTIC APPROACH

The history, if obtainable, may be particularly helpful. A premonitory headache supports a diagnosis of meningitis, encephalitis, or intracerebral or subarachnoid hemorrhage. A preceding period of confusion or delirium points to a diffuse process such as meningitis or effects of endogenous or exogenous toxins. The sudden apoplectic onset of coma is particularly suggestive of ischemic or hemorrhagic stroke affecting the brain stem or of subarachnoid hemorrhage or intracerebral hemorrhage with intraventricular rupture. Lateralized symptoms of hemiparesis or aphasia prior to coma occur with hemispheric masses.

The physical examination is critical, quickly accomplished, and diagnostic. The issues are three: (1) Does the patient have meningi-

Table 444–1 ■ CAUSES OF COMA WITH NORMAL COMPUTED TOMOGRAPHIC SCAN RESULT

Meningeal
   Subarachnoid hemorrhage (uncommon)
   Bacterial meningitis
   Encephalitis
   Subdural empyema
Exogenous toxins
   Sedative drugs/barbiturates
   Anesthetics/γ-hydroxybutyrate*
   Alcohols
   Stimulants
      Phencyclidine†
      Cocaine/amphetamine‡
   Psychotropic drugs
      Cyclic antidepressants
      Phenothiazines
      Lithium
   Anticonvulsants
   Opioids
   Clonidine§
   Penicillins
   Salicylates
   Anticholinergics
   Carbon monoxide/cyanide/methemoglobinemia
Endogenous toxins/deficiencies/derangements
   Hypoxia/ischemia
   Hypoglycemia
   Hypercalcemia
   Osmolar
      Hyperglycemia
      Hyponatremia
      Hypernatremia
   Organ system failure
      Hepatic encephalopathy
      Uremic encephalopathy
      Pulmonary insufficiency (CO_2 narcosis)
Seizures
   Prolonged post-ictal state
   Spike wave stupor
Hypo-/hyperthermia
Multifocal disorders presenting as metabolic coma
   Disseminated intravascular coagulopathy (DIC)
   Sepsis
   Pancreatitis
   Vasculitis
   Thrombotic thrombocytopenic purpura (TTP)
   Fat emboli
   Hypertensive encephalopathy
   Diffuse micrometastases
Brain stem ischemia
   Basilar artery stroke
   Brain stem or cerebellar hemorrhage
Conversion/malingering

*General anesthetic, similar to γ-aminobutyric acid; recreational drug and body building aid characterized by rapid onset, rapid recovery, often with myoclonic jerking and confusion; deep coma (2–3 hours; GCS = 3) with maintenance of vital signs.

†Coma associated with cholinergic signs: lacrimation, salivation, bronchorrhea, and hyperthermia.

‡Coma after seizures or status, i.e., a prolonged post-ictal state.

§An antihypertensive agent active through the opiate receptor system; overdose frequent when used to treat narcotic withdrawal.

tis? (2) Are there signs of a mass lesion? (3) Is this a diffuse syndrome of exogenous or endogenous metabolic cause?

IDENTIFY MENINGITIS. Although not invariably present and having varying sensitivity in regard to cause (very common with acute pyogenic meningitis and subarachnoid hemorrhage, less common with indolent, fungal meningitis), the presence of signs of meningeal irritation on examination is the central clue to the diagnosis. Missing these signs results in time-consuming additional tests such as CT scanning and the loss of a narrow therapeutic window of opportunity. Passive neck flexion should be carried out in all comatose patients unless head trauma is likely to have occurred. When the neck is passively flexed, attempting to bring the chin within a few finger-breadths of the chest, patients with irritated meninges will reflexively flex one or both knees. This sign (Brudzinski's reflex) is usually asymmetrical and not dramatic, but any evidence of knee flexion during passive neck flexion requires

that the spinal fluid be examined. Is a CT required prior to lumbar puncture in this setting? In the absence of lateralized signs (such as hemiparesis) indicating a superimposed mass lesion, a spinal puncture should be performed immediately. Although rare cases of herniation after lumbar puncture in children with bacterial meningitis have been reported, the urgency of diagnosis and treatment at the point of coma is paramount. The time required for CT scanning may cause a fatal therapeutic delay. An alternative approach is to obtain blood cultures and immediately initiate antibiotic therapy with subsequent lumbar puncture; CSF cell count, glucose level, and protein content are unchanged, and Gram's stain and culture often produce positive findings despite a short period of antibiotic treatment.

SEPARATE STRUCTURAL FROM METABOLIC CAUSES OF COMA. Structural and metabolic causes of coma can be distinguished by neurologic examination: As the evaluation and potential treatment modalities for structural versus metabolic coma are widely divergent and the disease processes in both are often rapidly progressive, initiating the evaluation in a medical or surgical direction may be life-saving. This task is accomplished by focusing on three features of neurologic examination: the motor response to a painful stimulus, pupillary function, and reflex eye movements.

The functioning of the motor system provides the clearest indication of a mass lesion. Elicitation of a motor response requires that a painful stimulus to which the patient will react be applied. The arms should be placed in a semiflexed posture and a painful stimulus applied to the head or trunk. Strong pressure on the supraorbital ridge or pinching of skin on the anterior chest or inner arm is most useful; nail bed pressure makes the interpretation of upper limb movement difficult.

The evolution of neurologic signs from an expanding hemispheric mass lesion is illustrated in Figure 444–1. Hemispheric masses at their early stage (early diencephalic, i.e., compromising the brain above the thalamus) will produce appropriate movement of one upper extremity toward the painful stimulus. The contralateral arm will reflect a hemiparesis. This lateralized motor movement in a comatose patient establishes the working diagnosis of a hemispheric mass. As the mass expands to involve the thalamus (late diencephalic) the response to pain is now reflex arm flexion associated with extension and internal rotation of the legs (decorticate posturing); asymmetry of the response in the upper extremities will be seen. With further brain compromise at the midbrain level, the reflex posturing now changes in the arms so that both arms and legs respond by extension (decerebrate posturing); at this level the asymmetry tends to be lost. With further compromise to the level of the pons, the most frequent finding is no response to painful stimulation although spinal movements of leg flexion may occur. The classic postures illustrated in Figure 444–1, and particularly their asymmetry, strongly support a mass lesion as cause. However, these motor movements, especially early in coma, are most frequently fragments of abnormal, asymmetrical flexion and extension in the arms rather than the complete decorticate and decerebrate postures illustrated in the figure. A small amount of asymmetrical flexion or extension of the arms in response to painful stimulus carries the same implications as the full-blown postures.

Metabolic lesions do not compromise the brain in a progressive level-by-level manner as do hemispheric masses and rarely produce the asymmetrical motor signs typical of masses. Reflex posturing may be seen, but it lacks the asymmetry of decortication from a hemispheric mass and is not associated with the loss of pupillary reactivity at the stage of decerebration.

PUPILLARY REACTIVITY. Functioning of the pupils reflects the structural integrity of the midbrain. If the pupils constrict to a bright light, the midbrain is intact, and if they do not, the midbrain has been compromised. In mass lesions, the loss of pupillary reactivity from a hemispheric mass is asymmetrical, with the pupil homolateral to the mass losing reactivity before its contralateral fellow. A midbrain pupil may be large and unreactive if the descending sympathetic pathways in the brain stem have not been compromised but are more commonly at midposition (5 mm), reflecting both parasympathetic (third nerve) and sympathetic (brain stem) injury.

In metabolic coma one feature is central to the examination: Pupillary reactivity is present. This reactivity is seen both early in coma when an appropriate motor response to pain may be retained, and late when no motor responses can be elicited. The reaction is

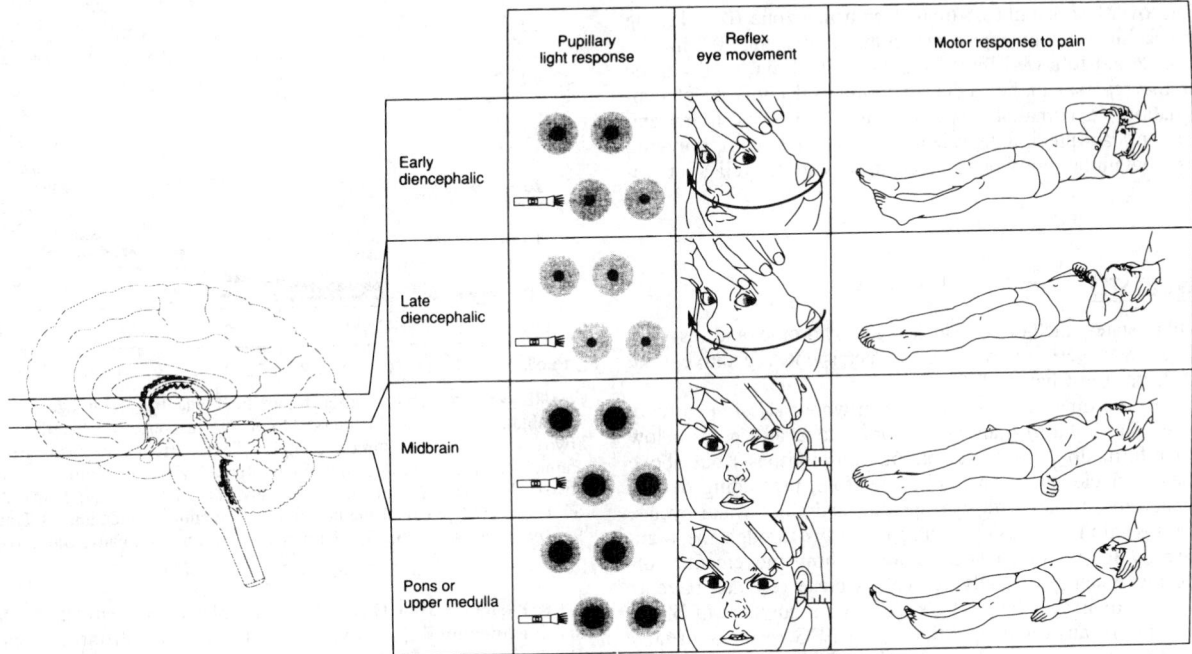

	Pupillary light response	Reflex eye movement	Motor response to pain
Early diencephalic			
Late diencephalic			
Midbrain			
Pons or upper medulla			

FIGURE 444–1 ■ The evolution of neurologic signs in coma from a hemispheric mass lesion as the brain becomes functionally impaired in a rostral caudal manner. Early and late diencephalic levels are levels of dysfunction just above (early) and just below (late) the thalamus. (Aminoff MJ, Greenberg DA, Simon RP: Clinical Neurology. Appleton and Lange, 1996.)

lost only when coma is so deep the patient requires ventilatory and blood pressure support.

REFLEX EYE MOVEMENTS. The presence of inducible lateral eye movements reflects the integrity of the pons (vestibular nucleus, pontine gaze center, and sixth cranial nerve moving the eye laterally). The medial longitudinal fasciculus traverses the dorsal pons to connect with the third cranial nerve (moving the eye medially). This system may first be compromised at the midbrain level, with loss of medial eye movement in the eye homolateral to the mass, but becomes clearly impaired by pontine dysfunction when no eye movements are inducible. These eye movements ("reflex eye movements," Figure 444–1) are brought about by passive head rotation to stimulate the semicircular canal input to the vestibular system (doll's-eyes maneuver), or by inhibition of function of one semicircular canal by infusion of ice water against the tympanic membrane (caloric testing).

In metabolic coma, reflex eye movements may be lost or retained. Lack of inducible eye movements with the doll's eyes maneuver, in the setting of preserved pupillary reactivity, is virtually diagnostic of drug toxicity. Caloric testing is not useful in drug-induced coma as it may produce any of the following: delayed downward ocular deviation, ipsilateral adduction with incomplete contralateral abduction, ipsilateral abduction with contralateral adduction, or no response. With metabolic coma of non-drug-induced origin such as organ system failure or electrolyte or osmolar disorders, reflex eye movements are preserved.

Brain stem mass lesions are a special case. These lesions are most commonly vascular. Reflex lateral eye movements, the pathways for which traverse the pons and midbrain, are particularly affected, and the reflex postures of decortication and decerebration typical of brain stem injury are common findings. Lesions restricted to the midbrain (e.g., embolization to the top of the basilar artery) will be manifest by sluggish or absent pupillary reflexes with or without impaired medial eye movements (third cranial nerve). With lesions restricted to the pons (e.g., intrapontine hypertensive hemorrhage), reactive but very small pupils—pinpoint or pontine pupils—will be seen, reflecting focal impairment of descending sympathetic fibers through the brain stem with preservation of sympathetic fibers in the third cranial nerve. Ocular bobbing (spontaneous symmetrical or asymmetrical rhythmic vertical ocular oscillations) may be seen.

Multifocal disorders may present as metabolic coma. A number of syndromes of multifocal vascular disease are characterized by diffuse brain dysfunction that appears to be a metabolic encephalopathy. Hypertensive encephalopathy, due in part to multifocal arterial spasm, produces a subacute encephalopathy with seizures and is characterized in adults by blood pressures above 250/150 mm Hg; (MRI) scanning may show prominent posterior white matter edema. Other subacutely evolving diffuse vascular syndromes without neuroimaging signatures include disseminated intravascular coagulation (DIC), endocarditis, the encephalopathy of sepsis, thrombotic thrombocytopenic purpura, fat emboli syndrome, diffuse small-vessel vasculitis, pancreatic encephalopathy, and venous thrombosis (particularly affecting the superior sagittal sinus).

CONSIDER SEIZURES. The diagnosis of a seizure is usually obvious from history or observation, and the return to an agitated confusional state and then consciousness that occurs over a few minutes solves any diagnostic problem. However, prolonged alteration in consciousness after an unwitnessed seizure may produce diagnostic confusion. Such prolonged post-ictal states follow seizures affecting an acutely or chronically impaired brain. Acute brain impairment occurs with encephalitis but also with multifocal vascular disease, such as hypertensive encephalopathy, acute metabolic impairment of brain function (such as hypo- or hypernatremia, hypo- or hyperglycemia), or drug toxicity complicated by seizures. In a post-ictal state the examination will detect reactive pupils and inducible eye movements (in the absence of overtreatment with anticonvulsants) and may detect upgoing toes; if the onset of the seizure was in a focal motor area of the cortex, there may be a prolonged hemiparesis ("Todd's paresis"). Non-convulsive seizures, particularly spike wave stupor, may occur in a patient without a history of epilepsy. The diagnosis is made by electroencephalogram (EEG).

Emergency management of the patient with a decreased level of consciousness includes assurance of airway adequacy and support of ventilation and of circulation. Withdraw blood for determination of serum glucose and electrolyte levels, hepatic and renal function, prothrombin and partial thromboplastin times, complete blood count, and drug screen. Administer 25 g of dextrose intravenously (IV) (typically 50 mL of 50% dextrose) to treat possible hypoglycemic coma. The glucose level is poorly correlated with the level of consciousness in hypoglycemia with coma, stupor, and confusion reported with blood glucose concentrations of 2–28, 8–59, and 9–60 mg/dL, respectively. As administration of dextrose alone can precipitate or worsen Wernicke's encephalopathy in thiamine-deficient patients, administer 100 mg of thiamine intravenously. A possible opiate overdose should be treated with naloxone (0.4–1.2 mg IV). The specific benzodiazepine antagonist flumazenil (0.2 mg IV repeated once and followed by 0.1 mg IV to 1–3 mg total) can be given for the reversal of benzodiazepine-induced coma or of conscious sedation. In coma of unknown cause, however, flumazenil administration can precipitate seizures in patients with polydrug overdoses containing both benzodiazepines with tricyclics or cocaine.

COMA-LIKE STATES

Coma-like states include the locked-in syndrome and psychogenic unresponsiveness, as well as the persistent vegetative state and brain death (see Chapter 446).

Locked-in syndrome patients are those in whom a lesion (usually hemorrhage or an infarct) transects the brain stem at a point below the reticular formation (therefore sparing consciousness) but above the ventilatory nuclei of the medulla (therefore, precluding death). Such patients are awake, with eye opening and sleep-wake cycles, but have transection of the descending pathways through the brain stem necessary for volitional vocalization or limb movement. Voluntary eye movement, especially vertical, is preserved, and patients open and close their eyes or produce appropriate numbers of blinking movements in answer to questions. The EEG result is usually normal, reflecting normal cortical function. The mortality rate is high (40–70%), and most patients who recover are left with major deficits. Recovery to independence can occur, however, over weeks to 3 to 4 months. Early recovery of lateral eye movements has been suggested as a particularly positive prognostic feature. Magnetic stimulation of motor cortex producing motor evoked potentials may be an additional positive prognostic feature. Survival in the locked-in state has lasted as long as 18 years.

Psychogenic unresponsiveness is a diagnosis of exclusion. The neurologic examination shows reactive pupils and no reflex posturing to pain. Eye movements during the doll's eyes maneuver show volitional override rather than the smooth uninhibited reflex lateral eye movements of coma. Ice water caloric testing will either arouse the patient because of the discomfort produced or induce cortically mediated nystagmus rather than the tonic deviation typical of coma. The slow conjugate roving eye movements of metabolic coma cannot be imitated and, therefore, exclude psychogenic unresponsiveness. In addition, the slow, often asymmetrical, and incomplete eye closure that follows passive eyelid opening of a comatose patient cannot be feigned. These signs, therefore, exclude psychogenic coma. On the other hand, conscious patients usually exhibit some voluntary muscle tone in the eyelids during passive eye opening. The EEG finding in psychogenic unresponsiveness is normal wakefulness with reactive posterior rhythms on eye opening and eye closing.

Table 444–2 ■ PROBABILITY (PERCENTAGE) OF RECOVERING INDEPENDENT FUNCTION FROM COMA AFTER CARDIAC ARREST

SIGN	DAYS AFTER CARDIAC ARREST			
	0	1	3	7
From Levey et al. (N = 210)				
No verbal response	13	8	5	6
No eye opening	11	6	4	0
Unreactive pupils	0	0	0	0
No spontaneous eye movements	6	5	2	0
No caloric response	5	6	6	0
Extensor posturing	18	0	0	0
Flexor posturing	14	3	0	0
No motor response	4	3	0	0
From Edgren et al. (N = 131)				
No eye opening to pain	31	8	0	0
Absent or reflex motor response	25	9	0	0
Unreactive pupils	17	7	0	0

Data from Levey DE et al: Predicting the outcome from hypoxic coma. JAMA 523: 1420, 1985. Copyright 1985, American Medical Association. Data from Edgren E et al: Assessment of neurological prognosis in comatose survivors of cardiac arrest. Lancet 343:1055, 1994. © by The Lancet Ltd., 1994.

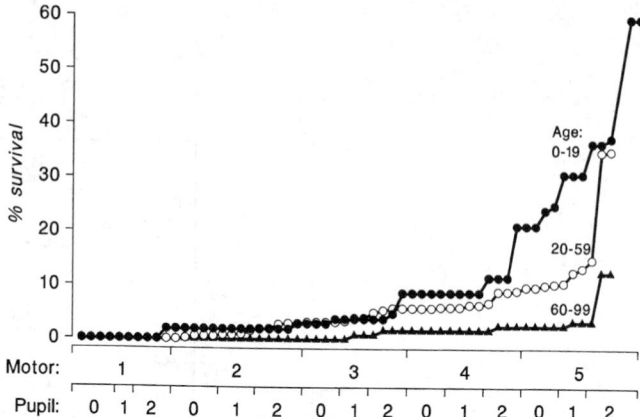

FIGURE 444–2 ■ Survival after traumatic coma based on age and clinical examination results at 24 hours. Motor: No response (one), reflex extension (two), reflex flexion (three), complex flexion (four), localizes pain (five). Pupils: No reactivity (zero), unilateral reactivity (one), bilateral reactivity (two). (Manelak AN, et al: Predicting survival from head injury 24 hours after injury: A practical method with therapeutic implications. J Trauma 41: 91–99, 1996, © 1996, The Williams & Wilkins Company, Baltimore.)

PROGNOSIS IN COMA. In coma after cardiac arrest, the prognosis for meaningful recovery can be assessed from clinical signs. Brisk, small-amplitude, mainly vertical eye movements are seen in patients with ischemia-induced electrographic status epilepticus and are predictive of a fatal outcome. In cardiac arrest patients without the complicating issue of seizures, return of pupillary reactivity and purposeful motor movements within the first 72 hours is highly correlated with a favorable outcome (Table 444–2). Rare late recoveries have been reported, however.

The outcome after traumatic head injury is more difficult to assess and includes an additional prognostic factor: age. Young patients (less than 20 years) are over three times more likely to survive than those above age 60. On examination at 24 hours, an absent motor response to pain combined with an absent pupillary response is a strong predictor of mortality, whereas localization of a painful stimulus with preserved pupillary reactivity is a highly favorable finding, especially in the young (Fig. 444–2). Unexpected late recoveries are not infrequent.

Plum F, Posner JB: Contemporary Neurology Series, vol. 19. 3rd ed. The Diagnosis of Stupor and Coma. Philadelphia, FA Davis, 1980. *The classic monograph.*
Young GB, Ropper AH, Bolton CF: Coma and Impaired Consciousness: A Clinical Perspective. New York, McGraw-Hill, 1998. *An extensive text of acute and critical care medical neurology.*

445 PERSISTENT VEGETATIVE STATE

Roger P. Simon

The term *persistent vegetative state* (PVS) characterizes the condition of 10,000–25,000 adults and 4000–10,000 children in the United States. Whereas coma represents a state lacking both wakefulness and awareness, in a vegetative state patients have awakened from coma but have not regained awareness. Wakefulness is manifested by eye opening and sleep-wake cycles.

The neuroanatomic characteristics of the vegetative state dictate that the reticular activating system of the brain stem be intact to produce wakefulness, but that the connections to the cortical mantle be interrupted, precluding awareness. These anatomic requirements for a vegetative state are satisfied most commonly by diffuse axonal injury, laminar necrosis of the cortical mantle, or thalamic necrosis. These pathologic alterations occur as the sequelae of a number of acute or chronic conditions affecting brain. Acute brain injury resulting in a vegetative state first produces coma, with the patient later awakening into the vegetative condition. Common causes include trauma with resultant diffuse axonal injury, hypoxia-ischemia secondary to cerebral hypoperfusion from cardiac arrest resulting in death of the selectively vulnerable neurons in the cortical mantle (laminar necrosis), bihemispheric infarctions, cortical injury following purulent meningitis or encephalitis, exposure to nervous system toxins (particularly carbon monoxide), and prolonged hypoglycemia. The sequelae of cerebral hypoperfusion may particularly affect hemispheric watershed areas and the thalamus; such thalamic necrosis was the major cause of the vegetative state of the widely reported patient Karen Quinlan.

A vegetative state may not always begin with coma but can develop as the end stage of neurodegenerative diseases of adults or children or accompany severe developmental abnormalities of the brain such as anencephaly.

Clinically, PVS patients have signs associated with an intact reticular formation: They open their eyes and have sleep-wake cycles, although these are irregular in timing. Their brain stem reflexes are intact: Pupils react and eye movements occur spontaneously and with the doll's-eyes maneuver. More complex brain stem reflexes are also seen, such as yawning, chewing, swallowing, and, uncommonly, making guttural vocalizations. The brain stem reflexes of arousal and startle are preserved as well, so that eye opening occurs with loud sounds and blinking may occur with bright lights. Tearing may be seen. Spontaneous roving eye movements are particularly characteristic; these are very slow movements of constant velocity, uninterrupted by saccadic jerks, and cannot be volitionally mimicked. These eye movements can be particularly distressing to family members as the patients appear to be looking about the room and at some point the roving eyes are pointed at the observer, who may perceive the patient to be "looking at" or following him or her throughout the room. The lack of quick directed saccadic eye movements in the presence of continual fixed velocity roving eye movements differentiates a willed response from reflex eye movements. The brain stem origin of the eye movements is further documented by their being readily redirected by the oculocephalic (doll's-eyes) reflex. The limbs may move but motor responses are only primitively purposeful, such as grasping an object that contacts the hand. Pain usually produces decorticate or decerebrate postures or fragments of these movements.

Results of brain imaging studies depict the sequelae of the causative injury but are not diagnostic of PVS. Findings of magnetic resonance (MR) spectroscopy have shown a decrease in the neuronal marker of *N*-acetylaspartate. Positron-emission tomography (PET) studies have shown decreased glucose utilization and cerebral blood flow, but such results in and of themselves are rarely diagnostic. Evoked responses are not useful.

The PVS is diagnosed after 1 month in a patient without detectable awareness of the environment. A vegetative state is termed persistent after 3 months if the brain injury was medical and after 12 months if the brain injury was traumatic. The determination as to when *persistent* equals *permanent* cannot be stated absolutely; to predict early in the vegetative state which patients will become persistently vegetative is particularly difficult in trauma. Lesions of the corpus collosum and dorsolateral brain stem seen on magnetic resonance imaging (MRI) between 6 and 8 weeks after trauma correlated with persistence of the vegetative state at 1 year.

Rare patients show late improvement but none regains normal function. Partial recovery to the level of communication and comprehension has been reported in 3% of patients after 5 years but improvement to independence in activities of daily living is even more rare. Although lack of awareness defines the vegetative state, patients may recover slightly beyond this criterion. Such minimally responsive patients present difficult ethical considerations for care.

Kampfl A, et al: Prediction of recovery from post traumatic vegetative state with cerebral magnetic-resonance imaging. Lancet 351:1763, 1998. *An attempt to use early MRI to predict recovery versus persistence of the vegetative state in traumatic brain injury.*

Medical Aspects of the Persistent Vegetative State. N Eng J Med 330:1499, 1994. *The consensus statement from the Multi-Society Task Force defining nomenclature, cause, evaluation, and prognosis. Includes the issue of late recoveries.*

Persistent vegetative state: Report of the American Neurological Association Committee on Ethical Affairs. Ann Neurol 33:386, 1993. *The American Academy of Neurology's position paper defining the persistent vegetative state and discussing the issues of withholding and withdrawing nutrition and hydration.*

Zeman A: Persistent vegetative state. Lancet 350:795, 1997. *A review from the United Kingdom including an extensive bibliography of clinical and ethical aspects and consensus statement from other bodies.*

446 BRAIN DEATH

Roger P. Simon

Irreversible cessation of cardiopulmonary function precludes function of the brain. The opposite is true as well. Therefore, death of the organism can be determined on the basis of death of the brain. Although some details may be dictated by local law, the standard criteria for the diagnosis of brain death are those established by the President's Commission report of 1981. This standard permits a diagnosis of brain death upon documentation of irreversible cessation of all brain function including those of the brain stem; the presence of seizures is not compatible with the diagnosis. The absence of hemispheric function is documented by unreceptivity and unresponsiveness, usually assessed in the setting of a painful stimulation; the patient does not rouse, groan, grimace, or withdraw limbs. Purely spinal reflexes may be maintained: deep tendon reflexes, plantar flexion reflex, plantar withdrawal, and tonic neck reflexes. Decorticate or decerebrate posturing is not compatible with the diagnosis. Absence of brain stem function is assessed by region. Lack of midbrain function is documented by the absence of a pupillary light reflex (most easily assessed by the bright light of an ophthalmoscope viewed through its magnifying lens when focused on the iris). Unreactive pupils may be either at midposition (as they will be in death) or dilated, as they often are in the setting of a dopamine infusion. Lack of pontine function is documented by the absence of a response to corneal stimulation and the absence of inducible eye movements: no eye movement toward the side of irrigation of the tympanic membrane with 50 cm³ of ice water. The oculocephalic response (doll's eyes) will always be absent in the setting of absent oculovestibular testing. Cessation of medullary function is documented by the apnea test: no ventilatory movements in the setting of maximum CO_2 stimulation. The test is performed by disconnecting the ventilator from the endotracheal tube. Oxygen can be supplied by diffusion from a cannula placed through the endotracheal tube (6 L/minute). In the absence of ventilation PCO_2 will passively rise 2–3 mm Hg/minute. As a PCO_2 of 60 mm Hg produces the maximum ventilatory stimulus required for the confirmation of apnea, a period of about 10 minutes will be required for the PCO_2 to reach that level from a normal baseline. A $PaCO_2$ greater than 60 mm Hg will adequately stimulate ventilatory drive within 60 seconds in a functioning brain.

Documentation of irreversibility requires that the cause of the coma be known and that it be adequate to explain the clinical findings of brain death. Irreversibility based on clinical criteria cannot be determined in the setting of sedative drugs or significant hypothermia (<32.2° C) or in the presence of shock and neuromuscular blockade.

Confirmatory tests may be useful. An isoelectric electroencephalogram (EEG) is frequently used. However, deep coma from sedative drugs or hypothermia below 20° C can produce EEG flattening. In addition, patients clinically brain dead may have residual EEG activity (alpha coma-like activity, low-voltage fast waves, or sleep-like slowing with spindle activity), which may persist for a number of days following a brain death diagnosis. The absence of cerebral blood flow is the most definitive confirmatory test and is most unequivocally demonstrated by angiography. The role of transcranial Doppler techniques in substantiating brain death is still unclear.

Sequential testing is necessary for a clinical diagnosis of brain death. The period of observation required is at least 6 hours for all cases and at least 24 hours in the setting of anoxic-ischemic brain injury.

With the confirmation of brain death, asystole usually occurs within days (mean = 4 days) even if ventilatory support is continued. Recovery after appropriate documentation of brain death has never been reported. Removal of the ventilator results in terminal rhythms, most often complete heart block without ventricular response, junctional rhythms, or ventricular tachycardia. Purely spinal motor movements may occur in the moments of terminal apnea (or during apnea testing in the absence of passive administration of oxygen): arching of the back, neck turning, stiffening of the legs, and upper extremity flexion.

Guidelines for the determination of death: Report of the medical consultants on the diagnosis of death to the President's Commission for the Study of Ethical Problems in Medicine and Biomedical and Behavioral Research. JAMA 246:2184, 1981. *The President's Commission report describing the equivalence of cardiac and brain death and providing criteria for each.*
Halevy A, Brody B: Brain death: Reconciling definitions, criteria and tests. Ann Intern Med 119:519, 1993. *A critique of the diagnostic criteria for brain death with attention to the issue of organ harvesting for transplantation.*

447 SYNCOPE

Roger P. Simon

Syncope is the phenomenon of loss of consciousness associated with loss of postural tone. The episode is caused by global impairment of blood flow to the brain; occasionally, hypoperfusion may be confined to the cerebral hemispheres or the brain stem, and involvement of either structure will produce unconsciousness. Syncope must be differentiated from seizures, which may be manifested similarly but have a different pathophysiology and therapy.

THE HISTORY

Because most spells of episodic loss of consciousness occur outside medical observation, the history is the most critical part of the evaluation. If multiple spells have occurred, their similarity should be established so that small pieces of history from one spell or another may be combined into a pathophysiologic profile. Each syncopal episode should be reviewed in detail, with attention to the three key elements: events and symptoms preceding the spell, what happened during the spell of unconsciousness, and the time course of regaining orientation once consciousness is regained. The 1st of these elements can be obtained from the patient, but the 2nd and frequently the 3rd cannot. Accordingly, information from a witness is essential to the evaluation and should be obtained by phone calls, interviews, or revisits scheduled to include persons who have witnessed one or more spells.

BEFORE THE SPELL. What position was the patient in when each spell began? Seizures or cardiac arrhythmias can develop with any body position, but vasovagal syncope very rarely and orthostatic hypotension never begins with the patient recumbent. Thus in patients with recurrent syncope, if even a single episode began in the recumbent posture, vasovagal and orthostatic etiologies are virtually excluded. What prodromal symptoms were appreciated before loss of consciousness? Symptoms of cerebral hypoperfusion should be sought, including lightheadedness, dizziness (but uncommonly vertigo), bilateral tinnitus, nausea, diffuse weakness, and finally dimming of vision from retinal hypoperfusion. This prodrome establishes the pathophysiology of the syncopal spell as that of cerebral hypoperfusion; such hypoperfusion may be of cardiac, orthostatic, or reflex cause. Loss of consciousness so rapid that a prodrome is absent may occur with seizures and with some cardiac arrhythmias such as asystole, which will cause loss of consciousness within 4 to 8 seconds in the upright position or within 12 to 15 seconds in the recumbent position. Palpitations during the prodrome occur with tachyarrhythmias but may also introduce vasovagal events. What was the activity of the patient immediately before the onset of symptoms? Extreme exertion (cardiac), an emotional or painful stimulus (vasovagal), a rapid change in posture (ortho-

static), and straining at urination (situational) are examples of help in identifying the etiology.

DURING THE EVENT. What events do witnesses describe as occurring during the episode of unconsciousness? Although body stiffening and limb jerking are well-known motor phenomena occurring during the loss of consciousness associated with generalized seizures, very similar motor movements can result from cerebral hypoperfusion. These motor movements occur especially if cerebral blood flow is not rapidly restored by termination of an arrhythmia or by falling to a recumbent posture in the setting of reflex syncope. Such muscle jerking is often multifocal and can be synchronous or asynchronous. In contrast to epileptic seizures, which generally produce tonic-clonic activity for at least 1 to 2 minutes, muscle jerking in syncope rarely persists longer than 30 seconds. If an arrhythmia continues or the patient is physically maintained upright (e.g., fainting in a phone booth or while sitting on a toilet), tonic stiffening of the body occurs (opisthotonos) and is then followed by jerking movements of the limbs. Occasionally, motor movements identical to a tonic-clonic seizure occur, and a mistaken diagnosis of epilepsy can be made. Urinary incontinence during the spell is frequently used to support or refute a diagnosis of epilepsy; however, fainting with a full bladder can result in incontinence, whereas seizures with an empty bladder will not. Tongue biting favors seizures.

AFTER THE EVENT. Over what time period were consciousness and orientation regained? This aspect of the history is the most useful in dealing with the differential diagnosis of seizures as the etiology for a syncopal-like spell. Recovery of orientation and consciousness following vasovagal or reflex-mediated syncope occurs simultaneously. Recovery of orientation following syncope of cardiac origin is proportional to the duration of the unconsciousness but is usually rapid (0 to 10 seconds); with periods of malignant arrhythmia producing unconsciousness of 2 minutes, confusion on waking is less than 30 seconds. Following seizures, however, the period of confusion, often with agitation, continues for 2 to 20 minutes following recovery of consciousness.

ETIOLOGY

REFLEX MEDIATED. VASOVAGAL SYNCOPE. Vasovagal spells, or simple faints, are the most common cause of syncope (Table 447–1). They occur in all age groups, are equally common in men and women, and may be more frequent in some families. Precipitating factors include pain (especially medical instrumentation), trauma, fatigue, blood loss, or prolonged motionless standing. Vagally mediated hypotension and bradycardia combine to produce cerebral hypoperfusion, with a resultant prodrome of lightheadedness, nausea, tinnitus, diaphoresis, salivation, pallor, and dimming of vision. Tachycardia may be the initial manifestation. The spells begin in the standing or sitting position, although during medical instrumentation (e.g., phlebotomy or intrauterine device insertion)

Table 447–1 ■ CAUSES OF EPISODIC LOSS OF CONSCIOUSNESS

	% PATIENTS IN EACH CATEGORY
Reflex mediated	
Vasovagal	18
Carotid sinus sensitivity	1
Situational	
Micturition, defecation, cough	5
Orthostatic hypotension	8
Medication-induced	3
Psychiatric/hyperventilation	2
Neurologic (seizures, TIAs, subclavian steal)	10
Cardiac	
Organic heart disease*	4
Arrhythmias**	14
Unknown***	34

*Aortic stenosis, hypertropic cardiomyopathy, pulmonary embolism, myxoma, myocardial infarction, coronary spasm, tamponade, aortic dissection.
**Sinus node disease, 2nd and 3rd degree heart block, pacemaker failure, drug-induced bradyarrhythmias, ventricular tachycardia, torsades de pointes, supraventricular tachycardia.
***Half would have neurocardiogenic syncope by tilt table testing.
Data from Linzer et al 1997, compiled from studies published 1980–1997 (prior to tilt table testing).

they can be induced with the patient horizontal. The patient loses consciousness and postural tone and falls with either flaccid or stiff limbs; eyes are open, often with an upward gaze. The patient is pale and diaphoretic and has dilated pupils. Tonic posturing or a few symmetrical or asymmetrical myoclonic jerks may occur, especially if the patient is maintained in a semiupright position. These jerking movements are not epileptic; concomitant electroencephalographic (EEG) recordings would show generalized slow waves. Consciousness is rapidly recovered when the patient becomes horizontal. Post-ictal confusion is absent. Symptoms of nervousness, dizziness, nausea, and urge to defecate may persist, and syncope can recur on standing.

SITUATIONAL SYNCOPE. Vagally mediated syncope can be induced by micturition, defecation, or swallowing or during episodes of glossopharyngeal neuralgia. Syncope during micturition occurs before, during, or after micturition in the upright position. Vagally mediated bradycardia is causative. The events are most frequent upon arising from the recumbency of sleep to urinate. Although much less common, a similar syndrome can occur with defecation. Brain stem reflexes triggering vagally induced bradyarrhythmias, with resultant syncope, can occur as a result of swallowing, with or without the association of severe pain in the tonsillar pillar, which may radiate to the ear (glossopharyngeal neuralgia). The pain can be prevented by carbamazepine, 400 to 1000 mg/day orally (see Chapter 484). In refractory cases, phenytoin (Dilantin), 300 mg/day, can be added.

Carotid sinus syncope results from vagal stimulation from the carotid sinus producing hypotension or bradycardia. The syndrome is uncommon, has a male preponderance, and affects patients mainly older than 60 years. Propranolol, digitalis, or methyldopa may predispose to carotid sinus syncope. Carotid sinus massage may be diagnostic and can be performed in an outpatient setting, but only in the absence of carotid bruits or a history of ventricular tachycardia, recent stroke, or myocardial infarction. Induction of asystole greater than or equal to 3 seconds, hypotension, or both constitute a positive test. False-positives are common, however, especially in the setting of contralateral carotid occlusion, because the ipsilateral massage transiently occludes the ipsilateral carotid and thereby prevents bilateral carotid blood flow. Symptomatic bradycardia can be treated by pacemaker implantation.

A non–vagally mediated situational syncope occurs with coughing (cough syncope). In predisposed patients the coughing increases intrathoracic venous pressure, which is transmitted to the intracranial veins; the resultant transient increase in intracranial pressure is adequate to impair blood flow. Spells can occur in any position. A prodrome is absent, and impaired consciousness lasts only a few seconds.

The term "neurocardiogenic syncope" has come into use to describe spells of cerebral hypoperfusion in the absence of a demonstrable cardiac cause or recognized vasovagal precipitants or situational triggers. Half of all patients with syncope of unknown cause may fall into this category. The mechanism of the peripheral vasodilation and hypotension is unclear; peripheral pooling of blood and activation of cardiopulmonary baroreceptors and mechanoreceptors or the renin-angiotensin system have been postulated. The prodrome (lightheadedness, tinnitus, visual dimming) and the pattern of recovery (simultaneous recovery of consciousness and orientation) are those of a vasovagal event. The patient's typical symptoms may be reproduced during head-up tilt table testing, e.g., tilting to 70 degrees for up to 45 minutes; sensitivity may be increased by the addition of an isoproterenol infusion to mimic catecholamine release. Of patients identified in this manner, a third have a vasodepressor response and two thirds have a cardioinhibitory response. A negative pregnancy test in women and an exercise stress test in older women and men are required by many centers before tilt table testing. With recurrent vasovagal syncope, including neurocardiogenic syncope, the bradycardia and hypotension can be treated with oral metoprolol (or other β-blockers), theophylline, disopyramide, or serotonin reuptake inhibitors. Cardiac pacing does not prevent hypotension or the consequent syncope.

CEREBROVASCULAR SYNCOPE. Loss of consciousness can be a component of a basilar artery transient ischemic attack, but unconsciousness alone is virtually never the initial sign. Other brain stem symptoms will always precede or accompany the syncope: Vertigo is most frequent, but diplopia or visual field disturbances,

hemifacial or perioral numbness, and dysarthria or ataxia are also common. Recovery of consciousness may require 30 to 60 minutes.

Subclavian artery stenosis may result in retrograde blood flow from the vertebral artery to one arm, with resultant brain stem hypoperfusion (subclavian steal syndrome). An asymmetry in upper extremity blood pressure averaging 45 mm Hg is nearly always present. Brain stem symptoms similar to those in basilar transient ischemic attacks occur and can include loss of consciousness; a subsequent stroke, however, is very rare. Syncope may also occur in up to 10% of patients with basilar artery migraine. It can have either a postural (orthostatic) manifestation or be associated with other basilar artery symptoms.

Neuropsychiatric syncope is a diagnosis of exclusion but is suggested by young age, frequent spells, multiple symptoms (dizziness, vertigo, lightheadedness, numbness), and duplication of the patient's symptoms by hyperventilation for 2 to 3 minutes with the mouth open. Whereas syncope and seizures occur with the eyes open, often with a gaze deviation, psychogenic events frequently begin with eye closing.

CARDIOGENIC SYNCOPE. Syncope that occurs during exercise or is associated with palpitations is particularly suggestive of a cardiac cause of syncope. A family history may be found in certain cases of prolonged QT interval syndrome. Cardiogenic syncope occurs in the setting of organic heart disease producing inflow (e.g., myxoma, constrictive pericarditis) or outflow obstruction (e.g., aortic or pulmonic stenosis, hypertrophic cardiomyopathy) or as the result of bradyarrhythmia or tachyarrhythmia. Premonitory symptoms may be those of cerebral hypoperfusion (faintness, tinnitus, and dimming of vision), but these symptoms may be absent with bradyarrhythmias because of the rapid fall in cardiac output and precipitous decline in cerebral blood flow resulting in abrupt loss of consciousness. Evaluation for arrhythmias should begin with a rhythm strip (with a 5% yield), followed by Holter monitoring for 24 hours (symptoms occur during the monitoring in approximately 20%). With recurrent events, long-term ambulatory loop electrocardiography (ECG) is useful in recording the rhythm during a spell, thus either confirming or excluding an arrhythmic etiology. This technique identifies another 25 to 50% of patients studied.

Intracardiac electrodiagnostic testing, in an attempt to induce arrhythmias, is used in patients with syncope and diagnosed organic heart disease or conduction block on ECG (especially in the elderly at risk for syncope-induced trauma); the yield is approximately 50%. Intracardiac electrodiagnostic testing is positive if the study demonstrates sustained monomorphic ventricular tachycardia, a sinus node recovery time greater than 1000 milliseconds, induced infra-Hisian block, or supraventricular tachycardia with hypotension.

ORTHOSTATIC HYPOTENSION. Postural hypotension can result in syncope that may be recurrent. The history confirms that the patients are in the upright posture during the spells, that the prodromal symptoms are those of cerebral hypoperfusion, and that symptoms are relieved with recumbency. The diagnosis is supported by noting a fall of 30 mm Hg or greater in systolic or a 10–mm Hg or greater fall in diastolic pressure between testing in the recumbent versus the upright posture. Many causes are known: drugs, polyneuropathies, or neurodegenerative disorders (see Chapters 451, 460, and 497).

SYNCOPE IN THE ELDERLY. The elderly often have multiple factors contributing to syncope, including situational, reflex, cardiac, cerebrovascular, and neurologic. Orthostatic syncope is particularly likely to occur 15 to 75 minutes after a meal or following rapid change of posture, even in the absence of neurologic or gastrointestinal disease. The postprandial systolic pressure reduction in non-syncopal elderly is approximately 14 mm Hg versus 24 mm Hg in those with a history of syncope. Medications with hypotensive side effects (even if administered at standard doses) commonly induce hypotension in the elderly; these drugs may include not only antihypertensive agents but also sedatives, antidepressants, and antianginal and antiparkinsonian medications; fluoxetine, haloperidol, and L-dopa are particularly notable. Protracted episodes of unresponsiveness lasting up to 4 hours occasionally occur in the elderly, especially while in the hospital. Investigations are not revealing. A disorder of the sleep cycle may be responsible.

ANCILLARY TESTING. Patients with a history of exercise-induced syncope, ischemic heart disease detected by history or ECG abnormalities, or auscultatory evidence of organic heart disease should be studied initially with echocardiography and then with exercise stress testing. A history suggestive of bradyarrhythmia (rapid loss of consciousness) or tachyarrhythmia (palpitations preceding the syncope) should be investigated with 24-hour Holter or long-term loop monitoring.

Routine EEG testing is not helpful unless the history suggests seizures; epilepsy is a clinical diagnosis, and even in epileptic patients a single EEG may be normal. When the history suggests seizures, particularly if prolonged confusion is a factor, interictal EEG abnormalities can be detected and are strongly supportive. Structural brain diseases are rarely a cause of episodic loss of consciousness; routine brain imaging studies are not indicated. Carotid Doppler studies may well show varying degrees of stenosis, especially in older patients, but because unconsciousness requires bihemispheric dysfunction, carotid stenosis alone does not cause syncope. Transcranial Doppler studies or magnetic resonance angiography of the basilar artery are indicated only if brain stem ischemic symptoms are present in addition to the loss of consciousness; moreover, false-positive tests are common, especially with increasing age.

PROGNOSIS IN SYNCOPE

The occurrence of syncope predicts a substantial risk for recurrence of syncope. Patients with cardiac causes have a higher mortality than do those with non-cardiac causes or those without a definable cause. However, syncope does not itself increase the risk of death inasmuch as mortality is associated with the underlying cardiac disease regardless of whether syncope has been a symptom. Congestive heart failure is the major cardiac risk factor for death.

Linzer M, et al: Diagnosing syncope. Ann Intern Med 126:989, 127:76, 1997. *A retrospective review of history, physical examination, and electrocardiography in an approach to unexplained syncope compiled by the Clinical Efficacy Assessment Project of the American College of Physicians.*

Calkins H, et al: The value of the clinical history and the differentiation of syncope due to ventricular tachycardia, atrioventricular block and neurocardiogenic syncope. Am J Med 98:365, 1995. *Reviews the diagnostic features of the history in 80 patients with syncope.*

448 DISORDERS OF SLEEP AND AROUSAL

Roger P. Simon ▪ Maria J. Sunseri

NEUROBIOLOGY OF SLEEP

The function of sleep has been speculated upon since at least pre-Homeric times, when Greeks believed they were "visited by dreams" representing messages from the Gods. Over 3000 years later, the precise function of sleep remains incompletely understood. Rest periods are known throughout all biologic systems. Sleep occurs in reptiles and birds, and nearly all mammals sleep and dream. Sleep is necessary for life; sleep deprivation in the rat results in weight loss in spite of increased food intake; metabolic

and thermoregulatory imbalance supervenes, and death occurs in about 1 month. Systemic functions such as effort and fatigue, as well as fever, induce sleep. Several sleep inducing factors such as the peptides isolated from the CSF of sleep-deprived goats have been described, but none have been fully characterized.

NEUROANATOMY/PHARMACOLOGY

Wakefulness is under the control of the reticular activating system (RAS) of the rostral brain stem that projects to thalamus and cortex. Inhibition of these projection systems are affected by modulatory neuronal groups in the pons and midbrain and result in sleep. A clearer anatomic and neuropharmacologic picture is available for the rapid eye movement (REM) stage of sleep during which most dreaming occurs. The tegmentum of the pons contains the REM sleep generator with modulation from the norepinephrine- and serotonin-containing neurons of the locus ceruleus and the dorsal raphe nucleus. Electrical events generated in the pontine reticular formation (pontogeniculoocipital waves—PGO) are propagated through the oculomotor and visual system during REM sleep simultaneously with rapid eye movements. PGO waves are suppressed by norepinephrine and serotonin neuronal systems suppress PGO waves and REM, while cholinergic neurons are stimulatory. PGO input can induce an action potential in neurons below threshold. Such PGO-facilitated activity in the visual system may play a role in the random imagery of dreaming.

SLEEP STAGES (BEHAVIORAL AND PHYSIOLOGIC CORRELATES)

Sleep stages in humans are defined electroencephalographically and behaviorally (Table 448–1). In *Stage I* sleep, patients are drowsy and may maintain some environmental awareness. The EEG loses its alpha rhythm (8–13 Hz), with theta (3–7 Hz) activity occurring; vertex potentials (negative deflections recorded from the midline) occur, especially in response to sensory stimuli. Slow lateral eye movements (EOG) occur, and spontaneous motor activity (EMG) is diminished. Stage I represents about 5% of normal sleep.

Stage II sleep is characterized by sleep spindles (12–14 Hz), vertex sharp waves, and K complexes (biphasic high-voltage slow waves often followed by a sleep spindle). Slow lateral eye movements may persist. EMG activity is further reduced. Stage II sleep represents 50 to 60% of sleep and increases with age.

Stage III and IV sleep are characterized by slow or delta waves (less than 4 Hz) and are, therefore, termed delta sleep or deep sleep. If 20 to 50% of the EEG is comprised of delta activity, the patient is in stage III sleep; if delta activity is 50% or greater, the sleep event is termed stage IV. Deep sleep constitutes 10 to 20% of sleep time (less with advancing age). EMG activity is again less active, and eye movements are not seen.

In *REM sleep,* the EEG is similar to that as seen in waking with low-voltage mixed frequencies. Abrupt rapid eye movements are characteristic. Ventilatory movements are irregular, as is heart rate. Penile erections occur, and there is an absence of EMG activity (muscular atonia). REM occupies 20 to 25% of sleep time. Patients awakening during REM report vivid dream imagery. Awakenings from non-REM sleep may also produce dream recall, but these dreams are without the intense detail of those occurring during REM.

What are the function(s) of dreams? PET studies show an increase in regional cerebral blood flow during REM sleep in the pontine tegmentum, left thalamus, bilateral amygdaloid complexes, the anterior cingulate cortex, and the right parietal opercular cortex. Cerebral blood flow is decreased in prefrontal cortex, parietal

Table 448–1 ▪ STAGES OF SLEEP

SLEEP STAGE	EEG	EYE MOVEMENTS	EMG ACTIVITY	IMAGERY
Wakefulness	Alpha and beta activity (low voltage fast)	Random, rapid	Active, spontaneous	Vivid, external
Non REM Sleep (NREM):				
Stage I (drowsiness)	Theta activity	Slow, rolling	Attenuated, episodic	Dulled
Stage II (light sleep)	Sleep spindles, K complexes	Slow/absent	Attenuated	Nonvivid
Stage III and IV (slow wave sleep)	Delta activity	Absent	Attenuated	
REM sleep	Low amplitude, irregular	Abrupt, rapid eye movements	Absent	Vivide, bizarre

cortex, and posterior cingulate cortex. Thus there is increased activity in the limbic system involved with basic emotions, and decreased activity in anatomic regions associated with executive functions. This pattern is compatible with the high emotional content of dreams. Both procedural (motor learning, e.g., typing) and declarative (episodic learning, e.g., recalling places/events) memory consolidation occur during REM sleep. REM sleep time increases following task training. Following episodic learning, memory consolidation is accomplished during slow wave sleep by a rapid reactivation of the hippocampal neurons previously activated by the place or event to be remembered. Alternately, it has been hypothesized that dream sleep functions as a random stimulator of the cortex to remove weak memories, permitting only stronger pieces of memory to be retained.

INSOMNIA

Insomnia is the perception of inadequate sleep, either in amount or quality, usually not associated with daytime sleepiness. The duration of sleep in a given patient is not an adequate measure of sleep adequacy, since normal sleep time can vary from as little as 4 to as many as 11 hours a day. This need for sleep time is relatively stable throughout adult life.

An approach to the complaint of insomnia begins with the history. Is the problem of recent onset or chronic? If new in onset, are there associated psychological, medical or medication changes? What is the character of the perceived impairment of sleep? Insomnia can be associated with impairment of sleep onset (getting to sleep), multiple awakenings during sleep (arousal), early awakenings or normal but non-refreshing sleep. Is there evidence of partial arousal (history often elicited from the bed partner), of breathing abnormalities or involuntary movements? Each have different differential diagnoses.

SITUATIONAL INSOMNIA. Such insomnias are usually of recent onset. They may be associated with exogenous events such as recognized or unrecognized life stresses, death of a family member or a friend, and stress at work or with endogenous depression. Alternatively, such insomnias can be caused by environmental changes, such as a new sleeping location or partner, shift work, or jet lag. Depression is known to produce REM potentiation, i.e., earlier onset of REM and longer lasting REM sleep. Stage IV sleep is suppressed. The normal balance of sleep stages is restored following non-pharmacologic and to a lesser extent following pharmacologic treatment of depression.

BEHAVIORAL INSOMNIA. Such patients have a chronic insomnia and a characteristic personality. They find the time of preparation for sleep one that induces rumination, emotional arousal, and increased autonomic activity. The focus on the inability to fall asleep becomes self-perpetuating.

Drug-related insomnia can be suggested by the temporal profile of the history of sleep disturbances. Caffeine use in beverages or as an unrecognized component of over-the-counter drugs can be a factor in sensitive patients, but others seem unperturbed by the drug even though their sleep may be fragmented. The history will be that of decreased ability to fall asleep.

Alcohol use, prior to sleep, has a dual effect. The induction of somnolence will hasten sleep onset but often at the price of an increasing exacerbation of sleep-related breathing abnormalities, and also the induction of sleep fragmentation and early awakening upon metabolic clearance of the drug. Multiple prescription medicines will affect sleep most often by arousal mechanisms. Corticosteroids, antidepressants, bronchodilators, and CNS stimulants are particularly notable. In addition, the withdrawal of short-acting sedatives, often prescribed for insomnia, may produce arousal.

A number of medical or neurologic conditions are associated with impaired sleep. These include pain, especially skeletal pain and arthritis. Cardiac and pulmonary conditions can produce frequent awakening because of shortness of breath and congestive heart failure (paroxysmal nocturnal dyspnea). Gastrointestinal disorders, especially those producing bowel hypermotility and nocturnal diarrhea, impair sleep. Eating disorders and hunger may produce arousal at night. Neurologic disorders may affect sleep, particularly those which impair normal movement during sleep. Thus, a patient following a stroke or a patient with advanced multiple sclerosis or Parkinson's disease may have disturbed sleep, as they are unable to turn in bed. Some headaches, such as cluster and hypnic headache,

characteristically awaken patients at night. The rare prion disorder of fatal familial insomnia is characterized by sleep impairment. Age alters sleep, with increased awakenings at the transition between non-REM and REM sleep; there is a decrease in slow wave sleep as well. The elderly frequently nap during the daytime, which may induce the presumption of inadequate sleep time since night time sleep will be shortened.

Arrival at altitude produces a usually transient insomnia in some persons. The altitude change is associated with hypoxia and altered ventilatory drive, resulting in periodic breathing and multiple awakenings. In particularly susceptible individuals, acetazolamide treatment may alter these arousals.

TREATMENT. The treatment of insomnia depends to a great degree upon its cause. Treatment of depression, elimination of stimulant drugs and providing an optimal sleep environment are general principals of sleep hygiene. Useful as well are, increasing daytime exercise but not exercise just prior to sleep; provision of a proper sleep environment (attention to optimal temperature, light, and ambient noise); the maintenance of a regular sleep time and schedule; avoidance of drugs and alcohol; "winding down" prior to sleep, i.e., quiet reading. If medications are used, they should be prescribed only briefly as tolerance develops to sedative drugs within several weeks. The choice of medications should address the type of insomnia, i.e., sleep onset or nocturnal awakening. For sleep onset, triazolam (Halcion) or zolpidem (Ambien) are rapidly acting, short half-life compounds. For sleep maintenance, longer acting drugs are more effective, such as, flurazepam (Dalmane) or quazepam (Doral). For patients with persistent insomnia, specific causes should be sought such as sleep apnea or periodic limb movements.

ABNORMAL AROUSALS

Abnormal arousals during sleep, resulting in the perception of inadequately restorative sleep, include sleep apnea (discussed below), restless leg syndrome, nocturnal myoclonus and periodic limb movements of sleep as well as chronic pain disorders (Table 448–2).

Restless leg syndrome occurs at the time of sleep onset and, therefore, interferes with the ability to fall asleep. Symptoms are reported variously as a need to move the legs or a deep sensory complaint in the lower extremities. Walking about, rubbing or moving the limbs briefly relieves the symptoms. Sinemet (beginning with 25/100, 30 minutes before bedtime) or bromocriptine (2.5–7.5 mg a few hours before sleep) is effective; clonazepam (1 mg q.h.s.), opiates or gabapentin may be helpful. *Periodic limb movements* often accompany restless leg syndrome. The movements are brief, repetitive dorsiflexion of the great toe or plantar flexion of the foot during stage 1–2 sleep and disappear with REM atonia. Clonazepam may be useful. *Myoclonus* involving body or limb jerking at the onset of sleep has been reported in nearly 80% of normal persons. The prolongation of these fragments of myoclonus during non-REM sleep constitute the phenomenon of *sleep myoclonus*, which does not usually require treatment.

PARASOMNIAS. These sleep-related phenomena are motor disorders with or without autonomic features during sleep that induce brief partial arousals. They are not associated with daytime sleepiness but are manifestations of disturbed mechanisms of sleep. They are most common in childhood but may be seen in adults.

Table 448–2 ■ SLEEP STAGE AND ASSOCIATED SLEEP DISORDER

SLEEP STAGE	SLEEP DISORDER
Pre-sleep	Restless leg syndrome
	Sleep onset myoclonus
NREM sleep (Stage I–II)	Periodic limb movements of sleep
	Sleep myoclonus
Deep sleep (Stage III–IV)	Sleepwalking
	Sleep terrors
REM sleep	Nightmares
	REM sleep behavioral disorder
Sleep/wake transition	Hypnagogic (sleep onset) and hypnopompic (on waking) hallucinations
	Sleep paralysis

Sleep walking occurs in over 10% of children, many of whom have a family history. The behavior occurs during stage III and IV sleep and may be fragmentary, such as merely sitting up in bed. Patients are difficult to arouse during the event and do not recollect it. Events usually occur in the first few hours of sleep and are brief (less than 10 minutes) but may be recurrent. *Sleep terrors* are often associated; they also occur in non-REM sleep, but include intense autonomic arousal, marked vocalization and motility, difficulty in arousing the patient and minimal recall of the episode. The spells may be attenuated by benzodiazepines. *Nightmares* are distinct from sleep terrors because of occurrence in REM sleep. Thus motility is limited, vocalization is much less intense, the patients are relatively easily aroused and vivid dream recall is evident.

REM behavioral disorder is an uncommon parasomnia affecting middle-aged or older men, or in patients with CNS degenerative disease especially involving the brain stem. The absence of REM atonia allows for motor behaviors that are often violent and may injure the patient or the bed partner. As is characteristic of REM disorders, there is vivid imagery reported upon awakening. Nocturnal seizures should be excluded. Brain stem lesions interrupting the pathways responsible for motor paralysis during dreaming have been hypothesized as a cause. Clonazepam is an effective treatment.

NARCOLEPSY. Narcolepsy is a disorder of excessive daytime sleepiness associated with abnormalities in REM sleep. It has its onset most often between the second and fourth decades. When fully expressed, the quartet of narcolepsy, cataplexy, hypnagogic hallucinations and sleep paralysis occurs.

Narcolepsy affects approximately 100,000 persons in the United States; there is no sex preponderance. A genetic predisposition is documented by the presence of the HLA allele, HLA DQB 1*0602 often with HLA DR2 in over 85% of narcolepsy-cataplexy patients. The penetrance is variable, as less than 5% of patients have affected family members. Narcoleptic hypersomnia occurs (as it does in normals) most often in settings of sedentary activity and with boredom, and can be alleviated to some degree by motor or intellectual stimulation. However, narcoleptic sleep attacks may also occur during conversation, meals, and while driving. Nearly 70% of patients have had automobile accidents or near accidents because of sleep attacks. The sleep episodes are brief and their frequency is little changed in patients following the first months of the disorder.

The diagnosis of narcolepsy is made on the basis of a typical and persistent history of excessive daytime sleepiness in the absence of underlying nocturnal sleep disorders producing daytime somnolence and is confirmed by the documentation of sleep onset REM (latency less than 15 minutes) and an abnormal multiple sleep latency test (MSLT). The MSLT studies sleep latency at 2-hour intervals during the day and documents (by EEG and EMG) the sleep type induced. Narcolepsy is diagnosed by mean sleep latency less than 5 minutes and the induction of REM at onset of two sleep events. These studies should be performed in a sleep laboratory, as standard EEGs are not adequately sensitive in documenting REM: false-positive results occur with depression, drug withdrawal, and sleep deprivation.

Narcolepsy may also be a rare symptom of central nervous system lesions in the region of the third ventricle and hypothalamus. Multiple disease processes have been associated with such symptomatic narcolepsy (which may include cataplexy).

Treatment of narcolepsy should begin with planned 15- to 20-minute naps as needed throughout the day. One to three such intervals is usually adequate, and each nap provides several hours of sleep-free performance. Exercise, avoiding heavy meals, and ingestion of caffeinated beverages are also effective.

Pharmacologic therapy has traditionally relied on stimulants (methylphenidate 5–60 mg or dextroamphetamine 5–50 mg daily). Complete relief of daytime sleepiness is rarely achieved, and side effects of irritability, restlessness, psychosis, and hypertension are of concern. Habituation may occur with chronic use, although drug holidays (1 day/wk) may decrease this risk. Alternative medications of different classes but similar CNS targets are now available, although their performance is not superior to the traditional stimulants. Modafinil (alpha-adrenergic agonist), 100 mg every morning to 200 mg every morning and at noon was effective in a recent controlled trial. The imidazole derivative mazindol and the mono-

amine oxidase inhibitor selegiline are also effective. Cylert (pemoline) is also commonly used.

CATAPLEXY. Cataplexy is eventually associated with narcolepsy in perhaps 70% of patients, although its onset may precede narcolepsy or not occur for a decade. A history of cataplexy is, therefore, useful to support a diagnosis of narcolepsy. The cataplectic phenomenon is that of emotion-induced, reflex muscular atonia, which spares respiratory muscles. Laughter is the most common inducer. The atonic phenomenon may be partial (dropping an object from the hand), generalized (buckling at the knees) or global (falling down). Most attacks last less than a minute, although prolonged atonic episodes have been described. Cataplexy, hypnagogic hallucinations, and sleep paralysis are fragments of events normally confined to REM sleep that appear during wakefulness. Atonia corresponds to the impairment of volitional movements that might otherwise occur during dreaming. The cellular group responsible has been defined in the narcoleptic dog to be that of a group of non-cholinergic neurons in the medial medulla that have high firing rates only during cataplectic events or rapid eye movement sleep.

Cataplectic attacks can be attenuated in most patients by clomipramine (10–150 mg/d). The antidepressants imipramine (10–150 mg/day) or desipramine (25–200 mg/day) are also effective. Cataplexy can rarely be the initial manifestation of a midbrain lesion.

SLEEP PARALYSIS. Sleep paralysis occurs in a quarter of narcoleptics but also occurs in non-narcoleptics as an isolated or recurrent phenomenon at the sleep-wake transition. Sleep paralysis is a frightening event with awareness of paralysis of all but the ventilatory and extraocular muscles. Hypnogogic and hypnopompic hallucinations may be associated (see Table 448–1). Both deep tendon reflexes and H reflexes are depressed during the event. The paralysis is limited to seconds to a few minutes. In the rare patient in whom this is a recurrent problem, 5HT reuptake inhibitors which suppress REM sleep (clomipramine) or fluoxetine (10–40 mg qd) have been prescribed. Hallucinations occur in a third of narcoleptics and are manifested as vivid dreams that occur at sleep/wake transitions and continue into the process of awakening. Patients are usually aware that the perceived events are hallucinations. Differential diagnosis includes peduncular hallucinosis (usually the result of emboli to the top of the basilar artery) or the vivid dreams that occurs as a side effect of anticholinergic or dopa-agonist medications (especially in patients with Parkinson's disease).

DISORDERS OF CIRCADIAN RHYTHM. Disorders of circadian rhythm are most commonly experienced in the setting of "jet lag" when a new sleep/wake cycle is required upon entering a distant time zone. Disordered sleep, impaired concentration, fatigue, decreased appetite, and irritability result. Symptoms are proportional to the number of time lines crossed and therefore do not occur even with long flights north to south. Eastward travel produces symptoms that are greater than those of western travel. Symptoms are also increased with age.

Circadian oscillations are the result of the CLOCK gene/gene product. Clock-induced proteins then feed back to inhibit their transcription resulting in circadian rhythms. The biologic clock is located in the superchiasmatic nucleus at the base of the hypothalamus. Loss of neurons in this region occur in Alzheimer's disease and may be responsible for "sundowning." The clock is modulated by light/dark cycles via pathways from the retina. The endogenous modulator is melatonin. Both metabolic and behavioral rhythms are regulated and linked; body temperature, for example, falls 1° C or more during the urge to sleep, with the lowest temperatures reached just prior to waking. Light and/or melatonin exposure might provide therapy for jet lag, but the relationship between the two is complex, with melatonin secretion being suppressed by light. Early evening ingestion of melatonin in the new time zone may attenuate jet lag: the optimal dose is uncertain. Tables for the dosing of bright light treatment as an adjustment for jet lag are published. The traditional use of short-acting benzodiazepines (zolpidem or temazepam) remains useful for sleep induction in new time zones.

SLEEP APNEA. *Obstructive sleep apnea* occurs in 2 to 5% of the adult American population and affects men and middle aged to elderly preferentially. The classic presentation is the patient with loud snoring who has multiple arousals or awakening during the night, gasping for breath. A hundred or more events per night may occur. The resultant sleep fragmentation produces daytime sleepiness and impaired occupational performance. Episodes are exacerbated by alcohol use at bedtime as well as sedative hypnotic drugs. The supine position for sleeping is the worst.

On physical examination, the patients are often obese. Crowding of the nasopharynx may be observable, induced by structural abnormalities, such as an edematous uvula, an enlarged tongue or tonsillar hypertrophy. The apneic spells must be 10 seconds or greater (average 20–30 seconds) in duration to be diagnostic, but may be considerably longer. The frequency must be greater than or equal to 5/hour recorded over 6 to 7 hours. The presence or absence of respiratory effort separates obstructive from central causes of sleep apnea.

Preventive treatments include weight loss and alcohol avoidance. Continuous positive airway pressure (CPAP) during sleep results in improvement in the vast majority of patients. Neurologic conditions inducing obstructive sleep apnea are mainly those producing weakness of the bulbar muscles: myasthenia gravis, the muscular dystrophies, ALS, and acid maltase deficiency as well as lower brain stem structural lesions or degenerative disorders.

Central sleep apnea results from impairment of central ventilatory control. These disorders account for less than 10% of sleep apneic patients. The syndrome is likely to be apnea at sleep onset in a non-obese patient with unremarkable snoring. Greater than five events per hour is abnormal. These apneic spells are briefer than those with obstructive sleep apnea. Any disease process affecting the caudal brain stem, where the ventilatory nuclei reside in the caudal medulla, may result in ventilatory impairment. Poliomyelitis was the classic disorder, but brain stem tumors, infections, ischemia, or autonomic dysfunction (Shy-Drager syndrome) or autonomic neuropathies (diabetic mellitus) predominates. Spinal cord lesions, including tumors and demyelinating disease, may interrupt pathways from the medulla to ventilatory muscles and produce apneic spells as well. The syndrome of Ondine's curse is one of intact volitional ventilation but impaired automatic breathing; in this syndrome, however, pathways for volitional ventilation from cortex through the corticospinal pathways are intact while the pathways for automatic breathing from medulla, which descend separately in the brain stem are impaired. Thus, apnea occurs with sleep. This syndrome can be seen with developmental, vascular, or degenerative processes affecting the brain stem. Examples include syringomyelia, spinocerebellar atrophy, unilateral or bilateral medullary strokes, or as the result of bilateral cervical cordotomies for pain. Complete impairment of automatic ventilation has often lead to tracheostomy and assisted ventilation. Many central sleep apnea patients can be successfully treated by bilevel positive airway pressure (BIPAP) ventilation. CPAP or BIPAP are also effective when central and obstructive sleep apnea coexist.

SLEEP DISORDERS IN AGING AND DEMENTIA. Increased daytime sleep with impaired nocturnal sleep is characteristic of late life. The phenomenon of "sundowning" is a most difficult problem for patient and caregiver. Sundowning episodes include nocturnal delirium with disordered thinking, perception, and agitation. Although the cause is unknown, Alzheimer's disease does result in degeneration of brain stem nuclei in the regions responsible for sleep regulation. Furthermore, degeneration of the superchiasmatic nucleus, responsible for circadian rhythms, occurs as well. In some patients, episodes of prolonged daytime, deep-sleep states occur during which the patient cannot easily be aroused.

Treatment of sleep disorders in Alzheimer's disease is difficult. The wisest approach is to begin with discontinuation of drugs that may exacerbate episodes of delirium. Infections, especially urinary tract infections, should be excluded, and any treatable metabolic disorders (congestive heart failure, chronic pulmonary disease) should be treated. Behavioral treatment consists of increasing daytime activity and decreasing daytime sleep. Bright light exposure during the day and a familiar surround at night are useful. Sedatives are often prescribed but they frequently exacerbate the confusional aspects of sundowning. Trazodone may be effective (50 mg at bedtime). Neuroleptics are a last resort.

Waterhouse J, Reilly T, Atkinson G: Jet-lag. Lancet 350:1611, 1997. *Review of melatonin and light therapy with suggested regimens.*

Hobson JA, Stickgold R, Pace-Schott EF: The neuropsychology of REM sleep dreaming. Neuroreport 16:R1, 1998. *Current thinking regarding the neuroanatomical and neuropsychology substrate in brain responsible for dreaming.*

Randomized trial of modafinil for the treatment of pathological somnolence in narcolepsy. US Modafinil in Narcolepsy Multicenter Study Group. Ann Neurol 43:88, 1998. *Data supporting modafinil as an alternative to stimulants for narcolepsy.*

449 DISORDERS OF COGNITION
Jeffrey L. Cummings

449.1 Diagnosis of Regional Cerebral Dysfunction

John M. Ringman ■ Jeffrey L. Cummings

Many neurologic disorders affect the cerebral hemispheres in a regionally specific, or *focal*, fashion. Defining the nature and extent of the resulting clinical syndrome is helpful not only in localizing brain lesions but also in establishing their etiologies, thus influencing medical management. Although recent developments in neuroimaging (e.g., magnetic resonance imaging) have greatly facilitated our ability to diagnose focal cerebral pathology, it is only through clinical examination that one can know when an imaging study is indicated in the management of a given patient. Additionally, only by defining specific deficits and preserved abilities can one appreciate the impact that a neurologic condition has on the patient's life. This information is crucial in determining an appropriate approach to treatment and rehabilitation.

Important clues regarding the etiology of a neurologic complaint may be obtained by taking a careful history. The rate of onset of symptoms, as well as the tempo of progression, can be helpful in distinguishing vascular events, which are normally abrupt, from space-occupying lesions, from which symptoms may evolve over days, weeks, or months. These rules have limits; many subacute or chronic processes (for example, arteriovenous malformations) may be initially manifested as a paroxysmal event such as a seizure or hemorrhage. Associated symptoms such as weight loss in the case of metastatic cancer or fever in the case of cerebral abscess should be specifically sought. A thorough general examination in addition to a neurologic examination may uncover an occult etiology.

Although routine neurologic examination may be adequate for determining the site of cerebral pathology in some cases, more complete mental status testing can define a deficit that would not otherwise have been appreciated. A carefully conducted mental status examination can provide information regarding regional hemispheric dysfunction similar to the information on motor and sensory abnormalities obtained from findings on routine neurologic examination. Mental status testing can occasionally uncover the only significant disturbances indicating a need for further work-up. Unfortunately, such testing is often omitted because of the time it takes, lack of expertise in interpretation, and unawareness of its importance. Many attempts have been made to circumvent these issues by developing brief, standardized, and well-validated bedside tests. The most commonly used such test is the Mini-Mental Status Examination (MMSE), a scale that samples attention, memory, language, calculation, and some visuospatial abilities. However, brief assessments such as the MMSE inevitably have limitations; the MMSE does not detect important but subtle cognitive changes that may be revealed by more extensive neuropsychological testing.

Such neuropsychological testing is helpful in some contexts, but it rarely contributes to the localization of a lesion not evident on bedside neurologic or mental status testing. Neuropsychological assessment is most useful when cognitive complaints are present despite a normal bedside examination, to delineate the strengths and weaknesses of a patient for planning rehabilitation, when normal aging must be distinguished from mild pathologic cognitive changes, or when a baseline value is needed to which subsequent change in cognitive performance can be compared. Care must be taken, however, when interpreting the results of neuropsychological tests because of the many factors (age, language, education, culture, etc.) that are known to affect performance, as well as the reliability and validity of the specific tests used.

The cerebral cortex may be divided into paired frontal lobes, temporal lobes, parietal lobes, and occipital lobes; some add a 5th, the limbic lobe. Further subdivisions are made on the basis of

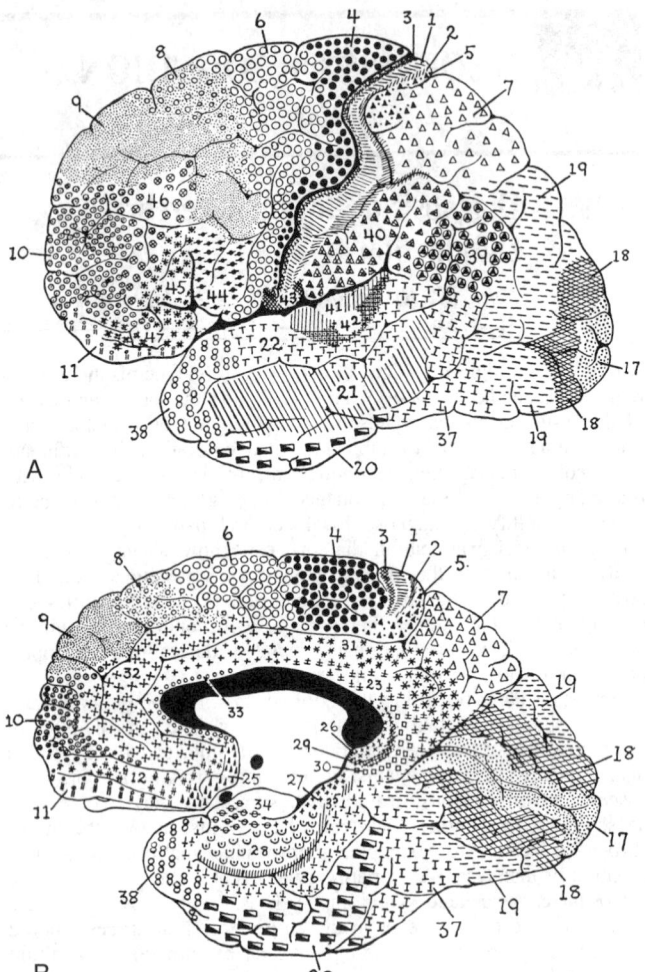

A

B

FIGURE 449-1 ■ Cortical areas as defined by Brodmann according to their cytoarchitectonic structure. See text for details.

cytoarchitecture (Brodmann areas, see Fig. 449–1) and connectivity. Those areas that most directly influence or are influenced by the external environment are called primary, or *isotypic,* cortex: the primary visual cortex (Brodmann area 17) in the occipital lobe, auditory cortex (41, 42) in the superior temporal gyrus, somatosensory cortex (3, 1, 2) in the anterior parietal lobe, and motor cortex (4) in the adjacent posterior frontal lobe. These areas project to and receive input from the adjacent *unimodal association* cortex. Higher processing of motor programs or sensory stimuli within a given modality occur here. These areas in turn project to and from the *heteromodal association* cortex, which occupies the posterior inferior parietal regions and the pre-frontal cortex. It is in these regions that information from different sensory modalities converges and can influence motor programs. An additional functional and anatomic unit, the limbic lobe, which includes portions of the frontal and temporal lobes, as well as subcortical structures, can also be distinguished. Figure 449–2 demonstrates the distribution of these functional cortical areas, and Figure 449–3 presents the gyral and sulcal landmarks that are alluded to in the rest of this chapter. In the following material we discuss the behavioral syndromes that arise when these structures are affected by focal disease processes.

FRONTAL LOBES

In humans the frontal lobes are the largest of the cerebral regions and represent almost one third of the total cortical surface area. The great development of the frontal lobes is the most salient neuroanatomic characteristic distinguishing humans from non-human primates and from other mammals. The specific role of the frontal lobes in cognition and behavior is controversial. On IQ tests

in which long-standing language, memory, and visuospatial skills are tested in a structured manner, subjects with extensive frontal lobe damage may perform well. However, in social and other real-life situations in which mental flexibility and planning are required, such subjects may be completely unable to cope. This ability to self-monitor behavior and choose an appropriate response in the context of ongoing internal and external events is among the frontal lobes' *executive* functions. Neuropsychological tests specifically designed to assess frontal lobe function may be helpful in revealing deficits that are otherwise silent.

Consisting of the primary motor area (Brodmann area 4) on the anterior bank of the central sulcus and all cortex anterior to it, different parts of the frontal lobe share the function of determining and organizing behavioral *output.* Projections from various regions of the frontal cortex descend to subcortical structures, including the spinal cord, brain stem nuclei, thalamus, and basal ganglia. Five separate circuits involving serial connections from parts of the frontal cortex to the striatum, globus pallidus, and thalamus with feedback to the cortex have been defined. Similar behavioral and cognitive syndromes may arise from lesions in distinct structures anywhere within a given circuit.

Anterior to isotypic area 4 are Brodmann areas 6 and 8. This region is the unimodal association cortex of the motor system and is referred to as *pre-motor* cortex. Its extension onto the medial bank of the superior frontal gyrus represents the *supplementary motor area.* The *motor* circuit arises from the primary sensorimotor cortex, pre-motor area, and supplementary motor area. Lesions along this circuit may result in weakness of contralateral extremity muscles or loss of coordination of fine finger movements. Lesions of the pre-motor area of the language-dominant hemisphere may cause a disturbance in the motor programs of speech, or cortical dysarthria. Unilateral stimulation of the supplementary area causes automatisms involving both sides of the body.

Broca's area (Brodmann areas 44 and 45) is in the inferior aspect of the pre-motor area, or the frontal *operculum.* Lesions in this area on the language-dominant side cause a characteristic language disturbance, or *aphasia,* characterized by loss of the orderly execution of language. In this *non-fluent* or *motor* aphasia, the patient's verbal output is sparse with short agrammatic phrases, word-finding abnormalities, and impaired repetition. Comprehension

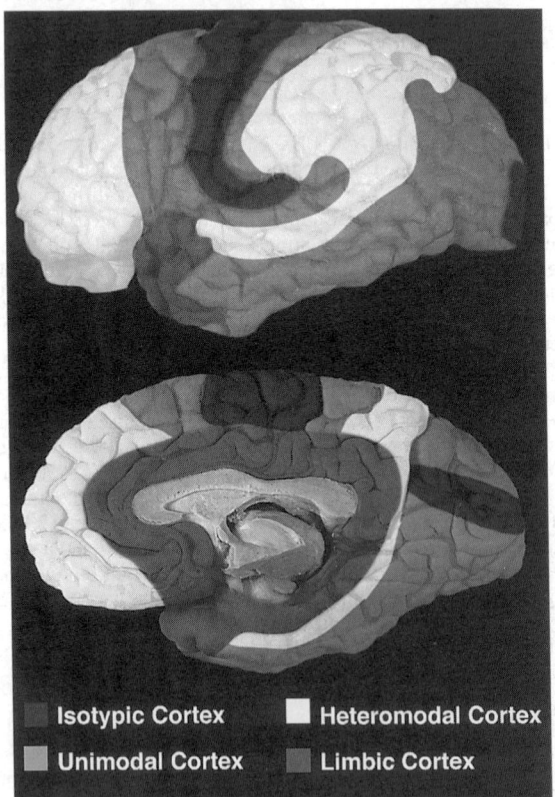

Isotypic Cortex   Heteromodal Cortex
Unimodal Cortex   Limbic Cortex

FIGURE 449–2 ■ Functional cortical regions defined according to their principal afferent and efferent projection patterns.

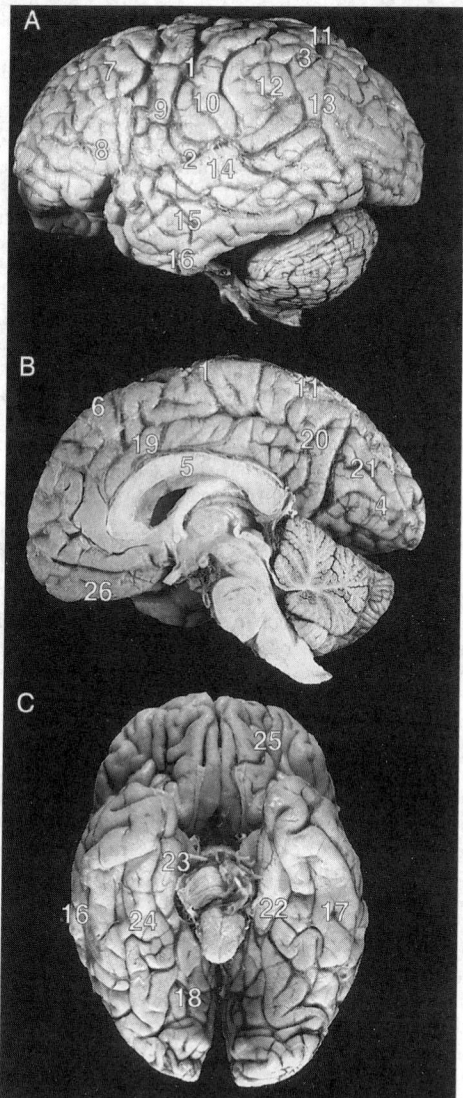

FIGURE 449-3 ■ *A* to *C,* The principal gyral and sulcal landmarks of the cerebral cortex shown in lateral, sagittal, and inferior views. 1, Central sulcus. 2, Sylvian fissure. 3, Intraparietal sulcus. 4, Calcarine sulcus. 5, Corpus callosum. 6, Superior frontal gyrus. 7, Middle frontal gyrus. 8, Inferior frontal gyrus. 9, Pre-central gyrus. 10, Post-central gyrus. 11, Superior parietal lobule. 12, Supramarginal gyrus. 13, Angular gyrus. 14, Superior temporal gyrus. 15, Middle temporal gyrus. 16, Inferior temporal gyrus. 17, Fusiform gyrus. 18, Lingual gyrus. 19, Cingulate gyrus. 20, Precuneus. 21, Cuneus. 22, Parahippocampal gyrus. 23, Uncus. 24, Occipitotemporal gyrus. 25, Orbital gyri of the frontal lobe. 26, Gyrus rectus.

The *dorsolateral pre-frontal* cortex includes Brodmann areas 9 and 10 on the convexity of the frontal lobe. The impairment in executive function arising from damage to this area is characterized by a memory retrieval deficit, reduced fluency of output, and an inability to think abstractly. The memory deficit is characterized by impaired spontaneous recall and preservation of recognition memory. Lesions on either side cause reduced verbal fluency (e.g., number of animals named in 1 minute), and patients with right-sided lesions have a reduced ability to produce varied figures. Subjects with lesions of the dorsolateral pre-frontal circuit have difficulty changing the cognitive set, impaired response inhibition, deficits in sustained attention, and perseveration. Such subjects have difficulty moving from one mode of response to another and tend to get stuck and repeat themselves verbally or through their performance. They exhibit *stimulus boundedness,* in which their behavior can be seen as a direct consequence of environmental influences. For example, when asked to copy a figure on paper, they might draw directly over the figure rather than next to it. The extreme form of this phenomenon is *utilization* behavior, in which objects within reach are automatically manipulated in the manner in which they are normally used, without regard for context. Depression is a common consequence of frontal lobe damage, particularly on the left side. Dorsolateral pre-frontal dysfunction is dramatic in frontotemporal lobar degeneration and also occurs in Alzheimer's disease. Frontal-subcortical circuit abnormalities are present in basal ganglia disorders. Tumors and thromboembolic events of the anterior branches of the middle cerebral artery may result in the dorsolateral frontal syndrome. Patients with chronic schizophrenia and depression may exhibit similar behavior, possibly a reflection of relative hypometabolism of the frontal lobes, which has been demonstrated on functional neuroimaging.

Damage to the *lateral orbitofrontal* cortex is frequently not evident on the usual neuropsychological testing. Instead, such lesions tend to be manifested as disturbed social behavior, including disinhibited, impulsive, and tactless responses. Idiopathic obsessive-compulsive disorder is associated with increased metabolism of the orbitofrontal cortex and the caudate nuclei. Acquired obsessive-compulsive behavior and occasionally mania may arise after damage to the orbitofrontal circuit. This area is prone to damage by closed head trauma and by meningiomas of the anterior cranial fossa. Such insults may be associated with *anosmia,* or a deficit in olfaction from damage to the underlying olfactory tracts.

The *medial frontal* portion of the frontal lobe contains the anterior cingulate gyrus. This cortical region mediates analysis of the emotional relevance of stimuli, and damage to it results in an apathetic state with reduced interest, lack of motivation, and decreased activity. The most profound form of this state, *akinetic mutism,* produces an awake, though motionless and mute patient and usually occurs when the damage is bilateral. Damage to the medial portion of the frontal lobes may result from vascular events affecting the distribution of the anterior cerebral artery.

Transcortical motor aphasia most commonly results from a lesion of the left medial frontal region. It may also be caused by a lesion that isolates Broca's area from the frontal heteromodal cortex, such as infarction of the watershed zone between areas perfused by the anterior and middle cerebral arteries. Like Broca's aphasia, it is non-fluent, but the ability to repeat verbal phrases is relatively preserved.

The frontal lobes serve a key role in determining, organizing, and executing behavior. Information regarding the external environment and its historical relevance is provided by more posterior portions of the cerebrum.

is relatively preserved, and patients with Broca's aphasia are often frustrated by their inability to speak. Lesions in Broca's area of the right hemisphere give rise to a deficit in executing prosodic elements of speech and music such as pitch and melody. Involvement of the motor and pre-motor areas by epileptic seizure activity may result in complex automatisms (coordinated, yet automatic-appearing movements), tonic contraversive head movements with tonic posturing of the contralateral limbs, and contralateral clonic movements.

Apraxia is loss of the ability to perform organized motoric acts despite relative preservation of strength, sensation, and comprehension. The brain has a hemispheric dominance for limb praxis such that lesions of portions of the pre-motor areas in the left hemisphere may cause an ipsilateral, or *sympathetic,* apraxia, as well as contralateral apraxia.

The frontal eye fields in area 8 and the supplementary eye fields govern eye movements and give rise to the *oculomotor* circuit. Electrical stimulation to this area elicits conjugate eye deviation toward the opposite side, and ablation causes ipsilateral gaze deviation.

PARIETAL LOBES

The central sulcus defines the anterior border of the parietal lobe. The parietal and temporal lobes are separated by a border defined by an imaginary line connecting the sylvian fissure with the occipital lobe. Brodmann area 3 lies along the posterior wall of the central sulcus and, along with areas 1 and 2, represents the isotypic primary somatosensory cortex. Areas 5 and 7 constitute the superior parietal lobule, which lies along the sagittal surface of the parietal lobe and is separated from the inferior parietal lobule by the intraparietal sulcus. The inferior parietal lobule is further divided into the supramarginal gyrus (Brodmann area 40) anteriorly and the angular gyrus (area 39) posteriorly. Situated between somatosensory, visual, and auditory cortical receiving areas, the bulk of the parietal lobe is involved in unimodal and heteromodal sensory processing. In the parietal and temporal lobes a marked functional asymmetry between the left and right hemispheres is evident. In part because of the arbitrary landmarks in the area, a number of behavioral syndromes have been loosely associated with the region of the parieto-temporo-occipital border.

Lesions of the primary somatosensory area cause loss of tactile sensation on the contralateral side of the body, the exact area involved depending on the portion of the somatotopic map affected. With such lesions, fundamental modalities such as contact, temperature, and pain sensation are generally retained, but the more highly processed somatosensation is impaired, such as decreased sensitivity to differences in intensity of a stimulus, loss of appreciation of the direction of movement of a stimulus, and poor two-point discrimination. This impairment results in forms of tactile deficits clinically identifiable as *astereognosis* (inability to recognize objects by touch) and *agraphesthesia* (inability to identify figures drawn into the palm). With unilateral lesions these deficits are most profound on the contralateral side of the body, but milder deficits may be appreciated ipsilaterally, especially when the lesion is in the right hemisphere. The most common aura associated with seizures originating from the parietal lobe is contralateral numbness and tingling. Although pain perception is not generally affected by primary sensory area lesions, painful experiences may occur when epileptic activity occurs in this region. Auras associated with epileptic foci in more posterior portions of the parietal lobe may consist of distortions in body schema and position, such as feeling as though an appendage is absent or an extra limb is present or the feeling of vertigo and other sensations of movement. Disorders of higher cognitive function associated with parietal lesions depend on the hemisphere involved. Because of the course of the optic radiations through the white matter, posterior parietal lesions may cause a contralateral inferior homonymous quadrantanopia.

Lesions of the left parietal lobe produce deficits in varied aspects of communication. Comprehension and semantics (word meaning) are typically most affected. Lesions of the parietal heteromodal cortex may result in *transcortical sensory* aphasia. This disorder is a fluent aphasia syndrome characterized by deficits in language comprehension and relatively spared repetition. Lesions of the left inferior parietal cortex may lead to *conduction aphasia,* in which repetition is impaired but spontaneous speech production and comprehension are spared. The lesion underlying this syndrome affects the arcuate fasciculus separating posterior language areas from anterior executive language areas.

Alexia, or the inability to read, is often accompanied by agraphia, the inability to write. In cases of alexia with agraphia, the lesion typically involves the angular gyrus of the left parietal lobe. Agraphia in the absence of any other language or praxis disturbance has been reported with lesions of the posterior middle frontal gyrus, with lesions of the superior parietal lobule, but most consistently with lesions of the supramarginal gyrus of the left hemisphere. The anatomy of alexia without agraphia, or pure word blindness, is better understood. This disorder is a *disconnection syndrome* in which afferents carrying processed visual information from the right hemisphere are affected, with the left angular gyrus isolated; the parietal lobe per se may not be damaged. *Anomia,* or difficulty recalling the names of objects, occurs with left angular gyrus or left temporal polar lesions. However, different forms of anomic aphasia are seen with lesions in various parts of the cerebral cortex and are frequent early signs in degenerative dementia. Anomia in itself is of little localizing value.

The tetrad of agraphia, right-left disorientation, finger agnosia (inability to identify specific fingers), and acalculia (inability to perform mathematic operations) constitutes Gerstmann's syndrome and occurs with damage to the left angular gyrus. A deficit in any one of these skills does not have specific localizing value. Only when all four coexist should one suspect angular gyrus involvement.

Apraxias in which subjects pantomime poorly or are unable to perform gestures on command occur with lesions of the left inferior parietal lobule, left pre-motor cortex, and corpus callosum. Performance is enhanced when the subject is given an actual object to manipulate. Parietal apraxia commonly occurs in association with conduction aphasia.

Lesions of the right parietal lobe are frequently characterized by *hemispatial neglect.* In this condition the subject does not attend to stimuli in the neglected sphere contralateral to the lesion. They may ignore the left half of the visual field, the left half of their bodies, auditory stimuli from the left hemispace, or anything in the left hemiuniverse. A milder form of neglect called extinction has been described; in extinction, subjects are capable of attending to contralateral stimuli but, when presented with stimuli simultaneously on both sides, respond only to the ipsilateral side. Neglect has been reported with damage to the right dorsolateral frontal lobe, cingulate gyrus, putamen, and thalamus, but most consistently with lesions of the right inferior parietal lobule. Neglect associated with frontal lobe damage may result in a decreased tendency to react with the contralateral limb. When acute, as when caused by a stroke, neglect may be severe but then tends to recover. Neglect may also occur transiently with left parietal lobe lesions but usually resolves.

Anosognosia, or the lack of knowledge of one's deficit, often accompanies hemispatial neglect arising from right parietal lesions. Subjects may deny their left hemiparesis, hemianesthesia, or hemianopia and as a result attempt to perform activities of which they are incapable. If they are aware of their deficit, they may exhibit anosodiaphoria, or relative lack of concern regarding their impairment.

Many studies have implicated a role for the parietal lobes, especially in the right hemisphere, in visuospatial functions. Specific tasks on which subjects with right parietal lesions have been shown to be more impaired include localization of points in space, estimation of line orientation, tests of topographic orientation, some tests of depth perception, and tests of facial discrimination. A common sequela of non-dominant parietal damage is difficulty dressing, which may be due to a combined hemibody neglect and spatial disorientation.

A convergence of information from electrophysiologic and ablation studies in animals is suggesting that visual information initially processed in the striate cortex (Brodmann area 17 in the occipital lobe) undergoes further processing in two separate pathways. A ventral pathway passing forward into the temporal lobes is concerned primarily with identifying visual stimuli, the so-called *what* pathway. The dorsal pathway that involves occipitoparietal connections plays a role in determining the location of visual stimuli, the so-called *where* pathway. These animal data conform to human neuropsychological studies implicating a role for the parietal lobes in visuospatial functions. Disorders of visual perception may occur with lesions at the occipitoparietal or occipitotemporal borders.

OCCIPITAL LOBES

The occipital lobes are the smallest of the cortical divisions and lie at the most caudal aspect of the cerebrum. The isotypic primary visual receiving area (Brodmann area 17) forms the lips of the calcarine sulcus on the medial aspect of the occipital lobes. The superior lip receives afferents representing the contralateral inferior visual field, and the inferior lip receives afferents from the contralateral superior visual field. The unimodal visual association areas 18 and 19 form concentric rings around area 17. Lesions of the occipital lobes are therefore manifested as changes in visual perception, and a homonymous visual field cut is frequently seen. In part because of the small size of the occipital lobes, isolated occipital lobe syndromes are relatively rare.

In complete cortical blindness, or blindness caused by bilateral destruction of the occipital lobes or their afferents, retention of pupillary responses reflects intact visual input to the brain stem. Denial of blindness, or *Anton's syndrome,* frequently occurs in association with damage to the visual cortex, as well as with more peripheral causes of blindness. Subjects with Anton's syndrome may bump into things when walking and frequently suffer from general intellectual impairment.

Hallucinations can occur as a result of occipital lobe injury by one of two mechanisms. *Release hallucinations* occur with visual loss of any etiology. When visual loss is cortical in origin, these hallucinations appear in the abnormal field and may be complex and continuous. *Ictal hallucinations* are rare and are a manifestation of seizures originating in the occipital lobes. Such hallucinations arising from area 17 generally consist of contralateral lights (or darkness) moving from the periphery to the center of the visual fields. Focal seizures arising from areas 18 or 19 may be motionless and pulsatile and may occur in both the ipsilateral and contralateral hemifields. More complicated visual hallucinations most likely originate in the temporal lobe.

When the occipitoparietal areas are damaged bilaterally, *simultagnosia* may occur. In this condition the subject is unable to attend to more than a small part of the visual field at once and consequently has difficulty understanding whole scenes. It may occur as part of the triad of *Balint's syndrome* along with optic ataxia (difficulty with visually guided arm movements) and sticky fixation (difficulty switching fixation from one object to another). Selective deficits in perception of movement may occur with occipital lobe lesions. Alexia without agraphia was described above as a disconnection syndrome in which the left angular gyrus is isolated from visual information. The most common cause is a lesion in the occipitoparietal white matter of the left hemisphere with concomitant involvement of the splenium of the corpus callosum and optic radiations. An associated right homonymous hemianopia is usually present.

Visual agnosia, or "a normal (visual) percept stripped of its meaning," may occur with more ventral occipital lobe damage. Agnosia has been subdivided into *apperceptive agnosia*, or a defect in perceiving all but the most basic aspects of visual stimuli such as color and movement, and *associative agnosia*, characterized by an inability to recognize stimuli despite completely intact visual perception (as demonstrated by the ability to draw the object). Patients with either type of agnosia can recognize objects through other sensory modalities. It is therefore necessary to assess language abilities, as well as the ability to recognize, in non-visual sensory modalities to characterize an agnosia. Visual agnosia is generally due to bilateral lesions in the occipitotemporal area affecting the inferior longitudinal fasciculus and is often associated with other visual disturbances. Visual agnosia has been described as resulting from lesions more anterior in the ventral visual pathway in the temporal lobes. *Achromatopsia*, or acquired color blindness, typically involves a single hemifield and is caused by a lesion of the contralateral occipitotemporal area. Prosopagnosia is the inability to recognize familiar faces visually, although it can also be manifested as an inability to distinguish individuals among a class of objects (e.g., a farmer unable to discriminate among his cows). The lesion is most frequently bilateral in the lingual and fusiform gyri of the ventral occipitotemporal area, although unilateral right-sided lesions can produce the syndrome. It is often associated with *environmental agnosia*, or the inability to recognize familiar places.

Infarction in the distribution of the posterior cerebral arteries is a frequent etiology of occipital lobe damage; head injury, tumors, and many other processes can affect the occipital lobes as well. Visual field defects, particularly those caused by lesions of the nondominant occipital lobe, are often overlooked by the patient.

TEMPORAL LOBES

The temporal lobe is bordered by the occipital lobes posteriorly and the sylvian fissure superiorly. Its lateral surface consists of the superior, middle, and inferior temporal gyri, which run longitudinally. The inferior surface is also composed of longitudinal gyri: the occipitotemporal gyrus and the more medial parahippocampal gyrus. The parahippocampal gyrus, as well as the underlying amygdala and hippocampus and the temporal pole, will be discussed below as limbic structures. The primary auditory area (Brodmann areas 41 and 42) is located within the sylvian fissure on a transverse portion of the superior temporal gyrus (Heschl's gyrus). Aside from this isotypic cortex, the temporal lobe consists mainly of paralimbic cortex and unimodal and heteromodal association cortex. The anterior temporal lobe connects with the orbitofrontal region via the uncinate fasciculus, and the posterior temporal lobe is connected with more lateral frontal lobe by the arcuate fasciculus. A portion of the optic radiations (Meyer's loop) courses through the temporal lobe such that temporal lesions can sometimes give rise to a contralateral superior quadrantanopia. Seizure

disorders frequently arise from pathology in the temporal lobes and adjacent structures.

Complete destruction of the primary auditory area unilaterally does not result in appreciable hearing deficits. Acute bilateral destruction (for example, by bilateral middle cerebral artery infarction) is rare and causes *cortical deafness*, or lack of a behavioral response to sounds of any kind. Over time this condition generally improves such that the subject can demonstrate some hearing but may have persistent *auditory agnosia*, or a deficit in the ability to recognize sounds. This condition also occurs with involvement of auditory association areas anterior to and sparing areas 41 and 42 and can be manifested as an inability to grasp the meaning of sounds such as car horns or a ringing telephone. Because of the proximity of areas important for language comprehension, auditory agnosia rarely exists without a concurrent language deficit. It is therefore important to assess language function when examining for auditory abilities. A condition termed *pure word deafness* in which patients are unable to understand spoken language but do not have a more general auditory agnosia or aphasia occasionally occurs. It is caused by bilateral lesions separating the primary auditory areas from the posterior association cortex. Usually such difficulty is associated with Wernicke's aphasia.

Lesions in the posterior superior temporal lobe of the left hemisphere cause Wernicke's aphasia, in which fluent paraphasic output and impairment in language comprehension are the predominant features. Patients also have impaired verbal repetition and some degree of alexia. Patients with this condition have intact motor output and persist in uttering nonsense phrases filled with *paraphasias* (incorrect word or letter substitutions) that retain grammatical structure. Unlike the frustration seen in patients with Broca's aphasia, those with Wernicke's aphasia are often oblivious to their deficit and therefore do not respond well to most forms of speech therapy. They are not aware that people do not understand them and may become alarmed as though believing that those around them are speaking in code.

A selective *amusia*, or the inability to recognize or appreciate pitch and melodies, may occur with right posterior temporal or inferior parietal lesions. Deficits resulting from right temporal lobe lesions are generally subtle and require specific testing for spatial orientation, fine visual discrimination, and odor discrimination.

Focal seizures arising from the temporal lobe may give rise to changes in ongoing language function and to sensory, emotional, or psychic phenomena. Auditory hallucinations arising from the superior temporal gyrus range from simple sounds to complex speech, whereas visual hallucinations arising from the temporal lobe are generally complicated scenes or visual memories. The psychic and visceral experiences that occur during seizures arising from limbic structures within the temporal lobes are discussed below.

LIMBIC LOBE

Situated between the neocortex and brain stem structures, the limbic lobe (from the Latin *limbus*, meaning edge or border) forms a ring on the medial surface of the cerebral hemisphere. It consists of the subcallosal gyrus anteriorly, includes the cingulate gyrus curving up and around the corpus callosum, and continues down the medial and inferior aspect of the temporal lobe as the parahippocampal gyrus. Some authors include the temporal poles, pyriform region of the frontal lobes, and portions of the insular cortex in the limbic lobe. The limbic cortex corresponds roughly to Brodmann areas 23, 24, 25, 28, and 35. As opposed to the six-layered neocortex, the cortex of the limbic lobe consists of a three-layered archeocortex (hippocampal formation and dentate gyrus), a three-layered paleocortex (parahippocampal gyrus), and a transitional juxtallocortex (cingulate gyrus). In mammals other than primates and in nonmammalian species, the limbic lobe makes up a much larger proportion of brain volume than it does in humans.

Convergence of data from anatomic investigations, animal studies, and observations in humans suggests that the limbic system plays a role in mediating the experience of emotions, visceral responses, and storage of memories. The limbic system has connections to most areas of the cortex and has intimate connections with the hypothalamus, the "head ganglion" of the autonomic nervous system. In animals, electrical stimulation of the anterior cingulate cortex and the orbital-insular-temporal cortex causes changes in blood pressure, gastrointestinal motility, pupillary dilatation, salivation, bladder contraction, and respiration. In humans, seizure activity in these same areas can cause similar autonomic changes, including orgasm. Lesions of the limbic lobe usually do not induce clinically evident autonomic changes, in part because of the independence of subcortical structures such as the hypothalamus in mediating autonomic reflexes.

Characteristic visceral and psychic phenomena occur with epileptic activity arising from limbic structures. Olfactory sensations, usually of an unpleasant nature, are classically associated with involvement of the uncus in the medial temporal lobe. Autonomic and gustatory sensations are seen with involvement of the opercular area within the sylvian fissure. Psychic sensations of déjà vu, jamais vu, dream-like states, and depersonalization may occur along with associated impairment in consciousness. Profound acute depression, fear, or extreme pleasure is sometimes seen. The temporal neocortex is intimately connected to the deeper limbic structures, so it is difficult to establish whether the observed seizure phenomena are due to limbic or neocortical involvement.

Lesions of the limbic lobe can produce profound deficits in memory. Bilateral anterior temporal dysfunction resulting from lobectomy or other conditions (such as blunt head trauma, stroke, or herpes encephalitis) can cause a severe deficit in the ability to form new memories. Less dramatic deficits in specific items are seen with unilateral lesions, verbal memories being more impaired with left-sided lesions and non-verbal memories such as that for faces being more impaired with right anterior temporal lobe lesions. Considerable debate has arisen over the specific structures that need to be involved to produce this memory deficit. Observations suggest that the hippocampus is required to store emotionally neutral declarative memories whereas the adjacent amygdala is necessary to store emotionally laden memories.

Aside from a memory deficit, bilateral lesions of the anterior temporal lobes can also induce *Klüver-Bucy syndrome*. First described in monkeys, this condition consists of hypersexuality, *hypermetamorphosis* (excessive exploratory behavior), emotional placidity, hyperorality, and agnosia.

ASYMMETRY OF CEREBRAL FUNCTION

Functional asymmetry of the cerebral cortex has been appreciated from the time of Broca's description of aphasia caused by a left hemisphere lesion. Since then, clinical observation and countless studies have confirmed a more important role of the left hemisphere in language production and comprehension in most individuals. Of right-handed subjects, 96 to 99% have left-sided speech representation and bilateral speech representation is rare. In people who are left-handed or of mixed handedness, the majority (70%) still have exclusively left hemisphere speech representation, with 15% having bilateral speech representation. Mild degrees of aphasia frequently result from injury to either hemisphere in left-handers, whereas the aphasia resulting from left hemisphere lesions in right-handed individuals is generally of greater severity and duration. This asymmetry applies more to expressive language inasmuch as some degree of comprehension can be demonstrated in the right hemisphere of strictly right-handed subjects. In addition to non-right-handed people, women as a group tend to exhibit less cerebral lateralization.

Right hemisphere superiority has been found in such tasks as somesthetic and visual recognition of shapes, perception of orientation and perspective, aspects of arithmetic ability, and perception and expression of emotional tone. The right hemisphere's abilities may be more difficult to demonstrate because it is difficult to completely remove language influences in neuropsychological testing.

DISCONNECTION SYNDROMES

Focal lesions can exert their effects in at least two ways. Direct damage to a neuronal structure that performs an operation will prevent that operation and thus impair the output of that region.

Alternatively, a lesion may destroy white matter tracts connecting two structures, thus impairing their interaction while leaving the structures themselves intact. The condition in which independent function of two structures is retained but their interaction is disturbed is referred to as a *disconnection syndrome.*

The most dramatic disconnection syndrome seen in humans occurs after surgical section or other damage to the corpus callosum. Patients who have undergone sectioning of the corpus callosum to control intractable epilepsy generally behave normally. In experimental situations in which stimuli are presented to a single hemisphere, however, they behave as though they have two separate minds. For example, an object placed in the left hand of a blindfolded callosotomized subject can only be sensed by that subject's right hemisphere. The subject may be able to select it out of a number of other objects and show other signs of recognition but is unable to name or verbally describe the object. Information regarding the object cannot reach the left hemisphere. When the object is placed in the right hand of such subjects, the information is available to the left hemisphere and they have no difficulty naming it. In a normal environment in which visual stimuli enter both visual hemifields and objects are palpated with both hands, the impairment may not be noticeable.

Other examples of disconnection syndromes are alexia without agraphia, sympathetic apraxia, and conduction aphasia, which have been described above.

CONCLUSION

The cerebral cortex has a modular organization with functionally related modalities connected in series. Focal damage or disconnection of a module results in a distinct signature syndrome. The hemispheres of humans have highly specialized modules.

The above discussion focuses mainly on the effects of lesions of the cerebral cortex and the underlying white matter. This presentation ignores the important contribution of subcortical structures in behavior. Lesions of the basal ganglia and thalamus may reproduce syndromes similar to those caused by lesions of the cortical areas to which they are connected, particularly in regard to the frontal lobes.

Acknowledgments

We would like to thank Michael Mega, M.D., Ph.D., for help in preparation of the illustrations for this chapter.

Cummings JL, Trimble MR: Neuropsychiatry and Behavioral Neurology. Washington, DC, American Psychiatric Press, 1995. *A handbook that contains information on both focal behavioral neurology and neuropsychiatric syndromes with a chapter devoted to treatment.*

Damasio H, Damasio AR: Lesion Analysis in Neuropsychology. New York, Oxford University Press, 1989. *Helpful in understanding the methodology of lesion studies.*

Heilman K, Valenstein E (eds): Clinical Neuropsychology, 4th ed. Oxford, Oxford University Press, 1995. *Discusses the phenomenology and anatomy of aphasias, apraxias, etc.*

Lezak MD: Neuropsychological Assessment. New York, Oxford University Press, 1995. *Helpful in understanding specific neuropsychological tests and contains an overview of much of the neuropsychological literature.*

Strub RL, Black FW: The Mental Status Examination in Neurology, 3rd ed. Philadelphia, FA Davis, 1993. *A useful and easily accessible approach to bedside testing.*

Penfield W, Jasper W: Epilepsy and the Functional Anatomy of the Human Brain. Boston, Little, Brown, 1954. *The classic description of the phenomenology of focal epilepsy and what it and electrical stimulation tell us about cortical localization.*

449.2   Amnesia and Aphasia

Mario F. Mendez ■ *Jeffrey L. Cummings*

AMNESIA

DEFINITIONS. Memory is the ability to store and recall new information. It is important to distinguish the different types and classifications of memory (Table 449–1). A basic differentiation is the distinction between short-term and long-term memory. Short-term memory involves holding information for a minute or less and is essentially synonymous with primary memory, immediate recall, and sustained attention. Long-term memory involves holding information for longer than a minute. Two types of long-term memory are distinguished: recent memory (secondary memory or new learning) and remote memory (tertiary memory or the retrieval of old

Table 449-1 ■ TYPES OF MEMORY

Temporal Classification
Short-term (primary or immediate) memory
   Working memory (the manipulation of short-term memory)
Long-term memory
   Secondary or recent memory
   Tertiary or remote memory
Explicit versus Implicit Classification
Explicit or declarative (factual) memory
   Episodic (unique characteristics)
   Semantic or generic (categorical membership)
Implicit memory
   Procedural
   Priming
Mechanistic Classification
Registration
Storage and encoding
Consolidation
Retrieval and recognition

established information). Amnesia refers to difficulty learning new information and is primarily concerned with recent memory.

Another classification scheme for memory is less familiar to clinicians but is becoming increasingly clinically relevant as we gain an understanding of brain function. Investigators make a distinction between explicit memory and implicit memory. *Explicit* memory is "declarative," factual, consciously recalled information that is either episodic (specific or unique event) or generic (category or class membership). *Implicit* memory, on the other hand, is not consciously recalled and usually involves the acquisition of skills rather than facts. Clinical amnesic disorders involve primarily explicit information of the episodic type.

In describing amnesia, other memory terms are commonly used. *Registration* refers to attending to information sufficiently to start memory storage. *Encoding,* or storage, refers to the actual process of creating memories. For information to be stored in long-term memory, a period sufficient for memory consolidation must also elapse. *Retrieval* refers to the recollection of established information and is usually tested by a process of recognition (e.g., choosing from among multiple-choice alternatives). *Anterograde amnesia* refers to ongoing memory difficulty and *retrograde amnesia* refers to loss of information stored before the brain insult. Retrograde amnesia ranges from seconds to months, most commonly occurs acutely after head injuries, and generally diminishes during the recovery period. Most amnesic disorders are primarily anterograde.

ETIOLOGY AND EPIDEMIOLOGY. Clinical amnesic disorders result from Alzheimer's disease and other dementias, anoxic or ischemic insults, traumatic brain injury, posterior cerebral artery distribution strokes, herpes encephalitis, thalamic and hypothalamic tumors, paraneoplastic syndromes, Wernicke-Korsakoff syndrome, bitemporal surgery, and epileptic seizures (Table 449–2). Amnesia is often the initial symptom of a dementia syndrome characterized by multiple cognitive deficits. When amnesia occurs in the absence of other cognitive deficits, it is often due to focal lesions in limbic structures (e.g., hippocampus or specific nuclei of the hypothalamus or thalamus).

PATHOPHYSIOLOGY. Amnesia implies injury to the limbic system in both hippocampi in the temporal lobes or in midline limbic structures such as the fornices, mamillary bodies, and mediodorsal nuclei of the thalamus. These structures process memory traces that will eventually be stored diffusely throughout the cortical association areas. Clinical amnesia usually requires bilateral damage in temporolimbic structures. Greater injury to the left hemispheric limbic structures can result in predominant verbal amnesia, and greater injury to the right hemisphere limbic structures can result in predominant visual amnesia. The frontal-subcortical circuits play an additional role in the facilitation of retrieval of old information, and frontal-subcortical circuit disorders result in a retrieval deficit syndrome characterized by poor recall but preserved recognition.

CLINICAL MANIFESTATIONS. Evaluation of memory complaints depends on a focused examination of memory ability. Many general screening mental status scales are insufficient for evaluating amnesia. This evaluation begins with an assessment of orientation, the ability of the patient to provide a history, and the patient's knowledge of current events. A common way to assess verbal

memory is a word list learning task. For the screening examination, a list of 3 or 4 words may suffice; however, for a more extended examination, a list of 10 or 16 words with multiple repetitions is preferable. In the 3- to 4-word tests, the examiner repeats the word list until the patients are able to repeat the words on their own; subsequently, the examiner asks them to recall the words after a 5-minute delay. Normal individuals learn all the words. In the longer word list tests, the examiner reads a list and asks the patient to immediately recall as many words as possible from the list. The examiner repeats this process three to five times. After an interval of 15 or more minutes, during which time the patient's attention is diverted to other tasks, the examiner tests the patient's spontaneous recall of the words. Normal individuals learn most of the list after three or four repetitions and spontaneously recall two thirds or more of the words on delayed recall. The examiner then checks recognition memory and retrieval by giving categorical and multiple-choice clues for the words that are not recalled. Normal patients recognize all of the words. The examiner screens visual memory by evaluating delayed recall of 3 or 4 figures previously drawn by the patient or 3 or 4 items previously hidden in the room. Finally, the examiner assesses remote memory by asking the patient to recall 3 or 4 past public events that have occurred during the individual's lifetime. Alternatively, patients must recognize photographs of famous people or recall the names of television programs. The main difficulty in interpreting remote memory tasks is determining the extent to which the past information was originally acquired.

DIAGNOSIS. "Memory loss" may result from deficits in attention or other cognitive process rather than from amnesia. An initial step in the differential diagnosis of a memory complaint is to exclude the presence of delirium or an acute confusional state. The normal functioning of memory presupposes normal arousal and attentional mechanisms. In general, patients with delirium will have prominent fluctuations in attention, as well as perceptual and other abnormalities.

In addition to delirium, clinicians need to distinguish neurologically based amnesia from the syndrome of "psychogenic amnesia." Patients with conversion reactions and other psychological mechanisms can manifest a memory disorder characterized by loss of remote memories and loss of personal identity or personal information. In sharp contrast to true amnesia, patients with psychogenic amnesia are able to incorporate and learn new information.

People may complain of mild memory loss related to the aging process. This age-associated memory impairment is not amnesia or dementia. Normal aging is associated with retrieval difficulties for proper names and recent events in some individuals older than 50 years. Criteria for age-associated memory impairment include memory difficulty sufficient to impair daily functioning, an otherwise adequate intellectual background, and the absence of dementia or a causative medical or psychiatric condition. In the elderly, this memory difficulty can be exaggerated in the presence of depression.

The most common amnesic syndrome is dementia. Worldwide, at least 7% of persons older than 65 years and nearly half of those older than 85 have some form of dementing illness, and about two

Table 449–2 ■ CAUSES OF AMNESIA

Alzheimer's disease and other dementias
Cerebrovascular
   Posterior cerebral artery and other strokes involving the hippocampi
   Infarction in the medial thalamic nuclei
   Ruptured anterior communicating artery aneurysms
Anoxic/ischemic encephalopathy or hypoglycemia
Head trauma
Encephalitides
   Herpes simplex and other infections
   Limbic and other paraneoplastic syndromes
Mass lesions involving the limbic system
Thiamine deficiency or Wernicke-Korsakoff syndrome
Epileptic seizures
Electroconvulsive therapy
Temporal lobe surgery
Transient global amnesia
Psychogenic amnesia

thirds of these have Alzheimer's disease. The presence of additional cognitive deficits such as aphasia, agnosia, or executive disturbances distinguishes amnesia in the context of dementia.

Most focal amnesic syndromes involve lesions in the temporolimbic region. Focal strokes can affect hippocampal structures from infarctions in the territory of the posterior cerebral arteries. Anoxia and ischemia are common causes of residual memory impairment, particularly after cardiopulmonary resuscitation. Traumatic brain injury is another common cause of amnesia because temporolimbic structures are injured bilaterally. The extent of post-traumatic (anterograde) amnesia is a good gauge of the severity of the head injury. Post-traumatic amnesia of less than 1 hour usually indicates a mild head injury, and post-traumatic amnesia of greater than 1 day indicates a severe head injury. Herpes simplex encephalitis, the most common sporadic form of infectious encephalitis, commonly damages the hippocampus and causes amnesia. Finally, complex partial and generalized seizures, as well as electroconvulsive therapy, can transiently disrupt hippocampal memory functions and cause amnesia.

A number of other important amnesias are also possible. Alcoholism with thiamine deficiency affects midline limbic structures and results in the Wernicke-Korsakoff syndrome. In addition to severe anterograde amnesia, patients with this syndrome often have difficulty retrieving remote or old information from the last few years. Acutely, they can manifest confabulation, or a false "filling in" of memory gaps. The Wernicke's encephalopathy aspect includes acute delirium, oculomotor paresis, nystagmus, and ataxia. Rupture of an anterior communicating aneurysm can also cause amnesia from ischemia of midline limbic structures, especially the fornix. Transient global amnesia is a transient memory impairment of uncertain etiology. It occurs in older persons and is suspected to result from a transient ischemic attack or, less likely, from epileptiform activity. Transient global amnesia is characterized by initial delirium, disproportionate anterograde amnesia, and retrograde amnesia for the proceeding few hours. It tends to last a few hours and then resolves without residual memory impairment.

TREATMENT AND PROGNOSIS. Recovery depends primarily on the cause of the memory difficulty. Patients with age-associated memory impairment can usually be reassured and taught simple memory aids and techniques such as writing things down and keeping a memory notebook. The memory of patients with depression often improves once the depression is treated. Some causes of amnesia, such as concussion or seizures, may resolve with recovery from the acute insult. Other patients, however, are left with at least some permanent impairment. In general, memory loss may be modestly improved with cognitive rehabilitation techniques. In the past, medications and dietary substances have had little effect on improving memory; however, the introduction of acetylcholinesterase inhibitors such as tacrine and donepezil can enhance memory function in patients with Alzheimer's disease. Future trials will show whether these "memory drugs" can enhance memory function in patients with other amnesic disorders.

APHASIA

DEFINITIONS. Language is the brain's use of symbols for communication. Language is the unique human ability to communicate through symbols, whether spoken or written language, Braille, musical notation, or most forms of sign language. Language is distinct from speech, the verbal expression of language. Aphasia is the loss or impairment of language caused by brain dysfunction.

ETIOLOGY AND EPIDEMIOLOGY. Aphasia is a common manifestation of brain disease. The aphasic syndromes disturb communication and can be severely disabling. The most common causes of focal aphasias are strokes. Nearly 500,000 strokes occur every year in the United States, and in up to 40% of these strokes the patients have aphasia. Two other common problems—intracranial neoplasm and traumatic brain injury—frequently produce language disturbances.

Neurodegenerative processes such as Alzheimer's disease also commonly produce aphasia as part of the multiple cognitive deficits that characterize the dementias. In Alzheimer's disease, patients usually progress from early word-finding difficulty to a transcortical

sensory aphasia (described below). In vascular dementia, various aphasia syndromes occur, depending on the location of the stroke. Most other dementia patients have decreased word list generation and poor naming ability. Finally, primary progressive aphasia is a syndrome featuring an insidious decline in language, either dysfluency or a semantic anomia, that usually progresses to a full dementia syndrome. Most patients with primary progressive aphasia have a frontotemporal dementia of Pick's disease.

PATHOPHYSIOLOGY. Aphasia can result from any lesion in the language areas of the brain. In about 95% of people, the principal language areas are located around the left sylvian fissure. The Wernicke-Geschwind model remains the best schema for organizing this perisylvian language system (Fig. 449–4). Broca's area (Brodmann area 44) in the anterior sylvian region is involved in the production of language. Wernicke's area (Brodmann area 22) in the posterior sylvian region is involved in the comprehension of language. In almost all right-handed persons the left hemisphere is dominant for language. Broca's, Wernicke's, or conduction aphasia develops in such individuals from focal lesions in the left perisylvian region, and transcortical aphasias develop from lesions outside the left perisylvian region. Most left-handed and ambidextrous persons are also left hemisphere language dominant, although they usually have additional language representation in the right hemisphere. In genetic left-handers, lesions on either side can cause aphasia, although the disability tends to be less severe and to improve.

CLINICAL MANIFESTATIONS. The language examination evaluates language fluency, auditory comprehension, repetition, word list generation, and naming, reading, and writing. In addition, evaluation of prosody, the inflection and melodic quality of speech, is an important part of the language examination. The examination begins by listening to the patient's spontaneous discourse. The six elements of fluency are words per minute (in English, normal is 100 ± 50), phrase length (4 or more words per phrase), effort in getting the words out, agrammatism or telegraphic output (absence of prepositions, conjunctions, and other "functor" words), dysprosody, and dysarthria. During the course of conversational speech, examiners should listen for the information content and the presence of paraphasic errors. Non-fluent aphasics may get their message across with a limited number of nouns or verbs. In contrast, fluent aphasics may produce long, effortless sentences devoid of meaning. Furthermore, fluent and conduction aphasics (on repetition) make paraphasic errors, e.g., word substitutions (verbal paraphasias), phonemic substitutions (literal paraphasias), and neologisms (new word formation). Finally, examiners should listen for prosody or the melodic, rhythmic, and inflectional elements that convey much of the emotional impact of speech.

The examination evaluates other elements of language in a systematic fashion. Tests of auditory comprehension include responses to simple commands, e.g., "close your eyes" or "touch your nose," followed by multiple-step commands, e.g., "point to the floor and then point to the window." The examiner also asks yes or no questions, e.g., "Are you sitting down?" "Is a hammer good for cutting wood?" "Does May come before June?" "If the lion was

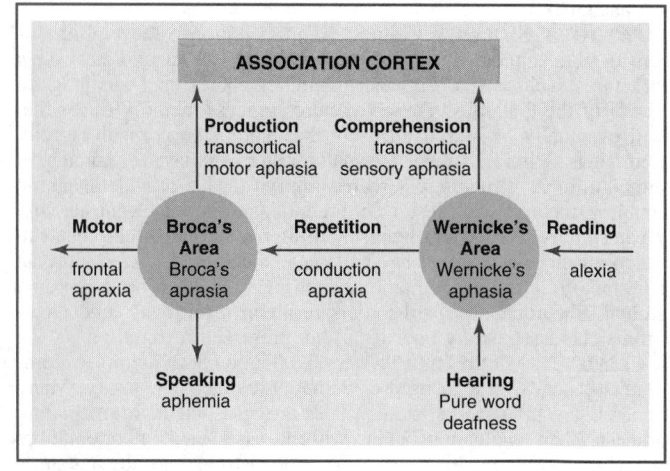

FIGURE 449–4 ■ Wernicke-Geschwind model of language.

killed by the tiger, which animal is dead?" The examiner can further evaluate the ability to comprehend relational phrases by placing several readily available items in front of the patient, e.g., keys, pens, coins. The patient is asked to "touch the keys with the pen" or to "point to the pen after pointing to the coin." In evaluating auditory comprehension with pointing commands, it should be remembered that motor weakness or apraxia may interfere with pointing. A test of repetition involves asking the patient to repeat "No if's, and's, or but's" and other grammatically intricate sentences. For word fluency, the examiner should listen for word-finding pauses and ask the patient to generate a list of as many animals as possible (or other category of items) in a minute. Normal subjects can list 18 ± 6 animals per minute without cueing. To assess naming, the examiner presents at least six common items (e.g., watch, ring, button, collar, nose, chin) and six lower-frequency items (e.g., eyelashes, eyebrows, lapel, shoelaces, sole or heel of a shoe, watch band or crystal) and asks the patient to name each item.

The language examination also includes an assessment of reading, comprehension of reading material, and writing. The examiner asks the patient to read aloud and perform various written commands comparable to the verbal commands. The examiner further requests the patient to write one sentence complete with punctuation by dictation and to compose and write one sentence of their own. Writing is disturbed in most of the aphasia syndromes, and the errors in writing typically parallel the errors in spoken language.

APHASIC SYNDROMES. The different language disorders or aphasias have different patterns of impaired language skills as outlined in Table 449–3.

BROCA'S APHASIA. Non-fluent verbal output characterizes Broca's aphasia. Spontaneous speech is sparse, effortful, dysarthric, dysprosodic, short in phrase length, and agrammatic. Decreased fluency occurs in the presence of relatively preserved comprehension (relational words such as "above" and "behind," however, may be poorly understood), abnormal repetition and naming, a disturbance in reading (particularly for relational words such as conjunctions), and impaired writing. Most patients with Broca's aphasia have right-sided weakness varying from mild paresis to total hemiplegia, and some have sensory loss as well. The neuropathology involves the left hemisphere frontal operculum containing Broca's area. Broca's aphasia must be distinguished from aphemia, a disorder of verbal output with preserved written language.

WERNICKE'S APHASIA. The most striking abnormality of Wernicke's aphasia is a disturbance in comprehension, which may range from a total inability to understand spoken language to a partial difficulty in decoding the spoken word. Wernicke's aphasia features a fluent verbal output with normal word count and phrase length; no abnormal effort, articulatory problems, or prosodic difficulties; and difficulty in repetition and word finding. The verbal output is often empty of content words and full of paraphasic substitutions and neologisms. Jargon aphasia refers to an extreme and unintelligible form of this type of output. Often no other neurologic defects

are evident, but a superior quadrantanopia may be present. The neuropathology involves the posterior superior temporal lobe of the left hemisphere. The disturbed auditory comprehension of Wernicke's aphasia helps distinguish it from the word salad of schizophrenia and the confused speech of delirium. Wernicke's aphasia must be distinguished from pure word deafness, a disorder of auditory input with preserved written language.

CONDUCTION APHASIA. Conduction aphasia features a prominent disturbance in repetition out of proportion to any other language disturbance. These patients have fluent verbal output and a preserved ability to comprehend. Paraphasias are common, particularly substitutions of phonemes, and naming is often limited by these paraphasic intrusions. Reading aloud is disturbed, but reading comprehension is normal. Most cases of conduction aphasia have neuropathology involving the arcuate fasciculus and other connections that run between Wernicke's area and Broca's area.

GLOBAL APHASIA. A severe language impairment in which all modalities—verbal fluency, comprehension, repetition, naming, reading, and writing—are impaired is known as global or total aphasia. Most patients have a right hemiparesis or hemiplegia, a right hemisensory deficit, and a right homonymous hemianopia. Global aphasia is usually caused by a complete middle cerebral artery territory infarction, although exceptions are noted, including cases of global aphasia without hemiparesis caused by multiple cerebral emboli to the left hemisphere.

TRANSCORTICAL APHASIAS. The major factor underlying these aphasias is relative preservation of the ability to repeat spoken language in the face of other language impairments. Transcortical motor aphasia resembles Broca's aphasia in its decreased verbal fluency but differs in the normal or nearly normal ability to repeat. Patients with this disorder struggle to utter words on spontaneous conversation but can easily say the same words on repetition. The neuropathology is most frequently located in the supplementary motor area of the left hemisphere or between that area and the frontal operculum. Transcortical sensory aphasia resembles Wernicke's aphasia in its fluent paraphasic output and decreased comprehension but differs in preservation of the ability to repeat. Patients with this disorder may echo or repeat everything that the examiner says. The most common site of neuropathology in transcortical sensory aphasia is the left posterior parietal region. Mixed transcortical (isolation) aphasia is a non-fluent aphasia with impaired comprehension and preserved repetition.

MISCELLANEOUS LANGUAGE-RELATED DISORDERS. Subcortical aphasias can be caused by infarcts in the left basal ganglia or the anterolateral nuclei of the thalamus. Basal ganglia aphasias most often show a combination of fluent, dysarthric speech accompanied by impaired auditory comprehension and a right hemiparesis. The thalamic aphasias resemble transcortical sensory aphasia. Anomia is a common residual deficit following improvement in other types of aphasia. Anomic patients have fluent verbal output and intact comprehension, but naming on confrontation is significantly disturbed.

Table 449–3 ■ **APHASIA SYNDROMES**

SYNDROME	SPONTANEOUS SPEECH	REPETITION	COMPREHENSIVE	NAMING	READING	WRITING	HEMIPARESIS	HEMISENSORY DEFECT	VISUAL FIELD DEFECT	NEUROPATHOLOGY IN LEFT HEMISPHERE
Broca's	Non-fluent	Poor	Good	Poor	Poor	Poor	Common	Rare	Rare	Posterior inferior frontal lobe
Wernicke's	Fluent, paraphasic	Poor	Poor	Poor	Poor	Poor	Rare	Variable	Variable	Posterior superior temporal lobe
Conduction	Fluent, paraphasic	Poor	Good	Variable	Good	Variable	Rare	Variable	Rare	Arcuate fasciculus region
Global	Non-fluent	Poor	Poor	Poor	Poor	Poor	Common	Common	Common	Combinations of the above three
Transcortical										
Motor	Non-fluent	Good	Good	Poor	Good	Poor	Common	Rare	Rare	Frontal, beyond Broca's area
Sensory	Fluent	Good	Poor	Poor	Poor	Poor	Rare	Common	Common	Parietal-temporal junction
Mixed	Non-fluent	Good	Poor	Poor	Poor	Poor	Common	Common	Common	Combination of the above two
Anomic	Fluent	Good	Good	Poor	Variable	Variable	Variable	Variable	Rare	Multiple sites
Subcortical										
Anterior	Non-fluent, paraphasic	Good	Good	Poor	Poor	Poor	Common	Rare	Rare	Putamen, globus pallidus
Posterior	Fluent, paraphasic	Good	Poor	Poor	Poor	Poor	Rare	Common	Variable	Thalamus

No specific causative location is known, although the neuropathology often involves the left hemisphere angular gyrus. Alexia, or reading impairment, most frequently occurs with the aphasias; however, isolated alexia with or without writing disturbances can result from lesions in the left visual occipital region or the left parietal lobe. Aprosody, or a disturbance in the affective intonation of communication, may result from right hemisphere lesions. Mutism accompanies a range of conditions from early non-fluent aphasias to focal lesions in the left supplementary motor area. Apraxia is common in aphasic patients, and acalculia commonly accompanies fluent aphasias.

TREATMENT AND PROGNOSIS. In addition to management of the underlying illness, treatment of aphasic patients includes speech and language therapy. Speech pathologists are professionals who are especially trained in the assessment and rehabilitation of aphasic patients. In addition to rote practice and rehearsal, special language therapy techniques are available, such as melodic intonation therapy. Drug treatments for language disturbances have had little success. In general, the prognosis of an aphasic patient depends on the type and severity of impairment. Fluent aphasics respond better to rehabilitation than do non-fluent aphasics. Finally, the clinician needs to be aware of the potentially treatable psychiatric disturbances that can accompany the aphasias, such as depression in patients with Broca's aphasia and paranoia in patients with Wernicke's aphasia.

Benson DF, Ardila A: Aphasia: A Clinical Perspective. New York, Oxford University Press, 1996. *An excellent review of current information on aphasia.*
Geschwind N: Disconnexion syndromes in animals and man. Brain 88:237, 585, 1965. *The classic description of the organization of brain-behavior relationships.*
Goodglass H, Kaplan E: The Assessment of Aphasia and Related Disorders, 2nd ed. Philadelphia, Lea & Febiger, 1983. *Describes the detailed evaluation of aphasia based on the Wernicke-Geschwind model.*
Schacter DL: Searching or Memory: The Brain, the Mind, and the Past. New York, Basic Books, 1996. *An excellent summary of current information on memory and its disorders.*
Squire LR: Memory and Brain. New York, Oxford University Press, 1987. *A comprehensive review of memory.*
Zola-Morgan SM, Squire LR: The primate hippocampal formation: Evidence for a time-limited role in memory storage. Science 250:288, 1990.

449.3 Alzheimer's Disease and Related Dementias

Tomoko V. Nakawatase
Jeffrey L. Cummings

Dementia is defined as an acquired persistent impairment in intellectual function with compromise in at least three of the following spheres of mental activity: (1) language, (2) memory, (3) visuospatial skills, (4) emotion or personality, and (5) cognition (abstraction, calculation, judgment). Dementia is acquired and must therefore be distinguished from congenital mental retardation syndromes. Most patients exhibit a decline in intellectual function over time. Delirium must be excluded before dementia can be identified. The most characteristic feature of delirium is impairment in attention with associated features of abrupt onset, short duration, impaired memory, incoherence of thought and conversation, hallucinations, disturbances of the sleep-wake cycle, and coexisting systemic medical illness or drug intoxication or withdrawal.

EVALUATION OF DEMENTIA

HISTORY. With the recent availability of approved pharmacologic agents for treatment of Alzheimer's disease, the clinician must not only recognize the dementia syndrome but also be able to define the specific etiology of the dementia. Evaluation of dementia starts with a detailed history of the initial problem from the patient and from family members or caregivers of the patient. Forgetfulness is a common complaint, and the onset, quality, and progression of the memory abnormalities require assessment. Memory disturbances associated with anxiety, depression, or fatigue or benign forgetfulness associated with aging must be considered before making a diagnosis of memory impairment secondary to a dementia. Other historical information relevant in the evaluation of dementia includes performance of activities of daily living such as the pa-

tient's ability to dress, groom, shop, and do household duties. A driving history is obtained and should include the number of recent accidents and episodes of getting lost while driving. Finally, behavioral disturbances must be considered, usually by obtaining the history from a family member or caregiver who lives with the patient. Neuropsychiatric disturbances such as apathy, hallucinations, delusions, sleep disorders, depression, agitation, or anxiety should be addressed in the interview.

The baseline intellectual and emotional functions of the patient should be determined before making a diagnosis of dementia. The highest educational level achieved, cultural background, occupational history, primary language, and other social history are taken into account. The past neurologic, psychiatric, and medical history, as well as current co-morbid illnesses, should be assessed and the current medications plus past use of psychotropic medications, alcohol, over-the-counter agents, and illicit drugs determined.

MENTAL STATUS EXAMINATION. The mental status examination begins with observation of the patient's appearance and behavior during the evaluation. Is the patient awake, attentive, and cooperative? Is the patient's speech fluent? Are any word-finding difficulties or paraphasic errors present? Is the patient properly dressed and groomed and socially appropriate?

Screening tests such as the Mini-Mental Status Examination (Table 449–4) can be used to determine a numerical cognitive baseline value; however, the clinician must understand the limitations of such tools. The test should be administered in a standardized fashion each time; variations reduce the comparability of serial scores. The Mini-Mental Status Examination may not be appropriate for a patient with a low educational level, one who speaks a foreign language, or a patient who comes from a different cultural background. It is insensitive to changes in the most mildly and most severely affected patients. Other scales such as the Geriatric Depression Scale, Katz's Scale for Activities of Daily Living, and the Neuropsychiatric Inventory may be helpful for assessing activities of daily living and behavioral changes. In patients who score in the normal range on the Mini-Mental Status Examination but historically complain of intellectual deficits as well as in diagnostically challenging cases, a formal neuropsychological evaluation conducted by a neuropsychologist provides more detailed information regarding the patient's cognitive ability. The results of neuropsychological testing may be compared with standardized scores of patients matched for age and level of education. Neuropsychological testing is rigorous and requires a cooperative, awake patient who can engage in paper and pencil tests for several hours. Patients with low education, aphasia, a primary language other than English, or moderately advanced dementias will not benefit from standard neuropsychological testing.

Table 449–4 ■ THE MINI-MENTAL STATUS EXAMINATION

	SCORE
Orientation: What is the month, day, date, year, season? Where are you, what floor, city, county and state? (score 1 point for each item correct)	10
Registration: state three items (ball, flag, tree) (score 1 point for each item that the patient registers **without** you having to repeat the words. You may repeat the words until the patient is able to register the words but do not give them credit. You must also tell the patient that he/she should memorize those words and that you will ask him/her to recall those words later).	3
Attention: Can you spell the word WORLD forwards, then backwards? Can you subtract 7 from 100, and keep subtracting 7? (100-93-86-79-72) (Do both items but give credit for best of the two performances).	5
Memory: Can you remember those three words I asked you to memorize? (Do not give clues or multiple choice).	3
Languages:	
Naming: Can you name (show) a pen and a watch?	2
Repetition: Can you repeat "No if's, and's, or but's"?	1
Comprehension: Can you take this piece of paper in your right hand, fold it in half, then put it on the floor? (score 1 point for each item done correctly)	3
Reading: Read and obey, "CLOSE YOUR EYES"	1
Writing: Can you write a sentence?	1
Visuospatial: Have patient copy intersecting pentagons	1
TOTAL	30

Different dementing processes involve disease-specific parts of the brain and produce identifiable patterns of neuropsychological deficits. They begin at one location, progress to other areas, and cause topographically linked deficits. The type of dementia may be partly surmised by the pattern of neuropsychological deficits manifested by the patient.

The physical examination should include a determination of blood pressure, auscultation for carotid bruits and cardiac murmurs, and a complete neurologic examination. The presence of focal neurologic deficits leads one to consider non–Alzheimer disease dementias; patients with Alzheimer's disease rarely exhibit focal neurologic deficits. The presence of rigidity and other extrapyramidal signs suggests a dementia related to Parkinson's disease, dementia with Lewy bodies, or vascular dementia. Gait abnormalities occur with normal-pressure hydrocephalus, Parkinson's disease, vascular dementia, progressive supranuclear palsy, or other subcortical dementias.

Laboratory studies should include electrolytes, calcium, blood urea nitrogen, creatinine, complete blood count, vitamin B_{12} level, thyroid-stimulating hormone, and syphilis serology. Apolipoprotein E-4 (apoE4) genotype increases the likelihood that the dementia syndrome is caused by Alzheimer's disease. A lumbar puncture is indicated if the serum serology is positive for syphilis or in cases of suspected central nervous system infections or demyelination. The diagnosis of Creutzfeldt-Jakob disease may be confirmed by specific protein detection in cerebrospinal fluid (CSF). CSF assays that support the diagnosis of Alzheimer's disease have become commercially available but do not provide pathognomonic results.

Radiologic studies helpful with diagnosis include magnetic resonance imaging (MRI) or computed tomography of the brain. In addition to tumors, subdural hematomas, and strokes, neuroimaging may be helpful when scans show focal atrophy in specific locations, such as frontotemporal atrophy in the frontotemporal dementias. Functional studies such as positron emission tomography (PET) or single-photon emission computed tomography (SPECT) may facilitate the diagnosis when structural imaging shows no abnormality. Parietal hypometabolism shown on PET or parietal hypoperfusion shown on SPECT or PET support the diagnosis of Alzheimer's disease. An electroencephalogram is helpful in cases of suspected Creutzfeldt-Jakob dementia, where periodic polyspike and wave abnormalities may be present.

DIFFERENTIAL DIAGNOSIS

Most of the many causes of dementia are rare and may be excluded with a thorough history and evaluation (Table 449–5). Of the dementias caused by degenerative disease, Alzheimer's disease is the most common. Although a definite diagnosis of Alzheimer's disease requires tissue examination at autopsy or biopsy, the diagnosis can be made with high accuracy by using clinical criteria. With the availability of disease-specific pharmacologic treatment with cholinesterase inhibitors, accurate diagnosis of the degenerative dementias is clinically important. Cholinesterase inhibitors can be expected to work only in the dementias with a deficit in cholinergic function, such as that found in Alzheimer's disease.

METABOLIC CAUSES OF DEMENTIA. Table 449–5 shows the principal metabolic conditions associated with dementia.

MEDICATION-INDUCED DEMENTIA. Most cases of medication-induced brain dysfunction are manifested as delirium; however, in a frail, elderly patient, inappropriate use of medications may cause dementia. Common offending medications include benzodiazepines, tricyclic antidepressants, conventional antipsychotics, monoamine oxidase inhibitors, barbiturates, cough suppressants, digitalis, and anticholinergics.

DEMENTIA ASSOCIATED WITH PSYCHIATRIC ILLNESS. The term *pseudodementia* has been used to describe dementia associated with a psychiatric illness. Most commonly, the term has been used in depressed patients whose cognitive impairment improves with resolution of the depression. Pseudodementia patients may have cognitive deficits including poor attention and concentration and impaired memory, but in most cases, the cognitive deficits are mild in comparison to the depression. Patients display depressed mood, blunted affect, and slowed responses or may answer with "I don't know" to direct questions. Patients may have hallucinations, self-deprecatory nihilistic delusions, paranoid ideation, or more anxiety than seen in depressed patients without cognitive impairment. Signs

Table 449–5 ■ MAJOR CAUSES OF DEMENTIA

Degenerative disorders	CNS infections
Alzheimer's disease	Prion diseaes (Creutzfeldt-Jakob
Frontotemporal dementia	Gertsmann-Straussler-Shenker,
Dementia with Lewy bodies	fatal familial insomnia)
Corticobasal ganglionic degener-	Encephalitis/chronic meningitis
ation	AIDS and AIDS-related infec-
Parkinson's disease	tions
Huntington's disease	Neurosyphilis
Progressive supranuclear palsy	CNS tumors
Conditions associated with anoxia	Cerebral effects of systemic malig-
Cardiac disease	nancies
Pulmonary insufficiency	Hydrocephalus
Postanoxia dementia	Vitamin deficiency states
Chronic renal failure	Thiamine (B_1)
Uremic encephalopathy	Cyanocobalamin (B_{12})
Dialysis dementia	Endocrinopathies
Hepatic diseases	Thyroid disturbances
Portal-systemic encephalopathy	Adrenal disease
Electrolyte abnormalities	Intoxication/toxicity
Hypernatremia	Medications
Hyponatremia	Alcohol
Hypercalcemia	Other toxins
Vascular dementia	Inflammatory disorders
Head trauma	
Dementia pugilistica	
Multiple contusions	
Subdural hematoma	
Myelin disorders	
Multiple sclerosis	
Adult-onset leukodystrophies	

of cortical impairment such as aphasia, agnosia, and apraxia are absent, and the dementia associated with depression usually resembles subcortical dementias such as dementia associated with subcortical vascular dementia.

CORTICAL DEGENERATIVE DISEASES. Table 449–6 presents the distinguishing features of the major degenerative dementias

ALZHEIMER'S DISEASE. Alzheimer's disease is the most common cause of degenerative dementia. The history of Alzheimer's disease began in 1907 with Alois Alzheimer's short medical report of a 56-year-old woman whose brain he evaluated. Five years before her death, the patient had rapidly progressive memory loss, became lost in her neighborhood and eventually in her own apartment, and had delusions about being killed. By the time that the patient was institutionalized, she was disoriented, had difficulty with language (reading, writing, and naming), and could not learn new material. Despite severe cognitive deficits, the neurologic examination was otherwise normal. Four and a half years after institutionalization, the patient was stuporous, lying in bed with her arms and legs held in flexion contractures. Autopsy revealed an atrophic brain without gross abnormalities. Sections stained with Bielschowsky silver stain showed neuronal changes that are now known as neurofibrillary tangles. Furthermore, Alzheimer demonstrated numerous "miliary foci" now called senile or neuritic plaques. Alzheimer emphasized the pre-senile nature of the dementia. His colleague Emil Kraepelin in a 1909 textbook proposed that this pre-senile dementia process be called Alzheimer's disease. As the identity of neuropathologic changes in "senile dementia" and in Alzheimer's-type pre-senile dementia was appreciated, the term "Alzheimer's disease" was extended to include both pre-senile and senile forms of the disease.

EPIDEMIOLOGY. With the increasing age of the population, Alzheimer's disease has become the most common degenerative brain disorder, with nearly 10% of the population older than 65 years being affected. In developed nations, Alzheimer's disease is the 4th leading cause of death after heart disease, cancer, and stroke. In the United States alone, approximately 4 million individuals have Alzheimer's disease.

GENETICS OF ALZHEIMER'S DISEASE. Studies of the incidence and patterns of transmission in families of patients with Alzheimer's disease show that relatives of affected individuals have an increased risk of the development of Alzheimer's disease when compared with members of the general population. Concordance rates among co-twins of monozygotic probands with Alzheimer's

Table 449-6 ■ DISTINGUISHING FEATURES OF COMMON PROGRESSIVE DEMENTIAS

DISEASE	SYMPTOMS/SIGNS	AGE AFFECTED	DURATION OF ILLNESS	NEUROLOGIC SIGNS
Alzheimer's disease	Amnestic memory loss early Getting lost Lack of awareness of one's illness Sleep-wake cycle disturbance Apathy	Greater than 65	Years, up to a decade	Normal until advanced stage
Familial Alzheimer's disease	Same as AD	From the 30s	Years	Normal until advanced stage
Frontotemporal dementia	Personality change Disinhibition Obsessions and compulsions "Alien stare" Amnestic memory loss later Visuospatial intact	45–65	Years	Normal until advanced stage
Lewy body dementia	Early falls Visual hallucinations Neuroleptic sensitivity Fluctuating course	Greater than 50	Months to years	Early extra-pyramidal signs With rigidity greater than tremor
Corticobasal ganglionic degeneration	Limb apraxia "Alien hand" Visuospatial deficits	Greater than 60	Years	Apraxia Rigidity Myoclonus
Vascular dementia	Retrieval memory loss Depression Slowness Step-wise progression	Greater than 65	Years	Focal neurologic deficits Rigidity and cogwheeling Gait abnormality
Normal pressure hydrocephalus	Retrieval memory loss Urinary incontinence Progressive gait difficulty Slowness Visuospatial infarct	Any age	Months	Gait abnormality Hyperreflexia (legs > arms) Babinski signs

disease are 40 to 60%, thus suggesting a strong but not absolute genetic influence on the disease.

Four genes have been linked to Alzheimer's disease (Table 449–7). Chromosome 21 carries the gene coding for the precursor of β-amyloid, amyloid precursor protein. This gene was cloned in 1987 after observing that dementia develops in a high proportion of individuals with Down syndrome (trisomy 21) who survive to adulthood and in whom Alzheimer disease–like pathology was present at autopsy. The subsequent discovery of mutations in the amyloid precursor protein gene in families with early-onset familial Alzheimer's disease suggested that overproduction of β-amyloid was associated with some cases of Alzheimer's disease.

The presenilin 1 (*PS1*) gene on chromosome 14 was localized in 1992 by using genetic linkage strategies in families with early-onset Alzheimer's disease. Approximately 25 different mutations in various areas of the protein have been found in white, Ashkenazi Jewish, Hispanic, and Japanese families. Another gene, presenilin 2 (*PS2*), was localized to chromosome 1 after evaluating several large Volga-German kindreds with autosomal dominant early-onset Alzheimer's disease. Mutations in *PS1* and *PS2* account for fewer than 2% of cases of Alzheimer's disease. Patients with *PS1* mutations have a characteristic early age of onset, between 35 and 60 years old. *PS2* mutations are found almost exclusively in families of Volga-German heritage. Most patients encountered in the clinic setting are probably not likely candidates for presenilin mutations testing, although *PS1* testing is available commercially. Chromosome 12 may harbor a causative mutation relevant to late-onset Alzheimer's disease and is currently under study.

ApoE is a plasma protein involved in cholesterol transport and is encoded by a gene on chromosome 19. It is synthesized primarily in the liver and is thought to be involved in repair of the nervous system after injury. ApoE genotype is an important contributor to susceptibility to Alzheimer's disease but is found in several other neurodegenerative diseases such as dementia pugilistica. Three common alleles, E2, E3, and E4, correspond to six phenotypes. The E4 allele has been identified as a risk factor for Alzheimer's disease, with the attributable risk estimated to be 45 to 60%. E4 homozygotes are at greater risk than E4 heterozygotes. ApoE4 is present in plaques and may facilitate amyloid accumulation in the brain.

CLINICAL MANIFESTATIONS. Historical information, as well as serial examination, is imperative for the diagnosis of Alzheimer's disease. The two principal approaches to a criterion-based diagnosis of Alzheimer's disease include the Diagnostic and Statistical Manual of Mental Disorders, 4th edition, and the criteria developed by the National Institute of Neurological and Communicative Disorders and Stroke and the Alzheimer's Disease and Related Disorders Association. Memory disturbance occurs early in the disease; patients have difficulty learning and remembering new material. Spatial and temporal disorientation also may occur early, with patients becoming lost in familiar surroundings. Aphasia, apraxia, and acalculia develop as the disease progresses, and apathy or paranoia may occur. Patients often have delusions of theft and spousal infidelity. Patients may wander, pace, open and close drawers repeatedly, and repeat the same questions. Sleep-wake cycle abnormalities may become evident; for example, a patient may be awake at night but think that it is daytime. Activities of daily living decline throughout the illness. Patients lose the ability to eat and groom themselves and have difficulty dressing. In the terminal stages of the disease, patients exhibit cognitive decline in virtually all intellectual spheres, motor abnormalities become evident, and both urinary and fecal incontinence develops.

DIAGNOSIS. In a patient with clinical findings suggesting Alzheimer's disease, other causes of dementia should be excluded by history, examination, and the laboratory studies described above. CSF evaluation for amyloid protein and tau protein can increase the likelihood of a diagnosis of Alzheimer's disease, but they are not sufficiently specific to be of routine value in screening or early diagnosis of Alzheimer's disease. Improvements in these tests in combination with quantitative MRI may ultimately allow early, specific testing. Presence of the apoE4 allele makes it very likely that the patient's dementia is produced by Alzheimer's disease. ApoE testing does not have predictive value for asymptomatic individuals.

TREATMENT. Treatment of Alzheimer's disease is multimodal,

Table 449-7 ■ GENETICS AND DEMENTIA

DISEASE	CHROMOSOME
Familial AD	1, 14, 21
Risk for sporadic AD	19
Frontotemporal dementia	17
Huntington's disease	14

tailored to each individual and modified with progression of the disease. Treatment may be divided into three areas: pharmacologic interventions targeting the specific pathophysiology of Alzheimer's disease, pharmacologic agents that ameliorate specific symptoms such as delusions and sleep abnormalities, and behavioral interventions, which may improve specific symptoms and improve the patient's activities of daily living.

Table 449–8 lists pharmacologic agents that may target the pathophysiology of the disease. Acetylcholinesterase inhibitors are available to increase the acetylcholine levels found to be decreased in the brains of patients with Alzheimer's disease. Currently, two agents, tacrine and donepezil, have been approved. Other cholinesterase inhibitors are being developed. Tacrine was the 1st drug marketed, and post-marketing studies have shown tacrine to be efficacious not only in improving cognition, as shown by a modest increase in Mini-Mental Status Examination scores, but also in improving the neuropsychiatric disturbances of patients with Alzheimer's disease such as apathy and anxiety. Donepezil has fewer side effects and requires no blood monitoring for hepatic dysfunction. It is given only once daily and is more widely used than tacrine. Acetylcholinesterase inhibitors should be used only in patients who have dementias with cholinergic deficits such as Alzheimer's disease, dementia with Lewy bodies, and Parkinson's disease and dementia. In general, they should be used early in the course of Alzheimer's disease. Vitamin E has been shown to slow progression of Alzheimer's disease, and epidemiologic evidence suggests that patients who have received estrogens or anti-inflammatory agents have a lower incidence of Alzheimer's disease. However, no prospective controlled clinical trials of estrogen or anti-inflammatory agents are available to guide their use in patients with Alzheimer's disease.

Pharmacologic agents that target specific problem behavior's are used for behavioral disturbances in Alzheimer's disease. Psychotropic agents such as tricyclics with anticholinergic effects are contraindicated in patients with Alzheimer's disease who have an underlying deficit in acetylcholine. In general, anticholinergic agents should not be used in any individual with dementia because these drugs may worsen cognition. Neuroleptic agents such as haloperidol may cause extrapyramidal side effects and thereby decrease the motor abilities of a patient with Alzheimer's disease. However, if the patient's delusions are severe and problematic for both the patient and caregiver, an antipsychotic agent is indicated. Haloperidol at low doses (with close monitoring of extrapyramidal signs) or newer agents such as risperidone, olanzapine, or quetiapine may be helpful. If the patient's primary problem is agitation, agents such as trazodone, divalproex, or carbamazepine may be helpful.

Behavioral interventions play an integral part in the management of patients with Alzheimer's disease. Controlling the environment by keeping the patient's home safe and easy to navigate may help these patients. An occupational therapist may evaluate the home to assess safety and provide recommendations to improve the patient's activities of daily living. Family members should also be educated concerning the patient's illness. Alzheimer's disease affects both the patient and the family. As the disease progresses, patients with Alzheimer's disease will lose insight into their disease and may show apathy and indifference while caregivers may become progressively distressed. Seeking ancillary help is imperative as the

caregiver burden increases. Attending support groups, arranging home help, and obtaining legal advice for finances, durable power of attorney, and conservatorships are an important part of managing the disease. The local chapter of the Alzheimer's Association and local Alzheimer's disease centers provide important resources. They are particularly helpful in devising strategies to return Alzheimer disease patients who wander from their homes. Such resources are essential for any caregiver's of patients with Alzheimer's disease.

FRONTOTEMPORAL DEMENTIA. HISTORY. In 1906, Arnold Pick described several elderly patients with progressive aphasia and identified a syndrome of progressive behavioral disorder in association with bilateral frontal lobe atrophy. Post-mortem correlations of focal atrophy were recognized, and the disease became known as Pick's disease. The syndrome was rarely reported and it was thought that Pick's disease could not be diagnosed in life. However, investigators in Lund, Sweden, Manchester, England, and elsewhere independently reported longitudinal studies of patients whose clinical characteristics were suggestive of frontal lobe dysfunction. The patients were demented, but the underlying pathology was distinct from that of Alzheimer's disease. A meeting between the Swedish and the British research teams led to adoption of the term *frontotemporal dementia* to describe these Pick's disease–like patients, and a consensus on the diagnosis of frontotemporal dementia was achieved. Three conditions are included within the frontotemporal dementia syndrome: Pick's disease, frontotemporal atrophy without Pick-type pathology, and frontotemporal atrophy with motor neuron disease.

EPIDEMIOLOGY. Frontotemporal dementia may account for as many as 20% of patients with pre-senile dementia secondary to primary cerebral degeneration. The possibility that frontotemporal dementia may be confined exclusively to the north of England and to southern Sweden was raised until more recent reports of similar patients from the United States and many other parts of the world. Frontotemporal dementia is probably underrecognized. Behavioral problems are the early cardinal features of the disease; many patients are not evaluated for dementia in the initial phases of the illness.

GENETICS OF FRONTOTEMPORAL DEMENTIA. In about 50% of cases of frontotemporal dementia, a family history of a similar disorder is present. Patients with familial frontotemporal dementia have been associated with Pick-type histology or histologic alterations characterized by microvacuolar changes without Pick bodies. Formal investigations of these families have been rare; in one, the histologic change appeared uniform, with all affected patients showing microvacuolar or Pick-type histology, but the clinical features of the individuals were variable. Analysis of the mutation responsible for some families with frontotemporal dementia has linked the disease to chromosome 17 and localized it to the tau protein gene.

CLINICAL CHARACTERISTICS. The onset of frontotemporal dementia is usually insidious and may manifest as subtle personality and affective changes. The pathologic process starts in the frontal and temporal lobes, and patients subsequently have symptoms of depression, anxiety, and disinhibited behavior often prompting psychiatric evaluation. Patients most commonly exhibit a change in

---

Table 449–8 ■ RECOMMENDED SPECIFIC PHARMACOLOGIC TREATMENTS

Alzheimer's disease	1. Cholinesterase inhibitor **Tacrine (Cognex)** (Available in 10, 20, 30, 40 mg tablets, start at 10 mg po QID and increase to 20 mg QID, then 30 mg QID, then 40 mg QID every six weeks. Must check ALT levels every two weeks for first four months, then every month for two months then every three months if AST normal). **Donepezil (Aricept)** (Available in 5 and 10 mg tablets, start at 5 mg po, then increase to 10 mg po QD after one month). 2. Vitamin E (Available in 400 and 1000 IU capsules, recommended dose, total of 2000 IU/day)
Dementia with Lewy bodies	Cholinesterase inhibitors (same as AD)
Vascular dementia	Aspirin 325 mg po QD or Ticlopidine 250 mg po BID (Must check CBC every two weeks for first three months, then consider CBC every three months). Clopidogrel (75 mg QD)
Parkinson's disease with dementia	Cholinesterase inhibitor (same as AD)

personality and a breakdown in social behavior. They become apathetic and lacking in initiative, judgment, and foresight, and they neglect their personal responsibilities to the point of mismanagement of their personal and professional affairs. They may dress bizarrely, wearing incongruous combinations of clothes that clash in color, make inappropriate remarks in public, and acquire compulsions and repetitive behavior. Hyperorality and selective food fads may develop, with patients having cravings for sweets and shoving large quantities of food in their mouth at one time. Memory, language, and visuospatial skills are preserved early in the illness, but with progression, the disease process may involve the posterior aspects of the brain and cause parietal lobe dysfunction.

TREATMENT. Cholinesterase inhibitors are not useful in frontotemporal dementia. Serotonergic agents may be useful in controlling behavior.

DEMENTIA WITH LEWY BODIES. Five years after Alzheimer described the pathologic hallmarks of the disease that has come to bear his name, another German neuropathologist, Friedrich Lewy, observed eosinophilic inclusions, which have been named Lewy bodies, in subcortical neurons of patients with Parkinson's disease. More recently, investigators have published reports of patients with prominent neuropsychiatric symptoms, dementia, and autopsy-proven cortical Lewy bodies. Dementia with Lewy bodies accounts for 15 to 25% of all degenerative dementias; it shares clinical and pathologic features with Alzheimer's disease and is regarded by some as an Alzheimer disease variant. The clinical features of dementia with Lewy bodies include the presence of dementia, fluctuations in cognition, visual hallucinations, and parkinsonian motor signs. Dementia with Lewy bodies may be similar to the dementia of Alzheimer's disease, with cortical features of visuospatial disturbance, language deficits, executive impairment (poor planning, impaired set shifting, disturbed sequencing), and memory loss. However, dementia with Lewy bodies has variable features that reflect subcortical deficits, as well as a combination of cortical and subcortical features. The visual hallucinations of dementia with Lewy bodies are usually well formed and recurrent and most commonly involve animals, children, or "small people." Parkinsonian motor features are present in about 80% of patients with Lewy body dementia, and unlike Parkinson's disease, these signs typically respond poorly to levodopa therapy. Other symptoms that may support the diagnosis of dementia with Lewy bodies include multiple falls, delusions and non-visual hallucinations, and neuroleptic sensitivity.

The key pathologic feature of dementia with Lewy bodies is the presence of cortical Lewy bodies, most commonly located in the neocortical (frontal and temporal) and paralimbic (insula and anterior cingulate) regions. Amyloid plaques may be found, but neurofibrillary tangles are rare. Neurotransmitter deficits in patients with dementia and Lewy bodies mostly involve the cholinergic and the dopaminergic systems. The cholinergic deficit appears to be more severe than that of Alzheimer's disease, and this deficit, combined with relative preservation of the serotonergic system, may account for the propensity of these patients to have visual hallucinations. Because of the marked cholinergic deficit, cholinesterase inhibitors (tacrine and donepezil) may be beneficial. Patients are very sensitive to neuroleptic medications; cholinesterase inhibitors may serve as 1st-line therapy for the neuropsychiatric as well as the cognitive symptoms of dementia with Lewy bodies. As in Alzheimer's disease, tricyclics and other anticholinergic agents should be avoided.

CORTICOBASAL GANGLIONIC DEGENERATION. Corticobasal ganglionic degeneration is a relatively rare degenerative disorder characterized by rigidity, focal dystonias, myoclonus, supranuclear gaze palsy, cortical sensory loss, postural action tremor and instability, severe apraxia, and "alien hand" phenomena (actions of the hand not consciously directed by the patient). Corticobasal ganglionic degeneration is typically associated with asymmetrical posterior cortical atrophy, most often affecting the right hemisphere. Visuospatial deficits and marked apraxias, with posturing or levitation of one arm more than the other, help distinguish this disorder from the other dementias. Pathologically, the condition is characterized by atrophy of the frontal and parietal cortex with cortical cell loss, gliosis, and in some cases, the presence of Pick cells, as well as degeneration of the substantia nigra, locus caeruleus, thalamus, subthalamic nucleus, red nucleus, lentiform nucleus, and midbrain tegmentum. In contrast to Alzheimer's disease, the temporal and hippocampal regions are spared. No specific treatment has been discovered, although depression is common and may respond to pharmacotherapy.

VASCULAR DEMENTIA. Vascular dementia is the 2nd most common dementia of the elderly in the United States. The terminology used for vascular dementia is variable because the syndromes and causes of vascular dementia are also variable. Vascular dementia may result from strategically placed single infarcts, multiple infarcts, small vessel disease with subcortical infarctions and ischemia, hypoperfusion, amyloid angiopathy, and brain hemorrhage. Many clinicians use the terminology "multi-infarct dementia" interchangeably with vascular dementia.

The clinical features of patients with vascular dementia vary, but a few generalizations are applicable to most patients. When compared with Alzheimer's disease, patients with vascular dementia tend to have an earlier age of onset, more men are affected than women, and the duration of survival after the onset of mental status changes is shorter. Historically, cognitive dysfunction may develop abruptly, and patients may experience stepwise deterioration or have a history of transient neurologic symptoms and transient ischemic attacks. Patients with vascular dementia often have risk factors of hypertension, diabetes, hyperlipidemia, and cigarette smoking. Clinically, patients may have focal signs on neurologic examination, most commonly limb rigidity, spasticity, hyperreflexia, extensor plantar responses, and gait disturbance. Features of pseudobulbar palsy, including emotional lability, dysarthria, and dysphagia, are often present. On neuropsychological assessment patients may show deficits in frontal executive tasks, orientation, and memory. The memory disturbance is usually of the retrieval type; patients are able to register information but have difficulty spontaneously recalling it. Categorical clues or multiple choices help patients retrieve stored material. Neuropsychiatrically, patients show evidence of depression, psychosis, and personality changes.

The diagnosis of vascular dementia is facilitated by brain imaging demonstrating moderate to severe ischemic white matter changes subcortically or focal cortical infarctions in strategic locations. Vascular dementia is treated by stroke prevention strategies: antihypertensives, cigarette cessation, and anticoagulants such as aspirin, clopidogrel, or ticlopidine. Warfarin (Coumadin) is used only in those specific limited circumstances where controlled trials have demonstrated its effectiveness in preventing embolic brain infarction. The combination of Alzheimer's disease with cerebrovascular disease is common, and these patients have a poor prognosis; however, they may benefit from cholinesterase inhibitors.

SUBCORTICAL DEGENERATIVE DISEASES

PARKINSON'S DISEASE. Parkinson's disease is a degenerative disorder with loss of substantia nigra neurons producing a movement disorder manifested by tremor at rest, limb rigidity, masked facies, and disturbances of gait, posture, and equilibrium. The cognitive deficits of Parkinson's disease were not as well described as the motor abnormalities of the disease in the writings of James Parkinson, after whom the disease was named. In his writings, Parkinson specifically denied the presence of mental changes, although he detailed the presence of neuropsychiatric abnormalities. Charcot, on the other hand, indicated that Parkinson's disease involved a progressive decline in memory and other cognitive abilities. The reported prevalence of dementia in patients with Parkinson's disease varies widely but is thought to be in the range of 35 to 55%. The principal features of the dementia of Parkinson's disease include slowing of cognition, failure to initiate activities spontaneously, poor word list generation, a retrieval deficit–type memory disturbance, and executive dysfunction.

A variety of pharmacologic agents are available for the treatment of Parkinson's disease, including dopamine agonists, dopamine precursors, monoamine oxidase inhibitors, and catechol O-methyltransferase inhibitors. These therapies improve the motor symptoms of the disease but afford little or no cognitive benefit. Most patients with clinically evident dementia have cholinergic deficits, and cholinesterase inhibitors may be useful.

HUNTINGTON'S DISEASE. Huntington's disease is a familial disorder characterized by chorea, dementia, and personality changes. In his original paper in 1872, George Huntington noted that "as the disease progresses the mind becomes more or less impaired, in many amounting to insanity, while in others mind and body gradually fail until death relieves them of their sufferings." Early signs of the disease include personality changes of irritability, apathy, and untidiness, which usually begin in mid-life. Depression is common and leads to suicide in up to 8% of males and 6% of females. The neuropsychiatric features are often manifested before the chorea. The dementia that occurs is similar to that of other subcortical dementias and includes retrieval memory deficit, slowing of cognition, and decreased verbal fluency. As the disease progresses, other areas of cognition decline, including concentration, judgment, executive skills, and visuospatial abilities.

No specific treatment of Huntington's disease is available.

PROGRESSIVE SUPRANUCLEAR PALSY. In 1963, Steele, Richardson, and Olszewski described several patients manifesting a syndrome characterized by supranuclear gaze paresis, pseudobulbar palsy, axial rigidity, and dementia. The syndrome became known as progressive supranuclear palsy and was found to begin in the 6th or 7th decade of life, more commonly in males than females, at a prevalence rate of approximately 1.4/100,000.

Neurologically, patients initially have postural instability and are subject to falls and gait abnormalities. Axial rigidity develops, and patients have difficulty looking down on the ground when they ambulate, thus leading to falls. Dysarthria and hypophonia may develop and eventually lead to mutism. Pseudobulbar palsy is manifested by a mask-like facies, exaggerated palatal and gag reflexes, drooling, and dysphagia. Paresis of vertical gaze, especially downgaze, is a common early sign. The neuropsychological profile of these patients includes apathy, slowness, and personality changes. Cognitive decline tends to be mild until late in the disease, when characteristic features of a subcortical dementia develop, including slowness of thought process, apathy, depression, forgetfulness, and an impaired ability to manipulate acquired knowledge. No treatment of progressive supranuclear palsy has been developed.

SUMMARY

Evaluation of a patient with dementia involves a detailed history from the patient and caregivers, laboratory and imaging data to exclude treatable causes, and serial assessment to show decline in cognition and change in behavior. The diagnosis of dementia is a clinical one that cannot be based on any one test. The specific etiology of the degenerative dementia should be determined because pharmacologic agents specific for Alzheimer's disease are available. The behavioral disturbances of dementia should be addressed with pharmacologic and behavioral interventions. Caregiver burden is high, and so caregiver assessment should be included at each evaluation.

Folstein MF, Folstein SE, McHugh PR: A practical method for grading the cognitive state for the clinician. J Psychiatr Res 12:189, 1975. *A useful diagnostic screening tool. The authors found that out of a possible total score of 30, the mean score for dementia was 9.7, that for depression with cognitive impairment was 19.0, and the mean score for uncomplicated affective depression was 27.6.*

McKeith IG, Kosaka K, Perry EK, et al: Neurology 47:1113, 1996. *The most comprehensive literature on Lewy body dementia, including the neuropathologic processing of brain tissue for diagnosis.*

Small GW, Rabins PV, Barry PP, et al: Diagnosis and treatment of Alzheimer disease and related disorders: Consensus Statement of the American Association for Geriatric Psychiatry, the Alzheimer's Association, and the American Geriatrics Society. JAMA 278:1363, 1997. *A detailed consensus statement for Alzheimer's disease and future directions.*

450 PSYCHIATRIC DISORDERS IN MEDICAL PRACTICE

R.B. Schiffer

At various times, most people experience anxiety, depression, sleep disturbance, or somatic preoccupation. Such symptoms are usually transient, and their causes are often evident—an upcoming examination, a new job, marriage, divorce, or work or family problems. In these instances, the physician has no difficulty in reassuring the patient that the symptoms are transient and situational. When these symptoms persist or when they occur in situations that have no clear precipitants, however, they should arouse the physician's concern. To determine whether someone has a psychiatric illness, the following questions must be considered: (1) Do the signs and symptoms fit a psychiatric diagnosis? For example, when patients say they are sad or depressed, do their symptoms meet the diagnostic criteria for a diagnosis of depression? (2) Is there a family history of similar symptoms? Many psychiatric illnesses tend to have a genetic or familial basis. (3) Is the longitudinal pattern of the symptoms consistent with the natural history of a psychiatric disorder? Emotional symptoms associated with specific situations are usually classified as reactions to the situation; they do not usually become psychiatric disorders. (4) Are the symptoms incapacitating? (5) Do delusions and hallucinations exist? Delusions and hallucinations in the absence of other medical causes always indicate major psychiatric illness. Illusory phenomena can occur with sleep deprivation or with certain intoxications or fever. However, their occurrence in a patient with a clear state of consciousness points to the presence of major psychiatric illness.

The separation of psychiatric disorders from normal emotional reactions depends on a careful history, a mental status evaluation, and a knowledge of psychiatric syndromes. If the findings of the history and mental status evaluation do not fit into any defined psychiatric syndrome, the physician should not make a psychiatric diagnosis but should observe and re-evaluate the patient. In many cases, the symptoms resolve. If the symptoms continue, the physician may recognize a clear psychiatric syndrome.

A 1995 World Health Organization collaborative study indicates that diagnosable (ICD-10) psychiatric morbidity is common among consecutive clinic attendees in general medical ambulatory settings in both developed and underdeveloped countries. General medical physicians can expect one in four of the patients they see to have active, diagnosable psychiatric disease. The most common diagnoses in medical settings are depression, generalized anxiety disorder, somatoform disorders, substance abuse, and personality disorders. Only about half of diagnosable psychiatric disorders in general medical ambulatory settings are recognized by the physicians caring for the patients. Most of these disorders have substantial psychosocial morbidity, and they are all treatable. This section emphasizes clues to recognition and initial therapy of the major psychiatric syndromes.

SYNDROMES

Depression and Suicidality

DIAGNOSIS AND CLINICAL FEATURES. Since the advent of the third version of the American Psychiatric Association's *Diagnostic and Statistical Manual of Mental Disorders* (DSM-III) in 1979, the depressive disorders have been diagnosed by descriptive criteria. This publication marked a major advance in psychiatric diagnostics since it required diagnoses to be substantiated by observable clinical data. Several depressive spectrum disorders are included in the current edition of the DSM (DSM-IV). The core clinical features of the depressive disorders, however, are included in the diagnostic criteria for a major depressive episode and for dysthymia (Table 450–1). These disorders tend to recur. When the pattern of recurrence is one of depressive syndromes only, the disorder is called a unipolar depressive disorder. When manic-like episodes are included (see later), the disorder is called a bipolar disorder.

The symptoms of depression are variable for each individual and sometimes are difficult to recognize. Behavior and cognition can be affected, as well as mood and affect. Some people experience depression as a slowing of thought and movement. For some, forgetfulness and difficulty concentrating are prominent features. Others experience agitation and even psychotic experiences when the disorder is severe. This variability of clinical features among patients can be used as a basis for classifying a major depressive episode into subtypes—agitated, psychotic, and others.

Table 450–1 ■ DIAGNOSTIC CRITERIA FOR DEPRESSIVE DISORDERS

Major Depressive Episode
1. At least five of the following symptoms have been present during the same 2-week period and represent a change from previous functioning; at least one of the symptoms is either depressed mood or loss of interest or pleasure.
   A. Depressed mood most of the day, nearly every day
   B. Markedly diminished interest or pleasure in all, or almost all, activities most of the day, nearly every day
   C. Significant weight loss or weight gain when not dieting or decrease or increase in appetite nearly every day
   D. Insomnia or hypersomnia nearly every day
   E. Psychomotor agitation or retardation nearly every day; observable by others
   F. Fatigue or loss of energy nearly every day
   G. Feelings of worthlessness or excessive or inappropriate guilt (which may be delusional) nearly every day
   H. Diminished ability to think or concentrate, or indecisiveness, nearly every day
   I. Recurrent thoughts of death, recurrent suicidal ideation without a specific plan, or a suicide attempt or a specific plan for committing suicide
2. A. It cannot be established that an organic factor initiated and maintained the disturbance.
   B. The disturbance is not a normal reaction to the death of a loved one.
3. At no time during the disturbance have there been delusions or hallucinations for as long as 2 weeks in the absence of prominent mood symptoms (i.e., before the mood symptoms developed or after they have remitted).
4. Not superimposed on schizophrenia, schizophreniform disorder, delusional disorder, or psychotic disorder; no other specific diagnosis.

Dysthymia
1. Depressed mood for most of the day for at least 2 years.
2. Presence, while depressed, of two or more of the following:
   A. Poor appetite
   B. Insomnia or hypersomnia
   C. Low energy or fatigue
   D. Low self-esteem
   E. Poor concentration or difficulty making decisions
   F. Feelings of hopelessness
3. During the 2-year period, the person has never been without the symptoms for more than 2 months at a time.
4. No major depressive episode has been present during the first 2 years of the disturbance.
5. There has not been an intermixed manic episode.
6. The disturbance does not occur during the course of a psychotic disorder.
7. The symptoms are not caused by the physiologic effects of a substance.
8. The symptoms cause significant distress or functional impairment.

ETIOLOGY. Occurrences of major depressive episodes clearly cluster in families. In general, increased rates of both bipolar and unipolar disorders are present among first-degree relatives of patients with a bipolar disorder, and increased rates of unipolar depressive disorder are present among first-degree relatives of those with unipolar disorders. Such relatives have lifetime risks ranging from 10 to 20% for major depressive disorders, with perhaps a higher risk for depressive spectrum disorders. This degree of increased risk is around three to five times that of the normal population. Twin and adoption studies are consistent with a genetic contribution to major depressive disorders, but such studies suggest that other factors are important as well. Recent techniques of molecular genetics, such as genomic mismatch scanning, repeat expansion detection, and mitochondrial DNA analysis, have not increased the current understanding of mechanisms in the genetics of affective disturbance. It is probable that multiple vulnerability genes operate in different families by different mechanisms and through complex interactions with life events.

PATHOPHYSIOLOGY. In the 1960s, hypotheses were first presented about an association between catecholamine metabolism (norepinephrine, epinephrine, dopamine) and depression. Subsequent neurochemical hypotheses invoked abnormalities of indolamine (serotonin) metabolism in depressive disorders. These neurochemical theories of affective disturbances derived largely from pharmacologic observations in the 1950s that suggested that catecholamine and indolamine depleters such as reserpine could cause depression, whereas drugs that upregulate catechole and indole metabolism (the tricyclic antidepressants) were therapeutic in depressed patients. These early neurochemical hypotheses for depression postulated that decreased availability of norepinephrine or serotonin at transmitter-specific synapses in the brain was associated with depression and that increased levels of these substances were associated with mania. Subsequent studies have generally supported the hypothesis that catecholamine and indolamine metabolism are important in mood states. Almost all drugs with antidepressant properties affect catecholamine and indolamine availability at the synapse in the central nervous system (CNS).

Evidence also suggests that neuroendocrine function is altered in many people with major depressive disorders. Overactivity of the hypothalamic-pituitary-adrenocortical axis has been the most prominent of these neuroendocrine disturbances. This overactivity is reflected in increased levels of circulating cortisol among depressed patients compared with controls, in addition to increased levels of cerebrospinal fluid cortisol, increased excretion of urinary free cortisol, and cortisol resistance to dexamethasone suppression. These findings have been the basis for the dexamethasone suppression test (DST) for the diagnosis of depression. Results of DST are positive if the patient fails to suppress plasma cortisol levels to less that 5 μg/dL between 8 and 24 hours after an oral dose of 1 mg dexamethasone given at 11:00 P.M. the night before. The DST is not useful for the diagnosis of depression because it has a false-negative rate of nearly 50%. In addition, its results can be abnormal in the setting of intercurrent systemic or other psychiatric illness, which limits the specificity of the test. However, the test can be useful for monitoring the treatment of patients who have an abnormal DST response. Moreover, it is a favorable prognostic sign for the prevention of depressive relapse if the DST reverts to normal during the treatment course.

Patients with affective disorders often have a disturbance of circadian rhythm reflected in abnormal sleep patterns. Complaints of difficulty falling asleep and early morning wakening are reliable clinical indicators of depression. Electroencephalographic (EEG) studies have demonstrated a relative absence of slow-wave sleep (stages 3 and 4) in depressed individuals and a shortened period between sleep onset and the first dreaming period (REM latency). These disturbances of sleep improve when the mood disturbance improves.

INCIDENCE AND PREVALENCE. Lifetime prevalence rates for major depressive disorders are 15 to 20%; the exact prevalence varies because of methods of ascertainment and diagnosis. Point prevalence rates for major depression in urban United States populations range from 2 to 4% for men and 4 to 6% for women. Depressive spectrum disorders provide additional affective disorder risk, and patients with chronic medical illness are at additional risk for the development of depressive spectrum illness.

SUICIDE RISK. Suicide is a uniquely human behavior for which we have only a limited psychobiologic understanding. Completed suicides are common in the United States, accounting for some 30,000 deaths each year. A much greater number of people attempt suicide, with variable degrees of intentionality. The most powerful associated features for completed suicide are current depression, alcohol abuse, and chronic medical illness. Suicide rates are highest for men over the age of 69 years, and rates are higher among whites and Native Americans than among other racial groups.

Most people who commit suicide have seen a physician within the previous month. Analysis of the preceding visits often provides evidence that covert and implicit clues were conveyed about suicidality. When there is any suspicion about suicide potential, it is important to ask patients directly. Risk factor assessment for degree of suicidal risk is not an easy algorithm. The presence and quality of depression are important. When associated depressive symptoms are more severe, or when they include features of agitation or delusional ideas, the risk for suicide is greater. Older age, male gender, and intercurrent alcohol abuse are risk factors. Social isolation is a powerful risk factor, as is chronic painful medical illness. Consultation with a psychiatrist is essential for high-risk patients.

PROGNOSIS AND TREATMENT. The diagnosis of a depressive disorder is the beginning of therapy. Depressed patients are usually relieved when their suffering is recognized and they are permitted to discuss it. The treatment plan must be individualized. A psychotherapeutic strategy (discussed later) should be considered for each patient before drug selection. It is the standard of care to initiate administration of an antidepressant drug at the time of diagnosis.

In general, follow-up ambulatory visits should be scheduled on a regular basis and more frequently than for other medical treatments. If improvement has not begun in 4 to 8 weeks, psychiatric consultation should be carefully considered.

DRUGS FOR DEPRESSION. Antidepressant drugs available in the United States (Table 450–2) vary in their structure and function.

SELECTIVE SEROTONIN REUPTAKE INHIBITORS. The selective serotonin reuptake inhibitors (SSRIs) marked an important advance in antidepressant pharmacology because they are more specific in their neurochemical effects on the CNS than other agents. SSRIs are the initial therapy for depressive illness. They block the reuptake of serotonin at presynaptic membranes, with relatively little effect on noradrenergic, cholinergic, histaminergic, or other neurochemical systems. As a result, they are associated with fewer side effects than the tricyclic antidepressants. Additional advantages of the SSRIs over the older tricyclic antidepressants include the ability to initiate treatment at target dose for most patients and once-daily dosing. For sertraline, the dose is 50 mg once daily for almost all patients. The dosage can be increased to 100 mg/day after 3 weeks if there is no evidence of symptom improvement. The dose can be increased to 150 or 200 mg/day, but this usually has little additional antidepressant efficacy. As an alternative, paroxetine can be started at 20 mg once daily and increased at similar intervals to 50 mg. Although plasma levels are available in some laboratories for these drugs and their metabolites, large clinical trials suggest that measurement of plasma levels is not a useful guide to clinical response.

TRICYCLIC ANTIDEPRESSANTS. The tricyclic antidepressants are thought to affect depressed mood by inhibiting synaptic reuptake of both norepinephrine and serotonin. Some of them, such as desipramine and nortriptyline, have a relatively greater effect on norepinephrine reuptake systems. Others, such as amitriptyline, have a broader effect on serotonin systems. As a group, however, the tricyclic antidepressants have the disadvantage that they affect neurochemical systems not thought to be essential for antidepressant efficacy, including the histaminergic, adrenergic, and acetylcholinergic systems. Tricyclic antidepressants have a wide range of side effects, including postural hypotension, cardiac tachyarrhythmias, urinary retention, and constipation. These drugs are considered second-line agents for the treatment of depression, to be used in patients in whom treatment with the SSRIs fails or in patients who have special complicating medical conditions, such as spastic bladder emptying or parkinsonism. In these latter situations, certain side effects of the tricyclic agents provide neurologic improvement.

MONOAMINE OXIDASE INHIBITORS. The monoamine oxidase (MAO) inhibitors used in psychiatric practice (see Table 450–2) are irreversible inhibitors of both forms (A and B) of brain MAO. As such, they block intracellular deamination of biogenic monoamines, including norepinephrine, serotonin, and dopamine. The clinical use of these drugs is limited by their potentially dangerous interactions with dietary tyramine or other agents with sympathomimetic or serotonergic properties. Use of these drugs should generally be initiated by psychiatrists.

ATYPICAL ANTIDEPRESSANTS. *Amoxapine* is an antidepressant with some dopamine-blocking properties. It is associated with some risk for extrapyramidal side effects. This drug has a theoretical advantage in depressed patients with psychotic features.

Trazodone and nefazodone inhibit the reuptake of serotonin (5-HT) at the synapse and have antagonism for a serotonin receptor subtype (5-HT2). The absence of prominent anticholinergic side effects is a specific advantage for nefazodone. Trazodone has some sedating properties, which makes it useful in agitated patients with disturbed sleep, particularly elderly persons.

Venlafaxine is a phenylethylamine antidepressant that inhibits reuptake of both serotonin and norepinephrine. It is selective for these two neurochemical systems, showing little in vitro binding to cholinergic, histaminergic, or dopaminergic receptors.

Table 450–2 ■ DRUGS FOR DEPRESSION (BY STRUCTURAL GROUP)

DRUG	TRADE NAME	INITIAL DOSE RANGE	TARGET DOSE RANGE	SIDE EFFECTS	COMMENTS
Tricyclics					
Imipramine	Tofranil	10–75 mg	100–300 mg	Dry mouth, constipation, postural hypotension, tachyarrhythmia	
Desipramine	Norpramin	10–75 mg	100–200 mg		
Amitriptyline	Elavil	10–50 mg	100–300 mg		
Trimipramine	Surmontil	25–75 mg	200–300 mg		
Nortriptyline	Pamelor	10–50 mg	75–150 mg		
Protriptyline	Vivactil	10–30 mg	20–50 mg		
Doxepin	Sinequan	25–75 mg	75–300 mg		
Tetracyclic					
Maprotiline	Ludiomil	25–75 mg	100–300 mg		
Selective Serotonin Reuptake Inhibitors					
Fluoxetine	Prozac	10–20 mg/day	10–80 mg/day	Nervousness, insomnia, tremor, agitation, headache, weight loss	
Sertraline	Zoloft	50 mg/day	50–200 mg/day		
Paroxetine	Paxil	20 mg/day	20–50 mg/day		
Fluvoxamine	Luvox	50 mg/day	50–300 mg/day		
Monoamine Oxidase Inhibitors					
Phenelzine	Nardil	15–45 mg	45–75 mg	Hypertensive crises; sedation, tremor	Patients taking these drugs must be on a tyramine-free diet
Tranylcypromine	Parnate	10–20 mg	20–30 mg		
Atypical or Nontricyclics					
Amoxapine	Asendin	25–75 mg	100–300 mg		
Trazodone	Desyrel	25–75 mg/day in divided doses	300 mg/day in divided doses	Priapism	Helpful as second drug for sleep disturbance
Nefazodone	Serzone	100 mg BID		Headache and drowsiness sometimes associated	As effective as imipramine
Venlafaxine	Effexor	25 mg TID	200–275 mg/day, TID dosing	Hypertension	Serotonin/norepinephrine reuptake inhibitor; may be effective in treatment resistant depression
Mirtazapine	Remeron	15 mg/day	30–45 mg/day	Somnolence, weight gain	Increase at 1–2 wk intervals
Bupropion	Wellbutrin	100 mg BID	300 mg/day, TID dosing	Affects dopamine and norepinephrine reuptake	May be especially helpful in atypical depression
Psychostimulants					
Dextroamphetamine	Dexedrine	2.5 mg	5–10 mg		Abuse potential must be considered
Pemoline	Cylert	18.75 mg	37 mg BID		
Methylphenidate	Ritalin	2.5 mg BID	10 mg TID		

Bupropion is a novel monocyclic compound in that it inhibits the reuptake of dopamine but has little effect on other adrenergic systems.

Mirtazapine is a newly approved tetracyclic piperazinoazepine, which is an analogue of mianserin, an antidepressant that has been available in Europe. It is a presynaptic α_2 blocker that increases the release of both norepinephrine and serotonin. It also blocks $5HT_2$ and $5HT_3$ receptors, as well as histamine H_1 receptors. Common side effects include weight gain, dizziness, dry mouth, and constipation. It should not be used as the initial treatment of depression but is a reasonable alternative for patients who do not respond to SSRIs.

Bipolar Disorders

Bipolar disorders (previously called manic-depressive disorders) are the most homogeneous psychiatric diagnostic grouping: marked swings in mood from major depressive episodes to major manic episodes. There is usually a return to normal behavior between episodes. There is little difficulty in recognizing the illness if one looks at the longitudinal course. If patients are examined only briefly, however, at a particular moment in time, manic excitement can be confused with schizophrenic psychosis. The severe depressive phase of bipolar illness can also be misconstrued as a catatonic state.

DIAGNOSTIC CRITERIA AND CLINICAL SIGNS AND SYMPTOMS. The manic phase of bipolar disorder is characterized by an expansive euphoric mood in which the patient is subject to grandiose plans and ideas. Despite this expansiveness and grandiosity, patients who are frustrated or disagreed with often become irritable and sometimes aggressive. The patient can be psychotic in the manic phase, with delusions and hallucinations consistent with grandiosity; persecutory delusions, (i.e., feelings of being controlled) may also be present. At times it is difficult to distinguish an excited schizophrenic patient from a manic one. One must examine the longitudinal course of the illness until either a depressive episode occurs or the course deteriorates after remission of the acute symptom to diagnose a schizophrenic process. In all instances, it is crucial to rule out metabolic and other medical disorders, particularly in older patients. The major diagnostic criteria are listed in Table 450–3.

The average age at onset of bipolar disorder is about 30 years, but about 20% of patients have an onset before the age of 20. In women, onset of the condition has a bimodal distribution, with one peak falling between 20 and 30 years and the other far earlier, but the age at onset of bipolar illness overlaps enough so that the differential diagnosis of a psychotic illness in a young person is difficult and may change as the clinical picture evolves over time. Almost half of patients with bipolar disorders have at least two or

---

Table 450–3 ■ MAJOR DIAGNOSTIC CRITERIA FOR A MANIC EPISODE

A distinct period of abnormally and persistently elevated, expansive, or irritable mood, lasting at least 1 week (or any duration if hospitalization is necessary).
During the period of mood disturbance, at least three of the following symptoms have persisted (four if the mood is only irritable) and have been present to a significant degree:
1. Inflated self-esteem or grandiosity
2. Decreased need for sleep (e.g., feels rested after only 3 hours of sleep)
3. More talkative than usual or feels pressure to keep talking
4. Flight of ideas or subjective experiences that thoughts are racing
5. Distractibility (i.e., attention too easily drawn to unimportant or irrelevant external stimuli)
6. Increase in goal-directed activity (either socially, at work or school, or sexually) or psychomotor agitation
7. Excessive involvement in pleasurable activities that have a high potential for painful consequences (e.g., engaging in unrestrained buying sprees, sexual indiscretions, or foolish business investments)

The mood disturbance is sufficiently severe to cause marked impairment in occupational functioning or in usual social activities or relationships with others to necessitate hospitalization to prevent harm to self or others.
The symptoms are not due to the direct effects of a substance (e.g., drugs of abuse, medication) or a general medical condition (e.g., hyperthyroidism).

---

three episodes of illness, and as many as a third experience seven or more episodes of illness once the pattern has started. Each episode of illness, whether manic or depressive, can last from 4 to 13 months; some go on to chronicity, and some cease much sooner. The course of the illness has been modified substantially with the advent of lithium therapy, diminishing both the severity and the frequency of the episodes. Shorter durations are usually related to the effectiveness of treatment. Although some patients rapidly alternate between extremes over 2 to 4 days, most episodes have a longer duration, and a manic phase frequently follows a depressive phase. In contrast to the situation in schizophrenia, chronicity is not a major problem with manic-depressive illness, being as low as 1% in some studies. Mortality with bipolar illness averages 2 to 2.5 times the expected rate for that age; 8 to 10% of patients commit suicide.

EPIDEMIOLOGY AND PATHOPHYSIOLOGY. The lifetime risk for development of bipolar illness ranges from 0.6 to 0.9%. The annual new-case incidence per hundred thousand is 9 to 15 in men and 7.4 to 32 in women. The risk increases with a family history of bipolar illness. The genetic pattern in bipolar illness is uncertain but suggests autosomal dominance with incomplete penetrance. There is a 72% concordance in monozygotic twins and a 19% concordance in same-sex dizygotic twins. Both the course of illness and the response to treatment are similar among related patients. In one well-studied Amish family, an abnormal gene was localized to chromosome 11. Other families with equally strong genetic patterns have not possessed this particular chromosomal localization.

The pathophysiology of bipolar illness, to the extent that it is known, is similar to the biology of the major depressive disorders.

DIAGNOSIS AND TREATMENT. The treatment of bipolar disorders has three distinct aspects: the manic episode, the major depressive episode, and long-term maintenance therapy. Before any specific therapy is begun, an adequate medical work-up is necessary to ensure that the patient has a primary affective illness. A patient in an acute manic state is typically delusional, grandiose, and hyperactive; in this condition, he or she appears similar to any patient with psychosis. In the first episode, one cannot differentiate this state by its clinical features from the first episode of schizophrenia or a psychosis due to physical illness. The differential diagnosis with the first episode rests on a careful history, family history, and physical and laboratory examination. Patient history, family history, and the nature of onset of the illness are important. Patients with their first psychotic episode should be evaluated by a psychiatrist.

The treatment of the acute manic phase is usually undertaken in the hospital, since it is imperative to protect patients from their own misdeeds (e.g., spending inordinate amounts of money or making embarrassing speeches). If family members are supportive, however, and believe they can control the situation, treatment can be started outside the hospital. Lithium is not useful for the acute management of mania, and if the patient is severely agitated, sedation is necessary. Neuroleptics are not used in the long-term treatment of bipolar illness, but benzodiazepines, particularly lorazepam, can effectively control most acute manic states. If the agitation cannot be controlled with medication, the clinician should obtain psychiatric consultation to consider using electroconvulsive therapy (ECT) to control manic excitement. Manic excitement creates a medical emergency; patients can die of exhaustion.

Although general physicians rarely initiate treatment of acute mania, they often have patients who are taking lithium. Lithium effectively prevents relapses in most bipolar illnesses; it is slightly more effective in preventing manic than depressive episodes. Its use should be considered with any repetitive affective disturbance.

Before lithium therapy is begun, a complete blood cell count, urinalysis, electrolytes, creatinine level, blood urea nitrogen level, thyroid studies, and a baseline electrocardiogram and EEG should be obtained. Chronic medical illnesses, especially renal insufficiency, can contraindicate use of the agent. Lithium carbonate is available in 300 mg tablets or capsules, and a 300-mg slow-release tablet is also available. The starting dose of lithium carbonate in acute mania is generally 300 mg three or four times per day. Lithium has a half-life of 24 to 36 hours, and it takes at least 4 days to achieve a steady state. Its specific therapeutic effectiveness is not evident until at least 4 to 10 days after institution of therapy. The dosage should be adjusted upward by a full or half tablet after the serum level is checked during this time period. Lithium does not work immediately for acutely agitated or manic patients but

Motor Tension
Trembling, twitching, or feeling shaky
Muscle tension, aches, or soreness
Restlessness
Easy fatigability
Autonomic Hyperactivity
Shortness of breath or smothering sensations
Palpitations or accelerated heart rate (tachycardia)
Sweating or cold, sweaty hands
Dry mouth
Dizziness or lightheadedness
Nausea, diarrhea, or other abdominal distress
Flashes (hot flashes) or chills
Frequent urination
Trouble swallowing or "lump in throat"
Vigilance and Scanning
Feeling keyed up or on edge
Exaggerated startle response
Difficulty concentrating or "mind going blank" because of anxiety
Trouble falling or staying asleep
Irritability

should nonetheless be started early in anticipation of maintenance use. It is necessary to monitor the serum level of lithium; adequate levels for acute illness are in the range of 0.8 to 1.4 mEq/L. For maintenance therapy, satisfactory responses accompany blood levels of 0.4 mEq/L. Dose and blood level, however, should be titrated against clinical effectiveness for each patient. Once maintenance levels are reached, patients usually can be maintained for long periods with minimal surveillance. Doses usually are given twice daily, because absorption from the gastrointestinal tract is rapid and the drug peaks in the serum within 1 to 2 hours. Elevation of serum lithium levels to more than 2 mEq/L is toxic and represents a medical emergency requiring immediate hospitalization and possibly hemodialysis. Side effects in the long-term use of lithium include the development of mild leukocytosis, hypothyroidism, diabetes insipidus, and renal tubular damage. Many patients have a tremor that can be embarrassing and that occasionally interferes with activities.

Antiepileptic drugs have increasingly been used as alternative or adjunctive therapy in patients with bipolar disorders or related disturbances of emotional stability. Carbamazepine can be used as an alternative for those who cannot tolerate lithium's side effects or who fail to respond to lithium. Antimania doses of carbamazepine are similar to those used for epilepsy and range from 600 to 1600 mg/day on a thrice daily schedule, aiming for a serum level of 6 to 12 μg/mL. Valproic acid is also effective in doses from 800 to 1800 mg/day, also on a thrice-dialy schedule aiming for a serum level above 50 μg/mL. Preliminary evidence suggests that lamotrigine, gabapentin, and topiramate may also have efficacy in the suppression of recurrence of bipolar disorder.

PROGNOSIS. Manic or depressive episodes produce major disruptions of psychological, social, and vocational function. Divorce and job loss are very real possibilities. Even when there is improvement with SSRIs or tricyclic antidepressants, long-term supportive psychotherapy is usually indicated. Moreover, the symptoms of some bipolar patients do not fully resolve; chronic symptoms often produce permanent psychosocial deterioration. Most bipolar patients, however, have a relapsing course and are free of symptoms between episodes. Their long-term functional outcome depends on the frequency and severity of their affective episodes and their response to treatment. The management of all bipolar patients involves careful surveillance for early signs of affective instability; prompt treatment can minimize long-term psychosocial disruption.

Anxiety Disorders

The anxiety disorders occur at any age and are associated with a variety of distressing symptoms, including nervousness, sleeplessness, hypochondriasis, and somatic complaints. It is useful clinically to consider the anxiety disorders in two different patterns: (1) chronic, generalized anxiety, and (2) episodic, panic-like anxiety. Episodic anxiety is often context dependent, such as the performance anxiety of a musician before an audience. When panic attacks occur, however, they are qualitatively different from generalized

anxiety. The patient typically experiences sudden onset of intense fear, arousal, and even respiratory distress without provocation. Panic attacks are often confused with systemic medical illness, such as angina pectoris or epilepsy. There is also a spectrum of related mental disorders, which includes anxious features, such as the phobias and post-traumatic stress disorder.

INCIDENCE AND PREVALENCE. Lifetime prevalence rates for DSM diagnosable anxiety disorders are as high as 30% for women and 19% for men. Point prevalence rates are in the range of 2 to 6% for generalized anxiety and 1% for panic disorder. The anxiety disorders may be the most common psychiatric disorders in general medical practice.

PATHOPHYSIOLOGY. Like the depressive disorders, the anxiety disorders cluster in families. Twin studies more clearly indicate a shared familial risk for panic disorder than for generalized anxiety. The underlying neurophysiology and neurochemistry of the anxiety disorders implicate overactivity of noradrenergic systems projecting from the locus caeruleus into forebrain regions.

DIAGNOSIS AND CLINICAL MANIFESTATION. Diagnostic criteria for generalized anxiety disorder (from DSM-IV) emphasize the presence of unrealistic or excessive worry and apprehension about two or more life circumstances, for a period of 6 months or longer, during which the person has been bothered more days than not by these concerns. At least six symptoms from Table 450–4 must be present during these periods.

Panic attacks are characterized by the sudden onset of intense apprehension, fear, or a sense of impending doom. These attacks are often spontaneous, and they may overlap with the more generalized anxiety disorder described earlier. The diagnostic criteria for panic disorder (from DSM-IV) are included in Table 450–5.

TREATMENT. Drugs for anxiety and panic are presented in Table 450–6. In acute anxiety or panic disorder, the efficacy of pharmacologic agents as measured by panic-free rates is high, with success rates in the range of 50 to 70%. Many patients require ongoing treatment, others have symptoms despite treatment. Sustained use of benzodiazepines and tricyclic antidepressants is equally effective in patients with panic disorder. They are the first-line therapies for panic disorder and its variants. A representative initial dosing regimen is imipramine, 10 mg thrice daily, or alprazolam, 0.5 mg twice daily. Alprazolam dosing may need to be increased to 6 to 8 mg/day unless sedation ensues at lower doses. The MAO inhibitors and the SSRIs have also been demonstrated to have efficacy in panic disorder.

For generalized or chronic anxiety, the antidepressants have much less efficacy. The short-term relief afforded by almost any benzodiazepine is dramatic in generalized anxiety, which accounts for the tremendous market size these drugs as a class have attained

Table 450–5 ■ DIAGNOSTIC CRITERIA FOR PANIC DISORDERS

One or more panic attacks (discrete periods of intense fear or discomfort) have occurred that (1) were unexpected (i.e., did not occur immediately before or on exposure to a situation that almost always caused anxiety) and (2) were not triggered by situations in which the person was the focus of others' attention.
Either four attacks have occurred within a 4-week period or one or more attacks have been followed by a period of at least a month of persistent fear of having another attack.
At least four of the following symptoms developed during at least one of the attacks:
Shortness of breath (dyspnea) or smothering sensations
Dizziness, unsteady feelings, or faintness
Palpitations or accelerated heart rate (tachycardia)
Trembling
Sweating
Choking
Nausea or abdominal distress
Depersonalization or derealization
Numbness or tingling sensations (paresthesia)
Flashes (hot flashes) or chills
Chest pain or discomfort
Fear of dying
Fear of "going crazy" or of doing something uncontrolled
During at least some of these attacks at least four of the symptoms developed suddenly and increased in intensity within 10 minutes of the beginning of the first symptom noticed in the attack.

in the United States. Habituation and addiction come close behind the initial relief properties of benzodiazepines, however, so caution should be exercised. If there is any situational quality to the generalized anxiety symptoms, other therapeutic measures should be considered before benzodiazepines are prescribed. Reassurance may be tried, relaxation exercises, hypnosis, and a variety of other psychotherapies. Environmental alterations may be considered at home or at work, depending on the individual's specific anxiety symptoms. When a psychopharmacologic intervention is prescribed, it should be given for a defined period of 1 to 4 weeks. The situation should be reassessed by the physician. Antihistamines such as diphenhydramine, 25 mg three times a day, can be tried for some patients. Buspirone is a non-benzodiazepine anti-anxiety agent that sometimes provides relief at doses of 5 mg twice a day initially (see Table 450–6). The benzodiazepines presented in Table 450–2 are all effective in many patients. Lorazepam is often the first used, since it is relatively short acting (half-life of 10 to 15 hours) and easier to titrate in elderly or medically ill patients. Because its half-life is shorter than drugs such as diazepam, lorazepam must be taken at least twice and often three times per day. A dosage of 0.5 mg twice daily is the initial regimen for most patients. The dose should be increased by 0.5 mg/day at 3-day intervals until target symptoms resolve or sedative side effects supervene. Elderly patients should always be watched carefully for gait ataxia. For all patients on maintenance benzodiazepine dosing, there should be constant surveillance for opportunities to taper or reduce the dosing regimen.

The Somatoform Disorders

The somatoform disorders are a heterogeneous group of disorders that share the common feature of mimicry of medical disease. The mimicry may involve an exaggeration of severity or disability accompanying actual medical illness, or it may consist entirely of simulation. A partial listing of these disorders derived from the DSM-IV is presented in Table 450–7. Several evolving disorders are "somatoform" in whole or in part but are not strictly classified in the somatoform disorders category.

DIAGNOSIS AND CLINICAL FEATURES. CONVERSION DISORDER. The essential feature of a conversion disorder is the presence of a symptom or deficit affecting voluntary motor or sensory function that suggests a neurologic or general medical condition. Conversion phenomena typically do not conform to known anatomic systems but instead follow the individual's unconscious conceptualization of neurologic function. Conversion disorders may be episodic, as in conversion seizures, or chronic and persistent, as in the case of sensory loss or weakness. To make a valid diagnosis of conversion, two features should be established: the failure of the disorder to respect known neuroanatomy and neurophysiology should be recognized, and some positive association with unintentional psychological motivation should be understood.

FACTITIOUS DISORDER. In a factitious disorder, the production of the symptom or sign is more deliberate. The individual may self-administer a drug or other material to create actual physical signs. The motivation for these actions may be unconscious, although the action itself is deliberate.

Munchausen's syndrome is perhaps the best known of the factitious disorders. It is defined as a repetitious pattern of medical attention–seeking behaviors in which the individual has dramatic but untruthful complaints. The somatic complaints typically involve systemic organ systems, such as abdominal pain or hemorrhage.

MALINGERING. Malingering refers to the production of false or grossly exaggerated physical or psychological symptoms when both the symptom production and the motivation are consciously understood by the patient. In the case of malingering, the secondary gain or environmental reinforcement for the behavior is usually transparent. These environmental reinforcers typically include relief from arduous duty or responsibility, as in military training, or the prospect of significant financial reward, as in litigation.

CHRONIC FATIGUE SYNDROME. In the mid-1980s reports began to appear in the United States of a syndrome of pathologic fatiguability. Unconscious psychological factors are almost certainly important contributors in some patients with this syndrome. Other contributors, including immune system dysfunction, orthostatic hypotension, and endocrinologic systems, are under investigation.

PATHOGENESIS. There are as yet no credible neurobiologic explanations for the somatoform disorders. They must be understood as psychological phenomena, with variable levels of self-awareness in each individual as to the factitious nature of the disorder. Freud and his colleagues believed that symptoms could be produced by a process of dissociation—the expulsion from consciousness of a painful memory or feeling and its replacement by a physical symptom. The advantage to the patient of the conversion disorder was

Table 450–6 ▪ DRUGS FOR ANXIETY AND PANIC

DRUG	TRADE NAME	INITIAL DOSE	TARGET DOSE RANGE	SIDE EFFECTS	COMMENTS
Sedative Hypnotics					
Chloral hydrate	Noctel	500 mg	500–1000 mg	Sedation; overdose risk	Seldom appropriate
Meprobamate	Miltown	200 mg TID	1200–1600 mg		
Antihistamines					
Diphenhydramine	Benadryl	25 mg PO QHS	50 mg	Dry mouth, mental confusion	Most useful at bedtime for associated sleep disturbance
Hydroxyzine	Atarax				
Benzodiazepines					
Lorazepam	Ativan	0.5 mg PO	2–10 mg, TID dosing		Also effective for generalized anxiety
Diazepam	Valium	5 mg PO	5–10 mg BID	Addictive	Abuse potential in many
Triazolam	Halcion	0.125 mg	0.25–0.5 mg HS		
Chlordiazepoxide	Librium	5 mg BID	10–30 mg		
Temazepam	Restoril	7.5 mg HS	15–30 mg		
Alprazolam	Xanax	0.25 mg BID	2–8 mg/day	Ataxia, drowsiness	
Clorazepate	Tranxene	7.5 mg HS	15–60 mg/day		
Flurazepam	Dalmane	15 mg HS	30–60 mg	Ataxia, drowsiness	Abuse potential
Oxazepam	Serax	10 mg BID	60–120 mg/day		
Clonazepam	Klonopin	0.25 mg QD	1–3 mg/day	Sedation, ataxia	Long duration of action permits once-daily dosing
Buspirone	Buspar	5 mg BID	20–30 mg/day	Nervousness, headache	No dependence with prolonged use
Zolpidem	Ambien	10 mg HS	10 mg HS	Habituation, drowsiness	Most useful on an as-needed basis
Beta Blockers					
Propranolol	Inderal	20 mg BID	Individualize 40–120 mg/day	Bradycardia, mental confusion	Does not block the fear component of anxiety or panic

Table 450–7 ■ THE SOMATOFORM DISORDERS

DISORDER	FEATURES
Somatization disorder	Chronic, multisystem disorder characterized by complaints of pain, gastrointestinal and sexual dysfunction, and pseudoneurologic symptoms. Onset is usually early in life, and psychosocial and vocational achievements are limited.
Conversion disorder	Syndrome of symptoms or deficits mimicking neurologic or medical illness in which psychological factors are judged to be of etiologic importance.
Pain disorder	Clinical syndrome characterized predominantly by pain in which psychological factors are judged to be of etiologic importance.
Hypochondriasis	Chronic preoccupation with the idea of having a serious disease. The preoccupation is usually poorly amenable to reassurance.
Body dysmorphic disorder	Preoccupation with an imagined or exaggerated defect in physical appearance
Other Somatoform-Like Disorders	
Factitious disorder	Intentional production or feigning of physical or psychological signs when external reinforcers (e.g., avoidance of responsibility, financial gain) are not clearly present.
Malingering	Intentional production or feigning of physical or psychological signs when external reinforcers (e.g., avoidance of responsibility, financial gain) are present.
Dissociative disorders	Disruptions of consciousness, memory, identity, or perception judged to be due to psychological factors.

the protection afforded from the psychic pain, since this pain had been connected to or symbolized by a physical symptom. This protection afforded from the psychological pain and stress is referred to as the primary gain of the somatoform illness. The primary gain is usually not readily discernible, since the patient is almost always unaware of it.

The secondary gain associated with a conversion illness refers to the clearly visible financial gain or relief from responsibility conferred by the sick role. Such gains may be seen in many guises, such as disability pensions, relief from work, enhanced attention from family and physicians, and litigation payouts.

INCIDENCE AND PREVALENCE. Good epidemiologic data about the somatoform disorders are lacking. Cross-sectional studies of patients attending general neurologic clinics indicate high prevalence rates of 15 to 20% in these populations. Disorder-specific and population-based studies are not available for these disorders.

TREATMENT. The long-term goal of treatment for the somatoform disorders is to enable the patient to convert from a medical into a psychiatric patient. This process requires patience and flexibility on the part of the physician. General medical interventions may be invoked initially, including biologic tests, medical rehabilitation, and pharmacotherapy. These interventions may make sense if an underlying medical disease is present or if the patient adamantly views the illness as a physical one. The danger of biologic interventions is that they may strengthen the conviction on the part of the patient that the illness is physical.

If a pharmacologically accessible symptom complex, such as anxiety or depression, accompanies the conversion phenomena, it may be helpful to initiate psychopharmacologic treatment. It is unclear how often the treatment of associated emotional symptoms results in improvement of conversion symptoms, but this approach is clearly effective on occasion.

Character Disorders

Behavior includes more than cognition and emotion. Action and style are additional dimensions of behavior that are essential to success and satisfaction in life. Sustained dysfunctional patterns of coping with the world are called *character disorders.* Each person has an enduring set of behavioral traits with which he or she faces life's challenges. These predispositions are for the most part not context dependent nor are they easily changed from one point in

time to another. These traits manifest themselves in style and action. An individual is typically unaware of these style qualities since they are formed in childhood as enduring aspects of the personality. Some individuals demonstrate clusters of maladaptive traits that cause recurrent psychosocial difficulties. These clusters of maladaptive traits are called character disorders or personality disorders. We have many names for such character qualities, including honesty, timeliness, reliability, aggressiveness, and submissiveness. A number of character disorders are listed with tables of qualifying features in DSM-IV (Table 450–8). In DSM-IV, these disorders are classified as Axis II disorders as opposed to the Axis I classification of the more overt major psychiatric disorders. The clinical descriptive research that underlies and validates these disorders as distinct clinical entities is more limited than it is for the Axis I disorders. The personality disorders have a spectrum of severity, with poorly specified boundaries and thresholds. It makes clinical sense to think of "personality styles" on occasions when the severity of maladaptive traits is less. The personality disorders also differ from the Axis I disorders in that they have to do with interpersonal relatedness more than they do with the intrapsychic symptoms of a single individual. It is difficult to imagine the diagnosis of a passive-aggressive personality style in a setting that did not include other people. Often the best clue to the diagnosis of character pathology is the pattern of behavior the patient shows in relating to the physician.

TREATMENT. Personality disorders are difficult to recognize and to treat. Patients are not consciously aware of the data that validate the diagnoses, and they are typically sensitive when dysfunctional patterns of behavior are clarified. Psychopharmacology is not indicated for these disorders. The goal of management is to help the patient to increase his or her awareness of the dysfunctional interpersonal traits so that conscious control of their adverse effects can increase. Although longer-term psychotherapies must be performed by psychiatric clinicians, general medical physicians can often provide initial clarifying intervention.

Schizophrenic Disorders

Schizophrenia and some forms of affective disorders constitute the major psychotic illnesses. (*Psychosis* is defined as the presence of hallucinations or delusions.) Schizophrenia most often starts in late adolescence. The course is usually marked by a decline in

Table 450–8 ■ CHARACTER DISORDERS

PERSONALITY TYPE	CHARACTERISTIC BEHAVIOR PATTERNS
Paranoid	Distrust and suspiciousness
Schizoid	Detachment from social relationships, with a restricted range of emotional expression
Schizotypal	Eccentricities in behavior and cognitive distortions; acute discomfort in close relationships
Antisocial	Disregard for rights of others; a defect in the experience of compunction or remorse for harming others
Borderline	Instability in interpersonal relationships, self-image, and affective regulation
Histrionic	Emotional overreactivity, theatrical behaviors, and seductiveness
Narcissistic	Persisting grandiosity, need for admiration, and lack of empathy for others
Avoidant	Social inhibition, feelings of inadequacy, and hypersensitivity to negative evaluation
Dependent	Submission and clinging behaviors
Obsessive-compulsive	Rigid, detail-oriented behaviors, often associated with compulsions to perform tasks repetitively and unnecessarily

psychosocial functioning, with a tendency for the patient to become downwardly mobile in social strata. Physicians encounter two principal groups of schizophrenic patients: an acute, florid psychotic illness and a chronic illness with less florid symptoms.

DIAGNOSTIC CRITERIA AND CLINICAL SIGNS AND SYMPTOMS. Table 450–9 lists diagnostic criteria for schizophrenia. With schizophrenia, the greater the number of delusions and hallucinations present, the more likely the person is to progress to a chronic psychotic condition. Other prominent symptoms of schizophrenia are incoherence and the inability to communicate in a logical and goal-directed fashion.

When these psychotic features last for a 6-month period (demonstrating a deterioration from a previous level of functioning), schizophrenia is defined as a more chronic disorder. When the duration of symptoms is shorter than 6 months, it is inadvisable to use the diagnosis of schizophrenia. With the first episode of psychotic illness, one should consider an affective disorder or a systemic medical illness as diagnostic possibilities. Psychotic episodes due to toxic drug reactions, sleep deprivation, and medical causes invariably last less than 6 months.

In the past, many subtypes of schizophrenia were described, but their predictive validity has been poor except for catatonia and paranoia. Catatonic symptoms involve either markedly retarded motor behavior (often to the point of no voluntary movement; the patient retains any posture into which he or she is passively placed) or markedly agitated motor behavior. The paranoid forms of schizophrenia also show some unique features in that the paranoid delusions are often the only major symptoms and they tend to remain stable over time.

EPIDEMIOLOGY. The prevalence of schizophrenia in the general population is about 1% for lifetime risk, or an incidence of about 0.5 in 1000 person-years. The prevalence rate is eight times as great in the lower as in the higher socioeconomic environments. Because the parents of schizophrenics have a social class distribution similar to that of the general population, the lower position of the patients appears to be a result of the illness rather than the cause of it.

Seventy per cent of schizophrenics become ill between the ages of 15 and 35. The illness affects males and females in equal proportion over the entire lifespan. The age of peak onset risk is 15 to 24 years in males and 25 to 34 years in females. There are slight ethnic differences, with a higher incidence in Scandinavian countries and in nonwhites.

PATHOPHYSIOLOGY. The pathophysiology of schizophrenia is unknown, and an anatomic origin of the symptoms has yet to be determined. Nevertheless, a number of conditions (e.g., trauma, seizure disorders, and Huntington's disease) can produce schizophrenia-like hallucinations and delusions. Many experts have reported a higher than normal incidence of nonlocalizing neurologic abnormalities in schizophrenia, changes that are not present in other psychiatric conditions.

Twenty-five per cent of hospitalized schizophrenic patients show abnormally slow EEG tracings using standard recording techniques. Computed tomographic and magnetic resonance imaging studies have shown lateral ventricle and third ventricle enlargement, widened cortical sulci, cerebellar atrophy, cerebral asymmetry, and decreased brain density. Although the implications of these findings are unclear, the findings correlate with increased cognitive disturbance, poorer premorbid adjustment, and longer duration of illness.

Strong evidence implicates genetic factors in schizophrenia. Ten to 15% of the offspring of schizophrenic parents have the disease. Furthermore, the coincidence of schizophrenia in monozygotic twins is roughly 60%. Additional evidence for a genetic factor comes from studies of children of schizophrenic parents who are raised by either their natural or adoptive nonschizophrenic parents: the chances of development of the disease are identical in both instances, regardless of the environment. Despite these findings, family factors have been implicated in other ways. In families with much highly charged emotional interaction, schizophrenic patients seem to do very poorly. Less emotionally stimulating environments appear to allow schizophrenic persons to function better.

PROGNOSIS AND TREATMENT. Prognosis in schizophrenia is poor, and there is no specific therapy. During a 25- to 30-year period, about one third of patients show some recovery or remission, and the remainder either have major residual symptoms or require long-term hospitalization. The major symptomatic treatment is antipsychotic medication. An overview of available drugs for psychosis is presented in Table 450–10.

The initial pharmacologic therapy of psychosis should begin with the administration of one of the newer, "atypical" antipsychotic drugs. This group of drugs includes olanzapine, risperidone, quetiapine, and clozapine. Clozapine cannot be considered a first-line therapy because of hematopoietic and hepatic side effect risks, which are discussed in more detail later. These agents are termed *atypical* because of their side effect spectrum, which differs significantly from that of the older, traditional antipsychotic agents such as haloperidol and chlorpromazine. The newer drugs as a group have less acute motor system side effects than the older drugs and may have less long-term risk for the development of tardive dyskinesias. These agents may be more efficacious for the negative psychotic symptoms of schizophrenia, such as apathy and anergia.

Typical initial regimens include risperidone, 2 mg twice daily, increasing to 6 to 10 mg/day total dose after 1 week if tolerated. Antipsychotic efficacy is usually seen in this target dose range for risperidol, with a 4- to 6-week delay for some effects. An alternative is olanzapine, which can be administered once daily. A starting dose for olanzapine is 5 mg daily, increasing by 5-mg increments at weekly intervals to the 15- to 20-mg range if symptoms do not improve and side effects are tolerable. The aggressiveness of the dosing regimen is dictated to some extent by the quality and severity of the psychotic symptoms. Because all the antipsychotic drugs have a time delay for onset of efficacy, additional psychotropic agents are sometimes added during the early days of treatment. For example, a benzodiazepine such as alprazolam, 0.25 mg thrice daily, may be added when agitation and sleep disturbance are severe. The most frequent limiting factor in the dosing of antipsychotic drugs is the appearance of extrapyramidal side effects, including dystonia, akathisia (restlessness), and parkinsonism.

An additional risk in the use of antipsychotic drugs is the development of tardive dyskinesia. Tardive dyskinesia is a syndrome of involuntary movements, usually choreoathetoid, that can affect the mouth, lips, tongue, extremities, or trunk. Although usually associated with use of neuroleptics for 6 months or more, tardive dyskinesia can occur with shorter administration. Patients receiving neuroleptics should be periodically evaluated for these abnormal

---

Table 450–9 ■ SCHIZOPHRENIA AND OTHER PSYCHOTIC DISORDERS

Characteristic Symptoms

At least two of the following, each present for a major portion of time during a 1-month period (or less if successfully treated):

1. Delusions
2. Hallucinations
3. Disorganized speech (e.g., frequent derailment "jumping from one topic to another or incoherence)
4. Grossly disorganized or catatonic behavior
5. Negative symptoms (i.e., affective flattening, alogia, or avolition)

(Note: only one characteristic symptom is required if delusions are bizarre or hallucinations consist of a voice keeping up a running commentary on the person's behavior or thoughts, or involve two or more voices conversing with each other.)

Social/Occupational Dysfunction

For a significant portion of the time since the onset of the disturbance, one or more major areas of functioning (e.g., work, interpersonal relations, or self-care) are markedly below the level achieved before the onset (or when the onset is in childhood or adolescence, failure to achieve expected level of interpersonal, academic, or occupational achievement).

Duration

Continuous signs of the disturbance persist for at least 6 months. This 6-month period must include at least 1 month of characteristic symptoms as described above (i.e., active-phase symptoms) and may include periods of prodromal or residual symptoms. During these prodromal or residual periods, the signs of the disturbance may be manifested by only negative symptoms or two or more of the characteristic symptoms present in an attenuated form (e.g., odd beliefs, unusual perceptual experiences).

Schizoaffective and Mood Disorder Exclusion

Schizoaffective disorder and mood disorder with psychotic features have been ruled out because either (1) no major depressive or manic episodes have occurred concurrently with the active-phase symptoms, or (2) if mood episodes have occurred during active phase symptoms, their total duration has been brief in relation to the duration of the active and residual periods.

Substance/General Medical Condition Exclusion

The disturbance is not due to the direct effects of a substance (e.g., drugs of abuse, medication) or a general medical condition.

Table 450-10 ■ **DRUGS FOR PSYCHOSIS**

CLASS	GENERIC NAME	TRADE NAME	ACUTE DOSE PER 24 HR	MAINTENANCE DOSE	SIDE EFFECTS
Phenothiazine Aliphatic	Chlorpromazine	Thorazine	25–1000 mg PO 25–400 mg IM	25–400 mg PO	EPMD, hyperprolactinemia
Phenothiazine Piperazine	Perphenazine	Trilafon	8–64 mg PO 15–30 mg IM	12–24 mg PO	EPMD
	Fluphenazine	Prolixin	2.5–40 mg PO 5–20 mg IM	12.5–50 mg IM decanoate weekly	
	Trifluoperazine	Stelazine	1–5 mg PO		
Phenothiazine Piperidine	Thioridazine	Mellaril	25–800 mg PO	25–300 mg PO	EPMD; retinal degenerative risk above 300 mg/day
	Mesoridazine	Serentil	50–400 mg PO	200–400 mg PO	
Butyrophenone	Haloperidol	Haldol	2–25 mg PO 6–30 mg IM	1–15 mg PO 25–200 mg IM decanoate monthly	EPMD; can cause a dysphoria side effect at low to moderate doses
Thioxanthene	Chlorprothixene	Taractan	30–100 mg PO	100–300 mg	
	Thiothixene	Navane	2–5 mg PO	5–10 mg PO	Intramuscular form available
Dibensoxazepine	Loxapine	Loxitane	50–250 mg PO	60–100 mg	
Dihydroindole	Molindone	Moban	50–225 mg PO	20–200 mg	Less likely to reduce seizure threshold
Benzisoxazole	Risperidone	Risperdal	2–4 mg PO	2–20 mg	Low incidence of extrapyramidal effects
Dibenzodiazepine	Olanzapine	Zyprexa	5–15 mg PO	5–10 mg PO	Fewer extrapyramidal effects; fatal agranulocytosis; sedating
	Clozapine	Clozaril	200–400 mg	200–600 mg	
Diphenylbutylpiperidine	Pimozide	Orap	10–30 mg	10–30 mg	
Phenylindole	Quetiapine	Seroquel	25 mg BID	300–400 mg/day	Low incidence of extrapyramidal effects

EPMD = Extrapyramidal movement disorders.

movements. A frequent early sign consists of involuntary movements of the tongue. The symptoms may decrease with an increase of the medication, but such improvement usually is only temporary and may lead to a vicious circle of worsening chorea and increased drug dosages. The cause of tardive dyskinesia is not known, but it is believed to represent the development of dopaminergic hypersensitivity in extrapyramidal motor systems.

The natural history of schizophrenia (even in treated patients) is of two major types: (1) an episodic, relapsing course with each episode resulting in a lower level of psychosocial functioning, and (2) a gradual, slow decline in functional ability. Both courses eventually result in a progressive loss of psychosocial capacities. Psychosocial treatment efforts in schizophrenia have taken a rehabilitative, or psychoeducational, approach in which the family is educated about the problems of schizophrenia and issues of living are openly confronted.

DRUGS FOR PSYCHOSIS. Drugs that affect dopaminergic function by blocking mesolimbic dopamine receptors have the demonstrated ability to improve a variety of psychotic symptoms. The older antipsychotic drugs demonstrated broad-spectrum dopamine receptor–blocking properties, affecting all receptor subtypes, and both nigrostriatal neurons (substantia nigra pars compacta, A9) and limbic dopaminergic neurons (ventral tegmental area, A10). Consequently, these drugs have many motor system side effects. A new generation of antipsychotic agents is now appearing that has variable effects on dopamine receptor subtypes as well as effects on other neurochemical systems such as serotonin. Some comments on selected agents in this class of new antipsychotic drugs follow.

Risperidone. Concomitant blockade of D_2 receptors in the basal ganglia has been presumed to underlie the production of extrapyramidal syndromes by traditional antipsychotic drugs. More recently, psychopharmacologic research has turned to agents that might simultaneously block D_2 and serotonin (5-HT_2) receptors. Some evidence suggests that such agents have fewer extrapyramidal side effects. They may be more broadly effective for the negative symptoms of schizophrenia compared with traditional antipsychotic drugs. In vitro evidence indicates that risperidone has affinity for 5-HT_{2A} receptors that is 20-fold higher than for D_2 receptors.

Clozapine. Clozapine was developed in Austria and Germany in the 1960s. Because of its tricyclic-like structure, it was hoped that it might be an antidepressant. Instead, it turned out to be an antipsychotic drug with no extrapyramidal side effects. Clozapine is a dibenzazapine with atypical properties and side effects. It possesses strong anticholinergic properties in addition to serotonin-blocking properties. It produces proportionally greater suppression of mesolimbic as opposed to striatal dopamine systems. Clozapine blocks D_2 receptors, as do other antipsychotic drugs, but it also produces a relatively greater blockade of D_1 systems, which may account for its altered pattern of efficacy and the absence of tardive dyskinesia as a side effect.

Unfortunately, clozapine can cause fatal agranulocytosis. An overview of available reports indicates that agranulocytosis occurs in 0.05 to 2% of patients given clozapine, which is higher than rates among patients given other antipsychotic drugs. The agranulocytosis does not appear to be dose related. In most cases, there is a several-week prodrome of declining peripheral white blood cell count, but this is not always true. Stopping administration of the medication does not always prevent progression to agranulocytosis. Most cases occur within 3 months of treatment initiation. Weekly monitoring of hematologic function is indicated for all patients receiving clozapine.

Olanzapine. Olanzapine blocks 5-HT_2 receptors in addition to a spectrum of dopamine receptor subtypes, including D_1, D_2, and D_4. It also has some anticholinergic and α1-blocking properties. This spectrum of pharmacologic properties generates fewer extrapyramidal side effects than most older antipsychotic drugs.

Quetiapine. Quetiapine has actions and uses similar to clozapine. It is associated with a lower incidence of agranulocytosis. Because of reports of cataracts associated with prolonged use, semiannual slit lamp examinations are recommended for patients taking quetiapine.

GENERAL APPROACH TO PSYCHOPHARMACOLOGY

Some general clinical guidelines should be followed in the use of all psychotropic drugs. In selecting an agent for administration, one should also select the symptom targets of the therapy, such as agitation, sleep disturbance, or weight loss. By selecting certain symptom targets in advance, the therapy is rendered as rational as possible. In addition, the clinician should establish clinical guideposts by which to judge the efficacy of the therapy. If the targeted symptoms fail to improve after some defined period, the therapy should be stopped or changed, or consultation should be sought.

DOSING AND TIMING. The two most common errors made by nonpsychiatrists in the use of psychopharmacologic agents are inadequate dosing and insufficient waiting time for effect. In using all of these agents, one first increases dosing of the selected drug either to a predetermined total daily target or to a maximal tolerated dose. Second, one waits for a predetermined time, usually 4 to 6 weeks for antidepressant and antipsychotic drugs, to allow evidence of clinical efficacy to emerge.

CLINICAL FAMILIARITY. Effective use of these drugs, as for other pharmacologic agents, requires practical expertise that comes only from experience. Clinicians should not attempt to become familiar with all psychopharmacologic drugs equally but should develop experience-based familiarity with one or two from each category.

A GENERAL APPROACH TO PSYCHOTHERAPY

Up to 90% of the total scope of ambulatory psychiatric morbidity is treated by primary care physicians and other nonpsychiatric physicians. At present, there is no generally accepted model by which to bring psychotherapeutic skills into the general medical setting. With the revolution in care delivery systems that is sweeping across the United States, it does not seem likely that mental health practitioners will be transplanted into general medical settings in any substantial way. It has been argued persuasively for decades that nonpsychiatric physicians in fact do perform various forms of psychotherapy on a regular basis through the relationships they already have with their patients.

THE THEORY OF THE THERAPEUTIC RELATIONSHIP. The patient comes to the physician out of an experienced need. There is almost always a felt need for help, which may be more or less developed and conceptualized, depending on the individual patient. It is from this fundamental need for assistance that the possibility of a therapeutic relationship arises. Nonpsychiatric physicians may underestimate the emotional depth and potential psychotherapeutic power of this therapeutic relationship. Such a relationship already exists in nascent form with many of their patients and constitutes an underused therapeutic tool.

PSYCHOTHERAPEUTIC STRATEGIES. There are fundamental psychotherapeutic skills that are universal across successful therapies regardless of specialty. These skills include empathy, sensitivity to emotional cues, the capacity to listen actively, and the ability to intervene with corrective information at acceptable time points. No rule reserves these skills to psychiatric physicians. Several general technical approaches can be used.

COGNITIVE/BEHAVIORAL THERAPY. Behavioral therapy is a psychotherapy based on the general principle that interventions should be focused on behaviors, thoughts, and emotions that are actually present at a given time. Such a hypothesis underlies most of our educational endeavors and is readily understandable to most physicians. Key elements of this psychotherapeutic technique are clarification, education, and emotional support. This strategy commends itself as a first-line therapeutic strategy for most mild psychiatric problems. Such an approach is similar to the approach physicians use for other diagnostic and therapeutic problems. These cognitive strategies therefore carry with them a comfort level for nonpsychiatric clinicians, which is a great help to those engaged in psychotherapeutic work.

PSYCHODYNAMIC THERAPY. Psychodynamic psychotherapy refers to more time limited versions of psychotherapy, which derive from psychoanalytic theory. One of the basic concepts of psychoanalytic theory is that of intrapsychic determinism. This principle asserts that psychological events are not produced randomly or by chance but by causal forces operating, often unconsciously, within the individual. These causal forces generally include the basic human drives, sexuality and aggression, as well as the life experience and early development of the individual.

Freud allowed his patients to think and speak freely during his sessions with them, while he listened intently for clues about meanings and motivations that were not quite consciously understood by the patients. He described resistances that the patients demonstrated to keep painful feelings and conflicts from emerging into conscious life, and he wrote about transference, the application to the physician of emotional attachment behaviors that derive from other areas of the patient's life experience. One of the major advantages of this perspective is that it permits the clinician to take full account of the strengths of individuals as they have expressed themselves across their entire life course. The technical skills most important in this technique include active listening, empathic connecting with the patient, and the ability to make interpretive connections to previous life events.

FAMILY THERAPY. A family-oriented psychological therapy is explicitly directed at the group system in which a patient lives or works, as opposed to the patient as an individual. Usually a family therapy is being performed whenever the physician brings more than the patient into the examination room. Couples therapy is a form of family psychotherapy and is the most common sort of family therapy performed by nonpsychiatric clinicians. In a family therapy, the physician addresses some difficulty in the interpersonal system. The relationship patterns of the system must be considered and the positive strengths identified. The problem must be amenable to definition within such a relationship system. The simplest metaphor to use for family therapy in medical settings is the system-wide impact of the medical illness being experienced by the identified patient.

A rough guideline to set a work plan for a medical psychotherapy might consider the following technical points:

Diagnosis: Define the problem with some psychosocial dimension that makes sense to the patient and family.
Work plan: Set an initial number of talking visits, specifying frequency and duration of each visit.
Strategy: Consider the overview strategies outlined here, and consider which might be best applicable to the situation at hand.
Consultation: Be prepared to request a psychiatric consultation.

American Psychiatric Association: Diagnostic and Statistical Manual of Mental Disorders, 4th ed. Washington, DC, 1994, pp 317–391. *The standard diagnostic lexicon for psychiatric illness.*

Andreasen NC: Understanding the causes of schizophrenia. N Engl J Med 340(8):645–647, 1999.

Balint M: The Doctor, His Patient and the Illness. London, Pitman, 1964. *A classical perspective on the psychiatry of relatedness in general medicine.*

Collaborative Working Group on Clinical Trial Evaluations: Adverse effects of the typical antipsychotics. J Clin Psychiatry 59 (Suppl. 12):17–22, 1998. *A current review of new drugs for severe mental illness.*

Fogel BS, Schiffer RB, Rao SM: Neuropsychiatry. Baltimore, Williams & Wilkins, 1996. *A multiauthored overview by designated experts of available knowledge on the neural substrate of behavior.*

Freud S: The Standard Edition of the Complete Psychological Works. (Trans James Stacker.) London, Hogarth Press, 1966. *The historical standard from which many of our current ideas about psychiatric illness and psychotherapy derive.*

Gabbard GO (ed): Treatments of Psychiatric Disorders, 2nd edition. Washington, American Psychiatric Press, 1995. *An excellent and encyclopedic summary of psychopharmacologic and behavioral therapies.*

Hirshfeld RMA, Russell JM: Assessment and treatment of suicidal patients. N Engl J Med 337:910–915, 1997. *An excellent review of suicidality and its assessment.*

Kessler RC, McGonagle KA, Zhao S, et al: Lifetime and 12-month prevalence of DSM-III-R psychiatric disorders in the United States: Results from the National Comorbidity survey. Arch Gen Psych 51:8–19, 1994. *An epidemiologic study that provides background information about frequency in psychiatric illness.*

Mayou R, Bass C, Sharpe M: Treatment of Functional Somatic Symptoms. Oxford, UK, Oxford University Press, 1995. *An excellent summary of current knowledge on somatoform illness and its treatment.*

Mortensen PB, Pedersen CB, Westergaard T, et al: Effects of family history and place and season of birth on the risk of schizophrenia. N Engl J Med 340(8):603–608, 1999.

Pincus HA, Tanielian TL, Marcus SC, et al: Prescribing trends in psychotropic medications: Primary care, psychiatry, and other medical specialties. JAMA 279:526–531, 1998. *An overview of recent trends in prescribing psychotropic medications in primary care practices.*

Shapiro D: Neurotic Styles. New York, Basic Books, 1965. *A classic work characterizing character disorders and their behavioral predispositions.*

Ustun TB, Sartorius N (eds): Mental Illness in General Health Care. New York, John Wiley & Sons, 1995. *An empirical survey of behavioral problems encountered in general medical settings—current and comprehensive.*

■ PATHOPHYSIOLOGY AND MANAGEMENT OF MAJOR NEUROLOGIC SYMPTOMS

451 AUTONOMIC DISORDERS AND THEIR MANAGEMENT

Clifford B. Saper

Disorders of the autonomic nervous system are of great importance to internal medicine because they can be manifested as disorders of virtually any organ system in the body. Furthermore, central regulation of the autonomic response is closely tied to neuroendocrine control, and both are often involved by central nervous system disorders. This chapter discusses disorders of the peripheral autonomic nervous system and disorders of central integration of autonomic control (Table 451–1). Aspects of neuroendocrine disease are discussed in Chapters 235, 236, and 237.

DISORDERS OF PERIPHERAL AUTONOMIC FUNCTION

The peripheral autonomic nervous system consists of three main divisions: the *parasympathetic* division, which includes the outflow from the cranial nerves and the low lumbar and sacral spinal cord; the *sympathetic* division, which comprises the autonomic outflow from the thoracic and high lumbar segments of the spinal cord; and the *enteric* nervous system, which includes neurons that are intrinsic to the wall of the gut. Details of the organization of the peripheral autonomic nervous system are covered in basic anatomy and physiology texts.

Knowledge about the different neurotransmitter and receptor types associated with the peripheral autonomic nervous system has resulted in the availability of a wide range of drugs to modify autonomic responses. Some key autonomic drugs and their clinical uses are listed in Table 451–2. These drugs are covered in detail in clinical pharmacology texts.

Pandysautonomias

ACUTE PANDYSAUTONOMIA. Widespread failure of the autonomic nervous system may evolve acutely or subacutely as part of a parainfectious inflammatory polyneuropathy (of the Guillain-Barré type). In rare cases, the autonomic neuropathy predominates and, when severe, may be life threatening. Wide swings in blood pressure and heart rate occur but usually reverse themselves in a few minutes. Generally, putting the patient into the Trendelenburg position is sufficient to maintain cerebral perfusion during hypotensive periods. Cardiac arrhythmias of all types may occur, presumably as a result of the instability of autonomic innervation of the cardiac conducting system. These arrhythmias must be treated gingerly because the underlying conduction abnormality may change very rapidly.

TETANUS. A similar subacute pandysautonomia is also seen in severe cases of tetanus. Tetanus toxin, elaborated by *Clostridium tetani* organisms in an infected wound, is transported by autonomic as well as motor axons back to the spinal cord, where it is taken up by and inactivates the terminals of inhibitory interneurons. Treatment of the motor manifestations of tetanus by paralyzing and sedating the patient does little to abate the autonomic storm. Up to 40% of patients with tetanus in an intensive care environment may suffer cardiac arrest as a result of arrhythmias. They are generally easily resuscitated with standard measures.

CHRONIC AUTONOMIC NEUROPATHY. The axons of the peripheral autonomic nervous system are generally of small caliber and thinly myelinated or unmyelinated. Certain polyneuropathies that have a predilection for small-diameter axons can result in autonomic changes. *Amyloid neuropathy* often includes a major autonomic component that may be manifested as a gastrointestinal motility disorder or orthostatic hypotension. Similarly, *diabetic neuropathy,* although it is often dominated by sensory or motor complaints, may cause widespread autonomic failure. The neuropathy of *acute intermittent porphyria* or certain toxic agents such as *Vacor* (a rat poison) may have a prominent autonomic component.

Table 451–1 ■ DISORDERS OF THE AUTONOMIC NERVOUS SYSTEM

Peripheral Autonomic Disorders	Genitourinary disorders
Pandysautonomias	Incontinence
Acute pandysautonomia	Urinary retention
Tetanus	Spastic bladder
Chronic autonomic neuropathy	Impotence
Familial dysautonomia	**Disorders of Central Autonomic Integration**
Idiopathic autonomic insufficiency (Shy-Drager syndrome)	Emotional disorders
Regional dysautonomia	Panic disorder
Horner's syndrome	Psychosomatic illness
Paraspinal tumors	Cardiac arrhythmias
Somatosympathetic dysreflexia	Thermoregulatory disorders
Complex regional pain syndrome	Poikilothermia
Disorders of specific autonomic functions	Paroxysmal hypothermia
Pupillary disorders	Hyperthermia and fever
Horner's syndrome	Neuroleptic malignant syndrome
Oculomotor paresis	Feeding disorders
Cardiovascular disorders	Hyperphagia and obesity
Glossopharyngeal neuralgia	Hypophagia and inanition
Carotid sinus hypersensitivity	Disorders of fluid and electrolyte regulation
Sweating disorders	Hypernatremia, hyperosmolality, and absence of thirst
Hyperhidrosis	Hyperdipsia, hyponatremia, and water intoxication
Anhidrosis	Paroxysmal hyponatremia
Gastrointestinal disorders	Central reproductive disorders
Disorders of motility	Arousal disorders
Vomiting	Hypersomnolence
	Insomnia

Table 451–2 ■ SYSTEMIC EFFECTS OF SOME COMMONLY USED AUTONOMIC DRUGS

RECEPTOR TYPE	DRUG TYPE (EXAMPLE)	TISSUE	EFFECT
Muscarinic cholinergic	Antagonist (atropine)	Pupil	Mydriasis
		Salivary gland	Dry mouth
		Bronchi	Dilation
		Heart	Tachycardia
		Gut	Decreased motility and secretion
α-Adrenergic	Antagonist (phenoxybenzamine)	Blood vessels	Vasodilation
α_1-Adrenergic	Agonist (phenylephrine)	Blood vessels	Vasoconstriction
	Antagonist (prazosin)	Blood vessels	Vasodilation
β-Adrenergic	Agonist (isoproterenol)	Heart	Increased rate and contractility
β_1-Adrenergic	Antagonist (metoprolol)	Blood vessels	Decreased rate and contractility
β_2-Adrenergic	Agonist (terbutaline)	Bronchi	Dilation

Acute poisoning with *organophosphate insecticides* that block acetylcholinesterase results in a hypercholinergic state, including miosis and cardiac slowing, that lasts for several days. The neuropathy that follows several weeks later does not usually have a strong autonomic component. Other peripheral neuropathies that may have an autonomic component are listed in Table 451–3.

DEGENERATIVE DYSAUTONOMIA. Recessively inherited *familial dysautonomia* of the Riley-Day type is most commonly seen in Ashkenazi Jewish children. Symptoms referable to the autonomic nervous system and relative indifference to pain are present from birth.

Pure autonomic failure may develop as a chronic degenerative condition in middle age or late adult life as a result of loss of neurons in the autonomic ganglia, as well as in the pre-ganglionic cell groups in the medulla and spinal cord. The initial complaint is often orthostatic hypotension, but signs or symptoms of pupillary, gastrointestinal, genitourinary, sweating, or other autonomic abnormalities are elicited by history and physical examination.

Pure autonomic failure is distinguished from non-neurologic causes of orthostatic hypotension by the lack of compensatory tachycardia, which indicates impairment of either the peripheral or central components of the baroreceptor reflex. Severe autonomic neuropathy affecting the glossopharyngeal or vagus nerves may also impair the baroreceptor response but is typically associated with other evidence of sensory or motor neuropathy. Other cardiovascular signs include loss of sinus arrhythmia and absence of normal overshoot in diastolic blood pressure during phase IV of the Valsalva maneuver. An abnormally accentuated blood pressure response to intravenous infusion of norepinephrine is consistent with widespread denervation supersensitivity. A detailed list of tests of autonomic failure is provided in Table 451–4.

Autonomic failure may be associated with *Parkinson's disease* in

Table 451–3 ■ PERIPHERAL NEUROPATHIES THAT MAY HAVE AN AUTONOMIC COMPONENT

Autonomic symptoms often prominent
  Guillain-Barré syndrome
  Amyloid neuropathy
  Diabetic neuropathy
  Acute intermittent porphyria
  Vacor (rat poison)
Autonomic symptoms may occur
  Renal failure
  Toxic neuropathies
    Vinca alkaloids
    Perhexiline maleate
    Thallium
    Arsenic
    Mercury
    Organic solvents
    Acrylamide
  Vasculitis
    Systemic lupus erythematosus
    Rheumatoid arthritis
    Mixed connective tissue disease
  Thiamine deficiency
  Leprosy
  Hereditary autonomic neuropathies
  Fabry's disease

about 10 to 20% of patients. These patients show Lewy bodies and loss of pigmented neurons in sympathetic ganglia as well as in the brain. This combination must be distinguished from a superficially similar disorder characterized by degeneration of central autonomic control nuclei, *the Shy-Drager syndrome*. The Shy-Drager syndrome is part of a spectrum of *multiple systems atrophy* in which evidence of cerebellar and extrapyramidal involvement is generally present but not evidence of peripheral autonomic degeneration on formal testing (see Table 451–4). Loss of neurons is seen in the basal ganglia, substantia nigra pons, cerebellum, inferior olives, and brain stem autonomic nuclei, but not in autonomic ganglia. No Lewy bodies are present, but glial fibrillary inclusions may be found. The clinical significance of this distinction is that the movement disorder in patients with Parkinson's disease shows a good response to L-dopa/carbidopa, but in multiple systems atrophy the response is poor. Carbidopa, however, can worsen blood pressure control in both conditions by blocking decarboxylase in sympathetic ganglion cells.

Orthostatic hypotension is generally the most disabling aspect of autonomic degeneration. Treatment with elastic stockings or even entire lower body suits can improve standing blood pressure by limiting blood pooling in the lower part of the body. Treatment with fludrocortisone, a mineralocorticoid (0.1 mg once to three times a day), expands intravascular blood volume and causes an elevation in blood pressure in all positions. Midodrine is the prodrug of a direct sympathetic agonist. A starting dose of 10 mg three times a day may increase blood pressure in all positions. In patients treated with either drug, the head of the bed should be elevated in recumbency to minimize hypertensive effects on the brain. L-Dihydroxyphenylserine is a promising new drug that is a synthetic precursor of norepinephrine. It has shown encouraging results in some, but not all trials and may require residual sympathetic neuronal function to be useful.

Regional Dysautonomia

The segmental organization of the sympathetic nervous system can result in regional disturbances of function. The most common of these disturbances is caused by injury to the cranial sympathetic innervation arising from the superior cervical ganglion, or *Horner's syndrome*. Miosis, ptosis, and anhidrosis may occur if the ascending sympathetic fibers are injured below the level at which they enter the skull with the internal carotid artery. Damage to sympathetic fibers along the course of the intracranial carotid artery produces only oculosympathetic paresis (Raeder's syndrome). Unfortunately, this difference is only of marginal value clinically inasmuch as a Horner syndrome produced by extracranial lesions is often incomplete. Lesions of the central descending sympathoexcitatory pathway, which runs through the lateral portions of the brain stem from the hypothalamus to the spinal cord, may produce a central Horner syndrome characterized by miosis and ptosis, as well as loss of sweating over the entire ipsilateral half of the body. Postganglionic Horner's syndrome can be differentiated from pre-ganglionic or central lesions by pharmacologic testing (see Table 451–4). The most common cause of Horner's syndrome is atherosclerotic disease affecting the vasa nervorum originating in the carotid artery. However, Horner's syndrome may also be seen when an intrathoracic or cervical tumor involves the sympathetic chain. Hence evaluation of Horner's syndrome should include ra-

Table 451-4 ■ TESTS OF AUTONOMIC FUNCTION*

TEST	INTERPRETATION
Pupillary responses	
4% cocaine	Pupillodilatation indicates release of normal catecholamine stores.
1% hydroxyamphetamine	Pupillodilatation indicates denervation supersensitivity.
1% phenylephrine	
0.1% epinephrine	
0.1% pilocarpine	Pupilloconstriction indicates denervation supersensitivity.
2.5% methacholine	
Sweating responses	
Thermal sweating	Regional absence of sweating indicates sympathetic cholinergic denervation.
Galvanic skin response	Increased conductivity under mild stress indicates normal adrenergic innervation.
1:1000 pilocarpine	Intradermal injection causes axon reflex sweating.
1:10,000 acetylcholine	
Axon reflex	
1:1000 histamine	Intradermal injection normally causes wheal and flare.
Cardiovascular responses	
Orthostatic challenge	Pulse normally increases and diastolic blood pressure falls <15 mm Hg.
Carotid sinus massage	Normally causes fall in blood pressure and heart rate.
R-R interval	Normally increases during inspiration (sinus arrhythmia).
Valsalva maneuver	Longest to shortest R-R interval ratio normally is ≥1.4.
Cold pressor test	Immersing hand in ice water normally increases blood pressure and heart rate.
Plasma catecholamines	Normally increase response to standing or stress.
Norepinephrine infusion 0.05 μg/kg/min	Diastolic blood pressure increase ≥20 mm Hg indicates supersensitivity.
Genitourinary, rectal responses	
Cremasteric reflex	Stroking skin of thigh normally causes testicular retraction.
Anal wink reflex	Scratching perianal skin normally causes anal sphincter contraction.
Bulbocavernosus reflex	Squeezing glans penis or clitoris normally causes anal sphincter contraction.

*For details see McLeod and Tuck, 1987.

diographic or magnetic resonance examination of the pulmonary apices and paracervical area.

Paraspinal tumors at lower levels along the sympathetic chain may cause loss of sweating over the involved dermatomes. This deficit can be appreciated by running the handle of a tuning fork down the skin in the paraspinal region. The smooth movement is interrupted by the dry skin at the level of the lesion. Occasionally, compression of a mid-thoracic spinal root, which carries visceral sensory fibers, by a disk or tumor may be manifested as abdominal pain.

Stimulation of pain fibers at any level results in both local (spinospinal) and generalized (spinobulbospinal) *somatosympathetic reflex responses,* including sweating, vasoconstriction, and pupillodilatation. In patients with pre-existing spinal cord transection, a noxious stimulus below the level of the transection may produce either local sympathetic reflex responses (segmental sweating) or more generalized spinal reflex patterns (e.g., hypertension with bladder overfilling). It is important in paraplegic patients to investigate sympathetic responses for evidence of occult disease that might cause pain in an intact individual.

Following injury to peripheral nerves, aberrant regeneration may result in severe pain, a condition known as *complex regional pain syndrome.* Normally innocuous sensory stimulation, such as covering the affected limb with a sheet or with clothing, may cause excruciating burning pain associated with variable autonomic changes. Atrophic changes in the skin and bone may reflect abnormal sympathetic innervation or disuse. It was once thought that the chronic pain may be due to *reflex sympathetic dystrophy* caused by aberrant regeneration of sympathetic efferent fibers. Although regional sympathetic block alleviates pain in some patients, injection of placebo has similar effects, and removal of the affected sympathetic ganglion rarely produces permanent relief.

Disorders of Specific Autonomic Functions

PUPILS. Anisocoria, or asymmetry of pupillary size, may reflect a deficit of sympathetic innervation of the smaller pupil (causing miosis) or parasympathetic innervation of the larger one (causing mydriasis). Because both oculosympathetic and oculomotor (parasympathetic) innervation participates in lid elevation, ptosis, if present, generally indicates the abnormal eye. Anisocoria may be long-standing and of little clinical significance, but pupillary asymmetry of recent onset should be evaluated by a neurologist. Impair-

ment of sympathetic innervation of the iris (pupillodilator) muscle is not always accompanied by ptosis or a sweating deficit (Horner's syndrome). The pupilloconstrictor fibers travel in the dorsomedial part of the oculomotor nerve, where they may be selectively affected by temporal lobe herniation or by an aneurysm of the posterior communicating artery. Pharmacologic testing may aid in identification of the pupillary abnormality (see Table 451-4). A common factitious cause of a unilateral dilated pupil is instillation of atropinic eyedrops; the situation is exposed when the pharmacologically dilated pupil does not respond even to strong solutions of pilocarpine. Another common cause of a large, poorly reactive pupil is *Adie's syndrome,* an idiopathic condition involving degeneration of the ciliary ganglion. The pupil usually shows sector paralysis and constriction with accommodation, and it dilates and responds to light after a period in complete darkness. The abnormal pupil responds briskly to 0.1% pilocarpine (see Table 451-4), and concomitant loss of tendon reflexes is seen in most cases.

CARDIOVASCULAR. The baroreceptor reflex is an important protective response that induces bradycardia and peripheral vasodilatation to counteract an acute increase in blood pressure—or the reverse response during hypotension. The afferent fibers for the response run in the glossopharyngeal (carotid sinus) and vagus (aortic depressor) nerves, whereas the efferent response includes both parasympathetic and sympathetic components. Injury to the glossopharyngeal or carotid sinus nerves in the neck (often by a tumor) can cause episodic attacks of hypotension and bradycardia, often manifested as syncope. In most cases, an associated pain or paresthesia is located in the cutaneous distribution of the glossopharyngeal nerve (in the external auditory meatus or the pharynx), known as *glossopharyngeal neuralgia.* The situation is analogous to tic douloureux, which is characterized by intermittent volleys of firing in the affected nerve. Atropine or a transvenous pacemaker may prevent the bradycardia associated with the attacks, but loss of vasoconstrictor tone sometimes results in symptomatic hypotension despite these maneuvers. Anticonvulsants, including phenytoin, carbamazepine, or gabapentin, may prevent the attacks. Dosages are titrated for the individual patient but are often much lower than those required to treat epilepsy.

Carotid sinus syncope (see Chapter 447) is a condition seen most commonly in elderly individuals with carotid atherosclerosis. Even mild pressure over the carotid bulb, such as a tight shirt collar, can produce a full-blown carotid sinus response resulting in syncope. The diagnosis is made by gently compressing the carotid artery below the angle of the jaw while the electrocardiogram is monitored. Facilities for cardiac resuscitation must be immediately available in case the compression results in sinus arrest. Vigorous massage should be avoided because it may dislodge an embolus and result in a transient or even permanent neurologic deficit. Treatment of carotid sinus hypersensitivity is the same as that for glossopharyngeal neuralgia.

SWEATING. Human sweat glands are innervated by both noradrenergic sympathetic fibers (mediating emotional responses) and cholinergic sympathetic fibers (thermal sweating). Certain somatosympathetic reflexes can produce generalized or regional sweating in response to innocuous or noxious somatosensory stimuli. *Hyperhidrosis,* or pathologically increased sweating, can be generalized, or it can be focal, most commonly involving the palms of the hands and the soles of the feet. Drugs that interrupt α-adrenergic transmission (phenoxybenzamine, 10 mg three times daily) or muscarinic transmission (propantheline, 15 mg three times daily) may be effective, particularly in combination. In extreme cases, regional sympathectomy has been performed.

Idiopathic anhidrosis may be segmental or generalized. This rare condition is sometimes associated with Adie's syndrome (Ross syndrome), but in other cases no other signs of autonomic impairment are noted. In some patients the impairment is pre-ganglionic and in others post-ganglionic, as judged by the axon reflex sweating response (see Table 451–4). In most recorded patients, the deficits have been stable and did not go on to involve other autonomic functions.

GASTROINTESTINAL. Disorders of intestinal motility, which may be due to damage to the parasympathetic innervation of the gut or to dysfunction of the enteric nervous system itself, are discussed in Chapter 132. Specific abnormalities of esophageal contraction and colonic tone have been noted in patients suffering from depression and may predict response to antidepressant medication.

Vomiting is a neurally mediated gastrointestinal reflex that is coordinated by neurons in the medullary reticular formation. Chemical emetic agents such as certain narcotics or dopaminergic agonists act at the area postrema, a chemosensory zone on the 4th ventricular surface of the medulla, to elicit the vomiting reflex. Local dopaminergic connections are thought to mediate the response, and antidopaminergic drugs such as prochlorperazine may act at the level of the area postrema to suppress vomiting. Intractable vomiting without any gastrointestinal abnormalities has been reported in certain patients with tumors involving the medullary cell groups controlling vomiting or their connections. Treatment of the tumor with steroids and radiation therapy generally results in improvement.

GENITOURINARY. The urinary bladder is composed of interlacing smooth muscle fibers of the detrusor covered by an internal mucous membrane and an outer serosa. The detrusor is innervated by parasympathetic neurons located in the intermediolateral column at the 2nd through 4th sacral segments. Additional motor neurons located in the ventral horn at the same levels constitute Onuf's nucleus. Their axons run through the pelvic nerve to innervate striated accessory muscles of micturition (including the external urethral sphincter) in the pelvic floor. Neurons of Onuf's nucleus are strikingly preserved in motor neuron disease but are lost along with autonomic pre-ganglionic cells in Shy-Drager syndrome. The internal sphincter at the bladder neck is innervated via the hypogastric nerve by sympathetic pre-vertebral pelvic ganglia whose preganglionic innervation arises from the intermediolateral column at the T12-L1 level.

Bladder relaxation during filling and subsequent coordination of micturition are under control of Barrington's nucleus and the adjacent pontine reticular formation, near the locus caeruleus. Brain stem control of micturition is, in turn, under voluntary regulation by areas within the cerebral sensory and motor cortex. When bladder fullness is sensed and the environmental conditions are appropriate, micturition is initiated by Barrington's nucleus, under forebrain control. External sphincter pressure decreases and thereby results in reflex relaxation of the internal sphincter and contraction of the bladder.

Forebrain impairment results in loss of voluntary control of micturition but does not otherwise affect the complex sensory and motor program that results in normal voiding. Incontinence in such patients can be managed with adult diapers or external urinary collection devices without the risk of frequent urinary tract infections or damage to the upper urinary tract. Injury to the bulbospinal pathway from Barrington's nucleus to the sacral intermediolateral column, however, causes major disruption of coordinated bladder function. Immediately following spinal cord injury is a period of spinal shock, during which the bladder does not undergo reflex contraction as it fills. Such patients require urinary catheterization to prevent vesical and renal damage.

One to 2 weeks after injury, spinal reflex control of the bladder returns. Some patients can induce reflex bladder emptying by somatosensory stimulation, such as stroking the skin over the thigh. The spastic bladder reflexively contracts at a lower volume and, because detrusor action is not coordinated with sphincter opening, rarely empties completely. Injury to sensory nerves supplying the bladder may also cause overfilling and incomplete emptying, thus indicating the importance of sensory feedback in bladder control. Patients with significant post-void residual urine are at increased risk for urinary tract infections, but bladder overfilling with elevated pressures above 40 cm H_2O may ultimately be a greater problem. Elevations in pressure above 40 cm H_2O may require continuous or intermittent catheterization to prevent damage to the upper urinary tract.

Pharmacologic intervention aimed at augmenting or suppressing autonomic motor responses of the bladder or internal sphincter has only limited value. Bethanechol, a cholinergic agonist (10 to 15 mg three times daily), is used to augment bladder contraction to improve emptying. It is most effective in combination with an α-adrenergic blocker, such as terazosin (1 to 10 mg daily), that simultaneously reduces pressure at the internal sphincter. Baclofen may be used to decrease spastic contraction of the external sphincter. Drugs that have atropinic properties, including a surprising variety of antiarrhythmic, antihistamine, neuroleptic, and antidepressant medications, may inhibit bladder contraction and result in overfilling and urinary retention (Table 451–5).

Erectile function in males is under parasympathetic control by the same sacral levels as the urinary system. Sensory afferent fibers travel via the pudendal nerve, whereas parasympathetic motor fibers run in the pelvic nerve. Sympathetic innervation via the hypogastric nerve contracts the seminal vesicles during ejaculation and closes the bladder neck to prevent retrograde emission. Although supraspinal influences are of great importance, reflex erection and ejaculation can occur in patients after spinal injury. Neurogenic impotence can result either from damage to the descending pathways relaying forebrain influence from the hypothalamus to the sacral pre-ganglionic neurons or from injury to the sensory or parasympathetic motor innervation of the penis. A variety of drugs that block either parasympathetic or sympathetic function can interfere with erectile function (Table 451–6). Because erections normally occur several times nightly during periods of rapid eye movement sleep, it is possible to document organic disorders of erection by measuring penile tumescence overnight. Disorders and treatment of male sexual function are considered in Chapter 247.

DISORDERS OF INTEGRATIVE CONTROL OF THE AUTONOMIC NERVOUS SYSTEM

ORGANIZATION OF CENTRAL AUTONOMIC AND ENDOCRINE REGULATION. The autonomic nervous system is under three levels of central control. The *pre-ganglionic* neurons located

Table 451–5 ■ **SOME COMMONLY PRESCRIBED DRUGS THAT MAY IMPAIR URINARY FUNCTION**

Antiarrhythmics	Antiparkinsonian agents
Atropine	Amantadine
Disopyramide	Dopa/carbidopa
Antihistamines	Bromocriptine
Diphenhydramine	Benztropine
Neuroleptics	Trihexyphenidyl
Haloperidol	Antispasmodics
Chlorpromazine	Baclofen
Antidepressants	
Amitriptyline	
Imipramine	

Table 451–6 ■ SOME COMMONLY PRESCRIBED DRUGS THAT
MAY IMPAIR ERECTILE FUNCTION

Drugs causing impotence	Drugs causing priapism
Parasympatholytics	Chlorpromazine
Atropine	Thioridazine
Amitriptyline	Trazodone
Sympatholytics	Prazosin
Methyldopa	Dopa/carbidopa
Guanethidine	
Clonidine	
Propranolol	
Prazosin	
Vasodilators	
Hydralazine	
Diuretics	
Hydrochlorothiazide	
Antihistaminergic	
Cimetidine	

in the medulla and the spinal cord provide the final common pathway for central autonomic control. Each of these neurons integrates the input from many sources, including afferents from higher levels of the nervous system and local reflex responses. A series of *brain stem and spinal* cell groups coordinate *reflex control* of the autonomic nervous system. These nuclei receive cranial (parasym-

pathetic) and spinal (sympathetic) afferent information and control a variety of important reflexes (e.g., swallowing, maintaining blood pressure, initiation of voiding). Both the pre-ganglionic neurons and the brain stem reflex neurons are under the control of *forebrain integrative* cell groups that coordinate autonomic function with behavior and with endocrine control.

The hypothalamus is the most important area for integration of behavior with autonomic responses and with neuroendocrine control of the anterior and posterior pituitary glands (Fig. 451–1). Because the hypothalamus consists of tightly packed, interwoven pathways and cell groups, it is unusual for an injury to selectively involve a single functional system. Nevertheless, considerable progress has been made in determining the anatomic substrates for specific integrative functions, and disorders of these systems are occasionally encountered (Table 451–7). In addition, autonomic dysfunction is a frequent concomitant of emotional disorders.

Emotional Disorders

Portions of the insular and cingulate areas of the cerebral cortex and the amygdala are believed to regulate autonomic responses to emotional stress. In healthy individuals, stress can induce sympathetic responses such as pupillodilatation, dry mouth, and increases in blood pressure. In patients with *panic disorder* (see Chapter

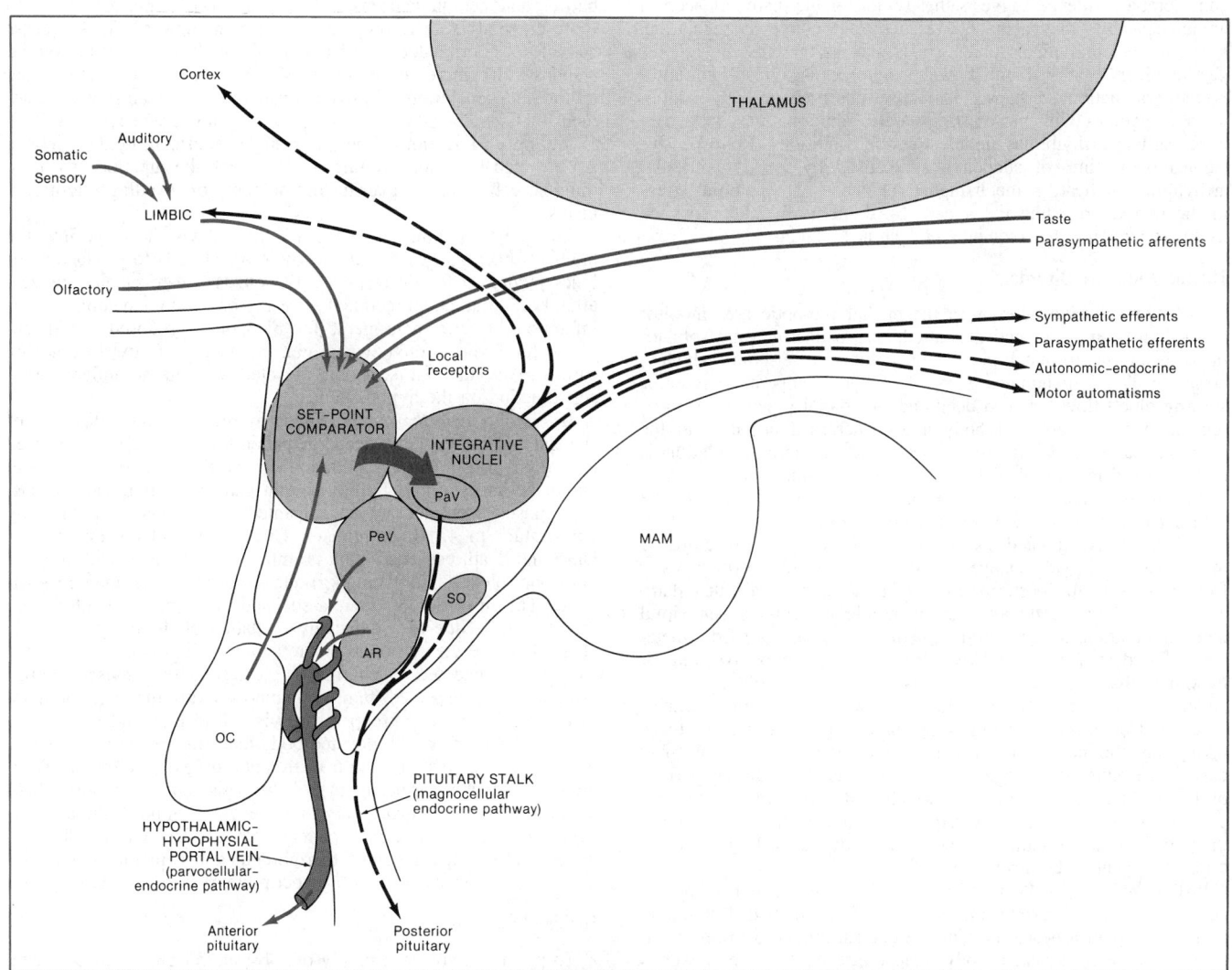

FIGURE 451–1 ■ Schematic illustration of the functional organization of the hypothalamus. General and visceral sensory, limbic, and local interoceptive (e.g., osmolality and temperature) information is compared against a homeostatic set-point by integrative cell groups in the preoptic area and tuberal hypothalamus. Efferent autonomic responses from the paraventricular nucleus (PaV) and lateral hypothalamic area are then integrated with anterior pituitary control via the periventricular (PeV) and arcuate (AR) nuclei and posterior pituitary control via the supraoptic (SO) and paraventricular nuclei, and with behavioral regulation exercised mainly by the lateral hypothalamic area. MAM = mamillary body; OC = optic chiasm. (Amended from Saper CB: Hypothalamus. *In* Pearlman AL, Collins RC (eds): Neurobiology of Disease. New York, Oxford University Press, 1989, p. 197.)

Table 451–7 ■ REGIONAL HYPOTHALAMIC SYNDROMES

REGION	NORMALLY REGULATES	DISORDERS
Preoptic	Blood volume, pressure, and electrolytes	Paroxysmal hyponatremia
		Essential hypernatremia
	Thermoregulation	Paroxysmal hypothermia
Tuberal	Gastrointestinal tract and feeding	Hyperphagia (ventromedial lesions)
		Hypophagia (lateral lesions)
	Reproduction	Hypogonadism
	Emotions	Rage responses
Posterior	Arousal	Hypersomnolence
	Descending autonomic and motor pathways	Poikilothermia

241), such autonomic responses can become overwhelming and convince the patient that a serious organic problem exists. Positron emission tomography studies show increased metabolism in the structures of the medial temporal lobe and the insular cortex during panic attacks. After eliminating the possibility of pheochromocytoma (see Chapter 241), anxiolytic or antidepressant drugs are usually found to be helpful.

Some individuals under chronic emotional stress are subject to a variety of syndromes involving disruption of autonomic control of the internal organs. Although *psychosomatic illness* is often thought to be non-organic and may respond to psychotherapeutic drugs, considerable evidence suggests that some organic disorders seen in anxious patients may also be caused by autonomic dysregulation. For example, individuals under stress may suffer erosive gastritis, gastric ulcers, and irritable bowel syndrome as a result of autonomic dysfunction. Perhaps the most serious problems are encountered in patients with pre-existing cardiac abnormalities, who may have cardiac arrhythmias under stressful conditions. Retrospective studies of victims of sudden death caused by lethal ventricular arrhythmias indicate a much higher incidence of behavioral stress in the period preceding the attack. β-Adrenergic blockers may be useful in reducing the frequency of such arrhythmias.

Thermoregulatory Disorders

Thermoresponsive neurons in the medial pre-optic area monitor brain temperature and activate autonomic, endocrine, and somatomotor responses to match body temperature to a set-point, which is normally 37° C in humans. Control of body temperature requires shifting blood flow between deep and superficial vascular beds and regulating conservation of body fluids (increased urination in the cold, increased sweating in the heat). Hence thermoregulation is tightly linked to control of blood pressure, volume, and electrolyte composition, which are also regulated by neurons around the anteroventral tip of the 3rd ventricle (see below).

Poikilothermy, defined as fluctuation in body temperature of more than 2° C with changes in ambient temperature, may result from lesions in the posterior hypothalamus or midbrain that damage hypothalamic pathways for autonomic as well as behavioral thermoregulation. Relative poikilothermy can also result from metabolic disorders such as sedative drug ingestion, hypoglycemia, or hypothyroidism, and a mild form is often seen in old age. Such patients are dangerously susceptible to lowered environmental temperature. Conversely, patients with relative poikilothermy or those taking anticholinergic drugs that prevent thermal sweating may experience dangerously elevated body temperatures during periods of hot weather. *Heat stroke,* in which body temperature may exceed 42° C, is often fatal and requires prompt treatment by cooling the patient in an ice bath and expanding body fluids. Death is often a result of ventricular arrhythmia.

PAROXYSMAL HYPOTHERMIA. Occasionally patients are encountered who suffer episodic attacks during which thermoregulation proceeds in a nearly normal fashion but around a lowered set-point. During an attack, a body temperature of 32° C or lower is maintained for a period of several days to 2 weeks. Attacks occur up to several times per year and may be accompanied by fatigue, malaise, somnolence, hypoventilation, hypotension, cardiac arrhythmias, lacrimation, ataxia, and asterixis. In some patients, the serum sodium level may decrease in tandem with the body temperature, to levels of 110 mEq/L or even lower. Attacks subside spontaneously and are followed by heat conservation measures to bring body temperature up to the normal set-point. Nearly all such patients have a hypothalamic abnormality involving the thermoregulatory pre-optic area, which suggests that the attacks may represent an "inverted" fever response. Anticonvulsants have not been effective in such attacks, but cyclooxygenase inhibitors such as aspirin may be useful in some patients.

FEVER AND HYPERTHERMIA. During a systemic immune response, circulating cytokines such as interleukin-1 and tumor necrosis factor may trigger macrophages in the meninges and along penetrating blood vessels at the borders of the brain to produce prostaglandins. These lipid mediators can cross the blood-brain barrier and act on neurons in the ventromedial pre-optic area to reset the body's thermoregulatory set-point upward. This process activates a coordinated set of autonomic, endocrine, and behavioral responses that increase thermogenesis and conserve heat. Drugs that inhibit the generation of prostaglandins are the mainstay of treatment of fever, but the wisdom of treating low-grade fever (<38.5° C) during an infectious illness has engendered considerable debate. An elevated body temperature may improve the function of certain immune cells while impairing the defenses of invading microorganisms.

Any physical injury to the brain that allows the entry into the brain of macrophages or activates microglial cells to produce cytokines induces a febrile response as well. Hence fever may be seen after head trauma, intracranial surgery, or cerebral hemorrhage or infarction. "Central neurogenic fever" is often proposed as a mechanism for fever of unknown origin, but in few if any documented cases is the thermal set-point elevated without an inflammatory signal acting on the hypothalamus.

Malignant hyperthermia is an autosomal dominant disorder of skeletal muscle that can occur in patients who have been exposed to certain drugs. During induction of anesthesia, particularly with halothane and succinylcholine, certain patients sustain sudden massive muscle contractions accompanied by a rapid rise in body temperature to 42° C or greater. Circulatory and respiratory collapse and death can ensue unless immediate treatment with intravenous dantrolene (1 to 10 mg/kg) and supportive measures are instituted. This disorder is often associated with muscle central core disease and is due to a defect in regulation of the calcium release channel in muscle sarcoplasmic reticulum. The disorder is genetically heterogeneous, so pharmacologic testing of a muscle biopsy sample from suspected family members (with the caffeine-halothane contracture test) preoperatively is still recommended.

Muscular rigidity and elevated body temperature can occasionally be seen during treatment with neuroleptic drugs or following withdrawal of dopaminergic agonists. The pathogenesis of this *neuroleptic malignant syndrome* is not understood, although it may reflect a febrile response in a patient with parkinsonian rigidity and drug-induced impairment of thermoregulation. Treatment with dopaminergic agonists such as bromocriptine can reverse the process.

Feeding Disorders

To provide a constant supply of substrate for energy metabolism, it is necessary to balance body requirements against the daily intake of nutrients and body stores of glycogen, fat, and protein. The discovery of leptin, a hormone made by fat cells in times of excess metabolic substrate, has led to unraveling of many of the neural pathways and molecular signaling mechanisms that drive food intake. Neurons in the region around the median eminence, which lacks a blood-brain barrier, are activated by circulating leptin.

These cells give rise to a complex web of pathways that use peptide neurotransmitters to drive autonomic, endocrine, and behavioral responses, which result in the regulation of feeding and body weight.

HYPERPHAGIA AND OBESITY. Lesions in the region of the ventromedial nucleus of the hypothalamus, which sits in the heart of this web of pathways, can result in massive overeating and obesity. A defect in the leptin gene or its receptor can result in leptin insensitivity, which also causes hyperphagia and obesity. Each of these conditions has been reported in humans, but they are rare causes of human obesity.

The *Kleine-Levin syndrome* is a poorly understood disorder in which patients, typically adolescent boys, have episodic attacks of somnolence, often sleeping up to 20 hours per day. When awake, they appear dull and often confused and consume enormous quantities of food. Attacks may last up to 2 weeks and can recur several times per year. Pathologic verification of the site of the lesion in typical cases is lacking, but a similar syndrome may be seen acutely in encephalitis involving the hypothalamus.

The *Prader-Willi syndrome,* a congenital disorder caused by a deletion in chromosome 15, is characterized by mental retardation, hypogonadism, and hyperphagia, often with massive obesity. The cause of the overeating is not known.

HYPOPHAGIA AND INANITION. Large lesions in the region of the lateral hypothalamic area at the level of the ventromedial nucleus result in aphagia, which may recover to hypophagia and regulation around a new, lower body weight set-point. Such lesions, which must be bilateral, are usually devastating, and selective impairment of eating on this basis has rarely been reported in adults. More often, patients with hypothalamic damage and inanition are somnolent and show a variety of endocrine abnormalities. No evidence of injury to the hypothalamus has been found in anorexia nervosa.

Children may demonstrate a quite different response to congenital hypothalamic tumors or malformations. The diencephalic syndrome of infancy is characterized by profound emaciation despite good feeding and linear growth. Affected children are often exceptionally good natured. The difference from adults with similarly placed tumors probably reflects the capacity for plasticity and the formation of new neuronal connections during development.

Central Disorders of Fluid and Electrolyte Regulation

The medial pre-optic area around the anteroventral tip of the 3rd ventricle plays a critical role in regulating blood pressure, volume, and electrolyte composition. Endocrine control (mineralocorticoids and especially vasopressin), autonomic regulation (control of blood flow in different vascular beds, innervation of sweat glands and kidney, especially the juxtaglomerular apparatus controlling renin release), and behavioral response (drinking) all play important roles in this process. Disorders of the release of vasopressin by neurons whose cell bodies are located in the supraoptic and paraventricular nuclei are discussed in Chapters 102.1 and 238. Coordinated central disorders of fluid regulation are rare.

HYPERNATREMIA, HYPEROSMOLALITY, ABSENCE OF THIRST. Neurogenic hypernatremia is a rare disorder marked by impairment of the normal responses to osmolar stimuli. Hence a deficit in the vasopressin response to increased sodium and osmolality is present, as well as an absence or relative deficiency of thirst. The vasopressin response to hypovolemia may be maintained, and the preservation of habitual drinking of water (often related to meals) may be sufficient to maintain serum osmolality under normal conditions. During hot weather, when loss of water is increased through evaporation of sweat, patients often fail to increase their water consumption adequately and may suffer attacks of fatigue, fever, muscle cramps and tenderness, and even myoglobinuria (associated with hypokalemia). With serum sodium in excess of 180 mEq/L, patients may experience confusion or even become stuporous, and some may die.

The hypothalamic injury giving rise to essential hypernatremia has been accurately localized in only a few cases, but in all of these cases it seems to involve the pre-optic area in the region of the anteroventral 3rd ventricle. Treatment consists of training the patient to drink adequate amounts of fluid, particularly during hot weather. Spironolactone, chlorpropamide, and thiazide diuretics have been used to reduce serum sodium and increase potassium.

HYPERDIPSIA, HYPONATREMIA, AND WATER INTOXICATION. Excessive water drinking in the absence of either hypovolemia or serum hyperosmolality is termed primary hyperdipsia and must be distinguished from the compensatory hyperdipsia of diabetes insipidus, diabetes mellitus, and polyuric renal failure. In the absence of inappropriate vasopressin secretion, symptoms of water intoxication such as stupor, delirium, or convulsions are infrequent. Most severe hyperdipsia occurs in persons who have psychiatric disturbances. We have seen only one case of primary hyperdipsia, that being in a patient who had suffered an attack of encephalitis involving the hypothalamus during childhood.

PAROXYSMAL HYPONATREMIA. Many patients with paroxysmal hypothermia (see above) suffer simultaneous hyponatremia, which may be sufficiently severe (serum sodium, <110 mEq/L) to cause symptoms of confusion or even convulsions. The serum sodium concentration is regulated around the reduced set-point but may respond to fluid restriction.

Central Reproductive Disorders

Reproductive hormonal control, behavior, and the associated autonomic responses are controlled by neurons in the pre-optic area close to those that regulate fluid and electrolyte control and by cells in the ventromedial hypothalamus close to neurons that regulate feeding. Although this contiguity may seem anomalous, reproductive capacity is closely tied to nutritional status (and leptin is a main regulator of both). In addition, sexual function and fetal maintenance rely on control of blood flow in specific vascular beds, which must be coordinated with control of body temperature and fluid balance. The change in body temperature that accompanies ovulation and the fluid shifts seen in the perimenstrual period in women are examples of this integration.

Reproductive endocrine disorders are covered in Chapters 247 and 250. Male erectile function, which is dependent on sacral parasympathetic innervation of the penis, may be affected by diseases of the peripheral autonomic nervous system (see above), as well as psychogenic factors acting at the level of the forebrain. Diagnosis and treatment of male sexual dysfunction are discussed in Chapter 247.

Arousal Disorders

The function of the autonomic nervous system is to augment the activity of various organ systems to deal with perturbations in internal homeostasis. Of all the body's organs, the single most important one to activate during an external threat is the brain. The ascending activating system, which runs from the brain stem reticular formation to the diencephalon, increases the responsiveness of the forebrain to external stimuli and may be considered a cerebral component of the autonomic system. Chapters 444, 445, and 447 describe the details of altered states of consciousness. We will briefly discuss disorders associated with lesions of the ascending arousal system. Sleep disorders are discussed in Chapter 448.

HYPERSOMNOLENCE. Following lesions of the ascending activating system at the level of the rostral brain stem, typically the level of consciousness is acutely impaired. After a few weeks, the forebrain recovers spontaneous wake-sleep cycles. Prolonged sleep-like stupor lasting longer than a few weeks is seen only when lesions involve the posterior diencephalon. It is not clear whether this continued somnolence results from injury to the thalamus, to the hypothalamus, or to the connections of these structures. Methylphenidate, amphetamine, and bromocriptine have been used in these patients, with some anecdotal reports of success.

INSOMNIA. Sleep is an active process requiring the participation of hypnogenic influences arising from the lower brain stem and serotoninergic neurons in the midbrain raphe. We have seen one patient in whom destruction of the medulla below the level of the ascending activating system resulted in a chronically wakeful state. Lesions of the pre-optic area may also cause a decrease in sleep that may be distinct from any deficit in thermoregulation.

Blok BF, Willemsen AT, Holstege G: A PET study on brain control of micturition in humans. Brain 120:111, 1997. *A careful study of central nervous system pathways controlling micturition in humans.*
Elmquist JK, Ahima RS, Elias CF, et al: Leptin activates distinct projections from the dorsomedial and ventromedial hypothalamic nuclei. Proc Natl Acad Sci U S A 95:

741, 1998. *A review of the central nervous system pathways activated by leptin and controlling feeding.*

Elmquist JK, Scammell TE, Saper CB: Mechanisms of CNS response to systemic immune challenge: The febrile response. Trends Neurosci 20:565, 1997. *A review of the mechanisms of fever and neuroimmune interactions.*

Freeman R, Miyawaki E: The treatment of autonomic dysfunction. J Clin Neurophysiol 10:61, 1993. *A review of treatment of autonomic disorders.*

Lefkowitz RL, Hoffman BB, Taylor P: Neurohumoral transmission: The autonomic and somatic motor neuron systems. *In* Gilman AG, Rall TW, Nies AS, Taylor P (eds): The Pharmacological Basis of Therapeutics. New York, Pergamon, 1990, p 84. *A thorough review of peripheral autonomic organization and neurotransmission.*

Loewy AD, Spyer KM: Central Regulation of Autonomic Functions. New York, Oxford Press, 1990. *A comprehensive series of reviews on the central components of the autonomic nervous system.*

Low PA: Clinical Autonomic Disorders. Little, Brown, Boston, 1993, pp 1–800. *A comprehensive reference volume on autonomic disorders.*

Low PA, Gilden JL, Freeman R, et al: Efficacy of midodrine vs placebo in neurogenic orthostatic hypotension. A randomized, double-blind multicenter study. JAMA 277: 1046, 1997. *A controlled trial of a new therapy for orthostatic hypotension.*

McLeod JG, Tuck RR: Disorders of the autonomic nervous system: Part 1. Pathophysiology and clinical features. Ann Neurol 21:419, 1987. *A review of autonomic physiology and pathophysiology.*

McLeod JG, Tuck RR: Disorders of the autonomic nervous system: Part 2. Investigation and treatment. Ann Neurol 21:519, 1987. *A guide to pharmacologic testing and treatment of autonomic dysfunction.*

Saper CB: "All fall down": The mechanism of orthostatic hypotension in multiple systems atrophy and Parkinson's disease. Ann Neurol 43:149, 1998. *A review of the central nervous system pathways controlling blood pressure and their involvement in neurologic disorders.*

452 DISORDERS OF MOTOR FUNCTION

Robert C. Griggs

452.1 Motor Symptoms

Robert C. Griggs

WEAKNESS. It is axiomatic that patients typically have motor signs before motor symptoms and, conversely, sensory symptoms before sensory signs. Thus patients with even severe weakness may not report symptoms of weakness. Somewhat paradoxically, patients who complain of "weakness" often do not have confirmatory findings on examination that document the presence of weakness.

Weakness, when actually a symptom of neurologic disease, is frequently caused by diseases of the motor unit (see Chapters 468, 497, 505, and 511) and is usually reported by a patient in terms of a loss of specific functions, e.g., difficulties with tasks such as climbing stairs, rising from a chair, sitting up, lifting objects onto a high shelf, or opening jars. Symptoms may also reflect the consequences of weakness such as frequent falls or tripping. Such symptoms can be remarkably quantitative. A patient with leg muscle weakness who is falling even as infrequently as once a month almost invariably has severe weakness of knee extensor muscles and can be shown on examination to have a knee extension lag: the inability to fully lift the leg against gravity and to lock the knee.

The symptom of "weakness" without findings of weakness on examination is not usually the result of neuromuscular disease but can be a sign of neurologic disease outside the motor unit or more commonly a symptom of disease outside the nervous system altogether (Table 452–1).

FATIGUE. The complaints of "fatigue," "tiredness," and "lack of energy" are even less likely than the symptom of "weakness" to reflect definable neurologic disease. With the exception of neuromuscular junction disorders such as myasthenia gravis, fatigue is rarely a complaint of diseases of the motor unit. Fatigue can be a sign of upper motor neuron disease (corticospinal pathways) and is a common complaint of established multiple sclerosis and other multifocal central nervous system disease. Similarly, any process that produces bilateral corticospinal tract or extrapyramidal disease

Table 452–1 ■ DISORDERS THAT COMMONLY PRESENT WITH "WEAKNESS"

Disorders of the motor unit
  Upper motor neuron lesions—spasticity
  Basal ganglia disorders—rigidity
General medical conditions
  Heart failure
  Respiratory insufficiency
  Renal, hepatic, other metabolic disease
  Alcoholism and other toxin-related disease
Psychiatric and behavioral disorders
  Depression
  Malingering

can produce fatigue. Examples include motor neuron disease, spinal cord disease in the cervical cord region, and Parkinson's disease. Finally, as one would expect, disorders that impair sleep may include fatigue as a complaint.

"Fatigue," like "weakness," is much more often than not a sign of disease outside the central and peripheral nervous system. Depression and other psychiatric and behavioral disorders, as well as the medical illnesses associated with a complaint of weakness, are all frequent causes of fatigue.

The chronic fatigue syndrome, as well as many cases of fibromyalgia (see Chapter 306), have fatigue as a dominant, disabling symptom. These disorders are defined in part by the absence of consistent neurologic findings and the absence of demonstrable pathology in the nervous system.

SPONTANEOUS MOVEMENTS. Muscle tremors, jerks, twitches, cramps, and spasms are all frequent symptoms. The cause of spontaneous movements can reside at any level of the nervous system. In general, movements that occur in an entire limb or in more than one muscle group concurrently are caused by central nervous system disease. Those confined to a single muscle are likely to be a reflection of disease of the motor unit (including the motor neurons of the brain stem and spinal cord). When spontaneous movements of a muscle are associated with severe pain, patients often use the term "cramp." *Cramp* is a medically defined disorder that reflects the intense contraction of a large group of motor units. Leg cramps are frequent in normal persons and particularly common in older patients. They are occasionally a sign of an underlying disease of the anterior horn cell, nerve roots, or peripheral nerve but are usually benign. When severe, cramps can produce such intense muscle contraction that muscle injury is produced and muscle enzymes (e.g., creatine kinase) are elevated in the blood.

The rare muscle diseases in which an enzyme deficiency interferes with substrate utilization as fuel for exercise (e.g., McArdle's disease) are often associated with severe, exercise-provoked muscle *contractures.* These contractures are electrically silent by electromyography, in contrast to the intense motor unit activity seen with cramps. They must not be confused with the limitation of joint range of motion resulting from long-standing joint disease or long-standing weakness—also termed contractures.

The intense muscle contractions of *tetany* are often painful. Usually a reflection of hypocalcemia, tetany can occasionally be seen without demonstrable electrolyte disturbance. Tetany results from hyperexcitability of the peripheral nerves. Similarly, in the syndrome of *tetanus* produced by a clostridial toxin, intensely painful, life-threatening muscle contractions arise from hyperexcitable peripheral nerves. A number of toxic disorders such as strychnine poisoning and black widow spider toxin produce similar neurogenic spasms.

MUSCLE PAIN. Acute muscle pain in the absence of abnormal muscle contractions is an extremely common symptom. When such pain occurs following strenuous exercise or in the context of an acute viral illness (e.g., influenza), it probably reflects muscle injury. In such patients the serum creatine kinase level is often raised. It is uncommon for this frequent and essentially normal sign of muscle injury to be associated with weakness or demonstrable ongoing muscle pathology.

Chronic muscle pain is a common symptom but is seldom related to a definable disease of muscle (see Chapter 306).

EPISODIC AND INTERMITTENT WEAKNESS. The complaint of attacks of severe weakness or paralysis occurring in a patient with baseline normal strength is an uncommon symptom. This symptom

Table 452–2 ■ CHARACTERISTIC GAIT DISORDERS

SPECIFIC DISORDER	LOCATION OF LESION(S)	CHARACTERISTICS
Spastic gait	Bilateral corticospinal pathways within thoracic or cervical cord, or in the brain	Legs stiff, feet turning inward "scissoring"
Hemiparetic gait	Unilateral central nervous system—cervical cord or brain	Affected leg circumducted, foot extended, arm flexed
Sensory ataxia	Posterior columns of spinal cord or peripheral nerve	Wide-based, high steps; Romberg sign present
Cerebellar ataxia	Brain stem or cerebellum	Wide-based; Romberg sign absent
Parkinsonian gait	Basal ganglia	Shuffling, small steps
Dystonic gait	Basal ganglia; also corticospinal pathways	Abnormal posture of arms, head, neck
Gait disorder of the elderly	Multifactoria: bihemispheric disease; spinal cord disease; impaired proprioception; muscle weakness	Stooped posture, wide-based; often retro-pulsion
Steppage gait	Distal muscle weakness	High steps ("steppage")
Antalgic gait	Non-neurologic, reflects disease of joints, bones, or soft tissue	Minimizes pain in hip, spine, leg
Hysterical gait	Psychiatric or behavioral disorder	Reeling side to side; associated astasia-abasia;* bizarre arm and trunk movements

*Astasia-abasia describes the severe difficulty maintaining standing balance with little or no comparable difficulty when sitting.

is typical of the periodic paralyses and may also be seen with episodic ataxias and myotonic disorders (see Chapter 505). All of these disorders are ion channelopathies. These channelopathies (e.g., the calcium channelopathy hypokalemic periodic paralysis) are rare but treatable disorders (see Chapter 505). Episodic weakness is also seen in patients with neuromuscular junction disorders such as myasthenia gravis and the myasthenic syndrome. Occasionally, patients with narcolepsy complain of intermittent paralysis as a reflection of *sleep paralysis* (see Chapter 448).

LOSS OF BALANCE. Unsteadiness of gait is a common symptom. When associated with the complaints of dizziness or vertigo, disease of the labyrinth, the vestibular nerve, the brain stem, or the cerebellum is a probable cause. When unsteadiness and loss of balance are unassociated with dizziness, particularly when the unsteadiness appears to be out of proportion to other symptoms of the patient, a widespread disorder of sensation or motor function is likely.

ABNORMAL GAIT AND POSTURE. The ability to stand and to walk in a well-coordinated, effortless fashion requires the integrity of the entire nervous system. Relatively subtle deficits localized to one part of the central or peripheral nervous system will produce characteristic abnormalities. Specific gait disturbances are categorized in Table 452–2.

453 MAJOR SENSORY SYMPTOMS
Michael J. Aminoff

Clinical sensory disturbances may reflect dysfunction at any point along the pathways from the peripheral sensory receptors to or within the central nervous system (CNS). Disorders of the special senses are considered elsewhere in the text and are not considered further here.

Cutaneous sensation is subserved by at least two distinct systems. Pain and temperature appreciation and aspects of tactile sensation are subserved by one system. The sensory receptors consist of naked nerve endings, from which impulses are conducted by either unmyelinated C fibers (1–2 μm) at a velocity of 0.5 m/sec or small (5 μm), thinly myelinated (A delta) fibers at a velocity of 30 m/sec. The cell bodies of these axons are in the dorsal root ganglia, and impulses pass along the central processes of these neurons to the spinal cord, where they synapse in the dorsal horn. Axons of the second-order sensory fibers cross to the contralateral anterior or anterolateral part of the contralateral spinal cord and ascend to the ventral posterolateral nucleus of the thalamus, from which third-order neurons project to the sensorimotor cortex.

A second sensory system subserves crude and light touch, position sense, and tactile localization or discrimination. The involved sensory receptors are cutaneous mechanoreceptors and receptors in joints, tendons, and muscles (muscle spindles). The afferent pathways consist of large myelinated fibers that pass to the spinal cord via the dorsal root ganglia and ascend in the ipsilateral posterior and, to a lesser extent, the posterolateral columns of the cord to reach the posterior column nuclei (gracile and cuneate nuclei) in the medulla oblongata, where they synapse with second-order neurons. The fibers from these neurons cross and then ascend in the medial lemniscus to synapse in the contralateral ventral posterolateral nucleus of the thalamus, from which third-order neurons project to the cortex.

Sensory symptoms have been divided into negative and positive ones. Negative symptoms are ones in which there is a loss of sensation, such as a feeling of numbness. Positive symptoms, by contrast, consist of sensory phenomena that occur without normal stimulation of receptors and include paresthesias and dysesthesias. *Paresthesias* may include a feeling of tingling, crawling, itching, compression, tightness, cold, or heat, and are sometimes associated with a feeling of heaviness. The term *dysesthesias* is used correctly to refer to abnormal sensations, often tingling, painful or uncomfortable, that occur after innocuous stimuli, while *allodynia* refers to the perception as painful of a stimulus that is not normally painful. Paresthesias and dysesthesias may be difficult to distinguish from pain by some patients. *Hypesthesia* and *hypalgesia* denote a loss or impairment of touch or pain sensibility, respectively, and *hyperesthesia* and *hyperalgesia* indicate a lowered threshold to tactile or painful stimuli, respectively, so that there is increased sensitivity to such stimuli.

With the use of a wisp of cotton, a pin, and a tuning fork, the trunk and extremities are examined for regions of abnormal or absent sensation. Certain instruments are available for quantifying sensory function, such as the computer-assisted sensory examination, which is based on the detection of touch, pressure, vibratory, and thermal sensation thresholds.

Alterations in pain and tactile sensibility can generally be detected by clinical examination. It is important to localize the distribution of any such sensory loss in order to distinguish between nerve, root, and central dysfunction. Similarly, abnormalities of proprioception can be detected by clinical examination, when patients will be unable to detect the direction in which a joint is moved. In severe cases, there may be pseudoathetoid movements of the outstretched hands, sensory ataxia, and, sometimes, postural and action tremors.

NEUROLOGIC CAUSES OF SENSORY DISTURBANCES

PERIPHERAL NEUROPATHIES AND NEURONOPATHIES. Disorders of peripheral nerves commonly lead to sensory disturbances that depend upon the population of affected nerve fibers. Some neuropathies are predominantly large-fiber neuropathies. Appreciation of movement and position are impaired, and paresthesias are common. Examination reveals that vibration, position, and movement sensations are impaired, and movement becomes clumsy and ataxic. Pain and temperature appreciation are relatively preserved. The tendon reflexes are lost early. In other neuropathies, it is the small fibers especially that are affected; spontaneous pain is common and may be burning, lancinating, or aching in quality. Pain and temperature appreciation are disproportionately affected in these neuropathies, and autonomic dysfunction may be present. Examples of small-fiber neuropathies include certain hereditary disorders, Tangier disease, and diabetes. The distribution of sensory loss should indicate the site of pathology and provide a clue to the underlying neurologic disorder. Most sensory neuropathies are characterized by a distal distribution of sensory loss, whereas sensory neuronopathies are characterized by sensory loss that may also involve the trunk and face, and which tends to be particularly severe. Sensory changes in a radiculopathy will conform to a root territory; in cauda equina syndromes, sensory deficits involve multiple roots and may lead to saddle anesthesia and loss of the normal sensation associated with the passage of urine or feces. A peripheral nerve lesion will lead to sensory loss in the distribution of a single nerve or nerve branch. Sensory loss sometimes suggests the discrete involvement of several different nerves (mononeuritis multiplex), while in other cases there is a symmetric distal sensory loss that does not conform to the territory of any individual nerves but, rather, suggests diffuse involvement of multiple nerves (polyneuropathy). The further evaluation of peripheral nerve lesions is considered in Chapters 497.

SPINAL CORD LESIONS. Lesions of the *posterolateral columns* of the cord, such as occur in multiple sclerosis, vitamin B$_{12}$ deficiency, and cervical spondylosis, lead often to a feeling of compression in the affected region and to a Lhermitte sign (paresthesias radiating down the back and legs on neck flexion). Examination reveals an ipsilateral impairment of vibration and joint position senses, with preservation of pain and temperature appreciation. Conversely, lesions of the *anterolateral region* of the cord (as by cordotomy), or *central lesions* interrupting fibers crossing to join the spinothalamic pathways (as in syringomyelia) lead to an impairment of pain and temperature appreciation with relative preservation of vibration and joint position sense, and of light touch.

Based upon the above, certain characteristic sensory syndromes occur with cord lesions. Lateral hemisection of the cord (*Brown-Séqard syndrome*) leads to ipsilateral pain, hyperesthesia, and impaired vibration and joint position sense below the level of the lesion, and contralateral impairment of pain and temperature appreciation. Patients with a central cord lesion that interrupts fibers crossing in the cord develop a *syringomyelic syndrome,* affecting the involved segments, with impairment of pain and temperature appreciation but preservation of vibration and joint position senses and the ability to localize touch. In patients with a severe transverse myelitis or complete cord transection, all sensation is lost below the level of the lesion although spinal reflex activity is preserved except in the acute stage of spinal shock. Examination of the patient typically shows a *"sensory level"* that provides an approximate guide to the location of the cord lesion.

Motor deficits may also be present and help to localize the lesion. Upper motor neuron dysfunction from cervical lesions lead to quadriplegia, whereas more caudal lesions lead to paraplegia; lesions below the level of the first lumbar vertebra may simply compress the cauda equina, leading to lower motor neuron deficits from a polyradiculopathy, and impairment of sphincter and sexual functions.

BRAIN STEM LESIONS. Because the ascending sensory pathways follow different courses in the brain stem, characteristic neurologic syndromes occur, depending upon the site of pathology. *Lateral medullary lesions* (Wallenberg syndrome) typically lead to a crossed sensory deficit, with loss of pain and temperature appreciation on the ipsilateral face (because of damage to the descending root of the trigeminal nerve) and contralateral side of the body. Proprioceptive pathways are spared. With *lesions of the medial lemniscus,* by contrast, contralateral appreciation of touch and proprioception is impaired, but pain and temperature sensation is unaffected. In the *rostral brain stem,* the spinothalamic and lemniscal pathways converge, and a lesion affecting them results in loss of all sensation contralaterally. With lesions at the level of the *thala-mus* or more rostrally, all sensory modalities are lost on the side opposite the lesion. Spontaneous pain is common and diverse cutaneous stimuli may cause unpleasant painful sensations (*Dejerine-Roussy syndrome*). The presence of weakness, cranial neuropathies, and ataxia help to localize the lesion.

CORTICAL LESIONS. Lesions of the sensory cortex cause loss of all sensations on the opposite side of the body and may also lead to the Dejerine-Roussy syndrome. Discrete lesions may lead to an impairment of cortical sensory function when primary sensory modalities are preserved. Patients are unable to recognize objects by touch, localize stimuli, discriminate simultaneous touch of two neighboring points, or recognize the position of body parts. There is loss of the ability to estimate size, weight (abarognosis) or shape (astereognosis). In some patients with cortical lesions but no overt loss of sensation, there is neglect of sensation from one side when the two sides are stimulated simultaneously.

NONORGANIC SENSORY DISTURBANCES

Sensory disturbances may occur on a non-organic basis. Such sensory loss has a distribution that is difficult to explain anatomically, tending to conform instead to bodily regions that are deemed distinct by patients. Sensory loss, for example, may involve an entire limb with a border that runs circumferentially around the junction of the limb with the trunk. Similarly, impairment of vibration on one side but not the other of a bony midline structure such as the skull is hard to explain on an organic basis, because bone would be expected to conduct vibration to both sides. Moreover, the transition between an area of non-organic sensory loss and adjacent areas with normal sensation is typically abrupt, whereas an area of abnormal sensation is usually interposed in patients with sensory loss that has an organic basis. Again, sensory loss may extend exactly to the midline, whereas organic sensory loss of peripheral origin tends to stop about 1 to 2 inches before the midline because of overlap with the innervation on the opposite side. In patients with non-organic sensory loss, function is often preserved despite sometimes dramatic sensory findings. Despite an apparent loss of position sense, for example, there is typically no clumsiness or ataxia, and the gait is unaffected.

454 HEADACHES AND OTHER HEAD PAIN

F. Michael Cutrer ■ *Michael A. Moskowitz*

Headache is a very common complaint encountered not only by primary care physicians but also by practitioners in almost every specialty of medicine and surgery. Over 90% of the population experience headache of one type or another at least once during life. The very common occurrence of headache sometimes leads to an underestimation of its potential importance as a symptom. Although headaches may be associated with minor trauma or febrile illness, they may also result from potentially life-threatening central nervous system disease. Fortunately, most patients with recurrent or chronic headaches suffer from a primary headache disorder for which no ominous underlying source can be found. Although reassuring, this lack of identifiable cause does not diminish either the patient's suffering or economic loss.

PATHOPHYSIOLOGY. A headache signifies activation of the primary afferent fibers that innervate cephalic blood vessels, chiefly meningeal or cerebral blood vessels. Most nociceptive fibers innervating these structures arise from pseudounipolar neurons located within the trigeminal ganglia (1st division), although some may be located within the upper cervical ganglia as well. Stimuli activating these fibers are quite variable and can range from direct mechanical traction by a tumor to chemical irritation caused by central nervous system infection or subarachnoid blood. In patients with so-called *secondary headache disorders,* headaches result from an identifiable structural or inflammatory source. In these patients, treatment of the primary abnormality often results in resolution of the headache. However, the overwhelming majority of patients with chronic headaches have *"primary headache disorders"* such as migraine or tension headache in which the physical examination and laboratory studies are generally normal. With the absence of an identifiable cause, the mode of trigeminal activation in migraine has been hotly debated. Traditional theories have been dominated by two points of view. The *vasogenic theory,* based on the work of Harold Wolff and colleagues, held that intracranial vasoconstriction was responsible for the symptoms of migraine aura and that headache resulted from a rebound dilation and distention of cranial vessels and activation of perivascular nociceptive axons. This theory was based on observations that (1) extracranial vessels distend and pulsate during a migraine attack in many patients, thus implying that cranial vessels might be of primary importance; (2) stimulation of intracranial vessels in awake patients results in an ipsilateral headache; and (3) substances that cause vasoconstriction such as ergot alkaloids abort headache, whereas vasodilators such as nitrates can provoke an attack. The alternative hypothesis, the *neurogenic theory,* identified the brain as the generator of migraine and held that the susceptibility in any individual to migraine attacks reflects thresholds intrinsic to the brain. The vascular changes occurring during migraine are thus the result rather than the cause of the attack. Supporters of the neurogenic hypothesis pointed to the observation that migraine attacks are often accompanied by a range of neurologic symptoms both focal (in the aura) and vegetative (in the prodrome) that cannot be explained simply by vasoconstriction within a single neurovascular distribution. It is likely that elements of both traditional theories explain some of the pathophysiology of migraine and other primary headache disorders. In fact, recent imaging studies (magnetic resonance imaging [MRI] and positron emission tomography) and genetic studies confirm that migraine and related headaches are disorders of neurovascular regulation.

Recent clinical and experimental observations suggest that the brain, although usually insensate, can activate or sensitize (directly or indirectly) trigeminal nerve fibers within the meninges. In some forms of migraine, endogenous neurophysiologic events in the neocortex (such as occur during the aura) may promote the release of nociceptive substances (e.g., potassium, protons, and arachidonate metabolites) from the neocortex into the interstitial space. Within the Virchow-Robin spaces, the released substances accumulate to levels sufficient to activate or sensitize the trigeminovascular fibers that surround the pial vessels supplying the draining neocortex. Under steady-state conditions, the brain vigorously maintains the equilibrium of its extracellular environment, and ions or transmitters normally released from cellular compartments are rapidly taken up in glia and neurons at rates that keep the levels of these ions, transmitters, and neuromodulators constant. Blood vessels provide a backup mechanism for clearance that is not invoked under normal conditions. However, before the onset of headache, mechanisms associated with spreading oligemia may enhance release of the various substances, block uptake and inactivation—thereby increasing extracellular levels—and overwhelm the normal clearance mechanisms. The substances released may discharge or sensitize small unmyelinated nociceptive fibers and either provide the trigger for headache or sensitize perivascular afferents to blood-borne or other as yet unidentified factors. The headache latency (20 to 40 minutes) observed in migraine may reflect the time needed for extracellular levels to exceed a threshold for axonal depolarization. Consistent with these notions, unilateral headaches tend to occur on the side corresponding to the dysfunctional hemisphere.

In this formulation, the brain becomes a master switch, a transducer. Triggering events, such as those associated with emotional stress, fatigue, bright lights, and too little (or too much) sleep, modulate activity within brain regions physically contiguous to the meningeal vessels innervated by the trigeminal nerve. In susceptible individuals, these events may provide a sufficient trigger for subsequent neurophysiologic events that lead to chemical activation of meningeal fibers. The photophobia, nausea, and vomiting associated with migraine are probably related to the consequences of meningeal irritation because symptoms such as these occur during meningeal infection or when blood enters the subarachnoid space. This pathogenetic framework for migraine is consistent with currently understood principles of neurobiology and the physiology of pain. However, some of the details will require revision as data emerge

from additional experimental studies in humans and animals. In all likelihood, migraine and other headaches arise from a combination of genetic and environmental factors. Some are intrinsic to the brain, others to blood vessels or to circulating substances. In each case the pain develops from trigeminal activation in sensitized axons as a consequence of actual or threatened tissue injury.

PRIMARY HEADACHE DISORDERS

MIGRAINE. Migraine is the 2nd most common primary headache disorder and has a prevalence of about 12%. It affects women disproportionately (approximately 17.6% of women versus 6% of men in the United States) and commonly afflicts the population during the most productive years of life (peak prevalence, 25 to 45 years).

CLINICAL FEATURES. Migraine falls into two categories: (1) migraine without an aura (previously called common migraine), which occurs in about 85% of patients, and (2) migraine with an aura (previously called classic migraine), which occurs in about 15% of patients. Migraine patients both with and without an aura may report prodromal symptoms that begin 24 to 48 hours before a headache attack. These symptoms can include hyperactivity, mild euphoria, lethargy, depression, craving for certain foods, fluid retention, and frequent yawning. Prodromal symptoms should not be confused with the migraine aura that consists of transient episodes of focal neurologic dysfunction appearing 1 to 2 hours before the onset of a migraine headache and resolving within 60 minutes. The aura symptoms may be of different types. More than a single symptom type may be present within a given aura. Typical aura symptoms include (1) homonymous (rarely monocular) visual disturbance, classically an expanding scotoma with a scintillating margin; (2) unilateral paresthesias or numbness, often affecting the distal ends of the extremities or the perioral region of the face; (3) unilateral weakness; and (4) dysphasia or other language disturbances. Sometimes aura symptoms localize to the brain stem and may include vertigo, dysarthria, tinnitus, fluctuating hearing loss, diplopia, bilateral weakness, ataxia, bilateral paresthesias, and a decreased level of consciousness. *Basilar migraine* is the diagnosis in patients in whom brain stem symptoms predominate. One must be aware that these symptoms can also occur with anxiety and hyperventilation. In many patients, basilar attacks are intermingled with more typical migraine attacks. Dizziness is frequently reported as a feature of an otherwise typical attack of migraine without an aura.

The headache phase of an attack is similar in migraine with or without an aura. It typically consists of 4 to 72 hours of unilateral throbbing head pain of moderate to severe intensity that is worsened by routine physical exertion and associated with nausea, photophobia, and phonophobia. *Complicated migraine* or *migraine with a prolonged aura* refers to migraine attacks associated with aura symptoms lasting for more than 1 hour, but less than 1 week, and in which neuroimaging studies are normal. If symptoms persist for greater than 1 week or result in neuroimaging abnormalities, migrainous infarction is likely. In general, migrainous infarction develops in the context of stereotypic aura symptoms.

Status Migrainosus. Migraine attacks that persist for longer than 72 hours despite treatment are classified as *status migrainosus.* During *status migrainosus,* headache-free periods of less than 4 hours (sleep not included) may occur. Status migrainosus is usually associated with prolonged analgesic use and may require in-patient treatment with detoxification.

GENETICS OF MIGRAINE. A higher than expected prevalence of migraine has been observed in the relatives of migraine patients. In one large family study drawn from the general population, the risk of migraine in relatives of migraineurs was three times higher than the risk among controls. Furthermore, data from large twin registries have consistently revealed higher concordance rates for migraine in monozygotic twins than in dizygotic pairs. One large study of over 2500 monozygotic and 5000 dizygotic twin pair estimated that 40 to 50% of susceptibility to migraine is genetically based. Although migraine is widely thought to reflect an autosomal dominant condition, segregational analysis has failed to identify any single mendelian pattern of transmission.

Familial Hemiplegic Migraine. Perhaps the most compelling genetic evidence to date comes from the identification of specific gene loci for familial hemiplegic migraine. Familial hemiplegic migraine is an autosomal dominant disorder characterized by transient hemiplegia during the aura phase of a migraine attack. This rare migraine subtype has been linked to point mutations in the gene *CACNL1A4* located on chromosome 19p13 in 50% of affected families. More recently, another genetic mutation in a group of families with familial hemiplegic migraine has been assigned to chromosome 1q31, thus implying genetic heterogeneity. Except for cerebellar atrophy in cases of disease that can be mapped to 19p13, no obvious clinical distinctions can be noted between affected families with and without this abnormal gene. The defective gene codes for the α1-subunit of a brain-specific p/q calcium channel that is coupled to neurotransmitter release and expressed throughout the human brain. Although the mutant channel may disrupt ion permeability, selectivity, or both, it is entirely unclear how sustained neurologic deficits and migraine result from a defect in an ion channel that operates (i.e., opens and shuts) in milliseconds.

MIGRAINE TREATMENT. Migraine therapy includes both non-pharmacologic and pharmacologic interventions. *Non-pharmacologic treatment* includes behavior modification techniques such as the avoidance of triggering factors (e.g., the ingestion of particular foods or food additives, strong smells, or glaring light) and establishment of regular meals and consistent sleeping patterns. Other techniques to minimize the effects of environmental stress, such as biofeedback, relaxation training, rational motive therapy, self-hypnosis, and meditation, are also sometimes helpful.

Pharmacologic treatment of migraine includes abortive therapy given to shorten the attack or decrease headache severity. In patients with infrequent and uncomplicated attacks, abortive medications are often sufficient. If migraines cause disability more than 3 days per month, daily prophylactic treatment may be taken to decrease the frequency and, less often, the severity of attacks. If taken at the time of attacks, prophylactic agents are usually ineffective, and agents used for treatment during an attack provide little protection against subsequent attacks. The use of analgesic medications more than 3 days per week (including over-the-counter formulations) may increase headache frequency and severity. In some cases, intermittent migraine progresses to a syndrome of daily severe headaches despite the use of escalating prophylactic medication or analgesics. Only non-steroidal anti-inflammatory drugs (NSAIDs) and ergotamine are used both during an attack and preventively.

Patients should be provided with a variety of treatments that may be taken in a manner appropriate to the severity of their symptoms. *Mild attacks* may be treated with simple analgesics such as acetaminophen (suggested dose, 650 to 1000 mg) or NSAIDs (aspirin, 900 to 1000 mg, ibuprofen, 1000 to 1200 mg, naproxen, 500 to 825 mg, and ketoprofen, 100 to 200 mg). Mild to moderate attacks during pregnancy may be treated with acetaminophen. *Moderate headaches* may respond to the combination of acetaminophen, isometheptene mucate (a mild vasoconstrictor), and dichloralphenazone (a mild sedative). Infrequent headaches of moderate to severe intensity may be treated with butalbital, a barbiturate, combined with caffeine, aspirin, or acetaminophen. Oral opiates have little place in the treatment of chronic, recurrent, primary headaches and should be avoided until alternatives, including NSAIDs and serotonin agonists such as dihydroergotamine or sumatriptan, have been considered. They may be the only viable option during pregnancy or in patients with severe vascular disease, however. If so, they should be used with caution, and the risks associated with opiate use, including rebound headaches and dependency, should be discussed with patients before treatment is initiated.

Ergotamine is the longest established antimigraine agent. It can be effective if the associated nausea and peripheral vasoconstriction can be tolerated. Ergotamine (2 mg sublingually, 1–2 mg orally) is typically most effective if given early in the migraine attack. Potential problems of ergotamine therapy include overuse, which can result in chronic daily headaches; with extreme excessive use, the gangrene-like complications of ergotism may result.

In the past decade a number of new abortive agents have been developed. *Moderate to severe* attacks may be treated outside the hospital with oral or intranasal formulations of 5-hydroxytryptamine such as 5-HT$_{B/D}$ receptor agonists like sumatriptan (25 or 50 mg orally, 20 mg intranasally, 6 mg subcutaneously), dihydroergotamine (1 to 2 mg intranasally), and more recently, new 2nd-generation sumatriptan-like drugs such as naratriptan, zolmitriptan, and rizatriptan, which are similar to sumatriptan in efficacy and mechanism. They may have a faster onset of action and fewer coronary vasoconstrictor properties. Nevertheless, patients with uncontrolled hypertension or those with a history of coronary artery disease or angina should not be given these drugs.

Very severe attacks sometimes require the administration of intravenous or intramuscular agents in the emergency department. Dihydroergotamine, an injectable hydrogenated ergot, has less potent peripheral arterial vasoconstrictive effects than ergotamine and is usually effective even when given well into an attack. Dihydroergotamine may be administered subcutaneously or intravenously. Given intravenously, dihydroergotamine causes less nausea than ergotamine does, but an antiemetic is still required before intravenous use. Meperidine, an opioid analgesic, is frequently administered intramuscularly, especially in combination with an antiemetic, to treat severe migraine attacks. With alternatives now available, the use of parenteral opioids should be limited to patients with infrequent, severe attacks for whom other treatments are contraindicated. The recent identification of 5-HT$_{1D}$ and 5-HT$_{1F}$ receptor binding proteins on trigeminovascular nerves may be relevant to next-generation abortive treatments of migraine. For patients who are non-responsive or have contraindications to vasoactive abortive agents, intravenous neuroleptics may be given to treat severe or prolonged migraine attacks. Intravenous chlorpromazine, 10 mg, may be used in this setting and repeated in 1 hour if no response is seen. The hypotension that sometimes accompanies the use of intravenous chlorpromazine may be avoided by administering 500 mL of normal saline intravenously before chlorpromazine (10 mg). Alternatively, intravenous prochlorperazine (10 mg over 5 min) can be given without prior saline infusion and repeated after 30 minutes.

PREVENTIVE TREATMENT OF RECURRENT MIGRAINE. In general, preventive treatment is recommended (1) if headaches limit work or normal daily activity 3 or more days per month, (2) if the symptoms accompanying headache are severe or prolonged, and (3) if previous migraine was associated with a complication (e.g., cerebral infarction). Preventive treatment is largely empirical, and the drugs currently used were discovered serendipitously while being developed for the treatment of other disorders. Increased appetite and weight gain are common side effects of most prophylactic agents. Treatment should be initiated at low doses and gradually titrated to headache improvement or the onset of side effects. Groups 1 to 5 are generally considered 1st-line agents and tend to be associated with either fewer or less potentially serious side effects.

The prophylactic agents fall into seven groups and include:

1. β-Adrenergic blockers: propranolol (40 to 240 mg), atenolol (50 to 150 mg), nadolol (20 to 80 mg), timolol (20 to 60 mg) and metoprolol (50 to 300 mg)
2. NSAIDs: aspirin (1000 to 1300 mg), naproxen (480 to 1100 mg), ketoprofen (150 to 300 mg)
3. Tricyclic antidepressants: amitriptyline (10 to 120 mg), nortriptyline (10 to 75 mg)
4. Calcium channel antagonists: verapamil (120 to 480 mg), flunarizine (5 to 10 mg)
5. Anticonvulsants: divalproex sodium (750 to 1000 mg), gabapentin (900 to 1800 mg)
6. Serotoninergic drugs: methysergide (4 to 8 mg), cyproheptadine (8 to 20 mg)
7. Monoamine oxidase inhibitor: phenelzine (30 to 60 mg)

Unfortunately, comparative data on migraine prophylactic treatments are sparse, and the decision to use one versus another is currently most often based on the practitioner's experience with one or more of the medications or the presence of co-morbid illnesses, which would be either an indication or contraindication to the use of one or more of the available antimigraine treatments.

CLUSTER HEADACHE. Cluster headache, which is much less common than either tension-type headache or migraine, affects 0.4 to 2.4 persons per 1000 in the general population. Unlike migraineurs, patients with cluster headaches usually seek medical consultation because of the intense pain that accompanies their attacks. As a result, physicians encounter cluster headache more commonly than would be predicted from its prevalence. The condition is more common in men than in women (male-to-female ratio, 6:1) and usually begins in the 3rd through the 6th decades of life. Although cluster headaches may cease during pregnancy, like migraine, attacks seldom correlate with menses.

CLINICAL FEATURES. Cluster headaches consist of recurrent episodes of unilateral, orbital, supraorbital, or temporal head pain usually accompanied by ipsilateral autonomic signs, including conjunctival injection, lacrimation, rhinorrhea, nasal congestion, ptosis, miosis, eyelid edema, and facial sweating. The attacks last from 15 minutes to 3 hours and occur as infrequently as every other day to as frequently as eight attacks per day. The syndrome derives its name from the characteristic clusters, or periods of frequent headache, that last from weeks to months separated by periods of months or years of headache-free remission. Chronic symptoms without remission may develop in about 10% of patients. During a cluster period, the headache attacks often assume a temporal cyclicity, with occurrence at almost the same time every day. Exposure to small amounts of nitrates or alcohol may trigger an acute attack during a cluster period.

PATHOGENESIS. The etiology of cluster headaches is not defined. Like other vascular headaches, they are presumed to develop from events that ultimately activate the trigeminovascular system. In the complete form of the disease, patients with cluster headache manifest pain referred to the 1st and 2nd trigeminal divisions, sympathetic dysfunction (Horner's syndrome), sympathetic activation (sweating of the forehead and face), and parasympathetic activation (lacrimation and nasal congestion). This constellation of symptoms and signs is best explained best by the presence of a single lesion at the point at which fibers from the ophthalmic and maxillary trigeminal division converge with projections from the superior cervical and sphenopalatine ganglia. This plexus is located within the cavernous sinus, and narrowing of the cavernous carotid artery has been observed in selected cases of cluster headache.

GENETICS. Genetic factors were not recognized as especially important in cluster headache until two separate groups recently reported an increased concordance of cluster headache in monozygotic twins. Moreover, studies of relatives of patients with cluster headache have found an increased frequency 13 times higher than expected by chance.

TREATMENT. During cluster headaches, oxygen inhalation (100%) delivered at a rate of 8 L/minute for 15 minutes through a loose-fitting face mask is a safe and effective treatment for acute attacks, particularly in patients younger than 50 years who have episodic cluster headaches. Patients who respond to oxygen usually do so within 10 minutes. Oxygen inhalation does not cause nausea and is not contraindicated in patients with coronary artery disease or peripheral vascular disease. Ergotamine tartrate, the classic treatment of cluster headache, is effective and well tolerated by many patients. Because of more rapid absorption, sublingual administration is generally preferred to oral administration. Intranasal dihydroergotamine reduces the severity of cluster headaches, but not their duration. Subcutaneous administration of sumatriptan (6 mg) is usually successful in alleviating acute cluster headaches and reduces both pain and conjunctival injection within 15 minutes in most patients. However, middle-aged males, who make up a large proportion of cluster headache sufferers, are at increased risk for coronary artery disease. Vasoconstrictive medications such as ergotamines and sumatriptan should be used with caution for cluster headache in such patients. Verapamil is often effective in cluster headache as a prophylactic agent. It has relatively few side effects when compared with other prophylactic agents. Another double-blind trial found it to be as effective as lithium. Prophylactic medication dosages are usually tapered and then discontinued within 3 to 6 weeks after recurrent cluster headaches cease. Ergotamine tartrate was for many years the only prophylactic agent used for cluster headache. It is effective and well tolerated in doses of 2 to 4 mg/day given either orally or by suppository. The ergot derivative methysergide is effective in about 70% of episodic cases. Retroperitoneal, pleural, or pericardial fibrosis is a severe potential side effect of long-term use. Patients with cluster headache usually require treatment for less than 2 to 3 months, so methysergide can

be used with more safety than in migraine. Lithium carbonate, which was effective in chronic cluster headache in over 20 open-label clinical trials, may also be beneficial in the episodic form of the disease. Because of the narrow range between toxic and therapeutic doses, it is important to monitor the serum lithium level 12 hours after the last dose. The usual therapeutic range is from 0.3 to 0.8 mmol/L, but low lithium levels may still be therapeutic. NSAIDs and thiazide diuretics may increase serum lithium levels. Average daily doses of lithium carbonate, from 600 to 900 mg, should be titrated according to the serum lithium level. Corticosteroids are frequently used to treat both the episodic and the chronic forms of cluster headache, even though evidence for their effectiveness is largely limited to open trials. Prednisone is frequently used in dosages of 60 to 80 mg/day for 1 week, followed by a taper in dosage over a period of 2 to 4 weeks.

TENSION-TYPE HEADACHE. Tension-type headache is the most common of the primary headache disorders, with a lifetime prevalence between 30 and 78%. Tension-type headaches are more common in females than in males and most often begin in the 2nd decade of life. In both sexes, the prevalence decreases with increasing age, and socioeconomic factors do not contribute to risk. Although no studies have been conducted in twins, genetic factors are not as prominent in the condition as in migraine or other headache syndromes.

PATHOPHYSIOLOGY. Tension-type headache is not well understood and defies a single or simple pathophysiologic explanation. In one model, headache pain is viewed as the sum of nociceptive input onto brain stem neurons from vascular structures, myofascial and muscular sources, and descending supraspinal modulation. The relative importance of these three factors varies among patients and among attacks in the same patient.

CLINICAL FEATURES. Tension-type headache occurs in episodic and chronic forms, which differ in their response to treatment and possibly in their pathophysiology. Pericranial muscle spasm or tenderness may or may not be present in either form. Episodic tension-type headache consists of recurrent attacks of tight, pressing (band-like), bilateral, mild to moderate head pain that last from minutes to days. Tension-type headaches do not worsen with routine physical exertion and are not associated with nausea, although photophobia or phonophobia may be present. In the chronic form, characteristic tension-type headaches occur at least 15 days per month.

TREATMENT. Episodic tension-type headaches usually respond to simple analgesics such as acetaminophen (650 to 1000 mg) or to NSAIDs such as aspirin (900 to 1000 mg), ketoprofen (12.5 to 50 mg), ibuprofen (200 to 800 mg), and naproxen (250 to 500 mg). More severe, episodic tension-type headaches may respond to higher doses of NSAIDs or to combination remedies that contain isometheptene mucate or butalbital. Frequent use of analgesics can increase the number of headaches, so caution is advised whenever analgesic use regularly exceeds three days per week. Chronic tension-type headaches occasionally require prophylactic treatment. Tricyclic antidepressants decrease both the frequency and the severity of attacks; amitriptyline is the drug of choice. Amitriptyline's use may be limited by sedation, dry mouth, or other anticholinergic side effects. To avoid these side effects, therapy should be started at low doses (10 mg) given at bedtime and increased slowly until either satisfactory improvement is achieved or intolerable side effects appear. Doxepin, maprotiline, and fluoxetine are other antidepressants that are sometimes effective in chronic tension-type headache.

CHRONIC DAILY HEADACHE. The term chronic daily headache may be applied to any headaches occurring more than 15 days per month for at least 1 month. By this definition the term includes several clinically distinct syndromes, including cluster headache, hemicrania continua, chronic paroxysmal hemicrania, and chronic tension-type headache. Chronic daily headache is often used more narrowly to include headaches that occur on a daily or almost daily basis (more than 4 days per week), have features of both migraine and tension-type headache, and are frequently but not always associated with overuse of analgesic medications. Patients meeting these criteria account for a major proportion of those seen in headache specialty clinics and are often the most difficult headache patients to treat. The typical patient with chronic daily headache is a woman in her 30s or 40s with a history of either episodic migraine or tension-type headache beginning in the teens or 20s. Over a period of months to years, the patient's headaches gradually increase in both severity and frequency to the point where consecutive headache-free days are rare. The headaches are often of two types. More frequent headaches are of mild to moderate intensity and have a pressure-like or mildly throbbing quality and mild photophobia or phonophobia but no associated nausea or vomiting. The duration of these milder headaches is variable and ranges from a couple of hours to constant (although waxing and waning). Superimposed are severe attacks that occur as frequently as three times per week and as infrequently as once or twice per month. The more severe attacks are usually, but not always throbbing and may be associated with nausea, photophobia, phonophobia, and sometimes vomiting. Severe attacks may be preceded by a migrainous aura. Quite often the patient exhibits features of depression or anxiety. Frequently the patient is taking one or more daily analgesics, sometimes in an effort to preempt a headache. Chronic daily headaches are referred to as *transformed migraine* when the migrainous component is prominent. When headaches begin without antecedent migraine or tension-type headache but with many features of tension-type headache, they are often labeled new daily persistent headaches. Chronic daily headache is often accompanied by other paroxysmal symptoms that are frequently as distressing as the head pain. These symptoms may include dizziness (both vertiginous and non-specific forms), tinnitus, extreme phonophobia, fluctuating fatigue or mood alteration, and feelings of depersonalization. It is unclear whether these symptoms are fragments of underlying migraine or a mood disorder. They often, but not always resolve with improvement in the headaches.

Medication overuse is the most common exacerbating factor in chronic daily headache, and withdrawal of the overused medication usually improves the condition. The medications most often overused include butalbital combinations, ergotamines, oral analgesics containing caffeine in combination with acetaminophen or NSAIDs, and opiate combinations. However, chronic daily headache may develop in the absence of medication, and it does not always improve after analgesic withdrawal.

LESS COMMON PRIMARY HEADACHE SYNDROMES. CHRONIC PAROXYSMAL HEMICRANIA. Chronic paroxysmal hemicrania is an uncommon syndrome with many features of cluster headache, including severe intensity, unilateral orbital/temporal location, and autonomic signs (e.g., conjunctival injection, tearing, rhinorrhea) ipsilateral to the pain. It is shorter in duration (5 to 20 minutes) than cluster headache and has a higher attack frequency (generally above five per day). The syndrome is more predominant in females and may be responsive to indomethacin (150 mg/day or less).

HEMICRANIA CONTINUA. Hemicrania continua is an unusual headache syndrome in which constant unilateral head pain of moderate to severe intensity underlies unprovoked brief episodes of sharp jabbing pain in a similar location.

BENIGN COUGH HEADACHE. Benign cough headache consists of severe bilateral head pain of sudden onset that follows coughing or other Valsalva maneuvers. It is a benign disorder that responds to indomethacin in about 90% of cases. However, the diagnosis of benign cough headache requires the exclusion of structural lesions with MRI because cough headache may sometimes result from posterior fossa tumors or the Arnold-Chiari malformation.

EXERTIONAL/ORGASMIC HEADACHE. In some individuals, exertion or various types of exercise may trigger bilateral throbbing or pressure-like headaches that persist for several minutes up to 48 hours. Headaches may also develop during sexual activity, including coitus and less frequently masturbation. These headaches usually begin with bilateral non-throbbing pain that escalates as sexual excitement increases and reaches a crescendo at orgasm. Both exertional and orgasmic headaches may occur in the absence of intracranial disorders; however, in rare cases, coital headache may be associated with unruptured cerebral aneurysms. The possibility of aneurysm should be excluded. Exertional headache can sometimes be prevented by ingestion of ergotamine or indomethacin before the planned exertion.

HYPNIC HEADACHES. Hypnic headaches constitute a rare primary headache syndrome of the elderly (mean age of onset, 60 years or older). Hypnic headaches, which persist for 15 to 60 minutes and typically awaken patients from sleep about the same time each night, are in some ways similar to cluster headaches. However, unlike cluster headache, hypnic headaches are more diffuse, are often bilateral and throbbing, and are not associated with the autonomic symptoms of cluster headache. The differential diagnosis includes temporal arteritis and mass lesions. After exclusion of organic disease with an imaging study and erythrocyte sedimentation rate (ESR), treatment with low-dose lithium (30 mg every night) or caffeine may induce remission. If headaches return, careful titration of the dosage upward may be necessary. Lithium should be used with caution in older patients, especially in the presence of dehydration, renal disease, and diuretic or NSAID therapy.

SECONDARY HEADACHE DISORDERS

Headache may be the initial complaint in a host of central nervous system and systemic abnormalities (see Table 454–1 for the differential diagnosis of secondary headache disorders). Many of the disorders are given detailed consideration in other chapters. However, a few of the most prominent abnormalities that may result in chronic headache are discussed briefly.

GIANT CELL ARTERITIS. Giant cell arteritis (temporal arteritis) is an inflammatory vasculitis involving branches of the temporal arteries. It most often affects individuals older than 60 years and can result in rapid and permanent loss of vision secondary to granulomatous occlusion of the posterior ciliary or central retinal arteries. Features suggestive of temporal arteritis include (1) orbital or frontotemporal head pain described as dull and constant with superimposed jabbing sensations; (2) aggravation of pain by cold temperatures; (3) pain in the jaw or tongue pain upon chewing (jaw

---

Table 454–1 ■ SECONDARY HEADACHE DISORDERS

Headaches Associated with Cranial Vascular Abnormalities
Subarachnoid hemorrhage
Intracerebral, epidural, and subdural hematoma
Unruptured vascular malformation
   Arteriovenous malformation
   Saccular aneurysm
Carotid or vertebral artery dissection
Carotidynia
Cerebral intra-arterial occlusion
Venous thrombosis
Arterial hypertension
Headaches Associated with Non-vascular Intracranial Disorders
Intracranial neoplasms
High- and low-pressure headaches
Inflammatory disorders
   Temporal (giant cell) arteritis
   Tolosa-Hunt syndrome
   Intracranial sarcoidosis
Intracranial infection
   Acute meningitis
   Meningoencephalitis
   Brain abscess
Headaches Associated with Systemic Abnormalities
Systemic infection, viral, bacterial, treponemal, etc.
Substance-induced headaches, exposure and withdrawal
Metabolic disturbance
   Hypoxia, altitude sickness, sleep apnea
   Hypercapnia
   Hypoglycemia
   Dialysis
Head and Facial Pain Associated with Disorders of Cranial Nerves
Neuralgias
   Trigeminal neuralgia
   Glossopharyngeal neuralgia
   Occipital neuralgia
Herpes zoster
Head and Facial Pain Associated with Disorders of Other Cranial Structures
Glaucoma
Sinusitis
Temporomandibular joint disease
Dental pain
Neck abnormalities

claudication); (4) accompanying constitutional or musculoskeletal symptoms such as weight loss, anemia, and polymyalgia rheumatica; (5) elevated liver function tests; and (6) decreased visual acuity, visual field cuts, pale or swollen optic disk, retinal splinter hemorrhages (anterior ischemic neuropathy) or a pale retina, and cherry-red spot (central retinal artery infarction).

The ESR, which should be measured in all suspected patients, is elevated in 95% of cases. Definitive diagnosis is made by biopsy of the temporal artery, which can be obtained within 48 hours after initiation of treatment with steroids. When the diagnosis is suspected, prompt treatment with corticosteroids is necessary to avoid visual loss, which often becomes bilateral (75% of cases) after unilateral loss.

TREATMENT. In patients with an elevated ESR, intravenous methylprednisolone, 500 to 1000 mg every 12 hours for 48 hours, should be followed by oral prednisone, 80 to 100 mg/day for 14 to 21 days, with a gradual taper over 12 to 24 months. The tapering rate should be guided by serial ESR measurements.

SUBSTANCE-INDUCED HEADACHES. Headaches may occur with acute exposure or as a result of withdrawal from many types of substances (Table 454–2).

HEADACHES ASSOCIATED WITH INCREASED INTRACRANIAL PRESSURE. Headache may occur when an alteration in intracranial pressure causes compression or traction on pain-sensitive vascular, meningeal, or neural structures in the apex or base of the brain. Most commonly, these headaches are bilateral and frontotemporal, although their location is variable. Causes of elevated intracranial pressure include mass lesion, blockage of cerebrospinal fluid (CSF) circulation, hemorrhage, hypertensive encephalopathy, venous sinus thrombosis, hyperadrenalism or hypoadrenalism, altitude sickness, tetracycline, and vitamin A intoxication. In most instances, the source of the headache and raised pressure are identifiable. Treatment of the underlying condition generally improves the headache.

INTRACRANIAL TUMOR. One of the most common concerns of patients seeking evaluation of chronic headaches is that their headache represents a space-occupying lesion such as a tumor or large vascular abnormality. Fortunately, the overwhelming majority of chronic headaches do not arise from a tumor or other structural lesion. Headaches in brain tumor patients are usually dull and bifrontal, although they tend to be worse on the side of the tumor. They are more often qualitatively similar to tension-type headache than to migraine and tend to be intermittent and of moderate intensity. They are accompanied by nausea about half the time and are usually resistant to common analgesics. "Classic" brain tumor headache (i.e., progressive and beginning in the morning) is not typical. Factors that should increase suspicion of an intracranial tumor include papilledema, new neurologic deficits, initial attack of prolonged headache occurring after the age of 45, previous malignancy, cognitive abnormality, or altered mental status.

IDIOPATHIC INTRACRANIAL HYPERTENSION. Idiopathic intracranial hypertension (pseudotumor cerebri) is a syndrome composed of headache, papilledema, and transient visual symptoms that occur in the absence of CSF abnormalities, except for elevated intracranial pressure. The syndrome is not associated with hydrocephalus or

another identifiable cause. In adults, females have an 8 to 10 times higher incidence than males. The prototypic patient is an overweight woman of childbearing age. The diagnosis is made by lumbar puncture (CSF pressure, >250 mm Hg; normal CSF composition) after excluding a mass lesion by neuroimaging. Visual field testing often reveals an enlarged blind spot. Spontaneous recovery may eventually occur, but treatment to reduce intracranial pressure is usually indicated to prevent visual loss. Simple measures such as weight reduction should be attempted whenever appropriate. Drug therapies are usually attempted next and include medications such as acetazolamide and furosemide, which are aimed primarily at reducing CSF production. Furosemide, a potent loop diuretic, must be given with potassium supplementation and may cause hypotension. If drug treatment is ineffective, repeated lumbar punctures may sometimes be useful, although frequent lumbar puncture is not without a risk of complications such as post–lumbar puncture headache, spinal epidermoid tumor, or infection. If other treatments fail, surgical options include optic nerve fenestration and ventricular-peritoneal shunting of CSF.

HEADACHE ASSOCIATED WITH DECREASED INTRACRANIAL PRESSURE. Decreased intracranial pressure (below 50 to 90 mm H_2O) (usually caused by a decrease in CSF volume) is commonly associated with dull, throbbing, sometimes severe headaches that are probably caused by reduced brain buoyancy and subsequent traction on pain-sensitive meningeal and vascular structures.

Low-pressure headaches often become more intense upon standing or sitting upright and may be relieved by lying down. They may be accompanied by dizziness, visual symptoms, photophobia, nausea, vomiting, and diaphoresis. Although low-pressure headaches may begin spontaneously, they most commonly follow lumbar puncture. Other possible etiologies include intracranial surgery, ventricular shunting, trauma, and various systemic medical conditions such as severe dehydration, post-dialysis status, diabetic coma, uremia, or hyperpnea. If the headache is prolonged, the possibility of a persistent CSF leak may be investigated by radioisotope cisternography or computed tomographic myelography. Post–lumbar puncture headaches can be caused by excessive leakage of CSF through a dural tear caused by the lumbar puncture needle. Headaches follow 10 to 30% of lumbar punctures and occur twice as frequently in women as in men. The headache may begin minutes to several days after the lumbar puncture and can persist up to 2 weeks. Treatment strategies include corticosteroids, oral fluid or salt intake, intravenous fluids, CO_2 inhalation, and methylxanthines such as theophylline (300 mg three times per day), caffeine (500 mg intravenously), or intrathecal autologous blood patch.

HEAD AND FACIAL PAIN ASSOCIATED WITH DISORDERS OF CRANIAL NERVES

Trigeminal neuralgia, also known as *tic douloureux*, usually occurs in older patients. The sharp, often electric shock–like pain of trigeminal neuralgia occurs in a rapid series of jabs (lasting seconds to minutes) in one or more division of the trigeminal nerve. The volleys of jabbing may be provoked by stimulation of areas on the face quite discrete from the site of pain and are usually followed by brief refractory periods. When trigeminal neuralgia occurs in persons younger than 40 years, a specific cause can often be found, such as demyelination (multiple sclerosis, especially when bilateral) and compression by vascular abnormalities or tumors (myeloma, metastatic carcinoma, cholesteatoma, chordoma, acoustic neuromas, trigeminal neuromas). In the elderly, trigeminal neuralgia has a prevalence of 155 per million and a female-to-male ratio of 3:2. Among older individuals with trigeminal neuralgia, microvascular compression of the trigeminal nerve root is often present. Because of the association with structural lesions (demyelinative or neoplastic), the initial work-up should include MRI studies, which detail the cerebellopontine angle and the entry foramen (V_I superior orbital fissure, V_{II} foramen rotundum, V_{III} foramen ovale). In the absence of a structural cause, treatment usually consists of administering drugs such as carbamazepine (400 to 1200 mg), valproate (500 to 1500 mg), phenytoin (200 to 500 mg), baclofen (40 to 80 mg), or clonazepam (2 to 6 mg). Therapy with any of these agents must be initiated slowly.

Table 454–2 ■ SUBSTANCES INDUCING HEADACHE

After Acute Exposure

Alcohol	Indomethacin
Amphotericin B	Monosodium glutamate
Azithromycin	Nifedipine
Carbon monoxide	Nitrates/nitrites
Cimetidine	Ondansetron
Cocaine/crack	Phenylethylamine
Danazol	Ranitidine
Diclofenac	Reserpine
Dipyridamole	Tyramine
Estrogen/birth control pills	Timolol ophthalmic drops
Fluconazole	Verapamil

Following Withdrawl after Chronic Use

Alcohol
Barbiturates
Caffeine
Ergotamine
Opiate analgesics

Glossopharyngeal neuralgia is characterized by paroxysmal pain within the distribution of the vagus and glossopharyngeal nerves. The pain is paroxysmal, unilateral, and sudden in onset and has a jabbing or briefly persistent (square wave) quality. The pain is most often felt in or around the ear, tongue, jaw, or larynx and can be triggered by swallowing, talking, chewing, clearing the throat, yawning, or tasting spicy food or cold liquids. Although pain is usually followed by a brief refractory period, attacks may occur over 20 times per day and may awaken sufferers from sleep. The intermittent pain may be superimposed on a dull, constant pain in the same area. Rarely, the pain of glossopharyngeal neuralgia is followed by bradycardia, syncope, or asystole, presumably resulting from the intense glossopharyngeal outflow and vagal efferent discharge. The usual cause of glossopharyngeal neuralgia appears to be microvascular compression, although abscess and tumor are sometimes associated. Medical treatment is similar to that for trigeminal neuralgia and includes slow introduction of carbamazepine (400 to 1200 mg) or baclofen (40 to 80 mg).

International Headache Society, Headache Classification Committee: Classification and diagnostic criteria for headache disorders, cranial neuralgias and facial pain. Cephalalgia 8(Suppl. 7):1, 1988. *Systematic classification of headache disorder.*

Olesen J, Tfelt-Hansen P, Welch KMA (eds): The Headaches. New York, Raven Press, 1993. *A multiauthored comprehensive text covering the basic and clinical aspects of all headache syndromes.*

Silberstein D, Goadsby PJ (eds): Headache. Boston, Butterworth-Heinemann, 1997. *A series of in-depth summaries of various primary and secondary headache syndromes.*

455 OTHER SPECIFIC PAIN SYNDROMES

Michael C. Rowbotham

THE TRANSITION FROM ACUTE TO CHRONIC PAIN. Although trauma, infection, inflammation, and tissue degeneration severe enough to cause acute pain are universal experiences, only a small minority of acute pains evolve into severe, unremitting, and disabling chronic pain. For example, about 2 to 5% of traumatic peripheral nerve injuries persist as severe neuropathic pain, and 10% of cases of acute herpes zoster go on to become established post-herpetic neuralgia.

The factors determining which acute pains become chronic remain incompletely understood. These factors can be grouped into four categories: persistent tissue-damaging disease, abnormal function of the nervous system, damage to the nervous system, and psychological factors. Chronic pain is to be expected when tissue destruction and inflammation are ongoing. In this situation, the nervous system is serving its normal function of signaling pain in response to tissue injury. Chronic pain caused by abnormal function of the nervous system is exemplified by disorders such as complex regional pain syndrome, type I (CRPS I, formerly called reflex sympathetic dystrophy). In this disorder, sensory nerves may be abnormally sensitive to their usual stimuli and also generate impulses in response to sympathetic nervous system activity. Furthermore, the central nervous system responds in a pathologically amplified manner to all sensory input from the region, no matter how it was generated. Damage to the nervous system promotes pain persistence in two ways. Chronically injured peripheral nerves may spontaneously generate impulses that are perceived as dysesthetic or painful. In addition, deafferentation causes reorganization within the central nervous system leading to hyperactivity in some central nervous system neurons and abnormal response patterns in others. Psychological factors, depression, disability compensation, and litigation may be suspected as the primary etiology in some patients with chronic pain. Such factors may explain a substantial proportion of pain severity, pain persistence, and failure to respond

to therapy. However, malingering, factitious disorders, and severe somatoform disorders are seldom the reason for complaints of chronic pain when no other etiology can be proved.

The above-described factors underlying the transition from acute to chronic pain have been verified from detailed longitudinal studies of acute herpes zoster. Herpes zoster most often strikes healthy elderly individuals and is extremely painful in a high percentage of patients. Age, severity of acute zoster pain, number of skin lesions, rash location, extent of peripheral sensory nerve injury, and specific psychosocial variables all emerge as independent factors predicting pain persistence in the form of post-herpetic neuralgia. The elderly may be more likely to suffer from post-herpetic neuralgia because of slower resolution of zoster-associated inflammation, greater tissue destruction, and enhanced susceptibility to permanent neural injury.

POST-HERPETIC NEURALGIA. Acute herpes zoster, or "shingles," represents recrudescence of the varicella-zoster virus. Herpes zoster may be sufficiently painful to be adequately controlled only by regional local anesthetic blockade and parenteral medications. The cutaneous rash is not the only source of herpes zoster pain; the intense inflammation and destruction of the peripheral nerve apparatus and surrounding tissues from the nerve root to the skin are also responsible for pain in patients with herpes zoster.

Post-herpetic neuralgia is defined by the persistence of pain after new lesions have ceased and healing of the skin is complete. A useful definition of post-herpetic neuralgia requires persistence of pain for 3 months after skin healing because pain resolves slowly in many patients as inflammation subsides and as tissues heal in the initial few months after final crusting of the skin lesions. Once the pain has persisted for a year, spontaneous remission from post-herpetic neuralgia pain is very unlikely. Over 1 million new cases of herpes zoster occur each year; the prevalence of post-herpetic neuralgia in the United States is about 200,000. The chronic pain of post-herpetic neuralgia probably involves a variety of pain mechanisms, including persistent "irritability" of sensory nerve fibers and deafferentation-induced changes in the central nervous system.

Patients with post-herpetic neuralgia collectively describe three components to their discomfort: (1) a *constant*, deep, aching, bruised, or burning sensation; (2) a spontaneous, recurrent, *lancinating*, shooting, or electric shock–like pain; and (3) an *allodynic* (pain from a usually non-painful stimulus), superficial, sharp, radiating, burning, tender, dysesthetic, or "itch"-like sensation evoked by wearing clothing or by gentle touch. Nearly all patients with post-herpetic neuralgia describe constant pain, and 90% will describe allodynia. Lancinating pain tends to fade over the initial year after herpes zoster. Pathologically, although the viral reactivation affects only a single dorsal root ganglion and dermatome, the area of pain and allodynia to gentle touch may cover a much larger band of skin.

The essence of established post-herpetic neuralgia is the chronicity of the pain and its resistance to therapy. Because the syndrome is common, strikes frequently in the healthy elderly population, and has a relatively stereotyped symptom complex, many clinical trials of new therapies for chronic neuropathic pain have been carried out in the post-herpetic neuralgia population. Double-blind controlled trials have provided evidence of efficacy for topical agents in the form of capsaicin cream and local anesthetic patches, oral opioids, tricyclic antidepressants, and the anticonvulsant medication gabapentin. The majority of patients will require more than one type of medication to adequately control their pain. A minority are refractory to all currently available medications. Neurolytic nerve blocks and destructive surgical approaches rarely provide long-term relief. Spinal stimulation and intrathecal medication pumps are occasionally indicated but require expert multidisciplinary evaluation.

COMPLEX REGIONAL PAIN SYNDROME (REFLEX SYMPATHETIC DYSTROPHY AND CAUSALGIA). CRPS has two forms, CRPS I and CRPS II. CRPS I replaces the term reflex sympathetic dystrophy and describes a pain syndrome that usually develops after an initiating noxious event, is not limited to the distribution of a single peripheral nerve, and is apparently disproportional to the inciting event. CRPS I is associated at some point with evidence of edema, changes in skin blood flow, abnormal sweating (sudomotor activity) in the region of the pain, and (or) allodynia or hyperalgesia. The affected site is usually the distal aspect of an extremity with a distal-to-proximal gradient. CRPS II (formerly causalgia) is the same syndrome in patients with demonstrable peripheral nerve injury. The name change was intended to reduce misunderstanding about the etiology and treatment of these disorders. Reflex sympathetic dystrophy as a diagnostic label was flawed because it implied that the problem was a reflexive response to an insult. Not all patients have dystrophy, and a few have dystrophy but no pain. Inclusion of the word "sympathetic" suggested that the sympathetic nervous system caused the pain and implied by extension that sympathetic blockade would relieve the pain. Although animal and some human studies suggest that CRPS I and II are disorders of augmented adrenergic responsiveness in peripheral tissues rather than abnormally increased sympathetic efferent activity, many patients who meet the definition of CRPS do not experience pain relief from blockade of the sympathetic nervous system. In addition, sympathetic blocks may relieve pain through actions unrelated to sympathetic efferents because the available techniques for blocking the sympathetic nervous system are not fully selective. For example, local anesthetic blocks of the sympathetic chain may also relieve pain by spread to sensory nerves, by systemic redistribution of local anesthetic, and by placebo effects.

Symptoms of CRPS may begin gradually in the days or weeks after an injury or may be manifested within a few hours. In unusual cases, the full syndrome occurs only after conservative treatment of a traumatic injury fails and more invasive procedures commence. The disorder has been described to progress in stages, each of which were originally thought to last 3 to 6 months. Stage I, the "acute" stage, is heralded by pain that seems more severe than usually caused by the initial injury, has a prominent burning or aching component, and is increased by dependency of the affected part, any physical contact, or emotional upset. Protection of the affected area, often with pronounced reluctance to mobilize it, is an early and obvious feature. Edema, warmth or coolness, and increased hair and nail growth may be apparent. Subtle bony changes may be present on radiographs. Stage II, the "dystrophic" stage, is notable for a change from edema to induration, cool hyperhidrotic skin, and livedo reticularis or cyanosis. Hair loss and ridged, cracked, or brittle nails may be apparent. Diffuse osteoporosis or periarticular demineralization may be visible on radiographs. Bone scans typically show increased uptake when physical manifestations of this severity are present. Magnetic resonance imaging (MRI) is probably more sensitive than either x-ray or radionuclide studies and demonstrates bone marrow abnormalities consistent with CRPS. In addition, MRI of the painful area may uncover a reversible and previously unrecognized source for the continuing pain, such as a ligamentous tear in a wrist joint. Stage III, the "atrophic" stage, is associated with proximal spread of pain and irreversible tissue damage. The skin is thin and shiny, digits are wasted, and flexion or Dupuytren's contractures may occur. Radiographs are invariably abnormal, often with ankylosis.

In practice, the above progression does not always occur. Some patients may progress rapidly to stage III, whereas others may have long-standing pain but only mild visible manifestations. Recognizing a patient in stage II or stage III is not difficult, but by this point nearly all will suffer long-term dysfunction even with aggressive treatment. When the physical examination is minimally abnormal, diagnostic assessment requires special care. Some patients with CRPS have the full range of physical findings early in the course of the disorder, but with therapy the tissue abnormalities resolve even though pain continues. These patients should be considered to have a "residual" form of CRPS that is relatively unresponsive to further treatment. Other patients have never had physical findings unequivocally supportive of CRPS but had been labeled as suffering from CRPS only because no other explanation for the pain could be found.

What constitutes appropriate treatment for CRPS is not agreed upon. The treating physician should recognize that CRPS is a syndrome, not an independent disease entity, and that a reversible cause (usually orthopedic) for continuing symptoms can occasionally be found. Unlike post-herpetic neuralgia, few well-designed, prospective, controlled clinical trials have studied any therapy for

CRPS. Overall, treatment outcomes are disappointing, with a high burden of continuing symptoms and disability. Extremely aggressive and invasive therapies should be avoided in favor of a conservative, multidisciplinary approach that combines physical therapy, medication management, individual and group counseling and education, and judicious use of local anesthetic nerve blocks. Surgical sympathectomy and other destructive procedures are seldom of long-term benefit, especially after more than 2 years of symptoms. Techniques using intrathecal pumps and spinal stimulators require expert multidisciplinary consultation, a thorough diagnostic evaluation for a reversible disorder that could be maintaining the pain, and an adequate trial of more conservative therapies.

FIBROMYALGIA SYNDROME AND MYOFASCIAL PAIN SYNDROME. Fibromyalgia syndrome has an estimated overall population prevalence as high as 1%. It remains an etiologic enigma. The current American College of Rheumatology classification for fibromyalgia syndrome requires widespread pain on both sides of the body and pain both above and below the waist. Pain must be present for at least 3 months. Examination for tender points should be positive in at least 11 of the 18 recognized sites. No specific laboratory abnormalities are seen. More than 75% of patients also complain of symptoms such as morning stiffness, chronic fatigue, and sleep disturbance. The disorder is most common in women in their 3rd to 5th decades.

Hypotheses about the etiology of fibromyalgia syndrome are varied. Evidence of abnormal muscle histology, metabolism, strength, and function is inconsistent. Studies of substance P levels, serotonin, growth factors, N-methyl-D-aspartate receptors, and experimental pain models have led other investigators to question whether general hypersensitivity of the central nervous system is the primary problem. Neuroendocrine studies have attempted to link symptoms of fibromyalgia syndrome with abnormal physiologic responses to stress.

Current therapy includes non-pharmacologic approaches such as exercise-based programs and cognitive-behavioral therapies. Both tricyclic and selective serotonin reuptake inhibitor–type antidepressants have proved beneficial in clinical trials. Prednisone is not effective, and limited prospective trials of opioids have not convincingly shown improvements in either pain or function. Anxiolytics combined with non-steroidal anti-inflammatory drugs have limited evidence in their favor. Of note is the diminishing effect of active medications versus placebo in trials lasting up to 6 months.

Myofascial pain syndromes are very common. Some authors use the term to refer to patients with widespread pain of unknown etiology, thus blurring distinction from fibromyalgia syndrome. The term is better used to refer to regional musculoskeletal pain disorders. Many represent a chronic phase of sports or overuse injuries, and associated but subtle joint or ligamentous degeneration may be present concomitantly. Physical examination should demonstrate trigger points that reproduce the ongoing pain complaint. Treatment should begin with a physical therapy approach that improves functional mechanics, prevents reinjury, provides general and regional reconditioning, and non-invasively treats trigger points. Medications and trigger point injections should be considered adjuncts. Some experts believe that opioids, anxiolytics, and muscle relaxants should be completely avoided.

Backonja M, Beydoun A, Edwards KR, et al: Gabapentin for the symptomatic treatment of painful neuropathy in patients with diabetes mellitus: A randomized controlled trial. JAMA 280:1831, 1998.

Fields HL: Pain. New York, McGraw-Hill, 1986.

McCain GA: Fibromyalgia and myofascial pain syndromes. In Wall PD, Melzack R (eds): Textbook of Pain. Edinburgh, Churchill Livingstone, 1994, pp 475–491.

Perl ER: Causalgia and reflex sympathetic dystrophy revisited. In Boivie J, Hansson P, Lindblom U (eds): Touch, Temperature, and Pain in Health and Disease. Progress in Pain Research and Management, vol 3. Seattle, IASP Press, 1994, pp 231–248.

Rowbotham M, Harden N, Stacey B, et al: Gabapentin for the treatment of postherpetic neuralgia: A randomized controlled trial. JAMA 280:1837, 1998.

Veldman PH, Reynen HM, Arntz IE, Goris RJ: Signs and symptoms of reflex sympathetic dystrophy: Prospective study of 829 patients. Lancet 342:1012, 1993.

Watson CPN (ed): Herpes Zoster and Postherpetic Neuralgia. Amsterdam, Elsevier, 1993.

■ DEVELOPMENTAL DISORDERS

456 NEUROCUTANEOUS SYNDROMES

A. James Barkovich ■ Ruben I. Kuzniecky

The neurocutaneous syndromes are congenital disorders characterized by dysplastic and neoplastic lesions primarily involving the nervous system and skin. Of the more than 40 syndromes involving abnormalities that can be characterized under this topic, the most important are neurofibromatosis, tuberous sclerosis, and Sturge-Weber and von Hippel-Lindau syndromes.

NEUROFIBROMATOSIS TYPE 1. Neurofibromatosis encompasses a wide spectrum of syndromes with neurocutaneous lesions. Although at least eight variants have been described, only two are well-recognized, genetically distinct entities: NF-1 and NF-2. NF-1 corresponds to the classic disorder described by von Recklinghausen, with a prevalence of 1 in 3000 births. Although it is an autosomal dominant disease, approximately 50% of cases are clinically sporadic with a high mutation rate.

PATHOLOGY AND PATHOGENESIS. Neurologically important lesions in neurofibromatosis include neurofibromas, plexiform neurofibromas, optic nerve gliomas, and astrocytomas of the brain and spinal cord. Hamartomas and meningiomas may also develop.

Molecular genetic studies have demonstrated that the majority of mutations in NF-1 occur in the parental germline. The NF-1 gene is located on chromosome 17q and encompasses about 350 kilobases of genomic DNA that expresses a protein designated as neurofibromin. Neurofibromin appears to be expressed in most tissues and functions as a tumor suppressor compound. Although pathogenic mutations in NF-1 are identified in approximately 75% of clinical cases, there does not appear to be any correlation between particular genotypes and phenotypes.

CLINICAL MANIFESTATIONS. Although NF-1 is a congenital disease, most manifestations appear during childhood and adult life. Clinical criteria for the diagnosis include (1) six or more café au lait macules larger than 5 mm in pre-pubescent patients and more than 15 mm in post-pubescent individuals, (2) two or more neurofibromas of any type or one plexiform neurofibroma, (3) axillary or inguinal freckling, (4) sphenoid bone dysplasia, (5) optic glioma, (6) Lisch nodules (iris hamartomas), and (7) a family history of NF-1. The diagnosis is made when at least two or more of the above criteria are present. Other manifestations may include learning difficulties, epilepsy, and mental retardation. Important complications may include scoliosis, gastrointestinal neurofibromas, pheochromocytomas, and renal artery stenosis.

DIAGNOSIS. The diagnosis is based on clinical criteria, sometimes supplemented by neuroimaging findings such as cerebellar, basal ganglia, and brain stem hamartomas, optic pathway gliomas, vascular dysplasia, and nerve sheath tumors.

TREATMENT AND PROGNOSIS. The majority of patients with NF-1 do not require treatment. Subcutaneous neurofibromas may be painful or disfiguring and can be excised surgically. Intraspinal and intracranial tumors are approached surgically. Optic nerve gliomas may be treated with radiation, but treatment may not affect the outcome. Brain imaging studies may be indicated in individual patients according to the clinical situation. Genetic counseling is important and must be provided to all patients and families in whom NF-1 is present.

NEUROFIBROMATOSIS TYPE 2. NF-2, or central neurofibromatosis, is an autosomal dominant syndrome with high penetrance. The prevalence of this disorder is much less lower than that of NF-1, with approximately 1 in 50,000 individuals having the disorder.

PATHOLOGY AND PATHOGENESIS. The classic pathologic abnormality in NF-2 is bilateral 8th nerve schwannomas. However, multiple meningiomas and multiple other schwannomas are also common features of NF-2. In addition, spinal cord ependymomas, meningioangiomatosis, and cerebral microhamartomas can occur.

NF-2 differs from NF-1 in its molecular genetics. The NF-2 gene is located on chromosome 22q. The gene product (merlin) is a cytoskeletal protein. The precise function of this protein is not known.

CLINICAL MANIFESTATIONS. Although skin lesions may be present in up to 30% of patients with NF-2, the diagnosis is based on the presence of the following criteria: (1) bilateral 8th nerve schwannomas detected by MRI; or (2) unilateral 8th nerve schwannoma, either first-degree relative with NF-2 or multiple meningiomas, and either neurofibroma, other schwannoma, glioma, or juvenile subcapsular lenticular opacity.

The mean age of onset of symptoms in patients with NF-2 is approximately 22 years. Cutaneous lesions such as café au lait macules and neurofibromas can be seen in up to 70% of cases, and approximately 40% of cases have cataracts, often evident in childhood.

TREATMENT AND PROGNOSIS. Treatment is related to the complications of the illness. Surgical treatment may be indicated in patients with intramedullary spinal tumors. Surgical treatment of schwannomas and meningiomas may be indicated in patients with compression of adjacent structures. Family members should be screened regularly with hearing tests and contrast-enhanced MRI. Genetic counseling should be provided to affected families.

TUBEROUS SCLEROSIS. Tuberous sclerosis complex is a genetic disease with hamartomatous lesions involving multiple organs at different stages in the course of the disease. The disease may occur as a familial autosomal dominant syndrome or in sporadic form with a high rate of spontaneous mutations. The incidence of this disorder is 1 in 10,000 to 50,000.

PATHOLOGY AND PATHOGENESIS. Tuberous sclerosis complex affects tissues from different germ layers. Cutaneous and visceral lesions, including adenoma sebaceum, cardiac rhabdomyomas, and renal angiomyolipomas may occur. The central nervous system (CNS) lesions seen in this disorder include hamartomas of the cortex, hamartomas of the ventricular walls, and subependymal giant cell tumors, which typically develop in the vicinity of the foramina of Monro.

Molecular genetic studies have defined at least two loci for tuberous sclerosis complex. In TSC-1 the abnormality is localized on chromosome 9q34, but the nature of the gene remains unclear. In TSC-2 the gene abnormalities are on chromosome 16p. This gene encodes tuberin, a guanosinetriphosphatase-activating protein. The specific function of this protein is not known. New mutations are frequent.

CLINICAL MANIFESTATIONS. The classic clinical criteria for diagnosis include mental subnormality, epilepsy, and skin lesions. However, refined criteria for diagnosis have been established and include primary criteria such as hypomelanotic skin macules (ash leaf spots, sometimes visible at birth), shagreen patches, facial angiofibromas and subungual fibromas, and imaging evidence of multiple calcified subependymal nodules, cortical tubers, or multiple retinal astrocytomas. Neurologic manifestations clinically apparent in most patients are seizures and mental retardation. Retinal hamartomas can be seen ophthalmoscopically in about half of the patients.

Diagnosis of this condition is usually clinical and confirmed by identification of calcified or uncalcified hamartomas on imaging studies.

TREATMENT AND PROGNOSIS. Treatment is directed at the complications of the disease, in particular, epilepsy. The degree of MRI-based abnormalities may correlate with the degree of neurologic disability. Neurosurgical intervention may be indicated for epilepsy under certain circumstances and for symptomatic treatment of complications such as hydrocephalus. Serial cardiac and renal ultrasound may be indicated in some patients. Because the disorder is autosomal dominant, genetic counseling is of paramount importance in familial cases.

STURGE-WEBER SYNDROME. Sturge-Weber syndrome is a sporadic, non-inherited abnormality, even though a few familial cases have been reported. The true incidence and prevalence of this disorder is poorly established, although reports have indicated that it occurs in fewer than 5 in 100,000 births.

The hallmark of this disorder is the presence of a capillary angiomatosis of the pia mater. Associated cerebral cortical calcifications are usually seen in a pericapillary distribution and are progressive.

CLINICAL MANIFESTATIONS. The hallmark of this disorder includes the presence of facial vascular nevi (port-wine stain), epilepsy, cognitive deficits, and less frequently, hemiparesis or hemiplegia, hemianopia, or glaucoma. The majority of patients have epilepsy, and there appears to be a correlation between the degree of epilepsy, the developmental status, and the presence of hemiparesis. However, seizures never develop in some patients with Sturge-Weber syndrome. A forme fruste of the syndrome has also been described without the usual skin lesion.

DIAGNOSIS. The diagnosis is usually made in the presence of a facial nevus and imaging confirmation of intracranial pathology. MRI with contrast may be indicated in some patients, particularly in those with the forme fruste of the disorder and those in whom surgery is contemplated. Although in most cases the intracranial lesion is ipsilateral to the facial nevus, contralateral and bilateral lesions have been described.

TREATMENT. Treatment is aimed at the epilepsy in most cases. Surgical excision of epileptogenic areas corresponding to the abnormality has been successful in some individuals. When the disorder is characterized by early intractable epilepsy and infantile hemiplegia, hemispherectomy can improve both seizures and neurodevelopmental outcome.

VON HIPPEL-LINDAU DISEASE (CNS ANGIOMATOSIS). von Hippel-Lindau disease is an autosomal dominant disorder caused by a defective tumor suppressor gene at chromosome 3p25-p26 and characterized by retinal angiomas, brain and spinal cord hemangioblastomas, renal cell carcinomas, endolymphatic sac tumors, pheochromocytomas, papillary cystadenomas of the epididymis, angiomas of the liver and kidney, and cysts of the pancreas, kidney, liver, and epididymis. Both sexes are affected equally. The diagnosis is established if patients have more than one CNS hemangioblastoma, one hemangioblastoma with a visceral manifestation of the disease, or one manifestation of the disease and a known family history.

CLINICAL MANIFESTATIONS. Symptoms typically begin during the 3rd or 4th decade. Retinal inflammation with exudate, hemorrhage, and retinal detachment from the retinal angiomas typically antedates the cerebellar complaints, but this order is not constant. Moreover, the ocular findings are non-specific and the retinal detachment may mask the underlying lesion. Headache, vertigo, and vomiting result from the cerebellar tumor. Other findings such as dysdiadochokinesia, dysmetria, and Romberg's sign are common. It is rare for patients to be initially seen with symptoms of spinal cord or visceral lesions. Rarely, patients may have hearing loss from tumors of the endolymphatic sac.

TREATMENT AND PROGNOSIS. Treatment is symptomatic. Retinal detachments and tumors are treated by laser therapy. Large brain tumors, renal cell carcinomas, pheochromocytomas, epididymal tumors, and endolymphatic sac tumors are treated surgically; smaller CNS tumors may be treated by gamma knife. A high index of suspicion and repeated imaging studies are necessary to detect the tumors before they metastasize or become unresectable.

Short M, Richardson E, Haines J, Kwiatowski D: Clinical, neuropathological and genetic aspects of the tuberous sclerosis complex. Brain Pathol 5:173, 1995. *A thorough, up-to-date overview of the tuberous sclerosis complex.*

Von Deimling A, Krone W, Menon A: Neurofibromatosis type 1: Pathology, clinical features and molecular genetics. Brain Pathol 5:153, 1995. *A thorough, up-to-date overview of the disease.*

457 MALFORMATIONS OF CORTICAL DEVELOPMENT

A. James Barkovich ■ *Ruben I. Kuzniecky*

Malformations of cerebral cortical development are a heterogeneous group, all resulting from disturbed development of cells that normally participate in formation of the cerebral cortex. The known causes include intrauterine infection, intrauterine ischemia, and chromosomal mutations. When small areas of the brain are involved, epilepsy typically develops in the 1st or 2nd decade, and patients have minor static neurologic dysfunction and normal intellect. Those with involvement of larger areas of the brain often have mental retardation and more severe neurologic dysfunction in addition to epilepsy. The diagnosis is established by magnetic resonance imaging (MRI), which can identify most of the groups. We will describe the most common malformations in each group.

FOCAL CORTICAL DYSPLASIA. Focal cortical dysplasia is caused by abnormal neuronal and glial proliferation. It is characterized by the histologic features of cortical dyslamination, neuronomegaly, and dysplastic "balloon cells." Affected patients often have intractable partial epilepsy that correlates with the anatomic location of the lesion. If extensive regions of the brain are involved, patients may have neurologic impairment such as mental subnormality and hemiparesis. The diagnosis can be made with cranial MRI by detecting focal abnormal gyral thickening, blurring of the cortical–white matter junction, and signal changes. Management includes medical control of seizures, but surgical resection is often necessary for complete remission.

LISSENCEPHALY. The term *lissencephaly* (smooth brain) describes a group of disorders caused by abnormal migration of neurons to the cerebral cortex. Lissencephaly is diagnosed in childhood; most patients have severe developmental delay, microcephaly, intractable seizures, and premature death. Two major groups ("classic" and "cobblestone") based on MRI morphology are recognized. Most children with classic lissencephaly have mutations of chromosome 17p13.3 or Xq22; some patients with the former have the Miller-Dieker syndrome, whereas those with the latter are often born to mothers with band heterotopia (double cortex). MRI shows a smooth cortex with minimal sulcation. Cobblestone lissencephaly is less common but is most frequently seen in patients with congenital muscular dystrophy.

BAND HETEROTOPIA. Band heterotopia is an X-linked (Xq22) disorder mostly affecting females; males with mutations at this locus occasionally have band heterotopia, but most have classic lissencephaly. The clinical manifestations of band heterotopia are variable; seizures and mild to severe developmental delay are most common. MRI studies are diagnostic for the condition and demonstrate a band of gray matter beneath a nearly normal cortex (Fig. 457–1). The thickness of the band correlates with the ultimate neurologic outcome. Management consists of seizure control and genetic counseling. For proper counseling, the mother of a child with band heterotopia should undergo brain MRI even if asymptomatic.

SUBEPENDYMAL NODULAR HETEROTOPIA. Subependymal nodular heterotopia is a disorder characterized by multiple bilateral gray matter nodules in the walls of the lateral ventricles. It is often X-linked (Xq28), with males much more severely affected. Clinical features include seizures starting at any age and variable degrees of mental impairment (generally mild in females and severe in males). Diagnosis is achieved by MRI, which demonstrates the typical gray matter nodules. Treatment consists of antiepileptic agents for seizures and genetic counseling.

POLYMICROGYRIA-SCHIZENCEPHALY COMPLEX. Polymicrogyria is caused by failure of cortical organization; it may result from in utero injury or, presumably, from mutation. Schizencephaly is thought to represent a more extensive injury or mutation in which the entire cerebral mantle is affected. Clinical features include developmental delay, pyramidal signs, motor speech dysfunc-

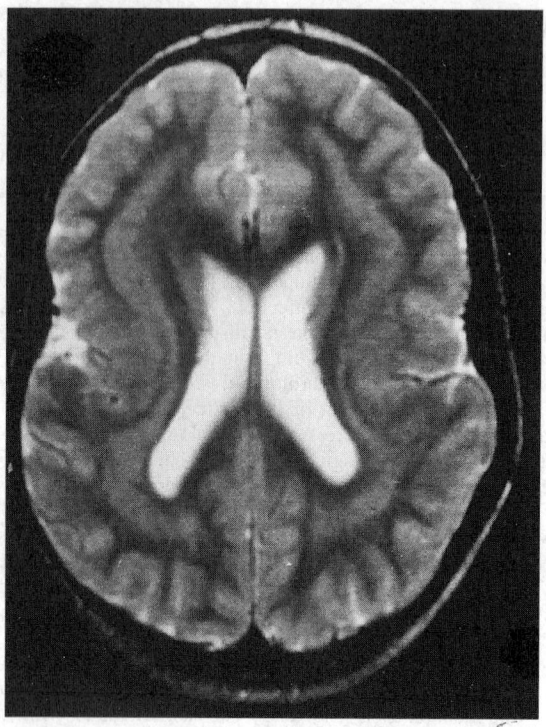

FIGURE 457–1 ■ A T2-weighted magnetic resonance image shows band heterotopia in a young woman.

tion, and epilepsy; in general, the clinical condition is more severe in schizencephaly. More severe signs and symptoms are related to more extensive or bilateral lesions. The diagnosis is established by MRI. Polymicrogyria is characterized by small gyri with shallow intervening sulci, whereas schizencephaly is characterized by gray matter–lined clefts that extend through the entire hemisphere from the subarachnoid space to the lateral ventricle. Treatment is medical and directed at the seizures. Resective surgery is performed in those rare patients in whom seizures are medically refractory and well localized to the region of polymicrogyria.

Barkovich AJ, Kuzniecky RI, Dobyns WB, et al: A classification scheme for malformations of cortical development. Neuropediatrics 27:59, 1996. *A rational classification of these disorders based on embryology, morphology, and genetics of the disorders.*
Dobyns WB, Andermann F, Andermann E: X-linked malformations of cortical development. Neurology 47:331, 1996. *A thorough discussion of the many malformations of cortical development that are the result of mutations of the X chromosome.*

458 CONGENITAL ANOMALIES OF THE CRANIOVERTEBRAL JUNCTION, SPINE, AND SPINAL CORD (INCLUDING SYRINGOMYELIA)

A. James Barkovich ■ Ruben I. Kuzniecky

Developmental anomalies of the vertebral bodies (i.e., hemivertebrae, butterfly vertebrae, non-segmentation of two or more adjacent vertebrae [Klippel-Feil anomaly], and transitional vertebrae) are frequently encountered on radiographs of patients with pain in the neck or back. Most are asymptomatic unless they lead to scoliosis or to accelerated degenerative changes of the spine, in which case they may cause pain or neurologic symptoms. Neurologic disability

is likely if the anomalies compress neural structures or alter cerebrospinal fluid (CSF) flow.

CHIARI MALFORMATIONS. *Chiari I malformations* are defined as ectopia of the cerebellar tonsils more than 5 mm below the foramen magnum. This abnormality is often incidental and asymptomatic. When clinical manifestations develop, they may include headaches accentuated by straining or cough, lower cranial neuropathies, downbeat nystagmus, ataxia, posterior column signs, or dissociated anesthesia of the trunk and extremities. Although the malformation is congenital, symptoms often begin in the 3rd and 4th decades or even later. It is often difficult to separate symptoms of neural compression at the craniocervical junction from those of associated syringohydromyelia or syringobulbia (see below). Similar signs and symptoms may result from multiple sclerosis or from other causes of neural compression of the craniocervical junction, including bony anomalies, metabolic bone diseases causing invagination of the skull base, and tumors. Definitive diagnosis is made by magnetic resonance imaging (MRI), which shows the compressed tonsils extending through the foramen magnum into the cervical subarachnoid space (Fig. 458–1). Treatment is surgical, by bony decompression of the craniocervical junction.

Chiari II malformations (sometimes called Arnold-Chiari malformations) are characterized by caudal elongation of the cerebellum and lower brain stem through the foramen magnum. Open spinal dysraphism (myelomeningocele) and hydrocephalus are almost always present. Brain stem dysfunction may develop secondary to intrinsic malformation or compression of neural structures at the C1 level. Other brain anomalies are common, in particular, anomalies of the corpus callosum and gray matter heterotopia. Treatment is surgical and aimed at repair of the myelomeningocele, relief of hydrocephalus, and occasionally, cervical bony decompression. The prognosis is dependent on the level (better for sacral, worse for thoracic) and extent of the myelomeningocele and on the severity of associated brain anomalies.

TETHERED SPINAL CORD. In the tethered spinal cord, the filum terminale is anomalous and results in either a lack of normal ascent of the conus medullaris to the L1 vertebral level or an ischemic or metabolic disturbance of the most caudal portions of the spinal cord. Associated spinal anomalies are commonly present, including diastematomyelia (split cord malformation), spinal lipomas, dermal sinuses, and fibrolipomas of the filum terminale. An increased incidence of cord tethering is present in patients with anorectal malformations (anomalies of the genitourinary tract and

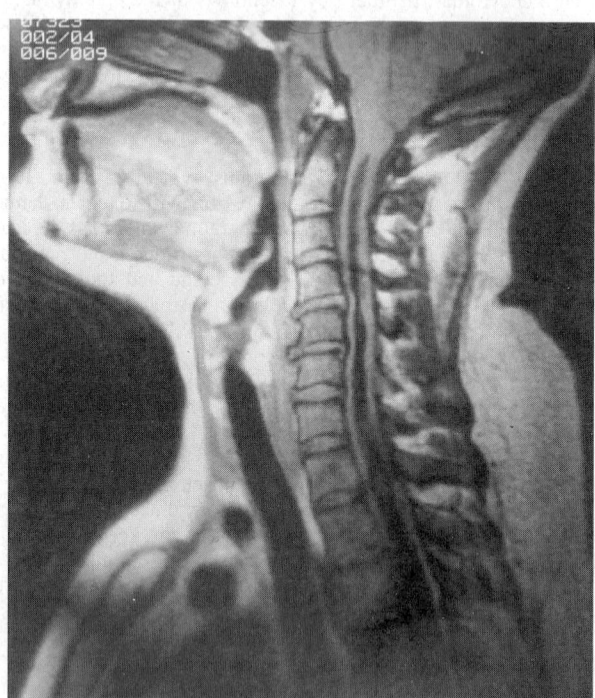

FIGURE 458–1 ■ Sagittal MRI shows low, pointed cerebellar tonsils (Chiari I malformation) and dilated central canal of the spinal cord (syringohydromyelia).

lower gastrointestinal tract). Patients typically have urinary incontinence in conjunction with lower extremity weakness and spasticity. Males may manifest impotence. Symptoms may occur at any age but typically develop in childhood or adolescence during periods of rapid growth. Cutaneous anomalies such as focal hypertrichosis, hemangiomas, and nevi may be seen over the lumbar spine. The differential diagnosis includes multiple sclerosis, tumors in the region of the conus medullaris, and lumbosacral hypogenesis. Definitive diagnosis is made by MRI, which shows diminished pulsations of the spinal cord, a low conus medullaris (below the bottom of the L2 vertebral body), or a thickened (more than 1 mm in diameter at the L5-S1 level) and fat-containing filum terminale. Treatment consists of surgical release of the tethered cord. If surgery results in adequate untethering, symptom progression is typically arrested, and in some patients, symptoms may improve.

SYRINGOHYDROMYELIA. DEFINITION AND PATHOGENESIS. Syringohydromyelia (see Fig. 458–1) is a condition in which the central canal of the spinal cord (hydromyelia), the substance of the spinal cord (syringomyelia), or the brain stem (syringobulbia) is expanded by the presence of fluid under pressure. Most experts believe that syringes form as a result of alterations in CSF flow that cause variations in pressure in different parts of the subarachnoid space. The variations in pressure create hydrostatic forces that drive CSF into the spinal cord. Causes of these alterations in CSF pressure include bony narrowing of the foramen magnum, as in achondroplasia or basilar invagination, Chiari I and II malformations, intramedullary and extramedullary tumors, and subarachnoid scarring secondary to trauma, hemorrhage, or infection. In patients with Chiari II malformations, hydrocephalus may result in syrinx formation. Rostral or caudal extension of the cyst may subsequently result from rapid changes in intraspinal pressure, such as those caused by coughing, straining, or sneezing.

CLINICAL MANIFESTATIONS. Symptoms of syringohydromyelia most commonly begin in late adolescence or early adulthood and progress irregularly with long periods of stability. In most instances the syrinx affects the cervical spinal cord. Classically, patients have asymmetrical segmental weakness and atrophy of the hands and arms, loss of upper limb deep tendon reflexes, and dissociated sensory loss (with impaired perception of pain and temperature but preservation of light touch and proprioception) in the neck, arms, and upper part of the trunk. In the legs, muscle tone is increased and the reflexes hyperactive. Some patients experience deep pain in the neck and arms. However, the clinical manifestations are dependent on the cross-sectional and vertical extent of cord involvement; symptoms may be unilateral or confined to the lower extremities. Extension into the medulla may cause nystagmus or lower cranial neuropathies. Moreover, symptoms from the syrinx may be difficult to differentiate from those of the associated craniocervical junction anomaly. When the syrinx is post-traumatic, symptoms develop after a latent period that can be more than 20 years. Ascending and descending levels of weakness or sensory impairment typically develop in affected patients.

The diagnosis is made by MRI (see Fig. 458–1), which defines the extent of the syrinx. In addition, MRI may show the associated craniocervical junction lesion, arachnoidal scarring, or tumor that is the cause. Electromyography reveals active and chronic denervation in the muscles of affected extremities. Nerve conduction studies are typically normal because the lesion is located central to the dorsal root ganglia. CSF is normal unless an inflammatory or neoplastic process is the cause.

If possible, treatment is directed at the cause of the syrinx. In patients with Chiari II malformations, adequate shunting of the lateral ventricles may result in collapsing the syrinx. Syringohydromyelia in patients with spinal tumors is treated by surgery. Patients with altered CSF dynamics caused by narrowing of the craniocervical junction are treated by bony foramen magnum decompression, sometimes accompanied by dural grafts to increase the size of the subarachnoid space. Patients with arachnoidal scarring are typically treated by insertion of a syringopleural or syringoperitoneal shunt. Treatment of patients with benign extramedullary tumors and craniocervical junction lesions may result in arrest of the process and long-term symptom relief. In patients with arachnoidal scarring, the relief is often only transient.

Klekamp J, Raimondi AJ, Samii M: Occult dysraphism in adulthood: Clinical course and management. Childs Nerv Syst 10:312, 1994. *A large series reviewing the many clinical features, with suggestions for management of patients with tethered cord.*

Menezes AH: Primary craniovertebral anomalies and the hindbrain herniation syndrome: Database analysis. Pediatr Neurosurg 23:260, 1995. *A thorough review of the cause, manifestations, and treatment of this anomaly.*

Milhorat TH, Johnson RW, Milhorat RH, et al: Clinicopathological correlations in syringomyelia using axial magnetic resonance imaging. Neurosurgery 37:206, 1995. *A landmark article on the understanding of the varied clinical features in affected patients.*

■ THE EXTRAPYRAMIDAL DISORDERS

459 INTRODUCTION

Joseph Jankovic

The term *extrapyramidal* refers to the anatomic and functional characteristics that distinguish the basal ganglia–regulated motor system from the pyramidal (corticospinal) and cerebellar systems. Extrapyramidal movement disorders are descriptively divided into *hypokinesias,* characterized by poverty and slowness of movement; *hyperkinesias,* manifested by abnormal involuntary movements; and miscellaneous motor disturbances (Table 459–1). Before discussing the clinical, pathophysiologic, and therapeutic aspects of the different movement disorders, it is important to review the anatomic and functional organization of the basal ganglia.

FUNCTIONAL AND NEUROCHEMICAL ANATOMY OF THE BASAL GANGLIA

The six paired nuclei that constitute the basal ganglia include the caudate nucleus, putamen, globus pallidus (or pallidum), nucleus accumbens, subthalamic nucleus, and substantia nigra (Fig. 459–1).

Table 459-1 ■ MOVEMENT DISORDERS

HYPOKINESIAS	HYPERKINESIAS	MISCELLANEOUS
Parkinsonism	Tremor	Ataxia
Hypomimia	Dystonia	Gait disorders
Dysarthria	Chorea	Hyperekplexia
Sialorrhea	Athetosis	Hemifacial spasm
Micrographia	Ballism	Myokymia
Shuffling gait	Tics	Stiff-person syndrome
Other signs of brady-	Myoclonus	Psychogenic
kinesia and rigidity	Sterotypy	
	Akathisia	
	Restless legs	
	Paroxysmal dyskine-	
	sias	

The caudate nucleus and putamen, although separated by the internal capsule, share cytoarchitectonic, chemical, and physiologic properties; they are often referred to as the *corpus striatum,* neostriatum, or simply striatum. The striatum is a highly inhomogeneous structure composed of subregions termed striosomes and matrix. The limbic system provides major input to the striosomes, whereas neocortical areas primarily project to the matrix. Although the internal capsule separates the internal segment of the globus

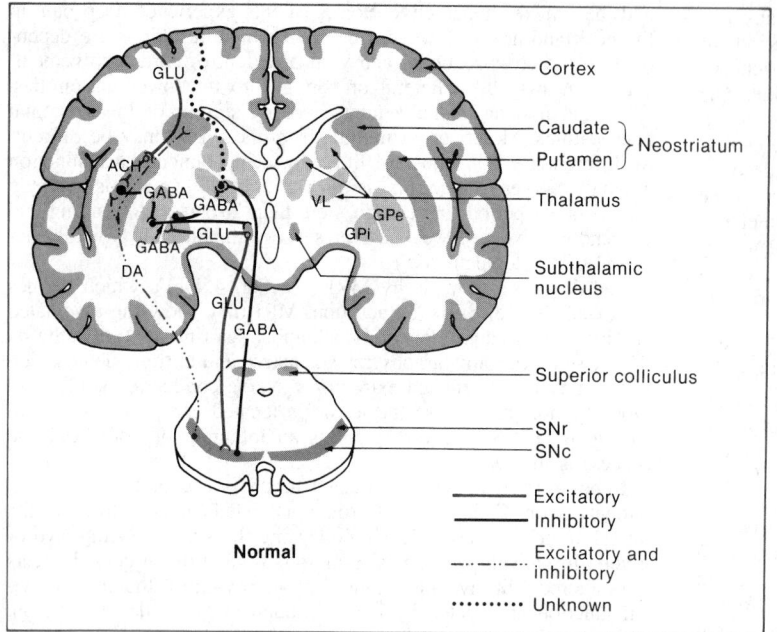

Normal

FIGURE 459–1 ■ Anatomy of the basal ganglia and their connections. ACH = acetylcholine; GABA = γ-aminobutyric acid; GLU = glutamate; GP = globus pallidum (e = external, i = internal); DA = dopamine; SN = substantia nigra (c = compacta, r = reticulata); VL = ventrolateral.

pallidus and the pars reticulata of the substantia nigra, evidence suggests that these nuclei should also be regarded as a single functional structure. The term *lenticular nucleus* refers to the putamen and globus pallidus combined because of their lens-like shape.

Recent anatomic and physiologic data suggest a complex organization of the basal ganglia and related structures (see Fig. 459–1). According to this schema, the sensorimotor, association, and limbic cortical areas provide anatomically and functionally segregated input to the dorsal (the caudate and putamen) and ventral (nucleus accumbens, not shown) striatum. The somatosensory, motor, and pre-motor cortical areas project mainly to the putamen, and the posterior parietal and temporal and frontal association cortical areas project largely to the caudate and nucleus accumbens. The anatomy is consistent with the concept that the putamen is primarily concerned with motor function and the caudate is more involved with emotional and cognitive processes. The corticostriatal afferents are mediated by the excitatory neurotransmitter glutamic acid. The other major striatal afferents originate in the substantia nigra pars compacta, which provides major dopaminergic inhibitory input to the basal ganglia via the nigrostriatal pathway. Other inhibitory input to the striatum arises from the brain stem raphe nuclei (serotonergic) and from the locus ceruleus neurons (noradrenergic). The striatum is composed largely of cholinergic neurons, and some excitatory cholinergic projections to the striatum originate in the midline intralaminar thalamic nuclei.

The striatal nuclei project somatotopically to the external and internal segments of the globus pallidus and the pars reticulata of the substantia nigra complex. The striatal efferents use the inhibitory neurotransmitter γ-aminobutyric acid (GABA). The subthalamic nucleus regulates the output of the basal ganglia to the thalamus by modulating the inhibitory GABAergic afferents from the external segment of the globus pallidus and the excitatory glutamatergic efferent projections to the globus pallidus (internal segment)–substantia nigra pars reticulata complex. The efferent inhibitory GABAergic projections from the internal segment of the globus pallidus terminate in the thalamus. The thalamic nuclei in turn project to the supplementary motor area of the cortex and the primary motor cortex.

MOVEMENT DISORDERS

Single-cell recordings in behaving animals and other studies have demonstrated that one of the primary roles of the basal ganglia is to scale the movement amplitude and velocity rather than initiate movements. Besides their crucial role in the execution of movement, the basal ganglia also seem to be involved in the preparation for movement.

In addition to impaired voluntary movements, dysfunction in the basal ganglia can also cause a variety of abnormal involuntary movements. Correlations between the various types of abnormal movement and sites of experimental and pathologic lesions have provided helpful insight and better understanding of the function of the basal ganglia. The remainder of this section is organized according to the major categories of movement disorders into hypokinetic (parkinsonian), hyperkinetic, and miscellaneous movement disorders (see Table 459–1).

HYPOKINESIAS (PARKINSONIAN DISORDERS). Bradykinesia is clinically manifested by slowness of automatic and spontaneous movements and an impaired ability to initiate voluntary movements (akinesia). This typical parkinsonian symptom presumably results from loss of the inhibitory dopamine input to the striatum and hypoactivity of the neurons in the external segment of the globus pallidus. This process in turn causes functional disinhibition (excitation) of the subthalamic nucleus, which induces an increase in neuronal activity in the internal segment of the globus pallidus, thereby raising the tonic inhibitory output from the basal ganglia (internal segment of the globus pallidus) to the thalamus and to the cortical projection areas (Fig. 459–2). The altered activity in the "motor" circuit is manifested by increased movement time, which becomes particularly prolonged when a parkinsonian patient performs sequential movements.

Rigidity, another cardinal sign of parkinsonism, is demonstrated clinically by increased resistance against passive movement of a body part, usually associated with the "cogwheel" phenomenon. A parkinsonian patient perceives rigidity as a feeling of joint stiffness and muscle tightness. The pathophysiologic mechanisms of rigidity have been attributed to pallidal disinhibition resulting in increased suprasegmental activation of normal spinal reflex mechanisms.

Postural instability resulting from loss of righting reflexes can cause propulsion (tendency to fall forward) and retropulsion (tendency to fall backward). It is one of the most disabling symptoms of Parkinson's disease. The mechanism of postural instability is unknown, but it has been attributed primarily to involvement of the pallidum. Other hypokinetic manifestations are listed in Table 459–1.

HYPERKINESIAS (ABNORMAL INVOLUNTARY MOVEMENTS). Tremor is a rhythmic oscillatory movement produced by alternating or synchronous contractions of opposing muscle groups. Tremors

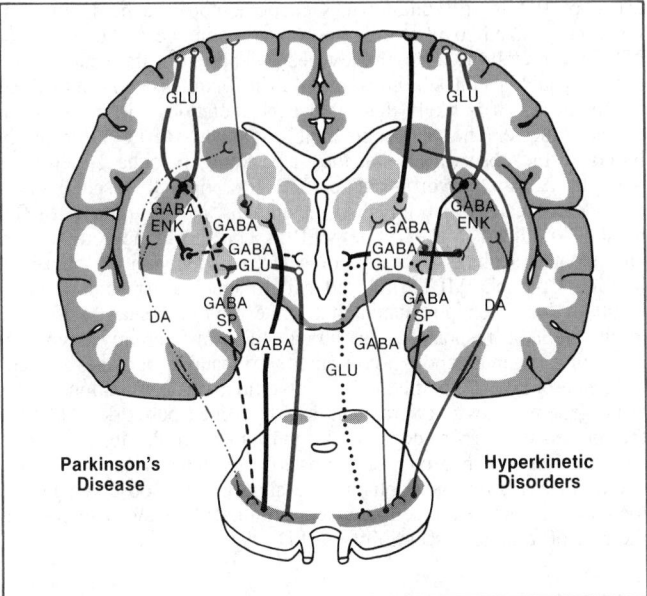

FIGURE 459–2 ■ Functional organization of the basal ganglia in parkinsonian disorders and hyperkinetic movement disorders. ACH = acetylcholine; GABA = γ-aminobutyric acid; GLU = glutamate; DA = dopamine; ENK = enkephalin; SP = substance P.

are divided into rest or action tremors; the latter are further subdivided into postural or contraction tremors (e.g., arms outstretched in front of the body or in a "wing-beating" position) and kinetic or intention tremors (e.g., during target-directed movement, such as the finger-to-nose maneuver). *Rest tremor*, usually asymmetrical at onset, is the typical tremor of Parkinson's disease. When it involves the hands, it causes a supinating-pronating oscillatory (pill-rolling) movement at approximately 4- to 6-Hz frequency. Parkinsonian tremor also often involves the legs, feet, lips, tongue, chin, and voice but almost never affects the head or neck. *Postural tremor*, with frequency ranging between 4 and 12 Hz, is most typically seen in patients with essential tremor. *Kinetic (intention) tremors* are slow and more irregular movements with a rate of 1.5 to 3 Hz. Kinetic tremors usually indicate an abnormality of the cerebellum or its outflow pathways (dentate nucleus, superior cerebellar peduncle, and contralateral red nucleus).

Dystonia is produced by involuntary, sustained (tonic) or spasmodic (rapid or clonic), patterned, and repetitive muscle contractions, frequently causing twisting (e.g., torticollis), flexing or extending (e.g., retrocollis), and squeezing (e.g., blepharospasm, writer's cramp) movements or abnormal postures. Dystonia is usually constant but occurs in some cases only during particular activities. Examples of task-specific dystonias include writer's or typist's cramp and inversion of a foot while running. As dystonia progresses, the involuntary contractions also appear at rest. A characteristic feature of dystonia is that the spasms lessen in intensity with "sensory tricks" such as touching one side of the face to maintain a primary position, thereby counteracting involuntary torticollis. Dystonia can fluctuate in intensity and is exacerbated by stress, fatigue, activity, or a change in posture. It subsides during sleep, relaxation, and hypnosis. These features and the bizarre nature of dystonic patterns are sometimes wrongly attributed to psychogenic causes. About half of patients with dystonia have a coexistent postural tremor, identical to essential tremor. The anatomic substrate for dystonia is unknown. Clinicopathologic studies of patients with secondary dystonias most often implicate the putamen and the rostral brain stem in their genesis.

Chorea consists of continuous, abrupt, rapid, brief, flowing, unsustained, irregular and random jerk-like movements. Choreic patients frequently mask the abnormal movements by voluntary semi-purposeful activities. A characteristic feature of chorea is the inability to maintain voluntary sustained contraction. Examples include an inability to sustain manual grip or tongue protrusion and the dropping of objects. Muscle stretch reflexes are usually "hung

up" and "pendular." Affected patients typically have a peculiar irregular and dance-like gait. The pathogenesis of chorea is unknown. Some findings point to abnormalities in caudate function. A selective loss of the GABA-enkephalin striatal neurons projecting to the external segment of the globus pallidus, found in Huntington's disease, results in excessive inhibition of subthalamic nucleus neurons.

The movement disorders of athetosis (see Chapter 463), ballism (see Chapter 463), myoclonus (see Chapter 464), tics (see Chapter 464), and stereotypies (see Chapter 464) are discussed in later chapters of this section.

Hallett M: Physiology of basal ganglia disorders: An overview. Can J Neurol Sci 20: 177, 1993. *An excellent review of current understanding of the basal ganglia connections in the normal and diseased brain.*

Jankovic J, Tolosa E (eds): Parkinson's Disease and Movement Disorders. Baltimore, Williams & Wilkins, 1998. *A comprehensive review of hypokinetic, hyperkinetic, and miscellaneous movement disorders.*

Parent A, Cicchetti F: The current model of basal ganglia organization under scrutiny. Mov Disord 13:199, 1998. *A critical review of the current model of basal ganglia circuitry and its limitations in explaining the mechanisms of surgical treatment of Parkinson's disease. The role of the subthalamic nucleus in relation to bradykinesia and its excitatory projections not only to the globus pallidus but also to other structures is emphasized.*

460 PARKINSONISM

Joseph Jankovic

Parkinsonism is a clinical syndrome dominated by four cardinal signs: tremor at rest, bradykinesia, rigidity, and postural instability. Less prominent manifestations concern the mood and intellect, autonomic function, and the sensory system (Table 460–1). The average age at onset, is 55 years, with about 1% of persons 60 years or older having the disease. Men are affected more frequently than women by a ratio of 3:2. At least two major subtypes of Parkinson's disease (PD) have been identified: One subtype is characterized by tremor as the dominant parkinsonian feature, and the other is dominated by postural instability and gait difficulty. The *tremor subtype* of PD is associated with relatively normal mental status, earlier age at onset, and slower progression of the disease than is the *postular instability–gait difficulty subtype*, which shows more bradykinesia, dementia, and a more rapidly progressive course.

Resting tremor and bradykinesia are the most typical parkinsonian signs and are virtually synonymous with the diagnosis. Bradykinesia accounts for most of the associated parkinsonian symptoms and signs: general slowing down of movements and activities of daily living, lack of facial expression (hypomimia or masked facies), staring expression resulting from a decreased frequency of blinking, impaired swallowing causing drooling (sialorrhea), hypokinetic and hypophonic dysarthria, monotonous speech, small hand-

Table 460–1 ■ NON-MOTOR DISTURBANCE IN PARKINSON'S DISEASE

Neurobehavioral Abnormalities in Parkinson's Disease
Personality changes (apathy, lack of confidence, fearfulness, anxiety, emotional lability and inflexibility, social withdrawal, dependency)
Dementia (tip-of-the-tongue phenomenon [partial anomia], spatial disorientation, paranoia, psychosis, hallucinations)
Bradyphrenia (slow thought processes, loss of concentration, difficulty with concept formation)
Depression
Sleep disturbance
Sexual dysfunction
Psychiatric side effects of therapy
Other Non-motor Manifestations of Parkinson's Disease
Autonomic dysfunction (orthostatic hypotension, respiratory dysregulation, flushing, "drenching sweats," constipation, sphincter and sexual dysfunction)
Sensory symptoms (paresthesias, pains, akathisia; visual, olfactory, and vestibular dysfunction)
Seborrhea, pedal edema, fatigue, weight loss

Table 460-2 ■ CAUSES OF THE PARKINSON SYNDROME

Primary (Idiopathic) Parkinsonism
Parkinson's disease
Juvenile parkinsonism
Secondary (Acquired, Symptomatic) Parkinsonism
Infectious: postencephalitic, slow virus
Drugs: neuroleptics (antipsychotic, antiemetic drugs), reserpine, tetrabena-
    zine, α-methyldopa, lithium, flunarizine, cinnarizine
Toxins: MPTP, CO, Mn, Hg, CS_2, methanol, ethanol
Vascular: multi-infarct, hypotensive shock
Trauma: pugilistic encephalopathy
Other: parathyroid abnormalities, hypothyroidism, hepatocerebral degenera-
    tion, brain tumor, normal-pressure hydrocephalus, syringomesencephalia
Heredodegenerative Parkinsonism
Autosomal dominant Lewy body disease
Huntington's disease
Wilson disease
Hallervorden-Spatz disease
Olivopontocerebellar and spinocerebellar atrophy
Familial basal ganglia calcification
Familial parkinsonism with peripheral neuropathy
Neuroacanthocytosis
Multiple-System Degeneration (Parkinsonism-Plus)
Progressive supranuclear palsy
Multiple-system atrophy
    Shy-Drager syndrome
    Striatonigral degeneration
    Olivopontocerebellar atrophy
Parkinsonism-dementia-ALS complex
Corticobasal ganglionic degeneration
Alzheimer's disease
Hemiatrophy-parkinsonism

MPTP = 1-methyl-4-phenyl-1,2,3,6-tetrahydropyridine; ALS = amyotrophic lateral sclerosis.

writing (micrographia), difficulties with repetitive and simultaneous movements, difficulty in arising from a chair and turning over in bed, shuffling gait with short steps, decreased arm swing and other automatic movements, and start hesitation and freezing. Freezing, manifested by a sudden and often unpredictable inability to move, is one of the most disabling of all parkinsonian symptoms.

Several disorders other than PD can cause at least part of the parkinsonian syndrome (Table 460–2). Non-PD parkinsonian disorders can be distinguished clinically from PD by the presence of atypical findings, absence or paucity of tremor, and poor response to levodopa. The last feature may be partly explained by the fact that post-synaptic dopamine receptors are preserved in PD but decreased in the other parkinsonian syndromes.

PARKINSON'S DISEASE

Pathogenesis

The most typical pathologic hallmarks of PD are (1) neuronal loss with depigmentation of the substantia nigra and (2) Lewy bodies, which are eosinophilic cytoplasmic inclusions in neurons consisting of aggregates of normal filaments. These abnormalities are most prominent in the ventrolateral region of the substantia nigra that projects to the putamen. At least an 80% loss of dopaminergic neurons in the substantia nigra and the same degree of dopamine depletion in the striatum must appear before clinical symptoms of PD become evident.

Motor symptoms of PD result chiefly from degeneration of the nigrostriatal pathway, which causes a deficiency of dopamine in the putamen and, to a lesser degree, the caudate nucleus. The cognitive deficits and some neurobehavioral symptoms have been attributed to degeneration of the dopaminergic mesocortical and mesolimbic pathways, and, the associated autonomic dysfunction may be partly caused by dopamine depletion in the hypothalamus. Besides dopamine deficiency, impairment of the other neurotransmitters may be responsible for some of the associated findings. For example, degeneration of the noradrenergic locus ceruleus may contribute to the "freezing" phenomenon and to depression. Degeneration of the cholinergic nucleus basalis probably relates to the dementia that eventually affects about a third of all PD patients.

Although several hypotheses are currently being investigated, the

cause of PD is still unknown. Genetic factors are being increasingly recognized to play an important role in the pathogenesis of PD. Two mutations have already been identified in the gene coding for α-synuclein on chromosome 4q in families with autosomal dominant PD. It is likely that other gene mutations will be found in the near future. The "environmental" hypothesis of PD is primarily based on the observation that the meperidine analogue 1-methyl-4-phenyl-1,2,3,6-tetrahydropyridine (MPTP), originally used by heroin addicts, causes parkinsonism in humans and in animals. MPTP must be oxidized to a pyridine MPP^+ species to be neurotoxic, and antioxidants such as deprenyl (a selective monoamine oxidase B inhibitor) prevent MPTP-induced experimental parkinsonism. As a result, it has been postulated that some environmental MPTP-like toxin might be responsible for human PD. An alternative hypothesis is that an endogenous toxin such as dopamine damages susceptible neurons. During the process of oxidative deamination, dopamine generates hydroxyl radicals and hydrogen peroxide, which in the presence of iron deposits in the brain, could lead to lipid peroxidation and neurotoxicity, possibly by interfering with mitochondrial oxidative metabolism. The abnormalities observed in mitochondrial complex I activity have stimulated renewed interest in the role of genetic susceptibility in PD.

Treatment

The finding that deprenyl prevents MPTP-induced parkinsonism stimulated interest in antioxidative therapy as a means of retarding the progression of PD. Some, but by no means all studies have found that deprenyl slows the development of motor disability when used in the early stages of PD. Deprenyl may also provide moderate symptomatic relief. After starting deprenyl therapy, many patients report improvement in their energy level and bradykinetic symptoms. The effect may be due to deprenyl's ability to increase striatal concentrations of dopamine by blocking its metabolism by monoamine oxidase. Addition of one of the anticholinergic drugs, such as trihexyphenidyl, may provide further symptomatic relief, particularly in younger patients and patients in whom tremor predominates. Associated depression, present in many parkinsonian patients, can be treated with tricyclic antidepressants such as amitriptyline or nortriptyline. Because the anticholinergics, including the tricyclics, can produce undesirable psychological symptoms, as well as other side effects such as dry mouth, blurring of vision, and urinary hesitancy, amantadine may offer a useful alternative, particularly in elderly patients. Amantadine, however, although helpful in controlling both tremor and bradykinesia, can also cause adverse effects, including livedo reticularis, ankle edema, exacerbation of congestive heart failure, and mild anticholinergic side effects. Its beneficial effects may wane after a few months.

Many neurologists favor the use of combinations of deprenyl, anticholinergics, and amantadine until they no longer provide satisfactory control of parkinsonian symptoms. At that point many authorities believe that dopamine agonists, which stimulate dopamine receptors directly, should be used as the initial dopaminergic therapy. When used as monotherapy, dopamine agonists provide only modest improvement in parkinsonian symptoms, but the improvement may be sufficient to delay the introduction of levodopa by several months or years and thus delay the onset of levodopa-related complications (see below). Support is also growing for the notion that dopamine agonists have a neuroprotective effect. This concept is suggested by the following observations: (1) by stimulating dopamine autoreceptors, dopamine agonists presumably decrease dopamine turnover and thus reduce oxidative stress; (2) dopamine agonists have been demonstrated to scavenge hydroxyl, superoxide, and nitric oxide radicals and induce up-regulation of the free radical scavenging enzyme superoxide dismutase; (3) certain dopamine agonists enhance the growth and survival of cultured dopaminergic neurons; and (4) dopamine agonists exert a levodopa-sparing effect. Furthermore, because levodopa "primes" for the development of dyskinesia, the use of dopamine agonists before levodopa seems to be a prudent practice. As symptoms increase, dopamine agonists must be combined with levodopa.

In 1997, three new dopamine agonists, cabergoline, pramipexole, and ropinirole, were added to bromocriptine and pergolide. Cabergoline, a potent D_2-agonist with a half-life of about 65 hours, has not, however, been approved for the treatment of PD in the United States. Pramipexole differs from ergot dopamine agonists such as bromocriptine and pergolide by its preferential affinity for the D_3-

receptor subtype. In contrast, ropinirole is a relatively pure D_2-receptor agonist. The non-ergoline structure of the new agonists pramipexole and ropinirole may have a potential advantage in their side effect profile in that the new drugs appear to be associated with a lower risk for such complications as peptic ulcer disease, vasoconstrictive effects, erythromelalgia, and pulmonary and retroperitoneal fibrosis. Similar to the earlier dopamine agonists pergolide and bromocriptine, the new dopamine agonists may cause nausea, vomiting, anorexia, malaise, orthostatic hypotension, and psychiatric reactions, particularly hallucinations, and they may exacerbate levodopa-induced dyskinesias. Not only have dopamine agonists been found to have beneficial symptomatic effects in the treatment of early PD, these drugs also smooth out the motor fluctuations associated with chronic levodopa therapy. No comparative trials have been performed to determine which of the dopamine agonists have the best efficacy–adverse effects ratio. When patients continue to be troubled by their parkinsonian symptoms despite deprenyl, anticholinergics, amantadine, and a dopamine agonist, levodopa combined with carbidopa, a peripheral dopa decarboxylase inhibitor, is added to the antiparkinsonian regimen. The starting dosage of carbidopa/levodopa is 25 mg/100 mg (controlled release) twice daily, to be gradually increased to three times per day. The dosage is then adjusted, depending on the severity of symptoms and occupational demands. Some patients require as much as 25 mg/250 mg four or five times daily; others tolerate only smaller doses. Although levodopa can suppress tremor, it is most useful in controlling bradykinesia and rigidity. Postural instability may be ameliorated by levodopa in early PD, but not in advanced stages of the disease. Levodopa should be used with caution in those with prominent psychosis or dementia, peptic ulcer disease, and cardiac arrhythmias.

About 15% of parkinsonian patients fail to improve with levodopa from the onset of therapy. Most of these non-responders probably have a form of post-synaptic parkinsonism rather than PD. Failure to respond to levodopa should also suggest the possibility of a wrong diagnosis, drug interaction (concomitant use of dopamine receptor blocking agents such as antipsychotic and antiemetic drugs), and pharmacokinetic reasons such as insufficient dosage, slow stomach emptying, and competition for absorption in the small intestine and at the blood-brain barrier by amino acids in protein meals. Almost all patients who initially improve begin to experience levodopa-related complications some time between 3 and 8 years after onset.

Patients with PD lose their response to levodopa because of (1) natural progression of the disease and (2) development of complications as a result of chronic levodopa therapy. Although nonneuronal elements may participate in the conversion of levodopa to dopamine, the surviving striatal dopaminergic terminals progressively lose their capacity for conversion of levodopa to dopamine, and motor fluctuations and symptomatic deterioration subsequently develop. The post-synaptic dopamine receptors also seem to play an important role in the pathogenesis of motor fluctuations.

The most challenging problem in managing PD is treating levodopa complications. Thanks to carbidopa and similar agents, gastrointenstinal side effects, chiefly nausea and vomiting, are seldom troublesome. The most common central side effects of levodopa therapy include psychiatric problems, dyskinesias (seen in about 80% of patients after 3 years of therapy), and clinical fluctuations (seen in about 50% of patients after 5 years of therapy). The most common form of clinical fluctuation is the wearing-off effect, characterized by end-of-dose deterioration and recurrence of parkinsonian symptoms as a result of shorter (sometimes only 1 to 2 hours) duration of benefit after a given dose of levodopa. Slow-release preparations of levodopa (e.g., Sinemet CR, Madopar CR) prolong the plasma (and presumably brain) levels and may be useful in treating or preventing motor fluctuations. Deprenyl may prolong the duration of benefit from each levodopa dose.

Another strategy designed to prolong levodopa response takes advantage of the inhibition of catechol *O*-methyltransferase (COMT) by drugs such as tolcapone and entacapone. Although tolcapone has both central and peripheral effect, unlike entacapone, which inhibits only peripheral COMT, it is not clear whether this difference will produce a different clinical pharmacologic effect. Tolcapone has a longer half-life (2 hours versus 1 hour) and can be administered three times per day, whereas entacapone requires more frequent administration (e.g., 200 mg four to six times per day), usually taken with each dose of levodopa. Although this pharmacologic action of the COMT inhibitors may prolong the "on" time without markedly increasing dyskinesias, most studies do report a higher frequency of levodopa-induced dyskinesia in patients treated with COMT inhibitors. Tolcapone may also cause potentially serious liver abnormalities, so liver function must be monitored every 2 weeks.

Because the onset of levodopa-induced complications seems to be related to the duration of levodopa therapy (as well as to the loss of dopaminergic striatal terminals), some authorities delay initiating levodopa therapy until the patient's symptoms begin to interfere with normal activities. Once levodopa treatment is initiated, the dose should be maintained as low as possible (Fig. 460–1).

The renewed interest in surgical treatment of PD has been stimulated in part by improved understanding of the functional anatomy underlying motor control, as well as refinement of methods and techniques in neurosurgery, neuroradiology, and neurophysiology. Stereotactic thalamotomy is still occasionally used in an attempt to ameliorate disabling tremor. This traditional procedure is being replaced by pallidotomy and high-frequency deep brain stimulation, with the stimulating electrode stereotactically implanted in one of the three target nuclei: thalamus, subthalamic nucleus, or globus pallidus (internal segment). Both the ablative and stimulating procedures have been found to be particularly effective in smoothing out motor fluctuations and eliminating levodopa-induced dyskinesias. Surgical transplantation of fetal substantia nigra into the striatum remains under investigation.

As with all progressive, disabling diseases, psychological support of patients and families offers important help. Patients should be encouraged to learn about their disease (by reading educational material provided by national and local support organizations) and, above all, to remain physically and socially active.

SECONDARY PARKINSONISM

POST-ENCEPHALITIC PARKINSONISM. A variety of movement disorders, including parkinsonism, later developed in many individuals who survived the acute febrile illness and encephalopathy during the pandemics of encephalitis lethargica (von Economo's encephalitis) between 1919 and 1926. Although the virus or viruses responsible for encephalitis lethargica were never isolated, infections caused by Coxsackie, Japanese B, and western equine encephalitis viruses have since been identified as being complicated by parkinsonism. In general, post-encephalitic parkinsonism has a slower progression and is more sensitive to levodopa therapy.

DRUG-INDUCED PARKINSONISM. Drugs that deplete the presynaptic stores of dopamine, such as reserpine and tetrabenazine (an investigational drug not available for general use in North America), and drugs that block dopamine receptors, such as antipsychotic and antiemetic agents, can cause a parkinsonian syndrome clinically indistinguishable from idiopathic parkinsonism (PD). The same drugs can also cause a variety of other movement disorders such as akathisia, dystonic reactions, and various tardive syndromes (e.g., tardive stereotypy, tardive dystonia, and tardive akathisia).

VASCULAR PARKINSONISM. Cerebrovascular disease accounts for only a small proportion of parkinsonism. Single strokes rarely cause parkinsonian findings, although multiple small infarctions involving the striatum can produce the syndrome. Brain imaging is helpful in the diagnosis. One form of vascular parkinsonism is the so-called "lower body parkinsonism," manifested chiefly by gait disturbance with short steps, "freezing," and difficulties turning. (Chronic communicating, "low-pressure" hydrocephalus causes a similar clinical picture.) Patients with vascular parkinsonism may have dementia, hyperactive reflexes, and urinary incontinence, but tremor is rare. Levodopa therapy usually fails, probably because ischemia damages the striatal post-synaptic receptors. The diagnosis is suggested by these atypical findings in patients with a history of stroke risk factors.

HEREDODEGENERATIVE PARKINSONISM

Very few parkinsonian patients have a family history suggesting a specific pattern of inheritance. With such a history, the differen-

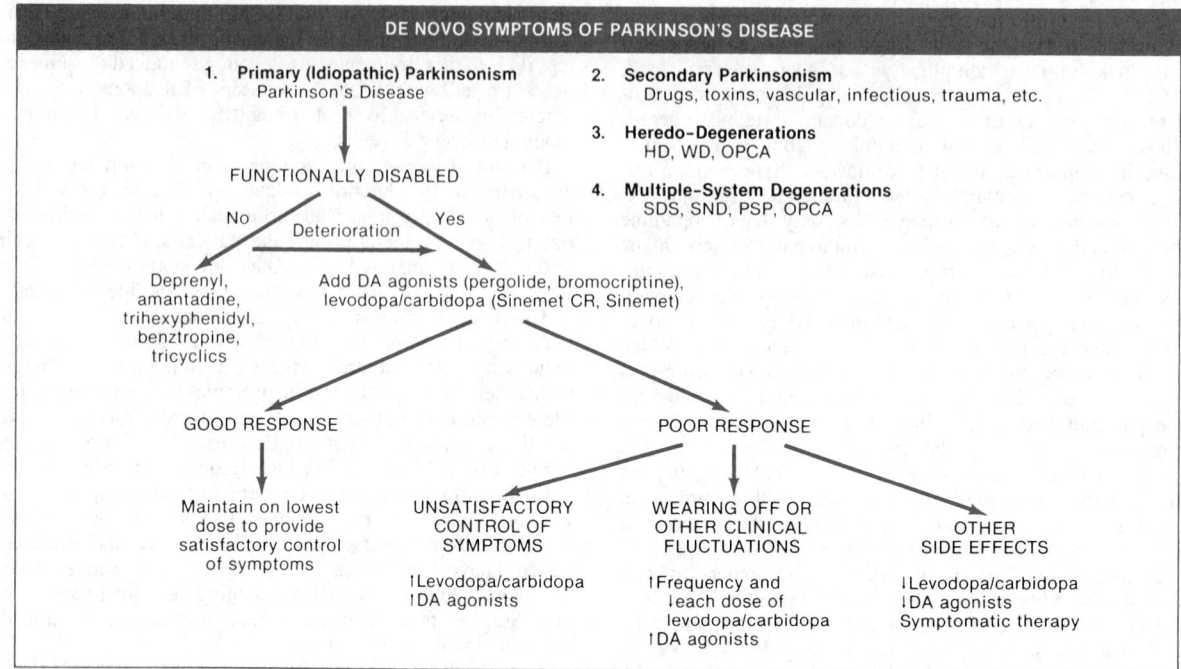

DE NOVO SYMPTOMS OF PARKINSON'S DISEASE

1. **Primary (Idiopathic) Parkinsonism**
   Parkinson's Disease

2. **Secondary Parkinsonism**
   Drugs, toxins, vascular, infectious, trauma, etc.

3. **Heredo-Degenerations**
   HD, WD, OPCA

4. **Multiple-System Degenerations**
   SDS, SND, PSP, OPCA

FUNCTIONALLY DISABLED

No — Deterioration — Yes

Deprenyl, amantadine, trihexyphenidyl, benztropine, tricyclics

Add DA agonists (pergolide, bromocriptine), levodopa/carbidopa (Sinemet CR, Sinemet)

GOOD RESPONSE

POOR RESPONSE

Maintain on lowest dose to provide satisfactory control of symptoms

UNSATISFACTORY CONTROL OF SYMPTOMS
↑Levodopa/carbidopa
↑DA agonists

WEARING OFF OR OTHER CLINICAL FLUCTUATIONS
↑Frequency and ↓each dose of levodopa/carbidopa
↑DA agonists

OTHER SIDE EFFECTS
↓Levodopa/carbidopa
↓DA agonists
Symptomatic therapy

FIGURE 460–1 ■ Diagrammatic representation of a therapeutic approach to patients with parkinsonism. DA = dopamine; HD = Huntington's disease; OPCA = olivopontocerebellar atrophy; PSP = progressive supranuclear palsy; SDS = Shy-Drager syndrome; Sinemet CR = controlled-release levodopa carbidopa; SND = striatonigral degeneration; WD = Wilson disease.

tial diagnosis should include one of the heredodegenerative disorders (see Table 460–2).

HALLERVORDEN-SPATZ DISEASE. This rare condition is manifested by childhood- or adult-onset progressive dementia, bradykinesia, rigidity, and spasticity, variously combined with dystonia, choreoathetosis, ataxia, seizures, amyotrophy, and retinitis pigmentosa. Most reported cases have suggested an autosomal recessive inheritance. Neuropathologically, iron accumulates in the globus pallidus and substantia nigra, accompanied by axonal swelling and neuronal degeneration in the basal ganglia, corticospinal tract, and cerebellum. Cysteine, found to be increased in the globus pallidus, possibly chelates iron and thereby causes the generation of free radicals and subsequent neuronal degeneration. Magnetic resonance imaging (MRI) of patients with Hallervorden-Spatz disease shows marked hypointensity on T2-weighted images in the internal segment of the globus pallidus and the pars reticulata of the substantia nigra. Typically, but not always, a central spot of hypointensity surrounded by a circumscribed region of hyperintensity gives the appearance of an "eye of the tiger." These MRI changes are indicative of heavy iron deposition. The disorder is also referred to as "neurodegeneration with brain iron accumulation type 1."

FAMILIAL BASAL GANGLIA CALCIFICATIONS. Calcium may accumulate in the basal ganglia in association with hypoparathyroidism or as a result of a familial disorder, sometimes referred to as Fahr's disease. Affected patients exhibit parkinsonism, chorea, dementia, and palilalia. Brain imaging may detect basal ganglia calcification in clinically unaffected relatives.

OLIVOPONTOCEREBELLAR AND SPINOCEREBELLAR ATROPHY. The combination of parkinsonism and cerebellar ataxia characterizes olivopontocerebellar degeneration or atrophy, a heterogeneous group of neurodegenerative disorders most often inherited in an autosomal dominant pattern, but occasionally occurring sporadically. In addition to the parkinsonism-ataxia complex, patients with olivopontocerebellar atrophy often exhibit marked dysarthria, neuro-ophthalmologic signs, and a variable degree of upper and lower motor neuron signs (see Chapter 466).

MULTIPLE-SYSTEM DEGENERATION (PARKINSONISM-PLUS)

Approximately 10 to 15% of all patients with parkinsonian findings have a more widespread disorder classified clinically as "parkinsonism-plus syndrome" and pathologically as a "multiple-system degeneration." Besides parkinsonism, such patients suffer from additional findings that may include supranuclear ophthalmoparesis (progressive supranuclear palsy), dysautonomia (Shy-Drager syndrome), ataxia (olivopontocerebellar atrophy), laryngeal stridor (striatonigral degeneration), apraxia and alien hand (corticobasal gaglionic degeneration), dementia (Alzheimer's disease with parkinsonism and diffuse Lewy body disease), and a combination of dementia and motor neuron disease (parkinsonism–dementia–amyotrophic lateral sclerosis complex). The cause of all forms of this syndrome is unknown.

PROGRESSIVE SUPRANUCLEAR PALSY. Progressive supranuclear palsy accounts for about 8% of all parkinsonian patients evaluated in a PD clinic. Progressive supranuclear palsy has its onset in the 7th decade, about 10 years after the usual onset of PD. Initial symptoms consist of a gradual onset of postural instability, unsteady gait, and supranuclear vertical ophthalmoparesis, initially expressed by impairment in downward gaze. Patients may complain of difficulty seeing. Later, upward and then lateral conjugate gaze also become impaired, but until the advanced stage, the external ophthalmoparesis can be overcome by labyrinthine stimulation via the oculocephalic maneuver. Patients with progressive supranuclear palsy often exhibit axial rigidity, nuchal dystonia, and a rigid-dystonic facial expression. Mild to moderate dementia is a late sign; tremor almost never occurs. Neither the hypokinetic rigidity nor the other changes respond to antiparkinsonian drugs.

Pathologically, progressive supranuclear palsy is characterized by selective neuronal loss and gliosis affecting the midbrain tegmentum and tectum, the internal segment of the globus pallidus, the subthalamic nucleus, the vestibular and dentate nuclei, the basal nucleus of Meynert, and the pedunculopontine nucleus. Neurofibrillary tangles, somewhat different from those in Alzheimer's disease, and granulovacuolar degeneration involve nerve cells in these areas.

SHY-DRAGER SYNDROME. When patients with atypical parkinsonism (usually without tremor) complain of orthostatic lightheadedness, incontinence, sexual impotence, and other autonomic symptoms, the diagnosis of Shy-Drager syndrome should be considered (see Chapter 451).

Jankovic J, Marsden CD: Therapeutic strategies in Parkinson's disease. *In* Jankovic J, Tolosa E (eds): Parkinson's Disease and Movement Disorders, 3rd ed. Baltimore,

Williams & Wilkins, 1998, pp 191–220. *A comprehensive review of current antiparkinsonian therapies.*

Quinn N: Multiple system atrophy. *In* Marsden CD, Fahn S (eds): Movement Diseases-3. London, Butterworth-Heinemann, 1994, p 262. *A clinicopathologic correlation of a large series of cases of Shy-Drager syndrome, olivopontocerebellar atrophy, and striatonigral degeneration.*

Santacruz P, Uttl B, Litvan I, Grafman J: Progressive supranuclear palsy. A survey of the disease course. Neurology 50:1637, 1998. *This study showed that early onset, presence of falls, slowness, and early downward-gaze palsy correlated with rapid progression.*

Stacy M, Jankovic J: Differential diagnosis of Parkinson's disease and the other parkinsonian syndromes. Neurol Clin 10:341, 1992. *A survey of most of the secondary forms of parkinsonism.*

maps to chromosome 2p in four families. Mov Disord 13:972, 1998. *A genetic study of four large families with autosomal dominant essential tremor showing a linkage to chromosome 2p22–25.*

Jankovic J, Beach J, Pandolfo M, Patel P: Familial essential tremor in four kindreds: Prospects for genetic mapping. Arch Neurol 54:289, 1997. *A detailed description and genetic characterization of four large families with essential tremor.*

Pollak P, Benabid AL, Krack P, et al: Deep brain stimulation. *In* Jankovic J, Tolosa E (eds): Parkinson's Disease and Movement Disorders, 3rd ed. Baltimore, Williams & Wilkins, 1998, pp 1085–1102. *A comprehensive review of the experience with thalamic, subthalamic, and pallidal stimulation in the treatment of severe tremors and Parkinson's disease.*

461 TREMORS

Joseph Jankovic

Essential tremor is the most common type of tremor encountered in developed countries. The tremor is inherited in an autosomal dominant pattern with high penetrance. Affected patients lack the hypokinetic features and rigidity of Parkinson's disease, discussed in the preceding chapter. Essential tremor typically produces flexion-extension oscillation of the hands at the wrists or adduction-abduction movements of the fingers when the arms are outstretched in front of the body. Although frequently referred to as "benign essential tremor," it may be partially disabling, often causing spilling of liquids and interfering with handwriting. Essential tremor also frequently involves the head and voice, which helps differentiate it from parkinsonian tremor. Another useful distinguishing feature is the occurrence of essential tremor during maintenance of posture; parkinsonian tremor is usually present when the affected body part is at relative rest. Parkinsonian patients, however, often exhibit postural tremor, and patients with essential tremor may have tremor at rest, thus suggesting an overlap between Parkinson's disease and essential tremor.

The frequency of essential tremor ranges from 4 to 12 Hz, and the oscillation may be produced by either alternating or synchronous contractions of antagonistic muscles. Some forms occur only during a specific activity, such as writing or holding an object in a particular position. Such *focal task-specific tremors* may be associated with task-specific dystonias ("occupational cramps") or with generalized essential tremor and dystonia. Nearly half of all patients with essential tremor show evidence of an associated dystonia. The nature of the link is unknown.

Essential tremor has many variants, including isolated head, voice, tongue, facial, and chin tremors and orthostatic tremor. Although considered a variant of essential tremor, orthostatic tremor usually does not respond to propranolol; clonazepam, however, provides satisfactory control in most patients. Rarely, focal tremor may be induced by trauma to the affected body part. This peripherally induced tremor is often associated with focal dystonia and reflex sympathetic dystrophy.

Essential tremor is an autosomal dominant disorder with a relatively high penetrance. Although no gene mutation has been identified, two loci, 3q13 and 2p22-p25, have been linked to the disease. Genetic heterogeneity in essential tremor is very likely given the different familial patterns characterized by either pure essential tremor or essential tremor in combination with dystonia or parkinsonism.

β-Adrenergic blocking drugs (e.g., propranolol at 80 to 240 mg/day) are the most effective agents in the treatment of essential tremor. Modest doses of alcohol also reduce the tremor in most instances, but this approach to treatment is impractical. Other occasionally useful drugs include primidone (starting dosage, 25 mg at bedtime; the daily dosage can be gradually increased to 750 mg/day), lorazepam, and alprazolam. Patients with a disabling essential tremor that does not respond satisfactorily to medications sometimes improve with local injections of botulinum. Thalamotomy is used as a last resort, but high-frequency thalamic stimulation is gaining wider acceptance as a treatment of disabling tremors unresponsive to pharmacologic therapy.

Higgins JJ, Loveless JM, Jankovic J, Patel P: Evidence that a gene for essential tremor

462 DYSTONIAS

Joseph Jankovic

DEFINITION. Dystonia is a syndrome dominated by involuntary, sustained (tonic) or spasmodic (rapid or clonic), patterned, and repetitive muscle contractions frequently causing twisting (e.g., torticollis), flexing or extending (e.g., writer's cramp, retrocollis), and squeezing (e.g., blepharospasm) movements or abnormal postures. Dystonia is frequently associated with other movement disorders, particularly tremor, myoclonus, and parkinsonism. Dystonia is diagnosed in about 1 in 3000 people, but the true prevalence is probably much higher.

CLASSIFICATION. Dystonia may vary in severity, and it may progress as follows: task-specific dystonia (occurring only during a specific activity such as writing or typing) progressing to action dystonia (present only during activity, not necessarily specific activity), progressing to overflow dystonia (involving adjacent muscles), progressing to dystonia at rest (present even during rest), and ultimately progressing to fixed postures (joint contractures). Dystonia is exacerbated by stress, fatigue, activity, or a change in posture and is relieved by sleep, relaxation, hypnosis, and a variety of sensory tricks. Whereas most dystonias are continuous, some occur paroxysmally and some have marked diurnal variations (Fig. 462–1). Partly because of fluctuations in severity, sometimes influenced by the emotional state of the patient, dystonia is often mistakenly attributed to psychogenic causes.

Dystonia can be classified according to its *distribution* as focal, segmental, multifocal, generalized, or unilateral (hemidystonia).

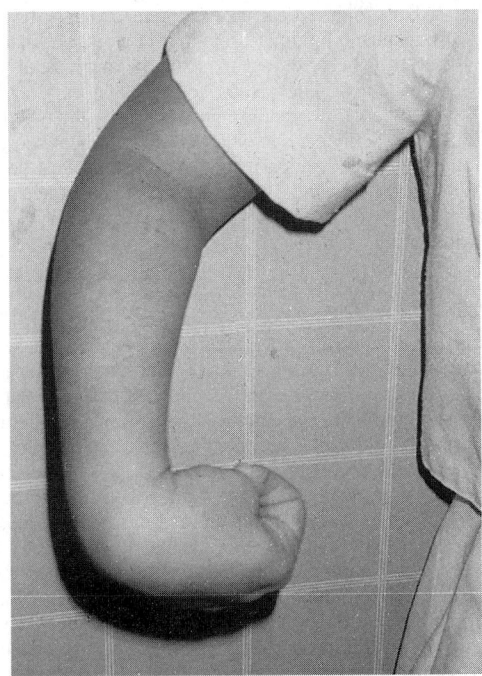

FIGURE 462–1 ■ Focal dystonia of the distal right arm.

Most childhood-onset dystonias begin focally, usually in one foot; other body parts become involved later, eventually resulting in generalized dystonia. In contrast, adult-onset dystonias tend to remain focal or segmental. Examples of focal dystonia include blepharospasm, oromandibular dystonia, torticollis, spasmodic dysphonia, and occupational (e.g., writer's, typist's, pianist's) cramps (see Fig. 462–1). Blepharospasm is categorized as a *focal* dystonia when it occurs alone (essential blepharospasm). In addition, blepharospasm is often associated with dystonic movements in the adjacent facial, oromandibular, laryngeal, and neck muscles. This *segmental dystonia* is sometimes referred to as Meige's syndrome, but the term *cranial-cervical dystonia* is more descriptive.

The most common form of dystonia is *cervical dystonia.* According to the position of the head, cervical dystonia can be categorized as torticollis, laterocollis, anterocollis, retrocollis, or a combination of these abnormal postures. A 3:2 female preponderance is noted, and the onset is usually in the 5th decade. Local pain is reported by about half the patients, and radiculopathy complicates cervical dystonia in about 20%. Half of all patients with cervical dystonia have an associated head-neck tremor. The tremor can be dystonic, seen only when the patient attempts to keep the head straight; essential, in which case the tremor persists irrespective of the position of the head; or a combination of dystonic and essential. About half the patients report a movement disorder such as tremor or dystonia in family members. The cause of most cervical dystonias is unknown. In 15% of cases, however, cervical dystonia can be attributed to either local trauma or exposure to neuroleptic drugs.

PATHOGENESIS. The pathoanatomy of dystonia is unknown, but studies suggest functional involvement of the basal ganglia, particularly the putamen, and the brain stem. Brain imaging and autopsy examinations usually yield normal findings. Post-mortem biochemical analyses have found evidence of enhanced noradrenergic transmission in the rostral brain stem.

PRIMARY DYSTONIA

Primary dystonia accounts for 90% of cases. Primary dystonias with onset in childhood have previously been termed *dystonia musculorum deformans.* Childhood-onset dystonias are often inherited, usually in an autosomal dominant pattern; about half of adult-onset cases seem to have a genetic basis. Other members of the family may have only partial manifestations, such as clubfoot, scoliosis, torticollis, writer's cramp, bruxism, or essential tremor. Genetic dystonia seems to have a higher prevalence among Ashkenazi Jews, but dystonias in both Jewish and non-Jewish individuals have been linked to a marker in the q32–q34 region of chromosome 9. Because a 3–base pair deletion in a gene coding for a novel adenosine triphosphate binding protein in the 9q34 locus termed *torsinA* has recently been shown to result in the loss of a pair of glutamic acid residues, gene testing for this abnormal *DYT1* gene can be carried out in individuals with dystonia. Other genetic dystonias include an X-linked dystonia, which has been described in some Filipino families. A dopa-responsive dystonia has been linked to a marker on chromosome 14, and several independent mutations in the guanosine triphosphatase–cyclohydrolase 1 *(GCH1)* gene have been identified.

SECONDARY DYSTONIA

Occasionally, a specific and potentially treatable cause of dystonia can be identified (see Fig. 462–1). One of the most important examples is *Wilson disease,* described in detail in Chapter 220. Neurologic symptoms are the initial manifestations in about 50% of patients with this autosomal recessive disorder, which appears during their 2nd or 3rd decade.

Tardive dystonia is a persistent form of dystonia caused by exposure to dopamine receptor blocking drugs such as major tranquilizers (e.g., chlorpromazine, thioridazine, fluphenazine, thiothixene, haloperidol, loxapine, amoxapine) and certain antiemetics (e.g., prochlorperazine, metoclopramide) (Fig. 462–2). Levodopa can also cause intermittent dystonia (and focal dystonia may be the initial symptom of Parkinson's disease). In all drug-induced dystonias, the offending drug should be withdrawn or the dosage reduced whenever possible. In contrast to focal, segmental, or generalized

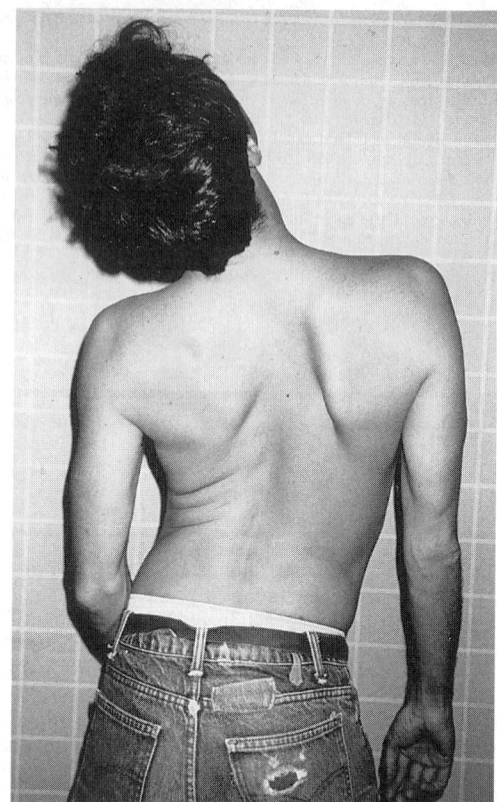

FIGURE 462–2 ■ Truncal dystonia in a manic-depressive patient with tardive dystonia secondary to a variety of antipsychotic drugs.

dystonia, hemidystonia is associated with an identifiable cause in most cases, including subcortical infarction, arteriovenous malformation, abscess, tumor, and other lesions, some of which can be treated surgically. Many other causes of secondary dystonia are possible, but only a few are amenable to therapy.

TREATMENT. Treatment consists of supportive therapy (e.g., relaxation techniques, prostheses), medications, botulinum toxin injections, and surgery. Anticholinergic drugs are sometimes beneficial. Trihexyphenidyl, the most frequently used anticholinergic, must be started in low doses and slowly increased to tolerance, perhaps up to 60 mg/day. Some children can tolerate such high doses, but anticholinergic side effects usually limit adult tolerance to 20 to 25 mg daily or less. In advanced cases, dopamine-depleting and dopamine receptor blocking drugs may be added. Muscle relaxants (e.g., diazepam or lorazepam), baclofen, and carbamazepine sometimes provide benefit. About 10% of patients with childhood or adolescent dystonia improve with levodopa, and therefore levodopa should be tried in all childhood and some adult-onset dystonia. Diurnal fluctuations with exacerbation of the movement disorder toward the end of the day are typical in this form of dystonia. In patients with refractory focal dystonia and, less often, segmental dystonia, injection of the paralysis-inducing botulinum toxin into the contracting muscles provides effective, albeit temporary relief. Such approaches are best left to those with experience in this treatment.

Patients who are socially and occupationally disabled by dystonia despite optimal medical therapy, including botulinum toxin, can sometimes be helped surgically. Surgical procedures include orbicularis myectomy for blepharospasm, cervical rhizotomy for neck dystonia, and thalamotomy, pallidotomy, or deep brain stimulation of the subthalamic nucleus or pallidum for hemidystonia or generalized (predominantly distal) dystonia. Such procedures are effective in a majority of patients but are associated with both potentially serious complications and high rates of symptom recurrence, thus making them a last resort.

Berardelli A, Rothwell JC, Hallett M, et al: The pathophysiology of primary dystonia. Brain 121:1195, 1998. *A review of physiologic abnormalities in patients with dystonia.*

Fahn S, Bressman S, Marsden CD: Classification of dystonia. Adv Neurol 78:1, 1998. *A comprehensive review of a new classification of dystonia.*

Jankovic J, Brin M: Therapeutic applications of botulinum toxin. N Engl J Med 324:

1186, 1991. *A critical review of studies using botulinum toxin in different dystonic and other disorders.*

Jankovic J, Fahn S: Dystonic disorders. *In* Jankovic J, Tolosa E (eds): Parkinson's Disease and Movement Disorders, 3rd ed. Baltimore, Williams & Wilkins, 1998, pp 513–551. *Comprehensive review of the clinical aspects and treatment of dystonia.*

Ozelius LJ, Hewett JW, Page CE, et al: The early onset torsion dystonia gene *[DYT1]* encodes an ATP-binding protein. Nat Genet 17:40, 1997. *A clinical-genetic study identifying torsinA as the mutated protein in primary, autosomal dominant dystonia.*

463 CHOREAS, ATHETOSIS, AND BALLISM

Joseph Jankovic

HUNTINGTON'S DISEASE

Huntington's disease (HD), an autosomal dominant disorder with complete penetrance, is the phenotype of an expanded triplet repeat sequence of a novel gene located at chromosome 4p16.3. Dementia and various emotional and psychiatric disturbances are prominent. The estimated prevalence of HD in the United States is 4 to 8 per 100,000 persons. Although about 10% of HD cases begin before age 20 years, the peak age at onset is in the fourth and fifth decades. Juvenile HD often first manifests with progressive parkinsonism, dementia, and seizures. In contrast, adult HD often starts with the insidious onset of clumsiness and adventitious, fidgety, random, brief movements. Initially, these purposeless movements may be incorporated into and masked by normal intentional acts, delaying the recognition of chorea. Chorea often begins distally, but as the disease progresses, it becomes generalized and can interrupt voluntary movements. Characteristically, patients with HD have difficulty in maintaining tongue protrusion or a steady grip, and their gait is often irregular, hesitant, unsteady, and dancelike. Other motor symptoms include dysarthria, dysphagia, and postural instability.

Neuropsychological symptoms may precede motor changes. They may consist of personality changes, apathy, social withdrawal, agitation, impulsiveness, depression, mania, paranoia, delusions, hostility, hallucinations, or psychosis. Cognitive changes are manifested chiefly by loss of recent memory and impaired judgment. Progressive motor dysfunction, dementia, and incontinence eventually lead to institutionalization and death. The duration of illness from onset to death is about 15 years for HD in adults and 8 to 10 years for the juvenile variant.

HD is regarded as truly an autosomal dominant disease in that homozygotes do not appear to differ clinically from typical heterozygotes. The mutation responsible for the disease consists of an unstable enlargement of the CAG repeat sequence in the 5' end of a large (210 kb) gene, IT15. This gene, located at 4p16.3, encodes a protein, called *huntingtin*. The expanded CAG repeat alters huntingtin by elongating a polyglutamine segment near the NH_2-terminus. Whereas the number of repeats varies between 10 and 29 copies in unaffected individuals, the HD gene contains 36 to 121 of such repeats. The intermediate-sized CAG repeats range from 30 to 35. Several studies have demonstrated that the number of repeats inversely correlates with the age at onset ("anticipation"). The rate of disease progression is generally faster in paternally transmitted HD independent of the CAG repeat length. Analyzing DNA for the expansion of trinucleotide repeats has provided a means for a reliable diagnostic test.

Postmortem changes in HD brains include neuronal loss and gliosis in the cortex and the striatum, particularly the caudate nucleus. The affected areas contain neuronal intranuclear inclusions and dystrophic neurites, but it is not yet clear whether these abnormalities result from or cause cell death and how they relate to the genetic mutation. It has been postulated that polyglutamine-tract expansion in the mutated huntingtin protein accumulate in the nucleus, forming insoluble amyloid-like fibrils, and these aggregates somehow interfere with normal cellular metabolism.

Chorea seems to be primarily related to the loss of striatal neurons projecting to the lateral globus pallidus (GPe), whereas rigid-akinetic symptoms correlate with the additional loss of striatal neurons projecting to the medial globus pallidus (GPi). Loss of medium-sized spiny neurons, which normally constitute 80% of all striatal neurons, is associated with a marked decrease in γ-aminobutyric acid (GABA) synthesis. Acetylcholine activity declines, presumably reflecting a degeneration of cholinergic striatal interneurons. Neuropeptides are markedly altered in HD: levels of substance P, cholecystokinin, and met-enkephalin decrease, but somatostatin, thyrotropin-releasing hormone, neurotensin, and neuropeptide Y levels increase. The number of dopamine, acetylcholine, and serotonin receptors is lowered in the striatum.

Reliable clinical diagnosis depends on the combination of chorea, emotional disturbances, progressive dementia, and a family history suggestive of autosomal dominant inheritance. Because spontaneous mutations are rare, lack of family history raises questions of paternity or misdiagnosis.

Treatment is symptomatic. The psychosis may improve with neuroleptic agents, such as haloperidol, pimozide, fluphenazine, and thioridazine, but these drugs can induce tardive dyskinesia and other adverse effects and should be used only if absolutely necessary. Monoamine-depleting drugs, such as reserpine (0.25 to 8 mg/day) and tetrabenazine (an investigational drug not available for general use in North America), may relieve chorea, do not cause tardive dyskinesia, and may be as effective as the dopamine-blocking drugs. Unfortunately, these drugs can cause or exacerbate depression, sedation, akathisia, and parkinsonism. Anxiolytics and antidepressants may be useful in some patients. Genetic aspects of HD should be discussed openly with patients to provide them and their relatives with nondirective counseling. The fact that presymptomatic individuals are in a position to determine their own disease status prior to having children places an unusually heavy burden on families with HD.

OTHER CHOREIC DISORDERS

Besides HD, other rare, genetically transmitted choreas include *benign hereditary chorea*, a nonprogressive chorea with childhood onset, and *paroxysmal choreoathetoses*. *Senile chorea* is a rare symptom complex in which chorea begins after age 60 years and is unaccompanied by the neurobehavioral symptoms or family history of HD. Some patients have been reported to have pathologic changes identical to those of HD; others have had predominant degeneration of the putamen rather than the caudate. *Neuroacanthocytosis*, also referred to as "chorea-acanthocytosis," usually presents in the third or fourth decade of life with a combination of self-mutilation manifested by lip and tongue biting, generalized chorea, lingual dystonia, and motor and phonic tics. Other features include seizures, amyotrophy, areflexia, and elevated levels of serum creatine phosphokinase. Wet blood or Wright-stained fast-dry smears reveal more than 15% of red blood cells as acanthocytes. Neuroimaging usually demonstrates caudate atrophy. The condition most often has a pattern of autosomal recessive inheritance. *Sydenham's chorea*, now uncommon, has an autoimmune basis, most often appearing as a consequence of infection with group A streptococcus. Unlike arthritis and carditis, which occur soon after such infection, chorea and various neurobehavioral symptoms may be delayed for 6 months or longer. Chorea appearing during pregnancy (chorea gravidarum), with use of birth control pills, or during the course of systemic lupus erythematosus probably has a similar pathogenesis.

ATHETOSIS

Athetosis is a slow form of chorea characterized by twisting, writhing movements. It most often accompanies static encephalopathy due to cerebral palsy, kernicterus, prematurity, glutaric aciduria, poststroke hemiplegia, and other causes of early life brain damage. In some cases, the movement disorder becomes progressive after decades of no apparent change. Athetosis usually does not respond to pharmacologic therapy.

BALLISM

Ballism is a form of forceful, flinging, high-amplitude, coarse chorea. Because the involuntary movement usually affects only one side of the body, the term hemiballism is used. The condition is often preceded by hemiparesis associated with a hemorrhagic or ischemic stroke involving the contralateral subthalamic nucleus (STN) or adjacent structures. Less common causes of hemiballism include abscess, arteriovenous malformation, cerebral trauma, hyperosmotic hyperglycemia, tumor, and multiple sclerosis. Most of these lesions involve the STN, but hemiballism has been described occasionally in patients with lesions outside the STN. Dopamine-blocking and -depleting drugs, used in the treatment of chorea, benefit most patients with hemiballism, but the disorder usually subsides spontaneously within several weeks. Occasional examples of prolonged disabling and medically intractable hemiballism can be treated with contralateral thalamotomy or pallidectomy.

Albin RL: Selective neurodegeneration in Huntington's disease. Ann Neurol 38:835–836, 1995. *Using neuropeptide immunochemistry, the investigators conclude that chorea correlates with damage to the striatal projections to GPe, whereas parkinsonian signs observed in some patients with HD result from additional damage in the projections to the GPi.*

DiFiglia M, Sapp E, Chase KO, et al: Aggregation of huntingtin in neuronal intranuclear inclusions and dystrophic neurites in brain. Science 277:1990–1993, 1997. *Using an antiserum against the NH₂-terminal of huntingtin, the authors found intense labeling localized to neuronal intranuclear inclusions in brains of three juvenile and six adult patients with HD.*

Jarman PR, Davis MB, Hodgson SV, et al: Paroxysmal dystonic choreoathetosis: Genetic linkage studies in a British family. Brain 120:2125–2130, 1997. *Assignment of locus for PDC to chromosome 2q; candidate gene: chloride/bicarbonate exchanger.*

464 TICS, MYOCLONUS, AND STEREOTYPIES

Joseph Jankovic

TICS

Tics are involuntary, abrupt, sudden, isolated, brief movements *(motor tics);* sounds produced by nose, mouth, or throat *(vocalphonic tics);* or sensations *(sensory tics).* Motor tics may be simple (e.g., eye blinking, nose twitching, head jerking) or complex (e.g., repetitive touching, jumping, kicking, pelvic gyrations). Similarly, vocalphonic tics may be simple (e.g., throat clearing, grunting, sniffing) or complex (e.g., echolalia, palilalia, coprolalia). Characteristics of tics include suppressibility, increase with stress and excitement, decrease with distraction and concentration, suggestibility, waxing and waning, and possible persistence during sleep.

The most common cause of tics is the *Gilles de la Tourette syndrome,* a genetic disorder dominated by tics and a variety of behavioral manifestations. Transient tics of childhood and persistent simple tics probably represent fragmentary forms of Tourette's syndrome. The following criteria are diagnostic:

1. Both multiple motor and one or more phonic tics must be present, although not necessarily concurrently
2. The tics occur many times, nearly every day or intermittently through a period of more than a year
3. The anatomic location, number, frequency, complexity, type, and severity of tics change over time
4. Onset is before age 21 years
5. Involuntary movements and noises cannot be explained by other medical conditions

Because of the fluctuating, heterogeneous, and often bizarre manifestations, affected patients frequently have their illness misdiagnosed by physicians and are mistreated by schoolmates, teachers, co-workers, and strangers.

Epidemiologic studies suggest that most cases of Tourette's syndrome are genetic, occurring in up to 1% of boys and with penetrance approaching 100%, particularly in males. A few cases may be nongenetic, triggered or caused by neuroleptic agents, carbon monoxide poisoning, head trauma, viral encephalitis, cocaine abuse, or opiate withdrawal. Many affected patients suffer from obsessive-compulsive disorder and have problems with attention and learning. Sleep disorders include parasomnias, bedwetting, and interruption by tics.

Therapy varies. Because most patients experience waxing and waning of symptoms and a generally favorable natural course, reassurance and behavioral therapy may be sufficient in mild cases. Drugs are indicated when tics cause physical discomfort or social embarrassment. Judicious use of dopamine receptor blocking drugs, such as fluphenazine, pimozide, and haloperidol, may reduce the frequency and severity of tics and ameliorate impulsive and aggressive behavior. These drugs, however, cause sedation, depression, and weight gain. Furthermore, tardive dyskinesia is a potentially serious complication of chronic neuroleptic therapy. Clonazepam, clonidine, fluoxetine, and clomipramine seem to be particularly helpful in the treatment of obsessive-compulsive disorder and other behavioral problems frequently associated with Tourette's syndrome.

MYOCLONUS

Myoclonus is a jerklike movement produced by a sudden, rapid, and brief contraction (positive myoclonus) or a muscle inhibition (negative myoclonus). *Segmental myoclonus* usually involves either the branchial structures, innervated by the lower cranial nerves and upper cervical nerve roots, or other body parts innervated by the spinal roots and nerves; it consists of rhythmic (1 to 3 Hz) contractions caused by a lesion of the brain stem or spinal cord. *Palatal myoclonus* results from acute or chronic lesions involving the anatomic triangle linking dentate, red, and inferior olivary nuclei. *Generalized myoclonus* is believed to reflect discharges arising from the brain stem reticular formation and is categorized as physiologic, essential, epileptic, or symptomatic. Two forms of myoclonus are associated with sleep: physiologic sleep myoclonus, occurring normally during initial phases of sleep, and nocturnal myoclonus, now called *periodic movements of sleep,* often associated with *restless legs syndrome* as well as with abnormal involuntary movements while the person is awake.

Causes of generalized myoclonus include acute and prolonged hypoxia and ischemia; various metabolic, infectious, and toxic factors; and exposure to neuroleptic drugs (tardive myoclonus). Myoclonus can be associated with familial chorea and dystonia and with many neurodegenerative disorders, including parkinsonism, progressive myoclonus epilepsy, and a variety of rare heredodegenerative disorders. Multifocal myoclonus often develops in the late stages of Creutzfeldt-Jakob disease and, less frequently, Alzheimer's disease.

The specific pathogeneses of myoclonus are unknown. Clonazepam, lorazepam, valproate, carbamazepine, and 5-hydroxytryptophan have been reported to have antimyoclonic activity. Clonazepam, at a dosage of 1 to 9 mg/day, is the drug of first choice, but the development of adverse effects, such as drowsiness, ataxia, and sexual dysfunction, often limits its usefulness.

STEREOTYPIES

The term *stereotypy* denotes a continuous or intermittent, involuntary, coordinated, patterned, repetitive, rhythmic, purposeless, but seemingly purposeful and ritualistic movement. Stereotypies may be simple (e.g., chewing movement, foot tapping, body rocking) or complex (e.g., complicated rituals, sitting down and arising from a chair). They can be volitionally suppressed. Stereotypies can accompany a variety of human behavioral disorders, such as anxiety, obsessive-compulsive disorders, Tourette's syndrome, schizophrenia, akathisia, autism, and mental retardation. Stereotypies and self-stimulatory or self-injurious behavior constitute the most recognizable symptoms in mentally retarded and autistic patients.

Tardive dyskinesia, a persistent movement disorder caused by exposure to dopamine receptor blocking drugs, is a frequently encountered stereotypy. Many other tardive movement disorders can result from the use of dopamine receptor blocking drugs (neuroleptics) (Table 464–1). The term *akathisia* describes the combination of stereotypy and a sensory component, such as an inner feeling of restlessness. The disorder particularly affects the lower extremities ("restless legs") and often is worse at night, causing insomnia, and it may be associated with periodic movements of sleep (see Chapter 448). Elderly women appear to be at particularly high risk for

Table 464–1 ■ NEUROLEPTIC-INDUCED MOVEMENT DISORDERS

ACUTE DISORDERS	CHRONIC DISORDERS
Dystonic reaction	Tardive dyskinesia
Parkinsonism	Stereotypic: oral-facial-lingual-masticatory
Akathisia	Trunk-pelvic
Neuroleptic malignant syndrome	Respiratory
	Choreic: limbs
	Tardive dystonia; tics; myoclonus; tremor; akathisia; parkinsonism

tardive dyskinesia. The mechanism of the disorder is poorly understood but is believed to result from the development of supersensitive dopamine receptors caused by chronic neuroleptic blockade. Prevention is the best treatment for the drug-induced movement disorders. Whenever possible, drugs other than the neuroleptics should be used for psychiatric or gastrointestinal problems. When no alternative exists, the dosage and duration of exposure should be kept at a minimum. Spontaneous remissions of tardive dyskinesia occasionally follow withdrawal of the offending agent. Dopamine-depleting drugs, such as tetrabenazine or reserpine, are the most effective drugs in its symptomatic treatment.

Jankovic J: Tardive syndromes and other drug-induced movement diseases. Clin Neuropharmacol 18:197–214, 1995. *A comprehensive review of clinical and pharmacologic features of tardive dyskinesias and other movement disorders produced by dopaminergic or antidopaminergic drugs.*
Jankovic J: Tourette syndrome: Phenomenology and classification of tics. Neurol Clin 15:267–275, 1997. *A critical review of current knowledge about the motor and behavioral aspects of Tourette's syndrome.*
Kurlan R: Tourette's syndrome and "PANDAS": Will the relation bear out? Neurology 50:1530–1534, 1998. *A critical review of the current concepts of post-streptococcal movement disorders, including tics.*
Ondo W, Jankovic J: Restless legs syndrome. *In* Appel SH (ed): Current Neurology, vol 17. Amsterdam, IOS Press, 1998, pp 207–236. *A comprehensive review of the clinical features and treatment of restless legs syndrome, a common neurologic movement disorder.*

■ DEGENERATIVE DISEASES OF THE NERVOUS SYSTEM

465 INTRODUCTION

Eva L. Feldman

Substantial progress has been made in recent years in our understanding of neurodegenerative diseases. Advances in molecular genetics have clarified the interrelationships between several degenerative diseases and have facilitated early disease diagnosis and improved disease classification. This section deals with several degenerative diseases in which a single gene has been identified as the cause of the disorder. These diseases include the hereditary ataxias, spastic paraplegia, and motor neuron diseases. Other major neurodegenerative diseases in which single genes are implicated are Alzheimer's disease (see Chapter 449.3) and Huntington's disease (see Chapter 463), whereas the degenerative disorder Parkinson's disease (see Chapter 460) is more likely polygenic.

An important common mutation mechanism in single-gene disorders involves the expansion of the normal genome by runs of three DNA bases, known as *trinucleotide repeats*. The trinucleotide repeat diseases can be inherited as autosomal dominant, recessive, or X-linked disorders. Individuals in successive generations are often more severely affected at a younger age. This phenomenon, known as *anticipation*, occurs as the unstable trinucleotide repeats expand between parents and offspring. Trinucleotide repeats can occur within the coding region (exons) or noncoding regions (introns) of genes. It is not yet known why genomic expansion leads to disease, although location of the mutation (i.e., in a coding or noncoding region) is likely important. For example, trinucleotide repeat disorders in which genomic expansion occurs in the coding region appear to represent adult-onset, gain-of-function disorders. These include the spinocerebellar ataxias. In contrast, if the repeat is located in a noncoding region, the disorder frequently occurs at a younger age, represents a loss of function, and involves multiple organs. Friedreich's ataxia is an example of a trinucleotide repeat occurring in a noncoding region. Table 465-1 lists the neurodegenerative diseases with trinucleotide repeats discussed in Chapters 466 and 468.

Table 465–1 ■ TRINUCLEOTIDE REPEAT DISEASES

DISEASE	CHROMOSOME:GENE	TRIPLET REPEAT	NORMAL SIZE REPEAT	EXPANDED REPEAT SIZE
Friedreich's ataxia	9q13:frataxin	GAA	7–22	200–>900
SCA1	6p23–24:ataxin-1	CAG	6–39	40–81
SCA2	12q23–24:ataxin-2	CAG	15–29	35–59
SCA3 and MJD	14q24.3–qter:ataxin-3	CAG	12–40	67–200 (SCA3) 66–84 (MJD)
SCA6	19p13:calcium channel	CAG	4–16	21–27
BSMA	Xq11–12:androgen receptor	CAG	11–33	40–66

MJD = Machado-Joseph disease; BSMA = bulbospinal muscular atrophy.
Adapted from Wasielewski PG, Scharre DW, Mendell JR: Inherited neurological disorders: Relevant considerations and new aspects. *In* Joynt RJ, Griggs RC (eds): Clinical Neurology, Vol. 1, pp 1–48. Philadelphia, Lippincott–Raven, 1997.

466 | HEREDITARY CEREBELLAR ATAXIAS AND RELATED DISORDERS

Eva L. Feldman

The hereditary cerebellar ataxias are progressive disorders that can begin in childhood or adulthood. The most common progressive inherited ataxia in children is Friedreich's ataxia. A less common disorder producing childhood ataxia, ataxia/telangiectasia, is further described in Chapter 272. In the adult ataxias, at least seven late-onset cerebellar disorders have been identified, now classified as spinocerebellar ataxia (SCA) types 1 through 7.

FRIEDREICH'S ATAXIA

DEFINITION AND ETIOLOGY. Friedreich's ataxia is a trinucleotide repeat disorder affecting the central and peripheral nervous systems and many other organs. A GAA unstable expansion on the long arm of chromosome 9 disrupts the protein frataxin, whose function is not yet known. In unaffected persons, the normal length of the GAA repeat is 10 to 21 copies. In individuals with Friedreich's ataxia, expansion results in between 200 to 900 copies. Disease severity correlates with number of copies and explains the different disease phenotypes. Higher numbers of copies correlate with more severe neurologic deficits. Friedreich's ataxia is thus far unique among the trinucleotide repeat disorders: it is an autosomal recessive disorder with no anticipation.

INCIDENCE AND PREVALENCE. The estimated carrier frequency is 1 in 100 with a disease prevalence of 1 per 50,000.

PATHOLOGY. At autopsy, patients with Friedreich's ataxia have atrophic spinal cords with loss of neurons in Clarke's columns and the dorsal root ganglia. Spinocerebellar tracts, pyramidal tracts, dorsal column tracts, and peripheral nerves are all degenerated with minor cell loss in the brain stem and cerebellum. Cardiac ventricular hypertrophy with chronic interstitial fibrosis of the myocardium is frequently present.

CLINICAL MANIFESTATIONS. The clinical diagnosis of Friedreich's ataxia is made when patients meet the following criteria: (1) onset during puberty; (2) progressive ataxia with loss of lower extremity deep tendon reflexes; (3) presence of Babinski's sign (extensor plantar responses); and (4) 5 or more years of disease and a family history compatible with autosomal recessive inheritance, often involving only a single patient in a family. Other common clinical features include nystagmus, dysarthria, stocking-glove neuropathy, and pes cavus with weakness in the lower extremities. Patients frequently have cardiomyopathy and skeletal abnormalities, such as kyphosis and scoliosis; and diabetes mellitus develops in a small percentage.

DIAGNOSIS. Diagnosis of Friedreich's ataxia is made by positive genetic testing in a patient with appropriate clinical signs and symptoms. Other diagnostic entities that can give a similar clinical picture include vitamin B_{12} deficiency, abetalipoproteinemia, and a selective defect in vitamin E absorption.

TREATMENT AND PROGNOSIS. No treatment, other than sup-portive measures, is currently available. The disorder is progressive, and patients are usually nonambulatory by their mid-20s. Patients occasionally have a much more benign course and atypical clinical features. The major cause of death is heart failure as a result of hypertrophic cardiomyopathy. The average age at death is 37 years.

SPINOCEREBELLAR ATAXIA TYPES 1 TO 7 AND MACHADO-JOSEPH DISEASE

DEFINITION AND ETIOLOGY. Before the advent of molecular genetics, classification of the autosomal dominant spinocerebellar ataxias was difficult, and it was a source of controversy. Recent advances in genetics have permitted these disorders to be divided into seven syndromes (SCA 1 to 7). Four of these ataxias are trinucleotide-repeat diseases.

SCA 1 to 3 and 6 are trinucleotide-repeat disorders, involving expansion of a CAG repeat coding for a polyglutamine tract within the normal gene product. In SCA 1 to 3, the function of the disrupted protein, known as ataxin, is unknown. In SCA 6, the CAG repeat disrupts the function of a voltage-dependent calcium channel found in the Purkinje cells of the cerebellum. SCA 6 is thus considered a channelopathy.

Chromosomal location is known for SCA 4 (16q24-ter), SCA 5 (centromeric region of 11), and SCA 7 (3p12.21.1). The gene and mutation for each disorder have not yet been identified. In SCA 5 and 7, the documented presence of anticipation suggests that these will prove to be trinucleotide triplicate-repeat disorders.

INCIDENCE AND PREVALENCE. The estimated carrier frequency is 1 to 10 per 100,000 in Europe. Data are not yet available for the incidence and prevalence of SCA 1 to 7.

PATHOLOGY. At autopsy, patients with SCA have olivopontocerebellar atrophy with loss of neurons in the inferior olives and the pons. Degeneration of spinocerebellar tracts, pyramidal tracts, and posterior column tracts occurs. Depending on the SCA type, neuronal loss is noted in the spinal cord (anterior horn cells), midbrain, basal ganglia, and cerebral and cerebellar cortex. In SCA 3 and Machado-Joseph disease, the cerebellar cortex and olives remain intact.

CLINICAL MANIFESTATIONS. The predominant clinical feature of these disorders is ataxia, followed by dysarthria and ophthalmoplegia. Other cerebellar signs include titubation, dysdiadochokinesia, and dysmetria. With increasing ataxia, patients can become nonambulatory. Additional clinical signs include dementia, optic atrophy, retinal pigmentary degeneration, deafness, dysphagia, extrapyramidal and pyramidal findings, and peripheral neuropathy. The extrapyramidal features include masked facies, cogwheel rigidity, dystonia, athetosis, and chorea. Pyramidal dysfunction includes limb spasticity (especially in the legs), hyperreflexia, and a Babinski response. The predominant clinical features of each disorder are presented in Table 466–1.

Machado-Joseph disease (MJD) and SCA 3 are allelic disorders. MJD was initially described in families of Azorean decent. Ataxia and ophthalmoplegia are common clinical features in MJD in each of the 3 MJD phenotypes. Distinguishing characteristics for MJD types 1 to 3 include the following:

1. Type I: Early onset (mean age, 24 years) with marked pyramidal and extrapyramidal dysfunction
2. Type II: Later onset (mean age, 40 years)
3. Type III: Latest onset (mean age, 47 years) with predominant weakness and amyotrophy

Table 466–1 ■ CLINICAL FEATURES OF THE SPINOCEREBELLAR ATAXIAS

DISEASE	AGE AT ONSET (yr)	ATAXIA	DYSARTHRIA	OPHTHALMOPLEGIA	OTHER SIGNS
SCA 1	30–40	+	+	+	Nystagmus, optic atrophy, pyramidal tract signs, dementia
SCA 2	Early 30s	+	+	+	Muscle cramps, slow saccades, peripheral neuropathy
MJD	20–40	+	+	+	
SCA 3	Mid-30s	+	+	+	
SCA 4	40	+	−	−	Sensory axonal neuropathy
SCA 5	Mid-30s	+	+	−	
SCA 6	20–40	+	+	−	Distal sensory loss
SCA 7	Mid-20s	+	+	+	Pigmentary retinal degeneration, pyramidal tract signs

MJD = Machado-Joseph disease.

DIAGNOSIS. Diagnosis of SCA 1 to 3, SCA 6, and MJD is made by positive genetic testing in a patient with appropriate clinical signs and symptoms. Magnetic resonance imaging shows olivopontocerebellar atrophy. Other diagnostic entities that can give a similar clinical profile include alcoholism (see Chapter 489) and paraneoplastic cerebellar syndromes.

TREATMENT AND PROGNOSIS. No specific therapy is currently available for the spinocerebellar ataxias. As with all neurodegenerative disorders, treatment is supportive and is aimed at maximizing and retaining function. These disorders are progressive but are not necessarily the cause of death, depending on the SCA type as well as the age at onset in individual cases. Patients with SCA 1 are usually nonambulatory about 10 years after appearance of the initial symptoms, and restrictive pulmonary disease and progressive weakness develop. The major cause of death in SCA 1 is usually pneumonia.

Conner KE, Rosenberg RN: The genetic basis of ataxia. *In* Rosenberg RN, Prusiner SB, DiMauro S, Barchi RL (eds): The Molecular and Genetic Basis of Neurological Disease, 2nd ed. Boston, Butterworth-Heinemann, 1997, pp 503–544. *A concise, lucid guide to understanding the genetics of ataxia.*

Harding AE: Cerebellar and spinocerebellar disorders. *In* Bradley WG, Daroff RB, Fenichel GM, Marsden CD (eds): Neurology in Clinical Practice, vol II, 2nd ed. Boston, Butterworth-Heinemann, 1996, pp 1773–1790. *An excellent description of the clinical manifestations of the spinocerebellar ataxias.*

Wasielewski PG, Scharre DW, Mendell JR: Inherited neurological disorders: Relevant considerations and new aspects. *In* Joynt RJ, Griggs RC (eds): Clinical Neurology, vol 1. Philadelphia, Lippincott-Raven, 1997, pp 1–48. *A reader-friendly review that incorporates succinct clinical descriptions with the known molecular genetics of the ataxias.*

467 HEREDITARY SPASTIC PARAPLEGIAS

Eva L. Feldman

DEFINITION AND ETIOLOGY. Pure hereditary spastic paraplegia (HSP), also known as Strumpell's disease, is usually an autosomal dominant disorder (70 to 80% of reported cases), although clear evidence also exists for autosomal recessive and X-linked inheritance. Three different loci are known for autosomal dominant HSP: (1) the spastic paraplegia 3 locus: 14q11.2–q24.3; (2) the spastic paraplegia 4 locus: 2p21–p24; and (3) the spastic paraplegia 6 locus: 15q11.1. Although the exact genes and mutations remain undefined, anticipation as well as CAG repeat expansions are present in HSP patients linked to 2p21–p24. It is likely, therefore, that one or more forms of HSP, like the spinocerebellar ataxias, represent trinucleotide repeat disorders.

INCIDENCE AND PREVALENCE. In the Cantabria region of Spain, a careful epidemiologic study revealed a prevalence of 10 cases of HSP per 100,000 individuals.

PATHOLOGY. At autopsy, patients with HSP have axonal degeneration of the pyramidal tracts and dorsal column tracts with lesser involvement of the spinocerebellar tracts. The neurons of origin are intact. The peripheral nervous system is unaffected.

CLINICAL MANIFESTATIONS. Patients with HSP meet the following clinical criteria: (1) progressive gait disturbance, (2) spasticity of lower extremities, and (3) hyperreflexia, frequently grade 4, with Babinski's sign (extensor plantar responses). Although patients can experience weakness of their lower extremities, spasticity is usually the disabling component of HSP. Patients have a slow, stiff gait, they trip easily, and they are unable to run. Other clinical features include pes cavus (30 to 50%); decreased vibratory sensation; and urinary frequency, urgency, and hesitancy.

DIAGNOSIS. Diagnosis of HSP is made when patients meet clinical criteria. Magnetic resonance imaging may show spinal cord atrophy; cerebrospinal fluid analysis and nerve conduction studies are normal. The differential diagnosis includes other genetic conditions, spinal cord disease from structural lesions, multiple sclerosis, and vitamin deficiencies or retroviral infections (Table 467–1).

TREATMENT AND PROGNOSIS. No specific treatment is currently available. Symptomatic therapy is aimed at decreasing disability and preventing complications, such as contractures. The

Table 467–1 ■ DIFFERENTIAL DIAGNOSIS OF HEREDITARY SPASTIC PARAPLEGIAS

Hereditary
  Dopa-responsive dystonia
  Spinocerebellar ataxias
  Adult-onset adrenoleukodystrophy
  Friedreich's ataxia
Structural lesions of the spinal cord
  Cervical spondylosis
  Tumor
  Arteriovenous malformation
  Syringomyelia
Multiple sclerosis
  Primary lateral sclerosis
Vitamin B_{12} or E deficiency
Infections
  HTLV-1
  HIV
  Tertiary syphilis

HTLV-1 = human T-lymphotropic virus type 1; HIV = human immunodeficiency virus.

main class of drugs used are the antispastic agents, such as baclofen. Oral baclofen improves spasticity but may worsen weakness. Preliminary reports have suggested improved therapeutic response with intrathecal baclofen. No controlled clinical trials have addressed this issue. Most patients become nonambulatory at between 60 and 70 years of age.

Reid E: Pure hereditary spastic paraplegia. J Med Genet 34:499–503, 1997. *A recently completed review of the subject citing virtually every key reference.*

468 MOTOR NEURON DISEASES

Eva L. Feldman

Motor neuron diseases are a heterogeneous group of disorders that selectively affect upper or lower motor neurons or both (Table 468–1). Upper motor neurons are large cerebral and bulbar motor neurons whose dysfunction leads to decreased strength, spasticity, and hyperreflexia. Lower motor neurons are located in the ventral spinal cord, and when they are affected by lesions they produce decreased strength, tone, and reflexes accompanied by fascicula-

Table 468–1 ■ THE MAJOR MOTOR NEURON DISEASES

Hereditary
Autosomal dominant
  Familial amyotrophic lateral sclerosis (FALS)
Autosomal recessive
  Spinal muscular atrophy
    Type I. Acute, infantile (Werdnig-Hoffmann disease)
    Type II. Late infantile
    Type III. Juvenile and adult types (Kugelberg-Welander disease)
X-Linked
  Bulbospinal muscular atrophy (Kennedy's syndrome)
Acquired
Acute: anterior poliomyelitis
Chronic:
  Sporadic ALS
  Postpoliomyelitis syndrome, motor neuron loss associated with spinocerebellar degeneration, multisystem atrophy, Creutzfeldt-Jakob disease
ALS-like syndromes:
  Motor neuron disease with gammopathy or paraproteinemia, heavy metal intoxication, hexoseaminidase-A deficiency, paraneoplastic motor neuronopathy
Primary lateral sclerosis (rare)

tions and atrophy. Pure upper motor neuron disorders are most commonly acquired, whereas pure lower motor neuron disorders are frequently inherited. The most common acquired motor neuron disease, amyotrophic lateral sclerosis, usually includes dysfunction of both upper and lower motor neurons. Recent advances in the molecular genetics of hereditary motor neuron diseases has improved their classification and led to advances in defining potential etiologies underlying acquired motor neuron disorders.

HEREDITARY MOTOR NEURON DISEASES: SPINAL MUSCULAR ATROPHIES

The spinal muscular atrophies are hereditary, progressive motor neuron disorders that can begin in utero, during infancy, in childhood, or in adulthood. This section focuses on spinal muscular atrophy (SMA) types 1 to 3 and bulbospinal muscular atrophy, also known as Kennedy's syndrome. The genetic characteristics of these disorders are defined; they are also more frequently diagnosed than the other spinal muscular atrophies: distal hereditary motor neuropathy types I and II, upper limb–predominant hereditary motor neuropathy (type V), proximal spinal muscular atrophy, and scapuloperoneal syndromes due to spinal muscular atrophies (see Table 468–1).

DEFINITION AND ETIOLOGY. SMA 1 to 3 represent the first class of neurologic disorders in which a developmental defect in neuronal apoptosis is the most likely cause of the disease. Linkage to chromosome 5q13 led to the identification of two genes involved in SMA, the neuronal apoptosis inhibitor protein (NAIP) and survival motor neuron (SMN) genes. Homozygous deletions in exons 7 and 8 are present in the telomeric copy (SMNt) of SMN. Individuals with homozygous deletions of SMNt are more severely affected and their disease is classified as SMA 1 or Werdnig-Hoffmann disease. Mutations that convert SMNt to the centromeric copy result in a milder disease phenotype. These individuals have SMA 2 (late infantile) and 3 (Kugelberg-Welander disease). Deletions of exons 5 and 6 of NAIP or complete absence of the gene occurs in 45 to 65% of patients with SMA 1 and in 20 to 40% of individuals with SMA 2 and 3. NAIP mutations may modify the severity of SMA.

INCIDENCE AND PREVALENCE. The estimated carrier frequency of a SMNt mutation is 1 in 50. SMA 1 (Werdnig-Hoffmann disease) has a cumulative incidence of disease of 1 in 8000 births.

PATHOLOGY. At autopsy, patients with SMA have atrophic spinal cords with loss of α-motor neurons and evidence of motor neuron degeneration and gliosis. Ventral roots are atrophic, and muscle groups supplied by these motor neurons and roots are atrophied and show microscopic evidence of denervation and reinnervation. Before genetic testing was available, muscle biopsies were the main diagnostic tool used to confirm the clinical diagnosis of SMA 1 to 3.

CLINICAL MANIFESTATIONS. The onset of SMA 1 (Werdnig-Hoffmann disease), by definition, occurs either in utero or within the first 3 months of life. Infants present with severe diffuse weakness, hypotonia, reduced or absent reflexes, and tongue fasciculations. The usual cause of death is respiratory failure; 50% of infants die by age 7 months and 95% by 17 months.

Individuals with SMA 2 (late infantile form) and 3 (Kugelberg-Welander disease) are less severely affected than those with SMA 1. SMA 2 is considered an intermediate phenotype. The onset occurs in children younger than 18 to 24 months. These children may never stand or walk, develop early scoliosis and respiratory insufficiency, and have a shortened lifespan. SMA 3 is the mildest phenotype, with onset frequently in later childhood or even in the teen years. These individuals have proximal, symmetrical weakness but stand and walk independently. With time, slow and mild loss of function usually takes place. Death occurs in adulthood, and whether SMA 3 shortens an individual's lifespan remains uncertain.

DIAGNOSIS. Diagnosis of SMA 1 to 3 is made by genetic testing in a patient with appropriate clinical signs and symptoms. Ninety-five per cent of affected individuals have SMN deletions. Carrier testing can only currently be performed by linkage analysis. Electromyography and muscle biopsy reveal evidence of denervation but are unnecessary if a molecular diagnosis is established.

They are often performed before the diagnosis has been considered. Both cerebrospinal fluid (CSF) analysis and serum creatine kinase level are normal.

It is important to distinguish SMA 1 from infantile botulism, which can present with a similar clinical picture. Electromyography with high-frequency repetitive nerve stimulation shows a decrement in botulism but not in SMA. Examination of the stool for botulinum can confirm the diagnosis of infantile botulism. SMA 2 and 3 can be distinguished from chronic inflammatory demyelinating polyneuropathy by the presence of normal CSF protein and normal nerve conduction studies in SMA. SMA 3 and the hereditary motor sensory neuropathies (Charcot-Marie-Tooth disease) can be clinically similar. In addition to genetic testing, key diagnostic differences lie in normal nerve conduction studies in individuals with SMA 3 compared to abnormal studies in individuals with hereditary motor sensory neuropathies.

TREATMENT AND PROGNOSIS. No treatment is currently available. In SMA 2 and 3, children benefit from passive and active physical therapy, lightweight braces, and, if necessary, surgery to correct scoliosis.

BULBOSPINAL MUSCULAR ATROPHY

DEFINITION AND ETIOLOGY. Bulbospinal muscular atrophy (BSMA) was first described in 1968 by Kennedy and colleagues, and consequently it is also called Kennedy's syndrome. BSMA is a trinucleotide-repeat disorder with a CAG expansion encoding for a polyglutamine tract in the first exon of the androgen receptor gene, on chromosome Xq11–12. It is not known why disruption of the androgen receptor gene alters the function of bulbar and spinal motor neurons. It is of interest that other disorders of androgen receptors result in testicular feminization but spare motor neurons. This suggests that BSMA may be due to a gain or change in function of the androgen receptor on motor neurons.

INCIDENCE AND PREVALENCE. BSMA is an X-linked recessive disorder. Incidence and prevalence have not been defined, but it is commonly held that BSMA is the most common form of adult-onset SMA.

PATHOLOGY. At autopsy, patients with BSMA have findings similar to those of SMA 3. Mild brain stem and cord atrophy with loss of α-motor neurons is seen, as is evidence of motor neuron degeneration and gliosis. Muscle biopsy reveals denervation and reinnervation in affected muscle groups.

CLINICAL MANIFESTATIONS. The mean onset of BSMA is 30 years with a range of 15 to 60 years. Gynecomastia occurs in 50% of affected individuals. Individuals present with facial, tongue, and proximal weakness. Dysphagia, dysarthria, and masseter muscle weakness are common. Weakness is symmetrical and slowly progressive over decades; patients only become dependent on canes or walkers in the fifth or sixth decade of life. Fasciculations are present largely in the face, and tendon reflexes are reduced or absent. Individuals frequently experience a mild postural tremor and a mild loss of vibratory sensation. No upper motor neuron signs are present.

DIAGNOSIS. Diagnosis of BSMA is made when a patient with appropriate clinical signs and symptoms has positive genetic test results. A direct correlation exists between disease severity and size of the CAG expansion; individuals affected at a younger age and more severely have longer polyglutamine tracts. The absence of upper motor neuron signs distinguishes BSMA from amyotrophic lateral sclerosis. Electromyography and a muscle biopsy are often performed, because creatine kinase levels are frequently elevated (up to 10-fold), and they reveal evidence of chronic denervation. This differentiates BSMA from muscular dystrophy and other myopathies.

TREATMENT AND PROGNOSIS. No specific treatment is available. Clinical trials are exploring the value of hormones. Currently, therapy consists of supportive care, such as ambulatory aids.

AMYOTROPHIC LATERAL SCLEROSIS

DEFINITION AND ETIOLOGY. Sporadic amyotrophic lateral sclerosis (ALS) accounts for approximately 80% of all cases of acquired motor neuron disease, whereas the remaining 20% of patients have either only lower motor neuron signs or a familial form of ALS (FALS).

The 80% of patients that have sporadic ALS present with spasticity, hyperreflexia, and Babinski's sign (upper motor neuron signs) in the setting of progressive muscle wasting and weakness (lower motor neuron signs).

Autosomal dominant FALS is an adult-onset disease that is clinically and pathologically indistinguishable from sporadic ALS. An ALS locus was first reported in 1991 on human chromosome 21q. In 1993, protein cytosolic copper-zinc superoxide dismutase (SOD1) was reported to be mutated in several FALS families, and more than 50 missense mutations in SOD1 have been identified in patients with FALS. However, SOD1 mutations account for only approximately 20% of cases of FALS. The importance of the SOD1 defect is that other cases of FALS, as well as sporadic ALS, are clinically identical to SOD1 cases, suggesting a common mechanism of disease.

SOD1 is a metalloenzyme with active sites for both copper and zinc. SOD1 detoxifies the superoxide anion to form hydrogen peroxide, which in turn is converted to water. Nitric oxide may also combine with superoxide to form peroxynitrite, which is non-enzymatically converted to hydroxyl radicals. These reactive oxygen species can cause oxidative degradation of proteins and lipids and lead to cell death. FALS is due to a gain of an adverse function of the mutated SOD1 protein. Mice that overexpress mutant SOD1 develop a denervating illness that resembles ALS despite normal or increased levels of SOD1 activity. The severity of the abnormality correlates with the levels of mutant SOD1; the higher the level of SOD1, the more widespread and lethal the disease.

The relationship between SOD1 mediated FALS and sporadic ALS is not known. However, research on FALS has led to the theory that sporadic ALS may represent an acquired age-associated change in SOD1 function with resultant oxidative injury to the nervous system. Other suggested etiologies for sporadic ALS include alterations in glutamate excitotoxicity or neurotoxicity, abnormal accumulations of neurofilaments, and altered neurotropism.

INCIDENCE AND PREVALENCE. ALS has an estimated annual incidence of 2 per 100,000 with a worldwide prevalence of 4 to 6 per 100,000.

PATHOLOGY. At autopsy, patients with ALS have brain stem and spinal cord atrophy with loss of motor neurons and associated extensive gliosis. In the cortex, large pyramidal cell loss leads to degeneration of the corticospinal tracts and gliosis of the lateral spinal cord columns. As with other denervating disorders, loss of ventral nerve roots, with microscopic evidence of denervation and reinnervation in affected muscle groups, is seen.

CLINICAL MANIFESTATIONS. ALS is a disorder of upper and lower motor neurons. This combination results in a complex clinical syndrome. Painless, progressive weakness is the usual presenting sign and symptom of ALS. Usually focal in onset, weakness then spreads to contiguous muscle groups. Weakness is accompanied by muscle atrophy. Head "ptosis" due to weakness of neck extensor muscles with head droop is often present in ALS. Individuals frequently experience muscle cramps. Spasticity is common, and patients may complain of spontaneous clonus. With more long-standing disease, foot and hand deformities are seen due to tendon imbalance and secondary joint contractures.

ALS can present with bulbar dysfunction, although more commonly bulbar signs and symptoms are seen in the presence of extremity and truncal weakness. Individuals experience dysarthria, or impaired speech, which may be flaccid or spastic or of a mixed flaccid-spastic quality. Dysphagia with choking is common and places patients at a high risk of aspiration. The absence of spontaneous swallowing results in sialorrhea, or drooling.

Weakness of respiratory muscles is common and is the presenting symptom in rare cases in ALS. Early in ALS, individuals complain of dyspnea with exertion and frequently sigh at rest. With disease progression, dyspnea at rest, inability to sleep in a supine position (orthopnea), sleep apnea, and morning headaches are present. Constitutional symptoms reflect loss of muscle mass and difficulties with swallowing and breathing. Individuals experience weight loss and frequently complain of fatigue.

Several aspects of neurologic function are usually spared in ALS. These include mentation, extraocular movements, bowel and bladder function, and sensation. Although they are rare, exceptions to

each of these have occurred. It has been reported that approximately 1 to 2% of patients with ALS have dementia and ophthalmoplegia, usually reflecting ocular apraxia. Although bladder function is usually reported as normal, detailed study of bladder function has revealed that nearly one-third of ALS patients experience urgency and obstructive micturition.

Debate continues about whether a disorder termed "primary lateral sclerosis" (PLS) is a subtype of upper motor neuron ALS or is a separate entity. In this rare condition, individuals present with a slowly progressive spastic paraparesis or quadriparesis, with no evidence of lower motor neuron involvement, either by clinical examination or diagnostic testing. Individuals with these presenting signs and symptoms should undergo the same diagnostic procedures and require similar treatment strategies as patients with sporadic ALS. Some patients with PLS have an autosomal recessive form of hereditary spastic paraplegia (see Chapter 467).

DIAGNOSIS. The El Escorial World Federation of Neurology criteria provide a set of guidelines for the diagnosis of ALS. In these criteria, the body is divided into four regions: (1) bulbar (jaw, face, palate, larynx, and tongue), (2) cervical (neck, arm, hand, and diaphragm), (3) thoracic (back and abdomen), and (4) lumbosacral (back, abdomen, leg, and foot). The diagnosis of definite ALS is made when upper and lower motor neuron signs are present in the bulbar region and two other spinal regions or in three spinal regions. Individuals with upper and lower motor neuron signs in two spinal regions alone are classified as having probable ALS; possible ALS is diagnosed if dysfunction is present in only one region or if an individual presents with only upper motor neuron signs in two regions or if lower motor neuron signs are rostral to upper motor neuron signs.

When the clinical findings suggest a diagnosis of ALS, nerve conduction studies with repetitive stimulation and electromyography (EMG) are performed to confirm lower motor neuron degeneration and to exclude disorders of the neuromuscular junction, such as myasthenia gravis, and of peripheral nerve and muscle. Neuroimaging of the brain and spinal cord is often needed to confirm the expected normal anatomy present in ALS and exclude structural pathologic processes. Routine clinical laboratory tests are necessary to exclude ALS-related syndromes. These tests include complete blood cell count and routine chemical analyses, thyroid studies, serum protein electrophoresis, serum immunoelectrophoresis with immunofixation, and measurements of serum VDRL, creatine kinase, erythrocyte sedimentation rate, antinuclear antibody, rheumatoid factor, and when clinically indicated hexosaminidase A and paraneoplastic antibodies. Additional tests may be warranted on the basis of the patient's clinical presentation.

The EMG, neuroimaging, and clinical laboratory tests exclude the most common ALS-related disorders: polyradiculopathy with myelopathy, post-polio syndrome, multifocal motor neuropathy, motor neuron disease with paraproteinemia, heavy metal intoxication, hexoseaminidase-A deficiency, paraneoplastic motor neuronopathy, and syringomyelia and syringobulbia. Table 468–2 presents a differential diagnosis of ALS based on anatomic classification of affected components of the nervous system.

TREATMENT AND PROGNOSIS. For direct disease treatment, the only drug currently available is riluzole (2-amino-6-[trifluoromethoxy]benzothiazole). Riluzole blocks glutamic acid release and may slow disease progression by disrupting glutamate-mediated neurotoxicity. Administered at 50 mg twice a day, riluzole is generally well-tolerated, although some patients experience nausea and general asthenia.

Combining the results of several clinical epidemiology studies, the mean disease duration between onset of symptoms and death in sporadic ALS ranges from 27 to 43 months, and the median duration from 23 to 52 months. The average 5-year survival is 25%. The mean disease duration of primary lateral sclerosis is much longer, with an average of 224 months between symptoms and death. The relentless progression and poor prognosis of ALS requires attentive, supportive care.

A multidisciplinary approach is essential and is best co-ordinated by a dedicated ALS nurse or other health-care professional. Symptomatic treatment of patients is frequently required for sialorrhea, pseudobulbar symptoms, cramps, and spasticity. A social worker should help the patient cope with a sense of general fear, anxiety,

Table 468–2 ■ THE DIFFRENTIAL DIAGNOSIS OF ALS CLASSIFIED BY ANATOMY OF THE NERVOUS SYSTEM

ANATOMIC SITE	POSSIBLE DISORDER
Muscle	Idiopathic inflammatory myopathy (especially IBM), distal myopathy, nemaline myopathy, isolated neck extensor myopathy, metabolic myopathy, oculopharyngeal dystrophy
Neuromuscular junction	MG, Lambert-Eaton myasthenic syndrome
Roots, plexus, nerve	Radiculopathy, diabetic polyradiculoneuropathy, infectious polyradiculopathy, plexopathies, mononeuropathies, motor neuropathies
Anterior horn cells	Spinal muscular atrophy, BSMA, monomelic amyotrophy, paraneoplastic motor neuropathy, progressive post-polio muscular atrophy, hexosaminidase deficiency
Spinal cord	Spondylotic myelopathy, syringomyelia, MS, adrenomyeloneuropathy, vitamin B_{12} deficiency, familial spastic paraparesis, HTLV-1 myelopathy
Central nervous system	Parkinson's disease, Creutzfeldt-Jakob disease, multisystem atrophy, Huntington's disease, brain-stem stroke, brain stem glioma, foramen magnum tumors
Systemic disorders	Hyperthyroidism, hyperparathyroidism

BSMA = bulbospinal muscular atrophy, HTLV-1 = human T-lymphotropic virus type 1, IBM = inclusion body myositis, MG = myasthenia gravis, MS = multiple sclerosis.
From Amyotrophic Lateral Sclerosis, by Hiroshi Mitsumoto, David. Copyright © 1997 by Oxford University Press, Inc. Used by permission of Oxford University Press, Inc.

and depression. A physical therapist should provide the patient with exercises for stretching and flexibility and recommend needed bracing and adaptive walking devices. An occupational therapist should arrange adaptive devices to improve functional independence. As swallowing function decreases and speech becomes more difficult, a speech pathologist is helpful to oversee barium-swallow tests and obtain augmentative communication devices. For patients who undergo percutaneous endoscopic gastrostomy (PEG), a dietitian assists in selection of proper feedings. Pulmonary specialists are often helpful in determining when non-invasive ventilation techniques, such as bilevel positive airway pressure (BiPAP), will be helpful for pulmonary symptoms and in assisting in the long-term care of patients who choose to become ventilator dependent.

Dubowitz V: Disorders of the lower motor neurone: The spinal muscular atrophies. In Muscle Disorders in Childhood, 2nd ed. Philadelphia, WB Saunders, 1995, pp 325–369. *Excellent clinical description that includes instructive pictures of affected individuals.*
Mitsumoto H, Chad DA, Pioro EP: Amyotrophic Lateral Sclerosis. Philadelphia, FA Davis, 1998. *A comprehensive guide to all aspects of ALS.*
Pestronk A: Neuromuscular Disease Center. St Louis, Washington University School of Medicine, Neuromuscular Disease Center, 1998. World Wide Web URL: http://www.neuro.wustl.edu/neuromuscular/ *Comprehensive collection of motor neuron disorders with key Web links to salient information on genetics, recent basic research, and therapy. This Website is user friendly, is updated continuously, and is invaluable for the clinician.*
Wang CH, Carter TA, Gilliam TC: Molecular and genetic basis of the spinal muscular atrophies. In Rosenberg RN, Prusiner SB, DiMauro S, Barchi RL (eds): The Molecular and Genetic Basis of Neurological Disease, 2nd ed. Boston, Butterworth-Heinemann, 1997, pp 787–796. *A concise, lucid guide to understanding the genetics of the spinal muscular atrophies.*

■ CEREBROVASCULAR DISEASES

469 CEREBROVASCULAR DISEASES— PRINCIPLES

William A. Pulsinelli

The family of cerebrovascular diseases can be classified according to whether they affect the brain's vascular supply either focally or diffusely (Fig. 469–1). The generic term *stroke* signifies the abrupt impairment of brain function caused by a variety of pathologic changes involving one (focal) or several (multifocal) intracranial or extracranial blood vessels. Approximately 80% of strokes are caused by too little blood flow (ischemic stroke), and the remaining 20% are nearly equally divided between hemorrhage into brain tissue (parenchymatous hemorrhage) and hemorrhage into the surrounding subarachnoid space (subarachnoid hemorrhage). In contrast, diseases that affect the heart or the systemic circulation cause generalized hypoperfusion and diffuse brain dysfunction or injury. Ischemic stroke and the hypoperfusion syndromes affecting the brain share much pathophysiology, and both processes are considered together in Chapter 470; hemorrhagic stroke is addressed in Chapter 471.

EPIDEMIOLOGY

The annual incidence and death rate for stroke have declined steadily in the United States throughout the 20th century and for most European countries and Japan since approximately 1960. In the United States, the 1% decrease in the annual mortality rate from stroke recorded since 1915 accelerated in the early 1970s to

approximately 5% per year. A recent analysis indicates that the stroke incidence has stabilized at approximately 0.5 to 1.0 per 1000 population. Incidence rates in western European countries are slightly higher (1.5 per 1000), but several eastern European countries and Japan have rates of 3 per 1000 based at least partly on environmental, dietary, and smoking habits. At these current rates, stroke remains the third leading cause of medically related deaths and the second most frequent cause of neurologic morbidity in developed countries.

Several other important facts about stroke incidence have emerged: incidence and death rate for stroke are higher among blacks than whites in the United States; approximately similar rates affect men and women, in contrast to the male predominance for myocardial infarction; and there is a strikingly higher incidence (20 to 30 per 1000) for those over age 75 years.

CEREBROVASCULAR ANATOMY

Because most strokes are caused by abnormalities within the cerebral circulation, an understanding of cerebrovascular anatomy helps in arriving at the correct diagnosis and determining the underlying pathogenesis and prognosis.

The brain is supplied by four major arteries: the left and right internal carotid and vertebral arteries (Fig. 469–2). The left common carotid artery arises from the aortic arch, but the other vessels originate from branches of the aorta. The right common carotid artery stems from the innominate artery, and the left and right vertebral arteries take off from their respective subclavian arteries.

INTERNAL CAROTID ARTERIES. Each common carotid artery bifurcates into an internal and external carotid artery in most individuals just below the angle of the jaw and approximately at the level of the thyroid cartilage (Fig. 469–2). The *internal carotid*

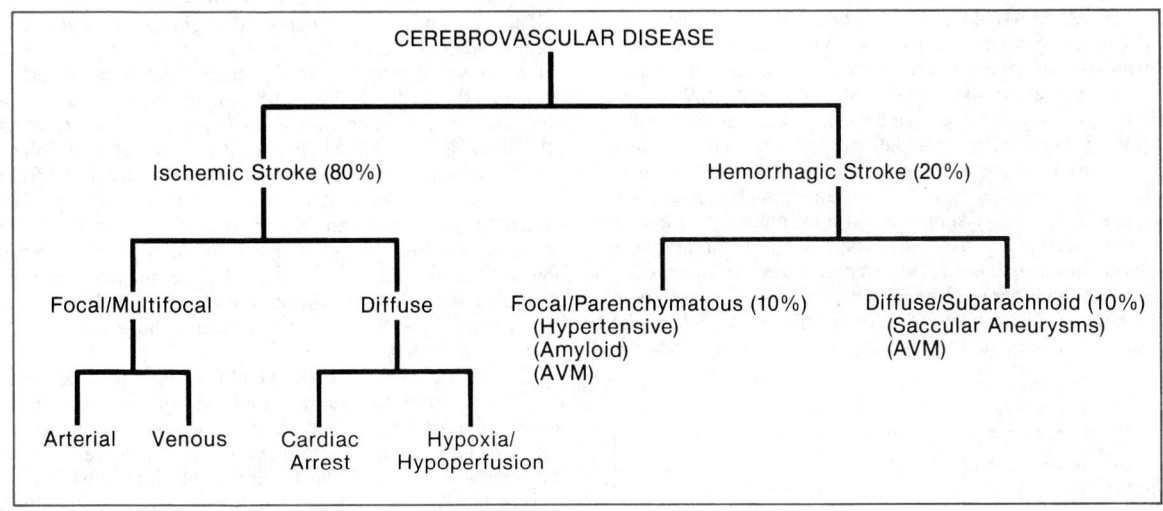

FIGURE 469-1 ■ Classification of cerebrovascular disease.

artery (ICA) enters the skull through the foramen lacerum and travels a short distance within the petrous portion of the temporal bone. It then enters the cavernous sinus before penetrating the dura and ascends above the clinoid processes to divide into the *anterior* and *middle cerebral arteries*. The portion of the internal carotid artery that lies between the cavernous sinus and the supraclinoid process forms an S shape and is sometimes referred to as the carotid siphon. The internal carotid artery gives off its first important branches at the supraclinoid level, the *ophthalmic, posterior communicating*, and *anterior choroidal arteries*, usually arising in that order. In approximately 10% of cases, the ophthalmic artery arises from the internal carotid artery within the cavernous sinus.

EXTERNAL CAROTID ARTERIES. Branches of the external carotid artery, important because they anastomose and provide collateral circulation to the internal carotid artery, include the *facial artery* and the *superficial temporal artery*. Both vessels anastomose with the *supratrochlear* branches of the ophthalmic artery. In instances of internal carotid artery occlusion below the level of the ophthalmic branch, the facial and superficial temporal arteries can supply blood through the ophthalmic branch to the distal internal carotid artery. The facial and superficial temporal arteries lie just beneath the skin, and their palpability can assist in diagnosing occlusion or stenosis of the ICA.

VERTEBRAL-BASILAR ARTERIES. Anatomic variation is considerably more common in the vertebral artery system than in the ICA. The vertebral arteries usually arise from the subclavian arteries (see Fig. 469–2), but their origins may migrate proximally to begin directly from the aortic arch or distally to form a common branch of the thyrocervical trunk. They enter the foramen of the sixth cervical vertebra or, much less commonly, the fourth, fifth, or seventh vertebral level. The vertebral arteries ascend through the transverse foramina and exit at C1, where they turn 90 degrees posteriorly to pass behind the atlantoaxial joint before penetrating the dura and entering the cranial cavity through the foramen magnum. The portion of the vertebral artery that loops behind the atlantoaxial joint is prone to mechanical trauma, and rotation of the head to approximately 60 degrees may cause arterial narrowing and reduce blood flow to the ipsilateral vertebral artery.

Intracranially, the vertebral arteries lie lateral to the medulla oblongata and then course ventrally and medially, where they unite at the medullopontine junction to form the *basilar artery*. The basilar artery bifurcates at the pontomesencephalic junction into the *posterior cerebral arteries* (PCAs).

In up to 20% of individuals, the right or left vertebral arteries terminate before reaching the basilar artery, leaving the latter to be supplied inferiorly by a single vessel. Intracranial branches of the vertebral arteries include medial branches, which unite to form the *anterior spinal artery*, and lateral branches to the dorsolateral medulla and posterior cerebellum, called the *posterior inferior cerebellar arteries*.

CIRCLE OF WILLIS. The *circle of Willis* (see Fig. 469–2) is formed by the union at the base of the brain of both anterior cerebral arteries via the *anterior communicating artery* and the middle cerebral arteries with the posterior cerebral arteries on each side via the *posterior communicating arteries* (see Fig. 469–2). Anomalies of the circle of Willis occur frequently; in large autopsy series of normal individuals, more than half showed an incomplete circle of Willis. The most common sites for such abnormalities, which usually present as hypoplasia or atresia, are the posterior communicating arteries (22%) and the anterior cerebral arteries (10%).

FIGURE 469-2 ■ Extracranial and intracranial arterial supply to the brain. Vessels forming the circle of Willis are highlighted in dark red. Abbreviations for intracranial and extracranial arteries are as follows: ACA = anterior cerebral artery; MCA = middle cerebral artery; PCA = posterior cerebral artery; E-I anast = extracranial-intracranial anastomosis; ICA = internal carotid artery; ECA = external carotid artery; CCA = common carotid artery; Ant. Comm. = anterior communicating artery; Post. Comm. = posterior communicating artery; SCA = superior cerebellar artery; AICA = anterior inferior cerebellar artery; PICA = posterior inferior cerebellar artery. (Modified from Lord R: Surgery of Occlusive Cerebrovascular Disease. St. Louis, C.V. Mosby Company, 1986; with permission.)

ANTERIOR CEREBRAL ARTERIES. The *anterior cerebral arteries* (ACAs) pass medially above the optic chiasm and head rostrally toward the interhemispheric fissure, where they arch caudally to lie just dorsal to the corpus callosum (Fig. 469–3). In approximately 10% of normal individuals, the A1 segment of the ACA (the portion between the middle cerebral and anterior communicating arteries) is atretic or absent, leaving its distal portion to be supplied by the opposite ACA via the anterior communicating artery. Branches of the ACA supply the frontal poles, the superior surfaces of the cerebral hemispheres where their distal branches anastomose with those of the middle cerebral artery, and all of the medial surfaces of both cerebral hemispheres with the exception of the calcarine cortex. Cortical areas served by the ACA include the motor and sensory cortex of the legs and feet, the supplementary

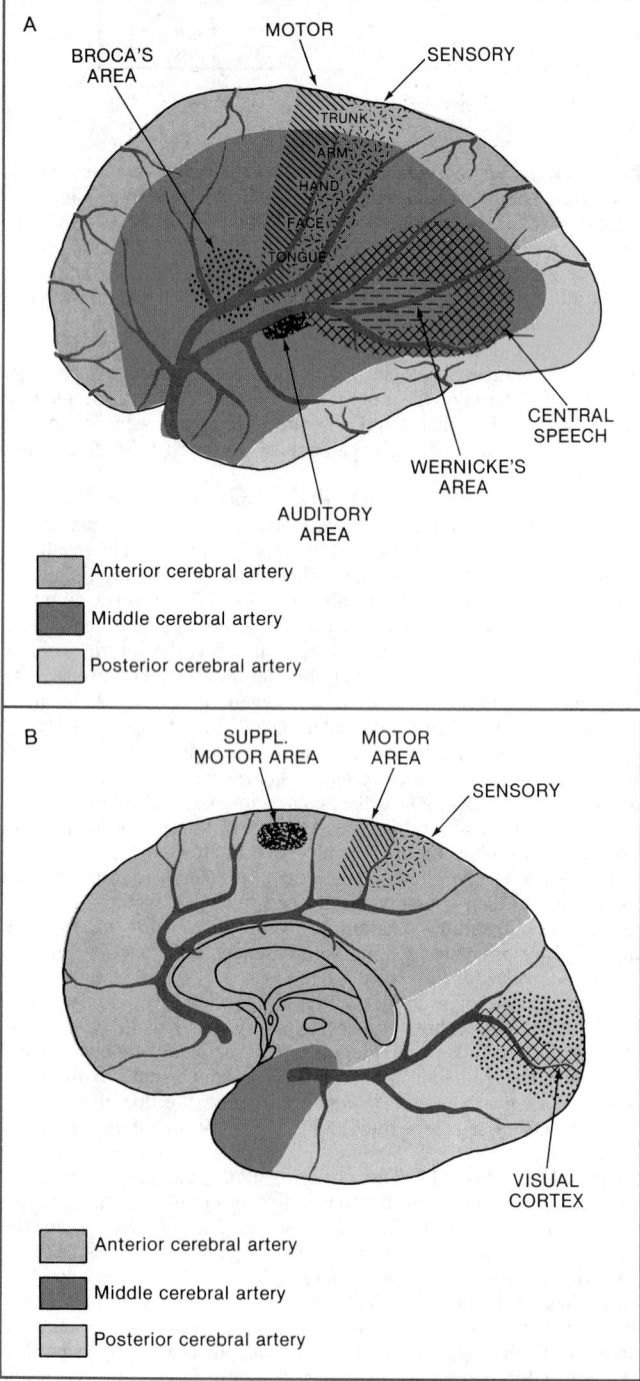

A

BROCA'S AREA

MOTOR

SENSORY

TRUNK
ARM
HAND
FACE
TONGUE

CENTRAL SPEECH

WERNICKE'S AREA

AUDITORY AREA

■ Anterior cerebral artery
■ Middle cerebral artery
■ Posterior cerebral artery

B

SUPPL. MOTOR AREA

MOTOR AREA

SENSORY

VISUAL CORTEX

■ Anterior cerebral artery
■ Middle cerebral artery
■ Posterior cerebral artery

FIGURE 469–3 ■ Lateral *(A)* and medial *(B)* views of the cerebral hemisphere showing the surface distributions of the anterior, middle, and posterior cerebral arteries.

motor cortex, and the presumed cortical micturition center lying in the paracentral lobule (Figs. 469–3 and 469–4).

The A1 and A2 segments (the portion between the anterior communicating artery and the genu of the corpus callosum) give off many small branches that penetrate the anterior perforated substance of the brain. These small penetrating branches include all of the *anterior* and some of the *medial lenticulostriate* arteries. Usually, there is a dominant medial striate vessel called the *recurrent artery of Heubner,* which arises in most instances from the A1 segment of the ACA. This artery penetrates the perforated substance of the brain and, along with the other small perforators, supplies (see Fig. 469–4) the anterior and inferior portions of the anterior limb of the internal capsule, the anterior and inferior head of the caudate nucleus, the anterior globus pallidus and putamen, the anterior hypothalamus, the olfactory bulbs and tracts, and the uncinate fasciculus.

ANTERIOR CHOROIDAL ARTERY. The *anterior choroidal artery* arises from the supraclinoid portion of the internal carotid artery in most persons. It travels caudally and medially over the optic tract, to which it provides a few small branches, and enters the brain via the choroidal fissure. Many important brain structures receive blood flow from the anterior choroidal artery; these include portions of the anterior hippocampus, uncus, amygdala, globus pallidus, tail of the caudate nucleus, lateral thalamus, geniculate body, and a large portion of the most inferior, posterior limb of the internal capsule (see Fig. 469–4).

MIDDLE CEREBRAL ARTERY. The *middle cerebral artery* (MCA) provides flow to most of the lateral surface of the cerebral hemispheres and is the vessel most frequently involved in ischemic stroke (see Figs. 469–3 and 469–4). As the main MCA trunk passes laterally toward the sylvian fissure, it gives rise to some of the *medial* and all of the *lateral lenticulostriate* arteries. These arteries irrigate (see Fig. 469–4) the putamen, the head and body of the caudate nucleus, the lateral globus pallidus, the full vertical extent of the anterior limb of the internal capsule, and a superior portion of the posterior limb of the internal capsule. The MCA then extends into the sylvian fissure, where it branches into several smaller arteries grouped into a superior division, which feeds the cortical surface above the fissure, and an inferior division, which supplies the cortical surface of the temporal lobe. The territory of the MCA includes the major motor and sensory areas of the cortex, the areas for contraversive eye and head movement, the optic radiations, auditory sensory cortex, and, in the dominant hemisphere, the motor and sensory areas for language.

POSTERIOR CEREBRAL ARTERIES. Blood flow to both *posterior cerebral arteries* (PCAs) derives primarily from the basilar artery (70% of the time) and from the ICA (10% of the time). In the remaining 20%, one PCA is supplied by the ICA and the other by the basilar artery. The PCAs pass dorsal to the third cranial nerves and across the cerebral peduncles and then ascend upward along the medial edge of the tentorium, where they branch into anterior and posterior divisions. The anterior division (see Figs. 469–3 and 469–4) supplies the inferior surface of the temporal lobe, where its terminal branches anastomose with branches of the MCA. The posterior division supplies the occipital lobe, where its terminal branches anastomose with both the ACA and the MCA. In its most proximal course along the base of the brain, the PCA gives off several groups of penetrating arteries commonly referred to as the thalamogeniculate, the thalamoperforating, and the posterior choroidal arteries. The red nucleus, the substantia nigra, medial parts of the cerebral peduncles, the nuclei of the thalamus, the hippocampus, and the posterior hypothalamus receive blood from these penetrating branches (see Fig. 469–4).

BRAIN STEM BLOOD FLOW. At all rostrocaudal levels of the brain stem, the ventral medial portion is supplied by short paramedian vessels; the ventrolateral portion by short circumferential branches from the vertebral or basilar arteries; and the dorsolateral portion and cerebellum by long circumferential branches, which include the *posterior inferior cerebellar* arteries, which arise from the vertebral arteries, and the *anterior inferior* and *superior cerebellar* arteries, which arise from the basilar artery (Fig. 469–5).

The pyramids, the inferior olives and medial lemnisci, the medial longitudinal fasciculi, and the emerging fibers of the hypoglossal nerve (see Fig. 469–5A) derive blood from the vertebral arteries. Longer branches from the vertebral arteries and posterior ICAs supply the spinothalamic tracts, the vestibular nuclei, the sensory nuclei of the fifth cranial nerve, the descending fibers of the sym-

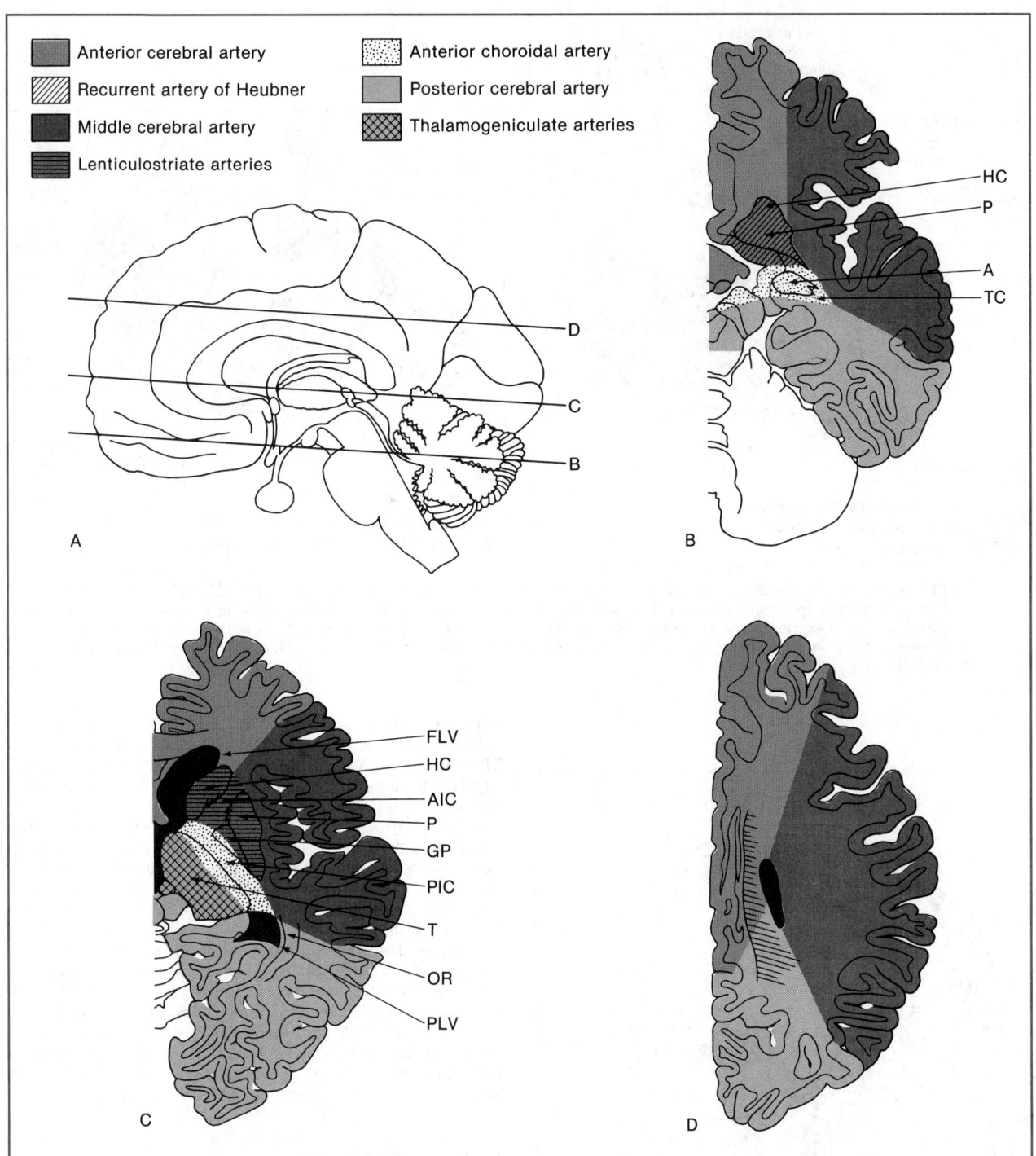

FIGURE 469–4 ■ Arterial supply of deep brain structures. *A,* Sagittal view of the brain showing the computed tomographic (CT) planes through which views B, C, and D were taken. *B,* CT plane through the head of the caudate nucleus (HC), putamen (P), amygdala (A), tail of the caudate nucleus (TC), hypothalamus, temporal lobe, midbrain, and cerebellum. *C,* CT plane through the frontal horn of the lateral ventricle (FLV), head of the caudate nucleus (HC), anterior and posterior limbs of the internal capsule (AIC, PIC), putamen (P), globus pallidus (GP), thalamus (T), optic radiations (OR), and posterior horn of the lateral ventricle (PLV). *D,* CT plane through the centrum semiovale. (Modified from De Armond S, et al: Structure of the Human Brain, A Photographic Atlas, 3rd ed. New York, Oxford University Press, 1989; with permission.)

pathetic nervous system, the restiform body, and the emerging fibers of the vagus and glossopharyngeal nerves. The most cephalad and dorsal segment of the medulla includes the vestibular and cochlear nuclei, which, along with the posterior portion of the cerebellum, receive flow from the posterior inferior cerebellar artery.

The basilar artery gives rise to perforating branches as it spans the ventral midline pons and midbrain (see Fig. 469–5B). These short perpendicular branches distribute blood to the paramedian structures, including the corticospinal tracts, the pontine reticular

nuclei, the medial lemnisci, the medial longitudinal fasciculi, and the pontine reticular nuclei. The *anterior ICA* feeds blood to the lateral pons, including the emerging seventh and eighth cranial nerves, the trigeminal nerve root, the vestibular and cochlear nuclei, and the spinothalamic tracts. It also branches to the most dorsal and lateral of these structures on its dorsal course toward the cerebellum.

At the midbrain level, the basilar artery lies in the midline in the peduncular fossa. Short branches pass laterally and dorsally to both sides to supply the cerebral peduncles, the emerging fibers of the

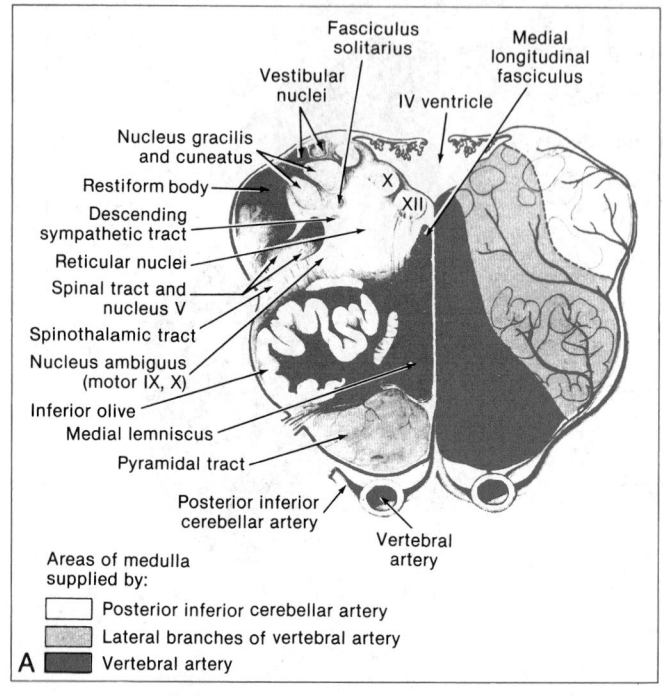

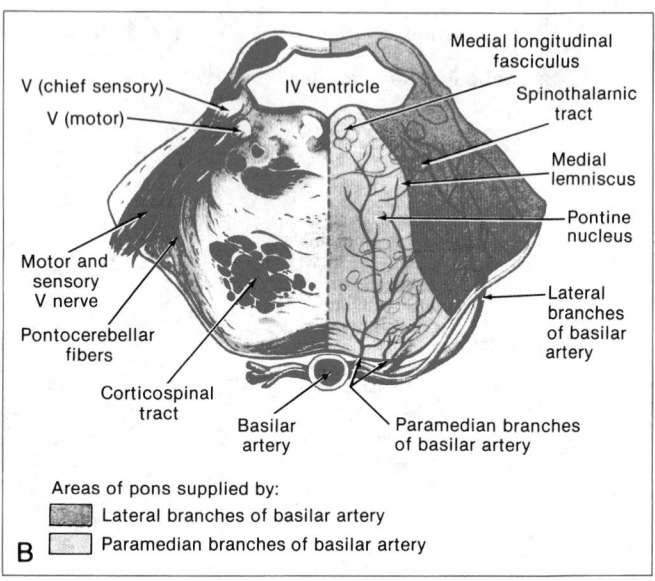

FIGURE 469-5 ■ *A,* Cross-section of the medulla oblongata at the level of the hypoglossal nuclei (XII). Short branches of the vertebral and anterior spinal arteries supply the medial medulla. Longer circumferential branches, including the posterior inferior cerebellar artery, supply the lateral portions of the medulla. *B,* Cross-section of the midpons. The medial portion receives the blood supply from short, perforating basilar artery branches. More laterally, the blood supply comes from lateral basilar artery branches.

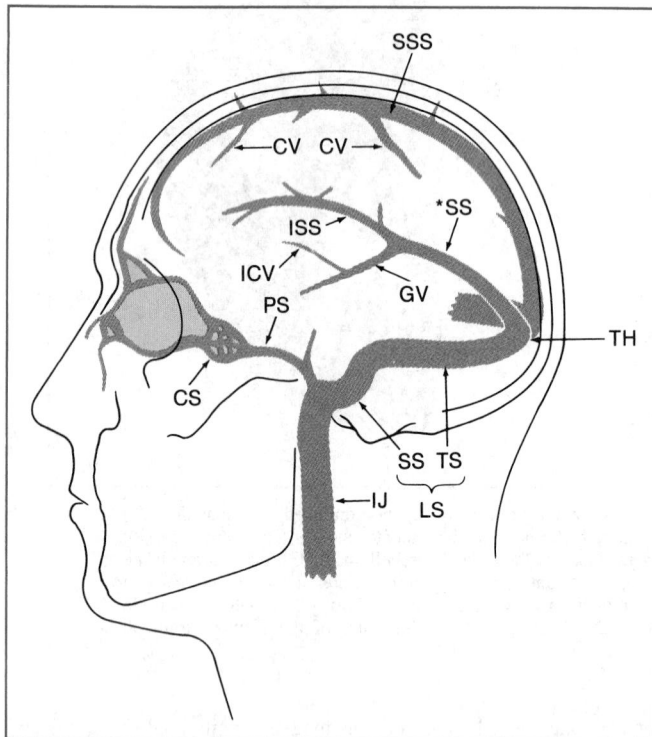

FIGURE 469-6 ■ Venous drainage of intracranial structures. SSS = superior sagittal sinus; CV = cortical veins; ISS = inferior sagittal sinus; ICV = internal cerebral vein; GV = great vein of Galen; *SS = straight sinus; TH = torcular herophili; PS = petrosal sinus; CS = cavernous sinus; TS = transverse sinus; SS = sigmoid sinus; LS = lateral sinus; IJ = internal jugular vein. (Reproduced with permission from Gates P, Barnett HJ, Mohr JP, et al [eds]: Stroke: Pathophysiology, Diagnosis and Management. New York, Churchill Livingstone, 1986.)

third nerve, medial portions of the red nuclei, the medial longitudinal fasciculus, the oculomotor nuclei, and the midbrain reticulum. The superior cerebellar arteries contribute to the dorsal midbrain supply, including that of the colliculi and the superior portion of the cerebellum on each side.

VENOUS DRAINAGE. The veins in the brain, unlike those in many other parts of the body, do not accompany the arteries (Fig. 469–6). Cortical veins drain into the superior sagittal sinus, which runs posteriorly between the cerebral hemispheres. Deeper structures drain into the inferior sagittal sinus and great cerebral vein (of Galen), which join at the straight sinus. The straight sinus runs posteriorly along the attachment of the falx cerebri and tentorium and joins the superior sagittal sinus at the torcular Herophili, from which the two transverse sinuses arise. Each transverse sinus passes laterally toward the petrosal bone to become the sigmoid sinus, which exits the skull into the internal jugular vein. Each cavernous sinus communicates with its contralateral twin and surrounds the ipsilateral carotid artery; both drain posteriorly into the petrosal sinuses, which in turn drain into the sigmoid sinus.

NORMAL PHYSIOLOGY

CEREBRAL METABOLISM AND BLOOD FLOW. The brain performs no mechanical work; nevertheless, the energy demands to support normal electrophysiologic brain activity in conscious humans equal, on a per weight basis, those of metabolically active tissues like the heart and kidney. Aerobic glucose metabolism provides the energy necessary to drive membrane ion pumps, synthesize, store, and release neurotransmitters, and maintain tissue structure. The normal, conscious human consumes approximately 160 μmol O_2 and 30 μmol glucose per 100 g of brain each minute (Table 469–1).

Approximately 10% of available blood glucose is extracted and phosphorylated by the brain in a single pass, yet only 80% of this glucose is used to generate energy. The 5:1 ratio of O_2 versus glucose consumption (see Table 469–1) indicates that approximately 20% of glucose carbons are not oxidized. Approximately 10% to 15% of glucose is metabolized to lactate, which may be lost to the circulation; the remainder is used for the synthesis of

Table 469–1 ■ METABOLIC ACTIVITY (NORMAL CONSCIOUS MAN)

	CONSUMED	SUPPLIED
	(100 g BRAIN/MIN)	
CBF	60 mL	–
O₂	156 μmol	350 μmol
Glucose	33 μmol	300 μmol

CBF = cerebral blood flow.

Table 469–2 ■ HUMAN HYPOXIC-ISCHEMIC THRESHOLD VALUES

	PaO₂ (torr)	CEREBRAL BLOOD FLOW (mL/100 g/min)	BLOOD GLUCOSE (mg/dL)
Normal	90	60	80
Stupor	30–40	20–30	25–30
Coma	20–30	15–20	20–25
Brain injury	<20	<15	<20

neurotransmitters, fats, and, to a small degree, proteins. Each mole of glucose metabolized by the brain through glycolysis and the mitochondrial respiratory chain therefore yields approximately 30 mol adenosine triphosphate (ATP) instead of the expected 38.

Unlike muscle or other tissues, the brain stores few glucose, glycogen, or other high-energy phosphate (ATP, phosphocreatine) reserves but instead relies on a sizable and well-regulated blood flow to satisfy its immediate needs for energy. Cerebral blood flow (CBF) averages 60 mL per 100 g of brain per minute in a normal, conscious human; in the absence of such flow, the brain has sufficient high-energy stores to support normal metabolic needs for only a few minutes. At normal arterial O₂ tensions and blood glucose concentrations, CBF delivers 350 μmol O₂ and 300 μmol glucose to 100 g of brain each minute (see Table 469–1). These values exceed the brain's normal consumption rates of O₂ and glucose by factors of approximately 2 and 10 respectively. The blood vascular reserves for both O₂ and glucose must be small, as is illustrated by the fact that all changes of synaptic activity, whether related to thinking, talking, or directing muscular activity, are tightly *coupled*, both temporally and anatomically, to an almost instantaneous, proportional increase in CBF. The anatomic segregation of the brain's functional activities results in an ever-changing mosaic of regional metabolic/blood flow values that reflect moment-to-moment changes in electrophysiologic activity.

The coupling of CBF to regional synaptic activity and metabolic activity represents only one of several important mechanisms regulating normal CBF. Changes in the respiratory rate or volume, which lead to even mild hypercapnia or hypocapnia, respectively, dilate or constrict cerebral resistance vessels, so that CBF shows a linear relationship to PaCO₂. This normal physiologic response to PaCO₂ is exploited clinically to treat cerebral herniation syndromes. Mechanical hyperventilation to a PaCO₂ of 20 to 25 mm Hg reduces CBF by approximately 40 to 45% and normal adult cerebral blood volume from 50 mL to approximately 35 mL. Although seemingly small, this 15-mL reduction often suffices to retard the progression of cerebral herniation. The response is short-lived,

however, and brain and blood HCO₃⁻ and H⁺ ions control blood vessel tone re-equilibrate within 30 to 60 minutes.

A complex system of neural pathways regulates CBF in response to normal and abnormal circumstances. Some of these neural pathways participate in autoregulation, a process that maintains CBF at a constant level despite wide fluctuations in cerebral perfusion pressure.

Because cerebral venous pressures closely approximate the intracranial pressure, autoregulation values usually are expressed in terms of mean arterial pressure.

Normal autoregulation has both upper and lower limits (Fig. 469–7); at mean arterial pressures above 150 mm Hg, blood flow increases and capillary pressure rises, while at mean arterial pressures below 50 mm Hg, CBF falls. Increased capillary pressure in hypertensive patients may be a factor in intracerebral hemorrhage and hypertensive encephalopathy. In patients with chronic hypertension, the upper and lower autoregulatory limits are shifted toward higher systemic pressures (Fig. 469–7). Consequently, too rapid therapeutic reduction of blood pressure to apparently normal levels carries the risk of further lowering cerebral blood flow in hypertensive patients with ongoing cerebral ischemia. Chronic treatment with antihypertensive agents readjusts the autoregulatory curve toward more normal values.

BLOOD-BRAIN BARRIER. Regulation within narrow limits of the extracellular ionic and molecular composition is more important for the normal function of the brain than for any other organ. Small changes in the extracellular concentrations of, for example, Na⁺ ions or the neurotransmitters glutamate or norepinephrine, greatly alter neuronal function. The blood-brain barrier is composed anatomically of unique endothelial cells that lack the usual transendothelial channels and that seamlessly abut one another (tight junctions). This anatomy protects the brain against the fluctuating composition of blood and minimizes the entry of potentially toxic compounds.

The entry of nutrients and egress of metabolic products cross the blood-brain barrier via simple diffusion, facilitated transport, or active transport. Lipid-soluble compounds rapidly diffuse across endothelial cell membranes, whereas polar compounds must be transported on special carrier molecules that are driven either by concentration gradients (facilitated transport) or through the expenditure of energy (active transport). Gas molecules such as O₂ and CO₂ freely diffuse across plasma membranes and rapidly equilibrate between blood and brain. Glucose, a highly polar molecule, enters the brain on a special carrier with a Km (7 to 8 mM) just slightly higher than the normal blood glucose concentration. The rate of brain glucose transport is normally two to three times faster than the metabolism of glucose, but since glucose uptake depends so highly on its concentration, a reduction of blood sugar to one third the normal amount, caused by either ischemia or hypoglycemia, may compromise normal metabolism (Table 469–2).

PATHOPHYSIOLOGY/PATHOLOGY OF CEREBRAL ISCHEMIA

A failed delivery of O₂ and glucose to the brain generates a cascade of events that vary qualitatively and quantitatively with the severity of the insult. The severity of cerebral ischemia, defined as the degree and duration of blood flow loss, largely determines whether the brain suffers only temporary dysfunction, irreversible injury to a few highly vulnerable neurons (selective ischemic necrosis), or damage to extensive areas involving all cell types (cerebral infarction).

TYPES OF CEREBRAL HYYPOXIA-ISCHEMIA. Cerebral hypoxia-ischemia can be conveniently divided into focal or multifocal ischemia from vascular occlusion, global ischemia from complete

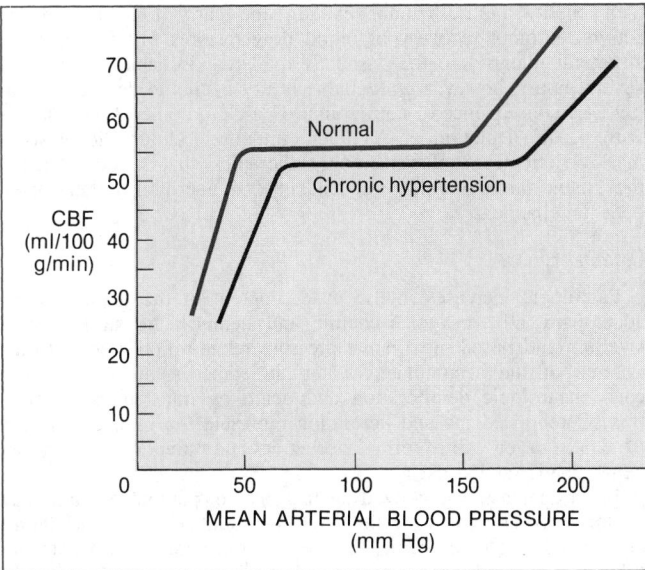

FIGURE 469–7 ■ Autoregulatory cerebral blood flow response to changes in mean arterial pressure in normotensive and chronically hypertensive individuals. Note the shift of the curve toward higher mean pressures with chronic hypertension.

failure of cardiovascular pumping, and diffuse hypoperfusion-hypoxia caused by respiratory disease or reduced perfusion pressure. *Focal cerebral ischemia,* resulting most frequently from embolic or thrombotic occlusion of extracranial or intracranial blood vessels, variably reduces blood flow within the involved vascular territory. Blood flow to the central zone of the ischemic vascular bed usually is severely reduced but rarely reaches zero because of partial filling from collateral blood vessels. In transition zones between normally perfused tissue and the severely ischemic central core, blood flow is moderately reduced. This rim of moderately ischemic tissue has been called the ischemic penumbra, and although brain cells in this region remain viable longer than do those in the ischemic core, they too will die if left deprived of adequate blood flow.

Focal cerebral ischemia sufficient to cause clinical signs or symptoms and lasting only 15 to 30 minutes causes irreversible injury to specific, highly vulnerable neurons. If the ischemia lasts an hour or longer, infarction of part or all of the involved vascular territory is inevitable. Clinical evidence of permanent brain injury from such ischemia may or may not be detectable, depending on the region and the amount of brain tissue involved (see Chapter 470).

Global cerebral ischemia, typically caused by cardiac asystole or ventricular fibrillation, reduces blood flow to zero throughout all of the brain. Global ischemia lasting more than 5 to 10 minutes is usually incompatible with recovery of consciousness in normothermic humans. Brain damage from more transient global ischemia, uncomplicated by periods of prolonged hypotension or hyperglycemia, is limited to specific populations of highly vulnerable neurons. This selective ischemic necrosis of neurons involves, for example, the CA1 pyramidal neurons of hippocampus, the cerebellar Purkinje cells, and the pyramidal neurons in neocortical layers 3, 5, and 6 (Table 469–3). While selective ischemic necrosis of neurons typifies transient global ischemia, such injury may also accompany prolonged hypoxemia, carbon monoxide poisoning, and focal cerebral ischemia of brief duration. Cardiac resuscitation complicated by prolonged hypotension or hyperglycemia may cause cerebral infarction, particularly in border zones that lie between the terminal branches of major arterial supplies.

Diffuse cerebral hypoxia, uncomplicated by cerebral ischemia, is limited to conditions of mild to moderate hypoxemia, since myocardial contractility and blood pressure fall with severe hypoxemia. As a consequence, pure cerebral hypoxia causes cerebral dysfunction but not irreversible brain injury. Individuals with pure cerebral hypoxia from altitude sickness, pulmonary disease, or severe anemia present with confusion, cognitive impairment, and lethargy. The onset of coma signals cardiovascular compromise and imminent brain damage. With relatively *acute* changes in arterial oxygen tension from normal to a PaO$_2$ of 40 mm Hg (see Table 469–2) or with a fall in the hemoglobin concentration below 7 g dL, compensatory increases of cerebral blood flow become inadequate, and clinical signs and symptoms of cerebral hypoxia develop.

NEUROPATHOLOGY OF CEREBRAL ISCHEMIA. Ischemic injury to the brain can be classified on the basis of cytopathologic criteria into four types. Cerebral *autolysis,* observed most frequently in brain-dead patients preserved on mechanical ventilators for several days, reflects enzymatic autodigestion of the tissue.

Cerebral *infarction,* usually caused by focal vascular occlusion, is characterized histopathologically by necrosis of neurons, glia, and, in some areas, endothelial cells. Cerebral infarcts are frequently described grossly as pale (anemic) or hemorrhagic (showing gross petechial bleeding). Most often, the hemorrhagic areas lie along border zones of partially perfused tissue and occur most

frequently with transient embolic occlusion followed by reperfusion of the infarcted vascular bed.

Transient arrest of the cerebral circulation (global ischemia) for a few minutes causes *selective ischemic necrosis of highly vulnerable neurons* (see Table 469–3).

The time required for histologic changes to reach their maximum in areas of cerebral infarction differs markedly from the time course of injury encountered in selective ischemic necrosis. Infarction usually requires only a few hours before histologic stains sharply outline the distinct margins between living and dying neurons and glia. By contrast, selective ischemic necrosis of neurons evolves more slowly and sometimes requires several days or more to reach its full extent.

Another distinctive neuropathologic lesion due to ischemia is *demyelination* of the central hemispheric white matter. Such injury is usually the consequence of carbon monoxide poisoning or other prolonged periods of moderately severe hypoxemia or cerebral hypoperfusion. Within these lesions, nerve cell axons are demyelinated, and oligodendroglial cells die off.

MOLECULAR MECHANISMS. In severely ischemic brain tissue, energy-rich compounds become depleted within seconds to a few minutes (see Table 469–2). Soon thereafter, the tissue begins to lose structural integrity. As energy-dependent membrane pumps fail, neuronal and glial cell membranes depolarize and allow the influx of Na$^+$ and Ca^{2+} ions and the efflux of K$^+$ ions. Elevated intracellular Ca^{2+} and other second messengers activate lipases and proteases, which in turn release membrane-bound free fatty acids and denature proteins. Depolarization of presynaptic terminals releases abnormally high concentrations of excitatory and inhibitory neurotransmitters, which may further exacerbate injury. If blood flow is restored in 15 to 30 minutes and no other complicating variables, such as hyperglycemia, are involved, most of these events are reversible, and only selectively vulnerable neurons die. If ischemia lasts hours or more, cerebral infarction develops.

In contrast to the rapid cascade of events caused by severe ischemia, moderate ischemia triggers poorly defined mechanisms that sacrifice electrophysiologic activity to preserve brain structure, at least temporarily. Acute reduction of blood flow below one half that of normal exceeds the capacity of compensatory mechanisms, such as an increased extraction of O$_2$ and glucose extraction by the tissue. The electroencephalogram (EEG) slows, and if ischemia is diffuse, the patient becomes confused, lethargic, or stuporous. The molecular mechanisms that induce this "anoxic anesthesia" are unknown. Depletion of whole tissue energy reserves is not an explanation, since these remain normal, partly as a consequence of the decreased energy demand normally used to maintain membrane ion pumps and EEG activity. With slightly greater ischemia, all synaptic activity ceases and the EEG becomes isoelectric. This too occurs before high-energy stores are depleted, indicating that generalized energy failure cannot explain the early loss of synaptic activity. Prompt recovery of blood flow restores full function and structural integrity to the tissue. If moderate ischemia persists for several hours, however, irreversible injury begins to develop, possibly as a consequence of compromised calcium homeostasis. Tissues with partial depletion of ATP and impaired calcium homeostasis may benefit from pharmacologic therapies that reduce calcium movement through voltage-dependent and neurotransmitter-dependent ion channels.

Cerebral Edema

Pathologic increases in the water content of the brain (edema) accompany all types of ischemic and hemorrhagic stroke. Brain swelling and raised intracranial pressure relate proportionally to the volume of the accumulated water; in some instances, they can cause neurologic deterioration and death by transtentorial herniation. Cerebral edema and herniation represent the immediate cause of death in one third of all ischemic and three quarters of all hemorrhagic fatal strokes.

Brain edema is categorized on the basis of pathophysiologic and anatomic criteria as intracellular or interstitial. Intracellular edema, also called cytotoxic edema, represents an accumulation of intracellular osmoles and water causing cell swelling at the expense of the interstitial brain volume. Intracellular edema develops rapidly in ischemic brain tissue as energy-dependent membrane ion pumps fail and Na$^+$ and other osmoles enter the cell from the interstitial and vascular compartments. Cell swelling occurs predominantly in

Table 469–3 ■ ORDER OF DECREASING NEURONAL VULNERABILITY TO ANOXIA

Hippocampus
    CA1, CA4 > CA3 > granule cells
Cerebellum
    Purkinje > stellate and basket > granule > Golgi cells
Striatum
    Small and medium-sized > large neurons
Neocortex
    Layers 3, 5, 6 > layers 2, 4

astrocytes, but neurons, oligodendroglial cells, and endothelial cells also are involved to a lesser degree. The osmolality of ischemic brain increases acutely from 310 mOsm to approximately 350 mOsm. The intracellular accumulation of water increases from a normal value of approximately 79% to 81% of brain weight, an addition insufficient in most instances to cause cerebral herniation. If cerebral circulation is re-established before permanent brain injury develops, intracellular brain edema resolves within a matter of hours without permanent sequelae.

Interstitial brain edema, also called vasogenic edema, occurs later than the intracellular form. Damage to blood-brain barrier endothelial cells allows macromolecules such as plasma proteins to enter the interstitial space, carrying with them osmotically bound water. Interstitial brain edema following cerebral infarction progressively worsens for 3 or 4 days after a stroke. Fluid accumulation within the vicinity of damaged endothelial cells and the zone of infarction can raise the local water content of brain by as much as 10%. Such large volume increases can lead to transtentorial herniation and similarly fatal consequences.

Barnett HJ, Mohr JP, Stein BM, et al (eds): Stroke: Pathophysiology, Diagnosis and Management, 3rd ed. New York, Churchill Livingstone 1998. *A comprehensive overview of all aspects of ischemic and hemorrhagic stroke.*
Caplan LR, Stein RW: Stroke: A Clinical Approach. Boston, Butterworth, 1986. *A pragmatic description of the diagnosis and treatment of stroke.*
Plum F, Pulsinelli WA: Cerebral metabolism in hypoxic-ischemic brain injury. *In* Asbury AK, McKann GM, McDonald IW (eds): Disease of the Nervous System, 2nd ed. Philadelphia, WB Saunders, 1992. *A contemporary review of the pathogenesis of ischemic injury to brain.*

470 ISCHEMIC CEREBROVASCULAR DISEASE

William A. Pulsinelli

470.1 Focal Ischemia

CLASSIFICATION

The clinical manifestations of focal ischemic stroke result from interference with blood circulation to the brain; the precise signs and symptoms depend on the region deprived of flow. For any brain region, however, focal ischemia can be classified into categories that have important clinical implications.

STROKE VERSUS TRANSIENT ISCHEMIC ATTACK. *Stroke* is defined as a neurologic deficit lasting more than 24 hours caused by reduced blood flow in a particular artery supplying the brain. The usual pathologic outcome is infarction. A *transient ischemic attack* (TIA) by contrast, is defined arbitrarily as a similar neurologic deficit lasting less than 24 hours. Originally, the defined time limit for TIAs was less than 1 hour, but this was subsequently expanded to the longer interval for practical purposes. Nevertheless, most TIAs resolve within an hour. Once a deficit has lasted longer than an hour, it is likely to be classified as a presumptive stroke and is often associated with permanent brain injury. Magnetic resonance imaging (MRI) brain scans frequently show cerebral infarction in areas affected by TIAs lasting longer than several hours. The relevant clinical distinction between a TIA and a stroke is whether the ischemia has caused brain damage (infarction or selective ischemic necrosis). Because no clear temporal threshold separates the two, decisions about the initiation of therapy and its type are unavoidably vague.

STABLE VERSUS UNSTABLE STROKES. *Unstable strokes* are those in which symptoms and signs either improve or deteriorate after the onset. Deciding the stability of a stroke may be difficult, since in theory all strokes require some period to reach a stable maximum or minimum. The decision depends on an accurate history, on the interval between onset of symptoms and the first examination, and, later, on the frequency and duration of observation. Two thirds of patients with anterior circulation strokes and a

higher number of those with vertebrobasilar strokes who are first examined within a few hours of onset fluctuate in their signs and symptoms during the first week.

The identification of patients with worsening signs and symptoms, frequently referred to as *progressing stroke* or *stroke in evolution,* is particularly important, since if the cause can be identified, treatment to limit brain damage may be possible. The pathogenesis of progression may involve one or a combination of factors. Clot propagation has been suggested, but little direct evidence supports this conclusion. Other equally, if not more important, causes for progressing stroke include compromise of cardiac output due to myocardial ischemia, cardiac arrhythmias, and congestive heart failure. Systemic hypotension and increased blood viscosity can adversely affect the course of acute cerebral ischemia, as can associated pneumogenic hypoxemia or systemic electrolyte imbalance. Progression of cerebral edema, which usually maximizes by 3 or 4 days, contributes to neurologic deterioration with large strokes but not with smaller ones. Bleeding into the infarct affects as many as 40% of patients but seldom causes new symptoms.

COMPLETE VERSUS INCOMPLETE STROKES. An important distinction is that made between a *complete* and an *incomplete* stroke. The terms refer to whether the affected vascular territory has been completely involved; if not, more brain remains at risk of additional focal ischemia, making treatment an urgent matter. The clinical distinction between complete and incomplete strokes can be difficult, especially soon after onset. As a practical matter, the distinction between a complete and an incomplete stroke is often based on the severity of functional loss, for example, hemiplegia versus hemiparesis.

CLINICAL MANIFESTATIONS AND VASCULAR SYNDROMES
(See Table 470–1)

INTERNAL CAROTID ARTERY. The carotid artery bifurcation and origin of the internal carotid artery (ICA) provide the most frequent sites for atherothrombosis of cerebral blood vessels. Symptoms from such severe stenoses closely resemble those caused by middle cerebral artery (MCA) disease (see below). Flow through the ophthalmic artery is often affected sufficiently to produce *transient monocular blindness* (also called amaurosis fugax). Severe bilateral ICA stenosis can sometimes cause cerebral hemispheric hypoperfusion and symptoms in *border zones* between the major vascular territories. Anterior circulation TIAs more frequently herald the presence of ICA disease than of intracranial atherosclerosis. Similarly, acute headache ipsilateral to an acutely ischemic hemi-

Table 470–1 ■ CLINICAL MANIFESTATIONS OF ISCHEMIC STROKE

OCCLUDED BLOOD VESSEL	CLINICAL MANIFESTATIONS
ICA	Ipsilateral blindness (variable)
	MCA syndrome (see below)
MCA	Contralateral hemiparesis, sensory loss (arm, face worst)
	Expressive aphasia (dominant) or anosognosia and spatial disorientation (nondominant)
	Contralateral inferior quadrantanopsia
ACA	Contralateral hemiparesis, sensory loss (worst in leg)
PCA	Contralateral homonymous hemianopsia or superior quadrantanopsia
	Memory impairment
Basilar apex	Bilateral blindness
	Amnesia
Basilar artery	Contralateral hemiparesis, sensory loss
	Ipsilateral bulbar or cerebellar signs
Vertebral artery or PICA	Ipsilateral loss of facial sensation, ataxia, contralateral hemiparesis, sensory loss
Superior cerebellar artery	Gait ataxia, nausea, dizziness, headache progressing to ipsilateral hemiataxia, dysarthria, gaze paresis, contralateral hemiparesis, somnolence

ICA = internal carotid artery; MCA = middle cerebral artery; ACA = anterior cerebral artery; PCA = posterior cerebral artery; PICA = posterior inferior cerebellar artery.

sphere more frequently signals occlusion of the ICA than of the intracranial vessels.

ANTERIOR CEREBRAL ARTERY. Occlusion of one anterior cerebral artery (ACA) distal to the anterior communicating artery produces motor and cortical sensory symptoms in the contralateral leg and, less often, proximal arm. Other manifestations of ACA occlusion include gait ataxia and sometimes urinary incontinence from damage to the parasagittal frontal lobe. Language disturbances, manifested as decreased spontaneous speech, may accompany a generalized depression of psychomotor activity. ACA occlusion does not typically cause paralysis of both legs, an acute syndrome more likely related to spinal cord disease or, rarely, occlusion of the superior sagittal sinus, which drains the medial surfaces of both cerebral hemispheres.

ANTERIOR CHOROIDAL ARTERY. Brain image analyses suggest a clinical syndrome associated with occlusion of this vessel. Affected patients suffer a hemiparesis involving the face, arm, and leg; variable hemisensory loss; and, in some instances, hemianopsia from optic tract ischemia. The syndrome is difficult to distinguish from MCA ischemia.

MIDDLE CEREBRAL ARTERY. Most ischemic strokes involve part or all of the territory of the MCA, usually caused by emboli from the heart or extracranial carotid arteries. Emboli may occlude the main stem of the MCA but more frequently produce distal occlusions of either the superior or the inferior branch. Occlusion of the superior branch causes weakness and sensory loss that are greatest in the face and arm; vision is spared, but an inferior quadrantanopsia may rarely coexist. Hemianopsias reported with MCA infarction more likely reflect visual inattention than true blindness, since deeply penetrating MCA branches supply only the dorsal, parietal half of the optic radiations. Voluntary gaze away from the side of the lesion may be impaired, but full-range oculocephalic or oculovestibular reflexes remain (see Chapter 444). In the dominant hemisphere, the deficit includes an expressive (Broca's) asphasia with impaired fluency, naming, and writing, but relatively preserved comprehension. In the nondominant hemisphere, unilateral neglect, anosognosia (unawareness of the deficit), and spatial disorientation may be prominent.

Occlusion of the inferior branches of the MCA infrequently produces sensory loss, most notably of integrated sensations, such as perception of shapes (stereognosis). In the dominant hemisphere, occlusion of the inferior division of the MCA causes receptive (Wernicke's) aphasia, with fluent speech characterized by jargon and paraphasias; comprehension, naming, reading, and writing are often abnormal.

The so-called deep MCA syndrome may occur from selective occlusion of the MCA main stem, causing ischemia in the territory of the lenticulostriate vessels but sparing the superior and inferior MCA branches. Collateral filling of the distal MCA cortical branches prevents cortical injury, but since the lenticulostriates are end arteries, infarction of the deep MCA territory evolves. Alternatively, the lenticulostriates may be occluded by local atherosclerotic or hypertensive vascular disease. Patients with occlusion of the lenticulostriate arteries experience internal capsular infarction accompanied by hemiparesis or hemiplegia unaccompanied by visual, language, or sensory disturbances.

Proximal occlusions of the MCA may affect both superior and inferior branches as well as perforating branches to the internal capsule, optic radiations, and basal ganglia. The result includes contralateral hemiplegia, hemianesthesia, dense homonymous hemianopsia, and global aphasia with dominant or anosognosia with nondominant hemisphere involvement.

POSTERIOR CEREBRAL ARTERY. Occlusion of the posterior cerebral artery (PCA) distal to its penetrating branches most frequently causes complete contralateral loss of vision or a superior or inferior quadrantanopsia, depending on whether the lower or the upper calcarine arteries are affected individually. Central (macular) vision may be spared because of collateral supply from the MCA. If only the calcarine cortex is involved, the patient is usually aware of the vision loss, but denial of unilateral or bilateral blindness can ensue if one or both adjacent parietal cortices are affected (see Chapter 449.1). Difficulty in reading (dyslexia) and performing calculations (dyscalculia) may follow ischemia of the dominant PCA territory.

Proximal occlusion of the PCA causes ischemia of penetrating branches (thalamogeniculate, thalamoperforating, posterior choroidal) to thalamic and limbic structures. The results include hemisensory disturbances that may chronically change to intractable pain on the defective side (thalamic pain). Memory dysfunction may result, especially with bilateral occlusions. With involvement of the subthalamic nucleus, wild, uncontrolled, flailing limb movements called hemiballism may develop (see Chapter 463).

VERTEBRAL AND BASILAR ARTERIES. Focal brain stem ischemia produces a group of so-called crossed syndromes in which contralateral dysfunction occurs below the lesion due to interruption of pyramidal, spinothalamic, and dorsal column pathways, whereas ipsilateral dysfunction affects cerebellar controls or peripheral nerve junctions whose nuclei lie within the infarct. Occlusion of a vertebral artery and interference with flow through the ipsilateral *posterior inferior cerebellar artery* cause the *lateral medullary syndrome,* consisting of severe vertigo, nausea, vomiting, nystagmus, ipsilateral ataxia, and ipsilateral Horner's syndrome. There is an ipsilateral loss of facial pain and temperature sense and a contralateral loss of the same sensory modalities in trunk and limb. Discrete lesions in the distribution of the *anterior inferior cerebellar artery* are less common.

The *superior cerebellar artery* supplies most of the cerebellar cortex. Occlusion of this vessel is the most common cause of *cerebellar infarction,* characterized initially by gait ataxia, headache, nausea, vomiting, dizziness, ipsilateral clumsiness, and dysarthria. Subsequent brain swelling may induce ipsilateral gaze paresis and/or nystagmus toward the side of the infarction; ipsilateral facial weakness is sometimes seen. With further progression, lethargy and stupor deepen, and contralateral hemiparesis sometimes develops. Cerebellar edema formation can obstruct the fourth ventricle, producing hydrocephalus, and can result in herniation of the cerebellum either upward across the tentorium or downward through the foramen magnum.

Vertebrobasilar ischemia often produces multifocal lesions, scattered on both sides and along a considerable longitudinal extent of the brain stem. Except for cerebellar infarction and the lateral medullary syndrome, the clinical syndromes of discrete lesions are thus seldom seen in pure form. *Vertebrobasilar ischemia* manifests with various combinations of symptoms such as dizziness (usually vertigo), diplopia, facial weakness, ataxia, and long-tract signs. Distinguishing mild vertebrobasilar ischemia from more banal causes of dizziness can be difficult; the solution lies in identifying other, more specific symptoms or signs of parenchymal brain stem disease. Rarely does a person with vertebrobasilar ischemia present with dizziness in the absence of other brain stem signs or symptoms.

Basilar artery occlusion produces massive brain stem dysfunction. The *locked-in state* is one possible consequence; in this condition, paralysis of the limbs and most of the bulbar muscles means that the patient can communicate only by moving the eyes or eyelids to command. Normal intelligence can often be demonstrated through codes involving eye movements (see Chapter 445). *Occlusion of the basilar apex* (or *top-of-the basilar*) is usually caused by emboli that lodge at the junction between the basilar artery and the two PCAs. The condition produces an initial reduction in arousal followed by blindness and amnesia (from interruption of flow into the PCAs) plus abnormalities of vertical gaze and pupillary reactivity (from tegmental damage).

DIAGNOSIS

HISTORY. The history should emphasize the precise onset of the clinical deficit and the course since onset (stable or unstable). Preceding TIAs are more likely to be associated with an ischemic than a hemorrhagic stroke. Headache more often occurs with hemorrhage and embolus than with atherothrombotic ischemic stroke. The possibility of other diagnoses (e.g., hypoglycemia or seizures) should be considered. The initial evaluation should include a thorough search for vascular disease risk factors (see later), since their presence will strengthen the likelihood of an ischemic stroke and influence eventual management.

PHYSICAL EXAMINATION. The neurologic examination serves to localize the lesion site, but the general medical examination more frequently provides clues to pathogenesis. Specific attention should be given to the cardiovascular examination and to evidence of hematologic disease. The arterial blood pressure in both arms, cardiac rhythm, and other cardiac abnormalities, such as murmurs or opening snaps, should be carefully recorded. The vascular examination should include gentle palpation of the carotid arteries and auscultation (with a bell-type stethoscope) of their course in the neck. Ophthalmoscopy can detect retinal cholesterol or platelet-fibrin emboli as well as evidence of chronic hypertensive or diabetic disease. The presence of retinal hypertensive changes can indicate that hypertension has been chronic rather than associated with TIA. Except with posterior circulation insufficiency or previous strokes, loss of consciousness or confusion should prompt consideration of other diagnoses.

LABORATORY EXAMINATION. HEMATOLOGIC TESTS. These include complete blood and platelet counts (to evaluate for polycythemia, thrombocytosis, bacterial endocarditis, and severe anemia). Blood should be taken to evaluate glucose, prothrombin time, partial thromboplastin time, and a lipid profile. In the elderly, determination of the erythrocyte sedimentation rate should be performed urgently to exclude giant cell arteritis; in the young, the presence of antiphospholipid antibodies helps to identify immune-related disease processes predisposing to stroke. Other blood tests (e.g., protein C, protein S, measurements of viscosity or platelet function, and tests for collagen vascular diseases) may be indicated in younger patients who lack obvious causes for their strokes. The rising incidence of syphilis in urban areas makes a serum VDRL desirable. Tests of renal function and serum electrolyte measurements help to establish systemic illnesses as well as the milieu in which subsequent diagnostic tests (e.g., contrast injection) and treatments might be offered.

CARDIOVASCULAR EXAMINATION. All stroke patients require a standard 12-lead electrocardiogram (ECG) and rhythm strip at presentation to exclude acute myocardial ischemia and arrhythmias. Authorities disagree about whether one should search with echocardiography for a cardiogenic source of emboli in acute focal stroke, since the yield is low in patients who have no history or physical evidence of cardiac disease. Our practice is to use transthoracic echocardiography or, preferably, transesophogeal echocardiography in patients with focal stroke who (1) are young; (2) have no detectable atherothrombosis of the appropriate extracranial vessel, regardless of age; and (3) have no detectable risk factors, including polycythemia or oral contraceptive use. In suitable patients, *stress testing* during convalescence may be recommended to evaluate possible ischemic cardiovascular disease.

BRAIN IMAGING. Brain imaging is the most important differential diagnostic test to identify other causes of focal neurologic dysfunction, such as neoplasms or subdural hematomas, and to distinguish ischemic from hemorrhagic stroke. Computed tomographic (CT) scanning, the most commonly used imaging technique, has limitations that must be considered. It cannot always detect cerebral infarction; the size, location, and age of the lesion affect the lesion's visibility. Infarcts less than 5 mm in diameter often escape detection, especially within the brain stem, where bone artifact can interfere with resolution. Further, only about 5% of strokes are visible on CT scan within the first 12 hours; detection increases to approximately 50% between 24 and 48 hours and approximately 90% by the end of 1 week.

Infarcts appear as hypodense areas on non–contrast-enhanced CT scans with increasingly well-demarcated margins as edema peaks between 3 and 5 days. Contrast-enhancing agents carry a small risk of neurotoxicity, and they may normalize the CT density of an otherwise small hypodense infarct, making the infarct less visible. Accordingly, one should use contrast-enhancing agents during the acute phase of the ischemic stroke only to seek out a mass lesion and only after a non-contrast scan has been obtained.

CT scans immediately delineate primary cerebral hemorrhage, but hemorrhagic conversions of an ischemic infarct usually develop only after 1 to 2 days. A few continue to appear for up to 4 weeks.

MRI is more sensitive than CT to changes in tissue structure and may provide a more accurate and earlier measure of cerebral infarction. MRI is more costly however, and, with the present equipment, requires more time to perform than CT; in addition, the need to exclude ferromagnetic materials from the MRI suite, as well as the difficulty in monitoring patients in the scanner, makes MRI unsuitable for many acutely ill patients. If the diagnosis remains in doubt, MRI may be used after the acute phase to verify infarction.

LUMBAR PUNCTURE. Lumbar puncture is no longer widely used to diagnose routine stroke because (1) noninvasive CT or MRI detects cerebral hemorrhage and (2) anticoagulation begun within 6 hours after a lumbar puncture risks causing a spinal epidural hematoma. A lumbar puncture is important, however, in diagnosing neurosyphilis or meningitis, as, for example, in patients with acute stiff neck who show no blood on brain imaging. If it is to be done in suspected stroke, it should be preceded by brain imaging and funduscopic examination to rule out raised intracranial pressure.

NONINVASIVE CEREBROVASCULAR EXAMINATION. Several noninvasive techniques help to evaluate the cerebrovascular supply. Indirect tests that examine blood flow in the periorbital or orbital circulation include *Doppler sonography* and *quantitative oculopneumoplethysmography*.

Direct examination of the common, internal, and external carotid arteries is best achieved with *duplex ultrasonography*. Duplex ultrasonography consists of B-mode ultrasonography, which produces a real-time image of the carotid vessels and a range-gaited pulsed Doppler that is visually guided by the B-mode image to measure the frequency shift associated with increased blood velocity through a stenotic lumen. The combination of the precise location of the Doppler frequency signal and the B-mode image provides the most accurate noninvasive method for analyzing disease of the extracranial circulation. Limitations of the technique include (1) access to only the portion of the carotid circulation that lies between the clavicles and the mandible (in approximately 10% of patients, the carotid bifurcation lies above the angle of the jaw, making ultrasonography difficult or impossible); (2) absorption of sound waves by calcium within a mural plaque, which may "shadow" and obscure a plaque on a distal vessel wall; and (3) echolucency of acute thrombi, which can be indistinguishable from flowing blood.

The direction and velocity of blood flow in the intracranial blood vessels originating from the circle of Willis can be examined with low-frequency *pulsed transcranial Doppler*. The intracranial blood vessels also can be examined on reconstructed CT or MRI images. An evolving technique involves the imaging of flowing blood using *magnetic resonance angiography*. The procedure produces images of the extracranial and intracranial blood vessels, as well as atherosclerotic abnormalities of the carotid bifurcation; some aneurysms can also be detected.

CEREBRAL ANGIOGRAPHY. Intracranial and extracranial *cerebral angiography* of elderly patients prone to ischemic stroke carries a 2 to 4% risk of producing a reversible neurologic deficit and a 0.5 to 1.0% risk of permanent neurologic deficits or death. Accordingly, angiography should be reserved for specific indications in which it may reveal abnormalities amenable to therapy. Examples include a search for fibromuscular dysplasia, arterial dissection, cranial arteritis, or as a preparation for cerebrovascular surgery. *Digital subtraction arteriography* permits use of smaller amounts of intravascular contrast material and may thus be of lower risk, especially in patients with marginal renal or cardiac function. *Digital subtraction venous angiography* is no longer widely used because of its unreliability in detecting plaque ulcerations and in differentiating carotid stenosis from complete occlusion.

OTHER TECHNIQUES. Methods for measuring cerebral blood flow in the clinical arena are still largely investigational; they include *positron emission tomographic (PET)* methods, usually using radiolabeled water or carbon dioxide, *single-photon emission computed tomography (SPECT)*, and radiolabeled and stable *xenon* inhalation techniques using CT imaging.

DIFFERENTIAL DIAGNOSIS OF ISCHEMIC STROKES AND TRANSIENT ISCHEMIC ATTACKS The clinical diagnosis of ischemic or hemorrhagic stroke relies primarily on the clinician's understanding of brain function and pathology. Deficits that evolve over weeks are usually caused by a brain mass, either *primary* or *metastatic brain tumor* or *brain abscess*. *Subdural hematoma* should be distinguishable from stroke by the hematoma's more prolonged course and its combination of diffuse and focal dysfunction.

TIAs may be confused with classic or complicated *migraine*, the former being associated with scintillating scotomata and the latter with hemiparesis or other focal deficits; some of the underlying pathophysiology may be ischemic for both TIAs and migraine, but evidence is accumulating that nonischemic electrical disturbances (spreading depression) may be involved in the pathophysiology of migraine.

Seizures can be confused with TIAs. Most seizures produce motor activity or positive sensory phenomena, whereas most strokes and TIAs produce weakness and sensory loss. Nevertheless, seizures can sometimes produce these negative symptoms. The postictal state following (unobserved) seizures is even more likely to imitate an ischemic deficit. Serial observations usually permit the differentiation of stroke from seizure, but rapid differentiation may be difficult and may interfere with early stroke treatment. As with migraine, strokes and seizures can coexist: A small proportion of strokes (about 10%), especially embolic strokes, are associated at onset with seizures.

Hemorrhagic stroke often enters the differential diagnosis for ischemic stroke. Although the anatomic locations of the two may differ, with hemorrhage seldom involving a discrete vascular territory, clinical differentiation can be uncertain, making the CT scan necessary. Other illnesses included in the differential diagnosis of vertebrobasilar ischemia include, as mentioned, nonspecific dizziness, Meniere's disease, or peripheral vestibulopathy.

CAUSES AND PATHOGENESIS (TABLE 470–2)

ATHEROSCLEROSIS. Atherosclerosis of extracranial and intracranial arteries accounts for approximately two thirds of all ischemic strokes and an even greater proportion of those affecting patients over the age of 60. Atherosclerosis causes strokes either by *in situ stenosis* or *occlusion* or by *embolization* of plaque thrombus material to distal cerebral vessels. In either case, the clinical and pathologic effects depend on the adequacy of collateral circulation to the affected vascular territory. It is not uncommon for unilateral or, more rarely, bilateral occlusion of the ICA to develop without neurologic symptoms, especially if the stenosis or occlusion develops slowly. In instances of marked stenosis or occlusion of extracranial arteries that is combined with intracranial atherosclerosis, cerebral perfusion sometimes can relate closely to small changes in blood pressure. One effect can be a worsening stroke deficit associated with orthostatic blood pressure changes that would otherwise be considered normal.

The more common effect of atherosclerosis is that a platelet-fibrin embolus detaches from a plaque and floats distally, where it occludes a smaller branch. Such emboli are likely to produce symptoms, since the more distal the occlusion, the less likely that collateral filling can prevent damage. In cases of artery-to-artery embolization, the embolus usually emanates from a plaque at the base of the aorta, the bifurcation of the common carotid artery, or at the point where the vertebral arteries originate from the subclavian arteries.

EMBOLI OF CARDIAC ORIGIN. Cerebral emboli of a cardiac source may account for up to one third of all ischemic strokes. Thrombus formation and the release of thromboemboli from the heart are promoted by arrhythmias and structural abnormalities of the valves and chambers.

MURAL THROMBI. Mural thrombi typically form under areas of dyskinetic myocardium damaged by *myocardial infarction.* Up to 35% of patients with recent anterior wall infarction harbor mural thrombi, and if not anticoagulated, nearly 40% of these will embolize systemically within 4 months after the myocardial infarction. *Cardiomyopathies* can also predispose to mural thrombi and embolization. In one study, systemic emboli were found in approximately 15% of patients with congestive or dilated cardiomyopathy, a subgroup of the condition that is usually caused by alcohol abuse or viral infections. Patients who also had atrial fibrillation had a higher incidence of embolism (33%) than did those without (14%). None of the cardiomyopathy patients receiving anticoagulation therapy experienced systemic emboli, however.

VALVULAR HEART DISEASE. Although less common than previously, *rheumatic heart disease* often gives rise to systemic embolization. In one series, 20 to 25% of patients with mitral stenosis developed systemic emboli, although most had coexisting atrial fibrillation.

Acute or subacute *infective endocarditis* produces vegetations on heart valves, and debris that can embolize into the cerebral circula-

Table 470–2 ■ CAUSES OF ISCHEMIC STROKE

ATHEROSCLEROSIS

EMBOLI OF CARDIAC ORIGIN

Mural thrombus
  Myocardial infarction (anterior wall sputum, akinetic segment)
  Cardiomyopathy (infectious, idiopathic)
Valvular heart disease
  Rheumatic heart disease
  Bacterial endocarditis
  Nonbacterial endocarditis (carcinoma, Libman-Sacks disease)
  Mitral valve prolapse
  Prosthetic valve
Arrhythmia (atrial fibrillation)
Cardiac myxoma
Paradoxical emboli

VASCULITIDES

Primary central nervous system vasculitis
Systemic necrotizing vasculitis (polyarteritis nodosa, allergic angiitis)
Hypersensitivity vasculitis (serum sickness, drug-induced, cutaneous vasculitis)
Collagen vascular diseases (rheumatoid arthritis, scleroderma, Sjögren's disease)
Giant cell (temporal arteritis, Takayasu's arteritis)
Wegener's granulomatosis
Lymphomatoid granulomatosis
Behçet's disease
Infectious vasculitis (neurovascular syphilis, Lyme disease, bacterial and fungal meningitis, tuberculosis, acquired immunodeficiency syndrome, ophthalmic zoster, hepatitis B)

HEMATOLOGIC DISORDERS

Hemoglobinopathies (sickle cell, HbSC)
Hyperviscosity syndromes (polycythemia, thrombocytosis, leukocytosis, macroglobulinemia, multiple myeloma)
Hypercoagulable states (carcinoma, pregnancy, puerperium)
Protein C or S deficiency
Antiphospholipid antibodies (lupus anticoagulant, anticardiolipin antibody)

DRUG RELATED

Street drugs (cocaine, crack, amphetamines, lysergic acid, phencyclidine, methylphenidate, sympathomimetics, heroin, pentazocine)
Alcohol
Oral contraceptives

OTHER

Fibromuscular dysplasia
Arterial dissection (trauma, spontaneous, Marfan syndrome)
Homocystinuria
Migraine
Subarachnoid hemorrhage or vasospasm
Other emboli (fat, bone marrow, air)
Moyamoya

tion. Many emboli are relatively small, but those associated with endocarditis caused by staphylococci, fungi, or yeast often are large enough to occlude proximal intracranial arteries. Systemic emboli are found in up to 30% of patients who die of infective endocarditis. Prompt recognition of the heart lesion plus the presence of fever, a murmur, petechiae, and other characteristics in patients with underlying valvular disease or intravenous drug use should prompt blood cultures and treatment with antibiotics to reduce the risk of embolism. Anticoagulation is not effective and may increase the risk of parenchymal bleeding. Infective endocarditis is associated with other forms of cerebrovascular disease, including cerebral hemorrhage, subarachnoid hemorrhage, and mycotic aneurysm, as well as cerebral abscess.

Embolization from heart valves also occurs in *nonbacterial endocarditis,* in which predominantly platelet-fibrin vegetations form on the heart valves and then embolize into the systemic circulation. This occurs commonly in association with cancer of the stomach, prostate, ovary, pancreas, and lung. In one autopsy series of patients with nonbacterial endocarditis, cerebral emboli were found in one third. Clinically, diffuse encephalopathy as well as focal stroke is observed; associated disseminated intravascular coagulation accompanies about 20% of cases.

Libman-Sacks (atypical verrucous) endocarditis is associated with systemic lupus erythematosus. Soft, friable vegetations form on the leaflets of any of the heart valves, not just the tricuspid valve, as believed earlier. Systemic (and cerebral) emboli are rare.

Mitral valve prolapse describes a billowing of the mitral leaflets into the left atrium during systole. Although usually asymptomatic, some patients experience palpitations or chest pain. The diagnosis is suggested by auscultatory and echocardiographic criteria, but normal standards are uncertain, making the true incidence unknown; it is estimated to be 6 to 10% in healthy young women. In part because of different diagnostic criteria, the role of mitral valve prolapse in cerebral embolism remains controversial: Several analyses of strokes in young adults suggest a disproportionately high representation of patients with mitral valve prolapse, but others indexed on patients with mitral valve prolapse suggest that systemic embolism is infrequent. Coexisting infective endocarditis or arrhythmia contributes to cerebral embolism.

Prosthetic heart valves carry a high risk of systemic (including cerebral) embolism; mechanical heart valves have a higher risk than biologic valves (e.g., porcine). The overall risk of embolism is roughly equivalent in anticoagulated patients with mechanical valves and in nonanticoagulated patients with biologic valves: 1 to 3% per year for aortic prostheses, and 3 to 5% per year for mitral substitutions.

ARRHYTHMIAS. *Atrial fibrillation,* with or without valvular disease, strongly increases the risk of embolic ischemic stroke, especially in patients over the age of 60. In one large series, the risk of ischemic stroke was 6 to 7% per year in nonanticoagulated patients. The risk is highest shortly after development of atrial fibrillation: Up to one third of emboli occur in the first month. Embolism can also accompany therapeutic cardioversion. About 35% of patients with nonvalvular atrial fibrillation sooner or later will have an ischemic stroke. In some, embolism underlies the stroke; in others, the fault lies in coexisting intrinsic cerebrovascular disease associated with coronary artery disease. Even thyrotoxic, nonvalvular atrial fibrillation is associated with a 10 to 12% risk of stroke. The one group without a strikingly increased risk is patients with isolated atrial fibrillation, unassociated with other clinical evidence of cardiopulmonary disease.

CARDIAC MYXOMA. Cardiac tumors are uncommon, occurring in about 0.05% of autopsies. *Myxomas* account for about 35% of all intracardiac tumors but are the ones most likely to embolize, from either overlying thrombus or the tumor itself. In one series, about one quarter of patients with autopsy-proven cardiac myxomas had clinical evidence of strokes. Aneurysms and intracranial hemorrhage were also reported. The coexistence of hemolytic anemia due to red blood cell trauma and lysis sometimes suggests a cardiac tumor, but firm diagnosis requires echocardiography or angiography.

PARADOXICAL EMBOLI. Emboli of venous origin have long been known to cross a patent foramen ovale into the systemic circulation. Studies using bubble echocardiography found that 40% of stroke patients under age 55 with a normal cardiac evaluation by history, examination, and ECG had a patent foramen ovale detected by bubble echocardiography.

VASCULITIDES. A group of disorders classified as vasculitides cause focal or multifocal cerebral ischemia through inflammation and necrosis of extracranial and/or intracranial blood vessels. The pathogenesis of vascular inflammation differs among these disorders, but all involve some deposition of humoral and cellular immune complexes and infiltration of polymorphonuclear and mononuclear cells in blood vessel walls. In most cases, the cause of the inflammatory response is unknown, but in others, infection, a postinfectious or neoplastic process, or a hypersensitivity immune reaction triggers the inflammation.

Segmental inflammation of cerebral blood vessels causes cerebral ischemia acutely at the site of involvement through platelet aggregation and/or clot formation or chronically through fibrinoid necrosis, which narrows the vessel lumen. Central nervous system (CNS) vasculitis, although a rare cause of stroke, is itself not uncommon and should enter the differential diagnosis whenever a young patient presents with a stroke or a patient of any age presents with a diffuse unexplained encephalopathy.

Symptoms of CNS vasculitis include cognitive disturbances, headache, and seizures (encephalopathy), which occur more frequently than with focal neurologic dysfunction. The diagnosis depends on the angiographic appearance of a "beadlike" segmental narrowing of cerebral blood vessels and/or the finding of character-

istic inflammatory histopathology in leptomeningeal and cortical biopsy specimens. Cerebral angiograms may appear normal in 20 to 30% of histologically positive cases. In addition, because of the segmental or "skip" nature of the inflammatory response, the histopathology may go undetected in the presence of a positive angiogram.

The diagnosis of CNS vasculitis is aided by the presence or absence of peripheral nervous system or systemic organ involvement and by identifying the underlying cause of the inflammation. Primary CNS vasculitis, Behçet's disease, Takayasu's arteritis, and temporal arteritis are notable for their infrequent involvement or noninvolvement of the peripheral nervous system. By contrast, the hypersensitivity and systemic necrotizing vasculitides frequently produce polyneuropathies.

Primary CNS arteritis, giant cell arteritis, and vasculitis associated with certain CNS infections deserve specific attention, since these may present initially or solely with neurologic signs and symptoms.

PRIMARY CNS ARTERITIS. Primary arteritis of the CNS, also called granulomatous arteritis of the CNS, causes headache and other encephalopathy-like symptoms in young or middle-aged individuals. The course is usually insidiously progressive but may wax and wane for periods of several months. It is a diagnosis of exclusion.

GIANT CELL VASCULITIS. Temporal arteritis and Takayasu's arteritis are characterized by a granulomatous vasculitis of medium-sized and large arteries. Temporal arteritis affects predominantly patients over the age of 60, causing constitutional symptoms such as fever, malaise, weight loss, and headache. In half the patients, symptoms consistent with polymyalgia rheumatica may coexist, including jaw, neck, and facial pain, as well as morning stiffness. Tenderness and pain over the temporal arteries and an elevated erythrocyte sedimentation rate are frequently, but not always, present. Biopsy of the superficial temporal artery provides the definitive diagnosis. Because of the segmental nature of the vasculitis, serial sections should be examined. Even then, typical features of fever, malaise, tender scalp vessels, and a grossly elevated sedimentation rate dictate the early initiation of corticosteroid therapy because of the high risk of acute ischemic blindness. A *dramatic* improvement in constitutional symptoms supports the diagnosis.

Takayasu's arteritis affects primarily young women and involves mainly the aortic arch, the large brachiocephalic arteries derived from the arch, and the abdominal aorta. Mononuclear infiltrates and fibrous proliferation produce progressive narrowing of the lumen of these vessels, causing reduced flow into the upper extremities (hence the name *pulseless disease*) and cerebral ischemia. Although initially diagnosed in Japanese women, it has been recognized in Western countries.

INFECTIOUS VASCULITIS. Bacterial, fungal, and viral infections can induce CNS vasculitis and cerebral ischemia (see Table 470–2). Neurosyphilis and its meningovascular complications have increased considerably in recent years (see Ch. 474) and should be considered in patients with atypical or unexplained cerebrovascular disease.

HEMATOLOGIC ABNORMALITIES. HEMOGLOBINOPATHY. Among the hemoglobinopathies, *sickle cell disease* is by far the most common cause of stroke. In sickle cell disease, a single substitution of the amino acid valine for glutamate at the sixth position of the β-globin molecule causes the mutant molecule HbSS to become highly insoluble and polymerize under deoxygenated conditions. The polymerization alters the erythrocyte's shape ("sickling") and decreases the cell's deformability, leading to increased blood viscosity, microvascular sludging, and microvascular infarction. Sickle cell disease also causes hyperplasia of fibrous tissue and muscle cells of the vascular intima, leading to stenosis and occlusion of some medium to large cerebral arteries.

Ischemic stroke occurs in approximately 15% of patients with HbSS and in a much smaller percentage of those with sickle cell trait (HbSA) or HbSC. At normal arterial oxygen saturations of 95 to 100% in HbSS, some sickling is present, and at 65% (i.e., just slightly lower than normal venous oxygen saturation), approximately 75% of erythrocytes sickle. Ischemic stroke arises most frequently in children, whereas hemorrhagic stroke is more common in adults with HbSS; subarachnoid hemorrhage in patients with sickle cell disease is frequently the result of a ruptured saccular aneurysm.

Small changes in oxygen tension, dehydration, acidosis, or infection can precipitate sickle cell crisis and stroke. Cerebral angiography causes an increased risk for patients with sickle cell disease. In instances when such angiography is necessary to evaluate the source of intracerebral hemorrhage, the level of HbSS should be reduced to less than 20% through transfusions.

HYPERVISCOSITY SYNDROME. Cerebral blood flow relates inversely to blood viscosity. The latter is directly proportional to the number of circulating red and white blood cells, the aggregation state, the number of platelets, and the plasma protein concentration. Blood flow is inversely proportional to the deformability of erythrocytes and blood velocity (shear rate). Patients with the hyperviscosity syndrome can have either focal neurologic dysfunction or, more frequently, diffuse or multifocal signs or symptoms, including headache, visual disturbances, cognitive impairment, and seizures.

Cellular hyperviscosity, associated with *polycythemia, thrombocytosis,* or *leukocytosis* of any cause, can reduce blood flow below threshold levels for cerebral dysfunction and injury. Hematocrits above 50%, white cell counts above 150,000/μL, and platelet counts in excess of 1 million/μL increase the risk of stroke.

Elevated plasma protein concentrations caused by *macroglobulinemia* or *multiple myeloma* elevate plasma viscosity and increase stroke risk. Approximately 25% of patients with macroglobulinemia experience some form of cerebral ischemia, and a lesser number of patients with multiple myeloma experience the hyperviscosity syndrome. Of the various forms of multiple myeloma, those with a predominance of immunoglobulin A (IgA) most frequently develop a hyperviscosity syndrome because this particular molecule is likely to form high-molecular-weight polymers.

HYPERCOAGULABLE STATES. Cancer, particularly the adenocarcinomas, pregnancy, and the puerperium have all been associated with hypercoagulable state that predisposes to arterial and venous thrombosis. Despite the fact that any one of several abnormalities—including elevations of fibrinogen levels, alterations of partial thromboplastin or prothrombin times, and platelet aggregation—occurs in the hypercoagulable state, no tests have been devised to diagnose it specifically.

PROTEIN C OR S DEFICIENCY. Proteins C and S are two naturally occurring anticoagulants synthesized in the liver via vitamin K–dependent mechanisms. Deficiencies of either are rare, dominantly inherited, and expressed phenotypically by incomplete penetrance. Homozygotes develop serious and frequently fatal clotting abnormalities at birth, whereas heterozygotes may show no signs of hypercoagulability. Proteins C and S act in concert to inactivate the activated coagulating Factors V and VIII; protein C also triggers the endogenous fibrinolytic pathways. Deficiencies in either are associated with ischemic vascular disease. Because of incomplete penetrance, the occurrence of thrombosis and stroke in the adult is extremely rare.

ANTIPHOSPHOLIPID ANTIBODIES. A strong epidemiologic association links a group of antiphospholipid antibodies to cerebral ischemia manifested clinically as atypical migraine, TIA, recurrent strokes, or ischemic encephalopathy. These antibodies bind to membrane phospholipids and include anticardiolipin antibody, the lupus anticoagulant, and antibodies causing a false-positive VDRL results. The pathogenetic relationship between the antibodies and enhanced cerebral thrombosis is unknown. The syndrome may manifest at any age but usually affects patients younger than 50 years. Antiphospholipid antibodies often accompany collagen vascular disease, especially systemic lupus erythematosus, as well as valvular heart disease. Circulating titers of phospholipid antibodies correlate poorly with either the incidence or the severity of cerebral ischemia.

DRUG-RELATED CAUSES OF STROKE. An extensive list of "street" drugs (see Table 470–2) has been associated with stroke, reflecting as much the social patterns of drug abuse as the unique properties of the drugs themselves. The sharing of nonsterile needles to inject many of these drugs intravenously (e.g., heroin, cocaine) may precipitate infectious processes (bacterial endocarditis, hepatitis B, mycotic aneurysms) that lead to strokes. Several of the drugs are potent vasoconstrictors and may initiate cerebral vasospasm. Others have been associated with cerebral vasculitis caused

either by immune responses to the primary drug or by hypersensitivity to contaminating adulterants. The intravenous injection of oral medications (pentazocine [Talwin], methylphenidate [Ritalin]) that have been crushed and suspended in water can cause cerebral microemboli owing to particles of talc and cellulose used as ingredients in the pills. The particles are thought to be trapped by pulmonary arterioles, causing local arteritis and later arteriovenous shunts that allow the microemboli to reach the CNS.

Over-the-counter cold remedies and nasal decongestants containing sympathomimetics such as ephedrine, phenylpropanolamine, and phenoxazoline have been associated with ischemic stroke. Cases have been reported following the prolonged use of oral cold medications as well as in patients who chronically overuse nasal decongestants.

The risk of ischemic and hemorrhagic stroke is increased from 4- to 13-fold among users of high-dose estrogen contraceptives. The coexistence of hypertension, prolonged use of the pill, smoking, a previous history of migraine, and age exceeding 35 years seems to enhance the risk of contraceptive-related stroke. A clear association between stroke and the newer low-dose estrogen contraceptives remains controversial, with a history of migraine raising greatest concern.

OTHER CAUSES OF STROKE. *Fibromuscular dysplasia* (or hyperplasia) describes areas of segmental nonatherosclerotic arterial narrowing, usually caused by fibroplasia and smooth muscle proliferation, that alternate with rings of medial thinning. The uncommon condition affects the carotid and vertebral arteries, usually at the level of the second cervical vertebra rather than at the origin of the vessels; it also affects the renal arteries and is associated with hypertension. Fibromuscular dysplasia predominates in women and occurs, on the average, in the sixth decade of life. It produces ischemic stroke both by the hemodynamic effects of stenosis and by thromboembolism. The condition is also associated with aneurysm formation and with arterial dissection. Angiography usually makes the diagnosis, although flow studies with MRI may prove useful. Because of its rarity, there is little information about treatment.

A *dissecting aortic aneurysm,* although uncommon, can occlude major branches of the aorta supplying the cranial circulation and produce ischemic strokes. Chest, back, or abdominal pain accompanying the stroke and differences in palpable pulses or in blood pressure in the limbs suggest the diagnosis. Emergency angiography is needed to confirm it.

Extracranial *dissections of the carotid artery* are increasingly recognized. Many follow relatively trivial trauma (e.g., pharyngeal injury with blunt objects in children, and neck torsion, sometimes from chiropractic manipulation, in adults). Some are associated with fibromuscular dysplasia, others with a variety of childhood conditions, including Ehlers-Danlos and Marfan syndromes and tuberous sclerosis. Pathologically, intraluminal blood enters the subintimal or medial vascular planes, and the lumen becomes progressively narrowed and thrombosed. Carotid artery dissections can sometimes be recognized clinically by intense ipsilateral pain. Angiography may be needed for diagnosis, but MRI is sometimes sufficient.

Homocystinuria is characterized by dislocated ocular lenses, bone deformities, a marfanoid appearance, mental retardation, accelerated atherosclerosis, and arterial or venous thromboses. Several different genetic defects can cause homocystinuria, but the most frequent is a deficiency of the enzyme cystathionine β-synthase. Approximately one third of affected individuals have one or more strokes by the age of 15 years. In some studies, heterozygous homocystinuria has been reported in up to one quarter of young persons who have suffered strokes. Moderately elevated plasma homocysteine levels without clinical signs of severe homocysteinemia or homocystinuria is also an independent risk factor for cerebrovascular disease. Treatment with pyridoxine or folic acid may limit disease progression.

Reactive vascular narrowing *(vasospasm)* causes ischemic strokes in two settings. One causes substantial disability in *subarachnoid hemorrhage* (see Chapter 471). Vasospasm also presumably explains ischemic strokes seen in a small number of patients with *migraine* headaches. Migraineurs develop ischemic strokes, either in conjunction with migraine (in which case they appear to result from a prolonged migraine attack) or remote from the attack (in which case more traditional stroke mechanisms, such as atherosclerosis, are likely to be responsible).

Fat emboli typically occur several days after trauma that includes fracture of long bones. Although focal ischemic strokes may occur, more typically the condition manifests with seizures and a diffuse encephalopathy consistent with disseminated embolization. Associated findings include petechiae, and fat emboli visible on funduscopic examination. Fat globules may be identified in urine or CSF.

Air emboli can occur with open heart surgery, in patients with pneumothorax, or in divers who ascend too rapidly to the surface. Air emboli cause altered mental status and seizures, but the changes are maximal immediately after the embolization. Segmental areas of pallor may be observed on the tongue, and there may be marbling of the skin and air emboli seen on funduscopic examination. When caused by sudden decompression, the condition is treated in a decompression chamber.

Moyamoya is a rare condition that is most common among the Japanese, in whom it has been reported to affect fewer than 0.1 per 100,000 of the general population. Diagnosis requires demonstration of bilateral terminal ICA occlusion that involves the origins of the MCA and ACA. An abnormal vascular network develops at the base of the brain that is believed to provide collateral circulation. The abnormal collateral channels appear on angiograms as a "smoky haze," hence the Japanese term *moyamoya*. The cause of the vascular occlusion is unknown, but it occurs most commonly in children (peak incidence at age 6 years), in whom it may be associated with ischemic stroke; in adults, it more commonly causes hemorrhage. A similar angiographic picture occasionally accompanies acute tonsillitis, atherosclerosis, meningitis, cancer, trauma, and radiotherapy.

A condition in which the walls of small arteries are thickened and disorganized, referred to by some as lipohyalinosis, was originally believed to underlie small; subcortical brain infarcts called *lacunes*. Traditional causes of stroke, including diabetes and hyperlipidemia, have appeared in these patients with almost the same frequency as in those with nonlacunar, ischemic stroke. Perhaps as a result, treatment recommendations, which initially differed for lacunar strokes, now parallel those for nonlacunar strokes.

PREVENTION AND TREATMENT OF STROKE

Currently, tissue plasminogen activator (tPA) given within 3 hours of symptom onset and aspirin given within 24 hours are the only generally accepted therapies for acute ischemic stroke. Even when other effective treatments become available, the physician's opportunity to treat and the utility of a particular pharmacotherapy will be hampered by time constraints; the evolution of irreversible brain damage occurs within several hours of focal vascular occlusion (see Chapter 469). Such considerations place a premium on preventing stroke.

The reduction of stroke risk factors, through therapy for hypertension, diabetes mellitus, smoking, atherosclerosis, and cardiac arrhythmias (Table 470–3) is largely responsible for the marked decline in the incidence of stroke during the past 30 to 40 years.

RISK FACTORS AND PRIMARY PREVENTION THERAPIES
(See Table 470–3)

Stroke risk factors have been determined on the basis of mathematical abstractions of epidemiologic data that imply an association or a cause-effect relationship. This section categorizes such risk

Table 470–3 ■ **PREVENTION OF STROKE**

Treatment of hypertension and diabetes mellitus
Smoking cessation
Limited alcohol intake
Control of diet and obesity
Thoughtful use of oral contraceptives
Antiplatelet drugs or anticoagulants for atrial fibrillation and selected acute myocardial infarctions
Antiplatelet drugs for symptomatic carotid or vertebrobasilar atherosclerosis
Endarterectomy for symptomatic carotid artery stenosis of 70–99% in selected patients with perioperative morbidity or mortality risk of <5–10%
Endarterectomy for symptomatic carotid artery stenosis of 50–69% in selected patients with perioperative morbidity or mortality risk of <6%
Endarterectomy for asymptomatic carotid artery stenosis of >60% in selected patients with perioperative morbidity or mortality risk of <3%

factors as *definite* or *presumed* and indicates whether they are related to *genetic* and *lifestyle* factors or to *disease processes*. Treatable risk factors are emphasized, and the expected outcome of such prophylactic therapy is presented.

DEFINITE GENETIC AND LIFESTYLE RISK FACTORS. HYPERTENSION. This is the most powerful risk factor for stroke. Even within relatively "normal" ranges of blood pressure, the risk of stroke increases by approximately 50% for every 5 mm Hg increase in diastolic pressure throughout the range of 70 to 110 mm Hg. All components of blood pressure (systolic, diastolic, mean) correlate with the incidence of stroke, and the elevation of the systolic pressure is probably a direct cause of stroke that is independent of the secondary complications of hypertension, such as atherosclerosis or arterial rigidity. The risk of stroke is approximately four times greater in patients with definite hypertension (160/95 mm Hg) than in normotensive individuals and is two times higher in so-called borderline hypertensive individuals. Antihypertensive therapy that lowers the diastolic pressure by as little as 6 mm Hg reduces stroke risk by nearly one quarter in as little as 2 to 3 years. Data from the Framingham Study indicate that the control of hypertension is as beneficial in reducing stroke risk in persons over 70 years of age as it is at earlier ages.

SMOKING. Smoking increases stroke risk two-fold to four-fold. Those who stop smoking substantially reduce their risk of stroke during a period of 2 to 5 years, but their level of risk may not return completely to that of nonsmokers.

AGE, GENDER, AND RACE. Age, gender, and race are all unalterable risk factors for stroke, but they may signal treatable disease processes. The incidence of stroke approximately doubles with each decade between ages 45 and 85. Unlike cardiovascular ischemia, in which the incidence in men is approximately three times that in women, stroke occurs only 1.3 times more often in men than in women. The stroke risk in US blacks is approximately 1.3 times that of whites. Some of the differences may be related to environmental or lifestyle factors, since southeastern blacks have a higher stroke rate than do northern ones. Similarly, the high incidence of stroke in the Japanese is not seen in their kindred living in Hawaii.

POSSIBLE GENETIC AND LIFESTYLE RISK FACTORS. CHOLESTEROL, LIPIDS, DIET, AND OBESITY. Several dietary factors and obesity may play a role in stroke incidence, but the evidence is inconclusive. Diet and obesity may predispose toward diabetes mellitus and cardiovascular disease, and such patients have a higher chance of dying of stroke than do age-matched controls. Despite the incontrovertible relationship between elevated blood cholesterol and lipids and coronary artery disease, no conclusive evidence currently links lipid abnormalities to stroke. Nevertheless, most authorities strongly advise stroke-prone patients to lower elevated cholesterol and triglyceride levels. Because of the relationships that link obesity with diabetes mellitus, elevated blood pressure, and lipid abnormalities, weight control also is recommended for stroke-prone patients.

ALCOHOL. Moderate alcohol consumption relates inversely to the incidence of atherosclerosis and coronary artery disease, and a similar reduction of stroke risk with moderate alcohol consumption has also been suggested but not proved. By contrast, binge drinking increases the incidence of both hemorrhagic and ischemic stroke, especially when combined with cigarette smoking. Much of the latter risk may be attributable to a combination of hemoconcentration and hypertension associated with heavy alcohol consumption.

ORAL CONTRACEPTIVES. Although formerly available high-dose estrogen oral contraceptives were related to stroke, the association is less clear for current preparations. Nevertheless, the combination of oral contraceptives with other risk factors, such as migraine, smoking, hypertension, and age greater than 35 years, may act in combination to raise stroke risk, and many recommend against oral contraceptives in such circumstances.

DEFINITE DISEASE-RELATED RISK FACTORS. HEART DISEASE. Rheumatic valvular disease plus atrial fibrillation increase the risk of stroke 17-fold. Chronic anticoagulation with warfarin to an International Normalized Ratio (INR) of 2.0 to 3.5 is recommended for such individuals. In patients with chronic atrial fibrillation without lesions of the heart valves (nonvalvular atrial fibrillation), the chance of stroke varies in concert with identifiable risk factors. Gender, age, hypertension, congestive heart failure, and prior arterial thromboembolism interact with nonvalvular atrial fibrillation to create risk profiles that vary between negligible to an 18% yearly increase in the risk of stroke. Because prophylactic treatment with antiplatelet drugs or warfarin carries a small but real risk of systemic/cerebral hemorrhage, treatment recommendations must weigh individual risk/benefit ratios. Therapy is unnecessary in men and women ≤ 60 years of age and older with nonvalvular atrial fibrillation who have none of three risk factors (hypertension, congestive heart failure, prior arterial embolism). Aspirin (325 mg/day) is recommended for all asymptomatic nonvalvular atrial fibrillation patients between the ages of 60 to 75 years. Men over the age of 75 years without additional risk factors may continue to receive aspirin, but woman over 75 years should be switched to warfarin therapy. Men and women of any age with nonvalvular atrial fibrillation and one or more of the three risk factors should receive chronic warfarin therapy to an INR of 2.0 to 3.0. Aspirin may be substituted if warfarin is contraindicated.

Valvular disease related to bacterial or nonbacterial endocarditis, myxomatous degeneration of the mitral valve, or other diseases causing mitral valve prolapse, mitral valve annulus calcification, and prosthetic heart valve replacements all predispose toward cerebral emboli. Chronic therapy with warfarin to an INR of 2.5 to 3.0 and aspirin (81 mg/day) is recommended in all patients with prosthetic heart valves. Patients with bacterial endocarditis should not undergo anticoagulation because of an increased risk of cerebral hemorrhage.

Myocardial infarction involving the anterior wall or septum is associated with a mural thrombus in up to 30% of patients, and of these, approximately 15% suffer a cerebral embolus within 2 years. Acute anticoagulation therapy with heparin, with later conversion to warfarin therapy, is recommended for patients with myocardial infarction involving the anterior or septal wall or in patients with an intramural thrombus detected by two-dimensional echocardiography. Anticoagulation should continue until the two-dimensional echocardiogram indicates resolution of the thrombus. Such therapy reduces the incidence of stroke by approximately 50%.

STROKE AND TIA. The occurrence of an initial stroke is a powerful predictor of recurrent stroke. Patients between the ages of 45 and 65 years have a 10- to 20-fold increased risk of having a recurrent versus an initial stroke. The comparative risk drops to 8-fold for those over the age of 65. The apparent decrease in the incidence of recurrent stroke with age reflects the marked increase in the incidence of an initial stroke in patients over the age of 65. The annual stroke risk following a TIA is 5% per year, which declines to 3% after 3 years. After the occurrence of amaurosis fugax, the annual risk of stroke is 1 to 2%.

Strong evidence derived from meta-analyses supports the use of prophylactic aspirin to protect against strokes in patients with prior strokes or TIAs. Similarly prophylactic antiplatelet therapy with ticlopidine or clopidogrel has also been shown to protect against such secondary events. The combination of low-dose aspirin (50 mg/day) and dipyridamole (400/mg sustained release) is twice as effective for stroke risk reduction than either drug alone. A decision to use antiplatelet or anticoagulant therapy in patients with prior strokes must take into account both the individual patient's risk of further functional loss and the risks of treatment.

ASYMPTOMATIC CAROTID STENOSIS. Individuals with asymptomatic carotid stenosis or carotid bruits have approximately a 1.5- to 2-fold increase in the risk of stroke compared with the general population. Cerebral infarction in this population, however, occurs as frequently in a vascular territory different from the stenotic artery as in the involved one. Asymptomatic carotid stenosis or bruit is a marker of cerebrovascular disease and signals an increased risk of stroke, but not necessarily one in the territory of the involved vessel. No large, randomized placebo-controlled trials have shown any efficacy of prophylactic antiplatelet therapy in patients with asymptomatic carotid stenosis or bruits.

Although prophylactic aspirin therapy in a healthy population of US physicians reduced the incidence of myocardial infarction, no change occurred in the incidence of ischemic stroke, and a slight increase was detected in the incidence of hemorrhagic stroke. Antiplatelet agents cannot be recommended for stroke prophylaxis in healthy individuals.

OTHER DISEASES. Diabetes mellitus is a risk factor independent of hypertension and is associated with an approximate three-fold increase in the risk of stroke. No present data indicate that normalization of the blood sugar level reduces the incidence of stroke. Polycythemia, sickle cell disease, migraine, CNS vasculitis, and several infectious diseases all somewhat increase the risk of stroke.

SURGICAL TREATMENT FOR THE PREVENTION OF STROKE

The role of *prophylactic surgery* in the prevention of ischemic stroke is only partly resolved. A multi-institutional, randomized trial of an external carotid artery–MCA middle cerebral artery anastomosis showed no benefit, and the procedure has been largely abandoned. *Carotid endarterectomy,* designed to remove stenotic plaques from diseased carotid arteries, was developed in the mid-1960s, and from 1971 until about 1984 the number of such operations steadily increased, despite controversy concerning its efficacy. Several multicenter trials in North America and Europe have examined the indications and efficacy of carotid endarterectomy versus medical therapy in symptomatic and asymptomatic carotid stenosis. Endarterectomy significantly reduces ipsilateral stroke in patients with recent stroke or TIA and angiographically proven 70 to 99% ipsilateral carotid artery stenosis provided the rate of perioperative morbidity and mortality is less than 5 to 10%. Results from the North American Symptomatic Carotid Endarterectomy Trial indicate that selected patients with symptomatic stenosis of 50 to 69% may benefit marginally from endarterectomy if the perioperative morbidity and mortality rate is below 6%. Patients with less than 50% stenosis are best treated medically. Endarterectomy significantly reduces ipsilateral stroke in patients with asymptomatic carotid artery stenosis of 60% or higher if perioperative morbidity and morality rates are less than 3%. This remarkably low rate of surgical morbidity and mortality is achieved by few surgeons and must be considered before endarterectomy is recommended in patients with asymptomatic carotid artery stenosis. The safety and efficacy of carotid artery angioplasty and stenting are currently under investigation.

Surgery for *subclavian steal* is almost never indicated. This steal is a radiographic finding associated with occlusion or severe stenosis of a proximal subclavian artery, resulting in retrograde flow in the ipsilateral vertebral artery. The finding is only rarely associated with symptoms of vertebrobasilar ischemia when the ipsilateral arm is exercised. In most cases, it is merely a radiographic curiosity.

MANAGEMENT AND TREATMENT OF ACUTE TRANSIENT ISCHEMIC ATTACK AND STROKE

Patients clinically diagnosed as having *acute cerebral ischemia* should be admitted to the hospital unless the deficit has existed for several days and is stable. The initial history and physical examination emphasize the rapid diagnosis of ischemic cerebral ischemia (TIA or stroke) and the exclusion of seizures, hypoglycemia, tumor, and other alternative diagnoses (Table 470–4). As already noted, a normal CT scan within the first several hours is consistent with an ischemic stroke. Admission is also advised for patients with *new-onset TIAs* or those in whom TIAs are occurring with markedly increasing frequency or severity (*crescendo TIAs*).

GENERAL MANAGEMENT. Once admitted, stroke patients should be maintained on bed rest for at least 24 hours to avoid postural hypotension. Since autoregulation (see Chapter 469) is usually ineffective in areas of ischemic brain, CBF declines if systemic blood pressure falls because of postural changes or volume restriction. Hypertension, if present, should be treated, but with limited stepwise reductions in blood pressure, for the same reason (see Table 470–4). If patients have bulbar dysfunction affecting chewing or swallowing, mouth feedings should be avoided to reduce the chance of aspiration. Virtually all patients should have intravenous catheters placed to facilitate urgent treatments. If oral feedings are restricted for prolonged periods, supplementation with intravenous thiamine becomes important to prevent Wernicke's disease; eventually, hyperalimentation or feeding by nasogastric or gastrostomy tube may be needed.

In the early days of an ischemic stroke, passive range-of-motion exercises to the affected limbs can help retain mobility and prevent contractures. Later, more intensive rehabilitation individualized to

Table 470–4 ■ EVALUATION OF ACUTE FOCAL NEUROLOGIC DYSFUNCTION

STABILIZE VITAL SIGNS

Establish and maintain airway
Nasal O₂
Repeat vital signs every 15 min
Treat temperatures > 100° F
Record but do not treat BP
    < 220/120
Blood lab (CBC with differential
    and platelet count, electrolytes,
    glucose, BUN, PT, PTT, ESR)
ECG with rhythm strip

↓

RECORD HISTORY

Time of symptom onset and
    course?
Anatomic localization?
Headache or meningeal
    symptoms?
Vascular risk factors?
Medications or illicit drug use?

↓

MEDICAL EXAMINATION

Cardiovascular examination (BP
    in both arms, cardiac murmurs
    and rhythm, auscultate neck
    for bruits, palpate peripheral
    pulses)
Hematologic (examine integument
    for coagulopathies)
General examination

↓

NEUROLOGIC EXAMINATION

Anatomic localization
Examine for head trauma,
    meningeal signs
Ophthalmoscopy for retinal emboli,
    hypertension, papilledema

↓

HEAD CT SCAN WITHOUT CONTRAST

Consider alternative diagnosis
    (seizures, migraine, hypo-
    glycemia, tumor)

HEMORRHAGIC STROKE	ISCHEMIC STROKE	OTHER FOCAL DISEASE
(see Ch. 420)		Brain tumor, brain abscess, encephalitis

↓

IDENTIFY ETIOLOGY AND TREAT

(see Table 470–6)

BP = blood pressure; BUN = blood urea nitrogen; PT = prothrombin time; PTT = partial thromboplastin time; ESR = erythrocyte sedimentation rate; ECG = electrocardogram; CT = computed tomography.

infusion over 60 minutes. Anticoagulants and aspirin are contraindicated for the first 24 hours after TPA therapy. Blood pressure must be monitored frequently during the first 24 hours and maintained below 185 mm Hg systolic and 110 mm Hg diastolic. The patient should be observed frequently for any sign of intracerebral or systemic hemorrhage. Despite a significant increase in intracerebral hemorrhage, mortality is unchanged and neurologic outcome is significantly improved at 3 months in patients treated with TPA. Aspirin (325 mg) should be given within 24 hours of symptom onset in patients who do not receive TPA and after 24 hours in those who do.

Controversy continues to surround acute anticoagulation of patients with ischemic stroke. Increasing data indicate that acute anticoagulation with intravenous heparin, low-molecular-weight heparins, and heparinoids provides no long-term benefit while increasing hemorrhagic complications in patients with cardioembolic stroke, lacunar stroke, or stroke of unknown etiology. However, patients with atherothrombosis of large intracranial or extracranial arteries show a positive benefit/risk ratio from early anticoagulation. Our practice is to give intravenous heparin to patients who present within 24 hours of symptom onset and who have signs of unstable or progressing atherothrombotic stroke of large intra- or extracranial arteries. Heparin is administered intravenously on a weight-based dose schedule by constant infusion without a bolus injection. The activated partial thromboplastin time is monitored every 6 hours until it reaches 1.5 to 2 times control values. Intravenous heparin is maintained for 3 to 7 days while a decision is made about long-term prophylaxis therapy with either antiplatelet drugs or warfarin.

Despite underlying bleeding into the blood vessel wall, patients with vascular dissections are often treated with heparin in an effort to maintain patency of the vascular lumen and limit the likelihood of embolism; no proof of benefit exists. Patients with lacunar strokes were previously considered not to be helped by heparin, but some authorities have modified that view in recent years.

Patients whose strokes are attributed to emboli of cardiac origin

Table 470–5 ■ MANAGEMENT OF ACUTE FOCAL BRAIN ISCHEMIA

GENERAL

Initial BP > 220/120, systemic organ failure: Reduce BP by 20–25%; IV nitroprusside or parenteral β-blocker
Initial BP > 220/120, no systemic organ failure: Reduce BP by 10–15%; oral ACE inhibitor or calcium channel blocker
Initial BP < 220/120: No antihypertensive therapy for 72 hr; then do not reduce below 160–170/90–100 for 1 wk
Maintain blood glucose between 75–200 mg/dL
Vigorous treatment for temperature >100° F

TRANSIENT ISCHEMIC ATTACK	STROKE
Atherothrombotic	**Atherothrombotic**

ASA, 325–1300 mg/day
Ticlopidine, 250 mg bid
Clopidogrel, 75 mg/day
	Complete/nonprogressing
	    ASA, 325–1300 mg/day
	    Ticlopidine, 250 mg bid
	    Clopidogrel, 75 mg/day
	Incomplete/progressing
	    Heparin to APTT of 1.5–2.0
	    times control for 3–7 days, then
	    ASA

Cardioembolic	**Cardioembolic**

Heparin to APTT of 1.5–2.0 times control
Warfarin to INR of 2.0–3.0
	Nonhemorrhagic, small infarct
	    Heparin/warfarin at 48 hr
	Nonhemorrhagic, large infarct
	    Heparin/warfarin at 5–7 days
	Hemorrhagic infarct
	    Heparin/warfarin at 2–4 wk

Lacunar	**Lacunar**
ASA, 325–1300 mg/day Ticlopidine, 250 mg bid Clopidogrel, 75 mg/day	ASA, 325–1300 mg/day Ticlopidine, 250 mg bid Clopidogrel, 75 mg/day

BP = blood pressure; ACE = angiotensin-converting enzyme; ASA = aspirin; APTT = activated partial thromboplastin time; INR = international normalized ratio.

improve gait, speech, dexterity, and ability to manage activities of daily living become important. Patients often benefit from brief, intensive rehabilitation in specialized hospitals before being sent home. All patients on bed rest should be encouraged to flex and extend their ankles periodically to reduce the chances of deep venous thrombosis, and all should also take occasional deep breaths to combat atelectasis.

PHARMACOTHERAPY (Table 470–5). Patients who present within 3 hours of ischemic stroke onset and who meet specific inclusion and exclusion criteria (Table 470–6) should be considered for intravenous thrombolytic therapy. Tissue plasminogen activator (TPA) in a dose of 0.9 mg/kg (maximum dose 90 mg) is given intravenously, 10% as a bolus and the remaining 90% by

Table 470–6 ■ INCLUSION AND EXCLUSION CRITERIA FOR USE OF INTRAVENOUS TISSUE PLASMINOGEN ACTIVATOR IN STROKE

INCLUSION CRITERIA
≥18 years of age
Clinical diagnosis of ischemic stroke
Persistent neurologic deficit
Baseline CT scan showing no evidence of intracranial hemorrhage
Initiation of tPA therapy within 3 hr of symptom onset
EXCLUSION CRITERIA
Rapidly improving or minor symptoms such as isolated ataxia or sensory symptoms
CT scan showing possible intracranial hemorrhage or large infarct (sulcal effacement, mass effect, edema)
History of seizure at stroke onset
Stroke or serious head trauma within ≤3 mo
History of intracranial hemorrhage, arteriovenous malformation, or aneurysm
Symptoms consistent with subarachnoid hemorrhage
Major surgery or serious trauma within ≤2 wk
Gastrointestinal or urinary tract hemorrhage within ≤3 wk
Systolic BP > 185 mm Hg; diastolic BP > 110 mm Hg; aggressive treatment required to lower BP below specified limits prior to tPA therapy
Glucose <50 mg/dL or >400 mg/dL
Arterial puncture at noncompressible site or lumbar puncture within ≤1 wk
Platelet count <100,000/mm³
Heparin within ≤48 hr and associated with elevated APTT
Oral anticoagulants associated with elevated PT > 15 sec or INR > 1.5
Pregnancy

tPA = tissue plasminogen activator; CT = computed tomography; BP = blood pressure; APTT = activated partial thromboplastin time; PT = prothrombin time; INR = international normalized ratio.

are frequently treated acutely with heparin. Chronic oral anticoagulation is usually started concurrently, but debate surrounds the use of heparin until oral anticoagulation takes effect. Some advocate heparin because of concern about early re-embolization and the possibility that warfarin (Coumadin) sometimes enhances coagulability during the first 6 to 8 hours of therapy; others worry about the risks of hemorrhage into the initial stroke. It seems clear that the risk of bleeding is greater for larger infarcts. A reasonable course is to begin administering heparin and then begin administering warfarin after a CT scan at 48 hours reveals a small nonhemorrhagic infarct or at 5 to 7 days for a large nonhemorrhagic infarct (see Table 470–6). Evidence of a hemorrhagic infarct should delay anticoagulation by 4 to 6 weeks. Heparin is generally not given to patients with bacterial endocarditis in whom embolization to the brain has occurred, since evidence suggests an increased risk of bleeding in such cases. Although not intended to reduce cerebral ischemia, low-dose heparin or heparinoids should be used in contraindication-free immobile patients to reduce the chance of peripheral thrombophlebitis.

Patients with stable, complete strokes or those admitted with new-onset or crescendo TIAs are often placed on *aspirin* therapy prophylactically at admission. It is advisable to observe these patients in the hospital for several days until the situation has stabilized. Numerous drugs with neuroprotective properties in animal models of stroke, such as glutamate receptor antagonists, sodium, potassium, and calcium channel blockers, antioxidants, anti-inflammatory compounds, and growth factors are now in Phase I to III clinical trials. Of these, lubeluzole, started within 6 hours of symptom onset and continued for 5 days, was the first such drug to produce a small but significant neurologic improvement in a Phase III acute stroke trial. A follow-up Phase IV trial of lubeluzole is currently under way in patients treated with TPA. Ultimately, effective stroke treatment may use multiple drugs.

OUTCOME AND REHABILITATION

About 10 to 15% of patients with ischemic stroke die, some because of brain swelling or neurologic dysfunction directly related to the stroke (e.g., impaired respiration with medullary infarctions), but most because of systemic complications, such as myocardial infarction, pulmonary embolism, and pneumonia. Several studies show an association of stroke with subendocardial necrosis. Most large population studies report that about one fifth of patients who survive stroke require long-term institutionalization and one third to one half of the remaining are left with various disabilities. Most functional recovery takes place during the first 3 months, but some continued slow improvement is possible.

Probably because of overlapping risk factors, the leading cause of death in patients who survive the initial stroke is myocardial infarction, underscoring the importance of cardiac evaluation. Patients who have had one stroke are at increased risk of having additional ones, particularly when the first stroke is attributed to emboli of cardiac origin.

VENOUS STROKE

Although considerably less common than arterial cerebrovascular disease, venous occlusions can cause massive damage and death. As with ischemic strokes from arterial disease, the primary mechanism of brain damage is reduction in capillary blood flow, in this instance because of increased outflow resistance. Back-transmission of high pressure into the capillary bed usually results in early brain swelling from edema and superimposes a potentially severe degree of hemorrhagic infarction in subcortical white matter.

The most dangerous form of venous disease arises when the superior sagittal sinus is occluded, but obstruction of a transverse sinus or one of the major veins over the cerebral convexity (e.g., vein of Labbé) also can produce significant damage. Venous occlusions occur most commonly in association with coagulopathies, often in the puerperal period or in patients with disseminated cancer, and sometimes as a result of contiguous disease, such as infection or cancer. The transverse sinus can be occluded as a consequence of inner ear infections (see Chapter 473), producing a once common condition called otitic hydrocephalus.

With *superior sagittal sinus obstruction,* veins draining into the sinus from the superior and medial surfaces of both cerebral convexities are commonly obstructed; thus, in its early stages, the condition can result in bilateral weakness and sensory changes in the legs. This bilaterality should alert the clinician to the possibility of sinus thrombosis. Brain swelling and bilateral involvement can produce lethargy or stupor early in the course. Seizures occur more often with venous than with arterial occlusion, possibly because of the irritating effect of parenchymal blood on the cortex.

The differential diagnosis of venous obstruction can include traditional arterial strokes but more often extends to diffuse processes such as herpes simplex encephalitis and meningitis. Diagnosis depends on the recognition of impaired venous flow. Increasingly, this is detected by loss of flow artifact on MRI. On contrast CT scans, a nonenhanced triangular area surrounded by contrast in the posterior sinus (the empty delta sign) should suggest the diagnosis. Because MRI is not infallible, angiography is still the definitive diagnostic procedure, but attention must be directed to films showing the venous phase.

The management of venous sinus thrombosis increasingly relies on the use of heparin anticoagulation, even in the presence of superimposed parenchymal hemorrhage. Venous occlusions are serious and often fatal, but acute anticoagulation started as soon as the diagnosis is recognized appears to lessen substantially the morbidity and mortality of the condition. Anticonvulsants should be used as needed to control seizures and limit concomitant increases in CBF that might otherwise aggravate brain swelling and bleeding. Nonanticoagulated superior sagittal sinus occlusion that is not complicated by infection is associated with a mortality rate of 25 to 40%. Uncontrolled series suggest that early heparin therapy can reduce the mortality and morbidity rates by more than half.

470.2 Diffuse Ischemia

Brief diffuse cerebral ischemia causes syncope without any permanent sequelae (see Chapter 469). Prolonged diffuse ischemia by contrast, has devastating consequences. The most common cause is cardiac asystole or other forms of overwhelming cardiopulmonary failure. Aortic dissection and global hypoxia or carbon monoxide poisoning can cause a similar picture.

Diffuse hypoxia-ischemia typically kills neurons in the hippocampus, cerebellar Purkinje cells, striatum, and cortical layers 3, 4, and 6. Clinically, it results in unconsciousness: coma followed often by the eyes-open vegetative state. If patients do not regain consciousness within 2 or 3 days, the prognosis for return of independent function becomes poor. Early absence of pupillary light reflexes, corneal reflexes, and reflex eye movements predict a poor outcome. Patients lacking all of these responses even within the first day of hypoxic-ischemic coma have less than a 5% chance of resuming independent activities within 1 year (see Chapter 444). Even if consciousness is regained, such patients often suffer long-term impairment of memory and sometimes a variety of sensorimotor syndromes consistent with lesions located in a boundary zone distribution.

Other than prompt and aggressive efforts to restore cardiovascular circulation, no treatments have been found to help patients who are comatose after cardiac arrest. A randomized, multi-institutional trial of barbiturates was without benefit, and corticosteroids may even be harmful. In young patients hypoxic because of drowning, evidence suggests that hypothermia may prolong resistance to ischemic damage, but therapeutic hypothermia in adults can induce cardiac arrhythmias and has not yet been tested. Chronically unconscious patients have not been shown to benefit from either physical or electrical stimulation programs.

Barnett HJ, Mohr JP, Stein BM, et al (eds): Stroke: Pathophysiology, Diagnosis and Management, 3rd ed. New York, Churchill Livingstone, 1998. *A comprehensive text of the diagnosis and management of ischemic and hemorrhagic stroke.*
North American Symptomatic Carotid Endarterectomy Trial Collaborators: The benefit of carotid endarterectomy in symptomatic patients with moderate and severe stenosis. N Engl J Med. In press, 1999. *The final article in this series, which establishes the guidelines for endarterectomy in symptomatic carotid artery atherosclerosis.*
Guidelines for carotid endarterectomy. Stroke 29:554, 1998. *A statement for health care professionals from a special writing group of the Stroke Council of the American Heart Association.*
Guidelines for thrombolytic therapy. Circulation 94:1167, 1996. *Detailed guidelines for the use of tPA in acute ischemic stroke.*
The Publication Committee for the Trial of ORG 10172 in Acute Stroke Treatment Investigators: Low molecular weight heparinoid, and outcome after acute ischemic stroke. JAMA 279: 1265, 1998. *Multicenter Phase III trial of heparinoids in acute ischemic stroke.*
Practice parameter: Stroke prevention in patients with nonvalvular atrial fibrillation. Neurology 51:671, 1998. *Report of the Quality Standards Subcommittee of the American Academy of Neurology creating a practice standard.*
Stroke Prevention in Atrial Fibrillation Investigators: Stroke Prevention in Atrial Fibrillation III study: Patients with nonvalvular atrial fibrillation at low risk of stroke during treatment with aspirin. JAMA 279:1273, 1998. *Summary of multi-institutional study identifying the stroke risk factor profiles of atrial fibrillation and the benefits of aspirin versus warfarin therapy.*

471 HEMORRHAGIC CEREBROVASCULAR DISEASE

William A. Pulsinelli

Approximately 20% of all strokes consist of intracranial hemorrhages, half into the subarachnoid space and half within the brain itself. The acute rise in intracranial pressure from arterial rupture causes loss of consciousness in about half of patients, and many of these die of cerebral herniation (see Chapter 444). Because hemorrhage into the subarachnoid space or brain parenchyma causes less tissue injury than does ischemia, however, patients who survive often show a remarkable recovery.

Like ischemic stroke, hemorrhagic stroke can be thought of as diffuse (subarachnoid or intraventricular) or focal (intraparenchymal). Subarachnoid hemorrhage (SAH) is caused by rupture of surface arteries (aneurysms, vascular malformations, head trauma), with blood usually limited to the cerebrospinal fluid (CSF) space between the pial and arachnoid membranes (Table 471–1). Intracerebral hemorrhage is most frequently caused by the rupture of arteries lying deep within the brain substance (hypertensive hemorrhage, vascular malformations, head trauma), but in some instances the force of blood from ruptured surface arteries can penetrate the brain parenchyma. Blood within the cerebral ventricles results either from reflux of subarachnoid blood through the fourth ventricular foramina or by extension from a site of intraparenchymal hemorrhage.

Table 471–1 ■ CAUSES OF SPONTANEOUS INTRACRANIAL HEMORRHAGE

Arterial aneurysms
   "Berry" aneurysm
   Fusiform aneurysm
   Mycotic aneurysm
   Aneurysm with vasculitis
Cerebrovascular malformations
Hypertensive-atherosclerotic hemorrhage
Hemorrhage into brain tumor
Systemic bleeding diatheses
Hemorrhage with vasculopathies
Hemorrhage with intracranial venous infarction

471.1 Aneurysmal Subarachnoid Hemorrhage

EPIDEMIOLOGY

Rupture of a saccular or "berry" aneurysm causes approximately 80% of all SAHs, 5% are caused by mycotic aneurysm rupture, and an even smaller percentage reflects bleeding from atherosclerotic, neoplastic, or dissecting cerebral aneurysms. The incidence of aneurysmal SAH is approximately 10 per 100,000 population, with 80% occurring in persons 40 to 65 years old, 15% in those 20 to 40 years old, and 5% in those below 20 years of age. Women are slightly more likely than men (3:2) to suffer rupture of a cerebral aneurysm, especially during pregnancy.

ETIOLOGY AND PATHOGENESIS

SACCULAR ANEURYSMS. The pathogenesis of saccular aneurysms reflects a combination of congenital, acquired, and hereditary factors. Congenital defects in the muscle and elastic tissue of the arterial media, seen at autopsy in 80% of normal vessels of the circle of Willis, gradually deteriorate as they are exposed over time to the hemodynamic stresses of pulsatile blood flow. These defects lead to microaneurysmal dilatations (smaller than 2 mm) of the circle of Willis arteries in 15 to 20% of the population. Larger (>5 mm) aneurysms are found in 5% of the population, characteristically distributed at the arterial bifurcations. Eighty per cent are located in the anterior, carotid artery–derived, arterial circulation; the rest lie along the bifurcations of vertebrobasilar arteries (Fig. 471–1).

The remarkably high incidence of wall defects in the media of normal vessels, the high frequency of incidental microaneurysms, and the tendency for aneurysms to enlarge with time and rupture imply that both congenital and acquired factors influence the pathogenesis of rupture. On the other hand, the relative rarity of SAHs (10 per 100,000 population) suggests that other factors, possibly genetic, may predispose to aneurysm formation. A modest incidence of familial saccular aneurysms as well as their association with polycystic kidney disease, Ehlers-Danlos syndrome, and other connective tissue disorders, implicates hereditary factors. Although hypertension per se is not a significant risk factor for aneurysmal SAH, aneurysms have been known to rupture under conditions associated with a sudden rise in blood pressure, including extremes of emotional excitement and physical exertion such as coitus and athletic events.

FUSIFORM ANEURYSMS. Fusiform or ectatic aneurysms acquire their name from the spindle-shaped dilatation and elongation that occur in large arteries at the site of arteriosclerotic narrowing. These aneurysms develop most frequently in the basilar artery but also may affect the internal, middle, and anterior cerebral arteries of individuals with widespread arteriosclerosis and hypertension. They rarely rupture and are difficult to treat when they do because their shape and stiff walls preclude easy surgical clipping. Progressive dilatation and the tortuous elongation of the vessel cause neurologic dysfunction most frequently by compressing surrounding

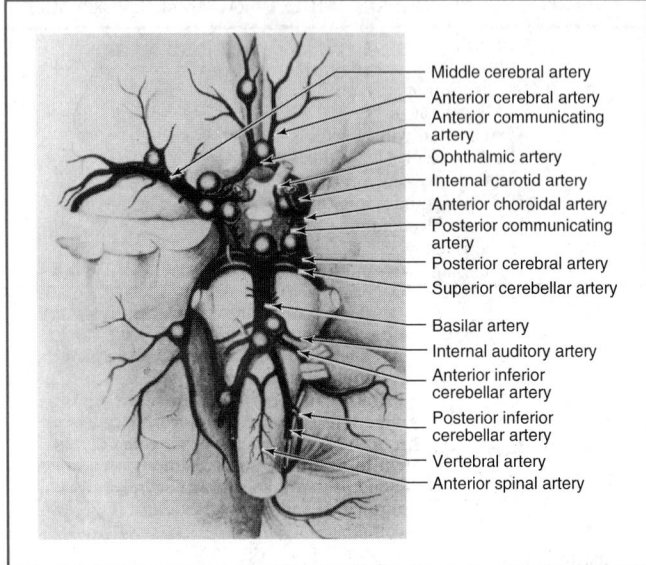

FIGURE 471–1 ■ The common sites for berry aneurysms to develop at the bifurcation of arteries on the undersurface of the brain.

structures. Typically, ectatic aneurysms of the basilar artery compress cranial nerves V, VII, and VIII, causing facial pain, hemifacial spasm, and hearing loss with vertigo, respectively. Fusiform aneurysms may initiate the features of cerebellopontine angle tumors, or they may mimic pituitary and suprasellar mass lesions.

MYCOTIC ANEURYSMS. Mycotic cerebral aneurysms are caused by septic degeneration of arterial wall muscle and elastic tissue. They form in distal cerebral arteries at the point where small septic cardiogenic emboli lodge. They are frequently multiple and can be found in either the anterior or the posterior cerebral circulation.

CLINICAL PRESENTATION

Prodromal signs and symptoms frequently precede the catastrophic rupture of saccular aneurysms. Focal headaches occasionally signal compression of pain-sensitive structures from an expanding aneurysm, in which case the headache is usually progressive. They also may generate "sentinel" leaks of sudden, focal head pain. Such sentinel headaches are frequently severe and may be accompanied by nausea or vomiting or may cause meningeal irritation. Despite the similarity of these headaches to common migraine, most patients can distinguish between the two. Patients with suspected sentinel headache should have computed tomographic (CT) scans and, if these are negative, lumbar punctures to exclude active bleeding.

Compression of the oculomotor nerve by an expanding aneurysm of the posterior communicating artery at its junction with either the internal carotid or the posterior cerebral artery and, less frequently, of the superior cerebellar artery can cause ipsilateral ophthalmoparesis, ptosis, and pupillary dilatation with loss of the pupillary light reflex. Orbital pain frequently accompanies these signs. The clinical picture may resemble diabetic involvement of cranial nerve III, but the latter usually spares the pupil. Other compression syndromes from cerebral aneurysms include amnesia combined with varying degrees of cranial nerve III paresis and quadriparesis from large, strategically placed, basilar-tip aneurysms. Giant (larger than 2.5 cm) aneurysms of the internal carotid artery lying within the cavernous sinus can cause unilateral ophthalmoplegia and orbital pain by compressing cranial nerves III, IV, VI, and the first division of V. Giant aneurysms of the supraclinoid portion of the internal carotid artery can produce unilateral vision loss or field defects through compression of the optic nerve or tracts.

Rupture of saccular aneurysms into the subarachnoid space seldom is associated with focal signs or symptoms. Nearly half of

patients so affected lose consciousness, at least transiently, as intracranial pressure exceeds cerebral perfusion pressure. Approximately 10% of patients remain in coma for several days, depending on the location of the aneurysm and the amount of bleeding. Patients who remain conscious and those who awaken from coma commonly recall the sudden onset as producing the "most excruciating headache" of their life. Rupture of an intracranial aneurysm in the absence of headache is rare, and some reported cases probably reflect amnesia for the event.

In addition to the frequent change in the level of consciousness, acute SAH causes meningeal irritation, nuchal rigidity, and photophobia, symptoms that can require several hours to develop. Subhyaloid retinal hemorrhages occur in 20 to 30% of patients as a result of increased intracranial pressure, raised retinal venous pressure, and dissection of blood along the optic nerve sheath. Blood pressure is frequently elevated, and body temperature usually rises, particularly during the early days after bleeding as subarachnoid blood products produce a chemical meningitis. Focal neurologic dysfunction is not a prominent feature of SAH unless there is associated compression by the aneurysm of surrounding brain structures, the jet of blood dissects directly into a clinically relevant brain region, or vasospasm occurs as a complication (see later).

LABORATORY EXAMINATION

Serum electrolytes should be measured at the time of hospital admission to serve as a baseline for detecting later complications. A complete blood count, including platelets and clotting times, should be obtained to evaluate possible infection or hematologic or clotting abnormalities. The electrocardiogram (ECG) may show various abnormalities, including heightened T waves, shortened PR intervals, peaked or inverted T waves, and increased U waves. These ECG abnormalities and subsequent arrhythmias have been attributed to multifocal myocardial necrosis caused by elevated levels of circulating catecholamines.

CT scans reveal subarachnoid blood within the basal cisterns in about three quarters of patients within 48 hours of bleeding. Magnetic resonance imaging (MRI) has a lower index of accuracy. Detection of intracranial blood on the CT scan, however, becomes more difficult with time as blood and its breakdown products become isodense. Blood localized to the basal cisterns, the sylvian fissure, or the intrahemispheric fissure more frequently indicates rupture of a saccular aneurysm, whereas blood lying over the convexities or within the superficial parenchyma of the brain is more consistent with either the rupture of an arteriovenous malformation (AVM) or a mycotic aneurysm. The amount and location of blood within the subarachnoid space relate directly to an aneurysm's location and the likelihood of subsequent vasospasm (see later). Importantly, an early CT scan also allows a baseline evaluation of ventricular size to compare against possible later hydrocephalus. A contrast-enhanced CT scan may aid in the identification of an AVM and some large (more than 1 cm) aneurysms but should be obtained only after a noncontrast study has been completed, since contrast agents may obscure detection of subarachnoid blood.

If the CT scan fails to show blood, a lumbar puncture is diagnostic. To avoid puncture of the venous plexus lying on the anterior wall of the spinal canal, the spinal needle should be advanced slowly, with frequent removal of the trocar to detect first entry of the subarachnoid space. A traumatic lumbar puncture usually can be distinguished from SAH by the failure of the latter to show a decrease in the red blood cell (RBC) count between the first and last tubes of CSF (Table 471–2). In addition, in the presence of

Table 471–2 ■ "TRAUMATIC TAP" OR SUBARACHNOID HEMORRHAGE?

PARAMETER	"TRAUMATIC TAP"	SPONTANEOUS SUBARACHNOID BLEED
Xanthochromia	Absent	Onset: 4–6 hr Duration: approximately 6 wk
Red blood cell count (serial tubes)	Decreasing	Constant
Blood clot formation	Rapid	Slower

bloody fluid, one of the CSF samples should be centrifuged immediately and the supernate examined for the presence of hematin or xanthochromia by visual inspection and testing the fluid with a benzidene (Hemoccult) stick. RBCs in the spinal canal begin to lyse within 2 to 3 hours, and the centrifuged supernate then appears pink. Later (10 hours) as the hemoglobin is converted to bilirubin, the fluid takes on a yellow tinge. The CSF pressure is usually elevated and may remain so for many days. Spinal fluid samples taken within the first 24 hours often show a white blood cell (WBC) count consistent with the normal circulating WBC/RBC ratio (around 1:1000); later samples contain increased polymorphonuclear and mononuclear cells secondary to chemical meningitis caused by breakdown products of subarachnoid blood. The CSF blood glucose level is usually normal early, but as chemical meningitis develops, the level may decline, but rarely to less than 40 mg/dL. The protein content of the CSF is usually elevated, consistent with contamination by blood (1 mg/dL fluid for every 1000 RBCs).

Cerebral angiography remains the definitive study to detect the source of SAH. In instances in which the diagnosis of aneurysmal SAH is certain, the timing and need for a cerebral angiogram should be determined by surgical considerations (see later). When diagnostic doubt exists, angiography should be performed immediately. Because as many as 33% of patients with aneurysmal SAHs harbor multiple cerebral aneurysms, both carotid and vertebral arteries should be examined. (Among patients with multiple cerebral aneurysms, almost 50% have identically placed aneurysms in the left and right circulation, so-called mirror aneurysms.) Cerebral angiography fails to detect the source of bleeding in 10 to 20% of cases. Such patients are thought to have a better prognosis, with only a 1 to 2% annual chance of recurrent SAH. Failure to detect the source of bleeding can result from obliteration of an aneurysm through clotting; because bleeding was caused by rupture of a small, superficial venous angioma; or when hemorrhage has occurred from a spinal cord aneurysm or AVM. The presence of back pain or spinal cord symptoms at onset should prompt a search for a spinal source of hemorrhage. Repeat cerebral angiography is indicated 3 to 4 weeks later when the initial angiogram is negative and no other clues to the bleeding site can be found.

Cerebral angiography is recommended immediately in patients who have septic endocarditis and SAHs to search for possible mycotic aneurysms. Since 25% of patients with subacute bacterial endocarditis and evidence of systemic embolism harbor one or more cerebral mycotic aneurysms, they should also undergo cerebral angiography.

LATE MEDICAL AND NEUROLOGIC COMPLICATIONS

The medical complications of SAH include cardiac myonecrosis and arrhythmias attributed to abnormal levels of circulating epinephrine. Symptomatic hyponatremia may also develop from secretion of atrial natriuretic factor by the heart leading to salt and water wasting.

Late neurologic complications include *rebleeding* from the same aneurysm, cerebral *vasospasm* and its ischemic consequences, *hydrocephalus* caused by blockage of CSF outflow pathways, and occasionally *seizures*. Aneurysmal rerupture is suggested by new headache or neurologic worsening but can be diagnosed firmly only if a second CT scan or lumbar puncture shows the presence of new blood in the subarachnoid space. Approximately 30% of patients with aneurysmal SAH rebleed during the first month, the incidence being highest during the first 2 weeks after the initial bleed. Patients with unclipped aneurysms who survive their initial bleed for more than 1 month have a 2 to 3% yearly risk of rebleeding.

Cerebral vasospasm as diagnosed by cerebral angiography is defined as an abnormal narrowing of cerebral arteries. Vasospasm has been reported in up to 75% of patients with SAH, 50% of whom have strokelike neurologic signs and symptoms. The peak onset for vasospasm is between days 3 and 14, but the complication can develop as late as 3 weeks after SAH. Arteries forming the circle of Willis and their major branches are the initial site of involvement, with more distal arteries becoming involved later. The amount and location of blood detected within the basal cisterns on CT scans correlate with the incidence and location of vasospasm.

The molecular mechanisms causing cerebral vasospasm are un-

known but probably involve release of vasoactive amines and polypeptides, which pathologically influence vascular smooth muscle contraction. Vasospastic vessels show medial necrosis within the first few weeks, and later medial atrophy, subendothelial fibrosis, and intimal thickening.

Communicating hydrocephalus may develop as early as the first or second week after SAH. Patients with more extensive bleeding are more likely to experience the complication, but its incidence correlates with the amount of blood on CT images less clearly than does the development of vasospasm. RBCs and their breakdown products cause hydrocephalus by obstructing CSF outflow pathways at the level of the fourth ventricle and through the pacchionian granulations lining the venous sinuses. Seldom does communicating hydrocephalus require surgical treatment early after SAH.

Seizures are infrequent but occasionally complicate SAH. Seizures usually signal cortical damage either from bleeding into the neocortex or from ischemic necrosis.

TREATMENT

SACCULAR ANEURYSMS. The definitive therapy for a ruptured saccular aneurysm consists of surgical clipping of the aneurysm to prevent rebleeding. Medical therapy aims to reduce the risk of rebleeding and cerebral vasospasm and to prevent other medical complications before and after surgical intervention. Patients should be kept quiet on bed rest, with the administration of appropriate analgesics for the treatment of headache and gentle sedation. Stool softeners minimize straining with subsequently increased intracranial pressure. Hypertension should be treated, but not aggressively, since some of the elevated pressure may represent a normal compensatory mechanism to maintain cerebral perfusion pressure in the face of increased intracranial pressure or cerebral arterial narrowing. Systolic pressures 160 to 170 mm Hg and diastolic pressures of 90 to 100 mm Hg are acceptable. The voltage-regulated calcium channel antagonist nimodipine should be given orally in a dosage of 60 mg every 4 hours for 21 days. Although it does not reduce the frequency of vasospasm, nimodipine lowers by one third the incidence of cerebral infarction in patients suffering SAH and cerebral vasospasm.

The effects of cerebral vasospasm can also be partly overcome by raising cerebral perfusion pressure through plasma volume expansion and pressor agents, usually phenylephrine or dopamine. Such measures, however, can raise the risk of rebleeding and should be undertaken only in patients with surgically clipped saccular aneurysms.

The optimal time to clip a ruptured saccular aneurysm remains controversial. Several studies show that patients with a Hunt grade (Table 471–3) of 1 to 3 do best if the aneurysm is clipped within 24 to 36 hours of the onset of bleeding. Otherwise, an increasingly accepted approach is to operate either within the first 3 days or after days 10 to 14. The logic relates to the timing of intrinsic rebleeding and the onset of cerebral vasospasm. Because the incidence of aneurysmal rebleeding is highest during the first 2 weeks after SAH and the mortality rate associated with each bleed approaches 40 to 50%, the aneurysm should be clipped as soon as possible. Nevertheless, undertaking aneurysmal surgery in the presence of active vasospasm has consistently been associated with poor neurologic outcomes. As a result, most surgeons avoid operat-

Table 471–3 ■ HUNT CLASSIFICATION OF PATIENT'S CONDITION

GRADE	CONDITION
0	Unruptured aneurysm
1	Asymptomatic or minimal headache and slight nuchal rigidity
1A	No acute meningeal or brain reaction but with fixed neurologic deficit
2	Moderate to severe headache, nuchal rigidity; no neurologic deficit other than cranial nerve palsy
3	Drowsiness, confusion, or mild focal deficit
4	Stupor, moderate to severe hemiparesis, possible early decerebrate rigidity and vegetative disturbances
5	Deep coma, decerebrate rigidity, and moribund appearance

ing during days 3 to 10, when maximal cerebral vasospasm is likely. In a patient whose aneurysm is clipped early, preliminary studies suggest that lysing blood clots in the basal cisterns with fibrinolytic drugs, followed by washing the blood out, may reduce subsequent vasospasm. Aneurysmal clipping should be delayed until 10 to 14 days after the last documented SAH in patients who present to the hospital after 3 days, who have active vasospasm on early cerebral angiograms, or who fall initially into a poor clinical grade (Hunt 4 and 5). In instances of delayed surgical intervention, most authorities recommend repeating cerebral angiography before surgery to rule out the continued presence of vasospasm. Some neurosurgeons also recommend postoperative angiography to verify proper clip placement and obliteration of the aneurysm.

MYCOTIC ANEURYSMS. Unruptured mycotic aneurysms should be treated with antibiotics appropriate for the infecting organism and followed angiographically. Single aneurysms and those in surgically accessible areas should be considered for prompt surgical clipping.

PROGNOSIS

The mortality rate from aneurysmal SAH amounts to a daunting 50 to 60% after 1 year. Almost 50% of such patients die before reaching the hospital, and most of the remaining die during the first month. An equally high mortality rate accompanies each episode of rebleeding. Approximately 25% of survivors have persistent neurologic deficits.

Unruptured cerebral aneurysms detected incidentally during cerebral angiography bleed at a yearly rate of 1 to 3%. Aneurysm size is strongly associated with the likelihood of rupture, so that saccular aneurysms less than 5 mm should be followed carefully, aneurysms between 5 and 10 mm can be considered for surgical clipping, and those larger than 10 mm should be clipped at the earliest convenience. The experience of the surgical team critically affects decisions and outcome concerning such treatment.

471.2 Hemorrhage from Vascular Malformations

CLASSIFICATION AND EPIDEMIOLOGY

Congenital vascular malformations of the brain and spinal cord fall into five categories according to vessel size and type. *Venous angiomas,* the most common cerebrovascular malformations, are composed entirely of veins and usually lie close to the brain's surface. Hemorrhage from a venous angioma is uncommon and rarely fatal. Nevertheless, these lesions have gained considerable attention, since they are readily detected by CT scans. They seldom produce seizures or headaches. A cerebral *varix* is a single dilated vein and rarely causes clinical symptoms.

Telangiectasias are uncommon vascular anomalies composed of tangles of small, capillary-like vessels. They are usually located deep in the brain (diencephalon, brain stem, cerebellum) and rarely produce symptoms. Because of their strategic location, hemorrhage from these small vessels can occasionally be fatal.

Cavernous angiomas are large sinusoidal channels served by large feeding arteries and veins. Many of the channels thrombose, and the remainder have low blood flow, which makes their visualization on angiograms difficult. They are readily detected by CT scan and rarely bleed, but they can cause headaches and seizures.

The most common symptomatic vascular anomaly is the *arteriovenous malformation.* AVMs are composed of tangles of arteries connected directly to veins without intervening capillaries. The resulting vessels are thin walled because of poorly developed elastic and muscle tissue within the media. The large arteries, which feed the AVM, usually show hypertrophy of the media and thickening of the endothelium. Brain tissue is usually absent from the AVM but, when present, is nonfunctional. AVMs can be located anywhere in the brain and can produce headaches, seizures, focal neurologic deficits, and intracranial hemorrhage. Intracranial hemor-

rhage from vascular malformations accounts for 1% of all strokes and 10% of all SAHs. The prevalence of AVMs among the general population is uncertain, but autopsy studies of unselected patients indicate that 4 to 5% harbor some form of vascular malformation, of which only 10 to 15% produce symptoms. Familial cases of AVMs are rare, indicating that the problem reflects sporadic abnormalities in embryologic development.

CLINICAL PRESENTATION

Most AVMs manifest with intracranial hemorrhage, a lower proportion causing seizures or progressive neurologic disability as first symptoms. The initial hemorrhage tends to occur during the second through fourth decades, with the risk of rebleeding averaging approximately 6 to 7% the first year, 2% after 5 years, and 1 to 2% thereafter. The decline in the incidence of rebleeding with time may reflect the spontaneous thrombosis of arterial feeders. The initial and subsequent hemorrhages are associated with a 10% chance of death. If the rebleeding rate of 1 to 2% is maintained for life, a young individual who has a hemorrhagic AVM faces a 50 to 60% chance of an incapacitating or fatal subsequent hemorrhage during a normal lifespan.

AVMs can bleed into the subarachnoid space, into the brain parenchyma, or into the ventricular system. Focal neurologic signs and symptoms depend on the severity of the bleeding and the extent to which brain parenchyma has been destroyed. Bleeding into the subarachnoid space is usually less severe than with saccular aneurysms, and blood tends to localize over the cerebral convexities rather than in the basal cisterns. The incidence of cerebral vasospasm with AVM hemorrhage appears less than for aneurysm SAH, perhaps because less blood accumulates around the large arteries at the base of the brain. No explanation has been provided for the observation that small AVMs (<2.5 cm) tend to bleed more frequently than do large AVMs (>5 cm).

Approximately 30% of patients who harbor an AVM have seizures, of which about 50% have a focal onset. Focal neurologic deficits independent of seizures also develop, resulting from vascular thrombosis and brain tissue hypoperfusion caused by either vascular compression or a "steal" syndrome. Shunting of blood through arteriovenous fistulas may draw blood away from normal brain tissue, causing hypoperfusion and dysfunction of the brain proximal to the AVM. With treatment of the AVM, either through surgical resection or by embolization of the feeding arteries, some of these focal neurologic signs may improve or disappear. Approximately 10% of patients with AVMs have a history of headache, the location of which seldom coincides with the site of the AVM. Some AVM-associated headaches closely resemble migraine, but unlike migraine, most AVM-associated headaches rarely alternate between the two sides of the head.

LABORATORY EXAMINATION

The laboratory evaluation for intracranial hemorrhage from an AVM is similar to that described for aneurysmal SAH. CT scanning with contrast is diagnostic in approximately 85% of patients. MRI is equally, if not more, effective in diagnosis. Angiography remains the definitive test to identify the AVM and delineate its feeding arteries and draining veins. Because approximately 10% of AVMs are associated with saccular aneurysms, four-vessel angiography is indicated even if the AVM is defined by unilateral carotid injection. In addition, extracranial or contralateral arteries occasionally supply intracranial AVMs and should be considered in the angiographic evaluation.

TREATMENT

Uncertainties concerning the natural history of unruptured AVMs, as well as the efficacy and complications associated with newer forms of interventional therapy, make it difficult to define a simple set of guiding therapeutic principles. Generally speaking, unruptured AVMs that manifest with either seizures or headache may be treated conservatively, especially in patients older than 55 to 60 years. In such patients, hypertension should be controlled, platelet antiaggregating agents and anticoagulants avoided, and anticonvulsants given to control the seizures.

Interventional therapeutic options include surgical resection of the AVM, embolization of the feeding arteries, and radiation-induced thrombosis. Various considerations, including age, degree of neurologic dysfunction, and location of the AVM, must be considered when choosing treatment. The present custom is to treat younger patients (<55 years) more aggressively, resecting surgically accessible AVMs, since removal of the AVM and *all* its arterial feeders is curative. In older patients or in these in whom the AVM lies in language-vulnerable areas or deep in the brain, use of focused gamma x-rays or proton beam radiation is safer but only effective in lesions less than 3 cm in diameter. Embolization of the feeding arteries is rarely recommended as the sole interventional therapy, since such an approach totally obliterates the arterial feeders in only about 40% of cases. Arterial embolization is frequently used in conjunction with either surgery or focused radiation therapy.

471.3 Focal Cerebral Hemorrhage

Focal hemorrhage occurs spontaneously in three common settings: hypertension, ruptured AVMs, and amyloid (or congophilic) angiopathy. Additional contributing causes are excessive anticoagulation, systemic bleeding diatheses, and trauma.

EPIDEMIOLOGY

In the United States, primary intracerebral hemorrhage occurs with an incidence of about 12 per 100,000 population, a rate similar to that for SAH but only 10% that for ischemic stroke. Age-adjusted rates for men are about 50% higher than for women, and rates for blacks are over twice those for whites. As with ischemic stroke, the incidence appears to be declining; excluding hemorrhage associated with anticoagulation, the rate in Rochester, Minnesota, fell from about 15 per 100,000 in 1945 to 5 per 100,000 in the early 1970s. The incidence of hypertension also declined in frequency during the same period, but no conclusive data link the two trends.

PATHOLOGY

The pathologic picture of primary intracerebral hemorrhage typically consists of a large confluent area of blood that clots and then weeks later begins slowly to be phagocytosed; after several months, the only residuum may be a small, collapsed cavity lined by hemosiderin-containing macrophages. Although hemorrhages may destroy brain tissue locally, histologic examination suggests that displacement of normal brain tissue and dissection along fiber tracts account for much of the pathology.

PATHOGENESIS

Hypertension can produce hemorrhages throughout the brain, but they usually occur in four central locations: external capsule–putamen, internal capsule–thalamus, central pons, and cerebellum (Fig. 471–2). A smaller number arise in the subcortical white matter, especially in the polar regions of the frontal, temporal, and occipital lobes. Bleeding producing central hemorrhages is believed to result from rupture of microaneurysms in small, intracerebral arteries (50 to 150 μm in diameter). The pathology of the microaneurysms includes replacement of normal lining endothelium, media, and elastic tissue with fibrous tissue and fat. Similar changes can lead to necrotic vascular degeneration, which, along with microaneurysms, predisposes to hemorrhage. A strong relationship links microaneurysms to hypertension; in one autopsy series, microaneurysms were found in 46 of 100 hypertensive brains and in 85% of hypertensive persons with hemorrhages, but in only 7 of 100 normotensive brains.

Amyloid (or congophilic) angiopathy is a pathologic diagnosis, increasingly encountered in the elderly. Unrelated to generalized amyloidosis and occasionally hereditary, the condition often appears in the brains of patients with Alzheimer's disease and has

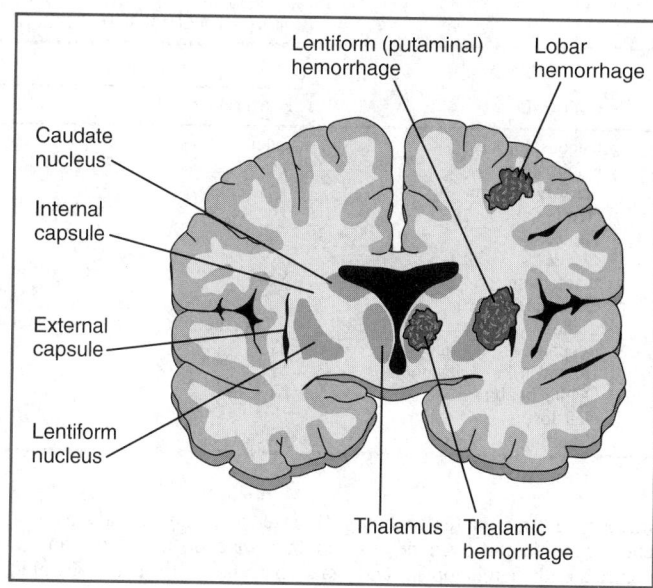

FIGURE 471–2 ■ A coronal section through the cerebral hemispheres illustrating thalamic, putaminal, and lobar subcortical hemorrhages.

been associated with nonhypertensive hemorrhages in the cerebral polar and white matter areas (see Fig. 471–2). It is rare in patients under age 55. Amyloid deposits, chemically related to those in Alzheimer plaques, are seen in the media and adventitia of medium- and small-sized arteries. Multiple small hemorrhages may be associated with the condition.

Anticoagulation, fibrinolysis, and other hematologic abnormalities can be associated with intracerebral hemorrhages. Warfarin anticoagulation has been implicated in about 10% of primary intracerebral hemorrhages. With the less aggressive programs of low-dose warfarin anticoagulation (target prothrombin time ratio of 1.2 to 1.5) now used for peripheral venous disease and to prevent arterial embolism, the rate of intracranial bleeding in one recent study had fallen to under 1% with 2 years of treatment. Data from large-scale studies of fibrinolysis (e.g., tissue plasminogen activator [tPA]) in acute myocardial infarction indicate that at a total tPA dose no greater than 100 mg, the rate of symptomatic intracerebral hemorrhage is only about 0.5% (although in one small series, it was 5%); at higher doses of 150 mg, the rate rises to about 1.5%. Cerebral hemorrhages occur in *leukemia, polycythemia, hemophilia,* and other clotting abnormalities, and they also occur in patients using *amphetamines* and *cocaine.*

Although *trauma* causes intracerebral (as well as subarachnoid) hemorrhage, the diagnosis is usually aided by the history and by coexistent external signs of trauma, SAH, and, on CT scan, multifocal inhomogeneous hemorrhages and areas of decreased density (see Chapter 490).

CLINICAL PRESENTATION

Large cerebral hemorrhages usually produce catastrophic, acute syndromes. The onset is often associated with physical (or emotional) activity; onset during sleep is rare. Common early features include alterations in consciousness, headache, nausea, and vomiting. Although uncommon, seizures occur, possibly reflecting cortical irritation by blood. With the increasing ability to recognize less dramatic hemorrhages by using CT and MRI, neurologists now realize that hemorrhages also can produce less severe dysfunction that may be indistinguishable clinically from ischemic stroke. Clinical evolution over hours is common and usually attributed to secondary brain swelling.

The clinician should be able to recognize common hemorrhagic syndromes (Table 471–4) to anticipate dangerous brain swelling and provide appropriate medical and supportive management.

PUTAMINAL HEMORRHAGE (35 TO 50%). Patients with massive putaminal hemorrhages (Fig. 471–3) become lethargic or co-

Table 471–4 ■ CLINICAL FEATURES OF COMMON HYPERTENSIVE HEMORRHAGES

| CLINICAL | SITE OF HEMORRHAGE | | | |
	Putaminal	Thalamic	Pontine	Cerebellar
Unconsciousness	Later	Later	Early	Late
Hemiparesis	Yes	Yes	Quadriparesis	Late
Sensory change	Yes	Yes	Yes	Late
Hemianopic	Yes	Yes	No	No
Pupils				
Size	Normal	Small	Small	Normal
Reaction	Yes	Yes or no	Yes or no	Yes
Gaze paresis				
Side	Contralateral, sometimes ipsilateral	Contralateral	Ipsilateral	Ipsilateral
Response to calorics	Yes	Yes	No	Yes or no
Downward eye deviation	Yes	No	No	
Ocular bobbing	No	No	Sometimes	Sometimes
Gait lost	No	No	Yes	Yes
Vomiting	Occasional	Occasional	Often	Severe

matose within minutes to hours of onset and concurrently experience contralateral weakness (including that of the face) and a contralateral hemianopsia and gaze paresis (with eyes deviated toward the side of the hemorrhage).

THALAMIC HEMORRHAGE (10 TO 15%). Some patients with thalamic hemorrhages lose consciousness early in the clinical course, but those who are awake often experience contralateral hemiparesis, sensory changes, and homonymous hemianopsia (the last often clearing quickly).

PONTINE HEMORRHAGE (10 TO 15%). Traditional teaching held that coma always accompanied the onset of pontine hemorrhage, but refined imaging shows that this is not always the case with smaller hemorrhages. In a comatose patient, small, reactive pupils are common, oculovestibular responses are lost early, and vomiting often occurs at onset. Patients usually have quadriplegia and bilateral extensor posturing.

CEREBELLAR HEMORRHAGE (10 TO 30%). Because cerebellar hemorrhage initially spares the brain stem, consciousness is usually preserved in the early stages. Occipital headache is usually the first symptom, followed by unsteady gait, clumsiness, nausea, and vomiting, which may be severe and repetitive. Motor weakness is seldom prominent at onset, but with progression and brain stem com-

pression, contralateral hemiparesis and caloric-resistant ipsilateral gaze paresis help to localize the lesion to the posterior fossa. Pupillary reactions are usually preserved. Further deterioration in arousal can result from several sources: extension into or compression of the brain stem, herniation of cerebellar tissue downward through the foramen magnum or upward across the tentorium, or hydrocephalus caused by obstruction of CSF flow into or out of the fourth ventricle. Prompt recognition and treatment of cerebellar hemorrhage by this stage can be life saving.

LOBAR CEREBRAL HEMORRHAGE. Lobar hemorrhages typically occur with amyloid angiopathy. The clinical presentation depends on the actual location of the hemorrhage, but there are some common features. Most patients are elderly; headache, nausea, and vomiting probably occur with about the same frequency but less intensity as in deep, hypertensive hemorrhages. Coma and seizures are less common, possibly because the bulk of the hemorrhage is comparatively small and located in subcortical white matter.

LABORATORY EXAMINATION

Noncontrast CT scans demonstrate areas of hemorrhage as zones of increased density and rule out infarction (Fig. 471–3). Spontane-

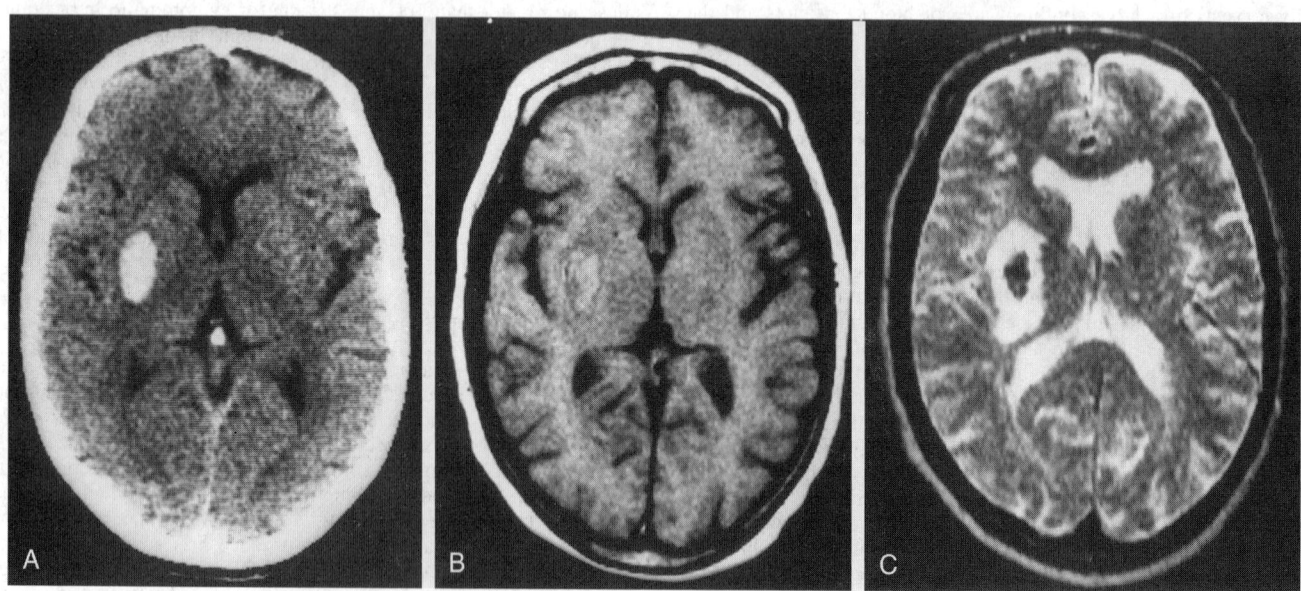

FIGURE 471–3 ■ Hypertensive putaminal hemorrhage shown on CT at 24 hours (A), T_1-weighted magnetic resonance image (MRI) at 72 hours (B), and T_2-weighted MRI at 72 hours (C). Uniform hyperdensity on CT distinguishes primary hemorrhage from hemorrhagic and nonhemorrhagic infarction (compare with Fig. 419–1). The relative, though mild, hyperintensity on the T_1-weighted MRI image distinguishes hemorrhage from the hypointensity of nonhemorrhagic infarction; T_1-weighted MRI scans within 24 hours (not available for this patient) typically display more marked hyperintensity than at 72 hours. The core of the hematoma appears hypointense on the T_2-weighted MRI scan at 72 hours; T_2-weighted MRI scans within 12 hours (not available) typically show hyperintensity of greater degree than do concurrent T_1-weighted images. The rim of hyperintensity in C probably represents edema fluid. (Reproduced with permission from Zimmerman RD, et al.: AJNR 9:47-57, 1988.)

ous hemorrhages typically display homogeneous areas of increased density and a mass effect, whereas hemorrhagic infarctions are characterized by areas of increased density (blood) interspersed with areas of decreased density (infarction). CT does not always distinguish reliably between a primary intraparenchymal hemorrhage and a hematoma resulting from a ruptured aneurysm. Similarly, some primary intracerebral hemorrhages dissect into the ventricular or subarachnoid system, inducing secondary intraventricular hemorrhage or SAH.

The MRI picture of hemorrhage depends on the precise sequence used and the age of the hemorrhage. The advantages and disadvantages of MRI in this condition remain incompletely described, particularly in the early hours after onset. One advantage of MRI is its ability to detect small hemorrhages, especially in the brain stem. Cerebral angiography is seldom used to evaluate acute hemorrhages, except those attributed to mycotic aneurysms being evaluated for surgical intervention.

TREATMENT

The management of acute parenchymal hemorrhage is supportive, but vigilance for transtentorial or foramen magnum herniation must be exercised, particularly with cerebellar hemorrhages. Incipient herniation is initially treated with hyperventilation (which takes advantage of the vasoconstricting effect of hypocapnia; see Chapter 469) and osmotic agents (e.g., mannitol), but both of these interventions lose effectiveness with time. Corticosteroids have not been effective in treating brain edema from cerebral hemorrhage, and since they carry added risks (e.g., immunologic compromise, gastrointestinal hemorrhage), they are not advocated.

Direct surgical evacuation of acute spontaneous cerebral hemorrhage seldom is justified, occasional cerebellar hemorrhages providing a possible exception. What few comparative studies are available suggest that acute surgical evacuation of hematomas from the cerebral hemispheres does not substantially improve mortality and considerably increase the risk of severe residual neurologic disability if the patient survives. With the cerebellum, lateral ventricular shunting appears to produce results as good as or better (fewer neurologic residua) than surgical removal of hematomas, although lesions more than 3 cm in diameter that continue to compress the brain stem after the shunt is placed occasionally benefit from evacuation.

As with ischemic strokes, blood pressure should not be lowered precipitously in patients with acute cerebral hemorrhage, since parenchymal blood and edema formation are likely to compress the tissue vascular bed and increase vascular resistance; an abrupt and steep reduction in systemic blood pressure could lower perfusion pressure below the critical threshold, thereby superimposing ischemic on hemorrhagic damage.

PROGNOSIS

The prognosis with intraparenchymal hemorrhage is surprisingly good in patients who survive the acute illness, but the mortality rate is higher (30 to 40%) than for ischemic stroke (10 to 20%). As with ischemic stroke, recent studies show that about 20% of patients who survive hemorrhage require institutionalization; in contrast to ischemic stroke, however, most of the remaining survivors of hemorrhage achieve a good status or complete recovery. Age and large hemorrhage size are associated with a worse prognosis, and prognosis after extensive brain stem hemorrhage is guarded. In contrast to SAH, the risk of recurrent hemorrhage is relatively low, the exception being that AVMs can rebleed at rates approaching 2% annually within the first several years of the initial bleed.

PROPHYLAXIS

Epidemiologic data strongly suggest that control of hypertension reduces the risk of hypertensive intraparenchymal hemorrhage. Careful control of anticoagulation and avoidance of other agents known to be associated with hemorrhage (e.g., amphetamines)

should reduce the risk of hemorrhage. At present, there is no way to control the risk of bleeding from amyloid angiopathy.

471.4 Hypertensive Encephalopathy

Hypertensive encephalopathy is a syndrome that accompanies markedly elevated blood pressures. Clinically, the disorder is characterized by symptoms of increased intracranial pressure (headache, nausea, vomiting, visual blurring) and of focal neurologic dysfunction, along with seizures and progressive stupor and coma. Retinal changes characteristic of severe hypertension are common and often include hemorrhages or papilledema, but arteriolar narrowing may be the only abnormality.

The cause of neurologic dysfunction is not clearly established. One theory, largely discounted, was based on observed retinal vasospasm and suggested that similar intracerebral vasospasm caused focal ischemia and resultant neurologic dysfunction. More recent evidence rests on the observation that with severe hypertension the upper limit of cerebral arterial autoregulation is exceeded, and blood flow rises passively with further increases in systemic blood pressure. Coincidentally, progressively higher pressures are transmitted into the capillary system, causing movement of plasma and even some cellular elements from blood into surrounding brain tissue. Resulting local and diffuse edema is postulated to cause the focal and diffuse neurologic changes.

Uremia uncomplicated by hypertension can produce a similar clinical picture, but this is easily excluded by determining the blood urea nitrogen and creatinine values. Other complications of hypertension to be considered in the differential diagnosis include hemorrhagic and ischemic stroke. Focal signs predominate in these conditions, whereas they are accompanied by prominent signs of diffuse dysfunction in hypertensive encephalopathy. Increased intracranial pressure from obstructive hydrocephalus, brain tumor, or subdural hematoma, particularly if pressure is transmitted into the fourth ventricle, can elevate blood pressure and slow the pulse. Usually, the absence of retinal changes suggesting chronic hypertension and the presence of signs reflecting the underlying neurologic diagnosis differentiate such neurogenic hypertension from hypertensive encephalopathy.

Hypertensive encephalopathy is a medical emergency. Treatment should be directed to acute, deliberate lowering of blood pressure (e.g., with intravenous nitroprusside), while avoiding hypotensive or even normal levels. In most patients with chronic hypertension, the upper and lower limits of autoregulation are shifted upward, and if systemic pressure is lowered below the lower limit of the patient's intrinsic autoregulation (which can rise as high as 120 mm Hg), cerebral ischemia can result. When associated with pregnancy (eclampsia), hypertensive encephalopathy usually responds well to prompt delivery of the fetus. Hypercapnia, by dilating cerebral blood vessels, can exacerbate the effects of hypertensive encephalopathy, and seizures also are associated with further increases in cerebral blood flow and capillary pressure. Both should be avoided by controlled ventilation, when required, with anticonvulsants such as intravenous diazepam, 10 to 20 mg given slowly in repeated doses as needed to control seizures, and followed by phenytoin or carbamazepine.

Brown RD Jr, Wiebers DO, Forbes G, et al: The natural history of unruptured intracranial arteriovenous malformations. J Neurosurg 68:352, 1988. *A follow-up study of 168 patients to define the natural history of clinically unruptured intracranial AVMs.*

Dias MS, Sekhar LN: Intracranial hemorrhage from aneurysms and arteriovenous malformations during pregnancy and the puerperium. Neurosurgery 27:855, 1991. *A review article discussing risks and medical and surgical management.*

Juvela S, Heiskanen O, Potanen A, et al: The treatment of spontaneous intracerebral hemorrhage: A prospective randomized trial of surgical and conservative treatment. J Neurosurg 70:755, 1989. *A randomized trial of 52 patients with brain hemorrhage showing that although surgery saves lives, it does not improve function.*

Kassell NF, Torner JC, Haley EC, et al: The International Cooperative Study on the timing of aneurysm surgery. Part I: Overall management results. J Neurosurg 73:18, 1990. *This article summarizes the results of the International Cooperative Study on saccular aneurysms and documents the status of medical management in the 1980s.*

Kassell NF, Torner JC, Jane JA, et al: The International Cooperative Study on the timing of aneurysm surgery. Part 2: Surgical results. J Neurosurg 73:37, 1990. *This article describes 3521 patients from 68 centers with ruptured saccular aneurysms. It presents a contemporary discussion of the diagnosis of SAH, prevention of rebleeding, vasospasm, and early versus late surgical intervention.*

▪ INFECTIONS AND INFLAMMATORY DISORDERS OF THE NERVOUS SYSTEM

472 INTRODUCTION

Joseph R. Berger ▪ *Avindra Nath*

The central nervous system (CNS) can be infected by all the major groups of animal viruses. The spectrum of viruses ranges from the large, complex DNA herpesviruses to small, relatively simple viruses with DNA or RNA genomes, such as the papovaviruses and retroviruses. Also included in this section are prions, which are not conventional viruses but unique transmissable agents that cause an encephalopathy. The neurologic manifestations of viral infections are also diverse, extending from the acute febrile encephalitides to chronic progressive neurodegenerative disorders. *Neuroinvasive* refers to a virus that has the ability to enter the nervous system, but this does not necessarily mean that it causes any symptoms. A *neurotropic* virus is one that infects cells within the nervous system, and a *neurovirulent* virus causes clinically recognizable neurologic symptoms. Factors such as patient age and immune status, viral dose, and, in some instances, route of entry influence the ability of the virus to affect the nervous system.

Most viral infections are asymptomatic, and nervous system involvement is an uncommon complication of a relatively common systemic infection. The nervous system in these instances is a bystander to the systemic infection. Extension of infection to the CNS may be considered accidental and may even preclude survival of the virus and its transmission to a new host. For example, the polioviruses cause enteric infections in which replication in the gut and fecal-oral transmission determine the essential survival and transmission of the organism; extension of infection to anterior horn cells of the spinal cord devastates the host but does not contribute to the "life cycle" of the virus. By contrast, the neurotropic herpesviruses, including herpes simplex virus type 1 and varicella zoster virus, cause a latent infection in the sensory ganglia, where they may reside for extended periods. Occasionally, the virus becomes reactivated, causing a productive infection and resulting in neurologic symptoms. Even in the case of the herpesviruses, however, CNS complications, such as acute herpes encephalitis, are "accidental" and not essential in the organism's adaptive strategy. By contrast, rabies is an illness in which CNS infection plays a central role in the life cycle of the virus: involvement of the brain produces "rabid," biting behavior that actually contributes to virus transmission.

Viruses most commonly enter the nervous system through hematogenous spread. Virus in the blood may circulate as free virions (e.g., enteroviruses) or may be cell associated. For example, human immunodeficiency virus (HIV) associates with CD4 lymphocytes and Colorado tick fever with red blood cells. The virus may enter through the choroid plexus and spread through cerebrospinal fluid pathways or, alternatively, invade the brain by crossing the blood-brain barrier. Another mechanism of viral spread to the nervous system is by means of neurons. Rabies virus, some of the herpesviruses, and poliovirus are transported along peripheral nerves to the CNS. Initial symptoms may be focal. Once the virus enters the brain, it may spread transneuronally throughout the CNS at synaptic and nonsynaptic sites, producing more diffuse clinical changes. Within the nervous system, some viruses do not discriminate among neurons and glial or endothelial cells, whereas others infect selective targets. For example, JC virus infects oligodendrocytes and astrocytes but not neurons, whereas herpesvirus type 1 infects predominantly neurons. Such selectivity is often determined by

cell-surface molecules, principally glycoproteins, that serve as receptors for viruses, allowing their specific attachment and subsequent entry into cells. Different cell types also vary in their capacity to support virus-directed metabolism and replication. Virus-cell interactions can assume a number of courses. *Abortive infection* results in little or no change in the cell and no viral replication. *Productive infection* is characterized by a full replication cycle with production of virions. If the infection results in cell death, it is called a *cytopathic infection*. If there is a prolonged release of low level of virions without cell death, it is termed *persistent infection*. In *latent infection*, the viral genome resides quiescently in the cell but retains the capacity to reactivate subsequently. *Transforming infection* causes increased and characteristically abnormal cell proliferation and thereby oncogenic transformation of the cells, usually in the absence of virus replication. *Restricted* or *defective infection* may result in nonproductive infection or production of incomplete particles but may nonetheless cause varying degrees of cell alteration and viral antigen expression.

Neural injury and dysfunction accompanying viral infections may be due to direct infection of the cells (e.g., neuronal death caused by herpes simplex virus or oligodendroglial cell death caused by JC virus). The infected cells may also be targeted by antigen-specific host responses (e.g., lysis of infected cells by cytotoxic T lymphocytes). However, dysfunction of uninfected cells may result from toxic effects of viral products released from the infected cells (best characterized for HIV infection) or nonspecific host responses that lead to the production of neurotoxic substances (e.g., nitric oxide and quinolinic acid) and cytokines (tumor necrosis factor-α) by activated glial cells or invading mononuclear cells. The relative importance of these factors in individual infections depends on both the interactions of the invading organism with the cells it infects and the profile of host cell responses that it elicits. This balance is highly variable from one virus to the next and strongly influences the time course, morbidity, and degree of recovery from each infection.

Diagnostic approaches to viral diseases depend on the clinical setting and specific agents involved. The arsenal of available diagnostic methods is steadily growing. For many acute infections, the time-honored serologic techniques assessing host antibody responses in serum and at times cerebrospinal fluid remain the most useful and cost-effective. Although some infections elicit diagnostic tissue reactions (e.g., Negri bodies in rabies), for most infections, newer techniques have displaced simple histopathology in identifying infection in tissue, including detection of viral antigens using specific antibodies and of viral nucleic acids using in situ hybridization. More direct identification of viruses in blood or other clinical specimens by culture isolation generally remains difficult and costly, but the introduction of the polymerase chain reaction gene amplification technique to clinical virology is rapidly expanding the diagnostic capability of the laboratory.

Efforts to combat viral disease consist of prevention through active, or at times passive, immunization. In the case of rabies only, active immunization may be given after exposure to the virus. Effective drug therapy is available for most neurotropic herpesviruses, and antiviral treatment can temporarily retard progression of HIV infection. Promise exists for more effective treatments for infection by these viruses as well as for the development of chemotherapeutic agents that will act selectively against other important viruses causing neurologic diseases.

Johnson RT: Viral Infections of the Nervous System. Philadelphia: Lippincott-Raven, 1998. *An excellent introduction to the general principles of viral infection of the nervous system.*

Tsai T: Arboviral infections in the United States. Infect Dis Clin North Am 5:73, 1991. *A general review of arboviral infections, including clinical and epidemiologic aspects.*

473 PARAMENINGEAL INFECTIONS

Roger P. Simon

Parameningeal central nervous system (CNS) infections include those that affect brain parenchyma directly (brain abscess), those that produce suppuration in potential spaces covering the brain and spinal cord (epidural abscess and subdural empyema), those that produce occlusion of the contiguous venous sinuses and cerebral veins (cerebral venous sinus thrombosis), and remote infectious processes (bacterial endocarditis and sepsis) that result in diffuse, multifactorial involvement of the CNS.

BRAIN ABSCESS

Brain abscess is an uncommon disorder accounting for only 2% of intracranial mass lesions. CNS abscesses are circumscribed, enlarging, focal infections that produce symptoms and findings similar to those of other space-occupying lesions, such as brain tumors. Brain abscesses, however, often progress more rapidly than tumors and more frequently affect meningeal structures.

CAUSE. Infections resulting in brain abscess originate in or extend from extracerebral locations. Although the most frequent predisposing factors have changed over the past decades and vary with a hospital's population and referral base, the most common (Table 473–1) are blood-borne metastases from unknown sources and from lung or heart, direct extension from parameningeal sites (otitis, cranial osteomyelitis, sinusitis), recent or remote head trauma or neurosurgical procedures, and infections associated with cyanotic congenital heart disease. Blood-borne infections seed the brain via hematogenous spread and produce abscesses in brain regions in proportion to the blood flow; accordingly, parietal lobe abscesses predominate. Extension of infection from otitis and mastoiditis involves contiguous brain regions of the temporal lobe and cerebellum, whereas abscesses resulting from sinusitis affect the frontal and temporal lobes. Until recently the most common cause of brain abscess in urban hospitals was toxoplasmosis occurring in immunodeficiency states as a result of co-infection with the human immunodeficiency virus (HIV). With the widespread use of trimethoprim/sulfamethoxazole (as prophylaxis for *Pneumocystis carinii*), protease inhibitors, and retroviral drugs, these abscesses are currently rare.

PATHOLOGIC CHARACTERISTICS. Clinical and experimental data indicate that most brain abscesses evolve over a number of stages, beginning with vascular seeding of brain parenchyma, producing early cerebritis during the first 1 to 3 days. Inflammatory infiltrates of polymorphonuclear cells, lymphocytes, and plasma cells follow within 24 hours. By 3 days, the surrounding area shows a marked increase in perivascular inflammation. The late cerebritis phase develops approximately 4 to 9 days after infection,

Table 473–2 ■ BRAIN ABSCESS: PRESENTING FEATURES IN 43 CASES

Headache	72%
Lethargy	71%
Fever	60%
Nuchal rigidity	49%
Nausea, vomiting	35%
Seizures	35%
Ocular palsy	27%
Confusion	26%
Visual disturbance	21%
Weakness	21%
Dysarthria	12%
Stupor	12%
Papilledema	10%
Dysphasia	9%
Hemiparesis	9%
Dizziness	7%

Chan CH, Johnson JD, Hofstetter M, et al: Brain abscess: A study of 45 consecutive cases. Medicine 65:415, 1986. © 1986, The Williams & Wilkins Company, Baltimore.

during which time the center becomes necrotic, containing a mixture of debris and inflammatory cells. Neovascularity is maximal at this time. Early reactive astrocytes surround the zone of infection and proceed to early capsule formation between approximately 10 and 13 days. At this time, the necrotic center shrinks slightly, and a well-developed peripheral fibroblast layer evolves. The late capsule stage continues to evolve between 14 days and 5 weeks, with continual shrinking of the necrotic center and a relative decrease in the inflammatory cells. The capsule thickens as reactive astrocytes proliferate.

BACTERIOLOGIC CHARACTERISTICS. The pathogenic organisms vary considerably, depending on the clinical circumstances. The most commonly isolated pathogens are aerobic and microaerobic streptococci and gram-negative anaerobes such as *Bacteroides* and *Prevotella* spp. Less commonly, gram-negative aerobes and *Staphylococcus* spp. are isolated (Table 472–1). *Actinomyces, Nocardia,* and *Candida* spp. are less frequent offenders. Infection is often polymicrobial. Culture-negative abscesses from surgical specimens occur in 30% of antibiotic-treated patients and in 5% of patients operated on before antibiotic administration.

CLINICAL PRESENTATION. Signs of infection may be minimal or absent. Almost half of affected patients maintain a normal body temperature, and fewer than a third show a peripheral white cell count above 11,000/μL. Neck stiffness is rare in the absence of increased intracranial pressure.

Otherwise, the presenting features resemble those of any expanding intracranial mass (Table 473–2). A headache of recent onset is the most common symptom, representing distortion or irritation of pain-sensitive structures within the cranial vault, especially those of the great venous sinuses and the dura mater about the base of the brain. If the process continues untreated, isolated headache will increase in severity and become accompanied by focal signs such as hemiparesis or aphasia, followed by obtundation and coma. The period of evolution may be as brief as hours or as long as many days to weeks with more indolent organisms. Seizures may occur with abscesses involving the cortical gray matter.

CEREBROSPINAL FLUID EXAMINATION. Cerebrospinal fluid (CSF) examination is not useful in diagnosis because the findings range from normal to those of purulent meningitis, depending on the walling off of the brain abscess or its closeness to CSF compartments (Table 473–3). More important, because abscesses often expand rapidly, lumbar puncture may aggravate impending transtentorial herniation. If possible, the procedure should not be performed until after brain imaging, which may eliminate the need for CSF analysis.

NEUROIMAGING. Contrast enhanced computed tomography (CT) and magnetic resonance imaging (MRI) are useful for diagnosis of brain abscesses and for monitoring of response to therapy. MRI is especially useful for posterior fossa abscesses, as it provides an artifact-free view of the brain stem and cerebellum. In addition, MRI with intravenous gadolinium contrast is superior in demonstrating cerebritis, surrounding edema, the extent of mass

Table 473–1 ■ SUMMARY OF UCSF CASES ACCORDING TO TIME PERIODS*

	1970–1974	1975–1980	1981–1986	TOTAL
Number of cases	22	33	47	102
Etiology	2(9)	4(12)	13(28)	19(19)
Local infection				
Cardiac	6(27)	6(18)	5(11)	17(17)
Surgery	1(4)	7(2)	8(17)	16(16)
Trauma	2(9)	1(3)	6(13)	9(9)
Pulmonary	4(18)	4(12)	1(2)	9(9)
Immunocompromise	2(9)	2(6)	2(4)	6(6)
Other	1(4)	4(12)	0(0)	5(5)
Unknown	4(18)	4(12)	13(28)	21(21)
Organisms	16(73)	27(82)	34(72)	77(75)
Aerobic				
Anaerobic	5(23)	8(24)	7(15)	20(20)
Multiple	5(23)	8(24)	7(15)	20(20)
None cultured	6(27)	6(18)	14(30)	26(25)
Deaths	9(41)	3(9)	2(4)	14(14)

*Figures in parentheses indicate percentages.
From Mampalam TJ, Rosenblum ML: Trends in the management of bacterial brain abscesses: A review of 102 cases over 17 years. Neurosurgery 23:451, 1988.

Table 473–3 ■ SUMMARY OF LUMBAR FLUID CHANGES ASSOCIATED WITH BRAIN ABSCESS*

		NUMBER OF PATIENTS	PER CENT
Pressure			
<200 mm		38	38
200–300 mm		35	35
>300 mm		26	26
	Total	99	
White cells per mm³		61	29
<5			
5–100		81	38
>100		71	33
	Total	213	
Protein (mg per dL)		26	24
<50			
50–100		38	35
>100		44	41
	Total	108	
Glucose (mg per dL)		89	79
>40			
<40		23	21
	Total	112	

*Most of these data were obtained before brain imaging was widely available.
From Fishman RA: Cerebrospinal Fluid in Diseases of the Nervous System. Philadelphia, WB Saunders, 1980, p. 264.

effect, or associated venous thrombosis. MRI with or without gadolinium is preferable to CT for demonstrating multiple lesions.

The evolution of the abscess can be followed radiologically. In the early cerebritis stage, CT images reveal a low-density lesion with partial ring enhancement. In the late cerebritis and early capsule stages, well-formed ring-enhancing lesions are seen. The ring enhancement is typically thin walled and uniform, with subtle medial thinning adjacent to the ventricular system. Thick, non-uniform, or nodular enhancement should raise suspicion of an alternative cause. Delayed contrast CT scans show diffusion of contrast material into the lucent center. In the late capsule stage, well-formed ring enhancement may be seen with no delayed diffusion of contrast. Other ring-enhancing lesions that may mimic the image of brain abscess include primary and metastatic tumor, a resolving infarct or hematoma, and, rarely, demyelinating disease.

TREATMENT. Pyogenic brain abscesses are treated with antibiotics combined with surgical aspiration or excision. Aspiration offers the advantage of identifying the infecting organism and may be performed stereotactically with CT guidance while the patient is under local anesthesia; excision requires craniotomy. Surgical therapy is required when significant mass effect is present, when the abscess adjoins the ventricular surface (raising the possibility of catastrophic rupture into the ventricular system), when abscesses arise in the posterior fossa (with the potential of brain stem compression), or when abscesses reach a large size (>3-cm diameter) or become refractory to medical therapy. In selected cases antibiotics alone are appropriate, as in the case of surgically inaccessible, multiple abscesses (seen in 10% of patients), or abscesses in the early cerebritis stage. If the causal organism is not identified, antibiotic coverage should be directed toward the most likely organisms (streptococci and anaerobes). A suggested regimen includes penicillin G, 3–4 million units given intravenously (IV) every 4 hours, and metronidazole, 7.5 mg/kg given IV or orally every 6–8 hours. If staphylococcal and aerobic gram-negative infection is suspected (e.g., because of a history of trauma or intravenous drug abuse), nafcillin plus cefotaxime or ceftriaxone is recommended. Concomitant corticosteroid therapy may attenuate edema surrounding abscesses and may be warranted if the abscess produces life-threatening mass-effect.

The resolution of abscesses can be followed by serial CT or MRI. Antibiotics must be continued until the abscess cavity resolves completely, usually in 6 to 8 weeks, although in surgically treated patients it may be 4 weeks. A failure to demonstrate abscess shrinkage in 4 weeks constitutes an antibiotic failure; a surgical procedure should then be performed. Of note is the fact that the ring enhancement may persist after clinical and CSF normalization.

PROGNOSIS. The current mortality rate is 5 to 15%, depending on location and the nature of preexisting illness. Outcome correlates inversely with the abscess size and the degree of neurologic dysfunction at presentation, but less well with age, cause, number of abscesses, or corticosteroid use.

SPINAL EPIDURAL ABSCESS

Infection within the epidural space about the spinal cord is an uncommon but readily diagnosable and treatable potential cause of paralysis and death. Its incidence is 0.5 to 1.0 per 10,000 hospital admissions in the United States, but the frequency is substantially increased in the intravenous drug-using population.

CLINICAL PRESENTATION. Patients are usually systemically ill with fever (to 38° to 39° C) in virtually all acutely evolving cases and in the majority of those with a subacute evolution. The initial feature is acute or subacute neck or back pain, with focal percussion tenderness a prominent sign in the great majority; stiff neck and headache are common. As the infection progresses over hours, days, or weeks, radicular pain occurs; the site varies with the location of the abscess. The pain can be mistaken for sciatica, a visceral abdominal process, chest wall pain, or cervical disk disease. If the condition goes unrecognized at this stage, the symptoms can rapidly evolve, over a few hours to a few days, to produce weakness and finally paralysis occurring distal to the spinal level of the infection. In this clinical setting, spinal epidural abscess should be assumed, systemic antibiotics begun, and urgent neuroradiologic confirmatory diagnostic procedures pursued.

The differential diagnosis includes compressive and inflammatory processes involving the spinal cord (transverse myelitis, intervertebral disk herniation, epidural hemorrhage, metastatic tumor), which can usually be differentiated clinically by the absence of systemic infection. Transverse myelitis, however, may be associated with fever; the most useful differential feature is its rapid evolution to maximum deficit within 24 hours or less. Other infectious processes that may produce back or neck pain or tenderness must be excluded (bacterial meningitis, perinephric abscess, disk space infection, bacterial endocarditis). Spinal subdural empyema can cause a similar syndrome but is much less frequent.

CAUSE. Infections of the epidural space originate from contiguous spread or via hematogenous routes from a distant source. Cutaneous sites of infection are the most common remote sources, especially in intravenous drug users. Abdominal, respiratory tract, and urinary sources are also common. Osteomyelitis may be a cause of either direct extension or hematogenous spread, especially when associated with sepsis. Contiguous spread of infection occurs, most commonly from psoas abscesses, decubitus ulceration, perinephric and retropharyngeal abscesses, surgical sites, or epidurally placed catheters. Whether or not spread can result from pelvic infections via spinal veins remains unsettled. Minor back trauma has been implicated in producing a hematoma near the spine, which is subsequently seeded via hematogenous sources.

PATHOPHYSIOLOGIC CHARACTERISTICS. The anatomic features of the epidural space dictate the location of the abscess; the frequency of epidural infections is proportional to the volume of the epidural space. Because the size of the intravertebral canal remains relatively constant while the circumference of the spinal cord changes, abscess formation is maximal in the thoracic and lumbar regions and least at the cervical spine enlargement. Further, as the dura mater about the cord is adherent to the vertebral column anteriorly, more epidural abscesses lie posteriorly and because no anatomic barriers separate spinal segments in the posterior epidural space, such abscesses usually extend over three to five or more vertebral segments.

As the epidural space is not confined rostrocaudally, there is no clear abscess cavity or focal mass to provide a situation of simple compression for spinal cord compromise in epidural abscess. Clinical signs often are substantially greater than would have been predicted from the anatomic extent of pus or granulation tissue found at surgical exploration. Further, in many instances, no frank compression is found at surgery or on post-mortem examination. The spinal cord dysfunction is likely to reflect toxic processes secondary to inflammation, as well as venous thrombosis, thrombophlebitis, ischemia, and edema.

BACTERIOLOGIC CHARACTERISTICS. Causative organisms can be identified by culture or Gram's stain from pus obtained at exploration (90% of cases), blood culture (60 to 90% of cases), or CSF (20% of cases). *Staphylococcus aureus* accounts for most infections, followed by streptococci and gram-negative anaerobes. Tuberculous abscesses remain common, representing as many as 25% of cases in high-risk populations.

DIAGNOSIS. CSF examination is often performed because of associated fever and meningeal signs. The fluid usually is non-specifically abnormal, containing normal or decreased glucose levels, an elevated protein content (400 to 500 mg/mL), and a lymphocytic pleocytosis (22 to 150/mm³). Spinal fluid cultures yield organisms in about 25% of cases and Gram's stain results are rarely positive. Almost 90% of patients show a peripheral blood leukocytosis.

Plain spine radiographs, with attention to the area of percussion tenderness, may show osteomyelitis/diskitis, a compression fracture, or a paravertebral mass. Gadolinium-enhanced MRI is the study of choice for the evaluation of a suspected epidural abscess because of its superior ability to demonstrate the craniocaudal extent of the extradural soft tissue mass, associated mass effect upon the cord or cauda equina, and potential signal abnormalities within the disks, vertebral bone marrow, and spinal cord. The addition of an intravenous gadolinium contrast agent better defines central necrosis suggestive of abscess rather than cellulitis. If MRI is unavailable or technically impossible, CT with myelography usually provides adequate information. A normal plain CT alone does not exclude the diagnosis.

TREATMENT. The disease is fatal in the absence of antibiotic therapy. Unless culture result and sensitivities dictate otherwise, penicillinase-resistant penicillin (nafcillin, 12 g/day, or oxacillin, 12 g/day) should be started empirically as antistaphylococcal treatment for presumed bacterial infection. Considering the severity of the disease, most authorities would provide additional gram-negative coverage with a third-generation cephalosporin, a quinolone, or an aminoglycoside. For confirmed *Staphlyococcus aureus* abscesses, penicillinase-resistant penicillin is the treatment of choice; however, some consider the addition of rifampin (300 mg every 12 hours) because of its ability to penetrate the abscess cavity. Therapy should be continued intravenously for 3 to 4 weeks in the absence of osteomyelitis and 6 to 8 weeks with associated osteomyelitis. Surgical decompression was once thought to be mandatory in all cases; now early diagnosis by CT or MRI scans allows for effective medical therapy prior to occurrence of neurologic complications. Medical management of cervical epidural abscess requires close neurologic monitoring because of the small space available for abscess expansion and the high potential for quadriparesis. If blood culture findings are negative, needle aspiration or laminectomy may be necessary to determine the causative organism.

PROGNOSIS. The chance of partial or complete recovery relates inversely to the amount of neurologic dysfunction at the time of diagnosis. Patients without findings other than pain recover without deficit. Approximately half the patients with some weakness have complete resolution, and nearly half the patients with paralysis of less than 36 hours' duration show some return of motor function. In tuberculous epidural abscess recovery of motor function has been reported even after paralysis lasting for weeks.

VENOUS SINUS THROMBOSIS SECONDARY TO INFECTION

Thrombosis of cerebral veins or sinuses may occur in the absence of a demonstrable cause, but also may occur in the setting of hematologic disorders or coagulation abnormalities or may result from local or contiguous infectious processes. The infection-related syndromes are dealt with here.

Venous drainage from the brain begins with venules and veins that drain into the great venous sinuses. The venous sinus system itself lacks valves, permitting retrograde propagation of clots or infections emanating from structures such as those located in the central portion of the face or the middle ear.

Septic Cavernous Sinus Thrombosis

The cavernous sinuses comprise the most caudal dural venous chambers at the skull base. The paired structures lie on either side of the pituitary fossa, immediately above the midline sphenoid sinus. The cavernous sinus encloses the "cavernous portion" of the internal carotid artery; the third, fourth, and sixth cranial nerves en route to the apex of the orbit; and the ophthalmic and maxillary branches of the trigeminal nerve, which supply sensation to the forehead, periocular regions, cornea, and malar area of the face. Septic cavernous sinus thrombosis most commonly results from extension of infections involving the neighboring sphenoid and ethmoid sinuses, the central portion of the face, or the pharynx or tonsils.

Presenting symptoms are headache or lateralized facial pain, followed in a few days to weeks by fever, and involvement of the orbit, producing proptosis and chemosis secondary to obstruction of the ophthalmic vein. Paralysis of oculomotor nerves follows rapidly. Sensory dysfunction in the first and second divisions of the trigeminal nerve and a decrease in the corneal reflex are less obvious. Further involvement of the contiguous orbital contents follows, with mild papilledema and decreased visual acuity, sometimes progressing to blindness. Extension to the opposite cavernous sinus or to other intracranial sinuses with cerebral infarction, or increased intracranial pressure secondary to impaired venous drainage can result in stupor, coma, and death.

The differential diagnosis includes carotid cavernous sinus fistula (diagnosed by ocular bruit and an afebrile state); idiopathic granulomatous involvement of the cavernous sinus (the Tolosa-Hunt syndrome) or orbital pseudotumor (diagnosed by relative sparing of the orbital contents); and orbital cellulitis (infection localized to the orbit but sparing the structures of the cavernous sinus). Some overlap often occurs between involvement of these contiguous structures of the orbit and the cavernous sinus.

The CSF is abnormal in almost all cases, sometimes with a profile resembling that of purulent meningitis or parameningeal infection.

The most common causative organism is *Staphylococcus aureus,* with streptococci and pneumococci less common; anaerobic infection has been reported. Radiologic evaluation includes sinus imaging, with attention to the sphenoid and ethmoid sinuses. MRI (with and without intravenous gadolinium contrast) can often demonstrate venous thrombosis by illustrating the lack of the normal "flow void" within vascular structures. Cranial CT scans, employed with or without intravenous contrast material, are less helpful but may show a subtle increase in size and enhancement in the thrombosed sinus. MR angiography may demonstrate extrinsic narrowing of the intracavernous portion of the internal carotid artery.

Treatment relies on early diagnosis and consists of the prompt drainage of infected paranasal sinuses as well as specific antistaphylococcal agents, such as nafcillin or oxacillin, given intravenously. Heparin anticoagulation may reduce morbidity from associated brain ischemia, but this treatment remains controversial in cases involving infection.

Lateral Sinus Thrombosis

Septic thrombosis of the lateral sinus results from acute or chronic infections of the middle ear. The symptoms consist of ear pain followed by headache, nausea, vomiting, and vertigo, evolving over several weeks. On examination, most patients are febrile. An abnormality on the otologic examination is nearly invariable; mastoid swelling may be seen. Sixth cranial nerve palsies can occur, but other focal neurologic signs are rare. Papilledema occurs in half the cases, and elevated CSF pressure is present in most, especially with occlusion of the right lateral sinus (which is the major venous conduit from the superior sagittal sinus). The CSF is usually normal, although a parameningeal inflammatory profile may be seen.

Treatment includes intravenous antibiotics to cover staphylococci and anaerobes (nafcillin or oxacillin with penicillin or metronidazole). Surgical drainage (mastoidectomy) may be required. Increased intracranial pressure seldom needs direct treatment unless vision is compromised. The outcome is usually favorable.

Septic Sagittal Sinus Thrombosis

Septic sagittal sinus thrombosis is an uncommon condition that occurs as a consequence of purulent meningitis, infections of the ethmoid or maxillary sinuses spreading via venous channels, compound infected skull fractures, or, rarely, neurosurgical wound infections. Symptoms include manifestations of elevated intracranial pressure (headache, nausea, and vomiting) that evolve rapidly to stupor and coma. Seizures and hemiparesis may result from cortical infarction. The rate of progression, severity of symptoms, and prognosis are all related to the location of thrombosis involving the sinus. When only the anterior third of the sinus is obstructed, symptoms are less intense and evolve more slowly. If the thrombosis progresses to involve the middle and posterior thirds of the sinus, deterioration progresses more rapidly and outlook for recovery declines.

CSF abnormalities accompany well over half the cases. The opening pressure is increased in proportion to the extent of the sagittal sinus involvement, and a pleocytosis usually reflects the association of a meningeal or parameningeal process.

Radiologically, septic sagittal sinus thrombosis may be excluded by visualization of the normal sagittal sinus during the venous phase of cerebral angiography; the diagnosis can usually also be made by MRI, which demonstrates an abnormal increase in signal intensity (absent flow void) within the affected venous sinus. Contrast-enhanced CT scanning may reveal a contrast void lying at the junction of the transverse and sagittal sinuses (the region of the torcular); this so-called delta sign is an intraluminal clot surrounded by contrast material.

Intravenous antibiotics should be directed at organisms recovered from the meningeal process or the meningeal site. *Staphylococcus aureus* (including the methicillin-resistant strains), β-hemolytic streptococci, pneumococci, and gram-negative aerobes such as *Klebsiella* spp. are the most common organisms. Initial antibiotic treatment should include nafcillin and a third-generation cephalosporin. Vancomycin can be used for antistaphylococcal coverage in patients with significant β-lactam allergy. Associated paranasal sinusitis should be drained surgically. Heparin use has been little tested in septic venous thrombosis, but experience with non-infected sinus thrombosis has shown it to reduce both morbidity and mortality rates appreciably.

Neurologic Complications of Infectious Endocarditis

Neurologic complications occur in one third of patients with bacterial endocarditis and triple the general mortality rate of the disease. Most of these complications derive from valvular vegetations. Cerebral (but not systemic) emboli are more common in cases of mitral valve endocarditis, for reasons unknown. The time of embolization during the course of endocarditis depends upon the virulence of the organism and whether it produces acute or subacute disease. With acute endocarditis (predominantly staphylococci or enterococci), embolization occurs early, often during the first week, whereas in subacute disease (predominantly viridans group streptococci, or enterococci) emboli occur over the full course of treatment and occasionally after treatment is completed. Cerebral emboli are distributed in the brain in proportion to cerebral blood flow. Therefore, most emboli lodge in the branches of the middle cerebral artery peripherally, with resultant hemiparesis. Focal seizures may result.

Whether or not warfarin anticoagulation decreases the risk of embolization remains a controversial issue. This therapy was administered in an earlier period to decrease platelet fibrin vegetations that sequestered the bacteria from the body's defenses. Current evidence suggests that a high rate of hemorrhagic intracerebral complications results from warfarin anticoagulation in native valve endocarditis, but not in prosthetic valve endocarditis. The reason for the difference is unknown. Nevertheless, most authorities believe that patients already receiving chronic anticoagulation therapy at the time of diagnosis of endocarditis should be maintained on such therapy.

Mycotic aneurysms complicate endocarditis in 2 to 10% of cases and are more common in acute than subacute disease. The middle cerebral artery is most commonly involved; aneurysms are located distally in the vessel, differentiating them from congenital berry aneurysms. The process by which the aneurysmal dilatation occurs remains in dispute, although embolization of infectious vegetations is accepted as the inciting event. Aneurysmal rupture results in an 80% mortality rate, and early diagnosis is therefore important. Whom to subject to angiography is uncertain. However, clinical or radiologic evidence of cerebral or other embolization defines the high-risk group. Other suggested indications for angiography include severe headache (presumably the result of aneurysmal leakage). When an unruptured aneurysm is identified by angiography, it may resolve with antibiotic therapy alone. Such patients need follow-up imaging to document an interval decrease in aneurysm size. Otherwise, surgical therapy requires excision of the infected portion of the artery. Patients with proximal mycotic aneurysms have a greater risk of perioperative stroke than do those with distal involvement.

Small brain abscesses may complicate the course of endocarditis, but macroscopic abscesses are rare and most occur in the setting of acute, rather than subacute, endocarditis. Multiple microabscesses, however, can result in a diffuse encephalopathy similar to that seen in sepsis. Such lesions may escape detection on CT scanning and are not amenable to surgical drainage. Antibiotic treatment of the primary disease is indicated.

A CSF pleocytosis occurs in 70% of patients with neurologic complications, but in an unknown number of patients in whom the CNS is clinically spared. The CSF profile may be that of a purulent meningitis (polymorphonuclear leukocyte predominance, elevated protein level, and low glucose level) or that of a perimeningeal infection (lymphocytic predominance, modest protein level elevation, and normal glucose level). A hemorrhagic component may be seen. Purulent CSF is associated with signs of meningeal irritation and infection with a virulent organism.

Subdural Empyema

Empyema is infection in a preformed space, in this case that separating the dura and arachnoid. Subdural empyema is responsible for one fifth of localized intracranial infections and results from direct or indirect extension from infected paranasal sinuses via a retrograde thrombophlebitis or, less frequently, untreated chronic otitis. Unilateral empyema is most common, as the falx prevents passage across the midline, but bilateral or multiple concurrent empyemas occur. Cortical venous thrombosis or brain abscess develops in approximately one fourth of cases; purulent meningitis is a less common accompaniment.

Symptoms initially reflect those of chronic otitis or sinusitis, as well as lateralized headache (a universal feature), fever, and obtundation. Vomiting, meningeal signs, and focal neurologic abnormalities (hemiparesis or seizures) usually follow. If the disease remains untreated, obtundation progresses, and the septic mass and swelling of the underlying brain soon lead to venous thrombosis or death from herniation. The major differential diagnosis is that of meningitis. Nuchal rigidity and obtundation occur in both, but papilledema and lateralizing deficits are more common in empyema. The result of lumbar puncture, obtained because of the suspicion of meningitis, reveals an elevated intracranial pressure accompanied by an increased protein content and a polymorphonuclear pleocytosis with usually a normal glucose concentration in the CSF. Contrast-enhanced CT or MRI can be diagnostic of empyema, showing an extra-axial, crescent-shaped mass with an enhancing rim lying just below the inner table of the skull over the cerebral convexities or the interhemispheric fissures. MRI better detects underlying parenchymal edema as well as the infection itself.

Treatment requires both prompt surgical drainage of the empyema cavity and high-dose intravenous antibiotics directed toward organisms found at the time of craniotomy. The bacteriologic characteristics of subdural empyemas are similar to those of sinusitis and cerebral abscess, discussed earlier. Anticonvulsants should be administered prophylactically, as seizures are common.

If cortical infarction from venous thrombosis does not occur, the prognosis is surprisingly favorable, although in one third of patients chronic epilepsy results.

Cranial Epidural Abscess

Infections of the epidural space coexist most often with subdural empyema and less frequently with chronic sinusitis or otitis alone. Symptoms and signs are headache and fever with focal neurologic abnormalities due to the coexistent subdural empyema or brain abscess. The diagnosis is made with MRI or contrast-enhanced CT scan (which demonstrate a peripherally enhancing lenticular-shaped lesion in the epidural space), and the abscess is treated by surgical drainage followed by systemic antibiotics. In uncomplicated cases, the prognosis is excellent.

Malignant External Otitis

Malignant external otitis is a necrotizing osteitis, that occurs in elderly patients with diabetes. The associated organism, *Pseudomonas aeruginosa*, is part of the normal flora of the external ear. In this case, it produces an external otitis that fails to respect normal anatomic boundaries. The result consists of a rapidly evolving syndrome of ear pain, facial swelling, osteomyelitis of the base of the skull, and purulent meningitis accompanied by multiple cranial nerve palsies. Urgent treatment with antipseudomonal penicillin or a third-generation cephalosporin combined with an aminoglycoside or ciprofloxacin, as well as surgical débridement and drainage, is essential. The mortality rate is high.

Brain Abscess

Haimes AB, Zimmerman RD, Morgello S, et al: MR imaging of brain abscesses. AJR 152:1073, 1989. *Review of MRI and differential diagnosis of brain abscesses.*

Maniglia AJ, Goodwin WJ, Arnold JE, et al: Intracranial abscesses secondary to nasal, sinus, and orbital infections in adults and children. Arch Otolaryngol Head Neck Surg 115:1424, 1989. *Review of association of sinus disease with brain abscesses.*

Patel KS, Marks PV: Management of focal intracranial infections: Is medical treatment better than surgery? J Neurol Neurosurg Psychiatry 53:472, 1990. *Discussion of the issue of non-surgical management.*

Yang SY, Zhao CS: Review of 140 patients with brain abscess. Surg Neurol 39:290, 1993. *Clinical features, bacteriologic characteristics, imaging, and treatment.*

Spinal Epidural Abscess

Darouiche RO, Hamill RJ, Greenberg SB, et al: Bacterial spinal epidural abscess: Review of 43 cases and literature survey. Medicine (Baltimore) 71:369, 1992. *A large recent series addressing the issue of medical versus surgical treatment.*

Hanigan WC, Asner NG, Elwood PW: Magnetic resonance and the nonoperative treatment of spinal epidural abscess. Surg Neurol 34:408, 1990. *Non-operative cases presented and criteria reviewed.*

Khanna RK, Malik GM, Rock JP, Rosenblum ML: Spinal epidural abscess: Evaluation of factors influencing outcome. Neurosurgery 39:958, 1996. *Outcome prediction based on clinical and radiographic features.*

Kuker W, Mull M, Mayfrank L, et al: Epidural spinal infection: Variability of clinical and magnetic resonance findings. Spine 22:544, 1997. *MRI imaging reviewed in 13 patients; frequent associated diskitis noted.*

Nussbaum ES, Rigamonti D, Standiford H, et al: Spinal epidural abscess: A report of 40 cases and review. Surg Neurol 38:225, 1992. *A neurosurgical series.*

Redekop GJ, Del MR: Diagnosis and management of spinal epidural abscess. Can J Neurol Sci 19:180, 1992. *Review of 25 recent cases: presentations, treatment, outcome.*

Teman AJ: Spinal epidural abscess: Early detection with gadolinium magnetic resonance imaging. Arch Neurol 49:743, 1992. *Early imaging addressed.*

Venous Sinus Thrombosis Secondary to Infection

DiNubile MJ, Boom WH, Southwick FS: Septic cortical thrombophlebitis. J Infect Dis 161:1216, 1990. *Fourteen-year experience from a single center.*

Garcia RD, Baker AS, Cunningham MJ, Weber AL, et al: Lateral sinus thrombosis associated with otitis media and mastoiditis in children. Pediatr Infect Dis J 14:617, 1995. *Clinical findings and literature review.*

Neurologic Complications of Infectious Endocarditis

Davenport J, Hart RG: Prosthetic valve endocarditis 1976–1987: Antibiotics, anticoagulation, and stroke. Stroke 21:993, 1990. *Anticoagulation in prosthetic valve endocarditis readdressed.*

Eidelman LA, Putterman D, Putterman C, Sprung CL: The spectrum of septic encephalopathy. JAMA 275:470. 1996. *The component of the encephalopathy due to sepsis alone reviewed.*

Jones HJ, Siekert RG: Neurological manifestations of infective endocarditis: Review of clinical and therapeutic challenges. Brain 112:1295, 1989. *Two-decade experience: review of central and peripheral nervous systems in addition to imaging and treatment.*

Roder BL, Wandall DA, Espersen F, et al: Neurologic manifestations in *Staphylococcus aureus* endocarditis: A review of 260 bacteremic cases in nondrug addicts. Am J Med 102:379, 1997. *Time of presentation, native valve but not valvular vegetations as risks for embolization and increased mortality rate.*

Van der Meulen JHP, Weststrate W, van Gijn J, Habbema JDF: Is cerebral angiography indicated in infective endocarditis? Stroke 23:1662, 1992. *Routine angiography not indicated.*

Subdural Empyema

Bok AP, Peter JC: Subdural empyema: Burr holes or craniotomy? A retrospective computerized tomography–era analysis of treatment in 90 cases. J Neurosurg 78:574, 1993. *Surgical treatment reviewed.*

Dill SR, Cobbs CG, McDonald CK: Subdural empyema: Analysis of 32 cases and review. Clin Infect Dis 20:372, 1995. *Retrospective (1970–1992) review of 32 cases: presentation, treatment, and outcome from sinusitis, trauma, and surgical cases.*

Pathak A, Sharma BS, Mathuriya SN, et al: Controversies in the management of subdural empyema: A study of 41 cases with review of literature. Acta Neurochir 102:25, 1990. *A recent large series and literature review.*

Weingarten K, Zimmerman RD, Becker RD, et al: Subdural and epidural empyemas: MR imaging. AJR 152:615, 1989. *MRI described.*

Cranial Epidural Abscess

Krauss WE, McCormick PC: Infections of the dural spaces. Neurosurg Clin North Am 3:421, 1992. *Epidural and subdural infections and treatment reviewed.*

Malignant External Otitis

Amorosa L, Modugno GC, Pirodda A: Malignant external otitis: Review and personal experence. Acta Otolaryngol Suppl 521:3, 1996. *Clinical features and imaging addressed.*

Johnson MP, Ramphal R: Malignant external otitis: Report on therapy with ceftazidime

and review of therapy and prognosis. Rev Infect Dis 12:173, 1990. *A review of clinical and therapeutic aspects.*

474 NEUROSYPHILIS
Roger P. Simon

The recent incidence of primary and secondary syphilis in the United States peaked in 1990 and has declined precipitously since (less than 10,000 reports in 1997). Current cases cluster in the intercity populations of the southeastern United States. If untreated, in approximately 7% of patients with primary syphilis infection some form of symptomatic neurosyphilis develops.

PATHOPHYSIOLOGIC CHARACTERISTICS. Each of the neurologic manifestations of syphilis is the consequence of a chronic, insidious meningeal inflammatory process caused by treponemal invasion of the central nervous system (CNS). An inflammatory response in the cerebrospinal fluid (CSF) occurs in at least one third of asymptomatic persons with syphilis, and in a third of these, if untreated, will progress to symptomatic neurosyphilis. CSF abnormalities peak at 13 to 18 months after the primary infection; if the CSF examination yields a normal result 5 years after the primary infection, the risk of development of symptomatic neurosyphilis drops to 1%.

CLINICAL SYNDROMES. The clinical manifestations of neurosyphilis are divided into acute syphilitic meningitis, cerebrovascular syphilis, syphilitic dementia (general paresis), and tabes dorsalis. These entities may overlap clinically, however, and two syndromes may coexist, as in "taboparesis." These clinical subtypes of neurosyphilis each develop in a predictable time frame after the primary infection (Fig. 474–1), as meningeal inflammatory process evolves. Symptomatic syphilitic meningitis is the earliest manifestation of nervous system syphilis. The meningeal inflammation later extends to involve the cerebral blood vessels and, when symptomatic, results in cerebrovascular neurosyphilis, usually seen within the first 5 years after primary infection. The so-called parenchymal forms of neurosyphilis (paresis and tabes) develop after a more protracted interval of 10 to 20 years or, rarely, longer.

ACUTE SYPHILITIC MENINGITIS. Symptomatic meningeal syphilis occurs during the first months to 2 years after the primary infection, with 10% of cases occurring coincident with a secondary rash. The course is subacute. Headache is common, and asymmetrical cranial nerve abnormalities are prominent (especially those involving auditory function, facial strength, eye movements, and unilateral or bilateral papilledema due to involvement of the optic nerve). Patients are afebrile; meningeal signs are often present, and some patients are confused. The CSF usually contains syphilitic antibodies and shows a lymphocytic pleocytosis. Accurate diagnosis is important, as mild symptoms may resolve without treatment and leave the patient at risk for progression to the irreversible deficits associated with the later forms of neurosyphilis.

CEREBROVASCULAR SYPHILIS. Over time (generally 3 to 5 years) the meningeal inflammatory process evolves to compromise the cerebral arteries traversing the subarachnoid space and cause a diffuse vasculitis. The symptoms now are those of a subacute encephalopathy with confusion, personality changes, and intellectual decline. This stage is usually then followed by the emergence of focal deficits resulting from occlusion of specific vessels; branches of the middle cerebral artery are most often involved, but any cerebral or spinal vascular bed may be affected alone or in combination. These ischemic lesions evolve over a period of several hours or days. The resulting syndrome differs from thromboembolic stroke because of the associated encephalopathy, the multifocal pattern, and the subacute time course. Diagnosis is confirmed by finding an inflammatory spinal fluid with a positive syphilis serologic result; angiography is not necessary for diagnosis, but if performed demonstrates vasculitis of medium-sized arteries. Areas of ischemia imaged by computed tomography (CT) or magnetic

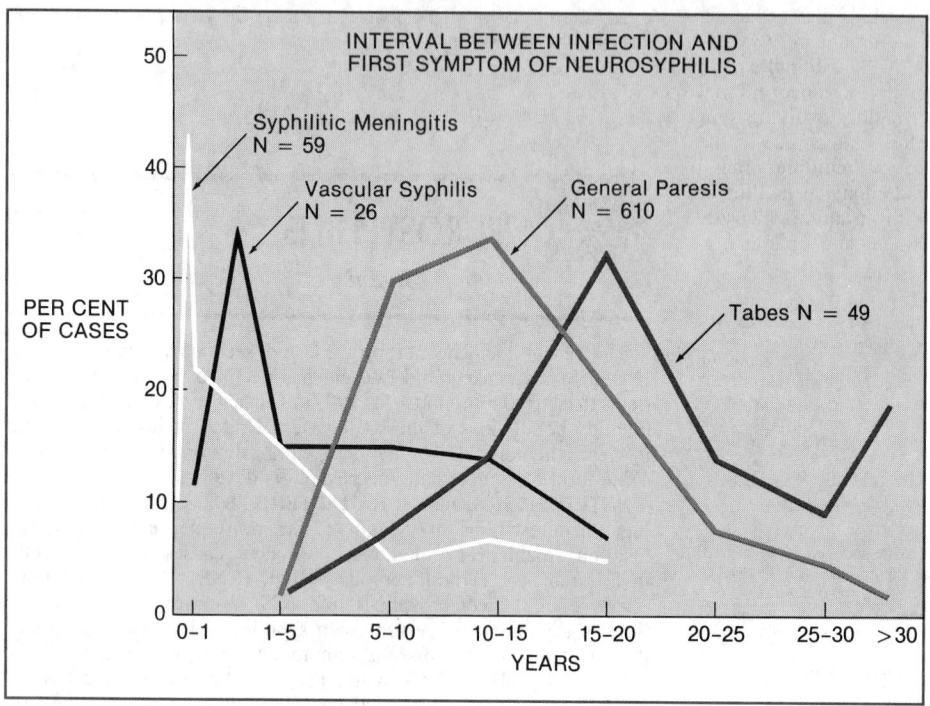

FIGURE 474–1 ■ Interval between primary and symptomatic neurosyphilis by type (meningeal, vascular, paretic, tabetic), abstracted from the literature and presented as percentage of total cases within type. (From Simon RP: Neurosyphilis. Arch Neurol 42:606, 1985. Copyright 1985, American Medical Association.)

resonance imaging (MRI) in association with the characteristic CSF findings suggest the diagnosis.

SYPHILITIC DEMENTIA. Dementia paralytica, or general paresis of the insane, is caused by the diffuse meningoencephalitic form of neurosyphilis. This disorder presents 5 to 15 years or more after the primary infection. General paresis affects men four to seven times more frequently than women, perhaps because the infectivity of *Treponema pallidum* declines during pregnancy.

The clinical pattern of syphilitic dementia can mimic that of many forms of dementia. The colorful descriptions of grandiose delusional states and psychosis are well known, but these conditions were uncommon even in the pre-penicillin era. Then, as now, a simple dementing illness predominated. In advanced cases, tremors of the hands, tongue, and lips resulted, producing a striking dysgraphia and dysarthria.

Several features differentiate syphilitic dementia from dementia of other causes. Syphilitic dementia has a relatively early onset, most commonly beginning between ages 30 and 50, and it progresses rapidly if untreated, being fatal within months to a few years. An inflammatory CSF is always found, and the blood and CSF serologic findings always contain diagnostic syphilitic antibodies.

TABES DORSALIS. The term *tabes dorsalis* denotes a myeloneuropathy that characteristically follows the primary infection by 10 to 20 years. The primary lesions affect either the proximal dorsal root entry zones or the dorsal root ganglia. As with paresis, a marked male predominance (7:1), was noted in the pre-penicillin era.

The classic triad of symptoms includes lightning pains, sensory ataxia, and urinary disturbance. The most common and earliest signs include pupillary abnormalities, lower extremity areflexia, and Romberg's sign. Lightning pains are transient, agonizing, shooting pains most common in the legs but potentially arising in any region of the body. Characteristic is an early loss of vibration and position sense attributed to secondary degeneration of the posterior columns of the spinal cord. The proprioceptive impairment engenders a wide-based, unsteady gait that is exacerbated by elimination of visual input (eye closure): Romberg's sign. Bladder hypotonia with overflow incontinence results from deafferentation of the lower sacral sensory nerve roots. Rectal incontinence is uncommon; genital sensory and autonomic impairment eventually results in impotence. Peripheral autonomic impairment, along with loss of peripheral nociceptive afferent fibers, is responsible for the development of trophic (Charcot) joint deformities and distal extremity ulcers.

Of the pupillary abnormalities, half have the classic Argyll-Robertson pattern, being small, irregular, bilateral and reacting poorly to light but constricting briskly to accommodation (the phenomenon of light-near dissociation). Other pupillary abnormalities in tabes dorsalis include unilateral mydriatic pupils with loss of pupillary light reflex.

CEREBROSPINAL FLUID EXAMINATION. A chronic inflammatory response in the CSF (Table 474–1) accompanies each of the clinical syndromes of neurosyphilis; this leukocytosis, in conjunction with a positive syphilis serologic result on the CSF, both establishes the diagnosis of active neurosyphilis and monitors the response to therapy. The absence of a CSF inflammatory response excludes a diagnosis of active neurosyphilis and therefore precludes a clinical response to antibiotic therapy. As with any chronic men-

Table 474–1 ■ CSF FINDINGS IN VARIOUS NEUROSYPHILITIC SYNDROMES

Syndrome	OP	WBC	Glu	Prot	Gamma globulin*	VDRL	
						Blood	CSF
Meningitis	170	154 (94% L)	29	95		1:64	1:4
Cerebrovascular	192	58 (87% L)	41	119	IgG index 0.93	1:512	1:16
Paresis		220	49	305	IgG index 1.99	1:128	1:8
Tabes dorsalis (active)		62		140		1:16	1:28
Tabes dorsalis (inactive)		2	76	43		1:16	1:2

*Normal IgG index = 0.23 to 0.64.

OP = opening pressure; WBC = white blood cell; Glu = glucose; Prot = protein; VDRL = Veneral Disease Research Laboratory; CSF = cerebrospinal fluid; L = lymphocytes; IgG = immunoglobulin G.

From Simon RP, Bayne LL: Neurosyphilis. In Martin J, Tyler K (eds): Infections of the Central Nervous System (Contemporary Neurology Series, Vol. 41). Philadelphia, FA Davis, 1993; pp. 237–256.

Table 474–2 ▪ **CEREBROSPINAL FLUID (CSF) RESPONSE TO PENICILLIN TREATMENT***

	ADMISSION	DAY 7	DAY 21	6 MONTHS
Opening pressure, mm CSF	120			Normal
Cells/mm³	207 (94% L)	100 (100% L)	24 (100% L)	0
Glucose, mg/dL	51	66	54	66
Protein, mg/dL	50 (14.4% gamma globulin)	38	48	34
Serology (VDRL) CSF	1:2	1:1	—	—
Blood	1:64	1:64	1:64	1:64

*Meningovascular syphilis treated with aqueous penicillin G, 24 million units/d for 21 days.
Data from Holmes MD, Brant-Zawadski MM, Simon RP: Clinical manifestations of meningovascular syphilis. Neurology 34:553, 1984.

ingitis, the gamma globulin fraction of the protein content is commonly elevated; oligoclonal bands may be present.

The possibility of a negative serologic result in neurosyphilis is unclear in the classic literature because of the use of the relatively insensitive Wassermann test and the unrecognized inclusion of nonsyphilitic syndromes of cerebrovascular disease and viral meningitis. When the clinical diagnosis was characteristic, however, only rare cases showed a negative CSF serologic result (even with the Wassermann reaction): In 100 paretic patients reported by Merritt in 1946, the CSF Wassermann test result was positive in every case. Wilson also reported universal CSF positivity in 77 cases of paresis. Theoretically, a negative CSF Venereal Disease Research Laboratory (VDRL) test finding might occur in the presence of severe immunosuppression, as a prozone phenomenon, or, in an early case, as a manifestation of the CSF inflammatory response preceding seropositivity. This last situation may explain occasional recent reports of false-negative results or delayed conversions in early meningeal syndromes.

The role of the more sensitive treponemal test (fluorescent treponemal antibody [FTA]) in the CSF remains uncertain because of a high false-positive response and decreased sensitivity (75%); without supporting clinical or laboratory data, the diagnostic value of a reactive CSF FTA result is unknown. An additional confirmatory test is to inject CSF into rabbit testes; a reactive testicular swelling and recovery of spirochetes prove treponemal infectivity.

TREATMENT. Because neurosyphilis of all clinical types is associated with a CSF inflammatory response, the CSF cell count provides the best monitor for the effectiveness of therapy, with any protein level elevation resolving more slowly. Normalization of the spinal fluid is the required endpoint of antibiotic therapy; once the CSF remains normal, clinical relapses do not occur.

Penicillin is the drug of choice; antimicrobial resistance does not occur. Various regimens from 12 to 24 million units/day have been suggested, but it is not clear that the higher doses improve the clinical outcome. Spirocheticidal levels (0.03 IU/mL, 0.018 mg/mL) in CSF occur with 12 million units/day of intravenous (IV) penicillin in four divided doses; the Center for Disease Control currently recommends 18–24 million units/day for 10 days. Intramuscular benzathine penicillin does not result in therapeutic levels in the CSF and therefore should not be used for treatment of neurosyphilis. Some regimens include probenecid to increase concentrations in CSF by decreasing reabsorption of penicillin through the choroid plexus. Probenecid, however, also decreases parenchymal penicillin concentrations by competing for uptake at membrane transport sites.

The optimal duration of penicillin treatment for neurosyphilis is uncertain. Complete normalization of CSF is uncommon during the usual 2- to 3-week course of intravenous treatment, but the CSF progressively improves to normal over the next weeks to months (Table 474–2). Proof of adequate treatment requires a normal cell count and a falling protein content at 6 months.

HUMAN IMMUNODEFICIENCY VIRUS (HIV) INFECTION IN NEUROSYPHILIS. Neurosyphilis and HIV-associated disease may coexist, as both are consequences of sexual promiscuity or intravenous drug abuse. Syphilitic syndromes in these patients do not differ in either time course or clinical presentation from those in the pre–acquired immunodeficiency syndrome (AIDS) era. Cases identified as "penicillin-resistant" may merely have coexistent HIV-induced CSF pleocytosis that is not altered by penicillin therapy. In addition, the occasional recovery of treponemes after penicillin treatment for syphilis in HIV-coinfected patients was similarly observed in the pre-AIDS era. A recent comparison of syphilitic

patients with or without HIV co-infection found no difference from those with the classically reported illness in clinical presentation, course of disease, serologic expression, or effect of treatment.

The treatment of neurosyphilis in HIV-co-infected patients is identical to that in patients without the retrovirus disease; intravenous penicillin should be used in spirocheticidal doses, and the CSF should be monitored as an index of therapy. As noted, when the inflammatory response is due partly to syphilis and partly to HIV infection, only a portion of the pleocytosis will disappear, leaving a new plateau of CSF cellularity. The Centers for Disease Control and Prevention recommend that patients co-infected with HIV and syphilis for more than 1 year have an examination of their CSF, whether or not they have neurologic symptoms.

Flood JM, Weinstock HS, Guroy ME, et al: Neurosyphilis during the AIDS epidemic. San Francisco, 1985–1992. J Infect Dis 177:931, 1998. *Retrospective report of clinical features, presentation CSF findings, and response to treatment of 117 patients; meningeal and meningovascular presentations were most common.*

Gourevitch MN, Selwyn PA, Davenny K, et al: Effects of HIV infection on the serologic manifestations and response to treatment of syphilis in intravenous drug users. Ann Intern Med 118:350, 1993. *No difference was found in presentation, course, response to treatment, and serologic findings with or without HIV coinfection.*

Hook EW III: Management of syphilis in human immunodeficiency virus–infected patients. Am J Med 93:477 1992. *Reviews management issues in the HIV coinfected.*

Merritt HH, Adams RD, Solomon HC: Neurosyphilis, 2nd ed. New York, Oxford University Press, 1946. *The classic descriptive work of the pre-penicillin era.*

Musher DM, Hamill RJ, Baughn RE: Syphilis in the presence of human immunodeficiency virus infection. Ann Intern Med 113:872, 1990. *A critique of the association of syphilis and HIV infection.*

Simon RP: Neurosyphilis. Arch Neurol 42:606, 1985. *A review of the clinical syndromes, CSF findings and serologic diagnostic criteria.*

475 ACUTE VIRAL MENINGITIS AND ENCEPHALITIS

Avindra Nath ▪ *Joseph R. Berger*

DEFINITIONS. The term *viral meningitis* refers to infection of the leptomeninges, *viral encephalitis* refers to infection of the brain parenchyma, and *viral meningoencephalitis* is sometimes used when both meninges and brain parenchyma appear to be infected, although viral encephalitis is almost always accompanied by meningeal inflammation. When the spinal cord and brain are involved, the term *viral encephalomyelitis* may be used. The nonspecific term *aseptic meningitis* refers to an inflammatory process of the meninges accompanied by a predominantly mononuclear cell pleocytosis and not caused by pyogenic bacterial infection. Although viral infections are the most common cause of aseptic meningitis, infections by other types of organisms, chemical irritation of the meninges, carcinomatous meningitis, and reactions to certain medications can cause a similar clinical picture and cerebrospinal fluid (CSF) profile. Acute central nervous system (CNS) infections caused by a variety of viruses are considered together because of their largely indistinguishable clinical features. Viral infections causing more distinct neurologic symptoms and signs are described separately in subsequent sections.

ETIOLOGIES. Many viruses can cause acute encephalitis or meningitis (Table 475–1), others may result in subacute or chronic encephalitis (Table 475–2). Enteroviruses are the most common cause of aseptic meningitis. They are small, non-enveloped RNA viruses of the picornavirus family with numerous serotypes. More than 50 have been associated with meningitis or encephalitis. Japanese encephalitis virus is the most common cause of encephalitis worldwide in humans. It has a high morbidity and mortality rate. Although an effective vaccine has been available since 1960, only small populations in Asia have been vaccinated.

Arboviruses include agents of several families that are transmitted by mosquitoes or ticks. More than 15 different arboviruses have been associated with encephalitis in various areas of the world. In the United States, the most important are California encephalitis (most cases involve the La Crosse subtype), eastern and western equine encephalitis, St Louis encephalitis, and Colorado tick fever. Less common in the United States are Venezuelan equine encephalitis and Powassan encephalitis.

Herpes simplex virus, type 1 (HSV-1), causes severe encephalitis, usually with characteristic focal features, whereas HSV-2 causes aseptic meningitis in association with genital herpes. Lymphocytic choriomeningitis virus, an arenavirus, is a sporadic cause of meningitis and occasionally of encephalitis. The human immunodeficiency virus may cause aseptic meningitis, usually at the time of

seroconversion. Adenoviruses are respiratory viruses that only rarely cause meningitis or severe childhood encephalitis. Cytomegalovirus and varicella zoster virus cause encephalitis, but only in immune-compromised individuals.

The acute neurologic disease associated with measles, vaccinia, or rubella infections is usually a sequel to infection termed *postinfectious encephalomyelitis*. The encephalitis that may also be postinfectious encephalomyelitis occasionally occurs with influenza and parainfluenza virus infections.

EPIDEMIOLOGY. Viral meningitis and encephalitis are relatively common disorders. In one study in Rochester, MN, for example, the incidence of aseptic meningitis was nearly 11 per 100,000 person-years, and that of viral encephalitis was more than 7 per 100,000 person-years. This finding was compared with a rate of 8.6 episodes of bacterial meningitis. In general, a specific cause is identified in only about 10 to 15% of cases of meningitis and encephalitis in the United States.

Each virus causing CNS infection has its own epidemiologic pattern (see Table 475–1). Because of the predominance of enteroviruses and arboviruses, the overall incidence of viral meningitis and encephalitis peaks in the late summer. Enteroviruses are transmitted by the fecal-hand-oral route. They often involve young children, with rapid spread in families or social groups. The geographic and seasonal incidence of arbovirus infection relates to the life cycle of arthropod vectors and animal reservoirs and their contact

Table 475–1 ■ VIRUSES ASSOCIATED WITH ACUTE CENTRAL NERVOUS SYSTEM INFECTIONS

	SEASON	MORTALITY (%)	MORBIDITY (%)
Non-arthropod viruses			
RNA viruses			
Picornaviruses (enteroviruses)	All year (tropics); summer and fall (temperate regions)		
Polioviruses			
Coxsackieviruses, group A			
Coxsackieviruses, group B			
Echoviruses		0	Rare
Enteroviruses 70, 71		Rare	Rare
Togaviruses			
Rubella	Spring	Rare	Rare
Arenavirus			
Lymphocytic choriomeningitis	Winter	Rare	Rare
Rhabdovirus			
Rabies	All year	>95	
Orthomyxoviruses	Winter and spring		
Influenza			
Parainfluenza			
Paramyxoviruses	Winter and spring		
Measles			
Mumps			
Retroviruses	All year		
Human immunodeficiency virus, type 1		100	
DNA viruses	All year		
Herpesviruses			
Herpes simplex, type 1		15	60
Adenoviruses		Rare	Rare
Arthropod-borne viruses			
RNA viruses			
Togaviruses			
Eastern equine encephalitis	Summer	50	30
Western equine encephalitis	Summer	5	30
Venezuelan equine encephalitis		10	<5
Flaviviruses			
Mosquito-borne encephalitis viruses			
Japanese encephalitis (Asia)	Summer	30	30
St Louis encephalitis	Summer and fall	<10	10
Murray Valley encephalitis (Australia, New Guinea)		20	40
West Nile virus			
Tick-borne encephalitis viruses			
Russian spring summer encephalitis	Spring and summer		
Louping ill (British Isles)			
Powassan virus (Canada, Northern US)	Spring and summer	<5	Rare
Kyassanur Forest virus (India)	Summer	Rare	Rare
Bunyaviruses			
California encephalitis	Spring and summer		
La Crosse virus		Rare	Rare
Snowshoe hare virus (Canada)			
Jamestown canyon virus			
Orbivirus			
Colorado tick fever	Spring and summer	Rare	Rare

Table 475–2 ■ VIRUSES ASSOCIATED WITH SUBACUTE OR CHRONIC NERVOUS SYSTEM INFECTION

	NEUROLOGIC SYNDROME
RNA viruses	
Togavirus	
Rubella	Progressive rubella panencephalitis
Paramyxovirus	
Measles	Subacute sclerosing panencephalitis
Retroviruses	
Human immunodeficiency virus, type 1	HIV dementia
Human T cell lymphotropic virus, type 1	HTLV-I associated myelopathy
DNA viruses	
Herpesviruses	
Herpes simplex, type 2	Mollaret's meningitis
Human herpes virus, type 6	(?) Subacute encephalitis
Varicella-zoster	Herpes zoster, subacute encephalitis
Epstein-Barr	Subacute encephalitis
Cytomegalovirus	Ventriculitis and encephalitis
Papovaviruses	
JC virus	Progressive multifocal leukoencephalopathy

with humans. Eastern equine encephalitis virus is limited largely to the Atlantic and Gulf coasts, whereas western equine encephalitis virus is confined to the western two-thirds of the country, with the highest incidence west of the Mississippi River Valley. The latter virus causes many more human infections than does the eastern virus, but only 1 in 100 infected persons develops encephalitis. St Louis encephalitis virus causes disease in both rural and urban areas over a large part of the United States. In the rural areas, the virus has the same pattern as western equine encephalitis virus, but in urban areas, more explosive outbreaks can occur. In recent years, the La Crosse subtype of the California encephalitis virus has been related every year to cases spread widely over the United States, particularly in the east and Midwest, mostly in children. Colorado tick fever occurs in the Rocky Mountain area: about 18% of infected patients develop meningitis, but encephalitis is rare. Venezuelan encephalitis has spread into Florida and the southwestern states and produces an influenza-like illness in most of those infected; however, about 3% develop acute meningitis or encephalitis. Powassan virus is a rare cause of encephalitis in Canada and along the northern border of the United States.

Lymphocytic choriomeningitis virus is the major zoonotic (an infection in man which is naturally transmitted from any vertebrate animal) virus causing meningitis and encephalitis. Humans acquire the infection by contact with dust or food contaminated by excreta of the common house mouse. Human disease is more common in winter, when the natural host tends to move indoors. Lymphocytic choriomeningitis virus has also been found in hamsters, and human infections have been traced to both laboratory and pet hamsters.

Mumps virus spreads by the respiratory route, with infection occurring throughout the year, but with the incidence increasing during the spring. Although mumps virus infects both sexes equally, meningitis develops in males three times more frequently than in females. Japanese encephalitis is geographically the most widely distributed of all the arthropod-borne viruses.

PATHOGENESIS. Events leading up to the development of the acute viral encephalitides and meningitides can be divided into three stages. The first involves exposure of an external body surface to the virus, usually with local replication of the "inoculum." In the case of enteroviruses, the infecting virus is contained in body fluids or excreta from infected persons and transferred by direct contact or within contaminated environmental materials. On ingestion, the virus replicates within the Peyer's patches of the lamina propria of the lower intestinal tract. The arboviruses, by contrast, are introduced by an arthropod bite. The next stage involves systemic viremia and amplification of virus in visceral organs: a secondary viremia may lead to invasion and replication within the nervous system or meninges. With the exception of rabies virus and the neurotropic herpesviruses, viruses that cause acute encephalitis or meningitis typically reach the nervous system hematogenously. This factor accounts for the widespread distribu-

tion of cerebral dysfunction associated with most of the encephalitides.

In viral encephalitis, infection of neurons, glial cells, and even vascular endothelium leads to cell dysfunction and sometimes cell death. Inflammatory responses follow. Clinical symptoms and signs depend on the distribution of infection and on both the direct effect of the virus and the secondary inflammatory reactions in the tissue. The relative contribution of each to brain dysfunction depends on the particular infecting virus. The remarkable degree of recovery in many patients suggests that secondary inflammatory and immune responses often predominate.

CLINICAL MANIFESTATIONS. Most acute viral encephalitides and meningitides produce similar symptoms, with variations depending on the particular virus. Often CNS manifestations are preceded or accompanied by fever, malaise, or myalgia; gastrointestinal disturbance; respiratory symptoms; or rash. These are followed by headache, photophobia, stiff neck, and other signs of meningeal irritation, usually with an intensity milder than that of bacterial meningitis.

When encephalitis exists, evidence of diffuse or, less commonly, focal brain dysfunction accompanies or overshadows signs of meningeal irritation. Patients characteristically exhibit altered attention and consciousness, ranging from confusion to lethargy or coma. Motor function may be abnormal, with weakness, altered tone, or incoordination, reflecting dysfunction of the cortex basal ganglia or cerebellum. Severe cases may cause difficult-to-control generalized or focal seizures. Some patients exhibit myoclonus or tremor. Hypothalamic involvement may lead to hyperthermia or hypothermia, autonomic dysfunction with vasomotor instability, or diabetes insipidus. Abnormalities of ocular motility, swallowing, or other cranial nerve functions are uncommon. Spinal cord infection is usually inconspicuous but can result in flaccid weakness, with acute loss of reflexes in the most severe cases. Focal symptoms other than seizures are usually minor and are overshadowed by generalized brain dysfunction; some patients may show hemiparesis, visual disturbance, or sensory loss. Focal involvement of limbic structures is particularly characteristic of rabies encephalitis.

The time course of acute viral meningitis and encephalitis varies. The onset may occur within a matter of hours or evolve more slowly over a few days. Usually, maximum deficit appears within 1 to 4 days.

LABORATORY FINDINGS. When viral encephalitis is suspected, if major focal signs are present, computed tomographic scan should be performed first. Examination of the CSF is essential. The presence of 10 to 1000 mononuclear cells per cubic millimeter (pleocytons) is characteristic. On occasion, early examination may show acellular fluid or predominance of polymorphonuclear leukocytes, but the typical mononuclear pleocytosis soon evolves. The pressure may be elevated, whereas the glucose level is characteristically normal or only modestly reduced. The protein content is usually elevated (50 to 100 mg/dL). Although not part of the routine examination, immunoglobulin concentration and oligoclonal bands may be observed. An increased protein content and pleocytons may persist for weeks or months after convalescence; oligoclonal bands can be detected for an even longer period.

Systemic laboratory findings vary, depending on the etiologic agent. Generally, the white blood cell count is not elevated, but either elevations or depressions can be seen, usually with a lymphocytic predominance. Involvement of salivary glands or pancreas in mumps may elevate the serum amylase level.

Neurodiagnostic tests usually reveal nonspecific abnormalities, with notable exception in the case of herpes simplex encephalitis (see Chapter 426). CT and magnetic resonance imaging (MRI) are usually normal early in the course of the nonherpetic viral encephalitides, but diffuse cerebral edema and multifocal areas of parenchymal injury with contrast enhancement may appear in the more severe cases. The greatest value of these neuroimaging procedures lies in excluding alternative diagnoses.

DIAGNOSIS. With a few exceptions, the neurologic and laboratory findings accompanying the acute viral meningoencephalitides are insufficiently distinct to allow an etiologic diagnosis, and it may even be difficult to distinguish these disorders from a number of nonviral diseases. The epidemiologic setting (e.g., time of year, exposure to insects, the local community) and accompanying systemic manifestations may be helpful in presumptive diagnoses. Thus, involvement of the nervous system by mumps virus is usually suspected from associated clinical parotitis or pancreatitis, although the neurologic disease can be the sole or presenting clinical manifestation; conversely, a certain history of previous mumps eliminates this diagnostic possibility. Several enterovirus infections produce a rash, which usually accompanies the onset of fever and persists for 4 to 10 days. In infections by coxsackievirus A5, 9, and 16, and echovirus 4, 6, 9, 16, and 30, the rash is typically maculopapular and nonpruritic and may be confined to the face and trunk or may involve extremities, including the palms and soles. Echovirus 9 infections can cause a petechial rash resembling meningococcemia. Herpangina, characterized by gray vesicular lesions on the tonsillar fossae, soft palate, and uvula, can accompany group A coxsackie infection. In coxsackievirus A16 and, rarely, other group A serotype infections, a vesicular rash may involve hands, feet, and oropharynx. As discussed below, the encephalitis related to Epstein-Barr virus occurs in the setting of acute mononucleosis. The principally postinfectious encephalitides related to measles and varicella follow overt systemic diseases with characteristic rashes.

Because no specific treatment exists for acute viral meningitis and encephalitis (except those caused by herpes) in immune-competent patients, and the signs and symptoms are often nonspecific, exclusion of other diagnoses becomes important. The following disorders are potentially confusing diagnostically: partially treated bacterial meningitis; rickettsial infections; Lyme disease; meningitis caused by a variety of nonpyogenic organisms, including *Mycobacterium tuberculosis* and *Cryptococcus neoformans* and other fungi; parameningeal bacterial infections; brain abscess; subacute bacterial endocarditis; and the cerebral vasculitides. Among noninfectious causes, trimethoprim-sulfamethoxazole, nonsteroidal analgesics, OKT3 antibody given for immunosuppression, intravenous immunoglobulin, and certain other drugs may occasionally cause aseptic meningitis reaction. Without a cerebrospinal fluid examination, the differential diagnosis becomes even broader, encompassing additional toxic and vascular diseases. Most alternative diagnoses can be suspected or eliminated by the history, the CSF profile, or brain imaging.

Despite the absence of effective treatment, specific virologic diagnosis is useful both for prognosis in the individual patient and for epidemiologic implications for the populations at risk. Diagnosis usually relies on serology, although direct detection of the organism in the CSF, blood, or stool may sometimes be achieved. Selection of tests and their interpretation depend on the particular organism. Almost all acute viral syndromes occur in the setting of a first encounter with the agent, which then results in lasting immunity. In these cases, seroconversion documented by a four-fold or greater rise in antibody titer between acute and convalescent sera is a principal means of diagnosis, although virus-specific IgM antibodies provide a rapid and accurate method of early diagnosis. A notable exception is herpes simplex encephalitis, in which antibody titers must be more cautiously interpreted (see Chapter 385). Attempts at direct viral isolation are of limited value in clinical management and must be tailored to the suspected agent. Arboviruses and enteroviruses can be isolated from the blood but are seldom recoverable at the time of clinically evident meningitis or encephalitis. During the acute disease, coxsackieviruses and echoviruses are most readily isolated from stool or CSF and, in some cases, throat washings. Lymphocytic choriomeningitis virus can be isolated from blood or CSF. Mumps virus may be isolated from saliva, throat washings, or CSF. HSV-2 may be cultured from the CSF or identified in genital lesions. Polymerase chain reaction (PCR) screening of CSF undoubtedly will improve specific diagnosis in the future.

VACCINATION. Effective vaccines are available for polio, measles, mumps, and rubella and illnesses related to these viruses have declined dramatically in countries with effective vaccination strategies. Similarly, vaccination against Japanese encephalitis has been effective in controlling the infection in Asia. A vaccine against varicella has recently been introduced. Rabies is the only infection in which the vaccine may be given after exposure to the virus.

TREATMENT. Effective antiviral therapy is available against HSV-1, cytomegalovirus, and varicella, the latter two cause enceph-alitis in immune-compromised patients only. In immunosuppressed patients, long-term therapy may be necessary. Several antiretroviral drugs are also available that provide temporary control of the virus, as drug-resistant strains of HIV frequently emerge. Treatment of acute viral encephalitis and meningitis (except herpes) is directed at symptom relief, supportive care, and prevention and management of complications. Strict isolation is not essential, although when enteroviral infection is suspected, precautions in handling stools and careful hand-washing practice should be instituted. Persons with measles, chickenpox, rubella, or mumps virus infections should observe the usual precautions of isolation from susceptible individuals. Arboviruses are not characteristically spread from person to person because they require an intermediate insect vector.

The headache and fever of meningitis can usually be managed with judicious doses of acetaminophen. Severe hyperthermia (>40°C) may require vigorous therapy, but mild temperature elevations may serve as a natural defense mechanism and are best left untreated. Patients with severe encephalitis often become comatose. Because, however, some may achieve remarkable recovery, vigorous support and avoidance of complications are essential. Meticulous care in an intensive care unit setting with respiratory and nutritional support is indicated.

Although seizures sometimes complicate encephalitis, prophylactic anticonvulsants are not routinely recommended. If seizures develop, they can usually be managed with phenytoin and phenobarbital. If status epilepticus ensues, appropriately vigorous therapy should be instituted to prevent secondary brain injury and hypoxia (see Chapter 433). Similarly, secondary bacterial infections should be sought and promptly treated. Steroids should probably generally be avoided in the treatment of encephalitis because of their inhibitory effects on host immune responses.

PROGNOSIS. Full recovery from viral meningitis usually occurs within 1 to 2 weeks of onset, although some patients describe persistence of fatigue, lightheadedness, and asthenia for months. The prognosis of encephalitis depends on its cause (see Table 475–1). Arbovirus encephalitides have variable mortality rates. Eastern equine encephalitis has the highest mortality rate of all arboviruses, whereas California virus has the lowest. The mortality rates for most viral encephalitides are greater in children younger than 4 years and in the elderly. Nonfatal encephalitis caused by eastern, western, and St Louis viruses has a relatively high rate of neurologic sequelae. Encephalitis associated with mumps or lymphocytic choriomeningitis virus is rarely associated with death, and sequelae are infrequent. The most common sequela following mumps meningoencephalitis is sensorineural deafness. Hydrocephalus from aqueductal stenosis has been reported as a late sequela of mumps meningitis and encephalitis in children.

McKendall RR, Stroop WG: Handbook of Neurovirology. New York, Marcel Dekker, 1994. *A useful text on pathogenesis, epidemiology, and clinical manifestations of viral infections. Has chapters on all major viral groups.*

476 POLIOMYELITIS

Avindra Nath ■ Joseph R. Berger

DEFINITIONS. Poliomyelitis (acute anterior poliomyelitis, infantile paralysis) is an acute illness caused by the three strains of poliovirus. The disease selectively destroys the motor neurons of the spinal cord and brain stem, resulting in flaccid asymmetrical weakness. Until recently one of the most feared of all human infectious diseases, poliomyelitis is now almost entirely preventable by vaccination.

ETIOLOGY. The three antigenically different strains of poliovirus (types 1, 2 and 3) are classified in the genus Enterovirus within the family Picornaviridae. The majority of cases are caused by type 1 strain. These are small (approximately 27 nm), roughly spherical particles, with icosahedral symmetry, containing a single-stranded RNA core surrounded by a protein capsid. Lacking a lipid envelope, the polioviruses are resistant to lipid solvents and are stable at low pH.

INCIDENCE, PREVALENCE, AND EPIDEMIOLOGY. In the United States the number of cases of paralytic poliomyelitis has fallen to just a few cases yearly due to the widespread use of an effective vaccine. In countries with low immunization rates, paralytic polio continues to occur, with high rates in sub-Saharan Africa, southern Asia, and countries engaged in war. It has a seasonal incidence in temperate zones but a more even distribution throughout the year in tropical areas. Poliovirus is acquired by the oral route and subsequently replicates in the oropharynx and lower gastrointestinal tract. It may be secreted for a week or two in saliva and for more prolonged periods in feces, which provides the major avenue of host-to-host transmission. Spread of polioviruses is greatly influenced by standards of hygiene, and greatest dissemination occurs within families or other crowded circumstances.

Paralysis is an unusual complication of poliovirus infection. During an epidemic, only 1 to 2% of infections result in neurologic symptoms and signs; another 4 to 8% of infected persons suffer nonspecific (minor) illness. Although polio occurs most commonly in preschool children, a number of other factors cause an increase in the incidence of paralytic disease, including advanced age, recent strenuous exercise, tonsillectomy, pregnancy, and impairment of B-lymphocyte (antibody) defenses. Immunity to each of the three types of poliovirus is lifelong, but infection with one strain does not protect against subsequent infection by another. In the United States, the incidence of poliomyelitis due to live-attenuated strains, although extremely rare, is now similar to that of wild-type virus occurring in non-immunized subjects.

PATHOGENESIS AND PATHOLOGY. Polioviruses selectively infect specific neuronal populations, inducing highly stereotyped pathologic processes; in this manner they contrast with most of the viruses causing acute encephalitis or meningitis.

The poliovirus invades the nervous system only after prior systemic replication. An initial alimentary phase with local replication in the intestinal mucosa and spread to the local lymphatics is followed by viremia, which seeds the nervous system. In addition, the virus may replicate in the skeletal muscle and be transported via the peripheral nerves to the spinal cord. This is similar to the myotropic nature of other enteroviruses, and may account for the myalgia that precedes the onset of weakness. Convalescent poliomyelitis is characterized by loss of motor neurons and denervation atrophy of their associated skeletal muscles.

CLINICAL MANIFESTATIONS. Acute poliomyelitis is separated into two distinct phases: "minor illness" and "major illness." The minor illness coincides with viremia and consists of fever, headache, and sore throat, which resolve within 1 to 2 days. In some patients, this is followed by the major illness, which is characterized by abrupt onset of fever, headache, vomiting, and meningismus. Cerebrospinal fluid (CSF) pleocytosis is present at this stage. The symptoms of aseptic meningitis resolve within 5 to 10 days. Asymmetrical muscle weakness is the hallmark of the illness. It is typically preceded by intense myalgia. Proximal muscles are more commonly involved, and legs more often than arms. In mild cases, paralysis affects only parts of muscles rather than selective peripheral nerve or nerve root distributions. Sensory changes are lacking. The paralysis may render one limb useless yet entirely spare the contralateral arm or leg. About 50% of patients develop acute urinary retention. The trunk musculature is least commonly affected. The affected muscles are flaccid, and the deep tendon reflexes may be absent. Atrophy develops rapidly, usually beginning within a week in paralyzed muscles and progressing over the ensuing weeks. The motor deficit rarely progresses for more than 3 to 5 days.

About 10 to 15% of cases affect the lower brain-stem motor nuclei. Involvement of the ninth and tenth cranial nerve nuclei leads to paralysis of pharyngeal and laryngeal musculature (bulbar poliomyelitis). Parts of the facial muscles can be involved, either unilaterally or bilaterally. Less often, the tongue and muscles of mastication become paralyzed. External oculomotor weakness occurs rarely. The pupils are spared. Direct involvement of the brainstem reticular formation can disrupt breathing and swallowing and produce serious disturbances in cardiovascular control. Poliomyelitis seldom causes permanent functional paralysis of the bulbar muscles, probably because of the relatively small size of the motor

units served by brain-stem nuclei and because overwhelming disease in these critical segments is often fatal.

DIAGNOSIS AND DIFFERENTIAL DIAGNOSIS. Because of its rarity in the United States, poliomyelitis may present diagnostic difficulties. Its early phases must be differentiated from other acute meningitides, and when paralysis ensues, a major differential diagnosis is postinfectious polyneuropathy or Guillain-Barré syndrome. However, almost no other acute disease produces headache, stiff neck, fever, and asymmetrical flaccid paralysis without sensory loss coupled with an increase in white blood cells in the CSF. Rarely, coxsackievirus and echoviruses have been reported to cause encephalitides with prominent but not extensive motor neuron symptoms and signs. Acute intermittent porphyria may cause a motor polyneuropathy somewhat similar to postinfectious polyneuropathy. At times, acute transverse myelitis may be confused with poliomyelitis, but findings of a sensorimotor spinal level at the appropriate spinal cord segment usually serves to separate an inflammatory cord transection from diffuse anterior horn cell involvement. Diagnosis can be established by isolation of virus from blood or CSF or by serologic evidence of acute poliovirus infection. In the rare cases related to vaccine strains, viral isolates can be distinguished in the laboratory.

TREATMENT. No specific treatment is available, but supportive care is important in reducing pain during the acute attack and in maintaining vital functions to ensure survival. Bedrest and treatment of pain are recommended during the myalgic phase. Important measures include preventing contractures, maintaining airway and cardiovascular stability, and preventing excessive calcium mobilization and bed sores.

PROGNOSIS. Death in poliomyelitis is usually the result of bulbar involvement and is attributable to respiratory and cardiovascular impairment. Mortality has been considerably reduced with modern management of respiratory insufficiency. Patients who survive an episode of acute paralytic poliomyelitis usually recover considerable motor function. Generally, motor improvement begins within the first weeks after onset, and 60% of eventual recovery is achieved by 3 months.

THE POSTPOLIO SYNDROME. A number of patients with previous poliomyelitis develop further motor deterioration later in life. In some, this relates simply to musculoskeletal decompensation or other factors but does not involve new weakness. However, other persons suffer a true loss of strength, termed *postpolio syndrome*. This disorder is characterized by an insidiously slow but gradually progressive weakness beginning 30 or more years after an attack of poliomyelitis. Most commonly it adds to the weakness of already affected muscles; less often weakness develops in muscles previously thought to be normal. This weakness is often accompanied by fasciculations, and additional atrophy may develop. Muscle biopsy shows type grouping consistent with chronic denervation-reinnervation. Overall, the prognosis is good, with slow progression of further weakness, which only rarely leads to a severe increase in disability or to death. The most likely pathogenesis consists of senescence of the surviving expanded motor units. This development must be distinguished from motor neuron disease of a more malignant variety, which has also been described many years after acute poliomyelitis, but which appears to be much less common than the more gradual and benign postpolio syndrome. In all cases it is imperative to exclude coincidental unrelated disease.

PREVENTION. Poliomyelitis can be prevented by either live-attenuated or killed polio vaccines. These are now given routinely in Western cultures, although the practice of immunization has relaxed as the threat of development of paralytic poliomyelitis has become less conspicuous. If this trend is not reversed, a resurgence of the disease can be expected. An important consequence of accurate diagnosis of poliomyelitis is the prompt institution of local vaccination programs for communities at risk, including cultures in which vaccination is avoided for religious or other reasons.

Windebank AJ, Litchy WJ, Daube JR, et al: Late effects of paralytic poliomyelitis in Olmsted County, Minnesota. Neurology 41:501, 1991. *A study characterizing the long-term clinical sequelae of a population sample with previous poliomyelitis.*

McComas AJ, Quartly C, Griggs RC: Early and late losses of motor units after poliomyelitis. Brain 120:1415, 1997. *Demonstrates that denervation progresses in patients with prior poliomyelitis in both clinically affected and unaffected muscles at rates that exceed those of normal aging.*

477 The Herpesviruses

Joseph R. Berger ■ *Avindra Nath*

477.0 Introduction

ETIOLOGY. The members of the family of Herpesviridae are large, enveloped viruses with double-stranded linear deoxyribonucleic acid in their core. They are icosadeltahedral in shape, dictated by their 162 capsomeres. Antigenic differences, including those between herpes simplex virus, types 1 and 2 (HSV-1 and HSV-2), permit identification by monospecific antibodies using immunocytochemical techniques. Knowledge of their DNA sequences has permitted the development of polymerase chain reaction (PCR) methods for their detection.

Herpesviruses have been detected in a wide range of hosts, including man, primates, horses, cattle, pigs, and chickens. Since the recognized onset of the acquired immunodeficiency syndrome (AIDS) epidemic in 1981, three new members of the family of human herpesviruses, human herpesviruses 6, 7, and 8 (HHV-6, HHV-7, and HHV-8), have been described, nearly doubling the number of recognized herpes viruses known to affect humans. Currently, three human herpesviruses (HSV-1, HSV-2, and herpes varicella-zoster virus [VZV]) are known to be neurotropic. A herpesvirus related to HSV-1, the simian herpesvirus, is also neurotropic, and in rare instances it may affect humans.

The survival and transmission of these herpesviruses is predicated on the latency that they establish in the nervous system. The initial peripheral viral infection is followed by retrograde axoplasmic transport to nervous system ganglia. Each of these viruses can then establish a latent infection of sensory ganglia that may subsequently reactivate to release progeny virus into the territory of the ganglion's epithelial innervation via orthograde axoplasmic transport. The most feared and best recognized neurologic complication of the herpesviruses is HSV encephalitis, a consequence of HSV-1 infection. Aseptic meningitis, radiculitis, and sacral autonomic dysfunction occur with HSV-2. The neurologic complications of VZV include encephalitis, myelitis, radiculopathy, and cerebral vasculitis.

Epstein-Barr virus (EBV), cytomegalovirus (CMV), and HHV-6, -7 and -8 are lymphotropic. Neurologic disease has been associated with all but HHV-7, about which little is currently known. The neurologic complications of EBV typically occur in the setting of a recent bout of infectious mononucleosis, whereas those associated with CMV generally occur in the setting of impaired immunity, as in AIDS and organ transplant recipients. The importance of HHV-6 as a trigger for neurologic disease remains uncertain at present. Prompt diagnosis of infections by these viruses is important because they are now amenable to selective antiviral drug therapy.

477.1 Herpes Simplex Virus, Types 1 and 2

INCIDENCE. Although HSV encephalitis is the most common identified cause of severe, sporadic viral encephalitis in the United States, it remains uncommon. Its estimated annual incidence is 1 in 250,000 to 500,000 persons. HSV encephalitis accounts for approximately 20% of the reported cases of encephalitis in the United States. Some HSV encephalitis may go unrecognized, and in a percentage of cases the infection undergoes spontaneous resolution. Therefore, prevalence figures probably underestimate the true number. The disease afflicts persons of all ages, with peaks of incidence in late childhood and middle age. There is no seasonal incidence of HSV encephalitis; it occurs throughout the year. Case-to-case transmission does not occur. Although immunologic mechanisms are important in HSV latency and its peripheral reactivation, the appearance of HSV encephalitis is not related to immunosuppression. However, the clinical expression of the illness may be modified if cell-mediated immunity is impaired.

HSV-1 is a ubiquitous organism. More than 90% of adults have serologic evidence of exposure. Immunocytochemical staining and PCR have confirmed that at least 75% of the population harbors latent HSV in the trigeminal ganglia at the time of death. Recurrent cold sores resulting from viral reactivation have been estimated to occur in one-fourth of adults. Although as many as 10% of patients with HSV encephalitis may have cold sores at the time of their illness, this number is not different from that for individuals hospitalized with other severe debilitating diseases. Although HSV encephalitis may occur as a primary infection in a person never previously infected with the virus, it is more likely that it results from reinfection by a new strain of virus or from reactivated virus.

CLINICAL MANIFESTATIONS. HSV encephalitis may be explosive at onset. The condition may progress to a state of altered consciousness accompanied by speech abnormalities and motor weakness in a matter of hours from onset of the illness. Typically, however, the onset is subacute, with fever, headache, and malaise preceding the development of neurologic deficits. Both diffuse and focal cerebral dysfunction is observed. Fever, often high, is seen in up to 90% of patients with HSV encephalitis. In as many as 10%, fever may be absent, particularly at the time of presentation. Therefore, HSV encephalitis warrants consideration even in afebrile patients who present with an altered mental status. The most common forms of presentation include severe headache, focal or generalized convulsions, and alterations in behavior and consciousness. Disorientation, dysphasia, and hemiparesis may be observed. Motor paralysis is present in fewer than 50% of affected individuals. Occasionally, patients are initially referred for psychiatric consultation because of delusions, agitation, personality changes, disorientation, or dysphasia. Without treatment, the mortality of HSV encephalitis is high (>70%), with major permanent morbidity in many survivors. Milder forms of the illness exist but are rarely correctly identified.

In the setting of immunosuppression, particularly in patients with AIDS, HSV encephalitis may present in a more benign and desultory fashion. The illness may be characterized by unexplained meningitis with few focal neurologic findings. A high index of suspicion is therefore required to establish the diagnosis. HSV has also been associated with focal brain-stem encephalitis.

PATHOLOGY. The characteristic gross and microscopic pathologic findings of herpetic infection, particularly its anatomic localization, distinguishes HSV encephalitis from other encephalitides. Although often asymmetrical, the disease is usually bilateral and afflicts the medial temporal and inferior lobes and related "limbic" structures, including the hippocampus, amygdaloid nuclei, olfactory cortex, insula, and cingulate gyrus. Necrosis with petechial hemorrhage is often so intense that the disease was once called *acute necrotizing encephalitis*. Microscopically, hemorrhagic necrosis with mononuclear inflammation characterizes involved areas, with neurons and glia often containing Cowdry type A intranuclear inclusions during the acute phase of infection. Perivascular cuffing, neuronophagia, and diffuse microglial hyperplasia are observed. Although gray matter is predominantly affected, the infection extends into the white matter as well. In addition to the necrosis and inflammation of the neural tissues, leptomeningeal infiltration by lymphocytes, plasma cells, and large mononuclear cells is also seen. In the immunosuppressed host, the inflammatory infiltrate may not be as intense.

DIAGNOSIS. Among the differential diagnoses of HSV encephalitis are pyogenic, tuberculous and fungal meningitis, brain abscess, brain neoplasm, vasculitis, and demyelinating disease. CSF examination is of paramount importance in detecting the presence of other infectious meningitic processes and in the definitive diagnosis of HSV encephalitis. Brain abscess seldom presents with the behavioral abnormalities so often evident in HSV encephalitis, and radiographic findings are often very helpful in distinguishing between the two conditions. Cerebral neoplasms tend to evolve slowly and are not accompanied by fever.

Neuroimaging with head computed tomographic (CT) scanning or magnetic resonance imaging (MRI) is generally regarded as the initial diagnostic measure when evaluating a patient suspected of having HSV encephalitis. However, CT scanning is relatively insensitive. At least 40% of patients with early HSV encephalitis have normal CT scans. The MRI is much more sensitive and often reveals highly characteristic abnormalities, including the virtually pathognomonic increased signal abnormalities on T2-weighted sequences in the medial temporal and insular cortical regions and inferior frontal cingulate gyri. The lesions are often bilateral. General anesthesia may be required to perform the MRI owing to agitation and a poor level of cooperation on the part of the patient. The MRI can also detect alternative pathologic processes, such as brain abscess, vasculitis, or demyelination, which may present in a similar fashion.

Brain biopsy, once regarded as the definitive diagnostic tool for HSV encephalitis, has been largely supplanted by the widespread introduction of CSF PCR for HSV. The employment of brain biopsy for the diagnosis of HSV encephalitis is not infallible and has been steeped in controversy. Arguments previously propounded for its broad application included its sensitivity and specificity in comparison to other diagnostic measures and its value in detecting other potentially treatable illnesses with similar presentations. The controversy has resulted from concerns about the morbidity and mortality associated with the procedure, the possibility of false-negative biopsy samples, and the benign nature of antiviral therapy. The application of CSF PCR for HSV has essentially rendered moot the argument in favor of brain biopsy. CSF PCR for HSV has a high specificity and sensitivity. Brain biopsy should be reserved for individuals with significant mass effect from necrotizing encephalitis in whom lumbar puncture represents a significant risk or in individuals for whom a high index of suspicion of HSV encephalitis remains despite a negative CSF PCR for HSV. Brain biopsy specimens should be subjected to histologic study, immunocytochemical analysis, electron microscopy, PCR, and viral culture.

Examination of the CSF reveals a mononuclear pleocytosis typically between 50 to 150 leukocytes (lymphocytes or mononuclear cells) per cubic millimeter (median, 130 cells/mm³) in more than two-thirds of patients. Occasionally, pleocytosis is not present. HSV encephalitis may result in hemorrhagic CSF. Red blood cells may be seen in the CSF, and the centrifugal fluid may appear xanthochromic. The protein content is usually slightly elevated; the median CSF protein is 80 mg/dL; however, the CSF protein is normal in 20%. The glucose level is normal or only slightly reduced. Like MRI, CSF analysis may also be useful in establishing alternative diagnoses, such as bacterial or fungal infection. Although PCR for HSV is very sensitive, attempts to isolate HSV by culture from the CSF are seldom successful. In the Collaborative Study of HSV Encephalitis, CSF was normal in 3% of biopsy-confirmed cases.

The use of blood serologic analysis for the diagnosis of HSV encephalitis is not useful. Most persons have been exposed to HSV at some time in their lives and demonstrate antibody levels. Fluctuations in the titer of antibody to HSV are commonly observed. A less than fourfold rise in titer is essentially meaningless. Additionally, in some confirmed cases of HSV encephalitis, the antibody titers to HSV fail to rise.

TREATMENT. The first antiviral therapy demonstrated to be effective for HSV encephalitis was vidarabine. Acyclovir, however, has proved to be a more potent agent in the treatment of HSV encephalitis. It is administered by intravenous infusion as 10 mg/kg given over at least an hour every 8 hours for 10 days. This agent selectively interacts with two herpesvirus-coded enzymes, thymidine kinase and DNA polymerase, giving it specificity for the herpes viruses. It is excreted by the kidney and should be administered cautiously in patients with impaired renal function. Toxic reaction is rare and includes phlebitis, rash, elevation of transaminase levels, and gastrointestinal disturbances. Neurotoxicity may be manifested by tremors, hallucinations, seizures, and altered consciousness.

HSV encephalitis is a medical emergency because of its characteristically aggressive course. Antiviral therapy with intravenous acyclovir should be administered at the time the diagnosis is considered. Treatment is best rendered in an intensive care unit. If the diagnosis cannot be confirmed, acyclovir should be discontinued.

In the presence of cerebral edema with impending brain herniation, high-dose corticosteroid therapy (4 to 6 mg of dexamethasone every 4 to 6 hours) should be given. Although a theoretical concern exists that corticostenosis will slow viral clearance, treatment of the accompanying vasogenic edema is imperative.

PROGNOSIS. The age of the patient and the level of consciousness at the time of institution of therapy determine the outcome. The best survival is observed in young individuals (younger than 30 years) with only lethargy at the time of the institution of

antiviral therapy. Patients with minor neurologic deficits may recover without severe long-term sequelae and return to normal function if antiviral therapy is instituted early. Relapse has been observed in rare patients despite seemingly adequate antiviral treatment. This relapse usually occurs within a few weeks of the resolution of the initial stage of the acute illness and often results in severe sequelae. The pathogenetic mechanisms for relapse are unknown.

477.2 Neurologic Complications of Genital Herpes

Herpetic infections below the umbilicus are typically caused by HSV-2. However, up to 15% of genital herpes may result from HSV-1 infection, presumably as a consequence of orogenital sexual practices. In one study, HSV-1, rather than HSV-2, accounted for 15% of all genital herpetic infections. When it is the consequence of HSV-2 infection, genital herpes recurs within 1 year in 80 to 90% of patients following the initial infection, whereas HSV-1 genital infections recur in only 55% in the first year of infection. Similarly, oral herpes may result from HSV-2 infection. HSV-2 is associated with intense burning, stinging, or itching pain at the site of skin blistering. Both the initial infection and recurrences may be complicated by radicular pain. The latter may result in pain radiating into the buttock, groin, genitalia, or lower extremities. This radicular pain may be misinterpreted as being the result of a lumbar disk problem when it occurs as a prodromal symptom (before the outbreak of the blistering rash) or when it occurs in the absence of an obvious rash. HSV-2 may also be associated with aseptic meningitis, autonomic (bowel, bladder, and sexual) dysfunction, and, rarely, myelitis. These neurologic complications are more common in the presence of primary genital herpes, but they may also be seen at the time of recurrence.

Symptoms of meningitis occur in approximately one-fourth of patients with primary genital herpes but rarely necessitate hospitalization. The CSF reveals mononuclear pleocytosis, mild elevation of protein, and normal or slightly reduced glucose. Clearing without residua occurs in 4 to 10 days on average. The demonstration of HSV-2 in the CSF by viral culture or PCR establishes the causal relationship. HSV-2 is the chief causative agent of Mollaret's meningitis, a recurrent aseptic meningitis with low-grade fever, headache, and myalgia. In approximately 50% of patients, transitory neurologic symptoms or signs may accompany the meningeal irritation. The CSF reveals mixed pleocytosis with leukocytes, lymphocytes, and endothelial cells (Mollaret cells) as well as an increased γ-globulin fraction. The disease remits spontaneously in several days. Careful history may indicate that the patient has concurrent genital herpes with the attacks. CSF PCR has demonstrated HSV-2. The prophylactic administration of acyclovir prevents attacks in affected patients.

The autonomic manifestations of urinary retention, constipation, and sexual impotence in association with genital herpes are less common than meningitis. Typically, these abnormalities occur in the setting of primary infection. Symptoms and signs of a sacral sensory radiculopathy sometimes accompany the autonomic changes. A direct herpetic infection of sacral autonomic structures may explain the autonomic dysfunction, but the exact pathogenesis remains uncertain. The autonomic dysfunction is reversible and generally clears in tandem with the resolution of skin and mucous membrane lesions. HSV-2 should be considered in anyone with complaints of isolated bladder, bowel, or sexual dysfunction. A thorough inspection of the genitalia may disclose ulcerations; viral culture of lesions is diagnostic. Rising antibody titers to HSV-2 may also be supportive of the diagnosis. In rare instances, transverse myelitis may be observed in association with HSV-2 infection. In adults, HSV-2 rarely produces encephalitis, although in newborns it is a major cause of meningoencephalitis. In the newborn, HSV-2 results in multiorgan systemic disease that is accompanied by herpetic lesions of the skin, eye, and mucous membranes.

In patients with frequent recurrent attacks of genital herpes, early, self-initiated treatment of recurrent lesions with oral acyclovir can be given, beginning therapy at the onset of prodromal symptoms. Alternatively, particularly if recurrences are frequent or associated with debilitation, daily prophylactic administration of acyclovir may be warranted.

477.3 Neurologic Complications of Herpes Varicella-Zoster Virus Infections

VZV is distantly related to HSV, sharing only minor antigen cross-reaction. It is the cause of chickenpox and shingles. Postviral encephalomyelitis may follow chickenpox. The estimated incidence of postviral encephalomyelitis with primary VZV infection has been estimated at 10 cases per 100,000. It has also been associated with Reye's syndrome. Herpes zoster (HZ), a dermatomal cutaneous infection, is the result of reactivation of the VZV that normally lies latent in sensory ganglia following an attack of varicella that generally occurs during childhood. In addition to its cutaneous manifestations, HZ is accompanied by neuritic symptoms and may be complicated by an array of neurologic sequelae.

EPIDEMIOLOGY. The annual incidence of herpes zoster (shingles, HZ) is estimated to be 3.4 cases per 1000 persons. Unlike varicella, HZ occurs throughout the year, with neither significant clustering of cases nor seasonal or yearly preponderance. Case exposure in HZ is rarely identified. The most important factors that influence its incidence are age and immunosuppression. HZ is rare in childhood. Its frequency is relatively constant between the ages of 20 and 50 years (approximately 2.5 cases per 1000 persons annually), and thereafter its incidence is doubled in those between ages 50 and 60 years and redoubled in those between ages 80 and 90 years. Impaired cell-mediated immunity in Hodgkin's disease and other lymphoreticular malignancies, the administration of cytotoxic drugs and corticosteroids, radiation therapy, or infection with human immunodeficiency virus (HIV), predisposes to the development of HZ. Occasionally, a history of neoplasm, radiation exposure, or physical injury in the proximity of the affected dorsal root ganglion or nerve is elicited. Immunosuppression predisposes to spread of virus beyond the ganglion nerve–dermatome unit into the central nervous system or systemically. It is likely that widespread introduction of varicella vaccination will decrease this incidence of both chickenpox and HZ.

PATHOLOGY AND PATHOGENESIS. Considerable evidence has indicated that VZV is latent in ganglionic satellite cells rather than neurons. Once latent virus reactivates, it can spread within the sensory ganglion and travel centrifugally over the peripheral nerve processes, eventually seeding the skin and producing a dermatomal vesicular rash. Cell-mediated defenses, rather than humoral immunity, are critically involved in protecting the host during HZ. Pathologically, acutely infected dorsal root ganglia and nerve show the presence of a mononuclear inflammatory response, neuronal degeneration with intranuclear Cowdry type A inclusion bodies, and HZV infection of local satellite cells. In more severe cases, dorsal root ganglia above and below the primarily affected ganglion also show active herpetic infection.

CLINICAL MANIFESTATIONS. Prodromal sensory symptoms include dermatomal pain, itching, or paresthesias, often preceding by 2 to 5 days the eruption of the segmental rash. The early pain of HZ may be confused with other types of neuropathic or visceral pain. Rarely, no rash appears, but the role of VZV is suggested by a rise in antibody titers (*zoster sine herpete*). Typically, the rash of HZ involves one dermatome and remains unilateral. Fifty per cent of rashes occur over the trunk, particularly from the third thoracic to the second lumbar segments. *Zona* refers to the circling or belt-like lesions on the trunk. Twenty per cent of HZ involves the head, usually in the distribution of the first (ophthalmic) division of the trigeminal nerve. Other cranial nerves may be affected. Approximately 15% of HZ rashes involve the arms, and a similar number involves the legs. A small focus of satellite skin lesions may occur at other locations. The rash itself initially consists of erythematous macules that vesiculate over 12 to 24 hours. New vesicles may appear over 2 days. Typically, the vesicular fluid develops a purulent appearance within 72 hours, and within 1 week these pustules

begin to dry. Crusting takes place by 10 to 12 days, and the crusts generally fall off in 2 to 3 weeks. In the immunocompromised host, this time course may be protracted. In uncomplicated cases, the rash heals with a variable degree of superficial scarring, at times leaving areas of hypopigmentation or depigmentation. These affected skin regions may be anesthetic. More severe cases may leave denervation of a large segment involving one or several dermatomes. HZ in patients younger than 50 years should suggest the possibility of an underlying immunosuppressive condition, in particular, AIDS.

The ophthalmic division of the trigeminal nerve is the cranial nerve most commonly affected. This is not surprising, as VZV latency may be demonstrated in the trigeminal ganglia of more than 80% of elderly persons. HZ in this location may be complicated by spread to orbital structures, resulting in acute and long-term ocular sequelae. Spread of cutaneous rash along the bridge of the nose to its tip should be taken as a signal of impending ocular infection (*herpes zoster ophthalmicus,* HZO), prompting early ophthalmologic consultation. This complication is more common in immunosuppressed patients; HZO occurs in 5 to 15% of all HIV-seropositive patients. Facial palsy, with or without accompanying loss of taste on the anterior two-thirds of the tongue, may accompany either otic HZ (Ramsay Hunt syndrome), with rash confined to a segment of the ear, or the second and third cervical dermatomes (cervical collar HZ). Occasionally, infection of the ninth and tenth or fifth cranial nerve may precede facial weakness. As with other motor syndromes (see below), weakness is often delayed for a variable period after appearance of the rash. Eighth nerve dysfunction with sensorineural hearing loss or vertigo occurs in the same setting as facial palsy but with less frequency. HZ may rarely cause facial palsy in the absence of rash (zoster sine herpete). HZ of the ninth and tenth cranial nerves is unusual and may be overlooked without a careful search for the pharyngeal rash or ipsilateral laryngeal or pharyngeal palsy.

HZ of the extremities or trunk can also be complicated by segmental motor weakness, the motor loss usually corresponding to the involved cutaneous dermatome. Weakness characteristically develops from a few days to 2 weeks after the onset of rash. Onset is characteristically abrupt, occurring over hours to 1 or 2 days with little or no subsequent deterioration. Weakness resolves in about 85% of cases, but may leave a permanent paralysis within the myotome.

An unusual complication of HZ that is more frequently observed in the immunosuppressed host is myelitis. This complication results from direct involvement of the spinal cord by HZ and is typically most severe at the level of the rash, although it may extend to higher levels. The most common clinical manifestations are motor weakness and bladder dysfunction generally occurring as the rash resolves. Reflex abnormalities and sensory loss below the level of the rash may be observed. In severe cases, the lesion may result in clinical findings suggestive of cord transection. Alternatively, a Brown-Séquard syndrome may be observed. Other signs include mild or transient asymmetrical reflexes, Babinski's signs, and sensory disturbance. Spinal MRI is essential in excluding other possible etiologies.

At least three types of brain involvement may complicate HZ: diffuse encephalitis, focal parenchymal infection, and vasculitis. Headache, stiff neck, and mild diffuse encephalitis often accompany acute HZ but are difficult to distinguish from the effects of fever, sepsis, narcotic analgesics, and other underlying medical problems. Most such patients recover fully. In more severe diffuse encephalitis, chances for recovery may also be good if other complications of the disease do not intervene. The clinical picture is that of acute or subacute lethargy or delirium accompanied by CSF pleocytosis with few focal features.

Focal VZV encephalitis is a rare central nervous system (CNS) complication of VZV most often observed in immunosuppressed patients. The cerebral lesions of focal VZV encephalitis chiefly involve the white matter. This encephalitis may occur long after the rash. Its clinical and radiographic appearance may be mistaken for progressive multifocal leukoencephalopathy. Brain biopsy is essential for diagnosis, allowing identification of Cowdry type A inclusions or of VZV antigens or nucleic acids.

Cerebral vasculitis is the most common serious postzoster CNS complication. Affected patients characteristically develop delayed contralateral hemiplegic strokes following trigeminal ophthalmic division HZ. The onset of cerebral dysfunction can occur as long as 6 months after rash, with a mean interval of 7 weeks. Pathologic studies reveal inflammation or occlusion of the internal carotid artery and its major branches ipsilateral to the rash. More widespread cerebral vasculitis following HZ in other locations has also been reported. The pathogenesis is not well understood. Viral nucleocapsids and viral antigens can be found within affected vessels, suggesting a direct infection of arterial walls. These vessels are innervated by VZV-infected ganglia. Inflammation and thrombosis undoubtedly contribute to the pathogenesis. Arteriographic evidence of vasculitis or occlusions in the involved vessels and the clinical setting usually allow diagnosis.

Postherpetic neuralgia is a disabling consequence of HZ. The incidence of postherpetic neuralgia ranges between 15 and 75%. Its frequency depends on the clinical definition of the syndrome and the patient population studied. Pain persisting for more than 1 year is present in approximately 3 to 5% of patients following HZ. Age is an important factor in the appearance of postherpetic neuralgia. It develops almost exclusively in persons older than 50 years. Over the age of 60 years, about one-half of patients develop postherpetic neuralgia. The pain has been characterized as two types: (1) a steady burning or boring pain and (2) paroxysmal pain with a lancinating quality. Both types may occur together and be aggravated by touch, including the simple contact of clothing. Treatment strategies include the use of amitriptyline, carbamazepine, gabapentin, topical capsaicin, and transcutaneous nerve stimulators. Success with these treatments is generally limited.

DIAGNOSIS. Characteristic dermatomal distribution and the evolution of the vesicular rash of HZ are diagnostic. Occasionally, HZ may be confused with HSV infection. Features helpful in distinguishing between the two include the dermatomal distribution of HZ and the association with scarring and postherpetic pain. In both HZ and HSV, cells obtained from the base of the lesion, air-dried and stained with Wright or Giemsa stain (Tzanck test) reveal multinucleated giant cells. Fluid scraped from the base of the vesicle and examined by direct fluorescent antibody technique may rapidly establish the diagnosis or viral cultures may be employed. The diagnosis of zoster sine herpete remains difficult. Thorough evaluation for an occult rash is of paramount importance. In many instances, this diagnosis remains presumptive due to a failure to apply a thorough diagnostic evaluation.

TREATMENT. The goals of therapy of HZ are to suppress the acute infection, prevent the spread of the infection to the nervous system, and prevent postherpetic neuralgia. The available means to accomplish these goals consist of using antiviral drugs to interrupt viral replication and corticosteroids to modify local inflammatory responses. Aggressive therapy is warranted in the immunosuppressed patient and in those with involvement of the ophthalmic division of the trigeminal nerve. Systemic therapy in these patients consists of intravenous acyclovir (10 mg/kg of body weight three times a day for 7 days). In the immunosuppressed host, particularly in patients with AIDS, oral maintenance for secondary prophylaxis should be employed. A regimen of acyclovir, 800 mg given three to five times a day, reduces recurrence rates. Famciclovir, 500 mg three times a day, may prove to be an effective alternative. Except in immunosuppressed patients and those with HZ ophthalmicus, an oral regimen of acyclovir may be employed. Acyclovir, 800 mg five times daily, decreases the acute pain and shortens healing time. The use of concomitant corticosteroid therapy to prevent postherpetic neuralgia remains controversial. The role of antiviral therapy in cerebral vasculitis or the other neurologic complications of HZ remains uncertain. However, the presence of viral antigen in the affected sites provides ample justification for their use. Similarly, few data are available on the value of the administration of corticosteroids for these complications.

477.4 Neurologic Complications of Cytomegalovirus, Epstein-Barr Virus, and Simian Herpes Virus Infection

CYTOMEGALOVIRUS

Human cytomegalovirus (CMV) is a ubiquitous herpesvirus acquired throughout life. In children, CMV is an important and rela-

tively common cause of congenital neurologic deficit. In the United States, 60 to 80% of adults have serologic evidence of infection. Primary infection is usually asymptomatic in young, healthy adults but may be associated with a transient mononucleosis-like syndrome. CMV results in major neurologic disability in the setting of immunosuppression, particularly in AIDS. In addition to retinitis, CMV may involve the brain, spinal cord, and peripheral nerves.

CMV ENCEPHALITIS. CMV encephalitis in AIDS has several presentations. The most typical presentation is subacute diffuse encephalopathy evolving over weeks, which is characterized by headache, impaired cognition and sensorium, apathy, and social withdrawal. Neurologic examination reveals abnormal mentation and variable motor features, including hyperreflexia, ataxia, and weakness. CMV ventriculitis is characteristically present and is often associated with cranial neuropathies, nystagmus, and progressive ventricular enlargement. Other features may suggest brain stem encephalitis, including internuclear ophthalmoplegia, cranial nerve palsies, gaze paresis, ataxia, and tetraparesis. On rare occasions, CMV may present as a cerebral mass lesion. Other presentations include cerebral infarction resulting from CMV vasculitis, acute subarachnoid hemorrhage, and intracerebral hemorrhage. Virtually all patients with CMV encephalitis have systemic CMV infection. CMV myelitis, polyradiculitis, and multifocal neuritis may also be seen with CMV encephalitis. Distinctive retinal lesions can often be seen ophthalmoscopically (see Chapter 386).

Cerebral imaging studies are of limited sensitivity and low specificity in patients with CMV encephalitis. Ependymal or meningeal enhancement, as well as areas of focal infarction or necrosis, may be visualized. Progressive ventricular enlargement should suggest CMV ventriculitis. CSF findings are variable. Most patients have protein elevation. Glucose levels may be normal or decreased. Leukocytes may be absent, but seizure pleocytosis is usual. Marked pleocytosis with polymorphonuclear leukocytes may occur in patients with CMV ventriculitis. CMV can rarely be cultured from CSF or detected by PCR.

NECROTIZING MYELITIS. Necrotizing myelitis due to CMV in HIV-infected patients is most commonly seen in association with polyradiculitis. Occasional cases of necrotizing myelitis in the absence of a typical polyradiculitis syndrome have been described, presenting with acute or progressive paraplegia and disturbances of urinary and rectal sphincter functions. Reflexes are preserved or enhanced in the legs unless concurrent neuropathy is present. A sensory level may be demonstrable.

POLYRADICULOMYELITIS. Neuromuscular pathology due to CMV has been found in approximately one-fourth of patients dying of AIDS, predominantly localized to perineurial and epineurial regions. CMV polyradiculomyelitis in HIV-infected patients presents subacutely over days to a few weeks. Initial symptoms of paresthesias or dysesthetic pain localized to perineal and lower extremity regions are followed by a rapidly progressive paraparesis with hypotonia and diminished or absent lower extremity reflexes. Urinary retention is characteristic, and rectal sphincter incontinence is common. Variable sensory findings are overshadowed by the motor features. Babinski's signs and diminished sensation below a discrete level across the trunk may indicate an associated myelitis. With time, symptoms progress by ascending to involve the upper limbs and sometimes the cranial nerves. The CSF usually reveals polymorphonuclear pleocytosis and prominent elevation of protein levels. Hypoglycorrhachia is often present. Spinal MRI may be normal or may reveal enhancement of the conus medullaris, cauda equina, meninges, and nerve roots. Electrophysiologic studies reveal axonal neuropathy with evidence of acute denervation. Variable slowing of nerve conduction may also be present.

The appearance of acute cauda equina syndrome in a patient with AIDS is suggestive of CMV when polymorphonuclear pleocytosis is present in CSF; however, the syndrome is not pathognomonic. Other conditions that may produce a cauda equina syndrome in AIDS patients include lymphomatous meningitis, syphilis, toxoplasmosis, other herpesviruses, and cryptococcal or bacterial meningitis. Progressive multifocal motor and sensory neuropathy that evolves over weeks to months has also been seen with CMV infection. Paresthesia and dysesthesia are quickly followed by prominent motor weakness, which involves both upper and lower limbs asymmetrically. Neurogenic atrophy may be prominent.

Nerve biopsy reveals necrotizing neuritis with mononuclear and polymorphonuclear infiltrates and cytomegalocytes localized around endoneurial capillaries in nerve trunks and roots. Necrotizing arteritis may be present

CMV neurologic complications should be treated with ganciclovir or foscarnet; however, the evidence of their efficacy in these conditions is chiefly limited to case reports and small series. The emergence of CMV strains resistant to both agents has been observed, and CMV encephalitis has developed in the presence of maintenance ganciclovir therapy for CMV retinitis.

EPSTEIN-BARR VIRUS

Epstein-Barr virus (EBV), the cause of infectious mononucleosis, is distributed worldwide. Its acquisition is dependent on population density and socioeconomic status. Individuals in areas of high population density and lower social strata acquire the virus in early childhood. However, seroepidemiologic studies indicate that virtually all persons are infected by EBV by age 30 years.

Neurologic manifestations occur in 1 to 5% of patients with primary EBV infection and may be the only prominent clinical manifestations. The most common neurologic disorder associated with infectious mononucleosis is meningoencephalitis. This complication is rare in early childhood and most often is observed in persons between the ages of 15 and 25 years. Onset may be gradual over several days or explosive. Fever, headache, mild stiff neck, confusion, lethargy, seizures, and hyperreflexia are the most typical features. On occasion, focal neurologic features, including hemiparesis, focal seizures, and cerebellar and brain stem findings, may be detected. The prognosis of EBV meningoencephalitis is excellent, with complete resolution anticipated in 1 to 2 weeks.

SIMIAN HERPES (B VIRUS, HERPESVIRUS SIMIAE)

B virus is a close relative of the human herpes simplex viruses. Serologic studies in monkeys have demonstrated high rates of infection and, on rare occasion, transmission to man has been reported by contamination, typically occurring in a research laboratory. Between 1973 and 1985, 25 cases of B virus were reported in man. The mortality rate was 72% and severe neurologic sequelae were observed in the majority of the survivors. Human-to-human transmission has been reported in a household contact. Human B virus infection most commonly presents as rapidly ascending encephalomyelitis.

Fodor PA, Levin MJ, Weinberg M, et al: Atypical herpes simplex virus encephalitis diagnosed by PCR amplification of viral DNA from CSF. Neurology 51:554–559, 1998. *As many as one fifth of patients with herpes simplex virus encephalitis have mild or atypical disease.*

478 RABIES

Avindra Nath ■ Joseph R. Berger

DEFINITION. Rabies is a viral infection with nearly worldwide distribution that affects principally wild and domestic animals; however, it also involves humans, in which case it results in devastating, almost invariably fatal encephalitis.

ETIOLOGY. Rabies virus is a bullet-shaped, enveloped, single-strand RNA virus classified in the Rhabdoviridae family (*rhabdos,* Greek for "rod") and Lyssavirus genus (*lyssa,* Greek for "frenzy"). It has particular neurotropic properties, and unlike many of the other viruses causing acute encephalitis, it appears to require central nervous system (CNS) infection as an essential part of its life cycle.

PATHOGENESIS. Viral transmission to both animals and humans characteristically results from the bite of a rabid animal, although cases of transmission by aerosol in the laboratory or in a bat cave and by transplanted infected corneal tissue have also been recorded.

Once the virus breaches the protective epithelium, it reaches the CNS via peripheral nerves, exploiting retrograde axoplasmic transport. The interval between the bite and the onset of disease ranges from days to a year or more, but in most cases it lasts 1 to 2 months. This delay may relate to amplification of the virus in peripheral tissues, particularly skeletal muscle, before it gains access to the CNS through motor and sensory nerves. During this delay, the virus can be eliminated by host immune mechanisms. Indeed, it is this delay that affords an opportunity for prophylactic postexposure immunization after the rabid animal bite. Once virus enters peripheral and CNS pathways, immune defenses are unable to suppress further replication and spread of infection, which includes axoplasmic transport and, perhaps, transsynaptic transmission.

The CNS is involved in the subsequent transmission of the virus by infected animals in two essential ways: (1) infection of certain brain regions causes characteristic behavioral changes in the rabid animal, leading to increased biting activity; and (2) antegrade or centrifugal transport of the virus from the brain to highly innervated areas (e.g., salivary glands, cornea, and skin) leads to virus shedding. In concert, these two aspects of infection ensure transmission and survival of the virus in the wild. They also have practical diagnostic implications for the human disease. The characteristic altered behavior in humans often results in a distinct clinical picture that distinguishes rabies from other viral encephalitides. Antegrade virus transport also affords a means of diagnosing rabies by isolation from saliva or immunohistochemical staining of infected cutaneous nerves innervating hair follicles. Humoral immune responses and neutralizing antibodies generated by rabies vaccine are most effective in tempering the virus; cell-mediated immune responses play only a minor role.

PATHOLOGY. Pathologic findings include both nonspecific and specific abnormalities. A considerable discrepancy often occurs between the degree of pathologic change, particularly neuronal loss, and the severity of antemortem clinical findings. Nonspecific changes include perivascular mononuclear infiltrates and microglial activation, although inflammation may be scant in relation to the widespread distribution of infected cells detected immunohistochemically. Similarly, neuronal destruction is less prominent than the abundance of viral antigen, which is located principally in neurons but also in astrocytes. More specific changes include the presence of Negri bodies, which are eosinophilic neuronal intracytoplasmic inclusion bodies composed of viral nucleoprotein. Negri bodies are pathognomonic of rabies virus infection. At autopsy, infection is usually widespread in the brain, but the brain stem, spinal cord, hippocampus, basal ganglia, cortex, and other structures are also prominently involved. The relation of virus infection of neurons and the attendant inflammatory reaction to the clinical manifestations remains incompletely understood. Rabies infection of neurons may alter their membrane properties or synaptic transmission. Patients eventually manifest widespread brain dysfunction with impairment of respiratory and autonomic control owing to brain stem involvement, which leads to death.

EPIDEMIOLOGY. The epidemiology of rabies varies in different parts of the world, falling into two patterns. In *sylvatic rabies,* infection is maintained in wildlife reservoirs. Thus, in the United States, rabies is endemic in the striped skunk in the midwestern states and in California, in the raccoon in the southeastern and mid-Atlantic states (and now invading northern Kentucky), in the red fox in northern New York and adjacent regions of Canada, and in the gray fox in parts of the southwestern states; bat rabies has a wide geographic range. Similarly, in western Europe, human rabies is rare, and it more often results from direct contact with wildlife than from contact with domestic dogs or cats. This pattern contrasts with that in much of Asia, Africa, and Latin America, where *urban rabies* is maintained as an epizootic infection in the domestic dog, and human disease is far more common. Viral strains differ among various animal hosts.

CLINICAL MANIFESTATIONS. After an incubation period averaging 1 to 2 months, clinical rabies usually begins with a prodromal phase of nonspecific symptoms of malaise, fever, and headache, but more specific local symptoms are present at the site of the original bite. These include itching, paresthesia, or other sensations that begin in the area of the healed wound and then spread to a wider region, reflecting ganglioneuritis. No accompanying sensory loss is present.

Within a few days, the full-blown illness begins, taking one of two forms: encephalitic (*furious*) or paralytic (*dumb*) rabies, perhaps depending on the source and strain of the infecting virus. In its initial phase, encephalitic rabies is often distinguished from other viral infections by irritability and hyperactivity of a number of automatic reflexes. Periods of lucidity may alternate with confusion and seeming intense anxiety precipitated by internal or external stimuli. Hydrophobia, with reflexive intense contraction of the diaphragm and accessory respiratory and other muscles, is induced on attempts to drink, or even by the mere sight of water. Similarly, blowing or fanning air on the chest may induce intense laryngeal, pharyngeal, or other muscle spasms (aerophobia). High fever persists throughout the illness. Patients may also have spontaneous inspiratory spasms and autonomic dysfunction (hypersalivation, non-reactive pupils, and piloerection). Seizures are rare.

Paralytic rabies is less common and is often misdiagnosed. Patients present with weakness, usually beginning in the bitten extremity and spreading to involve all four limbs and the facial muscles early in the course. Both consciousness and sensory function are spared. Areflexia often suggests Guillain-Barré syndrome. As the disease progresses, it may converge with the encephalitic form and be accompanied by irritative phenomena. Both forms evolve into lethargy and coma with prominent respiratory and cardiovascular dysfunction. Tachycardia, bradycardia, ectopic heart rhythms, and irregular breathing patterns such as cluster or periodic respirations. Patients die of respiratory failure or cardiovascular collapse within a mean interval of 4 to 7 days from onset. Intensive supportive care may extend survival in rare cases. Rare patients with partial vaccine-induced immunity have been reported to survive with intensive care.

DIAGNOSIS. Rabies is usually suspected on the basis of a history of animal bite or other exposure. But in as many as one-third of cases, no such history is obtained. Definitive antemortem diagnosis is established by immunohistochemical identification of rabies virus antigen in hair follicle nerve endings of biopsied skin, usually obtained from the nape of the neck. Isolation of virus from saliva or the presence of antirabies antibodies in blood in the absence of vaccination or in the cerebrospinal fluid may also be used to establish diagnosis. Postmortem diagnosis is usually made by immunohistochemical examination of the brain.

The differential diagnosis depends on the clinical presentation and the epidemiologic setting. In the case of paralytic rabies, diagnosis is most often confused with Guillain-Barré syndrome, poliomyelitis, or other neuropathies or myelopathies, whereas the encephalitic form must be differentiated from other viral and infectious encephalitides, tetanus, and toxic encephalopathies. In geographic regions where vaccine is prepared using neural tissue (still the practice in many regions of the world with the highest rates of rabies), allergic encephalomyelitis remains a principal differential diagnosis.

TREATMENT AND PREVENTION. Established CNS disease cannot be cured. Disease prevention relies on public health measures to reduce animal reservoirs and on postexposure immune prophylaxis to abort viral penetration of the CNS after a rabid bite or other contact. Although clinical rabies is a rare disease in United States and western Europe, the need to consider active prophylaxis is a common clinical issue. The physician first determines the type of possible exposure: an open wound or disrupted mucous membrane exposed to saliva may warrant postexposure prophylaxis, whereas contact of saliva with intact skin may not. The first step in management is to administer prompt local wound care, thoroughly washing the wound with soap and water, then applying iodine or 70% ethanol. The epidemiologic setting is important in determining the likelihood that the biting animal might be rabid and often requires consultation with local health authorities to ascertain which animals carry rabies in the geographic setting. In the absence of previous vaccination, both passive (rabies immune globulin of human origin) and active (diploid cell vaccines) immunizations are administered. Rabies immunoglobulin should be injected in and around the wound and should not be administered into the same limb in which the vaccine is given. Safe, tissue culture–derived vaccines are now available, which have a low incidence of major adverse reactions in contrast to those seen with earlier, nerve tissue–derived vaccines.

Fishbein DB, Robinson LE: Rabies. N Engl J Med 29:1632, 1993. *An outstanding review of the epidemiology and management of rabies and rabies exposure.*

Hemachudha T, Phuapradit P: Rabies. Curr Opin Neurol 10:260–267, 1997. *A valuable review of the clinical neurologic aspects of rabies.*

479 SLOW VIRUS INFECTIONS

479.1 Human Immunodeficiency Virus (see also Chapter 411)

Joseph R. Berger ■ Avindra Nath

INCIDENCE AND EPIDEMIOLOGIC CHARACTERISTICS. Neurologic disease occurring with human immunodeficiency virus (HIV) infection is common, debilitating, and life-threatening. In 40 to 70% of all persons infected with HIV, symptomatic neurologic disease will develop. Neurologic disease typically occurs in the setting of profound immunosuppression, but it may herald acquired immunodeficiency syndrome (AIDS) in 10–20% of HIV-seropositive persons. Findings of autopsy studies suggest a higher frequency of neurologic disease than those of clinical studies. In some series, neuropathologic abnormalities have been observed in more than 90% of patients dying with AIDS. Careful neurologic examination, even in the absence of specific complaints by the HIV-infected patient, frequently finds evidence of central or peripheral nervous system dysfunction.

SPECTRUM OF NEUROLOGIC DISEASE. The spectrum of neurologic disorders that complicates HIV-1 is extremely diverse. Any part of the neuraxis may be affected. Classification of these neurologic illnesses can be divided broadly into those occurring as a direct result of HIV-1 (primary) and those that result from other identifiable causes (secondary), which are typically the consequence of immunosuppression. Primary HIV-associated disorders include encephalopathy, myelopathy, peripheral neuropathy, and myopathy. Common secondary complications, chiefly the result of severe abnormalities of cellular immunity, include cerebral toxoplasmosis, cryptococcal meningitis, cytomegalovirus (CMV) infection, and progressive multifocal leukoencephalopathy (PML). Other secondary neurologic disorders include primary (usually primary central nervous system lymphoma) and metastatic neoplasms, drug related neurologic complications, metabolic-nutritional disorders, and cerebrovascular complications.

Multiple neurologic illnesses frequently coexist in a patient with AIDS. Also, common neurologic disorders unrelated to HIV-1, such as migraine headache, alcoholic and diabetic peripheral neuropathies, and herniated vertebral disks with associated cervical and lumbar radiculopathies, should always be considered in the differential diagnosis of the patient with AIDS presenting with neurologic symptoms.

HIV DEMENTIA

EPIDEMIOLOGIC CHARACTERISTICS. HIV dementia (also referred to as AIDS dementia complex, subacute encephalitis, HIV encephalopathy, multinucleate giant cell encephalitis, and HIV-1-associated cognitive/motor complex) increases in frequency in advanced stages of AIDS. The onset and progression of HIV dementia are variable. Dementia usually occurs late in HIV disease, after the patient has had other AIDS defining illnesses at a time when CD4 lymphocyte counts are below 200/mm³. Occasionally, dementia may be the first AIDS defining illness. The neurologic deficits usually progress insidiously, although rapid progression may occur. Retrospective studies have reported the prevalence of HIV dementia during the late stages of HIV disease in the range of 7.5% to 27%. HIV dementia is estimated to occur annually in between 7% and 14% of patients after the diagnosis of AIDS.

CLINICAL FEATURES. The symptoms of HIV dementia can be subdivided into three main categories: cognitive, motor, and behavioral. The primary cognitive symptom is forgetfulness, associated with slowed mental and motor abilities. Impaired concentration is common and patients often complain of difficulty in reading. Lower extremity weakness and impaired balance are among early motor signs. Other features of the illness that may be observed include abnormal smooth ocular pursuit, tremors of the upper extremities, impaired coordination, and increased motor tone. The most commonly observed behavioral symptoms are apathy and social withdrawal, which are often mistakenly diagnosed as depression. Occasionally organic psychosis, such as acute mania, may be a primary manifestation of HIV dementia.

Early in the course of HIV dementia, symptoms and signs may be too subtle to establish a definitive clinical diagnosis. Neuropsychological tests are useful in demonstrating early cognitive dysfunction and also provide quantitative markers of disease progression. With advanced disease, the cognitive impairment becomes more obvious. Psychomotor retardation and marked behavioral abnormalities are generally observed. Clinical features at this stage of the illness may include paraparesis from concomitant HIV-associated myelopathy, incontinence, and seizures. The Memorial Sloan Kettering staging system for HIV dementia classifies patients' condition from normal (grade 0) to end-stage vegetative state (grade 4). Subclinical dementia (grade 0.5) presents a diagnostic challenge. Individuals so classified typically present with equivocal cognitive complaints, accompanied by a relatively normal neurologic examination result. Whether individuals with equivocal features of HIV dementia invariably progress to a more severe form of dementia remains uncertain.

DIAGNOSTIC STUDIES. There are no laboratory or neuroimaging study results that are specific for HIV dementia. This disorder is currently a diagnosis of exclusion. Formal neuropsychological testing is important in determining the nature and extent of cognitive impairment. Blood and cerebrospinal fluid (CSF) studies (e.g., Venereal Disease Research Laboratory [VDRL] test, cryptococcal antigen, microbiologic cultures are essential to screen for systemic infections. CSF abnormalities are frequently present in HIV dementia: elevated total protein concentration (usually <65 mg/dL), mild pleocytosis (<20 mononuclear cells/mm³), increased total immunoglobulin fraction, and presence of oligoclonal bands. However, these CSF abnormalities are also seen in neurologically asymptomatic patients with HIV infection. Elevations of CSF markers of immune activation, such as β_2-microglobulin, neopterin, and quinolinic acid, correlate with the presence of HIV dementia.

Radiologic studies are necessary for excluding other infectious or neoplastic processes and provide information supporting the diagnosis of HIV dementia. Neuroimaging study results generally show a variable amount of cerebral atrophy, ventricular enlargement, and diffuse or multifocal white matter abnormalities (Fig. 479–1).

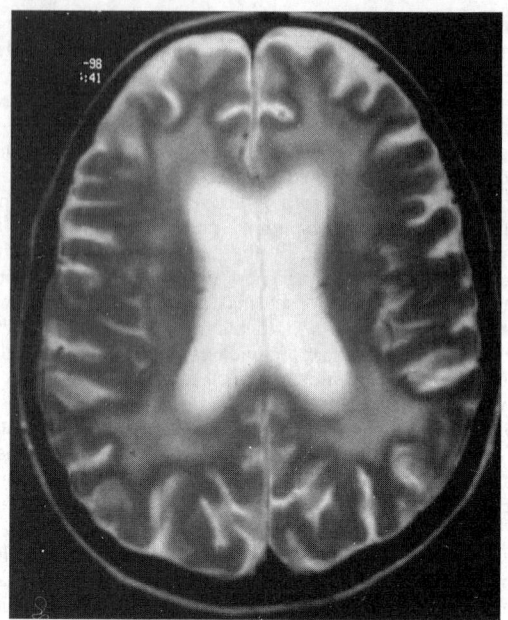

FIGURE 479–1 ■ MRI of the brain in HIV dementia in a 44-year-old woman. This T2-weighted image reveals bilaterally symmetrical, confluent, hyperintense signal abnormalities in the white matter. Sulcal widening and central atrophy are also apparent. MRI = magnetic resonance imaging; HIV = human immunodeficiency virus.

These findings are non-specific. A significant correlation occurs between the extent of cerebral atrophy, particularly central atrophy, indicated on brain magnetic resonance imaging (MRI) scans and the severity of HIV dementia. The clinical features of HIV dementia suggest predominantly subcortical abnormality: psychomotor slowing, bradykinesia, impaired manual dexterity, postural instability, gait abnormalities, rigidity, facial masking, and hypophonia.

PATHOLOGY. A spectrum of neuropathologic abnormalities has been described in patients with HIV dementia, including multinucleate giant cell and other inflammatory cell infiltration, reactive gliosis, and diffuse white matter pallor. The most important pathologic features are multiple foci of microglia, macrophages, and multinucleate giant cells (Fig. 479–2). Substantial neuronal loss may be seen. The pathologic alterations in the brain of patients with HIV dementia are often less prominent than their clinical symptoms would predict. Even in the face of severe dementia, microglial nodules and non-specific white matter pallor may be

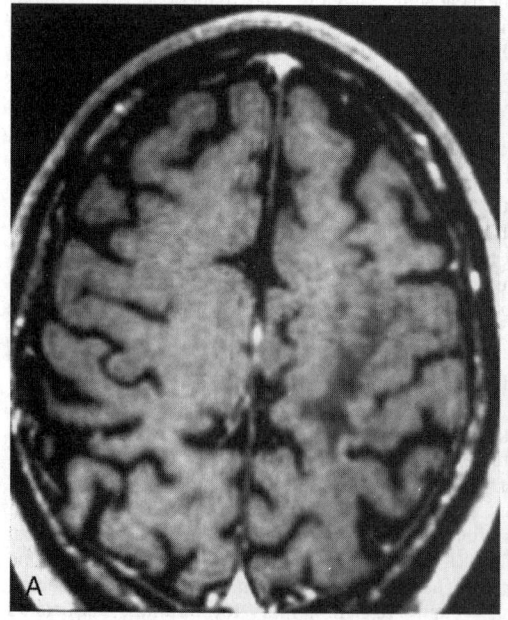
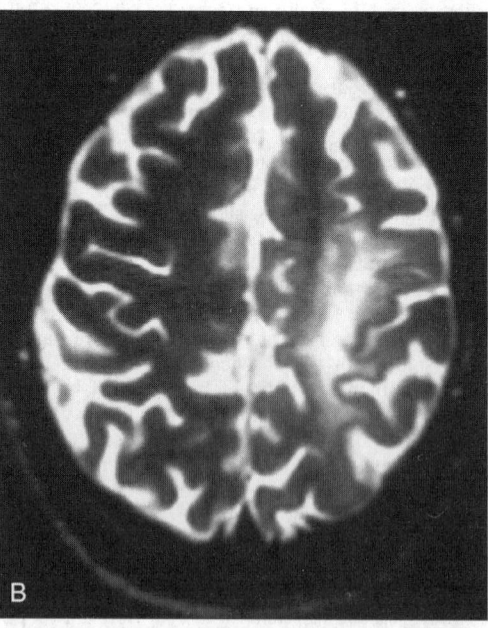

FIGURE 479–2 ■ Result of cranial magnetic resonance image of PML. The T1-weighted image (A) shows a hypointense signal abnormality of the left frontal lobe white matter. On T2-weighted sequence imaging (B), the lesion is hyperintense. PML = progressive multifocal leukoencephalopathy.

the only pathologic findings observed. At autopsy, HIV-associated vacuolar myelopathy is not often present in patients with HIV dementia and may account for some associated neurologic deficits including a spastic-ataxic gait, impaired vibratory and position sense in distal lower extremities, and bladder and bowel incontinence (see below).

PATHOGENESIS. The identification of HIV as the pathogenetic agent in AIDS made this an obvious candidate as the cause of HIV dementia. Although HIV invasion of the central nervous system may occur early after primary infection, it is uncertain what mediates the passage of the virus into the brain. HIV may be carried into the brain by infected peripheral monocytes, may be transported by infected T cells through a disrupted blood-brain barrier, or may directly penetrate endothelial cells. Although the virus does not infect neurons in any substantial quantity, there is a correlation between brain viral load and dementia. The mechanism by which the HIV affects the brain is not clear. The following are among the several possibilities (1) a cascade of events initiated by HIV protein products, resulting in release of cytokines and chemokines from infected brain microglial cells, leading to dysfunction and death of neurons; (2) activation of the N-methyl-D-aspartate (NMDA) receptors, similar to that described in other neurodegenerative disorders. Support for this hypothesis is provided by experiments showing that the neurotoxicity induced by some viral proteins can be blocked in vitro by N-methyl-D-aspartate antagonists and glutamate depletion.

TREATMENT. Although the pathogenesis of HIV dementia remains obscure, HIV clearly plays an important role, either by direct or indirect mechanisms. The reverse transcriptase inhibitors zidovudine and didanosine in relatively high doses have been demonstrated to be benefical for this HIV dementia. Anecdotal reports suggest a very beneficial response to highly active antiretroviral therapy. Several experimental agents are under investigation in the treatment of HIV dementia including pentoxifylline (tumor necrosis factor antagonist) and memantine (an N-methyl-D-aspartate antagonist).

HIV-ASSOCIATED MYELOPATHY

CLINICAL FEATURES. Patients with HIV-associated vacuolar myelopathy generally report a slowly progressive painless gait disturbance with leg stiffness. This disorder is most often seen in advanced AIDS and may not be recognized as a significant contributor to a person's bedridden status without careful neurologic examination. Lower extremity sensory complaints and sphincter abnormalities are variably present. Neurologic signs include spastic paraparesis, poor tandem gait, hyperreflexia of both upper and lower extremities, presence of Babinski and Hoffmann's signs, and mild sensory impairment. The sensory examination indicates that vibratory and position sense is disproportionately affected in comparison to pinprick, temperature, and light touch. A discrete sensory level is unusual and should suggest other causes of the myelopathy. HIV myelopathy is seen in up to 40% of cases at autopsy. A wide spectrum of causes of myelopathy in HIV infection has been observed (Table 479–1), and these need to be considered in the differential diagnosis.

Laboratory studies for HIV-infected persons with myelopathy, as a matter of routine, should include serum vitamin B_{12} levels and syphilis and human T-lymphocyte virus 1 HTLV-1 serologic analysis. Magnetic resonance imaging (MRI) of the spine is essential. A lumbar puncture with CSF analysis that includes viral cultures and polymerase chain reaction for cytomegalovirus, herpes simplex, and herpes zoster-varicella is warranted when abnormal meningeal enhancement or intramedullary signal abnormality is observed in the absence of mass effect or when the MRI finding is normal. With the demonstration of an intra- or extra-axial mass lesion, particularly with spinal block, a biopsy should be strongly considered. Typically the spinal MRI is normal in HIV-associated vacuolar myelopathy, but hyperintense signal abnormalities may be observed within the substance of the thoracic cord. Like that of HIV dementia, the diagnosis of HIV-associated vacuolar myelopathy is one of exclusion.

PATHOLOGIC CHARACTERISTICS AND PATHOGENESIS. The pathologic findings of HIV myelopathy include vacuolization of myelin sheaths, due to the accumulation of foamy macrophages and

Table 479–1 ■ DISEASE OF THE SPINAL CORD WITH HIV INFECTION

Infectious
Viral
 HIV
 Cytomegalovirus
 Herpes simplex, types 1 and 2
 Herpes zoster-varicella
 HTLV-1
 Measles
 PML
Bacterial
 Mycobacterium tuberculosis
 Pseudomonas cepacia
 T. pallidum
 Mixed with epidural abscess
Fungal
 Nocardia
 Cryptococcus
 Aspergillus
 Other
Parasitic
 Toxoplasma gondii
Neoplastic
 Primary CNS lymphoma
 Metastatic lymphoma
 Astrocytoma/glioma
 Plasmacytoma
Vascular
 Necrotizing vasculitis
 Disseminated intravascular coagulation
Metabolic
 Vitamin B_{12} deficiency

HIV = human immunodefficiency virus; HTLV-1 = human T-lymphotropic virus 1; PML = progressive multifocal leukoencephalopathy; CNS = central nervous system.
Adapted from Dal Pan G, Berger JR: *In* Berger JR, Levy RM (eds): AIDS and the Nervous System, 2nd ed. Philadelphia, Lippincott-Raven, 1997.

microglia, with relative preservation of axons. The specific role of HIV infection in the pathogenesis of this condition remains uncertain. A clinically and pathologically identical myelopathy has been described in a small number of immunocompromised persons without HIV infection. Clinical and pathologic similarities to subacute combined degeneration of the nervous system due to vitamin B_{12} deficiency suggest that HIV-associated vacuolar myelopathy may be the result of metabolic abnormalities in pathways requiring vitamin B_{12}. However, vitamin B_{12} levels are typically normal in HIV-associated vacuolar myelopathy, and the lesions predominate in the thoracic rather than the cervical cord as seen in subacute combined degeneration from B_{12} lock.

TREATMENT. Antiretroviral therapy is not of clear benefit in the management of this disorder, although anecdotal reports suggest that a rare patient may experience improvement after aggressive antiretroviral therapy. Symptomatic therapy includes antispasticity agents, such as baclofen and gabapentin; management of sphincter dysfunction; and physical therapy. The possibility that the disorder is a consequence of metabolic abnormalities has led to experimental trials with high-dose methionine.

HIV-ASSOCIATED PERIPHERAL NEUROPATHIES

EPIDEMIOLOGIC CHARACTERISTICS. A broad spectrum of peripheral neuropathies is seen in patients with HIV infection. The most common are a distal symmetrical polyneuropathy and inflammatory demyelinating polyradiculoneuropathy (Table 479–2). Once the CD4 count is below 200 cells/mm^3, peripheral neuropathy is estimated to occur with a 5% annual rate in HIV-infected persons. As many as 50% of HIV-infected persons experience peripheral neuropathy during their lifetime.

DISTAL SYMMETRICAL POLYNEUROPATHY (DSP). DSP is the most common form of neuropathy seen with HIV infection. Patients usually have complaints of numbness, burning, and paresthesias of both feet. These symptoms are often so severe that patients experience contact hypersensitivity and difficulty with walking. Involvement of both upper extremities and distal weakness may occur later in the course of DSP. Neurologic examination

Table 479–2 ■ SPECTRUM OF PERIPHERAL NEUROPATHIES IN HIV INFECTION

Distal symmetrical polyneuropathy
HIV-related
Neurotoxic drugs
Vitamin B$_{12}$ deficiency
Inflammatory demyelinating polyneuropathy
Autoimmune
CMV
Mononeuropathy multiplex
Autoimmune
Vasculitic
CMV
Progressive polyradiculopathy
CMV
Lymphoma
Autonomic neuropathy
Motor neuron disease(?)
Sensory neuronopathy(?)

HIV = human immunodeficiency virus; CMV = cytomegalovirus.
Adapted from Simpson DM, Tagliati: *In* Berger JR, Levy RM (eds): AIDS and the Nervous System, 2nd ed. Philadelphia, Lippincott-Raven, 1997.

reveals sensory loss to pain and temperature in a stocking and glove distribution, increased vibratory thresholds, and diminished or absent ankle reflexes. DSP is relatively uncommon early in the course of HIV disease but becomes frequent with advancing immunosuppression. Clinical or electrophysiologic abnormalities consistent with DSP are detected in approximately 35% of patients with AIDS. A "dying back" neuropathy affecting all fiber types, with prominent macrophage infiltration of peripheral nerve, is present in most patients dying with AIDS. The specific pathogenesis remains uncertain. Some investigators have suggested that cytokines may interfere with nerve growth factors, resulting in this peripheral neuropathy, thus providing a rationale for the investigation of therapeutic agents such as nerve growth factors and anticytokines in DSP. Among the symptomatic therapies for the pain and paresthesias of DSP are topical capsaicin and anticonvulsants, such as gabapentin and carbamazepine. Although widely employed in the therapy of DSP, the tricyclic antidepressant amitriptyline and the sodium-channel blocker mexiletine were not of benefit in a recent study.

TOXIC NEUROPATHY. Many conditions other than HIV infection may cause DSP, including vitamin deficiencies (e.g., pyridoxine, vitamin B$_{12}$), diabetes mellitus, and alcoholism. Peripheral neurotoxins such as dapsone, vincristine, isoniazid, and particularly the antiretroviral nucleoside analogues didanosine (ddI), zalcitabine (ddC), and stavudine (d4T) may cause DSP. Individuals with neuropathy prior to the initiation of neurotoxic therapy are more susceptible to the development of severe, symptomatic neuropathy after drug administration. It is difficult to differentiate clinically therapy-related neuropathy from that resulting from HIV alone. Numbness, tingling, and pain are present both in HIV-associated neuropathy and in nucleoside analogue–associated neuropathy. Similarly, both predominantly affect the distal extremities, most severely in the lower limbs, whereas the upper extremities may be relatively spared until late stages of disease. The onset of symptoms may provide useful information, as HIV-associated DSP may take weeks to months to develop, whereas nucleoside analogue neuropathy tends to evolve more rapidly. A clinical benefit of withdrawal of the offending agent is diagnostically useful. However, a "coasting period" of symptom intensification, lasting 4 to 8 weeks, may occur before improvement after drug cessation. Patients will often tolerate drug reintroduction at lower doses.

INFLAMMATORY DEMYELINATING POLYRADICULONEUROPATHY (IDP). IDP presents with acute or chronic progressive weakness, areflexia, and minor sensory complaints, similar to those of Guillain-Barré syndrome or chronic IDP observed in seronegative patients. IDP generally occurs early in the course of HIV disease and may be the presenting clinical disorder at the time of seroconversion. Cerebrospinal fluid pleocytosis is commonly found in HIV-infected patients with IDP, whereas HIV-negative patients with IDP tend to have acellular cerebrospinal fluid. IDP is likely mediated by an autoimmune mechanism, and has responded, in uncontrolled series, to immunomodulating treatment, including use of corticosteroids, plasmapheresis, and administration of intrave-

nous immunoglobulin. Prospective trials are required to determine whether HIV-infected subjects with IDP respond to therapy similarly to seronegative patients. When IDP occurs late in the course of HIV disease, in the setting of advanced immunosuppression, CMV may be the primary cause.

MONONEUROPATHY MULTIPLEX. Mononeuropathy multiplex results in multifocal, asymmetrical, cranial, or peripheral nerve lesions, including facial or laryngeal palsy, wrist or foot drop, and other neuropathic symptoms. In the early stages of HIV infection, mononeuropathy multiplex is usually limited to one or a few nerves and resolves spontaneously without treatment. In advanced HIV disease, particularly when CD4 counts fall below 50 cells/mm³, this neuropathy may progress rapidly to quadriparesis. When the neurologic deficits are diffuse and confluent, mononeuropathy multiplex may be mistaken for distal symmetrical polyneuropathy, inflammatory demyelinating polyradiculoneuropathy, or progressive polyradiculopathy. Some patients experience improvement with the anti-CMV agent ganciclovir.

PROGRESSIVE POLYRADICULOPATHY. Progressive polyradiculopathy is characterized by rapidly progressive lower extremity and sacral paresthesias, flaccid paraparesis, areflexia, sensory loss, and urinary retention. Cerebrospinal fluid examination reveals a marked pleocytosis, containing hundreds to thousands of polymorphonuclear leukocytes. A cerebrospinal fluid culture for CMV yields positive findings in only 50% of these patients, although there is considerable clinical and pathologic evidence that most cases of AIDS-associated progressive polyradiculopathy result from primary CMV infection of nerve roots. Approximately one half of patients with this disorder will experience neurologic improvement or stabilization after therapy with ganciclovir or foscarnet. It is important to treat progressive polyradiculopathy with anti-CMV therapy early in the course of disease before irreversible nerve root necrosis occurs. Less common causes of AIDS-associated progressive polyradiculopathy are neurosyphilis, leptomeningeal lymphoma, and tuberculosis.

MYOPATHY. HIV-associated myopathy may occur at any stage of HIV infection. Proximal muscle weakness, manifested by difficulty in rising from a chair or climbing stairs, is the predominant presenting symptom. Myalgia is present in 25–50% of affected patients but is non-specific. Weight loss is commonly observed.

The most sensitive serologic test for HIV myopathy, as in other primary muscle diseases, measures creatine kinase (CK) level. The CK level is elevated in more than 90% of patients with myopathy, with a median two-fold increase. An elevated CK level with or without myalgia is not by itself diagnostic of myopathy. The presence of proximal muscle weakness, preferably with supportive electrophysiologic and pathologic data, is needed to establish the diagnosis. The most common finding of muscle biopsy in HIV-associated myopathy is scattered myofiber degeneration with occasional associated inflammatory infiltrates.

The pathogenesis of HIV-associated myopathy is unknown, but it is likely an autoimmune phenomenon. Among the opportunistic infections that may affect muscles in AIDS are *Toxoplasma gondii,* CMV, microsporidia, *Cryptococcus neoformans, Mycobacterium avium intracellulare,* and *Staphylococcus aureus.*

Zidovudine has been implicated as a cause of myopathy; however, the degree to which it contributes to underlying HIV-associated myopathy, and the occurrence of distinguishing histopathologic features remain uncertain. The initial management of patients with significant limb weakness and objective evidence of myopathy includes zidovudine dose reduction or withdrawal. Subsequent improvement has been reported in 18 to 100%. In those patients with persistent weakness, prednisone therapy may improve strength without severe adverse effects.

MASS LESIONS IN THE BRAIN IN AIDS. Intracranial mass lesions are among the most common neurologic consequences of HIV infection, accounting for as many as 50% of these neurologic complications. HIV-associated intracranial mass lesions include three distinct categories—opportunistic infections, neoplasms, and cerebrovascular diseases—although cerebrovascular disease does not typically produce masses unless associated with cerebral edema. Toxoplasma encephalitis, the most common cause of intracranial mass lesions in AIDS, occurs in 3 to 10% of patients with AIDS in the United States and in up to 50% of patients with AIDS in Europe and Africa. Primary central nervous system lymphoma (PCNSL), the second most common cause of AIDS-related intracranial mass lesions in the developed world, occurs in up to 2% and may be increasing in frequency. Other causes of intracranial mass lesions in AIDS include tuberculous abscesses and tuberculomas, cryptococcal abscesses and cryptococcomas, *nocardia* abscesses, syphilitic gummas, *candida* abscesses, and other infectious disorders, metastatic tumors, and cerebrovascular disease when accompanied by edema.

The proper management of an HIV-infected patient with an intracranial mass lesion requires a working knowledge of the various causes of intracranial mass lesions observed with HIV and their relative frequencies, clinical and radiographic manifestations, associated therapeutic options, and prognosis. Considerable controversy surrounds the appropriate initial measures to diagnose these lesions. Recently proposed practice parameters developed by the American Academy of Neurology are outlined in Figure 479–1.

American Academy of Neurology: Practice parameters for mass lesions in AIDS. Neurology 50:21–26, 1998.

Berger JR, Levy RM (eds): *AIDS and the Nervous System*, 2nd Ed. Philadelphia, Lippincott-Raven, 1997.

479.2 Human T-Lymphotropic Virus Type 1

Joseph R. Berger, M.D.
▪ *Avindra Nath, M.D.*

INTRODUCTION. The history of the recognition of the neurologic manifestations associated with the human T-lymphotropic virus type 1 (see also Chapter 388) dates to the 1897 observations of Strachan, who described a spastic paraparesis in people living in the West Indies. A variety of terms were used to refer to this illness, including *tropical spastic paraparesis* (TSP), *neuritis,* and *Jamaican neuropathy.* In 1985, Gessain and colleagues recognized a correlation between seropositivity for the retrovirus HTLV-1 and TSP. Shortly after, a myelopathy endemic in southern Japan was recognized as the equivalent of TSP. This myelopathy has subsequently been referred to as HTLV-1–associated myelopathy (HAM). In November 1988, the United States Food and Drug Administration began screening blood donors for the presence of antibodies to HTLV-1.

EPIDEMIOLOGIC CHARACTERISTICS. Among volunteer blood donors in the United States, the seroprevalence of HTLV-1/2 is 0.016%. Certain populations have much higher seroprevalence rates, including prostitutes (3.7%), long-term chronic hemodialysis patients (6.2%), and parenteral drug abusers (7–10%). The seroprevalence in endemic areas, such as in the Caribbean basin, certain regions of Central and South America, southern Japan, Seychelles, Melanesia, and equatorial regions, may approach 15%. Only a small percentage of individuals infected with HTLV-1 ultimately have HAM. The lifetime incidence of HAM varies; estimates of the percentage of infected persons who will ultimately have HAM have ranged from 1 in 100 to 1 in 500. The prevalence of the disease in HTLV-1 endemic areas varies from 8.6 to 128/100,000, and the incidence from 0.04 to 3.0/100,000.

CLINICAL COURSE. HAM can begin at any time between the ages of 20 and 70 years. A female preponderance has been noted with ranges from 1.5:1 to 3.5:1. The onset of the illness is insidious, and it usually progresses slowly over many years. A young age of onset and infection after blood transfusion are associated with more rapid progression. Low and midback pain is common. Pain and paresthesias of the lower extremities also commonly accompany spastic lower extremity weakness. Urinary frequency, urgency, and incontinence accompany a spastic bladder. Complaints of constipation are frequent. Examination reveals brisk reflexes not only in the lower extremities, but also frequently in the upper extremities. Babinski's and Hoffmann's signs are elicitable. A sensory level may be detected. Hypesthesia to pinprick and light touch in distal lower extremities, wasting of the intrinsic muscles of the hands and lower extremities, and depressed ankle jerks may suggest an associated peripheral neuropathy. Optic neuropathy and intention tremor have also been reported. In 10 years, 30% of patients with HAM are bedridden and 45% require crutches to ambulate.

Other neurologic disorders possibly associated with HTLV-1 infection include polymyositis and myasthenia gravis. Non-neurologic disorders associated with HTLV-1 include adult T-cell leukemia or lymphoma, monoclonal gammopathy, cryoglobulinemia, pulmonary alveolitis, uveitis, Sjögren's syndrome, arthropathy, vasculitis, and ichthyosis.

PATHOLOGIC CHARACTERISTICS. Pathologic examination of the spinal cords of patients with HAM reveals moderate to severe atrophy. Meningomyelitis is most intense in the lower thoracic cords with inflammatory changes that correlate with disease duration. The inflammatory infiltrates surround parenchymal vessels and adjacent tissue. Long-standing disease shows hyalinized blood vessels, meningeal fibrosis, and glial scars. There is a predominance of CD8 cells overexpressing class I major histocompatibility complex (MHC).

LABORATORY AND RADIOGRAPHIC FINDINGS. Laboratory studies reveal HTLV-1 antibodies by both enzyme-linked immunosorbent assay (ELISA) and Western blot. A polyclonal gammopathy and abnormal multilobulated T cells in blood and cerebrospinal fluid (CSF) may be observed. CSF examination shows a lymphocytic pleocytosis, increased protein level, and increased immunoglobulin G (IgG) level. CSF-to-serum ratios of antibody to HTLV-1 exceed 1, suggesting production of antibody in the central nervous system. Magnetic resonance imaging (MRI) of the spinal cord may show a hyperintense signal abnormality of the affected cord on T2-weighted image. Cranial periventricular, white matter hyperintensities on T2-weighted MRI are seen in 75% of patients. Somatosensory and visual evoked potentials may be abnormally prolonged.

TREATMENT. Systemic corticosteroids are a most effective treatment, but their efficacy wanes over months to years. A variety of other strategies have been employed with varying success. Zidovudine and other antiretrovirals have been of limited value. Most therapies have attempted to modify the immune response, including danazol (Danocrine) (an anabolic steroid), intravenous immunoglobulin, zidovudine, cyclophosphamide, plasmapheresis, and antibodies to the α-chain of interleukin 2 receptor.

Levin MC, Jacobson S: HTLV-I associated myelopathy/tropica spastic paraparesis (HAM/TSP): A chronic progressive neurologic disease associated with immunologically mediated damage to the central nervous system. J Neurovirol 3:126, 1997.

479.3 Subacute Sclerosing Panencephalitis and Progressive Rubella Panencephalitis

Avindra Nath
▪ *Joseph R. Berger*

Subacute sclerosing panencephalitis (SSPE) is caused by measles virus. It usually affects children, but its onset can extend into young adulthood. Patients usually have a history of measles within the first 2 years of life, and it is speculated that such early host exposure allows emergence of persistent defective virus replication. As a result of effective vaccination strategy against measles virus, its incidence has markedly decreased in recent years.

SSPE usually begins with cognitive and behavioral changes; it progresses to include motor dysfunction with prominent myoclonus, choreoathetosis, dystonia, and rigidity. Its course progresses over 1 to 3 years to rigid quadriparesis and a vegetative state. The condition is more common in rural settings and affects males more often than females. The electroencephalogram (EEG) reveals periodic complexes with synchronous bursts of two or three slow waves per second, recurring at 5- to 8-second intervals in the myoclonic stage. Computed tomography (CT) scan of the brain shows generalized atrophy. The cerebrospinal fluid (CSF) protein, glucose, and cell levels are usually normal; CSF is characterized by a high immunoglobulin concentration, oligoclonal bands, and intrathecal synthesis of antibody to measles virus antigens. Serum measles antibody titers are also high. These findings are usually sufficiently characteristic for diagnosis; brain biopsy is rarely needed for definitive diagnosis in atypical cases. Gray matter is most prominently involved. The pathologic features of SSPE includes gliosis, loss of myelin, and perivascular infiltrates of lymphocytes and plasma cells in white and gray matter. Neuronal cell loss is noted in later stages of the illness. Intranuclear Cowdry type A inclusions containing viral nucleocapsids are noted in both neurons and glia. Measles RNA can be detected in the brain by polymerase chain reaction.

Measles virus may also cause a subacute encephalitis in the immunocompromised host. The prominence of cognitive and motor dysfunction in these patients resembles that of SSPE, but the clinical setting, its subacute onset and more rapid evolution, and the presence of generalized seizures rather than myoclonus are distinctive. Brain abnormalities include abundant intranuclear inclusions, but inflammation is minimal, and neither serum nor CSF antibody titers against measles virus are high. For this reason, brain biopsy is usually needed for diagnosis.

Progressive rubella panencephalitis is a rare disorder resembling SSPE but caused by rubella virus. It presents as a complication of either the congenital rubella syndrome or, more typically, after childhood rubella. A hiatus of years separates early infection from the onset of neurologic deterioration, which is characterized by behavioral changes, cognitive impairment, cerebellar ataxia, spasticity, and sometimes seizures. Myoclonus is a less prominent feature than it is in SSPE. The EEG result shows generalized slowing. The course of illness is similar to that of SSPE, progressing to coma, brain stem involvement, and death in 2–5 years. Serology or isolation of the virus from brain or peripheral blood lymphocytes confirms the cause.

With the advent of widespread measles and rubella immunization, these disorders have been nearly eliminated in the United States. There is no established specific treatment for SSPE or progressive rubella panencephalitis.

Wolinsky JS: Subacute sclerosing panencephalitis, progressive rubella panencephalitis, and multifocal leukoencephalopathy. *In* Waksman B (ed): Immunologic Mechanisms in Neurologic and Psychiatric Disease. New York, Raven Press, 1990. p 259. *An excellent review of the pathogenesis of SSPE and subacute rubella encephalitis.*

479.4 Progressive Multifocal Leukoencephalopathy

Joseph R. Berger
■ *Avindra Nath*

CAUSE AND PATHOGENESIS. Although descriptions of progressive multifocal leukoencephalopathy (PML) date to 1930, it was first crystallized as a distinct entity by Aström, Mancall, and Richardson in 1958 on the basis of its distinct pathologic features of demyelination, abnormal oligodendroglial nuclei, and giant astrocytes. Subsequently, this demyelinating disease was demonstrated to be associated with infection of oligodendrocytes by JC virus (JCV), a papovavirus widely distributed among humans. JC virus exhibits a neurotropism exclusive to glial cells. PML was the first demyelinating disease to be unequivocally associated with a viral infection.

EPIDEMIOLOGIC CHARACTERISTICS. Serologic studies indicate that by 5 years, approximately 10% of children have antibody to JCV and by age 10 years, 40 to 60%. Despite the wide dissemination of JC virus infection, PML is rarely observed in the absence of underlying cellular immunosuppression. It is also rarely observed in childhood. Until the acquired immunodeficiency syndrome (AIDS) epidemic, PML was most commonly observed in patients with lymphoproliferative disorders. In a review published in 1984 (Brooks and Walker), lymphoproliferative disorders were associated with 62.2% of PML cases; myeloproliferative diseases, 6.5%; carcinomatous disease, 2.2%; 10.9% of a variety of acquired immunodeficiency states; and 5.6% of cases with no underlying disease. Since the inception of the AIDS epidemic in 1981, AIDS has been the disorder associated with PML in the majority of cases. The dramatic increase in the incidence of PML in the past decade is due to the fact that approximately 5% of AIDS patients develop PML.

PATHOLOGIC CHARACTERISTICS. The cardinal feature of PML is demyelination, typically multifocal, but occasionally unifo-

cal. These lesions may occur in any location in the white matter but have a predilection for the parieto-occipital regions. The lesions range in size from 1 mm to several centimeters; larger lesions may reflect the coalescence of multiple smaller lesions. The other histopathologic hallmark of PML is the presence of hyperchromatic, enlarged oligodendroglial nuclei and of enlarged bizarre astrocytes with lobulated hyperchromatic nuclei. Electron microscopic examination reveals the JC virions, which measure 28 to 45 nm in diameter and appear singly or in dense crystalline arrays in oligodendroglial cells and, less frequently, in reactive astrocytes.

SIGNS AND SYMPTOMS. The clinical hallmark of PML is the presence of focal neurologic symptoms and signs associated with radiographic evidence of white matter disease in the absence of mass effect. The most common initial symptoms include weakness, speech abnormalities, and cognitive disturbances, each seen in approximately 40% of patients. Although rare in the non-AIDS patient, headache may occur in as many as one third of patients with AIDS. Gait disturbances, sensory loss, and visual impairment all occur in approximately 20% to 30%. Seizures and brain stem symptoms are less common. Signs noted on physical examination parallel the reported symptoms, with weakness, typically a hemiparesis, detected in over half the patients at the time of presentation. Gait abnormalities, cognitive problems, and language disorders (dysarthria and dysphasia) are observed in about one quarter of patients at presentation. Limb and trunk ataxia reflecting cerebellar involvement is detected in as many as 10% but may occasionally result from severe impairment in position sense (sensory ataxia). Neuro-ophthalmic symptoms occur in 50% of patients with PML and are the presenting manifestation in 30–45%. The most common visual deficit is homonymous hemianopsia or quadrantanopia due to lesions of the optic radiations. Cortical blindness is seen in as many as 5–8% of patients at the time of diagnosis. Other neuro-ophthalmic manifestations include optic agnosia, alexia without agraphia, and ocular motor abnormalities. Sensory disturbances occur with PML but are distinctly less common than impairment of strength or visual function.

DIAGNOSIS. The diagnosis of PML may be strongly suggested by the clinical manifestations and the radiographic imaging result. When the former are coupled with a positive JC viral polymerase chain reaction (PCR) finding in the cerebrospinal fluid (CSF), the diagnosis of PML is virtually certain. However, unequivocal confirmation requires brain biopsy.

Computed tomography (CT) of the brain reveals hypodense lesions of the affected white matter that generally have a "scalloped" appearance as an involvement of the subcortical arcuate fibers lying directly beneath the cortex. Cranial magnetic resonance imaging (MRI) shows a hyperintense lesion on T2-weighted images in the affected regions (Fig. 479–2) and, generally, a hypointense lesion on T1-weighted image. Contrast enhancement is seen in approximately 5–10% of pathologically confirmed cases of PML with either brain imaging technique. The enhancement observed is typically faint and at the periphery of lesions. In patients without AIDS, the lesions of PML have a predilection for the parieto-occipital lobes, but in AIDS patients the lesions are more often seen in the frontal lobes. Involvement of the basal ganglia, external capsule, and posterior fossa structures (cerebellum and brain stem) is also seen.

The result of routine analysis of CSF is not diagnostic; the CSF protein may be elevated. CSF PCR for JC virus is of great value in diagnosis; although not always positive, it is highly specific.

PROGNOSIS. PML usually progresses to death with a mean survival of 6 months. In a small proportion (<19%) of patients with AIDS-asssociated PML, survival may exceed 12 months; partial or nearly complete clinical and radiographic recovery may be noted. Factors associated with a more benign course include presence of PML as the heralding manifestation of AIDS, high or climbing CD4 T-lymphocyte counts, contrast enhancement of the lesions on radiographic studies, and any clinical or radiographic evidence of recovery.

TREATMENT. There is no effective therapy for PML. Although cytosine arabinoside prevents JC viral replication in vitro, a randomized, double-blind trial in which it was administered either intrathecally or intravenously in patients with AIDS-associated PML demonstrated no benefit. Because of their antiviral activity, presumably the result of their ability to stimulate natural killer (NK) cells, interferons have been proposed as potential therapeutic agents in the treatment of PML and one retrospective study appears to demonstrate an improved survival rate among persons receiving α-interferon. However, its efficacy remains to be established. Since the introduction of highly active antiretroviral therapy, the survival rate in AIDS-associated PML has appeared to improve. The evidence for spontaneous recovery in untreated patients makes it difficult to assess the results of experimental treatments in small or uncontrolled treatment trials.

Berger JR, Levy RM, Flomenhoft D, Dobbs M: Predictors for prolonged survival in AIDS-associated PML. Ann Neurol 44:341–349, 1998.

Berger JR, Pall L, Lanska D, Whiteman M: Progressive multifocal leukoencephalopathy in patients with HIV infection. J Neuro Virol 4:59, 1998.

Brooks BR, Walker DL: Progressive multifocal leukoencephalopathy. Neurol Clin 2: 299, 1984.

Hall CD, Dafni U, Simpson D, et al: Failure of cytosine arabinoside therapy for human immunodeficinecy virus-1 associated progressive multifocal leukoencephalopathy. N Engl J Med 338:1345, 1998.

479.5 Prion Diseases

Joseph R. Berger
■ *Avindra Nath*

INTRODUCTION. Several human diseases have been attributed to a unique infectious protein referred to as the *prion*. The prototypical human illness is Creutzfeldt-Jakob disease (CJD), subacute spongiform encephalopathy. Other prion illnesses of humans include kuru, Gerstmann-Straussler-Scheinker syndrome, and familial fatal insomnia. Prion-related illnesses are unique in that they may be hereditary, may occur spontaneously, or may be acquired by contamination by the agent. The appearance of variant CJD in association with the outbreak of bovine spongiform encephalopathy, postulated to be the result of contamination of beef, has greatly increased interest in a group of illnesses that is relatively rare.

This group of neurologic illnesses has been referred to by the term "slow infection" introduced by Bjorn Sigurdsson in 1954 when describing scrapie, a prion illness of sheep. The characteristics of slow infections include (1) a very long period of latency lasting for several months to several years; (2) a protracted course after clinical signs have appeared, generally ending in death; and (3) limitation of the infection to a single host species and anatomic lesion in only organ or tissue system. Slow viral illnesses can be classified into those that are the consequence of conventional, identifiable viruses (progressive multifocal leukoencephalopathy [PML], subacute sclerosing panencephalitis [SSPE], progressive rubella encephalitis) and those associated with unconventional infectious agents, namely, prions.

The prion protein (PrP) generally exists as a membrane-bound sialoglycoprotein that is a normal cellular constituent distributed chiefly, although not exclusively, in the brain. Neurons, in particular, contain high concentrations of cellular PrP (PrP^C) and the protein appears to be developmentally regulated. The gene for PrP is located on the short arm of chromosome 20 in humans. Prion diseases are the result of an abnormal isoform of PrP^C referred to as PrP^Sc. Whereas PrP^C exists as an α-helical structure, PrP^Sc consists of β-pleated sheets and arises from post-translational changes in the conformation of PrP^C. Unlike PrP^C, PrP^Sc resists proteolytic digestion and spontaneously aggregages to produce rodlike or fibrillary particles (scrapie-associated fibrils, prion rods) that can be isolated from brains of animals and humans with this class of illness.

KURU. In 1957, Gadjusek and Gibbs described a progressive dementing illness referred to as *kuru* in the Fore linguistic tribal group of the eastern highlands of Papua, New Guinea. Kuru affected as many as 1% of the population at its peak, with women and children chiefly affected. Kuru has been linked to ritualistic cannibalism. Since the cessation of the practice of cannibalism, it has virtually disappeared. A veterinarian recognized that the transmission, pathologic characteristics, and clinical features of this illness strongly resembled those of an illness in sheep referred to as *scrapie*. Subsequent studies demonstrated that kuru could be passed to primates by inoculation with human tissue. This line of investigation was continued with CJD, which also displayed a similar passage to primates after their inoculation with human CJD patients' brains.

The initial stage of the illness is characterized by headaches and joint pains. The ambulant phase that subsequently develops is characterized by ataxia, postural instability, dysarthria, and intervening intention tremors. A sedentary phase is characterized by worsening tremor and ataxia, myoclonus, choreoathetosis, dementia, and emotional lability. Eventually, the person is essentially bedridden with severe dysarthria, ataxia, and dementia.

CJD. In the 1920s, Creutzfeldt and Jakob independently described six patients with a progressive dementing illness. Three of these individuals were subsequently demonstrated to have a disorder that conforms to CJD as currently defined. The illness is seen worldwide with an estimated incidence of about 0.5 to 1.0 case per million per year. The vast majority of cases are sporadic in nature. Five to 15% of cases are estimated to be familial, with an autosomal dominant pattern of inheritance. Certain populations have higher rates of familial disease, including descendants of Jewish populations from Libya and North Africa. In this population, the annual incidence is as high as 31.3 per million. The illness may also occur in an iatrogenic fashion. It has been reported in recipients of supplemental growth hormone prepared from pooled human pituitary glands. Curiously, only a minority of the recipients of contaminated batches of human growth hormone contracted the illness. It has also been reported after cadaver corneal and dura mater transplantations received from patients with CJD or an unexplained dementia. It has also followed the use of stereotactic intracerebral depth electrodes.

The clinical manifestations of CJD are protean and it is frequently incorrectly diagnosed initially. Prodromal symptoms are reported in as many as one fourth of patients. These symptoms include altered sleep patterns and appetite, weight loss, changes in sexual drive, and complaints of impaired memory and concentration. Behaviorial changes are frequently detected early by family members. Spells of disorientation, hallucinations, and emotional lability may be observed. Typically, the patient has a rapidly progressive dementia associated with myoclonus. The dementia is generally global in nature. Myoclonus occurs in approximately 90% of patients. It is generally provoked or aggravated by tactile, auditory, or visual startle. There are a number of distinctive presentations. An apopleptic, abrupt onset is seen in 10 to 15% of patients. Other distinctive presentations include seizures, autonomic dysfunction, and lower motor neuron disease, suggesting amyotrophic lateral sclerosis. A wide variety of visual abnormalities may be observed, including visual agnosia; supranuclear palsies; nystagmus; Balint's syndrome, characterized by the inability to look at objects on command (psychic paralysis of visual fixation), to grab objects accurately (optic ataxia), or to recognize more than one object at a time visually (simultagnosia); distorted visual perceptions; and cortical blindness. Cerebellar ataxia is seen in up to one third of patients. Pyramidal and extrapyramidal manifestations are frequently observed; pre-terminally, they are observed in approximately 50 to 66% of patients. The latter often manifest with parkinsonian features including hypokinesia and rigidity. Hyperreflexia, spasticity, and extensor plantar reflexes are also seen. Lower motor neuron disease is detected in less than 1% at disease onset, but may ultimately affect up to 10% of patients.

The recently described variant form of CJD that may be linked to bovine spongiform encephalopathy generally occurs in younger individuals who have psychiatric manifestations and ataxia. Dementia develops late. Similary, the clinical presentation of CJD associated with cadaver pituitary growth hormone differs from classic CJD as the patients are younger and have an illness reminiscent of kuru.

The clinical tetrad supporting the diagnosis of CJD consists of a subacute progressive dementia, myoclonus, typical periodic complexes indicated on electroencephalography (EEG), and a normal cerebrospinal fluid. Findings of computed tomography and magnetic resonance imaging of the brain are normal, except in late stages of the disease, at which time rapidly progressive brain atrophy may be observed. Magnetic resonance imaging of the brain may also show a hyperintense signal abnormality of the basal ganglia or, more rarely, abnormalities such as hyperintense signal abnormality of the occipital cortex. The EEG hallmark of CJD is the pattern of periodic sharp wave complexes consisting of generalized slow background activity interrupted by bilaterally synchronous sharp wave complexes occurring at intervals of 0.5 to 2.5

seconds and lasting for 200 to 600 milliseconds. The classic EEG pattern is seen in 75 to 95% of established cases but may not be present in the early or terminal phases of the illness. Although the cerebrospinal fluid (CSF) is generally completely normal, a mild elevation in protein level may be seen. A CSF test for the protein 14-3-3 is commercially available and, in the appropriate clinical context, is highly specific and sensitive for CJD. Although brain biopsy with immunostaining for PrP^{Sc} is the gold standard for establishing the diagnosis, the positive CSF test result and clinical picture are adequate for diagnosis in most cases.

To date, there is no effective therapy for CJD. The disease is inexorably progressive. Death typically occurs within 1 year of the onset of symptoms with a reported range of 1 to 130 months. The median survival is 4.5 months and the mean is 8 months. Illness of more than 2 years' duration has been reported in 5 to 10% of patients. The clinical course has been divided into phases characterized by an initial slow intellectual and behavioral deterioration followed by a stepwise or progressive downhill course. Ultimately, a more slowly progressive terminal stage intervenes.

Gross pathologic examination shows brain atrophy. The pathologic hallmarks are generally maximal in the cortex but are also seen in basal ganglia, thalamus, and cerebellum. They include spongiform changes (small round vacuoles) within the neuropil resulting from cystic dilatation of neurons and focal necrosis of cellular membranes, neuronal loss, and hypertrophy and proliferation of glial cells. No inflammation is observed. Amyloid plaques are often observed. They are congophilic and composed of 10-nm fibrils. These plaques are stained with antibodies to protein.

Although the illness is not communicable in the conventional sense, there is a risk of handling materials contaminated with the prion protein. Gloves should be worn when handling blood, CSF, and other body fluids. Instruments must be disinfected by steam autoclaving for 1 hour at 132° C, by steam autoclaving for 4.5 hours at 121° C (1.5 psi), or by immersion in 1 *N* sodium hydroxide for 1 hour at room temperature.

GERSTMANN-STRAUSSLER-SCHEINKER SYNDROME. Gerstmann-Straussler-Scheinker syndrome is an autosomal dominant disorder that is considered a variant of CJD. Progressive cerebellar dysfunction dominates the clinical picture, typically developing in midlife. The initial features include unsteady gait, clumsiness, and incoordination. Dyarthria and nystagmus are also observed. Dementia often occurs later in the course of the illness. Other features include gaze palsies, deafness, blindness, loss of muscle stretch reflexes, and extensor plantar reflexes.

Gerstmann-Straussler-Scheinker syndrome (GSS) has been associated with distinct mutations in the PrP gene, most commonly a leucine-for-proline substitution at codon 102. Other mutations have included a valine-for-alanine substitution at codon 117 and a point mutation in codon 198. Variations in the clinical presentation may be related to difference in the genetic mutations. For instance, ataxia predominates in the codon 102 mutation, whereas the other two mutations are associated with ataxia and dementia.

The pathologic examination finding reveals widespread amyloid plaque formation. The spinocerebellar tracts are commonly atrophic.

FATAL FAMILIAL INSOMNIA. Fatal familial insomnia (FFI) is an autosomal dominant disorder first described by Medori and colleagues in 1992. Although the hallmark of FFI is intractable insomnia, patients may also have features indistinguishable from CJD. Sympathetic hyperactivity includes hypertension, hyperthermia, hyperhidrosis, and tachycardia. Other autonomic and endocrine disturbances are frequently observed, including a loss of the normal circadian rhythm of melatonin, prolactin, and growth hormone. Corticotropin (adrenocorticotropic hormone) secretion is decreased, although corticosteroid release is increased. Dysarthria and motor system abnormalities, which include myoclonus, tremor, ataxia, hyperreflexia, and spasticity, are also observed. Mentation may be normal, but most patients have mild memory impairment and attention deficits. Hallucinations and unexpected gross body movements during dream (rapid eye movement [REM]) sleep are also observed. The illness is rapidly progressive.

Pathologic changes include atrophy and gliosis of specific thalamic nuclei, cerebellar cortex, and inferior olives. Spongiform changes of the brain are rare. The PrP gene in these patients reveals an asparagine-for-aspartate mutation in codon 178, similar to that in some familial cases of CJD. To date, FFI has not been successfully transmitted to an animal host. As with other prion diseases, no specific treatment exists.

■ NEUROLOGIC DISORDERS ASSOCIATED WITH ALTERED IMMUNITY OR UNEXPLAINED HOST-PARASITE ALTERATIONS

480 NEUROLOGIC COMPLICATIONS IN THE IMMUNOCOMPROMISED HOST

Richard A. Rudick

Immunodeficient states induced by a variety of intrinsic or exogenous mechanisms greatly reduce central nervous system (CNS) natural resistance to infection (for discussion of mechanisms, see Chapter 266). Many well-known and a few uncommon causes of immunocompromise exist, some examples being genetically related immunodeficiency disorders (see Chapter 223); splenectomy; administration of immune suppressants to facilitate renal, bone marrow, or other organ transplants or to protect against severe autoimmune disorders; chemotherapy or radiation therapy for cancer or allied disorders; and the intrinsic capacity of human immunodeficiency virus, type 1 (HIV-1), to destroy CD4 lymphocytes. Each of these conditions predisposes to serious infections of the CNS, and some can foster primary or secondary lymphoma production in the brain or, rarely, the spinal cord.

In transplant recipients, hospital-acquired bacterial species provide the major early risk (see Chapters 266 and 267). Early on, severe immunosuppression of any kind also commonly reactivates herpesviruses, most frequently herpes simplex virus, herpes varicella-zoster virus, and cytomegalovirus (see Chapter 477.4). Sooner or later, with continued immunosuppression, nosocomial bacterial and mycotic infections may arise (see Chapter 267).

Among cancer patients (e.g., those with Hodgkin's disease or hairy cell leukemia), as well as in persons with certain hematologic disorders or other less common conditions, splenectomy may be indicated, which increases the risk of bacterial meningitis (see Chapter 151). Other immunosuppressed patients are similarly at risk for either bacterial or fungal infections of the brain and meninges. Progressive multifocal encephalopathy (see Chapter 479.4) appears as a complication of acquired immunodeficiency syndrome (AIDS), but the condition also may arise in patients suffering from other forms of severe immunosuppression or it may occur sporadically. Potential CNS immunologic complications of AIDS, among which differentiation between toxoplasmosis and lymphoma may be difficult, are discussed in Chapters 364 and 486.

Cohen BA: Neurologic complications of HIV infection. Primary Care 24:575–595, 1997. *Reviews neurologic syndromes in AIDS patients, with emphasis on infectious etiology.*

Ferrante P, Caldarelli-Stefano R, Omodeo-Zorini E, et al: Comprehensive investigation of the presence of JC virus in AIDS patients with and without progressive multifocal leukoencephalopathy. J Med Virol 52:235–242, 1997. *Reviews 12 cases of progressive multifocal leukoencephalopathy among 64 patients with AIDS. Free JC viral DNA in CSF was characteristic of the patients with PML.*

481 REYE'S SYNDROME

Richard A. Rudick

DEFINITION. Reye's syndrome is a form of hepatic encephalopathy with fatty infiltration of the liver, markedly raised intracranial pressure, and brain edema. The illness follows one of several common viruses or hepatotoxicity from commonly used drugs.

ETIOLOGY AND PATHOGENESIS. Reye's syndrome appears to be due to an abnormality of mitochondrial fatty acid metabolism. Entry of fatty acids into mitochondria or β-oxidation itself may be impaired. Biochemical manifestations of Reye's syndrome, regardless of the precipitant, include hypoglycemia, hepatic accumulation of fatty acids, fatty acyl co-enzyme A (CoA), and acyl carnitines. Accumulated products further injure mitochondria, further impairing β-oxidation. Reye's syndrome usually follows a viral infection. The syndrome most commonly follows influenza A, influenza B, or varicella-zoster. Little evidence links the precipitating viral infection directly to either the central nervous system (CNS) or hepatic involvement. A toxic origin is proposed for both types of involvement. Additionally, epidemiologic studies strongly support a link between the use of aspirin and Reye's syndrome. A causal relationship is suggested by a dramatic decline in Reye's syndrome in the United Kingdom and the USA following effective public education about the hazards of aspirin for children.

Hepatic dysfunction results in various metabolic derangements, including hyperammonemia, lactic acidemia, and elevated levels of serum free fatty acids. These metabolic derangements have been implicated in the pathogenesis of brain swelling and increased intracranial pressure that dominate the clinical course in severe cases. The precise mechanism of mitochondrial impairment remains to be clarified.

INCIDENCE. Reye's syndrome occurs most commonly among children between 1 and 15 years of age, but it has been reported in adolescents and has been recognized increasingly in adults. Inner city black infants may be especially at risk for the disease. Prospectively derived incidence figures for the most susceptible age groups were as high as 6.2 per 100,000 children. They are now much lower.

PATHOLOGY. The liver shows a noninflammatory, panlobular, hepatocellular accumulation of lipid droplets and both histochemical and ultrastructural evidence of inflammation. At postmortem examination, swelling of astrocytic foot processes and ultrastructural changes in mitochondria similar to those seen in hepatic mitochondria may be found in the greatly swollen brain.

CLINICAL MANIFESTATIONS AND COURSE. Reye's syndrome is a biphasic disorder. As symptoms of the initial viral illness begin to improve, intractable vomiting appears in association with lethargy or delirium. Early diagnosis is confirmed by the findings of non-icteric hepatic dysfunction, an elevated arterial blood ammonia level, and serum transaminase levels that exceed three times normal levels. Hepatic enlargement is present in about one-half of the cases. Children younger than 1 year often show hypoglycemia. Signs of CNS deterioration include the development of generalized seizures, deepening obtundation, and transtentorial herniation. The cerebrospinal fluid (CSF) is under increased pressure but is acellular, with otherwise normal constituents.

DIAGNOSIS. Diagnosis rests on the clinical findings and appropriate biochemical abnormalities. Liver biopsy usually is not necessary. CNS infection, inborn errors of metabolism, such as ornithine transcarbamoylase deficiency and systemic carnitine deficiency, and the presence of known hepatotoxins, including valproate, salicylates, and paracetamol, must be actively excluded. A childhood syndrome, distinguishable from Reye's syndrome only by the absence of hepatic involvement and a high incidence of acute convulsions, can follow either banal viral infections or immunizations.

TREATMENT. Affected patients require intensive care monitoring until the course of the disease is well established. Hypoglycemia and electrolyte abnormalities must be corrected. Many authorities suggest hydration with solutions of high glucose content. Appropriate measures should be taken to monitor intracranial pressure continuously in more severely affected patients, as judicious control of intracranial hypertension contributes to a favorable outcome. Mortality is about 10%.

Belay ED, Bresee JS, Holman RC, et al: Reye's syndrome in the United States from 1981 through 1997. N Engl J Med 340(18):1377, 1999.

Monto AS: The disappearance of Reye's syndrome: A public health triumph. N Engl J Med 340(18):1423, 1999. *This paper and the accompanying editorial document explain the nearly complete elimination of this disease.*

Ede RJ, Williams R: Reye's syndrome in adults. Br Med J 296:517, 1988. *Although uncommon, such cases do occur, and management is different from that required for children.*

Pranzatelli MR, DeVivo DC: Pharmacology of Reye syndrome. Clin Neuropharmacol 10:96, 1987. *A comprehensive review that includes detailed recommendations for medical management.*

▪ THE DEMYELINATING DISEASES

482 MULTIPLE SCLEROSIS AND RELATED CONDITIONS

Richard A. Rudick

This section discusses diseases that primarily affect central nervous system (CNS) myelin; demyelinating peripheral neuropathies are discussed in Chapters 499 and 500. CNS myelin is an elaborate extension of the oligodendrocyte cell membrane. A single oligodendrocyte myelinates as many as 20 or 30 different CNS axonal segments, each over a length of 1 mm or less. Oligodendrocyte membrane extensions wrap around the axons in a concentric fashion to form the myelin sheath. Tightly compacted mature myelin consists of parallel layers of bimolecular lipids apposed to layers of hydrated protein. Lipids, including cerebroside, phospholipids, and cholesterol, constitute 75% of myelin's dry weight. Myelin proteins include proteolipid protein, myelin basic protein, myelin-associated glycoprotein, and a number of less abundant proteins detectable by electrophoretic separation. Active myelin synthesis starts in utero and continues for the first 2 years of life; slower synthesis continues during childhood and adolescence. Turnover of mature myelin continues at a slower rate throughout life. Both developing and mature forms of myelin are readily susceptible to injury by the diseases described in this section.

Table 482–1 ■ DISEASES OF MYELIN

Idiopathic, presumably autoimmune (this chapter)
  Recurrent or chronically progressive demyelination (multiple sclerosis
    and its variants)
  Monophasic demyelination (may be first clinical episode of multiple
    sclerosis)
      Optic neuritis
      Acute transverse myelitis
  Acute disseminated encephalomyelitis; acute hemorrhagic leukoencepha-
    lopathy
      Following infection, with or without exanthem
      Following vaccination
Viral infections (see Chs. 475–478)
  Progressive multifocal leukoencephalopathy
  Subacute sclerosing panencephalitis
Nutritional disorders (see Ch. 489)
  Combined systems disease (vitamin B_{12} deficiency)
  Demyelination of the corpus callosum (Marchiafava-Bignami disease)
  Central pontine myelinolysis
Anoxic-ischemic sequelae (see Ch. 470)
  Delayed postanoxic cerebral demyelination
  Progressive subcortical ischemic encephalopathy
Leukodystrophies (this chapter)
  Primarily affecting CNS myelin
    Adrenoleukodystrophy (Schilder's disease)
    Pelizaeus-Merzbacher disease
    Spongy degeneration
    Others (Alexander's disease, Canavan's disease)
  Central peripheral nervous system
    Metachromatic leukodystrophy
    Globoid cell (Krabbe's disease)

Table 482–1 classifies the several forms of myelin diseases. Acquired disorders are separated from developmental abnormalities. Multiple sclerosis (MS) and its variants are by far the most common diseases in this group. Viral infections, nutritional disorders, and anoxic-ischemic sequelae are discussed in Chapters 469 to 471, 475 to 478, and 489. The leukodystrophies are uncommon but instructive disorders, because recent genetic and biochemical advances have elucidated the mechanisms that cause many of these conditions.

MULTIPLE SCLEROSIS

DEFINITION. MS is a disorder of unknown cause, defined clinically by typical symptoms, signs, and disease progression, and characterized pathologically by scattered areas of inflammation, demyelination, and axonal injury affecting the brain, optic nerves, and spinal cord. The first symptoms of MS usually occur between the ages of 15 and 50 years. Individual bouts of inflammatory demyelination may be accompanied by clinical symptoms, termed *relapses*, followed in most cases by some degree of recovery, producing the classic relapsing-remitting course seen early in the disease. Diagnosis requires intermittent or progressive CNS symptoms buttressed by evidence for two or more CNS white matter lesions and occurring in an appropriately aged patient who lacks an alternative explanation, such as recurrent strokes or systemic lupus erythematosus. The diagnosis is based on clinical features; currently available laboratory tests support the diagnosis but are not directly diagnostic.

ETIOLOGY. The initiating cause or causes of MS are unknown, but it is now widely believed that the pathogenesis involves immune-mediated inflammatory demyelination and axonal injury. Pathologic examination of brain affected by MS shows the hallmarks of an immunopathologic process: perivascular infiltration by lymphocytes and monocytes; class II MHC antigen expression by cells in the lesions; chemokines, lymphokines, and monokines secreted by activated cells; and the absence of overt evidence of infection. Additional evidence of an autoimmune pathogenesis includes (1) immunologic abnormalities in blood and cerebrospinal fluid (CSF) of MS patients, notably selective intrathecal humoral immune activation, lymphocyte subset abnormalities, and a high frequency of activated lymphocytes in blood and CSF; (2) an association between MS and certain MHC class II allotypes; (3) the clinical response of MS patients to immunomodulation—patients tend to improve with immunosuppressive drugs and worsen with interferon-gamma (IFN-γ) treatment, which stimulates the immune response; and (4) similarities between MS and experimental allergic encephalomyelitis (EAE)—an animal model in which recurrent episodes of inflammatory demyelination can be induced by inoculating susceptible animals with myelin proteins, such as myelin basic protein or proteolipid protein.

Epidemiologic studies suggest environmental and genetic factors in the etiopathogenesis of MS. The uneven geographic distribution of the disease and the occurrence of several point-source epidemics have suggested environmental factors. Migration studies have further suggested that exposure to undefined environmental factors prior to adolescence is required for subsequent development of MS. Intense study over the past 30 years has failed to establish an infectious cause, but studies continue to evaluate the possibility that one or more ubiquitous viruses may trigger the disease, leading to an autoimmune process in susceptible individuals.

A genetic influence is well-established by excess concordance in monozygotic (compared with dizygotic) twins, clustering of MS in families, racial variability in risk, and associations with class II MHC allotypes. Recent population-based genetic studies have identified approximately 8 to 10 uncharacterized candidate genetic loci. The genetic basis of MS is currently believed to result from the net effect of interactions between a number of currently uncharacterized susceptibility and, possibly, resistance genes. Immunologic, epidemiologic, and genetic evidence supports the concept that exposure of a genetically susceptible individual to an environmental factor or factors during childhood (perhaps any one of many common viruses) leads eventually to immune-mediated inflammatory demyelination.

INCIDENCE, PREVALENCE, AND EPIDEMIOLOGY. The annual incidence rate for MS ranges in different populations from 1.5 to 11 per 100,000 persons. Several studies suggest that the incidence rate has increased over time. For example, data from Olmsted County, MN, suggests a gradual increase in annual incidence during the past century from about 1.2 per 100,000 between 1905 and 1914 to about 6.2 per 100,000 between 1975 and 1984. In all studies, the highest age- and gender-specific rates occur in women between ages 20 and 40 years.

Worldwide prevalence differs according to geography. Distribution of MS has been well studied in North America, Northern Europe, Australia, and New Zealand. In both hemispheres, MS is more common in the temperate zones, decreasing toward the equator. The prevalence of MS in the northern United States, Canada, and northern Europe is at least 100 per 100,000 population; in certain regions, the prevalence of MS exceeds 300 per 100,000 persons, compared with less than 5 per 100,000 persons in the tropics. Regional heterogeneity has been reported within high prevalence zones, and several reports describe MS clusters in small areas. In the Faroe Islands, for example, a well-reported outbreak of MS occurred during the 20 years following the start of World War II, suggesting the effects of an unidentified environmental factor.

PATHOLOGY. Brain, optic nerves, and spinal cord from MS patients contain scattered areas of myelin loss ranging in size from 1 mm to several centimeters in diameter. The concept that MS spares axons has been refuted by recent evidence of axonal pathologic lesions topographically related to inflammatory foci. Confocal immunofluorescent microscopy has demonstrated abundant transected axons in the regions of inflammatory demyelination. The borders between histologically normal tissue and demyelinated zones are usually well-demarcated, but they may shade from normal to thinning before bare axons occur. Some areas show diffuse partial myelin loss. Although plaques may occur in any myelinated area of the CNS, the most commonly affected regions include optic nerves, periventricular cerebral white matter, and cervical spinal cord.

The earliest event in development of the MS lesion is breakdown of the blood-brain barrier, followed by perivenular mononuclear infiltrates, and quickly thereafter by circumscribed areas of myelin breakdown. Macrophages invariably occupy sites of active demyelination and appear necessary for myelin loss. B lymphocytes and plasma cells surround small CNS blood vessels, and T lymphocytes and monocytes infiltrate CNS parenchyma. Products of the immune response, including immunoglobulins, interleukins, interferons, and tumor necrosis factor, accompany the acute MS lesion. Tissue edema reaches a maximum after about 1 month, after which lesions evolve over several months into permanently demyelinated gliotic scars depleted of oligodendrocytes. After the initial events, immature oligodendrocytes appear and presumably participate in remyelination. As a rule, however, the evidence for oligodendrocyte proliferation and remyelination is insufficient to explain the remarkable clinical recovery observed in many patients.

LABORATORY ABNORMALITIES. CEREBROSPINAL FLUID. Immune activation within the CNS is a cardinal feature of MS. Increased CSF immunoglobulin levels, reflecting the presence of intrathecal humoral immune activation, appear in 80 to 90% of MS patients. CSF γ-globulin normally represents less than 13% of total CSF protein, but in MS patients, the proportion often rises much higher. After gel electrophoresis of CSF γ-globulin, separate, discrete "oligoclonal" bands (OCB) can be detected in 70 to 80% of patients. The sensitivity for detecting OCB can be increased by separating CSF by isoelectric focusing or by staining the gels or nitrocellulose blots with anti-immunoglobulin antibodies. As with most diagnostic tests, however, as the sensitivity of the method increases, the specificity decreases; CSF OCB are also observed in patients with CNS infections or inflammatory diseases and occasionally in patients with tumors or strokes. Increased CSF levels of free κ light chains develop less frequently than OCB, but they are more specific for MS than are IgG abnormalities.

The amount of antibody synthesis within the CNS can be quantified by measuring the CSF and serum IgG and albumin levels and calculating a CSF IgG synthesis rate. CSF protein is normal or only slightly elevated in MS; levels greater than 75 mg/dL require an alternative explanation. CSF cell count is nearly always fewer than 50 mononuclear cells per microliter; cell counts of more than 100 cells/μL require a search for an infectious cause. Myelin destruction releases myelin basic protein (MBP) into CSF, which can be detected by radioimmunoassay. The MBP level correlates to some extent with disease activity and lesion location; none is detectable in normal individuals or during quiescent periods in MS patients. MBP levels rise in association with acute attacks or rapid disease progression. This rise serves as an index of disease activity but is not specific to MS; myelin injury from other causes, such as acute brain infarction, increases CSF MBP.

In the presence of slight mononuclear pleocytosis and normal protein levels, the presence of oligoclonal bands, selectively increased IgG levels, and free κ light chains provide strong support for the diagnosis of MS, providing that CNS syphilis, subacute sclerosing panencephalitis, chronic meningitis, CNS Lyme disease, human T lymphotropic virus type 1 (HTLV-1) myelopathy, or other infectious diseases have been excluded.

SENSORY EVOKED POTENTIALS. Myelin allows rapid propagation of the nerve action potential. Myelin loss from any cause slows conduction velocity or causes conduction block. Conduction along sensory pathways can be measured by inducing a response to a visual, auditory, or somatosensory stimulus. Measurement of the latency after stimulus of the visual evoked potential (VEP) is used most widely (see Chapter 442). In most laboratories, the normal VEP latency is less than approximately 105 msec. Increased latency indicates an abnormality in the optic nerve on that side. Evoked potentials are considered extensions of the clinical examination, allowing for objective measurement of lesions within specific pathways. They have not proved useful for monitoring progression of disease or response to therapy.

IMAGING PROCEDURES. Computed tomographic (CT) brain scans sometimes reveal hypodense regions in white matter, but the imaging modality is relatively insensitive and usually shows no abnormalities. For these reasons, magnetic resonance imaging (MRI) has largely supplanted CT scanning. Head MRI scans show abnormalities in more than 85% patients with clinically definite MS. Typical lesions (Fig. 482–1) are multifocal, appear hyperintense on intermediate and T2-weighted MRIs, and occur predominantly in the periventricular cerebral white matter, corpus callosum, cerebellum, cerebellar peduncles, brain stem, and spinal cord. Usually MRI reveals many more hyperintense lesions than clinically anticipated. Intravenous paramagnetic agents, such as gadolinium, demonstrate acute lesions, which appear hyperintense on T1-weighted images. Serial studies have demonstrated that gadolinium enhancement appears and disappears in a given lesion in about 4 weeks. MRI is used widely to confirm a diagnosis of suspected MS and to rule out other conditions. MRI abnormalities are not specific for MS,

particularly in patients older than 50 years, who commonly develop nonspecific MRI signal changes of uncertain significance. The specificity of MRI lesions for MS increases with lesions 6 mm or more in diameter that are adjacent to the lateral ventricles, particularly when accompanied by brain stem, cerebellar, and spinal cord lesions. Use of MRI as a research tool to measure treatment effect or disease progression is rapidly evolving. Whether or not such studies are cost-effective for measuring clinical progress is debatable. Newer magnetic resonance-based techniques, such as magnetization transfer imaging, may allow differentiation between inflammation and demyelination. Such a distinction may become important as future therapies evolve.

CLINICAL MANIFESTATIONS. ONSET, COMMON CLINICAL MANIFESTATIONS, AND COURSE. Women are affected more frequently than men, with a 3:2 ratio. Symptom onset occurs between ages 20 and 50 years and peaks at approximately age 30 years. Occasionally, children younger than 12 years and adults older than 50 years present with their first symptom. MS produces myriad neurologic symptoms and signs, depending on the anatomic sites of involvement. In younger patients, the disease usually starts with a subacute or acute onset of focal neurologic symptoms and signs, most often reflecting disease in optic nerves, pyramidal tracts, posterior columns, cerebellum, central vestibular system, or medial longitudinal fasciculus. Older individuals commonly present with insidiously progressive myelopathy, manifest as some combination of progressive spastic leg weakness, axial instability, and bladder impairment. In a large group of MS patients studied at the University of Western Ontario in the 1970s (Table 482–2), approximately 30% of patients presented with visual symptoms, 30% with sensory symptoms, 20% with gait or balance disturbance, and the remaining 20% with various other symptoms. In general, as the disease progresses, new symptoms and signs appear, old symptoms and signs recur, and residual symptoms increase.

Visual symptoms include monocular visual loss, oscillopsia, or diplopia. Gait disorder results from spastic leg weakness, axial instability, and lower extremity sensory loss. Spasticity consists of increased muscle tone, hyperreflexia, and limb spasms, accompanied by weakness and loss of dexterity. Spasticity in MS patients almost always affects the lower more than the upper extremities. Upper extremity impairment includes sensory loss resulting in a clumsy hand, cerebellar ataxia, or, less commonly, spastic weakness. Bladder dysfunction includes urinary urgency with urge incontinence or hesitancy and incomplete emptying. Neuropsychological problems are common, including depression, emotional lability, and cognitive impairment.

Increased body temperature by as little as 0.5°C transiently reduces neurologic function in some patients. In the setting of increased ambient temperature, strenuous physical activity, or fever, patients may experience transient worsening of symptoms. This results from slowed axonal conduction induced by heating, and the new symptoms disappear within hours of regaining normal body temperature.

At least 70% of patients improve in the days to months following their initial bout, with the degree of improvement ranging from slight to virtual disappearance of the neurologic dysfunction. Although most patients experience exacerbations and remissions early in the course of the illness, as time goes by, recovery from individual bouts decreases, fixed impairment and disability remain, and the course becomes chronically progressive. About 30% of patients experience chronically progressive problems from the onset of disease, especially those older than 45 years. Ten years after onset, about half of all patients are still able to carry out their household and employment responsibilities. Fifteen years after onset, about half require a cane to walk. Approximately 25 years after onset, at least half are unable to walk, even with assistance. By contrast, some individuals, perhaps as many as a third, occupy the extremes of either avoiding disability altogether or having unusually severe limitations, becoming bedridden within months of onset. The average interval from clinical onset to death is 35 years; terminal events result from sepsis from urinary tract infection or decubitus ulcers, aspiration pneumonia, or suicide.

FACTORS AFFECTING THE CLINICAL COURSE. The only predictable factor in MS is its unpredictability in the individual patient. It has become clear, however, that certain features carry a relatively

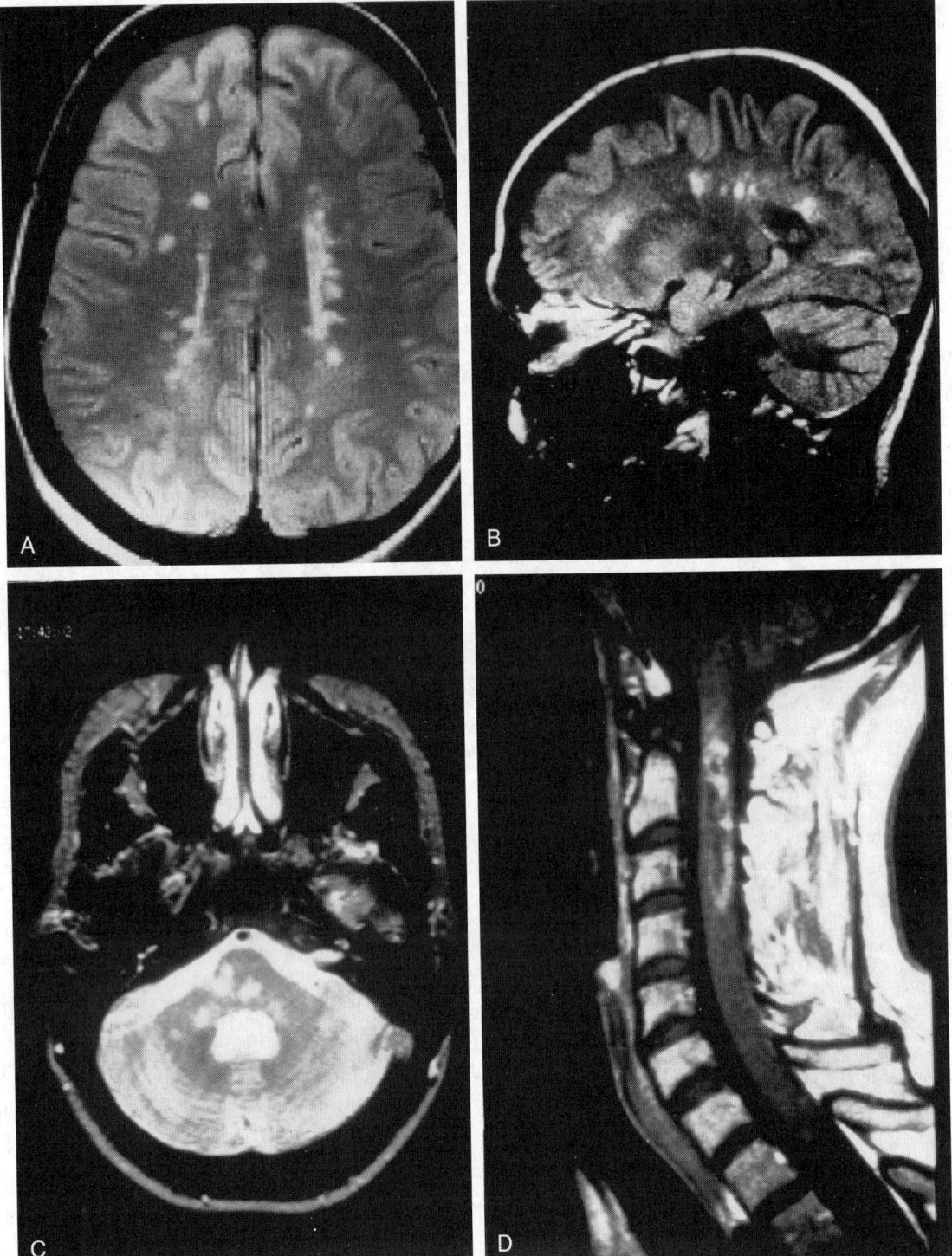

FIGURE 482–1 ■ Magnetic resonance imaging of brain and spinal cord from a patient with clinically definite multiple sclerosis. *A*, transverse section just above the bodies of the lateral ventricles. Note the numerous high-signal lesions adjacent to the bodies of the lateral ventricles in the deep cerebral white matter. *B*, Sagittal proton-density image showing ovoid lesions extending from the lateral ventricles into the deep cerebral white matter. *C*, T2-weighted section through the brain stem and cerebellum at the level of the middle cerebellar peduncles showing numerous high-signal lesions in the pons, cerebellar peduncles, and cerebellum. *D*, T1-weighted sagittal image through the cervical spinal cord lesion with gadolinium enhancement as signified by high signal around the periphery of the lesion. (Courtesy of Barbara Banger, M.D., Cleveland Clinic Foundation Department of Neuroradiology.)

poor prognosis. These include progressive disease from onset, preponderance of motor and cerebellar signs, and a near diagnostically abnormal head MRI at first presentation. Conversely, favorable indicators include a high degree of recovery after the first attack, predominance of sensory symptoms, and benign condition 5 years after symptom onset.

Several studies have found that infections of almost any type increase the risk for exacerbation. This is thought to result from immune system activation, with an associated increase in MS disease activity. As with numerous autoimmune diseases, MS disease activity decreases during pregnancy but increases somewhat in the postpartum period. The overall progression of MS, however, is not affected by one or more pregnancies.

DIAGNOSIS. Despite increasing reliance on sophisticated brain

Table 482–2 ■ INITIAL SYMPTOMS IN MS PATIENTS*

SYMPTOM	PERCENTAGE OF CASES
Sensory disturbance in one or more limbs	33
Disturbance of balance and gait	18
Visual loss in one eye	17
Diplopia	13
Progressive weakness	10
Acute myelitis	6
Lhermitte's sign	3
Sensory disturbance in face	3
Pain	2

*From Paty DW, Poser CM: Clinical symptoms and signs of multiple sclerosis. In Poser CM (ed): The Diagnosis of Multiple Sclerosis. New York, Thieme and Stratton, 1984, p. 27.

imaging, CSF analysis, and electrophysiologic tests, the diagnosis of MS is based on clinical features supplemented by laboratory tests, rather than the reverse. The Schumacher criteria have been widely used for diagnosis of MS. Clinically definite MS exists when an appropriate clinical history is supported by (1) objective abnormalities of CNS function in the neurologic examination; (2) examination or history indicating involvement of two or more areas of the CNS; (3) CNS disease predominantly reflecting white matter involvement; (4) involvement of the CNS following either a pattern of two or more episodes, each lasting more than 24 hours and occurring a month or more apart, or a slow or stepwise progression of signs and symptoms over at least 6 months; (5) patient age between 10 and 50 years; and (6) signs and symptoms that cannot be better explained by another disease process. These criteria are based entirely on clinical features. Laboratory testing plays an increasingly important role in documenting multicentric CNS lesions and eliminating alternative diagnoses. This is reflected in diagnostic criteria developed more recently that incorporate sensory evoked potentials and MRI to identify disseminated lesions, and CSF IgG abnormalities to support the diagnosis (Table 482–3).

Two common errors confound the diagnosis of MS. The first occurs in a patient with clear neurologic disease who has an alternative diagnosis (Table 482–4). Certain clinical or laboratory "red flags" are useful in alerting the clinician about a possible diagnostic error in this situation (Table 482–5). The two most useful red flags include disease that could be explained by a single lesion in the nervous system and the absence of a clinical remission. In a patient with localized disease, the working assumption must be that a definable, non-demyelinating structural lesion exists. Depending on the clinical features, diagnostic testing should be used to rule out brain or spinal cord tumor, arteriovenous malformation, cervical spondylosis with cord compression, cervical or thoracic disk herniation, Chiari malformation, brain abscess, or a parenchymal mass

Table 482–3 ■ WASHINGTON COMMITTEE CRITERIA FOR DIAGNOSIS OF MULTIPLE SCLEROSIS*

CATEGORY	ATTACKS	CLINICAL EVIDENCE		PARA-CLINICAL EVIDENCE†	CSF OB/IgG
Clinically definite MS					
1	2	2			
2	2	1	and	1	
Laboratory-supported definite MS					
1	2	1	or	1	+
2	1	2		1	+
3	1	1	and	1	+
Clinically probable MS					
1	2	1			
2	1	2			
3	1	1	and	1	
Laboratory-supported probable MS					
1	2				+

OB = oligoclonal bands.
*From Poser CM, et al: New diagnostic criteria for multiple sclerosis: Guidelines for research protocols. Ann Neurol 13:277, 1983.
†MRI or evoked potential studies.

Table 482–4 ■ CONDITIONS COMMONLY MISTAKEN FOR MULTIPLE SCLEROSIS

Vascular diseases
    Small-vessel cerebrovascular disease
    Vasculitis
Structural lesions
    Craniocervical junction tumor, malformation of base of skull
    Anomaly
    Posterior fossa tumor or arteriovenous malformation
    Spinal cord tumor or cervical spondylosis
Degenerative diseases
    Motor system disease
    Spinocerebellar degeneration
Infections
    HTLV-1 infection
    HIV myelopathy or HIV-related cerebritis
    Lyme disease
Other conditions
    Vitamin B_{12} deficiency
    Sjögren's syndrome
    Sarcoidosis
    Nonspecific MRI abnormalities

from sarcoidosis. MRI is the most sensitive differential screening procedure and currently eliminates the need for CT scanning or myelography in almost all cases.

Degenerative, infectious, or neoplastic diseases must be considered in patients with a steadily progressive course. Disorders that can be incorrectly diagnosed as MS include spinocerebellar degeneration, cervicomedullary syringomyelia, basilar invagination, motor neuron disease, HTLV-1 myelopathy, human immunodeficiency virus (HIV)-related myelopathy or brain infection, and neoplasms such as parenchymal lymphoma. Spinocerebellar degeneration and motor neuron disease are suspected by symmetrical neurologic impairment restricted to characteristic neural systems and by the absence of CSF inflammatory change or response to corticosteroids.

Progressive myelopathy should prompt testing for HTLV-1 and HIV, as well as for very-long-chain fatty acids, to rule out adrenoleukodystrophy (ALD). On rare occasions, CNS lupus or vitamin B_{12} deficiency may be clinically indistinguishable from MS. These disorders should be ruled out by determining antinuclear antibodies and vitamin B_{12} levels at the time of diagnosis.

Small-vessel cerebrovascular disease should be considered in hypertensive patients, particularly in those lacking CSF abnormalities typical of MS. MRI may help distinguish MS from small-vessel cerebrovascular disease; MS patients more commonly have lesions adjacent to the brain ventricles and involvement of the corpus callosum.

The second common type of diagnostic error occurs in patients with no definable neurologic disease. Patients commonly acquire an MS diagnosis because of nonspecific neurologic symptoms, such as weakness, fatigue, or tingling, at times accompanied by minimal nonspecific signal changes on brain MRI. The absence of objective neurologic signs at any time, patterns of weakness or sensory loss that fail to conform to known neuroanatomic systems, and disability out of proportion to objective clinical findings raise the suspicion of psychogenic illness. One must be open-minded, however, because MS can begin with sensory symptoms, fatigue, or other nonspecific symptoms. In many cases, it is necessary to follow the patient over time before an accurate diagnosis can be made.

TREATMENT. EDUCATION. MS patients and their families need information about MS after a diagnosis has been made. Typical questions include the following: (1) "What will happen to me?" One of the major psychological burdens for an MS patient is

Table 482–5 ■ RED FLAGS IN THE DIAGNOSIS OF MULTIPLE SCLEROSIS*

Syndrome that could be explained by localized disease
Steadily progressive disease, absence of clinical remission
Absence of oculomotor, optic nerve, sensory, or bladder involvement
Normal cerebrospinal fluid

*Modified from Rudick RA, Schiffer RB, Schwetz K, et al: Multiple sclerosis: The problem of incorrect diagnosis. Arch Neurol 43:578, 1989.

uncertainty about the future course of the illness. The physician should acknowledge the unpredictable course but emphasize the spectrum of severity and the significant proportion of patients who remain neurologically intact for many years. (2) "How can I control my illness?" Most patients have beliefs about what will improve or worsen their MS. The patient's need for control over the disease can often be focused on healthy life-styles, such as fitness programs or appropriate diet. (3) "When should I call you?" Patients should be advised to call when necessary but should be routinely seen at 6- or 12-month intervals. This allows ongoing assessment of neurologic impairment and results in a gradual decline in the need for telephone calls. (4) "Will my children get this?" The lifetime risk to a child of a mother with MS is 3 to 5%; this is a 30- to 50-fold increase over that for the general population, but still a small risk. (5) "Can I have a baby?" Pregnancy has a predictable effect on the pattern of MS, as discussed above. It appears that breast-feeding has little if any effect on the frequency, timing, or severity of postpartum exacerbations, and the bulk of evidence suggests that the overall course of MS, including the eventual degree of disability, is unaffected by one or more pregnancies. Women with mild to moderate disability should plan pregnancies primarily on the basis of issues other than MS.

SYMPTOM PHARMACOTHERAPY. Spasticity may be reduced by a combination of physical measures and antispastic drugs. The γ-aminobutyric acid (GABA)-agonist baclofen is the drug of choice, but its dosage should be individualized because it is effective over a wide dose range. Baclofen therapy should be instituted slowly to avoid sedation or weakness, and it must not be stopped abruptly, as its withdrawal can cause confusional states or seizures. Diazepam may be used as an adjunct to baclofen, particularly for patients with nocturnal spasms causing sleep disturbance. Even a small dose of diazepam may potentiate the benefits of baclofen. Tizanidine, an α-adrenergic agonist, is an alternative to baclofen. The antispastic effects of tizanidine are generally not accompanied by increased weakness, but drowsiness and orthostatic hypotension may limit its use in individual patients. Tizanidine may be cautiously added to baclofen when additional baclofen causes undue sedation or weakness. Dantrolene is another antispastic drug that can be used in patients who do not respond well to baclofen, tizanidine, or diazepam or cannot tolerate the sedation that sometimes complicates the use of these drugs. Dantrolene exerts its effects at the muscle; consequently, motor weakness almost always accompanies dantrolene's antispastic effect. Dantrolene should be used cautiously in patients with myocardial disease, and it occasionally causes toxic hepatitis. Patients with severe spasticity not effectively managed with the above measures may benefit from intrathecal baclofen, administered continuously at a rate of 200 to 800 µg/day via a fully implantable infusion pump.

Dystonic spasms consist of brief, recurrent, painful posturing of one or more extremities, not associated with altered consciousness or urinary incontinence. Dystonic spasms are easily controlled with carbamazepine or phenytoin. Ataxia is difficult to treat pharmacologically. Intention tremor may respond to clonazepam, which should be instituted slowly to avoid sedation. Clonazepam therapy should be initiated at a dose of 0.5 mg at bedtime and increased gradually to an end-point of sedation or effective control of tremor. One or more tonic-clonic seizures occur in about 5% of MS patients. A single motor seizure predicts a subsequent seizure in an MS patient and should be treated with an adequate dose of phenytoin. Bladder symptoms require urinalysis, culture, and measurement of postvoid residual volume. In the absence of a urinary tract infection or urinary retention greater than 100 mL, anticholinergic agents, such as oxybutynin or propantheline, are effective. Urinary tract infection or urinary retention greater than 100 mL requires urologic evaluation. Fatigue in MS, when disabling and not caused by depression, can be treated effectively with amantadine, 100 mg twice a day. Pemoline is effective for some individuals who have not responded to amantadine.

Heat sensitivity results from conduction failure in partially demyelinated CNS fibers. Patients may benefit from cool showers or air conditioning. Dramatic deterioration can accompany fever in patients with advanced MS, and elevated body temperatures should be treated aggressively, with specific infections being managed with appropriate antibiotics.

Pain syndromes consist of trigeminal neuralgia or atypical facial pain, paroxysmal limb paresthesias presenting as brief tic-like pain, burning dysesthesias, Lhermitte's phenomenon, and chronic back pain, due in most cases to mechanical stress caused by ataxia and weakness. Trigeminal neuralgia or disagreeable paresthesias may respond to carbamazepine or alternatively to amitriptyline, phenytoin, or baclofen. If medical therapy fails, trigeminal rhizotomy is an alternative. Chronic low back and leg pain are usually alleviated with nonsteroidal anti-inflammatory drugs and physical therapy. A proper walking aid, ankle-foot orthosis, or proper seating is critical. Coexistent herniated disks should be ruled out in the MS patient with radicular pain, particularly when an ankle or knee tendon reflex is absent.

Depression or emotional distress is often underrecognized and inadequately treated. Depression is particularly common when the illness is first diagnosed or when it worsens substantially. Depression lowers quality of life, impairs social relationships and job performance, and should be treated aggressively with psychiatric referral or antidepressant drugs. For depressed MS patients with anxiety and insomnia, amitriptyline is effective and inexpensive. For patients with coexisting bladder symptoms, imipramine is useful because its α-adrenergic properties may improve bladder dysfunction. For older patients or patients with memory impairment, a tricyclic antidepressant with less anticholinergic activity, such as desipramine or nortriptyline, or a serotonin reuptake inhibitor may be better tolerated. Emotional lability, which is distressing and socially disabling for some MS patients, may improve with low doses of amitriptyline.

Cognitive dysfunction may be difficult to recognize clinically but should be suspected in any MS patient with poor work performance, family disruption, or noncompliance with medical or rehabilitative therapies, particularly when the explanation for the problem is unclear. Neuropsychological tests are important to address the problem and should include sensitive measurements of complex attention and information processing, learning and recent memory, concept formation, and problem solving. No effective drug therapy is available, although patients often can learn compensatory strategies and may benefit from cognitive rehabilitation.

DISEASE PHARMACOTHERAPY. Numerous trials of drugs have been directed at improving the long-term course of MS or shortening the course of acute exacerbations. Nearly all current experimental therapy trials include MRI measures of outcome, and measures of clinical outcome have improved.

CORTICOSTEROID THERAPY. Recent evidence suggests that intravenous methylprednisolone has a more rapid onset of action and better efficacy than corticotropin or other steroid preparations in limiting acute exacerbations. A recent study suggested that bimonthly pulses of IV methylprednisolone therapy might slow the inexorable deterioration in patients with secondary progressive MS, but the effects were found to be modest. Excessive or injudicious use of steroids gradually lessens their value, and most patients eventually become unresponsive to steroids. For major clinical exacerbations, intravenous methylprednisolone, 500 or 1000 mg/day for 3 days, can be administered safely in an outpatient setting, followed by prednisone, 60 mg in a single morning dose for 3 days, tapering off over 12 days.

IMMUNOMODULATORY THERAPY. Two forms of recombinant beta interferon (IFN-β), interferon β-1a (Avonex) and interferon β-1b (Betaseron), have been approved for use in relapsing remitting MS patients. IFN-β therapy reduces the frequency and severity of MS relapses, slows disability progression, reduces the number and volume of new MRI lesions, and slows the progressive accumulation of T2 MRI lesions. Based on the results of controlled clinical trials, Betaseron is administered at a dose of 8,000,000 IU every other day by subcutaneous injection, whereas Avonex is administered at a dose of 6,000,000 IU/week by IM injection. Adverse effects include transient flu-like symptoms after each injection with both preparations, inflammatory reactions at the injection sites with Betaseron, and development of neutralizing antibodies after months of therapy, observed more commonly with Betaseron than with Avonex. Glatiramer acetate (Copaxone) is available for patients with relapsing remitting MS. Glatiramer acetate is a polypeptide consisting of basic amino acids. It was synthesized as a molecular mimic of MBP and is thought to inhibit cellular immune reactions to myelin. Glatiramer acetate is administered as a daily subcutaneous injection. Its principal documented beneficial effect is about a

30% reduction in the relapse rate, and its principal side effect is swelling and redness at the injection site. Various drugs that suppress the immune system have been reported to show partial efficacy. These include cyclophosphamide, cyclosporine, azathioprine, and methotrexate. Methotrexate, administered orally at a dose of 7.5 mg/week, was found to reduce the proportion of patients with chronic progressive MS who worsened during a 2-year treatment period compared with placebo-treated patients. This dose results in minimal apparent toxicity. Cyclophosphamide and cyclosporine have some reported benefit but are limited by toxicity. Evidence indicates that azathioprine reduces the rate of exacerbations, but the relative and ultimate benefits of azathioprine and IFN-β have not been determined. Currently, it is safest to restrict immunosuppressive drugs to centers operating within the context of controlled protocols.

MULTIPLE SCLEROSIS VARIANTS

NEUROMYELITIS OPTICA (DEVIC'S DISEASE). Neuromyelitis optica is a syndrome characterized by partial or complete transverse myelopathy and optic neuritis. Loss of vision and paraplegia may occur in either order, and the two major components of the disease may be widely separated in time. The syndrome of neuromyelitis optica may occur as the result of acute disseminated encephalomyelitis, systemic lupus erythematosus, or sarcoidosis, as well as during the course of typical MS or in isolation without apparent cause. In the latter case, it is considered a variant of MS.

CONCENTRIC SCLEROSIS. Concentric sclerosis is a rare form of demyelinating disease characterized by rapidly progressive demyelination. It appears to be a variant of rapidly progressive MS. Clinically, the disease begins with the acute or subacute onset of altered behavior, difficulty in communication, mutism, apathy, and headache. CSF is usually normal. Imaging shows extensive lesions in cerebral white matter. Concentric sclerosis may be suspected clinically but can be diagnosed only by its characteristic histopathology. Alternating bands containing demyelinated and partially demyelinated axons radiate concentrically. Oligodendrocyte loss characterizes the bands of demyelination.

MONOPHASIC DISORDERS RELATED TO MULTIPLE SCLEROSIS

OPTIC NEURITIS. Optic neuritis denotes acute or subacute partial or complete loss of vision in one or both eyes due to inflammation. Almost all patients with inflammatory optic neuritis experience pain in, around, or behind the affected eye, followed within a day or two by visual loss. Visual loss of varying intensity progresses for as long as 1 week. Optic neuritis is classified as retrobulbar neuritis when the lesion is in the posterior two-thirds of the optic nerve and as papillitis when the lesion is in the anterior portion of the optic nerve. The latter leads to an ophthalmoscopic appearance similar to that of acute papilledema resulting from increased intracranial pressure, but it differs from the latter in that visual acuity is markedly reduced in papillitis. Visual fields in optic neuritis reveal a central or cecocentral scotoma of varying degree. Color vision is impaired, and a deafferent Marcus Gunn pupil may be present. With retrobulbar optic neuritis, ophthalmoscopic examination remains normal for the first 2 to 3 weeks, after which the disk becomes pale, with loss of small vessels. Visual function almost always recovers to some degree, usually within weeks. Blindness as the result of optic nerve demyelination of MS seldom occurs.

The syndrome of optic neuritis can be caused by several diseases, of which MS is by far the most common. Other causes include tobacco-nutritional amblyopia, Leber's hereditary optic neuropathy, vasculitis, optic nerve compression on any basis, neurosyphilis, ischemic optic neuropathy, pernicious anemia, or sarcoidosis. Optic neuritis is usually easily differentiated from optic nerve ischemia, which has an abrupt onset, affects older individuals, and results in field cuts consistent with retinal artery occlusions. Compressive optic neuropathy causes slowly progressive visual loss. Vasculitis or sarcoidosis can usually be distinguished by characteristic funduscopic features and by the presence of uveitis.

Many patients with idiopathic isolated optic neuritis eventually develop MS; the reported frequency in several series has varied from 13 to 85%, according to the length of follow-up. The presence of CSF OGB or brain MRI abnormalities significantly increases the risk of early conversion to MS. Patients with idiopathic monosymptomatic optic neuritis who have periventricular MRI abnormalities have about a 35% chance of developing MS within 2 years and an 85% chance of developing MS within 5 years.

More rapid, but not necessarily greater, total visual recovery occurs by treating optic neuritis with intravenous methylprednisolone. A 3-day course of intravenous methylprednisolone followed by a prednisone taper within 8 days of the onset appears to reduce by about 50% the likelihood of conversion from idiopathic optic neuritis to MS during 2 years of follow-up.

ACUTE TRANSVERSE MYELITIS. Acute transverse myelitis denotes rapidly developing paraparesis or paraplegia as the result of spinal cord dysfunction. Abrupt or rapidly developing back or radicular pain may be followed by ascending paresthesias and weakness beginning in the feet. Urinary and fecal retention or incontinence is common. Progression varies from minutes, resembling infarction, to steady or stepwise progression over several days. Progression over days may occur with both spinal cord compression due to a tumor and MS. It is also common to observe patients with sensory symptoms below a particular dermatome corresponding to the spinal cord level of involvement, with or without ataxia and variable degrees of leg weakness. It may be difficult to distinguish idiopathic transverse myelitis from compressive myelopathy. Therefore, the syndrome of acute transverse myelitis demands immediate diagnostic evaluation.

Of the several disorders that can produce an acute transverse myelopathy (Table 482–6), the most important to rule in or out immediately are compressive lesions, including spinal or epidural abscess, tumor, herniated intervertebral disk, or injury; vascular occlusion due to arteritis, aortic dissection, aortic surgery, or arteriovenous malformation; varicella-zoster infection; and autoimmune disease including MS. In many instances, a careful history suggests the cause and the appropriate approach. The evaluation must include an immediate imaging procedure, such as MRI, with attention to the level of involvement to rule out spinal cord compression. Cord compression from metastatic tumor may present acutely even though the tumor has been present for weeks or longer. Central herniated intervertebral disks may cause acute cord compression without producing local pain. Rapidly progressing myelopathy in a previously healthy person should always raise the question of spontaneous epidural, subdural, or intraparenchymal abscess or bleeding, the latter occurring from an arteriovenous malformation or as a complication of anticoagulation or blood dyscrasia. About one-third of patients with idiopathic transverse myelitis give a history of an antecedent upper respiratory or flu-like illness. Transverse myelitis may also follow several other infectious illnesses, such as mycoplasmal infection or measles.

Transverse myelitis and slowly progressive myelopathy are common manifestations of MS, either as a first clinical manifestation or a late development. However, a syndrome suggesting complete cord transection rarely occurs. As with optic neuritis, CSF OGB or an abnormal brain MRI suggestive of MS makes clinically definite MS likely.

Proper treatment requires an expeditious diagnosis. When cord

Table 482–6 ■ ACUTE OR SUBACUTE TRANSVERSE MYELOPATHY

Associated with infection
  Bacterial
    Spinal epidural abscess
    Intramedullary abscess
  Viral, e.g., varicella-zoster
  Postviral, e.g., rubella with disseminated encephalomyelitis
Compression
  Tumor, especially metastatic
  Trauma
  Herniated intervertebral disk
Vascular
  Acute extradural, subdural, or parenchymal hemorrhage
  Dissecting aortic aneurysm
  Arteritis
  Systemic lupus erythematosus
Idiopathic

compression is present, surgical decompression and treatment with antibiotics or with corticosteroids are needed immediately. Treatment may halt progression but may not restore lost function. In idiopathic transverse myelopathy, MS, or cord compression, corticosteroids may reduce edema and lead to earlier restitution of function, although the effect on long-term outcome is uncertain. The treatment of choice for idiopathic transverse myelitis is intravenous administration of methylprednisolone. With severe disease, bladder catheterization, ventilatory support, and proper protection from compression neuropathies are necessary. Prognosis varies widely, with recovery ranging from almost none at all to complete, depending on the degree of acute necrosis.

LEUKODYSTROPHIES

The leukodystrophies (see Table 482–1) are uncommon dysmyelinating diseases in which myelin formation or maintenance is impaired by a genetically determined biochemical defect. The leukodystrophies affect individuals from the first months of life to the 20s. A biochemical effect is known for several, but they are not yet curable.

PEROXISOMAL DISORDERS (E.G., ADRENOLEUKODYSTROPHY). Adrenoleukodystrophy (ALD) includes two genetically determined disorders that cause dysfunction of adrenal glands and nervous system myelin. There are two distinct types of ALD: the X-linked form and a recessive form, termed *neonatal ALD*. Neonatal ALD is characterized by early and severe psychomotor retardation, seizures, retinopathy, hepatomegaly, and dysmorphic features occurring in infants of either sex.

The X-linked form of ALD is phenotypically heterogeneous, even though the disease is associated with a common biochemical defect. The two common patterns of X-linked ALD are the childhood form and adrenomyeloneuropathy. In the childhood form, boys develop normally until age 4 to 8 years, when they manifest behavioral changes with progressive cognitive decline leading over years to a chronic vegetative state. Young men with adrenomyeloneuropathy experience progressive paraparesis and bladder dysfunction. Almost all such ALD patients have adrenal insufficiency, although the degree varies considerably. Less common phenotypes of X-linked ALD include adrenal insufficiency without nervous system involvement, progressive dementia in adults, and an asymptomatic state in males with the same metabolic deficiency as affected relatives. Occasionally, female heterozygotes develop neurologic disturbances that resemble MS. The basis for clinical heterogeneity, despite a common metabolic defect, is unknown. Tissues and body fluids of patients with X-linked ALD contain high levels of unbranched, saturated, very-long-chain fatty acids. Fatty acids accumulate because of deficient peroxisomal catabolism, although the precise nature of the enzyme defect is not clear. The gene for X-linked ALD has been mapped to chromosome Xq28.

The diagnosis of X-linked ALD may be suspected in males with the clinical features described above. CSF shows inflammatory changes that may be identical to those seen in MS, although the CSF protein is usually higher in ALD. MRI shows symmetrical lesions in the posterior parietal and occipital white matter. Endocrine testing reveals primary adrenal insufficiency. The diagnosis is confirmed by demonstrating increased levels of very-long-chain fatty acids in blood, tissue, or cultured fibroblasts. Most female heterozygotes can be identified using these methods as well. A DNA probe is available for gene screening, and prenatal diagnosis is possible through biochemical and genetic screening of amniocytes.

Pathologic examination shows widespread demyelination in CNS and peripheral myelin, with numerous lipid lamellar inclusions throughout the tissue. Many lesions exhibit cellular infiltration with lymphocytes and macrophages, suggesting an inflammatory component to pathogenesis.

Treatment of X-linked ALD consists of adrenal hormone replacement and dietary restriction of long-chain fatty acids. Preliminary evidence suggests that bone marrow transplantation may slow progression of the disease, but there is no other specific treatment at present.

PELIZAEUS-MERZBACHER DISEASE. This is an extremely rare, chronic familial disease that has been generally classified among the leukodystrophies. The nosology of the disorder has been revolutionized by identification of the genetic defect in the myelin proteolipid (PLP; lipophilin) protein gene that accounts for the majority of cases. Extensive CNS myelin destruction is associated with myelin breakdown products staining bright red with the usual fat stains (resulting in the synonym *sudanophilic leukodystrophy*). Pelizaeus-Merzbacher disease is inherited as an X-linked recessive trait and primarily affects males. The condition begins in infancy and progresses slowly to produce extensive, diffuse, symmetrical disturbances of myelin associated with gliosis within the cerebrum and cerebellum. The peripheral nervous system is not affected.

Pelizaeus-Merzbacher disease is caused by mutations in the PLP gene. This seminal discovery came from extensive characterization of jimpy mutant mice, that exhibit X-linked dysmyelination. It was soon reported that the jimpy defect was associated with mutations in the PLP structural gene, specifically a mis-spliced primary RNA transcript that deleted 74 base pairs from the mature mRNA. In the mid-1980s, it became apparent that the Pelizaeus-Merzbacher mutation was located in the same region of the X chromosome as the PLP gene. Since that time, numerous reports of PLP mutations in Pelizaeus-Merzbacher families have appeared, and Pelizaeus-Merzbacher disease is now associated with point mutations throughout the coding region of the PLP gene in all seven exons. Surprisingly, duplication of a normal gene can produce the same disease, as can complete deletion. The association of multiple genotypes including mutations, duplications, and deletions underscores the importance of gene dosage of PLP for physiologic homeostasis of oligodendrocytes; it seems to be equally deleterious to have a mutant PLP, to have a complete lack of PLP, and to have excessive wild-type PLP. The exact pathogenesis of cases classified as Pelizaeus-Merzbacher disease remains unknown. No treatment is available.

METACHROMATIC LEUKODYSTROPHY. Metachromatic leukodystrophy (MLD) is the most common leukodystrophy. MLD is a lysosomal storage disease caused by deficiency of arylsulfatase A. Patients develop diffuse dysmyelination, usually starting in the first 10 years of life. The process leads to dementia, convulsions, cranial nerve abnormalities, and, finally, severe spasticity or rigidity. Death usually occurs after 2 to 4 years. Juvenile and adult-onset cases have been reported. In the adult form of MLD, patients' mental deterioration progresses to severe dementia with pyramidal tract and cerebellar signs. The diagnosis is suspected in an infant or child with progressive dementia, convulsions, and spasticity, and in a young adult with progressive dementia, particularly in the presence of absent tendon reflexes and elevated CSF protein levels.

The arylsulfatase A gene has been cloned and characterized. Nearly all patients have deficient arylsulfatase A enzyme activity, resulting in accumulation of sulfatides in lysosomes within central and peripheral nervous system tissue. Occasionally, arylsulfatase A activity is low, but the individual remains unaffected. This is termed *pseudodeficiency*. An increased urinary excretion of sulfatide and reduced arylsulfatase A activity in venous blood or cultured fibroblasts is diagnostic. Pathologically, sulfatides (which stain metachromatically) accumulate in oligodendrocytes and Schwann cells and within myelin lamellae. Sulfatides also collect within neurons, liver, gallbladder, kidneys, and spleen. Some evidence suggests that bone marrow transplantation may slow or halt progression of MLD.

GLOBOID CELL LEUKODYSTROPHY (KRABBE'S DISEASE). Globoid cell leukodystrophy is characterized biochemically as deficient galactocerebroside β-galactosidase activity. The disease affects infants in the first 2 to 3 months of life and is transmitted as an autosomal recessive trait. Rare instances occur in late infancy or in adulthood. The activity of galactocerebroside β-galactosidase can be determined in serum, peripheral leukocytes, or fibroblasts. Neuropathologic examination reveals marked loss of myelin throughout the brain, with the presence of round or oval mononuclear cells the size of large glia or as large, irregular multinucleated cells, termed *globoid cells*, containing galactocerebroside. Infants with the disorder usually progress to a vegetative state within their second year of life. Late-onset cases present with progressive motor impairment and, less frequently, visual failure. No treatment is known.

Multiple Sclerosis

Anderson DW, Ellenberg JH, Leventhal CM, et al: Revised estimate of the prevalence of multiple sclerosis in the United States. Ann Neurol 31:333, 1992. *The estimated number of MS cases in the United States was 350,000.*

Ebers GC, Sadovnick AD: The geographic distribution of multiple sclerosis: A review. Neuroepidemiology 12:1, 1993. *Synthesizes available epidemiologic information. A combination of both genetic and environmental factors appears to explain the available data on MS and geography.*

Goodkin DE, Rudick RA, Ross JS: The use of brain magnetic resonance imaging in multiple sclerosis. Arch Neurol 51:505, 1994. *Provides an overview of the use of MRI in MS patients.*

Prineas J, Kwon E, Goldenberg P, et al: Multiple sclerosis: Oligodendrocyte proliferation and differentiation in fresh lesions. Lab Invest 61:489, 1989. *Elegantly describes and illustrates the tissue alterations produced by MS.*

Ransohoff RM, Tuohy VK, Lehmann PV: The immunology of multiple sclerosis: New intricacies and new insights. Curr Opin Neurol Neurosurg 7:242, 1994. *Reviews recent advances in our understanding of immunopathogenesis.*

Rudick RA: Helping patients live with multiple sclerosis: What primary care physicians can do. Postgrad Med 88:197, 1990. *Provides practical management strategies for primary physicians caring for MS patients and their families.*

Rudick RA, Birk KA: Multiple sclerosis and pregnancy. *In* Goldstein PJ, Stern BJ (eds): Neurological Disorders of Pregnancy, 2nd ed. Mount Kisco, NY, Futura Publishing, 1992, p 165. *Reviews the relationship between pregnancy and MS, with emphasis on reproductive and pregnancy counseling.*

Rudick RA, Cohen JA, Weinstock-Guttman B, et al: Management of multiple sclerosis. N Engl J Med 337:1604–1611, 1997. *Review of current drug therapies that favorably influence the disease course.*

Trapp BD, Peterson J, Ransohoff RM, et al: Axonal transections in the lesions of multiple sclerosis. N Engl J Med 33:278–285, 1998. *Demonstrates extensive transection of axons in lesions in MS brain.*

Runmarker B, Andersen O: Prognostic factors in a multiple sclerosis incidence cohort with 25 years of follow-up. Brain 116:117, 1993. *Describes favorable prognostic indicators, including a high degree of recovery after first exacerbation, predominance of sensory symptoms, and benign condition 5 years after symptom onset.*

Schumacher G, Beebe G, Kibler R, et al: Problems of experimental trials of therapy in multiple sclerosis: Report by the panel on the evaluation of experimental trials of therapy in multiple sclerosis. Ann NY Acad Sci 122:552, 1965. *Defined clinical criteria that are still valid for the diagnosis of MS.*

Optic Neuritis

Beck RW, Cleary PA, Anderson MM, et al: A randomized, controlled trial of corticosteroids in the treatment of acute optic neuritis. N Engl J Med 326:581, 1992. *Reports that treatment of optic neuritis with intravenous methylprednisolone improved the rate of visual recovery but not the extent of eventual return of vision.*

Beck RW, Cleary PA, Trobe JD, et al: The effect of corticosteroids for acute optic neuritis on the subsequent development of multiple sclerosis. N Engl J Med 329:1764, 1993. *Found that treatment with intravenous MP reduced the likelihood of progression from optic neuritis to clinically definite MS within 2 years by 50%.*

Optic Neuritis Study Group: The clinical profile of optic neuritis: Experience of the optic neuritis treatment trial. Arch Ophthalmol 109:1673, 1991. *Provides definitive clinical and laboratory features of 448 patients with acute optic neuritis studied according to a comprehensive standardized protocol.*

Transverse Myelitis

Ropper AH, Poskanzer DC: The prognosis of acute and subacute transverse myelopathy based on early signs and symptoms. Ann Neurol 4:51, 1978. *Reviews the experience of a large general hospital with an excellent description of the clinical findings and follow-up.*

Tippett DS, Fishman PS, Panitch HS: Relapsing transverse myelitis. Neurology 41:703, 1991. *Describes patients with recurrent episodes of transverse myelitis, no evidence of brain stem or forebrain lesions, and absence of CSF oligoclonal bands. This is probably a variant of MS.*

Leukodystrophies

Aubourg P, Blanche S, Jambaque I, et al: Reversal of early neurologic and neuroradiologic manifestations of X-linked adrenoleukodystrophy by bone marrow transplantation. N Engl J Med 322:1860, 1990. *Suggests a benefit from bone marrow transplantation.*

Gieselmann V, von Figura K: Advances in molecular genetics of metachromatic leukodystrophy. J Inherit Metab Dis 13:560, 1990. *Reviews the genetics of MLD.*

Krivit W, Shapiro E, Kennedy W, et al: Treatment of late infantile metachromatic leukodystrophy by bone marrow transplantation. N Engl J Med 322:28, 1990. *Suggests a benefit from bone marrow transplantation.*

Moser HW, Bergin A, Cornblath D: Peroxisomal disorders. Biochem Cell Biol 69:463, 1991. *Provides a comprehensive overview of the biochemical abnormalities underlying ALD.*

Moser HW, Moser AB, Naidu S, Bergin A: Clinical aspects of adrenoleukodystrophy and adrenomyeloneuropathy. Dev Neurosci 13:254, 1991. *Provides an authoritative overview of clinical features.*

Moser HW, Moser AB, Smith KD, et al: Adrenoleukodystrophy: Phenotypic variability and implications for therapy. J Inherit Metab Dis 15:645, 1992. *Provides the largest experience with bone marrow transplants and suggests that results are encouraging.*

Seitelberger F: Pelizaeus-Merzbacher's disease. *In* Vinken P, Bruyn G (eds): Handbook of Clinical Neurology, vol 10. Amsterdam, North-Holland, 1970, p 150. *An excellent review of this and related degenerative diseases of myelin.*

Wanders RJ, Tager JM: Peroxisomal fatty acid beta-oxidation in relation to adrenoleukodystrophy. Dev Neurosci 13:262, 1991. *Provides the present state of knowledge regarding the organization of peroxisomal fatty acid oxidation with emphasis on X-linked adrenoleukodystrophy.*

483 CENTRAL NERVOUS SYSTEM COMPLICATIONS OF VIRAL INFECTIONS AND VACCINES

Richard A. Rudick

Central nervous system (CNS) signs arising during the course of systemic infection usually reflect CNS invasion by the inciting organism. Less frequently, systemic infections or use of certain vaccines gives rise to CNS abnormalities that do not reflect direct infection of nervous tissue, but rather result from presumed autoimmune or toxic mechanisms. Several reasonably distinct patterns of involvement have been delineated. Two of these, *acute disseminated encephalomyelitis* (ADEM) and *acute necrotizing hemorrhagic encephalopathy* (ANHE), appear to be mediated by immune mechanisms and have a peripheral nervous system counterpart, acute inflammatory polyneuropathy, or the Guillain-Barré syndrome. The remainder, Reye's syndrome, acute toxic encephalopathy, and acute cerebellar ataxia of childhood, are likely to be toxic in origin.

ACUTE DISSEMINATED ENCEPHALOMYELITIS

DEFINITION AND NOMENCLATURE. Acute disseminated encephalomyelitis is an uncommon acute inflammatory disease of the CNS that occurs following viral infections or vaccination. ADEM is thought to be immune mediated. Brain and spinal cord involvement is usually widespread but may at times be limited to discrete areas such as the optic nerves or a single spinal cord level. Various names have been used to describe this syndrome (Table 483–1), but the term ADEM is appropriately descriptive. The classic features of ADEM (Table 483–2) include an antecedent event, commonly a viral illness, which, after a latent period, is followed by acute onset of multifocal or diffuse CNS signs, the potential for extensive or even complete recovery, and pathologic evidence of perivascular inflammation and demyelination.

ETIOLOGY AND PATHOGENESIS. Table 483–3 lists the principal events preceding ADEM, although many cases occur without a known precipitant. Of the various viral infections, ADEM occurs more frequently with RNA viruses that bud from infected cells. Viral infections associated with exanthems, such as measles, rubella, and varicella, are particularly common antecedents, but the disease also follows mumps, influenza, herpes simplex, or viruses causing banal, nonspecific upper respiratory infections. The syndrome has been observed after vaccination for rabies, rubella, pertussis, influenza, or vaccinia, or in association with various medications. Neurologic manifestations usually occur 6 to 10 days after the exanthem, viral symptoms, or vaccination.

A compelling analogy links the ADEM complicating rabies vaccination with the animal disorder *experimental allergic encephalo-*

Table 483–1 ■ **TERMINOLOGY: ACUTE DISSEMINATED ENCEPHALOMYELITIS (ADEM)**

ADEM
Postinfectious encephalomyelitis
Postvaccinial encephalomyelitis
Acute perivascular myelinoclasis
Acute demyelinating encephalomyelitis
Postvaccinial microglial encephalitis
Disseminated vasculomyelinopathy
Perivenous encephalitis
Immune-mediated encephalomyelitis
Necrotizing form
Acute necrotizing hemorrhagic encephalopathy
Acute hemorrhagic encephalitis
Acute hemorrhagic leukoencephalitis
Hemorrhagic perivenous encephalitis
Hurst's disease
Hemorrhagic immune-mediated encephalomyelitis

Table 483–2 ■ CARDINAL FEATURES OF ACUTE DISSEMINATED
ENCEPHALOMYELITIS

Preceding event, usually viral illness
Latent period followed by acute onset of multifocal or diffuse CNS signs
Potential for full recovery
Pathologic features of perivascular inflammation and demyelination; vessel
damage and hemorrhage variable

myelitis (EAE). Inoculation of susceptible animals with brain homogenates, purified myelin components, or peptides containing en-
cephalitogenic sequences of myelin proteins can induce acute CNS
perivascular inflammation and demyelination that is histologically
identical to the pathologic findings observed in ADEM. In animals
with EAE, neurologic signs appear 10 to 14 days after sensitization
to myelin antigens in association with humoral and cellular immune responses to the inciting CNS antigen. Furthermore, in some
forms of EAE, the disease can be transferred to healthy animals by
injecting T lymphocytes from immunized animals, suggesting that
this cell type is of primary importance in the pathogenesis. In some
forms of EAE, pathogenic antibodies appear to play a primary role.
ADEM complicating rabies vaccination is considered a human form
of EAE. ADEM was observed in as many as one of every 600
individuals following rabies vaccination using inactivated inoculum
of fixed rabies virus propagated in animal brain. The complication
of rabies vaccination called "neuroparalytic accident" was caused
by vaccine contamination with CNS antigens. Both complement-
fixing antibody and specific lymphocyte proliferative responses to
crude and purified CNS antigens have been measured in blood of
patients receiving rabies vaccine, with the most abnormal responses
in patients with neuroparalytic accidents. Current rabies vaccines
derived from virus grown in human diploid cells appear to be
essentially free of neural complications.

ADEM following viral infection may also be immune mediated.
Lymphocytes that proliferate in the presence of myelin basic protein (MBP), complement-fixing antibodies to neural tissue, and humoral factors with demyelinating activity have been described. Encephalitis is relatively frequent following measles (1:1000 cases),
but little evidence is available to implicate invasion of the CNS by
measles virus as an obligate prerequisite. Theoretical data support
the possible importance of sequence similarities between measles
virus or other viral antigens and CNS proteins, such as MBP and
proteolipid protein. Very early in the course of measles ADEM,
specific proliferative responses to MBP are apparent in the lymphocytes of children, and measurable quantities of MBP are released
into CSF. These findings support the hypothesis that acute measles
transiently alters the immune system, which in some persons results
in a breakdown of tolerance to CNS antigens. Despite the usual
absence of CNS symptoms, this process appears to occur frequently, as reflected by a high incidence of abnormal-appearing
electroencephalograms (EEGs). Both EEG abnormalities and clinical ADEM can occur after vaccination with live-attenuated measles
virus but at a markedly lower frequency, with ADEM arising in
about 1 in 1 million vaccinated persons.

INCIDENCE. Valid incidence figures for ADEM are difficult to
derive. Encephalitis complicates about 1 in 1000 cases of measles.
ADEM following other childhood viral illnesses or vaccinations is
uncommon. Most adult cases of ADEM have no identifiable antecedents.

Table 483–3 ■ PRINCIPAL CONDITIONS PREDISPOSING TO
ACUTE DISSEMINATED ENCEPHALOMYELITIS

Infections
  Measles
  Varicella-zoster
  Influenza
  Rubella
  Mycoplasma pneumoniae
  Respiratory viruses
  Epstein-Barr
Vaccines: smallpox, measles, rabies (Semple vaccine)

PATHOLOGY. Characteristic lesions typically occur around venules within the white matter of brain and spinal cord. Leptomeninges contain lymphocytes, plasma cells, and occasional polymorphonuclear cells early in the course. Shortly thereafter, a
perivenular mononuclear inflammatory infiltration is seen. Myelin
in this distribution becomes fragmented and, eventually, entirely
absent. There is relative axonal sparing. This primary lesion can
occur throughout the neuraxis but tends to be most prominent in
the centrum semiovale of the cerebrum and in the pontine white
matter. Repair occurs through remyelination. In certain cases, large,
confluent demyelination can take on a superficial resemblance to
the plaques of multiple sclerosis, differing primarily in that all
lesions reflect a similar time of onset.

CLINICAL MANIFESTATIONS. In adults, neurologic symptoms
often first suggest the illness. With the childhood exanthems, CNS
symptoms usually begin about 5 days after the onset of the rash.
The clinical disorder can resemble any of the acute encephalitides.
Typically, nonspecific symptoms of fever, headache, anorexia, and
vomiting are rapidly followed by meningeal signs, altered consciousness, and focal signs referable to brain, spinal cord, optic
nerves, or spinal roots. About half of patients experience one or
more generalized seizures. Neurologic signs consist of some combination of pyramidal tract dysfunction, cranial nerve signs, movement disorders, sensory system dysfunction, cerebellar signs, and
loss of muscle stretch reflexes. Stupor, delirium, or coma develops
in severe cases. The EEG is abnormal, with widespread slowing of
background rhythms. The cerebrospinal fluid (CSF) in children almost invariably shows modest mononuclear pleocytosis of 20 to
200 cells/mm³ (occasionally higher). The fluid contains a slight
elevation of protein content, a normal glucose level, and a raised
MBP. Tests for oligoclonal bands are usually negative. After several days, magnetic resonance imaging (MRI) characteristically
demonstrates scattered white matter lesions, at least some of which
enhance with paramagnetic agents during the acute phases of the
disease.

The duration of active CNS disease varies from days to weeks,
often with a protracted convalescence. The overall mortality is
about 20%. About 90% of survivors recover completely or nearly
completely, although severe deficits can persist.

DIAGNOSIS. Diagnosis in ADEM is by exclusion. The most important consideration is CNS infection. In pathologic series of cases
of clinically diagnosed ADEM occurring during the course of mass
vaccination programs, postmortem examination showed that the
majority of patients had other illnesses, including potentially treatable CNS infections. In the setting of a recent exanthem, viral
illness, or vaccination, ADEM may be suggested. Differentiation
from an initial episode of multiple sclerosis (MS) (see Chapter 482)
can be difficult. Gadolinium enhancement of all areas of T2 hyperintensity on brain MRI scans suggests that the lesions are all of
recent onset. This finding suggests ADEM rather than an acute
presentation of MS.

TREATMENT. Treatment consists of supportive care, including
the use of anticonvulsants and, when necessary, intensive care
monitoring. Although sometimes used clinically, neither corticosteroids nor other immunosuppressive drugs have established efficacy.

ACUTE NECROTIZING HEMORRHAGIC ENCEPHALOPATHY

Acute necrotizing hemorrhagic encephalopathy (ANHE) is considered the hyperacute form of ADEM. As with ADEM, many
names have been applied to this syndrome (see Table 483–1).
ANHE is thought to have an immunopathogenesis similar to that of
ADEM. Typically, the illness arises spontaneously or after an uneventful upper respiratory illness. Sudden headache precedes the
neurologic symptoms, which include seizures and rapid progression
from lethargy to coma in a matter of a few hours to several days.
Major focal neurologic abnormalities are common and may suggest
lateralized cerebral involvement. Systemic signs and symptoms include fever and marked peripheral leukocytosis. The accompanying
CSF pleocytosis usually shows a preponderance of polymorphonuclear cells and sometimes evidence of hemorrhage. More than 80%
of all recognized cases of ANHE are fatal, although these findings
may be biased by the case selection. The brain is usually swollen,
with bilateral but asymmetrical petechial hemorrhages scattered
throughout the white matter. Microscopic lesions resemble hyperacute forms of EAE. The clinical differential diagnosis includes

ADEM and acute viral encephalitis, especially herpes simplex encephalitis (see Chapter 477.1). Computed tomography or MRI may be diagnostically helpful in selected cases. Therapy is supportive.

Griffin DE: Monophasic autoimmune inflammatory diseases of the CNS and PNS. Res Publ Assoc Res Nerv Ment Dis 68:91, 1990. *A review of advances in unraveling parainfectious nervous system disease.*
Kesselring J, Miller DH, Robb SA, et al: Acute disseminated encephalomyelitis—MRI findings and the distinction from multiple sclerosis. Brain 113:291, 1990. *Multifocal white matter lesions indistinguishable from those seen in multiple sclerosis in most patients with acute disseminated encephalomyelitis.*
O'Riordan JI: Central nervous system white matter diseases other than multiple sclerosis. Curr Opin Neurol 10:211–214, 1997. *This article discusses the essential differences between acute disseminated encephalomyelitis and classic multiple sclerosis.*

■ THE EPILEPSIES

484 THE EPILEPSIES

Timothy A. Pedley

DEFINITION

Epilepsy is a term applied to a group of chronic conditions whose major clinical manifestation is the occurrence of *epileptic seizures*—sudden and usually unprovoked attacks of subjective experiential phenomena, altered awareness, involuntary movements, or convulsions.

Although a diagnosis of epilepsy requires the presence of seizures, not all seizures imply epilepsy. Seizures are a relatively common symptom of brain dysfunction, and they may occur during the course of many acute medical or neurologic illnesses in which brain function is temporarily deranged (*acute symptomatic seizures*)

Table 484–1 ■ POTENTIAL CAUSES OF ACUTE SYMPTOMATIC SEIZURES

Medical conditions
  Metabolic derangements
    Hyponatremia (<120 mEq/L)—especially acute
    Hypernatremia (>150–155 mEq/L)—especially acute
    Hypoglycemia (<40 mg/dL)
    Hyperglycemia (>400 mg/dL)
    Hyperosmolality (>320 mOsm/L)
    Hypocalcemia (<7 mg/dL)
    Respiratory alkalosis—acute
  Drug-induced seizures
    Isoniazid, penicillins
    Theophylline, aminophylline
    Lidocaine
    Meperidine
    Ketamine, halothane, enflurane, methohexital
    Amitriptyline, maprotiline, imipramine, doxepin, fluoxetine
    Haloperidol, trifluoperazine, chlorpromazine
    Ephedrine, phenylpropanolamine, terbutaline
    Methotrexate, BCNU, asparaginase
    Cyclosporine
    Cocaine (crack), phencyclidine, amphetamines
    Alcohol (withdrawal)
  Illnesses
    Eclampsia
    Hypertensive encephalopathy
    Liver failure
    Polyarteritis nodosa
    Porphyria
    Renal failure
    Sickle cell disease
    Syphilis
    Systemic lupus erythematosus
    Thrombotic thrombocytopenic purpura
    Whipple's disease
Neurologic conditions
    Angiitis of the nervous system
    Meningitis
    Encephalitis
    Acute head trauma (impact seizures)
    Stroke
    Brain abscess
    Brain tumor

(Table 484–1). Such seizures are most often self-limited and do not persist after the underlying disorder has resolved. Seizures can also occur as a reaction of the brain to physiologic stress, sleep deprivation, fever, and alcohol or sedative drug withdrawal. Occurrence of seizures in such everyday settings is exceptional and implies an increased seizure susceptibility (lowered seizure threshold). This may reflect poorly understood genetic factors that determine an individual's intrinsic resistance to minor physiologic, metabolic, or toxic insults. Finally, isolated seizures also sometimes occur for no discoverable reason as unprovoked events in presumably healthy people. None of these kinds of seizures represents epilepsy.

ETIOLOGY

Epilepsy can arise from a variety of conditions and pathophysiologic mechanisms. About 70% of adults and 40% of children with new-onset epilepsy have partial (focal) seizures (Fig. 484–1A). In most of these, it is not possible to identify a specific cause, although the focal nature of the seizures generally implies a cerebral injury or lesion (so-called cryptogenic epilepsy) (see Fig. 484–1B). The most common specific lesions are hippocampal sclerosis, gangliogliomas and glial tumors, cavernous malformations, neuronal migrational defects (cortical dysplasia) and hamartomas, encephalitis, cerebral trauma and hemorrhage. Not all patients with cerebral pathology have epilepsy; how a particular lesion or injury causes a region of brain to become epileptogenic is still poorly understood.

Although specific mendelian (e.g., tuberous sclerosis, hyperglycinemia, Lafora's disease), chromosomal (e.g., Down syndrome), and mitochondrial (e.g., MELAS) genetic diseases account for only about 1% of epilepsy cases, heritable factors are important in a much higher percentage, especially in children. Forms of epilepsy that are demonstrably more heritable than others (e.g., childhood absence epilepsy, juvenile myoclonic epilepsy) are increasingly referred to as *idiopathic* or *primary* epilepsies. Common features include a variable family history, generalized spike-wave abnormality on electroencephalogram (EEG), and onset in childhood or adolescence.

Family history, cerebral injury, and neurologic disease are all risk factors for epilepsy, and the magnitude of the increased risk relative to the population at large can be specified for a number of different conditions that predispose to seizures. In many patients, several factors coexist, and the development of epilepsy reflects the interaction of acquired brain pathology and genetic predisposition.

CLASSIFICATION AND CLINICAL MANIFESTATIONS

Although a number of different classification schemes have been proposed to describe seizures and the various types of epilepsy, the most widely used today are those of the International League Against Epilepsy (ILAE).

Classification of Epileptic Seizures

Seizures are classified by their clinical manifestations (semiology) supplemented by EEG data (Table 484–2). There are many different kinds of seizures, each with characteristic behavioral changes and electrophysiologic alterations that usually can be detected by EEG recordings. The particular manifestations of any single seizure depend on several factors: (1) whether most or only a part of the cerebral cortex is involved at the beginning; (2) the functions of the cortical areas where the seizure originates; and (3)

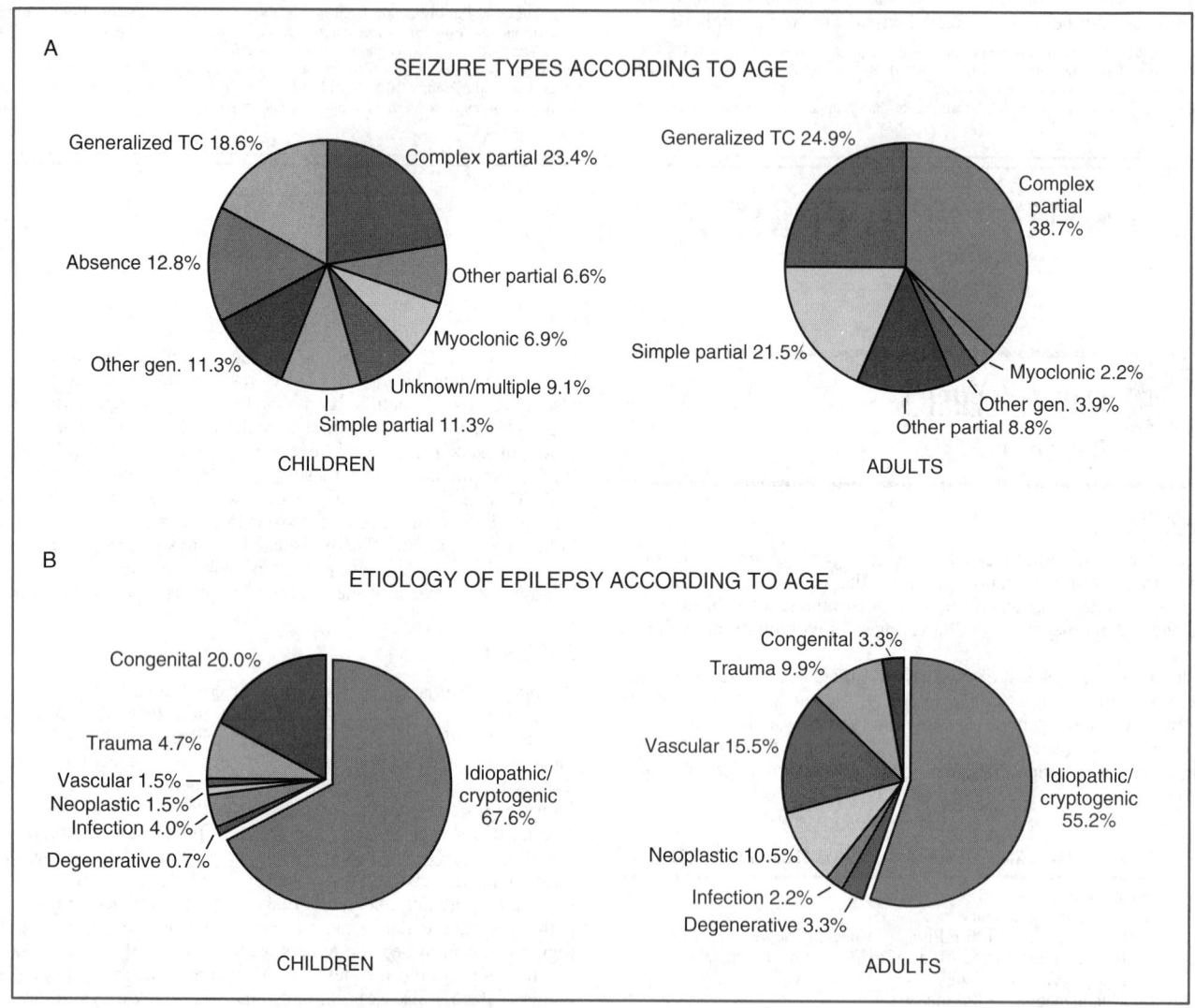

FIGURE 484–1 ■ *A,* Proportion of seizure types as a function of age for newly diagnosed cases of epilepsy in Rochester, Minnesota, 1935–1984. *B,* Etiology of epilepsy in all newly diagnosed cases in Rochester, Minnesota, 1935–1984. TC = tonic-clonic. (Modified from Hauser et al. Epilepsia 34:453–468, 1993.)

the subsequent pattern of spread within the brain. The International Classification reflects these considerations in two important ways. First, it divides seizures into two fundamental types: those with onset limited to part of one cerebral hemisphere (*partial* or *focal* seizures) and those that involve the cerebral cortex diffusely from the beginning (*generalized* seizures). Second, the International Classification recognizes that seizures are dynamic and evolving and that patients show variations in seizure pattern depending on the extent and manner of spread of the electrical discharge. Thus, simple partial seizures can evolve into complex partial seizures, and either simple or complex partial seizures can evolve into secondarily generalized tonic-clonic convulsions.

PARTIAL SEIZURES. The initial events of a seizure, described either by the patient or by an observer, are usually the most reliable indication to determine whether a seizure begins focally. *Simple* partial seizures result when the ictal discharge occurs in, and remains limited to, a circumscribed area of cortex. This is often referred to as the *epileptogenic focus.* Consciousness is not depressed, and patients can interact normally with their environment except for limitations imposed by the seizure on specific localized brain functions. Many symptoms or phenomena can be the expressions of simple partial seizures. Subjective sensory and psychoillusory phenomena are referred to collectively as *auras* and affect about 60% of patients with focal epilepsy. Sensory symptoms such as localized paresthesias, numbness, vertigo, auditory hallucinations, and unformed visual hallucinations occur with sei-

zures beginning in the corresponding primary sensory areas. Psychoillusory symptoms arise from ictal discharges in limbic and association cortex and include dysmnesic symptoms, such as feelings of familiarity (*déjà vu*) and unfamiliarity (*jamais vu*); dreamy states, feelings of unreality and depersonalization; time distortion; emotional symptoms such as fear or depression; visual illusions such as multiple images (polyopsia) or distortions of size (micropsia and macropsia); and hallucinatory phenomena, such as unpleasant smells, stereotyped visions, or familiar voices. Autonomic symptoms reflect ictal involvement of limbic structures that lie in the mesial temporal or frontal lobe and project to the hypothalamus and brain stem. Examples of autonomic phenomena include an epigastric rising sensation (especially common with seizures beginning in the mesial temporal lobe), nausea, lightheadedness, pallor or flushing, pupillary dilation, piloerection, salivation, and urinary incontinence.

Simple partial seizures with motor signs begin with *clonic* (rhythmic jerking) or *tonic* (stiffening) movements of a discrete body part. Because of their large cortical representation, muscles of the face and hand are often involved. When the seizure discharge begins in the primary motor cortex and spreads to involve the rest of the precentral gyrus, clonic movements progress in an orderly sequence (*"jacksonian march"*) that reflects the homunculus representation (e.g., thumb to fingers to face to leg). More often, however, ictal discharges involve supplementary or other secondary motor areas of the frontal lobe and produce contralateral flexion and elevation of the arm, contralateral turning of the head and eyes, and tonic extension of the ipsilateral arm (the so-called fencer's posture). Other simple partial motor signs include speech arrest, vocalizations, and eye blinking.

Simple partial seizures may be followed by a transient neurologic abnormality reflecting postictal depression of the epileptogenic cortical area. Thus, focal weakness may follow a simple partial motor seizure, numbness a sensory seizure, and blindness or amblyopia an occipital lobe seizure. These reversible neurologic deficits are collectively referred to as *Todd's paralysis* and rarely last for more than 48 hours. Similarly, prompt examination of a patient after a seizure may reveal transient focal abnormalities that provide useful clues to the site of seizure origin.

Complex partial seizures impair consciousness and produce unresponsiveness. In temporal lobe seizures, loss of consciousness results when the ictal discharge spreads bilaterally to involve both hippocampal and amygdala areas, the parahippocampal gyri and, to some extent, the entorhinal cortex and subfrontal, especially septal, regions. About 70 to 80% of complex partial seizures arise from the temporal lobe, and more than 65% of these originate in mesial temporal lobe structures, especially the hippocampus, amygdala, and parahippocampal gyrus. Remaining cases of complex partial seizures arise mainly from the frontal lobe, with smaller percentages originating in the parietal and occipital lobes. Many complex partial seizures evolve from simple partial seizures; consciousness becomes impaired as the seizure progresses. Complex partial seizures preceded by an olfactory aura are referred to as *uncinate fits* because of their origin in or near the uncus of the medial temporal lobe. Uncinate fits may have a higher association with brain tumors than other types of complex partial seizures.

The typical complex partial seizure of temporal lobe origin consists of a motionless stare accompanied by alteration of conscious-

Table 484–2 ■ INTERNATIONAL LEAGUE AGAINST EPILEPSY CLASSIFICATION OF EPILEPTIC SEIZURES AND SYNDROMES

Classification of seizures
I. Partial (focal) seizures
   A. *Simple partial seizures* (consciousness not impaired)
     1. With motor signs (including jacksonian, versive, and postural)
     2. With sensory symptoms (including visual, somatosensory, auditory, olfactory)
     3. With psychic symptoms (including dysphasia, hallucinatory, and affective changes)
     4. With autonomic symptoms
   B. *Complex partial seizures* (consciousness is impaired)
     1. Simple partial onset followed by impaired consciousness
     2. With impairment of consciousness at onset
     3. With automatisms
   C. Partial seizures evolving to secondarily generalized seizures
II. Generalized seizures nonfocal origin
   A. Absence seizures
   B. Myoclonic seizures; myoclonic jerks (single or multiple)
   C. Tonic-clonic seizures
   D. Tonic seizures
   E. Atonic seizures
III. Unclassified epileptic seizures

Classification of epileptic syndromes
I. Idiopathic epilepsy syndromes (focal or generalized)
   A. Benign neonatal convulsions
   B. Benign partial epilepsy of childhood
   C. Childhood absence epilepsy
   D. Juvenile myoclonic epilepsy
   E. Idiopathic epilepsy, otherwise unspecified
II. Cryptogenic or symptomatic epilepsy syndromes (focal or generalized)
   A. West's syndrome (infantile spasms)
   B. Lennox-Gastaut syndrome
   C. Epilepsia partialis continua
   D. Temporal lobe epilepsy
   E. Frontal lobe epilepsy
   F. Post-traumatic epilepsy
   G. Other symptomatic epilepsies, otherwise unspecified
III. Other epilepsy syndromes of uncertain or mixed classification
   A. Neonatal seizures
   B. Febrile seizures
   C. Reflex epilepsy
   D. Adult nonconvulsive status epilepticus
   E. Other unspecified

ness followed by *automatisms* (repetitive purposeless complex movements) and, often, dystonic positioning of the arm or hand *contralateral* to the seizure discharge. Oroalimentary automatisms are most common and include lip smacking, swallowing, and sucking and chewing movements. Gestural automatisms, such as fumbling, picking at clothes or objects, hand wringing, and patting movements, are also frequently encountered and are typically expressed maximally in the limbs *ipsilateral* to the epileptogenic temporal lobe. There may be clumsy perseveration of ongoing motor tasks, such as eating, drawing, walking, or washing dishes. Some patients show a degree of residual ability to react to their environment during the seizure, although their behavior is typically inappropriate. Complex partial seizures usually last 45 to 90 seconds and are followed by a period of confusion and disorientation lasting several more minutes. Without EEG recording, it is difficult to determine when the ictal state ends and postictal behavior begins. Characteristically, patients are amnesic for details of the seizure that occurred after the aura. There may be transient postictal aphasia when the seizure involves the dominant temporal lobe.

Complex partial seizures of frontal lobe origin are atypical and often differ dramatically from those originating in the temporal lobe. Although there are many variations, frontal lobe complex partial seizures tend (1) to begin and end abruptly; (2) to be brief with few, if any, postictal symptoms; (3) to express prominent, but often bizarre, motor manifestations, such as asynchronous thrashing or flailing of arms and legs, pelvic thrusting, pedalling leg movements, and loud vocalizations, all of which can at first suggest psychogenic attacks; and (4) to show minimal or nonlocalizing changes with scalp EEG recordings.

Psychomotor, temporal lobe, and *limbic* seizures are terms that have been used in the past to describe many of the ictal behaviors now classified as complex partial seizures, but they are not synonymous. Not all complex partial seizures arise from the temporal lobe, nor do all involve the limbic system. Some temporal lobe and limbic phenomena reflect unilateral ictal discharges and may not be associated with the significant alteration of awareness that invariably occur with complex partial seizures. Finally automatisms (the "psychomotor" element) are not uniformly present in complex partial seizures.

GENERALIZED SEIZURES. Generalized seizures begin diffusely and involve both cerebral hemispheres simultaneously from the outset. They lack clinical and EEG features that indicate a localized cerebral origin. Generalized seizures are subdivided mainly on the basis of the presence or absence and character of ictal motor manifestations. These features, in turn, depend on the extent to which subcortical and brain stem structures participate in the ictal discharge.

Generalized tonic-clonic seizures (*grand mal convulsions*) are characterized by abrupt loss of consciousness with bilateral tonic extension of the trunk and limbs (*tonic phase*), often accompanied by a loud vocalization as air is forcefully expelled across tightly contracted vocal cords (the "*epileptic cry*"), followed by bilaterally synchronous muscle jerking (*clonic phase*). In some patients, a few clonic jerks precede the tonic-clonic sequence; in others, only a tonic or a clonic phase is seen. Urinary incontinence is common, fecal incontinence rare. The actual ictus does not usually last more than 90 seconds. The postictal phase is marked by transient deep stupor followed in 15 to 30 minutes by a lethargic, confused state with automatic behavior. As recovery progresses, many patients complain of headache, muscle soreness, mental dulling, lack of energy, or mood changes lasting as long as 24 hours.

Generalized tonic-clonic seizures result in a number of striking but transient physiologic changes, including blood hypoxia and lactic acidosis, elevated plasma catecholamine levels, and increased concentrations of serum creatine kinase, prolactin, corticotropin, cortisol, β endorphin, and growth hormone. Complications include oral trauma, vertebral compression fractures, shoulder dislocation, aspiration pneumonia, and sudden death, which may be related to acute pulmonary edema, cardiac arrhythmia, or suffocation.

Absence seizures (petit mal seizures) occur mainly in children and are characterized by sudden, momentary lapses in awareness (the absence attack), staring, rhythmic blinking, and, often, a few small clonic jerks of arms or hands. Behavior and awareness return immediately to normal. There is no postictal period and usually no recollection that a seizure has occurred. Most absence seizures last less than 10 seconds. Longer absences are accompanied by automatisms, usually of a perseverative type, in about 70% of cases. Absence seizures commonly coexist with generalized tonic-clonic or myoclonic seizures. Untreated, absence seizures can occur hundreds of times each day.

Lapses of awareness that have a more gradual onset, do not resolve as abruptly, and are accompanied by autonomic features or loss of muscle tone are referred to as *atypical absence seizures*. These occur most often in children with mental retardation, and they do not respond as well to antiepileptic drug treatment. Typical and atypical absence seizures must also be distinguished from complex partial seizures manifested only by brief lapses of consciousness because cause, treatment, and prognosis differ among these three seizure types.

Myoclonic seizures manifest as rapid, recurrent, brief muscle jerks that can occur bilaterally, synchronously or asynchronously, or unilaterally without loss of consciousness. The myoclonic jerks range from small movements of the face or hands to massive bilateral spasms that simultaneously affect the head, limbs, and trunk. Repeated myoclonic seizures may seem to crescendo and terminate in a generalized tonic-clonic convulsion. Although they can occur at any time, myoclonic seizures often cluster shortly after waking or while falling asleep.

Atonic seizures ("drop attacks") occur most often in children with diffuse encephalopathies and are characterized by sudden loss of muscle tone that may result in falls with self-injury. Sometimes the loss of muscle tone is limited or fragmentary, producing, for example, only a head drop.

MISCELLANEOUS SEIZURE TYPES. Some seizures are designated by unique or unusual features. *Gelastic* seizures can be either complex partial or generalized nonconvulsive seizures in which pathologic laughter unaccompanied by any emotional content is a conspicuous feature of the epileptic event. *Cursive* seizures are complex partial seizures in which running is a prominent symptom. *Reflex* seizures are attacks precipitated by a specific stimulus, such as touch, a musical tune, a particular movement, reading, stroboscopic light patterns, or complex visual images.

Epileptic Syndromes

Some epileptic disorders are characterized by sufficiently reproducible aggregations of historical data, seizure patterns, associated clinical signs and symptoms, EEG findings, biochemical abnormalities, and imaging results that distinct *epileptic syndromes* can be defined. Furthermore, classifying the kind of epilepsy a patient has or identifying a person's specific epileptic syndrome is more important than describing seizures. This is because such a diagnosis has implications for diagnostic evaluation, treatment, genetic counseling, and prognosis.

The most widely used classification scheme is the 1989 revision of the ILAE Commission on Classification and Terminology (see Table 454–2). This classification separates major groups of epilepsy first on the basis of whether seizures are partial (*localization-related [focal] epilepsies*) or generalized (*generalized epilepsies*), and second by cause (*idiopathic, symptomatic,* or *cryptogenic epilepsy*). Subtypes of epilepsy are grouped by age and, in the case of focal epilepsies, by the anatomic location of the presumed site of seizure onset.

FEBRILE SEIZURES. Febrile seizures are the most common cause of convulsions in children, affecting between 3 and 5% of all children in the United States and Europe under the age of 5 years. Most febrile seizures occur between the ages of 6 months and 4 years, although they sometimes occur in children as old as 6 or 7 years. About 30% of children have more than one attack; chance of recurrence is greatest if the first seizure occurs before 1 year of age or if there is a family history of febrile seizures. Although most affected children have no long-term consequences, febrile seizures increase the risk of epilepsy development later. This risk is low for most children, about 2 to 3%, but it approximates 10 to 13% in those who have had prolonged or focal seizures, who have a family history of afebrile seizures, or who were neurologically abnormal before the first febrile seizure. Febrile seizures are not associated

with, nor do they cause, mental retardation, below average IQ, poor school performance, or behavior problems. Prophylactic treatment is generally not indicated because of the benign prognosis. If treatment is considered at all, rectal administration of diazepam only during febrile illnesses is effective, safe, and preferable to chronic therapy using phenobarbital.

BENIGN PARTIAL EPILEPSY OF CHILDHOOD WITH CENTRAL-MIDTEMPORAL SPIKES (ROLANDIC EPILEPSY). This is one of the most common epileptic syndromes of childhood, representing about 15% of all pediatric epilepsies. Seizures usually begin between the ages of 4 and 13 years; affected children are otherwise normal. Most have seizures principally or only at night. Because sleep promotes secondary generalization, parents report only tonic-clonic convulsions; any focal signature is usually missed. In contrast, seizures occurring during the day are typically focal and express themselves with twitching of one side of the face, speech arrest, drooling, and paresthesias of the face, gums, tongue, and inner cheeks. Seizures may progress to include hemiclonic movements or hemitonic posturing. EEGs show a distinctive pattern of stereotyped epileptiform discharges over the central and midtemporal regions. Prognosis is invariably good, and seizures disappear by mid to late adolescence. Outcome is not affected by treatment, but carbamazepine prevents recurrent attacks.

CHILDHOOD ABSENCE (PETIT MAL) EPILEPSY. This disorder begins most often between the ages of 4 and 12 years in children who are neurologically and intellectually normal. Absence attacks can often be precipitated by hyperventilation. The EEG is diagnostic, showing stereotyped 3-Hz spike-wave discharges in association with a typical spell (Fig. 484–2). Generalized tonic-clonic seizures occur in 30 to 50% of cases. Ethosuximide (10 mg/kg/day or, in older children, 250 mg two or three times daily) and valproate (15 to 30 mg/kg/day) are equally effective against absence seizures; valproate is preferable if generalized tonic-clonic seizures coexist.

JUVENILE MYOCLONIC EPILEPSY. This is one of the most frequently encountered types of idiopathic generalized epilepsy. It begins most often between the ages of 8 and 20 years in otherwise healthy individuals. When fully developed, the syndrome is characterized by morning myoclonic jerks, generalized tonic-clonic seizures that occur just after awakening, normal intelligence, a family history of similar seizures, and an EEG that shows generalized 4- to 6-Hz spike-wave and polyspike-wave discharges. Valproate controls attacks in over 80% of cases, but indefinite treatment is required in most cases because of the high rate of seizure relapse after attempted drug withdrawal.

LENNOX-GASTAUT SYNDROME. This term is used for a heterogeneous group of early childhood epileptic encephalopathies that have in common physical brain abnormalities, mental retardation, uncontrolled seizures, and an EEG pattern that shows generalized 1.5- to 2.5-Hz sharp slow-wave discharges ("slow spike-and-wave pattern"). No treatment is consistently effective; management is best directed by specialists in the field.

TEMPORAL LOBE EPILEPSY. This is the most common epileptic syndrome of adults, accounting for at least 40% of epilepsy cases. Seizures begin in late childhood or adolescence, and there is often a history of febrile seizures. Virtually all patients have complex partial seizures, some of which secondarily generalize. Epigastric or visceral auras are frequent. Interictal EEGs usually show epileptiform discharges over the anterior temporal region (Fig. 484–3). Most patients with temporal lobe epilepsy have impaired memory, and some show a decrease in either verbal or visuospatial skills, depending on whether the epileptogenic temporal lobe is dominant or nondominant.

Temporal lobe epilepsy arises most often from mesial temporal limbic structures, typically in association with a characteristic lesion known as *hippocampal sclerosis*. Hippocampal sclerosis refers to variable but selective neuronal loss, especially in the CA1 (Sommer's sector), CA3, and dentate gyrus regions of the hippocampus (Fig. 484–4). Secondary gliosis occurs, and corresponding atrophy of the hippocampal formation can be recognized on magnetic resonance imaging (MRI) brain scans (see later). Neurons in the hippocampal CA2 region (resistant zone) and granule cell layer are relatively spared. In 20% of cases, temporal lobe epilepsy is caused by other structural lesions, such as cavernous malformations, hamartomas, cortical dysplasia, glial tumors, and scars related to previous head injuries or encephalitis. Frontal or occipital lesions may

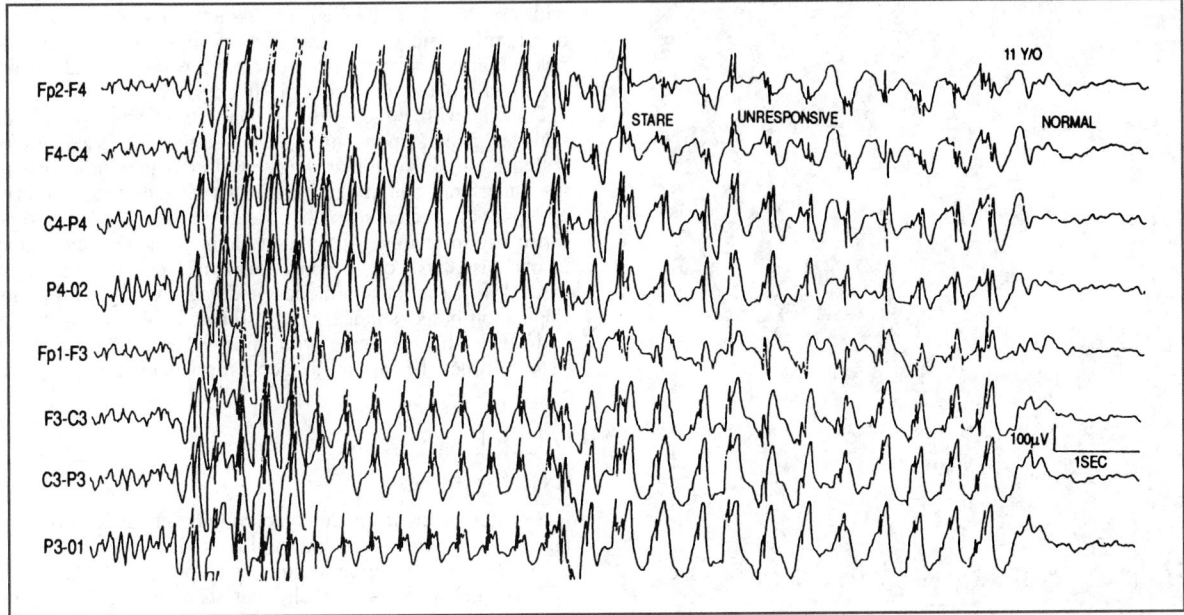

FIGURE 484–2 ■ Childhood absence epilepsy. The EEG shows the typical pattern of generalized 3-Hz spike-wave complexes associated with a clinical absence seizure.

give rise to temporal lobe seizures because of rapid spread of the ictal discharge into mesial temporal lobe structures.

Antiepileptic drugs are usually successful in suppressing secondarily generalized seizures, but over 50% of patients continue to have partial seizures. In drug-resistant cases, temporal lobectomy is the treatment of choice.

POST-TRAUMATIC EPILEPSY. The chance of development of post-traumatic epilepsy relates directly to the severity of the head injury. After penetrating wounds and other severe head injuries, for example, about one third of patients have seizures within 1 year. Severe head injuries are defined by the presence of a cerebral contusion, intracerebral or intracranial hematoma, unconsciousness or amnesia lasting more than 24 hours, or persistent abnormalities on neurologic examination, such as hemiparesis or aphasia. Although most patients experience seizures within 1 to 2 years of injury, new-onset seizures may still appear 5 or more years later. Two thirds of patients with post-traumatic epilepsy have partial or secondarily generalized seizures. Mild head injuries (e.g., uncomplicated brief loss of consciousness, no skull fracture, absence of focal

neurologic signs, no contusion or hematoma) do not increase the risk of seizures to a clinically significant degree.

Impact seizures (a generalized convulsion occurring at the time of, or immediately after, the injury) and early seizures (those occurring within the first 1 to 2 weeks) represent acute reactions of the brain to the trauma. Seizures beginning after 10 to 14 days reflect an increased risk of post-traumatic epilepsy development.

Early seizures should be treated with phenytoin. To minimize complications from seizures occurring during acute management, phenytoin should also be given prophylactically for 1 to 2 weeks to patients who have sustained severe head injuries. In the absence of overt attacks, phenytoin use should be discontinued after 2 weeks because no data indicate that antiepileptic drugs prevent the development of later epilepsy.

EPILEPSIA PARTIALIS CONTINUA. This term refers to continuous focal seizures involving part or all of one side of the body. In adults, epilepsia partialis continua occurs with severe strokes, primary or metastatic brain tumors, metabolic encephalopathies (especially hyperosmolar nonketotic hyperglycemia), encephalitis, and

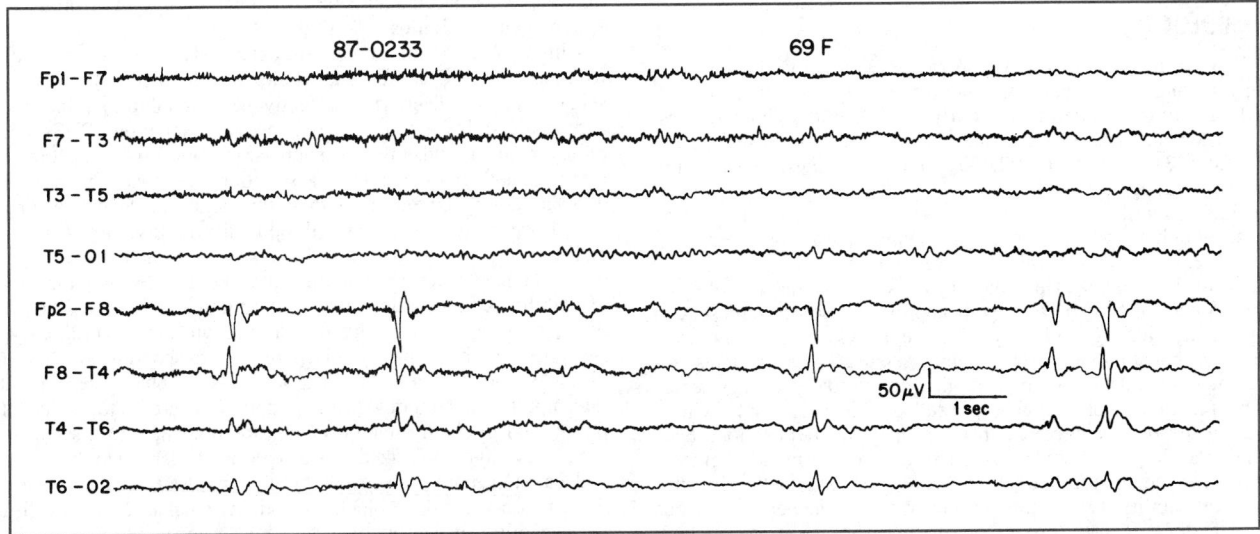

FIGURE 484–3 ■ Temporal lobe epilepsy. Epileptiform discharges are seen focally over the right temporal lobe (bottom four lines), and there is intermixed irregular slow-wave activity not seen on the other side.

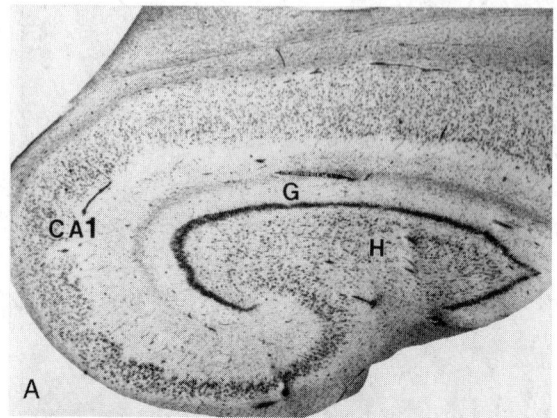

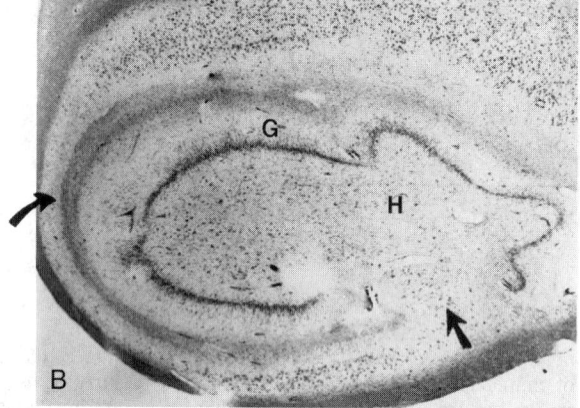

FIGURE 484-4 ■ Normal hippocampus *(A)* and hippocampus from a patient with temporal lobe epilepsy showing changes typical of hippocampal sclerosis *(B)*. Note loss of pyramidal cells in CA1 region *(curved arrow, left)*. CA4 *(straight arrow, right)*, and the hilus (H) of the dentate gyrus. The CA2 region (pyramidal cells lying to the left of arrow on right) and granule cell layer (G) are characteristically less affected. (Courtesy of Dr. Robert S. Sloviter. Departments of Pharmacology and Neurology, University of Arizona, Tucson, AZ.)

subacute or rare chronic inflammatory diseases of the brain (Rasmussen's encephalitis; Kozhevnikov's Russian spring-summer encephalitis; Behçet's disease). Antiepileptic drugs are usually ineffective, as are corticosteroids and antiviral agents. Fortunately, seizures remit spontaneously in some cases. IVIg has offered short-term benefit in some patients with Rasmussen's encephalitis but functional hemispherectomy is usually necessary.

EPIDEMIOLOGY

Epilepsy affects about 45 million people worldwide. Incidence is highest among young children and the elderly, and men are affected slightly more often than women (1.5:1). In the United States, age-adjusted annual incidence rates based on 1990 census figures range from 31 to 57 per 100,000 population. Cause and seizure type vary with age.

Excluding febrile seizures or those related to an acute illness, the lifetime likelihood of someone experiencing at least one seizure is about 10%. The risk of epilepsy development, however, is lower, about 3 to 4%, emphasizing that not all seizures lead to epilepsy. In fact, about 30% of persons with unprovoked seizures present to the physician having had only a single attack, almost always a generalized tonic-clonic seizure. Other seizure types, such as absence, myoclonic, and complex partial, are virtually always recurrent by the time a physician is consulted. Because people with a single seizure do not have epilepsy and may not require long-term antiepileptic drug treatment, it is important to determine whether a first unprovoked seizure is likely to lead to further attacks. Unfortunately, the ability to do this is imperfect. Nonetheless, various clinical features identify groups of patients who are at low or high relative risk for further seizures, and this helps in making treatment decisions and advising patients. The high-risk group consists of individuals with a history of significant brain injury or lesion and

an abnormal EEG. For these patients, recurrence risk at 2 years is about 65%. By contrast, recurrence risk is only 24% in persons with an idiopathic generalized seizure, a normal EEG, and a negative family history for seizures or epilepsy. After a second seizure, risk of further seizures rises to over 80%. A second seizure, therefore, is a reliable indication of epilepsy.

Persons with epilepsy have increased mortality rates compared with the general population. Most of this increased risk occurs in patients with symptomatic epilepsy in whom mortality relates to the underlying condition. In patients with idiopathic or cryptogenic epilepsy, the increased risk of death is related mainly to accidents, especially drowning. Autopsy and clinical series have demonstrated an increased risk of sudden unexplained death, presumably due to cardiac arrhythmia, pulmonary edema, or myocardial infarction. Population-based studies have estimated the risk of sudden unexplained death in patients with epilepsy as 1:1000 to 1:2000, more than 20 times the rate in the general population.

PATHOGENESIS

Cellular Physiology

Seizures result from the synchronous interactions of large populations of neurons that intermittently discharge in abnormal patterns. Because of the large number of processes that regulate cortical excitability, it is unlikely that there is a single epileptogenic mechanism. Nonetheless, neurophysiologic studies in a variety of experimental preparations have shown that "epileptic" neurons share a number of properties. although the total expression of these varies according to the particular model.

Intracellular recordings from neurons in an epileptogenic focus show recurring high-voltage, long-duration depolarizations with superimposed high-frequency bursts of action potentials. The extracellular current flow generated by these *paroxysmal depolarizing shifts* (PDSs) results in the interictal EEG spike or sharp wave, the characteristic epileptiform discharge that signifies susceptibility to seizures. PDS generation involves several mechanisms, including increased excitability resulting from changes in intrinsic voltage-dependent membrane currents, newly active excitatory circuits, and attenuation or loss of effective postsynaptic inhibition and other inhibitory processes, as well as increased effectiveness of excitatory synapses. In neurons showing "epileptic" patterns of behavior, ordinary synaptic inputs may elicit exaggerated or pathologically amplified responses. Activation of the *N*-methyl-D-aspartate (NMDA) type of glutamate receptors potentiates cellular excitability and leads to sustained neuronal depolarization and calcium influx. Prolonged NMDA receptor activation and excessive accumulation of intracellular calcium also result in neuronal toxicity and may lead to cell death ("epileptic brain damage") following severe repetitive seizures or status epilepticus. In some areas of cortex, the hippocampus for example, subsets of neurons that normally fire in bursts may serve as pacemaker cells for other groups of neurons during epileptogenic activities.

Although it is not known in detail what causes the transition from an interical to an ictal state, development of experimental seizures reflects decreasing effectiveness of inhibitory mechanisms accompanied by increasing evidence of excitation. PDSs become more frequent and involve ever larger numbers of neurons and more distant areas of cortex, a situation that results in progressive depolarization of neurons both within and outside the original focus. During frequent interictal epileptiform discharges and especially during seizures, extracellular potassium and intracellular calcium concentrations increase and contribute to the overall excitability of the epileptic neuronal aggregate. During the seizure itself, neurons are tonically depolarized and fire continuously in a sustained, high-frequency discharge (corresponding to the tonic phase of the seizure). The seizure ends as phasic repolarizations interrupt the continuous firing pattern (the correlate of the clonic phase) and gradually restore membrane potentials to normal or to a temporary hyperpolarized state (postictal depression). Phenytoin and carbamazepine are effective anticonvulsants because they produce a use-dependent block of sodium channels, thereby limiting the capability of neurons to fire at high-frequency rates. The benzodiazepines and barbiturates exert their anticonvulsant effect by enhancing post-synaptic GABA-mediated inhibition through an effect on the chloride ionophore.

In the focal epilepsies, abnormal neuronal behavior originates in and may remain confined to a restricted area of the cortex. The brain possesses powerful mechanisms to suppress and restrain abnormal electrical behavior. Typically during focal interictal discharges or focal seizures, areas surrounding the epileptogenic cortex are inhibited (surround inhibition), as is the homotopic contralateral cortex and areas of the thalamus and brain stem. Only when these restraining influences are overcome does a seizure spread and become secondarily generalized.

In temporal lobe epilepsy, certain neurons within the dentate gyrus of the hippocampus have been identified as being especially vulnerable to injury. Selective loss of mossy cells and of neurons containing somatostatin and neuropeptide Y results in deafferentation of the normally powerful GABA inhibitory neurons within the dentate gyrus, rendering them nonfunctional. As a result, the granule cells of the dentate gyrus become disinhibited and respond with abnormal synchronous bursts to cortical stimuli. Subclinical electrographic seizures develop and further damage vulnerable cell populations, creating a self-enhancing cycle of cell loss, impaired control of hippocampal excitability, and, eventually, clinical seizures associated with the pathologic picture of hippocampal sclerosis. How other lesions (e.g., tumors or cavernous malformations) cause focal epilepsy is not well understood.

The thalamus plays a critical role in generating generalized seizures and the generalized spike-wave EEG patterns that accompany them. The bilateral synchrony of generalized seizures and the rhythmicity of spike-wave discharges appear to depend on two main factors—a unique set of ionic conductances, including a T-type calcium current, which enable neurons in the thalamic nucleus reticularis to function as pacemaker control cells; and the special anatomy and pharmacology of the thalamocortical system. The substantia nigra also is critical to the expression of generalized convulsions, especially the tonic phase; GABA-ergic inhibitory transmission in the substantia nigra plays a regulatory role in the propagation of both primary and secondarily generalized seizure discharges. Because there are no consistent, demonstrable pathologic changes in the brains of patients with idiopathic generalized epilepsy, susceptibility to these seizures most likely results from inherited biochemical, membrane, or neurotransmitter defects that result in abnormal excitability within the involved circuits.

Genetics and Gene Defects

Among the more than 40 individual epileptic syndromes described in humans are at least 10 in which genetic factors appear to be prominently involved. Twin studies have confirmed strong genetic determinants in many types of seizure disorders, especially such ones as childhood absence epilepsy, juvenile myoclonic epilepsy, benign rolandic epilepsy, and idiopathic grand mal seizures. The role of genetic factors is quite complicated, however. For example, children of parents with either localization-related or generalized forms of epilepsy experience seizures at increased rates, although the difference is greatest for children of parents with the various types of idiopathic generalized epilepsy. Thus, there seems to be some degree of sharing of genetic susceptibilities in both the idiopathic and symptomatic epilepsies, and a major challenge facing investigators today is to clarify how different genes alter an individual's *susceptibility* to seizures and epilepsy in the presence of acquired brain pathology or as a reaction to acute or subacute cerebral dysfunction. Additionally, some inherited disorders, such as tuberous sclerosis and neurofibromatosis, are associated with brain lesions that in turn give rise to symptomatic epilepsies (see Chapters 456 and 457). Thus, although mutations in single genes account for some familial diseases that cause epileptic seizures as well as a few rare epileptic syndromes, in most cases multiple

genes determine the various neuronal functions that alter seizure threshold and predispose to development of clinically evident epilepsy. In most types of epilepsy, it remains to be determined to what degree abnormalities of single genes, or concordance of key overlapping genes, determine the phenotypic expression of any given epileptic condition.

Because of these considerations, there is most likely a continuum between idiopathic and symptomatic epilepsies, with the development of epilepsy deriving from the complex interrelation of genetic factors and brain pathology. In any given patient, therefore, the *relative* contribution of genetic or acquired pathologic factors determines whether the epilepsy presents as an idiopathic disorder or a symptomatic one. The failure thus far to identify a genetic component in post-traumatic epilepsy or in seizures following stroke most likely reflects the relatively small genetic "load" in these situations compared with the magnitude of acquired factors.

Animal models have defined several "epilepsy genes" and their encoded proteins, and gene defects have also now been specified in some rare forms of human epilepsy as well. A major problem in a complex disorder like epilepsy, however, is that the number of genes that encode molecules that regulate cortical excitability directly through membrane and synaptic functions, as well as the second messenger cascades that indirectly regulate membrane proteins involved in signal transduction, is very large.

Linkage studies have defined specific gene loci for several human epilepsies (Table 484–3): two autosomal recessive progressive myoclonic epilepsies (Unverricht-Lundborg disease and the form of neuronal ceroid lipofuscinosis known as Batten's disease); an autosomal dominant idiopathic generalized epilepsy (benign familial neonatal seizures); one type of idiopathic partial epilepsy (autosomal dominant nocturnal frontal lobe epilepsy); and two disorders of cortical malformation in which seizures are a prominent feature (the Miller-Dieker form of lissencephaly, and one type of tuberous sclerosis) (see Chapter 457). The defective gene in Unverricht-Lundborg disease encodes cystatin B, a ubiquitous inhibitor of cysteine protease, a lysosomal enzyme that cannot at present be related easily to any known epileptogenic mechanism, although programmed neuronal cell death may be involved. An abnormal potassium-channel gene results in the syndrome of benign familial neonatal seizures.

DIAGNOSIS

Accurate diagnosis is the cornerstone of rational management. The diagnostic evaluation has three objectives: (1) to determine whether the patient has epilepsy; (2) to classify the seizures and type of epilepsy accurately and determine whether the clinical data fit a particular epilepsy syndrome; and (3) to identify, if possible, a specific underlying cause.

History

A detailed and accurate history is imperative and the single most important factor in diagnosis. Because patients usually have only limited awareness of their behavior during a seizure, additional information usually must be obtained from family members or other close observers. The historical summary should provide a clear description of the patient's seizures, including details of any aura, the neurologic status between attacks, any reproducible precipitants, and relevant risk factors for epilepsy, such as a family history of seizures or a history of severe head trauma, encephalitis or meningitis, and febrile seizures (Table 484–4). In children and

Table 484–3 ■ HUMAN EPILEPSY GENES AND GENE DEFECTS

SYNDROME	GENE LOCATION	GENE PRODUCT
Unverricht-Lundborg disease	21q22.3	Cystatin B
Nocturnal frontal lobe epilepsy	20q13.2-q13.3	α4 subunit, nicotinic acetylcholine receptor
Benign familial infantile convulsions	20q13.2-13.3	Voltage-gated K^+ channel
Batten's disease	16	Unknown deletion (loss of function?)
Lissencephaly (Miller-Dieker)	17p13.3	Subunit, platelet-activating factor
Tuberous sclerosis (TSC2)	16	rasGAP-like signaling molecule

Table 484-4 ■ ESSENTIAL FEATURES OF THE SEIZURE HISTORY

Date and circumstances of first attack
First consistent event in the seizure: Is there an aura? Are initial symptoms and signs focal of lateralizing?
Subsequent evolution of the seizure, in sequence
Postictal manifestations (e.g., Todd's paralysis)
Is there more than one seizure type?
Average rate of occurrence; longest seizure-free interval since onset
Seizure precipitants (alcohol, sleep deprivation, particular stimuli, stress)
Is there a pattern to seizure occurrence (circadian, catamenial)?
Has there been a change in characteristics of the seizure?
Symptoms of neurologic or systemic disease between seizures: Are these static, intermittent, or progressive?
Risk factor for epilepsy (e.g., family history, cerebral injury)

young adults, one should inquire about gestation, birth, postnatal course, and early development. If a patient has been treated previously, it is important to learn what drugs were used, the doses and blood levels that were achieved, and therapeutic or adverse effects.

Physical Examination

Although the physical examination is normal in most patients with epilepsy, abnormal findings, when present, can be helpful in two ways. First, physical signs may point to an underlying neurologic or systemic disorder of which the seizures are a part. Neurocutaneous syndromes, for example, are commonly associated with seizures and may be suggested by café-au-lait spots, a facial angioma, hypopigmented macules, axillary freckling, and shagreen patches (see Chapter 456). Second, focal neurologic signs indicate localized cerebral pathology. Asymmetry in the size of the hands, feet, or face signifies a longstanding abnormality of the cerebral hemisphere contralateral to the smaller side. Absence seizures can be triggered in untreated patients by having them hyperventilate for 2 to 3 minutes.

Laboratory Tests

ELECTROENCEPHALOGRAPHY. EEG is the most important diagnostic test for epilepsy. EEG findings are useful and sometimes essential for establishing the diagnosis, classifying seizures correctly, identifying epileptic syndromes, and making therapeutic decisions. In combination with appropriate clinical findings, *epileptiform* EEG patterns termed *spikes* or *sharp waves* strongly support a diagnosis of epilepsy. In patients with seizures, focal epileptiform discharges indicate focal epilepsy, whereas generalized epileptiform activity indicates a generalized form of epilepsy. The particular pattern of epileptiform activity, defined by the morphology, spatial distribution, repetition rate, and other characteristics of the discharges, assists in identifying a particular type of epilepsy or epileptic syndrome. A note of caution is warranted, however. Most EEGs are obtained between seizures, and interictal abnormalities alone can never prove or refute a diagnosis of epilepsy. Epilepsy can be definitively established only by recording a characteristic ictal discharge during a representative clinical attack. Unfortunately, this is uncommon during routine EEG recordings. A further factor that can confound interpretation of interictal EEGs is the occurrence of similar epileptiform abnormalities in about 2% of normal people; many of these, especially in children, are asymptomatic markers of a genetic trait. Finally, epileptiform-like waveforms or artifacts can be misinterpreted and erroneously considered to be evidence of seizure susceptibility.

About 40 to 50% of patients with epilepsy show epileptiform abnormalities on their initial EEG. The chance of capturing epileptiform activity is enhanced by sleep deprivation for 24 hours before the test and by the patient's sleeping during a portion of the EEG recording. Serial EEGs increase the yield of positive tracings. A small number of persons with epilepsy, however, continue to have normal interictal EEGs despite all efforts to record an abnormality.

Specialized epilepsy centers in tertiary referral hospitals include monitoring units equipped with simultaneous EEG and closed-circuit television capability as well as computer-assisted detection and analysis systems. These facilities have greatly improved management of selected patients by giving physicians the means to distinguish epileptic from nonepileptic paroxysmal events, to make precise electrical-clinical correlations, and to localize epileptogenic foci for resective surgery.

NEUROIMAGING STUDIES. Brain MRI complements EEG findings by identifying structural brain pathology that may be causally related to the development of epilepsy. Properly performed MRI can detect the vast majority of epileptogenic cerebral lesions. Hippocampal sclerosis, defects of neuronal migration, gangliogliomas and some gliomas, and cavernous malformations are readily seen with MRI. It is important to obtain a complete imaging study that includes both T1- and T2-weighted images in coronal and axial planes. Imaging in the coronal plane perpendicular to the long axis of the hippocampus has improved detection of hippocampal atrophy and gliosis (Fig. 484-5), findings that correlate with the pathologic picture of mesial temporal sclerosis and an epileptogenic temporal lobe. An even more sensitive measure of hippocampal atrophy compares volume measurements of a patient's hippocampus with similar quantitative data obtained in normal controls. Gadolinium infusion does not improve detection of cerebral lesions associated with epilepsy, although it often aids in differentiating among types of cerebral pathology.

An MRI scan should be obtained in all patients suspected of epilepsy over the age of 18 years and in all children with partial seizures (except those with benign focal epilepsy of childhood), abnormal neurologic findings, or focal slow-wave abnormalities on EEG.

In contrast to MRI, positron emission tomography (PET) and single photon emission computed tomography (SPECT) offer functional views of the brain. These techniques use physiologically active, radiolabeled tracers to image the brain's metabolic activity (PET) or blood flow (SPECT). For example, about 70% of patients with temporal lobe epilepsy show focal hypometabolic areas on interictal PET scans that correspond to the epileptogenic focus. Abnormalities using PET or SPECT are often demonstrated even when MRI scans are normal. These procedures are reserved for research-level studies or for specialized epilepsy centers rather than routine diagnosis.

BLOOD TESTS. Routine blood tests rarely offer diagnostic assistance in otherwise healthy patients with epilepsy. Serum electrolytes, liver function tests, and an automated blood cell count may be useful, however, as baseline studies before antiepileptic drug therapy is begun. Blood tests are necessary and frequently informa-

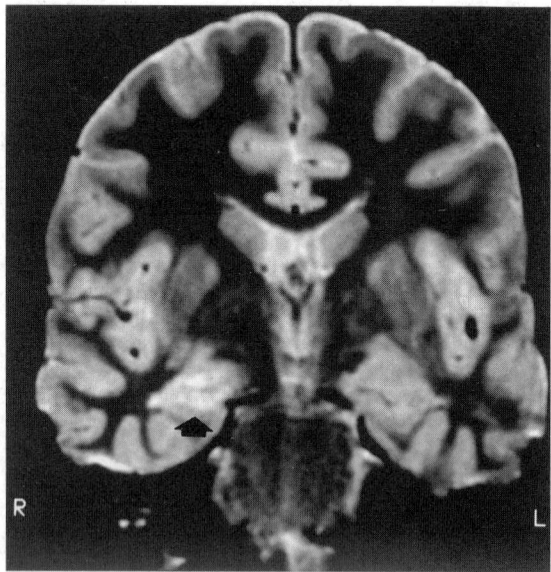

FIGURE 484-5 ■ Coronal MRI scan at the level of the anterior temporal lobe showing changes consistent with right-sided hippocampal sclerosis. The right hippocampal formation (*arrow*) is atrophic compared with the left and shows signal changes (white areas) indicating gliosis. (Courtesy of Dr. Stephen Chan, Division of Neuroradiology, Columbia-Presbyterian Medical Center, New York, New York.)

tive in older patients with acute or chronic systemic disease. Consideration should be given to obtaining blood or urine samples from adolescents and young adults with unexplained generalized seizures to screen for substance abuse, especially cocaine.

LUMBAR PUNCTURE. Lumbar puncture is mandatory if there is any suspicion of meningitis or encephalitis. It is otherwise unnecessary and need not be performed routinely. Repeated generalized seizures and convulsive status epilepticus can increase cerebrospinal fluid protein content slightly and produce a pleocytosis of up to 100 white blood cells (WBCs) per cubic millimeter for 24 to 48 hours. Cerebrospinal fluid pleocytosis should be attributed to seizures *only in retrospect;* infection or intracranial inflammatory processes should always be assumed first.

ELECTROCARDIOGRAM. An electrocardiogram (ECG) should be obtained in any young person with a first generalized seizure if there is a family history of arrhythmia, sudden unexplained death, or episodic unconsciousness. An ECG should also be obtained in any patient with a history of cardiac arrhythmia or valvular disease.

DIFFERENTIAL DIAGNOSIS

Not every paroxysmal event is a seizure, and misidentification of other conditions as epilepsy leads to ineffective, unnecessary, and potentially harmful treatment. In addition, misdiagnosis accounts for a substantial portion of patients whose spells have not responded to antiepileptic drug treatment.

A variety of conditions can be confused with epilepsy, depending on the age of the patient and the nature and circumstances of the attacks (Table 484–5). It is not always possible to distinguish among various diagnostic possibilities on clinical grounds alone, and admission to a specialized monitoring unit is frequently necessary.

Nonepileptic paroxysmal disorders have in common the occurrence of sudden, discrete events characterized by abnormal or inappropriate behavior, variable responsiveness, changes in muscle tone, and various postures or movements. These conditions are far more common and variable in their presentation in children than in adults. Many of the disorders simulating epilepsy in childhood can be viewed as transient "developmental" conditions that require no treatment other than reassurance.

Syncope (see Chapter 447) refers to the symptom complex that results when there is a transient, global reduction in cerebral perfusion with associated hypoxia. Loss of consciousness lasts only a few seconds, uncommonly a minute or more, and recovery is rapid. If the cerebral hypoxia is sufficiently severe, the syncopal episode may include brief tonic posturing of the trunk or a few clonic jerks of the arms and legs (*convulsive syncope*). Similarly, some forms of *migraine* can be mistaken for seizures, especially if the headache

Table 484–5 ▪ NONEPILEPTIC EPISODIC DISORDERS IN ADOLESCENTS AND ADULTS

Movement disorders
Myoclonus
Paroxysmal choreoathetosis
Episodic ataxias
Hyperekplexia (startle disease)
Migraine
Confusional
Vertebrobasilar
Syncope and cardiac arrhythmias*
Behavioral and psychiatric disorders
Psychogenic seizures*
Hyperventilation syndrome*
Panic disorder*
Dissociative states ("fugue states")
Episodic dyscontrol
Narcolepsy and sleep apnea
Automatic behavior syndrome
Partial cataplexy
Transient ischemic attacks
Transient global amnesia*
Acute confusional states
Alcoholic blackouts*
Hypoglycemic attacks

*Most commonly encountered.

is atypical or mild. Basilar artery migraine, a rare variant seen most often in adolescents and young adults, can include lethargy, mood changes, confusion and disorientation, vertigo, bilateral visual disturbances, and alteration or loss of consciousness.

Psychogenic seizures frequently cause intractable "epilepsy" in adults and may represent 20% or more of cases referred to an epilepsy monitoring unit. Many patients with psychogenic seizures have epilepsy as well. Definitive diagnosis requires video EEG documentation, although a history of atypical and nonstereotyped attacks, emotional or psychological precipitants, psychiatric illness, complete lack of response to antiepileptic drugs, and repeatedly normal interictal EEGs suggests the possibility of psychogenic seizures. *Panic attacks* and anxiety attacks with hyperventilation can superficially resemble partial seizures with affective, autonomic, or special sensory symptoms. Prolonged hyperventilation results in muscle twitching or spasms (tetany), and affected patients may faint.

Episodic dyscontrol is a poorly defined entity consisting of intermittent periods of inappropriately violent and destructive behavior that is out of character for the patient. Nonspecifically abnormal EEGs have been reported in children with the episodic dyscontrol syndrome, but most affected adults have little evidence of a structural brain disorder.

MEDICAL TREATMENT

The First Seizure

Patients with their first epileptic seizure should be screened for symptoms and signs of an acute medical or neurologic illness. Brain imaging need not be done emergently unless there is a high likelihood of an acute cerebral lesion or the patient remains obtunded. Most patients recover rapidly after an isolated seizure, so several hours of observation are usually sufficient to assess the clinical progress, obtain additional relevant information, and review the results of laboratory tests. Hospitalization is not necessary provided that there is no suspicion of an underlying illness and a responsible family member or friend can observe the patient closely at home. If these criteria cannot be met, or if there is uncertainty about them, hospitalization is indicated. If the patient is sent home, there should be a clear plan for follow-up and re-evaluation.

Whether an antiepileptic drug should be prescribed after a first seizure is a matter of controversy. Antiepileptic drugs reduce the risk of relapse following a first unprovoked generalized tonic-clonic seizure, but early treatment does not appear to affect long-term prognosis, especially with regard to such important issues as severity of epilepsy or the chance of entering a prolonged remission. Chronic treatment of all first seizures would expensively overtreat 75% of the patients. The decision to treat should be based on the physician's estimate of the risk of further seizures, the consequence to the patient of recurrent seizures, a reasonable expectation that the patient will comply with the treatment regimes, and the risk of adverse effects from antiepileptic drug therapy (10 to 30%). Patients are at relatively low risk for further seizures if they have a normal EEG, normal physical examination, no history of significant cerebral injury, a normal brain imaging study, and absence of a family history of epilepsy. Patients should be treated after a first seizure only if they have two or more of these risk factors. Nevertheless, the final decision about treatment must always be individualized and take into account the potential psychological, vocational, and physical consequences of further seizures for each patient.

Selection of Antiepileptic Drugs

The treatment of epilepsy has three main objectives: (1) to eliminate seizures or reduce their frequency to the maximum extent possible, (2) to avoid chronic drug-related adverse effects, and (3) to assist the patient in maintaining or restoring normal vocational and psychosocial adjustment. Although each of these goals is possible, no available medical treatment can permanently eliminate ("cure") epilepsy. Furthermore, less than 50% of adults treated for chronic partial and secondarily generalized seizures become seizure-free for more than 12 months with currently available drugs.

Table 484-6 ■ DRUGS USED IN TREATING DIFFERENT TYPES OF SEIZURES

TYPE OF SEIZURE	DRUGS
Simple and complex partial	Carbamazepine, phenytoin, valproate, gabapentin, lamotrigine, tiagabine, topiramate
Secondarily generalized	Carbamazepine, phenytoin, valproate, gabapentin, lamotrigine, tiagabine, topiramate
Primary generalized seizures	
Tonic-clonic	Valproate, carbamazepine, phenytoin, lamotrigine
Absence	Ethosuximide, valproate, lamotrigine
Myoclonic	Valproate, clonazepam
Tonic	Valproate, felbamate, clonazepam

Drugs used to treat seizures are listed in Table 484–6. Carbamazepine, phenytoin, primidone, and phenobarbital are equally effective in suppressing partial and secondarily generalized seizures. In individual patients, however, failure to respond to one drug does not preclude a good response to another. Valproate is somewhat less effective against complex partial seizures than either carbamazepine or phenytoin, but it is of comparable efficacy against secondarily generalized seizures. Despite similar pharmacologic potency, these drugs differ substantially in terms of side effects and pharmacokinetic properties. Thus, tolerability and ease of dosing schedule determine the particular choice of drug for an individual patient.

Cost may be another consideration. Phenytoin and extended release forms of carbamazepine have long half-lifes and can be given only twice daily. Drugs that must be administered more often increase problems with compliance for some patients. Concern about phenytoin's occasional undesirable cosmetic effects (gingival hypertrophy, hirsutism, and coarsening of the facial features) makes carbamazepine the drug of choice for many patients, especially younger ones. Primidone and phenobarbital have a high incidence of sedative and cognitive side effects and are rarely recommended as initial therapy.

Valproate is the drug of first choice for generalized-onset seizures. It can be used effectively as monotherapy in 80% of patients even when several types of generalized seizures coexist. Lamotrigine is a reasonable alternative and may have fewer side effects. Phenytoin and carbamazepine are only slightly less effective against generalized tonic-clonic seizures, but they may exacerbate absence and myoclonic seizures which frequently accompany generalized tonic-clonic seizures. Ethosuximide is as effective as valproate in treating typical absence seizures and, because of fewer side effects, is the drug of choice when no other seizure type coexists. Clonazepam prevents myoclonic seizures, but its benefit does not persist in some patients.

Drug Dosage and Pharmacokinetic Principles

Table 484–7 gives the usual dose and relevant pharmacokinetic data for each of the most commonly used antiepileptic drugs. After absorption, a drug is distributed between the plasma and various tissue compartments. Because most antiepileptic drugs are fractionally bound to serum proteins, an equilibrium exists between the

Table 484–7 ■ ANTIEPILEPTIC DRUGS: DOSAGE AND PHARMACOKINETIC DATA

DRUG	USUAL DOSAGE (PER 24 hr)	BIO/ AVAILABILITY (%)	PROTEIN BOUND (%)	CLEARANCE (mL/kg/min)	URINARY EXCRETION (UNCHANGED %)	VOLUME OF DISTRIBUTION (Ls/kg)	HALF-LIFE (hrs)	"THERAPEUTIC" CONCENTRATIONS
Carbamazepine*	Adult: 800–1600 mg / Child: 10–40 mg/kg/day	75–85	74	1.3 (postinduction) (very variable)	<1	0.8–2.0	11–22†	6–12 µg/mL
Ethosuximide	Adult: 750–1500 mg / Child: 10–75 mg/kg/day	>90	0	0.19 (higher in children)	18	0.62–0.69	45–60 (mean in children: 36)	40–100 µg/mL
Felbamate	Adult: 2400–3600 mg / Child: 15–45 mg/kg/day	—	25–35	—	50	0.70	18–24	20–60 µg/mL
Gabapentin	Adult: 900–3600 mg	51–59	<3	—	90–100		5–8	>2 µg/mL
Lamotrigine	Adult: 75–200 mg / Child: 1–5 mg/kg	>90	55	0.04	10	1.1	30 (14–50)	4–15 µg/mL
Phenobarbital	Adult: 90–180 mg / Child: 2–6 mg/kg/day	100	45–50	0.062 (higher in children)	25	0.54–0.70	99 (shorter in children)	15–40 µg/mL
Phenytoin	Adult: 300–400 mg / Child: 4–12 mg/kg/day	90	90	Capacity limited $V_{max} = 5.9$ mg/kg/day $K_M = 5.7$ µg/mL	2	0.78	6–42 (concentration dependent)	10–20 µg/mL
Primidone‡	Adult: 750–1250 mg / Child: 6–12 mg/kg/day	92	19	0.59–0.94	42	0.64–0.72	8–15	5–12 µg/mL
Topiramate	200–400 mg	>80%	9–17%	—	70%	—	16–30	2–20 µg/mL
Tiagabine	32–56 mg	90%	95%	—	<1%	—	5–13	100–200 µg/mL
Valproate	Adult: 1000–3000 mg / Child: 10–70 mg/kg/day	100	93 (concentration dependent)	0.11	2	0.19	14–20	50–120 µg/mL

*The carbamazepine metabolite carbamazepine-10,11-epoxide is also pharmacologically active: values given are for the parent compound.
†The half-life of carbamazepine is considerably longer when the drug is first introduced, prior to autoinduction of hepatic microsomal enzymes.
‡Primidone's primary metabolites, phenobarbital and phenylethylmalonamide, are also pharmacologically active; values given are for the parent compound.
Blood levels for lamotrigine, felbamate, topiramate and tiagabine and gabapentin have not been firmly established. These values are only estimates based on initial clinical trials and personal experience.

plasma concentrations of protein-bound and free (unbound) drug. Only unbound drug is capable of crossing the various lipoprotein membranes that surround brain receptor sites, making only this portion of the total drug concentration available to produce the desired effect. Antiepileptic drug blood levels that are routinely determined by laboratories reflect total plasma drug concentrations (bound plus unbound fractions). When protein binding is altered by disease (e.g., uremia), physiologic state (e.g., pregnancy), or other drugs (e.g., valproate), determining the unbound fraction provides a more accurate reflection of the drug's concentration in the brain's extracellular space. Measuring free levels can be helpful whenever there is a discrepancy between the total plasma concentration and the expected clinical effect.

A drug's *half-life* is a measure of the rate at which a drug is eliminated through metabolism or excretion. Drug half-life determines the dosing interval for antiepileptic drugs; to minimize fluctuations in plasma concentrations, this should amount to less than one third to one half the drug's half-life at steady state. *Steady state* refers to the equilibrium that is established between drug intake and clearance. The time it takes for a drug to achieve steady-state conditions is determined by its half-life. For practical purposes, steady state is reached at an interval equal to five times the drug's half-life. Because a drug continues to accumulate in the body until steady state is reached, plasma drug levels are reliable only when they are measured under steady-state conditions. Similarly, time to steady state determines how rapidly the dose of any antiepileptic drug can be increased. Phenytoin is an exception because of its nonlinear kinetics. Phenytoin's half-life is dose-dependent, which means that steady-state concentration at one dose cannot be used to predict directly the steady-state concentration at a higher dose. For example, phenytoin's half-life is about 24 hours at plasma concentrations of 10 to 20 μg/mL. However, its half-life increases to 36 hours (or more) at concentrations of 25 μg/mL.

Blood levels are useful in the treatment of epilepsy, but optimal levels for some patients fall either above or below usual recommended levels. Some patients, for example, consistently have side effects at low or "therapeutic" concentrations, whereas others benefit from "toxic" levels without experiencing side effects. Blood levels, therefore, should never be the goal of treatment. A level in the low to mid-therapeutic range is a reasonable target when initiating treatment, but subsequent dose adjustments should be based on the patient's clinical progress, seizure frequency, and appearance of drug-related side effects. Blood levels should be obtained when control of seizures is achieved or when toxic side effects appear. Noncompliance is the most common reason that a therapeutic drug level is not achieved using recommended dosing schedules. Blood levels can detect drug interactions in patients taking two or more drugs and determine hepatic or renal effects on drug elimination.

Initiating Antiepileptic Drug Therapy

Treatment should start with a single drug chosen according to the patient's type of seizure, as well as consideration of adverse effects, required dosing schedule, and cost. With the exception of phenobarbital and phenytoin, administration of antiepileptic drugs should be started in low doses to minimize acute toxicity and then increased to a maintenance schedule according to the patient's tolerance and the drug's pharmacokinetics. Most common side effects are temporary, and these are minimized if the dose is built up slowly. Nausea can be minimized by taking the medication with meals. Sedation may be less likely if a higher dose is given at bedtime.

If therapeutic blood levels need to be achieved rapidly, drugs for which loading doses are practical, such as phenytoin, valproate, or phenobarbital, should be given. Other drugs can gradually be substituted, if necessary, once seizures are controlled.

All antiepileptic drugs can produce adverse effects. The most common side effects are *dose related* and typically occur when the drug is first given or when the dose is increased. Dose-related side effects usually correlate with blood concentrations of the drug or its major metabolites. *Idiosyncratic* reactions create the most serious and life-threatening side effects of antiepileptic drugs. All antiepileptic drugs can cause similar idiosyncratic reactions, including rash, Stevens-Johnson syndrome, agranulocytosis, thrombocytopenia, aplastic anemia, and hepatic failure. Idiosyncratic reactions are not dose related, and no laboratory test can identify individuals specifically at risk for them. Routine blood monitoring at set intervals is costly and ineffective. Minor elevations in liver SGOT and SGPT occur in about 25 to 30% of patients with epilepsy, and these neither correlate with clinical symptoms nor predict development of hepatitis or liver failure. Isolated elevations in GGT levels seem to have little use as an indication of clinically significant liver dysfunction in persons with epilepsy. Nearly 20% of patients taking carbamazepine experience a benign leukopenia with WBC counts below 4000/mL. A few patients have WBC counts that drop transiently below 2500/mL. The risk of developing aplastic anemia is not increased in this group, nor is there an increased rate of infections or other possible complications that might be attributed to leukopenia.

When Initial Treatment Fails

Monotherapy results in satisfactory control of seizures (over 90% reduction) in about 60% of patients. Of patients in whom the first drug was ineffective, about half respond to an alternative drug used alone. Of the remaining, less than 50% have improved control by addition of a second drug. Gabapentin, lamotrigine, topiramate, and tiagabine have been approved as adjunctive therapy in patients with partial and secondarily generalized seizures. They are useful additions to phenytoin, carbamazepine, or valproate when these drugs fail as monotherapy. Although the new drugs have a number of desirable features and generally better therapeutic indices compared with more familiar agents, it is still too soon to predict what their ultimate place will be in the treatment of epilepsy. For example, felbamate, another relatively new drug, has already proved to be too toxic (causing aplastic anemia and liver failure) for routine use, and concern has risen recently about visual field defects attributed to vigabatrin.

Pregnancy Concerns

Epilepsy should not discourage a woman from becoming pregnant: well over 90% of women taking antiepileptic drugs have healthy babies. Nonetheless, epilepsy affects the pregnancy in many ways, and it is important that women be informed before conception about possible problems and the steps that can be taken to minimize these. Overall, women with epilepsy demonstrate 1.5 to 3 times higher rates of complications of pregnancy regardless of treatment. These include increased risks of intrapartum bleeding, toxemia, abruptio placentae, premature labor, and stillborn births. About 35% of women with epilepsy experience increased seizures during pregnancy. This is mostly due to falling antiepileptic drug levels associated with a variety of physiologic changes that promote increased volume of distribution and clearance. Thus, antiepileptic drug levels should be followed closely during pregnancy, especially after the first trimester.

In the general population, *major fetal malformations* (cardiac defects, cleft lip or palate, neural tube defects, including spina bifida and anencephaly) occur in about 2% of pregnancies. This risk is increased to 4 to 6% in infants born to women with epilepsy who have taken a single antiepileptic drug during pregnancy. Valproate increases the chance of neural tube defects by 1.5%, and carbamazepine may also raise this specific risk by 0.5%, especially if there is a family history of neural tube defects. Use of two or more drugs carries a 10% risk of major fetal malformations.

Minor anomalies (nail hypoplasia, hypertelorism, low-set ears, prominent lips, broad-based nose) are also increased in infants of mothers with epilepsy, but this seems to reflect both genetic and drug-related factors. Such anomalies occur at increased rates independent of treatment status, although antiepileptic drug therapy increases the risk further to a slight degree. It was formerly thought that particular profiles of these anomalies could be attributed to specific drugs (e.g., fetal hydantoin syndrome or fetal valproate syndrome), but recent data indicate that all antiepileptic drugs can produce similar anomalies. The cosmetic effects of most anomalies lessen with age, and many may be virtually undetectable by late adolescence.

Virtually all antiepileptic drugs promote a hemorrhagic diathesis in newborns. Intramuscular vitamin K, which is given routinely to babies, is occasionally inadequate to prevent hemorrhage. Therefore, oral vitamin K, 10 mg/day, should be prescribed for the mother during the last month of pregnancy.

The risk of neural tube defects is reduced, perhaps eliminated, by preconceptive use of folic acid, 1 mg/day. Ultrasonography and amniocentesis done at 18 to 19 weeks of gestation have a nearly 95% accuracy rate in experienced hands of identifying neural tube defects and other major malformations. Serum α-fetoprotein determinations can detect neural tube defects but have a 25% false-negative rate.

All major antiepileptic drugs have been associated with congenital malformations. On the other hand, frequent convulsions or status epilepticus can lead to a miscarriage or damage the fetus as a result of hypoxia and reduced placental blood flow. There is no "best" antiepileptic drug, and, as in other patients, the drug of choice for women with epilepsy who wish to become pregnant is the one that is most appropriate to the seizure type and that produces optimal control with the fewest side effects. Although management issues for women with epilepsy of child-bearing age are complex, and adverse pregnancy outcomes are increased compared with the general population, sufficient evidence-based information is available to allow understandable concerns to be addressed rationally with improved maternal and fetal health.

SURGICAL TREATMENT

Surgical intervention should be considered when seizures fail to respond to antiepileptic drugs and when they continue to disrupt patients' quality of life. Advances in surgical techniques and improved methods of identifying epileptogenic brain areas have made surgical treatment an option for more patients with uncontrolled seizures today than ever before. In 1985, for example, there were about 500 operations for epilepsy in the United States; in 1990, there were more than 1500, and in 1998 nearly 5000.

In the past, there was considerable disagreement about when to refer patients for surgery, and many physicians viewed it as a therapy of last resort. As a result, until recently, the average time from epilepsy diagnosis to operation was about 20 years. Currently, increasing numbers of neurologists believe that it is possible to identify patients who are likely to benefit from surgery earlier in the course of their illness, and that minimizing the delay between onset of seizures and successful intervention provides better seizure control, psychosocial outcome, and quality of life.

Few patients benefit from further attempts at medical treatment if seizures are not controlled with two trials of high-dose monotherapy using appropriate drugs and one trial of rational combination therapy. These steps can be accomplished within 1 to 2 years. At that point, the detrimental effects of continued seizures, often exacerbated by drug toxicity, warrant referral to a specialized epilepsy center.

The most common type of epilepsy surgery, and the one with which there is the greatest experience, is *focal cortical resection*. Surgery should be considered for any patient with focal seizures whose attacks remain disabling despite optimal medical therapy. Three criteria identify the ideal patient for resective surgery: (1) the seizures begin in an identifiable and localized area of cortex; (2) the surgical excision can encompass the epileptogenic region; and (3) the required resection does not impair neurologic function. These requirements are met most often by patients with temporal lobe epilepsy or other focal epilepsies associated with a demonstrable cerebral lesion (e.g., cavernous malformation, ganglioglioma). Over 70% of such patients become seizure-free, and about 90% have sufficiently fewer seizures to substantially improve their quality of life. The outcome is less favorable for patients undergoing nonlesional extratemporal resections: About 45% of patients become seizure-free; another 35% have worthwhile improvement.

Two other surgical procedures are used much less often and only for highly selected cases of persons with longstanding, uncontrolled seizures, usually beginning in childhood. *Corpus callosotomy* is indicated for intractable atonic and secondarily generalized tonic-clonic seizures such as occur in severe epileptic encephalopathies like the Lennox-Gastaut syndrome. *Hemispherectomy* is an effective operation for children with severely incapacitating unilateral seizures associated with hemiatrophy, hemiparesis, and a useless hand (infantile hemiplegia syndrome).

PROGNOSIS OF EPILEPSY

About 60 to 70% of people with epilepsy achieve a 5-year remission of seizures within 10 years of diagnosis. About half of these patients eventually become seizure-free. Factors favoring remission include an idiopathic form of epilepsy, a normal neurologic examination, and an onset in early to middle childhood (excluding neonatal seizures).

Thirty per cent of patients, usually with severe epilepsy starting in early childhood, continue to have seizures and never achieve a remission. In the United States, the prevalence of intractable epilepsy cases approximates 1 to 2 per 1000 population.

Discontinuing Antiepileptic Drugs

Because epidemiologic studies have shown that many patients with epilepsy become seizure-free for an extended period, a number of investigators have attempted to identify which patients can discontinue antiepileptic drugs without a high risk of relapse. Successful drug withdrawal is most likely if initial seizure control was readily achieved using monotherapy, there were relatively few seizures before remission, and the EEG and neurologic examination are normal just before drugs are discontinued. In addition, longer seizure-free intervals (4 years rather than 2) reduce the likelihood of relapse. Conversely, risk of relapse is high if seizure control was difficult to establish and required polytherapy, if there were frequent generalized tonic-clonic seizures before control was achieved, and if the EEG demonstrates moderate or severe disturbances of background activity or active epileptiform activity at the time drug withdrawal is considered.

STATUS EPILEPTICUS

Various types of status epilepticus take either convulsive or nonconvulsive forms. *Convulsive status epilepticus* is a medical emergency that requires timely and appropriate treatment to minimize serious systemic and neurologic morbidity. Like self-limited seizures, convulsive status may be either idiopathic and of generalized onset or secondary to bilateral spread from a focal epileptogenic brain area. *Nonconvulsive status* presents as a new-onset sustained confusional state.

Convulsive status epilepticus is the first manifestation of epilepsy in about 10% of cases; over 50% of patients with status epilepticus do not have a history of epilepsy. An acute precipitating factor or specific cause, such as metabolic abnormalities, drug abuse, hypoxia, infection, stroke, or tumor, can be identified in 50 to 65% of patients with status epilepticus. The mortality rate approaches 30% in adults, but death usually relates to the underlying condition. Status epilepticus itself accounts for death in less than 10% of cases.

Treatment protocols are designed to eliminate seizure activity and to identify and treat any underlying medical or neurologic disorder. Initial management focuses on ensuring adequate oxygenation and maintaining blood pressure (Table 484-8). There must be unimpeded access to the circulation, and cardiac function must be monitored continuously. Diagnostic studies should be initiated concurrently with blood obtained for antiepileptic drug levels, blood cell count, and routine chemistries. Brain imaging is necessary, but control of seizures must be the first priority. Lumbar puncture must be performed if meningitis is strongly suspected. If, however, focal neurologic signs point to a mass lesion, antibiotics should be given and a CT scan obtained first. In adults, thiamine (to avoid precipitating Wernicke's encephalopathy) followed by glucose should be administered to counteract hypoglycemia unless an adequate glucose concentration has been demonstrated.

Table 484-8 presents the recommendations of the Epilepsy Foundation for treating status epilepticus. A benzodiazepine, either diazepam (10 mg, repeated once) or lorazepam (4 to 8 mg) should be given, followed immediately by intravenous phenytoin or fosphenytoin, 20 mg/kg, at a rate not exceeding 50 mg/min. If seizures continue, an additional 5 mg/kg of phenytoin or fosphenytoin should be given. About 80% of patients respond to this protocol. If status is refractory, the patient should be admitted to an intensive care unit and anesthetized with intravenous pentobarbital, 5 mg/kg, followed by 25 to 50 mg every 25 to 50 minutes as necessary to produce a burst-suppression pattern on continuously monitored EEG. Maintenance doses are 1 to 3 mg/kg/hr. Ventilatory assistance and vasopressors are invariably required. Alternatively, midazolam drip (0.2 mg/kg followed by 0.75 to 10 μg/kg/min) can be used to induce anesthesia. Midazolam is cleared more rapidly and has less hypotensive effect than either phenobarbital or pentobarbital.

Table 484-8 ■ PROTOCOL FOR TREATING STATUS EPILEPTICUS

TIME (min)	ACTION*
0–5	Diagnose status epilepticus by observing continued seizure activity or one additional seizure.
	Give oxygen by nasal cannula or mask; position patient's head for optimal airway patency; consider intubation if respiratory assistance is needed.
	Obtain and record vital signs at onset and periodically thereafter; control any abnormalities as necessary; initiate ECG monitoring.
	Establish an IV in one or both arms using catheter; draw venous blood samples for glucose level, serum chemistries, hematology studies, toxicology screens, and determinations of antiepileptic drug levels.
	Assess oxygenation with oximetry or periodic arterial blood gas determinations.
6–9	If hypoglycemia is established or a blood glucose determination is unavailable, administer glucose; in adults, give 100 mg of thiamine first, followed by 50 mL of 50% glucose by direct push into the IV; in children, the dose of glucose is 2 mL/kg of 25% glucose.
10–20	Administer either 0.1 mg/kg of lorazepam at 2 mg/min or 0.2 mg/kg of diazepam at 5 mg/min by IV. If diazepam is given, it can be repeated if seizures do not stop after 5 min; if diazepam is used to stop the status, phenytoin should be administered immediately to prevent recurrent status.
21–60	If status persists, administer 15–20 mg/kg of phenytoin by IV no faster than 50 mg/min in adults and 1 mg/kg/min in children. Monitor ECG and blood pressure during the infusion. Phenytoin is incompatible with glucose-containing solutions: the IV should be purged with normal saline before the phenytoin infusion.
>60	If status does not stop after 20 mg/kg of phenytoin administration, give additional doses of 5 mg/kg to a maximal dose of 30 mg/kg.
	If status persists, give 20 mg/kg of phenobarbital by IV at 100 mg/min. When phenobarbital is given after a benzodiazepine, the risk of apnea or hypopnea is great, and assisted ventilation is usually required.
	If status persists, give anesthetic doses of drugs such as pentobarbital. Ventilatory assistance and vasopressors are virtually always necessary.

*Time starts at seizure onset.
ECG = electrocardiogram; IV = intravenous line.
From Dodson WE, DeLorenzo RJ, Pedley TA, et al: Treatment of convulsive status epilepticus: Recommendations of the Epilepsy Foundation of America's working group on status epilepticus. JAMA 270:854, 1993.

Nonconvulsive status epilepticus is difficult to diagnose and is frequently unrecognized. It presents most often in middle-aged or elderly persons without a history of seizures. Onset is generally abrupt, with a fluctuating confusional state that can last for days to weeks. Although clouding of consciousness occurs to a varying degree, the absence of stupor or coma contributes to misdiagnosis. Nonconvulsive status epilepticus may be mistaken for psychosis because of the abrupt development of bizarre behavior, inappropriate affect, paranoia, delusions, and catatonia. Alternatively, memory loss, confusion, and mood changes may predominate and suggest a metabolic or toxic encephalopathy or dementia. Some patients have recurrent episodes.

Diagnosis depends on demonstration of seizure discharges in the EEG in association with symptoms. Most patients show continuous or nearly continuous 1- to 2.5-Hz generalized spike-wave activity similar to generalized absence status ("spike-wave stupor") that occurs in children. Rarely, however, the EEG ictal activity is localized, usually to the frontal or temporal lobes, indicating that in these patients the nonconvulsive status is a form of continuous partial seizure activity. Intravenous diazepam (5 to 10 mg) or lorazepam (1 to 2 mg) suppresses epileptiform EEG abnormalities and produces dramatic improvement in the patient's mental state. Long-term seizure control is achieved using valproate, phenytoin, or carbamazepine.

A specific cause cannot be identified in most cases. Sometimes, however, nonconvulsive status results from electrolyte imbalance, drug toxicity (e.g., lithium), or a focal cerebral lesion (e.g., frontal lobe infarction).

PSYCHOSOCIAL ISSUES

Epilepsy and its effects result from multiple interacting factors, of which seizures are only a part. The extent of a patient's disability or quality of life may relate more to physical limitations caused by neurologic abnormalities, psychological factors, or adverse drug effects than to the seizures themselves. This observation is underscored by patients who become seizure-free after surgery but who remain disabled and unable to find employment, establish relationships, or become independent in other ways. Not the least of epilepsy's disabling aspects is the episodic nature of the condition: periods of relative well-being are punctuated by unpredictably occurring attacks that impose their own limitations, create embarrassment, and reinforce negative stereotypes. Recurrent seizures, despite treatment, are graphic reminders of medicine's failure. Adults experience discrimination at work and loss of mobility because they cannot drive.

The treatment of epilepsy can be effective only when interacting medical, psychological, and environmental factors are addressed successfully. Areas of psychosocial difficulty should be identified early in the course of treatment and an appropriate plan of management developed. This often requires a multidisciplinary approach to disabilities that have social, educational, vocational, and psychological dimensions. The physician must be sensitive to these issues, even if they are not voiced explicitly. In fact, psychosocial concerns may be the major focus of most follow-up visits. The physician has a special responsibility to educate society as well as the patient and family in order to counter the many misperceptions, myths, and prejudices that are ascribed to epilepsy.

Berg AT, Shinnar S: The risk of seizure recurrence following a first unprovoked seizure: A quantitative review. Neurology 41:965, 1991. *A meta-analysis of the most important articles to evaluate the development of and risks for epilepsy after a first unprovoked seizure.*

Brodie MJ, Dichter MA: Antiepileptic drugs. N Engl J Med 334:168, 1996. *A practical but critical review of commonly used antiepileptic drugs, their pharmacokinetics, and their use in treating patients with epilepsy.*

Devinsky O: A Guide to Understanding and Living with Epilepsy. Philadelphia, FA Davis, 1994. *This is a sensitive, well-written and informative review of epilepsy and its impact on quality of life that is suitable for patients and their families.*

Dodson WE, DeLorenzo RJ, Pedley TA, et al: Treatment of convulsive status epilepticus: Recommendations of the Epilepsy Foundation of America's working group on status epilepticus. JAMA 270:854, 1993. *A consensus report describing the epidemiology, pathogenesis, morbidity and mortality, treatment, and prognosis of status epilepticus.*

Durner M, Zhou G, Fu D, et al: Evidence for linkage of adolescent-onset idiopathic generalized epilepsies to chromosome 8—and genetic heterogeneity. Am J Hum Genet 64:1411, 1999.

Engel J Jr, Pedley TA (eds): Epilepsy: A Comprehensive Textbook. Philadelphia, Lippincott-Raven Press, 1997. *A multi-authored three-volume textbook that covers all aspects of epilepsy, from the basic molecular, cellular, and neural biology to details of medical and surgical management.*

Hauser WA, Hesdorffer DC: Epilepsy: Frequency, Causes and Consequences. New York, Demos, 1990. *An encyclopedia of facts about all aspects of epilepsy.*

Hauser WA, Annegers JF, Kurland LT: Incidence of epilepsy and unprovoked seizures in Rochester, Minnesota: 1935–1984. Epilepsia 34:453, 1993. *This ambitious study provides the best available data about seizure incidence and complements an earlier prevalence study by the same investigators.*

Hauser WA, Rich SS, Lee JR-J, et al: Risk of recurrent seizures after two unprovoked seizures. N Engl J Med 338:429, 1998. *A prospective study that demonstrates the sharp increase in risk for further seizures that follows a second unprovoked seizure. This complements the analysis of Berg and Shinnar.*

Lowenstein DH, Alldredge BK: Status epilepticus. N Engl J Med 338:970, 1998. *A review of current concepts of managing status epilepticus with treatment regimens that include fosphenytoin, midazolam, and propofol.*

Musicco M, Beghi E, Solari A, et al: Treatment of first tonic-clonic seizure does not improve the prognosis of epilepsy. Neurology 49:991, 1997. *An important multicenter, randomized investigation of the effect of treatment after a single seizure on the prognosis for development of epilepsy.*

Sloviter RS: The functional organization of the hippocampal dentate gyrus and its relevance to the pathogenesis of temporal lobe epilepsy. Ann Neurol 35:640, 1994. *The most coherent hypothesis and review of supporting experimental and clinical data linking the development of mesial temporal sclerosis to temporal lobe epilepsy.*

■ CENTRAL NERVOUS SYSTEM TUMORS AND STATES OF ALTERED INTRACRANIAL PRESSURE

485 INTRACRANIAL TUMORS

Nicholas A. Vick

More than 18,000 new cases of primary brain tumors are treated each year in the United States. Metastases are even more frequent and contribute considerably to suffering and death from systemic cancer. The diversity of brain tumors makes it important to attend to what is characteristic about each histologic type. Biologic specificity guides therapy to some extent now, and will be the key to successful treatment in the future.

The classification of brain tumors is a subject with confusing terminology. This text employs the simple approach of classifying brain tumors into *metastatic, primary extra-axial,* and *primary intra-axial* (Table 485–1). These categories include all of the primary brain tumors listed in the World Health Organization classification (Table 485–2), and adds pituitary and metastatic tumors. Although obviously simple, it follows practical clinical thinking. This chapter deals with the general biology, clinical features, and treatment of brain tumors as an overall problem. The following chapter describes the particular behavior of the most important subtypes in accordance with the outline of Table 485–1.

GENERAL CONSIDERATIONS

"Is it benign or malignant?" is invariably the first question asked by patients, families, and physicians when confronted with a diagnosis of brain tumor. About a third of primary brain tumors can be called benign. Meningiomas and acoustic neuromas are good examples. They grow slowly, often can be removed completely, and rarely recur.

The concept of malignancy in the central nervous system (CNS) has a different meaning from that which applies to systemic cancers. The term "malignant" has nothing to do with metastasis out of the CNS, which is extraordinarily rare. It has everything to do with anatomic location and the possibility of complete surgical removal. Unless a tumor can be completely excised to the last cell, all intracranial neoplasms are potentially malignant in that they may recur, and often do.

Table 485–1 ■ COMMON BRAIN TUMORS IN ADULTS WITH PERCENTAGE INCIDENCE BY CATEGORY*

METASTATIC	PRIMARY EXTRA-AXIAL	PRIMARY INTRA-AXIAL
Lung (37)	Meningioma (80)	Glioblastoma (47)
Breast (19)	Acoustic neuroma (10)	Anaplastic astrocytoma (24)
Melanoma (16)	Pituitary adenoma (7)	Astrocytoma (15)
Colorectum (9)	Other (3)	Oligodendroglioma (5)
Kidney (8)		Lymphoma (2)
Other (11)		Other (7)

*These figures, given in parentheses, can be extremely variable from one center to another, depending on referral pattern. They are given here as general estimates based upon many published series.

Table 485–2 ■ WORLD HEALTH ORGANIZATION CLASSIFICATION OF BRAIN TUMORS*

A. Astrocytic tumors
  1. Astrocytoma
    a. Fibrillary
    b. Protoplasmic
    c. Gemistocytic
  2. Pilocytic astrocytoma
  3. Subependymal giant cell astrocytoma (ventricular tumor or tuberous sclerosis)
  4. Astroblastoma
  5. Anaplastic (malignant) astrocytoma
B. Oligodendroglial tumors
  1. Oligodendroglioma
  2. Mixed oligoastrocytoma
  3. Anaplastic (malignant) oligodendroglioma
C. Ependymal and choroid plexus tumors
  1. Ependymoma
    Variants:
    a. Myxopapillary ependymoma
    b. Papillary ependymoma
    c. Subependymoma
  2. Anaplastic (malignant) ependymoma
  3. Choroid plexus papilloma
  4. Anaplastic (malignant) choroid plexus papilloma
D. Pineal cell tumor
  1. Pineocytoma (pinealcytoma)
  2. Pineoblastoma (pinealoblastoma)
E. Neuronal tumors
  1. Gangliocytoma
  2. Ganglioglioma
  3. Ganglioneuroblastoma
  4. Anaplastic (malignant) gangliocytoma and ganglioglioma
  5. Neuroblastoma
F. Poorly differentiated and embryonal tumors
  1. Glioblastoma
    Variants:
    a. Glioblastoma with sarcomatous component (mixed glioblastoma and sarcoma)
    b. Giant cell glioblastoma
  2. Medulloblastoma
    Variants:
    a. Desmoplastic medulloblastoma
    b. Medullomyoblastoma
  3. Medulloepithelioma
  4. Primitive polar spongioblastoma
  5. Gliomatosis cerebri

*This is one of several formal schemes that are based on neuropathologic criteria. Metastasis is not considered, and one can get no sense of a given tumor as a *clinical* problem, as suggested by the simple classification in Table 485–1.

INITIAL EVALUATION

SYMPTOMS AND SIGNS. Brain tumors present in two patterns, not necessarily mutually exclusive. One consists of nonfocal symptoms of *increased intracranial pressure,* such as headaches, nausea, vomiting, confusion, and lethargy. The other consists of symptoms or signs of *focal brain dysfunction,* such as hemianopia, hemiparesis, cranial nerve palsies, or focal seizures (Table 485–3). Such signs of focal brain dysfunction may have convincing localizing value even before an image of the brain is made by computed tomography (CT) or magnetic resonance imaging (MRI). Some tumors that arise in neurologically "silent" areas, such as the parietal or frontal association cortices, may produce only nonfocal gen-

Table 485-3 ■ FOCAL CLINICAL MANIFESTATIONS OF BRAIN TUMORS

Frontal lobe	Temporal lobe	Sella/optic nerve/pituitary
Generalized seizures	Complex partial (psychomotor) seizures	Endocrinopathy
Focal motor seizures (contralateral)	Generalized seizures	Bitemporal hemianopia
Expressive aphasia (dominant side)	Behavioral changes	Monocular visual defects
Behavioral changes	Olfactory and complex visual auras	Pons/medulla
Dementia	Corpus callosum	Cranial nerve dysfunction
Gait disorders, incontinence	Dementia (anterior)	Ataxia, nystagmus
Basal ganglia	Behavioral changes (posterior)	Weakness, sensory loss
Hemiparesis (contralateral)	Asymptomatic (mid)	Spasticity
Movement disorders rare	Thalamus	Cerebellopontine angle
Parietal lobe	Sensory loss (contralateral)	Deafness (ipsilateral)
Receptive aphasia (dominant side)	Behavioral changes	Loss of facial sensation (ipsilateral)
Spatial disorientation (nondominant side)	Language disorder (dominant side)	Facial weakness (ipsilateral)
Cortical sensory dysfunction (contralateral)	Midbrain/pineal	Ataxia
Hemianopia (contralateral)	Paresis of vertical eye movements	Cerebellum
Occipital lobe	Pupillary abnormalities	Ataxis (ipsilateral)
Hemianopia (contralateral)	Precocious puberty (boys)	Nystagmus
Visual disturbances (unformed)		

eralized symptoms of headache, confusion, behavioral change, or, eventually, a seizure, despite growing to a considerable size. Although the capacity to reach early diagnosis by CT or MRI has greatly reduced the numbers of patients in whom symptoms of increased intracranial pressure represent initial complaints, examples still remain, especially in association with fast-growing tumors and in children. The latter are particularly likely to have tumors in the posterior fossa that tend to obstruct spinal fluid pathways earlier than do supratentorial tumors. The tempo with which a brain tumor grows also influences the presenting symptoms. Despite the fixed space within the skull (once infantile sutures have closed), the human brain possesses a remarkable capacity to make room for a slowly growing tumor (Fig. 485-1). Because of this, and even allowing for the relative rapidity of growth of aggressive brain tumors, such as glioblastomas, the patient usually appears better clinically than might be expected from the degree of abnormality seen on CT or MRI scan.

DIFFERENTIAL DIAGNOSIS. Patients who present with symptoms and signs of increased intracranial pressure or a first convulsive seizure need to be hospitalized. Diagnosis and treatment measures must be started at once; it may be unsafe to wait. Those who present with focal neurologic impairment and who do not have symptoms of increased intracranial pressure may reasonably be evaluated in the outpatient setting for other conditions that are often considerations in the differential diagnosis of brain tumor

(Table 485-4). The tempo of evolution of symptoms and signs of focal neurologic impairment, much more than their severity, governs urgency of evaluation. The tempo also strongly influences diagnostic considerations. Although an occasional brain tumor may manifest with such rapid onset of hemiparesis or aphasia that a stroke is mimicked, most do not. Associated aspects of the history, such as recent head trauma, previous episodes of reversible neurologic impairment, or recent infection and fever, should direct attention to diagnostic alternatives such as subdural hematoma, multiple sclerosis, or cerebral abscess. Simply stated, it is the careful history, not the neurologic examination, that usually points to the alternative diagnoses.

IMAGING AND OTHER DIAGNOSTIC PROCEDURES

Brain imaging by MRI or CT scans is an indispensable component of the modern diagnosis of the presence, but not the type, of brain tumors. One type of tumor can look like another or even resemble a non-neoplastic mass lesion, such as a brain abscess, fungal infection, parasitic invasion, demyelinating disease, or stroke. For definitive diagnosis and adequate treatment planning, one must obtain a tissue diagnosis whenever possible. This can be made either by direct surgical biopsy or, in the case of some non-neoplastic conditions, by judging CT or MRI responses to particular therapies.

MRI is almost always superior to CT scanning in diagnosing intracranial mass lesions. MRI outlines posterior fossa structures and tumors with a clarity that CT cannot achieve because of x-ray distortions caused by the bony structure of that region. In several types of tumor, particularly the low-grade gliomas, MRI may show extensive brain infiltration in cases that fail to produce any image abnormality on CT or, at most, show a vague area of low density. Although either MRI or CT should be used with contrast enhancement in cases of suspected brain tumor, the passage of such contrast agents beyond the blood-brain barrier into the tissue does not necessarily imply the presence of a histologically malignant tumor. For example, although malignant gliomas almost always show contrast enhancement, so do meningiomas, which are entirely benign if they can be fully removed surgically.

CT scans done without contrast enhancement are of little value in the diagnosis of brain tumors or other mass lesions. Although it is true that hemorrhage, calcifications, hydrocephalus, and shift can

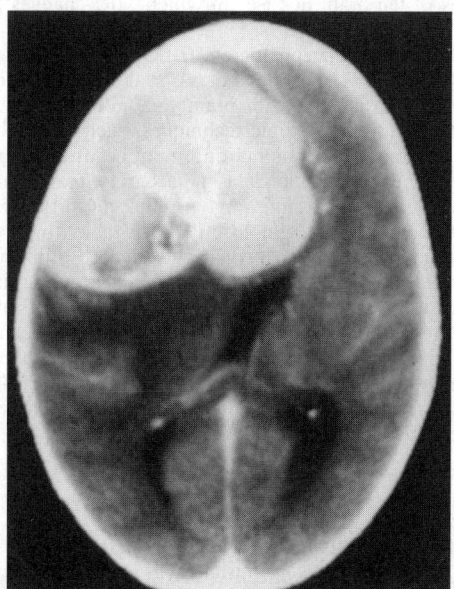

FIGURE 485-1 ■ CT scan with contrast of a meningioma in a patient who presented with mild cognitive deficits, illustrative of the size a slow-growing tumor can attain in the brain. The tumor was completely resected.

Table 485-4 ■ THE MAIN DIFFERENTIAL DIAGNOSES OF BRAIN TUMORS

Hematomas, especially in tumors that have a tendency to bleed, such as melanoma
Abscesses, including fungal
Granulomas
Parasitic infections, such as cysticercosis
Vascular malformations, especially those without arteriovenous shunts
Solitary large plaques of multiple sclerosis
Progressive strokes (rare)

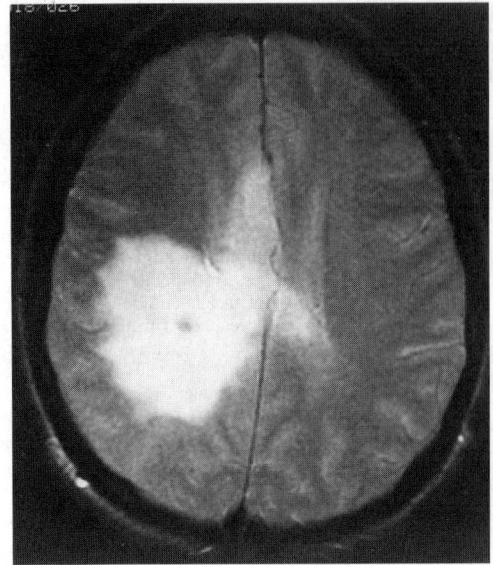 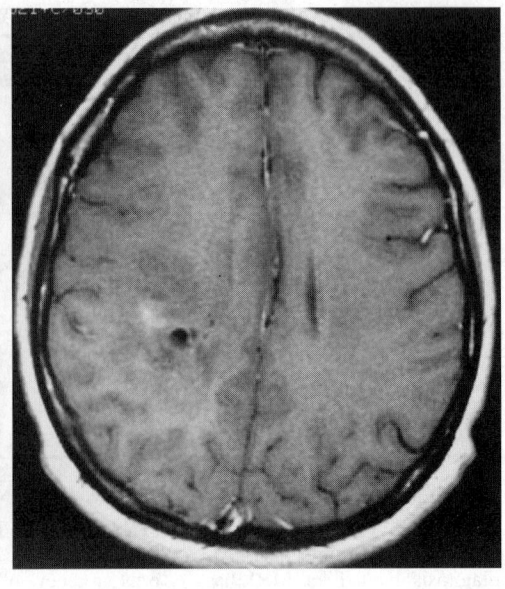

FIGURE 485-2 ▪ Low-grade astrocytoma as imaged by MRI. On the left, T2-weighted image; on the right, T1-weighted image, gadolinium contrast with minimum enhancement. The images are typical of this tumor, which is being detected with increasing frequency in seizure patients by MRI. Many are invisible on CT scans.

be well seen on a non-contrast CT scan, the interpretation of even these conditions is tentative because each can have an underlying causative structural abnormality, such as a brain tumor, which may fail to appear on a non-contrast CT study. Allergy to CT dye is rare and is readily manageable. Currently available non-ionic CT dyes have an extremely low incidence of side effects. Currently used CT dyes carry little risk of causing renal dysfunction in normally hydrated patients who are not known to have kidney disease.

MRI initially provided two types of images, designated T1 and T2. For brain tumors, the former generally showed a well-demarcated area of low density, and the latter showed bright whiteness that encompassed a more extensive region owing to the signal of the surrounding brain edema (Fig. 485-2). With the availability for general usage in 1988 of gadolinium contrast for MRI, a new set of criteria of usage and differential diagnostic considerations in brain imaging have quickly evolved (Table 485-5). T1 gadolinium imaging is the most precise way to image a brain tumor, and patients can often be followed up during and after treatment with that type of study alone. Such an approach is easier for patients because it reduces the length of time otherwise spent on T2 scanning. Now and then, T2 images are useful. For example, T2 images, besides showing the extent of edema, also delineate the demyelinating effects of radiation on white matter. FLAIR images (see Chapter 443), a variant of T1, are even better for this.

Cerebral angiography seldom is used in the diagnosis of brain tumors. In a few circumstances, neurosurgeons, in preparation for surgery, require a more precise knowledge of the pattern and position of blood vessels, which can be obtained only by angiography. The procedure is also used to embolize highly vascular meningiomas or to study cerebral dominance by injection of barbiturate into the carotid artery (the Wada test) in left-handed individuals who are to have surgery near language areas. Preoperative determination of cerebral localization helps surgeons to plan the extent of surgery and to avoid creation of postoperative language deficits in the patient.

Examination of the spinal fluid has limited indication in the diagnosis of brain tumors. One is to rule out an inflammatory disorder mimicking a brain tumor. Another is to establish the diagnosis of benign intracranial hypertension in patients with uninformative MRIs (see Chapter 488). In addition, spinal fluid cytology may be useful for determining instances of malignant meningitis secondary to metastatic neoplasms in association with spinal spread of medulloblastoma in some children and in identifying primary lymphomas of the brain in cases in which MRI changes are ambiguous.

The routine electroencephalogram (EEG) has no role in the diagnosis of brain tumors and does not assist in the choice of anticonvulsant drugs for patients with brain tumor. However, specialized intraoperative neurophysiologic techniques, such as depth electrode studies and intraoperative monitoring, may be useful in identifying and removing epileptogenic areas adjacent to brain tumors or to avoid resection of critical brain regions adjacent to tumors.

Positron emission tomography (PET) is able to quantify biochemical functions, such as oxygen and glucose utilization, within tumors as well as in normal brain tissue. PET scanning is a powerful research tool of limited availability for routine clinical purposes. Its spatial resolution is inferior to that of both CT and MR. In patients with brain tumors who develop recurrent symptoms after radiation therapy, PET can differentiate, with about 70% accuracy, radiation-induced injury from tumor recurrences. These disorders often appear identical on MRI.

TREATMENT

PREOPERATIVE CONSIDERATIONS AND MEDICAL MANAGEMENT. In almost every instance in which a brain tumor is suspected on the basis of the combined results of history, physical findings, and imaging studies, the *first consideration is its surgical resectability.* Exceptions exist, such as in a case of multiple brain metastases in a patient with known systemic cancer. Patients with

Table 485-5 ▪ T1 GADOLINIUM MRI CHARACTERISTICS OF BRAIN TUMORS

Metastases	These are remarkably variable. Some enhance brightly and solidly with gadolonium. Others are in ring configuration. Many are invisible with contrast CT.
Acoustic neuromas	These are invariably intensely contrasted by gadolinium, even more reliably than by CT.
Meningiomas	Same as for acoustic neuromas.
Pituitary adenomas	These always enhance less than the normal pituitary gland. MRI is superior in every way to CT, especially when thin slices and magnified views are ordered.
Glioblastoma	These are almost always in ring configuration.
Anaplastic astrocytomas	These are sometimes solidly bright; they are often patchy, may be noncontrasting, and may look like low-grade astrocytoma.
Low-grade astrocytomas	These do not enhance. They are often invisible by CT or are imaged only as vague low density.
Oligodendrogliomas	These generally do not enhance unless anaplastic and are often invisible on CT unless they are calcified.
Primary brain lymphomas	These usually exhibit homogeneous enhancement and are smoothly rounded. Periventricular location is common. They are multiple in about a fourth of cases. This lesion does not often look like glioblastoma but is easily mistaken for metastases if multiple.

single brain metastases, defined by MRI, may be candidates for surgical resection of the metastasis, depending on the systemic medical status. It is unproductive to embark on an extensive systemic evaluation in the search for an unknown primary cancer in patients with a single resectable presumed brain metastasis. If a primary tumor is not quickly revealed by a careful medical evaluation, with special attention to skin (for melanoma), breasts, and lungs, the pathologic diagnosis of the brain tumor needs to be disclosed by resection or, if unresectable owing to its position, by biopsy.

Although small meningiomas or acoustic neuromas usually do not require treatment to reduce intracranial pressure, in the majority of brain tumor patients it is appropriate to start administration of dexamethasone promptly. The purpose is to reduce intracranial pressure, which accompanies the majority of brain tumors, and to relieve neurologic symptoms caused by peritumoral brain edema (Fig. 485–3). The long biologic half-life of dexamethasone and steady action on the brain have made it the steroid of choice for treating patients with brain tumors. It should be started with an oral dose of 24 mg, followed with 8 mg twice daily. It is well absorbed by mouth, and its action by that route is almost as rapid as when given intravenously. If focal neurologic symptoms are due to peritumoral vasogenic edema, dexamethasone induces improvement within 48 hours and usually sooner. If there is no benefit, the neurologic symptoms are likely to be due to damage of the brain tissue by the tumor and not to edema.

Edema associated with brain tumors is due chiefly to abnormally fenestrated endothelium in the tumor, which permits excess flow of fluid from capillaries into the neoplasm. Normally, solutes are transported through capillaries into brain by dissolving in and diffusing through the cerebral endothelium, a phenomenon dependent on lipid solubility and molecular size. Endothelial cells also possess some facilitated or carrier-mediated processes that are stereospecific, saturable, and independent of lipid solubility and molecular size. In brain tumors, these selective properties of the blood-brain barrier are overwhelmed by increased bulk flow and hydraulic conductivity through the defective endothelium. The result is vasogenic edema, and it is this reaction that dexamethasone so greatly reduces.

In instances of extreme intracranial pressure, the speed and action of dexamethasone are not sufficient to reduce the brain swelling quickly enough to prevent complications. In such instances, hyperosmotic solutions of mannitol must be given. The usual dosage is 0.5 to 2.0 g/kg, given intravenously over 15 minutes, followed by additional boluses of 25 g as needed. The osmotic action of mannitol occurs within minutes. Clinical improvement may be dramatic. It is unusual for brain tumor patients preoperatively to decompensate so severely from increased intracranial pressure that

intubation becomes necessary. Nevertheless, this does occur. In such cases the arterial partial pressure of carbon dioxide ($PaCO_2$) must be decreased by passive hyperventilation to approximately 25 mm Hg. The effect constricts the cerebral vasculature and promptly induces a major reduction of intracranial pressure, which can be life-saving.

About 20% of brain tumor patients develop seizures at some time, even if they do not have seizures at the time of diagnosis. It is conventional but not clearly effective to treat all patients with supratentorial tumors with anticonvulsants before surgery. Most patients with acoustic neuromas or other posterior fossa tumors have a low probability of convulsive seizures and do not need such drugs. Phenytoin is the best initial drug because it can be administered either intravenously or orally, unlike either carbamazepine or valproic acid, which can only be used orally. An intravenous drug is especially useful for continuation during the perioperative period. If required, patients may be switched easily to alternative oral drugs later. Phenytoin should be started orally, given 1000 mg over 12 hours, or intravenously, with 1000 mg given over 1 hour. Thereafter, the usual dosage is 300 to 400 mg/day, administered in one dose or split between breakfast and dinner, along with dexamethasone. Periodic blood levels need to be checked to adjust the dosage to ensure concentrations of 10 to 20 mg/mL.

SURGERY. Although complete excision of a brain tumor is the ultimate goal in every case, this is not always possible. Even potentially curable tumors, such as meningiomas or acoustic neuromas, may reside in positions that make complete resection technically impossible. Malignant gliomas lack microscopic boundaries, even though they may appear by imaging studies to have well-defined limits. How much surgical success can be achieved with these tumors depends on several factors, including the tumor's proximity to indispensable areas, the skill and experience of the neurosurgeon and the preoperative level of neurologic function. The combination of current standards of neurosurgical anesthesia, the capacity to control intracranial pressure, and the recent addition of intraoperative imaging to other operative tools, such as the operating microscope, have greatly increased the surgeon's capacity for well-chosen radical resection. Radical operations on tumors involving language areas, sensorimotor regions, the basal ganglia, corpus callosum, and brain stem are generally avoided. However, partial removal in these areas by stereotaxic methods may be surprisingly effective. MRIs facilitate such surgery by showing that the tumor has pushed aside critical brain structures and that a macroscopic tumor edge can be delineated. It has been repeatedly shown that resection of the maximal amount of tumor consistent with functional preservation provides patients with better and longer lives.

A number of tumors cannot be even partially resected because they invade indispensable areas of the brain. Most are intra-axial tumors, such as the gliomas. Although imaging techniques may produce a characteristic picture suggestive of a particular histologic diagnosis, treatment planning demands a tissue diagnosis. All brain regions may be approached by MR-guided stereotactic biopsy. The tissue specimens are small, but they are almost invariably adequate to establish a diagnosis. Morbidity, chiefly hemorrhage, occurs in about 2% of cases. Patients usually need to remain in the hospital for less than 48 hours. Open biopsies of brain tumors are not justifiable. If the skull and dura are to be opened, the surgeon should be prepared to do a gross total resection or, at least, a major removal of as much tumor as is consonant with preservation of neurologic function.

Deep leg vein thrombophlebitis leading to pulmonary embolism is a recurrent postoperative problem only partially helped by prophylactic application of compression boots. Early passive exercises and mobilization are imperative. The staff must monitor and maintain anticonvulsant levels to prevent postoperative seizures. Dexamethasone should be administered at adequate levels for at least 5 days to minimize surgically induced brain edema.

RADIATION THERAPY. All forms of external-beam radiation, whether γ-photons emitted from ^{60}Co sources or x-rays generated from linear accelerators, act similarly. They produce fast-moving electrons and free radicals in biologic tissue that interrupt chemical

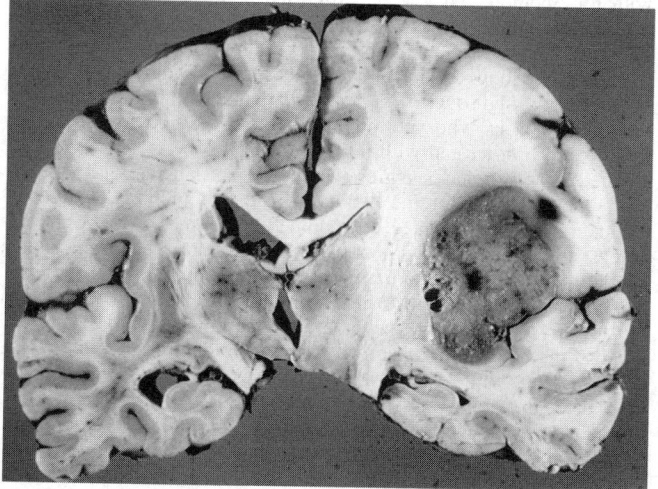

FIGURE 485–3 ■ Gross coronal pathologic specimen of a solitary metastasis from a non–small cell lung carcinoma to the right cerebral hemisphere. The tumor is well circumscribed. It causes marked edema that greatly expands the cerebral white matter. Metastatic tumors such as this can often be surgically resected.

bonds between DNA base pairs. Affected cells either die or become so altered that their mitotic rate is greatly diminished. Radiation therapy is given in small daily fractions to build to a total dose. It appears safer and more effective to do this than to give larger fractions over shorter periods. Hyperfractionation, defined as two (or more) doses during a day, does not seem to be worthwhile. Therapeutic brain irradiation with particulate radiation, such as neutrons, has been attempted experimentally at facilities with cyclotrons. Such densely ionizing radiation has shown no therapeutic advantage over x-rays. Interstitial (implanted) radiation therapy (brachytherapy) is usually given in the form of $^{125}I_3$ or $^{192}Ir_4$ in "seeds" placed by stereotactic techniques. This method permits localized high-dosage radiation with sharp edges and sparing of the adjacent brain. Considerable controversy exists about the utility of interstitial radiation therapy, but it can be effective in well-selected patients. Other non-operative radiosurgical techniques include the "gamma knife" and linear accelerators adapted to provide focused therapeutic beams. Efficacy has been shown for metastases but not for gliomas.

The complications of radiation therapy are often reported as infrequent, perhaps 2 to 5% of cases. These figures are unrealistically low if one includes effects on long-term survivors. They reflect the fact that most irradiated patients with brain tumor die before brain injury appears. A high percentage of patients receiving whole-brain radiation develop dementia or impaired mobility. Often, postradiation neurologic damage may not become fully developed for several years. Local field rather than whole-brain radiation has reduced the incidence of dementia in long-term survivors. Dementia is a considerable problem in children who survive radiation therapy for medulloblastoma. The incidence may reach 50% or more in those who survive treatment for 5 years.

External-beam radiation therapy has value in controlling the growth of malignant gliomas and metastatic brain tumors. It doubles median survival time for both types of tumors. Radiation therapy may be useful for recurrent meningiomas and acoustic neuromas, but they are usually better handled by reoperation. Primary brain lymphomas are so responsive to radiation therapy that many neurologists and radiation therapists continue to use it alone despite the fact that chemotherapy may prove to provide superior initial treatment. It has already been mentioned that solitary brain metastases are best managed by surgical resection before radiation therapy.

CHEMOTHERAPY. Chemotherapy for brain tumors has had a disappointing record. The reasons are many, but inadequacy of drug delivery, tumor cell heterogeneity, and inherent resistance are among the important ones. Almost all efforts have been directed toward the primary brain tumors, especially the gliomas. Established brain metastases, however, respond about as well as systemic metastases do in many cancers, especially breast and small cell lung cancer. Carmustine, the most frequently used drug, remains the most effective non-experimental agent available to treat the malignant astrocytomas. The combination of procarbazine, lomustine, and vincristine has an unusually beneficial effect against oligodendrogliomas. No more than 10% of patients with malignant astrocytomas have meaningful and durable responses to chemotherapy, whether it is given immediately after radiation therapy (when its effect is especially hard to assess) or at the time of recurrence. Efforts to improve response to chemotherapy by delivering drugs through the carotid artery have not been successful.

The pharmacokinetics of drugs used in brain tumor chemotherapy are not well understood. Knowledge about their ability to gain adequate concentration within the tumors is minimal, and almost nothing is known about chemosensitivity. Nonetheless, occasional remarkable responses to chemotherapy do occur in patients with gliomas. Among other primary intra-axial brain tumors, primary brain lymphoma has a reasonably good response rate. The drugs used are those given regularly for systemic lymphoma. Patients with primary brain lymphoma do better with chemotherapy added than with radiation therapy alone. On average, 3- to 4-year survivals can now be expected. Of the gliomas, oligodendroglioma has been the most responsive to drug treatment.

Several additional forms of medical treatment for brain tumors have been attempted. These include slow release of carmustine from implanted biodegradable polymers, which has been shown to have modest benefit. Interferons, other biologic response modifiers, angiogenesis inhibitors, gene therapy, and radionuclides coupled with monoclonal antibodies are still experimental. New biologic knowledge, such as the sequential genetic events that influence the malignant transformation and progression of brain tumors, will be required before new medical treatments become practical realities.

Posner JB: Neurologic Complications of Cancer. Philadelphia, FA Davis, 1995. *A true masterpiece about metastasis to the nervous system.*

Levin VA: Cancer in the Nervous System. New York, Churchill Livingstone, 1996. *Essential in its breadth and scope for primary gliomas.*

Kleihues P, Cavenee WK: Pathology and Genetics of Tumours of the Nervous System. Lyon, France, International Agency for Research on Cancer, 1997. *An ideal source of current knowledge in this field, with direct relevance to clinical thinking and patient care.*

Bigner DD, McLendon RE, Brunner JM: Russell and Rubinstein's Pathology of Tumors of the Nervous System, 6th ed. London, Arnold, 1998. *The masterful new revision of this great classic text.*

486 SPECIFIC TYPES OF BRAIN TUMORS AND THEIR MANAGEMENT

Nicholas A. Vick

METASTATIC TUMORS

All systemic cancers are capable of metastasizing to the intracranial contents and skull, although some do so more readily than others. The most frequent are lung, breast, and melanoma. This is not surprising, because they are among the most common cancers. In many instances, brain metastases produce symptoms before the primary tumor is suspected. Furthermore, the primary cancer may not be found without considerable effort.

Patterns of metastasis to the nervous system have some variability, but none is truly characteristic. Non–small cell carcinoma of the lung and renal carcinoma tend to be associated with single metastases, whereas small cell carcinoma of the lung, breast carcinoma, and melanoma often generate multiple secondary deposits. The metastases may be miliary in melanoma. T1 gadolinium magnetic resonance imaging (MRI) scans are critical in the imaging of brain metastases (Fig. 486–1). *Multiple metastases* may be revealed with this method, whereas T2 MRI and contrast computed tomography (CT) may show only one or, in rare instances, none. For multiple metastases, whole-brain irradiation is the best form of treatment so long as the patient's systemic condition indicates a potential for high-quality survival. Patients with widespread systemic metastasis who are unlikely to survive more than a few months are best treated with dexamethasone alone.

The major benefit of aggressive surgery in patients with a single brain metastasis is for the quality of life that remains. Studies of evaluation of performance are compelling. Some of the best outcomes are in patients with non–small cell lung carcinoma and a single metastasis to the brain. Surgical removal of both tumors sometimes leads to a protracted remission from the disease. With most brain metastases, however, 2-year mortality is similar between surgical patients and those who receive radiation therapy alone. Most patients with systemic metastases die of the systemic illness and not of the brain metastasis.

Metastases to the dura and meninges are relatively common. Meningeal carcinomatosis produces headache, cranial nerve palsies, and stiff neck. These symptoms are due to the presence of tumor cells within the spinal fluid and to small deposits on the meninges around cranial nerves, at the base of the brain, and on spinal roots. The diagnosis is made by cytologic examination of large-volume spinal fluid specimens. As many as three or more spinal taps may be needed to find cancer cells in some cases. The spinal fluid

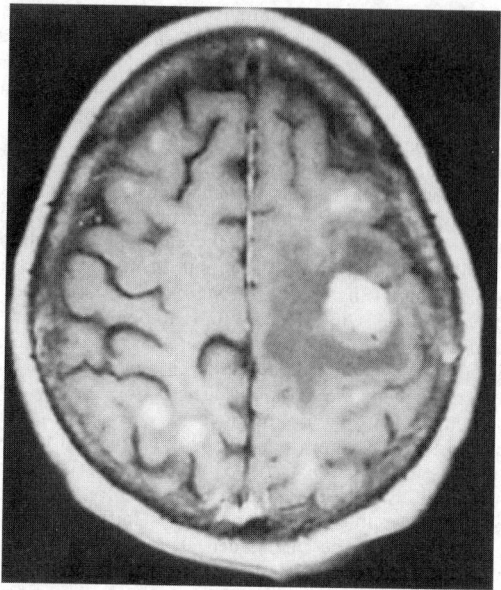

FIGURE 486–1 ▪ MRI scan, T1 gadolinium, of multiple metastases from breast carcinoma. The tumors were not visible on CT, even after giving a contrast agent.

protein level is generally elevated, and the glucose concentration may be low. The latter changes are sufficiently characteristic, in the absence of evidence of infection, to suggest the diagnosis. T1 gadolinium MRI scanning may image the small deposits in the meninges. They are especially evident in the cauda equina, even in the absence of clinical symptoms referable to lumbosacral nerve roots. The treatment of meningeal carcinomatosis includes irradiation of the brain and spinal cord, which usually provides benefit but rarely long remission. In patients with limited systemic metastases, intrathecal chemotherapy with methotrexate through an Ommaya reservoir is appropriate; patients occasionally show an impressive response. Most do not, however, and the effective treatment of meningeal carcinomatosis remains a difficult problem. In the future, the still-experimental treatment of meningeal carcinomatosis with isotope-emitting radionuclides coupled to monoclonal antibodies may replace intrathecal chemotherapy.

Table 486–1 lists some key features of metastatic brain tumors.

PRIMARY EXTRA-AXIAL TUMORS

Meningiomas, acoustic neuromas, and pituitary adenomas are the most frequent in this category, which, by definition, includes tumors that are not of the brain itself but of its coverings, the cranial nerves, and the adjacent structures. These primary "extra-axial" tumors differ from brain tumors in many ways. They are not of neuroectodermal origin, they are histologically unrelated, and most are truly benign because they can be cured by excision. They exert effects on the brain by pressure and only occasionally by actual invasion.

Meningiomas, which are growths of the fibroblast-like cells of the dura and arachnoid villi, account for about 15% of all primary brain tumors. They occur more often in women. The biologic explanation is unknown, but the finding has stimulated interest in the presence of progesterone receptors in the tumors. Meningiomas may occur many years after radiation delivered to the head, in which setting they may be multiple. A relationship to head trauma

Table 486–1 ▪ METASTATIC BRAIN TUMORS

These tumors affect 10% of cancer patients (and still another 20% have dural meningeal involvement).

At least 50% are multiple.

If solitary (the only metastatic lesion in the body), surgery clearly provides best results in most cases. Surgery may be the best approach even if other metastases are present in patients in good condition.

Radiation therapy is useful palliation but not curative. Long-term survivors may have consequential side effects such as dementia.

has never been convincingly documented. A few are familial. Such cases, as well as most apparently sporadic examples, are associated with a loss of a portion of chromosome 22, similar to that which characterizes neurofibromatosis type 2.

Most meningiomas arise as solitary tumors in characteristic sites, such as over the cerebral convexities, attached to the sagittal sinus, or at the base of the brain attached to the dura of the sphenoid sinus, the olfactory grooves, or the region of the sella. In some of these areas, they may be difficult to remove completely without excessive risk, and they may recur slowly but repeatedly. Many grow so slowly that serial CT or MRIs suggest no enlargement over many years. This slow growth sometimes permits the brain to accommodate them with modest symptoms even when they reach a large size (see Fig. 434–1). Many are detected incidentally. Small, asymptomatic meningiomas are often best watched by imaging studies at intervals; in the elderly, even large, asymptomatic ones may not require surgery.

Acoustic neuromas consist of distinctive growths of Schwann cells (schwannoma) of the eighth cranial nerve. Almost all are unilateral and not apparently familial. Bilateral acoustic neuromas are rare, familial, and diagnostic of neurofibromatosis type 2. This autosomal dominant condition occurs with nearly 100% penetrance in successive generations and derives from a gene deletion on chromosome 22.

Acoustic neuromas grow on the nerve into a round mass just as it emerges from the acoustic canal into the cerebellopontine angle. Some produce symptoms when they are small and confined within the canal. Others may go unsuspected until they grow to rather large size, filling the cerebellopontine angle and compressing the brain stem. Acoustic neuromas greatly surpass in frequency any other tumor of cranial nerves. Partial or complete nerve deafness is characteristic and is usually the first symptom. As acoustic neuromas grow, they sequentially affect the fifth and then the seventh cranial nerves on the same side. When large, they cause cerebellar ataxia on the same side and, ultimately, symptoms of brain stem dysfunction. MRI scans accurately detect even very small acoustic neuromas. All patients who develop hearing loss in the middle years of life should be considered to have an acoustic neuroma until proved otherwise. Audiometry alone is suggestive but not diagnostic; caloric tests of labyrinthine function almost always show abnormalities, but the most efficient physiologic study is the auditory evoked response. Current microsurgical techniques yield remarkably good results, usually preserving the seventh nerve and, occasionally, hearing as well.

Pituitary Adenomas

These tumors may cause endocrine symptoms, such as hypothyroidism, amenorrhea, galactorrhea, infertility, acromegaly, or Cushing's syndrome (see Chapter 237). With the exception of these hormonal impairments, early symptoms, if any, are usually limited to nonspecific headaches. As pituitary adenomas enlarge, they erode the sella turcica and extend above it to compress the optic nerves, eventually causing bitemporal visual field defects. Rarely, hemorrhages into large pituitary tumors can cause *pituitary apoplexy,* producing a characteristic syndrome of sudden-onset headache, partial ophthalmoplegia, and blindness in one or the other eye. Emergency surgical decompression must be applied to preserve vision.

Current endocrinologic and MRI techniques facilitate the diagnosis of pituitary tumors, especially if 1-mm cuts and magnified views through the sella are obtained. Medical treatment with bromocriptine may be effective but is slow in yielding results. The drug must be continued indefinitely. Only surgical removal can produce a cure. The safety and efficiency of transsphenoidal pituitary surgery warrant its consideration in all patients, including those with microadenomas that are confined to the sella and larger tumors that, in the past, could be approached only by a subfrontal craniotomy. Radiation therapy may be required in occasional patients who have large and incompletely removed adenomas.

Less common primary extra-axial tumors include *craniopharyngiomas,* related *suprasellar epidermoid cysts,* and *Rathke cleft cysts.* Although they reflect congenital abnormalities of the brain and most frequently become symptomatic in childhood, as many as one third of these tumors can first appear in adulthood, some as late as the sixth decade. In adults, craniopharyngiomas may compress the frontal lobes and occasionally cause dementia. Such tumors are almost always benign and surgically curable if they can be separated from adjacent parasellar structures, optic nerves, and hypothalamus. Pineal region tumors include *pineocytomas* and *pineoblastomas* derived from pineal parenchymal cells, as well as *teratomas* and *germinomas*. These two groups appear with about equal frequency, have the capacity to be biologically aggressive, and are difficult to manage surgically. Characteristic symptoms and signs include increased intracranial pressure, paresis of upward gaze, pupillary dysfunction, convergence nystagmus, and hydrocephalus due to obstruction of cerebrospinal fluid outflow pathways. Precocious puberty occurs in young males, the result of destruction of the pineal by germinomas. The true pineal tumors may cause delayed puberty. Intracranial *chordomas*, tumors of residual notochordal tissue, are rare and usually arise within the skull at the base of the brain, on the clivus. They are regionally invasive and rarely can be controlled even with aggressive surgery and radiation therapy. *Lipomas* occur chiefly in midline structures, especially over the corpus callosum. *Arachnoid cysts* can arise anywhere on the surface of the brain; some grow to remarkable size. Most arachnoid cysts are incidental, cause no symptoms, and are best left alone. Arachnoid cysts, as well as the other extra-axial tumors mentioned, are less frequent and important than meningiomas and acoustic neuromas (see Table 485–1).

PRIMARY INTRA-AXIAL TUMORS

This group includes astrocytomas, oligodendrogliomas, ependymomas, medulloblastomas, less common neuroectodermal tumors, and primary brain lymphoma. They share the quality of direct, invasive involvement of the substance of the brain, making them rarely curable by surgical excision. Accordingly, gliomas are fundamentally malignant, although some may behave in an indolent manner.

Astrocytomas are the most common gliomas. Their cause is unknown, with familial examples constituting only 1% of cases. Astrocytomas have occurred as a late consequence of radiation to the head or skull. The most aggressive variant, *glioblastoma multiforme,* accounts for more than 50% of all primary brain tumors. Glioblastoma (astrocytoma IV) is distinguished pathologically from the less aggressive *anaplastic astrocytoma* (astrocytoma III) on histopathologic grounds, and the two have important clinical differences. Glioblastoma is more common, is more characteristic of older age groups, and has a median survival time of less than 1 year, even with aggressive treatment with surgery, radiation therapy, and chemotherapy. By contrast, patients with anaplastic astrocytoma have a median survival time of slightly more than 2 years. Age is an important variable for both of these tumors: The younger the patient, the better the prognosis. Glioblastoma in children, for example, has a median survival of more than 2 years. In adults, men are affected more often than women. Anaplastic astrocytomas and glioblastoma occur in multicentric locations in about 5% of cases. In these instances, they may be mistaken for multiple cerebral metastases or for primary brain lymphoma on imaging studies.

Glioblastomas and anaplastic astrocytomas produce a similar clinical picture, and CT or MR images may be somewhat alike (Fig. 486–2). In most instances, the onset is relatively rapid and is heralded by seizures, headaches, and focal neurologic deficits. A minority of patients with these tumors have relevant histories of seizures with onset years before; one assumes that such malignant growths evolve from long-existing, low-grade astrocytomas. Sequential genetic alterations occur in astrocytomas as they become more aggressive. Loss of chromosome 10 is characteristic of glioblastoma cells and may occur subsequent to loss of chromosome 17, which is common in lower-grade astrocytomas. The latter is likely related to a mutation of a tumor suppressor gene, p53, on this chromosome.

Low-grade astrocytomas can pursue a highly variable course, and many of them do not progress to malignancy. Indeed, some are extremely indolent in their growth, so that the median survival time of patients with low-grade astrocytomas is 7 years from the time of diagnosis. This prognosis means little in individual cases, however, because the course of these tumors is, as noted before, highly variable. In some patients, low-grade astrocytomas transform to glioblastoma within a few years, whereas other astrocytomas can remain indolent for 10 years or more. Many low-grade astrocytomas spread too extensively before diagnosis can be made to allow surgical resection (see Fig. 485–2). By contrast, smaller, more favorably situated ones sometimes can be totally removed and the patient apparently cured. Paradoxically, astrocytomas associated with large cysts have a much better prognosis. This favorable circumstance occurs most often in the cerebellum in children and young adults but also in the cerebral hemispheres. Brain stem astrocytomas cannot be operated on except in rare instances in which they are exophytic. Most infiltrate the brain stem and enlarge it. In a similar way, optic nerve astrocytomas, an uncommon cause of vision loss that chiefly affects children, enlarge the optic nerves and may erode the optic foramina. They grow slowly, are sometimes associated with neurofibromatosis, and are often best left untreated until MRI scanning documents unequivocal tumor growth or vision deteriorates. What to do at that point is controversial. Many authorities withhold radiation treatment for low-grade astrocytomas, at least until all other approaches fail and for as long as the quality of life can be maintained. Two important reasons support this position. One is that little well-controlled evidence indicates that radiation greatly shrinks these tumors, eradicates them, slows their growth, or prevents their conversion into malignant astrocytomas. The other, as already remarked upon, is that radiation damages the normal brain, producing selective neuronal injury, areas of radiation necrosis, or both.

Oligodendrogliomas are the most "benign" of the gliomas, although some develop anaplastic features. Their clinical manifestations usually are indistinguishable from those of low-grade astrocytomas. Seizures are an important early symptom. Oligodendrogliomas occur chiefly in the cerebral hemispheres and especially in the frontal lobes. Many contain flecks of calcium, demonstrable by brain imaging. Complete surgical resection is the therapeutic goal, but this often cannot be realized because of the size and location of the tumors. Despite their slow growth, most oligodendrogliomas respond well to chemotherapy. As many as 80% improve with a regimen that combines procarbazine, lomustine, and vincristine. This response to chemotherapy seems to be superior to that observed with radiation therapy alone. Oligodendroglioma is the primary intra-axial tumor most likely to bleed spontaneously. In addition, anaplastic oligodendrogliomas tend to spread through the spinal fluid to the meninges. A few of these tumors eventually become so anaplastic that they histologically and clinically resemble glioblastomas.

Medulloblastomas occur chiefly in the region of the fourth ventricle and principally affect children and young adults. They cause characteristic symptoms of cerebellar and brain stem dysfunction.

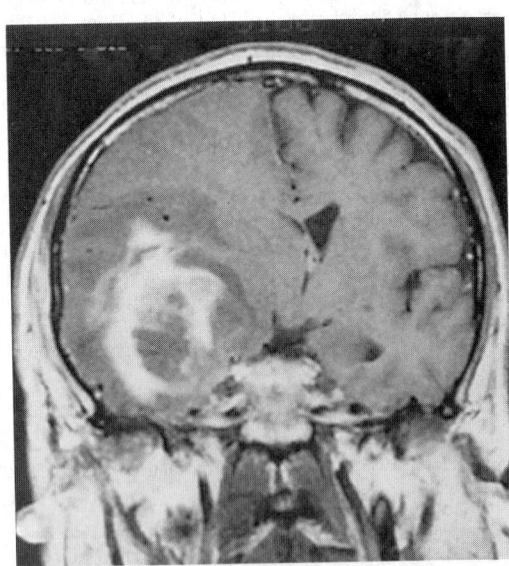

FIGURE 486–2 ■ MRI scan, T1 gadolinium enhanced, of a temporal lobe glioblastoma, showing typical ring configuration of contrast with central necrosis and marked mass effect.

In children, aggressive surgery and radiation therapy yield a 5-year survival of 50%, but many children treated in this manner suffer serious, permanent postradiation intellectual deficits. Several reports indicate that chemotherapy with cyclophosphamide and vincristine improves survival, and other drugs are being tried.

Medulloblastoma is characterized by an amplification of the c-myc oncogene and abnormalities of chromosome 17. Medulloblastomas arising in the cerebral hemispheres resemble, or may be the same as, primitive neuroectodermal tumors (PNET). These tumors are radiosensitive, like medulloblastomas of the fourth ventricle and cerebellum, and at times respond temporarily to aggressive chemotherapy.

Gangliogliomas are composed of neoplastic astrocytes and abundant dysmorphic neoplastic neurons. They occur chiefly in the temporal lobes of children and young adults, have an unusually slow growth rate, and may have a good prognosis even when untreated. Some are associated with tuberous sclerosis.

Primary brain lymphoma is increasing in frequency among both the acquired immunodeficiency syndrome (AIDS) and, for unknown reasons, the non-AIDS populations. These growths involve the brain diffusely, producing infiltrating and often multicentric tumors that tend to lie deep in the brain and adjacent to ventricular surfaces. Almost all of these tumors are B-cell derived; the eye is the only other extranodal site that is regularly involved concomitantly. Only rare patients go on to develop systemic lymphoma, and that occurs late in the disease. Primary brain lymphoma is fundamentally unresectable. Steroids are an important component of treatment; dexamethasone is uniquely chemotherapeutic for this tumor. Median survivals of 3 years can now be expected with the addition of multidrug chemotherapy to radiation therapy.

Rare intra-axial brain tumors include *choroid plexus papillomas and carcinomas,* which are even less common than the benign but troublesome *colloid cysts* of the third ventricle. The last-mentioned lesion may cause hydrocephalus by blocking the outflow of cerebrospinal fluid from the lateral ventricle. *Capillary hemangioblastomas* arise in the cerebellum and elsewhere. They are sometimes associated with an autosomal dominant inherited disorder that includes retinal angiomatosis as well as cysts and tumors of the pancreas, kidneys, and adrenals (von Hippel–Lindau disease). Some of these cerebellar capillary hemangioblastomas secrete erythropoietin and cause polycythemia.

Vascular malformations of the brain often can be mistaken for gliomas. They frequently manifest with nonhemorrhagic symptoms such as seizures. They sometimes resemble brain tumors in appearance on CT or MRI, and some, especially of the capillary variety (which lack large arteriovenous shunts), cannot be imaged by cerebral angiography. Many of these abnormalities lie in the brain stem and thalamus; because they are indistinguishable from brain tumors on even the best imaging studies, they may undergo biopsy as a diagnostic step, with devastating results. Vascular malformations of the brain involving large-caliber vessels are readily diagnosed by CT or MR images even without cerebral angiography.

Abscesses and *granulomas* of the brain cannot usually be distinguished from tumors by CT or MRI alone. If systemic evaluations fail to suggest a proper diagnosis, reliable management demands that biopsy be used. Even in the non-AIDS population, surprising alternatives to the clinical and radiologic diagnosis of a brain tumor are regularly revealed by biopsy.

Bigner DD, McLendon RE, Brunner JM: Russell and Rubinstein's Pathology of Tumors of the Nervous System, 6th ed. London, Arnold, 1998. *The masterful new revision of this great classic text.*

Kleihues P, Cavenee WK: Pathology and Genetics of Tumours of the Nervous System. Lyon, France, International Agency for Research on Cancer, 1997. *An ideal source of current knowledge in this field, with direct relevance to clinical thinking and patient care.*

Levin VA: Cancer in the Nervous System. New York, Churchill Livingstone, 1996. *Its breadth and scope make this an essential text about primary gliomas.*

Posner JB: Neurologic Complications of Cancer. Philadelphia, FA Davis, 1995. *A true masterpiece about metastasis to the nervous system.*

487 SPINAL TUMORS

Nicholas A. Vick

Tumors that cause nerve root or spinal cord compression can be paravertebral, extradural, intradural, or intramedullary. Most of those causing spinal cord compression are extradural and metastatic. Extradural neoplasms originate in the vertebral body surrounding the spinal cord, and they compress spinal roots or the spinal cord without invading them. Intradural neoplasms also cause symptoms by compressing spinal roots or cord without invasion, but unlike extradural neoplasms, the majority are benign and slow growing. Intramedullary neoplasms cause symptoms both by invading and compressing spinal structures; the tumors may be either benign or malignant.

PARAVERTEBRAL TUMORS. Neoplastic lesions that begin in or metastasize to the paravertebral space often cause serious and perplexing neurologic problems. They may extend longitudinally within the paravertebral space and progressively compress or invade nerve roots. They may grow through an intervertebral foramen and compress the spinal cord or radicular arteries that supply the spinal cord. If the tumor is more lateral than the immediate paravertebral space, the brachial, lumbar, or sacral plexus may be compressed, causing symptoms similar to root compression, but with a different pattern of sensory and motor loss. The symptoms of extravertebral tumor begin insidiously with severe, unremitting pain, often with a burning quality localized just lateral to the spine and radiating in a bandlike pattern in the distribution of the involved dermatomes. If the lesion involves abdominal or thoracic roots, motor and sensory changes are usually not appreciated by either the patient or the examiner. Autonomic changes may be a prominent or the only neurologic sign. Hyperhidrosis occurring in a band coinciding with the site of the pain strongly suggests the diagnosis. When the tumor involves cervical or lumbar roots, the pain may soon be followed by numbness in fingertips or toes, with accompanying weakness and reflex diminution, depending on the roots involved. Autonomic changes, including anhidrosis or hyperhidrosis, may affect the arm or leg. Horner's syndrome or diaphragmatic paralysis often accompanies cervical or upper thoracic paravertebral tumors. The diagnosis is best established by magnetic resonance (MR) scans of the level suggested by the clinical findings.

The differential diagnosis of paravertebral tumor includes disorders that cause paravertebral pain with or without compression of nerve roots. *Myofascial pain syndrome* causes low back or neck paravertebral pain with referred pain into arms or legs. On examination one often finds an area of exquisite muscle tenderness on a taut band of muscle. Relief of pain often can be accomplished by injecting the trigger point with saline solution or a local anesthetic. Temporary relief of pain after such injection does not imply that structural disease is absent; the trigger points may be a reaction to spinal or nerve root disease. In myofascial syndromes, autonomic, sensory, or motor changes are not usually present. Disease of kidneys and other viscera lying in the retroperitoneal space may cause aching pain similar to that caused by paravertebral tumors, but it is usually not radiating in quality or associated with autonomic, motor, or sensory changes. Percussion of the involved viscera reproduces the pain, which is described as a dull ache rather than a neurogenic burning pain. Chronic pain after a thoracotomy (*postthoracotomy pain*) probably results from entrapment of nerve roots at the time of surgery, perhaps with neuroma formation. Such pain can sometimes be relieved by paravertebral anesthetic blocks.

The management of paravertebral masses depends on the diagnosis. In patients known to have cancer, particularly lymphomas or carcinomas of the breast or lung, the tumor can be assumed to be metastatic and should be treated with radiation therapy; if it is of a responsive type, chemotherapy should be undertaken. If the patient has no history of cancer, a biopsy is required; depending on the site of the lesion, resection may be attempted both to establish a diagnosis and to decompress the nerve roots.

EXTRADURAL TUMORS. These compress spinal roots and spinal cord in one of three ways. Usually they arise in vertebrae surrounding the spinal cord and grow into the epidural space. Less often, they arise in the paravertebral space and grow through the intervertebral foramen to compress the cord laterally. Rarely, they arise in the epidural space itself without involving either vertebral or paravertebral structures. Most extradural tumors are metastatic (e.g., carcinoma of the breast, lung, prostate, or kidney). Some arise de novo in the vertebral bodies (e.g., chordoma, osteogenic sarcoma, myeloma, chondrosarcoma). A minority are benign (e.g., osteoma, osteoid osteoma, angioma). Because extradural tumors usually destroy bone before causing spinal cord compression, local pain is almost always the first symptom and may precede either radicular pain or other symptoms of spinal cord compression by weeks or months. As with other causes of spinal cord compression, extradural neoplasms first cause symptoms in a distal location and later in a proximal location. Even thoracic and cervical tumors generally cause weakness and numbness in the legs before trunk and upper extremity muscles are involved. The diagnosis of extradural spinal cord compression must be suspected by a history of pain followed by signs and symptoms of spinal cord dysfunction. It must be confirmed by radiographic study. About 85% of patients suffering from extradural spinal cord compression have bone lesions at the site of compression on plain radiographs. MRI establishes the site and degree of spinal cord compression and is superior to computed tomography (CT) for imaging of this lesion.

The differential diagnosis of extradural neoplasms includes inflammatory disease of bone and epidural abscess (e.g., vertebral tuberculosis, bacterial osteomyelitis), acute or subacute epidural hematomas, herniated intervertebral disks, spondylosis, and, very rarely, extramedullary hematopoiesis (in patients with severe and chronic anemia). MRI often distinguishes these from tumor, but sometimes a definitive diagnosis requires biopsy of the lesion either via decompressive laminectomy or by percutaneous needle biopsy.

Most neoplasms that cause extradural spinal cord compression are malignant and progress rapidly. Once spinal cord symptoms begin, paraplegia may develop in hours. Paraplegia is usually irreversible, whereas treatment often can correct mild to moderate spinal cord dysfunction. Early diagnosis and effective emergency treatment of extradural spinal cord compression are mandatory. Therapy should begin with corticosteroids (dexamethasone, 50 mg given intravenously) to decrease spinal cord edema, followed at once by 40 mg/day in divided doses, by mouth. Radiation therapy should be started the same day for patients known to have cancer, and as quickly as possible in those who first must have diagnostic studies to establish a tissue diagnosis. If effective chemotherapeutic agents are available, they should be used with dexamethasone and radiation therapy. In a few patients in whom radiation therapy and chemotherapy are ineffective, resection of the vertebral body involved by tumor may delay or prevent the development of paraplegia. Benign extradural tumors require surgery.

INTRADURAL EXTRAMEDULLARY TUMORS. Most intradural tumors are benign. Meningiomas and neurofibromas are by far the most common. Teratomas, arachnoid cysts, and lipomas are rare. *Meningiomas* occur in middle-aged and elderly women, predominantly in the thoracic region. Another common site is at the foramen magnum. Meningiomas are benign, slow growing, and usually located on the posterior aspect of the spinal cord. Pain is usually the first symptom, but in about 25% of cases, the first symptoms are those of spinal cord compression. Paresthesias and sensory changes beginning distally in the lower extremities are frequent and are often mistaken for peripheral neuropathy. As the disease progresses, however, corticospinal tract signs betray the spinal origin. Even when spinal cord signs and symptoms are obvious, the lack of pain may lead one to suspect a degenerative or demyelinating disease, such as multiple sclerosis, rather than a neoplasm. MRI with contrast enhancement is usually diagnostic. The treatment of spinal cord meningiomas is surgical removal.

Neurofibromas usually arise from the dorsal root and radicular pain is often the first symptom, preceding signs of spinal cord compression by months or years. When spinal cord compression develops, it progresses slowly. Some patients with spinal neurofibroma suffer from neurofibromatosis (usually type 1). The diagnosis may be suspected either by a positive family history or by the cutaneous signs of the disease. A neurofibroma may extend on either side of the intervertebral foramen, involving the root both in the paravertebral space and within the spinal canal. The diagnosis is established by MRI. Surgical removal usually leads to complete recovery.

Occasionally, *metastatic tumors* involving the leptomeninges present with intradural mass lesions. Pain is almost always prominent, and spinal cord compression develops more rapidly than with the more benign intradural tumors. In addition, malignant cells are frequently found in the spinal fluid. The spinal fluid glucose level may be decreased and the protein level elevated. The treatment of intradural malignant neoplasms is radiation therapy and chemotherapy. Complete surgical removal is almost never possible. Because the tumor usually seeds the entire subarachnoid space, radiation therapy, if it is to have more than a temporary effect, must either be delivered to the entire neuraxis or be supplemented by chemotherapy.

INTRAMEDULLARY TUMORS. The most common intramedullary spinal tumors are astrocytomas (usually low grade) and ependymomas. Other tumors that occasionally cause intramedullary spinal lesions are hemangioblastomas, lipomas, and hematogenous metastases. Pain is an early symptom of most intramedullary tumors, and signs of spinal cord dysfunction progress rapidly or slowly, depending on the growth characteristics of the tumor. Intramedullary tumors are often associated with a syrinx that may produce its own symptoms of spinal dysfunction. The so-called characteristic signs of intramedullary spinal cord lesions (dissociated sensory loss, sacral sparing, and early onset of bladder and bowel dysfunction) are not reliable enough clinically to distinguish intramedullary from extramedullary lesions; that diagnosis is established by MRI. In some patients with long-standing benign intramedullary lesions, plain radiographs of the spine may show widening of the spinal canal and erosion of the pedicles. The differential diagnosis of intramedullary tumors includes intramedullary abscesses and syringomyelia without tumor. A definitive diagnosis is established by biopsy. Successful surgical removal of intramedullary tumors is possible, particularly with ependymomas and hemangioblastomas. Highly skilled and experienced surgeons are needed to remove the tumors without causing an increase in neurologic symptoms. If the tumor cannot be totally excised, postoperative radiation therapy may delay its recurrence.

Byrne TN, Benzel E, Waxman SG: Diseases of the Spine and Spinal Cord. New York, Oxford, 2000. *Covers what is important to know; an excellent resource for the clinician.*

488 INTRACRANIAL HYPERTENSION AND HYPOTENSION

Nicholas A. Vick

Cerebrospinal fluid (CSF) pressure in excess of 250 mm CSF is usually a manifestation of serious neurologic disease. Intracranial hypertension is most often associated with rapidly expanding mass lesions, CSF outflow obstruction, or cerebral venous congestion. A variety of systemic and central nervous system disorders may be accompanied by an increase in intracranial pressure (ICP), however (Table 488–1). Lumbar CSF pressure may not accurately reflect ICP. In patients with intracranial mass lesions and brain herniation, lumbar CSF pressure may be normal or even low despite grossly elevated supratentorial CSF pressure. Kinking of the aqueduct of Sylvius by adjacent mass lesions, diencephalic–temporal lobe transtentorial herniation, and cerebellar compression of the fourth ventricle, with or without herniation of the cerebellar tonsils into the foramen magnum, can impede the free transmission of CSF into the lumbar subarachnoid space.

Table 488–1 ■ PATHOGENESIS OF INCREASED INTRACRANIAL PRESSURE

PERTURBATION	PROXIMATE CAUSE	CLINICAL EXAMPLE
Increased dural sinus venous pressure	Sinus compression or occlusion	Sagittal sinus thrombosis
		Otitic hydrocephalus
		Brain tumors
	Increased sinus blood flow	CO_2 retention
		Arteriovenous malformation
	Increased peripheral venous pressure	Internal jugular vein occlusion
		Superior vena cava syndrome
		Congestive heart failure
Increased CSF outflow resistance	Ventricular outflow obstruction	Brain tumors
	Obliteration of the cisternal and/or convexity subarachnoid space	Aqueductal stenosis
		Meningitis
		Extradural or subdural masses
	Plugging of the arachnoid villi	Cerebral masses or edema
		Subarachnoid hemorrhage
		Infectious polyneuritis
		Spinal cord tumors
Increased rate of CSF formation	Increased choroidal CSF formation	Choroid plexus papilloma
	Increased extrachoroidal CSF formation	Hypo-osmolality
		Cerebral edema
Unknown	Increased cerebral volume	
	Increased sagittal sinus pressure	Benign intracranial hypertension
	Increased CSF outflow resistance	

CSF = cerebrospinal fluid.

Table 488–2 lists the principal symptoms and signs associated with intracranial hypertension. Headache is produced by traction on pain-sensitive cerebral blood vessels or dura mater at the base or, less often, the vertex of the brain. Signs reflect the presence of impending herniation with intermittent vascular compression, midline shift, or axial distortion of the brain stem. In the absence of such shifts, increased ICP alone may be asymptomatic. *Papilledema* is the most reliable sign of ICP, although it fails to develop in many patients with increased ICP. This is particularly true in the elderly. Retinal venous pulsations, when present, imply that CSF pressure is normal or not significantly elevated, but their absence is not helpful diagnostically. Patients with increased ICP often complain of worsening symptoms, particularly headache, in the morning, perhaps because plateau waves (spontaneous elevations of ICP) occur more commonly during sleep.

The initial treatment of any patient with increased ICP whose neurologic status is deteriorating is aimed at reducing the volume of the intracranial contents in an attempt to prevent brain damage (Table 488–3). If ICP approaches the systolic blood pressure, the cerebral perfusion pressure decreases and irreversible ischemia may develop. The definitive treatment of intracranial hypertension is ultimately determined by the nature of the underlying pathologic process.

Table 488–2 ■ SYMPTOMS AND SIGNS OF INTRACRANIAL HYPERTENSION

Common
Headache
Tinnitus
Vomiting (with or without nausea)
Visual obscurations, visual loss, photopsias
Papilledema
Diplopia
Lethargy and increased sleep
Psychomotor retardation
Pain on eye movement
Less Common
Hearing distortion or loss
Vertigo
Facial weakness
Shoulder or arm pain
Neck pain or rigidity
Ataxia
Paresthesias of extremities
Anosmia
Trigeminal neuralgia

IDIOPATHIC INTRACRANIAL HYPERTENSION

Idiopathic intracranial hypertension is a syndrome of increased ICP unaccompanied by localizing neurologic signs, intracranial mass lesion, or CSF outflow obstruction in an alert, otherwise healthy-looking patient. Such patients are almost always obese and most often are women. Idiopathic intracranial hypertension (also called pseudotumor cerebri or benign intracranial hypertension) can be associated with a variety of systemic and iatrogenic disorders (Table 488–4). The cause is usually unknown. Chronically increased ICP may give rise to the "empty sella syndrome," which refers to a radiographically globular enlargement of the sella turcica, an incompetent diaphragma sellae, and a compressed but functioning pituitary gland.

The diagnosis of idiopathic intracranial hypertension is one of exclusion. Intracranial masses (tumors, hematomas, infections) and CSF outflow obstruction must be excluded by computed tomography (CT) or magnetic resonance imaging (MRI). Magnetic resonance angiography is necessary to rule out dural venous sinus thrombosis. Lumbar puncture, which is usually deferred until CT or MRI has revealed a normal or small ventricular system, is required to confirm the diagnosis. Lumbar CSF pressure is elevated, frequently above 300 mm CSF, but the composition of the fluid is normal; the protein content is usually in the low-normal range, below 20 mg/dL.

PATHOPHYSIOLOGY. In most cases of idiopathic intracranial hypertension, the cause is unknown. Chronically elevated ICP implies an increase in dural sinus venous pressure, an increase in CSF outflow resistance, an increase in the rate of CSF formation (if it ever really occurs), or some combination of these factors. One or more of these mechanisms must elevate the CSF pressure. Pathoge-

Table 488–3 ■ EMERGENCY TREATMENT OF IMPENDING HERNIATION IN ACUTELY DECOMPENSATING PATIENTS

THERAPY	DOSAGE OR PROCEDURE	ONSET (DURATION OF ACTION)
Hyperventilation	Lower $PaCO_2$ to 25 to 30 mm Hg	Seconds (minutes)
Osmotherapy	Mannitol, 0.5 to 2.0 g/kg IV over 15 min followed by 25 g as needed	Minutes (hours)
Corticosteroids	Dexamethasone, 50 mg IV push, followed by 50 mg daily in divided doses	Hours (days)

Table 488–4 ■ SYSTEMIC AND IATROGENIC DISORDERS ASSOCIATED WITH BENIGN INTRACRANIAL HYPERTENSION

Commonly Prescribed Drugs
   Nalidixic acid
   Nitrofurantoin
   Phenytoin
   Sulfonamides
   Tetracycline
   Vitamin A
Endocrine and Metabolic Disorders
   Addison's disease
   Cushing's syndrome
   Hypoparathyroidism
   Menarche, pregnancy, oral contraceptives
   Obesity and irregular menses
   Steroid therapy or withdrawal
Hematologic Disorders
   Cryoglobulinemia
   Iron deficiency anemia
Miscellaneous Disorders
   Dural venous sinus obstruction or thrombosis
   Head trauma
   Internal jugular vein ligation
   Systemic lupus erythematosus
   Middle ear disease

netic hypotheses that postulate an increase in brain bulk consequent to an increase in cerebral blood volume or in brain water content (interstitial brain edema) do not provide an adequate explanation. The constancy of obesity, often extreme, has suggested the possibility of a disorder of the hypothalamus. But no data have emerged to support this idea. Despite decades of knowledge of the association with obesity, the link remains completely obscure. The strikingly greater incidence in women than in men (4:1) is also unexplained but surely important in some way.

CLINICAL MANIFESTATIONS. Most patients complain of headache. Other common early symptoms include nausea and vomiting, visual disturbances, retro-ocular pain, diplopia, tinnitus, and vertigo. Bilateral papilledema, the cardinal feature, is almost always present and may be associated with peripapillary retinal hemorrhages, exudates, or both. Vision loss, the only serious complication of idiopathic intracranial hypertension, may occur either early or late in the course of the disease but is seen less than feared. Transient obscurations of vision do not predict subsequent failure of vision. Characteristically, visual field testing reveals enlarged blind spots. Quantitative visual field testing should be performed at monthly intervals early in the disease. Diplopia, caused by unilateral or bilateral abducens palsy, may develop as a false localizing sign. The remainder of the neurologic examination is almost always normal. It is important to distinguish pseudopapilledema—an anomalous elevation of the optic disc—from true papilledema, which is prima facie evidence of increased ICP. Anomalous elevation of the disk may be associated with identifiable hyaline bodies (drusen).

In some instances, idiopathic intracranial hypertension is a self-limited disease in which CSF pressure returns to normal as clinical symptoms remit over several months. However, clinical improvement is not always accompanied by a reduction in CSF pressure, and there is a vexing subgroup of patients whose pressure remains persistently elevated after neurologic signs and symptoms have resolved. The course of such cases implies that clinical symptoms may be independent of the absolute magnitude of CSF pressure and that chronically raised ICP may be totally asymptomatic. In addition, despite persistently elevated CSF pressure, patients do not become hydrocephalic. The ventricular system remains small or no larger than normal. This finding suggests that whatever mechanism "resets" CSF pressure above normal does not predispose to the development of communicating hydrocephalus and that the two conditions are biologically unrelated.

TREATMENT. Unfortunately, no convincing evidence exists that any of the frequently recommended treatments are regularly efficacious. The high rate of spontaneous remission complicates the eval-

uation of various therapies. At present, four general approaches to symptomatic treatment are used: (1) repeated lumbar puncture, (2) pharmacologic treatment, (3) ventriculosystemic or lumboperitoneal shunting, and (4) incision of the optic nerve sheath.

Frequent (i.e., alternate-day) large-volume lumbar punctures may provide relief of symptoms and document the occurrence of remission. Either it is beneficial or remission occurs independently during the period of treatment. Corticosteroids and diuretics have been the mainstay of medical treatment, and both are effective, or, again, the disease remits during the period of treatment. Dexamethasone, furosemide, and acetazolamide are often tried. CSF shunting procedures are not without risk, and their long-term efficacy remains to be established. Incision of the optic nerve sheath for the relief of papilledema is the treatment of choice for patients whose visual fields are deteriorating. Surprisingly, in some patients, headache and papilledema on the contralateral side are relieved as well as the ipsilateral papilledema.

HYDROCEPHALUS

Hydrocephalus refers to the net accumulation of CSF within the cerebral ventricles and their consequent enlargement. Although acute obstructive hydrocephalus usually produces a sudden increase in intraventricular pressure, CSF pressure is frequently normal (or low) in patients with chronic hydrocephalus. It is customary to distinguish between "noncommunicating" and "communicating" hydrocephalus; the former is produced by lesions that obstruct the intracerebral CSF circulation at or proximal to the foramina of Luschka and Magendie, the latter by obstruction of the basal cisterns or convexity subarachnoid space in such a way that the ventricular system communicates with the spinal subarachnoid space but CSF cannot drain through the arachnoid villi into the superior sagittal sinus. Because both "noncommunicating" and "communicating" types of hydrocephalus are obstructive and both are treated by shunts, the distinction really has less meaning than that usually ascribed to it. Perhaps the important distinction should be between obstructive and nonobstructive hydrocephalus. Ventricular dilatation associated with severe cerebral atrophy, sometimes called hydrocephalus ex vacuo, is the best example of nonobstructive hydrocephalus.

DIAGNOSIS. Hydrocephalus is easily diagnosed by MRI. The diagnosis must take into account the increase in ventricular volume that accompanies normal aging and the presence or absence of cerebral atrophy. Enlargement of the temporal horns and an inability to visualize the sylvian and interhemispheric fissures or cerebral sulci, plus the presence of periventricular lucencies (CT) or periventricular hyperintensity (MRI), favor the diagnosis of hydrocephalus. A normal or small fourth ventricle in the presence of enlarged lateral and third ventricles suggests aqueductal stenosis.

ACUTE VERSUS CHRONIC HYDROCEPHALUS. Sudden, complete ventricular outflow obstruction leads to acute hydrocephalus, coma, and, if untreated, death; partial obstruction is more common and only moderately less dangerous (Table 488–5). Chronic hydrocephalus in an adult is most often caused by aqueductal stenosis or the complications of subarachnoid hemorrhage. Other reported causes

Table 488–5 ■ CAUSES OF HYDROCEPHALUS

Acute
   Cerebellar hemorrhage/infarction
   Colloid cyst of the third ventricle
   Exudative meningitis
   Head trauma
   Intracranial tumor or hematoma
   Spontaneous subarachnoid hemorrhage
   Viral encephalitis
Chronic
   Aqueductal stenosis
   Ectasia and elongation of the basilar artery (rare)
   Granulomatous meningitis
   Head trauma
   Hindbrain malformations
   Meningeal carcinomatosis
   Brain and spinal cord tumors
   Spontaneous subarachnoid hemorrhage
   Syringomyelia

and associations are listed in Table 488–5. In many instances, the cause of symptomatic chronic hydrocephalus ("normal-pressure hydrocephalus") cannot be determined. Unequivocally asymptomatic hydrocephalus is found in approximately 4% of patients over the age of 60 who consult neurologists.

CLINICAL MANIFESTATIONS. A patient with acute obstructive hydrocephalus may have severe headache, lethargy, signs of increased ICP, papilledema, abducens palsy, and signs of the causative lesion. Hyperactive reflexes and bilateral extensor plantar responses are almost invariably present. Ventricular CSF pressure is markedly increased, but if CSF pathways are blocked, this increase may not be transmitted to the lumbar subarachnoid space. Patients with chronic communicating hydrocephalus, including normal-pressure hydrocephalus, have a progressive dementia characterized by forgetfulness and psychomotor retardation, an unsteady gait, and urinary incontinence. Bilateral pyramidal and extrapyramidal signs may be present. Some patients have a parkinsonian appearance. The lumbar CSF pressure is usually normal or nearly normal, although overnight recording of ventricular CSF pressure may reveal intermittent waves of elevated pressure.

TREATMENT. Acute hydrocephalus responds dramatically to ventricular drainage and CSF diversion. Treatment of the primary lesion is the treatment of choice, although temporary ventricular decompression or ventriculosystemic shunt may be necessary in some cases. Ventricular shunting has also been used for patients with chronic communicating hydrocephalus. Unfortunately, not all patients respond, or response may be delayed for weeks or months; moreover, there are no reliable clinical or neuroradiologic predictors of shunt response. Recent onset and mild dementia remain better predictors than does isotope cisternography. Absence of cerebral atrophy and temporary improvement after lumbar puncture seem to correlate with benefit from a shunt operation.

INTRACRANIAL HYPOTENSION

CSF pressure measured at a lumbar puncture site, with the patient in the lateral decubitus position, normally ranges from 70 to 200 mm CSF (5 to 15 mm Hg). Low or zero lumbar CSF pressure can be recorded under several circumstances, as indicated in Table 488–6. Symptoms of the first two or three circumstances in Table 488–6 are likely to be dominated by the underlying illnesses. The remainder of the circumstances tend to cause a consistent syndrome characterized by severe, throbbing frontal and occipital headache, which usually appears within 30 seconds after the patient assumes an erect posture and subsides completely when he or she lies flat. Associated complaints may include dizziness, nausea, stiff neck, photophobia, and, rarely, diplopia due to an associated abducens

Table 488-6 ■ CAUSES OF ABNORMALLY LOW (0–50 mm) CEREBROSPINAL FLUID (CSF) PRESSURE

Dehydration-hypovolemia
Cranial-intraspinal CSF block
Post-CNS surgery
CSF fistula
Post–lumbar puncture drainage
Spontaneous-idiopathic; dural nerve sheath tear

nerve palsy. The disorder often arises 1 to 21 days after lumbar puncture. The pathogenesis is as for lumbar puncture headache (see Chapter 442).

Rare cases of CSF hypotension may occur spontaneously, producing symptoms similar to those already described in previously healthy persons. The onset can be acute or subacute and is occasionally associated by history with mild trauma, such as a fall on the buttocks or a slight bump to the head. The cause usually remains unknown, although isotope cisternography sometimes reveals spontaneous rupture of a dural nerve sheath. Diagnosis can be difficult because measuring a low CSF pressure in the lumbar subarachnoid space can give the false impression of missing the thecal sac. Treatment is symptom oriented; spontaneous recovery usually requires days to a few weeks. When post–lumbar puncture symptoms are persistent or disabling, an epidural "blood patch" is indicated. The actual need for blood patches is far less than the frequency with which the procedure is done by worried physicians for impatient sufferers of post–lumbar puncture headache. The procedure involves the injection of 10 mL of the patient's own blood into the epidural space to seal a presumed dural leak. Rarely, in long-lasting cases, surgical exploration has exposed the dural leak, which must be sutured. In patients suffering from either lumbar puncture–induced or spontaneous intracranial hypotension, MRI of the brain may reveal intense enhancement of the meninges. Occasionally, subdural effusions develop. The process is benign and clears when the intracranial hypotension resolves.

Lyons HK, Meyer FB: Cerebrospinal fluid physiology and the management of increased intracranial pressure. Mayo Clin Proc 65:684, 1990. *A superb review with excellent references.*

Pannullo S, Reich JB, Krol G, et al: MRI changes in intracranial hypotension. Neurology 43:919, 1993. *A description of patients with intracranial hypotension and meningeal enhancement on MRI.*

Radhadkrishnan K, Ahlskog JE, Garrity JA, et al: Idiopathic intracranial hypertension. Mayo Clin Proc 69:169, 1994. *An outstanding discussion of the problem.*

Ropper AH, Kennedy SK: Neurological and Neurosurgical Intensive Care, 3rd ed. Rockville, MD, Aspen Publishers, 1993. *An excellent resource with well-chosen references on all aspects of the treatment of intracranial hypertension.*

■ NUTRITIONAL DISORDERS OF THE NERVOUS SYSTEM

489 NUTRITIONAL DISORDERS OF THE NERVOUS SYSTEM

John C. M. Brust

Neurologic disease is associated with deficiency of certain nutrients. In developing countries, such deficiency is usually the result of starvation or restricted diet. In developed countries, the major causes are alcoholism and, less often, malabsorption syndromes, chronic illness with cachexia, food faddism, psychiatric disease, infantile malnutrition, and, rarely, genetic disorders. The most clearly defined nutritional disorders of the nervous system are associated with deficiency of particular vitamins—organic compounds required for normal metabolic functions but not synthesized in the body. Vitamins are either water-soluble or fat-soluble, and deficiency of fat-soluble vitamins is a feature of malabsorption disorders (e.g., unavailability of bile acids, pancreatic insufficiency, sprue). With the exception of cobalamin, deficiency of water-soluble vitamins is usually secondary to inadequate intake. Such malnutrition seldom produces selective avitaminosis, and the resulting neurologic symptoms and signs therefore reflect multiple deficiencies.

Excessive intake of certain fat-soluble vitamins can be toxic. Symptomatic hypervitaminosis is less often encountered with water-soluble vitamins, which are much more rapidly excreted.

WATER-SOLUBLE VITAMINS

Thiamine (Vitamin B₁)

Thiamine in the body is converted to thiamine pyrophosphate, which is a co-enzyme at a number of steps in glucose metabolism. Although the adult daily requirement seldom exceeds 2 mg, limited body storage means that inadequate intake can produce symptomatic deficiency in only a few weeks or months. In developing countries thiamine deficiency most often produces beri-beri, with cardiac high-output failure and sensorimotor polyneuropathy. In North America and Europe, thiamine deficiency most often affects alcoholics and causes the Wernicke-Korsakoff syndrome; it probably contributes to other neurologic disorders as well.

Wernicke's syndrome evolves over days to weeks and has three features that may occur alone or together: (1) abnormal eye movements, which begin with nystagmus and lateral rectus or horizontal gaze paresis and progress to complete ophthalmoplegia, usually with pupillary sparing; (2) ataxia of gait and stance, often accompanied by lower-limb intention tremor and dysmetria (the arms are usually not affected, and dysarthria is usually absent); and (3) altered mentation, the earliest signs of which are inattentiveness, mental slowing (abulia), and impaired memory. If patients are not treated they become lethargic, and their condition progresses to coma and death. In patients who die of Wernicke's syndrome, pathologically characteristic lesions—loss of neuronal processes, gliosis, and sometimes endothelial proliferation and petechiae—involve the medial thalamus and hypothalamus, midbrain periaqueductal gray matter, and floor of the fourth ventricle. In the cerebellum neuronal loss affects especially Purkinje cells and is maximal in the vermis.

The diagnosis of thiamine deficiency is supported by decreased levels of erythrocyte transketolase, but if Wernicke's syndrome is a serious consideration, treatment must not be delayed. To minimize permanent neurologic residua, thiamine (50 to 100 mg) plus other water-soluble vitamins are given parenterally. The therapeutic response is often dramatic. Eye movements sometimes begin to improve within a few hours, and except for residual nystagmus may be normal within 1 or 2 weeks. Ataxia tends to improve less completely; more than half of patients are left with a broad-based, unsteady gait. More serious are lasting mental symptoms. Drowsiness, inattentiveness, and apathy tend to clear with treatment, but an amnestic disorder often persists, termed Korsakoff's syndrome, in which both anterograde and retrograde memory loss occur—sometimes accompanied by confabulation—which is out of proportion to additional mental abnormalities. Once established, the memory disorder is permanent in the majority of patients.

In alcoholics and others with low thiamine stores, administration of glucose can precipitate Wernicke's syndrome. Patients receiving parenteral glucose (e.g., for parenteral alimentation or in an acute setting for diagnosis and treatment of unexplained seizures or coma) should also be given parenteral thiamine (and other water-soluble vitamins).

Eighty per cent of patients with Wernicke-Korsakoff disease have peripheral neuropathy, and many alcoholics have peripheral neuropathy without other neurologic symptoms or signs. The earliest symptoms are sensory in nature, with paresthesias or pain in the feet and later the hands. Absent ankle tendon reflexes and impaired distal vibratory and pain sensation usually precede proprioceptive loss or weakness, but progression to a severe sensorimotor disorder can occur, with proximal as well as distal weakness in addition to vagal symptoms (e.g., hoarseness, dysphagia) and autonomic signs (e.g., tachycardia, postural hypotension). The neuropathy is axonal in origin, with secondary demyelination, and although its cause is very likely nutritional, the relative contributions of thiamine and other vitamins are uncertain.

Similarly, many alcoholics manifest cerebellar vermal degeneration without other clinical or histologic evidence of Wernicke-Korsakoff syndrome, raising the possibility that cerebellar degeneration, although more likely nutritional than toxic in origin, may be less related than Wernicke-Korsakoff syndrome to thiamine deficiency per se.

Optic neuropathy in alcoholics—formerly called "tobacco-alcohol amblyopia"—is also nutritional in origin, but the particular deficiencies are uncertain. Bilateral visual loss, usually with central or centrocecal scotomas, may evolve subacutely with swollen optic disks. Improvement follows treatment with multivitamins, but residual visual impairment and temporal disk pallor are often present. The term "Strachan's syndrome" refers to the combination of optic neuropathy and polyneuropathy in patients subjected to starvation.

In experimental animals, ethanol is directly toxic to neurons, but whether such observations are relevant to humans (i.e., whether there is such a thing as "alcoholic dementia") is controversial. It is notable that non-alcoholics with thiamine deficiency and beri-beri do not develop Wernicke-Korsakoff disease, raising the possibility that excessive ethanol plus nutritional deficiency can produce a pathologic condition that neither insult would cause alone.

Alcoholic myopathy can be either chronic, with progressive proximal weakness, or acute, with rhabdomyolysis, severe muscle weakness and pain, and myoglobinuria causing renal failure. Serum creatine kinase levels are elevated, and electromyography reflects myopathy. Such patients are often malnourished, but direct toxicity is probably more important than nutritional deficiency. Other factors, most importantly hypokalemia, are often present and contribute to the muscle necrosis and myoglobinuria. Symptoms sometimes begin or accelerate during a binge, and improvement follows abstinence. Alcoholic cardiomyopathy, a low-output state distinguishable from beri-beri heart disease, is often coexistent.

Marchiafava-Bignami disease, which occurs almost exclusively in alcoholics, is defined by characteristic demyelinating lesions of the corpus callosum. Early symptoms are usually mental in nature, with depression, paranoia, psychosis, or dementia. Major motor seizures are common, and hemiparesis, aphasia, abnormal movements, and ataxia may progress to coma and death over a few months. Computed tomography (CT) and magnetic resonance imaging (MRI) can detect the lesions, and in a few cases clinical improvement has been accompanied by regression of the CT or MRI abnormalities. The cause of Marchiafava-Bignami disease, including the role—if any—of nutritional deficiency, is unknown.

Niacin

Niacin, also called nicotinic acid, is converted in the body to nicotinamide adenine dinucleotide (NAD) or nicotinamide adenine dinucleotide phosphate, which are coenzymes in tissue respiration. Deficiency of niacin or its precursor tryptophan causes pellagra, a characteristic triad of dermatologic, gastrointestinal, and neurologic symptoms. An erythematous and later hyperpigmented rash appears on light-exposed areas. Glossitis and enteritis can be severe, with nausea, vomiting, and watery or bloody diarrhea. Neurologic abnormalities include altered mentation (irritability, insomnia, and fatigue progressing to depression, impaired memory, dementia, psychosis, delirium, or coma), sensorimotor polyneuropathy, myelopathy, seizures, cerebellar ataxia, parkinsonism, retinitis, and optic atrophy. A pathologic characteristic is widespread CNS neuronal chromatolysis. In developed countries, pellagra is most often encountered in alcoholics, in whom additional nutritional deficiencies are likely to be present. Treatment is with niacin or nicotinamide plus other vitamins. Response is usually rapid, but mental abnormalities can be permanent.

Niacin is used to treat hyperlipidemia, and large doses are associated with flushing, vomiting, diarrhea, hepatic dysfunction, lactic acidosis, delirium, and retinal maculopathy. In 1989, an epidemic of eosinophilia, myalgia, myopathy, peripheral neuropathy, and impaired memory affected several thousand people taking L-tryptophan obtained in health food stores. Most cases were traced to a single Japanese product, implicating a contaminant rather than the L-tryptophan itself.

Pyridoxine (Vitamin B₆)

Vitamin B₆ consists of pyridoxine, pyridoxol, and pyridoxamine, each of which is converted in the body to pyridoxal phosphate, a co-factor for several enzymes. Pyridoxine deficiency causes seizures and sensorimotor polyneuropathy and probably contributes to the neurologic manifestations of pellagra. More common than dietary deficiency of pyridoxine are conditions of pyridoxine dependency. Neonates and infants may develop seizures that respond to pyridoxine in doses several times the daily requirement. Isoniazid inhibits an enzyme that converts pyridoxine to its active form, and hydralazine converts pyridoxine to an inactive hydrazone; patients receiving either of these drugs can develop peripheral neuropathy or even CNS symptoms unless supplemental pyridoxine is given.

Severe sensory polyneuropathy affects persons taking pyridoxine in megadoses (2 to 6 g/day for 2 to 40 months; doses in excess of 100 mg/day are never indicated and are unwise, as the lower limit of toxicity has not been defined). Improvement follows pyridoxine withdrawal but typically requires months to years.

Cobalamin (Vitamin B₁₂)

Deficiency of cobalamin damages the entire neuraxis, with combinations of polyneuropathy, myelopathy ("combined systems disease," "subacute combined degeneration"), encephalopathy, and, less often, optic neuropathy. More than a third of patients with documented cobalamin deficiency have neurologic symptoms and signs, which are often the first symptoms and signs to appear. Some patients have earlier fatigue, glossitis, anorexia, vomiting, weight loss, generalized weakness, or syncope secondary to severe anemia. In the great majority, the earliest neurologic symptoms are sensory, with paresthesias and numbness in the hands and feet and gait ataxia secondary to proprioceptive loss. Sensory loss is secondary to peripheral neuropathy, myelopathy, or both. With progression, leg weakness and impaired manual dexterity are noted. Hyperactive tendon reflexes and extensor plantar responses reflect corticospinal tract involvement; decreased tendon reflexes also occur, reflecting peripheral neuropathy. Mental symptoms, which rarely occur without other neurologic abnormalities, include memory loss, personality change, dementia, and paranoid psychosis with hallucinations ("megaloblastic madness"). Less frequent symptoms include impotence, urinary incontinence, decreased visual acuity, and anosmia.

Pathologic features include swelling and vacuolization of myelin sheaths in the central nervous system, initially affecting the dorsal columns of the spinal cord and then the corticospinal tracts; eventually, over months or years, these become widespread and diffuse. The pathologic basis of the peripheral neuropathy is less clear.

Because pernicious anemia most often affects elderly patients, in whom a high frequency of Alzheimer's disease and gait unsteadiness can be anticipated, it is an easy diagnosis to overlook. Moreover, more than one-fourth of patients with cobalamin deficiency and neurologic symptoms have normal hematocrit readings, mean erythrocyte volumes, or both, and neurologic abnormalities tend to be more severe in these patients than in those with anemia or macrocytosis. Hypersegmented polymorphonuclear leukocytes are often present, but their identification may require the expertise of a hematologist. Furthermore, some patients with clinically significant cobalamin deficiency have low normal serum cobalamin levels. The diagnosis in such instances can be confirmed by the presence of increased serum levels of methylmalonic acid and homocysteine. Conversely, in subjects with falsely low serum cobalamin levels— a not uncommon occurrence—clinically significant cobalamin deficiency can be excluded by finding normal serum levels of these metabolites, elevations of which, in the absence of renal disease and folate deficiency, are highly specific for cobalamin deficiency.

Treatment of cobalamin deficiency is with vitamin B₁₂, which, in patients with pernicious anemia or malabsorption, is given intramuscularly. With treatment, improvement may take 3 months to begin and may then continue over months or even years. Most patients either make a complete neurologic recovery or improve. Normal hematocrit levels rise, and normal mean erythrocyte volumes fall within the normal range. Serum methylmalonic acid and homocysteine levels fall.

Nitrous oxide oxidizes cobalamin, rendering inactive the cobalamin-dependent enzyme methionine synthase. Chronic recreational use of nitrous oxide can produce the symptoms and signs of subacute combined degeneration in the presence of normal serum cobalamin levels (or precipitate such symptoms in subjects with low levels).

The diagnosis and management of cobalamin deficiency is further discussed in Chapter 163.

Folic Acid

By donating a methyl group to cobalamin, folic acid becomes available to participate in DNA synthesis; folate supplementation in patients with cobalamin deficiency probably accounts for some, but

not all, cases of neurologic impairment in the absence of anemia. Folate deficiency results in megaloblastic anemia, but little evidence is available to suggest that it causes either central or peripheral nervous system disease. Also questionable are claims that folate ingestion interferes with the antiepileptic action of phenytoin or barbiturates.

Folate supplementation during pregnancy prevents the occurrence of neural tube defects, such as spina bifida and anencephaly, and the U.S. Public Health Service recommends a daily dose of 0.4 mg of folic acid for "women . . . capable of becoming pregnant." Doses above 1.0 mg/day might complicate the diagnosis of cobalamin deficiency.

As noted, either cobalamin or folate deficiency results in elevated blood levels of homocysteine, and such levels constitute a risk factor for occlusive vascular disease. Studies are currently under way to test whether folate and cobalamin supplementation reduces the risk of stroke or myocardial infarction in subjects who are not folate- or cobalamin-deficient but who have high blood homocysteine levels.

Other Water-Soluble Vitamins

Because other deficiencies are nearly always present, the role of riboflavin, pantothenic acid, or biotin deficiency in neurologic or other disease is difficult to determine. Anecdotal reports and animal experiments suggest a possible relationship to sensory polyneuropathy and myalgia. Ascorbic acid deficiency causes bleeding, which can affect either the peripheral or the central nervous system.

FAT-SOLUBLE VITAMINS

Vitamin A (Retinol)

Retinol is necessary for the integrity of epithelial tissue and the retina. Deficiency, associated with malnutrition, malabsorption, liver disease, myxedema, diabetes mellitus, or renal failure, causes visual loss secondary to both retinal and corneal damage.

Hypervitaminosis A, most often affecting adolescents taking excessive dosage for acne, causes increased intracranial pressure which, if prolonged, can result in visual loss.

Vitamin D (Calciferol, Cholecalciferol)

Synthesized in the skin, vitamin D is further metabolized in the liver and kidney to its active form, 1,25-dihydroxycholecalciferol. Deficiency is associated with malnutrition, lack of sunlight, malabsorption, liver disease, renal failure, and phenytoin or barbiturate administration; several hereditary disorders are also characterized by vitamin D resistance. Hypovitaminosis D causes rickets in children and osteomalacia in adults. Severe bone disease can produce spinal cord or nerve root symptoms, and hypocalcemia causes tetany and altered mentation. Myopathic weakness is described.

Hypervitaminosis D, from excessive vitamin D intake, malignant or granulomatous disease, hyperparathyroidism, or other endocrinopathy, causes life-threatening hypercalcemia with bone, kidney, and neurologic disease; symptoms include weakness, lassitude, impaired memory, dementia, depression, paranoia, hallucinations, delirium, and coma. Treatment includes saline administration, furosemide diuresis, and sometimes corticosteroids.

Vitamin E (Tocopherols, Tocotrienols)

Vitamin E reduces peroxide production, and deficiency occurs in malabsorption disorders, including biliary atresia and cystic fibrosis. In the hereditary disorder abetalipoproteinemia (Bassen-Kornzweig syndrome), steatorrhea, acanthocytosis, decreased serum levels of cholesterol and triglycerides, retinitis pigmentosa, ophthalmoplegia, peripheral neuropathy, and spinocerebellar degeneration with ataxia, amyotrophy, and dorsal column and pyramidal signs are seen. Another hereditary disorder, isolated vitamin E deficiency, clinically resembles Friedreich's ataxia. A hereditary abnormality of vitamin E absorption is the cause. A number of oral and parenteral preparations of vitamin E are available for treatment.

Although vitamin E is readily available in health food stores, toxic symptoms related to its use are not recognized.

Vitamin K (Phytonadione, Menaquinones)

Neurologic symptoms in vitamin K deficiency are the result of bleeding. Intracranial hemorrhage may occur in the setting of trauma or hemorrhagic disease of the newborn.

Healton EB, Savage, DG, Brust JCM, et al: Neurologic aspects of cobalamin deficiency. Medicine 70:229, 1991. *A review of 189 patients, covering symptoms, signs, diagnosis, and the frequency of neurologic disease without anemia.*

Kaydon HV: The neurologic syndrome of vitamin E deficiency: A significant cause of ataxia. Neurology 43:2167, 1993. *A review of an underrecognized association.*

Serdaru M, Hausser-Hauw C, LaPlane D, et al: The clinical spectrum of alcoholic pellagra encephalopathy. Brain 111:829, 1988. *A review of 22 cases in which diagnosis was often needlessly delayed.*

U.S. Department of Health and Human Services: Recommendations for the use of folic acid to reduce the number of cases of spina bifida and other neural tube defects. MMWR 41:1, 1992. *Guidelines in the prevention of a major teratogenic disorder.*

Victor M, Adams RD, Collins GH: The Wernicke-Korsakoff Syndrome, 2nd ed. Philadelphia, FA Davis, 1989. *A classic monograph.*

■ INJURY OF THE HEAD AND SPINAL CORD

490 HEAD INJURY

Gabrielle F. Morris ■ *Lawrence F. Marshall*

GENERAL CONSIDERATIONS

Traumatic brain injury (TBI) is a major public health problem; it represents the leading cause of mortality in patients aged 0 to 45 years and accounts for a third of all injury-related deaths in this country. Each year in the United States, TBI results in 72,000 deaths and an additional 210,000 cases of serious morbidity. Mild degrees of head injury lead to more than 2 million emergency room evaluations. These patients are also susceptible to cognitive and behavioral sequelae. Closed head injury produces brain injury through a variety of mechanisms. Although TBI can occur in isolation, it is usually accompanied by additional organ-system injury. Spinal and brain injury frequently coexist.

MECHANISM OF BRAIN DAMAGE

The initial impact to the brain can immediately cause variable degrees of abnormality; the impact also initiates a cascade of events that, if left uninterrupted, may result in more severe tissue injury and even death. *Primary injury* that initially appears modest and compatible with good recovery may, in many cases, later give way to development of new hematomas or expansion of existing ones, or ischemic brain damage as a result of systemic factors; this is termed *secondary injury*. Hypotension and hypoxia are the most frequent; these factors are looked for and treated aggressively.

The pathology of head injury includes a spectrum of changes. Underlying almost all nonpenetrating brain trauma is diffuse axonal injury, a condition in which axons are either sheared at the time of impact or degenerate soon after because of irreversible traumatic or ischemic damage to the fibers. Superimposed on such white matter changes are hematomas, which are either focal collections of blood or less discretely defined hemorrhages admixed with injured brain tissue. Hematomas can occur on the external surface of the dura (epidural hematoma), under the dura but above the brain surface (subdural hematoma), or within the brain substance (intraparenchymal hematoma or contusion). Hemorrhage may also occur diffusely in the subarachnoid space. In mild and moderate head injury, the frequency of surgical hematomas is low. As the degree of neurologic injury increases, however, the severity of diffuse axonal injury rises in almost direct proportion, as does the frequency of intracranial hematomas. Molecular abnormalities due to regional anoxia plus direct trauma contribute to neuronal injury. Trauma results in the release of an excess of excitatory amino acids as well as inflammatory mediators and free radicals, into the contused or ischemic areas, inducing tissue edema and increased intracranial pressure due to brain swelling.

PRIMARY DAMAGE

Primary traumatic damage to the brain can be separated into several basic processes: diffuse axonal injury, intracranial hematoma and contusion, and subarachnoid hemorrhage. Diffuse axonal injury (DAI) always occurs in severe head injury and has a predilection for the brain stem, corpus callosum, and deep white matter. Experimental studies suggest that minor degrees of DAI probably occur in patients who suffer only a *concussion* (i.e., a transient loss of consciousness usually associated with no or minimal residua). With more severe head trauma, the number of areas and the severity of DAI increase proportionately.

Traumatic subarachnoid hemorrhage can theoretically occur anywhere along the surface of the brain and tends to be distributed differently than nontraumatic subarachnoid hemorrhage. The presence of traumatic subarachnoid hemorrhage is associated with a higher morbidity and mortality. It is not yet clear whether this hemorrhage itself is deleterious or whether it is a marker for severity of injury.

Epidural hematomas often result from moderate-impact injuries: a baseball striking the head, an assault producing only a transient loss of consciousness, or a fall from a horse. Epidural hematomas characteristically follow fractures of the temporal bone associated with laceration of the middle meningeal artery. In some instances, the hemorrhage may follow a fracture and, in the process, tear one of the major draining venous sinuses of the brain. The "classic" presentation is actually only demonstrated in a minority of cases and is described as a transient loss of consciousness followed by a period of lucidity and then a rather abrupt period of deterioration. Some persons lose consciousness immediately following impact, whereas some show rather abrupt deterioration without a history of initial loss of consciousness. The early detection of epidural hemorrhages is of utmost importance because most affected patients do not initially have irreversible brain damage. Thus, prompt surgical evacuation can be associated with favorable outcome.

Subdural hematomas are divided into two subgroups—acute and chronic—based on timing of presentation; these manifest as distinct syndromes. An *acute subdural hematoma* almost always signifies severe brain injury and is associated with substantial diffuse axonal injury and brain contusion. Most such patients are unconscious from impact, and half die. Typically, these lesions are caused by laceration of the bridging veins that drain blood from the brain's surface into the venous sinuses or from cortical vein laceration. Subdural hematomas are especially likely following assaults, falls (e.g., in alcoholic and elderly patients), and motor vehicle accidents in which the head decelerates suddenly on impact. The frequency of subdural hematomas increases with age, presumably

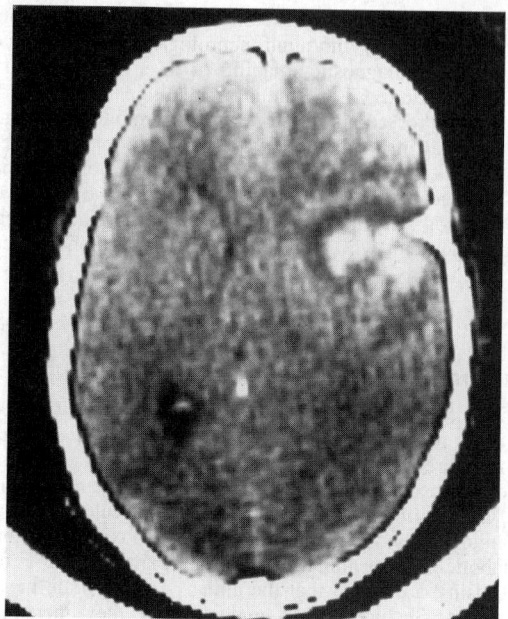

FIGURE 490–1 ■ Brain contusion.

because age-associated brain atrophy more readily allows the expansion of such venous bleeding. Given the severity of initial brain injury, it is not surprising that these patients tend to fare poorly. Prompt surgical evacuation via craniotomy alleviates mass effect and improves outcome, particularly in patients who show little other associated brain injury.

Chronic subdural hematomas usually become symptomatic between 1 and 6 weeks following injury and are not infrequently located bilaterally. They often follow trivial injuries, such as striking the head on a door with no associated loss of consciousness. Indeed, the inciting event is so minor that it is often not specifically recalled. Patients with chronic subdural hematoma tend to be older (>age 60 years) or have diseases causing brain atrophy (e.g. alcoholism and dementia). Headache, worse in the morning, somnolence or confusion, mild focal weakness, difficulty in writing, and unsteadiness are common complaints. Due to the more gradual accumulation of blood in an enlarged subdural space, which occurs as a process of age-related shrinkage of the brain, chronic subdural hematoma may reach a substantial size (>100 mL) before the patient seeks medical attention. Small chronic subdurals may resolve spontaneously, and for the remainder, treatment is relatively straightforward. The hematoma is evacuated via one or two strategically placed twist drill or burr holes with dural puncture. Many surgeons leave a subdural drain in place for 24 to 48 hours and keep the patient in a flat, supine position. This method is successful in approximately 90% of patients. Craniotomy is only necessary in those patients whom burr hole drainage has failed.

Intraparenchymal hemorrhage or *contusion* can occur anywhere throughout the brain, but usually occurs in characteristic regions of the frontal and temporal poles, where the brain overlies the bony ridges of the skull base. Figure 490–1 demonstrates a contusion. Contusions vary in size and act as mass lesions. Adjacent areas of secondary tissue edema are admixed, and the combination frequently enlarges, particularly in the first 24 hours after injury. Surgery for appropriately-sized (>25 mL) and accessible lesions may improve outcome. Medical maneuvers to control intracranial hypertension should be instituted.

PREHOSPITAL CARE AND INITIAL RESUSCITATION

Head injuries often occur under circumstances that traumatize other organ systems. When high velocity impact is the mechanism of injury, fractures of the long bones and injuries to the chest and abdomen are common. Even moderate hypotension can convert a reversible brain injury to one in which ischemic brain damage is ir-

reversible. Accordingly, immediate and adequate restitution of blood pressure and intravascular fluid volume, as well as early steps to prevent and treat hypoxia, represent essential preventive measures.

Utilization of the Glasgow Coma Scale (GCS), shown in Table 490–1, provides a simple and reproducible means for serially assessing the head-injured patient. This examination, which assesses the patient's ability to respond to pain, to speak, and to open the eyes, when performed in concert with examination of the pupils, serves as an excellent field guide to the severity of injury. Patients who cannot follow commands, do not open the eyes in response to noxious stimuli, and fail to utter words or comprehensible sounds are considered to be in a coma (GCS ≤8). All four limbs must be tested for responsiveness, either to verbal command or to pain, so as not to overlook focal neurologic deficits, such as hemiparesis, paraparesis, or quadriparesis. Changes in pupillary responsiveness suggest brain stem compression, which must be detected early and dealt with promptly if treatment is to be successful. However, the GCS does not specifically address the patient's state of alertness, and this should be recorded in the initial and subsequent assessments.

Attention must also be paid to the patient's systemic status. The frequency of shock and hypoxia increases in proportion to the severity of injury. Comatose or stuporous patients are at substantial risk for aspiration and are unable to protect their own airway. Hypoxia occurs in association with approximately 10 to 20% of all severe head injuries. If the prehospital provider is skilled, early controlled intubation, often at the scene of the injury, is highly recommended.

It has been clearly shown that the presence of hypotension doubles the mortality of severe head injury. Search for sources of hemorrhage is essential and should include the less obvious ones, such as scalp lacerations and pelvic fractures. Fluid resuscitation should begin at the scene, although the difficulties in administering large amounts of fluid under these conditions are obvious. Intravenous fluids should be given promptly, if possible, at the scene of the injury. Even with modern paramedic systems, shock treatment in the field is often inadequate. New strategies such as hypertonic saline or pressor agents are being considered.

COMPUTED TOMOGRAPHIC SCANNING

The availability of rapid-sequence computed tomographic (CT) scanning has revolutionized the care of the head-injured patient. The urgency of scan acquisition varies with the severity of injury and is based on clinical judgment. Patients with focal neurologic deficits or severe injuries (GCS ≤8) should undergo CT scanning as soon as airway and hemodynamic stability are ensured. To minimize the risks of transportation and movement, patients whose

Table 490–1 ■ GLASGOW COMA SCALE

The Glasgow Coma Scale is a practical means of monitoring changes in level of consciousness, based upon eye opening and verbal and motor responses. The responsiveness of the patient can be expressed by summation of the figures. The lowest score is 3, the highest is 15.

Eyes open	Spontaneously (eyes open does not imply awareness)	4
	To speech (any speech, not necessarily a command)	3
	To pain (should not use supraorbital pressure for pain stimulus)	2
	Never	1
Best verbal response	Oriented (to time, person, place)	5
	Confused speech (disoriented)	4
	Inappropriate (swearing, yelling)	3
	Incomprehensible sounds (moaning, groaning)	2
	None	1
Best motor response	Obeys commands	6
	Localizes pain (deliberate or purposeful movement)	5
	Withdrawal (moves away from stimulus)	4
	Abnormal flexion (decortication)	3
	Extension (decerebration)	2
	None (flaccidity)	1
	Total Score	

condition is deteriorating must be accompanied by a physician, and even stable but seriously injured patients require that, at a minimum, an experienced emergency room or trauma nurse be present at all times. Supervised respiratory assistance should ensure adequate ventilation during transport and during the scan.

The results of CT scans heavily influence subsequent management. If a surgical lesion is demonstrated, the patient should be taken to the operating room immediately. Otherwise, severe traumatic injuries are best treated in an intensive care unit, with lesser injuries being handled in units that provide close observation.

Several findings on the CT scan, other than intracranial hematomas, merit close attention and warn of possible deterioration. Compression or absence of the mesencephalic cisterns indicates a significant increase in intracranial volume and increases the risk of death. This is true even in patients whose clinical examination at the time suggests only a moderately severe injury. Unilateral or bilateral hemispheric swelling almost always predicts the likelihood of dangerous intracranial hypertension.

SERIAL ASSESSMENT

Close observation, with particular attention to the development of tachypnea and bradycardia, is important. Table 490–2 lists signs that portend potential intracranial catastrophe. An increase in systolic blood pressure of 15 mm Hg or more, or a decline in heart rate of 15 beats/minute often gives the first hint of the development of an intracranial mass lesion.

Tachypnea holds particular importance. Respiratory rates greater than 20/minute are abnormal in patients older than 15 years and may indicate an increase in intracranial pressure or the development of pulmonary failure or infection. Similarly, increasing headache is often present but overlooked; it may reflect rising intracranial pressure. The use of continuous flow sheets in an intermediate care setting or in a neurologic observation unit assists in monitoring the course and detecting subtle changes in vital signs, GCS, and level of alertness.

MANAGEMENT

General Concepts

The presence of head injury must be presumed until proven otherwise in all patients who present with an altered sensorium or a history of loss of consciousness following trauma. At a minimum, patients must undergo thorough neurologic examination complemented by either diagnostic imaging or a sufficient period of in-hospital observation. CT scanning is the screening procedure of choice. Criteria for admission for serial neurologic evaluations include the following: advanced age, presence of multiple organ system injuries, abnormal CT scan, and persistently diminished level of consciousness. Conversely, discharge home can be considered in neurologically normal patients with a normal CT scan who have a reliable adult who can monitor their condition for deterioration.

Intensive Care of the Patient with Severe Head Injury

The overriding objective in the care of the severely head-injured patient is to prevent further insults to the traumatized brain. The situation requires meticulous attention to detail and continuous vigilance to detect and counteract deterioration in hemodynamic, pulmonary, and neurologic function. The brain's vulnerability to secondary injury extends beyond shock and hypoxia. Fever increases the metabolic rate of the tissue by approximately 13% for each degree Celsius, a demand that the already injured brain may not be able to meet. Seizures are a major threat; they increase tissue energy requirements and markedly increase cerebral blood flow, accentuating any existing increase in the intracranial pressure.

An approach that includes both the avoidance of systemic insults to the brain and the treatment of intracranial hypertension is illustrated in Table 490–3. Most severe head injuries are accompanied by increased intracranial pressure (ICP). Compression of the mesencephalic cisterns detected by CT scanning can also be seen in moderate head injury and signifies an elevation of ICP. In addition to maintaining adequate cerebral perfusion, it is crucial to lower elevated ICP. Mortality can be dramatically reduced with rapid intervention for intracranial hypertension, and continuous monitoring of ICP is therefore required in these patients. The monitoring of intracranial pressure requires neurosurgical intervention and the availability of an intensive care unit. Invasive monitoring is difficult in patients with a coagulopathy.

The treatment of traumatic *intracranial hypertension* (defined as an ICP greater than 20 mm Hg) is central to the intensive care of the critically brain-injured patient. This goal is in conjunction with keeping the cerebral perfusion pressure concomitantly greater than 60 mm Hg. Note that cerebral perfusion pressure management should not supersede ICP management. The cornerstone of manage-

Table 490–2 ■ SIGNS OF POTENTIAL INTRACRANIAL CATASTROPHE AND WHAT THEY MAY SIGNIFY

SIGNS	CHANGES	POTENTIAL MEANING
Respiration	Rate > 20	Pulmonary edema or pneumonitis
Pulse	Change > 10/min or heart rate <60	Each may indicate elevated ICP with transtentorial herniation
Blood pressure	Change in systolic > 15 mm Hg or widening pulse pressure	
Headache*	Is it increasing?	Often indicates increased ICP
Pupils	Enlargement Asymmetry Irregular shape (oval) Decrease in reactivity Change from preresuscitation	
Motor	Decrease of 1 point on GCS New focal deficit	Increased mass effect New hemorrhage Recurrent hemorrhage
Level of consciousness	Abrupt decrease	Increased ICP Seizures Hypotension
	Transient	Seizures Hypoxia
	Progressive decrease	Rehemorrhage Brain stem involvement Septicemia Electrolyte imbalance Vasospasm Hydrocephalus

*All changes except headache may occur in both awake and unconscious patients. GCS = Glasgow coma scale; ICP = intracranial pressure.

Table 490-3 ■ INTENSIVE CARE UNIT MANAGEMENT OF SEVERE HEAD INJURY AND INTRACRANIAL HYPERTENSION

1. Head elevated 30 degrees and in neutral plane
2. Intubation with controlled ventilation to an arterial PCO_2 of 30–35 mm Hg
3. Good pulmonary toilet
4. Maintain fluid balance with normal saline (0.9%)
5. Maintain systolic arterial pressure between 110 and 160 mm Hg
6. Maintain cerebral perfusion pressure >60 mm Hg (CPP = MAP − ICP)
7. Adequate sedation
8. Muscle relaxants prn (must use sedation concurrently)
9. Maintain normothermia
10. Adequate anticonvulsant therapy
11. Ventricular drainage for intracranial hypertension
12. Mannitol 0.25 mg/kg if No. 11 fails or is not available
13. Hypnotic for elevated ICP in patients with diffuse or hemispheric swelling

ment is to adjust baseline ventilation to maintain an arterial carbon dioxide pressure ($PaCO_2$) in the range of 35 to 37 mm Hg, permitting brief periods of hyperventilation to respond to sudden increases in ICP. Levels of extreme hyperventilation may exacerbate cerebral ischemia by excessive vasoconstriction. Head-of-bed elevation is provided to 30 degrees. Prevention of venous outflow obstruction is attained by keeping the head aligned without rotation. Maintainence of intravascular volume is accomplished by providing balanced salt solutions, and by avoiding dextrose and water, or hypotonic solutions. Avoidance of hyperglycemia is wise, as studies have suggested a deleterious impact on experimental models of head injury. The osmotic diuretic agent mannitol is often used in intermittent therapy for ICP elevations and cerebral swelling.

Sedation and pain relief are essential in the initial phases of treatment. Morphine sulfate, given by continuous infusion of 2 to 8 mg/hour, is the least complicated and most effective regimen. Muscle relaxation with short-acting agents is occasionally helpful in patients in whom ICP is difficult to control, but these agents should not be used prophylactically.

Anticonvulsants have a limited but important role in acute traumatic head injury. Phenytoin given for the first 7 days after injury reduces the incidence of seizures during that period. No study has shown a protective effect when medication was continued beyond the first week.

LONG-TERM CONSEQUENCES OF SEVERE HEAD INJURY

Severe head injury often causes serious long-term intellectual and behavioral impairment. Unfortunately, some patients survive only in a persistent vegetative state (2 to 3%) or with severe disabilities (approximately 20%) requiring long-term supportive care. Recovery with the ability to return to near-normal activities is not unusual. Common long-term deficits are seen in recent memory, abstract thinking, and rapid information processing. Depression, fatigue, and impetuosity accentuate these cognitive deficits. Incomplete recovery of motor function is relatively uncommon and is less socioeconomically important. Many rehabilitation programs have been developed to assist the severely head-injured patient in the management of these problems. Counseling of the family is essential. Divorce, suicide, and spouse abuse can be reduced in frequency by early intervention.

MINOR HEAD INJURY

Minor head injury is defined as brain injury that results in a GCS score of 13 to 15, with a return to a normal level of consciousness and general mentation within 24 hours. It is not infrequent for patients to manifest cognitive and behavioral sequelae following minor head injury even in the absence of a defined period of unconsciousness. The majority of such patients have normal CT scans. These patients characteristically experience early post-traumatic problems with recent memory, concentration, and abstract thinking. In most instances, such problems subside within the first 1 to 6 months following minor injury. Approximately 15% have residual unremitting cognitive deficits. Age is a specific risk factor, and many elderly persons develop chronic dizziness and

disequilibrium after even minor trauma. Such patients are classified as having a *post-traumatic* or *post-concussive syndrome.*

Many patients with minor head injuries suffer transiently from insomnia, depression, and headache. Early support and reassurance from the physician often improve these symptoms. If headache persists for more than 60 to 90 days, propranolol, 30 to 60 mg given in three divided doses, may bring relief.

MODERATE HEAD INJURY

Patients who have not been rendered comatose but have a depressed level of consciousness for several hours or days following injury are classified as having suffered moderate head injuries (GCS 9 to 12). Approximately 10% of these patients have or will develop surgical hematomas. Many of these patients suffer measurable cognitive and behavioral difficulties over the long term. Nevertheless, many eventually return to gainful employment. Even so, the potential for social disruption is high, and traits of impetuousness and heightened irritability often create socioeconomic problems. Depression is frequent and may respond to tricyclic antidepressants. Intervention, using a variety of psychological services has a more favorable impact if carried out early.

Bullock R, Chesnut RM, Clifton G, et al: Guidelines for the Mangement of Severe Head Injury. Park Ridge, IL, American Association of Neurological Surgeons, 1995. *This text provides an evidence-based comprehensive literature review and provides guidelines useful to the intensivist in treating traumatic brain injury.*

Foulkes MA, Eisenberg HM, Jane JA, et al: Report on the traumatic coma data bank. J Neurosurg 75(suppl):51, 1991. *Outcome data and much more are described in a cohort of 1030 head-injury victims treated from onset in a multicenter trial.*

Marshall SB, Marshall LF, Vos H, et al: Neuroscience Critical Care: Pathophysiology and Patient Management. Philadelphia, WB Saunders, 1990. *Particular emphasis on assessment of the neurologically impaired patient, modern neuroradiology, and intensive care.*

Narayan RK, Wilberger JE Jr, Povlishock JT (ed): Neurotrauma. New York, McGraw-Hill, 1996. *An extensive, current text that incorporates the modern management concepts in head injury.*

Ropper AH (ed): Neurological and Neurosurgical Intensive Care, 3rd ed. New York, Raven, 1993. *A well-edited volume that contains an excellent, detailed chapter on head injury by Chesnut and Marshall.*

Temkin NR, Dikmen SS, Wilensky AJ, et al: A randomized, double-blind study of phenytoin for the prevention of post-traumatic seizures. N Engl J Med 323:497, 1990. *A series of 404 patients with serious head trauma were randomly assigned treatment with phenytoin or placebo within 24 hours of injury; significant reduction in seizure incidence (p < .001) occurred only between drug loading time and day 7.*

491 SPINE AND SPINAL CORD INJURY

Gabrielle F. Morris ■ *William R. Taylor* ■ *Lawrence F. Marshall*

Spinal cord injury (SCI) is a devastating problem that disproportionately affects young males, thereby resulting in huge costs to the individual patients and to society in terms of lost work productivity. Though the incidence has diminished somewhat recently to 35 per 1 million persons, there remain 250,000 Americans with long-term sequelae of SCI each year. The resultant morbidity causes an immediate, dramatic, and often permanent change in lifestyle and occupation. The most common etiology of SCI is an injury to the spinal column that disrupts the stability of the spine. The two most often coexist, yet either has the potential to occur in isolation.

To understand the pathophysiology and to formulate rational treatment plans, dual-axis parallel thinking is requisite. Both the spinal column and the spinal cord must be assessed and treated in concert at each stage. Manipulation of one aspect of treatment can directly affect the other; for example, when traction is applied for reduction of an unstable fracture, the spinal cord is at risk when any motion occurs.

NATURE OF THE INJURY

About half of all serious spinal injuries affect the cervical level of the spine, with nearly 50% of such patients rendered quadriplegic as a result. Injuries are also common at the thoracolumbar junction and in the lumbar spine with resultant nerve root injury. The three following major abnormalities result in damage to the tissue: (1) destruction from direct trauma; (2) compression by bone fragments, hematoma, or disk material; and, less frequently, (3) ischemia as a result of mechanical impingement of spinal arteries. Postinjury edema of spinal soft tissue and the cord itself accentuates these changes.

Spinal cord injuries can be categorized as complete or incomplete on the basis of the quantity of residual neurologic function. Acute, complete injuries most often produce *spinal shock*, with loss of all sensorimotor functions, including flaccidity and loss of reflexes at and below the level of injury. A few such cases may involve sustained priapism. Less severe injuries can produce a *central cord syndrome* resulting from ischemia or hematomas of the cervical cord (Fig. 491–1). These result in a clinical syndrome characterized by weakness in the distal upper extremities combined with impaired or lost pain and temperature sensations in the arms, but with sparing of touch and, often, of all functions below the cervical cord level. The upper extremity weakness generally improves in such cases. Other patterns of cord injury may produce an anterior spinal artery syndrome or a partial hemisection (Brown-Séquard syndrome), producing distal weakness and proprioceptive loss ipsilateral to the cord damage accompanied by contralateral pain and temperature impairment.

In the presence of one spinal axis injury, the incidence of a second non-contiguous fracture is 15%. It is imperative to search for this possibility and to document the integrity of the spinal column from occiput to sacrum.

EMERGENCY MANAGEMENT

For the patient, crucial elements in treatment arise at the accident scene or within the first few hours at the hospital. After that time, experienced neurosurgeons or spine-trained orthopedists provide the majority of patient care, supplemented, if possible, by resources of a tertiary care center.

At the accident site, three major concerns are paramount: (1) maintenance of ventilation, (2) protection against shock, and (3) neck immobilization to prevent further spinal cord damage. Damage to high thoracic or cervical spinal levels creates the immediate risk of ventilatory failure due to acute paralysis of intercostal and abdominal muscles, the diaphragm, or a combination thereof. Unrestricted movement of the neck risks converting a partial injury to a complete one, making nasotracheal intubation preferable to standard peroral intubation. Tracheostomy or cricothyroidotomy should be avoided if possible, because these procedures often put pressure on the vertebral column.

Severe hypotension often follows cervical injury because the lesion interrupts the descending sympathetic pathways; bradycardia characteristically accompanies the low blood pressure. Such neurogenic hypotension can be distinguished from hypovolemic shock by the tachycardia of the latter. In either case, the legs should be elevated gently to improve venous return and fluids delivered in amounts sufficient to counter both the traumatic and neurogenic aspects of the problem. Severe hypotension during the early minutes or hours after injury is itself a potential cause of spinal cord damage.

The neck and spine should be immobilized as gently as possible at the injury site, using a carrying board, sandbags and adhesive tape, or a Philadelphia collar. Soft collars are ineffective. The head is best maintained in a neutral position but should not be forced into such an attitude lest the maneuver induce further spinal cord damage.

HOSPITAL CARE

The medical care of spinal cord injuries is a specialty unto itself. Such patients often are critically ill owing to a combination of systemic injuries, blood and fluid loss, various fractures, and infections. Considerable expertise is required for the accurate interpretation of spinal radiographs. The treating physician must not accept as normal plain radiographs that do not demonstrate all of the cervical vertebrae. An overlooked spine injury can be catastrophic if, for example, an odontoid fracture or an injury to C7 results later in sudden instability. Patients with cervical fracture-dislocations usually are placed in skeletal traction with skull fixation before definitive surgical repair is undertaken. In patients with injury to the thoracic or lumbar spine, traction is of no benefit.

There is no treatment that reverses the devastation of acute SCI. Treatment is focused on preventing secondary injury by the following means: (1) appropriate immobilization; (2) maintenance of spinal cord perfusion (mean arterial blood pressure should be maintained above 80 to 85 mm Hg with volume resuscitation, cautiously supplemented with pharmacologic pressors); and (3) high doses of methylprednisolone. When therapy can be initiated within the first 3 hours after injury, the initial dose is given as a bolus at 30 mg/kg over 15 minutes followed by 45 minutes of waiting. From 2 to 24 hours, a continuous infusion is given at 5.4 mg/kg/hour. The earlier the protocol is initiated after injury, the higher the likelihood for improvement. Treatment should be instituted in the field. If the bolus cannot be initiated until 3 to 8 hours after injury, the continuous infusion is maintained for 47 hours instead of 24 hours. With a delay of greater than 8 hours following injury, methylprednisolone administration results in worse outcome and should not be given.

Other management includes use of a rotating bed to reduce the risk of decubitus ulcer formation, chest physiotherapy to minimize lung complications, and cardiac and fluid-electrolyte monitoring. Pneumatic antiembolism stockings and early mobilization reduce

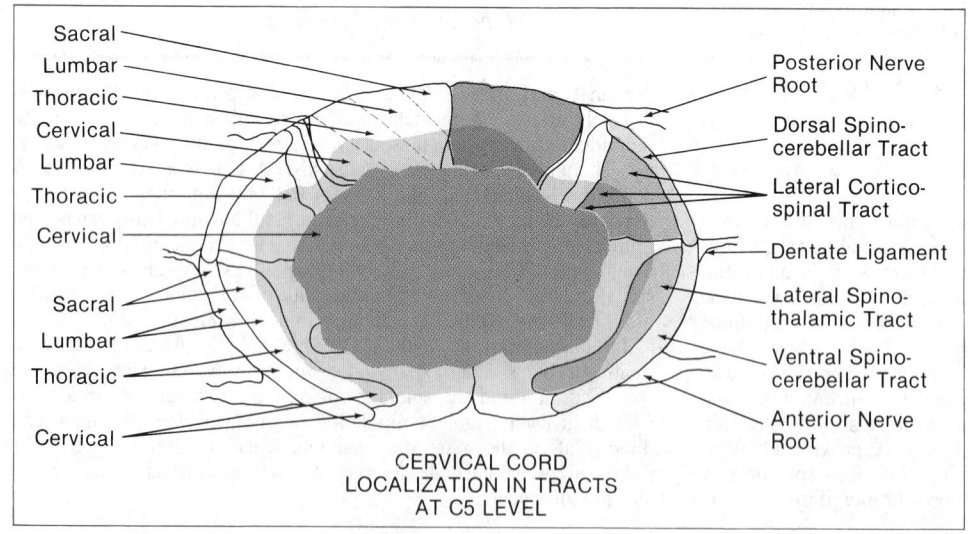

CERVICAL CORD
LOCALIZATION IN TRACTS
AT C5 LEVEL

FIGURE 491–1 ■ Diagrammatic description of the spinal pathways at the lower cervical level showing the usual distribution of the contusion-hemorrhage that causes a central cord syndrome.

the frequency of deep venous thrombosis (DVT). Increasingly in patients who cannot be mobilized rapidly for rehabilitation, low-molecular-weight heparin is being given to prevent DVT. Vena caval filters should also be considered for severely injured immobilized patients. Nearly all patients with SCI require prolonged urinary bladder catheterization. Immediate steps to prevent infection must be initiated; if possible, indwelling catheters should be replaced by intermittent catheterization at 4- to 6-hour intervals. Acidification of the urine with vitamin C or cranberry juice helps to reduce the incidence of infection.

Trauma patients require early nutrition to feed the demands of wound healing and the efforts of rehabilitation. Early enteral nutritional support is preferred. Subsequently, every effort should be made to provide appetizing food and adequate vitamins.

Autonomic dysfunction complicates the convalescence of more than half of patients who suffer severe SCI above the midthoracic level. Disconnected distal autonomic pathways can induce a variety of troublesome phenomena, including systemic hypertension, reflex sweating, skin flushing, headache, and painful flexor spasms of the lower extremities. Bladder distention and infection frequently trigger such acute-onset reflex dysautonomia and require urgent treatment. Patients are often unaware of a change in urinary bladder function. Diazepam (5 to 10 mg given three times a day) or baclofen (10 to 60 mg given in divided doses) given long term may be useful for the treatment of reflex spasms. The continuous intrathecal administration of baclofen by an indwelling pump is another approach that prevents disabling reflex spasms.

PHYSICAL AND OCCUPATIONAL THERAPY AND REHABILITATION

Almost all patients with SCI require prolonged postacute care. Those with complete transections have suffered a devastating injury with life-long functional and psychiatric consequences. Early physical and emotional therapy are crucial. Early range of motion prevents contractures, diminishes the risk of venous thrombosis, protects the skin, and boosts morale. The significant improvements

in stabilization techniques of the last several years have facilitated early patient mobilization. This enables patients to begin rehabilitation therapy earlier and reintegrate into their lifestyle more quickly. A comprehensive and individualized therapeutic plan is essential. Patients and family members must be counseled in detail about probable changes in lifestyle. All of these features are best carried out in experienced SCI centers that can provide assistance in home modification, driver retraining, and vocational rehabilitation. Depression following an initial period of denial occurs in almost all patients and may be masked by jocularity. Psychiatric intervention is essential if depression is severe or persistent. Narcotic addiction is also occasionally a problem that may require intervention. If the rehabilitation team moves quickly to provide emotional as well as physical management, many patients with SCI injury can return to a competitive place in society. Most of the injured do best if a single physician organizes the long-term approach to issues related to urinary tract function, skin care, sexual problems, and emotional-vocational needs.

An HS: Synopsis of Spine Surgery. Baltimore, Williams & Wilkins, 1998. *This pocket-sized manual provides a rapid overview for the clinician managing spinal cord injuries.*

Bracken MB, Shepard MJ, Hellenbrand KG, et al: A randomized, controlled trial of methylprednisolone or naloxone in the treatment of acute spinal cord injury. N Engl J Med 322:1405, 1990. *The first study to clearly demonstrate the efficacy of pharmacologic treatment for spinal cord injury.*

Bracken MB, Shepard MJ, Holford TR, et al: Administration of methylprednisolone for 24 or 48 hours or tirilazad mesylate for 48 hours in the treatment of acute spinal cord injury: Results of the Third National Acute Spinal Cord Injury Randomized Controlled Trial. JAMA 277:1597–1604, 1997. *A report of pharmacologic therapy with new agents, which also reaffirms the usefulness of methylprednisolone.*

Chiles BW III, Cooper PR: Acute spinal cord injury. N Engl J Med 334:514–520, 1996. *A concise update of the modern management of spinal cord injury.*

Cooper PR: Management of posttraumatic spinal instability. *In* Neurosurgical Topics. Park Ridge, IL, American Association of Neurological Surgeons, 1990. *An excellent compendium of the biomechanics of spinal injury, radiographic identification, and therapeutic options for stabilization.*

Menezes AH, Sonntag VKH (ed): Principles of Spinal Surgery. New York, McGraw-Hill, 1996. *This well-edited two volume text serves as an encyclopedic reference for spinal diseases, including neurotrauma.*

■ Mechanical Lesions of Nerve Roots and Spinal Cord

492 SPINAL ANATOMY

Michael J. Aminoff

The individual vertebrae are separated by intervertebral disks that serve to cushion the spine during various physical activities. Each disk consists of a thick outer fibrous portion called the annulus fibrosus within which is a soft, gelatinous, inner central portion called the nucleus pulposus, which is a remnant of the notochord. Posterior to the vertebral bodies, the vertebral arches (composed of paired pedicles anteriorly and laminae posteriorly) and transverse processes enclose the spinal cord in the spinal canal, and the posterior spinous process projects posteriorly, as shown in Figure 492–1. Paraspinal muscles help to support the spine.

The intervertebral disks are not pain-sensitive, but pain may arise from the ligaments connecting the vertebrae, facet joints, vertebral periosteum, outer layer of the annulus fibrosus, and spinal nerve roots. The paraspinal muscles are also pain-sensitive and are probably the most common source of neck or back pain.

The spinal canal contains the spinal cord and the spinal and autonomic roots. Its size varies at different levels and between different individuals. It tends to be more spacious in the cervical and lumbar regions than the thoracic. A congenitally narrow spinal canal (spinal stenosis) predisposes to neurologic dysfunction as a consequence of minor degenerative changes or disk protrusion. Such stenosis is common in both the cervical and lumbar regions.

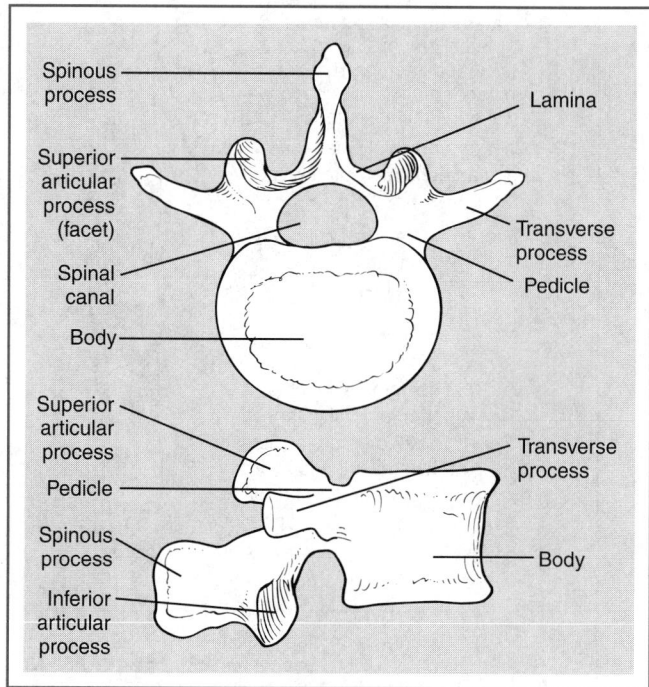

FIGURE 492–1 ■ Vertebral anatomy.

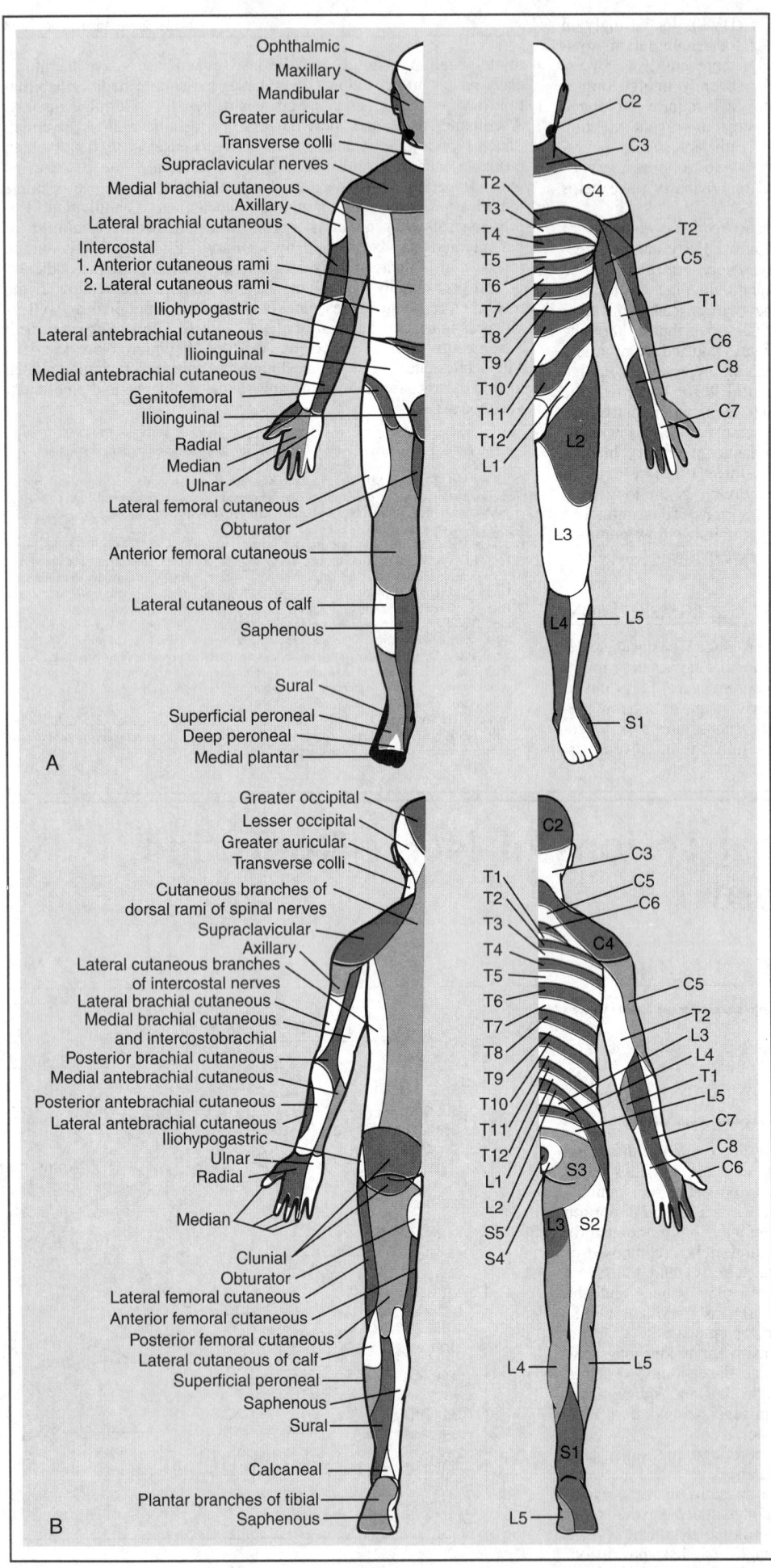

Ophthalmic
Maxillary
Mandibular
Greater auricular
Transverse colli
Supraclavicular nerves
Medial brachial cutaneous
Axillary
Lateral brachial cutaneous
Intercostal
1. Anterior cutaneous rami
2. Lateral cutaneous rami
Iliohypogastric
Lateral antebrachial cutaneous
Ilioinguinal
Medial antebrachial cutaneous
Genitofemoral
Ilioinguinal
Radial
Median
Ulnar
Lateral femoral cutaneous
Obturator
Anterior femoral cutaneous
Lateral cutaneous of calf
Saphenous
Sural
Superficial peroneal
Deep peroneal
Medial plantar

C2
C3
C4
T2
T3
T4
T5
T6
T7
T8
T9
T10
T11
T12
L1
T2
C5
T1
C6
C8
C7
L2
L3
L4 — L5
S1

A

Greater occipital
Lesser occipital
Greater auricular
Transverse colli
Cutaneous branches of dorsal rami of spinal nerves
Supraclavicular
Axillary
Lateral cutaneous branches of intercostal nerves
Lateral brachial cutaneous
Medial brachial cutaneous and intercostobrachial
Posterior brachial cutaneous
Medial antebrachial cutaneous
Posterior antebrachial cutaneous
Lateral antebrachial cutaneous
Iliohypogastric
Ulnar
Radial
Median
Clunial
Obturator
Lateral femoral cutaneous
Anterior femoral cutaneous
Posterior femoral cutaneous
Lateral cutaneous of calf
Superficial peroneal
Saphenous
Sural
Calcaneal
Plantar branches of tibial
Saphenous

C2
C3
C5
C6
C4
T1
T2
T3
T4
T5
T6
T7
T8
T9
T10
T11
T12
L1
L2
S5
S4
S3
L3
S2
C5
T2
L3
L4
T1
L5
C7
C8
C6
L4 — L5
S1
L5

B

FIGURE 492–2 ■ Cutaneous innervation. The segmental (dermatomal) distribution is shown on the left side of the body, and the peripheral nerve distribution on the right side of the body. *A*, Anterior view. *B*, Posterior view.

In adults, the cord ends as the conus medullaris at about the level of the first lumbar vertebra; below this level, the spinal canal is occupied by the descending nerve roots that comprise the cauda equina. The cervical cord segments are at approximately the same level as the cervical vertebral bodies; the thoracic cord segments are generally one or two levels higher than the corresponding vertebral segments, and much of the lumbar and sacral cord is found between T10 and L1. Thus, the nerve roots in the cauda equina have to descend in the subarachnoid space before exiting at their various foramina. The absence of a C8 vertebral body but presence of a C8 spinal segment means that roots above C8 exit above the corresponding vertebral body, whereas the remaining nerve roots exit below their respective vertebral bodies.

Thirty-one paired spinal nerves emerge from the spinal cord: 8 in the cervical region, 12 in the thoracic, 5 in the lumbar, 5 in the sacral, and 1 in the coccygeal. Each spinal nerve has both anterior and posterior roots that connect it with the cord. The fibers in the posterior roots originate primarily in the dorsal root ganglia, which are situated distally along the posterior roots, shortly before these unite with the anterior roots and usually within the entrance of the bony intevertebral foramen. The axons in the anterior roots arise mainly from cells in the anterior and lateral gray columns of the spinal cord.

Shortly after passing through the intervertebral foramina, the spinal nerves divide into anterior and posterior rami. The posterior rami supply the skin over the back of the neck and the trunk and the paraspinal musculature. The anterior rami innervate the antero-lateral trunk and the limbs. It is the anterior rami that contribute to the limb plexuses, where the fibers are reorganized to form the various peripheral nerves to the extremities: the brachial plexus to the arms and the lumbar and sacral plexuses to the legs.

The pattern of any motor or sensory deficits is helpful in localizing a lesion involving the cord or nerve roots. A *myotome* designates a group of muscles that have a common innervation from the same segment of the spinal cord and thus from the same nerve root. Most muscles belong to more than one myotome because they typically are innervated by two or more adjacent cord segments and nerve roots. The designation *dermatome* refers to the cutaneous territory innervated by a single nerve root. Adjacent dermatomes overlap considerably. Figure 492–2 illustrates the distinction between the segmental (dermatomal) and peripheral innervation of the skin.

In the remaining chapters of this section, the clinical findings in various mechanical disorders of the cord and roots are discussed. Their pathophysiologic basis, which is discussed in those chapters, can be considered only by reference to the anatomy summarized here.

493 NECK AND BACK PAIN

Michael J. Aminoff

Neck or back pain is one of the most common reasons for medical consultation, but it is usually short lived and responds to symptomatic measures. Most patients with acute neck or back pain, with or without radicular symptoms, have musculoskeletal or degenerative disorders that do not require specific treatment and often are self-limiting. However, the possibility of more serious abnormalities that require specific treatment should always be excluded. Among young patients (less than 40 years) presenting with low back pain, almost 90% have had more than one attack of pain, and most attacks have lasted for less than 2 weeks. Approximately 85% of patients with low back pain cannot be given a definitive diagnosis. Similarly, approximately one third of adults in the general population report neck pain within the previous year, the prevalence increasing with advancing age; almost 14% report chronic neck pain (i.e., pain exceeding 6 months in duration).

TYPE OF PAIN AND ASSOCIATED FINDINGS

Local pain and tenderness may occur from irritation of nerve endings at the site of pathology, such as in the vertebral periosteum. Similarly, degeneration or protrusion of intravertebral disks causes pain by compression of nerve endings in the annulus fibrosus or posterior longitudinal ligaments. Pain of muscle or ligamentous origin or related to a herniated disk is usually alleviated by recumbency. By contrast, the pain of vertebral metastases is often aggravated by recumbency and may be relieved by sitting up.

Referred pain arises from deep structures and is felt at a distant site within the same spinal segment. It often has a deep aching quality and is sometimes accompanied by tenderness at the site of referral. Pain may be referred to the spine from pelvic or abdominal viscera and is usually not affected by the position of the spine. Pain may also be referred from the spine to other regions. For example, disease of the upper lumbar spine may lead to pain in the groins or anterior thighs, and of the lower lumbar spine may cause pain in the buttocks and back of the thighs.

Musculoskeletal pain typically follows unaccustomed exercise, but occasionally occurs spontaneously, often on awakening in the morning. It may relate to spasm of paraspinal muscles as a result of injury or structural abnormality of the spine. Chronic neck pain is a well-recognized complication of whiplash injuries. Trigger points may be present and define certain myofascial pain syndromes. The pain is exacerbated by activity or movement and relieved by rest. Range of motion may be restricted by pain or muscle spasm. Localized tenderness is common. In the absence of a history of injury and of any significant neurologic findings, detailed investigation is usually unrewarding. Patients can be managed conservatively. There is no agreement as to the optimal duration of immobilization or bed rest. Physical therapy is often recommended for the treatment of acute low back pain, but the extent of any benefit is unclear. There is little evidence that traction, ultrasound, diathermy, or manipulation is helpful. Nonsteroidal analgesics are usually sufficient to relieve pain, but in severe cases narcotics may be required; in patients with chronic pain, tricyclic antidepressant drugs are often helpful. Muscle relaxants may relieve painful muscle spasm.

Radicular pain may occur from compression, angulation, or stretch of nerve roots, as by disk protrusion, degenerative spinal disease, or metastatic deposits. Less commonly, radicular pain occurs in certain medical disorders such as diabetes mellitus. The pain has a dermatomal distribution but may also be felt in muscles supplied by the affected root. It is usually sharp in character. Coughing, sneezing, and straining typically exacerbate the pain by increasing intraspinal pressure, as do maneuvers that stretch the nerve roots. Examination may reveal sensory changes in the dermatomal distribution of the affected root, weakness and atrophy in a myotomal distribution, and depression of tendon reflexes subserved by the affected root, but examination is often normal. In patients with weakness, not all muscles within the myotome are necessarily affected. *Cauda equina syndromes* are typically associated with bilateral radicular pain; saddle anesthesia and sphincter dysfunction are common, and examination reveals bilateral root dysfunction.

Spinal cord disease, especially compression of the long tracts, may lead to an unpleasant sensation in the extremities that also is enhanced by increased intraspinal pressure or movements that stretch the cord (such as neck flexion or straight leg raising). Neck or back pain may also be conspicuous. The associated signs vary with the extent of the lesion and speed of its development. Acute cord compression, as from an epidural hemorrhage, is associated with pain and the rapid onset of a paraparesis or quadriparesis that may not be reversed by decompressive surgery. By contrast, a gradually evolving compressive lesion may be painless and leads to a slowly progressive deficit that often recovers following decompression. Laterally placed lesions lead to a Brown-Séquard syndrome, posterior lesions to bilateral posterior column dysfunction with impaired position and vibration appreciation, anterior lesions to weakness, and intramedullary lesions to a dissociated sensory loss, with impairment of pain and temperature appreciation and preservation of posterior column sensation.

CLINICAL EVALUATION

History

Patients often first note the onset of neck or back pain when awakening in the morning, commonly following unaccustomed activity. The character and distribution of the pain are helpful in determining the probable underlying cause (Table 493–1) and thereby the further approach to its investigation. A history of cancer raises the possibility of metastatic disease, whereas local symptoms, such as rectal bleeding, suggest an undiagnosed neoplastic lesion that may have spread to involve the spine. Malignancies that frequently involve the spine are metastatic cancer of the breast, prostate, lung, kidney, colon, and thyroid gland; multiple myeloma; and Hodgkin's and non-Hodgkin's lymphoma. A past history of structural spinal disorder suggests a mechanical cause for pain, of a coagulopathy suggests a hemorrhagic cause, of osteoporosis suggests compression fracture, and of subarachnoid infection or inflammation suggests an arachnoiditis. Whiplash injuries occur in more than 1 million people annually in the United States and may be responsible for acute or chronic neck pain. A history of fever, sweats, diabetes mellitus, sickle cell disease, intravenous drug use, immunodeficiency states, recent penetrating injuries or surgical procedures, or intravenous injections suggests the possibility of an infection involving the spine, disk, or epidural space. Herpes zoster may lead to cutaneous pain over the neck or back, and the diagnosis is often uncertain until the characteristic skin rash develops. Spinal tuberculosis is common in many parts of the world and typically affects the lower thoracic and upper lumbar region, which are unusual sites for degenerative disk disease. Other causes of spinal osteomyelitis include staphylococcal infection, which may be suggested by primary disease of the skin, respiratory tract, or urinary tract. Spinal epidural abscess may lead to acute cord compression in addition to back pain and fever if diagnosis is delayed.

Forced flexion or extension movements of the neck from trauma may lead to significant injury or compression fractures. Compression fractures of the vertebrae occur especially in patients with osteoporosis, and thus most commonly in patients who are elderly, have a family history of osteoporosis, or a history of chronic corticosteroid usage or immobility. Fractures are also especially likely in patients with osteomalacia or Paget's disease and may lead to complications particularly in patients with ankylosing spondylitis, diffuse idiopathic skeletal hyperostosis, and spinal stenosis. Minor cervical trauma may lead to pain and significant deficits in patients with rheumatoid arthritis. Injury may also lead to epi- or subdural hemorrhage or hematomyelia, which is typically heralded by severe pain overlying the site of bleeding (see Chapter 491). Ankylosing spondylitis usually causes early morning stiffness and back pain, relieved by activity.

Primary tumors of the spine and spinal cord are uncommon and are overshadowed by the more frequent occurrence of secondary tumors including lymphoma, myeloma, and cancer. Among the features suggesting malignancy are constant unremitting pain in atypical or multiple sites, pain that is unrelated to activity or posture, the presence of systemic or constitutional symptoms, and an elevated erythrocyte sedimentation rate, especially in patients aged 55 years or older.

Examination

Examination commonly reveals spasm of the paraspinal muscles and limitation of spinal movements. Local tenderness may also be present. Spinal compression should be suspected when neck flexion leads to pain in the thoracic or lumbar region or when Lhermitte's sign is positive. Focal tenderness over a spinous process suggests vertebral involvement by tumor or infection. In patients with low back pain, the examination should include maneuvers that stretch different nerve roots: hip flexion with the knee extended stretches the L5 and S1 roots and may reproduce pain in the back, buttocks,

Table 493–1 ■ CAUSES OF BACK PAIN

	COMMON	LESS COMMON
Mechanical		
Degenerative	Disk protrusion	
	Osteoarthritis	
	Facet syndrome	
	Spinal stenosis	
Congenital	Spinal stenosis	Spondylolisthesis
		Spondylolysis
		Transitional vertebra
		Other structural anomalies
Deformity	Scoliosis	
Muscle	Myofascial syndrome	
	Spasm	
Metabolic	Osteoporosis	Paget's disease
		Gout
Trauma	Compression fracture	
	Lumbosacral/sacroiliac strain	
	Subluxation	
	Muscle injury	
Tumors	Metastatic disease	Benign bone/neural tumors (e.g., meningioma, osteoid osteoma, hemangioma)
	Multiple myeloma	Osteosarcoma
Inflammatory disease	Ankylosing spondylitis	Enteropathic arthropathy
	Arachnoiditis	Psoriatic arthropathy
	Rheumatoid arthritis	
Infections	Herpes zoster	Disk infections
		Epi- or subdural abscess
		Meningitis
Referred pain		Aortic aneurysm
		Cardiac/pericardial disease
		Pelvic or retroperitoneal disease
		Pulmonary/pleural disease
		Visceral disease
Non-organic disease	Anxiety	
	Conversion reaction	
	Psychosis	
	Litigation-related	
	Malingering	
	Chronic pain syndrome	
	Substance abuse	

and posterior thighs, whereas hip extension with the leg straight and the patient prone ("reverse straight-leg-raising sign") stretches the upper lumbar roots and may cause pain in the anterior thigh or medial calf region. Neurologic examination is important, and the presence of any deficits mandates further evaluation. The distribution of any abnormalities suggests the likely site of pathology.

General physical examination is also important in patients with back pain and should include rectal and pelvic examination. When pain is referred to the back and relates to visceral disease, abdominal palpation may reproduce it.

Investigations

In general terms, imaging procedures are not required in patients with uncomplicated neck or back pain of less than 1 month's duration. Imaging studies of the neck or back are required when clinical examination reveals a likely cause, such as a fracture, or when pain does not respond to conservative measures over several weeks. They are important in patients at particular risk for a neoplastic or infectious cause for pain. Imaging studies, especially computed tomography or MRI, may also be helpful in confirming spinal osteomyelitis or tuberculosis and in guiding bone biopsy. Further evaluation will depend upon the nature and extent of the underlying pathology. The presence of a focal or progressive neurologic deficit, or of pain in uncommon sites (such as the lower thoracic region), also requires investigation, usually by MRI. However, many asymptomatic middle-aged or elderly subjects have MRI abnormalities of the spine, and the clinical relevance of any structural abnormalities may therefore be uncertain. Electrophysiologic studies, particularly electromyography and nerve conduction studies, are sometimes helpful in showing the functional significance of anatomical abnormalities and are additionally important as a means of diagnosing a radiculopathy.

Children with low back pain generally require further investigation. Acute pain may relate to developing scoliosis, disk disease, or spondylolisthesis. Diskitis may also be responsible.

MANAGEMENT

If a cervical fracture is suspected following trauma, the neck is immobilized and radiographed (see Chapter 491). Acute hemorrhage may require evacuation, and infection requires antimicrobial therapy and, in some instances, drainage. Even in the absence of confirmatory evidence, a trial of antituberculous therapy may be necessary in those at high risk of spinal tuberculosis, such as the elderly, the immunocompromised, and those who have come from high-risk areas such as the Indian subcontinent.

Patients with ankylosing spondylosis may respond to nonsteroidal anti-inflammatory agents, and should also participate in a vigorous activity program to maintain spinal movement.

If MRI reveals a structural lesion, surgical treatment may be necessary. In the absence of clinical or imaging findings that suggest substantial underlying structural disease, patients with acute pain are treated symptomatically. This involves immobilization, analgesics, and eventually increasing mobilization. There is no agreement as to the optimum duration of bed rest for back pain, but 2 or 3 days is usually adequate. Local heat may help to relieve discomfort.

Many patients with chronic neck or back pain have no surgically remediable lesion, and a multidisciplinary approach is then necessary to ensure that symptoms eventually resolve and that patients are successfully rehabilitated. This may include the use of analgesic, nonsteroidal anti-inflammatory agents, or tricyclic drugs (taken at night), but patients should be encouraged to remain active. The chronic neck pain that sometimes follows whiplash injury has been attributed by some to psychological factors or related to pending litigation, but doubt can be cast on this view, which should not influence management.

Bovim G, Schrader H, Sand T: Neck pain in the general population. Spine 19:1307, 1994. *Epidemiological study.*

Carette S: Whiplash injury and chronic neck pain. N Engl J Med 330:1083, 1994. *Editorial review.*

Deyo RA, Rainville J, Kent DL: What can the history and physical examination tell us about low back pain? JAMA 268:760, 1992. *Clinical review.*

494 INTERVERTEBRAL DISK DISEASE

Michael J. Aminoff

The intervertebral disk that is placed between two adjacent intervertebral bodies consist of a soft, gelatinous, inner nucleus pulposus (a remnant of the notochord) that serves as a shock absorber between adjacent vertebral bodies. It is surrounded by thick fibrous tissue called the annulus fibrosus. With advancing years, the nucleus becomes harder, less resilient, and more susceptible to trauma. Tears tend consequently to develop in the annulus, through which a portion of the nucleus pulposus may herniate. Herniation is generally in a lateral direction and may lead to compression of the nerve roots as they enter the intervertebral foramina, but sometimes occurs centrally, so that either the spinal cord or cauda equina is compressed. In some instances, the protruded disk material loses its continuity with the nucleus pulposus, and becomes a free fragment within the spinal canal.

Disk herniations occur most commonly in the lumbosacral or cervical region. The early recognition of thoracic disk herniations is important, however, because there is only limited space in the thoracic portion of the spinal canal and delay in diagnosis may lead to an irreversible myelopathy.

Pain is common in patients with a herniated intervertebral disk. Neck or back pain may be accompanied by stiffness. Radicular pain may also occur, sometimes before the onset of axial pain. It does not necessarily affect the entire dermatomal territory and may be poorly localized by patients. Patients with cervical disk herniations generally hold their neck stiffly and are most comfortable when recumbent. Pain may be exacerbated by lateral flexion. With lumbar disk herniations, low back pain is accompanied by stiffness, is exacerbated particularly by extension or rotation of the spine, and is relieved by recumbency. With either cervical or lumbar disk herniation, any maneuver that increases intraspinal pressure, such as coughing or sneezing, further exacerbates the pain. Stretch of the compressed roots also aggravates it. Thus passive straight leg raising while the patient is recumbent typically reproduces the pain of an L5 or S1 root lesion, and the femoral stretch test often exacerbates the symptoms of an L4 radiculopathy. In patients with cervical disease, palpation of the brachial plexus and supraclavicular fossa is often painful. A reduced or absent tendon reflex provides objective evidence of root involvement.

There is no agreement concerning the optimal treatment for a herniated disk. Bed rest is often prescribed, but the optimal duration is unclear. Many physicians now recommend rest for 2 or 3 days compared with the 2 weeks that was previously advised. Some authors recommend a brief dose of corticosteroids by mouth, but such an approach has not been validated by extensive clinical trials. Others recommend epidural or subarachnoid injection of corticosteroids, but this is not advised because of the risk of infection or inflammation.

LUMBOSACRAL DISK DISEASE

Protrusion of an intervertebral disk may lead to a radiculopathy. Approximately two thirds or more of all compressive root lesions involve the lumbosacral roots. The L5 and S1 roots are involved most commonly. Multiple lumbosacral radiculopathies may occur with protrusion of a single intervertebral disk that compresses the roots as they descend in the cauda equina. Lumbosacral polyradiculopathies may also result from spinal stenosis, and, in rare instances, from lateral disk protrusion, but bilateral involvement is then often asymmetric.

An L5 or S1 radiculopathy is usually associated with low back pain and sciatica. An L5 root lesion leads to a foot drop, and an S1 lesion to weakness of plantar flexion and eversion. S2 radiculopathies are often bilateral, probably because the sacral fibers are more medially situated in the cauda equina and thus liable to midline compression. With involvement of sacral fibers, disturbances of bladder and bowel function are important complications. Table

Table 494–1 ■ DIAGNOSIS OF LOWER LUMBAR AND SACRAL RADICULOPATHY

	PAIN	WEAKNESS (SELECTED MUSCLES)	SENSORY LOSS	REFLEX LOSS
L4	Across thigh and medial leg to medial malleolus	Quadriceps Thigh adductors Tibialis anterior	Medial leg	Knee
L5	Posterior thigh and lateral calf, dorsum of foot	Extensor digitorum brevis and longus Peronei	Dorsum of foot	
S1	Buttock and posterior thigh, calf and lateral foot	Extensor digitorum brevis Peronei Gastrocnemius Soleus	Sole or lateral border of foot	Ankle
S2–4	Posterior thigh, buttocks and genitalia	Gastrocnemius Soleus Abductor hallucis Abductor digiti quinti pedis Sphincter muscles	Buttocks, anal region, and genitalia	Bulbocavernosus Anal

494–1 summarizes the findings in the most common lumbar and sacral radiculopathies.

A successful response to surgical treatment is common when symptoms correlate with objective physical signs and with an associated structural abnormality that is visualized by imaging. A central disk prolapse may lead to bilateral sciatica and to early sphincter involvement; early investigation is therefore warranted when either of these features is present.

Lumbar spinal stenosis is an important cause of disability in middle-aged or elderly patients. Superimposed minor disk disease then leads to symptoms that may be disabling. The disorder can be either congenital or acquired. The congenital disorder is caused by a reduction in the normal dimensions of the spinal canal and also occurs in achondroplastic dwarfs. Acquired lumbar stenosis is due usually to degenerative disease of the spine, and is typically associated with hyperplasia, fibrosis, and cartilaginous changes in the annulus, posterior longitudinal ligament, and ligamentum flavum. Spondylolisthesis (the anterior or posterior displacement of one vertebral body on the next) or spondylolysis, a defect in the pars interarticularis, may contribute to spinal stenosis, as may other anatomic abnormalities. Acquired stenosis may also relate to injury, bony overgrowth such as occurs in Paget's disease, ankylosing spondylitis, rheumatoid arthritis, and diffuse idiopathic skeletal hyperostosis. Patients present with pain that is brought on by activity and released by rest or leaning forward. The pain involves the lower back and one or both legs, typically in a radicular distribution, and may be accompanied by numbness or weakness. Examination often reveals no abnormality, except perhaps for a depressed knee or ankle reflex. If examination is performed after activity, a radicular motor or sensory deficit is sometimes found. Straight leg raising may be normal. MRI is the most sensitive technique for detecting the disorder. Conservative treatment with nonsteroidal anti-inflammatory medications and exercise to reduce lumbar lordosis are sometimes beneficial. In many cases, however, surgical intervention is the only means of relieving intolerable symptoms.

An *acute cauda equina syndrome* occurs after spinal trauma or central lumbosacral disk protrusions. Patients may present with bilateral sciatica and saddle anesthesia; disturbances of bladder or bowel function are common and are characterized by frequency, retention, or incontinence. The normal sensation associated with the passage of urine or feces may be lost; impotence is common. Examination reveals bilateral root dysfunction and, often, perianal anesthesia and a lax anal sphincter. Investigations involve urgent imaging to define any surgically remedial lesion.

CERVICAL DISK DISEASE

The cervical nerve roots occupy about 30% of the space in the intervertebral foramina that they traverse, accompanied by radicular vessels. The first cervical root exits between the occiput and the C1 vertebra and the subsequent cervical roots exit above their correspondingly numbered vertebra except for the C8 root, which exits between the C7 and the T1 vertebrae (because there is no C8 vertebra). Roots may be compressed by a protruded intervertebral disk or by pathology involving the facet joint or joints of Luschka. Disk herniation is the most common cause, and occurs especially at the C5–6 and C6–7 levels, affecting the C6 and C7 roots, respectively. The mechanism through which these various disorders cause radicular pain is not known. The pain, which often is attributed to compression, angulation, or stretch of the nerve roots, generally subsides with time even though the anatomic abnormality persists and the root therefore remains distorted. Most patients complain of neck or arm pain. Associated paresthesias are often localized poorly. Weakness is sometimes conspicuous. Table 494–2 summarizes the clinical features of the most common cervical radiculopathies.

Although there is considerable variation in the clinical findings between different patients, single root involvement can generally be diagnosed by clinical means. Weakness in a myotomal distribution is assessed by evaluating different muscles supplied by the same nerve root but by different peripheral nerves in order to exclude more distal pathology. Motor and sensory function in the lower extremities, and gait, is also evaluated in order to detect evidence of cord compression.

The Spurling test helps to localize symptoms to the cervical

Table 494–2 ■ DIAGNOSIS OF CERVICAL RADICULOPATHY

	PAIN	WEAKNESS (SELECTED MUSCLES)	SENSORY LOSS	REFLEX LOSS
C5	Neck, shoulder, and interscapular region; lateral arm	Deltoid Spinati Rhomboids	Lateral border of shoulder and upper arm	Biceps (Brachioradialis)
C6	Shoulder; lateral forearm and first 2 digits	Biceps Brachioradialis Extensor carpi radialis	Lateral forearm and first 2 digits	Brachioradialis (Biceps)
C7	Interscapular region, posterior arm, mid forearm	Triceps Extensor carpi and digitorum Flexor carpi radialis	Midforearm and middle digit	Triceps
C8	Medial forearm and hand	Extensor carpi and digitorum Flexor digitorum (sublimis and profundus) Flexor carpi ulnaris	Medial forearm and hand, and 5th digit	Finger flexors (Triceps)
T1	Medial arm to elbow	Intrinsic hand muscles	Medial arm to elbow	

spine. The extended neck is rotated and flexed to the side of symptoms, and careful pressure is then applied to the top of the head in a downward direction. An exacerbation of pain or numbness in the extremity supports a diagnosis of cervical root disease. The maneuver should be discontinued if symptoms are reproduced or exacerbated in this way.

Plain radiographs of the cervical spine may be abnormal, but such abnormalities are commonly encountered in asymptomatic subjects. Electromyography is often therefore important in showing the functional relevance of any anatomic abnormalities detected by imaging studies. MRI is the most useful imaging approach because it gives good delineation of soft tissues.

Treatment is individualized. Many patients improve without surgical treatment and can therefore be managed conservatively. Surgical decompression is necessary in patients with severe pain that is unresponsive to 10 to 12 weeks of conservative measures and in those with a progressive neurologic disturbance.

Cervical spondylosis is a common cause of dysfunction in patients older than 55 years of age. Typically, there is bulging or herniation of intervertebral disks, with osteophytes and ligamentous hypertrophy, sometimes accompanied by subluxation. The underlying primary pathology is usually degenerative disease of the intervertebral disks. This is followed by reactive hyperostosis, with osteophyte formation related to the disk and adjacent vertebral bodies, as well as the facet joints and joints of Luschka. Other associated pathologic factors include thickening of the ligamentum flavum, disk herniation, and a congenitally narrow spinal canal. Ischemia of the cord or roots from compression or distortion of small blood vessels may contribute to the neurologic deficit.

Cervical spondylosis can be categorized by the anatomic location of pathology. The lateral syndrome is characterized primarily by radicular pain and focal neurologic deficits that reflect root dysfunction; gait is usually unaffected. By contrast, the medial syndrome is associated with signs of cord involvement, and especially with pyramidal tract findings in the legs and a gait disturbance. Many patients have both root and cord involvement (combined syndrome). Thus, pain in the neck may be accompanied by a root deficit in one arm, clumsy hand, spastic paraparesis, and gait disturbance. A common presentation is with a spastic paraparesis. Sudden quadriplegia or paraplegia after trivial injuries or a fall in an elderly person is often also due to spondylotic myelopathy. In all of these syndromes, neck movement may exacerbate symptoms. Patients with cervical dystonia often have severe degenerative disease of the spine and are at greater risk of developing spondylotic myelopathy.

Examination often reveals a lower motor neuron deficit in one or both upper limbs, and a pyramidal tract deficit in the legs. Sensory changes are also present in a distribution that depends upon the site of involvement. When sensory findings are inconspicuous, the differential diagnosis of spondylotic myelopathy includes amyotrophic lateral sclerosis. The difficulty in diagnosis is compounded by the common occurrence of degenerative changes in the cervical spine in asymptomatic elderly persons and their coexistence in those with other neurologic disorders. Other causes of spastic paraparesis occurring in middle-aged or elderly persons always have to be excluded. Involvement of the hands in patients with spondylotic myelopathy may either be of the lower motor neuron type in patients with involvement of the C8–T1 segments, or of upper motor neuron type in patients with more rostral pathology. Extreme lateral herniation of a cervical disk may occasionally lead to vertebral artery compression and thus to ischemia in the posterior circulation.

Plain radiographs show disk space narrowing, osteophyte formation, and variable spondylolisthesis. Plain radiographs of the cervical spine in flexion and extension, and surface coil MRI are particularly helpful in diagnosing spinal canal stenosis (anteroposterior canal diameter of less than 11 mm), herniated disks, and intradural pathology. MRI also indicates whether the most prominent compression is anterior or posterior in patients with cervical spondylosis, thereby helping to guide treatment.

Surgical decompression is generally advised in patients with progressive neurologic dysfunction or a fixed deficit of less than 12 months' duration. The value of surgery, however, is uncertain. Surgery may involve either an anterior or posterior approach. The value of various surgical approaches is difficult to determine because the natural history of the disorder is unclear, methods of assessing outcome are not standardized, and postoperative compli-

cations are often not stated. The most optimistic figures suggest that between 15 and 30% of patients do not benefit from surgery, and several older studies indicate that up to 25% of patients worsen following laminectomy. A summary of the literature suggests that between 25 and 75% of patients improve following surgery, and between 5 and 50% worsen following it. Given the uncertainties of the natural history, it is not clear whether benefit relates to surgery or occurs despite it. Regardless of the difficulty in determining its precise value, surgery is now so widely accepted as a therapeutic option that it is difficult to withhold it in patients who are deteriorating despite conservative measures.

Measurement of cervical mobility is helpful in selecting patients who are more likely to deteriorate, because patients with spinal hypermobility are more likely to deteriorate without surgery. Patients without major deficits or whose disorder is non-progressive should be treated conservatively and followed over time. Those with a greater level of disability when first seen are usually referred for surgical treatment, which is also indicated to arrest a progressive course.

Surgical treatment includes posterolateral or anterolateral approaches, as well as laminectomy, foraminotomy and neurolysis, which may be combined with osteophyte excision. The *posterior approach* allows good visualization of affected nerve roots and facilitates removal of any constricting material and allows enlargement of the intervertebral foramen. In patients with diffuse spinal stenosis, laminectomy is the preferred approach, but does not reduce any dynamic forces affecting the cord and may increase cervical mobility, which is associated with an increased risk of neurologic complications. A few patients develop increased radicular or cord deficits following surgery by this approach.

The *anterior approach* permits easier decompression of roots and cord and removal of disk material. In patients with cervical spondylotic myelopathy, herniated disks and osteophytic spurs are indications for surgery by this approach. Fusion is favored by some surgeons, but the need for it is uncertain. Cord or root damage following surgery by the anterior approach occurs in a few instances and other complications have also been described, including esophageal perforation, damage to various nerves (brachial plexus, superior laryngeal nerve, hypoglossal nerve, and sympathetic nerves), epidural hemorrhage, and damage to major blood vessels.

Bernhardt M, Hynes RA, Blume HW, White AA: Cervical spondylotic myelopathy. J Bone Joint Surg 75A:119, 1993. *Review.*
Braakman R: Management of cervical spondylotic myelopathy and radiculopathy. J Neurol Neurosurg Psychiatr 57:257, 1994. *Review.*
Budway R, Senter HJ: Cervical disc rupture causing vertebrobasilar insufficiency. Neurosurgery 33:745, 1993. *Case report and review.*
Ellenberg MR, Honet JC, Treanor WJ: Cervical radiculopathy. Arch Phys Med Rehabil 75:342, 1994. *Clinical review.*
Hardin JG, Halla JT: Cervical spine and radicular pain syndromes. Curr Opin Rheumatol 7:136, 1995. *Review of recent literature.*
Rowland LP: Surgical treatment of cervical spondylotic myelopathy: Time for a controlled trial. Neurology 42:5, 1992. *Reviews the still unanswered questions about the indications for surgery.*

495 INFLAMMATORY DISORDERS INVOLVING THE SPINAL CORD

Michael J. Aminoff

Inflammatory disorders involving the spinal cord are considered in Chapters 473 and 482, and only brief additional comment is made here on aspects related specifically to the cord because surgically remedial lesions must always be excluded by appropriate imaging studies. It is particularly important to exclude a compressive lesion before the neurologic deficit is irreversible in patients with inflammatory disorders affecting the cord directly.

Compression of the spinal cord or nerve roots may occur in consequence of inflammatory diseases. Cord or root involvement may occur in spinal osteomyelitis or tuberculosis, acute or chronic meningitis, inflammatory diseases such as sarcoidosis, and the connective tissue diseases. When the inflammatory process involves the subarachnoid space, root involvement is often multifocal and difficult to explain on the basis of a lesion at one site or level. *Spinal arachnoiditis* may follow the introduction of blood or foreign substances into the intrathecal space, but in some instances arises without obvious precipitating cause. It has sometimes followed epidural steroid therapy or related procedures. It is characterized by neck or back pain, often accompanied by radicular pain at the level of involvement. Cord involvement occurs less commonly but in severe cases may lead to paraplegia. The diagnosis is established by imaging studies, which sometimes reveal evidence of associated cord cavitation. The spinal fluid typically shows an increased protein concentration; in some instances there may be a mild pleocytosis and a reduced glucose concentration. There is no specific treatment other than lysis of adhesions and opening of subarachnoid cysts for spinal arachnoiditis unless an infective organism can be identified.

Acute disseminated encephalomyelitis is an acute monophasic neurologic illness that develops a few days after viral infection (e.g., with measles or herpes zoster) and certain bacterial infections (e.g., with *Mycoplasma pneumoniae*). Patients present with symptoms of encephalitis or myelitis. The myelitis is manifested by a flaccid paralysis of one or more limbs, most commonly the legs, variable sensory loss that may produce a sensory level, and loss of sphincter function. The tendon reflexes are often depressed initially, but the plantar responses are extensor. The cerebrospinal fluid typically shows a lymphocytic pleocytosis and an increased protein concentration. In severe cases, spinal cord necrosis occurs and may be associated with a fatal outcome (acute necrotizing hemorrhagic leukoencephalomyelitis). In patients who succumb, pathologic examination reveals perivenular mononuclear cell infiltration with demyelination; cord lesions are typically subpial in location.

Multiple sclerosis is a disorder characterized by involvement of different regions of the central white matter at different times by an inflammatory process. The disorder commonly begins in young adult life and may follow either a chronic progressive or a relapsing and remitting course. Clinical onset is usually with the acute development of a focal neurologic deficit that worsens progressively over several days and then shows partial or complete remission over several weeks or longer. After a variable interval (from a few days to many years), another attack occurs. With succeeding attacks, remission is often incomplete, so that patients are left with a neurologic deficit that becomes increasingly severe as further attacks occur. In most patients, signs of a progressive myelopathy become increasingly conspicuous with advancing disease; other features are described in Chapter 482. The diagnosis is suggested clinically by a history indicating involvement of different parts of the CNS at different times, and by clinical examination that reveals multifocal white matter disease. MRI of the brain and spinal cord may provide corroborative evidence of diffuse white matter disease, and electrophysiologic studies may similarly show involvement of different afferent systems, thereby confirming the multifocal nature of the disease. Cerebrospinal fluid typically shows an increased IgG content with the presence of oligoclonal bands of IgG. There may also be a mild pleocytosis during exacerbations of the disease. Pathologically, there are areas of demyelination that are initially perivenular in location. Eventually, the spinal cord may become atrophic. Further details of the clinical course, cause, and treatment of the disease are provided in Chapter 482.

Devic's disease refers to an acute myelopathy accompanied by a retrobulbar or optic neuritis. It is unclear whether it is a distinct entity as opposed to a form of multiple sclerosis or acute disseminated encephalomyelitis (see Chapter 482).

Progressive necrotizing myelopathy may occur at any age but is seen especially in young adults, usually after an infectious illness, or in patients with a known malignancy (usually small-cell cancer of the lung or lymphomas such as Hodgkin's disease). Typically, patients present with pain in the back or legs, sometimes accompanied by paresthesias. The legs then become weak and eventually paralyzed. The tendon reflexes are often lost initially, but, after a variable interval, spasticity and hyperreflexia develop. Sensory deficits may be conspicuous, and sphincter disturbances are usual. The disorder follows a progressive course leading eventually to respiratory disturbances and bulbar signs. A somewhat similar disorder

has been described in patients with spinal vascular malformations under the eponym of Foix-Alajouanine syndrome. There is no specific treatment. Pathologic examination shows necrotic areas in the cord, especially in the thoracic region; in long-standing cases the cord is atrophic.

The designation *transverse myelitis* (see Chapter 482) is used for an intrinsic lesion that interrupts most of the large tracts across the greater part of the horizontal extent of the cord at the level of the lesion. The term implies an inflammatory process, but in most instances this has not been clearly established. Transverse myelitis may certainly occur as a feature of multiple sclerosis or Devic's disease, but it usually represents an isolated event occurring after viral infections and in other contexts where the cause is less clear or unknown. Patients typically present with back pain, leg weakness, sensory disturbances below the level of the lesion, and sphincter dysfunction, especially urinary retention. Onset is usually acute or subacute, from a few hours to several days, but the disorder sometimes evolves over several weeks. Weakness is typically associated initially with flaccidity and hyporeflexia, but spasticity and hyperreflexia subsequently develop. A sensory level may be present over the trunk and a band of hyperesthesia sometimes occurs just above this level. High-dosage corticosteroid treatment has been advocated for acute transverse myelitis. Although there are no controlled clinical trials, methylprednisolone 500 mg every 12 hours for 3 days followed by a tapering schedule of prednisone is often used. The prognosis is variable. About one third of patients show no recovery whatsoever; this is especially likely when onset is abrupt, the deficit is severe, or pain is conspicuous at onset. Nevertheless, some patients with a severe transverse myelitis may make a good recovery, and there is no means of accurately predicting the outcome at an early stage.

An acute transverse myelitis sometimes occurs in heroin addicts and usually involves the thoracic cord, although occasionally it has affected other regions. Its cause is uncertain, but the speed of onset suggests a vascular etiology. An acute myelitis may rarely occur in various connective tissue diseases, especially systemic lupus erythematosus. Other causes of an acute cord lesion must always be excluded, including iatrogenic myelopathies (e.g., following irradiation or after intrathecal administration of methotrexate), vitamin B_{12} deficiency, and the myelopathies discussed earlier.

Brammah, TB, Jayson MI: Syringomyelia as a complication of spinal arachnoiditis. Spine 19:2603, 1994. *Case report.*

Kriss TC, Kriss VM: Symptomatic spinal intradural arachnoid cyst development after lumbar myelography. Spine 22:568, 1997. *Case report and review.*

McLain RF, Fry M, Hecht ST: Transient paralysis associated with epidural steroid injection. J Spinal Disord 10:441, 1997. *Case report.*

Mok CC, Lau CS, Chan EY, Wong RW: Acute transverse myelopathy in systemic lupus erythematosus: Clinical presentation, treatment, and outcome. J Rheumatol 25:467, 1998. *Review of clinical series of cases.*

Pascuzzi RM, Shapiro SA, Rau AN, et al: Sarcoid myelopathy. J Neuroimaging 6:61, 1996. *Case report.*

496 VASCULAR DISORDERS INVOLVING THE SPINAL CORD

Michael J. Aminoff

The spinal cord is supplied by the anterior and paired posterior spinal arteries, which are fed by segmental vessels at different levels. The posterior spinal arteries receive numerous feeders along their length. The anterior spinal artery, by contrast, is supplied by only a limited number, but usually by three or more vessels in the cervical and upper thoracic region, one in the midthoracic region between T4 and T8, and caudally by a single large vessel, the artery of Adamkiewicz, which usually arises from a segmental artery between about T9 and L2, most commonly on the left side. The anterior and posterior spinal arteries give off branches that form a fine network around the spinal cord, from which radially oriented branches supply much of the white matter and the posterior horns of the gray matter. The central or sulcocommissural arteries are the main branches at the anterior spinal artery. They originate in varying number at each segmental level, in the anterior longitudinal fissure, and supply one or other lateral half of the cord. Through these vessels, blood is supplied to the gray matter and the innermost portions of the white matter.

The venous drainage of the cord is similarly organized into interconnecting anterior and posterior systems. An anteromedian group of intrinsic veins empties through the central veins into the anterior median spinal vein in the anterior longitudinal fissure. This venous system drains particularly the capillaries of the gray and white commissures, the medial columns of the anterior horns, and the anterior funiculi. The rest of the cord drains through radially oriented veins that connect with the posterolateral venous system running longitudinally on the surface of the cord. The veins on the surface of the cord drain by the medullary veins through the intervertebral foramina, converging there with the radicular veins that drain the nerve roots and with communications from the anterior and posterior epidural and paravertebral plexuses.

ISCHEMIC MYELOPATHIES

Ischemia may contribute to the neurologic deficit that occurs in patients with space-occupying lesions, and those with post-traumatic or postirradiation myelopathies. Wasting of the intrinsic muscles of the hands may result from compression of the anterior spinal artery in patients with lesions of the foramen magnum.

Disease of the abdominal aorta may cause an ischemic myelopathy. Aortic occlusion, dissecting or nondissecting aortic aneurysms, inflammatory aortitis, and emboli involving the aorta may all lead to cord dysfunction, as may surgery involving the aorta, especially in the region of the site of origin of the artery of Adamkiewicz. Imaging studies, such as aortography and mediastinal angiography, can also lead to an ischemic myelopathy. Aortic coarctation of the adult type may cause cord ischemia below the narrowed segment, and neurogenic intermittent claudication may occur because of diversion of blood from the cord by retrograde flow in the anterior spinal artery to bypass the narrowed region. In classic coarctation, a cervicothoracic myelopathy may result from cord compression by enlarged collateral vessels or from a steal phenomenon, and rupture of aneurysmally distended vessels may lead to subarachnoid hemorrhage. Management involves surgical treatment of the coarctation.

Severe hypotension from any cause has been associated with an ischemic myelopathy. The cord is involved particularly in the watershed regions where the anterior spinal artery is most remote from segmental feeding vessels. Some authors regard the midthoracic region as being especially vulnerable to such ischemia.

When acute ischemia leads to a transverse myelopathy, patients present with the sudden onset of a flaccid areflexic paraplegia or quadriplegia, analgesia and anesthesia below the level of the lesion, and retention of urine and feces. Back pain is sometimes conspicuous at the level of the lesion. Curiously, occlusion of the spinal arteries by atherosclerotic or inflammatory processes, by emboli from the heart, or by fragments of nucleus pulposus is rare. Rapid exposure to high altitude or decompression of divers may lead to nitrogen emboli. Pathologic involvement of the posterior spinal arteries is so rare that many authors doubt it can be recognized clinically. The syndrome attributed to it consists of ipsilaterally impaired vibration and postural sense below the level of the lesion, with segmental anesthesia and areflexia. An ipsilateral pyramidal tract deficit, mild and usually transient, also occurs if the lateral funiculus is affected. Anterior spinal artery occlusion, by contrast, is well described and leads to a sudden, severe back pain, sometimes associated with radicular pain; this is followed by the rapid onset of a flaccid paraplegia or quadriplegia, with urinary and fetal retention. With recovery from spinal shock, an upper motor neuron syndrome develops below the level of the lesion, and neurogenic atrophy occurs in muscles supplied from the infarcted segments. A dissociated sensory loss is characteristic, with impairment of temperature and pain appreciation but relative sparing of light touch and joint position sense. The prognosis for recovery is poor, especially if improvement fails to occur within the first 36 to 48 hours.

Venous infarction of the cord occurs most commonly in association with an arteriovenous malformation but occasionally in association with sepsis, malignant disease, or vertebral disorders. Sudden back pain heralds the onset of weakness and sensory loss in the legs, with accompanying retention of urine and feces. The deficit may progress over the next few days to that of an acute transverse myelopathy, and a fatal outcome is not uncommon.

Embolism of nucleus pulposus material has been reported particularly in women, who present with acute neck or back pain followed, within a few minutes, by rapidly progressive limb weakness and sensory loss to all modalities. The cervical region is affected most commonly. Infectious complications may lead to death. Diagnosis in life is usually difficult, but autopsy reveals characteristic emboli in the spinal vessels. The manner in which the fibrocartilage of the nucleus pulposus enters into the circulatory system is unclear.

NEUROGENIC INTERMITTENT CLAUDICATION

The development of pain or a neurologic deficit after exercise or with certain postures that extend the lumbar spine, and their relief by rest or change in posture (leaning forward), has been designated *neurogenic intermittent claudication*. This may involve either the spinal cord or the cauda equina. In contrast to the intermittent claudication of peripheral vascular disease, symptoms typically begin in part of a lower limb and then spread, often in a radicular distribution. Moreover, peripheral vascular disease is typically associated with reduced or absent peripheral pulses, a proximal arterial bruit, and cutaneous evidence of an impaired circulation.

Examination may reveal no abnormalities unless performed while the patient is symptomatic, when motor, sensory or reflex changes may be found. Imaging studies confirm the presence of spinal stenosis or a structural abnormality involving the cord or cauda equina. The most common cause of intermittent claudication of the cord is probably a spinal vascular malformation.

HEMORRHAGE

Hematomyelia (hemorrhage into the spinal cord) or spinal subarachnoid hemorrhage may occur from trauma, spinal vascular malformations, intradural spinal neoplasms, coarctation of the aorta, or ruptured spinal aneurysms. It may be associated with connective tissue diseases, blood dyscrasias, or anticoagulant therapy. In some instances, no cause can be identified.

Spinal subarachnoid hemorrhage is heralded by the onset of sudden severe pain that begins at the site of bleeding but spreads rapidly to the rest of the back and, with cervical lesions, to the head. Dysfunction of the cord or nerve roots may result from compression by blood or blood clot and leads to weakness, sensory disturbances, and impaired sphincter function. Signs of meningeal irritation are present. A spinal bruit or cutaneous vascular malformation suggests the spinal origin of the hemorrhage. CT scan confirms the presence of blood in the subarachnoid space, and MRI may reveal a spinal vascular malformation. When the MRI is unrevealing, myelography is undertaken using a large volume of contrast medium and with the patient examined in both prone and supine positions. The prognosis reflects the cause and severity of the hemorrhage. Decompressive surgery may be necessary. An underlying spinal vascular malformation requires angiographic definition followed by occlusion of feeding vessels by embolization or surgery. Neoplastic lesions may necessitate surgical treatment, while blood dyscrasias, anticoagulant-induced hemorrhage, or connective tissue diseases require appropriate medical management.

Intramedullary hemorrhage also leads to a neurologic deficit, but pain may be less conspicuous, especially if the hemorrhage remains confined within the spinal cord. Further evaluation is as for spinal subarachnoid hemorrhage.

Spinal subdural hemorrhage may occur spontaneously or after trauma or lumbar puncture, especially in patients with blood dyscrasias or receiving anticoagulant drugs. Sudden severe back pain is followed by a compressive myelopathy or cauda equina syndrome. CT scan or MRI is helpful in identifying the underlying lesion. Complete recovery may follow early evacuation of the hematoma, whereas an irreversible neurologic deficit can result from delaying surgery. The risk of spinal subdural hemorrhage is reduced in patients with predisposing hematologic disorders by correcting the underlying abnormality by transfusion prior to lumbar puncture. In patients with thrombocytopenia, platelet transfusion should be considered before lumbar puncture when the platelet count is less than 20,000/mm³ or is dropping rapidly.

Spinal epidural hemorrhage results most commonly from trauma but also occurs in patients with epidural vascular malformations or tumors or with hemorrhagic disorders. It sometimes occurs spontaneously or following spinal tap or epidural anesthesia, especially in patients receiving anticoagulant drugs. Sudden severe back pain, sometimes accompanied by radicular pain, is usually the presenting feature and is enhanced by activities that increase the pressure in the vertebral venous plexus. A cord or cauda equina syndrome then develops after a variable interval. Clinical distinction of epidural from subdural hemorrhage may be impossible. MRI is helpful in detecting the hemorrhage, defining its anatomic site, and distinguishing it from other epidural lesions. Urgent evacuation is necessary to prevent irreversible neurologic damage.

SPINAL VASCULAR MALFORMATIONS

A variety of vascular malformations occur in relation to the spinal cord and meninges. Arteriovenous malformations (AVMs), the most common and clinically important, consist of an abnormal communication between the arterial and venous systems, without intervening capillaries. Telangiectasias and cavernous malformations are uncommon and usually asymptomatic although hemorrhage occasionally leads to a focal neurologic deficit.

Most spinal AVMs are located in the thoracolumbar region, are extramedullary, are supplied by vessels that do not supply the cord, and are so situated that the arteriovenous shunt is actually dural in location. By contrast, 20 to 30% of AVMs are located in the cervical or upper thoracic segments and these are often intramedullary, are supplied by vessels contributing to the anterior spinal circulation, have multiple feeding vessels, and consist of an arteriovenous shunt that is usually of large volume.

Spinal AVMs may present with a subarachnoid hemorrhage or, more commonly, with a myeloradiculopathy. Spinal subarachnoid hemorrhage occurs from about 10% of all spinal AVMs and has an overall mortality of about 15%; approximately half of the survivors of the first hemorrhage will have another unless the underlying malformation is treated. The myeloradiculopathy is typically of gradual onset and progression, but sometimes follows a relapsing and remitting course. Initial symptoms consist most commonly of

pain or sensory disturbances, but by the time of diagnosis many patients have developed a more severe neurologic deficit characterized by weakness, sensory deficits, pain, and impaired sphincter function. Symptoms of neurogenic claudication of the cord or cauda equina are common. With thoracolumbar malformations, examination typically reveals a mixed upper and lower motor neuron deficit in the legs, and a sensory disturbance. With cervical lesions, a mixed motor deficit in the arms is associated with an upper motor neuron deficit in the legs and sensory changes below the level of the lesion. The presence of a spinal bruit is helpful in suggesting the diagnosis, but its absence does not exclude it. The myeloradiculopathy may progress with rapidity and cause severe disability unless the underlying malformation is treated. It probably relates to cord ischemia; venous hypertension causes a reduction in the arteriovenous pressure gradient across the spinal cord and thus a reduction in intramedullary blood flow. An acute onset or exacerbation of symptoms, however, may relate to intramedullary hemorrhage or to intravascular thrombosis. Radicular symptoms presumably relate to ischemia or compression of nerve roots.

MRI permits easy visualization of the spinal cord, but sometimes fails to detect a vascular malformation, in which case myelography should be undertaken when the diagnosis is suspected. The characteristic finding is of serpiginous defects in the column of contrast material as a result of vascular impressions. The examination should be performed using a large volume of contrast medium, and with the patient screened in the prone and supine positions. Spinal angiography is important in defining the anatomic features of the AVM and the normal blood supply to the spinal cord, but is not indicated when myelography fails to suggest an AVM. Depending upon the angiographic findings, either surgical excision, embolic occlusion of feeding vessels, or both, can be undertaken. Treatment may not be possible for AVMs that are anterior to or within the spinal cord and are fed by the anterior spinal artery or one of its feeding vessels. However, interventional radiologic procedures involving the embolization of some of the feeding vessels may still be possible in such circumstances.

Aminoff MJ: Spinal vascular disease. *In* Critchley E, Eisen A (eds): Spinal Cord Disease. London, Springer, 1997, pp 423–442. *Review of clinical features, pathology, and treatment.*

Nelson PK, Setton A, Berenstein A: Vertebrospinal angiography in the evaluation of vertebral and spinal cord disease. Neuroimaging Clin North Am 6:589, 1996. *Review of role of angiography.*

Porter RW: Spinal stenosis and neurogenic claudication. Spine 21:2046, 1996. *Review of clinical and pathologic features and treatment.*

■ DISEASES OF THE PERIPHERAL NERVOUS SYSTEM

497 GENERAL APPROACH TO NERVE DISEASE

John W. Griffin

The peripheral nervous system, through its motor, sensory, and autonomic divisions, serves as a major interface between the central nervous system and the environment. Diseases of the peripheral nervous system, termed *peripheral neuropathies,* are among the most prevalent neurologic conditions. They range in severity from the mild sensory abnormalities found in up to 70% of patients with longstanding diabetes to fulminant, life-threatening paralytic disorders such as the Guillain-Barré syndrome. Differential diagnosis of

peripheral nerve disease can be challenging because the catalogue of disorders that can produce neuropathies is extensive. Although a wide variety of symptoms and signs can result from diseases of the peripheral nervous system, the spectrum of underlying cellular abnormalities is limited, so that only a few clinical or pathologic features are specific to individual neuropathies. Nevertheless, the recent past has seen rapid advances in diagnosis and therapy. An increasing number of nerve diseases are now amenable to treatment, and the peripheral nervous system has a much greater capacity for regeneration and repair than the central nervous system, so that functional improvement is a realistic goal for a lengthening list of neuropathies.

Differential diagnosis in the peripheral nervous system begins with classification of the *clinical features* of the neuropathy and uses elucidation of the *underlying pathophysiologic* characteristics, primarily as reflected in electrodiagnostic tests, as a differential tool. On these bases, the specific laboratory tests that are likely to prove useful can be defined.

FA Davis, 1992. *A highly readable but succinct monograph aimed especially at the general physician.*

498 PATHOPHYSIOLOGY OF PERIPHERAL NEUROPATHIES

John W. Griffin

Normal function of myelinated nerve fibers depends on the integrity of both the axon and its myelin sheath. Nerve action potentials jump from one node of Ranvier to the next. This rapid saltatory conduction depends on the insulating properties of the myelin sheaths. The simplest type of nerve injury is transection of the axon. The axon distal to the site of transection degenerates while that proximal to the injury survives and has the potential for regeneration. As the axon degenerates the myelin in the distal stump is also broken down and cleared. Axonal degeneration due to a focal nerve injury occurs, for example, in severe compression and in focal ischemic injury to nerves. In the symmetrical polyneuropathies, the underlying abnormality is usually a slowly evolving type of axonal degeneration that involves the ends of long nerve fibers first and preferentially. With time, the degenerative process involves more proximal regions of long fibers, and shorter fibers are affected. This pattern of *distal axonal degeneration* or *"dying back"* of nerve fibers results from a wide variety of metabolic, toxic, and heritable causes. The resulting clinical picture includes early loss of the tendon reflex at the ankle, and weakness that initially involves the intrinsic muscles of the feet, the extensors of the toes, and the dorsiflexors at the ankle; the motor signs are accompanied by distally predominant loss of large-fiber sensory modalities such as vibratory sensibility in the toes. With progression, the hands are similarly involved, and the process may spread more proximally up the legs and arms. The resulting pattern of sensory loss is frequently termed a *stocking-and-glove* pattern. Recovery from axonal degeneration requires nerve regeneration, a notoriously slow process.

Demyelination of a peripheral nerve at even a single site can block conduction, resulting in a functional deficit identical to that seen after axonal degeneration. In contrast to repair by regeneration, however, repair by remyelination can be quite rapid. Autoimmune attack on the myelin sheath occurs in the *inflammatory demyelinating* neuropathies and in some neuropathies associated with paraproteinemias. Inherited disorders of myelin are the other major category of demyelinating neuropathy. Uncommon causes include some toxic, mechanical, and physical injuries to nerve. Although these examples have nearly pure demyelination, many neuropathies have an admixture of both axonal degeneration and demyelination. This mixed pathologic spectrum reflects the mutual interdependency of the axons and the myelin-forming Schwann cells.

On the basis of the clinical features alone, it is difficult to predict whether a patient has a predominantly axonal or demyelinating pattern of peripheral nerve injury. Electrodiagnostic tests—nerve conduction studies and electromyography—provide tools for assessing the relative contributions of axonal loss and demyelination. Nerve conduction studies are done by stimulating individual nerves with electrodes at two sites, one proximal to the other, and measuring the velocity of conduction of the action potential between those two sites. In addition, for both sensory and motor nerves, the amplitude of the evoked response can be determined. In general, axonal degeneration decreases the amplitude of the evoked action potential out of proportion to the degree of reduction in conduction velocity, whereas demyelination produces prominent reductions in conduction velocities.

Griffin JW, Hoffman PN: Degeneration and regeneration in the peripheral nervous system. *In* Dyck PJ, Thomas PK, Griffin JW et al (eds): Peripheral Neuropathy, 3rd ed. Philadelphia, WB Saunders, 1993, pp 361–376.
Schaumburg HH, Berger AR, Thomas PK: Disorders of Peripheral Nerve. Philadelphia,

499 IMMUNE-MEDIATED NEUROPATHIES

John W. Griffin

GUILLAIN-BARRÉ SYNDROME (ACUTE INFLAMMATORY DEMYELINATING POLYNEUROPATHY)

The Guillain-Barré syndrome (GBS) is usually characterized by weakness or paralysis affecting more than one limb, usually symmetrically, associated with loss of tendon reflexes and with increased spinal fluid protein without pleocytosis. Since the advent of polio vaccination, GBS has become the most frequent cause of acute flaccid paralysis throughout the world. In the 1960s, the pathologic substrate of many cases of GBS was shown to be lymphocytic infiltration of the spinal roots and peripheral nerves, with macrophage-mediated demyelination and a variable degree of secondary axonal degeneration. On this basis, GBS became virtually synonymous with *acute inflammatory demyelinating polyneuropathy* (AIDP) (Table 499–1). At the present time it seems preferable to retain the clinical term *GBS*, because it is becoming increasingly clear that a small proportion of cases in North America and Europe, and a large proportion of cases in other regions, especially in the developing world, are characterized by noninflammatory acute axonal degeneration. These cases are clinically indistinguishable and have similar spinal fluid profiles. They are termed the axonal forms of GBS.

GBS is almost certainly an immune-mediated disorder. It follows some type of infectious disorder in approximately 60% of cases. The best documented antecedents include infection with *Campylobacter jejuni*, infectious mononucleosis, cytomegalovirus, herpesviruses, and mycoplasma. *C. jejuni* is often associated with more severe "axonal" cases and most likely sensitizes the immune system to antigens shared between the organism and the peripheral nerve.

CLINICAL MANIFESTATIONS. The initial symptoms often consist of tingling and "pins-and-needles sensations" in the feet and may be associated with dull low-back pain. By the time of presentation, which usually occurs within hours or ten days after first symptoms, weakness has usually developed. The weakness is usually most prominently in the legs, but the arms or cranial musculature may be involved first. Tendon reflexes are lost early, even in regions where strength is retained. Because the spinal roots are usually prominently involved, GBS can involve short nerves (axial and intercostal as well as cranial nerves) as well as long ones. Weakness progresses, with the nadir reached within 30 days, and usually by 14 days. Progression can be alarmingly rapid, so that critical functions such as respiration can be lost within a few days or even a few hours.

The potential for respiratory insufficiency, as well as swallowing difficulty and autonomic dysregulation, underlies the life-threatening nature of GBS. In the past, mortality was as high as 15%. With modern critical care and the therapies outlined below, mortality has fallen to about 2%. The first aspect of management is prompt and accurate initial diagnosis. At the time of presentation, a high index of clinical suspicion is necessary. No laboratory test is specific for GBS, but careful electrodiagnostic testing can usually identify at least mild abnormalities during the early stages. Although elevation of the spinal fluid protein level is characteristic, it usually rises only after the first week, not within the first few days when the diagnosis may be uncertain. At the earliest stages, the differential diagnosis includes non-neuropathic conditions such as spinal cord

Table 499–1 ■ GUILLAIN-BARRÉ (GBS) SYNDROME AND RELATED IMMUNE-MEDIATED NEUROPATHIES

DISORDER	TYPE	CLINICAL CHARACTERISTICS	PATHOPHYSIOLOGY	TREATMENT
Guillain-Barré syndrome	Acute inflammatory demyelinating polyneuropathy	Prominent or predominant motor involvement of acute onset	Demyelination, lymphocytic infiltration	Plasmapheresis; intravenous immunoglobulin (IVIg); corticosteroids alone ineffective
	Fisher syndrome	Ataxia, ophthalmoparesis, and areflexia of acute onset	Antibodies against the ganglioside GQ1b	(Probably) plasmapheresis or IVIg
	Axonal GBS	Motor-sensory or pure motor forms	Noninflammatory axonal degeneration predominates; strongly associated with antecedent *Campylobacter jejuni* infection	(Probably) plasmapheresis or IVIg
Chronic inflammatory demyelinating polyneuropathy		Slower onset of weakness and sensory loss; may be recurrent	Widespread demyelination with remyelination, secondary axonal loss; may occur in association with monoclonal gammopathy	Corticosteroids, plasmapheresis, IVIg
Multifocal motor neuropathy		Stepwise involvement of individual nerves; nearly pure motor involvement	Focal demyelination of motor fibers	IVIg or cytotoxic agents (corticosteroids and plasmapheresis ineffective)

diseases (for example, transverse myelitis) and acute neuromuscular junction or muscle diseases.

TREATMENT. Because of the potential for rapid deterioration, patients with a presumptive diagnosis of GBS usually require hospitalization for observation. Monitoring should include frequent measurement of the vital capacity and ability to swallow. Intensive-care observation and insertion of an airway should be initiated early, before declining ventilatory strength, autonomic dysregulation, or fatigue due to unproductive coughing erupts into an acute emergency. Such early intervention largely prevents life-threatening crises. Most of the reduction in mortality in GBS derives from modern intensive care.

Two treatments are of benefit. *Plasmapheresis*—the exchange of the patient's plasma for albumin—was the first treatment definitively shown to shorten the time to recovery. Infusion of high doses of *human immunoglobulin* intravenously also produces benefit. These treatments are equally effective and there is no added benefit to combining them. The choice of modality should be individualized. In patients with limited venous access, gamma globulin is easier to administer. The use of corticosteroids alone is not beneficial. Whether either plasmapheresis or intravenous immunoglobulin is useful in the axonal variants of GBS is undetermined.

Thorough education of the patient about the possibility of rapid deterioration and about the overall favorable prognosis is an important early step. While able to breathe and speak, patients should be instructed in a communication system with nurses and family so that they will be able to make themselves understood if intubation and respiratory support are required.

The prognosis for GBS varies with age, severity, and the extent to which axonal degeneration exceeds demyelination. A middle-aged patient who requires respiratory assistance, and who receives plasmapheresis early in the course, on the average resumes walking about 3 months later (6 months without plasmapheresis). Indeed, many recover much more promptly than that. Relapses, if they occur, should be re-treated with plasmapheresis or gamma globulin.

Arnason BGW, Soliven B: Acute inflammatory demyelinating polyradiculopathy. *In* Dyck PJ, Thomas PK, Griffin JW, et al (eds): Peripheral Neuropathy, 3rd ed. Philadelphia, W.B. Saunders, 1993, pp 1437–1497.

Hartung H-P, Stoll G, Toyka KV: Immune reactions in the peripheral nervous system. *In* Dyck PJ, Thomas PK, Griffin JW, et al (eds): Peripheral Neuropathy, 3rd ed. Philadelphia, W.B. Saunders, 1993, pp 418–444.

McKhann GM, Cornblath DR, Griffin JW, et al: Acute motor axonal neuropathy: A frequent cause of acute flaccid paralysis in China. Ann Neurol 33:333, 1993. *Describes a large epidemic of a GBS variant occurring in an underdeveloped country.*

Ropper AH, Wijdicks EFM, Truax BT: Guillain-Barré Syndrome. Philadelphia, F.A. Davis, 1991. *A thorough analysis of all aspects of the disorder.*

van der Meché FGA, Schmitz PIM, Dutch Guillain-Barré Study Group: A randomized trial comparing intravenous immune globulin and plasma exchange in Guillain-Barré syndrome. N Engl J Med 326:1123, 1992.

Yuki N, Yoshino H, Sato S, et al: Severe acute axonal form of Guillain-Barré syndrome associated with IgG anti-GD$_{1a}$ antibodies. Muscle Nerve 15:899, 1992.

CHRONIC INFLAMMATORY DEMYELINATING NEUROPATHY

Chronic inflammatory demyelinating neuropathy (CIDP), sometimes referred to as chronic GBS, bears similarities to the clinical, pathologic, and laboratory pictures seen in acute GBS. It differs primarily in the time course and in the absence of identifiable antecedent events. The differences in response to therapy, however, suggest that the precise immunopathogenetic mechanisms are likely to differ.

CLINICAL MANIFESTATIONS. CIDP can occur at any age. The usual picture is one of slowly evolving weakness beginning in the legs, with widespread areflexia and loss of large-fiber (vibratory) sensibility on examination. In the more rapidly evolving cases of CIDP, the distinction from GBS is arbitrary. In general, in patients with acute GBS the nadir is reached within 4 weeks, while in patients with CIDP more time is required. The diagnosis is supported by prominent demyelinating features on nerve conduction studies and by elevation of the protein level of the spinal fluid.

TREATMENT. Blinded trials showed that, unlike GBS, most cases of CIDP respond to corticosteroids alone. Some patients with CIDP respond to plasmapheresis and with intravenous gamma globulin. In most instances the first choice of therapy is with corticosteroids, using the lowest dosage required to achieve and maintain an adequate response. Plasmapheresis, while simple and safe, usually must be repeated every several weeks to maintain a response and entails substantial expense. Nevertheless, this form of therapy is valuable in patients who do not respond to corticosteroids or in whom unacceptable corticosteroid doses are required or side effects supervene.

Dyck PJ, O'Brien PC, Oviatt KF, et al: Prednisone improves chronic inflammatory demyelinating polyradiculoneuropathy more than no treatment. Ann Neurol 11:136, 1982.

Dyck PJ, Prineas J, Pollard J: Chronic inflammatory demyelinating polyradiculoneuropathy. *In* Dyck PJ, Thomas PK, Griffin JW, et al (eds): Peripheral Neuropathy, 3rd ed. Philadelphia, W.B. Saunders, 1993, pp 1498–1517.

MULTIFOCAL MOTOR NEUROPATHY

An uncommon related disorder, *multifocal motor neuropathy,* occurs as "pure motor" multiple mononeuropathy. A patient may describe, for example, development of unilateral wristdrop (radial nerve involvement) followed by footdrop on the other side (peroneal nerve involvement). In addition, tendon reflexes may be lost outside the distribution of weakness, but the sensory examination is normal even in weak limbs. The pathologic characteristic, inflammatory demyelination, resembles that seen in CIDP, but is highly focal and largely spares sensory nerve fibers. A characteristic electrodiagnostic feature is the presence of *conduction block,* a reflection of the focal demyelination. The spinal fluid protein is usually normal. A nonspecific but helpful laboratory finding, noted in about 70% of cases, is markedly increased Igm, anti-GM ganglioside antibodies in the serum. Multifocal motor neuropathy is noteworthy because it can be confused with more ominous disorders such as amyotrophic lateral sclerosis, but responds favorably to intravenous immunoglobulin as well as to cytotoxic therapy. Neither corticosteroids nor plasmapheresis brings improvement.

Chaudhry V, Corse AM, Cornblath DR, et al: Multifocal motor neuropathy: Response to human immune globulin. Ann Neurol 33:237, 1993.

Pestronk A, Cornblath DR, Ilyas AA, et al: A treatable multifocal motor neuropathy with antibodies to GM₁ ganglioside. Ann Neurol 24:73, 1988.

NEUROPATHIES ASSOCIATED WITH MONOCLONAL GAMMOPATHIES

Peripheral neuropathy occurs in some monoclonal gammopathies, both the benign type and myeloma. Monoclonal proteins of IgM, IgG, and IgA types are all associated with neuropathy. In some instances the monoclonal protein has been shown to cause the neuropathy. For example, some IgM monoclonal proteins react with sugars found on a specific Schwann cell protein, the *myelin-associated glycoprotein* (MAG). The monoclonal protein intercalates into the myelin lamellae, producing a distinctive pathologic feature, abnormally wide spacing between adjacent myelin lamellae, and consequent demyelination. The neuropathy can be reproduced in experimental animals (chickens) by passive transfer of the monoclonal IgM from patients. A few other nerve epitopes have been defined with which specific paraproteins react. However, for most of the IgG and IgA monoclonal proteins the mechanism of nerve injury is not known.

CLINICAL MANIFESTATIONS. The clinical picture of the neuropathy varies. The IgM monoclonal antibodies with "anti-MAG" reactivity typically produce neuropathy with prominent large-fiber sensory loss and sensory ataxia, as well as milder weakness. The electrodiagnostic tests indicate demyelination, albeit admixed with nerve fiber loss. In other cases with IgM monoclonal proteins there is a distinctive picture that includes scleroderma-like skin changes, hepatomegaly, and endocrine abnormalities, as well as neuropathy (the POEMS syndrome described below). Other individuals with monoclonal proteins have a clinical picture identical to CIDP, and still others have distally predominant axonal degeneration.

Identification of a monoclonal protein does not necessarily mean that the protein is the cause of the neuropathy. Most of the monoclonal proteins found in patients with neuropathy are classed as monoclonal gammopathies of unknown significance, a group alternatively termed benign monoclonal gammopathies because there is no evidence of multiple myeloma at the time of presentation. The incidence of such monoclonal proteins increases with age. Especially in older patients, before the presumption is accepted that the paraprotein causes the neuropathy, it is important to exclude other causes of neuropathy, such as diabetes or alcoholism.

Three disorders should be specifically sought in individuals with paraproteins and neuropathy: (1) There is a special association of neuropathy with solitary plasmacytomas, often osteosclerotic. The POEMS syndrome—polyneuropathy, organomegaly, endocrinopathy (hirsutism, testicular atrophy), monoclonal IgM protein, and skin pigmentation—is highly associated with osteosclerotic myelomas. A skeletal radiographic survey is essential in patients with monoclonal proteins and neuropathy. (2) Cryoglobulinema, with or without monoclonal gammopathy, can produce neuropathy, and the possibility should be excluded. (3) The monoclonal proteins may result in amyloid deposition in nerve and thus produce neuropathy indirectly. Amyloid deposition is particularly associated with excretion of light chains in the urine. The distinctive neurologic picture of amyloidosis often suggests the possibility of amyloid neuropathy (see below). Unlike most other neuropathies, there is a predilection for involvement of small sensory and autonomic nerve fibers, so that the history may include painless injuries to the feet or hands and evidence of autonomic dysfunction, including impotence and orthostatic hypotension. Definitive diagnosis of immunoglobulin-associated amyloidosis is by histology. Fat pad aspiration and muscle biopsy may be useful before undertaking biopsy of rectal ganglia or peripheral nerve.

The one category of paraproteinemic neuropathies in which treatment is clearly beneficial is that of the solitary plasmacytomas.

Excision and radiation of the plasmacytoma can be curative. In other paraproteinemic neuropathies, some reports suggest modest benefit from plasmapheresis or other forms of therapy in neuropathies associated with benign monoclonal gammopathies. In general, however, the degree of improvement is insufficient for the nuisance and expense of therapy. The effort is better focused on gait training and protection from falls. No therapy has been shown to slow progression of amyloid neuropathy associated with paraprotein

Kyle RA, Dyck PJ: Osteosclerotic myeloma (POEMS syndrome). *In* Dyck PJ, Thomas PK, Griffin JW, et al (eds): Peripheral Neuropathy, 3rd ed. Philadelphia, W.B. Saunders, 1993, pp 1288–1293.

Kyle RA, Dyck PJ: Amyloidosis and neuropathy. *In* Dyck PJ, Thomas PK, Griffin JW, et al (eds): Peripheral Neuropathy, 3rd ed. Philadelphia, W.B. Saunders, 1993, pp 1294–1309.

Kyle RA, Dyck PJ: Neuropathy associated with the monoclonal gammopathies. *In* Dyck PJ, Thomas PK, Griffin JW, et al (eds): Peripheral Neuropathy, 3rd ed. Philadelphia, W.B. Saunders, 1993, pp 1275–1287.

IMMUNE-MEDIATED ATAXIC NEUROPATHIES

In this category there are three disorders: *carcinomatous sensory neuropathy, sensory ganglionitis associated with features of Sjögren's syndrome,* and *idiopathic sensory ganglionitis.* All three are characterized clinically by subacute or slowly developing proprioceptive sensory loss leading to gait ataxia and inability to localize arms and/or legs. Patients show rombergism: They can stand with feet together and eyes open, but fall when they close their eyes, reflecting loss of kinesthetic sensibility. Tendon reflexes usually disappear, but strength remains. Pathologic changes in all three disorders include lymphocytic infiltration of the dorsal root ganglia, with destruction of the primary sensory neurons and associated degeneration of their central and peripheral processes. Large sensory neurons are predominantly affected, leaving pain and thermal sensibilities relatively intact. Electrodiagnostic studies document the absence of sensory nerve action potentials and preservation of motor responses. Spinal fluid protein may be normal or contain increased protein. Modest pleocytosis often accompanies the carcinomatous disorder.

The possibility of occult carcinoma underlying an immunogenic (paraneoplastic) ataxic neuropathy adds urgency to differential diagnosis. The most frequent associations include small cell carcinoma of the lung, breast carcinoma, and ovarian carcinoma. In addition to clinical screening for these possibilities, a useful serologic test is the anti-Hu antibody, which reacts with a 37-kD neuronal nuclear protein. Although the presence of anti-Hu antibodies is neither perfectly sensitive nor specific, their association with ataxic neuropathy strongly suggests underlying carcinoma. It should be noted that carcinoma has also been associated with other types of neuropathy, including bland, slowly evolving, sensory motor neuropathy. However, this type of neuropathy is usually an accompaniment of advanced stages of cancer and is rarely a presenting manifestation. The evaluation for occult carcinoma is directed toward those uncommon patients with pure sensory ataxic neuropathy.

Another group of patients with a similar clinical and pathologic picture have features of Sjögren's syndrome, including keratoconjunctivitis sicca and elevated antinuclear antibody titers (Chapter 263). Surprisingly, these patients only occasionally have joint disease or other extraglandular manifestations of Sjögren's syndrome, and most will not have sought medical attention before neuropathy develops. Affected patients are likely to have associated autonomic insufficiency, including pupils that are large and are more reactive to accommodation than to light (Adie's pupils).

A third group of patients with idiopathic sensory ganglionitis have no associated systemic disease. Because this group of disorders often have a very acute onset, they may be misdiagnosed as Guillain-Barré syndrome. This group is referred to as *idiopathic sensory neuronopathy.*

Unfortunately, cytotoxic or corticosteroid therapy only rarely benefits any of these sensory ganglionitis disorders. The gait ataxia produces substantial early disability, but relearning through gait training, rehabilitation, and physical therapy allows a large proportion of affected individuals to resume daily activities.

Griffin JW, Cornblath DR, Alexander E, et al.: Ataxic sensory neuropathy and dorsal root ganglionitis associated with Sjogren's syndrome. Ann Neurol 27:304, 1990.

McLeod JG: Paraneoplastic neuropathies. *In* Dyck PJ, Thomas PK, Griffin JW, et al (eds): Peripheral Neuropathy, 3rd ed. Philadelphia, W.B. Saunders, 1993, pp 1583–1590.

Windebank AJ, Blexrud MD, Dyck PJ, et al: The syndrome of acute sensory neuropathy: Clinical features and electrophysiologic and pathologic changes. Neurology 40: 584, 1990.

VASCULITIC NEUROPATHIES

Peripheral nerves have extensive collateral circulation and are relatively invulnerable to occlusion of large peripheral arteries. By contrast, they are susceptible to focal interruption of circulation within the individual nerve fascicles due to small blood vessel diseases. As a result, many types of systemic vasculitis affect the peripheral nerves. They are one of the most frequently damaged organ systems in polyarteritis nodosa and are frequently involved in rheumatoid arteritis. Sjögren's syndrome, and the vasculitides associated with infections such as hepatitis B, Lyme disease, and HIV. They are less frequently affected in Wegener's granulomatosis because of its restricted regional involvement. The peripheral nerves can be the predominant site of vasculitis, producing a syndrome referred to as vasculitis restricted to the peripheral nervous system. This disorder offers special diagnostic challenges, because the usual footprints of systemic inflammatory disease, including elevated sedimentation rate, are often absent.

CLINICAL MANIFESTATIONS. The clinical manifestations of all of these vasculitic neuropathies reflect the patchiness of the underlying disease. The characteristic picture consists of multiple mononeuropathy, often evolving in a stepwise fashion, so that wristdrop from radial nerve palsy may occur on one side followed by footdrop on the other, with patchy areas of subjective numbness or sensory loss appearing elsewhere on the extremities. The asymmetry and the length-independence of the nerves involved suggest small vessel disease of nerve. In the absence of diabetes mellitus, vasculitis becomes the prime diagnostic consideration. Evaluation of multiple mononeuropathy includes screening of patients to detect evidence of systemic vasculitis in the skin, kidneys, eyes, and other organs. Ultimately, vasculitis is a histologic diagnosis, and if no other organ involvement is identified, combined nerve and muscle biopsy is needed to establish diagnosis.

Treatment of vasculitic neuropathies consists of treatment of the underlying vasculitis. In a neuropathy apparently restricted to the peripheral nervous system, corticosteroids may be tried initially, but most patients require cytotoxic therapy comparable to that used for polyarteritis.

Said G, Lacroix-Ciaudo C, Fujimura H, et al: The peripheral neuropathy of necrotizing arteritis: A clinicopathological study. Ann Neurol 23:461, 1988.

500 HEREDITARY NEUROPATHIES

John W. Griffin

Heritable neuropathies rank among the most prevalent inherited neurologic diseases. Because many occur in midlife and because the family history is often previously unrecognized, the heritable disorders constitute an important aspect of differential diagnosis, of nerve disease.

CHARCOT-MARIE-TOOTH DISEASE

DEFINITION. The eponymic designation, *Charcot-Marie-Tooth* (CMT) disease, identifies a group of heritable disorders of peripheral nerves that share clinical features, but differ in their pathology and the specific genetic abnormalities, as shown in Table 500–1. One group of disorders, classed together as CMT type I (CMT I), is characterized pathologically by abnormalities of peripheral myelination and, at a molecular level, by abnormalities of specific pro-

teins found in the myelin sheaths or Schwann cells. The CMT II group is characterized by axonal degeneration.

PATHOGENESIS. Most forms of CMT disease reflect an autosomal dominant trait, but some similar clinical phenotypes overlap different genetic abnormalities. Several gene abnormalities can cause CMT I (Table 500–1). Three specific gene abnormalities have been identified. The most prevalent is duplication of a segment of chromosome 17 that encodes the peripheral myelin protein-22 (PMP-22) gene. A chromosome 1-linked form is due to an abnormality of another myelin protein, termed P_0. Recently a sex-linked form has been related to abnormalities of the connexin-32 gene. The gene defects in the axonal forms are not yet known.

PATHOLOGY. The pathology of the demyelinating forms of CMT is characterized by excessive numbers of Schwann cells forming concentric rings around nerve fibers. Termed *onion bulbs* because of their appearance on microscopic examination, the wrappings often lead to a palpable and visible increase in the size of certain nerves, such as the ulnar nerve at the elbow or the greater auricular nerve running from the posterior margin of the sternocleidomastoid muscle to the base of the ear. Because of the increase in the size of the nerves, the demyelinating forms of CMT disease are termed *hypertrophic neuropathies.*

CLINICAL MANIFESTATIONS. All forms of CMT disease tend to occur in the second to fourth decades with insidiously evolving footdrop. On examination, there is distal wasting of the intrinsic muscles of the feet, the anterior tibial group, and the calves. A variable degree of impaired large-fiber sensory function is reflected in elevated vibratory thresholds in the toes. Tendon reflexes are lost, at least at the ankles. Typically a foot deformity exists, with high arches *(pes cavus)* and *hammer toes,* reflecting long-standing muscle imbalance in the feet. Upon specific questioning, affected individuals often recall that they were never athletic, that they could not run, jump, or ice skate as well as their peers. Often they report frequent ankle sprains. In general, these problems attract little concern on the part of patients or their families, reflecting the lifelong nature and slow evolution of the disease. Patients can frequently identify several other family members who have similar foot deformities. The most useful diagnostic test lies in the identification of the clinical features in other family members. Even mild or subclinical forms of the disease are usually identified readily on detailed news require examination.

TREATMENT. Most patients with CMT disease enjoy a nearly full spectrum of occupational and daily activities, and they have a normal lifespan. The footdrop can be relieved by appropriate bracing of the ankle. Occasionally, however, the disease produces much greater deficits. Genetic counseling and education of affected individuals and their families is important, both for reassurance and to preclude unnecessary diagnostic evaluation of affected members in future generations.

AMYLOID NEUROPATHIES

All forms of amyloid neuropathy are due to extracellular deposition of the fibrillary protein, amyloid, in peripheral nerve and sensory and autonomic ganglia, as well as around blood vessels in nerves and other tissues. The nonhereditary type of amyloidosis associated with monoclonal immunoglobulins has been described above. Many of the forms of heritable amyloidosis, at one time classified by geographic origin of the first families recognized, have been shown by molecular genetic techniques to represent a variety of point mutations in the transthyretin (prealbumin) gene. The most frequent variant transthyretin protein results from substitution of methionine for valine at position 30 in the molecule. In all forms of amyloidosis, the precise means by which amyloid deposition injures nerve remains unresolved. Mechanical distortion of neurons in the sensory and autonomic ganglia and of nerve fibers, as well as vascular involvement due to amyloid deposition around blood vessels, may both contribute to nerve damage.

CLINICAL MANIFESTATIONS. In all forms of amyloidosis the outstanding abnormalities affect the small sensory and autonomic fibers. Involvement of small fibers responsible for pain and thermal sensibilities leads to loss of the ability to perceive mechanical and thermal injury and tissue damage. As a result, painless injuries present a major hazard of this disorder; in advanced stages they can lead to chronic infections or osteomyelitis of the feet or hands, and

Table 500–1 ■ CHARCOT-MARIE-TOOTH (CMT) AND RELATED HERITABLE NEUROPATHIES

DISORDER	TYPE	CLINICAL FEATURES	PATHOPHYSIOLOGY	INHERITANCE	GENE DEFECT
CMT I		Slowly evolving motor-sensory neuropathies with high arches, hammer toes, hypertrophic nerves	Demyelination and remyelination with onion bulbs		
	a			Dominant	Duplication of a segment of chromosome 17 encoding PMP-22
	b			Dominant	Point mutation in the myelin protein P_0
	x			Sex-linked	Mutation in connexin 32
CMT II		Similar, without hypertrophic nerves	Distally predominant axonal degeneration	Dominant	Unknown
CMT III (Dejerine-Sottas disease)		Early onset, severe motor-sensory neuropathy	Severe hypomyelination with onion bulbs	Recessive	Mutation in P_0

the need for amputation. The autonomic dysfunction produces orthostatic hypotension, impotence, and, in late stages, bladder and bowel incontinence. Until the late stages, strength, touch-pressure sensibility, and vibratory sensation are usually preserved. In some of the heritable forms (as well as in immunoglobulin-associated amyloidosis), median nerve entrapment may occur because of amyloid deposition.

Diagnosis of systemic amyloidosis is made by histologic demonstration of amyloid in biopsy of nerve, muscle, fat aspirate, or other tissue. The heritable forms are normally autosomal dominant, so that the diagnosis may be suggested by family history. The specific genetic abnormality can be identified by molecular genetic analysis. No definitive treatment for any form of amyloid neuropathy is available, but education in prevention of injury to anesthetic limbs can preserve function.

501 METABOLIC NEUROPATHIES

John W. Griffin

DIABETIC NEUROPATHIES

Diabetes is the most frequent cause of peripheral neuropathy worldwide. Incidence figures depend on the employed definition; at least some peripheral nerve abnormalities can be detected in about 70% of patients with longstanding diabetes, and symptomatic neuropathy affects 5 to 10%. The diabetic neuropathies include a variety of clinical forms, including symmetric polyneuropathies, and a variety of forms of individual nerve injury (Table 501–1).

DIABETIC POLYNEUROPATHY

Diabetic polyneuropathy is symmetric and usually distally predominant, beginning with sensory loss in the feet. It is the most frequent of the diabetic neuropathies. It is uncommon at the time of

Table 501–1 ■ DIABETIC NEUROPATHIES

Diabetic polyneuropathies
Rapidly reversible physiologic dysfunction associated with hyperglycemia
Symmetric polyneuropathy
  Sensorimotor neuropathy
  "Small-fiber" neuropathy, with autonomic dysfunction, reduced pain sensibility, spontaneous burning pain
Diabetic mononeuropathies and plexopathies
Diabetic third nerve palsy
Diabetic fourth nerve palsy
Diabetic truncal neuropathy
Diabetic lumbosacral plexopathy (proximal diabetic neuropathy)

diagnosis of diabetes, but its prevalence increases with duration of diabetes. The precise pathogenesis remains a matter of controversy, but a signal recent advance has been the demonstration that, like the ocular and renal complications, diabetic neuropathy can be reduced in incidence and in severity by maintaining blood sugar levels close to normal. This effect of "tight control" is consistent with the hypothesis that hyperglycemia itself contributes to nerve damage. The complications of hyperglycemia that injure nerves may include one or more of the following: abnormalities of nerve vasculature and blood flow, leading to angiopathic injury; metabolic effects of abnormalities in polyol pathways; and nonenzymatic glycosylation of nerve proteins.

CLINICAL MANIFESTATIONS. The neuropathy is usually asymptomatic at the onset, a stage during which abnormalities in sensation and reflexes may be detected on routine examination. The symptomatic phase usually begins insidiously, but some cases have an abrupt onset, and in a small percentage of patients this appears to be precipitated by the institution of insulin. Unlike most other neuropathies, in diabetes small-fiber sensibility as well as large-fiber sensation are typically reduced, resulting in elevated pin, thermal, and vibratory thresholds. The small-fiber dysfunction is often manifested by spontaneous neuropathic pain. This includes bothersome *dysesthesias*—unpleasant sensations evoked by normally innocuous stimuli, such as the bedsheets on the toes at night. There may be continuous burning or throbbing pain, and walking often is distressing ("It feels like I'm walking on coals."). In addition, sudden intense "lightning" pains may affect the feet and legs.

Some degree of autonomic insufficiency is frequent in diabetic neuropathy. Manifestations include loss of the normal sinus arrhythmia; failure of blood pressure restoration and cardiac acceleration on standing, sometimes producing orthostatic hypotension; impotence; constipation; and a particularly distressing symptom, diabetic diarrhea, with unpredictable loose stools and fecal incontinence. In some patients, these "small-fiber" abnormalities, including neuropathic pain, loss of pin and thermal sensibility, and autonomic dysfunction, dominate the clinical picture.

The diagnosis of diabetic polyneuropathy is straightforward in established diabetics with typical clinical pictures. Electrodiagnostic studies, usually unnecessary, document neuropathy, and spinal fluid protein is frequently moderately elevated. Conversely, diabetic neuropathy is the most *overdiagnosed* cause of peripheral nerve disease. In general, the diagnosis of diabetic neuropathy can comfortably be made only in the setting of longstanding diabetes, usually insulin-requiring. If only recent mild hyperglycemia is present, the diagnosis of diabetic polyneuropathy should be regarded as suspect. In addition, diabetic neuropathy alone seldom results in severe painless weakness.

TREATMENT. The approach to management of diabetic hyperglycemia is outside the scope of this chapter, but there is increasing reason to think that primary prevention as well as slowing of the progression of established diabetic neuropathy is abetted by correction of blood sugar to as nearly normal values as possible ("tight control"; see Chapter 267). Once the diagnosis of diabetic polyneuropathy is established, no other specific treatment for the neuropathy is currently available. Symptomatic management includes use of tricyclic antidepressants or anticonvulsants such as gabapentin or carbamazepine for the spontaneous neuropathic pain. Full therapeutic doses are required, and the dosage must be slowly increased to minimize side effects such as dizziness. Opiates are usually contraindicated.

The major goal in management of diabetic polyneuropathy is prevention of the cycle of painless injury, ulceration, cellulitis, and osteomyelitis, that underlies much of the functional disability produced by this disorder and that contributes to an ultimate requirement for amputation. The loss of pain sensibility on examination should trigger increased vigilance. Painless injuries can largely be prevented by education, avoidance of physical and thermal hazards to the feet, well-fitting shoes, and frequent inspections of the feet. Erythema or injury is treated promptly with removal of the aggravating factor, such as an ill-fitting shoe. Cessation of weight bearing until healing occurs can minimize ulceration. Meticulous skin and nail care are required.

One of the most distressing aspects of the autonomic neuropathy is impotence. Exclusion of other causes, particularly offending medications, as well as behavioral strategies are important. A variety of methods are helpful to some patients. Other genitourinary disturbances include retrograde ejaculation and disordered micturition. Milder cases of diabetic diarrhea may respond to agents such as diphenoxylate.

MONONEUROPATHY AND MULTIPLE MONONEUROPATHIES

Diabetes also can cause a variety of mononeuropathies and multiple mononeuropathies. They probably represent vascular insufficiency or infarction in nerve, presumably caused by disease of the small blood vessels. Their onset is typically abrupt and often painful.

CLINICAL MANIFESTATIONS. A stereotyped disorder is *diabetic third nerve palsy,* characterized by sudden inability to adduct the eye or open the lid. Unlike third nerve compression from intracranial masses or carotid aneurysms, the pupil is typically spared. The sixth nerve, the femoral nerve, or other major nerves of the extremities, may be similarly involved.

In another characteristic syndrome, termed *diabetic lumbosacral plexopathy* or *proximal diabetic neuropathy,* affected persons develop pain in the hip with asymmetric weakness of the proximal leg muscles over days to a few weeks. The disorder often occurs in a setting of recent severe (> 10%) loss of body weight and frequently appears to be a "femoral" neuropathy, with quadriceps weakness and loss of the tendon reflex at the knee. Careful examination, however, usually discloses more widespread involvement of muscles innervated by the lumbosacral plexus, typically including the hamstring and gluteus muscles. Although the complaints may be referable to one side, mild abnormalities often affect the contralateral side. In addition, evidence of more symmetric polyneuropathy, with reduced tendon reflexes of the ankles, elevated sensory thresholds, and often weakness of toe extension and ankle dorsiflexion, may exist. The limited pathologic data available suggest that this is a consequence of small vessel disease in the lumbosacral plexus, perhaps amplified by associated atherosclerotic disease in the aortic bifurcation. In any event, the prognosis is surprisingly favorable; pain decreases, and strength returns to the affected muscles within weeks to months. At the onset this disorder can be confused with intraspinal disease or polyradiculopathy. Diabetic lumbosacral plexopathy is sometimes called diabetic amyotrophy, but this term is best avoided, because it has also been applied to a syndrome of widespread muscle wasting that occasionally develops in diabetics in association with a period of weight loss. A final noteworthy mononeuropathy is *diabetic truncal neuropathy.* Patients have pain in the distribution of one or more intercostal nerves, often associated with hypesthesia and numbness. Like the other diabetic mononeuropathies, recovery over months is the rule.

Dyck PJ, Karnes JL, Daube J, et al: Clinical and neuropathological criteria for the diagnosis and staging of diabetic polyneuropathy. Brain 108:861, 1985.

Johnson PC, Doll SC, Cromey DW: Pathogenesis of diabetic neuropathy. Ann Neurol 19:450, 1986.

Max MB, Culnane M, Schafer SC, et al: Amitriptyline relieves diabetic neuropathy pain in patients with normal or depressed mood. Neurology 37:589, 1987.

HEPATIC NEUROPATHY

Polyneuropathy is sufficiently uncommon in chronic liver disease that other underlying causes that can affect both liver and peripheral nerves (alcoholism, primary biliary cirrhosis) should be sought.

THYROID DISEASE

Myxedema neuropathy is usually a minor manifestation of myxedema, but areflexia and distal sensory loss can be seen. Cerebellar ataxia and behavioral changes usually predominate.

UREMIC NEUROPATHY

This peripheral neuropathy is associated with chronic renal insufficiency. Electrophysiologic abnormalities routinely occur when creatinine clearance is less than 10% of normal, but the severity and rate of progression of symptomatic uremic polyneuropathy vary widely. The syndrome usually consists of distally predominant, symmetric, motor-sensory polyneuropathy. In some patients, there is marked motor predominance, so that footdrop and leg weakness are major manifestations. In others, paresthesias and, occasionally, burning dysesthesias are early symptoms. In either event, loss of tendon reflexes, initially at the ankle, is characteristic. Electrophysiologic and pathologic studies indicate that both distal axonal degeneration and demyelination occur in uremic neuropathy, but the precise underlying mechanisms remain uncertain.

An important outcome of the past 30 years' experience with dialysis and renal transplantation is recognition that this peripheral neuropathy is both preventable and treatable by amelioration of the renal insufficiency. While both approaches are helpful, renal transplantation produces much better preservation of peripheral nerve function.

PORPHYRIC NEUROPATHY

The intermittent porphyrias, considered fully in Chapter 219, are important diagnostic considerations in acute neuropathies. The most prevalent of these disorders, acute intermittent porphyria (AIP), is associated with recurrent episodes of neuropathy, which are typically acute or subacute in onset. Paresthesias and dysesthesias of the extremities occur and in severe episodes are associated with rapidly evolving weakness or paralysis, mimicking the axonal form of Guillain-Barré syndrome, often associated with bladder dysfunction and constipation. The associated CNS effects may contribute to alterations in level of consciousness as well as hysteria-like or psychotic behavior, potentially delaying recognition of the emergent nature of the neuropathy. During acute attacks, most patients with AIP have increased excretion of porphobilinogen and delta-aminolevulinic acid in the urine. This simple diagnostic assay should be considered in any patient with acute paralytic neuropathy. The treatment of acute porphyria attacks is described in Chapter 219.

CRITICAL CARE NEUROPATHIES

The term "critical care neuropathy" is often used in patients following a severe medical illness, complicated by sepsis, and requiring prolonged intensive care. In a small proportion of patients, the only process that can be defined is axonal degeneration. Many of the cases that follow use of muscle relaxants and corticosteroids now appear to reflect primary changes in the muscle rather than the nerves ("quadriplegic myopathies"). The etiology is unclear, and no effective therapy other than time and adequate nutrition is known. Most affected persons recover completely.

502 TOXIC NEUROPATHIES

John W. Griffin

A wide array of environmental, occupational, recreational, and pharmaceutical agents can produce peripheral nerve disease. For

Table 502–1 ■ PHARMACEUTIC NEUROTOXINS

Amiodarone
Antiretrovirals (ddI, ddC)
Chloramphenicol
Cisplatin
Clioquinols
Dapsone
Disulfiram (Antabuse)
Ethambutol
Ethionamide
Gold
Hydralazine
Isoniazid
Metronidazole and misonidazole
Nitrofurantoin
Penicillamine
Perhexiline
Phenytoin (rare)
Pyridoxine (in excessive amounts)
Stilbamidine
Suramin
Thalidomide
Vincristine/vinblastine

agents in which the period of exposure is limited, the diagnosis is often suggested by subacute neuropathy. Most, although not all, neurotoxins produce distal axonal degeneration. The picture typically includes distally predominant sensory loss, loss of tendon reflexes at the ankles, and distal weakness. With continued exposure, the symptoms may progress more proximally; even after the offending agent is withdrawn, progression sometimes may continue, a phenomenon termed *coasting*. Nevertheless, withdrawal represents the optimal treatment. Tables 502–1 and 502–2 list important pharmaceutical and environmental toxins.

Persons with pre-existing nerve disease may be unusually susceptible to neurotoxins. For example, those with Charcot-Marie-Tooth disease can experience devastating toxic reactions to standard level chemotherapeutic doses of vincristine. In all toxic neuropathies the key to treatment lies in prompt recognition and withdrawal.

Schaumburg HH, Berger AR, Thomas PK: Disorders of Peripheral Nerve, 2nd ed. Philadelphia, F.A. Davis, 1992.

ALCOHOL-NUTRITIONAL NEUROPATHY

Polyneuropathy in persons with chronic alcoholism usually occurs in a setting of associated nutritional deficiency (see Chapter 456). Most persons with alcoholic neuropathy have evidence of multifactorial nutritional deficiency, but in some, nutritional background seems adequate, and the direct contribution of alcohol cannot be excluded. The pathology of alcohol-nutritional neuropathy is that of a bland "dying back" disorder affecting both sensory and

Table 502–2 ■ INDUSTRIAL AND ENVIRONMENTAL NEUROTOXINS

Metals
Arsenic
Lead
Mercury
Thallium
Substance abuse
Alcohol
Glue (hexacarbons) inhalation
Nitrous oxide inhalation
Industrial poisons
Acrylamide
Carbon disulfide
Cyanide (chronic)
Dichlorophenoxyacetic acid
Dimethylaminopropionitrile
Ethylene oxide
Hexacarbon (n-hexane) (glue sniffer, occupational exposure to solvents, glues, or glue thinner)
Organophosphorus esters (triorthocresyl phosphate, leptophos, mipafox, trichlorphon)
Polychlorinated biphenyls
Tetrachlorbiphenyl
Trichloroethylene (trigeminal neuropathy)

motor fibers. The initial symptoms are pain and paresthesias, beginning on the soles of the feet, sometimes evolving to burning feet and severe hyperpathia and often associated with aching and tenderness of the calves. Weakness is seldom severe and invariably distal, and tendon reflexes are lost first at the ankles. Treatment with nutritional supplementation, including thiamine and multivitamins, and cessation of alcohol ingestion are highly beneficial in the early stages of the disease. In advanced cases the disease may continue to progress for a period after initiation of therapy, and recovery may be incomplete.

503 NEUROPATHIES ASSOCIATED WITH INFECTIOUS DISEASES

John W. Griffin

HUMAN IMMUNODEFICIENCY VIRUS (HIV) INFECTION

A variety of nerve diseases can accompany HIV infection (see also Chapter 479). The *Guillain-Barré syndrome* (GBS) and *chronic inflammatory peripheral neuropathy* (CIDP) tend to occur early in HIV infection, when CD4 counts are 250 to 500, and before development of AIDS. They presumably reflect early immune dysregulation. They are distinguished by the frequent presence of pleocytosis, an uncommon finding in seronegative GBS and CIDP. Their course and response to treatment are similar to those observed in seronegative patients.

Cytomegalovirus (CMV) infection of nerve occurs in the setting of clinically evident AIDS and in association with systemic CMV infection. CMV can produce multiple mononeuropathy associated with focal infection of endothelial cells of the nerve, macrophages, and Schwann cells. A dramatic and potentially treatable disorder is *CMV polyradiculopathy*. It develops in persons with AIDS and is characterized by abrupt pain in the back and legs with rapidly progressing paraparesis and areflexia. A distinctive finding is polymorphonuclear pleocytosis, usually associated with markedly increased spinal fluid protein. Cytologic examination sometimes can identify CMV inclusions in spinal fluid. The differential diagnosis includes herpesvirus-associated transverse myelopathies. Prompt diagnosis of CMV polyradiculopathy is important, because some patients respond well to antiviral therapy with ganciclovir or foscarnet.

The most prevalent neuropathic complication of HIV infection is *sensory neuropathy of AIDS*. In advanced AIDS, affected patients typically complain of pain on the soles of the feet and discomfort while walking. Neuropathic pain may be intense, associated with loss of small and large-fiber sensory modalities, with a variable, usually mild, degree of motor impairment. Typically the reflexes are lost at the ankle but exaggerated at the knees. This pattern reflects both neuropathy and a CNS disease such as vacuolar myelopathy. Pathologic studies of the sensory neuropathy have shown noninflammatory distally predominant axonal degeneration of sensory fibers. Both large and small fibers are lost. The pathogenesis is unknown, but the disease does not appear to be produced by local productive HIV infection within the nerves themselves. The treatment is symptomatic.

Griffin JW, Wesselingh SL, Griffin DE, et al: Peripheral neuropathies in HIV infection: Similarities and contrasts with the central nervous system. In HIV, AIDS, and the Brain. Association in Research on Nervous and Mental Disease Proceedings, Vol 92. New York, Raven Press, 1994.

LYME DISEASE (BORRELIOSIS)

Neuropathic consequences can predominate in some patients with Lyme disease (see Chapter 368). The geographic area of the patient as well as history of the characteristic antecedent rash may suggest the diagnosis. The neuropathy is usually a multiple mononeuropathy, with a high predilection of facial nerve involvement, mimicking idiopathic Bell's palsy.

LEPROUS NEUROPATHY (See Chapter 360)

The clinical manifestations of leprosy are virtually exclusively those of peripheral neuropathy and its sequelae. Although WHO has set a target for eradication of active leprosy by the year 2000, at least 2.5 million individuals with residual disease will remain worldwide. In all forms of leprosy, infection of the skin with *Mycobacterium leprae* and destruction of cutaneous nerve fibers are the primary events. The major classes, *lepromatous* and *tuberculoid,* differ in the extent of postimmune response to the organism.

In *lepromatous leprosy,* no effective cellular immune response is mounted, and large numbers of bacilli reside within the skin, where they infect predominantly the Schwann cells of intracutaneous nerves. With time, Schwann cells throughout the peripheral nervous system are affected, with a striking distribution of nerve fiber damage related to environmental temperatures. Organisms proliferate in the nerve fibers in the coolest regions of the skin, such as the ears, the lateral area of the face, and the digits, before they affect warmer areas covered with clothing. The resulting cutaneous sensory loss includes strikingly selective loss of pain sensibility.

The other major form of the disease, *tuberculoid leprosy,* is characterized by an active inflammatory response to the organism with much of the nerve damage probably resulting from the immune response. Tuberculoid disease and the intermediate form, *borderline disease,* produce a less stereotyped, more patchy and asymmetric neuropathy.

Painless injuries and painless traumatic joint diseases are the major sequelae of both forms of leprosy. Recent data have shown that chemotherapy for leprosy is associated with regeneration of nerve fibers. In general, however, nerve fibers do not successfully reinnervate the skin, so that cutaneous anesthesia and its complications persist. In addition to chemotherapy, education and protection from painless injuries, as described for diabetic polyneuropathies, can substantially modify the outcome.

Miko TL, Le Maitre C, Kinfu Y: Damage and regeneration of peripheral nerves in advanced treated leprosy. Lancet 342:521, 1993.
Sabin TD, Swift TR, Jacobson RR: Leprosy. *In* Dyck PJ, Thomas PK, Griffin JW, et al (eds): Peripheral Neuropathy, 3rd ed. Philadelphia, W.B. Saunders Company, 1993, pp 1354–1379.

504 ENTRAPMENT AND COMPRESSIVE NEUROPATHIES

John W. Griffin

The peripheral nerves are vulnerable to chronic compression or entrapment in a variety of sites. The most frequently encountered are median nerve compression at the wrist within the carpal tunnel *(carpal tunnel syndrome);* median nerve compression in the upper forearm; ulnar nerve compression in the hand *(cubital tunnel syndrome),* wrist, or at the elbow *(tardy ulnar nerve palsy);* tibial nerve compression behind the medial malleolus *(tarsal tunnel syndrome);* and peroneal nerve compression over the lateral fibular head. Because of its prevalence, carpal tunnel syndrome deserves specific comment.

CARPAL TUNNEL SYNDROME

Entrapment of the median nerve at the wrist reflects the limited available space for the median nerve because of the surrounding bone, joint, and ligaments, as well as the tendons and synovium passing through the canal. Repetitive motion of the fingers is a highly publicized exacerbating element, but other precipitating factors that should be considered include trauma, osteoarthritis, ganglionic cysts, myxedema, and rarely, amyloid deposition. Mild symptoms typically involve paresthesias of the first three digits, often occurring overnight and relieved by shaking or elevating the hands. In more severe disease, objective sensory loss in the median nerve distribution, weakness of median-innervated muscles such as the abductor pollicis brevis, and prolongation of nerve conduction across the carpal tunnel (prolonged distal latency) are characteristic. The diagnosis is supported by identification of *Tinel's sign,* in which tapping the carpal tunnel elicits paresthesias in the median nerve distribution, and by paresthesias produced by sustained flexion of the wrist.

The treatment of carpal tunnel syndrome requires consideration of the relationship between symptoms and occupational or recreational activities. Treatment begins with splinting of the wrist in slight dorsiflexion during sleep, thereby increasing the cross-sectional area of the carpal tunnel. Injection of corticosteroids into the carpal tunnel and use of potassium-sparing diuretics are helpful in some patients. More severe carpal tunnel syndrome is treated surgically by release of the carpal ligament.

BELL'S PALSY

Unilateral facial paralysis of acute onset frequently occurs on an idiopathic basis (Bell's palsy). The etiology and pathophysiology remain unknown. The diagnosis is one of exclusion: facial nerve palsies also occur in the setting of *herpes zoster oticus,* in which they are typically associated with otalgia and varicelliform lesions affecting the external ear, ear canal, or tympanic membrane. Facial paralysis of a lower motor neuron type can be caused by *infiltrative disease in the meninges,* such as carcinomatous meningitis, and by *inflammatory diseases* such as sarcoidosis and Lyme disease. *Primary tumors of the facial nerve* can occur with apparently rapidly developing facial paralysis, although often in retrospect more subtle facial asymmetry had developed over a longer period. Facial paralysis can also occur in primary *CNS disease* affecting the pontomedullary junction, such as multiple sclerosis. Facial palsy has been noted in individuals with HIV infection, particularly in the early stages shortly after initial infection.

These considerations excluded, most cases of facial paralysis reflect idiopathic Bell's palsy. Patients typically notice facial paralysis on inspection in the mirror in the morning, and the disorder appears to come on overnight in many instances. Onset of facial paralysis may be heralded or accompanied by pain behind the ear (in the region of the stylomastoid foramen). The severity of paralysis varies widely. The prognosis can to some extent be predicted by electrophysiologic examination of the facial nerve after the first several days. In most cases, prognosis is quite favorable. Some believe that a course of oral corticosteroids with rapid tapering may improve the prognosis and is widely used, but this has never been verified. In severe cases, protection of the cornea from drying and injury is essential.

TRIGEMINAL NEURALGIA (TIC DOULOUREUX)

Trigeminal neuralgia is a recurring pain syndrome in which episodes of abrupt stabbing pain involve the second or third divisions of the trigeminal nerve. This and other painful cranial neuralgias are discussed in Chapter 455.

■ DISEASES OF MUSCLE (MYOPATHIES)

505 GENERAL APPROACH TO MUSCLE DISEASES

Richard J. Barohn

INTRODUCTION

Diseases of skeletal muscle, termed *myopathies,* are disorders in which there is a primary structural or functional impairment of muscle. Myopathies therefore do not include diseases of the central nervous system (CNS), lower motor neurons (motor neuron disease), peripheral nerves, or neuromuscular junction that secondarily produce muscle weakness. Myopathies can be differentiated from other disorders of the motor unit by characteristic clinical and laboratory findings. In addition, the disorders of muscles can be categorized and subdivided so that it is generally possible to recognize a particular myopathy on the basis of its distinctive features.

Myopathies can be broadly classified into hereditary and acquired disorders (Table 505–1).

ORGANIZATION AND STRUCTURE OF MUSCLE

A single *motor unit* consists of four components: (1) a motor neuron, (2) its peripheral axon and terminal branches, (3) the neuromuscular junctions at each terminal nerve ending, and (4) all of the skeletal muscle fibers innervated by the axon. The number of muscle fibers innervated by a single motor unit varies from muscle to muscle. Muscles subserving finely coordinated movements, such as ocular muscles, can have fewer than 10 muscle fibers in a motor unit. Powerful proximal limb muscles have large motor units with 1000 or 2000 fibers innervated by a single motor neuron. Individual fibers from different motor units intermingle randomly in the muscle. The muscle also contains connective tissue and blood vessels. All of these tissues can be affected in certain myopathic disorders.

The muscle fibers consist of thick and thin filaments (myofibrils) that are arranged in repeating units, or *sarcomeres,* limited by Z disks. The *thin filaments* (actin, troponin, and tropomyosin) are anchored to the Z disks and interdigitate between the *thick filaments* (myosin) in the central region (A band) of the sarcomere. The myofibrils are associated with transverse (T) tubules, sarcoplasmic reticulum (SR), glycogen, and mitochondria. The head of each myosin molecule acts as a cross-bridge between myosin and actin. T tubules are inward projections of the muscle fiber surface membrane and serve to propagate the action potential into the muscle fiber. The SR contains calcium and partially surrounds the T tubules. The depolarization of T tubules triggers the opening of calcium channels and the release of calcium from the SR into the myofilament space. Calcium then binds to troponin on the thin filaments, which acts on tropomyosin to allow repeated binding of

the myosin cross-bridges to actin. The conformational change in the myosin-actin cross-bridge moves the thin filaments toward the center of the sarcomere and the Z disks are pulled closer together, producing muscle fiber contraction. This contraction is an energy-dependent process that requires adenosine triphosphate (ATP), which is split by an ATPase on the cross-bridge.

The myofibrils and associated constituents are surrounded by the sarcolemmal membrane and basal lamina (Fig. 505–1). A great deal of attention has been focused on this aspect of muscle as a number of muscular dystrophies are now known to be due to genetic defects in this region. The sarcolemmal components are known as the *dystrophin-glycoprotein complex* (DGC). The DGC is a transsarcolemmal complex of proteins and glycoproteins that link the subsarcolemmal cytoskeleton to the extracellular matrix. The role of the DGC is to provide structural support to the sarcolemma during muscle contraction and stretch. In addition, the DGC may have a role in the regulation of intracellular calcium concentration and in signal transduction.

Dystrophin was the first well-characterized protein in the DGC. Dystrophin is a rod-shaped molecule on the cytoplasmic side of the skeletal and cardiac sarcolemma. It consists of an amino-terminal domain that binds to the cytoskeletal thin actin filaments. The midrod domain and the carboxy-terminal domain are important in linking dystrophin to the other glycoproteins of the DGC. These DGC components are the *dystroglycan* complex (α, β), the *sarcoglycan* complex (α, β, γ, δ), and the *syntrophin complex* (α, β1, β2). The exact relationships among all of the components of the DGC are still under investigation.

Closely adherent to the extracellular portion of the sarcolemma is the basal lamina, which is composed of collagen types I and IV, heparin sulfate proteoglycan, entactin, fibronectin, and laminin. *Laminin* is a heterotrimer composed of α, β, and γ chains held together by disulfide bonds. *Merosin* is the collective name for laminins that share a common α2 chain. α-Dystroglycan binds to laminin, anchoring the basal lamina to the sarcolemma.

Integrins are another group of transmembrane proteins distinct

Table 505–1 ■ CLASSIFICATION OF MYOPATHIES

Hereditary
 Muscular dystrophies
 Congenital myopathies
 Myotonias and channelopathies
 Metabolic myopathies
 Mitochondrial myopathies
Acquired
 Inflammatory myopathies
 Endocrine myopathies
 Myopathies associated with systemic illness
 Drug induced/toxic myopathies

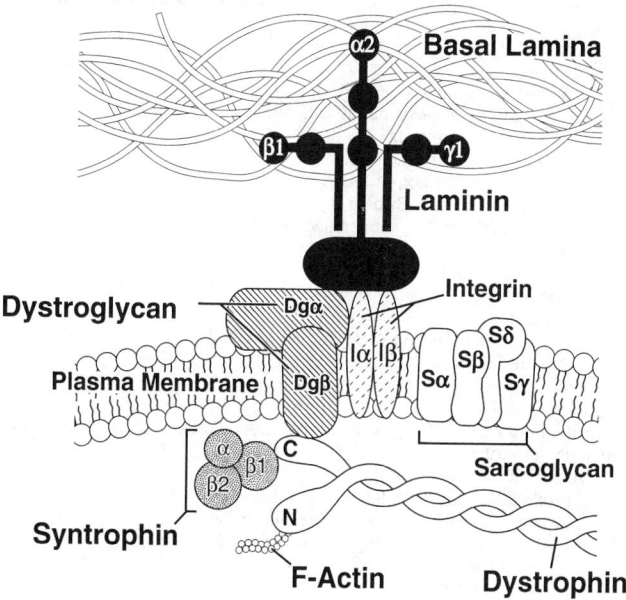

FIGURE 505–1 ■ The dystrophin-glycoprotein complex and related proteins.

from the DGC that link the extracellular matrix to the sarcolemma. Integrins also bind merosin to skeletal muscle, and this interaction appears to be as important as the α-dystroglycan linkage in providing structural stability. Integrins are also important in transducing signals from the extracellular matrix to the cell.

CLINICAL ASSESSMENT

The most important aspect of evaluating a patient with a myopathy is the information obtained from the history. After taking the history, the physician should formulate a reasonable preliminary diagnosis that places the patient into one of the categories in Table 505–2. The findings on the physical examination, in particular the pattern of weakness, help further define the diagnosis. The results of the laboratory studies (blood tests, electromyogram, muscle biopsy, molecular studies) serve to confirm the preliminary diagnosis arrived at from the history and physical examination.

HISTORY. Symptoms of muscle disease can be divided into "negative" and "positive" complaints.

NEGATIVE SYMPTOMS. The most common symptom of a patient with muscle disease is *weakness*. If the weakness is in the legs, patients will complain of difficulty in climbing stairs and rising from a low chair or toilet or from the floor. When the arms are involved, patients notice trouble lifting objects (especially over their head) and washing or brushing their hair. These types of symptoms in the arms and legs point to proximal muscle weakness, which is probably the most common site of weakness in a myopathic disorder (see later). However, occasional patients with myopathies can complain of poor hand grip (difficulty in opening jar tops and turning door knobs) or tripping due to ankle weakness caused by distal muscle weakness. Some myopathies involve "proximal" cranial muscles, and patients complain of a change in speech (dysarthria) or swallowing (dysphagia), droopy eyelids (ptosis), and rarely double vision (diplopia).

It is important to determine the *tempo* of the disease. Patients should be asked whether the weakness is present all of the time or is intermittent. Myopathies can present with either fixed weakness (muscular dystrophies, inflammatory myopathies) or episodic periods of weakness with normal strength interictally (periodic paralysis due to channelopathies, metabolic myopathies due to certain glycolytic pathway disorders). Muscle disorders can have acute (less than 4 weeks), subacute (4 to 8 weeks), or chronic (more than

Table 505–2 ■ USING THE HISTORY AND PHYSICAL EXAMINATION TO DIAGNOSE MYOPATHIES

History
- Symptoms
  - Negative
    - Weakness
      - Symptoms of proximal, distal, or cranial weakness
      - Constant or episodic
      - Monophasic or relapsing
      - Progressive or non-progressive
      - Acute, subacute, chronic
    - Fatigue and exercise intolerance
  - Positive
    - Pain—myalgias
    - Cramps
    - Contractures
    - Stiffness/inability to relax muscle—myotonia
    - Dark red urine
- Age at onset
- Family history
- Precipitating factors: Drug or toxin exposure; exercise; diet; temperature

Neurologic Examination
- Distribution of weakness
  - Proximal—"limb-girdle"
  - Proximal arms/distal legs—"scapuloperoneal"
  - Proximal (quadriceps) legs/distal (finger & wrist flexors) arms— "inclusion body myositis"
  - Distal—"distal myopathy"
  - Ocular or pharyngeal
  - Neck extensors
- Atrophy or enlargement
- Myotonia or stiffness

8 weeks) periods over which the weakness evolves. Of course, the disorders with episodic weakness have acute weakness that can return to normal strength within hours or days. The tempo of the disorders with persistent weakness can vary from (1) acute or subacute in some inflammatory myopathies (dermatomyositis and polymyositis), (2) to chronic slow progression over years (most muscular dystrophies), or (3) to fixed weakness with little change over decades (congenital myopathies). Finally, both constant and episodic myopathic disorders can have symptoms that may be monophasic or polyphasic (relapsing). For example, a myositis can occasionally have an acute monophasic course and return to normal strength within weeks or months. Patients with channelopathies or metabolic myopathies can have recurrent attacks of weakness over many years, whereas a patient with acute rhabdomyolysis due to a toxin such as cocaine may have a single episode.

Although weakness may be the most reliable symptom of a patient with a myopathy, many patients who complain of generalized global "weakness" or *fatigue* do not have a disorder of muscle, particularly if the neurologic examination is normal. Fatigue is a non-specific symptom. On the other hand, abnormal fatigability after exercise can result from certain metabolic and mitochondrial myopathies, and it is important to define the duration and intensity of exercise that provoke it.

POSITIVE SYMPTOMS. Muscle pain (*myalgia*) is another nonspecific complaint that accompanies some myopathies. Myalgias may be episodic (e.g., metabolic myopathies) or nearly constant (e.g., inflammatory muscle disorders). However, muscle pain is surprisingly uncommon in most muscle diseases, and limb pain is more likely to be due to bone or joint disorders. It is rare for a muscle disease to be responsible for vague aches and discomfort in muscle regions in the presence of normal neurologic examination and laboratory study findings.

A specific category of muscle pain is the involuntary muscle *cramp*. Cramps are usually localized to a particular muscle region and last from seconds to minutes. Usually they are benign, occurring in normal individuals, and do not reflect an underlying disease process, and in particular are seldom a feature of a primary myopathy. Cramps can occur with dehydration, hyponatremia, azotemia, and myxedema, and in disorders of the motor neuron (especially amyotrophic lateral sclerosis) or nerve.

Muscle contractures are uncommon but can superficially resemble cramps. They usually last longer than cramps and are provoked by exercise in patients with glycolytic enzyme defects. They can be distinguished from cramps with needle electromyography (see later)—contractures are electrically silent whereas cramps are associated with rapid firing motor unit discharges. Muscle contractures should not be confused with fixed *tendon contracture* (see later).

Myotonia is the phenomenon of impaired relaxation of muscle after forceful voluntary contraction. Patients can complain of muscle stiffness or persistent contraction in almost any muscle group, but particularly involving the hands and eyelids. They will note difficulty releasing their hand grip after a handshake, unscrewing a bottle top, or turning a doorknob. If they shut their eyes forcefully, they have difficulty opening their eyelids. With repeated exercise, the myotonia improves: the so-called warm-up phenomenon. Paramyotonia is the paradoxical phenomenon in which exercise makes the myotonia worse. Myotonia is due to repetitive depolarization of the muscle membrane. Exposure to cold worsens myotonia and paramyotonia.

If a patient complains of exercise-induced weakness and myalgias, he or she should be asked whether the urine has ever turned dark or red during or after these episodes, indicating *myoglobinuria*. Myoglobinuria follows excessive release of myoglobin from muscle during periods of rapid muscle destruction (*rhabdomyolysis*).

Other crucial points in the history concern the *age at onset* of symptoms. Did the weakness (or other symptoms) first manifest at birth or was onset in the first, second, third, or later decade? Identifying the age when symptoms began can provide important clues to the diagnosis. For example, of the muscular dystrophies, symptoms in Duchenne type muscular dystrophy usually are noted by age 3, whereas most facioscapulohumeral and limb-girdle dystrophies begin in adolescence or later. Disorders such as myotonic dystrophy and oculopharyngeal dystrophy may not become symptomatic until middle age or later. Of the inflammatory myopathies, dermatomyositis occurs in children and adults, polymyositis rarely occurs in children but can appear at any decade in the adult years, and inclusion body myositis is a myositis of the elderly.

The *family history* is obviously of great importance in correctly diagnosing the hereditary myopathies. A detailed family pedigree (tree) should be obtained to look for autosomal dominant, recessive X-linked, and vertical maternal (mitochondrial) patterns of transmission. Identifying a particular hereditary pattern not only can help in correctly diagnosing the disorder, but also is of importance in genetic counseling.

Finally, *precipitating factors* should be explored in the history. Is the patient taking legal or illegal drugs or exposed to toxins that can produce a myopathy? Does exercise provoke attacks of weakness, pain, or urine discoloration, raising the possibility of a glycolytic pathway defect? Are episodes of weakness associated with or preceded by a fever, a feature of carnitine palmitoyl transferase deficiency? Does the ingestion of a carbohydrate meal precede weakness, suggesting a channelopathy? Does cold exposure precipitate muscle stiffness, a characteristic finding in myotonic myopathies?

SIGNS ON NEUROLOGIC EXAMINATION. In order to determine whether a particular muscle group is weak, it is important to know what muscles to test and how to grade muscle power at the bedside. In examining the upper limbs, it is necessary to assess shoulder abduction, adduction, and external and internal rotation; elbow flexion and extension; wrist flexion and extension; and finger and thumb extension, flexion, and abduction. Muscle groups that should be tested in the lower extremities include hip flexion, extension, abduction, and adduction; knee flexion and extension; ankle dorsiflexion; plantar flexion, inversion, and eversion; and toe extension and flexion. Neck flexors should be assessed in the supine and neck extensors in the prone position. Finally, cranial nerve muscles such as eyelids, extraocular muscles controlling eye movements, upper and lower facial muscles of expression, tongue, and palate should be examined. All muscle groups should be tested bilaterally, and preferably against gravity. Knee extension and hip flexion should be tested in the seated position, knee flexion should be tested prone, and abduction should be tested in the lateral decubitus position. If testing against gravity is not done, the presence of substantive muscle weakness can escape recognition.

Assessment of muscle strength is usually based on the Medical Research Council of Great Britain (MRC) grading scale of 0 to 5:

5—Normal power
4—Active movement against gravity and resistance
3—Active movement against gravity
2—Active movement only with gravity eliminated
1—Trace contraction
0—No contraction

In addition to manual muscle testing, muscles should be inspected for *atrophy* or *hypertrophy*. Atrophy of proximal limb muscles is common in long-standing myopathies. However, certain myopathies have atrophy in specific groups that corresponds to severe weakness in those muscles and is a clue to the diagnosis. Atrophy around the periscapular muscles may be associated with scapular winging. Selective atrophy of the quadriceps muscles and forearm flexor muscles is highly suggestive of inclusion body myositis. Distal myopathies may have profound atrophy in anterior or posterior lower leg compartments. Muscles can become diffusely hypertrophic in some myotonic conditions such as myotonia congenita. Muscle hypertrophy can also occur in disorders such as amyloidosis and sarcoidosis and in hypothyroid myopathy. In Duchenne type and Becker's muscular dystrophy, the calves can become enlarged, but this is usually the pseudohypertrophy of the muscle due to replacement with connective tissue and fat. Focal muscle enlargement may indicate a neoplastic or inflammatory process, ectopic ossification, tendon rupture, and rarely partial denervation of various causes.

Tendon contractures (as distinct from the episodic muscle contractures of metabolic myopathy) can occur in many myopathies of long duration. However, contractures developing early in the course of the disease, especially at the elbows, can be a clue to Emery-Dreifuss dystrophy and Bethlem myopathy.

Muscle twitches or fasciculations can be noted on inspection. However, fasciculations are generally not a manifestation of a muscle disease but occur in the setting of denervation or as a benign process.

It is important to watch the patient perform functional activities: walking (to look for a wide-based waddling gait with hyperlordosis, which is a sign of pelvic muscle weakness); rising from a chair, from a squat, or from a seated position on the floor (*Gowers' sign*); or climbing stairs (noting whether there is a need to use the arms, another sign of proximal weakness in the lower extremities). The inability to walk on the heels or toes can indicate weakness in the anterior and posterior distal leg muscles, respectively. Observe the patient talk and smile to determine whether there is facial weakness. Is there the so-called horizontal smile, indicating lower facial muscle weakness? Is the patient unable to close the eyes completely when asked to do so, indicating upper facial muscle weakness? Are the upper eyelids lowered so that they touch the pupil, indicating ptosis? Is the speech nasal, indicating palatal muscle involvement?

Finally, if the patient complains of muscle stiffness, the examiner should attempt to elicit *myotonia*. This can be done by asking the patient to squeeze the examiner's finger and then observing whether the patient has an inability to relax the hand grip. Additionally, the muscles can be directly percussed with a reflex hammer. Observe for a slow persistent contraction and delayed relaxation. The muscles that can be most easily percussed to look for myotonia are the thenar and wrist/finger extensor muscle groups. Facial myotonia can also be observed after forceful voluntary eye closure. The patient will be unable to open the eyes easily after this maneuver.

Other aspects of the neurologic examination need to be assessed in all potential myopathy patients to ensure that they are not involved. The sensory examination result should be normal in muscle disease. Reflexes are usually preserved early in the disease process. Once the myopathy is advanced and the muscles are extremely weak, reflexes can become hypoactive or unelicitable. Evidence of upper motor neuron damage (spasticity, extensor plantar responses, clonus) is only present in myopathies if there is coincidental central nervous system (CNS) disease.

PATTERN OF WEAKNESS. Once the muscles have been inspected and tested for power, and functional activity has been observed, an attempt should be made to place the patient in one of the *patterns of muscle weakness* that can occur in myopathic disorders. The various patterns of muscle weakness can be divided into six broad groups:

1. The most common pattern in muscle disease is weakness that is exclusively or predominantly in proximal muscles of the legs and arms, or the so-called limb-girdle distribution. Neck flexor and extensor muscles can also be affected. This pattern of weakness can be seen in many hereditary and acquired myopathies and therefore is the least specific in arriving at a particular diagnosis. It is not known why most myopathic disorders selectively involve proximal muscles.

2. The pattern of *distal* weakness in the upper extremities (extensor muscle group) or lower extremities (anterior or posterior compartment muscle groups) (Table 505–3). Selective weakness and atrophy in distal extremity muscles are more often features of neuropathies but are uncommonly due to a primary muscle disease. When this pattern of weakness is determined to be due to a myopathic rather than a neuropathic disorder, a diagnosis of distal myopathy is appropriate.

3. The pattern of proximal upper extremity weakness of the periscapular muscles and distal lower extremity weakness of the anterior compartment—the *scapuloperoneal* pattern (Table 505–3). The scapular muscle weakness is usually accompanied by scapular winging. When this pattern is associated with facial weakness, it is highly suggestive of facioscapulohumeral dystrophy. Other hereditary myopathies can be associated with a scapuloperoneal syndrome, for example, scapuloperoneal dystrophy, Emery-Dreifuss dystrophy, acid maltase deficiency, and some congenital myopathies.

4. The pattern of distal upper extremity weakness in the distal forearm muscles (wrist and finger flexors) and proximal lower extremity weakness involving the knee extensors (quadriceps). This pattern is essentially pathognomonic for *inclusion body myositis*. In addition, the weakness is often asymmetrical between the two sides, a pattern that is uncommon in most myopathies.

Table 505-5 ■ MYOPATHIES WITH PROMINENT NECK EXTENSOR WEAKNESS

Table 505-3 ■ MYOPATHIES THAT CAN HAVE PROMINENT DISTAL WEAKNESS

Late adult onset distal myopathy type 1 (Welander)
Late adult onset distal myopathy type 2 (Markesbery/Udd)
Early adult onset distal myopathy type 1 (Nonaka)
Early adult onset distal myopathy type 2 (Miyoshi)
Early adult onset distal myopathy type 3 (Laing)
Desmin myopathy
Myotonic dystrophy
Facioscapulohumeral dystrophy*
Scapuloperoneal dystrophy*
Oculopharyngeal dystrophy
Emery-Dreifuss humeroperonal dystrophy*
Inflammatory myopathies
    Inclusion body myositis
Metabolic myopathy
    Debrancher deficiency
    Acid-maltase deficiency*
Congenital myopathy
    Nemaline myopathy*
    Central core myopathy*
    Centronuclear myopathy

*Can occur in a scapuloperoneal pattern.

5. Predominant involvement of ocular or pharyngeal muscles (Table 505-4). The combination of ptosis, ophthalmoplegia without diplopia, and pharyngeal weakness should suggest the diagnosis of oculopharyngeal dystrophy, especially if the onset is in middle age or later. Ptosis and ophthalmoplegia without prominent pharyngeal involvement are hallmarks of many of the mitochondrial myopathies. Ptosis and facial weakness without ophthalmoplegia or pharyngeal weakness are common features of myotonic dystrophy. Therefore, the presence of ocular or pharyngeal muscle involvement can suggest a particular muscle disorder. Patients with ocular or pharyngeal involvement can also have the typical pattern of limb-girdle weakness.

6. Prominent neck extensor weakness. Some myopathic conditions have such a dramatic degree of weakness of the neck extensor muscles that the term "dropped head syndrome" is used (Table 505-5). The neck flexors may or may not be weak. Neck extensor weakness can also occur with myopathies such as those with a limb-girdle pattern of weakness. Prominent neck extensor weakness is common in two other neuromuscular diseases: amyotrophic lateral sclerosis and myasthenia gravis.

These six patterns of myopathy have limitations, but are useful in narrowing the differential diagnosis. Neuromuscular diseases other than myopathies can also present with one of these weakness patterns. For example, although proximal greater than distal weakness is characteristic of myopathies, patients with acquired demyelinating neuropathies (Guillain-Barré syndrome and chronic inflammatory demyelinating polyneuropathy) often have proximal as well as distal muscle involvement. Such neuropathies will have the additional finding of sensory and reflex loss. Ocular, pharyngeal, and proximal limb weakness is characteristic of neuromuscular junction transmission disorders such as myasthenia gravis. However, these patients will also have diplopia, weakness that fluctuates, and addi-

Table 505-4 ■ MYOPATHIES WITH PTOSIS OR OPHTHALMOPLEGIA

Ptosis Usually Without Ophthalmoplegia
    Myotonic dystrophy
    Congenital myopathies
        Centronuclear myopathy
        Nemaline myopathy
        Central core myopathy
    Desmin storage myopathy
Ptosis with Ophthalmoplegia
    Oculopharyngeal muscular dystrophy
    Oculopharyngodistal myopathy
    Mitochondrial myopathy

Table 505-5 ■ MYOPATHIES WITH PROMINENT NECK EXTENSOR WEAKNESS

Isolated neck extensor myopathy
Polymyositis
Dermatomyositis
Inclusion body myositis
Carnitine deficiency
Myotonic dystrophy
Congenital myopathy
Hyperparathyroidism

tional laboratory findings that will lead to the correct diagnosis. Table 505-6 summarizes the key distinguishing clinical points among disorders of muscle, anterior horn cell, peripheral nerve, and neuromuscular junction.

Associated Organ Involvement or Systemic Illness

Involvement of organs or tissues other than muscle can provide additional diagnostic clues. Cardiac disease can be associated with myotonic dystrophy, dystrophinopathies, Emery-Dreifuss dystrophy, and certain types of periodic paralysis. Hepatomegaly can occur in sarcoidosis and in the myopathies associated with deficiencies of acid maltase, debranching enzyme, and carnitine. Intrinsic pulmonary involvement can be seen in some of the inflammatory myopathies and sarcoidosis. Evidence of a diffuse systemic disorder can indicate a collagen-vascular disease, amyloidosis, sarcoidosis, endocrine myopathies, or mitochondrial disorders.

LABORATORY STUDIES FOR THE EVALUATION OF MYOPATHY

SERUM ENZYMES OF MUSCLE ORIGIN. *Creatine kinase* (CK) occurs in high concentration in the sarcoplasm of skeletal and cardiac muscle. The MM isoenzyme of CK predominates in skeletal muscle, MB occurs primarily in cardiac muscle, and BB is mainly in brain. When skeletal muscle is injured CK can leak into the blood. Therefore, an elevated serum CK level is present in many muscle diseases. However, the absence of an elevated serum CK level does not rule out a myopathy, particularly in patients with severe muscle atrophy. In addition, the elevation of serum CK level does not necessarily imply that the muscle is the primary site of abnormality. The CK level is often elevated in normal individuals for days after strenuous voluntary exercise. Involuntary prolonged muscle contraction from a generalized motor seizure or tetany can elevate CK level. Serum CK level is above the normal range in some African individuals, in individuals with large muscles, and after minor muscle trauma (e.g., electromyography). Finally, other neuromuscular disorders such as motor neuron disease can produce up to a five-fold increase in CK level. Serum CK level is normal in peripheral neuropathies and neuromuscular junction disorders.

Other enzymes that can be released from injured skeletal muscle include aspartate aminotransferase (AST [SGOT]), alanine aminotransferase (ALT [SGPT]), and lactate dehydrogenase (LDH). These enzymes also occur in high concentration in the liver. The serum CK level is the most sensitive for muscle disease and it is rarely necessary to measure for these other enzymes. Levels of enzymes such as AST and ALT are elevated in hepatic disease and since they are often measured in large screening chemical panels, their elevation should prompt CK measurement to determine whether the source is muscle or liver. If a patient with an inflammatory myopathy is treated with a drug that may have hepatotoxicity as a side effect, it is not sufficient to measure ALT and AST levels; the liver-specific enzyme γ-glutamyl transferase (GGT) should be followed.

In general, CK isoenzymes are not helpful in myopathy evaluations. CK-MM level elevations are typical of muscle disease, but CK-MB level is also elevated in myopathies and does not indicate that cardiac disease is present.

ELECTROMYOGRAPHY (EMG). EMG is the electrophysiologic assessment of the neuromuscular system. It consists of nerve conduction study (NCS) and needle electromyography.

The basic principle of EMG is that a moving wave of electronegativity from either nerve or muscle is measured with a recording device. For NCS, a nerve is depolarized with an electrical

Table 505-6 ■ CLINICAL FINDINGS DIFFERENTIATING MUSCLE FROM NERVE DISEASE

	MYOPATHY	ANTERIOR HORN CELL DISEASE	PERIPHERAL NEUROPATHY	NEUROMUSCULAR JUNCTION DISEASE
Distribution	Usually proximal, symmetric	Distal, asymmetric and bulbar	Distal, symmetric	Extraocular, bulbar, proximal limb
Atrophy	Slight early, marked late	Marked early	Moderate	Absent
Fasciculations	Absent	Frequent	Sometimes present	Absent
Reflexes	Lost late	Variable, can be hyperreflexic	Lost early	Normal
Pain	Diffuse in myositis	Absent	Variable, distal when present	Absent
Cramps	Rare	Frequent	Occasional	Absent
Sensory loss	Absent	Absent	Usually present	Absent
Serum creatine kinase	Usually elevated	Occasionally slightly elevated	Normal	Normal

stimulator and the electrical potential is measured over the muscle (for motor NCS) or nerve (for sensory NCS). The recorded motor and sensory nerve potentials are measured for amplitude, latency, and conduction velocities. Both the motor and sensory NCSs usually have normal results in myopathies, but results are generally abnormal in neuropathies. In needle EMG, a needle electrode is inserted directly into the muscle. The electrical activity from the muscle is observed at rest and when the patient voluntarily contracts the muscle. The potentials recorded from the needle are viewed on a screen and the examiner also listens to the auditory pattern.

ABNORMAL EMG ACTIVITY AT REST. In a normal individual, there is no recorded electrical activity from a muscle when it is at rest. Electrical activity at rest is abnormal. Spontaneous rhythmic discharges of single muscle fiber are called *fibrillations* or *positive sharp waves* and occur when there has been a disconnection between the nerve and the muscle it innervates. Fibrillations occur more often in nerve diseases but can occur in active myopathies. Since a fibrillation represents the discharge of a single muscle fiber, it cannot be detected on the clinical examination but can only be observed on needle EMG.

Myotonia is the abnormal spontaneous discharge of muscle that occurs in some myopathies, such as myotonic dystrophy, myotonia congenita, periodic paralysis, and acid maltase deficiency. On EMG, myotonia consists of high-frequency repetitive discharges that spontaneously increase and decrease in amplitude and frequency and have the sound of a dive-bomber or motorcycle. Myotonia represents repeated muscle fiber depolarization due to an irritable muscle membrane and indicates a myopathy. A third spontaneous electrical phenomenon, the complex repetitive discharge, is usually the result of nerve disease. The complex repetitive discharge differs from myotonia in that it starts and stops abruptly and does not wax and wane in frequency and amplitude. It sounds like a jack hammer.

Fasciculations are to be distinguished from fibrillations and myotonia. A fasciculation represents a spontaneous discharge of a motor unit, which is a group of muscle fibers of the same histochemical type under control of a single anterior horn cell, and thus innervated by the same axon. These can be observed clinically as a small muscle twitch or movement. Electrically a fasciculation is a large-amplitude potential that consists of the simultaneous involuntary depolarization of a group of muscle fibers. Although they do not necessarily imply neuromuscular disease and occur in many normal patients, fasciculations can occur in diseases of the motor neuron or nerve. Neither clinical nor electrical fasciculations are a feature of muscle disorders.

EMG ACTIVITY WITH MOVEMENT. When the patient voluntarily contracts the muscle, individual *motor unit action potentials* are assessed. Motor units are normally triphasic potentials, and a normal motor unit recorded with the EMG needle consists of about 10 or more muscle fibers innervated by the same axon that are simultaneously depolarizing. Individual motor units are analyzed for their amplitude, duration, and number of phases. In addition, the firing rate and recruitment pattern of the voluntary motor units are noted.

Two abnormal motor unit patterns that can be observed suggest that the disease is either "neuropathic" or "myopathic." Neuropathic

motor unit potentials are increased in amplitude (>5 mV), and duration (>10 milliseconds), and are polyphasic. In addition, for a given degree of voluntary effort, few motor units are recruited and the ones that are fire too rapidly (>15-20 Hz). This indicates a loss of motor units with a compensatory increased firing rate in the remaining units, a pattern known as *decreased recruitment*. Myopathic motor unit potentials are small, brief polyphasic potentials (<4 milliseconds). In a myopathy, multiple small motor units are recruited with only minimal voluntary effort. This myopathic pattern occurs because the number of motor units is normal but there are fewer functioning muscle fibers within each unit, and therefore more units are required to generate a degree of force. These so-called neuropathic and myopathic needle EMG patterns are generalizations, and there are many examples of denervating illness that produces myopathic potentials, and vice versa. In addition, the EMG result can be normal in a patient with a myopathy.

However, if the needle EMG examination finding shows evidence of myopathic motor units this adds further data that the patient may indeed have a myopathy. In addition, multiple muscles can be sampled with needle EMG. Needle EMG can be useful in confirming the clinical phenotype of muscle involvement established on the neurologic examination. EMG can also provide a clue as to which muscles have had recent or ongoing muscle injury and can be a guide as to which muscle to biopsy.

THE MUSCLE BIOPSY. A muscle specimen can be obtained through either an open or a closed (needle or punch) biopsy procedure. Whether an open or punch biopsy procedure is performed, the tissue must be processed in a laboratory that is skilled in the evaluation of muscle and experienced in the specialized techniques needed for the assessment of the tissue. Fixed muscle is of little value for diagnosis.

Muscles that are moderately weak should undergo biopsy. Biopsy specimens should generally not be taken from severely weak (MRC grade 2 or less) muscles. Muscles that have recently been studied by needle EMG often have artifacts from the procedure.

Biopsy specimens are analyzed by light and electron microscopy, biochemical studies, and molecular genetic studies. In most instances, light microscopic observations are sufficient to make a pathologic diagnosis. Muscle tissue examination under light microscopy is primarily performed by using frozen specimens. The tissue is examined for muscle fiber size, shape, fiber type distribution, presence of fiber degeneration (necrosis), and regeneration. Structural changes such as central nuclei, disorganization of myofibrils and sarcoplasm (e.g., target fibers, ring fibers, central cores), and vacuoles can be observed with light microscopy. Connective tissue and blood vessels are examined for inflammation, and it is determined whether there are increased collagen and fat. The myosin ATPase stains at alkaline (pH 9.4) and acidic (pH 4.3 and 4.6) pH distinguish the types 1 and 2 fibers. *Type 1 fibers* (slow-twitch, fatigue-resistant, oxidative metabolism) stain lightly at alkaline and darkly at acidic pHs. *Type 2 fibers* (fast-twitch, fatigue-prone, glycolytic metabolism) stain darkly at alkaline and lightly at acidic pHs. Oxidative enzyme stains (reduced nicotinamide-adenine dinucleotide [NADH] dehydrogenase, succinate dehydrogenase, cytochrome-c oxidase) are useful for identifying myofibrillar and mitochondrial abnormalities. Qualitative biochemical enzyme stains can be performed for phosphorylase and phosfructokinase. Immunologic techniques can stain for muscle proteins that are deficient in some muscular dystrophies.

The muscle biopsy result can be useful in order to establish whether there is evidence of either a neuropathic or a myopathic disorder. A neuropathy can produce denervation atrophy with small angular fibers, groups of atrophic fibers, and, as a result of reinnervation, groups of fibers of the same histochemical type and target fibers. These features should not be present in a myopathy. Typical myopathic abnormalities include central nuclei, both small and large hypertrophic round fibers, split fibers, and degenerating and regenerating fibers. Inflammatory myopathies produce mononuclear inflammatory cells in the endomysial and perimysial connective tissue between fibers and occasionally around blood vessels. The atrophy of fibers located on the periphery of a muscle fascicle, perifascicular atrophy, is a common finding in a particular inflammatory myopathy, dermatomyositis. Any long-standing chronic myopathy can produce an increase in connective tissue and fat. Mitochondrial disorders are suggested by identification of ragged-red fibers on the Gomori's stain and various abnormal staining patterns on the oxidative stains. The enzymatic stains can demonstrate a non-specific type 1 fiber predominance in a number of myopathies.

Electron microscopy (EM) evaluates ultrastructural components of muscle fibers. In most myopathic disorders EM is not required to make a pathologic diagnosis; findings detected by EM are seldom of importance. However, EM is important in the study of certain disease states with abnormal light microscopic findings: congenital myopathies (e.g., nemaline rod, central core) and mitochondrial disorders.

In the evaluation of metabolic and mitochondrial myopathies, a portion of the muscle tissue can be processed for biochemical analysis to determine the specific enzyme defect. Western blot determinations from muscle tissue can be performed for certain muscle proteins (e.g., dystrophin).

MOLECULAR GENETIC STUDIES. The specific molecular genetic defect is known for an increasing number of myopathies. Molecular genetic testing is important for both diagnosis and carrier detection.

OTHER TESTS. Electrolyte, endocrine, and immunologic tests are indicated to establish specific medical diagnoses. A decrease in the serum creatinine level is a useful indicator of diseased muscle mass.

Forearm exercise testing in patients with a suspected metabolic myopathy is often performed to determine whether there is a defect in the glycolytic enzyme pathway. After vigorous exercise, serum lactate and ammonia levels are measured. In disorders such as phosphorylase deficiency (McArdle's disease), the characteristic elevation of serum lactate level after exercise is absent.

Urine analysis can detect the presence of myoglobinuria. This should be suspected if the urine test result is positive for blood but no red blood cells are seen.

Quantitation of urinary creatinine excretion is useful to determine whether there is a decrease in muscle mass but requires that the patient be on a meat-free diet and must be done over a period of 72 hours or more.

Imaging and spectroscopy studies include computed tomography, magnetic resonance imaging, and ultrasound. Muscle imaging is seldom useful to diagnose a myopathy. However, in selected patients undergoing muscle biopsy in whom it is unclear from the neurologic examination and needle EMG results which muscle to select for biopsy, an imaging procedure may be helpful.

Dubowitz V: Muscle Biopsy: A Practical Approach. London, Bailliere Tindall, 1985. *A treatise on the histologic characteristics of normal and abnormal muscle from a clinical perspective. It antedates most of the recent molecular discoveries regarding myopathies.*

Engel AG, Franzini-Armstrong C (eds): Myology, 2nd ed. New York, McGraw-Hill, 1994. *A multiauthored two-volume book on the anatomic, physiologic, and biochemical characteristics of skeletal muscle and the clinical aspects of muscle disease.*

Griggs RC, Mendell JR, Miller RG: Evaluation and Treatment of Myopathies. Philadelphia, FA Davis, 1995. *A concise monograph on the subject.*

Preston DC, Shapiro BE: Electromyography and Neuromuscular Disorders: Clinical-electrophysiologic Correlations. Boston, Butterworth-Heinemann, 1998. *The most up-to-date and readable text on EMG.*

Walton J, Karpati G, Hilton-Jones D (eds): Disorders of Voluntary Muscle, 6th ed. Edinburgh, Churchill Livingstone, 1994. *A single-volume text that is intermediate in size and detail between the first two books.*

506 MUSCULAR DYSTROPHIES

Richard J. Barohn

Muscular dystrophies are inherited myopathies characterized by progressive muscle weakness and degeneration and subsequent replacement by fibrous and fatty connective tissue. Historically, muscular dystrophies were categorized by their distribution of weakness, age of onset, and inheritance pattern. Advances in the molecular understanding of the muscular dystrophies has defined the genetic mutation and abnormal gene product for many of these disorders (Table 506–1).

DYSTROPHINOPATHIES

The dystrophinopathies include X-linked disorders resulting from mutations of the large dystrophin gene located at Xp21. Dystrophin is a large 427-kd subsarcolemmal cytoskeletal protein that along with the other components of the dystrophin-glycoprotein complex (DGC) provides support to the muscle membrane during contraction. The large size of the gene (2.4 megabases) accounts for the high mutation rate. Large deletions, several kilobases to over 1 million base pairs, can be demonstrated in approximately two thirds of patients; duplications occur in 5% of cases, and the remainder are small mutations that are not readily detectable. Mutations disrupting the translational reading frame of the gene result in near-total loss of dystrophin (Duchenne type muscular dystrophy), whereas in-frame mutations result in the translation of semifunctional dystrophin of abnormal size or amount (Becker's muscular dystrophy).

DUCHENNE TYPE MUSCULAR DYSTROPHY. GENETIC CHARACTERISTICS. The incidence of Duchenne dystrophy is 1 in 3500 male births, and the prevalence approaches 1 per 18,000 males. One third of the cases result from a new mutation. Most Duchenne dystrophy patients have a frame-shift mutation and total dystrophin deficiency. Dystrophin deficiency weakens the sarcolemma, permitting the influx of calcium-rich extracellular fluid, which then activates intracellular proteases and complement, leading to fiber necrosis. There is also a secondary reduction of the other components in the DGC in the muscle membrane. Normal dystrophin is required for assembly and integrity of the DGC.

CLINICAL FEATURES. Duchenne dystrophy presents as early as 2–3 years with delays in motor milestones and difficulty in running. The proximal muscles are the most severely affected early (limb-girdle pattern) and the course is relentlessly progressive. Patients begin to fall frequently by age 5–6 years, have difficulty in climbing stairs by age 8 years, and are usually confined to a wheelchair by age 12. Joint contractures commonly appear between 6 and 10 years. Calf hypertrophy is often present early, but after ambulation is lost all muscles atrophy; paraspinal muscle weakness leads to progressive kyphoscoliosis. The proximal tendon reflexes (biceps, quadriceps) disappear by the age of 10, although gastrocnemius reflexes are often preserved until late in the disease. Respiratory function gradually declines and decreased vital capacity can be detected after the age of 10. Most patients die of respiratory complication in their 20s. Cardiac muscle is also affected, and although patients are generally asymptomatic, congestive heart failure and arrhythmias can occur late in the disease. Up to 90% of Duchenne dystrophy patients have an abnormal electrocardiogram (ECG), with tall right precordial R waves and deep left precordial Q waves. Echocardiography shows either hypokinesis or dilatation of ventricular walls. The smooth muscle of the gastrointestinal tract is also involved and intestinal pseudo-obstruction occurs. The average intelligence quotient (IQ) of affected boys is one standard deviation below the normal mean, suggesting central nervous system involvement. Whether intellectual impairment is related to the loss of dystrophin at various synapses in the brain is unknown.

LABORATORY. A dystrophin gene deletion (or rarely a duplication) can be detected by analysis of DNA from leukocytes (by the polymerase chain reaction) in a blood sample in approximately two thirds of patients. The DNA from a muscle sample can be similarly tested, but it is no more specific than leukocyte DNA

Table 506–1 ■ MUSCULAR DYSTROPHIES

DISEASE	MODE OF INHERITANCE	GENE MUTATION LOCATION	PROTEIN
X-linked MD			
Duchenne/Becker's	XR	Xp21	Dystrophin
Emery-Dreifuss	XR	Xq28	Emerin
Limb-Girdle MD			
LGMD 1A	AD	5q22-34	Not known
LGMD 1B	AD	1q11-21	Not known
LGMD 1C	AD	3p25	Caveolin-3
LGMD 2A	AR	15q15	Calpain-3
LGMD 2B†	AR	2p12	Dysferlin
LGMD 2C	AR	13q12	γ-Sarcoglycan
LGMD 2D	AR	17q12	α-Sarcoglycan
LGMD 2E	AR	4q12	β-Sarcoglycan
LGMD 2F	AR	5q33	δ-Sarcoglycan
LGMD 2G	AR	17q11	Not known
LGMD 2H	AR	9q31	Not known
Congenital MD			
With CNS involvement			
Fukuyama CMD	AR	9q31-33	Fukutin
Walker-Warburg CMD	AR	9q31-33	? Fukutin
Muscle-eye-brain CMD	AR	1	Not known
Without CNS involvement			
Merosin-deficient classic type	AR	6q2	Laminin-2 (merosin)
Merosin-positive classic type	AR	?	Not known
Integrin-deficient CMD	AR	12q13	Integrin α7
Distal MD			
Late-adult-onset 1A (Welander)	AD	2p15	Dynactin
Late-adult-onset 1B (Markesbery/ Udd)	AD	2p	Not known
Early-adult-onset 1A (Nonaka)	AR	9p1-q1	Not known
Early-adult-onset 1B‡ (Miyoshi)	AR	2q12-14	Dysferlin
Early-adult-onset 1C (Laing)	AD	14	Not known
Other MD			
Facioscapulohumeral	AD	4q35	Not known
Oculopharyngeal	AD	14q11	Poly(A) binding protein 2
Myotonic dystrophy—Type 1	AD	19q13	Myotonin-protein kinase
Myotonic dystrophy—Type 2	AD	3q	Not known
Myofibrillar myopathy	AD	11q21-23	αβ-crystallin
Myofibrillar myopathy	AD	2q35	Desmin
Bethlem myopathy	AD	21q22	Collagen VI

MD = muscular dystrophy; LGMD = limb-girdle muscular dystrophy; CNS = central nervous system; CMD = congenital muscular dystrophy; XR = X-linked recessive; AD = autosomal dominant; AR = autosomal recessive.
†Probably same condition as Miyoshi distal MD.
‡Probably same condition as LGMD 2B.

analysis. If the patient falls into the one third of patients in whom a deletion cannot be detected, a muscle biopsy is required to demonstrate dystrophin deficiency by either Western blot or immunostaining. The muscle biopsy will also demonstrate typical features of a muscular dystrophy: fiber size variability, fiber necrosis, and regeneration, and replacement with connective tissue and fat.

The serum creatine kinase (CK) levels are markedly elevated at birth (20 to 100 times normal). The CK level remains elevated but tends to decline over the course of the disease, when there is severe loss of muscle mass. The electromyogram (EMG) shows fibrillation potentials and myopathic motor units. EMG and muscle biopsy are not necessary in Duchenne dystrophy if the diagnosis can be established by molecular studies of lymphocytes.

BECKER'S MUSCULAR DYSTROPHY. Becker's dystrophy is a milder form of dystrophinopathy and varies in severity, depending upon the gene lesion. It is less common than the Duchenne type with an incidence of 5 per 100,000 and prevalence of 2.4 per 100,000. The pattern of weakness resembles that of Duchenne dystrophy, but it is less severe and the mean age of onset of symptoms is later, between 5 and 15 years. Calf hypertrophy is often prominent and patients may complain of exercise-induced calf pain as an early symptom. Patients usually remain ambulatory after age 15 and the average time when a wheelchair is required is at age 30. Children with Duchenne dystrophy cannot lift their head fully against gravity (Medical Research Council of Great Britain [MRC] grade <3), whereas outlier children and those with Becker's dystrophy retain this ability. Cardiac abnormalities are similar to these described for Duchenne dystrophy. Most Becker's dystrophy patients experience slow progression; death may occur from respiratory or cardiac complications after age 40.

Most Becker's dystrophy patients have a non-frame-shift mutation, so that a reduced amount of an abnormal dystrophin is produced, resulting in a milder syndrome than Duchenne dystrophy. DNA analysis from blood leukocytes will show a Xp21 deletion in about 60%. Results of immunostaining and Western immunoblot for dystrophin on muscle extracts reveal the protein is not absent, as in Duchenne dystrophy, but is reduced in amount or abnormal in size.

Serum CK level is moderately elevated and the needle EMG shows electrophysiologic signs of a myopathy, similar to the findings in Duchenne dystrophy.

OTHER DYSTROPHINOPATHIES. Other, milder dystrophinopathy phenotypes include exercise intolerance associated with myalgias, muscle cramps, or myoglobinuria; minimal limb-girdle weakness or quadriceps myopathy; asymptomatic elevation of the serum CK level; cardiomyopathy with only mild muscle weakness; and fatal X-linked cardiomyopathy without muscle weakness. The different dystrophin phenotypes are determined by the site of the mutation in the dystrophin gene and the effect or lack of effect of the mutation on the expression of the cardiac isoform of dystrophin.

FEMALE CARRIERS. The mothers of affected children who also have a family history of Duchenne or Becker's muscular dystrophy, and the daughters of males with a dystrophinopathy are obligate carriers of the mutated dystrophin gene. Mothers and sisters of isolated Duchenne or Becker's dystrophy patients are at risk for being carriers. There is a 50% chance that males born to carrier females will inherit the disease, and 50% of the daughters born will become carriers themselves. Female carriers are usually asymptomatic, but rarely they may demonstrate moderate limb-girdle weakness.

CK level is elevated in about 50% of female carriers. A more accurate method of carrier detection is to look for a Xp21 deletion, which will be present if the affected males in the family are among the 60% who have a dystrophin gene deletion (or duplication). If a deletion is not present, linkage analysis on families can be performed. Genetic testing can be done for prenatal diagnosis on amniotic fluid cells or chorionic villi.

TREATMENT. No treatment prevents the progression of Duchenne dystrophy to wheelchair confinement and death. Controlled trials with prednisone 0.75 mg/kg/day in Duchenne dystrophy have demonstrated moderate improvement in strength and delay in progression into a wheelchair or braces; prednisone also delays respiratory compromise. Side effects of therapy include weight gain, growth delays, and changes in behavior. The use of prednisone is tolerated in the majority of Duchenne dystrophy patients. Gene therapy for the dystrophinopathies and other muscular dystrophies with known genetic mutations is still in pre-clinical stages. Trials of myoblast transfer from the normal fathers of Duchenne dystrophy patients to their affected sons found no effect.

EMERY-DREIFUSS DYSTROPHY. Emery-Dreifuss dystrophy is another X-linked disorder. This muscular dystrophy is characterized by the clinical triad of (1) early contractures of the elbows, ankles, and posterior cervical muscles; (2) slowly progressive muscle weakness usually in a scapulohumeroperoneal distribution; and (3) cardiomyopathy with atrial conduction defects.

The early elbow contractures are often an important phenotypic key to the diagnosis. Although Emery-Dreifuss dystrophy usually begins in childhood, most patients remain ambulatory into their third or fourth decade. The serum CK level is either normal or only moderately elevated. The muscle biopsy shows a range of myopathic changes but fewer dystrophic features than that for Duchenne or Becker's dystrophy. Electrocardiography can show sinus bradycardia, prolongation of the PR interval, or more severe degrees of conduction block. The cardiac conduction defects are potentially lethal and often require a pacemaker.

The family history may suggest an X-linked disorder. The mutated gene in the Xq28 region codes for a protein product, emerin. Emerin is a 254-amino-acid protein that localizes to the nuclear membranes of skeletal, cardiac, and smooth muscle fibers. The function of emerin is unknown. The definitive diagnosis can be made from either leukocyte DNA analysis or immunostaining muscle or skin tissue for emerin. The normal emerin perinuclear staining pattern in these tissues will be absent in Emery-Dreifuss dystrophy.

Bethlem myopathy clinically resembles Emery-Dreifuss dystrophy with a similar pattern of weakness and early contractures. However, Bethlem myopathy has no cardiac involvement and the inheritance pattern is autosomal dominant. At least some cases of Bethlem myopathy are due to a mutation of α_1 and α_2 subunits of collagen VI located on chromosome 21q.

THE RIGID-SPINE SYNDROME. Rigid-spine syndrome is a heterogeneous disorder in which muscle contractures involve the spine as well as other joints. Because of the severe contractures it must be distinguished from Emery-Dreifuss and Bethlem myopathy. In most cases the disease is sporadic and manifests in infancy with hypotonia, proximal weakness, and delayed motor milestones. Throughout the first decade the child experiences progressive severe limitation of spine mobility and scoliosis as well as elbow and knee contractures. The spinal deformities continue until about 7–13 years, at which time the disease appears to stabilize. Serum CK level is mildly elevated. Muscle biopsies demonstrate non-specific myopathic features. Genetic localization is unknown.

LIMB-GIRDLE MUSCULAR DYSTROPHIES (LGMDs). LGMDs include a large number of hereditary muscular dystrophies with a limb-girdle pattern of weakness. LGMDs are either autosomal recessive (the majority) or dominant and thus are clinically distinguished from the dystrophinopathies by an equal occurrence in both sexes. When LGMD occurs in early childhood, resembling Duchenne dystrophy, it has been termed *severe childhood recessive muscular dystrophy* (SCARMD). Milder phenotypes can resemble Becker's dystrophy. The laboratory features (serum CK, EMG, muscle biopsy) are consistent with a muscular dystrophy. Until recently, all LGMDs were lumped together. During the past decade, the gene mutation identification and the resulting protein defect have been established for many LGMD kindreds so that there

are already at least 10 subtypes, and the list continues to grow. The less common autosomal dominant forms have been labeled type 1 (LGMD 1A, 1B, 1C, etc.), and the autosomal recessive disorders are type 2 (LGMD 2A, 2B, etc.). There remain kinships with an LGMD disorder that still are not linked to a chromosomal locus.

AUTOSOMAL RECESSIVE LGMD. A number of the autosomal recessive LGMDs are due to defects in one of the sarcoglycan components of the DGC, termed sarcoglycanopathies (LGMD 2C, 2D, 2E, 2F).

The protein mutated in LGMD 2C, α-sarcoglycan, was previously known as *adhalin*—Arabic for "muscle." These disorders may account for as many as 20% of the muscular dystrophies that have a Duchenne type or Becker's muscular dystrophy phenotype. LGMD 2C and 2D usually begin in childhood; LGMD 2E and 2F have a more variable age of onset even within families. These LGMDs are not associated with intellectual impairment or cardiac abnormalities, in contrast to the dystrophinopathies.

The sarcoglycans are important components of the DGC, but the exact role of these proteins is unknown. A deficiency in one of the sarcoglycans results in a destabilization of the entire sarcoglycan complex. Results of muscle biopsies show normal dystrophin; however, immunostaining for each of the sarcoglycans is absent or diminished regardless of the primary sarcoglycan mutation.

Two other autosomal recessive LGMDs have known protein mutations that are not part of the DGC. LGMD 2A with an age of onset between 3 and 30 years (mean 13) is due to genetic mutation producing a deficiency of the muscle-specific proteolytic enzyme *calpain-3*. Calpains are non-lysosomal intracellular cysteine proteases. In LGMD 2B patients weakness develops between ages 13 and 35 and CK levels are elevated up to 200 times normal. The LGMD 2B mutation localizes to a region on 2p13 that codes for a protein recently named *dysferlin*. Dysferlin shares amino acid sequence homology with *C. elegans* spermatogenesis factor FER-1. LGMD 2B is also of interest because affected individuals can have one of two distinct phenotypes: limb-girdle or a distal myopathy pattern (see the discussion of distal muscular dystrophy). How a mutation in the same protein can result in such dissimilar clinical presentation is unclear. In addition, the mechanism by which either calpain-3 or dysferlin deficiency produces muscle disease is unknown.

AUTOSOMAL DOMINANT LGMD. The autosomal dominant LGMDs all have onset in childhood or early adult life. Linkage to chromosome locations is known for LGMD 1A and 1B; the molecular defect for LGMD 1C produces a protein deficiency of *caveolin-3*. Caveolins may act as scaffolding proteins on which caveolin-interacting lipids and proteins are organized. Caveolin-3 is not considered part of the DGC, although it is localized by immunostaining to the sarcolemma.

DIFFERENTIAL DIAGNOSIS OF LIMB-GIRDLE SYNDROMES. All patients with limb-girdle syndromes need to be investigated by EMG and muscle biopsy. In those with a positive family history, the differential diagnosis includes inherited metabolic myopathies (e.g., acid maltase deficiency or a lipid storage myopathy); morphologically distinct congenital myopathies or their late-onset variants (e.g., nemaline, central core, and myotubular myopathies); or the anterior horn cell disease, spinal muscular atrophy. In sporadic cases of a limb-girdle syndrome the differential diagnosis includes the same diseases, and also inflammatory myopathies (polymyositis, inclusion body myositis, or sarcoidosis confined to muscle), endocrine myopathies, sporadic Duchenne dystrophy, Duchenne or Becker's dystrophy manifesting in female carriers, other dystrophinopathies, and sporadic Emery-Dreifuss dystrophy before the appearance of joint contractures or cardiomyopathy.

CONGENITAL MUSCULAR DYSTROPHIES. The congenital muscular dystrophies (CMDs) are a group of autosomal recessive disorders with perinatal onset of hypotonia and proximal weakness; they have dystrophic muscle biopsy findings. The infants often have joint contractures of the elbows, hips, knees, and ankles (arthrogryposis). CMDs can be broadly divided into those without and those with clinical evidence of central nervous system involvement (severe mental retardation, seizures, and visual loss due to cerebro-ocular dysplasia). However, many patients without severe brain disease clinically, or the so-called classic type, usually have cerebral hypomyelination indicated on magnetic resonance imaging. The CMDs with significant brain and eye involvement generally produce progressive courses and death by age 10–12. Classic type

CMDs without clinical central nervous system involvement have a more benign outlook, with a non-progressive course; those affected may eventually walk independently.

Fifty per cent of classic type CMD is associated with a deficiency of the basal lamina protein α_2 *laminin,* also known as *merosin.* Merosin is bound to the DGC anchoring the basal lamina to the sarcolemma. Merosin-negative CMD can be diagnosed by immunostaining of muscle or skin. Other CMDs without clinical central nervous system (CNS) involvement are associated with a deficiency of integrin, a transsarcolemma protein that is not part of the DGC. The *Fukuyama-type* CMD, occurring primarily in Japan, is associated with mutations in the gene encoding for a protein named *fukutin.* The same genetic defect probably accounts for the Walker-Warburg cerebral-ocular dysplasia syndrome. Fukutin is not associated with the sarcolemma and appears to be a secreted protein, but its function is unknown.

FACIOSCAPULOHUMERAL DYSTROPHY. The inheritance of facioscapulohumeral dystrophy is autosomal dominant with high penetrance and variable expression within families. Affected family members may be unaware of their mild deficits, making examination of relatives of suspected patients very important. The incidence of facioscapulohumeral dystrophy is 1/20,000.

The disease presents in childhood or adult life. It involves the facial muscles early and then descends to the scapular stabilizers (serratus anterior, rhomboid, trapezius, latissimus dorsi), the muscles of the upper arm (biceps, triceps), and the anterior leg muscles. Early physical signs include failure to bury the eyelashes, an expressionless face, winging of the scapulas when the arms are raised, and prominent indentation of the anterior axillary folds. The deltoids are relatively spared compared to other proximal arm muscles. Distal muscle weakness occurs first in the tibialis anterior and may result in foot drop, leading to a scapuloperoneal pattern of weakness. Later, wrist and finger extensor weakness may develop. The rate of progression and the extent to which pelvic girdle and forearm muscles are eventually affected vary considerably between and within different families. In general, cases with early onset have a worse prognosis. Some patients experience a late exacerbation of weakness after years of little or slow progression. Approximately 20% of these patients eventually will require a wheelchair. There is no muscle hypertrophy, although a "trapezius hump" due to an upward movement of the unstable scapula may be mistaken for muscle hypertrophy. In addition, the marked biceps/triceps atrophy with relative preservation of the forearm muscles can produce the so-called Popeye arms. Joint contractures are uncommon.

The serum creatine kinase (CK) level is normal or shows mild elevation. The muscle biopsy shows moderate myopathic changes compared to those of other dystrophies. Occasionally a prominent mononuclear inflammatory infiltrate can be present, causing some confusion with polymyositis. However, these patients have no response to immunosuppressive therapy. A variant is associated with sensorineural hearing loss, and retinal telangiectasis and painless blindness (*Coats' disease*).

Facioscapulohumeral dystrophy has been linked to the telomeric region of chromosome 4q35. Although the gene has not been isolated, a deletion in this region is present in virtually all facioscapulohumeral dystrophy patients.

Scapuloperoneal muscular dystrophy is an autosomal dominant disorder that can resemble facioscapulohumeral dystrophy, but without facial weakness. In these families, there is no linkage to chromosome 4q35.

MYOTONIC DYSTROPHY. Myotonic dystrophy is an autosomal dominant multisystem disorder that affects skeletal, cardiac, and smooth muscle and other organs, including the eyes, the endocrine system, and the brain. This is the most common muscular dystrophy with an incidence of 13.5 per 100,000 live births and a prevalence of 3 to 5 per 100,000. Myotonic dystrophy can occur at any age with the usual onset of symptoms in the late second or third decade. However, some affected individuals may remain symptom free their entire life. A severe form with onset in infancy is known as *congenital myotonic dystrophy.* The severity is generally worse from one generation to the next.

Typical patients exhibit facial weakness with temporalis muscle wasting, frontal balding, ptosis, and neck flexor weakness. Extremity weakness usually begins distally and progresses slowly to affect the limb-girdle muscles proximally. Weakness is a more common symptom than muscle stiffness or myotonia, although patients may complain of the inability to relax the fingers after a hand grip. However, percussion myotonia can be produced on examination in most cases, especially in thenar and wrist extensor muscles. Patients may be areflexic, but the sensory examination is normal.

Associated manifestations include posterior subscapular cataracts, testicular atrophy and impotence, intellectual impairment, and hypersomnia due to both central and obstructive sleep apneas. Respiratory muscle weakness may be severe with impairment of ventilatory drive. Elevated serum glucose levels occurs as a result of end-organ unresponsiveness to insulin, but frank diabetes mellitus rarely develops. Involvement of the smooth muscle in the gastrointestinal tract can produce dysphagia, reduced gut motility, and chronic pseudo-obstruction. Cardiac conduction defects are common and can produce sudden death. Pacemakers may be necessary and annual electrocardiograms are recommended. Chronic hypoxia can lead to cor pulmonale. Affected females can have a high rate of fetal loss.

The serum CK level is normal or mildly increased. Muscle biopsies show excessive number of central nuclei, type 1 atrophy, and other non-specific myopathic changes. Fiber necrosis and increased connective tissue are not present. EMG shows myopathic motor units in addition to myotonic potentials.

The molecular defect of myotonic dystrophy is an abnormal expansion of CTG repeats in a protein kinase gene on chromosome 19q13.2. Affected individuals have more than 50 CTG repeats, and the severity of the disease directly correlates with the size of the expanded triplet repeat. The diagnosis can be established by documenting an increased number of CTG expansions in leukocytes from a blood sample. Marked expansion of the CTG repeat usually occurs in children of mothers with myotonic dystrophy, accounting for anticipation and the severe phenotype of congenital myotonic dystrophy. The protein kinase encoded by this gene has been termed *myotonin.* How the gene defect and the abnormal expression of myotonin cause tissue injury and myotonia is not known.

Recently, a second myotonic dystrophy locus was mapped to chromosome 3q. Clinical features of this large autosomal family were indistinguishable from those of the 19q-linked disorder.

Myotonic dystrophy patients rarely have myotonia that is so symptomatic that it requires treatment. Phenytoin is the safest drug for myotonia, as quinine, tocainide, and mexiletene can exacerbate cardiac arrhythmias and should be avoided. Annual ECGs are recommended and a pacemaker may be necessary. Positive-pressure ventilation devices may assist patients with sleep apnea. Sedatives and opiates should be used with caution as they can exacerbate ventilatory drive abnormalities. Myotonic dystrophy patients are at risk for pulmonary and cardiac complications during general anesthesia. Braces can assist patients with foot drop. Cataracts can be surgically removed when they become symptomatic.

Proximal myotonic myopathy (PROMM) is an autosomal dominant disorder that can clinically and histologically resemble myotonic dystrophy. However, proximal extremity weakness is significant, distal muscles are often normal, and patients usually complain of myotonia and myalagias. Patients with PROMM may have less cardiac muscle or other organ involvement. The exception to this rule is that many PROMM patients have cataracts that are indistinguishable from those in myotonic dystrophy. In some kindreds, PROMM has been localized to the 3q, the second myotonic dystrophy locus; in others the gene locus is unknown.

DISTAL DYSTROPHIES. Although a number of myopathies can have prominent distal weakness (see Table 505–3) some genetically distinct entities are considered as distal muscular dystrophies. There are two late-adult-onset autosomal dominant forms. *Welander distal dystrophy* occurs in Scandinavia and presents between the fourth and sixth decades with selective weakness and atrophy of the forearm extensor and intrinsic hand muscles and then involves the anterior leg and small foot muscles. In patients homozygous for the dominant gene, the onset is earlier and proximal muscles are also affected. *Markesbery/Udd distal dystrophy* has been observed in English and Finnish patients and initially involves the anterior tibial muscles and later the distal upper extremities. Two varieties of autosomal recessive distal muscular dystrophies with early-adult onset in the late second or early third decade have been described.

In the *Nonaka* form weakness begins in the anterior tibial muscles, whereas in the *Miyoshi* variety, the posterior gastrocnemius muscles are selectively affected first. An autosomal dominant childhood and early-adult-onset distal myopathy has been described by Laing. Serum CK level can be elevated in all of these disorders, but in Miyoshi myopathy the CK level is dramatically increased up to 200 times normal. Muscle biopsy result shows variable degrees of dystrophic changes, and rimmed vacuoles are common in all but Miyoshi myopathy. All of these disorders have progressive courses and over time can involve proximal muscles with the loss of ambulation. Chromosomal linkage has been found in each of these disorders (Table 506–1). Miyoshi myopathy and limb-girdle muscular dystrophy 2B are both associated with a 2p13 mutation in the *dysferlin* gene.

Myofibrillar myopathy (also known as *desmin* myopathy) is a heterogeneous group of muscular dystrophies that can present with either distal or limb-girdle patterns of weakness. Most kindreds are autosomal dominant, but sporadic cases occur. Cardiomyopathy is common. The muscle biopsy findings show vacuoles, cytoplasmic inclusions, and accumulations of desmin and other proteins such as dystrophin and β-amyloid precursor protein. Myofibrillar myopathy is probably not a single disorder, as some kindreds have a molecular defect in the $\alpha\beta$-crystallin chaperone protein on 11q21-23; others have a mutation in the desmin gene on 2q35; and one family has linkage to chromosome 12.

OCULOPHARYNGEAL MUSCULAR DYSTROPHY. The disease oculopharyngeal muscular dystrophy, inherited as an autosomal dominant disorder, presents in the fifth or sixth decade with progressive ptosis followed by dysphagia. Later, all external ocular and other extremity muscles may become affected. Diplopia does not develop. Extremity weakness is usually in a limb-girdle pattern, but some variants have significant distal involvement. In most patients the disease progression is slow. Death can result from aspiration pneumonia or starvation if adequate nutrition is not addressed. Patients may require surgical correction (cricopharyngeal myotomy) for achalasia or a gastric feeding tube. The serum CK level is normal or slightly increased. Muscle biopsy discloses non-specific myopathic changes with rimmed vacuoles in the muscle fibers, and the electron microscopy reveals 8.5-nm intranuclear filaments.

The molecular genetic defect is an increased expansion of a triplet GCG repeat on chromosome 14q11 within the *poly(A) binding protein 2* gene (*PABP2*). The function of *PABP2* and the means by which a mutation of this protein leads to muscle disease are unknown. Oculopharyngeal dystrophy appears to be more common in patients of French-Canadian or Hispanic ancestry.

Abn AH, Kunkel LM: The structural and functional diversity of dystrophin. Nat Genet 3:283, 1993. *A concise and comprehensive account of what is currently known about the dystrophin gene and dystrophin.*

Barohn RJ, Amato AA, Griggs RC: Overview of distal myopathies: From the clinical to the molecular. Neuromuscul Disord 8:309–316, 1998. *A good review of the currently recognized forms of distal dystrophies.*

Brown RH: Dystrophin-associated proteins and the muscular dystrophies: A glossary. Brain Pathol 6:19, 1996. *Review of the evolving terminology of these disorders.*

Duggan DJ, Gorospie JR, Fanin M, et al: Mutations in the sarcoglycan genes in patients with myopathy. N Engl J Med 336:618, 1997. *Provides data on the frequency of the various sarcoglycan deficiencies in patients with myopathy.*

Muntoni F, Sewry CA: Congenital muscular dystrophy: From rags to riches. Neurology 51:14, 1998. *An editorial review of advances in this area.*

Nagano A, Koga R, Ogawa M: Emerin deficiency at the nuclear membrane in patients with Emery-Dreifuss muscular dystrophy. Nat Genet 12:254, 1996. *Identifies the location of the protein deficiency in Emery-Dreifuss dystrophy.*

507 MORPHOLOGICALLY DISTINCT CONGENITAL MYOPATHIES

Richard J. Barohn

Congenital myopathies are distinguished from dystrophies in three respects. First, these disorders have characteristic morphologic alterations demonstrated on light and electron microscopy. Second, as the name implies, congenital myopathies usually present at birth with hypotonia and subsequent delayed motor development. Finally, most congenital myopathies are relatively non-progressive with more benign outcomes than occur in the muscular dystrophies. However, there are exceptions to all three generalizations. Onset can occur in childhood and even in early adulthood, and some congenital myopathies have a severe course and fatal outcome. Moreover, as the molecular genetic defects of the congenital myopathies become known, distinguishing between these disorders and muscular dystrophies becomes more difficult.

The four best recognized congenital myopathies are discussed later, and others are listed in Table 507–1. Common clinical findings in these conditions include reduced muscle bulk (no hypertrophy); slender body build and a long, narrow face, with skeletal abnormalities (high-arched palate, pectus excavatum, kyphoscoliosis, dislocated hips, pes cavus); and absent or reduced muscle stretch reflexes. Most patients have a limb-girdle weakness phenotype, although distal weakness can occur in some families (see Table 505–3). Serum creatine kinase (CK) is moderately elevated or normal and the electromyographic (EMG) usually shows a myopathic pattern, but may be normal. Inheritance patterns are variable.

CENTRAL CORE MYOPATHY. Central core myopathy is characterized by discrete zones (cores) of myofibrillar disruption in the center of muscle fibers. This is demonstrated on the oxidative enzyme stain, which reveals an absence of enzyme within the cores. Electron microscopy confirms the presence of cores along the length of muscle fibers. Central core myopathy is autosomal dominant, but sporadic cases occur. The disorder is associated with a mutation on chromosome 19q13.1 in the *ryanodine receptor gene*. Malignant hyperthermia patients also have mutations in this gene and thus the disorders may be allelic. Although not all central core myopathy patients are susceptible to malignant hyperthermia, and vice versa, patients with central core are at a high risk for malignant hyperthermia, and anesthetic precautions are necessary. The mechanism by which defects in the ryanodine receptor gene lead to these disorders is unknown.

Some families have multiple small *minicores* that do not extend the entire length of the muscle. These minicore myopathies are not associated with the ryanodine receptor gene and it is unclear whether those affected are at risk for malignant hyperthermia.

NEMALINE MYOPATHY. The histologic characteristic of nemaline myopathy, a congenital myopathy, is the presence of rods, or nemaline (*nema* = Greek "thread") bodies, within muscle fibers. Rods are similar to Z-disk material and are strongly immunoreactive for α-actinin. Clinically, the myopathy can present as a severe neonatal form with respiratory (diaphragm) involvement that is generally fatal within the first year of life or as a mild static or slowly progressive condition present from birth or early childhood. Nemaline myopathy can occur as an autosomal recessive or dominant condition. Most autosomal recessive families have been linked to 2q; nebulin is the likely candidate gene. Some autosomal dominant families have been linked to a mutation in the α-tropomyosin gene on 1q. Other cases are sporadic. Note that the presence of rods in muscle does not necessarily imply a congenital myopathy, as these structures can be seen in human immunodeficiency virus–related myopathy and occasionally in other inflammatory myopathies.

CENTRONUCLEAR (MYOTUBULAR) MYOPATHY. The histo-

Table 507–1 ■ MORPHOLOGICALLY DISTINCT CONGENITAL MYOPATHIES

Central core myopathy
Nemaline (rod) myopathy
Centronuclear (myotubular) myopathy
Severe X-linked recessive form
Milder autosomal recessive and dominant forms
Congenital fiber-type disproportion
Multicore/minicore myopathy
Fingerprint body myopathy
Sarcotubular myopathy
Reducing body myopathy
Trilaminar myopathy
Hyaline myopathy with focal lysis of myofibrils
Myofibrillar myopathy

logic hallmark of centronuclear (myotubular) myopathy is the presence of large central nuclei within many muscle fibers. Since this feature superficially resembles embryonic muscle, the term *myotubular myopathy* has also been used, although centronuclear myopathy is not due to an arrest of myotubes. As with nemaline myopathy, there are severe neonatal presentations and static or slowly progressive forms with onset from birth to adulthood. Ptosis and ophthalmoparesis occur commonly in all forms of centronuclear myopathy and may distinguish these patients from those with congenital myopathies. Otherwise, the clinical features are similar. The severe infantile form is usually X-linked recessive and is associated with respiratory insufficiency. Most die in infancy, but a few patients survive into childhood, usually with major disabilities. The molecular defect is a mutation in the *myotubularin* gene on Xp28. Myotubularin is a phosphatase important in muscle cell growth and differentiation. The genetic defects are unknown for the milder autosomal recessive and dominant forms.

CONGENITAL FIBER-TYPE DISPROPORTION. The distinguishing morphologic finding in congenital fiber-type disproportion is an increased number of small type I muscle fibers. Of all the congenital myopathies, congenital fiber-type disproportion is the most poorly understood and characterized. Most patients have onset at birth with hypotonia and have a relatively benign, non-progressive course. The genetic defect is unknown.

Fardeau M, Tonmé FMS: Congenital myopathies. In Engel AG, Franzini-Armstrong C (eds): Myology, 2nd ed. New York, McGraw-Hill, 1994, p 1487. *A comprehensive, well-illustrated review.*

Wallgren-Pettersen C: Genetics of the nemaline myopathies and the myotubular myopathies. Neuromuscul Disord 8:401, 1998. *A review of the current molecular understanding of these disorders.*

508 METABOLIC MYOPATHIES

Richard J. Barohn

Metabolic myopathies (see also Chapters 202 to 204) include (1) glucose/glycogen metabolism disorders; (2) lipid metabolism disorders; and (3) mitochondrial disorders. A fourth group involving the utilization of adenine nucleotides is more controversial (Table 508–1).

GLUCOSE/GLYCOGEN METABOLISM DISORDERS

Glucose and its storage form glycogen are essential for the short-term, predominantly anaerobic energy requirements of muscle. Disorders of glucose and glycogen metabolism (grouped under the term *glycogenoses*) have two distinct clinical presentations. One group of disorders has *dynamic* manifestations with exercise intolerance, pain, cramps, and myoglobinuria (Types V, VII, VIII, IX, X, XI). The second, *static* group is associated with fixed weakness without features of exercise intolerance or myoglobinuria (Types II, III, IV). Occasionally there is overlap between the two groups. Of the 11 distinct glycogenoses, only glucose-6-phosphate (Type I) and liver phosphorylase (Type VI) deficiencies do not affect muscle. The glycogenoses that affect muscle are usually transmitted as autosomal recessive traits, except for phosphoglycerate kinase, which is X-linked.

GLYCOGENOSES WITH EXERCISE INTOLERANCE/MYOGLOBINURIA. MYOPHOSPHORYLASE (TYPE V), PHOSPHOFRUCTOKINASE (PFK, TYPE VII), PHOSPHORYLASE B KINASE (PBK, TYPE VIII), PHOSPHOGLYCERATE KINASE (PGK, TYPE IX), PHOSPHOGLYCERATE MUTASE (PGM, TYPE X), LACTATE DEHYDROGENASE (LDH, XI) DEFICIENCIES. The common clinical features of the glycogenoses with exercise intolerance/myoglobinuria are exercise intolerance in childhood followed by exertion-induced muscle pain, and myoglobinuria in the second or third decade. Many patients note a "second wind" phenomenon after a period of brief rest so that they can continue the exercise at the previous level of activity. The muscle pain is caused by electrically silent contractures and is not associated with adenosine triphosphate (ATP) depletion; their mechanism

Table 508–1 ■ METABOLIC AND MITOCHONDRIAL MYOPATHIES

Glycogen metabolism deficiencies
  Type II   α-1,4 Glucosidase (acid maltase)
  Type III   Debranching
  Type IV   Branching
  Type V   Phosphorylase* (McArdle's disease)
  Type VII   Phosphofructokinase* (Tarui's disease)
  Type VIII Phosphorylase B kinase*
  Type IX   Phosphoglycerate kinase*
  Type X   Phosphoglycerate mutase*
  Type XI   Lactate dehydrogenase*
Lipid metabolism deficiencies
  Carnitine palmitoyl transferase*
  Primary systemic/muscle carnitine deficiency
  Secondary carnitine deficiency
    β-Oxidation defects
    Medications (valproic acid)
Purine metabolism deficiencies
  Myoadenylate deaminase deficiency*
Mitochondrial myopathies
  Pyruvate dehydrogenase complex deficiencies (including Leigh's syndrome)
  Progressive external ophthalmoplegia (PEO)
  Kearns-Sayre syndrome
  Mitochondrial encephalopathy with lactic acidosis and strokelike episodes (MELAS)
  Myoclonic epilepsy and ragged red fibers (MERRF)
  Mitochondrial neurogastrointestinal encephalomyopathy (MNGIE)
  Mitochondrial depletion syndrome
  Leigh's syndrome and neuropathy, ataxia, retinitis pigmentosa (NARP)
  Succinate dehydrogenase deficiency*

*Deficiency can produce exercise intolerance and myoglobinuria.

is not understood. Strength examination, serum creatine kinase (CK) level, and electromyographic (EMG) findings between attacks are usually normal early in the disease but may become abnormal with advancing age. After episodes of severe myoglobinuria with rhabdomyolysis, needle EMG can show myopathic units and fibrillations. If the needle EMG is performed during a "cramp" (see the discussion of muscle contracture in Chapter 505), there will be electrical silence. After the forearm exercise test, venous lactate level fails to rise in myophosphorylase, PFK, and PGK deficiencies, and only rises partially in PBK, PGM, and LDH deficiencies. The muscle biopsy shows scattered necrotic and regenerating fibers, especially after an episode of rhabdomyolysis. There is usually a modest accumulation of glycogen in the subsarcolemmal and intermyofibrillar areas indicated on light and electron microscopy.

Histochemical stains are readily available for some of these disorders (myophosphorylase, PFK), but definitive diagnosis requires biochemical analysis to document the enzyme deficiency. Molecular genetic mutations have been identified for all the glycogenoses except PBK deficiency.

Fatal infantile variants have been identified in myophosphorylase and PFK deficiency. In PFK deficiency hyperuricemia and gout occur in some cases, and there is mild hemolytic anemia caused by a partial erythrocyte enzyme defect. PGK mutations result either in severe hemolytic anemia and neurologic deficits but no myopathy or in a myopathy with only the features described earlier. PBK deficiency can manifest as a dynamic disorder with exercise intolerance or can present in infancy or childhood with weakness and delay in motor milestones. LDH deficiency is associated with a rash because M-lactate dehydrogenase is the dominant form of the enzyme expressed in skin.

Although no specific treatment is available for these disorders, aerobic exercise training and a high-protein diet have been proposed as sensible strategies.

GLYCOGENOSES WITH FIXED WEAKNESS AND NO EXERCISE INTOLERANCE. α-1,4-GLUCOSIDASE (ACID MALTASE, TYPE II), DEBRANCHING ENZYME (TYPE III), BRANCHING ENZYME (TYPE IV) DEFICIENCIES. α-Glucosidase, also known as *acid maltase,* is a lysosomal enzyme that breaks down glycogen to glucose; however, its role in carbohydrate metabolism is not fully defined. When its level is deficient, glycogen accumulates within lysosomes as well as freely in the cytoplasm of cells. There are three clinical variants. The *infantile type (Pompe's disease)* presents in early infancy with generalized and rapidly progressive weakness and heart, tongue, and liver enlargement. There is widespread glycogen excess in tissues, including lower motor neurons. Death results from cardiorespiratory failure before the age of 2 years. The *childhood (juvenile) type* presents in infancy or early childhood as a myopathy. Weakness is more proximal than distal, and there may be calf enlargement simulating muscular dystrophy. Glycogen excess is less marked and confined to muscle. The heart, but not the liver, may be involved. Death results from respiratory failure before age 20. The *adult type* presents between the second and seventh decades of life, either with slowly progressive limb muscle weakness that mimics limb-girdle dystrophy or with a scapuloperoneal presentation. These patients often experience insidious ventilatory insufficiency leading to respiratory failure. The adult form does not affect the heart or liver. In all three types the serum CK level is moderately increased. The EMG result in affected muscles shows myopathic changes and excessive abnormal electrical irritability, including myotonic discharges, particularly in paraspinous muscles. However, there is no clinical myotonia. The muscle biopsy demonstrates a vacuolar myopathy with high glycogen content and acid-phosphatase reactivity in the vacuoles. The diagnosis is confirmed by demonstrating α-glucosidase deficiency in either muscle, skin fibroblasts, or lymphocytes. Mutations have been identified in the α-glucosidase gene on chromosome 17q21. Therapy is primarily supportive, particularly for respiratory insufficiency.

Danon's disease has clinical and histologic features similar to those of the adult form of α-glucosidase deficiency, including glycogen accumulation, but no enzyme deficiency can be identified.

DEBRANCHING ENZYME DEFICIENCY (TYPE III). Debranching enzyme deficiency is a rare disease that can affect liver, heart, or skeletal muscle; it most commonly presents in childhood as hepatomegaly with fasting hypoglycemia that spontaneously resolves by adulthood. Patients less frequently have a disabling myopathy affecting both proximal and distal muscles that can appear in childhood or (more commonly) in adult life. Affected patients can experience exercise intolerance and there may be a depressed lactate response indicated by forearm testing, but myoglobinuria is rare. The CK level is elevated and the EMG shows myopathic changes and abnormal electrical irritability. The gene for the enzyme maps to chromosome 1p21.

BRANCHING ENZYME DEFICIENCY (TYPE IV). Deficiency of the branching enzyme has manifestations in many organs. The disease presents in infancy with progressive liver and cardiac dysfunction, which lead to death in the first years of life. Muscle weakness is variable; if weakness is present, the tongue is severely affected.

DISORDERS OF FATTY ACID METABOLISM

Lipids are essential for the aerobic energy needs of muscle during sustained exercise. Serum long-chain fatty acids are the primary lipid fuel for muscle metabolism. They are transported into the mitochondria as carnitine esters and are metabolized via β-oxidation. Carnitine palmitoyl transferase (CPT) I converts cytoplasmic acyl–coenzyme A (CoA) to acylcarnitine, which is then transported into the mitochondria by carnitine acyl-transferase in exchange for carnitine. CPT II on the inner mitochondrial membrane reconstitutes acyl-Co A. A deficiency of carnitine, CPT, or the enzymes of β-oxidation can lead to impaired muscle lipid metabolism.

As with glycogen pathway defects, the myopathic manifestations of fatty acid metabolism can consist of a dynamic exercise intolerance with myoglobinuria or static weakness with a lipid storage myopathy. A lipid storage myopathy can be caused by primary carnitine deficiency or by another defect of fatty acid oxidation with secondary carnitine deficiency. In addition, some disorders of lipid metabolism can produce multiorgan metabolic crises with hepatic failure and altered mental status (Reye's syndrome). Most lipid disorders occur sporadically; they are believed to be autosomal recessive.

CARNITINE PALMITOYL TRANSFERASE DEFICIENCY. CPT is present in two forms: Types I and II. Deficiency of CPT I may present in infancy or childhood with hepatic dysfunction. It causes a Reye's syndrome–like illness with hypoketotic hypoglycemia, encephalopathy, hyperammonemia, and liver dysfunction. Deficiency of CPT II typically causes exertional myalgias and myoglobinuria. This is the most frequently definable metabolic defect presenting with myoglobinuria. These attacks are distinct from those associated with glycolytic defects in that they occur after prolonged exercise, fasting, febrile illness, or other provocations that may increase muscle dependence on free fatty acids. Unlike patients with McArdle's disease, those with CPT deficiency tolerate brief, intense exercise and have no second wind phenomenon. Muscle strength and CK level are normal at rest. Fasting may provoke an increase in CK level; the normal ketosis does not develop. Serum and muscle carnitine levels are typically normal. The EMG is normal except for myopathic changes following episodes of rhabdomyolysis. Ammonia and lactate levels rise normally after forearm exercise. Muscle biopsy results are usually normal except for evidence of muscle myopathic injury after rhabdomyolysis. Diagnosis requires assay of CPT activity in muscle. Care must be taken with these assays to differentiate between measured CPT I activity and CPT II activity. CPT I activity is preserved in the muscle form of the disease and normally constitutes at least half of the total measured CPT activity. Although there is no specific treatment, increasing carbohydrate intake and meal frequency prevents episodes of rhabdomyolysis. The disorder is autosomal recessive, and mutations in the CPT II gene on chromosome 1p32 have been identified.

CARNITINE DEFICIENCY. Primary carnitine deficiencies may present as a generalized systemic illness or as a disorder confined to muscle. In the systemic form, there is impaired transport of carnitine into multiple tissues, which results from non-functional high-affinity carnitine receptors. Patients have a myopathy with cardiac involvement, as well as episodes of hepatic dysfunction with hypoketotic hypoglycemia and altered mental status. Abnormal lipid storage is seen on the muscle biopsy. Carnitine level is reduced in serum, muscle, and other tissues. There is no urinary excretion of organic acids to suggest a secondary metabolic illness. Patients with this condition improve with carnitine supplementation.

Primary muscle carnitine deficiency usually presents in childhood as a limb-girdle myopathy. Patients have diminished muscle uptake of carnitine and a fixed lipid-storage myopathy, but normal serum carnitine level. Carnitine replacement in these patients has been of inconsistent benefit.

SECONDARY CARNITINE DEFICIENCY. Most carnitine deficiencies are secondary to enzyme defects in β-oxidation (e.g., acyl-CoA dehydrogenase deficiencies), mitochondrial dysfunction, renal disease, impaired metabolism of medication such as valproic acid, or other metabolic disorders. Defects in lipid metabolism lead to accumulation of acyl-CoA molecules, which are converted to acylcarnitines, which are more readily excreted in the urine. This process leads to a negative carnitine balance and ultimately to carnitine deficiency. Impaired metabolism of valproic acid may similarly lead to excretion of valproylcarnitine and secondary carnitine deficiency. Most of these illnesses present in early childhood or infancy with Reye's syndrome–like episodes. Some surviving adults experience a lipid storage myopathy with the clinical phenotype of a limb-girdle syndrome. Muscle biopsy findings reveal lipid storage. Free carnitine level is diminished, but that of esterified carnitine may be increased, especially after oral supplementation of depleted carnitine stores. Abnormal urinary excretion of organic acids is a critical clue to differentiate these disorders from primary carnitine deficiency. Different metabolic blocks in fatty acid metabolism lead to the excretion of distinct urinary acylcarnitine species. These can be distinguished by mass spectroscopy to identify specific enzyme deficiencies. Carnitine supplementation produces variable results, but some patients have reduced frequency and severity of metabolic attacks. Some cases of multiple flavin-dependent dehydrogenase deficiency respond to riboflavin.

DISORDERS OF PURINE NUCLEOTIDE METABOLISM: MYOADENYLATE DEAMINASE DEFICIENCY

Myoadenylate deaminase (MAD) is an enzyme in the purine nucleotide cycle. MAD provides a short-term supply of adenosine triphosphate (ATP) in muscle by catalyzing the conversion of adenosine monophosphate (AMP) to inosine monophosphate (IMP) through the removal of ammonia. If MAD is absent, less ATP is formed. MAD deficiency has been found in patients with exertional muscle pain and occasionally myoglobinuria. The forearm exercise test result shows a normal rise in lactate level but no increase in ammonia level. Muscle biopsy tissue has absent staining for MAD. The gene for MAD is on chromosome 1p13-21 and is mutated in most patients with MAD deficiency. However, the frequency of this mutation in the "normal" population is high and patients without symptoms may have biochemical evidence of MAD deficiency. Therefore, it is still unclear whether or not MAD deficiency results in a metabolic myopathy or whether the enzyme deficiency is coincidental.

MITOCHONDRIAL MYOPATHIES

Mitochondrial myopathies produce slowly progressive weakness of limb-girdle or external ocular and other cranial muscles and abnormal fatigability on sustained exertion. Some affect multiple organs or systems, in addition to muscle.

In many mitochondrial myopathies a substantial proportion of the muscle fibers contains subsarcolemmal and intermyofibrillar accumulations of structurally and functionally abnormal mitochondria. These fibers appear "ragged-red" in the trichrome stain and may fail to react for cytochrome-c oxidase (CCO). Other laboratory features frequently seen in mitochondrial myopathies are an elevated serum lactic acid level on exertion or at rest, as well as modestly elevated CK level and a myopathic EMG. Interestingly, the level of cerebrospinal fluid (CSF) protein is often elevated.

Mitochondrial DNA encodes for 22 transfer RNAs (tRNAs), two ribosomal RNAs (rRNAs), and 13 messenger RNAs (mRNAs). The 13 mRNAs are translated into polypeptide subunits of the respiratory chain complex. A mutation in a mitochondrial tRNA gene can impair the proper translation of the 13 mitochondrial mRNAs. However, the 13 proteins encoded by the mitochondrial genome account for less than 5% of mitochondrial proteins; the majority are encoded by nuclear DNA and are translated in the cytoplasm and transported into mitochondria.

Mitochondrial diseases can arise from mutations in nuclear or mitochondrial DNA. During fertilization all of the mitochondria are contributed by the mother; thus, all mutations of mitochondrial DNA either are maternally transmitted or arise de novo in the maternal ovum or in early embryonic life. However, since the majority of mitochondrial proteins (95%) are encoded from nuclear genes, mitochondrial disorders can also have autosomal/dominant and even X-linked hereditary patterns.

From a biochemical standpoint, mitochondrial disorders can be due to defects proximal to the respiratory chain (involving substrate transport and utilization) or within the respiratory chain. Viewed in this way, the derangements of lipid metabolism can be considered "mitochondrial" dysfunctions. Acetyl-CoA feeds into the mitochondria to enter the Krebs cycle and the respiratory chain. However, the lipid disorders generally do not have structural defects of mitochondria or a "mitochondrial myopathy" phenotype. Among exceptions are substrate utilization abnormalities due to pyruvate dehydrogenase complex defects, which can produce an X-linked Leigh's syndrome or subacute necrotizing encephalomyopathy. Although the muscle biopsy may show ragged red fibers, the central nervous system abnormalities overshadow the neuromuscular abnormalities.

The classic mitochondrial disorders are due to biochemical defects in the mitochondrial respiratory chain that can involve coenzyme Q and the five distinct enzyme complexes: Complex I (reduced nicotinamide-adenine dinucleotide–[NADH]-coenzyme Q oxidoreductase); Complex II(succinate-dehydrogenase); Complex II (coenzyme Q-cytochrome-C oxidoreductase), Complex IV (cytochrome-C oxidase), and Complex V (adenosine triphosphatase [ATPase] synthetase). Defects in the electron transport complexes are associated with marked clinical, biochemical, and genetic heterogeneity. The reasons for this are that each complex is composed of multiple subunits, different subunits of a given complex are encoded by different genes, some subunits of a given complex are encoded by mitochondrial rather than nuclear DNA, and some subunits are tissue specific.

SPECIFIC MITOCHONDRIAL DISORDERS AFFECTING MUSCLE. PROGRESSIVE EXTERNAL OPHTHALMOPLEGIA. Severe ptosis and progressive external ophthalmoplegia (PEO) are clinical hallmarks of mitochondrial disease. Ptosis is often the presenting

symptom and is generally first noted in childhood. As the ophthalmoplegia progresses, it often becomes complete. Patients do not have diplopia. A limb-girdle weakness pattern may occur with varying degrees of severity. Thus, the term "oculocraniosomatic" was initially used to describe these disorders. The muscle biopsy reveals characteristic ragged-red fibers, and electron microscopy shows structurally abnormal mitochondria with "parking-lot" paracrystalline inclusions.

PEO due to mitochondrial disease is associated with single or multiple mitochondrial DNA deletions. Patients with single mitochondrial deletions have the *Kearns-Sayre syndrome,* which includes a variety of multisystem abnormalities. Some of the associated conditions in the Kearns-Sayre syndrome are retinitis pigmentosa, heart block, hearing loss, short stature, ataxia, delayed secondary sexual characteristics, peripheral neuropathy, and poor ventilatory drive. The syndrome presents before age 20. The Kearns-Sayre syndrome is due to single large mitochondrial deletions; it is sporadic and occurs with no family history of the disorder.

Patients with PEO who have multiple mitochondrial deletions have an autosomal dominant inheritance patterns. These patients usually have a later onset of symptoms than those with sporadic single deletions, often accompanied with various degrees of encephalomyopathy and neuropathy. In autosomal dominant PEO a nuclear gene defect somehow leads to communication errors between the nuclear and mitochondrial genomes, resulting in multiple mitochondrial deletions as mitochondrial DNA replicates. The mitochondrial deletions increase over time so that when they reach a critical number, clinical symptoms develop. Autosomal dominant kinships with PEO have been localized to both chromosomes 10q22-23 and 3ql4-21. In addition, maternally inherited kinships due to point mutations in mitochondrial tRNA have been reported, further emphasizing the genetic heterogeneity of the disorder.

MYOCLONIC EPILEPSY AND RAGGED RED FIBERS (MERRF). Patients affected by myoclonic epilepsy and ragged-red fibers have varying symptoms of myoclonus, generalized seizures, ataxia, dementia, sensorineural hearing loss, optic atrophy, as well as limb-girdle weakness. Some patients also have a sensorimotor peripheral neuropathy, cardiomyopathy, and cutaneous lipomas. Ptosis and ophthalmoparesis are usually not present. Most patients have a point mutation in the mitochondrial DNA encoding for tRNA, and the disease is maternally inherited.

MITOCHONDRIAL ENCEPHALOMYOPATHY WITH LACTIC ACIDOSIS AND STROKELIKE EPISODES (MELAS). MELAS patients have normal early development, experience migraine-like headaches and strokes before age 40, and have lactic acidosis. Other features frequently include dementia, hearing loss, and episodic vomiting, ataxia, and coma, as well as diabetes. Ptosis and ophthalmoparesis are uncommon. MELAS is inherited maternally and is caused by mitochondrial DNA mutation encoding for tRNA.

MITOCHONDRIAL NEUROGASTROINTESTINAL ENCEPHALOMYOPATHY (MNGIE). The disorder MNGIE is associated with sensorimotor polyneuropathy, leukoencephalopathy indicated on magnetic resonance imaging (MRI) of the brain, and chronic intestinal pseudo-obstruction. Patients have distal as well as proximal weakness, ptosis, and ophthalmoplegia. This is also referred to as the polyneuropathy, ophthalmoplegia, leukoencephalopathy, and intestinal pseudo-obstruction (POLIP) syndrome. There are multiple mitochondrial DNA deletions similar to those found in autosomal dominant PEO. MNGIE has been localized to chromosome 22q13 in some families.

MITOCHONDRIAL DNA DEPLETION SYNDROME. Mitochondrial DNA depletion syndrome presents at birth or shortly afterward and is characterized by generalized hypotonia and weakness. Other features can include cardiomyopathy, renal tubular defects, seizures, and liver failure. Infants experience respiratory failure and many die within the first year of life. Histologically there are many cytochrome-c oxidase–negative fibers as well as ragged-red fibers and abnormal mitochondria. This disorder is autosomal recessive. Mutations of nuclear genes important in regulating the mitochondrial genome are thought to be responsible for the mitochondrial DNA depletion. The severity of the depletion correlates with the clinical severity. There is also a benign infantile form in which the hypotonic infants can survive and appear normal by age 2 or 3 years.

LEIGH'S SYNDROME. Patients usually present in infancy or early childhood with altered mental status, generalized weakness or hypotonia, vomiting, ataxia, ptosis and ophthalmoplegia, seizures, and respiratory failure. The disease is generally fatal. The molecular genetic characteristics are heterogenous: Some disorders are X-linked and due to defects in the pyruvate dehydrogenase complex; others are maternally inherited and due to point mutations in the mitochondrial ATPase 6 gene; still others are sporadic with large mitochondrial DNA deletions. In some families, mitochondrial ATPase 6 mutations can result in neuropathy, ataxia, and retinitis pigmentosa (the NARP syndrome).

MITOCHONDRIAL MYOPATHIES ASSOCIATED WITH RECURRENT MYOGLOBINURIA. Recurrent myoglobinuria provoked by exercise is uncommon in mitochondrial disorders. Between attacks, the patient's condition is normal. This is a genetically heterogenous group of disorders: multiple mitochondrial DNA deletions (autosomal recessive inheritance), mitochondrial point mutations (maternal inheritance), and nuclear DNA mutations encoding for succinate dehydrogenase (Complex II).

Engel AG, Franzini-Armstrong C (eds): Myology, 2nd ed. New York, McGraw-Hill, 1994. *Chapters by DiMauro and Tsujino, Engel and Hirschhorn. Zierz, DiDonato, Morgan-Hughes, Penn, Victor and Sieb, Kaminski and Ruff, and Lehmann-Horn. Engel, Ricker, and Rüdel review the metabolic myopathies.*

DiMauro S, Hirano M, Bonilla E, De Vivo DC: The mitochondrial disorders. *In* Berg BO (ed): Principles of Child Neurology. New York, McGraw-Hill, 1996, pp 1201–1232. *Review by leading authorities on the mitochondrial disorders.*

509 CHANNELOPATHIES (NON-DYSTROPHIC MYOTONIAS AND PERIODIC PARALYSES)

Richard J. Barohn

The myotonias are categorized into dystrophic (see the discussion 506) and non-dystrophic disorders. The non-dystrophic myotonias and the periodic paralyses are caused by mutations of various ion channels in muscle (Table 509–1). The term *channelopathies* is often used to describe this group of disorders.

CHLORIDE CHANNELOPATHIES

Myotonia congenita is due to point mutations in the muscle chloride channel gene on chromosome 7q35. There are autosomal dominant and recessive forms that are allelic. The autosomal dominant form (Thomsen's disease) and the autosomal recessive form (Becker's myotonia) are both benign and are associated with muscle hypertrophy and action, percussion, and electrical myotonia. Cold increases the myotonia, and sustained exercise improves it (warm-up phenomenon). There is no involvement of the heart or other organs. Thomsen's disease patients are not weak, but those who have Becker's myotonia congenita have fluctuations in strength and may experience limb-girdle weakness. Myotonia congenita patients seldom complain of pain, a feature that distinguishes them from those who have proximal myotonic myopathy (PROMM). The membrane defect consists of a markedly reduced chloride conductance with resulting hyperexcitability and after-depolarization that produces involuntary myotonic potentials. Many patients do not require treatment, but drugs such as quinine, procainamide, phenytoin, and mexiletine may be effective in reducing symptomatic myotonia.

SODIUM CHANNELOPATHIES

Several autosomal dominant disorders are due to point mutations in the voltage-dependent sodium channel (*SCN4A*) gene on chromosome 17q23-25. All have symptoms beginning in the first decade that continue throughout life, and there is considerable clinical overlap between the disorders. *Paramyotonia congenita* (Eulenburg's disease) patients have paradoxical myotonia, in that myotonia increases with repetitive movements. This is often best observed on repeated forced eye closure: After several attempts the patient cannot open the eyelids. Muscle stiffness is worsened by cold temperature. The myotonia can be treated with sodium-channel blockers such as mexiletine.

Hyperkalemic periodic paralysis is characterized by attacks of weakness lasting 1 or 2 hours. Attacks are precipitated by fasting, by rest after exercise, or by ingestion of potassium-rich foods or compounds. During attacks patients are areflexic with normal sensation and there is no ocular or respiratory muscle weakness. The serum potassium level may or may not be increased during the attack, and therefore a more appropriate term may be *potassium-sensitive periodic paralysis*. Strength is generally normal between

Table 509–1 ■ CHANNELOPATHIES AND RELATED DISORDERS

DISORDER	CLINICAL FEATURES	PATTERN OF INHERITANCE	CHROMOSOME	GENE
Chloride channelopathies				
Myotonia congenita				
Thomsen's disease	Myotonia	Autosomal dominant	7q35	*CLC1*
Becker's disease	Myotonia and weakness	Autosomal recessive	7q35	*CLC1*
Sodium channelopathies				
Paramyotonia congenita	Paramyotonia	Autosomal dominant	17q13.1-13.3	*SCNA4A*
Hyperkalemic periodic paralysis	Periodic paralysis with myotonia and paramyotonia	Autosomal dominant	17q13.1-13.3	*SCNA4A*
Potassium-aggravated myotonias				
Myotonia fluctuans	Myotonia	Autosomal dominant	17q13.1-13.3	*SCNA4A*
Myotonia permanens	Myotonia	Autosomal dominant	17q13.1-13.3	*SCNA4A*
Acetazolamide-responsive myotonia	Myotonia	Autosomal dominant	17q13.1-13.3	*SCNA4A*
Calcium channelopathies				
Hypokalemic periodic paralysis	Periodic paralysis	Autosomal dominant	1q31-32	Dihydropyridine receptor
Schwartz-Jampel syndrome (chondrodystrophic myotonia)	Myotonia; dysmorphic	Autosomal recessive	1p34.1-36.1	Unknown
Rippling muscle disease	Muscle mounding/stiffness	Autosomal dominant	1q41	Unknown
Anderson's syndrome	Periodic paralysis, cardiac arrhythmia, distinctive facies	Autosomal dominant	Unknown	Unknown
Brody's disease	Delayed relaxation, no EMG myotonia	Autosomal recessive	16p12	Calcium ATPase
Malignant hyperthermia	Anesthetic-induced delayed relaxation	Autosomal dominant	19q13.1	Ryanodine receptor

EMG = electromyogram; ATPase = adenosine triphosphatase.

attacks, but some patients can have mild interictal limb-girdle weakness. Some families with potassium-sensitive periodic paralysis also have either myotonia or paramyotonia. Episodes of weakness are rarely serious enough to require acute therapy; oral carbohydrates or glucose may improve weakness. Treatment options to prevent attacks include thiazide diuretics, β-agonists, and preventive measures such as a low-potassium, high-carbohydrate diet and avoidance of fasting, strenuous activity, and cold.

Sodium-channel myotonias are a group of potassium-sensitive disorders due to molecular defects in the sodium channel but not characterized by periodic paralysis or paramyotonia phenotypes. These include *acetazolamide-responsive myotonia, myotonia fluctuans* (myotonia that fluctuates on a daily basis), and *myotonia permanens.*

CALCIUM CHANNELOPATHIES

Hypokalemic periodic paralysis is due to abnormal muscle membrane excitability arising from mutations in the muscle calcium channel α_1 subunit on chromosome 1q31-32. The α_1 subunit contains the *dihydropyridine receptor,* which acts as a pore for conducting calcium ions in the T tubule. The mutation produces a reduction of the calcium current in the T tubule. During attacks there is an influx of potassium into muscle cells and the muscles become electrically inexcitable. Patients have an increased sensitivity to the effects of insulin on potassium flux. However, the mechanism through which the shift in potassium from the extracellular to the intracellular space is associated with the functional impairment of the calcium-channel dihydropyridine receptor is unknown.

Hypokalemic periodic paralysis is an autosomal dominant condition. It is the most frequent form of periodic paralysis and is more common in males with a reduced penetrance in females. Attacks begin by adolescence and are aggravated by exercise, sleep, stress, alcohol, or meals rich in carbohydrates and sodium. The episodes last from 3 to 24 hours. A vague prodrome of stiffness or heaviness in the legs can occur, and if the patient performs mild exercise a full-blown attack may be aborted. Rarely, ocular, bulbar, and respiratory muscles can be involved in severe attacks. Early in the disease patients have normal interictal examination findings except eyelid myotonia (about 50%). Later, attack frequency can lessen, but many patients have proximal weakness; in occasional patients this weakness produces severe incapacity.

Preventive measures include a low-carbohydrate, low-sodium diet and drugs such as acetazolamide, dichlorphenamide, spironolactone, and triamterene. Acute attacks are treated with oral potassium every 30 minutes until strength improves; the cardiogram must be monitored. In severe episodes, particularly in patients with gastrointestinal symptoms, parenteral potassium may be necessary.

OTHER FORMS OF PERIODIC PARALYSIS, CHANNELOPATHIES, MUSCLE STIFFNESS

Andersen's syndrome is an autosomal dominant disorder with periodic paralysis (hypo-, hyper-, or normo-), distinctive facial features (hypertelorism, short stature, low set ears), prolonged QT interval, and life-threatening ventricular arrhythmias. The genetic defect is unknown.

Rippling muscle disease is an autosomal dominant disorder characterized by localized transient swelling or rippling of muscle induced by percussion or exercise. Patients complain of tightness in the thighs or upper arms. A pedigree has been localized to chromosome 1q41, but the molecular defect is unknown.

Brody's disease is characterized by exercise-induced impaired relaxation and stiffness, but with no abnormalities indicated by muscle percussion or on electromyogram (EMG). The disorder is autosomal recessive and due to mutations in the sarcoplasmic reticulum calcium adenosine triphosphatase (ATPase) gene of type 2 muscle fibers located on chromosome 16p12.

Schwartz-Jampel syndrome is an autosomal recessive disorder of early childhood adenosine triphosphatase characterized by chondrodystrophy, short stature, bone and joint deformities, hypertrichosis, blepharophimosis, and muscle stiffness. There is delayed muscle relaxation clinically resembling myotonia, but the EMG shows non-variable (non-myotonic) continuous high-frequency electrical activity.

Malignant hyperthermia is characterized by severe muscle rigidity, fever, and tachycardia precipitated by depolarizing muscle relaxants and inhalational anesthetic agents such as halothane. The symptoms usually occur during surgery but can first be noticed in the post-operative period. Patients may have had previous anesthesia without symptoms. During attacks creatine kinase (CK) level is markedly elevated and myoglobinuria develops. The disorder is due to excessive calcium release by the sarcoplasmic reticulum calcium channel, the ryanodine receptor. Some patients have mutations in the ryanodine receptor gene on chromosome 19q13, which is the same gene mutated in central core disease. However, malignant hyperthermia appears to be genetically heterogeneous, and other families have been localized to different chromosomes. The symptoms are treated with dantrolene, and at risk-patients should not be given known provocative anesthetic agents. The occurrence of malignant hyperthermia in one member of a family should prompt consideration as to whether other family members could also be at risk.

Neuromyotonia, or *Isaacs' syndrome,* is an autoimmune disorder with antibodies directed against voltage-gated potassium channels (VGKCs) on peripheral nerves. Therefore, although this is not a primary myopathy, it is an acquired channelopathy that has a major secondary effect on muscle activity. Inactivation of these channels makes the motor nerve hyperexcitable and produces continuous muscle fiber activity that persists even during sleep. Clinically, there is involuntary muscle activity with stiffness, twitches, fasciculations, and continuous small, undulating movements of the overlying skin (myokymia). Patients also may experience excessive sweating and a peripheral neuropathy, and stiffness. The EMG documents the myokymic potentials and very high-frequency bursts (150 to 300 Hz) of spontaneous motor activity, termed *neuromyotonia.* Some cases are associated with neoplasms: thymoma (with or without myasthenia gravis), small cell lung carcinoma, and lymphoma. The CK level can be mildly elevated, cerebrospinal fluid (CSF) shows elevated protein and oligoclonal bands, and VGKC antibodies are present in serum. Treatment consists of immunosuppressive agents, symptomatic therapy with phenytoin or carbamazepine, or removal of the malignancy. An autosomal dominant form of neuromyotonia exists; it is associated with ataxia or a hereditary peripheral neuropathy.

STIFF-PERSON SYNDROME. Stiff-person syndrome, an acquired autoimmune condition, presents as severe muscle stiffness of proximal, and especially paraspinous, muscles. The muscle spasms produce hyperlordosis and all movements are slow and laborious. There is excess motor unit activity due to autoantibodies to glutamic acid decarboxylase, which is a major enzyme in the synthesis of γ-aminobutyric acid (GABA), and this results in disinhibition in the central nervous system. CK level is elevated and the EMG shows continuous motor unit activity at rest that the patient cannot voluntarily suppress. Some patients also have antibodies to islet cells and develop diabetes mellitus. Symptomatic treatment consists of diazepam; immunosuppressive treatment can markedly improve the condition.

EVALUATION OF PERIODIC PARALYSIS

In any patient initially being evaluated for an attack of periodic paralysis with hypo- or hyperkalemia, secondary causes need to be excluded (Table 509–2). In the primary forms of periodic paralysis, the serum potassium level decreases or increases but may be within the normal range during attacks; it is normal between attacks. By contrast, in secondary periodic paralysis caused by potassium wastage or retention the serum potassium level is always markedly reduced or elevated during and even between attacks (see also Chaper 102.3).

Thyrotoxic periodic paralysis resembles hypokalemic periodic paralysis. It is most common in Asian and Latin American young male adults. β-Adrenergic blocking agents reduce the frequency and severity of attacks, but the ultimate treatment is directed against the thyrotoxicosis.

During an attack of periodic paralysis, potassium levels should be measured every 15 to 30 minutes to determine the direction of change when muscle strength is worsening or improving. An electrocardiogram is useful to demonstrate the changes of hypo- or

Table 509–2 ■ SECONDARY CAUSES OF PERIODIC PARALYSIS

Hypokalemic
  Thyrotoxic
  Primary hyperaldosteronism (Conn's syndrome)
  Renal tubular acidosis (e.g., Fanconi's syndrome)
  Juxtaglomerular apparatus hyperplasia (Barter's syndrome)
  Gastrointestinal potassium wastage
  Villous adenoma
  Laxative abuse
  Pancreatic non-insulin-secreting tumors with diarrhea
  Non-tropical sprue
  Barium intoxication
  Potassium-depleting diuretics
  Amphotericin B
  Licorice
  Corticosteroids
  Toluene toxicity
  p-Aminosalicyclic acid
  Carbenoxalone
Hyperkalemic
  Addison's disease
  Hypoaldosteronism
  Excessive potassium supplementation
  Potassium-sparing diuretics
  Chronic renal failure

hyperkalemia. The CK level is usually elevated during an attack. Between attacks the CK level is generally normal. Routine EMG is normal between attack, but the compound motor action potential may decline in amplitude after exercise (exercise test) and may show a reduction of amplitude and corroborate the presence (but not the cause) of periodic paralysis. Muscle biopsy between attacks may demonstrate vacuoles or tubular aggregates within fibers. The biopsy need not be performed during an attack to see these changes. Provocative testing for hypokalemic periodic paralysis consists of giving oral or intravenous glucose with or without insulin; for hyperkalemic periodic paralysis it consists of giving repeated doses of oral potassium. This should always be performed under close supervision with cardiac monitoring and intravenous access.

Grimaldi LME, Martino O, Braghi S, et al: Heterogeneity of autoantibodies in stiff man syndrome. Ann Neurol 34:57, 1993. *Reviews the evidence for the autoimmune pathogenesis of the disease.*

Hudson A, Ebers GC, Bulman DE: The skeletal muscle sodium and chloride channel diseases. Brain 118:547, 1995. *A review focusing on sodium and chloride channelopathies.*

Ptacek LJ, Johnson KJ, Griggs RC: Genetics and physiology of the myotonic disorders. N Engl J Med 328:482, 1993. *Review of dystrophic and non-dystrophic myotonias.*

Ptacek LJ, Tawil R, Griggs RC, et al: Dihydropyridine receptor mutations cause hypokalemic periodic paralysis. Cell 77:863, 1994. *Describes calcium-channel mutations in hypokalemic periodic paralysis.*

Ricker K. Moxley RT, Rohkamm R: Rippling muscle disease. Arch Neurol 46:405, 1989. *A good description of an uncommon disease.*

Shillito P, Molenaar PC, Vincent A, et al: Acquired neuromyotonia: Evidence for autoantibodies directed against K+ channels of peripheral nerves. Ann Neurol 38: 714, 1995. *Established the autoimmune basis for acquired neuromyotonia and identified antibodies to the voltage-gated potassium channel in affected patients.*

510 INFLAMMATORY AND OTHER MYOPATHIES

Richard J. Barohn

INFLAMMATORY MYOPATHIES (See Chapter 256)

Inflammatory myopathies include a heterogeneous group of acquired, non-hereditary disorders (Table 510–1) that are characterized by muscle weakness and inflammation indicated by muscle biopsy. Most have elevated creatine kinase (CK) levels, myopathic electromyographic (EMG) findings, and a limb-girdle distribution of weakness. Occasionally inflammatory myopathies have distal, focal, or other selective involvement of particular muscles. Most inflammatory myopathies are considered idiopathic; although the cause is unknown, an autoimmune origin is suspected. They may be caused by or related to specific bacterial, parasitic, or viral infections. This section focuses on the common idiopathic inflammatory myopathies.

IDIOPATHIC INFLAMMATORY MYOPATHY. The three major categories of idiopathic inflammatory myopathy are *dermatomyositis, polymyositis,* and *inclusion body myositis.* The incidence of these disorders is approximately 1 in 100,000. These inflammatory myopathies are clinically, histologically, and pathogenically distinct (Table 510–2).

CLINICAL MANIFESTATIONS. Polymyositis and dermatomyositis are both characterized by the onset of symmetrical weakness subacutely over weeks or several months. The earliest and most severely affected muscle groups are the neck flexors, shoulder girdle, and pelvic girdle muscles. Distal extremity weakness can also often be demonstrated, although involvement is seldom as severe as in the proximal muscle weakness. Both polymyositis and dermatomyositis occur more often in females. Polymyositis is generally an adult disorder, with onset usually after the age of 20. Dermatomyositis can present in children or adults and there appears to be a bimodal age of distribution with peaks at 5–24 years and 45–64 years of age. Myalgias can occur in up to one third of patients, but muscle pain and tenderness are rarely chief complaints. Patients complaining of myalgia who do not have demonstrable weakness are more likely to have polymyalgia rheumatica or fibromyalgia rather than polymyositis. In up to 30% of both polymyositis and dermatomyositis patients, esophageal muscles are affected, leading to dysphagia.

The characteristic rash of dermatomyositis may accompany or precede the onset of muscle weakness. The presence of the rash often allows dermatomyositis to be appropriately diagnosed early. The typical skin manifestations include a heliotrope rash (purplish discoloration of the eyelids often associated with periorbital edema); Gottron's sign (papular, erythematous, scaly lesions over the knuckles); a macular, erythematous, sun-sensitive rash on the face, neck, and anterior chest (V sign), on the shoulders and upper back (shawl sign), and on the elbows and knees; periungual erythema due to dilated capillary loops with thrombi or hemorrhage. These skin changes can occur at all ages; children frequently experience subcutaneous calcifications that can be extremely painful. Subcutaneous calcinosis is uncommon in adults.

Inclusion body myositis presents with an insidious onset of

Table 510–1 ■ CLASSIFICATION OF INFLAMMATORY MYOPATHIES

Idiopathic
  Polymyositis
  Dermatomyositis
  Inclusion body myositis
  Overlap syndromes with other connective tissue disease (scleroderma, systemic lupus erythematosus, mixed connective tissue disease, Sjögren's syndrome, rheumatoid arthritis, polyarteritis nodosa)
  Sarcoidosis and other granulomatous myositis
  Behçet's syndrome
  Inflammatory myopathies and eosinophila
    Eosinophilic polymyositis
    Diffuse fasciitis with eosinophilia
  Focal myositis
  Myositis ossificans
Infections
  Bacterial: *Staphlococus aureus,* streptococci, *Escherichia coli, Yersinia* spp., *Legionella* spp., gas gangrene *(Clostridium welchii),* leprous myositis, Lyme disease *(Borrelia burgdorferi)*
  Viral: acute myositis following influenza or other viral infections (adenovirus, coxsackievirus, echovirus, parainfluenza virus, Epstein-Barr virus, arbovirus, cytomegalovirus), retrovirus-related myopathies (HIV, HTLV-1),* hepatitis B and C
  Parasitic: trichinosis *(Trichinella spiralis),* toxoplasmosis *(Toxoplasma gondii),* cysticercosis, sarcosporidiosis, trypanosomiasis *(Taenia solium)*
  Fungal: candida, cryptococcus, sporotichosis, actinomycosis, histoplasmosis

*HIV = human immunodeficiency virus; HTLV-1 = human T-lymphocyte virus 1.

Table 510–2 ■ IDIOPATHIC INFLAMMATORY MYOPATHIES: CLINICAL AND LABORATORY FEATURES

	SEX	TYPICAL AGE AT ONSET	RASH	PATTERN OF WEAKNESS	CK LEVEL	MUSCLE BIOPSY	RESPONSE TO IS THERAPY	COMMON ASSOCIATED CONDITIONS
Dermatomyositis	F > M	Childhood and adult	Yes	Proximal > distal	Increased (up to 50× normal)	Perimysial and perivascular inflammation; CD4⁺ T cells, B cells; MAC, Ig, C deposition on vessels	Yes	Myocarditis, interstitial lung disease, vasculitis, other connective tissue diseases, malignancy
Polymyositis	F > M	Adult	No	Proximal > distal	Increased (up to 50× normal)	Endomysial inflammation CD8⁺ T cells, macros	Yes	Myocarditis, interstitial lung disease, other connective tissue diseases; ?malignancy
Inclusion body myositis	M > F	Elderly (>50 yr)	No	Proximal = distal; Predilection for finger/wrist flexors, knee extensors	Increased (<10× normal)	Endomysial inflammation; CD8⁺ T cells, macros; rimmed vacuoles; amyloid deposits; EM: 15–18 nm tubulofilaments	No	Neuropathy

Macros = macrophage; IS = immunosuppressive; MAC = membrane attack complex; Ig = immunoglobulin; C = complement; F = female; M = male; CK = creatine kinase.

slowly progressive proximal and distal weakness. The slow evolution of the disease process contributes to the delay in diagnosis, averaging 6 years from the onset of symptoms. Inclusion body myositis typically begins after age 50 and is the most common inflammatory myopathy in the elderly. Males are more commonly affected than females. These patients have a distinctive pattern of muscle involvement with early weakness and atrophy of the quadriceps (knee extensors), volar forearm muscles (wrist and finger flexors), and tibialis anterior (ankle dorsiflexors) muscles. Involvement of these muscle groups is frequently asymmetrical, in contrast to the symmetrical weakness in dermatomyositis and polymyositis. Patients have difficulty making a fist because of finger flexor weakness. Some degree of shoulder and hip girdle weakness is often present as well. Facial weakness and dysphagia occur in nearly one third and one half of patients, respectively. Although most patients have no sensory symptoms, evidence for a distal sensory peripheral neuropathy can be detected in up to 30% of patients through clinical examination and electrophysiologic testing. Muscle stretch reflexes at the knees are often decreased, particularly when quadriceps atrophy is severe. Although myalgias do not occur, as the quadriceps muscles progressively weaken and genu recurvatum develops, patients frequently complain of knee pain.

ASSOCIATED MANIFESTATIONS. Cardiac involvement, resulting in congestive heart failure and conduction defects, and interstitial lung disease can develop in a minority of polymyositis and dermatomyositis patients. Arthralgias are frequent in both conditions. Vasculitis of the gastrointestinal tract, kidneys, lungs, and eyes can complicate dermatomyositis (but not polymyositis), particularly in children. There is an increased incidence of malignancy in older adults with dermatomyositis, but the frequency varies in different studies from 6 to 45%. The most common malignancies are lung, breast, ovary, gastrointestinal tract, and myeloproliferative disorders. The malignancy risk with polymyositis is lower but may be slightly higher in elderly adults than expected in the general population. The search for a malignancy need not go beyond a comprehensive history and physical examination (including stool occult blood), chest radiograph, pelvic examination and mammogram in women, and prostate examination for men. Inclusion body myositis patients do not have associated pulmonary, cardiac, or malignant disorders. However, in one third of these patients a distal sensory neuropathy may develop and dysphagia can occur.

LABORATORY FEATURES. The EMG in all three disorders will usually demonstrate brief myopathic motor units, increased recruitment, and fibrillation potentials, particularly in the most involved muscles. Inclusion body myositis patients will often show a mixed pattern on EMG with both brief myopathic and long-duration, polyphasic neuropathic units. The serum CK level is usually significantly increased in dermatomyositis and polymyositis. Rarely it can be normal. Inclusion body myositis patients have only slight elevations of CK level, and normal enzyme levels are not uncommon. The erythrocyte sedimentation rate (ESR) is normal in most patients with polymyositis and dermatomyositis and is seldom ele-

vated in inclusion body myositis. An elevated ESR suggests a different or coincidental disease. Antinuclear antibodies can be detected in polymyositis and dermatomyositis patients and do not necessarily imply a systemic connective tissue disease. At least 50% of patients with interstitial lung disease and inflammatory myopathy have muscle-specific serum antibodies directed against transfer ribonucleic acid synthetase, so-called Jo-1 antibodies. Other muscle-specific antibodies have less clear significance. Antibodies directed against the nuclear protein Mi-2 are seen in 10–20% of dermatomyositis patients, who may have an acute onset, a florid rash, and a good response to therapy.

A muscle biopsy should be performed in all suspected inflammatory myopathy patients to establish the diagnosis. The muscle histology in all three of these disorders usually show inflammation and muscle fiber necrosis, but there are differences. The inflammation in dermatomyositis is predominantly perivascular and located in perimysial connective tissue between muscle fascicles. The inflammatory infiltrate is composed primarily of macrophages, B cells, and CD4⁺ (T-helper) cells. However, the pathologic hallmark in dermatomyositis is *perifascicular atrophy,* which may be present in the absence of inflammation. In addition, small muscle microinfarcts can occur and immunostaining can demonstrate the deposition of the C5b-9 complement membrane attack complex (MAC) and other complement components on small blood vessels. Electron microscopy reveals small intramuscular blood vessels that have endothelial hyperplasia and cytoplasmic inclusions. This leads to a loss of the number of capillaries. These histologic features are not observed in either polymyositis or inclusion body myositis. In polymyositis, inflammation is in the endomysial connective tissue and there is cellular invasion of non-necrotic muscle fibers. The inflammatory cells consist primarily of activated CD8⁺ (cytotoxic) T cells and macrophages. The inflammation seen in inclusion body myositis is also endomysial with a predominance of CD8⁺ T lymphocytes. However, the hallmark of inclusion body myositis on light microscopy is the presence of muscle fibers with one or more rimmed vacuoles lined with granular material and occasionally eosinophilic cytoplasmic inclusions. Additional findings are amyloid deposition in muscle fibers, as well as other "Alzheimer-characteristic" proteins such as β-amyloid precursor protein, prion protein, apolipoprotein E, ubiquitin, and τ protein. Electron microscopy demonstrates 15- to 21-nm cytoplasmic and intranuclear filaments.

PATHOGENESIS. The histologic features and immunologic studies suggest that dermatomyositis is a humorally mediated microangiopathy, which leads to ischemic damage of muscle fibers. The perifascicular atrophy is probably a reflection of hypoperfusion of muscle fascicles in a watershed distribution. Polymyositis is most likely a human leukocyte antigen (HLA)-restricted, antigen-specific, cell-mediated immune response directed against muscle fibers. The antigen to which this autoimmune attack is generated is not known. Although a viral cause has been suggested, there is no conclusive evidence supporting this theory. One exception may be the polymyositis that develops in patients infected with human immunodeficiency virus (HIV) and human T-lymphocyte virus-1 (HTLV 1) (see later). Finally, although inclusion body myositis may be a primary inflammatory myopathy, another explanation is that it is a primary degenerative myopathic disorder such as a dystrophy with secondary inflammation. This theory is supported by the poor response to immunosuppressive therapy (see later), the accumulation of the "Alzheimer-characteristic" proteins, and the presence indicated on electron microscopy of filaments that are seen in other muscular dystrophies.

TREATMENT. Immunotherapy can improve strength and function in dermatomyositis and polymyositis. In contrast, inclusion body myositis is usually refractory to immunosuppressive therapy. There is still some controversy whether or not patients with inclusion body myositis should be given a trial of therapy, but results are nearly always disappointing. It should be remembered that the best measure of response to therapy is the demonstration of improved muscle strength. Neither the lowering of serum CK level in a persistently weak patient nor its elevation in a strong patient without weakness should be the primary determinant of successful or unsuccessful therapy. The serum CK level declines in an inclusion body myositis patient on corticosteroid therapy, but patients do not get stronger.

The first line of therapy for dermatomyositis and polymyositis patients is the corticosteroid prednisone. Although no controlled trials are available, it is generally believed that high-dose prednisone reduces morbidity rate and improves muscle strength and function in these disorders. Typically, the starting prednisone dose is 1 to 2 mg/kg/day given as a once a day dose each morning. After strength has improved (often in 2 to 4 weeks of daily prednisone), the patient can sometimes be switched to alternate-day dosing. Some authorities keep patients on daily prednisone longer and make a more gradual change to alternate-day therapy. Objective clinical improvement is usually evident within 3 to 6 months. High-dose prednisone is maintained until patients regain normal strength or until improvement in strength has reached a plateau. At this point, the prednisone dose can be slowly tapered by 5 mg every 2 weeks. However, prednisone therapy should not be discontinued too soon, and most adult patients require therapy for many years. While the patient is on prednisone, side effects of corticosteroid therapy should be monitored. Patients should be placed on supplemental calcium and vitamin D for prevention of steroid-induced osteoporosis. Post-menopausal women should receive estrogen supplements and patients with abnormal bone density measurements should be given bisphosphonates.

Second line agents are added when patients do not significantly improve after 3 to 6 months of high-dose prednisone or there is an exacerbation during the taper. Short courses of intravenous methylprednisolone (1 g/day for 3 or 4 days) may also be helpful. The most frequently employed second line agents are the cytotoxic drugs methotrexate and azathioprine. The usual dose of azathioprine is 2–3 mg/kg given orally. Over 10% of patients have an idiosyncratic systemic reaction to azathioprine (fever, abdominal discomfort), which resolves promptly on stopping the drug. Oral methotrexate is given 15–20 mg 1 day each week. Higher methotrexate doses can be administered parenterally. Patients on either drug need to have careful monitoring of liver enzyme levels and blood counts. Because inflammatory myopathy patients frequently have elevated transaminase enzyme levels that are due to muscle destruction, liver-specific γ-glutamyl transpeptidase level should be measured. Intravenous immunoglobulin (IVIG) has been demonstrated to improve the strength in dermatomyositis patients in a controlled trial. The induction dose of IVIG is 2 g/kg over 2 to 5 days, followed by monthly maintenance doses of 0.4 to 1 g/kg. It is unclear whether IVIG is effective in polymyositis. As is true with all immunomodulating agents, IVIG is probably not beneficial in inclusion body myositis. Other forms of therapy in refractory polymyositis and dermatomyositis cases include cyclosporine, cyclophosphamide, and chlorambucil. Plasmapheresis and leukopheresis are not effective treatments. There are case reports of patients responding to total-body radiation.

In patients with residual proximal weakness on prednisone, the issue of possible weakness caused by "steroid" myopathy can arise. Chronic prednisone use infrequently produces clinically significant weakness (see the discussion of toxic myopathies), and in most

instances persistent weakness is due to the underlying disease. A repeat EMG or muscle biopsy may be useful in documenting an active inflammatory myopathy.

Once subcutaneous calcifications develop, they generally do not respond to therapy. Oral calcium-channel blocking agents such as diltiazem have been reported to reduce calcinosis in some dermatomyositis patients.

PROGNOSIS. Most patients with polymyositis and dermatomyositis respond to therapy. Approximately two thirds of patients respond but still have some residual weakness, and about one third return to normal strength. A few patients are refractory to all forms of therapy. Poor prognostic features are the presence of malignancy, increased age, associated interstitial lung disease or cardiomyopathy, and late or previous inadequate treatment. The 5-year survival rate is approximately 75% in adults, and the mortality rate in children is very low.

Although inclusion body myositis does not respond to therapy, life expectancy is normal. Many patients remain ambulatory, although they frequently require a cane or wheelchair for long distances. However, some patients become severely incapacitated and require a wheelchair within 10 to 15 years. Many patients with so-called steroid-resistant or refractory polymyositis, in fact, have inclusion body myositis. It is important to establish the true diagnosis in these patients so that they do not remain on ineffective, potentially harmful therapy.

OTHER IDIOPATHIC INFLAMMATORY MYOPATHIES. OVERLAP SYNDROMES. The term *overlap syndromes* denotes a group of disorders in which an inflammatory myopathy occurs in association with another well-defined connective tissue disorder. These include scleroderma, systemic lupus erythematosus, Sjögren's syndrome, rheumatoid arthritis, mixed connective tissue disease, and polyarteritis nodosa. Clinical and histologic features of either dermatomyositis or polymyositis can develop in up to 10% of each of these disorders. Some suggest the myositis associated with overlap syndromes is more responsive to immunosuppressive treatment than dermatomyositis and polymyositis.

EOSINOPHILIC POLYMYOSITIS. Eosinophilic polymyositis usually occurs as part of the hypereosinophilic syndrome. Peripheral eosinophilia in the absence of parasitic infection is associated with a multisystemic disorder of muscle, peripheral nerve, lung, heart, skin, and central nervous system. Endomysial inflammation in muscle is composed predominantly of eosinophils. Response to immunosuppressive therapy is inconsistent and in general the prognosis is poor.

DIFFUSE FASCIITIS WITH EOSINOPHILIA. In diffuse fasciitis with eosinophilia, also known as Shulman's syndrome, peripheral eosinophilia is associated with painful scleroderma-like skin changes, contractures, myalgia, arthralgias, and fever. However, unlike eosinophilic polymyositis, the heart, lungs, and other organs are not involved. Laboratory features include hypergammaglobulinemia, elevated erythrocyte sedimentation rate, and occasionally elevated CK level. Full-thickness biopsy from the skin to muscle is required to demonstrate the thickened fascia infiltrated by eosinophils and lymphocytes. The inflammation can invade the adjacent underlying muscle. Although the disorder is most likely autoimmune, it shares clinical and histologic features with the *eosinophilic myalgia syndrome* due to the ingestion of tryptophan. However, in Shulman's syndrome patients have no known toxic exposures. The prognosis is good and patients usually respond rapidly to corticosteroid treatment. Relapses are infrequent.

GRANULOMATOUS MYOPATHY WITH AND WITHOUT SARCOIDOSIS. Patients with sarcoidosis can have asymptomatic granulomas in the muscle or an elevated CK level. Occasionally they have nodular swellings of subcutaneous tissues and underlying muscle. These lesions have histopathologic features indicative of sarcoid. Patients can also experience focal muscle pain or a generalized limb-girdle weakness pattern reflecting muscle involvement by sarcoid granulomas. Symptomatic patients are usually treated with corticosteroids but respond poorly.

Giant cell or granulomatous myopathy can occur in the absence of sarcoidosis. Most of these patients also have myasthenia gravis or thymoma. Myocarditis can be part of the disease process. These patients generally improve with corticosteroids.

BEHÇET'S SYNDROME. Behçet's syndrome, a multisystem disorder, usually has mucocutaneous and ocular manifestations but may rarely be associated with myositis and myocarditis. The myositis can be focal or generalized and there is a predilection for the calves. The myositis often responds to immunosuppressive therapy.

FOCAL MYOSITIS. Focal myositis is an uncommon disorder that can develop at any age. It presents as a solitary, painful, and rapidly expanding skeletal muscle mass and must be distinguished from sarcoidosis, Behçet's disease, polyarteritis nodosa, or muscle tumors (sarcoma or rhabdomyosarcoma). The leg is the most common site of involvement, but it can occur in any region. Serum CK level is usually normal. Biopsy of the lesions show mononuclear inflammatory cells in the endomysium with muscle fiber necrosis. The myositis usually resolves spontaneously or with treatment. In rare cases focal myositis is the heralding sign of typical polymyositis.

INFECTIOUS MYOSITIS. VIRAL. An acute viral myositis can occur in the setting of an influenza viral upper respiratory infection. In addition to typical influenza-associated myalgias, these patients have proximal weakness, elevated CK level, and myopathic motor units indicated on EMG. The disorder is self-limited but when severe is often associated with myoglobinuria and occasionally with renal failure. A similar syndrome can complicate infections with coxsackie virus, parainfluenza virus, mumps, measles, adenovirus, cytomegalovirus, hepatitis B virus, herpes simplex virus, Epstein-Barr virus, respiratory syncytial virus, and echovirus.

An inflammatory myopathy can occur in the setting of human immunodeficiency virus (HIV) infection, in either the early or later acquired immunodeficiency virus (AIDS) stages of infection. The clinical presentation is similar to that of polymyositis and inflammation is present in muscle biopsy findings. Interestingly, nemaline rod bodies appear to be more common in these specimens than other inflammatory myopathies. Although patients may improve with corticosteroid therapy, an alternative treatment in this setting is intravenous immunoglobulin. The disorder must be distinguished from the toxic myopathy due to zidovudine (AZT), which is non-inflammatory and associated with mitochondrial abnormalities. AZT myopathy responds to dose reduction.

The neurologic manifestation of HTLV-1 infection typically consists of spastic paraparesis, but myositis can also develop. The clinical presentation and course are those of an indolent polymyositis that is poorly responsive to immunosuppressive therapy.

Evidence of viral antigens is difficult to demonstrate in both HIV and HTLV-1 myositis. HIV and HTLV-1 viral infections may indirectly trigger an autoimmune response by causing secondary cross-reactivity with specific muscle antigens, altering the expression of self-antigens on muscle fibers, or producing the loss of self-tolerance.

BACTERIAL. *Pyomyositis* refers to focal or multifocal abscesses associated with bacterial infection of muscle. Pyomyositis is more common in the tropics, in developing countries, and among intravenous drug users. It usually arises as an extension of an infection in adjacent tissues or from hematogenous spread. The most common organisms involved are *Staphylococcus aureus, Streptococcus* spp., *Escherichia coli, Yersinia* spp., and *Legionella* spp. Treatment consists of antibiotics and, in severe infections, incision and drainage of abscesses.

FUNGAL. Fungal infections of muscle can occur rarely, usually in immunocompromised individuals. Candidiasis is the most common fungal myositis. Diffuse muscle pain, weakness, and fever are associated with a papular erythematous rash.

PARASITIC INFECTIONS. Trichinosis is the most common parasitic disease that can produce a diffuse inflammatory myositis and can be confused with idiopathic polymyositis. Ingested larvae from undercooked pork migrate to muscle, and patients develop fever, myalgias, weakness, myocarditis, and central nervous system manifestations. There are a peripheral eosinophilia, elevated CK level, and antibodies against *Trichinella spiralis* that can be demonstrated 3 to 4 weeks after infection. Therapy consists of thiabendazole; in severe cases corticosteroids may be indicated.

An inflammatory myopathy can also occur in the course of cysticercosis (*Taenia solium*) and toxoplasmosis (*T. gondii*).

Amato AA, Barohn RJ: Idiopathic inflammatory myopathies. Neurol Clin 15:615, 1997. *An up-to-date review of the idiopathic inflammatory myopathies.*

MYOPATHIES DUE TO ENDOCRINE SYSTEMIC DISORDERS, TOXINS, AND MYOGLOBINURIA

Fatigue can be a symptom of any endocrine disorder, but objective muscle weakness due to a myopathy is less common. The serum CK level is often normal except in hypothyroidism. The EMG is normal or has myopathic motor units but generally without spontaneous electrical activity. The histologic alterations in muscle are often non-specific, such as type 2 fiber atrophy. Fiber necrosis and regeneration are uncommon. Muscle symptoms improve with successful treatment of the underlying endocrinopathy.

ADRENAL/GLUCOCORTICOID DISORDERS. Excess corticosteroids can result from endogenous Cushing's disease or can be due to exogenous glucocorticoid administration. Iatrogenic corticosteroid myopathy (or atrophy) is the most common endocrine-related myopathy. However, muscle weakness is rarely the presenting manifestation of Cushing's disease, and in virtually all instances of corticosteroid myopathy other factors contributing to weakness are also present. Women are more susceptible to corticosteroid atrophy than men, and divided daily doses are more toxic than single or alternate daily doses. Muscle biopsy shows type 2 muscle fiber atrophy, and serum CK level and EMG are normal. Therapy consists of reducing the corticosteroid dosage to the lowest possible level. Exercise and adequate nutrition prevent and may improve weakness. Muscle strength returns to normal within 1 to 4 months after therapy is stopped. Acute quadriplegic myopathy associated with high doses of intravenous glucocorticoids is discussed later.

Addison's disease (adrenal insufficiency) is often associated with fatigue, but objective signs of myopathy are rare. Electrolyte disturbances can produce weakness and simulate a periodic paralysis (see earlier and Table 509–2).

THYROID DISORDERS. Patients with *hyperthyroidism* often have some degree of weakness, but this is rarely the presenting manifestation of thyrotoxicosis. Weakness is predominantly proximal, especially in the shoulder region, and there may be atrophy. Weakness of extraocular muscles and proptosis occur in *Graves' disease*. Thyrotoxic periodic paralysis is described earlier. *Hypothyroid myopathy* is associated with proximal weakness and myalgias, muscle enlargement, slow relaxation of the reflexes, and marked (up to 100-fold) increase of the serum CK level.

PARATHYROID DISORDERS. *Hyperparathyroidism* (with hypercalcemia and hypophosphatemia) can be associated with proximal weakness, atrophy, and pain, especially in the setting of osteomalacia. Patients may also experience hoarseness, dysphagia, and neck extensor weakness. *Hypoparathyroidism* (with hypocalcemia and hyperphosphatemia) is usually not associated with a myopathy; however, paresthesias and tetany with Chvostek's sign and Trousseau's phenomenon can occur in hypocalcemic patients.

PITUITARY DISORDERS. *Acromegaly* can be associated with mild proximal weakness, but usually not until late in the disease. Muscles can look enlarged despite being weak. Weakness as a result of nerve, root, or spinal cord compression is a more likely cause of weakness. Panhypopituitarism results in weakness and fatigability, but this probably reflects the combined influence of thyroid and adrenal deficiencies.

DIABETES MELLITUS. Progressive, painless proximal weakness in a diabetic patient is seldom if ever the result of diabetes-related myopathy. Asymmetrical, usually painful proximal leg weakness can occur from an ischemic radiculoplexopathy ("amyotrophy"). Rarely, acute muscle infarction can develop in quadriceps or hamstring muscles. These patients complain of severe pain, tenderness, and swelling. Magnetic resonance imaging of the thigh shows changes consistent with a muscle infarct. The syndrome resolves spontaneously over weeks.

VITAMIN DEFICIENCY. *Vitamin E deficiency* as a result of malabsorption can produce a myopathy along with gait ataxia and neuropathy. *Vitamin D deficiency* (from decreased intake or impaired absorption or metabolism) may also lead to chronic muscle weakness.

OTHER ELECTROLYTE DISTURBANCES. *Hypermagnesemia* can produce acute generalized weakness probably from neuromuscular junction dysfunction. *Hypomagnesemia* results in muscle and nerve hyperexcitability with Chvostek's sign and Trousseau's phenomenon.

SYSTEMIC AMYLOID MYOPATHY. The most common neurologic complication in various types of amyloidosis is a predominantly sensory-autonomic neuropathy. Amyloid deposition in muscle is frequent, but the muscle involvement is usually subclinical.

Occasionally, amyloidosis presents or is associated with an overt myopathy characterized by muscle enlargement, macroglossia, stiffness, exertional muscle pain, and proximal or diffuse weakness. Electromyography shows myopathic features in proximal muscles with or without changes of neuropathy distally. The amyloid deposits, identified by their metachromasia and affinity for Congo red stain, appear between and around the mural elements of the small vessels and extend into the interstitial spaces, where they tightly surround individual muscle fibers.

MYOSITIS OSSIFICANS The *localized form* of myositis ossificans appears as a tender swelling after trauma to a muscle. After a few months this becomes hard and ossified. Therapy consists of excision. The *generalized form* is an autosomal dominant disease with variable expressivity that begins in childhood, involves many muscles, and causes progressive rigidity of body parts. The initial lesions appear in fascia and dermis and are associated with inflammation, hemorrhage, and connective tissue proliferation. Cartilage and bone formation occur at a later stage. Other congenital malformations (microdactyly of the great toe, exostoses, absence of upper incisors or of ear lobules, and hypogenitalism) are found in most patients. There is no effective therapy.

TOXIC MYOPATHIES

Many drugs have been associated with muscle damage; common ones are listed in Table 510–3. Most can produce proximal weakness, elevated CK level, myopathic EMG results, and abnormalities indicated on muscle biopsy findings. Symptoms generally improve on stopping the medication. Several drugs have can produce an inflammatory myopathy on muscle biopsy, including penicillamine and cimetidine. Zidovudine (AZT) causes a mitochondrial myopathy. A number of drugs can produce a necrotizing or vacuolar myopathy, including amiodarone, colchicine and chloroquine, and cyclosporine. Emetine (ipecac) produces proximal weakness and a myofibrillar myopathy. Isoretinoic acid, a vitamin A analogue used for acne, infrequently causes myalgias, elevation of the serum creatine kinase level, and reversible muscle damage.

Some drugs can produce an acute, rapidly progressive disorder with rhabdomyolysis and myoglobinuria. The hypocholesterolemic drugs and alcohol fall in this group. Clofibrate, gemfibrozil, lovastatin, simvastatin, pravastatin, and niacin can all produce a rapidly

Table 510–3 ■ TOXIC MYOPATHIES

Inflammatory	Malignant hyperthermia
Cimetidine	Halothane
D-Penicillamine	Ethylene
Procainamide	Diethyl ether
L-Tryptophan	Methoxyflurane
L-Dopa	Ethyl chloride
Non-inflammatory necrotizing or vacuolar	Trichloroethylene
	Gallamine
Cholesterol-lowering agents	Succinylcholine
Chloroquine	Mitochondrial
Colchicine	Zidovudine
Emetine	Myotonia
ε-Aminocaproic acid	2,4-*d*-chlorophenoxyacetic acid
Labetalol	Anthracene-9-carboxycyclic acid
Cyclosporine and tacrolimus	Cholesterol-lowering drugs
Isoretinoic acid (vitamin A analogue)	Chloroquine
	Cyclosporine
Vincristine	Myosin loss
Alcohol	Non-depolarizing neuromuscular blocking agents
Rhabdomyolysis and myoglobinuria	
Cholesterol-lowering drugs	Intravenous glucocorticoids
Alcohol	
Heroin	
Amphetamine	
Toluene	
Cocaine	
ε-Aminocaproic acid	
Pentazocine	
Phencyclidine	

progressive myopathy with weakness and pain, and myoglobinuria. An acute necrotizing myopathy associated with myoglobinuria occurs in chronic alcoholics after a bout of drinking. Hypokalemia caused by sweating, vomiting, diarrhea, and renal wastage may act as a precipitating factor. The hypokalemia may be followed by hyperkalemia as myoglobinuria and renal failure develop.

Illicit drugs such as heroin, cocaine, amphetamines, and pentazocine can produce rhabdomyolysis through direct toxic effects status epilepticus, or prolonged loss of consciousness, immobility, and secondary pressure.

ACUTE QUADRIPLEGIC MYOPATHY. Also known as critical illness myopathy, acute quadriplegic myopathy develops in a patient in the intensive care setting and is often discovered when a patient is unable to be weaned off a ventilator. The cause of the diffuse weakness is the prolonged daily use of either (often both) high-dose intravenous glucocorticoids (usually methylprednisolone) or non-depolarizing neuromuscular blocking agents (e.g., vecuronium). Patients often have had sepsis and multiorgan failure. Serum CK level is moderately elevated and the EMG shows myopathic units and fibrillations. On nerve conduction studies, motor amplitudes are small, and occasionally a decremental response can be seen on repetitive stimulation. The diagnosis can be confirmed by the muscle biopsy, which shows the loss of myosin thick filaments on electron microscopy. Treatment is supportive after discontinuing the offending agents. Strength recovers over a period of weeks or months; patients can usually be weaned off the ventilator.

A number of anesthetic agents can precipitate malignant hyperthermia in predisposed individuals (see earlier). *Neuroleptic malignant syndrome* with muscular rigidity, altered mental status, and hyperthermia is due to central dopaminergic blockade from neuroleptic. Although there is not a direct effect on muscle, the rigidity can produce rhabdomyolysis with myoglobinuria.

Focal muscle injury can be caused by injection of certain drugs, particularly pentazocine and meperidine. Muscle necrosis is followed by fibrous connective tissue replacement and induration.

MYOGLOBINURIA

Acute muscle destruction, or rhabdomyolysis, can produce a brown discoloration of urine by myoglobin. Myoglobin, a 17,000-molecular-weight protein that contains the heme moiety, is present in muscle at a concentration of 1 g/kg. Small amounts of myoglobin not sufficient to discolor urine are excreted in various necrotizing myopathies. The visible discoloration of urine by myoglobin indicates both massive and acute muscle destruction and warns of impending renal damage. The pigment has to be distinguished from hemoglobin. If there is no hematuria, a positive benzidine test result strongly suggests myoglobinuria. However, myoglobinuria itself can induce microhematuria, and certain identification of myoglobin must be made specifically.

Muscle pain, swelling, and weakness precede overt myoglobinuria by a few hours. In addition to myoglobin, phosphate, potassium, creatine, and muscle enzymes are released into the circulation. Serum CK level can be more than 1000 times normal. The heme pigment in the glomerular filtrate and casts in the tubules cause proteinuria, hematuria, and tubular necrosis. Renal failure is more likely if hypotension, acidosis, and hypovolemia coexist. With increasing renal insufficiency, hyperphosphatemia, hypocalcemia, tetany, and life-threatening hyperkalemia appear. Death may result from renal or respiratory failure. If patients are supported successfully, the myoglobinuria and proteinuria disappear in 3 to 5 days. The marked hyperenzymemia decreases gradually, and muscle strength returns relatively slowly after major attacks. EMG abnormalities (fibrillations and myopathic units) can persist for several months. The muscle biopsy shortly after an attack shows large numbers of necrotic fibers. Later biopsy reveals many regenerating fibers. Persistent weakness in patients recovering from myoglobinuria often reflects cervical or lumbar plexopathies.

Myoglobinuria can have many causes. The various metabolic and toxic causes have been discussed. Massive ischemia of muscle from any cause, crush injuries, prolonged pressure, or persistent contraction and rigidity (such as those caused by status epilepticus, malignant hyperthermia, and neuroleptic malignant syndrome) can all produce rhabdomyolysis and myoglobinuria. Infectious causes include viral and bacterial infections. Rarely, myoglobinuria can occur secondary to another myopathy, such as dystrophinopathies or idiopathic inflammatory myopathy.

The acute episode is treated by rest, maintenance of adequate urine flow by hydration and diuretics, and alkalinization of the urine with sodium bicarbonate. Other measures consist of treatment

of the renal insufficiency as required and removal of the offending cause if possible.

Barohn RJ, Jackson CE, Rogers SJ, et al: Prolonged paralysis due to nondepolarizing neuromuscular blocking agents and corticosteroids. Muscle Nerve 17:647, 1994.
Hirano M, Ott BR, Raps EC, et al: Acute quadriplegic myopathy: A complication of treatment with steroids, nondepolarizing blocking agents, or both. Neurology 42: 2082, 1992. *Provides insight into this common but underdiagnosed myopathy.*

■ DISEASES OF THE NEUROMUSCULAR JUNCTION

511 DISORDERS OF NEUROMUSCULAR TRANSMISSION

Andrew G. Engel

DEFINITION AND BASIC CONCEPTS. Disorders of neuromuscular transmission can be acquired or inherited and are associated with abnormal weakness and fatigability on exertion. In each disorder the safety margin of neuromuscular transmission is compromised by one or more specific mechanisms. These mechanisms involve acetylcholine (ACh) synthesis or packaging of ACh quanta (6,000 to 10,000 molecules) into synaptic vesicles, the exocytotic release of ACh quanta from the nerve terminal by nerve impulse, and the efficiency of the released quanta to generate a post-synaptic depolarization. The efficiency of the released quanta depends on the geometry of the synaptic space, the density of post-synaptic ACh receptors (AChRs), and the kinetic properties of the AChR ion channel. The depolarization induced by a single quantum gives rise to a miniature end-plate potential (MEPP); that induced by a larger number of quanta released by nerve impulse generates an end-plate potential (EPP). The EPP amplitude must exceed a critical threshold to activate the voltage-sensitive sodium channels around the end-plate and thereby generate a muscle fiber action potential. Neuromuscular transmission fails when the EPP fails to reach this critical threshold.

Table 511–1, shows a classification of currently recognized defects of neuromuscular transmission. Botulism is described in Chapter 336, the others in this chapter. The congenital syndromes are discussed in the indicated references.

MYASTHENIA GRAVIS (MG). Myasthenia gravis is an acquired autoimmune disorder in which pathogenic autoantibodies induce AChR deficiency at the motor end-plate. The safety margin of neuromuscular transmission is compromised by the small amplitude of the MEPP and consequently of the EPP. Circulating AChR antibodies are present in 80 to 90% of the cases, and immunoglobulin G (IgG) and complement components are deposited on the post-synaptic membrane. AChR deficiency results from complement-mediated lysis of the junctional folds, accelerated internalization and destruction of AChR cross-linked by antibody (modulation), and, to a lesser extent, antibodies blocking the binding of ACh to AChR.

CLINICAL FEATURES. The incidence is 2 to 5 per year per million and the prevalence 13 to 64 per million. The female to male ratio is 6:4. The disease may present at any age, but the incidence in women peaks in the third decade and in men in the sixth or seventh decade.

MG can involve either the external ocular muscles selectively or the general voluntary muscle system. The symptoms may fluctuate from hour to hour, from day to day, or over longer periods. They

Table 511–1 ■ CLASSIFICATION OF DISORDERS OF NEUROMUSCULAR TRANSMISSION

Autoimmune
Myasthenia gravis
Lambert-Eaton myasthenic syndrome
Congenital
Pre-synaptic defects
Defect in ACh resynthesis or packaging*
Paucity of synaptic vesicles and reduced quantal release*
Synaptic defect
Congenital end-plate AChE deficiency*,§
Post-synaptic defects: increased response to ACh
Slow-channel syndromes‡
Post-synaptic defects: decreased response to ACh
Low-affinity fast channel syndromes*,‖
Mode-switching kinetics of AChR*,‖
AChR deficiency without kinetic abnormality*
Partially characterized syndromes
Congenital myasthenic syndrome resembling LEMS†
Familial limb-girdle myasthenia*
Benign CMS with facial malformations*
Toxic
Botulism
Drug-induced
Organophosphate intoxication

*Autosomal recessive inheritance.
†Autosomal recessive inheritance suspected.
‡Dominant inheritance.
§Mutations in collagenic tail subunit of end-plate AChE.
‖Mutations in AChR subunit genes.
ACh = acetylcholine; AChE = acetylcholinesterase; AChR = acetylcholine receptor; CMS = congenital myasthenic syndrome.

are provoked or worsened by exertion, exposure to extremes of temperature, viral or other infections, menses, and excitement. Ocular muscle involvement is usually bilateral, asymmetrical, and typically associated with ptosis and diplopia. Weakness of other muscles innervated by cranial nerves results in loss of facial expression, everted lips, a smile that resembles a snarl, jaw drop, nasal regurgitation of liquids, choking on foods and secretions, and a slurred, hypernasal speech with a reduced volume. Abnormal fatigability of the limb muscles causes difficulty in combing the hair, lifting objects repeatedly, climbing stairs, walking, and running. Depending on the severity of the disease, dyspnea can appear on moderate or mild exertion or be present even at rest. The abnormal fatigability can be demonstrated by asking the patient to look up without closing the eyes for a minute, to count loudly from 1 to 100, to hold the arms elevated forward to the horizontal position for a minute, or to perform repeated deep knee bends. The tendon reflexes remain normally active even in weak muscles. Atrophy of masseter, temporal, facial, or tongue muscles, and less often of other muscles, occurs in about 15% of patients.

Initially, the symptoms are purely ocular in 40%, are generalized in 40%, and involve only the extremities in 10%, and only the bulbar or bulbar and eye muscles in another 10%. Subsequently, the weakness can spread from ocular to facial to lower bulbar muscles and then to torso and limb muscles, but the sequence may vary. Proximal limb muscles are affected more than distal ones. In the most advanced cases the weakness is universal. By the end of the first year, the ocular muscles are affected in nearly all patients. The symptoms remain ocular in only 16%. In nearly 90% of those in whom the disease becomes generalized, this occurs within the first year after the onset. Progression is most rapid within the first 3 years, and more than half of the deaths caused by MG occur in that period. Spontaneous remissions lasting from weeks to years can occur. Long remissions are uncommon, and most remissions occur during the first 3 years.

Two thirds of patients with MG have thymic hyperplasia and 10 to 15% have thymoma. In a few with thymoma myocarditis or giant cell myositis also develops. In about 10% the MG is associated with another autoimmune disease, such as hyperthyroidism, polymyositis, systemic lupus erythematosus, Sjögren's syndrome, rheumatoid arthritis, ulcerative colitis, pemphigus, sarcoidosis, pernicious anemia, or Lambert-Eaton myasthenic syndrome.

A clinical classification of MG originally proposed by Osserman, based on the distribution and severity of symptom, is still useful: group 1, ocular; group 2A, mild generalized; group 2B, moderately severe generalized; group 3, acute fulminating; group 4, late severe.

Transient Neonatal MG. Circulating AChR antibodies can be detected in most infants born to myasthenic mothers, but only 12% of such children have MG, usually during the first few hours of life. The findings are feeble cry, feeding and respiratory difficulty, general or facial weakness, and ptosis. The mean duration is 18 days. There is no relation between the severity of MG in mother and that in infant. The disease is caused by the transfer of AChR antibodies from mother to infant.

DIAGNOSIS. Diagnosis is based on the results of the characteristic history, physical examination, anticholinesterase tests, and laboratory studies. The latter include electromyelogram (EMG) studies, tests for AChR antibodies, and, in selected cases, microelectrode studies in vitro of neuromuscular transmission and ultrastructural and cytochemical studies of the end-plate.

Anticholinesterase Tests. Edrophonium given intravenously acts within a few seconds, and its effects last for a few minutes. One to two milligrams of the drug is injected intravenously over 15 seconds. If no response occurs in 30 seconds, an additional 8 to 9 mg is injected. The evaluation of the response requires objective assessment of one or more signs, such as degree of ptosis, range of ocular movements, and force of the hand grip. Possible cholinergic side effects of the drug include fasciculations, flushing, lacrimation, abdominal cramps, nausea, vomiting, and diarrhea. The drug must be given cautiously to patients with cardiac disease, for it may cause sinus bradycardia, atrioventricular block, and, rarely, cardiac arrest. Atropine is used to reverse toxicity. Intramuscular neostigmine, 0.5 to 1.0 mg, acts maximally in about 30 minutes, and its effects last up to 2 hours, allowing a more leisurely evaluation of changes in clinical status.

Electromyography. Supramaximal stimulation of a motor nerve at 2 to 3 Hz results in a 10% or greater decrement of the amplitude of the evoked compound muscle action potential from the first to the fifth response. The test result is positive in nearly all patients, provided that two or more distal and two or more proximal muscles are examined. The decrement is caused by a normally occurring decrease in the number of quanta released from the nerve terminal, and hence in the amplitude of the EPP, at the beginning of low-frequency stimulation. In MG the EPP amplitude is already reduced by the AChR deficiency, and the additional decrease during stimulation blocks transmission at an increasing number of endplates. Single-fiber EMG compares the timing of action potentials in pairs of closely adjacent muscle fibers in the same motor unit during a willed contraction. In MG the low amplitude and relatively long rise time of the EPP cause abnormally long interpotential intervals and intermittent blocking of action potential generation at some fibers.

Serologic Tests. The usual AChR antibody test measures the binding of antibody to AChR labeled with radioactive α-bungarotoxin. The toxin itself is attached irreversibly to the ACh binding site of AChR. The antibody binding test result is positive in nearly all adults with moderately severe or severe MG, in 80% with mild generalized MG, and in 50% with ocular MG, but in only 25% of

those in remission. The test is less reliable in juvenile than in adult MG. In a few patients only antibodies that block the binding of ACh to AChR can be detected. The antibody titer correlates only loosely with disease severity, but in individual patients a >50% decrease in titer for more than 12 months is nearly always associated with sustained clinical improvement. Striated muscle antibodies also occur in MG patients. Their role remains unknown, but they often are associated with thymoma.

Other Diagnostic Studies. Immune deposits can be localized at the MG end plate in cryostat sections even when circulating AChR antibodies cannot be detected. C3 localization is technically the easiest and most convenient way to confirm the suspected diagnosis.

DIFFERENTIAL DIAGNOSIS. The differential diagnosis includes neurasthenia, the Miller-Fisher variant of inflammatory polyneuropathy, oculopharyngeal dystrophy, mitochondrial myopathies involving the external ocular or other cranial and limb muscles, intracranial mass lesions compressing cranial nerves, congenital and drug-induced myasthenic syndromes, and other disorders of neuromuscular transmission listed in Table 511–1. Neurasthenia is recognized by the finding on motor testing that the patient "gives way" when individual muscle strength is tested. Laboratory tests for MG are negative. In myopathies involving the ocular muscles, the weakness does not fluctuate, diplopia is seldom a symptom, the muscle biopsy result may show distinct morphologic abnormalities, and findings of pharmacologic and laboratory tests for MG are negative. Drug-induced and other myasthenic syndromes are considered later.

THERAPY. Anticholinesterases, alternate-day prednisone treatment, azathioprine, cyclosporin A, thymectomy, intravenous immunoglobulin, and plasmapheresis are currently used to treat MG. Anticholinesterases are useful in all clinical forms of the disease. Pyridostigmine bromide (Mestinon) (60-mg tablets) acts for 3 to 4 hours, and neostigmine bromide (15-mg tablets) for 2 to 3 hours. The former drug has fewer muscarinic side effects and is therefore more widely used. One half to four tablets of pyridostigmine bromide are given every 4 hours in the daytime. This medication is also available in 180-mg "time-span" tablets for use at bedtime and as a syrup for children and patients requiring nasogastric feeding. If troublesome muscarinic side effects occur, these can be treated with 0.4 to 0.6 mg atropine given orally two or three times daily. Postoperatively or in critically ill patients intramuscularly injectable pyridostigmine bromide (the dose is one thirtieth of the oral dose) and neostigmine methylsulfate (the dose is one fifteenth of the oral dose) can be used.

Progressive weakness despite increasing amounts of anticholinesterases signals the onset of a cholinergic or myasthenic crisis. Cholinergic crises are associated with muscarinic effects, such as abdominal cramps, nausea, vomiting, diarrhea, miosis, lacrimation, increase in bronchial secretions, diaphoresis, and bradycardia. In a myasthenic crisis the muscarinic effects are not conspicuous, and 2 mg edrophonium given intravenously improves rather than worsens the weakness. In practice, however, the two types of crises often are difficult to distinguish, and overmedication of a myasthenic crisis can convert it into a cholinergic crisis. Therefore, patients who have increasing difficulty with respiration, feeding, or handling of secretions and who are not responding to relatively high doses of anticholinesterases are best treated by drug withdrawal, tracheal intubation or tracheostomy, support with respirator, and intravenous feeding. Refractoriness to drug therapy usually disappears after a few days.

In patients with generalized disease not responding adequately to modest doses of anticholinesterases, other forms of therapy must be employed. Thymectomy increases the remission rate and improves the clinical course of MG. Although controlled clinical studies of thymectomy according to age, gender, severity, and duration of disease have never been carried out, there is general agreement that the best response occurs in young women with hyperplastic thymus glands and high antibody titer. Thymoma represents an indication for thymectomy because the tumor is often locally invasive. Magnetic resonance imaging readily detects mediastinal tumors.

Alternate-day prednisone treatment induces remission or significantly improves the disease in more than half the patients. The treatment is relatively safe provided that one institutes the usual precautions for patients taking corticosteroid therapy. With an average dose of 70 mg on alternate days, the average time for significant improvement is 5 months. After the improvement reaches a plateau the dose must be lowered gradually over several months to establish the minimum maintenance dose.

Azathioprine in doses of 2–3 mg/kg/day also induces remissions or measurable improvement in more than half the treated patients. The earliest time for improvement is 3 months and often 12 months or longer. Surveillance to detect side effects (pancytopenia, leukopenia, serious infection, and hepatocellular injury) must be maintained during therapy. Azathioprine as an adjunct to alternate day prednisone reduces the maintenance dose of prednisone required, lessening side effects. Cyclosporin A, [controversial], can be used in cases refractory to prednisone and azathioprine.

Plasmapheresis is indicated in severe generalized or fulminating MG refractory to other forms of treatment. Daily exchanges of 2 liters of plasma result in objective improvement and lower the AChR antibody titer in a few days. Plasmapheresis, however, is expensive and does not confer greater long-term protection than immunosuppressants alone.

Intravenous immunoglobulin therapy at a dose of 400 mg/kg for 5 consecutive days may improve severe MG within 2 to 3 weeks of the start of therapy. The mean duration of the response is 9 weeks in patients also treated with corticosteroids and 5 weeks in those who are not.

LAMBERT-EATON MYASTHENIC SYNDROME. Lambert-Eaton myasthenic syndrome is an acquired autoimmune disease in which pathogenic autoantibodies cause a deficiency of voltage-sensitive calcium channels at the motor nerve terminal. The deficiency restricts calcium ingress when the terminal is depolarized by nerve impulses and thereby reduces the probability of quantal release. Among patients above 40 years 70% of men and 30% of women have an associated carcinoma, usually a small-cell carcinoma of the lung. The syndrome may predate tumor detection by up to 3 years. Non-neoplastic cases have an association with other autoimmune disorders, human leukocyte antigens B8 and DRw3 (HLA-B8 and DRw3), and organ-specific autoantibodies.

Patients have weakness and fatigability of proximal limb and torso muscles with relative sparing of extraocular and bulbar muscles. The lower limbs are more severely involved than the upper ones. On maximal voluntary contraction the force produced by a weak muscle increases for a few seconds and then again decreases. The tendon reflexes are hypoactive or absent in most patients. Autonomic manifestations (dry mouth, impotence, decreased sweating, orthostatic hypotension, or altered pupillary reflexes) occur in one half of the patients.

On EMG, the amplitude of the compound muscle action potential evoked by a single nerve stimulus from rested muscle is abnormally small. Repetitive stimulation at 2 Hz induces a further decrement, but stimulation at frequencies higher than 10 Hz or voluntary exercise for a brief period markedly facilitates the response so that the evoked potential attains normal amplitude.

Anticholinesterases are only slightly effective. Guanidine hydrochloride (10 mg/kg/day) or 3,4-diaminopyridine (1 mg/kg/day) increases quantal release from the nerve terminal and relieves the symptoms. However, the former drug has severe toxic side effects, and the latter is not yet available in clinical practice. Optimal treatment of non-neoplastic cases consists of modest doses of alternate-day prednisone and 2–3 mg/kg/day of azathioprine.

DRUG-INDUCED MYASTHENIC SYNDROMES. The drug-induced myasthenic syndromes are uncommon in clinical practice. Tetracycline, polymyxin, and aminoglycoside antibiotics, antiarrhythmic agents (procainamide, quinidine), β-adrenergic blockers (propranolol, timolol), phenothiazines, lithium, trimethaphan, methoxyflurane, and magnesium given parenterally or in cathartics reduce the safety margin of neuromuscular transmission. However, overt myasthenic symptoms do not usually appear unless an overdose of the drug is administered or the renal or hepatic elimination of the drug is impaired. The same drugs and inhalation anesthetic agents also can potentiate neuromuscular blocking agents used during surgical procedures and both may worsen or unmask pre-existing disorders of neuromuscular transmission. Calcium-channel blocking drugs can worsen the transmission defect in the Lambert-Eaton myasthenic syndrome.

Succinylcholine, a depolarizing blocking drug, is used to induce muscle relaxation during anesthesia. A single dose of the drug sufficient to cause transient apnea is eliminated by plasma pseudocholinesterase in 2 to 10 minutes. In approximately 1 of 2500 patients receiving the drug, prolonged apnea occurs and persists up to several hours. Most of these patients have an autosomal recessive abnormality of the plasma pseudocholinesterase. In some genetic variants the plasma pseudocholinesterase activity is abnormally low; in others the enzyme shows increased sensitivity to inhibition by dibucaine. Curare and related agents used during surgery and in critically ill patients to induce muscle relaxation produce non-depolarizing blockade of the neuromuscular junction. Their use in patients with myasthenia gravis and the congenital myasthenias is associated with profound and prolonged weakness.

ORGANOPHOSPHATE INTOXICATION. Organophosphate insecticides irreversibly inhibit cholinesterases. Poisoning occurs by accident or when the compounds are ingested with suicidal intent. The accumulation of ACh at central, muscarinic, and nicotinic cholinergic synapses is associated with alterations in sensorium, convulsions, coma, severe muscarinic side effects, cramps, fasciculations, and muscle weakness from a depolarization block as well as desensitization of AChR at the neuromuscular junction. Therapy consists of gastric lavage with more than 100 liters of water, followed by the use of activated charcoal and oral cathartics, respiratory support, and anticonvulsants as needed. Atropine, 1 to 2 mg intramuscularly every hour, can be used to control the excessive secretions. Pralidoxime (1 g intravenously, repeated in 20 minutes if necessary) has been used with variable success.

Engel AG, Franzini-Armstrong C (eds): Myology, 2nd ed. New York, McGraw-Hill, 1994. *Chapters by Engel and Magleby ably discuss the detailed anatomic and physiologic characteristics and clinical dimensions of neuromuscular transmission.*

Engel AG, Ohno K, Wang HL, et al: Molecular of congenital myasthenic syndromes: Mutations in the acetylcholine receptor. Neuroscientist 4:185, 1998. *A review of the current status of the congenital myasthenias.*

Gutmann L, Besser R: Organophosphate intoxication: Pharmacologic, neurophysiologic, clinical, and therapeutic considerations. Semin Neurol 10:46, 1990. *A lucid analysis of the pathophysiologic basis of the symptoms and a reliable guide to therapy.*

O'Neill JH, Murray MF, Newsom-Davis J: Lambert-Eaton myasthenic syndrome: A review of 50 cases. Brain 3:577, 1988. *A comprehensive review of the clinical and basic scientific aspects of the disease.*

PART XXVI

EYE, EAR, NOSE, AND THROAT DISEASES

Table 512–1 ▪ **VISUAL ACUITIES REQUIRED FOR COMMON DAILY TASKS**

20/20	Physiologic vision
20/30–20/100	Driver's license, varies by state
20/50	Newspaper print
20/70	Large print *Reader's Digest*
20/100	Write a check
20/200	Legally blind
20/400	Paper currency

GENERAL APPROACH TO VISUAL LOSS

Physiologic visual acuity is remarkably consistent among healthy humans. Diminished visual acuity warrants careful ophthalmic examination to identify the cause. In persons with appropriate vision, routine ophthalmic examination can detect asymptomatic pathology.

Evaluation of Ocular Function

Although human vision is most frequently quantified by line letter *acuity,* vision also comprises color, motion, contrast, brightness, field, and depth perception. These latter qualities are less frequently evaluated during screening because there is greater variation among humans. Visual acuity, however, is limited by retinal anatomy and remains remarkably consistent among individuals. Normal acuity describes accurate resolution of a flat object that subtends an angle of 1 degree on the human retina. The "20/20" line on a visual acuity chart consists of letters that, when held 20

feet from the subject, subtend an angle of 5 degrees; each individual segment of those letters subtends an angle of 1 degree and must be resolved to identify the letter. Letters half that size, held at half that distance, subtend the same angle (10/10 visual acuity). When a subject demonstrates an inability to resolve printed forms subtending 1 degree of arc, vision is substandard and leads to functional disability (Table 512–1). The cause may lie anywhere along the visual pathway from the tear film to the visual cortex of the occipital lobe (Fig. 512–1).

Whether a chief complaint or an incidental finding, poor visual acuity should prompt complete ophthalmic evaluation. Examination of *pupillary response* provides the most objective measure of ocular function. The swinging light test for *relative afferent pupillary defect* (RAPD, Marcus Gunn pupil) is performed by alternately illuminating the pupils while examining the direct (ipsilateral) and consensual (contralateral) response. An optic nerve or, rarely, a

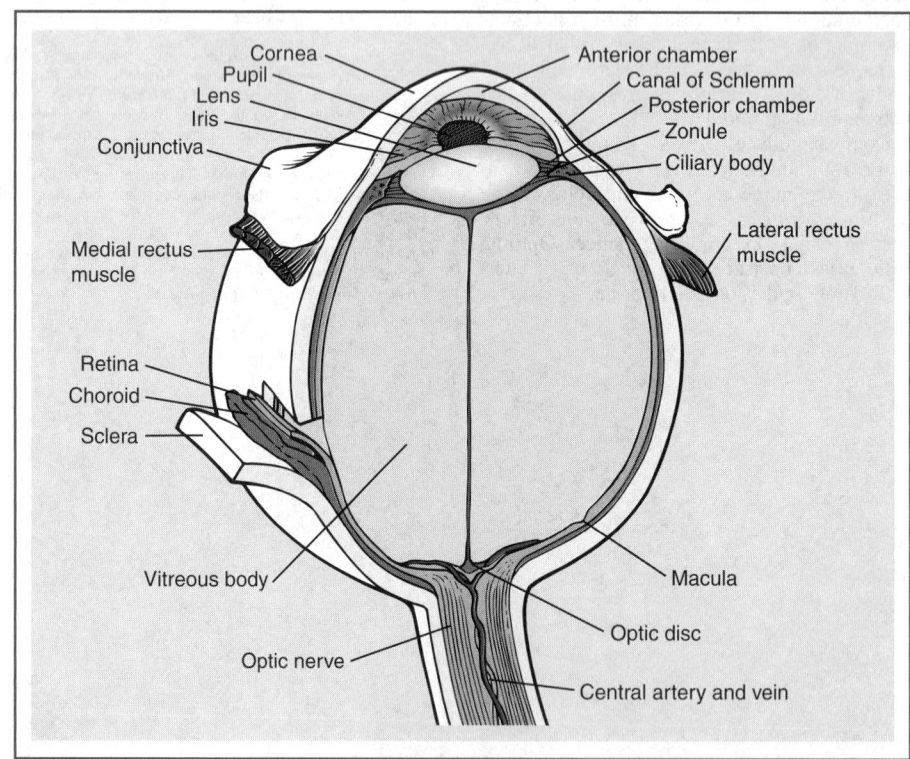

FIGURE 512–1 ▪ Anatomy of the eye.

Table 512–2 ■ DIFFERENTIAL DIAGNOSIS OF SUDDEN VISUAL LOSS

Unilateral	Bilateral
Amaurosis fugax (carotid artery stenosis)	Eclampsia
Central retinal artery occlusion	Cavernous sinus thrombosis
Occipital lobe infarct	Vertebrobasilar infarct
Temporal arteritis	Trauma
Non-arteritic anterior ischemic optic neuropathy	
Hemorrhage	
Preretinal (high altitude, Valsalva)	
Vitreous	
Aqueous (hyphema)	
Trauma	

central nervous system lesion interfering with afferent conduction will produce a paradoxical dilation of the involved side on direct illumination. Anterior segment pathology, including dense cataract and posterior segment pathology, does not produce RAPD. Severe amblyopia may occasionally produce RAPD. *Confrontational visual fields* are performed independently in each eye to detect gross quadrantic defects. *Color vision* testing plates are used as a sensitive indicator of optic nerve function. Extraocular motility is assessed for nerve or muscle abnormalities.

Intraocular tension may be determined most accurately by applanation tonometry in which an applanation prism is used to depress the cornea. Increased intraocular tension may indicate glaucoma, whereas decreased intraocular tension may indicate retinal detachment or a ruptured globe. *Ocular alignment* is determined by corneal light reflex and cover tests using prisms. *Binocular function* may be assessed using polarized glasses and targets at distance and near.

Sudden visual loss is commonly due to circulatory conditions or trauma (Table 512–2). Prompt evaluation is critical, although the condition may be irreversible.

Topographic Evaluation

Topographic evaluation of the eye begins with external examination with attention to exophthalmos or enophthalmos and lid contour and lesions. The orbital rim and regional lymph nodes are palpated. The globe is balloted for resistance to retropulsion.

Slit lamp biomicroscopy proceeds in orderly fashion to evaluate lid contour, lesions, and lashes. The conjunctiva, sclera, and cornea are examined for injection, discharge, and inflammation. The anterior chamber is examined for proteinaceous exudate (flare) and inflammatory or red blood cells. The lens and anterior vitreous are examined.

Gonioscopy may be performed using various mirrored lenses to view the angle structures and evaluate angle closure and neovascularization. Dilated fundus examination with an indirect ophthalmoscope provides a panoramic view of the fundus. Specific attention is paid to the optic nerve head, retinal vessels, and macular region. The peripheral retina is best seen with scleral depression.

Ancillary Studies

Numerous electrophysiologic and radiographic tests may be used to complement the ophthalmic physical examination. Automated perimetry utilizing static stimuli of variable intensity has replaced manual visual field testing in most offices. Computerized statistical analysis allows for more accurate comparison between serial examinations. Electroretinography may help distinguish specific retinal diseases, and measurement of visual evoked potentials may assess visual cortex function.

Among the more common imaging studies is fluorescein angiography of the retina and choroid. Fluorescein solution is injected intravenously into the antecubital fossa while timed photographs are taken through light filters. A-scan ultrasound is used to determine the axial length of an eye, most commonly to determine the appropriate power of implanted intraocular lenses in patients undergoing cataract extraction. B-scan ultrasound provides excellent intraocular imagery when the fundus cannot be viewed directly. Ultrasound biomicroscopy can provide detailed images of the anterior segment. Computed tomography is preferred to evaluate orbital

structures, whereas magnetic resonance imaging produces greater detail for optic nerve and central nervous system lesions.

Refractive Error

The most frequent cause for suboptimal visual acuity is refractive error: the refracting power of the eye is poorly suited for that particular eye. Patients with refractive errors are said to be ametropic; those eyes with properly suited refracting apparati are emmetropic. *Myopia* is a common condition in which the refracting power of the eye at rest is too great in relation to the axial length of the eye; the focused image of an object held at infinity lies anterior to the retina. *Physiologic myopia*, which is more common than pathologic myopia, results from a mismatch between the refracting power of the optical elements of the eye and the axial length of the globe when neither of these components lies outside the normal range. The refracting power of a normal human eye is approximately 65 diopters (D), with the cornea and tear film contributing 45 D and the crystalline lens contributing 20 D. The average axial length of the human eye is approximately 24 mm. Physiologic myopia usually ranges from -0.5 to -8.0 D, and the eye appears normal on physical and radiographic evaluation. Onset begins in the second decade and may progress through the third decade. Physiologic myopia is not thought to be heritable, but there appears to be an increased frequency of the disorder among higher socioeconomic groups and among those with greater academic training. Although the cause is not clear, several laboratory and epidemiologic studies indicate that prolonged accommodation as experienced through extensive reading may contribute to progression of physiologic myopia; well-lighted reading conditions may mitigate this effect.

Physiologic myopia is usually treated with spectacle or soft contact lens correction. Radial keratotomy (RK) decreases the refracting power of the central cornea by using radial incisions in the peripheral cornea to weaken it, allowing the peripheral cornea to bow slightly and the central cornea to flatten. Because of increased risk of rupture, difficult prediction of refractive result, and lessening of surgical effect with time, this procedure appears to be falling out of favor with most ophthalmologists. Photorefractive keratectomy (PRK) uses laser energy to ablate the anterior surface of the central cornea, directly creating a new refractive surface. Newer techniques involve surgical removal of an anterior corneal flap, stromal ablation, and replacement of the flap. Other investigations involve intracorneal lenses (epikeratophakia) and intracorneal rings to alter the central corneal curvature reversibly. Because physiologic myopia tends to progress into the third decade of life, a minimum of 6 months of stable refractive error should be demonstrated before a refractive procedure is performed.

Pathologic myopia is a heritable condition in which the eye is abnormally long; the refracting apparatus is usually normal. Refractive error in pathologic myopia is usually greater than -8.0 D. Peripapillary atrophy is common: the internal scleral surface of the elongated globe is incompletely covered by retina and retinal pigmented epithelium, and a white or yellow crescent or ring of bare sclera may be seen around the optic nerve. The optic discs may be tilted, making estimation of optic nerve cupping difficult. An outpouching of the posterior globe (posterior staphyloma) with broad areas of retinal pigmented epithelium alteration may be seen. Patients with pathologic myopia are predisposed to retinal tears and holes, retinal detachment, subretinal bleeding, and choroidal neovascularization. Pathologic myopia may be associated with systemic disorders, including trisomy 21, Cornelia de Lange syndrome, Stickler's syndrome, and Marfan syndrome. Dilated fundus examination should be performed at frequent intervals, and patients should be alerted to symptoms of retinal detachment (flashing lights, floaters). Pathologic myopia may be managed with spectacles or contact lenses. Refractive procedures are less successful in pathologic myopia due to high refractive errors and posterior segment anomalies. Surgical and laser procedures may be required to treat retinal and choroidal lesions.

Hyperopia is an ametropic condition in which the refracting power of the eye is insufficient to bring the focused image of an object held at infinity onto the retina; the image lies posterior to the retinal plane. Hyperopia is the normal condition in infants and young children. Adolescent and adult hyperopia is not usually associated with anatomic abnormalities of the posterior segment. Many patients with hyperopia are able to overcome their refractive deficiency by accommodating even when viewing at distance. Accommodation is an active process in which parasympathetic stimulation of the circular ciliary muscle relaxes the lens zonules, allowing the lens to relax into a more spherical conformation. The ability to accommodate diminishes with age. Emmetropes rely on accommodation to focus at near; they require near correction as they lose the ability to accommodate, usually entering the sixth decade (presbyopia). Hyperopes, however, may require near correction earlier in life because much of their accommodative power is used to offset the distance refractive error, and small decreases in accommodative ability may be symptomatic (hyperopic presbyopia).

In addition to blurred vision, hyperopia may incite headaches in young adults because increasing effort is required to focus at intermediate distances. Hyperopia is managed with periodic cycloplegic refraction and spectacle or contact lens correction. Excimer laser treatment of hyperopia is under investigation.

Astigmatism is a condition in which the corneal surface is asymmetrical: light is refracted differently along different meridians. In regular astigmatism, the steepest corneal meridian lies 90 degrees away from the flattest corneal meridian, a configuration similar to the shape of a football. Regular astigmatism can usually be corrected with cylindrical and spherical spectacle lenses or with rigid contact lenses. Irregular astigmatism may produce an array of corneal configurations, usually owing to corneal ectasias (keratoconus, keratoglobus, pellucid marginal degeneration) or corneal scarring. Irregular astigmatism is not correctable with spectacles but may be correctable with rigid contact lenses.

OPHTHALMIC DISORDERS USUALLY NOT ASSOCIATED WITH SYSTEMIC DISEASE

Congenital

Oculogenesis is initiated between 22 and 25 days of gestation when the neural tube begins to close and the optic pits first appear; retinal vascularization is completed shortly after birth, as is uveal pigmentation. As a result, there are many systemic congenital syndromes with protean ocular manifestations. The congenital disorders limited to the eye and discussed here may be treatable or may have catastrophic consequences if not detected early.

Strabismus

Normal development of visual pathways depends on simultaneous and appropriate retinal stimulation in early childhood. *Amblyopia,* or incomplete visual development, may be categorized according to cause as strabismic, anisometropic, or deprivational. Amblyopia may be minimized or prevented by early diagnosis and intervention.

Misalignment of the eyes, or *strabismus,* causes disparate images to be cast simultaneously on the two retinas. Diplopia is avoided by suppressing one of the images. Alternating images may be suppressed, in which case excellent vision may develop in each eye, but binocular vision will not develop. More frequently, however, one eye is constantly suppressed, preventing normal visual development in that eye.

Esotropia, in which the eyes are deviated inward, is the most common strabismus of childhood. Congenital esotropia may not manifest until 3 or 4 months of age and is therefore often termed *infantile esotropia.* There is usually a large angle deviation; cross fixation, in which each inward-turned eye is used to view the contralateral visual field, is not uncommon. Infantile esotropia must be distinguished from pseudostrabismus, in which a broad nasal bridge and prominent epicanthal folds create an illusion of esotropia by obscuring the nasal sclera; in this condition, however, corneal light reflexes will be symmetrical, and (later) alternate cover testing will show no movement. Abduction should be demonstrated to differentiate congenital bilateral sixth cranial nerve palsies. Family history of strabismus confers an increased risk, but no inheritance pattern has been determined. Infantile esotropia is most frequently seen in otherwise normal children, but it occurs with

increased frequency in several systemic conditions including cerebral palsy, prematurity, hydrocephalus, and trisomy 21. Cycloplegic refraction should be performed, and patching of one eye may be needed; however, surgery is almost always required to straighten the eyes. Binocular vision can rarely be produced.

Anisometropia is a condition in which the refractive states of the two eyes differ. One eye may focus a clear image on the retina without accommodation while the contralateral image is blurred, leading to unilateral amblyopia. Children may squint the affected eye. Cycloplegic refraction, spectacle or contact lens correction, and occlusive and/or pharmacologic penalization of the favored eye may reverse visual loss if instituted before 9 years of age.

Deprivational or occlusive amblyopia may be caused by any opacity along the visual axis. Blepharoptosis may result from dysgenesis of the levator palpebrae and may require early surgical intervention. Capillary hemangioma, the most common eyelid tumor of childhood, may produce ptosis by mechanical effects. These benign, red, elevated lesions may appear within the first few weeks of life and generally involute by age 10. Indications for treatment with intralesional corticosteroid injection include pupillary occlusion and induced refractive error. Most congenital cataracts incompletely occlude the pupil and permit normal vision to develop. Complete congenital leticular opacification, however, may cause amblyopia if not removed within the first few weeks of life.

Glaucoma

The clinical triad of epiphora, photophobia, and blepharospasm is characteristic of congenital glaucoma. It is thought to result from an anomalous aqueous outflow apparatus and may be seen in isolation or with other ocular and systemic abnormalities. *Congenital open-angle glaucoma* produces a large eye (buphthalmos) and megalocornea. Examination under anesthesia is required to evaluate the optic nerve head and anterior chamber angle. Medical therapy may provide temporary benefit, but early surgical intervention is indicated.

The rudimentary stump of iris present in congenital *aniridia* produces glaucoma within the first decade by blocking aqueous outflow through the trabecular meshwork. Congenital aniridia is inherited in an autosomal dominant pattern; 13% of cases are sporadic. Patients with congenital sporadic aniridia are at risk for Wilms' tumor and the WAGR syndrome (*W*ilms' tumor, *a*niridia, *g*enitourinary anomalies, and mental *r*etardation). Congenital glaucoma may be seen with any of the anterior segment dysgeneses. Genetic investigation and counseling is advised.

Leukocoria

A white pupil may result from anterior or posterior segment pathology (Table 512–3) and requires prompt and thorough ophthalmic investigation. *Leukocoria* is the most frequent presenting sign in patients with retinoblastoma, the most common intraocular malignancy of childhood. *Retinoblastoma* may be inherited or sporadic and bilateral or unilateral. Calcification is commonly demonstrated radiographically, and involved eyes are usually normal in size. Early, aggressive intervention with irradiation and/or surgery may be sight saving and lifesaving. Any disorder that produces congenital leukocoria may be confused with retinoblastoma. The *retinal telangiectasia* of Coats' disease produces unilateral leukocoria through exudative retinal detachment; 85% of patients are boys, and the disease is not heritable. Calcification is uncommon. Treatment consists of vascular ablation and management of retinal detachment.

Persistent hyperplastic primary vitreous (PHPV) is associated with unilateral microphthalmos in otherwise normal infants. Leukocoria is produced by a retrolenticular vascularized membrane or by induced cataract. Calcification is rare. Although visual prognosis is poor, early vitrectomy/lensectomy may prevent amblyopia and

Table 512–3 ■ **DIFFERENTIAL DIAGNOSIS OF LEUKOCORIA**

Retinoblastoma
Cataract
Persistent hyperplastic primary vitreous
Retinopathy of prematurity (retrolental fibroplasia)
Coats' disease (retinal telangiectasia)
Retinal detachment
Toxocariasis

glaucoma. *Familial exudative vitreoretinopathy* is an autosomal dominant, bilateral peripheral retinal disorder that produces retinal exudation and detachment. Incomplete vascularization of the temporal retina is seen in full-term, otherwise healthy infants. Severity may be asymmetrical, and prognosis is variable.

Congenital cataracts are relatively common and are seen in 1 in 2000 live births. Cases may be found in association with other ocular or systemic disorders or may be isolated; one third of cases are inherited (usually autosomal dominant). Intrauterine chemical or radiation insult and TORCH infections have been implicated. Severity is variable and relates to morphology and cause. Metabolic disorders such as galactosemia may produce total, bilateral lenticular opacity resulting in nystagmus and irreversible amblyopia; focal cataracts may be less visually devastating. Traumatic cataracts may result from child abuse.

Genetic

Hereditary disorders primary to the eye are far too numerous to address. Many ophthalmic syndromes and diseases that are not commonly considered hereditary exhibit patterns of inheritance in a minority of cases. The following representations highlight some of the more common and more interesting entities that demonstrate familial patterns in a majority of cases.

Mitochondrial Transmission

Among the ophthalmic disorders inherited through mitochondrial DNA are *Leber's hereditary optic neuropathy* and *chronic progressive external ophthalmoplegia*. Leber's hereditary optic neuropathy became the first human disease for which mitochondrial inheritance was definitively demonstrated. Symptoms are limited to subacute, bilateral, progressive loss of vision. Males are affected in 60 to 90% of cases. Onset occurs in the second and third decades. Vision is generally reduced to 20/200 or worse sequentially in the two eyes over a period of months. Clinical findings include optic disc hyperemia with telangiectatic, tortuous retinal vessels; optic nerve pallor (atrophy) is seen in the late stages. Treatment is limited to use of low vision aids.

Chronic progressive external ophthalmoplegia frequently presents as bilateral blepharoptosis in the first and second decades. The paralysis is called "external" because the extraocular muscles are primarily involved; the iris dilator, iris sphincter, and ciliary muscles are spared. Vision is usually spared, although funduscopic examination reveals deterioration of the retinal pigmented epithelium in the macular region. The condition may occur in isolation or with cardiac conduction abnormalities and arrhythmias—the Kearns-Sayre syndrome. Muscle biopsy specimens demonstrate ragged red fibers. Systemic corticosteroids are contraindicated because they have reportedly precipitated hyperosmermolar non-ketotic coma in patients with Kearns-Sayre syndrome.

Autosomal Dominant Transmission

The corneal dystrophies are bilateral, inherited disorders that may produce pain and visual loss or may go entirely unnoticed. Autosomal dominant transmission is the rule. Corneal dystrophies are characterized by particular layer of corneal involvement, material deposition, age at onset, and treatment of symptoms.

Recurrent corneal erosions commonly result from *map-dot-fingerprint dystrophy*, the most common of corneal dystrophies. Severe pain is produced on wakening and appears out of proportion to clinical signs. This epithelial basement membrane disorder produces patterned irregularities for which it is named. Epithelial cells are stripped away with seemingly trivial trauma as with lid opening on wakening. Clinical symptoms first appear in middle age. Methods of treatment range from hypertonic saline drops to mechanical anterior corneal puncture to excimer laser ablation. *Reis-Buckler dystrophy*, striking in the first or second decade, may also produce epithelial erosion. Scarring of Bowman's layer in the anterior cornea may require lamellar or penetrating (full-thickness) corneal transplantation.

Corneal stromal dystrophies rarely produce epithelial erosion but may cause decreased visual acuity. The focal, hyaline deposits of *granular dystrophy* produce modest visual disturbance and may recur in a corneal graft. *Lattice dystrophy* is characterized by amyloid deposition in the anterior stroma and may or may not be associated with systemic amyloidosis. Recurrence in a corneal graft is common. *Macular dystrophy* produces large, confluent areas of acid mucopolysaccharide in patients with a metabolic defect in the production or breakdown of keratan sulfate. Macular dystrophy is the only common corneal dystrophy that shows autosomal recessive transmission.

Thickened protuberances of Descemet's membrane, corneal edema, and painful subepithelial bullae are characteristic of *Fuchs' endothelial dystrophy*. Visual acuity is worse after sleep, when prolonged lid closure limits evaporation from the corneal surface. Transmission is autosomal dominant, but sporadic cases are seen. Temporizing treatment may include hypertonic solutions and bandage contact lenses. Definitive treatment requires penetrating keratoplasty.

Autosomal Recessive Transmission

Retinitis pigmentosa (RP) is a group of photoreceptor dystrophies in which damage to rods predominates. Nyctalopia (night blindness) and gradual, progressive loss of peripheral vision are invariably present. Although the appearance of the fundus varies greatly, signs include attenuation of retinal vessels, waxy pallor of the optic disc, and "bone spicule" pigmentation of the peripheral fundus in a majority of cases (Color Plate 17G).

Prevalence in the United States is approximately 1 in 400. Approximately 35% of RP cases show autosomal recessive transmission, about one fifth are autosomal dominant, about 10% are X-linked recessive, and about 35% are sporadic. Hundreds of genetic defects have been identified. Perimetry may be useful to document progression, but an electroretinogram (ERG) is required for definitive diagnosis. The ERG demonstrates progressive loss of rod photoreceptor function; cones are affected to a variable degree.

Spotty pigmentation of the fundus may be seen with a number of treatable disorders, including infectious and inflammatory chorioretinitis, vascular occlusions, drug toxicity, and retinal detachment. RP associated with congenital deafness is called Usher's syndrome.

Because there is no current treatment for RP, patient education is critical. In most cases, the disease is slowly progressive over decades. Central visual acuity may remain surprisingly good despite severe constriction of the visual field. Patients whose visual field is reduced to 20 degrees are considered legally blind in most states. Low vision aids are useful in many cases. Genetic counseling should be provided. Vitamin supplementation is under investigation, and some authorities advise limiting light exposure with the use of tinted glasses.

Leber's congenital amaurosis is considered by some authorities to be a variant of RP. Infants are usually brought to medical attention within the first 6 months of life when nystagmus develops or delay of visual maturation is otherwise evident. Transmission is autosomal recessive. Affected patients do not respond to visual stimuli on examination, and pupils show variable reactivity. Fundus findings range from normal to heavily spiculed. Multiple, small, white choroidal foci may be seen. The ERG demonstrates generalized photoreceptor dysfunction. No treatment is currently available.

Gyrate atrophy of the choroid is another autosomal recessive degeneration of the fundus. Progressive visual loss and night blindness begin in the first decade. Severely constricted visual fields are present in adults with the disease. The peripheral fundus appearance may be dramatic showing geographic areas of retinal pigmented epithelial (RPE) dropout and choroidal atrophy with hyperpigmented borders. The central retina may become involved later as these patches become confluent. The disease is associated with defects in ornithine aminotransferase, which result in elevated serum levels of ornithine. The ERG is abnormal early in the disease. Diagnosis is based on fundus findings and serum ornithine levels. Treatment requires dietary restriction of arginine. Differential diagnosis includes pathologic myopia, choroideremia, RP, and other causes of chorioretinal atrophy.

X-Linked Transmission

Choroideremia may be confused with gyrate atrophy due to its similar fundus appearance. It is an X-linked recessive condition that results in progressive atrophy of the choriocapillaris beginning in the first decade. The midperiphery is first involved with slow progression anteriorly to the ora serrata and posteriorly to the optic nerve. Hyperpigmented areas are generally not seen. Night blindness is often the presenting symptom, whereas visual acuity gradually decreases to the 20/200 level by the fourth decade. Female carriers are asymptomatic but may show subtle fundus signs.

Nearly all forms of congenital *dyschromatopsia* demonstrate X-linked recessive transmission. Three distinct cone photoreceptor subtypes provide color perception in most humans. The pigment of each subtype demonstrates specific peak wavelength absorption. Patients lacking red cones are said to demonstrate protanopia, whereas those lacking green cones are labeled deuteranopes. Congenital tritanopia, or absence of blue cones, is extremely rare and shows autosomal dominant inheritance.

Most cases of color blindness represent a relative deficiency or abnormality of one of the cone populations rather than a total absence. Genetic defects in coding for cone pigments usually result in subtle shifts in peak wavelength absorption such that color matching responses in affected individuals are incongruous with normal subjects but color differences are perceived nonetheless. Blue-yellow confusion is seen more frequently in acquired dyschromatopsia and may herald optic nerve disease.

Exogenous Infections

Exogenous ocular infections may involve any of the ocular or periocular tissues. Signs and symptoms reflect focality, chronicity, and the infectious pathogen. Treatment may range from modifications in hygiene to surgical debridement.

Inflammation of the eyelids may produce itching and redness of one or both eyes (Color Plate 18*F*). *Anterior blepharitis* primarily involves the eyelash follicles, which are located within the anterior lamella of the eyelid. *Staphylococcus aureus* is the most common infectious agent. If untreated, the condition becomes chronic and may lead to corneal and conjunctival inflammation. Patients are advised to clean the eyelids and eyelashes rigorously using a cotton-tipped applicator or washcloth daily. Ophthalmic antibiotic ointment (bacitracin or erythromycin) is more effective than eye drops to treat the lid margin. *Seborrheic blepharitis* is an anterior blepharitis in which crusting and oily material may envelope individual cilia. Treatment focuses on eyelid hygiene.

The inflammation of *meibomianitis* localizes to the posterior lamella, where the meibomian gland orifices exit the tarsal plate. Slit lamp examination reveals inspissated glands from which white material may be expressed with manual pressure to the eyelid. Vision may be impaired, and the conjunctiva may be inflamed by hyperviscous secretions that enter the tear film. Treatment requires daily eyelid hygiene. Warm, dilute solutions of baby shampoo and a clean washcloth may be used to massage the eyelid margin. Some patients may improve with oral tetracyclines, and half of patients may have rosacea (see Chapter 522).

Acute, focal infection of a meibomian or Zeiss gland is called a *hordeolum.* Commonly termed a *stye,* a hordeolum may be painful and may produce blepharoptosis when it occurs in the upper lid. Hordeola are usually self-limited infections, but they may progress to preseptal cellulitis in which the surrounding lid tissue becomes erythematous, edematous, and warm. Hordeola usually respond to warm compresses over a period of days, whereas preseptal cellulitis requires systemic antibiotics (see later).

Chalazion (Color Plate 18*E*) describes a chronically inspissated meibomian gland. Glandular secretions become fossilized within the tarsal plate, producing a firm, non-mobile subcutaneous nodule. Extravasation into adjacent soft tissue may produce chronic granulomatous inflammation with enlargement of the chalazion, internal or external erosion, spontaneous drainage, or focal cellulitis. Conservative treatment involves warm soaks with or without antibiotic ointment. Incision and curettage is usually reserved for very large lesions or those persisting despite more than 1 month of conservative treatment. Recurrent, isolated chalazia may respond to local corticosteroid injection, although hypopigmentation and tissue necrosis may occur. Multiple chronic chalazia may respond to systemic antibiotics. Chalazia may increase in size during pregnancy. Chronic, non-responsive chalazia, especially when accompanied by loss of eyelashes, must be evaluated to exclude *sebaceous cell carcinoma.*

Periocular cellulitis may involve deep orbital structures or may be confined to preseptal tissues. In either case, it may produce warm, erythematous eyelid edema and associated pain. Fever and leukocytosis is not uncommon. A history of an insect bite or other skin perforation is frequently elicited in cases of *preseptal cellulitis,* whereas ethmoidal sinusitis is the leading risk factor for *orbital cellulitis.* Treatment is critically dependent on proper diagnosis.

Clinical signs of *preseptal cellulitis* are limited to external soft tissues as described. Decreased visual acuity, relative afferent pupillary defect, limited ocular motility, and pronounced chemosis herald postseptal involvement. In the presence of orbital signs, computed tomographic scans of the orbit and sinuses should be obtained. If untreated, *orbital cellulitis* may extend intracranially.

Preseptal cellulitis is treated with oral antibiotics in an outpatient setting. First-generation cephalosporins are generally effective against *Streptococcus pneumoniae* and staphylococcal species. *Haemophilus influenzae,* found in pediatric patients, produces a characteristic violaceous discoloration. Infants and young children with preseptal cellulitis are admitted for intravenous antibiotics. Orbital cellulitis requires hospital admission with intravenous antibiotics in all age groups. Lack of clinical improvement in 24 to 36 hours may suggest another process. *Orbital pseudotumor* in adults and *rhabdomyosarcoma* in children must be excluded.

Acute dacryocystitis (Color Plate 18*G*) produces pain, redness, and swelling of the lacrimal sac. Patients may experience purulent discharge from the lacrimal punta, and secondary conjunctivitis is common. Symptoms of chronic dacryocystitis may be limited to epiphora. Both are associated with nasolacrimal duct obstruction. Digital massage of the lateral nasal wall may cause a mucopurulent reflux through the lacrimal punctum. Initial treatment with oral antibiotics may quell any acute inflammation, but definitive treatment usually requires dacryocystorhinostomy with intubation of the nasolacrimal system.

Conjunctivitis is a frequent complaint in which patients experience redness, itching, and foreign body sensation, with discharge ranging from watery to hyperpurulent. It must be differentiated from a corneal abrasion (Color Plate 17*F*) and other causes of a red, painful eye (Table 512–4). The great majority of cases are caused by viral infections that may begin unilaterally and progress to involve both eyes. Viral conjunctivitis is caused most frequently by adenovirus species. Transmission is by direct contact with an infected individual. *Epidemic keratoconjunctivitis* caused by adenovirus subtypes 7, 11, and 18 may spread rapidly through a school, summer camp, or physician's office. Patients diagnosed with viral conjunctivitis should be isolated from other patients; examining rooms and waiting areas should be disinfected.

Viral conjunctivitis produces inferior palpebral conjunctival follicles evident on slit lamp examination. There may be copious watery discharge, but mucopurulent discharge is uncharacteristic. Conjunctival hemorrhage suggests an alternate pathogen. Preauricular lymphadenopathy may be present, and a history of upper respiratory tract infection is common. Vision may be compromised by immune infiltration of the corneal stroma. The disease is self-limited, and treatment is aimed at patient comfort. Cool compresses may be used. Patients are advised to wash their hands frequently. When viral conjunctivitis has been diagnosed, antibiotic solutions and ointments are not required, and topical corticosteroids are contraindicated. Although viral particles may be recovered from infected individual for up to 2 to 3 months, most patients are believed to be contagious for 1 to 2 weeks.

Bacterial conjunctivitis (Color Plate 18*H*) represents fewer than 5% of all cases. Staphylococcal species present as chronic mild mucoid discharge and crusting and may be associated with chronic blepharitis or dacryocystitis. Symptoms may improve with erythromycin or bacitracin ointment, but treatment should be targeted at underlying infectious sources. Acute bacterial conjunctivitis caused by *Haemophilus* or streptococcal species may be seen in epidemic or isolated form. Transmission may be through direct contact or through fomites. Moderate purulent discharge is seen. There may be mild edema of the conjunctiva (chemosis) and lids. Slit lamp examination of the inferior palpebral conjunctiva reveals a fine papillary response. The disease is usually self limited but responds well to broad-spectrum antibiotic solutions, including gentamicin and Polytrim (polymyxin B and trimethoprim).

Hyperacute purulent conjunctivitis caused by *Neisseria gonorrhoeae* is transmitted through sexual contact. Copious green pus is produced, and the lids are often extremely edematous. Preauricular lymphadenopathy is common. Immediate intervention is critical to prevent perforation of corneal ulcers caused by bacterial exotoxins.

Table 512-4 ■ DIFFERENTIAL DIAGNOSIS OF COMMON CAUSES OF INFLAMED EYE*

FEATURE	ACUTE CONJUNCTIVITIS	ACUTE IRITIS†	ACUTE GLAUCOMA‡	CORNEAL TRAUMA OR INFECTION
Incidence	Extremely common	Common	Uncommon	Common
Discharge	Moderate to copious	None	None	Watery or purulent
Vision	No effect on vision	Slightly blurred	Markedly blurred	Usually blurred
Pain	None	Moderate	Severe	Moderate to severe
Conjunctival injection	Diffuse; more toward fornices	Mainly circumcorneal	Mainly circumcorneal	Mainly circumcorneal
Cornea	Clear	Usually clear	Steamy	Change in clarity related to cause
Pupil size	Normal	Small	Moderately dilated and fixed	Normal or small
Pupillary light response	Normal	Poor	None	Normal
Intraocular pressure	Normal	Normal	Elevated	Normal
Smear	Causative organisms	No organisms	No organisms	Organisms found only in corneal ulcers due to infection

*Other less common causes of red eyes include endophthalmitis, foreign body, episcleritis, and scleritis.
†Acute anterior uveitis.
‡Angle-closure glaucoma.

Gram stain and culture of the conjunctiva should be performed. Copious irrigation with saline solution is required to dilute the exotoxins. Systemic antibiotics are required. Third-generation cephalosporins may be given intramuscularly or intravenously. Adjunctive topical treatment with ciprofloxacin, gentamicin, or bacitracin may be useful.

Adult inclusion conjunctivitis is produced through sexual transmission of *Chlamydia trachomatis*. This chronic conjunctivitis produces conjunctival follicles in association with preauricular lymphadenopathy and is refractory to many antibiotic regimens. If untreated, the disease may linger for many months. Systemic treatment with erythromycin or azithromycin is required. *Trachoma* is a chronic cicatricial conjunctivitis resulting from repeated infection with particular chlamydial subspecies. Endemic in many developing countries, it is the world's leading cause of corneal blindness. The superior palpebral conjunctiva develops white, linear scars, and limbal pitting may be seen. Trichiasis, inverting of the eyelashes, eventually leads to corneal vascularization and opacification. Treatment requires systemic erythromycin or tetracycline.

Allergic conjunctivitis is commonly associated with atopy, hay fever, and allergic rhinitis. Itching is usually the prominent symptom, although foreign body sensation is common as well. Watery discharge occurs. Supportive treatment includes cool compresses and topical vasoconstrictors or antihistamines such as naphazoline or levocabastine.

Keratitis caused by herpes simplex virus usually represents secondary ocular infection (Color Plate 17A). Primary infection may go unnoticed or may be limited to a periocular vesicular dermatitis or blepharoconjunctivitis. Viral particles may lie dormant within the trigeminal ganglion indefinitely or may reinfect the corneal epithelium or stroma. Herpes simplex epithelial keratitis produces a characteristic dendritic epithelial defect and is believed to represent active viral infection. Treatment is with topical trifluridine or oral acyclovir. Isolated stromal manifestations are believed to represent immunologic activity against the virus. Treatment with topical corticosteroids reduces the risk of permanent corneal opacification. Prophylactic topical antiviral agents (e.g., trifluridine) are given during treatment with corticosteroids.

Bacterial keratitis may present as a minor peripheral corneal opacity or a large central suppurative ulcer. Symptoms include pain, redness, photophobia, and decreased vision. Fluorescein staining reveals an epithelial defect with underlying opacity. Gross or microscopic epithelial trauma is the primary risk factor. The risk of bacterial keratitis is five times greater in contact lens wearers and increases among those who sleep with lenses in place. Gram-positive cocci are the most common pathogens; *Pseudomonas* is most common in patients who wear contact lenses. Identification of the pathogen requires Gram stain and culture of corneal scrapings. Empirical treatment with topical fluoroquinolones is advised by some ophthalmologists in less severe cases. Administration of these agents as frequent as every 15 minutes is not uncommon. More severe cases require hospital admission and topical application of fortified antibiotic solutions every 10 to 15 minutes. Systemic antibiotics are not routinely administered. Perforation may be treated

with bandage contact lens, cyanoacrylate (crazy glue), or penetrating keratoplasty. Fungal infection, suspected after injury with vegetable matter, many require early surgical débridement.

Endophthalmitis, or inflammation of the intraocular cavity, may be exogenous or endogenous and infectious or sterile. Exogenous infectious endophthalmitis follows surgical or non-surgical penetrating trauma. Incidence is estimated at 0.1% after intraocular surgery and 5% after penetrating injury. The primary symptom is decreased vision. Vitritis and anterior uveitis are evident on examination. Corneal, conjunctival, retinal, and choroidal involvement are variable. Toxin-producing gram-positive species and gram-negative species produce rapid onset necrosis of the vitreous and other intraocular structures. *Propionibacterium acnes* and *Staphylococcus epidermidis* are indolent organisms causing more subtle presentations.

Endophthalmitis requires sampling of the aqueous and vitreous for Gram stain and culture. *P. acnes* and *S. epidermidis* may require injection of intravitreal antibiotics. More virulent infections require pars plana vitrectomy with intravitreal corticosteroids and intravenous antibiotics. Prognosis is variable and depends on the specific pathogen. Indolent infections may result in excellent postoperative vision. Aggressive pathogens can completely destroy intraocular tissues within several hours, eliminating all useful vision.

Idiopathic Inflammatory and Autoimmune

Ocular or periocular tissues may be the primary focus of isolated idiopathic or autoimmune inflammation. Pain is a common symptom. Vision is variably reduced. Treatment is aimed at reducing symptoms and limiting tissue destruction because the underlying cause is poorly understood.

Keratoconjunctivitis sicca, commonly called dry eye syndrome, results from deficiency of any of the tear film layers. Symptoms include gritty, foreign body sensations, burning, photophobia, and decreased visual acuity. The cornea and conjunctiva may stain with fluorescein, although rose bengal staining is more sensitive. Idiopathic inflammation of the lacrimal and salivary glands resulting in keratoconjunctivitis sicca and xerostomia is called Sjögren's syndrome (Chapter 291) and is more common in women. Secondary complications include recurrent corneal erosion, keratitis, and corneal opacification. Artificial tears, often administered six to eight times a day, and lubricating ointments at night are the mainstays of treatment, often in combination with temporary or permanent punctal occlusion.

Episcleritis is inflammation immediately underlying the conjunctiva. Pain, if present, is mild. Sectoral hyperemia, distinguished from conjunctivitis by radially oriented vessels that do not move with the conjunctiva, is dramatically reduced with instillation of phenylephrine 2.5% or 10%. Episcleritis is self-limited, although topical non-steroidal anti-inflammatory medications such as flurbiprofen or diclofenac may hasten resolution. In contradistinction to scleritis, episcleritis is not usually related to systemic rheumatoid disease.

Scleritis frequently presents as severe pain and redness. It may be associated with systemic disease or may be seen in isolation. Vision may be reduced when the posterior sclera is involved. There may be diffuse or sectoral hyperemia that is non-mobile and does not blanch with phenylephrine instillation. Scleral thinning may occur, but perforation is rare. Uveitis and keratitis may occur secondarily. Diagnostic evaluation includes ultrasonography and/or magnetic resonance imaging as well as laboratory tests to identify infectious or autoimmune connective tissue disease. Treatment may require topical or oral non-steroidal anti-inflammatory medications or corticosteroids. Refractory cases may require cytotoxic drugs.

Mooren's ulcer is a progressive, idiopathic peripheral corneal thinning thought to be an autoimmune phenomenon. The condition may be unilateral or bilateral, and pain is common. Perforation is rare except with trauma. Topical corticosteroids, mucolytics, and cytotoxic agents have been used. Bandage contact lenses and conjunctival recession or advancement have also been used with variable success.

Ocular cicatricial pemphigoid is a vesicular conjunctivitis named for its relentless destruction of the ocular surface. Involvement before age 60 is rare. Initial symptoms of foreign body sensation and burning reflect chronic conjunctivitis. Ruptured epithelial bullae destroy conjunctival goblet cells, leading to profound dry eye. The conjunctival fornices may be obliterated. Mild trauma or surgery may increase inflammation. Patients with ocular cicatricial pemphigoid demonstrate antibodies to the conjunctival basement membrane, and other mucous membranes may be affected. Dapsone is the first-line treatment, although it is contraindicated in patients with glucose-6-phosphate dehydrogenase deficiency. Cytotoxic medications or corticosteroids may be helpful.

Non-specific, idiopathic orbital inflammation has been called *orbital pseudotumor.* The inflammation may involve the lacrimal gland (dacryoadenitis), extraocular muscles (myositis), orbital fat, sclera, or optic nerve sheath (optic perineuritis). Inflammation primarily involving the orbital apex produces painful external ophthalmoplegia, the so-called Tolosa-Hunt syndrome. Pain is the most frequent symptom in orbital pseudotumor, although many cases present with proptosis and limitation of ocular movements; visual acuity may be reduced. Orbital computed tomography or magnetic resonance imaging is generally required to exclude mass lesions; biopsy may be indicated in atypical cases. A dramatic response to systemic corticosteroids within 24 hours is common. A poor clinical response should suggest an alternative diagnosis. Corticosteroids must be tapered slowly over months to prevent recurrence. Irradiation may be required if corticosteroids cannot be discontinued successfully.

Patients with *iritis* complain of pain, photophobia, and blurred vision. Greater than 50% of cases are unrelated to systemic disease. There may be a perilimbal conjunctival injection, and slit lamp examination demonstrates inflammatory cells and protein exudate (flare) in the anterior chamber. Initial episodes are usually treated symptomatically with prednisolone acetate 1% suspension four times a day and cycloplegic drugs (atropine 1% daily, cyclopentolate 2% twice daily). Repeat episodes require systemic evaluation for autoimmune and infectious causes.

Central serous retinopathy presents unilaterally as acutely decreased visual acuity and metamorphopsia in young to middle-aged adults. Patients are usually well educated and employed in stressful occupations. Visual acuity may range from 20/40 to 20/200. Fundus examination demonstrates a central, serous deviation of the neurosensory retina. Fluorescein angiography is useful in diagnosis. The disease is self-limited, although permanent visual deficits have been reported. Focal laser treatment reduces duration of symptoms but does not improve final outcome.

Neoplastic

Neoplasms primary to the eye and adnexa are vast. External lesions may be categorized as pigmented or non-pigmented. Orbital tumors may be intraconal or extraconal. Primary intraocular tumors are far outnumbered by metastatic foci.

Capillary hemangioma, the most common eyelid tumor, is a pediatric lesion that manifests in the first several weeks of life. The so-called strawberry nevus enlarges over several months but generally begins to involute after 1 year of age. Complications include

ptosis, astigmatism, and amblyopia. There may be orbital involvement. Large tumors may require intralesional corticosteroid injection, and systemic corticosteroids are now being used with greater frequency. Laser treatment has been successful in several cases.

Rhabdomyosarcoma is the most common primary orbital malignancy of children. Proptosis, ptosis, and lid ecchymosis are most common on presentation; visual loss is variable. History of incidental trauma may be misleading. Orbital computed tomography may be useful, but biopsy is required for definitive diagnosis. Systemic evaluation for metastases (including chest radiography, lumbar puncture, and bone marrow biopsy) should be initiated emergently. Survival rates exceeding 90% have been achieved with focal irradiation (4000–6000 cGy) and systemic chemotherapy.

Basal cell carcinoma, the most common eyelid malignancy, is most frequently seen on the lower eyelids of elderly patients. Lesions are typically pearly, umbilicated nodules, although morphology varies widely and includes deeply pigmented tumors. Excision with clear surgical margins is generally curative. Basal cell carcinoma rarely metastasizes, and local recurrence can be treated with excision. Caruncular lesions may extend into deep tissues and therefore warrant orbital imaging before surgery.

Squamous cell carcinoma occurs much less frequently than basal cell carcinoma but carries the risk of metastasis. Squamous cell carcinoma is found most frequently on the lower lid where actinic exposure is greatest. Advanced cases may involve the orbit and sinuses and require systemic evaluation. Surgical excision is required.

Sebaceous cell carcinoma may arise from any of the sebaceous glands of the eyelids. Chronic chalazia that destroy local lid architecture should raise the possibility of sebaceous cell carcinoma, as should chronic unilateral blepharitis. The tumor is aggressive and requires excisional surgery. Metastasis is not uncommon. Sebaceous cell carcinoma associated with visceral malignancy is termed *Muir-Torre syndrome.*

Malignant melanoma of the conjunctiva may arise de novo, from nevi, or in areas of *primary acquired melanosis* (PAM). Unilateral conjunctival pigmentation in lightly pigmented persons may exhibit cellular atypia, in which case the individual is at risk for melanoma. Conjunctival melanoma may be pigmented or amelanotic. Tumor thickness of greater than 0.8 mm portends a greater likelihood of metastasis. Early local excision with cryotherapy is often curative. Intraocular malignant melanoma is the most common primary intraocular tumor. Malignant melanoma arises in the choroid or ciliary body and may extend through the sclera to involve the conjunctiva. Choroidal malignant melanoma may arise de novo or from a previously identified choroidal nevus. Tumor thickness greater than 3 mm, breadth greater than 10 mm, or rapid enlargement suggests malignant melanoma. The liver is the most common site of metastasis, and liver enzymes are the most sensitive screening tool. In cases without metastases, treatment is controversial and may involve focal radiation, laser ablation, excision, or enucleation.

Retinoblastoma, the most common intraocular malignancy of childhood, may be inherited as an autosomal dominant trait or may be sporadic. Genetic study of retinoblastoma, a prototypic genetic malignancy, gave rise to the Knudson two-hit hypothesis. Normal development relies on a tumor suppresser gene located on the long arm of chromosome 13. One normal allele is sufficient to suppress tumorigenesis. Familial retinoblastoma may result from autosomal dominant transmission of one defective allele, in which all the cells in the body are affected. Bilateral or multicentric disease is common in this situation, and the abnormal gene is passed on to future offspring. Sporadic retinoblastoma results from mutations during embryogenesis. Mutation early in embryogenesis will affect all the cells in the body, and a de novo germline defect is created. Bilateral or multicentric disease is common in this situation. Late mutation in embryogenesis produces non-transmissible, unilateral, unifocal disease. In any of these settings, the second allele suffers somatic mutation in a developing retina cell. Patients most frequently present with leukocoria or strabismus, and 90% are diagnosed by age 3. Bilateral or multicentric disease indicates a germline mutation. Enucleation is required in most cases, and optic nerve extension is the most significant prognostic factor. Radiation, laser ablation, cryotherapy, and chemotherapy may be used in bilateral cases to treat the second eye. Survivors are at risk for other malignancies, including osteogenic sarcoma.

Intraconal orbital tumors generally produce axial proptosis and decreased vision. Orbital *cavernous hemangioma,* the most common orbital tumor, is a benign, vascular endothelial neoplasm that may be intraconal or extraconal. Orbital images reveal a well-circumscribed tumor. Significant pain should suggest another diagnosis. Excision is indicated only when vision becomes compromised.

Primary optic nerve tumors include *meningioma* and *glioma.* Optic nerve meningiomas are slow growing tumors seen in middle-aged individuals; women are affected more often than men. Vision may be reduced or may be normal. Characteristic computed tomographic images reveal primary involvement of the neural sheath. Serial examinations and images are performed to detect posterior progression. Threat of chiasmal involvement is the primary indication for excision, although this is somewhat controversial. Optic nerve glioma may be seen in children with von Recklinghausen's disease or tuberous sclerosis. Bilateral optic nerve glioma is pathognomonic for neurofibromatosis type I. Isolated optic nerve glioma in adults is rare but is often lethal.

Degenerative

Cataract, or opacification of the crystalline lens, is the leading cause of blindness in the world and the leading cause of visual loss in Americans older than age 40. Prevalence of cataract in the United States has been estimated at 50% for persons older than age 75. The great majority of cases represent normal aging changes in which progressive yellowing of the lens nucleus (nuclear sclerosis) and hydration of the lens cortex are seen. Genetic predisposition to senile cataract has been hypothesized but not proven. Prolonged exposure to ultraviolet radiation has been shown to be cataractogenic. Surgical extraction is required to improve vision; there is no known medical treatment.

Nearly all patients older than age 50 demonstrate some degree of degenerative lens changes when examined by slit lamp. Visual disability depends on the extent of lenticular changes as well as on the visual demands of the patient. Very rarely is cataract extraction medically indicated. Mature, swollen cataracts may induce phacomorphic glaucoma by narrowing the anterior chamber angle. Hypermature, liquefied cataracts may leak lens protein and thereby cause phacoantigenic uveitis. In the majority of cases, however, elective cataract extraction serves to restore lost vision. There is no urgency in most cases, and patients who are told they must have cataract surgery in the absence of disabling visual complaints should beware.

Congenital cataracts may be associated with metabolic disease, result from intrauterine TORCH infections, or may be familial. Traumatic cataracts result from hydration after penetrating injury to the lens. Some cataracts may be characteristic in color or location, such as the sunflower cataract of Wilson's disease or the posterior subcapsular cataract often resulting from systemic corticosteroid use.

Cataract extraction with intraocular lens implantation has become a very successful procedure in the developed world. Potential complications include cystoid macular edema, astigmatism, retinal detachment, and endophthalmitis. Current methods of surgery include small, self-sealing incisions performed under local (retrobulbar) or topical anesthesia. Prognosis for visual recovery is excellent barring any concomitant eye disease such as diabetic retinopathy, glaucoma, or macular degeneration.

Glaucoma is best defined as atrophy of the retinal ganglion cell layer in the presence of elevated intraocular pressure. The classic clinical triad consists of elevated intraocular tension, atrophic cupping of the optic nerve head, and characteristic visual field loss. Normal tension glaucoma has been described. Elevated intraocular pressure has not been clearly defined as causative. Many experts view glaucoma as a vascular optic neuropathy, whereas others favor an endogenous toxin etiology. Early in the disease, findings are variable and the diagnosis is difficult to make; many patients are categorized as "glaucoma suspects" based on one or more risk factors and should be examined every 4 to 6 months. Risk factors include family history of glaucoma, increasing age, diabetes mellitus, obesity, and ocular trauma. Glaucoma is the leading cause of blindness among African-Americans.

Primary open-angle glaucoma, the most common glaucoma, occurs in 15% of individuals older than age 80. The anterior chamber angle anatomy appears normal, but aqueous outflow is reduced.

Progressive visual field loss begins in the periphery and occurs so insidiously that affected individuals may be unaware until late in the disease course. Intraocular tension measurement is an effective, if imperfect, screening method, and all adults should be screened. Medical treatment attempts to reduce aqueous production by the ciliary body or to increase outflow through the trabecular meshwork or uvea. Topical β-blockers, carbonic anhydrase inhibitors, miotics, and prostaglandins may be additive in their effects. Refractory cases may require laser or cryoablative procedures. Filtering surgery produces a subconjunctival outflow conduit in advanced cases.

Angle-closure glaucoma constitutes an ophthalmic emergency. Patients present with a red, painful eye. Nausea and vomiting are common. The pupil is usually fixed in a mid-dilated position, and the cornea appears cloudy due to pressure-driven edema. The iris is bowed forward by posterior accumulation of aqueous humor, thereby sealing off the anterior chamber angle. Risk factors include narrow anterior chamber angles, for which the contralateral eye may provide diagnostic clues. Emergent treatment (Table 512–5) requires topical administration of a β-adrenergic antagonist, an α-adrenergic agonist, and carbonic anhydrase inhibitors. Systemic pressure-lowering medications include carbonic anhydrase inhibitors, glycerol, isosorbide, and mannitol. Definitive treatment requires peripheral iridotomy, usually performed with a laser after the initial crisis is resolved. The contralateral eye is treated prophylactically on an elective basis. Chronic angle closure may result from prolonged intraocular inflammation and secondary fibrosis of the anterior chamber angle.

Secondary glaucomas arise in the setting of mature cataract, intraocular inflammation, or gross anatomic distortion. Inflammatory debris may clog the trabecular meshwork in uveitis. Angle recession glaucoma may follow blunt trauma up to several years after the inciting event. Congenital glaucoma may be primary or may result from malformation such as aniridia causing mechanical dysfunction of the trabecular meshwork. Retinal ischemia from diabetic retinopathy or vascular occlusion may cause neovascularization of the anterior chamber angle leading to neovascular glaucoma. Treatment requires panretinal laser photocoagulation.

Age-related macular degeneration (Color Plate 17*H*) is an idiopathic atrophy of the photoreceptors and retinal pigmented epithelium. Many of the pathologic changes seen in age-related macular degeneration may be observed as normal aging changes in individuals with excellent visual acuity. These findings do not necessarily portend an ominous progression, and the term age-related macular degeneration should be reserved for individuals with visual loss. Amsler grid home monitoring (Fig. 512–2) is advised to detect acute visual field loss and metamorphopsia, which is focal image distortion often caused by focal retinal elevation.

Non-exudative ("dry") macular degeneration presents as painless, progressive loss of central vision. Pigmentary mottling is seen in the macular area of the fundus, and drusen are evident. Drusen are lipofuscin deposits beneath the retinal pigmented epithelium basement membrane. Drusen may be discrete (hard), indistinct (soft), or confluent. Focal retinal pigmented epithelium detachment is common. There is no known treatment for non-neovascular age-related macular degeneration. There is some suggestion that ultraviolet radiation may be causative, but this theory is not proven. Antioxidant vitamins may retard onset and progression; low vision aids may be extremely useful.

Table 512–5 ▪ **MEDICAL TREATMENT OF ACUTE ANGLE-CLOSURE GLAUCOMA**

1. Systemic
   A. Acetazolamide, 500 mg orally in one dose
   B. Isosorbide, 50–100 mg orally in one dose, *or* mannitol, 1–2 g/kg intravenously over 1 hour
2. Topical (administered at 5-minute intervals)
   Beta blocker (e.g., timolol 0.5%) one drop, repeat every 15 minutes × 4
   *Pilocarpine 1–2%, one drop, repeat every 15 minutes × 4
3. Place patient in supine position
4. Refer to ophthalmologist
5. Definitive treatment requires peripheral iridotomy

*Not given to aphakic or pseudophakic patients.

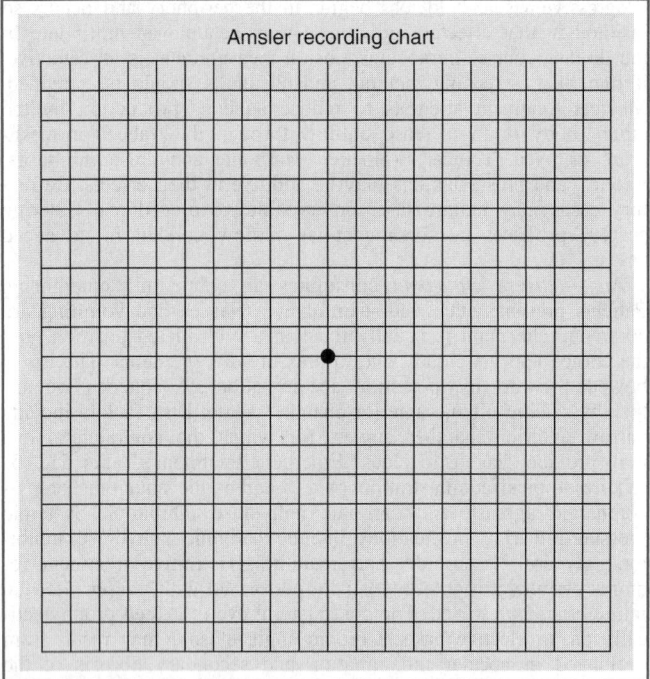

Amsler recording chart

FIGURE 512–2 ■ The Amsler grid is used daily to monitor progression of macular degeneration. Patients are instructed to fixate on the central dot and observe for any distortion or absence of the vertical or horizontal lines. Positive findings may suggest subretinal neovascularization or detachment.

Choroidal neovascularization is the main complication of age-related macular degeneration. Breaks in Bruch's membrane permit the choriocapillaris access to the subretinal space. Submacular hemorrhage is common in these cases. Lesions of appropriate size and location may be prophylactically treated with photocoagulation to decrease the likelihood of severe visual loss, and surgical excision of subretinal membranes is indicated in some cases.

Retinal detachment, or separation of the neurosensory retina from the retinal pigmented epithelium, may be classified as tractional, exudative, or rhegmatogenous. Tractional retinal detachments are most commonly associated with severe, proliferative diabetic retinopathy or follow non-diabetic vitreous hemorrhage. Tractional membranes form from organized hemorrhage and drag the retina as they contract. Exudative elevations are seen with malignant hypertension, posterior inflammation, or choroidal disease. Serous fluid accumulates in the subretinal space and produces a smooth, domed dependent detachment. Rhegmatogenous retinal detachment results from a break in the retina secondary to intraocular involutional changes or trauma.

Rhegmatogenous detachments are by far the most common among healthy individuals. Symptoms include acute decrease in acuity, photopsia (flashing lights), and floaters. There may be associated vitreous hemorrhage, and greater than 90% of cases demonstrate red blood cells in the vitreous (Shafer's sign). Retinal breaks may occur from trauma, posterior vitreous detachment, or retinal atrophy. The vitreous gradually liquefies (sineresis) in middle-aged to elderly individuals and remains firmly adherent to the retina anteriorly. Vitreous traction can produce a tear allowing liquefied vitreous to access the subretinal space. Trauma can produce a similar scenario in younger individuals. Approximately 25% of rhegmatogenous retinal detachments are found in patients with lattice degeneration of the retina, which is present in 10% of adults. Focal vitreous liquefaction occurs over the lattice lesions, whereas the vitreous is firmly attached at the lesion's perimeter. Atrophic retinal holes can also lead to rhegmatogenous detachment.

Not all rhegmatogenous retinal detachments require immediate intervention. Acute, symptomatic cases must be repaired, although the timing of surgery depends on the threat or presence of macular involvement and the condition of the eye. Patients with vitreous hemorrhage should adhere to strict bed rest with the head elevated to optimize visualization of the fundus. Asymptomatic or chronic detachments may be observed in some cases. Surgical treatment requires identification and closure of the break(s), usually through scleral buckling procedures, with or without intraocular surgery, and cryotherapy to induce a chorioretinal adhesion in the area of the break. Other procedures include retinopexy (intraocular gas injection) and laser photocoagulation. *Proliferative vitreoretinopathy* is a rare but potentially devastating complication of retinal breaks in which fibrovascular proliferation distorts the retina and intraocular surface.

Actinic exposure of the conjunctiva and cornea may cause degenerative changes. *Pingueculae* are yellowish elevations of the interpalpebral conjunctiva in which the substantia propria demonstrates elastotic degeneration: ultraviolet radiation–damaged fibroblasts produce altered collagen. Lesions encroaching on the nasal or temporal cornea and demonstrating identical histopathologic findings are known as *pterygia.* Programmed degeneration of the cornea may be seen in *keratoconus.* The central cornea is thinned, resulting in a conical shape. Keratoconus has been associated with atopy and eye rubbing. Patients present with severe astigmatism, usually in the second decade, which may progress until age 30. Rigid contact lenses correct astigmatism in many cases; others require penetrating keratoplasty, which has been very effective in these cases. Calcium deposition at the level of the corneal epithelial basement membrane is seen clinically as *band keratopathy.* Usually seen in the elderly or in degenerated eyes, band keratopathy may be amenable to chelation with edetic acid.

Vascular

Infarction of the optic nerve head is called anterior ischemic optic neuropathy. Many cases relate to vasculitides, whereas others are non-arteritic (idiopathic). Patients present with acute, painless, unilateral loss of vision. Most patients are between 50 and 75 years old. Other risk factors include a small optic disc with very little cupping, hypertension, and diabetes mellitus. Disc edema may be sectoral. Visual field loss is usually altitudinal, and sectoral atrophy ensues; 25% of patients will suffer contralateral disease. Optic nerve sheath fenestration has not been shown effective in acute cases but may be useful in rare cases that progress over days.

Systemic Effects of Ocular Medications

Many ophthalmic solutions may produce systemic side effects even when administered in small doses. Manual punctal occlusion after instillation of drops helps to limit systemic uptake through the nasal mucosa (and helps to increase ocular penetration). *β-Adrenergic antagonists* are among the most commonly prescribed ophthalmic solutions. Patients with asthma may experience bronchospasm or bradycardia; others may experience lethargy. *Epinephrine* may be administered as the pro-drug dipivefrin, which is converted to its active form by corneal enzymes, thereby virtually eliminating any systemic effects. The miotic drug *pilocarpine* is a direct-acting parasympathomimetic and causes few systemic effects. *Echothiophate,* however, is an acetylcholinesterase inhibitor and may produce cholinergic symptoms, including diarrhea and hypersalivation. Concomitant administration of succinylcholine should be avoided. *Atropine* and other muscarinic antagonists may be used to paralyze the ciliary muscle and dilate the pupil. Systemic effects may include tachycardia and fever. Severe cases may be treated with physostigmine. The α-adrenergic medication *phenylephrine* may produce rapid hypertension when given as a 10% topical solution. *Carbonic anhydrase inhibitors* may be administered topically and do not seem to carry the risk of central nervous system effects and aplastic anemia seen with systemic administration.

COMMON OPHTHALMIC MANIFESTATIONS OF SYSTEMIC DISEASES

Congenital

Systemic non-hereditary congenital disorders with frequent ocular manifestations include *Sturge-Weber* syndrome and prematurity. Sturge-Weber syndrome (encephalofacial angiomatosis) is defined as diffuse choroidal hemangioma and facial nevus flammeus (port wine stain). The fundus is diffusely red, the so-called tomato catsup fundus. Histologically, the lesions represent cavernous hemangiomas. Children may remain asymptomatic, although retinal detachment is a common complication in adults. Glaucoma is common in children and may require surgical filtration.

Premature and low-birth-weight infants who receive supplemental oxygen therapy are at risk to develop *retinopathy of prematurity* (ROP), an incomplete vascularization of the peripheral retina that may progress to retinal neovascularization, retinal detachment, and blindness in its most severe form. Previously called retrolental fibroplasia, it may produce leukocoria and be confused with retinoblastoma. Normal retinal vascularization begins at 16 weeks' gestation and is completed at 40 weeks' gestation. Although retinopathy of prematurity may rarely occur even in full-term infants, those at greatest risk weigh less than 1250 g at birth or have a gestational age of less than 28 weeks. The pathophysiology of retinopathy of prematurity has not been fully elucidated.

Initial examination of low-birth-weight infants should be performed before the child is discharged from the neonatal intensive care unit at approximately 4 weeks of age. Subsequent examinations to identify progression depend on the initial findings. The international classification of retinopathy of prematurity reflects degree and location of fibrous proliferation and provides guidelines for intervention. Approximately 8% of infants who weigh less than 1250 g at birth will require treatment. Of the infants who ultimately require treatment, more than 90% do so between 34 and 42 weeks after conception. Observation may be adequate in many cases in which spontaneous regression is seen. When treatment is required, laser or cryoablation of peripheral retinal tissue is usually adequate. More severe cases require pars plana vitrectomy and scleral buckling.

Genetic

The list of genetic abnormalities that exhibit ocular signs and symptoms is staggering. *Sickle cell disease* (see Chapter 169) is one of the more common causes of retinal vascular occlusive disease. Patients with SC disease are at greatest risk for ocular complications. Like arterioles elsewhere in the body, peripheral retinal vessels may become occluded, producing focal infarction. Subsequent neovascularization may result in vitreous hemorrhage and retinal detachment. Neovascular fronds may undergo spontaneous regression or may require photocoagulation. Characteristic comma-shaped conjunctival vessels may be noted on slit lamp evaluation.

Trisomy 21 has been associated with strabismus, myopia, keratoconus, and cataract. Optometric and surgical interventions are based on the severity of systemic and ocular abnormalities. *Kearns-Sayre syndrome,* a mitochondrial cytopathy demonstrating autosomal dominant inheritance, results in progressive external ophthalmoplegia. Diplopia is not common, and there is no known treatment. Either *ocular albinism* or *oculocutaneous albinism* may present as foveal hypoplasia, poor vision, and nystagmus. The former results from a decreased number of melanosomes and shows X-linked transmission. The latter results from decreased melanin granules within each melanosome and shows autosomal recessive transmission. Photophobia is common. Low vision aids may be of some help. *Marfan syndrome* (Chapter 215) is associated with many findings common to connective tissue disorders, including high myopia, lenticular subluxation, cataract, and colobomas. Lensectomy may be required. Inheritance is autosomal dominant.

Multisystem congenital hamartomatous diseases have been called *phakomatoses* (Greek, meaning "mother spot"). *Von Hippel-Lindau disease,* or *angiomatosis retinae,* is transmitted in autosomal dominant fashion. Early photocoagulation of retinal capillary hemangiomas may prevent exudation and retinal detachment. Cerebellar and visceral hemangiomas are common, and patients are at risk for renal cell carcinoma and pheochromocytoma. The ocular hamartomas of *von Recklinghausen's neurofibromatosis* (Chapters 456 and 522) include optic nerve glioma (astrocytic hamartoma), iris Lisch nodules, and plexiform neurofibromas of the eyelids. The optic nerve tumors are slowly progressive, producing painless loss of vision and proptosis. Approximately 50% of patients with neurofibromatosis develop optic nerve gliomas; bilateral tumors are pathognomonic for neurofibromatosis type 1. Lisch nodules are not seen in neurofibromatosis type 2. *Tuberous sclerosis* (Chapter 456)

is less frequently associated with optic nerve gliomas, but retinal glial hamartomas are seen in combination with angiofibromas of the eyelids. Transmission is autosomal dominant.

Endogenous Infections

Systemic infection may cause uveitis, enophthalmitis, retinitis, or choroiditis. Systemic severity often does not correlate with ocular activity. Ophthalmic manifestations may lead to diagnosis or may occur late in the disease.

Tuberculosis (see Chapter 358) involves the uvea in approximately 1% of pulmonary cases. Iridocyclitis and diffuse choroiditis are the most common manifestations. Symptoms include painless progressive visual loss. Small yellow choroidal lesions may be seen, and retinal periphlebitis may occur secondarily. Intermediate- and second-strength purified protein derivative testing may be positive. Clinical response to a 3-week trial course of isoniazid strongly suggests tuberculosis.

Ocular complications of acquired *syphilis* (see Chapter 365) occur in approximately 5% of patients with secondary syphilis, although symptoms may occur during any stage of the disease. Nearly any ocular structure may be involved. The more common presentations include anterior uveitis, neuroretinitis, and the syphilitic Argyll Robertson pupil in which miotic pupils react poorly to light but briskly to accommodation. Congenital syphilis produces "salt and pepper" pigmentation of the fundus.

Nerve fiber layer infarcts seen clinically as "cotton wool" spots are the most common ocular manifestation of the *acquired immune deficiency syndrome* (AIDS) (see Chapter 415). In combination with retinal hemorrhage, these lesions may mimic cytomegalovirus retinitis, another common finding in patients with AIDS. Additional ocular findings in AIDS include opportunistic infections of the retina, choroid, and optic nerve as well as cranial nerve palsies. Kaposi's sarcoma may occur in the lids, orbit, or conjunctiva.

Cytomegalovirus retinitis may present as subacute unilateral visual loss or vitreous "floaters" in immune compromised patients. Large areas of hemorrhagic infarction are seen with minimal vitritis (Color Plate 18A). Intravenous gancyclovir or foscarnet is the mainstay of treatment. Intravitreal administration is under investigation. Even with aggressive treatment, recurrences are seen in up to 50% of cases. Herpes zoster and herpes simplex viruses may produce fulminating necrosis of the retina, *progressive outer retinal necrosis,* in patients with AIDS.

Until recently, ocular *toxoplasmosis* (see Chapter 425) was thought to represent reactivation of congenital disease in nearly all cases; however, studies now suggest that many cases of toxoplasmosis retinitis are acquired after birth. Symptoms include reduced vision and floaters. The typical retinal fundus lesion comprises an active yellow satellite adjacent to an old chorioretinal scar with a dense overlying vitritis, the so-called headlight-in-the-fog. Antibody titers, even in undiluted serum, are significant. Treatment requires systemic combinations of pyrimethamine, clindamycin, sulfonamides, prednisone, and folinic acid. These regimens are moderately efficacious and potentially toxic; treatment is therefore limited to severe intraocular inflammation that threatens the macular area. The toxoplasmosis fundus lesions seen in AIDS patients may differ morphologically from those seen in non-AIDS patients.

Idiopathic Inflammatory and Autoimmune

Autoimmune diseases may produce incidental ocular findings or may have their greatest effects in ocular tissues. Dysthyroid ophthalmopathy commonly called *Graves' ophthalmopathy* (Chapter 239) may be seen in hyperthyroid, euthyroid, or hypothyroid individuals. Inflammation of the extraocular muscles and orbital fat causes proptosis, corneal exposure, and limited ocular motility. Optic neuropathy may result from extreme proptosis with stretching of the nerve or from compression at the orbital apex. Lid retraction is common. Patients present with pain, decreased vision, and vascular congestion. Active inflammation may be treated with systemic corticosteroids or external-beam irradiation in conjunction with aggressive topical lubrication. Emergent surgical decompression may be required when the optic nerve is threatened, but it may not reduce (and may aggravate) inflammation. Surgical decompression of severe proptosis is usually deferred until inflammation is controlled and the clinical examination is stable for several months. Active inflammation generally subsides after 1 to 12 months. Secondary surgeries to correct chronic exposure, diplopia, lid malposition, and proptosis may then be considered.

Sarcoidosis (see Chapter 81) is a common cause of intraocular inflammation among Americans of African descent, and chronic uveitis is seen in 25% of sarcoid patients. Sarcoid may also involve the optic nerve, cranial nerves, and lacrimal glands. Anterior uveitis is treated topically with prednisolone acetate in decreasing doses, depending on degree of inflammation, and with daily cyclopegics (cyclopentolate 2%, atropine 1%). Posterior uveitis and neurologic manifestations require systemic corticosteroids.

Uveitis accompanies many autoimmune diseases and there is often no correlation between ocular and systemic inflammatory activity. *Ankylosing spondylitis* (see Chapter 287) causes acute, recurrent anterior uveitis in 25% of patients. Anterior uveitis or conjunctivitis is seen in nearly all patients with *Reiter's syndrome* (see Chapter 287). Two to 12 per cent of patients with *inflammatory bowel disease* (see Chapter 135) develop anterior uveitis, which is also commonly found in patients with *psoriatic arthritis* but not with psoriasis alone (see Chapters 287 and 522). Symptoms include decreased vision and photophobia. Treatment with topical corticosteroids is usually sufficient to control the ocular disease.

Chronic anterior uveitis may severely reduce vision in patients with *juvenile rheumatoid arthritis* (see Chapter 286). The ocular disease may be insidious and devastating; routine examinations are critical. Pauciarticular juvenile rheumatoid arthritis carries an 80 to 90% risk of uveitis, and uveitis is rarely seen in patients with systemic onset. Girls have a fourfold higher risk of uveitic involvement compared with boys. Patients are usually symptom-free on diagnosis and must be carefully screened for eye involvement. Cataract often results from inflammation or from corticosteroid treatment. Early intervention with topical corticosteroids may delay progression, and oral or intravenous corticosteroids may be required in advanced cases. Megadose pulsed intravenous corticosteroids may be equally efficacious whereas minimizing systemic side effects.

Vogt-Koyanagi-Harada syndrome (uveomeningeal syndrome) may produce anterior or posterior uveitis in darkly pigmented individuals. Decreased vision is the primary ocular symptom. Periocular vitiligo and whitening of the lashes (poliosis) may be seen. Chorioretinitis may lead to exudative retinal detachment. Early treatment with topical or systemic corticosteroids may delay or prevent severe visual loss.

Stevens-Johnson syndrome, an idiosyncratic vesicular mucocutaneous eruption (see Chapter 522), may be triggered by medications or infectious agents. Adolescents are most frequently affected. Conjunctival involvement may lead to cicatrization and obliteration of the fornices with secondary entropion, loss of mucus-producing goblet cells, and corneal opacification. Aggressive lubrication in the acute stage may mitigate these sequelae. Reconstructive grafting with mucous membranes and amniotic membranes may be helpful. Penetrating keratoplasty alone is rarely successful.

Metabolic

Systemic metabolic diseases demonstrate protean ocular findings. Select metabolic diseases may be evident only in the eye. In either case, ocular findings can assist in diagnosis and ongoing evaluation.

Diabetic retinopathy (see Chapter 242) is a leading cause of blindness in the United States. Selective loss of pericytes in the retinal capillaries leads to microaneurysm formation, exudation, capillary obliteration, and neovascularization. Twenty years after diagnosis, virtually all patients with juvenile-onset diabetes and two thirds of those with adult-onset diabetes have some degree of retinal involvement. Onset and progression of retinal findings are delayed in patients with tight glycemic control, as demonstrated by the Diabetes Control and Complications Trial.

Diabetic retinopathy has been classified as non-proliferative or proliferative (Color Plate 18*B*). Non-proliferative disease, also called background diabetic retinopathy, manifests as microaneurysms, intraretinal hemorrhages, subretinal exudation, venous bleed-

ing, and intraretinal vascular abnormalities. Macular edema, the most frequent cause of visual loss, is common in this stage. Macular edema meeting the criteria of the Early Treatment Diabetic Retinopathy Study is treated with focal laser photocoagulation. This study concluded that focal laser photocoagulation reduced the incidence of moderate visual loss by 50% in patients who demonstrated clinically significant macular edema, defined as (1) retinal thickening within 500 μm of the fovea, (2) subretinal exudates within 500 μm of the fovea with adjacent retinal thickening, or (3) an area of retinal thickening of greater than 1 disc diameter, any part of which lies within 1 disc diameter of the fovea.

Retinal ischemia is thought to be the primary stimulus to proliferative diabetic retinopathy in which extraretinal fibrovascular tissue grows along the posterior vitreous scaffold. Neovascularization at the optic disc or elsewhere may lead to vitreous hemorrhage and acute loss of vision. Fibrous organization produces tractional detachment of the retina. Proliferative disease meeting the criteria set forth in the Diabetic Retinopathy Study is treated with panretinal laser photocoagulation. This multicenter, randomized study determined that panretinal laser photocoagulation reduced the incidence of severe visual loss from 16 to 6% in patients at high risk for vitreous hemorrhage. These patients were defined by (1) neovascularization of greater than one third of the optic nerve head, (2) neovascularization elsewhere associated with vitreous hemorrhage, (3) any degree of neovascularization of the disc associated with vitreous hemorrhage, or (4) any two of the following: retinal hemorrhages in four quadrants, venous beading in two quadrants, or intraretinal microvascular anomalies in one quadrant. Advanced cases may require pars plana vitrectomy with peeling of preretinal fibrovascular membranes.

Diabetics are at increased risk to develop painless, isolated cranial nerve palsies, most frequently involving cranial nerves III or VI and generally resolving in 6 to 8 weeks. Multiple cranial nerve palsies should prompt thorough and rapid investigation including magnetic resonance imaging of the brain. In the setting of acute hyperglycemia, accumulation of lenticular sorbitol may lead to lenticular swelling. Secondary refractive errors may linger for 6 to 8 weeks after glycemic control is realized; spectacle prescriptions may change dramatically over this period, and changes should be delayed until the examination stabilizes.

Accumulation of copper in the posterior cornea may aid in the diagnosis of *Wilson's hepatolenticular degeneration* (see Chapter 220), although its appearance usually lags neurologic symptoms. The characteristic Kayser-Fleischer ring fades after treatment. The so-called sunflower cataract is seen less frequently in such cases.

Corneal clouding and retinal degeneration are seen to varying degrees in specific mucopolysaccharidoses and are absent in others. *Tay-Sachs* and *Niemann-Pick* (Chapter 208) diseases are known for the appearance of a foveal cherry-red spot owing to ganglioside accumulation within perifoveal ganglion cells, which form a layer that is absent over the fovea and thickest in the adjacent macula. Pseudoxanthoma elasticum (Chapter 218) is often associated with its characteristic angioid streaks (Color Plate 17*C*). *Gyrate atrophy* of the retina and choroid occurs in the presence of increased serum ornithine caused by ornithine aminotransferase deficiency. Progressive geographic atrophy eventually involves the macula. Corneal, conjunctival, and retinal crystalline deposits may be seen in *cystinosis.* Vision is usually unaffected, but corneal involvement may cause photophobia. Conjunctivitis, iritis, and scleritis experienced during attacks of gout (see Chapter 299) usually abate with systemic control.

Neoplastic

Metastatic ocular disease and systemic neoplastic proliferations involving the eye are far more common than primary ocular malignancy. Pediatric metastases tend to involve the orbit, whereas the vascular choroid is usually affected in adults. Choroidal metastases are seen most commonly with adenocarcinoma of the breast in women; primary lung tumors are the leading cause in men. Together, breast and lung carcinoma account for 70% of ocular metastases. Left eye involvement surpasses right eye involvement by a ratio of 3:2 because of the direct connection between the aorta and the left common carotid artery. Decreased visual acuity is the leading symptom. In the case of breast carcinoma, nearly 70% of patients already carry the diagnosis when choroidal disease is detected. In contrast, choroidal metastases from lung disease may be the initial finding in 90% of cases. Disfiguring surgery should be limited to patients with severe pain.

Ocular findings in *multiple myeloma* (Chapter 181) include uveal protein-filled cysts and retinal hemorrhages second to hyperviscocity. Orbital involvement is rare, but periocular osteolytic lesions may be seen. Patients should undergo ophthalmic examination at the time of diagnosis. External-beam radiation may be dramatically effective. Although B-cell *lymphoma* (Chapter 179) of the large cell variety is the most common lymphoma to involve the eye, it involves the eye with much less frequency than does leukemia. *Leukemic* ocular disease (Chapter 177) may masquerade as a chronic, unilateral "uveitis" or may cause white-centered retinal hemorrhages similar to the Roth spots (Color Plate 17E) seen in infectious endocarditis (Chapter 326). Focal irradiation may augment systemic treatment with either entity.

Vascular

Because the retinal vasculature is uniquely accessible for direct visual inspection, nearly all systemic vascular diseases manifest ocular changes. Chronic *hypertension* (Chapter 55) produces characteristic retinal vascular findings that can be used to identify and assess progression of the disease. Arterial narrowing, nicking at arteriovenous crossings, nerve fiber layer infarcts, and intraretinal hemorrhages characterize hypertension. Arteriolar sclerosis heightens the arterial light reflexes. Moderately sclerosed arterioles demonstrate "copper wiring," whereas severely sclerosed vessels show "silver wiring." Acute hypertension may produce optic nerve edema and serous retinal detachments that shift dramatically with patient repositioning. These detachments usually resolve without significant sequelae if blood pressure is brought under control. Papilledema (Color Plate 17B) must be differentiated from benign causes of pseudopapilledema, such as optic disc drusen (Color Plate 17D).

Hypertension may be implicated in retinal vascular occlusions. *Branch retinal vein occlusion* may cause macular edema and decreased visual acuity or may be asymptomatic. Occlusion typically occurs at an arteriovenous crossing where a common adventitia binds the vessels together and causes compression of the venule wall by the sclerotic arteriole. Sectoral hemorrhages are seen. Photocoagulation may help to resolve macular edema but rarely improves functional outcome. Neovascularization is a rare complication, and most eyes maintain a favorable prognosis. *Central retinal vein occlusion* (Color Plate 18D) is a more severe disease entity. Ischemic and non-ischemic varieties are recognized and may be most accurately differentiated by electroretinogram. The characteristic fundus appearance includes dilated tortuous vessels in all quadrants, as well as variable degrees of retinal hemorrhage. Non-ischemic occlusion may result from hyperviscocity, whereas ischemic occlusion is thought to represent arteriolar impingement on the central retinal vein at the level of the lamina cribrosa. Neovascularization of the iris or retina, occurring in up to 52% of cases, usually occurs 3 months after the initial insult. Panretinal photocoagulation should be deferred until neovascularization is detected.

In contrast to venous occlusive disease, *central retinal artery occlusion* (Color Plate 18C) is not generally associated with systemic hypertension. Emboli result most commonly from carotid stenosis (Chapter 470), but endocarditis and cardiac thromboemboli are other potential sources. Unilateral sudden loss of vision is typical. Amaurosis fugax, or transient unilateral visual loss, may precede frank occlusion and warrants urgent carotid evaluation. Fundus examination reveals a characteristic "cherry-red spot" that reflects diffuse opacification of the infarcting macula contrasted to the hyperpigmented fovea. A relative afferent pupillary defect is present. An acute reduction in intraocular pressure by means of ocular massage, anterior chamber paracentesis, or systemic carbonic anhydrase inhibitors may dislodge a proximal embolus, allow reperfusion of the fovea, and return some useful vision if performed within several hours of onset. *Branch retinal artery occlusion* may go unnoticed by the patient despite a permanent visual *scotoma* (visual field defect).

Temporal arteritis (see Chapter 295) is an important cause of visual loss among the elderly. Symptoms include sudden, unilateral loss of vision. Headache, jaw claudication, scalp tenderness, weight loss, and malaise are common. Visual loss may result from arteritis

Table 512-6 ■ SYSTEMIC MEDICATIONS WITH OCULAR EFFECTS

AGENT	EFFECT
Chloroquine	Dyschromatopsia, visual field defects
Hydroxychloroquine	Dyschromatopsia, visual field defects
Thioridazine	Blurred vision
Chlorpromazine	Blurred vision
Digoxin	Yellow vision
Ethambutol	Optic neuritis
Amiodarone	Corneal whirls, pigmentary retinopathy
Corticosteroids	Glaucoma, cataract
Plaquenil	Pigmentary maculopathy
Tamoxifen	Retinopathy
Neuroleptics	Nystagmus
Compazine	Oculogyric crisis
Vitamin A	Pseudotumor cerebri

or associated central retinal artery occlusion. The erythrocyte sedimentation rate (ESR) is elevated. Systemic corticosteroids (prednisone, 1–2 mg/kg/day) should be initiated as soon as the diagnosis is suspected, and temporal artery biopsy should be performed within 7 days after beginning treatment. Corticosteroids are tapered slowly over months, and many patients require perpetual low-dose corticosteroid treatment as guided by following the ESR. If the disease is not treated, approximately 65% of patients lose vision in the contralateral eye.

Orbital involvement in *Wegener's granulomatosis* (Chapter 294) usually indicates extension from nasal or sinus mucosa and may produce proptosis. Ocular vasculitis may cause inflammation in any of the ocular tissues. Retinal involvement in *polyarteritis nodosa* (Chapter 293) is usually limited to the small vessels, although central retinal artery occlusion can occur. Cranial nerve palsies are not uncommon. The occlusive vasculitis of *Behçet's disease* (Chapter 298) produces retinal vasculitis and iridocyclitis in patients aged 20 to 40. Hypopyon (layering of leukocytes within the anterior chamber) can be seen in one third of cases. Topical corticosteroids are used to treat anterior disease, whereas systemic corticosteroids and cytotoxic agents may be required for posterior disease.

Ocular Effects of Systemic Medications (Table 512-6)

Patients taking systemic medications may require periodic surveillance to identify ocular toxicity. *Chloroquine* and *hydroxychloroquine* may cause decreased color vision and visual field defects at high dose. Chloroquine toxicity is thought to occur after a cumulative dose of 300 g, whereas hydroxychloroquine may cause symptoms after long-term maintenance of 750 mg/day. The fundus may show a typical bull's eye pattern, and corneal whirls may be seen. Symptoms are not reversible and may progress after cessation.

Pigmentary maculopathy may present as blurred vision in patients taking *thioridazine* or *chlorpromazine*. Approximately 800 mg/day of the former or 1200 mg/day of the latter are believed sufficient to cause toxicity. Patients should be examined every 6 months.

Any of the commonly used antituberculous medications may cause optic neuropathy, although *ethambutol* carries the greatest risk. Pupillary response, color vision, acuity, and visual fields are the clinical parameters used to assess optic nerve function.

Cornea verticillata may be seen in patients taking *amiodarone* due to lysosomal accumulations within the epithelial basement membrane. *Fabry's disease* produces similar changes, as can other medications. Corneal whirls are usually reversible when caused by drug toxicity, and they rarely interfere with vision.

Systemic *corticosteroids* carry the same ocular side effects as do topical corticosteroids, including glaucoma and posterior subcapsular cataract.

Albert DM, Jakobiec JA (eds): Principles and Practice of Ophthalmology: Clinical Practice. Philadelphia, WB Saunders, 1994.

Miller NR, Newman NJ (eds): Walsh and Hoyt's Clinical Neuro-Ophthalmology. 5th ed. Baltimore, Williams & Wilkins, 1998.

Spencer WH (ed): Ophthalmic Pathology: A Textbook and Atlas, 4th ed. Philadelphia, WB Saunders, 1996. *Several comprehensive texts.*

513 NEURO-OPHTHALMOLOGY

Robert W. Baloh

The mechanistic understanding of vision impairment along with disturbances of pupillary and oculomotor control lies close to the heart of diagnosing neurologic disorders.

VISION

One of the most difficult diagnostic problems is vision loss that cannot be explained by obvious abnormalities of the eye. To evaluate such a patient properly the examining physician must be familiar with the anatomy and physiology of the afferent visual system. The afferent visual pathways cross the major ascending sensory and descending motor systems of the cerebral hemispheres and in their anterior portion are intimately related to the vascular and bony structures at the base of the brain. Not surprisingly, localization of lesions within the afferent visual pathways has great localizing value in neurologic diagnosis.

Anatomy of the Visual Pathways

Light entering the eye falls on the retinal rods and cones, which transduce the stimulus into neural impulses to be transmitted to the brain. The distribution of visual function across the retina takes a pattern of concentric zones increasing in sensitivity toward the center, the fovea. The fovea consists of a "rod-free" central grouping of approximately 100,000 slender cones. The ganglion cells subserving these cones send their axons directly to the temporal aspect of the optic disk, forming the papillomacular bundle. Axons originating from ganglion cells in the temporal retina must curve above and below the papillomacular bundle, forming dense arcuate bands.

The arteries supplying the optic nerve and retina derive from branches of the ophthalmic artery. The central retinal artery approaches the eye along each optic nerve and pierces the inferior aspect of the dural sheath about 1 cm behind the globe to enter the center of the nerve. The artery emerges in the fundus at the center of the nerve head, from which it nourishes the inner two thirds of the retina by superior and inferior branches. Anastomotic branches derived from the choroidal and posterior ciliary arteries, the ciliary system, supply the choroid, optic nerve head, and the outer retinal layers, including the photoreceptors. In about 10% of the population, the macula is supplied by a retinociliary artery, a branch of the ciliary system. Venous drainage from the retina and nerve head flows primarily via the central retinal vein, whose course of exit from the eye parallels that of the entry of the artery.

What each eye "sees" is termed its visual field (Fig. 513–1). The nasal side of the left retina and the temporal side of the right see the left side of the world, and the upper half of each retina sees the lower half of the world. Behind the eyes the optic nerves pass through the optic canal to form the optic chiasm. In the chiasm, nerves from the nasal half of each retina decussate and join the fibers from the temporal half of the contralateral retina. From the chiasm, the optic tracts pass around the cerebral peduncles to reach the lateral geniculate ganglia. The orientation of the visual field is rotated 90 degrees in the lateral geniculate such that images from the inferior visual field project to the medial half, whereas images from the superior visual field project to the lateral half. The geniculo-localcarine radiation initially fans out into superolateral and inferolateral projections, the passing around the lateral ventricle and for a short distance into the temporal lobe (Meyer's loop) before turning posteriorly to reach the striate cortex of the occipital lobe. In the occipital lobe, the striate cortex (Area 17) lies along the superior and inferior bands of the calcarine fissure, with macular fibers projecting most posteriorly to the occipital pole and more peripheral retinal projections lying more anteriorly.

Localization of Lesions within the Visual Pathways

Monocular vision loss is due to a lesion of one eye or optic nerve. Binocular visual loss, on the other hand, can result from

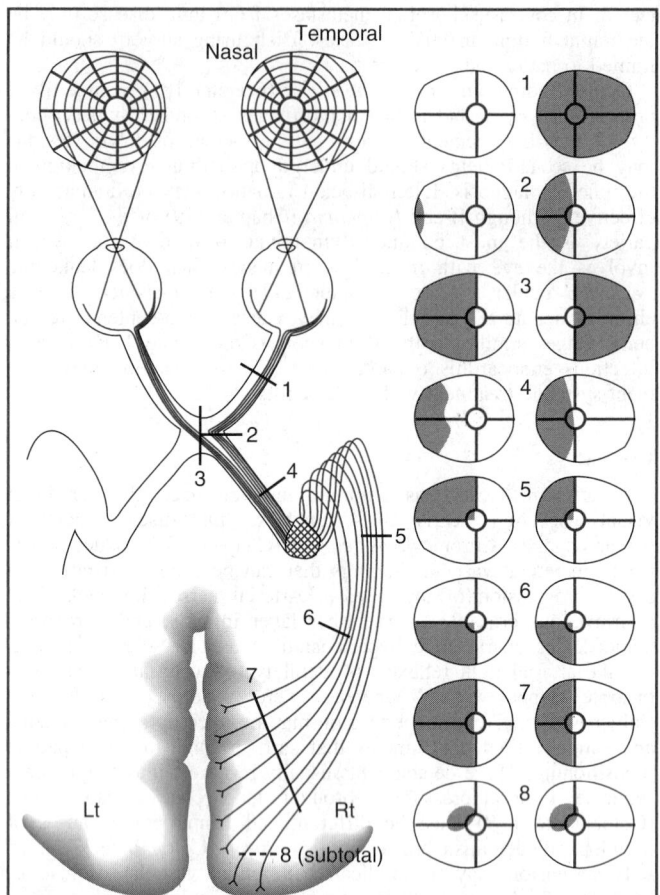

FIGURE 513–1 ■ Visual fields that accompany damage to the visual pathways. 1. Optic nerve: Unilateral amaurosis. 2. Lateral optic chiasm: Grossly incongruous, incomplete (contralateral) homonymous hemianopia. 3. Central optic chiasm: Bitemporal hemianopia. 4. Optic tract: Incongruous, incomplete homonymous hemianopia. 5. Temporal (Meyer's) loop of optic radiation: Congruous partial or complete (contralateral) homonymous superior quadrantanopia. 6. Parietal (superior) projection of the optic radiation: Congruous partial or complete homonymous inferior quadrantanopia. 7. Complete parieto-occipital interruption of optic radiation: Complete congruous homonymous hemianopia with psychophysical shift of foveal point often sparing central vision, giving "macular sparing." 8. Incomplete damage to visual cortex: Congruous homonymous scotomas, usually encroaching at least acutely on central vision.

disease located anywhere in the visual pathways from the corneas to the occipital poles. Lesions involving the optic chiasm produce nonhomonymous visual abnormalities (e.g., the bitemporal hemianopia illustrated by Lesion 3 in Fig. 513–1). Optic tract abnormalities are comparatively rare but produce characteristic visual changes. The fibers serving identical points in the homonymous half fields do not fully commingle in the optic tract, so lesions damaging this structure produce incongruous homonymous hemianopia. Lesions of the geniculate nuclei, optic radiations, or visual cortex produce congruent hemianopic field defects that may go unrecognized unless the hemianopia intrudes on macular vision. Post-geniculate visual loss can be differentiated from pregeniculate visual loss by (1) a normal funduscopic appearance, (2) intact pupillary light reactions, and (3) appropriate lesions on brain imaging.

Examination of the Afferent Visual System

Visual function is most commonly assessed by "best corrected visual acuity." If the visual acuity is not normal, then it must be determined whether acuity can be improved with lenses or at least with the use of a pinhole. The normal reference is a recognition of letters at an idealized 20 feet, and acuity charts are designed with even larger letters that normally are recognized at proportionally greater distances. Thus, if one reads letters at 20 feet no better than those normally perceived at 40 feet, vision is recorded as 20/40.

Small visual charts that are easily carried in the physician's case permit quick and fairly accurate bedside appraisals of acuity.

Visual fields can be tested at the bedside by confrontation, and rough estimates of their integrity can be made even in patients with reduced alertness. The fields should be tested individually for each eye because the pattern of visual field defects can provide important localizing information. A quick screen of the visual fields can be made by having the patient fixate on the examiner's nose and identify the number of fingers flashed in each of the four visual field quadrants. With practice and a cooperative subject, accurate confrontation fields can be obtained that outline even scotomas. Ophthalmoscopic examination permits direct visualization of the retina, and optic disk. Corneal, lenticular, or vitreous opacities severe enough to produce visual symptoms almost always can be detected with the ophthalmoscope.

Common Causes of Visual Loss

Eye

The cause of monocular vision loss due to ocular and retinal lesions often can be detected with ophthalmoscopic examination or with measurement of intraocular pressure. *Glaucoma* caused by impaired absorption of the aqueous humor results in a high intraocular pressure that usually produces gradual loss of peripheral vision, "halos" seen around lights, and, occasionally, pain and redness in the affected eye. Diagnosis comes from the tonometric measurement of a high intraocular pressure and may be suspected by palpating an abnormally firm globe and observing a deep, pale optic cup and attenuated blood vessels. *Retinal tears and detachments* give rise to unilateral distortions of the visual image seen as sudden angulations or curves of objects containing straight lines (metamorphopsia). *Hemorrhages* into the vitreous humor or *infections* or *inflammatory lesions* of the retina can produce scotomas that resemble those resulting from primary disease of the central visual pathway.

Binocular vision loss due to retinal disease in younger subjects is often due to *heredodegenerative conditions.* Vascular diseases, diabetes, and age-related macular degeneration are causes in older patients. In most *pigmentary retinal degenerations,* visual loss begins peripherally and slowly proceeds centrally. By contrast, *macular degenerations* impair central vision early in their course. Most of the retinal degenerations produce characteristic and recognizable ophthalmoscopic appearances.

Optic Nerve

Acute or subacute monocular vision loss due to optic nerve disease is most commonly produced by demyelinating disorders, vascular obstruction, or neoplasm. Demyelinating disease of the nerve head (*optic neuritis* or *papillitis*) produces disc edema along with loss of central vision in the affected eye only; subjectively unrecognized scotomas sometimes may be found in the other eye. Demyelination in the optic nerve behind where the retinal vein emerges (*retrobulbar neuritis*) initially leaves a normal-looking disc but a central or paracentral scotoma. With chronic demyelinating disorders, the optic disc becomes pale and atrophic. More than 50% of patients who initially present with optic neuritis go on to develop typical symptoms and signs of multiple sclerosis. Intraocular arterial occlusion may produce either central visual loss or an altitudinal field defect (*ischemic optic neuropathy*). The common causes of transient monocular vision loss and their differential features are listed in Table 513–1. *Tumors* invading the optic nerve or space-occupying lesions compressing it anywhere between the orbit and the chiasm cause gradually decreasing central vision or a sector defect of the peripheral visual field. With such chronic lesions, the affected optic nerve becomes visibly atrophic.

Acute binocular vision loss due to bilateral optic nerve disease is most often caused by demyelinating disease or by toxic or nutritional factors. In younger persons and those lacking a clear history of toxic exposures, demyelinating lesions overwhelmingly predominate. Symptoms are of abrupt or subacute onset with visual blurring, which may progress rapidly to blindness within hours or days. There may be pain about the eyes, particularly with movement.

Papilledema is disc edema due to increased intracranial pressure. Vision is normal except under one of two circumstances: (1) acute transient episodes of amaurosis lasting a few seconds and attributable to acute increases in intracranial pressure (plateau waves) and (2) progressive loss of peripheral vision with longstanding, severe

Table 513–1 ■ COMMON CAUSES OF TRANSIENT MONOCULAR VISION LOSS

CATEGORY/ (TYPICAL DURATION)	CAUSES	DIFFERENTIAL FEATURES
Thromboembolism (1–5 min)	Atherosclerosis	Other atherosclerotic vascular disease, associated crossed hemiparesis, angiography (carotid atheromata)
	Cardiac	Valvular disease, mural thrombi, atrial fibrillation, recent MI
	Blood dyscrasia	Blood tests + for sickle cell anemia, macroglobulinemia, multiple myeloma, polycythemia, etc.
Vasospasm (5–30 min)	Migraine	Ipsilateral headache, other classic aura, and family history
Vascular compression (few sec)	Increased intracranial pressure	Precipitated by position change, Valsalva maneuver, or pressure waves
	Tumor	Associated slowly progressive monocular visual loss
Vasculitis (1–5 min)	Temporal arteritis	Associated headache, polymyalgia rheumatica, palpable temporal artery, elevated sedimentation rate

papilledema, owing to compression of the optic nerve head. Table 513–2 gives the main differential points between papilledema and optic neuritis. Subacute or chronic binocular vision loss due to optic nerve disease can result from *toxic* and *nutritional* causes or *inherited optic atrophies.* The latter sometimes accompany spinocerebellar degeneration but may selectively affect the optic nerve. With either cause, visual loss is painless and primarily affects central vision; ophthalmoscopy shows optic atrophy.

Chiasm and Optic Tract

Patients with lesions of the optic chiasm or optic tract are often unaware of visual impairment until the deficit encroaches on central vision in one or both eyes. Intrinsic or extrinsic neoplasms and parachiasmal arterial aneurysms are the most common lesions in this location. Gliomas that arise within the chiasm or optic tract are rare in adulthood. Extrinsic lesions compressing the chiasm or tract include *dysgerminomas, craniopharyngiomas, pituitary adenomas, meningiomas* and large *aneurysms* of the carotid or basilar artery. The diagnosis rests on finding the characteristic visual field abnormalities (bitemporal hemianopa for chiasm and incongruous homonymous hemianopa for optic tract lesions) and identifying the lesion with computed tomography (CT) or magnetic resonance imaging (MRI). Pituitary apoplexy due to acute hemorrhage into the gland can result in sudden vision loss; prompt neurosurgical intervention under steroid coverage is required for most patients.

Table 513–2 ■ DIFFERENTIATION OF OPTIC NEURITIS FROM PAPILLEDEMA

	OPTIC NEURITIS	PAPILLEDEMA
Central-cecocentral vision loss	Present	Absent
Distribution	Usually unilateral	Usually bilateral
Ocular pain on movement	Present	Absent
Direct light reflex	±Reduced	Intact
CT and MRI scan of head	White matter plaques	Tumor, venous occlusion, etc.
Visual evoked responses	Abnormal	Normal
Lumbar puncture pressure	Normal	Elevated

Visual Radiations and Occipital Cortex

Lesions involving the postgeniculate visual pathways most often result from *vascular damage, traumatic injuries, neoplasms* or, rarely, *inflammatory* or *degenerative disorders* involving the cerebral white matter. Their localization can be deduced by the resulting visual field defects. Vascular disease of the occipital lobes is the most common cause of homonymous visual field defects in the middle-aged and elderly population. *Anton's syndrome* refers to cerebral visual loss with denial of visual defect. Affected patients not only deny the fact that they are blind but confabulate details of their visual environment from memory. Anton's syndrome results from bilateral lesions involving the parieto-occipital lobes or in the setting of a metabolic encephalopathy. *Tumors* are rarely confined to the limits of the occipital lobes; therefore neurologic deficits with occipital tumors are rarely only visual.

PUPILLARY CONTROL

The neuromechanisms that control pupil size and reactivity are complex, yet they can be evaluated by simple clinical procedures. The diameter of the pupil is determined by the antagonistic actions of the iris sphincter and dilator muscles with the latter playing a minor role. If the sphincter muscle is severed or ruptured, it does not retract toward one quadrant but rather continues to function except in the altered segment. Therefore, the pupillary response can be evaluated even in the presence of significant damage to the iris.

Anatomy and Localization of Lesions within Pupillary Pathways

The size of the pupil is governed by tonic balance between sympathetic and parasympathetic innervation of the muscles of the iris. Sympathetic stimulation dilates the pupil, and parasympathetic stimulation constricts it. In the normal resting state, light entering the eye provides the major stimulus governing the size of the pupil (Fig. 513–2). Light activates the retinal rods and cones with maximal sensitivity in the macular area. The optic nerve fibers follow the crossed and uncrossed visual pathways to the pregeniculate portion of the optic tracts, where the receptor fibers for light diverge to the pretectal nucleus located at the midbrain diencephalic junction. Interneurons project from this nucleus, to the Edinger-Westphal nuclei atop the midbrain third nerve nuclear complex of either side. From that point paired parasympathetic efferents leave the midbrain in third nerves, travel in the interpeduncular space across the petroclinoid ligament and edge of the tentorium, traverse the cavernous sinus, and then enter the orbit through the superior orbital fissure. In the orbit, the parasympathetic efferents synapse in the ciliary ganglion, from which ciliary nerves enter the eye to reach the pupillary muscles.

The principal sympathetic control of the pupil originates in the ventral lateral hypothalamus (first-order neuron), from which fibers descend ipsilaterally through the brain stem tegmentum and thence to the cervical cord, where they synapse with the preganglionic neurons in the intermedial lateral column of the upper three thoracic segments. Preganglionic fibers (second-order neurons) emerge with the ventral roots of C8, T1, and T2, and ascend in the neck to synapse in the superior cervical ganglion adjacent to the base of the skull. Postganglionic (third-order neurons) pupillary fibers accompany the internal carotid artery through the skull, leaving it to follow the ophthalmic branch of the trigeminal nerve to reach the pupillodilator muscle of the eye.

Sympathetic paralysis of the eye with ptosis, anhidrosis, and miosis (Horner's syndrome) can result from lesions anywhere along the course of the pathway described above. The diagnosis can sometimes be made by identifying associated signs in the brain stem or neck or along the carotid artery.

Examination of the Pupil

The pupillary response to light should be examined in a dimly lighted room, where the pupils are naturally dilated. First, the size and symmetry of the pupils are assessed by shining a dim light onto the face from below so that both pupils are seen simultaneously in the indirect illumination. To test light reactivity, gaze is directed at a distant object (so that constriction due to convergence is minimal) and first one and then the other pupil is illuminated with a bright light source. If a pupil reacts poorly to direct light, it

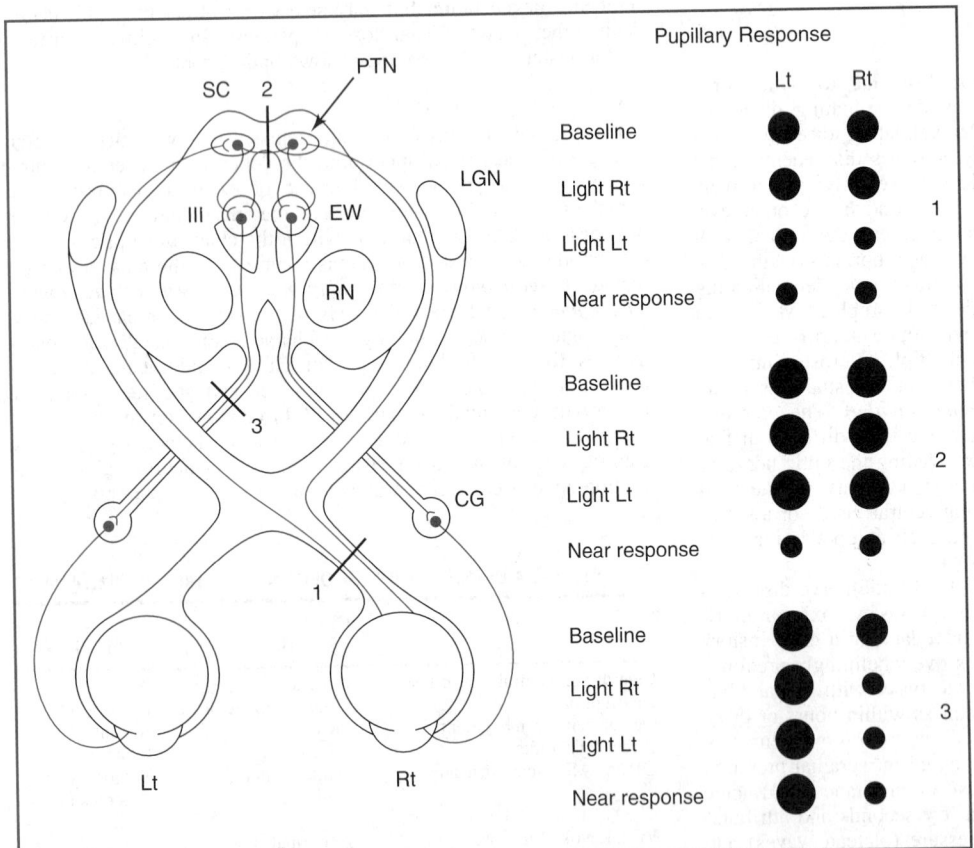

FIGURE 513–2 ■ Pupillary responses associated with lesions of the (1) optic nerve, (2) pretectum, and (3) oculomotor nerve. Baseline is obtained with fixation on a distant target and the near response with a target in front of the nose. SC = Superior colliculus; PTN = pretectal nucleus; EW = Edinger-Westphal nucleus; LGN = lateral geniculate nucleus; RN = red nucleus; CG = ciliary ganglion.

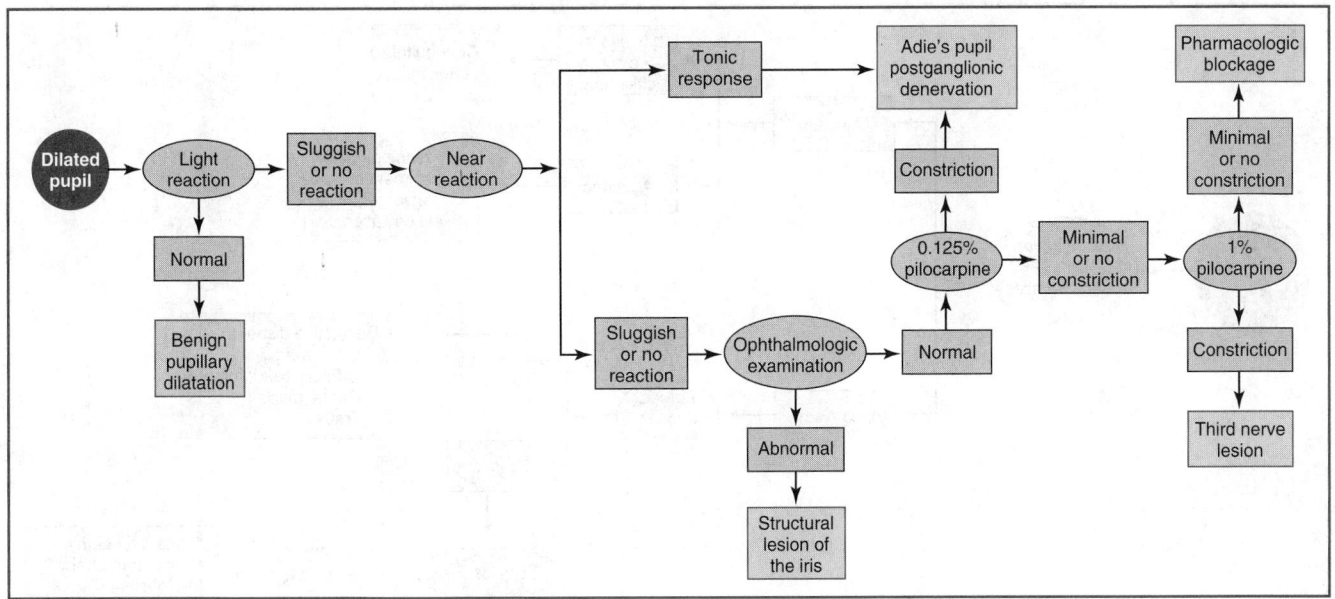

FIGURE 513–3 ■ Use of pilocarpine to help differentiate between different causes of a dilated pupil.

is observed as the opposite eye is illuminated (consensual response). Pupils that react poorly to light should be tested for reactivity to the near reflex by first having the patient gaze at a distant object and then quickly fixate on an object just in front of his nose. Light-near dissociation refers to a pupil that does *not* react to light but does accomodate by constricting to a near target.

Common Causes of Pupillary Abnormalities

With so-called benign pupillary dilatation or *physiologic anisocoria,* there is a longstanding difference in the size of the two pupils with normal reflex reactions; the disparity remains constant during constriction and dilatation. Lesions compressing or damaging the pretectal region interrupt the afferent light reflex bilaterally to produce dilated and light-fixed pupils (e.g., Lesion 2, Fig. 513–2). Pupillary constriction to the near response is preserved until late stages. Tumors of the pineal gland (e.g., dysgerminomas) and *localized infarctions* are the most common lesions in this location. *Adie's tonic pupil* is a medium-to-large (3 to 6 mm) pupil that constricts little or not at all to light and very slowly to accommodation but constricts with the instillation of dilute pilocarpine (0.125%) (Fig. 513–3). The abnormal pupil can be associated with diminished or absent deep tendon reflexes in the extremities. The condition usually affects one eye (occasionally both), is more common in woman 25 to 45 years of age, and carries no serious implications. Its cause is unknown. Unexplained unilateral or bilateral dilated pupil as an isolated finding can result from the *accidental or intentional instillation of mydriatic drugs.* Transdermal scopolamine is a common cause. Failure of the pupil to constrict promptly with pilocarpine (1%) gives the diagnosis if the history is unclear. Interruption of the emerging third nerve in the ventral midbrain or along the proximal part of its course produces a dilated pupil 6 to 7 mm in diameter. Important causes of compression of the third nerve in this region are *aneurysms, neoplasia,* and *brain herniation* due to increased intracranial pressure. In nearly all cases, the pupillary involvement is associated with other signs of third nerve involvement (see below).

The causes of *Horner's syndrome* are numerous because of the long course of sympathetic innervation to the eye. It is unlikely that a patient with a central nervous system lesion will present with an isolated Horner's syndrome. The most common lesions producing Horner's syndrome involve the ascending second-order neuron in the neck or the extracranial postganglionic neuron; *malignant tumors in the apex of the lung* are most common. Dissection of the carotid artery is another serious cause; it should be considered in a patient with Horner's syndrome and ipsilateral neck pain. *Argyll-Robertson pupils* are small (1 to 2 mm), unequal, irregular, and fixed to light; they constrict minimally to accommodation. Their principal cause is tertiary neurosyphilis.

OCULOMOTOR CONTROL

Abnormal eye movements can result from disturbances at several levels. Disconjugate eye movements result from lesions of the individual ocular muscles, the myoneural junctions, the oculomotor nerves and their three paired nuclei in the brain stem, and the internuclear medial longitudinal fasciculus (MLF) that yokes the eyes in horizontal movements. Supranuclear lesions typically produce disorders of conjugate gaze (gaze palsies).

Anatomy and Localization of Lesions within the Oculomotor Pathways

Nuclear and Internuclear Pathways

The abducens (sixth) nerve supplies the lateral rectus muscle. Selective involvement of the abducens nerve anywhere along its pathway leads to isolated weakness of abduction of the affected eye. Destruction of the abducens nucleus in the brain stem leads to a conjugate gaze paralysis (ipsilateral) because, in addition to oculomotor neurons, the nucleus contains interneurons destined for the contralateral medial rectus nucleus. The trochlear (fourth) nerve supplies the contralateral superior oblique muscle, which intorts and depresses the eye. Patients with superior oblique weakness note an increase in diplopia with head tilt toward the side of weakness and often tilt the head in the opposite direction. At rest there is slight upward deviation of the involved eye, and downward movement is impaired when the affected eye is turned in. Patients typically complain of diplopia when reading or when going down stairs. The third (oculomotor) cranial nerve supplies the remaining ocular muscles. Involvement of the third nerve nucleus in the midbrain always produces at least some bilateral oculomotor weakness; the superior rectus division of the nucleus supplies the contralateral superior rectus muscle (all other divisions supply ipsilateral muscles). Peripheral third nerve paralysis can result from lesions damaging the structure anywhere from its course within the ventral midbrain to where it enters the orbit via the superior orbital fissure. When complete, a third nerve palsy produces a widely dilated pupil, severe ptosis, and an externally deviated eye held in position by the unopposed contraction of the lateral rectus muscle. In such conditions, the continued trochlear action reveals itself by intorsion of the eye when the subject attempts to look down.

The MLF interconnects the abducens nucleus in the pons with the contralateral oculomotor nuclear complex in the midbrain. It terminates cephalad in the interstitial nucleus in the rostral midbrain and can be traced as far caudad as the thoracocervical region

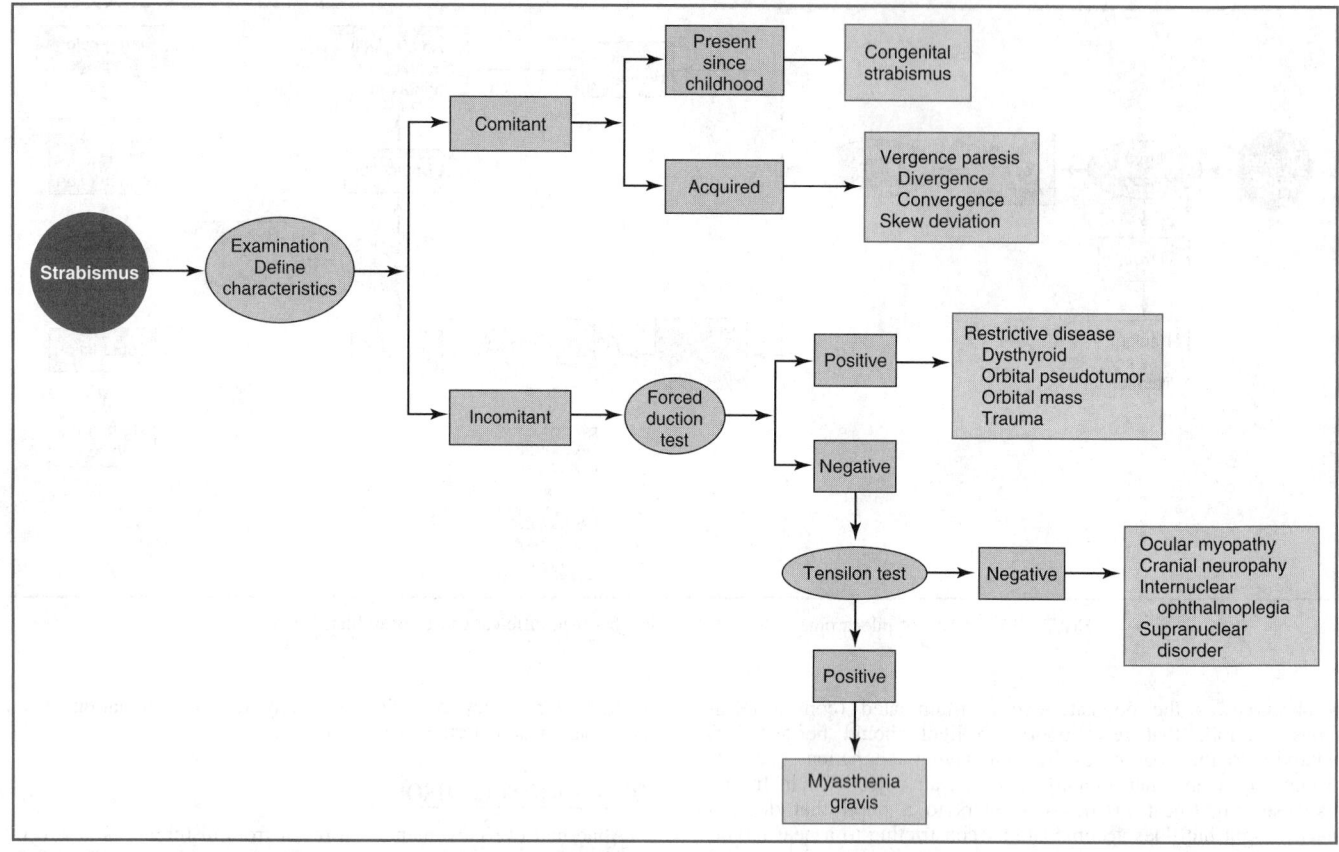

FIGURE 513–4 ■ Diagnostic tests that help differentiate between common causes of strabismus.

of the spinal cord (coordinating nuchal-ocular control). Lesions involving the MLF characteristically produce an internuclear ophthalmoplegia (INO) with which the eyes are conjugate in the primary position but disconjugate on lateral gaze. With a fully developed INO on lateral gaze away from the side of the lesion, the contralateral eye abducts and shows nystagmus, whereas the ipsilateral adducting eye does not move nasally because of failure of ascending impulses to reach the medial rectus division of the third nerve nucleus. Adduction for convergence is usually relatively maintained.

Supranuclear Pathways

The pathway descending from the frontal eye fields in the frontal lobe regulates rapid voluntary eye movements *(saccades)*. A signal from the frontal eye field activates a burst of firing in the contralateral horizontal gaze center in the paramedian pontine reticular formation. This high frequency burst (or pulse) of neuronal firing is transmitted directly to the nearby sixth nerve nucleus and via the MLF to the contralateral third nerve nucleus. For voluntary vertical gaze, both frontal eye fields send signals to the vertical gaze center in the pretectum (the interstitial nucleus of the MLF). Acute lesions involving a frontal or parietal eye field (e.g., hemorrhage or infarction) result in transient inability to direct the eyes contralaterally. Vertical eye movements are not affected by unilateral lesions. Bilateral damage to the frontal eye fields or their descending pathways may produce the inability to move the eyes voluntarily (horizontal or vertical) despite preserved reflex eye movements, a condition called *oculomotor apraxia*. Lesions involving the horizontal gaze center in the pons produce an ipsilateral paralysis of conjugate gaze and tonic deviation of the eyes to the contralateral side. Lesions of the pretectum selectively impair vertical gaze with the vertical upgaze center being slightly rostral and dorsal to the vertical downgaze center.

Pathways descending from the temporo-occipital and frontal regions of the two hemispheres subserve slow visual tracking or *smooth pursuit movements*. The exact location of these descending pursuit pathways is not completely known, but there are strong projections to the ipsilateral pons and cerebellar flocculus. Lesions of the temporo-occipital and frontal region, pons, and cerebellum impair smooth pursuit and optokinetic slow phases when the target moves ipsilateral to the lesion. The *convergence* center is located in the rostral-dorsal midbrain near the vertical gaze center. Lesions in this region typically impair convergence and voluntary vertical gaze. Pathways for cortical control of vergence have not been identified. The other supranuclear oculomotor control system, the *vestibulo-ocular reflex,* and its examination are discussed in Chapter 517.

Examination of Eye Movements

Fixation and gaze holding are tested by having the patient look center, right, left, up, and down. Each position should be held steady and unwavering with the observer carefully documenting abnormal movements or ocular disconjugacies. Each supranuclear oculomotor control system is examined separately. *Saccades* are tested by having the patient fixate alternately on two targets such as the examiner's finger and nose; the speed and accuracy are noted. *Smooth pursuit* is tested by slowly moving a target back and forth and up and down and observing the patient's ability to produce smooth tracking movements. It the target velocity is low, normal subjects should be able to pursue without requiring catch-up saccades. *Convergence* is tested by having the patient follow a target moving from far to near. The degree of convergence depends to some extent on the cooperation of the patient. A clear sign that the patient is attempting to converge is simultaneous pupillary constriction.

Common Causes of Abnormal Oculomotor Control

Strabismus (ocular misalignment)

A comitant (same in all directions of gaze) strabismus present since childhood is usually a benign *congenital disorder*. Latent congenital strabismus can become manifest in adulthood in association with a systemic illness. An acquired skew deviation (vertical displacement of the ocular axes) indicates a lesion within the otolith-ocular pathways (usually brain stem). Incomitant strabismus can result from restrictive disease of the orbit or from abnormal muscle or oculomotor nerve function. The presence of mechanical restriction is confirmed by the use of forced duction testing (Fig. 513–4). (After a topical anesthetic is applied to the eye, the ophthalmologist grasps the muscle insertion with a large blunt-toothed forceps. Failure of the eye to deviate fully in the pulled direction implies restriction.) Common causes of *orbital restrictive disease* include dysthyroid ophthalmopathy, orbital pseudotumor, trauma, and orbital mass lesions. Variable strabismus that increases with fatigue suggests *myasthenia gravis* (see Ch. 511). A Tensilon test can usually confirm the diagnosis (Fig. 513–4). If both restrictive disease and myasthenia gravis have been excluded, most patients with incomitant strabismus have processes affecting the oculomotor nuclei, their fascicles, or the cranial nerves themselves. Common causes of an *isolated third nerve palsy* in an adult include aneurysm, small vessel occlusive disease (including diabetes mellitus), trauma, and neoplasm. Typically, but not always, third nerve lesions due to vascular disease spare the pupil. Vascular disease and trauma are by far the most common causes of *isolated trochlear nerve palsies*. The abducens nerve is particularly vulnerable to isolated traumatic involvement because of its long pathway outside the brain stem. Lesions that produce increased intracranial pressure can lead to abducens nerve dysfunction regardless of the location and produce a "false localizing sign." Other common causes of *isolated sixth nerve palsy* are vascular disease, trauma, and neoplasm. About one fourth of cases with cranial nerve palsies (third, fourth, or sixth nerves) remain undiagnosed.

Internuclear Ophthalmoplegia (INO)

INO may be unilateral or bilateral, partial or complete, depending on the location of the lesion and the degree of damage to the MLF. *Demyelinating* and small *vascular lesions* are the most common cause of unilateral INO unaccompanied by other ocular palsies or brain-stem signs. Larger brain-stem lesions that damage one or more oculomotor nuclei plus the MLF often produce combinations of disconjugate eye movements coupled with nuclear oculomotor palsies. Myasthenia gravis can produce an ophthalmoparesis resembling INO owing to the greater involvement of the medial rectus compared with the lateral rectus. Demyelinating diseases are by far the most common causes of bilateral INO involvement.

Disorders of Conjugate Gaze

As noted earlier, infarction of the frontal cortex results in transient contralateral gaze paresis. Tumors and infarction of the paramedian pontine reticular formation produce ipsilateral horizontal gaze paralysis. With the so-called locked-in syndrome (secondary to basilar artery thrombosis), voluntary horizontal eye movements are absent; the patient's only remaining motor functions are vertical eye and lid movements. Lesions of the pretectum typically affect only vertical eye movements, although the descending pathways from the frontal eye fields to the horizontal gaze centers in the pons can also be affected. With the *dorsal midbrain syndrome* (Parinaud's syndrome), patients present with a conjugate up-gaze paresis. When they attempt to make upward saccades, they develop convergence retraction nystagmus. As noted earlier, impaired convergence and light-near dissociation of the pupillary reflexes are also part of the syndrome. The most common causes of the dorsal midbrain syndrome include tumors of the pineal gland (dysgerminomas), hydrocephalus, and localized infarction.

Nystagmus

Spontaneous nystagmus can be congenital or acquired. *Congenital nystagmus* typically has a high frequency and variable wave form (usually pendular) and is highly fixation-dependent. It typically remains horizontal in all positions of gaze. The lifelong history and lack of symptoms confirm the diagnosis. Spontaneous nystagmus due to a *peripheral vestibular* lesion (i.e., in the labyrinth or vestibular nerve) usually has combined horizontal and torsional components. (Table 513–3). The nystagmus resolves within a few days of the acute lesion. Acquired persistent spontaneous

Table 513–3 ■ KEY DISTINGUISHING FEATURES OF PERIPHERAL AND CENTRAL TYPES OF SPONTANEOUS AND POSITIONAL NYSTAGMUS

TYPE OF NYSTAGMUS	PERIPHERAL (END ORGAN AND NERVE)	CENTRAL (BRAIN STEM AND CEREBELLUM)
Spontaneous	Unidirectional, fast phase away from lesion, combined horizontal torsional, inhibited with fixation	Bidirectional or undirectional; often pure horizontal, vertical, or torsional; *not* inhibited with fixation
Static positional	Direction-fixed or direction-changing, inhibited with fixation	Direction fixed or direction-changing, *not* inhibited with fixation
Paroxysmal positional	Vertical-torsional, occasionally horizontal-torsional, vertigo prominent, fatigability, latency	Often pure vertical, vertigo less prominent, no latency, nonfatigable

nystagmus indicates a lesion in the brain stem and/or cerebellum. The latter is often purely vertical, horizontal or torsional. Spontaneous *downbeat nystagmus* is commonly seen with lesions of the cerebellum or cervicomedullary junction (e.g., Arnold-Chiari malformation).

Gaze-evoked nystagmus is always in the direction of gaze and is usually present with and without fixation. It is most commonly produced by ingestion of *drugs* such as phenobarbital, phenytoin, alcohol, and diazepam. It can also occur in patients with such varied conditions as myasthenia gravis, multiple sclerosis, and cerebellar atrophy. Asymmetric horizontal gaze-evoked nystagmus indicates a structural brain-stem or cerebellar lesion (particularly at the cerebellopontine angle), with the lesion usually being on the side of the larger amplitude nystagmus. *Rebound nystagmus* is a type of gaze-evoked nystagmus that either disappears or reverses direction as the eccentric gaze position is held. When the eyes are returned to the primary position, nystagmus occurs in the direction of the return saccade. Rebound nystagmus occurs in patients with cerebellar atrophy and focal structural lesions of the cerebellum; it is the only variety of nystagmus thought to be specific for cerebellar involvement. *Disconjugate gaze-evoked nystagmus* most commonly results from lesions of the MLF (see above), but it can also occur with other lesions of the brain stem involving the oculomotor nuclei. Positional nystagmus is discussed in Chapter 517.

Other Ocular Oscillations

Ocular bobbing consists of a fast conjugate downward eye movement followed by a slow return to the primary position. The phenomenon accompanies severe displacement or destruction of the pons or, less often, metabolic CNS depression. *Ocular myoclonus* consists of continuous rhythmic pendular oscillations, most often vertical, with a rate of 1 to 3 beats per second; often it accompanies palatal myoclonus and has a similar pathogenesis. *Square wave jerks* and *ocular flutter* consist of brief, intermittent, horizontal oscillations (back to back saccades) arising from the primary gaze position. These types of ocular oscillation are most commonly seen with cerebellar disease but can also accompany more diffuse central nervous system disorders. *Opsoclonus* consists of rapid, chaotic, conjugate, repetitive, saccadic eye movements (dancing eyes). Opsoclonus accompanies cerebellar dysfunction, with the most chaotic varieties associated with brain-stem encephalitis or the remote effects of systemic neoplasm, especially neuroblastoma in children. *Ocular dysmetria* refers to over- and undershooting of saccadic eye movements often followed by multiple attempts at refixation. It reflects cerebellar dysfunction.

Burde RM, Savino PJ, Trobe JD: Clinical Decisions in Neuro-ophthalmology, 2nd ed. St. Louis, CV Mosby, 1992. *Liberal use of flow charts to help the clinician answer the question, "Given the symptom and signs, what is the disease?"*

Glaser JS: Neuro-ophthalmology, 2nd ed. Hagerstown, MD, Harper & Row, 1990. *An excellent one-volume didactic introductory text.*

Leigh RJ, Zee DS: The Neurology of Eye Movement, 3rd ed. New York, Oxford University Press, 1999. *A monograph that gives the clinical and physiologic details of modern investigations on ocular motor control.*

514 DISEASES OF THE MOUTH AND SALIVARY GLANDS

Troy E. Daniels

More than 200 primary lesions or diseases occur in the oral mucosa, gingiva, teeth, jaws, and minor or major salivary glands. In addition, secondary abnormalities of the oral mucosa or salivary glands can be caused by systemic diseases or drugs. This chapter briefly discusses the most common or important of the mucosal and salivary gland diseases because they may be observed during physical examination and are often part of a systemic process. It will provide a basis for developing a differential diagnosis and guiding treatment and referral. More complete coverage of these and other topics will be found in the references cited at the end of the chapter.

ORAL MUCOSAL DISEASES

Acute Ulcerations

Painful short-term ulcerations are usually caused by mechanical trauma, immunologic mechanisms, and bacterial or viral infections (Table 514–1). Soon after formation, ulcers in the mouth become covered by a white to gray pseudomembrane, analogous to the scab that forms on dry epidermis. Pseudomembrane-covered ulcers are distinguished from the white hyperkeratotic lesions described below by their clinical features of pain, a flat surface, and an erythematous periphery. Traumatic ulcers characteristically are located on the tongue or inside the cheeks or lips, are close to the chewing surfaces of the teeth, and have irregular borders.

Aphthous Ulcers

These idiopathic recurrent ulcers, which afflict about 20% of the population, are found on all areas of the oral mucosa except the hard palate, gingiva, and vermilion. They are well-defined circles and may be single or multiple. There are three clinical forms: (1) minor, which are flat and < 1 cm in diameter, and last only 5 to 10 days; (2) major, which have raised borders, are > 1 cm, and often last for weeks or months; and (3) herpetiform, which are usually clusters of very small ulcers that resemble recurrent herpetic lesions but are not preceded by vesicles and do not occur on keratinized mucosa. A viral pathogenesis has not been established for any of these forms. Lesions clinically identical to minor aphthous ulcers occur in Behçet's syndrome (see Chapter 298). Aphthous ulcers are occasionally associated with macrocytic anemias or gluten-sensitive enteropathy and may become more frequent and severe in association with human immunodeficiency virus (HIV) infection (Table 514–2).

Minor or herpetiform aphthous ulcers may not require treatment. Topical steroids, such as fluocinonide ointment in Orabase, can reduce the severity and duration of the lesions only if used with prodromal symptoms or early signs. Major aphthae usually require treatment by topical or systemic corticosteroids and occasionally are biopsied to exclude neoplasia.

Viral Ulcers

Several types of virus (most commonly herpes virus type 1, the cause of herpes simplex) may cause oral mucosal vesicles that last only a few hours or days and then become shallow ulcers. In the initial infection by herpes simplex virus, usually in children, numerous vesicles may appear on any oral mucosal site (primary herpetic gingivostomatitis), accompanied by malaise, headache, fever, and cervical lymphadenopathy. Patients previously exposed to this virus may develop recurrent lesions, most commonly as clusters of small vesicles on the lips (herpes labialis); only a few will develop intraoral recurrent herpes, as clusters of vesicles on the keratinized mucosa of the gingiva or hard palate. Such lesions tend to recur at the same site, but less frequently with age.

Similar mucosal vesicles may also accompany the initial infection by the varicella-zoster virus in children with chicken pox (see

Chapter 383), and unilateral lesions may occur if herpes zoster (see Chapter 522) affects branches of the trigeminal nerve. Uncommonly, oral mucosal lesions may be caused by different types of coxsackievirus (see Chapter 389), appearing on any oral site in hand-foot-and-mouth disease or on the soft palate or pharynx in herpangina. After infection by the measles (rubeola) virus, small ulcers (Koplik's spots) form on the inside of the cheeks 1 to 2 days before development of the skin rash (see Chapter 381)

Erythema Multiforme

In this potentially recurrent mucocutaneous disease, painful oral mucosal ulcerations develop rapidly in as many as half of the patients. The lesions may be confined to the mouth, with no skin involvement. The affected patients, usually young adults with minimal or no systemic symptoms, have irregularly shaped ulcers that can be small and few or involve large areas of the mucosa; the most common site is the lower labial mucosa. These lesions can be distinguished from those of primary herpes by the absence of oral vesicles and systemic symptoms or by the presence of characteristic skin lesions (see Chapter 522). A major variant of this disease is Stevens-Johnson syndrome in which ocular, genital, and other lesions may accompany the oral lesions.

Table 514–1 ■ ORAL MUCOSAL ULCERS

TYPE/DISEASE	CLINICAL FEATURES
Insidious Onset, Chronic	
Multiple or bilateral	Shallow ulcers on mucosa, skin, or both
Pemphigus vulgaris	Begin as short-duration blisters
Mucous membrane pemphigoid	Begin as short-duration blisters
Lichen planus	Bilaterally symmetric lesions (associated with hyperkeratoses and/or erythema)
Lupus erythematosus	Asymmetric lesions, with or without systemic lupus (associated with hyperkeratoses and/or erythema)
Drug reaction	Variable lesions; appropriate history of drug use
Epidermolysis bullosa	Begin as blisters; life-long history
Solitary	Indurated or cratered ulcers
Squamous cell carcinoma	Most common on tongue, oropharynx, lip, mouth floor
Adenocarcinomas, various	Most commonly on palate, cheeks, mouth floor
Tuberculosis	Usually painful
Actinomycosis	Often associated with draining sinus
Deep mycoses (particularly histoplasmosis, coccidioidomycosis)	Associated with systemic infection
Midline granuloma	Associated with necrosis, may perforate palate
Acute Onset, Often Self-Limiting	
Clusters	Usually small and shallow ulcers; history of blisters
Primary herpes simplex	Any oral mucosal site, associated with fever, malaise
Recurrent herpes simplex	Only on gingiva, hard palate, or lip (keratinized mucosa)
Varicella-zoster	Unilateral lesions along neural distribution
Herpangina	Usually on oropharynx
Measles (rubeola)	Precede skin rash; associated with fever, malaise
Solitary or multiple (without clustering)	Variable, usually without history of blisters
Traumatic ulcers	Usually solitary; history of trauma
Recurrent aphthae	Circular, often multiple, only on nonkeratinized mucosa
Behçet's syndrome	Oral lesions similar to recurrent aphthae
Erythema multiforme	Multiple lesions, often involve lower labial mucosa; can be recurrent or chronic
Drug reaction	Appropriate history of drug use
Necrotizing sialometaplasia	Usually on palate
Primary syphilis	Solitary, indurated, painless, any site
Gonorrhea	Painful, surrounded by erythema, any site

Table 514-2 ■ ORAL LESIONS ASSOCIATED WITH HIV INFECTION

Kaposi's sarcoma
Candidiasis
    Pseudomembranous
    Hyperplastic
    Erythematous
Other opportunistic fungal infections (e.g., histoplasmosis or coccidioidomycosis)
Epithelial lesions
    Aphthous ulcers (increased frequency, duration, or size)
    Virus-associated epithelial hyperplasias
        Hairy leukoplakia
        Oral wart
        Focal epithelial hyperplasia (Heck's disease)
        Condyloma acuminatum
    Herpes zoster
Exaggerated forms of gingivitis and inflammatory periodontal disease
Decreased salivary gland function
Parotid gland enlargement (benign lymphoepithelial lesion)
Non-Hodgkin's lymphoma

Venereal Infections

Primary syphilis may present as a solitary, indurated, painless ulcer on the oral mucosa that resolves spontaneously in 4 to 6 weeks (see Chapter 362). Uncommonly, *Neisseria gonorrhoeae* may cause oral ulcers, usually in the pharynx, that may be confused with oral ulcers of other causes.

Oral Squamous Cell Carcinoma

About 4% of all cancers occur in the mouth, commonly as squamous cell carcinomas of the mucosal epithelium. Oral carcinoma occurs usually in the fifth decade or beyond, in men twice as frequently as in women, and associated with long-term use of tobacco in > 80% of case (Table 514-1).

Oral carcinoma usually presents as a chronic, indurated, cratered ulcer, but early lesions of squamous cell carcinoma may appear as white or red macules (Table 514-3). About 15% of oral carcinomas arise within a pre-existing white plaque (leukoplakia). The overall 5-year survival is approximately 50%, but early treatment of small, localized lesions can lead to survival rates as high as 90%.

Other Chronic Ulcerations

Several mucocutaneous diseases can cause chronic multifocal oral mucosal lesions composed of ill-defined areas of erythema and ulceration. They are among the most difficult oral lesions to diagnose and are discussed below with the red lesions (Table 514-3) Several microbial infections can lead to indurated, chronic oral mucosal ulcerations with moderate symptoms.

Table 514-3 ■ WHITE AND RED ORAL MUCOSAL LESIONS

White Lesions (Plaques)
Squamous cell carcinoma (early)
Frictional keratosis
Leukoplakia (idiopathic)
Smokeless tobacco–associated lesions
Nicotine stomatitis (palate)
Lichen planus (reticular and plaque types)
Pseudomembranous candidiasis (thrush)
Hyperplastic candidiasis (candidal leukoplakia)
Hairy leukoplakia (HIV-associated; usually on lateral tongue)
Geographic tongue
Mucous patch or condyloma latum of secondary syphilis
Pseudomembrane-covered ulcers (see Table 514-1)
Red Lesions (Macular, Maculopapular)
Squamous cell carcinoma (early)
Erythroplakia (epithelial dysplasia)
Erythematous (atrophic) candidiasis
Median rhomboid glossitis
Mucocutaneous diseases (see Table 514-1)
Angular cheilitis
Telangiectasias and purpuras
Kaposi's sarcoma (blue to purple color)

White Lesions

White plaques are commonly found in the mouth but, like ulcerations, have a wide variety of causes and outcomes (Table 514-3). The term "leukoplakia" applies to a white plaque that does not rub off and whose appearance does not indicate another disease. Leukoplakia can occur in any area of the mouth and usually exhibits benign hyperkeratosis on biopsy. On long-term follow-up, 2 to 6% of these lesions will undergo malignant transformation into squamous cell carcinoma. Areas of leukoplakia with a corrugated surface or mixed with areas of erythema are often found in the lower labial or buccal vestibule of those who use smokeless tobacco.

Frictional keratoses are often found posterior to the lower molar teeth as irregular white plaques and on the buccal mucosa as white lines adjacent to the dental occlusion. Unlike leukoplakia, these lesions rarely become malignant.

Lichen Planus

Oral lesions of lichen planus occur in about 1% of the population, usually as multiple, bilaterally symmetric reticular white plaques, with or without adjacent areas of erythema (atrophy or erosion) or ulcers. The presence of mucosal atrophy, erosion, or ulceration usually causes pain or sensitivity to certain foods. Most lesions can be adequately controlled by frequent topical application of fluocinonide or clobetasol ointment mixed with an equal weight of Orabase for periods of several weeks to several months, although recurrence is common.

Oral Candidiasis

This fungal disease has three clinical forms: pseudomembranous (thrush), erythematous (atrophic), and hyperplastic (candidal leukoplakia). Pseudomembranous candidiasis, usually of relatively short duration, occurs on any site and consists of white fungal plaques that can be rubbed off, leaving a red or bleeding base. Lesions of hyperplastic candidiasis are white, have fungal hyphae within the surface layers of hyperkeratotic epithelium, do not rub off, and are most often found on the anterior buccal mucosa or on the tongue. Erythematous candidiasis is discussed below with the red lesions. All forms of oral candidiasis represent overgrowth or superficial infection by *Candida* species from the oral flora, induced by a variety of causes including suppression of bacterial flora by systemic antibiotics, chronic salivary dysfunction, uncontrolled diabetes mellitus or anemia, and immunosuppression (especially in HIV-infected patients).

Hairy Leukoplakia

This lesion is a white plaque occurring most frequently on the lateral surfaces of the tongue bilaterally in immunosuppressed persons, usually HIV-infected. *Candida* may be present in the surface layers, but the lesion is not eliminated by effective antifungal therapy, and it contains large quantities of Epstein-Barr virus. Its diagnosis should be followed by an HIV antibody test.

Geographic Tongue

Also called "benign migratory glositis," this benign idiopathic condition affects the dorsal tongue of about 2% of the population. It is characterized by well-defined areas of atrophied filiform papillae bordered by arcs of normal or hyperplastic filiform papillae and by changes in the location of these lesions over time. Treatment is usually not necessary.

Secondary Syphilis

Secondary syphilis may manifest as a well-defined white plaque on the labial or palatal mucosa, called "condyloma latum" (or "split papule," because of their lobulated periphery).

Red Lesions

Solitary red macules or plaques ("erythroplakia") are less common in the mouth than white lesions but should be viewed with concern because they may exhibit microscopic dysplasia or represent carcinoma in situ (see Table 514-3). They may be associated with areas of leukoplakia. However, a red macule occurring in the midline of the posterior dorsal tongue, classified as median rhomboid glossitis, is an idiopathic but uniformly benign condition that is often associated with localized overgrowth of *Candida* species.

Erythematous (Atrophic) Oral Candidiasis

This chronic condition is characterized by erythema and atrophy of the filiform papillae on the dorsal tongue or by patchy or ill-defined erythema on the palate, tongue, or buccal mucosa. It is accompanied by symptoms of oral mucosal burning and sensitivity to certain foods and is often associated with salivary hypofunction. Patients who wear removable dentures often have mucosal erythema confined to the denture-bearing area.

Topical nystatin or clotrimazole or systemic ketoconazole can resolve these lesions and are administered for several weeks or months. In patients who have salivary hypofunction and remaining natural teeth, topical antifungal preparations containing sucrose or glucose must be avoided to prevent dental caries; slow oral dissolution of vaginal nystatin tablets is safe and effective. Systemic antifungal drugs may not be effective in patients with salivary hypofunction. Effective treatment significantly improves oral symptoms, regardless of the cause of the candidiasis. Treatment of denture-associated candidiasis requires concurrent treatment of the denture.

The treatment end point is reached when mucosal burning symptoms cease, the patient can again tolerate acidic or spicy foods, and papillae on the dorsal tongue have returned to normal; this recovery takes from 2 to 12 weeks. Recurrence is common in patients with chronic salivary hypofunction or immunosuppression, which necessitates recurring or long-term treatment using a topical antifungal drug that does not contain sucrose or glucose and provides sufficient duration of mucosal contact, e.g., vaginal tablets.

Angular Cheilitis

Erythema or crusting of the labial angles is usually caused by *Candida*. It is usually associated with intraoral candidiasis and in such cases topical treatment of the angular cheilitis with nystatin or clotrimazole should be accompanied by intraoral or systemic antifungal treatment as described above.

Mucocutaneous Diseases

The mucocutaneous diseases of pemphigus vulgaris, mucous membrane pemphigoid, atrophic or erosive lichen planus, and lupus erythematosus can cause similar-appearing oral lesions. Their diagnosis requires examination of a biopsy specimen by routine histopathology and usually also by direct immunofluorescence to identify characteristic deposits of immunoglobulins and complement components.

The first lesions of pemphigus vulgaris usually are oral mucosal vesicles that rapidly rupture, leaving painful erosions or ulcerations. These are followed by development of skin lesions. Rarely, the lesions remain confined to the mouth.

Lesions of mucous membrane (cicatricial) pemphigoid are usually confined to the oral mucosa or conjunctivae and occur in patients over age 50. They begin as vesicles that quickly rupture, leaving ulcers that are chronic but only moderately symptomatic. Use of topical fluocinonide or clobetasol for several months, as described above for lichen planus, will sometimes be sufficient to treat the oral lesions, but some patients also need systemic treatment (see Chapter 522).

Oral mucosal lesions of lupus may occur in patients who have systemic lupus erythematosus (SLE), in patients who do not have SLE but later develop that disease, or in patients who do not develop SLE. In this latter group, the lesions of mucosal lupus may be analogous to the skin lesions of chronic discoid lupus. Lesions of oral lupus are usually solitary or bilaterally asymmetric. They take the form of reticular hyperkeratotic figures associated with erythema, often resembling atrophic lichen planus. The lesions can be controlled by topical fluocinonide or intralesional triamcinolone.

Lesions of Kaposi's sarcoma associated with HIV infection often appear first on the oral mucosa, especially the palate. They begin as macules with a blue or purple color, at which time they need to be distinguished from purpura. Later, they spread radially and expand vertically.

Pigmentations

Brown or gray-black macules on the oral mucosa are relatively common and may be caused by localized increase in melanin production, proliferation of melanin-producing cells, or deposition of

Table 514–4 ■ PIGMENTATIONS OF THE ORAL MUCOSA (BROWN OR GRAY-BLACK IN COLOR)

Increased Melanin Production (Flat Lesions)
Oral melanotic macule
Ephelis (vermilion border)
Systemic diseases: Addison's disease, von Recklinghausen's disease of skin, Albright's syndrome, Peutz-Jeghers syndrome
Proliferation of Melanin-Producing Cells (Flat or Raised Lesions)
Pigmented cellular nevi (benign and premalignant types)
Atypical melanocytic hyperplasia, melanoma in situ, radial growth phase of melanoma
Malignant melanoma
Nonmelanin Pigmentation
Amalgam tattoo
Focal deposition of systemically distributed metal (lead, bismuth, mercury, others) usually at sites of chronic inflammation
Systemically administered drugs (chloroquine, minocycline, ketoconazole, cyclophosphamide)

local or systemically distributed pigmented substances (Table 514–4). Mucosal pigmentation may occur after long-term administration of chloroquine, minocycline, ketoconazole, or cyclophosphamide. Malignant melanoma can occur at any oral mucosal site but develops most frequently on the mucosa or gingiva covering the maxilla. Diagnosis of any of these conditions is usually established by biopsy and knowledge of relevant underlying conditions.

ORAL SOFT TISSUE TUMORS

In addition to the malignant neoplasms just described, a variety of oral benign soft tissue tumors are usually treated by excisional biopsy.

Connective Tissue Hyperplasias

The most common oral soft tissue tumors are small, pedunculated masses of hyperplastic fibrous connective tissue covered by normal-appearing mucosa (Table 514–5). Solitary lesions are usually found on the inside of the cheeks or lips. Similar lesions may be present at the border of an ill-fitting denture or may occur in clusters on the hard palate under an ill-fitting denture ("palatal papillomatosis"); the latter is often associated with erythematous candidiasis.

Generalized enlargement of the gingiva (gingival hyperplasia) may be caused by chronic administration of phenytoin, cyclosporine, and many of the calcium channel blocking drugs (e.g., dilti-

Table 514–5 ■ ORAL SOFT TISSUE TUMORS

Connective Tissue Hyperplasia (Normal-Appearing Overlying Mucosa)
Irritation fibroma
Denture-associated hyperplasia
Palatal papillomatosis
Generalized gingival hyperplasia
    Drug-induced (phenytoin, nifedipine, cyclosporine)
    Hereditary
Reactive Hyperplasia (Erythematous Overlying Mucosa)
Pyogenic granuloma/pregnancy tumor
Peripheral giant cell granuloma
Inflammatory gingival hyperplasia
Hyperplastic lingual tonsil
Epithelial Masses (Usually Irregular White Surface)
Papilloma/oral wart
Squamous cell carcinoma
Verrucous carcinoma
Focal epithelial hyperplasia (Heck's disease)
Condyloma acuminatum (venereal wart)
Keratoacanthoma (on lips)
Salivary Duct Obstruction (Minor Salivary Glands)
Mucocele/ranula (usually fluctuant)
Salivary stone (sialolith)
Subepithelial Neoplasms
Primary connective tissue or salivary gland tumors
Metastatic lesions, (especially in the mandible)
Lymphoma (especially in the palate or posterior mandible)
Focal or generalized leukemic infiltrates in the gingiva (especially with acute monocytic leukemia)

PLATE 17   EYE DISEASES

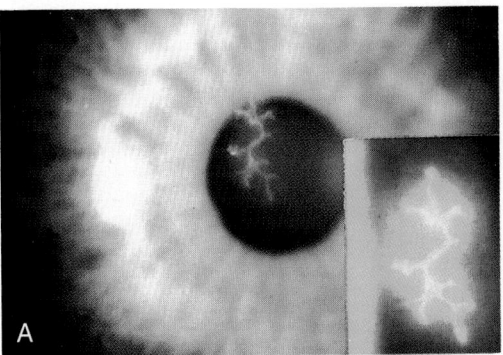

A, Herpes simplex corneal epithelial keratitis in diffuse light and (inset) in light passed through a cobalt blue filter after fluorescein staining.

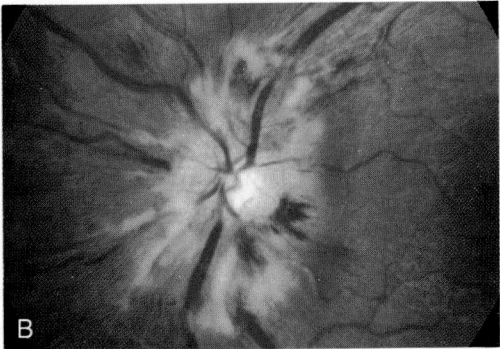

B, Papilledema in a young person. Note disk swelling, hemorrhages, and exudates, with preservation of the physiologic cup.

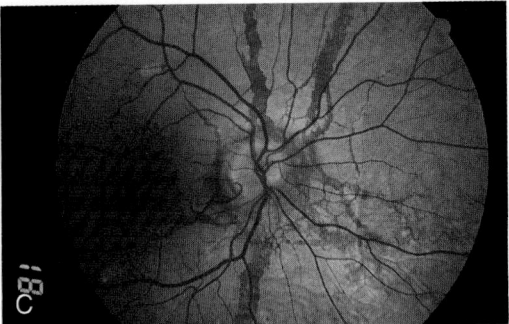

C, Angioid streaks in pseudoxanthoma elasticum. Breaks in the retinal pigment epithelium basement (Bruch's) membrane radial and circumferential to the disk indicate an underlying defect in elastic tissue formation.

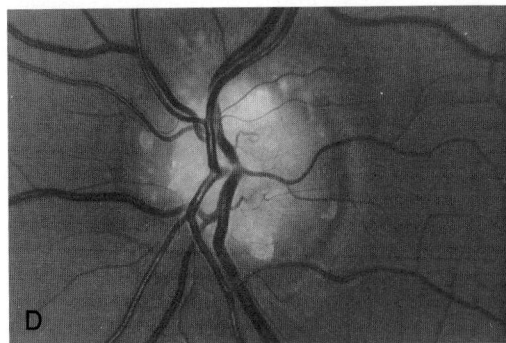

D, Optic disk drusen (also called hyaline bodies). Although obvious here, these calcified excrescences may be difficult to see in young persons, in whom the disk elevations they produce is mistaken for papilledema.

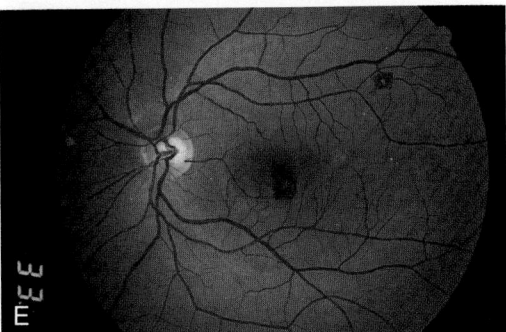

E, Roth's spots. Multiple white centered hemorrhages in a man with recurrent subacute bacterial endocarditis. White centered hemorrhages are also seen with leukemia and diabetes. The small white scars are probably the residua of previous episodes.

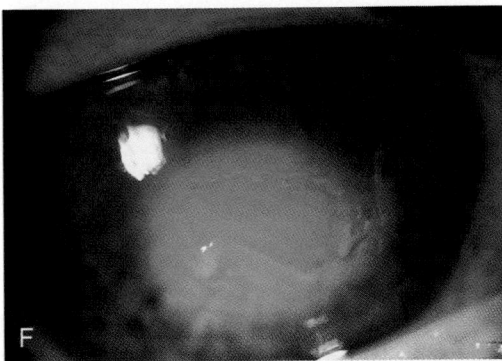

F, Corneal abrasion. Corneal epithelial defects are best observed with topical fluorescein stain under blue illumination. Pain is often out of proportion to clinical findings. Prophylactic topical antibiotics are required until the epithelium has healed. (Courtesy of Deborah P. Langston, M.D.)

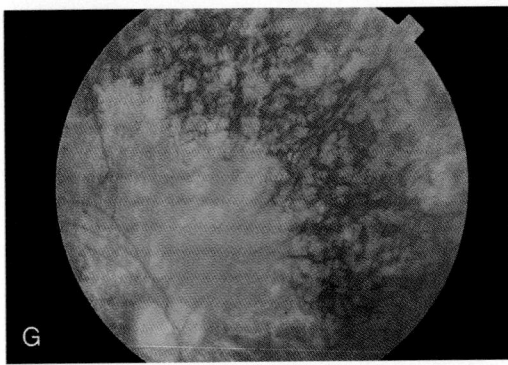

G, Retinitis pigmentosa. Fundus photograph shows "bone spicule" pigmentation of the midperipheral fundus, waxy pallor of the optic disk, and attenuated retinal vessels, the most consistent finding in RP. (Courtesy of John I. Loewenstein, M.D.)

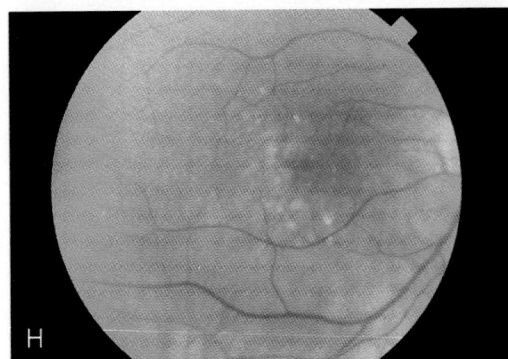

H, Age-related macular degeneration (ARMD). Fundus photograph of nonexudative ARMD shows discrete macular drusen, which are subretinal deposits of lipofuscin.

(A through E, Photographs taken by Harry Kachadoorian, C.R.A., University of Massachusetts Medical School, Worcester, MA.)

PLATE 18 EYE DISEASES

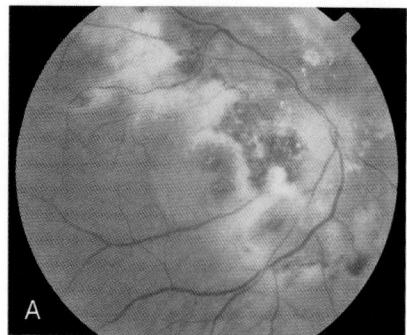

A, CMV retinitis. Fundus photograph shows retinal hemorrhage and exudate, the "cheese-pizza" fundus. CMV retinitis may be sectoral or diffuse. Early peripheral lesions may be asymptomatic. Patients at risk, therefore, require frequent examination. (Courtesy of John I. Loewenstein, M.D.)

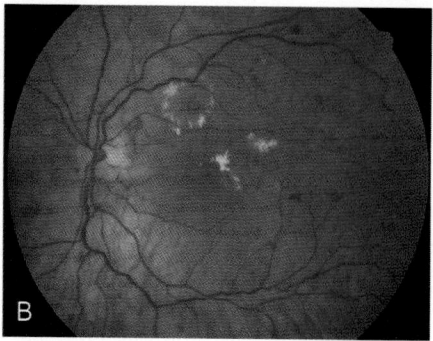

B, Diabetic retinopathy. Fundus photograph of background (nonproliferative) diabetic retinopathy demonstrates scattered dot and blot intraretinal hemorrhages and retinal exudates. A circinate exudate is seen surrounding a microaneurysm.

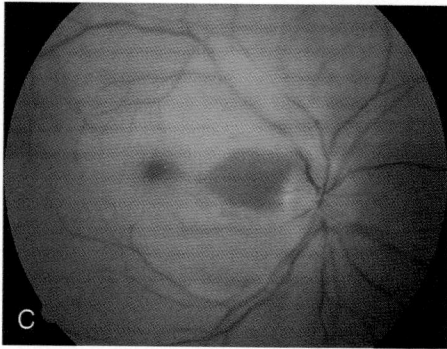

C, Central retinal artery occlusion. Fundus photograph shows diffuse retinal edema. The heavily pigmented fovea with its uniquely thin inner retina produces a "cherry red spot" against the dusky macula. A small area of retina adjacent to the optic disk is spared, owing to the presence of a cilioretinal artery.

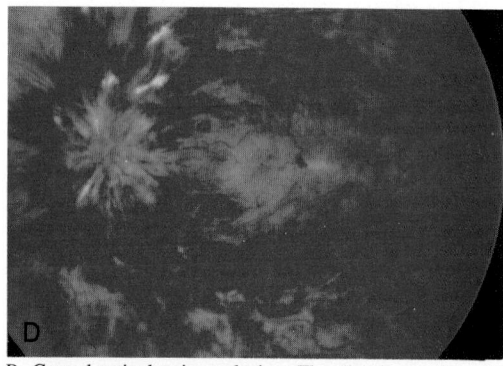

D, Central retinal vein occlusion. The disk is swollen with diffuse retinal hemorrhages and cotton-wool spots.

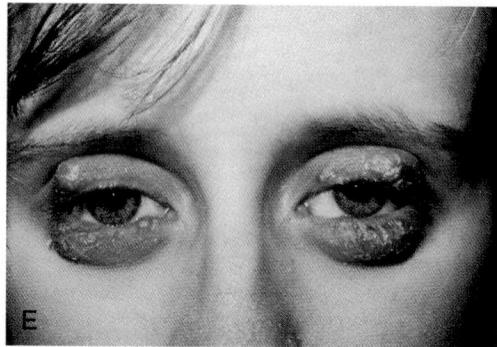

E, Chalazion. Inspissated secretions from an obstructed meibomian gland are extruded into surrounding tissue, causing chronic granulomatous inflammation. Pictured are multiple lipogranulomas involving all four eyelids. (Courtesy of Peter A.D. Rubin, M.D.)

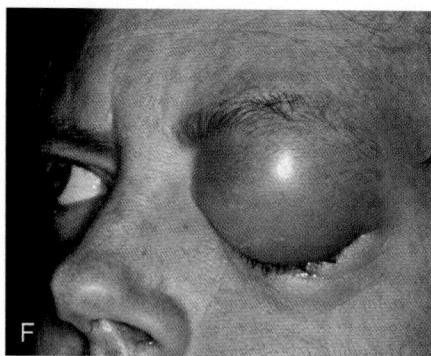

F, Eyelid abscess. Preseptal cellulitis, commonly resulting from minor penetrating trauma, may evolve into an abscess. Treatment requires incision and drainage followed by systemic antibiotics. (Courtesy of Peter A.D. Rubin, M.D.)

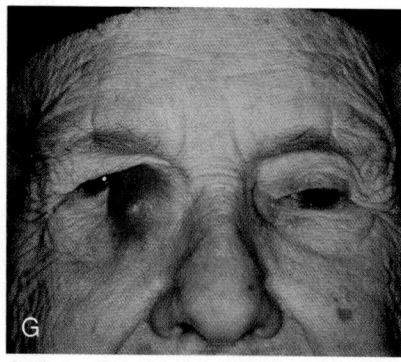

G, Acute dacryocystitis. External photograph shows erythema and edema in the region of the lacrimal sac. Pressure applied to the lesion produces purulent reflux through the canaliculi. Conservative treatment requires oral antibiotics and warm compresses. Pointing lesions such as the one pictured require incision and drainage. (Courtesy of Peter A.D. Rubin, M.D.)

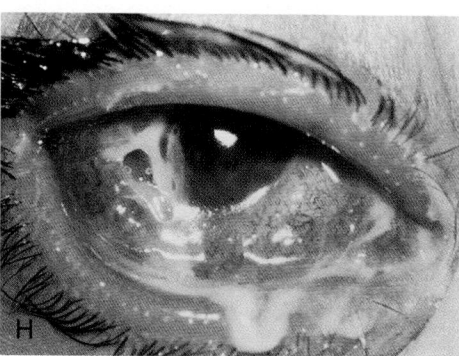

H, Bacterial conjunctivitis. Purulent discharge and conjunctival hyperemia suggest bacterial conjunctivitis. Viral conjunctivitis produces watery discharge, foreign body sensation, preauricular lymphadenopathy, and conjunctival follicles seen on slit lamp examination. (Reproduced with permission from the American Academy of Ophthalmology.)

azem, verapamil, or nifedipine). It can also be associated with a hereditary defect or be caused by an infiltration of white blood cells in some types of leukemia, especially acute monocytic leukemia. The drug-associated cases apparently represent an exaggerated response in susceptible patients to commonly occurring local irritants.

Reactive Hyperplasias

Small masses with surfaces that are ulcerated or only partially covered by normal-appearing mucosa usually represent reactive lesions in the form of pyogenic granulomas (whose frequency increases during pregnancy), peripheral giant cell granulomas, or lymphoid hyperplasia of the lingual or other tonsillar tissue. The granulomas are most often located on the gingiva. Rarely, such lesions may represent a metastatic neoplasm.

Epithelial Tumors

Small, white, wartlike epithelial masses are common and can occur in any area of the oral mucosa. They are occasionally classified as epithelial neoplasms, but most do not continue to grow. Human papillomavirus types 2, 6, 11, and 13 have been identified in some but not all of these wartlike lesions, which are usually classified generically as papillomas. A large wartlike lesion on the oral mucosa should raise the suspicion of verrucous carcinoma.

Mucus Retention Lesions (Mucoceles)

Mucoceles are small, chronic or recurring nodules that occur commonly on the inside of the cheeks and lips, the posterior palate, and the mouth floor. They are caused by injury to one of the many minor salivary glands, resulting in extravasation of mucus, which causes granulomatous inflammation or blockage of the excretory duct and leads to cyst formation. Both types of lesions require conservative surgical excision because simple incision and drainage usually is followed by recurrence.

SALIVARY GLAND DISEASES

Primary Diseases of Salivary Glands

Patients with enlargement of a major or minor salivary gland usually present a diagnostic challenge (Table 514–6). More than 20 types of benign or malignant salivary gland neoplasms may appear as unilateral enlargement of a major gland that is firm and nontender to palpation or as a firm submucosal nodule on the palate or the labial or buccal mucosa. Uncommonly, unilateral major gland enlargement may be reactive—e.g., benign lymphoepithelial lesion, or chronic sialadenitis from a sialolith or inadequately treated bacterial sialadenitis. Observation of any of these lesions should be followed by appropriate imaging and biopsy.

Unilateral major salivary gland enlargement that is markedly painful or tender to palpation and has a purulent exudate or nothing expressible from the duct suggests bacterial sialadenitis. Any exudate should be cultured, and initial treatment should be oral cephalexin or dicloxacillin.

Bilateral Salivary Gland Enlargement and Decreased Salivary Secretion Associated with Systemic Diseases

The best-known cause of bilateral salivary gland enlargement is infection by the mumps virus in children. However the incidence of mumps decreased in the United States by >90% after the introduction of an effective vaccine in 1967, and now there are only a few hundred to a few thousand cases per year. Uncommonly, a less acute, mumps-like illness may occur in adults in association with cytomegalovirus, influenza, or coxsackie A virus infection.

Sjögren's syndrome is characterized in about one third of patients by gradual development of firm, nontender or only slightly tender, bilateral enlargement of major salivary glands (see Chapter 291). The enlargement may slowly wax and wane. Salivary secretion decreases gradually, and, if hypofunction is severe and prolonged, the resulting dry mouth can impair speech and swallowing and be associated with rapidly progressive dental caries, symptomatic erythematous candidiasis, and difficulty in wearing dentures. In severe cases, the oral mucosa is dry and sticky, and saliva is not expressible from the major ducts. About one third of patients show signs of erythematous candidiasis (see above).

The salivary component of Sjögren's syndrome should be diagnosed from a labial salivary gland biopsy specimen containing at least five glands. Examination must show focal lymphocytic sialadenitis in most or all of the specimen and exclude nonspecific chronic sialadenitis or abnormalities indicative of another disease, such as noncaseating granuloma. A patient's symptoms of oral dryness (xerostomia) are important, but are subjective and caused by a wide variety of conditions (Table 514–7.) Results from salivary functional or imaging studies are not specific to Sjögren's syndrome.

Several chronic granulomatous diseases, such as sarcoidosis, tuberculosis, and leprosy, can cause bilateral enlargement and decreased function of salivary glands. The clinical and serologic features of sarcoidosis may closely mimic those of Sjögren's syndrome, and the distinction must be made by biopsy of a minor salivary gland.

A few adult patients with HIV infection, and most children who are infected in utero, develop major salivary gland enlargement and reduced salivary secretion that are caused by lymphocytic infiltration. Parotid gland enlargement usually represents a solid or cystic benign lymphoepithelial lesion (see Table 514–3).

Recurrent parotitis of childhood includes episodes of unilateral or bilateral parotid enlargement. During flares of this illness, salivary secretion may be reduced, but usually without prominent secondary symptoms or signs. This condition, of unknown cause, usually subsides after puberty. Some serologic evidence suggests an association with Epstein-Barr virus infection.

Asymptomatic Parotid Enlargement (Sialadenosis)

Parotid glands can develop bilateral, symmetric enlargement that is soft and nontender to palpation and not associated with salivary

---

Table 514–6 ■ CAUSES OF SALIVARY GLAND ENLARGEMENT

Usually Unilateral
Benign or malignant salivary gland neoplasms (more than 20 different histopathologic types)
Bacterial infection
Chronic sialadenitis (single gland)
Usually Bilateral and Associated with Salivary Hypofunction
Viral infection (mumps, cytomegalovirus, influenza, coxsackie A)
Sjögren's syndrome (benign lymphoepithelial lesion)
Chronic granulomatous diseases (sarcoidosis, tuberculosis, leprosy)
Recurrent parotitis of childhood
Human immunodeficiency virus infection/AIDS
Bilaterally Symmetric, Soft, Nontender, Parotid Only
Sialadenosis (asymptomatic parotid enlargment), idiopathic or associated with:

Diabetes mellitus	Chronic pancreatitis
Hyperlipoproteinemia	Acromegaly
Hepatic cirrhosis	Gonadal hypofunction
Anorexia/bulimia	Phenylbutazone use

Table 514–7 ■ CAUSES OF DECREASED SALIVARY SECRETION

Temporary
Effects of short-term drug use (e.g., antihistamines)
Virus infections (e.g., mumps)
Dehydration
Psychogenic causes (fear, depression)
Chronic
Effects of chronically administered drugs (especially antidepressants, MAO inhibitors, neuroleptics, parasympatholytics, some combinations of drugs for treating hypertension)
Systemic Diseases (with or without Gland Enlargement)
Sjögren's syndrome
Granulomatous diseases (sarcoidosis, tuberculosis, leprosy)
Amyloidosis
HIV infection
Diabetes mellitus (uncontrolled)
Graft-versus-host disease
Depression
Therapeutic radiation to the head and neck
Absent or malformed glands (rare)

hypofunction (see Table 514–6). Diagnosis is established by the clinical presentation and (if necessary to exclude sarcoidosis) a normal labial salivary gland biopsy. Usually, results of sialography and salivary scintigraphy are within normal limits. Biopsy of the affected glands is not indicated for diagnosis.

This chronic, noninflammatory, and non-neoplastic condition is usually associated with a variety of systemic diseases, including diabetes mellitus, hyperlipoproteinemia, hepatic cirrhosis, anorexia/bulimia, chronic pancreatitis, acromegaly, and gonadal hypofunction. It can also result from use of phenylbutazone or be a reaction to iodine-containing contrast media.

Impaired Salivary Secretion Without Gland Enlargement

The very common symptom of dry mouth (xerostomia) is most often a side effect of chronically administered drugs. Many classes of drugs reduce unstimulated salivary secretion through anticholinergic or other mechanisms (Table 514–7). At least initially, most of these drugs do not interfere with salivary production in response to gustatory, olfactory, or masticatory stimuli. Patients usually experience the symptoms soon after beginning to use the drug but will produce enough saliva during a meal for normal chewing and swallowing. The effects are dose-dependent and are produced by most tricyclic antidepressants, most neuroleptics, monoamine oxidase inhibitors, and all anticholinergics. A combination of drugs for treatment of hypertension may cause symptoms of dry mouth, but usually not to the extent of the drugs listed above.

Several systemic diseases affect salivary secretion. As noted above, most patients with Sjögren's syndrome, some with sarcoidosis, and a few patients with HIV infection experience symptoms of dry mouth to various degrees, with or without salivary gland enlargement. In addition, patients who have primary or secondary amyloidosis with salivary gland deposition may develop impaired secretion. Depressed patients who are not taking antidepressants apparently have decreased resting salivary secretion and complain more frequently of symptoms of dry mouth.

Irradiation of the head and neck region to treat a malignant tumor usually produces profound dry mouth before therapy is completed. Secretory capacity recovers only slightly in the months following treatment. Less severe dry mouth can accompany graft-versus-host disease following bone marrow transplantation; secretory capacity usually recovers when the reaction resolves.

Clinical Management of Patients with Impaired Salivary Secretion

Significant chronic salivary hypofunction from any cause produces a risk for dental caries in approximate proportion to the secretory impairment, but caries can largely be prevented if appropriate measures are taken as soon as the hypofunction begins. Remaining teeth should be protected by a comprehensive dental caries prevention program, monitored by a dentist, that includes daily application of an appropriate topical fluoride and removal of dental plaque, counseling on control of cariogenic dietary carbohydrates, and placement of appropriate dental restorations as necessary.

Symptomatic treatment of mild to moderately severe salivary hypofunction can include sialogogues such as sugarless hard candies or chewing gum, frequent sips of water, and use of saliva substitutes at night. Severe hypofunction, especially that following irradiation, can be improved by oral pilocarpine, 5 to 10 mg three times a day, if not contraindicated.

Chronic erythematous oral candidiasis is a frequent sequela of chronic xerostomia, and its treatment and retreatment, as noted above, will improve the patient's oral symptoms.

Daniels TE, Fox PC: Salivary and oral components of Sjögren's syndrome. Rheum Dis Clin North Am 18:571, 1992. *This review outlines the clinical features of the salivary component of Sjögren's syndrome and clinical management of patients with dry mouth.*

Greenspan JS, Greenspan D (eds): Oral Manifestations of HIV Infection. Chicago, Quintessence, 1995. *This volume of proceedings from an international workshop provides a comprehensive view of the oral manifestations of HIV infection, including their epidemiology, salivary and periodontal manifestations, and the pathogenesis and treatment of opportunistic mucosal infections.*

Regezi JA, Sciubba JJ: Oral Pathology: Clinical-pathologic Correlations, 3nd ed. Philadelphia, WB Saunders, 1999. *This useful and comprehensive text discusses and illustrates the clinical features, differential diagnosis, pathogenesis, and pathology of most diseases affecting the oral mucosa, jaws, and salivary glands.*

515 UPPER AIRWAY DISEASES

Kingman P. Strohl

The nose, ears, pharynx, and larynx are involved in such functions as conducting airflow to and from the lungs, taste, deglutition, speech, hearing, and smell. These chambered, highly specialized structures develop from the foregut and second through fourth branchial arches and are highly served by neural systems for motor control and sensation. Disease in any segment of the upper airway can have several functional consequences, and loss of any function can arise from both local processes and neural mechanisms. Because the larynx and pharynx act in series as the conducting airway to the trachea, bronchi, and the more distal gas-exchanging units of the lungs, dyspnea and air hunger result from swelling, encroachment, or neural dysfunction of these segments. Other presentations of upper airway disease include rhinorrhea and nasal obstruction, sneezing, postnasal and pharyngeal secretions, cough, dysphagia, changes in voice, swelling of the upper and lower jaw, hearing loss, tinnitus, snoring and apneas during sleep, epistaxis and pain.

Anatomic and functional assessments often reveal the cause of symptoms. For example, muffled speech and drooling in the presence of neck or jaw swelling indicate encroachment of the pharyngeal airway and require immediate assessment and monitoring of airway patency. Watching the patient with dysphagia while he/she drinks and eats may differentiate a neural from an anatomic process. Examining the upper airways requires an appreciation of the anatomic complexities of the area and a facility with the otoscope, tongue blade, tuning fork, and manual (gloved) palpation of the mouth. Knowledge of salivary gland and lymph node locations, bimanual examination of the floor of the mouth, and percussion of the teeth are needed to distinguish among periodontal abscess, mandibular swelling, fracture, or tumor. Referral to the appropriate specialist (orthodontist, oral surgeon, or otolaryngologist) saves time, prevents progression and complications, and/or avoids unnecessary procedures.

Clues to a systemic illness may arise from examining the upper airways in the absence of symptoms. Nasal polyps are associated with both aspirin-sensitive asthma and cystic fibrosis. Nasal ulceration, nasal drip, and sinusitis may be seen in chronic cocaine use and withdrawal as well as in pulmonary vasculitis, especially that of Wegener's granulomatosis (see Chapter 294) Parotid gland enlargement is associated with sarcoidosis, diabetes, amyloid, and collagen vascular diseases. Hereditary hemorrhagic telangiectasia (Osler-Weber-Rendu syndrome) presents to the internist with gastrointestinal bleeding and is characterized by dilated thin-walled capillaries and draining veins seen in the nose, lips, and mouth.

HEARING DEFICITS (see Chapter 517)

Otitis (also see Chapter 517)

Otitis media (Table 515–1) may occur at any age; however, the most frequent presentation is under age 10. Presenting symptoms include pain and conductive hearing loss, more often unilateral. In acute presentations, most patients acknowledge a preceding upper respiratory tract infection; symptoms improve with antibiotics. When the presentation is subacute or chronic, treatment should

Table 515–1 ■ OTITIS MEDIA

TYPE	MECHANISMS	TREATMENT
Acute	*Streptococcus pneumoniae,* and *Haemophilus influenzae;* rarely *Staphylococcus aureus, Streptococcus pyogenes, Proteus, Pseudomonas*	Oral antibiotics
Serous	Failure to clear fluid (Starling effect)	Antihistamines and decongestants
Chronic	Persistent eustachian tube obstruction (rarely tuberculosis)	Drainage tubes ± all of the above

include not only antibiotics but also consideration of mechanical factors, such as eustachian tube functional or anatomic obstruction and/or tympanic membrane rupture, which require surgical collaboration.

There are special concerns about otitis relevant to internal medicine. First, there may be serious complications from untreated or inadequately treated disease. Infection from the middle ear extending into the mastoid sinus and adjacent structures in the temporal bone may result in unilateral distal facial nerve palsy, osteomyelitis, infection of the basal structures of the skull, and/or intracranial extension, including dural abscess, brain abscess, and meningitis. Patients can present with sepsis and/or coma with increased intracranial pressure. Identification of the infecting organism is crucial. Problems in the inner ear may be addressed surgically after definitive intravenous antibiotic therapy. Second, the spectrum of organisms in immunocompromised hosts includes fungal infections (*Aspergillus* and *Candida*) that, if undetected, lead to complications. A third special circumstance is patients with longstanding endotracheal or nasogastric intubation. Nasal inflammation can block the eustachian tube and produce otitic and sinus infections with nosocomial organisms. Unexplained fever in the medical intensive care unit should involve examination of the upper airway and, occasionally, radiographic imaging and aspiration of the middle ear or sinuses for culture.

External otitis is characterized by severe pain edema, and discharge along the auditory meatus. In contrast to otitis media, the ear and the tragus are painful to the touch, and otoscopic examination is painful. Often there is a history of water in or trauma to the ear canal. Culture could reveal *Pseudomonas* organisms but usually is not needed. Treatment with topical broad-spectrum antibiotics combined with topical corticosteroids, so-called otic drops, resolves symptoms and results in cure in 3 to 5 days. Narcotic analgesics may be needed to manage pain. Oral antibiotics are indicated when regional lymphadenitis or erythema/cellulitis is present.

Infections of the external ear can present more severely in immunocompromised hosts and especially in diabetic patients, who have decreased host defenses and reduced sensation. This condition is sometimes called *"malignant" otitis* (see Chapter 473). Spread of infection from the ear inferiorly results in facial nerve paralysis (not to be dismissed as Bell's palsy); infection of the jugular foramen; involvement of the glossopharyngeal, vagus, and accessory nerves; and infection of the sheath of the jugular vein, with extension inferiorly and contralaterally into the neck and rostrally into the lateral sinus. Medial spread involves the middle ear and the mastoid, whereas anterior spread involves the temporomandibular joint. Broad-spectrum intravenous antibiotics should be instituted promptly. Surgical intervention is indicated to identify organisms when nerve involvement or foreign body obstruction is suspected.

With recurrent external otitis, a history of repetitive trauma or exposure to water (so-called *swimmer's ear*) is likely. In the former, counseling may be needed on proper ear hygiene; in the latter, over-the-counter ear drops containing an alcohol/glycerine mixture can be recommended for use after bathing or swimming.

RHINITIS (See Chapter 274)

Rhinitis comprises a group of disorders characterized by nasal itching, drip, and obstruction. These symptoms relate to irritation and inflammation of the mucosa and increased nasal secretions. Antigen challenge in susceptible hosts, histamine challenge, or activating nonmyelinated nerves with substance P can reproduce symptoms found in acute allergic reactions and acute rhinitis. Subacute and chronic symptoms and nasal obstruction result from the activation of mucosal prostanoids and cytokine networks to promote the nasal inflammatory response, recruit inflammatory cells, and promote healing. Acute insults take 3 to 5 days to resolve unless bacterial superinfection, concomitant eustachian tube or sinus obstruction, or repeated exposure to a causative noninfectious agent or allergen occurs. A persistent inflammatory state can develop in susceptible individuals and result in chronic symptoms, nasal polyps, and altered or decreased sense of smell (anosmia).

The most frequent cause of acute rhinitis is the common cold (see Chapter 375). An *upper respiratory tract infection* is commonly a self-limited illness. The severity of viral infections can be

attenuated by amantadine or similar agents if taken near the time of exposure. Antihistamines, decongestants, and cool mist relieve symptoms. Topical decongestants like oxymetrazoline, used as directed, relieve nasal obstruction; however, rebound congestion and the potential complications of chronic vascular constriction follow if therapy is prolonged beyond 1 week. Bacterial superinfection presenting as sinusitis or otitis should be suspected if recurrent fever, regional lymphadenopathy, persistent mucopurulent discharge, or persistent symptoms last longer than 5 days. In this situation, oral antibiotics are useful.

SINUSITIS

A mucopurulent discharge and a painful face suggest *sinusitis,* an inflammation of the lining of the paranasal sinuses. Most cases occur as a complication of the common cold or other upper respiratory tract infections, with occasional presentations due to extension of a periodontal infection under the maxillary sinus. Less than 1% of upper respiratory tract infections result in the clinical syndrome of acute sinusitis, and fewer meet the criteria for chronic sinusitis. Sinusitis is more common in adults, perhaps because the paranasal sinuses do not develop fully until the second and third decade of life. Bedside transillumination can suggest the presence of sinusitis. Normal light transmission to the frontal sinus from the supraorbital ridge or to the maxillary sinus through the hard palate excludes sinusitis; reduced or absent transmission is less helpful because considerable intraindividual anatomic variation exists. Radiographic evaluation is relatively sensitive. A coronal computed tomography image with bone window settings is the preferred test. Magnetic resonance imaging and ultrasonography have limited but specialized applications. Sinus aspiration and endoscopic sinuscopy may be necessary to recover organisms or to effect drainage. Surgical interventions are indicated for treatment failure, suppurative complications, diagnosis of nosocomial infection, and fever of unknown origin with sinus opacification.

Most causes of sinusitis are bacterial infections similar to those that produce otitis. The course of acute sinusitis is 3 to 4 weeks because of the anatomic difficulties in drainage. Decongestants improve nasal obstruction and may improve sinus drainage. The routine use of antihistamines is controversial because of concerns that mucociliary clearance may be impaired. Oral antibiotics are often prescribed. Occasionally, surgical interventions are used when disease is chronic and resistant to empiric therapy. Fungal sinusitis is uncommon and presents with a chronic course. *Aspergillus* is most common, but *Candida, Mucor,* and *Penicillium* organisms may be recovered from infected sinus aspirates. Invasive disease with eye, mouth, and brain extension occurs in patients with acquired immunodeficiency disease or on chemotherapy. Finally, *maxillary antrum tumors* produce a unilateral bloody nasal discharge that can be confused with sinusitis. Clues to a malignant process are the chronicity of symptoms, refractoriness to conventional therapy, and the presence of bony destruction of the antrum on radiographic examination.

MASSES, SWELLING, AND PAIN OF THE JAW
(See Chapter 514)

Occasionally the internist sees patients with swelling of the face and jaw. The differential diagnosis is based on careful history and examination. Duration of symptoms, presence of a fever, history of local trauma, orthodontic difficulties, shortness of breath, or dysphagia may help localize lesions and identify potential complications. The anatomic locations of the salivary glands and lymph nodes are distinct (Fig. 515–1). The site of swelling of the jaw is determined on physical examination by palpation, running the finger intraorally along the inner and outer borders of the mandible, and comparing the right and left sides. Inspection and tooth percussion with a metal rod localize periodontal processes.

Fracture of the lower jaw usually presents with a history of trauma, although sometimes minor in nature. Jaw fractures are treated like compound fractures because the teeth communicate with the oral cavity. Occasionally, soft tissue swelling from secondary infection obscures a fracture. *Aseptic necrosis* caused by a

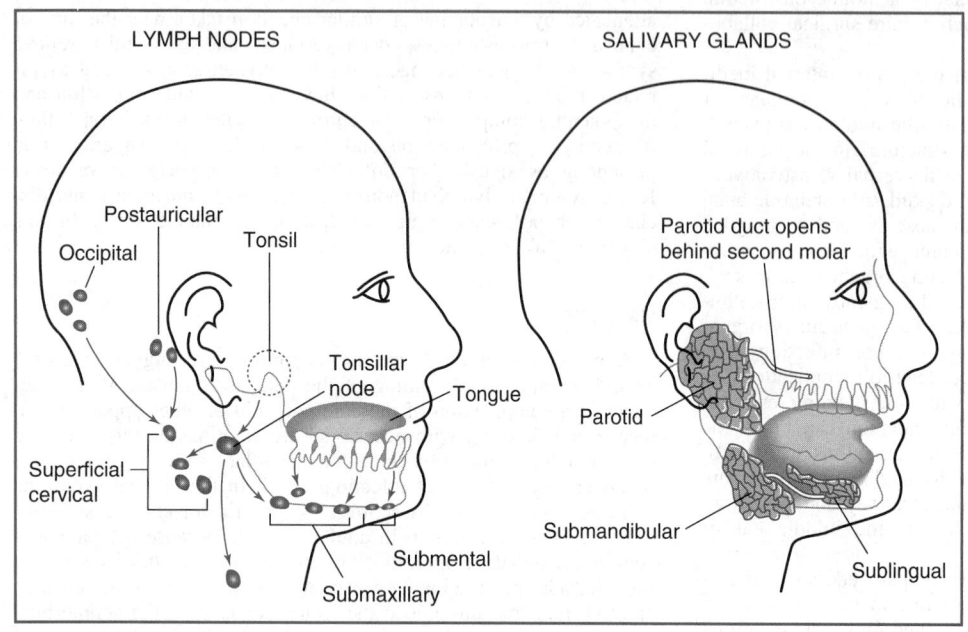

FIGURE 515–1 ■ Appropriate position of the lymph nodes *(left)* and the salivary glands *(right)*. Arrows indicate routes of lymphatic drainage.

vascular disease or a mandibular hairline fracture can also present with swelling and pain. *Periodontal abscess* results from poor dental hygiene or tooth trauma, particularly in the elderly, the diabetic, or the immunocompromised host. Complications result from periodontal abscess because infection can track rapidly along tissue planes to the basal structures of the skull and to the neck and mediastinum. *Ludwig's angina* (see Chapter 338) is an infection presenting with a painful swelling of the anterior floor of the mouth, drooling, and dysphagia. Left unrecognized or untreated, it can progress rapidly to respiratory obstruction. Intravenous antibiotics and corticosteroids must frequently be accompanied by surgical exploration and drainage.

Nonpainful swelling of the lower jaw suggests tumor of the bone or soft tissues. The most common nonmalignant tumor is an *epulis* (meaning "on the gum"), a granulomatous and fibrous tissue growth. Other growths include *osteoma, cyst, ameloblastoma* (a tumor of the cells that make enamel), and *malignant epithelioma.* Bilateral enlargement of the mandible occurs in *acromegaly, Paget's disease, osteitis fibrosa* from hyperparathyroidism, and *leontiasis ossea.* The last is a rare condition with jaw changes resembling acromegaly but without enlargement of the hands or feet.

Pain in the lower jaw without swelling is commonly due to *dental caries, periodontal disease,* or *temporomandibular dysfunction* (otomandibular syndrome). *Trigeminal neuralgia* presents with a unilateral dull pain, a distinct anatomic distribution, and a trigger zone for intense pain; neuralgia occurs in cranial nerve VII division II more than in III or I. In contrast, *herpes zoster* more commonly involves division I. Pain from cardiac angina also may be referred to the jaw and has been mistaken for periodontal disease.

DYSPHAGIA (see Chapter 124)

HOARSENESS

Simple hoarseness is the inability to pitch the voice and results from failure to use the larynx to produce tones. This change in voice occurs with voluntary acts, e.g., whispering, or with diseases affecting vocal cord motion and position. The most common cause of an acute onset of hoarseness is a bacterial or viral *infection.* Inhaled *irritants* (smoke or fumes) and *overuse* of the larynx present similarly. Inflammation and edema inhibit precise tension or closure of the cords. Treatment is rest and avoidance of irritants. Inhaled corticosteroids may produce cough and further irritation. Stridor suggests more than edema and inflammation of the vocal folds and warrants evaluation for extrinsic or intrinsic airway encroachment. Intermittent or recurrent hoarseness is usually associated with *smoking* and/or *allergy.*

Hoarseness persisting 2 weeks or more should be investigated by directly examining the laryngeal structures. Chronic hoarseness can result from benign and malignant processes, including *gastroesophageal reflux, laryngeal carcinoma* or *polyps, arthritis, hypothyroidism, goiter,* and infections *(tuberculosis, syphilis,* and *histoplasmosis).* Post-nasal drip is an uncommon cause. Chronic hoarseness due to malignancy in the chest, with entrapment of the left recurrent laryngeal nerve, and to pharyngeal or esophageal carcinomas, with entrapment of nerves or extrinsic compression, usually occurs after the primary tumor has declared itself by other symptoms. Hoarseness due to recurrent laryngeal nerve paralysis may present years after thyroid or parathyroid surgery, trauma to the neck, or goiter and is attributed to fibrosis and/or aging. Hoarseness following endotracheal intubation is common but should resolve within 3 to 5 days after removing the tube. Idiopathic, isolated unilateral, and bilateral vocal cord paralysis is rare. Treatment of chronic hoarseness is directed at the underlying cause. Nerve-grafting procedures can restore function in a paralyzed cord and laser therapy can be used for vocal folds entrapped after prolonged intubation, tracheostomy, or granuloma formation.

UPPER AIRWAY OBSTRUCTION

Presenting symptoms of pharnyeal or laryngeal obstruction are air hunger and stidor at rest or on exertion; the presentation may be acute or chronic. There may be signs of increased airway resistance with inspiratory chest retractions and active expiratory efforts. Assessment of the patient with symptoms at rest should focus first on restoring or assuring a patent airway before an examination. Most common misdiagnoses are asthma and heart failure, so that a failure to respond to empiric treatment should raise suspicion for an upper airway cause for dyspnea, wheezing, and hypercapnic respiratory failure.

Direct examination may precipitate complete airway closure and should be performed in a controlled setting like an emergency department. If the patient is stable, a flow-volume loop is one noninvasive test that will reveal the presence of flow limitation on inspiration or on both inspiration or expiration. A soft tissue lateral radiograph with the neck extended may localize the site of the obstruction.

Causes of acute obstruction include bacterial epiglottis, trauma, angioneurotic edema, allergic reactions, and foreign body aspiration. Chronic obstruction can be a presenting feature of neoplastic disease (sqamous cell carcinoma being the most common), cricoarytenoid arthritis, vocal cord polyps, bilateral vocal cord paralysis, goiter, and neurofibromatosis.

Glottic dysfunction, also called factitious asthma, is an uncommon disorder characterized by intermittent episodes of dyspnea and wheezing. The patient may present with hypercapnia but with a normal arterial-alveolar gradient, indicating that gas exchange in the distal airways and lung units is normal. Patients have complete resolution of symptoms in minutes to hours, a finding also inconsistent with asthma or heart failure. Recognition and subsequent treatment with assurance and medicinal restraint is coupled with stress reduction measures and, occasionally, antidepressant medications for better outcome, as measured by fewer presentations for assessment and/or hospitalizations.

SNORING (See Chapter 87)

Snoring is produced by vibrations of the soft tissues of the nasopharynx initiated by turbulent flow through a narrowed airway. Airway caliber is determined by anatomic factors, neuromuscular tone to skeletal muscle, and the pressure differences across the airway wall. Snoring occurs during sleep, a state in which postural tone to the skeletal muscles and reflex adjustments to respiratory loads are reduced. The airway closing at the level of the nasopharynx and/or oropharynx during sleep produces apnea (cessation of airflow) and is believed to represent an extension of the process that produces snoring. (see Chapter 87) Heavy snoring is terminated by changes in the sleep state or brief arousals from sleep. Repetitive arousals result in inadequate sleep and daytime sleepiness and increased sensitivity to central nervous system (CNS) depressants.

So common is snoring (30 to 50% of the population at age 50 report snoring) that it is the theatrical signature for sleep and the subject of social comment. Loud snoring, enough to be heard in the next room, is present in 5 to 10% of the population. In adults, examination reveals a reddened soft palate with or without anatomic narrowing of the nasal and oropharyngeal passages, micrognathia, or hypothyroidism. Other predisposing factors may include family history, obesity, respiratory depressants (alcohol and drugs), sleep restriction, nasal obstruction, and aging. Treatment is symptomatic for the bed partner, and one must first exclude hypothyroidism and then address predisposing factors. Medical therapy is directed toward weight loss, nasal decongestants, and drugs to reduce upper airway inflammation. Surgical therapy is directed at the naso-oropharynx with ablative or surgical procedures to reduce the size of the uvula or posterior palate. In children, tonsillar hypertrophy and craniofacial anomalies are more common, and surgical intervention is more successful.

Epidemiologic studies have suggested an association between snoring and increased risk of hypertension, myocardial infarction, and stroke, even when adjusted for obesity, smoking, and age. The link may be through the 17-fold increase in risk for apnea in people who report snoring. A clue to the presence of apnea is the bed partner reporting observed apneas or respiratory pauses followed by a loud snort during sleep. Multiple apneas (>10 per hour of sleep) during sleep may result in daytime symptoms, commonly excessive daytime sleepiness. Because snoring is very common, the trait by itself should not trigger a search for sleep apnea. Snoring, hypertension, or obesity alone is a poor indication for a detailed evaluation for sleep apnea. Snoring in combination with observed apneas, excessive daytime sleepiness, hypertension poorly controlled by medical therapy, and heart disease is a better indication for examining the patient during sleep to quantify the presence, type, number, and severity of respiratory disturbances during sleep.

Butler CC, Rollnick S, Kinnersley P, et al: Reducing antibiotics for respiratory tract symptoms in primary care: consolidating 'why' and considering 'how.' Br J Gen Pract 48:1865, 1998. *This review identifies consulting skills, guidelines and monitoring strategies, patient education, and use of anti-inflammatory drugs for recurrent and chronic sinusitis.*

Stewart MH, Siff JE, Cydulka RK: Evaluation of the patient with sore throat, earache, and sinusitis: An evidence based approach. Emerg Med Clin North Am; 17:153, 1999. *This article provides a window to the current literature regarding initial assessment of these common disorders.*

516 SMELL AND TASTE
Robert W. Baloh

Millions of people suffer from disorders of taste and smell, yet there is relatively little information available on how to evaluate or treat these patients. These disorders have been neglected because they are seldom fatal and, unlike abnormalities of vision and hearing, are not considered serious handicaps. Chemosensory disorders, however, often reduce the enjoyment and quality of life and are important to patients who suffer from them. Disorders of taste interfere with digestion because taste stimulants alter salivary and pancreatic flow, gastric contractions, and intestinal motility. Smell also contributes to the anticipation and ingestion of food because much of what we taste derives from olfactory stimulation during ingestion and chewing. The inability to detect noxious tastes and odors can result in food or gas poisoning, particularly in elderly subjects. In the extreme, chemosensory disorders can lead to overwhelming stress, anorexia, and depression.

ANATOMY

The sensory receptor for taste, the taste bud, is made up of 50 to 150 cells arranged to form a pear-shaped organ. The life span of these cells is 10 to 14 days, and they are constantly being renewed from dividing epithelial cells surrounding the bud. Taste buds are located on the tongue, soft palate, pharynx, larynx, epiglottis, uvula, and the upper one third of the esophagus. The taste buds located on the anterior two thirds of the tongue and on the palate are innervated by the chorda tympani branch of the seventh cranial nerve. The ninth cranial nerve innervates the posterior one third of the tongue. The ninth and tenth nerves innervate taste buds in the pharynx and larynx. Afferent signals from the taste buds project to the nucleus of the solitary tract in the medulla and then via a series of relays to the thalamus and postcentral somatosensory cerebral cortex (primary ipsilateral). Free nerve endings of the fifth cranial nerve are found on the tongue and in the oral cavity, and lesions involving these pathways also can alter taste perception.

Olfactory receptors lie in a roughly dime-sized area of specialized pigmented epithelium that arches along the superior aspect of each side of the nasal mucosa. Specialized bipolar sensory cells in this region thrust short receptor hairs into the overlying mucosa to detect aromatic molecules as they dissolve. As with taste buds, the specialized receptor portion of the bipolar neuron undergoes continuous renewal, turning over approximately every 30 days. Thin axons of the bipolar neurons course through small holes in the cribriform plate of the ethmoid bone to form connections in the overlying olfactory bulb on the ventral surface of the frontal lobe. From here, second- and third-order neurons project directly and indirectly to the prepiriform cortex and parts of the amygdaloid complex of both sides of the brain, representing the primary olfactory cortex.

PATHOPHYSIOLOGY OF CHEMOSENSORY DISORDERS

Disorders of taste and smell can be divided into local, systemic, and neurologic (Table 516–1). The taste buds and the specialized receptor portion of the bipolar olfactory cells are constantly being renewed, and the process of renewal can be affected by nutritional, metabolic, and hormonal states, therapeutic radiation, drugs, and age. For example, with interruption of mitosis by antiproliferative agents, a return of normal taste function takes a minimum of 10 days, while a return to normal olfactory function takes more than 30 days. Numerous local conditions such as colds and allergies, chronic sinusitis, and nasal polyposis can influence the sense of smell by restricting airway patency. Accidental blows to the head can shear the fine axons of the bipolar olfactory neurons, resulting in loss of smell. Lesions of the fifth, seventh *(chorda tympani),* and ninth nerves can lead to disordered taste sensation. Olfactory and gustatory disturbances can serve as important diagnostic signs for focal neurologic lesions (e.g., frontal lobe tumors). Hallucinations of smell and taste occur with epileptogenic lesions affecting the mesial temporal lobe and insular region, respectively. Finally, olfactory disturbances and hallucinations occur with a number of psychiatric illnesses (particularly depressive illness and schizophrenia).

EXAMINATION OF TASTE AND SMELL

Olfaction can be tested grossly at the bedside with a few easily recognized odors such as coffee, chocolate, and the roselike aroma

Table 516-1 ■ COMMON CAUSES OF LOSS OF TASTE AND SMELL

	TASTE	SMELL
Local	Radiation therapy	Allergic rhinitis, sinusitis, nasal polyposis, upper respiratory infection
Systemic	Cancer, renal failure, hepatic failure, nutritional deficiency (B_3, zinc), Cushing's syndrome, hypothyroidism, diabetes mellitus, infection (viral), drugs (antirheumatic and antiproliferative)	Renal failure, hepatic failure, nutritional deficiency (B_{12}), Cushing's syndrome, hypothyroidism, diabetes mellitus, infection (viral hepatitis, influenza), drugs (nasal sprays, antibiotics)
Neurologic	Bell's palsy, familial dysautonomia, multiple sclerosis	Head trauma, multiple sclerosis, Parkinson's disease, frontal tumor

of the compound phenylethyl alcohol. (Avoid nasal irritants.) Each nostril is tested separately to determine whether the problem is unilateral or bilateral. Gustatory sensation is typically tested with weak solutions of sugar, salt, and acetic acid, or vinegar. The patient must keep the tongue protruded and respond to questions either by nodding the head or pointing to names of the tastes written on cards. The anterior two thirds and posterior one third of the tongue should be tested separately.

COMMON CAUSES OF LOSS OF SMELL AND TASTE

The most frequently encountered causes of loss of smell are local obstructive disease, viral infections, head injuries that sever the neurons crossing through the cribriform plate, and normal aging. Patients can lose their sense of smell not only from chronic allergies and sinusitis but also from the nasal sprays and drops that they use to treat these conditions. The most common causes of loss of the sense of taste are viral infections and drug ingestion, particularly antirheumatic and antiproliferative drugs. Many of the systemic disorders listed in Table 516–1 probably have their effect by decreasing the rate of turnover of sensory receptors on the tongue and olfactory epithelia. Disturbances of smell and taste in malnourished patients may be due to specific deficiencies in vitamins and minerals, such as zinc. Viral illnesses such as influenza and viral hepatitis produce disorders of both taste and smell. Multifocal neurologic disorders such as multiple sclerosis can affect the central olfactory and gustatory pathways at multiple levels, and therefore abnormalities of taste and smell are common in such patients. Treatment of olfactory dysfunction due to nasal disease is aimed at opening the air passageways while preserving the olfactory epithelium. Intranasal steriods, antibiotics, and allergic therapies are useful in selected cases. Drugs known to affect taste or smell should be removed for a trial. Vitamin and mineral therapies are of unproven benifit.

Ackerman BH, Kasbekar N: Disturbances of taste and smell induced by drugs. Pharmacotherapy 17:482, 1997. *Reviews all the common drugs that affect taste and smell.*

Deems DA, Doty RL, Settle G, et al: Smell and taste disorders, a study of 750 patients from the University of Pennsylvania smell and taste center. Arch Otolaryngol Head Neck Surg 117:519, 1991. *A comprehensive look at the diagnosis and management of smell and taste disorders at a large university clinic.*

Schiffman SS: Taste and smell losses in normal aging and disease. JAMA 278:1357, 1997. *Extensive review of the literature on disorders of taste and smell in the elderly.*

517 HEARING AND EQUILIBRIUM

Robert W. Baloh

The neural pathways subserving hearing and those most important for equilibrium and spatial orientation are anatomically proximate in much of their course from their end organs in the inner ear to their termination in the superior portion of the temporal lobe. Because of the close anatomic linkage, disorders that affect hearing often affect equilibrium, and vice versa. For this reason they are considered together here. Despite their anatomic propinquity, how-

ever, substantial pathophysiologic differences make clinical examination of the two systems quite different. The auditory system is physiologically relatively isolated, so that its function and dysfunction can be tested independently of other neural systems. The vestibular system, in contrast, has many close physiologic links with other neural systems (particularly the cerebellum, oculomotor system, and autonomic nervous system) and can be tested only indirectly by noting secondary effects on these systems. Abnormalities of the auditory system lead to only a few well-defined and unique symptoms (i.e., hearing loss or tinnitus). Abnormalities of the vestibular system can cause symptoms that mimic disorders of the other neural structures. Such symptoms include dizziness, visual distortion (oscillopsia), imbalance, nausea, vomiting, and even syncope.

HEARING

Anatomy and Physiology of Hearing

In normal hearing, sound waves are transmitted from the tympanic membrane via the three ossicles of the air-filled middle ear (air conduction) to the oval window and the basilar membrane of the fluid-sealed cochlea. The ossicles serve to increase the gain from the tympanum to oval window about 18-fold, compensating for the loss that sound waves moving from air to fluid would otherwise suffer. In the absence of this system, sound may reach the cochlea by vibration of the temporal bone (bone conduction) but with much less efficiency (approximately 60 dB loss). Hair cells, tonotopically organized along the cochlear basilar membrane, detect the vibratory movement of that membrane and transduce vibration into nerve impulses. The nerve impulses are relayed via nerve cells that synapse at the base of hair cells and have their bodies in the spiral ganglion to the cochlear nucleus of the ipsilateral pontine tegmentum. The spiral cochlea mechanically analyzes the frequency content of sound. For high-frequency tones, only sensory cells in the basilar region are activated, whereas for low-frequency tones, all or nearly all sensory cells are activated. Therefore, with lesions of the cochlea and its afferent nerve, the hearing levels for different frequencies are usually unequal, typically resulting in better hearing sensitivity for low-frequency than for high-frequency tones. Within the brain stem, auditory signals ascend from the ventral and dorsal cochlear nuclei to reach the superior olivary nuclei of both sides. Thus nervous system lesions central to the cochlear nucleus do not cause monaural hearing loss and, conversely, unilateral central lesions do not cause deafness. From these structures the pathway projects by way of the lateral lemnisci to the inferior colliculi. Each inferior colliculus transmits to the other and to its ipsilateral medial geniculate body, which in turn sends the final projection to the transverse auditory gyrus lying in the superior portion of the ipsilateral temporal lobe.

The normal ear can detect sound frequencies ranging between 20 and 20,000 Hertz (Hz); the upper range drops off fairly rapidly with advancing age. The ear is most sensitive between 500 and 4000 Hz, which roughly corresponds to the frequency range most important for understanding speech. The hearing level in this range has several practical implications in terms of the degree of handicap and the potential for useful correction with amplification. A 30- to 40-dB hearing level in the speech range would impair normal conversation, whereas an 80-dB hearing level would make everyday auditory communication almost impossible (the social definition of deafness).

Conductive hearing loss results from lesions involving the external or middle ear. It is typically characterized by an approximately equal loss of hearing at all frequencies and by well-preserved speech discrimination once the threshold for hearing is exceeded. Patients with conductive hearing loss can hear speech in a noisy background better than in a quiet background because they can understand loud speech as well as anyone.

Sensorineural hearing loss results from lesions of the cochlea and/or auditory division of the eighth cranial nerve. With sensorineural hearing loss the hearing levels for different frequencies are usually unequal, typically resulting in better hearing for low- than for high-frequency tones. Patients with sensorineural hearing loss often have difficulty hearing speech that is mixed with background noise and may be annoyed by loud speech. Three important manifestations of sensorineural lesions are diplacusis, recruitment, and tone decay. Diplacusis and recruitment are common with cochlear lesions; tone decay usually accompanies eighth nerve involvement.

Central hearing disorders result from lesions of the central auditory pathways. As a rule, patients with central lesions do not have impaired hearing for pure tones, and they can understand speech as long as it is clearly spoken in a quiet environment. If the listener's task is made more difficult with the introduction of background noise or competing messages, performance deteriorates more markedly in patients with central lesions than in normal subjects.

Examination of Hearing

Bedside Test

A quick test for hearing loss in the speech range is to observe the response to spoken commands at different intensities (whisper, conversation, shouting). Tuning fork tests permit a rough assessment of the hearing level for pure tones of known frequency. The clinician can use his or her own hearing level as a reference standard. In the Rinne test, nerve conduction is compared with bone conduction by holding a tuning fork (preferably 512 Hz) against the mastoid process until the sound can no longer be heard. It is then placed 1 inch from the ear and, in normal subjects, can be heard about twice as long by air as by bone. If bone conduction is better than air conduction, the hearing loss is conductive, but care must be taken to assure that the bone conduction is not heard in the normal ear. In the Weber test, the tuning fork is placed on the patient's forehead or upper teeth. Normally this sound is referred to the center of the head. If it is referred to the side of unilateral hearing loss, the hearing loss is conductive; if it is referred away from the side of unilateral hearing loss, the loss is sensorineural.

Audiometry

Pure tone testing is the cornerstone of most auditory examinations. Pure tones at selected frequencies are presented via either earphones (air conduction) or a vibrator pressed against the mastoid portion of the temporal bone (bone conduction), and the minimal level that the subject can hear (threshold) is determined for each frequency. Two speech tests are routinely used. The *speech reception threshold* (SRT) is the intensity at which the patient can correctly repeat 50% of the words presented. The SRT is a test of hearing sensitivity for speech and should reflect the hearing level for pure tones in the speech range. The *speech discrimination test* is a measure of the patient's ability to understand speech when it is presented at a level that is easily heard. In patients with eighth nerve lesions, speech discrimination scores can be severely reduced, even when pure tone thresholds are normal or nearly normal; by comparison, in patients with cochlear lesions, discrimination tends to be proportional to the magnitude of hearing loss.

Brain stem auditory evoked responses (BAER) can be recorded from scalp electrodes at 0 to 10 msec (early), 10 to 50 msec (middle), and 50 to 500 msec (late) following a click (a high-frequency stimulus). The early potentials reflect electrical activity at the cochlea, eighth cranial nerve, and brain stem; the later potentials reflect cortical activity. Computer averaging of the responses to 1000 to 2000 clicks separates the evoked potential from background noise. Early evoked responses may be used to estimate the magnitude of hearing loss and to differentiate among cochlea, eighth nerve, and brainstem lesions.

Causes of Hearing Loss

Conductive Hearing Loss

The logic for identifying common causes of hearing loss is shown in Figure 517–1. The history, examination, and audiometry usually provide the key differential features. The most common cause of conductive hearing loss is *impacted cerumen* in the external canal. This benign condition is usually first noticed after bathing or swimming when a droplet of water closes the remaining tiny passageway. The most common serious cause of conductive hearing loss is inflammation of the middle ear, *otitis media,* either infected (suppurative) or noninfective (serous). Fluid accumulates in the middle ear, impairing the conduction of airborne sound to the cochlea. Since the air cavity of the middle ear is in direct connection with the mastoid air cells, infection can spread through the mastoid bone and, occasionally, into the intracranial cavity. Chronic otitis media with perforation of the tympanic membrane can result in an invasion of the middle ear and other pneumatized

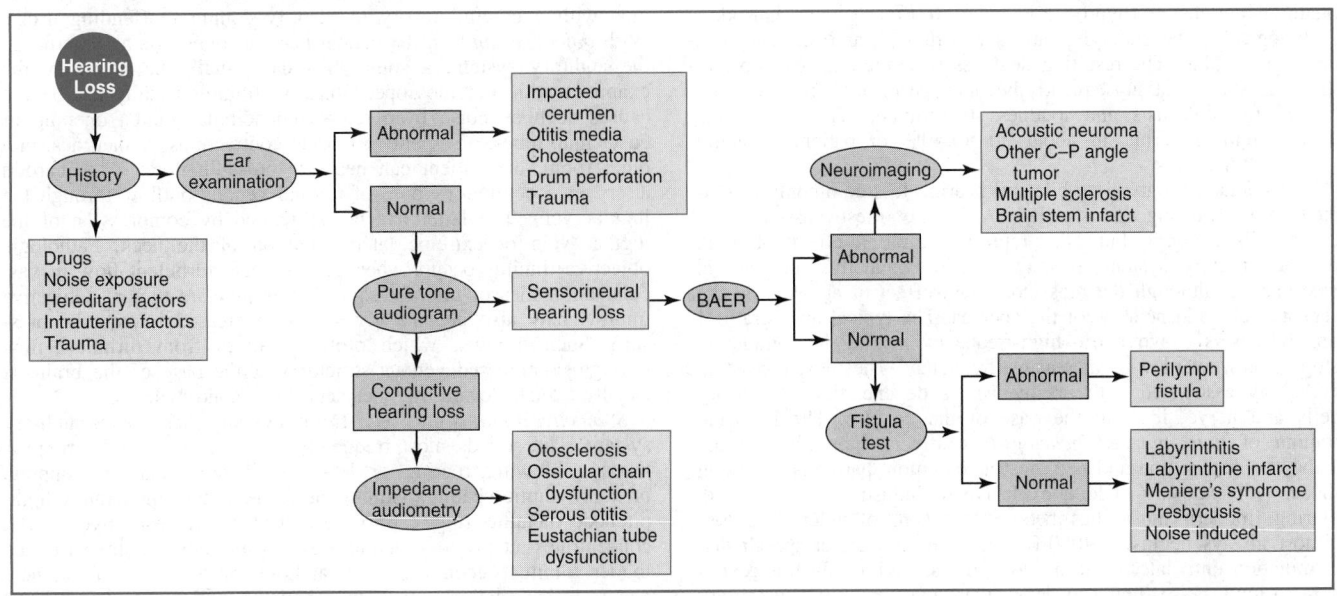

FIGURE 517–1 ■ Evaluation of hearing loss.

areas of the temporal bone by keratinizing squamous epithelium (*cholesteatoma*). Cholesteatomas can produce erosion of the ossicles and bony labyrinth, resulting in a mixed conductive sensorineural hearing loss. *Otosclerosis* commonly produces progressive conductive hearing loss by immobilizing the stapes with new bone growth in front of and below the oval window. The hearing loss is typically conductive, although in some persons the cochlea may be invaded by foci of otosclerotic bone, producing an additional sensorineural hearing loss. Otosclerosis usually stabilizes when the hearing level reaches 50 to 60 dB, and rarely progresses to deafness. Other common causes of conductive hearing loss include trauma, congenital malformations of the external and middle ear, and glomus body tumors.

Sensorineural Hearing Loss

Genetically determined deafness, usually from hair cell aplasia or deterioration, may be present at birth or may develop in adulthood. The diagnosis of *hereditary deafness* rests on the finding of a positive family history. In many instances the inheritance is through a recessive gene or a dominant gene with low penetrance, making it difficult to determine the genetic nature of the disorder. Mutations in cennexin 26, a key component of gap junctions in the inner ear, account for the majority of cases of inherited deafness identified so far. *Intrauterine factors* resulting in congenital hearing loss include infection (especially rubella); toxic, metabolic, and endocrine disorders; and anoxia associated with Rh incompatibility and difficult deliveries.

Acute unilateral deafness usually has a cochlear basis. *Bacterial or viral infections* of the labyrinth, *head trauma* with fracture or hemorrhage into the cochlea, or *vascular occlusion* of a terminal branch of the anterior inferior cerebellar artery all can extensively damage the cochlea and its hair cells. An acute idiopathic, often reversible, unilateral hearing loss strikes young adults and is presumed to reflect an isolated viral infection of the cochlea and auditory nerve terminals. Sudden unilateral hearing loss often associated with vertigo and tinnitus can result from a *perilymphatic fistula*. Such fistulae may be congenital or may follow stapes surgery or head trauma. *Drugs* cause acute and subacute bilateral hearing impairment. Salicylates, furosemide, and ethacrynic acid have the potential to produce transient deafness when taken in high doses. More toxic to the cochlea are aminoglycoside antibiotics (gentamicin, tobramycin, amikacin, kanamycin, streptomycin, and neomycin). These agents can destroy cochlear hair cells in direct relation to their serum concentrations. Some antineoplastic chemotherapeutic agents, particularly cisplatin, cause severe ototoxicity.

Subacute relapsing cochlear deafness occurs with *Ménière syndrome,* a condition associated with fluctuating hearing loss and tinnitus, recurrent episodes of abrupt and often severe vertigo, and a sensation of fullness or pressure in the ear. Recurrent endolymphatic hypertension (hydrops) is believed to cause the episodes. Pathologically, the endolymphatic sac is dilated, and the hair cells become atrophic. The resulting deafness is subtle and reversible in the early stages but subsequently becomes permanent and is characterized by diplacusis and loudness recruitment. The disorder is usually unilateral, but in about 20 to 40% of patients bilateral involvement occurs.

The gradual, progressive, bilateral hearing loss commonly associated with advancing age is called *presbycusis*. Presbycusis is not a distinct disease entity but rather represents multiple effects of aging on the auditory system. It may include conductive and central dysfunction, although the most consistent effect of aging is on the sensory cells and neurons of the cochlea. The typical audiogram of presbycusis is a symmetric high-frequency hearing loss gradually sloping downward with increasing frequency. The most consistent pathology associated with presbycusis is degeneration of sensory cells and nerve fibers at the base of the cochlea. The recurrent trauma of *noise-induced hearing loss* affects approximately the same cochlear region and is almost as common, particularly among those with exposure to loud explosive or industrial noises. Loud, blaring, modern music has become a recent offender. The loss almost always begins at 4000 Hz and does not affect speech discrimination until late in the disease process. With only brief exposure to loud, noise (hours to days), there may be only a temporary threshold shift, but with continued exposure, permanent injury be-

gins. The duration and intensity of exposure determine the degree of permanent injury.

Hearing loss from direct damage to the acoustic nerve in the petrous canal occasionally results from infection within or trauma to the surrounding bone; severe deafness of abrupt onset marks the event and is usually associated with acute vertigo due to concurrent vestibular nerve injury. Progressive unilateral hearing loss, that arises insidiously, initially in the high frequencies, and worsens by almost imperceptible degrees is characteristic of benign neoplasms of the cerebellopontine angle, such as *acoustic neuromas*. In about 10% of cases, the hearing loss can be acute, apparently owing to either hemorrhage into the tumor or compression of the labyrinthine vasculature.

Central Hearing Loss

Central hearing loss is unilateral only if it results from damage to the pontine cochlear nuclei on one side of the brain stem from conditions such as *ischemic infarction* of the lateral brain stem (e.g., occlusion of the anterior inferior cerebellar artery), a plaque of *multiple sclerosis*, or, rarely, invasion or compression of the lateral pons by a *neoplasm* or *hematoma*. Bilateral *degeneration* of the cochlear nuclei accompanies some of the rare recessive inherited disorders of childhood. As noted, clinically important unilateral hearing loss never results from neurologic disease arising rostrad to the cochlear nucleus. Although bilateral hearing loss could, in theory, result from bilateral destruction of central hearing pathways, in practice this is rare because involvement of neighboring structures in the brain stem or hemisphere would usually produce overwhelming neurologic disability.

Treatment of Hearing Loss

If an underlying disorder has not yet destroyed the auditory system and can be ameliorated medically or surgically, hearing may be improved or preserved. Most patients with otosclerosis respond to stapedectomy. Closure of a perilymph fistula may improve hearing. Antibiotic and decongestive treatment of otitis media should prevent permanent hearing loss. A low-salt diet and diuretics are effective in selective cases of Ménière syndrome, particularly if episodes are precipitated by premenstrual water retention. Hearing aids amplify sound, usually with the goal of making speech intelligible. Patients with conductive hearing loss require simple amplification, but those with sensorineural hearing loss often need frequency-selective amplification to make hearing aids useful. Recent advances in acoustic technology have markedly improved the outlook for the latter. Serial audiograms in patients with noise or ototoxic drug exposure are critical for prevention of permanent hearing loss.

Tinnitus

The evaluation of common causes of tinnitus (Fig. 517–2) begins with a careful history to identify common offending drugs. With *objective tinnitus,* the patient hears a sound arising external to the auditory system, a sound that can usually be heard by the examiner with a stethoscope. Objective tinnitus usually has benign causes such as noise from temporomandibular joints, opening of eustachian tubes, or repetitive muscle contractions. Sometimes, in a quiet room, the patient can hear the pulsatile flow in the carotid artery or a continuous hum of normal venous outflow through the jugular vein. The latter can be obliterated by compression of the jugular vein or extreme lateral rotation of the neck. Pathologic objective tinnitus occurs when patients hear turbulent flow in vascular anomalies or tumors (e.g., glomus jugulare tumor). Objective tinnitus may also be an early sign of increased intracranial pressure. Such tinnitus, which probably arises from turbulent flow through compressed venous structures at the base of the brain, is usually overshadowed by other neurologic abnormalities.

Subjective tinnitus can arise from sites anywhere in the auditory system. The sounds most frequently reported are metallic ringing, buzzing, blowing, roaring, or, less often, bizarre clanging, popping, or nonrhythmic beating. Tinnitus heard as a faint, moderately high-pitched, metallic ring can be observed by almost anyone who concentrates attention on auditory events in a quiet room. Sustained louder tinnitus accompanied by audiometric evidence of deafness occurs in association with both conductive and sensorineural hearing loss. Tinnitus observed with otosclerosis tends to have a roar-

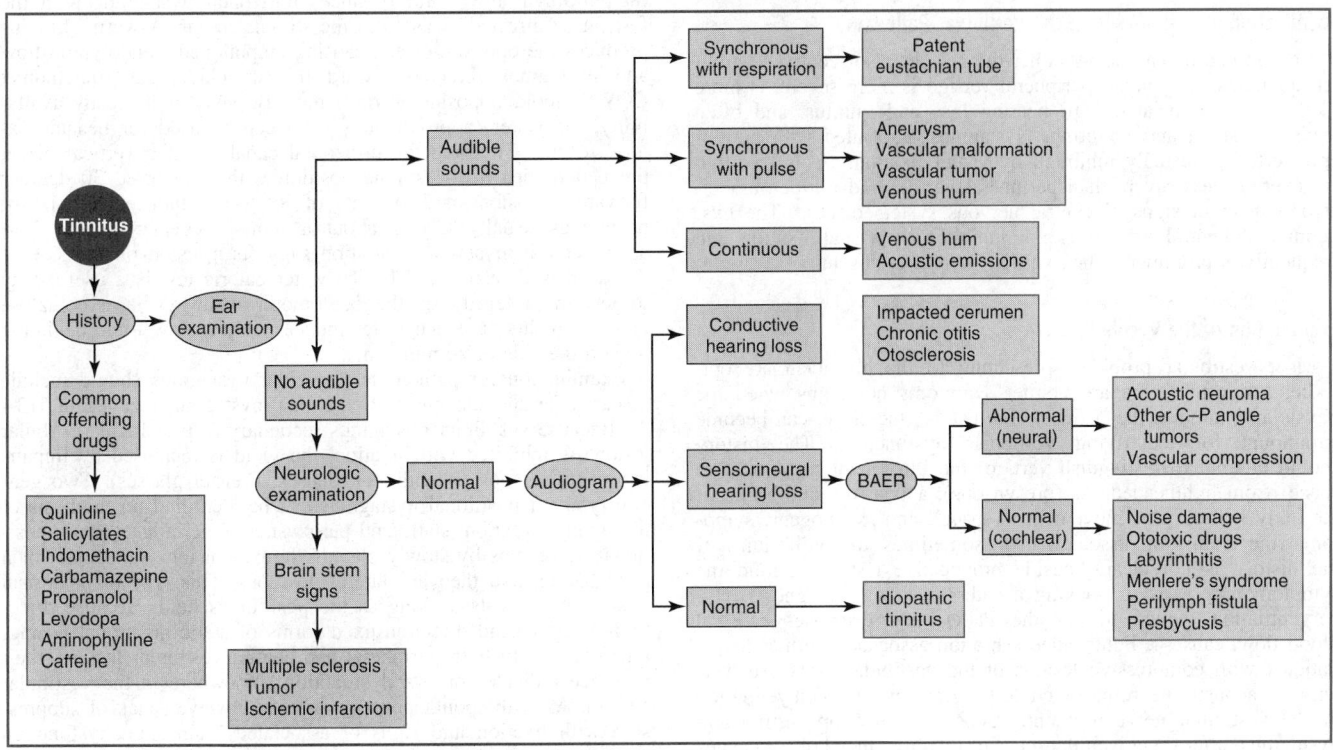

FIGURE 517–2 ■ Evaluation of tinnitus.

ing or hissing quality, while that associated with Ménière syndrome often produces sounds that vary widely in intensity with time and quality, sometimes including roaring or clanging. Tinnitus with auditory nerve lesions tends to be higher pitched and ringing in quality. Audiometric and brain stem–evoked response testing can help distinguish between lesions involving the conducting apparatus, the cochlea, and the auditory nerve. Tinnitus without observable deafness appears sporadically and for variable lengths of time in many persons without other evidence of an ongoing pathologic process.

Treatment of Tinnitus

Most patients with tinnitus can be helped by detailed interview together with the relevant examination and laboratory investigations followed by reassurance when appropriate. Often exacerbating factors such as chronic anxiety and depression can be treated. In patients with hearing loss and tinnitus, a hearing aid may improve tinnitus because the amplification of ambient sound may effectively mask the tinnitus. This mechanism probably explains the frequent observation that removal of cerumen from the external auditory canal to improve ambient hearing also improves tinnitus. Also, when cerumen is attached to the tympanic membrane, tinnitus may result from local mechanical effects on the conductive system. For patients who find their tinnitus most obtrusive when trying to sleep, a bedside FM clock radio tuned between stations can provide an effective masking sound that will switch itself off after the patient falls asleep. A careful drug history should be taken, and a drug-free trial period should be considered when possible. Some patients who notice that caffeine, alcohol, or nicotine exacerbates their tinnitus experience significant relief when these drugs are discontinued.

EQUILIBRIUM—VESTIBULAR SYSTEM

Anatomy and Physiology of the Vestibular System

The paired vestibular end organs lie within the temporal bones next to the cochlea. Each organ consists of three semicircular canals that detect angular acceleration and two otolith structures, the utricle and saccule, that detect linear acceleration (including gravitational). Like the cochlea, these organs possess hair cells that act as force transducers, converting the forces associated with head acceleration into afferent nerve impulses. The hair cells of the three semicircular canals, each of which is oriented at right angles to the others, are concentrated in the crista, where they are embedded in a gelatinous mass called the cupula. Movement of the head causes the endolymph to flow either toward or away from the cupula, bending the hair cells and, depending on the direction of endolymphatic movements, either exciting or inhibiting the afferent nerve firing. Because the afferent nerves arising from the semicircular canals are tonically active, the baseline activity can be increased or decreased depending on the direction of hair cell bending. Furthermore, the two sets of semicircular canals are approximately mirror images of each other, so that rotational movement of the head that excites one canal inhibits the analogous canal on the opposite side. The hair cells of the utricle and saccule are concentrated in an area called the macule. The macule of the utricle lies approximately in the plane of the horizontal canal, and the macule of the saccule is approximately in the plane of the anterior canal. The hair cells are embedded in a membrane that contains calcium carbonate crystals or otoliths; the density of otoliths is considerably greater than that of the endolymph. Linear accelerations of the head combine with the linear acceleration of gravity to distort the otolith membrane, thereby bending the underlying hair cells and modulating the activity of the afferent nerve terminals at the base of the hair cells.

The afferent vestibular nerves have their cell bodies in Scarpa's ganglion. The nerve fibers travel in the vestibular portion of the eighth cranial nerve contiguous to the acoustic portion. Fibers from different receptor organs terminate in different vestibular nuclei at the pontomedullary junction. There are also direct connections with many portions of the cerebellum, the greatest representation being in the flocculonocular lobe, the so-called vestibular cerebellum. Efferent fibers from the brain stem travel through the vestibular nerve to reach hair cells of the semicircular canals and macules. Efferent fibers are inhibitory in nature and, like the efferent fibers of the cochlea, may function to enhance inputs to which the brain attends. From the vestibular nuclei, second-order neurons make important connections to the vestibular nuclei of the other side, to the cerebellum, to motor neurons of the spinal cord, to autonomic nuclei in the brain stem, and, most importantly for the examining clinician, to the nuclei of the oculomotor system. Fibers from the vestibular nuclei also ascend through the brain stem and thalamus to reach the cerebral cortex bilaterally.

Localization of Lesions within the Vestibular Pathways

Vertigo can be caused by either the peripheral or central vestibular apparatus. In general, peripheral vertigo is more severe, is more likely to be associated with hearing loss and tinnitus, and often leads to nausea and vomiting. Nystagmus associated with peripheral vertigo is usually inhibited by visual fixation. Central vertigo is generally less severe than peripheral vertigo and is often associated with other signs of central nervous system disease. The nystagmus of central vertigo is not inhibited by visual fixation and frequently is prominent when vertigo is mild or absent.

Examination of the Vestibular System

Most vestibular problems presenting to the physician are episodic, and often there are neither symptoms nor signs when the physician examines the patient. The history, therefore, can become paramount for identifying vestibular dysfunction. The history should attempt to distinguish vertigo (the illusion of movement in space) from lightheadedness (presyncope), ataxia (disequilibrium of the body without true movement in space), and psychogenic symptoms (the feeling of dissociation or, sometimes, disequilibrium). If the history is not clear, bedside provocative tests to mimic the symptom may assist in making a pathophysiologic diagnosis. Hyperventilation, which lowers the $PaCO_2$ and decreases cerebral blood flow, causes a lightheaded sensation associated with syncope. Patients with compressive lesions of the vestibular nerve, such as with an acoustic neuroma or cholesteatoma, or with demyelination of the vestibular nerve root entry zone may develop vertigo and nystagmus after hyperventilation. Presumably, metabolic changes associated with hyperventilation trigger the partially damaged nerve to fire inappropriately.

Bedside tests of vestibulospinal function are often insensitive because most patients can use vision and proprioceptive signals to compensate for any vestibular loss. Patients with acute unilateral peripheral vestibular lesions may past point or fall toward the side of the lesion, but within a few days balance returns to normal. Patients with bilateral peripheral vestibular loss have more difficulty compensating and usually show some imbalance on the Romberg and tandem walking tests, particularly with eyes closed.

The vestibulo-ocular reflex can be tested at the bedside using the doll's-eye and head-thrust tests. In an alert human, rotating the head back and forth in the horizontal plane induces compensatory horizontal eye movements that are dependent on both the visual and vestibular systems. The doll's-eye test is a test of vestibular function in a comatose patient, since such patients cannot generate pursuit or corrective fast components. In this setting conjugate compensatory eye movements indicate normally functioning vestibulo-ocular pathways. Because the vestibulo-ocular reflex has a much higher frequency range than the smooth pursuit system, a qualitative bedside test of vestibular function can be made with the head-thrust test. It is performed by grasping the patient's head and applying brief, small-amplitude, high-acceleration head thrusts first to one side and then the other. The patient fixates on the examiner's nose and the examiner watches for corrective saccades, which are a sign of an inappropriate compensatory slow phase.

The caloric test uses a nonphysiologic stimulus to induce endolymphatic flow in the horizontal semicircular canal and horizontal nystagmus by creating a temperature gradient from one side of the canal to the other. With a cold caloric stimulus, the column of endolymph nearest the middle ear falls because of its increased density. This causes the cupula to deviate away from the utricle (ampullofugal flow) and produces horizontal nystagmus with the fast phase directed away from the stimulated ear. A warm stimulus produces the opposite effect, causing ampullopedal endolymph flow and nystagmus directed toward the stimulated ear (mnemonic: COWS—cold opposite, warm same). Because of its ready availability, ice water (approximately 0°C) can be used for bedside caloric testing. To bring the horizontal canal into the vertical plane, the patient lies in the supine position with head tilted 30 degrees forward. Infusion of 1 to 3 mL of ice water induces a burst of nystagmus usually lasting about a minute. Greater than a 20% asymmetry in nystagmus duration suggests a lesion on the side of the decreased response. The ice water caloric test is a useful way to test the integrity of the oculomotor pathways in a comatose patient. In this case, ice water induces only a slow tonic deviation toward the side of stimulation.

Examination for pathologic vestibular nystagmus should include a search for spontaneous and positional nystagmus (see Table 513–3). Because vestibular nystagmus secondary to peripheral vestibular lesions is inhibited with fixation, the yield is increased by impairing fixation (such as with +30 lenses, Frenzel glasses). Two general types of positional nystagmus can be identified on the basis of nystagmus duration: static and paroxysmal. One induces static positional nystagmus by slowly placing the patient into the supine, then right lateral, and then left lateral positions. This type of positional nystagmus persists as long as the position is held. Because direction-changing and direction-fixed forms of static positional nystagmus occur with both peripheral and central vestibular lesions, their presence indicates only a dysfunction somewhere in the vestibular system. As with spontaneous nystagmus, however, lack of suppression with fixation and signs of associated brain stem dysfunction suggest a central lesion.

Paroxysmal positional nystagmus (also called positioning nystagmus) is induced, after a brief delay, by a rapid change from erect sitting to supine head-hanging left, center, or right position (the so-called Dix-Hallpike test). It is initially high in frequency but dissipates rapidly (within 30 seconds to 1 minute). The most common variety of paroxysmal positional nystagmus, benign paroxysmal positional nystagmus, usually has a 3- to 10-second latency before onset and rarely lasts longer than 30 seconds. The nystagmus is always torsional with the upper pole of the eye beating toward the ground. It is usually prominent in only one head-hanging position, and a burst of nystagmus in the reverse direction occurs when the patient reassumes the sitting position. Another key feature is the severe vertigo and nystagmus that the patient experiences with the initial positioning, which, with repeated positioning, rapidly disappear (fatigability). Benign paroxysmal positional nystagmus is a sign of vestibular end-organ dysfunction (see below).

Electronystagmography (ENG), which is a technique for recording eye movements, allows precise quantification of both physiologic and pathologic nystagmus. A standard ENG test battery includes (1) tests of visual ocular control (saccades, smooth pursuit, and optokinetic nystagmus); (2) a careful search for pathologic nystagmus with fixation and with eyes open in darkness, and (3) measurement of induced physiologic nystagmus (caloric and rotational). ENG can be helpful in identifying a vestibular lesion and localizing it within the peripheral and central pathways.

Evaluating the "Dizzy" Patient

The history is key because it determines the type of dizziness (vertigo, light-headed, feeling of dissociation, disequilibrium), associated symptoms (neurologic, audiologic, cardiac, psychiatric), pre-

---

Table 517–1 ■ DISTINGUISHING BETWEEN VESTIBULAR AND NONVESTIBULAR TYPES OF DIZZINESS

	VESTIBULAR	NONVESTIBULAR
Common descriptive terms	Spinning (environment moves), merry-go-round, drunkenness, tilting, motion sickness, off-balance	Light-headed, floating, dissociated from body, swimming, giddy, spinning inside (environment stationary)
Course	Episodic	Constant
Common precipitating factors	Head movements, position change	Stress, hyperventilation, cardiac arrhythmia, situations
Common associated symptoms	Nausea, vomiting, unsteadiness, tinnitus, hearing loss, impaired vision, oscillopsia	Perspiration, pallor, paresthesias, palpitations, syncope, difficulty concentrating, tension headache

From Baloh RW, Honrubia V: Clinical Neurophysiology of the Vestibular System, 2nd ed. Philadelphia, FA Davis, 1990.

cipitating factors (position change, trauma, stress, drug ingestion), and predisposing illness (systemic viral infection, cardiac disease, cerebrovascular disease) (Table 517–1). The examination should include complete neurologic, head and neck, and cardiac assessments. When focal neurologic signs are found, neuroimaging usually leads to specific diagnosis. When vertigo is present without focal neurologic symptoms or signs, audiometry and electronystagmography aid in localizing the lesion to the labyrinth or eighth nerve. Patients with hyperventilation syndrome and/or acute anxiety should be identified after the history and examination so that needless tests are not obtained. A detailed cardiac evaluation (including Holter monitoring) often identifies the cause of episodic presyncopal light-headedness.

Common Causes of Vertigo (Figure 517–3)

Physiologic Vertigo

Physiologic vertigo includes common disorders such as *motion sickness, space sickness,* and *height vertigo.* In these conditions, vertigo (defined as an illusion of movement) is minimal or absent while autonomic symptoms predominate. With height vertigo, patients often experience acute anxiety and panic reaction. Individuals with motion sickness and space sickness typically develop perspiration, nausea, vomiting, increased salivation, yawning, and generalized malaise. Gastric motility is reduced and digestion impaired. Even the sight or smell of food is distressing. Hyperventilation is a common sign, and the resulting hypocapnia leads to changes in blood volume, with pooling in the lower parts of the body predisposing to postural hypotension and syncope. An unusual variant of motion sickness continues when the subject returns to stationary conditions after prolonged exposure to motion. Typically, affected patients report that they feel the persistent rocking sensation of a boat long after returning to solid ground. Rarely, the syndrome can last for months to years after exposure to motion and can even be incapacitating. The cause is unknown.

Physiologic vertigo can often be suppressed by supplying sensory cues that help to match the signals originating from different sensory systems. Thus, motion sickness, which is exacerbated by sitting in a closed space or reading (giving the visual system the miscue that the environment is stationary), may be improved by looking out at the environment and watching it move. Height vertigo, caused by a mismatch between sensation of normal body sway and lack of its visual detection, can often be relieved either by sitting or by visually fixating a nearby stationary object.

Benign Positional Vertigo (BPV)

BPV is by far the most common cause of vertigo. Patients with this condition develop brief episodes of vertigo (less than 1 min) with position change, typically when turning over in bed, getting in and out of bed, bending over and straightening up, or extending the neck to look up. BPV can result from *head injury, viral labyrinthitis,* and *vascular occlusion,* or it may occur as an isolated symptom (in about 50% of cases). The latter is particularly common in the elderly. This syndrome is important to recognize because in the vast majority of patients, the symptoms spontaneously remit. BPV does commonly recur, however. The diagnosis rests on finding characteristic fatigable paroxysmal positional nystagmus after a rapid change from the sitting to the head-hanging position (see above). BPV results from free-floating calcium carbonate crystals (normally attached to the utricular macule) that inadvertently enter the long arm of the posterior semicircular canal. The crystals move within the endolymph and displace the cupula. Consistent with this theory, the burst of paroxysmal positional nystagmus is in the plane of the posterior canal of the "down ear," and the positional nystagmus disappears after the ampullary nerve has been surgically resected from the posterior canal on the diseased side. If the history and physical findings are typical, a simple bedside positioning maneuver can remove the debris from the posterior semicircular canal in most patients (Fig. 517–4). If the history or findings are atypical, the condition must be distinguished from other causes of positional vertigo that may occur with tumors or infarcts of the posterior fossa.

Acute Peripheral Vestibulopathy ("Acute Labyrinthitis")

One of the most common clinical neurologic syndromes at any age is the acute onset of vertigo, nausea, and vomiting lasting for several days and not associated with auditory or neurologic symptoms. Most affected patients gradually improve over 1 to 2 weeks, but some develop recurrent episodes. A large percentage report an upper respiratory tract illness 1 to 2 weeks prior to the onset of vertigo. This syndrome occasionally occurs in epidemics (epidemic vertigo) may affect several members of the same family, and more often erupts in the spring and early summer. All of these factors suggest a viral origin, but attempts to isolate an agent have been unsuccessful, except for occasional findings of a herpes zoster infection. Pathologic studies showing atrophy of one or more vestibular nerve trunks, with or without atrophy of their associated sense organs, are evidence of a vestibular nerve site and, probably, viral cause for many patients with this syndrome (*viral neurolabyrinthitis*).

Ménière Syndrome

The typical clinical features of Ménière syndrome are described earlier. This disorder accounts for about 10% of all patients with vertigo. The diagnosis is based on documenting episodic severe attacks accompanied by fluctuating hearing levels on audiometric testing beginning in the low frequencies.

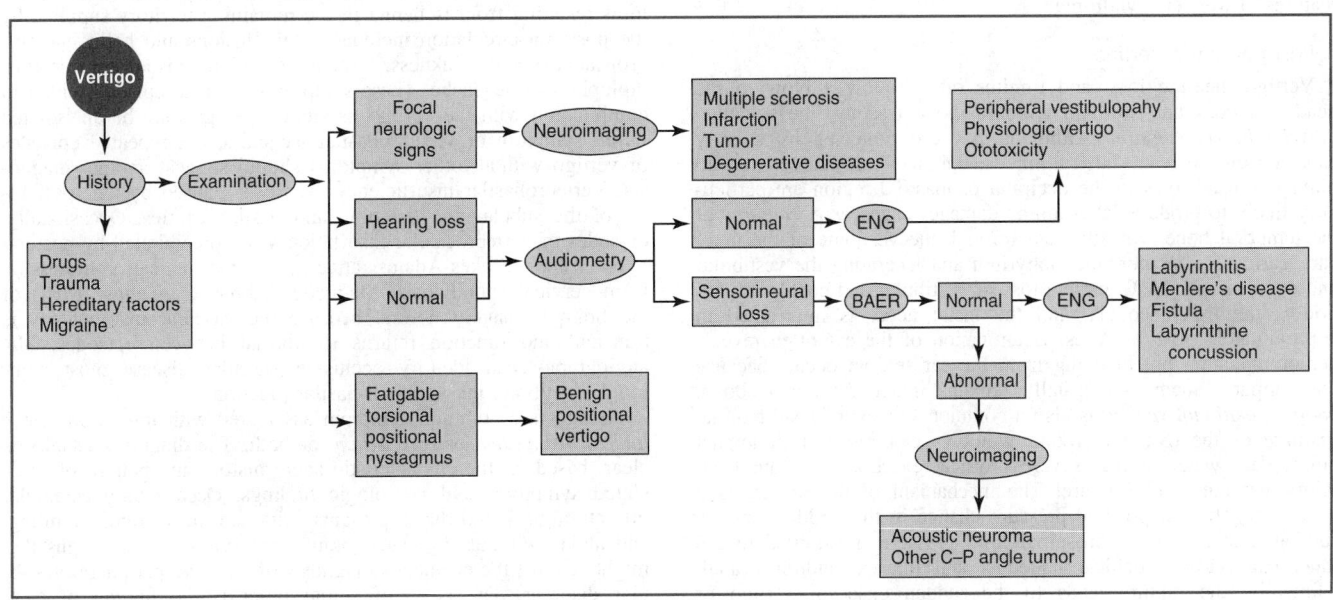

FIGURE 517–3 ■ Evaluation of vertigo.

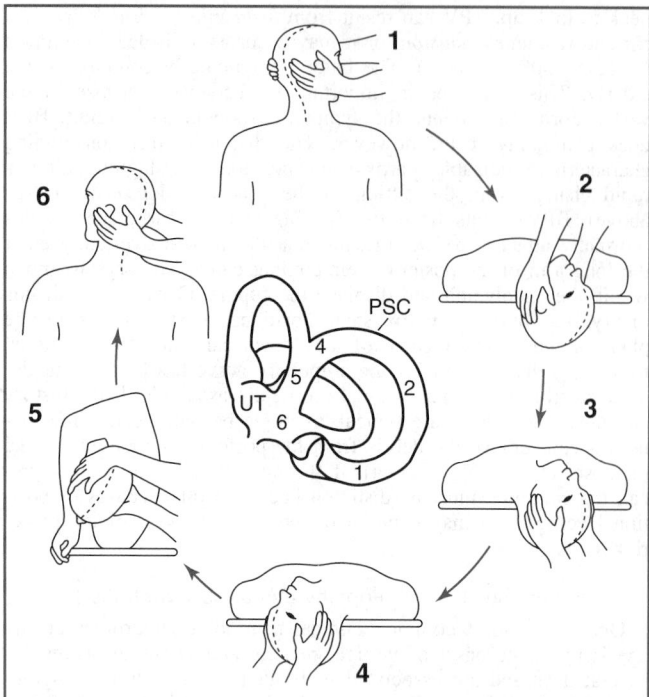

FIGURE 517-4 ■ Treatment maneuver for benign positional vertigo affecting the right ear. The procedure is reversed for treating the left ear. The numbers in the posterior semicircular canal (PSC) correspond to the position of the calcium carbonate crystals in each head position as they are moved toward the utricle (UT). Each position change is performed as rapidly as possible to accelerate the particles. Positions 2 and 3 are the same except that the therapist has moved from the front to the back of the patient to continue the maneuver easily. The entire sequence should be repeated until no nystagmus is elicited. (Courtesy of Carol A. Foster, MD, University of Colorado School of Medicine.)

Migraine

Vertigo is a common symptom with migraine. It can occur with headaches or in separate isolated episodes, and it can predate the onset of headache. So-called benign paroxysmal vertigo of childhood is often the first symptom of migraine. The mechanism of vertigo with migraine is not clear, but damage to the inner ear occurs in about one fourth of patients. A few develop typical features of Ménière syndrome.

Post-traumatic Vertigo

Vertigo, hearing loss, and tinnitus often follow a blow to the head that does not result in temporal bone fracture, the so-called *labyrinthine concussion.* Although they are protected by a bony capsule, the delicate labyrinthine membranes are susceptible to blunt trauma. Blows to the occipital or mastoid region are particularly likely to produce labyrinthine damage. *Transverse fractures* of the temporal bone typically pass through the vestibule of the inner ear, tearing the membranous labyrinth and lacerating the vestibular and cochlear nerves. Complete loss of vestibular and cochlear function is the usual sequela, and the facial nerve is interrupted in approximately 50% of cases. Examination of the ear often reveals hemotympanum, but bleeding from the ear seldom occurs because the tympanic membrane usually remains intact. As noted above, *benign positional vertigo* is also a common sequela of head trauma. *Fistulae* of the oval and round windows can result from impact noise, deep-water diving, severe physical exertion, or blunt head injury without skull fracture. The mechanism of the rupture is a sudden negative or positive pressure change in the middle ear or a sudden increase in cerebrospinal fluid pressure transmitted to the inner ear via the cochlear aqueduct and internal auditory canal. Clinically, the rupture leads to the sudden onset of vertigo or hearing loss, or both. Surgical exploration of the middle ear is warranted when there is a clear relationship between the onset of vertigo or hearing loss, or both, and the onset of severe exertion, barometric change, head injury, or impact noise.

Postconcussion Syndrome

The so-called postconcussion syndrome refers to a vague dizziness (rarely vertigo) associated with anxiety, difficulty in concentrating, headache, and photophobia induced by a head injury resulting in concussion. Occasionally, similar, less pronounced symptoms are associated with mild head injury judged to be trivial at the time. The cause is unknown, but animal studies indicate that small multifocal brain lesions (petechiae) commonly occur after concussive brain injury.

Other Peripheral Causes of Vertigo

Vertigo can be associated with *chronic bacterial otomastoiditis,* either from direct invasion of the inner ear by the bacteria or by erosion of the labyrinth by a cholesteatoma. Radiographic studies of the temporal bone readily identify these disorders. Just as *otosclerosis* can result in sensorineural hearing loss, it can also produce vertigo by involving the bony labyrinth. The typical audiometric findings of a combined conductive and sensorineural hearing loss should suggest this diagnosis. Several *drugs* that damage the auditory system, such as the aminoglycosides, may also damage the vestibular labyrinth. The patient may suffer acute vertigo, either along with or independent of hearing loss and tinnitus, if the toxic effect is asymmetric. More often there is a progressive symmetric loss of vestibular function leading to imbalance but not vertigo. Unfortunately, many patients being treated with ototoxic drugs are initially bedridden and unaware of the vestibular impairment until they recover from their acute illness and try to walk. Then they discover that they are unsteady on their feet and that the environment tends to jiggle in front of their eyes (*oscillopsia*). Younger patients adapt after weeks to the labyrinthine failure; older ones may be left permanently disabled. Usually there is no nystagmus (because of the symmetric involvement), but the patient is ataxic. Caloric and rotational tests during electronystagmography can document impairment or absence of vestibular function. The best treatment is prevention. If the drug is discontinued early during the course of symptoms, the disorder may stabilize or improve.

Vascular Insufficiency

Vertebrobasilar insufficiency is a common cause of vertigo in the elderly (see also Chapter 470). Whether the vertigo originates from ischemia of the labyrinth, brain stem, or both structures is not always clear because the blood supply to the labyrinth, eighth cranial nerve, and vestibular nuclei originate from the same source, the basilar vertebral circulation. Vertigo with *vertebrobasilar insufficiency* is abrupt in onset, usually lasting several minutes, and is frequently associated with nausea and vomiting. Associated symptoms resulting from ischemia in the remaining territory supplied by the posterior-circulation include visual illusions and hallucinations, drop attacks and weakness, visceral sensations, visual field defects, diplopia, and headache. These symptoms occur in episodes either in combination with the vertigo or alone. Vertigo may be an isolated initial symptom of vertebrobasilar ischemia, but repeated episodes of vertigo without other symptoms should suggest another diagnosis. Vertebrobasilar insufficiency usually is caused by atherosclerosis of the subclavian, vertebral, and basilar arteries. Occasionally, episodes of vertebrobasilar insufficiency are precipitated by postural hypotension, Stokes-Adams attacks, or mechanical compression from cervical spondylosis. Magnetic resonance imaging (MRI) of the brain is usually normal because the vascular insufficiency is transient and function returns to normal between episodes. MR angiography can identify occlusive vascular disease most commonly involving the vertebral-basilar junction.

Vertigo is a common symptom associated with *infarction of the lateral brain stem* or *cerebellum,* or both. The diagnosis usually is clear, based on the characteristic acute history and pattern of associated symptoms and neurologic findings. Occasionally cerebellar infarction or hemorrhage presents with severe vertigo, vomiting, and ataxia without associated brain stem symptoms and signs that might suggest the erroneous diagnosis of an acute peripheral vestibular disorder. The key differential point is the finding of clear cerebellar signs (extremity- and gait ataxia) and gaze-evoked nystagmus. Such patients must be watched carefully for several days because they may develop progressive brain stem dysfunction owing to compression by a swollen cerebellum.

Cerebellopontine-Angle Tumors

Most tumors growing in the cerebellopontine angle (e.g., *acoustic neuroma, meningioma, epidermal cyst*) grow slowly, allowing the vestibular system to accommodate so that they produce a vague sensation of disequilibrium rather than acute vertigo. Occasionally, however, episodic vertigo or positional vertigo heralds the presence of a cerebellopontine-angle tumor. In virtually all patients, retrocochlear hearing loss is present, best identified by an abnormal brain stem auditory evoked response. MRI with contrast is the most sensitive diagnostic study for identifying a cerebellopontine angle tumor.

Other Central Causes of Vertigo

Acute vertigo may be the first symptom of *multiple sclerosis,* although only a small percentage of young patients with acute vertigo eventually develop multiple sclerosis. Vertigo in multiple sclerosis is usually transient and often associated with other neurologic signs of brain stem disease, in particular, internuclear opthalmoplegia or cerebellar dysfunction. Vertigo may also be a symptom of *parainfectious encephalomyelitis* or, rarely, *parainfectious cranial polyneuritis.* In this instance, the accompanying neurologic signs establish the diagnosis. The *Ramsay-Hunt syndrome* (geniculate ganglion herpes) is characterized by vertigo and hearing loss associated with facial paralysis and, sometimes, pain in the ear. The typical lesions of herpes zoster, which may follow the appearance of neurologic signs, are found in the external auditory canal and over the palate in some patients. Rarely is herpes zoster responsible for vertigo in the absence of the full-blown syndrome. *Granulomatous meningitis* or *leptomeningeal metastasis* and cerebral or systemic *vasculitis* may involve the eighth nerve, producing vertigo as an early symptom. In these disorders cerebrospinal fluid analysis usually suggests the diagnosis. Patients suffering from *temporal lobe epilepsy* occasionally experience vertigo as the aura. Vertigo in the absence of other neurologic signs or symptoms is never caused by epilepsy or other diseases of the cerebral hemispheres.

Treatment of Vertigo

Treatment of vertigo can be divided into three general categories: specific, symptomatic, and rehabilitative. Specific therapies include antibiotics for bacterial or syphilitic labyrinthitis, anticoagulants for vertebrobasilar insufficiency, and surgery for acoustic neuroma. When possible, treatment should be directed at the underlying disorder. In most cases, however, symptomatic treatment is either combined with specific therapy or is the only treatment available (e.g., with acute peripheral vestibulopathy). Many different classes of drugs have been found to have antivertiginous properties, and in most instances the exact mechanism of action is uncertain. All of these agents produce potentially unpleasant side effects, and the decision on which drug or combination to use is based on their known complications and on the severity and duration of the vertigo. An episode of prolonged, severe vertigo is one of the most distressing symptoms that one can experience. Affected patients prefer to lie still with eyes closed in a quiet, dark room. Antivertiginous drugs with sedation such as Phenergan (25 mg four times daily [q.i.d.]) or diazepam (5 mg q.i.d.) may be helpful. Prochlorperazine suppositories (25 mg) may stop vomiting. In more chronic vertiginous disorders, when the patient is trying to carry on normal activity, less sedating antivertiginous medications such as meclizine (25 mg q.i.d.) or transdermal scopolamine (0.5 mg every 3 days) may provide relief. Vestibular rehabilitation exercises are designed to help the patient compensate for permanent loss of vestibular function.

Baloh RW: Dizziness, Hearing Loss and Tinnitus. New York, Oxford University Press, 1998. *Monograph reviewing basic and clinical aspects of auditory and vestibular function.*

Katz J: Handbook of Clinical Audiology, 4th ed. Baltimore, Williams & Wilkins, 1994. *Classic textbook and excellent reference source.*

Lanska DJ, Remler B: Benign paroxysmal positioning vertigo: Classic descriptions, origins of the provocative positioning technique, and conceptual developments. Neurology 48:1167, 1997. *How and why the positioning maneuver works.*

518 HEAD AND NECK CANCER

Adriane P. Concus ■ *Mark I. Singer*

Head and neck cancers, excluding those of cutaneous origin, comprise 3.5% of all new cancer diagnoses in the United States each year. Of these 42,000 cases, over 90% are squamous cell carcinomas of the upper aerodigestive tract. Despite newer approaches to treatment and decreased disease morbidity, long-term survival has not changed significantly over the past several decades. Head and neck cancers still have an overall 5-year survival of 60% and currently are responsible for just over 2% of cancer deaths annually in the United States.

Head and neck cancers carry enormous debilitating potential. Adverse effects on breathing, swallowing, and speech, along with disfigurement from either the tumor itself or its treatment, all too often lead to social isolation for head and neck cancer patients. A multidisciplinary approach, including input from otolaryngology, medical and radiation oncology, dentistry, social work, and speech therapy, provides the most comprehensive and effective care for head and neck cancer patients.

Head and neck cancers are staged according to the American Joint Committee on Cancer (AJCC) staging system using a T (primary tumor size), N (regional node), M (distant metastasis) classification system (Table 518–1). Each primary site has its own unique T-staging approach based on differences in anatomic structure, biologic behavior, and lymphatic drainage, but there is one common staging system for nodal and distant metastases. Head and neck cancers drain through cervical lymphatics, generally to successively contiguous ipsilateral nodes, although the base of tongue, tonsil fossae, and pharynx are common sites for bilateral nodal metastasis. For prognostic purposes and developing treatment plans, the neck is divided into five levels (Fig. 518–1). Level I, the submental and submandibular region, drains the anterior oral cavity. Level II, the jugulodigastric region, is the first echelon of nodes for the tongue, posterior oral cavity, and tonsil fossae. Hypopharynx and larynx cancers drain into level III, the midjugular nodes, and level IV, the low jugular chain. Level V, the posterior cervical triangle, drains the occiput and scalp as well as higher level neck nodes; patients with positive level V lymph nodes are very rarely cured of their disease. Carcinomas of the thyroid and parathyroids, which are covered elsewhere (see Chapters 239 and 264, respectively), are part of the differential diagnosis of any neck mass and must be considered in the evaluation of any complaint of dysphagia or hoarseness.

SQUAMOUS CELL CARCINOMA OF THE UPPER AERODIGESTIVE TRACT

Over 90% of head and neck cancers are primary squamous cell carcinomas of the upper aerodigestive tract. This complex anatomic area extends from the vermilion border of the lips to the level of the cricoid cartilage and includes the nose, paranasal sinuses, and nasopharynx. The upper aerodigestive tract is lined with stratified squamous and columnar epithelium, interspersed with minor salivary glands, lymph nodes, lymphatic and blood vessels, and nerves. The behavior of squamous cell carcinoma in different locations in the upper aerodigestive tract varies depending on the lymphatic drainage and anatomic barriers to spread such as fascia, fibroelastic membranes, perichondrium, and periosteum. For instance, true vocal cord cancers are typically contained within the larynx because of the poor lymphatic drainage of the glottis. The hypopharynx, in contrast, is an area rich in venous and lymphatic supply with few barriers to spread; squamous cell carcinoma arising in this location most frequently is advanced at detection and has the poorest prognosis of the upper aerodigestive tract malignancies. About half of upper aerodigestive tract squamous cell carcinoma occurs in the oral cavity and oropharynx, one third in the larynx, and the remainder in the hypopharynx, nasopharynx, and paranasal sinuses.

ETIOLOGY. Head and neck mucosal squamous cell carcinoma

Table 518–1 ■ AMERICAN JOINT COMMITTEE ON CANCER (AJCC) STAGING FOR HEAD AND NECK SQUAMOUS CELL CARCINOMA

LARYNX		ORAL CAVITY	OROPHARYNX	HYPOPHARYNX
Tis	Carcinoma in situ	Carcinoma in situ	Carcinoma in situ	Carcinoma in situ
T1	Tumor limited to one subsite of the larynx	Tumor ≤ 2 cm	Tumor ≤ 2 cm	Tumor ≤ 2 cm, limited to one subsite of the hypopharynx
T2	Tumor involving more than one subsite and/or impaired vocal cord mobility	Tumor > 2 cm and ≤4 cm	Tumor >2 cm and ≤4 cm	Tumor > 2 cm and ≤4 cm, involving more than one subsite
T3	Paralyzed vocal cord; involvement of pre-epiglottic or postcricoid areas (supraglottic primary)	Tumor > 4 cm	Tumor > 4 cm	Tumor > 4 cm, involving more than one subsite; paralyzed vocal cord
T4	Extension outside the larynx; cartilage invasion	Extension to soft tissues or bone outside the oral cavity	Invasion of adjacent bone or muscle	Invasion of adjacent bone/muscle/cartilage

N0	No cervical lymph nodes positive	M0	No distant metastasis
N1	Single ipsilateral lymph node ≤3 cm	M1	Distant metastasis present
N2a	Single ipsilateral lymph node >3 cm and ≤6 cm	Mx	Distant metastasis cannot be assessed
N2b	Multiple ipsilateral lymph nodes, each ≤6 cm		
N2c	Bilateral or contralateral lymph nodes, each ≤6 cm		
N3	Single or multiple lymph nodes >6 cm		

Stage	T	N	M
Stage I	T1	N0	M0
Stage II	T2	N0	M0
Stage III	T3	N0	M0
	T1–3	N1	M0
Stage IV	T4	N0–1	M0
	Any T	N2–3	M0
	Any T	Any N	M1

carcinogenesis is a multistep process of initiation, promotion, and progression reflected histologically by the transitions from the normal epithelial phenotype to dysplasia, carcinoma in situ, and invasive carcinoma. The most important predisposing risk factors for the development of primary head and neck squamous cell carcinoma is the use of alcohol and tobacco in all of its forms. Alcohol potentiates the carcinogenic effects of tobacco, and the use of the two together is more than additive in enhancing carcinogenesis.

Seventy-five per cent of head and neck cancer patients have a history of both tobacco and alcohol use.

Other associated etiologic agents include viruses. The human papillomavirus, in particular types 6, 11, 16, and 18, has been implicated in the development of upper aerodigestive tract squamous cell carcinoma. The Epstein Barr virus has been associated with nasopharyngeal carcinoma, as have dietary factors popular in southeast Asia where this type of carcinoma is most prevalent.

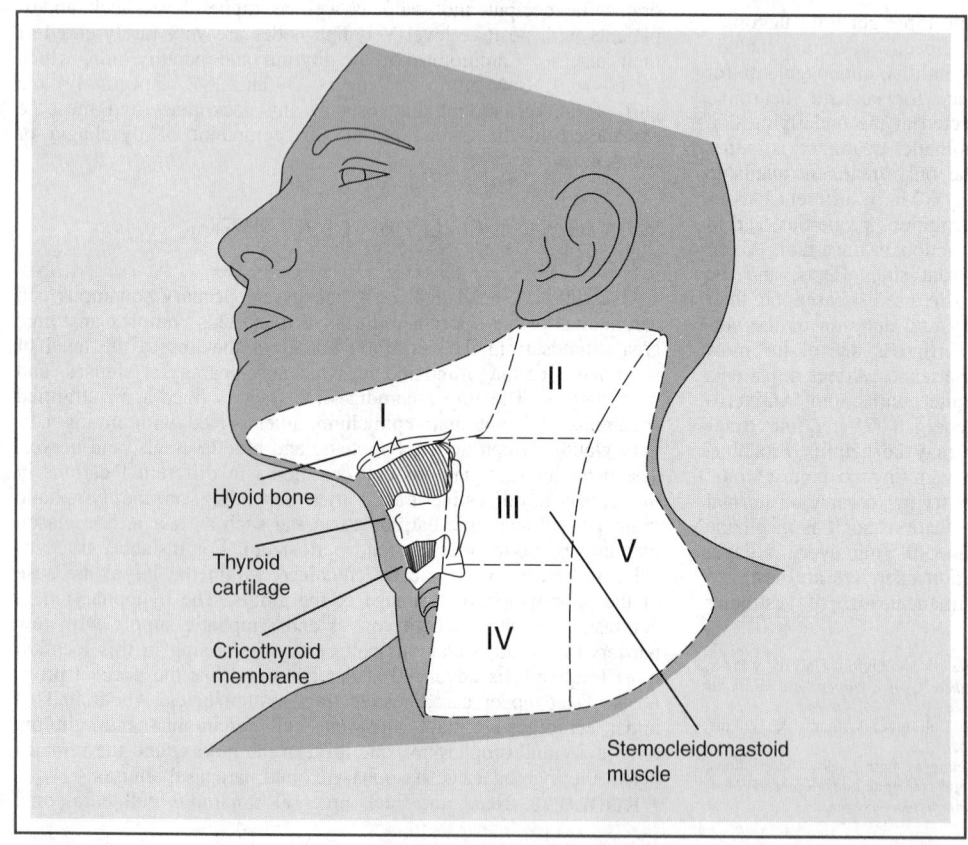

FIGURE 518–1 ■ Levels of the neck, as commonly subdivided for designation of nodal metastases. (Used with the permission of the American Joint Committee on Cancer (AJCC), Chicago, Illinois. The original source for this material is the AJCC Manual for Staging of Cancer, 4th ed. Philadelphia, Lippincott-Raven, 1992.)

Head and neck squamous cell carcinoma has a higher incidence in immunocompromised individuals, including those with human immunodeficiency virus (HIV) infection and those on chronic immunosuppression after organ transplantation. Familial studies also have suggested a genetic susceptibility. Cytogenetic changes, including loss of chromosomal heterozygosity, oncogene expression, and markers of dysregulated cell growth and proliferation are now being investigated as links in the carcinogenic process. Mutation of the *p53* tumor suppressor gene, the most common head and neck squamous cell carcinoma genetic abnormality, is found in 40 to 70% of patients and is associated with poorer response to treatment and worse prognosis.

The theory of field cancerization views the entire upper aerodigestive tract of a head and neck squamous cell carcinoma patient as "condemned mucosa," hypothesizing that chronic carcinogen exposure puts the entire area at risk for undergoing malignant transformation. Indeed, 4 to 7% of patients with a previous head and neck squamous cell carcinoma will develop a second primary squamous cell carcinoma each year, with a lifetime risk of 10 to 40%. Thus, a head and neck squamous cell carcinoma patient is a patient for life, requiring regular visits to exclude a second primary.

NATURAL HISTORY. Presenting symptoms for head and neck squamous cell carcinoma are varied and often related to the site of tumor origin. Tumors in the larynx or hypopharynx can cause hoarseness, dysphagia, odynophagia, stridor, and otalgia (ear pain referred from the pharynx by means of the glossopharyngeal nerve). An ill-fitting denture, non-healing "mouth sores," oral pain, or slurred speech may reflect an oral cavity tumor. Epistaxis, nasal obstruction, or headaches may be due to a paranasal sinus tumor. Unilateral serous otitis media in an adult is a nasopharyngeal neoplasm until proven otherwise. Other symptoms of head and neck cancers include trismus and cranial nerve palsies. Patients whose presenting compliant is an incidentally noted neck mass tend not to do as well because survival of those with nodal metastases at the time of diagnosis is half that of patients with stage I or II disease. Two thirds of patients with squamous cell carcinoma of the upper aerodigestive tract have regional nodal metastases at the time of diagnosis; 20% have distant metastases.

Head and neck squamous cell carcinoma spreads first through lymphatics to regional lymph nodes, mandating locoregional control as a goal of primary treatment. Distant systemic metastases occur most often in lung and bone, although liver, skin, brain, and other tissues also can be affected. Systemic metastases virtually never occur in the absence of regional lymphadenopathy. Hypercalcemia is seen in up to 25% of patients in far-advanced stages of the disease. Patients who die of head and neck squamous cell carcinoma succumb either to local tumor effects or to the effects of distant metastases.

DIAGNOSIS. The evaluation of a patient suspected of having an upper aerodigestive tract squamous cell carcinoma proceeds first to establish a tissue diagnosis. Lesions are varied in appearance. Early lesions can be as innocuous as an area of erythroplakia or, less often, leukoplakia. Larger tumors can be fungating, ulcerative, sessile, polypoid, or submucosal. Tumors in easily accessible areas can be sampled in the outpatient setting. Lesions in less accessible areas, such as the larynx or hypopharynx, usually require biopsy under general anesthesia. For staging purposes and because of the incidence of concurrent second primary lesions, a thorough endoscopic examination of the entire upper aerodigestive tract, typically done under general anesthesia with biopsies of all suspicious lesions, is indicated for all patients newly diagnosed with a head and neck squamous cell carcinoma.

Radiologic staging, usually with contrast medium–enhanced computed tomography (CT) or magnetic resonance imaging (MRI), helps assess the size, extent, and surgical resectability of a primary tumor and highlights the presence of suspicious nodal metastases that may not have been palpable on physical examination. Lymph nodes larger than 1 cm, those with irregular shape, and those with contrast ring enhancement or a heterogeneous appearance suggestive of central necrosis are radiologically suspicious for carcinoma. A routine chest radiograph screens for pulmonary metastases. Liver function tests or an abdominal ultrasound evaluation are sometimes included to screen for liver metastases.

Although still considered experimental, positron emission tomographic (PET) scanning identifies active tumor by highlighting metabolically active tissue and is particularly promising in the evalua-

tion of previously irradiated anatomy, whose signal characteristics on MRI or CT can be non-specific. For suspected laryngeal tumors, videostroboscopy can help document the current mobility of the vocal cords, the size and location of a laryngeal mass, and any impairment of vocal cord vibration, reflecting a submucosal process.

EVALUATION OF A NECK NODE. There is no substitute for a thorough head and neck examination in the evaluation of a neck mass. If a likely primary cancer is identified, that site is sampled and the neck node is presumed to be a metastasis from that primary site. If malignancy is suspected and no primary site is identified on physical examination, fine-needle aspiration (FNA) is indicated. In experienced hands, the specimen will give highly accurate histologic results (>95% sensitivity and specificity). CT or MRI can evaluate the size of the neck mass and possible invasion of adjacent structures and, in some cases, identify a primary source for the cancer. In particular, submucosal masses may not be apparent on physical examination but may appear as enhancing lesions on CT or MRI. If FNA identifies a malignant node but the primary source is still not identified, then direct laryngoscopy should be performed with directed random biopsies of the sites most likely to have neck metastases at the time of diagnosis and most likely to have a small focus of carcinoma hiding among redundant folds of tissue: the tonsil fossae, pyriform sinuses, nasopharynx, and base of tongue/vallecula. If no primary site is found, the tumor is considered a squamous cell carcinoma of unknown primary site and treated with radiation to the neck as well as to the upper aerodigestive tract, focusing on the same areas where random specimens have been taken. Salvage neck dissection may follow irradiation for residual carcinoma or neck mass.

Excisional biopsy of a neck node is virtually never indicated because fine-needle biopsy can give reliable results and because violation of the lymphatics may invite seeding of the neck with cancer. En bloc resection of the cervical lymphatic tissues (i.e., neck dissection) is the accepted oncologically sound treatment. The one exception to this rule is in the evaluation of lymphoma, for which excisional biopsy is performed to establish lymph node architecture, which is required for diagnosis and to direct treatment.

TREATMENT. The goal of treatment of head and neck squamous cell carcinoma is locoregional control of disease. Surgical extirpation and radiation remain the mainstays of treatment. Either surgery or irradiation can be used as the primary treatment modality for stage I and stage II squamous cell carcinoma in most anatomic locations. Surgery provides slightly better locoregional control, whereas irradiation provides better preservation of function, such as speech and swallowing. Surgical salvage of irradiation failures has slightly better success than irradiation salvage of surgical failures. Stage III and stage IV tumors are treated with both surgery and irradiation. Irradiation can be done preoperatively, but current philosophy favors postoperative irradiation to avoid the wound healing problems and alteration of lymphatic drainage patterns that irradiation may induce and to have better determination of the anatomic extent of the tumor. A study of 277 head and neck squamous cell carcinoma patients by the Radiation Treatment Oncology Group (RTOG) found a locoregional control advantage for postoperative irradiation compared with preoperative irradiation; survival rates over 10 years of follow-up were similar. Current indications for postoperative irradiation include multiple positive neck nodes, close or positive surgical margins, and perineural spread.

Ideal surgical treatment for squamous cell carcinoma of the oral cavity and pharynx is to remove the primary tumor en bloc with a 2-cm margin of normal tissue. For lesions abutting or invasive to bone, surgery should include cortical or segmental mandibulectomy or partial maxillectomy. Squamous cell carcinoma has a propensity for perineural spread; for advanced lesions, affected nerves, such as the lingual or hypoglossal, may need to be sacrificed. Because the glottic larynx has minimal lymphatic supply, early tumors of the glottis can be treated with more conservative surgical procedures. Vocal cord stripping, laser resection, and cordectomy have all been advocated for mid-cord Tis or T1 glottic squamous cell carcinoma. For slightly larger lesions and irradiation failures in anatomically favorable locations in the larynx, partial laryngectomy procedures have succeeded both in curing the cancer and preserving voice. The rare favorable T1 or T2 hypopharynx squamous cell carcinoma can be treated with partial pharyngectomy alone, but larger larynx and hypopharynx cancers require laryngectomy and (for hypopharynx involvement) partial or total pharyngectomy. The head and neck surgeon relies heavily on intraoperative frozen section biopsies of surgical margins to confirm complete removal of the tumor.

Principles of surgical treatment for regional lymph node metastases include en bloc resection of the draining nodal lymphatic areas. The standard radical neck dissection removes all nodal tissues of the neck and associated structures, including the spinal accessory nerve, internal jugular vein, and sternocleidomastoid muscle. Variations on this procedure, preserving one or more of these nonlymphatic structures (modified neck dissection), can be tailored to the individual case.

Treatment of the N0 neck for large squamous cell carcinoma primary tumors remains controversial. If the risk of occult positive nodal metastasis exceeds 20 to 30%, a selective neck dissection (removal of the first three or four echelons of nodal drainage, sparing other neck structures) is often included for staging purposes at the time of primary tumor resection. A pathologically N0 neck does not require further treatment. Alternatively, irradiation can be used to treat a neck considered at risk, with surgical treatment reserved for future recurrence. Primary sites with high rates of occult nodal metastasis include the anterior floor of mouth, the tongue, and hypopharynx.

Postoperative irradiation should start within 4 to 6 weeks after the surgical procedure. Typical postoperative irradiation delivers, in 180- to 200-cGy daily fractions, total doses to the primary site ranging from 6000 cGy for small lesions up to 7500 cGy for large bulky tumors. A dose of 5000 cGy to nodal drainage areas clinically free of disease is standard. Interstitial radioactive implants offer an alternative means of delivering extremely high doses of radiation to small tissue volumes; tongue lesions are particularly amenable to this mode of treatment.

In an effort to increase the total radiation dose for therapeutic purposes, changes in the standard daily radiation fraction schedule have been devised. Hyperfractionation reduces the dose of each individual fraction but reaches a higher total dose of radiation by giving two or more fractions per day. Overall duration of therapy is usually the same as for standard fractionation. Accelerated fractionation delivers the same total dose of radiation, compressed into a shorter period of time, typically with multiple fractions per day. Acute radiation effects sometimes require a 1- to 2-week break in the middle of treatment. Altered fractionation protocols have shown some improved locoregional control, but so far no survival advantage over standard fractionation.

Irradiation is the first choice of treatment for nasopharyngeal carcinoma, which has a propensity for earlier nodal metastasis and is more radiosensitive than other upper aerodigestive tract squamous cell carcinomas. Recent studies suggest an improved response using concomitant chemotherapy for advanced disease. Surgical treatment is reserved for selected recurrent cases that have failed other treatment modalities.

Side effects of surgical treatment for head and neck squamous cell carcinoma include impairment of function (swallowing, speech), due to loss of tissue and structures, and cosmetic defects. Modern surgical techniques with pedicled flaps and free tissue transfer can reconstruct deficits to improve functional and cosmetic outcome. Modified neck dissection has helped to limit cranial nerve deficits. Voice rehabilitation after total laryngectomy is achieved best with a tracheoesophageal stent prosthesis or esophageal speech. An electrolarynx offers a somewhat more cumbersome alternative.

Short-term effects from irradiation include mucositis and skin desquamation. The most disabling long-term side effect is xerostomia resulting from permanent damage to the major and minor salivary glands. The dry mouth is treated with hydration, salivary substitutes, and cholinergic agonists (pilocarpine). Xerostomia leads to changes in the microenvironment of the mouth, which can lead to dental carries and osteomyelitis. For this reason, extraction of partly diseased teeth is often recommended before the start of irradiation. Osteoradionecrosis and chondroradionecrosis are debilitating long-term effects that may require treatment with hyperbaric oxygen, mandibular replacement, or even laryngectomy. Other long-term effects of irradiation include thickening and fibrosis of

the skin and soft tissues, chronic serous otitis media, cataracts, sensorineural hearing loss, loss of taste, dysphagia, and ablation of remaining thyroid function.

Chemotherapy is currently used for palliation in recurrent, inoperable, or widely metastatic head and neck squamous cell carcinoma. Single-agent methotrexate, the historical gold standard, administered weekly yields a 30% response lasting up to 6 months in most studies. Cisplatin-based multiagent regimens have responses equivalent or superior to methotrexate. Many recent trials have addressed the role of chemotherapy in the primary treatment of head and neck squamous cell cancers. Studies of neoadjuvant, concomitant, and adjuvant chemotherapy for resectable head and neck squamous cell cancers suggest improved locoregional control and disease-free survival, highlighting the feasibility of organ preservation. Perhaps the best known of these trials is the Veterans Affairs Laryngeal Cancer Study Group, which enrolled 333 patients with advanced, resectable larynx cancer and randomized them to standard surgery with postoperative irradiation versus neoadjuvant chemotherapy, with responders proceeding on to more chemotherapy and definitive irradiation. After 8 years of follow-up, survival was the same in both arms of the study. There were more locoregional recurrences and fewer distant metastases in the chemotherapy/irradiation group. Of the patients randomized to the chemotherapy arm of the protocol, 60% had their larynges preserved. Multi-institutional phase III trials are in progress looking further into the usefulness of chemotherapy as an adjunctive primary treatment for head and neck squamous cell carcinoma. Because prolonged life expectancy has not been established, the use of chemotherapy in resectable disease is still considered experimental and should be administered only in formalized experimental protocols.

Second primary squamous cell carcinomas are the most common cause of death in patients previously treated for early stage head and neck squamous cell carcinoma. These second primary tumors have been prevented by vitamin A derivatives, the retinoids, which are known modulators of epithelial cell differentiation and have been shown to arrest, and even to reverse, the multistep process toward mucosal squamous carcinogenesis. In one study, 103 patients who were previously treated successfully for head and neck squamous cell carcinoma were randomized to 13-cis-retinoic acid (50–100 mg/m^2/day) versus placebo for 12 months. After 32 months of follow-up, the retinoid-treated group had only 4% incidence of second primary tumors compared with 24% in the placebo group. There was no effect in preventing recurrence of the original primary tumor. Side effects of the retinoids, including cheilitis, conjunctivitis, dry skin, and hypertriglyceridemia, limit the use of 13-cis-retinoic acid at these doses, but further studies are underway because this is promising chemoprevention of upper aerodigestive tract squamous cell carcinoma.

An adenovirus-mediated transfer of wild type p53 tumor suppressor gene has been effective in suppressing squamous cell carcinoma growth both in vitro, with human head and neck squamous cell carcinoma cell lines, and in vivo, in a mouse squamous cell carcinoma model. Molecular therapy for head and neck cancer may well revolutionize treatment for this frequently devastating group of diseases.

PROGNOSIS. Nodal metastasis at the time of diagnosis is the single most important prognostic factor and is associated with about a 50% reduction in 5-year survival compared with stage I and II disease (Table 518–2). Unfortunately, over 60% of patients with head and neck squamous cell carcinoma initially present with regional adenopathy and stage III or IV disease. Primary tumor site and size also have bearing on long-term prognosis. Larynx cancers have the most favorable prognosis, perhaps because these primary tumors are detected at an early stage due to hoarseness, the most

Table 518–2 ■ FIVE-YEAR DISEASE-FREE SURVIVAL, HEAD AND NECK SQUAMOUS CELL CARCINOMA, SELECTED SITES

	STAGE I	STAGE II	STAGE III	STAGE IV
Floor of mouth	68%	55%	28%	9%
Tonsil	>92%	71%	41%	21%
Base of tongue	82%	62%	48%	29%
Hypopharynx	59%	47%	28%	7%
Supraglottis	83%	67%	50%	25%
Glottis	>95%	80%	65%	45%

common symptom. By comparison, tumors of the hypopharynx present most often at an advanced stage, perhaps because they are not symptomatic until they have become large and invasive. Other features reflecting aggressive disease include extracapsular spread in involved lymph nodes, perineural spread of tumor, and intravascular invasion. Various histologic features including grade, differentiation, keratinization, and mitotic rate are frequently reported but do not correlate as strongly with prognosis. Recent work in molecular biology has introduced the possibility of molecular pathologic staging. In one study, mutations of the p53 tumor suppressor gene in the surgical margins and lymph nodes in histologically clean head and neck squamous cell carcinoma resections predicted recurrence at the resection margin within a mean follow-up period of 17 months, compared with no recurrences in the p53 negative margins.

Most treatment failures occur within the first 2 years. Follow-up every 4 to 8 weeks is therefore recommended for the first 2 years after treatment to screen for recurrence or new primary tumors. Routine chest radiographs should be obtained every 6 to 12 months. Patients are considered cured if they remain disease-free for 5 years, although continued follow-up at 6-month intervals is appropriate. In light of the high incidence of radiation-induced thyroid dysfunction, levels of thyroid-stimulating hormone should be monitored in such patients.

NON-SQUAMOUS CELL HEAD AND NECK CANCER

SALIVARY GLAND NEOPLASMS. Anatomically, the salivary glands consist of three paired major glands (parotid, submandibular, and sublingual) and nearly 1000 minor salivary glands lining the upper aerodigestive tract. Only 25 to 30% of salivary gland neoplasms are malignant, and over 50% of these malignancies occur in the parotid. Low-dose radiation exposure has been implicated as a risk factor, and tobacco may be a risk factor for epithelial salivary gland tumors. Exposure to wood dust and nickel refining are risk factors for minor salivary gland cancers of the sinonasal tract.

Most salivary gland malignancies present as incidentally noted masses. Facial nerve paresis or paralysis, pain, lymph node metastases, or other cranial nerve involvement at presentation are ominous signs. Fine-needle aspiration of salivary neoplasms gives accurate diagnostic information (77% sensitivity, 96% specificity) and guides therapy. Preoperative MRI or CT is indicated only if resectability or lymph node involvement is in question.

Acinic cell carcinoma and low-grade mucoepidermoid carcinoma are considered low-grade tumors (Table 518–3), whereas adenocarcinoma, adenoid cystic carcinoma, squamous cell carcinoma, carcinoma ex-pleomorphic adenoma, high-grade mucoepidermoid carcinoma, and undifferentiated carcinoma are high-grade histologies. Mucoepidermoid carcinoma is the most common malignancy of the parotid gland; adenoid cystic carcinoma is the most common malignancy of the submandibular and minor salivary glands. Each histologic cell type derives from a different part of the salivary gland unit and has its own unique biologic behavior. Carcinoma ex-pleomorphic adenoma, which is a malignant degeneration of a pleomorphic adenoma, is characterized by rapid growth in a mass that has been stable, sometimes for years. Adenoid cystic carcinoma tends to invade and travel along nerves; it can be insidious in its growth, and patients can live for many years before recurrence is detected. Unlike squamous cell carcinoma of the major salivary glands, which often spreads to the cervical lymphatics, the other histologic types spread to regional lymph nodes in only 10% of cases.

Treatment is primarily surgical, with excision of the entire gland for major salivary gland cancers or a wide cuff of normal tissue for minor salivary gland cancers. Great care is taken to preserve the facial nerve during parotidectomy unless the facial nerve is directly involved with tumor. Postoperative radiation is reserved for advanced disease or high-grade tumors. Overall 5-year survival is over 70%.

PARANASAL SINUSES. Cancer of the paranasal sinuses comprises only 3% of all upper aerodigestive tract malignancies. Of these, over half are squamous cell carcinomas, most commonly involving the maxillary antrum. Adenocarcinoma, the second most common histologic type, is found most often in the ethmoid sinuses. Minor salivary glands in the paranasal sinuses can also give rise to adenoid cystic carcinoma and mucoepidermoid carcinoma. Other epithelial-derived sinonasal tract malignancies are melanoma, esthesioneuroblastoma, and undifferentiated carcinomas. Soft tissue sarcomas, with rhabdomyosarcoma being the most common, and lymphoreticular malignancies are also found in the paranasal sinuses. Tumors that metastasize to the paranasal sinuses include renal cell carcinoma and breast and lung cancers. Malignant tumors virtually never involve the sphenoid or frontal sinuses.

Risk factors for paranasal sinus malignancies include occupational exposures such as woodworking, leather tanning, and nickel refining. Symptoms are often vague (nasal obstruction, epistaxis, nasal discharge, hyposmia, cheek or eye edema) and explain why these cancers frequently are not discovered until the symptoms have been present for several months and the tumors are at advanced stage. Cranial neuropathies are present in 34% of patients at presentation and are a poor prognostic sign.

Evaluation includes a careful physical examination with attention to the cranial nerves. Both CT and MRI are helpful, because the CT will highlight areas of bony erosion and the MRI will show soft tissue definition and separate tumor from mucus or normal adjacent tissue. Epithelial tumors are staged according to location, size, and extension to surrounding structures, such as the orbit and skull base. Mesenchymal tumors are staged according to histologic criteria.

Surgery is the treatment of choice, with irradiation reserved for the adjuvant setting for close surgical margins or invasion into adjacent structures. Modern skull base surgical procedures have succeeded in removing many paranasal sinus tumors that previously would have been deemed non-resectable. Chemotherapy is not of proven benefit, except for lymphoma and extramedullary plasmacytoma, where irradiation and chemotherapy are first choice treatments. Neck dissection is not done electively because only 10% of paranasal sinus squamous cell carcinomas have cervical nodal involvement and other histologic types have even less. The finding of positive neck nodes at the time of diagnosis is a poor prognostic sign but is not a contraindication for aggressive resection.

LYMPHOMA. Ten per cent of lymphomas present in the head and neck. Over half of these originate in the lymphatic tissues of Waldeyer's ring (palatine tonsils, base of tongue, nasopharynx). Cervical adenopathy is noted in 15% of patients with head and neck lymphomas at presentation. The remainder of head and neck lymphomas originate at extralymphatic sites, including the sinonasal tract, oral cavity, salivary glands, larynx, thyroid, and orbit.

Table 518–3 ■ SALIVARY GLAND CARCINOMAS: FREQUENCY AND 5-YEAR SURVIVAL

	% OF SALIVARY GLAND MALIGNANCIES	5-YR SURVIVAL
Low-Grade Tumors		
Acinic cell carcinoma	3%	85%
Low-grade mucoepidermoid carcinoma	20%	70%
High-Grade Tumors		
Adenocarcinoma	1–9%	60%
Adenoid cystic carcinoma	6–16%	62%
Squamous cell carcinoma	1%	25%
Carcinoma ex-pleomorphic adenoma	3–12%	40%
High-grade mucoepidermoid carcinoma	15%	47%
Undifferentiated carcinoma	2%	20%

The typical patient is male and in the sixth decate of life, although HIV-infected and other immunocompromised patients have a higher incidence of lymphoma at younger age. Thyroid and orbital lymphomas occur more often in women.

Presenting symptoms are similar to those of squamous cell carcinoma and include sore throat, dysphagia, airway or nasal obstruction, foreign body sensation, hoarseness, or an incidentally noted mass. Only 12% of patients with primary head and neck lymphoma have systemic symptoms of fever, weight loss, and night sweats.

Fine-needle aspiration is a useful diagnostic tool to distinguish lymphoma from other neoplasms and from benign lymphocytic hyperplasia. Because treatment of lymphoma depends on the number of sites involved above and below the diaphragm as well as histologic classification, open biopsy for formal tissue diagnosis is imperative. Lymphomas can be confused with undifferentiated carcinoma and melanoma; special tissue stains distinguish between these cancers. A full lymphoma staging evaluation (see Chapter 179) includes blood tests; CT or MRI imaging of the head and neck, chest, and abdomen; and bone marrow biopsy.

Treatment of head and neck lymphoma is with irradiation, chemotherapy, or a combination of the two. Three thousand to 4000 cGy is given for low-grade lymphomas and 4000 to 5000 cGy is given for intermediate- or high-grade lymphomas. Intermediate-grade early-stage lymphoma of the head and neck carries the best prognosis, with 5-year disease free survival reported as high as 100% with combined therapy. Lymphomas of the paranasal sinuses have the worst prognosis, with a propensity for central nervous system involvement and poor response to treatment; 5-year survival is less than 20%.

SOFT TISSUE MALIGNANCIES. Sarcomas involving the head and neck are rare. Malignant fibrous histiocytoma, the most common adult soft tissue sarcoma, occurs in association with previous irradiation. Angiosarcoma, an aggressive malignant tumor of vascular endothelial cell origin, is found in the scalp, neck, mouth, and maxillary antrum. It has a rapid onset but usually minimal symptoms. Hemangiopericytoma is a tumor arising from capillary connective tissues and can occur anywhere in the body; in the head and neck it has the same distribution as that of angiosarcoma. Chondrosarcomas of the larynx are typically low grade with a low potential for metastasis. Other soft tissue malignancies seen in the head and neck include rhabdomyosarcomas, fibrosarcomas, synovial sarcomas, and osteogenic sarcomas. Surgery is the treatment of choice for soft tissue sarcomas and in general the only modality affording the possibility of cure; irradiation is reserved for the adjuvant setting or palliation in non-resectable disease.

PARAGANGLIOMAS. Paragangliomas arise from neural crest cells located at the carotid body, the vagal body, and the jugulotympanic region and are called carotid body tumors, glomus vagales, glomus jugulares, and glomus tympanicum (limited to the middle ear). These tumors are typically extremely vascular and require embolization before surgical excision to minimize blood loss. Approximately 10% are hormonally active, excreting sympathomimetics that can precipitate hypertensive crises on the operating table. Surgery is the treatment of choice. Radiation therapy is used for palliation or in patients who are not surgical candidates.

Brennan JA, Mao L, Hruban RH, et al: Molecular assessment of histopathological staging in squamous-cell carcinoma of the head and neck. N Engl J Med 332:429–435, 1995. *A study detecting p53 in histologically negative surgical margins and lymph nodes as an indicator of occult disease.*

Clayman GL, Lippman SM, Laramore, Hong WK: Head and neck cancer. *In* Holland JF, Frei E, Bast RC, Maron DL (eds): Cancer Medicine, 4th ed. Baltimore, Williams & Wilkins, pp 1645–1710. *A thorough chapter on head and neck cancer, including nearly 800 references.*

Department of Veterans Affairs Laryngeal Cancer Study Group: Induction chemotherapy plus radiation compared with surgery plus radiation in patients with advanced laryngeal cancer. N Engl J Med 324:1685–1690, 1997. *Well-known clinical trial demonstrating similar survival in patients treated with total laryngectomy versus chemotherapy and radiation for advanced larynx cancer.*

Hong WK, Lippman SM, Itri LM, et al: Prevention of second primary tumors with isotretinoin in squamous cell carcinoma of the head and neck. N Engl J Med 323:795–801, 1990. *Clinical trial showing that retinoids can prevent the occurrence of second primary squamous cell carcinomas.*

McGuirt WF: The neck mass. Med Clin North Am 83:219–234, 1999. *A description of the proper evaluation of a neck mass, both malignant and benign.*

PART XXVII

SKIN DISEASES

519 STRUCTURE AND FUNCTION OF SKIN

Frank Parker

The skin is a dynamic organ containing a variety of tissues, cell types, and specialized structures, which together serve multiple functions important to health and survival. The skin interfaces with our dry, hostile environment and provides many functions crucial to survival, including protection against the elements (e.g., ultraviolet irradiation, mechanical and chemical injury, invasion by infectious agents, and prevention of desiccation and dehydration) and thermoregulation. The skin functions as a sensory receptor that monitors diverse environmental stimuli and plays an active role in immunologic surveillance. In many circumstances, the skin also actively reflects internal disease process.

The skin's variety of functions can be correlated with specific properties and anatomy of the epidermis and dermis. The epidermis differentiates to form enucleate cornified cells that act as a relatively impermeable protective barrier (stratum corneum) to the outward loss of body fluids and the inward penetration of various chemicals, allergens, and microorganisms. The lamellae of cornified stratum corneum surface cells, together with the brown pigment melanin, also help protect against the carcinogenic effects of ultraviolet radiation. Two anatomic features of the dermis play a vital role in thermoregulation: its unique massive microcirculatory system and its specialized cutaneous appendages, the sweat glands. Finally, the skin is important immunologically. Both epidermis (Langerhan's cells) and dermis (the epidermal-dermal junction structures) participate in a number of immunologic reactions that generate a variety of inflammatory skin diseases.

Skin problems are exceedingly common: Some 30% of Americans have dermatologic conditions requiring a physician's care. Fungal infections, other skin infections, and eczemas represent the most common problems. Furthermore, the health of the skin, the hair, and the nails are of cosmetic importance and can contribute to or detract from psychological well-being.

ANATOMIC CONSIDERATIONS

The skin is composed of two mutually dependent layers: the outer epidermis and the inner dermis, both cushioned on the fat-containing subcutaneous tissue, the panniculus adiposus (Figs. 519–1 and 519–2).

EPIDERMIS. The epidermis is a continuously renewing multilayered organ that constantly differentiates. The stratified structure contains two main zones of cells (keratinocytes): an inner region of viable cells known as the stratum germinativum and an outer layer of anucleate cells known as the stratum corneum, or horny layer. Three strata of cells are recognized in the germinativum: the basal, spinous, and granular layers, each representing progressive stages of differentiation and keratinization of the epidermal cells as they evolve into the dead, tightly packed stratum corneum cells on the skin surface.

The epidermis is derived from the mitotic division of the basal cells resting on the basement membrane (basal lamina), with the daughter cells moving outward to the surface, where they become polyhedral as they synthesize increasing quantities of keratin. These stratum spinosum cells attach to one another mechanically by desmosomes, which are complex modifications of the cellular membranes that impart a spinous or quill-like appearance to the cells. Desmosomes play a crucial role in maintaining the adherence of the epidermal cells to one another. They contain several intracellular proteins (i.e., desmoplakins, which are the paraneoplastic pemphigus autoantigens) and transmembrane proteins (desmogleins, which function as the pemphigus foliaceus and pemphigus vulgaris autoantigens). With further outward displacement the differentiating cells of the spinous layer become flattened, and refractile keratohyalin granules appear in the cytoplasm, accounting for the designation of granular layer that rests just below the stratum corneum. These granules are the site of active synthesis of filaggrin, which causes keratin filaments to aggregate in parallel array, forming the tough, "chemically resistant" internal structure of the stratum corneum cells.

The transformation from viable granular cells to anucleate, non-

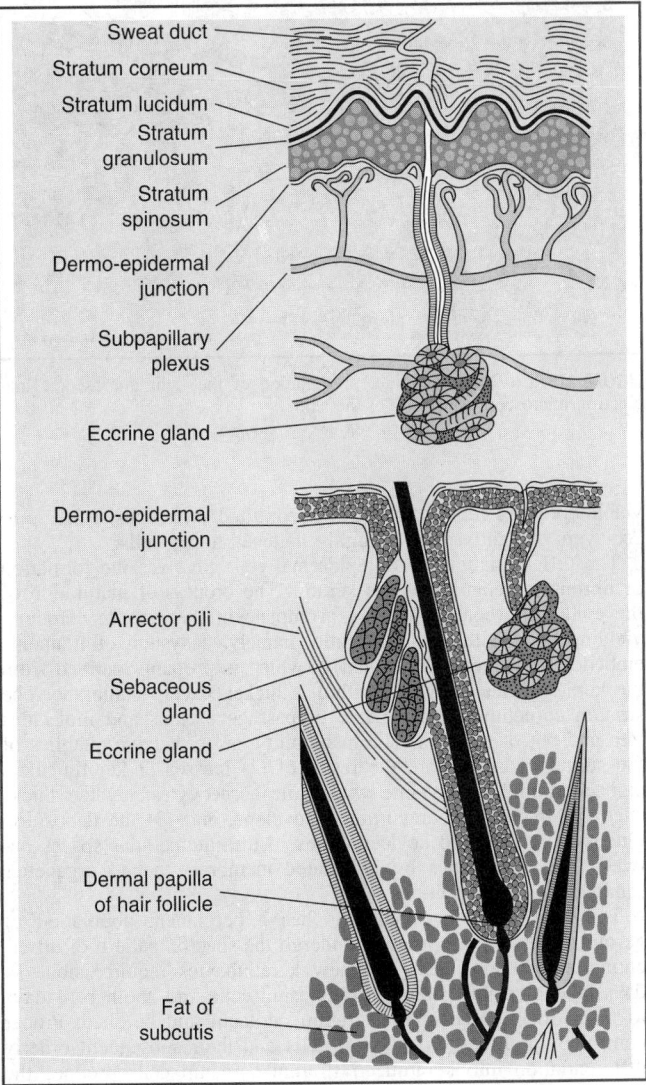

FIGURE 519–1 ■ Structure of the skin. (Adapted from the 17th edition of the *Cecil Textbook of Medicine* with the permission of Dr. Marie-Louise Johnson.)

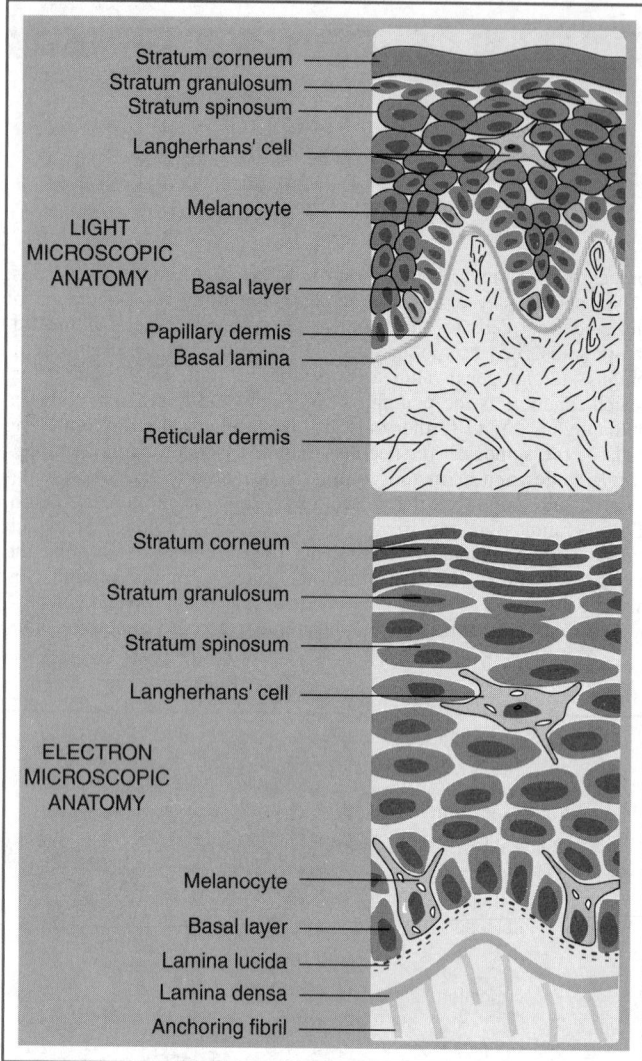

FIGURE 519–2 ■ Diagrammatic representation of the light microscopic and electron microscopic anatomy of the skin.

viable cornified cells is abrupt. The cornified layer consists of up to 25 layers of tightly packed, highly flattened horny cells.

The differentiation of the epidermal cells involves the formation of fibrous proteins known as keratin. The process of maturation of the epidermis (cornification) is complete in the stratum corneum, yielding cells with mature keratin, namely, a system of filaments embedded in a continuous matrix (which is probably derived from the keratohyaline granules) within a thickened cell membrane. The stratum corneum limits the rate of passage of ions and molecules into and out of the skin. The insolubility and protective qualities of the stratum corneum are the result of (1) masses of keratin fibers embedded in keratohyaline within the corneocytes, (2) the thickened cell membrane or cornified envelope, and (3) the deposition glucosylceramide and acylceramines in the intercellular spaces between the corneocytes by lamellated membrane bound organelles found in the upper spinous layer.

The basal layer of epidermis has a permanent population of germinal cells whose progeny undergo the specific pattern of differentiation just described. The new keratinocytes require about 14 days to evolve into stratum granulosum cells and another 14 days to reach the surface of the stratum corneum and be shed. Proper control of proliferation of basal cells and their subsequent orderly differentiation into keratinized stratum corneum cells produce the smooth, pliable surface of the skin. Alterations in the homeostatic state of cell division, defects in differentiation, or changes in exfoliation from the surface can lead to irregularities in the skin sur-

face, characterized as roughening, scaling, and hyperkeratosis (accumulation of excessive layers of stratum corneum).

Two other cell types are found in the epidermis: the melanocyte and the Langerhans' cell. Both are dendritic cells with cytoplasmic arms that stretch out to contact the keratinocytes in their vicinity. The melanocytes are pigment (melanin)-producing cells that are arrayed in the basal epidermal layer and hair follicles, whereas the Langerhans' cells are usually found in the suprabasal layers of the epidermis, and at times in the dermis. Each dendritic cell has a different origin and function.

Melanocytes evolve in the neural crest of the embryo and migrate to the skin in early embryonic life. These cells synthesize brown, red, and yellow melanin pigments that give the skin its distinctive coloration. Melanocytes contain submicroscopic organelles (melanosomes) that synthesize melanin. A specific enzyme, tyrosinase, found within the melanosome, oxidizes tyrosine to dihydroxyphenylalanine (DOPA) and then to DOPA quinone. Additional non-enzymatic oxidation and polymerization occur to form the final product, melanin. Two kinds of melanin are recognized: eumelanin (brown-black biochrome) and phaeomelanin (yellow-red biochrome that contains large quantities of cysteine). The genetic make-up of the individual determines which melanin is produced, thus providing the various colors and hues of skin and hair. Once melanosomes are fully melanized, the resulting granules are transported out the dendritic processes of the melanocyte and transferred into the adjacent epidermal cells or hair.

Langerhans' cells, derived from bone marrow, contain a unique submicroscopic racket-shaped organelle (Birbeck granule) that plays a major immunologic role in the skin (see Fig. 519–2). They contain surface receptors for immunoglobulins, and Ia-antigens, capturing external antigenic materials that contact the skin and circulating them to draining lymph nodes. Langerhans' cells thus play a central role in delayed hypersensitivity reactions of the skin (allergic contact dermatitis).

DERMIS. Beneath the epidermis lies the principal mass of the skin, the dermis, which is a tough, resilient tissue with viscoelastic properties. It consists of a three-dimensional matrix of loose connective tissue composed of fibrous proteins (collagen and elastin) embedded in an amorphous ground substance (glycosaminoglycans). At the microscopic level the collagen fibers resemble an irregular meshwork oriented somewhat parallel to the epidermis. Coarse elastic fibers are entwined in the collagenous fibers and are particularly abundant over the face and neck. This fibrous and elastic matrix serves as a scaffolding within which networks of blood vessels, nerves, and lymphatics intertwine and the epidermal appendages, sweat glands, and pilosebaceous units rest.

DERMOEPIDERMAL JUNCTION. The structures situated at the interface between the epidermis and dermis constitute an anatomic functional unit of complex membranes and lamellae laced by divergent types of filaments that together serve to support the epidermis, weld the epidermis to the dermis, and act as a filter to the transfer of materials and inflammatory or neoplastic cells across the junction zone. At the level of light microscopy, this boundary zone is seen as an undulating pattern of rete ridges (downward finger-like or ridgelike extensions of the epidermis) and dermal papillae (upward projections of the dermis into the epidermis) (see Fig. 519–2). Periodic acid–Schiff (PAS) staining discloses a thin uniform zone of intense reaction along this undulating junction that represents the basement membrane. Electron microscopic, immunoelectron microscopic, immunologic, biochemical, and genetic studies have elucidated the complexity of this region and are providing new insights into the pathogenesis of a variety of cutaneous diseases. Keratin filaments, hemidesmosomes, lamina lucida, lamina densa, anchoring filaments, and anchoring fibrils each function to maintain different levels of basement membrane adhesion (Fig. 519–3). A variety of inherited mechanobullous diseases (epidermolysis bullosa) as well as autoimmune bullous diseases (pemphigoid, herpes gestationis, bullous systemic lupus erythematosus) involve separation and bullous formation at various levels of the dermoepidermal junction.

CUTANEOUS APPENDAGES. Two to 3 million eccrine sweat glands distributed over all parts of the body surface participate in thermoregulation by producing hypotonic sweat that evaporates during heat or emotional stress (see Fig. 519–1). The combined output of these glands may exceed 1.5 L/hour. Each gland is a simple tubule with a coiled secretory segment deep in the dermis and a straight

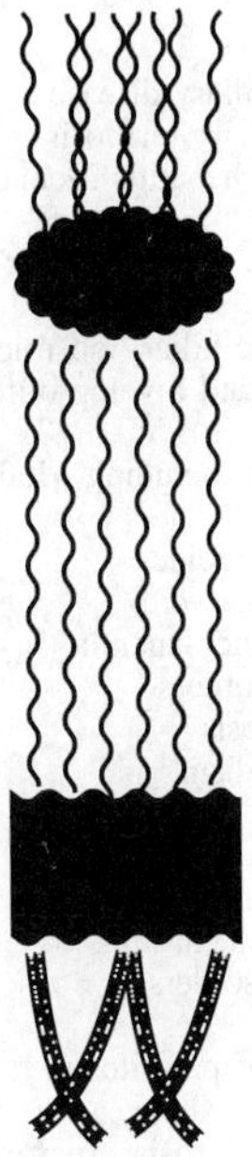

ELECTRON MICROSCOPIC STRUCTURE	MOLECULAR ORGANIZATION	DISEASES ASSOCIATED WITH GENETIC DEFECTS OR AUTOIMMUNE CONDITIONS
Keratins	Type 5 & 14 keratins	Epidermolysis bullosa simplex
Hemidesmosome	BP 230 kD BP 180 kD	Bullous pemphigoid Herpes gestationis Cicatricial pemphigus
Lamina lucida	Laminin, nidogen	
Anchoring filaments	Kalanin/nicein K-laminin	Junctional epidermolysis bullosa
Lamina densa	Type IV collagen	Alport's syndrome Goodpasture's syndrome
Anchoring fibrils	Type VII collagen	Dystrophic epidermolysis bullosa Bullous systemic lupus erythematosus

FIGURE 519–3 ■ Structures and diseases of the dermoepidermal junction.

duct extending up to the skin's surface. The glands respond to thermal stimulation and emotional stress.

Apocrine sweat glands in the axillae, circumanal and perineal areas, external auditory canals, and areolae of the breasts secrete viscid, milky material that accounts for axillary odor when bacteria degrade the secretion. Presumably, they are the vestigial remnants of lower species that communicate by cutaneous chemicals.

PILOSEBACEOUS APPENDAGES. Hair units, or pilosebaceous appendages, are found over the entire skin surface except on the palms, soles, and glans penis (see Fig. 519–1). Hair follicles consist of a shaft surrounded by an epithelial sheath continuous with the epidermis, the sebaceous gland, and the arrector pili smooth muscle. The bulb contains the proliferating pool of undifferentiated cells that gives rise to various layers comprising the hair and the follicle. The proliferating cells in the bulb differentiate into a hair consisting of keratinized, hard, imbricated, flattened cortex cells surrounding a central medullary space. The sebaceous glands are multilobular holocrine glands that connect into the pilosebaceous canal (hair canal) through the sebaceous duct. Germinative undifferentiated sebaceous cells at the periphery of each lobule of the gland generate daughter cells that move to the central areas of each acinus as they differentiate and form sebum (a complex oily substance composed of triglycerides and diglycerides, fatty acids, wax esters, squalene, and sterols). Most sebaceous glands adjoin a hair follicle, although some open directly on the skin surface. Sebaceous glands are also found normally in the buccal mucosa (Fordyce's spots), around the female areola (Montgomery's tubercles), on the prepuce (Tyson's glands), and in the eyelids (meibomian glands). The sebaceous glands and certain hair follicles are androgen-dependent target organs. Follicles particularly responsive to androgen stimulation are found over the frontal and vertex areas of scalp, beard, chest, axillae, and upper and lower pubic triangles.

Hair follicles are formed in early embryonic life, and no more develop after birth. Males and females have approximately the same number of hair follicles distributed over the body, but the degree of hairiness depends on two distinct features of hair growth—the *hair cycle* and the *hair pattern*. Hair growth consists of recurring cycles of growth, regression, and resting. The resting hair lies high in the follicle, where it forms a stubby hair bulb that is easily shed. Growth begins with a burst of mitotic activity, and the follicle grows downward to reconstitute a new hair bulb. The hair bulb cells divide rapidly and keratinize to form a new hair

shaft that dislodges the old resting club telogen hair. Regression provides a brief respite when mitosis ceases and the hair follicle pulls upward in the dermis as the hair shaft evolves into a resting club hair. In the adult scalp 85% of the hairs are in a growth state, 14% in a resting state, and 1% in regression. Considerable variation in timing of the hair cycle occurs from one region of the body to another, and the duration of growth determines the length of hairs.

Hair cycles also vary with the second important feature of hair growth, namely, hair pattern or the type of hair growing in each follicle. Two types of hairs are seen: vellus hair (fine, soft, short, non-pigmented, and common on "non-hairy" areas of the body) and terminal hair (coarse, long, pigmented, and found on hairy areas of the body).

Dramatic changes occur at puberty in both hair cycle and hair pattern mediated by either testosterone or dihydrotestosterone (DHT). The increased hairiness results from the conversion of vellus hair follicles to large terminal follicles. In the axillae and lower pubic triangle this conversion is mediated by testosterone and androstenedione. In other regions such as the beard, chest, upper pubic triangle, nostrils, and external ears, this conversion is mediated by DHT. Paradoxically, DHT also mediates the reverse process, namely, the miniaturization of large terminal follicles into vellus hairs. Such physiologic miniaturization occurs with the reshaping of the frontal hairline from a straight line to an M-shaped configuration at puberty; this process occurs in all men and in the majority of women.

Maternal androgens ensure full development and function of sebaceous glands at birth. The vernix caseosa covering the neonate is mostly sebum. Normally sebaceous glands atrophy after birth and until puberty, when androgens again stimulate their activity. Acne is often one of the earliest signs of puberty. Disorders of androgen excess in adult women (e.g., polycystic ovary syndrome) are also associated with increased sebaceous activity and acne. Estrogens in large amounts decrease gland size and secretion.

FUNCTIONS OF THE SKIN

PROTECTION. Several structures in the skin, including the stratum corneum, melanin, cutaneous nerves, and the dermal connective tissue, provide important survival functions. The skin protects against the loss of essential fluids, the entrance of toxic agents and microorganisms, and damage from ultraviolet radiation, mechanical shearing forces, and extreme environmental temperatures.

The stratum corneum serves as a low-permeability barrier that retards water loss from the inner epidermal hydrated layers and also shields against environmental damage. The barrier properties of the horny layer are of practical importance from several points of view: Excessive drying or inflammatory reactions in the skin (e.g., eczema) lead to roughness, scaling, and disruption of the normally compact layers of horny cells. These changes lead to increased transepidermal water loss and, if severe (as in generalized exfoliative dermatitis, erythroderma, or burns), can contribute to fluid and electrolyte imbalance. With breaks in the horny layer, external substances more readily gain entrance to the underlying epidermis. Thus, various chemical substances, including medications placed on injured skin, have a greater opportunity to be absorbed or to act as haptens or antigens, thereby increasing the possibility of allergic contact dermatitis. Allergic contact dermatitis becomes particularly common when topical antibiotics are applied to chronically inflamed skin. The disruption of the barrier also increases the chance of colonization of pathologic bacteria in the skin, especially in the presence of tissue fluid exudates, which serve as excellent culture media. Percutaneous absorption of various topical medications used in treating skin conditions can be enhanced by hydrating the stratum corneum with the use of occlusive plastic wraps.

The stratum corneum normally harbors a number of aerobic and anaerobic resident organisms (i.e., *Staphylococcus epidermidis,* diphtheroids, *Propionibacterium acnes,* and *Pityrosporon*). Breaks in the stratum corneum, poor hygiene, and excessive humidity with maceration (especially in intertriginous areas) all contribute to cutaneous infections such as impetigo, erysipelas, folliculitis, furunculosis, and ecthyma.

A second structural component that provides protection is the *melanocyte,* which produces melanin pigment. Melanin is a large polymer that has the unique capability of absorbing light over the broad range of 200- to 2400-nm wavelengths. It serves as an excellent screen against the untoward effects of solar ultraviolet radiation, such as aging and wrinkling of the skin and the development of cutaneous neoplasms. The importance of melanin is dramatically illustrated by the high incidence of skin cancers in sun-exposed areas of the body, particularly in light-skinned, blue-eyed, easily sunburned individuals and in albinos. Ultraviolet light exposure also causes aging and wrinkling of the skin. Neither sex nor race affects the number of melanocytes in the epidermis. Negroid skin contains the same number of melanocytes as white skin, but the pigmentation is more intense as a result of the synthesis of more melanin that is dispersed throughout the melanocytes and adjacent keratinocytes. Accordingly, black skin is much less likely to form skin cancers, and it ages more slowly than white skin.

Dermal nerves play an important role in bodily protection. Nerve endings are extensively distributed in the skin in two general morphologic types: free nerve endings and specialized endings (Pacini's and Meissner's corpuscles), which mediate many sensations, including pain, pressure, and itch. Loss of sensation (e.g., diabetic neuropathy) may result in deep traumatic ulcers (trophic ulcers) without the patient's awareness. Damage to the dermatomal nerves (e.g., herpes zoster) may result in prolonged burning pain and hypesthesias (postherpetic neuralgia).

Itch is mediated by cutaneous nerves. It may occur in conjunction with a number of dermatologic diseases or without clinically

Table 519–1 ■ SKIN DISEASES ASSOCIATED WITH ITCHING

Xerosis (dry skin)
Insect infestations (scabies, pediculosis, insect bites)
Dermatitis (atopic, contact, nummular) including poison ivy contact
Drugs (opiates, aspirin, quinidine)
Lichen planus
Urticaria
Dermatitis herpetiformis (burning itch)
Sunburn
Fiberglass dermatitis
Seborrheic dermatatis

Table 519–2 ■ PRURITUS ASSOCIATED WITH SYSTEMIC DISEASE

SYSTEMIC DISEASE	POSTULATED CAUSE
Uremia	Secondary hyperparathyroidism, high skin calcium concentration, proliferation of mast cells, xerosis

Obstructive biliary disease
  Primary biliary cirrhosis
  Cholestatic hepatitis secondary to drugs (chlorpropamide)
  Intrahepatic cholestasis of pregnancy
  Extrahepatic biliary obstruction
	High concentrations of bile salts in skin

Hematologic and myeloproliferative disorders
  Lymphoma including Hodgkin's disease
  Mycosis fungoides
  Polycythemia vera
  Iron-deficiency anemia
	Unknown

Endocrine disorders
  Thyrotoxicosis
  Hypothyroidism
  Diabetes
	Unknown

Carcinoid	Serotonin
Visceral malignancies Breast, stomach, lung	Unknown

Psychiatric disorders
  Stress
  Delusions of parasitosis
	Unknown

Neurologic disorders
  Multiple sclerosis (paroxysmal itching)
  Notalgia paresthetic—local itch of back, medial shaft scapula (local neuropathy)
Brain abscess
Central nervous system infarct
	Unknown

evident skin disease (pruritus) (Tables 519–1 and 519–2). Itch and pain are carried on unmyelinated C fibers found in the upper portion of the dermis of the skin, mucous membranes, and cornea. The afferent C fibers enter the dorsal horn of the spinal cord, synapse, cross the midline, and ascend the spinothalamic tracts to the thalamus. Then the impulse proceeds to the sensory area of the postcentral gyrus of the cortex. Cutting the spinothalamic tract, as in an anterolateral hemichordotomy, abolishes pain and itch. A variety of peripheral mediators stimulate the C fibers and induce itching. These mediators include histamine, trypsin, proteases, peptides (bradykinin, vasoactive intestine peptide, substance P—all potent histamine releasers), and bile salts. Prostaglandins are modulators of pruritus rather than primary mediators; they lower the threshold to itching evoked by both histamine and pain. Central modulators of pruritus, such as systemic morphine, cause itch while relieving pain by acting on central opiate receptors. Regrettably, no single pharmacologic agent effectively treats all kinds of pruritus.

Generalized itching in the absence of primary skin disease (pruritus) may be an important sign of internal disease (see Table 519–2). An important cause of pruritus is psychic stress. Some patients with psychogenic pruritus believe the itching is caused by invisible parasites in the skin. Such patients scratch until excoriations and prurigo papules (thickened papular areas of skin due to constant rubbing) evolve in areas that the patient can readily reach (extremities, scalp, upper back). Dry skin (xerosis) is a common cause of itching in older individuals. Certain drugs (aspirin, opiates) can cause itching without a visible rash. Patients with polycythemia vera display a unique form of itching triggered by sudden changes in temperature, especially when they emerge from a warm bath. The itch is prickly in nature and lasts minutes to hours.

The tough, viscoelastic properties imparted to the skin by the fibrous proteins (collagen and elastin) and amorphous ground substance that make up the dermis protect the skin against shearing forces. The viscous and elastic properties of the ground substance allow it to resist compression and accept molding, thus reducing point pressure on sensitive skin structures.

THERMOREGULATION. Thermoregulation is subserved concomitantly by the cutaneous vasculature and the sweat glands. A massive network of interconnecting musculocutaneous arteries and venules, as well as capillaries, arteriovenous shunts, and small venules, play a crucial role in the maintenance of body temperature. Most of the skin's blood resides in the large venous plexus, through which blood slowly moves close to the surface to dissipate heat. Equally important in thermoregulation is the formation of eccrine sweat, which provides cooling by evaporation from the skin's surface. Every gram of water that evaporates from the skin loses 580 calories of heat.

Blood flow through the skin is 10 to 20 times that required to supply needed metabolites and oxygen. Under basal conditions about 8.5% of the total blood flow passes through the skin, controlled primarily by the sympathetic nervous system. Blood flow can increase up to 3.5 L/min with exercise in a warm environment, thereby dissipating large amounts of heat. Both central (hypothalamic heating) and peripheral thermoreceptors stimulate sweating via the sympathetic nervous system, but in the case of sweat glands, acetylcholine is the postganglionic transmitter. Increase in body core temperature is the strongest stimulus for inducing sweating, whereas peripheral (cutaneous) thermoreceptors are only one tenth as effective in eliciting perspiration.

Response to cold begins when cool blood passes the hypothalamus, which elicits both heat conservation and production mechanisms. Sympathetic stimuli constrict cutaneous blood vessels, and hypothalamic impulses activate shivering, which increases heat production by as much as 50%. Conversely, when warm blood irrigates the hypothalamus, central heat production ceases, and cutaneous blood vessels dilate to allow heat loss from the skin surface. Vasodilatation also occurs reflexly through direct warming of the skin surface (in warm environments). In addition, stimulation of the hypothalamus produces sweating and increases evaporative heat loss. Periodic exposure to heat or to heat and work stresses (i.e., daily 1- or 2-hour exposures for 10 to 14 days) enhances the secretory capacity of the eccrine sweat glands (acclimatization).

The crucial role of cutaneous vasculature in thermoregulation and cardiovascular homeostasis can be reversed by widespread inflammatory conditions of the skin causing erythroderma. Diseases such as generalized dermatitis, psoriasis, drug reactions, and underlying lymphomas can cause generalized, inflammatory-based cutaneous vasodilatation that can divert 10 to 20% of cardiac output through the skin. To maintain blood pressure, cardiac output must increase; older individuals with impaired cardiac reserve can develop high-output failure accompanied by tremendous loss of body heat with wide swings in temperature and shivering.

THE SKIN AS AN ENDOCRINE ORGAN. Many metabolic activities of the skin are under hormonal regulation. Not only do sebaceous glands and certain hair follicles respond readily to androgens, but they are capable of many diverse steroid transformations, as described earlier.

DHT causes sebaceous glands to enlarge at puberty, stimulates the growth of certain hair (male sexual hair of the beard, chest, upper pubic triangle, nose, and ears), and generates the growth and development of the external genitalia. Drugs such as cimetidine and spironolactone have antiandrogenic activity and have been used to treat acne and hirsutism. In addition, thyroid hormones can regulate hair growth and alter the texture of the skin (fine, sparse hair and smooth, soft skin in hyperthyroidism; coarse hair and cool, rough, thick skin in hypothyroidism). Other hormones affect melanin pigment formation, melanocyte-stimulating hormone, and estrogen-stimulating skin pigmentation.

THE SKIN AS AN IMMUNOLOGIC ORGAN. The epidermis and the dermoepidermal junctional area participate actively in immunologic reactions. The skin includes immunologically important cells including keratinocytes, Langerhans' cells, and melanocytes as well as immunologic structures such as the lamina lucida and basal lamina that are involved in bullous reactions of the skin.

EPIDERMAL IMMUNOLOGICALLY IMPORTANT CELLS. The most important immunologic cell in the epidermis is the Langerhans' cell, comprising 2 to 5% of the total epidermal cell population. Langerhans' cells contribute to a number of immunologic reactions, including macrophage–T cell interaction, T and B lymphocyte interactions, graft-versus-host (GVH) reactions, and skin graft rejection. The Langerhans cell synthesizes and expresses Ia antigens (class II antigens, immune response gene-associated antigens) that are crucial in processing and presenting allergens to sensitized T lymphocytes critical in the elicitation of delayed hypersensitivity

contact dermatitis. Lymphokines, made by the Langerhans cells during these immunologic reactions, augment and enhance these processes and also contribute to the accompanying inflammatory response.

Keratinocytes participate in immunologic responses by expressing Ia antigens on their surfaces in such conditions as GVH reaction, mycosis fungoides, allergic contact dermatitis, lichen planus, and tuberculoid leprosy. In these conditions the keratinocytes make lymphokines, particularly interleukin-1, which provides a second signal supplementing macrophages (Langerhans' cells) in mitogen- and antigen-induced T-cell activation. In addition, epidermal cells make other cytokines, such as prostaglandin E2 and leukotrienes, that participate in inflammatory reactions in the skin. Keratinocytes are the immunologic target in the pemphigus group of diseases in which circulating autoantibodies against intercellular antigen of the epidermis and mucous membrane epithelium initiate intraepidermal acantholytic bullae.

THE DERMOEPIDERMAL JUNCTION. A variety of inflammatory diseases often characterized by bullous reactions seem to be mediated by immunoreactants, including IgG, IgA, and IgM, and complement deposition along the dermoepidermal junctional area. The anatomic site of blister formation correlates with the position of deposition of these immunoreactants. The antigens in several diseases have been isolated and partially characterized. The use of immunofluorescent techniques at the light microscopic and especially the ultrastructural level has been helpful in more precisely diagnosing these bullous conditions (Table 519–3).

INFLAMMATORY REACTIONS IN THE SKIN AND WOUND HEALING. Cutaneous inflammation reflects the sum of the effects of biologic products of cells (mast cells, infiltrating neutrophils, monocytes, macrophages, lymphocytes) as well as the effects of the products of the complement system, membrane-derived arachidonic acid metabolic pathways (prostaglandins and leukotrienes), and the Hageman factor–dependent pathways of coagulation, fibrinolysis, and kinin generation. Early phases of wound healing also encompass many of these reactions.

CUTANEOUS INFLAMMATION. Several pathophysiologic reactions initiate inflammation, including infectious, immunologic, and toxic processes that affect the epidermis or dermis, or both. Mast cells in the skin function not only as the sentinel cells in immediate-type hypersensitivity reactions but also as major effector cells in inflammatory reactions. They release (1) histamine, prostaglandin D2, and leukotrienes, which cause vascular dilatation and increased permeability, redness, swelling, pain, and itch; (2) chemotactic factors for eosinophils and neutrophils; (3) proteases that interact with the complement, kinin, and fibrinolytic pathways; and (4) heparin, which contributes to local angiogenesis. Degranulation of mast cells occurs in response to various antigens that cross-link IgE on the mast cell surface (immediate hypersensitivity reactions), to by-products of complement activation C3a and C5a (as occurs in leukocytoclastic vasculitides), and to radiocontrast media, aspirin, insect venom, and various physical stimuli. Circulating peripheral blood cells infiltrate local tissue sites in response to chemotactic factors released by mast cells and other infiltrating cells. Basophils release histamine and chemotactic substances, such as those involved in allergic contact reactions, bullous pemphigoid, erythema multiforme, and inflammatory responses. Neutrophils release myeloperoxidase, acid hydrolases, and neutral proteases that are active against microbes and cause tissue destruction (dermatitis herpetiformis, psoriasis, leukocytoclastic vasculitis, and bacterial infections of the skin). Eosinophils release major basic protein and peroxidase (allergic drug reactions in the skin, bullous pemphigoid). Lymphocytes release lymphokines that modulate immunologic and inflammatory responses (lichen planus, lupus erythematosus, allergic contact dermatitis, tuberculoid leprosy). Monocytes and macrophages engulf foreign proteins and microorganisms (granulomatous reactions in the skin such as sarcoidosis, deep fungus and acid-fast bacilli infections, and cutaneous foreign body responses). Both classic and alternate complement pathways release products that induce mast cell degranulation and induce inflammation. The activation of the system appears to contribute to inflammatory reactions in hereditary complement deficiencies causing lupus erythematosus–like syndromes or pyodermas, as well as necrotizing vasculitis.

Table 519–3 ■ IMMUNOFLUORESCENT CUTANEOUS FINDINGS IN IMMUNOLOGICALLY MEDIATED SKIN DISEASE

DISEASES	BIOPSY FINDINGS OF DIRECT IMMUNOFLUORESCENCE IMMUNOREACTANTS (DIF)	ULTRASTRUCTURAL LOCALIZATION OF IMMUNOREACTANTS	SITE OF BLISTER FORMATION ON ROUTINE LIGHT MICRO-SCOPIC PATHOLOGY	SERUM FINDINGS: INDIRECT IMMUNOFLUORESCENCE (IIF)
Bullous Diseases				
Pemphigus (all forms)	Deposits of IgG in intercellular areas between keratinocytes	Between keratinocytes	Suprabasilar in pemphigus vulgaris; substratum corneum in pemphigus foliaceus	IgG antibodies to intracellular areas of keratinocytes in 95% of patients
Bullous pemphigoid	IgG and/or complement (C) in BMZ	Lamina lucida and hemidesmosomes—upper part lucida and sub-basal cells	Subepidermal	IgG Ab to BMZ in 70%
Cicatricial pemphigoid	IgG and/or C in BMZ	Lamina lucida	Subepidermal	IgG antibodies BMZ in 10%
Herpes gestationis	Complement in BMZ—occasionally IgG	Lamina lucida—close to lamina densa	Subepidermal—sub-basal cell—above lamina densa	IgG antibodies BMZ in 20% (HG factor in 25%)
Dermatitis herpetiformis	IgA and C in dermal papillae (granular deposits)	Granular IgA associated with microfibril bundles in dermal papilla	Subepidermal in dermal papillae—papillar dermal microabscesses	No circulating antibodies
Epidermolysis bullosa acquisita	IgG, C3 in BMZ	Sublamina densa amorphous granular deposits	Subepidermal	Frequent IgG autoantibodies
Linear IgA bullous dermatosis in childhood	IgA and complement in linear deposition in BMZ	—	Subepidermal	No circulating antibodies
Connective Tissue Diseases				
Bullous Systemic LE	IgG, IgM, and complement in BMZ in involved and normal skin—linear homogenous	Just beneath lamina densa (basal lamina)	Subepidermal	Circulating antibodies to BMZ; ANA found in 90%
Discoid LE	IgG, other Ig, and C in lesional skin at BMZ	—	—	No circulating antibodies to BMZ, ANA titers normal
Systemic LE	IgG band at BMZ in normal skin (over 90% in sun-exposed areas)	—	—	Elevated ANA titers
Systemic sclerosis	Nucleolar IgG	—	Epidermal thinning and increased dermal collagen	ANA, speckled, 85%, centromere + in CREST syndrome
MCTD	IgG/IgM in BMZ in some patients; nuclear IgG in epidermis	—	—	Speckled ANA and ENA (extractable nuclear antigens)
Dermatomyositis	Negative	—	—	ANA often normal range

ANA = antinuclear antibody; BMZ = basement membrane zone; LE = lupus erythematosus; MCTD = mixed connective tissue disease.

WOUND HEALING IN THE SKIN. Healing proceeds temporally in three phases: substrate, proliferative, and remodeling. The initial substrate phase, encompassing the first 3 to 4 days after wounding, is so named because the cellular and other interactions lead to preparation for subsequent events. During this phase, vascular and inflammatory components prevail (vascular clotting in the severed vessels; leukocyte and macrophage chemotaxis into the area to ingest bacteria, débride the wound, and degrade collagen). The proliferative phase (10 to 14 days after wounding) results in regeneration of epidermis, neoangiogenesis, and proliferation of fibroblasts with increased collagen synthesis and closure of the skin defect. The final remodeling takes place over 6 to 12 months, during which time a more stable form of collagen is laid down to form a scar of progressively increasing tensile strength. In some instances so much collagen is deposited in the healing wound that an elevated hypertrophic scar (red, raised scar within the boundaries of the original wound) or keloid (scar tissue extending beyond the boundaries of original injury into surrounding normal tissue) is produced. Keloids occur most commonly over the anterior chest, upper back, and deltoid regions. They rarely regress, and they recur after excision.

THE COSMETIC IMPORTANCE OF SKIN. Aging alters virtually all the structures and functions of the skin. Environmental insults, especially chronic sun exposure, cause far greater damage to the skin than time itself.

Epidermal turnover rate decreases approximately 50% between the third and seventh decades. Concurrent loss of dermal elastic and collagen fibers accounts for the paper-thin, transparent quality of aged skin and the easy rupture of dermal vessels. An increasing cross-linkage of collagen and elastin accompanies aging, making the dermis more rigid and less able to withstand shearing forces. Aged skin, when "tented up," only slowly returns to its original form, whereas young skin readily snaps back. Sun-damaged aged skin shows microscopic collagen damage. Dermal collagen is replaced by amorphous basophilic staining material. This condition, termed *elastosis,* results in deep wrinkling and furrowing, especially over the face and back of the neck, and yellow papules and nodules in a reticular pattern on the face. Decreases in the number of functioning sebaceous and sweat glands contribute to the dryness of aged skin and to impaired thermoregulation in aged persons. Reduction in the vascular network in the skin surrounding hair bulbs and eccrine and sebaceous glands may be responsible for the atrophy of these appendages with age. A 50% reduction in the number of Langerhans' cells may account in part for the age-associated decrease in immune responsiveness and allergic contact dermatitis reactions in the elderly. Loss of enzymatically active melanocytes (10 to 20% per decade) causes irregular pigmentation of the skin and graying of the hair. Gradual reduction occurs in the number of body hairs, especially in the scalp, axillary, and pubic regions (related in part to decreased androgen production). Linear growth of nails also decreases by 30 to 50% between early and late adulthood. Often nails become brittle and thickened. A number of proliferative growths are associated with aging skin, including skin tags (acrochordon), cherry angiomata, seborrheic keratosis, lentigines, and sebaceous hyperplasia.

Arndt KA, LeBoit PE, Robinson JK, Wintroub BU: Cutaneous Medicine and Surgery. Philadelphia, WB Saunders, 1996.
Fitzpatrick TB, Johnson RA, Wolff K, et al: Color Atlas and Synopsis of Clinical Dermatology: Common and Serious Diseases, 3rd ed. New York, McGraw-Hill 1997. *Comprehensive texts of general dermatology.*

520 EXAMINATION OF THE SKIN AND AN APPROACH TO DIAGNOSING SKIN DISEASES

Frank Parker

THE DERMATOLOGIC HISTORY

A proper dermatologic history should initially address where the patient's skin condition first appeared. The patient should be asked to describe, in his or her own words, what the condition first resembled, any associated symptoms (e.g., pain, burning), and how the condition has progressed. The careful review of any medications, prescribed or over-the-counter, is critical. The relationship of the onset of the skin condition to the use of medications is particularly crucial in evaluating the possibility of a drug eruption or the development of an allergic contact dermatitis secondary to therapy. Any history of atopic diseases such as asthma, hay fever, and eczema should be sought. A careful family history of skin diseases can aid in the diagnosis of heritable dermatologic conditions. Many patients may have already tried a variety of therapies, topical or systemic, prescribed or over-the-counter; the effects of these therapies as well as any home remedies or "alternative" methods should be described.

A thorough social history is important, because some dermatoses may be related to occupational or recreational activities. Exposure to environmental elements such as sun, cold, and heat may provoke or exacerbate some skin conditions. The physician should also inquire about household and sexual contacts, particularly when a parasite or an infectious cause is being considered. Psychological stress, although seldom a sole cause of cutaneous conditions, can certainly exacerbate many dermatoses (e.g., acne, psoriasis, seborrhea, atopic dermatitis).

THE PHYSICAL EXAMINATION

Excellent lighting is paramount, and natural light usually serves as the best source, although fluorescent light may be used as well. Usually direct lighting is sufficient, although, in many cases, tangential lighting can aid in identifying subtle changes in many dermatoses (e.g., elevation or depression of lesions).

The examination should start with the hair and scalp and then move to the face and mucous membranes of the oral mucosae. Clues in the mouth (e.g., oral lesions of lichen planus) may help explain more distant cutaneous lesions. The back, chest, abdomen, and extremities, including palms, soles, and nails, should be examined. Skin generally covered by undergarments must also be examined because serious lesions, such as melanoma, can arise in these areas.

Signs of aging, nutritional status, trauma, and hygiene should be sought. Color changes related to underlying systemic conditions (e.g., jaundice with hepatobiliary conditions, cyanosis with various cardiopulmonary diseases, diffuse hyperpigmentation with Addison's disease, paleness with anemia) all are important.

In each region of the body, the physical examination includes three maneuvers: (1) observation for color or surface changes, which may often be preceded by use of an alcohol sponge to wipe off existing cosmetics, oil, or foreign material so the skin's natural color can be observed; (2) touching or light stroking to detect texture changes, warmth, and/or moisture, with an understanding that the smoothness or roughness of the skin depends on factors as normal keratinization, proper hydration of the stratum corneum, and normal cutaneous blood flow; and (3) palpation and stretching of the skin to determine its consistency and pliability, with the appreciation that elasticity depends on the normal structure and function of dermal connective tissue and ground substance and that certain infiltrates can be detected by palpation.

Because there are many hundreds of dermatoses, a logical process of elimination is required to narrow the possibilities, first to specific categories of diseases, then, it is hoped, to one final diagnosis. Dermatologic conditions are usually separated into specific morphologic categories (e.g., papulosquamous diseases) (see Chapter 522). Once a condition is determined to fit into a specific category, additional information such as history and laboratory data can help to eliminate other possibilities.

Three steps are involved in this systematic approach. First, the entire skin is examined for primary and secondary skin lesions (Table 520–1) that allow the examiner to place the patient in one of nine diagnostic groups (the second step) (Table 520–2) (Color Plates 15*A–F* and 16*A–F*). Many skin conditions are found in each group, but all of the conditions in a given group express the same primary and secondary lesions. The third step is to identify the patient's specific disease by looking for distinctive features, such as the distribution of skin lesions, any unusual shapes of the lesions, the arrangement of several lesions (annular, serpiginous, dermatomal), the dominant hue and color of the lesion, and its surface characteristics (particularly the appearance of scales or verrucous or vegetative changes).

STEP 1: DESCRIPTION OF PRIMARY AND SECONDARY SKIN LESIONS. Primary skin lesions are uncomplicated abnormalities that represent the initial pathologic change, uninfluenced by secondary effects such as infection, trauma, or therapy. Secondary lesions reflect progression of the disease or scratching or infection of the primary lesions. Most primary changes can also develop as secondary manifestations: for example, pustules may appear as primary lesions of folliculitis or as secondary lesions when scaling, itching lesions are scratched and infected. The challenge is to recognize the primary skin lesion so as to make the correct etiologic diagnosis.

The terminology used to describe primary and secondary skin changes (see Table 520–1) is the basic language of dermatology; if this terminology is not used correctly, it is difficult to arrive at the precise diagnosis of skin diseases. Each descriptive word is not only a short account of what is seen on the surface of the skin but also relays specific information about processes within the skin.

STEP 2: ASSIGNMENT OF THE LESION TO A MAJOR GROUP OF DISEASES. Each disease within a given group shares the same primary and secondary skin lesions. Some diseases have overlapping traits so they may be assigned to more than one group (see Table 520–2).

Table 520–1 ■ THE LANGUAGE OF DERMATOLOGY: PRIMARY AND SECONDARY SKIN LESIONS

Primary Skin Lesions

Macule—circumscribed flat change in skin color (e.g., café au lait spot)

Papule—solid elevated area with top; can be flat, pointed or rounded (e.g., acne)

Plaque—evolves from a confluence of papules leading to flat-topped, circumscribed elevations (e.g., psoriasis)

Scale—desiccated, thin plates of cornified epidermal cells that result from altered keratinization (e.g., ichthyosis)

Wheal—circumscribed, flat-topped, firm elevation of skin with a well-demarcated, palpable margin; results from tense edema in papillary dermis (e.g., urticaria)

Nodule—large, solid, deep-seated, raised mass in dermal or subcutaneous tissues; usually larger than 1 cm (e.g., erythema nodosum)

Vesicle/bulla—circumscribed, elevated lesion containing clear serous or hemorrhagic fluid; vesicles are <1 cm, bullae are >1 cm (e.g., herpes simplex and pemphigus vulgaris)

Pustule—a vesicle containing purulent exudate (e.g., folliculitis)

Atrophy—loss of epidermal or dermal tissue with some depression of skin surface and substance; epidermal atrophy leads to fine wrinkling of the skin surface (e.g., lichen sclerosis et atrophicus)

Secondary Skin Lesions

Lichenification—dry, leathery thickening of the skin with exaggerated skin markings (e.g., chronic eczema)

Scar—an area where fibrosis of the dermis or subcutaneous tissues results from an antecedent destructive process and replaces normal skin (e.g., healing wound)

Erosion—a moist, circumscribed, often depressed area that reflects loss of partial or full-thickness epidermis (e.g., ruptured bulla)

Fissure—a deep linear split in the skin extending through the epidermis (e.g., eczema)

Crust—dried, exudate of serum, blood, sebum, or purulent material on the surface of the skin (e.g., acute eczema)

Telangiectasia—dilated, small blood vessels in the skin (e.g., discoid lupus erythematosus and necrobiosis lipoidica diabeticorum)

Table 520–2 ■ MAJOR GROUPS OF DERMATOLOGIC DISEASES BASED ON THE CLINICAL MORPHOLOGY OF THE SKIN CONDITION

GROUP	CLINICAL MORPHOLOGY	EXAMPLES OF DISEASES IN THE GROUP
Eczema or dermatitis	Macules (erythema), papules, vesicles, lichenification, fine scaling, excoriations, crusting	Contact dermatitis, atopic dermatitis, stasis dermatitis, photodermatitis, scabies, dermatophytoses, exfoliative dermatitis, candidiasis
Maculopapular eruptions	Macules, erythema, papules	Viral exanthems, drug reactions, verruca vulgaris, Kawasaki's disease, vasculitic and purpuric eruptions
Papulosquamous dermatoses	Papules, plaques, erythema with unique scales	Psoriasis, Reiter's syndrome, pityriasis rosea, lichen planus, seborrheic dermatitis, ichthyosis, secondary syphilis, mycosis fungoides, parapsoriasis
Vesiculobullous diseases	Vesicles, bullae, erythema	Herpes simplex and zoster, hand-foot-and-mouth disease, insect bites, bullous impetigo, scalded skin syndrome, pemphigus, pemphigoid, dermatitis herpetiformis, porphyria cutanea tarda, erythema multiforme
Pustular diseases	Pustules, cysts, erythema	Acne vulgaris and rosacea, pustular psoriasis, folliculitis, gonococcemia
Urticaria, persistent figurate erythemas, cellulitis	Wheals and figurate, raised erythema, scaling	Urticaria, erythema annulare centrifugum, erysipelas, necrotizing fasciitis
Nodular lesions	Nodules and tumors, some associated with erosions and ulceration	Benign and malignant tumors—basal cell cancer, squamous cell cancer, rheumatoid nodules, xanthomas
Telangiectasia, atrophic, scarring, ulcerative diseases	Atrophic, sclerotic telangiectasia and ulcerative changes	Connective tissue diseases, radiation dermatitis, lichen sclerosus et atrophicus, vascular insufficiency (arterial and venous), pyoderma gangrenosum
Hypermelanosis and hypomelanosis	Increased and decreased melanin deposition in skin	Acanthosis nigricans, café au lait spots, vitiligo, tuberous sclerosis, xeroderma pigmentosum, chloasma, freckles

STEP 3: NARROWING THE POSSIBILITIES TO THE EXACT DIAGNOSIS. Of great importance in this step is the distribution of the skin disease, because many conditions have typical patterns or affect specific regions. For example, psoriasis commonly affects extensor surfaces, whereas atopic dermatitis commonly affects flexor surfaces of the extremities (Fig. 520–1). Photoreactions are confined to parts of the body exposed to sunlight. Involvement of the palms and soles is seen in erythema multiforme, secondary syphilis, some forms of psoriasis, and Rocky Mountain spotted fever. Contact dermatitis to exogenous allergens or irritants often presents as unusual patterns and distributions corresponding to the areas where the offending material came in contact with the skin.

An important clue in differentiating diseases lies in the shape of the individual lesions and the arrangement of several lesions in relation to each other. A linear arrangement of lesions may indicate a contact reaction to an exogenous substance brushing across the skin, a pathologic process involving a vascular or lymphatic vessel, or a cutaneous nevus. "Zosteriform" refers to lesions arranged along the cutaneous distribution of a spinal dermatome; these le-

sions are typically unilateral and denote herpes zoster or, occasionally, metastatic carcinoma of the breast or the dermatomal hemangiomatous growths of Sturge-Weber syndrome. "Annular" lesions are round to oval with an area of central clearing; annular macules are observed in drug eruptions, secondary syphilis, and lupus erythematosus. Resolving hives may also leave annular configurations, whereas annular lesions with scaling suggest dermatophytosis or pityriasis rosea. "Target lesions" are a special type of annular lesion in which an erythematous annular macule or papule develops a second red ring or a purplish papule or vesicle in the center; target lesions are seen in erythema multiforme. "Arciform" lesions form partial circles or arcs and may be seen in dermatophyte infections. "Polycyclic" patterns evolve when numerous annular lesions enlarge and run together. "Herpetiform" refers to a grouping of lesions such as occurs in herpes simplex or dermatitis herpetiformis.

"Umbilicated" vesicles are important diagnostic findings. Vesicular lesions with central delling or depression are suggestive of viral cutaneous infection, including herpes simplex, herpes zoster, vari-

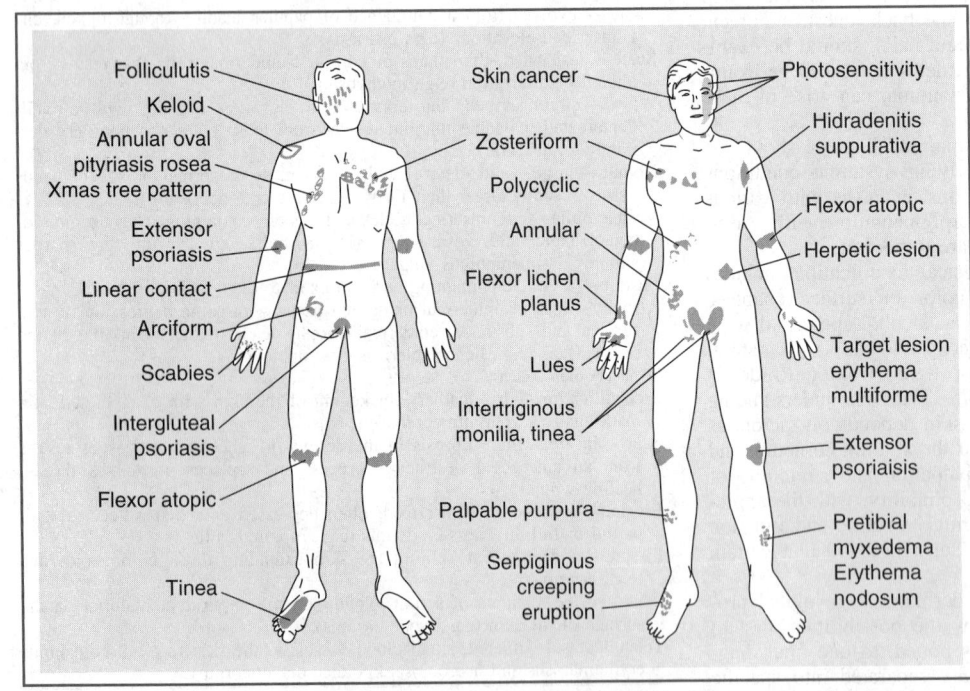

FIGURE 520–1 ■ Configurational and regional diagnostic aids for the diagnosis of primary and secondary skin lesions.

cella, and molluscum contagiosum (an umbilicated papular lesion). "Poikiloderma" refers to epidermal atrophy, reticulate hyperpigmentation, hypopigmentation, and erythema with telangiectasia; poikilodermatous skin lesions are typically seen in collagen vascular disease, cutaneous T-cell lymphoma (mycosis fungoides), and radiation skin damage. "Sporotrichoid or chancriform syndrome" describes nodular, ulcerative lesions on an extremity with satellite lymph nodes similar to the initial appearance of primary syphilis and sporotrichosis; primary skin inoculation of histoplasmosis, coccidioidomycosis, and blastomycosis may initially present in this manner, as may infection with *Nocardia* or *Mycobacterium marinum*.

Other physical features influence diagnoses. Dry, lichenified lesions suggest a chronic state, whereas wet, weeping, macerated lesions suggest acute reactions. Abscesses are soft and fluctuant, whereas nodules are usually firm. Redness caused by dilatation of superficial blood vessels blanches with pressure, whereas erythema caused by extravasated blood, as occurs in petechiae and purpuric lesions, does not blanch. Hues of brown to black usually indicate melanin, although some drugs cause brown-black pigmentation in the skin (e.g., minocycline). The variation in color from melanin is related to the depth of the pigment in the skin, with deeper pigment having a more blue-black color.

DIAGNOSTIC TESTS AND AIDS IN EXAMINATION OF THE SKIN

Certain aids and procedures, when combined with the history and physical examination, assist accurate diagnosis.

VISUAL AIDS. MAGNIFICATION. Magnification of skin lesions can detect the follicular plugging seen in discoid lupus erythematosus or fine telangiectasia in the pearly, opalescent borders of basal cell cancers.

TRANSILLUMINATION. Oblique lighting in a darkened room can help to detect slight degrees of elevation or depression of lesions as well as fine wrinkling or atrophy of the epidermis. The application of a penlight directly to nodular lesions in a dark room may give clues as to their density and make-up. Cystic lesions allow transmission of some light, whereas nodules composed of cellular infiltrates do not.

DIASCOPY. Firm pressure with a microscope slide against skin lesions differentiates the erythema of capillary dilatation from that of extravasated blood. Sarcoidosis, tuberculosis, and other granulomatous inflammatory reactions in the skin are suggested if diascopy of the lesions shows a characteristic "apple jelly" or glassy, fawn-colored appearance.

LONG-WAVE ULTRAVIOLET (UV) OR WOOD'S LIGHT EXAMINATION. Long-wave ultraviolet light (UVA) (360 nm) is useful in evaluating several conditions of the skin. Wood's light exaggerates the differences in the degree of pigmentation when the skin is examined with the lamp in a dark room. Melanin is a universal absorber of UV light, so decreased melanin shows more reflection (light color) and increased melanin less reflection (darker color). Pigment in the epidermis is exaggerated with UVA light, but pigment in the dermis is not, so a reasonable guess as to the site of melanin in the skin can be made. Wood's light may be the only means of recognizing the hypomelanotic ash leaf–shaped macules of tuberous sclerosis. The extent of vitiligo and melanotic nevi (which appear darker than surrounding normal skin) can also be determined. Some superficial fungal infections of the scalp fluoresce blue-green; erythrasma, a superficial intertriginous bacterial infection that produces a porphyrin, fluoresces a brilliant coral red; *Pseudomonas* infections may give off yellow-green color under a Wood's light.

CLINICAL TESTS. PATCH TESTS. Patch testing is used to validate a diagnosis of allergic contact sensitization and to identify the causative allergen. Because the entire skin of sensitized humans is allergic, the test reproduces the dermatitis in one small area where the allergen is applied, usually on the back. The suspected allergen is applied to the skin, occluded, and left in place 48 hours. A positive test reproduces a delayed hypersensitivity eczematous response at the test site from 48 hours up to a week later. Considerable experience is required to perform and interpret patch tests. Photopatch testing is performed to detect photocontact allergy. Suspected photoallergens are placed on the skin in two sets. One set of allergens is irradiated with appropriate wavelengths of light after the patches are in place on the skin for 24 hours; the second set of the same photoallergens is kept covered to serve as controls. Photoallergens cause an erythematous reaction that is evident 24 hours after exposure to light.

PHYSICAL CONTACT TESTING. Darier's sign is the development of an urticarial and flare reaction after vigorously rubbing cutaneous mast cell (urticaria pigmentosa) lesions of the skin. The rubbing degranulates the mast cells, releasing histamine.

Nikolsky's sign demonstrates disadherence of the epidermal cells to one another. Pushing, rubbing, or rotating normal skin near bullous lesions causes the epidermis to be dislodged, leaving a moist, glistening defect. This sign is present in various forms of pemphigus and in toxic epidermal necrolysis.

The Koebner phenomenon occurs in certain skin diseases that tend to evolve new skin lesions after traumatic injury in areas of apparently normal skin. Thus, psoriasis may evolve within surgical scars and after sunburn or in the wake of a drug reaction involving the skin. Lichen planus may also exhibit this phenomenon.

Pathergy, the development of pustular and ulcerative lesions at the site of needle puncture, is suggestive of Behçet's syndrome and pyoderma gangrenosum.

Hair-pull examination is done to assess hair loss in the scalp. It is often useful to pull vigorously on scalp hairs to determine whether there is an increased number of falling hairs (normally only one or two can be removed with a tug of a group of hairs between the thumb and forefinger); ascertain the ratio of anagen to telogen hairs; and examine the hairs under a microscope for various congenital malformations of the shaft. Normally 10 to 15% of scalp hairs are in their resting phase, but the percentage rises in naturally shed hair.

PARING HYPERKERATOTIC LESIONS TO DIFFERENTIATE WARTS FROM CALLUSES. After the hyperkeratosis is pared away, the wart displaces and obliterates epidermal ridges and small bleeding points, and black and red dots become visible. In calluses, the epidermal ridges are not interrupted, and no vessels are seen within the callus.

LABORATORY PROCEDURES. GRAM STAIN AND CULTURES. Gram stain for bacteria and bacteriologic cultures are important when the primary lesion is a pustule or furuncle or appears to be impetigo. When an unusual cutaneous infection is considered in an immunosuppressed patient, a skin biopsy specimen can be minced or ground in a sterile mortar and cultured for aerobic and anaerobic bacteria, including typical and atypical mycobacteria, deep fungi, and *Candida*. A more rapid method of screening for infectious agents in immunosuppressed patients (often the first sign of septicemia in such patients is pustules, nodules, or ulcerative lesions) is to perform frozen sections on a skin biopsy specimen taken from the lesion and to obtain Gram stains, acid-fast bacterial stains, and periodic acid–Schiff stains (to identify fungal and yeast elements). This approach may provide a diagnosis within a few hours.

EXAMINATION AND CULTURE FOR FUNGI AND CANDIDA. The presence of mycelia may be ascertained by applying 10% potassium hydroxide (KOH) to scale or exudative material scraped from suspected lesions and briefly heating the slide to dissolve the keratin. Hyphal elements can be observed by direct microscopic examination. Dermatophyte hyphae appear as long, branching, refractile, walled structures; *Candida* organisms appear as shorter, linear hyphae in association with budding yeast forms; tinea versicolor is seen as round yeast forms with short, club-shaped hyphae (so-called spaghetti and meatballs pattern). KOH examination of skin scrapings is mandatory to exclude tinea. A classic dictum is "if the skin lesion is scaly, scrape it."

TZANCK SMEAR. The microscopic examination of cells from the base of vesicles reveals the presence of giant epithelial cells and multinucleated giant cells in herpes simplex, herpes zoster, and varicella. Material is obtained from the base of a vesicle by gentle scraping with a scalpel and is spread on a glass slide and stained with Giemsa's or Wright's stain for the examination (Color Plate 14*C*).

SKIN BIOPSY. Lesions characteristic of the eruption (primary lesions) should be sampled. Lesions altered by scratching, infection, crusting, or lichenification are not likely to provide useful information. Clinical indications for biopsy include lesions thought to be malignant; lesions that fail to heal, increase in size, bleed easily, or

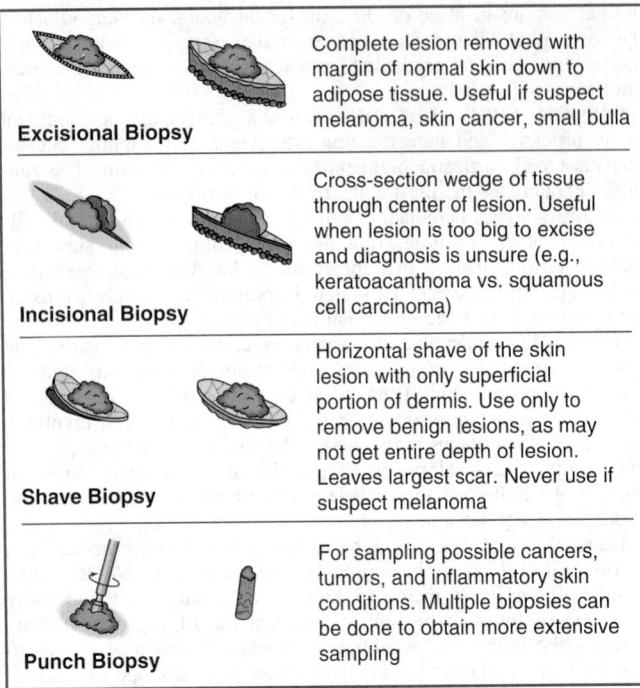

Excisional Biopsy		Complete lesion removed with margin of normal skin down to adipose tissue. Useful if suspect melanoma, skin cancer, small bulla
Incisional Biopsy		Cross-section wedge of tissue through center of lesion. Useful when lesion is too big to excise and diagnosis is unsure (e.g., keratoacanthoma vs. squamous cell carcinoma)
Shave Biopsy		Horizontal shave of the skin lesion with only superficial portion of dermis. Use only to remove benign lesions, as may not get entire depth of lesion. Leaves largest scar. Never use if suspect melanoma
Punch Biopsy		For sampling possible cancers, tumors, and inflammatory skin conditions. Multiple biopsies can be done to obtain more extensive sampling

FIGURE 520–2 ■ Methods of skin biopsy.

ulcerate spontaneously; tumors or growths of uncertain nature; and many inflammatory conditions, especially those for which the diagnosis is uncertain.

Four types of biopsies can be performed. The choice of technique determines the size and shape of the specimen obtained (Fig. 520–2). The procedure selected should secure the tissue most likely to contain the pathologic alterations and leave the smallest cosmetic defect (Table 520–3). For the most complete histopathologic assessment, an elliptical, full-thickness excision is best because, in one procedure, the entire lesion is removed and secured for diagnosis and the remaining defect is easily sutured. The excisional biopsy technique is indicated when malignant melanoma is

Table 520–3 ■ SOME GENERAL PRINCIPLES TO IMPROVE BIOPSY TECHNIQUES

Skin Biopsies and Various Skin Diseases

Shave biopsies can be used for pedunculated skin lesions.
An inflammatory dermatosis should not have a shave biopsy but rather a punch or incisional biopsy.
A pigmented lesion that is even slightly "atypical" or suggestive of a melanoma should be removed by an excisional biopsy if possible. Never perform a shave biopsy for suspicious pigmented lesions.
Non-pigmented tumors should be sampled from the thickest portion.
Ulcers should be sampled at the edge—not the center. Punch or incisional biopsy is preferred.
Vesicles or bullae should be sampled immediately adjacent to the blister edge. For immunofluorescence studies, it is preferable to sample some lesions, such as dermatitis herpetiformis, away from the blister, whereas other diseases, such as pemphigus, should be sampled from the blister edge.
If an infectious process is suspected, part of the biopsy specimen should be sent for culture and special stains.
Annular lesions should be sampled from the leading edge.

Mechanical Features About Skin Biopsies

Punch biopsy specimens smaller than 3 mm may not provide enough material to allow the pathologist to make a diagnosis.
Warn patients about residual scars after the biopsy. Shave biopsies leave circular scars; biopsies may form a keloid especially on the mid-chest, shoulder, and back.
Scalp biopsies bleed profusely. Use lidocaine with epinephrine and anesthetize the biopsy site 5–10 minutes before the biopsy is done.
Try to sample above the knees, especially in elderly patients with poor peripheral circulation or diabetes, because sampled areas on the lower leg heal slowly and often become infected.
Do not leave punch biopsies open; suture them.
Use soft sutures such as silk in body folds for patient comfort.

suggested or when a lesion is deep in skin or subcutaneous tissue and its orientation in surrounding tissue is relevant for diagnosis. A second procedure is the paramedian incisional biopsy, in which a thin but deep elliptical section is taken through the center of the lesion including normal skin at each end. This approach is especially useful in diagnosing large keratoacanthomas. A third biopsy method is the shave, or parallel incision, in which lidocaine is injected locally under the lesion to lift it above the skin surface and a scalpel (the knife horizontal to the skin surface) is used to "shave" off the protruding part of the skin and lesion. This technique is useful for diagnosing malignant and benign tumors when subsequent treatment by curettage and electrodesiccation is anticipated. It should never be used when melanoma is suspected, because the specimen obtained is too superficial for adequate histologic grading. Shave biopsy is convenient for removing superficial benign tumors such as seborrheic keratoses or skin tags. In the fourth technique, punch biopsy, the clinician uses a tubular blade to cut out a circular plug of skin by slightly rotating and pushing the cutting edge deep into the dermis. The specimen is clipped off at its base with scissors, and the defect can be readily closed with sutures. Punch biopsies are used to diagnose inflammatory diseases and tumors. If a first skin biopsy does not provide an answer, it is often necessary and appropriate to resample the area.

521 PRINCIPLES OF THERAPY

Frank Parker

The goals of therapy are to define and remove the cause of a disorder, restore the structural and functional integrity of the skin, and relieve symptoms such as itching, pain, or cosmetic disfigurement. The barrier function of damaged skin is impaired, but protection can be provided with dressings as well as by minimizing scratching and avoiding abrasive clothing, soaps, and chemicals. Removal of debris, such as excessive scale, hyperkeratoses, crusts, and infection, is also crucial. Topical and systemic medications, dressings, and other treatments can alter skin temperature and blood flow and thus favorably affect the metabolism of the skin.

TOPICAL MODES OF THERAPY

SOAKS AND WET DRESSINGS. Water, with or without various additives, can provide many benefits to the skin, including soothing comfort, antipruritic effects and increased rate of epidermal healing with hydration and débridement of crusts, dead skin, and bacteria.

BATHS. A bath is useful when the area of involvement is too large to apply compresses. Baths with whirlpool action are favored for débridement of large or deep ulcers. The tub should be one-half full and the soak should last no longer than 20 to 30 minutes to avoid maceration. Medicated baths can evenly distribute soothing antipruritic and anti-inflammatory agents to widespread lesions. Bath oil prevents drying by leaving a thin film of emollient on the skin. Warm baths cause vasodilation and may increase itching; cool baths constrict vessels and usually soothe pruritus. The best time to apply lubricants is immediately after the bath so that they may hold water in the hydrated stratum corneum.

WET DRESSINGS. Water and medication can be applied to the skin with dressings (finely woven cotton, linen, or gauze) soaked in solution. As water evaporates, the skin cools, and pruritus lessens. For maximal benefit from evaporation, dressings should be no more than a few layers thick and should be reapplied every few minutes for 15 to 30 minutes several times a day. Wet compresses, especially with frequent changes, provide gentle débridement of crusts, scales, and cutaneous debris. If the compresses are permitted to dry (wet to dry compresses) and become adherent, the débriding effect is increased but there may be further damage to the skin. Dried-out dressings should be re-moistened to facilitate removal. Wet compresses also leach water-binding proteins from the stratum corneum and epidermis and lead to later skin dryness, which is desirable for treating acute vesicular, bullous, oozing, or weeping conditions as well as for crusty, swollen, and infected skin.

Open wet dressings are applied directly to the skin, leaving the dressing exposed to the air to evaporate. Frequent reapplication débrides exudate, crust, and bacterial contamination and also dries out the skin, thus rapidly decreasing oozing and weeping.

Closed wet dressings, in which the moist fabric dressings are applied to the skin and covered with an impervious material such as plastic, oil cloth, or Saran wrap, may be useful when maceration and heat retention are required. For example, closed wet dressings may be appropriate when there is excessive keratin of the palms or soles or when an early abscess needs heat to localize the infection.

DRY DRESSINGS. Dry dressings protect the skin from dirt and irritants and can be used to apply medications, prevent scratching and rubbing by the patient or from clothing and sheets, and keep dirt away. Such dressings also prevent scratching and rubbing. In cases of neurodermatitis or stasis dermatitis, dry dressings often are left in place for several days. Soft casts or cast-like boots (e.g., Unna boot) serve the same purposes.

The medication most commonly added to baths and dressings is aluminium acetate, which coagulates bacterial and serum protein. As a 5% preparation it is known as Burow's solution, and it must be further diluted for use. Burow's solution can be readily made by dissolving tablets or powder packets in appropriate amounts of water. (One tablet or packet in 500 mL = 1:20 concentration.) Potassium permanganate and silver nitrate are seldom used because they stain the skin and may be absorbed if used over large raw areas of skin.

Wounds may also be cleansed and débrided by absorption beads or granules that absorb debris and exudate from wounds (Debrisan, DuoDerm granules), hydrogen peroxide, whirlpool treatments, and various enzymatic products, including trypsin/chymotrypsin, fibrinolysin, collagenase, and streptokinase. Antimicrobial agents are seldom applied by surface dressings because huge quantities would be required to reach therapeutic concentrations.

Occlusive dressings can treat acute wounds and chronic venous, diabetic, and pressure ulcers. In general, these materials provide good protection, help promote healing, and provide pain reduction of skin ulcerations.

TOPICAL MEDICATIONS. Most topical medications consist of two major agents, the active ingredient or specific medications, and the vehicle or base in which the active material is dissolved.

BASES OR VEHICLES. Bases come in a variety of forms. *Powders* promote dryness by absorbing evaporative moisture, and they reduce maceration and friction in intertriginous areas. Powders may be inert chemicals (corn starch, talcum) or contain medications. *Lotions* are suspensions of insoluble powders in water. As water evaporates on the skin surface, it collects and leaves a uniform film of powder behind. The addition of alcohol increases the cooling effect. *Creams* are emulsions of oil in water (more water than oil); they vanish into the skin because water evaporates and the residual oil is spread thinly and imperceptibly over the skin. *Ointments* consist of oils with variably smaller amounts of water added in suspension; they have a pleasant lubricating effect on dry or diseased skin, but they give a greasy feeling to the skin and clothing. Oils in bases provide a softening effect by forming an occlusive layer that traps water and retards evaporation. Thus, ointments with large amounts of oil give a more sustained, softening effect than creams or lotions. Some ointments containing large percentages of inert oil may be occlusive and retain heat, increase pruritus, and increase percutaneous absorption of active ingredients. The more

occlusive ointments should not be used on oozing or infected areas, because the resulting occlusion and warmth may increase bacterial growth. *Pastes* are mixtures of powder and ointment (e.g., zinc oxide paste). *Sprays* are propelled aerosols.

Selection of a base or emollient depends on the condition being treated and the needs of the patient. Lotions are useful for pruritic, oozing reactions. Petrolatum, by contrast, retains heat and promotes hydration and even maceration of the stratum corneum. Ointments are used most often on dry, scaling conditions in which endogenous hydration of the stratum corneum is defective.

ACTIVE AGENTS. *Topical corticosteroids* provide effective local anti-inflammatory and antipruritic effects. They cause immediate and profound cutaneous vasoconstriction, which prevents mobilization of polymorphonuclear leukocytes and monocytes into the reaction site, and also interfere with the inflammatory activities of already-present cells (e.g., mast cells). Topical corticosteroids are intrinsically active and have a rapid therapeutic effect. They slow the mitotic rate of fibroblasts, decrease collagen synthesis, and possibly enhance collagen catabolism.

All effective topical corticosteroids have the basic hydrocortisone structure. A 1% concentration of hydrocortisone ointment or cream serves as a norm for comparing potency of subsequently modified topical corticosteroids. By fluorinating hydrocortisone or adding acetonide, the potency of the corticosteroid is greatly enhanced (Table 521–1).

The potency of a preparation also relates to the concentration of active drug in the vehicle and the nature of the vehicle. Of the various types of vehicles used in corticosteroid preparations, ointments are the most efficient because they most effectively dissolve corticosteroids, and the occlusive nature of ointments increases stratum corneum permeability. Second in order of efficiency is acetone-alcohol gel, whereas creams and lotions are less useful.

The potency of corticosteroids corresponds closely to the degree of anti-inflammatory effectiveness as well as to the incidence and severity of associated side effects. Epidermal and dermal atrophy can be pronounced; decreased collagen synthesis and reduced stromal support for dermal blood vessels lead to telangiectasia, purpura, and striae. These changes are especially likely to occur in intertriginous occluded areas of the skin and on the face. Fluorinated corticosteroids can cause a perioral scaling, papular and pustular dermatitis, or facial redness, telangiectasia, and acne rosacea–like eruption. Potent topical corticosteroids applied for prolonged periods around the eyes can occasionally cause glaucoma and even cataracts. Topical corticosteroids can also predispose to or worsen skin infections such as folliculitis, tinea, and candidiasis. Systemic absorption of potent topical corticosteroids may transiently lower plasma cortisol levels when they are used with an occlusion over as little as 20% of the body.

Intermediate-potency corticosteroids are useful in most dermatologic conditions (Table 521–2). Ointments are useful for thickened skin or for dry, exposed areas whereas creams or gel preparations rapidly evaporate. Low-potency corticosteroids are used to treat the face and the thin and occluded skin of the groin and genital area. Lotions and gels are best for hairy areas. High-potency corticosteroid preparations should not be used to treat most dermatologic conditions; they generally should be reserved for areas of skin that have been substantially thickened by disease, such as dense plaques of psoriasis or chronic dermatitis.

Topical corticosteroids are usually applied once or twice a day.

Table 521–1 ▪ POTENCY RANKING OF SOME COMMONLY USED TOPICAL CORTICOSTEROIDS

POTENCY	GENERIC NAME	CLINICAL APPLICATION
Most potent	Clobetasol propionate cream and ointment 0.5%, halobetasol propionate cream and ointment 0.5%, betamethasone dipropionate cream and ointment 0.5%, clobetasol propionate cream and ointment 0.5%, halcinonide cream and ointment 0.1%, fluocinonide ointment 0.5%	Recalcitrant psoriasis, discoid lupus, recalcitrant lichen planus, nummular eczema
Intermediate potency	Triamcinolone acetonide 0.1%, betamethasone valorate cream 0.1%, amcinonide cream 0.17%	Dermatitis—allergic-contact, atopic eczema, neurodermatitis
Low potency	Hydrocortisone cream and ointment 2.5% and 1.0%, desonide cream and ointment 0.5%, locoid ointment 0.1%, dexamethasone sodium phosphate cream 0.1%	Intertrigo, pruritus ani, seborrheic dermatitis

Table 521–2 ■ GUIDELINES FOR SELECTING TOPICAL CORTICOSTEROIDS

LOCATION OR TYPE OF LESION	SUGGESTED POTENCY OF CORTICOSTEROID	SUGGESTED VEHICLE
Areas of Body		
Trunk, arms, legs	Intermediate or low	Ointment or cream
Palms, soles	Intermediate or high	Ointment
Scalp	Intermediate or low	Lotion, gel, aerosol
Intertriginous areas	Low	Cream, lotion
Face	Low	Cream, lotion
Area around eyes	Low	Cream or ophthalmic preparation
Ears	Intermediate or low	Cream, gel, or lotion
Types of Lesion		
Dry, scaling, fissuring, lichenified lesion	Intermediate	Ointment
Thickened, hyperkeratotic skin patches	High	Ointment
Oozing, weeping lesions	Intermediate	Lotion, cream
Ulcerative lesions	Do not use topical corticosteriods	

The stratum corneum acts as a reservoir and continues to release topical corticosteroid into the skin after the initial application. Chronic dermatoses become less responsive after prolonged use, but changing to another topical corticosteroid often overcomes this problem.

Intralesional corticosteroids, which dissolve in the tissues slowly over weeks to months, are used to shrink inflammatory acne cysts and hypertrophic scars and keloids. They are occasionally injected into unresponsive, localized dermatoses such as alopecia areata, granuloma annulare, discoid lupus erythematosus, psoriasis, and lichen simplex chronicus. Triamcinolone acetonide is the most widely used, and its maximal duration of action is 4 to 6 weeks. Triamcinolone hexacetonide is longer acting (6 to 8 weeks), whereas betamethasone (Celestone) and dexamethasone (Decadron) are of shorter duration (2 to 4 weeks). To avoid disfiguring atrophy, great care is necessary in using low concentrations (<5 mg/mL) and shaking the diluted material just before injection into the dermis.

Topical antibiotics help suppress bacteria in erosions or superficial infections and occasionally in chronic leg ulcers. Silver sulfadiazine preparations are particularly useful as an adjunct to currently accepted principles of burn wound care. Commonly used topical antibiotics are bacitracin, neomycin, clindamycin phosphate, erythromycin, and tetracycline hydrochloride. The last three are used to treat acne vulgaris. All topical antibiotics have the potential to sensitize, but neomycin is particularly prone to do so, especially after long-term use on chronic stasis dermatitis and leg ulcers. Mupirocin, a new topical antibiotic ointment, is particularly useful in treating staphylococcal and streptococcal infections of the skin, and it can treat nasal carriers of *Staphylococcus* when applied high into the nasal passages (with a cotton-tipped applicator) twice a day for 2 weeks.

Topical retinoids, including tretinoin (Retin A), adapalene (Differin), and tazarotene (Tazorac), are used primarily to treat comedonal acne vulgaris by normalizing keratinization. Clinical trials have demonstrated limited efficacy in amelioration of cutaneous signs of photoaging such as fine wrinkling, mottling, and, to a lesser extent, coarse wrinkling. Tazarotene is also approved to treat localized plaque-type psoriasis.

Topical antifungal agents include clotrimazole, econazole, and miconazole creams and lotions, commonly used twice daily. Topical agents useful against dermatophytes, but not *Candida,* include haloprogin and tolnaftate (Tinactin). Over-the-counter preparations, perhaps less effective against dermatophytes, are undecylenic acid and Verdefam. No topical preparations are useful against nail infections with these fungal organisms. Nystatin creams, oral suspensions, and vaginal tablets are effective against *Candida* infections in various areas of the body. Ketoconazole is a broad-spectrum imidazole antifungal agent highly effective against dermatophytes, *Candida,* and tinea versicolor. It is available in cream and oral forms.

Tars and anthralin are used for psoriasis. Crude coal tar increases the effectiveness of ultraviolet light (photosensitizer) and reduces the accelerated mitotic rate of keratinocytes in psoriasis. Tars are often incorporated into shampoos for control of seborrheic dermatitis and into bath oils for use in psoriasis. Anthralin, which is a synthetic coal tar derivative, must be started at the lowest concentrations (0.1%) and initially left on the skin for short periods of time (30 minutes) to avoid irritation.

Antiparasitic topical medications treat pediculosis capitis, pediculosis pubis, and scabies. The lice of pediculosis corporis live in the seams of clothes and bedding, which must be disinfected by washing or dry cleaning. One per cent gamma benzene hexachloride (lindane), crotamiton, and pyrethrin compounds (RID) are useful in treating pediculosis and scabies. Lindane is not suggested for children younger than 6 years of age or for pregnant or lactating women. Permethrin 5% (Elimite cream), a synthetic pyrethroid used for the treatment of scabies, has been particularly effective with one application, especially as some scabies organisms appear to be developing resistance to lindane. Other less effective therapies for scabies include 10% crotamiton (Eurax) and topical sulfur ointments (5% in Heb cream), but both require frequent applications.

Antiseptic cleaners are bacteriostatic or bactericidal agents used as local or generalized skin cleansers and or wound irrigations. Chlorhexidine is active against gram-positive and gram-negative bacteria and some fungi and yeasts. Antiseptic iodinated compounds slowly liberate iodine, which is effective against bacteria, fungi, yeasts, and viruses. One of the most frequently used preparations is povidone-iodine (Betadine).

Sunscreens help protect the skin from the acute and chronic effects of ultraviolet (UV) radiation. They are rated by their sun protective factor (SPF), which ranges from 3 to 50 and is the factor by which the product extends the period of exposure to reach the sunburn reaction that would have taken place without the sunscreen. The action of topical photoprotectives is to reduce penetration of photoactive non-ionizing radiation. Such protection can be achieved by either absorbing or reflecting the radiation. No sunscreen enhances tanning. Rather, partial sunblock permits melanin to be produced based on the inherent capacity of the partially protected skin to respond to the radiation transmitted. Topical photoprotectants can be divided into physical and chemical agents: physical agents or sunblocks (such as titanium dioxide or zinc oxide) reflect away ultraviolet radiation; chemical sunscreens bind to proteins in the outer layer of skin and absorb potentially harmful radiation. The wavelength of radiation absorbed (UVA or UVB) depends on the active ingredient, with the most common UVB agents containing esters of para-aminobenzoic acid (PABA; e.g., padimate O), whereas UVA screening products typically contain benzophenones or an anthralin. Most sunscreens are less effective in blocking UVA (320 to 400 nm) than UVB (290 to 320 nm), but newer broad-spectrum products also contain benzophenones or anthralin compounds and protect against both UVA and UVB. For complete protection or total blockage of UVB and UVA, physical sunscreens containing titanium dioxide, zinc oxide, or iron oxide are available as heavy creams or pastes.

The photoprotection conferred by clothing is proportional to the type of fabric, its color, and the tightness of the weave. In cases of extreme photosensitivity, specially designed sun protective clothing is available (e.g., Salumbra).

Topical scar and keloid treatments include silicone (Silastic) gel sheeting, which prevents and treats chronic hypertrophic and keloid scars when it is chronically bandaged to the scar for 12 to 24 hours per day for at least 2 months. Carbon dioxide or pulsed dye laser therapy, used alone or in concert with intralesional corticosteroids, is a promising modality for large, recalcitrant keloids.

SYSTEMIC MODES OF THERAPY FOR DERMATOLOGIC CONDITIONS

ANTIHISTAMINES. The most specific use antihistamines (Table 521–3) is to ameliorate or halt histamine-mediated disorders such as urticaria, angioedema, and allergic rhinitis. Antihistamines also suppress non–histamine-induced itching by soporific side effects. Antihistamines are of two types: the classic H_1-receptor blockers and the newer H_2-receptor blockers, which also decrease gastric acid secretion. H_1-receptor blockers have three limitations: (1) they do not block all the effects of histamine; (2) they provide only

Table 521–3 ■ ANTIHISTAMINES USEFUL FOR URTICARIA AND ANGIOEDEMA ARRANGED ACCORDING TO THEIR MOLECULAR CONFIGURATION

ANTIHISTAMINE GROUP	GENERIC NAME (PROPRIETARY NAME)
H$_1$-Receptor Antagonist	
Ethanolamines	Diphenhydramine (Benadryl)*
	Clemastine (Tavist)
Piperadines	Cyproheptadine (Periactin)
	Azatadine (Optimine)
Phenothiazines	Promethazine (Phenergan)
	Trimeperizine (Temaril)
Piperazines	Hydroxyzine (Atarax)
	Meclizine
Alkylamines	Chlorpheniramine (Chlor-Trimeton)†
Ethylenediamine	Brompheniramine (Dimetapp)
	Pyrilamine (Triaminic)
Miscellaneous	Fexofenadine (Allegra)
	Astemizole (Hismanal)
	Loratadine (Claritin)
H$_2$-Receptor Antagonist	Cetirizine (Zyrtec)
	Cimetidine (Tagamet)
	Ranitidine (Zantac)
H$_1$- and H$_2$-Receptor Antagonists	Doxepin (Sinequan)

*Safe with breast feeding.
†Safe in pregnancy.

limited protection against anaphylaxis because mediators other than histamine are involved in this reaction; and (3) they are not selective in their effects (i.e., they also have anticholinergic and sedative effects).

If response to one antihistamine is minimal, another from a different group should be added or substituted. Because blood vessels in human skin have H$_2$- as well as H$_1$-receptors, combined H$_1$- and H$_2$-receptor antagonists are effective in some cases of chronic urticaria otherwise unresponsive to H$_1$-receptor antagonists alone.

Antihistamines should be started in moderate doses until sufficient improvement or troublesome side effects develop. Generally, they are administered three or four times a day. Low doses should be given to elderly patients, who are more sensitive to central nervous system side effects such as confusion, dizziness, and syncope, as well as to urinary retention, dry mouth, and blurred vision. In children, paradoxically, antihistamines may induce hyperactivity.

SYSTEMIC CORTICOSTEROIDS. Systemic corticosteroids, which are used for a number of dermatologic conditions, have several drawbacks: (1) prolonged administration leads to adrenal suppression and susceptibility to infection; (2) many diseases such as psoriasis and atopic dermatitis may worsen after steroid withdrawal; (3) safer and simpler therapy is available for most common dermatoses. Systemic corticosteroids are used in three types of situations. First, patients severely ill with life-threatening diseases known to be responsive to corticosteroids (anaphylactic reactions, extensive erythema multiforme, acute exfoliative dermatitis, pem-

phigus vulgaris) should be started at high doses—80 to 100 mg daily. Second, patients with acute and severe but self-limited conditions are treated with corticosteroids to control or suppress episodes; examples include widespread poison ivy dermatitis, extensive sunburn, and acute generalized urticaria of known cause. Third, corticosteroids are used for patients with chronic dermatologic conditions that, because of periodic exacerbations, intermittently require low doses (15 to 20 mg) of prednisone together with supportive topical therapy. Examples include flares of chronic atopic dermatitis, pemphigoid, and some connective tissue diseases.

SYSTEMIC ANTIFUNGAL AGENTS. Three primary types of systemic antifungal agents are commonly used to treat dermatologic disease: (1) griseofulvin, (2) terbinafine (Lamisil), and (3) oral azoles, including ketoconazole, fluconazole, and itraconazole (Table 521–4). Griseofulvin is active against dermatophytes but not against tinea versicolor or *Candida*. It is fungistatic, entering the horny layer of the skin through the sweat and the nails by incorporation into the keratinizing cells of the nail matrix. The entire nail must grow out with griseofulvin incorporated into it before the tinea at the distal end of the nail is affected. The agent must be taken for many months before dermatophyte infections of the toenails disappear, although less time is required for infections of the fingernails and glabrous skin. Griseofulvin has rare side effects, including photo-sensitivity, urticaria, angioedema, headaches, gastrointestinal upset, and granulocytopenia. The drug may intensify underlying porphyria. Griseofulvin also decreases the activity of warfarin-like drugs so that patients taking these agents may require dosage adjustments. Possible hepatotoxicity is not well documented. This agent is effective in treating tinea capitus, onychomycosis, and tinea corporis too extensive for topical therapy and in treating superficial fungal infections in immunosuppressed patients. It remains the drug of choice for tinea capitis in children, but it is less commonly used for other indications, primarily due to the required long duration of therapy and high incidence of recurrent infections.

Terbinafine (Lamisil), a synthetic allylamine available in oral and topical formulations, is fungicidal and functions by inhibiting squalene epoxidase, which is vital to fungal sterol biosynthesis. Terbinafine is active against dermatophytes, but its efficacy against *Candida* has not been fully studied. Indications include fungal infection of the body, scalp, or nails. Potential side effects include gastrointestinal upset, transient taste disturbance, and rare cases of hepatobiliary dysfunction, which have prompted many to check baseline and mid-treatment liver function tests. Additionally, a variety of cutaneous reactions ranging from urticaria to Stevens-Johnson syndrome have been attributed to terbinafine. The incidence of medication interactions with terbinafine appears lower than with other antifungal agents, but drugs that affect cytochrome P-450 may alter terbinafine clearance.

Azole drugs are synthetic compounds that are classified as imidazoles (miconazole and ketoconazole) or triazoles (itraconazole and

Table 521–4 ■ THE ORAL ANTIFUNGAL AGENTS

AGENT (TRADE NAME)	TABLET STRENGTH	MECHANISM	ABSORPTION	MONITOR BLOOD LEVELS	SIDE EFFECTS
Griseofulvin (Gris-PEG)	250 mg	Static	Take with fatty meal, drink	No	Headache, gastrointestinal symptoms, erythema multiforme, rare leukopenia
Terbinafine (Lamisil)	250 mg	Cidal	Acid in stomach not necessary	Yes	Headache, gastrointestinal symptoms, rare taste disturbance, rare hepatitis
Itraconazole (Sporanox)	100 mg	Static	Acid in stomach is necessary	Yes	Nausea, vomiting, rare hepatitis, pruritus, edema
Fluconazole (Diflucan)	50, 100, 150, 200 mg	Static	Acid in stomach not necessary	Yes	Nausea, vomiting, rash, pruritus, rare hepatitis, Stevens-Johnson syndrome
Ketoconazole	200 mg	Static	Acid in stomach is necessary	Yes	Nausea, vomiting, pruritus, headache, adrenal insufficiency, decreased libido, gynecomastia

fluconazole) according to whether they contain two or three nitrogen atoms, respectively, in the five-membered azole ring. The antifungal effects of the azoles are due to their ability to inhibit ergosterol synthesis, which is critical for maintaining fungal membrane integrity. Ketoconazole and itraconazole, which are available only for oral use, require an acid environment for optimal absorption. Fluconazole is available in both oral and intravenous formulations. Ketoconazole is effective against tinea versicolor and *Candida.* Several instances of fatal hepatocellular toxicity have been recorded, so ketoconazole should be used only for extensive cutaneous dermatophyte infections unresponsive to griseofulvin or for extensive cutaneous *Candida* infections. Liver enzyme levels should be determined before starting treatment and monitored at monthly intervals during treatment. Because most cases of azole-related hepatitis occur during the first few months of treatment, monitoring with aminotransferase levels is especially important during this time. The role of itraconazole and fluconazole for treating superficial fungal infections remains uncertain, but it has been successful for treating tinea corporis and tinea cruris, onychomycosis, and cutaneous candidiasis with oral doses (150 to 200 mg once a week) for 2 to 4 months.

RETINOIDS. Retinoids are derivatives of natural vitamin A compounds. Two retinoids, isotretinoin and acitretin, are available to treat dermatologic conditions. Retinoids decrease epidermal cell proliferation and keratinization and inhibit sebaceous gland activity. Acitretin has been found to be useful in severe psoriasis, especially the erythrodermic and pustular forms, as well as in several forms of ichthyosis. Isotretinoin has proved to be especially useful in severe cystic acne, often inducing prolonged remissions for several years after the drug is given for the usual 3- to 4-month course. The retinoids have many side effects, including cheilitis, conjunctivitis, dryness and fragility of skin, congenital malformations (heart defects, hydrocephalus, microtia), osteophytic growths on the vertebrae, epiphyseal closure in growing youngsters, corneal opacities, night blindness, and elevations of very low-density and low-density lipoproteins. 13-*cis*-Retinoic acid (Accutane) should be given only for severe nodulocystic acne. When given in doses of 0.5 to 1.0 mg/kg for 4 to 5 months, acne clears in 85 to 95% of patients, and in about 85% of these patients clearance of their acne essentially continues indefinitely.

SYSTEMIC GOLD SALTS. Intramuscular gold has been useful in the treatment of autoimmune bullous disease, particularly pemphigus vulgaris, with remissions of 21 months or longer. Generally a total dose of 400 to 600 mg of gold must be given before bullae respond. Oral gold (Aurinotin) has not been used widely in dermatologic conditions.

SYSTEMIC ANTIBIOTICS. Cutaneous bacterial infections and conditions aggravated by bacterial overgrowth, such as acne vulgaris, acne rosacea, and acute dermatitis, usually involve *Staphylococcus aureus* or *Streptococcus pyogenes* (e.g., erysipelas, cellulitis, folliculitis, furunculosis, carbunculosis). Penicillins, cephalosporins, and erythromycins are commonly used to treat these conditions. Erythromycin and tetracyclines can control acne vulgaris and acne rosacea. Trimethoprim/sulfamethoxazole is used for pyodermas in patients allergic to penicillin or caused by methicillin-resistant *S. aureus.* Sulfone and sulfonamides are used most often to control dermatitis herpetiformis. Dapsone is most commonly used to treat leprosy but is also useful in treating cutaneous vasculitis, pyoderma gangrenosum, bullous forms of systemic lupus erythematosus, and brown recluse spider bites. Common side effects of dapsone are hemolysis and methemoglobinemia (especially in patients deficient in the enzyme glucose-6-phosphate dehydrogenase). Patients require frequent laboratory monitoring, including a complete blood cell count, differential, reticulocyte count, chemistry profile, and methemoglobin level.

ANTIMALARIAL AGENTS. Chloroquine, hydroxychloroquine, and quinacrine benefit patients with cutaneous lupus erythematosus, polymorphic light eruption, solar urticaria, and porphyria cutanea tarda. Antimalarial agents bind DNA, inhibit the LE cell phenomenon and antinuclear antibody reactions, block chemotaxis, and antagonize histaminic responses, all of which may be related to their therapeutic effects. Cutaneous and mucous membrane pigmentation, nausea, diarrhea, and cycloplegia are common toxic effects, but

retinopathy is the adverse reaction of greatest concern. Quinacrine does not cause retinopathy.

SYSTEMIC ANTIVIRAL AGENTS. Acyclovir, valacyclovir, famciclovir, and vidarabine can treat herpes simplex and zoster skin and systemic infections (see Chapter 385).

SYSTEMIC CYTOSTATIC DRUGS. Cytotoxic drugs such as methotrexate, cyclophosphamide, azathioprine, and hydroxyurea are used in a number of skin conditions when they cannot be controlled by more conventional means. For example, if psoriasis is generalized, severe, and life ruining, it may be treated with modest doses of methotrexate, azathioprine, or hydroxyurea. Life-threatening bullous diseases such as pemphigus vulgaris are occasionally treated with these agents rather than with high doses of corticosteroids. More recently, low-dose cyclosporine has been used for severe psoriasis.

ULTRAVIOLET LIGHT AS A THERAPEUTIC AGENT. UV light units are available in two wavelength ranges: UVB (the sunburn range of 238 to 320 nm) and UVA (long wavelength spectrum of 320 to 400 nm). UV phototherapy is used primarily to treat psoriasis and vitiligo but may also help patients with nummular and atopic eczema, pityriasis rosea, the pruritus of uremia, and mycosis fungoides. It is commonly used in combination with topical or oral psoralen, a drug that binds to DNA in the skin and sensitizes it to the effects of UVA. The long-term side effects of such therapy induce squamous and basal cell cutaneous carcinoma, but its role in causing melanoma is controversial. Used over many weeks to months, this approach is highly effective in controlling psoriasis. UVA light units are also employed by dermatologists and commercial suntan centers to cause tanning rather than burning. The ability of UVA to evoke a sunburn is 1000 times less than that of UVB. The unprotected cornea and retina can be damaged by UV light, so stringent guidelines for protecting the eyes must be observed.

522 SKIN DISEASES OF GENERAL IMPORTANCE

Frank Parker

THE ECZEMAS (DERMATITIS)

Eczematous dermatitis is an inflammatory response of the skin to multiple exogenous and endogenous agents, although often the cause is not clear (Table 522–1). Eczemas are defined by their clinical appearance and are subdivided either by their pattern of distribution or by etiologic factors (when known). Many eczematous processes are related to immunologic reactions.

The term *eczema* or *eczematous dermatitis* is applied to eruptions characterized histologically by epidermal intercellular edema, termed *spongiosis.* Eczemas can be acute, with marked spongiosis causing red papules and vesicles with oozing, weeping, and crusting; or they may be chronic, with redness, scaling, fissuring, and especially lichenification. Both acute and chronic forms of eczema

Table 522–1 ■ TYPES OF ECZEMA

Contact dermatitis
Photodermatitis
Atopic dermatitis
Stasis dermatitis
Nummular eczematous dermatitis
Lichen simplex chronicus
Seborrheic dermatitis
Xerotic eczema and eczema craquelé
Hand eczema
Exfoliative dermatitis (erythroderma)
Drug reactions
Infectious eczematoid dermatitis
Non-specific eczematous dermatitis
Fungal infections of the skin mimicking eczema

may affect the same patient, with the acute reactions progressing to oozing and crusting; with continued pruritus, the patient's rubbing and scratching convert the eczema to the chronic, dry, lichenified form. The hallmarks of all types of eczematous dermatitis are marked pruritus and varying degrees of erythema along with papules, vesicles, fine scaling, or lichenification. The histologic character of eczema is the same for the various types.

CONTACT DERMATITIS. There are two types of contact dermatitis, irritant and allergic. Irritant contact dermatitis is produced by substances that simply irritate or have a direct toxic effect on the skin, such as acids, alkalis, solvents, and detergents; no immunologic process is involved. Conversely, allergic contact dermatitis is a delayed-type hypersensitivity reaction that occurs in response to a wide variety of allergens commonly found in the environment. These allergens consist of low-molecular-weight substances that act as haptens and bind to proteinaceous components of the skin to form the sensitizing antigen. Sensitization develops 10 to 14 days after the first encounter; subsequent exposure elicits the eczematous response in 1 to 7 days (delayed hypersensitivity). Allergic contact dermatitis may develop shortly after the use of a new product or after many years of using an old product containing a potential allergen. If the cause of contact dermatitis can be identified, avoidance is curative.

The onset of irritant reactions after exposure to topical substance varies. Skin damage is evident within hours after contact with a strong irritant. Weaker irritants may require multiple applications and days or weeks before the development of the eczema (e.g., eczemas of the hands due to chronic exposure to water and detergents). Contact dermatitis accounts for more than 50% of all occupational illnesses (excluding injury): Approximately 70% is irritant and 30% allergic contact dermatitis.

Both irritant and allergic contact eczemas are initially confined to sites of contact. Allergic reactions to plants appear as linear, red, papular, and vesicular streaks where the plant brushes across the skin. Allergies to metals (especially nickel) cause eczematous reactions under rings or watchbands or on the lobes of ears (earrings). Dermatitis under a ring may also stem from trapped water and irritating soap residues.

The most common allergens causing allergic contact dermatitis are pentadecylcatechol (allergen in poison oak, ivy, and sumac as well as in cashews, mangos, and gingko trees), paraphenylenediamine (a substance in hair dyes that cross-reacts with benzocaine and hydrochlorothiazide), nickel, mercaptobenzothiazole and thiuram (components in rubber), and ethylenediamine (a preservative in many medications and also found in industrial dyes and insecticides). Other common sources of contactants include topical medications (neomycin, anesthetics such as benzocaine, topical antihistamines), preservatives (ethylenediamine, merthiolate), vehicles (propylene glycol), and cosmetics (fragrances, preservatives, paraphenylenediamines). A detailed history of the patient's occupation, hobbies, habits, clothing, cosmetics, and topical medications is necessary to identify the contactant; definitive diagnosis frequently requires patch testing.

The most common cause of irritant contact dermatitis is frequent hand washing. Allergic contact dermatitis, a Type IV delayed-type reaction (Chapter 270) to rubber gloves, is typically due to a component of rubber (e.g., thiuram, carba mix, or mercaptobenzothiazole) and less often to latex itself. Contact urticaria to latex, a Type I immediate-type reaction (Chapter 273), may trigger dermatitis and be complicated by allergic rhinitis and even anaphylaxis due to aerosolized latex protein carried by glove powder. Risk factors for potentially fatal latex sensitivity include having a history of multiple surgical procedures ($\geq$80% of spina bifida patients) and being a health care worker (8% of physicians, 10% of nurses, 13% of dental workers). Evaluation may include radioallergosorbent testing (RAST) to latex and patch or prick testing. Desensitization rarely helps, and often the only treatment is avoidance, usually by occupational adjustment.

Protective clothing is sometimes curative. Barrier creams are of little benefit. Acute, severe, generalized contact dermatitis is treated with a short (10- to 14-day) course of systemic steroids and wet dressings or baths. Milder eczematous reactions respond to topical steroids and systemic antihistamines, but an allergic contact dermatitis to either the vehicle or the active ingredient in topical steroids can complicate the clinical picture.

PHOTODERMATITIS. A variety of skin reactions, termed *photo-*

sensitivity reactions, may occur in response to exposure to ultraviolet (UV) light. Some appear as eczematous reactions, so-called photoallergic dermatitis, and may occur in response to topical as well as systemic substances in the presence of UV light. The distribution of the eczematous eruption in light-exposed areas is an important feature in the differential diagnosis, with the cheeks, nose, forehead, tips of ears, backs of hands, and forearms frequently involved.

Photoallergic dermatitis is immunologic. Absorption of a specific wavelength of ultraviolet light by a topical substance or a systemic drug (which is deposited in the skin from the vascular circulation) causes chemical conversion of the substance or drug to a hapten that binds cutaneous proteins to become a complete antigen capable of eliciting a Type IV delayed hypersensitivity reaction similar to an allergic contact dermatitis reaction. Photoallergic reactions appear only where the UV light hits the skin, even though the systemic drug or topical photoallergen is present in the skin all over the body—i.e., the reaction depends on UV light's hitting the skin with the allergen in it. Long-wavelength ultraviolet A (UVA) light usually generates these reactions. Because UVA light penetrates window glass, the reaction often results from indoor exposure. Drugs such as thiazides and phenothiazines can cause photoeczematous reactions, as can topically applied methyl coumarin, musk ambrette, halogenated salicylanilides, and sun-screening agents. Photopatch testing can identify substances causing these reactions. Oral and topical steroids relieve the inflammatory reaction, and avoidance of the offending material is often curative.

ATOPIC DERMATITIS. Atopic dermatitis, a chronic, eczematous condition of the skin, is often associated with a personal or family history of asthma, allergic rhinitis, and/or atopic eczema. Pruritus is prominent, and the consequent scratching and rubbing lead to lichenification, most typically in the antecubital and popliteal flexural areas. The eczema usually manifests itself after the first few months of life and appears on the face and extensor areas of the extremities as acute and subacute, red, vesicular, and oozing dermatitis. Many cases resolve spontaneously by puberty only to recur in adolescence and adulthood as a chronic dermatitis with scaling, dryness, and lichenification over the face, neck, upper chest, and characteristically the antecubital and popliteal fossae (flexural dermatitis). Atopic patients have a readily identifiable facies with diffuse erythema, perioral pallor, and a redundant crease or fold below the lower eyelids. The palms often have an increased number of skin markings, noticeable as fine cross-hatched lines. In atopic dermatitis, stroking the skin causes a white line, or white dermatographism, probably due to dermal edema and vasoconstriction.

The incidence of atopic dermatitis is increasing in industrialized countries, with up to 10% of babies suffering from atopic eczema. Up to 40% will "outgrow" their eczema and suffer no chronic disease; however, 60% will manifest some cutaneous problem related to atopic dermatitis as adults. The cause remains unknown, but atopic patients demonstrate excessive T-cell activation, specifically with increased helper T-cell (T_H2) cytokines such as interleukin 4 (IL-4) and IL-10, usually with elevated serum immunoglobulin E (IgE) level as well. Clinically, these patients have depressed cell-mediated immunity, which may account for their increased susceptibility to cutaneous infections by herpesvirus, vaccinia and molluscum contagiosum virus, and human papillomavirus. Abnormal neutrophil and monocyte chemotaxis may explain frequent staphylococcal infections, which also trigger flares of dermatitis; oral antibiotics often result in marked improvement.

Atopic individuals are often tense, resentful, aggressive, and restless, but whether these emotions trigger the diathesis or merely result from living with chronic, unremitting itching and skin inflammation is not certain. Regardless, the physician must help the patient meet the stresses of life.

Keratoconjunctivitis and stellate anterior subcapsular cataracts are associated with atopic eczema, particularly in patients with extensive skin changes. The conjunctivitis and keratitis usually start in childhood. The cataracts may also begin at a young age, often by age 20, and develop rapidly.

The treatment of atopic dermatitis is the same as for other eczematous eruptions and includes topical steroids, emollients, and systemic antihistamines. Refractory, severe disease in adults may require more potent immune modulators such as methotrexate, cyclosporine, or tacrolimus. In some children (less than 2 years of age), food allergy can cause atopic dermatitis, but dietary factors remain controversial. Skin tests or RAST tests help identify which foods may be responsible, but positive results must be confirmed with controlled food challenges and elimination diets. Allergic immediate skin testing and desensitization have been of little value.

Skin irritation must be avoided by wearing soft cotton clothing. Counseling, psychotherapy, and stress reduction sometimes help. The condition often worsens during the autumn and winter seasons when central heating and a dry environment dramatically decrease humidity. The frequent use of emollients is the best treatment for skin dryness, especially immediately after bathing, when the skin is hydrated. Given the extraordinarily high incidence of hand eczema in atopic patients (up to 70%), early occupational counseling should emphasize the need to avoid "wetwork." Topical corticosteroids are the most important means of controlling the inflammatory response; the least potent forms should be used, usually in an ointment base. Systemic steroids should be used only in short courses to overcome exacerbations not controlled by topical steroids.

STASIS DERMATITIS. An eczematous eruption occurs on the lower legs secondary to peripheral venous insufficiency, which increases hydrostatic pressure and capillary damage with extravasation of red blood cells and serum. These conditions trigger an inflammatory, brawny, edematous, red, and hyperpigmented petechial scaling or weeping reaction, usually around the medial malleolus or distal one third of the lower leg. Secondary allergic contact dermatitis frequently complicates the problem when neomycin is used chronically to treat accompanying stasis ulcers. Management consists of preventing venous stasis and edema with rigid external support in the form of supportive hose, or newer devices such as Circaid. Weight reduction and elevation of the extremity are helpful, particularly in obese patients. The eczema is treated with topical steroids and wet compresses when oozing and crusting are present, though care must be taken to prevent their application to ulcerated skin, as this treatment will delay wound healing. Occasionally, secondary infection of chronic stasis dermatitis leads to autosensitization dermatitis with acute inflammation in distant areas of the body. These secondary eczematous patches evolve on the face, neck, and extensor areas of the extremities. Topical steroids (occasionally oral steroids for severe reactions) control the reactions; antibiotics may be needed to halt cutaneous infection.

NUMMULAR ECZEMATOUS DERMATITIS. Nummular eczematous dermatitis is defined by recurrent coin-shaped patches predominantly on the extensor surfaces of the arms and legs, less often on the trunk. Minute patches of vesicles and papules spread to become scaling and thickened, occasionally clearing in the center so that they may resemble superficial fungal infections. Mild to severe pruritus accompanies the patches. Although the cause is unknown, many factors acting alone or in combination may contribute. Dry skin is frequent, and the disease reaches a peak in winter months. Irritating substances, such as wool and soap, and frequent bathing may contribute. The combination of topical steroids (usually of intermediate potency), 3% crude coal tar, and ultraviolet light treatments helps to control the persistent eczema.

LICHEN SIMPLEX CHRONICUS. Also known as *neurodermatitis,* lichen simplex chronicus is a chronic, pruritic, lichenified eczematous eruption that results from constant scratching. Pruritus often precedes the scratching, and rubbing induces lichenification, initiating a vicious cycle. In most patients it is a nervous habit. Patches of neurodermatitis commonly affect the nape of the neck, lower legs, groin, or other regions within easy reach of the hands. Occasionally, constant scratching results in scaling, thickened, excoriated papules and nodules. Treatment consists of explaining the cause and the need to stop rubbing. Topical steroids and oral antihistamines may be helpful. Steroids injected into the lesion break the itching cycle more successfully than topical oils. If practical and acceptable to the patient, localized extremity lichen simplex chronicus may be treated with occlusion under a medicated gauze bandage (Unna's boot). Smaller lesions may respond to topical steroids impregnated on an adhesive dressing (Cordran tape).

SEBORRHEIC DERMATITIS. Seborrheic dermatitis is characterized by erythematous, eczematous patches with yellow, greasy scales localized to hairy areas and regions of the skin with high

concentrations of sebaceous glands, especially the middle of the face, nasolabial folds, eyebrows, ear canals, retroauricular folds, and presternal areas. Dandruff is scaling of the scalp without inflammation. Severe cases can involve the axillae and groin region. Seborrheic dermatitis may appear in infants until about 6 months of age (cradle cap) and then disappear until after puberty. Patients with neurologic disorders, such as Parkinson's disease or stroke, may have a dramatic flare of their seborrhea. Although the cause of seborrhea is unknown, its association with emotional stress and neurologic disease suggests a central nervous system influence. Some studies suggest that the condition is related to excessive growth of yeast organisms (*Pityrosporon*) on the skin. It is sometimes difficult to differentiate seborrhea from psoriasis when the latter is localized to the scalp, ears, and face. Extensive, recalcitrant seborrhea may also signal infection with the human immunodeficiency virus regardless of CD4 counts or viral load and may therefore be one of the first cutaneous clues to this diagnosis.

Antiseborrheic shampoos containing tar, sulfur, salicylic acid, selenium sulfide, or pyrithione zinc provide the most useful treatment. The shampoo should be used daily, rubbed into the scalp, and left on for 5 minutes before rinsing. Inflammatory seborrhea that does not respond to shampoos alone may benefit from a topical steroid lotion or gel in hairy areas and from hydrocortisone cream in facial glabrous skin. Continual use of shampoo and topical steroids is required for control. Topical or oral ketoconazole helps in some patients.

XEROTIC ECZEMA AND ECZEMA CRAQUELÉ. The conditions xerotic eczema and eczema craquelé are characterized by chapping and symptomatic dryness that may lead to visible fissuring through the stratum corneum, giving crisscrossing cracks that resemble dried mud. Such changes occur most commonly in winter, and they respond to emollients and/or hydrocortisone ointments.

HAND ECZEMA. Hand eczema is most common in homemakers, cooks, food handlers, and medical personnel. The most common precipitators are constant exposure to mild primary irritants (soap, water), frequent hand washing, atopy, nummular dermatitis, and allergic contact dermatitis. Dyshidrotic eczema (pompholyx) is a relatively non-inflammatory, recurrent, pruritic vesicular eruption of the palms and soles of unknown cause; it differs from other hand eczemas in that the primary involvement is on the palm instead of the dorsum of the hands. The term *dyshidrotic eczema,* which suggests malfunction of the sweat ducts, is a misnomer; *pompholyx,* from the Greek meaning "bubble," is a more apt term. Emotional stress tends to be a trigger. Vesicles on the palms can also represent dermatophytid, an allergic reaction to a dermatophyte infection on the feet. If potassium hydroxide (KOH) examination of the feet yields a positive result, treatment of the fungus also resolves the palmar reaction.

Treatment of hand dermatitis involves avoidance of primary irritants such as soap, solvents, detergents, and frequent exposure to water. The use of cotton gloves with rubber gloves over them is helpful in protecting the hands in water. Emollients may help, but topical steroids are often required.

EXFOLIATIVE DERMATITIS (ERYTHRODERMA). Total-body cutaneous erythema, edema, scaling, and fissuring may occur as an idiopathic entity without preceding dermatologic or systemic disease, or it may result from a variety of cutaneous (atopic or contact dermatitis, psoriasis, seborrheic dermatitis, autosensitization, pityriasis rubra pilaris) or systemic disorders (mycosis fungoides, lymphomas, leukemias) or constitute a reaction to drugs (antibiotics, barbiturates, antiepileptic agents, gold). (Color Plate 14D). Other organ systems are affected by the general erythroderma and changes in the stratum corneum barrier function. The diffuse redness and warmth of the skin reflect vasodilatation and increased blood flow through the immense cutaneous vasculature; 5 to 8% of the total cardiac output may be directed to the dilated, inflamed cutaneous vasculature. Increased heat loss may lead to decreased core temperature, shivering, and swings in temperature; in older individuals with underlying cardiac disease, high-output heart failure may ensue. Oral steroids decrease the cutaneous inflammation and correct the associated abnormalities. In less acute situations, total-body applications of topical steroids with plastic sauna suit occlusion reverse the erythroderma.

OTHER ECZEMATOUS DERMATITIS. Occasionally, eczematous lesions will be drug-induced, such as a generalized eczematous rash that may occur after administration of penicillin. Classically, such reactions occur 10 or more days after first beginning the drug, but the eczema may begin sooner if the patient has been previously exposed; the rash clears after discontinuing the medication.

Infectious eczematoid dermatitis is a reaction to infected leg ulcers or linear infections and commonly occurs as an eczematous reaction near the site of the infection or other draining lesions. The eczematoid dermatitis clears with treatment of the infection.

Non-specific eczematous dermatitis is the name given to acute and chronic eczematous patches anywhere on the body, sometimes with severe itching. This definition is reserved for those cases in which no other cause of eczema can be determined.

FUNGAL INFECTIONS OF THE SKIN

Fungal infections, including dermatophytosis, candidiasis, and tinea versicolor, may be confused with eczema. Dermatophytes are a homogenous group of fungi that live on the keratin of the stratum corneum, nails, and hair and that frequently provoke a cutaneous inflammatory reaction with pruritus, redness, scaling, and vesiculation. Three general dermatophytes cause these infections: *Trichophyton, Microsporum,* and *Epidermophyton* species. Dermatophytosis of the trunk (tinea corporis) can be caused by several species (*T. rubrum* and *T. mentagrophytes* are most common), resulting in annular inflamed patches with elevated scaling and, at times, vesicular borders with a tendency to central clearing. The eruption may be widespread and may mimic nummular eczema. Extensive, red, scaling lesions with elevated serpiginous borders may occur in diabetic and immunosuppressed patients. Ringworm of the scalp appears as scaling areas of hair loss with black dots indicating breakage of hair shafts. Most infections are now due to *T. tonsurans* or *M. canis*. KOH preparations and cultures for fungi should be performed (using plucked hairs and scales from the affected areas). Tinea cruris infection in the groin appears as red patches with elevated serpiginous and scaling borders. The scrotum is seldom involved. Erythrasma is still another type of intertriginous erythema caused by a *Corynebacterium* sp. infection. It appears as velvety red patches with fine scale that, under Wood's light, fluoresce a diagnostic coral pink color. Erythromycin clears the infection. Tinea of the feet (pedis) and hands (manum) often present together. Infections of the feet appear in three forms: (1) interdigital maceration, scaling, and fissuring; (2) diffuse, dry scaling and mild erythema of the plantar surface, often extending onto the sides of the feet in a moccasin distribution, occasionally associated with dry scaling of one palm; (3) vesiculopustular lesions on the insteps of the feet. Involvement of the nails, onychomycosis, often accompanies hand and foot dermatophytosis.

Candidiasis, particularly that caused by *Candida albicans,* causes inflammatory skin reactions (Color Plate 14E). Intertriginous moniliasis occurs in the groin, perineum, gluteal folds, inframammary areas, axillae, and digital webs. Typically, the folds become macerated and erythematous with small satellite pustules, papules, and erosions around the periphery of the main lesion. Obesity, diabetes, and prior use of antibiotics may play a role. Chronic mucocutaneous candidiasis is a rare condition characterized by superficial *Candida* sp. infection of the skin, nails, and oral and genital mucosal surfaces complicating a variety of systemic immunodeficiencies (Chapter 400).

Tinea versicolor, a common superficial fungus infection caused by *Pityrosporon orbiculare,* is identified by scaling, red to brown or white oval patches over the neck, trunk, and upper arms (Color Plate 14F). As the name *versicolor* implies, the lesions vary in color. During the summer months when the skin is exposed to ultraviolet light, the lesions appear hypopigmented, as the infection prevents the involved skin from forming pigment. Examination of the lesion with KOH reveals budding yeast forms and club-shaped hyphae.

Either topical or systemic agents can treat fungal infections of the skin. If the dermatophytic or candidal glabrous skin infection is localized, econazole, miconazole, clotrimazole, ciclopirox, or terbinafine creams, ointments, and lotions are effective when applied two to three times a day for 3 to 4 weeks. Tinea versicolor also responds to these agents, but selenium sulfide, the 2% antidandruff shampoo, is less expensive and also effective. Application of the shampoo to the involved areas of skin for 10 minutes each night for 3 to 4 weeks clears the disease, although the hypopigmentation does not resolve until the patient is exposed to the sun. Regular shampooing with selenium sulfide reduces reinfection rates.

Scalp, nail, or follicular (as evidenced by pustular lesions) involvement or widespread, resistant fungal infections may require systemic agents. Newer fungicidal agents such as terbinafine (Lamisil) 250 mg/day for 2 weeks (body), 6 weeks (scalp or fingernails), or 12 weeks (toenails), as well as fungistatic azoles such as itraconazole are effective, but potential medication reactions require laboratory monitoring (Chapter 521). Griseofulvin, a fungistatic agent, is safe and effective, but treatment duration is longer, and recurrence rates higher than with the newer agents (Chapter 521). Other oral agents such as ketoconazole are used less frequently because of higher side effect profiles.

MACULOPAPULAR SKIN DISEASES

A diverse group of cutaneous and systemic conditions are characterized by widespread erythematous macules and papules (Table 522–2) (Color Plates 15A and 15C). Some of the conditions also have associated petechiae or purpura.

VIRAL EXANTHEMS. Because many viral exanthems are maculopapular, this group of skin diseases is often termed *morbilliform,* or measles-like. The clinical appearance of virus-induced erythema is not specific for a given etiologic agent; other signs and symptoms help to suggest a particular viral agent. Most viral exanthems are preceded by a prodrome of fever and constitutional symptoms. A history of previous exposure to infected individuals may be obtained. Incubation times vary from days to weeks depending on the virus. Drug history may also be important, especially with infectious mononucleosis, in which only 3% of patients have maculopapular or petechial eruption, but, with the administration of ampicillin, the frequency approaches 100%. In measles (rubeola) and rubella, the erythematous macules and papules begin on the face and spread to the trunk and extremities, fading with desquamation in 6 days in rubeola and on the third day in rubella. The rashes associated with enterovirus infection are most commonly rubella-like but occasionally are purpuric. Exanthem subitum (roseola infantum) displays fleeting, discrete, red papules surrounded by a whitish halo that begins on the trunk and then evolves on the neck. Erythema infectiosum (fifth disease) is an alarming-appearing red, slapped cheek rash over the face with reticulate maculopapular lesions on the extremities that clear in 3 to 6 days; mucous membranes are sometimes involved. In rubella, red spots occur on the soft palate. In measles, Koplik's spots, tiny gray-white papules on an erythematous base, are found on the buccal mucosa opposite the molars. An erythematous, maculopapular rash that begins peripherally on the palms and soles and then spreads to the trunk, often

Table 522–2 ■ **MACULOPAPULAR SKIN DISEASES**

Viral exanthems
  Measles (rubeola)
  Rubella
  Exanthem subitum (roseola infantum)
  Erythema infectiosum (fifth disease)
  Verruca vulgaris
  Molluscum contagiosum
Scarlatiniform eruptions
  Scarlet fever
  Kawasaki's syndrome
  Toxic shock syndrome
Drug reactions
Purpuric maculopapular skin lesions
  Non-palpable purpuras
    Actinic (senile) purpura
    Meningococcemia
    Gonococcemia
    Rocky mountain spotted fever
    Infectious endocarditis
  Palpable purpuras
    Vasculitis (see Table 522–3)
    Sepsis
    Cryoglobulinemia
    Drug reactions
    Carcinomas

with a petechial component, is seen in atypical measles, which is a hypersensitivity reaction to wild measles virus in a partially immune, vaccinated host.

Verruca vulgaris and molluscum contagiosum are two examples of viral infections that are confined to the skin and that elicit unique papular lesions. Wart papillomavirus induces various forms of warts: Common warts, which are dome-shaped papules with corrugated, hyperkeratotic surfaces; flat warts, which are slightly raised, smooth, flat-topped papules often on the hands and face; plantar warts, which are painful papules on the soles of the feet covered by a thick callus with black puncta within the lesion; and condylomata acuminata, or veneral warts, which are soft and moist and appear on genital areas. Molluscum contagiosum is caused by a DNA poxvirus that infects epidermal cells to induce smooth, dome-shaped, translucent papules with a central umbilication from which a cheesy core can be expressed. Verruca vulgaris lesions respond to a variety of nonspecific destructive techniques, including liquid nitrogen cryotherapy, salicylic and lactic acid combinations, cantharidin, and podophyllin. Molluscum contagiosum lesions are removed by curettage of the central core, liquid nitrogen freezing, or cantharidin application for short periods of time (15 to 30 minutes). It may be necessary to repeat the treatment every 2 weeks for several treatments.

SCARLATINIFORM ERUPTIONS. Scarlet fever, Kawasaki's syndrome, and toxic shock syndrome also present with erythematous macular and papular eruptions. Group A streptococcal pharyngitis or tonsillitis with a strain producing erythrogenic toxin initiates a confluent, papular eruption with sandpaper texture that begins on the neck and upper chest and evolves over the abdomen and extremities. The face is flushed, and circumoral pallor is prominent. Extensive desquamation occurs in 4 to 5 days. Punctate redness of the palate and strawberry tongue coexist.

Kawasaki's syndrome, a condition of unknown cause, displays a morbilliform or scarlatiniform eruption more prominent on the trunk than the face. Distinctive areas of magenta red discolorations of the palms and soles are associated with indurative edema of the hands and feet. The skin and mucous membrane changes occur within 3 to 4 days of the onset of fever. Palm, sole, and finger tip desquamation occurs 10 to 18 days after the onset of fever. Asymmetrical lymphadenopathy, especially in the cervical area, is seen in 75% of patients—hence the name *mucocutaneous lymph node syndrome*. This is a disease of young children and occasionally young adults, and 1 to 2% of these individuals experience coronary aneurysms or myocardial infarction, sometimes fatal.

Toxic shock syndrome (Chapters 324 and 327) is a serious condition arising from toxins elaborated by *Staphylococcus aureus,* or streptococcal infections, often in menstruating women using tampons but also in patients with post-surgical infections. The rash is an erythematous, macular, diffuse eruption that blanches readily with pressure followed by desquamation of the affected skin, in association with fever, strawberry tongue, hypotension, vomiting, and renal insufficiency. The rash often spares skin areas where clothing fits tightly with pressure on the skin, e.g., the waistline, where underwear elastic and belts press tightly.

DRUG REACTIONS. Drug reactions can mimic nearly all skin conditions. The most common eruptions, however, are hives and morbilliform rashes. Erythematous macules and papules usually begin within a week of initiating use of the drug and often become confluent. Unfortunately, no laboratory tests can identify a responsible drug, so reliance must be placed on the history. Often patients are taking several drugs. In trying to select the offending medication, factors to consider are the temporal relationship between the initiation of the drug and the rash and the probability that a given drug is likely to cause an eruption. Drugs most likely to cause maculopapular eruptions include trimethoprim-sulfamethoxazole, penicillin G, semisynthetic penicillins, ampicillin, quinidine, gentamicin sulfate, and blood products. Itching is common with drug reactions, and fever may occur. It is difficult to differentiate a maculopapular drug rash from viral exanthems except that viral prodromata and viral mucous membrane lesions are lacking in drug rashes.

The mechanisms of most cutaneous drug reactions are not understood. Only 10% of drug reactions have a clearly identified immunologic basis. Specific mechanisms of immunologically mediated drug reaction include immediate hypersensitivity (IgE or Type I–

mediated), cytotoxic antibody reactions (Type II), circulating immune complexes (Type III), and even Type IV delayed hypersensitivity. The mechanisms of non–immunologically mediated drug reactions include toxic overdose, idiosyncratic responses, drug interactions, and pharmacologic side effects.

Most cutaneous drug reactions remit within 2 to 3 weeks after the drug is stopped. Symptomatic therapy includes antihistamines, topical steroids, and occasionally systemic steroids.

PURPURIC MACULOPAPULAR SKIN LESIONS. Purpura represents extravasation of red blood cells outside the cutaneous vessels and, unlike erythema, cannot be blanched. Purpura can be classified as non-palpable (macular) and palpable (papular). Non-palpable purpura results from bleeding into the skin without associated inflammation of the vessels and indicates either a bleeding diathesis or fragile blood vessels. Non-palpable purpura can be petechial (macules < 3 mm) or ecchymotic (macules > 3 mm). Thrombocytopenia causes petechiae, whereas abnormalities in the clotting cascade commonly cause ecchymoses. Necrotic ecchymoses are found when thrombi form in dermal vessels and lead to infarction and hemorrhage, e.g., disseminated intravascular coagulation (DIC). Palpable purpura results from inflammatory damage to cutaneous blood vessels, as in vasculitis.

NON-PALPABLE PURPURAS. Non-palpable purpuras include thrombocytopenic conditions, senile or actinic purpura, hypergammaglobulinemic conditions, blood clotting abnormalities, Schamberg's disease, and disseminated intravascular coagulation. Actinic (senile) purpura, which is a common problem in older individuals, is the result of increased vessel fragility from connective tissue damage to the dermis caused by chronic sun exposure and aging. Minor trauma induces ecchymoses, usually on the dorsum of the hands and forearms. The skin in these areas is thin and fragile. Topical or systemic steroids can induce similar purpura. Other causes of vascular fragility of the skin include amyloidosis and the Ehlers-Danlos syndrome.

Schamberg's disease, or pigmented purpuric dermatitis, is an idiopathic capillaritis that causes petechial lesions of the lower legs (occasionally the arms and trunk) in association with hyperpigmentation. The lesions have the appearance of cayenne pepper. Occasionally Schamberg's disease is secondary to a drug reaction. Petechiae and purpura also occur in hypergammaglobulinemic purpura, which is a syndrome characterized by episodes of fever and arthralgias and appears to be the result of immune complex–mediated damage to small blood vessels.

In DIC (Chapter 186), uncontrolled clotting within blood vessels and diffuse thrombosis lead to hemorrhage, ecchymosis, and infarction. DIC occurs in association with bacterial sepsis (particularly meningococcemia), as a post-viral or post-streptococcal phenomenon (purpura fulminans), or in conjunction with malignancies such as prostatic carcinoma and acute myelocytic leukemia. The most distinctive hemorrhagic skin lesions are stellate (star-shaped) purpuric ecchymoses with necrotic centers. The center of the lesion is dark gray, indicative of necrosis and impending slough. Petechiae, hemorrhagic bullae, acral cyanosis, mucosal bleeding, and prolonged bleeding from wound sites can occur.

A variety of infectious diseases cause cutaneous petechiae, purpura, or ecchymoses. In meningococcemia (Chapter 329) the organisms produce acute vasculitis or local Schwartzman-like reactions with erythematous macules, petechiae, purpura, and ecchymoses on the trunk and legs. The lesions may become confluent, often with central necrosis. Patients with acute meningococcemia are ill with fever, malaise, headache, meningeal signs, and hypotension. The skin lesions of disseminated gonococcemia (Chapter 362) begin as tiny red papules and petechiae and then evolve into painful purpuric pustules and vesicles scattered on the distal extremities. Fever, polyarthritis, or monoarticular arthritis may be present. The rash of Rocky Mountain spotted fever (Chapter 371), appears between the second and sixth days of the illness, initially as small, erythematous macules that blanch on pressure, but then evolving into petechiae, purpura, and ecchymoses. The rash first occurs on the acral areas and then spreads up the extremities and trunk. Small areas of necrosis may occur on the fingers, toes, and ear lobes. Fever, severe headache, toxicity, confusion, and myalgias commonly occur. Infective endocarditis (Chapter 326) is associated with petechial and purpuric skin lesions. Petechiae appear in crops in the conjunctivae, buccal mucosa, upper chest, and extremities. Splinter hemorrhages (linear, red to brown streaks under the fingernails or

Table 522–3 ■ TYPES OF VASCULITIS AND ASSOCIATED SKIN LESIONS

TYPE OF VASCULITIS	BLOOD VESSELS INVOLVED	TYPE OF SKIN LESION
Leukocytoclastic or hypersensitivity angiitis: Henoch-Schönlein purpura, cryoglobulinemia, hypocomplementemic vasculitis	Dermal capillaries, venules, and occasional small muscular arteries in internal organs	Purpuric papules, hemorrhagic bullae, cutaneous infarcts
Rheumatic vasculitis: systemic lupus erythematosus; rheumatoid vasculitis	Dermal capillaries, venules, and small muscular arteries in internal organs	Purpuric papules; ulcerative nodules; splinter hemorrhages; periungual telangiectasia and infarcts
Granulomatous vasculitis Churg-Strauss syndrome	Dermal small and larger muscular arteries and medium muscular arteries in subcutaneous tissue and other organs	Erythematous, purpuric, and ulcerated nodules, plaques, and purpura
Wegener's granulomatosis	Small venules, arterioles of dermis, and small muscular arteries	Ulcerative nodules; peripheral gangrene
Periarteritis: classic type limited to skin and muscle	Small and medium muscular arteries in deep dermis, subcutaneous tissue, and muscle	Deep subcutaneous nodules with ulceration; livedo reticularis; ecchymoses
Giant cell arteritis: temporal arteritis, polymyalgia rheumatica, Takayasu's disease	Medium muscular arteries and larger arteries	Skin necrosis over scalp

toenails), Osler's nodes (2- to 15-mm, tender red nodules on the pads of the fingers and toes), and Janeway lesions (small, painless plaques and palpable, purpuric nodules on the palms or soles) may be seen. The skin lesions are related to immune complex vasculitis or septic emboli. Similar lesions may occur in association with atrial myxomas (Chapter 70) and cholesterol emboli (Chapters 67 and 112).

PALPABLE PURPURAS. Vasculitis and necrotizing angiitis characterize disorders in which there is segmental inflammation in the blood vessel wall with accumulation of neutrophils and fibrinoid necrosis. The vascular reaction is mediated by immune complexes. Papules with purpura result from extravasation of blood from the damaged vessels (Color Plate 13C). Although all sizes of blood vessels may be affected, the vasculitis in the skin involves venules. If the process is extensive or if large vessels are involved, skin necrosis and ulceration may occur. Depending upon the size of the affected blood vessels, at least five types of vasculitis may involve the skin. The size and type of vessels in the skin, in turn, determine the kind of morphologic lesion (Table 522–3).

In general, as the vasculitis involves progressively larger and more deeply situated vessels, the skin lesions become more nodular, with larger ulcerative or gangrenous processes. The term *granulomatous vasculitis* refers to angiitis associated with a histiocytic proliferation that also involves necrotizing granulomas in the connective tissue of multiple organs, causing rhinorrhea, sinusitis, cough, arthralgias, and ocular and neurologic symptoms (Churg-Strauss syndrome) (Chapter 292).

Necrotizing leukocytoclastic vasculitis can occur in a variety of settings including sepsis; connective tissue disease, especially systemic lupus erythematosus and rheumatoid arthritis; cryoglobulinemia, especially with hepatitis C; drug reactions; and, occasionally, underlying carcinomas, lymphomas, or leukemias. Circulating immune complexes have been demonstrated in patients with necrotizing angiitis. Immunoglobulins and complement are found in the affected vessel wall by direct immunofluorescence. The immune complexes lodge in the small vessel walls and activate the complement system, forming the anaphylatoxins C3a and C5a, which recruit neutrophils that induce inflammatory and necrotic damage to the vessel with accompanying fragmented nuclei of the neutrophils (so-called nuclear dust).

Several syndromes are associated with leukocytoclastic vasculitis, depending on the organ systems affected. Henoch-Schönlein syndrome (Chapters 106 and 292) occurs most often in children, frequently preceded by an upper respiratory infection and accompanied by arthralgias, abdominal pain, and renal vasculitis; IgA and complement are usually found in the involved vessels on direct immunofluorescence. Hypocomplementemic vasculitis is characterized by urticaria-like lesions, arthritis, facial and laryngeal edema, and low serum complement level; IgG and C3 are present in vessels taken from early skin lesions. Facial and laryngeal edema may also occur. A third form consists of purpura, arthralgia, weakness, and mixed cryoglobulinemia (mixed cryoglobulins contain IgG and IgM with anti-IgG or rheumatoid factor activity), which may be idiopathic or occasionally associated with systemic lupus erythematosus, infectious mononucleosis, lymphomas, or primary biliary cirrhosis.

If the vasculitis is idiopathic and cutaneous, the skin responds to prednisone (60 to 80 mg/day) or dapsone (100 to 150 mg/day). Systemic vasculitides may require prednisone and cyclophosphamide (2 mg/kg/day).

Necrotizing cutaneous vasculitis may occur with hepatitis B or hepatitis C, after intestinal bypass surgery for morbid obesity, or in patients with jejunal diverticula or other gastrointestinal conditions characterized by bacterial overgrowth. An arthritis-dermatitis syndrome associated with intestinal bypass surgery is characterized by polyarthritis and palpable purpura or purpuric nodules and pustules on the trunk, legs, feet, and arms. Antigenic components of the intestinal bacterial overgrowth lead to the formation of cryoprotein immune complexes that deposit in the skin and joints, causing a hypersensitivity vasculitis and non-deforming arthritis. Antibiotics such as chloramphenicol, sulfamethoxazole-trimethoprim, tetracycline, and metronidazole may improve the condition.

PAPULOSQUAMOUS SKIN DISEASES

Papulosquamous conditions include those that are both papular (even if only mildly elevated) and squamous or scaly (hyperkeratotic) (Table 522–4). They generally represent conditions in which the epidermis is thickened and the process of cornification is altered; concomitant dermal inflammation usually occurs.

PSORIASIS. Psoriasis is the prototypical papulosquamous condition, characterized by well-demarcated erythematous papules and plaques with silvery scale (Color Plate 12D). Psoriasis is, at least in part, genetically determined. It is usually a chronic condition of epidermal proliferation and dermal inflammation. Psoriasis begins most commonly in early adult life, but it may begin at any age. The disease may remain localized to just a few areas or may cause continuous generalized disease, occasionally resulting in total-body erythema and scale, termed *erythroderma.*

The pathogenesis of psoriasis is unknown, but it appears to be a multifactorial disease in patients who are genetically predisposed. There is an increased prevalence of psoriasis in individuals with human leukocyte antigens (HLAs) HLA BW17, B13, and BW37. Thirty per cent of patients have a family history of disease. The basic alteration represents an accelerated cell cycle in an increased

Table 522–4 ■ PAPULOSQUAMOUS SKIN DISEASES

Psoriasis
Reiter's syndrome
Pityriasis rosea
Lichen planus
Secondary syphilis
Pityriasis rubra pilaris
Pityriasis lichenoides et varioliformis acuta
Pityriasis lichenoides et varioliformis chronica
Mycosis fungoides

number of dividing epidermal basal cells, culminating in rapid epidermal cell proliferation. Cellular turnover is increased up to seven-fold, and the transit time from the basal layer to the top of the stratum corneum is 3 to 4 days rather than the usual 28. This rapid turnover of keratinocytes alters keratinization, resulting in thickened epidermis (seen as papules and plaques) and parakeratotic stratum corneum (silver scales). T lymphocytes play a role, but the exact mechanism underlying this benign proliferative reaction is unknown.

Classically, lesions of psoriasis are distributed symmetrically over areas of bony prominence such as elbows and knees. Frequently they may also be found periumbilically, in the intergluteal cleft, or even on the glans of the penis (a location that, if involved, can be very helpful in making the diagnosis). The palms and soles can be symmetrically involved with well-circumscribed plaques or even diffuse erythema with scale. The only discernible lesions may be very superficial pustules on the palms and soles with fine scale remaining after rupture. Nail involvement occurs in up to 50% of cases and can be a diagnostic clue. The nails may have small ice pick–like depressions on the surface of the nail plate; although some normal persons have one or two similar lesions, this finding is much more diffuse in psoriatic patients. Onycholysis (nail plate separation from the nail bed), which can also occur with a psoriatic plaque in the distal nail bed, may also cause a red-brown discoloration that is reminiscent of an oil stain under the nail.

When the individual silvery scales are plucked from psoriatic plaques, tiny pinpoint capillary bleeding may be seen (Auspitz's sign). Another helpful diagnostic sign is Koebner's phenomenon, in which trauma to the skin induces new skin lesions. Thus, scratches or surgical incisions elicit linear papulosquamous lesions that should alert the physician to the diagnosis. This phenomenon may also explain the high incidence of psoriasis on the elbows and knees. Other aggravating factors include streptococcal infections, emotional stress, overuse of alcohol, and drugs such as lithium or β-blockers.

There are several common variants of psoriasis: guttate psoriasis, in which numerous small papular lesions with silvery scaling evolve suddenly over the body, often 1 to 3 weeks after streptococcal pharyngitis; inverse psoriasis, in which plaques evolve in intertriginous areas and thus lack the typical silver scale because of maceration and moisture; and pustular psoriasis, a form of the disease in which superficial pustules may stud typical plaques, be confined to the palms and soles, or be associated with a rare generalized erythematous skin condition accompanied by fever and leukocytosis. Erythrodermic psoriasis with generalized erythema and scale covering the entire body may occur secondary to overvigorous therapy, a generalized Koebner phenomenon, a superimposed drug reaction, or withdrawal from oral corticosteroids. Erythroderma can be quite serious, even life-threatening, and often requires hospitalization. Psoriatic arthritis (Chapter 287) may be found in up to 10 to 15% of patients.

At times, Reiter's syndrome (Chapter 287) may be confused with psoriasis. The skin lesions of the two disorders are indistinguishable clinically and histologically. In Reiter's syndrome, pustular and hyperkeratotic papules and plaques commonly occur on the palms and soles (keratoderma blennorrhagicurn), and scaling, red patches evolve on the glans penis and within the groin (balanitis circinata). Reiter's syndrome is suggested by asymptomatic erosions on the tongue and buccal mucosa, urethritis, iritis or conjunctivitis, arthritis, and occasionally diarrhea.

The goal of therapy is to decrease epidermal proliferation and underlying inflammation. There is no curative agent for psoriasis, and treatment suppresses the condition only as long as it is administered. Topical therapy in some form is usually a mainstay of treatment. Intermediate- or strong-potency topical steroids may be used once or twice a day. Topical tar or anthralin preparations can be used and even compounded with topical steroids. UVB with tar or UVA with oral psoralens (PUVA) can provide excellent relief. Calcipotriene (Dovonex) when used twice a day as an ointment or cream is a "steroid-sparing" topical form of vitamin D that may be as effective as medium-potency steroids. Topical tazarotene (Tazorac) is the first topical retinoid to treat psoriasis.

Because of potential side effects, systemic therapy should be considered only in recalcitrant disease. Antimetabolites or antimi-

totic agents, including methotrexate, azathioprine, and hydroxyurea, are the most commonly used. Methotrexate is used in once-weekly low doses. Because these agents affect bone marrow and liver enzymes (in the case of methotrexate), laboratory monitoring is required. In addition, liver biopsies are usually performed in patients with cumulative doses of 1.5 to 2.0 g of methotrexate. Etretinate, a retinoid, is particularly useful in pustular and erythrodermic forms of psoriasis; it is being replaced by its active metabolite, acitretin, which is less lipophilic and has a shorter half-life. However, because some acitretin may be converted back to etretinate, particularly in the presence of alcohol, pregnancy must be avoided and blood counts, plasma triglyceride levels, and liver enzyme levels should be monitored.

PITYRIASIS ROSEA. Oval or round, tannish pink or salmon-colored, scaling papules and plaques appear rapidly over the trunk, neck, upper arm, and legs (Color Plate 12A). Several features of this self-limited papulosquamous condition are unique. The generalized eruption is preceded by a single lesion, termed the "herald patch," that is commonly misdiagnosed as "ringworm" or tinea corporis. The patch can occur anywhere but often appears on the neck or lower trunk area and precedes the general rash by several days to a week. The oval patches have an unusual fine, white scale located near the border of the plaques. The lesions follow skin cleavage lines, in a pattern likened to a Christmas tree. Itching can be quite prominent but is not invariable. The condition spontaneously resolves in 1 to 2 months. Recurrences are extremely rare, and the diagnosis of recurrent pityriasis rosea should lead the clinician to consider other possible papulosquamous conditions. Pityriasis rosea occasionally is preceded by a mild upper respiratory infection, and its greatest incidence is in the winter months, suggesting a viral cause. However, the disease does not occur endemically and is not transmitted person-to-person.

Such conditions as tinea corporis and guttate psoriasis may be considered in the differential diagnosis, but two possibilities should always be entertained: drug eruption and secondary syphilis. If the rash persists longer that 2 or 3 months or generalizes to involve the entire extremities, and especially the face, a drug reaction should be considered. Gold compounds, barbiturates, captopril, and clonidine can cause such a rash. Secondary syphilis should be suspected and a serologic test obtained if the rash involves palms and soles and if fever, coryza, or mucus membrane erosions (so-called mucus membrane patches) are present.

Treatment of pityriasis rosea is usually not necessary unless pruritus is present. Topical corticosteroids and antihistamines may relieve itching and decrease erythema. Ultraviolet light (UVB), given as three to five treatments to elicit a mild erythema reaction, often clears the rash.

LICHEN PLANUS. Lichen planus, an idiopathic, pruritic, inflammatory condition of the skin, is included in the papulosquamous group of disease because the primary lesion is a unique papule. The papules are flat topped (planus) and polygonal in configuration and have a lilac or purple hue. They may have visible scales on their surface, but more characteristic are subtle, fine white dots or white reticulated lines (Wickham's striae) surmounting the shiny, flat tops (resembling the appearance of a lichen). Wickham's striae are more visible under a hand lens after the application of a drop of mineral oil to the surface of the papule. The Koebner phenomenon occurs in lichen planus, so linear streaks of papules at the sites of skin trauma may be noted.

Although lichen planus can occur anywhere on the body, typical locations are the ankles, wrists, mouth, and genitalia. There may be only a few papules or innumerable ones in a generalized distribution. Mucus membranes are commonly involved, with the lesions appearing most frequently as asymptomatic white streaks in a reticulated pattern on the buccal mucosa, tongue, gums, or lips. In erosive lichen planus, blisters and erosions cause severe discomfort and herald a more prolonged course with resistance to treatment. Lichen planus may appear as violaceous annular lesions involving the male genitalia and, rarely, the legs and arms; it can also present as hyperkeratotic, follicular, scarring alopecia (lichen planopilaris). All lichen planus lesions leave residual hyperpigmented macules in their wake.

The cause of lichen planus is not known, but as many as 20 to 30% of patients have hepatitis C. Certain drugs such as thiazides, phenothiazines, gold, quinidine, and antimalarials can cause lichen planus–like, generalized eruptions. Also, some patients with chronic graft-versus-host disease may experience lichenoid lesions.

Treatment of lichen planus is at times unrewarding. Topical steroids, particularly ultrapotent steroids for short periods (2 to 3 weeks), can be very helpful. Sometimes ultraviolet light is useful to control pruritus. Mucous membrane lesions tend to be more difficult to treat, but corticosteroids and even "swish and spit" cyclosporine have been used with mixed results.

OTHER PAPULOSQUAMOUS LESIONS. *Secondary syphilis* presents with red or copper-colored scaling papules and plaques that are sometimes annular and are usually generalized and often include the palms and soles. Mucous membranes may be involved with white or red patches, and condyloma warts may be seen in the anal and genital areas (Chapter 365).

Pityriasis rubra pilaris presents with red, scaling plaques and patches with follicular horny excretions, especially on the dorsum of the hands and fingers. Diffuse, yellow hyperkeratoses may be seen on the palms and soles. The distribution is often diffuse, with rough scaling erythema involving the entire body with islands of normal skin. There may be lacy white plaques in the mouth. The lesions usually remit spontaneously in 2 to 4 years. Changes similar to those of psoriasis are sometimes seen.

Pityriasis lichenoides et varioliformis acuta appears as red, discrete, palpable papules that vacuolate and then become hemorrhagic, crust, scale, and leave a scar. The lesions may be scattered over the trunk and extremities and may resemble leukocytoclastic vasculitis. The lesions may resolve in a few months or persist for years.

Pityriasis lichenoides et varioliformis chronica presents as larger red, slightly scaling papules and plaques, which are usually nonpruritic. The lesions are usually on the trunk, but the mucous membranes may sometimes be involved. The lesions respond to UVB light treatments.

Mycosis fungoides (Chapters 179 and 196) presents with persistent, pruritic, red, thickened plaques with scales as seen with eczema, or with thick mica-like scales suggestive of psoriasis. The lesions, which may ulcerate, often appear first in the girdle area and tend to be scattered asymmetrically over the trunk and extremities (Color Plate 13*E* and 15*D*). There may be islands of normal skin within the reddened areas. Biopsy findings are diagnostic.

ICTHYOSIFORM DERMATOSES

The ichthyosiform dermatoses present at birth or in childhood. Lamellar ichthyosis, epidermalitic hyperkeratosis, and X-linked ichthyosis appear at birth. Ichthyosis vulgaris has its onset during childhood, tends to spare the flexural areas, and is associated with atopy (Color Plate 12*B*).

VESICULOBULLOUS DISEASES

Vesicles and bullae, when intact, are readily recognized primary skin lesions (Table 522–5). Crusts or superficial erosions are secondary lesions that suggest a preceding fluid-filled primary lesion. The causes of blistering disease includes bacterial and viral infections, contact dermatitis, and autoimmune and metabolic diseases. The pathogenesis of the blister formation is often helpful in understanding its anatomic location: Blisters occur either within the epidermis (intraepidermal) or at the dermoepidermal junction (subepidermal)

Intraepidermal vesicles or bullae usually contain clear fluid (but may become filled with purulent material secondarily) and have very thin roofs, so they are flaccid in appearance and are easily broken. At times the blisters are difficult to recognize, and only erosions, crusts, or the thin shreds of the epidermal blister roofs remain. Subepidermal blisters, on the other hand, have an epidermal roof and are tense and remain intact. Hemorrhagic fluid is common in subepidermal blisters because of their location close to dermal capillaries.

Biopsy of early vesicles or blisters is imperative in diagnosis. Immunofluorescence studies on biopsy material may differentiate certain immunologically mediated diseases. Pathologic studies are most informative when performed early, before therapy has been initiated.

INTRAEPIDERMAL VESICULOBULLOUS DISEASES. Pathologic

Table 522–5 ▪ VESICULOBULLOUS DISEASES

Intraepidermal vesiculobullous diseases
  Bullous impetigo
  Staphylococcal scalded skin syndrome
  Toxic epidermal necrolysis
  Herpes simplex
  Varicella (herpes zoster)
  Pemphigus diseases
    Pemphigus vulgaris
    Pemphigus vegetans
    Pemphigus foliaceus
    Pemphigus erythematosus
    Familial benign pemphigus
Dermal-epidermal vesiculobullous diseases
  Bullous pemphigoid
  Herpes gestationis
  Cicatricial pemphigoid
  Dermatitis herpetiformis
  Erythema multiforme (Stevens-Johnson syndrome)
  Porphyria cutanea tarda
  Bullous disease of renal disease
  Bullous disease in diabetics
  Epidermolysis bullosa
  Epidermolysis bullosa acquisita

processes involved in epidermal blister formation include spongiosis, primary cell damage, and acantholysis. In spongiosis, which is a common form of blister formation in eczematous processes, edema between cells of the prickle layer and liquefaction of cells gradually increase the size of the fluid spaces. Primary epidermal cell damage with fluid accumulation is seen in viral infections and friction damage. Blisters may also occur when cellular desmosomal attachments and intercellular cementing substances are immunologically or chemically altered, causing dyshesion, referred to as *acantholysis* (pemphigus).

Bullous impetigo, a subcorneal infection of the skin with staphylococcal and/or streptococcal organisms, causes large, fragile, clear or cloudy bullae that form thin, honey-yellow crusts and a delicate collarette-like remnant of blister roof after the blisters rupture (Color Plate 16*D*). Autoinoculation results in satellite lesions. The superficial epidermal blistering is caused by the toxic effects of an epidermal toxin elaborated by certain strains of these bacterial organisms.

A more serious variant of bullous impetigo is *staphylococcal scalded skin syndrome,* usually affecting infants and characterized by the formation of rapidly progressive, painful, erythematous patches in which large flaccid bullae evolve and shed as large sheets of skin, leaving a denuded, scalded-appearing surface. With only slight trauma the skin readily slides off, much as wet wallpaper slides off a wall. In contrast to localized bullous impetigo, in which the *Staphylococcus aureus* may be recovered in the skin lesions, the bullae of scalded skin syndrome are sterile, although a staphylococcal infection may be found in the conjunctiva, nose, or pharynx. The widespread intraepidermal blistering results from an epidermal toxin that is elaborated by specific strains of *Staphylococcus aureus* and hematogenously carried to the skin.

A somewhat similar condition, *toxic epidermal necrolysis,* occurs in adults, often secondary to drugs (e.g., ampicillin, allopurinol) and occasionally to *Staphylococcus* infections in an immunosuppressed patient. Toxic epidermal necrolysis is a reaction to a variety of antigenic materials that cause a suprabasilar split in the epidermis with necrosis of much of the overlying epidermis. Because of the more extensive destruction of epidermis and barrier stratum corneum layer (as opposed to staphylococcal scalded skin syndrome, in which the split is subcorneal), toxic epidermal necrolysis is often fatal and, when extensive, should be treated as a widespread burn. Toxic epidermal necrolysis also often involves the mucous membranes and therefore may be confused with Stevens-Johnson syndrome (see later).

Viral infections of the skin may cause vesicles and bullae by virtue of direct infection of the keratinocytes and the destructive effect on the cells. Vesicles caused by viruses often display two important characteristics: (1) They tend to occur in groups on an indurated erythematous base, and (2) they often take on an umbilicated appearance.

Herpes simplex infections (Chapter 365) cause vesicles. A complication of herpes simplex infection, *erythema multiforme,* is a hypersensitivity skin and mucous membrane reaction that evolves 1 to 2 weeks following herpetic recurrences as a result of a herpesvirus-containing immune complex reaction to the herpes antigen. Herpes infection is only one etiologic stimulus leading to erythema multiforme (see late). Diagnosis of herpes infections (including herpes-zoster and varicella-zoster) is made with a Tzanck test preparation of material taken from the roof of vesicles or by culture of the blister fluid (Color Plate 14*C*).

Varicella infection (Chapters 383), when initially encountered, causes chickenpox, a generalized pruritic eruption with widespread, delicate vesicles on an erythematous base; the lesions have been likened to a dew drop on a rose petal. They often become umbilicated, hemorrhagic, and pustular and may leave scars. Chickenpox lesions occur predominantly on the trunk but also involve the head, extremities, and mucous membranes of the mouth and conjunctiva. Successive crops of lesions evolve for a week.

Herpes zoster is a recrudescence of latent varicella virus in persons who previously had varicella. Zoster appears as grouped, umbilicated, and, at times, hemorrhagic vesicles and pustules on an erythematous base situated unilaterally along the distribution of cranial or spinal nerve roots. Several immediately adjacent dermatomes are frequently involved. Bilateral involvement is rare. Zoster is frequently associated with a prodrome of severe radicular pain in the involved areas. A common useful sign in making the diagnosis is dysesthesia of the dermatomal areas—the patient often bitterly complains that the rubbing of clothing on the area is intolerable. Most patients with herpes zoster are above 50 years of age, and cancer patients (especially those with lymphomas such as Hodgkin's disease) are particularly prone to this infection. In such patients or in immunocompromised individuals, cutaneous dissemination and visceral involvement of liver, lung, and central nervous system may occur. Treatment of herpes zoster is usually symptomatic with Burow's solution compresses, analgesics, and acyclovir (800 mg five times per day orally for 10 days), especially in immunocompromised patients. Post-herpetic neuralgia is common in individuals above age 50 (Chapter 383). Systemic corticosteroids may reduce acute herpetic pain; whether they reduce the risk of post-herpetic neuralgia is debatable. Capsaicin cream or oral amitriptyline can help treat post-herpetic pain.

Insect bites including flea and fire ant bites may also induce vesicles or bullae. The lesions are a response to injected toxins or foreign chemicals or proteins in the bite or an allergic reaction to them.

Pemphigus diseases cause blistering in the epidermis by virtue of the process of acantholysis. *Pemphigus vulgaris* and a variant, *pemphigus vegetans,* which heal with hypertrophic, "vegetative" surfaces, are acquired autoimmune diseases of the skin and mucous membrane. The superficial bullae evolve just above the basal layer, readily rupture, and leave denuded, bleeding, weeping, and crusted erosions over the body that do not heal. The oral mucosa is almost always involved and is frequently the presenting site. The painful erosions characteristically spill over the vermilion border of the lips and onto the skin. Lesions of the skin occur anywhere but often in pressure and friction areas. The blisters arise on normal-appearing skin. Untreated pemphigus vulgaris progresses slowly with extensive denudation, leading to fluid and electrolyte imbalance, sepsis, and death. Pain from mouth lesions prevents adequate food intake. A skin biopsy sample of early vesicles should be obtained for routine histologic examination. The edge of a bulla, including adjacent normal skin, should be examined by direct immunofluorescence to make the diagnosis. Immunofluorescence shows deposits of immunoglobulins (usually IgG) and/or C3 in the intercellular spaces around keratinocytes. Antibodies to the intercellular areas of the epidermis are found in the serum. Circulating antibodies to the epidermis are directed against several polypeptide components of the epidermal desmosomes. Their titers somewhat reflect disease activity, and they may contribute to the defective epidermal adhesion. High doses of systemic steroids (100 to 200 mg/day of prednisone over prolonged periods) usually control the disease. Methotrexate and other cytotoxic agents are useful as steroid-sparing

agents. Treatment with intramuscular gold often is successful and occasionally induces long-term remissions.

Pemphigus foliaceus is a less severe disease in which the acantholytic separation within the epidermis is in the upper portion of the prickle layer. *Pemphigus erythematosus* may be a localized variant of pemphigus foliaceus presenting with superficial blisters, erosions, and crusting and oozing over the scalp and face in a seborrheic dermatitis–like rash or often simulating the butterfly rash of systemic lupus erythematosus. Mucous membrane involvement is unusual in pemphigus foliaceus and pemphigus erythematosus, and lower doses of systemic steroids generally control these conditions. Immunofluorescent studies on skin from the edge of lesions reveal immunoglobulin and/or C3 in the intercellular areas of the upper portions of the epidermis.

Familial benign pemphigus, or Hailey-Hailey disease, is a dominantly inherited disorder with suprabasal cell acantholysis; the groups of bullae arise on erythematous skin in the flexural areas (neck, axillae, groin). Spreading erosions display vesicles and pustules at the borders with a moist, granular center. Warm weather and superficial bacterial infections seem to cause flares, and spontaneous exacerbations and remissions continue for years. Familial benign pemphigus differs from other forms of pemphigus in its genetic pattern, absence of mouth lesions, benign course, and absence of intercellular antibodies. Antibiotics, both topical and systemic, may improve acute flares of the disease. If *Candida* sp, infection is superimposed, topical antifungal agents are often of benefit. When chronic vegetating lesions are present, surgical removal with skin grafting may be useful.

DERMAL-EPIDERMAL VESICULOBULLOUS DISEASES. Separation of the epidermis from the dermis occurs in a variety of bullous diseases resulting from autoimmune and immunologic reactions, metabolic disturbances, and a number of inherited mechanicobullous conditions (see Table 522–5).

In *bullous pemphigoid,* which is an autoimmune disorder of the elderly, tense, large blisters occur on normal or erythematous skin, often in the groin, axillae, and flexural areas (Color Plate 13*A*). Only one third of patients have oral blisters. Healing usually occurs without scarring in some blisters while new lesions are evolving. Itching may be severe or absent. The skin biopsy result displays a subepidermal blister through the lamina lucida (at the electron microscopic level), and direct immunofluorescence reveals deposition of the IgG immunoglobulin and complement directed against an antigen in the lamina lucida. The prognosis is good, and the disease usually subsides after months or years. Widespread bullae require therapy with 40 to 60 mg/day of oral prednisone and occasionally with immunosuppressive agents. Large doses of erythromycin or tetracycline (2 g/day) can occasionally control the disease.

Another subepidermal blistering disease, *herpes gestationis,* is a rare autoimmune condition that occurs during pregnancy and the postpartum period. The name of the disease is misleading, for it is not associated with herpesvirus infection. The blisters develop at any time throughout the course of pregnancy, although they most often begin during the second and third trimesters and subside a few weeks post partum. Some patients may experience transient flares or recurrences with each menstrual period or following the use of oral contraceptives. There are recurrences with subsequent pregnancies. Herpes gestationis is a pruritic condition with numerous tense vesicles arising on both normal-appearing and erythematous areas of skin. Arcuate and polycyclic red plaques are seen with peripheral blistering. The lesions first appear on the abdomen and then spread to involve the entire integument. Skin biopsy findings are indistinguishable from those of bullous pemphigoid by light microscopy, and examination of perilesional skin by direct immunofluorescence reveals C3 and less often an IgG linear band just below the epidermis. There is an associated fetal mortality rate as high as 30%, and there is also an increased rate of premature live births. Transient vesiculobullous lesions may infrequently occur in some otherwise healthy infants of affected mothers. Occasionally the patients' intractable pruritus and extensive bullae respond to high-potency topical steroid ointments and diphenhydramine, but most patients require oral prednisone (20 to 60 mg/day) throughout pregnancy with intermittent tapering.

Erythema multiforme is an immunologic reaction in the skin and mucous membranes often mediated by circulating immune complexes that evolve in response to a number of antigenic stimulae (infections, drugs, connective tissue disease). As the name implies, the skin reaction is characterized by a variety of lesions, namely, erythematous plaques, blisters, and target or bull's-eye lesions (Color Plate 13*B*). When the mucus membranes of the mouth and eye are involved, the condition is called *Stevens-Johnson syndrome.* Typically the cutaneous lesions favor the extremities (often the palms) and are symmetrical. Target lesions are diagnostic and are recognized by a central, dark purple area or a blister surrounded by a pale, edematous, round zone, surrounded in turn by a peripheral rim of erythema. In Stevens-Johnson syndrome, the skin disease is more widespread, with blisters and painful erosions in the mouth and eyes. The patients look and feel ill, with fever, prostration, and difficulty in eating. On histologic examination, subepidermal separation is found in the blistering center of the target lesion, and when early lesions undergo biopsy, immunofluorescence reveals immunoglobulin and complement in the walls of the small dermal blood vessels; the inflammation and bullae form in response to vascular damage and leaking. In one half of cases, no cause is found for the reaction, but causes, especially drugs (penicillins, barbiturates, phenytoin, and sulfonamides) and infections (herpes simplex, streptococcal infections, *Mycoplasma pneumoniae*) should be sought in all cases. Recurrent herpes simplex infection is the most common cause of recurrent erythema multiforme. It is not clear whether medical therapy favorably alters the course of idiopathic erythema multiforme, although treatment of a precipitating infection is appropriate, and acyclovir may prevent recurrences of herpes-associated erythema multiforme. Stopping suspected drugs is also imperative. The value of systemic steroids in erythema multiforme and Stevens-Johnson syndrome is controversial. In addition intravenous (IV) fluids may be required in patients with severe oral involvement, and topical anesthetics (viscous lidocaine [Xylocaine]) may help to decrease mouth discomfort.

Cicatricial pemphigoid is an autoimmune condition with subepidermal IgG and linear deposits in the basement membrane zone. Scarring and blisters develop on the mucous membranes, and 25% of patients have blisters on the skin as well.

Dermatitis herpetiformis is associated with immunologic deposition of IgA in dermal papillae. The lesions are grouped and symmetrical with distributed vesicles and papules found on the scalp, scapulae, buttocks, elbows, and knees. The disease is associated with intense burning and itching. There is a high incidence of associated celiac sprue (Chapter 134).

Porphyria cutanea tarda (Chapter 219) is associated with tense bullae that leave scars in some exposed areas. *Bullous disease of renal disease* is associated with bullae on the extremities, whereas *bullous disease in diabetics* presents with large bullae on acral areas.

Epidermolysis bullosa is associated with splits above, below, and within the dermal-epidermal zone and is found in a variety of inherited conditions. It presents with tense blisters that erode and scar; severe forms may involve the mouth and esophagus.

Epidermolysis bullosa acquisita causes blisters below the lamina densa, where IgG and C3 deposits are found. Tense blisters lead to scars in pressure and trauma sites on the hands and feet as well as on the mucous membranes. A circulating antibody to sublaminal dense antigen is typically found.

Paraneoplastic pemphigus presents with cutaneous intraepidermal acantholytic bullae in association with lymphoma, thymoma, chronic lymphocytic leukemia, and Waldenström's macroglobulinemia. Lesions are severe, painful erosions on the oral pharynx, lips, conjunctiva, and skin.

PUSTULAR DISEASES OF THE SKIN

Pustules usually bring to mind infection, but not all pustular dermatoses are caused by pathogenic microorganisms (Table 522–6). Pustular conditions often occur in association with erythematous papules, cysts, and nodules and they may open to form crusts.

NON-INFECTIOUS PUSTULAR SKIN DISEASES. *Acne,* the most common pustular condition of the skin, is an inflammatory disorder affecting pilosebaceous units primarily over the face and upper trunk. Several pathogenic factors play a role as individuals enter puberty: Androgens stimulate the sebaceous glands and increase sebum production; abnormal keratinization and impaction in the pilosebaceous canal (comedones) obstruct sebum flow; proliferation of anaerobic bacteria, primarily *Propionibacterium acnes,* predis-

Table 522–6 ▪ PUSTULAR DISEASES OF THE SKIN

Non-infectious pustular skin diseases
  Acne
  Rosacea
  Perioral dermatitis
  Pustular psoriasis
  Miliaria pustulosa
Infectious
  Folliculitis, including hot tub folliculitis
Fungal infections
  Candidiasis
  Dermatophytes
  Deep fungal infections (blastomycosis, sporotrichosis, coccidioidomycosis)
Medication-induced pustules
  Lithium
  Corticosteroids
  Androgens
  Growth hormone
Systemic bacterial and fungal infections

poses to rupture of the pilosebaceous unit with extravasation into the surrounding dermis, resulting in sterile, inflammatory papules, pustules, and cysts; and these cysts later lead to disfiguring scarring. Other factors that may play a role in exacerbating acne include oil-based cosmetics, drugs (androgenic hormones, antiepileptics [phenytoin], high-progestin birth control pills, systemic corticosteroids when taken in high doses, and iodide- and bromide-containing agents), and endocrinologic conditions such as polycystic ovary disease and adrenal or ovarian tumors.

Therapy is usually successful in controlling the disease until the patient outgrows this condition. Topical agents, such as benzoyl peroxide and topical vitamin A preparations (such as tazarotene, adapalene), remove comedones and are particularly effective because their action allows sebum to flow freely onto the surface of the skin. Topical and oral antibiotics (tetracycline and erythromycin) are indicated in patients with inflammatory papules and pustules. Oral 13-*cis*-retinoic acid (Accutane), which decreases sebaceous gland size and sebum production, should be used primarily for severe cystic acne because in high daily doses it produces undesirable side effects and can be teratogenic. Spironolactone, the potassium-sparing diuretic, has antiandrogenic properties that have made it a useful adjunctive therapy in doses of 100 to 200 mg/day in women with difficult-to-control acne. Oral contraceptives may also benefit some women with moderate to severe acne, particularly if flares are correlated to menstrual cycles.

Rosacea is a chronic inflammatory disorder affecting the blood vessels and pilosebaceous units of the face in middle-aged individuals. Patients with rosacea have papules and pustules superimposed on diffuse erythema and telangiectasia over the central portion of the face. An important component is easy flushing and blushing of the face often accentuated when alcohol, caffeine, or hot spicy foods are ingested. Hyperplasia of the sebaceous glands, connective tissue, and vascular bed of the nose sometimes causes rhinophyma, which is a large, red, bulbous nose (Color Plate 12*C*). Ocular complications, which occur in a significant number of rosacea patients, include blepharitis, chalazion, conjunctivitis, and progressive keratitis that can lead to scarring and blindness.

Rosacea can usually be differentiated from adult acne by the lack of comedones and the prominent vascular (flushing/telangectasia) component. Other causes of a red face in adults such as the malar eruption of acute systemic lupus erythematosus and the heliotrope rash of dermatomyositis, seborrheic dermatitis, and perioral dermatitis must be considered. Rosacea and the eye complications usually respond well to tetracycline and/or oral metronidazole, but the antibiotic must be continued for life (at the lowest dose that suppresses the condition) because rosacea recurs when therapy stops. Topical antibiotics (metronidazole [MetroGel] or Noritate) can be helpful alone or in combination with low-potency topical steroids (e.g., hydrocortisone 1% lotion) once or twice a day; higher-potency steroids can actually worsen the disease.

Non-infectious causes of pustular disease include *perioral dermatitis,* which may be caused by potent topical steroids and is a variant of acne. It presents as perioral and periorbital red scaling patches, papules, and pustules.

Pustular psoriasis is a variant of psoriasis characterized by pustules localized to the palms and soles or generalized over the entire body. Patients often experience toxicity, with fever and leukocytosis.

Miliaria pustulosa is caused by an occlusion of sweat glands in hot environments. It presents as discrete red papules or pustules with a red base and is found principally over the trunk, especially the back.

INFECTIOUS CAUSES OF SKIN PUSTULES. *Folliculitis, a Staphylococcus aureus* infection of the hair follicle, appears as pustules with a red rim with hair emanating from the center of the pustule. Folliculitis typically occurs in hairy regions where clothing rubs (buttocks, thighs) or on the face. The key to diagnosis is finding a central hair in the pustule. Occasionally, the follicular infection can extend more deeply to form a larger, red, fluctuant nodule from one (furuncle) or more follicles (carbuncle). Systemic antibiotics such as erythromycin or dicloxacillin usually clear extensive infections; topical antiseptic cleansers such as povidone-iodine or chlorhexidine can resolve mild folliculitis and may be useful in preventing recurrences.

Hot tub folliculitis is a generalized, pruritic folliculitis caused by *Pseudomonas aeruginosa* that is acquired in contaminated hot tubs, whirlpools, or swimming pools. It usually begins 6 hours to 5 days after hot tub soaking and affects many people using the facility. It appears as a vesicular and then pustular eruption over the trunk, buttocks, legs, and arms but spares the head and neck (Color Plate 16C). *Pseudomonas* organisms can often be cultured from fresh pustules. In most instances, the folliculitis resolves within 7 to 10 days without specific treatment. Infected tubs and pools should be cultured for *Pseudomonas* sp. and disinfected.

Candidiasis appears as beefy red patches in intertriginous, moist areas characteristically surrounded by satellite pustules. Paronychia, a painful red swelling in the periungual regions of the finger, may also drain pus in which *Candida* organisms can be found with a KOH preparation. Topical agents such as clotrimazole and miconazole must be used two or three times a day for many weeks before the infection clears.

Dermatophytes can, at times, infect hair follicles and result in pustules, particularly in the beard (tinea barbae) and scalp (kerions). These lesions are readily confused with a bacterial folliculitis. Kerions appear as indurated, boggy, inflammatory plaques studded with pustules. These intense inflammatory reactions to superficial dermatophytes (especially *Trichophyton verrucosum*) respond to griseofulvin therapy, although a short course of oral corticosteriods is also useful.

Deep fungal infections such as blastomycosis, sporotrichosis, and coccidioidomycosis may cause pustules as well as verrucous, ulcerative papules and nodules. Sporotrichosis characteristically spreads up cutaneous lymphatics and appears as nodular, pustular lesions in a linear distribution.

Certain medications can lead to a follicular eruption, including lithium and hormonal/steroid preparations. A variant of hormonal folliculitis is seen in human immunodeficiency virus (HIV)-positive patients taking growth hormone or androgens; these lesions resemble corticosteroid-induced acne vulgaris (monomorphous, upper chest/back and proximal extremities) and respond to a decreased dosage of medication as well as to acne medications. Eosinophilic folliculitis is an extremely pruritic variant seen in HIV patients whose CD4 counts are typically below 200. Erythematous and urticarial papules and pustules present on the upper chest, back, and proximal extremities; they may be treated with potent topical steroids, antihistamines, and even itraconazole.

SYSTEMIC INFECTIONS CAUSING PUSTULES ON THE SKIN. A variety of septicemias including gonococcemia (Chapter 362), staphylococcal septicemia (Chapter 327), and *Candida* sp. septicemia (Chapter 400) (in immunosuppressed patients) cause pustular lesions associated with purpura.

URTICARIA, PERSISTENT FIGURATE ERYTHEMAS, CELLULITIS

Urticaria, persistent figurate erythemas, and cellulitis are skin lesions of disparate appearance and origin. The common feature is

Table 522–7 ■ URTICARIA, PERSISTENT FIGURATE ERYTHEMAS, AND CELLULITIS

Urticarial reactions
  Drugs
  Viral infectins
  Sinus and tooth infections
  Systemic parasites
  Pollens
  Injections (blood products and vaccinations)
  Light (solar urticaria)
  Cold (cold urticaria)
  Heat or exercise (cholinergic urticaria)
  Pressure or rubbing of the skin (dermatographism)
Urticaria-like skin lesions
  Erythema multiforme
  Juvenile rheumatoid arthritis
  Erythema marginatum
  Urticaria pigmentosa (mastocytosis)
Figurate erythemas
  Persistent figurate erythema
  Erythema repens
  Erythema annulare centrifugum
  Erythema chronicum migrans
Cellulitis
  Group A streptococcus
  Staphylococcus aureus
  Necrotizing fasciitis

a raised, edematous, red plaque with a sharply demarcated border (Table 522–7 and Color Plate 15E).

URTICARIAL REACTIONS. Urticaria, the most common condition in this group, appears as wheals, which are transient erythematous and edematous swellings of the dermis caused by a local increase in permeability of capillaries and small venules. This increased permeability results from histamine and other chemical substances released from cutaneous mast cells by Type I IgE hypersensitivity reactions, as well as by non-immunologic mechanisms (Chapters 20 and 224). Certain agents such as aspirin and opiates and some foods degranulate mast cells directly without an allergic mechanism. Other urticarial reactions are immunologically mediated by such allergens as infections (viral hepatitis, sinus and tooth infections), infestations (systemic parasites), drugs, pollens, and injections (blood products, vaccinations). Physical modalities including light (solar urticaria), cold (cold urticaria), heat or exercise (cholinergic urticaria), or pressure or rubbing of the skin (dermatographism) also cause hives. Hives are transient: Any given lesion persists <24 hours, although new ones may continuously evolve. Acute urticaria (i.e., lasting <6 weeks) often results from drugs, and the cause is frequently identified. The cause of chronic urticaria (lasting >6 to 8 weeks) is more difficult to identify.

Hives covering large areas and producing deep tissue swelling are termed *angioedema*. This condition can involve the tongue and throat and impinge upon the airway. In such patients, a careful history of use of medications (including over-the-counter drugs, especially cold tablets or medications containing aspirin) should be elicited. Infections such as sinusitis or apical abscess of teeth must be sought. In addition, physical types of urticaria should be considered: cholinergic urticaria is characterized by evanescent multiple, small wheals surrounded by a wide pink flare induced by heat and exercise; solar urticaria, by large plaques in sun-exposed areas; cold urticaria, by wheals that evolve with exposure to cold. Urticaria accompanied by fever and arthralgias occur in serum sickness reactions and in the prodromata of viral hepatitis. Occasionally, urticaria occurs in conjunction with internal conditions such as malignancies or connective tissue diseases. Hereditary angioedema, an autosomal dominant disorder, causes recurrent urticaria, angioedema, intestinal colic, and life-threatening laryngeal edema (Chapter 273).

If the cause of the urticaria cannot be found or avoided, symptomatic control is achieved with antihistamines or oral steroids. Acute angioedema or laryngeal edema requires rapid systemic treatment with epinephrine and diphenhydramine (Chapter 273).

Other urticaria-like skin lesions include erythema multiforme (see earlier); the skin lesions of juvenile rheumatoid arthritis (Chapter 286) (small, 2- to 3-mm, salmon-colored hives that last only a few hours and appear with fever spikes); and *erythema marginatum* (lesions found in 15% of patients with acute rheumatic fever) (Chapter 325). Urticaria pigmentosa (mastocytosis), a disease caused by increased accumulations of mast cells in the skin and, at times, in lymph nodes, liver, spleen, bones, and gastrointestinal tract (Chapter 280), presents with multiple tan to brown papular spots that urticate when rubbed as a result of the release of histamine from the mast cells. A skin biopsy specimen readily reveals increased numbers of mast cells in the dermis. When the lesions develop in early childhood, the condition is usually limited to skin, and the lesions resolve by puberty, leaving only hyperpigmented macules. If the skin lesions evolve in adulthood, there is a greater chance for systemic mast cell infiltration, and the skin lesions persist.

Hepatosplenomegaly, lymphadenopathy, and bone pain may occur. Patients may experience flushing, palpitations, headache, syncope, hypotension, abdominal pain, and diarrhea, all related to histamine and prostaglandin release from the mast cells.

FIGURATE ERYTHEMAS. Figurate erythemas are a group of uncommon conditions characterized by anular, polycyclic, and geographic erythematous skin lesions. These conditions, in contrast to the urticarial reactions, persist for many days or even years, moving slowly or rapidly over the skin surface (hence, the term sometimes used for these reactions, persistent figurate erythema). Usually, no specific cause is found for these lesions, but some may be associated with underlying malignancies. *Erythema repens,* characterized by a series of swirling wood grain–like red lines, is found in association with adenocarcinomas of the breast, lung, or gastrointestinal tract or with other fungal infections. *Erythema annulare centrifugum* is a slowly enlarging anular lesion that clears in the center with collarette scaling on the inner edge of the red rings. It is found, at times, with cutaneous dermatophyte infections, systemic *Candida* sp. infections, ingestion of blue cheese, parasitic bowel diseases, and autoimmune disorders. *Erythema chronicum migrans* is the unique anular skin lesion found in Lyme disease caused by a spirochete inoculated by infected tick bites (Chapter 366).

CELLULITIS. Although superficially resembling urticaria, cellulitis, an inflammatory infection of the dermis, is readily distinguished from hives by its persistent, slowly enlarging nature as well as pain and warmth (Color Plate 15*F*). Group A streptococci and *S. aureus* are most commonly responsible. *Erysipelas* is sometimes identified separately from cellulitis. It displays a sharply demarcated painful border and an orange-peel epidermal surface; a group A *Streptococcus* sp. is the usual cause. Patients usually feel ill and are febrile. Cellulitis on the lower legs in adults may develop from fissures between the toes from tinea pedis. Systemic antibiotics (erythromycin, dicloxacillin, or the cephalosporins) are the most commonly used drugs.

Necrotizing fasciitis is a specific form of cellulitis involving the deep fascial structures underlying the skin. These infections, which are caused by a mixture of aerobic and anaerobic gram-negative organisms, evolve rapidly in enclosed fascial spaces and are most common in diabetics and immunosuppressed patients. They must be diagnosed early by deep fascial biopsy and treated immediately with broad-spectrum antibiotics and surgical débridement.

NODULES AND TUMORS OF THE SKIN

Skin nodules and tumors (Table 522–8) can be classified as pigmented or non-pigmented, dermal or epidermal, benign or malignant. Neoplasms of epidermal differentiation are quite often recognized by their thickening of the upper cell layers of the skin, manifested as hyperkeratosis or scale. In contrast, lesions that are primarily located in dermis or subcutaneous fat may be smooth, dome shaped, lobulated, or solitary; they usually lack these epidermal changes. Vascular lesions may impart a violaceous or purple hue, and dermal nodules of some granulomatous processes may present with a classical "apple jelly" color.

Benign lesions tend to be small, symmetrical, and well circumscribed. Malignant lesions conversely tend to be larger, asymmetrical, and poorly circumscribed (Table 522–9). Even so, these generalizations are simply guidelines in evaluating skin tumors and nodules. Oftentimes, the most reliable way to make a diagnosis is by obtaining a biopsy specimen.

NON-PIGMENTED NODULES—BENIGN. *Warts* are benign epidermal growths. They may be classically verrucous, flat topped, or clustered. Warts are caused by many different varieties of the human papillomavirus (see the discussion of Maculopapular Lesions).

Table 522–8 ■ NODULES AND TUMORS OF THE SKIN

Non-pigmented nodules—benign
  Warts
  Sebaceous hyperplasia
  Solar (actinic) keratoses—perhaps pre-malignant
  Syringomas
  Follicular cysts
  Lipomas
  Neurofibromas
Non-pigmented nodules—malignant
  Basal cell carcinoma
    Nodular
    Superficial
    Sclerosing
    Pigmented
  Squamous cell carcinoma
    Bowen's disease
  Keratoacanthoma—possibly malignant
Pigmented nodules—benign
  Seborrheic keratoses
  Dermatofibromas
  Nevi (moles)
    Junctional nevi
    Compound nevi
    Intradermal nevi
Pigmented nodules—malignant
  Malignant melanoma
    Lentigo maligna melanoma
    Superficial spreading melanoma
    Nodular melanoma
    Acral lentiginous melanoma
Tumors and nodules of the hands
  Heberden's nodes (osteoarthritis)
  Rheumatoid nodules (rheumatoid arthritis)
  Granuloma annulare
  Multicentric reticulohistiocytosis
  Tophi (gout)
  Knuckle pads
  Gottron's papules (dermatomyositis)
Vascular tumors of the skin
  Hemangiomas
    Nevus flammeus
    Strawberry hemangiomas
    Cavernous hemangiomas
  Pyogenic granuloma
  Kaposi's sarcoma
Inflammatory nodules of the skin
  Erythema nodosum
  Subcutaneous fat necrosis
Nodules associated with metabolic diseases
  Xanthomas
  Xanthelasma
  Tophi (gout)

Sebaceous hyperplasia occurs generally on the face of an individuals above 50 years of age and in immunosuppressed transplantation patients. Individual lesions appear as slightly yellowish dermal papules of only a few millimeters in size without scale. Commonly the lesions are confused with basal cell carcinomas, as both may have a central dell and telangiectasias; biopsy is occasionally necessary to exclude a basal cell cancer. However, the yellow hue of sebaceous hyperplasia is quite distinctive. Sebaceous

Table 522–9 ■ CLINICAL FEATURES HELPFUL IN DISTINGUISHING BENIGN FROM MALIGNANT TUMORS

CLINICAL FEATURES	BENIGN	MALIGNANT
Configuration	Symmetrical sharp borders	Asymmetrical irregular borders
Rate of growth	Slow	Slow or rapid
Friability	No friability	Often friable
Bleeding or ulceration	Seldom bleed or ulcerate	Often bleed and ulcerate
Consistency	Firm or soft	Usually firm to hard
Color	Uniform color and pigmentation	Irregularity of color and pigmentation

hyperplasia requires no treatment other than removal for cosmetic purposes.

Solar (actinic) keratoses are erythematous papules or plaques with slightly irregular borders, usually with some degree of hyperkeratosis. They are found almost exclusively on sun-exposed skin, particularly the head, neck, dorsal forearms, and hands. If left untreated, a small number evolve into squamous cell carcinoma.

Syringomas are small flesh-colored papules that most commonly are found on the upper and lower eyelids of older individuals. They are often multiple and may be confused with other benign lesions such as warts and seborrheic keratosis. They are important only for their cosmetic appearance.

Follicular cysts (epidermal inclusion cysts) are often erroneously diagnosed as sebaceous cysts, but they contain essentially no sebaceous component histologically (Color Plate 15*B*). They are quite common, particularly on the head and neck as well as the trunk. Common presentation is in the form of a moderately firm dermal or subcutaneous nodule that will occasionally drain from a central pore. The material is "cheesy" in appearance and often somewhat foul smelling. Follicular cysts may also become intermittently inflamed and require drainage and antibiotics. A familial predisposition may exist. Bothersome cysts may be removed surgically once inflammation has subsided.

Lipomas are very common and may present in nearly any location. These subcutaneous collections of adipocytes are slow-growing neoplasms that usually increase in size over several years. Although typically asymptomatic, they may become tender, especially after recurrent trauma. A rare syndrome of multiple painful lipomas is Dercum's disease. Lipomas are also seen as part of Gardner's syndrome (Chapter 139).

Neurofibromas are dermal collections of neural cells that may present as soft, flesh-colored protruding nodules that, on compression, can be invaginated into what feels like a defect in the skin (buttonhole sign), or as deep, firm dermal or subcutaneous nodules (Color Plate 16*E*). Neurofibromas may be solitary; multiple neurofibromas, café au lait spots (light brown macules), and axillary freckling suggest von Recklinghausen's disease (Chapter 456).

NON-PIGMENTED NODULES—MALIGNANT. Basal cell carcinomas, squamous cell carcinomas, keratoacanthomas, and solar (actinic) keratoses are neoplasms of the epidermis. These lesions are much more common in skin exposed to sun and especially in persons who have lighter skin or are immunosuppressed or have a personal or family history of skin cancer.

Basal cell carcinomas, the most common type of skin cancer, arise from the basal layer of the epidermis. They may present as nodular, superficial, sclerosing (morphéaform), or pigmented forms, but many basal cell carcinomas have a mixed morphologic and/or histologic picture (Color Plate 12*E*). The natural history is gradual, local growth; if left untreated, however, they can cause tremendous local tissue destruction.

A nodular basal cell carcinoma is classically a pearly papule with telangiectasias, a rolled and waxy border, and occasional "rodent ulcer" central ulceration. As with many malignant skin lesions, patients will commonly complain that these lesions fail to heal. Stretching of the surrounding skin may accentuate the pearly or opalescent quality of the lesion. Superficial basal cell carcinomas are commonly found on the trunk or extremities and are often more reddish in appearance and can have some slight scale; a biopsy is sometimes needed to confirm the diagnosis because they can be confused with papulosquamous lesions. Sclerosing or morpheaform basal cell carcinomas frequently look like scars or lesions of scleroderma; their histologic margins often far exceed their clinical appearance, and a biopsy is usually needed to confirm the diagnosis. Pigmented basal cell carcinomas sometimes have rolled borders and an opalescent quality; they are often confused with melanoma, and biopsy is required for diagnosis.

Controlled cryotherapy, curettage and desiccation, scalpel excision, and fractionated radiation all achieve a cure rate of >90% when used properly on primary lesions. Mohs micrographic surgery, which uses serial excisions guided by frozen section histologic examination, should be considered for larger lesions, lesions that may be recurrent, lesions on the central face or preauricular area, or in cases, where tissue sparing is a concern.

Squamous cell carcinomas are malignant neoplasms of keratino-

cytic differentiation. They are less common than basal cell cancers but may be much more aggressive, occassionally metastasize, and even lead to death if not recognized and properly treated. Lesions are commonly found on sun-exposed skin, with a propensity for head, neck, upper extremities, and trunk. Usually they are firm, erythematous plaques or nodules with hyperkeratosis that sometimes can be quite dramatic, but they may be smooth or verrucous (Color Plate 12*F*). They are easily friable, crusted, and resistant to healing. Lesions are sometimes painful. Bowen's disease, which is squamous cell carcinoma in situ, may occur anywhere. Of particular interest is Bowen's disease that occurs on the penis (erythroplasia of Queyrat) of uncircumcised males and may present as an erythematous or velvety plaque.

Any lesion suspected to be squamous cell carcinoma should undergo biopsy (Color Plate 12*G*). Treatment is excision or curettage and dessication. Solar keratoses may be treated with liquid nitrogen or topical 5-fluorouracil (5-Fu).

Keratoacanthomas present on sun-exposed skin as flesh-colored to erythematous papules or nodules that grow quite rapidly over a period of about 6 weeks and develop a central hyperkeratotic crater (Color Plate 12*H*). They remain for 6 to 8 weeks and then resolve in about 8 weeks, scarring as they involute. Despite their usual natural course of involution, most of these lesions should be excised because of their unsightliness, propensity for scarring, and rare potential to metastasize.

PIGMENTED NODULES—BENIGN. *Seborrheic keratoses,* which are benign neoplasms of epidermal differentiation, appear on the face and trunk in middle age. These 2-mm to 5-cm, elevated, tan-to-brown or occasionally black, round to oval lesions give a verrucous, velvety, "stuck-on" appearance. No therapy is necessary unless they are of cosmetic concern, and then liquid nitrogen cryotherapy or curettage is effective.

Dermatofibromas are areas of focal dermal fibrosis accompanied by overlying epidermal thickening and hyperpigmentation. Clinically, they are firm, brown papules or nodules. A useful diagnostic test is the "dimple sign," in which pinching the lesion results in central dimpling of the overlying epidermis. Some dermatofibromas are dark brown in color and occasionally suggest melanoma, but fibromas are symmetrical and uniform in color. The lesions occur frequently on the lower extremities and less often on the arms. They may be multiple and are probably the result of a local inflammatory process, such as minor trauma or an inflamed hair follicle. Although therapy is usually not required, simple excision is curative.

Nevi or moles are benign accumulations of pigment-forming melanocytes. Nevi may be congenital or acquired, and most appear by 35 years of age, although some may appear later. Nevi may be junctional, compound, or intradermal, reflecting their natural history, evolution, and clinical appearance. *Junctional nevi* are macular, are light to dark brown, and are called junctional because the melanocytes are located at the dermoepidermal junction. *Compound nevi* are brown to dark brown and have flatter areas, which correspond to a junctional component, as well as a palpable portion; they evolve from junctional nevi and have melanocytes both at the dermoepidermal junction and in the dermis. Compound nevi are usually found in children and young adults. *Intradermal nevi* evolve from compound nevi and are usually sessile flesh-colored to brown papules. Melanocytes are found only within the dermis. Benign nevi are usually less than 6 mm in diameter, uniform in color, and symmetrical, with smooth borders. Occasionally, nevi darken in color or may itch, and new nevi may appear in pregnancy. Any symptomatic nevi or nevi that change raise the question of melanoma.

PIGMENTED NODULES—MALIGNANT. *Malignant melanoma* is the cutaneous neoplasm of melanocytes. Melanomas generally have features of asymmetry, irregular border, variegated color, and diameter greater than 6 mm (Table 522–10) (Color Plate 12*H*). The precise cause of melanoma is unknown, but sunlight and heredity are risk factors. Melanoma has been increasing during the past few decades. Suspicious lesions should be strongly considered for biopsy.

Lentigo maligna melanoma is a melanoma on the head and neck arising in a preexisting melanoma in situ. *Superficial spreading melanoma* may occur on any area of the body, with irregularly pigmented papules, nodules, and notched borders. *Nodular melanoma* refers to melanomas with nodular morphologic characteris-

A = Asymmetry of the lesion is due to irregular, random growth of the malignant cells associated with irregular surface topography and papules and nodules.

B = Borders of the tumors are irregular with notching and pigment "spilling" out beyond the edges.

C = Color variegation consists of browns, blacks, blues, and even shades of red and white. The variations in color represent different depths of invasion of pigment cells along with inflammatory reaction and immunologic response to the malignant cells.

D = Diameter or size of melanomas tends to be greater than 6 mm before they are recognized.

---

tics. *Acral lentiginous melanoma* refers to melanoma that occurs on acral skin.

Up to one third of melanomas may arise from existing nevi, so that a change in size, shape, and color or itching of a pigmented lesion (a common symptom in melanomas) should be carefully investigated. Early diagnosis is the key to survival. The deeper the melanoma, the more likely is metastasis. The depth of dermal invasion can be measured microscopically from the granular cell layer in the epidermis to the deepest penetration of melanoma cells into the dermis. Thin melanomas (<0.76 mm) enjoy a virtually 100% cure rate. If the depth is greater than 1.6 mm, only 20 to 30% survive for 5 years.

Any suspicious pigmented lesion must undergo biopsy, preferably by excision. Definitive surgical excision should be undertaken only after confirmation of melanoma is established histologically. In large lesions, it is acceptable to do incisional biopsy prior to definitive therapy. Suspicious pigmented lesions should never be shave-biopsied or shave-excised, nor should they be electrocauterized. Full-thickness tissue through the entire lesion is required for diagnostic and prognostic evaluation.

TUMORS AND NODULES OF THE HANDS. Nodules on the hands can present bilaterally in a number of arthritic conditions such as *osteoarthritis* (Chapter 302) (Heberden's nodes) and rheumatoid arthritis (Chapter 286). Rheumatoid nodules, which may be numerous and quite large, frequently occur on extensor surfaces, perhaps in sites with predilection for trauma. They are found more frequently in individuals who have more severe rheumatoid arthritis.

Granuloma annulare may also present as single to usually multiple nodules on the hands. When multiple lesions are present, they are frequently arranged in an anular configuration. Lesions are usually asymptomatic but may sometimes present with itching or other mild symptoms that are generally self-limited and do not require treatment. However, either topical or intralesional steroids are effective.

Multicentric reticulohistiocytosis (Chapter 305) often causes multiple nodules and hard reddish-brown to yellow papules and plaques over joints of the hands, particularly the fingers in confluent nodules around the nail folds. Additional lesions may be found elsewhere on the body. The accompanying arthritis may be quite severe and even disabling.

Tophi from *gout* may be either single or multiple and present as tender yellow or red papules. *Knuckle pads,* symmetrical erythmatous papules that present over the dorsal surfaces of finger joints, may result from chronic pressure such as regular pushups with the fists closed. *Gottron's papules* associated with dermatomyositis (Chapter 296) classically present with violaceous papules over the dorsal surface of finger joints (Color Plate 14*B*).

VASCULAR TUMORS OF THE SKIN. *Hemangiomas,* benign proliferations of dermal vessels, appear at or soon after birth as red, blue, or purple; flat; papular; or nodular lesions. Their appearance depends upon the number, size, and depth of the proliferating vessels. Thus, capillary angiomas are composed of small, superficial vessels causing *nevus flammeus* and *strawberry hemangiomas.* *Cavernous hemangiomas* are made up of larger and deeper vessels. Cavernous and strawberry angiomas often enlarge at an alarming rate over the first year or two and then usually involute by age 9 or 10. Cavernous hemangiomas are less likely to resolve and sometimes may be deeply situated. Large lesions located in strategic locations (around the eye and mouth) may require systemic steroids to try to shrink these tumors. Platelet consumption by large cavernous hemangiomas may occur in the *Kasabach-Merritt* syndrome.

Ordinarily hemangiomas require no therapy; watchful waiting allows them to resolve spontaneously, as the cosmetic result is usually superior to that obtained by therapeutic intervention. When large hemangiomas ulcerate, bleed, or impinge on vital structures or functions (e.g., around the ears, eyes, nose, mouth), oral steroids given over short periods of time in the dose of 1 to 2 mg/kg body weight shrink the tumor temporarily while awaiting the natural involution. Interferon α also has been used to shrink large hemangiomas that do not respond to steroids.

Pyogenic granuloma, a bright red, raspberry-like growth that can reach 1 cm in size, is friable and bleeds easily when traumatized. These lesions occur most often on arms, legs, fingers, and hands. They enlarge rapidly within weeks but have no malignant potential; they represent capillary hemangiomatous proliferation and follow injury or surgery. The term *pyogenic* is a misnomer, as no infectious process is involved. These lesions are treated with excision, curettage, and electrocauterization, or cryotherapy. Occasionally amelanotic melanomas may present as a pyogenic granuloma, so pathologic examination of pyogenic granulomas should be performed.

Kaposi's sarcoma (Chapters 196, 414 and 416) is a neoplasm of multifocal origin that presents as red-purple to blue-brown macules, plaques, and nodules of the skin and other organs. The cutaneous lesions (Color Plate 13*G*) may be firm or compressible, solitary or numerous, and may even appear initially as a dusky stain, especially about the toes.

Kaposi's sarcoma appears to be caused by human herpesvirus 8, which may transform a circulating precursor cell that, in tissues, develops into spindle cells. Kaposi's sarcoma is found in individuals who are immunosuppressed by HIV infection, and it also occurs endemically in tropical Africa and sporadically in Europe and North America. In HIV-infected patients, a single painless red nodule of the skin commonly identifies a profoundly immunocompromised state. The lesion in HIV-infected patients is an aggressive, often lethal tumor that can rapidly become generalized and involve mucous membranes, abdominal viscera, and lungs. In tropical Africa, the disease accounts for 3 to 9% of all malignancies and afflicts primarily blacks. The peak incidence is in the first decade, with most cases occurring in patients less than 20 years of age; survival is usually less than 3 years. Visceral involvement with marked adenopathy tends to predominate over cutaneous involvement. In Europe and North America, Kaposi's sarcoma lesions commonly affect older men, usually after their seventh decade, and appear primarily on the lower extremities. The lesions tend to be indolent and are associated with chronic lymphedema, which indicates tumor infiltration of the lymphatics. Average survival is about 10 years.

INFLAMMATORY NODULES OF THE SKIN. *Erythema nodosum,* an inflammatory reaction in subcutaneous fat, represents a hypersensitivity response to a number of antigenic stimuli. Well-localized, multiple, tender, red, deep nodules, 1 to 5 cm in size, usually develop bilaterally over the pre-tibial areas. They eventually involute, leaving yellow-purple bruises. Ulceration does not occur. Immunoglobulin and complement deposition has been found in deep blood vessels in early lesions, and in some patients circulating immune complexes have been detected. The localization of the painful nodules to the lower legs may relate to hemodynamic factors. Although no cause can be found in many patients, the following factors have been identified: drugs (especially oral contraceptives), pregnancy, inflammatory bowel disease, sarcoidosis, streptococcal infection, *Yersinia* sp. enterocolitis, deep fungus infections, and tuberculosis. If the cause cannot be identified and eliminated, symptomatic therapy with aspirin, nonsteroidal anti-inflammatory medications, potassium iodide, or short courses of systemic steroids may be useful.

Subcutaneous fat necrosis is a condition in which tender, red nodules occur on the lower legs and thighs in patients with pancreatitis or pancreatic carcinoma. The skin lesions may occur in the absence of signs associated with the internal carcinoma. Serum amylase and lipase values are elevated, and skin biopsy provides diagnostic findings.

Subcutaneous inflammatory nodules may be found in *rheumatoid arthritis* and in *acute rheumatic fever.* In addition to the fingers (see earlier), other common locations are over the knees and elbows.

NODULES ASSOCIATED WITH METABOLIC DISEASES AND MISCELLANEOUS CONDITIONS. *Xanthomas* are focal collections of lipid-containing histiocytes in the dermis and tendon sheaths. They appear as yellowish papules (eruptive xanthomas), plaques (xanthelasma), nodules (xanthoma tuberosum), and xanthomas in tendon and tendon sheaths (xanthoma tendinosum). Xanthomas often arise in association with inherited hyperlipoproteinemias (Chapter 206) or in several underlying metabolic diseases that alter lipoprotein metabolism, such as diabetes, hypothyroidism, cholestatic liver disease, pancreatitis, renal disease, and certain drug reactions (e.g., 13-*cis*-retinoic acid). Xanthelasma usually develops in the absence of hyperlipidemia, although hypercholesterolemia (and an increase in low-density lipoproteins) may be present.

Patients with gout occasionally have deposits in sodium urate in the skin, forming firm, hard papules and nodules (tophi) that may discharge whitish crystals in the pinnae of the ears and periarticular areas.

ATROPHIC SKIN CONDITIONS WITH SCARRING, INDURATION, ULCERATION, AND TELANGIECTASIAS

Connective tissue diseases are the most common conditions that lead to the spectrum of cutaneous changes in atrophic skin conditions (Table 522–11 and Color Plate 16*B*).

SCARRING. *Lupus erythematosus* may be localized to the skin (discoid lupus) or present as a systemic condition (Chapter 289). Discoid lupus skin lesions appear as red plaques with white, cohesive scales that often are accentuated in the follicular openings (follicular plugging). The plaques eventually atrophy, with depression and scarring along with hypopigmentation in the center of the lesions and a hyperpigmented rim. The lesions usually occur in sun-exposed areas and, when they involve the scalp, cause scarring alopecia. Systemic lupus erythematosus presents as an erythematous rash with a violaceous hue, accentuated in sun-exposed areas, especially the malar area, producing a butterfly configuration. Telangiectasias may also be prominent, and, at times, fine scaling is seen. Occasionally bullae, erosions, and ulcers also occur. Periungual telangiectasia is a prominent finding in systemic lupus as well as in other connective tissue diseases. Subacute lupus is a form in which psoriasiform skin patches are found on the face and trunk. Skin biopsy for both routine and direct immunofluorescence pathologic examination is useful in confirming the diagnosis.

Dermatomyositis (Chapter 296) findings include violaceous edema of the eyelids (heliotrope), flat-topped papules over the knuckles (Gottron's papules, Color Plate 14*B*), and reticulated patches of hy-

Table 522–11 ■ **ATROPHIC SKIN CONDITIONS WITH SCARRING, INDURATION, ULCERATION, AND TELANGIECTASIAS**

Scarring
    Lupus erythematosus
    Dermatomyositis
    Radiation
Dermal indurations (sclerosis)
    Scleroderma
    Lichen sclerosus et atrophicus
    Myxedema
Cutaneous ulcers
    Arterial insufficiency
    Venous insufficiency
    Sickle cell anemia
    Neurotrophic ulcers
    Pyoderma gangrenosum
    Ecthyma gangrenosum (*Pseudomonas* spp.)
Genital ulcers
    Herpes simplex
    Syphilis
    Chancroid
    Lymphogranuloma venereum
    Granuloma inguinale
    Behçet's syndrome
    Self-inflicted

per- and hypopigmentation, erythema, and telangiectasia (poikiloderma) found on the V of the neck, face, elbows, and knees.

X-radiation (Chapter 19) can cause chronic skin changes of atrophy, telangiectasias, irregular pigmentation, and eventually ulceration. Within these areas malignant changes may later appear.

DERMAL INDURATIONS (SCLEROSIS). *Scleroderma* is a condition in which excessive collagen is found in the dermis (Chapter 290). *Morphea* is localized scleroderma confined to the skin, whereas *systemic scleroderma,* or *progressive systemic sclerosis,* is a more extensive form in which fibrosis diffusely involves the skin as well as internal organs. Morphea lesions are asymptomatic, oval to irregular, whitish, firm, thickened patches with an erythematous border. The plaques are most often found on the trunk. The thickened skin in progressive systemic sclerosis is not sharply demarcated, but rather causes indurated, "hidebound" tight skin over the fingers, toes, and extremities (acrosclerosis). Thickening of the facial skin causes smoothness and loss of wrinkles except for furrowing around the mouth. Ulcerations followed by pitted scars occur on the finger tips. Telangiectasia may be prominent, appearing as periungual telangiectasias and multiple, small punctate macules on the face and hands (matlike telangiectasia). A variant of systemic scleroderma, the *CREST syndrome,* displays extensive telangiectasias over face and hands. Patients with *hereditary hemorrhagic telangiectasia* (Chapter 129) also display telangiectasia, particularly around the mouth and nose and on the fingers, as well as vascular malformations in the gastrointestinal tract and, at times, the lung. No cutaneous induration is found in this condition.

Lichen sclerosus et atrophicus, which may be confused with morphea, presents as porcelain white, atrophic, indurated plaques most commonly on the vulva or on the male genitalia (*balanitis xerotica obliterans*). At times it occurs as scattered patches on the trunk. Purpuric areas may also be seen within the lesions.

Myxedema (Chapter 239) may cause a doughy thickening of the skin from deposition of glycosaminoglycans in the dermis. Myxedema may be localized to the pre-tibial areas (pre-tibial myxedema) as firm, non-pitting plaques and nodules with accentuation of the follicular orifices giving a *peau d'orange* appearance.

CUTANEOUS ULCERS. Primary skin ulcers are caused by a wide variety of conditions. The location of the ulcers, the symptoms associated with them, and the rapidity of their appearance are important clues in diagnosing their various causes.

Ulcers of the extremities are frequently associated with vascular disease (Chapters 67–69) and diabetes mellitus (Chapter 242, Color Plate 16*F*). Sudden pain associated with numbness of an extremity and ulceration suggest arterial occlusion. Ulceration of digits associated with a purplish red color with dependency and pallor when the extremity is elevated suggests arteriosclerotic peripheral vascular disease. Brawny edema, brown discoloration, and dermatitis over the lower legs in association with ulcers around the malleoli are seen with venous insufficiency. Sickle cell anemia (Chapter 169) causes ulcerations in the lower third of the leg (Color Plate 16*A*). Areas of pressure and trauma, particularly on the foot, in patients with peripheral neuropathy are susceptible to neurotrophic ulcers (*mal perforans*), as in diabetes and leprosy. The skin around the ulcer is anesthetic and calloused. Pressure sores or decubitus ulcers occur in immobilized debilitated patients. Shearing forces, friction, moisture, and pressure contribute to the development of these sores. The sacral and coccygeal areas, ischial tuberosities, and greater trochanters are favored sites. The best treatment of pressure sores is prevention by frequently moving immobilized patients, keeping the skin clean, and using air mattresses (Chapter 8).

An unusual and dramatic ulcerative condition, *pyoderma gangrenosum,* often begins as an inflammatory nodule or pustule resembling a furuncle that breaks down, ulcerates, and gradually enlarges peripherally. Fully developed, the lesions are moderately deep, red, necrotic ulcers with undermined, violaceous, edematous borders. These lesions, which typically evolve on the lower legs, are postulated to represent a Shwartzman-like hypersensitivity reaction to a number of underlying internal conditions, including chronic ulcerative colitis or Crohn's disease (Chapter 135), rheumatoid arthritis, dysproteinemias, and occasionally leukemia or lymphoma. In over one half of the cases no cause is identified.

Ecthyma gangrenosum is characterized by ulcerative lesions, often in the body folds (anogenital and axillary areas), in immunosuppressed patients with *Pseudomonas septicemia.* The painless lesions begin as hemorrhagic bullous patches that become necrotic and ulcerate and are surrounded by considerable erythema with a central gray to black eschar. *Pseudomonas* can be cultured from these skin lesions.

Genital ulcers suggest venereal disease, including herpes simplex (see earlier), syphilis (indurated, painless, round ulcer with a clean base), chancroid (single or multiple, soft, painful, purulent ulcers with undermined erythematous edges), lymphogranuloma venereum (transient, painless skin ulcer with associated inguinal adenopathy), and granuloma inguinale (small nodules on genitalia which erode and become filled with velvety red granulation). Multiple genital ulcers also occur in *Behçet's syndrome* (Chapter 298) in association with oral ulcers and ocular disease (iridocyclitis). Erythema nodosum, arthritis, and neurologic and intestinal involvement may also occur. The oral and genital ulcers are small, painful aphthae. Occasionally sterile pustules and ulcers occur at the site of minor trauma such as blood sampling.

Geometric, bizarre-shaped, angular ulcers are characteristic of a self-inflicted, factitial cause.

HYPER- AND HYPOPIGMENTATION OF THE SKIN DISEASES

Disorders of melanin pigmentation can be classified as hypomelanoses (decreased or absent epidermal melanin) or hypermelanoses (increased epidermal or dermal melanin). Hyper- and hypomelanoses can be further subdivided into localized or generalized (total-body) alterations of pigmentation (Table 522–12).

LOCALIZED HYPERPIGMENTARY CONDITIONS. *Freckles (ephelides)*, which are light brown–red macules found in sun-exposed areas, are caused by increased melanin production in normal numbers of melanocytes. Freckles are more common in fair-complexioned individuals with red or sandy hair.

Lentigines are also hyperpigmented macules, but they occur because of increased numbers of melanocytes in the basal layer of the epidermis. Two types are recognized: lentigos that occur early in life and are congenital and actinic lentigines, which are acquired in middle age and are related to sun damage over the face, arms, and dorsum of the hands. Actinic lentigines are sometimes difficult to distinguish from early lentigo maligna on the face, but actinic lentigines have no malignant potential. The multiple lentigines syndrome is a rare, dominantly inherited condition characterized by hundreds of lentigines on the trunk, head, extremities, palms, and soles, and it is associated with electrocardiographic abnormalities—ocular hypertelorism, pulmonary stenosis, abnormal genitalia, retarded growth, and deafness (thus the acronym LEOPARD syndrome). Another dominantly inherited condition is Peutz-Jeghers

Table 522–12 ■ HYPERPIGMENTATION AND HYPOPIGMENTATION

Localized hyperpigmentation
  Freckles (ephelides)
  Lentigines
  Melasma (chloasma)
  Post-inflammatory hyperpigmentation
  Café au lait spots
  Xeroderma pigmentosum
Generalized hyperpigmentation
  Excessive melanocyte-stimulating hormone (MSH) or adrenocorticotropic
    hormone (ACTH)
    Addison's disease
    Cushing's disease after bilateral adrenalectomy
    Ectopic ACTH
    Small cell carcinoma of the lung
    Pancreatic carcinoma
  Scleroderma
  Systemic lupus erythematosus
  Hyperthyroidism
  Medications
  Arsenicals
  Hemochromatosis
  Biliary cirrhosis
Localized hypopigmentary changes
  Vitiligo
  Piebaldism
  Tuberous sclerosis
  Pityriasis alba
  Chemicals, principally phenol derivatives
Generalized hypopigmentation
  Albinism

syndrome (Chapter 139), distinctive for its numerous lentigines occurring around the mouth, eyes, hands, and feet in association with gastrointestinal polyps, gastrointestinal hemorrhage, and occasionally malignant degeneration of the polyps.

Melasma (chloasma) of the face usually affects women; the melanocytes produce more melanin than normal in response to hormonal factors (occurs during pregnancy or while on birth control pills) in association with ultraviolet radiation. This type of pigmentation occurs symmetrically over the malar eminences, forehead, and upper lip. The lesions may fade with delivery but often persist and are accentuated when birth control pills are used. Sunscreens are useful. Hydroquinone, a bleaching agent (2 to 4% creams), is controversial and may worsen the condition.

Post-inflammatory hyperpigmentation is macular pigmentation following inflammatory skin diseases (e.g., lichen planus typically causes brown to blue pigmentation).

Café au lait spots are light brown (coffee-with-cream hue) macules that occur on the trunk and extremities in neurofibromatosis (Chapter 456). Six or more such lesions, each greater than 1.5 cm in diameter, are diagnostic for this dominantly inherited disease, but 10% of the normal population have isolated café au lait spots. In Albright's syndrome (polyostotic fibrous dysplasia), three or four large, irregularly shaped (so-called coast-of-Maine configuration), hyperpigmented macules are usually found unilaterally distributed on the buttocks or cervical area.

Xeroderma pigmentosum is a rare, heterogenous group of diseases with hereditary deficiencies of enzyme systems that repair ultraviolet light–induced damage to keratinocyte and melanocyte DNA. This inability to maintain the integrity of DNA leads to extreme sun sensitivity and multiple freckles over the face, lips, conjunctivae, and extremities; the lesions evolve into variably sized, pigmented patches interspersed with hypopigmented areas. Keratoses, keratoacanthomas, basal and squamous cell cancers, and malignant melanomas evolve and frequently lead to early death. This entity should be considered whenever there is unexplained extreme sun sensitivity or excessive freckling in youngsters. This disease can be subtle in its initial presentation, and total avoidance of the sun from early life may prevent subsequent fatal skin cancers.

GENERALIZED HYPERPIGMENTATION. Diffuse brown hyperpigmentation is a feature of *Addison's disease* (Chapter 240) with accentuation of the pigment in body folds (palmar creases), pressure points (knuckles, elbows), and gingival mucus membrane. A similar diffuse hyperpigmentation is seen following adrenalectomy in patients with Cushing's disease due to a pituitary tumor, as well as in patients with pancreatic and lung carcinomas (Chapter 194). The generalized hypermelanosis results from overproduction of either melanocyte-stimulating hormone (MSH) or adrenocorticotropic hormone (ACTH), both of which share common amino acid sequences. Other conditions in which addisonian-like diffuse hyperpigmentation can be seen include scleroderma, lupus erythematosus, and hyperthyroidism.

Hyperpigmentation occurs with cyclophosphamide, busulfan, daunorubicin, and doxorubicin. Bleomycin can produce a distinctive linear "flagellate" pattern of hyperpigmentation, usually seen on the trunk. Antimalarials can cause a patchy slate-gray pigmentary alteration confined to cartilaginous structures (pseudo-ochronosis), and the acne medication minocycline can cause similar pigmentary deposition in the skin, nails, bones, and teeth. Amiodarone can also cause hyperpigmentation on the face.

In addition, inorganic trivalent arsenicals (found in insecticides and contaminated water) may also produce a generalized brown pigmentation, but in this instance the hypermelanosis is studded with small, scattered, depigmented macules (likened to rain drops on a dusty road) and punctate keratoses on the palms and soles. *Hemochromatosis* (Chapter 221) causes a metallic gray-brown generalized hyperpigmentation, and cutaneous changes are the presenting sign in 25 to 40% of patients. Similarly, brown generalized hyperpigmentation, which is accentuated in exposed areas, in association with pruritus, jaundice, and xanthoma, is typical of *biliary cirrhosis* (Chapter 157).

LOCALIZED PIGMENTARY CHANGES. *Vitiligo,* a circumscribed hypomelanosis of progressively enlarging amelanotic macules in a symmetrical distribution around body orifices and over bony prominences (knees, elbows, hands), is familial in 36% of cases. In one third of cases, some spontaneous repigmentation occurs, particularly in sun-exposed areas. White hairs are common in the vitiliginous areas. Although most patients with vitiligo are healthy, there is an increased association with certain autoimmune conditions such as thyroiditis, hyperthyroidism, Addison's disease, pernicious anemia, and diabetes mellitus. Melanocytes are absent from the vitiliginous macules. Circulating complement-binding anti-melanocyte antibodies have been found in some vitiligo patients. Treatment of vitiligo is frustrating. If an inflammatory border rims the patches of pigment loss, topical steroids may prove beneficial in slowing or halting progression of disease. In cases of extensive disease, chemical depigmentation with a bleaching agent (e.g., hydroquinone) of remaining normal skin may provide a superior cosmetic result. Repigmentation of localized or extensive disease may be attempted using psoralen plus ultraviolet A light (PUVA), but drawbacks of this modality include the need for multiple treatments and an increased risk of skin cancer.

Piebaldism is a dominantly inherited condition of localized hypopigmentation that resuts from a mutation in the c-*kit* proto-oncogene. Patients present with a characteristic white forelock and hypomelanosis on the extremities, anterior thorax, and central scalp, presumably representing mosaic patches of mutated neural crest cells. Waardenburg's syndrome also represents a congenital leukoderma and shares similar features, including a white forelock; however, these patients also typically demonstrate facial dysmorphism and sensorineural hearing loss.

Tuberous sclerosis is an autosomal dominant neurocutaneous disorder that includes localized hypopigmentation in almost all cases. The "ash-leaf macule," a distinctively shaped focal patch of pigment diminution typically on the trunk, is characteristic of this disease and is the earliest presenting cutaneous manifestation. Although up to 4% of the normal population has one hypopigmented macule, multiple lesions strongly suggest tuberous sclerosis (Chapter 456).

Pityriasis alba presents as oval hypopigmented macules on the cheeks, trunk, and extremities of children, particularly those with darker skin types, and likely represents a form of post-inflammatory pigment loss. This condition presents frequently in atopic children and can be differentiated from the superficial yeast infection tinea versicolor by a KOH examination. Infectious causes of localized pigment loss include the non-venereal treponemal infection *pinta*, which is endemic in areas of Central and South America.

Certain chemicals, particularly phenol derivatives, when applied to the skin, may cause permanent depigmentation. Hypomelanosis has been observed on the hands of black-skinned individuals wearing rubber gloves in which hydroquinine is used as an antioxidant.

GENERALIZED HYPOPIGMENTATION. (ALBINISM). Oculocutaneous albinism, which is an autosomal recessive disorder due to mutations affecting melanin biosynthesis, generally results in pigmentary absence or dilution of the hair, skin, and eyes. Type I represents mutations in the gene *tyrosinase*, whereas Type II results from defects in the pigment-related *P* gene. Mutations in this gene cause other diseases such as Prader-Willi and Angelman syndromes, as well as autosomal recessive ocular albinism.

REGIONAL DIAGNOSIS OF SKIN DISEASES—COMMONLY ENCOUNTERED PROBLEMS BY ANATOMIC REGION

Many skin diseases have a predilection for certain areas or regions of the body, often related to variations in the structure and function of the integument (Table 522–13).

DISORDERS OF THE NAILS

The nail is a plate of hard keratin synthesized from an invagination of the epidermis. The proximal nail fold houses the matrix of the nail, where basal cells rapidly proliferate and differentiate into the nail plate, which grows over the nail bed (Table 522–14). Nails grow continuously throughout life. The average fingernail grows 0.5 to 1.2 mm/week, whereas toenails grow at one half to one third

this rate. It takes a fingernail about 5.5 months and a toenail 12 to 18 months to regrow from the matrix, although rate of growth slows as the individual gets older.

SKIN DISEASES INVOLVING NAILS. In 10% of *lichen planus* patients, accentuated longitudinal nail ridging occurs with pterygium formation resulting from destructive focal scarring of the matrix. Early treatment with oral steroids is indicated. *Atopic eczema* and other eczematous entities may cause pitting, transverse striations, and onycholysis. Nail changes in *psoriasis* (see earlier) involve fingernails more frequently than toenails. *Onychomycosis,* or fungal infections of the nail, may be caused by dermatophyte (tinea unguium) or candidal infections. Infection of toenails is more frequent than of fingernails, but all nails may be involved. The nail plate is discolored, thickened, crumbly, and onycholytic with accumulation of debris. White superficial onychomycosis appears as white patches in the toenail plate as a result of organisms growing on the surface and barely penetrating the nail. Scrapings reveal hyphae upon KOH examination. An unusual condition, chronic mucocutaneous candidiasis, is caused by widespread *Candida albicans* infection leading to diffuse white thickening of all nails.

Topical antifungal therapy is ineffective. Terbinafine, itraconazole, griseofulvin, and ketoconazole are effective therapies (see earlier). In older individuals, toenail problems may never be totally eradicated because the nails grow so slowly. Residual fungal spores in shoes and environment no doubt cause frequent recurrences; topical antifungal powders may be helpful in long-term prophylaxis.

Paronychia, or painful, red swelling of the nail fold, can be either acute or chronic. Acute paronychia typically results from bacterial infection, whereas *C. albicans* usually underlies chronic infection. At times, a small abscess or purulent discharge is seen. This infection usually occurs in hands of those constantly exposed to a wet environment (bartenders, janitors). Therapy consists of avoidance of water and use of appropriate antibacterial or antifungal solutions two or three times a day for a month or so.

NAIL DISTURBANCES IN SYSTEMIC DISEASES. *Splinter hemorrhages* result from the extravasation of blood from longitudinally oriented vessels of the nail bed. Although often thought to be associated with bacterial endocarditis (Chapter 326), they are much more commonly associated with trauma. *Beau's lines* are nonspecific, appearing as transverse depressions across the nail plates following any severe disability that temporarily interferes with nail growth. Longitudinal pigmented bands occur most often in response to trauma or a nevus located in the matrix. *Yellow nail syndrome* exhibits yellow thickening of the nails with absence of the lunula and variable degrees of onycholysis accompanying pulmonary conditions such as bronchiectasis, pleural effusion, and chronic obstructive pulmonary disease. Lymphedema of the extremities may coexist. *Clubbing of the nails* (increased bilateral curvature of the nails with enlargement of the soft connective tissue of the distal phalanges resulting in the flattening of the obtuse angle formed by the proximal end of the nail and the digit) occurs most often with bronchiectasis, lung abscess, and pulmonary neoplasms. Cardiovascular disease and chronic gastrointestinal diseases (ulcerative colitis, sprue) are also associated with clubbing. Clubbing accompanied by bone pain and proliferative periostitis is termed *hypertrophic osteoarthropathy* (Chapters 196 and 197); this condition is most often associated with bronchogenic squamous cell carcinoma. Azidothymidine (zidovudine) (AZT) can cause black or blue discoloration of the nail plate in a longitudinal, horizontal, or diffuse pattern.

TUMORS OF THE NAIL. A variety of benign tumors occur around the nail unit. These include *periungual fibromas, myxoid cysts,* and *subungual exostoses.* Surgical removal is the only certain means of cure.

The most important malignant tumor involving the nails is melanoma, which appears as a pigmented area at the base of the nail or as a longitudinal pigmented streak in the nail. Leeching of pigment onto the proximal nail fold is known as Hutchinson's sign and is suggestive of melanoma. Melanoma must be distinguished from other causes of nail pigmentary alteration including trauma, medications, and nevi. A matrix biopsy is the only certain way to exclude a malignancy. Additionally, squamous cell carcinoma, Kaposi's sarcoma, and lymphoma can involve the nail unit.

Table 522–13 ■ REGIONAL DERMATOLOGY

REGION OF SKIN	TYPE OF SKIN GROUP	DISEASE PROCESS
Scalp	Papulosquamous and eczematous	Psoriasis, seborrheic dermatitis, tinea capitis, eczema (atopic, contact)
	Pustular	Folliculitis, kerion
	Nodular	Nevi, seborrheic keratosis, pilar cysts, verruca
	Atrophic and telangiectatic	Connective tissue disease, scleroderma, discoid lupus erythematosus
Face	Pustular	Acne, rosacea, folliculitis, tinea
	Papulosquamous and eczematous	Psoriasis, seborrheic dermatitis, contact dermatitis (cosmetics), atopic dermatitis, impetigo, lupus erythematosus, photodermatitis
	Vesicular	Herpes-zoster and herpes simplex, insect bites
	Nodular	Basal cell cancers, squamous cell cancers, melanomas, keratoacanthomas, nevi, actinic keratosis
Trunk	Papulosquamous and eczematous	Psoriasis, atopic and contact eczema, tinea versicolor, pityriasis rosacea, scabies
	Vesiculobullous	Pemphigus, bullous pemphigoid
	Maculopapular	Secondary syphilis, drug reaction, viral exanthems
	Nodular	Nevi, seborrheic keratosis, lipoma, basal cell cancer, keloid, neurofibroma, angiomas, melanoma
	Pustular	Acne
	Urticarial	Hives
Arms and forearms	Eczematous and papulosquamous	Contact dermatitis—plants; atopic dermatitis, lichen planus
	Nodular	Nevi, warts, seborrheic keratosis, actinic keratosis
	Atrophic telangiectatic	Scleroderma, dermatomyositis
Legs	Eczematous and papulosquamous	Contact dermatitis, stasis dermatitis, atopic dermatitis, psoriasis, lichen planus
	Nodular	Erythema nodosum, dermatofibromas, nevi, melanoma, Kaposi' sarcoma, lipoma
	Maculopapular	Vasculitis, Schamberg's disease, actinic purpura, pretibial myxedema
	Atrophic, telangiectatic, and ulcerative	Scleroderma, dermatostasis ulcers, arterial insufficiency
Genitalia and groin	Eczematous and papulosquamous	Contact dermatitis, seborrheic dermatitis, scabies, pediculosis pubis, psoriasis, Reiter's syndrome, erythrasma, tinea, candidiasis, lichen planus, intertrigo, lichen simplex chronicus
	Vesiculobullous	Herpes simplex, Stevens-Johnson syndrome
	Ulcerative and atrophic	Syphilis, chancroid, lymphogranuloma venereum, Behçet's syndrome
	Nodular	Verruca vulgaris, erythroplasia of Queyrat, squamous cell cancer, sebaceous cyst, molluscum contagiosum
	Pustular	Hidradenitis suppurativa
Hands	Eczematous and papulosquamous	Allergic contact and irritant contact dermatitis, dyshidrosis, pyoderma, tinea, dermatophytids, scabies, atopic, dermatitis, secondary syphilis
	Vesiculobullous, pustular	Erythema multiforme, hand-foot-and-mouth disease, porphyria cutanea tarda, psoriasis
	Nodular	Warts, squamous cells cancer, actinic keratosis, keratoacanthoma, pyogenic granuloma, granuloma annulare, synovial cysts
	Hypopigmented	Vitiligo
	Atrophic telangiectatic	Scleroderma, dermatomyositis
Feet	Eczematous and papulosquamous	Contact dermatitis, atopic dermatitis, tinea, psoriasis, lichen planus
	Vesiculobullous	Tinea, epidermolysis bullosa, erythema multiforme
	Nodules	Verruca, corn, nevus
	Atrophic telangiectatic	Scleroderma

HAIR LOSS (ALOPECIA) (FIGURE 522–1)

Hair loss can be due to physical and chemical forces and genetic predispostion. Autoimmune diseases and severe emotional stress also may lead to alopecia as well.

Physical exam should focus on the pattern of hair loss (i.e., is it patchy or diffuse). The presence of any underlying erythema or scale should be noted. Occurrence of alopecia in body locations other than the scalp maybe an important clue as to the cause. Some alopecia conditions heal with scarring, which sometimes serves as a useful characteristic to separate the various forms of alopecia.

NON-SCARRING ALOPECIA. LOCALIZED ALOPECIA. *Alopecia areata* is a fairly common form of alopecia that is almost always localized to discrete patches of alopecia on the scalp. Classic lesions are round-to-oval, well-circumscribed patches of hair loss with little or no underlying inflammation. Sometimes tiny hairs with tapered tops may be seen within the patches of alopecia, so-called exclamation point hairs. Alopecia that involves the occipital region and the area above the ears (ophiasis) portends a poor prognosis, as does alopecia of the eyebrows or lashes. Occasionally the entire scalp may be involved, and this is termed *alopecia totalis*. Total-body alopecia associated with alopecia areata is called *alopecia universalis*. Both the totalis and universalis variants have a poor prognosis.

Alopecia areata may have an autoimmune cause as it is occasionally associated with Hashimoto's thyroiditis as well as other thyroid gland dysfunction. It can also be found in patients with pernicious anemia.

Most patients with alopecia areata localized to the scalp have a very good prognosis. Hair usually regrows within a few months. Topical or intralesional steroids and PUVA have variable results.

Tinea capitis can be confused with alopecia areata. Tinea infection appears as one or more patches of hair loss with mild scaling and erythema. Additionally, broken hair shafts frequently leave residual black stumps (block dot ringworm). Griseofulvin is the drug of choice to treat tinea capitis.

Trichotillomania refers to traumatic, self-induced breaking, rubbing, plucking, and twisting of hairs that lead to alopecia. The scalp is usually affected, but the eyebrows and lashes may be involved as well. Patients with this condition may have underlying emotional or psychiatric problems.

Table 522–14 ■ POTENTIAL DEFECTS IN NAIL FORMATION

Brittleness—easy breaking of nail tips
Leukonychia—white discoloration of nails
Striations—Longitudinal ridges running parallel or perpendicular to the length of the nail
Onycholysis—separation of the nail plate from the bed
Onychogryphosis—hypertrophy and thickening of the nail
Onychomycosis—dystrophy, destruction of the nail due to yeast and fungal infections
Pitting—discrete pitlike depressions in the nail surface
Koilonychia—spoon-shaped deformity of the nails (concave nail with everted edges)
Pterygium formation—growth of cuticle onto the nail plate

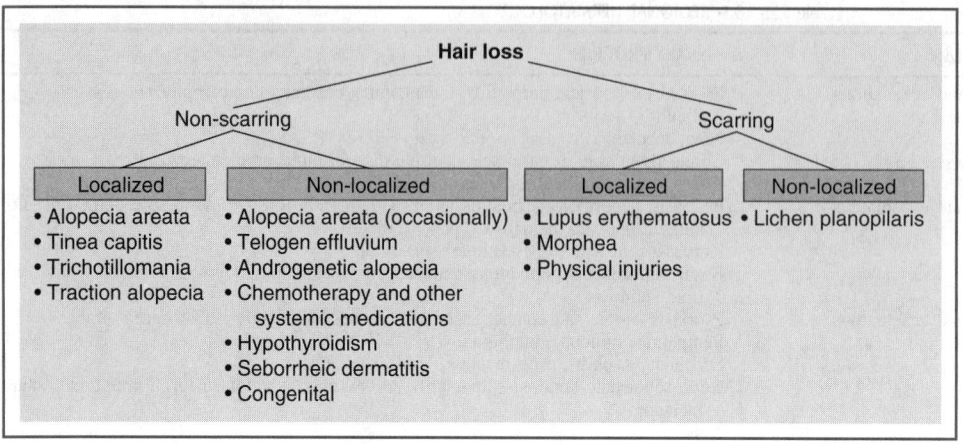

FIGURE 522–1 ■ An approach to the diagnosis of the cause of alopecia.

Traction alopecia may result from chronic tension on the hair, such as chronically pulling the hair back tightly. Traction alopecia usually occurs at the margin of the hairline and in women who overtighten the hairs when curling. This type of hair loss is usually non-scarring, but can go on to scar if done over long periods of time.

DIFFUSE OR GENERALIZED ALOPECIA. *Telogen effluvium* is a transient, reversible, diffuse hair loss of scalp hair that results from alterations in the normal hair cycle. Severe emotional and physiologic stress such as high fever, systemic illness or surgery, or crash diets may cause growing hairs to convert to resting hairs, which are subsequently shed. Certain drugs such as heparin, coumadin, allopurinol, amphetamines, β-blockers, and lithium are other causes. Pregnancy and oral contraceptives cause hairs to grow continually, rather than cycling at programmed times. After childbirth or discontinuation of oral contraceptives, growing follicles "catch up" by simultaneously resting. Shedding follows 2 to 4 months later. If the stress resolves, the hair generally regrows in 4 to 6 months. Diffuse hair loss may not be noticeable until there is greater than 50% scalp hair loss. Gentle pulling of the hair verifies the degree of shedding. A positive "hair pull" result occurs when five or more hairs easily are removed when about a dozen or so are gently pulled.

Androgenetic alopecia can occur in both males and females. In men, hair loss generally occurs in the frontal, vertex, and upper occipital regions of the scalp while sparing the posterior and lateral margins. The process may begin at any age after puberty, with temporal hair recession usually noted first. There is no actual loss of hair, but rather a conversion of thick terminal hairs to fine, unpigmented, "miniaturized" hairs. In women the pattern of hair loss is generally more diffuse with thinning throughout the scalp. Women with elevated androgen levels, as occur in masculinizing disorders, have a balding pattern similar to that of men.

Treatment of androgenetic alopecia may include topical minoxidil and surgical procedures to transplant hairs into areas of thinning. Recently finasteride (Propecia) has been released as a treatment for androgenetic alopecia in men; it blocks the enzyme 5-α-reductase, responsible for the peripheral conversion of testosterone to dihydrotestosterone. Dihydrotestosterone seems to induce the miniaturization of genetically predisposed hairs over the central and frontal scalp.

Toxic alopecia occurs if hair growth is disrupted. Newly synthesized hair shafts are weakened, and the hair breaks readily. Thinning may be extreme, occurring within a few weeks of an insult involving all 80% of growing follicles. Chemotherapeutic agents, especially doxorubicin and related agents, exert their effect on rapidly growing cells in the hair bulb and commonly cause hair damage in cancer patients receiving chemotherapy. Radiation therapy to the scalp area causes similar abnormalities. Retinoids and hypervitaminosis A cause hair loss through their interference with keratinization.

In *hypothyroidism,* diffuse hair loss over the scalp is associated with dry and brittle hair and loss of the lateral third of the eyebrows.

Seborrheic dermatitis with erythema and yellow, greasy scales throughout the scalp may be associated with mild, diffuse hair loss. Treatment with tar shampoos, selenium sulfide (Selsun) shampoos, and topical steroids may control the inflammatory process. Topical antifungal shampoos containing ketoconazole (such as Nizoral) can also be beneficial.

Diffuse hair loss can occur with many *congenital* syndromes associated with structural defects in the hair shaft. The hair may be sparse, fine, and wiry from early in childhood.

SCARRING ALOPECIA. Occasionally hair loss may be accompanied by permanent scarring of the scalp with permanent loss of hair follicles.

LOCALIZED SCARRING ALOPECIA. Systemic *lupus erythematosus* (Chapter 289) may cause diffuse, non-scarring alopecia of the scalp along with short, broken hairs in the frontal margin in 20% of patients. Discoid (skin-limited) lupus erythematosus causes oval scarring areas of alopecia. Typical plaques have an active erythematous margin, white atrophic center, telangectasias, and keratin-filled follicles.

Morphea (localized scleroderma) (Chapter 290) may occasionally involve the scalp. When it does, it causes localized scarring alopecia. Areas involved are generally firm, atrophic, ivory-colored, atrophic plaques. Margins of lesions may be erythematous, perhaps indicating active lesions. At times, morphea may be linear and even extend down onto the face, simulating a saber wound (en coup de sabre). Deep tissue deformity, even bony deformation, may result.

A number of *physical injuries* such as mechanical trauma, burns, and radiation dermatitis may also cause local scarring alopecias.

NON-LOCALIZED SCARRING ALOPECIA. *Lichen planus* involving the scalp may result in diffuse, patchy scarring alopecia (lichen planopilaris). Additional lesions of lichen planus may be found on more typical sites of the skin, mucous membranes, and nails.

HIRSUTISM (EXCESSIVE HAIR GROWTH) (see also Chapter 255)

Excessive hair growth, usually a complaint of females, may be due to either endocrinologic or nonendocrinologic conditions. When women are affected in those areas of the body that normally develop hair as a secondary sex characteristic in males, their hirsutism generally reflects treatable endocrinopathy, as these follicles respond to high concentrations of testosterone and can convert various androgens to dihydrotestosterone (Chapter 519).

NON-ENDOCRINE HIRSUTISM. *Ethnic or racial hirsutism* is characterized by excessive hair growth on the upper lip, beard area, chest, nipples, or lower abdomen in women without menstrual abnormalities or masculization. Type of hair, rate of hair growth, and distribution of hair over the body differ among the races, relating to variations in the sensitivity of follicles to circulating androgens. A male pattern of hirsutism is more common in females whose ancestors came from the southern parts of Europe. Asians and native Americans have less body hair. If serum testosterone, dehydroepiandrosterone, and androstenedione levels are normal, bleaching or shaving may make the hair less noticeable. Electrolysis permanently destroys hair follicles but is time-consuming and costly. Spironolactone, which has antiandrogenic properties, is also useful at 200 mg/day for decreasing hair growth although it is not formally approved for this purpose.

Certain *drugs* may increase hair growth. Androgenic or steroidal medications, such as anabolic steroids, corticosteroids, and contraceptives, may cause increased hair growth in the beard, chest, and groin areas. Drugs such as phenytoin, phenothiazines, cyclosporine, and minoxidil cause excess hair in both men and women anywhere on the body.

ENDOCRINE HIRSUTISM. A distinction must be made between hirsutism caused by increased androgen production with and that without virilization. In general, virilization is a sign of markedly elevated androgen levels derived from the adrenal glands or ovaries, especially adrenogenital syndrome, congenital adrenal hyperplasia, Cushing's disease or syndrome, Stein-Leventhal syndrome (polycystic ovarian syndrome), and occasionally malignant adrenal or ovarian tumors. Any woman with hirsutism and accompanying virilization should be tested for excess cortisol and androgen production.

Simple or idiopathic hirsutism denotes hirsutism in women in whom a specific diagnosis cannot be made and who have normal or slightly elevated adrenal or ovarian androgen level. Such patients have been successfully treated with cyclically administered birth control pills or with spironolactone.

PHOTOSENSITIVITY AND OTHER REACTIONS TO LIGHT

Certain wavelengths of light can induce a number of undesirable cutaneous reactions, including sunburn, skin aging, carcinogenesis, and a variety of photosensitivity reactions.

The solar spectrum that commonly affects human skin is in the ultraviolet light range (290 to 400 nm), which is subdivided into three bands designated as UVC (shorter than 290 nm), UVB (290 to 320 nm), and UVA, or long-wave ultraviolet light (320 to 400 nm). UVC does not reach the earth, being absorbed by ozone; UVB, or the sunburn spectrum, causes burning, tanning, aging, and carcinogenic changes in the skin. UVA is melanogenic and erythrogenic, but the amount of energy required to produce these effects is 1000 times greater than that for UVB. UVA causes skin reactions through window glass, and these wavelengths are often responsible for photoreactions in which chemical photosensitizers and UV radiation interact to cause inflammatory skin reactions.

The incidence of photoreactions depends on a number of factors such as the amount of light reaching the earth's surface, season of the year, latitude and weather conditions, and thickness of the ozone layer, as well as topographic features of the environment. Certain climatologic and environmental factors influence the amount of sunlight hitting the skin. For example, 50% of the daily ultraviolet light is emitted between 11:00 A.M. and 2:00 P.M.: Avoiding exposure during this time may minimize photoreactions. Sitting in the shade does not protect against UV exposure, because 50% of the ambient ultraviolet light is received; 90% of ultraviolet light penetrates clouds, so one can get sunburns even in the shade and on cloudy days.

DIRECT PHOTO EFFECTS ON THE SKIN. ACUTE EFFECTS. Sunburning and tanning are attributed primarily to UVB light, although prolonged exposure to UVA can produce mild burn and marked hyperpigmentation. The sunburn reaction produces a complex inflammatory process causing dyskeratotic cells, spongiosis, vacuolation of keratinocytes, and edema from capillary leakage, 12 to 24 hours after exposure. Occasionally, in addition to redness and pain, blisters may evolve. Prostaglandins may play a role in the burn reaction, as they are found in increased quantities in sunburned skin. Aspirin, indomethacin, or prostaglandin synthesis inhibitors can reduce the burn.

Three to four days after a sunburn, new melanin pigment is formed. Several cellular and molecular changes occur in the skin after each sunburn reaction, which, if repeated, may lead to the

chronic effects of UV light. A few days after UV light burning, epidermal mitosis and hyperplasia occur and DNA, RNA, and proteins in the skin are damaged.

CHRONIC EFFECTS. Degenerative changes of the skin consisting of wrinkling, telangiectasias, and keratoses result from chronic exposure to UV light. The skin may become furrowed and leathery and develop yellow papules and plaques due to degeneration of the dermal collagen. These changes are caused by both UVB and UVA radiation. Such changes can be minimized by daily topical applications of effective sunscreens. A number of malignant and premalignant skin lesions are associated with chronic sun exposure, including actinic keratoses, keratoacanthomas, basal cell and squamous cell carcinomas, and probably melanomas.

INDIRECT PHOTO EFFECTS ON THE SKIN. Photoreactions that occur when systemic or topical chemicals induce photosensitivity or when there is an underlying immunologic, biochemical, or genetic abnormality that predisposes to sun sensitivity are considered indirect reactions; that is, the sun alone does not cause photoreactions.

EXOGENOUS FACTORS CAUSING PHOTOSENSITIVITY. Chemical agents either taken systemically or placed topically on the skin can cause one of two general types of photoreactions: phototoxic and photoallergic. In photosensitivity reactions, the absorption spectrum of a given drug, substance, or chemical is maximal at a certain wavelength of light that induces molecular changes in the exogenous material. In most drug or chemical photosensitivity reactions, the wavelengths that evoke abnormal reactions are in the 320- to 400-nm (UVA) region. The reactions include acute, abnormal sunburn responses and eczematous and urticarial reactions.

Phototoxic reactions are non-immunologic cutaneous responses that occur when a drug or chemical in the skin absorbs enough light energy of a specific wavelength. The photosensitizer generates free radicals that damage cell membranes and lysosomes, inducing an exaggerated sunburn reaction, with intense redness, swelling, pain, and occasionally blistering. Most phototoxic agents absorb UVB light.

Photoallergic reactions to topical chemicals or internal drugs represent an acquired, immunogenically altered response to light. Absorption of specific wavelengths of light by chemicals or drugs causes changes in their chemical configuration so that these substances become haptens that bind to proteins in the skin to become a complete antigen capable of eliciting a Type IV delayed hypersensitivity immunologic response. The clinical manifestations of such photoallergic reactions are usually eczematous in nature (occasionally urticarial), evolving in exposed areas 24 hours after exposure to the sun. The action spectrum is generally long-range UVA light.

SYSTEMIC PHOTOSENSITIZERS. Drugs may cause either phototoxic or photoallergic reactions (Table 522–15).

TOPICAL AGENTS CAUSING PHOTOSENSITIVITY. Most topical photosensitizing agents respond to the UVA action spectrum. Drugs and chemicals that induce phototoxic contact reactions include coal tar derivatives, topical drugs (phenothiazines, sulfonamides), dyes (eosins, methylene blue), and plant derivatives (furocoumarins). The photosensitive properties of coal tar derivatives and furocoumarins (psoralens) are utilized in treating certain skin diseases with UV light.

When plants, vegetables, or fruits containing a phototoxic chemical cause phototoxicity, the reaction is referred to as a *phytophotodermatitis*. Photocontact dermatitis develops with contact with plants in the Umbelliferae family, such as figs, cow parsnip, fennel, parsley, parsnip, and gas plant. Phytophotodermatitis also occurs in individuals exposed to Persian limes and celery. Such reactions are caused by furocoumarin compounds that are found in the plant and readily penetrate the epidermis. Two things are needed for initiation of phytophotodermatitis: contact with a sensitizing furocoumarin and subsequent exposure to UV radiation greater than 320 nm. Phytophotodermatitis may take on unique clinical forms: berlock dermatitis presents as streaky erythema followed by hyperpigmentation in areas where perfumes containing oil of bergamot (a psoralen) are applied to the skin (e.g., on the neck); crisscross linear streaks of erythema, vesicles, and bullae that heal with hyperpigmentation where meadow grass or other related plants rub on the

Table 522–15 ■ SYSTEMIC PHOTOSENSITIZERS

NAME	TYPE OF PHOTOREACTION	ACTION SPECTRUM (nm)
Sulfonamides	Phototoxic and photoallergic	290–320
Sulfonylureas (tolbutamide, chlorpropamide)	Phototoxic	290–360
Chlorothiazides	Phototoxic and photoallergic	290–320 320–400
Phenothiazines	Phototoxic, urticaria eruption, gray-blue hyperpigmentation	290–400
Antibiotics (tetracyclines, griseofulvin, nalidixic acid)	Phototoxic and photoallergic bullae	320–400
Furocoumarins (psoralens)	Phototoxic	
Nonsteroidal anti-inflammatory agents	Phototoxic and photoallergic	Unknown
Anticancer drugs (DTIC, fluorouracil, methotrexate, vinblastin)	Phototoxic	Unknown
Estrogens, progestins, and other drugs	Phototoxic, melasma	?290–320
Chlordiazepoxide (Librium)	Photoallergic	290–360
Cyclamates	Phototoxic and photoallergic	290–360
Quinidine, quinine	Photoallergic	320–400

skin; and oil of the rind of a Persian lime causes erythema and pigmentation on the hands of bartenders.

Photoallergic contact dermatitis, a form of delayed eczematous reaction, evolves in some individuals after exposure to chemicals such as fragrances (methylcoumarin and musk ambrette), halogenated salicylanilides, sunscreens, and blankophores, or optical whitening agents, used in laundry soaps and bleaches. A number of perfumes (e.g., after-shave lotions, colognes) contain musk ambrette, a synthetic fragrance fixative that causes a photoeczematous reaction over the face and hands. Sunscreening agents containing aminobenzoic acid (PABA) esters and cinnamates that readily absorb UV light may cause eczematous reactions. A small number of individuals have persistent chronic eczematous dermatitis after all exposure to the photosensitizing agent has ceased—so-called persistent light reactivity; they even may react to artificial fluorescent light.

Identifying the cause of contact photoallergic reactions can be done by photopatch testing (Chapter 520). Treatment begins by eliminating the photosensitizing agent and minimizing exposure (avoiding sun and use of sunscreens). Topical or oral steroids may be needed to decrease the cutaneous inflammatory response.

ENDOGENOUS CONDITIONS ASSOCIATED WITH PHOTOSENSITIVITY. *Immunologic diseases characterized by photosensitivity* include connective tissue conditions such as lupus erythematosus, both discoid and systemic, and solar urticaria. Solar urticaria, hives with itching and burning, evolves within minutes of sunlight exposure and lasts an hour or more. *Biochemical conditions associated with photosensitivity* include porphyria cutanea tarda and erythropoietic protoporphyria.

Pellagra is caused by an inadequate diet and a deficiency of nicotinic acid. It is still seen occasionally with alcoholism, poor dietary intake in the elderly, and malabsorption. The carcinoid syndrome may also be associated with pellagra because tryptophan, the precursor of nicotinic acid, is diverted to serotonin production by the tumor. A scaly dermatitis affects sun-exposed parts of the skin, especially on the face, the neck, and the back of the hands, in association with diarrhea and dementia. Dietary replacement clears the skin and other signs of the disease.

OTHER PHOTOSENSITIVITY CONDITIONS. *Polymorphous light eruption* causes eczematous patches, red to violaceous papules or plaques, and urticarial lesions over the face, the nape and V of the neck, and the back of the hands. The rash characteristically arises hours to days after sun exposure. The onset is frequently in early summer with some degree of resistance being acquired with continued sun exposure. Recurrences each spring and summer are common, and the eruption remits during the winter. The disease is most frequent during the first half of life. The cause is unknown.

DERMATOLOGIC MANIFESTATIONS IN THE IMMUNOCOMPROMISED HOST AND IN ACQUIRED IMMUNODEFICIENCY SYNDROME

Immunosuppression causes an increase in benign and malignant skin growths as well as a variety of infections in the skin (Chapter 314). Cutaneous neoplasms such as squamous cell and basal cell carcinomas occur with a higher than expected frequency. Transplantation patients have a risk of skin cancer seven times greater than normal.

Any skin lesion, no matter how innocuous, should be carefully evaluated in the immunosuppressed host. The gross morphologic characteristics of infections are so frequently modified by the altered inflammatory response that early skin biopsy is essential for diagnosis. The array of potential pathogens is imposing in these patients, and even common infectious processes are greatly modified or obscured by immunocompromising illness. Skin infections are common, accounting for 22 to 33% of infections in immunosuppressed patients.

Microbial involvement of the skin and subcutaneous tissue can be grouped into two major categories in immunocompromised patients: *primary skin infections* include those occurring in non-immunocompromised hosts and those resulting from opportunistic agents that rarely cause skin infection in normal patients; and *disseminated systemic infections* metastatic to the skin from a noncutaneous portal of entry.

PRIMARY SKIN INFECTIONS. Typical primary skin infections, including group A streptococcal and *S. aureus* cellulitis, are frequent, although more unusual causes of cellulitis in granulocytopenic patients must also be considered (*Pseudomonas* spp., anaerobic bacteria). Skin biopsy of the cellulitic areas for Gram's stain and culture is often helpful.

Primary cutaneous infections by viruses and skin dermatophytes are also common. Warts caused by papillomavirus may be numerous and difficult to remove; malignant transformation has been documented. Herpes simplex infections may present as chronic, large, ulcerated lesions persisting for weeks to months, and there may be internal dissemination from cutaneous sites. Reactivation of herpes-zoster infections is common with systemic dissemination. Widespread dermatophyte infections of the skin appear as scaling, red patches that provide a portal of entry for bacterial infection.

Unusual opportunistic primary skin infections with atypical *Mycobacterium, Aspergillus, Rhizopus,* and *Candida* organisms cause cellulitis-like reactions that form a central pustule and eschar. Skin biopsy of such lesions with a portion of the biopsy specimen processed by frozen section and specially stained for acid-fast bacilli and fungi may identify the pathologic organisms rapidly.

DISSEMINATED INFECTION METASTATIC TO THE SKIN. Hematogenous dissemination of infection to the skin from distant primary sites frequently occurs in patients with impaired host defenses. Three groups of organisms are responsible: (1) *Pseudomonas* spp. and other gram-negative bacilli, (2) endemic systemic mycoses (*Histoplasma, Coccidioides* spp.), and (3) opportunistic fungi (*Aspergillus, Candida* spp., Mucoraceae). The range of cutaneous clinical presentations of these infections is varied and mimicked by (a) vesicles and bullae that become hemorrhagic, (b) gangrenous cellulitis with necrotic ulcerations, and (c) widespread, red, warm, fluctuant nodules with pustules and purpura. Prompt biopsy with frozen sections stained for bacterial and hyphal elements may provide rapid diagnosis. Skin biopsy specimens of the lesions should also be sent for appropriate cultures.

CUTANEOUS MANIFESTATIONS OF HIV INFECTIONS. Skin disease is common in patients with HIV (Chapter 414). Some dermatoses are characteristic, whereas others are just observed in a higher frequency or with atypical features. *Diseases characteristic of HIV infection* include Kaposi's sarcoma, oral hairy leukoplakia, bacillary angiomatosis (*Rochalimaea* sp. infection causing angiomatous proliferation resulting in red, raised nodular lesions with a scaling base), eosinophilic folliculitis (intensely pruritic follicular

Table 522-16 ■ CUTANEOUS DRUG REACTIONS

TYPE OF SKIN REACTION	DRUGS LIKELY TO CAUSE SKIN REACTION
Eczematous (allergic contact rection)	Antihistamines, neomycin, formaldehyde, sulfanamides
Photodermatitis	
Phototoxic	Chlorpromazine, psoralens, demeclocycline, doxycycline
Photoallergic	Promethazine, griseofulvin, chlorothiazide, hypoglycemic drugs
Exfoliative dermatitis	Carbamazepine, hydantoins, nitrofurantoin, isoniazid, gold, allopurinol, phenothiazines
Maculopapular eruption (exanthematous)	Penicillin, sulfonamides, hypoglycemic drugs, phenothiazines, allopurinol, phenytoin, quinine, gold salts, captopril, meprobamate
Papulosquamous reactions	
Psoriasiform, lichen planus, pityriasis rosea–like	Beta blockers, lithium (psoriasiform), thiazides, gold, phenothiazines, quinidine, antimalarials (lichen planus–like); gold (PR-like); others—dapsone, ethambutol, furosemide
Vesiculobullous reactions	Azapropazone, captopril, clonidine, furosemide, gold, psoralens, barbiturates, phenytoin, hydrochlorothiazide, penicillamine
Toxic epidermal necrolysis	Acetazolamine, allopurinol, barbiturates, carbamazepines, gold, hydantoin, nitrofurantoin, pentazocine, tetracycline, quinidine
Pustular—acneiform reactions	Androgen hormones, corticosteroids, iodides, bromides, hydantoin, lithium
Urticaria and erythemas	
Urticaria	May occur with anaphylaxis: penicillin, xenogenic sera, cephalosporins, sulfonamides, barbiturates, hydralazine, phenylbutazone, hydantoin, quinidine, x-ray contrast media
Erythema multiforme	Sulfonamides, hydantoin, barbiturates, penicillin, carbamazepines, allopurinol, amikacin, phenothiazides
Nodular lesions	
Erythema nodosum	Birth control pills, sulfonamides, diuretics, gold, clonidine, propranolol, furosemide, opiates, penicillin
Vasculitis reaction	Allopurinol, barbiturates, carbamazepine, chlorothiazide, cimetidine, gold, indomethacin, hydantoin, piperazine, sulfonamides
Telangiectatic and LE reactions	Procainamide, hydralazine, phenytoin, penicillamine, trimethadione, methyldopa, carbamazepine, griseofulvin, malidixic acid, oral contraceptives, propranolol
Pigmentary reaction	Anticonvulsants, antimalarials, antitumor agents (bleomycin, busulfan, cyclophosphamide, doxorubicin, melphalan), oral contraceptives, corticotropin, tetracyclines, phenothiazines, amiodarone
Other cutaneous reactions	
Fixed drug reaction	Phenolphthalein, barbiturates, gold, sulfonamides, meprobamate, penicillin, tetracyclines, analgesics
Alopecia	Alkylating agents, antimetabolites, heparin, coumarin, hydantoin, Accutane, gold, nitrofurantoin, propranolol, colchicine, allopurinol
Hypertrichosis	Anabolic agents, diazoxide, minoxidil, phenytoin

LE = lupus erythematosus; PR = pityriasis rosea.

papules on the head, neck, and extremities). *Diseases with increased frequency in HIV infection* include seborrheic dermatitis, yeast infections (especially thrush), drug reactions (morbilliform reactions especially to antibiotics), and pruritus.

DISEASES WITH ATYPICAL PRESENTATIONS IN HIV DISEASE. Molluscum contagiosum may appear as large 1- to 2-cm smooth to verrucoid papules and plaques on the face. Herpes simplex often appears as large chronic ulcerative lesions in anogenital and oral areas. Zoster may present as dermatomal or disseminated hyperkeratotic, scarring papules and plaques. Scabies may evolve into numerous hyperkeratotic pruritic plaques teaming with mites on KOH examination. Syphilis may appear with a typical primary genital ulcer, but secondary and tertiary lesions may evolve rapidly. Psoriasis and Reiter's disease may be more severe in HIV-infected patients, with widespread total-body involvement.

CUTANEOUS DRUG REACTIONS

Rashes are among the most common adverse reactions to drugs and occur in 2 to 3% of hospitalized patients. Any drug can potentially produce a rash, and over-the-counter preparations should be considered when defining drug reactions (Table 522–16).

Some of the most common drugs causing skin reactions in hospitalized patients are amoxicillin, trimethoprim-sulfamethoxazole, ampicillin, penicillin G, allopurinol, dipyrone, gentamicin sulfate, mefruside, nitrazepam, and barbiturates. Drugs least likely to cause allergic skin reactions include digoxin, antacids, promethazine, acetaminophen, nitroglycerin, aminophylline, propranolol, antihistamines, cromolyn, and emollient laxatives.

Fixed drug eruptions are unique reactions that appear in the same area of the skin each time the responsible drug is administered. These rashes appear as macular, eczematous, or even bullous, pink to dark-red patches occurring as few or many lesions. When the drug is stopped the lesions fade, leaving post-inflammatory hyperpigmentation. The lesions return in the same place within a few hours of taking the drug again. Nonsteroidal anti-inflammatory drugs may cause cutaneous reactions including vesiculobullous

photosensitivity reactions, serum sickness, erythroderma, fixed drug reactions, and toxic epidermal necrolysis.

The treatment of drug reactions is to withdraw the suspected agent. Once a drug reaction is suspected, all non-essential drugs should be stopped, and appropriate substitutes used for the necessary medications. An asymptomatic eruption may require no therapy, or a mild reaction with pruritus may be controlled with topical steroid applications and antihistamines. In severe conditions such as exfoliative dermatitis, oral steroids are often indicated. Most drug eruptions resolve in 1 to 2 weeks after withdrawal of the drug, but some take months to clear. Although an occasional reaction may be fatal (e.g., toxic epidermal necrolysis), patients with drug eruptions usually have an excellent prognosis.

DISTINCTIVE SKIN LESIONS IN BLACK SKIN

Highly pigmented skin makes it difficult to appreciate color changes, especially shades of red. In addition, black skin has distinctive ways of reacting to inflammation so that some common skin diseases may look atypical. It is normal to see longitudinal, pigmented bands under the nails, in the oral mucosa, and in the palmar creases. Black skin tends to lichenify readily with accentuation of the follicles, and follicular prominence in response to pruritic skin diseaes is common. In addition, post-inflammatory hyper- and hypopigmentation are frequently seen in skin diseases (i.e., dermatitis, discoid lupus erythematosus). The protection provided by the heavily melanized skin results in the very low incidence of skin cancers.

Keloids, which are exaggerated, fibroblastic reactions in response to skin wounds, present as nodules and plaques of hairless, shiny, hyperpigmented lesions; they are more common in black skin and occur most often on ears, neck, cheeks, pre-sternal, and shoulder areas. A variant, acne keloid, which is a deep, follicular acne process with firm papules and scarring masses over the nape of the neck, is almost exclusively seen in black skin. Laser treatment and silastic gel sheeting are sometimes beneficial.

Pseudofolliculitis barbae, an inflammatory, papular, pustular eruption on the neck, chin, and mandible, is due to coiled beard hairs that re-enter the skin. Scars and keloids result. The best treatment is to avoid close shaving and to grow a beard.

Dermatosis papulosa nigra presents as pigmented, pedunculated, and verrucous papules on the face. These lesions, which resemble seborrheic keratoses, evolve at puberty and increase in number with age. They have no malignant potential. The only treatment is removal with liquid nitrogen freezing or surgery, but these procedures should be done with great care as depigmented scars may result.

Disseminate and recurrent infundibulofolliculitis consists of dis-

crete, pruritic follicular papules that wax and wane over the chest, back, and buttocks. The condition defies all forms of therapy.

Arndt KA, LeBoit PE, Robinson JK, Wintroub BU: Cutaneous Medicine and Surgery. Philadelphia, WB Saunders, 1996. *A thorough up-to-date dermatology textbook.*

Braverman IM: Skin Signs of Systemic Disease, 3rd ed. Philadelphia, WB Saunders, 1998. *Excellent text for the internist. Thorough review of cutaneous manifestations of internal disease with useful table and color plates.*

Fitzpatrick TB, Eisen AZ, Wolff K, et al: Dermatology in General Medicine, 4th ed. New York, McGraw-Hill, 1993. *Comprehensive, detailed general dermatology textbook.*

Olsen EA: Disorders of Hair Growth: Diagnosis and Treatment. New York, McGraw-Hill, 1994. *Complete review of hair disorders.*

Scher RK, Daniel CR III: Nails: Therapy, Diagnosis and Surgery, 2nd ed. Philadelphia, WB Saunders, 1997. *The definitive textbook on nail disease. Very practical, with diagnostic and therapeutic algorithms.*

PART XXVIII

LABORATORY REFERENCE INTERVALS AND VALUES

523 REFERENCE INTERVALS AND LABORATORY VALUES*

Ronald J. Elin

Reference intervals are valuable guidelines for the clinician to assess health and disease, but they should not be used as absolute indicators of health and disease. For essentially every test, there is a significant overlap between the normal and diseased populations. Many factors may influence the determination of the reference interval. The method and mode of standardization are variables for the reference interval, particularly for immunologic and enzymatic tests. The selection of the "normal" population is also important because factors such as age, gender, race, diet, personal habits (e.g., alcohol consumption, smoking), and exercise may influence the reference interval for a given analyte. Last, the statistics chosen to define the reference interval are also a factor. These multiple variables for determining the reference interval indicate why there are differences among institutions for the same analyte.

The values in this chapter are primarily for adults in the fasting state. Values for other groups, when included, are clearly identified. For convenience, this chapter is divided into the following three sections: clinical chemistry, toxicology, and serology; hematology and coagulation; and drugs—therapeutic and toxic. The list includes reference intervals for the most common tests used in the practice of internal medicine. For more information about the reference interval for a given test or a test not included in the list, a recommended source is *Clinical Guide to Laboratory Tests,* third edition, edited by Dr. Norbert W. Tietz. This book contains literature citations for most of the tests listed in this chapter.

All laboratory values are given in conventional and international units. If the value and units for a reference interval are the same for conventional and international units, the interval is listed only

---

*The material in this chapter was partially extracted from Tietz NW (ed): Clinical Guide to Laboratory Tests. Philadelphia, WB Saunders, 1995. The material for the section on Therapeutic Drug Concentrations was partially extracted from Burtis CA, Ashwood ER (eds): Tietz Textbook of Clinical Chemistry. Philadelphia, WB Saunders, 1994. The main contributors to this section of the book are PC Painter, JY Cope, and JL Smith. Other sources are listed under references for this chapter.

PREFIXES DENOTING DECIMAL FACTORS

PREFIX	SYMBOL	FACTOR
mega	M	10^6
kilo	k	10^3
hecto	h	10^2
deca	da	10^1
deci	d	10^{-1}
centi	c	10^{-2}
milli	m	10^{-3}
micro	μ	10^{-6}
nano	n	10^{-9}
pico	p	10^{-12}
femto	f	10^{-15}

ABBREVIATIONS

AU	Arbitrary units
EU	Ehrlich unit
GD	General diagnostics
IFA	Immunofluorescent assay
IU	International unit (of hormone activity)
RIA	Radioimmunoassay
RID	Radial immunodiffusion
S	Substrate
U	International unit (of enzyme activity)

in the column for international units. The temperature for all enzyme assays listed in the chapter is 37° C. The pertinent prefixes denoting the decimal factors and abbreviations are listed above.

Burtis CA, Ashwood ER (eds): Tietz Textbook of Clinical Chemistry. Philadelphia, WB Saunders, 1994.

Conn RB (ed): Current Diagnosis, 9th ed. Philadelphia, WB Saunders, 1997.

Hardman JG, Limbird LE, Molinoff PB, Ruddon RW (eds): Goodman and Gilman's The Pharmacological Basis of Therapeutics, 9th ed. New York, McGraw-Hill, 1995.

Henry JB (ed): Clinical Diagnosis and Management by Laboratory Methods, 19th ed. Philadelphia, WB Saunders, 1996.

Tietz NW (ed): Clinical Guide to Laboratory Tests, 3rd ed. Philadelphia, WB Saunders, 1995.

Young DS: Effect of Drugs on Clinical Laboratory Tests, 4th ed. Washington, DC, AACC Press, 1995; Friedman RB, Young DS: Effects of Disease on Clinical Laboratory Tests, 3rd ed. Washington, DC, AACC Press, 1997. *If consideration is interference with or effects of disease on a clinical test, here are two references that are of value.*

CLINICAL CHEMISTRY, TOXICOLOGY, SEROLOGY

TEST	SPECIMEN	REFERENCE INTERVAL (CONVENTIONAL UNITS)	REFERENCE INTERVAL (INTERNATIONAL UNITS)
Acetoacetate Semiquantitative	Serum or plasma (fluoride/oxalate)	Negative (<1 mg/dL)	Negative (<0.1 mmol/L)
Acetone	Urine	Negative	Negative
Semiquantitative	Serum or plasma (fluoride or oxalate)	Negative (<1 mg/dL)	Negative (<0.17 mmol/L)
Quantitative Semiquantitative	Urine		Negative
Acid phosphatase (S:p-nitrophenylphosphate)	Serum		M: 2.5–11.7 U/L F: 0.3–9.2 U/L
Adrenocorticotropic hormone (ACTH)	Plasma (heparin)	0800 h: <120 pg/mL 1600–2000 h: <85 pg/mL	<26 pmol/L <19 pmol/L
Alanine aminotransferase (ALT, SGPT)	Serum	M: 10–40 U/L F: 7–35 U/L	0.17–0.68 μKat/L 0.12–0.60 μKat/L
Albumin Nephelometric, colorimetric	Serum	3.4–4.8 g/dL	34–48 g/L
Turbidimetric	CSF	<45 mg/dL	<450 mg/L
	Urine	<80 mg/d at rest <150 mg/d ambulatory	<80 mg/d <150 mg/d
Aldolase	Serum	1.0–7.5 U/L	0.02–0.13 μKat/L
Aldosterone	Plasma (heparin EDTA) or serum	Adult, average sodium diet supine: 3–16 ng/dL upright: 7–30 ng/dL	0.08–0.44 nmol/L 0.19–0.83 nmol/L
Alkaline phosphatase (S:4–NPP)	Serum	25–100 U/L	Adult (>20 y) 0.43–1.70 μKat/L
δ-Aminolevulinic acid (δ-ALA)	Serum	15–23 μg/dL	1.1–8 μmol/L
	Urine	1.5–7.5 mg/d	11.4–57.2 μmol/d
Ammonia nitrogen Resin or enzymatic	Serum or plasma (Na-heparin)	Adult 15–45 μg N/dL	11–32 μmol/L
	Urine, 24-h	140–1500 mg/d	10–107 mmol/d
Amylase (S:Beckmann, defined substrate)	Serum	27–131 U/L	0.46–2.23 μKat/L
	Urine, timed specimen		1–17 U/h
Angiotensin I	Peripheral venous plasma (EDTA)	<25 pg/mL	<25 ng/L
Angiotensin II	Plasma (EDTA) Arterial blood	10–60 pg/mL	10–60 ng/L
α_1-Antitrypsin (nephelometry)	Serum	78–200 mg/dL	0.78–2 g/L
Anion gap $[Na^+ - (Cl^- + HCO_3^-)]$	Plasma (heparin)	7–16 mEq/L	7–16 mmol/L
Arsenic	Whole blood (heparin)	0.2–2.3 μg/dL Chronic poisoning: 10–50 μg/dL Acute poisoning: 60–93 μg/dL	0.03–0.31 μmol/L 1.33–6.65 μmol/L 7.98–12.37 μmol/L
Ascorbic acid (see Vitamin C)	Urine, 24-h	5–50 μg/d	0.067–0.665 μmol/d
Aspartate aminotransferase (AST)	Serum	10–30 U/L	0.17–0.51 μKat/L
Base excess	Whole blood (heparin)	−2 to 3 mEq/L	−2 to 3 mmol/L
Bicarbonate	Serum	22–29 mEq/L	22–29 mmol/L
Bile acids, total	Serum, fasting	0.3–2.3 μg/mL	0.74–5.64 μmol/L
	Serum, 1-h postprandial	1.8–3.2 μg/mL	4.41–7.84 μmol/L
	Feces	120–225 mg/d	294–551 μmol/d
Bilirubin Total	Serum	0.3–1.2 mg/dL	5–21 μmol/L
	Urine		Negative
Conjugated (direct)	Serum	0–0.2 mg/dL	0–3.4 μmol/L
Calcium, ionized (iCa)	Serum	4.65–5.28 mg/dL	1.16–1.32 mmol/L
Calcium, total	Serum	8.6–10.0 mg/dL	2.15–2.50 mmol/L
	Urine, 24-h	100–300 mg/d	2.5–7.5 mmol/d
	CSF	4.2–5.4 mg/dL	1.05–1.35 mmol/L
Cancer antigen 125 (CA 125)	Serum	<35 U/mL	<35 kU/L
Carbon dioxide, partial pressure (PcO₂)	Whole blood, arterial (heparin)	M: 35–48 mm Hg F: 32–45 mm Hg	4.66–6.38 kPa 4.26–5.99 kPa
Carbon dioxide, total (Tco₂)	Serum or plasma (heparin)	23–29 mEq/L	23–29 mmol/L
Carcinoembryonic antigen (CEA)	Serum	Nonsmokers: <2.5 ng/mL	<2.5 μg/L
β-Carotene	Serum	10–85 μg/dL	0.19–1.58 μmol/L
Catecholamines, total	Urine, 24-h	<100 μg/d	<5.91 nmol/d
Ceruloplasmin	Serum	18–45 mg/dL	180–450 mg/L
Chloride	Serum or plasma (heparin)	98–106 mEq/L	98–106 mmol/L
	CSF	118–132 mEq/L	118–132 mmol/L
	Urine, 24-h	110–250 mEq/d	110–250 mmol/d
Cholesterol, total	Serum or plasma (EDTA)	Recommended: <200 mg/dL Moderate risk: 200–239 mg/dL High risk: ≥240 mg/dL	<5.18 mmol/L 5.18–6.19 mmol/L 6.22 mmol/L
Chorionic gonadotropin, β-subunit (β-HCG)	Serum or plasma (EDTA)	M and nonpregnant F: <5.0 mIU/mL	<5.0 IU/L
Complement Total hemolytic Complement activity	Serum	75–160 U/mL	75–160 kU/L
Copper	Serum	M: 70–140 μg/dL F: 80–155 μg/dL	10.99–21.98 μmol/L 12.56–24.34 μmol/L
	Erythrocyte (heparin)	90–150 μg/dL	14.13–23.55 μmol/L
	Urine, 24-h	3–35 μg/d	0.047–0.55 μmol/d

CLINICAL CHEMISTRY, TOXICOLOGY, SEROLOGY *Continued*

TEST	SPECIMEN	REFERENCE INTERVAL (CONVENTIONAL UNITS)	REFERENCE INTERVAL (INTERNATIONAL UNITS)
Coproporphyrin	Urine, 24-h	34–234 μg/d	51–351 nmol/d
	Feces, 24-h	<30 μg/g dry wt	<45 nmol/g dry wt
		400–1200 μg/d	600–1800 nmol/d
Corticosterone	Serum	0800 h: 130–820 ng/dL	4–24 nmol/L
		1600 h: 60–220 ng/dL	2–6 nmol/L
Cortisol	Serum or plasma (heparin)	0800 h: 5–23 μg/dL	138–635 nmol/L
		1600 h: 3–15 μg/dL	82–413 nmol/L
		2000 h: ≤50% of 0800 h	Fraction of 0800 h: ≤0.50
Cortisol, free	Urine, 24-h	20–90 μg/d	55–248 nmol/d
C-Peptide	Serum	0.78–1.89 ng/mL	0.26–0.62 nmol/L
C-Reactive protein	Serum	68–8200 ng/mL	68–8200 μg/L
Creatine kinase (CK)	Serum		M: 38–174 U/L
			F: 26–140 U/L
Isoenzymes, Fraction 2 (MB)	Serum	<4–6% of total (method-dependent)	Fraction of total: <0.04–0.06
Creatinine	Serum or plasma	M: 0.7–1.3 mg/dL	62–115 μmol/L
Jaffe, kinetic or enzymatic		F: 0.6–1.1 mg/dL	53–97 μmol/L
	Urine, 24-h	M: 14–26 mg/kg/d	124–230 μmol/kg/d
		F: 11–20 mg/kg/d	97–177 μmol/kg/d
Creatinine clearance (endogenous)	Serum or plasma, and urine	M: 90–139 mL/min/1.73 m²	0.87–1.34 mL/s/m²
		F: 80–125 mL/min/1.73 m²	0.77–1.20 mL/s/m²
Dehydroepiandrosterone (DHEA)	Serum	M: 1.8–12.5 ng/mL	6.2–43.3 nmol/L
		F: 1.3–9.8 ng/mL	4.5–34.0 nmol/L
11-Deoxycortisol (compound S)	Serum	12–158 ng/dL	0.3–4.6 nmol/L
Erythropoietin	Serum		5–36 U/L
Estrogens, total	Serum	M: 20–80 pg/mL	20–80 ng/L
		F, cycle:	
		1–10 d 61–394 pg/mL	60–200 ng/L
		11–20 d 122–437 pg/mL	
		21–30 d 156–350 pg/mL	160–400 ng/L
		Postmenopausal: ≤130 pg/mL	≤130 ng/L
		Follicular phase 60–200 pg/mL	60–200 ng/L
		Luteal phase: 160–400 pg/mL	160–400 ng/L
	Urine, 24-h	M: 15–40 μg/d	
		F: Preovulation: 4–25 μg/d	
		Ovulation: 28–100 μg/d	
		Luteal peak: 22–80 μg/d	
		Pregnancy, term: <45,000 μg/d	
		Postmenopausal: <20 μg/d	
Fat, fecal	Feces, 72-h	<7 g/d	
		fat-free diet: <4 g/d	
Fatty acids, nonesterified (free)	Serum or plasma (heparin)	8–25 mg/dL	0.28–0.89 mmol/L
Ferritin	Serum	M: 20–250 ng/mL	20–250 μg/L
		F: 10–120 ng/mL	10–120 μg/L
α₁-Fetoprotein	Serum	<10 ng/mL	<10 μg/L
Fibrinogen (see Hematology and Coagulation section)			
Folate	Serum	3–16 ng/mL	7–36 nmol/L
	Erythrocytes (EDTA)	140–628 ng/mL packed cells	317–1422 nmol/L packed cells
Follitropin (FSH)	Serum or plasma (heparin)	M: 4–25 mIU/mL	4–25 IU/L
		F: Follicular phase: 1–9 mIU/L	1–9 IU/L
		Ovulatory peak: 6–26 mIU/mL	6–26 IU/L
		Luteal phase: 1–9 mIU/mL	1–9 IU/L
		Postmenopausal: 30–118 mIU/mL	30–118 IU/L
	Urine, 24-h		M: 3–11 IU/d
			F: 2–15 IU/d
Gastrin	Serum	25–90 pg/mL	25–90 ng/L
Glucose	Serum	Adult: 74–106 mg/dL	4.1–5.9 mmol/L
		>60 y: 80–115 mg/dL	4.4–6.4 mmol/L
	Whole blood (heparin)	65–95 mg/dL	3.6–5.3 mmol/L
	CSF	40–70 mg/dL	2.2–3.9 mmol/L
Quantitative, enzymatic	Urine	<0.5 g/d	<2.8 mmol/d
Qualitative	Urine		Negative
Glucose, 2-h postprandial	Serum	<120 mg/dL	<6.7 mmol/L

Glucose, tolerance test (GTT), oral	Serum	mg/dL		mmol/L	
		Normal	Diabetic	Normal	Diabetic
	Fasting:	70–105	>140	3.9–5.8	>7.8
	60 min:	120–170	≥200	6.7–9.4	≥11
	90 min:	100–140	≥200	5.6–7.8	≥11
	120 min:	70–120	≥140	3.9–6.7	≥7.8

TEST	SPECIMEN	REFERENCE INTERVAL (CONVENTIONAL UNITS)	REFERENCE INTERVAL (INTERNATIONAL UNITS)
γ-Glutamyltransferase (GGT) (Szasz Method)	Serum	M: 2–30 U/L	0.03–0.51 μKat/L
		F: 1–24 U/L	0.02–0.41 μKat/L
Glycerol, free	Plasma	0.29–1.72 mg/dL	0.032–0.187 mmol/L
Growth hormone (HGH, somatotropin)	Serum	Adult, M: 0–4 ng/mL	0–4 μg/L
		F: 0–18 ng/mL	0–18 μg/L
		>60 y, M: 1–9 ng/mL	1–9 μg/L
		F: 1–16 ng/mL	1–16 μg/L

Table continued on following page

CLINICAL CHEMISTRY, TOXICOLOGY, SEROLOGY *Continued*

TEST	SPECIMEN	REFERENCE INTERVAL (CONVENTIONAL UNITS)	REFERENCE INTERVAL (INTERNATIONAL UNITS)
Haptoglobin (see Hematology and Coagulation section)			
HDL-cholesterol (HDLC) (5th percentile from Lipid Research Clinics)	Serum or plasma (EDTA)	M: >29 mg/dL F: >35 mg/dL	>0.75 mmol/L >0.91 mmol/L
Hemoglobin A$_{1c}$ (electrophoresis)	Whole blood (heparin, EDTA, or oxalate)	5.0–7.5% of total Hb	Fraction of Hb: 0.050–0.075
Homovanillic acid (HVA)	Urine, 24-h	1.4–8.8 mg/d	8–48 μmol/d
17-Hydroxycorticosteroids (17-OHCS)	Urine, 24-h	M: 3.0–10.0 mg/d F: 2.0–8.0 mg/d	8.3–27.6 μmol/d 5.5–22.1 μmol/d
5-Hydroxyindole acetic acid (5-HIAA)			
Qualitative	Fresh random urine		Negative
Quantitative	Urine, 24-h	2–6 mg/d	10.4–31.2 μmol/d
17-Hydroxyprogesterone (17-OHP)	Serum	M: 0.5–2.5 ng/mL F: Follicular: 0.2–1.0 ng/mL Luteal: 1.0–5.0 ng/mL Postmenopausal: ≤0.7 ng/mL	1.5–7.5 nmol/L 0.6–3.0 nmol/L 3.0–15.5 nmol/L ≤2.1 nmol/L
Immunoglobulin A (IgA)	Serum	40–350 mg/dL	400–3500 mg/L
Immunoglobulin D (IgD)	Serum	0–8 mg/dL	0–80 mg/L
Immunoglobulin E (IgE)	Serum	0–380 IU/mL	0–380 kIU/L
Immunoglobulin G (IgG)	Serum	650–1600 mg/dL	6.5–16 g/L
	CSF	0.5–5 mg/dL	5–50 mg/L
Immunoglobulin M (IgM)	Serum	55–300 mg/dL	550–3000 mg/L
Insulin (12-h fasting), immunoreactive	Serum	0.7–9.0 μIU/mL	5–63 pmol/L
Intrinsic factor (see Vitamin B$_{12}$)			
Iron	Serum	M: 65–175 μg/dL F: 50–170 μg/dL	11.6–31.3 μmol/L 9.0–30.4 μmol/L
Iron-binding capacity, total (TIBC)	Serum	250–450 μg/dL	44.8–80.6 μmol/L
Iron saturation	Serum	M: 20–50 F: 15–50	Fraction of iron saturation: 0.20–0.5 0.15–0.5
17-Ketogenic steroids (17-KGS)	Urine, 24-h	M: 5–23 mg/d F: 3–15 mg/d	17–80 μmol/d 10–52 μmol/d
Ketone bodies			
Qualitative	Serum	Negative (0.5–3.0 mg/dL)	Negative (5–30 mg/L)
	Urine, random		Negative
17-Ketosteroids, total (17-KS)	Urine, 24-h	M: 10–25 mg/d F: 6–15 mg/d	37–87 μmol/d 21–52 μmol/d
L-Lactate	Whole blood (heparin)	Venous: 8.1–15.3 mg/dL Arterial: <11.3 mg/dL	0.9–1.7 mmol/L <1.3 mmol/L
Lactate dehydrogenase (LDH)	Serum		208–378 U/L
LDH isoenzymes (Electrophoresis, agarose)	Serum	% Fraction 1: 18–33 Fraction 2: 28–40 Fraction 3: 18–30 Fraction 4: 6–16 Fraction 5: 2–13	Fraction of total: 0.18–0.33 0.28–0.40 0.18–0.30 0.06–0.16 0.02–0.13
Lead	Whole blood (heparin)	<25 μg/dL Toxic: ≥100 μg/dL	<1.21 μmol/L ≥4.83 μmol/L
	Urine	<80 μg/dL	<0.39 μmol/L
LDL-Cholesterol (LDLC)	Serum or plasma (EDTA)	Recommended: <130 mg/dL Moderate risk: 130–159 mg/dL High risk: ≥160 mg/dL	<3.37 mmol/L 3.37–4.12 mmol/L ≥4.14 mmol/L
Lutropin (LH)	Serum or plasma (heparin)	M: 1–8 mU/mL F: Follicular phase: 1–2 mU/mL Midcycle: 16–104 mU/mL Luteal: 1–12 mU/mL Postmenopausal: 16–66 mU/mL	1–8 U/L 1–12 U/L 16–104 U/L 1–12 U/L 16–66 U/L
	Urine		M: 9–23 U/d F: nonmidcycle, 4–30 U/d
Lysozyme	Serum, plasma	0.4–1.3 mg/dL	4–13 mg/L
Magnesium	Serum	1.3–2.1 mEq/L	0.65–1.05 mmol/L
	Urine, 24-h	6.0–10.0 mEq/d	3.00–5.00 mmol/d
Mercury	Whole blood (EDTA)	<5.0 μg/dL	<0.25 μmol/L
	Urine, 24-h	<20 μg/dL Toxic: >150 μg/L	<0.1 μmol/L <0.75 μmol/L
Metanephrine, total	Urine, 24-h	0.05–1.20 μg/mg creatinine	0.03–0.69 mmol/mol creatinine
Myelin basic protein	CSF		<2.5 μg/L
Myoglobin	Serum		M: 19–92 μg/L F: 12–76 μg/L
	Urine, random		Negative
Osmolality	Serum		275–295 mOsmol/kg
	Urine, random		50–1200 mOsmol/kg, depending on fluid intake After 12-h fluid restriction: >850 mOsmol/kg
	Urine, 24-h		~390–900 mOsmol/kg

CLINICAL CHEMISTRY, TOXICOLOGY, SEROLOGY *Continued*

TEST	SPECIMEN	REFERENCE INTERVAL (CONVENTIONAL UNITS)	REFERENCE INTERVAL (INTERNATIONAL UNITS)
Oxalate	Serum	1–2.4 μg/mL	11–27 μmol/L
		Ethylene glycol poisoning: >20 μg/mL	Ethylene glycol poisoning: >228 μmol/L
Oxygen (PO_2)	Whole blood, arterial (heparin)	83–108 mm Hg	11–14.4 kPa
Oxygen saturation	Whole blood, arterial (heparin)	95–98%	Fraction saturated: 0.95–0.98
Parathyroid hormone	Serum	Varies with laboratory	
		N-Terminal 8–24 pg/mL	8–24 ng/L
		C-terminal 50–330 pg/mL	50–330 ng/L
		Intact 10–65 pg/mL	10–65 ng/L
pH (37° C)	Whole blood, arterial (heparin)		7.35–7.45
Phosphorus, inorganic	Serum	2.7–4.5 mg/dL	0.87–1.45 nmol/L
		>60 y, M: 2.3–3.7 mg/dL	0.74–1.2 nmol/L
		F: 2.8–4.1 mg/dL	0.90–1.3 nmol/L
	Urine, 24-h	0.4–1.3 g/d	13–42 mmol/d
Porphobilinogen (PBG)	Urine, 24-h		
Quantitative	Urine, 24-h	0–2.0 mg/d	0–8.8 μmol/d
Qualitative	Urine, fresh random		Negative
Potassium	Serum	3.5–5.1 mEq/L	3.5–5.1 mmol/L
	Plasma (heparin)	3.5–4.5 mEq/L	3.5–4.5 mmol/L
	Urine, 24-h	25–125 mEq/d	25–125 mmol/d
Pregnanediol	Urine, 24-h	M: 0–1.9 mg/d	0–5.9 μmol/d
		F: Follicular: <2.6 mg/d	<8 μmol/d
		Luteal: 2.6–10.6 mg/d	8–33 μmol/d
		Postmenopausal: 0.2–1.0 mg/d	0.6–3.1 μmol/d
Progesterone	Serum	M: 0.13–0.97 ng/mL	0.4–3.1 nmol/L
		F: Follicular: 0.15–0.70 ng/mL	0.5–2.2 nmol/L
		Luteal: 2.0–25 ng/mL	6.4–79.5 nmol/L
Prolactin (hPRL)	Serum	M: 3.0–14.7 ng/mL	3.0–14.7 μg/L
		F: 3.8–23.2 ng/mL	3.8–23.2 μg/L
Prostate-specific antigen (PSA)	Serum, freeze	M: <4 ng/mL	<4 μg/L
Protein			
Total	Serum	6.4–8.3 g/dL	64.0–83.0 g/L
Electrophoresis (cellulose acetate)	Serum	Albumin: 3.5–5.0 g/dL	35–50 g/L
		α_1-Globulin: 0.1–0.3 g/dL	1–3 g/L
		α_2-Globulin: 0.6–1.0 g/dL	6–10 g/L
		β-Gobulin: 0.7–1.1 g/dL	7–11 g/L
		γ-Globulin: 0.8–1.6 g/dL	8–16 g/L
Total	Urine, 24-h		50–80 mg/d at rest
Total	CSF	Lumbar: 15–45 mg/dL	150–450 mg/L
Pyruvic acid	Whole blood (heparin)	0.3–0.9 mg/dL	0.03–0.10 mmol/L
Renin (normal diet)	Plasma (EDTA)	Supine: 0.2–1.6 ng/mL/h	0.2–1.6 μg/L/h
		Standing: 0.7–3.3 ng/mL/h	0.7–3.3 μg/L/h
Riboflavin (see Vitamin B₂)			
Sediment	Urine, fresh, random		
Casts			Hyaline: occasional (0–1) casts/hpf
			RBC: not seen
			WBC: not seen
			Tubular epithelial: not seen
			Transitional and squamous epithelial: not seen
Cells			RBC: 0–2/hpf
			WBC: M: 0–3/hpf
			F: 0–5/hpf
			Epithelial: few
			Bacteria:
			Unspun: no organisms/oil immersion field
			Spun: <20 organisms/hpf
Sodium	Serum or plasma (heparin)	136–146 mEq/L	136–146 mmol/L
	Urine, 24-h	40–220 mEq/d	40–220 mmol/d
Specific gravity	Urine, random		1.002–1.030
	Urine, 24-h		1.015–1.025
Testosterone, free	Serum	M: 50–210 pg/mL	174–729 pmol/L
		F: 1.0–8.5 pg/mL	3.5–29.5 pmol/L
Testosterone, total	Serum	M: 280–1100 ng/dL	9.7–38.2 nmol/L
		F: 15–70 ng/dL	0.5–2.4 nmol/L
	Urine	20–50 y,	
		M: 50–135 μg/d	173–470 nmol/d
		F: 2–12 μg/d	7–42 nmol/d
		>50 y,	
		M: 40–60 μg/d	139–210 nmol/d
		F: 2–8 μg/d	7–28 nmol/d
Thiamine (see Vitamin B₁)	Serum	0.10–0.54 μg/dL	2.9–16.1 nmol/L
Thyroglobulin (Tg)	Serum	3–42 ng/mL	3–42 μg/L
Thyroglobulin antibodies	Serum		<1:10
Thyroid microsomal antibodies	Serum		Nondetectable (hemagglutination) or <1:10 (IFA)
Thyrotropin (hTSH)	Serum or plasma	0.4–4.2 μU/mL	0.4–4.2 mU/L
Thyrotropin-releasing hormone	Plasma	5–60 pg/mL	5–60 ng/L

Table continued on following page

CLINICAL CHEMISTRY, TOXICOLOGY, SEROLOGY *Continued*

TEST	SPECIMEN	REFERENCE INTERVAL (CONVENTIONAL UNITS)	REFERENCE INTERVAL (INTERNATIONAL UNITS)
Thyroxine, free (FT$_4$)	Serum	0.8–2.4 ng/dL	10–31 pmol/L
Thyroxine (T$_4$), total	Serum	M: 4.6–10.5 μg/dL	59–135 nmol/L
		F: 5.5–11.0 μg/dL	71–142 nmol/L
Thyroxine-binding globulin (TBG)	Serum	15.0–34.0 μg/mL	15.0–34.0 mg/L
Thyroxine index, free	Serum		4.2–13.0
Transcortin	Serum	M: 18.8–25.2 mg/L	323–433 nmol/L
		F: 14.9–22.9 mg/L	256–393 nmol/L
Transferrin	Serum	200–400 mg/dL	2.0–4.0 g/L
		>60 y: 180–380 mg/dL	1.80–3.80 g/L
Transthyretin (prealbumin)	Serum	10–40 mg/dL	100–400 mg/L
Triglycerides (TG)	Serum, after ≥12-hr fast	Recommended: <250 mg/dL	2.83 mmol/L
Tri-iodothyronine, free	Serum	260–480 pg/dL	4.0–7.4 pmol/L
Tri-iodothyronine, total (T$_3$)	Serum	100–200 ng/dL	1.54–3.08 mmol/L
Tri-iodothyronine resin uptake test (T$_3$RU)	Serum	24–34%	24–34 AU (arbitrary units)
Urea nitrogen	Serum or plasma	6–20 mg/dL	2.1–7.1 mmol/L
	Urine	12–20 g/d	0.43–0.71 mol/d
Urea nitrogen/creatinine ratio	Serum		12/1–20/1
Uric acid (uricase)	Serum	M: 3.5–7.2 mg/dL	0.21–0.42 mmol/L
		F: 2.6–6.0 mg/dL	0.15–0.35 mmol/L
	Urine, 24-h	250–750 mg/d	1.48–4.43 mmol/d
Urinary sediment (see Sediment)			
Urobilinogen	Urine, 2-h	0.1–0.8 EU	0.1–0.8 U
	Urine, 24-h	0.5–4.0 EU	0.5–4.0 U
	Feces	75–275 EU/100 g	750–2750 U/kg
		75–400 EU/d	75–400 U/d
		40–280 mg/d	67–473 μmol/d
Uroporphyrin	Urine, 24-h	<50 μg/d	<60 nmol/d
	Feces, 24-h specimen	10–40 μg/d	12–48 nmol/d
	Erythrocytes (heparin or EDTA)		Negative
Vanillylmandelic acid (VMA)	Urine, 24-h	2–7 mg/d	10.1–35.4 μmol/d
Viscosity	Serum		1.10–1.22 centipoise
Vitamin A	Serum	30–80 μg/dL	1.05–2.8 μmol/L
Vitamin B$_1$ (Thiamine)	Serum	0–2 μg/dL	0–75 nmol/L
Vitamin B$_2$ (Riboflavin)	Serum	4–24 μg/dL	106–638 nmol/L
Vitamin B$_6$	Plasma (EDTA)	5–30 ng/mL	20–121 nmol/L
Vitamin B$_{12}$	Serum	200–835 pg/mL	148–616 pmol/L
Vitamin C	Plasma (oxalate, heparin, or EDTA)	0.5–1.5 mg/dL	28–85 μmol/L
Vitamin D$_3$, 1,25-dihydroxy	Serum	25–45 pg/mL	60–108 pmol/L
Vitamin D$_3$, 25-hyroxy	Plasma (heparin)	Summer: 15–80 ng/mL	37.4–200 nmol/L
		Winter: 14–42 ng/mL	34.9–105 nmol/L
Vitamin E	Serum	5.0–18.0 μg/mL	12–42 μmol/L
Zinc	Serum	70–150 μg/dL	10.7–22.9 μmol/L

HEMATOLOGY AND COAGULATION

TEST	SPECIMEN	REFERENCE INTERVAL (CONVENTIONAL UNITS)	REFERENCE INTERVAL (INTERNATIONAL UNITS)
Activated partial thromboplastin time (APTT)	Whole blood (Na citrate)		25–35 sec
Bleeding time (BT)			
Ivy	Blood from skin		Normal: 2–7 min
			Borderline: 7–11 min
Simplate (G-D)			2.75–8 min
Blood volume	Whole blood (heparin)		M: 52–83 mL/kg
			F: 50–75 mL/kg
Bone marrow	Bone marrow aspirate	% (mean)	Number fraction (mean)
Differential count			
Myeoblasts		0.3–5.0 (2.0)	0.003–0.05 (0.02)
Promyelocytes		1.0–8.0 (5.0)	0.01–0.08 (0.05)
Myelocytes:			
Neutrophilic		5.0–19.0 (12.0)	0.05–0.19 (0.12)
Eosinophilic		0.5–3.0 (1.5)	0.005–0.03 (0.015)
Basophilic		0.0–0.5 (0.3)	0.00–0.005 (0.003)
Metamyelocytes		13.0–32.0 (22.0)	0.13–0.32 (0.22)
Polymorphonuclear neutrophils		7.0–3.0 (2.0)	0.07–0.30 (0.20)
Polymorphonuclear eosinophils		0.5–4.0 (2.0)	0.005–0.04 (0.02)
Polymorphonuclear basophils		0.0–0.7 (0.2)	0.0–0.007 (0.002)
Lymphocytes		3.0–17.0 (10.0)	0.03–0.17 (0.10)
Plasma cells		0.0–2.0 (0.4)	0.00–0.02 (0.004)
Monocytes		0.5–5.0 (2.0)	0.005–0.05 (0.02)
Reticulum cells		0.1–2.0 (0.2)	0.001–0.02 (0.002)
Megakaryocytes		0.03–3.0 (0.1)	0.0003–0.03 (0.001)
Pronormoblasts		1.0–8.0 (4.0)	0.01–0.08 (0.04)
Normoblasts		7.0–32.0 (18.0)	0.07–0.32 (0.18)
Clot lysis, 37° C	Whole clotted blood		48–72 h

HEMATOLOGY AND COAGULATION *Continued*

TEST	SPECIMEN	REFERENCE INTERVAL (CONVENTIONAL UNITS)	REFERENCE INTERVAL (INTERNATIONAL UNITS)
Clot retraction screen	Whole blood (no anticoagulant)		Retraction begins at 1 h, maximum at 24 h
Clotting time, Lee-White, 37°C	Whole blood (no anticoagulant)		5–8 min
Differential count (see Bone marrow differential count or leukocyte differential count)			
Eosinophil count	Whole blood (EDTA); capillary blood	50–400 cells/μL (mm³)	50–400 × 10⁶ cells/L
Erythrocyte count (RBC count)	Whole blood (EDTA)	millions of cells/μL (mm³) M: 4.3–5.7 F: 3.8–5.1	×10¹² cells/L 4.3–5.7 3.8–5.1
Erythrocyte sedimentation rate (ESR), Wintrobe			M: 0–15 mm/h F: 0–20 mm/h
Ferritin (see Chemistry section)			
Fibrin degradation products (agglutination, Thrombo-Wellco test)	Whole blood: special tube containing thrombin and proteolytic inhibitor	<10 μg/mL	<10 mg/L
	Urine: 2 mL in special tube (see above)	<0.25 μg/mL	<0.25 mg/L
Fibrinogen	Plasma (Na citrate)	200–400 mg/dL	2.00–4.00 g/L
Glucose-6-phosphate dehydrogenase (G6PD) in erythrocytes	Whole blood (ACD, EDTA, or heparin)	12.1 ± 2.09 U/g Hb (1 SD)	0.78 ± 0.13 MU/mol Hb (1 SD)
Haptoglobin (Hp) RID	Serum; avoid hemolysis	26–85 mg/dL	260–1850 mg/L
Hematocrit (HCT, Hct) Calculated from MCV and RBC (electronic displacement or laser)	whole blood (EDTA)	M: 39–49% F: 35–45%	0.39–0.49 volume fraction 0.35–0.45 volume fraction
Hemoglobin (Hb)	Whole blood (EDTA)	M: 13.5–17.5 g/dL F: 12.0–16.0 g/dL	2.09–2.71 mmol/L 1.86–2.48 mmol/L
	Plasma (heparin, ACD)	<3 mg/dL	<0.47 μmol/L
	Urine, fresh, random		Negative
Hemoglobin electrophoresis	Whole blood (EDTA, citrate, or heparin)		Mass function
		HbA > 95% HbA₂ 1.5–3.5% HbF < 2%	HbA > 0.95 HbA₂ 0.015–0.035 HbF < 0.02
Leukocyte count (WBC count)	Whole blood (EDTA)	4.5–11.0 × 10³ cells/μL (mm³)	4.5–11.0 × 10⁹ cells/L
	CSF	0.5 mononuclear cells/μL	0.5 × 10⁶ cells/L

Leukocyte	Whole blood (EDTA)	%	Cells/μL (mm³)	Number fraction	Cells × 10⁶/L
Differential count					
Myelocytes		0	0	0	0
Neutrophils–bands		3–5	150–400	0.03–0.05	150–400
Neutrophils–segmented		54–62	3000–5800	0.54–0.62	3000–5800
Lymphocytes		23–33	1500–3000	0.25–0.33	1500–3000
Monocytes		3–7	285–500	0.03–0.07	285–500
Eosinophils		1–3	50–250	0.01–0.03	50–250
Basophils		0–0.75	15–50	0–0.0075	15–50

Leukocyte		%		Number fraction	
Differential count	CSF				
Lymphocytes		62 ± 34		0.62 ± 0.324	
Monocytes (includes pia-arachnoid mesothelial cells)		36 ± 20		0.36 ± 0.20	
Neutrophils		2 ± 5		0.02 ± 0.05	
Histocytes				Rare	
Ependymal cells				Rare	
Eosinophils				Rare	

TEST	SPECIMEN	REFERENCE INTERVAL (CONVENTIONAL UNITS)	REFERENCE INTERVAL (INTERNATIONAL UNITS)
Mean corpuscular hemoglobin (MCH)	Whole blood (EDTA)	26–34 pg/cell	0.40–0.53 fmol/cell
Mean corpuscular hemoglobin concentration (MCHC)	Whole blood (EDTA)	31–37% Hb/cell or gHb/dL RBC	4.81–5.74 mmol Hb/L RBC
Mean corpuscular volume (MCV)	Whole blood (EDTA)		80–100 fL
Methemoglobin (MetHb)	Whole blood (EDTA, heparin, or ACD)	0.06–0.24 g/dL	9.3–37.2 μmol/L
Plasma volume	Plasma (heparin)	M: 25–43 mL/kg F: 28–45 mL/kg	0.025–0.043 L/kg 0.028–0.045 L/kg
Platelet count (thrombocyte count)	Whole blood (EDTA)	150–450 × 10³/μL (mm³)	150–450 × 10⁹/L
Prothrombin consumption	Whole blood (no anticoagulant)		>30 sec
Prothrombin time, two-stage modified	Whole blood (Na citrate)		18–22 sec
RBC count (see Erythrocyte count)			
Red cell volume	Whole blood (heparin)	M: 20–36 mL/kg F: 19–31 mL/kg	M: 0.020–0.036 L/kg F: 0.019–0.031 L/kg
Reticulocyte count	Whole blood (EDTA, heparin, or oxalate)	0.5–1.5% of erythrocytes	0.005–0.015 (number fraction)
Sulfhemoglobin	Whole blood (EDTA, heparin, or EDTA)	≤1.0% of total Hb	<0.010 of total Hb (mass fraction)
Thrombin time	Whole blood (Na citrate)		Time of control ± 25 when control is 9–13 sec
Thromboplastin time, activated (see Activated partial thromboplastin time [APTT])			

DRUGS—THERAPEUTIC AND TOXIC

DRUG	SPECIMEN	REFERENCE INTERVAL (CONVENTIONAL UNITS)		REFERENCE INTERVAL (INTERNATIONAL UNITS)
Acetaminophen	Serum or plasma (hep or EDTA)	Therap:	10–30 μg/mL	66–199 μmol/L
		Toxic:	>200 μg/mL	>1324 μmol/L
Amikacin	Serum or plasma (EDTA)	Therap:		
		Peak	25–35 μg/mL	43–60 μmol/L
		Trough (severe infection)	4–8 μg/mL	6.8–13.7 μmol/L
		Toxic:		
		Peak	>35 μg/mL	>60 μmol/L
		Trough	>10 μg/mL	>17 μmol/L
ε-Aminocaproic acid	Serum or plasma (hep or EDTA); trough	Therap:	100–400 μg/mL	0.76–3.05 mmol/L
Amitriptyline	Serum or plasma (hep or EDTA); trough (>12 h after dose)	Therap:	120–250 ng/mL	433–903 nmol/L
		Toxic:	>500 ng/mL	>1805 nmol/L
Amobarbital	Serum	Therap:	1–5 μg/mL	4–22 μmol/L
		Toxic:	>10 μg/mL	>44 μmol/L
Amphetamine	Serum or plasma (hep or EDTA)	Therap:	20–30 ng/mL	148–222 nmol/L
		Toxic:	>200 ng/mL	>1480 nmol/L
Bromide	Serum	Toxic:	>1250 μg/mL	>15.6 mmol/L
Caffeine	Serum or plasma (hep or EDTA)	Therap:	3–15 μg/mL	15–77 μmol/L
		Toxic:	>50 μg/mL	>258 μmol/L
Carbamazepine	Serum or plasma (hep or EDTA); trough	Therap:	4–12 μg/mL	17–51 μmol/L
		Toxic:	>15 μg/mL	>63 μmol/L
Carbenicillin	Serum or plasma	Therap:	Dependent on minimum inhibitory concentration of specific organism	Same
		Toxic:	>250 μg/mL	>660 μmol/L
Chloramphenicol	Serum or plasma (hep or EDTA); trough	Therap:	10–25 μg/L	31–77 μmol/L
		Toxic:	>25 μg/L	>77 μmol/L
Chlordiazepoxide	Serum or plasma (hep or EDTA); trough	Therap:	700–1000 ng/mL	2.34–3.34 μmol/L
		Toxic:	>5000 ng/mL	>16.7 μmol/L
Chlorpromazine	Serum or plasma (hep or EDTA); trough	Therap:	50–300 ng/mL	157–942 nmol/L
		Toxic:	>750 ng/mL	>2355 nmol/L
Cimetidine	Serum or plasma (hep or EDTA); trough	Therap:	0.5–1.2 μg/mL	2–5 μmol/L
Clonazepam	Serum or plasma (hep or EDTA); trough	Therap:	15–60 ng/mL	48–190 nmol/L
		Toxic:	>80 ng/mL	>254 nmol/L
Clonidine	Serum or plasma (hep or EDTA)	Therap:	1.0–2.0 ng/mL	4.4–8.7 nmol/L
Clorazepate	Serum or plasma (hep or EDTA)	As desmethyldiazepam:		
		Therap:	0.12–1.0 μg/mL	0.36–3.01 μmol/L
Cocaine	Serum or plasma (hep or EDTA); on ice	Therap:	100–500 ng/mL	330–1650 nmol/L
		Toxic:	>1000 ng/mL	>3300 nmol/L
Codeine	Serum	Therap:	10–100 ng/mL	33–334 nmol/L
		Toxic:	>200 ng/mL	>668 nmol/L
Cyclosporine	Serum (12 h after dose)	Therap:	100–400 ng/mL	83–333 nmol/L
		Toxic:	>400 ng/mL	>333 nmol/L
Desipramine	Serum or plasma (hep or EDTA); trough (≥12 h after dose)	Therap:	75–300 ng/mL	281–1125 nmol/L
		Toxic:	>400 ng/mL	>1500 nmol/L
Diazepam	Serum or plasma (hep or EDTA); trough	Therap:	100–1000 ng/mL	0.35–3.51 μmol/L
		Toxic:	>5000 ng/mL	>17.55 μmol/L
Digitoxin	Serum or plasma (hep or EDTA) ≥6 h after dose	Therap:	20–35 ng/mL	26–46 nmol/L
		Toxic:	>45 ng/mL	>59 nmol/L
Digoxin	Serum or plasma (hep or EDTA) trough (≥12 h after dose)	Therap: CHF	0.8–1.5 mg/mL	1.0–1.9 nmol/L
		Arrhythmias:	1.5–2.0 ng/mL	1.9–2.6 nmol/L
		Toxic:	>2.5 ng/mL	>3.2 nmol/L
Diphenylhydantoin (see Phenytoin)				
Disopyramide	Serum or plasma (hep or EDTA); trough	Therap:		
		Arrhythmias:		
		Atrial	2.8–3.2 μg/mL	8.3–9.4 μmol/L
		Ventricular	3.3–7.5 μg/mL	9.7–22 μmol/L
		Toxic:	>7 μg/mL	>20.7 μmol/L
Doxepin	Serum or plasma (hep or EDTA); trough (≥12 h after dose)	Therap:	30–150 ng/mL	107–537 nmol/L
		Toxic:	>500 ng/mL	>1790 nmol/L
Ephedrine	Serum	Therap:	0.05–0.10 μg/mL	0.30–0.61 μmol/L
		Toxic:	>2 μg/mL	>12.1 μmol/L
Ethchlorvynol	Serum or plasma (hep or EDTA)	Therap:	2–8 μg/mL	14–55 μmol/L
		Toxic:	>20 μg/mL	>138 μmol/L
Ethosuximide	Serum or plasma (hep or EDTA); trough	Therap:	40–100 μg/mL	283–708 μmol/L
		Toxic:	>150 μg/mL	>1062 μmol/L
Fenoprofen	Plasma (EDTA)	Therap:	20–65 μg/mL	82–268 μmol/L
Flecainide	Serum or plasma (hep or EDTA); trough	Therap:	0.2–1.0 μg/mL	0.5–2.4 μmol/L
		Toxic:	>1.0 μg/mL	>2.4 μmol/L
Flurazepam	Serum or plasma (EDTA)	Therap:	not well defined	
		Toxic:	>0.2 μg/mL	>0.5 μmol/L
Furosemide	Serum (30 min after dose)	Therap:	1–2 μg/mL	3–6 μmol/L

DRUGS—THERAPEUTIC AND TOXIC *Continued*

DRUG	SPECIMEN	REFERENCE INTERVAL (CONVENTIONAL UNITS)		REFERENCE INTERVAL (INTERNATIONAL UNITS)
Gentamicin	Serum or plasma (EDTA)	Therap:		
		Peak (severe infection)	8–10 μg/mL	16.7–20.9 μmol/L
		Trough (severe infection)	<2–4 μg/mL	<4.2–8.4 μmol/L
		Toxic:		
		Peak	>10 μg/mL	>21 μmol/L
		Trough	>4 μg/mL	>8.4 μmol/L
Glutethimide	Serum	Therap:	2–6 μg/mL	9–28 μmol/L
		Toxic:	>5 μg/mL	>23 μmol/L
Haloperidol	Serum or plasma (hep or EDTA)	Therap:	6–245 ng/mL	16–652 nmol/L
		Toxic:	not defined	
Ibuprofen	Serum or plasma (hep or EDTA)	Therap:	10–50 μg/mL	49–243 μmol/L
		Toxic:	100–700 μg/mL	485–3395 μmol/L
Imipramine	Serum or plasma (hep or EDTA); trough (≥12 h after dose)	Therap:	125–250 ng/mL	446–893 nmol/L
		Toxic:	>500 ng/mL	>1784 nmol/L
Isoniazid	Serum or plasma (hep or EDTA)	Therap:	1–7 μg/mL	7–51 μmol/L
		Toxic:	20–710 μg/mL	146–5176 μmol/L
Kanamycin	Serum or plasma (EDTA)	Therap:		
		Peak	25–35 μg/mL	52–72 μmol/L
		Trough (severe infection)	4–8 μg/mL	8–16 μmol/L
		Toxic:		
		Peak	>35 μg/mL	>72 μmol/L
		Trough	>10 μg/mL	>21 μmol/L
Lidocaine	Serum or plasma (hep or EDTA); ≥45 min following bolus dose	Therap:	1.5–6.0 μg/mL	6.4–26 μmol/L
		Toxic:		
		CNS or cardiovascular depression	6–8 μg/mL	26–34.2 μmol/L
		Seizures, obtundation, decreased cardiac output	>8 μg/mL	>34.2 μmol/L
Lithium	Serum or plasma (hep or EDTA); (>12 h after last dose)	Therap:	0.6–1.2 mEq/L	0.6–1.2 nmol/L
		Toxic:	>2 mEq/L	>2 mmol/L
Lorazepam	Serum or plasma (hep or EDTA)	Therap:	50–240 ng/mL	156–746 nmol/L
Meperidine	Serum or plasma (hep or EDTA)	Therap:	400–700 ng/mL	1620–2830 nmol/L
		Toxic:	>1 μg/mL	>4043 nmol/L
Meprobamate	Serum	Therap:	6–12 μg/mL	28–55 μmol/L
		Toxic:	>60 μg/mL	>275 μmol/L
Methadone	Serum or plasma (hep or EDTA)	Therap:	100–400 ng/mL	0.32–1.29 μmol/L
		Toxic:	>2000 ng/mL	>6.46 μmol/L
Methaqualone	Serum or plasma (hep or EDTA)	Therap:	2–3 μg/mL	8–12 μmol/L
		Toxic:	>10 μg/mL	>40 μmol/L
Methotrexate	Serum or plasma (hep or EDTA)	Therap:	variable	variable
		Toxic:		
		Low-dose therapy (1–2 wk)	>9.1 ng/mL	>20 nmol/L
		High-dose therapy (48 h)	>227 ng/mL	>0.5 μmol/L
Methsuximide (*N*-desmethyl methsuximide)	Serum	Therap:	10–40 μg/mL	53–212 μmol/L
		Toxic:	>40 μg/mL	>212 μmol/L
Methyldopa	Plasma (EDTA)	Therap:	1–5 μg/mL	4.7–23.7 μmol/L
		Toxic:	>7 μg/mL	>33 μmol/L
Methyprylon	Serum	Therap:	8–10 μg/mL	43–55 μmol/L
		Toxic:	>50 μg/mL	>273 μmol/L
Morphine	Serum or plasma (hep or EDTA)	Therap:	10–80 ng/mL	35–280 nmol/L
		Toxic:	>200 ng/mL	>700 nmol/L
N-Acetylprocainamide	Serum or plasma (hep or EDTA); trough	Therap:	5–30 μg/mL	18–108 μmol/L
		Toxic:	>40 μg/mL	>144 μmol/L
Netilmicin	Serum or plasma (EDTA)	Therap:		
		Peak (severe infection)	8–10 μg/mL	17–21 μmol/L
		Trough (severe infection)	<4 μg/mL	<8 μmol/L
		Toxic:		
		Peak	>12 μg/mL	>25 μmol/L
		Trough	>4 μg/mL	>8 μmol/L
Nitroprusside	Serum or plasma (EDTA)	As thiocyanate:		
			6–29 μg/mL	103–499 μmol/L
Nortriptyline	Serum or plasma (hep or EDTA); trough (≥12 h after dose)	Therap:	50–150 ng/mL	190–570 nmol/L
		Toxic:	>500 ng/mL	>1900 nmol/L
Oxazepam	Serum or plasma (hep or EDTA)	Therap:	0.2–1.4 μg/mL	0.70–4.9 μmol/L
Oxycodone	Serum	Therap:	10–100 ng/ml	32–317 nmol/L
		Toxic:	>200 ng/mL	>634 nmol/L
Paraquat	Whole blood (EDTA)	Toxic:	0.1–1.6 μg/mL	0.39–6.2 μmol/L
	Urine	Occup exp:	0.3 μg/mL	1.17 μmol/L
		Toxic:	0.9–64 μg/mL	3.50–249 μmol/L
Pentazocine	Serum or plasma (EDTA)	Therap:	0.05–0.2 μg/mL	0.2–0.7 μmol/L
		Toxic:	>1 μg/mL	>3.5 μmol/L
	Urine	Toxic:	>3 μg/mL	>10.5 μmol/L

Table continued on following page

DRUGS—THERAPEUTIC AND TOXIC *Continued*

DRUG	SPECIMEN	REFERENCE INTERVAL (CONVENTIONAL UNITS)		REFERENCE INTERVAL (INTERNATIONAL UNITS)
Pentobarbital	Serum or plasma (hep or EDTA); trough	Therap:		
		Hypnotic	1–5 μg/mL	4–22 μmol/L
		Therap coma	20–50 μg/mL	88–221 μmol/L
		Toxic:	>10 μg/mL	>44 μmol/L
Phenacetin	Plasma (EDTA)	Therap:	1–30 μg/mL	6–167 μmol/L
		Toxic:	50–250 μg/mL	279–1395 μmol/L
Phencyclidine	Serum or plasma (hep or EDTA)	Toxic:	90–800 ng/mL	370–3288 nmol/L
Phenobarbital	Serum or plasma (hep or EDTA); trough	Therap:	15–40 μg/mL	65–170 μmol/L
		Toxic:		
		Slowness, ataxia, nystagmus	35–80 μg/mL	151–345 μmol/L
		Coma with reflexes	65–117 μg/mL	280–504 μmol/L
		Coma without reflexes	>100 μg/mL	>430 μmol/L
Phensuximide (both parent and *N*-desmethyl metabolites)	Serum or plasma (hep or EDTA)	Therap:	40–60 μg/mL	228–324 μmol/L
Phenylbutazone	Plasma (EDTA)	Therap: (not well defined)	50–100 μg/mL	162–324 μmol/L
		Toxic:	>100 μg/mL	>324 μmol/mL
Phenylpropanolamine	Serum	Therap:	0.05–0.10 μg/mL	0.33–0.66 μmol/L
		Toxic:	>5 μg/mL	>33.07 μmol/L
Phenytoin	Serum or plasma (hep or EDTA); trough	Therap:	10–20 μg/mL	40–79 μmol/L
		Toxic:	>20 μg/mL	>79 μmol/L
Primidone	Serum or plasma (hep or EDTA); trough	Therap:	5–12 μg/mL	23–55 μmol/L
		Toxic:	>15 μg/mL	>69 μmol/L
Procainamide	Serum or plasma (hep or EDTA); trough	Therap:	4–10 μg/mL	17–42 μmol/L
		Toxic:	>10–12 μg/mL	>42–51 μmol/L
		Also consider effect of metabolite, *N*-acetylprocainamide		
Propoxyphene	Plasma (EDTA)	Therap:	0.1–0.4 μg/mL	0.3–1.2 μmol/L
		Toxic:	>0.5 μg/mL	>1.5 μmol/L
Propranolol	Serum or plasma (hep or EDTA); trough	Therap:	50–100 ng/mL	193–386 nmol/L
Protriptyline	Serum or plasma (hep or EDTA); trough (≥12 h after dose)	Therap:	70–250 ng/mL	266–950 nmol/L
		Toxic:	>500 ng/mL	>1900 nmol/L
Quinidine	Serum or plasma (hep or EDTA); trough	Therap:	2–5 μg/mL	6–15 μmol/L
		Toxic:	>6 μg/mL	>18 μmol/L
Salicylates	Serum or plasma (hep or EDTA); trough	Therap:	150–300 μg/mL	1086–2172 μmol/L
		Toxic:	>300 μg/mL	>2172 μmol/L
Secobarbital	Serum	Therap:	1–2 μg/mL	4.2–8.4 μmol/L
		Toxic:	>5 μg/mL	>21.0 μmol/L
Theophylline	Serum or plasma (hep or EDTA)	Therap:	8–20 μg/mL	44–111 μmol/L
		Toxic:	>20 μg/mL	>110 μmol/L
Thiocyanate	Serum or plasma (EDTA)	Nonsmoker:	1–4 μg/mL	17–69 μmol/L
		Smoker:	3–12 μg/mL	52–206 μmol/L
		Therap, after nitroprusside infusion:	6–29 μg/mL	103–499 μmol/L
	Urine	Nonsmoker:	1–4 mg/d	17–69 μmol/L
		Smoker:	7–17 mg/d	120–292 μmol/L
Thiopental	Serum or plasma (hep or EDTA); trough	Hypnotic:	1–5 μg/mL	4.1–20.7 μmol/L
		Coma:	30–100 μg/mL	124–413 μmol/L
		Anesthesia:	7–130 μg/mL	29–536 μmol/L
		Toxic conc:	>10 μg/mL	>41 μmol/L
Thioridiazine	Serum or plasma (hep or EDTA)	Therap:	1.0–1.5 μg/mL	2.7–4.1 μmol/L
		Toxic:	>10 μg/mL	>27 μmol/L
Tobramycin	Serum or plasma (hep or EDTA)	Therap:		
		Peak (severe infection)	8–10 μg/mL	17–21 μmol/L
		Trough (severe infection)	<4 μg/mL	<9 μmol/L
		Toxic:		
		Peak	>10 μg/mL	>21 μmol/L
		Trough	>4 μg/mL	>9 μmol/L
Tocainide	Serum or plasma (hep or EDTA)	Therap:	4–10 μg/mL	21–52 μmol/L
Tolbutamide	Serum	Therap:	80–240 μg/mL	299–888 μmol/L
		Toxic:	>640 μg/mL	>2368 μmol/L
Valproic acid	Serum or plasma (hep or EDTA); trough	Therap:	50–100 μg/mL	347–693 μmol/L
		Toxic:	>100 μg/mL	>693 μmol/L
Vancomycin	Serum or plasma (hep or EDTA); trough	Therap:	5–10 μg/mL	3–7 μmol/L
		Toxic:	>80–100 μg/mL	>55–69 μmol/L
		(not sell established)		
Verapamil	Serum or plasma (hep or EDTA)	Therap:	100–500 ng/mL	220–1100 nmol/L
Warfarin	Serum or plasma (hep or EDTA)	Therap:	1–10 μg/mL	3–32 μmol/L

INDEX

Note: Page numbers in *italics* refer to illustrations; page numbers followed by t refer to tables. **Boldface** page numbers refer to main discussions.

ISBN 0-7216-7996-X

90071

TOPICAL TABLE OF CONTENTS